OPHTHALMOLOGY

SECOND EDITION

Edited by

Myron Yanoff, M.D.

Professor and Chair
Department of Ophthalmology
Drexel University College of Medicine;
Distinguished Senior Scientist Awardee
(Humboldt Awardee)
Philadelphia, Pennsylvania

Jay S. Duker, M.D.

Professor
Department of Ophthalmology
Tufts University School of Medicine;
Chairman
Department of Ophthalmology
Tufts-New England Medical Center;
Director
New England Eye Center
Tufts-New England Medical Center
Boston, Massachusetts

James J. Augsburger, MD

Professor and Chairman
Department of Ophthalmology
University of Cincinnati College of Medicine
Consultant in Ocular Oncology
Cincinnati Eye Institute
Cincinnati, Ohio

Dimitri T. Azar, M.D.

Associate Chief of Ophthalmology
Director of Cornea and Refractive Surgery
   Service
Massachusetts Eye and Ear Infirmary;
Associate Professor of Ophthalmology
Harvard Medical School
Boston, Massachusetts

Gary R. Diamond, M.D.

Professor
Department of Ophthalmology and
   Pediatrics
Medical College of Pennsylvania—
   Hahnemann University;
Division of Ophthalmology
St. Christopher's Hospital for Children
Philadelphia, Pennsylvania

Jonathan J. Dutton, M.D., Ph.D.

Clinical Professor
Department of Ophthalmology
University of North Carolina
Chapel Hill, North Carolina;
Atlantic Eye and Face Center
Cary, North Carolina

David Miller, M.D.

Associate Clinical Professor
Department of Ophthalmology
Harvard Medical School;
Staff Member
Department of Ophthalmology
Massachusetts Eye and Ear Infirmary
Boston, Massachusetts

Narsing A. Rao, M.D.

Professor of Ophthalmology and Pathology
Department of Ophthalmology
Doheny Eye Institute
USC, Keck School of Medicine
Los Angeles, California

Emanuel S. Rosen, M.D.

Consultant Ophthalmic Surgeon
Visiting Professor, Department of Vision
   Sciences
University of Manchester
Institute of Science and Technology
The Alexandra Hospital
Cheadle, Cheshire, United Kingdom

Alfredo A. Sadun, M.D., Ph.D.

Flora Thornton Chair of Vision Research
   and Professor of Ophthalmology and
   Neurosurgery
Department of Ophthalmology and
   Neurological Surgery
Doheny Eye Institute
USC, Keck School of Medicine
Los Angeles, California

Mark Sherwood, M.D.

Professor and Chairman
Department of Ophthalmology
University of Florida
Gainesville, Florida

Joel Sugar, M.D.

Professor, Director of the Cornea Service
Department of Ophthalmology and Visual
   Sciences
University of Illinois at Chicago Eye Center
Eye and Ear Infirmary
Chicago, Illinois

Janey L. Wiggs, M.D.

Assistant Professor of Ophthalmology
Department of Ophthalmology
Harvard Medical School
Boston, Massachusetts
Assistant Professor of Ophthalmology
Department of Ophthalmology
Massachusetts Eye and Ear Infirmary
Boston, Massachusetts

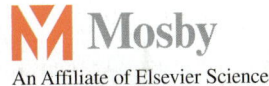
Mosby
An Affiliate of Elsevier Science

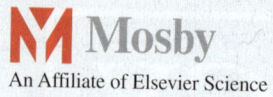

Mosby

An Affiliate of Elsevier Science

11830 Westline Industrial Drive
St. Louis, MO 63146

Ophthalmology
2nd Edition

NOTICE

Medicine is an ever-changing field. Standard safety precautions must be followed, but as new research and clinical experience broaden our knowledge, changes in treatment and drug therapy may become necessary or appropriate. Readers are advised to check the most current product information provided by the manufacturer of each drug to be administered to verify the recommended dose, the method and duration of administration, and contraindications. It is the responsibility of the treating physician, relying on experience and knowledge of the patient, to determine dosages and the best treatment for each individual patient. Neither the publisher nor the editor assumes any liability for any injury and/or damage to persons or property arising from this publication.

International Standard Book Number: 0-323-01634-0

Acquisitions Editor: Natasha Andjelkovic
Senior Managing Editor: Kathryn Falk
Publishing Services Manager: Patricia Tannian
Project Manager: Richard Hund
Book Design Coordinator: Teresa Breckwoldt
Cover Design: MW-Design

Printed in Spain

Last digit is the print number: 9 8 7 6 5 4 3 2 1

CONTRIBUTORS

JONATHAN J. DUTTON, MD, PhD 82-84, 95, 96
Clinical Professor, Department of Ophthalmology, University of North Carolina, Chapel Hill, North Carolina; Atlantic Eye and Face Center, Cary, North Carolina

DANIEL A. EBROON, MD 122
Assistant Professor and Director of Residency Training, Department of Ophthalmology, Northwestern University Medical School; Northwestern Memorial Hospital, Chicago, Illinois

ANTHONY ECONOMOU, DO, OD, FAOCO 230
Adjunct Professor, Department of Medicine, Oklahoma State University, College of Osteopathic Medicine; Attending, Department of Ophthalmology, St. Francis, St. John, Hillcrest, Southcrest Tulsa, Oklahoma

HOWARD M. EGGERS, MD 78
Professor of Clinical Ophthalmology, Department of Ophthalmology, Columbia University; Attending Ophthalmologist, Department of Ophthalmology, New York Presbyterian Hospital, New York, New York

TAREK M. EID, MD 237
Lecturer, Department of Ophthalmology, Tanta University, Tanta, Egypt; Ophthalmic Consultant, Department of Glaucoma and Cataract Units, Magrabi Hospital and Centers, Jeddah, Saudi Arabia

NORDELI ESTRONZA, MD 208
Private Practice, Attending Physician, Roanoke Neurological Associates; Attending Physician, Department of Neurology, Roanoke Memorial Hospital, Roanoke, Virginia

MAHER M. FANOUS, MD 225
North Florida Eye Center, PA, Private Practice, Gainesville, Florida

SAMIR G. FARAH, MD 22
Assistant Professor of Clinical Ophthalmology, Department of Ophthalmology, University of Balamand; Assistant Professor of Clinical Ophthalmology, Department of Ophthalmology, St. George Hospital University Medical Center, Beirut, Lebanon

AYAD A. FARJO, MD 56
Assistant Clinical Professor of Ophthalmology, Department of Ophthalmology and Visual Sciences, University of Iowa, Iowa City, Iowa

QAIS A. FARJO, MD 60
Clinical Assistant Professor, Department of Ophthalmology and Visual Sciences, University of Michigan, Ann Arbor, Michigan

DONALD C. FAUCETT, MD 91
Clinical Assistant Professor, Department of Ophthalmology, University of Mississippi Medical Center, Jackson, Mississippi

RONALD L. FELLMAN, MD 240
Associate Clinical Professor of Ophthalmology, University of Texas Health Science Center; Glaucoma Associate of Texas, Greenville Medical Tower, Dallas, Texas

I. HOWARD FINE, MD 47
Clinical Associate Professor, Casey Eye Institute, Department of Ophthalmology, Oregon Health Sciences University, Portland, Oregon; Clinical Associate Professor, Oregon Eye Surgery Center, Eugene, Oregon

YALE L. FISHER, MD 105
Clinical Professor of Ophthalmology, Department of Ophthalmology, New York Presbyterian Hospital; Attending Surgeon, Chief, Vitreoretinal Surgery, Department of Ophthalmology, Manhattan Eye, Ear, and Throat Hospital; Attending Surgeon, Department of Ophthalmology, New York Hospital-Cornell, New York, New York

GERALD A. FISHMAN, MD 110
Professor of Ophthalmology, Department of Ophthalmology and Visual Sciences, University of Illinois at Chicago, Chicago, Illinois

DAVID J. FORSTER, MD 161, 178
Clinical Associate Professor of Ophthalmology, Georgetown University, Washington, DC

JAMES A. FOUNTAIN, MD 170
Surgeon, Associated Vitreo-retinal and Uveitis Consultants; Consultant, Department of Ophthalmology, St. Vincent's Hospital, Indianapolis, Indiana

GREGORY M. FOX, MD 118
Assistant Clinical Professor, Department of Ophthalmology, University of Missouri, Columbia, Missouri; Retinal Surgeon, Department of Ophthalmology, St. Luke's Hospital, Kansas City, Missouri

SCOTT FRASER 210
Formerly Clinical Research Fellow, Glaxo Department of Ophthalmic Epidemiology, Institute of Ophthalmology, University College London, Moorfields Eye Hospital, London, England

JEFFREY FREEDMAN, MD 239, 242
Professor of Clinical Ophthalmology, Department of Ophthalmology, S.U.N.Y. Brooklyn; Professor of Clinical Ophthalmology, Department of Ophthalmology, S.U.N.Y. Downstate Medical Center, Brooklyn, New York

DEBORAH I. FRIEDMAN, MD 200, 208
Associate Professor, Department of Ophthalmology and Neurology, University of Rochester School of Medicine and Dentistry; Department of Ophthalmology and Neurology, Strong Memorial Hospital, University of Rochester, Rochester, New York

NEIL J. FRIEDMAN, M.D. 53
Clinical Faculty, Ophthalmology, Stanford University School of Medicine, Stanford, California; Private Practice, Palo Alto, California

ARTHUR FU, MD 131
Vitreoretinal Fellow, Department of Ophthalmology, California Pacific Medical Center, San Francisco, California

GREGG S. GAYRE, MD 93
Oculofacial Plastic and Reconstructive Surgery, Department of Ophthalmology, Kaiser Permanente, San Rafael, California

MICHAEL E. GIBLIN, FRANZCO 146
Visiting Medical Officer, Sydney Eye Hospital; Honorary Consulting Medical Officer, Royal Alexandra Hospital for Children, Sydney, Australia

JAMES W. GIGÁNTELLI, MD 87
Assistant Professor, Department of Ophthalmology and Otorhinolaryngology, University of Nebraska Medical Center; Attending Physician, Department of Ophthalmology, Omaha Veterans Affairs Hospital, Omaha, Nebraska

IVAN GOLDBERG, MB, BS, FRANZCO, FRACS 226
Save Sight Institute and Department of Ophthalmology, University of Sydney; Senior Consultant, Glaucoma Service, Sydney Eye Hospital; Vice President, Glaucoma Australia; President, Royal Australian and New Zealand College of Ophthalmology, Sydney, Australia

ROBERT ALAN GOLDBERG, MD 94
Associate Professor of Ophthalmology, Chief, Division of Orbital and Ophthalmic Plastic Surgery, Jules Eye Institute, University of California-Los Angeles School of Medicine, Los Angeles, California

DEBRA A. GOLDSTEIN, MD, FRCS(C) 64
Assistant Professor of Ophthalmology, Department of Ophthalmology, University of Illinois at Chicago, Chicago, Illinois

JOHN R. GONDER, MD, FRCS (C) 151
Associate Professor, Department of Ophthalmology, University of Western Ontario; Vitreoretinal Surgeon, Department of Ophthalmology, Ivey Eye Institute at London, Health Sciences Centre; Vitreoretinal Surgeon, Department of Ophthalmology, Ivey Eye Institute at St. Joseph's Health Centre; Vitreoretinal Surgeon, Department of Ophthalmology, London Regional Cancer Centre, London, Ontario, Canada

HARRY B. GRABOW, MD 42
Clinical Assistant Professor, Department of Ophthalmology, University of South Florida, Tampa, Florida; Attending Surgeon, Department of Surgery (Ophthalmology), Sarasota Memorial Hospital; Attending Surgeon, Department of Surgery (Ophthalmology), Doctors Hospital; Medical Director, Sarasota Cataract and Laser Institute, Center for Advanced Eye Surgery, Sarasota, Florida

JEFFREY P. GREEN, MD 94
Formerly Instructor of Ophthalmology Eye Plastics and Orbital Surgery Service, Massachusetts Eye and Ear Infirmary, Boston, Massachusetts

DONNA L. GREENHALGH, MBCHB, FRCA 45
Consultant Anesthetist, Department of Anesthetics, Wythenstiawe Hospital, Manchester, United Kingdom

CRAIG M. GREVEN, MD 135
Professor of Ophthalmology, Wake Forest University, Winston-Salem, North Carolina

NICOLE E. GROSS, MD 105
Retinal Fellow, Department of Ophthalmology, Manhattan Eye, Ear & Throat Hospital, New York, New York

RONALD L. GROSS, MD 233
Professor of Ophthalmology, The Clifton R. McMichael Chair in Ophthalmology, Department of Ophthalmology, Baylor College of Medicine; Professor of Ophthalmology, Department of Ophthalmology, The Methodist Hospital, Houston, Texas

SANDEEP GROVER, MD 110
Department of Ophthalmology & Visual Sciences, University of Illinois at Chicago, Chicago, Illinois

SEVGI GURKAN, MD 192
PGY-1, Department of Pediatrics, LAC/University of Southern California; PGY-1, Department of Pediatrics, Women's and Children's Hospital, Los Angeles, California

RUDOLF F. GUTHOFF, MD, PhD 148, 153
Chairman, Ophthalmological Department, Rostock University; Dean, Rostock University, Rostock, Germany; Secretary, European Society of Ophthalmic Plastic and Reconstructive Surgery (ESOPRS)

DAVID R. GUYER, MD 106
Professor and Chairman, Department of Ophthalmology, New York University School of Medicine; Attending, Department of Ophthalmology, Manhattan Eye, Ear, and Throat Hospital; Professor and Chairman, Department of Ophthalmology, Tish Hospital, New York University, New York, New York

ANTHONY B. HALL 35
Formerly Senior Registrar, Department of Ophthalmology, University of Leicester, Clinical Sciences Building, Leicester, United Kingdom

JULIA A. HALLER, MD 120
Associate Professor, Department of Ophthalmology, Johns Hopkins University School of Medicine; Associate Professor, Department of Ophthalmology, Johns Hopkins Wilmer Eye Institute, Baltimore, Maryland

NARESH MANDAVA, MD   106
Assistant Professor, Department of Ophthalmology, University of Colorado, Denver, Colorado

GEORGE E. MARAK, JR, MD   179
Clinical Professor, Department of Ophthalmology, Georgetown University Medical Center, Washington, DC

MICHAEL F. MARMOR, MD   100
Professor of Ophthalmology, Stanford University School of Medicine, Stanford, California

ADAM MARTIDIS, MD   125
Instructor, Department of Ophthalmology, Wills Eye Hospital, Philadelphia, Pennsylvania

ANDREW J. MAYS, MD   215
Assistant Professor of Ophthalmology, Department of Ophthalmology, University of Alabama at Birmingham, Birmingham, Alabama

MARK L. McDERMOTT, MD   57
Professor of Ophthalmology, Cornea and External Diseases, Kresge Eye Institute, Wayne State University; Attending Surgeon, Department of Ophthalmology, Detroit Medical Center, Detroit, Michigan

GERALD McGWIN, JR, MS, PhD   211
Associate Professor, Department of Epidemiology, School of Public Health, University of Alabama at Birmingham, Birmingham, Alabama

STEPHEN D. McLEOD, MD   62
Associate Professor of Clinical Ophthalmology, Vice Chairman for Clinical Affairs, Co-Director, Refractive Surgery Service, Department of Ophthalmology, University of California–San Francisco, San Francisco, California

ANDRE MERMOUD, MD   239
Head, Glaucoma Unit, Hopital Ophtalmique Jules Gonin, University of Lausanne, Lausanne, Switzerland

SANFORD M. MEYERS, MD   156
Ophthalmologist, Department of Surgery, Division of Ophthalmology, Lutheran General Hospital, Park Ridge, Illinois

WILLIAM F. MIELER, MD   123
Professor of Ophthalmology, Department of Ophthalmology, Baylor College of Medicine-Cullen Eye Institute, Houston, Texas

CLIVE MIGDAL, MD, FRCS, FRCPPHTH   232
Senior Lecturer, Imperial College; Head of Glaucoma Service, Western Eye Hospital, London, England

DAVID MILLER, MD   4, 6, 8-10, 13
Associate Clinical Professor, Department of Ophthalmology, Harvard Medical School; Staff Member, Department of Ophthalmology, Massachusetts Eye and Ear Infirmary, Boston, Massachusetts

RUSSELL MILLER, MD   5, 14
Formerly Researcher for Texas Tech University, Amarillo, Texas

ROBERT A. MITTRA, MD   123
Surgeon, Vitreo Retinal Surgery, P.A.; Clinical Assistant Professor, Department of Ophthalmology, University of Minnesota, Minneapolis, Minnesota

RAMANA S. MOORTHY, MD   170, 171, 182
Clinical Assistant Professor of Ophthalmology, Department of Ophthalmology, Indiana University School of Medicine; Active Staff, Department of Ophthalmology, St. Vincent's Hospital, Indianapolis, Indiana

MICHAEL G. MORLEY, MD   115
Assistant Clinical Professor of Ophthalmology, Department of Ophthalmology, Tufts University School of Medicine; Clinical Instructor, Department of Ophthalmology, Massachusetts Eye and Ear Infirmary, Harvard Medical School, Boston, Massachusetts

MARK L. MOSTER, MD   199
Professor of Neurology, Department of Neurology, Thomas Jefferson University; Chairman, Department of Neurosensory Sciences, Albert Einstein Medical Center; Active Attending, Department of Neurology – Ophthalmology, Wills Eye Hospital, Philadelphia, Pennsylvania

MARLENE R. MOSTER   237
Clinical Professor of Ophthalmology, Department of Ophthalmology, Thomas Jefferson University Hospital; Attending Surgeon, Glaucoma Service, Wills Eye Hospital, Philadelphia, Pennsylvania

SOMASHEILA I. MURTHY   167
Adjunct Faculty, Uvea and Ocular Immunology Services, L.V. Prasad Eye Institute, Hyderabad, Andhra Pradesh, India

ARVIND NEELAKANTAN, MD, FRCS, FRCOPHTH   222
Glaucoma Fellow, Department of Ophthalmology, University of Florida, Gainesville, Florida

ANN G. NEFF, MD   92
Assistant Professor of Clinical Ophthalmology, Department of Ophthalmology, Bascom Palmer Eye Institute, University of Miami School of Medicine; Assistant Professor of Clinical Ophthalmology, Department of Ophthalmology, Bascom Palmer Eye Institute, Ann Bates Leach Eye Hospital, Miami, Florida

SARAH M. NEHLS, MD   172
Resident, Department of Ophthalmology, Jules Stein Eye Institute, University of California-Los Angeles, Los Angeles, California

ANNA C. NEWLIN, MS, CGC   66
Genetic Counselor, Department of Medical Genetics, Evanston Northwestern Healthcare; Genetic Counselor, Center for Medical Genetics, Evanston Northwestern Healthcare, Evanston, Illinois

KENNETH G. NOBLE, MD   111
Associate Professor of Clinical Ophthalmology, Department of Ophthalmology, New York University Medical Center, New York, New York

COLM O'BRIEN, MD   218
Professor, Department of Ophthalmology, UCD/Mater Hospital, Dublin, Ireland

ANNABELLE A. OKADA, MD   176
Assistant Professor of Ophthalmology, Kyorin University School of Medicine, Tokyo, Japan

YVONNE A.V. OPALINSKI, MD   44
Formerly York Finch Eye Associates, Downsview, Ontario, Canada

MARK PACKER, MD   47
Assistant Clinical Professor, Casey Eye Institute, Department of Ophthalmology, Oregon Health Sciences University, Portland, Oregon; Oregon Eye Surgery Center, Eugene, Oregon

PAUL F. PALMBERG, MD   212
Professor of Ophthalmology, Department of Ophthalmology, Bascom Palmer Eye Institute; Professor of Ophthalmology, Department of Ophthalmology, Anne Bates Leach Eye Hospital, Miami, Florida

SURESH K. PANDEY, MD   40
Instructor, Department of Ophthalmology, John A. Moran Eye Center, University of Utah, Salt Lake City, Utah

GEETA PARARAJASEGARAM, PhD   159
Department of Pathology, Doheny Eye Institute, Los Angeles, California

KAY L. PARK, MD   160
Clinical Instructor, Department of Ophthalmology, Doheny Eye Institute, Los Angeles, California

TAMAR PEDUT-KLOIZMAN, MD   216
New England Eye Center, Tufts University School of Medicine, Boston, Massachusetts

JODY R. PILTZ-SEYMOUR, MD   231
Associate Professor of Ophthalmology, Department of Ophthalmology, University of Glaucoma Service; Director of Glaucoma Service, Scheie Eye Institute, Philadelphia, Pennsylvania

ALFIO PIVA, MD   195
Ophthalmology, Neurosurgery, Neurophthalmology Ophthalmic Plastic and Reconstructive Surgery, Department of Ophthalmology and Neurosurgery Hospital, Mexico San Jose, San Jose, Costa Rica

JOHN S. POLLACK, MD   123
Assistant Professor of Ophthalmology, Department of Ophthalmology, Rush Medical College, Chicago, Illinois

JONATHAN D. PRIMACK, MD   25
Assistant Professor of Ophthalmology and Visual Sciences, North Shore–Long Island Jewish Hospital Department of Ophthalmology, Albert Einstein College of Medicine; Director of Refractive Surgery, Department of Ophthalmology, Division of Cornea, External Disease, and Refractive Surgery, North Shore–Long Island Jewish Medical Center, Great Neck, New York

RONALD PRUETT, MD   126
Associate Clinical Professor, Department of Ophthalmology, Harvard Medical School; Surgeon, Department of Ophthalmology, Massachusetts Eye and Ear Infirmary, Boston, Massachusetts

CARMEN A. PULIAFITO, MD, MBA   102
Professor and Chairman, Department of Ophthalmology, Bascom Palmer Eye Institute, University of Miami School of Medicine; Medical Director, Anne Bates Leach Eye Hospital, Miami, Florida

JOSE S. PULIDO, MD, MS   127
Professor and Head, Department of Ophthalmology and Visual Sciences, University of Illinois-Chicago College of Medicine, Chicago, Illinois

PETER A. QUIROS, MD   207
Assistant Professor, Ophthalmology, Keck School of Medicine, University of Southern California, Los Angeles, California

NARSING A. RAO   167, 176, 180
Professor of Ophthalmology and Pathology, Department of Ophthalmology, Doheny Eye Institute, USC, Keck School of Medicine, Los Angeles, California

P. KUMAR RAO, MD   162
Assistant Professor, Department of Ophthalmology, Washington University School of Medicine; Barnes Retina Institute and Barnes Hospital, St. Louis, Missouri

RUSSELL W. READ, MD   169, 184
Assistant Professor of Ophthalmology and Pathology; Director, Uveitis and Ocular Inflammatory Diseases Service; Director, Ophthalmic Pathology Laboratory; Associate Scientist, Vision Science Research Center, University of Alabama, Callahan Eye Foundation Hospital, Birmingham, Alabama

FRANCO M. RECCHIA, MD   116
Fellow, Vitreoretinal Surgery, Associated Retinal Consultants, P.C., William Beaumont Hospital, Royal Oak, Michigan

CARL D. REGILLO, MD, FACS   141
Associate Professor of Ophthalmology, Thomas Jefferson University; Director, Clinical Retina Research, Retina Service, Wills Eye Hospital, Philadelphia, Pennsylvania

ELIAS REICHEL, MD   106, 107
Associate Professor, Department of Ophthalmology, Tufts University School of Medicine; Director, Vitreoretinal Service, New England Eye Center, Boston, Massachusetts

STEPHEN RHEINSTROM, MD   65
Visiting Associate Professor of Clinical Ophthalmology, Department of Ophthalmology, University of Illinois at Chicago; Attending Surgeon, Department of Ophthalmology, Michael Reese Hospital, Chicago, Illinois

FIONA O. ROBINSON, MB, BCH, BaO, MRCP, DO, FRCOphth   88
Consultant Ophthalmologist, Department of Ophthalmology, Kings College Hospital, London, England

HANNA RODRIGUEZ-COLEMAN, MD   105
Manhattan Eye, Ear, and Throat Hospital; New York Presbyterian Hospital Columbia-Cornell, Department of Ophthalmology, New York, New York

ADAM H. ROGERS, MD   113
Associate Professor of Ophthalmology, Department of Ophthalmology, New England Eye Center, Tufts University School of Medicine, Boston, Massachusetts

SHIYOUNG ROH, MD   101
Assistant Clinical Professor, Department of Ophthalmology, Tufts University School of Medicine, Boston, Massachusetts, Senior Surgeon, Department of Ophthalmology, Lahey Clinic Medical Center, Peabody, Massachusetts

EMANUEL S. ROSEN, B.Sc, MD, FRCSE, FROphth, FRPS   41
Visiting Professor, Department of Neural Sciences, University of Manchester Institute of Science and Technology (UMIST), Manchester, England

JAMES T. ROSENBAUM, MD   174
Professor and Chair, Division of Allergy, Immunology, and Rheumatology Disease, Department of Ophthalmology, Medicine, and Cell Biology, Oregon Health and Science University, Casey Eye Institute, Portland, Oregon

LISA F. ROSENBERG, MD   220
Associate Professor of Clinical Ophthalmology, Department of Ophthalmology, Feinberg School of Medicine, Northwestern University; Northwestern Memorial Hospital, Department of Surgery, Feinberg School of Medicine, Northwestern University, Chicago, Illinois

BRETT J. ROSENBLATT, MD   117
Resident, Wills Eye Hospital, Philadelphia, Pennsylvania

A. RALPH ROSENTHAL, MD   35
Visiting Professor, Department of Ophthalmology, Johns Hopkins Hospital, Baltimore, Maryland

MARK A. ROTHSTEIN, MD   17
Clinical Instructor, Department of Ophthalmology and Visual Sciences, Washington University, St. Louis, Missouri

JONATHAN B. RUBENSTEIN, MD   55
Professor of Ophthalmology, Ophthalmology, Rush Medical College, Chicago, Illinois

RICHARD M. RUBIN, MD   195, 201
Assistant Professor, Department of Ophthalmology, University of Texas Southwestern, Dallas, Texas

STEVEN E. RUBIN, MD   77
Clinical Associate Professor, Department of Ophthalmology, New York University School of Medicine, New York, New York; Chief, Pediatric Ophthalmology and Strabismus, Department of Ophthalmology, North Shore University Hospital, Manhasset, New York

PATRICK E. RUBSAMEN, MD   140
Retina Vitreous Consultants, Boca Raton, Florida

HOSSEIN G. SAADATI, MD   206
Department of Ophthalmology, Medical College of Wisconsin; The Eye Institute,, Froedtert Hospital, Milwaukee, Wisconsin

ALFREDO A. SADUN, MD, PhD
   186, 187, 189, 192, 195, 201, 206
Flora Thornton Chair of Vision Research and Professor of Ophthalmology and Neurosurgery, Department of Ophthalmology and Neurological Surgery, Doheny Eye Institute USC, Keck School of Medicine, Los Angeles, California

DARIN SAKIYALAK, MD   220
Clinical Instructor, Department of Ophthalmology, Faculty of Medicine, Siriraj Hospital, Mahidol University, Bangkok, Thailand

THOMAS W. SAMUELSON, MD   223
Clinical Associate Professor, Department of Ophthalmology, University of Minnesota; Attending Surgeon, Department of Ophthalmology, Phillips Eye Institute; Attending Surgeon, Department of Ophthalmology, Minnesota Eye Consultants, P.A., Minneapolis, Minnesota

GEORGE E. SANBORN, MD   152
Richard Retina Associates, Virginia Eye Institute, Richmond, Virginia

JEROME S. SARMIENTO, MD   8
Former Cornea Fellow, Cornea Consultants, Boston, Massachusetts

LISA A. SAXBY   28-34
Formerly Research Associate, Department of Ophthalmology, Royal Eye Hospital, Manchester, United Kingdom

SUSAN SCHNEIDER, MD   67, 150
Assistant Professor, Department of Ophthalmology, University of Cincinnati Medical Center; Attending Staff, Department of Ophthalmology, The University Hospital; Assistant Professor/Adjunct Attending Staff, Pathology and Laboratory Medicine, University of Cincinnati Medical Center; Director, Mary Knight Asbury Eye Pathology Laboratory, Department of Ophthalmology, University of Cincinnati Medical Center, Cincinnati, Ohio

HERMANN D. SCHUBERT, MD   99
Professor, Department of Clinical Ophthalmology and Pathology, Harkness Eye Institute, Columbia Presbyterian Medical Center, New York, New York

JOEL S. SCHUMAN, MD   216
Professor and Chairman, Department of Ophthalmology, The Eye and Ear Foundation, University of Pittsburgh, Pittsburgh, Pennsylvania

GARY S. SCHWARTZ, MD   50
Assistant Clinical Professor, Department of Ophthalmology, University of Minnesota, Minneapolis, Minnesota; Associated Eye Care, St. Paul, Minnesota

CLIFFORD A. SCOTT, OD, MPH   6, 10-12
Professor of Optometry, Chair, Department of Community Care and Public Health, New England College of Optometry, Boston, Massachusetts

JERRY SEBAG, MD, FACS, FRCOphth   144
Associate Clinical Professor of Ophthalmology, Doheny Eye Institute, Keck School of Medicine, USC, Los Angeles, California; Adjunct Associate Clinical Scientist, Schepens Eye Research Institute, Harvard Medical School, Boston, Massachusetts; Surgeon, Department of Ophthalmology, Hoag Memorial Hospital, Newport Beach, California; Consultant, Doheny Eye Institute, Keck School of Medicine, Los Angeles, California

ROBERT P. SELKIN, MD   63
Private Practice, Carolina's Eye Center, Charlotte, North Carolina

TAREK SHAARAWY, MD   239
Head, Department of Glaucoma, Memorial Research Institute of Ophthalmology, Giza, Egypt

PAUL A. SIEVING, MD, PhD   108
Director, National Eye Institute, National Institute of Health, Bethesda, Maryland

STEVEN T. SIMMONS, MD   230
Associate Clinical Professor, Department of Ophthalmology, Albany Medical College, Albany, New York; Co-Director, Glaucoma Consultants of the Capital Region, Slingerlands, New York

ARUNAN SIVALINGAM, MD   118
Clinical Associate Professor, Department of Ophthalmology, Jefferson Medical College of Thomas Jefferson University; Associate Surgeon, Department of Ophthalmology, Wills Eye Hospital, Philadelphia, Pennsylvania

STEPHEN G. SLADE, MD, FACS   20
Surgeon and Director, Laser Center of Houston; Memorial Hermann/Staff Ophthalmologist, Department of Ophthalmology, Houston, Texas

KENT W. SMALL, MD   109
Professor, University of California-Los Angeles, Jules Stein Eye Institute, Director Macular Disease Center, Director, Retina Research Lab, Los Angeles, California

WILLIAM E. SMIDDY, MD   130
Professor, Department of Ophthalmology, Bascom Palmer Eye Institute, University of Miami, Miami, Florida

JUSTINE R. SMITH, MBBS, PhD   174
Assistant Professor, Casey Eye Institute, Oregon Health and Science University, Portland, Oregon

M. FRAN SMITH, MD   213, 243
Associate Professor, Department of Ophthalmology, University of Florida; Chief, Department of Ophthalmology, Gainesville Veterans Administration Medical Center, Gainesville, Florida

H. KAZ SOONG, MD   56
Associate Professor of Ophthalmology, Department of Ophthalmology and Visual Sciences, W.K. Kellogg Eye Center, University of Michigan, Ann Arbor, Michigan

RICHARD F. SPAIDE   124
Clinical Associate Professor of Ophthalmology, New York University, New York, New York

THOMAS C. SPOOR, MD, FACS   193, 194
Professor Emeritus, Department of Ophthalmology and Neurosurgery, Wayne State University, Detroit, Michigan; Director, Department of Oculoplastic Orbital and Neuro-Ophthalmic Surgery, St. John Health System, Macomb Hospital, Warren, Michigan

KALLIOPI STASI, MD, PhD 24
Postdoctoral Fellow, Department of Ophthalmology, Mount Sinai School of Medicine, New York, New York

WILLIAM C. STEWART, MD 234
Department of Ophthalmology, University of South Carolina School of Medicine, Columbia, South Carolina; Director of Medical Affairs, Pharmaceutical Research Network, LLC, Charleston, South Carolina

ALAN SUGAR, MD 60
Professor and Associate Chair, Department of Ophthalmology and Visual Sciences, University of Michigan, Ann Arbor, Michigan

JOEL SUGAR, MD 58, 59, 66
Professor, Director of the Cornea Service, Department of Ophthalmology and Visual Sciences, The University of Illinois at Chicago Eye Center, Eye and Ear Infirmary, Chicago, Illinois

NANCY G. SWARTZ, MD 90
Assistant Professor, Department of Ophthalmology, Thomas Jefferson University Medical School; Assistant Surgeon, Department of Neuro-Ophthalmology, Wills Eye Hospital, Philadelphia, Pennsylvania

MYRON TANENBAUM, MD, FACS 97
Clinical Associate Professor of Ophthalmology, Bascom Palmer Eye Institute, University of Miami School of Medicine, Miami, Florida

WILLIAM S. TASMAN, MD 134
Chairman and Professor, Department of Ophthalmology, Jefferson Medical College; Ophthalmologist-in-Chief, Department of Ophthalmology, Wills Eye Hospital; Consulting Surgeon, Children's Hospital of Philadelphia; Attending Surgeon, Department of Ophthalmology, Chestnut Hill Hospital, Philadelphia, Pennsylvania

MATTHEW T.S. TENNANT, MD 118, 125
Wills Eye Hospital, Philadelphia, Pennsylvania

HOWARD H. TESSLER, MD 64
Professor of Ophthalmology, Department of Ophthalmology, University of Illinois at Chicago, Chicago, Illinois

ALLEN B. THACH, MD 164, 165, 183
Associate Professor of Clinical Surgery, Uniformed Services University of the Health Sciences, Bethesda, Maryland; Private Practice, Retinal Consultants of Arizona, Phoenix, Arizona

EDMOND H. THALL, MD, MS (OPTICAL SCIENCES) 5, 7, 13, 14
Riverton Memorial Hospital, Riverton, Wyoming

PAVIKA THAMMANO, MD 14
Commander, Royal Thai Navy, Staff Ophthalmologist, Naval Medical Department, Somdejphrapinklao Hospital; Refractive Surgery Specialist, TRSC International Lasik Center, Bangkok, Thailand

CARLO E. TRAVERSO, MD 222
Professor, Clinica Oculistica, Di.N.O.G., Università di Genova, Azienda Ospedale San Martino, Genova, Italy

MICHAEL T. TRESE, MD 145
Clinical Professor of Biomedical Sciences, Eye Research Institute, Oakland University, Rochester, Michigan; Chief, Pediatric and Adult Vitreoretinal Surgery, Department of Ophthalmology, William Beaumont Hospital, Royal Oak, Michigan

WILLIAM G. TSIARAS, MD 149
Chairman, Clinical Professor, Department of Ophthalmology, Brown University; Surgeon-in-Chief, Department of Ophthalmology, Rhode Island Hospital, Providence, Rhode Island

ELMER Y. TU, MD 65
Assistant Professor, Director, Refractive Surgery Service, Department of Ophthalmology, University of Illinois; Attending Physician, Department of Ophthalmology, University of Illinois Hospital, Chicago, Illinois

NANCY TUCKER, MD 89
Formerly Assistant Professor of Ophthalmology, McGill University and Université de Sherbrooke, Royal Victoria Hospital, Royal Victoria Hospital, Montreal, Quebec, Canada

MASAHIKO USUI, MD, PhD 176
Professor and Chairman, Department of Ophthalmology, Tokyo Medical University; Director and Professor, Department of Ophthalmology, Tokyo Medical University, Shinjuku-ku, Tokyo, Japan

SHAILAJA VALLURI, MD 171
Assistant Professor of Ophthalmology, Department of Ophthalmology, Indiana University School of Medicine; Assistant Professor of Ophthalmology, Department of Ophthalmology, Indiana University Hospital, Indianapolis, Indiana

JAMES F. VANDER, MD 133
Assistant Professor, Department of Ophthalmology, Thomas Jefferson University; Attending Surgeon, Department of Ophthalmology-Retina, Wills Eye Hospital, Philadelphia, Pennsylvania

GREGORY J. VAUGHN, MD 93
Formerly The Vaughn Institute, Atlanta, Georgia

BRIAN S. BOXER WACHLER, MD 27
Director, Boxer Wachler Vision Institute, Beverly Hills, California; Assistant Professor of Ophthalmology, Department of Ophthalmology, University of California-Los Angeles, Los Angeles, California

JONATHAN D. WALKER, MD 173
Assistant Clinical Professor, Department of Ophthalmology, Indiana University School of Medicine, Fort Wayne, Indiana

REBECCA S. WALKER, MD, FACS 231
Active Staff, Department of Ophthalmology, Grandview Hospital, Sellersville, Pennsylvania

FREDERICK M. WANG, MD 68
Clinical Professor, Department of Ophthalmology and Visual Science, Albert Einstein College of Medicine, Bronx, New York; Attending Surgeon, Department of Ophthalmology, New York Eye and Ear Infirmary, New York, New York; Attending Surgeon, Department of Ophthalmology, Montefiore Medical Center, Bronx, New York

LI WANG, MD, PhD 53
Research Associate, Department of Ophthalmology, Baylor College of Medicine, Houston, Texas

MING X. WANG, MD, PhD 63
Director, Wang Vision Institute, Research Associate Professor of Biomedical Engineering, Vanderbilt University, Nashville, Tennessee

ROBERT C. WANG, MD 168, 180
Texas Retina Associates, Dallas, Texas

DAVID V. WEINBERG, MD 143
Associate Professor of Ophthalmology, Department of Ophthalmology, Feinberg School of Medicine, Northwestern University, Chicago, Illinois

JOEL M. WEINSTEIN, MD 205
Associate Clinical Professor, Department of Ophthalmology and Visual Sciences, University of Wisconsin, University of Wisconsin Hospital, Madison, Wisconsin

JOHN J. WEITER, MD, PhD 101
Associate Clinical Professor, Department of Ophthalmology, Harvard University and Tufts University; Surgeon, Department of Ophthalmology, Massachusetts Eye and Ear Infirmary, Boston, Massachusetts

ELLIOT B. WERNER, MD 214
Clinical Professor of Ophthalmology, Department of Ophthalmology, MCP/Hahnemann University; Director, Glaucoma Service, Department of Ophthalmology, Hahnemann University Hospital, Philadelphia, Pennsylvania

LILIANA WERNER, PhD 40
Assistant Professor, Director of Research, David J. Apple MD Laboratories for Ophthalmic Devices Research; Department of Ophthalmology, John A. Moran Eye Center, University of Utah, Salt Lake City, Utah

PAUL F. WHITE, OD 12
Professor of Optometry, New England College of Optometry, Boston, Massachusetts

JANEY L. WIGGS, MD 1, 2, 212
Assistant Professor of Ophthalmology, Department of Ophthalmology, Harvard Medical School, Boston, Massachusetts; Assistant Professor of Ophthalmology, Department of Ophthalmology, Massachusetts Eye and Ear Infirmary, Boston, Massachusetts

CHARLES P. WILKINSON, MD 136
Professor, Department of Ophthalmology, Johns Hopkins University; Chairman, Department of Ophthalmology, Greater Baltimore Medical Center, Baltimore, Maryland

GEORGE A. WILLIAMS, MD 103
Clinical Professor of Biomedical Sciences, Eye Research Institute, Oakland University, Rochester, Michigan; Chairman, Department of Ophthalmology, William Beaumont Hospital; Director, Department of Ophthalmology, Beaumont Eye Institute, Royal Oak, Michigan

ZINARIA Y. WILLIAMS, MD 216
New England Eye Center, Tufts University School of Medicine, Boston, Massachusetts

WILLIAM J. WIROSTKO, MD 127
Assistant Professor, Department of Ophthalmology, Vitreoretinal Section, Medical College of Wisconsin, Milwaukee, Wisconsin

RICHARD WORMALD, MA, MB, BCh, MSc 210
Honorary Senior Lecturer, Department of Epidemiology and International Eye Health, Institute of Ophthalmology, University College London; Consultant Ophthalmologist, Glaucoma Service and Research and Development, Moorfields Eye Hospital, London, England

LAWRENCE A. YANNUZZI, MD 106
Professor, Department of Clinical Ophthalmology, College of Physicians and Surgeons, Columbia University School of Medicine; Vice Chairman, Department of Ophthalmology, Director of Retinal Research, Manhattan Eye, Ear, and Throat Hospital, New York, New York

ROBERT D. YEE, MD 202

Professor and Chairman of Ophthalmology, Department of Ophthalmology, Indiana University School of Medicine; Professor and Chairman of Ophthalmology, Department of Ophthalmology, University of Indiana Hospital, Indianapolis, Indiana

SONIA H. YOO, MD 26

Assistant Professor of Clinical Ophthalmology, Department of Ophthalmology, University of Miami School of Medicine; Assistant Professor of Clinical Ophthalmology, Department of Ophthalmology, Bascom Palmer Eye Institute, Miami, Florida

JOSHUA A. YOUNG, MD 16

Assistant Professor of Ophthalmology, Department of Ophthalmology, New York University School of Medicine, New York, New York

EHUD ZAMIR, MD 163

Assistant Professor of Uveitis and Ocular Inflammation, Ophthalmic Pathology Department of Ophthalmology, Hadassah-Hebrew University Medical School, Ein Kerem, Jerusalem, Israel

PAUL L. ZIMMERMAN, MD 181

Assistant Professor of Ophthalmology, Department of Ophthalmology, University of Utah Medical Center, John A. Moran Eye Center, Salt Lake City, Utah

RAYMOND ZIMMERMAN, MD 220

Private Practice Group, Affiliated Eye Surgeons, Phoenix, Arizona

PREFACE

We published the first edition of *Ophthalmology* in 1999. At that time, although excellent multivolume textbooks that attempted to cover all aspects of ophthalmology were available, no complete textbook of ophthalmology in a single volume existed. In preparing the first edition we had considerable discussion about whether to publish a single volume or to produce a two-volume textbook. Obvious pros and cons existed on both sides. In the end, we decided on a single volume. We found that there was wide acceptance to the final product.

Now, only 4 years later, we again find that enormous advances have taken place in ophthalmic technology, genetics, and immunology, along with other areas. For example, in the first edition, we described in detail the radial keratotomy procedure, but only mentioned LASIK in passing. In this edition we have several new chapters on LASIK, LASEK, and LTK. Electronic vision and wavefront testing are covered in greater detail. Other chapters new to this edition are tumors of the conjunctiva and cornea, nonpenetrating glaucoma surgery, and perspectives on aberrations of the eye. A new section on neuro-ophthalmic emergencies has also been added.

The color coding of the sections in the first edition proved highly successful, and we have again used this style in the second edition. We also carefully integrated the basic visual science with clinical information throughout and maintained an entire separate section dedicated to genetics and the eye. Despite the extensive use of color photographs, we offer this comprehensive book at a cost that is a fraction of the multivolume sets.

Once again, we do not intend the second edition of *Ophthalmology* to be encyclopedic, but we have tried to make it quite comprehensive. As an example, in dealing with surgery, the individual techniques continue to change so rapidly, so we do not emphasize the details of every surgical approach to ophthalmic disease but rather concentrate on those areas that are more generally accepted and less volatile, namely surgical indications, general principles of surgical techniques, and surgical complications. For in-depth discussions of current surgical techniques, a plethora of excellent books already exists, as well as books covering every ophthalmic subspecialty and anatomical area within the eye. An attempt is made to list key references for every entry while avoiding pages and pages of redundant references. The emphasis is on current information that is relevant to clinical practice superimposed on the broad framework that comprises ophthalmology.

With the publishing of this second edition, we must extend doubly our gratitude to our spouses, Karin and Julie, who have been most understanding and encouraged us throughout the long life of this project. We also are greatly indebted to the "Mosby Team" who spent so many hours in developing the final product. Specifically, we wish to thank Kathy Falk, Natasha Andjelkovic, and Richard Hund.

Myron Yanoff
Jay S. Duker

PREFACE TO THE FIRST EDITION

Over the past 30 years, enormous technologic advances have occurred in many different areas of medicine—lasers, molecular genetics, and immunology to name a few. This progress has fueled similar advances in almost every aspect of ophthalmic practice. The assimilation and integration of so much new information makes narrower and more focused ophthalmic practices a necessity. As a direct consequence, many subspecialty textbooks with extremely narrow focus are now available, covering every aspect of ophthalmic practice. Concurrently, several excellent multivolume textbooks detailing all aspects of ophthalmic practice have been developed. Yet there remains a need for a complete single-volume textbook of ophthalmology for trainees, non-ophthalmologists, and those general ophthalmologists (and perhaps specialists) who need an update in which they are not expert. *Ophthalmology* was created to fill this void between the multivolume and narrow subspecialty book.

This book is an entirely new, comprehensive, clinically relevant, single-volume textbook of ophthalmology, with a new approach to content and presentation that allows the reader to access key information quickly. Our approach, from the outset, has been to use templates to maintain a uniform chapter structure throughout the book so that the material is presented in a logical, consistent manner, without repetition. The majority of chapters in the book follow one of three templates: the disease-oriented template, the surgical procedure template, or the diagnostic testing template. Meticulous planning went into the content, sectioning, and chaptering of the book, with the aim of presenting ophthalmology as it is practiced rather than as a collection of artificially divided aspects. Thus, pediatric ophthalmology is not in a separate section but is integrated into relevant sections across the book. The basic visual science and clinical information, including systemic manifestations, is integrated throughout, with only two exceptions. We dedicated an entire section to genetics and the eye, in recognition of the increasing importance of genetics in ophthalmology. Optics and refraction are included in a single section as well, because an understanding of these subjects is fundamental to all of ophthalmology.

To achieve the same continuity of presentation in the figures as well as in the text, all of the artworks have been redesigned from the author's originals, maximizing their accessibility for the reader. Each section is color coded for easy cross-referencing and "navigation" through the book. Despite the extensive use of color in artworks and photographs throughout, the cost of this comprehensive book has been kept to a fraction of the multi-volume sets. We hope to make this volume more accessible to more practitioners throughout the world.

Although comprehensive, *Ophthalmology* is not intended to be encyclopedic. In particular, in dealing with surgery, we do not stress specific techniques or describe rarer ones in meticulous detail. The rapidly changing nature of surgical aspects of ophthalmic practice is such that the reader will need to refer to one or more of the plethora of excellent books that cover specific current techniques in depth. We concentrate instead on the areas that are less volatile but nevertheless vital: surgical indications, general principles of surgical technique, and complications. The approach to referencing is parallel to this: for every topic, all the key references are listed, but with the aim of avoiding pages of redundant references where a smaller number of recent classic reviews will suffice. The overall emphasis of *Ophthalmology* is current information that is relevant to clinical practice superimposed on the broad framework that comprises ophthalmology as a subspecialty.

Essential to the realization of this ambitious project is the team of Section Editors, each bringing unique insight and expertise to the book. They have coordinated their efforts in shaping the contents list, finding contributors, and editing chapters to produce a book that we hope will make a great contribution to ophthalmology.

We are grateful to the editors and authors who have contributed to *Ophthalmology* and to the superb, dedicated *Ophthalmology* team at Mosby.

Myron Yanoff
Jay S. Duker
July 1998

USER GUIDE

COLOR CODING

Ophthalmology is organized into 12 parts, which are color-coded as follows for quick and easy reference:

 PART 1: GENETICS AND OCULAR EMBRYOLOGY

 PART 2: OPTICS AND REFRACTION

 PART 3: REFRACTIVE SURGERY

 PART 4: THE LENS

 PART 5: CORNEA AND EXTERNAL DISEASE

 PART 6: STRABISMUS

 PART 7: ORBIT AND OCULOPLASTICS

 PART 8: RETINA AND VITREOUS

 PART 9: INTRAOCULAR TUMORS

 PART 10: UVEITIS AND OTHER INTRAOCULAR INFLAMMATIONS

 PART 11: NEURO-OPHTHALMOLOGY

 PART 12: GLAUCOMA

CONTENTS

PART 9: INTRAOCULAR TUMORS
JAMES J. AUGSBURGER

PART 12: GLAUCOMA, 1411
MARK SHERWOOD

GENETICS AND OCULAR EMBRYOLOGY

Janey L. Wiggs

CHAPTER 1

Fundamentals of Human Genetics

JANEY L. WIGGS

DNA AND THE CENTRAL DOGMA OF HUMAN GENETICS

The regulation of cellular growth and function in all human tissue is dependent on the activities of specific protein molecules. In turn, protein activity is dependent on the expression of the genes that contain the correct DNA sequence for protein synthesis. The DNA molecule is a double-stranded helix. Each strand is composed of a sequence of four nucleotide bases—adenine (A), guanine (G), cytosine (C), and thymine (T)—joined to a sugar and a phosphate. The order of the bases in the DNA sequence forms the genetic code that directs the expression of genes. The double-stranded helix is formed as a result of hydrogen bonding between the nucleotide bases of opposite strands.[1] The bonding is specific, such that A always pairs with T, and G always pairs with C. The specificity of the hydrogen bonding is the molecular basis of the accurate copying of the DNA sequence that is required during the processes of DNA replication (necessary for cell division) and transcription of DNA into RNA (necessary for gene expression and protein synthesis; Fig. 1-1).[2,3]

Gene expression begins with the recognition of a particular DNA sequence, called the promoter sequence, as a start site for RNA synthesis by the enzyme RNA polymerase. The RNA polymerase "reads" the DNA sequence and assembles a strand of RNA that is complementary to the DNA sequence. RNA is a single-stranded nucleic acid composed of the same nucleotide bases as DNA, except that uracil takes the place of thymine. Human genes (and genes found in other eukaryotic organisms) contain DNA sequences that are not translated into polypeptides and proteins. These sequences are called intervening sequences or introns. Introns do not have a specific function, and although they are transcribed into RNA by RNA polymerase, they are spliced out of the initial RNA product (termed heteronuclear RNA, or hnRNA) to form the completed messenger RNA (mRNA). The mRNA is the template for protein synthesis. Proteins consist of one or more polypeptide chains, which are sequences of specific amino acids. The sequence of bases in the mRNA directs the order of amino acids that make up the polypeptide chain. Individual amino acids are encoded by units of three mRNA bases, termed codons. Transfer RNA (tRNA) molecules bind specific amino acids and recognize the corresponding three-base codon in the mRNA. Cellular organelles called ribosomes bind the mRNA in such a configuration that the RNA sequence is accessible to tRNA molecules and the amino acids are aligned to form the polypeptide. The polypeptide chain may be processed by a number of other chemical reactions to form the mature protein (Fig. 1-2).[4]

Human DNA is packaged as chromosomes located in the nuclei of cells. Chromosomes are composed of individual strands of DNA wound about proteins called histones. The complex winding and coiling process culminates in the formation of a chromosome. The entire collection of human chromosomes, called the human genome, includes 22 paired autosomes and two sex chromosomes. Women have two copies of the X chromosome, and men have one X and one Y chromosome (Fig. 1-3).[5,6]

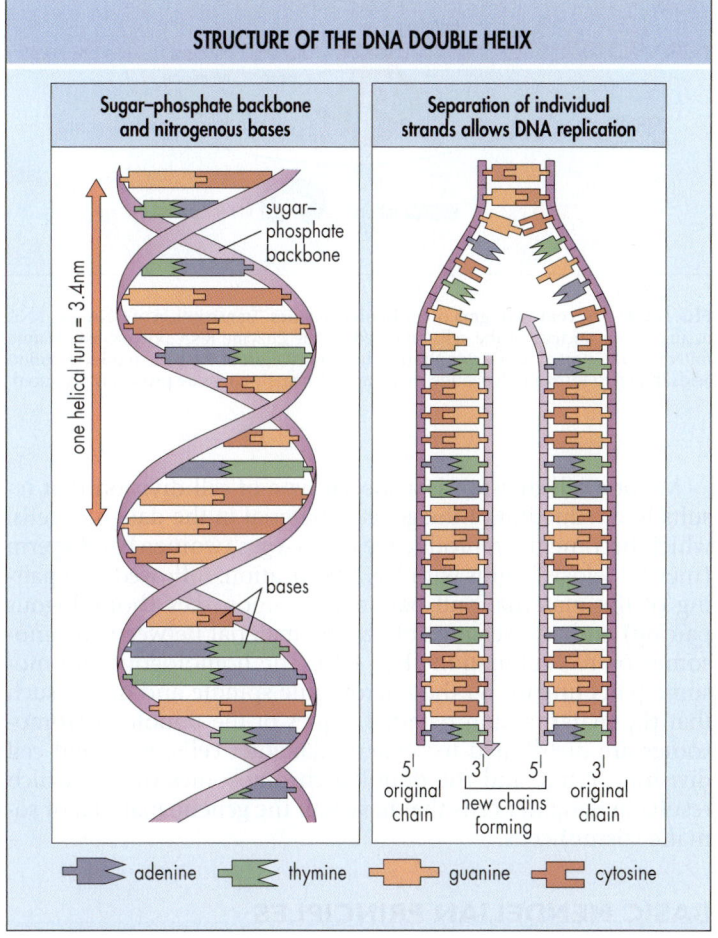

STRUCTURE OF THE DNA DOUBLE HELIX

Sugar–phosphate backbone and nitrogenous bases

Separation of individual strands allows DNA replication

one helical turn = 3.4nm

sugar–phosphate backbone

bases

5' original chain | 3' new chains forming 5' | 3' original chain

adenine   thymine   guanine   cytosine

FIG. 1-1 ■ **Structure of the DNA double helix.** The sugar-phosphate backbone and nitrogenous bases of each individual strand are arranged as shown. The two strands of DNA pair by hydrogen bonding between the appropriate bases to form the double-helical structure. Separation of individual strands of the DNA molecule allows DNA replication, catalyzed by DNA polymerase. As the new complementary strands of DNA are synthesized, hydrogen bonds are formed between the appropriate nitrogenous bases.

Mitosis and Meiosis

In order for cells to divide, the entire DNA sequence must be copied so that each daughter cell can receive a complete complement of DNA. The growth phase of the cell cycle terminates with the separation of the two sister chromatids of each chromosome, and the cell divides during mitosis. Prior to cell division, the complete DNA sequence, which comprises the entire human genome, is copied by the enzyme DNA polymerase in a process called DNA replication. DNA polymerase is an enzyme capable of the synthesis of new strands of DNA according to the exact sequence of the original DNA. Once the DNA is copied, the old and new copies of the chromosomes pair, and the cell divides such that one copy of each chromosome pair belongs to each cell (Fig. 1-4). Mitotic cell division produces a daughter cell that is an exact replica of the dividing cell.

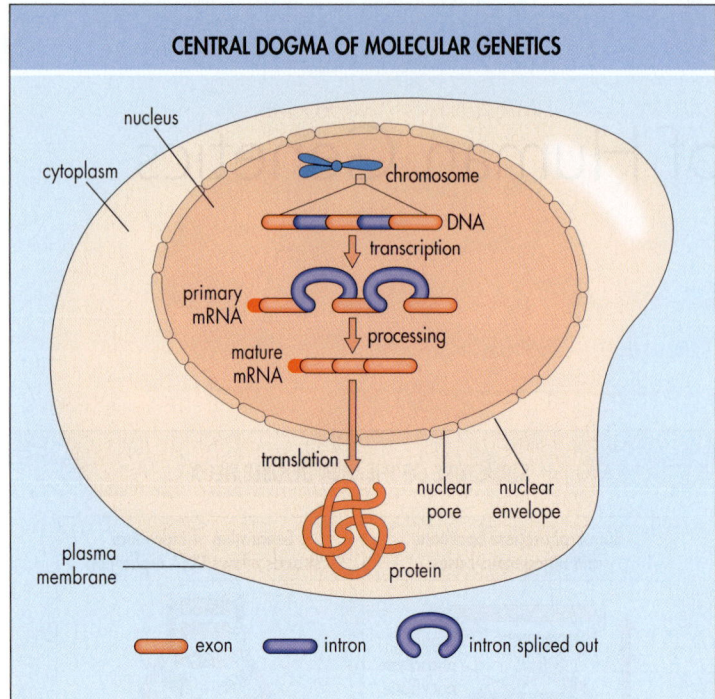

CENTRAL DOGMA OF MOLECULAR GENETICS

FIG. 1-2 ■ **The central dogma of molecular genetics.** Transcription of DNA into RNA occurs in the nucleus of the cell, catalyzed by the enzyme RNA polymerase. Mature mRNA is transported to the cytoplasm, where translation of the code produces amino acids linked to form a polypeptide chain, and ultimately a mature protein is produced.

Meiotic cell division is a special type of cell division that results in a reduction of the genetic material in the daughter cells, which become the reproductive cells—eggs (women) and sperm (men). Meiosis begins with DNA replication, followed by a pairing of the maternal and paternal chromosomes (homologous pairing) and an exchange of genetic material between chromosomes by recombination (Fig. 1-5). The homologous chromosome pairs line up on the microtubule spindle and divide such that the maternal and paternal copies of the doubled chromosomes are distributed to separate daughter cells. A second cell division occurs, and the doubled chromosomes divide, which results in daughter cells that have half the genetic material of somatic (tissue) cells.

BASIC MENDELIAN PRINCIPLES

Two important rules central to human genetics emerged from the work of Gregor Mendel, a nineteenth-century Austrian monk.[7] The first is the principle of segregation, which states that genes exist in pairs and that only one member of each pair is transmitted to the offspring of a mating couple. The principle of segregation describes the behavior of chromosomes in meiosis. Mendel's second rule is the law of independent assortment, which states that genes at different loci are transmitted independently. This work also demonstrated the concepts of dominant and recessive traits. Mendel found that certain traits were dominant and could mask the presence of a recessive gene.

A practical example of Mendel's two laws is seen in the inheritance of human eye and hair color. Blue eyes and blond hair are recessive traits, while brown eyes and hair are dominant traits. This means that for an individual to have blond hair and blue eyes, he or she must have two genes for blond hair and two genes for blue eyes (one from the mother and one from the father). An individual with brown eyes and brown hair may have two genes for brown eye color and two genes for brown hair color; however, because the brown genes are dominant, brown eyes may occur when an individual has one gene for brown eye color and one gene for blue eye color. A homozygous individual has two of the same genes (i.e., two blue eye-color genes or two brown eye-color

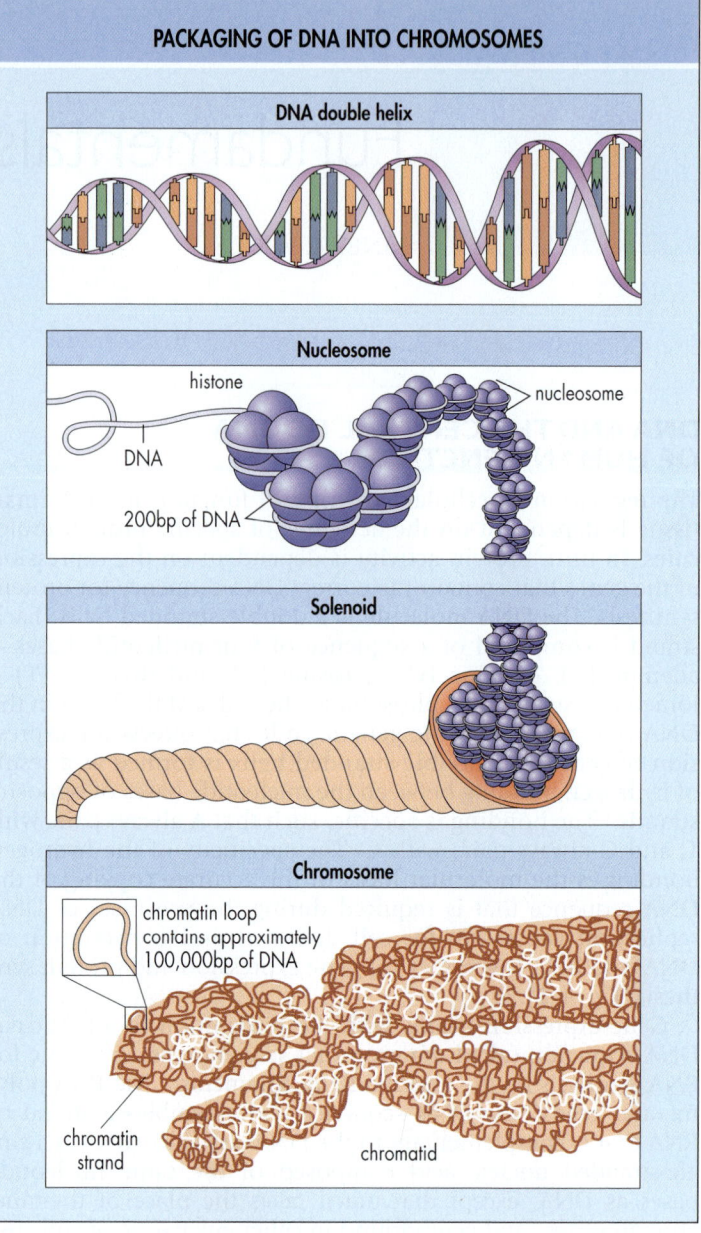

PACKAGING OF DNA INTO CHROMOSOMES

DNA double helix

Nucleosome

histone
nucleosome
DNA
200bp of DNA

Solenoid

Chromosome

chromatin loop contains approximately 100,000bp of DNA

chromatin strand
chromatid

FIG. 1-3 ■ **The packaging of DNA into chromosomes.** Strands of DNA are wound tightly around proteins called histones. The DNA-histone complex becomes further coiled to form a nucleosome, which in turn coils to form a solenoid. Solenoids then form complexes with additional proteins to become the chromatin that ultimately forms the chromosome.

genes), whereas a heterozygous individual has two different genes (i.e., one blue eye-color gene and one brown eye-color gene).

Mendel's rules on segregation and independent assortment are evident when the possible matings and offspring of individuals with blond or brown hair and blue or brown eye color are observed (Fig. 1-6). If two blond-haired, blue-eyed individuals mate, all their offspring will have blond hair and blue eyes, because these individuals must be homozygous, and the only genes available to the offspring are those for blue eyes and blond hair. If a blond-haired, blue-eyed individual mates with a brown-haired, brown-eyed individual who is homozygous for brown hair genes and brown eye genes, all the offspring from this mating will have brown hair and brown eyes because the brown genes are dominant. However, all these offspring will be heterozygous for genes at these loci, because they must have inherited recessive blue eye and blond hair genes.

The law of independent assortment becomes evident when the offspring of two individuals who are heterozygous for eye and hair color are examined. Among the offspring of this mating, 25% will have blue eyes, and 75% will have brown eyes (50% will be het-

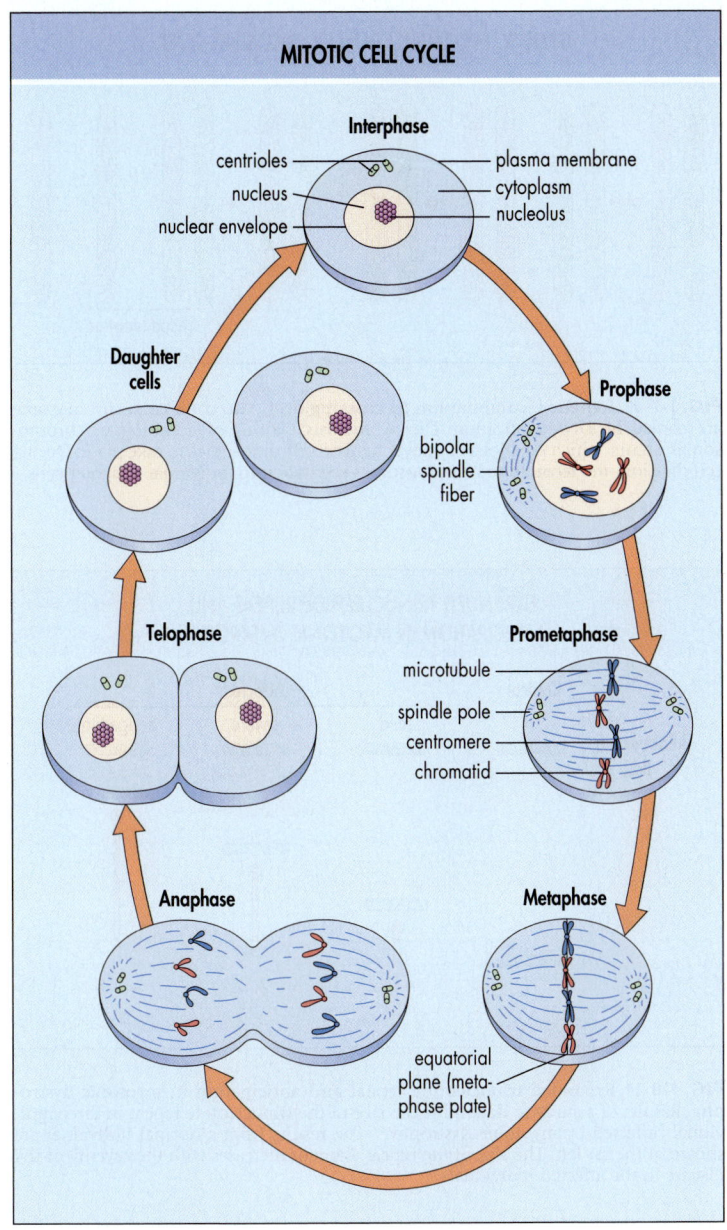

FIG. I-4 ▮▮ **The mitotic cell cycle.** During mitosis, the DNA of a diploid cell is replicated, which results in the formation of a tetraploid cell that divides to form two identical diploid daughter cells.

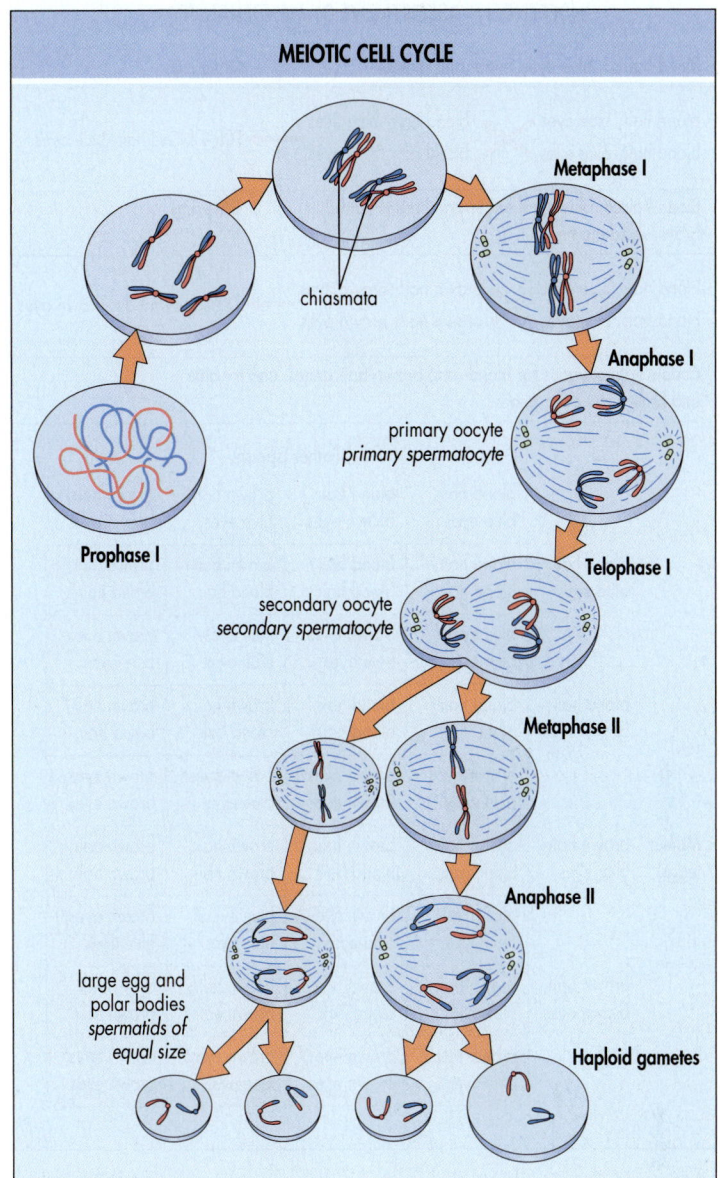

FIG. I-5 ▮▮ **The meiotic cell cycle.** During meiosis, the DNA of a diploid cell is replicated, which results in the formation of a tetraploid cell that divides twice to form four haploid cells (gametes). As a consequence of the crossing over and recombination events that occur during the pairing of homologous chromosomes prior to the first division, the four haploid cells may contain different segments of the original parental chromosomes. For brevity, prophase II and telophase II are not shown.

erozygous for eye color, and 25% will be homozygous for brown eye color). Similarly, 25% of the offspring will have blond hair, and 75% will have brown hair (again, 50% will be heterozygous for hair color, and 25% will be homozygous for brown hair color). However, the 25% of offspring with blue eyes will not necessarily have blond hair. Some offspring will have blond hair and blue eyes, and some offspring will have brown hair and blue eyes. This is because the eye color and hair color genes are located at distinct loci that segregate independently of each other. Independent segregation, or assortment, occurs because maternal and paternal chromosomes segregate randomly into gametes during meiosis, and because of the random recombination that occurs between homologous chromosomes when they pair during meiosis.

At the same time that Mendel observed that most traits segregate independently, according to the law of independent assortment, he unexpectedly found that some traits frequently segregate together. The physical arrangement of genes in a linear array along a chromosome is the explanation for this surprising observation. On average, a recombination event occurs once or twice between two paired homologous chromosomes during meiosis

(Fig. 1-7). Most observable traits, by chance, are located far away from one another on a chromosome, such that recombination is likely to occur between them, or they are located on entirely different chromosomes. If two traits are on separate chromosomes, or a recombination event is likely to occur between them on the same chromosome, the resultant gamete formed during meiosis has a 50% chance of inheriting different alleles from each loci, and the two traits respect the law of independent assortment. If, however, the loci for these two traits are close together on a chromosome, with the result that a recombination event occurs between them only rarely, the alleles at each loci are passed to descendant gametes "in phase." This means that the particular alleles present at each loci in the offspring reflect the orientation in the parent, and the traits appear to be "linked." For example, in Mendel's study of pea plants, curly leaves were always found with pink flowers, even though the genes for curly leaves and pink flowers are located at distinct loci. These traits are linked, because the curly-leaf gene and the pink-flower gene are located close to each other on a chromosome, and a recombination event only rarely occurs between them.

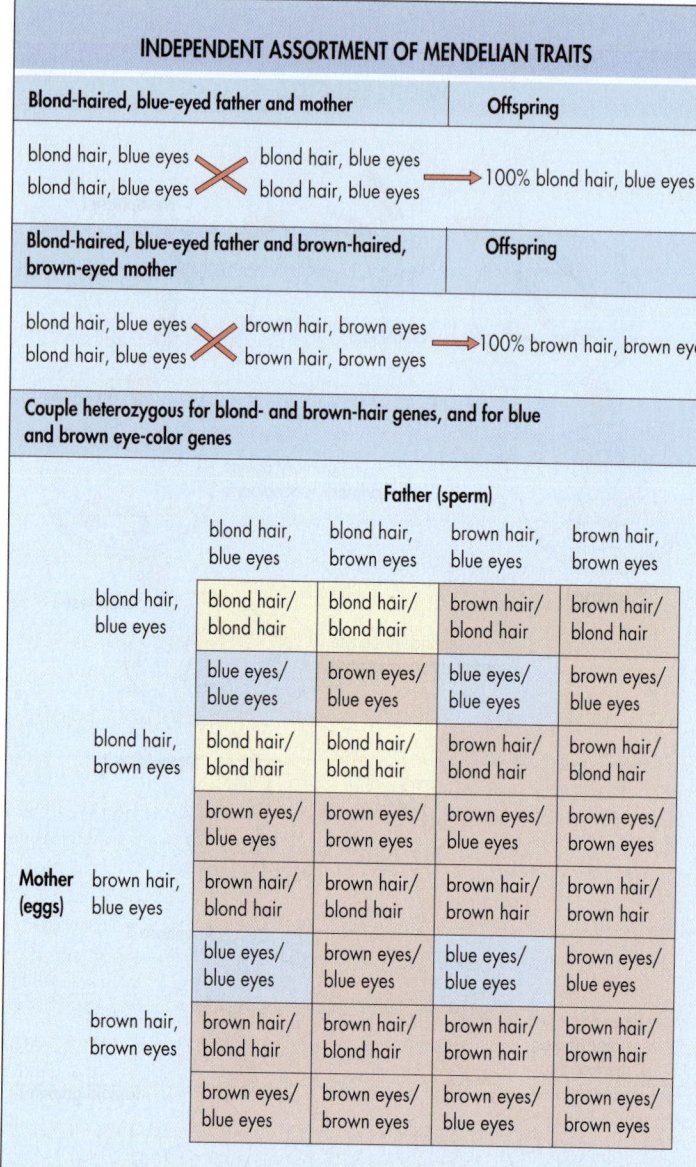

INDEPENDENT ASSORTMENT OF MENDELIAN TRAITS

Blond-haired, blue-eyed father and mother	Offspring
blond hair, blue eyes ✕ blond hair, blue eyes blond hair, blue eyes ✕ blond hair, blue eyes	→ 100% blond hair, blue eyes

Blond-haired, blue-eyed father and brown-haired, brown-eyed mother	Offspring
blond hair, blue eyes ✕ brown hair, brown eyes blond hair, blue eyes ✕ brown hair, brown eyes	→ 100% brown hair, brown eyes

Couple heterozygous for blond- and brown-hair genes, and for blue and brown eye-color genes

		Father (sperm)			
		blond hair, blue eyes	blond hair, brown eyes	brown hair, blue eyes	brown hair, brown eyes
Mother (eggs)	blond hair, blue eyes	blond hair/blond hair blue eyes/blue eyes	blond hair/blond hair brown eyes/blue eyes	brown hair/blond hair blue eyes/blue eyes	brown hair/blond hair brown eyes/blue eyes
	blond hair, brown eyes	blond hair/blond hair brown eyes/blue eyes	blond hair/blond hair brown eyes/brown eyes	brown hair/blond hair brown eyes/blue eyes	brown hair/blond hair brown eyes/brown eyes
	brown hair, blue eyes	brown hair/blond hair blue eyes/blue eyes	brown hair/blond hair brown eyes/blue eyes	brown hair/brown hair blue eyes/blue eyes	brown hair/brown hair brown eyes/blue eyes
	brown hair, brown eyes	brown hair/blond hair brown eyes/blue eyes	brown hair/blond hair brown eyes/brown eyes	brown hair/brown hair blue eyes/blue eyes	brown hair/brown hair brown eyes/brown eyes

FIG. I-6 ■ **Independent assortment of mendelian traits.** Shown are the results of a mating between a blond-haired, blue-eyed father and a blond-haired, blue-eyed mother; a mating between a blond-haired, blue-eyed father and a brown-haired, brown-eyed mother; and a mating between a couple heterozygous for blond and brown hair and for blue and brown eyes.

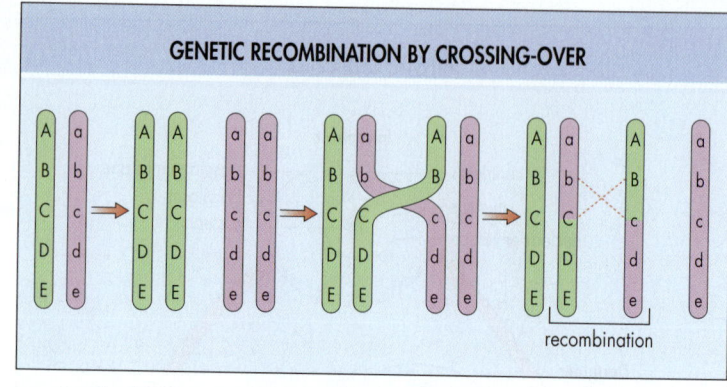

GENETIC RECOMBINATION BY CROSSING-OVER

recombination

FIG. I-7 ■ **Genetic recombination by crossing over.** Two copies of a chromosome are copied by DNA replication. During meiosis, pairing of homologous chromosomes occurs, which enables a crossover between chromosomes to take place. During cell division, the recombined chromosomes separate into individual daughter cells.

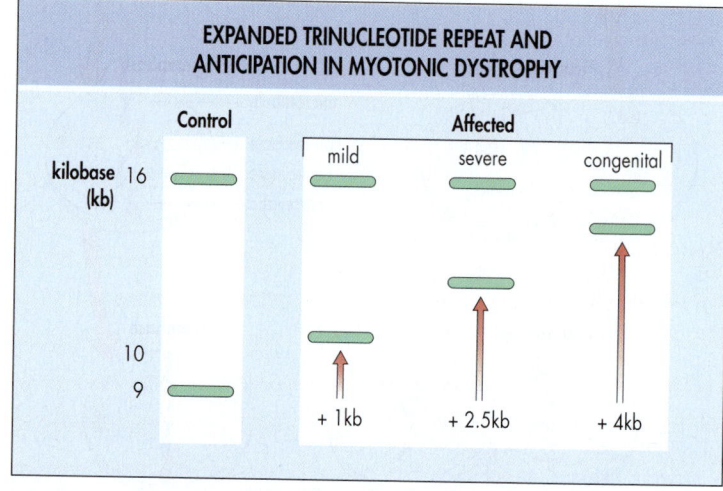

EXPANDED TRINUCLEOTIDE REPEAT AND ANTICIPATION IN MYOTONIC DYSTROPHY

Control   Affected
kilobase (kb)   mild   severe   congenital
16
10
9
+ 1kb   + 2.5kb   + 4kb

FIG. I-8 ■ **Expanded trinucleotide repeat and anticipation in myotonic dystrophy.** Results of a study to determine the size of the trinucleotide repeat in three individuals affected by myotonic dystrophy.[12] The results from a normal individual are shown at the far left. The size of the repeat element increases with the severity of the disease in the affected individuals.

Recombination and linkage are the fundamental concepts behind genetic linkage analysis.[8] The search for a gene responsible for a phenotypic trait (or disease) depends on the ability to observe linkage between the trait and mapped genetic markers. The identification of a marker that segregates with the trait (i.e., is linked genetically to the trait) defines the location of the gene for that trait, because the lack of recombination between the marker and the trait means that the gene responsible for the trait is located physically near the linked marker. The chromosomal locations of genetic markers are readily available to the public as a result of the successful efforts of the nationally funded Human Genome Project.[9] Once an approximate location of a gene responsible for a trait has been determined, analysis of rare recombination events between markers in the region and that trait can help further define the precise physical location of the gene on the chromosome. In this way, "positional cloning" of genes may be accomplished.[9,10]

MUTATIONS

Mutations are changes in the gene DNA sequence that result in a biologically significant change in the function of the encoded protein. If a particular gene is mutated, the protein product might not be made, or it might be produced but work poorly. In some cases, mutations create proteins that have an adverse effect on the cell (dominant negative effect). Point mutations (the substitution of a single base pair) are the most common mutations encountered in human genetics. Missense mutations are point mutations that cause a change in the amino acid sequence of the polypeptide chain. The severity of the missense mutation is dependent on the chemical properties of the switched amino acids and on the importance of a particular amino acid in the function of the mature protein. Point mutations also may decrease the level of polypeptide production because they interrupt the promoter sequence, splice site sequences, or create a premature stop codon.

Gene expression can be affected by the insertion or deletion of large blocks of DNA sequence. These types of mutations are less common than point mutations but may result in a more severe change in the activity of the protein product. A specific category of insertion mutations is the expansion of trinucleotide repeats found in patients affected by certain neurodegenerative disorders. An interesting clinical phenomenon, "anticipation," was understood on a molecular level with the discovery of trinucleotide repeats as the cause of myotonic dystrophy.[11,12] Frequently, offspring with myotonic dystrophy were affected more severely and at an earlier age than their affected parents and grandparents. Examination of the disease-causing trinu-

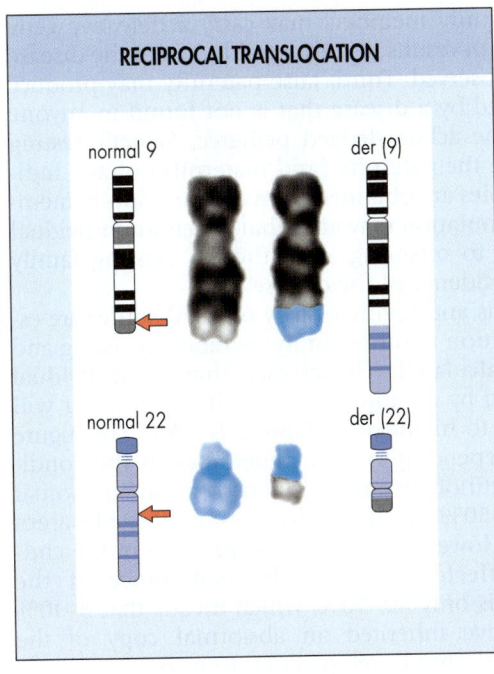

RECIPROCAL TRANSLOCATION

normal 9   der (9)

normal 22   der (22)

FIG. 1-9 ■ Reciprocal translocation between two chromosomes. The Philadelphia chromosome (responsible for chronic myelogenous leukemia) is shown as an example of a reciprocal chromosomal translocation that results in an abnormal gene product responsible for a clinical disorder. In this case, an exchange occurs between the long arm of chromosome 9 and the long arm of chromosome 22.

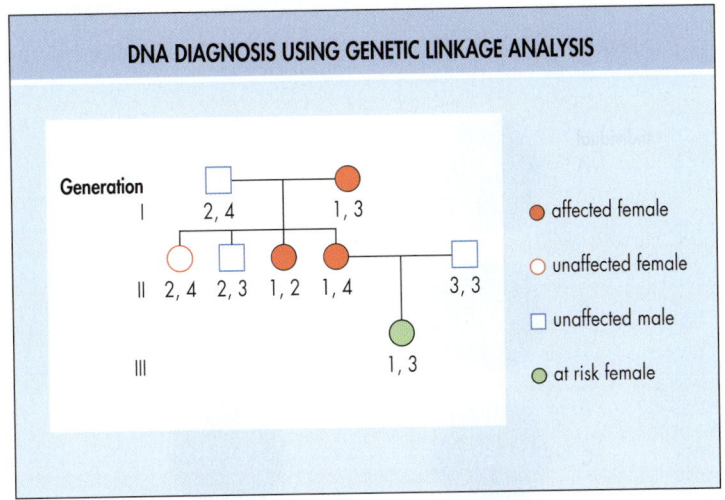

DNA DIAGNOSIS USING GENETIC LINKAGE ANALYSIS

Generation

I   2, 4   1, 3

II   2, 4   2, 3   1, 2   1, 4   3, 3

III   1, 3

● affected female
○ unaffected female
□ unaffected male
● at risk female

FIG. 1-10 ■ DNA diagnosis using genetic linkage analysis. This pedigree shows a mother and two daughters affected by a condition inherited as an autosomal dominant trait. Analysis carried out using a marker closely linked to the disease gene shows that allele 1 segregates with the condition. The daughter in the third generation has inherited this allele from her affected mother, which suggests that she has also inherited the disease gene and is therefore at risk for development of the condition.

cleotide repeat in affected pedigrees demonstrated that the severity of the disease correlated with the number of repeats found in the myotonic dystrophy gene in affected individuals. This phenomenon has been observed in a number of other diseases, including Huntington's disease (Fig. 1-8).

Chromosomal rearrangements may result in breaks in specific genes that cause an interruption in the DNA sequence.[13] Usually, the break in DNA sequence results in a truncated, unstable, dysfunctional protein product; occasionally, the broken gene fuses with another gene to cause a "fusion polypeptide product," which may have a novel activity in the cell. Often such a novel activity results in an abnormality in the function of the cell. An example of such a fusion protein is the product of the chromosome 9;22 translocation that is associated with many cases of leukemia (Fig. 1-9).[14]

DNA-BASED DIAGNOSIS

The use of molecular tools to demonstrate causative DNA mutations and identify individuals at risk for an inherited condition is called DNA-based diagnosis.[15] The goal of genetic diagnosis is early recognition of a disease so that intervention can be undertaken to prevent or reverse the disease process.[16] This was one of the goals of the Human Genome Project.[17] Two general approaches have been used to detect mutations in genes. The indirect approach uses genetic linkage analysis,[18] and the direct approach identifies specific changes in DNA sequence.

Linkage analysis can be used to diagnose any genetically mapped disorder. Segregation of genetic markers known to be linked to a gene responsible for a condition is used to determine whether an individual has inherited a chromosome that carries the abnormal gene. This method does not require physical isolation and sequencing of the gene. Linkage analysis is useful when large genes with many possible mutations are responsible for a disease (Fig. 1-10). Several important disadvantages of this approach must be recognized. First, analysis of DNA from multiple family members is required to identify the markers that segregate with the abnormal chromosome in each affected pedigree. Second, not all genetic markers provide useful information for this analysis. Some individuals may not be "informative" at a particular marker, and a definitive demonstration of the abnormal chromosome may not be possible. Third, recombination may occur between the genetic markers used for testing and the disease-causing mutation. Although the markers selected for the analysis are physically close to the disease gene, a rare recombination event may occur and result in a misdiagnosis be-

cause of an apparent separation between the genetic markers that define the normal and abnormal chromosomes.

Direct mutation analysis uses a variety of techniques based on the DNA sequence of a gene to identify the specific base-pair change that is responsible for the disease. Because this method does not rely on the segregation of genetic markers to identify the abnormal chromosome, multiple family members are not usually required. Also, potential errors caused by rare recombination events between the markers and the disease gene do not occur with this method, but there are several drawbacks to direct mutation analysis. The gene responsible for the disease must first be isolated and sequenced. Some genes are very large (e.g., the gene for retinoblastoma spans more than 200,000 kilobases of DNA sequence) and are difficult and time-consuming to sequence. Multiple mutations and novel mutations present in a single gene may require complete sequencing of the DNA for each diagnostic test.

In some disorders, the majority of stricken individuals are affected by the same mutation. For example, 70% of individuals affected by cystic fibrosis have the delta 508 mutation.[19] For disorders of this type, a simple screening test based on the particular mutation may be developed. This technique involves the synthesis of an oligonucleotide probe that hybridizes only to the mutated sequence. Such a probe, called an allele-specific oligonucleotide, is very useful when the DNA sequence that causes the genetic disease is known and the number of disease-causing mutations is limited (Fig. 1-11). Those patients whose DNA hybridizes with the normal sequence do not have the mutation, and those patients whose DNA hybridizes with the mutant sequence do have the mutation.

GENETIC COUNSELING

Genetic counseling has become an important part of any clinical medicine practice. In 1975, the American Society of Human Genetics adopted the following descriptive definition of genetic counseling[20]:

Genetic counseling is a communication process which deals with the human problems associated with the occurrence or risk of occurrence of a genetic disorder in a family. This process involves an attempt by one or more appropriately trained persons to help the individual or family to: (1) comprehend the medical facts including the diagnosis, probable course of the disorder, and the available management, (2) appreciate the way heredity contributes to the disorder and the risk of recurrence in specified relatives, (3) understand the alternatives for dealing with the

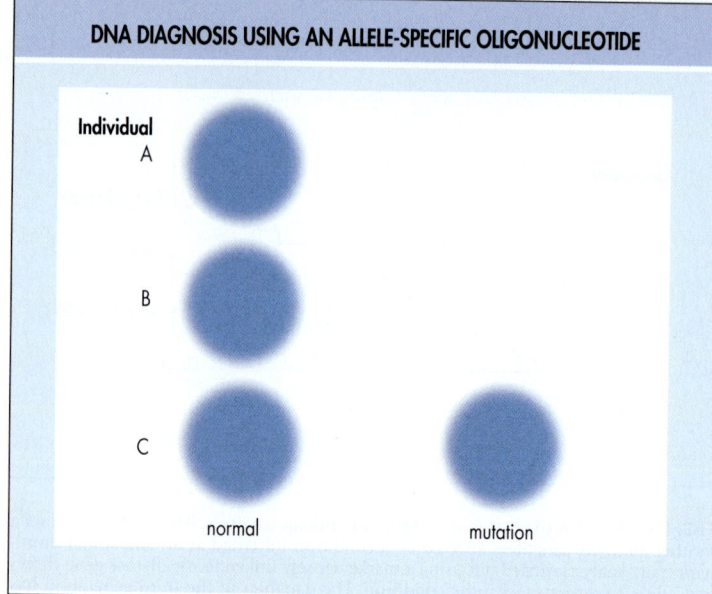

DNA DIAGNOSIS USING AN ALLELE-SPECIFIC OLIGONUCLEOTIDE

FIG. 1-11 ▉ **DNA diagnosis using an allele-specific oligonucleotide.** Oligonucleotides specific for mutations are synthesized, as well as oligonucleotides that correspond to the normal sequence. DNA purified from individuals to be tested is placed on a small "dot" on a piece of filter paper and allowed to hybridize (base pair) with the specific oligonucleotides. Individuals A and B are normal, as their DNA hybridizes with the normal sequence only and not with the mutant sequence. Individual C's DNA hybridizes with both the normal and the mutant sequences; hence, this individual has one normal gene and one mutant gene. Individual C is a carrier of the disease if it is a recessive condition or is affected by the disease if it is a dominant condition.

risk of recurrence, (4) choose a course of action which seems to them appropriate in their view of their risk, their family goals, and their ethical and religious standards and act in accordance with that decision, and (5) to make the best possible adjustment to the disorder in an affected family member and/or to the risk of recurrence of that disorder.

An accurate diagnosis is the first step in productive genetic counseling.[21] The patient-physician discussion of the natural history of the disease and of its prognosis and management is entirely dependent on the correct identification of the disorder that affects the patient. Risk assessment for other family members and options for prenatal diagnosis also depend on an accurate diagnosis. In some cases, appropriate genetic testing may help establish the diagnosis.

A complete family history of the incidence of the disorder is necessary to determine the pattern of inheritance of the condition. The mode of inheritance (i.e., autosomal dominant, autosomal recessive, X-linked, or maternal) must be known to calculate the recurrence risk to additional family members, and it helps confirm the original diagnosis (Fig. 1-12). A family history is recorded most easily as a pedigree using universally recognized nomenclature (Fig. 1-13). For the record of family information, the gender and birth date of each individual and his or her relationship to other family members are indicated using the standard pedigree symbols. It is also helpful to record the age of onset of the disorder in question (as accurately as this can be determined). The pedigree diagram must include as many family members as possible. Miscarriages, stillbirths, and consanguineous parents are indicated.

Occasionally, a patient may appear to be affected by a condition that is known to be inherited, but the patient is unable to provide a family history of the disease. Several important explanations for a negative family history must be considered before the conclusion is made that the patient does not have a heritable condition. First, the patient may not be aware that other family members are affected by the disease. Individuals frequently are reluctant to share information about medical problems, even with close family members. Second, many disorders exhibit variable expressivity or reduced penetrance, which means that other family members may carry a defective gene that is not expressed or results in only a mild form of the disease that is not readily observed. Third, false paternity may produce an individual affected by a disease that is not found in anyone else belonging to the acknowledged pedigree. Genetic testing can easily determine the paternity (and maternity) of any individual if blood samples are obtained from relevant family members. Fourth, a new mutation may arise that affects an individual and may be passed to offspring, even though existing family members show no evidence of the disease.

Once the diagnosis and family history of the disorder are established, risk prediction in other family members (existing and unborn) may be calculated. The chance that an individual known to be affected by an autosomal dominant disorder will transmit the disease to his or her offspring is 50%. This figure may be modified, depending on the penetrance of the condition. For example, retinoblastoma is inherited as an autosomal dominant trait, and 50% of the children of an affected parent should be affected. However, usually only 40–45% of the children at risk are affected, because the penetrance of the retinoblastoma trait is only 80–90%, which means that 5–10% of children who have inherited an abnormal copy of the retinoblastoma gene do not develop ocular tumors.

An individual affected by an autosomal recessive trait will have unaffected children unless he or she partners with another individual affected by the disease or with an individual who is a carrier of the disease. Two individuals affected by an autosomal recessive disease produce only affected offspring. (There are some rare exceptions to this rule. If the disease is the result of mutations in two different genes, it is possible for two individuals affected by an autosomal recessive trait to produce normal children. Also, in rare cases, different mutations in the same gene may compensate for each other, and the resultant offspring will be normal.) If an individual affected by an autosomal recessive disease partners with a heterozygous carrier of a gene defect responsible for that disorder, the chance of producing an affected child is 50%. Among the offspring of an individual affected by an autosomal recessive disease, 50% will be carriers of the disorder. If one of these offspring partners with another carrier of the disease, the chance of producing an affected child is 25%.

X-linked disorders are always passed from a female carrier who has inherited a copy of an abnormal gene on the X chromosome received from either her mother (who was a carrier) or her father (who was affected by the disease). Man-to-man transmission is not seen in diseases caused by defects in genes located on the X chromosome. Among sons born to female carriers of X-linked disorders, 50% are affected by the disease, and 50% of daughters born to female carriers of X-linked disorders are carriers of the disease. All the daughters of men affected by X-linked disorders are carriers of the disease.

Mitochondrial disorders are inherited by sons and daughters from the mother. The frequency of affected offspring and the severity of the disease in affected offspring depend on the number of abnormal mitochondria present in the egg that gives rise to the affected child. Diseased and normal mitochondria are distributed randomly in all cells of the body, including the female gametes. As a result, not all the eggs present in a woman affected by a mitochondrial disorder have the same number of affected mitochondria (heteroplasmy). Men affected by mitochondrial disorders only rarely have affected children, because very few mitochondria in the developing embryo are derived from the sperm used to fertilize the egg.[22]

With careful diagnosis and family history assessment, even sporadic cases of heritable disorders are identifiable. In such cases, an estimate of recurrence risk can be calculated using the available pedigree and clinical information and the statistical principle called Bayes' theorem. These individuals should be referred to clinical genetics services, such as those commonly found in hospital settings (Box 1-1).

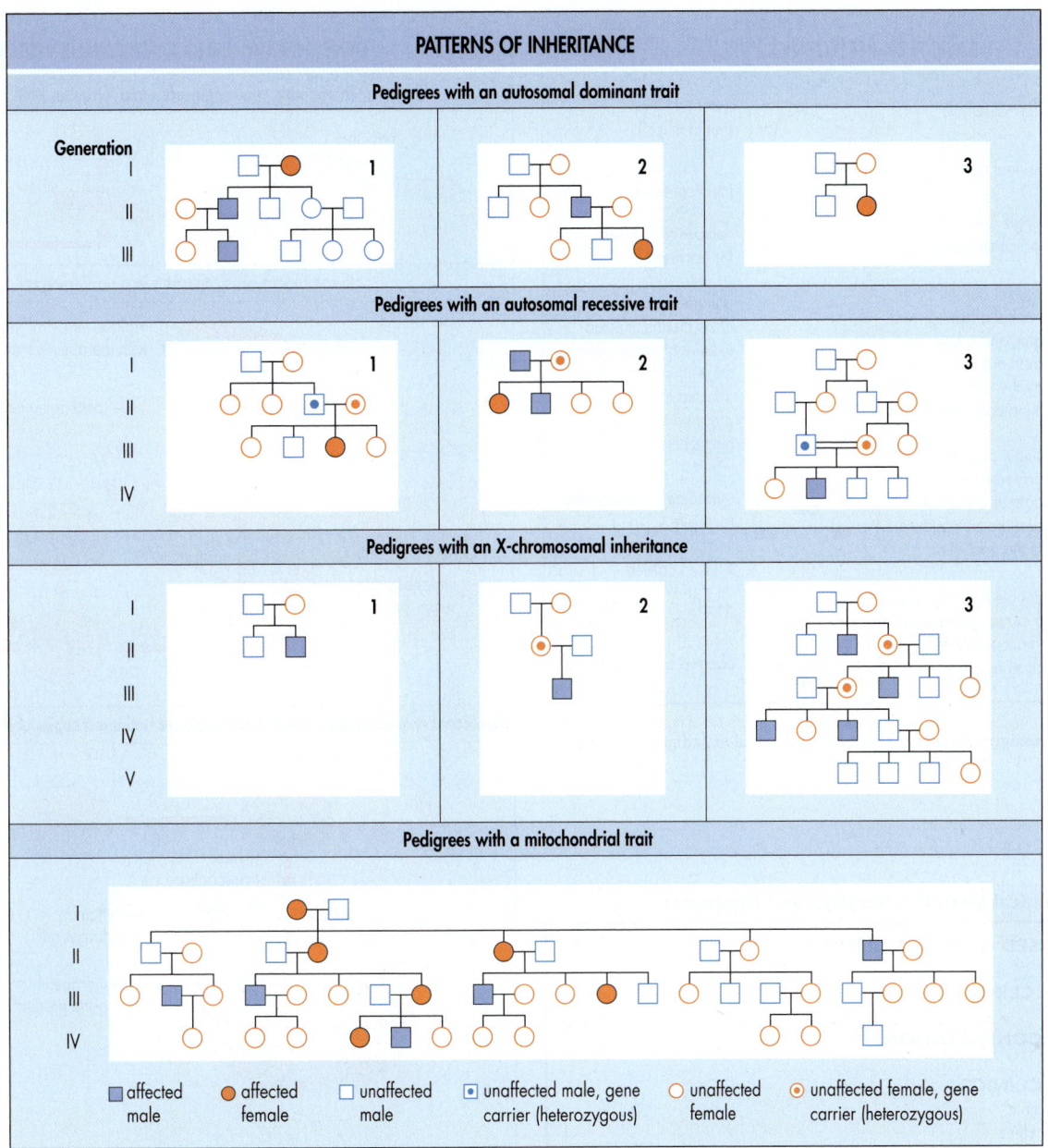

PATTERNS OF INHERITANCE

Pedigrees with an autosomal dominant trait

Generation
I   1   2   3
II
III

Pedigrees with an autosomal recessive trait

I   1   2   3
II
III
IV

Pedigrees with an X-chromosomal inheritance

I   1   2   3
II
III
IV
V

Pedigrees with a mitochondrial trait

I
II
III
IV

■ affected male   ● affected female   □ unaffected male   ⊡ unaffected male, gene carrier (heterozygous)   ○ unaffected female   ⊙ unaffected female, gene carrier (heterozygous)

FIG. 1-12 ■ **Patterns of inheritance.** For pedigrees with an autosomal dominant trait, panel 1 shows inheritance that originates from a previous generation, panel 2 shows segregation that originates in the second generation of this pedigree, and panel 3 shows an apparent "sporadic" case, which is actually a new mutation that arises in the most recent generation. This mutation has a 50% chance of being passed to offspring of the affected individual. For pedigrees with an autosomal recessive trait, panel 1 shows an isolated affected individual in the most recent generation (whose parents are obligatory carriers of the mutant gene responsible for the condition), panel 2 shows a pair of affected siblings whose father is also affected (for the siblings to be affected, the mother must be an obligate carrier of the mutant gene), and panel 3 shows an isolated affected individual in the most recent generation who is a product of a consanguineous marriage between two obligate carriers of the mutant gene. For pedigrees with an X-chromosomal trait, panel 1 shows an isolated affected individual whose disease is caused by a new mutation in the gene responsible for this condition, panel 2 shows an isolated individual who inherited a mutant copy of the gene from the mother (who is an obligate carrier), and panel 3 shows segregation of an X-linked trait through a multigeneration pedigree (50% of the male offspring are affected, and their mothers are obligate carriers of the disease). For pedigrees with a mitochondrial trait, the panel shows a large, multigeneration pedigree—men and women are affected, but only women have affected offspring.

GENE THERAPY

Mutations in the DNA sequence of a particular gene can result in a protein product that is not produced, works poorly, or has adopted a novel function that is detrimental to the cell. Gene therapy involves the delivery of a normal gene to the tissue that contains the flawed gene.[23] Theoretically, a normal copy of the gene can physically take the place of the flawed gene and restore the gene function of the cell. In practice, however, actually replacing the flawed gene with a normal gene is a difficult task.[24] Currently, the aim of gene therapy is to add a useful gene to the cell or tissue that suffers the consequences of the flawed gene. In some cases, the new gene may code for an entirely different protein whose function compensates for the protein encoded by the flawed gene. Useful genes may be delivered to specific tissues that require treatment using modified viruses as vectors.[25] Normally, certain types of viruses invade a host cell, are incorporated into the host genome, and express the viral genes required for replication of the virus. The mature virus eventually takes over the cell, with the result that the cell dies and releases new, infectious viral products that can infect adjacent cells. A general approach to gene therapy is to use an altered (recombinant) virus to carry the gene of interest to the desired tissue. Using genetic engineering techniques, the viral DNA is modified so that the viral genes required for virus proliferation are removed and the therapeutic gene is put in their place. Such a virus may invade the diseased tissue, become incorporated into

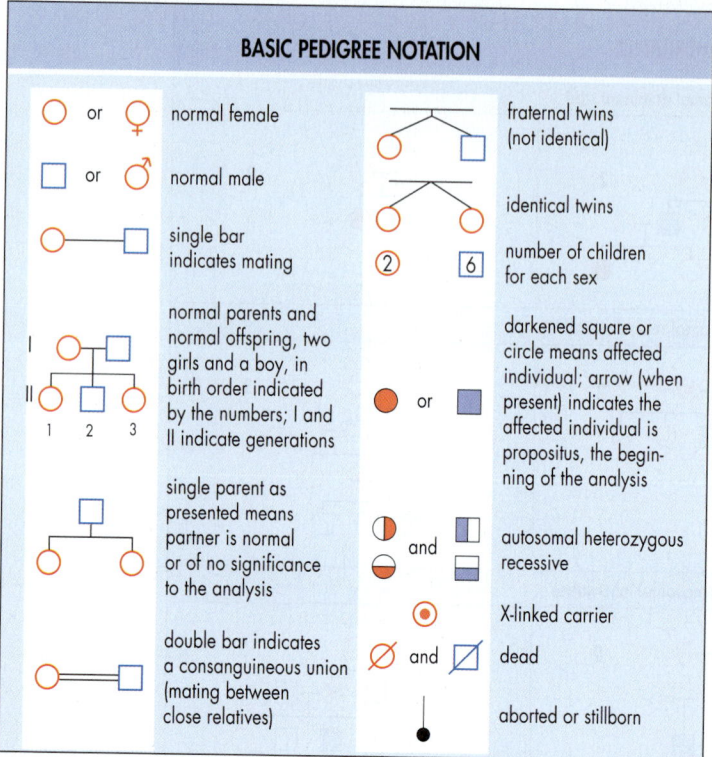

FIG. 1-13 ■ **Basic pedigree notation.** Typical symbols used in pedigree construction are defined.

BOX 1-1

Types of Clinical Genetics Services and Programs

CENTER-BASED GENETICS CLINIC

OUTREACH CLINICS

INPATIENT CONSULTATIONS

SPECIALTY CLINICS
- metabolic clinic
- spina bifida clinic
- hemophilia clinic
- craniofacial clinic
- other single-disorder clinics (e.g., neurofibromatosis 1 clinic)

PRENATAL DIAGNOSIS PROGRAM: PERINATAL GENETICS
- amniocentesis/chorionic villus sampling clinics
- ultrasound program
- maternal serum α-fetoprotein program

GENETIC SCREENING
- newborn screening program/follow-up clinic
- other population-screening programs (e.g., for Tay–Sachs disease)

EDUCATION/TRAINING
- health-care professional
- general public
- school system
- teratology information services

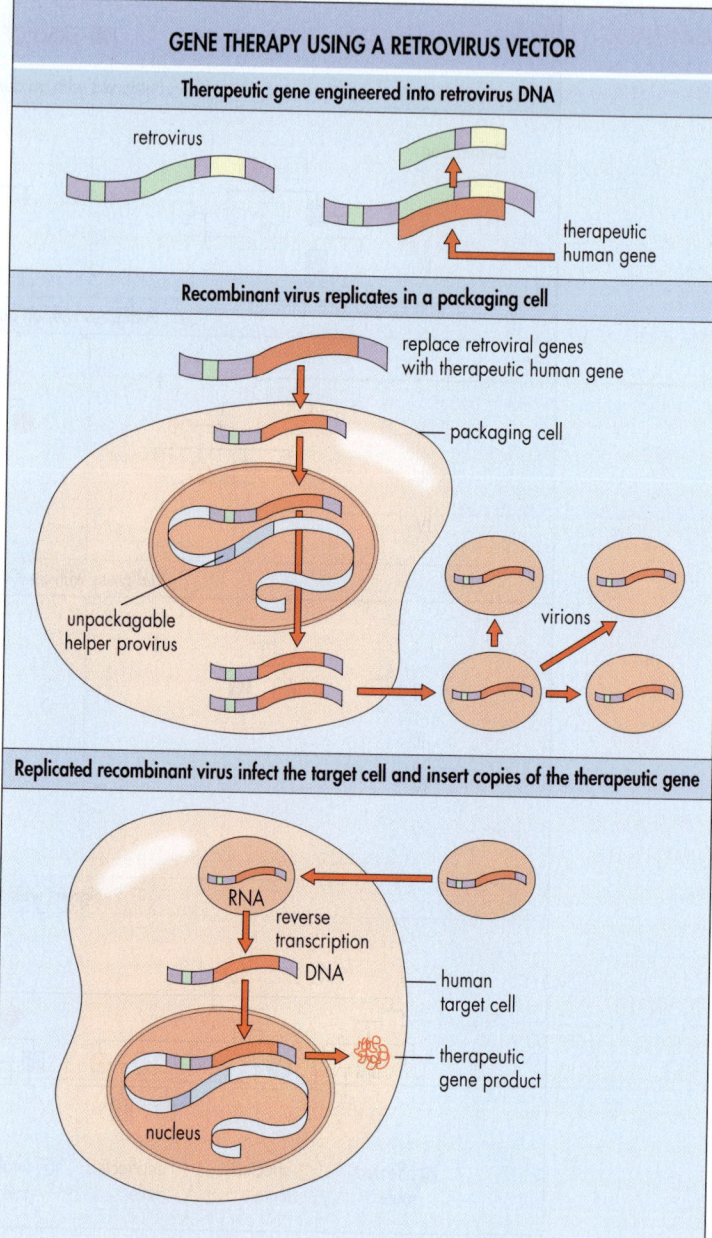

FIG. 1-14 ■ **Gene therapy using a retrovirus vector.** A therapeutic gene is engineered genetically into the retrovirus DNA and replaces most of the viral DNA sequences. The "recombinant virus" that carries the therapeutic gene is allowed to replicate in a special "packaging cell," which also contains normal virus that carries the genes required for viral replication. The replicated recombinant virus is allowed to infect the human diseased tissue, or "target cell." The recombinant virus may invade the diseased tissue but cannot replicate or destroy the cell. The recombinant virus inserts copies of the normal therapeutic gene into the host genome and produces the normal protein product.

Diseases caused by mutations that create a gene product destructive to the cell need to be treated using a different approach. In these cases, genes or oligonucleotides that may inactivate the mutated gene are introduced into the cell. This is called "antisense therapy," and it is proving to be a useful approach for diseases caused by the "gain of function mutations." A number of different viral vectors likely to be useful for gene therapy are currently under investigation. In addition, evaluation of nonviral mechanisms for the introduction of therapeutic genes into diseased tissue is ongoing.

In general, most of the current approaches to gene therapy are aimed at repairing the somatic cells of the particular tissue affected by the disease gene.[27] Gene delivery may be tailored to the somatic cells affected by the disorder. Gene therapy of ocular disorders benefits from the accessibility of the eye, the ability to visualize the diseased tissue, and the large number of specific

the host DNA, and express the desired gene. Because the modified virus does not have the viral genes required for viral replication, the virus cannot proliferate, and the host cell does not die (Fig. 1-14). A successful example of this approach has recently been demonstrated by the restoration of vision in a canine model of Leber congenital amaurosis using a recombinant adeno-associated virus carrying the normal gene (RPE65).[26]

gene defects known to be responsible for many inherited eye disorders.[28]

Specific treatment of the diseased cells does not affect the other cells of the body, which include the germline cells. Because the germline cells continue to carry flawed copies of the gene, the disease may still be passed to offspring of the affected patient. Gene therapy targeted to germline cells as well as the diseased somatic cells results in successful treatment of the disease in the affected individual and prevents transfer of the disease to any offspring.

REFERENCES

1. Watson JD, Crick FHC. Molecular structure of nucleic acids: a structure for deoxyribose nucleic acid. Nature. 1953;171:737–8.
2. Clayton DA. Structure, replication, and transcription of DNA. In: Leder P, Clayton DA, Rubenstein E, eds. Introduction in molecular medicine. New York: Scientific American; 1994.
3. Kelman Z, O'Donnel M. DNA replication: enzymology and mechanisms. Curr Opin Genet Dev. 1994;4:185–95.
4. Murray A, Hunt T. The cell cycle: an introduction. Oxford: Oxford University Press; 1994.
5. Bentley DR, Dunham I. Mapping human chromosomes. Curr Opin Genet Dev. 1995;5:328–34.
6. Gardiner K. Human genome organization. Curr Opin Genet Dev. 1995;5:315–22.
7. McKusick VA. Mendelian inheritance in man: catalogs of autosomal dominant, autosomal recessive, and X-linked phenotypes, ed 11. Baltimore: Johns Hopkins University Press; 1994.
8. McKusick VA. Medical genetics: a 40-year perspective on the evolution of a medical specialty from a basic science. JAMA. 1993;270:2351–6.
9. International Human Genome Sequencing Consortium. Initial sequencing and analysis of the human genome. Nature 2001;409:860–921.
10. Collins FS. Positional cloning moves from perditional to traditional. Nat Genet. 1995;9:347–50.
11. Harper PS, Harley WG, Reardon W, Shaw DJ. Anticipation in myotonic dystrophy: new light on an old problem. Am J Hum Genet. 1992;51:10–6.
12. Warren ST. The expanding world of trinucleotide repeats. Science. 1996;271:1374–5.
13. Shaikh TH, Kurahashi H, Emanuel BS. Evolutionarily conserved low copy repeats (LCRs) in 22q11 mediate deletions, duplications, translocations, and genomic instability: an update and literature review. Genet Med. 2001;3:6-13.
14. Rabbitts TH. Chromosomal translocations in human cancer. Nature. 1994;372:143–9.
15. Korf B. Molecular diagnosis. N Engl J Med. 1995;332:1218–20.
16. Caskey CT. Presymptomatic diagnosis: a first step toward genetic health care. Science. 1993;262:48–9.
17. Collins FS, Patrinos A, Jordan E, et al. New goals of the US Human Genome Project: 1998–2003. Science. 1998;282:682–9.
18. Ott J. Analysis of human genetic linkage, ed 2. Baltimore: Johns Hopkins University Press; 1991.
19. Bobadilla JL, Macek M Jr, Fine JP, Farrell PM. Cystic fibrosis: a worldwide analysis of CFTR mutations—correlation with incidence data and application to screening. Hum Mutat. 2002;19:575–606.
20. National Academy of Sciences. Genetic screening: programs, principles and research. Washington, DC: National Academy of Sciences; 1975.
21. Harper PS. Practical genetic counseling, ed 4. Oxford: Butterworth Heinemann; 1993.
22. Wallace DC. Mitochondrial DNA sequence variation in human evolution and disease. Proc Natl Acad Sci U S A. 1994;91:8739–46.
23. Friedmann T, Roblin R. Gene therapy for human genetic disease. Science. 1972;175:949–55.
24. Wolff JA, Malone RW, Williams P, et al. Direct gene transfer into mouse muscle in vivo. Science. 1990;247:1465–8.
25. Lee RJ, Huang L. Lipidic vector systems for gene transfer. Crit Rev Ther Drug Carrier Syst. 1997;14:173–206.
26. Acland GM, Aguirre GD, Ray J, et al. Gene therapy restores vision in a canine model of childhood blindness. Nat Genet. 2001;28:92–5.
27. Brenner MK. Human somatic gene therapy: progress and problems. J Intern Med. 1995;237:229–39.
28. Bennett J, Maguire AM. Gene therapy for ocular disease. Mol Ther. 2000;1:501–5.

2

Molecular Genetics of Selected Ocular Disorders

JANEY L. WIGGS

INTRODUCTION

Tremendous advances in the molecular genetics of human disease have been made in the past 10 years. Many genes responsible for inherited eye disease have been isolated and characterized, and the chromosomal location of a number of additional genes has been determined (Table 2-1). The goal of this work is to understand how mutated genes cause human ocular disease. This knowledge will lead to improved methods of diagnosis and treatment and will ultimately improve the prognosis for vision. The disorders discussed in this chapter represent the latest advances in human ocular molecular genetics and illustrate important principles of human genetics.

Mutations of DNA that occur in genes may result in the formation of a defective gene product. If the normal protein product of a mutated gene is necessary for a critical biological function, an alteration of the normal phenotype may occur. Many changes in phenotype are normal variations of human traits (for example, brown hair instead of blond hair). However, some changes cause severe cellular dysfunction, which may be the cause of a disease.

Although all inherited disorders are the result of gene mutations, the molecular consequences of a mutation are quite variable. The type of mutation responsible for a disease usually defines the inheritance pattern. For example, mutations that create an abnormal protein detrimental to the cell are typically autosomal dominant, because only one mutant gene is required to disrupt the normal functions of the cell. Mutations that result in proteins that have reduced biological activity (loss of function) may be inherited as autosomal dominant or autosomal recessive conditions, depending on the number of copies of normal genes (and the amount of normal protein) required. Disorders may be caused by mutations in mitochondrial DNA that result in a characteristic inheritance pattern. Also, mutations in genes carried on the X chromosome result in characteristic inheritance patterns.

DOMINANT CORNEAL DYSTROPHIES

The autosomal dominant corneal dystrophies are an excellent example of dominant negative mutations that result in the formation of a toxic protein. Four types of autosomal dominant dystrophies that affect the stroma of the cornea have been described:

- Groenouw's (granular) type I.[1]
- Lattice type I.[2]
- Avellino (combined granular-lattice).[3,4]
- Reis-Bücklers'.[5]

Although all four corneal dystrophies affect the anterior stroma, the clinical and pathological features differ. The granular dystrophies typically form discrete, white, localized deposits that may obscure vision progressively. Histopathologically, these deposits stain bright red with Masson trichrome and have been termed "hyalin." In lattice dystrophy, branching amyloid deposits gradually opacify the visual axis. These deposits exhibit a characteristic birefringence under polarized light after staining with Congo red. Avellino dystrophy includes features of both granular and lattice dystrophies. Reis-Bücklers' dystrophy appears to involve primarily Bowman's layer and the superficial stroma.

All four dystrophies have been mapped genetically to a common interval on chromosome 5q31.[6–9] Mutations in a single gene, big–h3, located in this region have been identified in affected families.[10] The product of this gene, keratoepithelin, is probably an extracellular matrix protein that modulates cell adhesion. Four different missense mutations, which occur at two arginine codons in the gene, have been found (Fig. 2-1). Interestingly, mutations at one of these arginine codons cause lattice dystrophy type I or Avellino dystrophy, the two dystrophies characterized by amyloid deposits. Mutations at the other arginine codon appear to result in either granular dystrophy or Reis-Bücklers' dystrophy. The mutation analysis of this gene demonstrates that different mutations within a single gene can result in different phenotypes.

The mutation that causes Avellino and lattice dystrophies abolishes a putative phosphorylation site, which probably is required for the normal structure of keratoepithelin. Destruction of this aspect of the protein structure leads to formation of the amyloid deposits that are responsible for opacification of the cornea. Consequently, the mutant protein is destructive to the normal tissue.

Meesmann's corneal dystrophy is an autosomal dominant condition that affects the corneal epithelium. The corneal changes consist of fine, punctate opacities in the epithelium and occasionally in Bowman's membrane (see Chapter 59).[11] The intermediate filament cytoskeleton of corneal epithelial cells is composed of cornea-specific keratins K3 and K12. Genetic linkage studies indicate that a gene responsible for this condition is located on the same region of chromosome 12q13 as the location of the K3 and K12 genes. Recently, heterozygous missense mutations in the genes that code for K3 and K12 have been discovered in affected pedigrees,[12] which are likely to be dominant negative or gain of function mutations that result in instability of the corneal epithelium.

ANIRIDIA, PETER'S ANOMALY, AUTOSOMAL DOMINANT KERATITIS

Some cellular processes require a level of protein production that results from the expression of both copies of a particular gene. Such proteins may be involved in a variety of biological processes. Certain disorders are caused by the disruption of one copy of a gene that reduces the protein level by half. Such a reduction is also called "haploinsufficiency."

Mutations in the Pax6 gene are responsible for aniridia, Peter's anomaly, and autosomal dominant keratitis (see Chapters 58 and 59).[13–15] Most of the mutations responsible for these disorders alter the paired-box sequence within the gene (Fig. 2-2) and result in inactivation of one copy of the Pax6 gene. The paired-box sequence is an important regulatory element that participates in regulation of the expression of other genes.[16]

TABLE 2-1

SELECTED GENES RESPONSIBLE FOR HEREDITARY OPHTHALMIC DISEASES

Location	Disease	Gene
Cornea	Dominant corneal dystrophies (lattice, macular, Avellino, Reis-Bücklers')	Keratoepithelin (5q31)
	Meesmann's corneal dystrophy	Keratin K3 (12q12–q13)
	Cornea plana (type 2 AR)	KERA (keratocan) (12q)
	Fuchs' endothelial corneal dystrophy	Collagen type VIII (1p34)
Anterior segment	Rieger's syndrome	PITX2 (4q25)
	Iridodysgenesis	FOXC1 (6p25)
	Aniridia Peters' anomaly	Pax6 (11q13)
	Juvenile open-angle glaucoma	Myocilin (TIGR) (1q25)
	Adult open-angle glaucoma	
	Congenital glaucoma	CYP1B1 (2p16)
	Glaucoma /nail-patella syndrome	LMX1B (9q34)
	Normal-tension glaucoma	Optineurin (10p15)
Lens	Zonular pulverulent cataract	Connexin 50 (1q21)
		γ-C-crystallin (2q35)
		Connexin 46 (13q11)
	Nuclear cataract	γ-D-crystallin (2q33)
	Coppock cataract	γ-E-crystallin (2q33)
	Dominant congenital cataract	BFSP2 (3q21-q22)
		α-A-crystallin (21q22)
	Congenital posterior	
	Polar cataract	α-B-crystallin (11q21)
	Congenital progressive	
	Polymorphic cataract	MIP AQP0 (12q)
	Zonular sutural cataract	β-A3-crystallin (17q11)
	Presenile cataract	LIM2 (19q)
	Cerulean-blue dot	β-B2-crystallin (22q)
	Dominant pulverulent	β-B1-crystallin (22q)
Retina	Retinoblastoma	RB1 (13q14)
	Tritanopia	Blue opsin (7q22)
	X-linked color blindness	Red cone opsin (Xq22-q28)
		Green cone opsin (Xq22-q28)
	Retinitis pigmentosa (AD)	Rhodopsin (3q21)
		RP1 (8p11)
		RGR (10q23)
		ROM1 (11q13)
		NRL (14q11)
		CRX (19q13)
		PRKCG (19q13)
	Retinitis pigmentosa (AR)	RPE65 (1p31)
		ABCA4 (1p21)
		CRB1 (1q31)
		USH2A (1q41)
		MERTK (2q14)
		SAG (arrestin) (2q37)
		Rhodopsin (3q21)
		PDE6B (4p16)
		CNG1 (4p14)
		PDE6A (5q31)
		TULP1 (6p21)
		RGR (10q23)
		NR2E3 (15q23)
		RLBP1 (15q26)
	Retinitis pigmentosa (X-linked)	RPGR (Xp11)
		RP2 (Xp11)
	Retinitis pigmentosa (digenic)	RDS (peripherin) (6p21)
		ROM1 (11q13)
	Usher's syndrome type I	Myosin VIIa (11q13)
	Congenital stationary night blindness	Rhodopsin (3q21)
		Rod transducin (alpha subunit) (3p21)
		Rod cGMP-phosphodiesterase (4p16)
	Oguchi's disease	Rod arrestin (2q37)
		Rhodopsin kinase (13q34)
	Sorsby's macular dystrophy	TIMP3 (22q12)
	Stargardt's disease	ABCR4 (1p21)
	Norrie's disease	Norrie's disease gene (Xp11)
	Leber's congenital amaurosis	RPE65 (1p31)
		Guanylate cyclase (17p13)
	Gyrate atrophy	Ornithine aminotransferase (10q26)
	Abetalipoproteinemia	Microsomal triglyceride transfer protein (4q22)
	Refsum's disease	Phytanoyl-CoA alpha-hydroxylase (10pter)
	Ocular albinism	OA1 (Xp22)
Neuro-ophthalmic	Leber's optic atrophy	Mitochondrial proteins
	Kjer AD optic atrophy	OPA1 (3q28)
	Kearns-Sayre syndrome	Mitochondrial DNA deletions
	Congenital extraocular fibrosis	ARIX (PHOX2A) (12cen)
	Duane's radial ray syndrome	SALL4 (20q13)

AD, Autosomal dominant; *AR,* autosomal recessive.

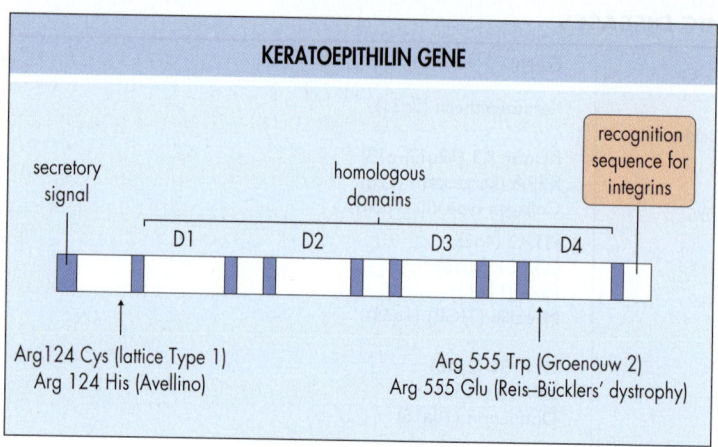

FIG. 2-1 ■ **Keratoepithelin gene.** Arrows point to the location of the reported mutations.

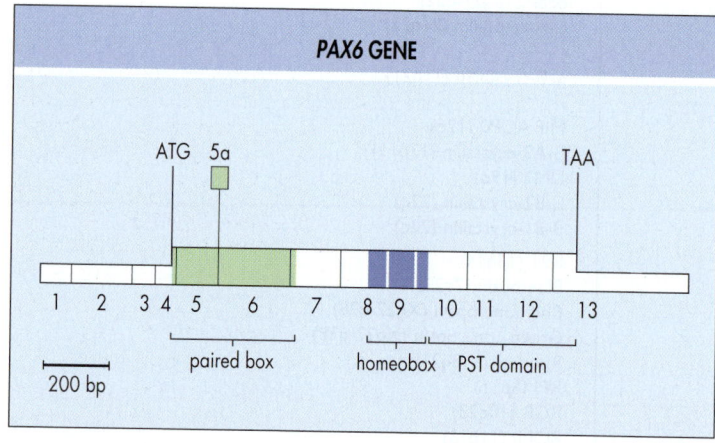

FIG. 2-2 ■ The *Pax6* gene. (Data with permission from Glaser T, *et al. PAX6* gene mutations in aniridia. In: Wiggs JL, ed. Molecular genetics of ocular disease. New York: Wiley-Liss; 1995:51–82.)

Losing half the normal paired-box sequence, and probably other regulatory elements of the *Pax6* gene, appears to be the critical event that results in the disease.[17] *Pax6* plays an important role in ocular development, presumably by regulation of the expression of genes that are involved in embryogenesis of the eye. A reduction in the amount of active gene product alters the expression of these genes, which results in abnormal development. The genes that code for the lens crystallin proteins are one class of genes developmentally regulated by *Pax6*.[18]

The clinical disorders caused by mutations in *Pax6* exhibit extensive phenotypic variability. Similar mutations may give rise to aniridia, Peters' anomaly, or autosomal dominant keratitis.[19] This spectrum of phenotypic abnormalities that results from mutations in one gene is termed "variable expressivity" and is a common feature of disorders that arise from haploinsufficiency. Possibly, the variability of the mutant phenotype results from the random activation of downstream genes that occurs when only half the required gene product is available.

RIEGER'S SYNDROME

Rieger's syndrome is an autosomal dominant disorder of morphogenesis that results in abnormal development of the anterior segment of the eye.[20] Typical clinical findings may include posterior embryotoxon, iris hypoplasia, iridocorneal adhesions, and corectopia (see Chapter 58). Approximately 50% of affected individuals develop a high-pressure glaucoma associated with severe optic nerve disease. The cause of the glaucoma associated with this syndrome is not known, although anomalous development of the anterior chamber angle structures is usually found.[21]

Genetic heterogeneity of Rieger's syndrome is suggested by descriptions of affected individuals who have a variety of chromosomal abnormalities, which include deletions of chromosome 4[22] and deletions of chromosome 13.[23] Genes for Rieger's syndrome have been located on chromosomes 4q25,[24] 13q14,[23] and 6p25.[25] Iris hypoplasia is the dominant clinical feature of pedigrees linked to the 6p25 locus, whereas pedigrees linked to 4q25 and 13q14 demonstrate the full range of ocular and systemic abnormalities found in these patients.

The loci of genes responsible for Rieger's syndrome on chromosomes 4q25 and 6p25 have been identified. The chromosome 4q25 gene (*RIEG1*) codes for a bicoid homeobox transcription factor.[26] Like *Pax6*, this gene is expressed during eye development and is probably involved in the processes that result in a normal eye. Future studies designed to investigate the interaction of this gene with other genes involved in eye development, such as *Pax6*, will be of great interest. The chromosome 6p25 gene, *FOXC1* (also called *FKHL7*), is a member of a fork-head family of regulatory proteins.[27] FOXC1 is expressed during ocular development, and mutations in the gene cause a loss of function or haploinsufficiency, resulting in a reduction in the active protein product.[28] The identification of other genes responsible for Rieger's syndrome and anterior segment dysgenesis is necessary to determine whether these genes are part of a common developmental pathway or represent redundant functions necessary for eye development.

JUVENILE GLAUCOMA

Primary juvenile open-angle glaucoma is a rare disorder that develops during the first two decades of life. Affected patients typically present with a high intraocular pressure, which ultimately requires surgical therapy.[29,30] Juvenile glaucoma may be inherited as an autosomal dominant trait. Large pedigrees have been identified and used for genetic linkage analysis. One gene responsible for this condition, myocilin (also known as TIGR, trabecular meshwork glucocorticoid response protein), is located on chromosome 1q23 (*GLC1A*).[31–34]

Myocilin has been shown to be expressed in the human retina, ciliary body, and trabecular meshwork.[35,36] In the retina, the gene is localized to a region that connects the inner and outer segments of the photoreceptors. The protein has several functional domains, including a region homologous to a family of proteins called olfactomedins. Although the function of the protein and the olfactomedin domain is not known, nearly all the mutations associated with glaucoma have been found in the olfactomedin portion of the protein (Fig. 2-3). Mutations in myocilin also have been associated with some cases of adult-onset primary open-angle glaucoma. It is unclear why mutations in this gene cause glaucoma and why some mutations cause juvenile-onset disease and others result in adult-onset disease. Patients with only one copy of the myocilin gene (because of chromosomal deletion removing the second copy of the gene) or without any functional myocilin (caused by homozygosity of a stop-codon polymorphism in the first part of the gene) do not develop glaucoma.[37,38] These results suggest that mutations in myocilin cause a gain of function or dominant negative effect rather than a loss of function or haploinsufficiency. Disruption of the myocilin gene in the mouse also supports this conclusion.[39]

CONGENITAL GLAUCOMA

Previous studies suggest that congenital glaucoma is largely an inherited condition that is genetically heterogeneous.[40] Pedigrees from a variety of ethnic origins affected by autosomal recessive forms of the disease have been reported. Cytogenetic abnormalities that involve a number of different chromosome have been described. Collectively, these results suggest that many different genes may be responsible for this condition.[41]

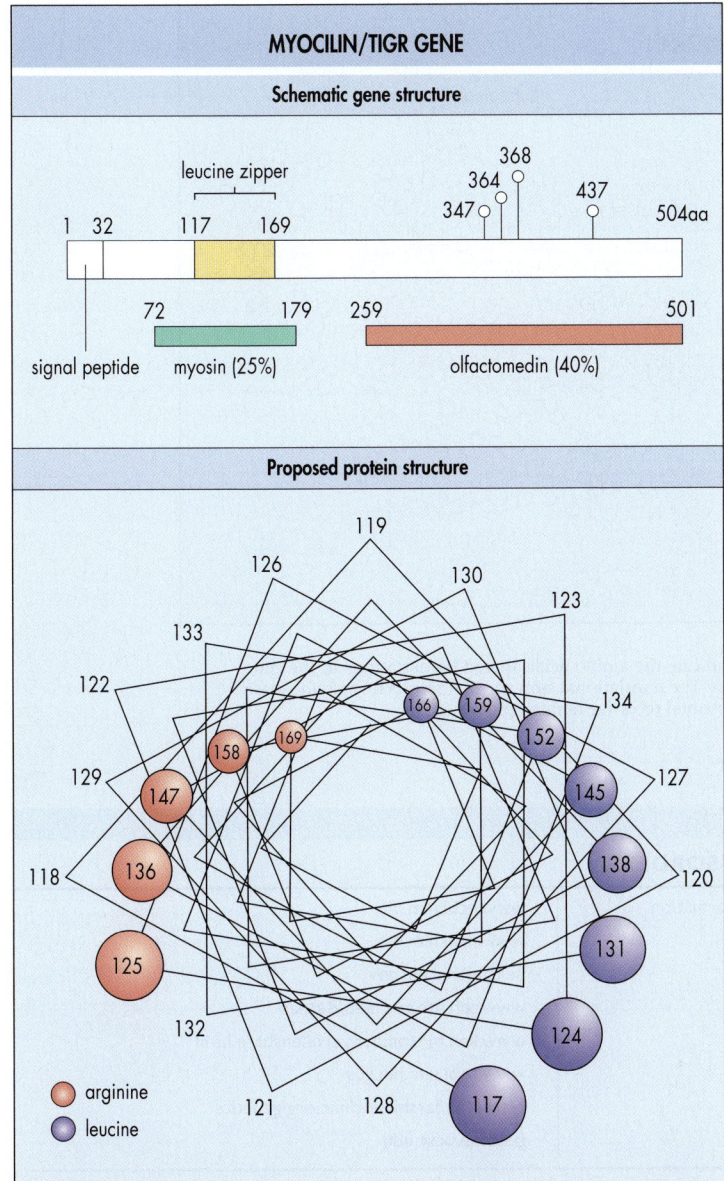

FIG. 2-3 ▌ Myocilin–trabecular meshwork glucocorticoid response (TIGR) protein gene. The myosin-like domain, the olfactomedin-like domain, and the leucine zipper are indicated. Amino acids altered in patients with juvenile- or adult-onset glaucoma are shown. (Data with permission from Orteto J, Escribano J, Coca-Prados M. Cloning and characterization of subtracted cDNAs from a human ciliary body library encoding TIGR, a protein involved in juvenile open angle glaucoma with homology to myosin and olfactomedin. FEBS Lett. 1997;413:349–53.)

Two genes responsible for autosomal recessive forms of congenital glaucoma have been located in the human genome (*GLC3A* at 2p21, and *GLC3B* at 1p36).[42] The responsible gene at the chromosome 2p21 location, *CYP1B1*, is a member of the cytochrome P-450 family of proteins.[43] Mutations in *CYP1B1* have been identified in patients with autosomal recessive congenital glaucoma from all over the world. Responsible mutations disrupt the function of the protein, implying that a loss of function of the protein results in the phenotype.[44] Several of the identified mutations are recurrent and are likely to be the result of founder chromosomes that have been distributed to many populations throughout the world.[45] Because the defects responsible for congenital glaucoma are predominantly developmental, cytochrome P-4501B1 must play a direct or indirect role in the development of the anterior segment of the eye.

NONSYNDROMIC CONGENITAL CATARACT

At least one third of all congenital cataracts are familial and are not associated with other abnormalities of the eye or with systemic abnormalities. Two forms of familial cataract inherited as autosomal dominant traits have been shown to be caused by abnormalities in human lens crystallin proteins.

Cerulean cataracts have peripheral bluish and white opacifications in concentric layers. Genes of one form of congenital cerulean cataract were mapped to a region of chromosome 22 that contains three β-crystallin genes.[46] Individuals affected by this form of cerulean cataract have a chain-terminating mutation in one of the β-crystallin genes, *CRYBB2*, which results in a reduction in the level of active protein product.[47] It is interesting to speculate how the loss of the normal levels of this protein results in the formation of the cataracts. Some investigators suggest that the lens proteins are not simply soluble, structural proteins but also may function as enzymes or be closely related to enzymes. Further work is necessary to resolve this intriguing problem.

The human γ-crystallin genes constitute a multigene family that contains at least seven highly related members. All seven of the γ-crystallin genes have been assigned to chromosome 2q34–q35.[48,49] Of the genes mapped to this region, only two of them, γ-C and γ-D, encode abundant proteins. Two of the genes, γ-E and γ-F, are pseudogenes, which means they are not expressed in the normal lens.[50] A pedigree affected by the Coppock cataract, a congenital cataract that involves primarily the embryonic lens, was shown to be linked genetically to the region that contains the γ-crystallin genes.[51] In individuals affected by the Coppock cataract, additional regulatory sequences have been found in the promoter region of the γ-E pseudogene.[52] This result implies that the γ-E pseudogene is expressed in affected individuals and that expression of the pseudogene is the event that leads to cataract formation.

A number of other genes have been associated with hereditary cataract (see Table 2-1). A useful collection of mutations and phenotypes can be found at LENSNET (http://ken.mitton.com/ern/lensbase.html) and OMIM (http://www.ncbi.nlm.nih.gov) (Table 2-2).

RETINITIS PIGMENTOSA

The molecular genetics of retinitis pigmentosa is exceedingly complex. Twenty-six genes responsible for retinitis pigmentosa had been identified, and an additional 14 genes had been mapped but not yet found.[53] Most of these genes are expressed preferentially in the retina, but some are expressed systematically. A useful resource listing genes responsible for various forms of retinal diseases, including retinitis pigmentosa, can be found at the RETNET website (http://www.sph.uth.tmc.edu/Retnet/).

The form of autosomal dominant retinitis pigmentosa caused by mutations in rhodopsin demonstrates how mutant proteins can interfere with normal cellular processes. Initially, one form of autosomal dominant retinitis pigmentosa was mapped to chromosome 3q24.[54] Using a candidate gene approach, the rhodopsin gene was identified as the cause of the disease in affected families.[55] Many of the first mutations detected in the rhodopsin protein were missense mutations located in the C-terminus of the gene (Fig. 2-4). To explore the pathogenic mechanisms of these mutations, transgenic mice were created that carried mutant copies of the gene.[56] Histopathological studies of these mice showed an accumulation of vesicles that contained rhodopsin at the junction between the inner and outer segments of the photoreceptors. The vesicles probably interfere with the normal regeneration of the photoreceptors, thus causing photoreceptor degeneration. Because the C-terminus of the nascent polypeptide is involved in the transport of the maturing protein, the accumulation of rhodopsin-filled vesicles is likely to result from abnormal transport of the mutant rhodopsin to the membranes of the outer segments.

Null mutations (mutations that cause a prematurely shortened or truncated protein) also have been found in the rhodopsin gene in patients who have autosomal recessive retinitis pigmentosa (see Fig. 2-4).[57] Mutations responsible for reces-

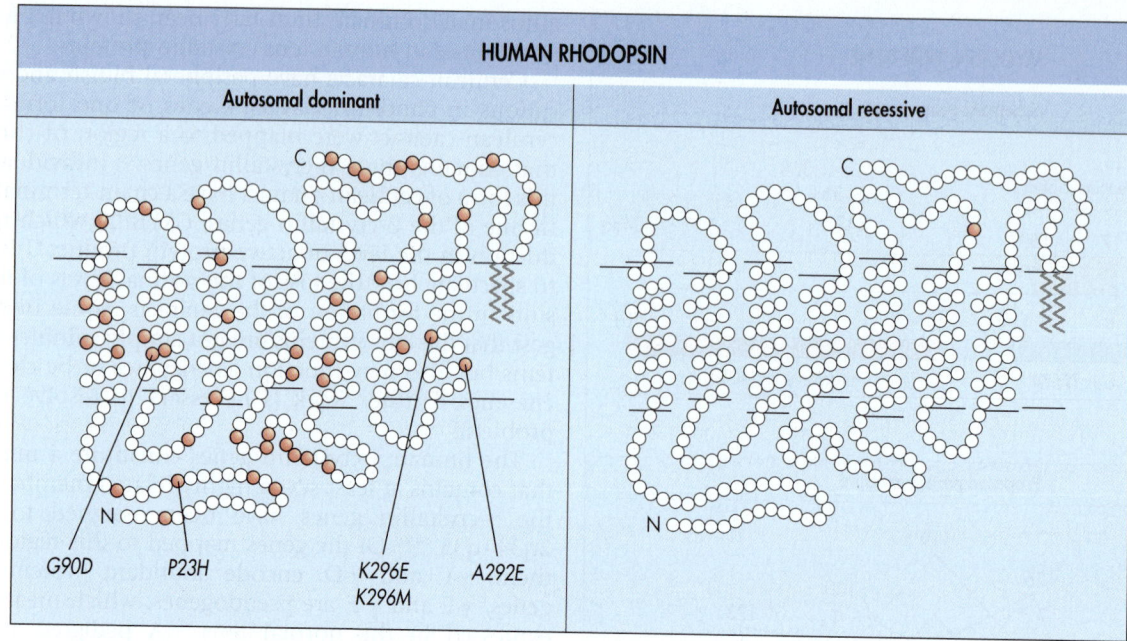

FIG. 2-4 ■ **Human rhodopsin mutations.** The red circles indicate the amino acids altered by mutations in the gene in patients who have autosomal dominant retinitis pigmentosa. The translational stop site that results from a nonsense mutation is indicated as a red circle in a patient who has autosomal recessive retinitis pigmentosa.

TABLE 2-2

WEB-BASED RESOURCES FOR INHERITED HUMAN OCULAR DISORDERS

NCBI	National Center for Biotechnology Information	www.ncbi.nlm.nih
OMIM	Online Mendelian Inheritance in Man	www.ncbi.nlm.nih
NEIBank	Expression databases	neibank.nei.nih.gov
RetNet	Retinal disease genes	www.sph.uth.tmc.edu/Retnet/
LENSNET	Lens disease genes	www.ken.mitton.com/ern/lensbase.html
GENES and DISEASE	Systemic inherited disorders	www.ncbi.nlm.nih.gov
Center for Medical Genetics	Gene and genetic marker maps	research.marshfieldclinic.org/genetics
UCSC	Human Genome Sequence	genome.ucsc.edu

sive disease typically cause a loss of biological activity, either because they create a defective protein product that has little or no biological activity or because they interfere with the normal expression of the gene (regulatory mutations). Most individuals heterozygous for autosomal recessive disorders are clinically normal. Unlike the missense mutations responsible for the dominant form of the disease, the null mutations in rhodopsin produce an inactive protein that is not destructive to the cell. Null mutations result in retinitis pigmentosa only when they are present in both copies of the gene. Mutations in just one copy of the gene (heterozygous individuals) do not have a clinically detectable phenotype.

One form of retinitis pigmentosa has been shown to be inherited as a digenic trait. Digenic inheritance is a newly described pattern of inheritance in humans. A disease inherited as a digenic trait develops only when mutations are found in each of two independent genes simultaneously. Digenic inheritance is an example of the complex interactions that occur between multiple gene products in polygenic inheritance (see later).

Three families affected by retinitis pigmentosa were found to have unusual features for a typically dominantly inherited disease[58]:

- The disease originated in the offspring of two unaffected individuals.
- Affected individuals transmitted the disease to less than 50% of their offspring.
- Many asymptomatic individuals were carriers of an identifiable mutation.

Mutation analysis of the peripherin gene and the *ROM1* gene showed that affected individuals had specific mutations in both genes. Individuals who had a mutation in one copy of either gene were unaffected by the disease (see Fig. 2-4). Mutant copies of *ROM1* and peripherin also may cause autosomal dominant forms of retinitis pigmentosa.[59,60] These results suggest that some mutant forms of peripherin and *ROM1* cause retinitis pigmentosa in a digenic pattern, whereas other mutations independently cause autosomal dominant forms of the disease.

STARGARDT'S DISEASE (MACULAR DEGENERATION)

Stargardt's disease is characterized by progressive bilateral atrophy of the macular retinal pigment epithelium (RPE) and neuroepithelium, with the frequent appearance of orange-yellow flecks distributed around the macula. The choroid is characteristically dark on fluorescein angiography. Stargardt's disease results in a loss of central acuity that may have a juvenile to adult onset; it is inherited as an autosomal recessive trait. In the simplest terms, this observation suggests that disruption of one copy of the gene is not sufficient to result in the disease phenotype. Inactivation of both copies of the responsible gene is necessary to cause the disease. Mutations in a photoreceptor cell–specific ATP-binding transporter gene (*ABCR*) have been found in patients affected by autosomal recessive Stargardt's disease.[61] Most of the mutations reported to date are missense mutations in conserved amino acid positions. All the individuals affected by Stargardt's disease have mutations in both copies of the gene.

The retina-specific ABC transporter responsible for Stargardt's disease is a member of a family of transporter proteins[62] and is expressed in rod photoreceptors, which indicates that this protein mediates the transport of an essential molecule either into or out of photoreceptor cells. Accumulation of a lipofuscin-like substance in Stargardt's disease may result from inactivation of this transporter protein.

Patients who have age-related macular degeneration (ARMD) also may demonstrate an accumulation of lipofuscin-like substance in the RPE and progressive atrophy of the macular RPE.[63] Various genetic forms of retinal degeneration with possible phenotypic overlap with ARMD have been identified; however, none of these genes is associated with a significant fraction of patients with ARMD.[64]

X-LINKED JUVENILE RETINOSCHISIS

Retinoschisis is a maculopathy caused by intraretinal splitting; the defect most likely involves retinal Müller cells.[65] Retinoschisis is inherited as an X-linked recessive trait. X-linked recessive disorders, like autosomal recessive disorders, result from a mutant gene that causes loss of a critical biological activity. Because men have only one X chromosome, one mutant copy of a gene responsible for an X-linked trait results in the disease. Usually, women are heterozygous carriers of recessive X-linked traits and do not demonstrate any clinical abnormalities.

Mutations in a gene located in the retinoschisis region on the X chromosome,[66] and expressed in the retina, have been found in a protein that is implicated in cell-cell interaction and may be active in cell adhesion processes during retinal development. Mutational analysis of the retinoschisis gene (XLRS1) in affected individuals from nine unrelated families showed one nonsense, one frameshift, one splice acceptor, and six missense mutations.[67] Presumably, these mutations all result in an inactive protein product.

NORRIE'S DISEASE

Norrie's disease is an X-linked disorder characterized by progressive, bilateral, congenital blindness associated with a dysplastic process of the retina that has been referred to as a "pseudoglioma" (see Chapter 120). The disease also may be associated with mental retardation and hearing defects.[68] Norrie's disease is inherited as an X-linked recessive trait, and a locus on the X chromosome has been identified using genetic linkage analysis.[69] Subsequent cloning and characterization of the Norrie's disease gene showed that the gene product has a tertiary structure similar to transforming growth factor-β.[70-73] This result suggests that the Norrie's disease protein is implicated in the regulation of neural cell differentiation and proliferation.[73]

SORSBY'S MACULAR DYSTROPHY

Sorsby's macular dystrophy is an autosomal dominant disorder characterized by macular edema, hemorrhages, and exudate.[74] The disease typically begins at about 40 years of age. Several missense mutations in the gene that codes for tissue inhibitor metalloproteinase-3 have been found in affected individuals.[75-77] This protein is involved in remodeling of the extracellular matrix. Inactivation of the protein may lead to an increase in activity of the metalloproteinase, which may contribute to the pathogenesis of the disease.

GYRATE ATROPHY

Hyperornithinemia results from deficiency of the enzyme ornithine ketoacid aminotransferase and has been shown to be the cause of gyrate atrophy, an autosomal recessive condition characterized by circular areas of chorioretinal atrophy.[78] Mutations in the gene for ornithine ketoacid aminotransferase mapped to chromosome 10q26 have been associated with the disease in affected individuals.[79,80] Most of the responsible mutations are missense mutations, which presumably result in an inactive enzyme. One mutation has been found in homozygous form in the vast majority of apparently unrelated cases of gyrate atrophy in Finland, an example of a founder effect that produces a common mutation in an isolated population.

Identification of the enzyme defect responsible for this disease makes it an interesting candidate for gene therapy. Previous studies indicated that a lower ornithine level, achieved through a strict low-arginine diet, may retard the progression of the disease.[81] Replacement of the abnormal gene, or genetic engineering to produce a supply of normal enzyme, may result in a reduction of ornithine levels without dietary restrictions.

COLOR VISION

Defective red-green color vision affects 2–6% of men and results from a variety of defects that involve the color vision genes. In humans, the three cone pigments—blue, green, and red—mediate color vision. Each visual pigment consists of an integral membrane apoprotein bound to the chromophore 11-cis retinal. The genes for the red and green pigments are located on the X chromosome, and the gene for the blue pigment is located on chromosome 7. The X chromosome location of the red and green pigment genes accounts for the X-linked inheritance pattern observed in red or green color vision defects.

The common variations in red or green color vision are caused by the loss of either the red or the green cone pigment (dichromasy) or by the production of a visual pigment with a shifted absorption spectrum (anomalous trichromasy). A single amino acid change (serine to alanine) in the red pigment gene is the most common color vision variation. Among Caucasian men, 62% have serine at position 180 in the red pigment protein, and 38% have alanine in this position. Men who carry the red pigment with serine at position 180 have a greater sensitivity to long-wavelength radiation than do men who carry alanine at this position.[82]

The red and green pigment genes are organized in a head-to-tail tandem array, and the DNA sequence of the genes is 98% identical. Such an arrangement of repetitive sequences predisposes to unequal recombination that may generate variant arrays in which entire repeat units are gained or lost. Unequal recombination also may generate genes that are red and green hybrids.[83] These hybrid genes are the cause of anomalous trichromasy. Most X chromosomes carry more than one green pigment gene, and occasionally, some of the green pigment genes are not expressed. It is possible, therefore, to have an abnormal green pigment gene but have normal color vision (Fig. 2-5).

Complete absence of the red and green pigment genes results in blue cone monochromasy. Two different types of mutations have been identified as the cause of this condition. First, unequal recombination may reduce the number of red and green pigment genes to one or two genes that are dysfunctional because of point mutations.[84] The second type of mutation that results in this condition is a deletion of the X chromosome that removes the locus control region that allows for normal expression of the red and green pigment genes. In this case, the red and green pigment genes are normal but are not expressed because of the absence or inactivity of the locus control region (see Fig. 2-5).[85]

RETINOBLASTOMA

A gene responsible for the childhood eye tumor retinoblastoma was identified in 1986 on chromosome 13q14.[86] The gene product is involved in regulation of the cell cycle.[87] Absence of

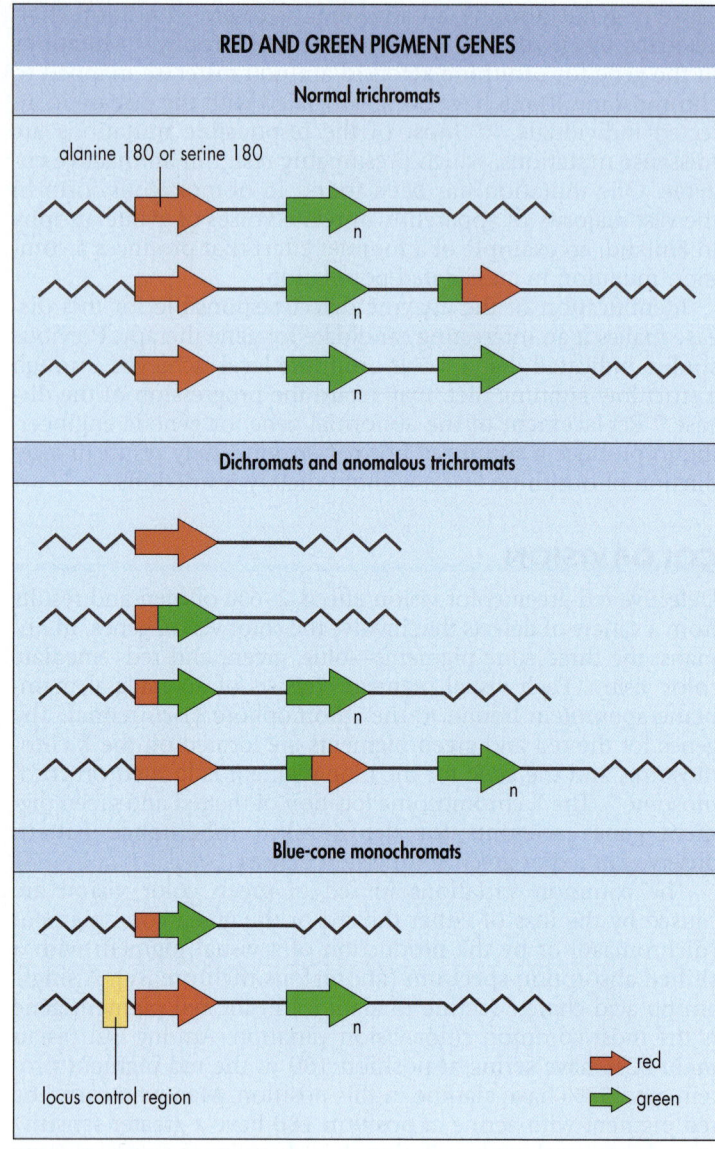

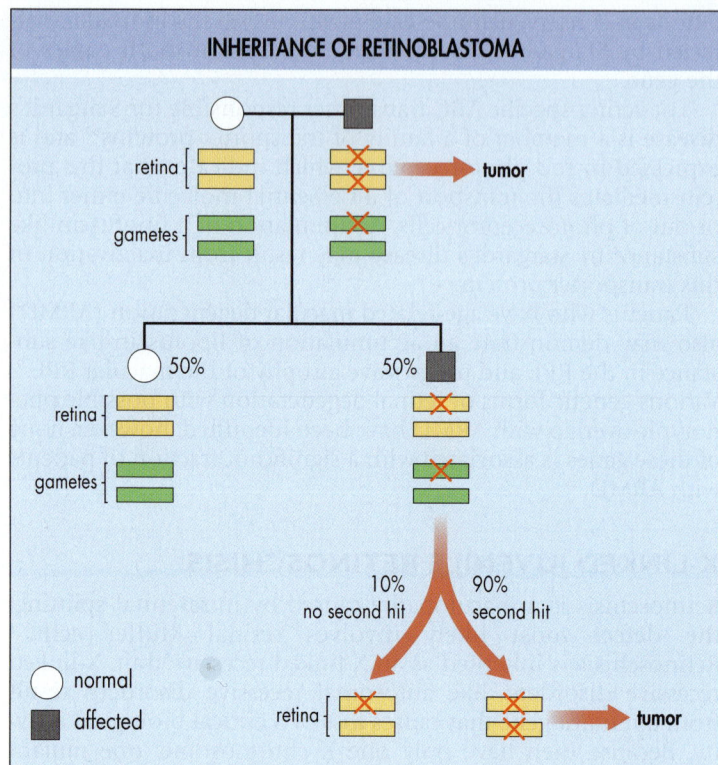

FIG. 2-5 ■ **Red and green pigment genes.** Shown for individuals who have normal and variant red and green color vision. (Data with permission from Nathans J. In the eye of the beholder: visual pigments and inherited variation in human vision. Cell. 1994;78:357–60.)

FIG. 2-6 ■ **Inheritance of retinoblastoma.** Individuals who inherit a mutation in the retinoblastoma gene are heterozygous for the mutation in all cells of the body. The "second hit" to the remaining normal copy of the gene occurs in a developing retinal cell and leads to tumor formation (see text for explanation).

this protein in an embryonic retinal cell results in the uncontrolled cell growth that eventually produces a tumor (see Chapter 146). Susceptibility to hereditary retinoblastoma is inherited as an autosomal dominant trait. Mutations in the retinoblastoma gene result in underproduction of the protein product or production of an inactive protein product.[88] A retinal cell that has only one mutant copy of the retinoblastoma gene does not become a tumor. However, inactivation of the remaining normal copy of the retinoblastoma gene is very likely in at least one retinal cell out of the millions present in each retina. Among individuals who inherit a mutant copy of the retinoblastoma gene, 90% sustain a second hit to the remaining normal copy of the gene and develop a tumor (Fig. 2-6).[89] Fifty percent of the offspring of individuals affected by hereditary retinoblastoma inherit the mutant copy of the gene and are predisposed to develop the tumor. Approximately 10% of individuals who inherit a mutant copy of the gene do not sustain a second mutation and do not develop a tumor. The offspring of these "carrier" individuals also have a 50% chance of inheriting the mutant copy of the retinoblastoma gene (see Fig. 2-6).

ALBINISM

Autosomal recessive diseases often result from defects in enzymatic proteins. Albinism is the result of a series of defects in the synthesis of melanin pigment.[90] Melanin is synthesized from the amino acid tyrosine, which is first converted into dihydroxyphenylalanine through the action of the copper-containing enzyme tyrosinase. An absence of tyrosinase results in one form of albinism. Mutations in the gene that codes for tyrosinase are responsible for tyrosinase-negative ocular cutaneous albinism. Most of the mutations responsible for this disease cluster in the binding sites for copper and disrupt the metal ion–protein interaction necessary for enzyme function.[91] Both copies of the gene for tyrosinase must be mutated before a significant interruption of melanin production occurs. Heterozygous individuals do not have a clinically apparent phenotype, which suggests that one functional copy of the gene produces sufficient active enzyme for the melanin level to be phenotypically normal (Fig. 2-7).

LEBER'S OPTIC NEUROPATHY

Mutations in mitochondrial DNA are an important cause of human disease. Disorders that result from mutations in mitochondrial DNA demonstrate a maternal inheritance pattern. Maternal inheritance differs from mendelian inheritance, in that men and women are affected equally, and only affected females transmit the disease to their offspring. The characteristic segregation and assortment of mendelian disorders depend on the meiotic division of maternal and paternal chromosomes found in the nucleus of cells. In contrast, mitochondrial DNA is derived from the maternal egg and replicates and divides with the cell cytoplasm by simple fission. A mutation that occurs in mitochondrial DNA is present in all cells of the organism, which includes the gametes. Female eggs have abnormal mitochondria that may be passed to offspring. Sperm contain mitochondria but do not transmit mitochondria to the fertilized egg. A man who carries a mitochondrial DNA mutation may be affected by the disease, but he cannot transmit the disease to his offspring.

Leber's hereditary optic neuropathy was one of the first diseases to be recognized as a mitochondrial DNA disorder.[92] For some time, clinicians had observed maternal inheritance of this

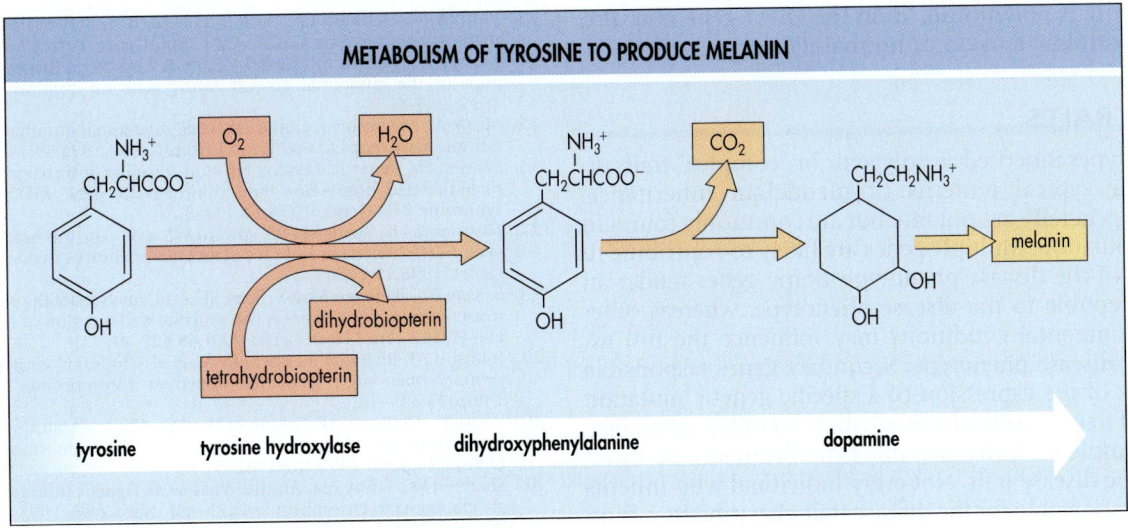

FIG. 2-7 ■ Metabolism of tyrosine to produce melanin. In the final step, dopamine is converted into an indole derivative that condenses to form the high-molecular-weight pigment melanin.

condition in affected families. In familial cases of the disease, all affected individuals were related through the maternal lineage, consistent with inheritance of human mitochondrial DNA.

Patients affected by Leber's hereditary optic neuropathy typically present in midlife with acute or subacute, painless, central vision loss that results in a permanent central scotoma and loss of sight. The manifestation of the disease varies tremendously, especially with respect to onset of visual loss and severity of the outcome. The eyes may be affected simultaneously or sequentially; the disease may progress rapidly, over a period of weeks to months, or slowly over several years; within a family, the disease may also vary among affected members. Several factors contribute to the variable phenotype of this condition. Certain mutations are associated with more severe disease. For example, the most severely affected patients who carry the 11778bp mutation may have no light perception, whereas the most severely affected patients who carry the 3460bp mutation may retain light perception.[93,94] Another important factor that affects the severity of the disease is the heteroplasmic distribution of mutant and normal mitochondria. Not all mitochondria present in diseased tissue carry DNA mutations. During cell division, mitochondria and other cytoplasmic organelles are distributed arbitrarily to the daughter cells. Consequently, the daughter cells are likely to have unequal numbers of mutant and normal mitochondria (Fig. 2-8). Because the diseased mitochondria are distributed to developing tissues, some tissues accumulate more abnormal mitochondria than others. Hence, some individuals have more abnormal mitochondria in the optic nerve and develop a more severe optic neuropathy.[95]

CONGENITAL FIBROSIS SYNDROMES

Congenital fibrosis of the extraocular muscles and Duane's syndrome are inherited forms of congenital fibrosis and strabismus. Five congenital fibrosis loci have been mapped (three for congenital fibrosis of the extraocular muscles, and two for variants of Duane's syndrome).[96] Recently, genes for congenital fibrosis of extraocular muscles type 2 (ARIX/PHOX2A)[97] and Duane's radial ray syndrome (SALL4)[98] have been identified. Interestingly, both these genes participate in developmental processes, suggesting that these syndromes are developmental defects of the ocular muscles or the nerve nuclei controlling the muscles.

AUTOSOMAL DOMINANT OPTIC ATROPHY

Of the inherited optic atrophies, autosomal dominant optic atrophy of the Kjer type is the most common. This disease results

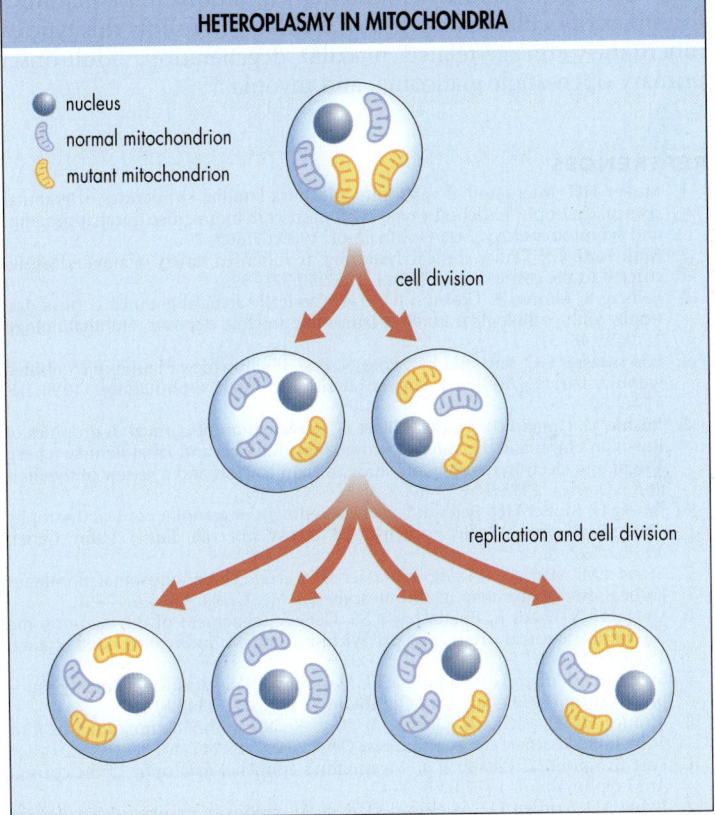

FIG. 2-8 ■ Heteroplasmy in mitochondria. Daughter cells that result from the division of a cell that contains mitochondria with mutant DNA may contain unequal numbers of mutant mitochondria. Subsequent divisions lead to a population of cells with different numbers of normal and abnormal mitochondria.

in a progressive loss of visual acuity, centrocecal scotoma, and bilateral temporal atrophy of the optic nerve. The onset is typically in the first two decades of life. The condition is inherited as an autosomal dominant trait with variable expressivity, and a locus was mapped to chromosome 3q28–q29.[99] Mutations in a gene located in this region, *OPA1*, have been found in a number of affected families.[100] The gene product is a dynamin-related GTPase that is targeted to mitochondria and may function to stabilize mitochondrial membrane integrity. It is interesting that this gene and the gene responsible for another optic atrophy, Leber's hereditary optic atrophy (see earlier), both function in the mitochondria, emphasizing the role of mitochondria in optic nerve function. A polymorphism in the *OPA1* gene may also be associated with low-tension or normal-tension glaucoma.[101]

COMPLEX TRAITS

Human phenotypes inherited as polygenic or "complex" traits do not follow the typical patterns of mendelian inheritance. Complex traits generally are not rare but are commonly found in the human population. Multiple genes are likely to contribute to the expression of the disease phenotype. Some genes render an individual susceptible to the disease phenotype, whereas other genes or environmental conditions may influence the full expression of the disease phenotype. Secondary genes responsible for modulation of the expression of a specific genetic mutation may be referred to as "modifier genes"; these modifier genes may be inherited completely independently from the gene directly responsible for the disease trait. Not every individual who inherits the mutation responsible for the disease trait also inherits a form of the modifier gene that is required for full expression of the disease. The digenic inheritance of retinitis pigmentosa that occurs via certain mutant alleles of peripherin and *ROM1* is an example of the simplest form of polygenic inheritance (see earlier). Certain conditions may require multiple genes or a combination of different genes and environmental conditions to be manifest. Examples of ocular disorders that are likely to follow this type of inheritance are age-related macular degeneration, adult-onset primary open-angle glaucoma, and myopia.[102]

REFERENCES

1. Moller HU. Inter-familial variability and intra-familial similarities of granular corneal dystrophy Groenouw type I with respect to biomicroscopical appearance and symptomatology. Acta Ophthalmol. 1989;67:669–77.
2. Klintworth GK. Lattice corneal dystrophy: an inherited variety of amyloidosis restricted to the cornea. Am J Pathol. 1967;50:371–99.
3. Folberg R, Alfonso E, Croxatto JO, et al. Clinically atypical granular corneal dystrophy with pathologic features of lattice-like amyloid deposits. Ophthalmology. 1988;95:46–51.
4. Rosenwasser GO, Sucheski BM, Rosa N, et al. Phenotypic variation in combined granular-lattice (Avellino) corneal dystrophy. Arch Ophthalmol. 1993;111:1546–52.
5. Kuchle M, Green WR, Volcker HE, et al. Reevaluation of corneal dystrophies of Bowman's layer and the anterior stroma (Reis-Bucklers and Thiel-Behnke types): a light and electron microscopic study of eight corneas and a review of the literature. Cornea. 1995;14:333–54.
6. Eiberg H, Moller HU, Berendt I, et al. Assignment of granular corneal dystrophy Groenouw type I locus to within a 2 cM interval. Eur J Hum Genet. 1994;2:132–8.
7. Stone EM, Mathers WD, Rosenwasser GO, et al. Three autosomal dominant corneal dystrophies map to chromosome 5q. Nat Genet. 1994;6:47–51.
8. Gregory CY, Evans K, Bhattacharya SS. Genetic refinement of the chromosome 5q lattice corneal dystrophy to within a 2 cM interval. J Med Genet. 1995;32:224–6.
9. Small KW, Mullen L, Barletta J, et al. Mapping of Reis-Bucklers' corneal dystrophy to chromosome 5q. Am J Ophthalmol. 1996;121:384–90.
10. Munier FL, Korvatska E, Djemai A, et al. Kerato-epithelin mutations in four 5q31-linked corneal dystrophies. Nat Genet. 1997;15:247–51.
11. Fine B, Yanoff M, Pitts E, et al. Meesmann's epithelial dystrophy of the cornea. Am J Ophthalmol. 1977;83:633–42.
12. Irvine AD, Corden LD, Swensson O, et al. Mutations in cornea-specific keratin K3 or K12 genes cause Meesmann's corneal dystrophy. Nat Genet. 1997;16:184–7.
13. Glaser T, Jepeal L, Edwards JG, et al. PAX6 gene dosage effect in a family with congenital cataracts, aniridia, anophthalmia and central nervous system defects. Nat Genet. 1994;7:463–71.
14. Hanson IM, Fletcher JM, Jordon T, et al. Mutations at the PAX6 locus are found in heterogeneous anterior segment malformations including Peters' anomaly. Nat Genet. 1994;6:168–73.
15. Mirzayans F, Pearce WG, MacDonald IM, et al. Mutation of the PAX6 gene in patients with autosomal dominant keratitis. Am J Hum Genet. 1995;57:539–48.
16. Ton CCT, Hirvonen H, Mira H, et al. Positional cloning and characterization of a paired box- and homeobox-containing gene from the aniridia region. Cell. 1991;67:1059–74.
17. Jordan T, Hanson I, Zaletayev D, et al. The human PAX6 gene is mutated in two patients with aniridia. Nat Genet. 1992;1:328–32.
18. Richardson J, Cvekl A, Wistow G. Pax-6 is essential for lens-specific expression of zeta-crystallin. Proc Natl Acad Sci U S A. 1995;92:4676–80.
19. Davis A, Cowell JK. Mutations in the PAX6 gene in patients with hereditary aniridia. Hum Mol Genet. 1993;2:2093–7.
20. Fitch N, Kaback M. The Axenfeld syndrome and the Rieger syndrome. J Med Genet. 1978;15:30–4.
21. Heckenlively JR, Isenberg SJ, Fox LE. The Rieger syndrome: a heritable disorder associated with glaucoma. Johns Hopkins Med J. 1982;151:351–5.
22. Ligutic I, Brecevic L, Petkovic I, et al. Interstitial deletion 4q and Rieger syndrome. Clin Genet. 1981;20:323–7.
23. Phillips JC, DelBono EA, Haines JL, et al. A second locus for Rieger syndrome maps to chromosome 13q14. Am J Hum Genet. 1996;59:613–9.
24. Murray JC, Bennett SR, Kwitek AE, et al. Linkage of Rieger syndrome to the region of the epidermal growth factor gene on chromosome 4. Nat Genet. 1992;2:46–9.
25. Mears AJ, Mirzayans F, Gould DB, et al. Autosomal dominant iridogoniodysgenesis anomaly maps to 6p25. Am J Hum Genet. 1996;59:1321–7.
26. Semina EV, Reiter R, Leysens NJ, et al. Cloning and characterization of a novel bicoid-related homeobox transcription factor gene, RIEG, involved in Rieger syndrome. Nat Genet. 1996;14:392–9.
27. Nishimura DY, Swiderski RE, Alward WL, et al. The forkhead transcription factor gene FKHL7 is responsible for glaucoma phenotypes which map to 6p25. Nat Genet. 1998;19:140–7.
28. Saleem RA, Banerjee-Basu S, Berry FB, et al. Analyses of the effects disease-causing missense mutations have on the structure and function of the winged-helix protein FOXC1. Am J Hum Genet. 2001;68:627–41.
29. Johnson AT, Richards JE, Boehnke M, et al. Clinical phenotype of juvenile-onset primary open-angle glaucoma linked to chromosome 1q. Ophthalmology. 1996;103:808–14.
30. Wiggs JL, DelBono AE, Schuman JS, et al. Clinical features of five pedigrees genetically linked to the juvenile glaucoma locus on chromosome 1q21–q31. Ophthalmology. 1995;102:1782–9.
31. Sheffield VC, Stone EM, Alward WLM, et al. Genetic linkage of familial open angle glaucoma to chromosome 1q21–q31. Nat Genet. 1993;4:47–50.
32. Wiggs JL, Haines JL, Paglinauan C, et al. Genetic linkage of autosomal dominant juvenile glaucoma to 1q21–31 in three affected pedigrees. Genomics. 1994;21:299–303.
33. Richards JE, Lichter PR, Herman S, et al. Probable exclusion of GLC1A as a candidate glaucoma gene in a family with middle-age-onset primary open-angle glaucoma. Ophthalmology. 1996;103:1035–40.
34. Stone EM, Fingert JH, Alward WLM, et al. Identification of a gene that causes primary open angle glaucoma. Science. 1997;275:668–70.
35. Kubota R, Noda S, Wang Y, et al. A novel myosin-like protein (myocilin) expressed in the connecting cilium of the photoreceptor: molecular cloning, tissue expression, and chromosomal mapping. Genomics. 1997;41:360–9.
36. Ortega J, Escribano J, Coca-Prados M. Cloning and characterization of subtracted cDNAs from a human ciliary body library encoding TIGR, a protein involved in juvenile open angle glaucoma with homology to myosin and olfactomedin. FEBS Lett. 1997;413:349–53.
37. Wiggs JL, Vollrath D. Molecular and clinical evaluation of a patient hemizygous for TIGR/MYOC. Arch Ophthalmol. 2001;119:1674–8.
38. Moon S-JK, Kim H-S, Moon J-I, et al. Mutations of the TIGR/MYOC gene in primary open-angle glaucoma in Korea. Am J Hum Genet. 1999;64:1775–8.
39. Kim BS, Savinova OV, Reedy MV, et al. Targeted disruption of the myocilin gene (MYOC) suggests that human glaucoma-causing mutations are gain of function. Mol Cell Biol. 2001;21:7707–13.
40. Morton NE. Heterogeneity in nonsyndromal congenital glaucoma (letter). Am J Med Genet. 1982;12:97–102.
41. Gencik A, Genickova A, Gerinec A. Genetic heterogeneity of congenital glaucoma. Clin Genet. 1980;17:241–8.
42. Sarfarazi M, Akarsu AN, Hossain A, et al. Assignment of a locus (GLC3A) for primary congenital glaucoma (buphthalmos) to 2p21 and evidence for genetic heterogeneity. Genomics. 1995;30:171–7.
43. Stoilov I, Akarsu AN, Sarfarazi M. Identification of three different truncating mutations in cytochrome P4501B1 (CYP1B1) as the principal cause of primary congenital glaucoma (buphthalmos) in family linked to the GLC3A locus on chromosome 2p21. Hum Mol Genet. 1997;6:641–7.
44. Stoilov I, Akarsu AN, Alozie I, et al. Sequence analysis and homology modeling suggest that primary congenital glaucoma on 2p21 results from mutations disrupting either the hinge region or the conserved core structures of cytochrome P4501B1. Am J Hum Genet. 1998;62:573–84.
45. Bejjani BA, Lewis RA, Tomey KF, et al. Mutations in CYP1B1, the gene for cytochrome P4501B1, are the predominant cause of primary congenital glaucoma in Saudi Arabia. Am J Hum Genet. 1998;62:325–33.
46. Kramer P, Yount J, Mitchell T, et al. A second gene for cerulean cataracts maps to the beta crystalline region on chromosome 22. Genomics. 1996;35:539–42.
47. Litt M, Carrero-Valenzuela R, LaMorticella DM, et al. Autosomal dominant cerulean cataract is associated with a chain termination mutation in the human beta-crystallin gene CRYBB2. Hum Mol Genet. 1997;6:665–8.
48. Tsui L-C, Breitman ML, Meakin SO, et al. Localization of the human gamma-crystallin gene cluster (CRYG) to the long arm of chromosome 2, region q33–q35. Cytogenet Cell Genet. 1985;40:763–4.
49. Shiloh Y, Donlon T, Bruns G, et al. Assignment of the human gamma-crystallin gene cluster (CRYG) to the long arm of chromosome 2, region q33–q36. Hum Genet. 1986;73:17–9.
50. Siezen RJ, Thomson JA, Kaplan ED, Benedek GB. Human lens gamma-crystallins: isolation, identification, and characterization of the expressed gene products. Proc Natl Acad Sci U S A. 1987;84:6088–92.
51. Lubsen NH, Renwick JH, Tsui L-C, et al. A locus of a human hereditary cataract is closely linked to the gamma-crystallin gene family. Proc Natl Acad Sci U S A. 1987;84:489–92.
52. Brankenhoff RH, Henskens HAM, vanRossum MWPC, et al. Activation of the gamma-E-crystallin pseudogene in the human hereditary Coppock-like cataract. Hum Mol Genet. 1994;3:279–83.
53. Wang Q, Chen Q, Zhao K, et al. Update on the molecular genetics of retinitis pigmentosa. Ophthalmic Genet. 2001;22:133–54.
54. Sheils D, Ryan C, Stevens K, et al. Autosomal dominant retinitis pigmentosa (ADRP): localization of an ADRP gene to the long arm of chromosome 3. Genomics. 1989;5:619–22.
55. Dryja TP, McGee TL, Reichel E, et al. A point mutation of the rhodopsin gene in one form of retinitis pigmentosa. Nature. 1990;343:364–6.
56. Li T, Snyder WK, Olsson JE, et al. Transgenic mice carrying the dominant rhodopsin mutation P347S: evidence for defective vectorial transport of rhodopsin to the outer segments. Proc Natl Acad Sci U S A. 1996;93:14176–81.
57. Rosenfeld PJ, Cowley GS, McGee TL, et al. A null mutation in the rhodopsin gene caused rod photoreceptor dysfunction and autosomal recessive retinitis pigmentosa. Nat Genet. 1992;1:209–13.

58. Kajiwara K, Berson EL, Dryja TP. Digenic retinitis pigmentosa due to mutations at the unlinked peripherin/RDS and ROM1 loci. Science. 1994;264:1604–8.

59. Kajiwara K, Hahn LB, Mukai S, et al. Mutations in the human retinal degeneration slow gene in autosomal dominant retinitis pigmentosa. Nature. 1991;354:480–3.

60. Bascom RA, Schappert K, McInnes RR. Cloning of the human and murine ROM1 genes: genomic organization and sequence conservation. Hum Mol Genet. 1993;2:385–91.

61. Anderson KL, Baird L, Lewis RA, et al. A YAC contig encompassing the recessive Stargardt disease gene (STGD) on chromosome 1p. Am J Hum Genet. 1995;57: 1351–63.

62. Allikmets R, Singh N, Sun H, et al. A photoreceptor cell-specific ATP-binding transporter gene (ABCR) is mutated in recessive Stargardt macular dystrophy. Nat Genet. 1997;15:236–46.

63. Allikmets R, Shroyer NF, Singh N, et al. Mutation of the Stargardt disease gene (ABCR) in age-related macular degeneration. Science. 1997;277:1805–7.

64. Stone EM, Sheffield VC, Hageman GS. Molecular genetics of age-related macular degeneration. Hum Mol Genet. 2001;10:2285–92.

65. Yanoff M, Kertesz Rahn E, Zimmerman LE. Histopathology of juvenile retinoschisis. Arch Ophthalmol. 1968;79:49–53.

66. Pawar H, Bingham EL, Lunetta KL, et al. Refined genetic mapping of juvenile X-linked retinoschisis. Hum Hered. 1995;45:206–10.

67. Sauer CG, Gehrig A, Warneke-Wittstock R, et al. Positional cloning of the gene associated with X-linked juvenile retinoschisis. Nat Genet. 1997;17:164–70.

68. Warburg M. Norrie's disease: a new hereditary bilateral pseudotumour of the retina. Acta Ophthalmol (Copenh). 1961;39:757–72.

69. Gal A, Stolzenberger C, Wienker T, et al. Norrie's disease: close linkage with genetic markers from the proximal short arm of the X chromosome. Clin Genet. 1985;27:282–3.

70. Chen Z-Y, Hendriks RW, Jobling MA, et al. Isolation and characterization of a candidate gene for Norrie disease. Nat Genet. 1992;1:204–8.

71. Berger W, Meindl A, van de Pol TJR, et al. Isolation of a candidate gene for Norrie disease by positional cloning. Nat Genet. 1992;1:199–203.

72. Berger W, van de Pol D, Warburg M, et al. Mutations in the candidate gene for Norrie disease. Hum Mol Genet. 1992;1:461–5.

73. Meitinger T, Meindl A, Bork P, et al. Molecular modeling of the Norrie disease protein predicts a cystine knot growth factor tertiary structure. Nat Genet. 1993;5:376–80.

74. Sorby A, Mason MEJ, Gardner N. A fundus dystrophy with unusual features (late onset and dominant inheritance of a central retinal lesion showing oedema, haemorrhage and exudates developing into generalized choroidal atrophy with massive pigment proliferation). Br J Ophthalmol. 1949;33:67–97.

75. Weber GHF, Vogt G, Pruett RC, et al. Mutations in the tissue inhibitor metalloproteinase-3 (TIMP-3) in patients with Sorsby's fundus dystrophy. Nat Genet. 1994;8:352–6.

76. Carrero-Valenzuela RD, Klein ML, Weleber RG, et al. Sorsby fundus dystrophy: a family with the ser181cys mutation of the tissue inhibitor of metalloproteinase 3. Arch Ophthalmol. 1996;114:737–8.

77. Felbor U, Stoher H, Amann T, et al. A novel ser156cys mutation in the tissue inhibitor of metalloproteinase-3 (TIMP3) in Sorsby's fundus dystrophy with unusual clinical features. Hum Mol Genet. 1995;4:2415–6.

78. Kennaway NG, Welber RG, Buist NRM. Gyrate atrophy of the choroid and retina with hyperornithinemia; biochemical and histologic studies and response to vitamin B$_6$. Am J Hum Genet. 1980;32:529–41.

79. Mitchell GA, Brody LC, Sipila I, et al. At least two mutant alleles of ornithine delta-aminotransferase cause gyrate atrophy of the choroid and retina in Finns. U S Natl Acad Sci. 1989;86:197–201.

80. Mitchell GA, Brody LC, Looney J, et al. An initiator codon mutation in ornithine-delta-aminotransferase causing gyrate atrophy of the choroid and retina. J Clin Invest. 1988;81:630–3.

81. Kaiser-Kupfer MI, deMonasterio FM, Valle D, et al. Gyrate atrophy of the choroid and retina: improved visual function following reduction of plasma ornithine by diet. Science. 1980;210:1128–31.

82. Merbs SL, Nathans J. Absorption spectra of human cone pigments. Nature. 1992;356:433–5.

83. Nathans J, Merbs SL, Sung C-H, et al. Molecular genetics of human visual pigments. Annu Rev Genet. 1992;26:403–24.

84. Nathans J, Maumenee IHG, Zrenner E, et al. Genetics heterogeneity among blue-cone monochromats. Am J Hum Genet. 1993;53:987–1000.

85. Winderickx J, Battisti L, Motulsky AG, et al. Selective expression of human X chromosome–linked green opsin genes. Proc Natl Acad Sci U S A. 1992;89: 9710–4.

86. Friend SH, Bernards R, Rogelj S, et al. A human DNA segment with properties of the gene that predisposes to retinoblastoma and osteosarcoma. Nature. 1986;323:643–6.

87. Weinberg RA. The retinoblastoma protein and cell cycle control. Cell. 1995;81: 323–30.

88. Dryja TP, Cavenee W, White R, et al. Homozygosity of chromosome 13 in retinoblastoma. N Engl J Med. 1984;310:550–3.

89. Knudson AG Jr. Genetics of human cancer. Annu Rev Genet. 1986;20:231–51.

90. Spritz RA. Molecular genetics of oculocutaneous albinism. Hum Mol Genet. 1994;3:1469–75.

91. Spritz RA, Strunk K, Giebel LB, et al. Detection of mutations in the tyrosinase gene in a patient with type 1A oculocutaneous albinism. N Engl J Med. 1990; 322:1724–8.

92. Wallace DC, Singh G, Lott MT, et al. Mitochondrial DNA mutation associated with Leber's hereditary optic neuropathy. Science. 1988;242:1427–30.

93. Johns DR, Smith KH, Savino PJ, et al. Leber's hereditary optic neuropathy. Clinical manifestations of the 15257 mutation. Arch Ophthalmol. 1993; 110:981–6.

94. Johns DR, Smith KH, Miller NR. Leber's hereditary optic neuropathy. Clinical manifestations of the 3460 mutation. Arch Ophthalmol. 1992;110:1577–81.

95. Brown MD, Voljavec AS, Lott MT, et al. Leber's hereditary optic neuropathy; a model for mitochondrial neurodegenerative diseases. FASEB J. 1992;6:2791–9.

96. Engle EC. Applications of molecular genetics to the understanding of congenital ocular motility disorders. Ann N Y Acad Sci. 2002;956:55–63.

97. Nakano M, Yamada K, Fain J, et al. Homozygous mutations in ARIX (PHOX2A) result in congenital fibrosis of the extraocular muscles type 2. Nat Genet. 2001;29:315–20.

98. Al-Baradie R, Yamada K, St Hilaire C, et al. Duane radial ray syndrome (Okihiro syndrome) maps to 20q13 and results from mutations in SALL4, a new member of the SAL family. Am J Hum Genet. 2002;71:1195–9.

99. Votruba M, Moore AT, Bhattacharya SS. Genetic refinement of dominant optic atrophy (OPA1) locus to within a 2 cM interval of chromosome 3q. J Med Genet. 1997;34:117–21.

100. Alexander C, Votruba M, Pesch UE, et al. OPA1, encoding a dynamin-related GTPase, is mutated in autosomal dominant optic atrophy linked to chromosome 3q28. Nat Genet. 2000;26:211–5.

101. Aung T, Ocaka L, Ebenezer ND, et al. A major marker for normal tension glaucoma: association with polymorphisms in the OPA1 gene. Hum Genet. 2002; 110:52–6.

102. Wiggs JL. Complex disorders in ophthalmology. Semin Ophthalmol. 1995; 10:323–30.

CHAPTER

3

Embryology of the Eye

NATHALIE F. AZAR • ELIZABETH A. DAVIS

INTRODUCTION

The development of the human eye is a complex series of orderly events that begins with the fertilization of the ovum and continues until the early postnatal period (Table 3-1). Although the tendency is to depict these changes in distinct stages, numerous events happen simultaneously. Not only may interrelations between ocular tissues influence their development, but one ocular tissue may induce the formation of another. Impairment or interruption of these events may result in congenital abnormalities of the eye. The earlier the disruption, the more severe the anomaly.[1]

OCULAR EMBRYOGENESIS

In general, there are three main stages in the prenatal development of the eye. The first period, called embryogenesis, involves the establishment of the primary layers of the developing embryo. After fertilization, the sequential formation of three cell masses—morula, blastula, and gastrula—occurs. Cells within the gastrula are repositioned to form three germinal layers. Each layer gives rise to specific ocular structures, as shown in Table 3-2. The inner layer becomes the endoderm, and the outer layer develops into the ectoderm. A linear opacity of ectodermal thickening (the primitive streak)[1] develops longitudinally over

TABLE 3-1

TIME LINE OF OCULAR EMBRYOGENESIS

Period After Conception	Event	Period After Conception	Event
22nd day	Optic groove appears	3rd month	Differentiation of precursors of rods and cones
25th day	Optic vesicle forms from optic pit		Ciliary body develops
26th day	Primordia of superior rectus, inferior rectus, medial rectus, and inferior oblique appear		Appearance of limbus
			Anterior chamber appears as a potential space
27th day	Formation of lens plate from surface ectoderm		Sclera condenses
	Primordium of lateral rectus appears		Eyelid folds lengthen and fuse
28th day	Embryonic fissure forms	4th month	Formation of retinal vasculature begins
	Cells destined to become retinal pigment epithelium acquire pigmentation		Beginning of regression of hyaloid vessels
			Formation of physiologic cup of optic disc
29th day	Primordium of superior oblique appears		Formation of lamina cribrosa
5th week	Lens pit forms and deepens into lens vesicle		Major arterial circle of iris forms
	Hyaloid vessels develop		Development of iris sphincter muscle
	Primary vitreous develops		Development of longitudinal ciliary muscle and processes of ciliary body
	Osseous structures of the orbit begin to develop		Formation of tertiary vitreous
6th week	Closure of embryonic fissure		Bowman's membrane forms
	Corneal epithelial cells develop interconnections		Canal of Schlemm appears
	Differentiation of retinal pigment epithelium		Eyelid glands and cilia form
	Proliferation of neural retinal cells	5th month	Photoreceptors differentiate
	Formation of secondary vitreous		Eyelid separation begins
	Formation of primary lens fibers	6th month	Cones differentiate
	Development of periocular vasculature		Ganglion cells thicken in macula
	Appearance of eyelid folds and nasolacrimal duct		Differentiation of dilator pupillae muscle
	Ciliary ganglion appears		Nasolacrimal system becomes patent
7th week	Migration of ganglion cells toward optic disc	7th month	Rods differentiate
	Formation of embryonic lens nucleus		Ora serrata forms
	Development of choroidal vessels from periocular mesenchyme		Migration of ganglion cells to form nerve fiber layer of Henle
	Three waves of neural crest migration:		Choroid becomes pigmented
	first wave: formation of corneal and trabecular endothelium		Circular ciliary muscle fibers develop
	second wave: formation of corneal stroma		Myelination of optic nerve
	third wave: formation of iris stroma		Posterior movement of anterior chamber angle
	Formation of tunica vasculosa lentis		Orbicularis muscle differentiation
	Sclera begins to form	8th month	Completion of anterior chamber angle formation
			Hyaloid vessels disappear
		9th month	Retinal vessels reach the temporal periphery
			Pupillary membrane disappears
		After birth	Development of macula

the dorsal surface of the embryo. Ectodermal cells from the anterior part of the primitive streak migrate laterally and cephalad in between layers of ectoderm and endoderm to form the intraembryonic mesoderm. The greater part of the brain and eye develops from the ectoderm anterior to the primitive streak, the

so-called neuroectoderm. The cells of the neuroectoderm divide and form the neural tube. During the folding of the neural tube, a ridge of cells (neural crest)[2–4] develops from the converging edges and migrates to the dorsolateral aspect of the tube (Fig. 3-1). Neural crest cells subsequently migrate and give rise to various structures within the eye and orbit. By the end of embryogenesis, the cranial end of the neural tube has developed into three primary brain vesicles—prosencephalon (forebrain), mesencephalon (midbrain), and rhombencephalon (hindbrain). The prosencephalon further divides into the telencephalon and diencephalon. The optic primordia (the optic grooves) form between these two structures.

After the third gestational week, the period of organogenesis begins, and the organization of the segregated cells into rudimentary organs takes place. The optic pits form as lateral outpouchings of the anterior end of the neural tube[5] and are attached to the forebrain by optic stalks. The optic pits subsequently enlarge to form the optic vesicles (Fig. 3-2).[6] Contact with the overlying surface ectoderm induces the formation of a thickened lens plate.[5–7] During the fourth week, the outer walls of the optic vesicles begin to invaginate and form a two-layered optic cup (see Fig. 3-2). Simultaneously, the lens plate undergoes invagination to form the lens vesicle (see Fig. 3-2).[8] A deep groove, the fetal fissure,[9–12] develops on the undersurface of each optic cup and extends to the most proximal portion of the optic stalk. Within this groove are mesodermal cells, which ultimately differentiate into the hyaloid vessels and the central retinal artery. Between the fifth and seventh weeks of gestation, the fetal fissure closes. Closure is first apparent centrally and proceeds anteriorly toward the margin of the optic cup and posteriorly toward the optic stalk. During the development of the optic cup and lens vesicle, the associated paraxial mesoderm gives rise to various vascular and orbital tissues (see Table 3-2).

Finally, a period of differentiation, which begins around the eighth gestational week, occurs before the eye is fully functional. For some ocular structures, such as the macula, differentiation is completed after birth.

In the following sections, the embryology of the retina, optic nerve, vascular system, vitreous, uvea, lens, chamber angle, iris, cornea, and sclera is discussed.

TABLE 3-2

DERIVATIVES OF EMBRYONIC TISSUES

Ectoderm	Neuroectoderm	Neural retina
		Retinal pigment epithelium
		Pigmented ciliary epithelium
		Nonpigmented ciliary epithelium
		Pigmented iris epithelium
		Sphincter and dilator muscles of iris
		Optic nerve, axons, and glia
		Vitreous
	Cranial neural crest cells	Corneal stroma and endothelium
		Sclera (see also mesoderm)
		Trabecular meshwork
		Ciliary muscles
		Choroidal stroma
		Melanocytes (uveal and epithelial)
		Meningeal sheaths of the optic nerve
		Schwann cells of ciliary nerve
		Ciliary ganglion
		Orbital bones (all midline)
		Inferior orbital room and lateral rim
		Cartilage
		Connective tissue orbit
		Muscular layer and connective tissue sheaths of all ocular and orbital vessels
	Surface ectoderm	Epithelium, glands, cilia of skin and lids, and caruncle
		Conjunctival epithelium
		Lens
		Lacrimal gland
		Lacrimal drainage system
		Vitreous
Mesoderm		Fibers of extraocular muscles
		Endothelial lining of all orbital and ocular blood vessels
		Temporal portion of sclera
		Vitreous

Reproduced with permission from Academy Manual.

NEURAL RETINA

Retinal development begins very early in gestation. By the time of invagination of the optic vesicle to form the optic cup, the inner retinal wall has divided into two zones—a superficial, marginal, non-nucleated zone and a deeper, primitive, nucleated zone (Fig. 3-3). The outermost layer of cells in the nucleated zone is lined by cilia, which project toward the outer layer of the optic cup, the future retinal pigment epithelium (RPE).[13,14]

Development of the retinal layers arises by mitosis of cells in the primitive zone, which occurs first in the posterior pole and

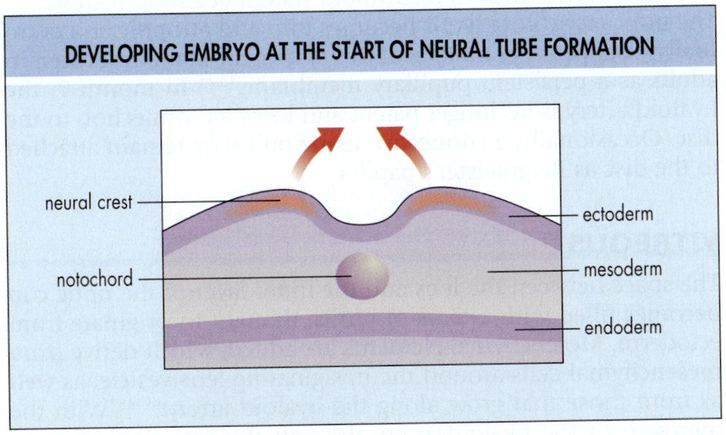

FIG. 3-1 ▊ Developing embryo at the start of neural tube formation.

DEVELOPING EMBRYO AT THE START OF NEURAL TUBE FORMATION

neural crest — ectoderm
notochord — mesoderm
— endoderm

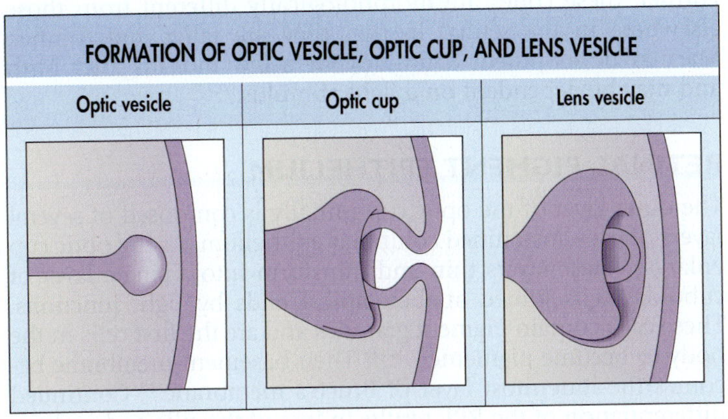

FIG. 3-2 ▊ Formation of the optic vesicle, optic cup, and lens vesicle.

FORMATION OF OPTIC VESICLE, OPTIC CUP, AND LENS VESICLE

Optic vesicle	Optic cup	Lens vesicle

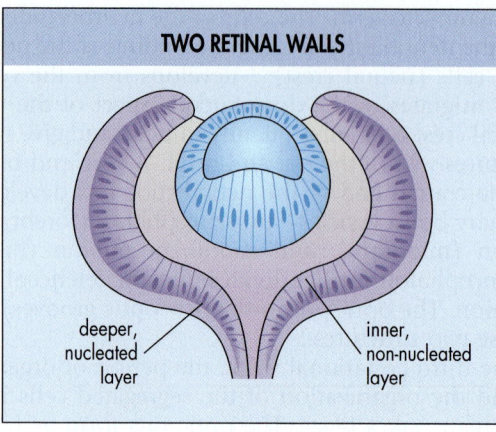

TWO RETINAL WALLS

deeper,
nucleated
layer

inner,
non-nucleated
layer

FIG. 3-3 ■ **The two retinal walls.** The inner retinal wall shows two zones—an inner, non-nucleated layer and a deeper, nucleated layer.

proceeds peripherally. Migration of nuclei from the marginal zone results in the formation of two nuclear layers in the posterior pole—the inner and outer neuroblastic layers.

The inner neuroblastic layer develops first and differentiates into cells of Müller, ganglion cells, and amacrine cells.[15-17] The outer neuroblastic layer gives rise to bipolar cells, horizontal cells, and precursors of the photoreceptors. The cells of Müller develop long, fibrous processes that extend to the inner and outer layers of the retina and form the inner and outer limiting membranes. The ganglion cells develop axons that grow toward the optic disc and form the nerve fiber layer of the retina. The amacrine cells arise from the deeper layers of the inner neuroblastic layer.

The formation of the layers of the retina begins with establishment of the ganglion cell layer.[18,19] Next, an acellular zone develops between the ganglion cells and the rest of the inner neuroblastic layer to form the inner plexiform layer. In the outer neuroblastic layer, the bipolar and horizontal cells become separated from the photoreceptor cells by the acellular outer plexiform layer. Together with the amacrine cells and the cells of Müller, the bipolar and horizontal cells make up the inner nuclear layer. The cell bodies of the photoreceptors compose the outer nuclear layer. Formation of the inner nuclear layer obliterates the nerve fiber layer of Chievitz, a transient layer of fibers that separates the inner and outer neuroblastic layers.[20]

Differentiation of the photoreceptors begins with replacement of the cilia in the nucleated zone by outer segments.[21] Cones appear first between months 4 and 6, followed by the rods in month 7.

Development of the macula has some unique features. Early in gestation, it may be differentiated by an increase in ganglion cells. The axons of these cells elongate such that the ganglion cell bodies become located more peripherally. The nearly horizontally positioned axons thus form the nerve fiber of Henle.

Only cones develop within the macula; no rods are present. Further, these cones are morphologically different from those elsewhere in the retina, in that they are taller and thinner. Macular development continues for a few months after birth and may be dependent on a light stimulus.[22,23]

RETINAL PIGMENT EPITHELIUM

The outer layer of the optic cup initially is composed of several layers of pseudostratified columnar epithelium. As the optic cup enlarges, these layers thin and transform into a single layer of cuboidal cells joined at their apical ends by tight junctions. These cells contain pigment granules and are the first cells in the body to become pigmented.[24-26] Their basement membrane becomes the innermost layer of Bruch's membrane.[27] Continued differentiation of the RPE results in loss of the cilia and replacement with apical villi.

OPTIC NERVE

The optic nerve forms within the optic stalk.[28-30] Vacuolization of cells in the optic stalk results in passages through which ganglion cell axons migrate. Glial cells develop from the inner layer of the optic stalk and separate the axons into bundles. The central axis of the optic nerve contains the hyaloid artery, which eventually develops into the central retinal artery. The outer layer of the optic stalk gives rise to the lamina cribrosa. In month 8, the lamina becomes permeated by collagen fibers from the sclera and choroid. The final tensile strength of the lamina is not achieved until several months after birth, through condensation of these fibers. A central layer of neural crest cells differentiates into the optic nerve sheath. Myelination, which begins in month 8, starts at the chiasm and proceeds toward the optic nerve base.[31-33]

VASCULAR SYSTEM

The development of the vascular system of the eye is a complex process that involves the appearance of vessels to meet the nutritional needs of metabolically active tissues and subsequent regression of those same vessels when tissue activity becomes more quiescent. In the early embryo, the internal carotid artery supplies a fine capillary plexus to the dorsal aspect of the optic cup (the dorsal ophthalmic artery). Soon thereafter, a second branch of the internal carotid artery forms to supply the medial aspect of the optic cup. This branch is called the ventral ophthalmic artery, and its anastomosis with the dorsal ophthalmic artery forms the annular vessel. An important branch of the dorsal ophthalmic artery, the hyaloid artery,[34-38] develops and passes through the embryonic fissure into the optic cup interior. Simultaneously, the orbital tissues are supplied by a branch of the internal carotid artery, the stapedial artery.

The venous system develops simultaneously with the arterial system. Two primary drainage systems, the supraorbital and infraorbital plexuses, are formed and surround the optic vesicle.

Once the hyaloid artery enters the optic cup, it extends toward and around the lens vesicle and anastomoses with the annular vessels. These vessels project a vascular meshwork across the lens to form the tunica vasculosa lentis.[39]

During week 6, the primitive dorsal ophthalmic artery is transformed into the definitive ophthalmic artery, and the ventral ophthalmic artery regresses; its only remnant is the posterior nasal ciliary artery. The ophthalmic artery branches become the central retinal artery, the temporal long posterior ciliary artery, and the short posterior ciliary artery.

The hyaloid artery develops branches that penetrate the inner retina and then become branches of the central retinal artery. These vessels arborize anteriorly from the peripapillary area to the peripheral retina. The nasal periphery is reached first at about month 6 of gestation. The temporal periphery is not reached until month 9 of gestation. Thus, the retinas of premature infants may be incompletely vascularized.

In the third trimester, the hyaloid system begins to regress.[40-42] The tunica vasculosa lentis becomes thin and atrophic and eventually disappears. Remnants of this system are sometimes seen in adults as a persistent pupillary membrane.[43,44] In month 7, the hyaloid artery is no longer patent and loses its connection to the disc. Occasionally, a connective tissue bud may remain attached to the disc as Bergmeister's papilla.

VITREOUS

The space between the lens and the inner layer of the optic cup becomes filled with a mass of fibrils, thought to originate from ectoderm. Mesenchymal elements are added, which derive from mesenchymal cells around the invaginating lens vesicle, as well as from those that grow along the hyaloid artery.[45-48] With the ingrowth of the hyaloid artery through the embryonic fissure, the primary vitreous is formed (Fig. 3-4).

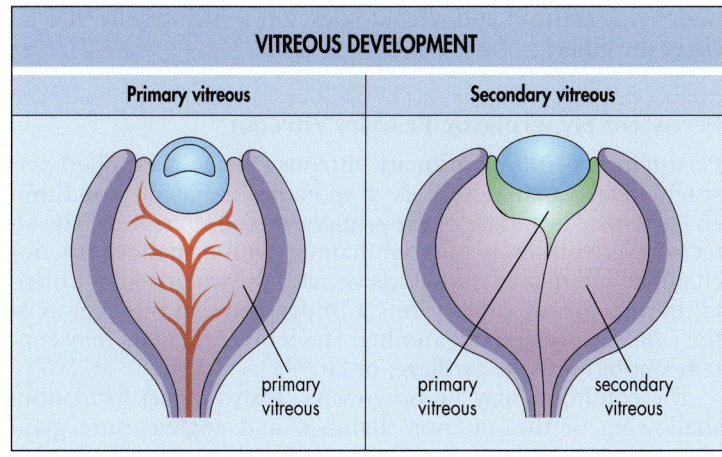

FIG. 3-4 ■ Vitreous development. The primary vitreous and hyaloid artery fill the optic cup. The primary vitreous retracts and the hyaloid artery regresses, while the secondary avascular vitreous develops.

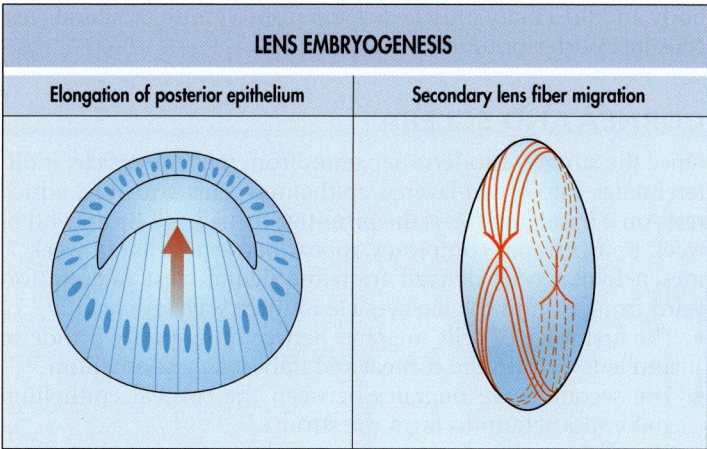

FIG. 3-5 ■ Lens embryogenesis. Elongation of the posterior epithelium results in obliteration of the lens lumen. Secondary lens fiber migration leads to the formation of the Y sutures.

Formation of the secondary vitreous is marked by the appearance of an orderly array of very fine, dense fibers. The secondary avascular vitreous surrounds the primary vitreous. An area of condensation between the primary and secondary vitreous forms the wall of the canal of Cloquet, in which the hyaloid artery runs. Regression of the tunica vasculosa lentis and hyaloid artery by the end of month 3 leads to retraction of the primary vitreous (see Fig. 3-4).

A condensation along the anterior border of the secondary vitreous results in the formation of the tertiary vitreous, the zonules of the lens.

UVEA

The primitive choroidal vasculature first appears as a plexus of endothelial blood spaces in close proximity to the outer layer of the optic cup; anastomoses of these at the rim of the cup form the annular vessel. Drainage occurs through the two venous networks, the supraorbital and infraorbital venous plexuses. In month 2, connections to the primitive choroidal vasculature are made by the posterior ciliary arteries. The large drainage sinuses consolidate into four vortex veins. In month 3, a definitive choriocapillaris emerges.[49-52] The sclera begins to condense and demarcates the outermost boundary of the choroid, the suprachoroidal space. Subsequently, distinct layers of the choroid begin to form. Posterior to the equator are three layers—large vessels, medium vessels, and choriocapillaris. Anterior to the equator, only two layers are present—medium vessels and choriocapillaris. The iris is supplied by the major arterial circle, a coalescence of branches of the anterior ciliary and long posterior ciliary arteries. The ciliary body receives recurrent branches from the greater arterial circle in the last trimester.

Melanosomes first appear in the lamina suprachoroidea and outer choroid of the posterior pole, but they are rarely evident before month 7. Precursors of melanocytes are of neural crest origin. The production of melanin proceeds anteriorly from the peripapillary area to the retinal periphery.

LENS

Lens formation begins when the optic vesicle contacts the surface ectoderm and induces the formation of a disc-shaped thickening, called the lens plate. This structure subsequently invaginates to form the lens vesicle, which separates from the surface epithelium at day 33 of gestation. The lens vesicle is lined by a single layer of cells surrounded by a basal lamina. The basal lamina later develops into the lens capsule. Cells in the posterior half of the vesicle undergo a transformation that involves a decrease in DNA synthesis and intracellular organelles, the ap-

pearance of crystallin proteins in the cytoplasm,[53] and cellular elongation that results in obliteration of the vesicle lumen (Fig. 3-5).[54,55] These cells make up the primary lens fibers.

Secondary lens fibers consist of the cytoplasm of anterior epithelial cells, which migrate toward the equator and then elongate. These fibers extend anteriorly and posteriorly around the primary lens fibers and meet centrally to form the lens sutures. The sutures are Y-shaped, being upright anteriorly and inverted posteriorly (see Fig. 3-5).

Continued production of secondary lens fibers changes the shape of the lens from spherical to elliptical. Nuclei of the deeper fibers are lost, and their chromatin and ribosomes disintegrate. The lenticular fibers continue to grow and differentiate into the postnatal period.[56]

CHAMBER ANGLE, IRIS, AND CILIARY BODY

In week 5, a group of neural crest cells at the peripheral posterior aspect of the cornea differentiates into the chamber angle, the trabecular meshwork, and Schlemm's canal.[57-62]

As the rim of the optic cup grows anteriorly, it advances around the edge of the lens to form the iris.[63] The stroma develops from neural crest cells, and the two epithelial layers form from the neuroectodermally derived optic cup rim. The anterior layer of epithelial cells becomes pigmented and is continuous with the pigment epithelium of the retina posteriorly. The posterior epithelium remains nonpigmented until month 5 and is continuous with the inner retinal layer of the optic cup.

The iris sphincter muscle arises from myofibrils in the anterior wall of the marginal sinus, a circular cavity that forms between the two layers of the optic cup.[64] Thus, this structure is of neuroectodermal origin. In month 7, blood vessels penetrate into the growing sphincter from the surrounding mesoderm and divide the muscle into bundles.

The dilator muscle begins to develop in month 6. Myofibrils form from the anterior layer of the iris epithelium and become oriented parallel to the plane of the iris. This muscle, too, is of neuroectodermal origin.

The ciliary body begins to form in month 3 as the margin of the optic cup folds just posterior to the rim of the advancing edge.[65-67] These folds form the two epithelial layers of the ciliary processes. The outer layer becomes pigmented, and the inner layer remains nonpigmented. The ciliary processes grow and by month 4 reach the equator of the lens. Fine filaments develop from surface cells of the processes and form the zonules of the lens. This portion of the ciliary body is called the corona ciliaris. In month 5, growth of a smooth region just posterior to the corona develops into the pars plana. The stroma of the ciliary body and the ciliary muscle develop from a group of neural crest cells just posterior to the cornea.

CORNEA AND SCLERA

Once the surface ectoderm separates from the lens vesicle, it differentiates into a two-layered epithelium. This structure, which rests on a basal lamina, is the primitive cornea.[68–71] By the end of week 6, junctional complexes appear between cells. In week 7, mesenchymal cells derived from the neural crest migrate forward from around the lens vesicle in three waves:

- The first wave of cells migrates between the surface ectoderm and lens to form the corneal and trabecular endothelium.[72–74]
- The second wave migrates between the corneal epithelium and endothelium to form the stroma.[75]
- The third wave migrates between the corneal endothelium and lens to form the iris stroma.

The corneal endothelium forms as a two-cell layer of cuboidal cells. In week 8, these cells produce a basement membrane, Descemet's membrane.[76,77]

In month 3, fibroblasts and collagen fibrils appear. The fibroblasts begin synthesis of the glycosaminoglycan ground substance. Keratan sulfate production becomes apparent in the cornea. Bowman's layer is first noted in month 4; it develops as an extension of filaments from the basal lamina of the epithelium. It is also around this time that tight junctions form between the apices of the endothelial cells. Subsequently, aqueous humor appears in the anterior chamber. Further development results in enlargement of the cornea and dehydration of its stroma to form a transparent structure.

Scleral formation begins in week 7 from a condensation of the anterior periocular mesenchyme, a derivative of neural crest cells.[78] In month 3, this condensation extends posteriorly to surround the posterior pole and optic nerve. Some of the scleral cells migrate between the optic nerve fibers to contribute to the formation of the lamina cribrosa.

SELECTED OCULAR DEVELOPMENTAL DEFECTS

Coloboma

Coloboma (Greek for mutilated) implies the absence of a particular ocular tissue and results from incomplete closure of the embryonic fissure around weeks 5–8 of gestation.[79] Colobomas are categorized as typical and atypical. Typical colobomas are located in the area of the embryonic fissure and thus are seen inferonasally. Atypical colobomas are found outside that area and therefore do not originate in a defect of fetal fissure closure. Colobomas have a wide variety of clinical presentations—they may be complete or partial; they may involve the iris, retina, choroid, or optic disc. Closure of the embryonal fissure starts at the equator and continues anteriorly and posteriorly. Any insult during the time of closure can create defects of varying sizes and locations. Colobomas may extend from the iris margin to the optic disc or may involve one or more defects along the fusional lines. Therefore, a coloboma of the iris may or may not involve a coloboma of the retinochoroid or the optic disc.

Typical colobomas are usually bilateral. Inheritance generally is autosomal dominant with variable penetrance and expressivity, although environmental factors can play a role.[80]

Colobomas that involve the choroid result in absolute scotomata, whereas those that affect the nerve may cause visual field defects not commensurate with the findings. Amblyopia is also a factor because of the associated myopic astigmatism.

The clinical appearance of colobomas is variable. Iris colobomas range from a notch in the pupillary margin to a whole sector of iris missing, which results in the "keyhole" appearance commonly described. Optic disc colobomas vary from large, excavated, inferonasal, chorioretinal defects to subtle changes in the RPE. Failure of the RPE to develop may lead to failure of the

underlying choroid and sclera to develop, which results in ectasia of the globe.

Persistent Hyperplastic Primary Vitreous

Persistent hyperplastic primary vitreous (PHPV; also called persistent fetal vasculature)[81] is a sporadic, unilateral condition characterized by failure of the primary vitreous to regress. The affected eye typically is microphthalmic, with a shallow anterior chamber and dilated, radial iris vessels. A vascularized, retrolental fibrous plaque often forms a bridge between one region of the ciliary processes and another. The retrolental mass may contain smooth muscle, cartilage, or fat.[82,83]

The condition may be progressive, with cataract formation, shallowing of the anterior chamber, and angle-closure glaucoma. Vitreous hemorrhage, retinal detachment, and phthisis bulbi may occur. Cataract extraction and vitrectomy often prevent the development of secondary glaucoma. Vision may remain poor because of the associated retinal dysplasia and glaucoma (see Chapter 145).

Anophthalmia

Anophthalmia denotes the complete absence of an eye because of a developmental defect; it is extremely rare. More commonly, a small cystic remnant is seen, and the term clinical anophthalmia is used. To differentiate true anophthalmia from clinical anophthalmia, histological sections of eviscerated orbital tissue are studied microscopically.

True anophthalmia results from failure of the optic pit to develop and form the optic vesicle.[84,85] This transpires early in the development of the embryo, usually during weeks 1–3 postconception. Anophthalmia may be unilateral or bilateral. Bilateral cases suggest an early teratogenic event. Most cases are sporadic, although hereditary transmission with chromosomal abnormalities have been reported.[86–88]

Microphthalmos

Microphthalmos is a continuation of a spectrum that begins with anophthalmia. The definition of microphthalmos is an eye that has an axial length less than 21mm in an adult or less than 19mm in a 1-year-old child. Microphthalmos may be isolated, or it may be associated with ocular or systemic abnormalities. Isolated microphthalmos may be sporadic or inherited, with a variable degree of visual deficit. Microphthalmos may be associated with microcornea, cataract, aniridia, PHPV, and systemic disease such as MIDAS (microphthalmos, dermal aplasia, sclerocornea) syndrome, among others.[89]

Microphthalmos results from an insult to the embryo after the outgrowth of the optic vesicle. If the insult occurs before complete invagination of the optic vesicle, an orbital cyst may result. This condition (microphthalmos with cyst) can present as progressive swelling from birth; the cyst may course along the optic nerve with free communication with the intraocular contents.[90] Very large cysts may require frequent aspiration or total excision.

REFERENCES

1. Duke-Elder S, Cook C. Normal and abnormal development. Part I. Embryology. In: Duke-Elder S, ed. System of ophthalmology, vol. 3. London: CV Mosby; 1963:23–4.
2. Johnston MC. A radio-autographic study of the migration and fate of cranial neural crest cells in the chick embryo. Anat Rec. 1966;156:143–56.
3. Noden DM. Periocular mesenchyme. Neural crest and mesodermal interactions. In: Jakobiec FA, ed. Ocular anatomy, embryology and teratology. Philadelphia: Harper & Row; 1982:97–119.
4. Beauchamp GR, Knapper PA. Role of the neural crest in anterior segment development and disease. J Pediatr Ophthalmol Strabismus. 1984;21:209–14.
5. Ozanics V, Jakobiec F. Prenatal development of the eye and its adnexae. In: Jakobiec FA, ed. Ocular anatomy, embryology and teratology. Philadelphia: Harper & Row; 1982:11–96.
6. Coulombre AJ. The eye. In: Dahaan U, ed. Organogenesis. New York: Holt, Rinehart & Winston; 1965:219–40.

7. Worgul BV. The lens. In: Jakobiec FA, ed. Ocular anatomy, embryology and teratology. Philadelphia: Harper & Row; 1982:677–731.

8. Marshall J, Beaconfield M, Rottery S. The anatomy of the human lens and zonules. Trans Ophthalmol Soc UK. 1982;102:423–39.

9. Geeraets R. An electron microscopic study of the closure of the optic fissure in the golden hamster. Am J Anat. 1976;145:411–32.

10. Suzuki T, Shirai S, Majima A. Morphological study on the mechanism of closure of the embryonic fissure. Acta Ophthalmol Soc Jpn. 1988;92:238–42.

11. Hero I. The optic fissure in the normal and microphthalmic mouse. Exp Eye Res. 1989;49:229–39.

12. Hero I. Optic fissure closure in the normal Cinnamon mouse. Invest Ophthalmol Vis Sci. 1990;31:197–216.

13. Hollenberg J, Spira AW. Human retinal development. Ultrastructure of the outer retina. Am J Anat. 1973;137:357–86.

14. Mund MI, Rodrigues MM. Embryology of the human retinal pigment epithelium. In: Zinn KM, Marmor MF, eds. The retinal pigment epithelium. Cambridge: Harvard University Press; 1979:45–52.

15. Rhodes RH. Ultrastructure of Müller cells in the developing human retina. Graefes Arch Clin Exp Ophthalmol. 1984;221:171–8.

16. Provis JM, Driell D, Billson FA, Russell P. Development of the human retina: patterns of cell distribution and redistribution in the ganglion cell layer. J Comp Neurol. 1985;233:429–51.

17. Driell D, Provis JM, Billson FA. Early differentiation of ganglion, amacrine, bipolar and Mueller cells in the developing fovea of the human retina. J Comp Neurol. 1990;291:203–19.

18. Provis JM. Patterns of cell death in the ganglion cell layer of the human fetal retina. J Comp Neurol. 1986;259:237–46.

19. Provis JM, Billson FA, Russell P. Ganglion cell topography in human fetal retina. Invest Ophthalmol Vis Sci. 1983;24:1316–20.

20. Smelser GK, Ozanics V, Rayborn M, Sagun D. The fine structure of the retinal transient layer of Chievitz. Invest Ophthalmol. 1973;12:504–12.

21. De Robertis E. Some observations on the ultrastructure and morphogenesis of photoreceptors. J Gen Physiol. 1960;43(Suppl):1–14.

22. Isenberg SI. Macular development in premature infant. Am J Ophthalmol. 1986;101:74–80.

23. Abramov I, Gordon J, Hendrickson A, et al. The retina of the newborn infant. Science. 1982;217:265–7.

24. Breathnach AS, Wyllie LM. Ultrastructure of retinal pigment epithelium of the human fetus. J Ultrastruct Res. 1966;16:584–97.

25. Moyer F. Development, structure, and function of the retinal pigment epithelium. In: Straatsma BR, Hall MO, Allen RA, Crescitelli F, eds. The retina. Berkeley: University of California Press; 1969:1–30.

26. Streeten BW. Development of the human retinal pigment epithelium and the posterior segment. Arch Ophthalmol. 1969;81:383–94.

27. Takei Y, Ozanics V. Origin and development of Bruch's membrane in monkey fetuses: an electron microscopic study. Invest Ophthalmol. 1975;14:903–16.

28. Rhodes RH. Development of the optic nerve. In: Jakobiec FA, ed. Ocular anatomy, embryology and teratology. Philadelphia: Harper & Row; 1982:601–38.

29. Kuwabara T. Development of the optic nerve of the rat. Invest Ophthalmol. 1975;14:732–45.

30. Sturrock RR. A light and electron microscopic study of proliferation and maturation of fibrous astrocytes in the optic nerve of the human embryo. J Anat. 1975;119:223–34.

31. Sturrock RR. Development of the meninges of the human embryonic optic nerve. J Hirnforsch. 1987;28:603–13.

32. Sturrock RR. A quantitative histological study of cell division and changes in cell number, in the meningeal sheath of the embryonic human optic nerve. J Anat. 1987;155:133–40.

33. Sturrock RR. An electron microscopic study of macrophages in the meninges of the human embryonic optic nerve. J Anat. 1988;157:145–51.

34. Hamming NA, Apple DJ, Gieser DK, Vygantas CM. Ultrastructure of the hyaloid vasculature in primates. Invest Ophthalmol Vis Sci. 1977;16:408–15.

35. Foos RY, Kopelow JM. Development of retinal vasculature in paranatal infants. Surv Ophthalmol. 1973;18:117–27.

36. Shakib M, De Oliveira F, Henkind P. Development of retinal vessels II. Earliest stages of vessel formation. Invest Ophthalmol. 1968;7:689–700.

37. Michaelson IC. The mode of development of the vascular system of the retina with some observations on its significance for certain retinal diseases. Trans Ophthalmol Soc UK. 1948;68:137–80.

38. Mutlu F, Leopold IH. The structure of the retinal vascular system of the human fetus eye. Arch Ophthalmol. 1964;71:531–6.

39. Sellheyer K, Spitznas M. Ultrastructure of the human posterior tunica vasculosa lentis during early gestation. Graefes Arch Clin Exp Ophthalmol. 1987;225:377–83.

40. Zypen E, Fankhauser F. Ultrastructure of the hyaloid canal and its retraction during gestation. Klin Monatsbl Augenheilkd. 1982;180:329–32.

41. Jack RL. Regression of the hyaloid vascular system: an ultrastructural analysis. Am J Ophthalmol. 1972;74:261–71.

42. Cogan DC. Development and senescence of the human retinal vasculature. Doyne memorial lecture. Trans Ophthalmol Soc UK. 1963;83:464–83.

43. Matsuo N, Smelser GK. Electron microscopic studies in the pupillary membrane: the fine structure of the white strands of the disappearance stage of the membrane. Invest Ophthalmol. 1971;10:108–19.

44. Renz BE, Vygantas CM. Hyaloid vascular remnants in human neonates. Ann Ophthalmol. 1977;9:179–84.

45. Kawamura M, Azuma N, Akiya S, Uemura Y. Morphologic studies on attachment of vitreous fibers in the developing human eye. Acta Ophthalmol Soc Jpn. 1988;92:351–8.

46. Balazs EA, Laurent TC, Laurent UBG. Studies on the structure of the vitreous body VI. Biochemical changes during development. Biol Chem. 1959;234:422–30.

47. Balazs EA, Toth LZ, Jutheden G, Collins BA. Cytological and biochemical studies of the developing chick vitreous. Exp Eye Res. 1965;4:237–48.

48. Balazs EA. Fine structure of developing vitreous. Int Ophthalmol Clin. 1975;15:53–63.

49. Sellheyer K, Spitznas M. The fine structure of a developing human choriocapillaris during the first trimester. Graefes Arch Clin Exp Ophthalmol. 1988;226:65–74.

50. Heimann K. The development of choroid in man. Ophthalmic Res. 1972;3:257–73.

51. Sellheyer K. Development of the choroid and related structures. Eye. 1990;4:255–61.

52. Ozanics V, Rayborn ME, Sagun D. Observations on the ultrastructure of the developing primate choroid coat. Exp Eye Res. 1978;26:25–45.

53. Thomson JA, Augusteyn RC. Ontogeny of the human lens crystallins. Exp Eye Res. 1985;40:393–410.

54. Coulombre JL, Coulombre AJ. Lens development: fiber elongation and lens orientation. Science. 1963;142:1489–90.

55. Coulombre JL, Coulombre AJ. Lens development IV. Size, shape, and orientation. Invest Ophthalmol. 1969;8:251–7.

56. Smelser GK. Embryology and morphology of the lens. Invest Ophthalmol. 1965;4:398–410.

57. Tripathi BJ, Tripathi RC. Neural crest origin of human trabecular meshwork and its implications for the pathogenesis of glaucoma. Am J Ophthalmol. 1989;107:583–90.

58. Kupfer C, Kupfer-Kaiser ML. Observations on the development of the anterior chamber angle with reference to the pathogenesis of congenital glaucoma. Am J Ophthalmol. 1979;88:424–6.

59. McMenamin PG. A morphologic study of the inner surface of the anterior chamber angle in pre and post natal human eyes. Curr Eye Res. 1989;8:727–39.

60. Anderson DR. The development of the trabecular meshwork and its abnormality in primary and infantile glaucoma. Trans Am Ophthalmol Soc. 1981;79:458–85.

61. Reme C, Urner U, Aeberhard B. The development of the chamber angle in the rat eye: morphologic characteristics of developmental stages. Graefes Arch Clin Exp Ophthalmol. 1983;220:139–53.

62. Ruano-Gil D, Costa-Vila J, Barastegui C. Arrangement of the sclero-corneal trabecular system in human fetuses. Acta Anat. 1986;127:233–6.

63. Rodrigues MM, Hackett J, Donohoo P. Iris. In: Jakobiec F, ed. Ocular anatomy, embryology and teratology. Philadelphia: Harper & Row; 1982:285–302.

64. Ruprecht WK, Wulle KG. Light and electron microscopic studies on the development of the human pupillary sphincter muscle. Graefes Arch Clin Exp Ophthalmol. 1973;186:117–30.

65. Sellheyer K, Spitznas M. Surface morphology of the human ciliary body during prenatal development: a scanning electron microscopic study. Graefes Arch Clin Exp Ophthalmol. 1988;226:78–83.

66. Mancel E, Hirsch M. Development of tight junctions in the human ciliary epithelium. Exp Eye Res. 1989;48:87–97.

67. Sellheyer K, Spitznas M. Differentiation of the ciliary muscle in the human embryo and fetus. Graefes Arch Clin Exp Ophthalmol. 1988;226:281–7.

68. Sellheyer K, Spitznas M. Surface differentiation of the human corneal epithelium during prenatal development. Graefes Arch Clin Exp Ophthalmol. 1988;226:482–8.

69. Sevel D, Isaacs R. A re-evaluation of corneal development. Trans Am Ophthalmol Soc. 1988;86:178–207.

70. Ben-Zvi A, Rodrigues MM, Krachmer J, et al. Monoclonal antibodies studies of corneal epithelial development in human eyes. Invest Ophthalmol Vis Sci Suppl. 1985;26:274.

71. Tisdale AS, Spur-Michaud SJ, Rodrigues MM, et al. Development of the anchoring sutures of the epithelium in the rabbit and human fetal corneas. Invest Ophthalmol Vis Sci. 1988;29:727–36.

72. Waring GO, Bourne WM, Edelhauser HF, Kenyon KR. The corneal endothelium: normal and pathologic structure and function. Ophthalmology. 1982;89:531–90.

73. Fitch JM, Linsenmayer TF. Monoclonal antibody analysis of ocular basement membrane during development. Dev Biol. 1983;95:137–53.

74. Hayashi K, Sueishi K, Tanaka K, Inomata H. Immunohistochemical evidence of the origin of human corneal endothelial cells and keratocytes. Graefes Arch Clin Exp Ophthalmol. 1986;224:452–6.

75. Ozanics V, Rayborn M, Sagun D. Observations on the morphology of the developing primate cornea. Epithelium: its innervation and anterior stroma. J Morphol. 1977;153:263–98.

76. Murphy C, Alvarado J, Juster R. Prenatal and postnatal growth of the human Descemet's membrane. Invest Ophthalmol Vis Sci. 1984;25:1402–15.

77. Wulle KG. Electron microscopy of the fetal development of the human corneal endothelium and Descemet's membrane of the human eye. Invest Ophthalmol. 1972;11:897–904.

78. Sellheyer K, Spitznas M. Development of the human sclera: a morphological study. Graefes Arch Clin Exp Ophthalmol. 1989;226:89–100.

79. Apple DJ, Rabb MF, Walsh PM. Congenital anomalies of the optic disc. Surv Ophthalmol. 1982;27:3–41.

80. Clavert A. Analysis of the anomalies of the optic cup and of the optic nerve induced by cyclophosphamide in a rabbit embryo. Excerpta Medica International Congress Series 297; 1973.

81. Goldberg MF. Persistent fetal vasculature (PFV): an integrated interpretation of signs and symptoms associated with persistent hyperplastic primary viteous (PHPV). LIV Edward Jackson memorial lecture. Am J Ophthalmol. 1997;124:587–626.

82. Font RL, Yanoff M, Zimmerman LE. Intraocular adipose tissue and persistent hyperplastic primary vitreous. Arch Ophthalmol. 1969;82:43–50.

83. Reese AB. Persistent hyperplastic primary vitreous. Am J Ophthalmol. 1955;40:317–31.

84. Mann I. Developmental abnormalities of the eye, 2nd ed. Philadelphia: JB Lippincott; 1957:60–98.

85. Heselberg C. Congenital bilateral anophthalmia. Acta Ophthalmol. 1951;29:183–9.

86. Ashley LM. Bilateral anophthalmos in a brother and sister. J Hered. 1947;38:174.

87. Hoefnagel D, Keenan ME, Allen FH, Hanover NH. Heredo-familial-bilateral anophthalmia. Arch Ophthalmol. 1963;69:760–4.

88. Joseph R. A pedigree of anophthalmos. Br J Ophthalmol. 1957;41:541–3.

89. Taylor D. Pediatric ophthalmology, 2nd ed. Blackwell Scientific Publications; 1997:208–9.

90. Waring GO, Roth AM, Rodrigues MM. Clinicopathologic correlation of microphthalmos. Am J Ophthalmol. 1976;82:714–21.

OPTICS AND REFRACTION

David Miller

CHAPTER 4

Visible Light

DAVID MILLER • STEPHEN K. BURNS

DEFINITION

- Visible light represents a small portion of the electromagnetic spectrum; wavelengths range between 400 and 700 nm.

KEY FEATURES

- The main source of visible light is the Sun.
- The Earth's atmosphere absorbs most of the light below 400nm.
- Visible light sensing by the eye depends upon
  a. The parameters of the light receptors
    – Unique size
    – Unique shape
    – Spectrum of sensitivity
    – Orientation as light guides
  b. The characteristics of the dioptric media

ASSOCIATED FEATURES

- Understanding the transformation of an optical image composed of visible light into an electronic image composed of visible light
  a. Processing of a 2D optical image into an electronic image
  b. Processing of a 3D optical image into an electronic image

ORIGIN OF VISIBLE LIGHT

Source

Clinical optics concerns the focusing or processing of visible light. Of course, visible light comes primarily from suns (stars); children are taught that this visible light also generates the energy necessary for life. The wavelengths of visible light ($4 \times 10^{-6} - 7 \times 10^{-6}$m) represent a minute fraction, about 1%, of the electromagnetic spectrum, which ranges from the shortest ionizing radiation (1×10^{-16}m) to the longest radiowaves (1×10^6m; Fig. 4-1).[1] Interestingly, visible light does not start out as such in the core of the Sun.

The Sun's core may be considered a furnace in which thermonuclear fusion takes place. Here, because of the crush of gravity, temperatures close to 16×10^6K are generated. In such a hot environment the elemental hydrogen protons fuse to produce helium nuclei and energy in the form of gamma rays. (The Sun converts 4×10^6 tons of matter into energy every second.) This resultant short-wavelength energy passes through about half a million miles (8×10^5km) of dense solar matter before reaching the Sun's surface.

During this long and slow journey, the photons lose energy and hence increase in wavelength. The radiation that leaves the Sun's surface primarily represents a spectrum of radiation between ultraviolet and infrared, with a small fraction of ionizing radiation in the form of x-rays with wavelengths of 10^{-10}m and γ-rays with wavelengths of 10^{-14}m. This ionizing radiation (part of the entire cosmic radiation) can destroy life, however the Sun also ejects huge amounts of matter (one million tons of hot electrons and protons every second), called the solar wind, which produces a vast shell around the Sun and prevents ionizing radiation from reaching the Earth. The fast-moving ions of the hot plasma of the solar wind are repulsed by the Earth's magnetic field.

Effect of Earth's Atmosphere

The Earth's atmosphere is held in position by the gravitational pull of the mass of the Earth. The potentially harmful ultraviolet and infrared radiation released from the Sun's surface is absorbed by ozone, carbon dioxide, and water vapor in the Earth's atmosphere (Fig. 4-2).[1] The Earth's temperature, which is a result of the temperature of the Sun's surface (6000K) and its distance from Earth (almost 100×10^6 miles [160×10^6km]), is responsible for the volume of atmospheric water vaporized from the oceans. Ozone and carbon dioxide result from photosynthesis and respiration. Thus early forms of life had to exist and produce these atmospheric gases before ultraviolet and infrared radiation could be absorbed and higher forms of life evolve.

It may seem incredible that only life-supporting visible light reaches the Earth from its origin in the solar core, although it may be argued that the process of evolution would have adopted life on Earth to any wavelength that reached Earth. The core-produced x-rays are filtered first by the outer layers of the Sun's matter. The Earth is 1/100th the diameter of the Sun and almost 100×10^6 miles (160×10^6km) away, and it receives only a tiny fraction of the radiation (about a billionth of the total).[2] The radiation that travels toward Earth is further filtered by the particles of the solar wind. In turn, this deadly solar wind is repelled by the Earth's magnetic field. Finally, the size and temperature of the Earth, as well as life on Earth, combine to produce an atmosphere that allows little more than visible light to pass through.

VISIBLE LIGHT SENSING

We have traced the origins of visible light from the Sun to the Earth's surface. Equally instructive are the mechanisms by which the biological molecule absorbs visible light and then informs the animal of that event. In a sense this represents the equivalent of Einstein's photoelectric effect. Rhodopsin is the biological molecule typically used for this purpose. Perhaps the earliest form of sensory rhodopsin, bacteriorhodopsin, is found in a primitive purple-colored bacterium, *Halobacterium halobium*.[3] It is not known how long this organism has inhabited the Earth. However, its preference for anaerobic conditions and a very salty environment may mean it developed at a time when little or no oxygen existed in the atmosphere and the sea contained high salt concentrations.

Bacteriorhodopsin is a complicated molecule that contains 248 amino acids in the opsin portions, which are linked to one retinal chromophore. Time-resolved spectroscopic measurements have determined that a *cis/trans* isomerization in the retinal portion of the molecule begins about 10^{-12} seconds after light stimulation. This is followed by deprotonation in the opsin portion at 10^{-5} seconds after stimulation.[4] This early rhodopsin absorbed light maximally at 495nm but responded to almost all

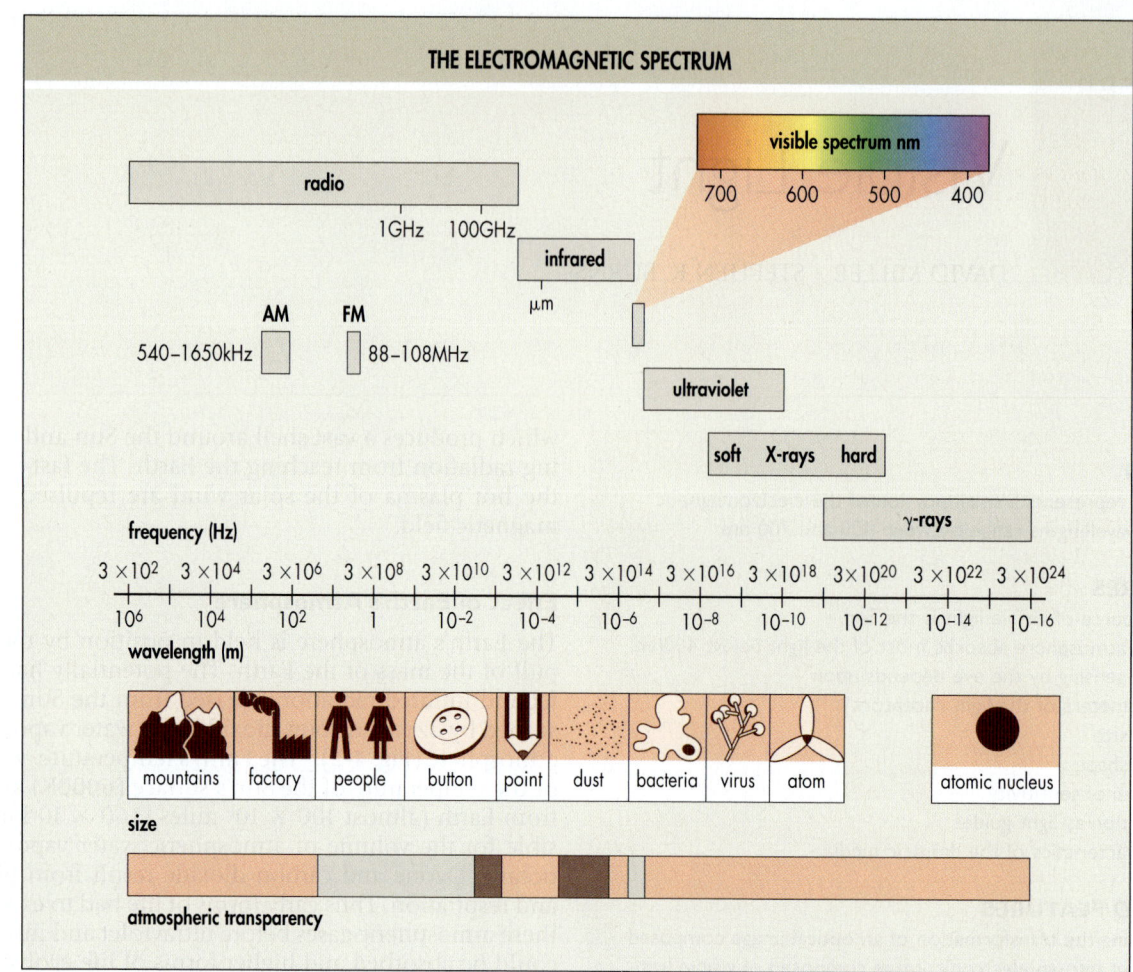

FIG. 4-1 ▌▌ **The electromagnetic spectrum.** The pictures of mountains, people, buttons, viruses, etc., are used to produce a real (i.e., visceral) feeling of the size of some of the wavelengths. (Adapted from Zeilik M. Astronomy: the evolving universe, ed 3. New York: Harper & Row; 1982.)

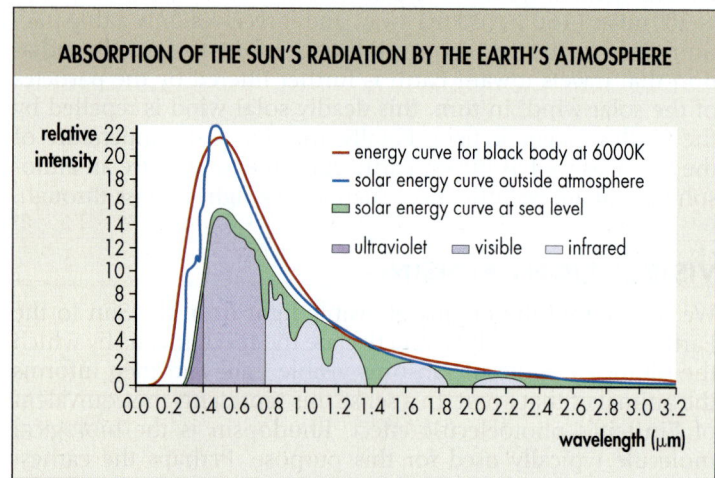

FIG. 4-2 ▌▌ **Absorption of the Sun's radiation by the Earth's atmosphere.** The white areas show the actual measured spectrum at sea level. Note the white areas of absorption are produced by ozone, water, and carbon dioxide. (Adapted from Zeilik M. Astronomy: the evolving universe, ed 3. New York: Harper & Row; 1982.)

visible light. Estimates suggest that the ancestor of human color pigment genes diverged from the rhodopsin gene about 800 million years ago and eventually resulted in a series of pigments with maximal absorption peaks in the blue, green, and red areas of the spectrum.[5] These specially adapted molecules are needed for accurate color vision.

Thus early animals used something akin to the original rhodopsin and a very simple optical system to see. For example, early worms and shellfish had light-sensing cells that lined a small cup-like structure. Such a system gives a sense of directionality, because each cell is shielded from light that approaches the cup from the nonseeing side. If the cup is made deeper and the sides are turned over, a lensless pinhole system is produced. Such a system is used by a very primitive swimming mollusk called *Nautilus*.[6]

Thus with visible light falling on the Earth, and rhodopsin already present, the stage was set for the development from simple light-sensing to natural or living optics.

VISIBLE LIGHT RECEPTORS AND THE OCULAR MEDIA

Life has existed on Earth for about 4 billion years. Primitive fish that had eyes resembling human eyes first appeared about 400 million years ago, so it might be said that ophthalmic optics originated at this time.[7-9] The living form of optics operates under the same rules and regulations as mechanical glass optics. Obviously, the various aspects of natural optics are linked closely to the dimensions of the wavelengths of visible light. Some of the basic elements of optics, using living optics examples, are introduced below.

Receptors

RECEPTOR SIZE AND SHAPE. The essential job of an optical system is to convert information about an object into an image. In natural optics, the image is formed on the retina and, therefore, it usually is much smaller than the object. Classically, the object has been considered as made up of a series of luminous points. For example, an object such as a tree does not contain points of light but can be thought of as reflecting points of light. The optical system converts the object points of light into image points. Because the image is smaller, the image points may be considered more densely packed.

Thus an image of high quality—also called an image of high resolution—demonstrates much detail. The finer and more tightly packed the receptors, the more detail is registered. The retinal receptor size and shape is influenced by a number of factors.

Because smaller receptors are better for resolution than larger receptors, what factor actually limits the smallness of a photoreceptor such as a retinal cone? The answer is diffraction. The smallest point focus of light is surrounded by a diffraction pattern. Thus very narrow receptors that receive a large diffraction pattern are wasteful. The size of the diffraction pattern, on the retina or on a screen, is known as an Airy disc. The diameter of this disc determines the distance between two resolvable points.

That is to say, the diameter of the Airy disc, D_λ, or the width of the central maxima, also is equal to the just resolvable distance between two intensity peaks when the minima of the interference patterns overlap (equation 4-1[10]; Fig. 4-3).[11,12]

Equation 4-1
$$D_\lambda = \frac{1.22 f \lambda}{p}$$

where 1.22 = constant for round pupil, λ = 550nm (average for visible light), f = focal length of system, and p = pupillary diameter.

For example, the size of the Airy disc image of a point of light for the human eye under photopic conditions may be determined as follows. If f = 17mm (focal length of eye), p = 4mm (average photopic pupil), l = 0.00055mm (median wavelength in visible spectrum of 0.0004–0.0007mm), then the diameter of the Airy disc, D_λ, is given by equation 4-2.

Equation 4-2
$$D_\lambda = \frac{(1.22)(17)(0.00055)}{4} = 2.8\mu m$$

Note that the size of the Airy disc can vary with the focal length of the eye, the wavelength of light, and the pupil size. Also note that 2.8μm is close to the size of the average foveal cone (1.5–2.0μm). In comparison, the eagle has a large photopic pupil (about 6mm); its foveal cones are thinner than those of the human and the eagle eye's resolution is finer.

Two other important optical concepts are buried in equation 4-1. First, note that f/p may be a key factor in determining the size of the Airy disc. The f/p ratio is called the f-number of the system. As p, the pupil diameter, decreases, the diameter of the diffraction pattern increases, and the resolution power lessens. The same occurs if the focal length increases, because this tends to widen the projection of the diffraction pattern. Thus a larger f-number suggests a degradation in resolution.

The second concept, the angle of resolution, is related closely to the Airy disc. The Airy disc is the physical distance, on the retina or a screen, between two points that are just resolvable. The angle of resolution, AS, is another way to describe just resolvable points in physical space (equation 4-3; see Fig. 4-3).

Equation 4-3
$$AS = \frac{1.22\lambda}{p}$$

where 1.22 = constant for a round pupil, p = pupil diameter, and l = 0.000550mm. The focal length of the system, f, is not used in equation 4-3.

The angle of resolution, AS, for two distant stars viewed by a healthy, average human eye with a pupil of 8mm in diameter is given by equation 4-4. However, it is known that the human eye can resolve two separate points in 1 minute or even less.[11] This discrepancy is explained as follows. The Raleigh criterion for resolution demands that the maxima of one point source must intersect the minima of the second point source (see Fig. 4-3),[13] which allows a patch of no light (high-contrast image) between the two maxima. However, in the case of the healthy young human eye, contrast determinations can be made for targets of

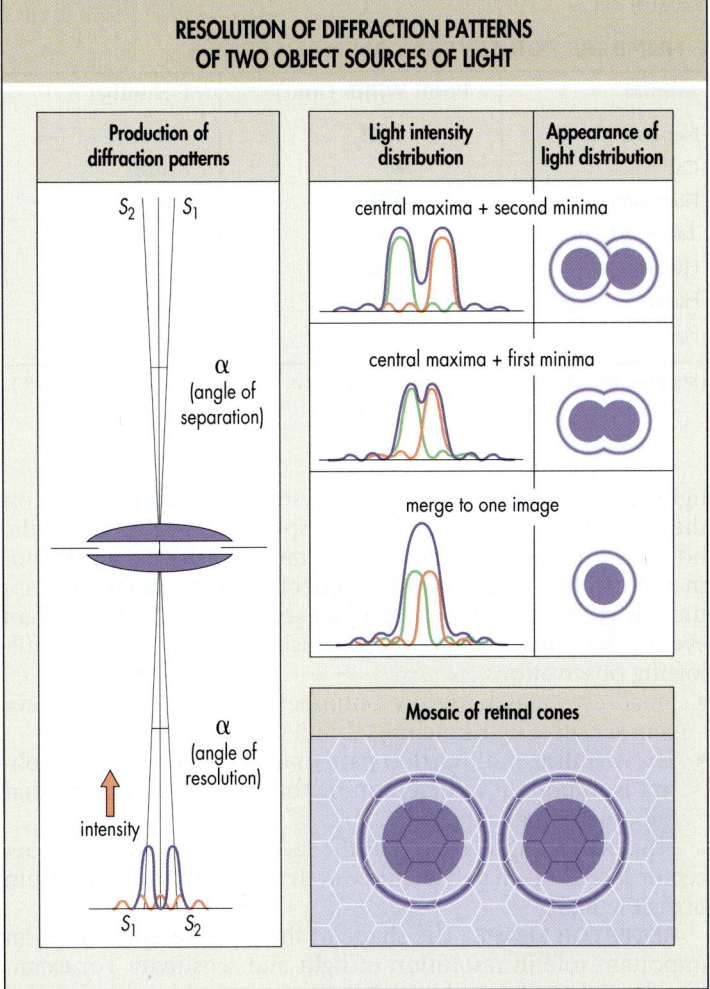

RESOLUTION OF DIFFRACTION PATTERNS OF TWO OBJECT SOURCES OF LIGHT

| Production of diffraction patterns | Light intensity distribution | Appearance of light distribution |

FIG. 4-3 ▮ Two object sources of light (S_1 and S_2) cannot be resolved if their diffraction patterns (Airy discs) overlap substantially. Two refraction patterns are produced by a circular aperture placed between two lenses, and resultant patterns of the light intensity distribution and appearance are shown: the central maxima of one diffraction pattern falls on the second minima of the diffraction pattern from the second source; the central maxima of one diffraction pattern falls on the first minima of the diffraction pattern from the second source, and the two images can just be resolved (Rayleigh's criterion); the two images merge as one. Mosaic of retinal cones with the diffraction pattern superimposed.

lower contrast. Thus many human eyes are able to distinguish two point sources or two black bars when the diffraction patterns overlap (see Fig. 4-3).

Equation 4-4
$$AS = \frac{(1.22)(0.00055)}{8} =$$
$$0.000084 \text{ radians} = 2.5 \text{ minutes}$$

For example, if it is assumed that the human separation criterion is one half the width of the Airy disc, then the angle of resolution is close to 1 minute of the arc. If the contrast enhancement known to be built into the neural processing of the human visual system is considered, it becomes apparent how some subjects have a resolution angle of less than 1 minute of arc.[10,14]

In conclusion, the resolution limit of natural optics is related to the size of the wavelengths within the spectrum of visible light.

LIGHT SENSITIVITY. When a firefly is seen in the distance, the number of photons collected by the eye from the firefly (per unit time) is distributed over the retinal image. Each image point is an Airy pattern. Thus the smaller the patterns, the more concentrated the pattern and the brighter is the image. It may be wondered whether animals that have small eyes, with a small focal length, or insects that have even smaller eye facets can collect light as well as the human eye does. From equation 4-1, if the

TABLE 4-1

F-NUMBERS FOR SEVERAL ANIMAL SPECIES

Animal	Pupil Width (mm)	F-Number
Net-casting spider	1.325	0.08
Cat	14	0.89
Flour moth	0.02	1.2
Tawny owl	13.3	1.3
Housefly	0.0025	2.0
Human	7–8	2.1–2.4
Pigeon	0.2	4.0

(Modified from Lythgoe JN. The ecology of vision. Oxford: Clarendon Press; 1979.)

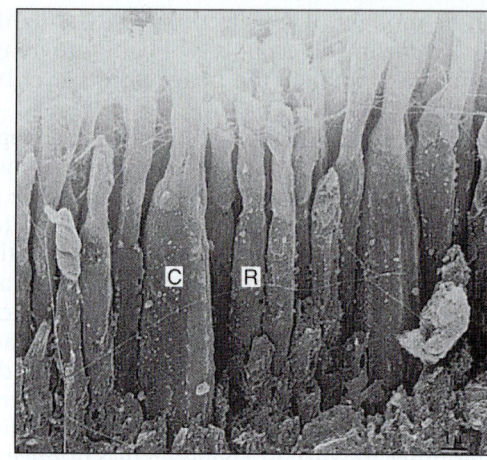

FIG. 4-4 ■ Scanning electron micrograph of photoreceptors that can be considered a light guide. *C, Cone; R, rod.* (From Prause JU, Jensen OA. Scanning electron micrograph of frozen-crack, dry cracked and enzyme digested retinal tissue of a monkey and man. Graefes Arch Klin Exp Ophthalmol. 1980;212:261–70.)

light-catching ability of an optical system depends primarily on the f-number (*f/p*), the small eyes of spiders and each facet of the housefly eye, theoretically, are even more sensitive than the human eye. Table 4-1 gives the f-number for some animal species[12]; the tiny eye of the net-casting spider sees dim objects better than eyes of the other animals. In conclusion, we can make the following observations.

- Small eyes may have low f-numbers and consequently have very sensitive light-catching abilities.
- The Airy disc or diffraction pattern from any point on the object is important in determining the density of photons that fall on a retinal area.

Thus we can appreciate that the level of sensitivity of the receptor is tied ultimately to the wavelength within the spectrum of visible light.

RECEPTOR SHAPE. The shape of the photoreceptor plays an important role in resolution of light and sensitivity. For example, the tighter the packing of receptors, the closer the focused points on the retina may be placed (actually, these are Airy patterns). Theoretical analysis shows that hexagonal cross-sections of close elements allow the tightest packing and, in fact, photoreceptors have such hexagonal cross-sections.[13,14] Of course, the tightness of the packing is related to the angle of resolution.

RECEPTOR AS A LIGHT GUIDE. A light guide (fiberoptic element) receives light at its entrance. Because the core of the guide has a higher index of refraction than the outer coating, or cladding, light that enters beyond the critical angle is not refracted but forced to reflect continually off the walls of the guide until it reaches the other end. (Critical angle refers to a refracting system, in which the incident ray is reflected instead of refracted.) As might be expected, at angles of entry close to the critical angle, a small amount of light may leak between closely packed light guides. The retinal cone acts as a light guide (Fig. 4-4).[15] The body of the cone has one index of refraction and the surrounding interstitium, although narrow, has a lower index of refraction. Recall that the index of refraction varies with wavelength. A second point to note is that as the diameter of the guide gets smaller, the wave nature of light plays a more important role in the functioning of the guide. For example, as the diameter of the guide approaches the light's wavelength, the waves of light that enter interfere more destructively with each other, which reduces the amount of light that reaches the other end. The interference pattern is known as a modal pattern.

Because diffraction is ultimately dependent on the wavelength, the limiting diameters of a light-guiding cone are related to the wavelength.[16-18] The second limiting factor is light crossover between receptors, which is related to the indices of refraction of the receptor and its surround, as well as to the closeness between receptors.[19,20] Both of these properties may be thought of as related to the wavelength of light.

In summary, the dimensions of receptors of about 2 μm in diameter and the separation between receptors of about 0.33 μm are related to the wavelength of visible light.

Dioptric Media

It seems obvious that dioptric media, or the optical elements of the eye, must be transparent. A perfectly transparent medium does not absorb or scatter light. Classically, pigments are described as absorbing visible light. The characteristic feature of a pigment molecule is a series of single and double bonds formed by the carbon atoms. The *pi* electrons of the double bond may be thought of as "free to wander" across the carbon backbone structure of the molecule, which increases their combined probability distribution over the entire molecule. This condition makes it easier to excite the *pi* electrons with the less-energetic visible wavelengths; ultraviolet, x-ray, and ionizing radiation have more energy than visible light. Transparent media have few or no pigment molecules. A good example of a medium transparent to visible light is the human ocular media,[21] which consists primarily of water.

When a beam of visible light passes through pure water, the water appears transparent because it contains no pigments and because the light waves scattered from each of the water molecules interfere destructively with one another in all directions except the forward direction. No light appears to have been scattered, because the scattered waves mutually cancel to give zero net scatter to the side. Water and glass interact with light in this way because their components are all of the same index of refraction and uniformly distributed. The transparent cornea may be thought of as made up of collagen fibers of one index of refraction embedded in a mucopolysaccharide (high water content) of a second index of refraction. However, because the distribution of the elements is in a uniform pattern, and because the collagen fibers are never more than the distance of one half a wavelength of visible light apart, the number of scattered waves is small. In reality the cornea is only 90% transparent (10% of the incident light is scattered). It is functionally transparent,[22] although not perfectly transparent. Once again, an important optical property (transparency) may be thought of as dependent on the wavelength of the incident light.

TRANSFORMATION OF A REAL IMAGE TO AN ELECTRONIC IMAGE

Light is visible because it can be detected in the retina. It produces changes in receptor cells in our eye. These changes stimulate nervous activity, which is processed by retinal nerve cells and conveyed to our brain. Electrical sensors can "see" light, too. There are two major classes of electrical light sensors, photovoltaic and photoconductive. The photovoltaic class generates electrical power, which is related to the power of the light incident to the sensor. Photoconductive devices conduct more elec-

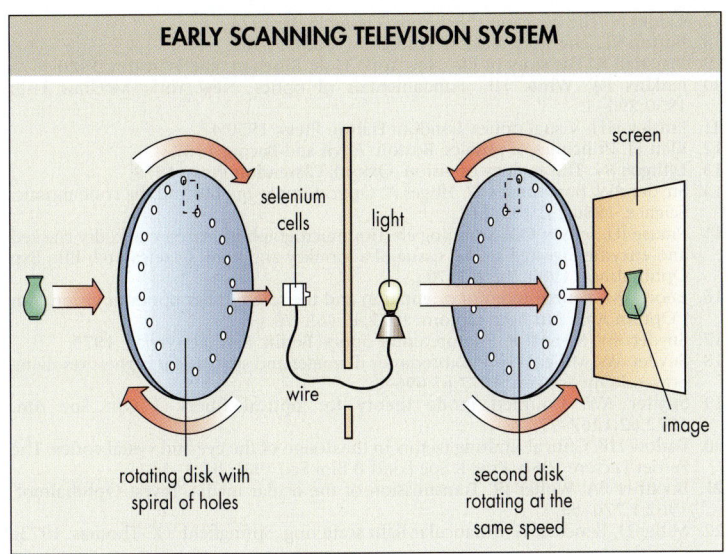

EARLY SCANNING TELEVISION SYSTEM

FIG. 4-5 ■ Example of early mechanical version of a scanning television system (Patented in 1884 by Paul Nipkow) (Courtesy Cinemedia Corporation) [http://www.cinemedia.net/SFCVRMItAnnex/maughton/nipkow_disk.gif]

tricity with increasing light. A solar cell is a photovoltaic device. The sensor which turns on the streetlights at night is usually a photoconductive device. Either type can produce an electrical signal which can be conveyed to a distant receptor.

The association between light and electricity has been known for a long time. Lightning is a spectacular example of light and electricity. Electricity can produce light related to the amount of electricity. The brightness of an electric arc or an incandescent filament of a electric lamp are both related to the current flow producing the light. Television, fax, and electronic cameras all depend on the ability to electrically and proportionally sense and create light.

Paul Nipkow invented mechanically scanned television and patented it in 1884 (Fig. 4-5). This system "scanned" a real image using a rotating disk pierced with a spiral of holes that presented a small portion of the image to a selenium photoconductive sensor. The sensor was connected to a light source that was observed through a second, synchronized, rotating disk which placed the received light in the right place in the image plane.

An electronic image differs from a real image in several ways. (1) The electronic image is sampled. It is made up of a finite number of little light spots, or picture elements called pixels, which are seen together as a continuous image but individually simply represent the light at a point in a real image. (2) The light provided by these (pixels) is made up of three different primary colors (red, blue, and green) which are perceived as nearly any color. (3) Finally, the information is not there all of the time but is presented repeatedly at a rate sufficiently fast that the image is seen as continuous. Electronic images are thus neither spatially nor temporally continuous. Although it is not essential to an electronic image, the information describing the individual pixels is conveyed serially or one at a time. By agreeing on a correspondence between the location of a pixel and the order that it is transmitted, it is unnecessary to transmit the location with the color and brightness information. This orderly sequence of analysis and synthesis describes a pattern known as a raster.

Solid state electronic image sensors have replaced mechanically scanned image sensors and electronically scanned sensors like Vidicon tubes with arrays of electrical sensors. Electronic image sensors have a photosensor for each pixel, while mechanically and electronically scanned sensors examine a portion of a photosensitive region large enough to accommodate the entire image. The first solid state image sensor was the charge-coupled device (CCD). CCDs represent the amount of light at a pixel by stored electrical charge. The pixels are arranged in rows and columns. The charge is collected by an individual pixel element

in each row. This charge is collected and transferred to the CMOS Imager, so called because it incorporates CMOS transistors and includes light sensors with individual transistor amplifiers and electronic switches. The switches can connect the selected sensor to an output amplifier. The switches usually are operated in an orderly sequence. Color filters can be placed in front of individual sensors so that they provide color information as well as a measure of the amount of light.

The information associated with an electronic image can produce a visible image in several ways. Probably the most common image presentation uses a cathode ray tube. In this tube, a beam of electrons excites a phosphor that produces light. Modern color cathode ray tubes incorporate a complex image plane with regions of three colored phosphors. The electron beam traces a raster, which corresponds to the raster used to scan the original image. When this original image is stored in an electronic memory, the date is read out in the order needed to display it on a standard raster. This is called a *bit-mapped image.* Liquid crystal displays (LCDs) are an important current technology. Individual pixels are implemented with tiny "light valves" that control the amount of light coming from that pixel. The light valves work by electrically shifting the polarization of light passing through a liquid crystal material. Polarized light passes through it and encounters a second polarizer which transmits only light aligned with it. The contrast ratio (brightest-to-dimmest light) is limited with a light valve. Contrast ratios between 200 and 500 are now available. Transmissive LCD displays can provide around 200 nits of illumination. Color LCDs are implemented by placing color filters in the path of the light valve.

LCDs work by controlling transmitted or reflected light. Plasma displays and light-emitting diode (LED) displays, like cathode ray tubes, provide light directly and are consequently quite bright. It is difficult to fabricate small pixels (0.3mm in a 15-inch cathode ray tube display) with these technologies. Plasma technology creates light from a glowing plasma which excites colored phosphors. Pixel dimensions can be made sufficiently small to realize large-format television (50-inch) displays. Conventional semiconductor LEDs are relatively large and are suitable only for very large displays (greater than 10 feet) but can be very bright (5000 nit). Organic LEDs (OLEDs) are evolving rapidly. Very small OLEDs can be fabricated. High-resolution ($852 \times 3 \times 600$ pixels) "microdisplays" (0.62-inch diagonal) are currently available.

Processing

An electronic image can be manipulated as data and offers tremendous opportunities to present or receive visual information which is beyond the power of physical optics. Moreover the current generation of computer technology is fast enough to process an image as we view it. This makes it possible to see subtle differences in light intensity by mapping shades to differences in color. Edges can be enhanced. Reference points can be marked, distances measured, and templates superposed. There is much promise in the computer-enhanced electronic image.

Stereoscopic Vision

We see the world through two eyes. Stereoscopic vision is of immense value to a surgeon. Most surgical microscopes provide a stereoscopic view. Stereoscopy requires acquiring and transmitting images for the left and right eye in the same amount of time required for transmitting a single image. This doubles the required bandwidth. Reducing the bandwidth with slower transmission produces unacceptable flicker and interrupted motion. The current generation of computer technology offers greatly increased bandwidth so we can anticipate economical, high-quality stereo imaging will become economically feasible. This suggests the practical possibilities for stereoscopically recording or viewing an image from an operating microscope.

SUMMARY

In conclusion, in this chapter a perspective for optics as well as a focus on an important common denominator in optics is given. The common theme is related to the properties of the tiny portion of the electromagnetic spectrum known as visible light. The wavelength of visible light is critical in understanding the structural dimensions of the optical systems of animal and human eyes. Electronic images are increasingly common and have unique characteristics and possibilities, which should be included whenever considering vision and visible light.

REFERENCES

1. Zeilik M. Astronomy: the evolving universe, ed 3. New York: Harper & Row; 1982.
2. Kippenhahn R. Light from the depths of time. New York: Springer-Verlag; 1986.
3. Oesterhelt D, Stoekenius W. Rhodopsin-like protein from the membrane of *Halobacterium halobium*. Nature New Biol. 1971;233:149–52.
4. Atkinson GH, Blanchard D, Lemaire H, *et al*. Picosecond time resolved fluorescence spectroscopy of K-590 in the bacteriorhodopsin photocycle. Biophys J. 1989;55:263–74.
5. Yokoyama S, Yokoyama R. Molecular evolution of human visual pigment genes. Mol Biol Evol. 1989;6:186–97.
6. Dawkins R. The blind watchmaker. New York: WW Norton; 1986:85–6.
7. Calder N. The life game. New York: Viking Press; 1974.
8. Burton VL. Life story. Boston: Houghton Mifflin; 1962.
9. Marshall K. The story of life. New York: Holt, Rinehart, and Winston; 1980.
10. Jenkins FA, White HE. Fundamentals of optics. New York: McGraw Hill; 1950:290–3.
11. Emsley HH. Visual optics. London: Hatton Press; 1950:47.
12. Blatt FJ. Principles of physics. Boston: Allyn and Bacon; 1987.
13. Lythgoe JN. The ecology of vision. Oxford: Clarendon Press; 1979.
14. Snyder AW, Bossomaier JR, Huges A. Optical image quality and the cone mosaic. Science. 1986;231:499–501.
15. Prause JU, Jensen OA. Scanning electron micrograph of frozen-crack, dry cracked and enzyme digested retinal tissue of a monkey and man. Graefes Arch Klin Exp Ophthalmol. 1980;212:261–70.
16. Enoch JM. Retinal receptor orientation and the role of fiber optics in vision. Am J Optom Arch Am Acad Optom. 1972;49:455–70.
17. Snyder AW, Menzal R. Photoreceptor optics. Berlin: Springer-Verlag; 1975.
18. Snyder AW, Miller WH. Photoreceptor diameter and spacing for highest resolving power. J Opt Soc Am. 1977;67:696–8.
19. Snyder AW. Coupled mode theory for optical fibers. J Opt Soc Am. 1972;62:1267–77.
20. Barlow HB. Critical limiting factors in the design of the eye and visual cortex: The Ferrier Lecture 1980. Proc R Soc Lond B Biol Sci. 1981;212:1–34.
21. Boettner EA, Wolter JR. Transmission of the ocular media. Invest Ophthalmol. 1962;1:776–83.
22. Miller D, Benedek G. Intraocular light scattering. Springfield: CC Thomas; 1973.

CHAPTER 5

Physical Optics for Clinicians

EDMOND H. THALL • RUSSELL MILLER • CHRISTOPHER CALVANO

DEFINITION

- Whereas geometrical optics considers light to be a series of rays, physical optics approaches problems in optics by treating light as a waveform.

KEY FEATURES

- Interference of light waves.
- Polarization of light waves.
- Diffraction effects of light waves.
- Scattering of light waves (effects on glare and contrast sensitivity).
- Understanding the quantum model of light waves.

ASSOCIATED FEATURES

- Lasers and light waves.
- Interaction of tissue and light waves (i.e., laser light).

ELECTROMAGNETIC WAVE

FIG. 5-1 ▮▮ Electromagnetic wave. An electromagnetic wave consists of an oscillating electric field perpendicular to an oscillating magnetic field. The direction of propagation is perpendicular to both the electric and the magnetic fields.

INTRODUCTION

Geometrical optics ignores the basic nature of light yet remarkably is able to explain many aspects of image formation, such as image location and magnification, based on the geometry of the paths that light follows when moving from object to image. However, many clinical phenomena can be understood only through knowledge of light's physical nature.

ELECTROMAGNETIC AND SCALAR WAVE MODELS OF LIGHT

Certain phenomena are best explained by modeling light as a wave. Maxwell showed that light behaved as an electromagnetic wave consisting of an electric field oscillating perpendicular to an oscillating magnetic field, with both fields perpendicular to the direction of propagation (Fig. 5-1).[1] Since the magnetic field oscillates in lockstep[2] with the electric field, it is often sufficient to consider only the electric field. In the scalar wave model, light is modeled as a single transverse wave (Fig. 5-2).

POLARIZATION

In both the electromagnetic and the scalar wave models, light is a transverse wave. In such waves, the direction of oscillation is always perpendicular to the direction of propagation. Nevertheless, the wave may oscillate in many different directions. A linearly polarized wave oscillates in a single plane (see Fig. 5-2).

Polarization may be achieved in several ways.[3] If light is reflected specularly from a plane surface, it is polarized partially—the direction of polarization is parallel to the reflecting surface.[4] If light is reflected at a specific angle (discovered by Brewster and named in his honor), the reflected light is polarized totally. The Brewster angle can be calculated using the following equation:

$$\Phi_B = \tan^{-1} n2/n1$$

Fresnel took Brewster's discovery further and calculated the degree of (partial) polarization produced by a reflecting surface at any angle of incidence. Fresnel's equations are somewhat complicated but can be found in any standard treatment of optics.[5]

Some materials have different refractive indices, depending on the direction of polarization; they are called birefringent because they have two different refractive indices. Light incident on such birefringent materials travels in different directions, depending on its polarization. Such materials separate a beam of light into two beams, each linearly polarized at right angles to each other.[6]

Dichroic materials absorb light linearly polarized in one direction and transmit light linearly polarized at right angles to this. These materials are commonly used in polarized sunglasses. Most reflecting surfaces in human surroundings are horizontally oriented, such as floors, automobile hoods, and so forth. Light reflected from a surface (and consequently at least partially polarized) is absorbed by dichroic materials in the lenses of polarized sunglasses. In sunglasses, the dichroic material is oriented to transmit vertically polarized light and absorb horizontally polarized light. Polarizing sunglasses reduce only reflected glare, and only when the reflecting surface is horizontal. Despite these limitations, polarization is a popular feature in sunglasses.

Several ocular structures are birefringent; these include collagen fibers in the cornea and iris and nerve fibers of the inner retina.[7] A number of attempts have been made to capitalize on this. An instrument is now available for clinical use that measures birefringence in the retinal nerve fiber layer as an indicator of thickness of that layer. However, the accuracy of nerve fiber

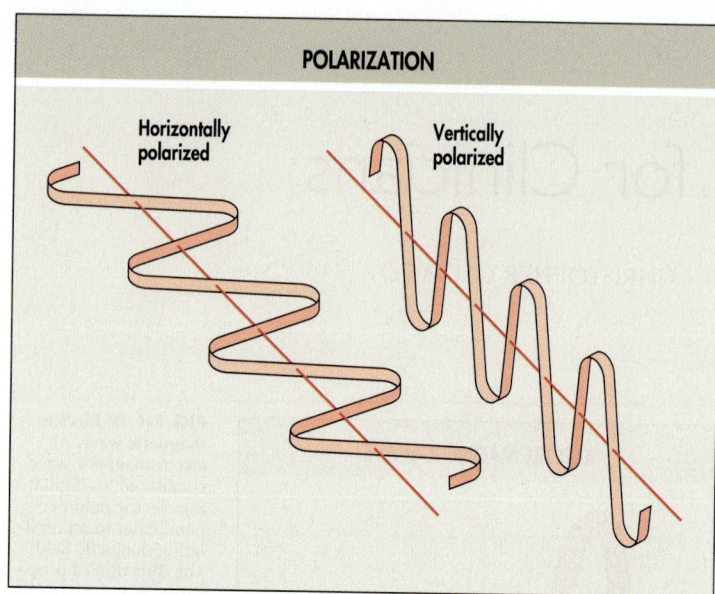

POLARIZATION

Horizontally polarized

Vertically polarized

FIG. 5-2 ▮ **Polarization.** Both transverse waves propagate in the same direction but oscillate in different planes. Here, only the scalar wave approximation is adopted, and only the electric field is shown.

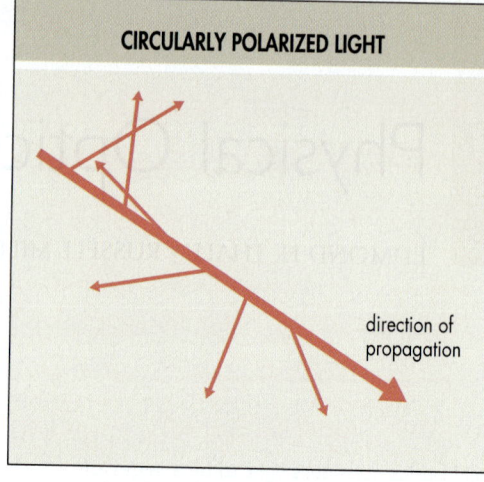

CIRCULARLY POLARIZED LIGHT

direction of propagation

FIG. 5-3 ▮ **Circularly polarized light.** In circularly polarized light, the electric field has a constant amplitude, and the plane of polarization rotates at a constant speed. The plane of polarization follows a corkscrew path as the wave travels.

layer measurements may be affected by birefringence in other ocular tissues, especially the cornea.

The potential for changes in other ocular structures to produce apparent changes in the nerve fiber layer should always be considered when interpreting data based on birefringence measurements. Recently, changes in nerve fiber layer thickness measured by birefringence were reported following LASIK. Whether the change in birefringence is the result of a decrease in nerve fiber layer thickness or a change in corneal birefringence is an open question, but one that can be easily resolved using laser keratectomy. Intraocular pressure increases only to 30mmHg during laser keratectomy. It is extremely unlikely that this would produce a change in the nerve fiber layer, so any apparent change would be an artifact.

Birefringence in the anterior segment is demonstrated easily using the circular polarizer furnished in some direct ophthalmoscopes to eliminate annoying corneal reflections. In circularly polarized light, the plane of polarization rotates uniformly (Fig. 5-3). If the anterior segment is focused on, instead of the retina, a dark Maltese-style cross is seen, with bright, iridescent colors between the arms of the cross. The dark cross is produced by Fresnel reflection at the corneal surface. The colors are probably produced by birefringence of the corneal and iris collagen.

Several attempts have been made to measure corneal topography using Fresnel reflection by the anterior corneal surface. When light is reflected from a surface, it is at least partially polarized. The degree of polarization is related to the angle between the light and the reflecting surface. In theory, it is possible to calculate corneal shape from measurements of the degree and direction of polarization of light reflected from the corneal surface. In practice, this has proved exceedingly difficult.

Birefringence has been used to detect defects in intraocular lenses. The birefringence is detected by placing the lens between two linear polarizers at right angles to each other. Any light transmitted appears as a readily recognizable bright spot that indicates a possible defect in the strength of the lens. These defects arise from various causes, such as heat produced when the haptics of a three-piece lens are inserted, or from heat generated during lathe cutting or polishing.

Polarization is the basis of the "Fly test" for stereopsis.[8] Two images are superimposed and slightly displaced. Each image linearly polarizes light, and the axes of polarization are perpendicular. The patient wears polarizing glasses so that each eye sees only one of the images. Because each image is slightly displaced, the observer perceives the image in front of the page. By wearing

the polarizing glasses upside down, each eye sees the opposite image, and the perception is that the image is below the page.

Projector charts and polarization can also be used to detect malingering in patients claiming unilateral vision loss. Again, the patient wears polarizers over each eye so that each eye sees only some of the letters on a line. The patient is instructed to keep both eyes open and read the chart. If the patient identifies all the letters on the 20/20 line, the unilateral vision loss is factitious.

INTERFERENCE

When two different light waves overlap, their amplitudes add. If two waves of equal amplitude are 180° out of phase, the amplitudes cancel out, and the net result is zero (Fig. 5-4).[9] If the waves are perfectly in phase, the amplitudes double, and the intensity (square of the amplitude) is four times greater than that of a single wave. Interference refers to the summation of amplitudes that always occurs when two waves overlap. When the waves are in phase, the interference is constructive, and when the waves are out of phase, the interference is destructive.

Imagine shining two identical flashlights illuminating the same spot on a wall. You would expect to see twice as much light, but if the waves from each light were perfectly out of phase, you would actually see no light at all. In practice, in order to observe interference effects, the waves must be coherent and polarized in similar directions. The light from two different sources always interferes either constructively or destructively, but you cannot observe the interference because the light from one source is not coherent with the other light.

Because of coherence requirements, interference can be observed only under certain conditions. An interference phenomenon widely used in clinical practice, but not widely appreciated, is the basis for antireflection coatings.[10] When light travels from one medium to another, a small amount of light is reflected at the interface between the two media. Anyone who has used a direct ophthalmoscope has experienced the annoying reflection from the corneal surface. In indirect ophthalmoscopy, reflection from the handheld lens may interfere with fundus visualization, particularly when the slit lamp is used. Patients often complain of reflections associated with spectacle lenses.

One way to reduce reflected light is to coat lenses with thin films. One type of antireflective coating consists of a thin film (one half wavelength thick, approximately 250nm) of material with a refractive index in between those of air and glass. Light is reflected from both the front and back surfaces of the film, but because the film is half a wavelength thick, the two reflections interfere destructively and reduce the amount of back-scattered light.

In practice, thin film coatings are much more complicated and usually consist of multiple layers of different materials. A simple one-layer antireflective coating may eliminate reflection

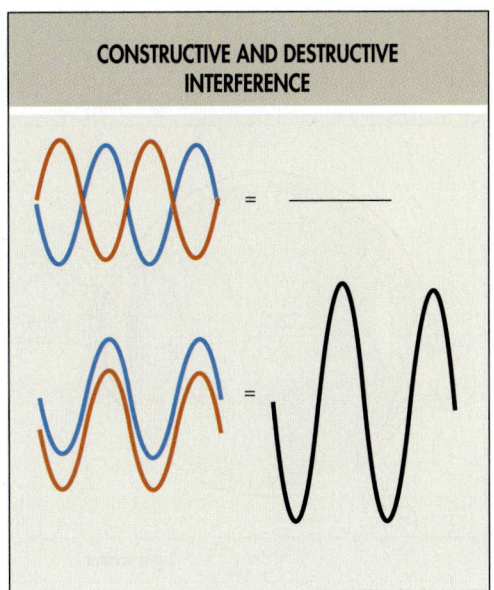

CONSTRUCTIVE AND DESTRUCTIVE INTERFERENCE

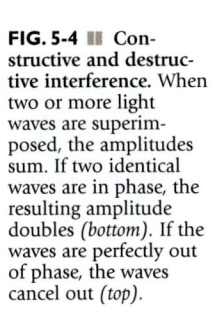

FIG. 5-4 ■ Constructive and destructive interference. When two or more light waves are superimposed, the amplitudes sum. If two identical waves are in phase, the resulting amplitude doubles (bottom). If the waves are perfectly out of phase, the waves cancel out (top).

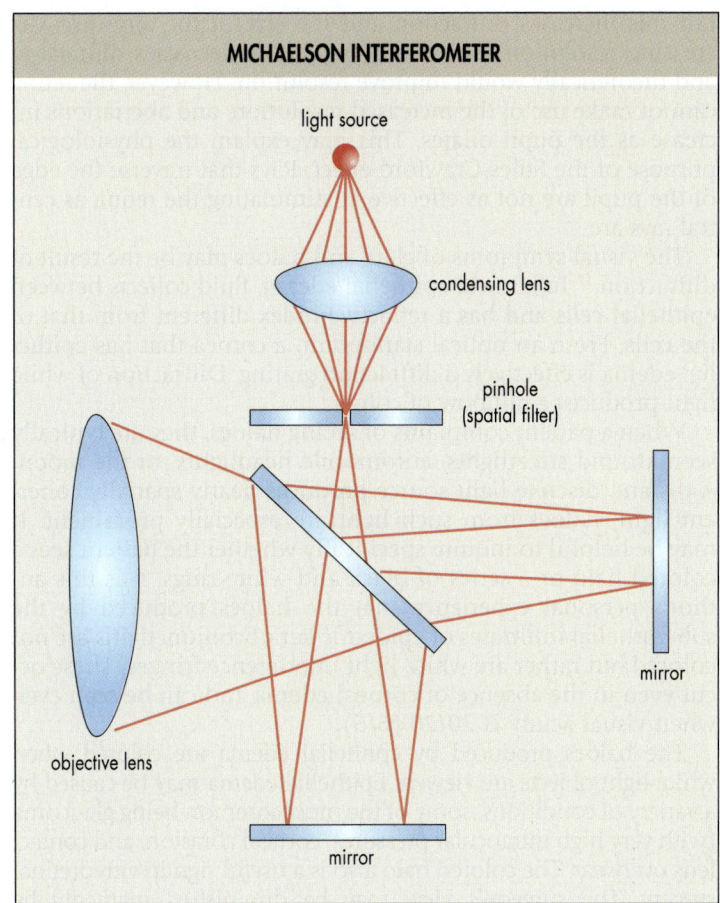

FIG. 5-5 ■ Michaelson interferometer is the basis of optical coherence tomography. A beam splitter divides one light beam into two, which travel different paths and then are recombined. If the light source has low coherence, interference fringes are observed only when the optical path length of each arm is nearly identical. Placing the eye in one path of the interferometer and varying the length of the other arm can measure the optical path length to various ocular tissues.

for only one wavelength of light. Multilayer coatings may reduce reflection significantly over a range of wavelengths. Single-layer coatings also are scratched easily and can be removed by routine lens cleaning. Additional layers are used to make the coatings more durable.

Thin films also occur clinically. The tear film consists of three layers: an outer oil layer, a middle aqueous layer, and an inner mucin layer. The oil layer constitutes a thin film that produces a colored interference pattern visible on slit-lamp examination.[11] The appearance of the interference pattern is similar to the iridescent colors produced by a layer of oil or gasoline on the surface of a puddle of water. Inability to elicit the interference pattern suggests a specific defect in the oil layer.

Sometimes a nearly transparent layer of inflammatory cells grows on the surface of an intraocular lens implant.[12] It may be difficult to see this layer with conventional slit-lamp illumination, but with placement of the slit beam at a slight angle to the visual axis, a rainbow of color caused by thin film interference may be appreciated. Cortical cells growing on the posterior capsule can produce a similar effect.

Interference is used to assess retinal function in patients with media opacity, especially cataract. A laser light source is split into two narrow beams that presumably pass through small, clear regions of the lens. Because the beams are coherent, they form interference fringes on the retina. The arrangement is essentially a modification of Young's two-slit experiment. The greater the separation of beams in the pupil, the narrower the interference fringes on the retina. The patient reports when he or she can see the fringes; the narrower the fringes the patient can detect, the better the potential acuity. To avoid a falsely low estimate of potential acuity, the patient must have a sufficiently large pupil to produce narrow fringes on the retina. Unfortunately, a falsely optimistic estimate of acuity can also be obtained in patients with macular edema or degeneration, because the test uses coherent light.

The most recent innovative clinical application of interference is optical coherence tomography (OCT).[13] The OCT scanner is basically a Michaelson interferometer (Fig. 5-5). The light source is a superluminescent diode, which has more coherence than white light but less than a laser diode. The limited coherence allows detection of interference effects over only a small optical path difference. By scanning the reference mirror, the optical path difference between various tissue layers can be measured.

When interpreting OCT images, it is important to realize that OCT measures optical path length, not physical length. Optical path length is physical length multiplied by refractive index.

OCT has also been used to measure axial length and corneal thickness. Just as the accuracy of ultrasound biometry depends on assumptions about the speed of light in ocular media, the accuracy of OCT measurements depends on assumptions about the refractive index of ocular tissues. Two corneas of identical thickness but with small differences in refractive index will appear to have different lengths when measured by OCT.

DIFFRACTION EFFECTS

Diffraction refers to the bending of light as it passes through an aperture; it was first observed independently by Hooke and Grimaldi in the mid-1600s.[14,15] Ultimately, diffraction limits the resolution of optical images. If an imaging system is well corrected, the image of a point source is an airy disc, and the radius of the central maximum is[16]:

$$r = \frac{1.22\lambda}{2\ n'Sin(u')}$$

For the average eye, the exit pupil diameter is about 3mm, and it is 18.5mm from the retina. Thus, for an eye of these dimensions, the airy disc has a radius of about 2μm or a diameter of 4μm. This corresponds roughly to the diameter of a photoreceptor. If the airy disc were considerably larger than a photoreceptor, the optics of the eye would limit vision, and the retina would have an unnecessarily large number of photoreceptors. Conversely, if the airy disc were much smaller than the diameter of a photoreceptor, the imaging capabilities of the eye would far exceed the retinal resolution. So it is not surprising that the resolution of the ocular media correlates with the retinal anatomy.

The calculation of ocular resolution assumes that the eye is essentially aberration free. Aberrations can be decreased by miosis, but this increases diffraction and the size of the airy disc, decreasing resolution. Conversely, mydriasis decreases diffraction and theoretically would improve resolution. However, the retina cannot make use of the increased resolution, and aberrations increase as the pupil dilates. This may explain the physiological purpose of the Stiles-Crawford effect. Rays that traverse the edge of the pupil are not as effective at stimulating the retina as central rays are.

The visual symptoms of glare and haloes may be the result of diffraction.[17] In corneal epithelial edema, fluid collects between epithelial cells and has a refractive index different from that of the cells. From an optical standpoint, a cornea that has epithelial edema is effectively a diffraction grating. Diffraction of white light produces a rainbow of colors.

When a patient complains of seeing haloes, they are typically seen around streetlights, automobile headlights, or the moon. A distant, discrete light source produces nearly spatially coherent light; haloes from such light are especially prominent. It may be helpful to inquire specifically whether the patient sees a colored halo or a series of black and white rings. It is this author's personal experience that the haloes produced by the subepithelial infiltrates of epidemic keratoconjunctivitis are not colored but rather are white-light interference fringes. These occur even in the absence of corneal edema and can be seen even when visual acuity is 20/20 (6/6).

The haloes produced by epithelial edema are colored when white-light objects are viewed. Epithelial edema may be caused by a variety of conditions, some of the most common being glaucoma (with very high intraocular pressure), corneal abrasion, and contact lens overwear. The colored halo also is a useful sign in vitreoretinal surgery. The surgeon's view may be diminished markedly by corneal epithelial edema or many other causes. Shining the light pipe on the working instrument gives a specular reflection that invariably has a colored halo around it if epithelial edema is present. A diminished view from epithelial edema can be overcome by removing the epithelium, but this can lead to postoperative complications such as corneal ulcer, especially in diabetics, who tend to re-epithelialize slowly. In the absence of a colored halo, the surgeon should consider other possible causes for the decreased view before removing the epithelium, perhaps unnecessarily.

Binary optical lenses combine refractive and diffractive effects. Some multifocal intraocular lenses use binary optical designs. In the early 1990s there was considerable interest in the use of diffractive optics for the correction of presbyopia. The diffractive part of the lens produced two images at different focal lengths. Some patients can tolerate the monocular diplopia and decreased image contrast. However, currently there is greater interest in more physiological approaches.

GLARE AND LIGHT SCATTER

In an ideal world, light would travel straight through a material, but in reality, a small amount of light is scattered in all directions.[18] Glare occurs when a defect in the ocular media scatters light, which decreases the contrast of the retinal image (Fig. 5-6).

Light scatter generally is caused by particles in the medium. There are two types of scatter: Rayleigh scatter is caused by particles smaller than the wavelength of incident light, and Mie scatter is caused by particles larger than the wavelength of light. In Rayleigh scatter, the amount of scatter is proportional to the fourth power of the wavelength of the incident light. In Mie scatter, the amount of scatter is directly proportional to the wavelength of the incident light.

Molecules of air result in Rayleigh scatter of sunlight. In Rayleigh scatter, blue light is scattered about 16-fold more than red. Consequently, the atmosphere acts as a blue-light filter. When the sun is overhead, sunlight traverses relatively little atmosphere, and the sun appears yellow. When the sun is low over the horizon, light must travel through more of the atmosphere, and more blue light is scattered, which gives the sun a red appearance.

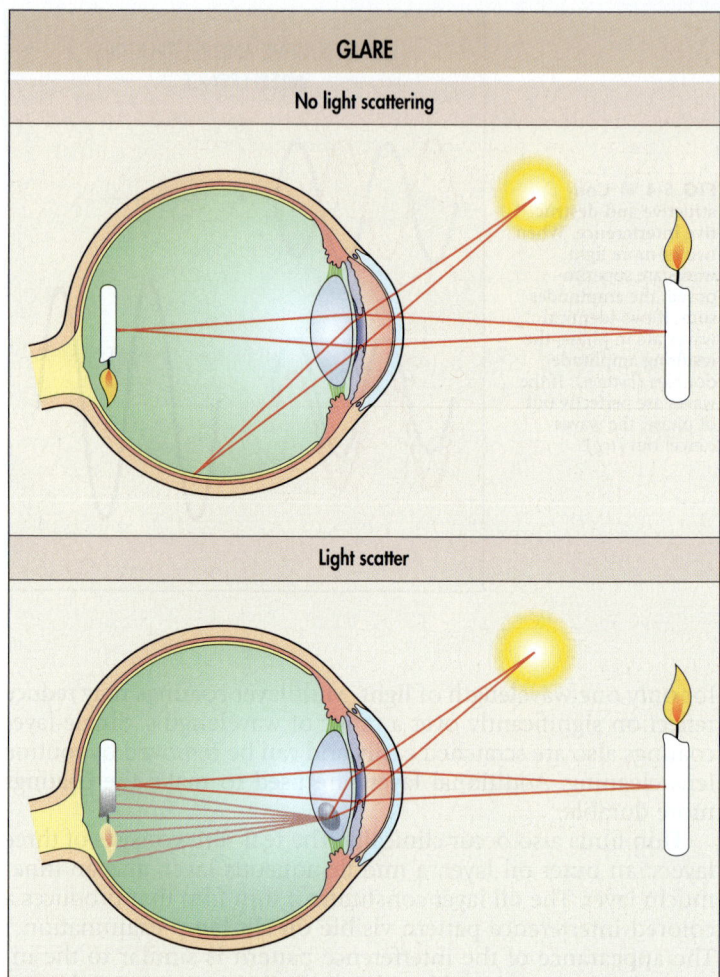

FIG. 5-6 ■ Glare. Without light scatter, light from an off-axis glare source does not overlap with the central retinal image. Light scatter by the ocular media, such as an early cataract, may decrease contrast in the central retinal image.

The same applies to scatter by the ocular media, especially the crystalline lens. As a person ages, light scatter by the lens increases, and fundus features appear more yellow and red. After cataract extraction, fundus details appear whiter. If a patient has had a cataract removed from one eye but has a cataract in the other eye, the optic nerve in the operated eye may appear atrophic by comparison to that in the phakic eye. This appearance may result from the difference in light scatter between the two eyes.

For several reasons, attempts have been made to measure the amount of light scattered by the crystalline lens. Such measurements may be able to verify whether a cataract is bad enough to explain a patient's visual loss or whether another cause is present. A fundamental problem is that only back-scattered light can be measured clinically. Back-scattered light is light that hits the lens and is scattered through the pupil and out of the eye. Back-scattered light does not reach the retina and therefore does not affect vision. Forward-scattered light hits the lens and is scattered, but it continues through the crystalline lens to reach the retina (and decrease vision). No definite relationship exists between forward- and back-scattered light.

Some investigators hoped that objective measurements of light scatter by the crystalline lens would provide a guideline for cataract surgery. However, the appropriateness of cataract surgery depends on the effect of a visual deficit on the patient's lifestyle, not on the degree of visual loss per se. A better use for light scatter measurements is to evaluate the efficacy of drugs intended to slow or prevent cataract formation.

The difficulty in performing useful light scatter measurements cannot be overstated. Generally, to be of value, the amount of light scattered in all directions must be measured for every possible direction of incident beam. The results of such measurements constitute the bidirectional reflection distribution function. No current commercial instrument can measure the bidirectional reflection distribution of crystalline lens light scatter.

A device that measures both Mie and Rayleigh scatter has been introduced to quantify both cells and flare in the anterior chamber. To date, the principal value of such measurements is to compare the efficacy of different treatment regimens.

QUANTUM MODEL OF LIGHT

Although the wave model is very useful, some phenomena can be explained only on the basis of a quantum or discrete model of light. When electrons change energy levels, they often absorb or emit a photon. An electron in an elevated energy level may drop to a lower energy level spontaneously or as a result of stimulated emission. If a photon of appropriate energy passes by an electron in a high-energy state, the photon induces the electron to drop to a lower energy level and give off a second photon. The two photons are identical in energy and phase.[19]

BASIC LASER PHYSICS

Stimulated emission is the basis of the laser. The word *laser* was originally an acronym for light amplification by stimulated emission of radiation. In any laser there is a working medium. Normally, in any working material there are more electrons in lower energy levels than in higher levels. By some means, which can vary depending on the type of laser, energy is added to the working material so that a preponderance of electrons are in a high-energy state, a condition referred to as a population inversion. Eventually, one electron spontaneously decays, producing a photon that passes by other electrons and stimulates them to emit more identical photons. Partially reflecting mirrors placed at the ends of the medium cause the photons to pass through the working material multiple times, yielding a chain reaction that produces a beam.[20]

LIGHT-TISSUE INTERACTIONS

Depending on the working material, photons of various wavelengths can be produced. To understand the clinical use of lasers, it is necessary to understand the various ways light interacts with tissue.

In photocoagulation, light energy is absorbed by tissue generating heat.[21] The heat denatures proteins, producing coagulation, much as the white of an egg coagulates when it is fried. To produce thermal effects, a tissue must absorb light; the more pigmented the tissue, the greater its absorption. The retina is largely transparent and does not absorb much light. However, the retinal pigment epithelium (RPE) and choroid do absorb light and produce heat that coagulates the adjacent retina. It can be difficult to photocoagulate the retina in patients with a blond fundus, because the choroid and RPE absorb less light. For similar reasons, producing a peripheral iridectomy using a thermal laser is more difficult in blue irides.

In photodisruption, a shock wave is generated by optical breakdown. Photodisruption is essentially a miniature lightning bolt. In lightning, high electric fields literally tear the electrons away from the molecules of air, generating an expanding plasma. When the lightning stops, the electrons recombine, and the contraction of the air produces an acoustic shock wave commonly called thunder. In photodisruption, a very high power density is produced in a very small region, causing the material in that region to break down into a plasma. A small spark is seen at the site of optical breakdown. Recombination of electrons with ions in the plasma produces an acoustic shock wave that can alter ocular tissues.[22]

Because the posterior capsule is largely transparent, photocoagulation cannot reliably produce a capsulotomy, so photodisruption is used instead. When performing a capsulotomy, the goal is to produce an optical breakdown behind the lens implant and capsule and let the acoustic shock wave tear the capsule. It is more difficult to perform a capsulotomy in patients with silicone implants, because optical breakdown of silicone occurs at lower power densities than does breakdown of polymethylmethacrylate. Often the optical breakdown occurs in the lens and not posterior to it. Optical breakdown in the lens implant produces a small pit that by itself is usually not visually significant, but severe pitting of the lens can decrease vision.

In photoablation, high power densities break chemical bonds and vaporize tissue, but with minimal thermal or acoustic effects. LASIK and photorefractive keratectomy are based on photoablation. It is often stated that each excimer laser pulse removes a precise amount of tissue. This, of course, is nonsense. Many factors affect the amount of tissue removed. The amount of energy delivered in each pulse varies, depending on factors associated with the laser and atmospheric conditions. The amount of tissue removed also varies with corneal hydration and probably other patient-specific factors.

REFERENCES

1. Wood RW. Physical optics, 3rd ed. New York: Optical Society of America; 1988: 1–41.
2. Born M, Wolf E. Principles of optics, 6th ed. New York: Pergamon; 1980:10–32.
3. Lipson SG, Lipson H, Thannhauser DS. Optical physics, 3rd ed. Cambridge: University Press; 1995.
4. Bass M, ed. Handbook of optics, 2nd ed. New York: Optical Society of America; 1995:5.1–5.31.
5. Hecht E. Optics, 3rd ed. Reading: Addison Wesley; 1997:111–21.
6. Jenkins FA, White EW. Fundamentals of optics, 3rd ed. New York: McGraw-Hill; 1990.
7. Fariza E, O'Day T, Jalkh AE, Medina A. Use of cross-polarized light in anterior segment photography. Arch Ophthalmol. 1989;107;608–10.
8. Michaels DD. Visual optics and refraction: a clinical approach, 2nd ed. St. Louis: CV Mosby; 1980:702–4.
9. Malacara D. Optical shop testing, 2nd ed. New York: Wiley; 1992:1–5.
10. Macleod A. Thin film optical filters, 2nd ed. New York: McGraw-Hill; 1989: 71–135.
11. Lamberts DW, MacKeen DL, Holly FJ, eds. The preocular tear film in health, disease, and contact lens wear. Yantis, Tex: Dry Eye Institute; 1986.
12. Okada K, Sagawa H. Newton rings on the surface of implanted lenses. Ophthalmic Surg. 1989;20:33–7.
13. Huang D, Swanson EA, Lin CP, et al. Optical coherence tomography. Science. 1991;254:1178–81.
14. Hooke R. Micrographia. New York: Dover; 1961.
15. Park DA. The fire within the eye. Princeton: Princeton University Press; 1997:190.
16. Smith G, Atchison DA. The eye and visual optical instruments. New York: Cambridge; 1997:656.
17. Ditchburn RW. Light. Mineola: Dover; 1991:1–17.
18. van de Hulst HC. Light scattering by small particles. New York: Wiley; 1957.
19. Eisberg R, Resnick R. Quantum physics of atoms, molecules, solids, nuclei, and particles. New York: Wiley; 1974.
20. Hecht J. Understanding lasers: an entry-level guide, 2nd ed. New York: Wiley–IEEE Press; 1994.
21. Mainster MA, Ho PC, Mainster KJ. Nd:YAG laser photocoagulators. Ophthalmology. 1983;90 (Suppl):48–54.
22. Mainster MA, Ho PC, Mainster KJ. Nd:YAG laser photodisrupters. Ophthalmology. 1983;90 (Suppl):45–7.

CHAPTER

6

Light Damage to the Eye

DAVID MILLER • CLIFFORD A. SCOTT

DEFINITION
- Structural or functional damage to the external or internal eye from thermal or photochemical effects of the absorption of light.

KEY FEATURES
- With age, many of the photoprotective mechanisms of the eye degrade.
- Cataract development and the risk of macular degeneration are accelerated by cumulative or excessive exposure to UV radiation.

ASSOCIATED FEATURES
- Reduction of environmental exposure and the use of absorptive lenses diminish the risk of light damage to the eye.
- Intake of antioxidant foods or dietary supplements may slow the development of cataracts and macular degeneration.

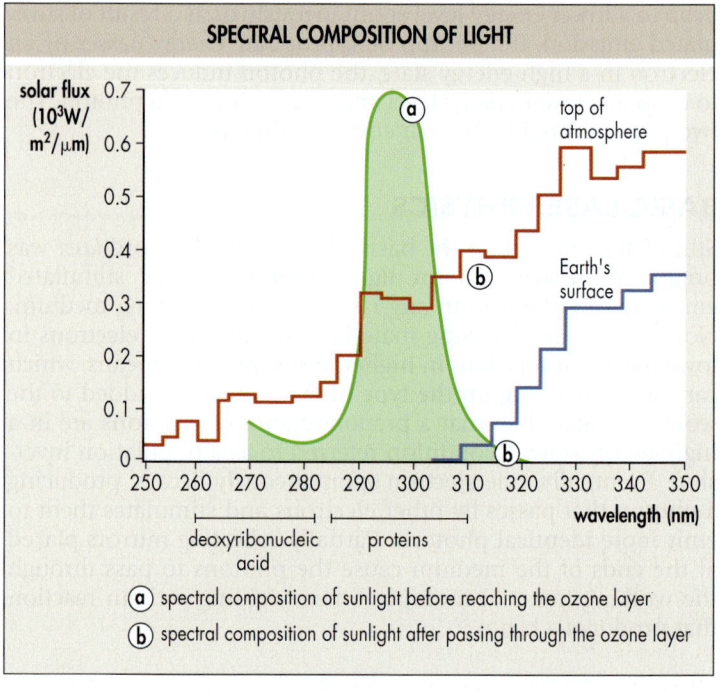

FIG. 6-1 ■ **Spectral composition of sunlight.** Before reaching ozone layer and after passing through the ozone layer. (Adapted from MacCracken M, Change J. Preliminary study of the potential chemical and climate effects of atmospheric nuclear explosion. UCRL 51653. San Francisco: Lawrence Livermore Laboratory, 1975 April 25:48.)

ULTRAVIOLET FILTRATION

The oxygen holocaust, a term invented by Margulis and Sagan,[1] describes that period in the evolution of life on Earth when the atmospheric oxygen content rose from 0.0001% to 21%. The source of such an atmospheric change was the evolution of photosynthesis by ancient green and purple bacteria, which seems to have started about 2 billion years ago. Of course, the change in environment destroyed most of the anaerobic microbes on Earth. Newly evolved resistant bacteria multiplied and ultimately developed the reactions of aerobic metabolism that prevail in life today.

A secondary effect of this "newly formed oxygen" was that as it rose into the upper reaches of the Earth's atmosphere, it reacted with incoming ultraviolet (UV) light from the sun and formed the ozone layer near the top of the atmosphere, about 30 miles (48.3 km) up. The ozone layer is important in two ways[2] (Fig. 6-1). First, it helps to stabilize the atmospheric oxygen level at 21% (excess oxygen is used to make more ozone); it has been suggested that many living organisms would not tolerate levels of atmospheric oxygen a few percent higher than 21%. However, it is the second effect of the ozone layer that is discussed in this chapter.

The ozone layer, only about 2–3mm in thickness, is produced in the stratosphere by a photochemical reaction fueled by UV-C radiation and/or lightning and spread by the stratospheric winds. This is ironic, because the ozone layer then filters out most of the potentially destructive UV light that arrives from the sun. Research that started in 1980 noted a 3–6% per decade decay in the ozone layer, notably in the Northern Hemisphere. This depletion of the ozone layer, thought to be caused by chlorine from industrial pollutants, leads to an approximate 1% increase in UV-B radiation that reaches the Earth's surface for every 1% reduction in ozone.[3]

Ultraviolet Profile

Of all the light energy that rains down on Earth, <10% may be considered to be UV radiation in the range 280–400nm.[4] The UV spectrum has been subdivided into the following categories:
- UV-A, 400–320nm (90% of UV radiation from the sun)
- UV-B, 320–280nm
- UV-C, 280nm and below

Although UV radiation with this profile has fallen on Earth from the time the ozone layer was established, forms of life still remain that can be damaged by UV radiation. Of course, the specific wavelength and dosage determine the specific organism's response. Thus bacteria may survive under the fluorescent light of the operating room (which has very small amounts of UV) but are destroyed by germicidal lamps (high amounts of short-wavelength UV radiation). Planck's equation states that the energy content (eV) of radiation of a certain wavelength is 1240/wavelength (nm). Normal human skin maintains health under average light conditions but can experience sunburn that is damage caused by prolonged exposure to high doses of UV radiation.

ULTRAVIOLET VULNERABILITY

UV radiation can be potentially damaging if a certain balance is upset. Groups vulnerable to ocular UV radiation damage are discussed in this chapter.

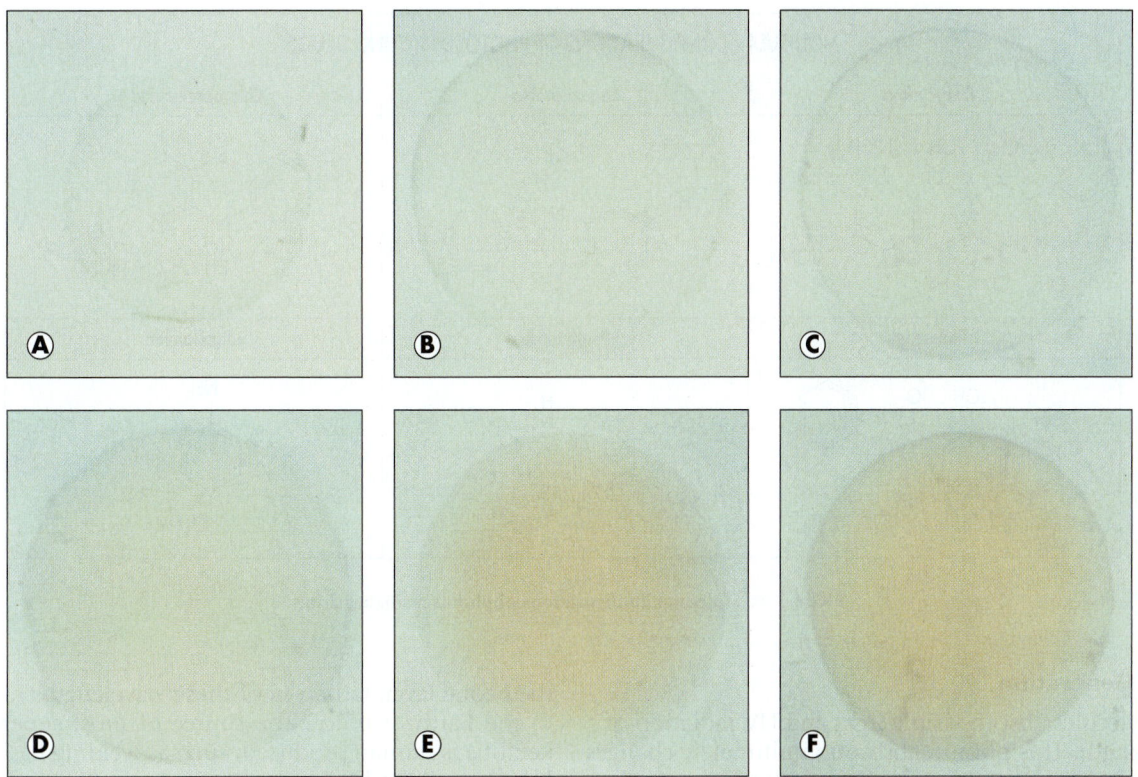

FIG. 6-2 ▓ Increasing yellow to brown coloration in human lenses. A, 6 months. B, 8 years. C, 12 years. D, 25 years. E, 47 years. F, 60 years. (Reproduced with permission from Lerman S. Phototoxicity: clinical considerations. Focal Points. San Francisco: American Academy of Ophthalmology. 1987;1–22.)

Older Individuals

Light damage to tissue ultimately depends on a series of photochemical reactions. The body, in turn, has a series of protective molecules that either filter out the harmful wavelengths or scavenge the harmful photometabolites. With increased age, it has been suggested that the concentration of some of these protective molecules decreases. As discussed later, age-related macular degeneration and cataract formation may be related to a combination of cumulative light exposure and a coincident decrease in protective biochemicals.

Lightly Pigmented Individuals

Studies have shown that patients whose irises are blue (lighter-pigmented eyes) have a significantly higher incidence of age-related macular degeneration than a control series of patients who have brown irises.[5] Also, age-related macular degeneration is almost unknown in the black African patient.

Aphakia

Results from the Framingham study suggested that nuclear sclerosis in the elderly protects the retina from age-related degeneration.[6] Lerman[7,8] has shown that the aging crystalline lens is an efficient filter against UV radiation and blue light (Fig. 6-2). Ham *et al.*[9] may have brought together the above information when they were able to produce retinal injury in aphakic monkeys using short-wavelength visible light.

Use of Photosensitizing Drugs

Chemical compounds with multiple cyclic rings (Fig. 6-3) that contain alternating double bonds are often photosensitizing agents. These agents are able to absorb UV radiation and short-wavelength visible light and then generate free radicals, which damage tissue. Compounds that fall into this group include phenothiazines, 8-methoxypsoralen (used in that treat-

ment of psoriasis), allopurinol, tetracyclines, and hematoporphyrins used for phototherapy. When these compounds deposit in the lens or retina, the tissues become more vulnerable to light damage.

Outer Segment Turnover

It appears that nature copes with the anticipated light damage to the discs that contain photopigment through the daily retinal pigment epithelium digestion of a portion of the outer segment. If a malfunction occurs in this digestive system as a result of genetics, malnutrition, or injury, then a buildup of photoreceptor disc metabolites results. Such a buildup may be related to drusen deposition and clinical age-related macular degeneration. Thus, some form of faulty, radiation-damage defensive system may be partially responsible for age-related macular degeneration.[10]

BIOCHEMICAL MECHANISM OF UV RADIATION DAMAGE

For photodamage to occur, tissue must contain a molecule that absorbs light. Tissue damage may occur in two ways: molecular fragmentation and free radical generation.

Molecular Fragmentation

Proteins, enzymes, and nucleic acids contain alternating double bonds. Such molecular configurations efficiently resonate with radiation of UV wavelength. An analogy is that of opera singers who break wineglasses by striking certain notes; they tap the glass to establish its resonating frequency and sing loudly in that frequency. The resonating frequency may be thought of as fitting snugly into the glass structure. The increased intensity of UV radiation, like a dynamite charge placed snugly in a rock crevice, breaks the molecular bonds. The new molecules may induce inflammation or neoplasm, or affect the immune system.

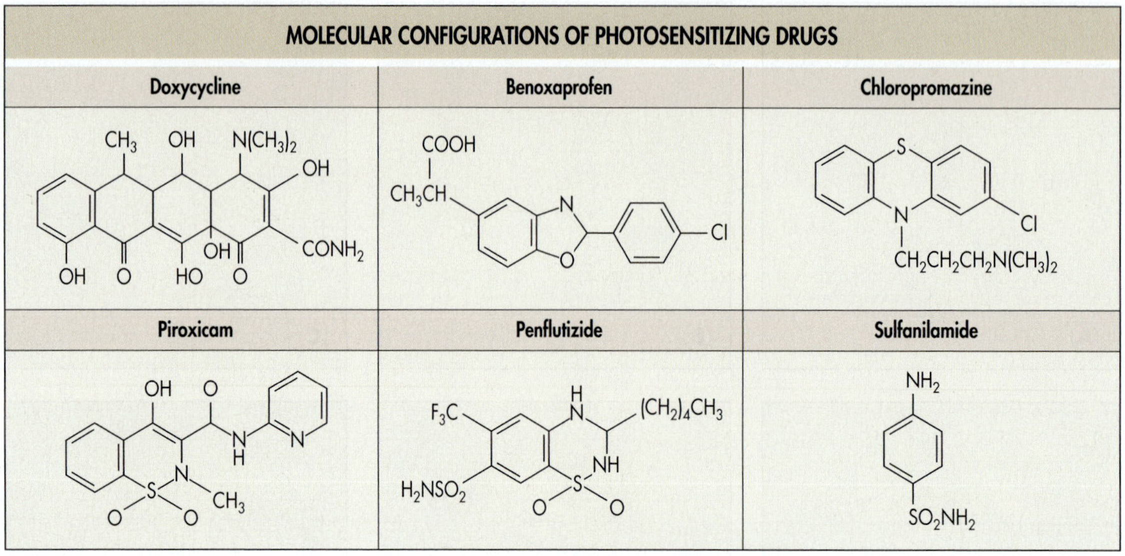

FIG. 6-3 ▮ Molecular configurations of photosensitizing drugs.

Free Radical Generation

Pigmented molecules absorb visible light and UV radiation of a specific wavelength. This photon absorption ultimately changes the energy level to the unstable triplet state. The molecule then ejects an electron, which usually combines with a neighboring molecule (often oxygen in cases of photodamage). When an oxygen molecule gains an extra electron, it is known as superoxide, one of a family of compounds called *free radicals*. These are, in truth, super oxidizers. Free radicals may disrupt cell membranes, mitochondrial membranes, and nucleic acids; depolymerize collagen and hyaluronic acid; and destroy tissue.

Free radical light damage to tissue requires three components. A light-absorbing molecule (dye, pigment), oxygen, and short-wavelength radiation. Fortunately, specialized molecules occur in the body to disarm any newly arrived free radical. These scavenger molecules (of which many exist) include the ubiquitous superoxide dismutase, vitamin C, vitamin E, glutathione peroxidase, and carotene. A shortage of these scavengers in the very young (premature infants), the old, or the nutritionally impaired can tip the balance toward greater vulnerability to light damage.

CLINICAL EXAMPLES OF OCULAR LIGHT DAMAGE

Lids

Caucasian skin, including eyelid skin, is subject to a multitude of changes induced by UV radiation.[11] The simple but annoying acute sunburn reaction falls at one end of the spectrum and is essentially a UV-B–induced response. Clouds do not filter out UV radiation and therefore do not prevent sunburn. Since UV radiation is reflected off sand and water, beach umbrellas do not provide full protection from UV damage.

The middle of the spectrum of common skin conditions induced by UV radiation includes epidermal keratoses, age spots, skin dryness, wrinkling, sebaceous hyperplasia, and comedones. On the far side of the spectrum of UV-B–induced damage are the malignant skin changes, which include basal cell carcinoma, squamous cell carcinoma, and malignant melanoma. Each of these conditions has an impressive statistical association with UV radiation.[12]

Cornea

UV damage to the cornea is both wavelength and intensity dependent.[13] For example, the most effective range of damaging wavelengths is 260–290nm,[14] but as a result of absorption by the ozone layer, radiation of these wavelengths rarely penetrates to the Earth's surface. The source of most superficial punctate keratitis is human produced, such as welding flashes, germicidal lamps, and sun lamps. At 270nm, only $0.005mJ/cm^2$ of energy produces a lesion; at 300nm, about $0.01mJ/cm^2$ produces a lesion; and at 320nm, $10.5mJ/cm^2$ (2000 times above the lowest threshold) does so. Thus, for short wavelengths, a very small amount of UV energy may produce a corneal lesion.[15] From a basic science viewpoint, the nucleic acids of the corneal epithelium maximally absorb these wavelengths, as do certain amino acids such as tryptophan. However, the clinician must not forget that the longer wavelength UV-B (320–400nm) also may produce corneal lesions, if the exposure is long enough. Snow blindness is a result of prolonged exposure to UV-B radiation reflected from the snow; fresh snow can reflect as much as 85% of the incident UV radiation.[16]

Clinically, superficial punctate keratitis appears about 8–12 hours after exposure. Pain probably arrives when the damaged epithelial cells desquamate, which produces the characteristic punctate fluorescein staining.

Chronic exposure to UV radiation is said to produce spheroidal degeneration of the cornea (Labrador keratitis and climatic droplet keratopathy). The incidence of this condition in the Eskimo population is about 14%.[17] Epidemiological evidence also suggests that chronic exposure to UV radiation produces or is associated with pterygium.[18]

Lens

The chemical components of the crystalline lens are particularly vulnerable to different parts of the electromagnetic spectrum. For example, short wavelength ionizing radiation is cataractogenic. The mechanism is probably a combination of the creation of overwhelming numbers of damaging free radicals, as well as molecular bond breakage.[19]

A number of important epidemiological studies show a connection between environmental levels of UV radiation and a higher incidence of cataract (primarily cortical cataract) formation.[20–24] Basic biochemical research has given further insight into the mechanism behind these changes. For example, lens exposure to UV-A and UV-B radiation results in lens enzyme changes. Specifically, exposure of rat lenses to $5mW/cm^2$ of UV radiation (wavelength, 360nm) almost totally destroys Na^+/K^+-adenosine triphosphatase activity in less than 24 hours. The lens of the gray squirrel is a favorite model because its yellow color is similar to that of the aging human lens. Exposure of such lenses to $1.5–2mW/cm^2$ UV radiation (wavelength, 365nm) produces

TABLE 6-1

ONSET OF PRESBYOPIA IN DIFFERENT REGIONS

Age (years)	Place	Latitude (°)	Author	Year Published
47	England	51–54	Ayrshire	1964
43	England	51–54	Turner	1958
45	New York	41–45	Duane	1912
50	Cleveland	38–42	Allen	1961
45	Japan	36–44	Kajiura	1965
43	Japan	36–44	Fukuda	1965
42	Japan	36–44	Ishihara	1919
43	California	32–42	Hamasaki	1956
45	Texas	26–36	Fitch	1971
41	Israel	32	Raphael	1961
40	South Africa	26–29	Coates	1955
37	India	10–30	Rambo	1960
39	Puerto Rico	18–18.5	Miranda	1977

(From Jacques PF, Chylak LT Jr, Hankinson SE, *et al.* Long-term nutrient intake and early age-related nuclear lens opacities. Arch Ophthalmol. 2001 Jul;119[7]:1009–19.)

significant aggregation of insoluble lens proteins. These large protein aggregates of insoluble lens proteins are responsible for the increased light scatter seen in the aging human lens and in human cataracts.[25] The mechanism for these changes is related to the formation of singlet oxygen by the radiation. Specifically, Goosey et al. showed that an inhibitor of singlet oxygen formation (sodium azide) completely prevented protein aggregation in the presence of UV radiation.[26] However, whereas high doses of antioxidant nutrient supplementation does not appear to affect the development or progression of cataracts, dietary intake of antioxidant foods is associated with a lower prevalence of nuclear lens opacities.[27,28]

Infrared (IR) radiation also has an effect on the lens. The higher frequency (lower wavelengths) of IR radiation closely matches the resonant frequency of water molecules. The development of glassblower's cataract has long been recognized as a clinical example of this relationship, in which lens water absorbs the radiation from the IR source and literally cooks the proteins that surround the lens.

Finally, it is important to mention the relationship between age of onset of presbyopia and geographic latitude (Table 6-1). Note that presbyopia occurs 5 years earlier in the tropics than in northern climates. Increased solar radiation has been suggested as the cause. In particular, the IR rather than the UV portion of the solar spectrum has been implicated because in a specific latitude the onset of presbyopia is earlier in coastal regions (less UV radiation) than in mountain regions.[29]

Retina

There is no doubt that prolonged illumination from the indirect ophthalmoscope, the operating microscope, or the sun can produce a level of light equivalent to the noonday sun at equinox and 40° latitude, which measures 12,800 foot candles (137,700 lux). Light measurements from different operating microscopes are in the range 5,120–28,160 foot candles (55,090–303,000 lux) at the surface of the patient's eye. Clearly, such intensity directed on a dilated pupil for a prolonged period may produce maculopathy.[30–32] Illumination from the indirect ophthalmoscope with a focusing lens may produce a focal energy on the retina equivalent to that produced by the sun.[33] It is not clear which specific wavelengths that emanate from these instruments produce the damage. This damage may result from a combination of wavelengths, since photochemical damage from short wavelengths is enhanced by an increase in the retinal temperature of 3–4°C.[9]

Age-related macular degeneration has been suggested as a manifestation of light toxicity.[9] Experimental visible wave-lengths (primarily blue light) can produce retinal damage to the monkey retina,[9] but these experimental lesions do not resemble age-related macular degeneration in humans in terms of clinical appearance. Bleached visual pigments (which become waste products [i.e., lipofuscin] and may have photocytotoxic effects in the retinal pigment epithelium[34]) maximally absorb blue and UV-A.[35] Enhanced choroidal pigmentation seems to protect against this degeneration.[36] To complicate matters further, epidemiological studies of age-related macular degeneration in the elderly are difficult to evaluate when cataract is present, since a cataract may filter out light harmful to the retina.

However, it is not known if the increased melanin works its protective effect as a light filter or as a metabolic agent. It seems as if any condition in which bleached visual pigments build up in the retina may promote light damage. The increased choroidal melanin in the African black patient may simply prevent the light reflected off the sclera from striking the vulnerable pigments on a second pass. With so many unanswered questions, further research is required in this area.

Finally, it seems appropriate to address the role of light toxicity in the causation of retinopathy of prematurity (see Chapter 116, Retinopathy of Prematurity). Certainly, strong evidence associates the use of oxygen therapy with the early development of the disease in the premature infant.[9] As noted above, the combination of oxygen, light, and the appropriate pigmented molecules may incubate damaging free radicals. Therefore light may enhance the damaging potential of oxygen. Interestingly, fluorescent lights were introduced into nurseries at about the same time as oxygen therapy for premature infants. The production of a high concentration of free radicals in an immature retina (perhaps devoid of protective agents [i.e., free radical scavengers]) may lead to the disease. One experimental study seems to support the hypothesis that light damage is involved in retinopathy of prematurity.[37] Again, further research is needed in this area.

In summary, the human eye is quite resistant to light damage. However, age, pigmentation, nutritional status, drugs taken, and genetic and biochemical makeup can make some patients more vulnerable to light damage.[38,39]

LIGHT PROTECTION
During Surgery

As noted earlier, light from the operating microscope has been shown to produce maculopathy during a prolonged cataract extraction (with or without an implant).[29–32] Thus a number of methods have been suggested to reduce the concentration of light that strikes the retina during surgery. For example, light can

TABLE 6-2

COMMONLY PRESCRIBED LENS TINTS

Lens Tint	Visible Light Transmission (%)	Uses
UV absorbing clear	90	Absorbs almost all UV up to 385nm
Amber	90	Enhances low light contrast
Light gray	35	Outdoor glare reduction
		Uniform color transmission
Standard gray sunglass	15	Uniform color transmission
Mirrored lenses (reflect rather than absorb light)	15	Uniform color transmission
		No optical advantage
Dark green	2	Shade 5 Welding goggles

be blocked by a small occluder disc placed on the cornea, directly over the pupil. A bubble of air may also be placed in the anterior chamber, which (optically speaking) neutralizes the corneal focusing power. However, the bubble also enhances the refractive power of the anterior surface of the intraocular lens. The combined neutralization and enhancement effects of the bubble substantially defocus the light that strikes the retina. Certain operating microscopes are equipped with an occluder disc that may be placed in the center of the path of the light that strikes the eye. This system produces an annulus of light with a dark center, which is incident upon the cornea. The most effective protective measure against maculopathy induced by operation light is to shorten the time of surgery.

Ultraviolet Filters in Intraocular Lenses

Currently, most intraocular lens manufacturers produce implants with UV filters. In general, these implants filter out all wavelengths of light <400nm, which not only protects the plastic of the implant from UV degradation, but appears to prevent decreases in visual function such as color vision and contrast sensitivity.[16,40]

Absorptive Lenses

In certain high-illumination situations, sunglasses allow better visual function in a number of ways (Table 6-2).

Improvement of Contrast Sensitivity

On a bright sunny day, illuminance from the sun is in the range 10,000–30,000 foot lamberts (34,260–103,000cd/m²). These high light levels tend to saturate the retina and therefore decrease finer levels of contrast sensitivity. The major function of a dark sunglass is to return the retina to a level of maximal contrast sensitivity (i.e., eliminate the "increased noise" of the retina).[41] Most dark sunglasses absorb 70–80% of the incident light of all wavelengths. (Light levels are often described in $\log^{10}$ units [i.e., 1, 2, 3 or −1, −2, −3; a $\log_{10}$ value of −1 reduces the light level by 90% and is equivalent to a sunglass that absorbs 90% of the incident light; a lens that absorbs 70% is equivalent to a $\log_{10}$ value of −0.84.)

Improvement of Dark Adaptation

Experiments have shown that a full sunny day at the beach (without dark sunglasses) may impair dark adaptation for over 2 days. Thus dark sunglasses (absorption of 70–80% of incident light) are recommended for prolonged periods in bright sun.[42]

Reduction of Glare Sensitivity

A number of sunglass modalities may reduce glare sensitivity. Polaroid sunglasses reduce the intensity of reflected light from

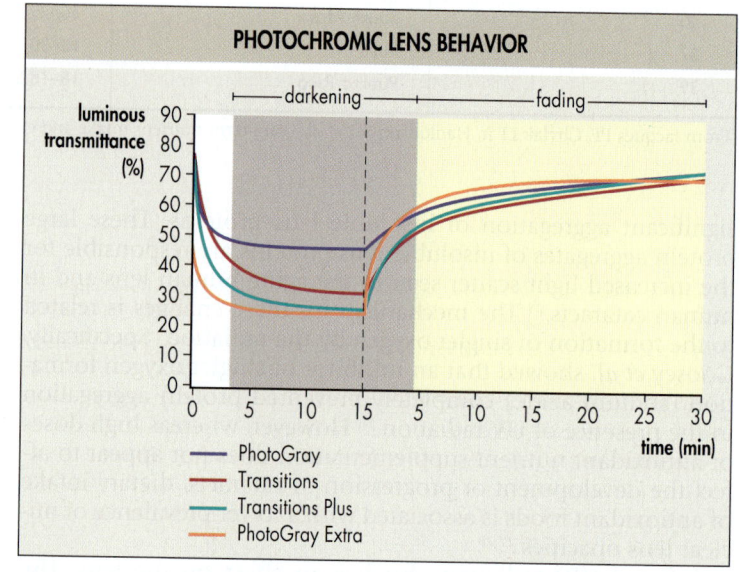

FIG. 6-4 ■ **The darkening and fading of four popular photochromic lenses.** Note that most darken maximally by 2–3 minutes and fade in 5 minutes. (Modified with permission from Young JM. Photochromics: past and present. Opt World. 1993;Feb.)

road surfaces, glass windows, lake and river surfaces, and metal surfaces. Thus dazzle and glare sources are reduced in intensity. Since light reflected from a horizontal surface produces light polarized in the horizontal plane, properly oriented Polaroid sunglasses may eliminate this component. For many activities, such as fishing or driving, reduction in surface glare improves overall visual comfort. However, polarized lenses eliminate the clue of reflection to a pilot scanning the skies for other aircraft. Graded density sunglasses are tinted deeply at the top and gradually become light toward the lens center. They effectively remove dazzle from glare sources above the line of sight (e.g., the sun). Wide temple sunglasses reduce glare from sources at the side.[41]

Improvement of Color Contrast

Orange sunglasses efficiently absorb wavelengths in the purple through blue-green range. All these colors appear as different forms of dark gray to the wearer. On the other hand, the wearer clearly sees the spectrum from green through yellow to orange to red. Colors appear slightly unreal, but color contrast improves. Patients who have conditions such as cataracts or corneal edema, for whom color contrast sensitivity has decreased, report improvements in color contrast using these sunglasses.[43]

Use of Photochromic Lenses

Photochromic lenses are either glass or plastic. When short-wavelength light (300–400nm or longer) interacts with glass photochromic lenses, they darken (Fig. 6-4). The chemical

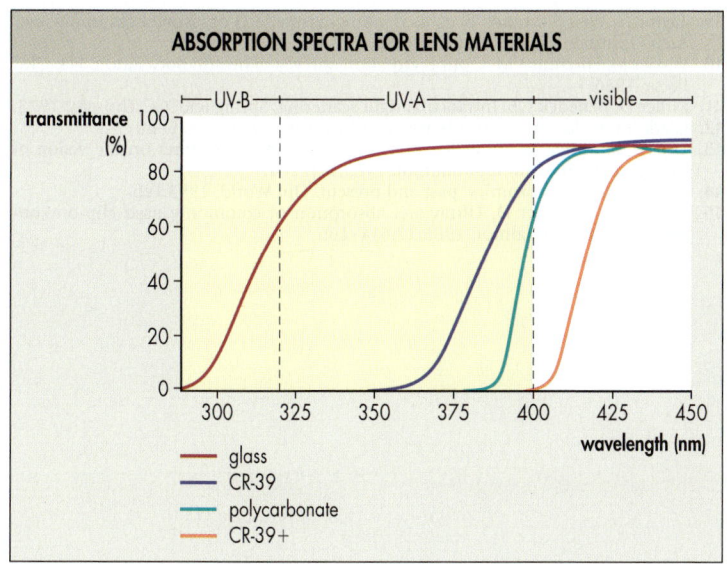

FIG. 6-5 Absorption spectra for crown glass, CR-39, CR-39+, and polycarbonate lenses.

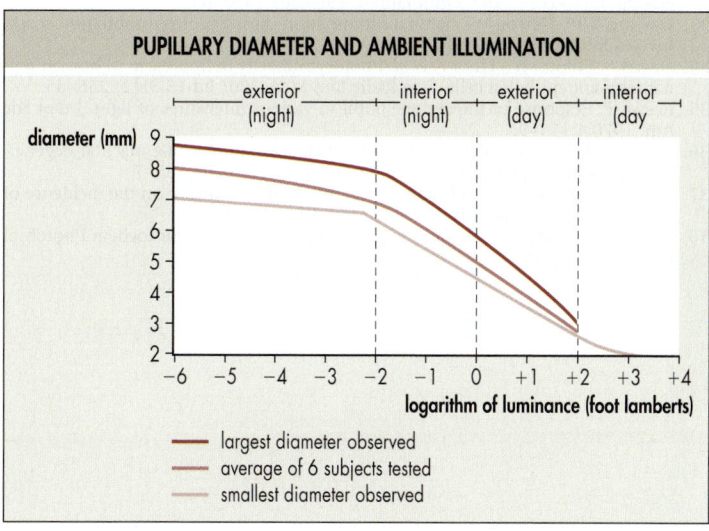

FIG. 6-6 Relationship between pupillary diameter and ambient level of illumination. (Modified with permission from Reeves P. Response of the average pupil to various intensities of light. J Opt Soc Am. 1970;4:135–9.)

reaction (i.e., the conversion of silver ions into elemental silver) is similar to the reaction that occurs when photographic film is exposed to light. In contrast to the chemical reaction in film sensitive to radiation of these wavelengths, that in photochromic lenses is reversible. With continued exposure to radiation of short wavelengths, the lens continually darkens to absorb about 80% of the incident light, and then lightens when the illumination falls to absorb about 20% of the incident light. These lenses take longer to lighten than to darken, but when darkened they are also excellent ultraviolet absorbers.[44] Plastic photochromic lenses are coated with an organic molecule from the generic molecular group indolinospironaphthoxazine, which changes shape and consequently light-absorptive properties when illuminated.

Ultraviolet Absorbing Lenses

Almost all dark sunglasses absorb most of the incident ultraviolet radiation, which is also true for certain coated, clear-glass lenses and the clear plastic lenses made of CR-39 (a commonly used clear plastic with a special coating) or polycarbonate. A study of the transmission spectra for nine inexpensive clip-on sunglasses showed that all but the blue-colored clip-ons remove over 90% of the UV.[45] Figure 6-5 shows the absorption curve for clear glass, CR-39, and clear polycarbonate.

It has been suggested that certain sunglasses, ironically, may produce light damage to the eye. The argument contends that the pupil dilates behind dark glasses. Thus sunglasses that do not absorb significant amounts of UV radiation actually allow more of it to enter the eye than when no sunglass is worn. Figure 6-6 shows that the pupil enlarges most under scotopic conditions. On a bright sunny day, irradiance is in the range 10,000–30,000 foot lamberts (34,260–103,000cd/m²) and the pupil constricts maximally. A dark sunglass (one that absorbs 80% of the incident light) reduces the level of light that strikes the eye to the range 2000–6000 foot lamberts (6,850–20,600cd/m²). Such levels are about ten times higher than those of an averagely lit room. At such light levels, the pupil is still constricted significantly.

REFERENCES

1. Margulis L, Sagan D. Microcosmos. New York: Summit Books; 1986.
2. MacCracken M, Change J. Preliminary study of the potential chemical and climatic effects of atmospheric nuclear explosion. UCRL 51653. San Francisco: Lawrence Livermore Laboratory, April 25. 1975;48.
3. Frederick JE. Yearly Review: Trends in atmospheric ozone and ultraviolet radiation: mechanisms and observations for the Northern Hemisphere. Photochem Photobiol. 1990;51:757–63.
4. Terrestrial Global Spectral Irradiance Tables for Air Mass 1.5. ASTM Document 138 RI E 44.02, Feb 1981.
5. Hyman LG, Lillienfeld AM, Ferris FL III, Fine SL. Senile macular degeneration. A case controlled study. Am J Epidemiol. 1983;118:350–4.
6. Sperduto TD, Holler R, Seigel D. Lens opacities and senile maculopathy. Am Arch Ophthalmol. 1981;99:1004–9.
7. Lerman S. Phototoxicity: clinical considerations. Focal Points. San Francisco: American Academy of Ophthalmology, 1987;1–22.
8. Lerman S. Radiant energy and the eye. New York: Macmillan; 1980.
9. Ham WT Jr, Mueller HA, Ruffolo JJ Jr, et al. Action spectrum for retinal injury from near ultraviolet radiation in the aphakic monkey. Am J Ophthalmol. 1982;93:299–306.
10. Li W, Yanoff M, Li Y, et al. Artificial senescence of bovine retinal pigment epithelial cells induced by near-ultraviolet in vitro. Mechanisms of Aging. 1999;110:137–55.
11. Bernhard JD. Light induced changes in the skin of the lid. In: Miller D, ed. Clinical light damage to the eye. New York: Springer-Verlag; 1987:127–44.
12. Urbash F. Photocarcinogenesis. In: Regan JD, Parrish JA, eds. The science of photomedicine. New York: Plenum Press; 1982:261–92.
13. Voerhoeff FH, Bell L, Walker CB. The pathological effects of radiant energy on the eye. An experimental investigation with a systemic review of the literature. Proc Am Acad Arts Sci. 1916;51:630–818.
14. Cogan DG, Kinsey VE. Action spectrum of keratitis produced by ultraviolet radiation. Arch Ophthalmol. 1946;35:370–6.
15. Pitts DG, Tredici TJ. The effects of ultraviolet on the eye. Am Ind Hyg Assoc J. 1971;32:235–46.
16. Miller D. Clinical light damage to the eye. New York: Springer-Verlag; 1987.
17. Norn MS. Spheroidal degeneration of cornea and conjunctiva. Prevalence among Eskimos in Greenland and Caucasians in Copenhagen. Acta Ophthalmol. 1978;56(4):551–62.
18. Cameron EE. Pterygium throughout the world. Springfield: CC Thomas; 1965.
19. Geeraets WJ, Harrel W, Guery D, et al. Aging anomalies and radiation effects on rabbit lens. Acta Ophthalmol. 1965;43:3–10.
20. Giblin FH, Chakrapani B, Reddy VN. High molecular weight aggregates in X-ray induced cataracts. Exp Eye Res. 1978;26:507–15.
21. Hiller R, Sperduto RD, Ederse F. Epidemiologic association with cataract. The 1971–72 natural health and nutrition examination survey. Am J Epidemiol. 1983;118:230–49.
22. Brilliant LB, Grosset NC, Ram PT, et al. Association among cataract prevalence, sunlight hours and altitude. Am J Epidemiol. 1983;118:2350–64.
23. Taylor H. The environment and the lens. Br J Ophthalmol. 1980;64:303–10.
24. Taylor H, West SK, Rosenthal FS, et al. Effect of ultraviolet radiation on cataract formation. N Engl J Med. 1988;319(22):1429–33.
25. Zigman S. Light damage to the lens. In: Miller D, ed. Clinical light damage to the eye. New York: Springer-Verlag; 1987:65–78.
26. Goosey JD, Zigler JS Jr, Kinoshita JH. Cross linking of lens crystalline in a photodynamic system. Science. 1980;208:1278–80.
27. No authors listed. A randomized, placebo-controlled, clinical trial of high-dose supplementation with vitamins C and E and beta carotene for age-related cataract and visual loss: AREDS report no. 9. Arch Ophthalmol. 2001 Oct;119(10):1439–52.
28. Jacques PF, Chylak LT Jr, Hankinson SE, et al. Long-term nutrient intake and early age-related nuclear lens opacities. Arch Ophthalmol. 2001 Jul;119(7):1009–19.
29. Miranda MN. The environmental factor in the onset of presbyopia. In: Stark L, Obrecht G, eds. Presbyopia. Recent research and reviews from the Third International Symposium. New York: Professional Press; 1987.
30. Calkins JL, Hochheimer BF. Retinal light exposure from operation microscopes. Arch Ophthalmol. 1974;97:2363–7.
31. Covard DM. Operating microscope light induced retinal injury. J Am Intraocul Implant Soc. 1984;10:438–43.

32. Irvine AR, Wood I, Morris BW. Retinal damage from the illumination of the operating microscope. Arch Ophthalmol. 1984;102:1358–64.

33. Dawson WW, Herron WL. Retinal illumination during indirect ophthalmoscopy. Invest Ophthalmol. 1970;9:89–95.

34. Davies S, Elliott MH, Floor E, *et al.* Photocytotoxicity of lipofuscin in human retinal pigment epithelial cells. Free Radic Biol Med. 2001 Jul 15;31(2):256–65.

35. Reeves P. Response of the average pupil to various intensities of light. J Opt Soc Am. 1970;4:135–9.

36. Weiter JJ, Delori FC, Wing GL, Fitch KA. Relationship of senile macular degeneration to ocular pigmentation. Am J Ophthalmol. 1985;99:185–7.

37. Glass P, Avery G. Effect of bright light in the hospital nursery on the incidence of retinopathy of prematurity. N Engl J Med. 1985;313:401–4.

38. Dillon J. The photophysics and photobiology of the eye. J Photochem Photobiol B. 1991;10:23–40.

39. Taylor H, West S, Munoz B, *et al.* The long-term effects of visible light on the eye. Arch Ophthalmol. 1992;110:99–104.

40. Waxler M, Hitchins VM. Optical radiation and visual health. Boca Raton, Fla: CRC Press; 1986.

41. Miller D, Benedek GB. Intraocular light scattering. Springfield: CC Thomas; 1973.

42. Clark BA. Color in sunglass lenses. Am J Optom. 1969;46:875–80.

43. Tupper B, Miller D, Miller R. The effect of 550nm cutoff filter on the vision of cataract patients. Ann Ophthalmol. 1985;17:72–4.

44. Young JM. Photochromics: past and present. Opt World. 1993;Feb.

45. Magnante D, Miller D. Ultraviolet absorption of commonly used clip-on sunglasses. Ann Ophthalmol. 1985;17:614–16.

7

Principles of Lasers

NEAL H. ATEBARA • EDMOND H. THALL

DEFINITION

- "Laser" is an acronym for *light amplification by stimulated emission of radiation*.

KEY FEATURES

- Lasers have had a greater impact on ophthalmology than on any other medical specialty, largely because the transparent nature of the ocular tissues allows laser light to reach many parts of the eye noninvasively.
- In modern ophthalmology, lasers are used to treat a wide range of ocular conditions, and their uses are some of the most commonly performed procedures in medicine.
- Lasers are also important in a growing number of diagnostic studies that promise to significantly enhance our understanding and clinical management of many disease processes in the eye.

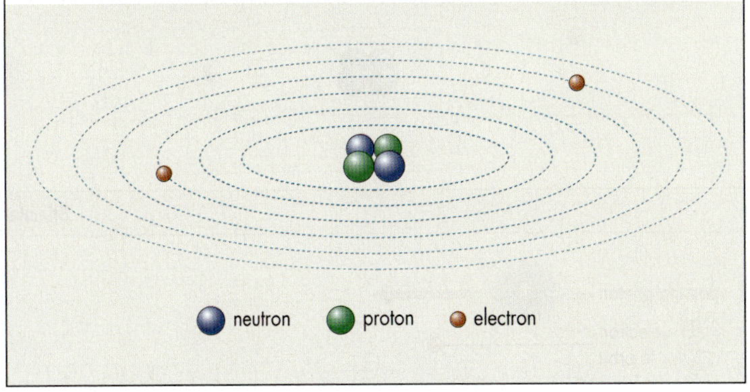

SIMPLE MODEL OF A HELIUM ATOM AT A SINGLE POINT IN TIME

neutron   proton   electron

FIG. 7-1 ■ **Simple model of a helium atom at a single point in time.** Electrons orbit a nucleus of protons and neutrons. Each orbit has a unique energy. The two electrons in this case occupy two different orbits. By gaining or losing energy the electrons can move to other, currently empty, orbits.

INTRODUCTION

The word *laser* is an acronym for *light amplification by stimulated emission of radiation*,[1] a term coined by Gordon Gould while a graduate student at Columbia University. Stimulated emission of a photon of electromagnetic radiation is the basic physical principle that makes lasers possible. This process was first predicted theoretically by Albert Einstein in 1917, but for many years it was believed that putting this theory into practice was not possible.

In the 1950s, Charles Townes first produced microwaves (radiowaves) using stimulated emission. His work proved that it was possible to produce electromagnetic radiation using stimulated emission. Once this had been established, several groups sought ways to produce shorter wavelengths of electromagnetic radiation (e.g., visible light) by stimulated emission, and in 1960 the first laser was built by Theodore Maiman using a ruby crystal medium.

The first laser system used in ophthalmology utilized a pulsed ruby laser coupled with a monocular direct ophthalmoscopic delivery system, first reported in 1961.[2] It was used to treat retinal breaks and proliferative diabetic retinopathy. In 1968, L'Esperance[3] developed the argon laser, which was technically superior to the ruby laser. The argon laser continues to be one of the types of lasers most frequently used in ophthalmology today.

LASER PHYSICS

In order to understand how lasers work, one must first review some basic physical principles, including the nature of photons, the nature of atoms, and how photons and atoms interact. Light may be viewed as being comprised of individual "wave packets" called photons. Each photon has a characteristic frequency, and its energy is proportional to its frequency.[4] Thus, a photon of blue light carries more energy than a photon of red light.

Although an atom may superficially resemble a miniature solar system, with negatively charged electrons that orbit a positively charged nucleus, there are significant differences. In our solar system, each planet stays in one stable orbit, whereas in an atom the electrons are capable of jumping between different orbits. Further, in our solar system, a planet may theoretically have any energy, but electron orbits are strictly constrained to discrete energy levels.[5]

Figure 7-1 simplistically depicts a helium atom at one particular instant showing the two electrons that orbit the nucleus and several other empty orbits that electrons could occupy. Each orbit has a unique energy, and to jump from one orbit to another an electron must either gain or lose energy. The amount of energy gained or lost by an electron when it changes orbits equals the energy difference between the two orbits. An atom is extremely dynamic, with electrons constantly absorbing and emitting photons and changing orbits.

The three basic ways for photons and atoms to interact include: (1) absorption, (2) spontaneous emission, and (3) stimulated emission. An electron can absorb a passing photon and jump into a higher energy orbit.[6] Absorption occurs only if the photon's energy exactly matches the difference in energy between the two electron orbits. Absorption begins with a photon and a low-energy electron and yields a higher energy electron with the elimination of the photon.

In spontaneous emission, an electron in a high-energy state spontaneously drops into a lower energy state and, in the process, creates a photon.[6] The photon created has an energy equal to the difference in energies between the two electron orbits. Spontaneous emission begins with a high-energy electron and yields a photon and a low-energy electron.

Spontaneous emission is a random process. At any moment, an electron in a high-energy state may drop into a lower state with the emission of a photon. Generally, electrons spend only a few nanoseconds in the high-energy state before this emission

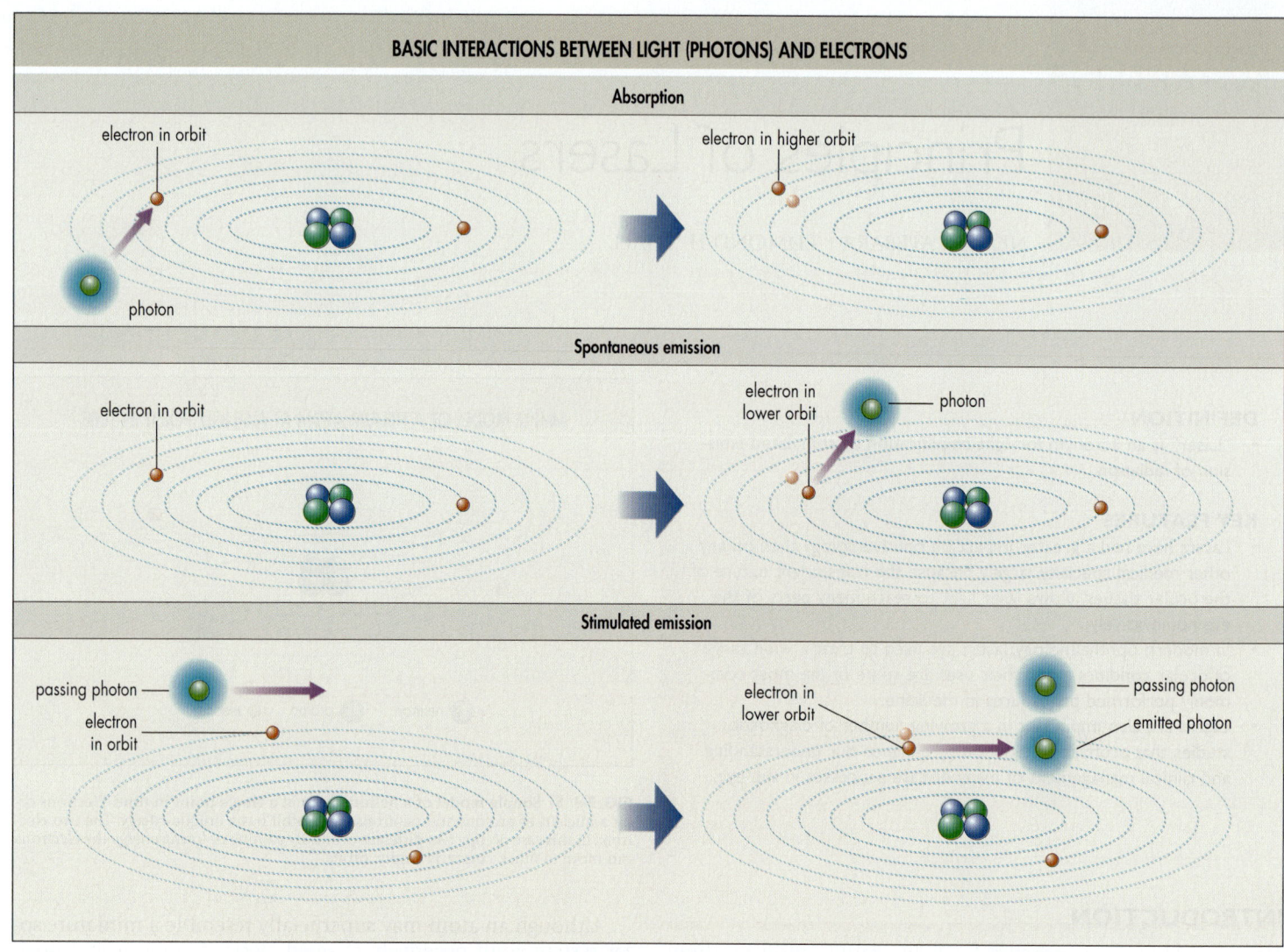

BASIC INTERACTIONS BETWEEN LIGHT (PHOTONS) AND ELECTRONS

FIG. 7-2 ▮▮ **Three basic interactions between light (photons) and electrons.** An electron absorbs a photon, which forces it to move to a higher energy orbit. In spontaneous emission a photon is produced by the electron, which then "falls" to a lower energy orbit. In stimulation, a photon passes by an electron and stimulates it to "fall" into a lower energy orbit and produce a second photon, coherent with the first figure.

occurs. Some high-energy states, however, are metastable. Electrons linger in these states for a lengthy few milliseconds before spontaneous emission occurs.[7]

In stimulated emission, a photon passes in the vicinity of a high-energy electron. The photon stimulates the electron to emit a photon and drop into a lower state. The stimulating photon must have an energy equal to the energy difference between the two electron orbits. Stimulated emission begins with a photon and a high-energy electron and yields two photons and a low-energy electron.

Stimulated emission is not a random process. The electron drops at the moment a passing photon stimulates the electron to drop and emit a photon. Importantly, the stimulating photon and the emitted photon will be identical in frequency and phase. In other words, the two photons are coherent.[8] Many ways exist to produce light, but stimulated emission is the only method known that produces coherent light, a property with many practical applications. Figure 7-2 illustrates these three processes—absorption, spontaneous emission, and stimulated emission.

HOW LASERS WORK

Gas lasers are the most widely used lasers in clinical ophthalmology. Atoms of the working gas, such as argon or krypton, are enclosed in a cylindrical tube, called the *laser cavity* (Fig. 7-3). Under natural conditions there are more electrons in lower energy orbits than higher energy orbits. Eventually one of the high-

energy electrons undergoes spontaneous emission, generating a photon. If this photon first encounters a low-energy electron (which is much more common at this point), it is merely absorbed. However, in the event that it encounters another high-energy electron, stimulated emission occurs.

To sustain a large number of stimulated emissions, there must be more electrons in high-energy states than low-energy states, a condition called *population inversion*. To produce a population inversion in the gas laser, the gas is pumped by a powerful light source or by an electric discharge that forces electrons to go into high-energy states.

Merely achieving a population inversion is not sufficient; it must be maintained, because most high-energy states decay in a few nanoseconds by spontaneous emission. However, when electrons are pumped into a metastable state the population inversion may be maintained for a longer period of time. With the majority of electrons in a high-energy metastable state, a photon generated by spontaneous emission is now more likely to produce a stimulated emission instead of merely being absorbed. The two coherent photons generated by a stimulated emission go on to produce more stimulated emissions, and a chain reaction begins.

In order to maintain the chain reaction of stimulated emissions, mirrors are placed at each end of the cavity, an arrangement called a *resonator*.[9] One mirror reflects totally and the other partially (see Fig. 7-3). Most of the coherent light generated is reflected back into the cavity to produce more stimulated emis-

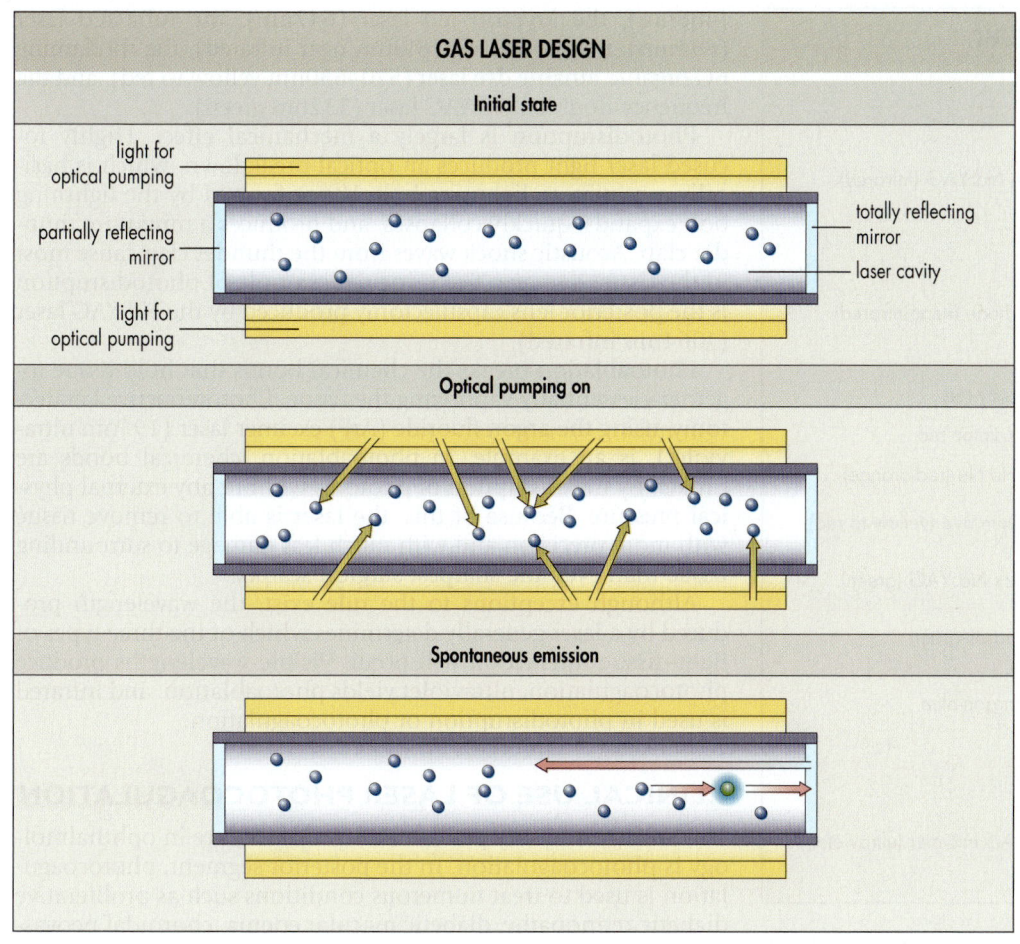

GAS LASER DESIGN

Initial state

light for optical pumping

partially reflecting mirror

light for optical pumping

totally reflecting mirror

laser cavity

Optical pumping on

Spontaneous emission

FIG. 7-3 ▮▮ **Gas laser.** A typical design consists of a gas-filled cavity, external optical pumping lights, and a resonator that comprises partially and totally reflecting mirrors. Without optical pumping, most of the gas atoms are in lower energy states and incapable of undergoing either spontaneous or stimulated emission. With optical pumping, photons from the external lights are absorbed by the gas atoms, which raises the energy of the atoms and makes them capable of undergoing spontaneous or stimulated emission. Ultimately, the majority of atoms are in excited states—a population inversion. One of the higher energy atoms spontaneously emits a photon that produces stimulated emissions as it passes by other high-energy atoms. By reflecting the photons back and forth across the cavity multiple times, a chain reaction of stimulated emissions is produced.

sions. The relatively small amount of light that is allowed to pass through the partially reflecting mirror produces the actual laser beam.

CONTINUOUS AND PULSED LASERS

Lasers emit light either continuously or in pulses. Although a pulsed laser produces only modest amounts of energy, the energy is concentrated into very brief periods, and so each pulse has a relatively high power (power is energy per unit time). Neodymium:yttrium–aluminum–garnet (Nd:YAG) and excited dimer (excimer) lasers are examples of pulsed lasers.

A continuous laser modality delivers more overall energy to a target tissue, but it does so over a relatively long time; thus the power is lower. Because clinical applications do not generally require high power (usually less than one watt), most ophthalmic lasers operate continuously with a shutter to control the specific exposure time and thereby allow more control over the energy delivered to the target tissue. Argon lasers, krypton lasers, diode lasers, and dye lasers are all examples of continuous laser modalities.

WHAT COLOR IS YOUR LASER?

The number of optical wavelengths that can be produced by lasers is rather limited, dependent on the particular metastable state of the working material. For instance, in the krypton ion, when an electron drops from its metastable state to a lower energy level, it produces light with a wavelength of 647nm (which corresponds to red light). Using different nonmetastable states, the krypton ion can produce several other wavelengths, but only at significantly lower powers. For practical reasons, only krypton lasers that operate at the 647nm wavelength are available commercially. The argon ion has two metastable states, and it therefore produces two prominent wavelengths of light at 488nm and 514nm, which correspond to blue–green and green, respectively.

Most commercial argon lasers allow the clinician to select either the green 514nm light or a mixture of blue–green 488nm and green 514nm light.

Some laser procedures demand peak wavelengths that do not correspond to the metastable state of any conventional working material. For instance, in the treatment of macular choroidal neovascularization using photocoagulation, xanthophyll pigment in the macula absorbs a significant amount of laser light, thereby increasing the risk of damage to the neurosensory retina and decreasing the amount of energy delivered to the abnormal blood vessels below. Xanthophyll pigment transmits light best at 577nm, but it is difficult to generate this wavelength with lasers.

Two ways exist to increase the number of available wavelengths: harmonic generation and employing organic dyes. In harmonic generation, laser light is passed through an optically nonlinear crystal,[10] which doubles its wave frequency. When light traverses any medium, a small amount of the light is absorbed. Typically, the absorption is linear in the sense that doubling the light intensity doubles the amount of energy absorbed. In a nonlinear medium, doubling the intensity does not double absorption; it increases it, by perhaps fourfold or more. Laser light causes such nonlinear crystals to vibrate, not only at the laser's frequency, but also at exact multiples of the laser's frequency, called harmonics. For instance, the middle A note on a piano has a frequency of 440 cycles per second; its harmonics include 880, 1320, 1760 cycles per second, and so on. Generally, this method of creating new wave frequencies is quite inefficient, and the harmonics generated have very low power. However, a nonlinear crystal has been found that efficiently doubles the frequency of the 1064nm output of an Nd:YAG laser, producing a 532nm wavelength, which is relatively close to the transmission window of xanthophyll (577nm).

Another method used to produce more wavelengths employs organic dyes.[11] As a result of their complex chemical structure, organic dyes provide a large number of metastable orbits that differ little in energy, so a variety of different wavelengths are available. Dye lasers may be tuned to the desired wavelength, allowing

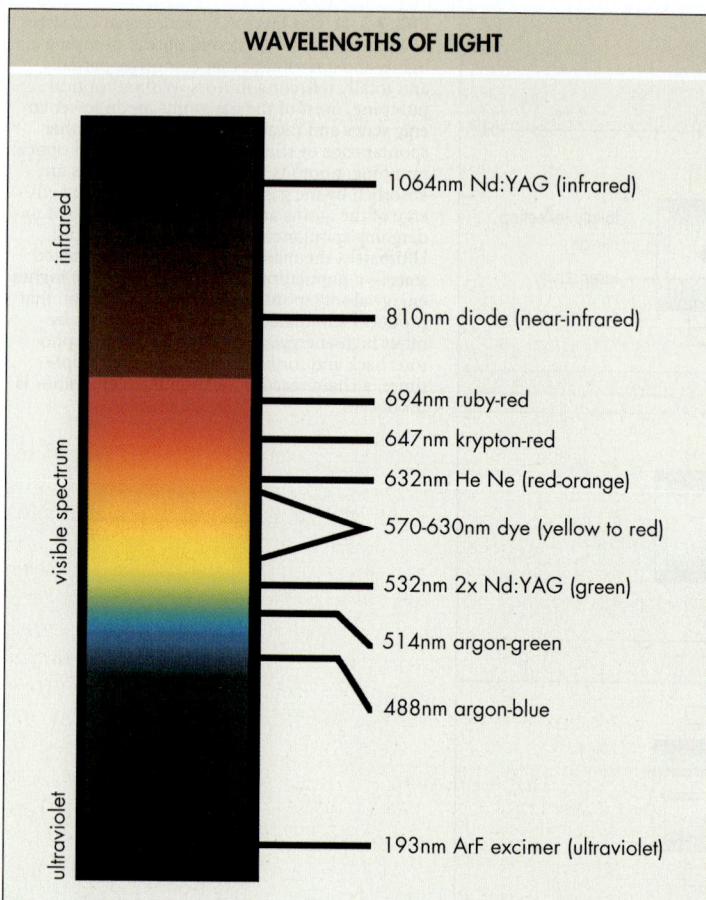

WAVELENGTHS OF LIGHT

infrared

1064nm Nd:YAG (infrared)

810nm diode (near-infrared)

visible spectrum

694nm ruby-red

647nm krypton-red

632nm He Ne (red-orange)

570-630nm dye (yellow to red)

532nm 2x Nd:YAG (green)

514nm argon-green

488nm argon-blue

ultraviolet

193nm ArF excimer (ultraviolet)

FIG. 7-4 ■ Wavelengths of light produced by the more commonly used ophthalmic lasers and where these wavelengths lie on the electromagnetic spectrum.

clinicians to select the optimum wavelength for each procedure. For example, the organic dye laser based on rhodamine 6G can be tuned continuously from 570nm to 630nm. The drawbacks of dye lasers are that they are the least efficient producers of laser energy and most expensive to manufacture. In fact, current tunable dye lasers utilize an argon laser to pump energy into the fluorescent dye. This complex system of two lasers increases the manufacturing cost and the likelihood of mechanical failure.

Figure 7-4 shows the different wavelengths of light produced by the more commonly used ophthalmic lasers and where these wavelengths lie on the electromagnetic spectrum.

CLINICAL USE OF LASERS

Notwithstanding the planet-destroying capabilities of the lasers depicted in Hollywood movies, real-life lasers are not death rays. Although lasers have been used to target or guide military weapons, no laser has become an effective weapon in its own right despite years of research. In fact, lasers are not particularly powerful (a penlight produces more light than any clinical laser) or efficient (it may require thousands of watts of power to produce a mere 1–2W of laser light). But despite low power and inefficiency, lasers are very useful, because they produce such a highly concentrated focus of coherent light.

Effective clinical use of lasers requires an understanding of the three basic light–tissue interactions as follows: (1) photocoagulation, (2) photodisruption, and (3) photoablation. In photocoagulation, laser light is absorbed by the target tissue or by neighboring tissue, generating heat that denatures proteins (i.e., coagulation). Clinical examples of photocoagulation include panretinal photocoagulation, argon laser trabeculoplasty, peripheral iridectomy, and thermal destruction of choroidal neovascular membranes. Types of lasers which produce photocoagulation include the argon green laser (514nm), the argon blue–green laser

(488nm), the krypton red laser (647nm), the ruby red laser (694nm), the diode laser (810nm near infrared), the rhodamine 6G organic tunable dye laser (570–630nm yellow to red), and the frequency-doubled Nd:YAG laser (532nm green).

Photodisruption is largely a mechanical effect. Highly focused laser light produces an optical breakdown, which is basically a miniature lightning bolt. Vapor formed by the lightning bolt expands, quickly collapses, and produces a miniature thunder clap. Acoustic shock waves from the thunder clap cause most of the tissue damage. The principal example of photodisruption is the posterior lens capsulectomy produced by the Nd:YAG laser (1064nm infrared).

Photoablation breaks the chemical bonds that hold tissue together—essentially vaporizing the tissue. Photorefractive keratectomy, using the argon fluoride (ArF) excimer laser (193nm ultraviolet), is an example. In photoablation, chemical bonds are broken by the absorption of photons, without any external physical pressure. Because of this, the laser is able to remove tissue with more precision and with much less damage to surrounding tissue than even the sharpest surgical scalpel.

Although exceptions to the rule exist, the wavelength produced by a laser generally determines which of the three types of light–tissue interaction will occur. Visible wavelengths produce photocoagulation, ultraviolet yields photoablation, and infrared is used in photodisruption or photocoagulation.

CLINICAL USE OF LASER PHOTOCOAGULATION

The most commonly performed laser procedure in ophthalmology is photocoagulation. In the posterior segment, photocoagulation is used to treat numerous conditions such as proliferative diabetic retinopathy, diabetic macular edema, choroidal neovascularization secondary to age-related macular degeneration, retinal breaks, and retinal detachments. In the anterior segment, photocoagulation is used to perform iridoplasty, iridectomy, trabeculoplasty, and cyclophotocoagulation.

In photocoagulation the surgeon controls the exposure time, the power, and the spot size. It is important that the surgeon has a clear understanding of how these parameters affect the lesions produced. An increase in exposure time (while all other parameters are maintained constant) modestly increases the lesion's diameter. A tenfold increase in exposure time roughly doubles lesion diameter. Longer exposure time also extends the damage deeper into the target tissue. Very brief exposure times, of the order 0.01–0.05 seconds, allow little time for heat to dissipate from the burn. A small area of intense damage may be produced, resulting in the perforation of delicate ocular structures such as Bruch's membrane or the neural retina.

An increase in power has a strong influence on lesion diameter. In fact, doubling the laser power almost doubles the size of lesion created. Such increases in laser power create more damage and can be painful to the patient. This can be avoided in some cases by increasing the exposure time rather than laser power.

Careful control of laser spot size is important in order to achieve the desired therapeutic effect. When working in sensitive areas such as the macula, a small spot size (such as 100µm) is preferred so as to minimize unnecessary damage to adjacent retinal tissue. In contrast, treatment of broader areas of tissue is facilitated by a larger spot, such as a 200-500µm spot size for panretinal photocoagulation.

Laser contact lenses may also affect the spot size. Whereas the Goldmann three-mirror lens will increase spot size only by a factor of 1.08, the Panfundoscope lens has a multiplication factor of 1.41. The Mainster wide-angle lens multiplies spot size by a factor of 1.47, and the QuadrAspheric lens by a factor of 1.92. If the spot size is increased, power needs to be increased, as well. However, because energy is concentrated in the center of the beam, it is best to raise power only modestly (no more than twofold at a time) and to use test burns to refine the power setting.

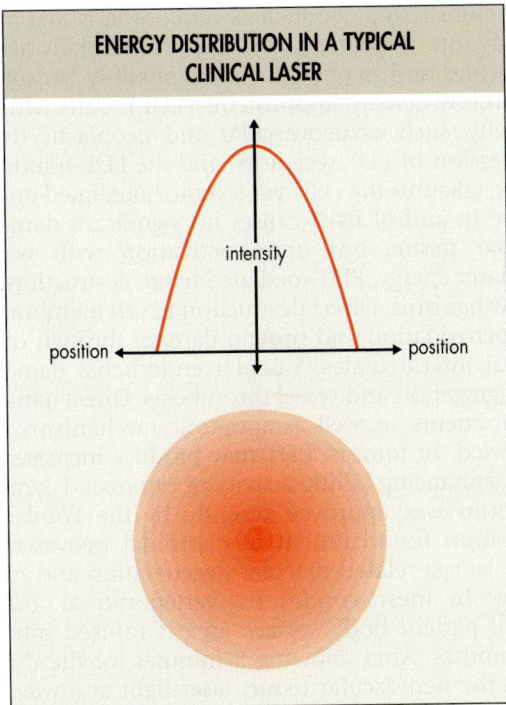

FIG. 7-5 ▮▮ **Energy distribution in a typical clinical laser.** Notice that the energy is concentrated in the center of the beam.

COMPLICATIONS FROM LASER PHOTOCOAGULATION

Laser Beam Profile

It is important for the laser surgeon to be aware of the laser beam profile, the way light energy is distributed over the beam's cross-section. In most photocoagulating lasers, the energy is concentrated in the center of the beam, with less energy at the edges (Fig. 7-5). Therefore, if excessive power is used during laser treatment of the retina, the center of the laser beam may cause water vaporization, possibly resulting in an inadvertent retinal hole. Also, the lower energy at the periphery of the laser beam may produce permanent tissue damage even though it does not produce a visible reaction. It is therefore important to realize that the area of laser damage may extend beyond the area of immediately visible reaction.

Effect of Off-Axis Astigmatism on the Laser Beam

When the peripheral retina is being treated, the aiming beam takes on an elliptical shape as a result of off-axis astigmatism. An elliptical laser beam profile has a higher power density, and this may result in complications such as inadvertent retinal holes. Tilting the lens will counteract this effect, producing a round laser beam and a more even laser beam profile.

Treatment of the Peripheral Retina

The retina thins in the periphery and, consequently, less power is required to treat this area. Laser photocoagulation of the peripheral retina is often more painful for the patient, especially in the horizontal meridians where the ciliary nerves enter the globe. Longer exposure times, lower laser power, or the administration of a local anesthetic may help minimize patient discomfort.

Photocoagulation in the Retinal Posterior Pole

Brief exposure times minimize the risk of inadvertent damage to the fovea that may arise from patient motion. Even when retrobulbar anesthesia is administered in order to produce ocular akinesia, a short exposure time is important because the patient is still capable of moving his or her head, thereby jeopardizing the procedure.

Photocoagulation Treatment of Macular Edema

Where the retina is thickened from edema more power is necessary to achieve a burn, because the retina is farther from the light-absorbing pigment in the retinal pigment epithelium (RPE) and choroid. The clinician must recognize the subtler, deeper burn that is the end point for focal treatment in patients who have macular edema.

CLINICAL USE OF THE YTTRIUM–ALUMINUM–GARNET LASER

The Nd:YAG laser works on the principle of photodisruption. Light is a type of electromagnetic field, and such fields produce forces on charged particles, including electrons. Typically, light energy causes electrons to oscillate as they travel around their nuclei. Extremely high electromagnetic field strengths, from a laser for example, can actually strip electrons from their nuclei, producing an entirely different physical state of matter called plasma.

Where the plasma forms, the chemical nature of the material is destroyed. The orderly array of molecules is fractured into a random mixture of electrons and protons in a process called optical breakdown. A similar effect occurs when a powerful electric field turns air into a plasma, forming a lightning bolt. After the high-intensity laser light passes, electrons and nuclei reunite, and the plasma collapses. An acoustic shock wave, analogous to a thunder clap, is produced. This acoustic shock wave is responsible for most of the physical damage to the ocular tissue produced by the Nd:YAG laser.

Optical breakdown requires electromagnetic fields so powerful they can be produced only by concentrating laser energy into very brief periods, thereby giving each pulse an extremely high power level. There are two ways of pulsing an Nd:YAG laser: Q-switching and mode locking. In Q-switching, a shutter in front of one of the mirrors in the laser cavity blocks laser light emission until a large population inversion has been established. The shutter is opened quickly, and the stored energy bursts forward in the form of a brief pulse that lasts about one millionth of a second. Q-switching is comparatively inexpensive and reliable but cannot produce pulses as short or powerful as mode locking.

In mode locking, electromagnetic energy in the laser cavity exists in various modes that depend on the length of the laser cavity and the construction of the resonator mirrors. In mode locking an optical element (Fabry–Perot interferometer) inside the cavity synchronizes the modes so all the light is emitted in extremely brief pulses. Most clinical Nd:YAG lasers today are Q-switched, because mode-locked lasers are more expensive and difficult to maintain.

The light produced by the Nd:YAG laser is infrared (1064nm), invisible to the clinician, so an ancillary aiming system, typically a red helium–neon (HeNe) laser, is necessary. Just as a prism causes blue light to bend more than red light, the optics of the patient's eye cause the red aiming beam to bend more than the Nd:YAG's infrared light. Consequently, the focus of the Nd:YAG laser rarely coincides precisely with the focus of the aiming beam (Fig. 7-6). Some lasers have an adjustment to compensate for this source of error, called chromatic aberration.

Performing an Nd:YAG laser capsulectomy in an eye with a silicone intraocular lens implant poses a particular challenge, because optical breakdown occurs in silicone at relatively low power. Therefore, damage to the intraocular lens may occur even when the laser is focused posterior to the implant. And if the capsule is in intimate contact with the implant, creating the capsulotomy is even more difficult. A corneal contact lens designed for laser capsulotomy causes the Nd:YAG laser beam to converge at a steeper angle, resulting in a more sharply focused beam of

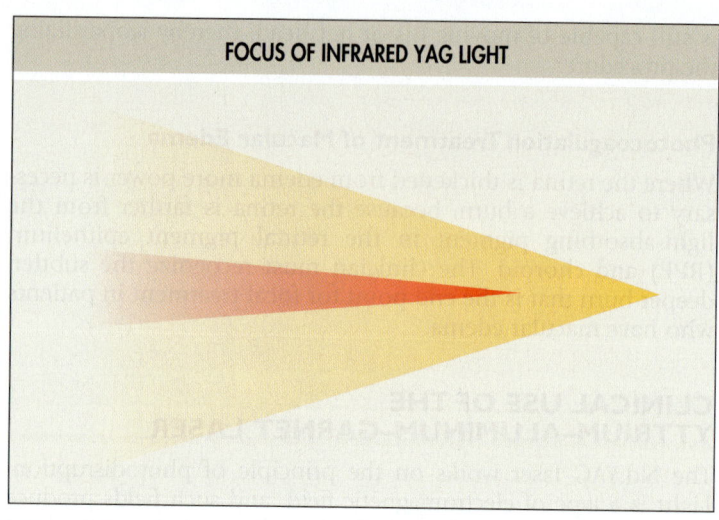

FOCUS OF INFRARED YAG LIGHT

FIG. 7-6 ◼ The focus of the infrared YAG light usually does not coincide with the aiming beam's visible red light.

light. This makes optical breakdown at sites outside the focal point less likely. Intraocular lenses made of polymethylmethacrylate (PMMA) and acrylic are less susceptible to optical breakdown than silicone lenses.

CLINICAL USE OF LASER PHOTOABLATION

Photoablation is the most recent light–tissue interaction to be exploited clinically. It is used to treat corneal pathology such as ulcers and scars, and its use in keratorefractive surgery has become a rapidly evolving field. The argon–fluoride (ArF) excimer laser produces electromagnetic energy with a wavelength of 193nm, in the extreme ultraviolet. With each pulse of the excimer laser, a large area of the cornea is ablated. With such a large area of tissue being treated at a time, it is important to have a uniform beam profile. When the excimer beam initially emerges from the laser cavity it has a Gaussian profile, with energy concentrated more heavily in the center of the beam. Beam-shaping optics are then used to create an even beam profile. However, these beam-shaping optics are, themselves, ablated slowly by the ultraviolet laser beam, and they must be replaced periodically.

Although the excimer laser removes approximately 0.1mm of corneal tissue on average with each pulse, irregularities in the corneal stroma and the presence of keratocytes in the stroma may cause uneven ablation, even when the beam profile is uniform. Further, corneal collagen density varies with a number of factors, including altitude, atmospheric pressure, relative humidity, patient age, and duration of the procedure. Fortunately, the microscopic irregularities that may be produced due to patient-specific corneal factors do not appear to affect final visual acuity to a great extent.

In older techniques of corneal ablation, the entire anterior surface of the cornea—including the epithelium and Bowman's membrane—would be ablated. In laser-assisted *in situ* keratomileusis (LASIK), a partial lamellar incision through the anterior corneal stroma is performed using a keratome. The anterior corneal surface is then temporarily displaced, exposing the corneal stroma to excimer laser treatment (Chapter 20). In this manner, the corneal surface contour may be reshaped by controlled removal of stromal tissue by the excimer laser, while keeping the corneal epithelium and Bowman's membrane intact.

PHOTODYNAMIC THERAPY

Photodynamic therapy (PDT) is a new laser technique for treatment of choroidal neovascularization and various tumors in the eye. In this technique, a special laser-activated dye is used to cause damage selectively to abnormal blood vessels, while minimizing damage to the nearby retinal tissue.

A photosensitizing dye such as verteporfin is first injected intravenously into the patient. The dye preferentially accumulates in neovascular and neoplastic tissue, possibly because the dye binds with low-density lipoproteins (LDL). Cells with high mitotic activity, such as neovascular and neoplastic tissue, have high expression of LDL receptors, and the LDL-bound dye may thereby be taken in the cells via receptor-mediated endocytosis.

The dye in and of itself causes no significant damage to the neovascular tissue, but upon activation with wavelength-matched laser energy, PDT-mediated tissue destruction occurs by several mechanisms. Direct destruction to cell membranes occurs via lipid peroxidation and protein damage through oxygen and free radical intermediates. Vascular endothelial damage causes platelet aggregation and vessel thrombosis. Direct damage to nuclear components, as well as apoptotic mechanisms, have also been reported. In tumors, PDT may produce increased levels of cytokines, enhancing killing activity of cytotoxic T-lymphocytes.

Verteporfin was approved recently by the Food and Drug Administration for treatment of choroidal neovascularization secondary to age-related macular degeneration and myopic degeneration. In these conditions, verteporfin at a dosage of $6mg/m^2$ of patient body surface area is infused intravenously over 10 minutes. After allowing 5 minutes for the dye to accumulate in the neovascular tissue, laser light at a wavelength of 689nm is then applied for 83 seconds at an intensity of $600mW/cm^2$, to give a total light dose of $50J/cm^2$.

The treatment of age-related macular degeneration with photodynamic therapy (TAP) investigation determined that verteporfin PDT reduces the risk of moderate vision loss, defined as a loss of at least three lines of visual acuity, compared with a placebo sham treatment, with 2 years of follow-up data.[12,13] However, patients often require repeat treatments after 3–4 months due to a recurrence of leakage from the choroidal neovascularization, as determined by fluorescein angiography. Patients must also avoid direct sunlight exposure for up to 5 days after injection with verteporfin, because sunlight can activate the dye, possibly resulting in PDT-mediated damage to the skin and retina. With more clinical experience in the use of PDT, our indications for its use in other ocular conditions will undoubtedly expand.

DIAGNOSTIC USE OF LASERS

Lasers also have several important diagnostic applications, including scanning laser ophthalmoscopy and optical coherence tomography.

Scanning Laser Ophthalmoscopy

In the scanning laser ophthalmoscope (SLO), developed by Robert Webb and George Timberlake,[14] a narrow laser beam illuminates the retina one spot at a time, and the amount of reflected light at each point is measured. As with natural light, the amount of light reflected back to the observer depends on the physical properties of the tissue which, in turn, define its reflective, refractive, and absorptive properties. Media opacities, such as retinal hemorrhage, vitreous hemorrhage, and cataract, also affect the amount of light transmitted back to the observer. Because the SLO uses laser light, which has coherent properties, the retinal images produced have a much higher image resolution than conventional fundus photography. Also, because only a single point on the retina is illuminated at any given time, the patient is not affected by a bright illumination source or flash. This allows for high-resolution, real-time motion images of the macula without patient discomfort.

Current SLOs use a single wavelength of laser light, so the images produced are monochromatic. SLO angiography can be performed after intravenous injection of fluorescein or indocyanine green in order to study retinal and choroidal blood flow. By varying the brightness of the scanning laser beam, the scanning

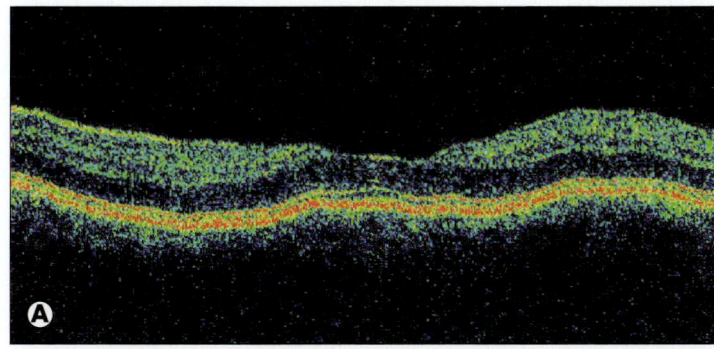

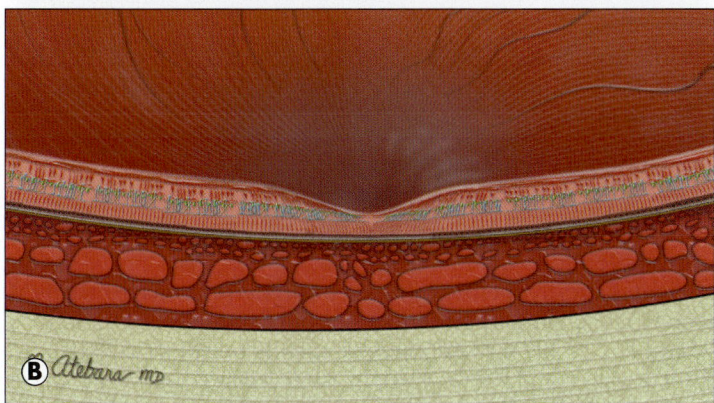

FIG. 7-7 ▊ **A,** Cross-sectional image of the macula using optical coherence tomography. There is sufficient resolution on this scan to demonstrate the various retinal layers, as depicted in the correlative illustration (**B**).

the retinal surface. When this occurs, the wave patterns of the measuring and reference beams are in precise synchronization, resulting in constructive interference. This appears as a bright area on the resulting cross-sectional image. However, some of the light from the measuring beam will pass through the retinal surface and will be reflected off deeper layers in the retina. This light will have traversed a longer distance than the reference beam, and when the two beams are brought back together to be measured by the photodetector, some degree of destructive interference will occur, depending on how much further the measuring beam has traveled. The amount of destructive interference at each point measured by the OCT is translated into a measurement of retinal depth and graphically displayed as the retinal cross-section.

OCT images are displayed in false color to enhance differentiation of retinal structures. Bright colors (red to white) correspond to tissues with high reflectivity, whereas darker colors (blue to black) correspond to areas of minimal or no reflectivity. The OCT can differentiate structures with a spatial resolution of only 10μm (Fig. 7-7).

CONCLUSION

In a relatively brief period, lasers have evolved from an obscure research novelty to an invaluable clinical instrument. The continual refinement of existing laser types, as well as the introduction of new laser technology, mark this area of ophthalmology as one of its most energetic and dynamic fields. The role of lasers in clinical ophthalmology has expanded continually, and this trend will doubtless continue.

laser ophthalmoscope also may be used to perform microperimetry, an extremely accurate mapping of the macula's visual field.

Optical Coherence Tomography

Optical coherence tomography (OCT) uses diode laser light in the near-infrared spectrum (810nm) to produce high-resolution cross-sectional images of the retina using coherence interferometry.[15] In coherence interferometry, a partially reflective mirror is used to split a single laser beam into two, the measuring beam and the reference beam. The measuring beam is directed into the patient's eye and onto the retina. Because many of the retinal layers are transparent to near-infrared light, the laser beam passes through the neurosensory retina to the RPE and the choriocapillaris. At each optical interface, some of the laser light is reflected back to the OCT's photodetector.

The reference beam, on the other hand, is reflected off of a reference mirror at a known distance from the beam splitter, back to the photodetector. The position of the reference mirror can be adjusted to make the path traversed by the reference beam equal to the distance traversed by the measuring beam to

REFERENCES

1. Halliday D, Resnick R, Walker J. Fundamentals of physics, ed 5. New York: Wiley; 1997:1042.
2. Zaret MM, Mreinin GM, Schmidt H, *et al.* Ocular lesions produced by an optical maser (laser). Science. 1961;134:1525.
3. L'Esperance FA. Ophthalmic lasers. St Louis: CV Mosby; 1989.
4. Reed BC. Quantum mechanics: a first course. Winnipeg: Wuerz; 1990:1–35.
5. Allen L, Eberly JH. Optical resonance and two-level atoms. New York: Wiley; 1975.
6. Halliday D, Resnick R, Walker J. Fundamentals of physics, ed 5. New York: Wiley; 1997:1043–4.
7. Hecht J. Understanding lasers: an entry level guide. Piscataway: IEEE; 1992:62–3.
8. Lipson SG, Lipson H, Tannhauser DS. Optical physics, ed 3. Cambridge: Cambridge University Press; 1995:423–5.
9. Siegman AE. Lasers, ed 2. Mill Valley, Calif: University Science Books; 1986:558–891.
10. Hecht J. Understanding lasers: an entry level guide. Piscataway: IEEE; 1992: 142–3.
11. Siegman AE. Lasers, ed 2. Mill Valley, Calif: University Science Books; 1986:295.
12. TAP Study Group. Photodynamic therapy of subfoveal choroidal neovascularization in age related macular degeneration with verteporfin. One-year results of 2 randomized clinical trials—TAP Report 1. Arch Ophthalmol. 1999;117:1329–45.
13. TAP Study Group. Photodynamic therapy of subfoveal choroidal neovascularization in age related macular degeneration with verteporfin. Two-year results of 2 randomized clinical trials—TAP Report 2. Arch Ophthalmol. 2001;119:198–207.
14. Timberlake GT, Mainster MA, Webb RH, *et al.* Retinal localization of scotomata by scanning laser ophthalmoscopy. Invest Ophthalmol Vis Sci. 1982;22:91–7.
15. Puliafito CA, Hee MR, Lin CP. Imaging of macular diseases with optical coherence tomography. Ophthalmology. 1995;102:217.

CHAPTER 8

Light Units

DAVID MILLER • JEROME S. SARMIENTO • STEPHEN K. BURNS

DEFINITIONS

- Light intensity can be defined either in general energy units or in operational terms, that is, in units that relate to the amount of light from optical and electronic images, as well the amount of light needed to damage the eye.
- Candles, candelas, watts, and joules are units that describe the intensity of light emitted from a light source.
- Illuminance is the blanket term covering luxes, phots, foot-candles, and lumens, which are light units describing the amount of light falling onto a surface.
- Luminance is the blanket term covering luxes, nits, stilbs, foot-lamberts, and candelas/area, which are units describing the amount of light coming from a surface.
- Joules and watts are the units used to describe the amount of light that causes eye damage (e.g., in laser treatment).

KEY FEATURES

- Lighting levels that damage the eye.
- Lighting levels used in laser treatment.

ASSOCIATED FEATURES

- Lighting levels needed for patients with cataracts and macular degeneration.

INTRODUCTION

A cursory attempt to understand light units may result in a high level of frustration. Candles, candelas, watts, and joules are all used to describe the intensity of light sources; luxes, phots, and foot-candles are used to measure light that falls on a surface (i.e., illumination); and light that comes off a surface is measured in luxes, nits, stilbs, foot-lamberts, and candelas/cm^2.

It was much simpler in 1760, when Lambert wrote his essay on photometry and the only standard source of artificial light was the candle. In the mid-1880s, John Herschel and his sister compared one star with another to measure the brightness of both. Using two telescopes, they kept the control star in focus and placed layers of muslin over the second telescope, until the star in question became as dim as the control; a star's brightness was thus given by its muslin index.

As science developed, more was learned about new light sources, new light sensors, and the wavelength composition of these new light sources. Thus, terms such as candles and the muslin index were used less. With each passing generation of light scientists, new units were developed to replace the older ones. Unfortunately, the new units were not accepted universally, and older books with older units continue to be used.

DEFINING LIGHT OPERATIONALLY

As clinicians, we must use the units that manufacturers and standards committees use to describe light levels that damage, com-fortable reading light levels, or projector chart light levels. In other words, the definitions are divided into operational categories.

Light Used to Produce Damage

Lasers or conventional light sources damage the eye if the density of energy (i.e., the energy distributed per unit area) exceeds a threshold level.

Light is a form of energy that is emitted as photons from a light source. The energy in an individual photon is given by Planck's equation, $E = hc/\lambda$. Light energy depends on the wavelength, λ. Short wavelengths (blue) contain more energy than long wavelengths (red). The basic unit of light energy is the lumen, which measures the total flow of photons or light energy produced by a light source. One lumen represents a power of 1/683 joule per second at a wavelength of 555nm (yellow–green). Energy is measured in joules or calories. One joule is approximately 0.24 calorie. One joule raises the temperature of 1g of water 0.24°C. Power is the flow of energy. One joule per second is 1 watt of power, so a lumen is 1/683 watt. A lumen measures the *total light* (the sum of energy from all the photons) emanating from a source. The luminous intensity of a real light source is measured in candles or candelas. The standard states: "The candela is the luminous intensity, *in a given direction,* of a source that emits monochromatic radiation of frequency 540×10^{12} hertz and that has a radiant intensity in that direction of 1/683 watt per steradian."[1] The candela measures the luminous intensity/steradian of light originating from a specific direction of a real source as if it were emerging from a point source at that origin. The number of candelas from a real source varies with direction but not with distance. The number of photons per second emitted does not change with distance from the source. The same number strikes a 1m radius sphere that completely surrounds the source as strikes a 2m radius sphere. The solid angle is independent of the distance. Light power from a 1 candela source is 1/683 watt/steradian. The total power is 1/683 watt $\times$ 4π = 4π lumens = 12.566 lumens. The total amount of light (photons/sec) emitted from a point source is constant, but the spatial density (photons/sec per unit area) decreases with the square of the distance. Light flux is measured in luxes, where 1 lux = 1 lumen/m^2. If you were to enclose a 1-lumen light source in a 1m radius sphere, the total amount of light striking the surface of the sphere would still be 1 lumen, but the density of the light at the surface would be 1 lumen divided by the area of the sphere (4πR^2 = 12.566m^2). So the illumination of the surface would be 1 lumen/12.566m^2 = 1/12.566 lux = 0.0796 lux. A 2m radius sphere would still receive 1 lumen of light, but this light would now be distributed over 50.265m^2. The surface illumination of the 2m radius sphere would be 0.0199 lux. The candela specifies light coming from a particular direction, measured as if it were coming from a point source in that direction. The lumen specifies the total amount of light. The lux specifies the amount of light illuminating a surface.

To create damage, the power from the light source needs to be concentrated in a small area and develop heat. Thus, it is the power density—power or work per unit area—that gives the best indication of the damage done. Another term for the power density that falls on a surface is irradiance. In terms of damage from laser light, it is the light incident on a surface (irradiance, or illumination) that is important, not the light reflected from the surface (radiance, or luminance).

For example, in panretinal photocoagulation for diabetic retinopathy, the irradiance or power density of the argon laser is about $22mW/0.04mm^2$, or $22mW/0.0004cm^2$ (spot size of $200\mu m$), delivered in bursts of 0.1-second duration each. Energy densities from this laser are very high: $22mW/0.0004cm^2 = 55,000$ watts/m^2 = 378,565,000 lumens/m^2 = 378,565,000 luxes. The damage is restricted to the area of the spot. A $200\mu m$ cube of tissue is essentially $8\mu g$ of water. The laser delivers 2.2 millijoules = 0.53 millicalorie to $8\mu g$ of tissue. If isolated, this would raise the temperature of $8\mu g$ of the water by 275°C, vaporizing it.

The indirect ophthalmoscope can produce retinal damage after a few minutes of steady illumination at its power density of $70mW/cm^2 = 700w/m^2 = 478,100$ luxes. This is $70mW/sec = 70$ millijoules or 16.8 millicalories delivered to a 1cm^2 area in 1 second. A 1cm^2 area $200\mu m$ deep contains about 20mg of tissue, and 16.8 millicalories would raise the temperature of 20mg of isolated water 0.84°C. Of course, the heated volume is not isolated, and some heat would be conducted away to the underlying tissue and circulating blood. But a substantial temperature rise would be expected in 10s of seconds from such an exposure. The slit lamp can produce the same damage in less time if the light is focused on the retina, because it emits 200mW/cm^2 ($2000w/m^2 = 1,366,000$ luxes).

The operating microscope emits $1000mW/cm^2 = 10,000w/m^2 = 6,830,000$ luxes. Compare this with the argon laser ($55,000w/m^2$), which is on for 0.1 second. With a moist, smooth corneal surface and clear crystalline lens in place, it may produce retinal damage in a short time. Fortunately, during cataract surgery, the cornea dries and becomes distorted once the eye has been entered via an incision. This, along with the presence of a cataract, diffuses the power density of the light on to the retina. However, once the implant is seated and the incision closed, the eye's focusing elements can concentrate the enormous light energy of the microscope light on to the retina. At that time, either an opaque disc must be placed on the corneal surface to obstruct the light, or an air bubble must be placed in the anterior chamber to defocus the light.

The yttrium-aluminum-garnet (YAG) laser delivers bursts of energy measured in millijoules. The unique effect of the YAG laser is achieved because a burst of one or more pulses is delivered in a billionth or a trillionth of a second and because the energy is concentrated at a point. The power levels of the YAG laser light are immense, since all the energy is delivered in a very short time and concentrated in a very small region. One millijoule delivered in 10^{-9} seconds corresponds to 1,000,000 watts/beam area. The focused beam further increases the power density. The beam power is so large that any material at the focal point of the laser breaks down, absorbs the energy, and is vaporized. These exceedingly high power levels affect transparent materials and even air.

Light Used to See

Since eyes see certain wavelengths of light better than others, light also can be described in terms relevant to the physiology of the eye. The devices used to describe indoor lighting are calibrated only for visible light and are further calibrated to the most sensitive wavelengths (i.e., green–yellow) to the retina. The lighting engineer divides the analysis of any lighting system into four categories:

1. Light source, described in watts or lumens; dimensions in watts.
2. Luminous intensity of a point source, described in candles or candelas; dimensions in watts/steradian.
3. Illumination, or light falling on a surface, described in luxes or lumens/m^2, foot-candles, or phots; dimensions in watts/ unit area.
4. Light reflected from the surface, described in candelas/m^2, foot-lamberts, meter-lamberts, or nits; dimensions in watts/ unit area.

Table 8-1 summarizes the categories, and illuminance and luminance are described in Boxes 8-1 and 8-2.

Electronic Vision

Television cameras have illumination requirements that are comparable to those of the human eye, typically between 10 and 200 luxes. Television and computer displays typically produce a maximal luminance of 250 candelas/m^2, or 250 nits. The dynamic range (the ratio of brightest to dimmest perceivable objects) of human vision is very large, around 10^8:1. Our environment commonly provides wide ranges of illumination. The ratio

---

BOX 8-1

ESSENTIAL COMPONENTS OF ILLUMINANCE

Illuminance is defined as the luminous flux on a surface per unit area. Illumination decreases as the distance from the source increases. For a point source, illumination decreases as the square of the distance from the source increases. The precise formulation for the decrease in illumination from a finite source is dependent on the nature of the source.

The inverse square law applies when:
- Illuminance is the luminous flux incident on a surface per unit area at the surface being illuminated without regard to the direction from which the light approaches.
- Use of the cosine correction to correct for changes in the illuminated area of a surface as a function of angle incidence guarantees that the measured value of illuminance is independent of the direction from which the light approaches the sensor.[1,4,8]

Units are foot-candles or lumens:
- 1 lm/m^2 = 1 lx = 1 meter-candle = 0.0929 foot-candle = .3183 cd/m^2
- 1 lm/ft^2 = 1 foot-candle = 10.764 lx
- 1 lm/cm^2 = 1 phot

BOX 8-2

ESSENTIAL COMPONENTS OF LUMINANCE

Luminance is defined as a luminuous flux per unit area per unit solid angle from a surface, whether reflected or emitted.

Luminance refers to light that emanates from a source or is reflected from a surface.

The inverse square law does not apply because it is the luminous intensity per unit area in a given direction.

1 foot-lambert is the luminance of a perfectly diffusing and reflecting surface illuminated by 1 candle at a distance of 1 foot.

Unit conversions:
- 1 lambert (L) = 1 candle/ft^2
- 1 foot-lambert = $(1/\pi)$lm/steradian/ft^2 = $(1/\pi)$candle/ft^2 = 0.00003426 candle/cm^2
- 1 candle/ft^2 = 1 lm/steradian/ft^2 = 0.001076 candle/cm^2
- 1 lm/W/m^2 = 1 candle/m^2 = 0.3142 millilambert = 0.2919 foot-lambert
- 1 lm/W/m^2 = 1 lambert

TABLE 8-1

SIMPLIFIED CATEGORIES OF LIGHT

Light Category	Description	Units
Light source	Total light from source	Lumens (lm)
Light source	Light/per unit solid angle from source	Candles, candelas (cd) 1 candle = 1.02 candelas
Illuminance (see Box 8-1)	Light incident on a surface	Luxes (lx; lm/m^2)
Luminance (see Box 8-2)	Light reflected from a surface	Luxes (lx; lm/m^2); lamberts; candelas (cd/m^2); nits; stilbs 1 cd/m^2 = 1 nit = 10^{-4} stilbs

of light available on a sunny noon to moonlight can be $10^7:1$. Television and computer images, like photography, have much more limited dynamic ranges. The contrast ratio of a modern liquid-crystal display is around 200–400.

ILLUMINANCE

Illuminance (E) is the light flux (lumens) incident on a surface and is measured in luxes (1 lux = 1 lumen/m^2 = 1 foot-candle/ 10.764). For example, a visual acuity wall chart is calibrated by measurement of the light that falls on it and should have an illumination in the range 480–600 luxes, or 44.6–55.74 foot-candles. A well-lit desk is illuminated by 20 foot-candles, or 215 luxes.

In the relationship between the point light source and the light incident on a surface, the intensity of the illuminance diminishes as the light is positioned farther away, according to Newton's inverse square law (the intensity of light is related inversely to the square of the distance from its source). The total amount of light from a source falling on a closed surface is the same no matter what the shape or distance of the surface. For example, consider a source of 1 lumen of light. The total light striking the surface of a 1m diameter sphere enclosing the 1-lumen source is the same as the total light striking the inside of a 2m sphere. But the density, measured in luxes, would be four times larger on the surface of the 1m sphere (1 lumen/πm^2 = 0.318 lux) than on the surface of the 2m sphere (1 lumen/$4\pi m^2$ = 0.0796 lux). The amount of light (candelas, lumens) is given by the density of light (nits or candles/m^2; luxes or lumens/m^2) multiplied by the total surface area it falls on. Thus, if E is the illuminance, I the point light source intensity, and d the distance, then $E = I/d^2$, where E is measured in luxes (lumens/m^2), I in lumens, and d in meters.

LUMINANCE

Luminance refers to light that leaves, is reflected, or is backscattered from a surface. Reflected light requires a few extra considerations, as different surfaces reflect light differently. Thus, white paper may reflect more than 90% of the incident light, and red paper much less. Of course, the amount of reflection also depends on the angle of incidence of the light and on the angle of observation. All combine to determine the luminance of the light that reaches the eye.

Photographers are particularly interested in reflected light, because they must adjust their camera lenses according to the light that is reflected from the subject and enters the camera. Since lighting engineers must be most rigorous, they use units such as nits, stilbs, and lamberts, which are direction dependent. Photographers use the lux (lumens/m^2), which has no directional consideration.

Ophthalmologists may want to calibrate the light of a visual acuity chart that is projected onto a screen, for which a light meter that measures reflected light in foot-lamberts may be used. The conversion factor for foot-lamberts into candelas/m^2 is

0.291. For example, the British standard for minimal luminance for an internally illuminated acuity chart (projected chart) is 411.1 foot-lamberts,[2] which is 411.1 × 0.291 = 120 candelas/m^2.

People who have normal sight need a luminance of about 70 candelas/m^2 (220 luxes), which is produced by varying the wattage of the lamp or adjusting the distance of the light from the printed page.

LIGHTING LEVELS FOR PATIENTS WITH EYE DISEASE

Cataracts

Opacity that results from cataracts may reduce the amount of light incident on the retina by 10–90%. Therefore, such patients require an increased luminance to read or do work. To read efficiently, a patient who has a cataract may (on average) need about double or triple the luminance required by a person of normal sight (about 70 candelas/m^2), which may be achieved by using a 75- or 100-watt incandescent bulb held at a distance of 1ft (0.3m) or less from the reading material.[3] A 100-watt bulb typically produces 1570 lumens, or 125 candelas, when new.

A patient who has a cataract may need about double or triple the average illuminance level (750 luxes) for a reading task, which would be 1500–2500 luxes (477–795 candelas/m^2).

Age-Related Macular Degeneration

Patients who have age-related macular degeneration have either a diminished number of photoreceptors within the macular area or photoreceptors that need higher levels of light energy to be stimulated. Logically, the luminance of reading material for these patients must be greater than 200 foot-candles (64 candelas/m^2, or 2152 luxes).

In the literature, the recommended illuminance on the printed page is in the range of 400–4000 luxes.[4] Understandably, the more serious the level of damage, the greater the illuminance needed. Also, the coefficient of reflectance and the color of the page both influence the amount of light (luminance) that finally reaches the patient.[5–8]

REFERENCES

1. Ferris FL, Sperduto RD. Standardized illumination for visual acuity testing clinical research. Am J Ophthalmol. 1982;94:97–8.
2. Bergem-Jansen PM. Ergonomic workplace design for a visually impaired person. In: Kooijman AC, Looijestijn PL, Welling JA, van der Wildt GJ, eds. Low vision. Washington DC: IOS Press; 1994:183–90.
3. Com AL, Koenig AJ. Foundations of low vision: clinical and functional perspectives. New York: American Foundation of Blind; 1996:137–8.
4. Faye EE, Hood CM. Low vision. Springfield: CC Thomas; 1975:42–5.
5. Cornelissen FW, Kooijman AC, School AJ, et al. Optimizing illumination for visually impaired persons; comparing subjective and objective criteria. In: Kooijman AC, Looijestijn PL, Welling JA, van der Wildt GJ, eds. Low vision. Washington DC: IOS Press; 1994:68–77.
6. Lagrow SJ. Assessing optimal illumination for visual response accuracy in visually impaired adults. J Vis Impairment Blindness. 1986;8:888–95.
7. Lehon LH. Development of lighting standards for the visually impaired. J Vis Impairment Blindness. 1980;74:249–53.
8. Taylor BN, ed. The international system of units. Special publication 330 (2001). Gaithersburg: National Institute of Standard and Technology; 2001:8.

CHAPTER 9

Optics of the Normal Eye

DAVID MILLER • PETER C. MAGNANTE

DEFINITION

The optics of the eye can best be understood in terms of the optical characteristics of its components, the cornea, pupil, crystalline lens, and retina, and how they function in combination.

KEY FEATURES

The quality and characteristics of the different optical components and the combination are described in the following terms.
- Chromatic aberration
- Spherical aberration
- Coma
- High-order aberrations
- Light scattering
- Retinal factors
- Resolution
- Focal length
- Depth of focus

ASSOCIATED FEATURES

Optical function is best described by a series of tests.
- Visual acuity
- Contrast sensitivity
- Modulation transfer function
- Wave-front testing
- Vernier testing
- Detection of fast-moving objects (flicker)
- Dark adaptation

INTRODUCTION

Eye clinicians define the abnormal eye by comparison with the normal. Thus the theoretical limits of the best quality, or threshold, image for the normal, emmetropic eye must be known. In this chapter the optical variables that determine the thresholds of image quality for distant objects for the human eye are discussed.

INDIVIDUAL OPTICAL ELEMENTS OF THE EYE

Corneal Factors

The cornea's anterior surface is approximately spherical with a radius of curvature that is typically 8mm. This surface is responsible for about two thirds of the eye's refractive power. The corneal stroma must be transparent for high-quality image formation on the retina, yet the normal human cornea scatters 10% of the incident light.[1] By comparison, the corneal stroma of the eagle is almost as transparent as glass.[2] This factor (along with the larger pupil size and finer cone diameter) is why the resolution of the eagle eye is better than 120 cycles per degree, which is equivalent to a Snellen acuity of 20/5 (6/1.5).[3]

The aspherical shape of the cornea's anterior surface affects the quality of the retinal image. Astigmatism is caused by this surface having different radii of curvature along different meridians. A survey of normal eyes shows that almost every human eye has a baseline corneal astigmatism of at least 0.25–0.50D.[4] Spherical aberration is caused by the corneal surface's radius of curvature changing (generally increasing) with distance from the center of the pupil to the pupillary margin. The amount of spherical aberration contributed by the cornea varies with pupillary aperture and individual corneal shape. For a pupil 4mm in diameter, spherical aberration varies from +0.21D to +1.62D, depending on the specific corneal form.[5]

Pupillary Factors

The iris, which gives the eye its color, expands or contracts to control the amount of light admitted to the eye. The pupil formed by the iris can range in diameter from 8mm in very dim light down to about 1.5mm under very bright conditions.[6] There is a strong association between visual acuity and pupillary diameter. For example, visual acuity has been shown to improve steadily as background illumination increases up to a value of $3400cd/m^2$.[7] Also, as the eye focuses on objects close at hand, the pupil gets smaller.

Retinal image quality, as determined by optical aberrations such as spherical aberration, tends to improve with decreasing pupil diameter, because optical aberrations decrease with decreasing pupil size. On the other hand, retinal image quality, as determined by diffraction, tends to improve with increasing pupil diameter. For most eyes the best retinal images are obtained when the pupil diameter is about 2.4mm, which is the diameter at which the effects of aberration and diffraction are balanced optimally. Thus the optimal pupillary size seems to be determined by several influences. In fact, Campbell and Gregory have shown that pupil size tends to be adjusted automatically to give optimal visual acuity over a wide range of luminance.[8]

Crystalline Lens Factors

The crystalline lens, which has about one third of the eye's refractive power, enables the eye to change focus. When the eye views nearby objects, the ciliary muscle changes the shape of the crystalline lens making it more bulbous and, consequently, optically more powerful. The lens of a young adult can focus over a range greater than 10D. Presbyopia, which begins at about 40 years of age, is the inability of the eye to focus (accommodate) due to hardening of the crystalline lens with age. When the eye can no longer accommodate at the reading distance, positive spectacle lenses of about 2–3D are prescribed to correct the difficulty.

The normal 20-year-old crystalline lens scatters about 20% of the incident light. The amount of scatter is more than double this in the normal 60-year-old lens.[9] Such scatter significantly diminishes contrast sensitivity.[10] Also, the normal 20-year-old lens absorbs about 30% of incident blue light. At age 60, this absorption increases to about 60% of the incident blue light.[11] The

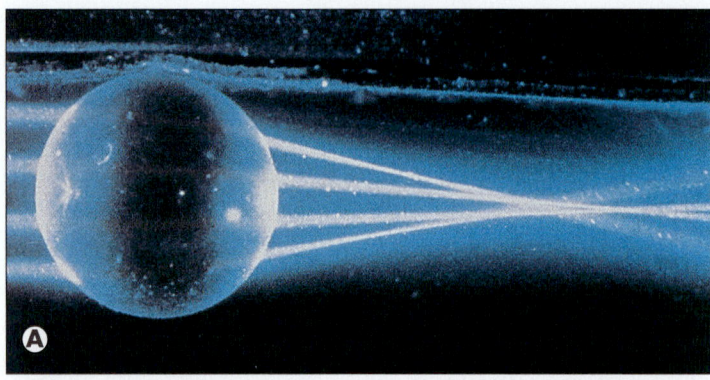

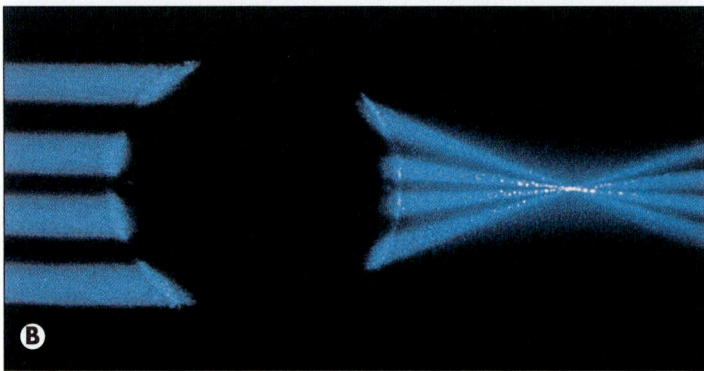

FIG. 9-1 ■ Spherical aberrations produced by lenses of the same shape. *A,* A glass lens. *B,* A fish lens. The variation in index of refraction is responsible for the elimination of spherical aberration in the fish lens. (From Fernald RD, Wright SE. Nature. 1983;301:618–20.)

increase of blue light absorption with age results in subtly decreased color discrimination, as well as decreased chromatic aberration.

The variation in index of refraction of the crystalline lens (higher index in the nucleus, lower index in the cortex) is responsible for neutralization of a good part of the spherical aberration caused by the human cornea. Figure 9-1 shows how this variation of index of refraction in the spherical fish lens almost eliminates its spherical aberration when compared with a spherical glass lens.[12]

Ocular Aberrations

CHROMATIC ABERRATION. Because the index of refraction of the ocular components of the eye varies with wavelength, colored objects located at the same distance from the eye are imaged at different distances with respect to the retina. This phenomenon is called axial chromatic aberration. In the human eye the magnitude of chromatic aberration is approximately 3D.[13] However significant colored fringes around objects generally are not seen because of the preferential spectral sensitivity of human photoreceptors. Studies have shown that humans are many times more sensitive to yellow-green light with a central wavelength at 560nm than to red or blue light.[5]

SPHERICAL ABERRATION. The variation of refractive power with pupil diameter, which causes light rays to focus at different distances from the retinal plane, is called spherical aberration. The eye's spherical aberration, in addition to depending on pupil diameter, depends on individual corneal contour, accommodative state, and the age of the lens.[14] For a normal photopic eye, spherical aberration may vary from approximately 0.25D to almost 2D.[5]

COMA. A comet-like tail or directional flare appearing in the retinal image, when a point source is viewed, is a manifestation of another aberration called coma. Because the eye is a somewhat nonaxial imaging device, and because the cornea and lens are not perfectly centered with respect to the pupil, coma generally is present in all human eyes.[15]

HIGHER ORDER ABERRATIONS. The eye's aberrations of even higher order than the so-called *primary aberrations,* which include astigmatism, spherical aberration, and coma, are now being measured with wave front sensors, and the data are being used to control photorefractive surgical lasers with the hope of achieving aberration-corrected vision.[16]

LIGHT SCATTERING. Another significant optical factor that degrades vision is intraocular light scatter. The mechanism of light scatter is different from the aberrations discussed above, each of which deviates the direction of light rays coming from points in object space to predictable and definite directions in image space. With light scattering, incoming light rays are deflected from their initial (i.e., prescattered) direction into random (postscattered) directions, which generally lie somewhere within a cone angle of approximately a degree or so. Therefore a dioptric value cannot be placed on the blur caused by light scatter. A glaring light worsens the effect of light scatter on vision. Thus a young, healthy tennis player may not see the ball when it is nearly in line with the Sun. Light scattering is the mechanism associated with most cataracts and causes significant degradation of vision due to image blur, loss of contrast sensitivity, and veiling glare.

Retinal Factors

An image may be considered as made up of an array of point-like regions. When a picture on the video screen is viewed with a magnifying glass, these small regions, called *pixels,* are seen clearly. Similarly, the elements that form a photographic image are the silver halide grains in the film's emulsion. Likewise, the pixel elements comprising a retinal image are the cone and rod photoreceptors. It is the finite size of these photoreceptors that ultimately determines the eye's ability to resolve fine details.

The finest details in a retinal image can be resolved only within the foveal macular area. This area is an elliptical zone of about 1.5mm in maximal width,[17] having an angular size of approximately 0.3 degrees about the eye's visual axis. It contains over 2000 tightly packed light-sensitive cones. The cones themselves have diameters of 1–2μm (a dimension comparable to 3–4 wavelengths of green light) and are separated by about 0.5μm.[18] Cone size is an important factor in determining the ultimate resolution of the human eye (Fig. 9-2). In much of the fovea no nerve fiber layer, ganglion cell layer, inner plexiform layer, or inner nuclear layer is present, and in the very center of the fovea no outer nuclear layer is present. Only the outer plexiform and cones exist.

Another important aspect of the cone receptors is their orientation. Each cone functions as a "light pipe" or a fiber optic, which is directed to the second nodal point of the eye (Fig. 9-3). This orientation optimally receives the light that forms an image and partially prevents this light from being scattered to neighboring cones.[19]

Another retinal factor that helps to improve vision is the configuration of the foveal pit, which is a small concavity in the retina. This recessed shape acts as an antiglare device in which the walls of the depression prevent stray light, within the internal globe of the eye, from striking the cones at the center of the depression. Finally, the yellow macular pigment may be considered to act as a blue filter that limits chromatic aberration and also absorbs scattered light, which is predominantly of shorter wavelength (i.e., the blue end of the spectrum).

Resolution and Focal Length Factors

A derivation of the theoretical diffraction-limited resolution of a normal emmetropic human eye must consider the eye's optimal pupil diameter, its focal length, which is associated with its axial length, and the anatomical size of the photoreceptors. A point object imaged by a diffraction-limited optical system has an an-

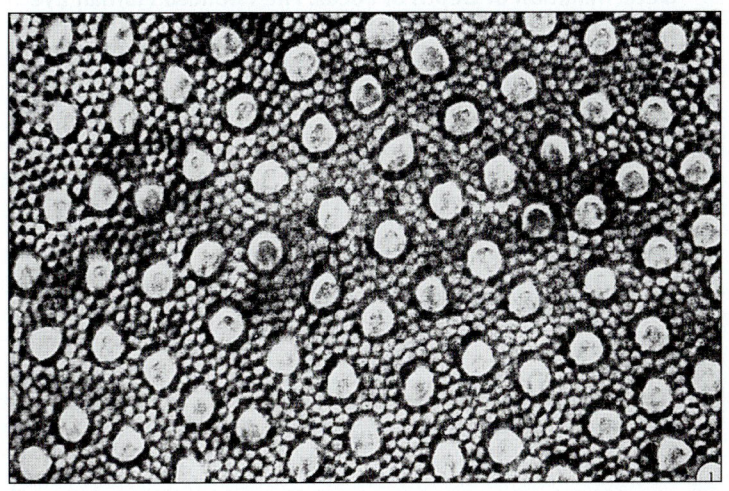

FIG. 9-2 ▌ **Retinal mosaic (rhesus monkey) in an area adjacent to the fovea.** The large circles are rods and the clusters of small circles are cones. This section gives a perspective of the different receptor sizes. (From Wassle H, Reiman HJ. The mosaic of nerve cells in mammalian retina. Proc R Soc Lond B. 1978;200:441–61.)

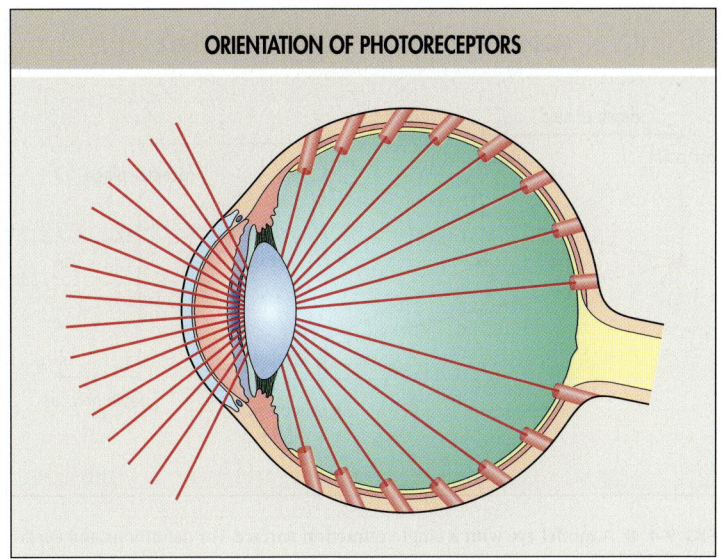

ORIENTATION OF PHOTORECEPTORS

FIG. 9-3 ▌ **Orientation of the photoreceptors.** They all point toward the second nodal point of the eye.

gular diameter in radians (diameter at one half the peak intensity of the Airy disc) given by equation (9-1).

Equation 9-1 $\text{Angular diameter} = \dfrac{1.22 \ (\text{wavelength})}{\text{pupil diameter}}$

In equation (9-1), let pupil diameter be 2.4mm which, for a normal eye, is the largest pupil diameter for which spherical aberration is insignificant, and let the wavelength be 0.00056mm (yellow-green light) to find the diffraction-limited angular diameter = 0.00028 radians (or, equivalently, 0.98 minutes of arc). Note that this angular diameter matches the angular resolution of an eye with 20/20 Snellen acuity, because the black-on-white bands of the letter E on the 20/20 line of the Snellen chart are spaced 1 minute of arc apart.

The spatial diameter in millimeters of the diffraction-limited Airy disc on the retina is found by multiplying the angular diameter, given by equation (9-1), by the effective focal length of the eye.

Equation 9-2 $\text{Spatial diameter} = (\text{angular diameter}) \times (\text{effective focal length})$

Using the angular diameter found from equation (9-1) and a value of 17mm for the eye's effective focal length (i.e., second nodal point to retina distance) in equation (9-2) results in the diffraction-limited spatial diameter = 0.0048mm (i.e., 4.8μm).

It is interesting to use our results to make a comparison with Kirschfield's estimate that about five receptors are needed to scan the Airy disc in order to obtain the maximal visual information available.[20] If we assume that the foveal cones are approximately 1.5μm in diameter and are separated by about a 0.5μm of space, then the distance between neighboring cones is 2.0m. We estimate the number of receptors covered by the Airy disc by calculating in equation (9-3) the ratio of the area of the Airy disc to the area occupied by a single cone.

Equation 9-3 $\text{Number of cones covered by Airy disc} = \dfrac{(\text{spatial diameter of Airy disc})^2}{(\text{distance between cones})^2}$

Using equation (9-3) we find that approximately six receptors are covered by the Airy disc in close accord with Kirschfield's estimate of five. Thus given an eye with maximal sensitivity to yellow light and an optimal pupil size of 2.4mm, we find that the human eye's 17mm effective focal length and, correspondingly, its 24mm axial length are properly sized to achieve optimal res-

olution for the cone sizes present. The higher resolution of the eagle's eye compared with the human's eye probably results from a larger pupil size-to-focal–length ratio, cones of smaller diameter, and a clearer cornea and lens.[2]

Depth of Focus

An optical system with a fairly large depth of focus enables a fixed-focus camera to give sharp pictures of both a mountain in the distance and a subject 6ft (1.8m) away, an insect or a small animal to see objects clearly from 30ft (9m) to 4 inches (10cm) away with no accommodation mechanism, and a presbyopic patient to read a newspaper through a pinhole with no reading correction. Depth of focus of an imaging system is defined to be the distance range (usually in millimeters) from the best-focused image distance where the resolution does not change or, equivalently, the blur caused by defocusing goes unnoticed. Depth of focus also can be expressed in diopters when the dioptric equivalent is the additional power needed for an optical system to change its focal length by an amount equal to the depth of focus. Depth of field, which is related to but different from depth of focus, is defined as the distance range that an object may move (toward or away from a fixed-focus optical system) and still be considered in focus.

In Figure 9-4, the eye is represented in a simplified form with only one refractive element. We define the following symbols.

O = The object which can move from infinity to a near point
p = Pupillary diameter
f = Focal length of the model eye
x = Distance from the retina where the object at the near point comes to focus
c = Photoreceptor size determining the eye's ultimate resolution
n = Refractive index of the model eye
$D_1 = n/f$, which is the dioptric power of the eye when an object is viewed at infinity
$D_2 = n/(f + x)$, which is the dioptric power of the eye when an object is viewed at the near point

The depth of focus may be expressed by equation (9-4).

Equation 9-4 $D_1 - D_2 = \dfrac{n}{f} - \dfrac{n}{f + x} = \dfrac{nx}{f(f + x)}$

Equation (9-5) is obtained by the method of similar triangles shown in Figure 9-4.

Equation 9-5 $\dfrac{c}{p} = \dfrac{x}{f + x}$

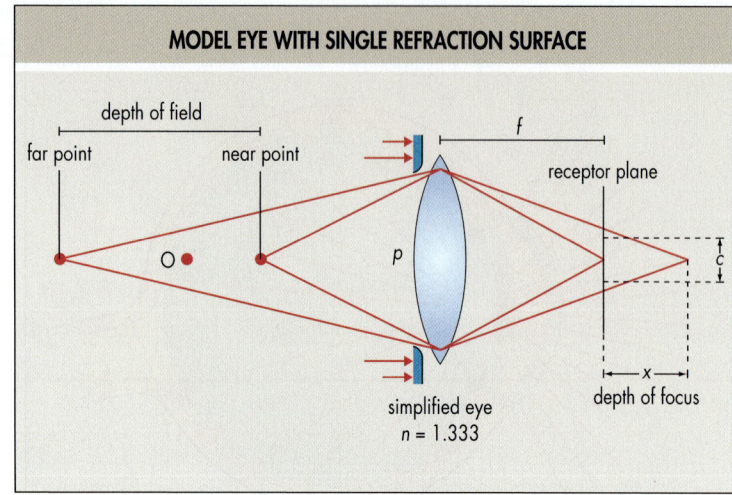

MODEL EYE WITH SINGLE REFRACTION SURFACE

depth of field

far point   near point

f

receptor plane

O •

p

depth of focus

x

c

simplified eye
n = 1.333

FIG. 9-4 ■ **A model eye with a single refraction surface.** For definitions and explanation, see text.

Substitution of equation (9-5) in equation (9-4) results in equation (9-6).

Equation 9-6
$$D_1 - D_2 = \frac{nc}{fp}$$

Equation (9-6) shows that the depth of focus ($D_1 - D_2$), in diopters, is proportional to the product of the index of refraction (n) and the limiting photoreceptor or grain size (c), and inversely proportional to the product of the focal length of the system (f) and the pupil size (p). Therefore a small pupillary aperture brings objects at a wide range of distances from the lens into focus. Associated with the smaller pupillary size may be a larger blur spot due to diffraction. However if the blur spot is no larger than the size of the receptor, the blur will be unnoticed. Examples based on equation (9-6) are shown in Box 9-1.

The examples of Box 9-1 use the reduced eye, where $f = 22.2$mm and $n = 1.33$. In the more accurate human schematic eye of Gullstrand, $f = 17$mm and $n > 1.33$, because the different indices of refraction of the cornea, aqueous, lens, and vitreous are taken into account. For comparison, a clinically orientated study of humans showed that pupils of diameter 1–2mm produced a mean depth of focus >4D.[21-23] The image-enhancing mechanism in the retina and brain may have helped to increase the subjects' perceived depth of focus in the clinical studies cited when compared with our calculated results found in Box 9-1.

The example in Box 9-2 shows that, even without a mammalian accommodation system, the fly theoretically can see objects from infinity to within <1mm. Of course, this theoretical range does not account for the degradation effect of diffraction on fine details. However, it may be assumed that the fly is most interested in large objects.

Depth of focus and visual acuity are quite different among the species. For example, although a human and a falcon[25] have a comparable depth of focus, the falcon has a much better acuity than that of humans. On the other hand the bat's eye, compared with those of the human and falcon, has a relatively large depth of focus of about 10D and relatively poor visual acuity.[26] As noted in equation (9-6), a larger retinal grain size implies larger depth of focus. However, it also implies reduced resolution.

PINHOLE OPTICS

Figure 9-5 shows an out-of-focus eye viewing a distant point source of light and how reducing pupil size with a pinhole (or a stenopeic slit) diminishes the size of the blurred retinal image. The diagram illustrates how a small aperture placed in front of the pupil of an out-of-focus eye (e.g., myopic or hyperopic) can improve visual acuity. The pinhole not only helps to reduce focus error and increase depth of focus, it also helps to correct both regu-

---

BOX 9-1

Determination of Depth of Focus. The Reduced Human Eye Model with One Refracting Surface

EXAMPLE 1
Conditions:
$p = 3$mm
$f = 22.2$mm (for reduced eye model with one refracting surface)
c = three cones (assume each cone is 1.5 μm in diameter and spacing between cones is 0.5 μm); the total cluster of three cones = 4.5 μm + 2 spaces = 5.5 μm
$n = 1.333$

Calculation of depth of focus:

Equation 9-7 $D_1 - D_2 = \dfrac{1.33 \times 0.0000055}{0.0222 \times 0.003} = 0.11D$

This figure falls within the experimental literature, which shows a range of depth of foci in human subjects from +0.04D to +0.47D.[23]

EXAMPLE 2
Conditions:
Example 1 is calculated for a resolution system of 1 minute of arc or the equivalent of 20/20 (6/6) visual acuity, and a high level of contrast. If the system's limit is 20/40 (6/12), the angle of resolution may be doubled to 2 minutes, which covers six cones or 11μm. Assume the eye has a 2mm pupil.

Calculation of depth of focus:

Equation 9-8 $D_1 - D_2 = \dfrac{1.33 \times 0.000011}{0.0222 \times 0.002} = 0.33D$

EXAMPLE 3
Conditions:
The system in Example 2 [i.e., 20/40 (6/12) resolution], but using a 1mm pinhole.

Equation 9-9 $D_1 - D_2 = \dfrac{1.33 \times 0.000011}{0.0222 \times 0.001} = 0.66D$

BOX 9-2

Calculation to Show the Depth of Focus for the Fly's Eye

In the compound eye of the fly the organization is based on ommatidia with separate groups of receptors (about eight) under each lens.[24]

Conditions:
$p = 26$μm
$f = 50$μm
$c = 2$μm
$n = 1.365$

Calculation of depth of focus:

Equation 9-10 $D_1 - D_2 = \dfrac{1.365 \times 0.000002}{0.00005 \times 0.000026} = 2100D$

---

lar and irregular astigmatism, as well as other higher order optical aberrations. Disadvantages of using a small-aperture system are increased diffraction blur and decreased retinal illuminance. For example, the diffraction blur caused by a 0.5mm pinhole will reduce noticeably the visual acuity of someone who tests normally as having 20/20 vision. Also, if a small aperture is used with a camera in order to take pictures indoors that have a large depth of field, bright lights will be needed to illuminate the scene.

On the other hand, a small-aperture lens can efficiently deliver good illuminance provided the lens has a correspondingly short focal length. The key parameter that governs the efficiency of illumination of an imaging system, as well as its theoretical optical resolution, is the size of the cone angle of the light from a point object which comes through the aperture and converges onto a point in the image plane. The term *numerical aperture*, or NA, which is used commonly to describe microscope objectives, is a measure of this cone angle. An alternate parameter (equivalent to

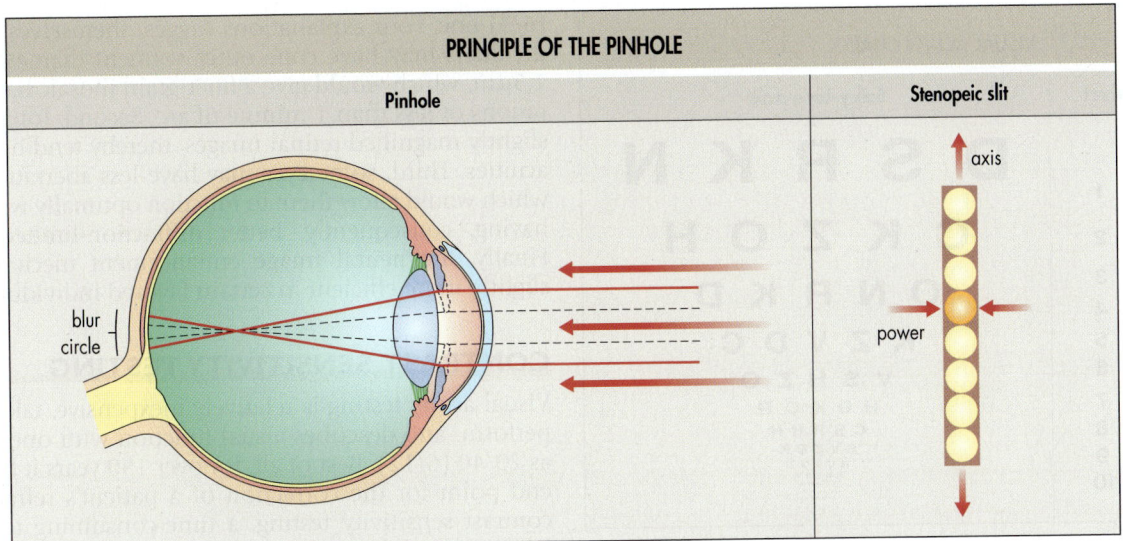

PRINCIPLE OF THE PINHOLE

| Pinhole | Stenopeic slit |

blur circle

axis

power

FIG. 9-5 ▌ **The principle of the pinhole.** A narrower pupillary aperture decreases the angle of the cone of light that produces the blur circle. Ultimately the blur circle, albeit dimmer, is the size of the limiting cluster of photoreceptors (i.e., pixel-size or grain-size equivalent). A stenopeic slit may be considered as a line of pinholes.

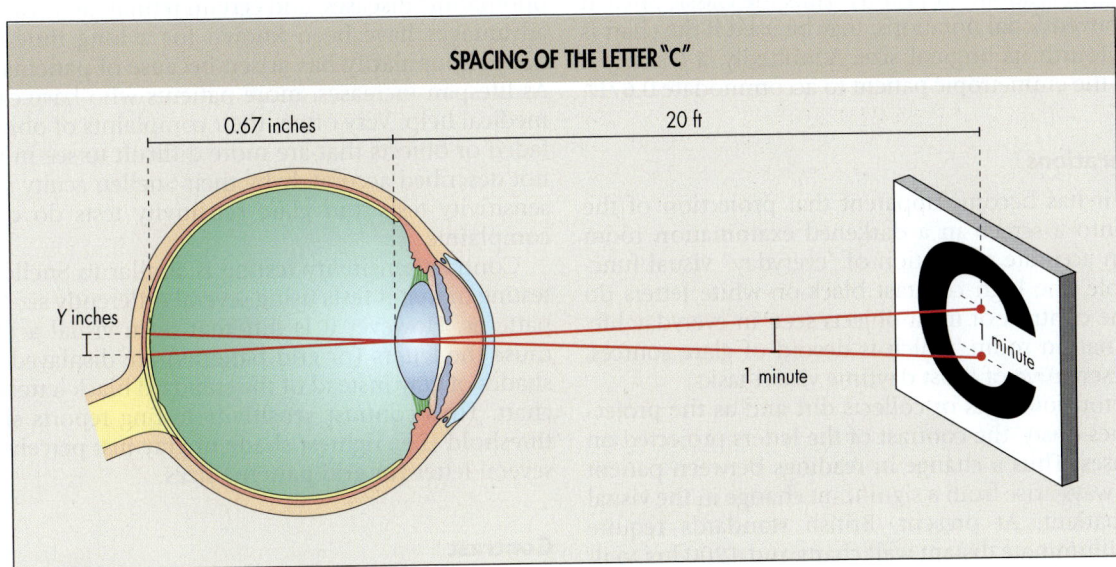

SPACING OF THE LETTER "C"

0.67 inches   20 ft

Y inches

1 minute

1 minute

FIG. 9-6 ▌ **Spacing of gap in the letter C.** This letter is used to determine the minimal separable spacing or resolution of the eye at the retina. The gap in the letter C subtending 1 minute, when imaged on the retina, has a dimension (Y) representing the resolution of the eye where tan (1 minute) = Y/0.67 (with Y in inches); therefore Y = 0.00019 inches (or 4.8m). The overall size of the letter is X = 0.349 inches, and the gap dimension is 0.070 inches (see text).

the cone angle), which is used commonly to describe photographic lenses, is the "speed" or "f-number" of the lens. The f-number is the ratio of the lens's focal length to its entrance aperture diameter. For example, an f/8 lens has a focal length that is 8 times greater than its aperture diameter. Note that the f-number may be the same for a hawk's eye as for the facet of an insect's eye.

VISUAL ACUITY TESTING

The idea that the minimal separation between two point sources of light was a measure of vision dates back to Hooke in 1679, when he noted, "'tis hardly possible for any animal eye well to distinguish an angle much smaller than that of a minute: and where two objects are not farther distant than a minute, if they are bright objects, they coalesce and appear as one."[27] In the early nineteenth century, Purkinje and Young used letters of various sizes for "judging the extent of the power of distinguishing objects too near or too remote for perfect vision." Finally, in 1863, Professor Hermann Snellen of Utrecht developed his classic test letters. He quantitated the lines by comparison of the visual acuity of a patient with that of his as-

sistant who had perfect vision. Thus 20/200 (6/60) vision meant that the patient could see at 20ft (6m) what Snellen's assistant could see at 200ft (60m).[28]

The essence of correct identification of the letters on the Snellen chart is to see the clear spaces between the black elements of the letter. Thus in Figure 9-6, the angular spacing between the bars of the C is 1 minute for the 20/20 (6/6) letter. The entire letter has an angular height of 5 minutes. To calculate the height, x, of a 20/20 (6/6) letter use equation (9-11).

Equation 9-11 $\tan (5 \text{ minutes}) = \dfrac{x \text{ feet}}{20}$

From equation (9-11), x = 0.0291 feet (0.349 inches). In like manner, the 20/200 (6/60) letter is 10 times taller, or 3.49 inches (8.87 cm) high.

Testing Distance

The Snellen acuity test traditionally is done at a distance of 20ft (6m). At this distance very little accommodation is required by the patient. For hospital patients, testing must often be carried

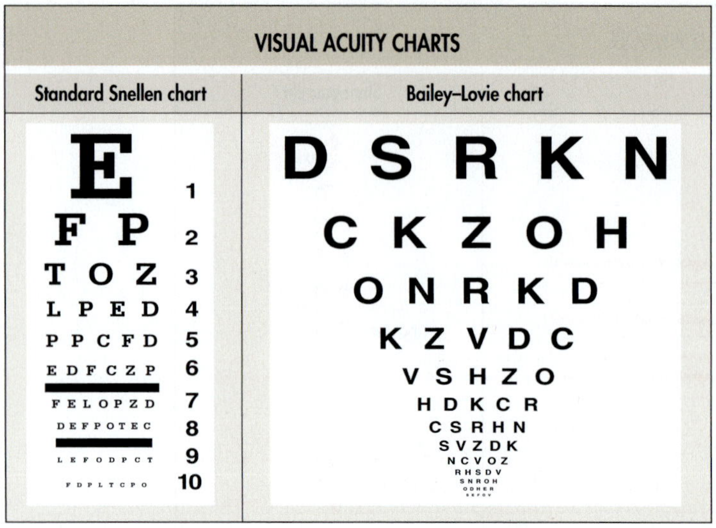

VISUAL ACUITY CHARTS

Standard Snellen chart	Bailey–Lovie chart

FIG. 9-7 ▪ **Visual acuity charts.** Standard Snellen and Bailey–Lovie charts.

out in a smaller room. If the doctor stands at the foot of the bed and the patient sits, propped up at the head of the bed, the distance between them is about 5ft (1.5m). Thus the classic Snellen chart, with its conventional notations, may be used if the chart is reduced to one fourth its original size. Admittedly, a test at 5ft (1.5m) requires the emmetropic patient to accommodate 0.67D.

Other Considerations

Over the years it has become apparent that projection of the Snellen chart onto a screen in a darkened examination room does not give an accurate replication of "everyday" visual function. For example, the high contrast black-on-white letters do not represent the contrast of most objects seen in everyday life. The dark examination room, which is devoid of glare sources, also is not representative of most daytime visual tasks.

As the projector bulb ages or collects dirt and as the projection lens becomes dusty, the contrast of the letters projected on the chart decreases. Thus a change in readings between patient visits may not always arise from a significant change in the visual status of the patient. At present, British standards require 480–600 lux to illuminate distant wall charts and 1200 lux to illuminate projected charts.[5]

As the letters become smaller on the Snellen chart, the number of letters per line increases. Thus one error per line means a different score for each line. It, therefore, is necessary to establish criteria by which it can be agreed that a patient has seen the line. Some clinicians credit a patient if more than one half the letters are identified correctly. Others require identification of all the letters before credit is given. Also remember that no orderly progression of size change exists from line to line. Thus a two-line change on the Snellen chart going from the 20/200 (6/60) line to the 20/80 (6/24) represents an improvement of visual acuity by a factor of 2.5, whereas a two-line change going from the 20/30 (6/9) line to the 20/20 (6/6) line represents an improvement by only a factor of 1.5.

Another problem is that the identification of different letters of the same size has been shown to vary in difficulty. Thus A and L are easier to identify than E. The Bailey–Lovie chart (Fig. 9-7), designed by two Australian optometrists[29] and modified by Ferris et al.[30] in 1982, uses 10 letters of similar difficulty with 5 different letters per line and has uniform size change between neighboring lines. Another approach is to use the Landolt ring test in which circles, each with an open gap, of decreasing size are used in successive lines, with the orientation of the gaps in the circles randomly changing.

The 20/20 (6/6) Snellen line represents the ability to see 1 minute of arc, which is close to the theoretical diffraction limit, but the occasional patient can see the 20/15 (6/4.5) or 20/10

(6/3) line. Four explanations suggest themselves. First, some individuals may have cone outer segment diameters of less than 1.5μm, which would give a finer-grain mosaic having cone separations of less than 1 minute of arc. Second, longer eyes provide slightly magnified retinal images, thereby tending to yield better acuities. Third, some eyes may have less aberration than others, which would allow them to function optimally with larger pupils having, consequently, better diffraction-limited performance. Finally, the neural image enhancement mechanisms may be slightly more efficient in certain favored individuals.

CONTRAST SENSITIVITY TESTING

Visual acuity testing is relatively inexpensive, takes little time to perform, and describes visual function with one notation, such as 20/40 (6/12). Best of all, for over 150 years it has provided an end point for the correction of a patient's refractive error. Yet contrast sensitivity testing, a time-consuming test born in the laboratory of the visual physiologist and described by a graph rather than a simple notation, recently has become a popular clinical test. It describes a number of subtle levels of vision not accounted for by the visual acuity test; thus it more accurately quantifies the loss of vision in cataracts, corneal edema, neuro-ophthalmic diseases, and certain retinal diseases. Although these advantages have been known for a long time, the recent enhanced popularity has arisen because of patients with cataracts. As lifespan increases, more patients who have cataracts request medical help. Very often, their complaints of objects that appear faded or objects that are more difficult to see in bright light are not described accurately by their Snellen acuity scores. Contrast sensitivity tests and glare sensitivity tests do quantitate these complaints.

Contrast sensitivity testing is similar to Snellen visual acuity testing in that it tests using several differently sized letters or grid patterns. However it is different from visual acuity testing, because the letters (or grid patterns) are displayed in six or more shades of gray instead of the standard black letters of the Snellen chart. Thus contrast sensitivity testing reports show a contrast threshold (i.e., lightest shade of gray just perceived) for each of several letter (or grid pattern) sizes.

Contrast

The components of a conventional newspaper photo consist of various regions associated with the scene where each region is filled in with a definite density of black dots depicting that region's contrast or level of gray. Such newspaper photos may have over 100 half-tone levels (i.e., densities of black dots) to represent the different contrast levels in the scene. A video engineer will describe the ability of an electronic display device to faithfully depict contrast levels by citing the display's gray-scale resolution. For example, a video monitor may be said to have 8-bit gray-scale resolution, which means that $2^8 = 256$ different levels of gray (ranging from white to black) can fill in the various regions that make up a picture on the monitor's screen.

Whereas a black letter on a white background is a scene of high contrast, a child crossing the road at dusk and a car looming in a fog are scenes of low contrast. The contrast of a target on a background is defined by equation (9-12).

Equation 9-12 $$\text{contrast} = \frac{\text{target luminance} - \text{background luminance}}{\text{target luminance} + \text{background luminance}}$$

As an example, suppose a photometer measures the luminance of a target at 100 units of light and the luminance of the background at 50 units of light. Substitution into equation (9-12) gives equation (9-13).

Equation 9-13 $$\text{contrast} = \frac{100 - 50}{100 + 50} = 0.33 \text{ (or 33\%)}$$

Contrast Sensitivity

Suppose the contrast of a target of a certain size is 0.33, which also may represent a particular older patient's threshold, which means that this patient cannot detect similar sized targets of lower contrast. The older patient's contrast sensitivity (CS) is the reciprocal of the contrast, namely CS = 3.0. On the other hand, a young, healthy subject viewing a target of the same size may have a contrast threshold of 0.01 with a corresponding CS = 100. Occasionally subjects (for certain size targets) have even better contrast thresholds. A subject could have a contrast threshold of 0.003, which converts into a CS of 333. In the visual psychology literature, CS often is described in logarithmic terms. For example, associated with CS = 10 is log(CS) = 1, with CS = 100 is log(CS) = 2, and with CS = 1000 is log(CS) = 3, and so on.

Targets

Both the visual scientist and the optical engineer use a series of alternating black and white bars as targets. The optical engineer describes the fineness of a target by the number of line pairs per millimeter (a line pair consists of a dark bar with a white space next to it). The higher the number of line pairs per millimeter, the finer is the target. For example, about 82 line pairs per millimeter imaged on the retina of an eye with a focal length of 21 mm is equivalent to a periodic black-white target in object space, where the white space between two black spaces subtends approximately a minute of arc (like the letter E of the Snellen chart viewed at 20 feet). Equivalently, with a Snellen chart viewed at 20 feet, 109 line pairs per millimeter on the retina is equivalent to the 20/15 (6/4.5) letters.

The visual scientist generally describes a periodic bar pattern in terms of its spatial frequency as perceived at the test distance—the units are cycles per degree (cpd). A cycle is a black bar and a white space. To convert Snellen units into cpd at the 20 ft (6 m) testing distance, the Snellen denominator is divided into 600 (180). For example, 20/20 (6/6) converts into 30 cpd. Likewise, 20/200 (6/60) converts into 3 cpd.

Sine Waves

So far, targets have been described as high-contrast dark bars of different spatial frequency against a white background. These also are known as square waves or Foucault gratings. However, in optics very few images can be described as perfect square waves with perfectly sharp edges. Diffraction tends to make most edges slightly fuzzy, as do spherical aberration and oblique astigmatism, particularly in the case of the optics of the eye. If the light intensity is plotted across a strongly blurred image of a Foucault grating, a sine wave pattern results. Sine wave patterns have great appeal, because they can be considered the essential elements from which any pattern can be constructed. The mathematician can break down any alternating pattern, be it an electrocardiogram or a trumpet's sound wave, into a unique sum of sine waves. This mathematical decomposition of patterns into sinusoidal components is known as a Fourier transformation. Joseph Fourier, a French mathematician, initially developed this waveform language to describe sound waves and vibrations. Fourier's theorem describes the way that any pattern may be written as a sum of sine waves that have various spatial frequencies, amplitudes, and phases.

Also, it is thought that the visual system of the brain may operate by breaking down observed patterns and scenes into sine waves of different frequencies. The brain then adds them up again to produce the mental impression of a complete picture. Fourier transformations may be the method the visual system uses to encode and record retinal images. It has been shown that different cells or "channels" occur in the retina, lateral geniculate body, and cortex that selectively carry different spatial frequencies.[31] So far, 6–8 channels have been identified. It also has been shown that all channels respond to contrast—the cortex shows a

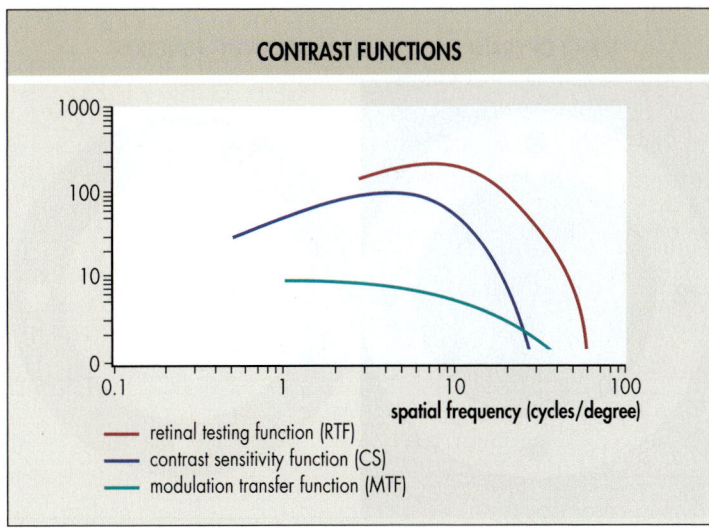

FIG. 9-8 ▓ **Contrast functions.** The human eye's contrast sensitivity (CS) function is the product of the contrast transfer function of the purely optical contribution, called the modulation transfer function (MTF), and the contrast sensitivity function of the purely neuroretinal contribution, called the retinal testing function (RTF). The MTF is magnified 10× in the graph. (Redrawn from Mainster MA. Contemporary optics and ocular pathology. Surv Ophthalmol. 1978;23:135–42.)

linear relationship between the amplitude of the neuronal discharge and the logarithm of the grating contrast. Consequently many contrast sensitivity tests are based on sine wave patterns rather than square wave patterns.

RECORDING CONTRAST SENSITIVITY

Figure 9-8 shows a number of functions, including the contrast sensitivity testing function for a normal subject. The shape of the human eye's contrast sensitivity function is different from that of inanimate optical imaging systems in which the function generally decreases continuously from very low to very high spatial frequencies. For the normal human eye, the contrast sensitivity generally increases from very low frequencies to about 6 cpd and then decreases with increasing frequency beyond 6 cpd. The decrease of the contrast sensitivity with frequency above 6 cpd is due to the influence of diffraction and aberrations, which make the detection of finer details more difficult. The increase of the contrast sensitivity with frequency up to 6 cpd is due to the retina–brain processing system, which is programmed to enhance our contrast sensitivity in the range of 2–6 cpd. Receptor fields, on-off systems, and lateral inhibition are the well-known physiological mechanisms that influence the different spatial frequency channels and are responsible for such enhancement. In Figure 9-8, the plot labeled retinal testing function (RTF) represents the retinal–neural system's contrast sensitivity performance.[32,34,35] A striking proof of brain enhancement of contrast is given in Figure 9-9.

Also shown in Figure 9-8 is the plot labeled modulation transfer function (MTF), which represents the sinusoidal components of the object-to-image transfer function for the purely optical portion of the visual system (cornea, lens).[33] The MTF is described more completely in the following section. There is a significant mathematical relationship among the three functions, which is expressed by equation (9-14), the so-called *Campbell–Green relation*,[33] and is illustrated in Figure 9-8. The Campbell–Green relation has been demonstrated in clinical studies.[36]

Equation 9-14   CS = RTF × MTF for all frequencies

Differences in the contrast sensitivity function are expected among different subject groups. For example, contrast sensitivity decreases with age, for which two factors appear to be responsible. First, the normal crystalline lens scatters more light with increasing age,[9] which thus blurs the edges of targets and degrades the contrast. Second, the retina–brain processing system, itself, loses its ability to enhance contrast with increasing age.

EFFECT OF BRAIN'S CONTRAST ENHANCEMENT FUNCTION

FIG. 9-9 ▌ Effect of brain's contrast enhancement function. One gray circle is seen against a black background and one against a white background. The brain's contrast enhancement function makes the gray look lighter against the dark background and darker against the light background.

The contrast sensitivity function also is an accurate method by which to follow certain disease states. For example, the contrast sensitivity function of a patient who has a cataract is diminished, as it is in another light-scattering lesion, corneal edema. Because the contrast sensitivity function is dependent on central nervous system processing, it is not surprising that conditions such as optic neuritis and pituitary tumors also characteristically have diminished contrast sensitivity functions.

The contrast sensitivity of patients also decreases as the illumination decreases.[37] Thus contrast sensitivity for a spatial frequency of 3cpd typically drops from 300 to 150 to 10 as the retinal luminance drops from 9 trolands to 0.09 trolands to 0.0009 trolands. (The troland is a psychophysical unit. One troland is the retinal luminance produced by the image of an object, the luminance of which is 1 lumen/m^2 [1 lux] for an area of the entrance pupil of 1mm^2.) Therefore when doing careful contrast sensitivity function comparisons, the illuminance of the test targets must be kept at the recommended value.

MODULATION TRANSFER FUNCTION TESTING

Optical engineers generally evaluate optical systems by the MTF test method, which is somewhat akin to contrast sensitivity testing. One MTF test method measures the image contrast of sinusoidal grating (or periodic bar) targets of known contrast over a range of spatial frequencies. The MTF is the ratio of image contrast to object contrast as a function of spatial frequency. In MTF graphs the MTF values are plotted along the vertical axis, and the spatial frequencies (e.g., cpd) are plotted along the horizontal axis. MTF values (vertical axis) generally decrease from 1.0 to 0 as spatial frequencies (horizontal axis) increase. The MTF evaluates only the optical image–forming capability of the human eye and not its retinal–neural capability.

Another and faster way to measure the MTF of the human eye uses a computerized instrument that quickly performs a Fourier transformation on the blurred retinal image of a fine point or line target and, thereby, obtains the amplitudes of the spatial frequency components.[38] The MTF is obtained simply by squaring these amplitudes. Campbell and Green determined the MTF of the normal human eye for various pupillary diameters and found that the largest (best) MTF functions were for pupil diameters in the range from 2.0–2.8mm.[33] Smaller pupil diameters produced the deleterious effects of increased diffraction, whereas larger pupil diameters showed the degrading effects of increased spherical and other aberrations.

MTF testing is conceptually similar to the methods used by electronic engineers when they evaluate audio amplifiers. The performance of an amplifier is evaluated by measurements of the output-to-input voltage ratio, or gain, for different sound frequencies. With optical systems the MTF gives more detailed information about the system's imaging capability than does a single-parameter value for optical resolution (e.g., imaged spot diameter). For example, two systems may have the same optical resolution but one, which has smaller MTF values at high frequencies, might be unable to form useful images of low-contrast fine objects whereas the other, which has larger MTF values at high frequencies, can form useful images of the same objects.

WAVE FRONT TESTING

Fast and precise methods for measuring the higher order aberrations of the eye are available due to the development of the Hartmann–Shack wave front sensor modified for ophthalmic use.[39] These devices project a narrow beam of light into the eye, which is imaged on the retina as a point source. Light scattered back from the point source leaves the eye at the pupillary plane as a wave front. The wave front is then imaged onto an square array of small lenses, which are spaced typically about 0.5mm apart. Each microlens in the array focuses a small region of the wave front as a spot on the image plane of a charge-coupled device (CCD) camera that is connected to a computer. The entire collection of focused spots forms a more-or-less regular pattern on the imager—the deviations of the pattern from perfect regularity actually are the manifestation of the aberrations. Analysis of the pattern of spots gives the emerging light rays' directions (i.e., wave front slope) as a function of the x and y coordinates in the pupillary plane. These data allow the actual wave front to be reconstructed mathematically. The wave front generally is represented in final form as a series of Zernike polynomials in which the coefficients represent the strengths of the various aberrations. Wave front information for an eye provides a basis to design and fabricate custom surfaces on corneal tissue[16] and on contact lenses.[40] These techniques hold the promise of providing aberration-corrected vision.

RETINA–BRAIN IMAGE PROCESSING

As discussed above, retina–brain systems may improve the contrast of the optical image placed on the retina. The different visual parameters in which retina–brain processing enhances the optical image are reviewed here. An anatomical basis exists for retina–brain image processing, because it has been shown that more than three ganglion cells are connected to each foveal cone. These ganglion cells probably amplify, enhance, and otherwise process the signals initially generated by the foveal cones.[41]

Vernier Acuity

The ability to line up three dots, or to align two lines into a single straight line, or to perceive a kink (discontinuity) in a straight line is known as vernier acuity. Optically speaking, the angular subtense of the smallest measurable opening is measured as two overlapping lines are slowly displaced from each other. Threshold values of less than 20 seconds of arc are obtained, which are far lower than the diffraction limit of resolution of the human eye. The only explanation is to credit the retina–brain system with being able to decipher this information. It is not clear whether this depends on the configuration of the retinal mosaic, the constantly changing information recorded by the normal micronystagmus of the eye, cortical processing, or all three factors. The famous Danish astronomer, Tycho Brahe, accurately plotted the orbits of many planets using only a protractor alignment device and his naked eye. Although he used no telescope, his readings were so accurate that his assistant Kepler was able to show that the orbits were elliptical, not circular. These calculations suggested that the Earth rotated around the Sun rather than the other way around.[42] To Newton the elliptical path of the planetary orbits suggested that the force of gravity (the apple experiment) also functioned in space. It could be said, therefore, that the precision of the vernier acuity of humans aided an early insight into the basics of astrophysics.

Fast-Moving Objects

In Stein and Slatt's book, *Hitting Blind,* one illustration shows four professional tennis players hitting the ball while looking somewhere else.[43] The implied message is that the speed of the ball is faster than the eye–motor system. Thus they cannot watch the ball until it arrives and then proceed with the appropriate motor response; consequently, the appropriate motor response must start well before the ball arrives. Once the player sees the ball leave his opponent's racquet, a trajectory is computed unconsciously and the appropriate motor response initiated. It is the "mind's eye," not the retinal image, that guides the player's movements.

Flicker

A human being can appreciate a flickering light until the frequency of the flicker exceeds threshold. Motion pictures that present frames at a speed of 48 or more frames per second produce no flicker. The same applies to video, in which the high frequency of alternating current (60 Hertz) abolishes any flicker. In the motion picture example, 48 discrete retinal images are produced each second. However, the retina–brain fuses these images into the perception of a smooth movement.

Dark Adaptation

Although only a portion of the light incident on the eye reaches the photoreceptors (i.e., there is loss from intraocular absorption and scatter), these receptors demonstrate a remarkable sensitivity—they can be triggered by one quanta of visible light. This exquisite sensitivity is dependent on two factors. First is the biological augmentation that follows the photoactivation of one molecule of rhodopsin. Photoactivation of one molecule of rhodopsin starts an impressive example of biological amplification, in which hundreds of molecules of the protein transducin activate a similar number of phosphodiesterase molecules which, in turn, hydrolyze a similar number of cyclic guanosine monophosphate (CGMP) molecules, which then trigger a neural signal to the brain. Second is the organization of rod receptors into large retinal function units when illumination is low. Thus the input from large groups of rods can converge onto a bipolar, and many bipolars can converge onto a ganglion cell, which produces an amplification effect. This is another example of enhancement of a weak optical image by retina–brain circuitry.

Other processes influenced by the retina–brain are stereopsis, Gestalt illusion, increased color contrast, the illusion of movement, and the enhanced ability to see a camouflaged object. The retinal image produced by the eye's dioptrics does not form the total basis of humans' views of the world around them. It is the retina–brain processing (which includes various psychological factors) that ultimately gives humans their perception of the surrounding world.

This concept is summarized by a story about one of the greatest baseball hitters of all time. In a letter to the editor of *Argus,* the monthly newspaper of the American Academy of Ophthalmology, Dr. Gerald Kara writes about examining Babe Ruth.[44] It seems that Ruth was amblyopic in his left eye, never having more than 20/200 (6/60) visual acuity in that eye. His right eye had a visual acuity of 20/15 (6/4.5). If an essentially one-eyed man was the greatest baseball player of all time, then there is certainly more to seeing than ocular dioptrics and basic stereopsis.

REFERENCES

1. Miller D, Benedek GB. Intraocular light scattering. Springfield: CC Thomas; 1973.
2. Miller D. The eye of the eagle. Eur J Implant Refractive Surg. 1991;3:71–3.
3. Reymond L. Spatial visual acuity of the eagle. *Aquila audax*: a behavioral, optical and anatomic investigation. Vision Res. 1985;25:1477–91.
4. Borish IM. Clinical refraction, vol 1, ed 3. Chicago: Professional Press; 1970: 83–114.
5. Bennett AG, Rabetts RB. Clinical visual optics, ed 2. London: Butterworths; 1988.
6. Kaufman SE, ed. IES lighting handbook, ed 4. New York: Illumination Engineering Society; 1966:2–10.
7. Foxell CAP, Stevens WR. Measurement of visual acuity. Br J Ophthalmol. 1955;39:513–33.
8. Campbell FW, Gregory AH. Effect of pupil size on visual acuity. Nature. 1960;208:191–2.
9. Hemenger RP. Intraocular light scatter in normal lens with age. Appl Opt. 1984;23:1972–4.
10. Owsley C, Sekuler R, Siemsen D. Contrast sensitivity throughout adulthood. Vision Res. 1983;23:689–99.
11. Said FS, Weale RA. The variation with age of the spectral transmissivity of the living human crystalline lens. Gerontologia. 1959;3:213–31.
12. Fernald RD. Vision and behavior in an African Cichlid fish. Am Sci. 1984;72:58–65.
13. Wald G, Griffin DR. The change in refractive power of the human eye in dim and bright light. J Opt Soc Am. 1947;37:321–36.
14. Glaser A, Campbell MC. Presbyopia and the optical changes in the human crystalline lens with age. Vision Res. 1998;38:209–29.
15. Iglesias I, Berrio E, Artal P. Estimates of the ocular wave aberration from pairs of double-pass retinal images. J Opt Soc Am A. 1998;15:2466–76.
16. MacRae S, Krueger R, Applegate R. Customized corneal ablation—the quest for SuperVision. Thorofare NJ: Slack; 2001.
17. Wassle H, Reiman HJ. The mosaic of nerve cells in mammalian retina. Proc R Soc Lond B Biol Sci. 1978;200:441–61.
18. Gregory RL. Eye and brain. New York: World University Library McGraw-Hill Book Company; 1973.
19. Enoch JM. Vertebrate rod receptors are directionally sensitive. In: Snyder A, Menzel R, eds. Photoreceptor optics. Berlin: Springer-Verlag; 1975:17–37.
20. Kirschfield K. The resolution of lens and compound eyes. In: Zettler F, Weiler R, eds. Neural principles of vision. Berlin: Springer-Verlag; 1976:354–69.
21. Miller D, Johnson R. Quantification of the pinhole effect. Surv Ophthalmol. 1977;21:347–50.
22. Miller D, Chang L, Miller R, *et al.* A crossed Polaroid pinhole device. Ann Ophthalmol. 1986;18:212–15.
23. Charman WN, Whitefoot H. Pupil diameter and depth of focus of the human eye as measured by laser speckle. Optica Acta. 1977;24:1211–6.
24. Stavenga DG. Refractive index of fly rhabdom. J Comp Physiol. 1974;91:417–26.
25. Reymond L. Spatial visual acuity of the falcon: a behavioral, optical and anatomic investigation. Vision Res. 1987;27:1859–74.
26. Green DG, Power MK, Banks MS. Depth of focus, eye size and visual acuity. Vision Res. 1980;20:827–35.
27. Ronchi L, Fontana A. Laser speckles and the depth of field of the human. Optica Acta. 1975;22:243–6.
28. Levene JR. Clinical refraction and visual science. London: Butterworths; 1977.
29. Bailey IL, Lovie JE. New design principles for visual acuity letter charts. Am J Optom Physiol Opt. 1976;53:740–5.
30. Ferris FL, Kassoff A, Bresnick GH, Wiley IL. New visual acuity charts for clinical research. Am J Ophthalmol. 1982;94:91–6.
31. Maffei L, Fiorentin A. The visual cortex as a spatial frequency analyzer. Vision Res. 1973;13:1255–67.
32. Mainster MA. Contemporary optics and ocular pathology. Surv Ophthalmol. 1978;23:135–42.
33. Campbell FW, Green DG. Optical and retinal factors affecting visual resolution. J Physiol. 1965;181:576–93.
34. Campbell FW, Robson JG. Application of Fourier analysis to the visibility of gratings. J Physiol. 1968;197:551–66.
35. Campbell FW, Gubisch RW. Optical quality of the human eye. J Physiol. 1966;186:558–78.
36. Balaram M, Ragavan A, Tung W, *et al.* Testing the Campbell-Green Equation using MTF and CS data from normal and cataractous eyes. Opt Soc Am Tech Dig Vis Sci Appl. 1998;1:82–5.
37. Van Nes FL, Bouman MA. Spatial modulation transfer in the human eye. J Opt Soc Am. 1967;57:401–6.
38. Magnante P, Fadden B. Instrument for MTF measurements of cataractous eyes. Opt Soc Am Technical Digest on Vision Science and Its Applications. 1997;1:76–9.
39. Liang J, Grimm B, Goelz S, Bille J. Objective measurement of wave aberrations of the human eye with the use of a Hartmann–Shack wave-front sensor. J Opt Soc Am A. 1994;11:1949–57.
40. Magnante P, Coletta N, Moore B. Aberration-correcting contact lenses to improve human vision. Opt Soc Am Tech Dig Vis Sci Appl. 2001;1:94–7.
41. Wassle H, Grunert U, Rohrenbeck J, Boycott BB. Cortical magnification factor and the ganglion cell density of the primate retina. Nature. 1989;341:643–6.
42. Zeilik M. Astronomy: the evolving universe, ed 3. New York: Harper & Row; 1982.
43. Stein H, Slatt B. Hitting blind. Don Mills: Musson Book Company; 1981.
44. Kara GB. Lost vision: Babe Ruth's legend. Argus. 1990;July:6.

Epidemiology of Refractive Errors

DAVID MILLER • CLIFFORD A. SCOTT

DEFINITION
- Presence of various refractive errors within demographic groups.

KEY FEATURES
- Age and emmetropization.
- Genetic predisposition.
- Effects of visual environment.

ASSOCIATED FEATURES
- Current research.
- Interventions.

PREVALENCE

Studies that tabulate the distribution of refractive errors often employed data on young army recruits,[1,2] which show the incidence of myopia to be about 10%. However, this group of healthy young men is not representative of the general population. A study in Sweden is only representative of Scandanavia—not of the United States! Stenstrom's[3] study in Uppsala, Sweden, consisted of clinic patients, colleagues, nurses, and cadet officers, which is a group more reflective of the general population. His study showed that about 29% of the population have low myopia (≤2D), 7% have moderate myopia (2–6D), and another 2.5% have high myopia (>6D). The great majority of his population (i.e., just under 70%) clustered between emmetropia and 2D of hyperopia, and the rest were high hyperopes and aphakes.

The spectacle-wearing population in a typical Western country provides a different focus on emmetropes. Bennett's[4] study on the distribution of spectacles dispensed in England indicated that from the distribution of refractions carried out by the average eye clinician, about 20% are myopic and about 75% require prescriptions between −0.50D and +8.00D. Subtraction of Stenstrom's estimate of the percentage of high hyperopes shows that about 65% of all refractive prescriptions are for presbyopes.

MYOPIA

Pathological Myopia

Curtin[5] estimated that 2–3% of the population has pathological myopia (a condition in which there is an enlargement of the eyeball with a lengthening of the posterior segment). This group primarily falls into Stenstrom's group of myopes of >6D. The term *pathological* is used because these patients show marked choroidal and retinal degenerative changes, a high incidence of retinal detachment, glaucoma, and increased occurrence of staphyloma development. At present, high myopia (>6D) is considered to be a sex-linked, recessive inherited disorder.[6] Fig. 10-1 illustrates the anatomy of the myopic crescent—note that as the eye enlarges, the sclera and choroid begin to show at the edge of the optic nerve (see Chapter 126).

Physiological or School Myopia

As noted by Stenstrom,[3] the vast majority of myopes are ≤2D; this type of myopia is called *physiological* or *school myopia*. The word *physiological* implies that this form of myopia is a normal, physiological response to a stress. In fact, substantial evidence exists that increased time spent reading from the early teen years to the mid-20s is related to the development of myopia.[7,8] One of the authors also observed that over 60% of the average medical school class is myopic. That the long-term use of atropine eyedrops in conjunction with wearing bifocals stabilizes myopia also lends credence to this proposition.[9]

However, near work is not the sole cause of physiological myopia. Racial and ethnicity studies show that myopia is more prevalent among Asians and Jews and less prevalent among African-Americans.[6] (The results of a study in Taiwan showed the incidence of myopia to be about 12% in children 6 years of age or less, 55% in children 12 years of age or less, 76% in children 15 years of age or less, and 84% in those over 18 years of age.[10]) Thus it appears that an inherited predisposition, linked with excessive close work during the student years, results in most of the cases of physiological myopia.

ASTIGMATISM

About 50% of full-term infants in their first years of life show astigmatism of over 1D.[11,12] This may arise from the influence of the recti muscles that pull upon the delicate infant sclera because the astigmatism seems to change in different gaze directions. Howland *et al.*[13] suggested that the high astigmatism helps the infant to bracket the position of best focus while it learns to accommodate. By adulthood, this high incidence of astigmatism has disappeared. Studies show that about 15% of the adult population have astigmatism >1D and only 2% have astigmatism >3D. It is possible that much of the high astigmatism in the latter group is related to some form of intraocular surgery (e.g., corneal transplants, cataract surgery, or repair of corneal lacerations).

PRESBYOPIA

Although presbyopia is age related, its age of onset varies around the world. For example, presbyopia develops earlier in people who live closer to the equator.[14,15] Specifically, the age of onset of presbyopia was noted to be 37 years in India, 39 years in Puerto Rico, 41 years in Israel, 42 years in Japan, 45 years in England, and 46 years in Norway (see Chapter 6). Further studies show the important variable to be ambient temperature rather than latitude. Thus, the higher the ambient temperature, the earlier the onset of presbyopia.

On the other hand, life expectancy is lower in developing countries, where the ambient temperatures are usually high. Thus, although presbyopia starts at a younger age in the developing world, fewer presbyopes are found in the general population. For example, in Haiti the prevalence rate of presbyopia is about 16% for the normal population, whereas in the United States it is 31%. The lower rate of presbyopia in Haiti is para-

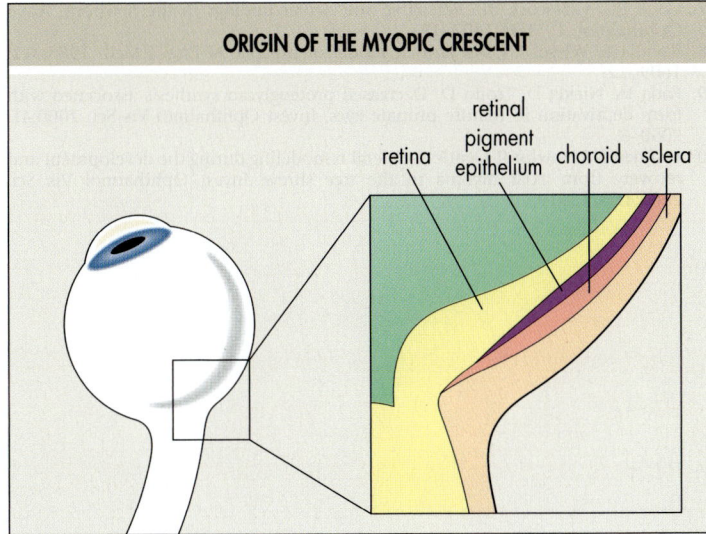

ORIGIN OF THE MYOPIC CRESCENT

retina / retinal pigment epithelium / choroid / sclera

FIG. 10-1 ▪ **Origin of the myopic crescent.** As the eye enlarges, the choroid and retina gradually pull away from the temporal optic nerve head. Thus, in extreme cases, sclera is seen. In less extreme enlargement, choroid or a rim of pigment epithelium can be seen.

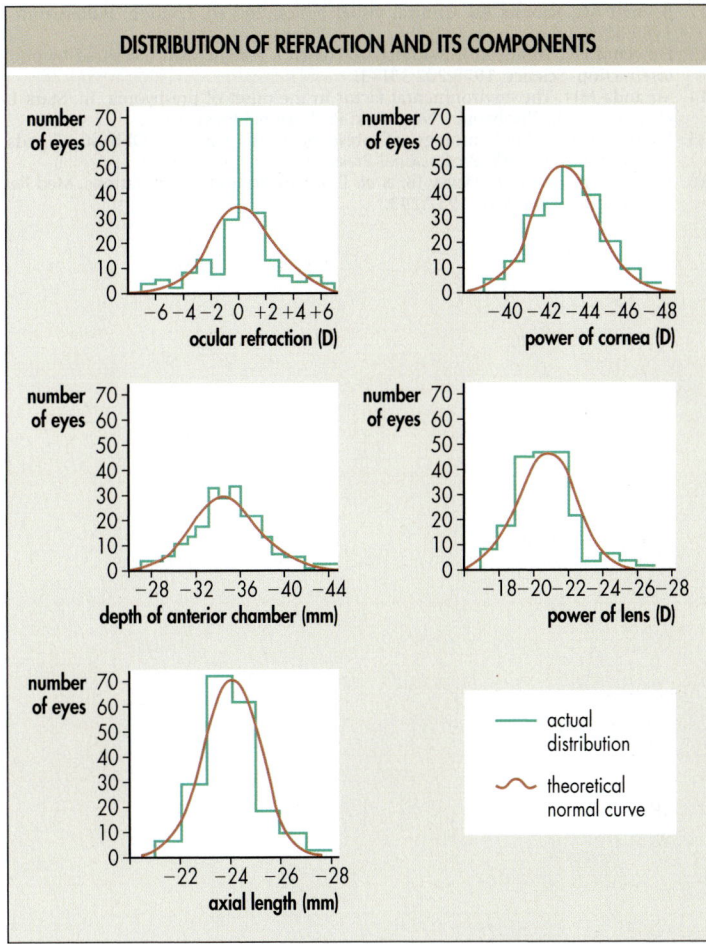

DISTRIBUTION OF REFRACTION AND ITS COMPONENTS

FIG. 10-2 ▪ Curves of distribution of refraction and its components in 194 eyes. (Adapted with permission from Sorsby A, Benjamin B, Davey JB, *et al.* Emmetropia and its aberrations. Med Res Counc Special Rep Serv. 1957; 293.)

doxical. It is due to the fact that the average life span in Haiti is much shorter than in Western countries. Seen in perspective, presbyopia accounts for about 65% of all people who wear glasses in the developed Western countries. Thus, it is of little surprise that the first spectacles produced some time in the 14th century were created for presbyopes.

COMPONENTS OF AMETROPIA

The overall refractive state of the eye is determined by four components:

- Corneal power (mean, 43D)
- Anterior chamber depth (mean, 3.4mm)
- Crystalline lens power (mean, 21D)
- Axial length (mean, 24mm)

Fig. 10-2 shows the distribution of total refraction and the four components just mentioned for 194 eyes.[16]

The most striking conclusion drawn from Fig. 10-2 is that, whereas each of the individual optical components may be considered to be randomly distributed, the overall refractive status does not show a normal distribution of refractive errors but shows a skew in the region of emmetropia. It seems that the various components cooperate to achieve a higher than expected incidence of refractive state between 0 diopter and +2 diopters.

This cooperation of components to produce a higher than expected incidence of emmetropia and lower hyperopia has been called *emmetropization*.[16] The process of emmetropization seems to be fully effective during the infantile growth of the eye. Specifically, the average sagittal diameter of the eye is approximately 18mm at birth. By the age of 3 years, the axial length increases to about 23mm. Such elongation of the eye theoretically yields a state of myopia of about 15D. Yet, during this period the data show that almost 75% of these young eyes are hyperopic.[17] Between 3 and 14 years of age, the elongation increases by, on average, an additional millimeter. Again, this should theoretically produce another 3D of myopia. Yet at 14 years of age, the average refractive state shows a strong clustering in the emmetropic neighborhood. Because the cornea and anterior chamber depth change very little during these periods of eye growth, it appears that the power of the crystalline lens changes to maintain emmetropia. It seems possible that the process is coordinated by the retina-brain complex, which might tune each component to ensure a sharp image. However, studies of infant monkeys that were raised in the dark or had the optic nerve sectioned suggest that emmetropization is largely programmed on a genetic basis.[18] The

experiments further showed that procedures that result in significant degradation of the retinal image, such as suture of the lids together or induction of a corneal opacity during the early growth period, influence the axial growth process. Surprisingly, these types of opacifications significantly increase the axial length and produce states of myopia of up to 12D. Such excessive image degradation seems to override the emmetropization process and result in high levels of axial myopia. The biological mechanism for this process seems to be a remodeling of posterior scleral tissue caused by a reduction in the synthesis of proteoglycans that is related to form deprivation.[19,20]

REFERENCES

1. Stromberg E. Uber refraktion und Achsenlange des menschlicken Auges. Acta Ophthalmol. 1936;14:281–93.
2. Sorsby A, Sheridan M, Leary GA. Vision, visual acuity and ocular refraction in young men. Br Med J. 1960;i:1394–8.
3. Stenstrom S. Untersuchungen uber die Variation und Kovariation des optischen Elemente des menschlichen Auges. Acta Ophthalmol. 1946;26(Suppl) (also English translation by Woolf D. Am J Optom. 1948;25:218–32).
4. Bennett AG. Lens usage in the supplementary ophthalmic service. Optician. 1965;149:131–7.
5. Curtin BJ. The myopias: basic science and clinical management. Philadelphia: Harper & Row; 1985.
6. Wold KC. Hereditary myopia. Arch Ophthalmol. 1949;42:225–35.
7. Angle J, Wissman DA. The epidemiology of myopia. Am J Epidemiol. 1980;111:220–31.
8. Hepsen IF, Evereklioglu C, Bayramlar H. The effect of reading and near-work on the development of emmetropic boys: a prospective, controlled, three-year follow-up study. Vision Res. 2001;41:2511–20.
9. Syniuta LA, Isenberg SJ. Atropine and bifocals can slow the progression of myopia in children. Binocul Vis Strabismus Q. 2001;16:201–2;227.
10. Luke LK, Yung–Feng S, Chong–Bin T, *et al.* Epidemiological study of ocular refraction amount school children in Taiwan. Invest Ophthalmol Vis Sci. 1996;6:1002.
11. Mohindra I, Held R, Gwiazda J, Brill S. Astigmatism in infants. Science. 1978; 202:329–31.

12. Bennett AG, Rabbits RB. Clinical visual optics, 2nd ed. London: Butterworths; 1989:50.
13. Howland HC, Atkinson J, Braddick O, French J. Astigmatism measured by photorefraction. Science. 1978;202:331–3.
14. Miranda MH. The environmental factor in the onset of presbyopia. In: Stark L, Obrecht G, eds. Presbyopia. New York: Professional Press; 1987.
15. Kleinstein RN. Epidemiology of presbyopia. In: Stark L, Obrecht G, eds. Presbyopia. New York: Professional Press; 1987.
16. Sorsby A, Benjamin B, Davey JB, *et al.* Emmetropia and its aberrations. Med Res Counc Special Rep Serv. 1957;293.
17. Cook RC, Glasscock RE. Refractive and ocular findings in the newborn. Am J Ophthalmol. 1951;34:1407–13.
18. Raviola E, Wiesel TN. An animal model of myopia. N Engl J Med. 1985;312:1609–12.
19. Rada JA, Nickla D, Troilo D. Decreased proteoglycan synthesis associated with form deprivation in mature primate eyes. Invest Ophthalmol Vis Sci. 2000;41:2050–8.
20. McBrien NA, Lawlor P, Gentle A. Scleral remodeling during the development and recovery from axial myopia in the tree shrew. Invest Ophthalmol Vis Sci. 2000;41:3713–19.

CHAPTER 11

Subjective Testing of Refraction

CLIFFORD A. SCOTT

DEFINITION
- The neutralization of an individual's refractive error using a variety of tests in which the patient's responses determine the lens power that best produces a sharply focused image on the retina.
- The selection of a prescription for corrective lenses that balances optical clarity with other important physical and psychological factors, such as equality of magnification, single vision, and comfort.
- The determination of the most appropriate form of optical correction based on the patient's visual needs and on environmental factors.

INTRODUCTION

Many people equate an eye examination with a refraction for glasses. The confusion is understandable because for the vast majority, especially those in the preretirement age group, eyeglasses or contact lenses resolve the main complaints they have about their eyes. Also, a refraction is almost always part of a comprehensive eye examination, not only to provide a prescription for corrective lenses but also to determine the best acuity that an eye is capable of achieving.

As the rest of this textbook attests, refraction is only one of the many methods used to determine the function and health of the visual system. Because of the value of the results, it is important to develop an efficient and accurate basic refractive technique that can be modified when unusual variations present themselves.

Although often relegated as a purely technical task in the spectrum of high-technology examination and treatment procedures that characterize contemporary ophthalmic practice, refraction provides relief for one of the world's most common physical defects. An understanding of the concepts used to identify and measure refractive errors is the basis for prescribing individual corrections that offer patients improved quality of life. Equally important, refraction is one of the few procedures that consistently provides doctors with immediate gratification for their knowledge and efforts.

HISTORICAL REVIEW

Spectacles were first described during the Middle Ages. In 1266, Roger Bacon magnified print in a book using a segment of a glass sphere. A painting completed in 1352 shows a prelate wearing lenses in a mounting. In the late fifteenth century, merchants sold spectacles to buyers who chose them on the basis of their own judgment of how vision improved. As the trade of lens making proliferated throughout Europe, it became organized into a guild. Although cylindrical lenses had been manufactured since 1827, it was not until Donders published his methods of refraction that correcting astigmatism became an exact science. In 1893, when American Optical developed the trial case of lenses, opticians, rather than spectacle peddlers, became the primary providers of

eye examinations.[1] Although instrument makers have dramatically improved the ability of examiners to provide accurate and repeatable lens prescriptions, most subjective techniques still rely upon a comparison of views through different lenses.

PURPOSE OF THE TEST

One of the most common reasons that patients seek eye care is to obtain correction of their refractive error. However, refraction is also a diagnostic tool used to differentiate decreased acuity caused by uncorrected or incompletely corrected refractive error from blurred vision related to eye disease.

In most cases, the final determination of the refractive correction is based upon the patient's appreciation of the lens power that provides the clearest vision at the desired viewing distance. This procedure, subjective refraction, is a time-honored combination of the technical skill required to select a lens that produces a sharply focused image on the retina tempered with the fine art of determining the best overall correction, incorporating other factors such as the balance between the two eyes, the patient's visual needs, the patient's age, and the rate of change of the refractive error. The concepts and procedures described here refer to neutralization of the refractive error with spectacles, but most of these principles and techniques also apply to correction using contact lenses.

UTILITY OF THE TEST

Subjective refraction is usually performed after an in-depth history has been obtained,[2] which includes ascertaining that clear vision has been achieved previously, describing visual symptoms and any relief provided with the current correction, and specific visual requirements related to work and avocations. It should be performed before any other test that might alter the patient's responses because of physical changes to the eye, including Goldmann tonometry and gonioscopy. Any examination procedure that uses bright lights, such as ophthalmoscopy or slit-lamp evaluation, can produce a photostress response. Refraction should be done either before performing these tests or after an appropriate recovery period.

Cycloplegic eyedrops can be used to eliminate accommodation during the examination. In most cases, the results of a cycloplegic refraction are not prescribed as a correction. Rather, this type of examination is used in select circumstances to determine the baseline refractive status of the eye. There are two common situations in which this is valuable.

- In young individuals who are suspected of accommodative spasm, especially when it is accompanied by esophoria or esotropia, it is important to prescribe the strongest plus power correction in order to relax accommodation. A follow-up examination, not under cycloplegia, is usually required to determine the maximum amount of lens power that can be tolerated in the natural state.
- Recent protocols for refractive surgery dictate that the cycloplegic refractive power of the eyes be determined prior to undergoing the procedure.[3]

PROCEDURE

Although a totally subjective test is possible, most examiners use a baseline starting point, such as an evaluation of the patient's previous eyeglasses, retinoscopy, or the results of an automated refraction, which they then refine to meet the patient's requirements. In general, the goal is to determine the maximum plus power correction that provides clear vision at far and a near correction that provides clear vision at the desired distances. Many methods have been developed to determine the "best" correction, any of which an adept refractionist can call upon to resolve a specific refractive quandary. For the purposes of this chapter, only the most widely accepted methods are described.

Instrumentation

As with most health care procedures, many levels of sophistication in the instruments are available to perform this technique. They range from highly automated scanners and analyzers that provide an objective measure of the eye's refractive error in seconds to the centuries-old method of placing loose lenses by hand into a trial frame worn by the patient. Each method has its proponents and, in particular situations, each method has its advantages.

Automated refractors analyze the focal power of emitted light from the eye and convert it into a dioptric correction. They are very fast, require minimum skill levels to operate, and are fairly accurate.[4] They are also very expensive. Certain high-end models have subjective refraction capability so that the correction can be refined in the instrument. Portable automated refractors are now available.

Most practitioners rely upon the manually operated refractor or Phoroptor that contains a battery of lenses arranged in wheels that can be positioned in front of the patient's eyes; the lenses can be changed quickly to provide a wide array of plus and minus spherical lenses as well as a range of cylindrical lenses, available in both minus cylinder and plus cylinder configurations, that can be rotated to the appropriate axis. Earlier in this century, when most ophthalmic lenses were manufactured in plus cylinder form, it made sense to use plus cylinder examination lenses that mimicked the final lens design as closely as possible.

Contemporary ophthalmic lenses are made in minus cylinder form, so it now may make sense to refract using minus cylinders.

A trial frame can be used to mount loose trial lenses in front of the patient's eyes. Trial frame refraction is a time-consuming procedure, and because of the thickness of individual lenses, especially at stronger powers, a power shift is induced when several lenses are stacked together. This error can be minimized by placing the strongest spherical lens in the rear well closest to the patient's eye. A variation of this technique is to use a clip-on trial lens holder which can be mounted on the patient's current glasses or on a "loaner" pair of glasses made up in a spherical power close to the patient's required correction. This works exceptionally well when the existing eyeglasses contain a strong spherical or cylindrical component. The most practical use of a trial frame or clip-ons is to allow the patient to experience the change in correction before investing in a new pair of glasses.

Monocular Subjective Refraction

There are three basic components in the operation of a spectacle lens: the spherical power, the astigmatic cylinder power, and the axis. An accurate determination of the spherical component is predicated on having fully corrected the astigmatic error to ensure that a point focus is obtained with the final correcting lens. Therefore, subjective examinations proceed in that order. In eyes with astigmatism, each of the principal meridians produces a linear image at its focal distance. In the space between foci, the interval of Sturm, the image has a progressive change in its elliptic profile and, at the focal distance of the dioptric average of the two principal powers, the image is round, the circle of least confusion. In an eye uncorrected for astigmatism, the best acuity occurs when the circle of least confusion falls upon the retina (Fig. 11-1). At all other points within the astigmatic pencil, the image is distorted along the principal meridians whereby each point source produces an oval image.[5] The oval images of two or more adjacent point objects overlap along one of the principal meridians and appear darker along their long axes. Some refractive techniques use this effect to neutralize subjectively the astigmatic focus.

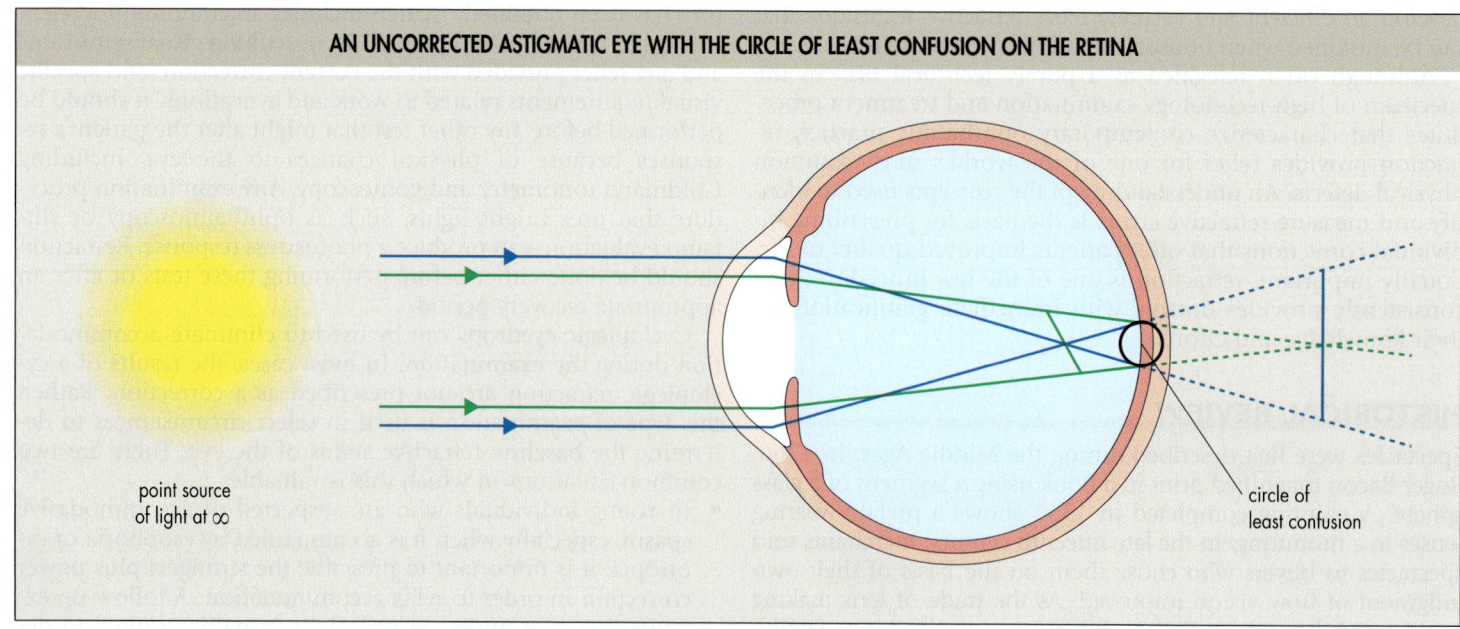

AN UNCORRECTED ASTIGMATIC EYE WITH THE CIRCLE OF LEAST CONFUSION ON THE RETINA

point source of light at ∞

circle of least confusion

FIG. 11-1 ■ **An uncorrected astigmatic eye with the circle of least confusion on the retina.** The horizontal and vertical focal lines are dioptrically equal in front of and behind the retina.

The "clock dial," a standard target in most ophthalmic projector systems, is a circular chart with radii drawn at 30° intervals. When the correct power toric lens is interposed along the appropriate axis, each image is circular and all of the radii appear equally dark (Fig. 11-2). The starting point of the test is to have sufficient plus lens power in the tentative correction so that the focal points of both principal meridians are anterior to the retina, yet are recognizable. This "fogging" technique serves to inhibit the natural accommodative response to blur; any focusing effort only further blurs the image. In practice, the initial starting sphere (obtained by omitting the minus cylinder from the net retinoscopy result, the previous spectacle correction, or the autorefraction result) is placed before the eye under test. For an eye correctable to 20/20 (6/6), sufficient plus lens power is added to blur the 20/40 (6/12) line of letters, usually at least 1.00D.

In eyes with more astigmatism, enough plus power must be added to fog the least myopic or the most hyperopic meridian. The clock chart is projected and the patient is asked, "Which, if any, spokes on the wheel are darker?" Because the details on the chart are standardized at the 20/30 level, incremental reductions in plus power are required until some of the lines are clear. If no astigmatism is present, all of the spokes remain equally blurred as plus power is reduced. In astigmatic eyes, the focal line produced by the flatter principal meridian is closer to the retina and appears darker or bolder. With high values of astigmatism, one or two lines are prominent, whereas at lower values several lines may initially appear equally dark. The center of the group is estimated by the patient. A direct method of communicating the correct axis is to have the patient point out the darkest meridian with a laser pointer.[6] The axis of the correcting minus cylinder is placed at 90° to this line.

Another simple method is to use the lowest clock time of the darkest line and multiply by 30. For example, if the vertical line was darkest, the patient would respond, "The 6 o'clock/12 o'clock line." The correcting cylinder should be placed at axis 180° (6 × 30). To maintain the refractive fog, a +0.25D sphere is added for each −0.50D of cylinder that is added. Minus cylinder lenses are then added in 0.25D increments until all the spokes are equally dark. When equality of the spokes is reported, the process should be continued until reversal occurs to ensure that the full cylinder power has actually been achieved.

Because the meridians on the clock chart are 30° apart, the true axis may lie between them. There are several other commonly used charts that can refine the axis more precisely. The sunburst chart has radii that are only 15° apart; however, it is of-

ten difficult to communicate the precise axis to the examiner because of fluctuations in response related to minor head movements. The Paraboline rotary slide (Fig. 11-3) has two symmetrical parabolic arcs whose asymptotic ends approximate the image of an arrowhead.[7] With the eye in a "fogged" state, the slide is rotated until both halves of the arrowhead appear equally dark. The axis can be read from a protractor projected onto the screen. Along the principal axes of the pattern is a cross of dotted lines, which is then used as described before to determine the correct cylinder power.

The Jackson Cross-Cylinder (JCC) test is perhaps the most commonly used method for subjectively determining the presence of astigmatism and for refining the power and axis of a refractive cylinder.[8] It relies on the principle of placing the circle of least confusion on the retina. A crossed cylinder is a lens whose principal powers are equal and opposite in sign. The standard power JCC has powers along its principal meridians of +0.37D and −0.37D to produce an astigmatic range of 0.75D. Each end of the minus axis is marked with a red dot, whereas the plus axis has white dots. The rotating handle in the manual

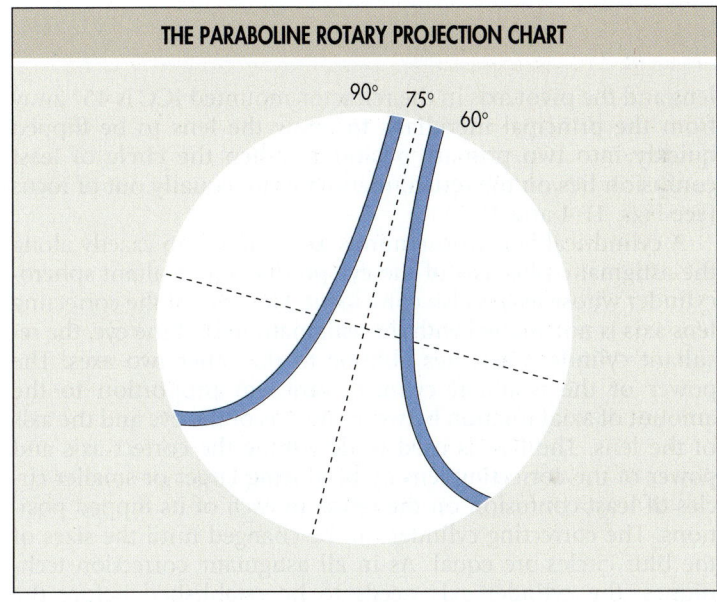

THE PARABOLINE ROTARY PROJECTION CHART

FIG. 11-3 ▮ **The Paraboline rotary projection chart.** The axis of the correcting lens is determined by rotating the slide until both arms of the pattern appear equally dark.

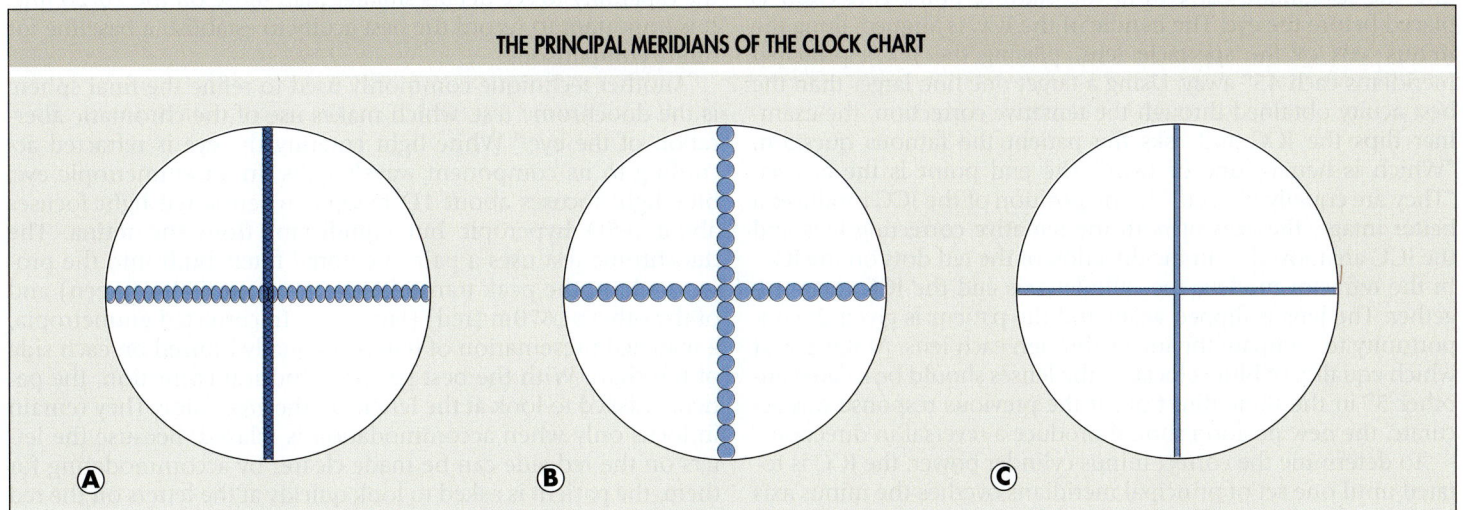

THE PRINCIPAL MERIDIANS OF THE CLOCK CHART

Ⓐ   Ⓑ   Ⓒ

FIG. 11-2 ▮ **The principal meridians of the clock chart. A,** As seen by an eye with uncorrected astigmatism in which each image appears as a vertical oval. The overlapping ovals make the vertical line darker. **B,** The same eye when the correct amount of cylinder is in place and the fogging lens has not been removed. Each image appears as a blurred circle so that all the lines appear equally dark. **C,** The same eye with the full spherocylindrical correction in place. Each image appears as a sharp point, giving an even, well-focused appearance to the chart.

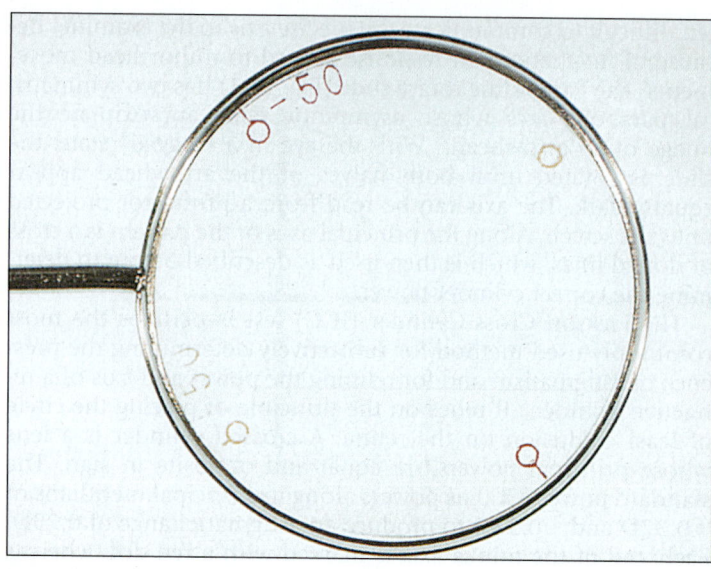

FIG. 11-4 ■ The handheld Jackson Cross-Cylinder. Note the red circles at the ends of the minus axis.

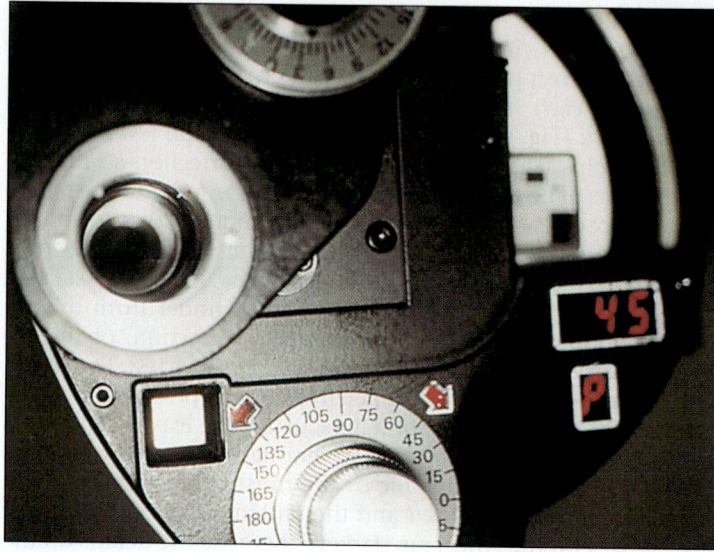

FIG. 11-5 ■ The refractor-mounted Jackson Cross-Cylinder in place to check for axis orientation of a cylinder axis 45°.

lens and the pivot axis in the refractor-mounted JCC is 45° away from the principal meridians to allow the lens to be flipped quickly into two primary positions. When the circle of least confusion lies on the retina, meridians are equally out of focus (see Figs. 11-4 and 11-5).

A cylindrical lens whose minus axis is lined up exactly along the astigmatic plus axis of the eye produces a resultant spherocylinder whose axis is also coincident. However, if the correcting lens axis is not aligned with the astigmatic axis of the eye, the resultant cylinder's axis lies oblique to the other two axes. The power of the resultant cylinder varies in proportion to the amount of axial rotation between the axis of the eye and the axis of the lens. The JCC is used to determine the correct axis and power of the correcting lens by producing larger or smaller circles of least confusion on the retina in each of its flipped positions. The correcting cylinder can be changed until the sizes of the blur circles are equal. As in all astigmatic correction techniques, the cylinder axis needs to be established before the power can be determined.

When the JCC is used to locate the correcting axis, the images are equally blurred when the principal meridians of the JCC are equally misaligned with the true correcting axis of the eye. To refine the astigmatic correction, the starting point correction is placed before the eye. The handle of the JCC is aligned along the minus axis of the spectacle lens, placing the JCC's principal meridians each 45° away. Using a target one line larger than the best acuity obtained through the tentative correction, the examiner flips the JCC and asks the patient the famous question, "Which is better—one or two?" The end point is the answer, "They are equally blurred." If one position of the JCC produces a better image, the axes of both the tentative correcting lens and the JCC are moved 5° in the direction of the red dots on the JCC. In the refractor models, the cylinder axis and the JCC rotate together. The lens is flipped again and the patient is given the opportunity to compare the image through each lens. At the axis at which equality of blur is located, the lenses should be rotated another 5° in the same direction. If the previous response was accurate, the new position should produce a reversal in direction.

To determine the correct minus cylinder power, the JCC is rotated until one set of principal meridians overlies the minus axis of the correcting lens. The handle of the manual JCC is now 45° away. On the refractor units, the position is marked by a click-stop detent. Using the same line of letters, the JCC is flipped and, again, the patient is asked to choose the better of the two images. If the JCC's minus axis, marked by the red dots, is

aligned with the cylinder axis, a cylinder of 0.25D more minus power is added to the correction. If the better image is produced when the plus axis, marked by the white dots, is aligned, the cylinder power is reduced by 0.25D. To ensure that the circle of confusion remains on the retina, for each 0.50D of cylinder that is added, a 0.25D sphere of the opposite power should be added. The procedure is repeated until the two images are equally blurred. Going one lens past to reversal ensures that the correct lens is selected.

Once the proper cylindrical correction has been established, the final sphere needs to be determined. One simple technique is to "refog" the eye using plus lenses to minimize the effects of uncontrolled accommodation. Obviously, this is more of an issue in younger individuals who have a large accommodative reserve. Using the line of expected best acuity, the power is reduced by 0.25D at a time with a sufficient intervening pause to allow the patient to attempt to interpret the letters. Once the letters are identified, the next smaller line is presented. If these letters are not clearly recognized, power is reduced by another 0.25D. If the letters are still not clear, the previous lens probably produces the sharpest unaccommodated focus. If the letters are seen, the process is repeated with the next smaller line. Many individuals have the capability to see details smaller than those on the 20/20 line. It is important to record the best acuity to establish a baseline for future comparisons.

Another technique commonly used to refine the final sphere is the duochrome test, which makes use of the chromatic aberration of the eye.[9] White light entering the eye is refracted according to its component wavelengths. In an emmetropic eye, blue light focuses about 1D myopic, whereas red light focuses about 0.5D hyperopic but equidistant from the retina. The duochrome test uses a pair of colored filters built into the projector chart, the peak transmission of one at 530m (green) and of the other at 670m (red) (Fig. 11-6). In corrected emmetropia, a matched presentation of letters is equally blurred on each side of the chart. With the best spherocylindrical correction, the patient is asked to look at the letters on the green side. They remain in focus only when accommodation is relaxed. Because the letters on the red side can be made clearer by accommodating for them, the patient is asked to look quickly at the letters on the red side and then back at the green and compare their clarity. If the letters on the green side are clearer, the correcting sphere is changed by 0.25D in the plus direction. If the letters on the red side are clearer, 0.25D is added in the minus direction. This test is sensitive enough for 0.25D to cause a reversal in clarity.

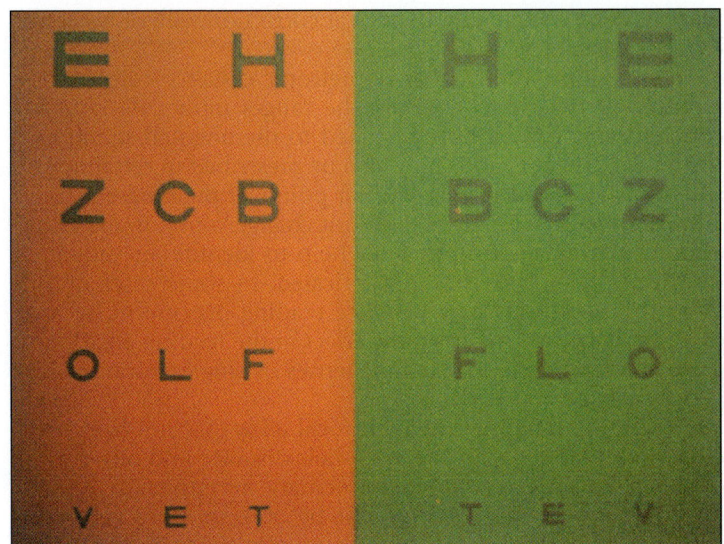

FIG. 11-6 ▪ When letters on the green side of the chart are clearer, more spherical plus power needs to be added.

Binocular Balance

The entire procedure is repeated for each eye to produce two monocular subjective prescriptions. Assuming that the patient has clear, single binocular vision, the effects of compensating for an existing heterophoria or the effects of summation of vision from both eyes may alter the lens powers chosen for the binocular subjective prescription.[10] The process is usually accomplished in two steps.

The first is to ensure that equal accommodative effort is present between the two eyes. If the best-corrected vision is approximately the same in each eye, vision is fogged with +0.75D lenses. Sufficient vertical prism is placed in front of each eye to produce two separate images of the isolated 20/40 (6/12) line. The patient is asked to compare the clarities of the upper line and the lower line. If they appear equally blurred, +0.25D is added to one eye and they are compared again. The other eye should now see slightly more clearly. The lens is removed and the process repeated for the other eye. Adjustments are made until the images are as equally blurred as possible. If there is no pair of lenses that produces an equality of blur between the two eyes, the pair that gives the slightly better image in front of the dominant eye is often preferred.

The best acuity line is then isolated on the chart. The fogging lenses are reduced from both eyes by 0.25D at a time, allowing sufficient time between stages for the patient to adjust to the lens change. In the same way as with the monocular subjective test, the lens power that gives best acuity without inducing accommodation is usually the final choice. The duochrome test offers an alternative method of determining the lens powers that produce a sharp unaccommodated retinal image.

The same technique can be employed with eyes that have a moderate discrepancy in best-corrected vision, either from amblyopia or from some other abnormality. The lens powers can be balanced using a larger line of letters, for example, the 20/80 (6/24) line, and then reduced to the best acuity, which is that of the better eye. This solves the dilemma of trying to determine the best monocular subjective correction in an eye with poor visual discrimination.

Binocular refraction is an infrequently used technique in which both eyes are fixating while the monocular refraction is measured. Most contemporary devices use some form of vectographic separation in which a polarized target is presented to each eye through interposing polarized analyzers with a different axis in front of each eye.[11] This has the advantage of mimicking the normal form of seeing, incorporating all of the patient's binocular efforts including horizontal and vertical phorias.[12] In addition, this method offers the only way to identify a cyclophoria in which the astigmatic axes of the eyes are different under binocular conditions than when observed monocularly.[13]

Trial frame confirmation of the final prescription is often overlooked but is an extremely valuable verification of the comfort and acuity of the new lens power. Although an examination room of length 20ft (6m) is considered to be the equivalent of optical infinity, .17D of accommodation is still required at that distance. It is psychologically reassuring for the patient to step out of the examination room and view the end of the hallway or, better still, the other side of the street through the new lenses. This small investment of time may save lengthy follow-up visits that could result from miscommunication in the examination room.

If the cylinder correction is similar to that of the patient's old glasses, it is relatively straightforward to have the patient handhold spherical trial lenses in front of the glasses and compare vision with and without the change in prescription. This is a simple way to determine which is the more satisfactory lens correction when there is a discrepancy between the monocular subjective and the binocular subjective tests. As the monocular subjective test's end point is best acuity and the binocular subjective test's end point is equality of accommodation, some patients may have a slight difference in right and left eye acuities through the binocular prescription. This refinement offers them the opportunity to observe the difference between the two corrections and to make a practical choice between them.

If there is some doubt about the visual comfort of the change, the lenses can be held in position with a clip-on lens holder while the patient takes the opportunity to walk around and adjust to the difference. In some cases, it may be beneficial to allow patients to borrow the lenses and holders overnight in order to evaluate the lens changes in their own environment. It is important to mark the right and left lenses and, if cylinders are required, to provide a sketch to help align the axis marks.

A similar procedure can be used when the change in correction is a spherocylinder. It is unwieldy to place and remove more than one lens in front of the patient's glasses. If the new cylinder axis is different from that of the old eyeglasses, a calculation of resultant cylinder axis and power is required to determine the appropriate lens to hold in front of the glasses. In such a situation, it is more practical to place the new correction in a trial frame and to let the patient alternately view at a distance through the trial frame and the old glasses. The trial frame interpupillary distance, the vertical lens position, and the pantoscopic angle should be adjusted correctly, especially with strong lens powers.

Near Refraction

The near correction is the distance correction with sufficient plus additional power (the "add") to satisfy individual needs for clear, comfortable single vision at a desired near point. Although there are normative tables for determining an add according to the patient's age, these simply function as benchmarks to help the examiner recognize a potential overcorrected or undercorrected condition.[14] This is an important time to listen to your patient. Although patients are notoriously inaccurate when estimating their working distances, the description of how they use their eyes at near helps to determine not only the strength of the lens power required for tasks at near but also the form in which the correction will be most effective. For example, a presbyope who requires a +2.00D add for reading may be very satisfied with a bifocal correction for most activities but may require a +1.25D add in single-vision lenses to work at a computer terminal.

One rule of thumb that has gained wide acceptance is that the near add at a given distance should allow half of the patient's accommodative amplitude to remain in reserve.[15] The amplitude is determined by measuring the closest point at which an individual can maintain focus through the distance correction. For a prepresbyope, this simply means measuring the distance at which a fine line of print can no longer be focused. This distance, measured in centimeters, is divided into 100 to convert it into amplitude of accommodation. A presbyope needs to place a plus lens over the distance correction to be able to see the fine print. The closest distance to which the print can be moved before blurring is again converted into diopters and the power of the interposed lens subtracted to give the amplitude (Box 11-1 and Fig. 11-7).

A clinical method commonly used to measure the near add is the Fused Cross-Cylinder test. A cross made up of multiple horizontal and vertical lines is presented to the patient at a distance of 40cm. A JCC with its minus axis vertical is placed in front of the distance correction. The patient is asked to compare the boldness of the horizontal and vertical lines of the cross. If no add is required, the lines are equally dark. If the horizontal lines are darker, plus power is added binocularly in 0.25D increments until the lines are equally black or until the vertical lines become more prominent. This lens power becomes the tentative add.[16]

The final add is determined by verifying that the add is appropriate for the patient's visual needs. The range of clear near vision is the linear distance between the far point of the near lens (usually the reciprocal of the add power) and the near point of accommodation through the add. Because the range of vision is inversely proportional to the power of the lens, many experienced refractionists prescribe the weakest add that meets the patient's demands.[17] For most individuals, having a larger range in which objects are clear overrides the desire to see extremely fine print at a close distance. It is often helpful to patients who are receiving their first presbyopic correction to have lenses held in place to demonstrate that their near correction will, of necessity, blur their distance vision.

In situations where an anisometropic distance correction is required, it is wise to measure the ranges monocularly to account for any optical effects related to the unequal strength of the lenses. Unequal adds may also be prescribed in certain other situations to keep the near and far points of the ranges at similar distances. As with any significant change, a trial frame evaluation of the new correction may help to identify any potential difficulties before glasses are fabricated. In some cases of anisometropia, bifocals may produce reading discomfort because of an induced vertical prismatic effect in the reading position of gaze. Specially designed slab-off lenses or single-vision reading glasses may be required.

Patients who require higher bifocal adds may not have sufficient accommodation to overlap their distance and near ranges of vision. This "dead zone" is problematic in certain jobs and avocations. An accountant may not be able to see a calculator clearly in its normal desktop position, and a violinist may have difficulty reading stand music. Although trifocals or progressive lenses may be satisfactory, special use lenses, such as low-add bifocals with a high segment line, may be required.

Computer users who must also read place a unique set of demands upon their glasses. The video screen is usually just below eye level at arm's length or slightly closer, whereas reading material and the keyboard are positioned lower and somewhat closer. It is often worthwhile to have patients adjust one of the computer terminals in the examiner's office to simulate their workstation conditions.[18] Eye-to-screen and eye-to-keyboard measurements can be used to determine the necessary add powers. Many presbyopic computer operators have occupational bifocals in which the top section of the lenses has the intermedi-

---

BOX 11-1

Calculated Near "Add" at Any Distance Should Keep Half of the Patient's Accommodative Amplitude in Reserve

With an extra +1.50D lens, the near point of accommodation is 40cm (2.50D).

The patient's amplitude is **1.00D** (2.50D − 1.50D).

For a working distance of 50cm, **2.00D** of accommodation is required.

Therefore, the patient's "add" for that distance should be +1.50D [**2.00D** − 1/2(**1.00D**)].

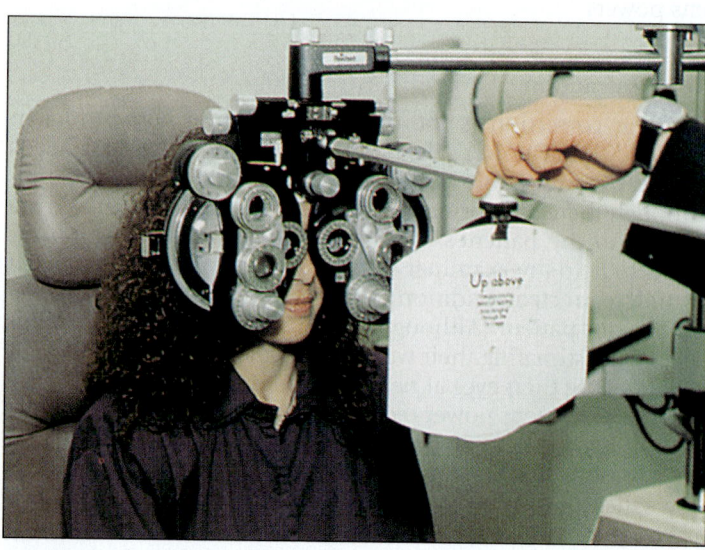

FIG. 11-7 ■ A near card is placed in front of the Phoroptor and slid back and forth to determine the closest distance at which the print can be seen before blurring takes place.

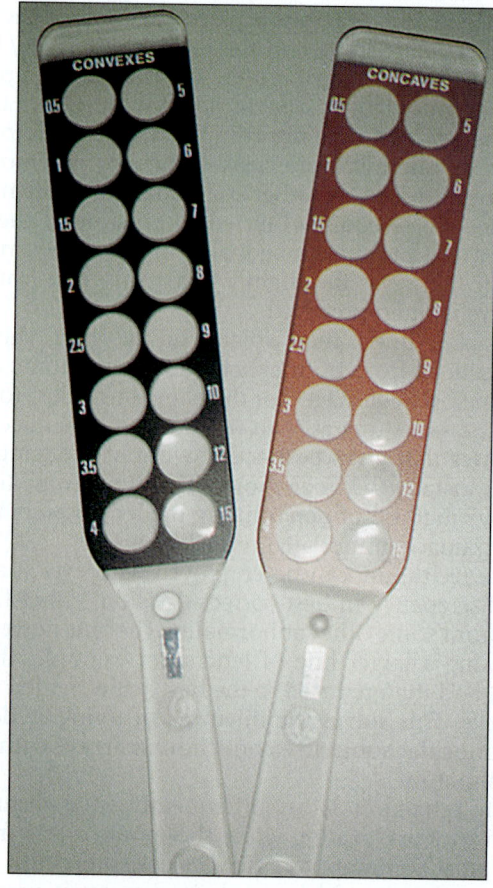

FIG. 11-8 ■ Plus and minus racks of spherical lenses used for retinoscopy screening. They are also useful to determine an approximate subjective spherical equivalent lens.

ate correction and the lower portion is set for the keyboard distance. When the operator leaves the workstation, these glasses are left at the terminal and a conventional correction is used.

ALTERNATIVE TESTS

Bedside examinations, nursing home visits, and equipment failure are examples of situations that require skill in trial frame refraction. When poorly controlled ambient lighting exists, retinoscopy is often, at best, an estimate. A retinoscopy rack, made up of a battery of spherical lenses (Fig. 11-8) arranged in ascending order of power, can be used to determine the subjective spherical equivalent. Using this power as the initial trial frame starting lens, a handheld JCC can be used to determine the presence of any astigmatism. The handle is positioned along a true oblique meridian (45° or 135°) so that the principal powers are along the horizontal and vertical meridians. The lens is flipped and the patient is asked whether either position is better. If not, the handle is repositioned horizontally so that the principal powers now lie along the 45° and 135° meridians and the procedure is repeated. If again there is no preference, there is no clinically significant astigmatism in that eye. If the patient indicates a preference in any of those positions, the JCC tests proceed as described earlier.

Some examiners locate the axis of a tentative cylinder by rotating the lens and asking the patient to indicate the position where vision is the clearest. For strong cylinders, this is an accurate and repeatable technique. However, for low-power cylinders there is a range of axis positions that produce clear vision for most observers.[19] A modification of this test to increase its accuracy is to rotate the lens until a small line of letters first blurs noticeably, then rotate the lens back in the opposite direction to first blur. The midposition is the correcting axis. This test is highly dependent upon an acutely observant patient.

One drawback of the JCC is its reliance on the patient's visual memory to determine preferences. Modifications of the refractor-mounted versions exist that use split prisms to produce a simultaneous presentation of both positions of the JCC. The lens and device can be rotated together until the images are equally

blurred to locate the cylinder axis. In the same way, the power can be determined by changing the correcting cylinder power until both images appear equal.

In situations where vision in an eye is very poor and no other instruments are available, the stenopeic slit can be used to screen for a high degree of astigmatism (Fig. 11-9). It functions as a series of pinholes along a meridian. Using a trial frame or clip-on device, the trial lens stenopeic slit is placed in the lens cell and slowly rotated. If there is a position that produces improved vision, it is treated as a principal meridian of the eye. Leaving the slit in place, spherical plus and minus lenses are positioned in front of it. A convenient method is to use the retinoscopy rack. When the lens power that gives the most improvement has been established, the stenopeic slit is rotated 90° and the procedure repeated. The two spherical lens powers are considered to be the correcting lens powers for each of the principal meridians. The powers are combined in a spherocylinder lens, which is placed in the trial lens cell. If vision is improved sufficiently, it may be possible to refine the correction using conventional methods.

REFERENCES

1. Gettes BC. Refraction. Boston: Little, Brown; 1965:343–5.
2. Amos JF. Patient history. In: Eskridge JB, Amos JF, Bartlett JD, eds. Clinical procedures in optometry. Philadelphia: JB Lippincott; 1991:3–16.
3. Azar D. Refractive Surgery. Stamford, Conn: Appleton & Lange; 1997:118–9.
4. Rosenberg R. Automated refraction. In: Eskridge JB, Amos JF, Bartlett JD, eds. Clinical procedures in optometry. Philadelphia: JB Lippincott; 1991:168–73.
5. Borish IM. Subjective testing of refraction. In: Miller D, ed. Optics and refraction. A user-friendly guide, Vol I. Textbook of ophthalmology. Chicago: Professional Press; 1975:9.4–9.6.
6. Borish IM. Subjective testing of refraction. In: Miller D, ed. Optics and refraction. A user-friendly guide, Vol I. Textbook of ophthalmology. New York: Gower Medical; 1991:9.8.
7. Borish IM. Clinical refraction. Chicago: Professional Press; 1970:722–3.
8. Polasky M. Monocular subjective refraction. In: Eskridge JB, Amos JF, Bartlett JD, eds. Clinical procedures in optometry. Philadelphia: JB Lippincott; 1991:180–2.
9. Borish IM. Clinical refraction. Chicago: Professional Press; 1970:736–9.
10. West D, Somers WW. Binocular balance validity: a comparison of five common subjective techniques. Ophthalmic Physiol Opt. 1984;4:155–9.
11. Grolman B. Binocular refraction. A new system. N Engl J Optom. 1966;17:118–29.
12. Eskridge JB. Rationale for binocular refraction. N Engl J Optom. 1971;123:160–6.
13. Rutstein RP, Eskridge JB. The effect of cyclodeviations on the axis of astigmatism. Optom Vis Sci. 1990;67:80–3.
14. Wold RM. The spectacle amplitude. Am J Optom. 1967;44:642–64.
15. Maxwell JT. Outline of ocular refraction. Omaha: Medical Publishing Co; 1937:169.
16. Carlson NB, Kurtz D, Heath DA, Hines C. Clinical procedures for ocular examination. Stamford, Conn: Appleton & Lange; 1996:188–90.
17. Morgan MW. Accommodative changes in presbyopia and their correction. In: Hirsch MJ, Wick RE, eds. Vision of the aging patient. Philadelphia: Chilton; 1960:101.
18. Scheiman M. Accommodative and binocular vision disorders associated with video display terminals: diagnosis and management issues. Am J Optom. 1996;67:531–9.
19. Carter JH. On the significance of axis error. Alumni Bull Pa Coll Optom. 1966; 20:6–8.

FIG. 11-9 ■ A stenopeic slit in place to check the power along the 130th meridian. Once the spherical power has been determined, the lens should be rotated 90° and the spherical power measured along the 40th meridian. The two powers can then be combined in a spherocylindrical lens.

CHAPTER 12

Contact Lenses

PAUL F. WHITE • CLIFFORD A. SCOTT

DEFINITION
- Contact lenses are visual devices that provide an artificial anterior refracting surface to the human eye and are used for corrective, cosmetic, and therapeutic purposes.

KEY FEATURES
- Lenses are made from various soft and rigid materials and are configured in a variety of designs.
- Special design lenses include disposable, colored, astigmatic, aphakic, presbyopic, and keratoconic.
- Initial fitting procedures should fulfill specific general and individual criteria.
- Follow-up care is essential to provide optimum vision, appearance, comfort, and tissue integrity.

ASSOCIATED FEATURES
- Corneal and conjunctival tissue problems.
- Common categories include superficial punctate keratopathy, edema, microcysts, infiltrates, hyperemia, neovascularization, polymegathism, blebs, and giant papillary conjunctivitis.
- Mechanical or physical problems include spectacle blur, flexure, visual flare, aberrations, magnification, accommodation, convergence, and tear fluid effects.

INTRODUCTION

Contact lenses have changed dramatically since their basic optical concept was described first by Leonardo da Vinci in the 16th century and later by René Descartes in the 17th century.[1,2] Many large textbooks are devoted exclusively to the subject of contact lenses; in this chapter an overview is presented.

About 32 million people in the United States wear contact lenses, constituting about 20% of those who use refractive correction.[3] The major use of contacts is to correct myopia, but contact lenses are also used to correct hyperopia, astigmatism, presbyopia, and aphakia. Rigid contact lenses are often the best type to correct for irregular corneal surfaces, as found in keratoconus, corneal trauma, and penetrating keratoplasty and, sometimes, after radial keratotomy. Soft contact lenses may be used as a therapeutic bandage for some conditions, such as bullous keratopathy and recurring corneal erosion, and also to improve comfort, vision, and wound healing in the immediate postoperative period after photorefractive keratectomy.[4]

GENERAL LENS AND MATERIAL TYPES

In terms of their overall lens diameter (LD), contact lens types are classified as
- scleral
- semiscleral (soft)
- corneal

Scleral LD is 23–25mm; the central optic zone diameter is 11.5–13.5mm, peripheral to which is an annular haptic area. The optic zone is fitted to clear slightly the underlying cornea and limbus, and the haptic area has a flatter curvature to align with the underlying sclera.[5] Either a diagnostic trial set is used when contact lenses are fitted or an impression is made of the ocular surface and a lens molded to conform with this. From their original production in the late 19th century up to the late 1950s, only scleral contact lenses were available. Originally, these were made of glass, but in the late 1930s a plastic called polymethyl methacrylate (PMMA) came into general use.[6] Although PMMA has many excellent properties as a contact lens material, it is almost completely impermeable to the gases, such as oxygen, that are essential for normal corneal metabolism. Some currently available scleral lenses are made from rigid gas-permeable (RGP) materials that allow oxygen permeation. Corneal rigid and semiscleral soft lenses are used by the vast majority of patients, but scleral lenses are preferable for some patients who have severe keratoconus, very irregular corneas, and ocular surface disorders such as occur in Stevens–Johnson syndrome.

The development of corneal contact lenses made from PMMA began in about 1950. The LD of these earlier corneal contact lenses was about 11.5mm, whereas contemporary LDs are usually in the range 8.5–9.5mm. In contrast to scleral lenses, corneal lenses are easier to fit because they cover much less of the ocular surface. The smaller area covered also allows better flow of preocular tear fluid and direct access to atmospheric oxygen for the ocular surface not covered by the contact lens. Early corneal contact lenses had a monocurve back surface, or base curve, but this did not allow appropriate conformation to the cornea, which flattens from the apex to the limbus.[7] Contemporary corneal contact lenses usually have bicurve or tricurve back surfaces, wherein the spherical secondary curves are flatter than the back curve toward the periphery of the lens. Aspheric back surface curvatures are sometimes used for better conformation to the aspheric cornea, whose elliptical shape has an eccentricity of about 0.5. Early corneal contact lenses often had a large center thickness; for example, a −3.00D lens had a center thickness of 0.30mm, which is about twice that of contemporary lenses. Since the mid-1970s, PMMA has been copolymerized with silicone and/or fluorocarbons and polyvinylpyrrolidone (PVP) and/or methacrylic acid (MAA) for use in contact lenses.[8] Silicone is highly permeable to oxygen, but it is flexible and hydrophobic, whereas PVP and MAA are hydrophilic. Almost all current corneal contact lenses are RGP materials, and the various brands are formulated with different percentages of PMMA or similar materials, silicone or fluorocarbons, and povidone or MAA. Accordingly, the resultant contact lenses have different characteristics of oxygen permeability, stability and/or flexure, and surface wetting and/or reactivity. These lenses are termed siloxane acrylates or fluorosiloxane acrylates.

The development of soft (hydrogel), semiscleral contact lenses began in the late 1960s and early 1970s.[9] The LDs of soft lenses fall in the range 12.5–15.5mm but most often are 13.5–14.5mm. These lenses are fitted to cover the cornea and limbus and to extend slightly onto the sclera. Soft lenses with LDs similar to those of corneal lenses move excessively, fold, and are uncomfortable.

With the appropriate LD, soft lenses wrap around the ocular surface, which makes them comfortable and easy to fit. The basic material of most soft lenses is hydroxyethyl methacrylate, which is able to absorb fluid.[10] When dehydrated, a soft lens is hard and brittle; after hydration, the lens swells and softens, its thickness and diameter increase, and its refractive index decreases. The combination of various percentages of hydroxyethyl methacrylate, povidone, MAA, and other monomers produces different fluid absorption capacity, strength, and surface reactivity. Low-fluid soft lenses absorb about 38% of their weight in fluid, medium-fluid lenses absorb about 55%, and high-fluid lenses absorb about 70%.

The U.S. Food and Drug Administration (FDA) gives each contact lens material a generic name.[11] In general, all hydrogel lens generic names have the suffix "filcon" and all nonhydrogel lenses, "focon." Hydrogel lenses are categorized into four groups by the FDA to enable the evaluation of effects of accessory products upon the lens material (Table 12-1). Lenses with less than 50% water content are considered to be "low water," and the others are known as "high water." Less reactive surfaces are termed "nonionic," and more reactive materials are labeled "ionic." Disinfection of low water content group 1 and 3 lenses can usually be done safely and effectively using thermal, chemical, or hydrogen peroxide systems. High water content group 2 and group 4 lenses generally should not be disinfected thermally, but chemical and hydrogen peroxide systems usually provide safe and effective disinfection for these.

The Dk (permeability) of hydrogel contact lenses is a function of the water content; materials of lower water content have lower Dk values and those of higher water content higher Dk values. Theoretically, Dk values are an absolute for any given material, but practically the values found by different researchers vary somewhat. A clinically useful approximation is to consider Dk values in three groups (Table 12-2).

It also is important to remember that Dk/L (central transmissibility) and $Dk/\overline{L}$ (average overall transmissibility) are dependent upon lens thickness (L) and are more important than Dk. Minimum center thicknesses for minus-powered soft lenses with different water contents are about 0.03mm for low water, 0.06mm for medium water, and 0.12mm for high water. Thus, the Dk/L is approximately the same, about 30×10^{-9}, for all lenses of minimum center thickness.[12]

In the term Dk, D stands for diffusion and k stands for solubility. The oxygen permeability of soft materials is almost entirely the result of solubility, whereas for RGP materials it is almost entirely the result of diffusion. When fully hydrated, RGP materials absorb less than 1% of their weight in fluid; RGP materials with a Dk less than 20 are low, 20–49 medium, 49–99 high, and over 100 very high. The better materials should have a balance of oxygen permeability, surface wettability and/or reactivity, and stability and/or flexure. Materials of medium Dk provide this best.

For over 20 years, manufacturers have tried to develop contact lenses that combine RGP and soft materials. The goal was to maintain the fit and comfort of soft lenses while significantly increasing the Dk/L. The gas permeability of such combinations comes from both the solubility (k) of soft and the diffusion (D) of RGP materials. In the past few years, silicone-hydrogel lenses have become available in Dk values over 100.

SPECIAL LENSES AND USAGE

Daily wear (DW) contact lenses are worn during the day; after removal, they are cleaned and disinfected. Extended wear (EW) contact lens were to be worn day and night for periods of 1–7 days, which had been the maximum continuous FDA-approved wearing period. They must then be removed, cleaned, and disinfected.[13] In 2001, the FDA approved a lens made from a silicone-hydrogel material for continuous wear of up to 30 days and nights. Since then a second silicone-hydrogel material and an RGP material have also been approved for continuous wear of up to 30 days and nights. Mandatory postmarketing surveillance is required as part of the approval in order to determine the true level of safety and efficacy under real-life conditions and for more patients than were involved in the research required for approval. For example, 5000 "subject years" are required to assess the incidence of microbial keratitis during a 1-year follow-up period. Conventional soft DW and EW lens materials are basically the same, and so too are their Dk/L values. Although these values are generally sufficient for DW, they are about one third of those required for EW.[14] The resultant EW hypoxia and insufficient soft lens hydration and cleanliness during sleep increase significantly the probability of infectious and inflammatory tissue reactions in relation to the continuous duration of wear. For example, microbial keratitis is 10–15 times more common with conventional EW lenses than with DW.[15] The vast majority of contact lens clinical researchers advise most patients against conventional soft lens EW, except for occasional periods of short duration. Some RGP materials have a high enough Dk/L value to satisfy the cornea's oxygen needs with EW; however, owing to problems such as binding and increased corneal distortion, only a small percentage of patients are fitted for RGP EW.

The Dk/L valves of silicone-hydrogels materials seem to be adequate for EW and researchers believe that it is safe for many patients to use them for EW. For example, one of the FDA-approved silicone hydrogels has a Dk of 140 and a water content of 24, whereas another has a Dk of 110 and a water content of 36. The lenses are treated in gas plasma–reactive chambers to transform the hydrophobic to hydrophilic surfaces, which are necessary for good in vivo wetting and resistance to deposit formation.

Disposable Contact Lenses

The use of disposable and programmed replacement soft contact lenses has grown enormously since their introduction in 1986.[16] They, too, are made from the same basic materials as conventional DW and EW soft lenses, and their Dk/L values are also insufficient for EW. Silicone-hydrogel lenses are also available for the programmed replacement regimen. Their uniqueness lies in the manufacturing techniques that produce lenses inexpensively and with relatively good reproducibility; this reduces the per lens cost to patients. Should patients replace their lenses daily, weekly, monthly, quarterly, semiannually, or annually? The answer is different for each patient and is determined by safety, efficacy, economic, and convenience factors.

Colored Lenses

Soft and rigid lenses can have very light tints to improve their visibility when off the eye and to aid the patient in handling

TABLE 12-1

PROPERTIES OF FOOD AND DRUG ADMINISTRATION GROUPS (FDAS) 1–4

Group	Water Content	Surface Reactivity
1	Low	Nonionic
2	High	Nonionic
3	Low	Ionic
4	High	Ionic

TABLE 12-2

USEFUL CLASSIFICATION OF Dk VALUES

Water (%)	Dk (permeability)
c. 38	c. 9
c. 55	c. 18
c. 75	c. 36

them. Soft and rigid lenses that alter the apparent eye color are available in cosmetic enhancement tints for people who have lighter eyes and opaque tints for people who have darker eyes. Such lenses typically have a clear central area of about 4mm for visual purposes and a clear annular peripheral area of about 1mm that overlies the sclera.

Contact Lenses for Astigmatism

Front surface toric rigid lenses and front or back surface toric soft lenses may be used for vision correction in patients who would have 0.75D or more of residual astigmatism if fitted with spherical lenses. Corneal rigid and semiscleral soft lenses rotate on the eye, and proper meridional orientation of the cylinder axis is established primarily by the incorporation of prism and/or thin zones (slab-off) in the lens. Back surface toric rigid lenses may be used to provide better physical matching for corneas that have 2D or more of keratometric astigmatism.[17] Such lenses also require a front surface toricity for vision correction; they are called bitoric lenses.

The amount of astigmatism that remains uncorrected when a contact lens is worn is referred to as residual astigmatism. Several potential reasons exist for residual astigmatism in an eye. Corneal toricity, which can be measured with a keratometer or other corneal surface analyzer, produces a corresponding amount of astigmatism. However, many individuals manifest a different amount of cylinder in their refractive correction. The difference can be ascribed to astigmatism produced by the internal refractive elements of the eye, specifically, the posterior cornea and the crystalline lens. The eyeglass cylindrical correction (referred back to the corneal plane) represents the total astigmatism of the eye. Reiterated differently, the internal astigmatism (A_I) is the difference between the total astigmatism (A_T) of the eye and the corneal astigmatism (A_C), that is, $A_I = A_T - A_C$.

A spherical base curve rigid lens neutralizes the corneal toricity.[18] Residual internal astigmatism occurs when the corneal cylinder has been neutralized. The cylinder present in the spherocylindrical overrefraction results from the internal astigmatism of the eye. Patients who have small amounts of uncorrected astigmatism are often symptom free and are left uncorrected. Individuals who have infrequent symptoms can manage successfully with a pair of spectacles that have the required residual astigmatic correction and that are worn in situations known to provoke eyestrain or blurred vision. Patients who cannot tolerate the uncorrected astigmatism can be refitted with an anterior toric rigid lens that incorporates the correcting cylinder. These lenses are difficult to fit in that they must be axis stabilized with a lens configuration designed to prevent lens rotation.

A toric base curve rigid lens is used to match the corneal toricity in cases in which a spherical base curve is unstable. As a result of the induced cylinder at the base curve–tear layer interface, a toric front surface is almost always required to provide accurate correction. Since the anterior surface power is determined by overrefracting the lens in situ, the correction for internal astigmatism is also incorporated, which results in a lens fit with no residual astigmatism.

Residual induced astigmatism from a toric base curve rigid lens may be corrected by designing a spherical power effect lens for that eye. Since the on-eye back surface cylinder power is about one third the cylinder power of the lens in air, an offsetting front surface cylinder of one third the toricity produces a lens whose total power on the eye is a sphere, irrespective of its rotation.[19] In the same way that a spherical base curve spherical power rigid lens works, the spherical power effect lens corrects only the corneal astigmatism, leaving any internal astigmatism uncorrected.

A spherical base curve soft lens drapes the anterior eye; as a result, the front surface of the lens assumes almost the same toricity as the cornea. A spherocylindrical overrefraction yields approximately the same cylinder power and axis as the spectacle correction. Toric soft lenses have become the method of choice to correct bothersome amounts of residual soft lens astigmatism.

A toric soft lens drapes the eye in the same way that a spherical soft lens does, so no appreciable lacrimal lens and no induced astigmatism occurs at the back surface interface. A toric lens that has the amount and axis of the spectacle cylinder (referred back to the corneal plane) corrects the total astigmatism of the eye. Meridional stabilization is achieved by a variety of lens designs that incorporate prism ballast, thin zones, and eccentric lenticulation.

Soft contact lens materials vary in their water content as well as in their stiffness. Some soft lenses are reputed to work better than others to mask corneal astigmatism. This tendency can be enhanced by using lenses in standard thicknesses rather than in ultrathin designs.

Contact Lens Asphericity

Both rigid and soft lenses can be manufactured with aspheric curves. Back surface aspheric lenses were originally designed to provide a closer approximation to the aspheric surface of the cornea. They are also used to provide a progressive "add" effect for use as multifocal lenses. Several different shapes have been used as aspheric base curves. Ellipses most closely represent the shape of the corneal contour. The variable used to select an ellipse is its rate of flattening, the eccentricity. The range of eccentricities is from zero, which represents a circle, to over 1.0. The greater the back surface eccentricity, the greater the amount of plus power that is produced in the midperipheral area of the lens. Often, manufacturers describe the asphericity of their lenses in terms of the amount of add produced.

Other forms of aspheric back curves include the sphere-aspheric, the biaspheric, the sphere-cone, and the offset periphery designs. Soft lenses can be produced with aspheric curves by a spin-cast technique, molding, or lathing. Front aspheric lenses are used to provide a continuous change in power from the center to the periphery of the lens. This gradual steepening produces a progressive multifocal effect in which plus power decreases from the center to the periphery.

Contact Lenses for Presbyopia

The 60-year-old concepts of alternating and simultaneous vision still provide the basis of contact lens design for presbyopia.[20] Most alternating vision bifocal lenses have a prism to stop lens rotation and small optic zone diameters, superior for distance and inferior for near. As with eyeglass multifocal lenses, it is intended that the patient's fixation alternates between the zones as needed for specific tasks. With simultaneous vision, the patient's pupils are covered partially and simultaneously with optic zones that contain both the required distant and near powers. One type of simultaneous lens design incorporates a small central zone and an annular zone that surrounds this. The central zone may have either the distance or near power; the annular zone has the opposite power. Newer simultaneous lens designs have a series of four or five concentric zones in which distance, near, or intermediate powers are alternated. The goal is to provide consistent pupillary coverage by these various powers as the lens moves or the pupil diameter changes. A second type of simultaneous design uses either front or back surface aspheric curvature to produce a somewhat progressive power change from the center to the periphery of the optic zone. The third type of simultaneous vision approach uses single vision lenses, with one eye given the distant and the other eye the near correction, that is, monovision. Generally, alternating vision is preferable with rigid corneal lens bifocals and simultaneous vision is preferable with soft lens bifocals. However, the exact positioning and movement required for good vision are not attained for many patients. Success is much greater with distant single vision contact lenses and reading glasses or with single vision monovision contact lenses. With monovision, usually the patient's dominant eye has the distance prescription and the other eye has the near prescription.[21] A fourth type of simultaneous vision uses the optical pinhole concept. A single power between the patient's distance and near corrections is used to focus vision. The pinhole increases the depth of focus so that all objects from infinity to a practical near distance are imaged adequately on the retina. Pinhole diameter is usually selected from 1.5 to 2.0mm to balance image clarity, brightness, and visual field. A narrow ring surrounded by a clear zone has been used to create the central pinhole to enhance brightness and field.

Contact lens wear places a demand on the ocular surface, which is not always accepted by presbyopes. The aging presbyopic eye, with its many changes of anatomy and physiology, is even less likely to accept this demand.[22] With aging, a reduction of the quantity and quality of the precorneal fluid typically occurs because of decreased lacrimal aqueous tear production and meibomian gland lipid tear production. Eyelid tonus decreases, which decreases spreading of precorneal fluid and may cause various degrees of ectropion. Pupil diameters decrease, and the pupillary response to stimuli becomes sluggish. The crystalline lens loses transparency, the retina's nerve fiber layer becomes thinner, some optic nerve fibers atrophy, and the macula may degenerate. These internal ocular changes simultaneously decrease the quantity and quality of light that reaches the retina and its ability to receive and transmit images properly.

Unusual Back Surfaces

Very unusual corneal topography, which can occur with keratoconus, after penetrating keratoplasty, and after radial keratotomy, requires specialized back surface configurations of rigid or soft lenses to conform better to the corneal shape. Specialized back surface configuration rigid lens designs are also available for orthokeratology.[23] This somewhat controversial procedure uses rigid lenses to reshape the cornea and to reduce myopia. Orthokeratology is safe in that it does not produce significant undesired corneal problems, but its efficacy to produce the desired corneal reshaping and myopia reduction is limited. In general, myopia is reduced by less than 2D, the results are not permanent, and so-called retainer lenses must be worn for many hours a week. Newer reverse geometry design lenses may prove to increase myopia reduction to 4 or 5 diopters. Wearing orthokeratology lenses during sleep is being investigated to determine whether this method provides safety and efficacy while eliminating the need to wear lenses during waking hours.

INITIAL FITTING

Two general methods exist to fit contact lenses. First, in the measurement and standard procedures used to determine the parameters, readings are taken of the corneal curvature using keratometry or videokeratography and measurements are made of the horizontal iris diameter, vertical palpebral aperture, and pupil diameter. These findings then are related to nomograms to determine the contact lens parameters to be ordered. Second, in the diagnostic lens procedure, the preceding measurements are made initially. Next, the appropriate lens is selected from the practitioner's contact lens trial set, inserted on the patient's eye, and allowed to settle for 15–20min. With corneal lenses this is necessary so that the initial lacrimation decreases; with soft lenses it is necessary because the temperature on the eye is greater than the ambient temperature, which forces fluid out of the lens (i.e., the lens must equilibrate).[24] Then the position, movement, and relationship between the back surface of the contact lens and the front surface of the eye are evaluated in relation to criteria for a good fit.

Corneal lenses are fitted for either superior positioning or intrapalpebral aperture positioning. For either of these (with pri-

mary fixation) the lens should be centered horizontally and its lower edge should be at least 1–2mm above the lower eyelid. The upper edge with a superior positioning lens should be under the upper eyelid, but not over the superior limbus, and with intrapalpebral positioning the upper edge should be just below the upper eyelid. With blinking, the lens should move 1–2mm, return to its original resting point, and remain there during the interphase between blinks.

The relationship between the back surface of the lens and the front surface of the cornea is evaluated after sodium fluorescein has been applied.[25] Fluorescein mixes with the preocular film between the lens and the cornea and, when activated with a "black light," it fluoresces with specific patterns. When the curves of the lens are very different from those of the cornea, the precorneal fluid is deeper and the fluorescence is a brighter yellowish green. Conversely, closer alignment of lens and corneal curves produces a shallow precorneal fluid, less fluorescence, and a bluish black appearance. For corneas that have less than 1.5D of astigmatism, the desired optic zone pattern is blue-black or a very mild, uniform yellow-green and the desired secondary zone pattern is a moderately bright yellow-green (Figs. 12-1 to 12-3).

Soft lenses should cover the cornea fully and be relatively centered around it; they should move 1–2mm with blinking. Fluorescein is not used with soft lenses as they absorb the dye. Direct evaluation with large-molecule diagnostic dyes (such as fluorexon) has not proved to be a significantly useful method for evaluating the relationship of posterior radius to cornea curve. Indirect methods of evaluation include keratometry, retinoscopy, and the subjective report of stability of vision.[26] The goal is to obtain a fit that provides a clear, consistent mire, retinoscopy reflex, refraction, and vision. A steep lens (too large a sag or vault) between blinks theoretically shows distorted or irregular keratometry mires, a central dark spot in the retinoscopy reflex, and blurred vision. Directly after blinks, these responses improve for a short time and then revert. A flat lens (too small a sag or vault) between blinks theoretically shows slightly distorted keratometric mires, an inferior dark spot in the retinoscopic reflex, and fairly good vision. Directly after blinks, these responses worsen for a short time and then improve. Poor keratometric mires, as well as poor retinoscopy reflex or vision, can result from a dry lens surface. The patient is asked to blink four or five times to help differentiate this condition from an improperly fitted lens.

The edge of the lens may provide information about the sag of the lens. An edge that turns away from the eye between blinks often indicates a flat lens. An edge that bears heavily against the cornea or bulbar conjunctiva often indicates a steep lens; also, using a slit lamp, blanching of the conjunctival vessels or conjunctival "drag" may be observed with a steep lens.

The position and movement of a soft lens provide information about the sag of the lens on the eye; clinically, these data are the most frequently used in this context. A lens that decenters or has excessive movement is often too flat, and the converse applies to a lens that is too steep. If lens position, movement, or back surface fitting relationship does not meet the criteria, trial lenses with different parameters are inserted and the evaluation is repeated. After the appropriate fit is attained, the necessary power is determined. This is done by computation or by refraction over the trial lens *in situ*.

After the spherical power of a contact lens has been calculated, the effect of vertex distance needs to be considered. In myopia, the strength of a spectacle correction lens is greater than the correction required at the corneal plane. Conversely, the power of a spectacle lens for hyperopia is less than the lens power required at the cornea. The effects are not significant until about 4D of correction is required. Tables that list the appropriate vertex compensation are readily available.

In fitting rigid lenses with a spherical base curve, the "lacrimal lens" fills in the space between the cornea and the back surface of the lens. Because the toricity of the cornea is

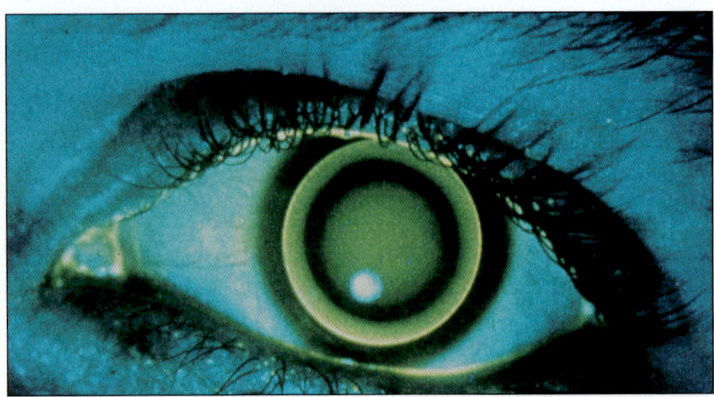

FIG. 12-1 ■ Fluorescein pattern of corneal contact lens fitted 1D steeper than "flat K." Note the central clearance.

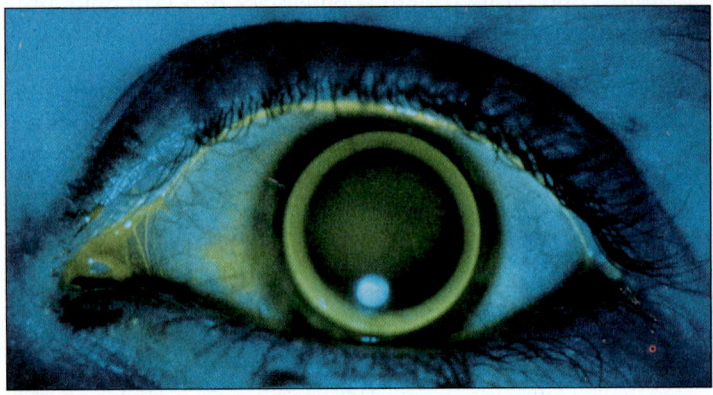

FIG. 12-2 ■ Fluorescein pattern of corneal contact lens fitted "on K." Note the central alignment.

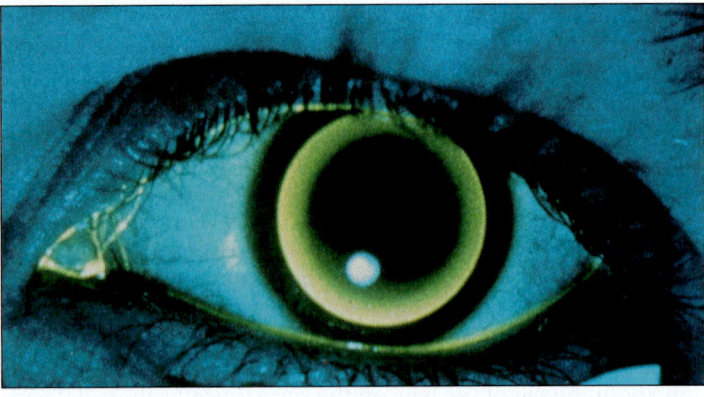

FIG. 12-3 ■ Fluorescein pattern of corneal contact lens fitted 1D flatter than flat K. Note the central touch.

filled in by the lacrimal lens, thus neutralizing the corneal cylinder, the flattest corneal meridian (flat K) becomes the reference for optical calculations.[27] Compared with the radius of flat K, a lens base curve is "on K" (i.e., the same radius as the flat meridian), "steeper than K," or "flatter than K." A lens on K has a plano power lacrimal lens; a steeper than K lens has a plus power lacrimal lens; and a lens that is flatter than K has a minus power lacrimal lens. A rule of thumb commonly used to compare dioptral adjustments from changes in base curve is that a 0.05mm change in radius produces a 0.25D change in overall refractive power.

In fitting soft contact lenses with a spherical base curve, little or no lacrimal lens exists because the back surface tends to drape the cornea.[28] Therefore very little neutralization of the corneal cylinder occurs. However, soft lenses that may be somewhat stiffer than most, because of their material and thickness, may manifest some mild lacrimal lens effects.

FOLLOW-UP CARE

A contact lens is a foreign, plastic object placed on the ocular surface; therefore, patients must be instructed properly in effective lens care and in the necessity of follow-up visits. These are more frequent during the earlier stages of wear, but visits at least annually are necessary for the duration of lens wear. Some problems may occur during the first few weeks, others during the first 6 months, and still others over years of wear. Follow-up examinations include evaluations of history, vision, lens fit, tissue integrity, patient compliance, and lens physical structure.

A contact lens may be considered to be an optical patch and bandage.[29] As a patch, it reduces the availability of oxygen to and the dissipation of carbon dioxide from the cornea. As a bandage, it creates pressure on the underlying tissues and reduces wetting of the ocular surface and dissipation of material from between the contact lens and the cornea. It may also become contaminated with organic and inorganic deposits and become scratched, chipped, or ripped. The patch effect creates different amounts of hypoxia and interference with the cornea's normal aerobic metabolic cycle. This leads to edema, decrease of glycogen reserves, and increase of lactic acid dehydrogenase.[30] The last decreases the cornea's pH, which may result in stromal and endothelial reactions. The bandage effect may lead to problems of desiccation, mechanical abrasion, and chemical reaction with solutions and toxins from the breakdown of trapped debris.

A large body of knowledge of basic science and clinical research has been gathered over the past 30 years concerning the corneal and conjunctival complications caused by contact lens wear. The following information is based on these data. For newer design contact lenses that combine silicone and hydrogel materials and have *Dk* values over 100, much less research and clinical history are available. This is discussed separately after the general discussion of corneal and conventional tissue problems.

Corneal and Conjunctival Tissue Problems

Given here are very brief discussions of the more common corneal and conjunctival tissue problems related to contact lens wear.

SUPERFICIAL PUNCTATE KERATOPATHY. Corneal staining occurs when sodium fluorescein is retained in gaps on the epithelial surface; these are caused by the absence, damage, displacement, or breakdown of cells. Staining related to contact lenses commonly results from mechanical trauma, exposure desiccation, metabolic interference, or chemical toxicity and/or hypersensitivity. Mild staining may be asymptomatic, but as the epithelial disruption increases, discomfort, pain, increased lacrimation, and photophobia are reported. With extensive and deeper epithelial disruption, fluorescein may enter the corneal stroma.

Mechanical trauma may be caused by a foreign body while it moves between the contact lens and the cornea; by a foreign body that wedges against the cornea; by a torn, scratched, or coated contact lens; or by fingernails during lens insertion or removal. Metabolic interference caused by hypoxia may break down or change the selective permeability of epithelial cells over a wide corneal area. Exposure desiccation with corneal lenses may result in staining around the 3 and 9 o'clock positions or inferior corneal areas. Chemical toxicity and/or hypersensitivity staining is most often a result of reactions against contact lens solutions or lens deposits and substances adherent to the deposits. Severe epithelial disorder associated with solution toxicity and/or hypersensitivity can result in pseudodendrites, which appear as raised gray epithelial plaques with serpentine shapes and light staining, or superior limbic keratoconjunctivitis, which is manifest as an inflammatory reaction of the superior cornea and adjacent bulbar conjunctiva (Fig. 12-4).[31] A deep or broad

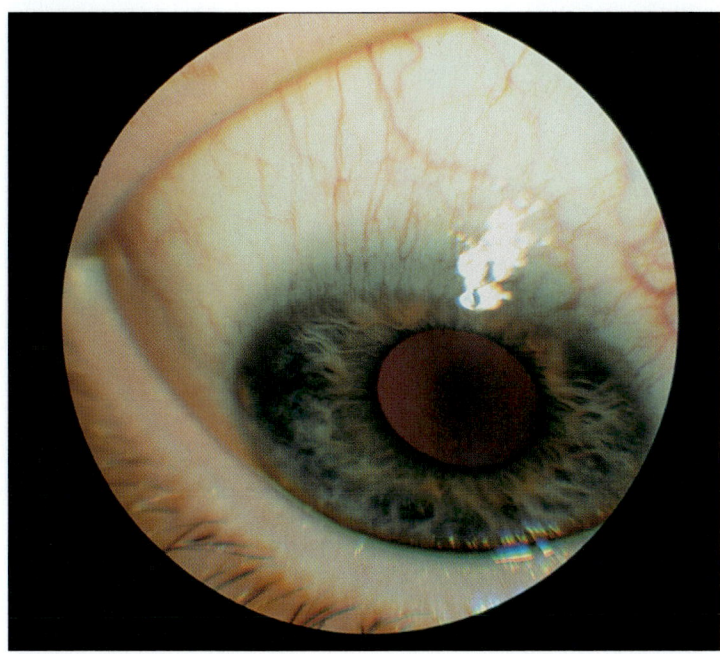

FIG. 12-4 ■ **Superior limbic keratoconjunctivitis.** This is most often caused by a reaction to thimerosal.

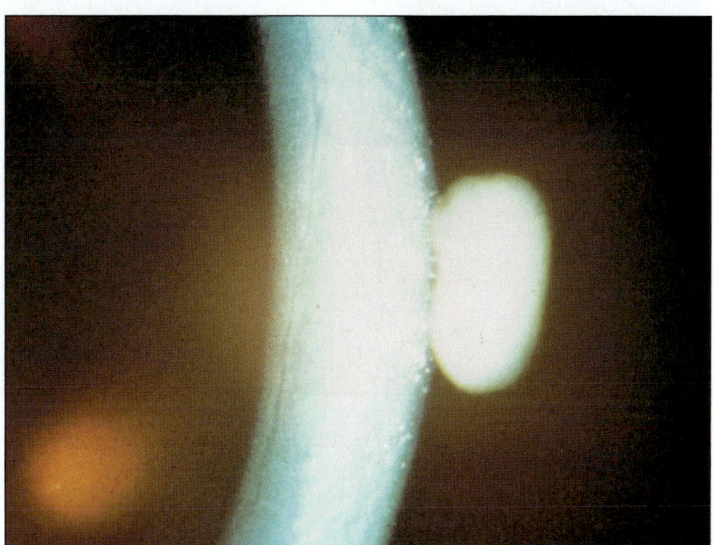

FIG. 12-5 ■ **Endothelial folds.** These folds often have a vertical orientation.

area of epithelial disruption reduces the epithelium's ability to function as a barrier to infection, which may lead to ulcerative keratitis. The incidence of microbial keratitis is very small with DW, RGP corneal or soft contact lenses but it is much greater with soft EW lenses, for which *Pseudomonas aeruginosa* is the pathogen most frequently involved.[32]

EDEMA. Hypoxia is the primary reason for corneal stroma edema induced by contact lens wear, but a hypotonic preocular tear film may also contribute. With PMMA or very low *Dk/L* RGP corneal lenses, edema is manifest as a gross, circumscribed, whitish gray area.[33] Termed *central circular clouding*, it appears around the point at which the center of the optic zone positions in primary fixation. To view it, a split-limbal technique is used with the slit-lamp biomicroscope; the area in question is viewed by the practitioner not looking through the microscope and against the black background of the pupil. As the central circular clouding moves from grade 1 to grade 3, the coloration deepens, the borders become more distinct, and the epithelium stains. With soft contact lenses, edema does not present clinically as central circular clouding but rather is detected by the appearance of striae in the posterior stroma when the corneal thickness has increased by about 6% and of endothelial folds when corneal thickness has increased by about 10% or more (Fig. 12-5).[34] Rigid or soft DW lenses seldom change corneal thickness to these degrees, with the exception of PMMA lenses, but the vast majority of patients who use soft EW lenses awaken with at least a 10% corneal thickness increase.[35] Striae are fine, grayish white, short lines in the posterior stroma. It is believed that these are the result of a refractive effect that arises from the fluid separation of vertically orientated collagen fibrils and posterior stroma. Endothelial folds appear as a "buckling" of the posterior corneal layers; when observed with specular reflection they appear as dark lines and with direct illumination as bright lines.

MICROCYSTS. Microcysts induced by contact lens wear are probably pockets of dead cellular material that form adjacent to intraepithelial sheets at the epithelium's basement membrane; these are clinical evidence of disorganized cell growth that results from significant hypoxia.[36] Microcysts viewed with a slit-lamp biomicroscope display reversed illumination; that is, the distribution of light within the microcysts is opposite to that of the background. They appear as small and irregularly scattered dots, which must be differentiated from dimple indentation and

vacuole fluid pockets. Microcysts very frequently accompany soft EW lens use but may not be manifest for the first several months. As microcysts work through the epithelial surface, corneal staining is seen. When soft lens EW is discontinued, the number of microcysts initially increases and then diminishes until elimination, over about 2 months.[37]

INFILTRATES. Infiltrates induced by contact lens wear are accumulations of white blood cells between the corneal stroma's collagen fibers; the accumulation occurs as a result of hypoxia, chemical toxicity and/or hypersensitivity, decomposition of debris trapped between the contact lens and cornea, denatured proteins, or exotoxins.[38] The infiltrates appear as white or whitish gray, single or multiple foci in the anterior stroma; more often, they are located toward the limbus. Small or few infiltrates may be asymptomatic, but greater infiltration causes discomfort, pain, photophobia, and lacrimation. Superior limbic keratoconjunctivitis is accompanied by many microinfiltrates in the superior cornea. In contact lens acute red eye syndrome, there are larger infiltrates on various segments of the peripheral cornea.[39] This syndrome is most often caused by soft EW lenses—patients awaken with cellular debris trapped behind an immobile lens. It is probable that decomposition of the debris releases enzymes and other necrotic wastes that then act as chemotoxic stimuli for cell migration from the adjacent limbal vessels, which are very hyperemic with this painful inflammation (Fig. 12-6).

HYPEREMIA AND NEOVASCULARIZATION. Sectorial hyperemia usually accompanies 3 and 9 o'clock desiccation staining and peripheral corneal infiltrates, ulcers, or abrasions. More generalized circumcorneal hyperemia may be caused by hypoxia and other inflammatory stimuli (e.g., chemical, osmotic, and physical). Adjacent to the limbus, a normal area of physiological edema occurs and within this is the normal corneal vasculature, which typically extends a little further onto the superior cornea. The rest of the cornea is avascular because its structure is too compact to allow vessel growth. However, degradation of corneal metabolism and its sequela of edema loosen the structure with the result that neovascularization may occur from secondary stimuli. Neovascularization related to contact lens wear involves the superficial vessels much more often than the deeper vessels.[39] It is uncommon for neovascularization induced by contact lenses to extend onto the cornea by more than 2–3mm. After proper management, the vessels

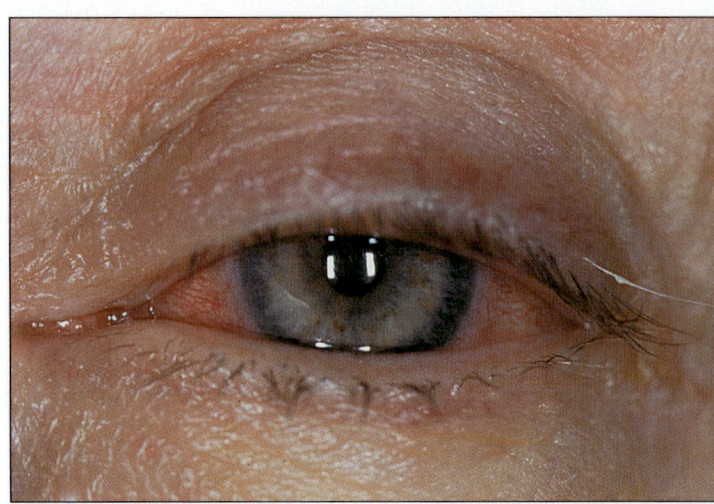

FIG. 12-6 ■ **Contact lens acute red eye.** This is often accompanied by pain and photophobia.

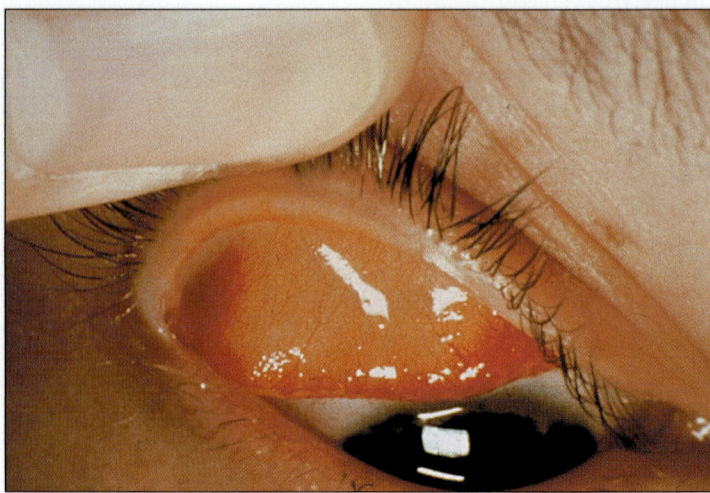

FIG. 12-7 ■ **Grade one giant papillary conjunctivitis.** Note the mild hyperemia and mucus.

empty, but the vessel wall remains. These ghost vessels appear as faint white lines when observed with indirect illumination, and they remain for years. Subsequent mild stimuli may refill the vessels with blood.

POLYMEGATHISM AND BLEBS. Sufficient hypoxia and chronic corneal acidosis can cause variation in endothelial cell size (polymegathism), as viewed with specular reflection and very high magnification.[40] After proper management to reduce or eliminate the causes, the endothelial mosaic usually normalizes. Endothelial blebs constitute intracellular edema that develops with sufficient hypoxia and acidosis; they usually occur in unadapted soft lens wearers and may be a precursor of polymegathism.[41] In specular reflection, blebs appear as black spots and resemble corneal guttae.

GIANT PAPILLARY CONJUNCTIVITIS. Papillary conjunctivitis induced by contact lens wear is usually termed *giant papillary conjunctivitis.*[42] It is caused primarily by mechanical irritation of the superior tarsal conjunctiva and secondarily by an autoimmune reaction to the patient's mucoproteins on the lens. Normal micropapillae have a diameter of less than 0.3mm, macropapillae have a diameter of 0.4–0.9mm, and giant papillae have a diameter of 1mm or greater. The enlarged papillae are collections of lymphocytes and plasma cells. In addition to the enlarged papillae, papillary conjunctivitis induced by contact lens wear is characterized by hyperemia, reduced transparency, and increased production of mucus by the tarsal conjunctiva (Fig. 12-7). Patients' symptoms include decreased comfort, increased lens movement, hazy vision, and itchiness. Signs and symptoms increase directly with the severity of papillary conjunctivitis.[43] Mast cell stabilizers may be used to reduce symptoms, but elimination of the causes is necessary. This requires improved care of the lenses, more frequent lens replacement, and reduced wearing time.

Silicone Hydrogel Lenses

The highly oxygen-permeable silicone hydrogel lenses have eliminated physiological changes resulting from hypoxia for a vast majority of patients. Overnight edema levels approximate those detected with no contact lens wear. Other hypoxia-related contact lens–induced tissue changes such as corneal striae, microcysts, and endothelial polymegathisms are rarely seen. Limbal redness, vascularization, and the myopic shift commonly observed with the wear of conventional soft EW lenses are reduced in incidence and severity.[44]

Microbial keratitis is the most serious and potentially sight-threatening complication from contact lens wear. It is hypothesized that hypoxia from EW with conventional soft lenses leads to severe metabolic stress in the closed-eye environment. This produces a thin, weakened, poorly metabolizing epithelium, which in turn allows pathogenic microorganisms to invade the cornea and cause microbial keratitis. The high oxygen transmissibility of those silicone hydrogel lenses maintains a healthy corneal epithelium. Thus the eye's defenses are not compromised and protect against infection. Microbial keratitis is of much lower incidence with silicone hydrogel lenses compared with conventional soft lenses worn for EW.[45]

The rates of inflammatory conditions between silicone hydrogel and conventional soft lenses worn for EW are similar. These inflammatory conditions include contact lens acute red eye, infiltrative keratitis, and contact lens peripheral ulcer. Some mechanically induced tissue changes are greater with silicone hydrogel lenses. These include giant papillary conjunctivitis, superior epithelial arcuate lesion, and corneal erosion.[46]

Mechanical or Physical Problems

The evaluation of a patient's overall vision during contact lens follow-up examinations involves not only the proper correction of spherical and astigmatic refractive errors but also other factors specific to contact lenses or to the difference between contact lenses and spectacles.

SPECTACLE BLUR. Contact lens wear can temporarily alter the prescription that a patient requires for spectacles.[47] This is the result of mechanical pressure applied to the corneal surface and both corneal edema. This so-called spectacle blur is found more often in association with rigid lenses, which produce greater mechanical pressure than soft lenses. Spectacle blur with soft lens wear is usually a result of corneal edema; it is often manifest as the need for increased minus or decreased plus power in both the contact lens and eyeglass prescriptions. The induced spectacle blur with rigid lenses is much less predictable, as both the spherical and cylindrical corrections needed in eyeglasses may vary in both the directionality and quantity of change required.[48] However, usually no change in the required contact lens power occurs because the lacrimal lens compensates optically for the induced corneal topographic changes.

FLEXURE. Flexure is the tendency of a contact lens, either rigid or soft, to bend in response to internal or external forces. Regular flexure produces a symmetrical change with primary meridians 90° apart. Usually, the resultant change in refraction can be corrected using conventional spherocylindrical lenses. Irregular flexure produces an alteration in lens shape and refraction for which no simple optical resolution exists.

Constant flexure, such as occurs with a spherical soft lens on a toric cornea, gives a consistent refractive measurement.

Intermittent flexure, such as occurs when a thin, spherical rigid lens is placed on a toric cornea, can vary in its presence and amount. The "plastic memory" of the lens and the capillary attraction of the cornea to the lens can cause fluctuations in the toricity of the contact lens. Intermittent flexure can occur in soft lenses when the base curve is steeper than the corneal curvature. The soft material can pucker in the center, which results in optical distortion that cannot be resolved with correcting lenses. The lid compresses the lens, forcing it against the cornea during a blink, and sharp vision may result until the lens memory causes a return to the steeper, but distorted, curve.

Irregular flexure commonly occurs when a soft lens dehydrates below its normal water content. This can happen if the lens is allowed to dry out when it is not being worn. It can also occur with the lens on the eye as a result of a drier than normal environment, incomplete or infrequent blinking, or simply alterations in the polymer structure caused by age, coating, and handling. It is less common for a rigid lens that is well cared for to have irregular flexure.

Rigid materials vary in their innate resistance to flexure. Lenses made of PMMA are very stable, even when produced in thin designs. Siloxane acrylate and fluorosiloxane acrylate, although used much more frequently for rigid lenses because of their gas permeability, have a greater tendency to flex on the eye. Other characteristics that influence rigid lens flexure are thickness and fit. A lens that has an average thickness is stabler than the same lens in a thin design. Empirically, it has been found that a lens fit approximately 0.15mm flatter than K tends to flex less than a lens fit on K or steeper than K.

Lid pressure may compress temporarily a soft lens that does not drape the cornea and so produce sharp vision. In between blinks, vision may distort again. With a flexible rigid lens, blinking may compress the steeper meridian to match the toricity of the cornea, which results in blurred vision. When the lens rebounds to its spherical shape between blinks, normal vision returns. Rigid lenses can also undergo flexure because of poor handling techniques. Holding a lens by its edges may flex the lens sufficiently to maintain some toricity when the lens is placed on the cornea.

Rigid lens flexure, which results from any of the situations discussed above, can produce residual induced astigmatism. A spherical base curve lens that flexes on the eye produces an astigmatic refraction at the base curve–tear layer interface. The corresponding front surface warpage produces an offsetting, but stronger, amount of induced astigmatism. Transient flexure is difficult to identify with the lens on the eye because of the continual rotation with blinking. Keratometry of the front surface of the lens may show an inconsistent reading in one meridian. A warped lens can be identified by analysis of the base curve using a radiuscope or other reflective analyzer. A toric base curve rigid lens may suffer from the same flexure problems, but these are more difficult to recognize because of the toric nature of the curves.

Soft lens flexure, whether in a spherical or in a toric lens, usually results from a lens whose base curve is too steep for the particular eye. The vault produces an irregular flexure in the center of the lens, which may be alleviated temporarily after the lid has compressed the lens during a blink. Shape memory causes the curve to rebound after the blink is completed. This condition can be identified by observing the retinoscopy reflex during a blink. The reflex changes from a well-delineated pupillary reflex to one that has central distortion. The keratometry reflex from the front of the lens also may show fluctuations during a blink.

VISUAL FLARE. Flare is the symptom of peripheral reflections that occur when the optic zone of the lens is smaller than the pupil.[49] Light can reflect from the junction between the base curve and secondary curve. Because the secondary curve is usually flatter than the base curve, more plus refraction through that zone results, which is often seen as a halo around objects. Flare can also be induced by junctions on front surface curves, such as lenticulars, but these usually occur peripheral to the back surface

junctions. A lens may malposition so markedly that the edge of the lens may infringe upon the pupil.

ABERRATIONS. In all spherical refraction systems, nonparaxial light rays are refracted more than the rays that follow the principal axis; this produces linear spherical aberration. The amount of aberration is related to the power of the lens system and the distance from the principal axis of the incident ray. Remarkably, the eye is corrected for spherical aberration. However, the asphericity of the cornea is neutralized by any lacrimal lens that may form beneath a contact lens.[50] Empirically, no observable decrement in vision seems to occur from this aberration. Early research is being done to use custom-shaped contact lens surfaces to correct the unique higher order-aberrations of each eye that can be determined using wave-front analysis technology.

Dispersion of the spectral wavelengths of light during refraction is termed chromatic aberration. All single-lens refraction systems suffer some degree of chromatic aberration, depending on the power and the index of the lens. Materials used in contact lenses are of relatively low index compared with those used for glass spectacle lenses. Chromatic aberration has not proved to be a clinical problem in the contact lens field.

MAGNIFICATION. Contact lenses and spectacles induce different magnifications,[51] which has practical application for high refractive errors. High hyperopes, especially aphakics, have significant magnification with their eyeglasses. For example, a +10.00D lens produces a magnification of 19%. The equivalent contact lens produces a magnification of 4%. This affects directly the ability to gauge depth but is of more significance when the strong correction is in one eye only. The magnification differences produced by high anisometropic corrections are usually minimized with contact lens wear.

This property can also be useful in cases of high astigmatism. The same principles of magnification apply unilaterally to each meridian of the correcting lens. In spectacle corrections, usually a large difference in the magnification occurs along the principal meridians, which produces a sensation of distortion. A contact lens produces less difference, with a corresponding reduction in distortion.

ACCOMMODATION AND CONVERGENCE. Lens effectiveness, which is a measure based on the distance of a correcting lens from the nodal point of the eye, produces a change in the amount of accommodation required to see at near with glasses compared with that with contact lenses. A myope who wears contact lenses must accommodate more than when wearing glasses. Conversely, a hyperope requires less accommodation with contacts than with spectacles.[52] This must be considered when an individual with marginal accommodative insufficiency, such as an incipient presbyope, is being fitted.

Convergence requirements are altered when a change is made from glasses to contact lenses. A myope, when converging through spectacles, has an induced base-in effect and has to converge more than is required with contact lenses. A hyperope, on the other hand, has a base-out effect when converging through glasses and requires less convergence effort than is required with contact lenses. Contact lenses, because they remain centered on the eye, do not induce any prismatic effect upon convergence.

FLUID EFFECTS. The optics of a contact lens are predicated on the transparency of the medium. Rigid lenses do not absorb measurable amounts of fluids, whereas the transparency of hydrogel lenses is dependent upon maintenance of the proper water content. As a hydrogel lens ages or is exposed to extreme conditions, the fluid content may diminish and affect the transmission of light. Often, this is observed in untinted lenses as a yellowish or gray cast when the lens is viewed against a white background. Such lenses should be replaced.

Loss of transparency within the cornea that is related to contact lens wear can also result from corneal edema. In rigid lens wear, fluid tends to accumulate in the area covered by the optic zone and is referred to as corneal central edema. As a result of the widespread use of gas-permeable materials, corneal central edema is now an infrequent occurrence. In soft lens wear, the edema tends to be more diffuse and spreads across the entire cornea. Most contemporary soft lens designs use a combination of gas permeability and thickness to create minimal corneal hypoxia.

Uneven surface-wetting characteristics cause uneven refraction of light and produce a degraded image. This can occur as a result of scratches, crazing of the even surface from chemical exposure, incomplete cleaning, or an insufficient or unstable tear film.

REFERENCES

1. da Vinci L. Codex of the eye. Manuscript D (circa 1508). For translation and illustration, see Hofstetter HW, Graham R. Leonardo and contact lenses. Am J Optom. 1953;30(1):41–4.
2. Descartes R. Methods of correcting vision. In: Descartes R, ed. Discours de la methode, 1636, Discours 7, La dioptrique, p 147 (in French). For translation and illustrations, see Enoch JM. Descartes' contact lens. Am J Optom. 1956;33(2):7–85.
3. Kanely J. Trends in lens care 1996. Rochester, NY: Bausch and Lomb; 1996:1–2.
4. McDonald MB, Kaufman HE, Frantz JM, et al. Excimer laser ablation in a human eye. Arch Ophthalmol. 1989;107:641–2.
5. Braff SM. Scleral lenses. J Am Optom Assoc. 1976;47:321–5.
6. Feinbloom W. A plastic contact lens chronicle. Am J Optom Arch Am Acad Optom. 1937;14:41.
7. Muth EP. Kevin Michael Tuohy, optician, the father of modern contact lenses. Opt Prism. 1987;7(Sept/Oct):42–8.
8. Bailey NJ. Neal Bailey's contact lens chronicle. Contact Lens Spectrum. 1987;2:29–34.
9. Wichterle O, Lim D. Hydrophilic gels for biological use. Nature. 1960;185:117–21.
10. Mandell RB. Contact lens practice, 4th ed, Ch 1. Springfield, IL: Thomas; 1988.
11. White P, Scott C. Contact lenses and solutions summary. Fort Washington, Pa: Cardinal Business Media, No 10, 2002.
12. White P, Scott C. Contact lenses and solutions summary. Fort Washington, Pa: Cardinal Business Media, No 10, 2002.
13. Lippman R. In: Bennett E, Weissman B, eds. FDA regulations: contact lens applications in clinical contact lens practice, Ch 71. Philadelphia: Lippincott; 1996:1–20.
14. Fatt I, Bieber MT. The steady-state distribution of oxygen and carbon dioxide in the in vivo cornea 1. The open eye in air and the closed eye. Exp Eye Res. 1968;7:103–9.
15. Schein O, Glynn R, Poggio E, et al. The relative risk of ulcerative keratitis among users of daily wear and extended wear soft contact lenses. N Engl J Med. 1989;32:773–80.
16. White P. Disposable and programmed replacement soft contact lenses. Contact Lens Spectrum. 1994;8(May):40–52.
17. Bailey NJ. Residual astigmatism with contact lenses. Arch Soc Am Ophthalmol Optom. 1959;11(1):37–41.
18. Sarver MD. Fluid lens power effect with contact lenses. Am J Optom. 1962;39(8):434–7.
19. Sarver MD. Calculation of the optical specifications of contact lenses. Am J Optom. 1963;40(1):20–8.
20. Harris MG, Sheedy JE, Gan CM. Vision and task performance with monovision and diffractive bifocal contact lenses. Optom Vis Sci. 1992;69(8):609–14.
21. Fleischman WE. The single vision reading contact lens. Am J Optom Physiol Opt. 1968;45:408–9.
22. White P, Watanabe R. Presbyopic contact lens care. Contact Lens Spectrum. 1996;10(Aug):34–40.
23. Carney L. Orthokeratology. In Guillon M, Ruben CM, eds. Contact lens practice. London: Chapman and Hall; 1994:877–88.
24. Andrasko G. The amount and time course of soft contact lens dehydration. J Am Optom Assoc. 1982;53:207.
25. Obrig TE. Contact lenses, 2nd ed. Philadelphia: Chilton; 1947:153.
26. Young G. Soft lens fitting reassessed. Contact Lens Spectrum. 1992;7(12):56–61.
27. Bennett ES. Basic fitting. In Bennett ES, Weissman BA, eds. Clinical contact lens practice. Philadelphia: Lippincott; 1991:1–22.
28. Caroline PJ, Norman CW. A blueprint for rigid lens design: part I. Contact Lens Spectrum. 1988;3(11):39–49.
29. White P. What is the safe duration of extended wear? Contact Lens Spectrum. 1990;4(Feb):6–63.
30. Tomlinson A. Oxygen requirements of the cornea. In Tomlinson A, ed. Complications of contact lens wear. St Louis: Mosby; 1992:3–20.
31. Kame RT. Limbal epithelial hypertrophy. Int Contact Lens Clin. 1987;14:453.
32. Mondino BJ, Weisman BA, Farb MD, Pettit TH. Corneal ulcers associated with daily-wear and extended-wear contact lenses. Am J Ophthalmol. 1986;102:58–65.
33. Korb DR, Exford JM. The phenomenon of central circular clouding. J Am Optom Assoc. 1968;39:223–30.
34. Holden BA, Mertz GW, McNally JJ. Corneal swelling responses to contact lenses worn under extended wear conditions. Assoc Res Vision Ophthalmol. 1983;24:218–26.
35. Zantos SG, Holden BA. Transient endothelial changes soon after wearing contact lenses. Am J Optom Physiol Opt. 1977;54:856–8.
36. Zantos SG. Cystic formations in the corneal epithelium during extended wear of contact lenses. Int Contact Lens Clin. 1983;10:128–35.
37. Madigan MC, Holden BA, Kwok LS. Extended wear of hydrogel contact lenses can compromise the corneal epithelium. Invest Ophthalmol Vis Sci. 1986;27(Suppl):140–7.
38. Gordon A, Kracher GP. Corneal infiltrates and extended-wear contact lenses. J Am Optom Assoc. 1985;56:198–201.
39. Silbert JA. The role of inflammation in contact lens wear. In Silbert JA, ed. Anterior segment complications of contact lens wear. New York: Churchill Livingstone; 1994:123–42.
40. Schoessler JP. Corneal endothelial polymegathism associated with extended wear. Int Contact Lens Clin. 1983;10:148–56.
41. Vannas A, Holden BA, Makitie J. The ultrastructure of contact lens induced changes. Acta Ophthalmol. 1984;62:320–33.
42. Allansmith MR, Greiner JV, Korb DR. Giant papillary conjunctivitis in contact lens wearers. Am J Ophthalmol. 1977;86:697–706.
43. Allansmith MR, Greiner JV, Covington HI. Surface morphology of giant papillary conjunctivitis in contact lens wearers. Am J Ophthalmol. 1978;85:242–9.
44. Holden BA. Extended wear: past, present, and future. Contact Lens Spectrum. 2002;1:32–7.
45. Fonn D, Dumbleton K, Jones L, et al. Silicone hydrogel material and surface properties. Contact Lens Spectrum. 2002;3:24–8.
46. Du Toit R, Sweeney D, Fonn D, Stern J. Managing silicone hydrogel complications. Contact Lens Spectrum. 2002;5:34–40.
47. Barr JT. Problem-solving with rigid lenses. Rev Optom. 1986;123(10):58–66.
48. Bennett ES. Immediate refitting with gas permeable lenses. J Am Optom Assoc. 1983;54:239–42.
49. Grohe RM, Bennett ES. Problem solving. In Bennett ES, Weissman BA, eds. Clinical contact lens practice. Philadelphia: Lippincott; 1991:1–16.
50. Bauer GT. Longitudinal spherical aberration of soft contact lenses. Int Contact Lens Clin. 1979;6(3):72–9.
51. Bennett AG. Optics of contact lenses, 2nd ed. Kent: Walter E English; 1956.
52. Alpern M. Accommodation and convergence with contact lenses. Am J Optom. 1949;26(9):379–87.

CHAPTER
13

Ophthalmic Instrumentation

DAVID MILLER • EDMOND H. THALL • NEAL H. ATEBARA

KEY FEATURES
- The ability of a transparent medium to bend a ray of light is the basis for most of the instruments used in ophthalmology today.
- Spherical lenses, prisms, mirrors, slit-shaped illumination, astronomical and Galilean telescopes, and a multitude of other optical components—both simple and complex—have been devised and manufactured for over two centuries in order to study the human eye and its function.

INTRODUCTION

In this chapter, the basic principles that underlie some of the more common instruments used in ophthalmology will be reviewed, including the following:

1. Keratometer and corneal topographer
2. Slit-lamp biomicroscope
3. Slit-lamp funduscopic lenses
4. Applanation tonometer
5. Optical corneal pachymeter
6. Specular microscope
7. Operating microscope
8. Retinoscope
9. Automated objective refractometer
10. Lensometer
11. Binocular indirect ophthalmoscope
12. Direct ophthalmoscope
13. Fundus camera
14. Magnifying devices

KERATOMETER AND CORNEAL TOPOGRAPHER

The keratometer and its cousin, the Placido disc corneal topographer, are among the most widely used, yet misunderstood, instruments in clinical practice today. The principle of the keratometer is simple enough. An illuminated target, usually a ring, is placed near the patient's eye. The cornea (with its overlying tear film) acts as a convex mirror to produce a virtual, erect, image of the ring. The size and position of the virtual image are measured (Fig. 13-1). The corneal radius of curvature may be estimated from this, provided several assumptions are valid. They are: (1) the position of the illuminated ring and image must be known to high precision, (2) the cornea is assumed to be spherical, (3) paraxial optics is assumed, and (4) the power of the back corneal surface is estimated. However, the information gained is, in and of itself, very little.

Because the image is erect and smaller than the object, it can be stated with certainty that the cornea is a convex surface. However, any smooth convex surface can produce an image identical to the mires produced by the cornea. The corneal shape

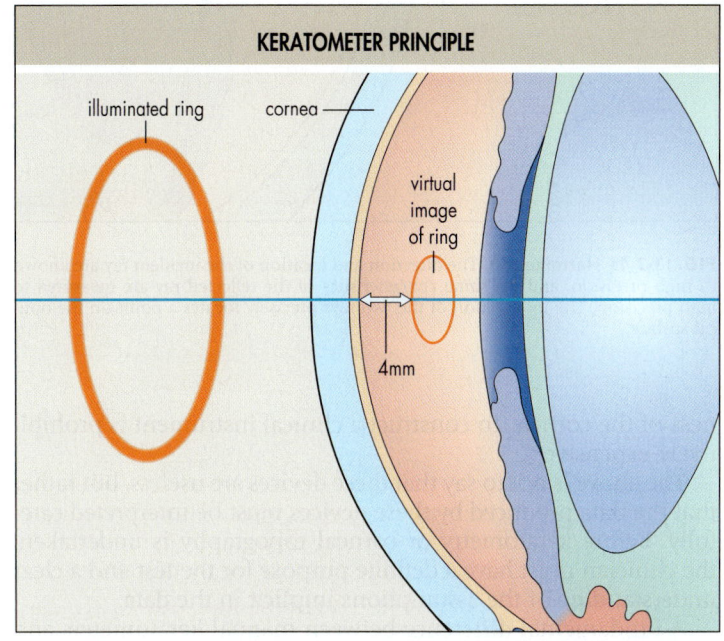

FIG. 13-1 ■ Keratometer principle. An illuminated ring is placed in front of the cornea, which acts as a convex mirror and produces a virtual image of the ring approximately 4mm behind the cornea.

could be spherical, paraboloid, hyperboloid, ellipsoid, or any other convex aspherical shape and would still produce images identical to those observed using the keratometer. A very fundamental problem in the design of the instrument is that it does not provide enough information to determine corneal shape accurately. The same is true for the Placido disc.

Perhaps the easiest way to understand the shortcomings of these instruments is to compare their characteristics with those of a technique commonly used in optical engineering to measure optical surfaces accurately, the Hartman test.[1] In the Hartman test a narrow beam of light from a precisely known position and direction is reflected from the surface to be measured. The position and direction of the reflected beam are measured precisely (Fig. 13-2). The intersection of the two beams precisely locates the position of one point on the mirror. The process is repeated point by point, until enough points have been measured to determine the overall shape of the surface.

The problem with the keratometer and the Placido disc is that the characteristics of only one of the two beams are known with certainty. Those of the reflected beam are known, but those of the incident beam could be any of an infinite number of possibilities depending on the corneal shape (Fig. 13-3). To determine the corneal shape that produces the image of the mire is not possible. Adding additional rings or data points does not solve the problem. No matter how many data points are sampled, the direction of the incident beam for each point is unknown.

Why not simply perform a Hartman test on the cornea? Researchers have tried this, but it is difficult because of the steep-

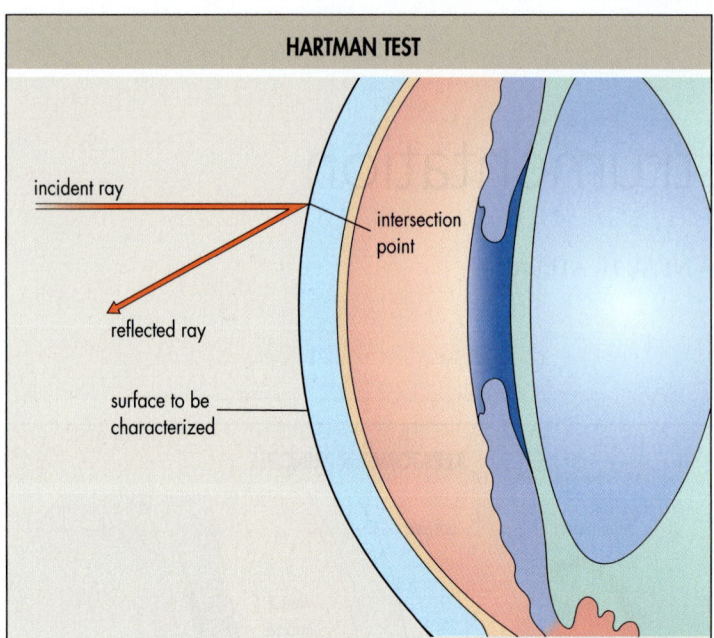

FIG. 13-2 ■ **Hartman test.** The direction and location of the incident ray are known to high precision, and the same characteristics of the reflected ray are measured to high precision. The intersection of the two rays precisely locates a point on the optical surface.

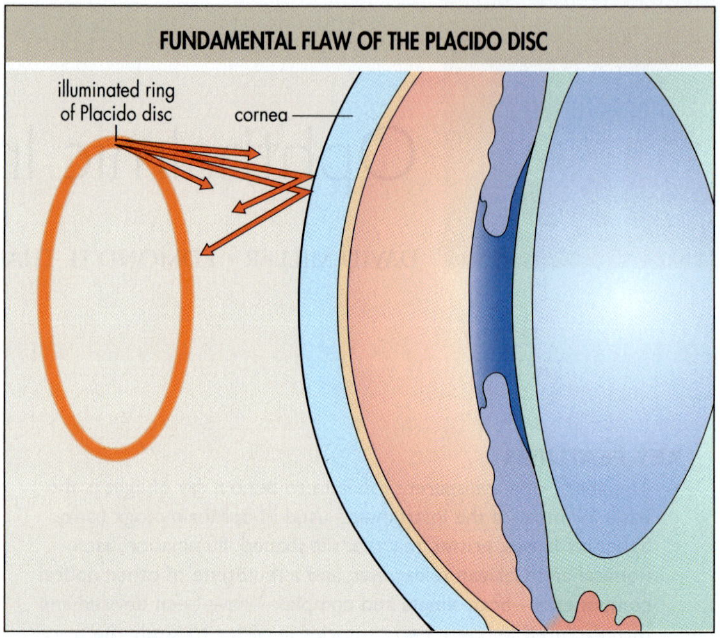

FIG. 13-3 ■ **Fundamental flaw of the Placido disc.** For the Placido disc and its many variants, the direction and location of the reflected ray are measured precisely, but the direction of the incident ray is unknown.

ness of the cornea. To construct a clinical instrument is prohibitively expensive.

The above is not to say that these devices are useless, but rather that the data produced by these devices must be interpreted carefully. Before keratometry or corneal topography is undertaken, the clinician must have a definite purpose for the test and a clear understanding of the assumptions implicit in the data.

A fundamental difference between manual keratometers and Placido disc corneal topographers is that the former use a Scheiner double-pinhole focusing system so that the position of the virtual image is known precisely. In Placido disc corneal topographers, each ring produces an image in a slightly different plane and the instrument cannot assess the position of each image (Fig. 13-4).

In keratometry, the assumption is that the cornea is spherical or toric. In general, the cornea is not spherical, so this assumption is known to be false. Nevertheless, this is the underlying assumption, in part because a sphere has a much simpler geometry than the true corneal surface. A sphere may be described completely by a single parameter (the radius), and a toroid may be described by three parameters (the two radii and an axis). The keratometer does not reveal the corneal shape, but it does describe the shape of a toric surface that would produce the same mires.

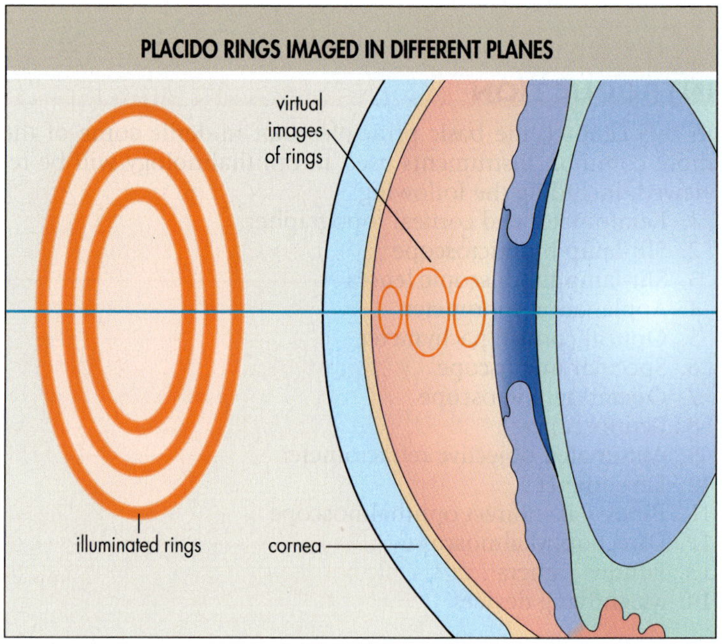

Clinical Use of Keratometric Information

For fitting rigid contact lenses this information is accurate enough, especially because keratometry is used to provide a starting point that is refined empirically. Multiple attempts over nearly half a century to automate the fitting process completely by relying on either keratometry or topography have failed.

Since the advent of IOLs, the keratometer has been used to measure corneal power, which requires additional assumptions. The keratometer and Placido disc topographers assess only the anterior corneal surface, but corneal power depends on both anterior and posterior surfaces and, to a much lesser degree, on thickness. The keratometer makes an assumption about the posterior corneal surface. Because the posterior surface has minus power, most keratometers compensate by using a smaller refractive index in the lens maker's formula. The typical, but not universal, formula is given in Equation 13-1, in which P is the

FIG. 13-4 ■ **Placido rings are imaged in different planes.** The virtual images of Placido rings do not lie in the same plane.

corneal power (D, diopters) and r is the radius (m).[2] This formula assumes a corneal refractive index of 1.3375 instead of Gullstrand's value of 1.376.

Equation 13-1
$$P = \frac{1.3375}{r}$$

Reliability of Keratometry for the Measurement of Corneal Power

The reliability depends to some extent on the formula used to calculate implant power. Many formulas are derived empirically or contain "fudge factors" that may compensate for erroneous assumptions inherent in the keratometer. Whatever the reason, keratometry appears to work reasonably well for the calculation of intraocular lens (IOL) power.

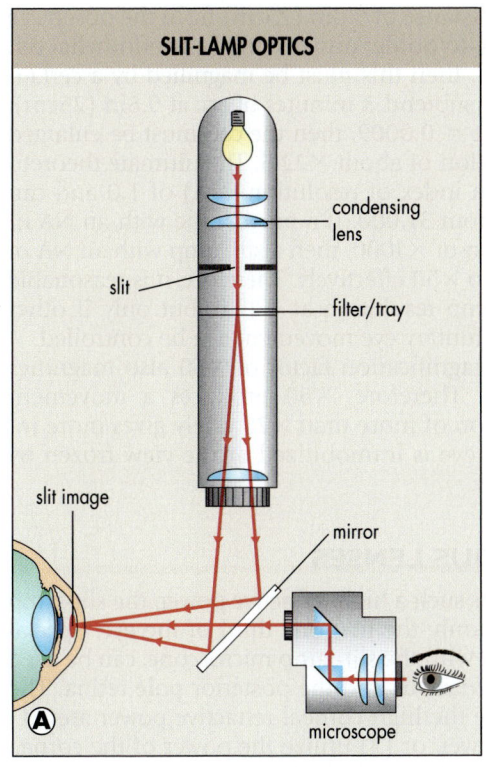

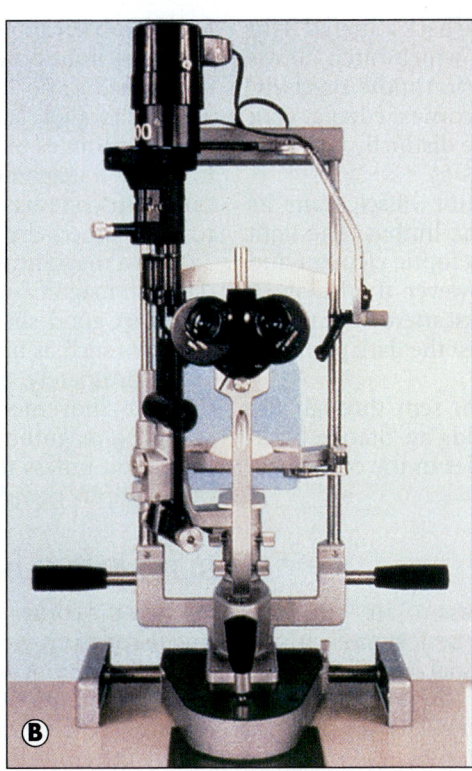

FIG. 13-5 ▪ **The slit lamp. A,** Some slit lamps first bring the light to a sharp focus within the slit aperture, and the light within the slit is focused by the condensing lens on to the patient's eye. The observation system of a modern slit lamp has many potential reflecting surfaces; antireflection coatings on these surfaces help reduce loss of light. **B,** Slit-lamp apparatus. (**A,** Modified from Spalton DJ, Hitchings RA, Hunter PA. Atlas of clinical ophthalmology. New York: Gower Medical; 1984:10.)

The interpretation of Placido disc corneal topography data is much more complicated. First, Placido disc topography does not use the Scheiner double pinhole, so even more assumptions are involved, which is why corneal topography companies constantly discuss improved algorithms. Fundamentally, every different algorithm is simply a different set of assumptions. Whether one set of assumptions is uniformly superior to another is difficult to establish. For this reason, corneal topography must be regarded as a developing technology.

SLIT-LAMP BIOMICROSCOPE

The slit lamp is the piece of equipment most frequently used by the ophthalmologist. With the addition of auxiliary lenses, it can give unique, magnified views of every part of the eye. With the use of auxiliary devices it can be used to make quantitative measurements, including intraocular pressure, endothelial cell counts, pupil size, corneal thickness, anterior chamber depth, and others, and to take photographs. Illumination and observation are discussed in this section.

Illumination

Although Purkinje, in 1823, attempted to develop a type of slit lamp by using one handheld lens to magnify and another handheld lens to focus strong oblique illumination,[3] it was not until almost 100 years later that a version of the slit lamp appeared that is recognizable today. By 1916, the slit lamp was composed of the newly developed bright Nernst lamp; the Gullstrand illumination system, which condensed the light onto a slit aperture and then projected the slit onto the eye; the rotatable Henker arm; and the Azanski stereomicroscope, which slid across a glass-topped table.[3] Because the transparent cornea only backscatters about 10% of incident light,[4] development of the bright lamp and a powerful condensing system was essential before the faint nuances of the cornea could be seen.

In the terminology of the visual physiologist, the brighter illumination allowed the observer to move farther along the contrast-versus-background intensity curve and exploit the heightened sensitivity of the arrays of retinal cones.[5] At present, the physiological limits of illumination may have been reached for both the doctor and the patient. Most patients are unable to endure bright

lights; illumination beyond a certain limit simply produces a noisy frenzy in the retinal circuitry and does not improve resolution. It is possible that a dim illumination system coupled with electronic light amplification may be used in the future.

Specifically, the modern slit lamp produces an intensity of about 200mW/cm². When operated at the rated voltage, halogen lamps have a higher luminance and color temperature than do conventional incandescent lamps. For slit-lamp work, a high color temperature (e.g., a greater amount of blue light) is useful. Because many of the ocular structures are seen via light scatter, and because the shorter wavelengths are scattered most, a light with a high blue component illuminates the structures best. The light is first brought to a focus at the slit aperture (Fig. 13-5),[6] and the light within the slit is focused by the condensing lens onto the patient's eye.

Improving Tissue Contrast

One of the great strengths of the modern slit lamp is the way in which contrast can be improved by various maneuvers:
- Optical sectioning: as the beam is narrowed, the scattered light of adjacent tissue is removed and greater detail of the optical section is seen.
- Tangential illumination: when the light is brought in from the side, highlights and shadows become stronger, and the texture (i.e., elevations and depressions) is seen better.
- Pinpoint illumination: the cells and flare in the anterior chamber in a patient who has iritis are best seen using a narrow beam focused into the aqueous, so that the black pupil becomes the background. The combination of the narrow beam and the dark pupillary background eliminates any extraneous light, which would reduce contrast. The same principle holds when the examiner pushes the lower lid up to examine the tear meniscus. For example, the stagnant cell pattern of an obstructed tear duct is best seen using a narrow beam, with the dark iris in the background.
- Specular reflection: in this technique the angle of observation is set to equal the angle of illumination. In this way, the structure of the front surfaces of the cornea (i.e., ulcers, dry areas) and the rear surfaces (endothelial pattern) may be assessed.
- Proximal indirect illumination: in this technique a moderately wide beam is directed to the areas adjacent to the area

89

of interest. Against a dark background, the backscattered light from the lesion yields a higher contrast, which often allows the observer to see the borders of the lesion more precisely. For example, using this technique subtle corneal edema, with its minute pools of fluid, stands out more distinctly against a dark pupil.

- Sclerotic scatter: with the slit illuminator offset from its isocentric position, light is directed to the limbus. The light then follows the cornea as if it were a fiberoptic element and reaches the other side of the limbus. However, if a lesion or particles within the cornea exist, the backscattered light from the lesion or particles is seen clearly against the dark pupillary background.
- Retroillumination from the fundus: light sent through the pupil to the fundus is reflected and yields an orange background. Holes in the iris or subtle wrinkles in the cornea become silhouetted and much easier to see.

Observation System

The observation system has many glass-to-air surfaces. Theoretically, 4% of the incident light may be lost at each surface by reflection, which results in a substantial light loss. If the elements are given antireflection coatings (as they are in all modern slit lamps), the total gain in brightness rises by 20% compared with that of an uncoated system.

Another feature of the slit lamp is that the observation system is really a microscope, but with a long working distance (i.e., about 3.9in [10cm]). Prisms take the divergent rays from the patient's eye and force them to emerge as parallel pencils from each eyepiece. Thus, a stereoscopic appreciation of the patient's eye is achieved without convergence of the observer's visual axis. Most slit-lamp microscopes offer magnifications between ×5 and ×50, with ×10, ×16, and ×25 being the most popular. The issue of resolution ultimately becomes an issue of diffraction limit. The working distance of the slit lamp (for the ×10 objective) is at least 100 times longer than that of the laboratory microscope. Therefore, the cone of light that emanates from the patient's eye and is captured by the slit-lamp objective is small relative to that of the microscope. This narrower cone yields a wider diffraction pattern. Because the ability to resolve two cells implies a distinct space visible between each cell, and because the image of each cell border has a diffraction fringe, tighter diffraction fringes allow the viewer to distinguish two separate cells that are closer together. Abbe, an optical physicist, was able to combine the factors of aperture size and working distance (i.e., the focal length for a microscope) into an index of resolution called the numerical aperture (NA).[5] The NA not only includes aperture size and working distance, but also index of refraction of the media (i.e., oil, water, or air) and the wavelength of illuminating light. However, these latter factors are relatively constant for most systems.

The NA of the slit lamp is substantially lower because the laboratory microscope's objective may be larger, its working distance smaller, or both. If the NA is known, the optimal magnification of an optical system may be calculated. The term *optimal magnification* is used here to define the limit beyond which further magnification yields no more information.

In the calculation of the magnification needed to see individual endothelial cells using slit-lamp specular reflection, the limitations are set by the resolution limit of the observer's eye. For example, if the 20/20 (6/6) Snellen letter represents the accepted resolution limit, and each bar of a 20/20 (6/6) "E" subtends 1 minute of arc, then the details of each endothelial cell must be magnified to subtend 1 minute of arc on the observer's retina. Although 1 minute of arc is the threshold, the lens designer often uses 3 minutes of arc to minimize fatigue. The two adjacent endothelial cells may be thought of as two outer cell borders that contain a common double cell border, a Snellen "E" with the open side closed. To calculate the magnification needed, convention assumes that the magnified image is positioned at the com-

fortable observation distance of 9.8in (25cm) from the observer's eye. Thus, if the border-to-border dimension of an endothelial cell is assumed to be 10m, then this must be magnified by a certain amount to allow it to subtend 3 minutes of arc at 9.8in (25cm). If tan 3 minutes of arc = 0.0009, then the cell must be enlarged to 225m, a magnification of about ×22.5. The ultimate theoretical microscope has an index of resolution (NA) of 1.0 and can magnify objects by about 31,000. If a microscope with an NA of 1.0 has a magnification of ×1000, then a slit lamp with an NA of 0.05 can magnify up to ×50 effectively. Therefore, it is reasonable to expect good slit-lamp resolution at ×22.5, but only if other variables such as involuntary eye movement can be controlled.

Unfortunately, a magnification factor of ×50 also magnifies fine eye movements. Therefore, ×50 produces a movement smear, so magnification of more than ×25 rarely gives more information unless the eye is immobilized or the view frozen by photography or video.

SLIT-LAMP FUNDUS LENSES

Because the cornea has such a high refractive power, the slit-lamp microscope can view only the first one third of the eye. Special lenses, in conjunction with the slit-lamp microscope, can be used to view the posterior vitreous and the posterior pole retina. The two ways to overcome the high corneal refractive power are: (1) nullify the corneal power, or (2) utilize the power of the cornea as a component of an astronomical telescope, in a manner similar to that exploited by the indirect ophthalmoscope.

The Goldmann contact lens (Fig. 13-6) and other similar lenses work in conjunction with the slit-lamp microscope to nullify the dioptric power produced by the corneal curvature and to bring the retina into the focal range of the slit-lamp microscope. These plano-concave contact lenses are placed on the cornea, forming virtual, erect, and diminished images of the illuminated retina near the pupillary plane, within the focal range of the slit-lamp microscope.

The Hruby lens is a powerful plano-concave lens, minus 58.6 diopters in power. It is held immediately in front of the cornea, forming a virtual, erect, and diminished image of the illuminated retina, near the pupillary plane, bringing it within focal range (Fig. 13-7).

The 60D, 78D, and 90D funduscopic lenses (Fig. 13-8) use a different approach to view the posterior vitreous and posterior pole retina. These lenses act as high-powered, biconvex, condensing lenses, projecting an inverted, real image in front of the lens, within focal range. This is the same optical principle used by the indirect ophthalmoscope; the higher the power of the lens, the lower the magnification of the image.

The Goldmann three-mirror contact lens (Fig. 13-9), as its name implies, incorporates three internal mirrors. The contact lens nullifies the refractive power of the patient's cornea, and the three mirrors then reflect light from the patient's midperipheral retina, peripheral retina, and the iridocorneal angle, respectively. The posterior pole of the fundus can be visualized, also, in a manner similar to that of the Goldmann posterior pole contact lens.

The panfundoscope contact lens and the Rodenstock contact lens are high-powered, spherical, condensing lenses, as are corneal contact lenses (Fig. 13-10). A real, inverted image of the fundus is formed within the spherical glass element, which is within the focal range of the slit-lamp microscope. Because the condensing lens is so close to the eye and has such a high power, the field of view is very wide, making these lenses specially suited for a wide-angle view of the posterior pole and midperipheral fundus.

GOLDMANN APPLANATION TONOMETER

The applanation tonometer (Fig. 13-11) is used to measure intraocular pressure. It relies on an interesting physical principle: for an ideal, dry, thin-walled sphere, the pressure inside a sphere

GOLDMANN FUNDUS CONTACT LENS

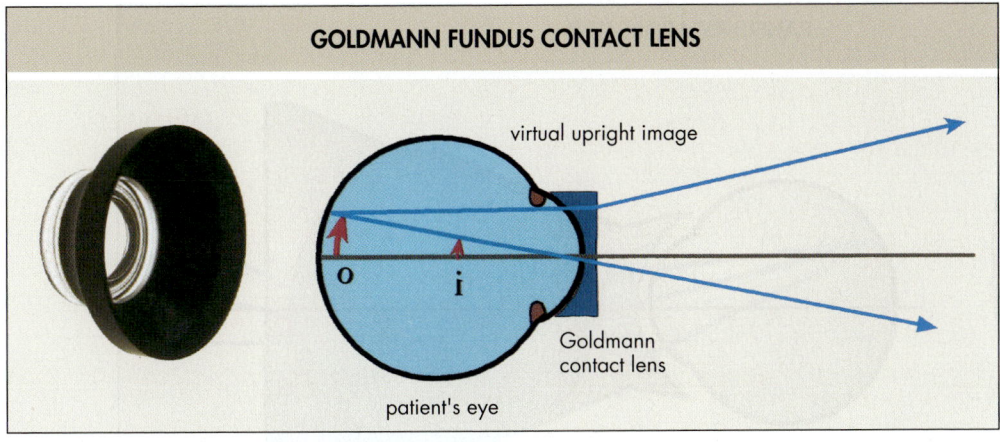

virtual upright image

o i

Goldmann
contact lens

patient's eye

FIG. 13-6 ▮ The Goldmann fundus contact lens, or any similar plano-concave contact lens, nullifies the refractive power of the cornea, thereby moving the retinal image close to the pupillary plane and into the focal range of the slit-lamp microscope. The image formed is virtual, erect, and diminished in size.

CONCAVE HRUBY LENS

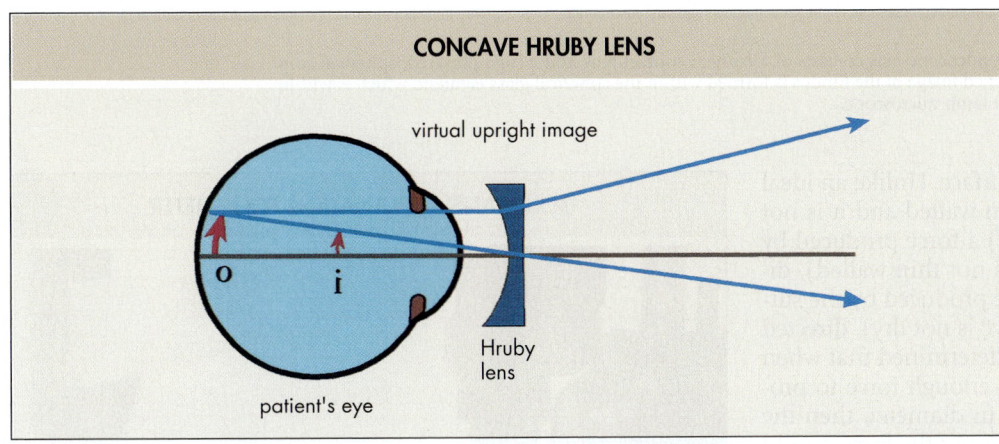

virtual upright image

o i

Hruby
lens

patient's eye

FIG. 13-7 ▮ The concave Hruby lens, when placed close in front of the patient's eye, forms a virtual, erect image of the illuminated retina that lies within the focal range of the slit-lamp microscope.

60D AND 90D LENSES

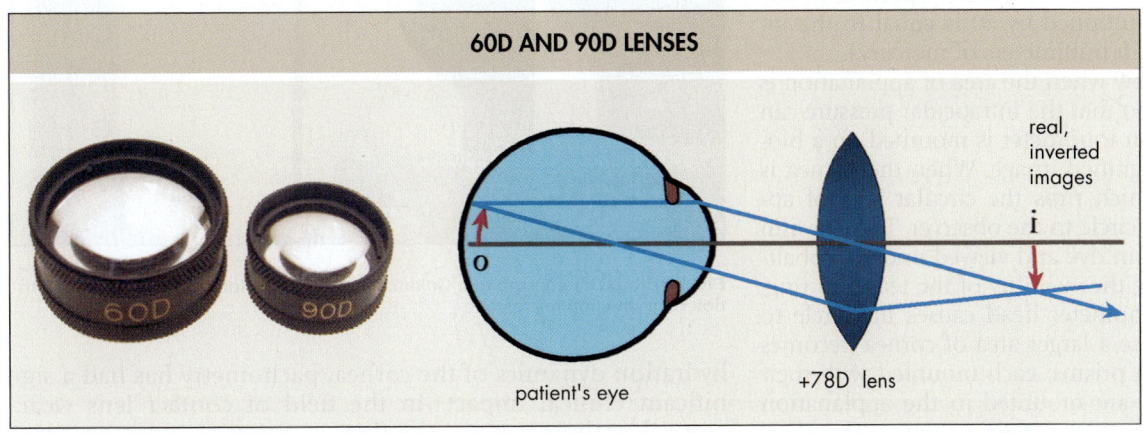

real,
inverted
images

o

i

patient's eye   +78D lens

FIG. 13-8 ▮ The 60D, 78D, and 90D lenses produce inverted, real images of the retina within the focal range of the slit-lamp microscope in a fashion similar to that employed by the indirect ophthalmoscope.

EFFECT OF GOLDMANN LENS AND MIRRORS

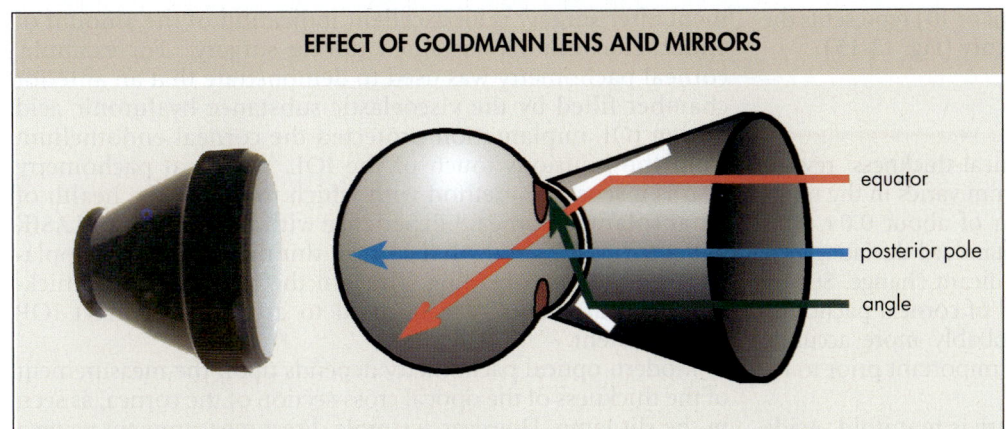

equator

posterior pole

angle

FIG. 13-9 ▮ The contact lens of the Goldmann lens nullifies the refractive power of the patient's cornea, while the three mirrors then reflect light from the patient's peripheral retina (orange ray) and iridocorneal angle (green ray). The posterior pole of the fundus also can be visualized in a manner similar to that of the Goldmann posterior pole contact lens (blue ray).

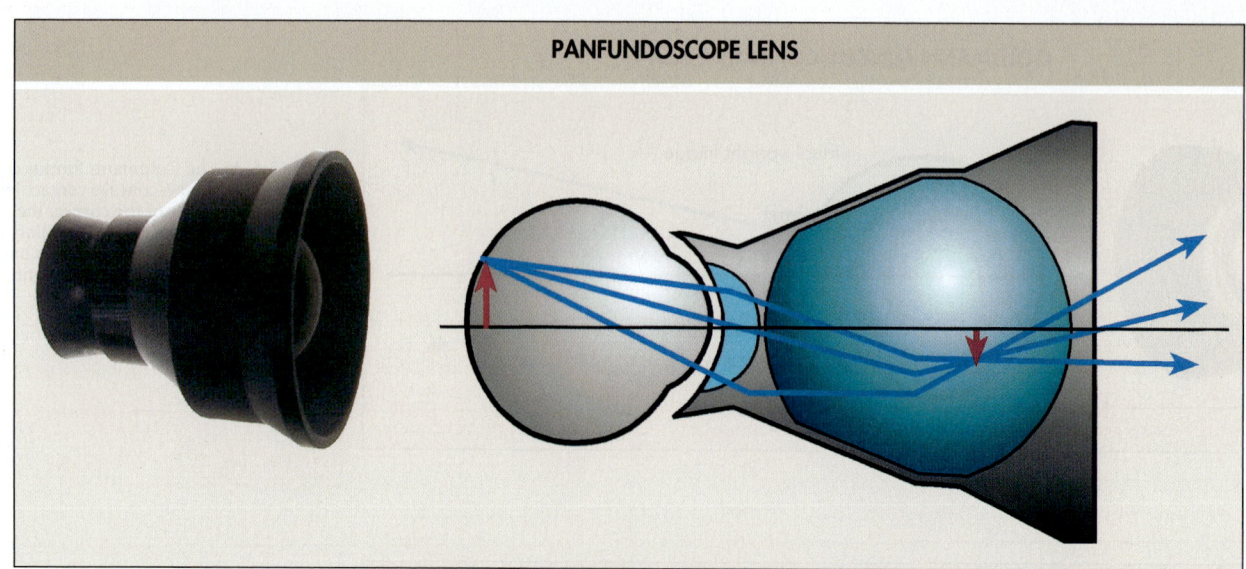

PANFUNDOSCOPE LENS

FIG. 13-10 ■ The panfundoscope lens consists of a corneal contact lens and a high-powered, spherical condensing lens. A real, inverted image of the fundus is formed within the spherical glass element, which is within the focal range of the slit-lamp microscope.

is proportional to the force applied to its surface. Unlike an ideal sphere, however, the human eye is not thin walled and it is not dry, producing two confounding forces: (1) a force produced by the eye's scleral rigidity (because the eye is not thin walled), directed away from the globe, and (2) a force produced by the surface tension of the tear film (because the eye is not dry), directed toward the globe (Fig. 13-12). Goldmann determined that when a flat surface is applied to the cornea with enough force to produce a circular area of flattening 3.06mm in diameter, then the force caused by scleral rigidity exactly cancels out the force caused by surface tension. Therefore, the applanating force required to flatten a circular area of cornea exactly 3.06mm in diameter is directly proportional to the intraocular pressure. Specifically, the force (measured in dynes) multiplied by 10 is equal to the intraocular pressure (measured in millimeters of mercury).

How does the observer know when the area of applanation is exactly 3.06mm in diameter so that the intraocular pressure can be measured? The applanation tonometer is mounted on a biomicroscope to produce a magnified image. When the cornea is applanated, the tear film, which rims the circular area of applanated cornea, appears as a circle to the observer. The tear film often is stained with fluorescein dye and viewed under a cobalt-blue light in order to enhance the visibility of the tear film ring. Higher pressure from the tonometer head causes the circle to have a wider diameter, because a larger area of cornea becomes applanated (Fig. 13-13). Split prisms, each mounted with their bases in opposite directions, are mounted in the applanation head, creating two images offset by exactly 3.06mm. The clinician looks through the applanation head and adjusts the pressure until the half circles just overlap one another (Fig. 13-14). At this point, the circle is exactly 3.06mm in diameter, and the reading on the tonometer (multiplied by a factor of 10) represents the intraocular pressure in millimeters of mercury (Fig. 13-15).

OPTICAL PACHYMETER

A review of the literature concerning corneal thickness[7] reveals that the average thickness of the central 3mm varies in the range 0.50–0.57mm, with a standard deviation of about 0.04. This means that a change of thickness of two standard deviations, or 0.08mm, is considered a statistically significant change. Such a statement indicates the precision required of corneal pachometry. Electronic corneal pachometry is probably more accurate than optical pachometry, and precision is important prior to refractive surgery procedures.

The value of optical corneal pachometry is manifold. Aside from providing information about the normal physiological

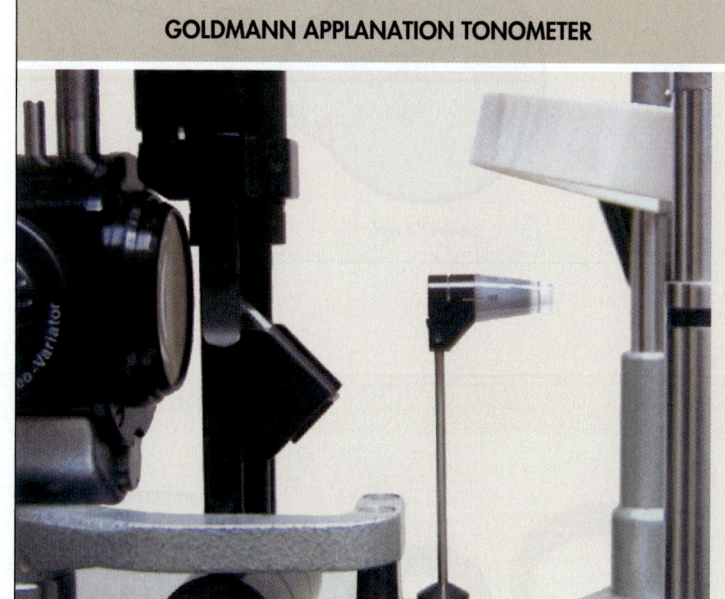

GOLDMANN APPLANATION TONOMETER

FIG. 13-11 ■ Photograph of a Goldmann applanation tonometer in working position on a slit-lamp microscope.

hydration dynamics of the cornea, pachometry has had a significant clinical impact. In the field of contact lens wear, corneal pachometry was the first quantitative objective parameter which differentiated a contact lens that fits well from a poorly fitting one.[8] Because corneal thickness is directly related to the health of the corneal endothelium, its measurement after surgery is an excellent indication of the amount of endothelial trauma sustained during surgery.[9] For example, corneal pachometry was used to demonstrate that an anterior chamber filled by the viscoelastic substance hyaluronic acid during IOL implantation protected the corneal endothelium from the injurious touch of the IOL.[10] Corneal pachometry also is a sensitive method with which to follow the health of a transplanted cornea.[11] Experience with post-operative LASIK patients has taught us that corneal thinning lowers the applanation tonometer reading. Thus, in the future, corneal thickness measurements may be used to arrive at a correct IOP measurement.

Modern optical pachometry depends upon the measurement of the thickness of the optical cross-section of the cornea, as seen in the slit lamp. However, a simple direct measurement using a ruler (a measuring reticule in the eyepiece of the slit lamp)

EFFECT OF FORCE ON CORNEA

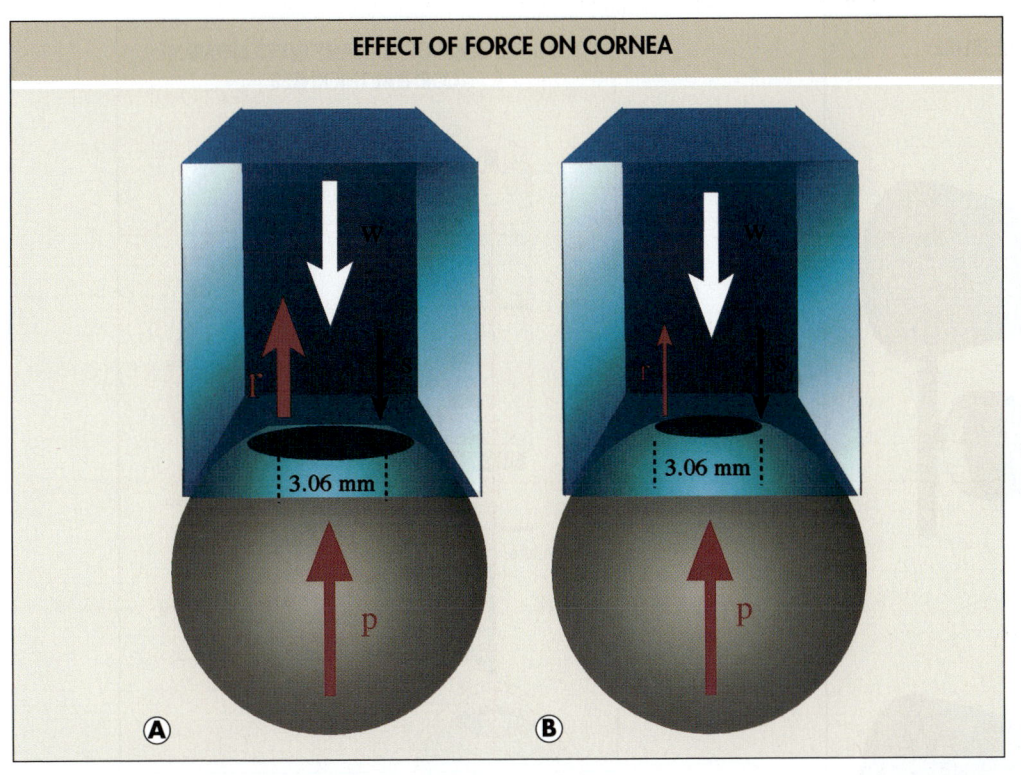

FIG. 13-12 ■ **A**, When a flat surface is applied to the cornea with enough force *(w)* to produce a circular area of flattening greater than 3.06mm in diameter, the force caused by scleral rigidity *(r)* is greater than that caused by the tear film surface tension *(s)*. **B**, When the force of the flat surface produces a circular area of flattening exactly 3.06mm in diameter, the confounding forces caused by scleral rigidity and tear film surface tension cancel each other. The applied force *(w)* then becomes directly proportional to the intraocular pressure *(p)*.

FLUORESCEIN-STAINED TEAR FILM

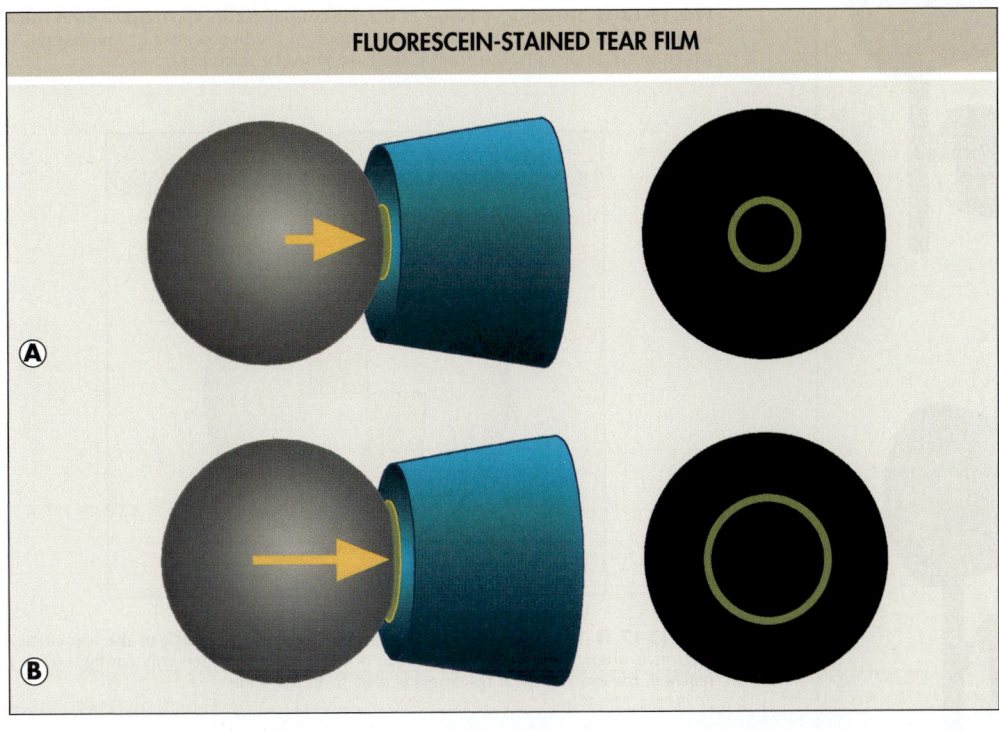

FIG. 13-13 ■ When viewed through a transparent applanation head, the fluorescein-stained tear film appears as a circular ring **(A)**. Greater applanation pressure causes the ring to increase in diameter **(B)**.

EFFECTS OF APPLANATION ON SPLIT-PRISM

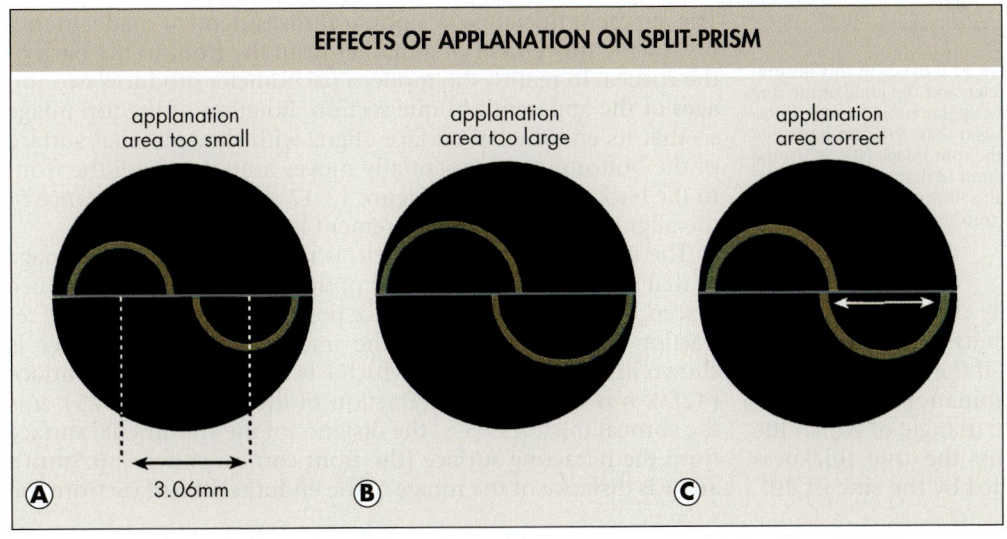

FIG. 13-14 ■ The split prism in the applanation head creates two images offset by 3.06mm, allowing greater ease in determining when the circular ring is exactly 3.06mm in diameter. When the area of applanation is smaller than 3.06mm, the arms of the semicircles do not reach each other **(A)**. When the area of applanation is greater than 3.06mm, the arms of the semicircles reach past each other **(B)**. When the area of applanation is exactly 3.06mm, the arms of the semicircles touch each other **(C)**. This is the end point at which the intraocular pressure can be measured.

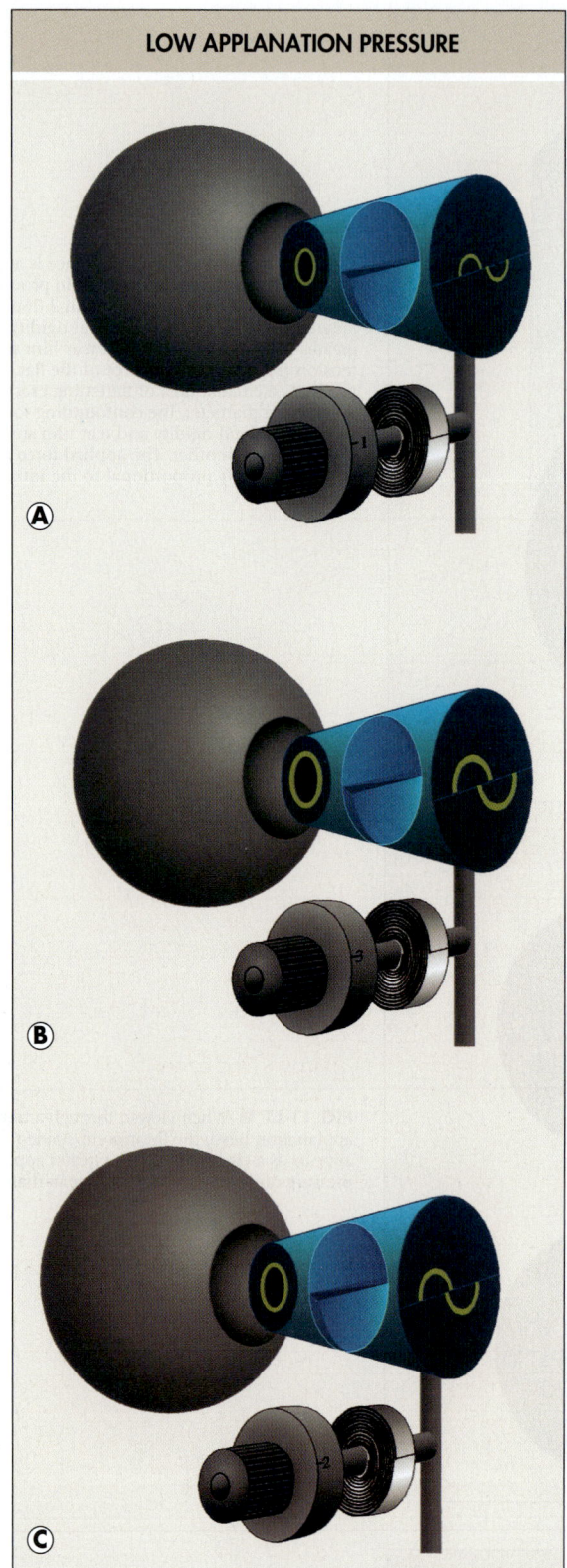

LOW APPLANATION PRESSURE

Ⓐ

Ⓑ

Ⓒ

FIG. 13-15 ▮ When the applanation pressure is too low (1.0 dynes in this illustration) the circular ring is smaller than 3.06mm in diameter, and the arms of the ring do not reach each other in the split image (**A**). When the applanation pressure is too high (3.0 dynes in the illustration) the circular ring is larger than 3.06mm in diameter, and the arms of the ring stretch past each other in the split image (**B**). When the applanation pressure creates a circular ring exactly 3.06mm in diameter, the arms of the ring just reach each other in the split image (**C**). In this illustration, the end point is reached at 2.0 dynes of applanation pressure, which corresponds to an intraocular pressure of 20mmHg.

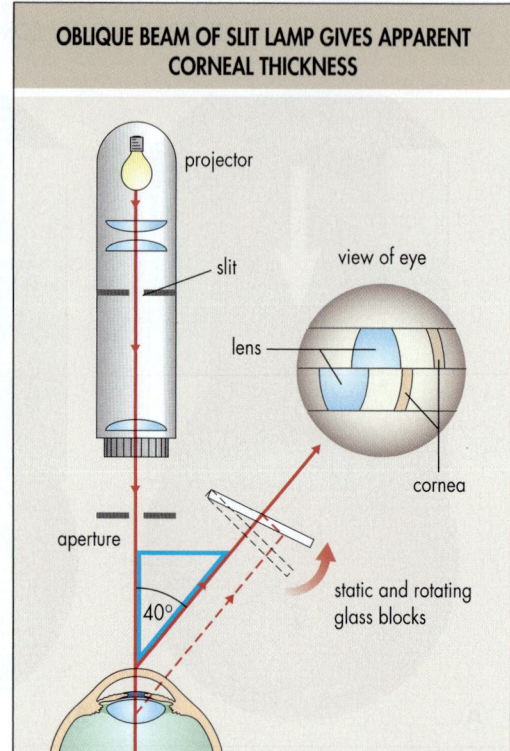

OBLIQUE BEAM OF SLIT LAMP GIVES APPARENT CORNEAL THICKNESS

projector

slit

view of eye

lens

cornea

aperture

40°

static and rotating glass blocks

FIG. 13-16 ▮ The oblique beam of the slit lamp gives an apparent corneal thickness. To calculate the real thickness, the length of the hypotenuse of the triangle, of which the oblique optical section is the base, must be calculated.

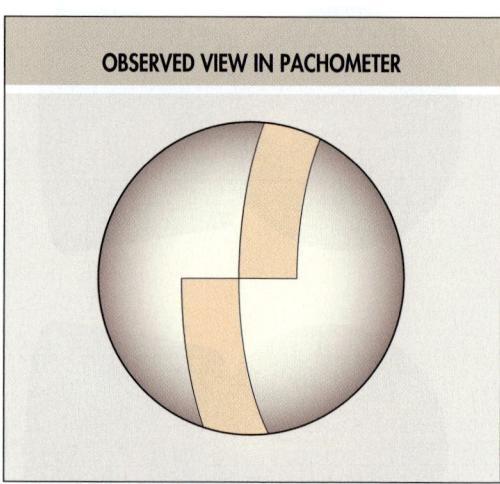

OBSERVED VIEW IN PACHOMETER

FIG. 13-17 ▮ The observed view in the pachometer. The back of the top corneal section is aligned with the front of the bottom section. When this configuration is reached, the exact corneal thickness is read from the scale.

across the corneal cross-section gives only the apparent value. Figure 13-16 shows that the slit lamp, with its oblique illumination, views an oblique slice of the cornea. If the observation microscope makes a 40° angle with the illumination system, then the real thickness is the hypotenuse of the triangle of which the oblique optical section is the base. Thus, the true thickness equals the oblique apparent section divided by the sine of 40°.

The apparent thickness is a physical measurement made, in theory, by the movement of a marker from the front to the back of the cornea. In reality, the modern pachometer produces two images of the apparent oblique section. Rotation of the top image so that its endothelial surface aligns with the epithelial surface of the bottom image essentially moves a marker from the front to the back of the cornea. Figure 13-17 shows the appearance of the alignment when a measurement is taken.

The endothelial surface, itself, is not seen. Instead, an image of that surface produced by the optics of the front of the cornea is seen. The effect of front-surface power and corneal index of refraction on the position of the image of the back surface is shown in Equation 13-2, in which F is the power of front surface (42D), n is the index of refraction of the cornea (1.3375), u is the corneal thickness (i.e., the distance of the endothelial surface from the refracting surface [the front corneal surface]; 0.5mm), and v is distance of the image of the endothelial surface from the

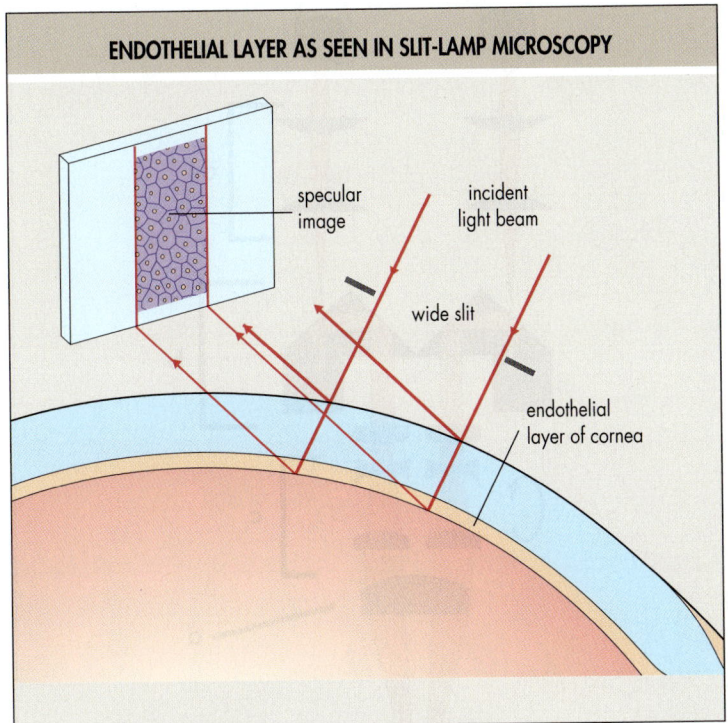

ENDOTHELIAL LAYER AS SEEN IN SLIT-LAMP MICROSCOPY

specular image

incident light beam

wide slit

endothelial layer of cornea

FIG. 13-18 ■ Endothelial layer as seen in slit-lamp microscopy. Note the wide angle between the illumination beam and the observation path needed to remove the bothersome surface reflection and stromal scatter from the view of the endothelial mosaic.

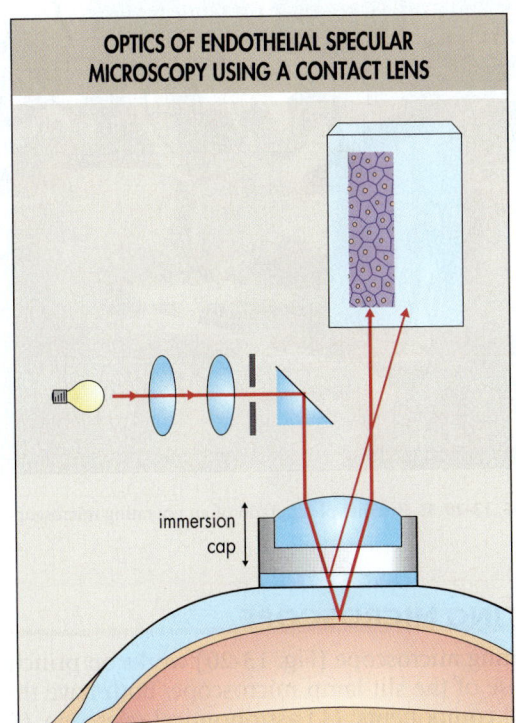

OPTICS OF ENDOTHELIAL SPECULAR MICROSCOPY USING A CONTACT LENS

immersion cap

FIG. 13-19 ■ Optics of endothelial specular microscopy using a contact lens. (Adapted from Bigar F. Specular microscopy of the corneal endothelium. In: Straub W, ed. Developments in ophthalmology, vol 6. Basel: Karger; 1982:1–88.)

refracting surface. Thus, for corneas of average curvature, the image of the endothelial surface is within 0.01mm of the real endothelial surface.

$$\frac{n}{u} + F = \frac{n}{v}$$

Equation 13-2

$$\frac{1.3375}{0.0005} + 42 = \frac{1.3375}{v}$$

$$v = 0.49mm$$

SPECULAR MICROSCOPE

It seems remarkable that just 8 years after Gullstrand unveiled his first model of the slit lamp in 1911,[12] Vogt described the endothelium in the living eye using a modified Gullstrand slit lamp.[13,14] The optics of the visualization of the endothelial mosaic produced by slit-lamp microscopy are shown in Figure 13-18.[14] A photograph of the endothelium in the enucleated rabbit eye was first produced by Maurice in 1968.[15] In 1975, 56 years after Vogt presented a painting of the endothelium in vivo, Laing et al. developed a camera to photograph the layer in the living, human subject.[16]

Optics of Endothelial Microscopy

A number of significant obstacles stand in the way of easy microscopic observation of the living corneal endothelium. First, the reflection from the front corneal surface interferes with a sharp view of the endothelium. Second, the intervening stromal layers backscatter light, which decreases the contrast of the endothelial details. In addition, the thicker and more edematous the stroma, the hazier the views of the endothelium. Finally, because of the small difference in index of refraction between the cornea (1.376) and the aqueous (1.336), only 0.02% of the incident light (for most angles of incidence) is reflected from the interface between corneal endothelium and aqueous.[17]

To eliminate the bothersome reflection from the front corneal surface, two approaches are used. An increase in the angle of in-

cidence moves the anterior reflection to the side, so it covers less of the specular reflection from the endothelium. This approach alone is used in the noncontact technique. If the cornea could be thickened artificially (without an increase in light scatter), this also would move the surface reflection further to the side. By using a contact lens that has a coupling fluid of index of refraction similar to that of the cornea, the surface reflection is eliminated and the corneal thickness may be assumed to include the contact lens thickness. The reflection from the surface of the contact lens replaces that of the corneal surface. However, because of the thickness of the contact lens, the surface reflection is moved well over to the side (Fig. 13-19).

Theoretically, some of the stromal backscatter could be removed by using both a Polaroid element, because some of the backscattered light is polarized, and a red filter, which eliminates the more heavily scattered light of short wavelength.[18] Unfortunately, these maneuvers also decrease the intensity of light from the endothelial sheet and require very long camera exposures. Thus, the only practical course against stromal backscatter is a wide angle of incidence (the stromal region is moved to the side) and a narrow slit beam (to narrow the stromal zone seen). Of course, a narrow beam also yields a narrow view of the endothelium. To overcome this latter problem, Koester[19] has developed a scanning endothelial microscope that captures a number of the narrow endothelial zones on the same film frame by scanning across a larger area of cornea.

The magnification needed to yield important details about the shape and size of the endothelial cells lies between a magnification of ×80 and ×250. Of course, a lower magnification photograph may allow an accurate count of the endothelium. In normal individuals the number of endothelial cells per square millimeter decreases with age, while the size of the cells increases with age.

When the cornea is injured, as in surgical or nonsurgical trauma, or subjected to the chronic insult of many years of contact lens wear, the cells vary in size and shape. This variability of size and shape of endothelial cells is known as polymegathism.

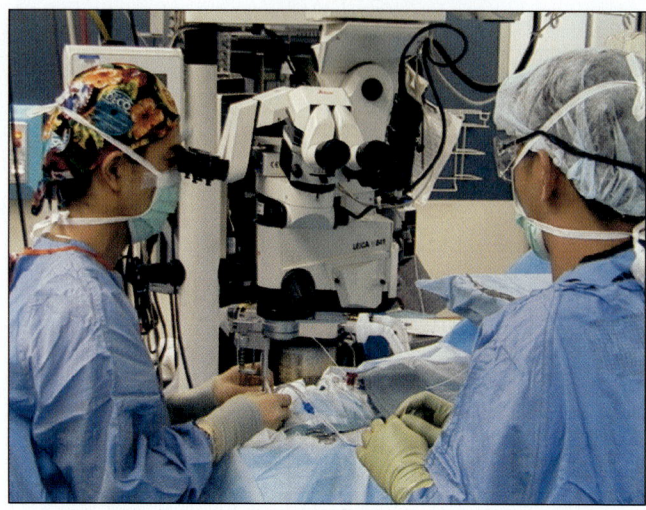

FIG. 13-20 ■ External photograph of an operating microscope.

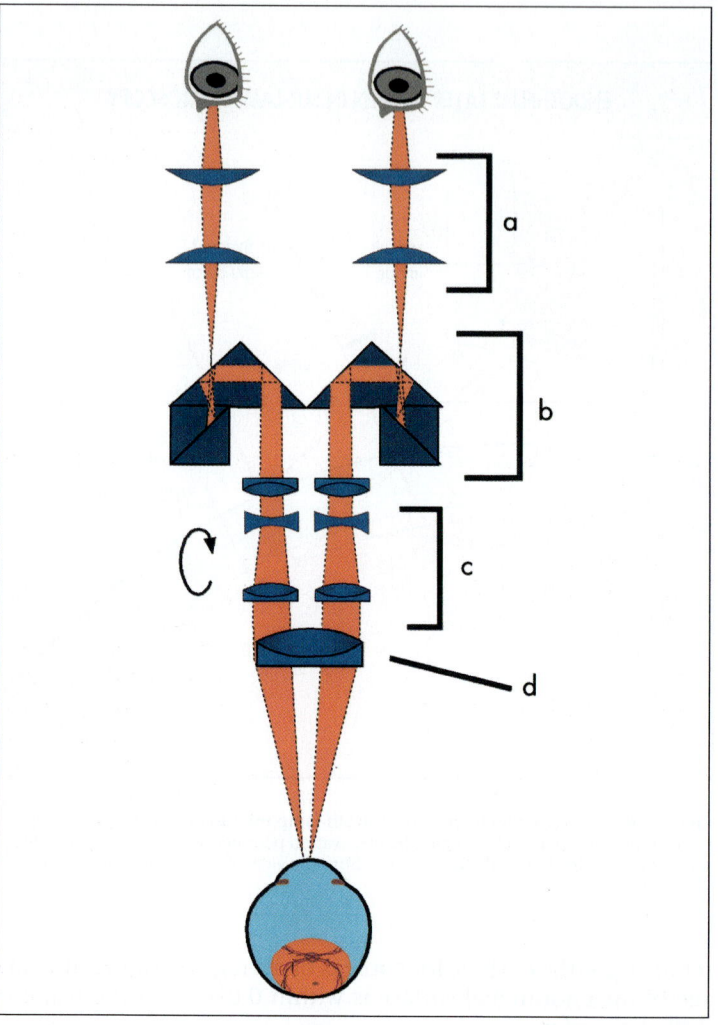

FIG. 13-21 ■ Schematic diagram of an operating microscope. The major components include: **(A)** the eyepiece, an astronomical telescope system, which provides most of the magnification, **(B)** an inverting prism, such as a Porro-Abbe prism, to correct for the inverted image produced by the eyepiece, **(C)** a magnification changer, such as a Galilean telescope system, in which different lenses can be introduced in order to change the degree of magnification; and **(D)** the objective lens, which adjusts the working distance. Two parallel optical systems, each a mirror image of the other, provide a stereoptic view of the patient's eye.

OPERATING MICROSCOPE

The operating microscope (Fig. 13-20) works on principles similar to those of the slit-lamp microscope. Both have the following optical components: (1) astronomical telescope, (2) inverting prism, (3) Galilean telescope, (4) objective lens, (5) light source, and (6) binocular viewing system (Fig. 13-21). Unlike the slit-lamp microscope, the operating microscope's illumination source is not slit shaped, and the working distance for the operating microscope (the distance from the objective lens to the patient's eye) is longer in order to accommodate the specific requirements of ocular surgery.

The working distance of this microscope is equal to the focal length of the objective lens. Commonly used objective focal lengths in ophthalmic surgery are 150mm, 175mm, and 200mm. Use of the proper working distance can greatly lessen back and neck strain on the surgeon, especially during lengthy operations: a difference of 25mm often can affect body comfort and the positioning of the surgeon's arms and hands.

The total magnification of the operating microscope is equal to the product of the magnifications of its various components. Because several different lenses are available for the objective and the eyepiece, magnification can be controlled. Smoothly variable magnification changers (zoom Galilean telescopes) are now incorporated into many operating microscopes. The 12.5× eyepiece is the most popular choice for ophthalmic surgery with magnification from 6× to 40×.

Various illumination systems are available, but the most important system for ophthalmic surgery is known as *coaxial illumination*. This system is especially useful for visualization of the posterior capsule and for vitreous surgery. Fiberoptic delivery systems reduce heat near the microscope and facilitate the changing of bulbs during surgery.

RETINOSCOPE

Every time a close-up photograph is taken of the face of a subject and a vivid red pupil (called *red eye*) is seen instead of the usual black pupil, the essence of retinoscopy is captured. The red reflex is produced when the flash lamp is positioned close to the optical axis of the camera.

The source of the red reflex is the aerial image of the blood-filled choroid, superimposed on the pupil. Because the image is very small, it is seen only if the optical systems of the subject's eye and the camera, respectively, are close to alignment. Because the aerial image cannot be in the plane of the pupil, it must always be out of focus when the plane of the face or eye is in sharp focus. Von Helmholtz realized that the origin of the reflex must be the fundus itself and developed the ophthalmoscope to focus on the

details of the fundus.[20,21] The position of the aerial image of the fundus, hence, is determined by the optical components of the eye. Therefore, determination of the position of the image can lead to determination of the refractive error of the eye. Cuignet, a French army ophthalmologist who measured the refractions of a large numbers of army recruits, must be credited with the development of a better way to define the position of the aerial image.[22] His method always brought the aerial image to the same location in space, at the examiner's eye, a principle employed by most contemporary retinoscopists. Subtraction of the dioptric-value equivalent of the "working distance" determined the power of the lens required to correct the refractive error.

Optics of Retinoscopy

The essence of retinoscopy is to illuminate the retina and then locate the image of the retina in space. Thus, the retinoscope combines a light source with an observation aperture (i.e., peephole). The position of the retinal image is called the *far point*. Its position in dioptric units is equal to the refractive error. Thus, the eye may be considered as an element in an optical bench. When the light rays that leave the eye are made visible, the far point can be located and the refractive error calculated. Unfortunately, a side-view analysis of the human eye as though it is on an optical bench cannot be done. However, with this side-view analysis in mind, the mechanism of retinoscopy can be understood.

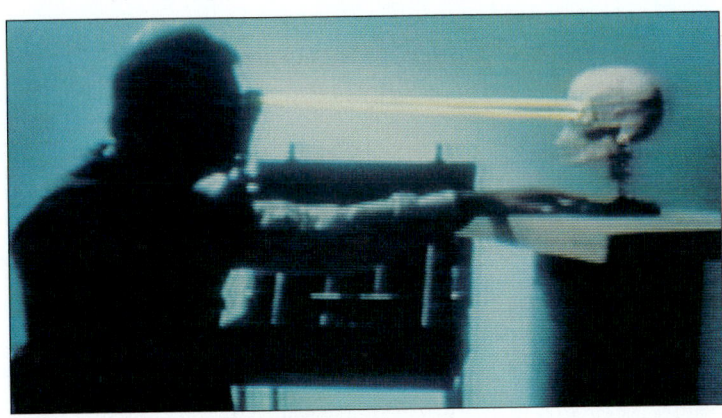

FIG. 13-22 ■ The far point of the myopic eye lies between the patient and the retinoscopist.

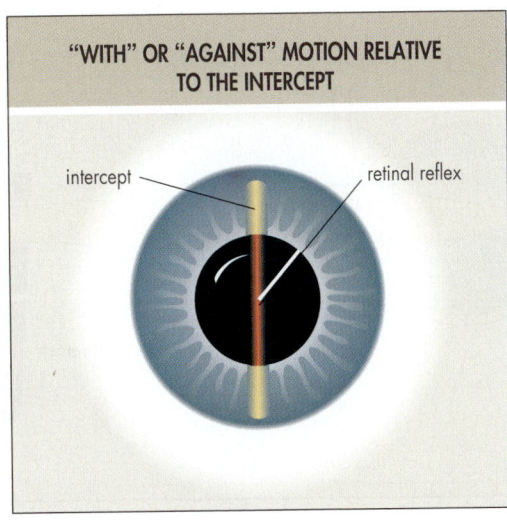

"WITH" OR "AGAINST" MOTION RELATIVE
TO THE INTERCEPT

intercept   retinal reflex

FIG. 13-23 ■ "With" or "against" motion is evaluated relative to the motion of the intercept. The intercept is the part of the retinoscopic beam (not acted upon by the dioptrics of the eye) that strikes the eye outside the pupil.

For the purposes of this description, it is assumed that a side-view analysis is possible. The retinoscopist places lenses in front of the patient's eye, so that the patient's far point is focused at the peephole of the retinoscope. For example, the emmetrope's far point is at infinity. If the retinoscopist works at a distance of 25in (66cm) from the patient (called the working distance), a +1.50D lens brings parallel light to a focus at 25in (66cm) from the patient's eye. In Figure 13-22, the far point of the myope lies between the examiner and the patient. A minus lens of the appropriate power brings the image to the peephole of the retinoscope. The refractive error equals the dioptric power of the minus lens needed less that of the working-distance lens (+1.50D). Thus, if a −5.00D lens is needed to bring the far point to the examiner, then the refractive error is −5.00D + 1.50D = −3.50D. The far point of the hyperope is theoretically behind the head of the patient. A plus lens of the appropriate power brings the far point to the peephole of the examiner. Thus, if a +5.00D lens is needed to bring the far point to the examiner, then the refractive error is 5.00D + 1.50D = +6.50D.

Neutrality

Cuignet found the position of the far point by using a version of the Foucalt knife-edge test. Imagine a thin, sharp knife that moves across the beam of light that leaves the patient's eye. If the knife edge passes across the point of focus, then the knife edge blocks all the light for an instant, after which all the light reappears; the edge of the peephole of the retinoscope may be considered such a knife edge. If the far point is brought to a focus at the peephole, then the focused light appears to vanish and reappear with a slight side-to-side motion of the peephole. This situation is called neutrality and represents the end point of retinoscopy. It is at this end point that the power of the lens in front of the patient's eye minus the +1.50D working lens yields the value of the refractive error.

With and Against Motion

The image that emerges from the patient's eye before neutrality is reached is significant. In a myopic eye, as the examiner moves the illumination light upward the retina is illuminated in an upward direction; the real, inverted image of the retina is focused between the patient and examiner; and the retinal image appears to move downward in a direction opposite to the movement of the retinoscope. This is called *against* motion. Minus lenses are placed in front of the patient's eye until the focus is brought to the plane of the peephole, at which point neutrality is seen. In a hyperopic eye, as the beam from the retinoscope moves upward, the retina is illuminated in an upward direction. The virtual, upright image of the retina appears illuminated in an upward direction. Because the image moves in the same direction as the retinoscope, the motion is called a *with* motion.

Plus lenses are placed in front of the patient's eye, the image is moved to the plane of the retinoscopic pinhole, and neutrality is seen.

With and against motion may be described in another way. In the case of a myope, as an edge (the peephole) is moved downward, light from the top of the retina is eliminated and against movement is created. In the case of the hyperope, as the edge (peephole) is moved downward, light is eliminated from the top of the retina, but now a with motion is perceived.

Other Clues

The retinoscopist must be aware of other subtle clues that differentiate fine with and against motions from neutrality. For example, the aerial image becomes larger, the closer it is to the examiner's eye. A closer aerial image also appears to move faster, because more of the closer image fills the peephole than does a smaller, more distant aerial image. A small movement of the peephole crosses a larger percentage of the aerial image and gives the appearance of a faster movement. The closer to neutrality, the faster is the movement of the reflex. In a similar vein, the brighter the reflex, the closer it is to neutrality. Here again, the closer the aerial image is to the retinoscopist (Newton's law), the brighter it is.

When a movement is termed *with* or *against*, it is with or against the movement of the portion of the retinoscopic beam that strikes the eye outside the pupil. This part of the light beam, not acted upon by the dioptrics of the eye, is called the intercept (Fig. 13-23).

Enhancement

The sleeve of the streak retinoscope may be moved to bring the light closer or move it further away from the condensing lens (Fig. 13-24). Of course, in the case of a hyperope (i.e., a relatively weak dioptric system), the more divergent are the rays from the retinoscope, which produces a broader intercept and illuminates a large retinal area. As the sleeve is moved, a narrower or wider intercept is produced. On the other hand, the greater the amount of hyperopia, the smaller the retinal image, and thus the less the retinoscopic reflex fills the pupil. If the finest intercept equals the size of the reflex, then the refractive error is about +5.00D. If the plane of the far point is very far from the pupil (i.e., a small amount of hyperopia), then sleeve movement does not bring the edges of the reflex within the pupil to equal the size of the intercept, a situation that occurs if the hyperopia is <1.00D. Incidentally, enhancement involves sleeve movement only, and not side-to-side movement or the use of trial lenses.

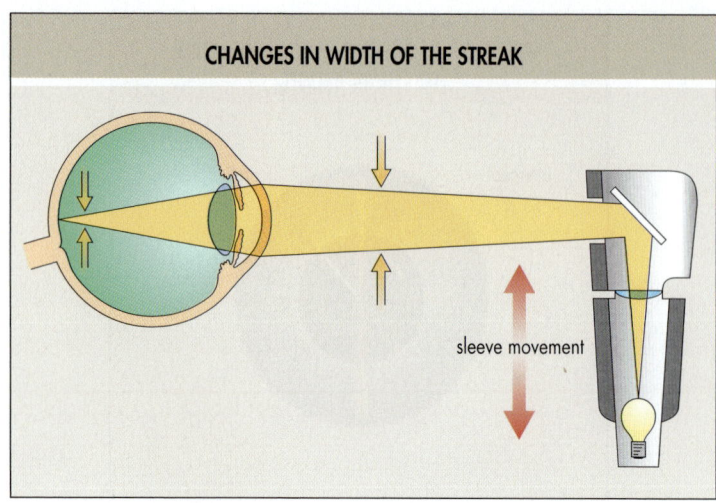

FIG. 13-24 ■ **Changes in width of the streak.** Changes in the distance between the bulb and the condensing lens narrow or widen the streak width. Such changes are accomplished when the sleeve of the retinoscope is moved up or down. When the width of the reflex equals that of the intercept, the refractive error is about +5.00D.

FIG. 13-25 ■ **Optics of a generic indirect ophthalmoscope.** Note the illumination beam enters the pupil of the patient in a different area of the pupil from that in which the observation beam exits. This configuration eliminates corneal reflection, which would confuse an automated evaluation of the fundus.

Myopia Estimation

If the initial retinoscopic movement is slow and dull, with movement, then high myopia is present. To estimate quickly the amount of myopia, without using trial lenses, simply move toward the patient, and simultaneously move the retinoscope slowly from side to side. As the far point is reached, the end point of neutrality is given. The distance from the patient is the far point and must be converted into diopters. Thus, if neutrality takes place at 7.5in (20cm), the amount of myopia is 5.00D (no working distance compensation is needed).

Astigmatism

To determine the presence of astigmatism, simply sharpen the streak and slowly rotate it to 360°. If little or no astigmatism exists, the retinoscopic streak reflex always is parallel to the intercept. A break phenomenon occurs when the reflex is not in perfect alignment with the intercept as the streak is rotated. The orientation of the streak reflex when it lies parallel to the intercept indicates the direction of one of the major meridians of the astigmatism. The examiner must find the lens of neutrality for a side-to-side movement along that meridian and establish neutrality for the meridian 90° away. For example, assume that the maximum break phenomenon is along the 90° meridian. Rotate the streak into a horizontal position and move the retinoscope up and down (along the 90° meridian). Imagine that a +4.50D sphere neutralizes the vertical movement. Now, rotate the streak vertically and move it side to side along the 180° meridian. With the +4.50D sphere in place, a −2.00D cylinder of axis 90° neutralizes the side-to-side movement. Subtraction of the +1.50D power of the working distance lens from the dioptric power of the sphere yields a +2.00D sphere with a −2.00D cylinder of axis 90°.

AUTOMATED OBJECTIVE REFRACTOMETER

Any clinician who has asked enough patients, "Is it better with lens 1 or lens 2?" must have dreamed of an automated refractor. After all, the eye is a partial optical bench. The fundus can be a serviceable target if illuminated. The cornea and lens make a passable aspherical focusing system. To complete the optical bench, a positive lens needs to be placed before the eye to form a real aerial image of the fundus, as in indirect ophthalmoscopy. Except that distances are not standardized and calibration is not present, an indirect ophthalmoscope has most of the essential elements of an objective refractor.

The first objective refractor based upon an ophthalmoscopic principle was probably that demonstrated by Schmidt–Rimpler

in 1877.[22] As with other ophthalmoscopes of that day, the examiner viewed the retina through a hole in a concave mirror, while the reflected light came into the patient's eye from a source located at the side. Schmidt–Rimpler modified his ophthalmoscope, using a trace of the lattice pattern placed directly onto its lamp. The retinal image of this lattice pattern provided the detail needed to set the focus. A positive lens, located at a fixed distance in front of the eye to be examined, formed a real, inverted image of the lattice, which could be visualized through the hole in the mirror. To use the Schmidt–Rimpler refractor, the separation between the mirror and the lens was varied until the lattice image was seen clearly by the examiner. The patient's refraction was derived as a correlate of this separation.

Objective Optometers

Objective optometers may be thought of as modified, table-bound, indirect ophthalmoscopes (Fig. 13-25). For the most part, early objective optometers were manual rather than automated instruments. Although an "electronic refractionometer" was reported by Dollins[23] as early as 1937, the development of the integrated circuit and various forms of electro-optical and electromechanical transducers rendered the use of the automatic objective optometer clinically practicable.

Modern instruments have two sources of light. First, the target is illuminated with visible light for fixation and accommodation control and, second, a low-intensity infrared or near-infrared source sends light into the patient's eye, which is "seen" by a sensor. The optometer must use "invisible" (or at least dim, unobtrusive) light for measurement to preclude an unwanted stimulus to accommodation and to allow comfortable fixation. These two (visible and infrared) systems usually are derived from a single incandescent lamp by the use of filters. For example, a cut-off filter of 800nm allows only infrared light to enter the system.

The area of retina irradiated by infrared radiation produces a real image within the optometer. This image is analyzed by photoelectric means using an infrared-sensitive device. The use of infrared for focus evaluation presents a few problems. For example, an examiner cannot calibrate the focusing system "by eye" but must use an indirect method. In terms of accuracy, the eye's chromatic aberration is a problem. Anyone familiar with the duochrome (red–green) test knows that the human eye focuses light of various wavelengths differently. Because the goal is to learn the eye's refractive error in visible (yellow) light, a correction factor of about 1.00D must be built into any infrared device.

Most objective optometers use one of three methods for focus analysis—the retinoscopic principle, Scheiner's disc principle, or the grating focus principle. Before instruments based upon each of these principles are discussed, it is valuable to consider some problems that had to be solved in the design of modern objective refractors.

Accommodation

Accommodation associated with the use of a target that is optically distant but objectively near may induce errors in the measurement of refraction. Modern devices use a fogging lens through which the fixation target is viewed. The subject hopefully learns that accommodation tends to make the visible target even more blurred and, therefore, relaxes accommodation. Occasional failure of accommodation to relax under a fog is presumed to occur because of an awareness that the target is not truly distant. This phenomenon has been termed *instrument myopia*.

Subject Alignment

It is almost paradoxical to request a subject to simultaneously look at a fixation target and not attempt to clear it by accommodation. These divergent responses are required, however, if refraction is to be measured accurately for foveal vision. Accordingly, when the examiner aligns the optometer with respect to the subject's pupil as the subject fixates the target, proper overall alignment must be ensured. At the same time, a fogging lens provides a disincentive to accommodate.

Focusing

Modern objective refractors are focused automatically, which eliminates the variability otherwise introduced by examiner accommodation. Automatic focusing for various meridians is accomplished swiftly, the number and locations of meridians actually scanned depending upon the method of image evaluation and upon the approach to refractive error analysis used in the particular instrument. The computational power of the microprocessors found in today's automated refractors allows refraction to be calculated within 10 seconds or less. This high speed tends to negate one of the major problems associated with older manual devices, such as momentary changes in fixation or accommodation, or both, that may take place during the course of measurement.

Instruments That Utilize the Retinoscopic Principle

Bausch and Lomb's Ophthalmetron was the first clinical automated refractor to utilize the retinoscopic principle.[24] No longer commercially available, this instrument used paired light sensors to register movement of the retinoscopic reflex. For example, if sensor 1 was stimulated before sensor 2, an analog of a retinoscopic "with" existed. Conditions that gave rise to a retinoscopic "against" caused sensor 2 to be stimulated first. In any event, a servomechanism found the focus in one meridian and attempted to maintain focus as each meridian was scanned in turn. The Ophthalmetron produced a graph that displayed the refraction in each meridian. Modern automated refractors are much more rapid and display refractive data directly in numeric form.

Instruments That Utilize Scheiner's Disc Principle

In the early seventeenth century, Fr. Christopher Scheiner observed that an in-focus candle is seen singly, whereas an out-of-focus candle is seen double when viewed through paired apertures separated by a distance slightly less than the diameter of the pupil. An automatic focusing device that uses Scheiner's disc principle divides the rays that emerge from a subject's eye into two bundles and then seeks the point at which these intersect. For example, a photoelectric sensing device might register an end point for a particular meridian under the condition that all

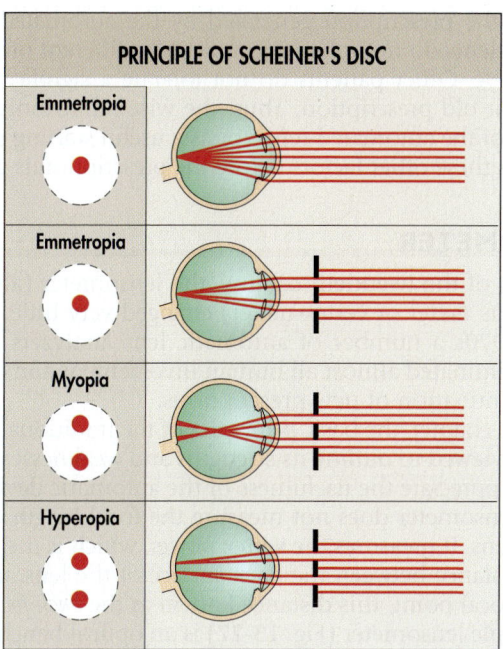

FIG. 13-26 ■ **Principle of Scheiner's disc.** Light enters the two pinholes and produces two images on the retina until the light is brought to a focus. (Adapted from Guyton DL. Automated clinical refraction. In: Duane T, ed. Clinical refraction, vol 1. Baltimore: Harper & Row; 1987:1–43.)

the light falls on one sensing element rather than two. The 6600 Autorefractor[23] is an example of an instrument that operates on Scheiner's principle (Fig. 13-26).

Instruments That Utilize the Grating-Focus Method

In the grating-focus method, an image of a luminous target grating is formed on the retina. The sharpness of the aerial image of the illuminated "retina grating" is assessed continuously, usually by a scanning process. A high-speed servomechanism varies the focusing lenses until the actual grating image is as sharp as a standard in-focus image provided by the device.

Characteristics of Contemporary Objective Refractors

The spherical range is between about −15D and +15D and the cylindrical range reaches about 6D. The accuracy (reliability) is about 0.25D at constant alignment. The minimum pupillary diameter is in the range 2–3mm, the vertex distance is about 12mm, and the measurement time is between 0.2 and 10 seconds.

Patient observation is carried out variously via optical eyepiece, observation window, or television monitor.

Possible Problems

A small percentage of patients cannot tolerate the prescription measured by the automated refractor. The reason for this may lie in the relationship between the illumination beam and the patient's pupil. As shown in Figure 13-25, the paths for illumination and observation must pass separately through different portions of the patient's pupil to avoid corneal reflection noise. Thus, a pupil larger than or equal to 3mm in diameter, along with no eye or head movement, is required for an accurate measurement. To add to this alignment problem, in some patients the eye's optics vary across different parts of the pupil. Spherical aberration, crystalline lens tilt, or abrupt changes in corneal power are responsible for this variation. Because most automated refractors send a very narrow illumination beam into the patient's eye, the ultimate refractive reading may be dependent on the particular part of the pupil illuminated. Thus, the patient who has variable optics across the pupil is apt to be given the wrong prescription. Finally, a series of human factors occur that may account for nonacceptance of the prescription generated by the automated refractor. Some patients do not tolerate significantly different prescriptions in each eye. Other patients do not tolerate a significant change from their old prescription. Thus, the wise refractionist uses the findings of the automated refractor as a useful starting point, and examines these other factors before the prescription is given.

LENSOMETER

For most of the twentieth century, the lensometer (also known as the lens meter or vertex meter) changed very little. However, in the 1970s a number of automatic lens analyzers appeared, which eliminated almost all human involvement and quickened the determination of new prescriptions.

In this chapter, the basic principles of the traditional lensometer are reviewed to outline its strengths and weaknesses, and thus help to appreciate the usefulness of the automatic devices.

The lensometer does not measure the focal length of the unknown lens. It measures the vertex power, which is the reciprocal of the distance between the back surface of the lens and its secondary focal point, this distance known as the *back focal length.*

A simple lensometer (Fig. 13-27) is an optical bench that consists of an illuminated, moveable target, a powerful fixed-field lens, and a telescope eyepiece focused to infinity.[25] The key element is the field lens; without this, to measure the merest 0.25D lens would require a lensometer of the optical bench type to be over 4m long. The fixed-field lens is situated so that its focal point is on the back surface of the unknown lens being analyzed which, in turn, sends parallel light to the observation telescope. Thus, the small movement of the target is amplified optically and in such a way that the distance between the target and field lens is always directly proportional to the power of the unknown lens (an example of Badal's principle). Such an arrangement allows the instrument's linear scale to read in diopters.

To determine the power of each principal meridian of an unknown lens, the lens simply is inserted into the lensometer, the principal meridian located, the target lines focused sharply, and the power recorded. The second target, set 90° from the first, is refocused and the new power recorded. Once the powers in the two principal meridians and the axes are known, the final prescription is calculated.

The automatic device rapidly measures the powers in all meridians, selects the meridians with the greatest difference in power between them, and designates these as the major meridians of the lens. The device is programmed to calculate the prescription and print out the result. The entire procedure, from spectacle insertion to printout, takes less than 1 minute.

The main advantage of the automated lensometer is its elimination of human error. In today's busy ophthalmic office, in which technicians and doctors juggle many mental tasks at the same time, a clear advantage exists to a device that does not need to be focused, have numbers written down, or require calculations to be made.

If an automated lensometer does not focus a sharp image, how does it work? It simply measures the deflection of a fixed number of light rays produced by the unknown lens. To do this, the direction of the rays must be known before they enter the lens. The easiest way to accomplish this is to have them all enter parallel to one another. Figure 13-28 shows a beam of collimated green light (which eliminates chromatic aberration) incident to the unknown lens. Thus, a circle of light of a known dimension strikes the lens. The refracted light is passed through a ring aperture to tailor the size of the new beam to the size of the board of light detectors. By deflection of the parallel beam in its unique manner, the unknown lens produces a new pattern (i.e., a smaller or larger circle or an ellipse), which is detected and carefully measured by an array of photodiodes. These measurements yield deflection information, which is fed into a small computer that calculates the lens parameters (powers, axis, adds, prisms), and a printer creates a record of the parameters. Because these devices measure ray deflections, if the lenses in the lensometer are tipped at all, the deflection is altered and erroneous results are produced.

Another small error arises in the measurement of the add of a bifocal. All automated lensometers are designed to measure the vergence of the light that exits a lens when parallel light enters it. However, light that enters the add when worn by a patient is typically divergent (i.e., originates at 16in [40cm] or the reading distance from the spectacle plane). The error is significant only in high-powered lenses, such as for an aphakic correction. To minimize this error, the distance and near powers are measured using the back surface of the lens (in the position usually occupied by the front surface).

Accurate measurements of the progressive multifocal lens presents a problem with many lensometers. The operator must first align the lens so as to measure the distance correction, bind then find and realign, and measure the area of the lens with the maximum add.

BINOCULAR INDIRECT OPHTHALMOSCOPE

The entire retina, if spread out and flattened, is about the size of a large postage stamp. The important structures themselves are rather small. For example, the optic nerve is 1.5mm in diameter and the major blood vessels are only 0.1–0.2mm in diameter.

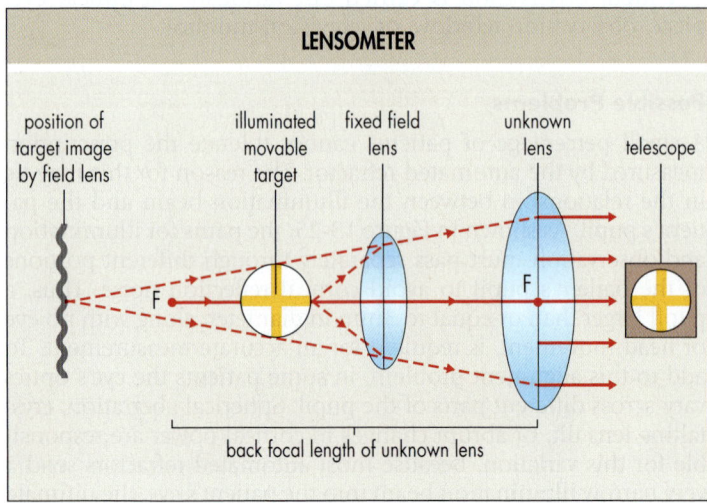

FIG. 13-27 ■ **The lensometer resembles an optical bench.** The moveable illuminated target sends light to the field lens, with the target in the end point position. Because the focal point of the field coincides with the position of the unknown lens, all final images are the same size (Badal principle).

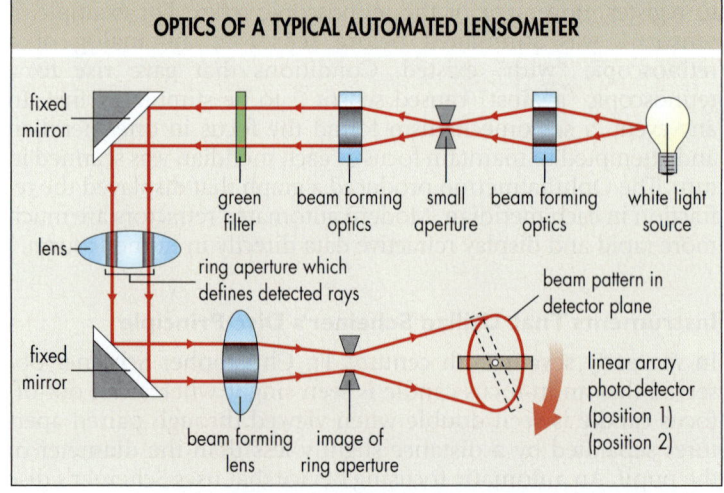

FIG. 13-28 ■ **Optics of a typical automated lensometer.** Parallel light strikes the unknown lens. The refracted light rays (which are confined to a pencil beam within an annulus) ultimately strike an array of electronic photoreceptors.

Significant papilledema, with an elevation of the nerve head of 3.00D, is equivalent to only a 1mm change in elevation. Most of the important red and yellow details, including blood vessels, hemorrhages, and exudates, are seen against the light red background of the blood-filled choroid. Subtle changes in the pinkish white backscattered light of the optic disc announce major glaucomatous or neuro-ophthalmic alterations. The presence of the corneal reflection and the usual backscattered light of the healthy cornea and lens make the evaluation of fundus changes even more difficult.

In the face of these obstacles, it seems almost miraculous that the examiner is able to make a significant number of diagnoses using the direct ophthalmoscope. Even more advantageous is the binocular indirect ophthalmoscope, which gives a wide field of view, a stereoscopic impression, and an image of high contrast. Of course, a small price must be paid for these advantages. The patient's pupil must be dilated, the instrumentation is larger, heavier, and more expensive, and the illumination is almost painfully bright for the patient.

Illumination System

Gullstrand evaluated the principles required of the illumination system to minimize bothersome reflection and backscatter. Gullstrand's solution required that the observation beam and the illumination beam be separated at the corneal and lens plane, to avoid corneal and lens reflection and scatter (Fig. 13-29). To separate both beams until they intersect at the retina, a dilated pupil is needed. The filament of the bulb is actually brought to a focus in a portion of the patient's pupil. To minimize the loss of light, the condenser lens also brings the observer's pupil to a focus in the patient's pupil. With patient and observer pupils conjugate, loss of light is minimized, and field of view is maximized.

Observation System

CONTRAST. Because the observation beam path is different from the illumination beam path, glare degradation from reflection and backscatter is minimized and subtle details are seen more easily. Of course, the observer must learn to tilt the handheld lens strategically to avoid reflection from the surface of the lens itself. This reflection is minimized (from about 4% of incident light to 1%) by a lens that has an antireflection coating.

INVERTED IMAGE. The handheld condenser lens creates a real, inverted aerial image of the illuminated patient's fundus, as expected from a positive lens. Thus, the examiner must learn to reorient details from where they appear to be to where they are located actually.

FIELD OF VIEW. Figure 13-30 illustrates how the handheld lens produces the aerial image of the fundus. Rays that pass through the nodal point of the patient's eye and the edge of the handheld lens determine the size of the field of view. The distance of the handheld lens from the patient's eye also determines the angular subtense of the patient's fundus caught by the lens. This distance is optimal if it equals the focal length of the lens. Thus, the field of view is determined by the expression d/F, where d is the diameter and F the focal length of the handheld lens.

For example, given equal diameters, stronger lenses (e.g., $F = 30D$, $f = 3.3cm$) provide larger fields of view. However, a weaker lens may be made with a larger diameter, because it is less vulnerable to spherical aberration. Thus, a 20D lens of 3cm diameter yields almost the same field of view as a 30D lens of 2cm diameter.

MAGNIFICATION. First, the magnification of the aerial image of the fundus is considered here. Figure 13-30 shows the chief ray that passes from the edge of the fundus view, through the nodal point of the eye, to the aerial image. For simplicity, assume the handheld lens is close to the patient's cornea. The ratio of the fundal object to the aerial image is proportional to the ratio of the focal length of the patient's eye to the focal length of the condenser lens, or inversely proportional to the power (F) of the eye (60D) and the handheld lens. Thus, for an emmetropic eye and a 20D lens, the magnification = 60D/20D = ×3; for a 30D lens, the magnification = 60D/30D = ×2.

Ultimately, the distance of this mildly magnified aerial image from the observer determines the total magnification. If the observer has a large amplitude of accommodation, the aerial image is brought closer and its overall magnification increased.

STEREOPSIS. The light beam that emerges from the patient's dilated pupils is directed through the handheld lens and into the two eyepieces (separation usually 15mm) of the binocular indirect ophthalmoscope. Prisms then redirect the two beams into the examiner's eyes. A smaller distance between the two eyepieces than the interpupillary distance reduces the stereopsis appreciated by an observer (interpupillary distance of 60mm) by about one fourth. However, axial magnification (which equals one fourth of the square of lateral magnification) augments the stereoscopic appearance. If the lateral magnification of a 20D lens is ×3, the axial magnification equals 9/4 or ×2.25. Thus, high-power, handheld lenses amplify small changes in retinal topography.

Finally, new variations of indirect ophthalmoscopy include the scanning laser ophthalmoscope and various analyzers of the optic nerve head (see Chapter 213).

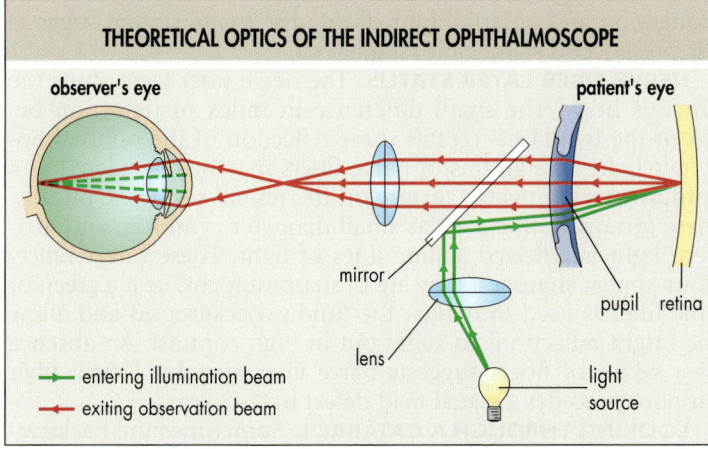

THEORETICAL OPTICS OF THE INDIRECT OPHTHALMOSCOPE

observer's eye | patient's eye

mirror

lens

pupil | retina

light source

→ entering illumination beam
← exiting observation beam

FIG. 13-29 ■ Theoretical optics of the indirect ophthalmoscope. The illumination beam enters a small part of the pupil and does not overlap with the observation beam, and thus minimizes bothersome reflection and backscatter.

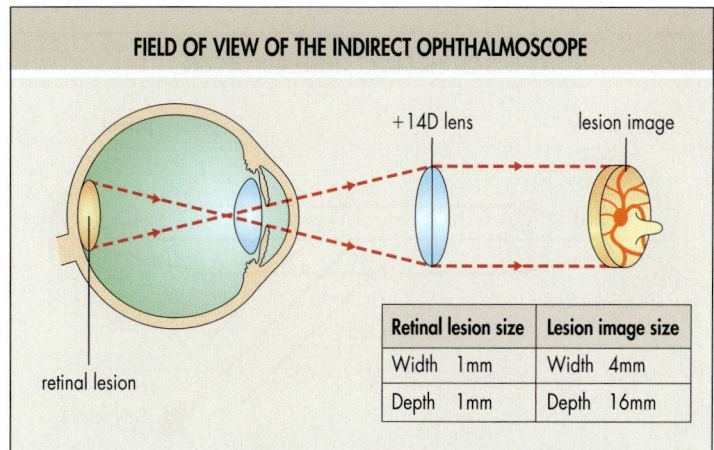

FIELD OF VIEW OF THE INDIRECT OPHTHALMOSCOPE

+14D lens | lesion image

retinal lesion

Retinal lesion size		Lesion image size	
Width	1mm	Width	4mm
Depth	1mm	Depth	16mm

FIG. 13-30 ■ Field of view, indirect ophthalmoscope. The focal length of the handheld lens determines the distance from the patient's eye at which to hold the lens. The tangent of the angle of field of view equals the lens diameter divided by the focal length.

DIRECT OPHTHALMOSCOPE

A thorough review of the origin of almost any important scientific development usually reveals that a number of people were involved in its discovery. Jan Purkinje published a complete technique of ophthalmoscopy in Latin in 1823.[26] During the next 25 years, a number of inventive people of different backgrounds, who include Kussmaul, Cumming, Brucke, and Babbage,[27] worked on the ophthalmoscope. In 1851 Helmholtz invented the first useable direct ophthalmoscope, which he described in a letter to his father.[20]

> I had to explain to my students that the theory of emission of the reflected light from the eye was discovered by Brucke. He was a hair's breadth from the invention of the ophthalmoscope. He failed to ask himself what optical image was formed by the rays reflected from the luminous eye.
>
> To obtain an optical image of the retina, he had only to devise an instrument in which his eye could be placed in line with rays of light entering and leaving the observed eye.

Optical Principles

In the 1970s, a camera company designed a flashbulb that fitted tightly onto a small, flat camera. To the chagrin of the company, the subjects in all the close-up shots had eerie red pupils. Optically speaking, this occurs when the axes of the light source and the observation system of the camera are almost coincident. The redness of the pupil is actually the unfocused image of the blood-filled choroid. This system of concentric illumination and observation is the very essence of the optics of the ophthalmoscope. Because the flashbulb company did not want to simulate the optics of the ophthalmoscope, the ultimate decision was to place the flashbulb on a stalk connector to keep it well out of line with the axis of the camera lens.

Figure 13-31 illustrates how the ophthalmoscope directs the light rays of illumination and observation in a concentric pattern—the essence of the observation system is a peephole. The lens and cornea of the patient's eye actually create the retinal image. Thus, the observer does not really see the retina of the patient, but an optical image of the retina.

To bring the red fundus reflex into sharp focus for the viewer, the modern ophthalmoscope has a disc of lenses, developed by Rekoss for Helmholtz only 1 year after the original discovery.[27] Because the compensating lens neutralizes the refractive error of both the physician and the patient, as well as the accommodation of each, its total power provides only a rough estimate of the patient's refractive state. However, one of the authors recently noticed that, in cases of astigmatism, the patient's foveal reflex is drawn out into a band that coincides with one of the major astigmatic meridians. A review of the literature demonstrated that this phenomenon was described originally in 1960.[28] Interestingly, the magnitude of a large amount of astigmatism may be estimated if the lens is focused on a blood vessel that travels parallel to the foveal reflex and then refocused on a vessel that travels perpendicular to the first vessel.

Probably the most important advance in direct ophthalmoscopy was the use of the halogen tungsten bulb,[29] which has a number of advantages over the older tungsten bulb. A quartz jacket can withstand higher temperatures than can the glass jacket; thus, the filament temperature may be raised higher than that in the conventional tungsten bulb, to produce an increased lumen output. Use of halogen vapor (bromine or iodine) within the quartz envelope extends the life of the filament and maintains an almost constant light output until the bulb's demise. In the ordinary incandescent lamp, tungsten particles evaporate from the hot filament and are carried by convection to the cooler bulb jacket; ultimately the filament is attenuated and a progressive black deposit formed on the jacket. In the new bulb, at high temperatures, tungsten atoms and halogen vapor form tungsten halide, which does not adhere to the jacket but returns by convection to rest on the filament. The heat of the filament chemically reduces the tungsten halide so that tungsten redeposits on the filament and halide vapor recirculates. Interestingly, the spectral output is similar to that of the traditional tungsten incandescent bulb, so that fundus details appear to have the same color as with the older bulbs.

The field of view of the new instruments also averages about 10° and is limited by the most oblique pencil of rays that can pass from the outer edge of the observer's pupil to the opposite outer edge of the patient's pupil. To enlarge the field of view of the direct ophthalmoscope the investigator's eye must be brought closer to the patient's eye with the patient's pupils dilated.

Because the enlargement capacity of any magnification lens usually is defined as one fourth of the lens power, the retinal image in the typical emmetropic eye of 60D may be considered to be magnified by 60/4, or ×15. In aphakic eyes, from which a 20D natural lens has been removed, the magnification for the observer is reduced to about 40/4 or ×10.

Extra Features of the Ophthalmoscope

BULB COLOR TEMPERATURE. An increase in the voltage directed to the bulb changes the color of the light from red to yellow. Clearly, the red light makes the nerve look healthier.

GREEN FILTER. Green filters in the ophthalmoscope make red tissue (blood vessels) and the pink tissue of the optic nerve appear gray. Use of a green filter often may differentiate the borders of the optic cup, which helps to determine the cup-to-disc ratio.

HIGH ASTIGMATISM. In a case of +2.00D of astigmatism (with the rule), the vertical dimension of the optic nerve is magnified and slightly out of focus. Thus, the combination of disc elongation and a partial blur of the disc margin often suggests the presence of significant astigmatism.

NERVE FIBER LAYER STATUS. The nerve fiber layer abuts the vitreous body. The small difference in index of refraction between the two layers creates some reflection of the ophthalmoscopic light. The groups of nerve fibers may be considered as a corduroy or corrugated texture on the retinal surface. Optically, these groups of fibers act as small-diameter cylinders, and incident light is reflected as fine lines of light. These linear reflections appear sharper if they are in sharpest focus, or if a green or blue filter is used to darken the fundus background and allow the bright reflections to stand out in high contrast. An absence of a sector of fibers suggests nerve fiber atrophy. Often, fiber dropout precedes a visual field defect by 1–2 years.

LOOKING THROUGH A CATARACT. Sometimes the backscatter from a cataract is not uniform and small clear areas are present. The small-diameter beam allows the observer to penetrate these clear areas and avoid the glare from the surrounding cataract that produces backscatter.

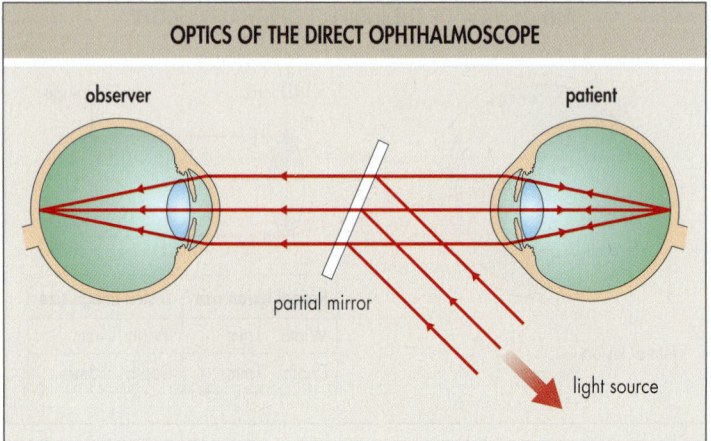

OPTICS OF THE DIRECT OPHTHALMOSCOPE

observer

patient

partial mirror

light source

FIG. 13-31 ■ Optics of the direct ophthalmoscope. By using a mirror (either half silvered or one that has a central aperture), the directions of the light of observation and the light incident to the patient are made concentric (coaxial).

CORNEAL REFLECTION. Gullstrand recognized the glare effect of the corneal reflection and described the principle of reflex in ophthalmoscopy in 1910.[30] The illumination and observation systems are concentric, as shown in Figure 13-31. In Gullstrand's solution, the illumination and observation systems are separated in the plane of the cornea and come together only at the retina. The embodiment of this principle is best seen in the indirect ophthalmoscope. For direct ophthalmoscopy, this principle works best when the ophthalmoscope is tipped and the patient's pupil dilated. Compromise solutions for smaller pupils are used in most of the present-day instruments, which do not give both optimal illumination and reflex-free observation. Use of polarization filters to remove reflections also has been suggested.[31] Unfortunately, a polarization system needs much higher levels of illumination and tends to constrict the natural pupil. When Helmholtz invented the ophthalmoscope, a prominent ophthalmologist of the day was said to remark that such introduction of a naked light surely must be harmful to the human eye.[20] Studies in the 1970s have raised this issue again. Whether the light from ophthalmoscopes, slit lamps, and operating microscopes results in permanent harm to the retinas of patients is unclear.[32,33] Studies suggest that the direct ophthalmoscope, with a standard bulb at design voltage, may be used safely for only about 1.5 minutes on each section of the retina that is observed.[34]

FUNDUS CAMERA

In 1851, Helmholtz's ophthalmoscope enabled ophthalmologists to view the living human fundus.[20] A mere 35 years later, Jackman and Webster published the first photographs of the human fundus *in vivo*.[35] Of course, those first pictures are not acceptable by today's standards—the disc looked like an irregular blotch and the retinal vessels could hardly be seen. These early pictures demonstrated that to capture the details of tissue so close to the cornea in a breathing, moving human being presented problems not ordinarily encountered in photography.

To best appreciate the technology of the present-day fundus camera, it might be helpful to see how each problem was solved historically.

Lighting

It is not difficult to obtain a photographic close-up using one of today's flashbulbs. Enough light is reflected from the subject to activate film of almost any sensitivity. In contrast, consider the feat accomplished by Howe in 1887 when he produced the first sharp photograph of a fundus.[36] His source of light was the hot Argand gas burner (similar to the Bunsen burner). The heat and glare of the flame was so intense that Howe was forced to use topical cocaine to keep his subject from squirming. It took another 35 years before Nordenson produced a camera that resembled today's models.[37] For illumination, they activated a carbon arc lamp, but the carbon arc was temperamental, noisy, lacked exposure control, and was not always bright enough. Cleverly placed reflectors and condensers did not always funnel enough carbon arc light through a smallish pupil or an eye that moved. Even if enough light managed to find a way through to the pupil, insufficient light always was reflected back to the film—the average fundus reflects only about 10% of the light back[38,39] (the optic nerve reflects more and heavily pigmented parts less). The solution of the illumination problem was solved partly by the arrival of the electronic flash. The stroboscopic flash was developed originally by Professor Harold Egerton of the Massachusetts Institute of Technology in 1931[40] to examine an engine's rapidly moving gears. The flashtube, filled with an inert gas (xenon or krypton), was ionized first by a trickle current and stimulated to glow by the release of a high voltage stored in a capacitor. Up to 10,000V may be released in a millisecond, to produce illumination as bright as 100,000 lu-

men seconds. (The average 100W bulb yields 2000 lumens in 1 second.) The life of such flashtubes is quite long—the average lamp produces 10,000 pictures before replacement. About 30 years after Egerton's first publication, Ogle and Rucker of the Mayo Clinic incorporated the electronic flash into the fundus camera.[41]

The present illumination system of the Zeiss fundus camera is shown in Figure 13-32.[42] Light from the incandescent lamp (for observation) and the flashlamp (for photography) is superimposed by means of the beam splitter, so that the light from the flash travels along the same path as that of the observation light. The lamp filaments are imaged in the vicinity of the holed mirror, which deflects the light toward the eye. The holed mirror is similar to the mirrors used in many retinoscopes, with a central hole to allow observation. In contrast to the retinoscope arrangement, the holed mirror in the fundus camera is imaged onto the plane of the patient's pupil by the objective lens, to ensure the necessary separation of illumination and observation pathways at the pupil. The objective lens corresponds to the condenser lens in the indirect ophthalmoscope; both lenses are designed with aspherical surfaces to provide the best possible image quality over a wide field of view.

The next illumination hurdle was to photograph through the natural pupil; this was achieved by observation of the fundus using infrared light, which does not stimulate the retina. In such a system, the infrared light penetrates the 4–5mm diameter pupil in a dark setting and is captured by a television camera after reflection from the retina. The television screen converts infrared information into a visible picture. Once the retina has been focused and framed, a powerful electronic flash takes a picture before the pupil constricts. It has been stated that 20–25 patients may be photographed in 1 hour using this television system, with only a 10% failure rate (blurred images).[43] Unfortunately, this natural pupil system cannot remain open long enough to be used under the continual flash assault needed for fluorescein angiography.

Bothersome Reflections

Anyone who has tried to evaluate subtle macular detail using a direct ophthalmoscope is familiar with the annoyance of corneal reflection. For example, Howe's early pictures clearly

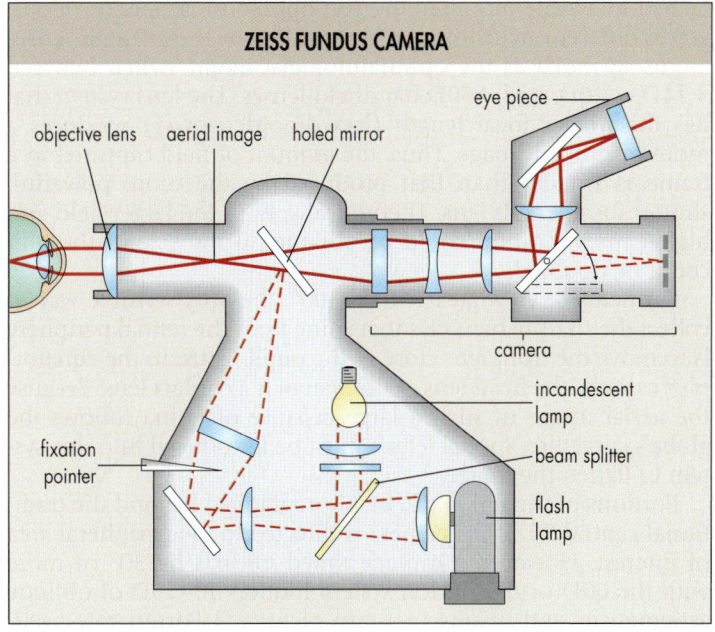

FIG. 13-32 ■ **Zeiss fundus camera.** See text for the description. (Adapted from American Academy of Ophthalmology. Home study course, optics and refraction. San Francisco: American Academy of Ophthalmology; 1990.)

showed corneal reflection that covered important retinal detail. This problem was solved ultimately by Gullstrand.[30]

Gullstrand's table-mounted ophthalmoscope embodied his principle that the illumination system should not intersect the cornea in the same area as the rays that come from the observation system. In the Zeiss system, this principle is satisfied by a mirror that has a central hole. The mirror reflects a circle of light through the pupillary periphery, while the fundus is viewed through the central hole of the mirror. Although such a system eliminates most ocular and camera lens reflections, bothersome reflections still are present. A well-designed camera can collect all the adversely reflected light and bring it to a point to become absorbed on a black absorption spot located on the front lens.[44]

The Observation System

Figure 13-32 illustrates all the elements of the fundus camera. As noted above, light from the incandescent lamp and that from the flashlamp are folded into a common path, which ultimately strikes the holed mirror and is reflected into the patient's eye. This illumination system and the observation system are very similar to those of the indirect ophthalmoscope. In the case of the fundus camera, light reflected from the patient's retina passes through the hole in the mirror and focuses a real image in the film plane of the camera. A beam splitter diverts a portion of the light directed to the camera and sends it to the eyepiece. In essence, the eyepiece is like a simple microscope. It receives the real image of the fundus and processes it such that parallel light exits for the observer.

Field of View

If the entire retina, fully illuminated, sends light rays out of the pupil then, even through a small pupil, theoretically a 180° aerial image of the retina can be reconstructed outside the eye. Because the rays from the equator exit the pupil at a very sharp angle, the collection of these rays can be accomplished only by a lens held very close to the pupil or a lens of very wide diameter. Put another way, the tangent of the angle that represents the field of view is made by the pupillary edge rays that strike the opposite edge of the observation lens (indirect ophthalmoscope lens or front camera lens). Of course, wide-diameter lenses produce a greater field of view, but they also introduce spherical aberration. The fundus camera is a single-lens reflex camera attached to a table-mounted indirect ophthalmoscope. To photograph different fields of view three different focal length lenses are used, much as the ophthalmologist might switch between +14D, +20D, and +30D handheld lenses. The lens system that has the longer focal length (less dioptric power) produces a more magnified image. Thus, the amount of field captured in a frame is smaller than that produced by the more powerful, shorter focal length lens. Theoretically, both the larger field and higher magnification could be obtained if the size of the film could be doubled.

For fields of view greater than 100°, the only sensible way to collect the sharply bent rays that come from the retinal periphery is to move the front lens close to the pupil. Thus, in the equator-plus camera, the front lens of the system is a contact lens. Because the aerial image of such a large expanse of retina follows the globe's curvature, special lenses must be introduced into this system to flatten the image.

Portions of the retina can be photographed beyond the traditional central 30° if the camera is directed to the peripheral area of interest. However, a camera aimed off axis by 30° or more with the 60D ocular optical system induces 10–15D of oblique astigmatism and results in fuzzy pictures.[45] Fortunately, well-designed fundus cameras anticipate off-axis photography and include a large range of cylindrical corrections with which to sharpen the peripheral views.

Fluorescein Angiography

In 1960, two third-year medical students, Norotny and Alvis, became the first investigators to perfect the technique of fluorescein angiography.[46] Their original photographs, taken after they had injected themselves with fluorescein, confirmed the early work of Flocks et al. on cats using a movie camera.[47] Subsequent photographs of patients who had diabetes showed leaking retinal circulation and were very clear, even by today's standards.

From an illumination point of view, a standard fluorescein angiographic series is very impressive. Peak emission of fluorescein occurs at 525nm, which is only 40nm longer than the peak excitation wavelength. For the best results, in terms of contrast, the system requires two narrow-band interference filters (barrier and excitation), the transmitted spectra of which do not overlap. Thus, a picture of the fundus taken just before the fluorescein arrives in the eye should be totally dark. Only a very restricted portion of the spectral output on the flashlamp excites the film and that portion only for a fraction of a second. Such a performance is impossible without very sensitive film, high-performance flashlamps, and a power supply that recharges and fires in less than 1 second. With such systems, up to 3 frames per second may be photographed. In addition, a motor drive is added that not only advances the film rapidly but also continually activates the swing-away mirror of the single-lens reflex camera for each exposure. Fortunately, modern video and computer image enhancement makes the task easier.

Stereoscopic Photography

Theoretically, a proper stereoscopic view of the fundus is obtained by two pictures of the fundus taken simultaneously at different angles. A similar effect is achieved if the pictures are not taken simultaneously. The Allen separator, which captures the fundus from two different angles, sequentially, not simultaneously, produces stereoscopic pictures. Such a system works well most of the time, but not if the eye moves between sequential pictures. To appreciate the height of papilledema or the depth of a glaucomatous cup, the stereoscopic pairs must be observed in a special stereoscopic viewer.

Camera and Film

Because a camera and film pack are attached to the back of the fundus camera, it is instructive to explore how these elements came into being.[48]

Of course, the elements of photography have been known for a number of centuries. In 1568, Professor Daniel Barbaro of the University of Padua described the first lens camera. He used a darkened room as his camera body. Light from the outside was funneled through a lens held against a hole in the curtain and brought to a focus on a sheet of white paper, held in the film plane. Obviously, the system did not give a permanent record of the events focused on the paper. The first successful attempt to capture a lighted image more permanently was accomplished by the German physicist, Johann Heinrich Schultz, in 1727. Schultz filled a glass flask with chalk, nitric acid, and silver and shook the mixture thoroughly, which created the light-sensitive transducer, silver nitrate. He then pasted stencils of opaque paper onto the flask and set it in the sun. Later, when he removed the stencils, he saw the image of the stencils traced on the surface of the mixture. It was another 100 years before the next important step—the first photographic plate—was accomplished by the fortuitous interaction of the two inventors of the hot-air engine, the Niepce brothers, and a painter by the name of Mande Daquerre.

By 1850, photographers made their own plates—a silver nitrate solution was mixed with collodion, a plate coated with the fresh mixture, and the picture shot before the plate dried. The gelatin-emulsion photographic film of today originated in the 1870s and was first marketed by an inventive entrepreneur named George

Eastman in 1888. Eastman's slogan for the Kodak system, "you press the button; we do the rest," involved selling the photographer a camera loaded with film. After the roll had been used, the photographer simply sent the camera with the film to the factory. The film was processed, and the prints and the camera (loaded with a fresh roll of film) were returned to the customer, all for $10 (U.S.).

The key to the photographic process is that when light strikes a crystal of silver halide, it converts some of the silver ions, which are clear, into atomic silver, which is black.[40] This reaction takes place primarily at the natural cracks of the crystal, which might be made up of millions of silver ions. The larger the crystal (the coarser the film grain), the more light is collected, and thus the more sensitive or faster the film. Film sensitivities or speeds are designated by the American Standards Association (ASA) number in the United States. For example, an ASA rating of 400 is 4 times faster or 4 times more light sensitive than a film of ASA 100. During chemical development, the partially decomposed silver halide crystals are converted into metallic silver.

The 35mm camera was introduced by the Leica Company soon after World War I. In time, a moveable mirror was incorporated into the small camera. The mirror was used to reflect (hence the name reflex camera) the image of the scene to be taken onto the viewfinder. Upon activation of the shutter button, the mirror swung out of the way, the focal plane shutter opened, the film was exposed, and the shutter closed. When the lever was cocked to advance the film to the next frame, the mirror was brought back into position and the aperture opened fully for optimal observation. The viewfinder in the single lens reflex uses a pentaprism which, along with the reflex mirror, takes the inverted image of the camera lens and reverts it. The final scene usually is depicted on a ground glass screen. The surface irregularities of the screen receive light and scatter it in many directions so that each point becomes an apparent source of light. The appropriate exposure, obtained via variation of the aperture diameter or shutter speed, is controlled automatically by a light meter in the latest models.

MAGNIFYING DEVICES

Angular Magnification

Most magnification devices ultimately produce parallel light and not real images. Devices that produce parallel light are described in terms of angular magnification, whereas lateral magnification devices produce images the sizes of which are comparable with the sizes of real objects.

Magnifying Glass

The first magnifying glass probably was invented by an unknown optician in about 1300 AD. Magnification produces an increase in the angular subtense of the retinal image, which can be achieved in a number of ways—when a child holds an object close to its eye, and when an adult (with little accommodation) looks at an enlarged object at a comfortable distance. By contrast, a magnifying glass creates a larger image of the close object, yet produces parallel light for the observer. Two basic concepts are involved in the magnifying glass. First, it is assumed that the enlarged angular subtense (in radians) of the retinal image equals the object size (y) divided by the power of the lens (F). Second, just as a patient's Snellen acuity is compared with that of someone who has normal vision, so the magnification angle y/F is compared with an object at a comfortable distance of 10in (25cm). In Figure 13-33, the relationship of y (object), $y1$ (image), and f (focal length) can be evaluated using similar triangles (Equation 13-3), and the magnification is given by Equation 13-4.

Equation 13-3
$$\frac{y}{f} = \frac{y1}{25}$$

Equation 13-4
$$\frac{y}{f} = \frac{y1}{25} = \frac{F}{4}$$

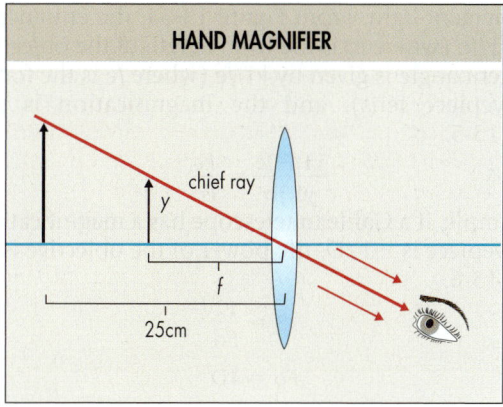

FIG. 13-33 ■ Optics of a magnifying glass. A virtual image is created at a distance of 25cm (see Equations 13-3 and 13-4).

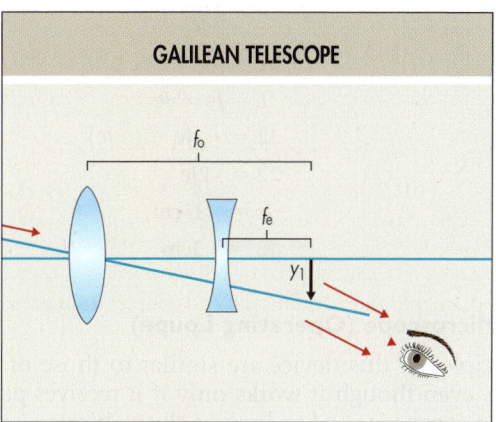

FIG. 13-34 ■ A Galilean telescope. Note the objective lens takes parallel light and places a real image at the focal point of the negative eyepiece. The eyepiece takes the incident convergent light and renders rays parallel.

For example, the angular magnification of a +8.00D lens = $F/4 = 8/4 = \times2$.

Galilean Telescope

The points on a distant object may be considered to produce parallel light. To enlarge the retinal image, the incident angle of the incoming rays of parallel light must be enlarged, yet the emergent rays must remain parallel. The true inventor of the telescope, Hans Lipershey, probably pointed a magnifying lens at a distant object. An image was produced at the focal point of the lens, which probably placed the image too close to the eye and strained his accommodation. He might have added a minus lens behind the magnifying glass to reproduce parallel light. As shown in Figure 13-34, to produce parallel light for the observer the initial image must be placed at the real focal point of the negative eyepiece; thus, the eyepiece receives convergent light and renders the rays parallel.

The Lipershey telescope originally was sold as a toy, called a spy glass, and had a magnification of ×3. About a year after its invention, Galileo learnt of it and unraveled the underlying principles. He then made a ×30 telescope and reported a number of astronomical observations, which popularized the device. Because it had a small field of view, he attached a low-powered spotting telescope for orientation. Ironically, these important scientific observations led to his downfall. His observation of the four moons of Jupiter that orbit that planet contradicted the church doctrine of the day, which decreed that every heavenly body moved around the Earth. Ultimately, he was sentenced to house arrest and suffered public humiliation.

To calculate the magnification of a telescope, the angle of incident parallel light is compared with the angle of the parallel rays of emergent light. From Figure 13-34, the entrance angle is given by $\gamma 1/fo$ (where fo is the focal length of the objective lens), the emergent angle is given by $\gamma 1/fe$ (where fe is the focal length of the eyepiece lens), and the magnification is given by Equation 13-5.

Equation 13-5
$$\frac{\gamma 1/-fe}{\gamma 1/fo} = \frac{Fe}{Fo}$$

For example, if a Galilean telescope has a magnification of ×3 and the eyepiece is −12D, the power of the objective is given by Equation 13-6.

Equation 13-6
$$3 = \frac{12}{Fo}$$
$$Fo = 4D$$

As another example, for a telescope of magnification ×3 and tube length (L), the distance between objective and eyepiece, of 22cm, fo and fe are given by Equation 13-7.

Equation 13-7
$$-3 = \frac{fo}{-fe}$$
$$-3fe = fo$$
$$L = fo - fe$$
$$22 = -3fe - (-fe)$$
$$22 = -2fe$$
$$-fe = -11cm$$
$$fo = 3.3cm$$

Simple Microscope (Operating Loupe)

The principles of this device are similar to those of a Galilean telescope, even though it works only if it receives parallel light and a microscope is used to look at close objects.

However, if a magnifying lens (Fw) is added, the focal length of which is the working distance, then the magnifying lens introduces parallel light to the telescope, as shown in Figure 13-35, and the total magnification is given by Equation 13-8.

Equation 13-8
$$\text{Magnification} = \frac{Fw}{4} \times \frac{Fe}{Fo}$$
Where Fe = dioptric power of eyepiece of telescope
Fo = dioptric power of objective of telescope

For example, for a loupe with a ×3 telescope and a +8D working lens (reading cap) the magnification = (8/4) ×3 = ×6.

Effects of Lens Aberrations

During the early days of the optics industry, a strong objective lens produced bothersome chromatic aberration. Newton, who was born the year Galileo died, realized that the main function of the objective lens of the telescope was simply to catch as much light as possible from the object and present it to the eye-piece for the real magnification. He replaced the objective lens with a mirror—mirrors do not produce chromatic aberration.

Before the days of aspherical lenses or multiple element lenses, the only way to correct spherical aberration was to use low-power lenses of small diameter (the amount of spherical aberration is related directly to the diameter and power of the lens). Today, high-powered lenses can be made in aspherical form and aberration can be eliminated.

REFERENCES

1. Malacara D. Optical shop testing, ed 2. New York: Wiley; 1992:367–96.
2. Doss JD, Hutson RL, Rowsey JJ, et al. Method for calculation of corneal profile and power distribution. Arch Ophthalmol. 1981;99:1261–5.
3. Tage GW, Safir A. The slit lamp; history, principles and practice. In: Duane TD, ed. Clinical ophthalmology, vol 1. New York: Harper & Row; 1980:1–44.
4. Feuk T, McQueen D. The angular dependence of light scattering by rabbit cornea. Invest Ophthalmol. 1987;10:294–8.
5. Slayter EM. Optical methods in biology. Huntington: Rob E Krieger Publishing; 1963:253–64.
6. Spalton DJ, Hitchings RA, Hunter PA. Atlas of clinical ophthalmology. New York: Gower Medical; 1984:10.
7. Mishima S. Corneal thickness. Surv Ophthalmol. 1968;13:57–96.
8. Miller D, Exford J. The effect of contact lenses on corneal thickness. Contact Lens. 1967;1:5–7.
9. Miller D, Dohlman CH. The effect of cataract surgery on the cornea. Trans Am Acad Ophthalmol Otolaryngol. 1970;74:369–74.
10. Miller D, Stegmann R. Use of Na-hyaluronate in human IOL implantation. Ann Ophthalmol. 1981;13:811–5.
11. Maumenee AE. Clinical aspects of the corneal homograft reaction. Invest Ophthalmol. 1962;1:244–52.
12. Gullstrand A. Demonstration der Nerstspattlempe. Heidelberg: Heidelberger Bericht; 1911.
13. Vogt A. Ober Sichtbarkeit des lebenden Hornhautendothels in Liehtbuschel der Gullstrandschen Spaltlamp. Klin Monatsbl Augenheilkd. 1919;63:233–4.
14. Vogt A. Lehrbuch und Atlas der Spaltlampen mikroskopie des lebenden Augen mit Anlestung zur Technik und Methodikder Untersuchung, vol 1. Berlin: Julius Spring; 1930.
15. Maurice DM. Cellular membrane activity in the corneal endothelium of the intact eye. Experientia. 1968;24:1094–5.
16. Laing RA, Sandstrom UM, Leibowitz HM. In vivo photomicroscopy of corneal endothelium. Arch Ophthalmol. 1975;93:143–5.
17. Laing RA, Sandstrom MM, Leibowitz HM. Clinical specular microscopy. I: Optical principles. Arch Ophthalmol. 1979;97:1714–9.
18. Bigar F. Specular microscopy of the corneal endothelium. In: Straub W, ed. Developments in ophthalmology, vol 6. Basel: Karger; 1982:1–88.
19. Koester CJ. Scanning mirror microscope with optical sectioning characteristics: applications in ophthalmology. Appl Opt. 1980;19:1749–57.
20. Rucker CW. A history of ophthalmology. Rochester: Whiting Printers and Stationers; 1971:57–62.
21. Von Helmholtz H. Ueber eine neue einfachste Form des Augenspiegel. Arch Physiol Heilbron. 1852;2:827–40.
22. Duke-Elder S. System of ophthalmology, vol 4. St Louis: CV Mosby; 1949:4391–3.
23. Guyton DL. Automated clinical refraction. In: Duane T, ed. Clinical refraction, vol 1. Baltimore: Harper & Row; 1987:1–43.
24. Safir A. Automatic measurement of the refractive properties of the eye. Med Res Eng. 1972;2:12–8.
25. Rubin M. Optics for clinicians. Gainesville: Triad Publications; 1974.
26. Albert DM, Miller WH. Jan Purkinje and the ophthalmoscope. Am J Ophthalmol. 1973;76:494–500.
27. Pearlman JT, Pearlman SJ, Engreen FE. Early efforts to view the human fundus. Doc Ophthalmol. 1973;34:317–25.
28. Kent PR. The foveal light reflex and its use as an objective test for astigmatism. Am J Optom Arch Am Acad Optom. 1960;37:304–8.
29. GTE Sylvania Lighting Center. Tungsten–halogen lamps. Sylvania Engineering Bulletin O-349. Danvers: GTE Sylvania Lighting Center; 1970.
30. Gullstrand A. Neue Methoden der reflexlosen Ophthalmopskiepie. Ber Disch Ophthalmol Ges. 1910;30:36–75.
31. Savell AL. The Cardell polarized ophthalmoscope. S Afr Refractionist. 1954;1:7–10.
32. Lanum J. The damaging effects of light on the retina: empirical findings. Theoretical and practical implications. Surv Ophthalmol. 1978;22:221–49.
33. Sperling HD. Are ophthalmologists exposing their patients to dangerous light levels? Invest Ophthalmol Vis Sci. 1980;19:989–95.
34. Calkins JL, Hochheimer BF. Retinal light exposure from ophthalmoscopes, slit lamps and overhead surgical lamps: an analysis of potential hazards. Invest Ophthalmol Vis Sci. 1980;19:1009–15.
35. Jackman WT, Webster JD. On photographing the retina of the living eye. Phil Photographer. 1886;23:275–80.
36. Howe L. Photography of the interior of the eye. Trans Am Ophthalmol Soc. 1885–7;4:568–78.
37. Nordenson JW. Augen kamera zum stationaren Ophthalmoskop von Gullstrand. Ber Disch Ophthalmol Ges. 1925;45:278–88.
38. Vos JJ, Munnik AA, Buogaard J. Absolute spectral reflectance of the fundus oculi. J Opt Soc Am. 1965;55:573–80.
39. Flower RW, McLeod DS, Pitts SM. Reflection of light from the ocular fundus. In: International Symposium on Ophthalmological Optics. Jap Soc Ophthalmol Optics. 1978:129–33.
40. Rhode FB, McCall FH. Introduction to photography. New York: McMillan; 1971:165.
41. Ogle KN, Rucker CW. Fundus photographs in color using a high speed flash tube in the Zeiss retinal camera. Arch Ophthalmol. 1953;49:435–40.
42. American Academy of Ophthalmology. Home study course, optics and refraction. San Francisco: American Academy of Ophthalmology; 1990.

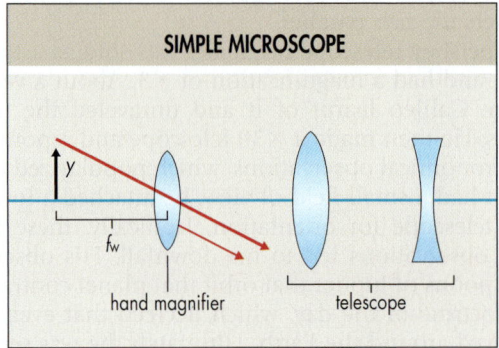

SIMPLE MICROSCOPE

hand magnifier   telescope

FIG. 13-35 ■ **A simple microscope.** A positive lens (working distance lens) is placed in front of a Galilean telescope. This lens takes light from an object located at its focal point and renders the rays parallel for the Galilean telescope part of the device.

43. Shimamoto S, Matsubara H, Itoi M. The fundus camera with an infrared TV system. In: International Symposium on Ophthalmological Optics. Jap Soc Ophthalmol Optics; 1978:141–5.
44. Leutwein K, Littman H. The fundus camera. In: Duane T, ed. Clinical ophthalmology, vol. 1. Hagertown: Harper & Row; 1981:1–16.
45. Busse BJ, Mittleman D. Use of the astigmatism correction device on the Zeiss fundus camera for peripheral retina photography. In: Justice J, ed. Ophthalmic photography. Int Ophthalmol Clin. 1976;16:63–75.

46. Novotny HR, Alvis DL. Methods of photographing fluorescein in the circulating blood in human retinal circulation. Circulation. 1961;24:82–90.
47. Flocks M, Miller J, Chae P. Retinal circulation time with the aid of fundus cinephotography. Arch Ophthalmol. 1966;61:1359–66.
48. Newhall B. The history of photography. New York: Museum of Modern Art; 1964.

14 Perspectives in Aberrations of the Eye

EDMOND H. THALL • PAVIKA THAMMANO • RUSSELL MILLER

DEFINITION
- Optical aberrations refer to specific defects in an optical system that diminish the resolution of an image. The eye, like any other optical system, suffers from a number of specific aberrations.

KEY FEATURES
- Understanding of the wave front concept.
- Understanding of wave front analysis.
- Understanding of irregular astigmatism.
- Understanding of the limitations of aberration theory.

ASSOCIATED FEATURES
- Understanding of the clinical methods of measurement.
- Understanding of the limits of retinal resolution.
- Understanding of the limits of corneal topography.
- Useful rules of thumb for clinicians.

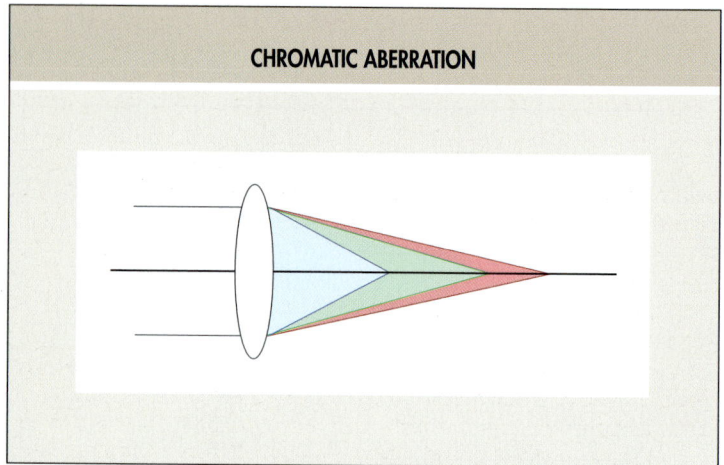

FIG. 14-1 ▒ **Chromatic aberration.** The refractive index of a material varies with wavelength. Consequently, blue light, green light, and red light focus in different locations. In this figure, chromatic aberration is greatly exaggerated for purposes of illustration.

INTRODUCTION

Aberrations of optical imaging systems and, specifically, aberrations of the eye have been studied for nearly 400 years. In the early 1600s, Galileo found empirically that apertures restricting the amount of light entering a telescope often improved the images.[1] In 1619, Scheiner described his own regular astigmatism by observing the change in the appearance of a needle oriented in different axes.[2] In 1611, Kepler described spherical aberration and the use of hyperboloidal lenses to correct it.[3]

Occasionally, aberrations are intentionally exaggerated for artistic effect, but aberrations decrease the contrast and amount of detail (i.e., resolution) and produce other undesirable effects in the image.[4] Consequently, a great deal of effort is devoted to reducing aberrations.

The average ophthalmologist is probably unaware of not only the amount work required to reduce aberrations but also the importance of doing so in even the simplest imaging systems. Today's plastic disposable cameras have been carefully designed and, depending on the manufacturer, consist of either three or four lenses that correct all the Seidel aberrations as well as some chromatic aberration. Obviously, disposable cameras do not yield the excellent images rendered by professional photographic equipment, but they are nevertheless sophisticated devices.

Reducing even a few aberrations produces noticeable benefits. By eliminating aberrations through careful design, some of today's toy telescopes and microscopes far outperform the best instruments used by Galileo, Hooke, van Leeuwenhoek, and generations of mariners.

There are two general ways to reduce aberrations. One method is to use multiple lenses instead of a single lens. The aberrations produced by one lens tend to cancel, or "balance," the aberrations of the other lenses so that the combination has less total aberration than any single lens. An example of this approach is the correction of chromatic aberration.

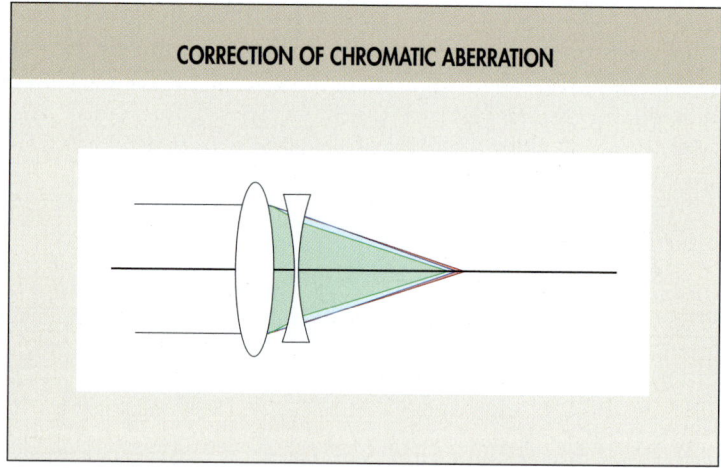

FIG. 14-2 ▒ **Correction of chromatic aberration.** Chromatic aberration can be reduced by replacing a single lens with two lenses constructed from different types of glass. The chromatic aberration of the first lens is largely canceled by the chromatic aberration of the second lens. The combination is referred to as an achromatic lens, although the term is somewhat misleading, because there is still some residual chromatic aberration.

The refractive index of a material varies with wavelength, so a single lens focuses blue and red light in slightly different locations, producing an effect called chromatic aberration (Fig. 14-1). The amount of chromatic aberration produced by a single lens is the product of its power and the dispersion of the material used to construct the lens. Thus, a lower-power negative lens made with high-dispersion glass can cancel the chromatic aberration of a higher-power plus lens made with low-dispersion glass (Fig. 14-2). By replacing a single lens with a combination of two lenses (with the same total power) constructed from different materials, chromatic aberration can be reduced greatly.

The same approach works for other aberrations. In general, each additional lens added to an optical system allows the correction of more aberration.[5] A quality camera lens usually consists of six to twelve individual lenses or elements and produces images containing more detail than film can record.[6] Thus, it is the film, not the lens, that limits the amount of detail that can be captured photographically.[7]

The multiple-lens approach is used clinically to correct refractive errors. A corrective lens is simply an additional lens added to the eye's optical system to correct aberrations. However, practical considerations largely limit corrective lenses to a single element, so only a few ocular aberrations are correctable. Ophthalmologists are quite familiar with the aberrations (i.e., refractive errors) that can be corrected by a single lens. The rest of the eye's aberrations are lumped into the single category of irregular astigmatism, which has been largely ignored by clinicians because of our limited ability to treat it.

However, the aberrations constituting irregular astigmatism have been thoroughly studied by optical engineers, who are able to correct these aberrations in other imaging systems.[8-10] The aberration theory developed by engineers is applicable to the eye, and basic researchers have produced a vast literature dealing specifically with the eye's aberrations. It is important for clinicians to realize that irregular astigmatism is in fact a subject that has been extensively studied and continues to be actively researched.

Aspherical surfaces provide another way to correct aberrations. In the seventh century AD, Ibn Sahl discovered that a lens with a hyperboloidal surface—not a spherical surface—was the most efficient way to focus sunlight to start a fire.[11] As mentioned earlier, Kepler and later Descartes and others showed that ellipsoidal and other forms of aspherical refracting surfaces could reduce many aberrations.[8] However, until recently, it was impossible to fabricate accurate aspherical refracting surfaces at an acceptable cost.[12] An accurately constructed spherical surface is superior to an inaccurately configured aspherical surface.[13]

In the past, owing to manufacturing limitations, the only shapes that could be accurately configured were spherical, cylindrical, and plano (flat), so all imaging systems were constructed using only these three shapes. In the last 30 years, it has become possible to produce a variety of aspherical surfaces, and many imaging systems now employ aspherical elements.

However, it is difficult to apply aspherical surfaces to the correction of ocular aberrations because the eye moves relative to the corrective lens, whereas in most imaging systems, the individual elements are fixed and carefully aligned with respect to one another. Progressive add lenses are aspherical, but they are used to correct presbyopia, not irregular astigmatism.

Placing the correction of irregular astigmatism in the cornea obviates problems associated with ocular movement. With the advent of narrow-beam, scanning excimer lasers, it may be possible to produce an accurate aspherical corneal surface that corrects some irregular astigmatism as well as the conventional refractive errors. However, the correction of irregular astigmatism requires not only a means of sculpting the cornea but also a means of measuring and analyzing irregular astigmatism.

Clinical correction of irregular astigmatism must be approached quantitatively. The irregular astigmatism in an eye must be accurately measured. Just as conventional refractive error is separated into spherical and cylindrical components, irregular astigmatism must be separated into its component parts.

Aberration theory is the branch of optics that deals with the measurement and analysis of irregular astigmatism. Aberration theory was not clinically relevant in the past, but because of developments in refractive surgery, it has come rather suddenly to the forefront of clinical optics. Unfortunately, most treatments of aberration theory are in the engineering literature, and these are of limited value to clinicians because of the unfamiliar terminology and highly mathematical style of presentation. This chapter presents aberration theory from a clinical perspective,

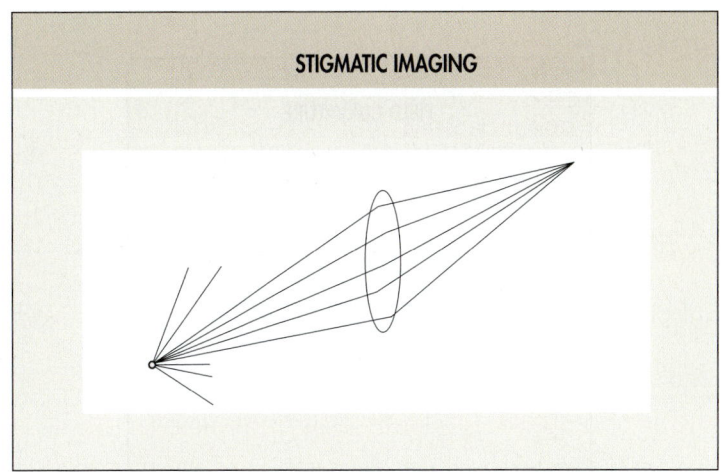

FIG. 14-3 ▌ **Stigmatic imaging.** Ideally, all rays from a single object point converge to a single image point. This ideal is never achieved in practice, but generally, the closer to stigmatic the image, the better the image quality.

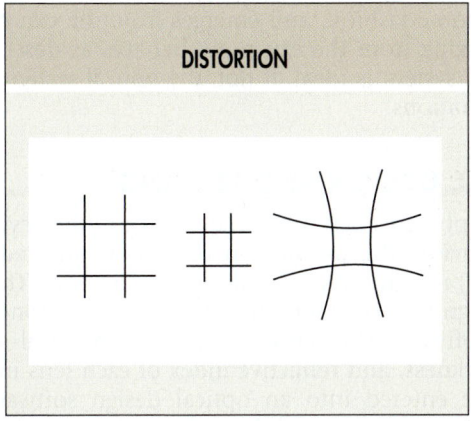

FIG. 14-4 ▌ **Distortion.** The object is on the left, and a distortion-free image is in the center. In the image on the right, straight lines in the object are imaged as curved lines. The image on the right is distorted.

with an emphasis on its application to refractive surgery. Enough mathematical detail is contained in the appendix to allow the interested reader to explore the subject further.

THE IDEAL OPTICAL IMAGING SYSTEM

Although the study of aberrations began in the early 1600s, the approach was largely qualitative. The study of aberrations was placed on a firm quantitative basis in the mid-1800s when Mobius and Hamilton independently developed the concept of the ideal optical system.[14,15] By definition, the ideal, rotationally symmetrical optical system has three characteristics.

1. Stigmatic imaging: All rays originating from a point source located *anywhere* in object space must converge to a perfect point in image space (Fig. 14-3).
2. Geometrical similarity: The image must be a "scale model" of the object. The image may be smaller than, larger than, or the same size as the object, but it cannot be distorted (Fig. 14-4). This requirement applies only to objects confined to any single plane perpendicular to the axis. Geometrical similarity places no restriction on image orientation. The image may be rotated or even inverted with respect to the object.
3. No field curvature: If the object is confined to a plane, the image must be confined to a plane (Fig. 14-5).

Note that the ideal imaging system is defined functionally, in other words, by what it does. Nothing has been said about the construction of the system. The optical system can be thought of as a "black box." Light enters through the entrance pupil, is redi-

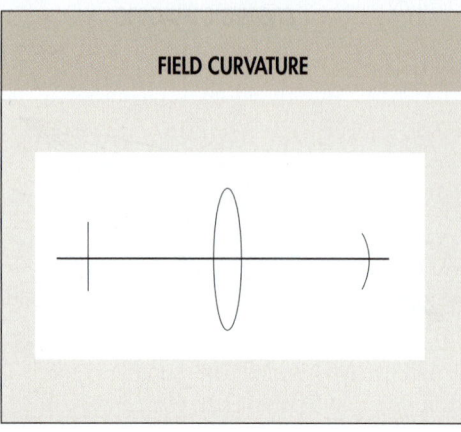

FIG. 14-5 ▪ **Field curvature.** The object is flat and perpendicular to the axis, but the image is curved. The ideal optical system would produce an image that is also flat and perpendicular to the optical axis.

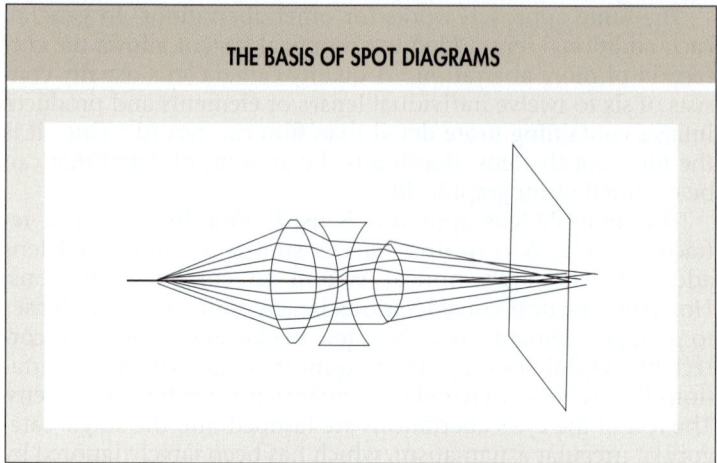

FIG. 14-6 ▪ **The basis of spot diagrams.** In reality, rays do not focus stigmatically (i.e., to a perfect point). An imaginary plane is located near the desired image point, and the intersection of each ray with the plane is plotted as a spot diagram.

rected in some fashion, and emerges from the exit pupil. If the light emerging from the exit pupil behaves as described above, the optical system is ideal. If not, the optical system has one or more aberrations.

OPTICAL DESIGN AND TESTING

Quite simply, an aberration is defined as any deviation from ideal behavior. The production of a well-corrected (i.e., low-aberration) imaging system is done in two stages. The first stage is the design process. Modern optical design is done using specialized software. The power, shape (if aspherical surfaces are used), thickness, and refractive index of each lens in an optical system are entered into an optical design software package. Hundreds of rays are traced through the theoretical system, and the aberrations are calculated. The design is modified and the aberrations are recalculated many times until a design with acceptably low levels of aberration is achieved.

After the design is completed, it must be fabricated. To ensure proper fabrication, the aberrations are measured and compared with the designer's theoretical prediction. If the measured aberrations exceed the theoretical aberrations by more than a small tolerance, the surfaces must be modified. The discipline of optical testing is devoted to measuring the aberrations of existing optical systems. Optical testing can be quite complicated; indeed, the problems with the Hubble telescope were the result of inadequate optical testing.

The clinical correction of irregular astigmatism requires some aspects of both design and testing. First, irregular astigmatism in an eye must be measured using some form of optical testing. Then correction of the aberrations must be planned using some sort of software that incorporates principles of optical design.

Aberration theory is used in both the design and testing stages. There are two general, complementary approaches to the study of aberrations: ray aberrations and wave aberrations. In a sense, ray aberrations are based on Snell's law, whereas wave aberrations are based on Fermat's principle.

RAY ABERRATIONS

Figure 14-6 shows a three-element optical system, an object point, and a plane in image space. The choice of object point and plane is completely arbitrary, but usually the plane is in the vicinity of, but not necessarily at, the image. Textbooks usually show the rays from the object point converging to a single image point (stigmatic imaging; see Fig. 14-3), and this is certainly the ideal situation, but in reality, owing to aberrations, rays rarely converge to a common point. Instead, rays cluster within a small area.

The exact path of a ray can be determined by applying Snell's law to each surface of an optical system. The point where the ray intersects the plane in image space can be precisely located (see Fig. 14-6). The process is repeated for many rays originating from the same image point, and the end result is a spot diagram showing the intersection of each ray with the plane. The transverse ray aberration is the displacement (expressed as a vector) of the actual ray from a reference point—either the chief ray or the desired image point.[16]

Usually spot diagrams are generated for several planes in front of, at, and behind the image, yielding a set of through-focus spot diagrams. Exact ray tracing is calculation intensive, and the production of spot diagrams is greatly facilitated by commercially available lens design software.

The advantage of the spot diagram is that it gives an immediate visual representation of the total amount of aberration present and the image quality. Generally, the smaller the spot diagram (at best focus), the fewer the aberrations and the better the image. Table 14-1 shows the spot diagrams associated with many aberrations.

Spot diagrams are especially useful for studying the effects of individual aberrations in isolation. Ophthalmologists are quite familiar with the conoid of Sturm, which is essentially a through-focus spot diagram of the aberration known clinically as regular astigmatism.

Spot diagrams are more difficult to interpret when several aberrations are present, as is usually the case in most optical systems, including the eye. When several aberrations are present, wave aberrations are easier to interpret.[17]

THE GEOMETRICAL WAVE FRONT

Wave aberrations are based on the concept of a geometrical wave front. Light radiates in all directions from a point source in a homogeneous medium (Fig. 14-7). Consider an imaginary circle (or sphere in three dimensions) centered on the object point (see Fig. 14-7). Although light travels with great speed, it requires some time to reach the circle, and that time is the same no matter which path (i.e., ray) the light follows. The circle is a geometrical wave front for the given object point.

In general, a geometrical wave front is any isochronic surface associated with a specific object point. Isochronic means equal time, and the amount of time required for light to travel from a specified object point to the wave front is equal for all rays. Note that wave fronts are associated with only one object point. Two different object points produce two distinct sets of wave fronts.

At the boundary between two optical media, light changes speed, which alters the shape of the wave front (see Fig. 14-7). No matter what the shape, the amount of time required for light

Text continued on p. 114

TABLE 14-1

ZERNIKE POLYNOMIALS UP TO THE EIGHTH ORDER AND THEIR ASSOCIATED SPOT DIAGRAMS

Zernicke Term	Spot Diagrams	Aberration Surfaces

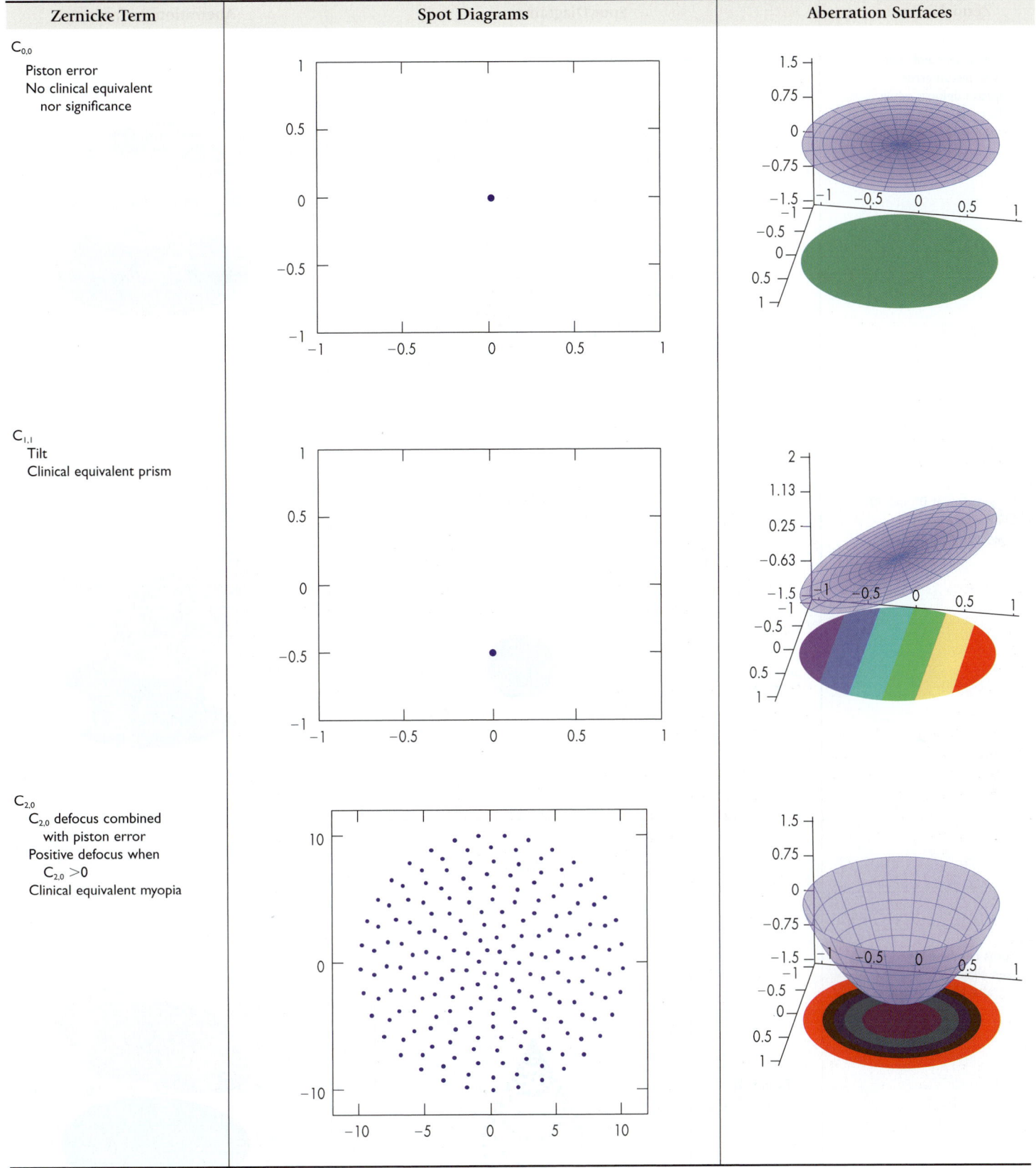

$C_{0,0}$

   Piston error
   No clinical equivalent
     nor significance

$C_{1,1}$
   Tilt
   Clinical equivalent prism

$C_{2,0}$
   $C_{2,0}$ defocus combined
     with piston error
   Positive defocus when
     $C_{2,0} > 0$
   Clinical equivalent myopia

Continued

TABLE 14-1

ZERNIKE POLYNOMIALS UP TO THE EIGHTH ORDER AND THEIR ASSOCIATED SPOT DIAGRAMS—cont'd

Zernicke Term	Spot Diagrams	Aberration Surfaces

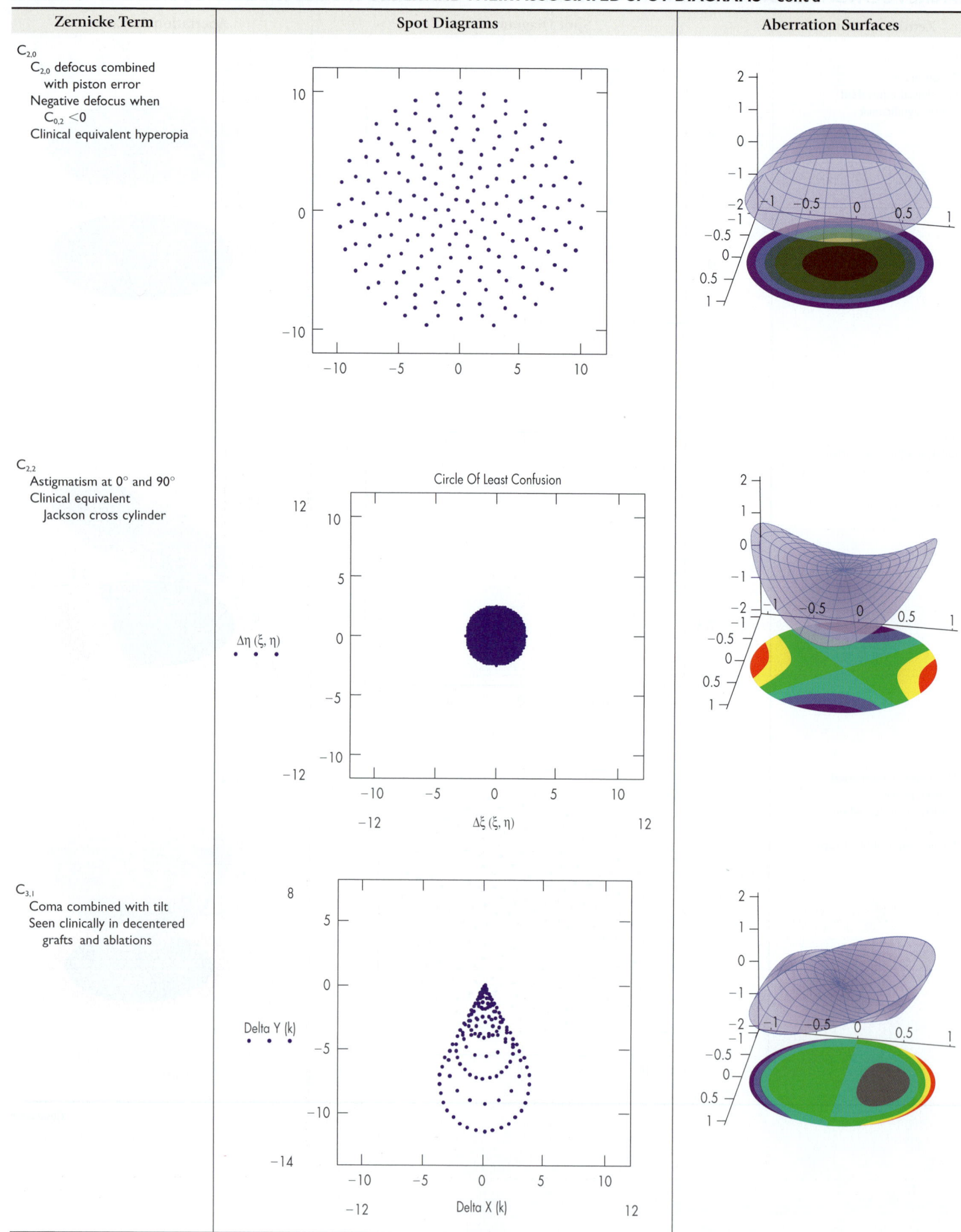

$C_{2,0}$
$C_{2,0}$ defocus combined with piston error
Negative defocus when $C_{0,2} < 0$
Clinical equivalent hyperopia

$C_{2,2}$
Astigmatism at 0° and 90°
Clinical equivalent Jackson cross cylinder

Circle Of Least Confusion

$\Delta\eta\ (\xi, \eta)$

$\Delta\xi\ (\xi, \eta)$

$C_{3,1}$
Coma combined with tilt
Seen clinically in decentered grafts and ablations

Delta Y (k)

Delta X (k)

TABLE 14-1

ZERNIKE POLYNOMIALS UP TO THE EIGHTH ORDER AND THEIR ASSOCIATED SPOT DIAGRAMS—cont'd

Zernicke Term	Spot Diagrams	Aberration Surfaces
$C_{3,3}$	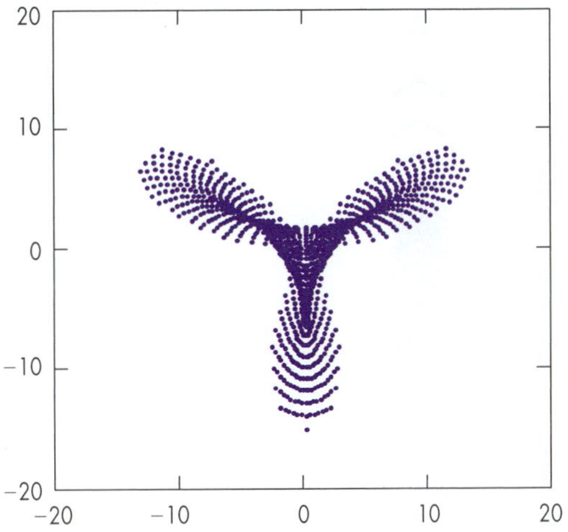	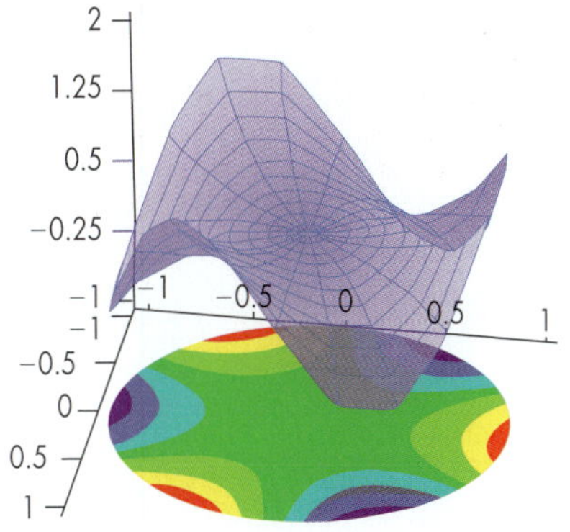
$C_{4,0}$ Spherical aberration combined with defocus and piston error Seen clinically in oblate corneas	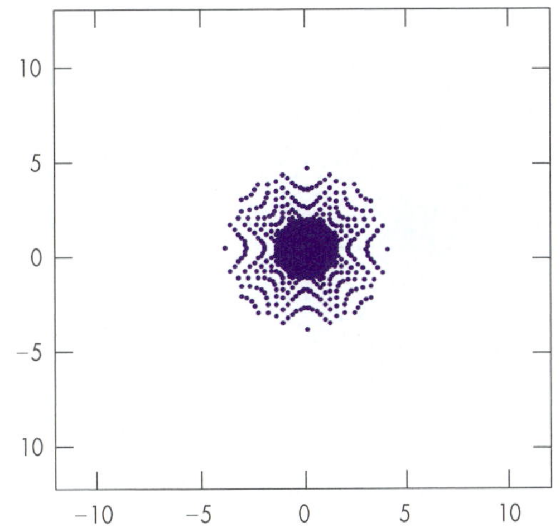	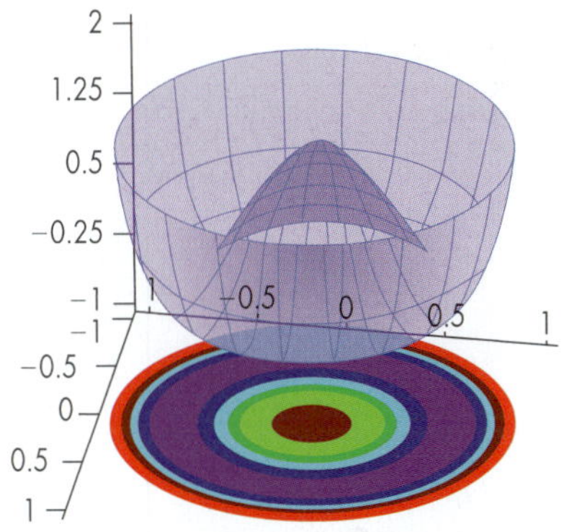
$C_{4,2}$	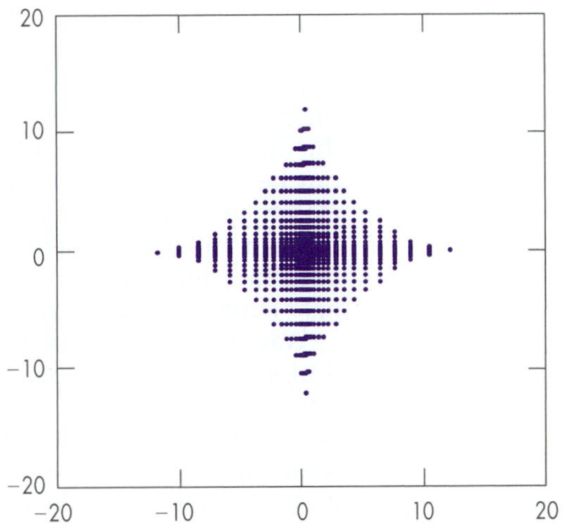	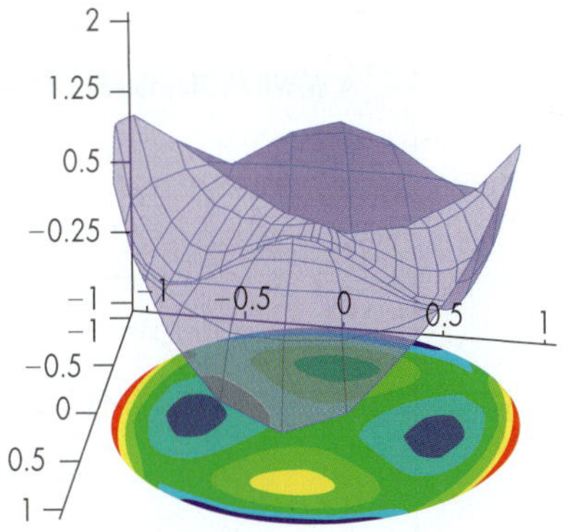

Continued

TABLE 14-1

ZERNIKE POLYNOMIALS UP TO THE EIGHTH ORDER AND THEIR ASSOCIATED SPOT DIAGRAMS—cont'd

Zernicke Term	Spot Diagrams	Aberration Surfaces
$C_{5,1}$	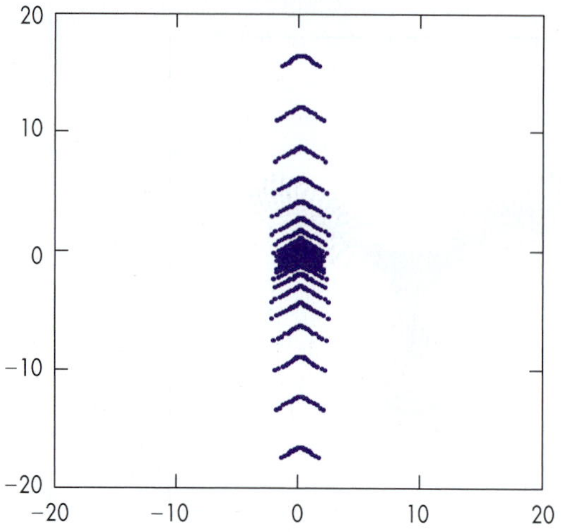	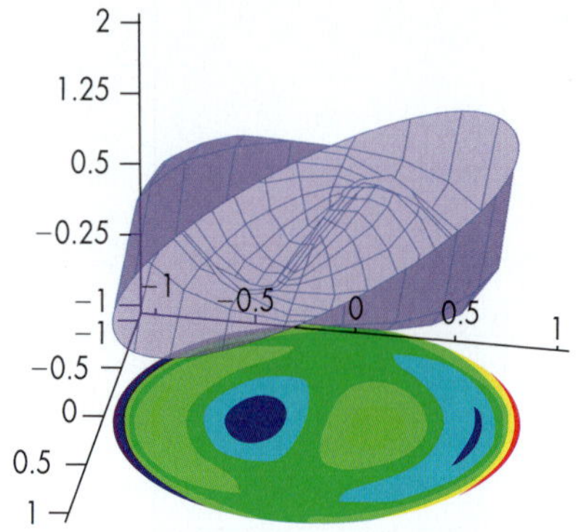
$C_{6,0}$	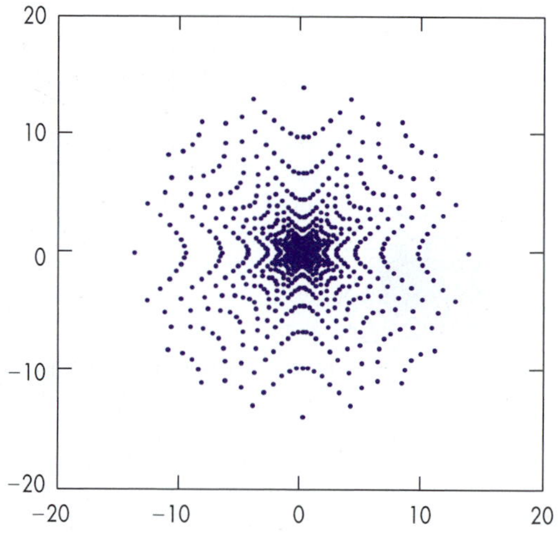	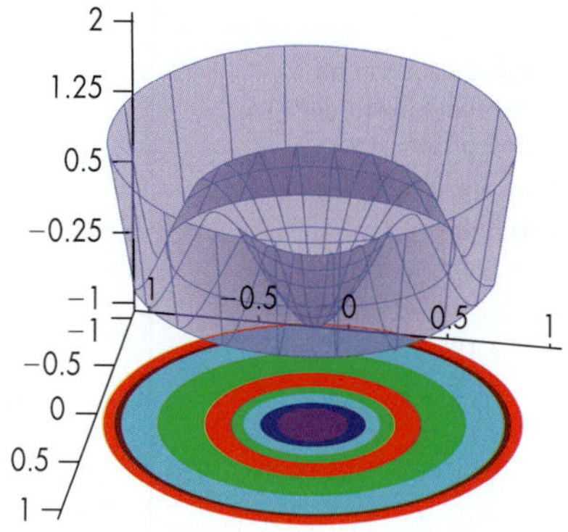

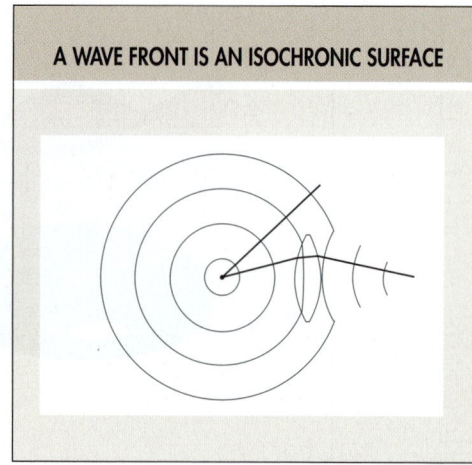

FIG. 14-7 ■ **A wave front is an isochronic surface.** All light from a single object point reaches the wave front simultaneously. The lens changes the shape of the wave front, ideally into converging spheres. Rays are perpendicular to the wave front.

to travel from the object point to the wave front is identical for all rays. Wave fronts and rays are closely related. Rays are always normal to the wave front. Thus, given the shape of the wave front, the direction of any light ray can be calculated. Conversely, given the direction of (several) light rays, the shape of the wave front can be calculated. Wave fronts and rays are two different but closely related ways of representing how light propagates through an optical system. A single ray represents one of many different paths light can follow, but a wave front represents all the light (from one object point) that traverses the optical system.

Wave fronts start as perfect spheres, and each surface of an optical system changes the shape of the wave front. If the wave front has the shape of a perfect sphere centered on the image point when it emerges from the optical system, the focus will be stigmatic. Otherwise, the focus will not be stigmatic, and one or more aberrations will be present.

WAVE ABERRATION

When a wave front emerges from a real optical system, it rarely has the ideal spherical shape, owing to the presence of aberrations. The wave aberration is the difference between the actual wave front and the ideal spherical wave front. Wave aberration is the difference between two surfaces; therefore, its surface is usually shaped somewhat like a potato chip.

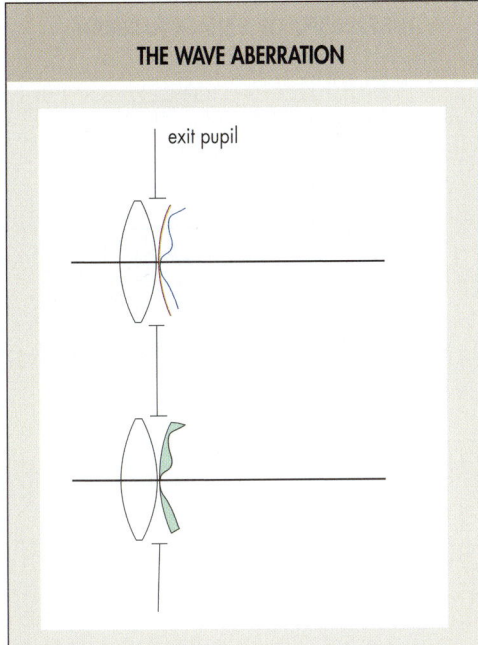

THE WAVE ABERRATION

exit pupil

FIG. 14-8 ■ **Wave aberration.** The reference sphere is centered on the desired image point and intersects the center of the exit pupil (shown in red on the top). An ideal optical system would produce an actual wave front that coincides with the reference sphere. A real optical system produces a wave front that does not coincide with the reference sphere (shown in blue on the top). The difference between the actual wave front and the reference sphere is the wave aberration (shown in green on the bottom).

Without belaboring the mathematics, some additional details are necessary to adequately define wave aberration. By convention, in wave aberration theory, there are three references: the desired image point, the exit pupil, and the reference sphere. Every optical system has an exit pupil. Clinically, the desired or intended image point is on the retina. The intended image point is the center of the reference sphere, and the radius of the reference sphere is the distance from the image point to the exit pupil's center (Fig. 14-8). The reference sphere represents the ideal, aberration-free wave front. For images at infinity, the reference sphere becomes a reference plane.

The shape of the actual wave front is either calculated using optical design software or measured. There are infinitely many wave fronts associated with one object point, but only one wave front intersects the center of the exit pupil, and the difference between this wave front and the reference sphere is the wave aberration.

WAVE FRONT ANALYSIS OF SPHERICAL AND CYLINDRICAL AMETROPIA

Clinically, wave aberrations are used primarily to describe irregular astigmatism, but any aberration of the eye can be analyzed using wave fronts. In myopia, the actual image is anterior to the intended image point; thus the actual wave front has a smaller radius than the reference sphere (see Fig. 14-8). The difference between the actual wave front and the reference sphere is a bowl-shaped surface (see Table 14-1). Hyperopia is much the same, except that the bowl is upside down. As one might expect, regular astigmatism produces a cylindrical wave front aberration, and the combination of either hyperopia or myopia with regular astigmatism produces a toroidal or spherocylindrical wave aberration.

WAVE FRONT ANALYSIS OF IRREGULAR ASTIGMATISM

Just as conventional refractive error is the sum of spherical and cylindrical components, total irregular astigmatism is the sum of individual aberrations. For instance, spherical aberration and coma are two important types of aberration. Spherical aberration is bowl shaped and similar to hyperopia and myopia, except that in spherical aberration the center of the bowl is flatter

and the sides are steeper than in myopia and hyperopia (see Table 14-1). Coma looks somewhat like a reclining chair (see Table 14-1). Many different amounts of total irregular astigmatism can be produced by combining spherical aberration and coma in different proportions.

CLASSIFICATION OF IRREGULAR ASTIGMATISM

The basic approach to irregular astigmatism is the same as the approach to conventional refractive errors. The total irregular astigmatism is measured and then expressed as the sum of individual aberrations. What are the basic aberrations that constitute irregular astigmatism? Seidel identified five different types of ray aberrations: spherical aberration, coma, distortion, field curvature, and astigmatism (not the same astigmatism that clinicians correct using cylinder). Later, Buchdahl[18] and Conrady[19] greatly extended the classification of ray aberrations. Wave aberrations were developed in the 1950s by Hopkins,[17] who initially based the classification on a form of Taylor's series expansion.[20] One advantage of Hopkins's approach was that certain wave aberrations exactly corresponded to the Seidel aberrations.

In the 1930s, Zernike[21] (inventor of the phase-contrast microscope) developed a polynomial expansion for the purpose of studying interference fringes. The Zernike polynomials have the mathematical property of orthogonality on a continuous unit circle, which was helpful in analyzing interference data when they were continuous over a circular aperture. Although not originally intended for aberration theory, Zernike polynomials were later applied to wave aberrations. Each polynomial represents one type of aberration. Zernike polynomials simplify the numerical analysis of aberrations, but none of the Zernike polynomials corresponds exactly to the Seidel aberrations. The Zernike system uses aberrations that are different from but related to the aberrations based on a Taylor's series.[22]

There is some debate as to which approach is best for clinical work, but in recent years, Zernike polynomials have predominated in the clinical literature and are becoming a de facto standard. Individual Zernike polynomials are grouped into orders (Table A-1 in appendix). In general, each order contains several individual aberrations; the higher the order, the more individual aberrations belonging to it.

Individual aberrations also have a property called parity, which may be either even or odd. The significance of parity is described later.

Pupil dependence is an important clinical property. Pure myopia and pure hyperopia are examples of pupil-independent aberrations. The amount of these errors does not change with pupil size. If refractive error changes with pupil size, additional pupil-dependent aberrations must also be present. In general, pupil dependence increases with higher-order aberrations.

CURRENT CLINICAL APPLICATIONS OF WAVE FRONT THEORY

Clinical application of aberration theory is a recent phenomenon. Much of the current interest in aberration theory is based on speculation rather than established clinical results. It is difficult to predict the ultimate impact of aberration theory on clinical practice, but the current clinical applications are in the area of fundus imaging and supernormal vision.

The fundus must necessarily be examined through the eye's optical system. By partially correcting ocular aberrations using adaptive optics techniques, remarkably detailed fundus images have been achieved.[23] The method is promising, but technical problems must be overcome before it can be implemented clinically.

The early success with fundus imaging has fueled speculation that by correcting irregular astigmatism, visual acuities on the order of 20/7.5 (6/2.25) can be achieved. This is highly speculative. It has not been established that adequate correction can be achieved routinely with refractive surgery or that improving the retinal image will result in better vision.

CLINICAL LIMITATIONS OF ABERRATION THEORY

Clinical application of aberration theory may be limited by several technical problems. Aberrations depend not only on the optical system but also on the object's location. An optical system capable of producing an aberration-free image for one object point will still have aberrations for other object points. In general, it is impossible to correct the aberrations of an optical system except for a few object points. Many articles in the clinical literature give the mistaken impression that the eye's aberrations can be completely eliminated. It is possible to reduce the eye's aberrations, but it is impossible to completely eliminate them.

Clinical Measurement of Aberrations

In order to apply aberration theory clinically, it is necessary to have the capability of reliably measuring ocular aberrations. Measurement of ocular aberrations presents some unique challenges. Many techniques of measuring the eye's aberrations have been described.[24-30] Currently, the two most popular methods for measuring aberration are based on the Hartman test or the Shack-Hartman test.

The Hartman test is basically an attempt to trace rays through the eye. Many individual beams of light parallel to the visual axis are directed through the pupil. When aberrations are present, the beams do not focus in a single spot. The distribution of rays on the retina form, in effect, a spot diagram that can be observed by indirect ophthalmoscopy and the aberrations determined. One disadvantage of the Hartman test is that it is a double pass system and cannot measure odd parity aberrations.

In the Shack-Hartman test, a low-intensity, narrow laser beam forms a small single spot on the fovea that acts like a point source. In the unaccommodated, emmetropic eye, the wave fronts from this point source emerge as flat planes. Since the image is at infinity, the ideal wave front is not a reference sphere but rather a reference plane. If aberrations exist, the wave fronts are not planes. The emerging wave front is sampled by passing through an array of small lenses (called lenslets or microlenses). Each microlens produces a small point image on a detector. The displacement or position of the image on the detector can be used to determine the overall shape of the wave front (Fig. 14-9). This approach can measure both odd and even parity aberrations.

Current clinical wave front sensors are laser based. A laser can measure aberrations at only one wavelength and thus cannot measure chromatic aberration, one of the eye's major optical defects. Moreover, the current systems utilize either red or infrared wavelengths, at which the eye has little or no sensitivity. Correction of monochromatic aberrations does not correct chromatic aberration, so the surgical correction of monochromatic aberrations may have limited value.[31-33] Chromatic aberration is also age dependent, declining with age. Beyond the sixth decade, chromatic aberration is equal to a third of its value in young adults.[34]

Aberrations change with accommodation because of changes in the position and alignment of the crystalline lens with respect to the pupil and cornea. Monochromatic wave front aberrations tend to increase with increasing levels of accommodation, but there is substantial individual variation in the actual change in wave front aberration. Overall optical quality of the eye is best at the resting point of accommodation. If an ideal correction is performed for the unaccommodated eye, it would not be perfect for the accommodated eye, and vice versa.[29,30,35-38]

Difficulties with chromatic aberration and accommodation can manifest as errors in spherical correction. At the 2001 meeting of the American Academy of Ophthalmology, one of the authors (EHT) had his right eye measured by every wave front system available. All the systems underestimated the myopia by at least 1D.

Even an optimally corrected eye may not stay that way due to aging changes. Aberrations increase with age due to changes in both the crystalline lens and the cornea. In younger patients, the aberrations of the cornea and lens tend to cancel each other, but this balance is lost with age.[39] The pupil becomes more miotic

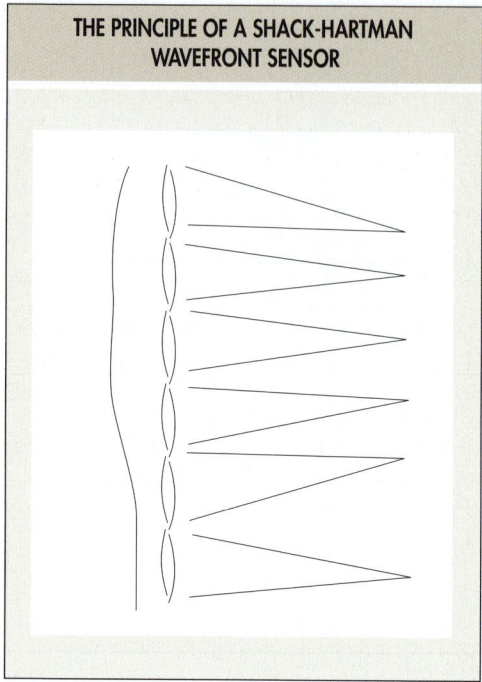

FIG. 14-9 ■ **The principle of a Shack-Hartman wave front sensor.** Each lenslet samples a small section of the wave front. Each segment of the wave front is focused to a point. The position of the point depends on the wave front shape.

with age, which may somewhat offset the increase in aberrations. It has been shown that the increase in wave front aberration with dilatation is more significant for higher-order aberrations in older patients, but no significant differences were found when the aberration coefficients for the natural pupil diameters were compared.[38,40-44]

Any local change in the tear film will affect ocular aberrations.[45,46] The effect is more prominent in individuals with anomalies of the tear film such as dry eye. Decreased blinking during wave front measurement may be a problem, especially in patients with tear film instability.

Aberrations, particularly coma, depend greatly on pupil centration.[38,47] The pupil center shifts as pupil size changes under the influence of lighting level and drugs.[37,38] Measurements of the aberrations of the eye have been performed with dilated pupils, and because of pupil center shifts, these measurements may differ from the those obtained with natural pupils.[28,37,38,48-50]

Misalignment of the eye during wave front measurement affects the accuracy of the measurement. Misalignment can also be a problem during treatment. Alignment is especially critical for higher-order aberrations.[39] Since none of the eye's optical elements is coaxial, it is not clear what constitutes correct alignment. Whether refractive procedures should be centered on the corneal axis or the visual axis remains an open question.

In order to get the benefits of correcting higher-order aberrations, the lower-order refractive errors of defocus and astigmatism, which are the most important optical defects of the eye, must be eliminated first. This may be difficult or perhaps impossible to achieve, however.[38]

In general, most of the techniques used to measure aberrations have difficulty when the total refractive error is large. Lower-order aberrations affect image quality much more than higher-order aberrations do. In the fabrication of quality optical systems, there is no point in measuring higher-order aberrations until the lower-order aberrations have been corrected. Consequently, the techniques for measuring higher-order aberrations usually assume that the optical system is already fairly well corrected. In the eye, this is often not the case.

In the aberrometer, for eyes suffering from large amounts of aberration, spot overlap can occur. This situation presents difficulties when analyzing the detected pattern.[38,51]

The Shack-Hartman wave front sensor assumes that the wave front is locally flat, which is true only when small amounts of higher-order aberrations are present. Under appropriate circumstances, only the displacement of spots is needed for computing the local slope of the wave front over each lenslet aperture. Classic analysis of data from a Shack-Hartman wave front sensor takes no account of the quality of individual spots formed by the lenslet array. The presence of blurred spots indicates a violation of the underlying assumption. There are two possibilities for the blurred spots. The first possibility is that the gross aberration is so large that the wave front is significantly curved over the area of a single microlens. The result is a blurry spot that is difficult to localize. The second possible cause of a blurred spot is a very high-order aberration that varies substantially over the aperture of a single microlens. Perturbations of the wave front within the lenslet aperture are too fine to be resolved by the wave front sensor using classic methods. Rather than displacing the spots laterally, these "microaberrations" scatter light and blur the spots formed by the aberrometer.[38] This second possibility is of theoretical interest but is probably not a problem in clinical use.

Aberration Terms

Technically, there are infinitely many aberrations. As a general rule, the higher the order of an aberration, the less its effect on image quality. Also, higher-order aberrations tend to have less effect on image quality for smaller pupils. How many aberrations have a clinically significant effect on visual function and how many aberrations should be connected in a custom ablation are unresolved questions.

In many studies of monochromatic aberration, the order of aberration terms has been very limited. For example, aberroscope studies do not go beyond the fourth order. Using the wave front sensor method, Liang and Williams determined aberration terms up to the 10th order. For 3mm pupils, they found that aberrations beyond the fourth order were small and had minimal effect on image quality. However, for large 7.3mm pupils, the fifth to eight orders made substantial contributions to the deterioration of image quality.[38]

Retinal Resolution

Even if the eye were aberration free, the retina places an absolute limit on visual function. Photoreceptor diameter and the spacing between adjacent photoreceptors determine the highest spatial frequency resolvable. The foveola is 0.35mm in diameter and has the highest packing density of cones. In the foveola, cones are long and narrow, with an average width of 1.5μm and a separation of about 0.5μm. The distance between the center of these tightly packed cones is about 2μm.[52] This contributes to resolution limit or, as it is usually called, the minimum angle of resolution of 30 seconds of arc, which is equivalent to a Snellen acuity of 20/10.[31,33,52,53]

Visual acuity is a far less sensitive measure of the benefits of correcting higher-order aberrations than is contrast sensitivity. This is because neural factors ultimately limit acuity even when improvements in retinal image contrast can continue to provide better vision at lower spatial frequencies. This in turn provides important improvements in the sharpness of vision, even if finer structure in the image cannot be resolved due to the grain of the mosaic.[23,33,53,54]

Although contrast sensitivity can be improved by correcting higher-order aberration, the aging eye has a decrease in contrast sensitivity that is not related to this higher-order aberration. Monochromatic wave front aberrations for a given pupil size increase with age, but older people have smaller pupils and benefit from a reduction in the effects of the wave front aberration. The age-related reduction in contrast sensitivity is due to a decrease in retinal illumination caused by a reduction in pupil diameter with age and a decrease in ocular transmittance from increasing light scatter and absorption at the lens. Moreover, some level of neural change may contribute to this decreased visual performance.

Pupil size decreases with age at all illuminance levels, which is called senile miosis. Senile miosis has the potential disadvantage of leading to lower retinal illuminance, thereby affecting visual performance under low light levels. However, a positive result is a reduction in the effects of the wave front aberration. Thus, all these factors might prevent aging eyes from benefiting from customized ablation.[41-44,55,56]

The normal eye has a mechanism to reduce the impact of aberration on the pupil, called the Stiles-Crawford effect, which results in improvement of retinal image quality.[57] The Stiles-Crawford effect is a phenomenon related to the directional sensitivity of retinal photoreceptors. This phenomenon is related to the orientation of photoreceptors. Each cone functions as a light pipe or fiber-optic, which is directed to the second nodal point of the eye. Parallel rays of light entering the pupil through its center are more effective in stimulating retinal cones than are those entering near the edge of a dilated pupil, reaching the retinal cones somewhat more obliquely. Hence, this could reduce the effect of aberrations associated with the margin of a dilated pupil.[58,59]

Limitations of Corneal Topography

Assuming that the wave aberration can be accurately measured, calculating the proper correction requires accurate corneal topography data as well. A complete review of corneal topography is beyond the scope of this chapter, but it is doubtful that current instruments have sufficient accuracy to take advantage of wave aberration data.

CLINICAL RULES OF THUMB

For those who are just beginning to become familiar with aberration theory, a few guidelines are helpful. Bear in mind that, like everything in medicine, there are exceptions to these "rules."

To overcome spherical aberration, the cornea should be steeper centrally and flatten toward the periphery. In many refractive procedures, the opposite is achieved. This leads to an increase in spherical aberration that is pupil dependent, leading to visual complaints exacerbated under low light conditions.

Misalignment tends to produce coma. Decentered intraocular lenses produce small amounts of coma. Decentered corneal grafts produce more coma. A lens implant and graft decentered in opposite directions produce the most coma. A decentered pupil can also produce coma. An off-axis ablation can create many aberrations, especially coma and tilt (i.e., prism).

SUMMARY

All forms of refractive error are aberrations. The first-order aberrations myopia, hyperopia, and regular astigmatism can be understood without sophisticated analytical methods. However, the analysis of irregular astigmatism requires advanced techniques. Until recently, there was no need to analyze irregular astigmatism in detail. However, because recent progress in imaging and refractive surgery may allow the correction of irregular astigmatism, aberration theory is now applicable to clinical practice. There are two ways to analyze aberrations—ray aberrations and wave aberrations. The latter way is more popular and in many ways easier. The clinical application of aberration theory is a recent phenomenon, and its ultimate clinical value is yet to be fully defined.

REFERENCES

1. King HC. The history of the telescope. New York: Dover; 1955:42.
2. Scheiner C. Oculus hoc est: fundamentum opticum. Oeniponti; 1619.
3. Kepler J. Dioptrice. 1611.
4. Smith WJ. Image formation: geometrical and physical optics. In: Driscoll WG, ed. Handbook of optics. Optical Society of America; 1978.
5. Stavroudis ON. The optics of rays, wavefronts, and caustics. New York: Academic Press; 1972.
6. Malacara D, ed. Methods of experimental physics. Vol 25. Geometrical and instrumental optics. New York: Academic Press; 1988.
7. Jenkins FA, White HE. Fundamentals of optics, 3rd ed. New York: McGraw-Hill; 1957.
8. Kingslake R. History of the photographic lens. New York: Academic Press; 1991.

9. O'Shea D. Elements of modern optical design. New York: Wiley; 1985.
10. Kingslake R. Optical system design. New York: Academic Press; 1988.
11. Park D. The fire within the eye. Princeton: Princeton University Press; 1999.
12. Smith WJ. Modern optical engineering, 3rd ed. New York: McGraw-Hill; 2000.
13. Naval Education and Training Program Development Center. Basic optics and optical instruments, rev ed. New York: Dover; 1969.
14. Synge JL. Hamilton's method in geometrical optics. J Opt Soc Am. 1937;27:75-82.
15. Synge JL. Hamilton's characteristic function and Brun's eiconal. J Opt Soc Am. 1937;27:138-44.
16. Hecht E. Optics, 3rd ed. New York: Addison-Wesley; 1998.
17. Hopkins HH. Wave theory of aberrations. Oxford: Oxford Clarendon Press; 1950:59-65.
18. Buchdahl HA. Optical aberration coefficients. New York: Dover; 1968.
19. Conrady AE. Applied optics and optical design, vol 1. New York: Dover; 1957.
20. Irons BM, Shrive NG. Numerical methods in engineering and applied science. New York: Wiley; 1987.
21. Zernike FZ. Tech Phys. 1935;16:454.
22. Welford WT. Aberrations of optical systems. New York: Adam Hilger; 1997.
23. Williams D, Yoon GY, Porter J, et al. Visual benefit of correcting higher order aberrations of the eye. J Refract Surg. 2000;16:554-9.
24. Walsh G, Charman WN, Howland HC. Objective technique for the determination of monochromatic aberrations of the human eye. J Opt Soc Am A. 1984;1:987-92.
25. Liang J, Grimm B, Golez S, et al. Objective measurement of wave aberrations of the human eye with the use of a Hartman-Shack wavefront sensor. J Opt Soc Am A. 1957;11:1949-57.
26. Novarro R, Losada MA. Aberrations and relative efficiency of light pencils in the living human eye. Optom Vis Sci. 1997;74:540-7.
27. He JC, Marcos S, Webb RH, et al. Measurement of the wave-front aberration of the eye by a fast psychophysical procedure. J Opt Soc Am A. 1998;15:2449-56.
28. Mrochen M, Kaemmerer M, Mierdel P, et al. Principles of Tscherning aberrometry. J Refract Surg Suppl. 2000;16:570-1.
29. Burns SA. The spatially resolved refractometer. J Refract Surg. 2000;16:566-9.
30. Artal P. Understanding aberrations by using double-pass techniques. J Refract Surg. 2000;16:560-2.
31. Thibos LN. The prospects for perfect vision. J Refract Surg. 2000;16:540-6.
32. Marcos S, Burns SA, Barriusop EM, Navarro R. A new approach to the study of ocular chromatic aberrations. Vision Res. 1999;39:4309-23.
33. Schwiegerling J. Theoretical limits to visual performance. Surv Ophthalmol. 2000;45:139-46.
34. Millodot M. Effect of the aberrations of the eye on visual perception. Vis Psychophys Physiol. 441-52.
35. Lopez-Gil N, Iglesias I, Artal P. Retinal image quality in the human eye as a function of the accommodation. Vision Res. 1998;38:2897-907.
36. He JC, Burns SA, Marcos S. Monochromatic aberrations in the accommodated human eye. Vision Res. 2000;40:41-8.
37. Atchison DA, Collins MJ, Wildsoet CF, et al. Measurement of monochromatic ocular aberrations of human eyes as a function of accommodation by the Howland aberroscope technique. Vision Res. 1995;35:313-23.
38. Atchison DA. Monochromatic aberrations. Optics Human Eye. 137-59.
39. Williams DR, Yoon GY, Guirao A, et al. How far can we extend the limits of human vision? In: Macae S. Customized corneal ablation: the quest for super vision. Thorofare, NJ: Slack; 2001:10-32.
40. Kaemmerer M, Mrochen M, Mierdel P, et al. Clinical experience with Tscherning aberrometer. J Refract Surg. 2000;16:584-7.
41. Calver RI, Cox MJ, Elliott DB. Effect of aging on the monochromatic aberrations of the human eye. J Opt Soc Am A. 1999;16:2069-78.
42. Oshika T, Klyce SD, Applegate RA, Howland HC. Changes in corneal wavefront aberrations with aging. Invest Ophthalmol Vis Sci. 1999;40(7):1351-5.
43. Atchison DA. The aging eye. Optics Human Eye. 221-33.
44. Winn B, Whitaker D, Elliott DB, Phillips NJ. Factors affecting light-adapted pupil size in normal human subjects. Invest Ophthalmol Vis Sci. 1994;33:1132-7.
45. Thibos LN, Hong X. Clinical applications of the Shack-Hartman aberrometer. Optom Vis Sci. 1999;76:817-25.
46. Tutt R, Bradley A, Begley C, Thibos LN. Optical and visual impact of tear break-up in human eyes. Invest Ophthalmol Vis Sci. 2000;41:4117-23.
47. Wilson MA, Simonet P. The Julius F. Neumueller Award in Optics, 1989: Change of pupil centration with change of illumination and pupil size. Optom Vis Sci. 1992;69:129-36.
48. Krueger RR. Technology requirements for Summit-Autonomous CustomCornea. J Refract Surg. 2000;16:592-601.
49. Fankhauser F, Kaemmerer M, Mrochen M, Seiler T. The effect of accommodation, mydriasis and cycloplegia on aberrometry. Invest Ophthalmol Vis Sci. 2000;41(suppl):S461.
50. Charman WN, Walsh G. The effect of pupil centration and diameter on ocular performance. Vision Res. 1998;28:659-65.
51. Hamam H. A quick method for analyzing Hartman-Shack patterns: application to refractive surgery. J Refract Surg. 2000;16(5):636-42.
52. Miller D. Optics of the normal human eye. In: Yanoff M, Duker JS, eds. Ophthalmology, 1st ed. London: Mosby; 1999:7.1-7.8.
53. Applegate RA. Limits to vision: can we do better than nature? J Refract Surg. 2000;16:547-51.
54. Rabin J. Luminance effects on visual acuity and small letter contrast sensitivity. Optom Vis Sci. 1994;71:685-8.
55. Guirao A, Gonzalez C, Redondo M, et al. Average optical performance of the human eye as a function of age in a normal population. Invest Ophthalmol Vis Sci. 1999;40:203-13.
56. Owsley C, Sekuler R, Siemsen D. Contrast sensitivity throughout adulthood. Vision Res. 1983;23:689-99.
57. Zhang X, Ye M, Bradley A, Thibos L. Apodization by the Stiles-Crawford effect moderates the visual impact of retinal image defocus. J Opt Soc Am A. 1999;16:812-9.
58. Hart WM. Entoptic imagery. In: Kaufman PL, ed. Adler's physiology of the eye, ed 10. Philadelphia: WB Saunders; 2001:373-88.
59. Charman WN. Limits on visual performance set by the eye's optics and the retinal cone mosaic. Optics Human Eye. 81-96.

APPENDIX: MATHEMATICAL CONSIDERATIONS

Any point in the exit pupil can be located by either Cartesian or polar coordinates. By convention, the origin of the coordinate system is at the center of the exit pupil. The direction of the positive x- and y-axes is shown in Figure A-1. In optics, when polar coordinates are used, the angle is measured from the positive y-axis and is positive in the clockwise direction. Note that this is contrary to standard mathematical conventions. The following equations convert between polar and Cartesian coordinates:

$$x = \rho\sin\theta \qquad \rho = \sqrt{x^2 + y^2}$$
$$x = \rho\cos\theta \qquad \theta = \arctan\left(\frac{x}{y}\right)$$

For example, a point with Cartesian coordinates (−0.5mm, −1mm) would have polar coordinates:

$$\rho = \sqrt{(-0.5mm)^2 + (1mm)^2} = 1.12mm$$
$$\theta = \arctan\left(\frac{-0.5}{-1.0}\right) = -116.57deg$$

Note that when using the arc tangent function, care must be exercised to ensure that the appropriate quadrant is identified.

The reference sphere is centered on the desired image point and intersects the center of the exit pupil. Every ray from the object point traverses a unique point in the exit pupil. Conversely, each point in the exit pupil identifies a unique ray in image space. At any given point in the exit pupil, the wave aberration is the directed distance, measured along the actual ray from the reference sphere to the wave front, multiplied by the refractive index of image space.

Therefore, for every point in the exit pupil, there is a unique scalar value for the wave aberration. The wave aberration can be expressed as a function:

$$W = f(x,y)$$

or, if polar coordinates are used:

$$W = g(\rho,\theta)$$

The exact form of the function $f(x,y)$ or $g(\rho,\theta)$ has yet to be determined. Since the wave aberration W must be continuous and differentiable, the function $f(x,y)$ or $g(\rho,\theta)$ can be expanded as a series. There are many different series expansions that could be used, and one common (but not necessarily the best) choice is the Zernike expansion.

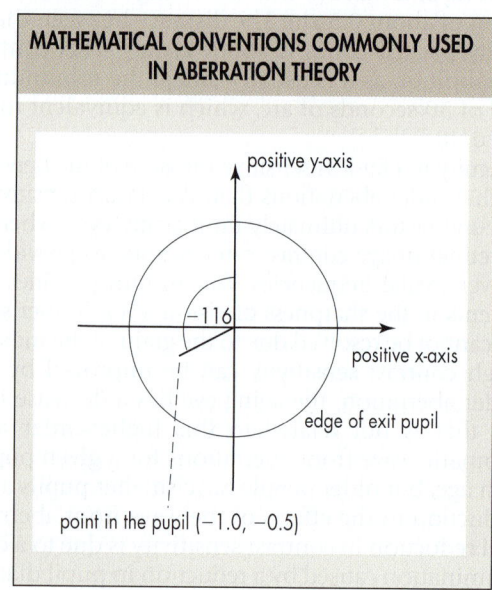

FIG. A-1 ▣ **Mathematical conventions commonly used in aberration theory.** The exit pupil is depicted as seen looking in the negative z direction. Angles are measured from the vertical y-axis, not the x-axis. Moreover, the angles are positive in the clockwise direction, also contrary to most mathematical conventions.

There are various ways to express the Zernike polynomials. The following approach is based on the senior author's notes from a course in aberration theory taught by Professor Roland V. Shack, PhD. The wave aberration can be expressed as:

$$W = g(\rho,\theta) = \sum_{t=0}^{\infty} \sum_{m=0}^{\infty} R_{nm}(\rho)\left(C_{nm}\cdot Cos(m\theta) + S_{nm}\cdot Sin(m\theta)\right)$$

where,

$$n = m + 2t$$

$$R_{nm}(\rho) = \sum_{q=0}^{t} (-1)^{t-q}\frac{(m + t + q)!}{(t - q)!(m + q)!q!}\rho^{(m + 2q)}$$

From the last equation, one may obtain the following intermediate results.

For t = 0, n = m and

$$R_{m,m}(\rho) = \rho^m$$

For t = 1, n = m + 2 and

$$R_{m+2,m}(\rho) = -[(m + 1) - (m + 2)\rho^2]\cdot\rho^m$$

and so forth for t = 2, 3, etc.

From these intermediate results, one can construct the Zernike polynomials (see Table A-1). The order of the polynomial is the sum n + m. Note that the orders are restricted to even integers: 0, 2, 4, etc. There are no first, third, or higher odd orders. Also, m and n are either both even or both odd. Therefore, the parity of the polynomial is even when n is even and odd when n is odd.

Thus, the wave aberration W = g(ρ,θ) can be expressed as follows:

$$W = g(\rho,\theta) = C_{0,0} + C_{1,1}\rho Cos\theta + S_{1,1}\rho Sin\theta + C_2(2\rho^2 - 1) +$$
$$C_{2,2}\rho^2 Cos2\theta + S_{2,2}\rho^2 Sin2\theta + \text{higher-order terms}$$

Only the values of the coefficients change from patient to patient.

Each individual Zernike polynomial can be considered a separate aberration. Table A-1 gives the Zernike polynomials in polar and Cartesian forms up to the eighth order. Table 14-1 shows the shape of the Zernike polynomials up to the eighth order and their associated spot diagrams. Note that aberrations with the same subscript (e.g., $C_{2,2}$ and $S_{2,2}$) have the same shape and are essentially identical, except that one is a rotated version of the other. Only one of the pair of aberrations is shown in the table.

In practice, the wave aberration is determined at many points in the exit pupil either by measurement or by calculation. The measured or calculated data are then fit to a curve using multiple linear regression. To perform the regression analysis, it is necessary to decide how many terms in the aberration expansion to use.

The Zernike polynomial expansion is not the only way to expand the aberration function. Hamilton expanded the aberration function in terms of rotationally invariant quantities. Each approach has advantages and disadvantages. Zernike polynomials are orthogonal on a continuous unit circle (but not a discretely sampled unit circle), and this property facilitates the regression analysis. However, Zernike polynomials consist of combinations of aberrations, as discussed in the next section on terminology issues.

TABLE A-1

ZERNIKE POLYNOMIALS TO THE EIGHTH ORDER

Order	Coefficient	Polar Form	Cartesian Form
0	$C_{0,0}$	1	1
2	$C_{1,1}$	$\rho Cos\theta$	y
	$S_{1,1}$	$\rho Sin\theta$	x
	$C_{2,0}$	$2\rho^2 - 1$	$2x^2 + 2y^2 - 1$
4	$C_{2,2}$	$\rho^2 Cos2\theta$	$y^2 - x^2$
	$S_{2,2}$	$\rho^2 Sin2\theta$	$2xy$
	$C_{3,1}$	$(3\rho^3 - 2\rho)Cos\theta$	$3y^3 + 3x^2y - 2y$
	$S_{3,1}$	$(3\rho^3 - 2\rho)Sin\theta$	$3x^3 + 3xy^2 - 2x$
	$C_{4,0}$	$6\rho^4 - 6\rho^2 + 1$	$6(x^2 + y^2)^2 + 6(x^2 + y^2) + 1$
6	$C_{3,3}$	$\rho^3 Cos3\theta$	$y^3 - 3x^2y$
	$S_{3,3}$	$\rho^3 Sin3\theta$	$3xy^2 - x^3$
	$C_{4,2}$	$(4\rho^4 - 3\rho^2)Cos2\theta$	$4y^4 - 4x^4 + 3x^2 - 3y^2$
	$S_{4,2}$	$(4\rho^4 - 3\rho^2)Sin2\theta$	$8x^3y + 8xy^3 - 6xy$
	$C_{5,1}$	$(10\rho^5 - 12\rho^3 + 3\rho)Cos\theta$	$10y^5 + 20x^2y^3 + 10x^4y\text{-}12x^2y - 12y^3+3y$
	$S_{5,1}$	$(10\rho^5 - 12\rho^3 + 3\rho)Sin\theta$	$10x^5 + 20x^3y^2 + 10xy^4 - 12x^3y\text{-}12x^3+3x$
	$C_{6,0}$	$20\rho^6 - 30\rho^4 + 12\rho^2 - 1$	$20y^6 + 60y^4x^2 + 60x^4y^2 + 20x^6 - 30y^4 - 60x^2y^2 - 30x^4+12y^2 + 12x^2 - 1$
8	$C_{4,4}$	$\rho^4 Cos4\theta$	$y^3 - 3x^2y$
	$S_{4,4}$	$\rho^4 Sin4\theta$	$3xy^2 - x^3$
	$C_{5,3}$	$(5\rho^5 - 4\rho^3)Cos3\theta$	$4y^4 - 4x^4 + 3x^2 - 3y^2$
	$S_{5,3}$	$(5\rho^5 - 4\rho^3)Sin3\theta$	$8x^3y + 8xy^3 - 6xy$
	$C_{6,2}$	$(15\rho^6 - 20\rho^4 + 6\rho^4)Cos2\theta$	$10y^5 + 20x^2y^3 + 10x^4y - 12x^2y - 12y^3 + 3y$
	$S_{6,2}$	$(15\rho^6 - 20\rho^4 + 6\rho^4)Sin2\theta$	$10x^5 + 20x^3y^2 + 10xy^4 - 12x^3y - 12x^3 + 3x$
	$C_{7,1}$	$(35\rho^7 - 60\rho^5 + 30\rho^3 - 4\rho)Cos\theta$	$35y^7 + 105y^5x^2 + 105x^4y^3 + 35x^6y - 60y^5 - 120y^3x^2 - 60x^4y + 30y^3 + 30x^2y - 4y$
	$S_{7,1}$	$(35\rho^7 - 60\rho^5 + 30\rho^3 - 4\rho)Sin\theta$	$35x^7 + 105x^5y^2 + 105y^4x^3 + 35y^6x - 60x^5 - 120x^3y^2 - 60y^4x + 30x^3 + 30y^2x - 4x$
	$C_{6,0}$	$70\rho^8 - 140\rho^6 + 90\rho^4 - 20\rho^2 + 1$	$70y^8 + 280y^6x^2 + 420x^4y^4 + 280x^6y^2 + 70x^8 - 140x^6 - 420x^4y^2 - 420x^2y^4 + 90x^4 + 180x^2y^2 - 20x^2 - 20y^2 + 1$

Even parity aberrations are shown in blue, and odd parity aberrations are shown in red.

TERMINOLOGY ISSUES

Various authors have used different terminology to describe aberrations. The current situation can be very confusing, because the same term is often used in different ways. Thus, there is presently an ongoing attempt to standardize terminology, but there is some resistance to this standardization. For one thing, it would be very expensive to convert existing software to a new standard. Nor would standardization necessarily solve the problem, because many textbooks on the subject already use differing terminology and will be used for years to come. This section addresses the terminology issues that in the authors' experience are most likely to cause confusion amongst clinicians.

There is only one zero-order aberration. Mathematically, it is a constant and can have any value: 1.26, −4, or whatever. Engineers refer to this as piston error, and it is clinically insignificant. It corresponds to no clinical entity and rarely arises in engineering work.

The aberration called defocus encompasses both myopia and hyperopia. The graph of myopia is bowl shaped, and the graph of hyperopia is an inverted bowl. Mathematically, the only difference is the algebraic sign of the coefficient. It may seem contrary to clinical convention, but positive defocus corresponds to myopia, and negative defocus is hyperopia.

Aberrations are frequently referred to by their coefficients. Thus, the $C_{4,0}$ may refer to the amount of spherical aberration present or to spherical aberration in general.

Technically, there is no Zernike polynomial that corresponds to defocus. The Zernike aberration $C_{2,0}$ representing defocus is actually a combination of defocus and piston error. In general, one weakness of the Zernike polynomials is that they represent combinations of aberrations. For instance, the Zernike polynomial for spherical aberration is actually a combination of spherical aberration, defocus, and piston error.

To refer to pure aberrations, a different polynomial expansion is used. The details of alternative expansions are not discussed here, but usually a subscripted "W" represents the coefficients. For example, $W_{2,0}$ represents pure defocus, $W_{4,0}$ represents pure spherical aberration, and so forth.

Aberrations are usually grouped into orders. Different schemes classify the orders in different ways. Usually, several individual aberrations belong to the same order, and the higher the order, the more aberrations belong to it. In the classification used here, there are only even-order wave aberrations. In some classifications of ray aberrations, there are only odd-order ray aberrations. Fourth-order wave aberrations correspond to third-order ray aberrations, sixth-order wave aberrations to fifth-order ray aberrations, and so on. The main significance of order is that, unless a large amount of a high-order aberration is present, the higher the order, the less the effect on the image.

DIMENSIONAL ISSUES

Wave aberration is defined as the optical path difference between the wave front and the reference sphere. Optical path difference is a length and may be expressed in any unit of length, such as meters or centimeters. Wave front aberrations are typically on the order of 10^{-6}m, so wave aberration is most often expressed in micrometers. By definition, a diopter is a reciprocal meter (m^{-1}). A wave aberration is fundamentally a length, and a diopter is fundamentally a curvature. It is therefore impossible to convert directly from diopters to wave aberration because they are expressed in fundamentally different units.

It is common but not universal practice to use normalized pupil coordinates. The physical pupil coordinates are divided by the pupil radius so that x and y vary between −1 and 1, and ρ

varies between 0 and 1. More importantly x, y, and ρ are dimensionless quantities. When the aberrations are used in practice, the physical coordinates must be converted to the normalized coordinates, and vice versa. Although it is not always necessary to use normalized coordinates for every wave expansion, it is necessary for the Zernike aberration expansion.

In alternative aberration expansions, each aberration is measured in different physical units. For instance, if the only aberration present is spherical aberration, in Cartesian coordinates:

$$W(x,y) = W_{4,0}(x^2 + y^2)^2$$

The variables x and y represent position in the pupil and are measured in units of length (typically millimeters). Thus, $(x^2 + y^2)^2$ has dimensions of length^4, typically mm^4. Thus, the coefficient $W_{4,0}$ must have units of length^{-3}, so that W has units of length. Typically, $W_{4,0}$ would have units of μm/mm^4. A similar analysis of coma would show that the coefficient has units of length^{-2}. In general, each coefficient has different physical units.

The coefficient for defocus has units of 1/length, and if length is measured in meters, this is equivalent to the diopter. Some authors believe that this means that there is an exact conversion between the aberration defocus and diopters. However, wave aberration changes with location of the reference sphere. Thus, if two eyes—one short, one long—had identical amounts of myopia, they would have different amounts of defocus aberration.

However, if one makes several reasonable assumptions, it is possible to arrive at a clinically useful rule of thumb relating diopters to micrometers of wave aberration. The mathematical representation of myopia is:

$$W(x,y) = W_{2,0}(x^2 + y^2),$$

where x and y represent coordinates of a point in the exit pupil. The center of the exit pupil has coordinates of x = 0 and y = 0. A point at the top edge of a pupil 3mm in diameter (radius 1.5mm) has coordinates x = 0 and y = 1.5mm. Since W is expressed in units of micrometers, and x and y have dimensions of millimeters, W_{20} has dimensions of μm/mm^2.

Consider an average eye with 1D of myopia. Let us assume that the exit pupil is 3mm in diameter and 19mm anterior to the retina (typical values). In an eye with 1D of myopia, the image forms about 0.33mm anterior to the retina. A marginal ray through the top of the pupil has a transverse ray aberration of:

$$-(1.5mm/19mm)(0.33mm) = -26.3\mu m$$

The negative sign indicates myopia.

The relationship between the wave aberration and the transverse ray aberration, Δy is[22]:

$$\Delta y = -(R/n)\, \partial W/\partial y$$

The refractive index of vitreous is n = 1.336, for defocus $\partial W/\partial y = W_{20}(2y)$, for a marginal ray y = 1.5mm, and R is the radius of the reference sphere, 19mm in this case. Thus,

$$-26.3\mu m = -(19/1.336)\, W_{20}(2 \times 1.5mm)$$

Thus, $W_{20} = 0.62\mu m/mm^2$. The total wave aberration for the marginal ray at the top of the exit pupil (coordinates x = 0, y = 1.5mm) is therefore:

$$W = W_{20}(x^2 + y^2) = 0.62\ \mu m/mm^2\ [(0mm)^2 + (1.5mm)^2] = 1.4\mu m$$

Thus, as a very rough rule, 1D of refractive error corresponds to approximately 1.4μm. Caution must be applied in using this rule, because it does not apply to large pupils or unusually long or short eyes.

REFRACTIVE SURGERY

Dimitri T. Azar

CHAPTER
15

Current Concepts, Classification, and History of Refractive Surgery

JUAN CARLOS ABAD • DIMITRI T. AZAR

DEFINITION
- Refractive surgery is an evolving field of ophthalmology focusing on the correction of refractive errors of the eye, including myopia, hyperopia, astigmatism, and presbyopia.

KEY FEATURES
- Realistic patient expectations.
- Stable preoperative refraction.
- Absence of ocular diseases.
- Adequate understanding of potential surgical complications, limitations, and alternatives.
- Avoidance of untested and unstable surgical procedures or procedures with high unpredictability and loss of best-corrected visual acuity.

ASSOCIATED FEATURES
- Alterations in optical aberrations after surgery.
- Reduced dependence on spectacles and contact lenses.

INTRODUCTION

Owing to the permanent nature of refractive surgery, one of its most important aspects is adequate patient selection and counseling. With increased exposure in the press and continual advertisements about the extreme precision of refractive surgery, it is not surprising that many potential refractive surgery candidates walk into the doctor's office with great expectations. A patient may meet all the medical and surgical requirements for refractive surgery but not be a good candidate because of unrealistic expectations or because of inadequate knowledge about the procedure, its risks and benefits, or alternatives.

Spectacles and contact lenses are reasonable alternatives to refractive surgical procedures. Not only is the accuracy of these forms of optical correction greater than that of refractive surgery, but they are totally reversible. Additionally, in refractive surgery, the variation in biomechanical properties and in corneal wound healing must be taken into account.

Although operating on a normal eye merely to free a patient of the need for glasses or contact lenses may seem aggressive, patients are generally delighted after successful refractive surgery. To achieve uniform satisfaction with newer refractive surgical procedures, they must be validated continuously through controlled and well-designed scientific investigations to ensure better predictability and reproducibility.

OPTICS FOR THE REFRACTIVE SURGEON

The successful performance of refractive surgery demands a thorough understanding of the optics of the human eye.[1] The eye's refractive power is determined predominantly by three variables: power of the cornea, power of the lens, and length of the eye.

In emmetropia, these three components combine to produce no refractive error. In an emmetropic eye, a pencil-like ray of light parallel to the optical axis and limited by the pupil focuses on the retina (the secondary focal point of an emmetropic eye; Fig. 15-1). The far point in emmetropia (defined as the point conjugate to the retina in the nonaccommodating state) is optical infinity.

Eyes with refractive errors have a mismatch of these variables. For example, an eye with an axial length in the upper range of normal may be myopic if the corneal steepness variable is also in the upper range of normal.

Myopia

Myopia is the most common visually significant refractive error, with a prevalence of nearly 25% for Caucasians and 13% for African Americans. The myopic eye brings a pencil of parallel rays of light into focus at a point anterior to the retina. This point, the secondary focal point of the eye, is in the vitreous (see Fig. 15-1). The far point of a myopic eye is between infinity and the anterior surface of the cornea. Rays that diverge from this point are brought to focus on the retina without the aid of accommodation. For the full correction of myopia, a distance corrective lens placed in front of the eye must have its secondary focal point coincident with the far point. The newly created optical system allows parallel rays that come from infinity to diverge as if they originated from the far point of the eye and thus focus on the retina. In refractive surgical procedures for myopia, the refractive power of the cornea, or the crystalline lens, is reduced so that parallel rays from infinity can also focus on the retina.

Hyperopia

The hyperopic eye brings a pencil of parallel rays of light into focus at a point behind the retina.[2] Accommodation of the eye may produce enough additional plus power to allow the light rays to focus on the retina. The far point of a hyperopic eye is behind the eye, or beyond infinity. For the full correction of hyperopia, a corrective lens placed in front of the eye must have its secondary focal point coincident with the far point. Parallel rays from infinity exit the corrective lens, converge toward the far point of the eye, and thus can focus on the retina without the aid of accommodation. Hyperopia affects approximately 40% of the adult population. In the prepresbyopic age group, low to moderate hyperopia is less visually significant than myopia is. The great majority of young hyperopes regard their eyes as being optically normal. They might experience an earlier onset of presbyopia, however. Older hyperopes or patients with high degrees of hyperopia that exceed their accommodative reserve require optical correction for clear distance vision. They can benefit from refractive surgical procedures in which the corneal curvature is steepened or the power of the crystalline lens is increased

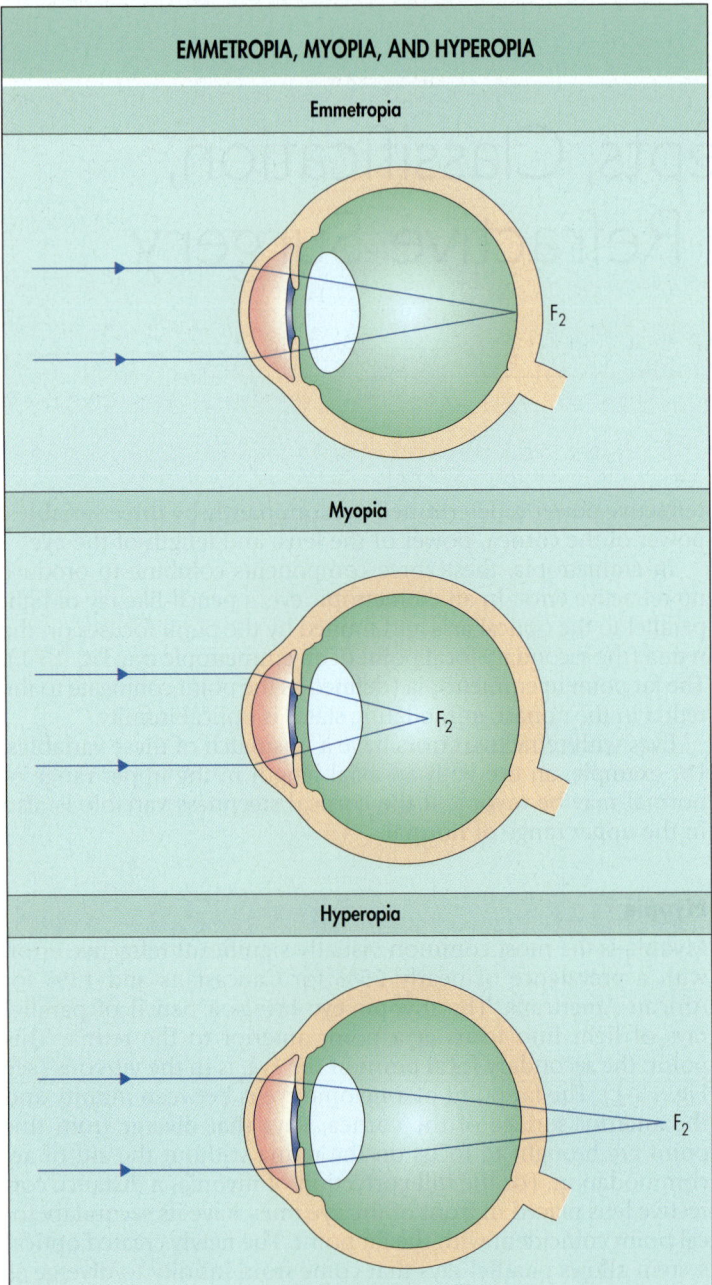

EMMETROPIA, MYOPIA, AND HYPEROPIA

Emmetropia

Myopia

Hyperopia

FIG. 15-1 ■ **Emmetropia, myopia, and hyperopia.** In emmetropia, the far point is at infinity, and the secondary focal point (F_2) is at the retina. In myopia, the far point is in front of the eye, and the secondary focal point (F_2) is in the vitreous. In hyperopia, the secondary focal point (F_2) is behind the eye. (Modified with permission from Azar DT, Strauss L. Principles of applied clinical optics. In: Albert DM, Jakobie FA, eds. Principles and practice of ophthalmology, vol 6, ed. 2. Philadelphia: WB Saunders; 2000:5329–40.)

to converge rays of light that emanate from distant objects onto the retina without the aid of accommodation.

Astigmatism

Astigmatism is caused by a toric cornea or, less often, by astigmatic effects of the crystalline lens. Astigmatism is regular when it is correctable with cylindrical or spherocylindrical lenses. Otherwise, the astigmatism is irregular (see Wave Front Deformation, later). Regular astigmatism is termed "with the rule" when the steepest corneal meridian is close to 90° and "against the rule" when the steepest meridian is close to 180°. When the astigmatism is regular but the principal meridians do not lie close to 90° or 180°, the astigmatism is called oblique. Depending on the spherical ametropia of the particular eye, astigmatism may be classified as simple or compound based on whether one or both meridians, respectively, are focused outside the retina. If one meridian focuses in front of the retina and the other meridian focuses behind it, the astigmatism is called mixed.

Astigmatism can be natural or surgically induced. Natural astigmatism is common; up to 95% of eyes may have some clinically detectable astigmatism. In the general population, 10–20% can be expected to have natural astigmatism greater than 1D, with an uncorrected visual acuity that might be considered unsatisfactory. Binocular spectacle correction of oblique astigmatism tilts each eye's view and may distort the perceived three-dimensional image. This spatial distortion disappears when one eye is occluded; it is minimized, at the expense of clarity, by rotation of the axis toward 90° or 180° to reduce the tilt, or by reduction of the cylinder power (Fig. 15-2).[3] When astigmatism is corrected at the corneal plane, such as with contact lenses or keratorefractive surgery, full correction reduces meridional magnification and eliminates the optical distortion.

Presbyopia

The mechanism of accommodation, suggested by von Helmholtz[4] in the 1850s, states that as the ciliary muscle contracts circumferentially, it relaxes the zonules and allows the crystalline lens to assume a more spherical configuration by virtue of its own elasticity. As the crystalline lens hardens with age, it is no longer able to attain the more spherical form, leading to the onset of presbyopia. An alternative theory of accommodation contends that the rounding of the central crystalline lens is due to the peripheral pulling of the radial fibers of the ciliary muscle, increasing the tautness of the equatorial zonules.[5] This latter theory states that the cause of presbyopia is the continuous growth of the crystalline lens throughout life with relaxation of the equatorial zonules and decrease of its pulling ability.

The age of onset of presbyopia depends on the refractive error. A myope always has clear vision of objects placed at or near his or her far point. A latent hyperope, in contrast, uses accommodative reserve for clear distance vision; as the amplitude of accommodation decreases with age, reading difficulties arise. The method of optical correction also affects the age of onset of presbyopia. When myopes focus on a near object through the distance prescription of spectacles, less accommodation is needed than with contact lenses or after keratorefractive surgery. Conversely, hyperopes have a decreased accommodative demand with contact lenses or keratorefractive surgery.

Presbyopia is an important aspect of informed consent for keratorefractive surgery patients. Patients older than 40 years who consider refractive surgery for myopia must appreciate the extent to which they exchange dependence on distance spectacles for dependence on near-vision spectacles. Surgically corrected presbyopic myopes will need reading glasses as they age, whereas before surgery, they could remove their spectacles to read.

Image Magnification

When an image of an object is formed, the linear magnification may be defined as the quotient of the sizes, measured perpendicular to the optical axis, of image and object. Axial magnification is measured in a similar fashion but parallel to the optical axis; it is the square of the linear magnification.[1] Angular magnification refers to the quotient of the angles subtended by the object's image when viewed with and without an optical aid.

Different optical aids create different angular magnifications. For viewing through spectacle minus lenses, a minification of roughly 2% per diopter occurs; this decreases dramatically when the same correction occurs at the corneal plane by either contact lenses or keratorefractive surgery. A patient with −20D who undergoes refractive surgery is expected to gain a line of best-corrected visual acuity by the elimination of image minification secondary to high-power spectacles. With high hyperopes, the effect is the opposite.

Cycloplegic Refraction

After the pupil has dilated, spherical aberration is produced as the rays of light hit the peripheral lens and are bent more than

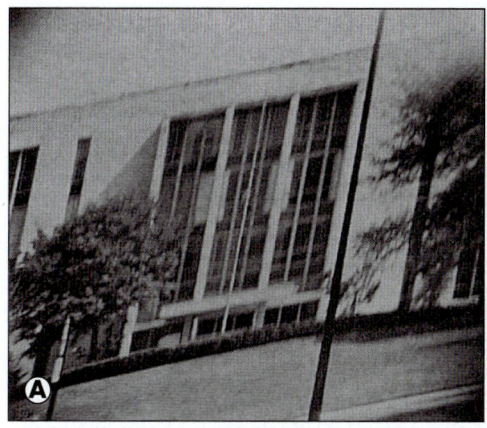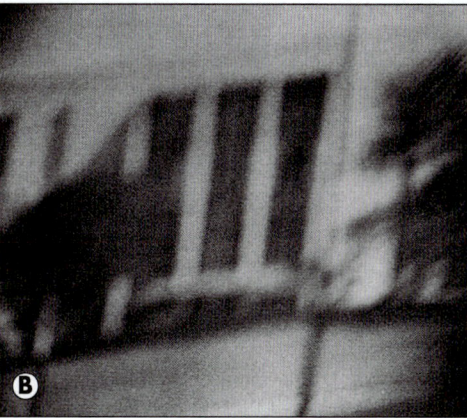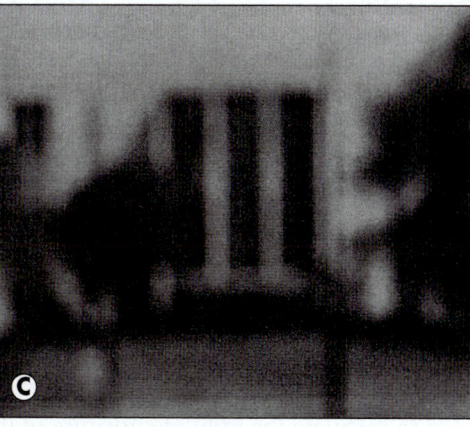

FIG. 15-2 ▪ Simulation of changes to astigmatic correction to reduce distortion. **A,** Distorted image from full specta-cle correction of oblique astigmatism. **B,** Decreased distortion obtained by a reduction of the cylinder power. **C,** Improved direction of distortion (vertical) as well as decreased amount of distortion obtained by rotation of the plus cylinder axis to 180° and reduction of the cylinder power. (Reprinted with permission from Guyton DL. Prescribing cylinders: the problem of distortion. Surv Ophthalmol. 1977;22:177–88.)

the central rays; this produces a myopic shift, which is partially counteracted by the asphericity where the cornea flattens toward the periphery. A cycloplegic refraction is an essential part of the evaluation of a refractive surgery candidate. With cycloplegia, or relaxation of the ciliary body, a hyperopic shift occurs, counteracted by the spherical aberration just described. The intensity of this shift depends on the accommodative tone and is quite pronounced in young individuals. It may be useful to measure the cycloplegic refraction through a 3–4mm aperture to account only for the accommodative tone; in this way, the effect of the peripheral cornea and the lens on the refraction is negated.

Pupil Size and Centration of Refractive Procedures

Rays of light from a single point source are refracted by the area of the cornea that overlies the entrance pupil. That area is called the corneal optical zone (see Central Cornea, later). The entrance pupil is the virtual image of the anatomical pupil formed by the magnifying effect of the cornea; it is larger and closer to the cornea than is the real pupil. The entrance pupil is conjugate to the anatomical pupil, so light rays refracted by the cornea and directed toward the entrance pupil pass through the anatomical pupil. Even if the pupil is eccentric, the pencil of light rays that reaches the fovea is limited by the entrance pupil (Fig. 15-3). The elusive visual axis is located within this bundle of light rays and does not correspond to the corneal light reflex or the geometrical apex of the cornea.[6] The foveal photoreceptors orient themselves toward the center of the pupil (Stiles-Crawford effect), even if the entrance pupil becomes eccentric.[7]

Another factor to consider when establishing the center for keratorefractive procedures is pupillary dilatation under mesopic or scotopic conditions. The pupil diameter might reach 6–8mm under decreased light conditions. The optical zone in a keratorefractive procedure is defined as the area of the central cornea that bears the refractive change caused by the surgery. There is a limit to the size of the optical zone in the different keratorefractive procedures: 3.0–5.5mm in radial keratotomy and 4.5–8.0mm in photorefractive keratectomy (PRK) and laser-assisted *in situ* keratomileusis (LASIK). As the pupil dilates beyond the edge of the optical zone, the rays of light are refracted differently in the midperipheral and the central cornea. This differential causes edge glare and haloes around objects, a phenomenon that is more pronounced at night or in cases of decentration of the optical zone. Some patients with particularly large pupils may have a mismatch between pupil size and optical zone diameter and should be warned before surgery about possible optical distortion under mesopic conditions.

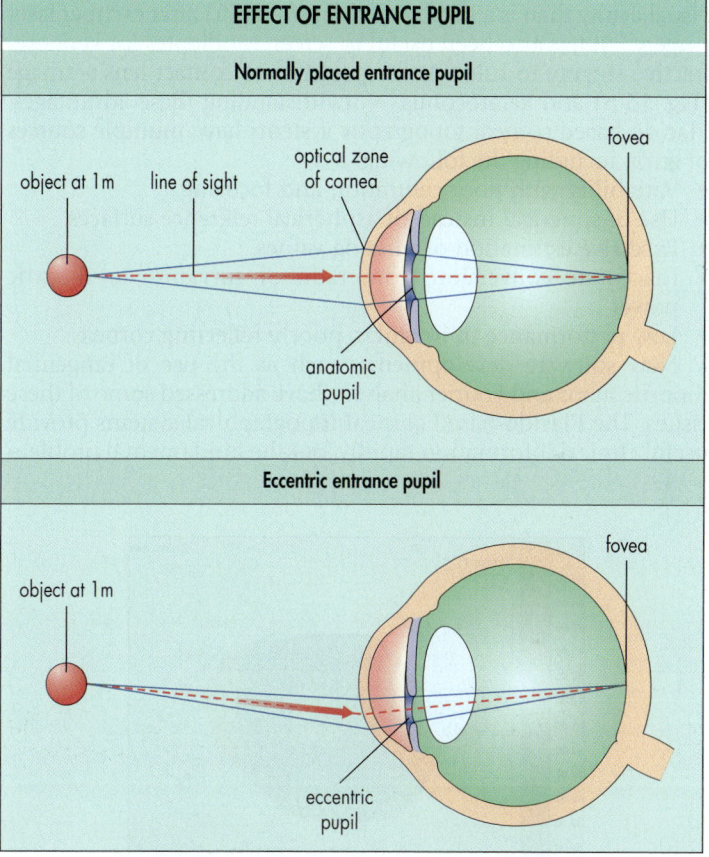

FIG. 15-3 ▪ **Effect of entrance pupil.** The optical zone of the cornea and the line of sight are limited by the entrance pupil. If the pupil becomes eccentric, the optical zone and the line of sight are limited by the new entrance pupil. Note that the new optical zone and line of sight are unrelated to the center of the cornea or the corneal light reflex. (Modified with permission from Uozato H, Guyton DL. Centering corneal surgical procedures. Am J Ophthalmol. 1987;103:264–75.)

The active reorientation of the photoreceptors toward the center of the pupil and the possibility of edge glare if the entrance pupil extends beyond the optic zone of the keratorefractive procedure favor the centration of keratorefractive procedures on the pupil instead of on the elusive visual axis. The same optical principles apply to anterior and posterior chamber intraocular lenses (IOLs).

It may be better not to use miotics to center the refractive procedure, because the center of the pupil may move in the nasal direction with miosis, which produces temporal edge glare when the pupil dilates after surgery.

Corneal Topographical Changes After Keratorefractive Procedures

Classic and automated keratometers are used to measure the radii of curvature of the cornea along two major axes of a circle approximately 3.0mm in diameter. The dioptric power of the cornea is calculated from the radii measurement, using the keratometric index.

To obtain information about the radius of curvature at corneal points other than those at 3.0mm, several corneal topographical systems have been developed. These provide a complete dioptric map of the central and peripheral cornea. Most available corneal topographical systems are based on Placido's disc, in which a series of concentric rings is projected onto the anterior corneal surface. The reduced and upright specular image is digitized and used to calculate the radii of curvature of the cornea at different points.[8] From the radii values, the dioptric power of the cornea is calculated and displayed in a color-coded scale.[9]

The use of corneal topography has enhanced the understanding of various keratorefractive procedures and has unveiled crucial information about regular and irregular astigmatism, optical zone sizes, centration, refractive change, regional healing patterns, and many other aspects of the refractive procedure (Fig. 15-4). An irregular corneal surface (intraoperative drift) is more deleterious to visual acuity than is a displaced ablation (shift) after excimer laser surgery.[10] It has also been useful to screen candidates for keratorefractive surgery to rule out the presence of contact lens warpage (Fig. 15-5) and keratoconus. Notwithstanding these advantages, Placido-based corneal topography systems have multiple sources of error, including the following:

- Variability with poor centration and focusing.
- Use of spherical instead of aspherical reference surfaces.
- Excessive estimation of missing values.
- Inaccurate conversion from radii of curvature to dioptric power.
- Low performance in irregular, poorly reflecting corneas.

New software developments, such as the use of tangential dioptric maps and Fourier analysis, have addressed some of these issues. The Placido-based corneal topographical systems provide useful clinical information rapidly, but the fundamental problem of calculating surface elevation from a projected set of rings seems inherent to all machines. Two new forms of corneal topography are commercially available today—rasterstereo videokeratography and slit-lamp scanning systems. The latter also allows calculation of the shape of the posterior surface of the cornea, the thickness of the cornea, the depth of the anterior chamber, and the anterior and posterior surfaces of the crystalline lens.

Wave Front Deformation

The principles of wave front deformation measurements come from astronomical optics. In a perfect optical system, all the refracted rays are focused on a single plane (wave front). Optical aberrations induce deformations on this plane and can be quantitated. They represent the optical performance of the entire visual system, not only the anterior surface of the cornea, as in most corneal topography machines. The lower-order optical aberrations (sphere and astigmatism) can be corrected with spherocylindrical glasses. The higher-order aberrations (spherical aberration, coma) correspond to what is clinically known as irregular astigmatism (Fig. 15-6). With the use of advanced lasers and wave front deformation measuring devices, the correction of these distortions of the human eye has been attempted.[11]

Intraocular Lens Calculation After Keratorefractive Surgery

When calculating the power of an IOL, two biological variables are measured—the effective corneal power, and the length of the eye. Because the shape of the cornea is modified by keratorefractive surgery, calculation of the effective corneal power using the traditional method of keratometry before cataract surgery has led to poor estimations of the IOL power required after surgery.

Two problems may be encountered in estimating corneal power after keratorefractive surgery. The first occurs after radial keratotomy (RK) or other peripheral corneal procedures with small optical zones, in which the ring measured by classic and automated keratometers falls in the midperipheral, steepened cornea outside the small, flattened optical zone, overestimating the effective

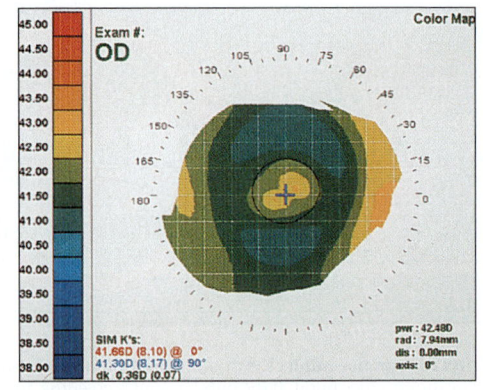

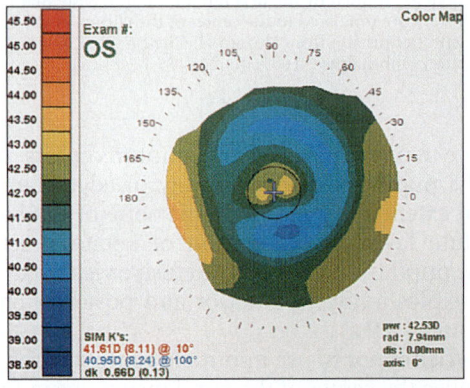

FIG. 15-4 ■ Corneal topography after refractive surgery in a 58-year-old man.

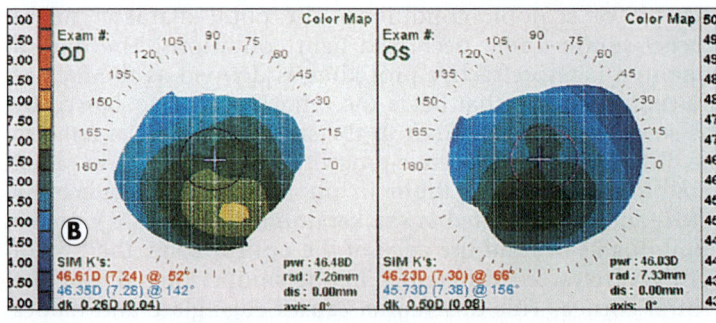

FIG. 15-5 ■ Corneal topography before refractive surgery in a 34-year-old woman who had used daily-wear soft contact lenses for 12 years. **A,** Despite not wearing contact lenses for 2 weeks prior to the appointment, the patient's corneal topographies were asymmetrical, with a pseudokeratoconus picture of the left eye. **B,** After 2 months, the topographical picture assumed a more normal pattern, and the refraction stabilized without using the contact lenses; refractive surgery was then undertaken.

corneal power. The second problem occurs in cases of PRK or LASIK for myopia, in which a decrease occurs in the central thickness of the cornea. The refractive index of the corneal tissue is 1.37. The keratometric index used in most keratometers to convert from radius of curvature to dioptric power is the slightly lower value of 1.3375, to account for the divergent posterior surface of the cornea. If the thickness of the cornea is decreased, the diverging power of the posterior surface of the cornea increases relative to that of the anterior surface, so the keratometric index should be even smaller than 1.3375. Current keratometers and computerized videokeratoscopes that use this value when the cornea has been thinned tend to overestimate the effective corneal power.

Different approaches, such as the use of computerized videokeratography with smaller rings and different software or of hard contact lens overrefraction using a standardized lens, have been suggested to calculate the effective corneal power after keratorefractive procedures. If the preoperative keratometric readings are known, the change in refraction at the corneal plane can be subtracted from those readings to calculate the postoperative effective corneal power.[12]

CLASSIFICATION OF REFRACTIVE PROCEDURES

New refractive techniques are being developed continually and the older techniques refined and simplified. The refractive power of an optical system, such as the eye, can be modified by changing the curvature of the refractive surfaces, the index of refraction of the different media, or the relative location of the different elements of the system.

Several classifications of keratorefractive surgery have been proposed, based on the mechanisms of action of the surgery[13] or on the type of surgery.[14] A simplified classification has been proposed in which the site of action of the surgery on the cornea—either over the optical zone or peripheral to it—is matched against the four different mechanisms of action of corneal surgery: addition, subtraction, relaxation, and coagulation-compression. The procedures that act on the optical zone are further subdivided into superficial or intrastromal (Table 15-1). The use of IOLs to correct the refractive error does not have as many variations as do keratorefractive procedures. The lenses can be inserted into a phakic or aphakic eye or into the anterior or posterior chamber to add or subtract from the refractive status of the eye. The management of presbyopia depends on the theory of its pathogenesis that the technique intends to correct; it may either render the crystalline lens more pliable or increase the tension of the equatorial zonules.

Cornea

Approximately two thirds of refraction occurs at the air-tear interface, which generally parallels the anterior surface of the cornea. The cornea is readily accessible, and its curvature can be modified as an extraocular procedure. Most keratorefractive procedures to date modify the radius of curvature of the anterior surface of the cornea.[15]

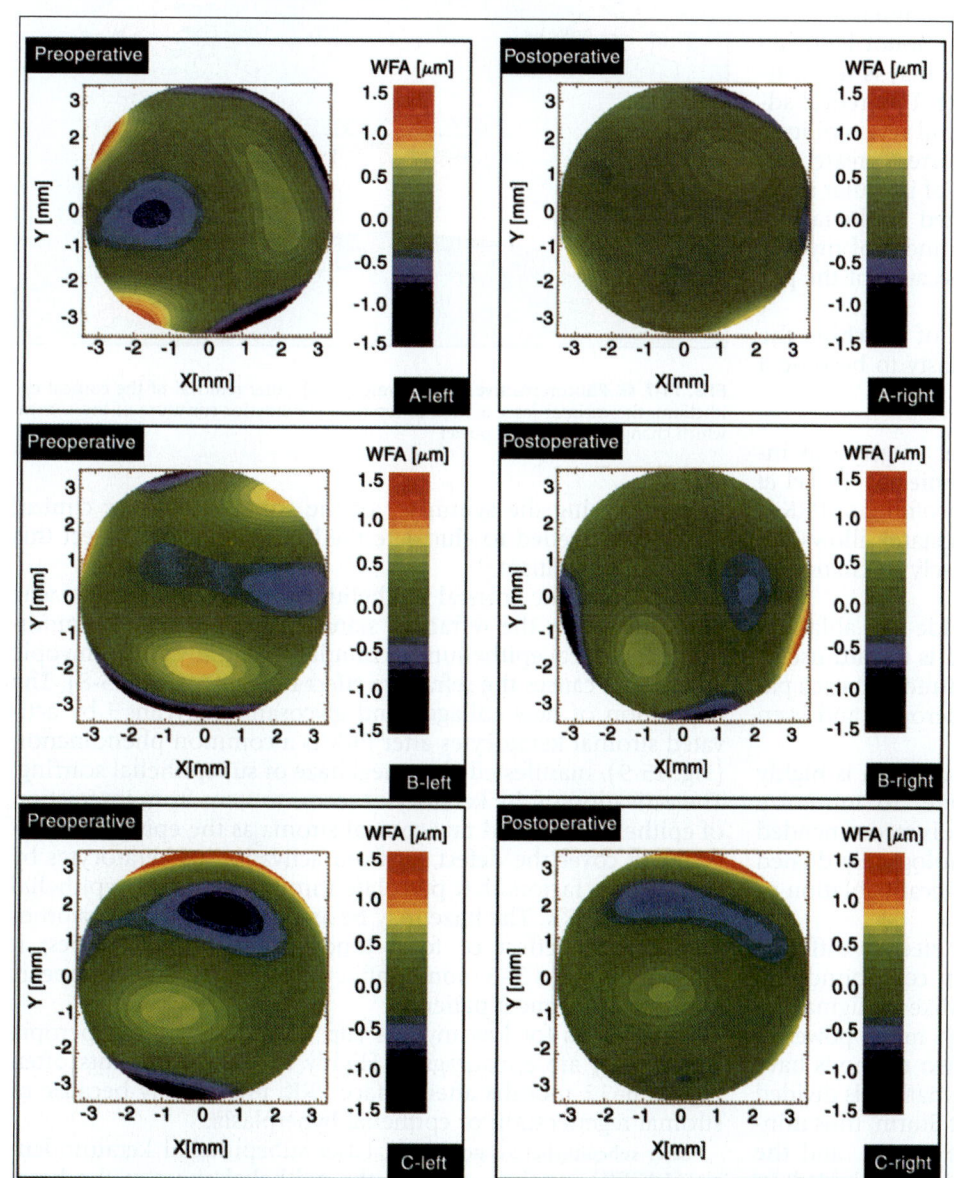

FIG. 15-6 ■ Wave front changes after refractive surgery. (From Mrochen M, Kraemmerer M, Seiler T. Wavefront-guided laser in situ keratomileusis: early results in three eyes. J Refract Surg. 2000;16:116–21.)

TABLE 15-1

PROPOSED CLASSIFICATION OF KERATOREFRACTIVE SURGICAL PROCEDURES

Optical Zone	Addition	Subtraction	Relaxation	Coagulation-Compression
Superficial	Epikeratophakia Synthetic epikeratophakia	PRK LASEK		Corneal molding
Intrastromal	Keratophakia Intracorneal lenses	LASIK Intrastromal laser Keratomileusis *in situ* BKS keratomileusis Classic keratomileusis	Lamellar keratotomy	
Peripheral cornea	Intracorneal ring segments	Wedge resection	Radial keratotomy Hexagonal keratotomy Arcuate keratotomy	Thermokeratoplasty Compression sutures Circular keratorrhaphy

BKS, Barraquer-Krumeich-Swinger; *LASEK*, laser subepithelial keratomileusis; *LASIK*, laser stromal *in situ* keratomileusis; *PRK*, photorefractive keratectomy.

CENTRAL CORNEA. Most procedures used to modify the corneal optical zone, or central cornea, change the relationship between its anterior and posterior surfaces; the thickness of the cornea is also modified. The central cornea may be modified either on the surface or intrastromally. If the intrastromal procedure involves either the blunt or sharp dissection of the corneal lamellae, it is called lamellar refractive surgery.

Corneal Surface: Addition

Epikeratophakia. Epikeratophakia (also known as epikeratoplasty and onlay lamellar keratoplasty) was introduced by Werblin *et al.*[16] It involves removal of the epithelium from the central cornea and preparation of a peripheral annular keratotomy. No microkeratome is used. A lyophilized donor lenticule (consisting of Bowman's layer and anterior stroma) is reconstituted and sewn into the annular keratotomy site. Theoretical advantages of epikeratophakia are its simplicity and reversibility.

Although this procedure can be used to correct greater degrees of myopia and hyperopia, complications of irregular astigmatism, delayed visual recovery, and prolonged epithelial defects are common. Its use for the general treatment of myopia and hyperopia has been abandoned, largely because of the potential loss of best-corrected visual acuity.

Synthetic materials[17] and improved means of attaching the lenticule to the cornea may allow epikeratoplasty to become a more useful refractive technique in the future.

Corneal Surface: Subtraction

Photorefractive keratectomy. Excimer laser corneal surgery was introduced as a precise tool for linear keratectomies by Trokel *et al.*[18] in 1983 but was later used for corneal reprofiling or PRK.[19] The 193nm ultraviolet laser (excimer or solid state) allows the anterior corneal surface to be reprofiled precisely to change its radius of curvature[20] (Fig. 15-7).

Three types of laser delivery are available: wide-area ablation, scanning slit, and flying spot lasers. The trend is toward use of the last, which allows customization of the treatment to each patient. Treatment of myopia, astigmatism, hyperopia, and even presbyopia has been attempted.

The depth of ablation necessary to correct myopia is highly dependent on the size of the treatment zone. To minimize haloes and edge glare in scotopic conditions, it is recommended that the optical zone be larger than the physiologically dilated pupil, which in certain cases may require significant ablation of the anterior stroma.

The excimer laser can be used to flatten or steepen differentially the corneal meridians and hence to treat compound myopic and compound hyperopic astigmatism. Mixed astigmatism can be treated by flattening the refractively more powerful meridian or by steepening the weaker one. Two methods have been used: the bitoric method, where the astigmatism is divided at the circle of least confusion of the conoid of Sturm, thus minimizing the total amount of ablation to the cornea, and the cross-cylinder method, where the astigmatism is divided in equal amounts, adding the spherical equivalent ablation and

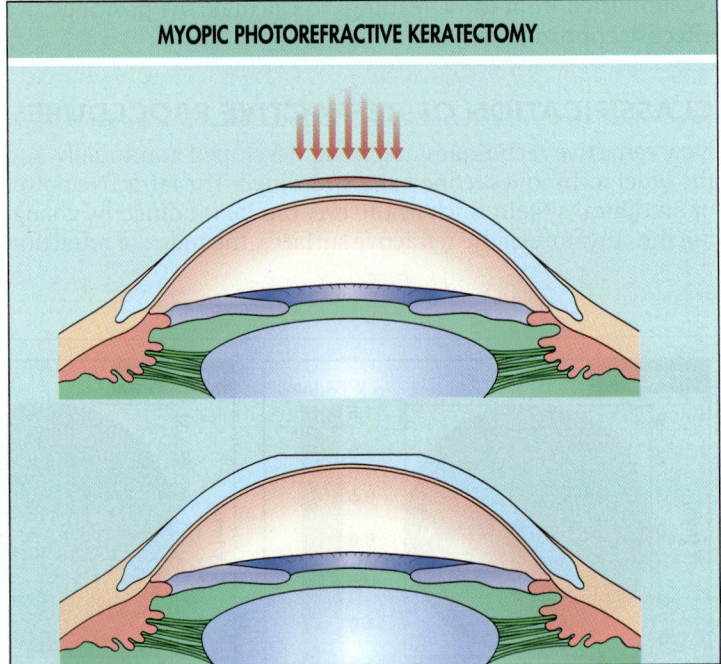

MYOPIC PHOTOREFRACTIVE KERATECTOMY

FIG. 15-7 ■ Photorefractive keratectomy (PRK). After removal of the corneal epithelium, the excimer laser is used to reprofile the anterior curvature of the cornea, which changes its refractive power.

thus increasing the symmetry of the ablation. Further clinical studies are needed to elucidate the best method to correct this form of astigmatism.[21]

After PRK, the corneal epithelium undergoes a hyperplastic phase in which the refractive status of the eye may be modified.[22] If corneal epithelium accumulates centrally after a myopic ablation, it causes the refractive effect to regress (Fig. 15-8). The deposition of new collagen and glycosaminoglycans[23] by activated stromal keratocytes after PRK is a common phenomenon (Fig. 15-9), manifested as corneal haze or subepithelial scarring. The activation of the keratocytes seems to stem from interaction of epithelial cells and raw corneal stroma as the epithelium migrates to cover the defect, or from activation of keratocytes by soluble tear factors that percolate through the initial epithelial defect after PRK. The haze may be associated with regression of the refractive effect or focal topographical abnormalities; it peaks in humans 3–6 months after the operation and disappears after 1 year for most patients.

PRK results for low myopia (up to 6D) and low hyperopia (up to 3D) are encouraging. Highly ametropic patients often regress 6–12 months after surface PRK, presumably because of stromal regeneration or epithelial hyperplasia.

Laser subepithelial keratomileusis. Laser subepithelial keratomileusis (LASEK) involves cleaving the epithelial sheet at the basement membrane with dilute alcohol, applying the laser as in

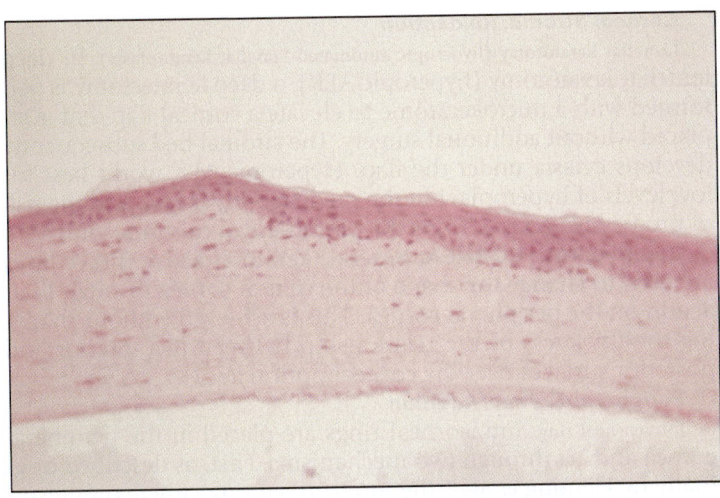

FIG. 15-8 ■ **Epithelial healing.** Light microscopic findings of rabbit cornea 1 week after superficial midperipheral annular keratectomy. Note the epithelial hyperplasia on the ablated area toward the right side of the microphotograph. (From Jain S, Chamon W, Stark WJ, et al. Intrastromal epithelial accretion follows deep excimer annular keratectomy. Cornea. 1996;15:248–57.)

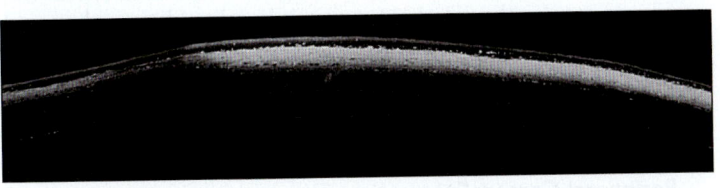

FIG. 15-9 ■ **Subepithelial haze.** Fluorescent microscope composite microphotograph 1 month after photorefractive keratectomy in a rabbit. The collagen at the base of the ablation was permanently stained with fluorescein to reveal a dark area of new connective tissue deposition between the stained area and the corneal epithelium.

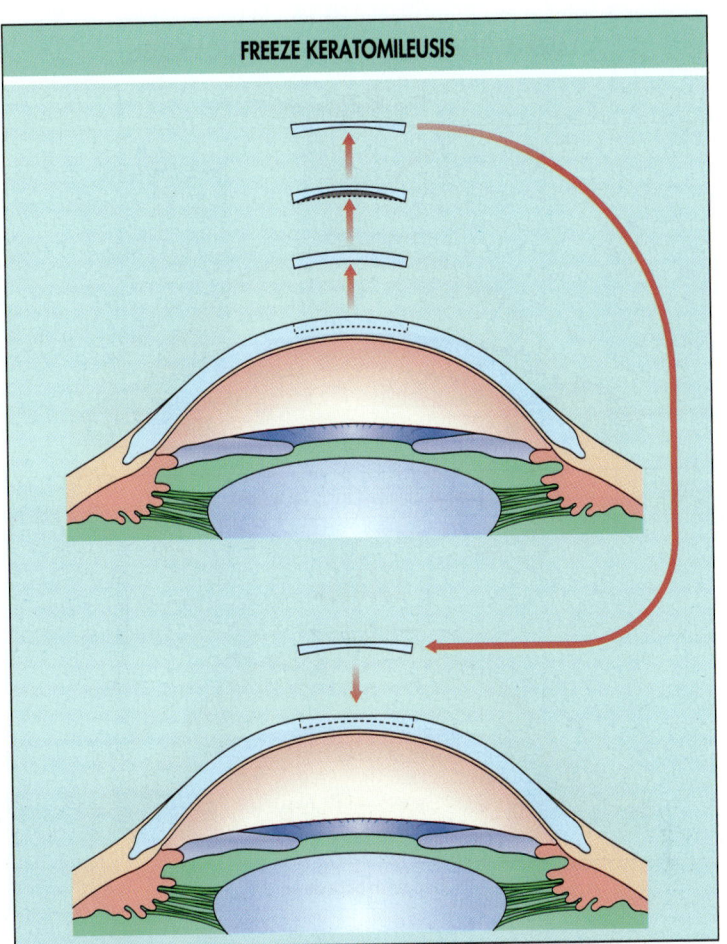

FREEZE KERATOMILEUSIS

FIG. 15-10 ■ **Freeze keratomileusis.** A disc of parallel sides is resected from the cornea with the microkeratome. After freezing the disc, a lenticule of predetermined power is removed from the stromal side with a lathe. The removed cornea is sutured back in place.

conventional PRK, and repositioning the epithelium afterward. There is some decrease in pain, quicker visual rehabilitation, and less haze than after classic PRK.[24]

Corneal Stroma: Subtraction

Keratomileusis. Keratomileusis refers to carving the cornea. Barraquer[25] first reported clinical results in 1964. Krwawicz from Poland reported on the resection of midstromal corneal tissue or stromectomy for the treatment of myopia in 1963, but he did not elaborate or develop the technique as extensively as Barraquer did.

Classic keratomileusis involves the excision of a lamellar button of parallel faces from the cornea with a microkeratome, freezing and reshaping the lamellar button, and replacing it in position with sutures (Fig. 15-10). The procedure was modified by Krumeich and Swinger, who reshaped the disc with a second microkeratome pass and did not have to freeze it, in a procedure known as BKS (Barraquer-Krumeich-Swinger) keratomileusis. Ruiz and Rowsey[26] made further modifications by applying the second microkeratome pass to the stromal bed instead of to the resected disc, in a procedure called in situ keratomileusis. Even though the refractive cut with the microkeratome gave a disc of parallel surfaces with no optical power, a dioptric effect was achieved because of the remodeling corneal tissue, as described by Barraquer[27] in the law of thickness. The development of a mechanized microkeratome, or automatic corneal shaper, provided a more consistent thickness and diameter of the corneal disc and improved the predictability of the procedure. This procedure is known as automated lamellar keratoplasty (ALK). The fact that the corneal cap does not have to be modified led to the use of a hinged flap instead of a free cap. This, in turn, led to sutureless repositioning of the flap, which simplified the procedure further.

Laser-assisted in situ keratomileusis. The exponential growth of LASIK refractive correction makes it the most commonly performed refractive surgery in the world today. The combination of a lamellar dissection with the microkeratome and a refractive ablation in the bed with the excimer laser was first performed in

rabbits by Pallikaris et al.[28] in a modification of Ruiz's keratomileusis in situ (Fig. 15-11). Buratto and Ferrari[29] first performed this procedure in humans after inadvertently obtaining a thin resection with the microkeratome while performing a modification of Barraquer's classic keratomileusis using the excimer laser instead of the cryolathe to modify the corneal cap.

LASIK is similar to PRK in that an excimer or ultraviolet laser is applied to the cornea to modify its radius of curvature. The difference is that in PRK the laser is applied directly to Bowman's layer, whereas in LASIK the laser is applied to the midstroma after a flap has been lifted from the cornea. The flap is replaced and adheres spontaneously, helped by the endothelial pump. In LASIK there is some degree of epithelial hyperplasia that causes regression of the effect, although to a lesser degree than in PRK.[30] No visually significant haze follows LASIK,[31] but when the flap is too thin or is ablated accidentally with the laser, haze may occur, suggesting that a critical amount of unablated flap keratocytes is needed to inhibit haze formation after routine LASIK. An additional factor to take into account after LASIK is the biomechanical response of the corneal lamellae after creation of the flap; there seems to be peripheral steepening and central flattening of the cornea.[32]

The disadvantages of LASIK include microkeratome malfunction and flap malposition. The optical principles discussed in the preceding section are similar for PRK and LASIK. The latter is more effective for higher degrees of myopia and hyperopia, and it is increasingly being used for lower corrections owing to its faster and less painful rehabilitation.[33]

Intrastromal laser ablation. Intrastromal, solid-state, picosecond lasers are more compact and portable than excimer lasers, but their development is in its early stages. An intrastromal ablation is made to flatten the central cornea, so the epithelium and Bowman's layer are spared and thus fewer keratocyte fibroblastic

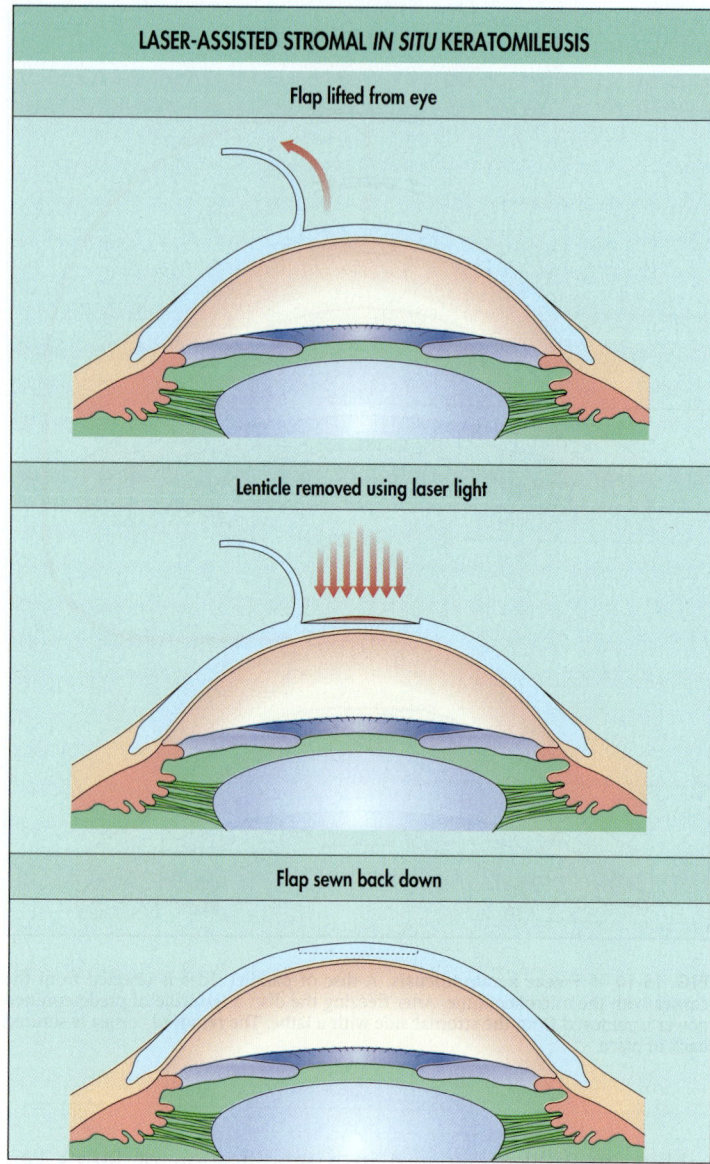

LASER-ASSISTED STROMAL *IN SITU* KERATOMILEUSIS

Flap lifted from eye

Lenticule removed using laser light

Flap sewn back down

FIG. 15-11 ▨ **Laser-assisted stromal *in situ* keratomileusis.** A flap with parallel sides is lifted using the microkeratome. The excimer laser is used to remove a lenticule of predetermined power from the exposed corneal stroma. The flap, with its intact epithelium, is then folded back, and as it drapes over the modified stromal surface, the refractive power of the anterior corneal surface is modified. The dotted area in the bottom panel corresponds to the lenticule that was removed. Usually, no sutures are required.

responses are seen. The anterior cornea of experimental animals collapses and flattens. Early human studies have failed to demonstrate similar collapse in the space created by the ablated tissue. Lifting a corneal flap similar to LASIK allows Bowman's layer to drape over the remodeled stroma, increasing the refractive effect.

Corneal Stroma: Addition

Keratophakia. Keratophakia is the technique by which a corneal lens is inserted to change the shape of the cornea and modify its refractive power.[34] A lamellar keratectomy is performed with a microkeratome on the recipient's cornea. A fresh or preserved donor cornea also undergoes a lamellar keratectomy. A stromal lens is created from the donor cornea and placed intrastromally in the recipient. A modification of this technique used in relatively thin corneas to safely perform a highly myopic or hyperopic ablation involves inserting a disc of a donor cornea under a LASIK flap to later change its refractive status with the excimer laser.

Intracorneal lenses. Intracorneal lenses may prove beneficial in the treatment of various refractive errors. Even presbyopia has been treated by the insertion of a small positive lens in the center of the cornea to create a multifocal effect. Hydrogel[35] and materials with a high index of refraction, such as fenestrated polysulfone, have been used.

Corneal Stroma: Relaxation

Lamellar keratotomy (hyperopic automated lamellar keratoplasty). In deep lamellar keratotomy (hyperopic ALK), a deep keratectomy is performed with a microkeratome to elevate a corneal flap that is replaced without additional surgery. The stromal bed subsequently develops ectasia under the flap. Hyperopic ALK works best for low levels of hyperopia, but the predictability is low, and the risk of progressive ectasia limits the usefulness of this procedure.

PERIPHERAL CORNEA. Several keratorefractive procedures are used to change the shape of the central cornea through their action on the peripheral cornea. This is achieved without changing the thickness or the relationship between the anterior and posterior surfaces over the corneal optical zone.

Peripheral Cornea: Addition

Intracorneal ring. Intracorneal rings are placed in the peripheral cornea and act through two mechanisms. First, as described originally by Fleming et al.,[36] the intracorneal ring either compresses or expands the peripheral cornea, changing the radius of curvature of the central cornea. The second mechanism takes advantage of the fact that the arc of the cornea (the distance from limbus to limbus) remains constant at all times, so when the anterior surface is lifted focally over the ring, a compensatory flattening of the central cornea occurs (Fig. 15-12). Intracorneal ring segments can be threaded into a peripheral midstromal tunnel. Recently, intracorneal rod segments have been placed in a radial fashion in the peripheral cornea to correct hyperopia. An advantage of intracorneal segments over other refractive surgical techniques is reversibility. The main drawback is the limited range of correction (up to −3D in myopia and up to +2D in hyperopia).

Peripheral Cornea: Subtraction

Wedge resection. The use of wedge resections and resuturing in the flat meridian, often with relaxing incisions in the steep meridian, was developed by Troutman. Although the procedure effectively decreases astigmatism, clinical results are highly unpredictable; this technique is therefore reserved for the correction of postkeratoplasty astigmatism of high degree.

Peripheral Cornea: Relaxation

Radial keratotomy. RK for myopia involves deep, radial corneal stroma incisions, which weaken the paracentral and peripheral cornea and flatten the central cornea (Fig. 15-13). Sato et al.[37] in Japan used anterior and posterior corneal radial incisions to treat keratoconus, astigmatism, and myopia. The procedure was abandoned because of the long-term complication of bullous keratopathy secondary to endothelial cell loss.[38] Anterior RK was performed by several ophthalmologists in the former Soviet Union in the early 1970s and was later popularized by Fyodorov and Durnev.[39] RK has been performed in the United States since 1978,[40] where many improvements in the technique have increased its safety and predictability and contributed to its popularity.

Patients with low or moderate myopia (up to 5D) achieve the best results with RK in terms of the highest levels of uncorrected visual acuity. Stability of refraction after RK is lower than with many other refractive surgical procedures. The 10-year prospective evaluation of RK revealed long-term instability of refractive errors—43% of eyes changed refractive power in the hyperopic direction by 1D or more (hyperopic shift) between 6 months and 10 years after surgery.[41] Shorter incisions (mini-RK)[42] improve stability outcomes. RK has been largely replaced by excimer laser procedures, although it remains a useful option in selected cases.

Hexagonal keratotomy. Proposed by Gaster and Yamashita in 1983, hexagonal keratotomy was first performed in humans by Mendez in 1985. This technique consists of making circumferential, hexagonal, peripheral cuts around a clear optical zone. It "uncouples" the central cornea from the periphery, which allows the cornea to bulge or steepen, thereby decreasing hyperopia. The procedure has been largely abandoned because of the complications of poor healing and irregular astigmatism.[43]

Astigmatic keratotomy. The first modern cataract extraction through a corneal incision, performed by David in France in 1747, introduced ophthalmologists to surgically induced astig-

INSERTION OF INTRACORNEAL RING

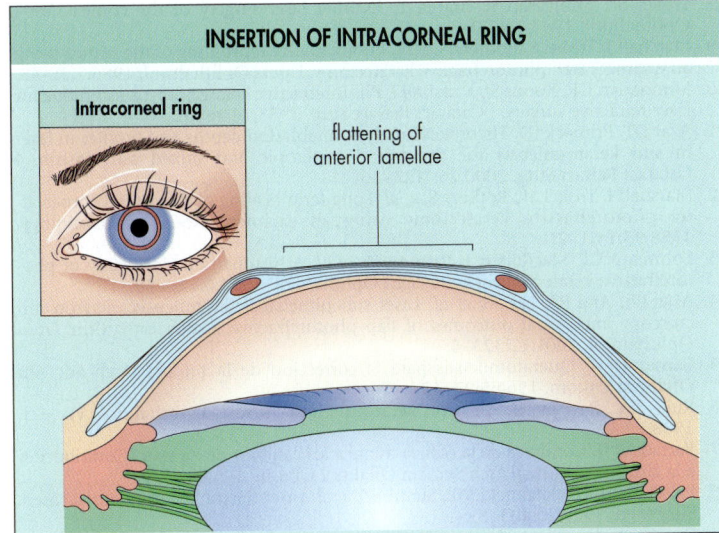

FIG. 15-12 ▮▮ **Intracorneal ring.** After a peripheral circular lamellar dissection, two polymethyl methacrylate ring segments of predetermined diameter and thickness are inserted. The midperipheral anterior lamellae are lifted focally by the ring segments, which results in a compensatory flattening of the central anterior lamellae and hence a decrease in the refractive power of the cornea.

RADIAL KERATOTOMY

Partial thickness incisions

Compensatory flattening of the central cornea

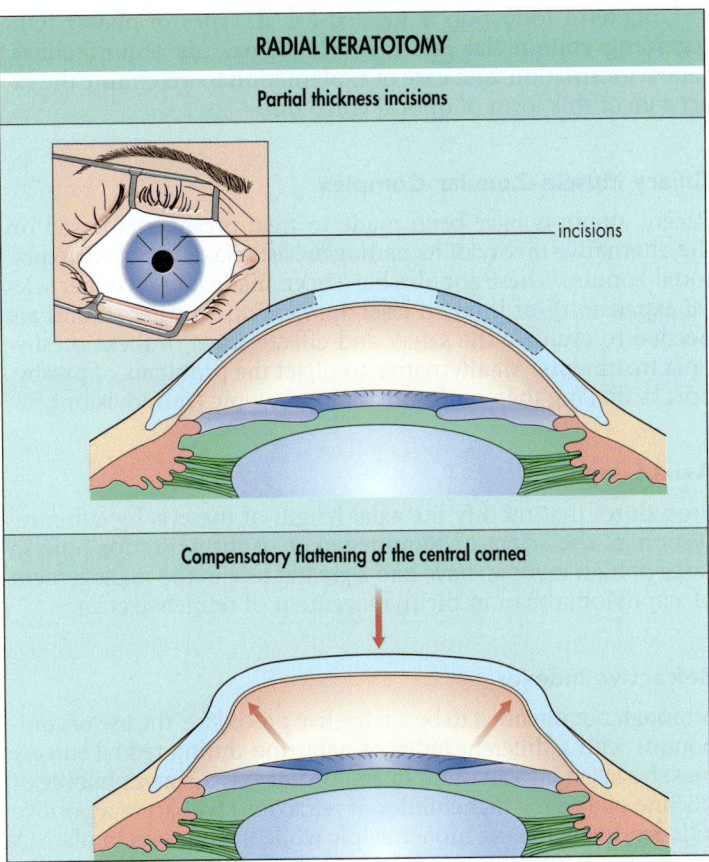

FIG. 15-13 ▮▮ **Radial keratotomy.** Partial-thickness incisions result in ectasia of the paracentral cornea and compensatory flattening of the central cornea.

matism. Several investigators in the latter part of the nineteenth century, including Snellen, Schiötz, and Bates, among others, attempted to correct corneal astigmatism with transverse relaxing corneal incisions. The first systematic study of the correction of astigmatism was performed by Lans[44] in 1898.

Astigmatic keratotomy involves making transverse cuts in an arcuate or straight fashion perpendicular to the steep meridian of astigmatism to produce localized ectasia of the peripheral cornea and central flattening of the incised meridian, thereby decreasing the astigmatism. For practical purposes, the change in the preoperative spherical equivalent is close to zero. The Ruiz procedure employed trapezoidal cuts, four transverse cuts inside two radial incisions. Although important in its time, astigmatic keratotomy is no longer in use because of poor predictability.

For cataract surgery, many issues have to be addressed with regard to natural astigmatism, such as wound location, incision length, sutures versus no sutures, and concurrent placement of arcuate keratotomy incisions. Limbal relaxing incisions have gained popularity because they are more comfortable for the patient than are arcuate or transverse midperipheral incisions.[45]

Peripheral Cornea: Coagulation-Compression

Thermokeratoplasty. Radial intrastromal thermokeratoplasty shrinks the peripheral and paracentral stromal collagen to produce a peripheral flattening and a central steepening of the cornea to treat hyperopia. Unable to produce satisfactory results with relaxing incisions, Lans used cautery to selectively steepen a corneal meridian in rabbits. It was not until 1914 that Wray performed the procedure in humans in a case of hyperopic astigmatism. The procedure was later modified to correct hyperopia and popularized by Fyodorov. Although an initial reduction in hyperopia was observed, the lack of predictability and significant regression are persistent problems.

Solid-state infrared lasers, such as the holmium:yttrium-aluminum-garnet (Ho:YAG) laser, have been used in a peripheral intrastromal radial pattern (laser thermokeratoplasty) to treat hyperopia of 2.50D and less.[46] However, the long-term effects and refractive stability of Ho:YAG laser thermokeratoplasty are unknown. A handheld radiofrequency probe to shrink the peripheral collagen has also been employed.

Circular keratorrhaphy. A suture placed in a circular fashion on the peripheral cornea to constrict the cornea and steepen the central cornea was first attempted by Krasnov in Russia in 1985 to treat hyperopia and aphakia. A similar technique was developed by Starling in the management of overcorrection after radial keratopathy. The principal problems are the development of irregu-

lar astigmatism by differential tension and loss of the effect as the suture elongates, and "cheese-wires" through the tissue.

Intraocular Lenses and Refractive Lensectomy

Extraction of the clear lens to correct high myopia was performed by Fukala[47] in Germany in 1890. The procedure was later abandoned because of an unacceptably high rate of complications. With more recent operative techniques, such as phacoemulsification, and better IOLs, there has been renewed interest in managing high refractive errors by clear lens extraction. The procedure seems more useful in high hyperopes[48] than in high myopes,[49] owing to the higher incidence of complications in the latter. For young patients, one drawback is the loss of accommodation. The use of a malleable material (silicone or collagen) to replace the crystalline lens could obviate this problem; such material might be used to treat presbyopia in the future.[50] The same result might be achieved with an accommodating or a multifocal IOL.[51]

PHAKIC INTRAOCULAR LENSES. The use of phakic IOLs was attempted first by Strampelli and Barraquer but abandoned at that time because of multiple complications. Improved IOLs have renewed interest in the procedure.

The iris-claw lens originally devised by Worst for the correction of aphakia was later modified by Fechner *et al.*[52] to correct high myopia in phakic patients. It is enclaved in the midperipheral, less mobile iris and presently requires a 6.0mm incision for its insertion.

The angle-supported phakic IOL was introduced by Baikoff and Joly[53] for the correction of myopia and has gone through several modifications. Long-term follow-up has reported progressive pupil ovalization with an older model.[54]

The posterior chamber phakic IOL was introduced by Fyodorov *et al.*[55] in 1990. It must accommodate to the space between the posterior iris and the crystalline lens. If it vaults too much, pigment dispersion and even papillary block glaucoma could result. If it lies against the anterior surface of the crystalline lens, cataract could result.

Long-term follow-up is needed for all types of phakic IOLs regarding endothelial cell loss, glaucoma, iris abnormalities, cataract formation, and ease of explantation to determine the exact role of this form of optical correction.

Ciliary Muscle–Zonular Complex

Recent attempts have been made to treat presbyopia based on the alternative theory of its pathogenesis: relaxation of the equatorial zonules. These zonules have been made taut by either scleral expansion[56] or infrared laser application. Further studies are needed to evaluate the safety and effectiveness of these presbyopia treatments. An alternative to offset the problems of presbyopia is making the nondominant eye myopic (monovision).[57]

Axial Length

Procedures that modify the axial length of the eye, by either resection of the sclera or reinforcement of the posterior pole in cases of high myopia, have had a greater role in the management of staphyloma than in the management of refractive error.

Refractive Indexes

Although not intended to be a refractive procedure, the use of compounds with a different index of refraction during retinal surgery must be taken into account. In an aphakic eye, a convex bubble of silicone oil (with a higher index of refraction) will act as a positive IOL, rendering the eye more myopic while the oil stays in place. A gas bubble, with a lower index of refraction, will act as a diverging IOL, rendering the eye hyperopic while the gas stays in place.

SUMMARY

A refractive procedure that is predictable, stable, safe, and titratable but also uses large optical zones and preserves or eventually treats presbyopia may not be far away. In the meantime, the refractive surgeon has to choose the procedure, from among all the techniques described here, that best fits each particular patient's needs. The patient should be made fully aware of all the risks and benefits, as well as all the optical alternatives to the proposed procedure.

REFERENCES

1. Azar DT, Strauss L. Principles of applied clinical optics. In: Albert DM, Jakobiec FA, eds. Principles and practice of ophthalmology, vol 6, ed 2. Philadelphia: WB Saunders; 2000:5329–40.
2. Donders RC, Moore WD. On the anomalies of accommodation and refraction of the eye. London: New Sydenham Society; 1864:415–7.
3. Guyton DL. Prescribing cylinders: the problem of distortion. Surv Ophthalmol. 1977;22:177–88.
4. von Helmholtz H. Uber die Akommodation des Auges. Graefes Arch Ophthalmol. 1855;1:1–89.
5. Schachar RA. Cause and treatment of presbyopia with a method for increasing the amplitude of accommodation. Ann Ophthalmol. 1992;24:445–52.
6. Uozato H, Guyton DL. Centering corneal surgical procedures. Am J Ophthalmol. 1987;103:264–75.
7. Bonds AB, MacLeod DIA. A displaced Stiles-Crawford effect associated with an eccentric pupil. Invest Ophthalmol Vis Sci. 1978;17:754–61.
8. Rowsey JJ, Reynolds AE, Brown R. Corneal topography: Corneascope. Arch Ophthalmol. 1981;99:1093–100.
9. Klyce SD. Computer-assisted corneal topography: high-resolution graphic presentation and analysis of keratoscopy. Invest Ophthalmol Vis Sci. 1984;25:1426–35.
10. Azar DT, Yeh PC. Corneal topographic evaluation of decentration in photorefractive keratectomy: treatment displacement vs intraoperative drift. Am J Ophthalmol. 1997;124:312–20.
11. Mrochen M, Kaemmerer M, Seiler T. Wavefront-guided laser in situ keratomileusis: early results in three eyes. J Refract Surg. 2000;16:116–21.
12. Gimbel HV, Sun R. Accuracy and predictability of intraocular lens power calculation after laser in situ keratomileusis. J Cataract Refract Surg. 2001;27:571–6.
13. Waring GO III. Making sense of keratospeak IV: classification of refractive surgery, 1992. Arch Ophthalmol. 1992;110:1385–91.
14. Barraquer JI. Cirugia Refractiva de la Cornea. Bogota, Colombia: Instituto Barraquer de America; 1989:67–85.
15. Barraquer JI. Queratoplastia Refractiva. Estudio Inform Oftalmol Inst Barraquer. 1949;10:2–10.
16. Werblin TP, Kaufman HE, Friedlander MH, et al. A prospective study of the use of hyperopic epikeratophakia grafts for the correction of aphakia in adults. Ophthalmology. 1981;88:1137–40.
17. Thompson KP, Hanna K, Waring GO III. Emerging technologies for refractive surgery: laser-adjustable synthetic epikeratoplasty. Refract Corneal Surg. 1989;5:46–8.
18. Trokel SL, Srinivasan R, Braren B. Excimer laser surgery of the cornea. Am J Ophthalmol. 1983;96:710–5.
19. Marshall J, Trokel S, Rothery S, et al. Photoablative reprofiling of the cornea using an excimer laser: photorefractive keratectomy. Lasers Ophthalmol. 1986;1:21–48.
20. Munnerlyn CR, Koons SJ, Marshall J. Photorefractive keratectomy: a technique for laser refractive surgery. J Cataract Refract Surg. 1988;14:46–52.
21. Azar DT, Primack JD. Theoretical analysis of ablation depths and profiles in laser in situ keratomileusis for compound hyperopic and mixed astigmatism. J Cataract Refract Surg. 2000;26:1123–36.
22. Marshall J, Trokel SL, Rothery S, et al. Long-term healing of the central cornea after photorefractive keratectomy using an excimer laser. Ophthalmology. 1988;95:1411–21.
23. Lohmann CP, MacRobert I, Patmore A, et al. A histopathological study of photorefractive keratectomy. Lasers Light Ophthalmol. 1994;6:149–58.
24. Azar DT, Ang RT, Lee JB, et al. Laser subepithelial keratomileusis: electron microscopy and visual outcomes of flap photorefractive keratectomy. Curr Opin Ophthalmol. 2001;12:323–8.
25. Barraquer JI. Queratomileusis para la correccion de la miopia. Arch Soc Am Oftalmol Optom. 1964;5:27–48.
26. Ruiz LA, Rowsey JJ. In situ keratomileusis. Invest Ophthalmol Vis Sci. 1988;29:392.
27. Barraquer JI. Conducta de la cornea frente a los cambios de espesor (Contribución a la cirugia refractiva). Arch Soc Am Oftalmol Optom. 1964;5:81–92.
28. Pallikaris IG, Papatzanaki ME, Stathi EZ, et al. Laser in situ keratomileusis. Lasers Surg Med. 1990;10:463–8.
29. Buratto L, Ferrari M. Excimer laser intrastromal keratomileusis: case reports. J Cataract Refract Surg. 1992;18:37–41.
30. Chayet AS, Assil KK, Montes M, et al. Regression and its mechanisms after laser in situ keratomileusis in moderate and high myopia. Ophthalmology. 1998;105:1194–9.
31. Chang S-W, Benson A, Azar DT. Corneal light scattering with stromal reformation after laser in situ keratomileusis and photorefractive keratectomy. J Cataract Refract Surg. 1998;24:1064–9.
32. Roberts C. Future challenges to aberration-free ablative procedures. J Refract Surg. 2000;16:S623–9.
33. Azar DT, Farah SG. Laser in situ keratomileusis versus photorefractive keratectomy: an update on indications and safety (editorial). Ophthalmology. 1998;105:1357–8.
34. Barraquer JI. Modificacion de la refraccion por medio de las inclusiones intracorneales. Arch Soc Am Oftalmol Optom. 1963;4:229–62.
35. Werblin TP, Blaydes JE, Fryczkowski AW, et al. Stability of hydrogel intracorneal implants in non-human primates. CLAO J. 1983;9:157–61.
36. Fleming JF, Reynolds AF, Kilmer L, et al. The intrastromal corneal ring: two cases in rabbits. J Refract Surg. 1987;3:227–32.
37. Sato T, Akiyama K, Shibata H. A new surgical approach to myopia. Am J Ophthalmol. 1953;36:823–9.
38. Yamaguchi T, Kanai A, Tanaka M, et al. Bullous keratopathy after anterior-posterior radial keratotomy for myopia and myopic astigmatism. Am J Ophthalmol. 1982;93:600–6.
39. Fyodorov SN, Durnev VV. Operation of dosaged dissection of corneal circular ligament in cases of myopia of a mild degree. Ann Ophthalmol. 1979;11:1185–90.
40. Bores LD, Myers W, Cowden I. Radial keratotomy—an analysis of the American experience. Ann Ophthalmol. 1981;13:941–8.
41. Waring GO III, Lynn MJ, McDonnell PJ, et al. Results of the prospective evaluation of radial keratotomy (PERK) study 10 years after surgery. Arch Ophthalmol. 1994;112:1298–308.
42. Lindstrom RL. Minimally invasive radial keratotomy: mini-RK. J Cataract Refract Surg. 1995;21:27–34.
43. Basuk WL, Zisman M, Waring GO III, et al. Complications of hexagonal keratotomy. Am J Ophthalmol. 1994;117:37–49.
44. Lans U. Experimentelle Untersuchngen über Astigmatismus durch nichtperforirende Corneawunden. Graefes Arch Klin Exp Ophthalmol. 1898;45:117–52.
45. Budak K, Friedman NJ, Koch DD. Limbal relaxing incisions with cataract surgery. J Cataract Refract Surg. 1998;24:503–8.
46. Koch DD, Kohnen T, McDonnell PJ, et al. Hyperopia correction by noncontact holmium:YAG laser thermal keratoplasty: U.S. phase IIA clinical study with 2-year follow-up. Ophthalmology. 1997;104:1938–47.
47. Fukala V. Operative Behandlung der hochgradigen Myopie durch Aphakie. Graefes Arch Ophthalmol. 1890;36:230–43.
48. Osher RH. Comments on clear lens extraction and intraocular lens implantation in normally sighted hyperopic eyes. J Cataract Refract Surg. 1994;19:122.
49. Cohn J, Robinet A, Cochener B. Retinal detachment after clear lens extraction for high myopia: seven-year follow-up. Ophthalmology. 1999;106:2281–4.
50. Haefliger E, Parel J-M, Ing E-G, et al. Accommodation of an endocapsular silicone lens (phaco-ersatz) in the non-human primate. Ophthalmology. 1897;94:471–7.
51. Javitt JC, Steinert RF. Cataract extraction with multifocal intraocular lens implantation: a multinational clinical trial evaluating clinical, functional, and quality-of-life outcomes. Ophthalmology. 2000;107:2040–8.
52. Fechner PU, van der Heijde GL, Worst JGF. The correction of myopia by lens implantation into phakic eyes. Am J Ophthalmol. 1989;107:659–63.
53. Baikoff G, Joly P. Comparison of minus power anterior chamber intraocular lenses and myopic epikeratoplasty in phakic eyes. Refract Corneal Surg. 1990;6:252–60.
54. Alió JL, de la Hoz F, Pérez-Santonja JJ, et al. Phakic anterior chamber lenses for the correction of myopia: a seven year cumulative analysis of complications in 263 cases. Ophthalmology. 1999;106:458–66.
55. Fyodorov SN, Suyev VK, Tumanyan ER, et al. Analysis of long-term clinical and functional results of posterior chamber intraocular lenses in high myopia. Ophthalmic Surg. 1990;4:3–6.
56. Fukasaku H, Marron JA. Anterior ciliary sclerotomy with silicone expansion plug implantation: effect on presbyopia and intraocular pressure. Int Ophthalmol Clin. 2001;41(2):133–41.
57. Sippel KC, Jain S, Azar DT. Monovision achieved with excimer laser refractive surgery. Int Ophthalmol Clin. 2001;41:91–101.

CHAPTER 16

Preoperative Evaluation for Refractive Surgery

JOSHUA A. YOUNG • ERNEST W. KORNMEHL

PREOPERATIVE WORK-UP
• Preoperative work-up consists of a sequence—screening, preoperative examination, and counseling.

PATIENT SELECTION
• Important factor that determines the likelihood of success in refractive surgery.
• Improper preoperative evaluation may result in:
  • Treatment of patients who should not be treated (e.g., those who have keratoconus).
  • Denial of treatment to some who show only transient abnormalities at the time of examination (e.g., corneal distortion because of contact lens wear).
  • Unnecessary prolongation of the postoperative course (e.g., patients affected by undiagnosed dry eye).

BOX 16-1

Systemic Contraindications to Photorefractive Keratectomy and Laser-Assisted *In Situ* Keratomileusis

IMMUNOLOGIC DISEASE
Autoimmune
Collagen vascular
Immunodeficiency

PREGNANCY OR NURSING

ABNORMAL WOUND HEALING
Keloids
Abnormal scars

DIABETES MELLITUS

INTERFERENCE FROM SYSTEMIC MEDICATIONS
Isotretinoin
Amiodarone hydrochloride

SCREENING

The purpose of screening is to eliminate patients who are clearly not candidates for refractive surgery. Areas of inquiry may include age and the type and degree of refractive error. Although all excimer lasers perform grossly the same tasks, their approved ranges of photorefractive keratectomy and laser *in situ* keratomileusis (LASIK) differ. Contact lenses must be removed prior to the preoperative examination (3 weeks for hard or rigid gas-permeable lenses and 7–14 days for soft contact lenses). In addition, patients must be asked to bring copies of old spectacle prescriptions if available or the old spectacles themselves so that refractive stability may be assessed.

PREOPERATIVE EXAMINATION

The preoperative examination consists of three parts—history, ophthalmic examination, and counseling.

HISTORY

Systemic Contraindications for Keratorefractive Surgery

The medical history interview must include questions about allergies, autoimmune disease, diabetes mellitus, pregnancy, thyroid disease, collagen vascular disorders, and abnormal wound healing (Box 16-1).

Autoimmune history is particularly important. Seiler *et al.*[1] reported one patient who was found to have unrecognized systemic lupus erythematosus after postoperative complications severe enough to require penetrating keratoplasty. Diabetes mellitus is a contraindication as well. Pregnancy is a contraindication for a number of reasons. First, pregnancy is believed to in-

duce refractive fluctuations. Although Hefetz *et al.*[2] reported no unexpected outcomes in 11 eyes of eight women who became pregnant shortly after undergoing photorefractive keratectomy (PRK), Sharif[3] reported a greater risk for corneal haze and myopic regression in women who become pregnant within 5 months of PRK. Second, postponement of surgery until after childbirth or weaning avoids fetal exposure (or infant exposure in the case of nursing mothers) to topical and systemic post–refractive surgery medications. Third, refractive surgery is delayed until after childbirth because of possible changes that occur in the tear layer during pregnancy (discussed subsequently). Thyroid disease and related orbitopathy are important in relation to the tear layer as well.

Abnormalities of wound healing, such as keloid formation, may lead to postoperative complications, which include corneal haze. Although anecdotal evidence suggests that keloid formers may not be at greater risk of complications,[4] it is advisable not to perform PRK on these patients. Anecdotal evidence suggests that keloid formation is not a contraindication to LASIK.[5]

Ophthalmic Contraindications

Ophthalmic contraindications (Table 16-1) fall into three categories—disorders that interfere with the tear layer, disorders that themselves may be exacerbated by photoablation, and abnormalities of corneal topography. Herpetic reactivation is a reasonable concern because ultraviolet exposure may initiate dendritic eruption, and the excimer laser, which uses ultraviolet radiation, may provide such a trigger. Indeed, anecdotal reports of herpetic reactivation after photoablation have been

TABLE 16-1

OPHTHALMIC CONTRAINDICATIONS TO PHOTOREFRACTIVE KERATECTOMY

	Relative Contraindications	Absolute Contraindications
Ocular surface disease	Mild dry eye • Lid disorders that affect the tear layer	Severe dry eye • Keratoconjunctivitis sicca; • Exposure keratitis; • Lid disorders that affect the tear layer
Disorders that may be exacerbated by photorefractive keratectomy	Herpes zoster ophthalmicus/herpetic keratitis (if inactive for >1 year—unproved)	Neurotrophic keratitis Herpes zoster ophthalmicus/herpetic keratitis (especially if active during the previous 6 months)
Abnormalities of corneal shape	Shape changes induced by contact lens Mild irregular astigmatism	Glaucoma Corneal ectasias • Keratoconus • Pellucid marginal degeneration • Keratoglobus High, irregular astigmatism
Prior ophthalmic surgery that involved the central cornea	Radial keratotomy (unproved) Penetrating keratoplasty, etc.	Radial keratotomy
Other ophthalmic disorders		Uveitis Diabetic retinopathy Progressive retinal disease

published.[6] Bialasiewicz et al.[7] described a patient who underwent phototherapeutic keratectomy for treatment of a herpetic scar, was noted subsequently to have stromal infiltration, and progressed to descemetocele and eventually to corneal perforation.

Opinions differ, however, as to whether photoablation may be implicated in herpetic reactivation. Fagerholm et al.[8] reported a series of 20 eyes in 20 patients for whom recurrence after photoablation occurred no more frequently than prior to ablation. Another indication that herpetic reactivation may be incidental to excimer exposure is that when reactivation does occur, it often does so several months after treatment.[6] Such recurrences may be related to topical corticosteroid therapy rather than to laser exposure itself.

Experimental work that involved a murine model demonstrated the shedding of virus after photoablation.[9] It is unclear whether this shedding is a result of excimer exposure or a result of mechanical irritation, as suggested by Tervo and Tuunanen.[10] Subsequent work by Dhaliwal et al.[11] with a rabbit model suggests that herpes simplex virus (HSV) shedding occurs following excimer exposure in both surface ablations and LASIK.

Moreover, some evidence suggests that HSV may be spread in the laser plume. Moreira et al.[12] exposed cell monolayers infected with HSV or adenovirus to excimer photoablation and demonstrated viral spread to sentinel dishes. Presence of vacuum aspiration influenced the direction of spread of the virus toward dishes in the direction of the vacuum.[12] Although it does not demonstrate evidence of spread in the clinical setting, this study raises concerns for the treating physician, staff, and other patients.

Glaucoma may be exacerbated indirectly by PRK. Corticosteroid responders may be difficult to manage after PRK. Although LASIK may be performed in the well-managed glaucoma patient, a decrease in central corneal thickness, resulting from photoablation or otherwise, will result in an apparent reduction in intraocular pressure as measured by applanation.[13,14]

Visual field defects have been documented in patients after LASIK.[15,16] Barotrauma and ischemia have been suggested as etiologies for post-LASIK optic neuropathy.

Topographic contraindications to PRK include keratoconus, pellucid marginal degeneration, and topographic abnormalities that signify irregular astigmatism. Patients known to have ectatic conditions such as keratoconus and pellucid marginal degeneration must not undergo photoablation for the obvious reason that ablation thins the cornea.

Ocular conditions that interfere with wound healing include previous radial keratotomy, neurotrophic corneas, and dry eye. Prior radial keratotomy is a relative contraindication to PRK and

LASIK. Success, as defined by the likelihood of achieving 20/40 (6/12) or better uncorrected visual acuity, is substantially lower in patients who have undergone radial keratotomy before PRK compared with patients who have not undergone refractive surgery previously.[17] However, in the light of anecdotal success in PRK after radial keratotomy,[18] radial keratotomy must remain no more than a relative contraindication. Anecdotal reports exist of success with LASIK after radial keratotomy, but well-controlled studies need to be carried out.

Even in the absence of recurrent corneal erosions, poor adherence of the epithelium resulting from epithelial basement membrane disease may interfere with the production and subsequent healing of the flap after LASIK. Complications associated with epithelial sloughing resulting from microkeratome use in patients with epithelial basement membrane dystrophy include flap distortion, interface epithelial ingrowth, flap keratolysis, and corneal scarring.[19]

The most important disorder of the tear layer is keratoconjunctivitis sicca. Unrecognized dry eye may substantially delay reepithelialization[20] and result in increased postoperative haze after PRK[21] and keratitis after LASIK. An inadequate tear volume may fail to dilute proteolytic enzymes such as plasmin and growth mediators such as epithelial growth factor.[21] Moreover, a decreased tear volume may result in decreased levels of tear immunoglobulins, lactoferrin, and lysozyme and thereby increase the susceptibility of the cornea to infection.[22]

A variety of conditions predispose the patient to dry eye. Hormonal causes of lacrimal insufficiency include pregnancy and menopause.[23] Infectious causes include syphilis, tuberculosis, trachoma, hepatitis B and C, and diffuse infiltrative lymphadenopathy syndrome associated with human immunodeficiency virus.[24] Lymphoma, amyloidosis, hemochromatosis, and sarcoidosis cause dry eye through infiltrative mechanisms.[24] Multiple sclerosis and seventh nerve cranial neuropathies may cause dry eye. Sjögren's syndrome causes dry eye but is unlikely to remain undetected in the thorough refractive preoperative evaluation. Also, many medications have been implicated in the incitement or worsening of dry eye (Box 16-2).[25] Depending upon the cause, dry eye is a readily treatable pathology. Seiler and McDonnell[20] recommend frequent use of nonpreserved artificial tears and temporary or permanent punctal plugs. Patients who have progressive retinal pathologies are also ruled out for refractive surgery. Similarly, patients who have myopic degeneration, uveitis, or visually significant cataracts are not suitable for refractive surgery.

Family ocular history is important, especially with regard to corneal ectatic disorders, progressive retinal disease, glaucoma, and cataracts.

OPHTHALMIC EXAMINATION

The preoperative ophthalmic examination consists of determining ocular dominance, pupil size measurement in dim light, manifest and cycloplegic refraction, topography, pachometry, slit-lamp examination, and dilated funduscopy (Box 16-3). Special care is required when manifest refraction is performed, with emphasis on an accurate measurement without accommodation. Proper fogging and binocular balance are central because it is ultimately only the value obtained by refraction that is entered into the excimer. Cycloplegic refraction with 1% cyclopentolate is mandatory because even the most careful refraction may fail to disclose an accommodative component.

A complete slit-lamp examination is necessary; special attention is paid to the lids, conjunctiva, and cornea. Eyelid malpositions, lagophthalmos, proptosis, and other external conditions that predispose the cornea to exposure must be recognized and treated before refractive surgery is attempted. Small interpalpebral fissures should be noted if LASIK is planned because of the difficulty of inserting the suction ring. Blepharitis and meibomian gland dysfunction are treated aggressively before photoablation to reduce the risk of bacterial superinfection, to improve the quality of the tear layer, and to prevent meibomian gland secretions and lash debris from becoming lodged in the interface between the flap and the corneal stroma.

Patients affected by significant corneal neovascularization that extends into the central 7mm of the cornea are excluded from treatment. Peripheral pannus may be associated with bleeding following the keratectomy. The tear meniscus must have a height of approximately 0.3mm and the tear-film breakup time must be at least 10 seconds.[22] Equivocal results or history of contact lens intolerance requires the ophthalmologist to perform vital staining (rose bengal) and a tear production test.

An accurate preoperative measure of pupillary diameter is necessary. Pupillometry is performed in both room light and dimmed light. Although a pupillary diameter exceeding 6mm is not a contraindication to photoablation if the procedure is to be performed with a laser that has large optical diameter capability, modification of the surgical plan is required. Pupil diameters may be assayed by directly measuring the pupil with a Rosenbaum card, although measurements so performed often overestimate pupil size.[26] Pupillometry may also be performed using a handheld infrared pupillometer.[27] Keratometry is measured to assess the power of the central cornea, to gauge the quality of the mires, and to provide a basis for later intraocular lens calculations. As part of a thorough examination, tonometry is performed to ascertain intraocular pressure.

Dilated funduscopy is performed to identify patients affected by progressive retinal disease; retinal holes, tears, or atypical lattice degeneration; unrecognized diabetic retinopathy; myopic degeneration; and other pathologies that preclude photoablative treatment.

ANCILLARY TESTING

Computerized Videokeratography

Computerized videokeratography is absolutely essential in the preoperative evaluation of patients for refractive surgery. It is the only way to uncover early or mild keratoconus.[28] The population of patients who seek refractive surgery seems to carry an increased incidence of keratoconus (3–5%), perhaps as much as 10 times that of an expected random sample of myopes.[28] These patients are probably a self-selected group for both keratoconus and dry eye because both pathologies manifest as contact lens intolerance.

It is likely that many patients who exhibit keratoconus-like patterns that are undetectable by other means and cause no symptoms (so-called keratoconus suspects) remain subclinical. Only long-term follow-up differentiates these patients from those who go on to progressive ectasia.[29] However, Seiler and Quurke[30] reported a case of a patient with forme fruste keratoconus progressing to frank ectasia following LASIK. Therefore, these patients should be avoided.

Corneal molding (warpage) is a transient corneal distortion produced primarily by rigid contact lens wear, but it may result from soft contact lens wear as well. Although transient, this distortion may persist for up to 5 months.[31] For this reason, it is advisable for a patient to discontinue contact lens wear before the preoperative examination—for at least 3 weeks for rigid lenses and 2–14 days for soft lens wearers. If topographic examination is suggestive of corneal molding, a longer period of contact lens cessation is warranted until the topography stabilizes.

Pachymetry

Pachymetry must be performed prior to LASIK. It is mandatory that there be at least 250μm of tissue in the bed after ablation.[32] If this important parameter is ignored, the patient is at risk for corneal ectasia and an unstable refraction. Controversy exists as to whether optical pachymetry as provided by the Orbscan device may be substituted for ultrasonic pachymetry. Although optical pachymetry has the advantage of providing an array of corneal thickness measurements throughout the cornea and therefore identifying areas of corneal thinning outside the central cornea, recommendations for minimum bed thickness have been based upon ultrasonic and not optical devices.[32] Furthermore, the Orbscan algorithm seems to produce readings that are consistently higher than those obtained by ultrasonic means.[33,34]

COUNSELING

Not all patients who meet medical and ophthalmic criteria for refractive surgery are necessarily good candidates for the procedure. Patients must be told that spectacles may be required for certain tasks such as driving at night. After surgery, patients should not expect to obtain perfect uncorrected distance acuity. Those who are dissatisfied with these projections are likely to be dissatisfied after surgery. Presbyopic myopes must be made aware that the removal of distance glasses to achieve a near addition is no longer possible after refractive surgery. However, if the patient's lifestyle permits and the patient is motivated sufficiently, monovision may be a possibility.

The preoperative evaluation of the patient for refractive surgery is lengthy and must be performed in an unrushed manner. However, it is time well spent because the best treatment for complications and disappointment is avoidance.

REFERENCES

1. Seiler T, Holschbach A, Derse M, et al. Complications of myopic photorefractive keratectomy with the excimer laser. Ophthalmology. 1994;101:153–60.
2. Hefetz L, Gershevich A, Haviv D, et al. Influence of pregnancy and labor on outcome of photorefractive keratectomy. J Refract Surg. 1996;12:511–12.
3. Sharif K. Regression of myopia induced by pregnancy after photorefractive keratectomy. J Refract Surg. 1997;13(Suppl):S445–6.
4. Tanzer DJ, Isfahani A, Schallhorn SC, et al. Photorefractive keratectomy in African Americans including those with known dermatologic keloid formation. Am J Ophthalmol. 1998;126:625–9.
5. Epstein R. Results of Internet poll on outcome of LASIK in keloid formers [letter]. J Refract Surg. 2000;16:380–1.
6. Vrabec MP, Durrie DS, Chase DS. Recurrence of herpes simplex after excimer laser keratectomy [letter]. Am J Ophthalmol. 1992;114:96–7.
7. Bialasiewicz AA, Schaudig U, Draeger J, et al. Descemetocele after excimer laser phototherapeutic keratectomy in herpes simplex virus–induced keratitis: a clinico-pathologic correlation. Klin Monatsbl Augenheilkd. 1996;208:120–3.
8. Fagerholm P, Ohman L, Orndahl M. Phototherapeutic keratectomy in herpes simplex keratitis. Clinical results in 20 patients. Acta Ophthalmol (Copenh). 1994;72:457–60.
9. Pepose JS, Laycock KA, Miller JK, et al. Reactivation of latent herpes simplex virus by excimer laser photokeratectomy. Am J Ophthalmol. 1992;114:45–50.
10. Tervo T, Tuunanen T. Excimer laser and reactivation of herpes simplex keratitis [letter; comment]. CLAO J. 1994;20:152–3, 157.
11. Dhaliwal DK, Romanowski EG, Yates KA, et al. Experimental laser-assisted in situ keratomileusis induces the reactivation of latent herpes simplex virus. Am J Ophthalmol. 2001;131:506–7.
12. Moreira LB, Sanchez D, Trousdale MD, et al. Aerosolization of infectious virus by excimer laser. Am J Ophthalmol. 1997;123:297–302.
13. Shah S. Accurate intraocular pressure measurement—the myth of modern ophthalmology? Ophthalmology. 2000;107:1805–7.
14. Chatterjee A, Shah S, Bessant DAR, et al. Reduction in intraocular pressure after excimer laser photorefractive keratectomy. Correlation with pre-treatment myopia. Ophthalmology. 1997;104:355–9.
15. Cameron BD, Saffra NA, Strominger MB. Laser in situ keratomileusis–induced optic neuropathy. Ophthalmology. 2001;108:660–5.
16. Bushley DM, Parmley VC, Paglen P. Visual field defect associated with laser in situ keratomileusis. Am J Ophthalmol. 2000;129:668–71.
17. Ribeiro JC, McDonald MB, Lemos MM, et al. Excimer laser photorefractive keratectomy after radial keratotomy. J Refract Surg. 1995;11:165–9.
18. Meza J, Perez-Santonja JJ, Moreno E, Zato MA. Photorefractive keratectomy after radial keratotomy. J Cataract Refract Surg. 1994;20:485–9.
19. Dastgheib KA, Clinch TE, Manche EE, et al. Sloughing of corneal epithelium and wound healing complications associated with laser in situ keratomileusis in patients with epithelial basement membrane dystrophy. Am J Ophthalmol. 2000;130:297–303.
20. Seiler T, McDonnell PJ. Excimer laser photorefractive keratectomy. Surv Ophthalmol. 1995;40:89–118.
21. Tervo T, Mustonen R, Tarkkanen A. Management of dry eye may reduce haze after excimer laser photorefractive keratectomy [letter]. Refract Corneal Surg. 1993;9:306.
22. Nelson JD. Diagnosis of keratoconjunctivitis sicca. Int Ophthalmol Clin. 1994;34:37–56.
23. Warren DW. Hormonal influences on the lacrimal gland. Int Ophthalmol Clin. 1994;34:19–25.
24. Fox RI. Systemic diseases associated with dry eye. Int Ophthalmol Clin. 1994;34:71–87.
25. Fraunfelder FT, LaBraico JM, Meyer SM. Adverse ocular reactions possibly associated with isotretinoin. Am J Ophthalmol. 1985;100:534–7.
26. Wachler BS, Krueger RR. Agreement and repeatability of infrared pupillometry and the comparison method. Ophthalmology. 1999;106:319–23.
27. Schnitzler EM, Baumeister M, Kohnen T. Scotopic measurement of normal pupils: Colvard versus Video Vision Analyzer infrared pupillometer. J Cataract Refract Surg. 2000;26:859–66.
28. Wilson SE, Klyce SD. Screening for corneal topographic abnormalities before refractive surgery. Ophthalmology. 1994;101:147–52.
29. Nesburn AB, Bahri S, Salz J, et al. Keratoconus detected by videokeratography in candidates for photorefractive keratectomy. J Refract Surg. 1995;11:194–201.
30. Seiler T, Quurke AW. Iatrogenic keratectasia after LASIK in a case of forme fruste keratoconus. J Cataract Refract Surg. 1998;24:1007–9.
31. Wilson SE, Lin DT, Klyce SD, et al. Topographic changes in contact lens–induced corneal warpage. Ophthalmology. 1990;97:734–44.
32. Seiler T, Koufala K, Richter G. Iatrogenic keratectasia after laser in situ keratomileusis. J Refract Surg. 1998;14:312–17.
33. Marsich MW, Bullimore MA. The repeatability of corneal thickness measures. Cornea. 2000;19:792–5.
34. Yaylali V, Kaufman SC, Thompson HW. Corneal thickness measurements with the Orbscan Topography System and ultrasonic pachymetry. J Cataract Refract Surg. 1997;23:1345–50.

17 Radial and Astigmatic Keratotomy

KERRY K. ASSIL • MARK A. ROTHSTEIN

HISTORICAL REVIEW

Incisional Keratotomy

The Dutch ophthalmologist Snellen[1] (1834–1908) proposed, in his 1869 thesis on the surgical correction of astigmatism, that incisions within the steep corneal meridian might affect astigmatic magnitude. In 1885, Schiøtz,[2] a Norwegian ophthalmologist, confirmed Snellen's hypothesis when he reported a significant degree of corneal flattening in a cataract patient after the placement of a corneal incision tangential to the steep meridian. Nearly a decade later, in 1894, Bates[3] made the seemingly casual observation that in patients who had corneal scars, flattening of the corneal surface occurred along the meridian of tangential scars.

Soon thereafter, in 1896, the Dutch ophthalmologist Lans[4] conducted extensive studies in rabbits and demonstrated that anterior surface corneal incisions resulted in corneal flattening within the meridian of the tangential incisions. Lans further demonstrated that deeper and longer incisions are associated with greater flattening and that steepening occurs in the meridian 90° away from the tangential incision.

The work of these early ophthalmic pioneers was largely ignored until the late 1930s, at which time Sato,[5] in Japan, noted that patients with keratoconus who experienced breaks in Descemet's membrane developed significant corneal flattening. In 1953, Sato et al.,[6] who then recognized only part of the role of the corneal endothelium, reported a comprehensive study of surgical approaches toward corneal flattening by the administration of numerous radial incisions on both the epithelial and endothelial corneal surfaces.

Nearly two decades later, in 1972, the Russian ophthalmologists Beliaev and Ilyina[7] demonstrated that externally placed radial incisions limited to the anterior corneal stroma also resulted in a flattened cornea. Their contemporaries, Durnev and Fyodorov,[8-10] reported that variation in the predetermined size of the central clear zone produced surgical variation that appeared to titrate the effect of the incisional procedure. Incisional keratotomy is now typically limited to astigmatic keratotomy at the time of cataract surgery, or two-incision radial keratotomy for patients with low-grade myopic astigmatism who are not good candidates for laser refractive surgery.

Radial Keratotomy Technique

Radial keratotomy predictive factors, surgical technique, instrumentation, and adjunctive technology continued to evolve during the 1980s and 1990s.[11-19] Solid-state ultrasonic pachymeters are used widely to provide surgeons with precise corneal thickness measurements, and coaxial microscopes are used to enable more precise determination of the surgical centration site and for diamond blade calibration.

It was recognized that age is a significant variable, accounting, on average, for slightly less than 1D of refractive effect per decade of age. It is also recognized that centripetally directed incisions (uphill, or Russian, method; Fig. 17-1) provide consistently deeper incisions than the centrifugal incisions (downhill, or American, method; Fig. 17-2) used in the surgical protocol of the Prospective Evaluation of Radial Keratotomy (PERK) study.[12,18-21] As described later in this chapter, a more refined incisional technique combines the safety of the centrifugal method with the efficacy of the centripetal method for radial keratotomy incisions (Fig. 17-3). This radial keratotomy procedure, known as the combined technique (Genesis method), optimizes safety and efficacy for the performance of radial keratotomy.[22-25] The ideal combined incision incorporates the advantages of both the Russian and American techniques; results in a safely performed, uniformly deep incision with slight undermining of the optical zone; and yields maximal corneal flattening for a radial incision.

CORNEAL WOUND HEALING AFTER INCISIONAL KERATOTOMY

The basic principles of corneal wound healing help explain many of the resultant effects of incisional keratotomy.

Phases of Normal Epithelial and Stromal Wound Healing

Immediately after an incision into the corneal stroma, an initial wound gape occurs that effectively generates new surface area, with a resultant central corneal flattening. Subsequently, the corneal epithelium and stroma undergo, over a period of a few hours to several years after surgery, a series of physiological and anatomical changes. These characteristic transformations of the normal wound healing process may be classified into one of the following phases: epithelial, stromal, cross-linking, and remodeling. These phases of wound healing occur in a chronological sequence of early postoperative (12–48 hours), intermediate postoperative (1–6 weeks), and late postoperative (2–6 months) periods (Table 17-1).

EPITHELIAL PHASE. The early epithelial stage of wound healing lasts 12–48 hours. As new basement membrane is deposited, the surface epithelium begins to slide and replicate, resulting in the formation of an epithelial plug that fills the cavity (Figs. 17-4 and 17-5). This concludes the epithelial phase of wound healing, although maturation of basement membrane adhesion complexes may require up to 6 weeks.

STROMAL PHASE. The stromal phase, also known as the keratocyte phase, lasts for several weeks (Fig. 17-6). The most important part of this phase is the migration of activated keratocytes into the wound. These keratocytes transform into myofibroblasts, which behave like smooth muscle cells; they serve to bridge the gap with secondary contraction and thus help to reapproximate the wound margins and pull the wound closed. The transformed myofibroblasts also synthesize and se-

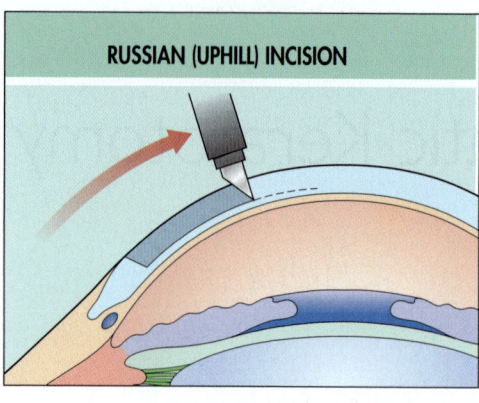

FIG. 17-1 ▮ Centripetal (Russian) radial incision technique.

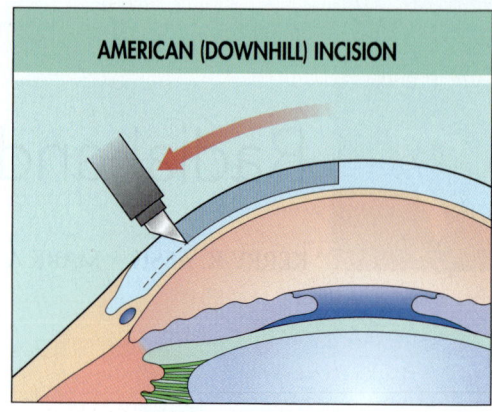

FIG. 17-2 ▮ Centrifugal (American) radial incision technique.

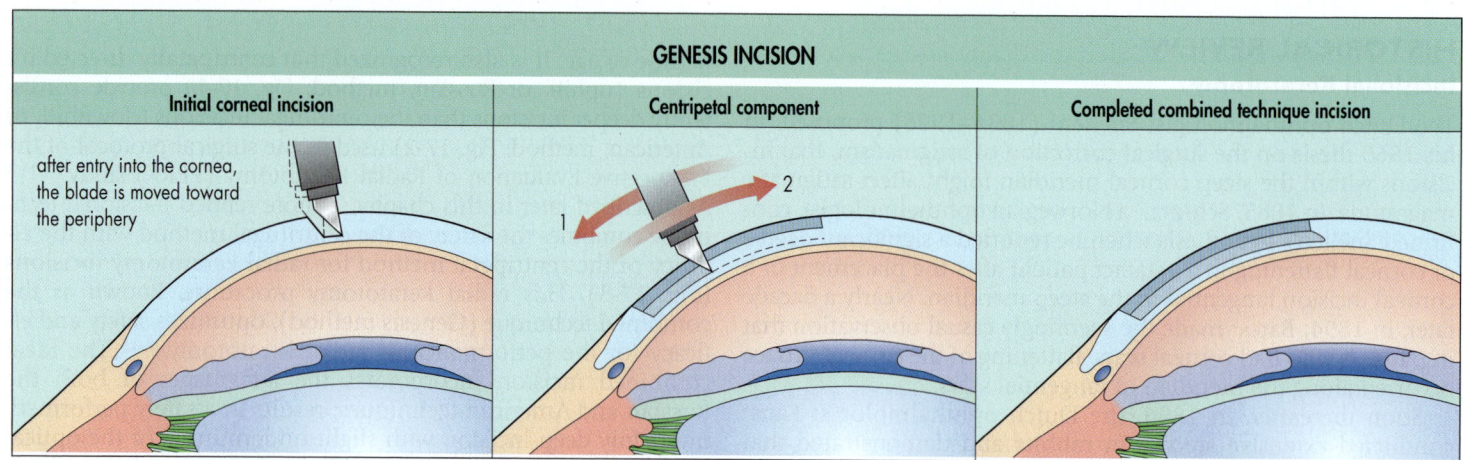

FIG. 17-3 ▮ **Combined technique (Genesis incision).** Initial corneal penetration of the diamond knife tip: It is important to enter at a slightly oblique angle, pause to ensure appropriate epithelial tissue penetration, and slightly undermine the optical zone before orienting the diamond blade perpendicularly and commencing the centrifugal (downhill) incision. Centripetal component of combined incision technique: The completed centrifugal (shallow) incision is followed by reversal of the incision direction in a centripetal motion, which creates a deeper second incision guided within the initial (shallow) groove. Completed combined technique incision: Note the relative depth and limits of the combined centrifugal and centripetal cuts.

TABLE 17-1

PHASES OF WOUND HEALING IN CORNEAL EPITHELIUM AFTER INCISIONAL KERATOTOMY

	Epithelial Phase (keratocyte)	Stromal Phase and Remodeling Phase	Cross-linking Phase
Relative chronology	Early (12–48 hours)	Intermediate (1–6 weeks)	Late (2–6 months and beyond)
Characteristics	Epithelial sliding	Keratocyte migration	Collagen synthesis
	Mitosis	Myofibroblast transformation	Collagen cross-linking
	Epithelial plug	Myofibroblast contraction	Collagen slippage
	Basement membrane synthesis	Collagen synthesis	
Comments	Nonsteroidal anti-inflammatory drugs and corticosteroids diminish wound healing by blunting the inflammatory response	Dipivefrin and pilocarpine stimulate regression of effect while pressure patching diminishes regression of effect	Vitamin C promotes collagen cross-linking

crete new collagen. This new tissue gradually extrudes and displaces the epithelial plug and serves as a permanent spacer; this maintains the corneal flattening achieved by the original wound gape at the time of the radial incision.

CROSS-LINKING AND INITIAL STABILIZATION PHASE. The collagen forms cross-links over a period of several months, which stabilizes and strengthens the wound and secures it in its partially contracted position.

REMODELING AND STRENGTHENING PHASE. The final phase of wound healing, the remodeling phase, lasts for many months after surgery (Fig. 17-7). Residual collagen synthesis and breakdown, as well as continued collagen cross-linking, occur

during this phase. These processes help to further strengthen the wound. Over the ensuing years, if mechanical trauma occurs, such as contact lens wear, chronic eye rubbing, or insufficient collagen cross-linking, the collagen layers may slip past one another, stretching the wounds and causing a hyperopic shift.

Postoperative Side Effects Related to Wound Healing

The previous section helps explain many of the side effects that follow radial keratotomy (Table 17-2). A common side effect is early visual fluctuation in the perioperative period, possibly as a result of overnight wound edema associated with lid closure and

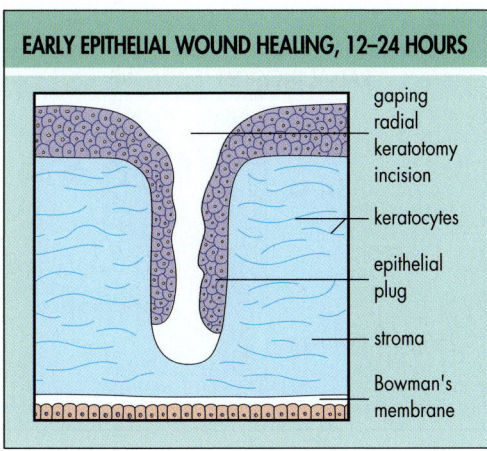

FIG. 17-4 ▪ **Early epithelial wound healing, 12–24 hours.** After an incisional wound to the epithelium and stroma, the epithelial cells migrate and replicate and move down into the groove during the first 12–24 hours after the incision.

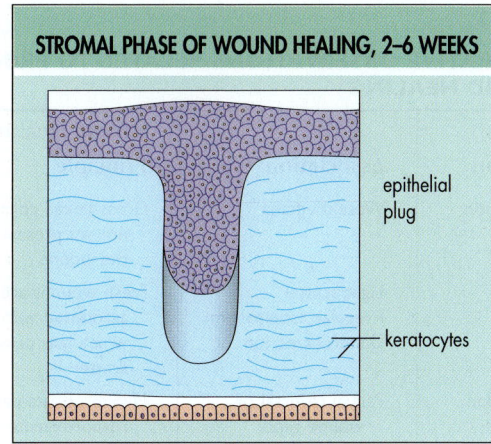

FIG. 17-6 ▪ **Stromal phase of wound healing, 2–6 weeks.** Keratocytes migrate into the wound cavity and then transform into myofibroblasts, which help to pull the wound closed while collagen is deposited and the epithelial plug is displaced.

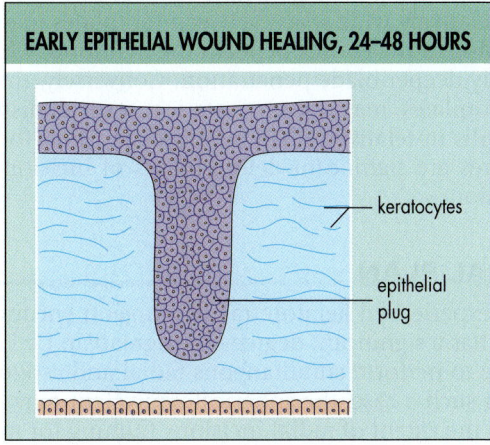

FIG. 17-5 ▪ **Early epithelial wound healing, 24–48 hours.** A complete epithelial plug forms within the wound 24–48 hours postincision.

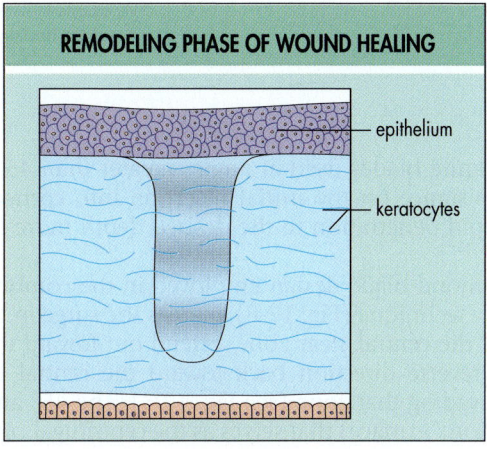

FIG. 17-7 ▪ **Remodeling phase of wound healing, 2–6 months.** This late phase of stromal healing includes the synthesis, breakdown, and cross-linking of collagen, which results in overall wound remodeling and strengthening.

wound expansion (relative gaping) and a greater degree of corneal flattening during the early-morning hours. As the corneal wound becomes more detumescent over the ensuing hours, the cornea steepens, with a regression toward myopia. Besides irregular astigmatism and altered asphericity, the phenomenon of glare may, in part, be associated with both edema and the prominent nature of the wound in the early period.

The early regression of effect is probably secondary to the keratocyte phase, as myofibroblast contraction provides partial reapproximation of the wound margins. These early responses tend to resolve as the wound matures. Late progression of effect may be secondary to collagen slippage. The interindividual variability in outcome after radial keratotomy thus may be accounted for, in part, by the variability in wound healing and the effect of age on the wounds.

INSTRUMENTATION

To maximize surgical outcome predictability, surgeons should adopt a standardized surgical protocol based on adjunctive technologies, standardized equipment, and instrumentation.

Solid-State Ultrasonography

To achieve reliable corneal pachymetry readings, intraoperative, real-time, solid-state ultrasonography is invaluable. The optimal ultrasonic pachymeter design includes a continuous display monitor, data memory, and solid-state probe tip that can pro-

vide sequential measurements without a foot pedal. It is advisable to conduct paracentral screening pachymetry during the preoperative evaluation to supplement intraoperative measurements and thus establish a rough map of corneal thickness.

Furthermore, to reduce perforation risk, intraoperative pachymetry for radial keratotomy is conducted at a 3mm central clear zone (1.5mm from the surgical centration point), over both the temporal and the thinnest paracentral cornea (as determined by screening pachymetry). These two loci often coincide.

Diamond Knife

Modern diamond knife blades generally are of high quality. However, it may be valuable to select a knife design that includes a protective housing to prevent blade chipping. Although diamond blades of thinner width are preferred because of less tissue resistance, a diamond blade that is too thin may be more prone to damage. Thicker diamond blades (≥200mm) may generate greater resistance and more variable depth of tissue penetration over the incision course. Additionally, incisions made using thicker diamonds could theoretically result in more prominent scarring. Although the authors' clinical experience supports this concept, it has not been documented clinically in a formal study.

DESIGN. The angle formed by the radial and enhancement diamond tip is 35–45°. A more acute angle using a pointed diamond blade renders the centrifugal incision susceptible to meander and the blade susceptible to chipping. More important,

TABLE 17-2

POSTOPERATIVE OBSERVATIONS RELATED TO PRINCIPLES OF WOUND HEALING

Patient Observation	Association	Wound Healing Principle
Early fluctuation	Wound edema	Cross-linked collagen not yet present in the wound
Glare	Light scatter Irregular astigmatism Undercorrection	Fresh wounds are associated with edema, which may cause light scatter
Early regression	Partial reversal of wound gape	Myofibroblasts partially reapproximate wound margins
Late progression	Progressive wound gape associated with mechanical trauma	Insufficient collagen cross-linking
Variability (individual)	Varied degree of postoperative regression	Diverse biomechanical properties of individual cornea Variations in overall wound healing response

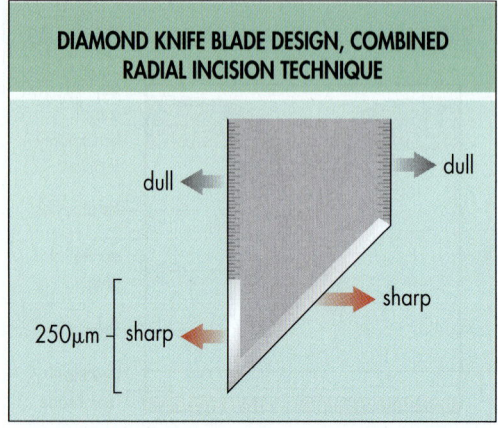

FIG. 17-8 ■ Diamond knife blade design for combined (Genesis) radial incision technique. The sharpened cutting edge extends only 250μm along the vertical edge from the pointed tip; the remainder of the vertical margin remains blunt. The angled margin of the knife is sharpened to provide a cutting edge along its entire length.

diamond knife blades used at angles greater than 45° meet increased resistance on the initial insertion into corneal stroma, making rapid penetration to the desired depth more difficult to achieve.

The diamond blade design employed in the combined radial keratotomy technique (Fig. 17-8) enables the surgeon to start the incision at the central clear zone, extend out toward the limbus, and then reverse direction back toward the central clear zone without invading that zone (see Fig. 17-3). The 45° angled margin (the "front" surface) that serves as the centrifugal cutting component is sharpened along its entire length. The vertical margin (the "back" surface) is ground sharp to a cutting edge for a distance of only 250μm from the blade tip (see Fig. 17-8). The blunt, superficial segment of the knife's vertical margin prevents unwanted invasion of the central clear zone margin during the final centripetal return to the central clear zone[23] (see Fig. 17-3). This diamond knife design was selected based on vector force analysis to optimize each of the two separate incision components, allowing the surgeon to incorporate the benefits of each into the combined incision technique. The ideal features of the centrifugal method—a linear groove and minimal risk of central clear zone invasion—are thus combined with the ideal features of the centripetal method—a uniformly deeper incision (for reproducible corneal flattening) and reduced risk of globe penetration.

FOOTPLATES. The diamond knife footplate is designed to maintain the diamond blade tip at a relatively uniform stromal depth over a broad range of angular deviation of the knife (relative to the corneal surface), which minimizes incision depth variations that can result from undesirable movement of the surgeon's hand. With knife footplates that make minimal radial corneal contact, the blade tends to maintain a constant and uniform depth within the stroma, even if the surgeon's hand rocks radially (Fig. 17-9). The footplates also are relatively broad to provide maximal lateral support (Fig. 17-10). As the surgeon's hand rocks from side to side, the footplates exert lateral compression on the cornea and thus maintain constant and uniform stromal penetration (see Fig. 17-10).

Footplate tips are curved and smoothly polished and thus offer minimal resistance against a dry epithelium. Finally, diamond knife footplates enable the diamond and cornea to be viewed simultaneously, a feature referred to as having a low profile. Footplates with such a combination of features are referred to as being of universal design.

Footplate spacing is a significant variable that affects incision depth. A relatively wide space between footplates may cause anterior bowing of the cornea beneath the diamond, which results in relatively deeper blade penetration. Conversely, more closely spaced footplates may cause posterior corneal displacement, which results in relatively shallow incisions. Thus, footplate design features are significant determinants of incision efficiency and precision.

SURGICAL PLAN

When an experienced keratorefractive surgeon encounters a patient who has a significant degree of astigmatism (>1.75D), it is reasonable to perform simultaneous radial and astigmatic keratotomy. In such a case, the spherical equivalent may be used to determine the extent of radial incisions (aiming for mild undercorrection), and the tangential (or arcuate) incisions are chosen to eliminate approximately two thirds of the astigmatism. In patients who have less than 1D of astigmatism, the radial marks are positioned to include the astigmatic meridian, because even a radial incision tends to provide slightly preferential flattening along a steep axis. In patients who have 1D or more of astigmatism, the steep axis of astigmatism is not incised radially so that if simultaneous or subsequent astigmatic keratotomy is required, that meridian is readily available.

GENERAL TECHNIQUES

Radial Keratotomy

Numerous valid protocols are available for the safe and effective delivery of incisional keratotomy. Since a review of each is beyond the scope of this chapter, the authors' personal perspective is offered to provide the reader with a clear overview.[22]

IMMEDIATE PREOPERATIVE PROTOCOL

Topical Antibiotics. Although there is no conclusive clinical evidence that prophylactic topical antibiotics diminish or prevent the incidence of keratitis, the low cost and convenience of these agents make them a good investment for the possible prevention of infectious complications. The selected antibiotics should have broad-spectrum efficacy against both gram-negative and gram-positive organisms. They may be administered approximately 30 minutes before the operation. Prophylactic antibiotic drops should not be given before the day of the operation, because they may enhance the survival and proliferation of resistant microorganisms, including fungi.

Miotic Pupil. It may be beneficial to administer pilocarpine 1%, because the miotic pupil enhances the patient's ability to view the operating microscope relatively undisturbed by the intensity of the filament light. Although the miotic pupil is often displaced nasally,

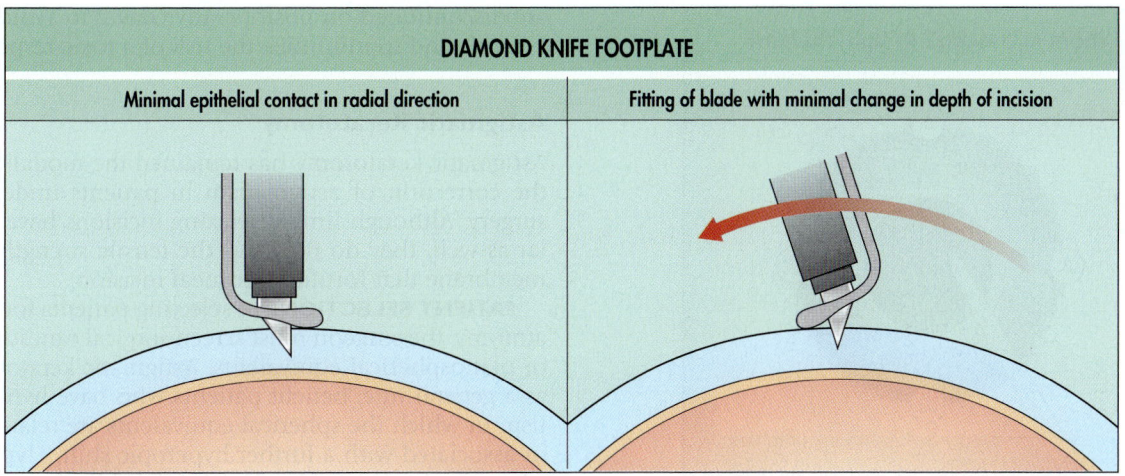

FIG. 17-9 ■ **Diamond knife footplate.** Footplate designed for minimal epithelial contact in the radial direction. These footplates counteract the effects of radial rocking of the surgeon's hand (as shown by the directional arrow), such that depth of stromal penetration of the diamond blade is unaffected.

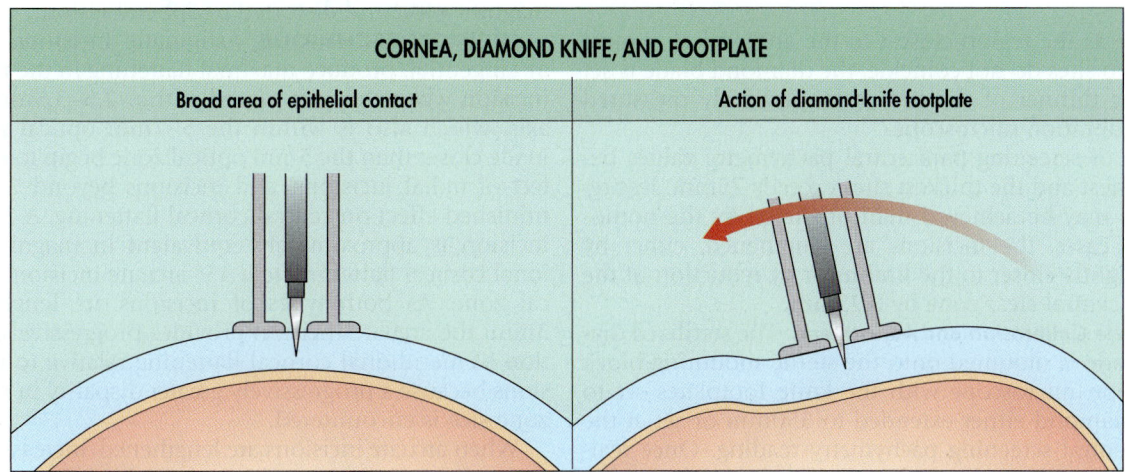

FIG. 17-10 ■ **The cornea, diamond knife, and footplate.** The broad area of epithelial contact in the lateral direction is shown. Action of a diamond knife footplate: the knife position shows that greater epithelial contact laterally counteracts the effects of radial rocking of the surgeon's hand (as shown by the directional arrow), such that a uniform depth of stromal diamond blade penetration is maintained.

this location may align more closely with the physiological visual axis. Hence, the miotic pupil may serve to reassure the surgeon of the relative accuracy of visual axis determination.

Topical Anesthetic. Topical lidocaine (lignocaine) 4%, two successive drops with a 10-minute interval, plus tetracaine (amethocaine) 0.5%, also two successive drops with a 10-minute interval, provide effective topical anesthesia. To minimize epithelial toxicity and desiccation, direct application of the anesthetic drops onto the corneal epithelial surface is avoided and the corneal surface is periodically moistened.

General Sedation. A sedative (e.g., diazepam 5mg orally, which may be repeated once if needed) serves not only as a significant anxiolytic but also as a muscle relaxant so that the eyelid speculum does not become unduly bothersome. It is optimal to administer the oral sedative approximately 20 minutes before the surgical procedure.

PREOPERATIVE PATIENT PREPARATION

Visual Axis Determination and Marking. A corneal light reflex used to guide procedure centration serves only to approximate the physiological visual axis location, since a coaxially aligned light reflex corresponds to the center of the corneal optical system and not the true visual axis. Studies have demonstrated this site to be associated most closely with the physiological visual axis.[26] To overcome errors introduced by parallax, the PERK study group recommended that the patient fixate on the micro-

scope light filament while the surgeon looks through one eyepiece and marks the epithelial surface that overlies the cornea inferior to the light filament reflex, opposite to the surgeon's sighting (open) eye. For example, if the surgeon views through the right eye, the mark is placed on the left lower border of the microscope filament reflex (Fig. 17-11). Globe decentration within the operative field also may introduce significant parallax-associated central clear zone marking decentration. An alternative technique is to use a coaxial light source mounted on or within the operating microscope optical system. This provides the patient with a light target that is nearly coaxial with the viewer. A third alternative is to center the epithelial mark over the entrance pupil.

For the visual axis to be marked, the administration of a drop of fluid over the corneal apex may enhance an otherwise dull corneal light reflex. A Sinskey hook is used to indent gently the epithelium that overlies the visual axis. If the epithelial indentation is not visualized readily, a Weck cell may be applied to the central epithelium, which enhances the central epithelial mark.

INTRAOPERATIVE CORNEAL PACHYMETRY. The paracentral corneal thickness (1.5mm from the visual center, at the 3mm central clear zone) is measured at both the temporal site and the thinnest paracentral site, as previously established by pachymetry at the screening examination. Most often, this thinnest paracentral site coincides with the paracentral temporal (or infer-

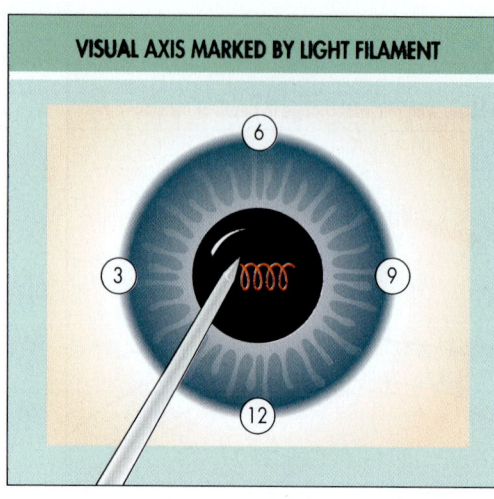

VISUAL AXIS MARKED BY LIGHT FILAMENT

FIG. 17-11 ■ Visual axis marked by light filament. Approximation of the visual axis relative to a paraxial light microscope filament image, which is the recommended method of visual axis marking adopted by the Prospective Evaluation of Radial Keratotomy study group.

otemporal) site as the region closest to the anatomical corneal center. If the two sites do not coincide, the diamond blade is set to 100% of the thinner of the two intraoperatively measured sites using a calibration microscope.

If the range of screening paracentral pachymetry values between the thinnest and the thickest sites exceeds 75mm, less refractive change may be achieved than predicted by the nomogram. In such cases, the incisions are lengthened, either by extension to slightly closer to the limbus or by reduction of the recommended central clear zone by 0.25mm.

Diamond Knife Calibration and Adjustment. The sterilized diamond knife blade is mounted onto the sterile mounting block of the calibration microscope with the knife footplates set to zero and the diamond either extended to 550mm or set at the thinnest paracentral screening pachymetry reading. Once real-time, intraoperative ultrasonic pachymetry is obtained, the diamond-tip extension is adjusted to the newly selected level. In this way, a minor adjustment is generally all that is needed, and it can be carried out in only a few seconds.

POSSIBLE ADVANTAGES OF THE COMBINED TECHNIQUE. The combined (Genesis) technique of radial incision was created to use the previously described special diamond knife design, which enables the surgeon to combine the ideal safety features of the centrifugally directed incision with the ideal efficacy of the centripetally directed incision (see Fig. 17-3). This centrifugal motion results in the formation of a groove of inconsistent depth that is relatively shallow at multiple locations. However, the critical function of this incision is to provide a linear safety groove to guide and confine the ensuing centripetal incision. At the termination of this centrifugal motion, the blade is maintained within the groove and the direction is reversed; the diamond blade is returned toward the central clear zone (see Fig. 17-3). This second motion deepens the groove evenly, but the blade design greatly reduces the risk of central zone invasion.

Incision sites are not routinely irrigated. When deemed necessary, irrigation may be carried out using a bent 27-gauge cannula with the stream directed from the central clear zone to the limbus; care is taken not to challenge Descemet's membrane. Self-sealing perforations are not irrigated.

IMMEDIATE POSTOPERATIVE PROTOCOL. At the termination of the procedure, diclofenac sodium and a triple anti-infective agent (dexamethasone–neomycin–polymyxin B) drops can be given, in addition to tobramycin, ciprofloxacin, ofloxacin, or norfloxacin (gram-negative coverage). This combination provides analgesic (diclofenac) and broad-spectrum antimicrobial coverage and a mild corticosteroid effect. The diclofenac drops

are discontinued on postoperative day 2 to avoid masking early keratitis and to minimize the risk of a toxic response.

Astigmatic Keratotomy

Astigmatic keratotomy has remained the modality of choice for the correction of astigmatism in patients undergoing cataract surgery. Although limbal relaxing incisions have become popular as well, they do not have the tensile strength of Descemet's membrane that fortifies a corneal incision.

PATIENT SELECTION. In selecting patients for astigmatic keratotomy, the surgeon must screen surgical candidates for myopic or planospherical equivalents. Astigmatic keratotomy does not, as a general rule, benefit patients who have hyperopic astigmatism in which the spherical equivalents are relatively unaffected or associated with a further hyperopic shift. Hyperopic subjects who experience extreme degrees of astigmatism and cannot tolerate both spectacles and contact lenses may, however, be candidates for astigmatic keratotomy.

Ideal candidates for astigmatic keratotomy, besides having a myopic or planospherical equivalent, are intolerant of contact lenses, because high-cylinder spectacles produce meridional magnification and distorted peripheral vision.

INCISION TECHNIQUE. Astigmatic incisions, either arcuate or tangential, produce maximal flattening in the meridian of the incision when they are placed within 2.5–3.5mm of the visual axis, which also is within the 5–7mm optical zone. Incisions made closer than the 5mm optical zone begin to simulate the effect of radial incisions, and incisions beyond 7mm have a diminished effect on central corneal flattening. A 3mm tangential incision is approximately equivalent in magnitude of meridional corneal flattening to a 45° arcuate incision at a 6mm optical zone. As both types of incisions are lengthened beyond 3mm, the arcuate incision provides progressively greater reduction of meridional corneal flattening relative to tangential incisions because a progressively greater disparity in effective optical zone size is encountered.

When arcuate incisions are lengthened, increasingly greater degrees of astigmatic correction are provided, up to an arc length of 90°. Beyond an arc length of 90°, no reliable additional flattening occurs. Stacking multiple rows of astigmatic incisions is neither productive nor advised. A pair of tangential incisions yields approximately 75% of maximal flattening, and two additional incisions yield approximately 25% additional flattening. Further incisions carried out at progressively smaller optical zones may result in global corneal flattening. Such incisions also may be associated with an increased incidence of irregular astigmatism.

VARIABLES AFFECTING SURGICAL OUTCOME. Just as with radial keratotomy, the effect of astigmatic keratotomy is influenced by wound healing and patient age. Some studies do not support this observation, but they generally have not accounted for other major variables such as control for apparent cyclotorsion or centration of the surgery with respect to the visual axis.

The recommended nomograms for the performance of tangential keratotomy, with some modifications, are those constructed by Dr. Richard Lindstrom, Dr. Lee Nordan, and Dr. Spencer Thornton. One modification to Lindstrom's nomogram (as recommended by Dr. Miles Friedlander) reduces the optical zone from 7 to 6mm, which provides more predictable results. Lindstrom's nomogram predicts the effect on a 30-year-old patient, with a calculated 2% per year age-related change in effect. Thus, on average, compared with the predicted effect for a 30-year-old patient, a 31-year-old patient experiences a 2% greater effect from the same incision, and a 29-year-old patient experiences a 2% smaller effect. Similarly, a 30-year-old patient achieves, on average, about half as much effect from the same incision as does an 80-year-old patient.

The standard distribution of effect that results from astigmatic keratotomy is greater than that observed for radial keratotomy. For this reason, the keratorefractive surgeon generally does not aim to eliminate the entire astigmatic error using a single procedure. The surgical objective of correcting approximately two thirds of the astigmatic error is advised, because this avoids a 90° rotation in the astigmatic axis induced by overcorrection, a condition that patients find annoying.

SURGICAL PROTOCOL. When astigmatic keratotomy is planned, careful attention to quantitative keratography (corneal topography) may be valuable, because paired incisions based on either the standard keratometer measurements or the refraction alone may be inaccurate. If a manifest refraction fails to yield the patient's potential acuity, irregular astigmatism may be present, and a topographical analysis is useful.

The preoperative surgical protocol for astigmatic keratotomy is similar to that for radial keratotomy. The visual axis is determined first, followed by selection of the appropriate optical zone, incision number, and length, as directed by the nomogram.

Axis of Astigmatism. When disparity occurs between corneal topography and clinical refraction, the surgeon must rely on sound clinical judgment on a case-by-case basis. In such circumstances, if topographical analysis demonstrates orthogonal astigmatism, the surgeon may abide by the manifest refraction, as this provides the physiological combined (lenticular plus corneal) astigmatism. Alternatively, in cases of nonorthogonal astigmatism (when the two steep hemimeridians differ by any angle other than 180°), if the spherocylindrical reconstruction of the topographical pattern is consistent with the refraction, the incisions are placed as indicated by the topographical map.

For example, if refraction indicates a steep axis at 90°, and the topographical map demonstrates one steep hemimeridian at 75° and the other at 285°, this "bent bow-tie" pattern of true astigmatism has as its spherocylindrical counterpart a refractive axis of 90°. In such a case, the most precise surgical outcome is achieved by the placement of incisions centered at 75° and 285°.

Alternatively, if in this example the surgeon cannot reconcile the manifest refraction with the topographical analysis, the cycloplegic refraction is evaluated for confirmation of either the manifest refraction or the topographical analysis. The cycloplegic refraction is not used as a primary source for surgical decisions in astigmatic keratotomy; however, because in the setting of astigmatism, a cycloplegic refraction may include peripheral (nonphysiological) corneal and lenticular astigmatism.

Once the desired axis of astigmatic correction has been determined, this needs to be translated onto the cornea. Because the astigmatic axis is defined so carefully with the patient in an upright position without sedation or a lid speculum, one must not estimate the surgical axis intraoperatively with the patient in a supine position or sedated or with a lid speculum in place. Cyclotorsional rotation of the globe may occur and introduce significant error.

To control for these sources of error, with the patient seated at the slip lamp, epithelial marks are placed on either the vertical or horizontal axis. Using the slit beam for centration and with the contralateral eye covered, the patient fixates first on the slit-lamp light source from straight ahead. Fixation on the slit-lamp filament at eye level and from head-on provides a virtual image of the light filament, which falls at the center of the corneal optical system and closely approximates the visual axis. The patient is asked to view straight ahead through the light and onto the horizon to minimize accommodation. The location of the 8mm-long slit beam is then adjusted, vertically (if a horizontal beam is projected) or laterally (if a vertical beam is projected), so that it intersects with the slit-lamp filament reflex. When the slit lamp enables the slit beam to be projected at a known axis, the epithelial mark may be placed directly at the desired surgical hemimeridian. The epithelium is abraded at the outer margins along the beam's long axis using either jeweler's forceps or a Sinskey hook.

After precisely marking true 90° or 180° at the slit lamp, the true visual axis is determined in the operating room under the operating microscope. With the 90° (or 180°) position determined precisely (reference axis), any desired axis may be marked using an axis marker and a surgical marking pen.

When arcuate incisions are carried out on patients who have orthogonal astigmatism, radial markers are quite useful in delineating the precise arc length to be incised. A four-incision radial keratotomy marker partitions the desired optical zone marking into 90° arcuate intervals, while a six-wing marker intersects the marking into 60° arcuate intervals and an eight-wing marker into 45° arcuate intervals.

In patients who have nonorthogonal astigmatism, the precise position to be incised is marked using a degree gauge marker and marking pen. For example, if paired 60° arcuate incisions are desired, centered at 75° and 285°, once the true vertical or horizontal axis has been established, a degree gauge marker (aligned relative to the marked reference axis) is used to mark the epithelium at the 45° and 105°, as well as the 255° and 315°, sites of the desired optical zone.

After appropriate marking of the astigmatic axis, pachymetry is carried out at the selected optical zone over the incision sites. The diamond blade is set at 100% of the measurement at the thinner of the two sites. With the globe fixated, the corneal marks are incised.

The use of guarded diamond knife blades, as for radial keratotomy incisions, is advisable. The conjunctiva is grasped close to the limbus, where it fuses with Tenon's capsule and enables stable fixation; this region also is anesthetized more deeply than are the posterior conjunctiva and sclera.

The preoperative and postoperative pharmacological care of astigmatic keratotomy patients is identical to that for radial keratotomy patients. The use of mydriatic agents is recommended during secondary enhancement procedures, as the previous incisions are observed more prominently against the mydriatic red reflex, which greatly reduces the risk of intersecting incisions and associated complications.

The keratorefractive surgeon is advised to exercise patience when secondary enhancements to astigmatic keratotomy are planned and performed. Because astigmatic keratotomy incisions require more time to stabilize than radial incisions do, any possible enhancement should be deferred for a minimum of 6 weeks after the primary procedure, regardless of the apparent initial results. A computerized videokeratography system is indispensable when the enhancement of an astigmatic keratotomy procedure is carried out. If the corneal topography map demonstrates persistent regular astigmatism in the original hemimeridian, a slit-lamp examination is likely to show the presence of either a too shallow or a shelved, nonperpendicular astigmatic incision. In either case, an adjacent incision properly placed in the same hemimeridian may remedy the problem of persistent regular astigmatism. Alternatively, if videokeratographical analysis demonstrates a shift in the axis of astigmatism, the presence of irregular astigmatism, or an undercorrection, the topographical map may serve as a guide to the surgeon when the original incision is elongated in the direction of the resultant steep zone.

Extreme caution is advised in treating astigmatic keratotomy patients who demonstrate overcorrection. If the resultant refractive error is one of hyperopic astigmatism, the original incisions may be reopened, the fibrous plug removed, and the wound margins reapproximated using a 10–0 nylon suture. Likewise, in the event that an astigmatic incision is placed incorrectly in the flat axis, the wound margins are reapproximated using a 10–0 nylon suture. Alternatively, if the residual refractive error is one of myopic astigmatism, further astigmatic incisions may be placed in the newly defined, steep hemimeridian. Such incisions are shorter than otherwise indicated, since the cornea now demonstrates an excessive response to the initial incisions and could respond in like fashion to any further astigmatic incisions.

Potential Complications of Refractive Keratotomy

SELF-LIMITED
Halo effect
Starburst effect
Diurnal visual fluctuation
Early regression

INTRAOPERATIVE
Marking
• inaccurate visual axis marking
Incisions
• incision invading optical zone
• incision beyond clear cornea
• intersecting incisions
Perforations
• corneal perforation
• lens capsule perforation
Associated with retrobulbar anesthetic
• optic nerve damage
• globe penetration/retinal detachment
Miscellaneous
• diamond blade chip

POSTOPERATIVE
Non sight-threatening complications related to refractive changes
• undercorrection
• overcorrection
• regression
• progression
• induced irregular astigmatism
Miscellaneous non sight-threatening complications
• contact lens intolerance
• epithelial basement membrane disorders
• epithelial inclusion cysts
• foreign particles within grooves
• epithelial iron lines
• diminished corneal strength
• endothelial cell loss
Sight threatening
• stromal melting
• infectious keratitis

THERAPY RELATED
Pharmacologic
• drug toxicity
Chronic corticosteroid
• cataracts
• glaucoma
Contact lens
• keratitis
• neovascularization
• late progression of effect
Retrobulbar injection
• optic atrophy
• globe penetration/retinal detachment

COMPLICATIONS OF INCISIONAL KERATOTOMY

Several million people have undergone radial and astigmatic keratotomy. Although serious complications of incisional keratotomy are both rare and easily avoided, it is important for any ophthalmic surgeon who plans to practice incisional keratotomy to become familiar with them (Box 17-1).

The best approach to the management of radial keratotomy complications is to avoid them by being aware of and understanding the potential causes. In the event of a complication, early recognition and prompt therapy avert a poor outcome in almost every case.

The complications associated with incisional keratotomy may be categorized into those that are self-limited side effects, those that occur intraoperatively, those that occur postoperatively, and those that are associated with adjunctive therapy.

A number of potential complications may develop intraoperatively as a result of deviations from prescribed surgical protocol or faulty surgical technique. Such complications can generally be avoided by diligent training, literature review, detailed preparation, and adherence to proper surgical protocols. In the unusual event that a complication does occur, sound judgment generally can remedy the problem.

Complications Related to Corneal Marking

Inaccurate marking of the visual axis may result in incisions that invade the optical zone, which leads to slightly increased glare and significant irregular astigmatism with monocular diplopia. The most common causes of incision decentration are improper estimation of the intraoperative visual axis, inadequate globe centration (which introduces errors of parallax) within the op-

erative field, and misalignment of the optical zone marker cross-hairs using the visual axis marking. As a result of the noncoaxial orientation of the microscope light source, the PERK study group recommendation to mark the visual axis provides the best approximation.

Coaxial light sources have been designed to reduce the inaccuracies of visual axis determination, as well as to enable the patient to maintain fixation during the procedure. To minimize errors of parallax, the surgeon should first view the globe under high magnification to ensure good globe centration in the field of view.

Complications Related to Corneal Incisions

INCISION BEYOND CLEAR CORNEA. Extension of incisions beyond the clear cornea onto the corneoscleral limbus or onto limbal vascular arcades must be avoided to prevent subsequent vascular ingrowth. Incisions that invade the limbus may render the patient intolerant to subsequent contact lens use because of the associated vascularization of the incision grooves. Fibrovascular ingrowth may result in corneal destabilization over time, with large diurnal fluctuation and progression of refractive effect.

OPTICAL ZONE INVASION. Optical zone invasion, as a result of spontaneous patient eye movement or lack of surgical control, represents one of the more worrisome potential complications of centripetal incisions. Patient education or globe fixation may reduce, but not entirely eliminate, the potential for optical zone invasion.

The combined (Genesis) incision technique was designed to address this and other potential complications. Because the up-hill margin of the blade cuts only along its distal portion, the diamond cannot produce deep incisions outside the previously incised groove. Thus, it is nearly impossible to incise the visual axis inadvertently when this technique is employed properly. Once the central zone has been reached and intentionally slightly undermined, however, continued pressure must not be applied against the optical zone as the diamond is lifted from the groove.

INTERSECTING INCISIONS. Intersecting incisions, which may lead to wound gape and poor healing, must also be avoided. In the event that such intersection does occur intraoperatively, interrupted 10–0 or 11–0 nylon sutures are used to reapproximate the gaping wound margins (Fig. 17-12). The knots are buried, and the sutures are left in place for 10–12 weeks, or until they loosen. When radial and transverse incisions cross, it is generally best to place a radial suture across the transverse incision margins adjacent to the radial incision.

Postoperative examination of patients who have unsutured intersecting incisions often reveals that the region of intersection is filled with an epithelial plug. An epithelial plug develops because the severe wound gape does not allow proper wound stabilization. Epithelial plugs also may be spontaneously extruded, which causes transient pain and photophobia and progressive stromal melting.

To treat patients experiencing complications caused by previously crossed incisions, first scrape the epithelium from within the wound using a fine spatula. Next, reapproximate the wound margins using 10–0 nylon. The knots are buried, and the sutures may be left in place for 4–6 months, or until they spontaneously loosen.

Complications Related to Corneal Perforations

With the advent of screening and real-time pachymetry, the availability of microscopes for precise diamond knife calibration, and the adherence to protocols suggesting incision of the thinnest corneal zones first and the use of diamonds not set at substantially more than 100% of paracentral pachymetry, the risk of corneal perforation has been reduced (Fig. 17-13). The

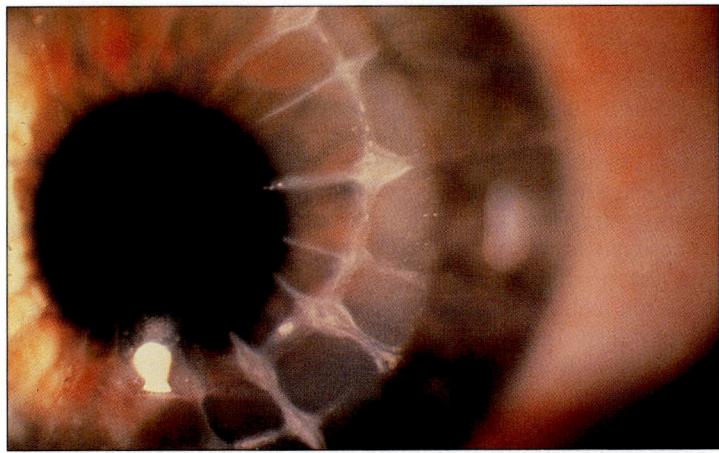

FIG. 17-12 ▮▮ **Intersecting incisions.** Pronounced wound gaping at the intersection of fresh incisions precludes the proper sequence of normal wound healing.

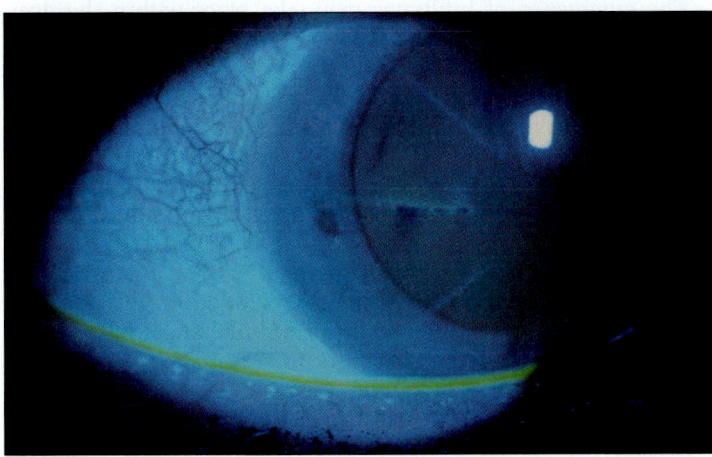

FIG. 17-13 ▮▮ **Corneal perforation.** The risk of corneal perforation has been minimized greatly through recent developments (see text). The horizontal slit shows mild leakage of fluorescein.

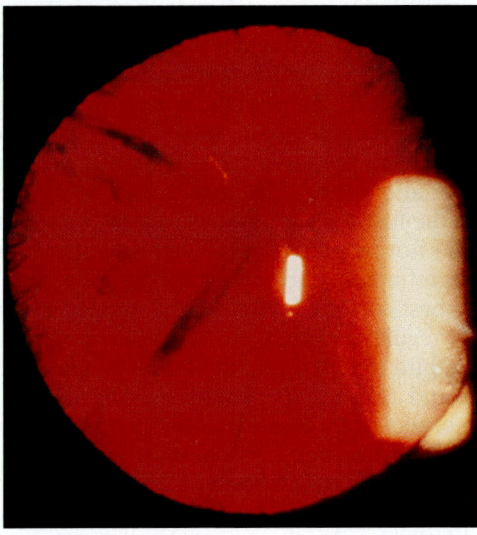

FIG. 17-14 ▮▮ **Lens capsule rupture.** On rare occasions, nonsealing perforations with lens capsule rupture have been reported. This occurred when diamonds were set at significantly greater than 100% of corneal thickness and firm pressure was applied to make the incision, and when radial keratotomies were performed using a metal knife.

best way to prevent the development of a self-sealing perforation into a more serious perforation is to operate on a relatively dry field so that any leakage of aqueous humor is detected readily.

A self-sealing perforation does not continue to leak, even when tested using a Weck cell. Self-sealing perforations spontaneously seal as the adjacent corneal stroma becomes edematous and tamponades the leak. A nonsealing perforation leaks on gentle compression using a Weck cell sponge and also leaks spontaneously.

Early recognition of a self-sealing perforation, by operating on a relatively dry field (no tear pooling within the cul-de-sac), prevents its extension into a nonsealing perforation. Patients who have self-sealing perforations are managed using cycloplegia (to dilate the pupil and prevent adherence of the iris to the self-sealing perforation site), as well as topical aqueous suppressants such as beta blockers, a loading dose of topical antibiotics such as polymyxin and ofloxacin every 5 minutes times three doses, and an ocular shield placed over the eye. The eye must not be patched, as this compresses the corneal apex, bows open the incisions, and retards healing. Likewise, the use of collagen shields is not recommended in such cases. Incision of the thinnest quadrant first greatly reduces the risk of a self-sealing perforation, as the cornea continues to thin throughout the procedure. If the diamond penetrates the globe on the first incision or on the centrifugally directed component of any incision, the operation may be terminated and completed at a later time, with repeated pachymetry and diamond calibration. The surgeon simply cannot determine intraoperatively the degree to which the diamond has been overextended or whether pathological corneal thinning exists.

If a self-sealing perforation occurs on the second phase of subsequent incisions (directed centripetally), the degree to which the diamond is overextended is probably minimal. In such an event, the surgeon may retract the diamond blade before proceeding. The micrometer on the knife handle is used to first retract the blade by 100mm, then advance the blade again by 80mm. The net retraction of 20mm is achieved more accurately in this manner than when an initial 20mm retraction is used.

In the event of a nonsealing perforation, it is prudent to place a single (or multiple) interrupted 10–0 or 11–0 nylon suture to seal the wound and prevent any of the sequelae of hypotony or of an open wound.

The evolution of the combined technique, the elimination of centrifugal-style incisions (for which diamonds are set at 120% or less of the paracentral corneal thickness), and the ability to calibrate precisely diamond knife blades that have safety features such as footplates have made the occurrence of nonsealing perforations uncommon (Fig. 17-14).

Postoperative Complications

PROGRESSIVE HYPEROPIA. Risk factors associated with postoperative progressive hyperopia include radial incisions that extend to the limbus, multiple enhancement procedures, peripheral redeepening procedures, lack of preoperative cycloplegic refraction (latent hyperopia), postoperative contact lens wear, and postoperative ocular massage. The surgeon may wish to consider these factors when patient management strategies are determined.

Progression of effect over time has become a less common occurrence. Previously, many patients who experienced significant progression of effect had undergone peripheral redeepening procedures, with repeated incisions that radiated from the midperiphery toward the limbus and with the blades set at the deeper midperipheral measurement. Furthermore, in those procedures, the incisions often extended *out* to the limbus. These redeepened and extended incisions were prone to ingrowth by fibrovascular tissue, which advances centripetally within the groove and provides an increased mass effect with progressive corneal flattening. The absence of cross-linked stromal collagen within this tissue also renders the wound unstable, with significant diurnal refractive fluctuation. The best treatment for such patients is to reopen the incisions, strip the fibrovascular tissue, and resuture the incisions. Other risk factors for progressive hyperopia include the performance of surgery without the prior discontinuation of contact lens wear and unsutured perforation sites.

INDUCED ASTIGMATISM. Another potential complication associated with any keratorefractive procedure is induced regular or irregular astigmatism, which may occur if fewer incisions are placed, if the incisions are placed asymmetrically about the visual axis or are of variable depth, or if the optical zone is decentered with respect to the visual axis. The great majority of these refractive aberrations are self-limited and spontaneously improve within the first 6 postoperative weeks. Thus, additional incisions should not be placed in the setting of irregular astigmatism until the refraction and surface topography have stabilized.

Decreased best-corrected visual acuity is associated most commonly with irregular astigmatism. Corneal topographical analysis is most helpful to determine the extent of persistent irregular astigmatism and to track its change over time. Further, in the event that subsequent incisions become necessary, topography is useful for determining their optimal location and placement.

CONTACT LENS INTOLERANCE. Contact lens intolerance is now less common after radial keratotomy. Newly designed rigid, gas-permeable lenses that have peripheral curves to match the patient's preoperative parameters are recommended to overcome postoperative lens intolerance. The risk of lens-associated corneal vascularization is reduced greatly by a shorter incision that does not extend to the limbus. The fibrovascular tracks within the incision sites are associated most often with chronic irritation and hypoxia from subsequent soft contact lens wear (Fig. 17-15). To diminish the risk of this complication, radial keratotomy incisions are stopped approximately 1mm short of the limbus. Chronic contact lens wear may also provide a direct compressive effect, with associated wound stretching and progressive hyperopia.

Sight-Threatening Complications

Two types of postoperative sight-threatening complications occur—corneal stromal melting and infectious keratitis.

STROMAL MELTING. Stromal melting often develops in patients who have crossed incisions. Thus, this complication can be prevented by taking great care to avoid crossed incisions during surgery. Corneal stromal melt is also associated with patients who have rheumatoid arthritis or other collagen vascular diseases and concomitant severe keratoconjunctivitis sicca with diffuse punctate epitheliopathy (Fig. 17-16). Patients affected by such advanced disease are not viable candidates for incisional keratotomy. For patients who have significantly diminished tear production, it may be necessary to perform punctal occlusion before considering incisional keratotomy.

INFECTIOUS KERATITIS. Although its incidence is lower than that observed in contact lens wearers, the most common sight-threatening complication associated with radial keratotomy is infectious keratitis. This disorder generally develops in the perioperative period, although delayed cases in association with contact lens wear have been reported. Indeed, the only two cases of keratitis reported in the PERK study occurred in association with postoperative contact lens wear.

It is possible to reduce the risk of infection by the perioperative administration of broad-spectrum prophylactic antibiotic drops. Prophylactic use of antibiotic drops before the day of surgery may be selected for resistant organisms. Preexisting blepharitis also must be ruled out during the preoperative ocular examination.

Sterile technique must be maintained during refractive keratotomy; this includes preparation of the surgical field using povidone-iodine and the use of sterile gloves and masks by ophthalmic personnel in the operation room. Patients must be instructed to avoid eye makeup and contaminated water, which includes that found in swimming pools and hot tubs, for 1 week after the surgical procedure. In the event of infection, early detection is important. Patients must have a follow-up examination by the second or third postoperative day.

The emergence of infiltrates may take place within the deep stroma with intact overlying epithelium. Acute infiltrates are probably of bacterial origin. In such patients, the epithelium over the incision site is opened, and samples are obtained from the side walls of the incision groove for the preparation of inoculation test cultures and smear stains. Samples are inoculated onto culture media of blood and chocolate agar for aerobic organisms, thioglycolate broth for anaerobic organisms, and Sabouraud's dextrose agar for fungi. Smears include Gram's stain and Giemsa stain.

Intensive, broad-spectrum antibiotic therapy is instituted. An appropriately aggressive protocol may include fortified cefazolin (50mg/ml), fortified tobramycin (14mg/ml), and fourth-generation fluoroquinolone-gatifloxacin on an hourly basis, with rotation every 20 minutes, while culture results are awaited. A combination of 0.4ml cefazolin (250mg/ml) and 0.4ml tobramycin (40mg/ml) mixed with 0.1ml lidocaine 2% may be administered further as a subconjunctival injection to the affected quadrant on a daily basis until culture results are available. Any epithelium that overlies the incisional groove is débrided gently for the first few days to enable high concentrations of antibiotic penetration into the deep stroma. In cases not responsive to antibacterial therapy, the possibility of a fungus or other atypical microorganism as an infective agent must be considered. Corticosteroids must not be used in the treatment of deep stromal keratitis. The scar eventually fades in most cases.

Complications Associated with Adjunctive Therapy

Radial keratotomy complications associated with adjunctive therapy include drug toxicity from the antimicrobial or the top-

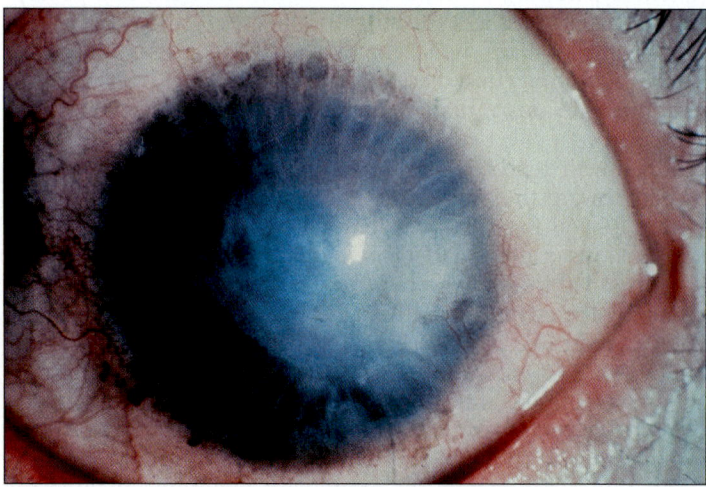

FIG. 17-15 ■ **Fibrovascular tracks.** The postoperative development of fibrovascular tracks within incision grooves is most often associated with chronic irritation or hypoxia.

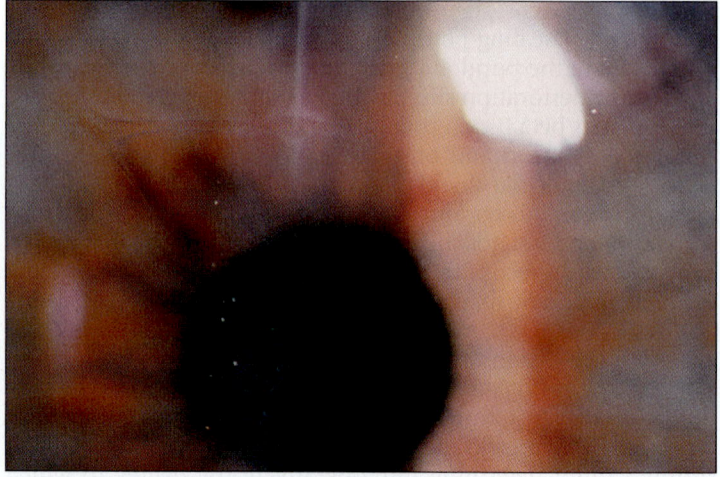

FIG. 17-16 ■ **Chronic stromal melting.** Serious complications as a result of chronic stromal melting may occur in the setting of crossed incisions.

ical corticosteroid medications. Infectious keratitis may develop with subsequent contact lens wear or chronic corticosteroid therapy. Corticosteroids also may be associated with cataracts, elevated intraocular pressure, or even infectious crystalline keratopathy. However, it is important to reiterate that radial keratotomy does not require prolonged topical corticosteroid therapy.

The ophthalmic surgeon also must consider that a certain number of patients who undergo radial keratotomy subsequently develop cataracts at some point in their lives. Conventional keratometry does not work in the intraocular lens calculation for these patients.[27,28] In such cases, the resultant change in refraction is measured and subtracted from the pre–radial keratotomy K value; this new value is assigned as the keratometry value for the lens calculation, and the post–radial keratotomy K values are ignored. Also, it may help to record the computerized videokeratography of the average corneal curvature of the 3mm central zone. If the surgeon obtains multiple K values by different methods in the same patient, the flattest K value should be used for intraocular lens calculation.

REFERENCES

1. Snellen H. Die Richtung der Hauptmeridiane des astigmatischen Auges. Graefes Arch Ophthalmol. 1869;15:199–207.
2. Schiotz HA. Ein Fall von hochgradigem Hornhautastigmatismus nach Staarextraction. Besserung auf operativem Wege. Arch Augenheille. 1885;15:178–81.
3. Bates WH. A suggestion of an operation to correct astigmatism. Arch Ophthalmol. 1894;23:9–13.
4. Lans LJ. Experimentelle Untersuch ungen uber Entstehung von Astigmatismus durch nicht-perforirende Corneawunden. Graefes Arch Ophthalmol. 1898;45:117–52.
5. Sato T. Treatment of conical cornea (incision of Descemet's membrane) [Japanese]. Nippon Ganka Gakkai Zasshi. 1939;43:544–55.
6. Sato T, Akiyama K, Shibata H. A new surgical approach to myopia. Am J Ophthalmol. 1953;36:823–9.
7. Beliaev VS, Ilyina TS. Scleroplasty in the treatment of progressive myopia. Vestn Oftalmol. 1972;3:60–3.
8. Durnev VV. Decrease of corneal refraction by anterior keratotomy method with the purpose of surgical correction of myopia of mild and moderate degree. In: Proceedings of the First Congress of Ophthalmologists of Transcaucasia. Tbilisi: The Congress; 1976:129–32.
9. Durnev VV, Ermoshin AS. Determination of dependence between length of anterior radial nonperforating incisions of cornea and their effectiveness. In: Transactions of the Fifth All-Union Conference of Inventors and Rationalizers in the Ophthalmology Field. Moscow: 976:106–8.
10. Fyodorov SN, Durnev VV. Anterior keratotomy method application with the purpose of surgical correction of myopia. In: Pressing problems of ophthalmosurgery. Moscow: 1977:47–8.
11. Waring GO III, Moffitt SD, Gelender H, et al. Rationale for and design of the National Eye Institute Prospective Evaluation of Radial Keratotomy (PERK) study. Ophthalmology. 1983;90:40–58.
12. Waring GO III, Lynn MJ, Nizam A, et al. Results of the Prospective Evaluation of Radial Keratotomy (PERK) study five years after surgery. Ophthalmology. 1991;98:1164–76.
13. Rowsey JJ, Balyeat HD, Rabinovitch B, et al. Predicting the results of radial keratotomy. Ophthalmology. 1983;90:642–54.
14. Salz JJ, Villasenor RA, Elander R, et al. Four-incision radial keratotomy for low to moderate myopia. Ophthalmology. 1986;93:727–38.
15. Buzard KA. Deepening of incisions after radial keratotomy using the "tickle" technique. Refract Corneal Surg. 1991;7:348–55.
16. Franks S. Radial keratotomy undercorrections: a new approach. J Refract Surg. 1986;2:171–3.
17. Deitz MR, Sanders DR, Marks RG. Radial keratotomy: an overview of the Kansas City study. Ophthalmology. 1984;91:467–78.
18. Merlin U, Bordin P, Rimondi AP, Sichirolo R. Factors that affect keratotomy depth. Refract Corneal Surg. 1991;7:356–9.
19. Assil KK, Schanzlin DJ, eds. Assistive technology for performing radial keratotomy. In: Radial and astigmatic keratotomy: a complete handbook for the successful practice of incisional keratotomy using the combined technique. Thorofare: Slack; 1994:23–34.
20. Melles GRJ, Binders PS. Effect of radial keratotomy incision direction on wound depth. Refract Corneal Surg. 1990;6:394–403.
21. Berkeley RG, Sanders DR, Piccolo MG. Effect of incision direction on radial keratotomy outcome. J Cataract Refract Surg. 1991;17:819–23.
22. Assil KK, Schanzlin DJ, eds. Radial keratotomy surgical technique and protocol. In: Radial and astigmatic keratotomy: a complete handbook for the successful practice of incisional keratotomy using the combined technique. Thorofare: Slack; 1994:87–110.
23. Assil KK, Kassoff J, Schanzlin DJ, Quantock AJ. A combined incision technique of radial keratotomy: a comparison to centripetal and centrifugal incision techniques in human donor eyes. Ophthalmology. 1994;101:746–54.
24. Assil KK. Genesis technique of radial keratotomy: initial clinical experience. Presented at the American Society of Cataract and Refractive Surgery Summer Symposium on Refractive Surgery, August 1993, Los Angeles.
25. Verity SM, Talamo JH, Chayet A, et al. The combined (genesis) technique of radial keratotomy: a prospective, multi-center study. Ophthalmology. 1995;102:1908–17.
26. Pande M, Hillman JS. Optical zone centration in keratorefractive surgery: entrance pupil center, visual axis, coaxially sighted corneal reflex, or geometric corneal center? Ophthalmology. 1993;100:1230–7.
27. Gimbel H, Sun R, Kaye GB. Refractive error in cataract surgery after previous refractive surgery. J Cataract Refract Surg. 2000;26(1):142–4.
28. Seitz B, Langenbucher A. Intraocular lens power calculation in eyes after corneal refractive surgery. J Refract Surg. 2000;16(3):349–61.

CHAPTER

18

Excimer Laser Photorefractive Keratectomy (PRK)

WILLIAM J. LAHNERS • DAVID R. HARDTEN

DEFINITION

- Photorefractive keratectomy (PRK) is a procedure in which the cornea is reshaped using an excimer laser. The procedure is designed to reduce the patient's dependence on glasses or contact lenses. The excimer laser has revolutionized the field of refractive surgery.

INTRODUCTION

The surgical treatment of myopia has made great strides over the last 15 years with the introduction and advancement of the excimer laser. The surgical treatment of astigmatism and hyperopia is also possible with the excimer laser. Its development has changed the face of refractive surgery more than any other technology in the history of ophthalmic surgery.

Ultraviolet radiation at the 193nm wavelength can remove precise amounts of tissue from the anterior cornea. This precision overcomes in a large part one weakness of incisional refractive keratotomy: a lack of predictability. Use of the excimer laser at 193nm for the treatment of low, moderate, and high myopia has now been well established.[1–6] The excimer laser can also be used to remove superficial anterior corneal scars[7–9] and to make hyperopic and astigmatic corrections.[10] Despite its promise in reshaping the cornea, the excimer laser is still unable to produce the perfect results that many expect with robotic laser surgery, and fortunately for the surgeon, there is still some surgical art required.[11,12]

More than 120 million Americans are currently dependent on glasses or contact lenses and may therefore be potential candidates for refractive surgical procedures, with even more potential candidates worldwide.[13] Patients with anterior corneal scars whose vision is not improved by contact lenses or glasses usually are treated with penetrating keratoplasty, and excimer laser scar removal may reduce the need for this procedure in some patients. Advances in technology that improve the safety and predictability of refractive surgical procedures consequently may benefit a large number of patients.

Excimer laser photorefractive keratectomy (PRK) appears to be most reproducible for patients with −1.5 to −8.0D of myopia.[2–6] Higher degrees of myopia can be corrected, but this may be associated with higher degrees of regression or corneal haze.[4,5] Hyperopic corrections have taken more time to develop but are now routine for low to moderate levels.[10] Low and moderate degrees of astigmatism can also be corrected with the excimer laser.[10]

HISTORY OF THE LASER

The acronym *laser* was given to this process by Schawlow and Townes[14] and stands for light amplification by stimulated emission of radiation. The first clinically useful laser, using ruby as the medium, was developed in 1960 by Maiman[15] and was used in ophthalmology as early as 1961.[16,17] In 1961, the first continuous laser was developed by Ali Javan, with semiconductor lasers appearing in 1962 and liquid dye lasers in 1966.[16,18] Over the next several years, other lasers such as gas, solid crystal, and tunable dye lasers were developed.

Excimer lasers began in 1975 at Kansas State University, when Velasco and Setser[19] noted that meta-stable rare gas atoms such as xenon (Xe) could react with halogens such as fluorine (F) to produce unstable compounds such as XeF under high pressures.[20,21] These compounds rapidly dissociated to the ground state of the individual molecules associated with the release of an energetic ultraviolet photon. These compounds could be made to undergo light amplification by stimulated emission when they were excited by an electron beam, with the argon-fluorine (ArF) molecule emitting light with a wavelength of 193nm.[22]

The word *excimer* (short for *excited dimer*) was first used to describe an energized molecule with two identical components.[23] The argon molecule does not actually form an excited dimer, and the term *rare gas halide* or *argon-fluorine* more accurately describes the medium, but the term *excimer* has persisted.

Taboada *et al.*[24,25] noted that the ArF laser could produce opacification of the cornea and fluorescein staining with indentation at energy levels greater than 27.5mJ/cm². Trokel *et al.*[26] were able to demonstrate that the 193nm laser could remove tissue very precisely in bovine cornea. About 0.25μm of corneal tissue was removed with each pulse of the ArF laser, with minimal damage to surrounding tissues.[27] The ablation thresholds, ablation rates, and healing patterns for different excimer wavelengths were described by Krueger and Trokel.[28–30] The ablation threshold for the cornea is the fluence at which tissue removal begins, which is approximately 50mJ/cm² for 193nm. Below this fluence level, the cornea experiences only photochemical changes.

Munnerlyn[30a] described that when using PRK to change corneal curvature at a small optical zone, less tissue removal was needed to create the same change in curvature as when using a larger zone. The relationship can be simplified to:

Depth of ablation (μm) =

$$[\text{diameter of optical zone (mm)}]^2 \times \tfrac{1}{3} \text{ power (D)}$$

For example, with a 6mm optical zone, 4D of myopia is corrected with a 48μm ablation depth. Early results showed clear corneas and good predictability of refractive effect in primate eyes. Blind human eyes were treated next, with promising clarity of the cornea and ability to change refraction.

Steepening of the cornea with the excimer laser to correct hyperopia was first introduced by L'Esperance *et al.*[31] A larger ablation zone than that used in myopic PRK was needed to correct hyperopia. The optical zone is a relatively small portion of the ablated area, centered within a furrow created in the midperipheral region of the cornea. The treatment of hyperopia has lagged behind that of myopia because of the greater difficulty of steepening the cornea than flattening it, as required for myopic correction.

FUNDAMENTALS OF LASER MECHANICS

The electromagnetic spectrum is composed of a broad range of wavelengths, from long radio waves to short gamma waves. In this chapter, we are interested in the optical wavelengths in the invisible ultraviolet range, 100–300nm. Each wavelength of the electromagnetic spectrum interacts with the cornea in a specific way. The cornea absorbs ultraviolet and infrared radiation, yet transmits radiation between 300 and 1300nm. Numerous wavelengths in the range of absorption by the cornea have been tested for PRK, including 193, 248, 3900, and 10,000nm. This chapter deals mainly with the 193nm ArF excimer laser, which is the most commonly used laser for corneal refractive surgery.

A collection of atoms, molecules, or ions with unique properties that can emit radiation in the optical part of the electromagnetic spectrum makes up the medium, which can be a gas, liquid, or solid. Commonly used gas media are krypton, carbon dioxide, and ArF, as used in the excimer laser. Most of the chamber is filled with an inert buffer gas such as helium or neon, which fills 88–99% of the cavity to mediate the transfer of energy. The argon constitutes 0.5–12% of the mixture, and the halogen gas such as fluorine constitutes only 0.5–1%.

In any laser, a source of energy must be present that can cause the atoms to undergo a transition from the ground state to the higher energy level (Fig. 18-1). In the excimer laser, electricity is used as the source of energy. The emitted light beam is reflected between two mirrors in the optical resonator. Other atoms are stimulated to a higher energy level by the light, and the light is amplified by reflecting back and forth in the resonator. This creates a much more powerful laser light.

The individual atoms must be stimulated to emit in phase instead of being allowed to emit randomly. This allows the atoms to gain benefits from constructive interference. The radiation that occurs has the same frequency, wavelength, and phase as the stimulating photon or wave.

INTERACTION OF CORNEAL TISSUE AND EXCIMER LASER ENERGY

A unique combination of properties makes excimer lasers appropriate for corneal surgery using 193nm wavelength light. Excimer lasers operate through a process known as ablative pho-

todecomposition. Most organic materials, including the cornea, have a very strong absorbance for ultraviolet radiation below 300nm. The higher the absorption of light of a given wavelength, the easier it is for that wavelength to destroy tissue (Fig. 18-2). The ultraviolet photons can directly break chemical bonds because of their high energy. Protein molecules are broken into fragments comprising two or three atoms by ultraviolet radiance. Much of the surplus energy within the system is blown clear of the illuminated area, which minimizes thermal damage to surrounding tissue (Fig. 18-3).

The macromolecules of the cornea, such as the proteins, nucleic acids, and proteoglycans, absorb the most energy when treated with light in the far ultraviolet region, with wavelengths less than 300nm. The water of the cornea absorbs light energy in both the middle infrared region near 3000–6000nm and the far infrared region above 10,000nm (Figs. 18-4 and 18-5).

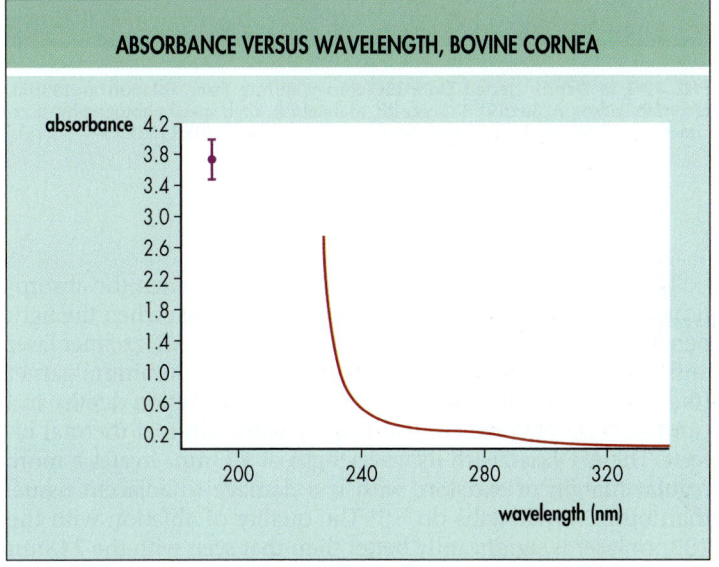

ABSORBANCE VERSUS WAVELENGTH, BOVINE CORNEA

FIG. 18-2 ■ **Absorbance versus wavelength for bovine cornea in the far ultraviolet spectrum.** The error bar indicates one standard deviation for measurement performed at 193nm. (From Puliafito CA, Steinert RF, Deutsch TF, *et al.* Excimer laser ablation of the cornea and lens. Experimental studies. Ophthalmology. 1985;92:741–8.)

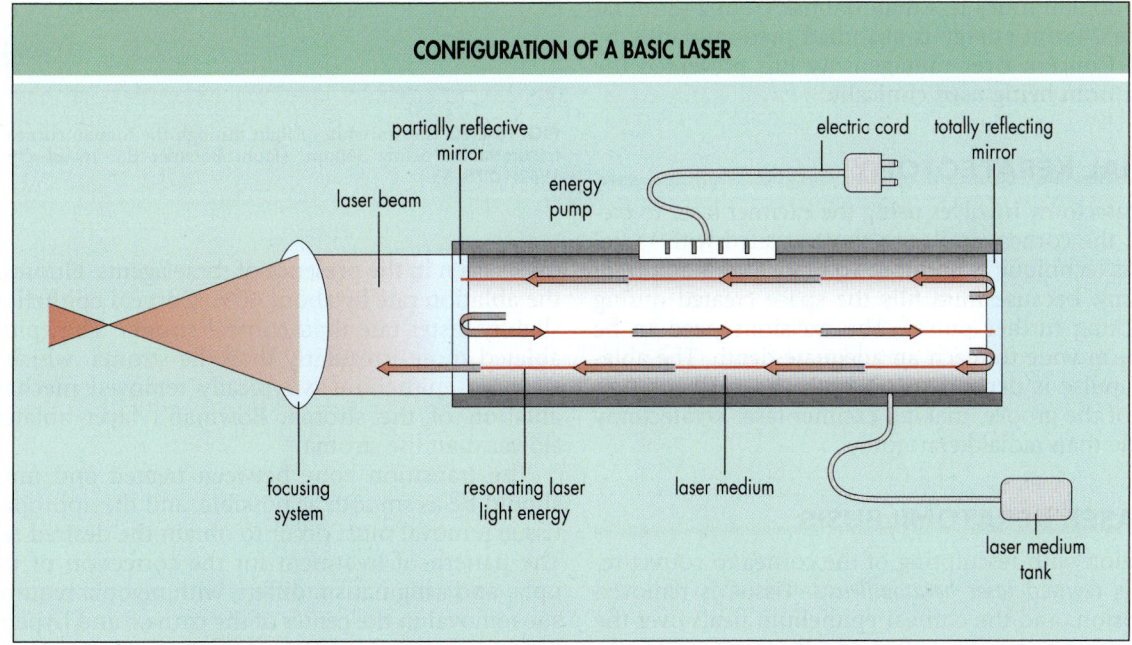

CONFIGURATION OF A BASIC LASER

FIG. 18-1 ■ **Schematic configuration of a basic laser.** Active laser medium is pumped into the laser cavity from a storage tank. Energy is then discharged into the cavity to stimulate the medium into higher-energy states. As the atoms decay to the lower-energy state, photons are discharged. These then resonate back and forth in the laser cavity and are reflected off the mirrors at the ends of the cavity. This allows amplification of the beam before it is allowed to exit from the partially reflective mirror. The beam is then shaped by various lenses for delivery to the corneal surface.

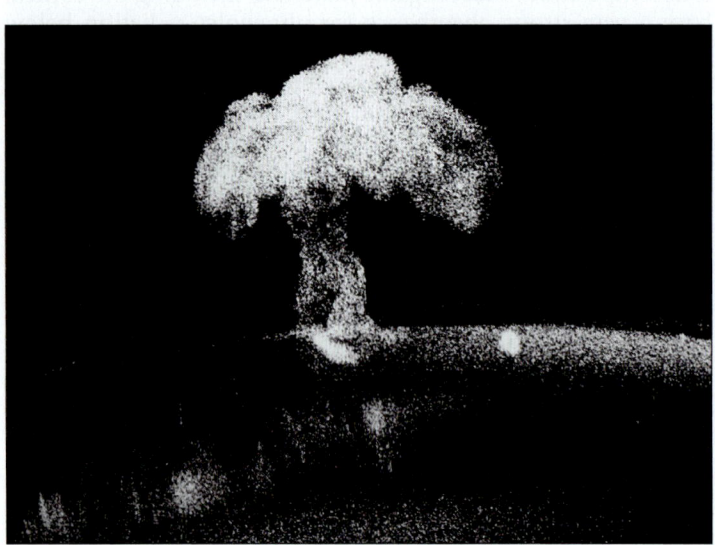

FIG. 18-3 ■ Debris ejected from the cornea during laser ablation at 193nm. (From Puliafito CA, Stern D, Krueger RR, Mandel ER. High speed photography of excimer laser ablation of the cornea. Arch Ophthalmol. 1987;105:1255–9.)

ABSORPTION SPECTRA FOR VARIOUS MOLECULES IN THE CORNEA

FIG. 18-4 ■ **Absorption spectrum for various molecules in the cornea.** The *x*-axis delineates wavelength. The *y*-axis indicates the relative absorption. The vertical dotted line represents the 193nm wavelength corresponding to the ArF excimer laser. At this point, there is a relatively high absorption for both collagen and keratan sulfate. (Adapted with permission from Brightbill FS. Corneal surgery: theory, technique, and tissue, 2nd ed. St. Louis: Mosby; 1993.)

The penetration depth of laser light is lower when the absorption of the light is higher. Thermal damage is least when the light penetrates minimally with total absorption. The ArF excimer laser and the fifth harmonic neodymium:yttrium-aluminum-garnet (Nd:YAG) ultraviolet laser have very small penetration depths and can therefore perform corneal surgery with minimal thermal effects. The ArF laser, with its wavelength of 193nm, creates a more regular margin of excision, with less damage to adjacent tissue, than other wavelengths do.[32-34] The quality of ablation with the 193nm laser is significantly better than that seen with the 248nm wavelength of the krypton-fluorine laser.[32,35]

Ultraviolet light with a wavelength of 193nm appears to have little if any mutagenic effect on corneal tissue.[36] The reaction of corneal tissue to ultraviolet light, as well as the effect of ultraviolet light on other tissue, may still have some potential for mutagenesis, however.[34-41] The risk of mutagenesis from 193nm light is 1000 to 10,000 times less than the risk from 248nm radiation, because 248nm energy is absorbed predominantly by nucleic acids.[39] Concern over mutagenicity has prevented the 248nm excimer from being used clinically.

LASER RADIAL KERATECTOMY

Laser radial keratectomy involves using the excimer laser to create incisions in the cornea similar to those created with radial keratotomy. This technique is no more accurate than traditional radial keratotomy, because fluid fills the space created during treatment, blocking further pulses. The excisions need to be greater than 30μm wide to reach an adequate depth. The ablation depth per pulse is dependent on both corneal hydration and the width of the groove, making excimer laser keratectomy less reproducible than radial keratotomy.

EXCIMER LASER KERATOMILEUSIS

Large-area ablation with resculpting of the cornea to correct refractive errors is termed *laser keratomileusis*. Tissue is removed with great precision, and the corneal epithelium heals over the ablated area to create a smooth surface. Ideally, this occurs without hyperplasia or a significant wound healing response.

Medications such as cocaine, oxybuprocaine, proxymetacaine, and pilocarpine do not appear to change the ablation rates of tissue. About 0.25μm of tissue is removed with each

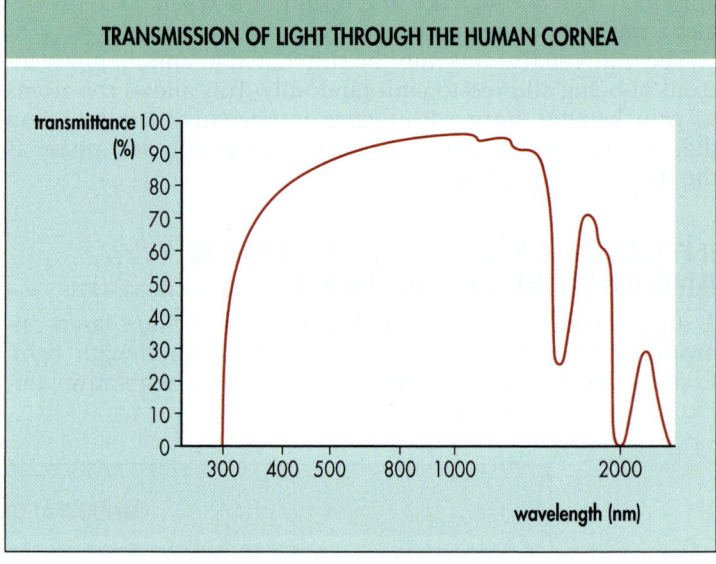

TRANSMISSION OF LIGHT THROUGH THE HUMAN CORNEA

FIG. 18-5 ■ **Transmission of light through the human cornea.** There is minimal transmittance below 300nm. (From Boettner EA. Invest Ophthalmol Vis Sci. 1962;1:776–83.)

pulse, even in the presence of these agents. Fluorescein decreases the ablation rate by about 40%. Corneal epithelium ablates at a slightly faster rate than corneal stroma. The epithelium is also ablated more irregularly than the stroma, which is the reason why the epithelium is typically removed mechanically before ablation of the stroma. Bowman's layer ablates about 30% slower than the stroma.

The transition zone between treated and untreated cornea should be as smooth as possible, and the appropriate pattern of tissue removal must occur to obtain the desired refractive effect. The pattern of treatment for the correction of myopia, hyperopia, and astigmatism differs, with myopia requiring greater tissue removal in the center of the cornea, and hyperopia requiring tissue removal from the periphery.[42] Moving slits, constricting and expanding diaphragms, ablatable masks, and computer-controlled application of the laser have been developed to create the appropriate ablation profiles.[43] Lenses can also be used to shape the beam to the desired configuration (Fig. 18-6).

MASKING TECHNIQUES

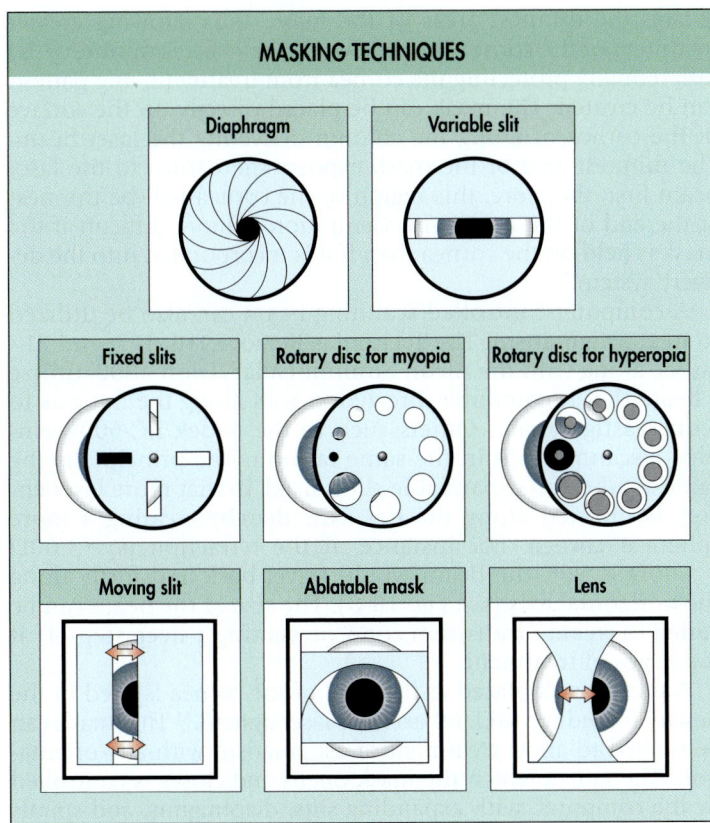

FIG. 18-6 ■ A variety of masking techniques can be used to control the delivery of laser energy to the eye.

DEPTH OF TISSUE REMOVAL

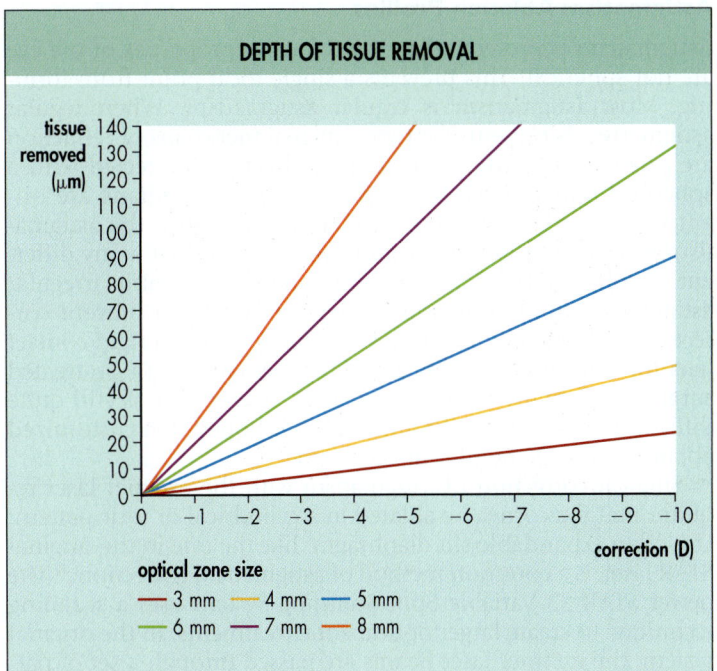

FIG. 18-7 ■ Illustration of the depth of tissue removal required to correct a myopic refractive error using various ablation zone diameters. (Munnerlyn CR, Koons SJ, Marshall J. Photorefractive keratectomy: a technique for laser refractive surgery. J Cataract Refract Surg. 1988;14:46–52.)

EXCIMER LASER SAFETY

Safety equipment for operating room staff includes safety glasses designed to block the wavelength of the 193nm excimer laser. The fluorine gas used in excimer lasers is extremely toxic in high concentrations, but at the concentrations typically used in laser surgery, it is less so. However, the operating room should have good ventilation to allow the rapid removal of fluorine gas in case of a leak. Undesirable effects of laser exposure are related to total exposure time, duration of the laser pulse, absorption by the body, and wavelength of the energy.

CURRENT INSTRUMENTATION

Several 193nm excimer lasers are commercially available for photorefractive and phototherapeutic keratectomy. Some of these lasers use a large beam diameter of 5–7mm, whereas others use a scanning technique to deliver a small spot or slit in a computer-controlled manner across the surface of the cornea. All systems include a computer control module with an interactive menu, allowing the development of an ablation protocol for each individual patient or refractive error. Proper positioning of the eye is important, so the excimer laser system should include a microscope with the ability to provide accurate alignment of the eye in all axes. Some lasers have a vacuum apparatus to remove particle debris from the ablation plume. Foot pedal and fingertip controls can be used by the surgeon to manipulate the position of the eye and ablating beam. Even though other wavelengths have been tried, the 193nm wavelength is totally absorbed by the cornea, causing the breakage of molecular bonds, making it uniquely applicable for corneal treatment[1] (see Figs. 18-2 and 18-4).

ABLATION PROFILES

In the United States, ablation profiles are regulated by the Food and Drug Administration and are restricted to those profiles used in studies leading to the approval of each instrument. As mentioned earlier, there are a variety of masking techniques to control the positioning of laser pulses. For instance, the VISX/STAR laser has an expanding diaphragm that the scanning beams are passed through, allowing a larger amount of ablation in the central cornea than in the periphery for the treatment of myopia.[8] For hyperopic ablations, the center is left untreated and the energy is preferentially directed to the midperipheral zones through a scanning system. For astigmatism, expanding slits are used for small zone treatments, and a scanning system is used for larger astigmatic treatments, both of which allow greater treatment along one meridian than another, creating a toric cut.

Other systems use an expanding ring, ablatable mask, rotating mask, or scanning spot of laser energy that preferentially directs energy to the center for myopia and the midperiphery for hyperopia[10] (see Fig. 18-6). Some authors now believe that for higher degrees of myopia, multiple treatment zones may be better.[44,45] These multizone recipes give a portion of the treatment using large zones of 6–7mm and various degrees of treatment with several smaller optical zones. This creates a more tapered approach for higher degrees of myopia, reducing the depth of cornea ablated as well as regression and haze. The trade-off in multizone treatment can be visual quality, especially under scotopic conditions. Despite these modifications, high myopia is more difficult to correct than low myopia.[4,5]

Myopia Ablation Profiles

As discussed earlier, the amount of tissue that must be removed to produce a certain refractive result is dependent on the optical zone size[46] (Fig. 18-7). The depth of the ablation required to achieve a given refractive result for myopia is approximated by the equation given earlier.

Smaller optical zones are associated with greater degrees of regression, night haloes, and haze.[47] Deeper ablations are associated with greater wound healing and regression, as well as haze. The optical zone size and depth need to be optimized to avoid the excessive wound healing seen in deep ablations and the excessive haloes, edge glare, and irregular astigmatism seen with small optical zones.[48] Larger zones have been shown to be beneficial at reducing scotopic visual complaints.

Astigmatism Ablation Profiles

Astigmatism is present when the refractive properties of the eye are not spherical. This prevents a single focal point from forming. Most astigmatism is regular astigmatism. When regular astigmatism is present, the two principal meridians of refraction are oriented 90° from each other and can be corrected with a spherocylindrical lens. If the two principal meridians are oriented at an angle other than 90° from each other, the astigmatism is termed bioblique or nonorthogonal. When many different meridians of refraction are present, the eye exhibits irregular astigmatism. Bioblique and irregular astigmatism prevent correction with a spherocylindrical lens and require a rigid contact lens for optical correction. Regular astigmatism can be treated surgically by many methods. Irregular astigmatism is still quite difficult to treat surgically, although it is hoped that customized ablations may be helpful in the future.

Surgical correction of astigmatism with the excimer laser requires that the cornea be ablated in a cylindrical or toric pattern. Use of an expandable slit diaphragm, like the one in the original STAR laser, is a common method of astigmatism correction.[49] The newer STAR S3 Variable Spot Scanning System uses a scanning technique to create larger optical zone treatments. In the original system, the excimer laser beams are passed through a set of parallel blades that gradually open as directed by the computer algorithm. The speed of opening depends on the amount of astigmatism to be corrected. The orientation of the blades depends on the orientation of the astigmatism. Deeper ablations occur in the center along the axis of the blades, with gradual transition to shallower ablations at the sides of the slit. Flattening occurs perpendicular to the long axis of the slits. No change in power occurs along the axis of the slits. Thus, for correction of astigmatism in a patient with the refractive error $-3.00D +3.00D \times 90°$, the slits would be oriented horizontally, thus flattening the vertical meridian (Fig. 18-8).

The spherical equivalent is shifted toward the hyperopic side in excimer laser treatment of astigmatism because tissue is removed, causing flattening of the cornea.[50] VISX adds a transition zone to the edge of the long axis to prevent an abrupt change in elevation at the end of the slits.

If the slits and the circular diaphragm open at the same time, an elliptical ablation occurs, correcting compound myopic astigmatism. The rate at which they open can be controlled independently and reflects the amount of myopia and the amount of astigmatism to be corrected. This ablation pattern corrects only regular astigmatism; it is not capable of correcting irregular astigmatism.

Another method of creating a toric ablation utilizes an ablatable mask, such as the system used by Summit. The laser first ablates the thinnest areas of the mask, thus allowing greater treatment of the cornea in areas where the mask is thinnest.[51] By differentially protecting the cornea from treatment, any pattern can be created. The mask can be placed directly on the surface of the cornea or along the column delivering the laser beam. The thinnest area of the mask exposes the cornea to the laser beam first; therefore, this region of the cornea will be thinnest at the end of the treatment. Centration is more difficult if the mask is held on the cornea than if it is incorporated into the delivery system.[52]

A computer-controlled scanning beam can also be utilized to treat astigmatism. The Technolas Keracor 116, 117, and 217 lasers, along with the Alcon-Summit LadarVision 4000, utilize a beam that is computer directed to scan along the flat axis to reduce astigmatism. Others such as the Nidek EC-5000 employ a scanning slit in the same fashion. The principle is the same as when an expandable slit is used, in that more laser energy is directed along the flat axis, thereby creating a more spherical cornea. For instance, if the refraction is $-3.00D +3.00D \times 90°$, the beam would travel back and forth along the horizontal axis (see Fig. 18-8). The size of the beam can be varied to create a transition zone, preventing a steep step-off at the edges of treatment.

A metal mask placed at the level of the cornea is used in the Aesculap-Meditec MEL 60 excimer laser system.[53] This mask can be rotated to allow treatment of astigmatism with any orientation. The rate at which the mask opens and closes is controlled by the computer, with expanding slits, diaphragms, and spirals allowing concurrent treatment of both myopia and astigmatism or hyperopia and astigmatism.

Hyperopia Ablation Profiles

These ablations use a variety of masking techniques to allow more laser pulses in the midperiphery, with blend zones toward the center and far periphery of the cornea. In some older systems, the beam was passed through multiple diaphragms, allowing a larger amount of ablation in the peripheral cornea than in the center.[8] Other broad-beam systems use an expanding ring, ablatable mask, or rotating mask. Smaller beam systems, such as scanning slit and spot systems, are directed preferentially to the midperiphery by complex computer programs. The amount of tissue that must be removed to produce a certain refractive result is dependent on the optical zone size.[46]

TRACKING SYSTEMS

Patient fixation is critical to the proper placement of laser ablation in all laser systems. As the technology has expanded, allowing the treatment of hyperopic astigmatism and the design of custom corneal treatments for higher-order ablations, the accuracy of laser placement has become more critical. This is especially true in lasers utilizing small scanning spot systems. All patients show evidence of saccadic movement, including small refixation movements, during periods of fixation. Patients also vary in their ability to cooperate with fixation.

Several laser manufacturers offer laser tracking systems to increase the accuracy of shot placement. Tracking systems may improve the quality of ablations and the accuracy of centration and provide greater smoothness.[54,55] Tracking systems vary in sampling frequency from 60Hz for camera-based systems such as in the VISX Active-Trak system to 4000Hz for the laser-radar system in the LadarVision 4000. The active tracking systems can be very useful in treating patients with head tremors, tics, and nystagmus.[56] Tracking is an excellent adjunct to laser vision correction, but it is no substitute for proper and attentive patient fixation. Tracking systems will undoubtedly assume greater importance as attempts are made at mapping the treatment of higher-order aberrations.

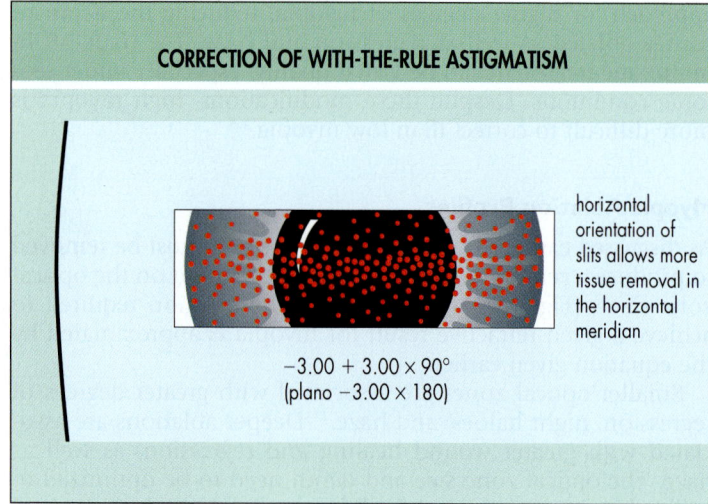

CORRECTION OF WITH-THE-RULE ASTIGMATISM

horizontal orientation of slits allows more tissue removal in the horizontal meridian

$-3.00 + 3.00 \times 90°$
(plano -3.00×180)

FIG. 18-8 ■ For correction of with-the-rule astigmatism, the slits are oriented horizontally, allowing flattening of the vertical meridian.

SURGICAL TREATMENT

Examination and Counseling

The risks and benefits for each individual patient should be assessed, as with all refractive surgical procedures. Visual acuity should be measured with a careful manifest and cycloplegic refraction, ocular dominance testing, and distance and near vision with and without correction. Anterior segment and posterior segment examinations should be performed to rule out other conditions that might adversely affect the surgical result. Pachymetry measurements are performed to make certain that the cornea is of normal thickness. Computerized topographical analysis can help screen for subclinical keratoconus or other corneal diseases.

Relative contraindications to laser treatment include advanced diabetes, collagen vascular disease, previous herpes (simplex or zoster) infection, severe dry eye, untreated blepharitis, neurotrophic cornea, peripheral ulcerative keratitis of any cause, and patients on the following medications: isotretinoin (Accutane), amiodarone (Cordarone), or sumatriptan (Imitrex).

The most important aspect of treating presbyopic patients is preoperative counseling. The patient's goals for increased spectacle independence must be fully understood. For example, a 20-year-old patient who has a result of plano in each eye with 20/20 uncorrected distance acuity will function well for all tasks, including near vision. A 50-year-old patient with the same results can have good distance function but will become significantly more dependent on correction for near vision. A careful understanding of the patient's goals and vocational demands will help prevent disappointment postoperatively. Target refraction should be carefully discussed with every patient, but this is critical in presbyopes.

Monovision should be carefully discussed with all presbyopes. Monovision success rates vary from 33–50%, so a trial in contact lenses is usually appropriate before laser vision correction. Generally, a 39-year-old pre-presbyope will not tolerate 3D of anisometropia to allow monovision. Even a 49-year-old presbyope will have difficulty accepting this condition. In general, a 40-year-old will tolerate −0.75 to −1.00D of anisometropia, a 50-year-old will tolerate monovision of −1.25 to −1.50D, and a 60-year-old will tolerate −1.50 to −1.75D of residual myopia in the nondominant eye. When attempting levels of anisometropia greater than this, it is mandatory to try the correction in contact lenses first to make certain that the patient is truly tolerant of this degree of anisometropia. Some patients may be at a level of myopia such that treating only the dominant eye and leaving the nondominant eye myopic would be appropriate.

Technique

There are many variations in the technique for excimer PRK. This section describes a typical technique, but it is important for each surgeon to keep his or her technique as consistent as possible and to monitor the results. Attention to consistency in technique as well as to ambient conditions such as temperature and humidity can have a profound effect on refractive results. The development of a personalized nomogram to allow for variations in individual technique, laser variations, and differences in altitude or climate is recommended. The cornea's state of hydration when treatment occurs plays a large role in the refractive result after excimer laser vision correction, including PRK and laser in situ keratomileusis (LASIK).

For PRK, the spectacle correction is adjusted to the corneal plane to take into account vertex distance. On some older systems, this must be done by looking at a chart or table; in newer systems, the computer software performs the calculation. If astigmatism is to be treated, the minus cylinder format is helpful, but in many systems, positive cylinder can be used if this is more convenient.

Preoperatively, the patient should receive anesthetic drops. It is important to perform the treatment as soon as possible after the drops are instilled to prevent exposure keratitis from poor blinking, which will dry and thin the cornea. This can lead to overcorrection or an asymmetrical ablation. Drying of the inferior half of the cornea, as often occurs after anesthetic drops have been instilled, can lead to increased thinning inferiorly (Figs. 18-9 and 18-10).

The patient is positioned under the microscope, carefully aligning the head to make sure that the iris plane is perpendicular to the laser beam. The eyelids are prepared with dilute povidone-iodine (Betadine) solution. The conjunctival fornices can be prepared with Betadine drop preparations or broad-spectrum antibiotic drops. A lid speculum is inserted to open the eyelids. Careful centration with the eye aligned in the x, y, and z planes is crucial. Centration on the pupil is preferred by some but continues to be an area of controversy.[57,58]

The epithelium is marked with a 7 or 8mm optical zone marker for myopia or a 9 or 10mm marker for hyperopia, again centering on the pupil. The epithelium is bluntly removed with a Tooke knife (Storz Ophthalmics, St. Louis, MO), a #64 or #69 Bard-Parker blade (Bard-Parker, Franklin Lakes, NJ), Visitec disposable excimer spatula (Visitec Company, Sarasota, FL), or rotating brush (Amoils Epithelial Scrubber; Innova, Inc., Toronto, Canada). Alcohol can also be used to loosen the epithelium. It is typically used as a 20% concentration of ethanol and is ap-

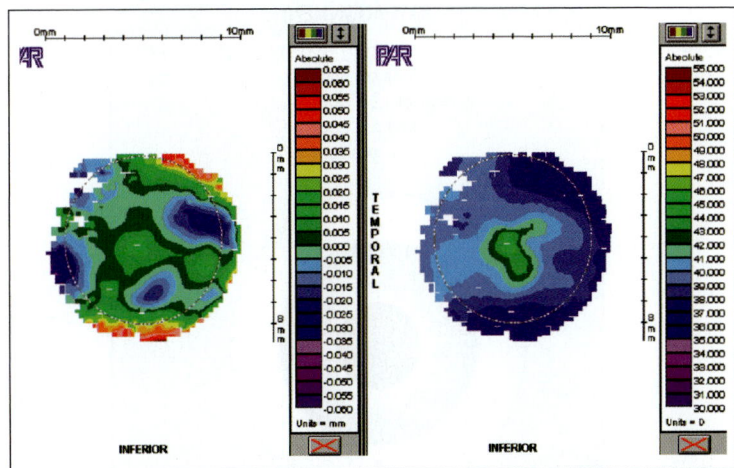

FIG. 18-9 ■ This patient has a poor blink reflex and, after the administration of anesthetic drops, has thinning of the inferior cornea. This can lead to greater tissue removal inferiorly and an asymmetrical ablation. Care must be taken to ensure even hydration.

FIG. 18-10 ■ Elevation topography of a patient with a poor blink reflex after the administration of anesthetic drops. Relative depression of the cornea can be seen inferiorly with irregular astigmatism.

plied for 20–30 seconds. The area of epithelial removal depends on the total ablation diameter, which is greater for the treatment of hyperopia. It is important to remove the epithelium totally, so that only Bowman's membrane remains. Any residual epithelium will create an uneven ablation and irregular astigmatism.

It is also possible to remove the epithelium with the excimer laser. The laser should be set to a depth of approximately 50μm, with the beam set to its widest aperture. The excimer laser is centered, and the ablation is begun. The microscope light is dimmed so that an area of fluorescence is seen where the epithelium is being ablated by the laser beam. The ablation is stopped when a change from a fluorescent pattern to a dark pattern is seen, indicating that the epithelium has been ablated. The epithelium may be more or less than 50μm deep. If there is still fluorescence across the whole area after a 50μm ablation has been performed, an additional depth of 25μm should be set for the laser, stopping the treatment when all the epithelium has been removed. It is often difficult to tell exactly when all the epithelium has been removed by visual clues alone.

When the epithelium is more adherent, such as in eyes that have had previous laser treatment, it may be helpful to use both the laser and scraping to remove the epithelium. This is also useful when it is difficult to see the change from a fluorescent to a dark pattern. This transition is more difficult to see on lasers operating at slower pulse rates. The laser is used first to remove 40μm of the epithelium with the largest optical zone. A blade or excimer spatula can then be used to bluntly remove the remaining debris, which essentially consists of the bottom half of the basal epithelial cell layer. This laser-scrape method is preferred by some in retreatments, but it may also be useful in primary cases of PRK. Each surgeon should use the method of epithelial removal that provides the most consistent hydration of the cornea.

Centration is rechecked after epithelial removal. The ablation should promptly follow epithelial removal to prevent drying, which can lead to increased haze and scarring.[59,60] Regardless of the epithelial removal technique used, it is important to make certain that the hydration status of the corneal stroma is uniform during the procedure. This can be assured by wiping a cellulose sponge wetted with artificial tears or balanced salt solution across Bowman's membrane. The amount of fluid added or removed also depends on the laser being used; greater hydration is typically used in lasers that have a vacuum method to remove ablated debris, such as the VISX/STAR. Consistency in hydration is crucial for all patients, but the level of hydration inevitably varies from surgeon to surgeon.

For astigmatic corrections, alignment on the proper axis must also be accomplished. This can be done by marking the patient's limbus at the 12 and 6 o'clock positions with gentian violet dye on a Sinsky hook at the slit lamp prior to the procedure (Fig. 18-11). If the procedure is performed off axis, significant reduction of effect will occur. The STAR S3 allows the projection of a vertical helium-neon laser along the midline axis of the patient's face to ensure proper facial positioning. The LadarVision 4000 allows intraoperative adjustment to limbal markings at 3 and 9 o'clock to ensure proper axis alignment to the globe itself, thus allowing the surgeon to overcome not just facial misalignment but ocular cyclotorsion as well.

The ultraviolet excimer lasers used for PRK have wavelengths outside the visible spectrum; therefore, an auxiliary aiming device that is coaxial to the ablating laser is required to make certain the laser is centered on the eye during treatment. Helium-neon lasers, laser diodes, or a coaxial aiming target are commonly used for this (Fig. 18-12). In automated systems with eye trackers, this is used only for initial alignment, but in manually controlled systems, it is used to align the eye during the entire procedure.

The ablation is begun, centered over the pupil with the patient looking at the fixation light. Eye movements should be minimized during the ablation to reduce irregular surfaces that can lead to an inaccurate optical correction. Various methods can be utilized to achieve proper fixation and centration, including patient fixation, forceps fixation, or the use of suction rings. Forceps or compression ring fixation should be avoided to prevent globe distortion. If the patient loses fixation, it is important to stop and regain centration before completing the ablation.

The use of an eye tracker may be helpful in maintaining centration.[55,61] A number of tracking systems are available from different manufacturers. The use of a tracking system does not obviate the need for patient fixation, however. Even with proper centration over the entrance pupil, poor laser placement results from poor fixation. Some systems utilize a suction handpiece that maintains centration as well as fixation.

The maintenance of uniform hydration is very important during ablation. If excess fluid is detected, the procedure should be paused and the excess fluid removed by using a spatula to "squeegee" the cornea or a cellulose sponge to dry the cornea, taking care to ensure even hydration (Fig. 18-13). If the cornea becomes too dry during the treatment, a cellulose sponge can be used to evenly hydrate the cornea. Excessive drying should be avoided, as it can dehydrate and thin the cornea. Inadequate tis-

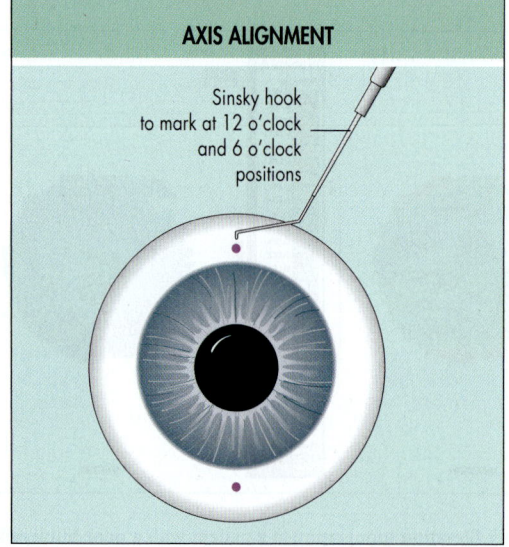

FIG. 18-11 ■ Axis alignment is crucial for accurate astigmatic ablations. A Sinsky hook can be used at the slit lamp to mark the 12 and 6 o'clock positions. If the ablation is performed off axis, significant reduction of effect will occur.

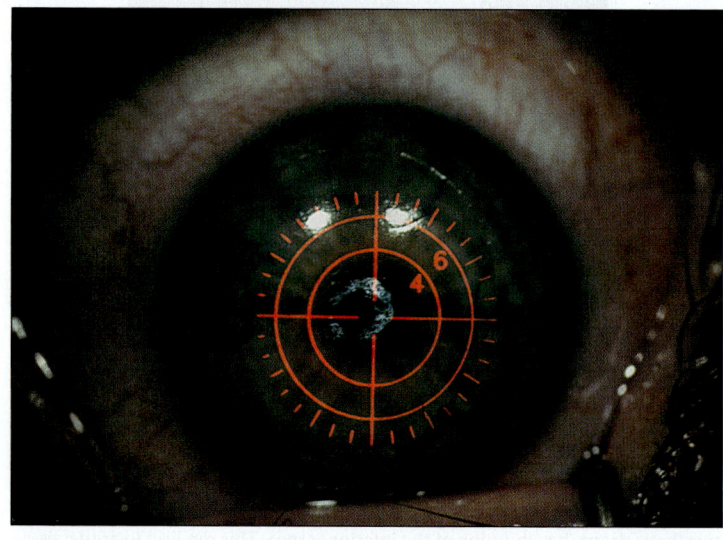

FIG. 18-12 ■ In the VISX/STAR laser system, an aiming target in the microscope system allows the surgeon to know where the laser energy is being directed.

sue hydration leads to more tissue ablated per pulse, resulting in an overcorrection. Fluid should not be allowed to collect centrally, as this can result in central island formation. Immediately following the ablation, a drop of antibiotic, steroid, and nonsteroidal medication can be placed on the eye. A bandage soft contact lens can be inserted to reduce pain after the procedure.

Moderate and High Myopia

Some unique aspects of treatment exist for the correction of moderate and high myopia. Some authors have abandoned moderate and high myopia treatment with surface PRK in favor of LASIK (see Table 18-3).[62,63] Helmy *et al.* demonstrated better accuracy of refractive results as well as a decreased incidence of complications in patients undergoing LASIK for myopia between −6 and −10D compared with those undergoing surface PRK. Fernandez *et al.*[63] showed similarly that LASIK outperformed PRK in moderate myopia.

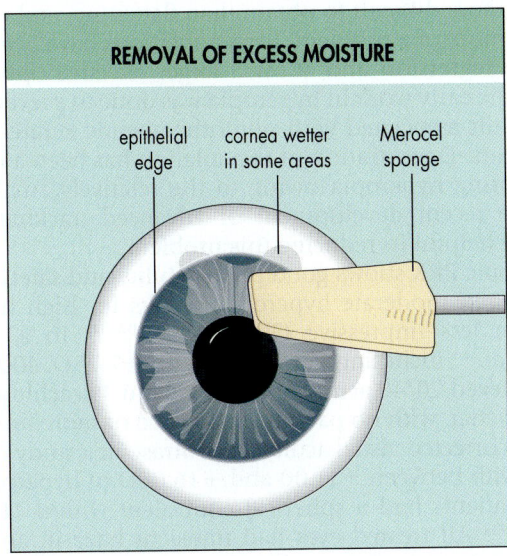

FIG. 18-13 ■ A Merocel sponge can be used to remove excess moisture in a uniform fashion. Maintaining proper central corneal hydration can improve results.

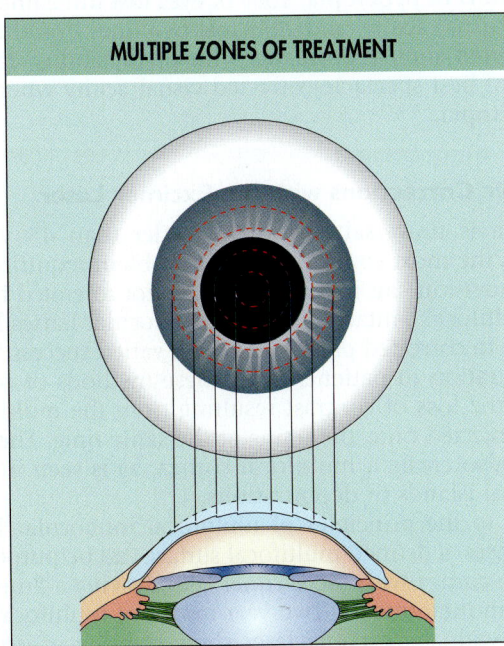

FIG. 18-14 ■ Multiple zones of treatment allow a more gradual transition of curvatures.

Others have begun to make various adjustments to the ablation profiles to correct high myopia. The multizone approach appears to have significant advantages over a monozone approach for higher degrees of myopia.[45] The multizone approach uses a combination of repetitive treatments. For example, to treat 12D of myopia, a 2D treatment at a 3mm optical zone would be used first, then 3D at a 4mm optical zone, 3D at a 5mm optical zone, and 4D at a 6mm optical zone (Fig. 18-14). In a study by Zato *et al.*,[63a] no significant difference in degree of correction or visual acuity was seen when comparing a one-zone ablation protocol to a multizone protocol. There was, however, a higher frequency of severe haze in the group treated with a single zone. Multizone treatments may increase optical aberrations. In low myopia, the incidence of haloes, hyperopic shift, and haze appears to be less with a 6mm zone alone than with a combination of 5 and 6mm zones.

POSTOPERATIVE MEDICATIONS AND FOLLOW-UP

If a bandage soft contact lens is used, it is left in place for 3–5 days until the epithelium has healed. Antibiotic, steroid, and nonsteroidal medications should be used four times a day. Nonsteroidal drops can significantly reduce the amount of postoperative pain after PRK.

As an alternative to a bandage soft contact lens, pressure patching can be used. Some studies have suggested slightly faster epithelial healing with pressure patching. Most patients, though, appreciate the ability to have binocular vision, which is not possible when patching is performed.

The antibiotic can be discontinued when the epithelium has healed. Steroid medications are used in a tapering regimen over the first 3–6 months. Typically, mild steroids are used six times a day for the first week and then four times a day for the rest of the first month; then the patient is tapered off steroids by 3 months. For some corneal scars or deeper ablations, the topical steroids may need to be continued for a longer period. If there is any increased haze, topical steroids should be reinstituted at a higher dosage to prevent scarring. The haze in hyperopic patients is less of a problem because of the midperipheral location. Patients should be monitored for steroid side effects such as intraocular hypertension. The corneal topography should be followed after these procedures.[64,65] Late-onset haze following PRK is defined as haze presenting 4–14 months postoperatively.[66] It has been linked to ultraviolet exposure, and for this reason, patients should be cautioned to always wear ultraviolet protection when outdoors for the first 2 years following PRK.

Attempts to use steroids to modify the refractive result after PRK have had mixed results.[67] After surface ablation, the patient should be slightly overcorrected at the 1-month examination. Regression can occur from proliferation of keratocytes, synthesis of extracellular matrix, and hyperplasia of the epithelium. Greater ablation depths are associated with greater haze and regression. If the patient has more than 1D of hyperopia, the steroids should be tapered rapidly. If the patient has some regression toward myopia, the steroids can be increased to try to maintain full effect.[68] Some studies suggest that steroids have minimal effect on the long-term outcome after PRK.[67] With the potential for steroid-related side effects, some believe that steroids should be used only in select patients.[69]

WOUND HEALING

With regard to wound healing after PRK, patients can be classified into three groups.[70] Most patients (85%) fall into the normal responder group, with a small amount of hyperopia at 1 month and a gradual regression toward emmetropia at 1 year. Inadequate responders account for a smaller number of patients (11%) and manifest early hyperopia with minimal regression over time. Aggressive healers are less common (4%) and display early hyperopia with aggressive regression toward myopia that is associated with significant subepithelial haze.[70]

The timing of PRK on the second eye depends on the speed of visual recovery in the first one, as well as on the patient's visual needs. The patient should have good function of the first eye before treatment of the second eye is performed.

RETREATMENT

Retreatment can reduce residual refractive error or correct irregular astigmatism caused by central islands or decentered ablations.[71] Excimer laser ablations can also be used to treat residual refractive errors after radial keratotomy.[72]

In a study by the Melbourne Excimer Laser Group,[72a] 58 eyes were retreated after myopic PRK. Eyes with higher degrees of myopia were more likely to require retreatment, as were eyes with concomitant correction of astigmatism. Corneal haze is not seen more frequently following retreatment for residual myopia than after original treatment. Results of retreatment were not as predictable as the results of primary treatment for low myopia. Sixty-nine percent of eyes were within 1.00D of emmetropia following retreatment, whereas 75% were within 1.00D of emmetropia after primary treatment by the same group. It is best to wait at least 6 months before considering retreatment with PRK.

When regression is seen with no or minimal haze, retreatment can be performed with good results.[73,74] When haze is present, retreatment is less predictable, with a higher incidence of overcorrection, regression, and haze.[75] Despite these problems, most patients experience a significant reduction in haze. LASIK is also effective in treating ametropias following PRK.[76]

RESULTS

Photorefractive Keratectomy for Myopia

The results and long-term stability of PRK for myopia and myopic astigmatism have been acceptable overall, and the results have improved as techniques, lasers, and nomograms have evolved based on the experience gained from early studies (Table 18-1).[44,45,77-111] When evaluating results, the typical factors examined are the proportion of eyes within 0.5–1.0D of emmetropia of the intended correction, the proportion of eyes with better than 20/25 or 20/40 uncorrected vision, and the proportion of eyes with loss of best-corrected visual acuity.

Looking at the results of these studies (see Table 18-1), several trends can be observed. PRK has demonstrated excellent refractive results, showing good predictability and safety. Results for low and moderate myopia are superior to results for high myopia. One early study of high myopia using the Chiron Technolas Keracor 116 laser showed that 41.5% of patients with between −0.25 and −10.00D of preoperative myopia were within 1D of emmetropia postoperatively.[90] In patients with more than −10.00D of myopia, only 13.8% were within 1D of intended correction. In another study of patients with myopia of −10.25D and higher, only 37% were within 1D of emmetropia at 1 year after treatment.

Loss of best-corrected visual acuity, a measure of safety, is typically 2–4% but rises significantly in studies treating high and very high myopia. In a study by McCarty et al.,[92] for eyes with more than −10.00D of myopia, 39% were within 1D of emmetropia at 1 year, with 2% having 20/20 or better uncorrected vision and 27% having better than 20/40 vision without correction. In this study, 22% of patients lost two or more lines of best-corrected vision. Early results at 6 months after PRK showed that 33% of patients with more than −10.00D of myopia had 20/40 or better vision without correction.[112] Thirteen percent of these eyes lost two or more lines of best-corrected acuity.

Regression of refractive error is typically seen within the first year after PRK. Few long-term studies are available to analyze long-term stability. In a study of 457 eyes treated with PRK using 4.5mm ablation zone diameters, the mean refractive error at 36 months was −0.25 ± 0.75D, which was not statistically different from the results at 24 months (−0.27 ± 0.74D).[88] Other studies, though, have suggested some regression occurring as long as 3 years after surgery. Significant regression with surface PRK is more common in higher myopes.

Typically, the treatment of astigmatism is combined with the treatment of myopic or hyperopic refractive errors. Astigmatism correction is generally more complicated than myopia or hyperopia correction because it involves both the amount and the orientation of the astigmatism. Results of treating astigmatism have been promising, especially in light of improvements in more recent results.[50,53,83,94,105] In general, results in those with low and moderate levels of astigmatism (up to 2D) have greater predictability and safety than do results in those with high astigmatism.

Photorefractive Keratectomy for Hyperopia

The treatment of hyperopia with excimer laser PRK has lagged behind that of myopia. Reproducible steepening of the cornea has been more difficult to obtain than flattening, and regression has been more of a problem. Larger ablations have been helpful to reduce regression and allow a larger effective optical zone. Much of the early work in hyperopia was done to prevent the hyperopic shift associated with phototherapeutic keratectomy for corneal scars. Decentration of the ablation has been a challenge when treating hyperopia owing to the relatively small optical zone. The recent development of advanced tracking systems should be helpful in reducing this problem.

Hyperopic PRK shows good predictability and safety in those with low and moderate hyperopia; results for high hyperopes have been less impressive (Table 18-2).[113-123] In a study by Pacella et al.[123] including hyperopia up to +7.75D, 100% of patients achieved 20/40 acuity or better and 46.4% achieved 20/20 acuity or better, with no patients losing two or more lines of best spectacle-corrected visual acuity. In contrast, in a study including patients with between +11.00 and +16.00D of hyperopia, only 37% of patients had a spherical equivalent within 1D of emmetropia.[124] All treated eyes had transient haze in an annular fashion, appearing 3–4 weeks after treatment. The haze was greater in patients with deeper ablations and increased up to 4 months after treatment. Significant loss of acuity under glare conditions was seen, especially in patients with higher degrees of treatment. In another study of patients with between +6.00 and +10.00D of hyperopia, 15% of eyes lost three lines of best-corrected visual acuity, and 22% lost two lines.[125] Other studies have reported similar problems with predictability, regression, and loss of best spectacle-corrected visual acuity when treating high hyperopia.[116,117]

Presbyopic Corrections with the Excimer Laser

Presbyopia is universal in patients older than 45 years and represents the most common optical problem requiring correction. Monovision can be used, but it is not tolerated by all patients. Multifocal contact lenses and intraocular lenses have also been used to corrected presbyopia, with varied success.[126,127] The main frustration in patients using these methods of correction has been the loss of contrast resulting from the multiple focal images projected onto the retina at the same time. The excimer laser can also create a multifocal cornea, as is seen in patients with central islands or decentrations.

Similar to the principles of multifocal intraocular lenses or contact lenses, a defined multifocal surface can be purposely created in the cornea with the excimer laser, leaving a 2mm area of steepness in the center.[127] Two-year results of multifocal corneal treatment with the excimer laser show stability of useful near acuity at the J3 level while preserving distance acuity.[128] Although these results are encouraging, a loss of contrast sensitivity and best-corrected acuity can occur. Multifocal PRK most likely

TABLE 18-1

RESULTS OF PHOTOREFRACTIVE KERATECTOMY FOR MYOPIA AND MYOPIC ASTIGMATISM

Author	Year	No. of Eyes	Follow-up (Months) [Mean]	Attempted Correction (D) [Mean]	±1D of Emmetropia (%)	≥20/40 VASC (%)	≥20/20 VASC (%)	Losing ≥2 Lines BCVA (%)
McDonald et al[77]	1991	7	12	−2 to −5	57	86		0
		10	12	−5 to −8	18	18		11
Gartry et al[78]	1991	120	8–18 (mean 12)	−1.5 to −4	50	61		NR
Seiler, Wollensak[79]	1991	26	12	−1.4 to −9.25	92	96		0
Tengroth et al[80]	1993	420	12	−1.5 to −7.5	86	91		NR
		194+	15		87	87		NR
Salz et al[81]	1993	71	12	−1.25 to −7.5	84	91		1.4
		12	24		92	100		0
Kim et al[82]	1993	135	12	−2.0 to −7.0	91	99		8.1
		67		−7.25 to −13.5	52	63		17.9
Brancato et al[83]	1993	146	12	−0.8 to −6	71	NR		1.4
		145	12	−6.1 to −9.9	35	NR		2.1
		39	12	−10 to −25	28	NR		7.7
Seiler[52]	1993	42	12	−1.25 to −3.0	97	100		0
		85	12	−3.1 to −6.0	92	97		0
		27	12	−6.1 to −9.0	44	60		7.4
Lavery[84]	1993	99	12	−1.25 to −9.6	93	84		1
Gimbel et al[85]	1993	52	15.5	−5.6 to 1.6	43	96		NR
		52	9	−5.9 ± 15	45	92		NR
Piebenga et al[86]	1993	21	36	−2.0 to −8.0	60	70		0
		25	24	−1.0 to −5.0	58	67		0
		70	12	−1.0 to −6.0	71	75		0
Talley et al[6]	1994	85	12	−1.0 to −7.5	93	98		1
FDA Study		544	12	−1.0 to −6.0	76	91		NR
Summit FDA Study		691	12	−1.0 to −6.0	79	86		1
VISX		691	24	−1.0 to −6.0	79	85		1
Dutt et al[87]		47	12	−1.5 to −6.1	80	94		0
Hamberg-Nystrom et al[88]	1996	457	36					
		457	24					
Shah, Hersh[89]	1996	45	6	−1.5 to −6.0		100	62 (20/40)	0
Kaskaloglu[90]	1996			−1.75 to −3.0	100			
		157		−3.25 to −6.0	64.1			
Talamo et al[91]	1995		6	−6.0 to −8.0	67	74		2
McCarty et al[92]	1996	645	12	−1.0 to −5.0	87	87	47 (20/20)	4
		645	12	−5.0 to −10.0	65	71	25 (20/20)	8
Hamberg-Nystrom et al[93]	1997	40	12	−1.0 to −6.0		100		
Ohashi et al[94]	1997	67	6	−1.0 to −7.50	72.5			0
Piovella et al[44]	1997	56	48	−5.75 to −24.5				
Wang et al[95]	1997	432	12	−1.25 to −6.0	83		72	
Williams[45]	1997	26	24	−6.0 to −10.0	77	89		
		33	24	−10.25 to −25.75	48	42		
Hersh et al[96]	1998	105	6	−9.23 mean	57	66	19	12
Ozdamar et al[76]	1998	20	24	−2.25 to −6.0	90	95		5
Pietila et al[97]	1998	226	12	−1.25 to −6.0	87	87	39	1
		104	12	−6.1 to −10.0	41	53	5	5
		39	12	−10.1 to −25.0	31	29	0	0
Shah et al[98]	1998	3218	12	−1.0 to −12.0	91	94	59	
Spadea et al[99]	1998	53		−8.0 to −17.0		45		
Steinert, Hersh[100]	1998	134	12	−6.0 to −12.0	68		42	
Tuunanen, Tervo[101]	1998	52	12	−1.5 to −6.0	87	88	58	
		4	12	−6.1 to −8.0	79	68	26	
		24	12	−8.1 to −11.50	67	68	33	
Gabrieli et al[102]	1999	76	18	−8.0 to −23.50		87		
Hadden et al[103]	1999	192	18	−6.0 to −10.0	94	94	59	
Lipshitz et al[104]	1999	30	12	−2.5 to −8.75	97	95	47	
		30	12	−2.5 to −8.75	87	96	53	
McDonald et al[105]	1999	414	12	−1.0 to −6.0	94	98	72	1.8
		211	12	−1.0 to −6.0	95	97	62	2.5
Pop, Payette[106]	1999	42	12	−10.0 to −27.0	48	85	56	
Wee et al[107]	1999	971	6	−1.0 to −6.0	74	93		0.4
			6	−6.0 to −15.25	50	75		3.4
Fisher et al[108]	2000	23		−2.8 to −5.5	100		74	10.5

BCVA, Best-corrected visual acuity; *NR,* not reported; *VASC,* visual acuity without correction.

TABLE 18-2

RESULTS OF PHOTOREFRACTIVE KERATECTOMY FOR HYPEROPIA AND HYPEROPIC ASTIGMATISM

Author	Year	No. of Eyes	Follow-up (Months) [Mean]	Attempted Correction (D) [Mean]	±1D of Emmetropia (%)	≥20/40 VASC (%)	≥20/20 VASC (%)	Losing ≥2 Lines BCVA (%)
Dausch et al[113]	1997	68	12	+2.0 to +8.25	81	97	40	1
Daya et al[114]	1997	45	6	+1.0 to +6.5	87	93		6.7
Jackson et al[115]	1997	25	6	+1.0 to +4.0			8	4
Pietila et al[116]	1997	34	12	+1.5 to +6.0	40	67		0.3
			12	+6.25 to +9.75	17	8		
Sener et al[119]	1997	15	12	+1.0 to +4.75	66			
			12	+5.0 to +9.75	0			
			12	Aphakia	0			
Venter[118]	1997	10		+1.75 to +4.0				
Carones et al[119]	1998	25	24	+1.0 to +4.0				0
Vinciguerra et al[120]	1998	67	12	+3.76 mean				
Corones et al[121]	1999	38		+1.0 to +8.0				
Haw, Manche[122]	2000	18	24	+1.13 to +4.0	83			0
Parcella et al[123]	2001	28	18	+1.0 to +7.75	93	100	46	0

BCVA, Best-corrected visual acuity; *VASC*, visual acuity without correction.

represents a treatment option for a few select patients who should be carefully screened.

Photorefractive Keratectomy for Treatment of Residual Myopia after Radial Keratotomy

Residual myopia after radial keratotomy has been a problem for patients who already have a maximum number of incisions or in whom further radial keratotomy may not be advantageous. PRK can be used to correct this residual myopia.[72,129-131] In one study, 25 eyes underwent PRK for residual myopia after radial keratotomy; 60% of the eyes were within 1D of emmetropia, and 53% achieved 20/40 or better uncorrected acuity. It appears that PRK after radial keratotomy is less predictable than in primary cases, but it still may be useful. Haze also appears to be a greater problem in patients undergoing PRK after radial keratotomy.[132,133]

In another study of 28 eyes treated with PRK for residual myopia after radial keratotomy, 75% of eyes had vision of 20/25 or better without correction, and 85% had 20/40 or better vision without correction.[129] No eyes lost more than one line of best-corrected vision. At 1 year, 90% were within 1D of emmetropia.

Topography

The cornea dramatically changes shape after PRK, going from a negative asphericity (prolate shape, with the center steeper than the periphery) to a positive asphericity (oblate shape, with the center flatter than the periphery). With increasing refractive correction, increasing amounts of positive corneal asphericity are seen. The measurement of this change is crucial to our understanding of the refractive effects induced by the excimer laser. Technology in the field of corneal surface mapping has been driven largely by the need for accurate information on the results of PRK. There are now techniques available that can provide information not only about corneal curvature but also about relative elevations of various points on the corneal surface.[134,135]

Corneal topography can also be used to screen for the presence of abnormal curvature conditions, such as keratoconus.[136] Patients suspected of having keratoconus have traditionally been excluded from refractive surgery because of the possibility of increasing corneal ectasia. Although some studies have reported success in treating these patients with PRK, others have reported progressive ectasia of the cornea with various laser techniques.[137,138] Most of

these patients have a high risk of ectasia with or without laser treatment and may develop progressive changes in their refractive error. It may be difficult to tell in any individual patient whether the laser treatment induces a quicker rate of progression of ectasia.

COMPLICATIONS

Complications can occur with any refractive surgical procedure. Under- and overcorrection can be seen, caused by improper surgical ablation, malfunctioning of the excimer laser, abnormal corneal hydration status, or excessive or inadequate wound healing response. It is crucial to maintain consistent hydration of the cornea, because excessive fluid on the cornea can result in an undercorrection. If desiccation of the corneal stroma is present, overcorrection and haze can occur. An enhanced wound healing response can lead to regression, resulting in an undercorrection and possibly scarring. No or minimal tissue healing can sometimes lead to an overcorrection.

Undercorrection

In cases of undercorrection with residual myopia, the simplest form of management is to use spectacles or contact lenses. Contact lens use can be highly successful after PRK. An attempt can be made to reduce wound healing in patients with mild residual myopia by using steroids; mixed results have been reported with this technique. Care must be taken to limit steroid use in these otherwise normal eyes to prevent steroid-related complications such as glaucoma and cataract formation.

Some patients with residual myopia have a thickened epithelial cell layer, and this epithelial hyperplasia results in steepening of the cornea and increased myopia. In one study, hyperplastic epithelium was removed in an attempt to reduce myopia in eight eyes. The myopia actually increased from a mean of −3.11D before epithelial débridement to −4.67D 12 months after epithelial cell removal, suggesting that increased wound healing played a larger role than epithelial hyperplasia did. This conclusion has been supported by the work of Moller-Pedersen et al.,[139] which showed that refractive regression is a manifestation of stromal keratocyte healing.

Systemic factors may also play a role in wound healing and regression after PRK. Zabel et al.[139a] reported complete regression in a woman who was later found to be 2 weeks pregnant at the time of the laser surgery.

TABLE 18-3

RESULTS OF STUDIES COMPARING PHOTOREFRACTIVE KERATECTOMY (PRK) AND LASER *IN SITU* KERATOMILEUSIS (LASIK)

Author	Year	No. of Eyes	Follow-up (Months) [Mean]	Attempted Correction (D) [Mean]	±1D of Emmetropia (%)	≥20/40 VASC (%)	≥20/20 VASC (%)	Losing ≥2 Lines BCVA (%)
Wang et al[144]	1997	432 PRK	12	−1.25 to −6.0	83		72	
		137 LASIK	12	−1.25 to −6.0	89		83	
Hersh et al[96]	1998	105 PRK	6	−6.0 to −15.0	57	46	19	11.8
		115 LASIK	6	−6.0 to −15.0	41	56	26	3.2
el Danasoury et al[145]	1999	26 PRK	12	−2.0 to −5.50			63	0
		26 LASIK	12	−2.0 to −5.50			79	0
El Maghraby et al[146]	1999	33 PRK	24	−2.5 to −8.0			36	
		33 LASIK	24	−2.5 to −8.0			61	
Fernandez et al[63]	2000	208	12	−1.0 to −3.0 (PRK)	92			
			12	−1.0 to −3.0 (LASIK)	95			
			12	−3.25 to −6.0 (PRK)	82			
			12	−3.25 to −6.0 (LASIK)	98			
Kasetsuwan et al[147]	2000	73 PRK	12	−1.50 −15.75	86	91		0
		74 LASIK	12	−1.50 −15.75	77	97		0
Pop, Payette[148]	2000	107 PRK	12	−1.0 to −9.5			86	0
		107						
Tole et al[149]	2000	308 PRK	6	−0.5 to −6.0			65	1
		314 LASIK	6	−0.5 to −6.0			80	1.4

BCVA, Best-corrected visual acuity; *VASC*, visual acuity without correction.

Residual myopia can also be managed by further refractive surgery, including radial keratotomy, PRK, or LASIK.[75,76] These methods can be used in patients who reject spectacles or contact lens correction.

Overcorrection

Overcorrection is a desired result in the first few months after PRK, as there is usually regression of 0.50–1.00D. If the patient has a greater degree of overcorrection than is expected at 1 month or longer after surgery, an attempt should be made to increase wound healing by tapering the steroids rapidly. If additional stromal remodeling occurs during this steroid taper, a decrease in the amount of hyperopia will occur. A rapid taper of steroids may induce corneal haze in some patients, so frequent monitoring is important. Also, as previously mentioned, refractive modulation with steroid therapy is not always successful.

Overcorrection often results from inadequate wound healing in the postoperative period. This wound healing can be increased by scraping the epithelium and underlying corneal stroma. In 19 eyes that were overcorrected after PRK, more than 2D of myopic refractive shift was seen when the epithelium was débrided and the underlying stroma scraped. The prescraping refractive error averaged +2.77D and was reduced to +0.68D 12 months after the epithelial débridement.

Corneal Scar Formation

Haze or scar formation can occur after any corneal injury, including PRK. This haze formation can be visually significant and can cause loss of best-corrected visual acuity. Corneal haze can occur relatively soon after PRK but can also be seen late after treatment.[27,66,140] In one study, five eyes of four patients developed localized scars after PRK.[140] Surgical removal of the scar with the excimer laser can be helpful in improving visual function in these patients. Frequent topical steroids are important in reducing recurrent scar tissue formation. Typical haze appears 1 month after treatment, reaches a maximum at 3–4 months, and fades to a level where it is difficult to detect by 1 year. Haze is more common in higher corrections, especially greater than 8D of myopia.[44,141] In one report, patients with brown irises were at higher risk for haze development.[142] Haze may be less common and less severe with lasers that use smaller scanning slits or spots,[105] although this has been disputed in other studies.[104] Laser *in situ* epithelial keratomileusis (LASEK) is currently being evaluated and may be associated with less haze than PRK with manual scraping of the epithelium, although long-term follow-up studies or comparative studies are not yet available.[143] LASIK is less likely to induce haze formation than is PRK, especially at higher levels of correction (Table 18-3).[63,96,144–149]

Late-onset haze is an unusual variant that appears 4–14 months postoperatively and can be quite severe.[66] This variant can require treatment with steroids, mitomycin C, or surgical intervention. It has a reported incidence of 1.8% and may be more common in higher myopic corrections. Because this late-onset haze has been linked to ultraviolet exposure, the use of ultraviolet-absorbing lenses (sunglasses) while outdoors should be protective.

The haze following hyperopic PRK is peripherally located.[115,116,122,123] Bowman's membrane remains intact in the center of the cornea, protecting this area from haze. Haze takes a second place to decentration in causing a decrease in best-corrected visual acuity following hyperopic ablations. If haze occurs in myopic eyes, it can be centrally located, leading to a decrease in best-corrected visual acuity.

Central Islands

Central islands have been reported after excimer laser treatment.[6] These small central elevations in the corneal topography may occur for a variety of reasons (Fig. 18-15). This phenomenon is seen exclusively in broad-beam delivery systems. Beam profile abnormalities, increased hydration of the central corneal stroma due to shock-wave formation, and plume effect have been implicated.[150] In one study using a PMMA model, all of the following were considered significant in the development of central islands: shock waves, plume effect, random eye movement, and beam diameter. A flat ablation beam may direct stromal fluid into the central area of ablation, and the hydrated tissue is ablated at a slower rate. This can lead to less tissue removal in the central 1–3mm of the cornea. Laser software can add extra pulses in the central cornea to compensate for this

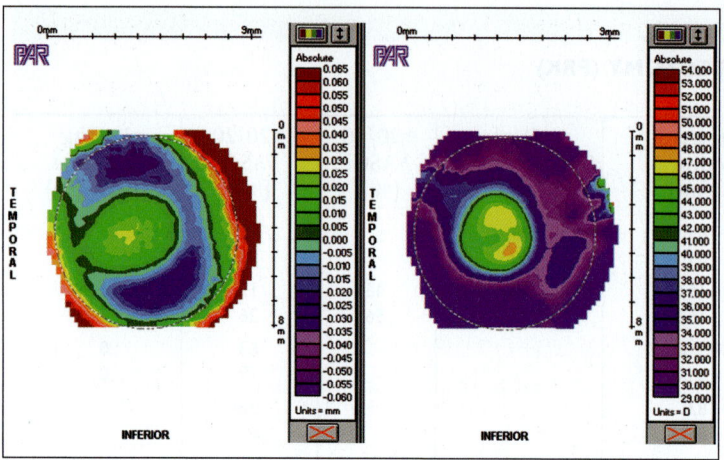

FIG. 18-15 ■ Central topographical elevation in a patient 6 months after a −6.00D myopic ablation. Often these central islands resolve over time, but retreatment is sometimes indicated. Maintenance of proper corneal hydration and additional central pulses can decrease the incidence of central islands.

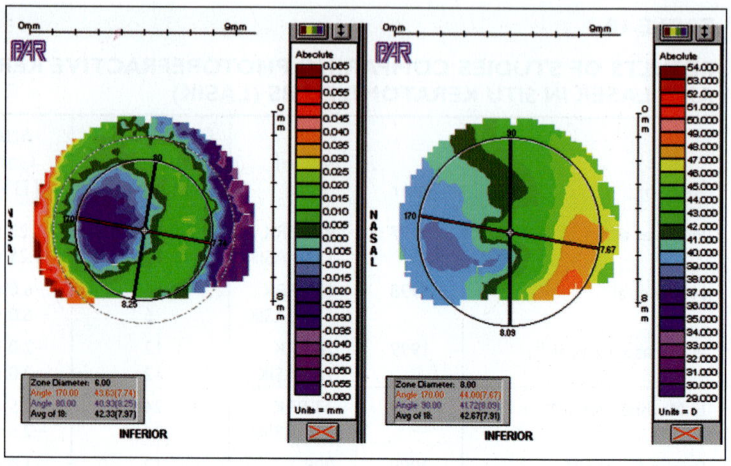

FIG. 18-16 ■ Decentration of this −5.50D myopic ablation led to a decrease in best-corrected visual acuity with haloes. Proper centration is crucial to a good result.

("anti–central island software"), but careful monitoring of the hydration of the central cornea is important. If excessive hydration of the central cornea is noted, the procedure should be paused to remove excess fluid.[150]

Central islands tend to resolve with time after PRK, probably owing to differential wound healing or epithelial hyperplasia.[151,152] Central islands can be associated with loss of best-corrected visual acuity due to the irregular astigmatism that they create.

Infectious Keratitis

Infectious keratitis can result in scarring, haze, and a decrease in vision. Appropriate culture and aggressive treatment with fortified broad-spectrum antibiotics should be used. After the offending organism or organisms are discovered, antibiotic therapy can be tailored accordingly. If topical nonsteroidal anti-inflammatory drugs are used without appropriate steroid coverage, an increase in polymorphonuclear leukocyte migration into the cornea can occur, causing inflammatory infiltrates. These are best treated by discontinuing the nonsteroidal anti-inflammatory drug and instituting frequent topical steroids.

Pain

Pain relief by the use of nonsteroidal anti-inflammatory agents appears to be modulated by reducing prostaglandin E_2 levels. When topical steroids are used along with nonsteroidals, leukocyte infiltration is diminished. Diclofenac appears to cause greater leukocyte infiltration than ketorolac does.

Decentration

Decentration of the refractive cut can result in glare, irregular astigmatism, and a decrease in best-corrected visual acuity (Fig. 18-16).[10,57,58,153,154] There is still some controversy about proper centration landmarks, but it appears that the treatment should be centered on the pupil, with the patient looking directly at the fixation light of the laser.[57,58,155] A carefully centered excimer ablation can result in a uniform topographical pattern.

Visual Aberrations

Glare and haloes at night are uncommon but can result in patient dissatisfaction in some cases.[154] In most cases, nighttime visual disturbances are temporary and resolve within the first 6 months postoperatively. Careful attention should be paid preoperatively to the scotopic pupil size and the patient's vocational requirements. Risk factors for night complaints that should be recognized preoperatively include large scotopic pupil size, large refractive errors, and high astigmatism. Treatment of large refractive errors results in a more pronounced transition area surrounding the ablation. High amounts of astigmatism cause the effective laser profile to decrease in diameter in the meridian of the negative cylinder. Glare in low-contrast situations can persist for longer than a year.[153] Low-contrast visual acuity is a more sensitive measurement of visual function after PRK. Loss of contrast sensitivity can occur, especially with the treatment of high myopia, but it usually returns to baseline values at 6–12 months postoperatively.

Endothelial Cell Loss

Endothelial cell damage does not appear to be a problem after PRK in patients with normal eyes.[156,157] In one study with a 2-year follow-up, there was no significant loss of endothelial cells following excimer laser treatment of myopia.[158] In this study, the loss of endothelial cells was no greater than the expected loss due to aging.

In patients taking antipsychotics, endothelial damage may occur.[159] A patient taking haloperidol sustained severe endothelial cell loss directly underneath the area of PRK.[159] Central endothelial cell density decreased from 3884 cells/mm² preoperatively to 955 cells/mm² 9 months postoperatively. The peripheral endothelial density remained normal in this case.

Recurrent Erosion Syndrome

Map dot fingerprint changes similar to those seen in anterior basement membrane dystrophy can occur following PRK.[160] These usually occur outside of the ablation zone in areas where the epithelium has been removed. Recurrent erosions can occur in areas adjacent to the ablation zone or, more rarely, in the treated zone.[160] Excimer laser phototherapeutic keratectomy appears to be an effective treatment for recurrent erosion syndrome.

Environmental Changes in Refractive Error

Hyperopic shift has been seen at high altitudes following radial keratotomy. These effects may be secondary to the hypoxic effects on the cornea. The refractive effects of PRK are stable in patients who are exposed to hypobaric and hypoxic environments.[161]

CONCLUSION

The excimer laser is a promising tool for refractive surgery. The techniques are still developing, and it is certain that there will be significant advances in the future. An increased understanding of the optics of refractive surgery and the corneal wound healing response may help us improve our results and modulate the patient's postoperative healing, thus furthering our goal of predictable, safe refractive surgery. The excimer laser is a highly complex surgical tool that requires attention to detail, an appropriate physician-patient relationship that includes careful patient counseling, and meticulous postoperative care to achieve high-quality results.

REFERENCES

1. Puliafito CA, Steinert RF, Deutsch TF, et al. Excimer laser ablation of the cornea and lens: experimental studies. Ophthalmology. 1985;92:741–8.
2. Gartry DS, Kerr Muir MG, Marshall J. Excimer laser photorefractive keratectomy: 18-month follow-up. Ophthalmology. 1992;99:1209–19.
3. Sher NA, Chen V, Bowers RA, et al. The use of the 193-nm excimer laser for myopic photorefractive keratectomy in sighted eyes: a multi-center study. Arch Ophthalmol. 1991;109:1525–30.
4. Sher NA, Barak M, Daya S, et al. Excimer laser photorefractive keratectomy in high myopia: a multi-center study. Arch Ophthalmol. 1992;110:935–43.
5. Sher NA, Hardten DR, Fundingsland B, et al. 193-nm Excimer photorefractive keratectomy in high myopia. Ophthalmology. 1994;101:1575–82.
6. Talley AR, Hardten DR, Sher NA, et al. Results one year after using the 193-nm excimer laser for photorefractive keratectomy in mild to moderate myopia. Am J Ophthalmol. 1994;118:304–11.
7. Campos M, Nielsen S, Szerenyi K, et al. Clinical follow-up of phototherapeutic keratectomy for treatment of corneal opacities. Am J Ophthalmol. 1993;115:433–40.
8. Sher NA, Bowers RA, Zabel RW, et al. Clinical use of the 193-nm excimer laser in the treatment of corneal scars. Arch Ophthalmol. 1991;109:491–8.
9. Steinert RF, Puliafito CA. Excimer laser phototherapeutic keratectomy for a corneal nodule. Refract Corneal Surg. 1990;6:352.
10. Dausch D, Klein R, Schröder E. Excimer laser photorefractive keratectomy for hyperopia. Refract Corneal Surg. 1993;9:20–8.
11. Krauss JM, Puliafito CA, Steinert R. Laser interactions with the cornea. Surv Ophthalmol. 1991;7(3):214–22.
12. Loertscher H, Mandelbaum S, Parrish RK, et al. Preliminary report on corneal incisions created by a hydrogen fluoride laser. Am J Ophthalmol. 1986;102:217–21.
13. Poggio EC, Glynn RJ, Schein OD, et al. The incidence of ulcerative keratitis among users of daily-wear and extended-wear soft contact lenses. N Engl J Med. 1989;321:779–83.
14. Schawlow AL, Townes CH. Infrared and optical masers. Phys Rev. 1958:112.
15. Maiman TH. Stimulated optical radiation in ruby masers. Nature. 1960;187:493.
16. Wilson J, Hawkes JFB. Lasers: principles and applications. New York: Prentice-Hall; 1987.
17. Wilson J, Hawkes JFB. Optoelectronics, an introduction. Cambridge: Simon & Schuster; 1989.
18. Siegman AE. Introduction to masers and lasers. New York: McGraw-Hill; 1971.
19. Velasco JE, Setser DW. Bound-free emission spectra of diatomic xenon halides. J Chem Phys. 1975;62:1990–1.
20. Searles SK, Hart GA. Stimulated emission at 281 nm XC. Br Appl Phys Lett. 1975;27:243–5.
21. Trokel SL. Development of the excimer laser in ophthalmology—a personal perspective. Refract Corneal Surg. 1990;6:357–62.
22. Hoffman JM, Hays AK, Tisone GC. High-power UV noble gas–halide lasers. Appl Phys Lett. 1976;28:538–9.
23. Steven B, Hutton E. Radiative lifetime of the pyrene dimer and the possible role of excited dimers in energy transfer processes. Nature. 1960;1986:1045–6.
24. Taboada J, Archibald CJ. An extreme sensitivity in the corneal epithelium to far-UV ArF excimer laser pulses. Proc Sci Progr Aero Med Assoc, San Antonio, TX, 1981.
25. Taboada J, Mikesell GW, Reed RD. Response of the corneal epithelium to KrF excimer laser pulses. Health Phys. 1981;40:677–83.
26. Trokel SL, Srinivasan R, Braren B. Excimer laser surgery of the cornea. Am J Ophthalmol. 1983;96:710–5.
27. Marshall WJ, Trokel SL, Rothery S. Long-term healing of the central cornea after photorefractive keratectomy using an excimer laser. Ophthalmology. 1988;95:1411–21.
28. Krueger RR, Trokel SL. Quantitation of corneal ablation by ultraviolet laser light. Arch Ophthalmol. 1985;103:1741–2.
29. Krueger RR, Trokel SL, Schubert HD. Interaction of ultraviolet laser light with the cornea. Invest Ophthalmol Vis Sci. 1985;26:1455–64.
30. Trokel SL. The cornea and ultraviolet laser light. In: Laser in der Ophthaologie. Stuttgart: Enke Verlag; 1988.
30a. Munnerlyn CR, Koons SJ, Marshall J. Photorefractive keratectomy: a technique for laser refractive surgery. J Cataract Refract Surg. 1988;14:46–52.
31. L'Esperance FA Jr, Warner JW, Telfair WB, et al. Excimer laser instrumentation and technique for human corneal surgery. Arch Ophthalmol. 1988;107:131–9.
32. Marshall J, Trokel S, Rothery S, et al. Photoablative reprofiling of the cornea using an excimer laser: photorefractive keratotomy. Lasers Ophthalmol. 1986;1:21–48.
33. Trokel SL, Srinivasan R, Braren BA. Excimer laser surgery of the cornea. Am J Ophthalmol. 1983;96:710–5.
34. Krueger RR, Trokel SS, Shubert H. Interaction of UV light with the cornea. Invest Ophthalmol Vis Sci. 1985;26:1455–64.
35. Reed RD, Taboada J, Midsell JW. Response of the corneal epithelium to krypton fluoride excimer laser. Health Phys. 1981;40:677–83.
36. Nuss RC, Puliafito CA, Dehm E. Unscheduled DNA synthesis following excimer laser ablation of the cornea in vivo. Invest Ophthalmol Vis Sci. 1987;28:287–94.
37. Clarke RH, Nakagawa K, Isner JM. The production of short-lived free radicals accompanying laser photoablation of cardiovascular tissue. Free Radic Biol Med. 1988;4:209–13.
38. Green HA, Margolis R, Boll J, et al. Unscheduled DNA synthesis in human skin after in vitro ultraviolet-excimer laser ablation. J Invest Dermatol. 1987;89:201–4.
39. Green H, Boll J, Parrish JA, et al. Cytotoxicity and mutagenicity of low intensity, 248 and 193 nm excimer laser radiation in mammalian cells. Cancer Res. 1987;47:410–3.
40. Rimoldi D, Miller AC, Freeman SE, Samid D. DNA damage in cultured human skin fibroblasts exposed to excimer laser radiation. J Invest Dermatol. 1991;96:898–902.
41. Seiler T, Bende T, Winckler K, Wollensak J. Side effects in excimer corneal surgery. DNA damage as a result of 193 nm excimer laser radiation. Graefes Arch Clin Exp Ophthalmol. 1988;226:273–6.
42. Waring GO. Development and evaluation of refractive surgical procedures. Part 1. Five stages in the continuum of development. J Refract Surg. 1987;3:142–57.
43. Hanna K, Chastang JC, Pouliquen Y, et al. A rotating slit delivery system for excimer laser refractive keratoplasty. Am J Ophthalmol. 1987;103:474.
44. Piovella M, Camesasca FI, Fattori C. Excimer laser photorefractive keratectomy for high myopia: four-year experience with a multiple zone technique. Ophthalmology. 1997;104(10):1554–65.
45. Williams DK. Multizone photorefractive keratectomy for high and very high myopia: long-term results. J Cataract Refract Surg. 1997;23(7):1034–41.
46. Munnerlyn CR, Koons SJ, Marshall J. Photorefractive keratectomy: a technique for laser refractive surgery. J Cataract Refract Surg. 1988;14:46–52.
47. Waring GO III, O'Connell MA, Maloney RK, et al. Photorefractive keratectomy for myopia using a 4.5 mm ablation zone. J Refract Surg. 1995;11:170–80.
48. Barraquer JI. Keratomileusis. Int Surg. 1967;48:103–17.
49. McDonnell PJ, Moreira H, Garbus J, et al. Photorefractive keratectomy to create toric ablations for correction of astigmatism. Arch Ophthalmol. 1991;109:710–3.
50. Campos M, Hertzog L, Garbus J, et al. Photorefractive keratectomy for severe postkeratoplasty astigmatism. Am J Ophthalmol. 1992;114:429–36.
51. Maloney RK, Friedman M, Harmon T, et al. A prototype erodible mask delivery system for the excimer laser: photorefractive keratectomy. Lasers Ophthalmol. 1986;1:21–48.
52. Seiler T. Photorefractive keratectomy: European experience. In: Thompson FB, McDonnell PJ, eds. Color atlas text of excimer laser surgery. The cornea. New York: Igaku-Shoin; 1993:53–62.
53. Dausch D, Klein R, Landesz M, Schroder E. Photorefractive keratectomy to correct astigmatism with myopia or hyperopia. J Cataract Refract Surg. 1994;20:252–7.
54. Taylor NM, Eikelboom RH, van Sarloos PP, et al. Determining the accuracy of an eye tracking system for laser refractive surgery. J Refract Surg. 2000;16(5):S643–6.
55. Mulhern MG, Foley-Nolan A, O'Keefe M, et al. Topographical analysis of ablation centration after excimer laser photorefractive keratectomy and laser in situ keratomileusis for high myopia. J Cataract Refract Surg. 1997;23(4):488–94.
56. Siganos DS, Evangelatou KA, Papadaki TG, et al. Photorefractive keratectomy in eyes with congenital nystagmus. J Refract Surg. 1998;14(6):649–52.
57. Amano S, Tanaka S, Shimizu K. Topographical evaluation of centration of excimer laser myopic photorefractive keratectomy. J Cataract Refract Surg. 1993;20:616–9.
58. Uozato H, Guyton DL. Centering corneal surgical procedures. Am J Ophthalmol. 1987;103:264–75.
59. Campos M, Trokel SL, McDonnell PJ. Surface morphology following photorefractive keratectomy. Ophthalmic Surg. 1993;24:822–5.
60. Maguen E, Nesburn AB, Papaioannou T, et al. Effect of nitrogen flow on recovery of vision after excimer laser photorefractive keratectomy without nitrogen flow. J Refract Corneal Surg. 1994;10:321–6.
61. Pallikaris I, McDonald MB, Siganos D, et al. Tracker-assisted photorefractive keratectomy for myopia of −1 to −6 diopters. J Refract Surg. 1996;12:240–7.
62. Salah T, Waring GO III, Maghraby AE, et al. Excimer laser in situ keratomileusis under a corneal flap for myopia of 2 to 20 diopters. Am J Ophthalmol. 1996;121:143–55.
63. Fernandez AP, Jaramillo J, Jaramillo M. Comparison of photorefractive keratectomy and laser in situ keratomileusis for myopia of −6 D or less using the Nidek EC-5000 laser. J Refract Surg. 2000;16(6):711–5.
63a. Zato MA, Matilla A, Gomez T, Jimenez V. Multizone versus monozone in the treatment of high and moderate myopia with an excimer laser. Ophthalmic Surg Lasers. 1996;27:S466–70.
64. Lin DT. Corneal topographic analysis after excimer photorefractive keratectomy. Ophthalmology. 1994;101:1432–9.
65. Corbett MC, O'Brart DP, Marshall J. Do topical corticosteroids have a role following excimer laser photorefractive keratectomy? J Refract Surg. 1995;11:380–7.
66. Lipshitz I, Loewenstein A, Varssano D, et al. Late onset corneal haze after photorefractive keratectomy for moderate and high myopia. Ophthalmology. 1997;104(3):369–73; discussion 373–4.
67. Moreira H, Garbus JJ, Fasano A, et al. Multifocal corneal topographic changes with excimer laser photorefractive keratectomy. Arch Ophthalmol. 1992;110:994–9.
68. Goggin M, Foley-Nolan A, Algawi K, O'Keefe M. Regression after photorefractive keratectomy for myopia. J Cataract Refract Surg. 1996;22:194–6.
69. Gartry DS, Muir MG, Lohmann CP, Marshall J. The effect of topical corticosteroids on refractive outcome and corneal haze after photorefractive keratectomy. A prospective, randomized, double-blind trial. Arch Ophthalmol. 1992;110:944–52.
70. Durrie DS, Lesher MP, Cavanaugh TB. Classification of variable clinical response after photorefractive keratectomy for myopia. J Refract Surg. 1995;1:341–7.
71. Seiler T, Derse M, Pham T. Repeated excimer laser treatment after photorefractive keratectomy. Arch Ophthalmol. 1992;110:1230–3.
72. Azar DT, Tuli S, Benson RA, et al. Photorefractive keratectomy for residual myopia after radial keratotomy. PRK After RK Study Group. J Cataract Refract Surg. 1998;24(3):303–11.

72a. Snibson GR, McCarty CA, Alfred GF, *et al.* Retreatment after excimer laser photorefractive keratectomy. The Melbourne Excimer Laser Group. Am J Ophthalmol. 1996;121(3):250–7.
73. Pop M, Aras M. Photorefractive keratectomy retreatments for regression. One-year follow-up. Ophthalmology. 1996;103:1979–84.
74. Higa H, Couper T, Robinson DI, *et al.* Multiple photorefractive keratectomy retreatments for myopia. J Refract Surg. 1998;14(2):123–8.
75. Gartry DS, Larkin DF, Hill AR, *et al.* Retreatment for significant regression after excimer laser photorefractive keratectomy. A prospective, randomized, masked trial. Ophthalmology. 1998;105(1):131–41.
76. Ozdamar A, Sener B, Aras C, *et al.* Laser *in situ* keratomileusis after photorefractive keratectomy for myopic regression. J Cataract Refract Surg. 1998;24(9):1208–11.
77. McDonald MB, Lui JC, Byrd TJ, *et al.* Central photorefractive keratectomy for myopia: partially sighted and normally sighted eyes. Ophthalmology. 1991;98:1327–37.
78. Gartry DS, Kerr Muir MG, Marshall J. Photorefractive keratectomy with an argon fluoride excimer laser: a clinical study. Refract Corneal Surg. 1991;7:420–35.
79. Seiler T, Wollensak J. Myopic photorefractive keratectomy with the excimer laser: one-year follow-up. Ophthalmology. 1991;988:1156–63.
80. Tengroth B, Epstein D, Fagerholm P, *et al.* Excimer laser photorefractive keratectomy for myopia: clinical results in sighted eyes. Ophthalmology. 1993;100:739–45.
81. Salz JJ, Maguen E, Nesburn AB, *et al.* A two-year experience with excimer laser photorefractive keratectomy for myopia. Ophthalmology. 1993;100:873–82.
82. Kim JH, Hahn TW, Lee YC, *et al.* Photorefractive keratectomy in 202 myopic eyes: one year results. Refract Corneal Surg. 1993;9:11–6.
83. Brancato R, Carones F, Trabucchi G, *et al.* The erodible mask in photorefractive keratectomy for myopia and astigmatism. Refract Corneal Surg. 1993;9:S125–30.
84. Lavery FL. Photorefractive keratectomy in 472 eyes. Refract Corneal Surg. 1993;9:98–100.
85. Gimbel HV, Van Westenbrugge JA, Johnson WH, *et al.* Visual, refractive and patient satisfaction results following bilateral photorefractive keratectomy of myopia. Refract Corneal Surg. 1993;9:5–10.
86. Piebenga LW, Matta CS, Dietz MR, *et al.* Excimer photorefractive keratectomy for myopia. Ophthalmology. 1993;100:1335–45.
87. Dutt S, Steinert RF, Raisman MB, *et al.* One-year results of excimer laser photorefractive keratectomy for low to moderate myopia. Arch Ophthalmol. 1994;112:1427–36.
88. Hamberg-Nystrom H, Fagerholm P, Tengroth B, Sjoholm C. Thirty-six month follow-up of excimer laser photorefractive keratectomy for myopia. Ophthalmic Surg Lasers. 1996;27:S418–20.
89. Shah SI, Hersh PS. Photorefractive keratectomy for myopia with a 6mm beam diameter. J Refract Surg. 1996;12:341–6.
90. Kaskaloglu M. Results of photorefractive keratectomy for myopia with the Technolas Keracor 116 excimer laser. J Refract Surg. 1996;12:S255–7.
91. Talamo JH, Siebert K, Wagoner MD, *et al.* Multicenter study of photorefractive keratectomy for myopia of 6.00 to 8.00 diopters. VISX Moderate Myopia Study Group. J Refract Surg. 1995;11:238–47.
92. McCarty CA, Alfred GF, Taylor HR. Comparison of results of excimer laser correction of all degrees of myopia at 12 months postoperatively. The Melbourne Excimer Laser Group. Am J Ophthalmol. 1996;121:372–83.
93. Hamberg-Nystrom HL, Fagerholm PP, Tengroth BT. Photorefractive keratectomy for low myopia at 6mm treatment diameter. A comparison of two excimer lasers. Acta Ophthalmol Scand. 1997;75(4):433–6.
94. Ohashi Y, Takahashi K, Yorii H. Photorefractive keratectomy for myopia and photoastigmatic keratectomy for astigmatism. J Refract Surg. 1997;13(5 suppl):S452–3.
95. Wang P, Liu S, Xia X, *et al.* [Photorefractive keratectomy to correct myopic astigmatism]. Hunan Yi Ke Da Xue Xue Bao. 1997;22(5):465–6.
96. Hersh PS, Steinert RF, Brint SF, *et al.* Photorefractive keratectomy versus laser in situ keratomileusis for moderate to high myopia. A randomized prospective study. Ophthalmology. 1998;105(8):1512–22; discussion 1522–3.
97. Pietila J, Makinen P, Pajari S, *et al.* Photorefractive keratectomy for −1.25 to −25.00 diopters of myopia. J Refract Surg. 1998;14(6):615–22.
98. Shah SS, Kapadia MS, Meisler DM, *et al.* Photorefractive keratectomy using the Summit SVS Apex laser with or without astigmatic keratotomy. Cornea. 1998;17(5):508–16.
99. Spadea L, Colucci S, Bianco G, *et al.* Long-term results of excimer laser photorefractive keratectomy in high myopia: a preliminary report. Ophthalmic Surg Lasers. 1998;29(6):490–6.
100. Steinert RF, Hersh PS. Spherical and aspherical photorefractive keratectomy and laser *in-situ* keratomileusis for moderate to high myopia: two prospective, randomized clinical trials. Summit Technology PRK-LASIK study group. Trans Am Ophthalmol Soc. 1998;96:197–221.
101. Tuunanen TH, Tervo TT. Results of photorefractive keratectomy for low, moderate, and high myopia. J Refract Surg. 1998;14(4):437–46.
102. Gabrieli CB, Pacella E, Abdolrahimzadeh S, *et al.* Excimer laser photorefractive keratectomy for high myopia and myopic astigmatism. Ophthalmic Surg Lasers. 1999;30(6):442–8.
103. Hadden OB, Ring CP, Morris AT, *et al.* Visual, refractive, and subjective outcomes after photorefractive keratectomy for myopia of 6 to 10 diopters using the Nidek laser. J Cataract Refract Surg. 1999;25(7):936–42.
104. Lipshitz I, Fisher L, Lazar M, *et al.* Bilateral comparison of photorefractive keratectomy for myopia using two excimer lasers. J Refract Surg. 1999;15(3):334–7.
105. McDonald MB, Deitz MR, Frantz JM, *et al.* Photorefractive keratectomy for low-to-moderate myopia and astigmatism with a small-beam, tracker-directed excimer laser. Ophthalmology. 1999;106(8):1481–8; discussion 1488–9.
106. Pop M, Payette Y. Multipass versus single pass photorefractive keratectomy for high myopia using a scanning laser. J Refract Surg. 1999;15(4):444–50.
107. Wee TL, Chan WK, Tseng P, *et al.* Excimer laser photorefractive keratectomy for the correction of myopia. Singapore Med J. 1999;40(4):246–50.
108. Fisher EM, Ginsberg NE, Scher KS, *et al.* Photorefractive keratectomy for myopia with a 15Hz repetition rate. J Cataract Refract Surg. 2000;26(3):363–8.
109. Matta CS, Piebenga LW, Deitz MR, *et al.* Five and three year follow-up of photorefractive keratectomy for myopia of −1 to −6 diopters. J Refract Surg. 1998;14(3):318–24.
110. Brancato R, Tavola A, Carones F, *et al.* Excimer laser photorefractive keratectomy for myopia: results in 1165 eyes. Refract Corneal Surg. 1993;9(suppl):95–104.
111. Sher NA, Hardten DR, Fundingsland B, *et al.* 193-nm Excimer photorefractive keratectomy in high myopia. Ophthalmology. 1994;101:1575–82.
112. Carson CA, Taylor HR. Excimer laser treatment for high and extreme myopia. The Melbourne Excimer Laser and Research Group. Arch Ophthalmol. 1995;113:431–6.
113. Dausch D, Smecka Z, Klein R, *et al.* Excimer laser photorefractive keratectomy for hyperopia. J Cataract Refract Surg. 1997;23(2):169–76.
114. Daya SM, Tappouni FR, Habib NE. Photorefractive keratectomy for hyperopia: six months results in 45 eyes. Ophthalmology. 1997;104(11):1952–8.
115. Jackson WB, Mintsioulis G, Agapitos PJ, *et al.* Excimer laser photorefractive keratectomy for low hyperopia: safety and efficacy. J Cataract Refract Surg. 1997;23(4):480–7.
116. Pietila J, Makinen P, Pajari S, Uusitalo H. Excimer laser photorefractive keratectomy for hyperopia. J Refract Surg. 1997;13(6):504–10.
117. Sener B, Ozdamar A, Aras C, *et al.* Photorefractive keratectomy for hyperopia and aphakia with a scanning spot excimer laser. J Refract Surg. 1997;13(7):620–3.
118. Venter JA. Photorefractive keratectomy for hyperopia after radial keratotomy. J Refract Surg. 1997;13(5 suppl): S456.
119. Carones F, Brancato R, Morico A, *et al.* Photorefractive keratectomy for hyperopia using an erodible disc and axicon lens: 2-year results. J Refract Surg. 1998;14(5):504–11.
120. Vinciguerra P, Epstein D, Radice P, *et al.* Long-term results of photorefractive keratectomy for hyperopia and hyperopic astigmatism. J Refract Surg. 1998;14(2 suppl):S183–5.
121. Corones F, Brancato R, Morico A, *et al.* Photorefractive keratectomy for hyperopia: long-term nonlinear and vector analysis of refractive outcome. Ophthalmology. 1999;106(10):1976–82; discussion 1982–3.
122. Haw WW, Manche EE. Prospective study of photorefractive keratectomy for hyperopia using an axicon lens and erodible mask. J Refract Surg. 2000;16(6):724–30.
123. Pacella E, Abdolrahimzadeh S, Gabrieli CB. Excimer laser photorefractive keratectomy for hyperopia. Ophthalmic Surg Lasers. 2001;32(1):30–4.
124. Dausch J, Klein R, Schroder E. Excimer laser photorefractive keratectomy for hyperopia. Refract Corneal Surg. 1993;9:20–8.
125. Anschutz T, Ditzen K. Hyperopia PRK results after 1 year. Presented at the ninth ESCRS, Paris, 1993.
126. Chipman RA. Image formation by multifocal lenses. In: Maxwell WA, Nordan LT, eds. Current concepts of multifocal intraocular lenses. Thorofare, NJ: Slack; 1991:37–52.
127. Holladay JT, van Dijk H, Lang A, *et al.* Optical performance of multifocal intraocular lenses. J Cataract Refract Surg. 1990;16:413–22.
128. Vinciguerra P, Nizzola GM, Bailo G, *et al.* Excimer laser photorefractive keratectomy for presbyopia: 24-month follow-up in three eyes. J Refract Surg. 1998;14(1):31–7.
129. John ME, Martinez E, Cvintal T. Photorefractive keratectomy for residual myopia after radial keratotomy. J Cataract Refract Surg. 1996;22:901–5.
130. Kwitko ML, Gow JA, Bellavance F, Woo G. Excimer photorefractive keratectomy after undercorrected radial keratotomy. J Refract Surg. 1995;11:S280–3.
131. Meza J, Perez-Santonja JJ, Moreno E, Zato MA. Photorefractive keratectomy after radial keratotomy. J Cataract Refract Surg. 1994;20:485–9.
132. Probst LE, Machat JJ. Conservative photorefractive keratectomy for residual myopia following radial keratotomy. Can J Ophthalmol. 1998;33(1):20–7.
133. Gimbel HV, Sun R, Chin PK, *et al.* Excimer laser photorefractive keratectomy for residual myopia after radial keratotomy. Can J Ophthalmol. 1997;32(1):25–30.
134. Belin MW, Zloty P. Accuracy of the PAR corneal topography system with spatial misalignment. CLAO J 1993;19:64–8.
135. Belin MW, Litoff D, Strods SJ, *et al.* The PAR corneal topography system. Refract Corneal Surg. 1992;8:88–96.
136. Maeda N, Klyce SD, Smolek MK. Comparison of methods for detecting keratoconus using videokeratography. Arch Ophthalmol. 1995;113:870–4.
137. Amoils SP. Photorefractive keratectomy using a scanning-slit laser, rotary epithelial brush, and chilled balanced salt solution. J Cataract Refract Surg. 2000;26(11):1596–604.
138. Speicher L, Gottinger W. [Progressive corneal ectasia after laser *in situ* keratomileusis (LASIK)]. Klin Monatsbl Augenheilkd. 1998;213(4):247–51.
139. Moller-Pedersen T, Cavanagh HD, Petroll WM, *et al.* Stromal wound healing explains refractive instability and haze development after photorefractive keratectomy: a 1-year confocal microscopic study. Ophthalmology. 2000;107(7):1235–45.
139a. Zabel RW, Sher NA, Ostror CS, *et al.* Myopic excimer laser keratectomy: a preliminary report. Refract Corneal Surg. 2990;6:329–34.
140. Meyer JC, Stulting RD, Thompson KP, Durrie DS. Late onset of corneal scar after excimer laser photorefractive keratectomy. Am J Ophthalmol. 1996;121:529–39.
141. Siganos DS, Katsanevaki VJ, Pallikaris IG. Correlation of subepithelial haze and refractive regression 1 month after photorefractive keratectomy for myopia. J Refract Surg. 1999;15(3):338–42.
142. Tabbara KF, El-Sheikh HF, Sharara NA, *et al.* Corneal haze among blue eyes and brown eyes after photorefractive keratectomy. Ophthalmology. 1999;106(11):2210–5.
143. Shah S, Sebai Sarhan AR, Doyle SJ, *et al.* The epithelial flap for photorefractive keratectomy. Br J Ophthalmol. 2001;85(4):393–6.
144. Wang Z, Chen J, Yang B. Comparison of laser *in situ* keratomileusis and photorefractive keratectomy to correct myopia from −1.25 to −6.00 diopters. J Refract Surg. 1997;13(6):528–34.
145. el Danasoury MA, el Maghraby A, Klyce SD, *et al.* Comparison of photorefractive keratectomy with excimer laser *in situ* keratomileusis in correcting low myopia (from −2.00 to −5.50 diopters). A randomized study. Ophthalmology. 1999;106(2):411–20; discussion 420–1.
146. El-Maghraby A, Salah T, Waring GO III, *et al.* Randomized bilateral comparison of excimer laser *in situ* keratomileusis and photorefractive keratectomy for 2.50 to 8.00 diopters of myopia. Ophthalmology. 1999;106(3):447–57.

147. Kasetsuwan N, Puangsricharern V, Pariyakanok L. Excimer laser photorefractive keratectomy and laser *in situ* keratomileusis for myopia and astigmatism. J Med Assoc Thai 2000;83(2):182–92.

148. Pop M, Payette Y. Photorefractive keratectomy versus laser *in situ* keratomileusis: a control-matched study. Ophthalmology. 2000;107(2):251–7.

149. Tole DM, McCarty DJ, Couper T, *et al.* Comparison of laser *in situ* keratomileusis and photorefractive keratectomy for the correction of myopia of −6.00 diopters or less. Melbourne Excimer Laser Group. J Refract Surg. 2001;17(1):46–54.

150. Oshika T, Klyce SD, Smolek MK, *et al.* Corneal hydration and central islands after excimer laser photorefractive keratectomy. J Cataract Refract Surg. 1998;24(12):1575–80.

151. Krueger RR, Saedy NF, McDonnel PJ. Clinical analysis of steep central islands after excimer laser photorefractive keratectomy. Arch Ophthalmol. 1996;114:377–81.

152. Abbas UL, Hersh PS. Late natural history of corneal topography after excimer laser photorefractive keratectomy. Ophthalmology. 2001;108(5):953–9.

153. Niesen UM, Businger U, Schipper I. Disability glare after excimer laser photorefractive keratectomy for myopia. J Refract Surg. 1996;12:S267–8.

154. Schallhorn SC, Blanton CL, Kaupp SE, *et al.* Preliminary results of photorefractive keratectomy in active-duty United States Navy personnel. Ophthalmology. 1996;103:5–22.

155. Fay AM, Trokel SL, Myers JA. Pupil diameter and the principle ray. J Cataract Refract Surg. 1992;18:348–51.

156. Mardelli PG, Piebenga LW, Matta CS, *et al.* Corneal endothelial status 12 to 55 months after excimer laser photorefractive keratectomy. Ophthalmology. 1995;102:544–9.

157. Trocme SD, Mack KA, Gill KS, *et al.* Central and peripheral endothelial cell changes after excimer laser photorefractive keratectomy for myopia. Arch Ophthalmol. 1996;114:925–8.

158. Rosa N, Cennamo G, Del Prete A, *et al.* Endothelial cells evaluation two years after photorefractive keratectomy. Ophthalmologica. 1997;211(1):32–9.

159. Nakaya-Onishi M, Kiritoshi A, Hasegawa T, *et al.* Corneal endothelial cell loss after excimer laser keratectomy, associated with tranquilizers. Arch Ophthalmol. 1996;114:1282–3.

160. Maguen E, Salz JJ, Nesburn AB, *et al.* Results of excimer laser photorefractive keratectomy for the correction of myopia. Ophthalmology. 1994;101:1548–56.

161. Mader TH, Blanton CL, Gilbert BN, *et al.* Refractive changes during 72-hour exposure to high altitude after refractive surgery. Ophthalmology. 1996;103:1188–95.

19 Automated and Manual Lamellar Surgical Procedures and Epikeratoplasty

SHU-WEN CHANG • DIMITRI T. AZAR

DEFINITION
- Lamellar refractive surgery comprises various surgical procedures that entail lamellar dissection of the cornea and reshaping the corneal stroma to correct refractive errors of the eye.

KEY FEATURES
- Usually employed to correct high myopia or hyperopia.
- The lamellar dissection is usually performed using a microkeratome with an oscillating blade.
- A lamellar lenticule is lifted and reshaped, replaced, or flapped to allow refractive correction.

ASSOCIATED FEATURES
Several procedures are encompassed in this category:
- Keratomileusis with freezing.
- Planar lamellar refractive keratoplasty.
- Keratomileusis *in situ*.
- Automated lamellar keratoplasty.
- Laser *in situ* keratomileusis.
- Epikeratoplasty.
- Synthetic epikeratoplasty.
- Deep lamellar keratoplasty.

HISTORICAL REVIEW

Lamellar refractive surgery has undergone a long evolutionary process. Lamellar refractive surgery for the correction of hyperopia and myopia (Fig. 19-1), also known as keratomileusis, was pioneered by Barraquer in the early 1960s.[1] Another lamellar procedure to correct aphakia, termed keratophakia, was introduced by Barraquer[2] as well. In 1977, Troutman and Swinger[3,4] introduced hyperopic lamellar procedures in the United States, and Swinger[5] performed the first myopic procedure in 1980. Swinger and Villasenor[5] contributed substantially to the surgical knowledge of keratomileusis in the United States, and Nordan[6] and Maxwell standardized it for consistent and systematic teaching.

Kaufman[7] introduced the onlay lamellar refractive procedure in 1979, initially termed epikeratomileusis and later epikeratoplasty (now the accepted term). Nonfreeze planar keratomileusis, which permitted operations without freezing, was described by Krumeich and Swinger in 1983.[8] In an effort to avoid the drawbacks of these techniques, keratomileusis *in situ* (see Fig. 19-2) has been developed and carried out. Combining this approach with excimer laser surgery led to laser *in situ* keratomileusis (LASIK), which is currently the method of choice to correct wide ranges of refractive errors (discussed in greater detail in Chapters 20 and 27). Lamellar refractive surgery has un-

dergone a long evolutionary process. However, for lamellar techniques to be the first choice for the correction of extreme refractive errors, the accuracy and optical performance must approach those of intraocular lens surgery.[9–11]

PREOPERATIVE EVALUATION AND DIAGNOSTIC APPROACH

Patient Selection for Lamellar Refractive Surgery

Generally, patients must be over 18 years of age and serial examination must reveal stable refraction and topography prior to surgery. Patients are screened for corneal disease—epithelial basement membrane disease, forme fruste keratoconus and/or corneal warpage detectable by routine corneal topography, and history of recurrent erosions or keratitis are considered relative contraindications. The patient must also be screened for retinal disease, which may have to be treated before surgery. Contact lens wear is discontinued for at least 1 week for soft lenses and for 3–4 weeks for hard lenses.

The patient must have adequate globe exposure and be cooperative enough for local anesthetic. All patients are informed thoroughly as to the nature of the procedure and must know what to expect intraoperatively and postoperatively.

Centration

No matter which corneal surgical procedure is performed, proper centration is critical to avoid postoperative complications such as irregular astigmatism and glare that may interfere with visual function. Different approaches to the precise site at which the procedure is centered are used. Although some investigators argue that the "visual axis" is the optimal site of centration, the preponderance of evidence indicates that the center of the entrance pupil is the optimal site on which to center keratorefractive procedures.[9, 10]

Various techniques have been described for corneal centration. Steinberg and Waring[11] utilized the light reflex as a reference point. This technique has been abandoned because most surgeons currently center treatment on the pupil and not on the corneal light reflex.

The Osher centration device is best used to center the treatment on the pupil (the corneal light reflex is ignored), which is valuable if the surgeon has no ocular dominance while the cornea is viewed binocularly. The fixation light in the Zeiss and Weck centration devices and the nonluminous fixation point in Thornton's methods are other examples of such devices.[10]

When lamellar refractive surgery, such as automated lamellar keratoplasty and laser-assisted *in situ* keratomileusis, is carried out, the center is sometimes marked using two concentric circles, one internal (3mm in diameter) and one external (10.5mm in diameter), attached by a line that touches the smaller circle tangentially to give a pararadial line. Alternatively, multiple pararadial lines may be used.

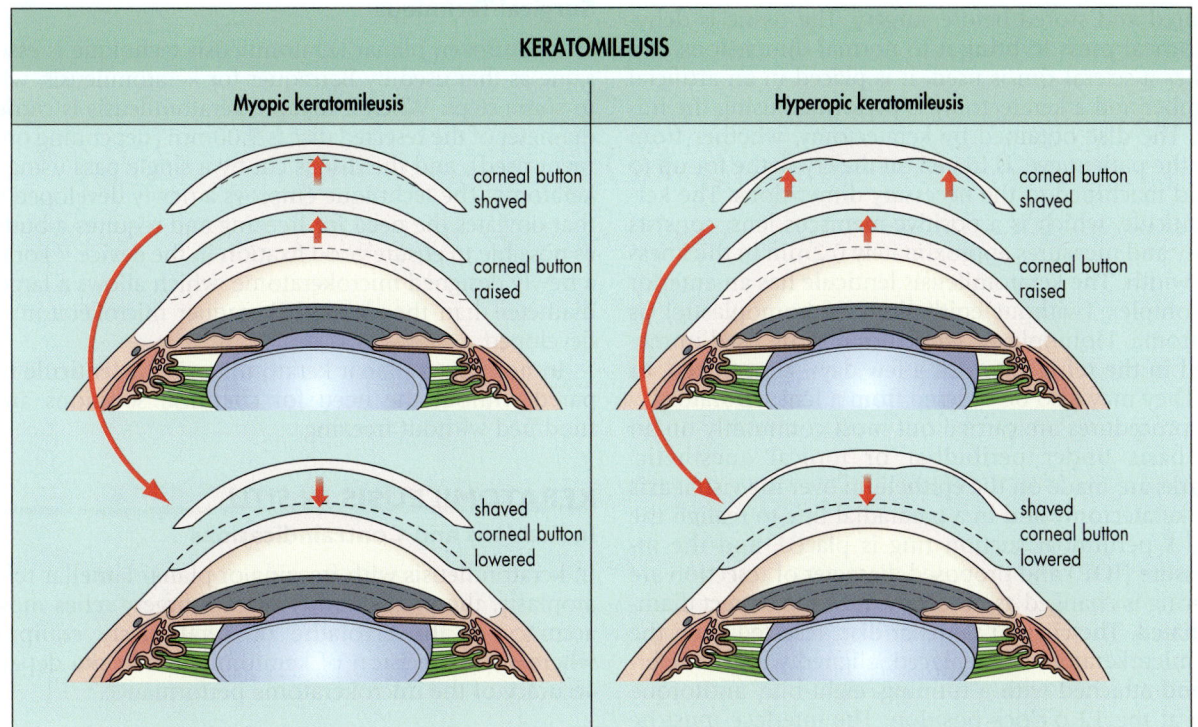

FIG. 19-1 ▮ **Keratomileusis.** In myopic keratomileusis, a corneal button is raised using a microkeratome, and it is re-shaped using a cryolathe (upper part). When the button is replaced, the central cornea is flattened (lower part). In hyperopic keratomileusis a cryolathe is used to reshape the stromal lenticule and increase central corneal curvature.

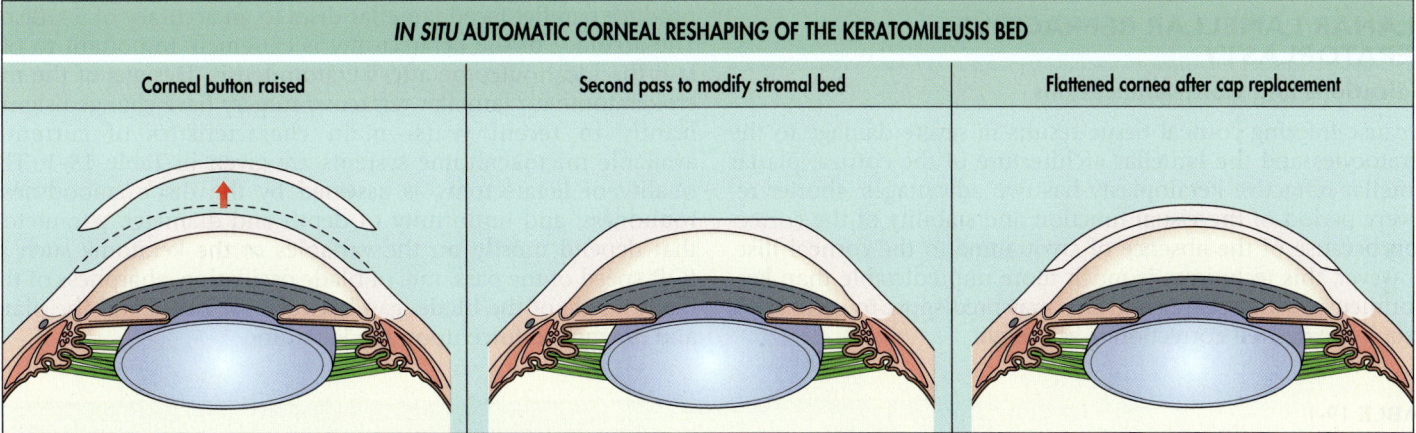

FIG. 19-2 ▮ *In situ* **automatic corneal reshaping of the keratomileusis bed.** A corneal button is raised using a microkeratome. A second pass modifies the stromal bed to allow corneal flattening after replacing the cap.

KERATOMILEUSIS WITH FREEZING

Indications and Contraindications

Keratomileusis with freezing was used to correct myopia surgically by as much as 16D with low predictability. Major disadvantages of keratomileusis with freezing include the following:

• Complexity of the technique
• Sophistication of the technical equipment itself—a microkeratome and a cryolathe
• Time required to attain sufficient expertise in using the two instruments
• Long recovery period because of the changes in the corneal tissue structure after freezing of the lenticule

Surgical instruments necessary for keratomileusis with freezing include a microkeratome to perform the lamellar keratectomy, a set of suction rings with which to fix the eye and guide the microkeratome, a microcomputer or calculator for the cryolathe procedure, the cryolathe itself, and the means to prepare the refractive lenticule.

Surgical Technique

CRYOLATHE. The Barraquer cryolathe consists of a Levin contact lens lathe modified with freezing circuits, digital micrometers, and other necessary alterations. After the microkeratome resection, the host cornea is turned on the cryolathe. During lathing, the corneal tissue, the head stock of the lathe on which the cornea is mounted, and the lathing tool are all brought to approximately −20°C. After the cornea has been reshaped, it is thawed and placed back in the host bed.

The Barraquer cryolathe is accurate but technically complex and expensive. Although the process of freezing enables the resected disc to be shaped precisely, it nonetheless results in death of the keratocytes and considerable postoperative corneal edema. Both of these factors contribute to a prolonged postoperative recovery period and to delayed epithelialization and epithelial ingrowth.

LENTICULE PRODUCTION. In autoplastic refractive procedures, the lenticule is prepared while the patient is on the operation table, whereas in homoplastic procedures, the lenticule is usually prepared and stored before surgery. The tissue is dehydrated in a corneal press to bring it to normal dimensions. If a cornea that has a scleral rim is used, it is placed in an artificial anterior chamber and a keratectomy is performed using the microkeratome. The disc obtained by keratectomy, whether from the donor or the patient eye, is frozen on the cryolathe for up to 2 minutes and machined to the necessary dimensions. The keratophakia lenticule, which is a positive-meniscus lens, consists of stroma only and measures approximately 0.2mm in thickness and 6mm in width. The keratomileusis lenticule has an anterior membrane complex (without epithelium, if homoplastic) as well as the stroma. Homoplastic lenticules may be used immediately, stored in the refrigerator for a few days, kept frozen, or lyophilized. They may also be ordered from a lens laboratory.

Refractive procedures are carried out most commonly on an ambulatory basis under peribulbar or topical anesthetic. Reference marks are made on the epithelium over the visual axis to center the keratectomy and in a pararadial line to realign the anterior cap. A perilimbal suction ring is placed, and the intraocular pressure (IOP) and proposed diameter of resection are verified. The ring is changed as necessary until the correct diameter is applanated. The circular lamellar disc, resected from the patient by a microkeratome, is replaced, aligned with the reference mark, and attached with a running, eight-bite, antitorque suture begun at the 12 o'clock position. The interface must be cleaned meticulously. The previously prepared keratophakic lenticule is placed into the interface using a spatula and centered over the visual axis. The suture is tied and the tension adjusted under keratometric control such that it is not too tight and a small gap is present for 360°.

PLANAR LAMELLAR REFRACTIVE KERATOPLASTY

Indications and Contraindications

Because freezing corneal tissue results in severe damage to the keratocytes and the lamellar architecture of the cornea, planar lamellar refractive keratoplasty has two advantages: shorter recovery period of the visual function and stability of the correction because of the absence of cryotrauma to the corneal disc. However, this technique is much more unpredictable than keratomileusis with freezing and also may predispose to corneal ectasia if the desired correction is very high.

Surgical Technique

The nonfrozen planar keratomileusis technique is essentially the same as that used by Barraquer for keratomileusis, with changes to some steps. When a myopic keratomileusis is carried out, the diameter of the resected disc is 9.00mm (depending on the equipment used), and the disc is cut by a single pass using the microkeratome. The technique employs a newly developed instrument that obviates the need for freezing and requires a button as large as possible to ensure good fixation in the device.[12] For this reason, a newly designed microkeratome, which allows a larger resection diameter than the classical Barraquer microkeratome, has been developed.

In nonfrozen planar keratomileusis the lenticule may be prepared without the need for chemical solutions and the disc modified without freezing.

KERATOMILEUSIS IN SITU

Indications and Contraindications

In keratomileusis with freezing or planar lamellar refractive keratoplasty, the predictability of the surgery relies mostly on the accuracy of the cryolathe or keratoplasty equipment used, whereas the precision of keratomileusis in situ depends on the accuracy of the microkeratome performance.

Microkeratome

The microkeratome has a high-speed oscillating blade; the principle of the carpenter plane is used to resect corneal discs of different diameters and thicknesses from either the patient or the donor cornea. Keratomes are microprecise machines that can produce parallel-faced lamellar discs to an accuracy of 5–10μm. The accuracy of the keratectomy is extremely important to obtain the ideal outcome after keratomileusis. Designs of the microkeratome for lamellar refractive surgery have changed significantly in recent years—main characteristics of currently available microkeratome systems are given in Table 19-1. The quality of keratectomy is assessed by the disc's smoothness, roundness, and uniformity of depth and diameter, parameters that depend mostly on the variables of the keratome such as IOP, speed of the pass, rate of blade oscillation, sharpness of the blade, angle of the blade, gap between the blade and the plate, and downward force upon the keratome.

TABLE 19-1

MAIN CHARACTERISTICS OF MICROKERATOME SYSTEMS

Type	Conventional Mechanical	Disposable	Water Jets	Laser Keratomes
Manual or automatic	Manual and automatic	Automatic	Automatic	Automatic
Advance rate (mm/s)	0.75–3.7	3.6	Unknown	Unknown
Cutting mechanism	• Stainless steel blade • Circular stainless steel blade • Natural diamond blade • Diamond blade • Sapphire blade	Stainless steel blade	Water jet	• Laser beam • "Point ablation" laser beam
Oscillations per minute	0–20,000	10,000–12,500	400–500 m/s	Not applicable
Flap diameter (mm)	3–10	10–10.5	3–9	Creates intrastromal bubbles and flaps; otherwise unknown
Blade angle	0–26°	26°	Not applicable	Not applicable
Eye fixation	Single, double, four or multiple suction rings/grip fingers	Single suction ring	Single suction ring/none	Computerized eye-tracking system/suction rings
Depth (μm)	1–500 (fixed or variable)	130–160 variable	Adjustable at factory or fixed	Infinitely adjustable or variable
Variable flap	Dependent on the machine type used	Yes	Yes	Unknown/not applicable
Power source	Electric, nitrogen gas pneumatic turbine	Electric	Electric	Electric
Composition	Stainless steel, titanium	Plastic	Titanium, various alloys	Not applicable

AUTOMATED LAMELLAR KERATOPLASTY

Indications and Contraindications

Keratomileusis *in situ* is a highly effective surgical technique. However, as mentioned previously, microkeratome speed and pressure are factors that result in lenticule properties different from the desired ones. In the search for a technique that excluded these effects, the Automated Corneal Shaper was developed. It is used in automated lamellar keratoplasty (ALK) and ensures accurate, regular, and predictable resections as it renders the procedure independent of human factors. Success depends on close attention to detail in the assembly, operation, and maintenance of the instrument. The device is designed to cut corneal lenticules of preselected thickness and diameter, which allows an increase in the accuracy and predictability of ALK. However, ALK is now replaced by LASIK for the most part.

Surgical Technique

INSTRUMENTATION. The shaper head has two parts, upper and lower, joined by a hinge that facilitates its assembly. After a blade has been placed between the two parts, the head is closed and fastened by a nut. A motor is connected to the upper body of the shaper head. The plates are essential to define the thickness of the tissues to be resected. Variation in the thickness of the plates results in various distances between the plate itself and the sharp edge of the blade, which allows prior adjustment of the resection thickness within a variation range as small as 5mm.

The fixation ring, which is of adjustable height, consists of two parts—one fixates the patient's eye and the other raises or lowers the level of corneal passage and thus varies the diameter of the resection. Three basic functions are fulfilled by the fixation ring:

- Fixes the ocular globe
- Increases the IOP up to >65mmHg (>8.6kPa) for the resection to be uniform and regular
- Serves as a guide for the passage of the shaper head

PROCEDURE. The technique described here is used for myopic, hyperopic, and homoplastic ALK. The setup and procedure until the corneal disc is removed are virtually identical for these situations. The pneumatic fixation ring is placed on the globe so that the eyeball is well exposed. When adequate IOP has been obtained, the resection diameter is graded using the applanation lens. The lens is lowered slowly until it rests horizontally (the cornea must be perfectly dry before the applanation lens is placed to avoid false applanation). The applanation lens used for the first resection is 7.2mm in diameter. As soon as the applanation lens is placed on the ring, its height has to be adjusted to make the applanation coincide with the inner circle marked on the surface of the lens. This is carried out using the regulating wrench of the ring. Once a given height of the ring has produced the applanation needed for the operation, the resection diameter equals the applanation diameter. The applanation lens and the adjustment wrench are removed.

The shaper is lowered to the horizontal position and inserted in the notch seen on the side of the handle. The shaper is pushed forward gently until a tooth of the largest pinion engages the first tooth of the dented rack. From this position the shaper may be moved readily and the resection carried out. When the pedal is pressed, the shaper slides and cuts the disc. It stops automatically when the large pinion reaches the end of the rack. The shaper then is removed back along the plane of its insertion. The ring is removed. The corneal bed is inspected after the corneal flap has been folded.

Myopic Automated Lamellar Keratoplasty. If the fixation ring had been removed, it has to be replaced to carry out the second resection; if not, only the applanation lens needs to be placed. The latter is selected, according to the calculation table used, before surgery and placed on a dry corneal bed. The height-regulating wrench is gyrated until the applanation ring touches the inner margin of the circle marked on the lens.

Afterwards, the wrench is removed and the shaper is positioned as already described. When the resection is completed, both the shaper and the ring are removed and the accuracy of the lenticule dimensions is checked. The interface and the disc are washed using a brush and saline solution, which prevents proliferation of cells on the interface and results in a much clearer cornea postoperatively. All excess fluid is removed by aspiration and the corneal bed is air dried. As soon as the disc is placed back, the anterior curvature of the cornea shows an applanation equivalent to the said correction.

Hyperopic Automated Lamellar Keratoplasty. No refractive resection is necessary for the correction of hyperopia. Once the corneal disc has been checked, the surgeon proceeds to wash the corneal bed, air-dry it, and replace the disc in the bed.

To replace the disc accurately, the surgeon must identify and check the epithelial and stromal sides. These must be identified throughout the surgery, from the moment the disc is removed from the microkeratome to when it is measured, cleaned, and stored.

To prevent the disc from folding, it is advisable to place it on a fenestrated spatula. Rotate the spatula and lower the disc toward the eye. With a Weck sponge in each hand, quickly rotate the disc to align it with the pararadial reference line. When placed back in the eye, the disc must have its original position. If instead of forming a straight line, the segments form an angulation, it is likely that the epithelial side is against the stroma. If this occurs, the disc must be removed, both the disc and the corneal surface washed again, and the disc repositioned. Air dry the edge of the disc and check for centration. Any air trapped under the disc must be pushed out gently using forceps. Once alignment and centration are verified, further manipulation of the disc is not required. Air may be used to enhance the cohesion of the disc to the corneal-stromal surface. Do not overdry the cornea with the air as this may cause corneal irregularities. After careful removal of the eyelid speculum, allow the lids to close and make sure that the disc is not displaced by the lid margins.

Homoplastic Automated Lamellar Keratoplasty. After the corneal disc has been obtained by the method described previously, it is discarded and a new one created from donor tissue. The primary procedure must be repeated using either a whole donor eye or an artificial anterior chamber for anterior donor sections. It is necessary to suture the donor disc to the recipient cornea because the alignment of the donor tissue cannot be duplicated precisely.

Suturing the Corneal Disc. Sutures may be placed once the corneal disc is positioned correctly. Usually, the material used is 10-0 nylon. An eight-bite, antitorque, running suture is placed—the needle takes 0.75mm from the disc and 1.0mm from the periphery, and the knot is buried peripherally. However, it has been established that sutures are not necessary. Various theories of why the cap stays in position have been proposed, which include surface tension, the inherent stickiness of glycoproteins, and the partial relative vacuum of the endothelial cell pump. Without sutures, induced astigmatism is less and the recovery time improves.

Postoperatively, the patient is given mild pain medication and asked to return to the clinic the next day. On this first visit, vision is tested and a slit-lamp examination is performed. The patient is started on a combination corticosteroid antibiotic four times a day for 5 days. The patient is allowed to resume normal activities but is instructed to avoid hits or trauma to the operated eye.

Intraoperative complications include corneal perforation, irregular keratectomy, errors in thickness or diameter, decentered keratectomy, incomplete keratectomy, destruction of the cap, and decentered refractive treatment. Postoperative complications include epithelial growth on the interface, irregular astigmatism, epithelial defect, deposits in the interface, infection, over- and undercorrection, glare, and haze.

Surgical procedures and postoperative care for keratomileusis using manual microkeratomes rather than automated ones are similar except for the setup for particular microkeratomes.

LASER *IN SITU* KERATOMILEUSIS

Experience with planar keratomileusis and the use of the excimer laser in the treatment of mild and moderate myopia resulted in the combination of these two techniques to take advantage of the high corrective capacity of keratomileusis and the excimer laser's precision in tissue removal. The aim was to overcome the technical difficulties associated with the refractive incision of both the cryolathe and the nonfrozen keratomileusis technique and thus to achieve an accurate, reproducible, and predictable surgical result.[13-17]

The excimer laser may be used to ablate corneal tissue from the resected corneal cap or on the corneal bed. The latter is termed laser-assisted *in situ* keratomileusis (LASIK), details of which are given in Chapter 20. The refractive results indicate that this technique may be valuable in the treatment of moderate and mild myopia. As laser software improves, the operation may be of benefit for higher degrees of myopia.

EPIKERATOPLASTY

Epikeratoplasty, or onlay lamellar keratoplasty, for aphakia and myopia is a surgical procedure in which a lens made of human corneal tissue is sutured onto the anterior surface of the cornea to change the anterior curvature, and hence refractive properties, of the cornea (Fig. 19-3). Technically, it demands less and is easier to learn than keratomileusis. Suitable methods of tissue preservation allowed manufacture of the graft lenticule, based on reproducible quality standards, by an off-site commercial firm, which improved the uniformity and quality of the lenticules. In addition, this eliminated the need to lathe at the time of surgery. Epikeratoplasty does not violate the optical zone, so it is partially reversible. Because the lenticule is attached to the host cornea peripherally and superficially, it may be removed easily.

The tissue lens, or lenticule, consists of Bowman's layer and anterior stroma of a donor cornea that has been frozen and lathed. Once the host cornea has been deepithelialized, a small peripheral keratotomy or keratectomy is made to fix the lenticule, held "tongue in groove," into the circumferential keratectomy, the host epithelium gradually covers the surface, and keratocytes slowly repopulate the donor tissue.[13-16,18,19] Although a simpler technique than keratomileusis with freezing, epikeratoplasty demands the surface of the cornea to be normal for its maintenance. The technique is less predictable than keratomileusis with freezing and requires a long time before total visual rehabilitation occurs. A donor cornea is used instead of the host cornea to achieve the correction of a refractive error.

Indications and Contraindications

Epikeratoplasty was performed initially in aphakic patients who were not good candidates for secondary intraocular lens (IOL) implantation.[8,17,20-22] Epikeratoplasty was used later in aphakic pediatric patients.[23-25] Compliance with optical and occlusive therapy is a major problem for the ophthalmologist and family of a unilaterally aphakic child. For such children, epikeratoplasty and secondary IOL implantation are the only alternatives to the abandonment of therapy. Generally, epikeratoplasty is recommended for children over the age of 1 year and is useful for cases of unilateral aphakia for which contact lenses are not possible because of intolerance or socioeconomic conditions that discourage successful contact lens use. Also, it is particularly useful for unilateral traumatic aphakia and may be used if corneal scars are present as long as the visual axis is not involved. In cases of bilateral aphakia for which spectacle therapy has been unsuccessful, epikeratoplasty may be used bilaterally to minimize the risk of amblyopia from optical noncompliance.

Epikeratoplasty for keratoconus was designed to reinforce the cornea and flatten the cone in keratoconus patients intolerant of contact lens wear and who do not have central or paracentral scarring within 1mm of the visual axis.[26-28] Exception may be made for those who have Down syndrome, for whom the advantages of an extraocular procedure may outweigh the disadvantages of a "less than perfect" visual result. Although correction can be attempted for any corneal steepness, some observers found that patients who had cones <60D seemed to benefit more from epikeratoplasty than those who had steeper cones. Vajpayee and Sharma[29] reported a postoperative spectacle-corrected visual acuity of 6/12 or better in 80% of patients using fresh or McCarey-Kaufman preserved, manually dissected donor lenticules. Epikeratoplasty was successfully expanded for other ectatic corneal disorders, such as keratoglobus[30,31] and pellucid marginal degeneration.[32]

Epikeratoplasty for myopia was developed for patients intolerant of spectacles and contact lenses who had severe myopia of up to 30D.[33,34] Its use has declined sharply because of associated problems, such as extended recovery period, unpredictability, instability of correction, and epithelial changes that often mandate removal of the lenticule.

Surgical Technique

DONOR LENTICULE. All epikeratoplasty lenticules used in the original studies were commercially prepared. The corneal tissues were supplied by eye banks and stored in McCarey-Kaufman medium for 4–14 days prior to processing. The donor tissue (Bowman's layer and anterior stroma) is stained with a temporary

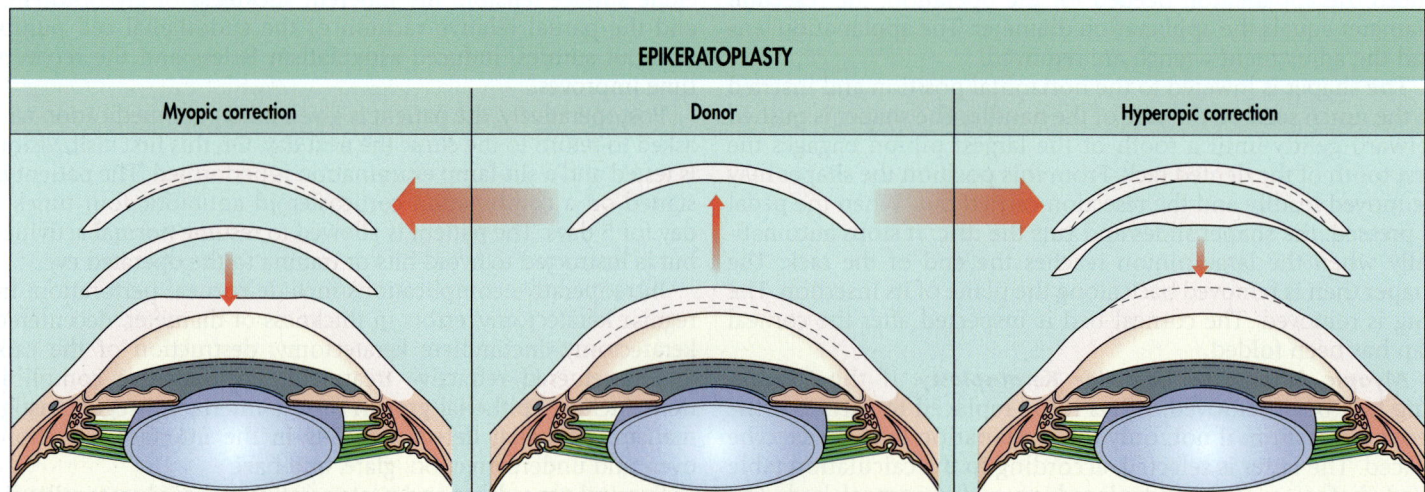

FIG. 19-3 ■ **Epikeratoplasty.** A preshaped donor lenticule is sutured to the recipient stromal bed to correct myopia and hyperopia.

dye to enhance visibility, lyophilized, lathed to a specified power (based upon the patient's spherical equivalent corrected to the corneal plane—with the exception of keratoconus, which was lathed to planopower), placed in a vacuum-sealed container, and shipped to the surgeon within 2 months of the date of manufacture (Fig. 19-4). Several modifications were explored in an attempt to improve epikeratoplasty. Erlich and Nordan[35] developed a nonkeratectomy version of the procedure in which a knife-edged lenticule was slipped into an angled slit made in the peripheral cornea and then sutured. Rostron et al.[36] worked with corneal tissue glues in an attempt to eliminate sutures from the procedure. Goosey et al.[37] reported 20 cases of myopic epikeratoplasty without a keratectomy in an attempt to avoid the astigmatism and scarring associated with the standard techniques. The most recent designs use an 8.5mm donor lenticule for aphakia and myopia and a 9.0mm lenticule for keratoconus.

RECIPIENT PREPARATION. In epikeratoplasty, first the visual axis is marked and the greater part of the corneal epithelium removed, except for a small central area that contains the visual axis mark and a small peripheral cuff.[38] Next, a Hessburg-Barron trephine (7.0mm for aphakia and 8.5mm for keratoconus) is centered on the visual axis and a keratotomy performed to 0.20–0.30mm in depth. After keratotomy, the central epithelium is removed, and an annular keratectomy approximately 0.5mm in diameter is made using Vannas scissors central to and continuous with the keratotomy, which allows fixation of the lenticule and migration of the host keratocytes into the acellular lenticule. After the keratectomy, a spatula is passed peripherally at the level of the base of the keratectomy to create a 360° lamellar pocket approximately 1.0mm peripheral to the initial keratotomy. The precarved lenticule, which has been hydrated in a balanced salt solution enhanced with an antibiotic such as gentamicin 100mg/ml for 20 minutes, is placed on top of Bowman's membrane. For the treatment of aphakia or myopia, the lenticule is sutured into the lamellar pocket. A 0.5mm oversize lenticule is used to flatten the host cornea in the management of keratoconus. However, a 1.5mm oversize graft is optimal for other epikeratoplasty treatments, to eliminate a flattened host cornea and the induction of undesirable refractive changes.

The preferred suture technique is to use 16 uninterrupted 10-0 nylon sutures. Some surgeons have advocated "no-stitch" techniques to reduce some of the problems induced by lenticule suturing.[39] Topical antibiotics (e.g., Polysporin ophthalmic ointment three times a day) are used until reepithelialization is complete.

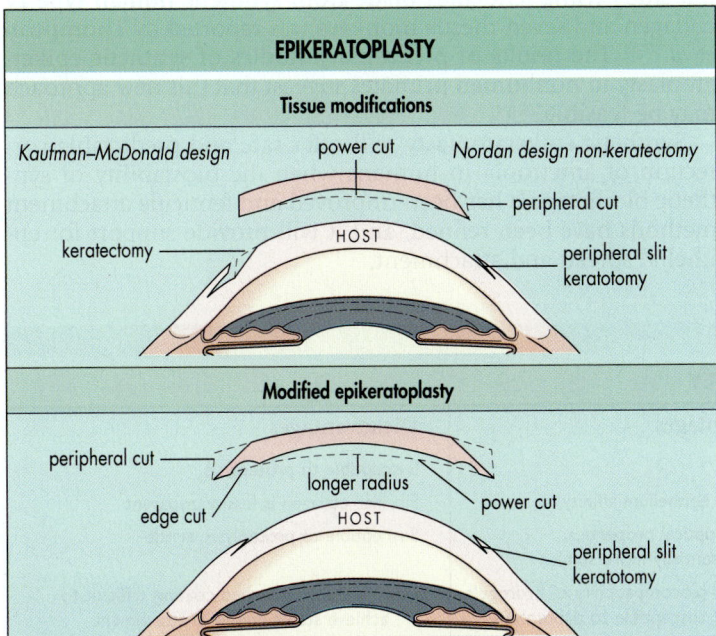

FIG. 19-4 ■ **Epikeratoplasty lens modifications.** The design was modified extensively away from a keratectomy to allow a tapered edge to be inserted into a keratotomy.

Topical corticosteroids (e.g., prednisolone acetate 1% three times a day) are used to prevent premature suture vascularization and loosening, particularly important after epikeratoplasty for keratoconus, in which early loosening and removal of sutures may result in the development of irregular astigmatism.

In uncomplicated cases, all sutures are removed after 2–3 weeks for pediatric aphakia and after 8 weeks for adult aphakia and myopia.[21,40-44] For keratoconus, better results may be obtained if the sutures are retained for 4–6 months.[45] However, vascularized sutures are removed promptly to avoid reduced prognosis or potential future penetrating keratoplasty.

Clinical Results and Complications

In addition to persistent epithelial defects, complications after epikeratoplasty include interface opacification, later interface scarring and opacification, infectious keratitis, sterile ulceration of the lenticule and recipient stroma, steepened recipient cornea, and endothelial changes (attenuation of cells, irregular shape, and decreased density with poor interdigitation). Other major complications of epikeratoplasty for keratoconus include persistent irregular astigmatism caused by premature removal or loosening of sutures and residual myopia.[45] Although secondary refractive procedures such as radial keratotomy[46] or relaxing incisions[47] have produced improvement in some cases, it is often best to proceed to penetrating keratoplasty in situations in which the visual results are suboptimal.[45] In developing countries, where there is a paucity of quality donor material, tissue unsuitable for penetrating keratoplasty because of poor epithelial quality, inadequate endothelial cell count, length of storage time, or other reasons can be used for epikeratoplasty. Vajpayee and Sharma[48] reported a shorter recovering time in epikeratoplasty using fresh, manually dissected corneas instead of cryolathed and lyophilized corneas.

Most large series report an anatomical success of 95% in epikeratoplasties for aphakic adults, with persistent epithelial defects and loss of graft clarity being the major reasons for graft failure. The two major functional limitations are the rate of recovery of best-corrected visual acuity (BCVA) and the relatively poor contrast sensitivity. The anatomical and refractive results for pediatric aphakia are similar to those for adult aphakia.[49-51] Anatomical success may be as high as 95%, and refractive success (within 3D of emmetropia) is achieved in approximately 75% of eyes. Pediatric aphakia remains the lead indication for the use of epikeratoplasty.

For myopic epikeratoplasty, early optimism was tempered by the results of most investigators.[52-54] The major postoperative problem is one of regression of refractive effect, defined as >2D of myopia shift more than 4 months postoperatively. For myopic epikeratoplasty, the procedure is not truly reversible. The recipient cornea may steepen in the range −2.40D[55] to −5.5D after lenticule removal. The low percentage of patients who achieve acceptable levels of uncorrected visual acuity, as well as the resultant poor contrast sensitivity in comparison with other keratorefractive techniques, makes epikeratoplasty a less important tool for the correction of myopia.

SYNTHETIC EPIKERATOPLASTY

Synthetic epikeratoplasty is an investigational procedure in which a biocompatible synthetic lenticule is attached to the anterior surface of a deepithelialized host cornea. Unlike the situation in keratophakia and keratomileusis (which require dissection and removal of a portion of the central cornea and a technically complex lathe procedure that depends on expensive equipment), in epikeratoplasty the need for a keratectomy on the central cornea is eliminated and the refractive correction is accomplished at less cost, with less technical complexity, and with fewer complications. Widespread commercial use of human donor tissue may cause ethical problems, and transmission of infectious agents is a risk. As with keratomileusis, the time for visual recovery is prolonged (many patients require up to 1 year to achieve BCVA). The refractive outcome of epikeratoplasty has poor predictability because of the possible distortions that occur when the lenticule is shaped and placed intraoperatively[56] and of postoperative cellular remodeling.[57] A lower BCVA after epikeratoplasty most commonly results from irregular astigmatism.[58,59]

A synthetic lenticule attached to the cornea may be ablated using an excimer laser system to adjust its optical power and refine the refractive error.[60] Because such ablation affects the acellular lenticule rather than the native recipient cornea, the patient's Bowman's layer may not be violated.

If the synthetic lenticule could be attached directly to Bowman's layer, additional benefits would accrue. Maintenance of an intact Bowman's layer may allow the whole procedure to be reversible. Confinement of the procedure to the area anterior to Bowman's layer would preserve the structural integrity of the cornea and minimize corneal stromal wound healing.[61]

A synthetic material suitable for epikeratoplasty should meet the following requirements:

- Optical clarity
- Support epithelial spreading and attachment
- Permeability to nutrients and metabolites[62]
- Biocompatibility and long-term stability

Two major types of proteolytic enzymes are present in the cornea:

- Collagenases released by keratocytes, which are capable of breaking down native interstitial collagen molecules
- Neutral proteases secreted by both keratocytes and epithelial cells, which break down denatured collagen so that it loses its typical helical structure

To ensure long-term refractive stability, the synthetic lenticule must be capable of withstanding erosion and breakdown caused by natural corneal enzymes.

Potential biomaterials for investigation include pure collagen, collagen synthetic copolymers, coated synthetics, and bioactive synthetics. The advantages and disadvantages for each group are summarized in Table 19-2.

A blown mixture of polypropylene and polybutylene microfibers has been employed to imitate the structure of the extracellular matrix.[63] Although this material does not contain collagen, it may support epithelial migration and attachment to its surface. However, this approach serves as an experimental device, and a suitable bioactive synthetic material still has to be developed.

Excimer Laser Ablation Characteristics

Results of excimer laser photorefractive keratectomy suggest that the excimer laser may be used for the precise ablation of synthetic lenticules. Because the photoablation would be performed in an acellular synthetic lenticule, the haze and collagen remodeling that occurs after photorefractive keratectomy may be avoidable. Therefore, modification of the lenticule surface could be repeated with minimal danger of corneal scarring or regression of the refractive effect.

Preliminary experiments suggest that synthetic biomaterials that contain collagen for epikeratoplasty could be shaped successfully using the excimer laser, to give a smooth surface, reproducible ablation depth, and minimal structural damage of the molecules adjacent to the ablation area.

Attachment of the Synthetic Lenticule to the Cornea

INTRASTROMAL POCKET. Albinet et al.[64] performed a 4mm circular keratotomy and inserted an oversize, synthetic, type IV lenticule (which measured about 7.5mm in diameter) into the corneal pocket created using a trephine and scalpel, but this procedure may induce unpredictable changes to the shape of the lenticule and cornea. For this reason, Waring and Hanna[65] introduced a rotating device derived from the trephine these authors used for penetrating keratoplasty. This instrument can be used to create an angled keratotomy in the cornea to seat a suitably designed synthetic epikeratoplasty lenticule.

LASER WELDING. Laser welding of tissue[66] or synthetic biomaterials[67] to the cornea has proved unsuccessful. Even with the application of adjunct biological solder, a reliable attachment was not achieved. Probably the dense, collagenous matrix of Bowman's layer and the relative paucity of connective tissue prevent a suitable attachment.

BIOLOGICAL ADHESIVES. Attempts to employ biological adhesives were reported by Robin et al.[68] in 1988, and later by Rostron et al.[36] The lenticule failed to epithelialize, presumably because of either the toxicity of the adhesive or the poor edge design of the lenticule. Collagen-based adhesives have been employed successfully in corneal surgery and so may be helpful in the future.

SUTURES. Most of the tested potential biomaterials were found to be unsuitable for suturing because the sutures cut through the lenticules like a cheese wire.

MOLECULAR LINKING. The most desirable attachment technique is that which avoids any damage to Bowman's layer and the corneal stroma. A possible approach for this may be to link the synthetic biomaterial to Bowman's layer molecularly. The biomaterial might be applied in liquid or gel form to the cornea, where it would polymerize and link to the collagen fibers of Bowman's layer. Polymerization and linkage may be supported by adjuvants such as lysyl oxidase or ultraviolet light.

Preliminary Study in the Monkey Eye

To test the feasibility of synthetic epikeratoplasty in vivo, an initial study using lenticules made from synthetic human type IV collagen and seven rhesus monkeys was reported by Thompson et al.[59-61] The results of preliminary studies of synthetic epikeratoplasty in nonhuman primates suggest that this new approach may be feasible.

Synthetic epikeratoplasty will offer safe and predictable correction of ametropia in humans when the biostability of synthetic biomaterials has been improved and lenticule attachment methods have been refined, and it will provide support for epithelial spread and attachment.

TABLE 19-2

POTENTIAL BIOMATERIALS FOR SYNTHETIC EPIKERATOPLASTY

Materials	Examples	Advantages	Disadvantages
Pure collagen	Cross-linked, human Type IV collagen (nonfibrillar)	Clear	Susceptible to proteolysis
	Cross-linked, bovine Type I or III collagen	Strong epithelium affinity	Fibrillar collagen is less transparent
Collagen synthetic copolymers	2-Hydroxyethylmethacrylate–collagen composites	Good optical properties, potentially more stable	Susceptible to proteolysis, brittle
Coated synthetics	Laminin-, fibrin-, or fibronectin-coated 2-hydroxyethylmethacrylate	Proved biocompatibility of hydrogels, not susceptible to proteolysis	Dependent on attached coating; difficult to achieve stable epithelial attachment
Bioactive synthetics	Blown synthetic microfibers	Resistant to proteolysis	Difficult to achieve stable epithelial attachment

Data from Thompson KP, Daniel J. Synthetic epikeratoplasty. In Azar DT. Refractive surgery. Hartford, CT: Appleton & Lange; 1997:405.

OTHER LAMELLAR SURGERIES

The inherent philosophy of lamellar keratoplasty (LK) is to replace only the diseased tissue and leave the remaining cornea intact. The surgery is usually used for tectonic purposes; however, new techniques and technology over the past 25 years have expanded the applications of LK in optical rehabilitation. Instrumentation such as viscoelastics, diamond knives, ultrasonic pachymetry, artificial anterior chambers, advanced microkeratomes, and the excimer laser have enhanced our ability to work more safely in the tedious microsurgical environment of the lamellar procedure. Advances in surgical techniques such as deep lamellar anterior keratoplasty and deep lamellar endothelial keratoplasty have expanded the application of lamellar surgery to endothelial replacement and have achieved visual results approaching those of penetrating keratoplasty while reducing the rate of rejection and improving the long-term graft stability.[69] As research continues, LK promises to be an increasingly important option for the corneal surgeon.

Microkeratome-Assisted Deep Lamellar Keratoplasty with a Hinged Flap

Azar et al.[70] described a technique of deep LK under a hinged host flap in selected patients with considerable corneal stromal disease and normal endothelium. This surgical technique involves performing LK by using a microkeratome to create a hinged anterior corneal flap, resecting or ablating the host stromal abnormalities, and transplanting a complementary donor stromal button (which is prepared using a microkeratome and an artificial anterior chamber). In theory, this approach may be valuable in corneal stromal dystrophies and stromal scarring secondary to traumatic, inflammatory, or infectious causes. It has two potential theoretical advantages: (1) the host epithelium and endothelium are preserved, which may reduce the risk of graft rejection, and (2) the superficial hinged corneal flap may reduce astigmatism and surface irregularities. Furthermore, the hinged corneal flap and preplaced alignment marks may allow improved postoperative reapposition. This may potentially create an optically smoother corneal surface with a reduced incidence of high astigmatism. The flap may be lifted at a later date and an excimer laser used to correct residual refractive errors. In addition, there is a theoretical benefit in dealing with vision-threatening complications, such as expulsive hemorrhage, as the hinged corneal flap can quickly secure the wound with less suturing. Nevertheless, clinical studies are needed to determine whether this technique indeed reduces graft-host interface problems, improves visual outcomes, or is potentially a practical alternative for traditional LK techniques.

Deep Lamellar Keratoplasty with Lyophilized Tissue

Coombes et al.[71] reported a technique of deep LK with lyophilized tissue in the management of keratoconus. Using a 30-gauge needle, air is injected into the corneal stroma, expanding its normal thickness two- to threefold. The recipient area is marked with a trephine and a vertical incision made with a diamond blade. Hydrodissection, with injection of balanced salt solution into the air-expanded central stromal island, is followed by lamellar dissection close to Descemet membrane (DM). Once the bulk of stroma has been removed, if a pre-DM plane has been defined by the air/hydrodissection, it is filled with viscoelastic through a small puncture. This allows the central posterior stromal fibers to be excised with scissors. If no pre-DM cleavage plane is created, lamellar dissection is performed as deeply as possible without perforation. If perforation occurs, because further lamellar resection is difficult, donor tissue is applied to the bed.

The rehydrated donor button is sutured in place with interrupted monofilament sutures (11-0 polyester or 10-0 nylon). Finally, the eyelids are closed with a temporary tarsorrhaphy suture until epithelialization is complete. In mentally ill or handi-

capped patients we use either a botulinum toxin ptosis or a bandage contact lens instead. Topical antibiotic ointment is used until epithelialization, and topical corticosteroid (betamethasone) is tapered over 2–3 months.

Endothelial Replacement without Surface Corneal Incisions or Sutures

The most vexing problem for the corneal surgeon is the unpredictability of corneal topography after penetrating keratoplasty. Currently, two approaches to lamellar replacement of the endothelium are used in the clinical setting. One approach uses the technique first described by Barraquer,[1] in which an anterior corneal flap is formed by a microkeratome to access the deep corneal stroma; the other approach uses a limbal pocket wound to access and replace the deep stromal tissue and endothelium.

In the flap technique, Jones and Culbertson[72] used a microkeratome to create a 480μm thick, 9.5mm diameter hinged flap that was then retracted, and a 7.0mm diameter trephine was used to resect the recipient stroma. A slightly larger 7.2mm diameter donor button was then sutured into place, the flap repositioned, and the flap also sutured into place. Busin et al.[73] have modified this technique and reported clinical results for six patients, and Azar[74] reported the results of the first patient treated with this approach. The flap approach to endothelial replacement has the distinct advantage of automated access to the middle and deep stroma and the creation of a possibly smoother interface than with manual dissection. Also, the techniques of trephination and transplantation with suturing of the donor posterior button are familiar territory to the corneal surgeon, and this approach gives easy access to other intraocular work, such as lens exchange, vitrectomy, and iridoplasty. However, the significant disadvantage of this approach is the use of sutures in the corneal tissue for the donor button and the surface flap. The compressive "donut" effect on the sutured edge of the donor-recipient interface would initially be transmitted from the interface to the surface of the flap. Also, the macrostriae and microstriae induced by peripheral flap sutures are well known to LASIK surgeons, and the flap created by this procedure would not be exempt from the same compressive forces. Finally, the loss of epithelium from the surface of the flap during its relatively prolonged retraction time increases the risk of infection, ulceration, and epithelial ingrowth into the interface. Whether the advantages of this automated approach outweigh the disadvantages of suturing with this technique remains to be seen.

REFERENCES

1. Barraquer JI. Special methods in corneal surgery. In: King JHJ, McTigue JW, eds. The cornea. Washington: Butterworths; 1965.
2. Barraquer JI. Keratomileusis for myopia and aphakia. Ophthalmology. 1981; 88:701–8.
3. Troutman RC, Swinger CA, Kelly RJ. Keratophakia: a preliminary evaluation. Ophthalmology. 1979;86:523–33.
4. Troutman RC, Swinger C. Refractive keratoplasty: keratophakia and keratomileusis. Trans Am Ophthalmol Soc. 1978;76:329–39.
5. Swinger CA, Barker BA. Prospective evaluation of myopic keratomileusis. Ophthalmology 1984;91:785–92.
6. Nordan LT: Keratomileusis. Int Ophthalmol Clin. 1991;31:7–12.
7. Kaufman HE. The correction of aphakia. Am J Ophthalmol. 1980;89:1–10.
8. Krumeich JH. Indications, techniques, and complications of myopic keratomileusis. Int Ophthalmol Clin. 1983;23:75–92.
9. Walsh PM, Guyton DL. Comparison of two methods of marking the visual axis on the cornea during radial keratotomy [letter]. Am J Ophthalmol. 1984;97:660–1.
10. Waring GO III. Refractive keratotomy for myopia and astigmatism. St Louis: Mosby-Year Book; 1992:721–74.
11. Steinberg EB, Waring GO III. Comparison of two methods of marking the visual axis on the cornea during radial keratotomy. Am J Ophthalmol. 1983;96:605–8.
12. Binder PS, Akers PH, Deg JK, Kavala EY. Refractive keratoplasty, microkeratome evaluation. Arch Ophthalmol. 1982;100:802–6.
13. Barraquer JI. Modification of refraction by means of intracorneal inclusions. Int Ophthalmol Clin. 1966;6:53–78.
14. Rich LF, Friedlander MH, Kaufman HE, et al. Keratocyte survival in keratophakia lenticules. Arch Ophthalmol. 1981;99:677–80.
15. Baumgartner SD, Binder PS. Refractive keratoplasty. Histopathology of clinical specimens. Ophthalmology. 1985;92:1606–15.
16. Samples JR, Binder PS, Zavala EY, et al. Epikeratophakia: clinical evaluation and histopathology of a non-human primate model. Cornea. 1984;3:51–60.

17. Binder PS, Zavala EY, Baumgartner SD, *et al.* Combined morphological effects of cryolathing and lyophilization on epikeratoplasty lenticules. Arch Ophthalmol. 1986;104:671–9.
18. Jaeger MJ, Berson P, Kaufman HE, Green WR. Epikeratoplasty for keratoconus: a clinicopathologic case report. Cornea. 1987;6:131–9.
19. Werblin TP, Kaufman HE, Friedlander MH, Granet N. Epikeratophakia: the surgical correction of aphakia. III. Preliminary results of a prospective clinical trial. Arch Ophthalmol. 1981;99:1957–60.
20. Werblin TP, Kaufman HE, Friedlander MH, *et al.* A prospective study of the use of hyperopic epikeratophakia grafts for the correction of aphakia in adults. Ophthalmology. 1981;88:1137–40.
21. Werblin TP, Kaufman HE, Friedlander MH, *et al.* Epikeratophakia: the surgical correction of aphakia. Update: 1981. Ophthalmology. 1982;89:916–20.
22. McDonald MB, Koenig SB, Safir A, *et al.* Epikeratophakia: the surgical correction of aphakia. Update: 1982. Ophthalmology. 1983;90:668–72.
23. Morgan KS, Werblin TP, Asbell PA, *et al.* The use of epikeratophakia grafts in pediatric monocular aphakia. J Pediatr Ophthalmol Strabismus. 1981;18:23–9.
24. Morgan KS, Asbell PA, McDonald MB, *et al.* Preliminary visual results of pediatric epikeratophakia. Arch Ophthalmol. 1983;101:1540–4.
25. Morgan KS, Stephenson GS, McDonald MB, Kaufman HE. Epikeratophakia in children. Ophthalmology. 1984;91:780–4.
26. Kaufman HE, Werblin TP. Epikeratophakia for the treatment of keratoconus. Am J Ophthalmol. 1982;93:342–7.
27. McDonald MB, Koenig SB, Safir A, Kaufman HE. Onlay lamellar keratoplasty for the treatment of keratoconus. Br J Ophthalmol. 1983;67:615–8.
28. McDonald MB, Safir A, Waring GO, *et al.* A preliminary comparative study of epikeratophakia or penetrating keratoplasty for keratoconus. Am J Ophthalmol. 1987;103:467.
29. Vajpayee RB, Sharma N. Epikeratoplasty for keratoconus using manually dissected fresh lenticules: 4-year follow-up. J Refract Surg. 1997;13:659–62.
30. Cameron JA. Epikeratoplasty for keratoglobus associated with blue sclera. Ophthalmology. 1991;98:446–52.
31. Cameron JA. Keratoglobus. Cornea. 1993;12:124–30.
32. Fronterre A, Portesani GP. Epikeratoplasty for pellucid marginal degeneration. Cornea. 1991;10:450–3.
33. Werblin TP, Klyce SD. Epikeratophakia. The surgical correction of myopia. I. Lathing of corneal tissue. Curr Eye Res. 1981;1:591–9.
34. McDonald MB, Klyce SD, Suarez H, *et al.* Epikeratophakia for myopia correction. Ophthalmology. 1985;92:1417–22.
35. Erlich MI, Nordan LT. Epikeratophakia for the treatment of hyperopia. J Cataract Refract Surg. 1989;15:661–666.
36. Rostron CK, Brittain PH, Morton DB, Roes JE. Experimental epikeratophakia with biological adhesive. Arch Ophthalmol. 1988;106:1103–6.
37. Goosey JD, Prager RC, Marvelli TL, *et al.* Epikeratophakia without annular keratectomy. Ann Ophthalmol. 1987;19:388–91.
38. Swinger CA. Surgical correction of myopia. In: Cornea, refractive surgery, and contact lenses. Transactions of the New Orleans Academy of Ophthalmology. New York: Raven Press; 1986.
39. Cotter JB. No-stitch aphakic epikeratoplasty. Refract Corneal Surg. 1992;8:27–32.
40. McDonald MB, Kaufman HE, Durrie DS, *et al.* Epikeratophakia for keratoconus: the nationwide study. Arch Ophthalmol. 1986;104:1294–300.
41. McDonald MB, Kaufman HE, Aquavella JV, *et al.* The nationwide study of epikeratophakia for aphakia in adults. Am J Ophthalmol. 1987;103:358–65.
42. McDonald MB, Kaufman HE, Aquavella JV, *et al.* The nationwide study of epikeratophakia for myopia. Am J Ophthalmol. 1987;103:375–83.
43. Morgan KS, McDonald MB, Hiles DA, *et al.* The nationwide study of epikeratophakia for aphakia in children. Am J Ophthalmol. 1987;103:366–74.
44. Morgan KS, McDonald MB, Hiles DA, *et al.* The nationwide study of epikeratophakia for aphakia in older children. Am J Ophthalmol. 1988;95:526–31.
45. Steinert RF, Wagoner MD. Long term comparison of epikeratoplasty and penetrating keratoplasty for keratoconus. Arch Ophthalmol. 1988;106:493–6.
46. Casebeer JC, Shapiro DR. Radio keratotomy in intact epikeratoplasty graft. Refract Corneal Surg. 1993;9:133–4.
47. Fronterre A, Portesani GP. Relaxing incisions with compression sutures to reduce astigmatism after epikeratoplasty. Refract Corneal Surg. 1990;6:413–17.
48. Vajpayee RB, Sharma N. Epikeratoplasty for keratoconus using manually dissected fresh lenticules: 4-year follow-up. J Refract Surg 1997;13:659–62.
49. Werblin TP, Pieffer RL, Patel AS. Synthetic keratophakia for the correction of aphakia. Ophthalmology. 1987;94:926–34.
50. Arffa RC, Marvelli TL, Morgan KS. Keratometric and refractive results of pediatric epikeratophakia. Arch Ophthalmol. 1985;103:1656–9.
51. Cheng KP, Hiles DA, Belgian AW, *et al.* Risk factors for complications following epikeratoplasty. J Cataract Refract Surg. 1992;18:270–9.
52. Choi YS, Choi SK. Trephination with a vacuum trephine in under correction of myopic epikeratoplasty. Korean J Ophthalmol. 1993;7:16–19.
53. Colin J, Sangiuolo B, Malet F, Volant A. Photorefractive keratectomy following undercorrected myopic epikeratoplasties. J Fr Ophtalmol. 1992;15:384–8.
54. Teichman KD. Combining epikeratoplasty and photorefractive keratectomy. J Cataract Refract Surg. 1991;17:867.
55. Nirankari VS. Corneal steepening after epikeratoplasty. Cornea. 1989;8:240–6.
56. Barrett C, Moore MB. A new method of lathing corneal lenticules for keratorefractive procedures. J Refract Surg. 1988;4:142–7.
57. Grabner C. Complications of epikeratophakia for the correction of phakia, myopia, hyperopia and keratoconus. Fortschr Ophthalmol. 1991;8:4–11.
58. McDonald MB. The future direction of refractive surgery. Refract Corneal Surg. 1988;4:158–67.
59. Thompson KP, Hanna KD, Gipson IK, *et al.* Synthetic epikeratoplasty in rhesus monkeys with human type IV collagen. Cornea. 1993;12:35–45.
60. Thompson KP, Hanna K, Waring GO, *et al.* Current status of synthetic epikeratoplasty. Refract Corneal Surg. 1991;7:240–8.
61. Thompson KP. Will the excimer laser resolve the unsolved problems with refractive surgery? Refract Corneal Surg. 1990;6:315–17.
62. Kim JH, Green K, Martinez, Paton U. Solute permeability of the corneal endothelium and Descemet's membrane. Exp Eye Res. 1971;12:231–8.
63. Trinkhaus-Randall V, Capecchi J, Sanmon L, *et al.* In vitro evaluation of fibroplasia in a porous polymer. Invest Ophthalmol Vis Sci. 1990;31:1321–6.
64. Albinet P, Romanet JH, Motrin M, *et al.* Epikeratoplastic sans suture ava lentille de collagene IV chez le singe: description de la technique chirurgicale. J Fr Ophtalmol. 1990;13:109–14.
65. Waring GP, Hanna KD. The Hanna suction punch block and trephine system for penetrating keratoplasty. Arch Ophthalmol. 1989:107:1536–9.
66. Keates RH, Fried S, Levy SN, Morris JR. Carbon dioxide laser use in wound healing and epikeratophakia. J Cataract Refract Surg. 1987;13:290–5.
67. Gailitis RF, Thomson KP, Ken QR, *et al.* Laser welding of synthetic epikeratoplasty lenticules to the cornea. Refract Corneal Surg. 1990;6:430–6.
68. Robin JB, Picciano P, Kusleika RS, *et al.* Preliminary evaluation of the use of mussel adhesive protein in experimental epikeratoplasty. Arch Ophthalmol. 1988;106:973–7.
69. Terry M. The evolution of lamellar grafting techniques over 25 years. Cornea. 2000;19:611–6.
70. Azar DT, Jain S, Sambursky R. A new surgical technique of microkeratome-assisted deep lamellar keratoplasty with a hinged flap. Arch Ophthalmol. 2000;118:1112–5.
71. Coombes AG, Kirwan JF, Rostron CK. Deep lamellar keratoplasty with lyophilised tissue in the management of keratoconus. Br J Ophthalmol. 2001;85:788–91.
72. Jones DT, Culbertson WW. Endothelial lamellar keratoplasty. Inrest Opthalmol Vis Sci 1998;39:576.
73. Busin M, Arffa RC, Sebastiani A: Endokeratoplasty as an alternative to penetrating keratoplasty for the surgical treatment of diseased endothelium. Ophthalmol 2000,107:2077–2082.
74. Azar DT, Jain S, Sambursky R, Strauss L. Microkeratome-assisted posterior keratoplasty. J Cataract Refract Surg 2001,27:353–356.

20 LASIK: Indications and Techniques

JOHN F. DOANE • STEPHEN G. SLADE

DEFINITION
- LASIK stands for laser *in situ* keratomileusis, in which an anterior flap of cornea is lifted with a keratome and an excimer laser is used to sculpt the stromal bed to change the refractive error of the eye.

KEY FEATURES
- LASIK is the most commonly used corneal refractive procedure.
- It can be used to treat wide ranges of refractive error.
- Laser sculpting can be used to treat near- and farsightedness and astigmatism.
- It can be used in conjunction with other refractive techniques for extremely large ametropia.
- In the near future, LASIK may be used to provide improved lines of acuity postoperatively.

ASSOCIATED FEATURES
- As in other corneal refractive surgeries, LASIK complications can result in a loss of best spectacle-corrected vision.
- Most complications can be managed to preserve vision.
- LASIK continues to evolve with improvements in technology and understanding.

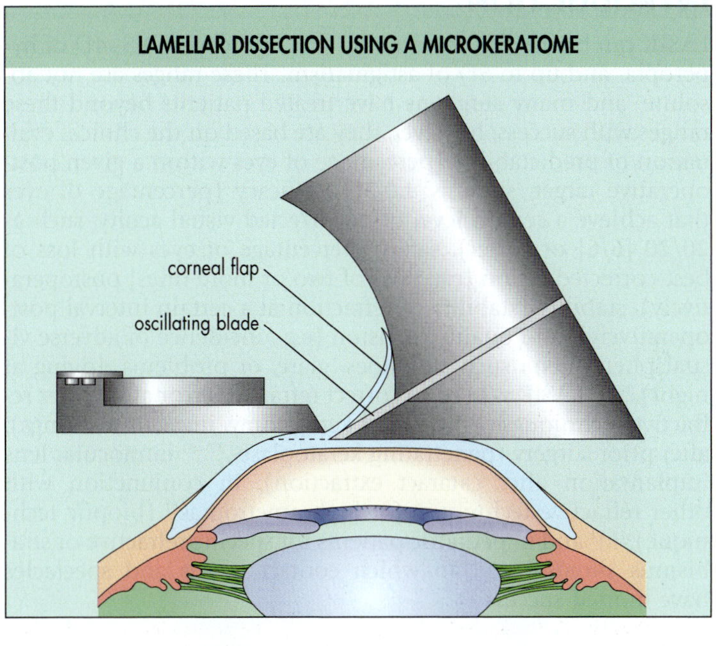

LAMELLAR DISSECTION USING A MICROKERATOME

corneal flap

oscillating blade

FIG. 20-1 ‖ **Lamellar dissection using a microkeratome.** The corneal flap is created by applanation of the cornea, which is carved in a similar fashion to using a carpenter's plane.

INTRODUCTION

Refractive lamellar corneal surgery has been used to correct myopia and hyperopia for more than 40 years, and for the majority of that time, it has been performed by relatively few centers.[1-5] Conceptually, refractive lamellar corneal surgery attempts to remove, add, or modify the corneal stroma so that the radius of curvature of the tear film–anterior corneal interface is altered as desired. Laser *in situ* keratomileusis (LASIK) has gained increasing popularity since 1995. Benefits of lamellar refractive surgery include:

- Ability to treat a large range of refractive error effectively.
- Relatively short visual rehabilitation period postoperatively.
- Relatively pain-free experience for patients.
- Less intense healing response, compared with other modalities.[6-11]

Disadvantages of lamellar surgery include the risk of serious side effects, a large capital outlay, and the technical expertise required to perform an acceptable lamellar keratectomy. Clinical outcomes of efficacy, predictability, safety, and stability for lamellar refractive surgery are available from numerous sources.[12-16]

HISTORICAL REVIEW

Corneal lamellar refractive keratoplasty has its roots in the work of Professor Jose Ignacio Barraquer, beginning in 1949 in Bogota, Colombia.[1,3-5] Barraquer developed myopic keratomileusis,

which used a cryolathe to shape the cornea and alter its refractive power. The term *keratomileusis* is derived from the Greek roots *keras* ("horn-like," referring to the cornea) and *smileusis* ("carving").[2] The main difficulties with myopic keratomileusis were the training and experience required to perform the keratectomy effectively and the complexity of managing the cryolathe. When a manual keratome is driven across the eye by hand, the thickness and evenness of the keratectomy are intimately dependent on the speed of the passage (Fig. 20-1). Any irregularity in this cut results in irregular astigmatism for the patient and a subsequent decrease in best-corrected vision.[2,12-16] Complications specific to myopic keratomileusis and lamellar keratoplasty include epithelial ingrowth in the stromal interface and induction of irregular astigmatism.[2,12-16] Good results were obtained initially by several investigators; however, the technique proved too difficult to master for a large number of surgeons.[13,14]

The concept that the corneal cap can be raised and central tissue removed from the bed, keratomileusis *in situ*, was first described by Krwawicz[17] in 1964 and subsequently by Pureskin[18] in 1967. Dr. Luis Antonio Ruiz, in Bogota, developed a microkeratome with gears that advanced the instrument across a geared track with an adjustable-height suction ring; this system made the automated lamellar keratoplasty (ALK) technique possible. This motorized advancement of the microkeratome allowed a constant-velocity passage that resulted in the resection of a lamellar disc of tissue of even thickness and a smoother corneal stromal bed. This substantial instrumentation breakthrough made lamellar corneal surgery more appealing to a larger number of surgeons.

Several reports that revealed relatively poor predictability, central haze, and regression with photorefractive keratectomy (PRK) for moderate myopia (−3 to −6D) and even more so for high myopia (>−6D),[6–11,19–25] along with the relatively wide predictability range and safety concerns for myopic ALK and keratomileusis *in situ*,[26,27] prompted researchers to substitute lasers for the keratome in the refractive correction step of the myopic ALK procedure.[28–36]

LASER *IN SITU* KERATOMILEUSIS (LASIK)

INTRODUCTION

LASIK can be used to correct 0.5–12D of myopia, 0.5–4D of hyperopia, and up to 8D of astigmatism. These ranges are not absolute, and many surgeons have treated patients beyond these ranges with success; however, they are based on the clinical evaluation of predictability (percentage of eyes within a given postoperative target, such as ±0.5D), efficacy (percentage of eyes that achieve a certain level of uncorrected visual acuity, such as 20/20 [6/6] or better), safety (percentage of eyes with loss of best-corrected vision [e.g., loss of two or more lines] postoperatively), stability (stability of refraction at a certain interval postoperatively), and quality of vision (e.g., incidence of adverse visual phenomena such as haloes, glare, or problems driving at night).[28–36] LASIK is used to correct refractive error after other refractive techniques (PRK, radial keratotomy, intracorneal rings), after prior surgery (penetrating keratoplasty,[37–40] intraocular lens implantation after cataract extraction), in conjunction with other refractive techniques for high ametropias[41] (bioptic technique),[42,43] and in pediatric patients for specific refractive or strabismus situations[44,45] in which contact lenses and spectacles have limited success.

PREOPERATIVE EVALUATION AND DIAGNOSTIC APPROACH

The minimum age for LASIK is typically 18 years. The exception to this is the few investigations of LASIK in the pediatric population as noted earlier. More important than age is the refraction stability of the patient, because this is one component of the long-term stability of the attempted correction. All patients are evaluated and selected for LASIK on the basis of how successful the outcome may be in comparison to that using other refractive surgical procedures such as radial keratotomy (rarely used as of mid-2003), PRK, or laser subepithelial keratectomy (LASEK). Last, patient education, evaluation of the patient's postoperative expectations, and informed consent must be addressed.

Prospective candidates for LASIK should undergo a complete ocular examination, which includes visual acuity testing, refraction, computerized videokeratography, wave front analysis if available, slit-lamp examination, retinal evaluation, eye dominance testing, and evaluation for monovision when appropriate. Patients who have keratoconus or active corneal or ocular disease or those who are pregnant or lactating should not undergo LASIK. A history of recurrent erosion syndrome is considered a relative contraindication, because an epithelial defect can occur during the keratectomy and lead to poor flap adhesion, with subsequent epithelial ingrowth and flap melting. Anterior basement membrane dystrophy can be treated by débridement to achieve acceptable basement membrane complex adhesion before LASIK, with successful results.

The refraction of the eye must be obtained. Manifest refraction, using the duochrome test and fogging techniques, and cycloplegic refraction can be utilized. The refraction is compared with prior spectacle corrections to assess the stability of refraction for the given eye. In addition, the wave front refraction can be a standard for comparison, and with the advent of custom laser vision correction, it may be the basis for the actual ablation. For patients who wear contact lenses, the lenses should be discontinued to allow the cornea to stabilize. Soft lenses should be removed at least 3 days prior to examination, and hard lenses at least 3 weeks. For those who wear rigid contact lenses, at least two examinations 3 days apart are obtained. A difference of 0.25D or less in refraction validates stability. Astigmatism is evaluated using refraction, keratometry, and videokeratography. The axis of the astigmatism noted on refraction should correlate with that found on keratometry and videokeratography and should be compared with the wave front refraction. If they do not correlate, lenticular and posterior corneal astigmatism must be considered, and clinical discretion should be used regarding treatment or nontreatment of the astigmatism.

Central corneal thickness is evaluated to assess the safe limits of corneal stromal removal. With each procedure, three central corneal measurements must be considered—flap thickness, depth of the ablation, and residual thickness of the stromal bed after the ablation. Clinical experience has shown that a flap 160μm thick affords sufficient safety, as it minimizes induced irregular astigmatism from too thin a flap. A thin stromal bed (<250μm) is postulated to have a greater likelihood of central ectasia, with unstable refraction status in the long term. The recommended maximal amount of tissue removal for a given eye can be calculated by subtracting the cap thickness and the suggested residual stromal bed thickness from the central pachymetry reading. For example, if the preoperative central corneal reading is 560μm and a 160μm flap is created, the preablation stromal bed measures 400μm, of which 150μm can be ablated to maintain a 250μm stromal bed. With 150μm of tissue removal, 12D of myopia reduction is expected, based on a 6mm maximal single ablation zone and assuming 14μm of tissue removal per diopter. Nevertheless, if the preoperative central corneal thickness is thinner and the ablation does not proceed beyond the stated 250μm stromal bed, less refractive error can be corrected to maintain long-term corneal stability.

As mentioned previously, 12–15D of myopic correction may be obtained with a single 6mm ablation zone. Multizone ablation has been used as an alternative to correct larger amounts of refractive error, since less tissue is removed than in single-zone ablation, but the overall optical zone is smaller, and scotopic vision may be compromised if the scotopic pupil is significantly larger than the optical zone of the ablation. When the astigmatic ablation is planned, the axis, magnitude, and impact of the cylinder correction on the spherical component must be taken into consideration. Most lasers tend to induce a given amount of hyperopic shift for each diopter of cylinder ablated (typically 0.2D of spherical hyperopic shift per diopter of cylinder treated) when the laser is operating in pure cylinder format, which must be considered when the spherical component of the treatment is planned. In LASIK, as with PRK and LASEK, the surgeon must formulate a personal nomogram. Lasers come with algorithms for the treatment of a specific refractive error, but clinical experience has shown that surgical technique, room conditions (humidity, temperature, air particulate matter), and laser components (quality of optics, gas mixture) directly impact the refractive result. The laser algorithm does not vary with any of these factors, but the nomogram formulated by the surgeon accounts for all these variables.

ANESTHESIA

In most cases, oral sedation with diazepam 5–10mg approximately 45 minutes before the procedure is advisable. The patient should be relaxed for the procedure but not overly sedated, because patient cooperation is necessary for proper fixation. Before the laser suite is entered, standard surgical skin preparation of the eyelids using an iodine-based solution is carried out. The patient is positioned under the laser in a supine position with the frontal surface of the cornea perpendicular to the laser beam aperture. One to two drops of a mild topical anesthetic, such as proparacaine, are instilled. The eyelashes are dried using a gauze sponge, and a fenestrated drape is placed to keep the lashes out of the surgical field. An eyelid speculum that affords maximal corneal exposure is then placed. No preoperative miotic is used.

SPECIFIC TECHNIQUES

Before preparation and draping of the patient in sterile fashion, the conjunctival cul-de-sacs are irrigated to remove debris and eyelid glandular secretions. It is important during the draping to create a clear path for microkeratome passage. Topical anesthetic is instilled in the eye.

Instrument Setup

The surgical success of LASIK requires proper cleaning, assembly, and testing of the microkeratome and accurate calibration and setup of the laser. To ensure that each member of the surgical team is responsible for every aspect of the procedure, each one carries out multiple checks along the way. Appropriate humidity, temperature, and air purification must be present in the laser room at all times. The laser is turned on and calibrated in accordance with the manufacturer's recommendations. Importantly, the laser cutting rate, or fluence, and the beam quality, or homogeneity, must meet acceptable operation standards.

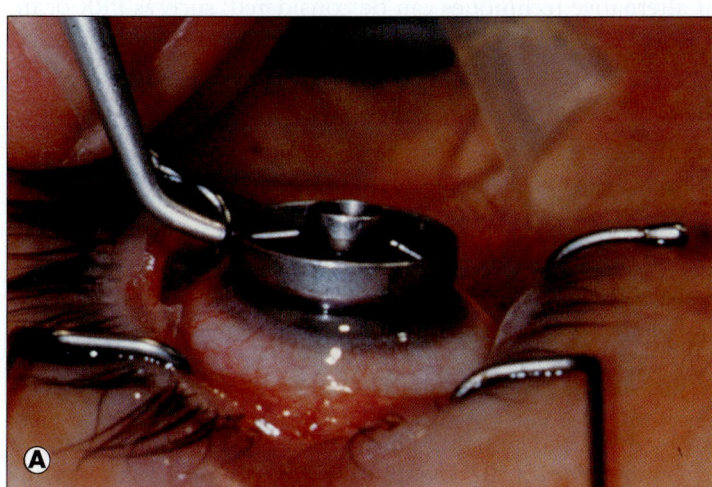
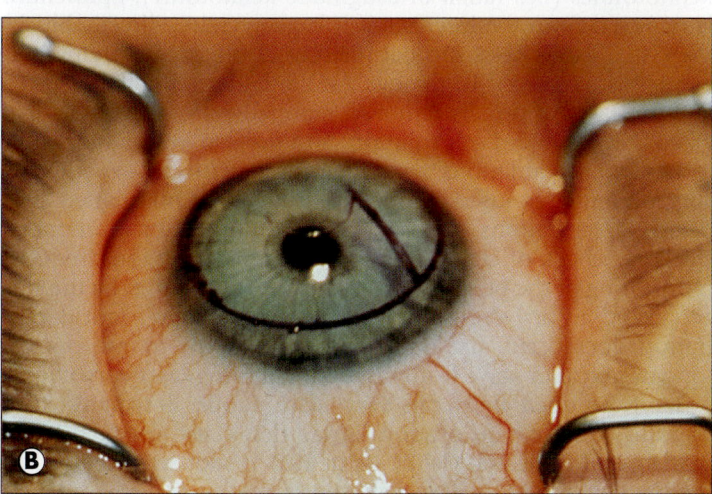

FIG. 20-2 ■ A Ruiz marker is impregnated with ink. **A,** It is used to outline a pararadial mark to enable orientation of the flap. **B,** A 9mm optical zone is outlined to help with proper placement of the suction ring.

Keratectomy

After the lid speculum has been placed, the corneal epithelium is marked with a commercially available lamellar surgery marker. The patient is instructed to look at the microscope light, and an inked marker is used to delineate the optical center, the orientation of the flap via a pararadial line, and a 9mm optical zone circle to center the circular suction ring (Fig. 20-2). A spacer device or depth plate (typically 130, 160, or 180μm) determines the thickness of the cut, and a microkeratome head of specified thickness can be preselected. The LASIK pneumatic suction ring is then placed onto the eye. The LASIK ring serves three useful functions—globe fixation, elevation of intraocular pressure (IOP) to create an even-thickness keratectomy, and provision of a geared track for advancement of the geared microkeratome head. After a vacuum to the pneumatic suction ring has been activated, and before passage of the microkeratome, the surgeon must verify that the IOP is sufficient (>65mmHg [8.6kPa]). This is achieved with a pneumotonometer or the Barraquer tonometer. Once an adequately high IOP is obtained, the corneal surface is irrigated with topical anesthetic solution to minimize epithelium disruption as the microkeratome is passed. The microkeratome is loaded into the dovetailed grooves on the suction ring and advanced (by activation of the surgeon-controlled foot pedal) to the stopper mechanism to create a hinge in the flap and then reversed. The vacuum is discontinued, and the LASIK suction ring is removed. As an alternative, femtosecond lasers are being developed to create the flap with focused laser energy instead of mechanical microkeratomes.[46]

Laser Ablation

Before lifting the flap and beginning the ablation, the surgeon and staff confirm that the laser settings are correct and position the patient's head so that the corneal surface is perpendicular to the ablation beam. The flap is lifted and folded out of the ablation field, the ablation is centered over the entrance pupil, and the active eye tracker is engaged (Fig. 20-3). As the ablation proceeds, the centration is monitored carefully. During the ablation, fluid can accumulate on the corneal surface and should be wiped dry with a single pass of a sponge or blunt spatula. As the ablation proceeds to the largest-diameter treatment zones, the corneal hinge is covered with a blunt instrument to prevent ablation of the back surface of the corneal flap.

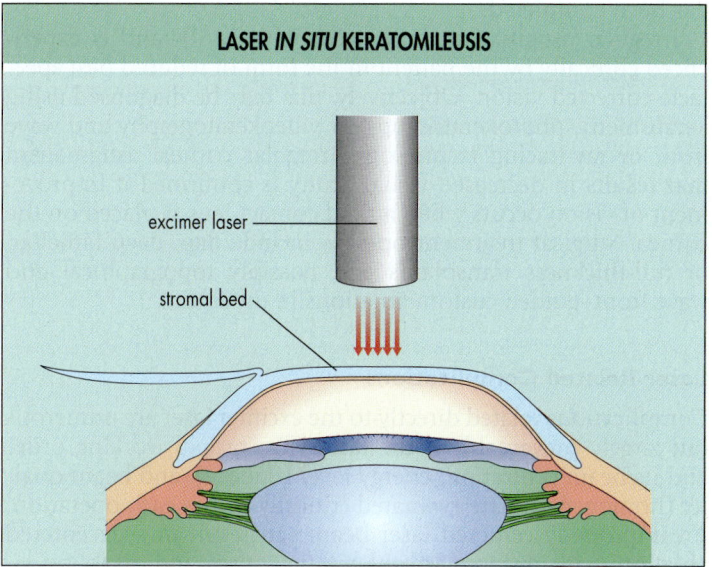

FIG. 20-3 ■ **Laser *in situ* keratomileusis.** Excimer laser ablation to the stromal bed after lamellar keratectomy.

Flap Repositioning

When the ablation is completed, the backside of the flap and the stromal bed are irrigated with balanced salt solution using a syringe and cannula. The flap is then positioned back onto the stromal bed using a blunt-tipped instrument. The cannula is placed underneath the flap, and irrigation is completed to clear any remaining debris from the interface. To confirm that the flap is in the proper position, an inspection is made to ensure that an equal gutter–keratectomy edge distance is present throughout the circumference. The interface is allowed to dry for 2–3 minutes. A stria test is completed by depressing the peripheral cornea using closed blunt-tipped forceps. When striae pass well into the flap for 360°, appropriate apposition has been achieved.

At this point, the procedure is completed by careful removal of the speculum and drape. The eye is re-examined to make certain the flap is in the proper position. Immediately after surgery, one drop of antibiotic and nonsteroidal anti-inflammatory agent is instilled. A shield is placed over the orbit, but no pressure patch is applied.

AVOIDANCE OF COMPLICATIONS

Although lamellar surgery techniques appear to be devoid of the complications associated with intraocular surgery,[47–57] they are dependent on the use of the microkeratome and a complete understanding of the excimer laser. Postoperative visual complications for lamellar surgery are analogous to those seen in many corneal procedures, such as glare, haloes, and decreased contrast sensitivity. Unusual complications such as vascular occlusion, macular hemorrhage, perforated globe, and microbial infection can also occur in association with these techniques, including LASIK.[58–67]

Microkeratome-Related Complications

Lamellar corneal surgery builds on the success of the previous steps in the operative sequence, so the quality of the keratectomy is the basis for a successful LASIK technique. Interruption of the movement or suction during resection can result in irregular resection and may necessitate abortion of the procedure. In this circumstance, the flap is repositioned and left to heal, in which case the patient does not experience any permanent impairment in vision. Reoperation 3 months later may be performed.

A free cap should not present a major problem for the patient or the surgeon. If an adequate diameter is achieved, it is appropriate to complete the ablation. During the ablation, the free cap should be placed in an antidesiccation chamber and replaced over the stromal bed in the proper orientation after the ablation has been completed.

Irregular astigmatism may occur with LASIK and is experienced clinically by the patient in the form of reduced best spectacle-corrected vision. Objectively, this may be diagnosed using keratometry, photokeratoscopy, or videokeratography and wave front or ray-tracing technology. Irregular corneal astigmatism that results in decreased visual acuity is confirmed if improvement of vision occurs when a rigid contact lens is placed on the cornea. Surgical treatment options include flap, deep lamellar, or full-thickness transplants and possibly topographical and wave front–guided custom ablations in the future.

Laser-Related Complications

Complications related directly to the excimer laser are numerous but largely preventable if the laser is in proper working order and its beam centration, energy level (fluence), and beam quality (homogeneity) are evaluated critically before each operation. An improperly centered laser beam can result in a decentered ablation, with induced irregular astigmatism and disabling visual side effects. Proper fluence can avoid over- and undercorrections, and good homogeneity can prevent an irregular ablation with associated irregular astigmatism and visual side effects.

Central islands can occur with LASIK when large-area ablation lasers are used. For the most part, however, they have become a thing of the past with the advent of scanning lasers. Such islands may be diagnosed by videokeratography, and the clinical significance depends largely on patient complaints. The use of scanning lasers largely avoids the central island phenomenon. The vast majority of central islands regress with time, so expectant observation is the typical management recommendation.[68]

Primary overcorrections of myopia are infrequent when an experienced surgeon uses LASIK and a tested nomogram. Refractions tend to regress over the first 1–3 months with LASIK, so the vast majority of early overcorrections are "on target" at the 3-month postoperative examination. If the overcorrection persists, videokeratography and pachymetry are checked and compared with preoperative values. The surgical record and laser parameters are checked to make certain that typing or data-entry errors are not the cause. If the overcorrection is disabling, the best surgical option is a hyperopic LASIK completed no sooner than at the 3-month postoperative visit.

Undercorrections are not uncommon, and the necessity for further treatment often depends on the patient's requirement for best unaided visual acuity. The patient record and laser treatment parameters are evaluated to rule out error. Before retreatment, the refraction should be stable (the overwhelming majority of patients are stable by 3 months), and videokeratography is used to rule out a central island with residual myopia or abnormal ablation pattern. Reoperation can be accomplished by lifting the flap several months or even years after the initial operation. The same nomogram as used for the initial procedure may be used in the retreatment. In cases in which insufficient stromal bed tissue remains for additional laser vision correction enhancements, ablation can be performed on the back of the flap[69] or alternative techniques can be considered, such as PRK or intracorneal rings.

Intraoperative Complications

Complications that may be attributed directly to the surgeon's technique include lamellar interface contamination, decentration of the ablation, and improper position of the keratectomy flap.

Several contaminants may come to rest in the lamellar interface during the procedure (e.g., talc, fibers, blood from micropannus, stainless steel fragments from the blade of the microkeratome, tear film secretions). Interestingly, most of these contaminants are of no visual consequence but are esthetically displeasing to observe at the slit lamp.

Epithelial cyst and ingrowth are a different matter and may occur by direct implantation during the procedure or, more likely, by ingrowth from the keratectomy edge or previously existing keratotomies (i.e., radial or astigmatic keratotomy). Epithelium is removed from the interface if it is progressive, directly blocks the visual axis, causes stromal melting of the flap, or induces irregular astigmatism. To remove the epithelium, the flap is lifted and the layer of cells is removed manually, the interface is irrigated with balanced salt solution, and the flap is replaced.[70]

Decentered ablations are uncommon with an experienced surgeon and are caused by poor technique or a misaligned laser beam. Decentrations are avoided or minimized by a preoperative laser check of centration, proper patient fixation, frequent monitoring of the beam position during the ablation by the surgeon, and an active eye tracking system. If a significant decentration does occur, the best approach may be to use custom topographical or wave front–assisted scanning laser correction.

Malpositioned flaps can vary from subtle Bowman's layer folds to complete dislocation. Striae that cause irregular astigmatism and decreased vision are treated as soon as noted by lifting the flap and repositioning it. For a markedly displaced flap, the stromal bed and the back surface of the flap are cleared of any epithelium, and the flap is repositioned. If the malposition persists because of poor adhesion, the stromal surfaces are cleared of epithelium again, and the flap is secured with anti-torque suturing. If a flap is completely lost, the patient is treated with prophylactic antibiotics and topical corticosteroids, since there is an increased risk of significant haze formation. A lamellar graft may be required if significant haze leads to vision loss.

Postoperative Infection

Intralamellar infection is extremely uncommon after LASIK.[63-67] If an infection does develop, it is treated aggressively. The flap is lifted, an isolate is obtained for culture and sensitivity testing, the interface is irrigated with a bactericidal solution, and fortified antibiotics are initiated. If the infection progresses despite these measures, the flap may be removed to maximize antibiotic-organism contact.

Other Complications

The incidence of dry eye symptoms has been studied extensively, and many consider dry eye a relative contraindication for LASIK.[71-73] Corneal ectasia after LASIK has caused growing concern among refractive surgeons.[74,75] It is agreed by most that forme fruste keratoconus is a relative if not a definite contraindication for LASIK.[76] A unique entity that has been identified after LASIK is diffuse lamellar keratitis. Its possible causes and management have been well studied.[77-82] Other complications have also been reported.[83,84]

VISUAL OUTCOMES

The typical postoperative care of a patient who has undergone LASIK is relatively simple. Generally, no pain occurs, but some foreign body sensation may be present immediately after surgery, which dissipates by 4 hours postoperatively. On the first postoperative day, the uncorrected visual acuity should be 20/40 (6/12) or better in the low and moderate myopia treatment ranges. On slit-lamp examination, the cornea is clear with intact epithelium. Proper flap apposition is checked, and stromal edema or interface debris is documented. The patient is placed on topical prophylactic antibiotics four times per day for the first week. Topical, preservative-free, lubricating drops are helpful in selected patients on an as-needed basis for the first several weeks after surgery. Topical corticosteroids may be used, but systemic analgesics are rarely necessary with LASIK. The patient may resume normal activities if the postoperative examination after 1 day is normal. The patient is cautioned not to rub the cornea and to avoid contact sports unless proper protection is worn. Final visual recovery may take several weeks or may be delayed if significant irregular astigmatism exists.

Accuracy of Excimer Laser Keratomileusis for Myopia and Astigmatism

Numerous clinical studies of LASIK have been published.[29-36,85-90] Accuracy appears to be greater for lower degrees of myopia. With the nomograms employed in the reported studies, the occurrence of greater than 1D deviation from intended correction was larger for higher degrees of myopia.[32,33,36,85,86] Significant rates of complications similar to those associated with other forms of lamellar surgery also were noted by many authors.[32,33,36,87,89,90]

FUTURE CONSIDERATIONS

The ultimate goal of refractive surgery is to obtain vision that is quantitatively and qualitatively better than that which can be obtained using spectacles or contact lenses with a procedure that is adjustable and reversible. The basic goal is for the postoperative uncorrected vision to equal or better the best spectacle-corrected preoperative vision. Until recently, no peer-reviewed

article had been published that reported the results of a technique, in terms of either short-term or longitudinal follow-up, that could even remotely match the results for spectacles or contact lenses with regard to efficacy for any level of myopia, with or without astigmatism. With the advent of customized wave front–guided ablation, the outcome in terms of unaided vision has improved remarkably over that achieved with conventional symmetrical laser ablation.[91-95]

LASIK is but one point on a continuum of work initiated by Barraquer almost 50 years ago. The reports to date are encouraging. Enthusiasm must be tempered by the fact that long-term results are not available. Additionally, the capital expenditure for a microkeratome, much less an excimer laser, poses a significant financial commitment, along with potential operative risks. LASIK is still in its early development, and continued refinements have occurred in microkeratomes, laser delivery systems, software, and nomograms that may improve the early results. Longer follow-up of current studies in progress and future controlled studies of LASIK will supply long-term data that will define these procedures' efficacy, predictability, safety, stability, and quality of vision, along with outcome reports on patient acceptance and satisfaction.[96]

REFERENCES

1. Barraquer JI. Oueratoplastia refractiva. Estudios Inform Oftal Inst Barraquer. 1949;10:2–21.
2. Bores L. Lamellar refractive surgery. In: Bores L, ed. Refractive eye surgery. Boston: Blackwell Scientific Publications; 1993:324–91.
3. Barraquer JI. Keratomileusis. Int Surg. 1967;48:103–17.
4. Barraquer JI. Results of myopic keratomileusis. J Refract Surg. 1987;3:98–101.
5. Barraquer JI. Method for cutting lamellar grafts in frozen corneas: new orientations for refractive surgery. Arch Soc Am Ophthalmol. 1958;1:237.
6. Campos M, Cuevas K, Garbus J, et al. Corneal wound healing after excimer laser ablation: effects of nitrogen gas blower. Ophthalmology. 1992;99:893–7.
7. Epstein D, Tengroth B, Fagerholm P, Hamberg-Nystrom H. Excimer retreatment of regression after photorefractive keratectomy. Am J Ophthalmol. 1994;117:456–61.
8. Lohmann C, Gartry D, Kerr Muir M, et al. Corneal haze after excimer laser refractive surgery. Objective measurements and functional implications. Eur J Ophthalmol. 1991;1:173–80.
9. Fagerholm P, Hamberg-Nystrom H, Tengroth B. Wound healing and myopic regression following photorefractive keratectomy. Acta Ophthalmol. 1994;72:229–34.
10. Gartry DS, Kerr Muir MG, Lohmann CP, Marshall J. The effect of topical corticosteroids on refractive outcome and corneal haze after photorefractive keratectomy. Arch Ophthalmol. 1992;110:944–52.
11. O'Brart DPS, Lohmann CP, Klonos G, et al. The effects of topical corticosteroids and plasmin inhibitors on refractive outcome, haze, and visual performance after photorefractive keratectomy. Ophthalmology. 1994;101:1565–74.
12. Maguire LJ, Klyce SD, Sawelson H, et al. Visual distortion after myopic keratomileusis: computer analysis of keratoscope photographs. Ophthalmic Surg. 1987;18:352–6.
13. Swinger CA, Barker BA. Prospective evaluation of myopic keratomileusis. Ophthalmology. 1984;91:785–92.
14. Nordan LT, Fallor MK. Myopic keratomileusis: 74 consecutive non-amblyopic cases with one year of follow-up. J Refract Surg. 1986;2:124–8.
15. Nordan LT. Keratomileusis. Int Ophthalmol Clin. 1991;31:7–12.
16. Barraquer C, Guitierrez A, Espinoza A. Myopic keratomileusis: short term results. Refract Corneal Surg. 1989;5:307–13.
17. Krwawicz T. Lamellar corneal stromectomy. Am J Ophthalmol. 1964;57:828–33.
18. Pureskin N. Weakening ocular refraction by means of partial stromectomy of cornea under experimental conditions. Vestn Oftal. 1967;80:19–24.
19. Wilson SE. Excimer laser (193) myopic keratomileusis: differential stability in lower and higher myopes. Refract Corneal Surg. 1990;6:383–5.
20. Sher NA, Barak M, Daya S, et al. Excimer laser photorefractive keratectomy in high myopia. Arch Ophthalmol. 1992;110:935–43.
21. Sher NA, Hardten DR, Fundingsland B, et al. 193 nm Excimer photorefractive keratectomy in high myopia. Ophthalmology. 1994;101:1575–82.
22. Carson CA, Taylor HR, for the Melbourne Excimer Laser and Research Group. Excimer laser photorefractive keratectomy in moderate and high myopia. Arch Ophthalmol. 1995;113:431–6.
23. Brancato R, Tavola A, Carones F, et al. Excimer laser photorefractive keratectomy for myopia: results in 1165 eyes. Refract Corneal Surg. 1993;9:95–104.
24. Serdarevic O, Vinciguerra P, Bottoni F, et al. Excimer laser photorefractive keratectomy for high myopia. ARVO abstracts. Invest Ophthalmol Vis Sci. 1992;33(4 suppl):763.
25. Ditzen K, Anschuetz T, Shroeder E. Photorefractive keratectomy to treat low, medium and high myopia: a multicenter study. J Cataract Refract Surg. 1994;20(suppl):234–8.
26. Bas AM, Nano HD. In situ myopic keratomileusis; results in 30 eyes at 15 months. Refract Corneal Surg. 1991;7:223–31.
27. Arena-Archilla E, Sanchez-Thorin JC, Naranjo-Uribe JP, Hernandez-Lozano A. Myopic keratomileusis in situ: a preliminary report. J Cataract Refract Surg. 1991;17:424–35.
28. Peyman GA, Badaro RM, Khoobehi B. Corneal ablation in rabbits using an infrared (2.9 microns) erbium:YAG laser. Ophthalmology. 1989;96:1160–9.
29. Pallikaris IG, Papatzanaki ME, Stathi EZ, et al. Laser in situ keratomileusis. Lasers Surg Med. 1990;10:463–8.

30. Burrato L, Ferrari M, Genisi C. Myopic keratomileusis with the excimer laser: one-year follow-up. Refract Corneal Surg. 1993;9:12–9.
31. Brint SF, Ostrick DM, Fisher C, et al. Six-month results of the multicenter phase I study of excimer laser myopic keratomileusis. J Cataract Refract Surg. 1994;20:610–5.
32. Bas AM, Onnis R. Excimer laser in situ keratomileusis for myopia. J Refract Surg. 1995;11(suppl):S229–33.
33. Salah T, Waring GO III, El Maghraby A, et al. Excimer laser in situ keratomileusis under a corneal flap for myopia of 2 to 20 diopters. Am J Ophthalmol. 1996;121:143–55.
34. Fiander DC, Tayfour F. Excimer laser in situ keratomileusis in 124 myopic eyes. J Refract Surg. 1995;11(suppl):S234–8.
35. Kremer FB, Dufek M. Excimer laser in situ keratomileusis. J Refract Surg. 1995;11(suppl):S244–7.
36. Guell JL, Muller A. Laser in situ keratomileusis (LASIK) for myopia ranging from −7 to −18 diopters. J Refract Surg. 1996;12:222–8.
37. Donnenfeld ED, Kornstein HS, Amin A, et al. Laser in situ keratomileusis for correction of myopia and astigmatism after penetrating keratoplasty. Ophthalmology. 1999;106:1966–74.
38. Webber SK, Lawless MA, Sutton GL, et al. LASIK for post-penetrating keratoplasty astigmatism and myopia. Br J Ophthalmol.1999;83:1013–8.
39. Vajpayee RB, Dada T. LASIK after penetrating keratoplasty. Ophthalmology. 2000;107:1801–2.
40. Rashad KM. Laser in situ keratomileusis for correction of high astigmatism after penetrating keratoplasty. J Refract Surg. 2000;16:701–10.
41. Davis EA, Hardten DR, Lindstrom RL. Laser in situ keratomileusis after intracorneal rings. Report of 5 cases. J Cataract Refract Surg. 2000;26:1733–41.
42. Zaldivar R, Davidorf JM, Oscherow S, et al. Combined posterior chamber phakic intraocular lens and laser in situ keratomileusis: bioptics for extreme myopia. J Refract Surg. 1999;15:299–308.
43. Guell JL, Vazquez M, Cris O, et al. Combined surgery to correct high myopia: iris claw phakic intraocular lens and laser in situ keratomileusis. J Refract Surg. 1999;15:529–37.
44. Wagner RS. Considerations and implications of LASIK in children. J Pediatr Ophthalmol Strabismus. 2000;37:325.
45. Goodman D. Strabismus: accommodative component treated by LASIK. Surv Ophthalmol. 1999;44:183–4.
46. Ratkay-Traub I, Juhasz T, Horvath C, et al. Ultra-short pulse (femtosecond) laser surgery: initial use in LASIK flap creation. Ophthalmol Clin North Am. 2001;14:347–55.
47. Barraquer C, Cavelier C, Mejia LF. Incidence of retinal detachment following clear-lens extraction in myopic patients. Arch Ophthalmol. 1994;112:36–9.
48. Coonan P, Fung WE, Webster RG Jr, et al. The incidence of retinal detachment following extracapsular cataract extraction: a ten year study. Ophthalmology. 1985;92:1096–101.
49. Lindstrom RL, Lindquist TD, Huldin J, Rubenstein JB. Retinal detachment in axial myopia following extracapsular cataract surgery. Trans New Orleans Acad Ophthalmol. 1988;36:253–68.
50. Rodriquez A, Gutierrez E, Alvira G. Complications of clear lens extraction in axial myopia. Arch Ophthalmol. 1987;105:1522–3.
51. McPherson A, O'Malley R, Bravo J. Retinal detachment following late posterior capsulotomy. Am J Ophthalmol. 1983;95:593–7.
52. Alio JL, Ruiz-Moreno JM, Artola A. Retinal detachment as a potential hazard in surgical correction of severe myopia with phakic anterior chamber lenses. Am J Ophthalmol. 1993;115:145–8.
53. Javitt JC, Street DA, Steinberg EP. National outcomes of cataract extraction: retinal detachment and endophthalmitis following outpatient cataract extraction. Cataract Patient Outcomes Research Team. Ophthalmology. 1994;101:100–5.
54. Javitt JC, Tielsch JM, Canner JK, et al. National outcomes of cataract extraction: increased risk of retinal complications associated with Nd:YAG laser capsulotomy. Ophthalmology. 1992;99:1487–98.
55. Colin J, Robinet A. Clear lensectomy and implantation of low-power posterior chamber intraocular lens for the correction of high myopia. Ophthalmology. 1994;101:107–12.
56. Javitt JC. Clear lens extraction for high myopia. Arch Ophthalmol. 1994;112:321–3.
57. Goldberg MF. Clear lens extraction for axial myopia. Ophthalmology. 1987; 94:571–82.
58. Iskander NG, Peters NT, Penno EA, et al. Postoperative complications of laser in situ keratomileusis. Curr Opin Ophthalmol. 2000;11:273–9.
59. Davis EA, Hardten DR, Lindstrom RL. LASIK complications. Int Ophthalmol Clin. 2000;40:67–75.
60. Ellies P, Pietrini D, Lumbroso L, et al. Macular hemorrhage after laser in situ keratomileusis for high myopia. J Cataract Refract Surg. 2000;26:922–4.
61. Holland SP, Srivannaboon S, Reinstein DZ. Avoiding serious corneal complications of laser assisted in situ keratomileusis and photorefractive keratectomy. Ophthalmology. 2000;107:640–52.
62. Areval JF, Ramirez E, Suarez E, et al. Incidence of vitreoretinal pathologic conditions within 24 months after laser in situ keratomileusis. Ophthalmology. 2000;107:258–65.
63. Kim EK, Lee DH, Lee K, et al. Nocardia keratitis after traumatic detachment of a laser in situ keratomileusis flap. J Refract Surg. 2000;16:467–9.
64. Gelender H, Carter HL, Bowman B, et al. Mycobacterium keratitis after laser in situ keratomileusis. J Refract Surg. 2000;16:191–5.
65. Dada T, Sharma N, Dada VK, et al. Pneumococcal keratitis after laser in situ keratomileusis. J Cataract Refract Surg. 2000;26:460–1.
66. Chung MS, Goldstein MH, Driebe WT, et al. Fungal keratitis after laser in situ keratomileusis: a case report. Cornea. 2000;19:236–7.
67. Tripathi A. Fungal keratitis after LASIK. J Cataract Refract Surg. 2000;26:1433.
68. Tsai YY, Lin JM. Natural history of central islands after laser in situ keratomileusis. J Cataract Refract Surg. 2000;26:853–8.
69. Maldonado MJ. Undersurface ablation of the flap for laser in situ keratomileusis retreatment. Ophthalmology. 2002;109:1453–64.
70. Doane JF, Slade SG. LASIK complications and management. In: Probst L, Machat J, Slade S, eds. The art of LASIK. Thorofare, NJ: Slack; 1998:417–26.
71. Yu EY, Leung A, Rao S, Lam DS. Effect of laser in situ keratomileusis on tear stability. Ophthalmology. 2000;107:2131–5.
72. Lee JB, Ryu CH, Kim J, et al. Comparison of tear secretion and tear film instability after photorefractive keratectomy and laser in situ keratomileusis. J Cataract Refract Surg. 2000;26:1326–31.
73. Linna TU, Vesaluoma MH, Perez-Santonja JJ, et al. Effect of myopic LASIK on corneal sensitivity and morphology of subbasal nerves. Invest Ophthalmol Vis Sci. 2000;41:393–7.
74. Seiler T, Quurke AW. Iatrogenic keratectasia after LASIK in a case of forme fruste keratoconus. J Cataract Refract Surg. 1998;24:1007–9.
75. Joo CK, Kim TG. Corneal ectasia detected after laser in situ keratomileusis for correction of less than 12 diopters of myopia. J Cataract Refract Surg. 2000;26:292–5.
76. Schmitt-Bernard CF, Lesage C, Arnaud B. Keratectasia induced by laser in situ keratomileusis in keratoconus. J Refract Surg. 2000;16:368–70.
77. Holland SP, Mathias RG, Morck DW, et al. Diffuse lamellar keratitis related to endotoxins released from sterilizer reservoir biofilms. Ophthalmology. 2000; 107:1227–33.
78. Doane JF. Diffuse interlamellar keratitis: sands of Sahara syndrome. In: Buratto L, Brint S, eds. LASIK: surgical technique and complications. Thorofare, NJ: Slack; 2000:581–90.
79. Steinert RF, McColgin AZ, White A, Horbaugh GM. Diffuse interface keratitis after laser in situ keratomileusis (LASIK): a nonspecific syndrome. Am J Ophthalmol. 2000;129:380–1.
80. Dada T, Sharma N, Vajpayee RB, et al. Sterile central disciform keratopathy after LASIK. Cornea. 2000;19:851–2.
81. Shah MN, Misra M, Wihelmus KR, et al. Diffuse lamellar keratitis associated with epithelial defects after laser in situ keratomileusis. J Cataract Refract Surg. 2000; 26:1312–8.
82. Haw WW, Manche EE. Late onset diffuse lamellar keratitis associated with an epithelial defect in six eyes. J Refract Surg. 2000;16:744–8.
83. Lee AG, Kohnen T, Ebner R, et al. Optic neuropathy associated with laser in situ keratomileusis. J Cataract Refract Surg. 2000;26:1581–4.
84. Paciuc M, Mendieta G, Naranjo R, et al. Oculocardiac reflex in sedated patients having laser in situ keratomileusis. J Cataract Refract Surg. 1999;25:1341–3.
85. Knorz MC, Liermann A, Steiner H, et al. Laser in-situ keratomileusis to correct myopia of −6 to −29 diopters. J Refract Surg. 1996;12:575–84.
86. Lindstrom RL, Hardten DR, Chu YR. Laser in situ keratomileusis (LASIK) for the treatment of low, moderate and high myopia. Trans Am Ophthalmol Soc. 1997;95:285–96.
87. Knorz MC, Liermann A, Jendritza B, et al. LASIK for hyperopia and hyperopic astigmatism—results of a pilot study. Semin Ophthalmol. 1998;13:83–7.
88. Siganos DS, Popescu CN, Siganos CS, et al. Seven years experience with LASIK for myopia. Oftalmologia. 1999;47:50–2.
89. Esquenazi S, Mendoza A. Two-year follow-up of laser in situ keratomileusis for hyperopia. J Refract Surg. 1999;15:648–52.
90. Lindstrom RL, Linebarger EJ, Hardten DR, et al. Early results of hyperopic and astigmatic laser in situ keratomileusis in eyes with secondary hyperopia. Ophthalmology. 2000;107:1858–63.
91. Knorz MC. TopoLink LASIK. Int Ophthalmol Clin. 2000;40:145–9.
92. Knorz MC, Jendritza B. Topographically guided laser in situ keratomileusis to treat corneal irregularities. Ophthalmology. 2000;107:1138–43.
93. Mrochen M, Kaemmerer M, Seiler T. Wavefront-guided laser in situ keratomileusis: early results in three eyes. J Refract Surg. 2000;16:116–21.
94. Panagopoulou SI, Pallikaris IG. Wavefront customized ablations with the WASCA Asclepion workstation. J Refract Surg. 2001;17:S608–12.
95. Arbelaez MC. Super vision: dream or reality. J Refract Surg. 2001;17:S211–8.
96. Miller AE, McCulley JP, Bowman RW, et al. Patient satisfaction after LASIK for myopia. CLAO J. 2001;27:84–8.

21

LASIK Complications

VOLKAN DAYANIR • DIMITRI T. AZAR

DEFINITION
- Despite the overwhelming success of LASIK, complications of LASIK may result in poor visual outcomes.

KEY FEATURES
- Preoperative complications may result from excessive anesthetics, conjunctival chemosis, or improper draping of the eyelashes.
- Intraoperative complications include poor suction, free cap, incomplete flap, buttonhole, thin flap, irregular flap, flap dislocation, and introcular penetration.
- Postoperative complications include decentration, central island, DLK, epithelial ingrowth, epithelial defect masquerade syndrome, flap striae, infections, and ectasia.

ASSOCIATED FEATURES
- Knowledge of potential LASIK complications will allow the surgeon to prevent several of these complications.
- Early recognition and management may reduce the impact of LASIK complications on visual outcomes.

INTRODUCTION

Laser *in situ* keratomileusis (LASIK) surgery enjoyed tremendous success in the past decade because of its high success rate but also because of rapid visual recovery, minimal pain, and relatively low rate of complications. Some LASIK complications may be very serious; others[1] may be inconsequential or easily avoidable.

PREOPERATIVE COMPLICATIONS

Anesthesia

LASIK is most commonly performed under topical anesthesia. Although 0.5% proparacaine is commonly used, other topical anesthetics include 0.5% tetracaine and 0.4% oxybuprocaine. The onset of anesthesia is less than 1 minute, and the duration is approximately 1 hour.[2] Topical anesthetics can cause superficial punctate keratopathy (SPK) or frank epithelial defects.[1] Placing a drop of anesthetic on the superior and inferior bulbar conjunctiva rather than directly on the cornea reduces the incidence of SPK. Having the patient close the eyelids after instillation of the anesthetic increases its contact with the ocular surface, which may reduce the need for additional medication. In contrast to SPK, a frank epithelial defect may require the use of a bandage soft contact lens to allow rapid wound healing.

Conjunctiva

Conjunctival chemosis may lead to poor coupling of the suction ring to the sclera. As the suction ring is applied on the chemotic conjunctiva, the suction may end prematurely, without raising the intraocular pressure for safe lamellar cutting.

Chemosis, sectoral or circumferential, may occur after peribulbar injections. One might try to massage the fluid away with a cannula or aspirate it with a needle, but the latter approach may run the risk of a subconjunctival hemorrhage. Chemosis can also result from repeated attempts at centering the suction ring, resulting in tissue edema as well as some subconjunctival hemorrhage. If the edema is excessive and the intraocular pressure is not sufficiently elevated (even after occlusion), the procedure should be postponed.

Raised conjunctival lesions such as nevi or conjunctival scars may also lead to pseudosuction. This problem can be dealt with by positioning the ring so that its opening does not overlap with the pathology or by using a ring with multiple suction holes.

Lashes, Drape, and Speculum

A properly draped and exposed eye is a prerequisite for uncomplicated LASIK surgery. The lids should be dried and an adhesive drape placed over the lids and lashes. The lashes must be completely covered by the drape so as not to interfere with the speed or continuity of the moving apparatus of the microkeratome.[3] The drape may loosen if the lids or lashes are wet. This may interfere with the movement of the microkeratome. It is also important to use an appropriate speculum to provide maximal exposure of the globe so that the suction ring and the microkeratome can be engaged easily.

INTRAOPERATIVE COMPLICATIONS

Suction-Related Problems

Suction-related problems may lead to irregular, small, and incomplete flaps. They may occur at the beginning of the surgery when enough suction cannot be obtained or during the surgery when suction is lost. In the first situation, the suction hole(s) should be checked with the gloved fingertip to exclude machine malfunction. Then the conjunctiva can be examined for chemosis or for any conjunctival lesion that might be occluding the suction holes. The uncommon complication of lost suction during surgery can theoretically arise from a power outage or a mechanical failure. Modern suction units have backup for power outage.

Free Cap

The size of the flap after a microkeratome pass depends on the amount of cornea protruding above the superior plane of the suction ring. If there is less tissue than necessary, there is a risk of free cap. The incidence of free cap is 0.1–1%.[3-6]

A flat cornea with a K value of <41D might lead to a free cap. It is important to measure the K values before surgery and, if necessary, to use a larger ring to compensate for the flatness of the cornea.[3] A large ring will engage more cornea, providing more tissue for the blade.

A free cap might also occur if suction is insufficient.[5] Application of suction on the cornea must always be followed by an intraocular pressure check by either a Barraquer applanation tonometer or a pneumotonometer. A pressure of at least 65mmHg, and preferably 85mmHg, is required to proceed with the surgery.[7] Low pressure will lead to less available tissue for cutting, resulting in a free or small cap.

A suction ring that is small for the cornea may also expose inadequate tissue, causing a free or small cap. Incorrect adjustment of the stopper device of the microkeratome may also result in a free or small cap.[8]

A free cap should be placed epithelial side down in a moist chamber to prevent desiccation. If the cap size compensates for the ablation zone, the surgery can proceed. Free caps of adequate size do well when ablation is performed, and postponing the procedure might risk other intraoperative complications.[5] It is important to position the cap correctly with the help of a drop of balanced salt solution (BSS) in the stromal bed and the preoperative aligning marks. Severe irregular and regular astigmatism may be produced if the cap ends up rotated relative to the original position.[7] A wet sponge might be the best instrument while handling the cap as this minimizes trauma to the cap. After repositioning, the cornea is air dried for 1–2 minutes and the cap is checked with the striae sign while gently pressing on the posterior lip of the LASIK cut with a blunt-tipped instrument. If the free cap does not stabilize on the wound, one can consider suturing the cap in place while bearing in mind that sutures will induce astigmatism. If the cap is too small, postponing the surgery is indicated.

Incomplete Flap

The incidence of incomplete flap in LASIK surgery is 0.3–1.2%, but the incidence of flap-related complications decreases as the surgeon becomes familiar with the microkeratome.[3–5] Reasons for an incomplete microkeratome pass include inadequate globe exposure due to the interference of eyelid, lashes, speculum, and/or drape and loss of suction during the pass. A suggested cause of premature blade stop, termed "galling," was a surface flaw in the blade or a resistance to the sliding of the blade within the microkeratome housing.[9] To avoid this problem, every blade should be inspected before installation, and the instrument should be serviced biannually.

Management of an incomplete flap depends on how far the microkeratome had advanced. One option is to proceed with the ablation by covering the undersurface of the incomplete flap with an instrument. In this case, the unablated hinge region may lead to astigmatism and visual complaints under scotopic conditions.

If the cut is within or at the periphery of the ablation zone (Fig. 21-1), postponing the surgery to a later date may be in the best interest of both patient and surgeon. Reports indicate that patients with an incomplete flap whose surgeries were postponed did better than those who had laser surgery immediately. The lat-

ter group had highly irregular astigmatism and were markedly symptomatic postoperatively.[5,10] It is usually agreed to recut at a 180μm depth in 2–3 months,[10] but recuts have been reported as early as 4 weeks after an incomplete flap.[9]

Buttonhole and Thin Flap

Buttonholes in the flap occur when the blade surfaces at the middle of the flap and then enters the cornea again to complete the pass. Thin flaps are encountered when the blade does not surface but travels close to the cornea surface. In one series, buttonhole complications had the worst outcome in terms of best spectacle-corrected visual acuity when compared with other intraoperative flap complications.[5] Buttonholes and thin flaps are encountered in 0.1–0.6% and 0.1–0.4% of LASIK cases, respectively.[3–6] The four major causes of buttonholes and flaps are as follows:

1. Steep corneas. Thin flaps and buttonholes occur more often in eyes with steep corneas[3] (Fig. 21-2). As the microkeratome is advanced, it creates a dimple in the center of the cornea, which may result in a buttonhole. If the dimpling is shallow, the flap may be thin.
2. Eyes with previous ocular surgery. The steep curvature and anterior displacement of a corneal graft and the conjunctival scarring of scleral buckle surgery may predispose an eye to a buttonhole.[5]
3. Eyes with K values below the thin flap or buttonhole range[3] may still have a buttonhole[11] because the power of the microkeratome is thought to decrease with increasing use. In cases with increased resistance to the oscillatory motion of the blade, the synchrony between the forward movement of the microkeratome and the cutting action of the blade may be lost. Then, with more pushing and less cutting, the flap may become progressively shallower and a buttonhole may eventually form.
4. The size of the intended flap and the intraocular pressure are thought to play a role in buttonhole formation.[6] A large flap requires a more applanated cornea. Flattening more cornea is thought to produce a central dimple that is opposed by the raised intraocular pressure. If the intraocular pressure is inadequate, a thin flap or buttonhole may form. Therefore, a large flap is believed to be more likely than a small flap to cause a buttonhole.

A thin flap of proper size with a hinge beyond the ablation zone should not change the course of the procedure. In case of a buttonhole, it is generally agreed that the ablation procedure should be abandoned[3,5,6,11] because it tends to decrease best spectacle-corrected visual acuity.[5] A waiting period of at least 3 months should be allowed and should include checking of the refraction stabilization. Retreatment with no-touch transepithelial photorefractive keratectomy (PRK) can be considered within 1–2 weeks in low refractive errors where there is superficial corneal scar and/or epithelial ingrowth associated with the buttonhole.[7]

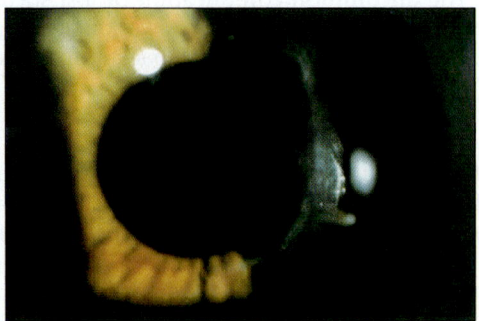

FIG. 21-1 ▌ Stromal scarring in an incomplete flap after aborted LASIK. (From Melki SA, Azar DT. LASIK complications: etiology, management, and prevention. Surv Ophthalmol. 2001;46:95–116, p 98.)

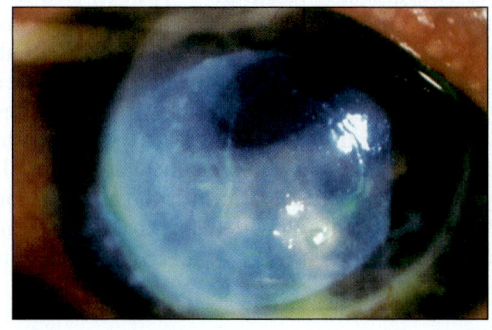

FIG. 21-2 ▌ Buttonhole in a steep cornea. (From Melki SA, Azar DT. LASIK complications: etiology, management, and prevention. Surv Ophthalmol. 2001;46:95–116, p 96.)

Irregular Flap

Irregular flaps occur when the cut of the microkeratome blade is not uniform throughout the flap; the incidence is around 0.1%.[4-6] Irregular flaps are also termed notched or bilevel flaps. In one case there was a bisected flap where the blade did not cut the middle part, resulting in superior and inferior half-flaps.[4] On examination, it was found that the blade had a defect in its middle. A leveled flap can also occur if the blade has a curve in it. Every blade must be inspected under the microscope for flaws before the installation.

Postponing the surgery about 3 months or waiting for stabilization of refraction is a safe option in the presence of an irregular flap.

Flap Dislocation

Intraoperative flap dislocation is a rare occurrence that may be encountered at the end of the surgery.[3] The patient may squeeze the eye and turn it upward while the speculum and drape are being removed, causing the flap to dislocate.

To prevent this problem, the drape may be removed while the speculum is in place. Then the eyelids are held open, and the speculum is lifted up and away from the globe and removed. The patient is instructed to close the eyelids as slowly as possible. The patient is instructed not to touch the eyelids. This may prevent flap dislocation by microtraumas and rubbing in the immediate postoperative period.[12] Dislocation of the flap may occur several weeks after surgery (Fig. 21-3). Techniques of flap repositioning during the intraoperative or postoperative period include flap refloating and smoothing, ironing, stretching, and suturing.

Intraocular Penetration

One of the most dreaded and rarest complications of LASIK is inadvertent intraocular penetration. If the microkeratome does not have a fixed-depth blade, it must be triple-checked for the tightness of the depth plate before engaging the microkeratome handle. With a loose or absent depth plate, the blade will make a cut of 900µm depth, making intraocular penetration inevitable.

Fortunately, modern microkeratomes have a fixed-depth blade, which rules out the possibility of intraocular penetration. However, surgery on an unrecognized thin or keratoconic cornea may still lead to penetration. Preoperative pachymetry and videokeratoscopy are valuable in avoiding this problem.

POSTOPERATIVE COMPLICATIONS

Decentration

A decentered ablation zone may go unrecognized during surgery, and result in irregular astigmatism. This decentration (Fig. 21-4) may cause visual symptoms such as halos, glare, and monocular diplopia as well as decrease in best spectacle-corrected visual acuity.[13] Decentration can be characterized as mild (0–0.5mm), mod-

erate (0.5–1.0mm), or severe (>1mm); the amount of decentration that causes a visual complaint varies with the patient.[14]

Several reasons have been postulated for the occurrence of decentration. Patients with high myopia have more decentration than those with lower myopia.[15,16] This might be attributed to the difficulty in focusing on the fixation light.

The eye tends to make rapid saccadic movements in which fixation is lost briefly. During longer ablations, as for high myopes, the eye tends to drift, losing fixation for a longer period. If the patient knows what will happen and cooperates with the physician, decentration decreases significantly.[16]

The type of fixation may also influence decentration. The amount of decentration is increased when fixation depends largely on the patient's cooperation as compared with the use of a suction mask or a tracker during ablation.[16,17]

Modern lasers used in LASIK incorporate real-time tracking devices. These systems detect changes in fixation and respond by moving the laser beam to the new location.[16] When fixation changes excessively, the system stops.

Once decentration has occurred, it may be very difficult to treat. There is no proven method of treating patients with symptomatic decentration. It might be best to postpone further LASIK treatment until customized topographical- or wavefront-guided ablations become available for such patients.

Central Island

A central island is defined as a well-circumscribed area of increased refractive power located in the central cornea and demonstrated by topography (Fig. 21-5). As the island becomes larger in size and in refractive power, the uncorrected visual acuity and best-corrected visual acuity tend to decrease.[18,19] Central islands are common in the early postoperative period, varying between 3.2% and 29%.[18,20,21] In time, central islands decrease slowly but significantly in both size and dioptric power. About one fourth of the cases are resolved by 6 months.[18]

Factors contributing to the central island formation include plume dynamics,[22] in which the debris created by ablation absorbs some of the incoming energy. This leads to less central ablation and hence a steeper central cornea. Another factor relates to the fluid dynamics of the cornea. Acoustic shock waves created when the laser beam hits the cornea[23] can drive the water in the cornea centrally, resulting in less central/paracentral ablation. The posterior stroma is more hydrated than the anterior.[24]

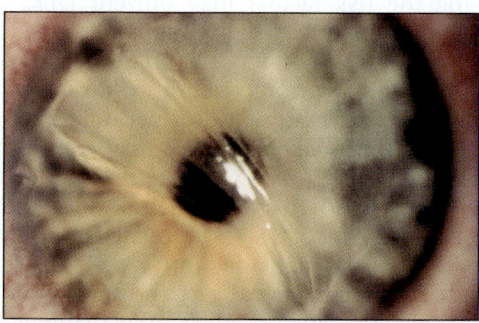

FIG. 21-3 ■ Traumatic flap dislocation, 3 weeks after LASIK. (Courtesy of Nada S. Jabbin, MD. In Melki SA, Azar DT. LASIK complications: etiology, management, and prevention. Surv Ophthalmol. 2001;46:95–116, p 99.)

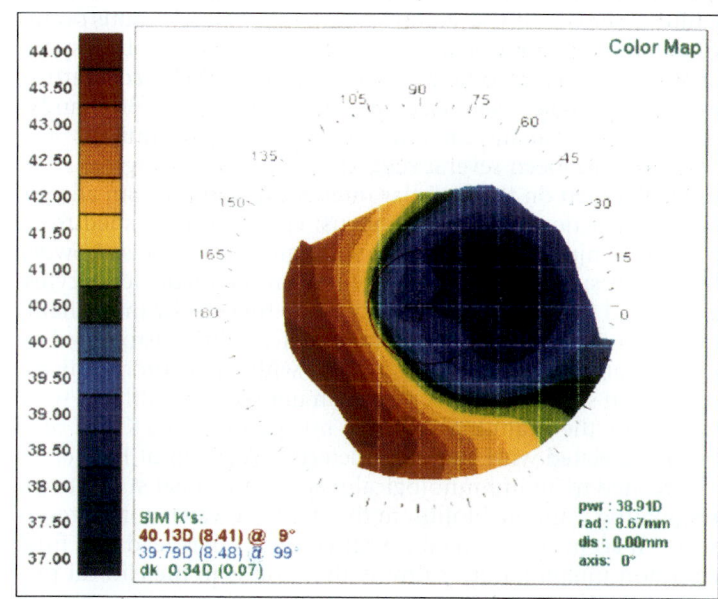

FIG. 21-4 ■ Superonasal decentration. (From Melki SA, Azar DT. LASIK complications: etiology, management, and prevention. Surv Ophthalmol. 2001;46:95–116, p 105.)

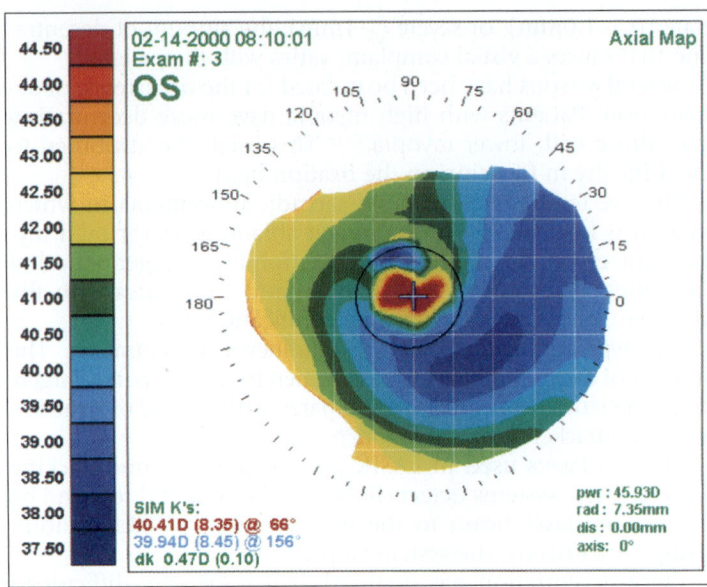

FIG. 21-5 ▌ Central island after LASIK. (From Melki SA, Azar DT. LASIK complications: etiology, management, and prevention. Surv Ophthalmol. 2001;46:95–116, p 105.)

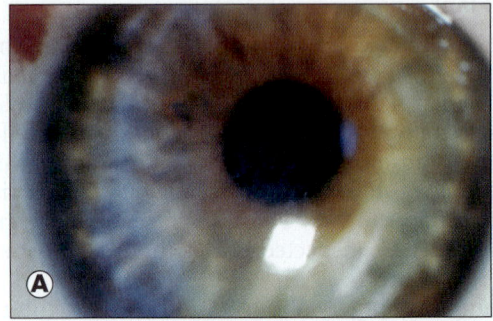
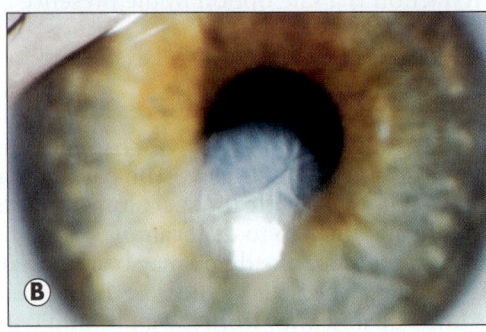

FIG. 21-6 ▌ Diffuse lamellar keratitis 2 days (A) and 5 days (B) fter LASIK. (From Melki SA, Azar DT. LASIK complications: etiology, management, and prevention. Surv Ophthalmol. 2001;46:95–116, p 109.)

Because the central cornea has the deepest ablation, the water accumulates most in the center,[25] resulting in less ablation centrally. Temporal degradation of the laser optics can lead to inhomogeneity of the laser beam itself, resulting in uneven ablation. Individual wound healing responses that are poorly understood may also contribute to the formation of central islands.

Some corneas with central islands acquire a smoother profile over time. Increased epithelial thickness in the midperiphery of the ablation zone and stromal remodeling contribute to the smoothing. There is no consensus on the follow-up period to be allowed before attempting to correct a symptomatic central island. Treatment should be tailored on an individual basis, taking the symptoms into account. A steep central island can be ablated by using an excimer laser in a PRK/PTK (phototherapeutic keratectomy) mode or in a topographically guided mode.[19,26,27]

Diffuse Lamellar Keratitis (Shifting Sands, Sands of Sahara)

Diffuse lamellar keratitis (DLK) is a serious complication of LASIK surgery. The first documented cases were characterized by white, granular, diffuse, culture-negative lamellar keratitis occurring in the first postoperative week.[28] Some cases resolved spontaneously, whereas others progressed and developed scarring with unfavorable visual outcomes (Fig. 21-6). "Shifting sands" and "sands of Sahara" are other names for this condition.

There have been several suggestions for the etiology of DLK. Any debris left on the lamellar interface may initiate an allergic or toxic reaction. Tear fluid; mucus; epithelial cells shed from cornea, conjunctiva, or skin; meibomian secretions; powder from gloves; metal particles or wax from the blade; leukocytes; and blood from a pannus are potential triggers for this inflammatory condition.[29,30] LASIK flap interface debris surrounded by inflammatory reaction was observed with the confocal microscope, and scattered bits of debris on unused sterile blades were seen with the scanning electron microscope.[31] DLK has also been associated with epithelial defects.[32] A group of DLK cases was related to an immunological reaction to a heat-stable toxin originating from the biofilm in the sterilizer water storage reservoir.[33] It seems that several causative agents may lead to a final common inflammatory pathway that results in the clinical picture of DLK.

DLK can be seen following LASIK or LASIK enhancement; a postoperative epithelial defect increases the risk considerably.[34] Symptoms may include discomfort, mild to moderate pain, for-

eign body sensation, tearing, and photophobia. A typical lamellar infiltrate has the following characteristics[28]:

- It is composed of white, granular opacities.
- It is confined to the plane of the lamellar cut; there is no anterior or posterior extension.
- There is no anterior chamber reaction.
- There is no overlying epithelial defect.
- The conjunctiva may be inflamed.

DLK has been staged for the purpose of treatment and prognosis.[35] The patient can progress from one stage to another quite rapidly. Patients with DLK should be monitored closely to detect progression (Box 21-1).

Stages 1 and 2 can be managed medically with prednisolone acetate 1% every hour and very careful daily inspection. The inflammation will be limited to about 10 days. Steroids can be tapered when the inflammation is under control and starts to improve.

If stage 3 is diagnosed, the flap is lifted. The bed and stromal side of the flap are irrigated with BSS and wiped with a semiwet surgical sponge. The flap is then placed and allowed to dry. Hourly prednisolone acetate 1% is the mainstay of treatment and is tapered as clinical improvement is seen.

When the stromal melting starts in stage 4, lifting the flap may not be as rewarding as in stage 3. If stage 4 is reached, it is still worthwhile to lift and wash the interface, as this will debulk the inflammation, but care should be taken not to add to the tissue loss. Postoperative treatment is identical with that in stage 3.

Minimizing the risk factors may prevent DLK. Powderless gloves, proper draping, preoperative removal of the tear fluid in the fornices by surgical sponge, irrigating the blade and microkeratome head with BSS prior to assembly, sterilizing the instruments immediately after surgery, and periodic microbiological control of the sterilizer water reservoir may contribute to a decreased incidence of DLK.

Johnson et al.[36] proposed a novel classification of DLK based on a retrospective review of 2711 eyes treated with LASIK in a 3-year period. The cases were divided into type I DLK (center sparing) or type II DLK (center involved) and then subdivided into A (sporadic—DLK not diagnosed in other patients treated on the same day) or B (cluster—other patients identified with DLK). Thus type IA, center sparing, sporadic; type IB, center sparing, cluster; type IIA, center involved, sporadic; and type IIB,

Stages of Diffuse Lamellar Keratitis

Stage 1: Fine, white or brown, granular, powdery haze that either spares the visual axis or involves it slightly. There is no loss of best spectacle-corrected visual acuity. This stage is the most common presentation of DLK on postoperative day 1 that can be observed with a careful slit-lamp examination. It may be seen in 1 in 25 to 1 in 50 cases.

Stage 2: White, granular infiltrate becomes more pronounced and starts to extend toward the center of the flap. As the inflammation moves centripetally, a "windblown sand" appearance becomes prominent. This stage can be seen on the first postoperative 3 days in about 1 in 200 cases. If the visual axis is involved, there may be a slight drop in visual acuity.

Stage 3: White, clumped infiltrate becomes more dense centrally with relative clearing in the periphery. The best spectacle-corrected visual acuity often declines by 1 or 2 lines. Stage 3 is seen in about 1 in 500 cases. The recognition of this stage is important in deciding whether to lift the flap to blunt the inflammatory process. Intervention at this stage seems to prevent permanent scarring.

Stage 4: Inflammation has built up so much that collagenases are breaking down the stroma. There are stromal melting, striae, and scarring, resulting in loss of best spectacle-corrected visual acuity and a hyperopic shift. Incidence is about 1 in 5000. Extracorneal involvement occurs as anterior chamber reaction, ciliary injection, and lid edema.[29]

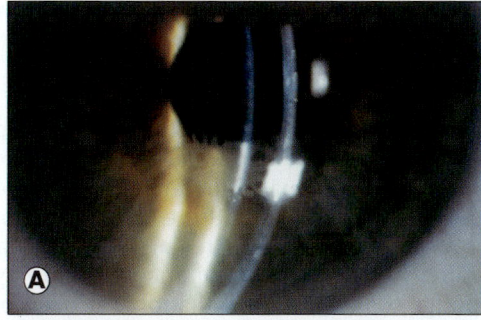
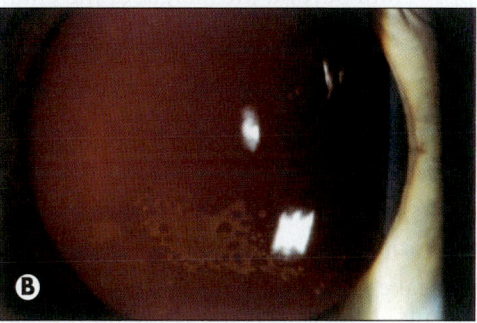

FIG. 21-7 ■ Epithelial ingrowth seen by slit-beam illumination *(A)* and retroillumination *(B)*. (From Melki SA, Azar DT. LASIK complications: etiology, management, and prevention. Surv Ophthalmol. 2001;46:95–116.)

center involved, cluster. The main outcome measures were incidence of DLK after LASIK, time to diagnosis, time to resolution, and changes in best spectacle-corrected visual acuity.

Thirty-six eyes (1.3%) developed DLK. Type I occurred in 58.3% of the 36 eyes (type IA, $n = 18$; type IB, $n = 3$), and type II, in 41.7% of the 36 eyes (type IIA, $n = 10$; type IIB, $n = 5$).[36] Of the 36 eyes, 14 (38.9%) developed DLK after an epithelial defect, representing an odds ratio of 13 times.[36] The mean time to resolution in type I was significantly shorter than in type II. Loss of two or more lines of best spectacle-corrected visual acuity occurred in two of five patients with type IIB and in no patients with type IA, IB, or IIA.[36]

Epithelial Ingrowth

Epithelial ingrowth is seen when epithelial cells proliferate in the lamellar interface, producing opacification of the interface and occasionally melting of the flap.[11,13] This can lead to irregular astigmatism and loss of best spectacle-corrected visual acuity. Epithelial ingrowth is usually detected within 1 month postoperatively in about 4.3% of cases.[30] There are conflicting reports on the likelihood of epithelial ingrowth in enhancement LASIK. Some authors report increased risk, whereas others report unchanged risk of epithelial ingrowth in LASIK retreatment compared with primary LASIK.[5,37] The high rate of bilaterality may indicate genetic predisposition.[37]

There are theoretically three ways in which epithelial cells can gain access to a flap interface: the microkeratome blade can mechanically drag epithelial cells into the interface, irrigation after photoablation can float epithelial cells onto the stroma, and cells of the surface epithelium can grow into the interface at the flap junction (Fig. 21-7). Clinically, ingrowth can be present either as an isolated epithelial island or as a sheet of epithelium continuous with the surface epithelium. The latter is by far the more frequent observation. A poorly adherent flap is considered a major risk factor.[38,39] Poor adhesion may be caused by an epithelial defect, basement membrane dystrophy, or excessive intraoperative hydration, allowing epithelial cells access to the interface.[38] Indeed, the epithelial plug found at the site of keratotomy during the wound-healing process has been observed, by *in vivo* confocal microscopy, to grow beneath the flap.[40]

Isolated epithelial islands are unlikely to cause a problem. If the ingrowth connects with the surface epithelium, it can continue growing and become more symptomatic as it encroaches on the visual axis and causes distortion on the flap surface. Photophobia, glare, decreased vision, and foreign body sensation are symptoms of epithelial ingrowth. A more serious complication of epithelial ingrowth is epithelial defect masquerade syndrome,[38] which may lead to melting of the flap.

Epithelial ingrowth can involve aggressive inflammation early in its course, mimicking infectious keratitis.[41] There are four clinical signs of epithelial ingrowth on slit-lamp examination: (1) epithelial pearls in the interface formed by dividing epithelial cells, (2) fluorescein pooling on the edge of the flap or fluorescein tracking under the flap, (3) fibrotic demarcation line at the leading edge of the epithelial sheet, and (4) keratolysis, or melting at the edge of the flap. As the epithelial sheet grows and settles in, remodeling along the sheet causes keratolysis due to epithelial-stromal interaction and release of proteolytic enzymes. Remodeling forms a sleeve into which the sheet grows. Even if the epithelial sheet is removed surgically, the sleeve will remain. This might explain the high rate of recurrence through the original site after removal of the sheet.[38]

All possible efforts must be made to prevent epithelial ingrowth. The bed should be irrigated and sponged before closing the flap. One should avoid excessive irrigation that might swell the stroma and contribute to poor flap adhesion. Allowing enough drying time and checking for adequate attachment of the flap at the end of the surgery can help prevent poor adhesion. Using a bandage contact lens in the first 24 hours may prevent partial lifting of the flap edge with blinking. When lifting a flap in enhancement LASIK, it is preferable to use a 0.12mm toothed forceps and not a spatula to lift the flap after breaking the interface. A spatula may carry epithelial cells onto the stroma.[42]

An epithelial ingrowth that has documented growth or causes visual disturbance should be treated. Asymptomatic epithelial nests can be observed.[41] The natural history of an epithelial ingrowth continuous with the surface epithelium is not known. If remodeling is an ongoing process and flap melting is a possibility, intervention should occur as soon as possible.[37]

Lifting of the flap is followed by scraping of both the bed and the cap with a no. 64 Beaver blade or a blunt epithelial PRK spatula and dry sponges. The flap is irrigated with BSS and the fluid collected through a suctioning lid speculum that minimizes reflux of the irrigation solution. The flap is repositioned and stroked with a semiwet sponge to obtain good apposition. A bandage contact lens is inserted to minimize flap edge lifting.[37,41–43]

A serious complication of epithelial ingrowth is the masquerade syndrome of a persistent epithelial defect. This syndrome was described by Azar et al.[38] If the epithelial growth recurs, the surgeon has three options. After the flap is lifted, irrigated, and scraped, the machine can be programmed for PTK so that each point on the bed and the cap receives one or two bursts of laser energy, ablating the remaining epithelial cells.[41,42] Another approach is to use ethanol after the scraping and irrigating. A sponge soaked in 50% ethanol is stroked on the bed and the cap, 1–2mm beyond the margin of the epithelial sheet, for about 20–40 seconds. Then the interface is irrigated with BSS.[43] Transient lamellar keratitis may follow ethanol treatment, but it is controllable with topical steroids. A third (theoretical) possibility is to use mitomycin C to get rid of the unwanted epithelial cells, although there is no reported study on this approach.

Infectious Keratitis

An intact corneal epithelium is an ideal barrier in holding back infectious agents. A breach in the epithelium always carries a risk of infectious keratitis. Bacterial or fungal keratitis is encountered rarely following LASIK, probably because the epithelium is almost intact after the procedure. However, infectious agents can be inoculated into the stromal bed during the procedure itself.

The risk of infectious keratitis after LASIK is 0.1–0.2%.[44,45] Most of these cases are caused by gram-positive bacteria. Symptoms may include pain, photophobia, watering, decreased visual acuity, ghost images, and halos. Slit-lamp examination may reveal ciliary injection, epithelial defect, anterior chamber reaction, and hypopyon. Stromal infiltrate may involve the LASIK interface and in more than one locus. In advanced cases, the flap may become necrotic and slough off. Fungal keratitis, although less common than the bacterial variety, should be in the differential diagnosis, especially if the infection is resistant to antibiotic treatment.[44]

The suspicion of infectious keratitis should prompt lifting the flap and scraping, staining, and culturing for bacteria, mycobacteria, and fungi. The stromal bed is washed with broad-spectrum antibiotics/antifungals. Treatment is modified according to the culture results.

Flap Wrinkles or Striae

Fine or gross wrinkling of the flap can be seen in 0.2–4% of LASIK cases.[3–5,13,17] This may result from undetected intraoperative misalignment of the flap on the stromal bed; excessive blinking and squeezing in the early postoperative period; or the difference in curvature between the posterior face of the flap and the stromal bed after ablation.[17,46,47] If the wrinkles are large and involve the visual axis, vision may be affected adversely.

Wrinkles resemble fingerprint lines against the red reflex upon slit-lamp retroillumination. However, if there are no visible lines in the presence of visual complaints, a fluorescein test may reveal the presence of subtle flap wrinkles by uneven pooling of the tear film.[48,49]

Symptomatic wrinkles warrant treatment. Our preferred treatment method is lifting the flap and irrigating both surfaces with BSS. Use of a hypotonic solution has also been recommended.[50] The flap is then repositioned and ironed with a Pineda iron after instilling a few topical anesthetic drops. Ironing away from the hinge is continued until an epithelial defect is formed at the center of the cap. Alternatively, a LASEK technique using alcohol to loosen the epithelium is used. The cornea is wetted with BSS. The deepithelialized flap absorbs more BSS. The swollen cap becomes more taut, helping the effort of ironing of the wrinkles. The epithelial flap is repositioned, and a bandage contact lens is applied. Sutures are not frequently used because of the risk of inducing astigmatism.[4,46]

Keratectasia

Since the introduction of incisional and ablative refractive corneal procedures, there has been great concern about iatrogenic keratectasia. The least amount of corneal thickness necessary to resist intraocular pressure and prevent anterior bulging is not known. Residual corneal thickness of <250μm has been associated with iatrogenic keratectasia.[51,52] There is agreement on leaving 250μm untouched posterior corneal stroma. Ablation below that limit may cause biomechanical weakening and the cornea may bulge forward. Measuring corneal thickness after reflecting the flap and even after the ablation will help provide a better estimate of the residual bed thickness. A study looking at the posterior corneal curvature demonstrated increased anterior bulging of the posterior surface in eyes that had <250μm residual bed thickness.[53] This may be due to the possibility that the repositioned flap does not contribute to the biomechanical stability of the cornea.

Another important cause of iatrogenic keratectasia is LASIK performed on unrecognized keratoconus suspects.[54,55] Videokeratographic clues to a keratoconus suspect include a K value of >47.2D, inferior steepening of >1.4D, and a difference of >1.9D between the K values of both eyes.

Iatrogenic keratectasia has been reported as early as 1 week postoperatively and as late as 2 years, at refractive errors as low as −4.0D spherical equivalent.[55–57]

REFERENCES

1. Melki SA, Azar DT. LASIK complications: etiology, management, and prevention. Surv Ophthalmol. 2001;46:95–116.
2. Liu JC, Steinemann TL, McDonald MB, et al. Topical bupivacaine and proparacaine: a comparison of toxicity, onset of action, and duration of action. Cornea. 1993;12:228–32.
3. Gimbel HV, Penno EE, van Westenbrugge JA, et al. Incidence and management of intraoperative and early postoperative complications in 1000 consecutive laser in situ keratomileusis cases. Ophthalmology. 1998;105:1839–47.
4. Lin RT, Maloney RK. Flap complications associated with lamellar refractive surgery. Am J Ophthalmol. 1999;127:129–36.
5. Stulting RD, Carr JD, Thompson KP, et al. Complications of laser in situ keratomileusis for the correction of myopia. Ophthalmology. 1999;106:13–20.
6. Tham VMB, Maloney RK. Microkeratome complications of laser in situ keratomileusis. Ophthalmology. 2000;107:920–4.
7. Wilson SE. LASIK: management of common complications. Cornea. 1998;17:459–67.
8. Marinho A, Pinto MC, Pinto R, et al. LASIK for high myopia: one year experience. Ophthalmic Surg Lasers. 1996;27(5 Suppl):S517–20.
9. Rao SK, Padmanabhan P, Sitalakshmi G, et al. Partial flap during laser in-situ keratomileusis: pathogenesis and timing of retreatment. Indian J Ophthalmol. 2000;48:209–12.
10. Holland SP, Srivannaboon S, Reinstein DZ. Avoiding serious corneal complications of laser assisted in situ keratomileusis and photorefractive keratectomy. Ophthalmology. 2000;107:640–52.
11. Leung ATS, Rao SK, Cheng ACK, et al. Pathogenesis and management of laser in situ keratomileusis flap buttonhole. J Cataract Refract Surg. 2000;26:358–62.
12. Buratto L, Ferrari M. Indications, techniques, results, limits, and complications of laser in situ keratomileusis. Curr Opin Ophthalmol. 1997;8(4):59–66.
13. Pérez-Santonja JJ, Bellot J, Claramonte P, et al. Laser in situ keratomileusis to correct high myopia. J Cataract Refract Surg. 1997;23:372–85.
14. Mulhern MG, Foley-Nolan A, O'Keefe M, et al. Topographical analysis of ablation centration after excimer laser photorefractive keratectomy and laser in situ keratomileusis for high myopia. J Cataract Refract Surg. 1997;23:488–94.
15. Cantera E, Cantera I, Olivieri L. Corneal topographic analysis of photorefractive keratectomy in 175 myopic eyes. Refract Corneal Surg. 1993;9(2 Suppl):S19–22.
16. Tsai YY, Lin JM. Ablation centration after active eye-tracker-assisted photorefractive keratectomy and laser in situ keratomileusis. J Cataract Refract Surg. 2000;26:28–34.
17. Condon PI, Mulhern M, Fulcher T, et al. Laser intrastromal keratomileusis for high myopia and myopic astigmatism. Br J Ophthalmol. 1997;81:199–206.
18. Tsai YY, Lin JM. Natural history of central islands after laser in situ keratomileusis. J Cataract Refract Surg. 2000;26:853–8.
19. Manche EE, Maloney RK, Smith RJ. Treatment of topographic central islands following refractive surgery. J Cataract Refract Surg. 1998;24:464–70.
20. Sano Y, Carr JD, Takei K, et al. Videokeratography after excimer laser in situ keratomileusis for myopia. Ophthalmology. 2000;107:674–84.
21. Knorz MC, Liermann A, Seiberth V, et al. Laser in situ keratomileusis to correct myopia of −6.00 to −29.00 diopters. J Refract Surg. 1996;12:575–84.
22. Noack J, Tonnies R, Hohla K, et al. Influence of ablation plume dynamics on the formation of central islands in excimer laser photorefractive keratectomy. Ophthalmology. 1997;104:823–30.
23. Krueger RR, Krasinski JS, Radzewicz C, et al. Photography of shock waves during excimer laser ablation of the cornea: effect of helium gas on propagation velocity. Cornea. 1993;12:330–4.

24. Lee D, Wilson G. Non-uniform swelling properties of the corneal stroma. Curr Eye Res. 1981;1:457–61.
25. Oshika T, Klyce SD, Smolek MK, *et al.* Corneal hydration and central islands after excimer laser photorefractive keratectomy. J Cataract Refract Surg.1998;24:1575–80.
26. Alió JL, Artola A, Rodriguez-Mier FA. Selective zonal ablations with excimer laser for correction of irregular astigmatism induced by refractive surgery. Ophthalmology. 2000;107:662–73.
27. Knorz MC, Jendritza B. Topographically guided laser in situ keratomileusis to treat corneal irregularities. Ophthalmology. 2000;107:1138–43.
28. Smith RJ, Maloney RK. Diffuse lamellar keratitis: a new syndrome in lamellar refractive surgery. Ophthalmology. 1998;105:1721–6.
29. Alió JL, Pérez-Santonja JJ, Tervo T, *et al.* Postoperative inflammation, microbial complications, and wound healing following laser in situ keratomileusis. J Refract Surg. 2000;16:523–38.
30. Farah SG, Azar DT, Gurdal C, *et al.* Laser in situ keratomileusis: literature review of a developing technique. J Cataract Refract Surg. 1998;24:989–1006.
31. Kaufman SC, Maitchouk DY, Chiou AG, *et al.* Interface inflammation after laser in situ keratomileusis: sands of the Sahara syndrome. J Cataract Refract Surg. 1998;24:1589–93.
32. Haw WW, Manche EE. Late onset diffuse lamellar keratitis associated with an epithelial defect in six eyes. J Refract Surg. 2000;16:744–8.
33. Holland SP, Mathias RG, Morck DW, *et al.* Diffuse lamellar keratitis related to endotoxins released from sterilizer reservoir biofilms. Ophthalmology. 2000;107:1227–34.
34. Shah MN, Misra M, Wihelmus KR, *et al.* Diffuse lamellar keratitis associated with epithelial defects after laser in situ keratomileusis. J Cataract Refract Surg. 2000;26:1312–18.
35. Linebarger EJ, Hardten DR, Lindstrom RL. Diffuse lamellar keratitis: diagnosis and management. J Cataract Refract Surg. 2000;26:1072–7.
36. Johnson JD, Harissi-Dagher M, Pineda R, *et al.* Diffuse lamellar keratitis: incidence, associations, outcomes, and a new classification system. J Cataract Refract Surg. 2001;27:1560–6.
37. Wang MY, Maloney RK. Epithelial ingrowth after laser in situ keratomileusis. Am J Ophthalmol. 2000;129:746–51.
38. Maloney RK. Epithelial ingrowth after laser in situ keratomileusis. Am J Ophthalmol. 2000;129:746–51.
39. Maloney RK. Epithelial ingrowth after lamellar refractive surgery [abstract]. Ophthalmic Surg Lasers. 1996;27(Suppl):S535.
40. Vesaluoma MH, Petroll WM, Pérez-Santonja JJ, *et al.* Laser in situ keratomileusis flap margin: wound healing and complications imaged by in vivo confocal microscopy. Am J Ophthalmol. 2000;130:564–73.
41. Helena MC, Meisler D, Wilson SE. Epithelial growth within the lamellar interface after laser in situ keratomileusis (LASIK). Cornea. 1997;16:300–5.
42. Walker MB, Wilson SE. Incidence and prevention of epithelial growth within the interface after laser in situ keratomileusis. Cornea. 2000;19:170–3.
43. Haw WW, Manche EE. Treatment of progressive or recurrent epithelial ingrowth with ethanol following laser in situ keratomileusis. J Refract Surg. 2001;17:63–8.
44. Sridhar MS, Garg P, Bansal AK, *et al.* Fungal keratitis after laser in situ keratomileusis. J Cataract Refract Surg. 2000;26:613–15.
45. Garg P, Bansal AK, Sharma S, *et al.* Bilateral infectious keratitis after laser in situ keratomileusis: a case report and review of the literature. Ophthalmology. 2001;108:121–5.
46. Lam DSC, Leung ATS, Wu JT, *et al.* Management of severe flap wrinkling or dislodgment after laser in situ keratomileusis. J Cataract Refract Surg. 1999;25:1441–7.
47. Probst LE, Machat J. Removal of flap striae following laser in situ keratomileusis. J Cataract Refract Surg. 1998;24:153–5.
48. Rabinowitz YS, Rasheed K. Fluorescein test for the detection of striae in the corneal flap after laser in situ keratomileusis. Am J Ophthalmol. 1999;127:717–18.
49. Carpel EF, Carlson KH, Shannon S. Fine lattice lines on the corneal surface after laser in situ keratomileusis (LASIK). Am J Ophthalmol. 2000;129:379–80.
50. Muñoz G, Alió JL, Pérez-Santonja JJ, *et al.* Successful treatment of severe wrinkled corneal flap after laser in situ keratomileusis with deionized water. Am J Ophthalmol. 2000;129:91–2.
51. Seiler T, Koufala K, Richter G. Iatrogenic keratectasia after laser in situ keratomileusis. J Refract Surg. 1998;14:312–17.
52. Wang Z, Chen J, Yang B. Posterior corneal surface topographic changes after laser in situ keratomileusis are related to residual corneal bed thickness. Ophthalmology. 1999;106:406–10.
53. Seitz B, Torres F, Langenbucher A, *et al.* Posterior corneal curvature changes after myopic laser in situ keratomileusis. Ophthalmology. 2001;108:666–73.
54. Schmitt-Bernard CFM, Lesage C, Arnaud B. Keratectasia induced by laser in situ keratomileusis in keratoconus. J Refract Surg. 2000;16:368–70.
55. Amoils SP, Deist MB, Gous P, *et al.* Iatrogenic keratectasia after laser in situ keratomileusis for less than –4.0 to –7.0 diopters of myopia. J Cataract Refract Surg. 2000;26:967–77.
56. Seiler T. Iatrogenic keratectasia: academic anxiety or serious risk? J Cataract Refract Surg. 1999;25:1307–8.
57. Muravchik J. Keratectasia after LASIK. J Cataract Refract Surg. 2000;26:629–30.

SAMIR G. FARAH • DIMITRI T. AZAR

CHAPTER
22
Management of LASIK Complications

DEFINITION
- The management of LASIK complications involves an appreciation of specific pathogenetic mechanisms, knowledge of appropriate interventional measures, and careful observation of surgical outcomes.

KEY FEATURES
- Serious microkeratome-related complications often require repositioning of the flap and postponing laser ablation.
- Laser-related complications and other postoperative complications require flap.

ASSOCIATED FEATURES
- Intraoperative complications include incomplete cuts, free cap, buttonholing, corneal perforation, poor coupling to the globe, epithelial defects, wound dehiscence, slicing, bleeding, decentration, edema, irregular ablation, central islands, interface debris, and flap wrinkles.
- Postoperative complications include overcorrections, undercorrections, sliding, dislodged flap, flap loss, diffuse lamellar keratitis (DLK), infectious keratitis, epithelial ingrowth, flap melt, regression, corneal ectasia, glare, and night vision problems.

FIG. 22-1 ■ Attempting to extend the flap using a blade is not advisable because of the risk of flap perforation. (From Melki SA, Azar DT. Eight pearls in prevention and management of LASIK complications. In: Melki SA, Azar DT, eds. 101 Pearls in refractive, cataract, and corneal surgery. Thorofare, NJ: Slack; 2001:23–32.)

INTRODUCTION

The majority of LASIK complications occur intraoperatively. Preoperative complications are related to the preparation for the procedure. Postoperative complications are almost always related to events that occurred during surgery. Many complications unique to LASIK are microkeratome related. With improvement in microkeratome technology, the incidence of LASIK complications has been substantially reduced and may decrease further as instrumentation becomes more sophisticated.[1] In one study,[2] the incidence of intraoperative complications decreased from 2.1% during the first 3 months to 0.7% during the last 9 months of the study, proving that the complication rates can be reduced as the surgical team gains experience. Most intra- and postoperative complications are common to myopic and hyperopic LASIK. Several complications may be prevented if the eye is examined on the slit lamp in the direct postoperative period.

This chapter summarizes the information obtained through an Advanced PubMed (National Library of Medicine) search for all articles reporting on LASIK complications as well as their management. The literature was searched using Medline (key word "LASIK" or "laser-assisted *in situ* keratomileusis") and using citations from the articles obtained.

This search revealed that LASIK is not simply a blend of photorefractive keratectomy (PRK) and keratomileusis.[2-14] Although effective methods are available to deal with many LASIK complications, others are still subject to investigation. A comprehensive awareness of the potential complications of LASIK and the numerous strategies to handle them is fundamental for surgeons performing the procedure.

INTRAOPERATIVE COMPLICATIONS
Microkeratome-Related Complications

These complications are related to the learning curve associated with microkeratome use. Experience with the Hansatome, Moria M-2, and new horizontal microkeratomes suggests that their use will significantly reduce the incidence of serious LASIK complications.

INCOMPLETE OR IRREGULAR CUT.[1,5,14-19] Incomplete flaps occur when the microkeratome blade comes to a halt before reaching the intended location of the hinge. Visual aberrations are most likely to occur when the new hinge results in scarring in proximity to the visual axis.

In cases in which the microkeratome head is jammed, the suction should be released, followed by careful removal of the suction-microkeratome complex from the eye.

If the exposed stromal bed is not large enough to allow adequate laser ablation, the flap should be repositioned and the laser procedure postponed. Irrigation of the flap-stromal interface is performed in a manner similar to that in uncomplicated LASIK. The flap is then flattened carefully and dried. Resuming forward cutting after stoppage may result in an irregular stromal bed and irregular astigmatism.

If the created hinge is beyond the visual axis, some surgeons may consider manually extending the dissection with a blade (Fig. 22-1). Caution is advised when attempting such a maneuver because of the risks of uneven bed creation and flap buttonhole formation.[1] When the laser ablation is performed, the flap should be protected from laser exposure. Placement of a metallic plate or a surgical sponge over the flap may prevent inadvertent laser ablation on the hinge and flap.

With irregular cuts, the surgeon should not proceed with the ablation, but the flap or fragments thereof should be carefully replaced and realigned to their original position using the gutter width as a landmark. The pieces should fit together like a jigsaw puzzle. Additional waiting/drying time is used, and a bandage contact lens overnight may be considered if the epithelium is rough.

A LASIK flap may be fashioned 3 to 6 months later, assuming there was an uneventful postoperative course. It is advisable to attempt a deeper and more peripheral cut during the retreatment. Factors to consider in setting the depth for the second pass include corneal thickness and amount of tissue ablation contemplated.

In more serious situations, it may be necessary to perform a lamellar keratoplasty at least 6 months after the initial operation.

FREE CAP. This may be due to inadvertent omission of the stopper or to the use of a thin suction ring on a flat cornea (Moria microkeratomes).[17,18,20–25] In instances when a free cap is not visible on the surface of the cornea, the microkeratome head should be carefully inspected and, if need be, disassembled because the cap is probably inside the instrument.

Preplaced corneal marks with gentian violet used for proper orientation and careful attention during retrieval of the cap from the microkeratome head allow favorable management of a free cap.[26] If the diameter of the exposed stroma is equal to or larger than the intended laser ablation zone, laser treatment may proceed as planned. The cap is then retrieved from the antidesiccation chamber and repositioned using the preplaced marks. Proper orientation is important. The width of the gutter should be observed and a blunt atraumatic Merocel sponge sweep may be used for this purpose.

Chatter marks from vibration along the edges of the bed due to blade oscillation can often be of assistance; in order to highlight them better, the surgeon should use high magnification. It is important that the cap is replaced, epithelial side up, on the stromal bed. It has been suggested that the free cap be floated on a bed of balanced salt solution (BSS) and allowed to adhere spontaneously to the stroma assisted by careful placement of a Merocel sponge at different gutter positions. The bed of BSS will slowly disappear by capillary action toward the dry Merocel sponge, assuring even wrinkle-free adherence of the free cap to the corneal stroma. Care must be taken in aligning the preplaced corneal marks. Cap and stromal adhesion should be ensured by allowing adequate time of contact; 5 to 8 minutes should be sufficient for this purpose. Performing the striae test to check for adherence may be valuable. A dry Merocel sponge is used to exert light pressure on the outer section of the gutter of resection. Good adhesion is manifest as formation of striae that radiate from the point of pressure toward the center of the cornea. Sutures are seldom necessary but may be placed in an antitorque, external compression, or interrupted fashion.[26] A bandage contact lens may be placed in order to protect the cap, especially if the epithelium has been damaged. Some surgeons prefer to avoid the use of a bandage contact lens if the epithelium is intact because the lens may dislocate the cap.[27] Slit-lamp evaluation of the cap should be performed.

The potential for cap loss is real if the patient does not exercise caution in the early postoperative period. Wearing eye shields at night and special protective polycarbonate eyewear for sports activities is helpful. The patient should also be advised against eye rubbing because of the potential of cap dislocation.

PERFORATED LENTICULE OR BUTTONHOLING. If the suction is broken during passage of the microkeratome, the blade will surface; an irregular cap with a cut through the central cornea may result.

If the intraocular pressure is too low during passage of the head, a thin or "donut-shaped" flap or cap is likely to be created; it will probably be small in diameter.

Nonuniform cutting speed[28] in case of a manually advanced microkeratome may also predispose to this complication.[6,14,17,25,29–33] Buttonholed flaps can provide a channel for epithelial cells to infiltrate the flap-stroma interface. There is also an increased risk of subepithelial scar formation in flaps with buttonholes. Steep corneas (>46D) have been compared with tennis balls that buckle centrally under applanating pressure, resulting in a central dimple missed by the blade leading to a buttonhole. Another theory is that higher keratometric values offer increased resistance to cutting when applanated, leading to upward movement of the blade. The latter is probably more applicable to keratomes with lower blade oscillation rates. Blunted blades, poor oscillation, and microflaws of blades have also been described as mechanical microkeratome problems that may lead to buttonholes.[34–36] Inadequate coupling of the blade to the cornea is often due to poor suction.[37,38] Another possible risk factor for flap buttonhole occurrence is previous ocular surgery.[2] A higher incidence of buttonholes with large flaps when using the Hansatome is reported. It is theorized that the larger area required for flattening may result in central dimpling if the intraocular pressure is not adequate.[39]

The safest way to proceed when a buttonholed flap is encountered is to avoid lifting the flap or immediately reposition the flap and abort the procedure. Epithelial debris should be gently irrigated out with BSS.

Although some advocate proceeding with scraping the epithelium and performing a PRK laser ablation within 2 weeks,[40] this approach may not be feasible in higher myopes because of the appearance of unexpected subepithelial haze.[41] A bandage contact lens should be used to protect the buttonholed flap from migration.

Most patients with buttonholes end up with no significant loss of vision after adequate healing has occurred, especially if uncomplicated by epithelial ingrowth (Fig. 22-2). Epithelial ingrowth after a buttonhole can be central or in the periphery.[27] Management of epithelial ingrowth of this type can be very frustrating. Often the only viable option is discarding what remains of the flap. Reepithelialization is then allowed to occur with subsequent performance of phototherapeutic keratectomy (PTK) later.

The long-term approach to these eyes may be (1) soft contact lenses, (2) gas-permeable contact lenses, (3) retreatment with LASIK 3 to 6 months later if adequate thickness remains, (4) PRK (high risk of haze and irregular astigmatism), and (5) complete flap removal with PTK.

CORNEAL PERFORATION (FULL-THICKNESS ANTERIOR CHAMBER ENTRY).[16] All LASIK surgeons should possess a good understanding of the mechanics, assembly, and calibration of the microkeratome being used.

This complication is almost always due to human error in placing the plate and controlling depth of cut in instruments such as the automated corneal shaper.

Anterior chamber penetration may occur during lamellar dissection[14,42,43] or through laser ablation.[44,45] Globe perforation may range from a simple corneal perforation to perforation with damage to the iris and crystalline lens with or without vitreous loss. Corneal perforation may result from excessively thin corneas, for instance, following old corneal wounds, ulcers, or previous refractive surgery.[44]

Most modern microkeratomes have an integrated plate; thus, the risk of corneal perforation is avoided. With these newer mi-

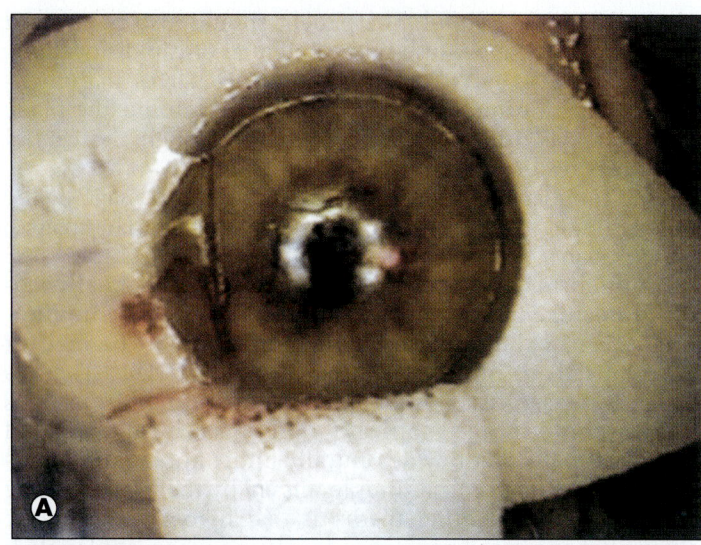

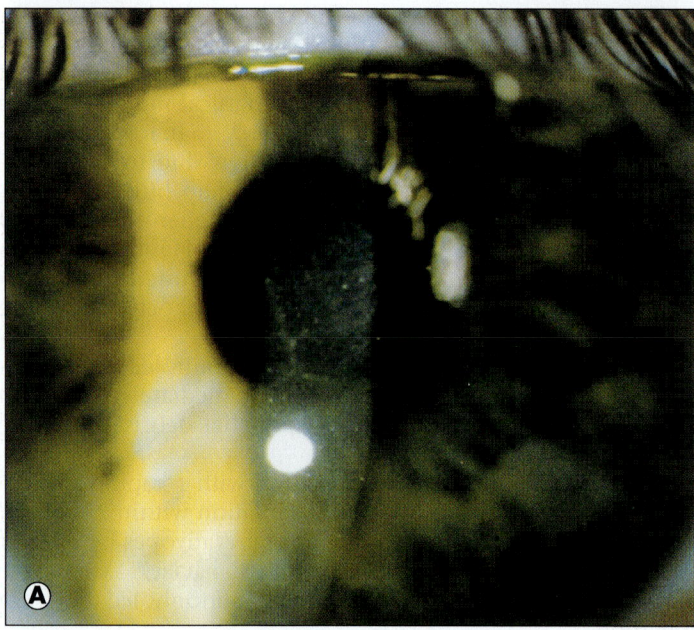

FIG. 22-2 ■ **A,** Corneal reflex showing irregular flap and stromal bed. (From Melki SA, Azar DT. Eight pearls in prevention and management of LASIK complications. In: Melki SA, Azar DT, eds. 101 Pearls in refractive, cataract, and corneal surgery. Thorofare, NJ: Slack; 2001:23–32.) **B,** Epithelial irregularity overlapping area of buttonholed flap without associated loss of visual acuity.

crokeratomes, perforation occurs only if the surgeon performs the lamellar cut on a very thin or irregular cornea or a cornea with advanced keratoconus. It is therefore mandatory to perform accurate pachymetry at several points on the cornea.

Immediate closure of the corneal wound with 10-0 nylon sutures should be performed. Further management depends on the severity of the damage caused to the globe. An ocular protective shield should be placed, and the patient is asked to try to relax and minimize straining and coughing. The patient should be transferred to the major operating room and given general anesthesia after ensuring adequate closure of the corneal entry site. Administration of local periocular anesthesia increases the potential risks of ocular damage during surgical repair of an open globe. Repair may involve corneal repair, iris repair, lensectomy with or without intraocular lens implantation, and anterior and/or posterior vitrectomy.

A contact lens may be necessary postoperatively. Aphakic contact lenses with or without an artificial pupil may be required. There may be a need for a secondary intraocular lens implantation (posterior chamber, iris-sutured, or trans-scleral sutured). In some instances a rotational or penetrating keratoplasty (PK) may be required for visual rehabilitation.

POOR COUPLING TO THE GLOBE

Inadequate Suction. Inadequate suction or total loss of suction is a potential source of serious problems during LASIK. The result maybe a thin or superficial flap, a buttonhole or interrupted flap, or an irregular flap.

If chemosis is induced from repeated suction ring placement, an incision in the conjunctiva may allow drainage of excess fluid; alternatively, blunt instruments such as a Merocel sponge, the handle of a swab, or a forceps can be used in an attempt to "milk" the fluid away from the limbus.

A better alternative is to wait 30 to 45 minutes and then try again. It is best to postpone the procedure for 1 to 2 days and allow the subconjunctival edema to reabsorb.

Inadequate Exposure. Microkeratome placement is more difficult in sunken globes and in eyes with narrow palpebral fissures and small corneas.[14] The use of the newer generation microkeratomes with the down-up flap has overcome this obstacle. By turning the head of the patient slightly to the opposite side or by exerting a gentle pull and tilt on the eye through the suction ring handle, these cases can be operated on easily. Other authors advise using a manual dissection[16] of the corneal flap or another refractive procedure.

PRK or laser subepithelial keratomileusis (LASEK) should be considered if appropriate when suction cannot be obtained. A lateral canthotomy may be indicated. Alternatively, it may be possible to operate without using a speculum. If a speculum is not used, one must ensure that the eyelashes and the eyelids do not overlap and cover the ring, especially the track. In small eyes, an axial length measurement performed preoperatively allows the surgeon to select the correct ring diameter for the operation (under the circumstances, the standard 11mm suction ring may not be suitable). A retrobulbar injection to cause proptosis of the globe has been suggested. This is a valid technique but may induce chemosis-related problems described previously, as can repeated attempts to place the ring. The patient with a prominent brow should be positioned with the chin raised slightly, as this will maximize exposure.[1]

CORNEAL EPITHELIAL DEFECT.[37,38,46] This complication is usually caused by microkeratome head passage over a dry corneal surface. In the event of detachment, the epithelium is repositioned if possible. A loose-fitting bandage contact lens is used to protect the epithelium, with antibiotic coverage to avoid secondary infection. These measures help in pain control as well as improving flap adherence and preventing epithelial cell ingrowth.[47-49] Nonsteroidal anti-inflammatory drug[49-54] drops may be used minimally (twice daily for 2 days maximum), as these will slow reepithelialization.

The bandage lens is removed as soon as epithelization is nearly complete. It should be thoroughly hydrated with artificial tears and a drop of anesthetic and floated on the corneal surface prior to gentle removal. Care should be taken to rule out an epithelial defect masquerade syndrome, a newly described, well-defined syndrome in which unrecognized epithelial ingrowth contributes to a persistent epithelial defect.[47]

Patients with a history of recurrent erosions[55,56] and/or anterior basement membrane dystrophy (ABMD) are at higher risk of developing epithelial abrasions with LASIK and would probably be better PRK candidates.[57-61]

WOUND DEHISCENCE. This complication may occur when a flap is being cut on a cornea-grafted eye. The high intraocular pressure exerted during the application of the suction ring is the cause. Several surgeons find LASIK a good treatment for the myopic and astigmatic refractive errors after a PK. Yet the time of surgery is still debatable. The consensus is to delay the LASIK procedure as much as possible after a PK. The presence of a good wound scar and the documentation of refractive and topographic stability for at least 3 months after removal of all keratoplasty sutures are good signs to do the surgery.[62] Surgeons should always warn their patient about this potential complication. In these cases, the same treatment as for corneal penetration may apply.

PIZZA SLICING.[63] This complication may occur when a flap is cut in an eye that had radial keratotomy (RK) with the incisions extending beyond the 8–9mm central area. Inadequate healing of the RK incisions causes a part of the flap to separate in a triangular shape. An epithelial plug in the incision almost always precipitates this complication. As a rule, always check the RK incisions under the microscope before cutting the flap.

CORNEAL BLEED.[37] This usually occurs when the microkeratome blade hits limbal vessels in case of a decentered flap or corneal pannus in contact lens wearers. Bleeding can be minimized in the following ways:

1. Apply a dry sponge to the bleeding area (if bleeding is localized) and exert slight pressure (sufficient to arrest it) or wick away the blood and simultaneously perform the ablation.
2. A Gimbel-Chayet sponge may be used to prevent the blood from oozing into the bed, as well as elevating the flap and keeping fat and debris in the tear film from coming into contact with the interface.
3. Leave the flap in position and wait until coagulation begins and bleeding diminishes.
4. Pressurized air can be used as a vasoconstrictor and to encourage coagulation.
5. In uncontrolled bleeding, the suction ring may be reapplied and pressure reactivated for the duration of the ablation; this will arrest bleeding until the end of treatment but should not be used longer than 30 seconds. A lower negative pressure would be better, which is available with some microkeratomes. A simple way of doing this is to perforate the suction tubing with a needle (the tubing will be discarded at the end of the surgery). Pressure can be instantly activated as needed by occluding the perforation.

Continuous oozing at the end of the procedure is stopped by flap replacement, irrigation, and smoothing, which closes the interface and tamponades the vessels.

THIN AND DECENTERED FLAPS.[4,40] If the flap is decentered and the area for ablation is adequate, the surgeon may proceed with laser treatment, possibly with a slight reduction in the optical zone. If this is not possible, the flap is repositioned and the operation repeated in 3 to 4 months. This is particularly important in hyperopic or astigmatic treatments and when a large ablation zone is planned.

The safest way to proceed when a thin or irregular flap is encountered is to reposition the flap and abort the procedure (see Fig. 22-2). It may be tempting to lift a thin flap and treat with the laser. If the thin flap has sufficient stromal tissue (i.e., sparing Bowman's layer) and is of sufficient size, laser ablation may be possible.[27]

In cases of thin, irregular, or decentered flaps, a deeper flap may be recut (20–60μm deeper) approximately 10–12 weeks later (after confirming a stable refraction) and the LASIK procedure completed. Three months seems to be the well-accepted time for reoperations. Although there have been reports of reoperations performed at earlier times, the risk of flap slippage during the reoperation may outweigh the benefits of early visual rehabilitation. A deeper properly placed flap during reoperation is essential, especially in hyperopic procedures requiring large ablation zones.[1]

Others advocate using a no-touch transepithelial PRK within 2 weeks of the initial irregular cut to prevent irregular astigmatism formation from the uneven ablation profile resulting from any late scar formation.[30,64] This technique seems reasonable, especially in low myopes. During the reoperation, one can perform transepithelial PRK to eliminate the scar. This is best performed in cases with a very superficial cut and within the first few weeks after the initial procedure.

EDEMATOUS FLAPS. Having an edematous flap precludes the possibility of having a hassle-free adhesion of the flap to the

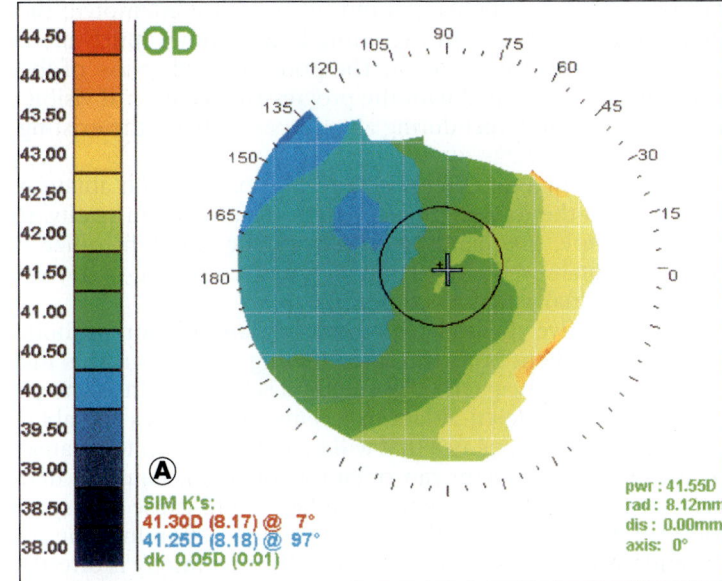

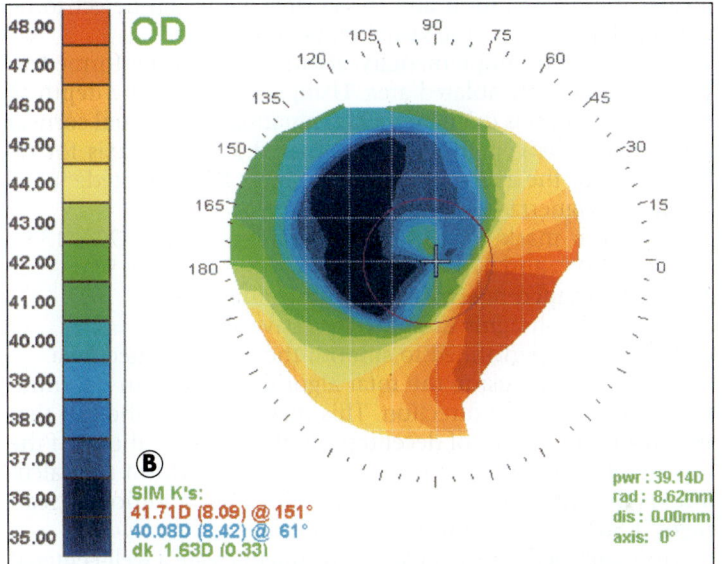

FIG. 22-3 ■ A, Temporal decentration after LASIK. B, Topographical pattern of pseudodecentration in a patient with lost LASIK cap. (From Johnson JD, Azar DT. Surgically induced topographical abnormalities after LASIK: management of central islands, corneal ectasia, decentration, and irregular astigmatism. Curr Opin Ophthalmol. 2001;12:309–17.)

stromal bed. Flap decentration or displacement may occur. This occurrence has been notorious enough to merit a name the "floating flap" phenomenon.[27]

Prolonged manipulation of the flap will traumatize the flap. Overzealous fluid irrigation under the flap is believed to be the culprit in producing an edematous flap.

Attempting to distend the flap gently with a nearly dry Merocel sponge or a blunt spatula to milk the flap may help. The use of the instruments such as the Pineda LASIK flap iron or the Caro island masher may be handy in flattening out these edematous corneas. In severe cases, suturing of the flap may be necessary in order to prevent flap migration. Aggressive use of topical steroids postoperatively may expedite the resolution of corneal edema.

Photoablation-Related Complications

DECENTRATION.[8,15,16,20,21,24,65–69] Significant decentration is defined as ablation center displacement from the pupil center by 0.5mm or more (Fig. 22-3). Decentration may be precipitated by a decentered laser beam prior to ablation (shift) or to eye drift during ablation (drift).[65,70] Decentration in LASIK may be precipitated by the higher amount of correction attempted; the duration of the treatment becoming longer allows much more time for patient drift to occur. The poor unaided vision of the high myopes combined with the progressive decrease in visibility of the fixation target during ablation exacerbates the existing fixation difficulties.[65]

Correction of a decentered ablation is possible with ablation correlated to the topography (topolink treatment). In reality, it is not as simple. Frequently, two—one on the top of the other—do not integrate well; there is often excessive removal of the tissue and residual astigmatism persists.

An alternative method for recentering an ablation without topolink treatment is to use a recentering system, such as the one devised by Vinciguerra. This method is based on the concept that with a decentered ablation, recentering requires the ablation of a larger, deeper area that will include the decentered area. In this way, the surgeon can obtain a correction equal to that originally expected. A decentered ablation will cause an asymmetry of the optical zone through excessive ablation in some areas and insufficient ablation in others. The asymmetry is directly proportional to the amount of decentration. Moreover, the greater the decentration and the greater the visual defect to be corrected, the greater the visual reduction.

A secondary complementary ablation can be performed to produce an evenly ablated area. Using algorithms, the depth of the new ablation is calculated. By evaluating a tangential corneal topography, the center of the decentered zone, the axis for retreatment, or the axis of decentration must be calculated.

The Vinciguerra system consists of:
1. A suction mask with blocking positions at 45°, 90°, 135°, 180°, 225°, and 270°.
2. A cross-shaped reference point for centration.
3. 7 to 10 diaphragms used for successive ablations.
4. PTK is then performed to smooth the newly ablated area.

Unfortunately, using the total algorithm results in decentration in the opposite direction. This may be due to the fact that the greater the degree of decentration, the less the validity of the topography. Therefore, it is more difficult to perform the calculations. In any case, it is easier to perform an additional treatment if 50% of the algorithm is used.

The combined treatment and retreatment create a well-centered ablation, the optical zone is wider, the ablation is deeper, and the final refraction outcome corresponds to the value originally expected. In order to do this, it is of the utmost importance to correlate the exact algorithm to the amount of decentration. All this produces a thinning of the cornea that is greater than the decentration of the initial error to be corrected and the initial optical zone used.

CENTRAL ISLANDS.[17,71-73] Central islands are diagnosed on corneal topography as central steep areas within the treatment zone and are defined by their width (≥2mm) and dioptric height (≥3 keratometric diopters) (Fig. 22-4). Central islands can cause irregular postoperative astigmatism, glare, ghosting and halo effect, loss of best-corrected visual acuity (BCVA), and monocular diplopia.

When faced with the diagnosis of a central island, always rule out iatrogenic keratectasia of the posterior corneal surface, especially in high myopia correction. Central islands should be treated conservatively as they may tend to resolve spontaneously, although not as successfully as with PRK, which forces the epithelium to undergo more extensive remodeling. Patient reassurance is needed pending possible laser retreatment. Statistics demonstrate that the incidence of central islands with broad-beam lasers is 80% in the first postoperative week, with a drop to 15% after 3 months and 5% after 6 months. When it persists for 6 months and more, one should consider treatment by laser ablation. Central islands are not seen with the flying spot laser. The amount of correction and diameter of the optical zone to be corrected depend

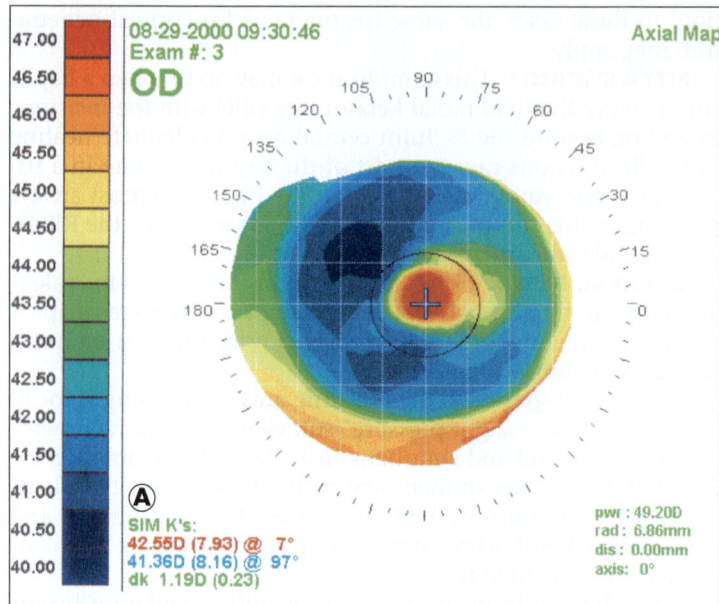

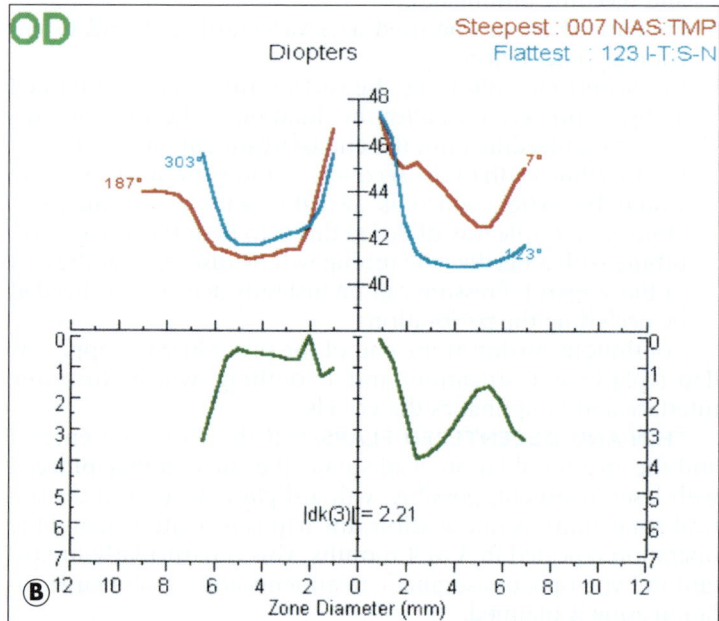

FIG. 22-4 ■ Central island after LASIK represented by axial topography (A) and profile map (B) showing approximately 5D island power. (From Johnson JD, Azar DT. Surgically induced topographical abnormalities after LASIK: management of central islands, corneal ectasia, decentration, and irregular astigmatism. Curr Opin Ophthalmol. 2001;12:309–17.)

on the corneal topography, according to Munnerlyn's formula. In order to avoid a hyperopic shift, the conservative approach is recommended. It is better to undercorrect slightly (Fig. 22-5). Treatment involves raising the original flap and then using laser ablation; treat with PRK or PTK mode centrally where the islands are found (see Fig. 22-5).

Wrinkles

Two types of flap wrinkles are described. Those that occur intraoperatively are due to malpositioning of a thin flap (undetectable intraoperative misalignment of the corneal flap on the stromal bed). These wrinkles may not be detected with the operating laser microscope. Surgeons should inspect the flap at the slit lamp immediately after surgery to ensure that flap wrinkles are not present.

The second type occurs in the early postoperative period and might be caused by eye rubbing or by the eyelid pressure dur-

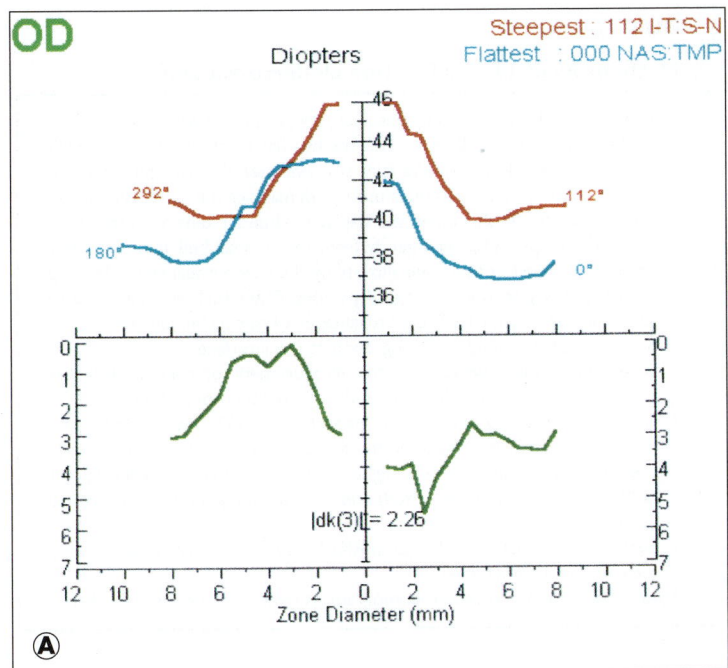

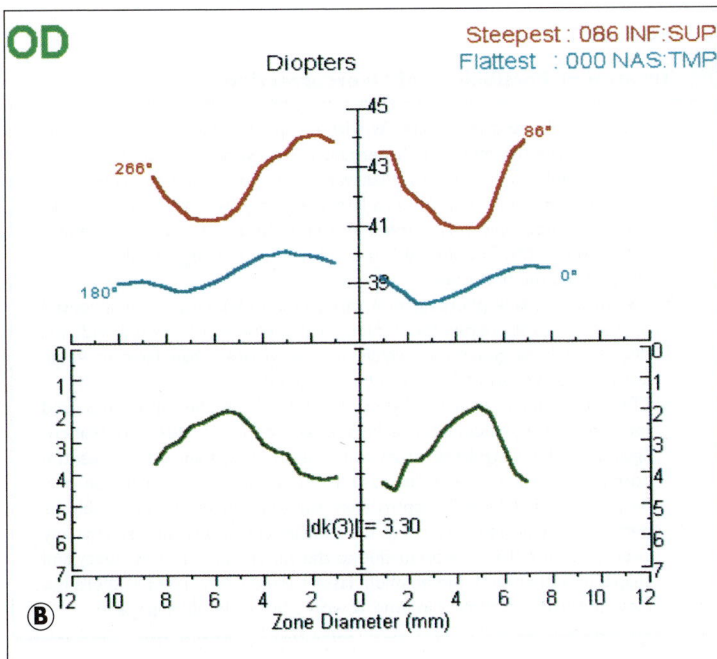

FIG. 22-5 ▪ LASIK-induced central island power profile prior to (A) and after (B) surgical management, showing a decrease in central island curvature. (From Johnson JD, Azar DT. Surgically induced topographical abnormalities after LASIK: management of central islands, corneal ectasia, decentration, and irregular astigmatism. Curr Opin Ophthalmol. 2001;12:309–17.)

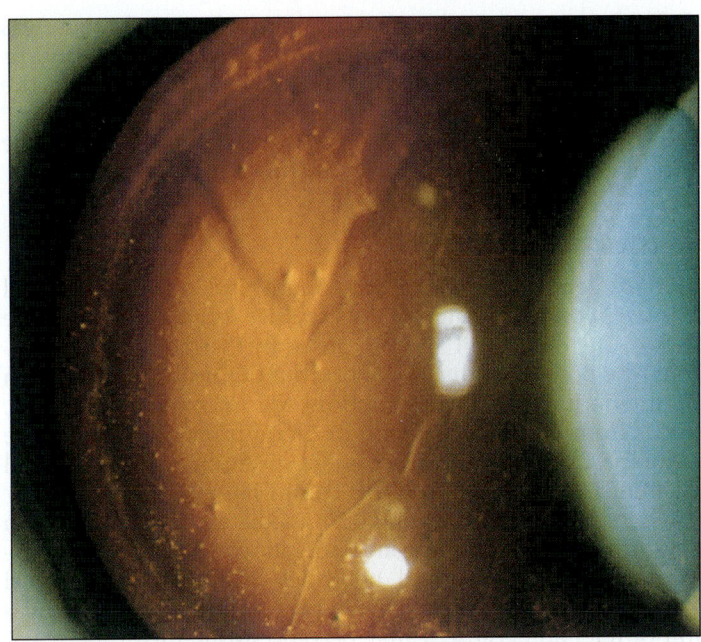

FIG. 22-6 ▪ Flap folds following LASIK causing topographical abnormalities that improved upon surgical ironing and smoothing of the flap. (From Johnson JD, Azar DT. Surgically induced topographical abnormalities after LASIK: management of central islands, corneal ectasia, decentration, and irregular astigmatism. Curr Opin Ophthalmol. 2001;12:309–17.)

ing blinking. Slight sliding or dislodgment of the flap almost always accompanies this type. After instillation of fluorescein dye in the eye, an uneven pattern of pooling in the tear film may be detected.[74]

The intraoperative management of flap wrinkles, striae, and folds is gentle replacement of the flap to its original neutral position. Gentle refloating of the flap may be attempted. This is followed by systematic sweeps of a moistened Merocel sponge to smooth to flap from the hinge out. A single-parallel-direction technique may be used in attempting to smooth out the flap, or a central-to-peripheral radial technique may be undertaken. Fluid in the flap-stroma interface should be eliminated. Air drying time should be at least 4 minutes to increase the likelihood of good adhesion. Mechanical hot air dryers may prove useful in this situation. Occasionally the Pineda or Caro LASIK flap irons

may be used to flatten the corneal irregularities. Usually epithelial wrinkling, striae, or folds disappear spontaneously within a few days.

Flap folds can induce irregular astigmatism with optical aberrations and loss of BCVA, especially if they involve the visual axis.[75-77] They are easily visualized as negative-staining lines with sodium fluorescein[74,78] or with retroillumination (Fig. 22-6).

A higher incidence of flap folds is usually found in higher myopes and is sometimes unavoidable. This is due to the reduced central convexity and stromal support resulting in flap redundancy that may be quite difficult to flatten. The latter is referred to as the "tenting" effect.[79] Folds and striae that have been neglected by the surgeon may be treated weeks or even months after the surgery, although the success rate declines with passing time.[80-84] The technique is the same except that after the flap has been lifted and refloated, folds typically appear much more prominent than they previously did at the slit lamp. The principle of flap centration and peripheral smoothing is the same, except that much more vigorous "ironing" with the smooth side of a spatula or forceps (Pineda iron) is required. The epithelial surface should be allowed to dry so that adequate traction with the smoothing instrument is achieved. Similarly, dry Merocel sponges on a dry corneal surface may be used. After this 8- to 12-minute process, the epithelium is usually in poor condition and a bandage contact lens is required.

The postoperative management of flap folds ranges from simple lifting and refloating of the flap to placement of sutures to stretch the flap in position. It is likely that the earlier a flap is attended to, the higher the chances of quick resolution.[79] Fixed folds probably occur when epithelial hyperplasia has time to form in the crevices formed by the folds. Flattening should aim at an even distribution of forces applied to the flap.[77,79-81] Instruments such as the Pineda or Caro LASIK flap iron can also be used to flatten isolated flaps at the slit lamp or under the operating microscope by gently pressing on them. Recalcitrant folds may respond well to placement of running antitorque sutures at the flap edge.[40] However, this may result in significant astigmatism. Another strategy is to make superficial epithelial incisions or frank epithelial débridement over the wrinkled area. This may relieve contractures that occur secondary to epithelial hyperplasia in longer standing folds. A technique was described using the red reflex as a way to better detect mild irregularities.[79] Other reported strategies include hydrating the flap with hypotonic saline (60–80%) or deionized water,[85] which may facilitate flattening. In extreme cases, removal of the corneal cap may be the most successful course of action.[27,40]

Interface Debris[14,29,65,66,86–88]

Interface debris may arise from conjunctival or skin epithelial cells swept on to the interface by excessive irrigation or excessive tearing. The debris can also be caused by the meibomian secretions, the powder of the gloves or from the swabs used to clean the interface, metal fragments from the microkeratome blade, mucus from the ocular surface, or blood from cut pannus. The use of the Chayet ring, the suction lid spectrum, and the Merocel has tremendously decreased this complication.

If debris is observed during or immediately after surgery, flap elevation and repositioning after irrigation are helpful, and perhaps both surfaces should be wiped with a moist Merocel sponge. The surgeon should avoid prolonged or repeated irrigation of the flap because it may become swollen with the attendant problems mentioned earlier.

Others

DESTRUCTION OF THE FLAP. If the corneal flap is irreversibly damaged during photoablation, a homoplastic flap will be necessary to replace the damaged tissue. If no homoplastic tissue is available and the cut surface is sufficiently smooth, the surgeon may proceed with the ablation, using a contact lens postoperatively to facilitate epithelialization. If the surface is moderately uneven prior to the refractive ablation, a standard PTK should be performed.

If the surface is extremely uneven, a number of options are available:

1. Extensive PTK can be performed, which requires a considerable amount of ablation.
2. A second very thin lamellar cut can be performed, using a plate of 70–80μm (if available); this allows the removal of the majority of irregularity. PTK is then performed, followed by the refractive ablation (the refractive calculation in such a case is very difficult). It is then necessary to use a lamella of homoplastic tissue because the corneal thickness has been considerably reduced.
3. The operation can be aborted, a contact lens applied, the epithelium allowed to regenerate, a transepithelial PTK performed, and then the refractive ablation.

UNEVEN ABLATION (IRREGULARITIES AND SMALL TRANSITION ZONE). Smoothing the ablated stromal bed with the excimer laser (PTK) can treat these types of complications. The real problem is whether the surgeon is really able to make an intraoperative diagnosis of a nonhomogeneous ablation. Actually, irregularities of the ablated surface can be highlighted intraoperatively only by using the Scheimpflug camera.

In the absence of wave front–guided custom ablation, a smoothing treatment is advisable in LASIK patients with visually significant interface irregularities. This technique is comparable to therapeutic photoablation: a wide ablation is used (9.0–10mm) as well as a masking fluid in order to obtain a better result with broad-beam lasers. Induction of hyperopia is highly unlikely.

The fluid must cover the entire corneal surface—no areas of dry cornea are allowed or the ablation will not be performed correctly. Another useful method is fluorescence under ultraviolet light to highlight the stromal areas that emerge from the masking fluid.

POSTOPERATIVE COMPLICATIONS

In a study[2] of 1026 eyes that underwent LASIK, the rate of postoperative complications averaged 3.1%.

BOX 22-1

Methods Available for Treating Undercorrection

1. Lifting the flap and reablating. This is usually performed within 3–4 months of the first treatment. By this time, the eye has reached refractive stability. The surgeon looks for the faint scar between the flap and the uncut cornea. A sharp Sinskey hook is used to demarcate the margin and incise the epithelium. At this point, the flap is held under tension with a fine-toothed forceps and peeled gently from the stromal bed. It is preferable to use the largest optical zone allowed by the new corneal hinge. The flap is then gently placed in its original position. The interface is hydrated to allow sutureless closure. The disadvantages of this technique are:
   a. Increased risk of epithelial ingrowth at the interface.
   b. Attention must be paid to the measurement of corneal thickness when evaluating the ablation depth to leave adequate residual bed.
2. Recutting a new flap (for myopias greater than 10D). This should be performed at least 6 months after the initial surgical treatment. The in situ operation is repeated with a slightly deeper cut than the primary cut (a 180μm plate is normally used) and entering peripheral to the original cut, if possible.
3. Surface photoablation technique (PRK). Postoperative haze is significantly greater than in virgin eyes.

Always use an undercorrected nomogram, as overcorrection is very likely.

BOX 22-2

Treatment Possibilities of Overcorrection

1. Lifting the flap and reablating. As with myopic retreatment, it is possible to repeat the treatment for hyperopic values within 2–3 months. It may be preferable to wait longer than with undercorrection to allow more time for regression. In addition, a larger flap may be necessary (recut) to allow the hyperopic correction and a recut should be done no sooner than 4–6 months. Therefore it is mandatory that the biggest flap diameter is fashioned the first time.
2. Hyperopic surface photoablation (hyperopic PRK). This is not a central procedure, so it creates fewer functional problems correlated with the degree of haze generated, which will be greater than haze in virgin corneas. Hyperopia of 1–3D can be corrected.
3. LTK with holmium laser (for hyperopia of 3–4D). A fiber-optic tip is used for contact (or noncontact) technique to produce localized corneal coagulation. The coagulated areas will create steepening of the central cornea with a subsequent decrease in the positive power. This can only be performed at least 3 months after surgery and should preferably be performed in an area external to the lamellar cut, as this will also limit any overcorrection that may occur due to the varied corneal consistency and shape. Treatment with the holmium laser should overcorrect as there is a clear tendency to regress in time. It works better in older patients.

Early Postoperative Complications

OVERCORRECTION AND UNDERCORRECTION.[14,17,20–23,38,65,89] Undercorrection is the most frequent complication after primary LASIK.[22,38,65,90–99]

It is usually diagnosed in the first few weeks postoperatively, and the refractive error stabilizes early thereafter. Several methods are available for treating undercorrection (Box 22-1). Overcorrection is most often seen after retreatments[100] and in elderly patients (>50 years). Under- and overcorrection are related to the ablation algorithm, nonaccurate nomograms, age, and the amount of myopia, astigmatism, or hyperopia to be corrected.[101,102] Several factors determine the maximum correction possible for high-myopia patients, including the total corneal thickness[15,65] (flap and residual bed thickness) and the diameter of the optical zone.[65] Often the full correction is not possible, which explains the undercorrected results in many high-myopia groups.

Overcorrection is disappointingly common after LASIK, especially in the hands of aggressive surgeons who are still adjusting their nomograms. Luckily, many of these cases have regression during the first year after surgery. Thus, patients are best monitored for at least 6–12 months postoperatively. Some cases, however, will be permanently overcorrected to clinically significant hyperopia. Retreatment should be considered 2 or 3 months later, waiting longer in high myopia for stabilization (Box 22-2).

SLIDING OR DISLODGED FLAP.[18,20,40,103–111] Flap displacement occurs most commonly in the first 24 hours after LASIK, before the epithelium has had time to heal over the lamellar entry site. The appropriate time to allow for flap adhesion intraoperatively is still debatable; recommended times vary between 3 and 5 minutes. Whatever the waiting time is, performing the flap striae maneuver at the end is recommended. This displacement can occur as late as many months after the procedure.[30,48,81,112,113] Mechanical displacement by lid action is the main culprit in the early period. It may also follow eyelid rubbing or squeezing. Larger diameter and thinner flaps are more prone to be displaced, especially if the hinge is small. The flap remains vulnerable to traumatic displacement several months after surgery.[102,112,114–123]

A dislodged flap is an emergency. It should be repositioned as soon as possible to prevent fixed folds and epithelial ingrowth. Failure to act promptly increases the likelihood of permanent striae formation with decreased visual quality. The flap should first be reflected and the interface (stromal bed and stromal aspect of the flap) carefully examined for epithelial cells or other debris. They should be aggressively scraped prior to repositioning the flap. A contact lens can be applied to provide added protection from further displacement.[48] Techniques described earlier to flatten any associated folds should be used. Additional time should be taken in smoothing and drying the flap. This is important to prevent epithelial cell migration from the healing periphery toward the flap interface under the tented folds.

Additional time should be allowed for smoothing and stretching the flap symmetrically into place. This can usually be achieved using moist Merocel sponges, allowing drying as smoothing proceeds to facilitate grasp on the flap, stretching of striae, and extending the flap so that it completely fills the bed. The gutter margins should be symmetrical and minimal. In cases in which striae formation is more pronounced, the edges must be ironed out to fill the peripheral groove and eliminate striae. This is a laborious procedure, taking several minutes, but it works even after several months. The surgeon should be aware that striae will initially remain visible but will disappear over 24 to 48 hours if the flap has been fully distended. The flap should be well lubricated for a couple of weeks. This will decrease the probability of friction causing further mischief. An eye shield may be suggested for an extended period of time. Rarely, sutures may be necessary to maintain flap position until the situation has stabilized.[12]

LOSS OF THE FLAP/CAP. Cap loss may occur intraoperatively or during the early or late postoperative period. Factors that may lead to the loss of the corneal cap include incomplete adherence of the cap to the stroma, eye rubbing, loosening and removal of the pressure patch, excessive blinking, and trauma.

Some patients fully tolerate LASIK with cap loss and recover well with no significant visual problems. The eye has a greater risk of developing pseudodecentration (see Fig. 22-3, *B*) and significant haze than with primary PRK. Haze is more common with deep ablations, in brown eyes, and in younger patients. If the haze is marked after several months, the surgeon may perform PTK with the excimer following complete removal of the epithelium with the placement of a homoplastic corneal cap, as described previously.

If the flap is not found, the corneal epithelium is allowed to grow centrally in a manner similar to that after other "superficial" keratectomy procedures such as PRK with possibly a more profound central applanation effect. A bandage contact lens is placed and surface is evaluated over a period of 3–4 days or until the cornea is fully reepithelialized. Any excimer laser treatment should be aborted and retreatment deferred until refractive stability is achieved. However, some authors advocate immediate suturing of a lamellar homograft to the stromal bed[27,124] whenever possible. A slightly smaller cap is produced to serve as a lamellar homograft to the recipient stromal bed. Prophylactic topical antibiotics and steroids should be given. Secondary enhancement procedures may be performed later.[124,125]

If the flap is found, it typically has been detached for a number of hours and has become very edematous, making it very difficult to distinguish the stromal face from the epithelial surface. The fine stromal granulation and occasionally the edges of the microkeratome cut can be used to identify the stromal side of the flap. Fluorescein may also be of assistance. If a bandage was used, the flap may actually be stuck to it. In this situation, the flap will be severely dehydrated. If the flap is found, its stromal surface and stromal bed must be carefully cleaned to remove debris or epithelial growth; the flap may then be repositioned to its original location. This is not simple as there are no marks and may be no landmarks.

Even when the flap has been found, cleaned, and oriented into position, it is highly unlikely that it will adhere without sutures. Running sutures are preferred instead of interrupted or compression sutures as the risk of epithelial ingrowth is less. If the flap is irreparably damaged, it must be discarded.

DIFFUSE LAMELLAR KERATITIS OR THE SHIFTING SANDS OF THE SAHARA.[126–138] Diffuse lamellar keratitis (DLK) is a diffuse inflammation in the interface without microbial cause. This sterile inflammation may appear within 24 hours or be delayed a few days after surgery.[139–142] Direct cultures from the interface after lifting the flap show no growth of bacteria or fungi. The course of this disorder can be highly variable, gradually disappearing, persisting, or increasing.

Although more common following primary LASIK, this complication can develop after LASIK retreatments.[24,141] When the surgeon is in doubt between DLK and bacterial keratitis, a culture taken from the interface after lifting the flap is highly recommended. Scrapings of the interface material have demonstrated neutrophils but no bacteria.

Topical steroids are the mainstay of treatment. They should be potent drops of dexamethasone and prednisolone, not fluorometholone. They must initially be administered with high frequency in addition to a prophylactic antibiotic cover. Antibiotic prophylaxis is necessary as infective keratitis cannot be ruled out even though the presentation is usually much more severe than nonspecific DLK. The fact that the response to steroids is extremely rapid suggests that this syndrome is of immune origin.

Milder forms of the syndrome resolve easily in 1 to 2 weeks with topical steroid drops alone. More severe forms of the syndrome have moderate to marked findings and are symptomatic with moderate to severely reduced vision. In these cases, the flap must be lifted, gently cleaned, and aggressive steroid treatment immediately started with the addition of topical antibiotics as prophylaxis. Topical steroids act specifically to prevent degranulation by the polymorphonuclear enzyme cells, limiting or preventing melting. In these cases, there may be a worsening of the clinical picture on day 2, stabilization by day 3, and the start of improvement by day 4 to 5.

Slit-lamp examination on a more or less daily basis is necessary for at least the first week. Generally speaking, if treatment is rapid and massive, there is improvement within 1 to 3 days after initiation with complete resolution in 1 to 2 weeks to 1 month at most. Improvement normally starts peripherally and progresses toward the center (Box 22-3).

INFECTIOUS KERATITIS.[143–154] Bacterial infection under a LASIK flap is rarely reported but remains one of the most vision-threatening complications. LASIK carries a significant risk of infection because the corneal stroma can be exposed to infective agents during lamellar surgery. Eyelashes, conjunctiva, drapes, speculum, microkeratome, and surrounding atmosphere are all sources of infection.[155–162]

Although complications such as epithelial ingrowth and interface inflammation can cause similar symptoms, a high index of suspicion should be maintained for infections and the patient treated accordingly.

When faced with this problem, the most important considerations are the need for early diagnosis, adequate microbiological sampling, and appropriate treatment. Lifting the flap for culture scrape, debulking and cleaning of the interface, and irrigation with antibiotics have a diagnostic and therapeutic effect. Corneal scraping through the flap may result in loss of the flap. Fortified topical antibiotics are then started.

Most of the reported cases had a final BCVA of 20/40 or better. It is reassuring to note that it is possible for these patients to attain an unaided acuity and final refraction compatible with an uncomplicated LASIK procedure. However, other patients have not fared well.[158,159,161]

Only one case[158] had a bilateral corneal infection, yet other reported cases were done simultaneously.[155,156,159]

Bacterial keratitis is one of the major concerns that the surgeon should consider and inform the patient about when deciding on simultaneous or sequential surgery. The augmented risk of bilateral simultaneous LASIK compared with sequential LASIK appears to be low.[163] It would appear that there is, as yet, insufficient evidence to compel surgeons to perform sequential rather than simultaneous surgery. On the other hand, LASIK should be performed under sterile operative conditions, as one would expect for intraocular surgery. A number of very prominent surgeons do not use gloves during LASIK and do not report infection as a complication. Despite this, the standard should be to wear powder-free surgical gloves. Typically, fluoroquinolone antibiotic is applied four times per day for 5–7 days after surgery.

EPITHELIAL INGROWTH.[16–18,20,22,65,68,86,164–170] Two types of epithelial ingrowth are identified. The epithelium may be introduced into the interface at the time the lamellar cut is performed or may grow in from the peripheral surface epithelium. If the epithelial tissue contains viable cells, these cells may proliferate and produce a nest of tissue within the interface. Most of the time, these cells have only limited proliferative potential; if so, a nest of cells may appear, stop expanding, and remain stable within the interface for years. Occasionally, the nest of cells will continue to expand and may produce more significant complications. In other cases it is clear from a visible track of cells that epithelium grew into the interface from the periphery.

The main risk factor for epithelial ingrowth is a deficient technique that results in a peripheral epithelial defect, poor flap adhesion, or a perforated corneal flap.

The frequency of this complication appears to be highly variable.[30] LASIK retreatments[120] may be associated with a higher risk of interface epithelial growth, especially if a spatula is inserted through the epithelium and used to break open the interface by sweeping. The epithelial tissue may adhere to the spatula and be transferred into the interface. It may be preferable to break open the interface temporally or inferiorly with a probe, grasp the temporal or inferior edge of the flap with a 0.12 forceps, and gently peel the flap back.

The treatment is dependent on the extent and location of the ectopic epithelial tissue. A small nest of epithelium that is present in the periphery can be left alone if it does not progress or affect visual acuity.

Treatment is indicated when the epithelial ingrowth exceeds 2.0 mm from the flap edge, if progression is observed, if melting occurs, if it affects visual acuity, or if it induces astigmatism. The specific treatment depends on the situation: if epithelial cells are present centrally, visual acuity is decreased because of the presence of cells, irregular astigmatism, and undercorrection. Cells must always be removed. Removal must be immediate to prevent extension of the cell mass and secondary stromal melting. If areas of epithelialization are peripheral and do not affect the refraction or keratometry, they can be monitored regularly by biomicroscopy and photography during the postoperative checks to ensure that the situation is stable and not progressive. In some cases, there may be spontaneous regression and disappearance of some moderately sized epithelial islands in the peripheral or paracentral zones. To evaluate whether there has been progression, the patient must simply be monitored 1 and 2 weeks and then 1, 2, and 3 months after surgery. If the ingrowth does not disturb the patient's vision and is in the outer 2.0 mm with a demarcation line, it is probably safer to leave it alone, considering that removal may create folds or irregular astigmatism.

Removal techniques consist of lifting the flap while the patient is lying under the microscope. A spatula (Suarez type) or chalazion curette is used to remove the epithelial island, which normally has a globular, cystic, almost encapsulated shape. The stromal bed must also be cleaned even though the epithelium is normally adherent to the underside of the flap. The instrument used to clean it must be cleaned after every stroke to avoid reintroducing epithelial cells. Irrigation and brushing may be used if there is any doubt about any removal of the epithelium. Paying close attention, the surgeon should be able to remove all the material with a single stroke, reducing the chance of leaving cells and recurrence. If more than one pass of the spatula is needed, the two surfaces should be gently scraped. Irrigation with abundant BSS to remove any residual cells and other debris from the interface should be done. It is advisable to direct the jet of irrigating BSS obliquely to the surface to be cleaned, using the flow to remove any occult cells or debris. Once cleaning has been completed, the flap edges are reapproximated.

The same applies on the stromal side of the flap. In some instances, few PTK pulses are applied. In the case of a sheath extending from the periphery, peeling is done.

FLAP MELT. In all reported cases, flap melting always developed over an area of epithelial ingrowth.[20,171] The incidence can be decreased by careful keratectomy with no epithelial damage, good irrigation of the stromal bed, ensuring strong adhesion with a minimal gap between flap edge and stromal bed, and early epithelial cell débridement when significant areas of ingrowth are present or progression or melt is observed. If a spontaneous epithelial defect occurs on the surface above a nest of epithelium, the ectopic epithelium should be removed.

The flap should be lifted. It may not be possible to do this smoothly due to tissue alterations. The flap undersurface and stromal bed must be cleaned and gently débrided with a smooth spatula; all debris, impurities, or epithelial nests must be removed. The flap is then smoothed and repositioned following irrigation of the stromal surfaces with BSS. A bandage contact lens is recommended if significant epithelial defects are present. Treatment continues with topical antibiotic and tear substitutes under strict follow-up.

Despite aggressive management, melting may still occur. There may be necrosis of the flap with extension and loss of anatomical integrity of the flap itself. This situation requires rapid removal of the flap to avoid infection or necrosis spreading to deeper stromal layers. The damaged flap may require replacement with a homoplastic flap.

Late Postoperative Complications

REGRESSION. Regression is a documented return in the direction of the original refractive error, recorded over several visits, 3 to 6 months after LASIK. Regression appears to be minimal after LASIK.[8,16,17,20,22,23,68,117]

Regression is reported to be more pronounced in hyperopic than in myopic LASIK.[172] The profile and size of the ablation and transition zone are incriminated. As the epithelium grows from the periphery, it encounters the sudden depression and tries to fill this depression by a hyperplastic response. This process reduces the power of the positive lens shape created by ablation and leads to regression and loss of effect.

Regression after LASIK was associated with increased corneal thickness and increased corneal steepening.[117] Potential mechanisms for regression of the refractive effect include nuclear sclerosis, stromal synthesis (wound healing),[173] compensatory epithelial hyperplasia (CEH), and iatrogenic keratectasia.

Some investigators argue that because of the absence of haze and the minimal formation of collagen after LASIK,[123] CEH appears to be the key mechanism in refractive regression.[117] This concept is endorsed by postoperative ultrasound corneal epithelial thickness measurements, which were found to be increased and which correlated highly with the postoperative regression.[174]

The corrective options are the same as those described for undercorrection. Again, in this case the flap lifting and reablation technique is advisable. Topical steroids may be useful to control haze. However, prior to considering enhancement, the surgeon must be sure that regression has stabilized and is not due to progressive ectasia. Corneal ectasia or iatrogenic keratoconus occurs when the quantity of stromal tissue remaining after the laser procedure is insufficient. It is of utmost importance that the flap and ablation depth not exceed 50% of the initial preoperative thickness, or, better still, the residual stroma should measure at least 250μm.

INDUCED OR IATROGENIC KERATECTASIA.[175–182] Iatrogenic keratectasia is a vision-threatening complication after LASIK. It is related to the weakening of the cornea's mechanical strength.

The corneal flap does not contribute to the biomechanics of the cornea. Most of the corneal stress is withstood by the residual thickness of the stromal bed only. Therefore, the question of a minimal thickness of the residual stroma arises. It is related to the upper limits of myopia correction by means of LASIK. The minimal thickness of residual stroma to withstand progressive ectasia has been derived from biomechanical measurements to be 250μm or 30% of the original thickness.

Clinically, there is a progressive deterioration in uncorrected visual acuity with a regression of the refractive effect (progressive myopic shift) and possible identification of the keratectasia on slit-lamp biomicroscopy.

Serial corneal topographies show progressive steepening of the central cornea. Most reported cases[181–184] had thin corneas on preoperative pachymetry, high myopia (>10D), and a residual postoperative stromal thickness of less than 250μm. Preoperative corneal pachymetry is mandatory on each case in order to make individual decisions about the ablation depth and subsequently the amount of myopia that could be corrected.[185] Even with adequate corneal thickness, this complication may still arise because of the inconsistencies in flap thickness with the current microkeratomes leading to deeper ablations than anticipated.

During the early postoperative period, it is not easy to differentiate topographically between a conventional central island that resulted from the ablation and a central keratectasia. The temporal evolution, however, will determine the nature of the central steep zone. The conventional central steep island tends to disappear within several months after surgery whereas the central keratectasia shows progression on topography.

If this serious complication occurs, PK is required because of loss of transparency of the deep stroma and poor optics.

NIGHT VISION PROBLEMS AND GLARE.[20,22,66,68,186] Distortion of vision in the form of glare and halos is one of the major concerns after LASIK. Glare and halo symptoms typically become worse at night when the pupil dilates and more peripheral light rays enter the eye from the untreated zone. The major contributor to glare and halo symptoms is the effective spherical aberration of the centrally flattened cornea.[187] Decentered ablations, small treatment zones, newly formed cataracts, and induced astigmatism are other important causes of night glare after LASIK.

With current LASIK techniques, patients with pupillary diameters larger than 6mm in scotopic conditions and those with high myopia are the most affected. These patients should be warned of this potential complication. In the early postoperative period, when in doubt about the cause of glare in the presence of wound healing and flap complications, the decrease or disappearance of glare in the affected eye while shining the pen light in the contralateral eye is a pathognomonic sign. Luckily, the majority of patients improve with time. With bilateral LASIK, the patient usually learns to ignore optical aberrations as a result of cortical integration.[27]

Increasing the optical zone is not always the answer as this means using an excessively deep ablation—a greater chance of inducing central islands—as in the case of a broad-beam laser. Patients with a disproportionately large pupil compared with the optic zone to be treated should be avoided. Phakic intraocular lenses for higher correction should be considered; however, large scotopic pupils might contraindicate these as well. Luckily, the majority of patients improve with time. Flying spot lasers with newer software may be used to enlarge the effective optic zone, even with a residual refractive error near emmetropia, if there is adequate residual corneal tissue for additional ablation.

REFERENCES

1. Melki SA, Azar DT. LASIK complications: etiology, management, and prevention. Surv Ophthalmol. 2001;46:95–116.
2. Stulting RD, Carr JD, Thompson KP, et al. Complications of laser in situ keratomileusis for the correction of myopia. Ophthalmology. 1999;106:13–20.
3. Gimbel HV, Penno EE, van Westenbrugge JA, et al. Incidence and management of intraoperative and early postoperative complications in 1000 consecutive laser in situ keratomileusis cases. Ophthalmology. 1998;105:1839–47.
4. Lin RT, Maloney RK. Flap complications associated with lamellar refractive surgery. Am J Ophthalmol. 1999;127:129–36.
5. Buratto L, Ferrari M. Indications, techniques, results, limits and complications of laser in situ keratomileusis. Curr Opin Ophthalmol. 1997;8(4):59–66.
6. Farah SG, Azar DT, Gurdal C, et al. Laser in situ keratomileusis: literature review of a developing technique. J Cataract Refract Surg. 1998;24:989–1006.
7. Pallikaris IG, Papatzanaki ME, Stathi EZ, et al. Laser in situ keratomileusis. Lasers Surg Med. 1990;10:463–8.
8. Melki SA, Azar DT. Eight pearls in prevention and management of LASIK complications. In: Melki SA, Azar DT, eds. 101 Pearls in refractive, cataract, and corneal surgery. Thorofare, NJ: Slack; 2001:23–32.
9. Slade SG, Updegraff SA. Advances in lamellar refractive surgery. Int Ophthalmol Clin. 1994;34:147–62.
10. Yoo SH, Azar DT. Laser in situ keratomileusis for the treatment of myopia. Int Ophthalmol Clin. 1999;39:37–44.
11. Trokel SL, Srinivasan R, Braren B. Excimer laser surgery of the cornea. Am J Ophthalmol. 1983;96:710–15.
12. Velasco-Martinelli EJ, Tarcha FA. Superior hinge laser in situ keratomileusis. J Refract Surg. 1999;15:S209–11.
13. Johnson JD, Azar DT. Surgically induced topographical abnormalities after LASIK: management of central islands, corneal ectasia, decentration, and irregular astigmatism. Curr Opin Ophthalmol. 2001;12:309–17.
14. Gimbel HV, Basti S, Kaye GB, Ferensowicz M. Experience during the learning curve of laser in situ keratomileusis. J Cataract Refract Surg. 1996;22:542–50.
15. Bas AM, Onnis R. Excimer laser in situ keratomileusis for myopia. J Refract Surg. 1995;11(Suppl):S229–33.
16. Pallikaris IG, Siganos DS. Laser in situ keratomileusis to treat myopia: early experience. J Cataract Refract Surg. 1997;23:39–49.
17. Knorz MC, Liermann A, Seiberth V, et al. Laser in situ keratomileusis to correct myopia of −6.00 to −29.00 diopters. J Refract Surg. 1996;12:575–84.
18. Marinho A, Pinto MC, Pinto R, et al. LASIK for high myopia: one year experience. Ophthalmic Surg Lasers. 1996;27(Suppl):S517–20.

19. Rao SK, Padmanabhan P, Sitalakshmi G, Rajagopal R. Partial flap during laser in-situ keratomileusis: pathogenesis and timing of retreatment. Indian J Ophthalmol. 2000;48:209–12.
20. Pérez-Santonja JJ, Bellot J, Claramonte P, *et al.* Laser in situ keratomileusis to correct high myopia. J Cataract Refract Surg. 1997;23:372–85.
21. Fiander DC, Tayfour F. Excimer laser in situ keratomileusis in 124 myopic eyes. J Refract Surg. 1995;11(Suppl):S234–8.
22. Guell JL, Muller A. Laser in situ keratomileusis (LASIK) for myopia from −7 to −18 diopters. J Refract Surg. 1996;12:222–8.
23. Salah T, Waring GO III, El-Maghraby A, *et al.* Excimer laser in situ keratomileusis under a corneal flap for myopia of 2 to 20 diopters. Am J Ophthalmol. 1996;121:143–55.
24. Argento CJ, Cosentino MJ. Laser in situ keratomileusis for hyperopia. J Cataract Refract Surg. 1998;24:1050–8.
25. Buratto L, Brint SF. LASIK principles and techniques. Thorofare, NJ: Slack; 1998:113–39,371–9.
26. Kim EK, Choe CM, Kang SJ, *et al.* Management of detached lenticule after in situ keratomileusis. J Refract Surg. 1996;12:175–9.
27. Buratto L, Brint S. Complications of LASIK. In: Buratto L, Brint S, eds. LASIK: surgical techniques and complications. Thorofare, NJ: Slack; 2000:177–264.
28. Kim YH, Choi JS, Chun HJ, Joo CK. Effect of resection velocity and suction ring on corneal flap formation in laser in situ keratomileusis. J Cataract Refract Surg. 1999;25:1448–55.
29. Brint SF, Ostrick DM, Fisher C, *et al.* Six-months results of the Multicenter Phase I Study of Excimer Laser Myopic Keratomileusis. J Cataract Refract Surg. 1994;20:610–15.
30. Wilson SE. LASIK. Management of common complications. Cornea 1998; 17:459–67.
31. Waring GO III, Carr JD, Stulting RD, *et al.* Prospective randomized comparison of simultaneous and sequential bilateral laser in situ keratomileusis for the correction of myopia. Ophthalmology. 1999;106:732–8.
32. Thompson V. Flap management during LASIK after radial keratotomy [letter]. J Refract Surg. 1997;13:128.
33. Leung AT, Rao SK, Cheng AC, *et al.* Pathogenesis and management of laser in situ keratomileusis flap buttonhole. J Cataract Refract Surg. 2000;26:358–62.
34. Lam DSC, Cheng ACK, Leung ATS. LASIK complications [letters]. Ophthalmology. 1999;106:1455–6.
35. Leung ATS, Rao SK, Cheng ACK, *et al.* Pathogenesis and management of laser in situ keratomileusis flap buttonhole. J Cataract Refract Surg. 2000;26:359–62.
36. Penno EA, Kaye G, van Westenbrugge J, *et al.* LASIK complications [authors' reply]. J Cataract Refract Surg. 1999;106:1456–7.
37. Davidorf J, Zaldivar R, Oscherow S. Results and complications of laser in situ keratomileusis by experienced surgeons. J Refract Surg. 1998;14:114–22.
38. Zaldivar R, Davidorf JM, Oscherow S. Laser in situ keratomileusis for myopia from -5.5 to -11.5 diopters with astigmatism. J Refract Surg. 1998;14:19–25.
39. Tham VMB, Maloney RK. Microkeratome complications of laser in situ keratomileusis. Am J Ophthalmol. 2000;107:920–4.
40. Lam DS, Leung AT, Wu JT, *et al.* Management of severe flap wrinkling or dislodgment after laser in situ keratomileusis. J Cataract Refract Surg. 1999;25:1441–7.
41. Polunin GS, Kourenkov VV, Makarov IA, *et al.* The corneal barrier function in myopic eyes after laser in situ keratomileusis and after photorefractive keratectomy in eyes with haze formation. J Refract Surg. 1999;15:S221–4.
42. Ansari EA, Morrell AJ, Sahni K. Corneal perforation and decompensation after automated lamellar keratoplasty for hyperopia. J Cataract Refract Surg. 1997;23:134–6.
43. Arevalo JF, Ramirez E, Suarez E, *et al.* Incidence of vitreoretinal pathologic conditions within 24 months after laser in situ keratomileusis. Ophthalmology. 2000;107:258–62.
44. Hori Y, Wantanabe H, Maeda N, *et al.* Medical treatment of operative corneal perforation caused by laser in situ keratomileusis. Arch Ophthalmol. 1999; 117:1422–3.
45. Joo CK, Kim TG. Corneal perforation during laser in situ keratomileusis. J Cataract Refract Surg. 1999;25:1165–7.
46. Smirennaia E, Sheludchenko V, Kourenkova N, Kashnikova O. Management of corneal epithelial defects following laser in situ keratomileusis. J Refract Surg. 2001;17:S196–9.
47. Azar DT, Scally A, Hannush SB, *et al.* Epithelial defect-masquerade syndrome after LASIK: characteristic clinical findings and visual outcomes. J Cataract Refract Surg. 2003 (in press).
48. Montes M, Chayet AS, Castellanos A, *et al.* Use of bandage contact lenses after laser in situ keratomileusis. J Refract Surg. 1997;13:S430–1.
49. Salz JJ, Reader AL 3rd, Schwartz LJ, *et al.* Treatment of corneal abrasions with soft contact lenses and topical diclofenac. J Refract Corneal Surg. 1994;10:640–6.
50. Cherry PM. The treatment of pain following excimer laser photorefractive keratectomy: additive effect of local anesthetic drops, topical diclofenac, and bandage soft contact. Ophthalmic Surg Lasers. 1996;27:S477–80.
51. Forster W, Ratkay I, Krueger R, *et al.* Topical diclofenac sodium after excimer laser phototherapeutic keratectomy. J Refract Surg. 1997;13:311–13.
52. Phillips AF, Hayashi S, Seitz B, *et al.* Effect of diclofenac, ketorolac, and fluorometholone on arachidonic acid metabolites following excimer laser corneal surgery. Arch Ophthalmol. 1996;114:1495–8.
53. Tomas-Barberan S, Fagerholm P. Influence of topical treatment on epithelial wound healing and pain in the early postoperative period following photorefractive keratectomy. Acta Ophthalmol Scand. 1999;77:135–8.
54. Tutton MK, Cherry PM, Raj PS, *et al.* Efficacy and safety of topical diclofenac in reducing ocular pain after excimer photorefractive keratectomy. J Cataract Refract Surg. 1996;22:536–41.
55. Heyworth P, Morlet N, Rayner S, *et al.* Natural history of recurrent erosion syndrome—a 4 year review of 117 patients. Br J Ophthalmol. 1998;82:26–8.
56. Puk DE, Probst LE, Holland EJ. Recurrent erosion after photorefractive keratectomy. Cornea. 1996;15:541–2.
57. Azar DT, Steinert RF. PTK in the management of PRK complications. phototherapeutic keratectomy, management of scars, dystrophies, and PRK complications. Baltimore: Williams & Wilkins; 1997:175–88.
58. Kozobolis VP, Siganos DS, Meladakis GS, *et al.* Excimer laser phototherapeutic keratectomy for corneal opacities and recurrent erosion. J Refract Surg. 1996;12:S288–90.
59. Lohmann CP, Sachs H, Marshall J, *et al.* Excimer laser phototherapeutic keratectomy for recurrent erosions: a clinical study. Ophthalmic Surg Lasers. 1996; 27:768–72.
60. O'Brart DP, Muir MG, Marshall J. Phototherapeutic keratectomy for recurrent corneal erosions. Eye. 1994;8:378–83.
61. Orndahl MJ, Fagerholm PP. Phototherapeutic keratectomy for map-dot-fingerprint corneal dystrophy. Cornea. 1998;17:595–9.
62. Forseto AS, Francesconi CM, Nose RAM, Nose W. Laser in situ keratomileusis to correct refractive errors after keratoplasty. J Cataract Refract Surg. 1999;25: 479–85.
63. Chung MS, Pepose JS, Manche EE. Management of the corneal flap in laser in situ keratomileusis after previous radial keratotomy. Am J Ophthalmol. 2001; 132:252–3.
64. Kapadia MS, Wilson SE. Transepithelial photorefractive keratectomy for treatment of thin flaps or caps after complicated laser in situ keratomileusis. Am J Ophthalmol. 1998;126:827–9.
65. Condon PI, Mulhern M, Fulcher T, *et al.* Laser intrastromal keratomileusis for high myopia and myopic astigmatism. Br J Ophthalmol. 1997;81:199–206.
66. Buratto L, Ferrari M, Genisi C. Keratomileusis for myopia with the excimer laser (Buratto technique): short term results. Refract Corneal Surg. 1993; 9(Suppl):S130–3.
67. Knorz MC, Wiesinger B, Lierman A, *et al.* Laser in situ keratomileusis for moderate and high myopia and myopic astigmatism. Ophthalmology. 1998;105: 932–40.
68. Kremer FB, Dufek M. Excimer laser in situ keratomileusis. J Refract Surg. 1995;11(Suppl):S244–7.
69. Vinciguerra P, Camesasca FI. Decentration after refractive surgery. J Refract Surg. 2001;17:S190–1.
70. Mulhern MG, Foley-Nolan A, O'Keefe M, Condon PI. Topographical analysis of ablation centration after excimer laser photorefractive keratectomy and laser in situ keratomileusis for high myopia. J Cataract Refract Surg. 1997;23:488–94.
71. Tsai YY, Lin JM. Natural history of central islands after laser in situ keratomileusis. J Cataract Refract Surg. 2000;26:853–8.
72. Kang SW, Chung ES, Kim WJ. Clinical analysis of central islands after laser in situ keratomileusis. J Cataract Refract Surg. 2000;26:536–42.
73. Johnson JD, Azar DT. Surgically induced topographical abnormalities after LASIK: management of central islands, corneal ectasia, decentration, and irregular astigmatism. Curr Opin Ophthalmol. 2001;12:309–17.
74. Rabinowitz YS, Rasheed K. Fluorescein test for the detection of striae in the corneal flap after laser in situ keratomileusis. Am J Ophthalmol. 1999;127: 717–18.
75. Carpel EF, Carlson KH, Shannon S. Folds and striae in laser in situ keratomileusis flaps. J Refract Surg. 1999;15:687–90.
76. Steinemann TL, Denton NC, Brown MF. Corneal lenticular wrinkling after automated lamellar keratoplasty. Am J Ophthalmol.1998;126:588–90.
77. Pannu JS. Wrinkled corneal flaps after LASIK [letter; comment]. J Refract Surg. 1997;13:341.
78. Vesaluoma M, Perez-Santonja J, Petroll WM, *et al.* Corneal stromal changes induced by myopic LASIK. Invest Ophthalmol Vis Sci. 2000;41:369–76.
79. Probst LE, Machat J. Removal of flap striae following laser in situ keratomileusis. J Cataract Refract Surg. 1998;24:153–5.
80. Hernandez-Matamoros J, Iradier MT, Moreno E. Treating folds and striae after laser in situ keratomileusis. J Cataract Refract Surg. 2001;27:350–2.
81. Lyle WA, Jin GJ. Results of flap repositioning after laser in situ keratomileusis. J Cataract Refract Surg. 2000;26:1451–7.
82. Carlson KH, Carpel EF. Epithelial folds following slippage of LASIK flap. Ophthalmic Surg Lasers. 2000;31:435–7.
83. Norden RA, Perry HD, Donnenfeld ED, Montoya C. Air bag–induced corneal flap folds after laser in situ keratomileusis. Am J Ophthalmol. 2000;130:234–5.
84. Munoz G, Alio JL, Perez-Santonja JJ, Attia WH. Successful treatment of severe wrinkled corneal flap after laser in situ keratomileusis with deionized water. Am J Ophthalmol. 2000;129:91–2.
85. Pannu JS. Incidence and treatment of wrinkled corneal flap following LASIK. J Cataract Refract Surg. 1997;23:695–6.
86. Kremer I, Blumenthal M. Myopic keratomileusis in situ combined with VISX 20/20 photorefractive keratectomy. J Cataract Refract Surg. 1995;21:508–11.
87. Hirst LW, Vandeleur KW. Laser in situ keratomileusis interface deposits. J Refract Surg. 1998;14:653–4.
88. Stein HM. Powder-free gloves for ophthalmic surgery. J Cataract Refract Surg. 1997;23:714–17.
89. Zadok D, Maskaleris G, Garcia V, *et al.* Outcomes of retreatment after laser in situ keratomileusis. Ophthalmology. 1999;106:2391–4.
90. Choi RY, Wilson SE. Hyperopic laser in situ keratomileusis: primary and secondary treatments are safe and effective. Cornea. 2001;20:388–93.
91. Jacobs JM, Sanderson MC, Spivack LD, *et al.* Hyperopic laser in situ keratomileusis to treat overcorrected myopic LASIK. J Cataract Refract Surg. 2001; 27:389–95.
92. Lindstrom RL, Linebarger EJ, Hardten DR, *et al.* Early results of hyperopic and astigmatic laser in situ keratomileusis in eyes with secondary hyperopia. Ophthalmology. 2000;107:1858–63.
93. Mulhern MG, Condon PI, O'Keefe M. Myopic and hyperopic laser in situ keratomileusis retreatments. Indications, techniques, limitations, and results. J Cataract Refract Surg. 2001;27:1278–87.
94. Agarwal A, Agarwal A, Agarwal T, *et al.* Laser in situ keratomileusis for residual myopia after primary LASIK. J Cataract Refract Surg. 2001;27:1013–17.
95. Patel NP, Clinch TE, Weis JR, *et al.* Comparison of visual results in initial and retreatment laser in situ keratomileusis procedures for myopia and astigmatism. Am J Ophthalmol. 2000;130:1–11.
96. Lyle WA, Jin GJ. Retreatment after initial laser in situ keratomileusis. J Cataract Refract Surg. 2000;26:650–9.
97. Rashad KM. Laser in situ keratomileusis retreatment for residual myopia and astigmatism. J Refract Surg. 2000;16:170–6.

98. Febbraro JL, Buzard KA, Friedlander MH. Reoperations after myopic laser in situ keratomileusis. J Cataract Refract Surg. 2000;26:41–8.

99. Brahma A, McGhee CN, Craig JP, et al. Safety and predictability of laser in situ keratomileusis enhancement by flap reelevation in high myopia. J Cataract Refract Surg. 2001;27:593–603.

100. Ozdamar A, Sener B, Aras C, Aktunc R. Laser in situ keratomileusis after photorefractive keratectomy for myopic regression. J Cataract Refract Surg. 1998; 24:1208–11.

101. Huang D, Stulting RD, Carr JD, et al. Multiple regression and vector analyses of laser in situ keratomileusis for myopia and astigmatism. J Refract Surg. 1999; 15:538–49.

102. Ditzen K, Handzel A, Pieger S. Laser in situ keratomileusis nomogram development. J Refract Surg. 1999;15:S197–201.

103. Iskander NG, Peters NT, Anderson Penno E, Gimbel HV. Late traumatic flap dislocation after laser in situ keratomileusis. J Cataract Refract Surg. 2001; 27:1111–14.

104. Lombardo AJ, Katz HR. Late partial dislocation of a laser in situ keratomileusis flap. J Cataract Refract Surg. 2001;27:1108–10.

105. Schwartz GS, Park DH, Schloff S, Lane SS. Traumatic flap displacement and subsequent diffuse lamellar keratitis after laser in situ keratomileusis. J Cataract Refract Surg. 2001;27:781–3.

106. Geggel HS, Coday MP. Late-onset traumatic laser in situ keratomileusis (LASIK) flap dehiscence. Am J Ophthalmol. 2001;131:505–6.

107. Patel CK, Hanson R, McDonald B, Cox N. Case reports and small case series: late dislocation of a LASIK flap caused by a fingernail. Arch Ophthalmol. 2001;119: 447–9.

108. Melki SA, Talamo JH, Demetriades AM, et al. Late traumatic dislocation of laser in situ keratomileusis corneal flaps. Ophthalmology. 2000;107:2136–9.

109. Recep OF, Cagil N, Hasiripi H. Outcome of flap subluxation after laser in situ keratomileusis: results of 6 month follow-up. J Cataract Refract Surg. 2000;26: 1158–62.

110. Ginsberg NE, Hersh PS. Effect of lamellar flap location on corneal topography after laser in situ keratomileusis. J Cataract Refract Surg. 2000;26:992–1000.

111. Lemley HL, Chodosh J, Wolf TC, et al. Partial dislocation of laser in situ keratomileusis flap by air bag injury. J Refract Surg. 2000;16:373–4.

112. Chaudhry NA, Smiddy WE. Displacement of corneal cap during vitrectomy in a post-LASIK eye. Retina. 1998;18:554–5.

113. Perez EP, Viramontes B, Schor P, et al. Factors affecting corneal strip stroma-to-stroma adhesion. J Refract Surg. 1998;14:460–2.

114. Leung AT, Rao SK, Lam DS. Traumatic partial unfolding of laser in situ keratomileusis flap with severe epithelial ingrowth. J Cataract Refract Surg. 2000;26:135–9.

115. Shakin EP, Fastenberg DM, Udell IJ, et al. Late dislocation of a corneal cap after automated lamellar keratoplasty and epithelial debridement for retinal surgery [letter]. Arch Ophthalmol. 1996;114:1420.

116. Yang B, Chen J, Wang Z. Enhancement ablation for the treatment of undercorrection after excimer laser in situ keratomileusis for correcting myopia. Chin Med J (Engl). 1998;111:358–60.

117. Chayet AS, Assil KK, Montes M, et al. Regression and its mechanisms after laser in situ keratomileusis in moderate and high myopia. Ophthalmology. 1998;105:1194–9.

118. Durrie DS, Aziz AA. Lift-flap retreatment after laser in situ keratomileusis. J Refract Surg. 1999;15:150–3.

119. Martines E, John ME. The Martines enhancement technique for correcting residual myopia following laser assisted in situ keratomileusis. Ophthalmic Surg Lasers. 1996;27:S512–16.

120. Perez-Santonja JJ, Ayala MJ, Sakla HF, et al. Retreatment after laser in situ keratomileusis. Ophthalmology. 1999;106:21–8.

121. Febbraro JL, Buzard KA, Friedlander MH. Reoperations after myopic laser in situ keratomileusis. J Cataract Refract Surg. 2000;26:41–8.

122. Ozdamar A, Aras C, Bahcecioglu H, et al. Secondary laser in situ keratomileusis 1 year after primary LASIK for high myopia. J Cataract Refract Surg. 1999;25: 383–8.

123. Park CK, Kim JH. Comparison of wound healing after photorefractive keratectomy and laser in situ keratomileusis. J Cataract Refract Surg. 1999;25:842–50.

124. Pallikaris I, Siganos D. LASIK complications and management. Cornea , 2nd ed. Thorofare, NJ: Slack; 1999:227–43.

125. Melki SA, Proano CE, Azar DT. Optical disturbances and their management after myopic laser in situ keratomileusis. Int Ophthalmol Clin. 2000;40(1):45–56.

126. Keszei VA. Diffuse lamellar keratitis associated with iritis 10 months after laser in situ keratomileusis. J Cataract Refract Surg. 2001;27:1126–7.

127. Probst LE, Foley L. Late-onset interface keratitis after uneventful laser in situ keratomileusis. J Cataract Refract Surg. 2001;27:1124–5.

128. Harrison DA, Periman LM. Diffuse lamellar keratitis associated with recurrent corneal erosions after laser in situ keratomileusis. J Refract Surg. 2001;17:463–5.

129. Peters NT, Iskander NG, Anderson Penno EE, et al. Diffuse lamellar keratitis: isolation of endotoxin and demonstration of the inflammatory potential in a rabbit laser in situ keratomileusis model. J Cataract Refract Surg. 2001;27:917–23.

130. Buhren J, Baumeister M, Kohnen T. Diffuse lamellar keratitis after laser in situ keratomileusis imaged by confocal microscopy. Ophthalmology. 2001;108: 1075–81.

131. Weisenthal RW. Diffuse lamellar keratitis induced by trauma 6 months after laser in situ keratomileusis. J Refract Surg. 2000;16:749–51.

132. Haw WW, Manche EE. Late onset diffuse lamellar keratitis associated with an epithelial defect in six eyes. J Refract Surg. 2000;16:744–8.

133. Shah MN, Misra M, Wihelmus KR, Koch DD. Diffuse lamellar keratitis associated with epithelial defects after laser in situ keratomileusis. J Cataract Refract Surg. 2000;26:1312–18.

134. Linebarger EJ, Hardten DR, Lindstrom RL. Diffuse lamellar keratitis: diagnosis and management. J Cataract Refract Surg. 2000;26:1072–7.

135. Holland SP, Mathias RG, Morck DW, et al. Diffuse lamellar keratitis related to endotoxins released from sterilizer reservoir biofilms. Ophthalmology. 2000;107:1227–33.

136. Steinert RF, McColgin AZ, White A, Horsburgh GM. Diffuse interface keratitis after laser in situ keratomileusis (LASIK): a nonspecific syndrome. Am J Ophthalmol. 2000;129:380–1.

137. Macaluso DC, Rich LF, MacRae S. Sterile interface keratitis after laser in situ keratomileusis: three episodes in one patient with concomitant contact dermatitis of the eyelids. J Refract Surg. 1999;15:679–82.

138. Peters NT, Lingua RW, Kim CH. Topical intrastromal steroid during laser in situ keratomileusis to retard interface keratitis. J Cataract Refract Surg. 1999;25:1437–40.

139. Haw WW, Manche EE. Sterile peripheral keratitis following laser in situ keratomileusis. J Refract Surg. 1999;15:61–3.

140. Fraenkel GE, Cohen PR, Sutton GL, et al. Central focal interface opacity after laser in situ keratomileusis. J Refract Surg. 1998;14:571–5.

141. Smith RJ, Maloney RK. Diffuse lamellar keratitis: a new syndrome in lamellar refractive surgery. Ophthalmology. 1998;105:1721–6.

142. Kaufman SC, Maitchouk DY, Chiou AGY, Beuerman RW. Interface inflammation after laser in situ keratomileusis. Sands of the Sahara syndrome. J Cataract Refract Surg. 1998;24:1589–93.

143. Kouyoumdjian GA, Forstot SL, Durairaj VD, Damiano RE. Infectious keratitis after laser refractive surgery. Ophthalmology. 2001;108:1266–8.

144. Kuo IC, Margolis TP, Cevallos V, Hwang DG. Aspergillus fumigatus keratitis after laser in situ keratomileusis. Cornea. 2001;20:342–4.

145. Gupta V, Dada T, Vajpayee RB, et al. Polymicrobial keratitis after laser in situ keratomileusis. J Refract Surg. 2001;17:147–8.

146. Rudd JC, Moshirfar M. Methicillin-resistant Staphylococcus aureus keratitis after laser in situ keratomileusis. J Cataract Refract Surg. 2001;27:471–3.

147. Levartovsky S, Rosenwasser G, Goodman D. Bacterial keratitis following laser in situ keratomileusis. Ophthalmology. 2001;108:321–5.

148. Garg P, Bansal AK, Sharma S, Vemuganti GK. Bilateral infectious keratitis after laser in situ keratomileusis: a case report and review of the literature. Ophthalmology. 2001;108:121–5.

149. Sridhar MS, Garg P, Bansal AK, Gopinathan U. Aspergillus flavus keratitis after laser in situ keratomileusis. Am J Ophthalmol. 2000;129:802–4.

150. Karp KO, Hersh PS, Epstein RJ. Delayed keratitis after laser in situ keratomileusis. J Cataract Refract Surg. 2000;26:925–8.

151. Chung MS, Goldstein MH, Driebe WT Jr, Schwartz B. Fungal keratitis after laser in situ keratomileusis: a case report. Cornea. 2000;19:236–7.

152. Read RW, Chuck RS, Rao NA, Smith RE. Traumatic Acremonium atrogriseum keratitis following laser-assisted in situ keratomileusis. Arch Ophthalmol. 2000;118:418–21.

153. Dada T, Sharma N, Dada VK, Vajpayee RB. Pneumococcal keratitis after laser in situ keratomileusis. J Cataract Refract Surg. 2000;26:460–1.

154. Chung MS, Goldstein MH, Driebe WT Jr, Schwartz BH. Mycobacterium chelonae keratitis after laser in situ keratomileusis successfully treated with medical therapy and flap removal. Am J Ophthalmol. 2000;129:382–4.

155. Webber SK, Lawless MA, Sutton GL, Rogers CM. Staphylococcal infection under a LASIK flap. Cornea. 1999;18:361–5.

156. Al-Reefy M. Bacterial keratitis following laser in situ keratomileusis for hyperopia. J Refract Surg. 1999;15:S216–17.

157. Kim H-M, Song J-S, Han H-S, Jung H-R. Streptococcal keratitis after myopic laser in situ keratomileusis. Korean J Ophthalmol. 1998;12:108–11.

158. Watanabe H, Sato S, Maeda M, et al. Bilateral corneal infection as a complication of laser in situ keratomileusis. Arch Ophthalmol. 1997;115:1593–94.

159. Reviglio V, Rodriguez ML, Picotti GS, et al. Mycobacterium chelonae keratitis following laser in situ keratomileusis. J Refract Surg. 1998;14:357–60.

160. Pérez-Santonja JJ, Sakla HF, Abad JL, et al. Nocardial keratitis after laser in situ keratomileusis. J Refract Surg. 1997;13:314–17.

161. Mulhern MG, Condon PI, O'Keefe M. Endophthalmitis after astigmatic myopic laser in situ keratomileusis. J Cataract Refract Surg. 1997;23:948–50.

162. Aras C, Ozdamar A, Bahçecioglu H, Sener B. Corneal interface abscess after excimer laser in situ keratomileusis. J Refract Surg. 1998;14:156–7.

163. Waring GO 3rd, Carr JD, Stulting RD, et al. Prospective randomized comparison of simultaneous and sequential bilateral laser in situ keratomileusis for the correction of myopia. Ophthalmology. 1999;106:732–8.

164. Haw WW, Manche EE. Treatment of progressive or recurrent epithelial ingrowth with ethanol following laser in situ keratomileusis. J Refract Surg. 2001;17:63–8.

165. Wang MY, Maloney RK. Epithelial ingrowth after laser in situ keratomileusis. Am J Ophthalmol. 2000;129:746–51.

166. Walker MB, Wilson SE. Incidence and prevention of epithelial growth within the interface after laser in situ keratomileusis. Cornea. 2000;19:170–3.

167. Wright JD Jr, Neubaur CC, Stevens G Jr. Epithelial ingrowth in a corneal graft treated by laser in situ keratomileusis: light and electron microscopy. J Cataract Refract Surg. 2000;26:49–55.

168. Leung AT, Rao SK, Lam DS. Traumatic partial unfolding of laser in situ keratomileusis flap with severe epithelial ingrowth. J Cataract Refract Surg. 2000; 26:135–9.

169. Maloney RK. Epithelial ingrowth after lamellar refractive surgery. Ophthalmic Surg Lasers. 1996;7:S535.

170. Helena MC, Meisler D, Wilson SE. Epithelial growth within the lamellar interface after laser in situ keratomileusis (LASIK). Cornea. 1997;16:300–5.

171. Castillio A, Diaz-Valle D, Gutierrez AR, et al. Peripheral melt of flap after laser in situ keratomileusis. J Refract Surg. 1998;14:61–3.

172. Ibrahim O. Laser in situ keratomileusis for hyperopia and hyperopic astigmatism. J Refract Surg. 1998;14:S179–82.

173. Helena MC, Baerveldt F, Kim W-J, Wilson SE. Keratocyte apoptosis after corneal surgery. Invest Ophthalmol Vis Sci. 1998;39:276–83.

174. Lohmann CP, Guell JL. Regression after LASIK for the treatment of myopia: the role of the corneal epithelium. Semin Ophthalmol. 1998;13:79–82.

175. Eggink FA, Beekhuis WH. Contact lens fitting in a patient with keratectasia after laser in situ keratomileusis. J Cataract Refract Surg. 2001;27:1119–23.

176. Lafond G, Bazin R, Lajoie C. Bilateral severe keratoconus after laser in situ keratomileusis in a patient with forme fruste keratoconus. J Cataract Refract Surg. 2001;27:1115–18.

177. Vinciguerra P, Camesasca FI . Prevention of corneal ectasia in laser in situ keratomileusis. J Refract Surg. 2001;17:S187–9.

178. Amoils SP, Deist MB, Gous P, Amoils PM. Iatrogenic keratectasia after laser in situ keratomileusis for less than −4.0 to −7.0 diopters of myopia. J Cataract Refract Surg. 2000;26:967–77.

179. Joo CK, Kim TG. Corneal ectasia detected after laser in situ keratomileusis for correction of less than –12 diopters of myopia. J Cataract Refract Surg. 2000;26:292–5.

180. McLeod SD, Kisla TA, Caro NC, McMahon TT. Iatrogenic keratoconus: corneal ectasia following laser in situ keratomileusis for myopia. Arch Ophthalmol. 2000;118:282–4.

181. Seiler T, Koufala K, Richter G. Iatrogenic keratectasia after laser in situ keratomileusis. J Refract Surg. 1998;14:312–17.

182. Seiler T, Quurke AW. Iatrogenic keratectasia after LASIK in a case of forme fruste keratoconus. J Cataract Refract Surg. 1998;24:1007–9.

183. Wang Z, Chen J, Yang B. Posterior corneal surface topographic changes after laser in situ keratomileusis are related to residual corneal bed thickness. Ophthalmology. 1999;106:406–10.

184. Geggel HS, Talley AR. Delayed onset keratectasia following laser in situ keratomileusis. J Cataract Refract Surg. 1999;25:582–6.

185. Price FW Jr, Koller DL, Price MO. Central corneal pachymetry in patients undergoing laser in situ keratomileusis. Ophthalmology. 1999;106:2216–20.

186. El Danasoury MA, Waring GO III, El Maghraby A, Mehrez K. Excimer laser in situ keratomileusis to correct compound myopic astigmatism. J Refract Surg. 1997;13:511–20.

187. El Danasoury A. Prospective bilateral study of night glare after laser in situ keratomileusis with single zone and transition zone ablation. J Refract Surg. 1998;14:512–16.

23 Laser Subepithelial Keratomileusis (LASEK)

DIMITRI T. AZAR • ROBERT T. ANG

DEFINITION

- Laser subepithelial keratomileusis (LASEK) is a surgical technique that combines features of photorefractive keratectomy (PRK) and laser *in situ* keratomileusis (LASIK) in which a corneal epithelial flap is elevated and replaced at the end of the procedure.

KEY FEATURES

- Following preplaced epithelial marking, dilute ethanol is applied and a hinged epithelial flap is created by peeling the loosened epithelium as a sheet. After laser ablation, the flap is repositioned over the ablated stroma.

ASSOCIATED FEATURES

- Although LASEK may not consistently provide immediate and complete epithelial coverage, the early results seem promising, especially for the potential applications in wave front–guided keratorefractive surgery.[1,2]

BOX 23-1

LASEK Indications and Contraindications

INDICATIONS

Thin corneal pachymetry
Epithelial irregularities (M/D/F changes)
LASIK complications in the contralateral eye
Predisposition to trauma
Low myopia
Irregular astigmatism (corneal topographical abnormalities not qualifying as keratoconus [Fig. 23-1])
Glaucoma suspects

CONTRAINDICATIONS

Patient concern about postoperative pain
Keratoconus
Glaucoma
Pregnancy
Hyperopia and hyperopic astigmatism

From Azar DT, Ang RT. Laser subepithelial keratomileusis: evolution of alcohol-assisted flap surface ablation. Int Ophthalmol Clin. 2002;42:89–97.

INTRODUCTION

In laser subepithelial keratomileusis (LASEK), loosening and replacing the corneal epithelium can be performed using several techniques.[1,3–8] Photorefractive keratectomy (PRK) and laser *in situ* keratomileusis (LASIK) are currently the most popular procedures in refractive surgery. PRK is a relatively safe procedure; its major limitations are postoperative pain, subepithelial haze, and prolonged visual rehabilitation. The epithelial removal done prior to laser ablation in PRK is believed to be the major factor contributing to these drawbacks.[2,9] LASIK offers more comfort, faster visual rehabilitation, and minimal haze, but it has its own set of complications, predominantly related to the flap. These include free caps, incomplete pass of the microkeratome, flap wrinkles, epithelial ingrowth, flap melt, interface debris, and diffuse lamellar keratitis.[1,2,9]

In selected patients for whom PRK would be the recommended procedure, such as patients with thin corneas, patients with lifestyles or professions that predispose to flap trauma including athletes in contact sports and military personnel, and patients with low myopia who are at a lower risk for subepithelial haze, laser epithelial keratomileusis (LASEK) may be a viable alternative.[1,2,9]

LASEK theoretically offers the advantage of avoiding the flap complications of LASIK and also addresses the drawbacks of discomfort and delayed recovery associated with conventional PRK. Epithelial sheet viability and adhesion are the basis for achieving the potential advantages of LASEK.[1–8] The indications and contraindications for LASEK are summarized in Box 23-1.

In patients with corneal pachymetry of 500μm or lower and in patients with asymmetric corneal curvature, the use of the Azar-Lu MEEI keratoconus classification (Fig. 23-1) is helpful in identifying patients with keratoconus in whom surgery should be avoided.[1]

PREOPERATIVE PREPARATION

Patients undergo routine preoperative evaluation in a manner similar to that for other refractive surgical procedures. These include uncorrected visual acuity (UCVA), best-corrected visual acuity (BCVA), manifest and cycloplegic refraction, ocular dominance, keratometry, tonometry, pachymetry, slit-lamp examination, aberrometry, and computerized videokeratography.[1,3,4,8]

SURGICAL TECHNIQUES

Several surgical techniques have been described including minor modifications of our original technique, which is illustrated in Figure 23-2. Camellin and Cimberle[3] and Vinciguerra and Epstein[4] have described similar techniques with encouraging results.

Thirty minutes before surgery, the eye receives trimethoprim sulfate 1mg/ml, polymyxin B 10,000 U/ml (Polytrim; Burroughs Wellcome, Research Triangle, NC) or ciprofloxacin (Ciloxan; Alcon Laboratories, Fort Worth, TX).[1,9]

A sterile drape is placed around the eye. Then one drop each of topical 0.5% proparacaine (Ophthetic; Allergan, Irvine, CA) and 4% tetracaine (formulated in the MEEI pharmacy) are instilled and a lid speculum applied. The cornea is marked with overlapping 3mm circles around the corneal periphery, simulating a floral pattern. In our early cases a 7mm optical zone marker (model E9011 3.0; Storz, St. Louis, MO) was used to delineate the area centered around the pupil. Gentle pressure was applied on the cornea while the barrel of the optical zone

M.E.E.I. KC Classification

Name_____   Patient ID #_____

		Score	Score			
KOD-KOS	< 1.9	0		0	< 1.9	KOS-KOD
	> 1.9	1		1	> 1.9	
KOD	< 47.2	0		0	< 47.2	KOS
	47.2-48.7	1		1	47.2-48.7	
	>48.7	2		2	>48.7	
ISOD	<1.4	0		0	<1.4	ISOS
	1.4-1.9	1		1	1.4-1.9	
	>1.9	2		2	>1.9	
≥ 2 Findings on hx (atopy, down), FH and exam (Fleisher, Vogt, Munson, nerves, scarring)	No	0		0	No	≥ 2 Findings on hx (atopy, down), FH and exam (Fleisher, Vogt, Munson, nerves, scarring)
	Yes	2		2	Yes	
Corneal Hydrops (by exam or hx) OD	No	0		0	No	Corneal Hydrops (by exam or hx) OS
	Yes	2		2	Yes	
	Total Score	OD	OS	Total Score		

SCORE	DIAGNOSIS
(Zero)	Normal
(1-3)	Suspect
(4-5)	Early KC
(6-9)	Advanced KC

Diagnosis_____OD   **Diagnosis_____OS**

FIG. 23-1 ■ The Azar-Lu Keratoconus Classification. (From Melki SA, Azar DT. LASIK complications: etiology, management, and prevention. Surv Ophthalmol. 2001;46:95–116.)

marker was filled with two drops of 18% ethanol (dehydrated alcohol, 1ml ampules; American Reagent Laboratories, Shirley, NY). In more recent cases an alcohol dispenser consisting of a customized 7mm semisharp marker (ASICO, Westmont, IL) attached to a hollow metal handle served as a reservoir for the 18% alcohol. Firm pressure is exerted on the central cornea and a button is pushed on the side of the handle, releasing the alcohol into the well of the marker. After 25 seconds, the ethanol is absorbed using a dry cellulose sponge (Weck Cell or Merocel; Xomed, Jacksonville, FL) to prevent alcohol spillage onto the epithelium outside the marker barrel.[1,9]

Modified Vannas scissors are inserted under the epithelium and traced around the delineated margin of the epithelium, leaving 2–3 clock hours of intact margin, preferably at the 12 o'clock position. The loosened epithelium is peeled as a single sheet using a blunt spatula or a Merocel sponge, leaving a flap of epithelium with the hinge still attached. The laser ablation is initiated immediately thereafter using an excimer laser. After ablation, a 30-gauge anterior chamber cannula is used to hydrate the stroma and epithelial flap with balanced salt solution. The epithelial flap is replaced on the stroma using the straight part of the cannula under intermittent irrigation. Care is taken to realign the epithelium flap using the previous marks and to avoid epithelial defects. The flap is then allowed to dry.

Topical medications are then applied: diclofenac sodium 0.1% (Voltaren Ophthalmic; Ciba Vision Ophthalmics, Duluth, GA) and tobramycin 0.3% dexamethasone 0.1% ointment (TobraDex; Alcon Laboratories) or diclofenac sodium 0.1% (Voltaren Ophthalmic; Ciba Vision Ophthalmics), ciprofloxacin (Ciloxan; Alcon Laboratories), and fluorometholone 0.1% (FML; Allergan America, Hormigueros, PR) drops.[1] A bandage contact lens (Soflens 66; Bausch & Lomb, Rochester, NY) is then placed.[9]

POSTOPERATIVE CARE

After the procedure, all patients are prescribed oral analgesics and instructed to take them only if needed. The postoperative regimen consisted of tobramycin-dexamethasone ointment (TobraDex; Alcon Laboratories) four times a day for 1 week and prednisolone acetate 1% (Pred Forte 1%; Allergan, Irvine, CA) four times a day for 2 weeks. Artificial tears are also prescribed (on an as-needed basis). The bandage contact lens is removed after complete reepithelialization (at postoperative days 3 and 4). Removal of the contact lens in the first postoperative day risks peeling the epithelial flap with the contact lens.[9]

RESULTS

Intraoperative Findings

After exposure to 18% ethanol for 25 seconds, the epithelium was successfully peeled as a single sheet leaving a 2–3 clock hour hinge.[1] The wound edge was sharply demarcated, and no residual islands of epithelium were grossly visible under the microscope. After laser ablation, the folded epithelium was repositioned and the flap edge closely reapproximated to the wound edge. No epithelial defects were visible in all cases prior to placement of the bandage contact lens.[1,9]

Postoperative Findings

One day after surgery, an epithelial defect was documented in 30 of the 55 (54.5%) cases that were followed up. On the third postoperative day, 25 of the 30 defects (83.3%) had completely healed, 2 cases still had a defect, and 3 cases did not return for postoperative check.[7] Twenty-five eyes (45.4%) had no defect on the first postoperative day. On day 3, a defect developed in 5 of these 25 (20%) eyes. Three resolved by 1 week; the other two

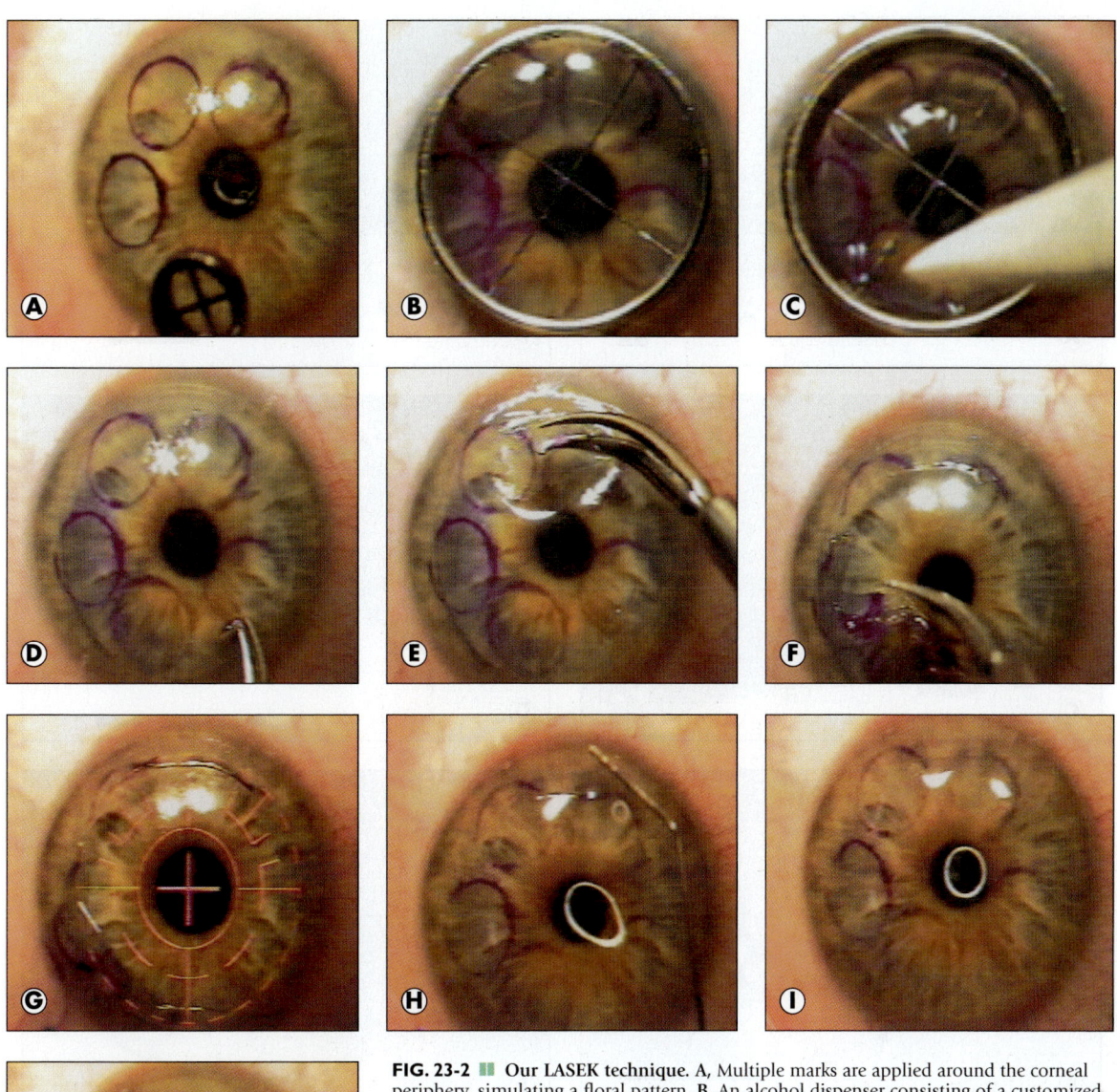

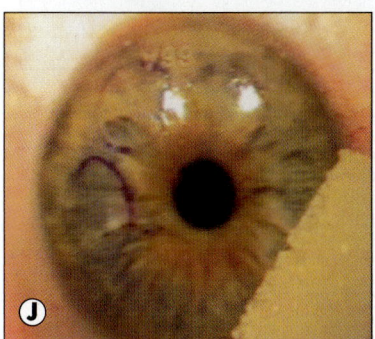

FIG. 23-2 ■ **Our LASEK technique. A,** Multiple marks are applied around the corneal periphery, simulating a floral pattern. **B,** An alcohol dispenser consisting of a customized 7 or 9mm semisharp marker attached to a hollow metal handle serves as a reservoir for 18% alcohol. Firm pressure is exerted on the cornea and alcohol is released into the well of the marker. **C,** After 25–30 seconds, the ethanol is absorbed using a dry cellulose sponge. **D** and **E,** One arm of a modified Vannas scissors (Azar scissors; note the knob at the tip of the lower arm) is then inserted under the epithelium and traced around the delineated margin of the epithelium, leaving a hinge of 2–3 clock hours of intact margin, preferably at the 12 o'clock position. **F,** The loosened epithelium is peeled as a single sheet using a Merocel sponge or using the edge of a jeweler's forceps, leaving it attached at its hinge. **G,** Laser ablation is performed. **H,** An anterior chamber cannula is used to hydrate the stroma and epithelial flap with balanced salt solution. The epithelial flap is replaced on the stroma using the cannula under intermittent irrigation. **I,** Care is taken to realign the epithelial flap using the previous marks and to avoid epithelial defects. The flap is then allowed to dry for 2–5 minutes. Topical steroids and antibiotic medications are then applied. **J,** A bandage contact lens is then placed. (From Feit R, Taneri S, Azar DT, *et al.* LASEK results. Ophthalmol Clin North Am. 2003;16:127–35.)

cases were not followed up. After the first postoperative week, all previous defects had healed and no reports of recurrent erosions were noted on subsequent visits.[1,2]

One day after LASEK, 32 of 55 (58.1%) patients complained of postoperative pain or took oral medications to relieve pain or discomfort.[1,2] At the 3-day follow-up, 24 of the 32 (75%) patients reported pain disappearance without medications, 6 still had pain, and 2 cases were not followed up. Of the 23 (41.8%) cases who did have pain and did not take medications on the first postoperative day, 6 patients reported pain on day 3. One week after LASEK, no further pain episodes were reported.[1,2]

On day 1, 25.4% had UCVA of 20/40 or better. This increased to 62.7% at day 3, reaching 100% by 1 week and 1 month. At 3 days 23.5% of patients achieved UCVA of 20/25 or better, improving to 80.4% at 1 month. A postoperative spherical equivalent of 0.50D was achieved in 75.6% of cases by 1 month.

A healing line in the epithelium was observed in 22 of 51 (43.1%) eyes at day 3. The line was still seen in three eyes (16.6%) at 1 week and totally disappeared at 1 month. Subepithelial punctate keratopathies (SPKs) appeared in eight subjects (15.6%) at day 3. Among these eight cases, one eye still had the SPK at 6-month follow-up. Eight additional cases of SPK were diagnosed from 1 week to 6 months postoperatively. Trace corneal haze was observed as early as 3 days in one eye but disappeared at 3 months. At 1 month, trace to slight corneal haze was noted in nine eyes. Of the nine, five cleared by 3–12 months postoperatively whereas two had persistent haze at 6 months. Five new cases of haze were reported at 3 months, four of which resolved after 6 months.[1,2]

Transmission Electron Microscopy

We examined several corneal epithelium specimens that were obtained from patients who underwent alcohol-assisted epithe-

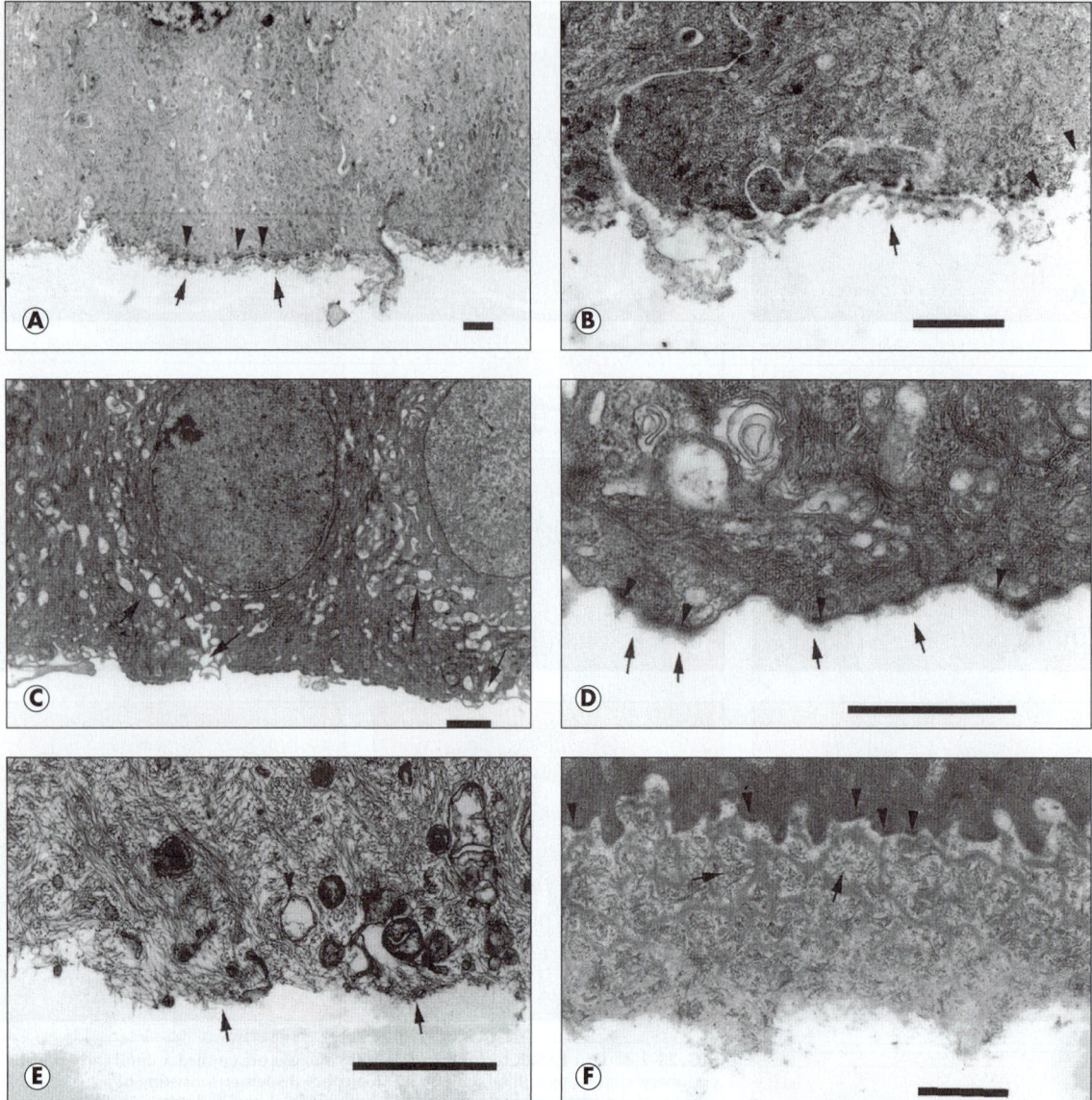

FIG. 23-3 ■ **A,** Low-magnification transmission electron micrograph of specimen. The epithelial cells were associated tightly with flattened superficial cell layers. **B–D,** Higher magnification transmission electron micrographs of the basal cells and basement membrane region. **B,** The irregular structure of the basement membrane was observed under the basal cell layer. **C,** The basal cells were attached to each other through desmosomes *(white arrowheads)*. **D,** The ultrastructure of the basement membrane was irregular *(black arrowheads)*, but hemidesmosomes were abundant and *intact (white arrowheads)*. (Bar, A: 10μm, B, C, D: 1μm.) (Reproduced from Chen CC, Chang JH, Lee JB, et al. Human corneal epithelial cell viability morphology after dilute alcohol exposure. Invest Ophthalmol Vis Sci. 2002;43(8):2593–602.)

lial removal prior to PRK.[1] The specimens were fixed in glutaraldehyde and processed in 0.1 M cacodylate buffer (pH 7.5). The samples were then postfixed in osmium tetroxide, dehydrated in graded alcohols, embedded in Epon 812, and oven-dried at 60°C for 48 hours. Sections 1m thick were stained with toluidine blue for orientation. Subsequently, ultrathin sections were obtained using a transmission electron microscope (Philips 410; Lico, Bedford, MA).

Electron microscopy showed variability in the histological appearance of the basement membrane zone. Most specimens showed intact epithelial cell layers (Fig. 23-3). Edematous cells and abnormal vacuoles were observed in other specimens. Higher magnification revealed variable configurations of the epithelial basement membranes including normal areas and areas of discontinuities and irregularities in the basement membrane. Basement membrane fragments were still attached to the epithelial basal cells in most specimens. Bowman's layer and corneal stroma were absent, indicating that the epithelial sheets separate from Bowman's layer with variable amounts of basal laminae attached to the basal epithelial cell layer. The ultrastructures of desmosomes and hemidesmosomes were normal in most specimens.

DISCUSSION

The main indications for LASEK are thin corneas and professions or lifestyles such as contact sports and the military that predispose to flap trauma.[1–9] Patients with low myopia who are at a lower risk for subepithelial haze may also benefit from LASEK. It is a simple, inexpensive procedure that involves the creation of an epithelial flap after exposure to 18% alcohol for 25 seconds and subsequent replacement of the flap after laser ablation.[1,2,9] It offers the potential advantage of avoiding LASIK-related flap complications and decreasing the epithelial healing time and postoperative pain associated with PRK.

Our LASEK technique evolved from PRK after alcohol-assisted epithelial removal. Abad *et al.*[5,6] showed that alcohol-assisted epithelial removal was a simple and safe alternative to mechanical epithelial removal before PRK. Applying 25% ethanol for 3 minutes, Stein *et al.*[5] were able to grasp, lift, pull apart, and split the corneal epithelium using two McPherson forceps. Similarly, Shah *et al.*[8] exposed the epithelium using a dry sponge. These early reports revealed that epithelial removal using 18–25% alcohol for 20–25 seconds was fast, easy, and safe to perform compared with mechanical débridement; that this concentration can produce sharp wound edges and a clean, smooth Bowman's layer; and that the central epithelium can be translocated in part or *in toto*.[7,8]

To study the effect of alcohol exposure and mechanical manipulation on corneal epithelium, we carried out electron microscopic studies of specimens obtained after conventional alcohol-assisted PRK. The images revealed that the epithelial cell layer is intact and the epithelial cells are still viable immediately after exposure to alcohol and surgical peeling. The presence of the basement membrane attached to the basal epithelial cell layer indicates that the point of separation was likely to be within the basement membrane or between the basement membrane and Bowman's layer. In addition, the adherence of the basement membrane to the basal layer of the epithelium is significant because it is believed that the basement membrane provides the stability and support that keep the epithelium intact even after manipulation. The preservation of the hemidesmosomes in the basal epithelial layer provides a structure that may promote the adhesion of a viable epithelium to the ablated stroma.

The Camellin LASEK technique differs slightly from our technique: a preincision is made using a Janach trephine (Como, Italy) and specialized microhoe, 20% alcohol solution is instilled using a small silicone irrigator, the corneal surface is dried after 30 seconds, and then the epithelium is detached using the short side of a hockey spatula and returned after laser ablation.[3] From our experience, we have learned that the technique may not require specialized instruments but requires several key steps for consistent epithelial flap creation and replacement. Pretreatment with 4% tetracaine prior to alcohol exposure was helpful in loosening the epithelium and lessening intraoperative discomfort. Placement of overlapping corneal marks was crucial in ensuring correct epithelial alignment and avoiding irregular epithelial placement and mismatch. We used an alcohol dispenser, but any optical zone marker with a barrel could be used to expose the epithelium to alcohol and avoid spillage. A jeweler's forceps to delineate the wound edge and locate the dissection plane and a dry, nonfragmenting, cellulose sponge to peel the epithelial sheet are easily available instruments that can be used to create the flap. The flap can be repositioned with an irrigating cannula under intermittent hydration using the preplaced corneal marks as a guide. No overlap of the flap and wound edge was observed, which would have been attributable to stretching of the flap during peeling or overexpansion due to generous hydration. A 5-minute waiting period was adequate to allow adhesion of the epithelial flap to the stroma. Although LASEK required approximately 10 additional minutes of surgical time, including 25 seconds for alcohol exposure, 1 minute for peeling, 2 minutes for flap repositioning, and 5 minutes drying time, it was easily performed and reproducible. The epithelial flap and hinge remained intact despite handling and manipulation with the irrigating cannula.

After treating 249 patients, Camellin and Cimberle[3] observed that intraoperative flap management was easy in 60% of cases, average in 28%, and difficult in 12%. No pain was experienced by 44% of their cases in the first 24 hours after surgery, and 80% of preoperative BCVA was achieved by 90% of their patients 10 days postoperatively. Vinciguerra and Epstein[4] reported only postoperative grittiness with no pain episodes in 432 eyes treated; 89% achieved refractive stability at 1–2 weeks. The 12-month mean spherical equivalent was -0.10 ± 0.7D. Haze was not found to exceed trace.

Using the techniques we have described,[1,2,9] sloughed epithelium was observed under the bandage contact lens in most patients with epithelial defect at day 1. Visual stability of 20/40 UCVA was consistently achieved after 1 week. This was consistent with the results of Camellin and Vinciguerra. SPK was observed in some patients, indicative of postrefractive surgery dry eye. The use of artificial tears was helpful in relieving dry eye discomfort. Trace to slight haze was noted in some patients but was found to disappear after several months. This may be due to the low myopic corrections in our study population, making it attractive to patients with low myopia who may want to avoid the risk of flap complications.[9]

The main limitation of LASEK reports is the very small study populations because of the relatively limited indications for this procedure. We have persistently offered it to our patients with low myopia, but most still prefer LASIK, with which the absence of postoperative pain and epithelial defect and fast visual rehabilitation can be more consistently achieved. Two patients initially had LASEK performed 6 years ago. One patient was lost to follow-up after 1 year. The other patient showed long-term stability of refractive outcomes 5 years after surgery.[9]

The main disadvantages of this procedure remain the unpredictable postoperative pain and epithelial healing. Even after ensuring that no epithelial defects were present at the end of each procedure, deepithelialized areas were still observed in more than half of the cases 1 day after surgery. This was accompanied by a similar number of reports of postoperative pain. Because pain is the most compelling drawback of PRK, rapid epithelial coverage is paramount to ensure the patient's comfort in the immediate postoperative period. LASEK cannot guarantee that it can achieve this consistently.[1,2,9]

REFERENCES

1. Azar DT, Ang RT, Lee JB, et al. Laser subepithelial keratomileusis: electron microscopy and visual outcomes of flap PRK. Curr Opin Ophthalmol. 2001;12: 323–8.
2. Azar DT, Ang RT. Laser subepithelial keratomileusis: evolution of alcohol assisted flap surface ablation. Int Ophthalmol Clin. 2002;42:89–97.
3. Camellin M, Cimberle M. LASEK technique promising after 1 year of experience. Ocul Surg News. 2000;18(14):1, 14–17.
4. Vinciguerra P, Epstein D. Laser epithelial keratomileusis (LASEK): one-year results of a new excimer refractive procedure. Presented in the 104th AAO Meeting; Dallas, TX; October 2000.
5. Abad JC, An B, Power WJ, et al. A prospective evaluation of alcohol-assisted versus mechanical epithelial removal before photorefractive keratectomy. Ophthalmology. 1997;104:1566–75.
6. Abad JC, Talamo JH, Vidaurri-Leal J, et al. Dilute ethanol versus mechanical debridement before photorefractive keratectomy. J Cataract Refract Surg. 1996;22: 1427–33.
7. Stein HA, Stein RM, Price C, Salim GA. Alcohol removal of the epithelium for excimer laser ablation: outcomes analysis. J Cataract Refract Surg. 1997;23:1160–3.
8. Shah S, Doyle SJ, Chatterjee A, et al. Comparison of 18% ethanol and mechanical debridement for epithelial removal before photorefractive keratectomy. J Refract Surg. 1998;14:S212–14.
9. Feit R, Taneri S, Chen CC, et al. LASEK techniques and outcomes. Ophthalmol Clin North Am. In press.

CHAPTER

24

Laser Thermal Keratoplasty and Conductive Keratoplasty

KALLIOPI STASI • DIMITRI T. AZAR • DOUGLAS D. KOCH

DEFINITIONS

- Laser thermal keratoplasty (LTK) is a procedure using laser energy to heat the cornea and increase its curvature.
- Conductive keratoplasty (CK) steepens the cornea using high radiofrequency currents.

KEY FEATURES

- LTK and CK steepen the central cornea by shrinking peripheral collagen.
- The corneal time-space heat distributions differ between LTK and CK, which may explain the greater stability of CK.

ASSOCIATED FEATURES

- Renewed interest in LTK has emerged because of the future potential of wave front-guided treatments.
- Despite the instability of corrections, LTK and CK have a major advantage of untouched central cornea.

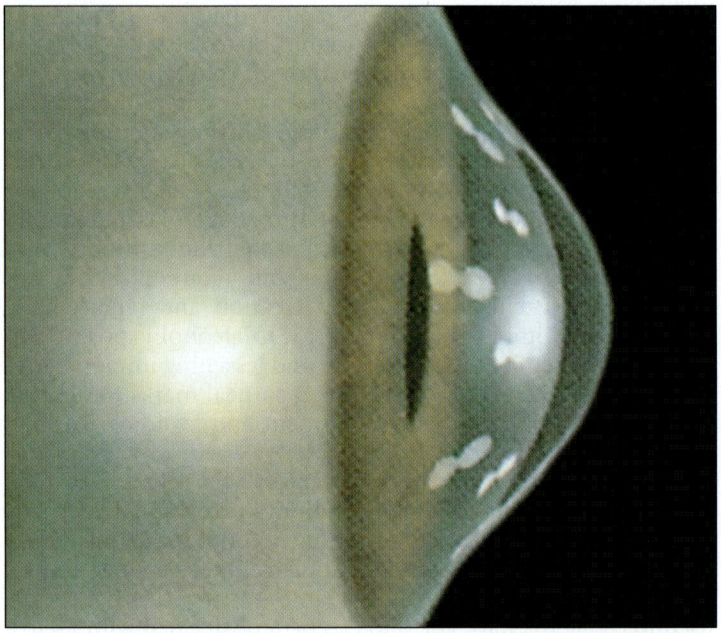

FIG. 24-1 ■■ Side view of the location of a 16-spot laser thermal keratoplasty application with the resultant corneal steepening.

INTRODUCTION

Laser thermal keratoplasty (LTK) and conductive keratoplasty (CK) are procedures aimed at altering the corneal curvature using laser energy to heat the peripheral corneal collagen. This results in shrinking of the peripheral and paracentral stromal collagen, flattening of the peripheral cornea, and steepening of the central cornea, the last of which offers a means of treating hyperopia and hyperopic astigmatism (Fig. 24-1). LTK has been plagued, however, by regression of the refractive effect. Improved understanding of the response of corneal collagen to heat and the availability of state-of-the-art heat delivery systems may result in a promising future for LTK and related thermal refractive surgical procedures.

Conductive keratoplasty (CK) delivers low-energy, high-frequency (radiofrequency) current to heat the peripheral collagen and shrink it, which results in seemingly more stable central steepening of the cornea (Fig. 24-2).

HISTORICAL REVIEW

The use of heat to alter the curvature of the cornea can be traced to 1879, when Gayet used cautery to treat keratoconus. That procedure remained popular until penetrating keratoplasty was popularized by Castroviejo in 1936.[1] In 1898, Lans[2] described a method to reduce astigmatism by changing the corneal curvature in rabbit eyes by applying electrocautery to the peripheral cornea. By 1933, three reports of successful correction of severe astigmatism using corneal cautery had been published.[3–5]

The discovery by Stringer and Parr[6] in 1964 of the shrinkage temperature of corneal collagen (55–58° C) led to renewed in-

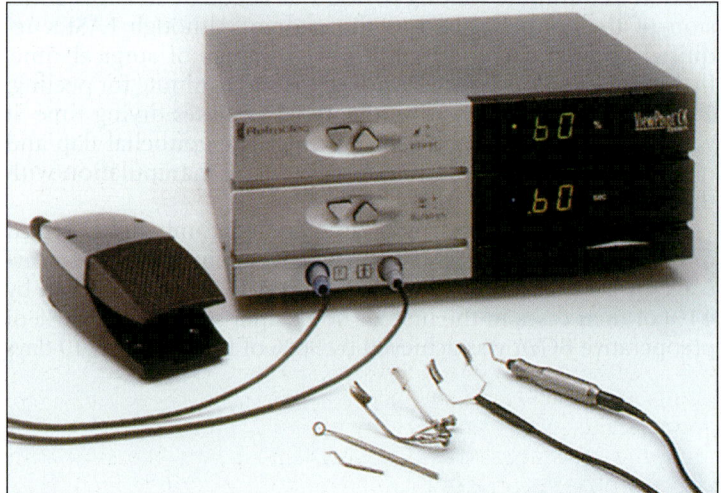

FIG. 24-2 ■■ The ViewPoint CK System from Refractec Inc.

terest in thermal keratoplasty. Over the past three decades, several nonlaser and laser devices have been tested.

In the early 1970s, a thermostatically controlled electric probe was used to flatten the central cornea in keratoconus patients by Gasset et al.,[7] who demonstrated excellent 1-year results in five patients. Other investigators reported a high incidence of regression and a case of total regression. Reported complications ranged from mild surface problems to corneal melting and stromal scarring.[8-10] Nowadays, this method is used only as a surgical adjunct during keratoplasty to flatten steep cones and improve the quality of the host trephination. In a later attempt to minimize the surface problems of the electric probe, a 1.6MHz radiofrequency probe (the Los Alamos probe) was designed to deliver thermal energy localized to a zone of 200–400μm inside the stroma, thus sparing the epithelium and endothelium.[11-13] Poor predictability and regression of the effect led to withdrawal of this probe in 1987.[14,15] In 1984, Fyodorov used a retractable wire probe heated to 600° C for 0.3sec, preset to penetrate the cornea at 95% depth, to perform deep coagulations in a radial pattern (radial keratoplasty) for the correction of hyperopia.[16] A retrospective review of 159 of Fyodorov's patients revealed unacceptably high unpredictability, regression, and serious complications (stromal necrosis, endothelial damage, and corneal decompensation).[17,18]

Fyodorov proposed a less invasive approach of laser coagulation of the cornea to overcome some of these problems. This was followed by the development and testing of CO_2 lasers for corneal thermal shrinkage. CO_2 lasers produced 10.6μm radiation with very shallow penetration in the corneal tissue (99% was absorbed in the first 50μm of the stroma).[19] A 1.54μm yttrium-erbium-glass laser was also tested. It created gray coagulation cones that extended to Descemet's membrane, but its penetration depth of at least 1mm risked endothelial and iris damage.[20] Efforts to find a laser with a penetration depth that approximates the corneal thickness led to the holmium:yttrium-aluminum-garnet (Ho:YAG) solid-state laser. Such a laser would have to emit light in the wavelength range of 1.9–2.3μm, and to achieve homogeneous coagulation throughout the corneal stroma, the laser beam would have to be focused so that the maximal energy occurs in the central stroma.[20] In contrast to the conical footprints of LTK, the CK approach using radiofrequency current results in a cylindrical thermal footprint extending to 80% depth.

CORNEAL RESPONSE TO HEAT

Heating can induce collagen shrinkage up to one third of its native length. Thermal energy disrupts the hydrogen bonds of the tertiary collagen structure (without altering the primary structure), allowing the collagen triple helix to unwind partially and form new cross-links between amino acids.[21] Heating human corneal collagen to temperatures of 55–58° C induces collagen shrinkage by approximately 7%.[21] Heating past the shrinkage temperature, into the 65–78° C range, results in relaxation of the contracted collagen secondary to hydrolysis of the heat-labile cross-links. The aging process increases the number of thermally stable cross-links, raising the temperature threshold for collagen relaxation. Further elevation of the temperature (beyond 78° C) eventually leads to collagen fibers necrosis.

Appropriate elevation of corneal collagen fiber temperature results in contraction and subsequent flattening of the area of heating. Central heating of the cornea (to the 4mm-diameter zone) results in central corneal flattening, decrease of the refractive power of the cornea, and a hyperopic shift. Peripheral heating of the cornea produces a beltlike effect of peripheral flattening with evident collagen stress lines emanating from each stromal burn, resulting in central steepening and increase of the refractive power of the eye (Fig. 24-3). In general, the greater the number of peripheral burns or radials, and the smaller the optical zone beyond the 4.5mm diameter, the greater the central steepening and the concomitant myopic shift (Fig. 24-4). For astigmatic corrections, peripheral heating along a single meridian (the flatter meridian) causes central steepening along the meridian of treatment (similar to a wedge resection). A compound treatment for hyperopia with astigmatism can be designed by treating more of

the cornea or closer to the visual axis along the flattest meridian of the cornea.[21]

The effect of corneal collagen contraction tends to decrease with time in both human and animal studies (Fig. 24-5), which might be explained by the production of new collagen by

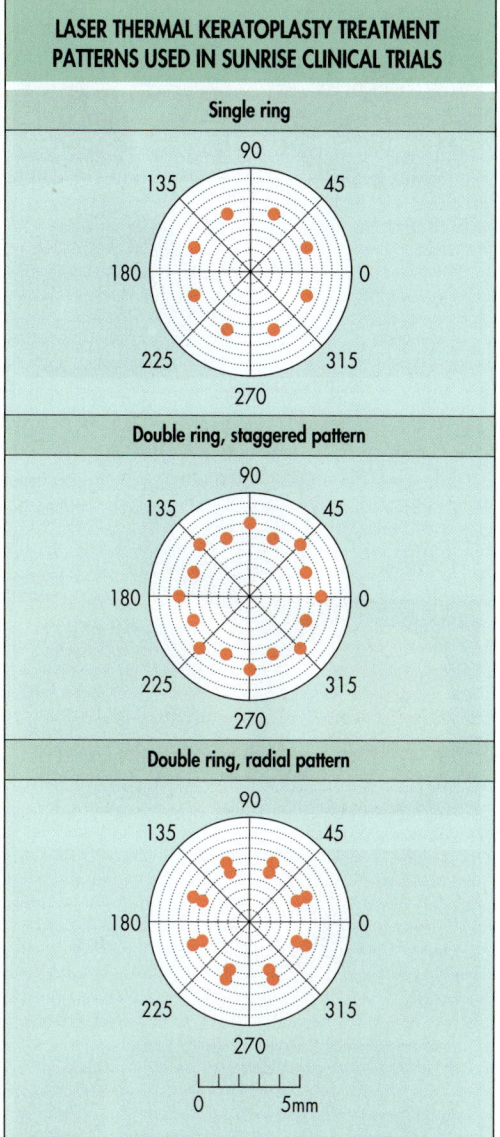

LASER THERMAL KERATOPLASTY TREATMENT PATTERNS USED IN SUNRISE CLINICAL TRIALS

Single ring

Double ring, staggered pattern

Double ring, radial pattern

0   5mm

FIG. 24-3 ■ Laser thermal keratoplasty treatment patterns used in some of the Sunrise clinical trials.

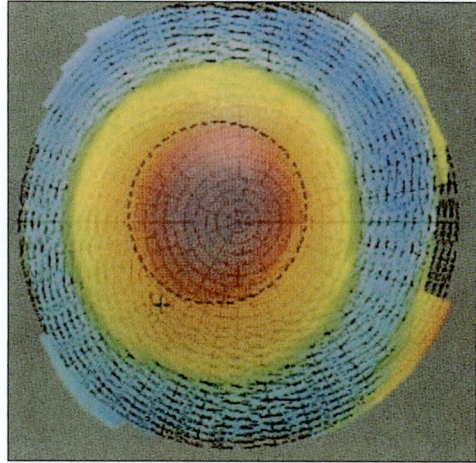

FIG. 24-4 ■ Corneal topography map after laser thermal keratoplasty, showing the optical zone of treatment.

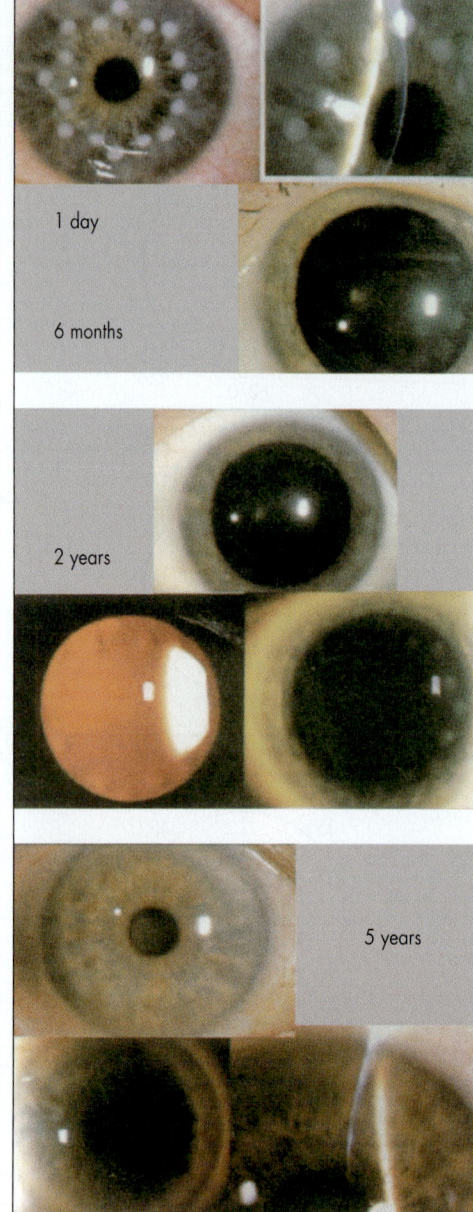

1 day

6 months

2 years

5 years

FIG. 24-5 ▮ Photographs of a cornea treated with laser thermal keratoplasty at different intervals after the procedure.

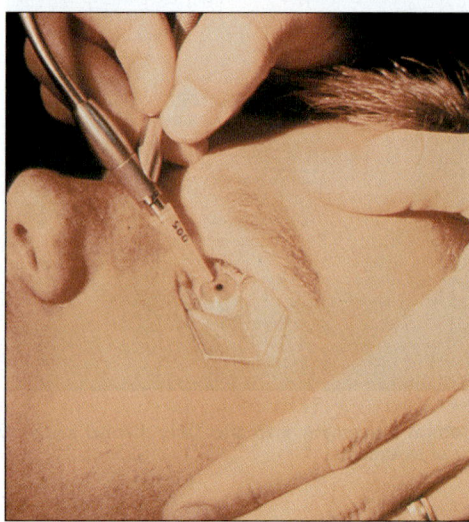

FIG. 24-6 ▮ Probe applied to the corneal surface.

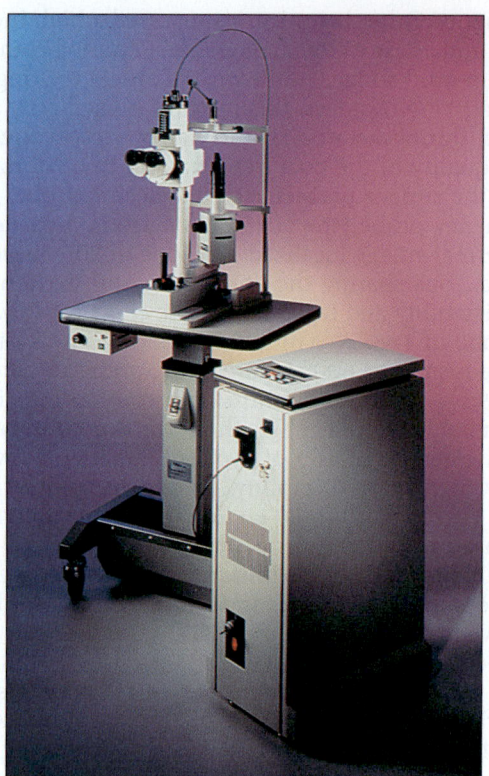

FIG. 24-7 ▮ Noncontact holmium:yttrium-aluminum-garnet laser (Sunrise Technologies). Left, the slit-lamp delivery system; right, the laser unit, which has a fiber-optic cable to transmit the energy to the delivery system. (Reproduced with permission from Sunrise Technologies, Fremont, CA.)

corneal fibroblasts.[21,22] At least three key factors are believed to play a role in achieving adequate refractive results: the collagen shrinkage temperature, the collagen stability, and the keratocyte response.[23] Because of the narrow temperature range for collagen shrinkage, thermal keratoplasty requires excellent control of corneal temperature. Normal corneal collagen appears to be very stable, with a probable half-life greater than 10 years, but the stability of thermally contracted collagen is not known.[24] Minimal wound healing with a minimal inflammatory and keratocyte wound healing response would probably require minimization of temperature levels.[21]

As the heating temperature increases, the likelihood of tissue destruction and an inflammatory response, with subsequent wound healing and remodeling, also increases. Normal energy levels from the noncontact Ho:YAG laser tested in rabbits produced the expected stromal scarring, but the endothelium appeared to be only minimally affected.[25] With a maximal energy of 32 spots treated with at least 20J/cm^2, the total endothelial loss was less than 1.2%.

HOLMIUM:YAG LASER THERMAL KERATOPLASTY AND CONDUCTIVE KERATOPLASTY

Ho:YAG laser devices provide adequate control to avoid overheating of the cornea past the shrinkage temperature, which could result in collagen relaxation and a wound healing response. The corneal penetration depth of this laser light, 480–530µm, is ideal for stromal heating with minimal damage to adjacent tissue. The beam produces a cone-shaped temperature profile, which leads to more pronounced shrinkage of the collagen fibrils in the anterior than the posterior stroma, resulting in better refractive correction and long-term stability.[26]

Two principal Ho:YAG laser delivery systems have been investigated:

1. The contact probe types previously manufactured by Summit Technology and Technomed (Fig. 24-6), and
2. The noncontact device manufactured by Sunrise Technologies (Fig. 24-7).

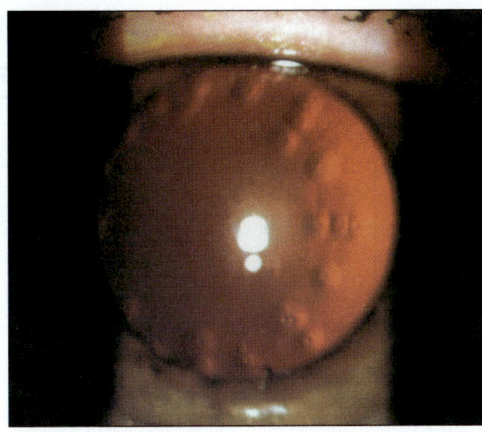

FIG. 24-8 ■ An eye immediately after undergoing conductive keratoplasty.

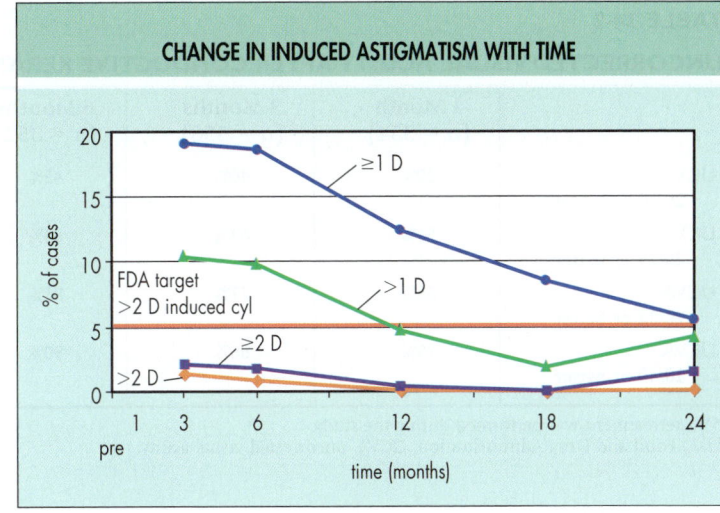

FIG. 24-9 ■ Change in induced astigmatism over time after laser thermal keratoplasty.

The CK approach is a contact method employing a disposable stainless steel tip that penetrates about 450μm into the corneal stroma. The eyelid speculum is attached to the probe to allow for the electrical return path (see Figs. 24-2 and 24-8).

These systems produce different corneal temperature-time-space distributions. The laser contact mode procedure almost certainly heats stromal collagen to a higher average temperature, because of the delivery of approximately twice as much energy per spot (19mJ × 25 pulses, versus 24–30mJ × 10 pulses), at three times the pulse repetition frequency (15Hz versus 5Hz), and in a higher irradiance (strongly versus weakly focused) geometry. The CK approach may seem more invasive, but the temperature distribution is such that the treated zone is cylindrical (which seems to be more favorable than the conical distribution of the laser approaches).

Contact Laser Thermal Keratoplasty

Contact Ho:YAG lasers were manufactured by Summit Technology Inc. (Waltham, MA, USA) and Technomed (Baesweiler, Germany). They consisted of solid-state infrared lasers emitting electromagnetic radiation with a wavelength of 2.06μm in 300μsec pulses at 15Hz repetition frequency and a pulse power of approximately 19mJ.[27] The lasers focally raise the stromal collagen temperature to approximately 60° C by delivering 25 pulses at each treatment location.

The energy is delivered to the corneal stroma through a quartz fiber-optic hand piece that is focused by a sapphire tip that provides a cone angle of 120°. The tip is applied to the corneal surface and is used to focus the laser energy to form a wedge-shaped collagen shrinkage zone that measures 700μm in diameter at the corneal surface and reaches a depth of approximately 450μm.[28]

SPECIFIC TECHNIQUES. In a typical treatment, each treatment location accommodates 25 pulses of 19mJ per pulse. For low hyperopia, one ring of eight applications is placed in the peripheral cornea, at a larger optical zone.[29] For higher hyperopia, a second ring of another eight applications is placed along the same radial meridians as the first eight spots but more peripherally. The probe is manually placed in contact with the cornea, after marking the locations for probe placement with an instrument similar to a radial keratotomy marker. In contact LTK, it is important to orient the hand piece perpendicular to the corneal surface during the treatment to obtain consistent coagulation profiles and to prevent decentration and irregular treatments. The epithelium generally sloughs at the treatment sites and is removed with a cotton tip. Patients generally have foreign body sensation for the first three postoperative days. For astigmatism treatment, two to four treatment spots are placed on either side of the flat meridian in a variable optical zone.[27]

CLINICAL OUTCOME. Several reports on the clinical outcome of using contact LTK devices for the treatment of hyperopia revealed important regression, poor predictability, and significant induced astigmatism[30-32,41-49] (Fig. 24-9). Treatment of astigmatism, with two coagulation spots placed on each side of the flat meridian in the 8.5mm zone, resulted in high regression.[33] Thereafter, astigmatism treatment was tried in rabbits[34] or human eye-banked eyes.[35] The efficacy of LTK on corneas that have already undergone photorefractive keratectomy (PRK) might be different from the treatment of primary hyperopia or astigmatism, because Bowman's layer is removed by PRK. Two reports showed that in eyes with hyperopia induced by PRK, LTK appeared to be considerably more successful than in eyes with primary hyperopia, even if the predictability of the method is low and astigmatism can be induced with the attempted spherical correction.[36,37]

Conductive Keratoplasty

CK uses a probe that heats the cornea through high-radiofrequency currents in eight peripheral locations (similar to LTK). Its major advantage is the greater stability of the refractive effect (Table 24-1).

In CK, topical anesthetics are applied, followed by insertion of the eyelid speculum (which acts as a return pathway for the electrical current) without an eyelid drape. The CK tip is inserted in premarked peripheral corneal spots, and the treatment is applied according to published nomograms.

For lower hyperopic corrections, eight spots are applied at the 6mm optical zone and eight spots are applied at the 7mm optical zone. For greater hyperopic corrections (+2–+2.50D), 24 spots are applied (eight additional spots at the 8mm optical zone). For even greater hyperopic corrections, 32 spots are applied (Table 24-2).

The efficacy, stability, and safety of CK have been established. It is not clear why there are major differences in the stability of CK and LTK. Further studies are needed to determine the basis for these differences.

TABLE 24-1

STABILITY OF CONDUCTIVE KERATOPLASTY (24-MONTH COHORT: ALL EYES TREATED)

	6–9 Months	9–12 Months	12–24 Months
Manifest reaction (n = 88)	0.04/month SD 0.13	0.04/month SD 0.13	0.03/month SD 0.04
Cycloplegic reaction (n = 79)	0.06/month SD 0.15	0.04/month SD 0.11	0.03/month SD 0.03

TABLE 24-2

UNCORRECTED VISUAL ACUITY AFTER CONDUCTIVE KERATOPLASTY (EYES TREATED WITH CURRENT NOMOGRAM)*

	1 Month (n = 354)	3 Months (n = 358)	6 Months (n = 352)	9 Months (n = 35)	12 Months (n = 354)	24 Months (n = 70)	FDA Target
UCVA 20/20 or better	29%	40%	45%	49%	54%	54%	—
UCVA 20/25 or better	51%	63%	64%	73%	74%	77%	—
UCVA 20/32 or better	68%	77%	81%	85%	88%	85%	—
UCVA 20/40 or better	79%	86%	90%	93%	92%	91%	85%

*No retreatment was performed during the study.
FDA, Food and Drug Administration; UCVA, uncorrected visual acuity.

Noncontact Laser Thermal Keratoplasty

TECHNICAL DESCRIPTION. Noncontact Ho:YAG LTK treatments are performed with the Sun1000TM Corneal Shaping System and the newer Sunrise Hyperion LTK System, both manufactured by Sunrise Technologies (Fremont, CA, USA). They both consist of the Ho:YAG laser console, a slit lamp, and a polyprism beam-splitting optical tower delivery system. The Corneal Shaping System emits pulses of infrared light (2.13m) with a pulse duration of 250μsec full width at half maximum intensity, a pulse repetition frequency of 5Hz, and adjustable pulse energy up to 300mJ.[38] The device projects a ring pattern of up to eight spots on the cornea with an adjustable diameter in the 3–8mm range. The system employs a fiber-optic noncontact delivery system mounted to a slit lamp to deliver up to eight simultaneous treatment spots. Each spot has a nominal spot diameter of 600μm (containing 90% of the energy per shot) and a nonuniform energy distribution within the spot. The Sunrise Hyperion LTK System is an improved device that produces the same kind of laser light.[39]

SPECIFIC TECHNIQUES. Topical anesthesia (tetracaine 1%) is applied, and a speculum is used to keep the eyelids open for 3 minutes to allow the tear film to dry. Epithelial drying can be achieved by blotting the cornea with a moist sponge. Centration is obtained by centering red helium neon (HeNe) laser tracer beams (wavelength 633nm) around the entrance pupil while the patient is focusing on a flashing yellow HeNe light fixation source (Hyperion System). The laser is focused on the surface of the cornea using calibrated green HeNe laser-focusing beams (wavelength 543nm).

In a typical treatment, each treatment location accepts 5–10 pulses to each spot simultaneously over a 1.4sec exposure time using a pulse frequency of 5Hz. The total pulse energy[15] varies in a linear manner for each level of pretreatment refractive error and ranges from 228mJ (for +0.75D correction) to 256mJ (for +2.50D correction). For hyperopia, two concentric eight-spots rings of 8mm and 7mm centerline diameters are placed, with spots of 0.6mm on radials (radial pattern, Fig. 24-10). The two rings are delivered in a centrifugal (inner to outer) pattern.[39] If retreatment is necessary, the pattern can be rotated to a location between the eight original spots. Postoperatively, antibiotic and nonsteroidal anti-inflammatory drops are administered four times daily until the epithelium heals.

CLINICAL OUTCOME

Hyperopia.[40,42–49] Early in vitro studies with fresh swine eyes[41] and human eye-bank eyes[25] revealed that at smaller treatment zones, factors such as spot size, spot number, and energy density play a role in the refractive outcome. In the United States, the Corneal Shaping System has been tested in animal eyes, in poorly sighted patients, and in an early series of sighted patients.[41–45] In those trials, the histological changes after laser

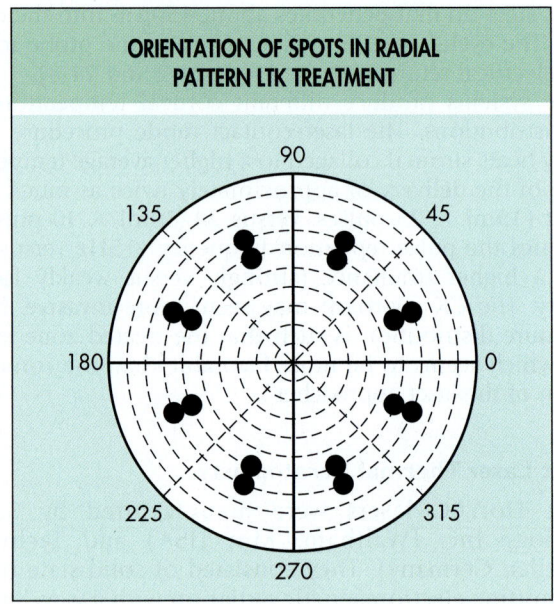

FIG. 24-10 ■ Orientation of the spots delivered in a radial-pattern laser thermal keratoplasty treatment.

treatments were studied,[27,28] and it was also found that a greater change in curvature was produced using two-ring treatment instead of one-ring treatment.[29]

Noncontact LTK treatments of hyperopic patients have been reported by several groups worldwide.[41–49] The phase I U.S. feasibility study began in November 1992, studying a total of 10 poorly sighted eyes. The phase IIa U.S. investigation started in September 1993, and 18 patients were enrolled. Thereafter, a change was made in the nomograms, and the Hyperion LTK System was used by the same company in both the explanted phase IIa U.S. study of 200 patients and the phase III U.S. study started in November 1997 that enrolled 200 additional patients.[47–49] The results in 612 eyes from 379 patients who participated in both phase IIa and phase III U.S. studies after 2 years follow-up have been presented by Aker and Brown.[39]

In this extended trial, the procedure appeared to be very safe, since no eyes lost more than two lines of best spectacle-corrected visual acuity. No laser-related adverse effects were reported during this clinical study, and the only adverse event reported was a transient increase in intraocular pressure. Corneal edema (0.2%) and pain (0.2%) were also reported. A mild foreign body sensation (an itchy, scratchy feeling requiring artificial tears) was observed in a small number of patients, mostly at the 1-month examination. The incidence of other symptoms (glare, photophobia, night vision difficulties, double vision) was ex-

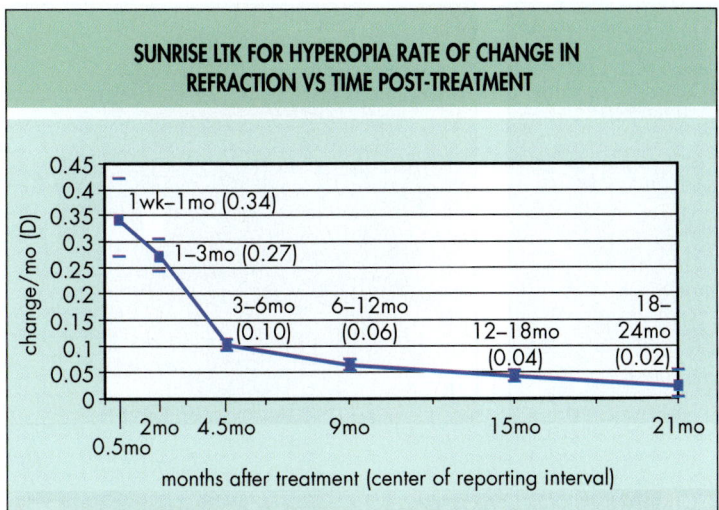

FIG. 24-11 ▪ Rate of change of refraction as a function of time elapsed after laser thermal keratoplasty. Parentheses enclose the rate of change per month at the reported interval. Horizontal lines indicate 95% confidence intervals.

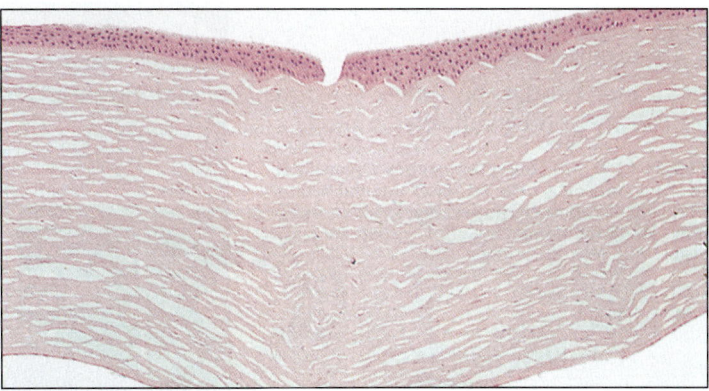

FIG. 24-12 ▪ Human cornea 6 weeks after laser thermal keratoplasty. Note the wedge-shaped area (apex toward the endothelium) of relatively homogeneous corneal stroma and acellularity.

tremely low. Astigmatism less than 2.00D was induced in 4.2% of individuals in the second year (see Fig. 24-9). Regarding efficacy, at the 2-year examination, 69.4% of patients showed improvement of distance uncorrected visual acuity (UCVA) by two or more lines, with the mean improvement in UCVA being 2.8 lines. Near UCVA improved by two lines in 56.3% of patients at 2 years post-treatment. At 2 years post-treatment 76.4% of the individuals showed an induced reduction in their manifest hyperopia of 0.50D or more, with a mean reduction of hyperopic correction of 0.79D.[49] No patients experienced a greater than 0.25D increase in hyperopia. Clinical outcomes were similar for both manifest and cycloplegic refraction.[49]

In that study, the attempted correction was emmetropia in the early post-treatment period (third–sixth month). Two years after treatment, the proportion of eyes within 1.0D of emmetropia was 62.5%, up from 10.9% preoperatively. The remaining 37.5% of eyes not within 1.0D of emmetropia at the 2-year post-treatment examination were all undercorrected by more than 1.0D, with 4.2% of eyes being undercorrected by more than 2.0D. A review of the study revealed that the initial nomogram was approximately 30% underpowered, so on average, patients were undercorrected during treatment. The mean rate of change per month improved over the post-treatment period (Fig. 24-11). Until the third postoperative month, the rate of refraction change was approximately 0.3D per month; thereafter, it declined to 0.1D per month and kept declining until the second postoperative year.

Retreatment was done in 10 patients participating in this expanded U.S. study by rotating the laser pattern to a location between the original spots, and this appeared to be safe and effective. International data on retreatment after undercorrection were collected by the authors by means of a questionnaire sent to eight physicians outside the United States. These physicians have not observed that the contact LTK procedure precludes the performance of subsequent ophthalmic procedures (PRK, laser *in situ* keratomileusis [LASIK]) or the use of contact lenses. The authors of this extended study concluded that noncontact LTK is a safe and effective method for the correction of +0.75–+2.50D of hyperopia, with a very low risk of potential complications or side effects.

Similar studies outside the United States also suggest that LTK is safe and effective for low hyperopia and has a low complication rate.[50,51] Good patient selection is the key to obtaining satisfactory results. Some authors think that the technique works best for up to +3.00D in older individuals with a central corneal thickness less than 525μm.

Myopia Overcorrection. Reports of noncontact LTK for treating overcorrection after myopic PRK,[52,53] LASIK,[54] and corneal lamellar cutting[55] found that LTK was more effective and stable than for primary hyperopia. This phenomenon may be attributed to the absence of Bowman's layer or to low central corneal pachymetry. The wedge-shaped area of heating is evident histologically (Fig. 24-12).

Laser Thermal Keratoplasty Overcorrection. LTK overcorrections have been treated with hyperopic LASIK.[56,57] Hyperopic LASIK after LTK is safe and effective, without vision-threatening complications, and is a good alternative for hyperopic regression. Predictability and efficacy are less than with primary LASIK for hyperopia, but the procedure is equally safe.

FUTURE DIRECTIONS

All studies of pulsed LTK in congenital hyperopia with a minimum of 1-year follow-up have shown that the amount of correction is limited to a maximum of 2.50D with contact and 2.0D with noncontact devices. A change of more than 4.0D was achieved only if the central cornea was thinned by previous ablative surgeries.[58] The fact that the effect of LTK with a pulsed laser depends strongly on the pulse repetition rate led to the idea of using a continuously emitting laser source, such as a diode, to achieve a more steady temperature rise and to avoid temperature peaks. Diode LTK can induce a more lasting refractive change than pulsed holmium LTK.[59,60] Trials in porcine eyes[61,62] have shown that diode LTK can provide defined and uniform coagulation resulting in sufficient refractive changes. Although the potential exists for endothelial cell damage, diode LTK appears to be superior to pulsed holmium LTK (Figs. 24-13 and 24-14). The first trial of the diode LTK technique in blind human eyes for treating hyperopia revealed that at a wavelength of 1.870μm, corneal endothelial damage was limited, and the procedure appeared to be safe and effective.[63] Regression occurred mainly in the first three postoperative months.

The most exciting direction of LTK is that of wave front-guided treatment. This has been shown to be possible via an adaptation to the currently available system, but it has not yet been approved by the Food and Drug Administration. The major advantage of this modification is that it is, theoretically, the only keratorefractive procedure for hyperopia wherein wave-front-guided treatment effects can be monitored and adjusted continuously during treatment. Energy adjustments during surgery may allow greater predictability, reduced astigmatism, and the ability to achieve a predetermined amount of overcorrection to ensure acceptable visual results for the longest possible duration.

This approach may also be used as an adjunct to other refractive procedures for hyperopia, including LASIK and CK. Real-time wave front-guided LTK will overcome several of the known limitations of LTK and may become an important adjunct procedure for the correction of hyperopia in the next decade.

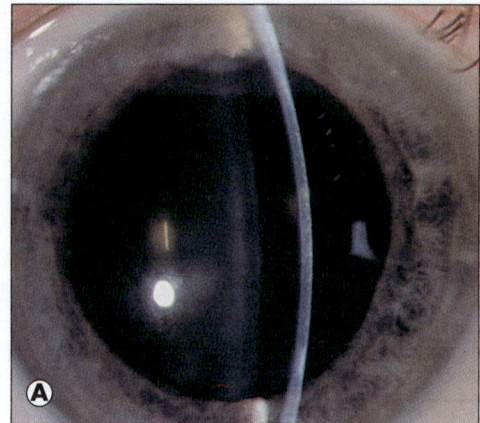 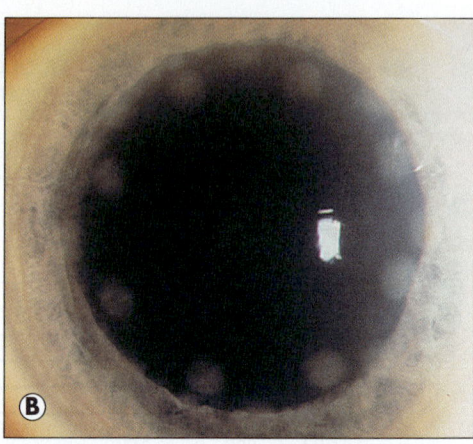

FIG. 24-13 ■ Slit-lamp photographs 2 years after two-ring noncontact Ho:YAG laser thermal keratoplasty. **A,** The spots are almost imperceptible with direct slit-beam illumination. **B,** The spots are readily visible with sclerotic scatter.

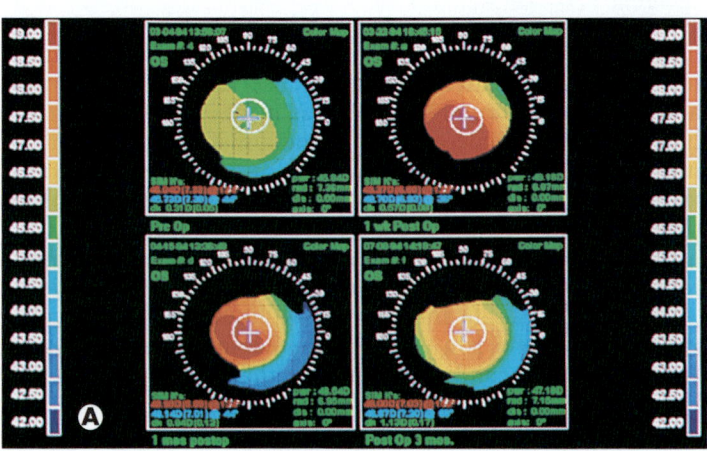 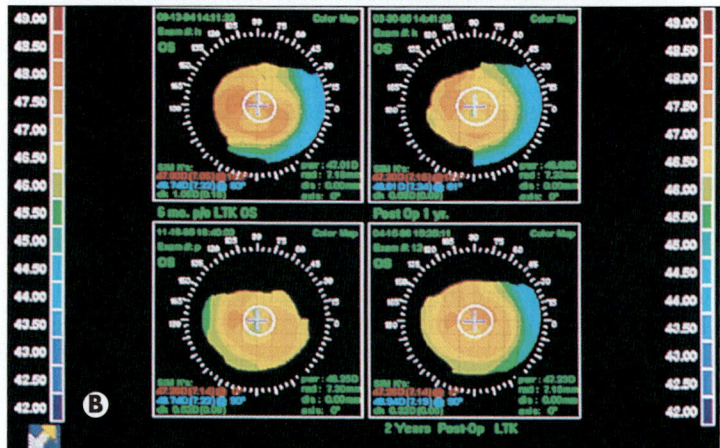

FIG. 24-14 ■ Computerized videokeratographs following noncontact Ho:YAG laser thermal keratoplasty with two-ring application. **A,** Intervals for the topographical maps from upper left to lower right are preoperative and 1 week, 1 month, and 3 months postoperatively. **B,** Intervals for the topographical maps from upper left to lower right are 6, 12, 18, and 24 months postoperatively. This patient showed an increase in corneal steepening of 2.12D and a change in subjective manifest refraction (spherical equivalent) of −1.75D. The postoperative topographical maps demonstrate surgically induced peripheral corneal flattening and central corneal steepening with excellent stability between 12 and 24 months. Note the large (approximately 5mm) central steepened zone.

REFERENCES

1. Gasset A. Changes in corneal curvature associated with thermokeratoplasty. In: Schachar RA, Levy NS, Schachar L, eds. Keratorefraction. Benison, TX: LAL Publishing; 1980.
2. Lans LJ. Experimentalle Untersuchungen uber Entstehung von Astigmatismus durch nicht-perforirende Corneawunden. Albrecht v Graefes Arch Ophthalmol. 1898;45:117–52.
3. Terrien F. Dystrophia marginale symetrique des deux cornees avec astigmatisme regular consequitif et guerison par la cauterisation ignee. Arch Ophthalmol. 1900;20:12.
4. Wray C. Case of 3 D of hypermetropic astigmatism cured by the cautery. Trans Ophthalmol Soc UK. 1914;34:109.
5. O'Connor R. Corneal cautery for high myopic astigmatism. Am J Ophthalmol. 1933;16:337.
6. Stringer H, Parr J. Shrinkage temperature of eye collagen. Nature. 1964;204:1307.
8. Gasset AR, Shaw EL, Kaufman HE, et al. Thermokeratoplasty. Trans Am Acad Ophthalmol Otolaryngol. 1973;77:441.
8. Keates RH, Dingle J. Thermokeratoplasty for keratoconus. Ophthalmic Surg. 1975;6:89.
9. Aquavella JV, Smith RS, Shaw EL. Alterations in corneal morphology following thermokeratoplasty. Arch Ophthalmol. 1976;94:2082.
10. Kenyon KR. Histological changes in Bowman's membrane associated with thermokeratoplasty. In: Schachar RA, Levy NS, Schachar L, eds. Keratorefraction. Benison, TX: LAL Publishing; 1980.
11. Rowsey JJ. Radio frequency probe keratoplasty. In: Schachar RA, Levy NS, Schachar L, eds. Keratorefraction. Benison, TX: LAL Publishing; 1980.
12. Rowsey JJ, Gaylor JR, Dahlstrom R, et al. Los Alamos keratoplasty techniques. Contact Intraocul Lens Med J. 1980;6:1.
13. Rowsey JJ, Doss JD. Preliminary report of Los Alamos keratoplasty techniques. Ophthalmology. 1981;88:755.
14. McDonnell PJ, Garbus J, Romero JL, et al. Electrosurgical keratoplasty: clinicopathological correlation. Arch Ophthalmol. 1988;106:235.
15. Rowsey JJ. Electrosurgical keratoplasty: update and retraction. Invest Ophthalmol Vis Sci. 1987;28:224.
16. Caster AI. The Fyodorov technique of hyperopia correction by thermal coagulation: a preliminary report. J Refract Surg. 1988;4:105.
17. Neumann A, Sanders D, Salz J. Radial thermokeratoplasty for hyperopia. II. Encouraging results from early laboratory and human trials. Refract Corneal Surg. 1989;5:52.
18. Neumann A, Sanders D, Raanan M, et al. Hyperopic thermokeratoplasty: clinical evaluation. J Cataract Refract Surg. 1991;17:830.
19. McCally R, Bargeron C, Green W, et al. Stromal damage in rabbit corneas exposed to CO_2 laser radiation. Exp Eye Res. 1983;37:543.
20. Seiler T. Ho:YAG laser thermokeratoplasty for hyperopia. Ophthalmol Clin North Am. 1992;5:773–80.
21. Ogawa GSH, Azar DT, Koch DD. Laser thermokeratoplasty for hyperopia, astigmatism and myopia. In: Azar DT, ed. Refractive surgery. Stamford, CT: Appleton & Lange; 1997.
22. Feldman ST, William E, Frucht-Pery J, et al. Regression of effect following radial thermokeratoplasty in humans. Refract Corneal Surg. 1989;5:288.
23. Koch DD, Berry MJ, Vassiliadis A, et al. Non-contact holmium:YAG laser thermal keratoplasty for treatment of hyperopia. In: Salz JJ, McDonnell PJ, McDonald MB, eds. Corneal laser surgery. St Louis: Mosby; 1995.
24. Smelser CK, Polack FM, Ozanies V. Persistence of donor collagen in corneal transplants. Exp Eye Res. 1965;4:349.
25. Moreira H, Campos M, Sawasch MR, et al. Holmium laser thermokeratoplasty. Ophthalmology. 1993;100:752.
26. Seiler T, Matallana M, Bende T. Laser thermokeratoplasty by means of a pulsed holmium:YAG laser for hyperopic correction. J Refract Corneal Surg. 1990;6:335.
27. Thompson VM, Seiler T, Durrie DS, et al. Holmium:YAG laser thermokeratoplasty for hyperopia and astigmatism: an overview. Refract Corneal Surg. 1993;9:S134.
28. Durrie DS, Schumer J, Cavanaugh TB. Holmium:YAG laser thermokeratoplasty for hyperopia. J Refract Corneal Surg. 1994;10:S277.
29. Yanoff M. Holmium laser hyperopia thermokeratoplasty update. Eur J Implant Ref Surg. 1995;7:89–91.
30. Tutton MK, Cherry PM. Holmium:YAG laser thermokeratoplasty to correct hyperopia: two years follow-up. Ophthalmic Surg Lasers. 1996;27(5 suppl):S521–4.
31. Tassignon MJ, Trau R, Mathys B. Le traitement de l'hypermetropie a l'aide du laser holmium laser thermokeratoplastie (LTK). Bull Soc Belge Ophtalmol. 1997;266:75.
32. Eggink CA, Bardak Y, Cuypers MHM, Deutman AF. Treatment of hyperopia with contact Ho:YAG laser thermal keratoplasty. J Refract Surg. 1999;15:16.
33. Thompson VM. Holmium:YAG laser thermokeratoplasty for correction of astigmatism. J Refract Corneal Surg. 1994;10:S293.
34. Lim KH, Kim WJ, Wee WR, et al. Holmium:YAG laser thermokeratoplasty for astigmatism in rabbits. J Refract Surg. 1996;12:190.
35. Bende T, Jean B, Derse M, et al. Holmium:YAG thermokeratoplasty: treatment parameters for astigmatism induction based upon spherical enucleated human eyes. Graefes Arch Clin Exp Ophthalmol. 1998;236:405.

36. Goggin M, Lavery F. Holmium laser thermokeratoplasty for the reversal of hyperopia after myopic photorefractive keratectomy. Br J Ophthalmol. 1997;81:541.

37. Eggink C, Meurs P, Bardak Y, et al. Holmium laser thermal keratoplasty for hyperopia and astigmatism after photorefractive keratectomy. J Refract Surg. 2000; 16:317.

38. Parel JM, Ren Q, Simon G. Noncontact laser photothermal keratoplasty. I. Biophysical principle and laser beam delivery system. J Refract Corneal Surg. 1994;10:511.

39. Aker AB, Brown CB. Hyperion laser thermokeratoplasty for hyperopia. Int Ophthalmol Clin. 2000;40(3):165.

40. Koch DD. Histological changes and wound healing response following noncontact holmium:YAG laser thermal keratoplasty. Trans Am Ophthalmol Soc. 1996;94:745.

41. Koch DD, et al. Ho:YAG laser thermal keratoplasty: in vitro experiments. Invest Ophthalmol Vis Sci. 1993;34(4 suppl):1246.

42. Koch DD, Kohnen T, Anderson J, et al. Histologic changes and wound healing response following 10-pulse noncontact holmium:YAG laser thermal keratoplasty. J Refract Surg. 1996;12:623.

43. Kohnen T, Husain SE, Koch DD. Corneal topographic changes after noncontact holmium:YAG laser thermal keratoplasty to correct hyperopia. J Cataract Refract Surg. 1996;22:427.

44. Koch DD, Abarca A, Villareal R, et al. Hyperopia correction by noncontact holmium:YAG laser thermal keratoplasty. Clinical study with two-year follow-up. Ophthalmology. 1996;103:731.

45. Kohnen T, Villareal R, Menefee R, et al. Hyperopia correction by noncontact holmium:YAG laser thermal keratoplasty: five-pulse treatments with 1-year follow up. Graefes Arch Clin Exp Ophthalmol. 1997;235:702.

46. Gezer A. The role of patient's age in regression of holmium:YAG thermokeratoplasty-induced correction of hyperopia. Eur J Ophthalmol. 1997;7:139.

47. Koch DD, Kohnen T, McDonnell PJ, et al. Hyperopia correction by noncontact holmium:YAG laser thermal keratoplasty. United States phase IIA clinical study with 1-year follow-up. Ophthalmology. 1996;103:1525.

48. Kohnen T, Koch DD, McDonnell PJ, et al. Noncontact holmium:YAG laser thermal keratoplasty to correct hyperopia: 18-month follow-up. Ophthalmologica. 1997;211:274.

49. Koch DD, Kohnen T, McDonnell PJ, et al. Hyperopia correction by non-contact holmium:YAG laser thermal keratoplasty. U.S. phase IIA clinical study with 2-year follow-up. Ophthalmology. 1997;104:1938.

50. Alio JL, Ismail MM, Sanchez Pego JL. Correction of hyperopia with noncontact Ho:YAG laser thermal keratoplasty. J Refract Surg. 1997;13:17.

51. Nano HD, Muzzin S. Noncontact holmium:YAG laser thermal keratoplasty for hyperopia. J Cataract Refract Surg. 1998;24:751.

52. Vinciguerra P, Kohnen T, Azzolini M, et al. Radial and staggered treatment patterns to correct hyperopia using noncontact holmium:YAG laser thermal keratoplasty. J Cataract Refract Surg. 1998;24:21.

53. Alio JL, Ismail MM, Artola A, et al. Correction of hyperopia by photorefractive keratectomy using noncontact Ho:YAG laser thermal keratoplasty. J Refract Surg. 1997;13:13.

54. Pop M. Laser thermal keratoplasty for the treatment of photorefractive keratectomy overcorrections. A 1-year follow-up. Ophthalmology. 1998;105:926.

55. Ismail MM, Alio HL, Perez-Santonja JJ. Noncontact thermokeratoplasty to correct hyperopia induced by laser in situ keratomileusis. J Cataract Refract Surg. 1998; 24:1191.

56. Ismail MM, Perez-Santonja JJ, Alio HL. Laser thermokeratoplasty after lamellar corneal cutting. J Cataract Refract Surg. 1999;25:212.

57. Portellinha W, Nakano K, Oliveira M, et al. Laser in situ keratomileusis for hyperopia after thermal keratoplasty. J Refract Surg. 1999;15(suppl):S218.

58. Attia W, Perez-Santonja JJ, Alio JL. Laser in situ keratomileusis for recurrent hyperopia following laser thermal keratoplasty. J Refract Surg. 2000;16:163.

59. Geerlng G, Koop N, Brinkmann R, et al. Continuous-wave diode laser thermokeratoplasty: first clinical experience in blind human eyes. J Cataract Refract Surg. 1999;25:32.

60. Geerling G, Brinkmann R, Koop N, et al. Laser thermokeratoplasty—experimental study in minipigs with a CW-IR laser diode. Invest Ophthalmol Vis Sci. 1996; 37:S65.

61. Brinkmann R, Koop N, Geerling G, et al. Diode laser thermokeratoplasty: application strategy and dosimetry. J Cataract Refract Surg. 1998;24:1195.

62. Wirbelauer C, Koop N, Tuengler A, et al. Corneal endothelial cell damage after experimental diode laser thermal keratoplasty. J Refract Surg. 2000;16:323.

63. Brinkmann R, Radt B, Flamm C, et al. Influence of temperature and time on thermally induced forces in corneal collagen and the effect on laser thermokeratoplasty. J Cataract Refract Surg. 2000;26:744.

25 Intrastromal Corneal Ring Segments for Low and High Myopia

DIMITRI T. AZAR • JONATHAN D. PRIMACK

DEFINITION
- Polymethyl methacrylate (PMMA) arcuate segments that are placed within the peripheral cornea to correct myopia.

KEY FEATURES
- Inner diameter of 6.8mm.
- Refractive effect is related to the thickness of the segments.
- Initial enthusiasm regarding beneficial effect in low myopia.
- Emerging role as adjunct treatment for high myopia and corneal ectasia.

ASSOCIATED FEATURES
- Surgical steps include intrastromal corneal ring segment channel formation, insertion of segments, and suturing of entry site.
- Surgical techniques are slightly modified for keratoconus and for combined intrastromal corneal ring segments and laser *in situ* keratomileusis.
- Reversibility and hyperacuity are potential advantages.

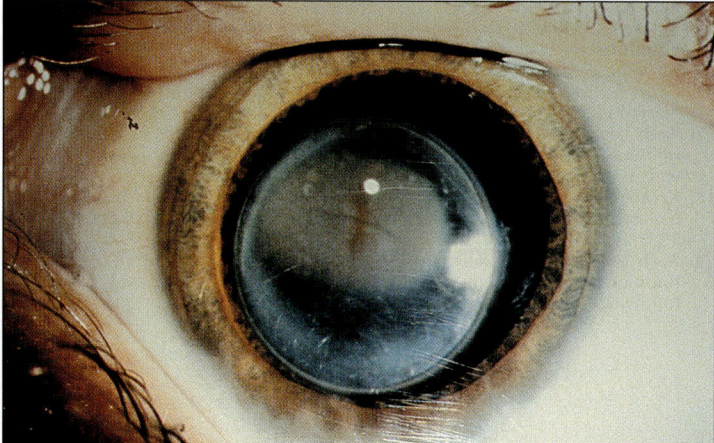

FIG. 25-1 ▌ Slit-lamp photograph of corneal opacity after implantation of a polysulfone intracorneal lens. (Courtesy of Stephen S. Lane, MD.)

INTRODUCTION

In 1949, Barraquer first proposed the use of alloplastic materials as a method to correct refractive errors. Several intracorneal implants, or inlays, made of various materials (hydrogels, polysulfones) have been evaluated in animal and human eyes for the correction of myopia, aphakia, or presbyopia. However, none of them are currently used routinely.[1] Among the materials that have been tested for use as intracorneal implants are polysulfone lenses, small diameter corneal inlays, and hydrogel lenses (Figs. 25-1 to 25-4).

Intrastromal corneal ring segments (ICRSs), or Intacs, are placed in the peripheral stroma at approximately two-thirds depth, outside the central optical zone, to reshape the anterior corneal surface while maintaining the positive asphericity of the cornea.[1–8] The first-generation design of Intacs was referred to as the 360° intrastromal corneal ring (ICR). The current design consists of two segments, each with an arc length of 150° (Fig. 25-5). Intacs are manufactured from polymethyl methacrylate (PMMA).[1]

Each Intacs segment has a hexagonal cross section that lies along a conic section. With a fixed outer diameter of 8.1mm and an inner diameter of 6.8mm, Intacs leave a large, clear central optic zone. Each segment has a small positioning hole at the superior end to aid with surgical manipulation once the segments have been inserted. The two segments are designated as clockwise and counterclockwise to correspond to their orientation within the intrastromal tunnel.[1]

Intacs change the arc length of the anterior corneal curvature. The refractive effect achieved is directly related to the thickness of the product. Placing the product in the periphery of the cornea causes local separation of the corneal lamellae, which results in shortening of the corneal arc length. This has a net effect of flattening the cornea, thereby correcting for myopia by lowering the optical power of the eye. Increasing the thickness of Intacs causes greater degrees of local separation and increased corneal flattening. Thus, the degree of corneal flattening—or correction—achieved by Intacs is directly related to thickness.[1]

The same effect can be observed by placing a pencil underneath a sheet of paper. With the added bulk of the pencil, the paper is no longer flat and is shorter. In much the same way, when Intacs are placed within the stromal layers of the cornea, they shorten the arc length across the optical zone.[1]

Intacs are available in the United States in three different thicknesses—0.25, 0.30, and 0.35mm—intended for the reduction or elimination of low myopia (Table 25-1). The initial enthusiasm regarding ICRSs for the correction of myopia has faded for multiple reasons, including a limited range of correction, induced astigmatism, and slow visual recovery. Although the future role of ICRSs in refractive surgery is unclear, they may evolve into an important therapeutic intervention in keratoconus patients.[9] Another potential application of ICRSs may be to minimize the risk of corneal ectasia following laser *in situ* keratomileusis (LASIK) in patients with high myopia.[10] Intacs are also available in thicknesses of 0.40 and 0.45mm to correct myopia up to −4.50D.

SURGICAL TECHNIQUE

Topical anesthetic and antibiotic drops are administered preoperatively. The operative eye is prepped with an antiseptic solution, and sterile drapes are placed appropriately. Peri- or retrobulbar anesthesia is unnecessary and could interfere with patient fixation during LASIK.

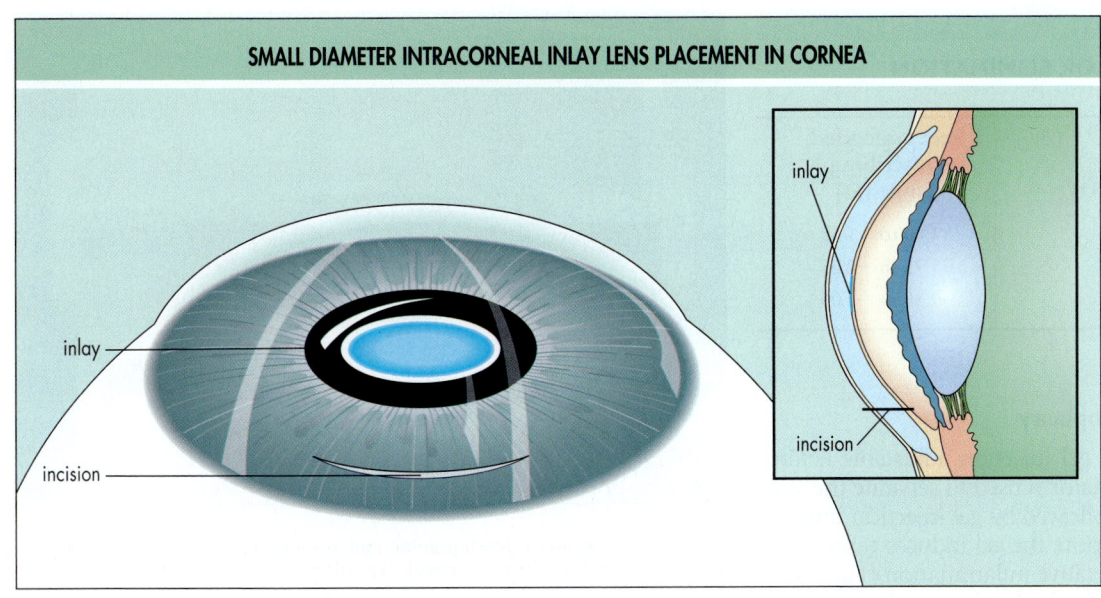

SMALL DIAMETER INTRACORNEAL INLAY LENS PLACEMENT IN CORNEA

inlay

incision

inlay

incision

FIG. 25-2 ▌ Schematic of small diameter intracorneal inlay lens placement in cornea. (Adapted with permission of Judy Gordon, MD, and Richard L. Lindstrom, MD.)

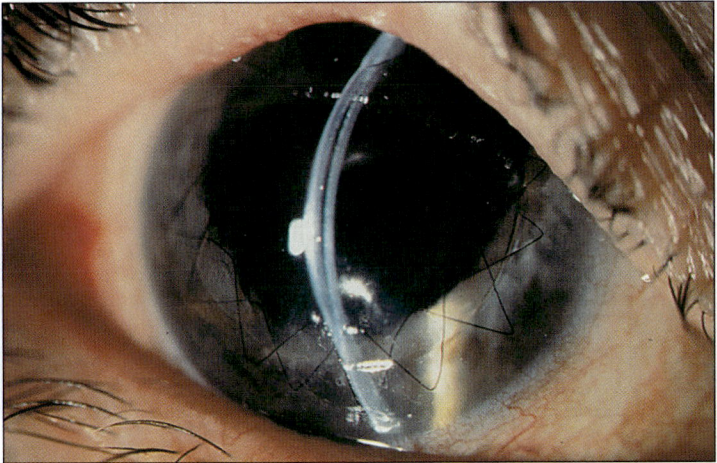

FIG. 25-3 ▌ Slit-lamp photograph of a hydrogel intracorneal lens in position in the patient's cornea. (Courtesy of Roger F. Steinert, MD.)

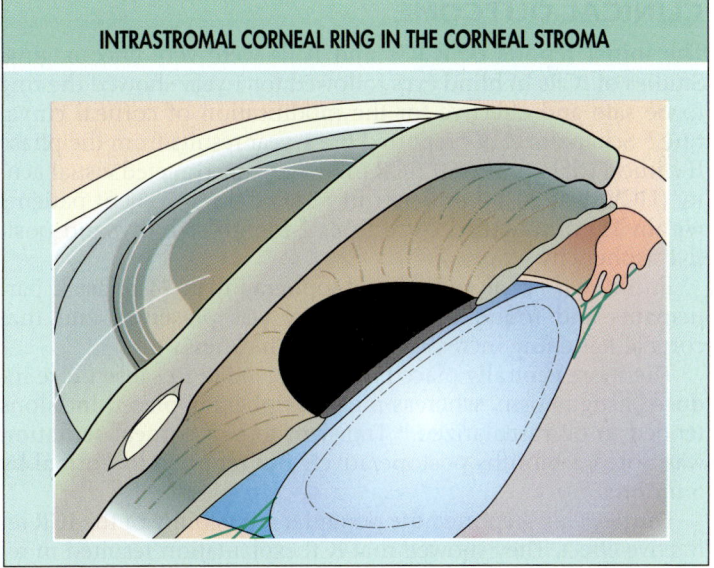

INTRASTROMAL CORNEAL RING IN THE CORNEAL STROMA

FIG. 25-4 ▌ Intrastromal corneal ring in the corneal stroma. (Original drawing courtesy of Thomas Loarie.)

ICRS Channel Formation

The center of the cornea is located, and an incision and placement marker (KeraVision, Fremont, CA) is applied to indicate where the PMMA segments and the superior, radial incision will ultimately lie.[1,8] Ultrasonic pachymetry is performed at the 12 o'clock incision site, and an approximately 1mm incision of 68% corneal thickness is created with a calibrated diamond knife. A modified Suarez spreader is used to perform a small lamellar dissection at the base of the incision, to create an entry pocket on either side. Next, a vacuum centering guide (KeraVision) is positioned on the globe and stabilized under suction. Specially designed 0.9mm dissectors are then introduced through the incision (clockwise and counterclockwise) to create stromal tunnels by blunt dissection (Fig. 25-6). Ideally, the channels are located at two-thirds corneal depth. Suction is then released, and the centering guide is removed.

Segment Insertion

Using forceps, the PMMA segments are introduced into the channels. In their final position, the segments are located 3mm apart superiorly. If necessary, the flap is refloated to eliminate any iatrogenically induced wrinkles. The incision site is hydrated and closed with 10-0 nylon sutures.[8] Figure 25-7 illustrates the appearance of the cornea following this procedure.

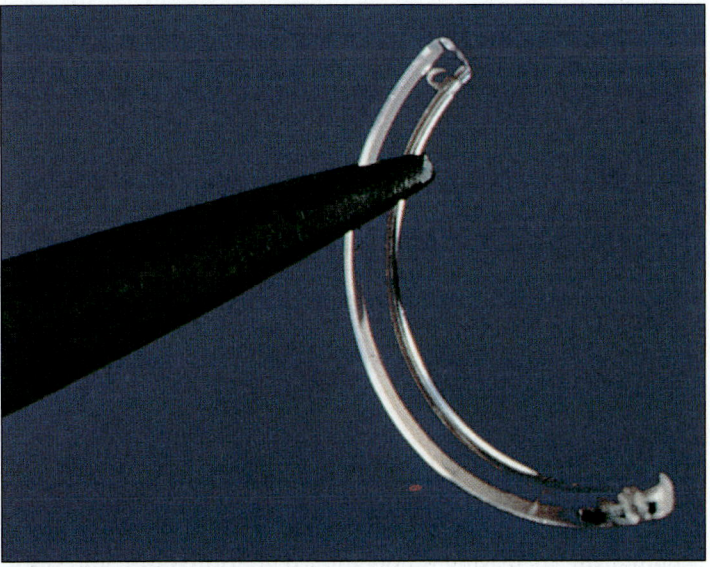

FIG. 25-5 ▌ A 150° intrastromal corneal ring segment. (Courtesy of Thomas Loarie.)

TABLE 25-1

INTACS FOR THE REDUCTION OR ELIMINATION OF LOW MYOPIA

Intacs Thickness (mm)	Predicted Nominal Correction (D)	Recommended Prescribing Range (D)
0.25	−1.03	−1.00 to −1.63
0.30	−2.00	−1.75 to −2.25
0.35	−2.70	−2.38 to −3.00

Gel Injection Adjustable Keratoplasty

A modification of ICRS surgery is gel injection adjustable keratoplasty. In this procedure, a delaminator is used to separate the stromal lamellae (Fig. 25-8). This is followed by gel injection into the stromal channel. After polymerization, the gel induces central flattening, without significant postoperative inflammation (Fig. 25-9). This procedure may have potential advantages over ICRSs, but it has not been approved by the U.S. Food and Drug Administration.

CLINICAL OUTCOME

The initial reports of ICRSs and ICRs were very encouraging. Studies of ICRs in blind eyes followed for 1 year showed the ring to be safe and effective for the modification of corneal curvature.[11] Schanzlin et al.[8] reported the 1-year results from the phase II clinical trial of the 360° ICR in 81 eyes: uncorrected visual acuity (UCVA) of 20/40 or better in 88% of cases, 73% of patients within 1D of intended correction, 2-month stability, and positive asphericity.

Burris et al.[3] analyzed corneal topography in 74 phase II participants and found that asphericity was preserved and that corneal flattening increased with ring thickness.

The more centrally placed incisions tended to cause more induced astigmatism, whereas more peripherally placed incisions tended to be vascularized.[11] Transient loss of corneal sensation was noted 2 months postoperatively but returned to normal by 6 months.[11]

Durrie et al.[12] reported the potential reversibility of the ICR refractive effect. They showed that ICR explantation resulted in return of corneal curvature and refractive error to preimplant values. Similar results were reported by Davis et al.[13] and Twa et al.[14]

POSTOPERATIVE CARE AND MANAGEMENT

Immediately following surgery, an antibiotic-steroid combination ointment or solution (0.1% dexamethasone–0.3% tobramycin or equivalent) is applied to the operative eye. Small epithelial defects are treated with lubricating drops, and bandage contact lenses are used for large defects. The segment placement and incision closure should be observed using slit-lamp examination. The operative eye is protected with a clear shield, and the patient should be given appropriate postoperative instructions.[1,15]

Foreign body sensation or "scratchiness" is common during the immediate postoperative recovery period. Symptoms of infection include dull, aching pain or discomfort, with or without photophobia, any time in the postoperative period. During recovery, eyes may feel dry the first 2–3 months. Expect vision to fluctuate during the first month.[1,15]

ICRSs FOR KERATOCONUS AND AFTER LASIK

ICRSs have been used to treat patients with keratoconus. The results are very encouraging, especially in terms of decreasing astigmatism, increasing topographical abnormalities, and minimizing the risk of further progression of corneal ectasia. Similarly, ICRSs have been used as an adjunct to LASIK surgery.

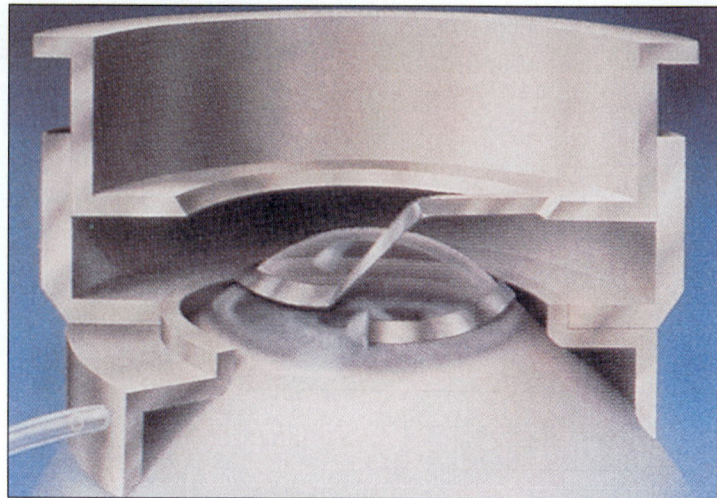

FIG. 25-6 ▌ Vacuum centering guide and stromal separator used to create the channel for the intrastromal corneal ring. (Reproduced with permission from Assil KK, Barrett AM, Fouraker BD, et al. One-year results of the intrastromal corneal ring in nonfunctional human eyes. Arch Ophthalmol. 1995;113:159–67.)

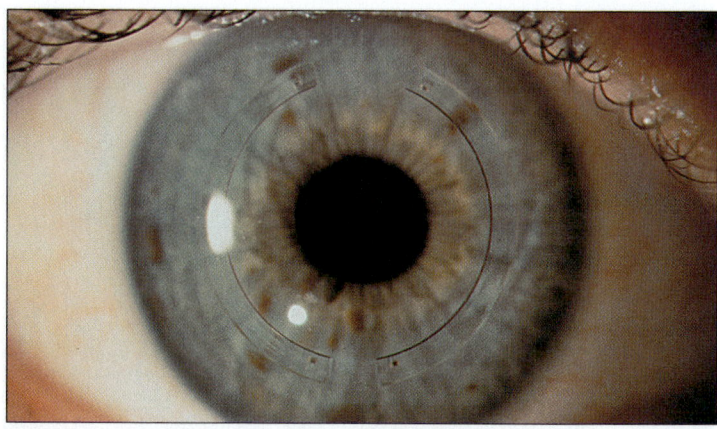

FIG. 25-7 ▌ Slit-lamp photograph of the intrastromal corneal ring segments in position in the patient's cornea. (Courtesy of Thomas Loarie.)

LASIK and ICRSs differ in several respects. LASIK is a more versatile technique that corrects low to moderately high levels of myopia (<10D) and myopic astigmatism (up to 5D).[16–18] In contrast, ICRSs are designed to treat only low levels of nearsightedness (up to 3D) without clinically significant astigmatism.[8,14] The dissimilarity between the underlying mechanisms responsible for the induced central corneal flattening suggests that the procedures could be additive. Using ICRSs as an adjunct to LASIK surgery carries several of the advantages of using ICRSs to treat keratoconus,[9] without further compromising corneal thickness and stability.

Eyes receiving both LASIK and ICRSs as sequential surgeries have been reported. We have implanted ICRSs in patients as a means of treating residual myopia 2 years after LASIK. Further excimer laser surgery might have been unsafe in these patients and may have increased the risk of keratoectasia.[19] Our first patient was a 38-year-old woman with a corneal thickness of 539μm who underwent LASIK on the right eye (OD) for a refractive error of −8.00 −0.50 × 75 (ablation depth 96μm). Three months postoperatively, the UCVA was 20/20− OD. Over the following year, however, regression occurred, with a resultant UCVA of 20/40 and a refractive error of −1.00 −0.75 × 18. Given the patient's low pachymetry value of 439μm and a theoretical flap thickness of 180μm, an ICRS procedure was offered as a means of treating the residual myopia. Three weeks after receiving 0.25mm ICRS OD, the patient's UCVA was 20/30 and her best spectacle-corrected visual acuity (BSCVA) was 20/20 with 11.75 −1.00 × 118. The sec-

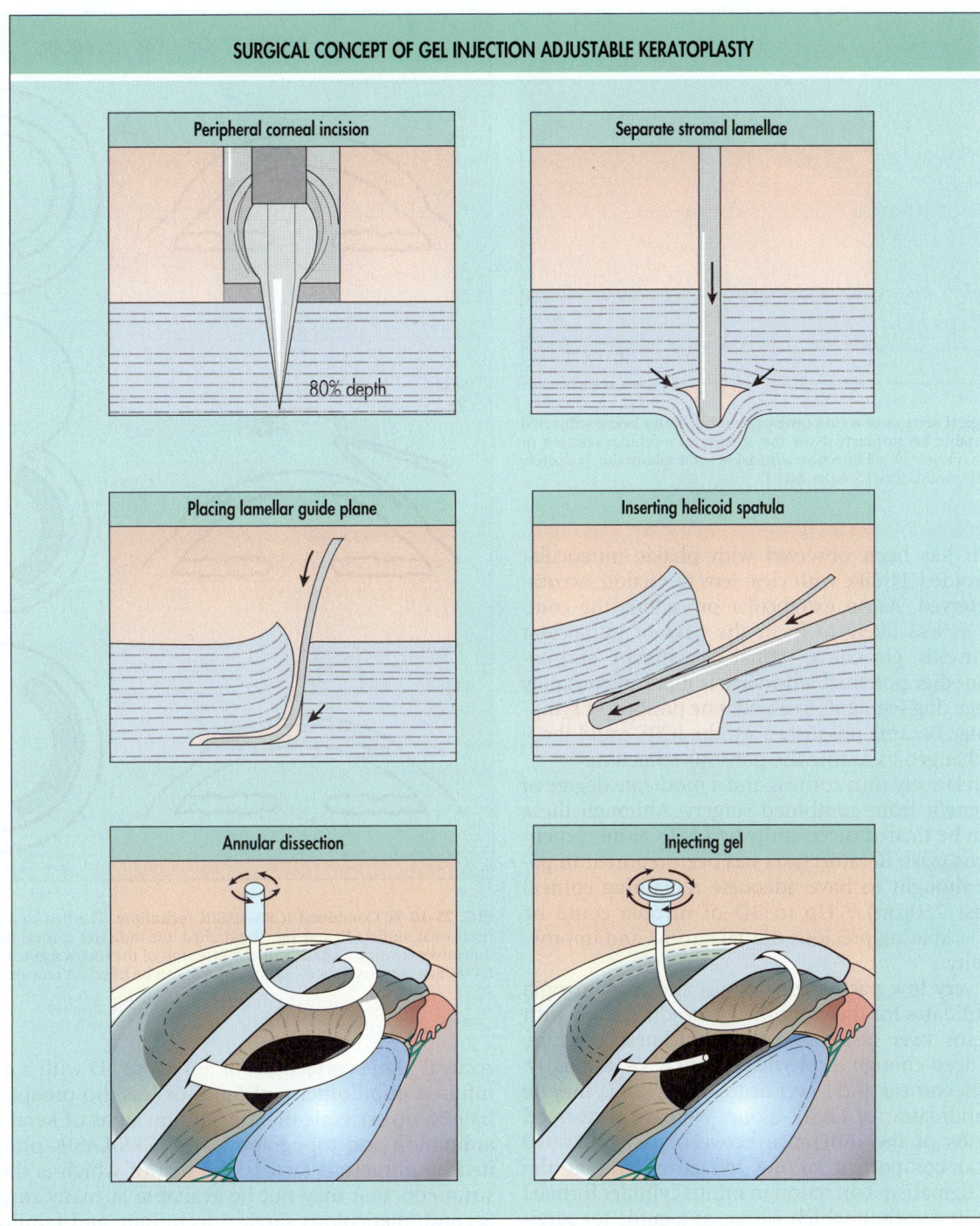

SURGICAL CONCEPT OF GEL INJECTION ADJUSTABLE KERATOPLASTY

Peripheral corneal incision

80% depth

Separate stromal lamellae

Placing lamellar guide plane

Inserting helicoid spatula

Annular dissection

Injecting gel

FIG. 25-8 ■ **Surgical concept of gel injection adjustable keratoplasty.** A 0.8mm peripheral corneal incision is made at a selected depth (50–80% of corneal thickness) with a diamond knife. The stromal lamellae are then separated with a blunt spatula, and the lamellar plane guide is placed. The helicoid spatula is inserted below the guide, and the annular dissection is performed. Last, the gel is injected. (Reproduced with permission from Simon G, Parel J-M, Lee W, Kervick GN. Gel injection adjustable keratoplasty. Graefes Arch Clin Exp Ophthalmol. 1991;229:418–24.)

ond patient was a 50-year-old woman who had undergone LASIK on the left eye (OS) for a refractive error of −6.75 −1.50 × 180. Several months after surgery, the patient regressed to −1.00 −1.50 × 180, with a BSCVA of 20/25+ and a UCVA of 20/150. The patient underwent relifting of the flap and a second laser ablation, which resulted in a UCVA of 20/20. One year later, regression resulted in a UCVA of 20/60 and a BSCVA of 20/20 with −0.75 −0.75 × 175. Orbscan revealed a central pachymetry of 467µm without signs of ectasia or irregularity. To prevent further corneal thinning, an ICRS procedure was offered as a means of treating the myopia. Six weeks after receiving 0.25mm ICRS OS, the patient's UCVA was 20/30− and her BSCVA was 20/20 with 11.50 −1.25 × 090.

Similar reports of sequential treatment have been published. Fleming and Lovisolo[20] reported a patient who received ICRS 10

months following LASIK that left a residual spherical equivalent (SE) of −3.375D. Four months after ICRS placement, the UCVA was 20/20. No flap complications occurred.

Eyes that received LASIK after ICRS have been reported only following explantation of the PMMA segments. Asbell et al.[21] described 10 patients who received LASIK following ICRS explantation. No complications were reported. Davis et al.[13] reported five patients who received LASIK following ICRS explantation for induced astigmatism and intraoperative complications. All patients experienced uneventful LASIK.

COMBINED LASIK AND ICRS

Combined LASIK and ICRS offers several theoretical advantages over other procedures used to correct high myopia. Early cataract

215

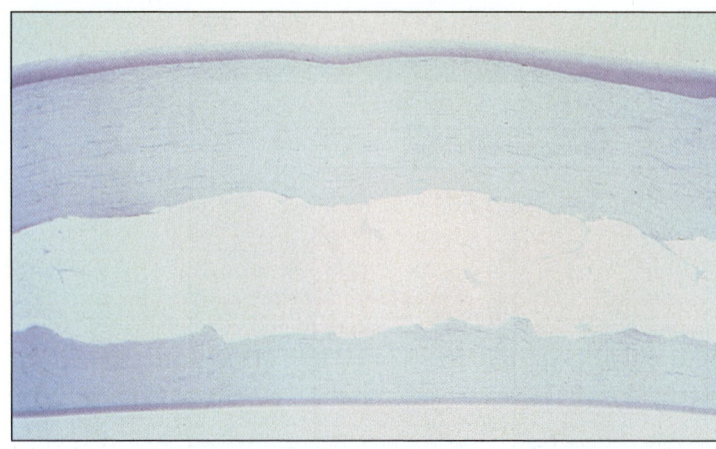

FIG. 25-9 ■ Histological section of a cat cornea 23 months after being subjected to gel injection adjustable keratoplasty. Note the absence of a cellular reaction or scarring in the tissue that lines the gel injection adjustable keratoplasty site. (Courtesy of Jean-Marie Parel, MD, and Gabriel Simon, MD.)

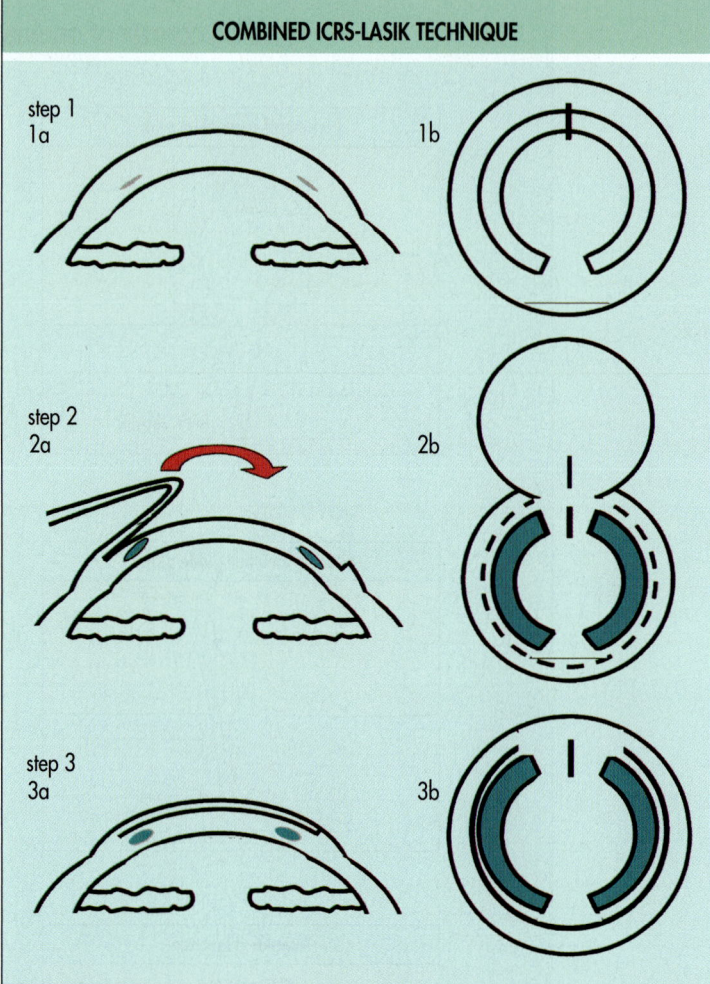

COMBINED ICRS-LASIK TECHNIQUE

step 1
1a
1b

step 2
2a
2b

step 3
3a
3b

FIG. 25-10 ■ Combined ICRS–LASIK technique. The first step to prepare the intrastromal tunnel (1a and 1b). The dashed line indicates corneal flattening (1a). Step 2 involves creating a LASIK flap and insertion of the Intacs segments (2a and 2b). The LASIK flap is repositioned (3a and 3b) and can be lifted for retreatment at a later time.

formation, which has been observed with phakic intraocular lenses, may be avoided. Unlike with clear lens extraction, accommodation is preserved. As an extraocular procedure, the combined technique is less likely to incur the risks of intraocular surgery such as uveitis, glaucoma, retinal detachment, and endophthalmitis. Another potential advantage is that surgeons may be able to exchange ring segments to ameliorate presbyopic symptoms. If this change became unsatisfactory, the ICRS could theoretically be re-exchanged to restore the previous refraction.[10,19]

Patients with relatively thin corneas and a moderate degree of myopia could benefit from combined surgery. Although these patients can often be treated successfully by LASIK alone, potential safety concerns exist. Keratoectasia has been reported in patients who were thought to have adequate remaining corneal thickness (at least 250μm).[22] Up to 3D of myopia could be treated with ICRSs, sparing precious central stroma and improving corneal stability.

Patients with very low pachymetry values and high myopia are not good candidates for the combined procedure. Even with the ICRS, concerns over residual corneal thickness preclude LASIK ablations deep enough to provide good UCVA. Similarly, patients with thick corneas and lower degrees of myopia may be more suitable candidates for LASIK alone. We have performed simple calculations of the difference between pachymetry/10 and the spherical component of the refractive error at the corneal plane (astigmatism correction in minus cylinder format) to generate the Δ10 constant, which we use as a guide for surgical options:

$$\Delta 10 = \frac{\text{pachymetry }(\mu m)}{10} -$$

spherical component of refractive error at the corneal plane

We consider performing LASIK without ICRS when Δ10 is greater than 44. When Δ10 is less than 42, we discourage keratorefractive surgery for fear of keratoectasia. We generally perform the combined ICRS-LASIK technique if preoperative calculations reveal a Δ10 value of 43 ± 1 (Fig. 25-10).

A problem associated with ICRS surgery is corneal flattening in the meridian of the ICRS incision (against-the-rule astigmatic shift). In our patients, induced astigmatism was also against the rule. For patients with high myopia undergoing ICRS-LASIK, we recommend performing 4–5D less of the LASIK ablation before placing the ICRS. This helps avoid a potential ICRS-induced overcorrection that could also result from a greater than expected flattening effect in the thinned stromal bed. One potential remedy for ICRS-induced astigmatism may be to incorporate any ICRS-induced refractive changes into a later LASIK retreatment.

Given the potential shortcomings of the combined procedure, we have narrowed our indications to myopic patients with

corneal plane corrections of −6 to −12D with a Δ10 of 43 ± 1, infrared pupillometry of 6mm or less, no preoperative glare or haloes, no systemic disease, and no signs of keratoconus on examination and topography. The ICRS-LASIK procedure is limited by numerous factors, the first of which is the need for instruments that may not be available at many surgical facilities. Second, meticulous surgical technique and familiarity with the procedures are important to prevent intraoperative complications such as anteriorly placed intrastromal channels that could preclude the performance of LASIK. Third, the ICRS component provides only an additional 3D of correction. This value could, theoretically, increase in a corneal bed made thinner by a corneal flap and deep LASIK ablation. Therefore, in high myopes, we recommend performing only 70–80% of the LASIK ablation at the initial surgical encounter. Last, astigmatism can be induced by the ICRS. Although this may be amenable to LASIK retreatment, the laser could induce astigmatism that becomes manifest upon ICRS removal or exchange.[19]

We believe that the combined procedure is not applicable to keratoconus patients, because LASIK corrections in such patients have led to ectasia.[22,23] Colin et al.[9] reported an increase in topographical regularity and decreased astigmatism after ICRS implantation in keratoconus patients. These patients, however, did not undergo lamellar surgery, which may cause corneal instability that is unaffected by the ICRS surgery. We therefore recommend that the combined procedure be avoided unless long-term results convincingly confirm the potential benefits.[19]

In summary, this combined technique is directed toward high and moderate myopes and may especially benefit those with relatively thin corneas. This combined procedure is relatively new, and its long-term results are still unknown.[19] Further studies are necessary to establish the efficacy, stability, and safety of ICRS-LASIK.

REFERENCES

1. Colin J, Cochener B. Intracorneal implants. In: Azar DT, ed. Intraocular lenses in cataract and refractive surgery. Philadelphia: WB Saunders; 2001:273–8.
2. Assil KK, Barrett AM, Fouraker BD, et al. One-year results of the intrastromal corneal ring in nonfunctional human eyes. Arch Ophthalmol. 1995;113:159–67.
3. Burris TE, Ayer CT, Evensen DA, et al. Effects of intrastromal corneal ring size and thickness on corneal flattening in human eyes. Refract Corneal Surg. 1991;7: 46–50.
4. Cochener B, Le Floch G, Colin J. Les anneaux intracorneens pour la correction des faibles myopies. J Fr Ophtalmol. 1998;21:191–208.
5. Fleming JF, Reynolds AE, Kilmer L, et al. The intrastromal corneal ring: two cases in rabbits. J Refract Surg. 1987;3:227–32.
6. Fleming JF, Wan WL, Schanzlin DJ. The theory of corneal curvature change with the intrastromal corneal ring. CLAO J. 1989;15:146–50.
7. Nosé W, Neves RA, Burris TE, et al. Intrastromal corneal ring: 12-month sighted myopic eyes. J Refract Surg. 1996;12:20–8.
8. Schanzlin DJ, Asbell PA, Burris TE, et al. The intrastromal corneal ring segments: phase II results for the correction of myopia. Ophthalmology. 1997;104:1067–78.
9. Colin J, Cochener B, Savary G, Malet F. Correcting keratoconus with intracorneal rings. J Cataract Refract Surg. 2000;26:1117–22.
10. Primack JD, Azar DT. A three-step approach combining LASIK and ICRS for correction of high myopia. Presented at the annual meeting of the American Society of Cataract and Refractive Surgery, Philadelphia, 2002.
11. Friedman NJ, Husain SE, Kohnen T, Koch DD. Investigational refractive procedures. In: Yanoff M, Duker JS, eds. Ophthalmology, 1st ed. London: Mosby; 1999:3.7.4–6.
12. Durrie D, Asbell PA, Burris TE. Reversible refractive effect of ICR. Presented at the annual meeting of the American Society of Cataract and Refractive Surgery, Seattle, 1996.
13. Davis EA, Hardten DR, Lindstrom RL. Laser in situ keratomileusis after intracorneal rings: report of 5 cases. J Cataract Refract Surg. 2000;26:1733–41.
14. Twa MD, Karpecki PM, King BJ, et al. One-year results from the phase III investigation of the KeraVision Intacs. J Am Optom Assoc. 1999;70:515–24.
15. Linebarger EJ, Song D, Ruckhofer J, Schanzlin DJ. Intacs: the intrastromal corneal ring. Int Ophthalmol Clin. 2000;40(3):199–208.
16. Lindstrom RL, Hardten DR, Chu YR. Laser in situ keratomileusis (LASIK) for the treatment of low, moderate, and high myopia. Trans Am Ophthalmol Soc. 1997;95:285–306.
17. Salah T, Waring GO III, El Maghraby A, et al. Excimer laser in situ keratomileusis under a corneal flap for myopia of 2 to 20 diopters. Am J Ophthalmol. 1996;121: 143–55.
18. Farah SG, Azar DT, Gurdal C, Wong J. Laser in situ keratomileusis: literature review of a developing technique. J Cataract Refract Surg. 1998;24:989–1006.
19. Primack J, Azar DT. A three-step procedure combining LASIK and ICRS. J Cataract Refract Surg. 2003 (in press).
20. Fleming JF, Lovisolo CF. Intrastromal corneal ring segments in a patient with previous laser in situ keratomileusis. J Refract Surg. 2000;16:365–7.
21. Asbell PA, Uçakhan ÖÖ, Durrie DS, Lindstrom RL. Adjustability of refractive effect for corneal ring segments. J Refract Surg. 1999;15:627–31.
22. Amoils SP, Deist MB, Gous P, Amoils PM. Iatrogenic keratectasia after laser in situ keratomileusis for less than −4.0 to −7.0 diopters of myopia. J Cataract Refract Surg. 2000;26:967–77.
23. McLeod SD, Kisla TA, Caro NC, McMahon TT. Iatrogenic keratoconus: corneal ectasia following laser in situ keratomileusis for myopia. Arch Ophthalmol. 2000;118:282–4.

CHAPTER

26 Phakic Intraocular Lenses

DIMITRI T. AZAR • SONIA H. YOO • FRANÇOIS MALECAZE • GEORGE BAIKOFF
• JEAN-LOUIS ARNÈ • THANH HOANG-XUAN

DEFINITION
• Phakic intraocular lenses (IOLs) are prosthetic devices introduced in the anterior or posterior chamber of phakic patients to correct the refractive error.

KEY FEATURES
• Three kinds of phakic IOLs have been tested: angle-supported anterior chamber IOLs, iris-fixated IOLs, and posterior chamber IOLs.
• The predictability and safety of these lenses are high.
• Their safety has not been established fully.

ASSOCIATED FEATURES
• Early models of AC and iris-supported phakic IOL were made of polymethyl methacrylate (PMMA). Newer lenses are foldable, as are PC phakic IOLs.
• Complications include glaucomas, iris atrophy, endothelial cell loss, and cataract formation.

INTRODUCTION

Treatment options for the surgical correction of mild to moderate degrees of myopia, astigmatism, and hyperopia include excimer laser photorefractive keratectomy (PRK) and laser *in situ* keratomileusis (LASIK). For cases of high myopia and hyperopia, however, these options are limited by a decreased predictability of postoperative results. For this reason, there has been a growing interest in the use of phakic intraocular lenses (IOLs) to correct refractive errors.[1] Phakic IOL implantation has the advantage of preserving the architecture of the cornea, arguably the healthiest part of a highly myopic eye; additionally, it may provide more predictable refractive results than surgical techniques that manipulate the corneal curvature.[1]

HISTORY OF PHAKIC LENSES

In the second half of the nineteenth century, the fundamentals of refractive surgery were introduced, accompanied by many of the discussions and controversies that still exist in the field today. Clear lens extraction for the correction of myopia was a concept introduced in the early 1800s, and the technique became increasingly popular from 1850 to 1900.[2] It was not until the end of the nineteenth century, however, that complications of this operation (e.g., retinal detachment and choroidal hemorrhages) began to be reported, and the technique largely fell out of favor.[1]

The 1950s saw the emergence of the idea of correcting myopia by inserting a concave lens into the phakic eye. At this time, Strampelli,[3] Barraquer,[4] and Choyce[5] experimented with anterior chamber angle-fixed lenses, which were eventually abandoned

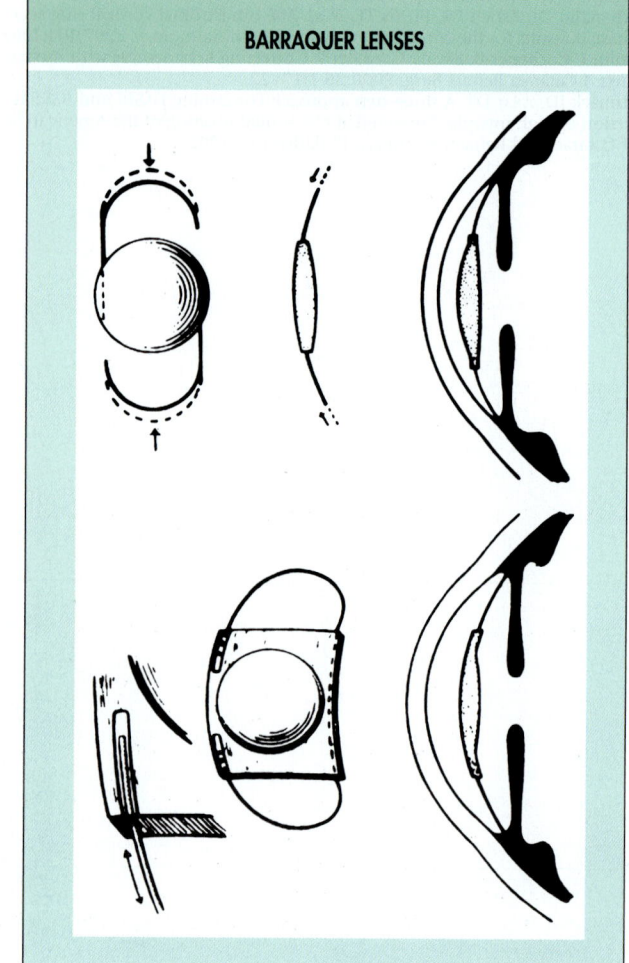

BARRAQUER LENSES

FIG. 26-1 ▌ Barraquer lenses.

owing to complications of corneal edema and chronic iritis (Fig. 26-1). In 1988, Baikoff presented his version of an anterior chamber angle-fixed IOL.[6] The Baikoff IOL is a single-piece, biconcave anterior chamber lens based on a multiflex Kelman anterior chamber IOL. It is made of polymethyl methacrylate (PMMA) containing an ultraviolet blocker. The lens is angulated posteriorly at 20°, and the optic is 5mm in diameter (Fig. 26-2). Complications of this lens included pupil block, endothelial cell loss, haloes and glare, iritis, implant rotation, retinal detachment, and iris retraction with pupillary ovalization.

Around the same time that the Baikoff lens was being developed, Worst and Fechner developed a biconcave anterior chamber lens fixed to the front of the iris,[7] based on experience with Worst's iris-claw lens for aphakic eyes (Fig. 26-3).[8] Complications with this style of lens included iritis, cystic wounds, glaucoma, difficulty with fixation of the IOL, retinal detachment, cataract forma-

BAIKOFF PHAKIC INTRAOCULAR LENSES

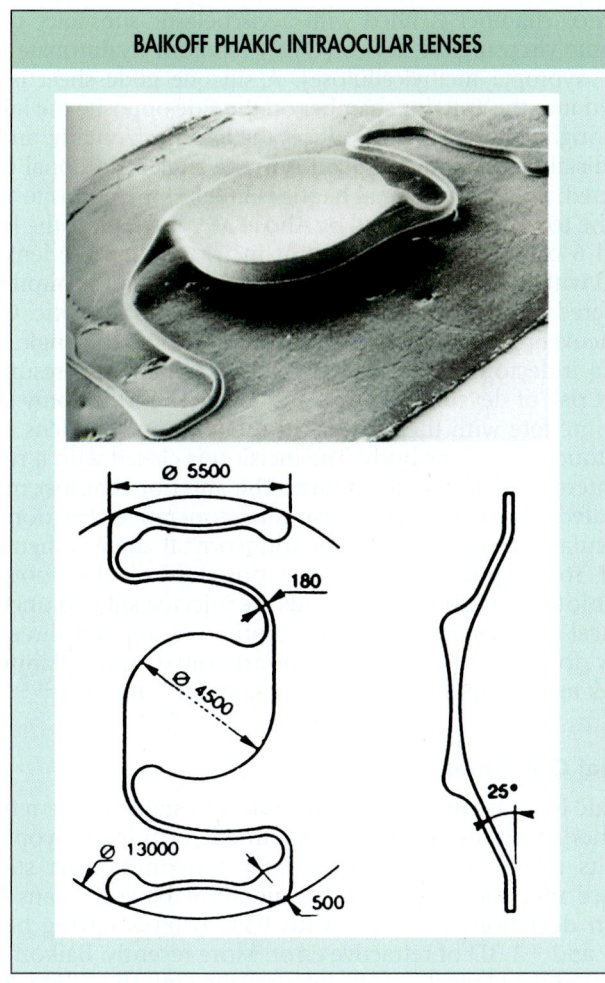

FIG. 26-2 ■ Baikoff Z-shaped anterior chamber phakic intraocular lenses.

WORST IRIS-CLAW LENS

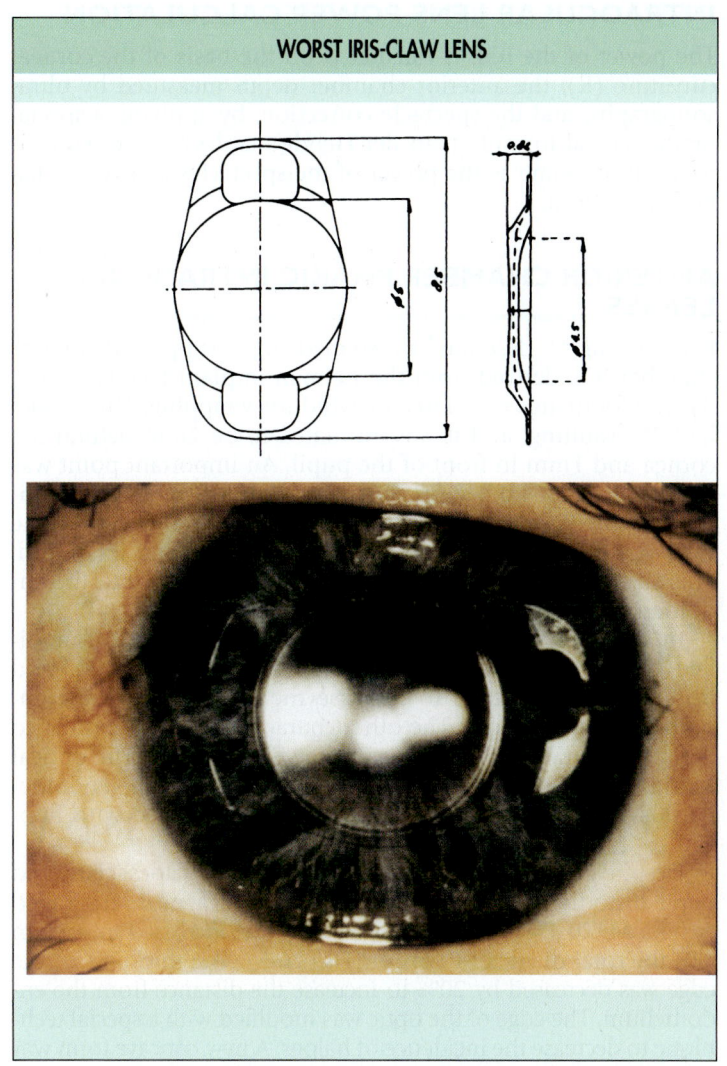

FIG. 26-3 ■ Worst iris-claw lens.

OPHTEC WORST (ARTISAN) PHAKIC INTRAOCULAR LENS

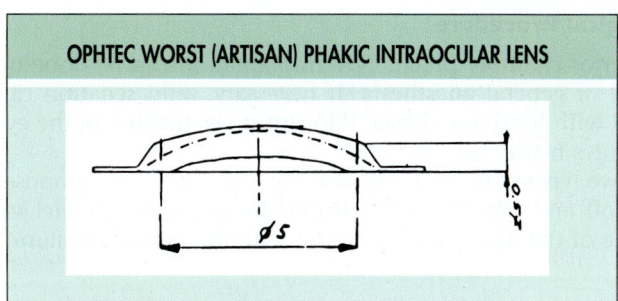

FIG. 26-4 ■ Ophtec Worst (ARTISAN) phakic intraocular lens of −10.00D. This style has been in use since 1992.

tion, and corneal decompensation from endothelial cell loss.[9] To minimize the possibility of IOL-cornea contact, in 1991 the biconcave design was changed to a convex-concave model with a lower shoulder and a thinner periphery (Fig. 26-4).

In the mid-1980s, the implantation of posterior chamber IOLs in phakic eyes was reported by Fyodorov *et al.*[10] In 1987, the Moscow Research Institute of Eye Microsurgery reported favorably on posterior chamber IOL implantation in phakic eyes to correct high myopia.[10] The original lens design was a collar-button type, with the optic located in the anterior chamber and the haptics behind the iris plane. Later, Chiron-Adatomed modified this design to produce a silicone elastomer posterior chamber lens. The concave posterior optic curvature, which closely approximates the anterior crystalline lens curvature, has a radius of 9.9mm. The anterior curvature is also concave. The optic diameter is 5.5mm, and the haptic thickness is 0.18mm. This lens design has been reported to have a high incidence of cataract formation after implantation.[11]

In 1993, Zaldivar, Davidorf, and Oscherow began implanting a plate posterior chamber phakic IOL (Staar Surgical Implantable Contact Lens [ICL]).[12] This lens design was modified from the one Fyodorov originated in 1986, using a one-piece silicone collar-button phakic IOL with a 500–600nm Teflon coat. Incorporation of a porcine collagen–HEMA copolymer into the lens material has improved the lens's biocompatibility. Phase I trials by the Food and Drug Administration were approved in February 1997 for the treatment of hyperopia with this posterior chamber phakic IOL.[13]

INDICATIONS AND CONTRAINDICATIONS

Patients enrolled in the above-mentioned studies had preoperative spherical equivalents (SEs) ranging from −5.00 to

−31.75D.[6,9,12–15] The Staar posterior chamber phakic IOL was also implanted for hyperopic patients with SEs ranging from +2.50 to +10.875D.[21] Inclusion criteria varied slightly from study to study, but the basic tenets were similar; namely, that the endothelial cell count was normal (at least 2500 cells/mm²) and the anterior chamber depth was adequate (≥3mm). Exclusion criteria included the presence of the following: inflammation of the anterior or posterior segment, chronic keratitis, corneal dystrophy, iris atrophy or rubeosis, aniridia, cataracts, vitreous pathology, retinal disease, microphthalmos, nanophthalmos, glaucoma, or previous intraocular surgery. For patients who received the posterior chamber phakic IOL, peripheral laser iridotomies were performed at least 4 days before surgery to decrease the incidence of postoperative pupillary block.

INTRAOCULAR LENS POWER CALCULATION

The power of the IOL is calculated on the basis of the corneal curvature (K), the anterior chamber depth measured by ultrasonography, and the spectacle correction, by applying a special mathematical formula (van der Heijde's tables).[16,17] Roughly, it is about the same as the power of the spectacles at a vertex distance of 12mm.

ANTERIOR CHAMBER PHAKIC INTRAOCULAR LENSES

Baikoff et al.[18,19] described a Z-shaped, angle-supported anterior chamber IOL derived from the Kelman implant (see Fig. 26-2, A). The footplates were large to avoid iris wrapping. This model had 25° vaulting, and it was estimated to be 2mm behind the cornea and 1mm in front of the pupil. An important point was to supply a wide range of power between −8 and −30D and diameters of 12, 12.5, 13, and 13.5mm to better fit the angle.[20] The total optic diameter was 4.5mm, and the real one was 4mm. This size was supposed to provide sufficient distance to the endothelium, but endothelial damage did occur.

In an attempt to minimize the complications, Baikoff modified his original design and lowered the vaulting to 20° and thinned the optic edge to increase the distance from the endothelium by 0.6mm.[21] The other characteristics were similar to the first-generation Baikoff lenses (see Fig. 26-2, B). The optical results were as good as with the earlier lenses, and the endothelial loss decreased.[22] Later, the surface was modified with fluorine to improve biocompatibility.[23,24]

Despite good anatomical and optical results, haloes, glare, and pupil distortion prompted Baikoff to design a new lens called NuVita MA20.[22] The real optic diameter was increased to 4.5mm and the total diameter to 5mm (Fig. 26-5). The thickness of the edge was decreased by 20% to increase the distance from the endothelium. The edge of the optic was modified with a special technique to decrease the incidence of haloes. A new concave form was given to the posterior surface to increase the distance from the natural lens. The anterior chamber phakic IOL can have a power between −7 and −20D and a length of 12, 12.5, or 13mm.

Surgical Procedure

Anterior chamber phakic IOL implantation can be done under local or general anesthesia. If necessary, mild sedation can be used with local anesthesia. Pilocarpine is instilled in the eye 30 minutes before surgery.[20,23,24]

Two types of incision can be done. The classic one, proposed by Baikoff and Joly,[25] is done temporally or nasally parallel to the plane of the iris, avoiding contact with the eyelid speculum. The anterior chamber is filled with a viscoelastic substance or ophthalmic viscosurgical device (OVD) (sodium hyaluronate or 2% hydroxypropyl methylcellulose). A silicone glide sheet is introduced into the anterior chamber on the side opposite the incision. The original procedure introduces the lens horizontally, and once the distal haptic of the implant is in the angle, additional OVD is injected; then the proximal haptic is fitted in the opposite angle.[19]

The technique proposed by Alio et al.[23] introduces the lens toward 6 o'clock from the superior incision. Then the lens is rotated with a lens dialer to the meridian in which the pupil is best centered in relation to the anterior chamber IOL optic. Careful maneuvers prevent damage to the structures of the angle.[19]

An iridectomy is helpful, especially for patients presumed to be at risk of developing pupillary block. The iridectomy should not interfere with the stability of the lens, and the lens should not touch the ciliary body. The incision is closed with a running or interrupted 10-0 nylon suture. The anterior chamber must be irrigated to remove OVD to avoid postoperative elevation of intraocular pressure (IOP).[19] The iridocorneal angle is then examined for a possible improper position of the footplates. Antibiotic or antibiotic-corticoids are injected subconjunctivally. Topical corticosteroids and antibiotics are applied three times daily for 4–6 weeks. Topical nonsteroidal anti-inflammatory drugs may be applied three times daily for 3 months.[22,23]

Visual Outcomes

Phakic IOLs are the most predictable and stable of the refractive methods for preserving the crystalline lens in high myopia. The results reflect an excellent accuracy.[19] A multicenter study in France reported that the first-generation Baikoff[21] lens had a mean deviation of −0.2D, with 95% of eyes having between −1.3 and +1.3D of refractive error. More recently, Baikoff et al.[22] reported new French multicenter results with the ZB5M. The SE averaged approximately −1D over 3 years, and no eye was overcorrected by more than +1D. Refraction stability was 87–91% within ±2D at 2 years, and it was 80% at 3 years. In a small subset, the average change in SE between 6 months and 3 years was −0.37D. The mean error in refractive correction, calculated as the difference between achieved and intended correction, was less than 1D over the entire study.[19]

The stability of this method is conditional on the stability of the myopia, which is one of the requirements for this surgery. Myopia can progress in some cases, sometimes severely,[22] but the changes in refraction due to the evolution of the myopia are usually slow.

Visual acuity recovery is rapid; the preoperative level is attained by the second postoperative day. Visual acuity in myopic eyes corrected with phakic IOLs increases by one Snellen line or more due to the retinal magnification induced by the IOL.[19]

The French multicenter study reported intermediate results with the ZB5M at 3 years of a 5-year trial.[22] Distance uncorrected visual acuity (UCVA) averaged 0.048 at baseline, improved to 0.5–0.52 over the first 2 years, and then declined to 0.45 at 3 years. Postoperative UCVA scores were 0.5 or greater in 37.8–57.1%, 0.8 or greater in 13.5–21.5%, and 1 or greater in 3.7–7.2%; the lowest percentages for UCVA were recorded at the 3-year follow-up examination for scores of 0.5 and 0.8 but not for 1. Distance best corrected visual acuity (BCVA) improved from 0.54 to 0.69 at the 3-year examination; only 2.1–8.3% of eyes lost two Snellen lines, and one eye (2.8%) lost three lines.

Complications

ELEVATION OF INTRAOCULAR PRESSURE. Elevation of IOP usually occurs during the early postoperative period and is transient. There are several causes. The most frequent, with a reported incidence of 2.4–29%,[18,20,22,23,26–29] is a result of postoperative steroid application in patients who may be sensitive to the medication. Inadequately removed OVD is an avoidable cause

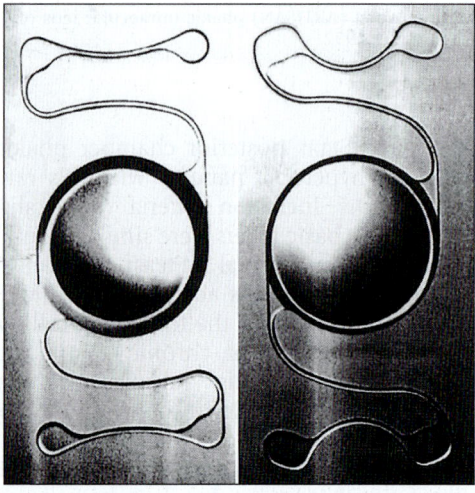

FIG. 26-5 ▪ Baikoff NuVita MA20.

of elevated IOP; it can be prevented with good cleaning of the anterior chamber at the end of surgery.

Only a few cases of pupillary block secondary to this surgery have been noted.[22] A thorough evaluation of the anterior chamber in every patient and an iridectomy in patients suspected to be at risk can be helpful. If pupillary block occurs, a peripheral iridotomy should be performed.

UVEITIS. Transient acute uveitis is usually secondary to iris trauma during surgery. The incidence of early postoperative uveitis is 2–13.3%[18,20,27–29] with first-generation Baikoff lenses and 2.3–4.56%[22,23] with the ZB5M. This complication is defined as an evident increase in the level of cell and flare counts above normal baseline levels observed by slit lamp. The inflammation can be so severe as to cause sterile hypopyon or lens explantation.[22,23] An oversized lens also has been reported as a cause of uveitis.[20]

Patients usually respond quickly to topical steroid treatment, with no delayed sequelae.[20,22,23] However, the presence of a phakic IOL in the anterior chamber can alter blood-aqueous barrier (BAB) permeability, as tested with the laser flare cell meter[30,31] and fluorophotometry.[32] These changes can continue for several years as a consequence of the IOL in the anterior chamber. The chronic inflammation may induce other complications such as glaucoma, cataract, or anterior synechiae.[31]

CATARACT. Care must be taken to avoid lens trauma during surgery. The miotics and OVD help maintain the distance from the lens, but the risk of cataract development remains after surgery. The phakic IOL is a foreign body that modifies not only the BAB but also the transmittance of the lens.[33] Decreased lens transmittance could be the result of surgery or of changes in BAB permeability. These changes cause metabolic disturbances that could decrease transmittance and speed cataract development.[32]

In short-term follow-up, the first-generation Baikoff lenses had a very low rate of cataract formation, 0–0.7%.[18,20,27–29] Reducing the vaulting in the ZB5M did not cause a higher incidence of cataract in the short term, but a long-term study by Alio et al.[23] reported an incidence of 4%. Cataract extraction with a posterior chamber IOL is often successful.[19]

PUPILLARY DISTORTION. Pupil ovalization is one of the most prevalent complications, with a reported incidence of 4–42%.[18,20,27–29,33] This wide range can be due to the subjective method used to quantify whether the deformation is significant. Alio et al.[23] defined significant pupil ovalization as pupil deviation in the meridian of the placement of the phakic IOL haptic that reaches the edge of the optic in at least one point. They found pupil ovalization in 6.08% of cases and lesser degrees of ovalization in 10.3%. The cause of pupillary distortion was thought to be an oversized lens and the force created by the haptics, but the possibility of a retractable fibrous membrane has also been proposed. The axis of the deviation usually coincides with the major axis of the lens.[23,34]

Another complication usually associated with pupil ovalization is iris atrophy; the reported incidence is 0–4.8%.[16,23] The atrophy usually occurs in the iris sector affected by ovalization. This atrophy can be severe and can lead to total sector iris atrophy.

HALOES AND GLARE. These symptoms can be very disturbing to the patient. The incidence has a clear relationship to the diameter of the pupil and of the optic zone of the phakic IOL. In darkness, with a mid-dilated pupil, the optical zone can be smaller than the pupil,[26] and this difference creates haloes. Pilocarpine 1% can be prescribed in patients who cannot tolerate the haloes.[16]

ENDOTHELIAL DAMAGE. The history of endothelial cell loss is linked to the history of lens design. With the continuous improvement in design and surgical technique since the first generation of lenses, there is now only minor cell loss, and this trend will probably continue. Nevertheless, we have to assume that there is some level of endothelial damage during any surgery in which an eye is opened. This loss was estimated as 300 cells/mm² by Perez-Santonja et al.[35] with the ZB5M phakic IOL. However, a permanent implant in the anterior chamber is

a continuous risk for progressive endothelial loss with cell abnormalities and marked pleomorphism.[28]

The largest studies were performed with the Baikoff lenses. The first generation of these lenses caused a large cell loss. The vaulting of 25° made the distance between the phakic IOL and the endothelium very narrow, and acellular zones corresponding to endothelial defects were probably due to contact between the cornea and IOL.[28,36] The mean loss with these lenses in the first year was 9–19%.[27,28,36–38] Bour et al.[36] reported that the peripheral endothelial density was slightly lower than the central density, owing to a smaller distance between the cornea and the phakic IOL.

The problems with excessive vaulting were minimized with the ZB5M (angle of 20°). The cumulative endothelial cell loss in the central cornea was 4.5%, 5.6%, and 5.5% and in the peripheral cornea was 4.2%, 4.4%, and 3.9% during the first, second, and third years, respectively.[22]

Alio et al.[23] reported 7 years of data with similar results. They did not report the difference between the peripheral and central cornea, but the cumulative endothelial cell loss was 5.53%, 6.83%, 7.5%, 7.78%, 8.33%, 8.7%, and 9.26% for each year of follow-up. The authors expressed concern about implanting patients at a young age and the long-term relative risks they might face. According to the data, it might be 20–30 years before reaching the lower limit of endothelial cell count (1500 cells/mm²), at which point the eye may have a decreased ability to sustain other types of surgery, including cataract extraction. The new lens ZSAL-4 was implanted in a small number of cases. The follow-up in these patients was only 2 years, but no differences were found between the ZSAL-4 and the ZB5M. No data are available for the NuVita MA20.

RETINAL DETACHMENT. Retinal detachment (RD) is a potential hazard of the phakic IOL. The reported incidence is very low, but Ruiz-Moreno et al.[39] reported a rate of 4.8% in a large study with ZB5M lenses. The incidence was significantly higher, 14.28%, in patients who had been treated before surgery with laser for predisposing lesions in the retina, versus only 3.94% in the nontreated group. However, the lesions that caused the RD were unrelated to the treated area. The incidence of RD in patients with predisposing lesions previously treated with laser confirmed the doubtful efficacy of such prophylactic treatment in these patients. However, RD can appear in a zone that was previously treated.[22] It is very difficult to say whether this incidence is induced by the phakic IOL or the myopia, because the incidence of RD in myopic patients is higher than that in the emmetropic population.[39] The mean time to develop RD was 17.4 months (range, 1–44 months).

These RDs were treated with classic procedures. The surgery was more difficult owing to poor visualization through the phakic IOL. In seven of the eight cases of Ruiz-Moreno et al.,[39] the surgery was successful, and the visual acuities changed from 0.4 before the RD to 0.27. Obviously, with the scleral buckle, new myopia was induced, with a mean of 1.7D. In these seven cases, it was not necessary to remove the lens to do the procedure. In one case, a proliferative vitreoretinopathy developed after RD recurrence. The lens had to be removed, and silicone oil was injected. Visual acuity fell to light perception, despite reattachment of the retina.

OTHER COMPLICATIONS. A small number of eyes have been reported with other complications of phakic IOLs, such as corneal edema,[22] expulsive choroidal hemorrhage,[21] flat anterior chamber,[18] and endophthalmitis.[40] Wound dehiscence, Urretz-Zavalia syndrome, and acute ischemic optic neuropathy have been reported as complications with the Fechner-Worst lenses, but they can also occur with angle-fitted lenses.[24,41]

IRIS-FIXATED PHAKIC INTRAOCULAR LENSES

The first iris-fixated lenses were sutured to the iris stroma with a Perlon stitch or a stainless steel suture. The claw fixation method rendered iris stitching unnecessary. Various lens designs with midperipheral fixation by a claw mechanism were tested before 1978, when Worst introduced his final conceptual model of the iris-claw lens for secondary lens implantation or as a standby lens in cases of posterior capsule rupture. Because of the good tolerance and refractive results, the iris-claw lens was used as a primary implant after intracapsular and extracapsular cataract extraction (about 12,000 implantations in the Netherlands up to 1990).[42,43] In 1986, the concept of the claw lens was applied to correct myopia in phakic patients. Initially, the iris-claw phakic IOL for myopia was biconcave (Worst-Fechner biconcave lens). The iris-claw lens is fixated to the anterior iris surface by enclavation of a fold of iris tissue into the two diametrically opposed "claws" of the lens. The fixation sites are located in the midperiphery of the iris, which is virtually immobile during pupillary movements.

In 1991, this lens was modified into a convex-concave design to increase the distance between the IOL and the corneal endothelium. Suppression of the prominent optical rim has also allowed a reduction in the prismatic effect, which may be responsible for haloes or glare. Initially called the Worst Myopia Claw Lens, the iris-claw phakic IOL is presently manufactured by Ophtec (Groningen, Netherlands) under the trade name ARTISAN Myopia Lens. The vaulted design (0.5mm) of the posterior face of the IOL ensures optimal space in front of the natural lens (about 0.8mm) and prevents aqueous flow blockage. It also accounts for the forward displacement of the human lens during accommodation, which is about 0.6mm maximum.[44]

The ARTISAN Myopia Lens has two different diameters for the optical part: 5.0 and 6.0mm for the lenses, with a power range of −3.0 to −23.5D and −3.0 to −15.5D, respectively (in 0.5D steps). The thickness of the IOL in the optical axis is 0.2mm, and the total height is about 1mm. It is a one-piece ultraviolet light–absorbing Perpex-CQ (polymethyl methacrylate) compression molded lens with an overall diameter of 8.5mm, a width of 5.0 or 6.0mm, and a total height of 0.9mm. The weight is 10mg in air (15.0D lens).[45]

In 1997, an iris-claw lens specially designed for the correction of aphakia was introduced. Hyperopic iris-claw lenses are also available (5mm diameter, power range +1.0 to +12.0D).[45]

Surgical Procedure

Preoperative application of topical pilocarpine results in miosis. Miosis is mandatory, as it forms a protection shield for the natural lens during the insertion and fixation of the iris-claw lens. A constricted pupil also facilitates proper centration of the lens. Although there is theoretically a very low risk of pupil block glaucoma (because the vaulted configuration of the ARTISAN Myopia Lens ensures a normal aqueous outflow), a peripheral iridectomy during surgery or an argon or yttrium-aluminum-garnet (YAG) laser iridotomy before surgery, particularly when a tunnel incision is performed, is recommended. Two marks can be made on the iris at 3 and 9 o'clock, using an argon laser, to facilitate proper IOL centration during surgery.[45]

Various incision techniques (e.g., corneal, scleral tunnel incision) can be used. The lens is usually implanted vertically, then rotated and centered in front of the pupil with the haptics at 3 and 9 o'clock (Fig. 26-6). Depending on the diameter of the ARTISAN Myopia Lens used—5.0mm or 6.0mm—the incision should be at least 5.2mm or 6.2mm, respectively, to avoid difficulties with IOL insertion.

Two types of puncture incisions can be used, depending on the entrapment technique of the iris: two small incisions of at least 1.5mm at 3 and 9 o'clock, when iris entrapment forceps are used, or two small incisions of at least 1.1mm at 10 and 2 o'clock, when iris entrapment needles are used (Fig. 26-7).

The anterior chamber is filled to capacity with the OVD material. It is mandatory to use high-viscosity sodium hyaluronate to maintain working space in the anterior chamber. Materials of lower viscosity (e.g., methylcellulose, hydroxypropyl methylcel-

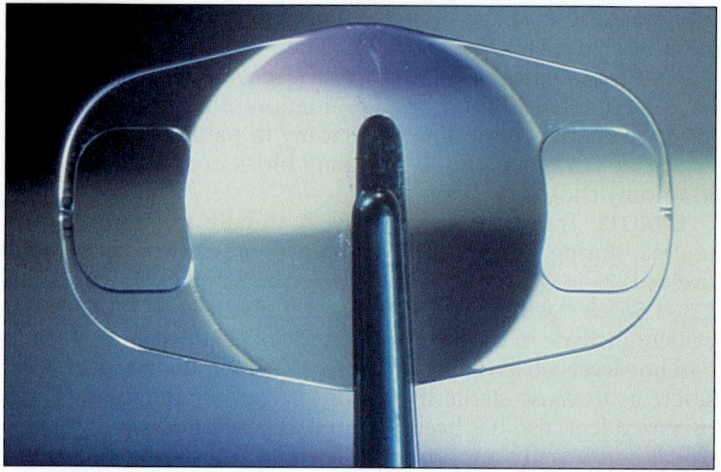

FIG. 26-6 ■ Worst-Fechner iris-claw lens. (Courtesy of Mrs. Anneke Worst.)

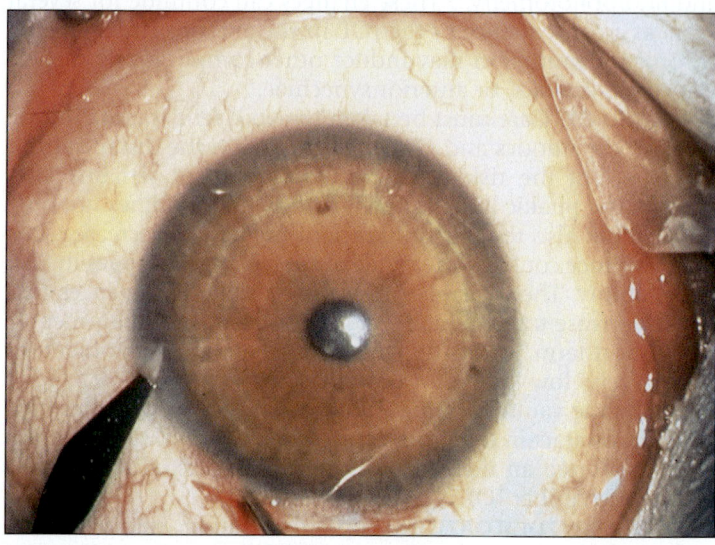

FIG. 26-7 ■ Corneal punctures are made to allow the iris entrapment needle or forceps to be passed. (From Hoang-Xuan T, Malecaze F. Iris-fixated phakic IOLs. In: Azar DT, ed. Intraocular lenses in cataract and refractive surgery. Philadelphia: WB Saunders; 2001:257–65.)

lulose) should be avoided. The OVD is injected through one of the puncture incisions to create a deep anterior chamber. If additional OVD material needs to be injected during surgery, care should be taken not to let it slip under the IOL. It should be used as a stabilizing agent that presses the implant onto the iris surface.[45]

Before entrapment of the haptics, OVD material is injected on top of the implant to protect the endothelium. The ARTISAN entrapment forceps and needles, which are specially designed for this procedure, should be used.

The IOL is introduced with the ARTISAN fixation forceps into the anterior chamber in a vertical position. This is necessary because of the size of the incision and because the claws otherwise tend to interfere with the insertion (Fig. 26-8). Then the IOL is rotated to the horizontal position, ready for fixation.

Pupillary miosis should be guaranteed during the insertion and fixation procedure. Use of an intraocular miotic facilitates proper centration of the IOL and reduces the risk of lens touch.

Centration and fixation of the IOL are probably the most critical steps of the procedure, and their accuracy influences the postoperative results. Centration of the IOL involves determining the x- and y-axes on the iris surface and defining the two fixation spots. The pupil is used as a reference for centration. Correct axial centration of the operating microscope prevents postoperative parallactic errors. These errors are likely to occur when the eye fails to remain in a central position.[45]

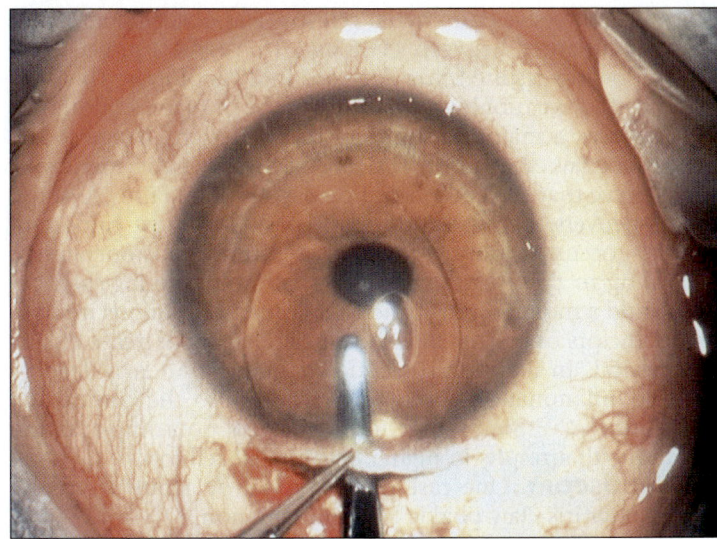

FIG. 26-8 ▮ The intraocular lens is introduced into the anterior chamber in a vertical position. (From Hoang-Xuan T, Malecaze F. Iris-fixated phakic IOLs. In: Azar DT, ed. Intraocular lenses in cataract and refractive surgery. Philadelphia: WB Saunders; 2001:257–65.)

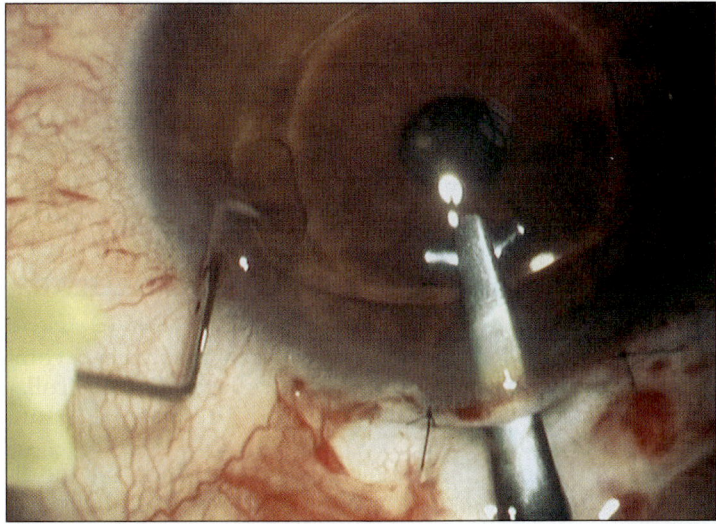

FIG. 26-9 ▮ Blunt ARTISAN iris entrapment needles can also be used to create a fold of midperipheral iris tissue through vertical movement of the needle. (From Hoang-Xuan T, Malecaze F. Iris-fixated phakic IOLs. In: Azar DT, ed. Intraocular lenses in cataract and refractive surgery. Philadelphia: WB Saunders; 2001:257–65.)

The enclavation spots also can be determined preoperatively by making two marks on the iris surface with the argon laser. Fixation is performed by gently creating an iris fold under the claw and then entrapping the iris fold in the claw. One should avoid pulling upward on the iris; rather, one should press the claw down onto the iris fold. Two specially designed instruments can be used: (1) ARTISAN iris entrapment forceps allow a 1mm fold of midperipheral iris tissue to be grasped, and the IOL claws are pressed over the forceps tips; (2) ARTISAN iris entrapment needles, which are blunt, allow the creation of a fold of midperipheral iris tissue through vertical movement of the needle, and the IOL claws are pressed over it (Fig. 26-9).

Although a prophylactic iridectomy or iridotomy is theoretically not necessary (the ARTISAN Myopia Lens is vaulted to encourage natural fluid flow), experience has shown that it can prevent pupil block glaucoma in certain cases (Fig. 26-10).

The number of stitches depends on the type of incision. Watertight wound closure is of paramount importance to prevent a shallow anterior chamber's leading to IOL-endothelial contact in the immediate postoperative period.

The OVD material should be completely removed after the wound has been almost completely closed to prevent a shallow

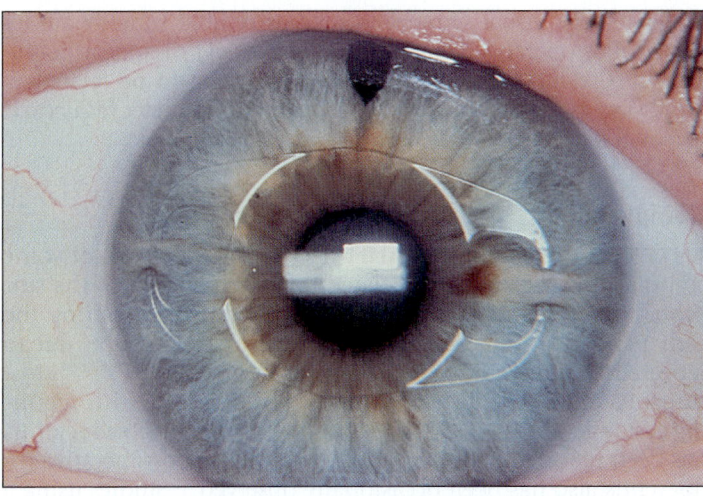

FIG. 26-10 ▮ Slit-lamp photograph of a Worst-Fechner iris-claw lens in position. Note the superior iridectomy. (Courtesy of Mrs. Anneke Worst.)

anterior chamber and contact between the IOL and the cornea. Incomplete removal of the OVD material may induce an early postoperative rise in IOP.

Nonsteroidal or steroidal anti-inflammatory drugs are usually prescribed for 2–4 weeks after surgery. Glaucoma drugs are not used on a regular basis. Patients also must be instructed not to rub their eyes after surgery.

It is critical to inform the patient of the necessity for regular follow-up. In particular, long-term evaluation of the corneal endothelium density using specular microscopy is recommended.

Visual Outcomes

Improvement in quality of vision and enlargement of visual field are common. In the earlier series of Fechner et al.[7] (62 eyes; preoperative SE −7.0 to −28.0D), 63% of eyes were within 1.0D correction. None deviated more than 20% from the predicted correction. In the series of Worst et al.[46] including 18 eyes (range, −8.0 to −18.0D), predictability of outcome was good: seven eyes needed no spherical correction postoperatively, and only two eyes deviated more than 2.0D from the aimed refraction. In the series of Fechner et al.[47] including 109 implanted eyes (preoperative mean SE −14.4D; range, −5.0 to −31.5D), 75 eyes (68.8%) were corrected within 1.0D of the desired refraction, and only 10 eyes (9.2%) deviated more than 2.0D from the aimed result. Landesz et al.[48] reported a 74.3% rate of postoperative SE refractive error within 1.0D of emmetropia in a series of 35 eyes (range, −6.0 to −28.0D). Menezo et al.[49] reported that 80.5% of eyes (90 eyes; range, −7.0 to −24.0D) were within 1.0D of emmetropia. Malecaze, in his unpublished series of 25 eyes (mean SE −13.43D; range, −8.00 to −17.25D) implanted with the ARTISAN Myopia Lens, found a 52% (13 eyes) and 84% (21 eyes) predictability value for 0.5D or less and 1.0D or less of aimed postoperative UCVA, respectively. Efficacy, defined as the ratio between postoperative UCVA and preoperative BCVA, was 0.80 in his series. Comparatively, efficacy was 0.73 for LASIK in 41 myopic eyes (preoperative mean SE −7.50D) in the hands of the same surgeon. Visual recovery was rapid, since mean UCVA was 0.46 ± 0.22D the first postoperative day.

There is a change in the retinal image size, which is increased by 20% compared with the image with spectacles.[16,17] Menezo et al.[50] found that 77 of 94 eyes (81.9%) gained two or more lines of BCVA compared with preoperative values. Malecaze (personal data) found that 16 of 25 eyes (64%) gained one line or more of BCVA postoperatively, and only one eye (4%) lost one line. According to this investigator, induced astigmatism was not a problem; it was 1.33 ± 0.88D and 1.00 ± 0.73D preoperatively and postoperatively, respectively.

Very rarely, visual symptoms such as double contour are reported. Postoperative glare and haloes usually disappear gradually.[48,50] The incidence of haloes did not seem to be related to pupil size, as measured with the Colvard Pupillometer (Malecaze, personal data).

Complications

ANTERIOR CHAMBER INFLAMMATION. The incidence of some complications seems to be related to the experience of the surgeon. Rare cases of exudative iritis were described during the early periods of some surgeons' learning curves, probably due to repeated traumatic attempts at iridic incarceration.[45,47,50] Most surgeons did not report any cases of postoperative iritis requiring systemic steroid therapy.[46,50] Early postoperative iridocyclitis has been reported in 6.4–16% of eyes.[47,51] Late postoperative iridocyclitis also has been occasionally observed.[52] Studies using a laser flare-cell meter showed contradictory results. Fechner *et al.*[47] reported no more inflammation than after a cataract extraction with posterior chamber implantation. Also, iris angiography did not show vascular leaks in some studies.[47,50]

Conversely, Pérez-Santonja *et al.*[52,53] showed chronic subclinical inflammation using a laser flare-cell meter 1–2 years postoperatively. Alio *et al.*[54] also reported elevated flare values 1 year following implantation of Worst-Fechner lenses, but their results were probably artifactual. Finally, fluorophotometry on 15 eyes implanted with the Worst-Fechner iris-claw lens showed prolonged breakdown of the BAB.

Pigment deposition on the corneal endothelium also was observed, suggesting a release from the iris induced by the phakic lens.[52]

GLAUCOMA. Postoperative glaucoma can be corticosteroid induced and usually resolves after discontinuation of steroid therapy. Secondary glaucoma can also occur if the OVD material has been inadequately removed. Only rare cases of temporary ocular hypertension have been reported.[50] In one case, the pupil dilated and could not be constricted,[45] and the phakic IOL had to be removed. One case of anterior ischemic optic neuropathy also occurred immediately after surgery, possibly due to simultaneous increased IOP and systemic hypertension.[55]

IRIS ATROPHY OR DISLOCATION. Pérez-Santonja *et al.*[52] observed iris atrophy at both fixation sites in 81% of eyes, lens instability in 9.3%, and delayed implant displacement secondary to iris fold perforation or haptic disincarceration in three eyes. Mertens and Tassignon[56] and Risco and Cameron[57] also reported one case of delayed detachment of the iris-claw haptic and IOL dislocation. Most reports, however, do not mention iris atrophy. Pupil deformation can also occur.

DECENTRATION. Implant decentration can be measured using a slit-lamp beam or a digital imaging system.[52,58] Patients report haloes that may be related to lens decentration in 23.4–56% of cases, but this rarely requires reintervention.[50,52,59]

ENDOTHELIAL CELL LOSS. There is some concern about the progressive decrease of corneal endothelial cell density. Various investigators have found an acceptable mean endothelial loss of 5.3–8.9% 1 year following iris-claw phakic lens implantation,[48,60] which is similar to results of posterior chamber IOL implantation.[61] Menezo *et al.*[50,59,62] noted endothelial cell loss of 7.63% and 17.9% at 2 and 5 years, respectively, without morphometric changes. They did not find any statistical significance in the biconcave versus convex-concave design of the iris-claw lens with respect to endothelial cell density. In a few cases, the endothelial cell count decreased because of corneal trauma during implantation.[45,63] Landesz *et al.*[64] implanted an opaque iris-claw lens in a phakic eye to correct acquired diplopia and found an 18.6% difference in mean endothelial cell density compared with the nonimplanted fellow eye 14 years after surgery.

Several reports, however, showed that some eyes developed unexplained endothelial cell loss following uncomplicated surgery.[47,52,65–67] Pérez-Santonja *et al.*[52] reported an endothelial cell loss of 17.6% at 2 years. According to Fechner *et al.*,[67] significant progressive endothelial cell loss was observed in 13.4% of eyes implanted between 1986 and 1991, and a projected 8-year follow-up resulted in a decrease in 27% of eyes. This may be related to eye rubbing or vaulting of the implant. Endothelial cell loss was a major reason behind the design change to the convex-concave shape of the ARTISAN Myopia Lens. Menezo *et al.*[59] believe that the endothelial damage is due mainly to surgical maneuvers, because they found that the most important changes occurred during the first 6 months postoperatively. According to these investigators, a shallower anterior chamber depth and a more powerful and therefore thicker minus implant are predictors of greater endothelial cell density decrease during this period. In addition, breakdown in the BAB may lead to chronic inflammation that is directly toxic to the corneal endothelium.[52,68,69] Some surgeons advocate a poor implantation technique that results in higher endothelial cell loss.[70]

FUNDUSCOPY. One case of flat retinal detachment was reported after iris-claw phakic lens implantation.[65] Cystoid macular edema was not observed, and the peripheral fundus is easily visualized through a dilated pupil.

OTHER COMPLICATIONS. Cystic wounds associated with subconjunctival fistulae requiring resuturing have been reported.[47,52,65] Intraoperative hyphema due to the iridectomy or excessive iris manipulation can occur, but it usually clears completely.[59] Pseudophakodonesis is not visible, except in nystagmic patients. Two cases of Urretz-Zavalia syndrome were reported,[47] due to insufficient removal of the OVD material associated with a frail iris. Viscoelastic injection associated with prolonged iris prolapse may damage the iris sphincter. Contact between the IOL and the natural lens has not been noted, and age-related cataracts can easily be extracted in patients with iris-claw phakic lenses.[71]

POSTERIOR CHAMBER PHAKIC INTRAOCULAR LENSES

The Staar Surgical ICL is made of a collagen copolymer, a compound combining acrylic and porcine collagen (<0.1% collagen). Its refractive index is 1.45 at 35°C. The material is soft, elastic, and hydrophilic.

The optical zone of the myopic lenses is 60m thick, and the diameter is 4.5–5.5mm, according to the power required. The optical zone diameter of the hyperopic lenses is 5.5mm. Available powers are −3 to −21D for myopic lenses and +3 to +17D for hyperopic lenses (Fig. 26-11). Several lengths are available: 11.0–12.5mm for hyperopic lenses, and 11.5–13mm for myopic lenses. The posterior surface is concave, to vault over the anterior capsule.[72]

Surgical Technique

Two weeks before surgery, laser iridotomies are performed. Two peripheral superior iridotomies are placed 80° apart to avoid the possibility of iridotomy occlusion by the haptics of the implant.

A combination of mydriatic topical medications (e.g., tropicamide 1%, phenylephrine 2.5%) is applied serially, beginning 1 hour before surgery. The anesthesia method is based on patient and surgeon preferences: general anesthesia, peribulbar injection, or topical anesthesia.

A superior puncture incision is made, and aqueous humor is replaced by a viscoelastic gel. A temporal corneal tunnel (width, 3.20mm; length, 1.75–2.00mm) is created. A narrow diamond blade allows a progressive opening of the anterior chamber. OVD material is injected. The implant can be inserted by two different techniques:

- With an injector.[72] The IOL is positioned in the lens insertion cartridge under direct visualization with the operating microscope. In the absence of a soft-tip injector, a small silicone sponge can be placed to protect the IOL from the hard injector arm. Because IOL insertion in the cartridge is complicated and time consuming, it must be performed before making the incision. The injector tip is placed in the tunnel, and the lens is in-

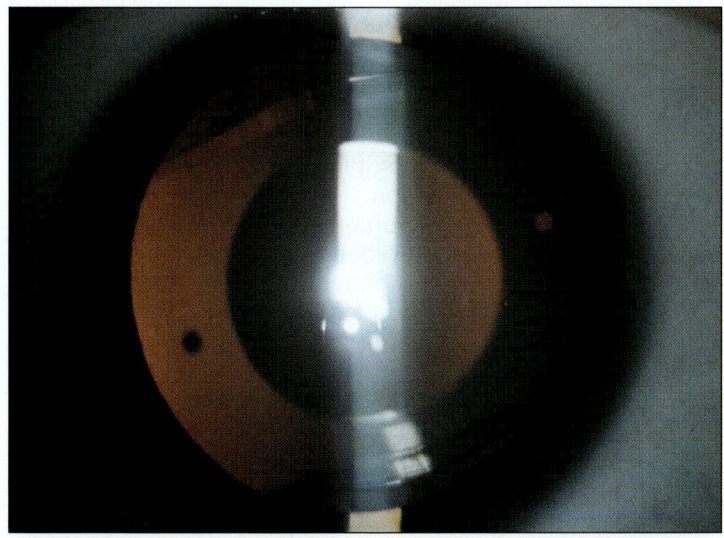
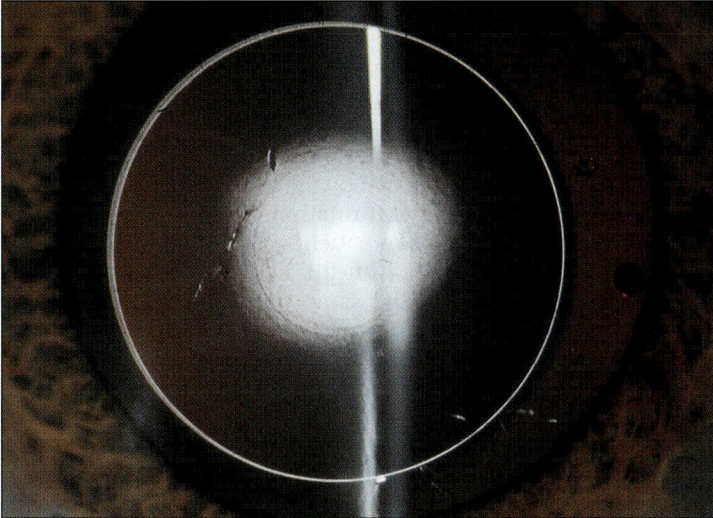

FIG. 26-11 ■ Staar Surgical posterior chamber phakic intraocular lenses. (From Arné JL, Hoang-Xuan T. Posterior chamber phakic IOL. In: Azar DT, ed. IOLs in cataract and refractive surgery. Philadelphia: WB Saunders; 2001:267–72.)

jected into the anterior chamber. As the IOL unfolds slowly, its progression must be controlled, ensuring proper orientation.

- With forceps.[72] The IOL is easy to fold between the jaws of a MacPherson forceps. The tip of the forceps is introduced into the entrance of the tunnel. Another MacPherson forceps held in the other hand grasps the sides of the implant. The first forceps is opened, regrasps the IOL a little further, and pushes it slowly. By repeating these maneuvers with the forceps, the IOL moves into the tunnel and can unfold in a controlled manner. The tip of the forceps must not enter the anterior chamber, to avoid contact with the crystalline lens.

While the IOL unfolds, its proper orientation must be checked. Then each footplate is placed one after the other beneath the iris with a specially designed, flat, nonpolished manipulator, without placing pressure on the crystalline lens. It is important to avoid touching the optic of an ICL in the middle, as this is the thinnest part. Then the OVD material is removed with gentle irrigation-aspiration, and acetylcholine chloride is injected. Steroid-antibiotic eyedrops are instilled. The patient receives 500mg of intravenous acetazolamide at the conclusion of the surgery and 4 hours later.[72]

Clinical Outcomes

PREDICTABILITY. Asseto et al.[73] implanted 15 lenses in 14 patients. Average follow-up was 7.00 ± 1.95 months. Mean SE was −15.3 ± 3.1D preoperatively and −2.0 ± 1.5D postoperatively. Only 31% of the eyes had less than 1.0D of residual myopia. However, an old model of lenses was used.

Rosen and Gore[74] operated on 16 myopic eyes (preoperative SE −5.25 to −14.50D). At 3 months after surgery, refraction ranged from −1.25 to +1.00D; 56.2% of the eyes were within 0.50D of emmetropia.

Zaldivar and Davidorf[75] analyzed the most important cohort including 124 eyes. Mean follow-up was 11 months (range, 1–36 months). Mean preoperative SE was −13.38 ± 2.23D (range, −8.50 to −18.63D). The target was emmetropia. Postoperative mean SE was −0.78 ± 0.87D (range, +1.63 to −3.50D); and 69% of eyes were within 1.00D and 44% within 0.50D of emmetropia.

Arné and Lesueur[76] implanted 58 eyes of 46 myopic patients. Follow-up ranged from 9 months to 2 years. Mean SE was −13.85 ± 4.61D (range, −8.00 to −19.21D) preoperatively and −1.22 ± 0.58D postoperatively; 56.9% of eyes were within 1.00D of emmetropia. Residual myopia was more than 2.00D in 15.5% of eyes.

There have been two studies on hyperopic posterior chamber phakic IOLs. Rosen and Gore[74] operated on nine hyperopic eyes (preoperative SE range, +2.25 to +5.62D). Three months postoperatively, the SE refraction ranged from −0.12 to +1.00D. Davidorf et al.[77] implanted a collagen-containing polymer phakic IOL into 24 eyes with hyperopia greater than 3.50D. Mean preoperative SE was +6.51 ± 2.08D (range, +3.75 to +10.50D). Mean postoperative SE was −0.39 ± 1.29D (range, +1.25 to −3.88D). Postoperatively 79% of eyes were within 1.00D and 58% within 0.50D of emmetropia. This compares favorably with the predictability obtained by the authors in their series of high myopic eyes.[75]

VISUAL ACUITY. In the series of Zaldivar et al.[75] on myopic eyes, preoperative BCVA was 20/40 or better in 80% of eyes and 20/20 or better in 5% of eyes. Postoperatively, UCVA was 20/40 or better in 93% of eyes and 20/20 or better in 19% of eyes. A gain of two or more lines of postoperative BCVA was attained in 36% of eyes; 7% lost one line, and 0.8% lost two lines.

In the series of Arné and Lesueur,[76] preoperative mean BCVA was 0.57, and postoperative mean UCVA and BCVA were 0.40 and 0.71, respectively. Postoperative UCVA was better than preoperative BCVA in 15.5% of eyes, unchanged in 15.5%, and worse in 68.9%. Mean efficacy, the ratio of postoperative UCVA to preoperative BCVA, was 0.84; 20.6% of eyes preserved the same BCVA, 77% gained one or more lines, and 3.4% lost two lines. Safety, the ratio between postoperative and preoperative BCVA, was 1.46.

Good efficacy and predictability have been demonstrated in all studies on the use of posterior chamber phakic IOLs for the treatment of high myopia. The marked gain in postoperative BCVA compared with preoperative best spectacle-corrected visual acuity in high myopes is largely due to elimination of the spectacle-induced image reduction.

Conversely, only 8% of hyperopic eyes operated on by Davidorf et al.[77] demonstrated a gain in postoperative BCVA compared with preoperative best spectacle-corrected visual acuity. In this series, 4% of eyes lost two or more lines of best spectacle-corrected visual acuity due to postoperative glaucoma.

STABILITY. Excellent stability has been demonstrated in all series. On 51 eyes followed by Zaldivar et al.,[75] refraction was −0.90D at 1 month, −0.91D at 6 months, and −0.83D at 12 months postoperatively.

QUALITY OF VISION. The level of patient satisfaction is very high. In the study of Arné and Lesueur,[76] 55.7% of the patients were very satisfied, 36.2% satisfied, and 6.9% moderately satisfied. No patient was dissatisfied.

The rate of subjective complaints, including glare and haloes, varies, depending on the series; it was 2.4% for Zaldivar et al.[75] and 55% for Arné and Lesueur.[76] The rate of haloes was higher when the size of the optical zone of the ICL was small. Mahrinho et al.[78] had to remove a silicone phakic IOL because of excessive glare.

In one study,[76] contrast sensitivity was tested preoperatively in myopic patients corrected with their contact lenses and 6 months after implantation of an ICL. The mean postoperative level without correction was higher than the mean preoperative level with correction, and the difference was statistically significant for each level of luminance.[72]

Complications

ENDOTHELIAL CELL DAMAGE. Although endothelial cell loss is a major concern with anterior chamber IOLs, it does not seem to present a problem with posterior chamber phakic IOLs. Fyodorov et al.[10] reported a mean decrease in endothelial cell density of 5% with their silicone posterior chamber phakic IOL, and Asseto et al.[73] found a mean endothelial cell loss of 4% with the Staar IOL. Arné and Lesueur[76] noted a mean endothelial cell loss of 2.1% 3 months after surgery with the same phakic IOL; it was 2.3% at 6 months, 2% at 1 year, and 2% at 2 years. In no case did endothelial cell loss exceed 3.8% at 1 year.[72,76]

INFLAMMATION. Subclinical inflammation has been reported as a frequent complication of the first model of silicone posterior chamber phakic IOLs. Two cases of postoperative uveitis also were reported with the Chiron-Adatomed silicone phakic IOLs.[78] Conversely, no inflammation was found with the Staar collagen-containing polymer IOL using laser flare fluorophotometry.[76] Six months postoperatively, flare remained at insignificant levels, even in an eye that had experienced an early but transient postoperative inflammatory reaction.

PIGMENTARY DISPERSION AND ELEVATED INTRAOCULAR PRESSURE. Pigmentary reaction was first reported by Asseto et al.[73] Pigment deposits on the periphery of the ICL optic is constant 1 year after surgery, but it has no visual consequence. In two cases,[13] pigmentary deposits that were not present preoperatively were seen in the angle in association with elevated IOP (Fig. 26-12). According to Zaldivar et al.,[75] this is a nonprogressive pigmentation.

Although contact and rubbing of the optic shoulder against the posterior surface of the iris are the major logical sources of pigmentary dispersion,[79] it also may be surgically induced, due to YAG iridotomies and the iridic trauma during implantation.[14] Pigmentary dispersion can be of some concern, because highly myopic eyes are, by their nature, at increased risk for glaucoma.[72]

Elevation of IOP can result from several mechanisms, including postoperative use of topical corticosteroids, narrowing of the angle (demonstrated by ultrasound biomicroscopy studies,[79] especially in hyperopic eyes), and pigmentary deposits in the angle.[75]

CATARACTOGENESIS. Cataract formation is one of the most crucial concerns for the future of posterior chamber phakic

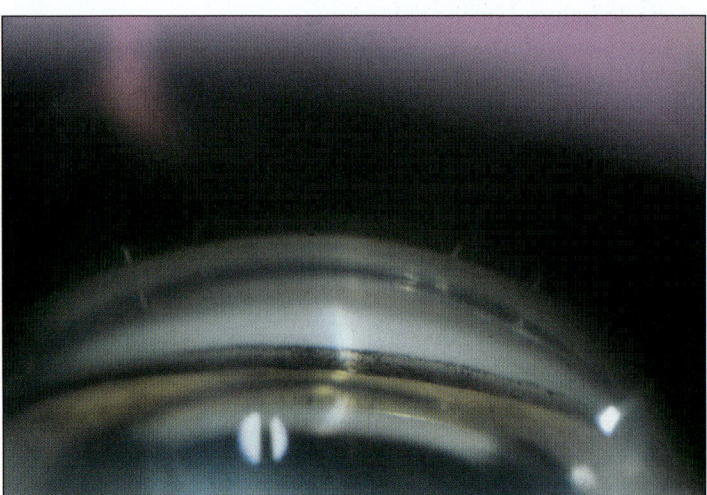

FIG. 26-12 ■ **Pigmentary deposits are seen in the angle in an eye with a posterior chamber phakic intraocular lens.** (From Arné JL, Hoang-Xuan T. Posterior chamber phakic IOL. In: Azar DT, ed. IOLs in cataract and refractive surgery. Philadelphia: WB Saunders; 2001:267–72.)

IOLs.[72] Trindade and Pereira[80] reported a case of significant cataract formation 6 months after uneventful implantation of an ICL. Finks et al.[81] reported on the occurrence of lens opacification in three eyes of two patients. Arné and Lesueur[76] observed two cases of anterior subcapsular opacities; one required removal of the ICL, followed by phacoemulsification and posterior chamber IOL implantation.

Cataract may form as a result of trauma to the crystalline lens during the implantation procedure. However, in most reported cases, the implantation was nontraumatic. Contact between the ICL and the central area of the crystalline lens was considered the cause of cataract formation in several cases.[72] Examination by ultrasound biomicroscopy[79] and Scheimpflug camera[76] can demonstrate this contact in case of insufficient vault. A study using very high frequency ultrasound on two eyes implanted with new posterior chamber phakic IOLs failed to show any contact between the implant and the natural lens, even during accommodation and light reflex.[82] The choice of a large implant appears necessary to obtain a greater axial vault, along with a larger space between the ICL and the central part of the crystalline lens. However, an excessive vault pushes the iris forward and favors narrowing of the angle, increased contact between the ICL and the posterior surface of the iris, and, consequently, pigmentary dispersion. Excessive vault also may induce contact between the haptics of the ICL and the periphery of the crystalline lens. Metabolic disturbances induced by the implant also may be partially responsible for cataract formation.

The treatment of cataract in patients implanted with posterior chamber phakic IOLs is not difficult. Explantation of the ICL is easily performed through the same unenlarged primary clear corneal incision. Phacoemulsification and posterior chamber IOL implantation can be done in a routine fashion.

CONCLUSION

Phakic IOL implantation for the correction of myopia and hyperopia seems to be an efficacious and predictable alternative to keratorefractive surgery, particularly for high refractive errors. Longitudinal, controlled multicenter trials are needed to determine the long-term safety of phakic IOLs.

REFERENCES

1. Yoo S. Phakic IOL implantation: comparison with keratorefractive surgical procedures. In: Azar DT, ed. Intraocular lenses in cataract and refractive surgery. Philadelphia: WB Saunders; 2001:239–44.
2. Seiler T. Clear lens extraction in the 19th century—an early demonstration of premature dissemination. J Refract Surg. 1999;15:70–3.
3. Strampelli B. Sopportabilita di lenti acriliche in camera anteriore nella afachia e nei vizi di refrazione. Ann Oftalmol Clin Oculist. 1954;80:5–82.
4. Barraquer JI. Anterior chamber plastic lenses. Results of and conclusions from five years experience. Trans Ophthalmol Soc UK. 1959;79:393–424.
5. Choyce DP. Discussion to Barraquer: Anterior chamber plastic lenses. Results of and conclusions from five years experience. Trans Ophthalmol Soc UK. 1959;79:423.
6. Baikoff G, Arne JL, Bokobza Y, et al. Angle-fixated anterior chamber phakic intraocular lens for myopia of −7 to −19 diopters [see comments]. J Refract Surg. 1998;14:282–93.
7. Fechner PU, van der Heijde GL, Worst JG. The correction of myopia by lens implantation into phakic eyes [see comments]. Am J Ophthalmol. 1989;107:659–63.
8. Los LI, Worst JG. Implant surgery. Something old and something new. Doc Ophthalmol. 1990;75:377–90.
9. Fechner PU, Haubitz I, Wichmann W, Wulff K. Worst-Fechner biconcave minus power phakic iris-claw lens. J Refract Surg. 1999;15:93–105.
10. Fyodorov SN, Zuev VK, Tumanyan ER. Modern approach to the stagewise complex surgical therapy of high myopia. Transactions of International Symposium of IOL Implantation and Refractive Surgery. 1987:274–9.
11. Brauweiler PH, Wehler T, Busin M. High incidence of cataract formation after implantation of a silicone posterior chamber lens in phakic, highly myopic eyes. Ophthalmology. 1999;106:1651–5.
12. Zaldivar R, Davidorf JM, Oscherow S. Posterior chamber phakic intraocular lens for myopia of −8 to −19 diopters [see comments]. J Refract Surg. 1998;14:294–305.
13. Sanders DR, Martin RG, Brown DC, et al. Posterior chamber phakic intraocular lens for hyperopia. J Refract Surg. 1999;15:309–15.
14. Krumeich JH, Daniel J, Gast R. Closed-system technique for implantation of iris-supported negative-power intraocular lens. J Refract Surg. 1996;12:334–40.
15. Davidorf JM, Zaldivar R, Oscherow S. Posterior chamber phakic intraocular lens for hyperopia of +4 to +11 diopters [see comments]. J Refract Surg. 1998;14: 306–11.
16. van der Heijde GL, Fechner PU, Worst JGF. Optische Konzequenzen der Implantation einen negativen Intraokularlinse bei myopen Patienten. Klin Monatsbl Augenheilkd. 1988;193:99–102.

17. van der Heijde GL. Some optical aspects of implantation of an IOL in a myopic eye. Eur J Implant Refract Surg. 1989;1:245–8.
18. Baikoff G, Joly P. Comparison of minus power anterior chamber lenses and myopic epikeratoplasty in phakic eyes. Refract Corneal Surg. 1990;6:252–60.
19. Galarreta Mira DJ, Yoo SH, Baikoff G, Azar DT. Anterior chamber phakic IOLs. In: Azar DT, ed. Intraocular lenses in cataract and refractive surgery. Philadelphia: WB Saunders; 2001:245–55.
20. Baikoff G. Phakic anterior chamber intraocular lenses. Int Ophthalmol. 1991;31:75–86.
21. Baikoff G. The refractive IOL in the phakic eye. Ophthalmic Pract. 1991;9:58–61, 80.
22. Baikoff G, Arne JL, Bokobza Y, et al. Angle-fixated anterior chamber phakic intraocular lens for myopia of −7 to −19 diopters. J Refract Surg. 1998;14:282–93.
23. Alio JL, de la Hoz F, Pérez-Santonja JJ. Phakic anterior chamber lenses for the correction of myopia: a 7-year cumulative analysis of complications in 263 cases. Ophthalmology. 1999;106:458–66.
24. Garrana RMR, Azar DT. Phakic intraocular lenses for correction of high myopia. Int Ophthalmol Clin. 1999;39:45–57.
25. Baikoff G, Joly P. Correction chirurgicale de la myopie forte par un implant de chambre antérieure dans l'oeil phak: Concept-résultats. Bull Soc Belge Ophtalmol. 1989;233:109–25.
26. Joly P, Baikoff G, Bonnet P. Mise en place d'un implant négatif de chambre antérieure chez des sujets phaques. Bull Soc Ophtalmol Fr. 1989;89:727–33.
27. Colin J, Mimouni F, Robinet A, et al. The surgical treatment of high myopia: comparison of epikeratoplasty, keratomileusis and minus power anterior chamber lenses. Refract Corneal Surg. 1990;6:245–51.
28. Mimouni F, Colin J, Koff V, et al. Damage to the corneal endothelium from anterior chamber intraocular lenses in phakic myopic eyes. Refract Corneal Surg. 1991;7:277–81.
29. Baikoff G. Etude comparative des complications des epikeratoplasties myopiques et des lentilles intraoculaires de chambre antérieure pour le traitement des myopies fortes. Ophtalmologie. 1991;5:276–9.
30. Perez-Santonja JJ, Iradier MT, Benitez del Castillo JM, et al. Chronic subclinical inflammation in phakic eyes with intraocular lenses to correct myopia. J Cataract Refract Surg. 1996;22:183–7.
31. Alio JL, de la Hoz F, Ismail MM. Subclinical inflammatory reaction induced by phakic anterior chamber lenses for the correction of high myopia. Ocul Immunol Inflamm. 1993;1:219–23.
32. Benitez del Castillo JM, Hernandez JL, Iradier MT, et al. Fluorophotometry in phakic eyes with anterior chamber lens implantation to correct myopia. J Cataract Refract Surg. 1993;19:607–9.
33. Eloy R, Parrat D, Tran Min Duc, et al. In vitro evaluation of inflammatory cell response after CF4 plasma surface modification of PMMA intraocular lenses. J Cataract Refract Surg. 1993;19:364–9.
34. Saragoussi JJ, Othenin-Girard P, Pouliquen Y. Ocular damage after implantation of minus power anterior chamber intraocular lenses in myopic phakic eyes: case reports. Refract Corneal Surg. 1993;9:105–9.
35. Perez-Santonja JJ, Iradier MT, Sanz Iglesias L, et al. Endothelial changes in phakic eyes with anterior chamber intraocular lenses to correct high myopia. J Cataract Refract Surg. 1996;22:1017–22.
36. Bour T, Piquot X, Pospisil A, et al. Repercussions endothéliales de l'implant myopique de chambre antérieure ZB au cours de la première année: etude prospective avec analyse statistique. J Fr Ophtalmol. 1991;14:633–41.
37. Baikoff G, Joly P, Bonnet PH. Evolution de l'endothelium corneen apres implant myopique. Ophtalmologie. 1991;5:525–6.
38. Saragoussi JJ, Cotinat J, Renard G, et al. Endothelium corneen et implants myopiques. Ophtalmologie. 1991;5:527–8.
39. Ruiz-Moreno JM, Alio JL, Perez-Santonja JJ. Retinal detachment in phakic eyes with anterior chamber intraocular lenses to correct severe myopia. Am J Ophthalmol. 1999;127:270–5.
40. Perez-Santonja JJ, Ruiz-Moreno JM, de la Hoz F. Endophthalmitis after phakic intraocular lens implantation to correct high myopia. J Cataract Refract Surg. 1999;25:1295–8.
41. Baikoff G, Samaha A. Phakic intraocular lenses. In: Azar DT, ed. Refractive surgery. Stamford, CT: Appleton & Lange; 1997:545–60.
42. Fechner PU. Die Irisklauen-Linse. Klin Monatsbl Augenheilkd. 1987;191:26–9.
43. Singh D, Singh IR. Use of the Worst-Singh lobster claw intraocular lens in children. Ophthalmic Pract. 1987;5:18.
44. de Vries FR, van der Heijde GL, Goovaerts HG. A system for continuous high-resolution measurement of distances in the eye. J Biomech Eng. 1987;9:32–7.
45. Hoang-Xuan T, Malecaze F. Iris-fixated phakic IOLs. In: Azar DT, ed. Intraocular lenses in cataract and refractive surgery. Philadelphia: WB Saunders; 2001:257–65.
46. Worst JGF, van der Veen G, Los LI. Refractive surgery for high myopia: the Worst-Fechner biconcave iris claw lens. Doc Ophthalmol. 1990;75:335–41.
47. Fechner PU, Strobel J, Wichmann W. Correction of myopia by implantation of a concave Worst-iris claw lens into phakic eyes. Refract Corneal Surg. 1991;7:286–98.
48. Landesz M, Worst JGF, Siertsema JV, et al. Correction of high myopia with the Worst myopia claw intraocular lens. J Refract Surg. 1995;11:16–25.
49. Menezo JL, Cisneros A, Hueso JR, et al. Long-term results of surgical treatment of high myopia with Worst-Fechner intraocular lenses. J Cataract Refract Surg. 1995;21:93–8.
50. Menezo JL, Avino JA, Cisneros AL, et al. Iris claw phakic intraocular lens for high myopia. J Refract Surg. 1997;13:545–55.
51. Harto MA, Menezo JL, Pérez L, et al. Correccion de la alta miopia con lentes intraoculares (Worst-Fechner) en ojos faquicos. Arch Soc Esp Oftalmol. 1992;62:267–74.
52. Pérez-Santonja JJ, Bueno JL, Zato MA. Surgical correction of high myopia in phakic eyes with Worst-Fechner myopia intraocular lenses. J Refract Surg. 1997;13:268–84.
53. Pérez-Santonja JJ, Iradier MT, Benitez del Castillo JM, et al. Chronic subclinical inflammation in phakic eyes with intraocular lenses to correct myopia. J Cataract Refract Surg. 1996;22:183–7.
54. Alio JL, de la Hoz F, Ismail MM. Subclinical inflammatory reaction induced by phakic anterior chamber lenses for the correction of high myopia. Ocul Immunol Inflamm. 1994;1:219–23.
55. Pérez-Santonja JJ, Bueno JL, Meza J, et al. Ischemic optic neuropathy after intraocular lens implantation to correct high myopia in a phakic patient. J Cataract Refract Surg. 1993;19:651–4.
56. Mertens E, Tassignon MJ. Detachment of iris claw haptic after implantation of phakic Worst anterior chamber lens: case report. Bull Soc Belge Ophtalmol. 1998;268:19–22.
57. Risco JM, Cameron JA. Dislocation of a phakic intraocular lens. Am J Ophthalmol. 1994;118:666–7.
58. Pérez-Torregrosa VT, Menezo JL, Harto MA, et al. Digital system measurement of decentration of Worst-Fechner iris claw myopia intraocular lens. J Refract Surg. 1995;11:26–30.
59. Menezo JL, Cisneros AL, Rodriguez-Salvador V. Endothelial study of iris claw phakic lenses: four year follow-up. J Cataract Refract Surg. 1998;24:1039–49.
60. Mathys B, Zanen A, Schrooyen M. Lentille de chambre antérieure négative d'un nouveau type dans la myopie élevée. Bull Soc Belge Ophtalmol. 1991;242:19–26.
61. Werblin TP. Long-term endothelial cell loss following phacoemulsification: model for evaluating endothelial damage after intraocular surgery. J Refract Corneal Surg. 1993;9:29–35.
62. Menezo JL, Cisneros AL, Cervera M, et al. Iris claw phakic lens—intermediate and long-term corneal endothelial changes. Eur J Implant Refract Surg. 1994;6:195–9.
63. Landesz M, Worst JGF, Siertsema JV, et al. Negative implant. Doc Ophthalmol. 1993;83:261–70.
64. Landesz M, Worst JGF, Van Rij G, et al. Opaque iris claw lens in a phakic eye to correct acquired diplopia. J Cataract Refract Surg. 1997;23:137–8.
65. Fechner PU, Wichmann W. Correction of myopia by implantation of minus optic (Worst iris claw) lenses into the anterior chamber of phakic eyes. Eur J Implant Refract Surg. 1993;5:55–9.
66. Pérez-Santonja JJ, Iradier MT, Sanz-Iglesias L, et al. Endothelial changes in phakic eyes with anterior chamber intraocular lenses to correct high myopia. J Cataract Refract Surg. 1996;22:1017–22.
67. Fechner PU, Haubitz I, Wichmann W, et al. Worst-Fechner biconcave minus power phakic iris claw lens. J Refract Surg. 1999;15:93–105.
68. Miyake K, Asakura M, Kobayashi H. Effect of intraocular lens fixation on the blood-aqueous barrier. Am J Ophthalmol. 1984;98:451–5.
69. Apple DJ, Brems RN, Park RB, et al. Anterior chamber lenses. Part I: Complications and pathology and review of designs. J Cataract Refract Surg. 1987;13:157–74.
70. Krumeich JH, Daniel J, Gast R. Closed-system technique for implantation of iris-supported negative-power intraocular lens. J Refract Surg. 1996;12:334–40.
71. Menezo JL, Cisneros AL, Rodriguez-Salvador V. Removal of age-related cataract and iris claw phakic intraocular lens. J Refract Surg. 1997;13:589–90.
72. Arné JL, Hoang-Xuan T. Posterior chamber phakic IOL. In: Azar DT, ed. IOLs in cataract and refractive surgery. Philadelphia: WB Saunders; 2001:267–72.
73. Asseto V, Benedetti S, Pesando P. Collamer intraocular contact lens to correct high myopia. J Cataract Refract Surg. 1996;22:551–6.
74. Rosen E, Gore C. Staar collamer posterior chamber phakic intraocular lens to correct myopia and hyperopia. J Cataract Refract Surg. 1998;24:596–606.
75. Zaldivar R, Davidorf JM, Oscherow S. Posterior chamber phakic IOL for myopia of −8 to −19 diopters. J Refract Surg. 1998;14:294–305.
76. Arné JL, Lesueur LC. Phakic posterior chamber lenses for high myopia: functional and anatomical outcomes. J Cataract Refract Surg. 2000;26:369–74.
77. Davidorf JM, Zaldivar R, Oscherow S. Posterior chamber phakic intraocular lens for hyperopia of +4 to +11 diopters. J Refract Surg. 1998;14:306–11.
78. Mahrinho A, Neves MC, Pinto MC, et al. Posterior chamber silicone phakic intraocular lens. J Refract Surg. 1997;13:219–22.
79. Trindade F, Pereira F, Cronemberger S. Ultrasound biomicroscopic imaging of posterior chamber phakic intraocular lens. J Cataract Refract Surg. 1998;14:497–503.
80. Trindade F, Pereira F. Cataract formation after posterior chamber phakic intraocular lens implantation. J Cataract Refract Surg. 1998;24:1661–3.
81. Fink AM, Gore C, Rosen E. Cataract development after implantation of the Staar collamer posterior chamber phakic lens. J Cataract Refract Surg. 1999;25:278–82.
82. Kim DY, Reinstein DZ, Silverman RH, et al. Very high frequency ultrasound analysis of a new phakic posterior chamber intraocular lens in situ. Am J Ophthalmol. 1998;125:725–9.

27 Refractive Aspects of Cataract Surgery

MARIA REGINA CHALITA • RONALD R. KRUEGER • BRIAN S. BOXER WACHLER

INTRODUCTION

The precise postoperative refractive outcome of cataract surgery became a main focus during the 1990s.[1] Small incision surgical techniques such as clear corneal or posterior limbal tunnel incisions,[2] combined with astigmatic keratotomy and the use of foldable intraocular lenses (IOLs), have led to early stable refractive results. Visual rehabilitation in most patients, however, is limited by residual refractive error. The common goal of modern cataract surgery is not only to perform a safe and flawless procedure but also to achieve postoperative emmetropia with improved uncorrected visual acuity.[3]

In this chapter, the history and principles of surgically induced astigmatism are described, as well as the devices and methods of measuring astigmatism. In addition, the astigmatic effects created and modified by incision parameters (size, configuration, construction, location, and closure) in cataract extraction are discussed, along with the use of transverse and arcuate keratotomy in cataract surgery. Issues concerning IOL calculation and selection to achieve spherical emmetropia are dealt with elsewhere in this book.

HISTORY

The mathematics for calculating surgically induced refractive changes was first described in 1849.[4] In 1975, Jaffe and Clayman[5] properly applied this method to analyze the relationship between cataract surgical technique and the refractive results in 1557 eyes undergoing cataract extraction. The wounds were closed using various techniques, including 10-0 monofilament nylon sutures that were either started at the 2:30 or 9:30 positions and tied at the 12 o'clock position (Troutman suture technique) or started at the 12 o'clock position and tied at the 2:30 or 9:30 positions (Willard suture technique). Knots tied superiorly were associated with with-the-rule (WTR) astigmatism, whereas knots tied close to the horizontal meridian were associated with against-the-rule (ATR) astigmatism. This early report facilitated an understanding of the dynamics of suture tension and corneal astigmatism in cataract surgery. It applied vector analysis using graph paper, rectangular coordinates, and the law of cosines and sines to determine surgically induced astigmatism. In 1979, Cravy[6] expanded the principles of Jaffe and Clayman by developing an approximate method for categorizing postoperative astigmatism as WTR or ATR to help guide suture removal and understand the dynamics of various types of wounds.

PRINCIPLES

The principles of corneal biomechanics are the foundation for understanding surgically induced refractive changes. Jaffe and Clayman[5] found that the steepness of the corneal meridian is related to suture knot placement; Cravy[6] emphasized that total central corneal power is conserved in cataract surgery, not decreased or increased, as long as tissue is neither added nor removed.

Using a corneoscope, Rowsey[7] established the principles that govern our ability to understand refractive power changes and coupling in the cornea. The first six of the ten "caveats" are listed here, as they are most applicable to the dynamics encountered in cataract surgery:

- The normal cornea flattens over any incision.
- Radial corneal incisions flatten the adjacent cornea and the cornea 90° away.
- The flattening effect of radial incisions on the cornea increases as incisions approach the visual axis.
- The cornea flattens directly over any sutured incision.
- The cornea flattens adjacent to loose limbal sutures, flattens 180° away, and steepens 90° away.
- The cornea steepens adjacent to tight limbal sutures, steepens 180° away, and flattens 90° away.

Wound slippage that results from a sutureless limbal cataract incision leads to the opposite curvature effect of central meridional flattening.

DEVICES FOR MEASURING ASTIGMATISM IN THE CLINIC

Manual Keratometer

By doubling a projected ring image onto the cornea, the keratometer best measures regular astigmatism in the central 3.0mm of the cornea. Irregular astigmatism and prolate to oblate corneal changes (from refractive surgery) are conditions in which the keratometer may not perform optimally.

Corneal Topography (Computerized Videokeratography)

This examination remains the gold standard for astigmatism measurement. Various technologies exist that analyze the curvature and elevation of the cornea, extending to the periphery. Many machines employ Placido disc imagery but differ in terms of the proprietary algorithms that process the Placido images. Some devices contain vector analysis software to measure surgically induced astigmatism based on simulated keratometry.

Van Loenen Keratoscope

The Van Loenen keratoscope (JedMed Inc., St. Louis, MO) is a simple, handheld device used to assess qualitatively the corneal shape by projecting rings along a translucent cylinder onto the cornea and observing their reflection (Fig. 27-1). In the clinic, this is done by the illumination and magnification of a slit-lamp microscope. Corneal astigmatism creates an oval Placido disc reflection, where the steep axis corresponds to the short axis of the oval. The Van Loenen keratoscope is useful in the clinic to assess higher degrees of astigmatism.

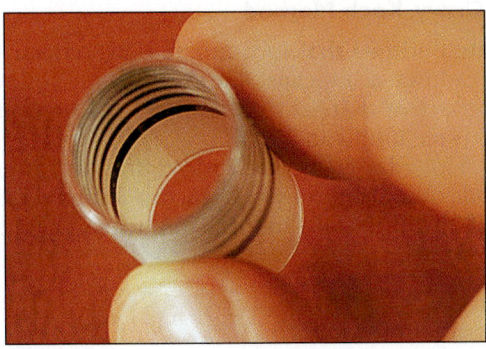

FIG. 27-I ▮▮ **Van Loenen keratoscope.** The concentric circles are projected onto the cornea with the aid of the slit lamp or operating microscope.

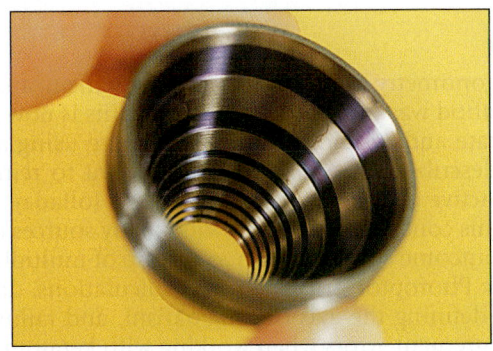

FIG. 27-2 ▮▮ **Maloney keratometer.** Constructed of metal, this keratoscope is used to assess qualitatively the intraoperative corneal curvature.

Corneoscope

Before corneal topography became commonplace, the corneoscope provided qualitative and quantitative measurements of corneal curvature out to the periphery. It is rarely used today.

DEVICES FOR MEASURING ASTIGMATISM INTRAOPERATIVELY

Terry Keratometer

This device, which also uses a doubling of a projected ring, attaches to the head of the operating microscope. In a study by Lindstrom and Destro,[8] the group of patients that had cataract wounds closed with the aid of the Terry keratometer experienced significantly better postoperative astigmatism control than did the group for which the keratometer was not used.

Van Loenen Keratoscope

This device, described earlier, can also be used to project rings onto the cornea intraoperatively using the illumination and magnification of the operating microscope.

Maloney Keratometer

Similar to the Van Loenen keratoscope, the Maloney keratometer (Storz, St. Louis, MO) differs in that it is manufactured from metal (Fig. 27-2). It is used to assess qualitatively corneal shape and astigmatism.

METHODS OF CALCULATING ASTIGMATISM

Simple Method

In this method, only magnitude is subtracted; axis is disregarded. It is invaluable to gain information about the final outcome of a procedure performed in patients who have minimal preoperative astigmatism. Because the axis is ignored, this method is inherently inaccurate. Compared with the vector

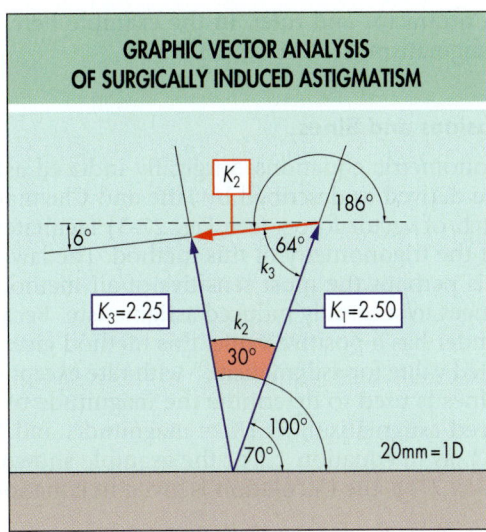

GRAPHIC VECTOR ANALYSIS OF SURGICALLY INDUCED ASTIGMATISM

FIG. 27-3 ▮▮ Graphic vector analysis of surgically induced astigmatism as plotted with a protractor. By drawing preoperative (K_1) and postoperative (K_3) astigmatism, surgically induced astigmatism (K_2) can be easily deduced (20mm = 1D; see text for details).

BOX 27-I

Example of Vector Method of Calculation

PREOPERATIVE	ASTIGMATISM
46.50D @ 035°	K_1:2.50D @ 035°
44.00D @ I25°	

POSTOPERATIVE	ASTIGMATISM
46.00D @ 050°	K_3:2.25D @ 050°
43.75D @ I40°	

See Figure 27-3.

---

method, the simple method grossly underestimates surgically induced astigmatism[9] and can produce errors in the range of 33–166%.[10] Hence, the simple method is not recommended.

Vector Method

Originally described by Stokes in 1849 and later by Jaffe and Clayman,[5] the vector method is perhaps the most straightforward method to incorporate both magnitude and direction. The vector method relies on geometrical principles and graphing of the direction and amplitude of preoperative and postoperative astigmatism (or cylinder) on paper to determine the surgically induced vector. Because the graph covers 360°, the axis must be doubled before drawing the vector on paper. Figure 27-3 demonstrates this method for determining corneal power. The method may be used for positive or negative cylinder as long as the preoperative and postoperative cylinders are of the same sign. By convention, the example uses the Jaffe and Clayman notations: K_1 (preoperative astigmatism), K_2 (surgically induced astigmatism), and K_3 (postoperative astigmatism).

For the example shown in Box 27-1, K_2, the surgically induced change, is to be determined. The astigmatism vectors are drawn using a protractor and denoting the magnitude with a convenient scale (see Fig. 27-3). The scale can be adjusted as long as consistency is maintained for each problem. A triangle is formed by creating a third side, which is K_2. The magnitude is measured with the millimeter scale and is found to be 1.25D. The axis is determined using the protractor after a dashed parallel line is drawn at the end of vector K_1 (186° in Fig. 27-3). The axis is always measured around K_1, not K_3. This value is halved to yield the surgically induced meridian of the astigmatism (93° in this example). Use of polar coordinate paper eliminates the need for a protractor and ruler. In the example here, surgically induced astigmatism is 1.25D @ 93°.

Law of Cosines and Sines

Using trigonometric equations, surgically induced astigmatism can also be derived as described by Jaffe and Clayman.[5] Even a rough sketch of vector forces (see Fig. 27-3) facilitates comprehension of the trigonometry of this method. The law of cosines and sines is perhaps the most sensitive of all methods used to detect changes in surgically induced astigmatism. Because all induced cylinder has a positive value, this method gives the highest calculated value for astigmatism,[11] with rare exceptions.[12] The law of cosines is used to determine the magnitude of the surgically induced astigmatism, K_2 (K = magnitude, and k = angle opposite K), as in equation 1. For the example shown in Figure 27-3 and Box 27-1, the calculation is given in equation 2.

Equation 1
$$K_2^2 = K_1^2 + K_3^2 - 2K_1K_3 \cos k_2$$

Equation 2
$$\begin{aligned} K_2^2 &= 2.5^2 + 2.25^2 - 2(2.5)(2.25) \cos 30° \\ &= 11.31 - 9.74 \\ &= 1.57 \\ K_2 &= 1.25D \end{aligned}$$

The law of sines is used to calculate the angle, as in equation 3, from which equation 4 is obtained. To determine the meridian of K_2: $70 - 64.2 = 5.8$; add 5.8 to 180 to yield 185.8° (see Fig. 27-3). This angle is halved to find the meridian of the surgically induced astigmatism: 92.9°. So, in the example above, surgically induced astigmatism is 1.25D @ 92.9°.

Equation 3
$$K_1/(\sin k_1) = K_2/(\sin k_2) = K_3/(\sin k_3)$$

Equation 4
$$\begin{aligned} k_3 &= [(\arcsin K_3)\,(\sin k_2)]/(K_2) \\ &= [(\arcsin 2.25)\,(\sin 30)]/(1.25) \\ &= \arcsin 0.9 \\ k_3 &= 64.2° \end{aligned}$$

Polar Values

Naeser[13] simplified the vector method by breaking down astigmatism into WTR and ATR components and formulating a single value, *KP*, which represents the polar value of net astigmatism (see equation 5, where *M* is magnitude of the astigmatism). Naeser points out advantages and disadvantages of this method. The single number represents the astigmatism and incorporates a balance between WTR and ATR astigmatism. However, a single value loses specificity, since different combinations of meridians and magnitudes may have the same polar value. Additionally, there may be a discrepancy between astigmatic magnitudes and polar values; some polar values may be 0 (45° meridian) when there is truly magnitude to the astigmatism.

Equation 5
$$KP = M \times (\sin^2\alpha - \cos^2\alpha)$$

Cravy Method

This method details the derivation of an astigmatism ratio. This ratio serves both as an indicator of wound apposition, suture placement, and tension and as a means of categorizing WTR or ATR astigmatism.[6] At best, this method yields approximate results, except when the preoperative and postoperative astigmatisms are not oblique.

Alpins Method

Alpins[10] introduced the concepts of targeted induced astigmatism, magnitude and axis of error, coefficient of adjustment, and index of success to measure the ability to achieve a desired outcome and refine surgical technique.

Holladay, Cravy, Koch Method

Ten steps are outlined that incorporate both refractive and keratometric readings as a means of measuring and following postoperative refractive changes.[14] Olsen[15] reported a slight modification of this technique in 1993.

In 1998, Holladay et al.[16] recognized that his former calculation method could be improved by incorporating the magnitude and axis of the surgically induced refractive change into the calculations.

Azar Sinusoidal Method

This method uses a single sinusoidal equation to calculate surgically induced refractive changes as applied to cataract and refractive surgery.[17]

Summary

Before trigonometry was applied to astigmatism analysis, the simple method was the standard; however, this is now known to be inaccurate and should not be used. Before using any of the methods described previously, it is important to remember to adjust refractive data for statistical analysis. Holladay et al.[18] introduced this concept in 2001, showing many sources of error in refractive outcome statistics, such as the use of multiple lens systems in the Phoroptor, errors in vertex calculations, difficulty in accurately defining the axis of astigmatism, and failure to consider measurement errors when working with keratometric data. They pointed out that refractive data must be adjusted for vertex distance before comparison to topographical or keratometric data. Descriptive statistics such as means, standard deviations, shape factor (ρ), standard error of the mean, and correlation coefficients can be calculated only after converting polar to Cartesian values.

Regardless of the method used, as long as surgeons take the time to understand the effects of their surgery by using astigmatism analysis, they will be more successful in achieving their surgical goals by modifying their plans as indicated by such analysis.

ASTIGMATISM IN EXTRACAPSULAR CATARACT EXTRACTION

Extracapsular expression of the nucleus requires an incision with a chord length of 9.0–11.0mm. These long incisions can induce initial large amounts of WTR astigmatism. Neumann et al.[9] reported aggregate surgically induced astigmatism of 1.29D at 3 months and 1.08D at 6 months. Minassian et al.[19] compared extracapsular cataract extraction (ECCE) with small incision phacoemulsification (phaco) and found that whereas the phaco group attained a good, stable level of visual acuity quickly (by the third postoperative week), the vision in the ECCE group continued to improve for up to 6 months. Analysis by multiple regression indicated that the poorer results with ECCE were due to higher levels of astigmatism after surgery.

Even with meticulous wound closure, these wounds are keratometrically unstable. The postoperative shift toward ATR astigmatism reflects wound slippage that occurs for as long as 2 years. This incorporates the premise of "coupling," in which an increase in corneal power in one meridian is accompanied by a decrease in the orthogonal meridian, with preservation of average corneal power. Although the corneal surfaces changed dramatically over time in the study by Talamo et al.,[20] the average corneal power determined by keratometry and by spherical equivalent manifest refraction showed a high degree of stability over 4 years (Fig. 27-4).

Another important point is determining the optimal time to remove sutures after ECCE. Talamo et al.[20] recommend suture removal at the 8–10 week visit if significantly more than 3D of WTR astigmatism is present 3–5 weeks postoperatively. Other authors have suggested removing sutures at 12 weeks postoper-

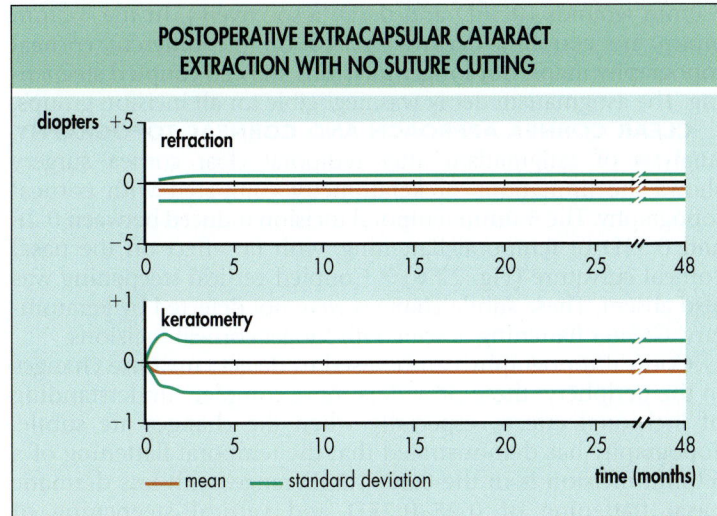

POSTOPERATIVE EXTRACAPSULAR CATARACT EXTRACTION WITH NO SUTURE CUTTING

FIG. 27-4 ■ Postoperative extracapsular cataract extraction course of manifest refraction and keratometry without suture cutting. Mean spherical equivalent refraction and keratometry (mean for all patients) correlate well and change little over time, which indicates that total central corneal refractive power is conserved through coupling, despite against-the-rule astigmatism drift. The upper and lower bars represent one standard deviation from the mean. (Adapted with permission from Talamo JH, Stark WJ, Jottesch JD, et al. Natural history of corneal astigmatism after cataract surgery. J Cataract Refract Surg. 1991;17:313–8.)

atively and prescribing glasses 1 month after suture removal. Beware that suture cutting may turn WTR astigmatism into unwanted ATR astigmatism over time.[21]

Preoperative astigmatism also has predictive value for postoperative astigmatism. Talamo et al.[20] showed that patients tend to have less postoperative than preoperative WTR astigmatism. Preoperative ATR astigmatism showed the opposite trend. These results imply that the cornea tends toward the original magnitude and direction of the initial astigmatism, except when more than 2D of ATR astigmatism exists preoperatively.

ASTIGMATISM IN PHACOEMULSIFICATION

Nuclear Expression versus Phacoemulsification

Phacoemulsification offers the advantage of cataract removal through a smaller wound, which decreases the surgically induced astigmatism and the decay of induced astigmatism compared with ECCE.[19] Lindstrom and Destro[8] showed that in a group of patients who had 6.5mm incision phacoemulsification, 5% had greater than 3D and 65% had less than 1D of astigmatism at 6–10 weeks postoperatively. This compared favorably with the results in the 10mm ECCE group: 24% with greater than 3D and 27% with less than 1D of astigmatism. The longer incision and increased number of sutures in ECCE undoubtedly result in the greater degree of astigmatism (Table 27-1).[8]

Wound Length with Sutured Closure

Sutures cause corneal steepening in the meridian of the suture. However, greater surgically induced astigmatism results with a longer wound, even when the same number of sutures is used. A 7mm long scleral pocket incision causes more postoperative keratometric cylinder than a 4mm wound (1.33D and 1.03D, respectively) up to 6 weeks postoperatively.[22] In a larger wound, more tissue can be affected by suture tension. Small wounds have less surgical edge surface area and, therefore, are more resistant to the mechanical forces of the sutures.

Sutured wounds that differ by 1.5mm are similar in the amount of surgically induced astigmatism. In a large cohort of 276 cases, Davison[23] found no difference for up to 1 year in patients who had 4.0mm and 5.5mm incisions using a standardized double "X" suture closure. At 1 year, the induced mean was

TABLE 27-1

COMPARISON OF SURGICALLY INDUCED CYLINDER BY VECTOR ANALYSIS FOR NUCLEAR EXPRESSION AND PHACOEMULSIFICATION

Study Group		Follow-up Visit	
		3 Months	6 Months
Phaco/silicone	Mean (SD)	1.29 (0.96)	1.08 (0.69)
	Range	0–3.25	0–2.67
Phaco/PMMA	Mean (SD)	1.06 (1.09)	1.06 (1.15)
	Range	1–7.42	0–7.42
ECCE/PMMA	Mean (SD)	2.27 (1.28)	1.74 (1.16)
	Range	0.5–7.0	0–4.61

The nuclear expression/polymethyl methacrylate (NE/PMMA) results are significantly different from those of the two phacoemulsification groups (by one-way ANOVA at 3 months, $p = 0.0001$; at 6 months, $p = 0.014$). No difference occurred between the phacoemulsification groups. (Adapted with permission from Lindstrom RL, Destro MA: Effect of incision size and Terry keratometer usage of postoperative astigmatism. J Am Intraocul Implant Soc. 1985;11:469–73.)

TABLE 27-2

EVALUATION OF ASTIGMATISM IN 4.0MM SUTURED CATARACT SURGERY WOUNDS

Study	Period		
	1 Week	4 Weeks	12 Weeks
Shepherd[24]	+0.13 (0.67)	+0.02	−0.22 (0.47)
Steinert et al.[11]	+0.07 (1.18)	+0.05 (1.11)	−0.21 (0.93)
Uusitalo et al.[25]	−0.35 (0.79)	−0.35 (0.07)	−0.53 (0.69)

Astigmatism decay over a 3-month period is similar for three studies that used the Cravy method (+, with-the-rule astigmatism; −, against-the-rule astigmatism).

0.3D and 0.2D of ATR astigmatism in the 4.0mm and 5.5mm groups, respectively.

The 4.0mm sutured incision allows for a short rehabilitation period. Not only is less astigmatism induced, but also less variability occurs in the amount of induction. Using the Cravy method, Shepherd[24] illustrated this with 4.0mm incisions. At 1 week, 0.13D of WTR astigmatism was induced, compared with 0.22D of ATR astigmatism at 3 months. Steinert et al.[11] showed similar findings for 4.0mm incisions. The work of Uusitalo et al.[25] also supports minimal decay in 4.0mm wounds. Table 27-2 shows the similarities of the three studies.

Larger wounds produce greater amounts of WTR astigmatism. In addition, the astigmatism induced by these wounds decays faster over time and requires more time for stabilization (Fig. 27-5).[24] Uncorrected visual acuity also parallels the amount of residual cylinder. Patients who have longer wounds must wait longer until they receive spectacles, and during that longer time, they have relatively reduced uncorrected visual acuity compared with patients who have shorter incisions. Longer sutured incisions prolong visual rehabilitation in patients.

Wound Length with Sutureless Closure

SCLERAL POCKET APPROACH. Sutureless closure offers the efficiency of decreased operating time as well as reduced material cost and less ocular tissue manipulation.

The ability to detect changes in astigmatism seems to be influenced by which instrument is used to evaluate the sutureless technique.[26,27] The difference map of corneal topography detected flattening along the wound and central and paracentral steepening.[26] Similar-sized incisions of 3.2mm, 4.0mm, and 5.0mm were evaluated for 6 months by Hayashi et al.[27]; for these incisions, an automated keratometer and corneal topography showed good consistency. The 3.2mm wound induced significantly less astigmatism (0.38D) compared with the 4.0mm and

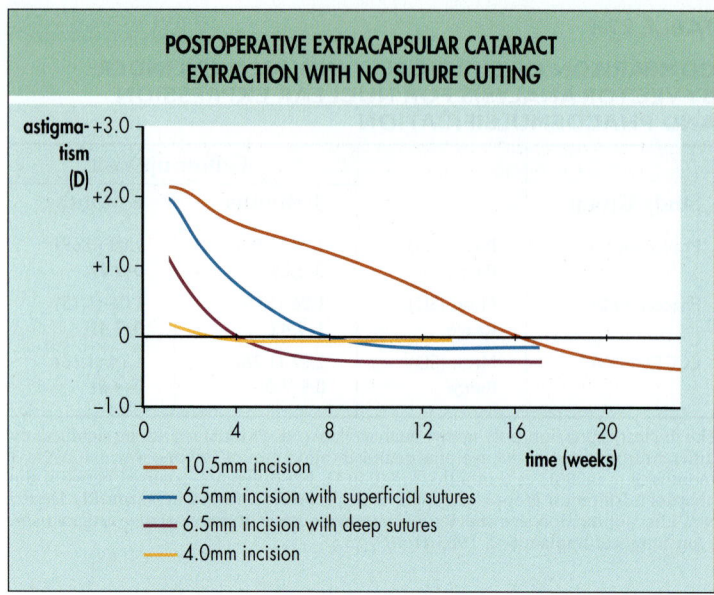

POSTOPERATIVE EXTRACAPSULAR CATARACT
EXTRACTION WITH NO SUTURE CUTTING

— 10.5mm incision
— 6.5mm incision with superficial sutures
— 6.5mm incision with deep sutures
— 4.0mm incision

FIG. 27-5 ▮ Degradation of postoperative induced astigmatism for various wound lengths. Longer incisions induce more astigmatism and require a longer period to reach stabilization. (Adapted with permission from Shepherd JR. Induced astigmatism in small incision cataract surgery. J Cataract Refract Surg. 1989;15:85–8.)

5.0mm wounds (0.56D and 0.6D, respectively). In the 3.2mm group, no coupling occurred based on the different corneal topography maps, but longer incisions showed coupled steepening. The astigmatism decay was negligible for all incision groups.

CLEAR CORNEA APPROACH AND CORNEAL TOPOGRAPHY. Analysis of astigmatism after temporal clear cornea surgery shows the limitations of keratometry compared with corneal topography. The 3.0mm temporal incision induced between 0.28 and 0.53D of temporal flattening, with no effect on the nasal corneal curvature (Fig. 27-6).[28] Coupled vertical steepening was also absent. These subtle changes were not detected by keratometry. Greater flattening is seen with longer corneal incisions.

Corneal topography can be used to detect curvature changes in the periphery; these provide a more complete understanding of incisional effects, especially when the changes are subtle. Topography has demonstrated that the temporal flattening of a 5.0mm incision is in the 0.50–1.75D range, with less dramatic nasal flattening of 0.25–0.75D and vertical steepening of 0.25–0.75D (Fig. 27-7).[29] Clear corneal entries do not induce equal and opposite coupling in curvature, especially in the periphery. The astigmatic influence of clear corneal incisions disproportionately affects the temporal meridian. Automated keratometry and corneal topography have shown good consistency in sutureless scleral incisions.[30]

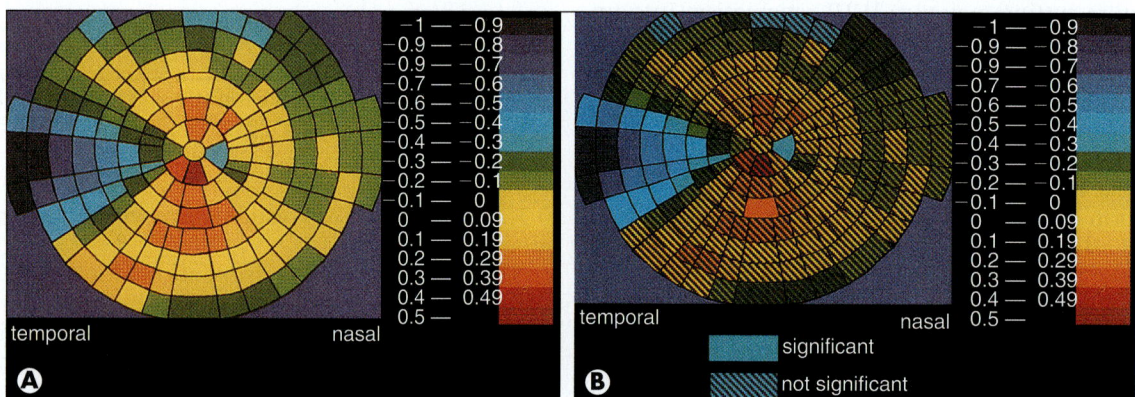

FIG. 27-6 ▮ Temporal 3mm incision. **A,** Surgically induced topographical change 1 month following temporal 3.0mm clear corneal cataract surgery. Note the temporal flattening. **B,** Paired Wilcoxon test results of significance ($p = 0.05$) for surgically induced topographical change 1 month following temporal 3.0mm clear corneal cataract surgery. Note the absence of vertical coupling. (Reprint permission granted by The American Journal of Ophthalmology; C. Vass, MD; and Ophthalmic Publishing Company. From Vass C, Menapace R. Computerized statistical analysis of corneal topography for the evaluation of changes in corneal shape after surgery. Am J Ophthalmol. 1994;118:177–84.)

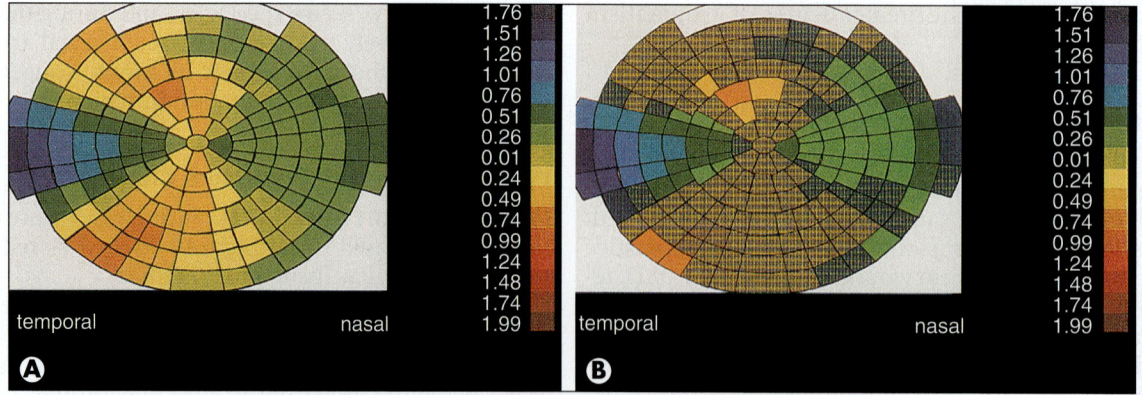

FIG. 27-7 ▮ Temporal 5mm incision. **A,** Surgically induced topographical change 3 months following temporal 5.0mm clear corneal cataract surgery. Note the nasal and temporal flattening. **B,** Paired Wilcoxon test results of significance ($p < 0.01$) for surgically induced topographical change 3 months following temporal 5.0mm clear corneal cataract surgery. Note the vertical coupling, which was not present in 3.0mm wounds. (Adapted with permission from Vass C, Menapace R, Amon M, et al. Batch by batch analysis of topographic changes induced by sutured and sutureless clear corneal incisions. J Cataract Refract Surg. 1996;22:324–30.)

Effects of Other Incision Types

FROWN INCISION. Singer[31] was the first to introduce this technique, which was named for its appearance to the surgeon during surgery (Fig. 27-8). Although the incision is curved, the arc length is either 6mm or 7mm, and the apex of the frown is 1.5mm posterior to clear cornea. A single horizontal vertical mattress suture of 10-0 nylon secures the central one third of the wound. This wound can accommodate insertion of a 6.0mm or 7.0mm diameter optic IOL. Of Singer's 62 cases, one patient had a self-resolving filtering bleb, and a second patient had a wound leak that required additional radial sutures.[31]

This technique has two advantages. First, it induces less surgical astigmatism compared with standard scleral pocket incisions (0.82D versus 1.30D at 1 year). Only 0.28D of ATR astigmatism was reported at 6 months postoperatively.[32] The second advantage is its high degree of stability. Although a modest degree of induced astigmatism results, there is only a minimal change in the actual amount of astigmatism induced. Therefore, this incision can be considered decay resistant. The curve of this incision integrates radial components, which are more stable than for a transverse and antifrown incision.

RADIAL TRANSVERSE INCISION. Siepser[33] developed this incision technique, which incorporates a "pita pocket" dissected through a radial incision (Fig. 27-9). The 3.5mm radial incision is made 1.5mm posterior to the vascular arcade. A 2.0mm microsclerotome is used to create pita pockets on both sides of the radial incision for the insertion of a 6.0mm diameter IOL. No sutures are used for closure. Lens insertion is technically more difficult, which explains the rate of conversions to other techniques (19/124). At 3 months postoperatively, 0.2D of cylinder was induced, and the wound stabilized at 1 week.

The architecture of this radial wound may preserve scleral support of the cornea. It is possible that a traditional horizontal incision disrupts the scleral fibers that maintain tension on the cornea over the length of the incision, thereby allowing the cornea to relax in that meridian. By suturing the wound, tension is put back on the cornea in that meridian. However, the suture does not prevent eventual slippage. The sutureless transverse radial incision allows for insertion of large, optic, rigid IOLs, but with insignificant long-term induced astigmatism.

THE "W" INCISION. Hennekes's[34] one-stitch "W" incision utilizes intrinsic scleral support for rapid stabilization (Fig. 27-10). The length of the "W" is 7.0mm, and its base is 2.0mm from the limbus. A single Vicryl suture is used to secure the apex of the central flap. This incision may be used in conjunction with filtering surgery for glaucoma or a pars plana approach for posterior segment surgery. One case of hypotony occurred in a series of 82 eyes.

Induced astigmatism was 1.18D at 1 week, 1.03D at 1 month, and 0.9D at 3 months. The increased surface area of the scleral triangular flap allows for more rapid wound healing and stabilization. The radial arms of the "W" provide additional support against wound slippage.

Effects of Suture Technique

The horizontal (tangential) closure induces less astigmatism than radial closures do. "Tight" and "loose" radial running sutures (four-cross shoelace) for 6.5mm scleral pocket incisions induce more initial WTR refractive cylinder than a horizontal figure-eight does.[35] Steinert et al.[11] showed that induced astigmatism in the first 1–2 weeks after a 6.5mm wound is dependent on suture technique. The horizontal closure is remarkably resistant to decay up to 6–12 months, whereas the running closure results in decay. For larger incisions, horizontal suture closure offers the

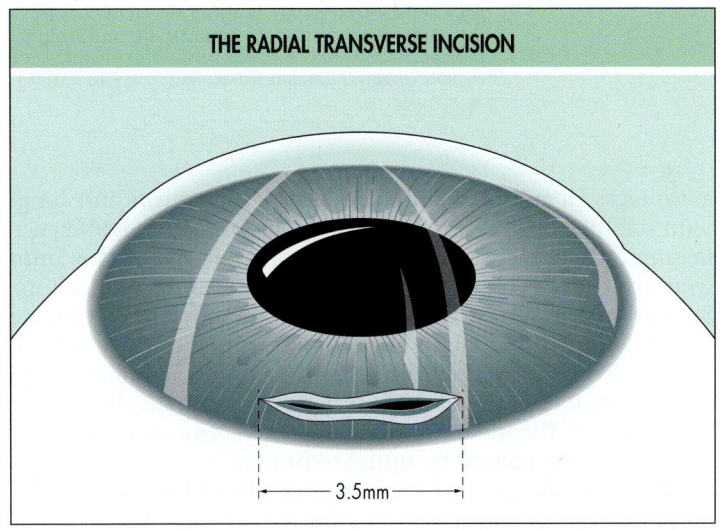

THE RADIAL TRANSVERSE INCISION

FIG. 27-9 ▮ Radial transverse incision. This wound is highly stable, but lens insertion is technically difficult. (Adapted with permission from Siepser SB. Sutureless cataract surgery with radial transverse incision. J Cataract Refract Surg. 1991;17:716–8.)

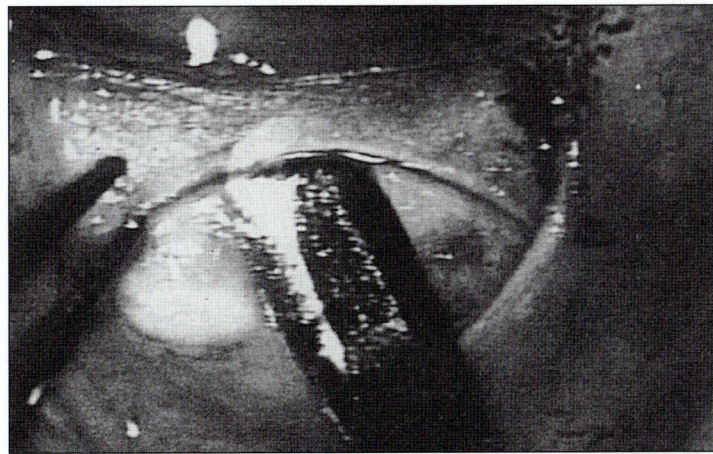

FIG. 27-8 ▮ Frown incision. This technique preserves scleral support, which helps prevent wound slippage, while being able to accommodate a rigid polymethyl methacrylate intraocular lens. (Adapted with permission from Singer JA. Frown incision for minimizing induced astigmatism after small incision cataract surgery with rigid optic intraocular lens implantation. J Cataract Refract Surg. 1991;17[suppl]:677–88.)

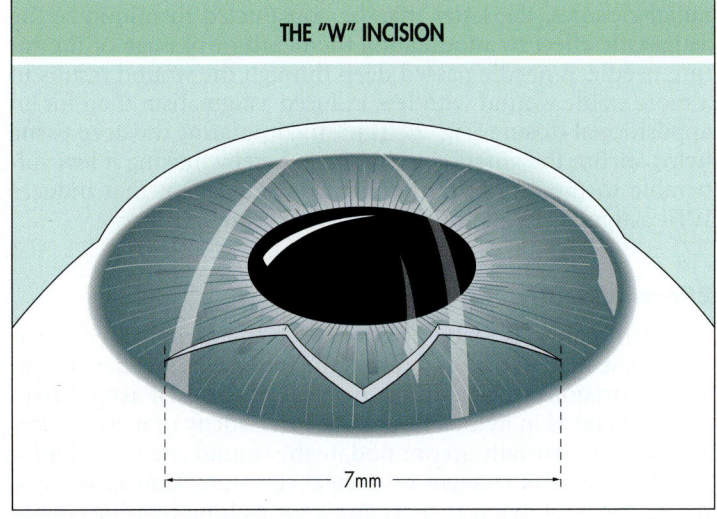

THE "W" INCISION

FIG. 27-10 ▮ "W" incision. This wound preserves scleral support and may be versatile for other concomitant surgical procedures. (Adapted with permission from Hennekes R. A high-stability, one-stitch W incision for cataract surgery. J Cataract Refract Surg. 1996;22:407–10.)

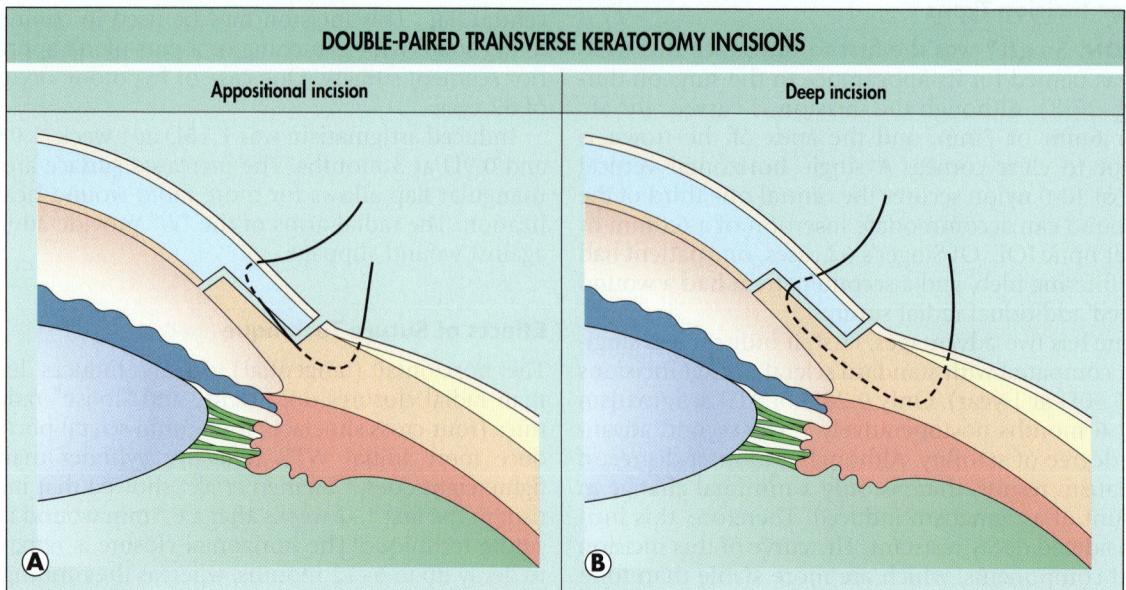

FIG. 27-11 ■ **Double-paired transverse keratotomy incisions. A,** Cross section of the scleral pocket incision closed with a continuous suture in apposition. Note that the suture passes within the wound space superficial to the internal layer of the scleral pocket. **B,** Cross section of the scleral pocket incision closed with a deeply placed suture. Note that the suture passes deep to the wound space and incorporates the internal layer of the scleral pocket. (Adapted with permission from Masket S. Deep versus appositional suturing of the scleral pocket incision for astigmatic control in cataract surgery. J Cataract Refract Surg. 1987;13:131–5.)

advantages of minimal initial induced astigmatism and long-term stability. Buzard and Shearing[36] demonstrated no difference in surgically induced astigmatism among 5.0, 6.0, and 6.5mm wounds with a central, one third width horizontal suture. Smaller 4.0mm wounds show no significant difference if they are closed with a horizontal suture or left sutureless.[37] A 4.0mm wound closed with a single vertical suture induces minimal astigmatism, as does a sutureless closure, as demonstrated by corneal topography.[38] The induced astigmatism of 3–4mm scleral pocket incisions is not affected by suture technique.[39]

The vector forces of a radial suture preferentially affect tissue and thus corneal curvature along the axis of the suture. The advantage of the horizontal (tangential) suture closure is that the horizontal vector forces have much less effect on the cornea, and hence less induced astigmatism. The reason for minimal decay compared with that found with radial closures may be the absence of significant induced astigmatism.

Although horizontal closures induce less astigmatism than radial closures, the latter may be constructed to minimize the astigmatic effect by modulating the depth of passage of the suture needle. A needle passed deep through the wound results in a more stable wound with less induced astigmatism than for an appositional closure (Fig. 27-11).[40] Incorporating the deep tissue helps anchor the anterior scleral flap, thereby making it less vulnerable to the intraoperative superior movement that induces WTR astigmatism and less prone to subsequent decay.

Effects of Suture Materials

Mersilene suture is made of nonbiodegradable polyester that is less elastic than nylon. As a result, the initial wound edema from scleral incisions causes almost twice as much WTR astigmatism in Mersilene as in nylon closures.[41] The elasticity of nylon allows the suture to partially accommodate the wound edema and minimize subsequent changes in corneal curvature. Conversely, it is the elasticity of nylon that accounts for its long-term instability in ECCE. The use of nylon sutures results in a slow drift to ATR astigmatism, and at 2 years postoperatively, there is a rapid ATR astigmatism change as a result of spontaneous rupture of the sutures. Mersilene does not rupture, but there is also a slow drift toward ATR astigmatism with its use.[42]

Other Operative Factors Affecting Astigmatism

INTRAOCULAR PRESSURE. IOP is a hidden variable that seldom receives much attention in terms of refractive effect. Securing the wound in a soft eye has been postulated to result in greater induced postoperative astigmatism, because greater tension is placed on the suture after the IOP increases to the normal range in the postoperative period. Trying to suture at physiological IOPs obviates this effect. A postsuture inflation technique is advocated that utilizes a snug first suture throw, followed by filling of the anterior chamber with balanced salt solution to give a pressure of 7–23mmHg, and then the final throws.[43]

INCISION DISTANCE FROM THE LIMBUS. A more posterior incision is believed to be more stable, as it minimizes any "slip" the cornea may experience from a more anterior (closer to the limbus) incision.[44] Posterior incisions benefit from greater scleral support, which counters wound slippage.

LENGTH OF SUTURE. Long sutures are thought to induce more steepening (with the incision) than short bites, because of the greater forces needed to secure the former.[45] For a given incision that can be closed adequately with a certain number of short sutures, fewer long sutures are required to close the same wound because the greater vector forces generated by each long suture oppose a wider amount of tissue margin.

POSTOPERATIVE CORTICOSTEROIDS. Manipulation of the duration of action of corticosteroids has been advocated to tailor the postoperative course to a desired astigmatic end point. Prolonged use of steroids in selected cases may allow great wound slippage to help treat preexisting WTR astigmatism. Likewise, a short course of postoperative steroids may help minimize astigmatic decay from a superior scleral pocket incision in a patient who has preoperative ATR astigmatism.

ASTIGMATIC KERATOTOMY IN PHACOEMULSIFICATION

Wound manipulation and adjustment of architecture are ways to modulate astigmatism. A near astigmatically neutral cataract extraction may be achieved with a small incision phacoemulsification. Incorporation of astigmatic keratotomy intraoperatively may then provide the surgeon with the most

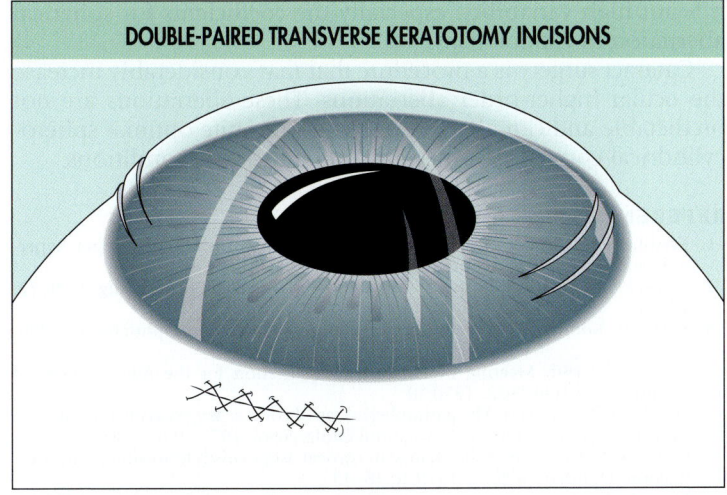

FIG. 27-12 ■ Schematic of cornea with double-paired transverse keratotomy incisions. This technique may be used to correct astigmatism intraoperatively or postoperatively. (Adapted with permission from Maloney WR, Grindle L, Senders D, Pearcy D. Astigmatism control for the cataract surgeon: comprehensive review of surgically tailored astigmatism reduction (STAR). J Cataract Refract Surg. 1989;15:45–54.)

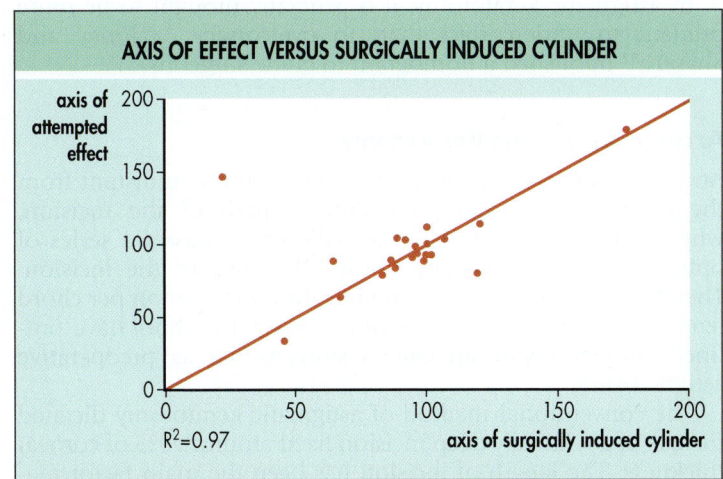

FIG. 27-13 ■ Scatterplot of the axis of the attempted effect versus the axis of the surgically induced cylinder. In patients who had 1.0–1.9D of preexisting astigmatism and who received double-paired keratotomy incisions, a high correlation existed between attempted and achieved axes of correction. (Adapted with permission from Maloney WF, Senders DR, Pearcy DE. Astigmatic keratotomy to correct pre-existing astigmatism in cataract surgery. J Cataract Refract 1990;16:297–304.)

TABLE 27-3

COMPARISON OF THE EFFECT OF TRANSVERSE ASTIGMATIC KERATOTOMY (TAK) AT 7.0MM, 6.0MM, AND 5.5MM OPTICAL ZONES (GROUPS 2, 3, AND 4, RESPECTIVELY)

Group	Preoperative Astigmatism (D)	Number of Eyes	TAK Optical Zone (mm)	Average Preoperative K (K_1) (D)	Average Postoperative K (K_2) (D)	Average Surgically Induced K (K_3) (D)	
						Total	TAK Only (estimate)
1	<1.00 (control)	105	—	0.53 0.43	0.82 0.63	0.78 0.57	— —
2	1.00–2.00	30	7.0	1.24 0.33	0.74 0.56	1.57 0.76	2.04 0.74
3	2.00–3.00	19	6.0	2.36 0.44	0.91 0.81	2.59 0.93	2.85 0.90
4	>3.00	12	5.5	3.62 0.63	1.76 1.00	3.49 1.60	3.52 2.10

Averages and standard deviations of preoperative and postoperative astigmatism, total change in astigmatism, and estimated change in astigmatism from TAK incisions alone are shown. (Adapted with permission from Hall GW, Campion M, Sorenson CM. Reduction of corneal astigmatism at cataract surgery. J Cataract Refract Surg. 1991;17:407–14.)

predictable and stable means of treating a patient for cataract and astigmatism.

Transverse Astigmatic Keratotomy

In addition to its use for postkeratoplasty astigmatism, trapezoidal astigmatic keratotomy was used by Lavery and Lindstrom[46] to correct astigmatism in cataract surgery. Later, their work showed that two transverse corneal incisions produced the greatest degree of flattening, and the radial component was not necessary. This led to the development of transverse astigmatic keratotomy (TAK), which is a method used to manage astigmatism during or after cataract surgery (Fig. 27-12).[44]

Critical factors that influence the amount of meridional flattening are:
- Diameter of the optical zone in which the incisions are made
- Length and depth of the transverse incisions
- Single versus dual paired incisions

Age, gender, and IOP are other factors that determine the way the cornea responds to relaxing incisions.

In 1989, Davison[47] evaluated both single and double pairs of 3.5mm transverse incisions tangential to a 7.0mm optical zone and to 7.0mm and 9.0mm optical zones, respectively. Patients who had preoperative WTR and ATR astigmatism in the single-pair group experienced a decrease of 1.3D and 1.1D, respectively. Patients who had the same preoperative WTR and ATR astigmatism in the double-pair group showed a more striking

decrease of 1.9D and 4.1D, respectively. Larger optical zones were associated with a decreased astigmatic effect from paired transverse incisions.[48] In addition, relaxing incisions placed at smaller optical zones cause increased irregular astigmatism.[49]

Although many patients experience a reduction of preoperative astigmatism, a tendency exists to cause overcorrection. For 1–2D of astigmatism, Maloney et al.[50] showed that paired 3.0mm incisions at the 7.0mm optical zone flattened the cornea on average by 1.96D, which led to overcorrection in 25% of patients; dual incisions at 7.0mm and 8.0mm optical zones led to a similar level of overcorrection. In patients who had greater than 2D of astigmatism, less overcorrection occurred. On average, 7% were undercorrected and 14% were overcorrected with single and dual paired incisions, respectively, and overcorrections occurred in both groups. Both single and double transverse pairs showed good correlation of intended and surgical axes (Fig. 27-13).[50] Placing more shallow incisions, Hall et al.[51] found overall undercorrection derived from 3mm double-paired transverse incisions. More importantly, they calculated the effect of TAK independent of the superior cataract incision by using 105 control patients who had 6.0mm scleral pocket incisions without TAK; on average, these patients had 0.78D of ATR astigmatism change. The flattening from the incision tended to negate the effect of TAK, which was done mostly for ATR astigmatism. At 7.0mm, 6.0mm, and 5.5mm optical zones, the average TAK flattening was 2.04D, 2.85D, and 3.52D, respectively (Table 27-3).[51]

In astigmatic keratotomy, it is generally thought to be more prudent to undercorrect than to overcorrect. Maloney and Shapiro[52] published a nomogram to guide surgeons.

Arcuate Astigmatic Keratotomy

An arcuate incision creates corneal relaxation equidistant from the optical center along the entire length of the incision, whereas a tangential incision actually encompasses a series of optical zones that increase toward the ends of the incision. Therefore, arcuate incisions provide greater relaxation per chord length than do transverse incisions. Several authors have outlined nomograms for arcuate incisions to manage preoperative astigmatism[53]

The conventional method of astigmatic keratotomy dictated the use of a relatively deep incision fixed around 90% of corneal thickness. The length of incision has been the main factor manipulated in controlling the degree of astigmatism correction. Based on patients who underwent astigmatic keratotomy with short incisions and developed undesirable corneal changes, Akura et al.[54] developed a new method. This method uses a relatively long incision (90° in length in regular astigmatism) covering the full arc of the steep area and controls the degree of astigmatic correction by varying the incision depth. They noted that controlling the level of correction by varying the incision depth allows the surgeon to use long incisions covering the entire steep area, minimizing the undesirable changes induced by conventional deep and narrow incisions and resulting in an ideal corneal sphericity after surgery.[54]

Cataract patients may experience an increased depth of focus after corneal relaxing incisions. Gills et al.[53] reported anecdotally good undercorrected near as well distance acuity in patients who had more than 2D of preoperative astigmatism. This effect may occur because residual steep areas, found on topography, contribute to a bifocal effect. Good uncorrected distance and near vision has also been noted after standard cataract extraction with residual myopic astigmatism.[55]

Limbal Relaxing Incisions

Limbal relaxing incisions were first described by Gills and Johnson[56] as a useful method to reduce astigmatism. These incisions are believed to produce more homogeneous coupling and less irregular astigmatism, since they are placed far from the center of the cornea. With a diamond blade set at $600\mu m$, a single 6.0mm incision placed anterior to the palisades of Vogt corrects up to 1D of astigmatism. For 1–2D of astigmatism, paired incisions placed at the steep axis may be used, and for 2–3D, each incision is extended to 8.0mm. For astigmatism greater than 3D, the limbal incisions may be combined with corneal relaxing incisions. These incisions may be used to prevent overcorrection, as their effect is weaker than that of corneal relaxing incisions.

FUTURE TRENDS

Until the 21st century, the methods used to evaluate and correct refractive errors were spectacles, contact lenses, IOLs, and refractive surgeries. But these methods allow the measurement and correction of only the spherical and cylindrical components of refractive errors. With the development of wave front sensing, the method of analyzing refraction and quality of vision has changed. Higher-order aberrations are of some importance in this new paradigm. How cataract surgery changes higher-order aberrations in the human eye is still not fully known. Mierdel et al.[57] published the first pilot study to evaluate the effects of cataract surgery on ocular higher-order aberrations. They found that the averaged Zernike coefficients exhibited no significant differences from normal values, except for the coefficient K_5 (astigmatism at 0° and 90°). However, coefficients showed a significant high variability, especially the coefficients for spherical aberration or astigmatism.

Cataract surgery is a procedure that may considerably increase the ocular higher-order aberrations. These aberrations are not predictable and can affect visual acuity, despite optimal spherocylindrical correction, especially under mesopic conditions.

REFERENCES

1. Kershner RM. Clear corneal cataract surgery and the correction of myopia, hyperopia and astigmatism. Ophthalmology. 1997;104:381–9.
2. Ernest PH, Neuhann T. Posterior limbal incision. J Cataract Refract Surg. 1996;22:78–84.
3. Koch MJ, Kohnen T. Refractive cataract surgery. Curr Opin Ophthalmol. 1999;10:10–5.
4. Stokes GG. 19th Meeting of the British Association for the Advancement of Science. 1849 Trans Sect. 1850;10.
5. Jaffe NS, Clayman HM. The pathophysiology of corneal astigmatism after cataract extraction. Trans Am Acad Ophthalmol Otolaryngol. 1975;79:615–30.
6. Cravy TV. Calculation of the change in corneal astigmatism following cataract extraction. Ophthalmic Surg. 1979;10:38–49.
7. Rowsey JJ. Ten caveats in keratorefractive surgery. Ophthalmology. 1983;90:148–55.
8. Lindstrom RL, Destro MA. Effect of incision size and Terry keratometer usage of postoperative astigmatism. J Am Intraocul Implant Soc. 1985;11:469–73.
9. Neumann AC, McCarty GR, Sanders DR, Raanan MG. Small incisions to control astigmatism during cataract surgery. J Cataract Refract Surg. 1989;15:78–84.
10. Alpins NA. A new method of analyzing vectors for changes in astigmatism. J Cataract Refract Surg. 1993;19:524–33.
11. Steinert RF, Brint SF, White SN, Fine IH. Astigmatism after small incision cataract surgery. Ophthalmology. 1991;98:417–24.
12. Pleger T, Skorpik C, Menapace R, et al. Long-term course of induced astigmatism after clear cornea incision cataract surgery. J Cataract Refract Surg. 1996;22:72–7.
13. Naeser K. Conversion of keratometer readings to polar values. J Cataract Refract Surg. 1990;16:741–5.
14. Holladay JT, Cravy TV, Koch DD. Calculating the surgically induced refractive change following ocular surgery. J Cataract Refract Surg. 1992;18:429–43.
15. Olsen T. Simple method to calculate the surgically induced refractive change. J Cataract Refract Surg. 1993;19:319.
16. Holladay JT, Dudeje DR, Koch DD. Evaluating and reporting astigmatism for individual and aggregate data. J Cataract Refract Surg. 1998;24:57–65.
17. Leiteman T, Proctor KS, Aran DT, Aran NF. Measuring surgically induced astigmatic and prismatic corrections. In: Aran DT, ed. Refractive surgery. Stamford, CT: Appleton & Lange; 1997:185–93.
18. Holladay JT, Moran JR, Kezevan GM. Analysis of aggregate surgically induced refractive change, prediction error, and intraocular astigmatism. J Cataract Refract Surg. 2001;27:61–79.
19. Minassian DC, Rosen P, Dart JK, et al. Extracapsular cataract extraction compared with small incision surgery by phacoemulsification: a randomized trial. Br J Ophthalmol. 2001;85:822–9.
20. Talamo JH, Stark WJ, Jottesch JD, et al. Natural history of corneal astigmatism after cataract surgery. J Cataract Refract Surg. 1991;17:313–8.
21. Storr-Paulsen A, Vangsted P, Perriard A. Long-term and modified course of surgically induced astigmatism after extracapsular cataract extraction. Acta Ophthalmol. 1994;72:617–21.
22. Brint SF, Ostrick M, Bryan JE. Keratometric cylinder and visual performance following phacoemulsification and implantation with silicone small-incision or poly(methylmethacrylate) intraocular lens. J Cataract Refract Surg. 1991;17:32–6.
23. Davison JA. Keratometric comparison of 4.0 and 5.5mm scleral tunnel cataract incision. J Cataract Refract Surg. 1993;19:3–8.
24. Shepherd JR. Induced astigmatism in small incision cataract surgery. J Cataract Refract Surg. 1989;15:85–8.
25. Uusitalo RJ, Ruusuvaara P, Jarvinen E, et al. Early rehabilitation after small incision cataract surgery. Refract Corneal Surg. 1993;9:67–70.
26. Martin RG, Senders DR, Miller JD, et al. Effect of cataract wound incision size on acute changes in corneal topography. J Cataract Refract Surg. 1993;19:170–7.
27. Hayashi K, Hayashi H, Nacao F, Hayashi F. The correlation between incision size and corneal changes in sutureless cataract surgery. Ophthalmology. 1995;102:550–6.
28. Vass C, Menapace R. Computerized statistical analysis of corneal topography for the evaluation of changes in corneal shape after surgery. Am J Ophthalmol. 1994;118:177–84.
29. Vass C, Menapace R, Amon M, et al. Batch by batch analysis of topographic changes induced by sutured and sutureless clear corneal incisions. J Cataract Refract Surg. 1996;22:324–30.
30. Olsen T, Dam-Johansen M, Bek T, Juortdal JO. Evaluating surgically induced astigmatism by Fourier analysis of corneal topography data. J Cataract Refract Surg. 1996;22:318–23.
31. Singer JA. Frown incision for minimizing induced astigmatism after small incision cataract surgery with rigid optic intraocular lens implantation. J Cataract Refract Surg. 1991;17(suppl):677–88.
32. Nielsen PJ. Induced astigmatism and its decay with a frown incision. J Cataract Refract Surg. 1993;19:375–9.
33. Siepser SB. Sutureless cataract surgery with radial transverse incision. J Cataract Refract Surg. 1991;17:716–8.
34. Hennekes R. A high-stability, one-stitch W incision for cataract surgery. J Cataract Refract Surg. 1996;22:407–10.
35. Werblin TP. Refractive stability after cataract extraction using a 6.5-millimeter scleral pocket incision with horizontal or radial sutures. J Refract Corneal Surg. 1994;10:339–42.
36. Buzard KA, Shearing SP. Comparison of postoperative astigmatism with incisions of varying length closed with horizontal sutures and with no sutures. J Cataract Refract Surg. 1991;17:734–9.
37. Ernest PH. Corneal lip incision. J Cataract Refract Surg. 1994;20:154–7.

38. Koch DD, Haft EA, Gay G. Computerized videokeratography analysis of corneal topographic changes induced by sutured and unsutured 4mm scleral pocket incisions. J Cataract Refract Surg. 1993;19:166–9.
39. Martin RG, Senders DR, Van der Karr MA, DeLuca M. Effect of small incision, intraocular lens surgery on postoperative inflammation and astigmatism. J Cataract Refract Surg. 1992;18:51–7.
40. Masket S. Deep versus appositional suturing of the scleral pocket incision for astigmatic control in cataract surgery. J Cataract Refract Surg. 1987;13:131–5.
41. Masket S. Comparison of suturing materials for closure of scleral pocket incisions. J Cataract Refract Surg. 1988;14:548–51.
42. Drews RC. Astigmatism after cataract surgery: nylon versus mersilene. J Cataract Refract Surg. 1995;21:70–2.
43. Pacifico RL, Morrison C. Astigmatically neutral sutured small incision. J Cataract Refract Surg. 1991;17:710–2.
44. Maloney WR, Grindle L, Senders D, Pearcy D. Astigmatism control for the cataract surgeon: comprehensive review of surgically tailored astigmatism reduction (STAR). J Cataract Refract Surg. 1989;15:45–54.
45. Eisner G. An introduction to operative technique, 2nd ed. New York: Springer Verlag; 1978:96–7.
46. Lavery W, Lindstrom RL. Clinical results of trapezoidal astigmatic keratotomy. J Refract Surg. 1985;2:70–4.
47. Davison JA. Transverse astigmatic keratotomy combined with phacoemulsification and intraocular lens implantation. J Cataract Refract Surg. 1989;15:38–44.
48. Osher RH. Paired transverse relaxing keratotomy: a combined technique for reducing astigmatism. J Cataract Refract Surg. 1989;15:32–7.
49. Guell JL, Manero F, Muller A. Transverse keratotomy to correct high corneal astigmatism after cataract surgery. J Cataract Refract Surg. 1996;22:331–6.
50. Maloney WF, Senders DR, Pearcy DE. Astigmatic keratotomy to correct pre-existing astigmatism in cataract surgery. J Cataract Refract Surg. 1990;16:297–304.
51. Hall GW, Campion M, Sorenson CM, et al: Reduction of corneal astigmatism at cataract surgery. J Cataract Refract Surg. 1991;17:407–14.
52. Maloney WR, Shapiro DR. Transverse astigmatic keratotomy: an integral part of small incision cataract surgery. J Cataract Refract Surg. 1992;18:190–4.
53. Gills JP, Martin RG, Thornton SP. Astigmatic keratotomy in the cataract patient. In: Gills JP, Martin RG, Thornton SP, eds. Surgical treatment of astigmatism. Thorofare: Slack; 1994:27–49.
54. Akura J, Matsuura K, Hatta S, et al. A new concept for the correction of astigmatism: full-arc, depth-dependent astigmatic keratotomy. Ophthalmology. 2001;107:95–104.
55. Bradburi JA, Hillman JS. Optimal postoperative refraction for good unaided near and distance vision with monofocal intraocular lenses. Br J Ophthalmol 1992;76:300–2.
56. Gills JP, Johnson DE. Limbal relaxing incisions help reduced astigmatism. Ophthalmol Times. 1996;Nov1:27.
57. Mierdel P, Kaemmerer M, Krinke HE, Seiler T. Effects of photorefractive keratectomy and cataract surgery on ocular optical errors of higher order. Graefes Arch Clin Exp Ophthalmol. 1999;237:725–9.

THE LENS

Emanuel S. Rosen

SECTION I BASIC SCIENCE OF THE LENS

CHAPTER

28

Anatomy

MICHAEL BOULTON • LISA A. SAXBY

DEFINITION
- The lens is a highly organized, transparent structure that has evolved to alter the refractive index of light entering the eye.

KEY FEATURES
- The lens comprises three parts, (1) the capsule, (2) the lens epithelium, and (3) the lens fibers.
- Capsule—an elastic acellular envelope that encloses the epithelium and the lens fibers.
- Lens epithelium—a single layer of cells beneath the anterior capsule which form new fiber cells at the equator.
- Lens fibers—constitute the main mass of the lens and form the basis of the nucleus and cortex and contain high concentrations of crystallin.

GROSS STRUCTURE OF THE ADULT LENS

The adult human lens is an asymmetrical oblate spheroid that does not possess nerves, blood vessels, or connective tissue. The biconvex shape results from the anterior surface being less convex than the posterior surface. The poles represent the center points of these two surfaces—the anteroposterior axis runs from the anterior pole to the posterior pole (polar axis). The equator represents the lateral region of the lens, where the anterior and the posterior surfaces meet. The equatorial axis is at right angles to the anteroposterior axis.[1-5]

The lens is located behind the iris and pupil in the anterior compartment of the eye. The anterior surface is in contact with the aqueous on the corneal side; the posterior surface is in contact with the vitreous and faces the retina. The anterior pole of the lens and the front of the cornea are separated by approximately 3.5mm.[4] The lens is held in place by the zonular fibers (suspensory ligaments), which run between the lens and the ciliary body. These zonular fibers, which originate from the region of the ciliary epithelium, are a series of fibrillin-rich fibers that converge in a circular zone on the lens. Both an anterior and a posterior sheet meet the capsule 1–2mm from the equator and are embedded into the outer part of the capsule (1–2µm deep). It also is thought that a series of fibers meets the capsule at the equator.[2,5]

Histologically the lens consists of three major components—capsule, epithelium, and lens substance (Fig. 28-1).

Capsule

The lens is ensheathed by an elastic acellular envelope, which serves to contain the epithelial cells and fibers as a structural unit and allows the passage of small molecules both into and out of the lens. The thickness of the capsule depends upon the region of the capsule being measured and the age of the individual (thickness increases with age).[2,4,5] The thickest region (up to 23µm) is located close to the equator on both the anterior and the posterior surfaces; the thinnest region is that of the posterior pole (4µm), while the equator (17µm) and the anterior pole (9–14µm) are of intermediate thickness (Fig. 28-2).[5] This basement membrane–like structure is continuously synthesized and represents one of the thickest basement membranes in the body. The capsule is produced anteriorly by the lens epithelium and posteriorly by the elongating fiber cells.

The lens capsule is composed of a number of lamellae stacked on top of each other. The lamellae are narrowest near the outside of the capsule and widest near the cell mass.[6] The anterior capsule also contains linear densities (Fig. 28-3). The major structural proteins (type IV collagen, laminin, heparin sulfate proteoglycan, and entactin) and a small amount of fibronectin are found within the lamellae.[7] Although the precise interactive role of these different components is not known, experiments using lens epithelial cells in culture have shown that collagen IV promotes cellular adhesion and fibronectin promotes migration.[8]

Epithelial Cells

The lens epithelium arises as a single layer of cells beneath the anterior capsule and extends to the equatorial lens bow. These cells have a cuboidal shape, being approximately 10µm high and 15µm wide. Their basal surface adheres to the capsule, whereas their anterior surface abuts the newly formed elongating lens fibers. Lens epithelial cells have large, indented nuclei and a normal array of organelles, which include smooth and rough endoplasmic reticulum, polysomes, ribosomes, lysosomes, mitochondria, and Golgi bodies. They also contain dense bodies and glycogen particles. The lateral membranes of epithelial cells (membranes in contact with the adjacent epithelial cells) are highly tortuous (Fig. 28-4). Adjacent cells are attached to each other by adhesion complexes located in the lateral membranes and include both desmosomes and tight junctions.[1,7,9,10] The desmosomes serve to not only to provide adhesion but also allow the transfer of mechanical stress across the cell sheet via the intermediate filament vimentin. Tight junctions regulate the movement of macromolecules through the extracellular space and, dependent on the number of interlinking strands, can exhibit varying degrees of permeability ranging from impermeable to partially permeable. In the lens this barrier does not appear to restrict the movement of small molecules such as ions and water. Direct communication between lens epithelial cells is via gap junctions that allow the passage of small molecules (less than 1500 Da) between cells. These junctions are composed of connexin 43.[1,9]

Cytoskeletal elements form a network that serves many important functions within the cell. This network provides structural support; controls cell shape and volume, intracellular compartmentalization, and movement of organelles; enables cell movement, distribution of mechanical stress, and chromosome movement during cell division. Lens epithelial cells are known to contain the three main groups of cytoskeletal elements, which are microfilaments (actin), intermediate filaments (vimentin),

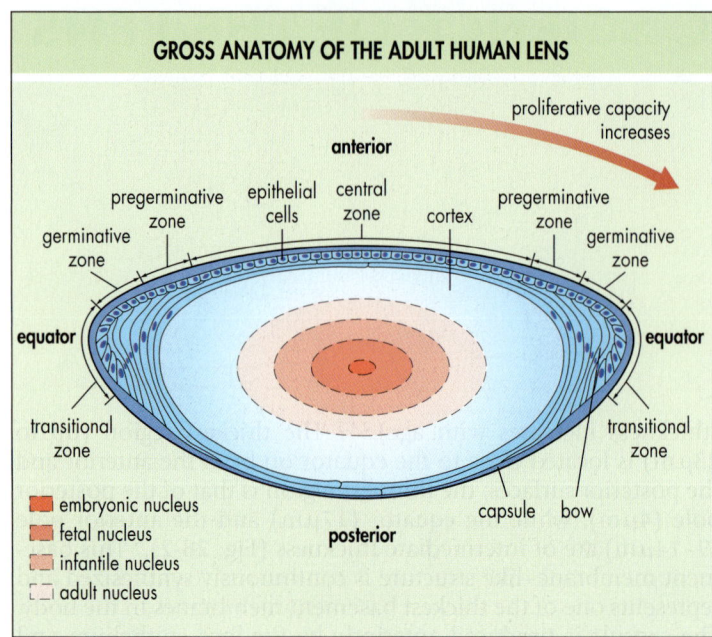

GROSS ANATOMY OF THE ADULT HUMAN LENS

FIG. 28-1 ■ **Gross anatomy of the adult human lens.** Note the different regions are not drawn to scale.

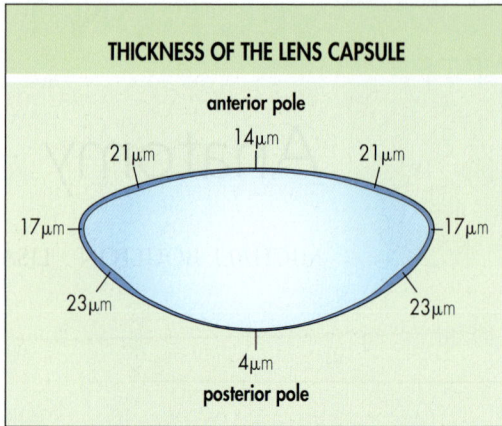

THICKNESS OF THE LENS CAPSULE

FIG. 28-2 ■ Changes in thickness of the adult lens capsule with location.

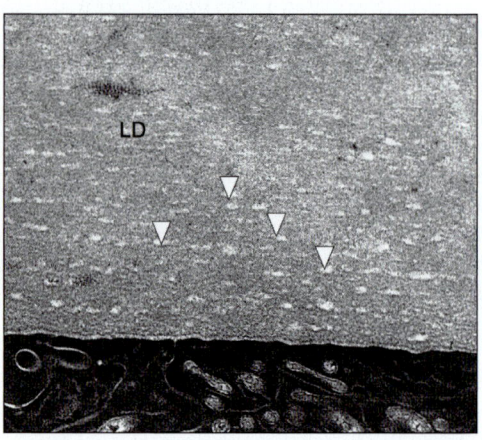

FIG. 28-3 ■ High-power transition electron micrograph of the lens capsule. The linear density (*LD*) exhibits a periodicity of about 60nm as a result of the axial banding of its constituent fibrils. Electron lucent "bubbles" (*arrowheads*) occur between the adjacent lamellae. (Courtesy of GE Marshall. From Phelps Brown N, Bron AJ. Lens structure. In: Phelps Brown N, Bron AJ, Phelps Brown NA. Lens disorders. A clinical manual of cataract diagnosis. Oxford: Butterworth-Heinemann; 1996:32–47.)

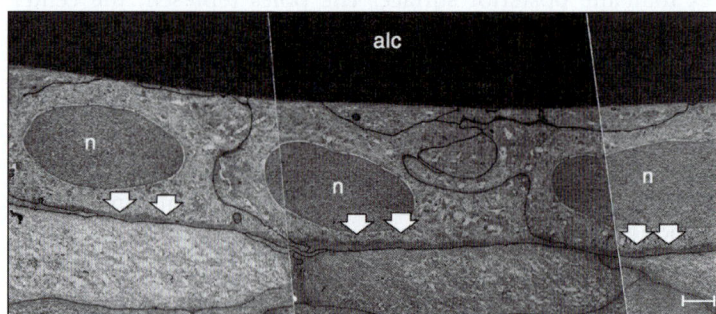

FIG. 28-4 ■ Transmission electron micrograph of lens epithelial cells from a young adult monkey. Montage showing nuclei (*n*), anterior lens capsule (*alc*), markedly indented lateral plasma membrane, apical ends of underlying elongating secondary lens fiber cells and perpendicularly sectioned polygonal arrays of actin bundles or geodomes (*arrows*) immediately subjacent to the apical membranes of lens epithelial cells. (Bar = 1.0μm.) (From Kuszak JR, Brown HG. Embryology and anatomy of the lens. In: Albert DM, Jakobiec FA, eds. Principles and practice of ophthalmology. Basic sciences. Philadelphia: WB Saunders; 1994:82–96.)

and microtubules (tubulin). The β- and γ-actins, which are often cell membrane–associated, normally localize with myosin to make polygonal arrays. Lens epithelial cells also express the proteins spectrin and α-actinin, which play an important role in connecting actin to cell adhesion receptors.[1,11,12] Lens epithelial cells are unique in that they contain vimentin and not cytokeratin, an intermediate filament normally associated with epithelial cells. It is thought that the cytokeratin expression is lost after early invagination of the lens placode. Microtubules composed of α- and β-tubulin are found in small numbers.

The proliferative capacity of epithelial cells varies according to their location (see Fig. 28-1) and is greatest at the equator. Most epithelial cells are found in the central zone, a region in which cells normally do not proliferate, although they may do so under pathological circumstances. Cells in this zone are the largest epithelial cells found in the lens. Cells in the pregerminative zone rarely divide, whereas those in the germinative zone constitute the stem cell population of the lens, and therefore are responsible for the formation of all new fibers and the subsequent increase in size and weight of the lens throughout life. Because cells in the germinative zone are dividing constantly, newly formed cells are forced into the transitional zone where they elongate and differentiate to form the fiber mass of the lens.[1,8] Although it is known that growth factors in the aqueous and vitreous regulate this proliferation and differentiation, the precise nature of these interactions is not understood fully.

Lens Substance

The lens substance, which constitutes the main mass of the lens, is composed of densely packed fibers with very little extracellular space. The adult lens substance consists of the nucleus and the cortex, two regions that often are histologically indistinct. Although the size of these two regions is age dependent, studies of lenses with an average age of 61 years indicate that the nucleus accounts for approximately 84% of the diameter and thickness of the lens and the cortex for the remaining 16%.[13] The nucleus is further subdivided into embryonic, fetal, infantile, and adult nuclei (see Fig. 28-1). The embryonic nucleus contains the original primary lens fiber cells that are formed in the lens vesicle. The rest of the nuclei are composed of secondary fibers, which are added concentrically at the different stages of growth by encircling the previously formed nucleus. The fetal nucleus contains the em-

bryonic nucleus and all fibers added to the lens before birth. The embryonic and fetal nuclei, together with all the fibers added until 4 years of age, compose the infantile nucleus. The adult nucleus is composed of all fibers added before sexual maturation. The cortex, which is located peripherally, is composed of all the secondary fibers continuously formed after sexual maturation and can be divided into the deep, intermediate, and superficial cortex. The region between the hardened embryonic and fetal nuclear core and the soft cortex (i.e., the fibers added to form the in-

FIG. 28-5 ■ **Light micrograph of elongating fibers of a rat lens (thick section along the equatorial axis).** The arrangement of fibers in radial cell columns and concentric growth shells is apparent. Note that while the fibers are generally hexagonal in cross-section, occasional pentagonal cross-sectional profiles are present. (Bar = 10μm.) (From Kuszak JR. The ultrastructure of epithelial and fiber cells in the crystalline lens. Int Rev Cytol. 1995;163:305–50.)

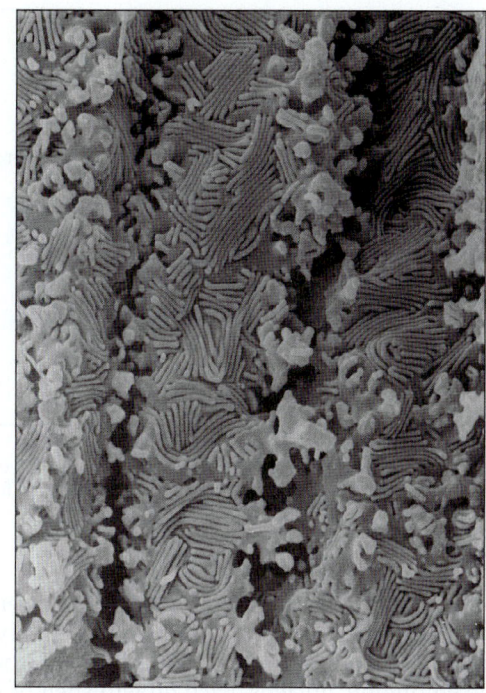

FIG. 28-6 ■ **Scanning electron micrograph of polygonal domains of furrowed membranes.** They are aligned at acute angles to the long axis of the fibers. (From Kuszak JR. The ultrastructure of epithelial and fiber cells in the crystalline lens. Int Rev Cytol. 1995;163:305–50.)

fantile and adult nuclei) sometimes is referred to as the epinucleus. The region between the deep cortex and adult nucleus is sometimes referred to as the perinuclear region.[1,9]

Fibers are formed constantly throughout life by the elongation of lens epithelial cells at the equator. Initially, transitional columnar cells are formed but, once long enough, the anterior end moves forward beneath the anterior epithelial cell layer and the posterior end is pushed backward along the posterior capsule. The ends of this U-shaped fiber run toward the poles of both capsular surfaces.[1–5] Once fully matured, the fiber detaches from the anterior epithelium and the posterior capsule. Each new layer of secondary fibers formed at the periphery of the lens constitutes a new growth shell. Lens fibers from these concentric shells are aligned so that radial cell columns extend from the center of the lens to the periphery (Fig. 28-5). In some regions, neighboring fibers fuse to maintain these columns and ensure that spaces do not develop between the fibers as the lens grows. The growth shell forming at any one time always has more of these fusion zones than the previous shell to ensure that the correct suture is formed. Because new fibers always are added at the periphery and older fibers are internalized, every fiber formed throughout life needs to be maintained and supported.[1,7,9]

The formation of a new fiber is associated with the production of components of the fiber cell membrane—major intrinsic protein 26 (MIP26 or MP26), lipids, phospholipids, and peripheral proteins. Lens fiber membranes contain similar amounts of proteins and lipids. The major sterol is cholesterol (50–60% of total lipid) and the major phospholipid is sphingomyelin (47–56% of the total phospholipid). The predominant saturated fatty acid is palmitate. The high levels of these three constituents result in a highly ordered membrane with very little fluidity.[14]

The newly formed lens fibers have a consistent hexagonal cross-sectional morphology with six faces, two of which are broad and four of which are narrow. These hexagonal fibers are approximately 2μm thick, 10μm wide, and up to 10mm long. More centrally located fibers lose their uniform shape and adopt an irregular polygonal profile in cross-section.[1,9] One study of adult lenses shows that fibers in the embryonic nucleus have an

average cross-sectional area of approximately 80μm², and those added to form the fetal, infantile, and adult nuclei and the cortex have cross-sectional areas of approximately 35, 14, 7, and 24μm², respectively.[13] Superficial elongating lens fibers still contain most of the organelles present in epithelial cells. As the fibers are internalized and elongate further, the cell nucleus is displaced anteriorly. The cell nucleus of the newest fiber, therefore, always is located more posteriorly, which results in the formation of a lens bow. Organelles also are lost and, as a result, the principal cytoplasmic components of a mature fiber cell are crystallins and the cytoskeleton.[2,3] The cytoskeletal components are almost the same as those found in the epithelial cells, except for an additional structure known as the beaded chain, the function of which is of potentially great interest because of its uniqueness to lens fibers. The cytoskeletal components are not distributed evenly throughout the fiber mass. Although actin is found in all fibers, vimentin, tubulin, and myosin are found only in cortical fibers. Beaded chains, which emerge in the differentiating fibers and are found in all mature fibers, may play a role in the loss of the nucleus.[11,12]

Lens fibers are held together by the interlocking of the lateral plasma membranes of adjacent fibers to form ball-and-socket and tongue-and-groove joints. These joints, which are found at regular intervals along the length of their membranes, are characterized by square array membranes. Once matured, fibers have polygonal domains of furrowed membranes along both their broad and narrow faces (Fig. 28-6). Both desmosomes and tight junctions are absent from mature lens fibers, although desmosomes are found between elongating fibers.[1,7,9] Of the protein found in lens fiber plasma membranes, 50–60% is MP26 (approximately 26kDa). Although this protein is thought to be the major gap junction protein, it has no sequence homology with well-known gap junction proteins. It is found also in other regions of the membrane, in which it is thought to promote cell–cell attachment. It has been suggested that MP70 (approximately 70kDa) may be the major gap junction protein, but this polypeptide is found only in the outer lens cortex. It is degraded to MP38 (approximately 38kDa) in the more internal regions of the lens.[11,14,15]

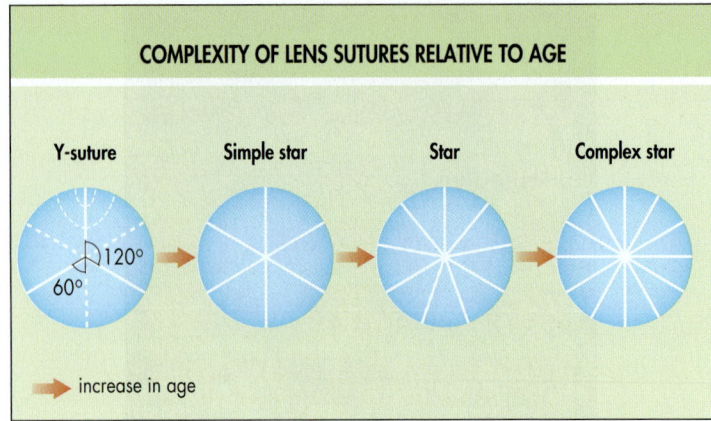

FIG. 28-7 ■ **Increase in complexity of lens sutures with age.** Dotted area represents the inferior suture pattern and is drawn only at the Y-suture stage for simplicity.

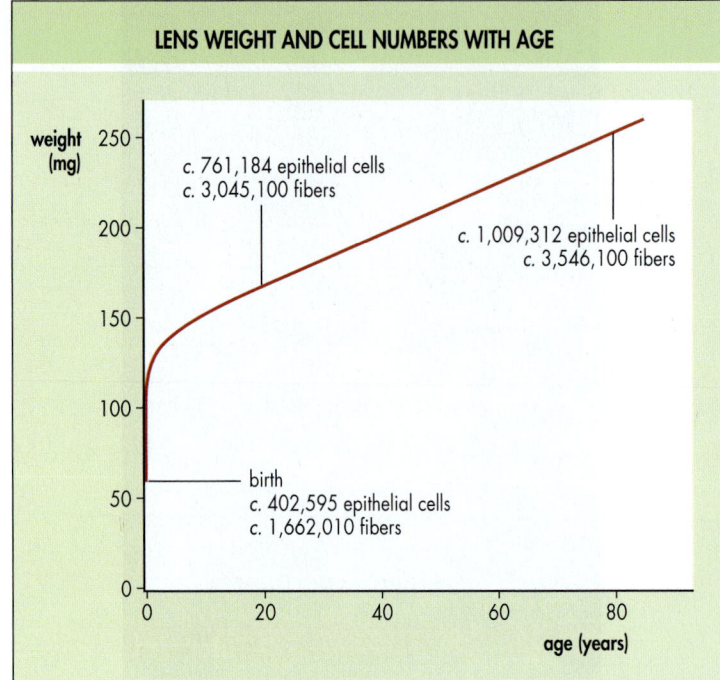

FIG. 28-8 ■ **Increase in lens weight and cell numbers with age.** Note the correlation between these two parameters. (Lens weight data from Phelps Brown N, Bron AJ. Lens growth. In Phelps Brown N, Bron AJ, Phelps Brown NA. Lens disorders. A clinical manual of cataract diagnosis. Oxford: Butterworth-Heinemann; 1996:17–31. Cell number data from Kuszak JR, Brown HG. Embryology and anatomy of the lens. In: Albert DM, Jakobiec FA, eds. Principles and practices of ophthalmology. Basic sciences. Philadelphia: WB Saunders; 1994:82–96.)

Sutures

Sutures are found at both the anterior and the posterior poles. They are formed by the overlap of ends of secondary fibers in each growth shell. No sutures are found between the primary fibers in the embryonic nucleus. Each growth shell of secondary fibers formed before birth has an anterior suture shaped as an "erect Y" and a posterior suture shaped as an "inverted Y." Each of these symmetrical sutures is composed of three branches, each 120 degrees apart. The anterior and the posterior suture are offset by 60 degrees. After birth, suture pattern complexity increases with increasing age, because of the addition of progressively more fibers and changes in both fiber length and shape (Fig. 28-7). Although discontinuous suture planes are formed after birth, the sutures remain symmetrical until sexual maturation. During childhood a "simple star" suture with six branches is formed. This changes to a "star" suture with nine branches during adolescence and finally to a "complex star" suture with 12 or more branches during adulthood. Observations of the adult lens indicate that these four different types of suture—Y, simple star, star, and complex star—are found in the fetal, infantile, and adult nuclei, and in the lens cortex, respectively. The formation of sutures enables the shape of the lens to change from spherical to that of a flattened biconvex sphere.[1,9,16]

The formation of the different suture patterns corresponds to the localization of the zones of discontinuity, which are found at both the anterior and the posterior of the lens. There are four of these zones, which originate at approximately 4, 9, 19, and 46 years of age. These zones are initiated at the edge of the lens and then internalized as more new fibers are added at the periphery. They represent regions of increased light scatter due to the loss of structural uniformity.[17]

GROWTH

The growth of the lens throughout life is a unique characteristic not shared with any other internal organ. The growth rate, which is greatest in the young, diminishes with increasing age. During an average lifespan the surface area of the lens capsule increases from 80mm² at birth to 180mm² by the seventh decade.[2,6] The rate of increase in cell numbers parallels the increase in both mass and dimensions of the lens, and therefore decreases dramatically after the second decade. Numbers of both epithelial cells and fibers increase by approximately 45–50% during the first two decades (Fig. 28-8). After this the increase in cell numbers is reduced, with the proportional increase in fibers being very small.[1]

MASS

The weight of the lens rapidly increases from 65mg at birth to 125mg by the end of the first year. Lens weight then increases at

approximately 2.8mg/year until the end of the first decade, by which time the lens has reached 150mg. Thereafter, the mass of the lens increases at a slower rate (1.4mg/year) to reach about 260mg by the age of 90 years (see Fig. 28-8).[18] The lenses of men are heavier than those of women of the same age, the mean difference being 7.9 ± 2.47mg (once adjusted for age).[19]

DIMENSIONS

The equatorial diameter of the human lens increases throughout life, although the rate of increase is reduced significantly after the second decade. The diameter increases from approximately 5mm at birth to 9–10mm in a 20 year old. The thickness of the lens increases at a much slower rate than does the equatorial diameter. The distance from the anterior to the posterior poles, which is 3.5–4mm at birth, increases throughout life, reaching up to 4.75–5mm (unaccommodated).[4,18] The thickness of the nucleus decreases with age, as the result of compaction, whereas cortical thickness increases as more fibers are added at the periphery. Because the increase in cortical thickness is greater than the decrease in size of the nucleus, the polar axis of the lens increases with age.[20] The radius of curvature of the anterior surface decreases from 16mm at the age of 10 years to 8mm by the age of 80 years as this surface becomes more curved. There is very little change in the radius of curvature of the posterior surface, which remains at approximately 8mm.

REFERENCES

1. Kuszak JR, Brown HG. Embryology and anatomy of the lens. In: Albert DM, Jakobiec FA, eds. Principles and practice of ophthalmology. Basic sciences. Philadelphia: WB Saunders; 1994:82–96.
2. Snell RS, Lemp MA. The eyeball. In: Clinical anatomy of the eye. Oxford: Blackwell Scientific; 1989:119–94.
3. Davson H. The lens. In: Physiology of the eye, ed 5. London: Macmillan Press; 1990:139–201.
4. Saude T. The internal ocular media. In: Ocular anatomy and physiology. Oxford: Blackwell Scientific; 1993:36–52.
5. Forrester J, Dick A, McMenamin P, Lee W. Anatomy of the eye and orbit. In: Forrester JV, Dick AD, McMenamin P, Lee WR. The eye: basic sciences in practice. London: WB Saunders; 1996:1–86.

6. Seland JH. The lens capsule and zonulae. Acta Ophthalmol. 1992;70 (Suppl 205):7–12.
7. Phelps Brown N, Bron AJ. Lens structure. In: Phelps Brown N, Bron AJ, Phelps Brown NA. Lens disorders: a clinical manual of cataract diagnosis. Oxford: Butterworth-Heinemann; 1996:32–47.
8. Olivero DK, Furcht LT. Type IV collagen, laminin, and fibronectin promote the adhesion and migration of rabbit lens epithelial cells. Invest Ophthalmol Vis Sci. 1996;34:2825–34.
9. Kuszak JR. The ultrastructure of epithelial and fiber cells in the crystalline lens. Int Rev Cytol. 1995;163:305–50.
10. Lo W, Harding CV. Tight junctions in the lens epithelia of human and frog: freeze-fracture and protein tracer studies. Invest Ophthalmol Vis Sci. 1983;24:396–402.
11. Zigler JS. Lens proteins. In: Albert DM, Jakobiec FA, eds. Principles and practice of ophthalmology. Basic sciences. Philadelphia: WB Saunders; 1994:97–113.
12. Rafferty NS, Rafferty KA. Lens cytoskeleton and after-cataract. Acta Ophthalmol. 1992;70(Suppl 205):34–45.
13. Taylor VL, Al-Ghoul KJ, Lane CW, *et al*. Morphology of the normal human lens. Invest Ophthalmol Vis Sci. 1996;37:1396–410.
14. Berman ER. Lens. In: Blakemore C, ed. Biochemistry of the eye. New York: Plenum Press; 1991:201–90.
15. Johnson KR, Sas DF, Johnson RG. MP26, a protein of intercellular junctions in the bovine lens: electrophoretic and chromatographic characterization. Exp Eye Res. 1991;52:629–39.
16. Kuszak JR. The development of lens sutures. Prog Retina Eye Res. 1995; 14:567–91.
17. Koretz JF, Cook CA, Kuszak JR. The zones of discontinuity in the human lens: development and distribution with age. Vision Res. 1994;34:2955–62.
18. Phelps Brown N, Bron AJ. Lens growth. In: Phelps Brown N, Bron AJ, Phelps Brown NA. Lens disorders. A clinical manual of cataract diagnosis. Oxford: Butterworth-Heinemann; 1996:17–31.
19. Harding JJ, Rixon KC, Marriott FHC. Men have heavier lenses than women of the same age. Exp Eye Res. 1977;25:651.
20. Cook CA, Koretz JF, Pfahnl A, *et al*. Aging of the human crystalline lens and anterior segment. Vision Res. 1994;34:2945–54.

MICHAEL BOULTON • LISA A. SAXBY

DEFINITION

- Lens function and transparency is dependent on the supply of appropriate nutrients to its different structures.

KEY FEATURES

- The metabolic needs of the adult lens are met by the aqueous and vitreous humors.
- There is continuous transport of ions into and out of the lens.
- Transport of molecules across the lens is dependent upon channels, pumps, transporters, charge, cell–cell coupling, and occluding junctions.

PERMEABILITY, DIFFUSION, AND TRANSPORT

After involution of the hyaloid blood supply to the lens (tunica vasculosa lentis), the metabolic needs of the lens are met by the aqueous and the vitreous humors. The capsule is freely permeable to water, ions, other small molecules, and proteins with a molecular weight up to 70kDa. The tight junctions between the epithelial cells do not restrict greatly the movement of molecules into the fiber mass. Epithelial cells and fibers possess a number of different channels, pumps, and transporters that enable transepithelial movement to and from the extracellular milieu. Because the extracellular space, especially in the cortex and nucleus, is narrow and tortuous, the existence of a network of gap junctions provides a hydrophilic passage that greatly increases the intracellular diffusion rate.[1] These junctions allow exchange of small molecules across epithelial–epithelial, epithelial–fiber, and fiber–fiber boundaries. However, because there is only a small amount of coupling between epithelial cells and the elongating fibers, and this predominantly is localized to the pregerminative, germinative, and transitional zones, it is thought that transport between epithelial and fiber cells also involves rapid endocytosis, particularly in the central region (Fig. 29-1).[2]

Transport of Ions

A lens cell contains large concentrations of negatively charged crystallins. As a result, a large number of positively charged cations enters the lens cell to maintain electrical neutrality, and therefore the osmolarity of the intracellular fluid becomes greater than that of the extracellular fluid. Because water enters the cell by osmosis, if this entry were not controlled the lens cells would swell and eventually burst. Fluid flow is minimized by the resting potential of the plasma membrane being set at a negative voltage using, principally, potassium (K^+)-selective channels. An equilibrium is reached when the electrical force that attracts these ions is balanced by the outward leak of K^+ down its concentration gradient. Any sodium (Na^+) that leaks into the cell down its electrochemical gradient is pumped out by Na^+,K^+-adenosinetriphosphatase (Na^+,K^+-ATPase). Because two K^+ ions are pumped into the cell as three Na^+ ions are

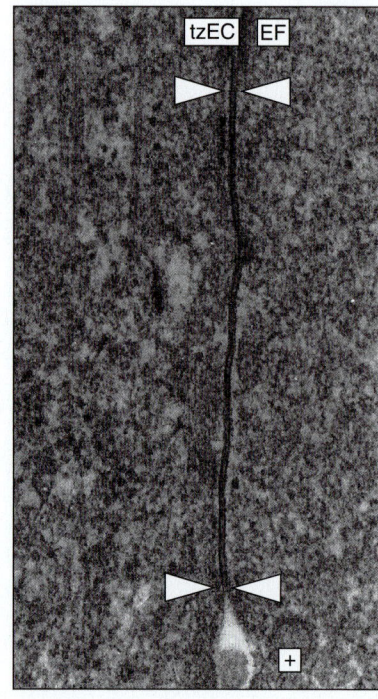

FIG. 29-1 ⬛ High-magnification transition electron micrograph of a thin-section of transitional zone epithelial cells (tzEC) and the underlying elongating fibers (EF). Occasional gap junctions *(arrowheads)* and clathrin-coated vesicles *(cross)* can be seen in these regions of the epithelial–fiber interface. (With permission from Kuszak JR, Novak LA, Brown HG. An ultrasound analysis of the epithelial–fiber interface [EFI] in primate lenses. Exp Eye Res. 1995;61:579–97.)

pumped out, the ATPase also helps control intracellular K^+ levels. Although the lens possesses nonselective cation channels, which allow the passage of both Na^+ and K^+, the role of these channels in the maintenance of the resting voltage is unclear. Chloride (Cl^-) is thought to be at equilibrium across the cell membrane and therefore its distribution is controlled by the resting voltage. Most Cl^- movement is thought to be via carrier mechanisms, although chloride channels have been found in the fiber plasma membrane.[1]

Levels of Na^+ are greatest in the posterior cortex and much lower in the remainder of the lens. The converse is true for K^+ levels, which are greatest in the anterior fibers. Because lens fibers extend from pole to pole, the Na^+ and K^+ concentration gradients must also exist within the fiber cytoplasm. The distribution of these two ions is controlled by a number of factors.
- Na^+,K^+-ATPase activity is greatest in the epithelial cells.
- Different isoforms of the Na^+,K^+-ATPase, which have different activities, are expressed in the epithelial cells and fibers.[3]
- The Na^+ and K^+ ions move asymmetrically across the lens. Na^+ ions influx through both the anterior and the posterior poles using Na^+-specific channels found in the fibers, diffuse through the lens down their concentration gradient, and are pumped out by the Na^+,K^+-ATPase in the epithelial layer.

The Na^+ ions removed are exchanged actively for K^+ ions, which diffuse through the lens down their concentration gradi-

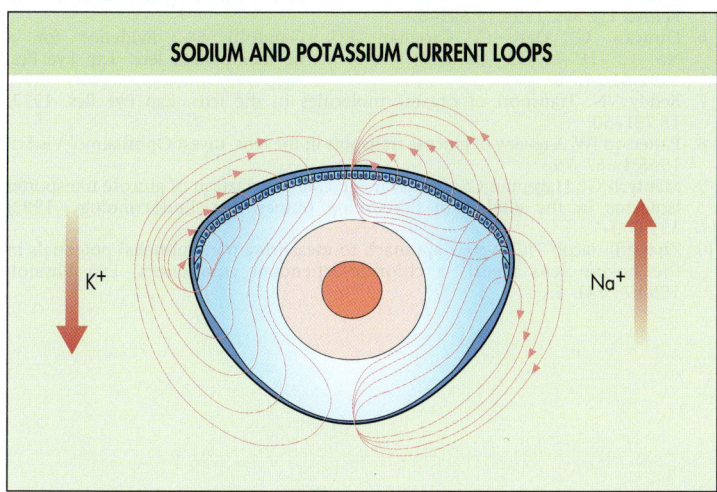

FIG. 29-2 ■ Sodium and potassium current loops. (Adapted from Patterson JW. Characterization of the equational current of the lens. Ophthalmic Res. 1998; 20:139–42.)

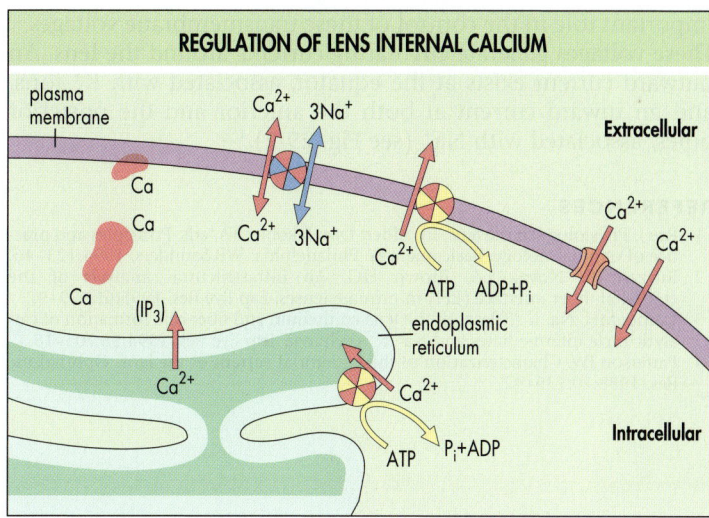

FIG. 29-3 ■ Regulation of lens internal calcium. Outline of the mechanisms involved in the regulation of lens internal calcium.

ent and leave through ion channels in both the epithelial cells and surface fibers. There is a net movement of Na^+ ions from posterior to anterior and of K^+ ions from anterior to posterior (Fig. 29-2).[4]

In the normal lens the intracellular concentration of calcium (Ca^{++}) is below 0.1% of that found in the ocular humors, which enables this cation to function as an intracellular messenger. High external Ca^{++} levels in the aqueous and vitreous humors play an important role in the control of membrane permeability to both Na^+ and K^+. Because the extracellular concentrations of Ca^{++} are high and the charge inside of the cell is negative, Ca^{++} moves down its electrochemical gradient to enter cells through nonselective cation channels and also by receptor-mediated endocytosis. The low intracellular concentration of Ca^{++} is maintained by several different mechanisms (Fig. 29-3). The most important of these is thought to be a calmodulin-regulated Ca^{++}-ATPase, found in the cell membranes of both epithelial cells and fibers, which actively pumps Ca^{++} out of the cell. A Na^+/Ca^{++} exchange mechanism, dependent upon the Na^+ gradient within the lens, also plays a significant role. For every three Na^+ ions transported in, one Ca^{++} ion is extruded. Also, Ca^{++} can be sequestered at binding sites in the plasma membrane and cytosol (e.g., by phospholipids, crystallins, and calmodulin-binding proteins). The endoplasmic reticulum, an organelle found in both the epithelial cells and surface cortical fibers, stores Ca^{++} by using a calmodulin-independent Ca^{++}-ATPase and a Ca^{++} channel gated by inositol 1,4,5-triphosphate to remove this cation from the cytoplasm.[1,5]

Although a pH gradient exists, which increases from the central nucleus to the peripheral layers, the intracellular pH of the lens is approximately 7.0. Lens cells need continually to extrude intracellular protons that are generated from lactic acid, as a result of anaerobic glycolysis, and by the continuous inward movement of positive ions from the extracellular space. The pH is regulated by mechanisms capable of increasing and decreasing intracellular acid levels. Molecules, especially proteins, with the capacity to act as buffers also play a role. Many of the transporters used are thought to be localized to the epithelial cells and the surface fibers. Lenses of various species also have been shown to possess a Na^+/HCO_3^- cotransporter, a Cl^-/HCO_3^- exchanger, a Na^+/H^+ exchanger,[1] and a $Na^+/Cl^-/H^+/HCO_3^-$ exchange system which is activated when intracellular pH levels fall.[6]

Amino Acid and Sugar Transport

Although amino acids can enter the lens across both the anterior and posterior surfaces, most amino acids are transported into the lens from the aqueous. Because the amino acid content of the lens is higher than that of the surrounding ocular fluids, this movement occurs against a concentration gradient by using an active transport process which is localized to the epithelial layer. At least three different carrier systems exist to transport amino acids of different charge (acidic, neutral, and basic). The lens contains most, if not all, amino acids and also can convert keto acids into amino acids. The lens acts as a "pump–leak" system: amino acids are "pumped" into the lens through the anterior capsule and passively "leak" out through the posterior capsule. It is thought also that the efflux of some amino acids involves mobile carriers. By balancing the rate of entrance and exit, a steady state concentration is maintained.[7]

The lens differentiates the optical isomers of sugars and usually transports the D-form (with the exception of L-arabinose). D-Glucose, which enters the lens by insulin-independent facilitated transport, is not found at concentrations that exceed those of the surrounding environment. Although glucose has the capacity to enter via both the anterior and the posterior surfaces, most enters from the aqueous humor. Transporters are found mainly in the fibers, although some also are present in epithelial cells.[1,8] Glut-1, one of the seven isoforms of mammalian facilitative glucose transporters characterized, is expressed in fibers. L-Glucose, which is not transported actively into the lens but slowly enters by passive diffusion, is found only in the epithelial cells and outer cortical regions.[9]

ELECTROPHYSIOLOGY

The membrane potential of an isolated human lens is approximately $-50mV$ at 20 years of age and decreases to $-20mV$ by the age of 80 years. This membrane potential exists because the inside of each cell is negative and the outside is positive. Three common K^+-selective channels occur, localized to the epithelial cells, which are thought to be responsible for much of this conductance and, as a result, set the negative resting potential. These channels generate three currents:

- An outwardly rectifying current, which contributes to membrane conductance at the resting voltage
- An inwardly rectifying current, important for setting the resting voltage
- A calcium activated current, function unknown

Although the intracellular voltage is very similar throughout the lens, the extracellular voltage changes from the center to the surface of the lens. As a result, transmembrane voltages are generated which vary as a function of depth.[1] The Cl^- distribution, which also varies as a function of depth, is thought to play an important role in the control of these transmembrane voltages.[10] These voltages generate circulating currents around the lens. An outward current exists at the equator, associated with K^+ ions, and an inward current at both the anterior and the posterior poles, associated with Na^+ (see Fig. 29-2).[4]

REFERENCES

1. Rae J. Physiology of the lens. In: Albert DM, Jakobiec FA, eds. Principles and practice of ophthalmology. Basic sciences. Philadelphia: WB Saunders; 1994:123–46.
2. Kuszak JR, Novak LA, Brown HG. An ultrastructural analysis of the epithelial–fiber interface (EFI) in primate lenses. Exp Eye Res. 1995;61:579–97.
3. Garner MH. Na, K-ATPases of the lens epithelium and fiber cell: formation of catalytic cycle intermediates and $Na^+:K^+$ exchange. Exp Eye Res. 1994;58:705–18.
4. Patterson JW. Characterization of the equatorial current of the lens. Ophthalmic Res. 1988;20:139–42.
5. Duncan G, Williams MR, Riach RA. Calcium, cell signaling and cataract. Prog Retinal Eye Res. 1994;13:623–52.
6. Duncan G, Dart C, Croghan PC, Gandolfi SA. Evidence for a Na^+–Cl^-–H^+–$HCO3^-$ exchange system in the mammalian lens. Exp Eye Res. 1992;54:941–6.
7. Reddy VN. Transport of organic molecules in the lens. Exp Eye Res. 1973; 15:731–50.
8. Patterson JW. A review of glucose transport in the lens. Invest Ophthalmol Vis Sci. 1965;4:667–79.
9. Mantych GJ, Hageman GS, Devaskar SU. Characterization of glucose transporter isoforms in the adult and developing human eye. Endocrinology. 1993; 133:600–7.
10. Zhang JJ, Jacob TJC. A new approach to measuring transepithelial potentials in the bovine lens reveals a chloride-dependent component. Exp Physiol. 1994;79:741–53.

CHAPTER
30

Biophysics

MICHAEL BOULTON • LISA A. SAXBY

DEFINITION
- The lens serves two major functions
  —Focusing visible light rays on the fovea, and
  —Preventing damaging ultraviolet radiation from reaching the retina.

KEY FEATURES
- Transparency is dependent on the highly organized structure of the lens and the dense packing of crystallin.
- Ability to change its focusing power by a process called accommodation.
- Accommodation occurs by increasing the curvature of the anterior surface, thereby changing the refractive index of the lens.

ASSOCIATED FEATURES
- Light transmission and elasticity of the lens decreases with age.

LIGHT TRANSMISSION

The cornea and lens act as spectral filters absorbing the more energetic wavelengths of the magnetic spectrum (i.e., ultraviolet [UV] radiation) that have the potential to damage the retina. The cornea absorbs wavelengths below 295nm while the lens absorbs strongly in the long UV-B (300–315nm) and the full UV-A (315–400nm) wavelengths. Both the cornea and the lens also absorb part of the infrared radiation at water bands at 980nm, 1200nm, and 1430nm. The transmission of visible light decreases with increasing age, a feature that arises largely from age-related changes and brunescence in the lens (Fig. 30-1).[1,2] The total transmittance of the young lens begins increasing rapidly at about 310nm and reaches 90% at 450nm, compared with the older lens (e.g., 63 years) which begins transmitting at 400nm but does not reach 90% total transmittance until 540nm. There are also spectral changes in transmission, with more short-wavelength radiation reaching the retina in the young eye when compared with the old eye (Fig. 30-1). In children under 5 years there is a transmission band centered around 320nm of about 8%. It is reduced by the age of 22 years to 0.1%, and by the age of 60 years no UV radiation reaches the retina except in aphakic eyes.

TRANSPARENCY

During the early stages of embryonic development the lens is opaque, but as development continues and the hyaloid vascular supply is lost, the lens becomes transparent. The young lens is transparent because of the absence of chromophores able to absorb visible light and the presence of a highly organized structure that gives minimal light scatter (less than 5% in the normal human lens). Although the epithelial cells contain large organelles that scatter light, the combined refractive index of this layer and the capsule is no different from the refractive index of the aqueous, so light scatter in this area is minimized. Because lens fibers form a hexagonal lattice and the amount of intercellular space is small, the differences in the refractive index between the plasma membranes of lens fibers and the cytoplasm are regularly placed throughout the lens. These membranes, therefore, do not cause turbidity but act as a diffusion grating. Although newly formed cortical fibers still contain all the organelles present in epithelial cells, these cells do not cause any significant light scatter because while they elongate they are not in the visual axis. Once the fibers have elongated fully and matured, these organelles have degenerated, so the amount of particulate matter in the cytoplasm has decreased and therefore the amount of scatter is minimized. Although crystallins form approximately 30% by weight of the lens fiber cytoplasm (the majority of the remaining 70% is water), they cause a minimal amount of scatter because they are packed in such a way that a high level of short-range spatial order exists. This is possible because of the nonspecific interactions between the different crystallin families, which ensure that a closely packed, even distribution of these proteins occurs within the cytoplasm. The scatter from two neighboring molecules tends to cancel out the refractive index fluctuation between protein molecules. Coupling of the epithelial layer, cortex, and nucleus allows the control of ion levels, water content, and pH needed to maintain lens transparency.[3,4]

REFRACTIVE INDICES

Light travels in straight lines. Refraction is the process whereby light rays are bent as they move from a medium of one refractive index to a medium of a different refractive index. Although light is refracted at the cornea, aqueous humor, lens, and vitreous humor, the major sites of refraction in the eye are the anterior surface of the cornea and the lens. Because the difference in refractive index is higher between the air–cornea than the aqueous–lens and lens–vitreous interfaces, the refractive power of the cornea (~40D) is considerably greater than that of the lens (<15D).[5]

A gradient of refractive index increases from 1.386 in the peripheral cortex to 1.41 in the central nucleus of the lens. Because both the curvature and refractive index of the lens increase from the periphery toward the center, each successive layer of fibers has more refractive power and, therefore, can bend light rays to a greater extent.[5] The anterior capsular surface of the lens has a greater refractive index than the posterior capsular surface (1.364–1.381 compared with 1.338–1.357). These values, however, do not alter from the center to the periphery of either capsular surface. It is possible that the difference in refractive index between the anterior and the posterior capsule is related to the thickness of these two surfaces.[6]

The change in refractive index from the surface of the lens to the center results from changes in protein concentration; the higher the concentration, the greater the refractive power. This increase must occur as a result of both packing and hydration properties, because protein synthesis in the nucleus is minimal.[1,3] The protein content of the adult human lens is highest in the nucleus

249

(approximately 37% of lens weight), when levels remain relatively constant across the central 3–4mm of the polar axis, but drop quite quickly at the peripheral 0.4–0.6mm of the lens (approximately 20% of lens weight in cortex) (Fig. 30-2). This change in protein content is even and continuous, which produces a refractive index free of significant discontinuities.[7] Because crystallins make up approximately 90% of the protein content of the lens, this group of proteins is primarily responsible for this variation across the lens. The γ-crystallins are attracted to each other, whereas the α-crystallins and β-crystallins repulse each other. Because the γ-crystallins are located primarily in the nucleus, their close packing helps to increase the refractive index in this region of the lens.[3] The increase in crystallin concentration also correlates with the change in water content of the lens; 80% of the fresh weight of the anterior cortex plus epithelium and 75% of the fresh weight of the posterior cortex is water. However, only 68% of the fresh weight of the nucleus is water.[8]

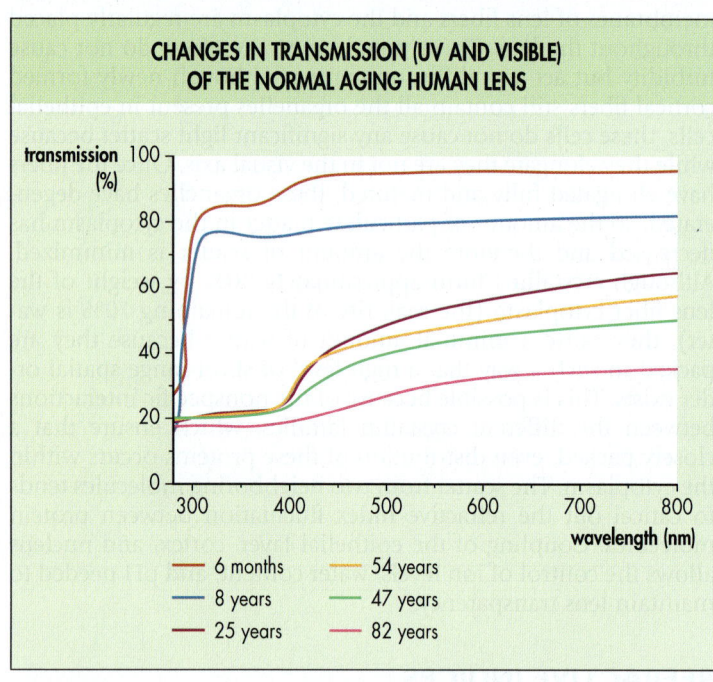

CHANGES IN TRANSMISSION (UV AND VISIBLE) OF THE NORMAL AGING HUMAN LENS

- 6 months
- 8 years
- 25 years
- 54 years
- 47 years
- 82 years

FIG. 30-1 ■ **Changes in transmission (UV and visible) of the normal aging human lens.** (From Lerman S. Lens transparency and aging. In: Regnault F, Hockwin O, Courtios Y, eds. Ageing of the lens. Amsterdam: Elsevier/North-Holland Biomedical Press; 1980:263–79.)

OPTICAL PERFORMANCE

When visible light passes through the lens it is split into all the colors of the spectrum. The different wavelengths of these colors result in different rates of transmission through the lens and some deviation. As a consequence, yellow light (570–595nm) normally is focused on the retina; light of shorter wavelengths, for example blue (440–500nm), falls in front because of the slower transmission and increased refraction compared with yellow light; and light of longer wavelengths, for example red (620–770nm) (Fig. 30-3), falls behind because of the faster transmission and less refraction. However, although the lens is not designed to correct this chromatic aberration, yellow is normally the ray of greatest intensity. Because the amount of dispersion between the red and the blue images is approximately 1.5–2D, very little reduction occurs in the clarity of the image that is formed on the retina. As the lens accommodates, refraction increases as a result of the increasing power of the lens and, therefore, the amount of chromatic aberration also increases.[5,9-11]

Light rays that pass through the periphery of an optical lens have a focal length shorter than that of light rays that pass through the center (Fig. 30-4). This occurs because the refractive power is greater at the periphery, so the light rays are refracted to a greater degree as they pass through this region. The lens of the human eye is designed to minimize this spherical aberration.

- Refractive index increases from the periphery to the center of the lens.
- Curvature of both the anterior and the posterior capsule increases towards the poles.
- Curvature of the anterior capsule is greater than that of its posterior counterpart.

As a result of these structural features the focal points of the peripheral and central rays are similar, which ensures that the reduction in the quality of the image is minimal. The pupil diameter also affects the amount of spherical aberration, because light rays do not pass through the periphery of the lens (unless the pupil is dilated). The optimal size of the pupil needed to minimize this imperfection is 2–2.5mm.[5,9-11]

Many other aberrations of the lens occur, but these are not as important as either chromatographic or spherical aberration. The refractive surfaces of the cornea and the lens are not precisely on the optical axis. As a result, the image is decentered, but because the amount of decentering is small, the formed image is not greatly affected. Coma, oblique astigmatism, and distortion

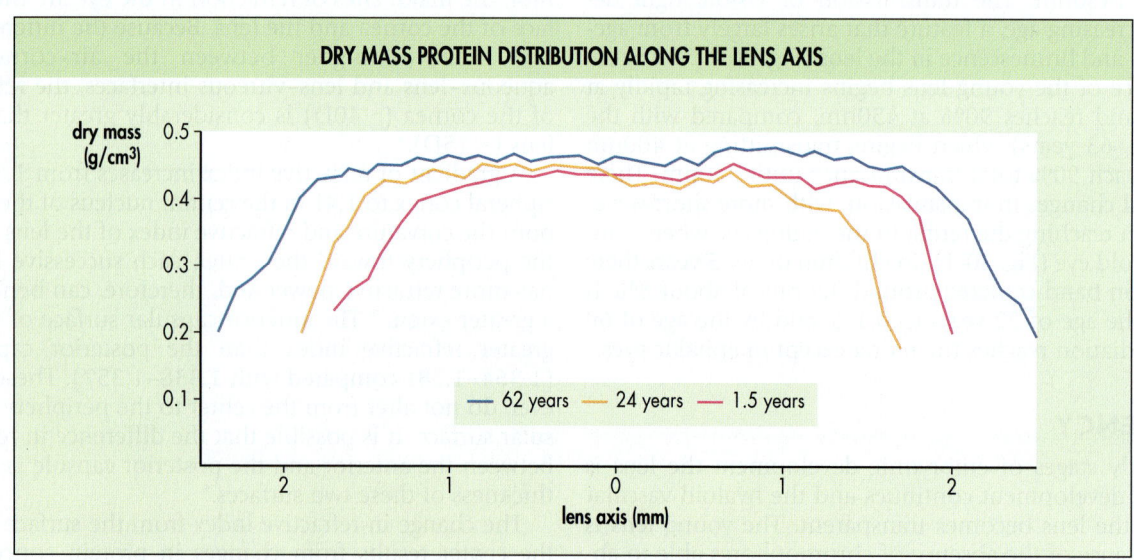

DRY MASS PROTEIN DISTRIBUTION ALONG THE LENS AXIS

- 62 years
- 24 years
- 1.5 years

FIG. 30-2 ■ **Dry mass protein distribution along the lens axis in three normal lenses of different ages.** (From Fagerholm PP, Philipson BT, Lindstrom B. Normal human lens—the distribution of protein. Exp Eye Res. 1981;33:615–20.)

of the image are all aberrations that affect the peripheral vision. Although the image formed at the peripheral retina is affected, the curvature of the retina neutralizes these aberrations to some extent.[5,9-11]

ACCOMMODATION

The lens, through its ability to change shape, has the capacity to change the focusing power of the eye. This process is known as accommodation and enables both distant and close objects to be brought to focus on the retina (see Fig. 30-4). At rest the ciliary muscle is relaxed and, therefore, the zonules pull on the lens, which keeps the capsule under tension. In this state the capsule is stretched and the lens flattens, enabling the eye to focus on distant objects (of approximately 20ft [6m] away). Light rays from these distant objects are almost parallel and, therefore, do not need to be refracted greatly to hit the fovea. By contrast, light rays from close objects are divergent and, therefore, are focused behind the retina with the lens in this shape. The lens accommodates these objects by increasing the curvature of the anterior surface, decreasing the radius of curvature from 10mm to 6mm. The increase in curvature of the anterior surface increases the refractive power, so that the light rays from close objects are refracted toward each other to a greater extent and, therefore, converge on the fovea. Because the front of the lens has moved forward, the depth of the anterior chamber decreases from 3.5mm to 3.2–3.3mm. Very little change occurs in the curvature of the posterior capsule, which remains at ap-

proximately 6mm (Fig. 30-5). The distance between the cornea and the posterior surface of the lens, therefore, changes very little or not at all. If the eyeball is relatively short or the lens does not have enough refractive power, the light rays converge behind the retina and the eye is unable to focus on close objects (hypermetropic or far sighted). If the eyeball is relatively long or the lens too strong, the opposite is true (myopic or near sighted).[12-15]

The change in lens shape results from the contraction of the ciliary muscle (by approximately 0.8mm in the young), which pulls the ciliary body forward and inward toward the center of the lens. The tension on the zonules is released and the capsule relaxes, the equatorial diameter shortens (by 0.26mm in the young), and the lens thickens and becomes more spherical as a result of the change in shape of the nucleus.[16] Accommodation is accompanied by a decrease in pupil size (miosis) and convergence of the two eyes. Light rays can pass only through the thickest central parts of the lens and the two images become fused. Accommodation, miosis, and convergence all are controlled by the third cranial nerve.[12-16]

The mechanisms of accommodation can be divided into both physical and physiological processes. Physical accommodation, a measure of the change in shape of the lens during the accommodative process, is measured in terms of the amplitude of accommodation using the unit diopter. It represents the difference between the contractility of the eye at rest and when fully accommodated and, therefore, a measure of the extent to which objects close to the eye can be focused. Physiological accommo-

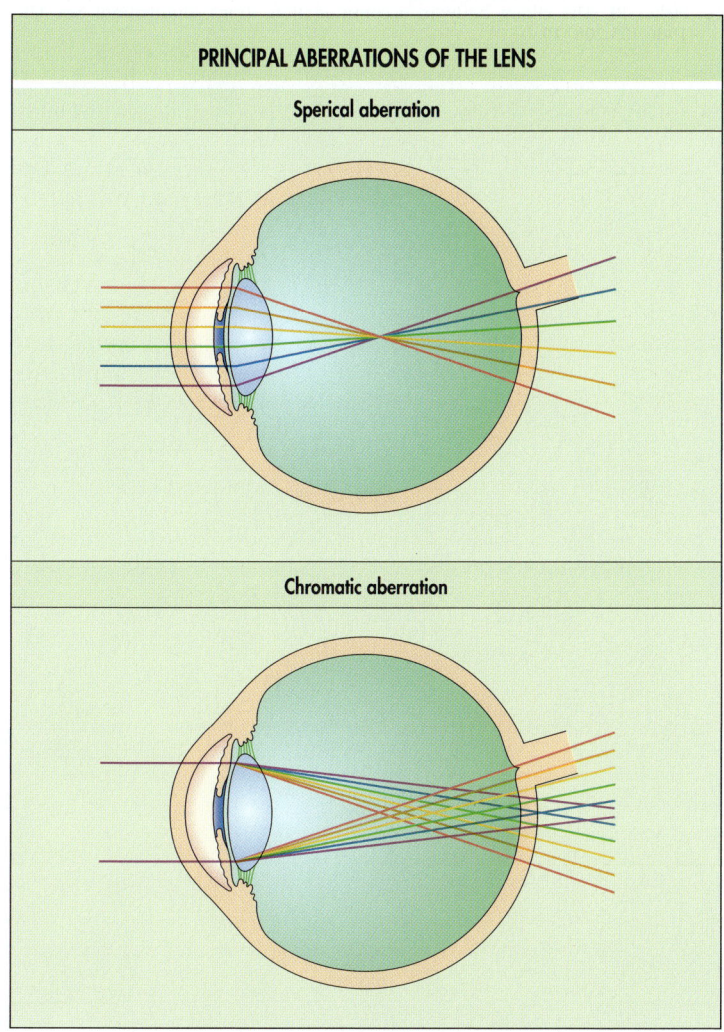

FIG. 30-3 ▪ Principal aberrations of the lens.

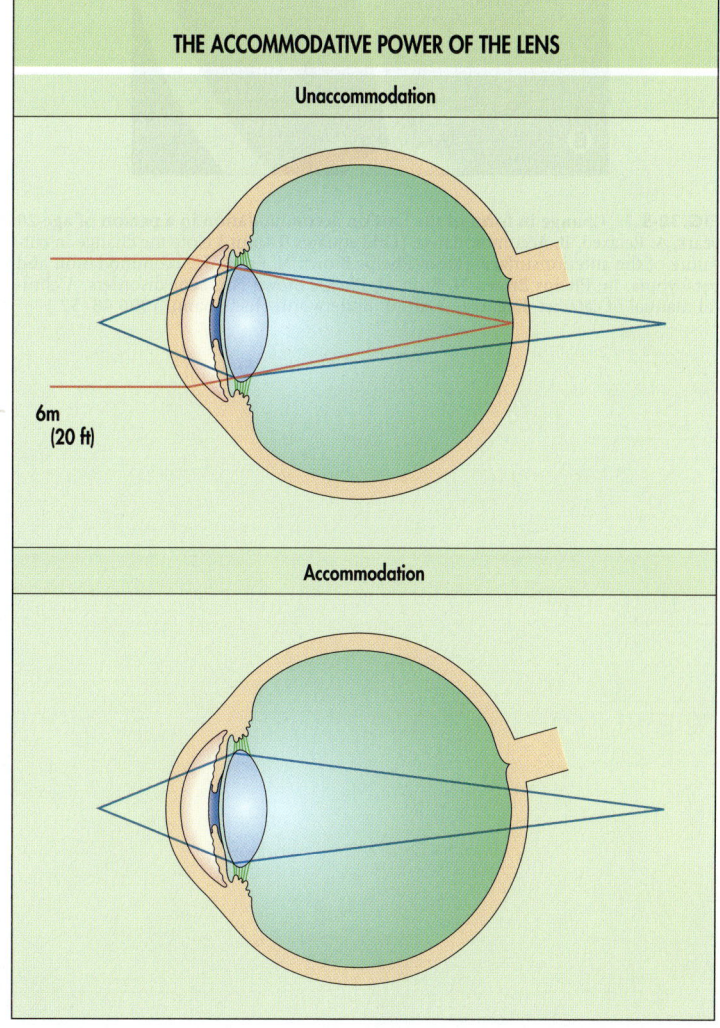

FIG. 30-4 ▪ **The accommodative power of the lens.** At rest the eye focuses on distant objects but needs to accommodate to focus on near objects.

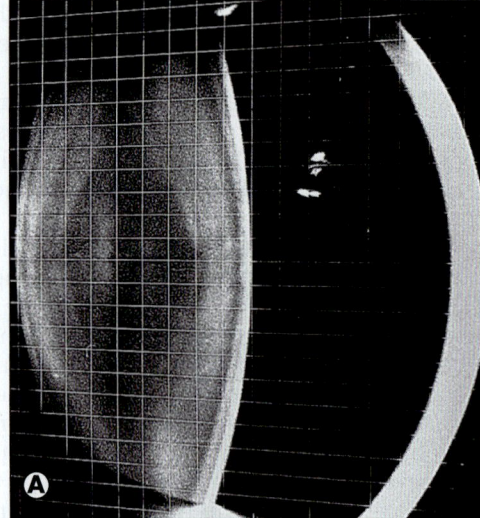

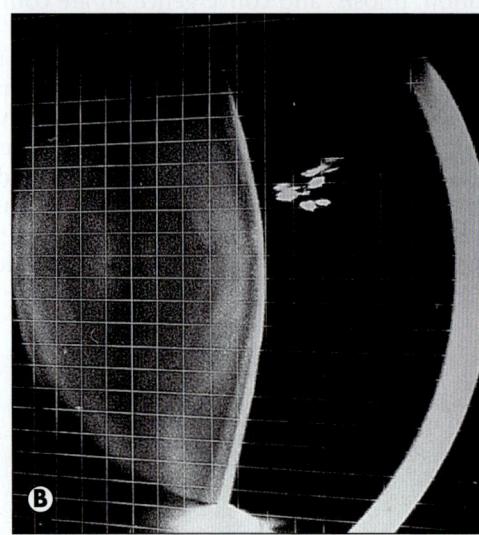

FIG. 30-5 ■ Change in form of the lens on accommodation in a person of age 29 years. A, Relaxed. **B,** Accommodated. (Grid squares 0.4mm.) Note the change in curvature of the anterior surface. (From Phelps Brown N, Bron AJ. Accommodation and presbyopia. In: Phelps Brown N, Bron AJ, Phelps Brown NA. Lens disorders. A clinical manual of cataract diagnosis. Oxford: Butterworth-Heinemann; 1996:48–52.)

dation, a measure of the force of ciliary muscle contraction per diopter, is measured with the unit myodiopter. The myodiopter increases during the act of accommodation.[13,16]

REFERENCES

1. Lerman S. Lens transparency and aging. In: Regnault F, Hockwin O, Courtios Y, eds. Ageing of the lens. Amsterdam: Elsevier/North-Holland Biomedical Press; 1980:263–79.
2. Zigman S. Photochemical mechanisms in cataract formation. In: Duncan G, ed. Mechanisms of cataract formation in the human lens. London: Academic Press; 1981:117–49.
3. de Jong WW, Lubsen NH, Kraft HJ. Molecular evolution of the eye lens. Prog Retina Eye Res. 1994;13:391–442.
4. Clark JI. Development and maintenance of lens transparency. In: Albert DM, Jakobiec FA, eds. Principles and practice of ophthalmology. Basic sciences. Philadelphia: WB Saunders; 1994:114–23.
5. Duke-Elder S. The refraction of the eye—physiological optics. In: Abrams D, ed. The practice of refraction, ed 10. Edinburgh: Churchill Livingstone; 1993:29–41.
6. Pierscionek BK. Refractive index of the human lens surface measured with an optic fibre sensor. Ophthalmic Res. 1994;26:32–5.
7. Fagerholm PP, Philipson BT, Lindstrom B. Normal human lens—the distribution of protein. Exp Eye Res. 1981;33:615–20.
8. Deussen A, Pau H. Regional water content of clear and cataractous human lenses. Ophthalmic Res. 1989;21:374–80.
9. Bennett AG, Rabbetts RB. Ocular aberrations. In: Clinical visual optics, ed 2. London: Butterworths; 1989:331–57.
10. Elkington AR, Frank HJ. Aberrations of optical systems including the eye. In: Clinical optics, ed 2. Oxford: Blackwell Scientific; 1991:75–82.
11. Moore DC. Geometric optics. In: Coster DJ, ed. Physics for ophthalmologists. Edinburgh: Churchill Livingstone; 1994:29–34.
12. Phelps Brown N, Bron AJ. Accommodation and presbyopia. In: Phelps Brown N, Bron AJ, Phelps Brown NA. Lens disorders. A clinical manual of cataract diagnosis. Oxford: Butterworth-Heinemann; 1996:48–52.
13. Duke-Elder S. Accommodation. In: Abrams D, ed. The practice of refraction, ed 10. Edinburgh: Churchill Livingstone; 1993:85–9.
14. Koretz JF. Accommodation and presbyopia. In: Albert DM, Jakobiec FA, eds. Principles and practice of ophthalmology. Basic sciences. Philadelphia: WB Saunders; 1994:270–82.
15. Saude T. The internal ocular media. In: Ocular anatomy and physiology. Oxford: Blackwell Scientific; 1993:36–52.
16. Fisher RF. The ciliary body in accommodation. Trans Ophthalmol Soc UK. 1986;105:208–19.

CHAPTER 31

Biochemistry

MICHAEL BOULTON • LISA A. SAXBY

DEFINITION
- Lens function is dependent on the metabolism of glucose to produce energy, protein synthesis, and a complex antioxidant system.

KEY FEATURES
- Glucose metabolism occurs largely by anaerobic glycolysis.
- The protein concentration is higher than that of any other tissue in the body.
- Protein synthesis occurs throughout life and predominantly involves the production of the crystallins and major intrinsic protein 26.
- Glutathione is found at high concentrations and helps protect the lens from oxidative damage.
- The lens has a complex antioxidant system, which protects against reactive oxygen species produced during photochemical reactions in the lens.

INTRODUCTION

Lens metabolism is a complex process and our understanding of lens biochemistry is still evolving. The lens, like most tissues, requires energy to drive thermodynamically unfavorable reactions. Adenosine triphosphate (ATP) is the principal source of this energy within the cell, because it has the capacity to release energy upon the hydrolysis of its high-energy phosphate bonds. The majority of ATP produced within the lens comes from the anaerobic metabolism of glucose. Other important components required by the lens include the reduced form of nicotinamide adenine dinucleotide phosphate (NADPH), which is produced principally by the pentose phosphate pathway and acts as a source of readily available reducing power used in the biosynthesis of many essential cellular components, such as fatty acids and glutathione. In addition to producing ATP and NADPH, these pathways also produce the building blocks needed to synthesize DNA, RNA, proteins (e.g., crystallins), and membrane components (e.g., phospholipids, sphingolipids, and cholesterol). Because the lens is susceptible to oxidative damage, it also must maintain sufficient antioxidant defenses to protect against the accumulation of this damage and the development of cataract. These aspects are discussed in detail in the following sections.

SUGAR METABOLISM

Approximately 90–95% of the glucose that enters the normal lens is phosphorylated into glucose-6-phosphate in a reaction catalyzed by hexokinase. Although this enzyme exists as three different isoforms (types I–III), only two have been found in the lens. Because type I has a greater affinity for glucose, it is found in the lens nucleus where glucose levels are low. Type II, which accounts for 70% of the total soluble lens hexokinase but has a

lower affinity for glucose, is found predominantly in the epithelium and cortex, where glucose levels are higher. Glucose-6-phosphate is used either in the glycolytic pathway (80% of total glucose) or in the pentose phosphate pathway (hexose monophosphate shunt; 10% of total glucose) (Fig. 31-1). Because hexokinase is saturated by the normal concentrations of glucose found in the lens, this enzyme is working to maximal capacity and, therefore, limits the rate of both glycolysis and the pentose phosphate pathway. Hexokinase is inhibited by high levels of glucose-6-phosphate, hydrogen (H^+), citrate, and ATP. Glycolysis also is regulated by phosphofructokinase, an enzyme that exists in either a type I or type II form. The inactive type I form can be converted into the catalytically active type II form. Phosphofructokinase activity is modified by ATP, with the result that activity is low when ATP is plentiful and high when ATP is scarce. Pyruvate kinase, a third enzyme which plays a role in the control of the glycolytic pathway, is inhibited by high levels of ATP, alanine, and fructose 1,6-biphosphate.[1,2]

Due to its avascularity and location in the ocular humors, the lens exists in a hypoxic environment with a partial pressure of oxygen as low as 5mmHg. This results in at least 70% of lens ATP being derived from anaerobic glycolysis, a relatively inefficient mechanism for the production of ATP (two net molecules of ATP per molecule of glucose). However, although only a very small amount, approximately 3% per molecule of glucose, of lens glucose passes into the tricarboxylic acid cycle (see Fig. 31-1), this aerobic metabolism generates 25% of lens ATP (36 net molecules of ATP per molecule of glucose). Glycolysis and the tricarboxylic acid cycle generate two energy-rich molecules, the reduced form of nicotinamide adenine dinucleotide (NADH) and the reduced form of flavin adenine dinucleotide ($FADH_2$). These donate their electrons to oxygen, which releases large amounts of free energy that is subsequently used to generate ATP. This cycle, which is restricted to the epithelial layer, also provides carbon skeleton intermediates for biosynthesis, such as amino acids and porphyrins.[1,3]

The bulk of the pyruvate produced by the glycolytic pathway is reduced to lactate in a reaction catalyzed by lactate dehydrogenase (see Fig. 31-1). Five lactate dehydrogenase isozymes are distributed throughout the lens, being concentrated mostly in the cortex. The formation of lactate results in the reoxidation of the cofactor NADH to NAD^+. Glyceraldehyde-3-phosphate dehydrogenase, an enzyme used in the glycolytic pathway, regulates the activity of lactate dehydrogenase by controlling the rate of conversion of glyceraldehyde-3-phosphate into 1,3-diphosphoglycerate and, therefore, the availability of NADH. Lactate, once generated, is not further metabolized and diffuses into the aqueous humor, where it can be present at quite high levels.[1–3]

Although the pentose phosphate pathway only utilizes approximately 10% of total lens glucose, its activity increases if glucose levels are increased above normal. The activity of phosphofructokinase and the concentration of the oxidized form of nicotinamide adenine dinucleotide phosphate ($NADP^+$) and ATP determine whether the glucose-6-phosphate follows the glycolytic pathway or the pentose phosphate pathway. The primary function of the pentose phosphate pathway is to produce

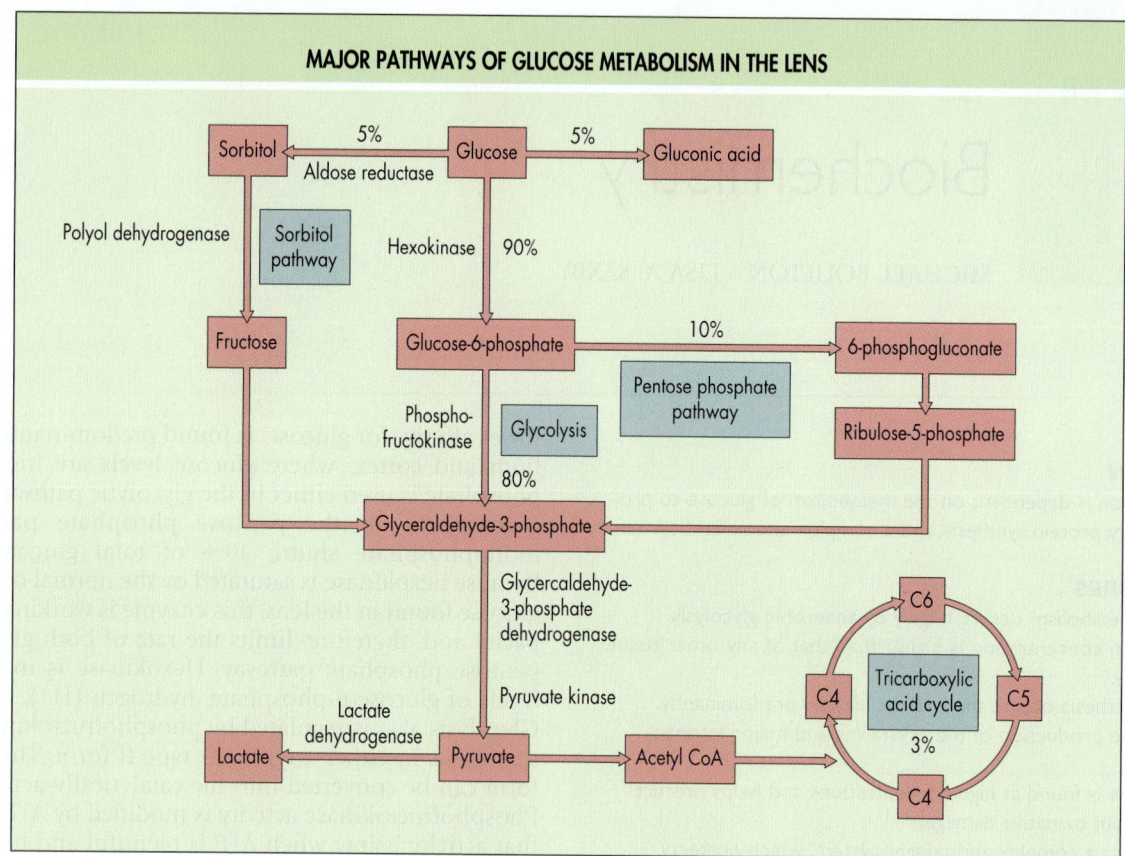

MAJOR PATHWAYS OF GLUCOSE METABOLISM IN THE LENS

FIG. 31-1 ■ **Overview of the major pathways of glucose metabolism in the lens.** Percentages represent the estimated amount of glucose used in the different pathways.

the reduced form of NADPH in vitro, a reducing equivalent used in the synthesis of fatty acids, the maintenance of reduced glutathione, and the conversion of glucose into sorbitol. The pathway also produces pentose sugars needed for the synthesis of nucleic acids and CO_2. The end products of this pathway are converted into glyceraldehyde-3-phosphate, which then enters the glycolytic pathway (see Fig. 31-1).[1-3]

The 5–10% of glucose that is not phosphorylated into glucose-6-phosphate either enters the sorbitol pathway or is converted into gluconic acid (see Fig. 31-1). Although the precise function of these pathways is still unknown, the activity of the sorbitol pathway increases if glucose levels are increased above normal. Glucose is converted into sorbitol by aldose reductase, an enzyme localized to the epithelial layer. This enzyme uses NADPH supplied by the pentose phosphate pathway as a cofactor. Sorbitol then is converted by polyol dehydrogenase into fructose, a suboptimal, but usable, substrate for glycolysis. This enzyme is inactive at low concentrations of sorbitol and metabolizes sorbitol into fructose only if sorbitol has accumulated. Because both sorbitol and fructose have the potential to increase osmotic pressure, and so cause water to enter cells, these sugars may help to regulate the volume of the lens.[1-3]

PROTEIN METABOLISM

The protein concentration within the lens is higher than that of any other tissue in the body. Because the lens grows throughout life, protein synthesis also must occur throughout life. Most of this synthesis is concerned with the production of the crystallins and major intrinsic protein 26 (MIP26). The availability of amino acids within the lens does not affect the rate of protein synthesis.[4] It has been presumed that protein synthesis occurs only in the epithelial cells and surface cortical fibers, which contain the organelles needed.[5] However this idea is controversial, because the nucleus of the rat lens has been shown to contain messenger RNA (mRNA) sequences for MIP26.[6] Evidence also

exists from many species that nuclear fibers contain small fragments of DNA and RNA which could be used for protein synthesis. Most protein synthesis, however, must occur in the outer regions of the lens.[2,4]

Because fibers are internalized continuously, most proteins once synthesized remain in the lens throughout life, although some protein turnover does occur in the epithelial layer. The majority of proteins are subject to posttranslational modifications; for example, plasma membrane proteins and some crystallins are phosphorylated. Lens proteins remain stable for long periods because the majority of the degradative enzymes normally are inhibited. The lens controls the breakdown of proteins by marking those to be degraded with a small 8.5kDa protein called *ubiquitin*. This system, which is ATP dependent, is most active in the epithelial layer. Lens proteins are broken down into peptides by endopeptidases and then into the constituent amino acids by exopeptidases. Neutral endopeptidase, previously called neutral proteinase, is activated by both calcium and magnesium, and is optimally active at pH 7.5 (the pH of the lens is approximately 7.0–7.2). The principal substrate of this enzyme is α-crystallin. The calpains (I and II), which mainly are localized in the epithelial cells and cortex, are used to degrade crystallins and cytoskeletal proteins. They are cysteine endopeptidases, the activities of which are regulated by calcium (Ca^{++}). Although calpain I requires only around 10μmol/l Ca^{++} for activation, calpain II requires 1mmol/l Ca^{++}. These enzymes are inhibited by calpastatin, a natural inhibitor found at higher concentrations than the calpains. The lens also contains a serine proteinase (with trypsin-like activity) and a membrane-bound proteinase.[2-4]

The main exopeptidase is leucine aminopeptidase, an enzyme which is optimally active at pH 8.5–9.0, which catalyzes the removal of amino acids from the N-terminal of peptides. The activity of this enzyme is controlled by the binding of metal ions at two binding sites found on each subunit; one site must contain zinc and on the other zinc, magnesium, or manganese

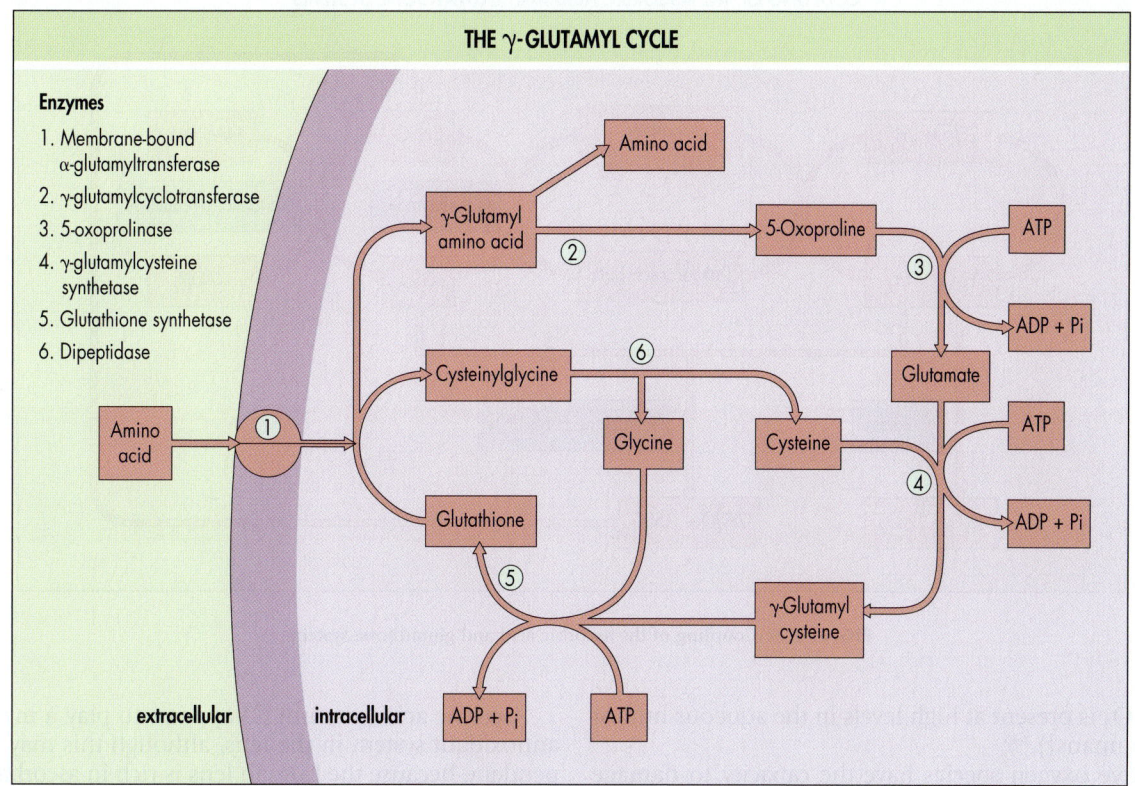

THE γ-GLUTAMYL CYCLE

Enzymes
1. Membrane-bound α-glutamyltransferase
2. γ-glutamylcyclotransferase
3. 5-oxoprolinase
4. γ-glutamylcysteine synthetase
5. Glutathione synthetase
6. Dipeptidase

FIG. 31-2 ■ **The γ-glutamyl cycle.** (From Harding JJ, Crabbe MJC. The lens: development, proteins, metabolism and cataract. In: Davson H, ed. The eye, ed 3. London: Academic Press; 1984:207–492.)

can confer activity. The ion bound to the second site affects the specific activity of the enzyme. An endogenous inhibitor of leucine aminopeptidase may be present in the lens. Aminopeptidase III, another endopeptidase found in the lens, has an optimal pH of 6.0 and as a result has a greater activity than leucine aminopeptidase in the normal lens.[2–4]

GLUTATHIONE

Glutathione (L-γ-glutamyl-L-cysteinylglycine) is found at high concentrations in the lens (3.5–5.5 μmol/g wet weight), especially in the epithelial layer (in which levels are higher than in the nucleus; the cortex contains an intermediate concentration). Glutathione has many important roles in the lens, including the following.[2,3,7]

- Maintenance of protein thiols in the reduced state, which helps to maintain lens transparency by preventing the formation of high–molecular-weight crystallin aggregates
- Protection of thiol groups critically involved in cation transport and permeability; for example, oxidation of the –SH groups of the Na⁺,K⁺-ATPase pump which results in an increased permeability to these ions
- Protection against oxidative damage (see later in the chapter)
- Removal of xenobiotics; glutathione-S-transferase catalyzes the conjugation of glutathione to hydrophobic compounds with an electrophilic center
- Amino acid transport

Glutathione has a half-life of 1–2 days and, therefore, is recycled constantly by the γ-glutamyl cycle; its synthesis and degradation occur at approximately the same rate (Fig. 31-2). Glutathione is synthesized from L-glutamate, L-cysteine, and glycine in a two-step process that uses 11–12% of lens ATP.[2,3,7] γ-Glutamylcysteine synthetase is the rate-limiting enzyme and L-cysteine the rate-limiting substrate for this synthesis.[8] Reduced glutathione also can be taken into the lens from the aqueous humor. A reduced glutathione transporter that allows the uptake of

glutathione by the lens epithelial cells has recently been characterized.[9] The breakdown of glutathione releases its constituent amino acids, which subsequently are needed to synthesize more glutathione.

Glutathione exists in both an oxidized form (GSSG) and a reduced form (GSH). At least 95% of lens glutathione is found in the reduced GSH form. Glutathione reductase, an enzyme that uses NADPH as a cofactor (provided by the pentose phosphate pathway) reduces GSSG into GSH (Fig. 31-3). Because this enzyme works at low substrate levels, any GSSG formed is converted rapidly into GSH.[2,3,7]

ANTIOXIDANT MECHANISMS

Reactive oxygen species is a collective term for highly reactive oxygen radicals (including free radicals) that have the potential to damage lipids, proteins, carbohydrates, and nucleic acids. Such radicals include the superoxide anion, the hydroxyl free radical, hydroperoxyl radicals, lipid peroxyl radicals, singlet oxygen, and hydrogen peroxide (H_2O_2). Reactive oxygen species generally have two origins in tissues; cell metabolism and photochemical reactions. Photochemical damage occurs when light is absorbed by a photosensitizer, a chromophore, which upon photoexcitation to photoexcited singlet state undergoes intersystem crossing and forms a transient excited triplet state. The excited triplet state is long lived, allowing for interaction with other molecules producing free radicals *via* electron (hydrogen) transfer, or singlet oxygen *via* transfer of excitation energy from the photosensitizer in the triplet state to molecular oxygen. The continuous entry of optical radiation into the lens, in particular the preferential absorption of shorter wavelengths (295–400nm), makes lens tissue particularly susceptible to photochemical reactions. The major ultraviolet (UV) absorbers in the lens are free or bound aromatic amino acids (e.g., tryptophan), numerous pigments (e.g., 3-hydroxykynurenine), and fluorophores. Reactive oxygen species also can enter the lens from the surrounding

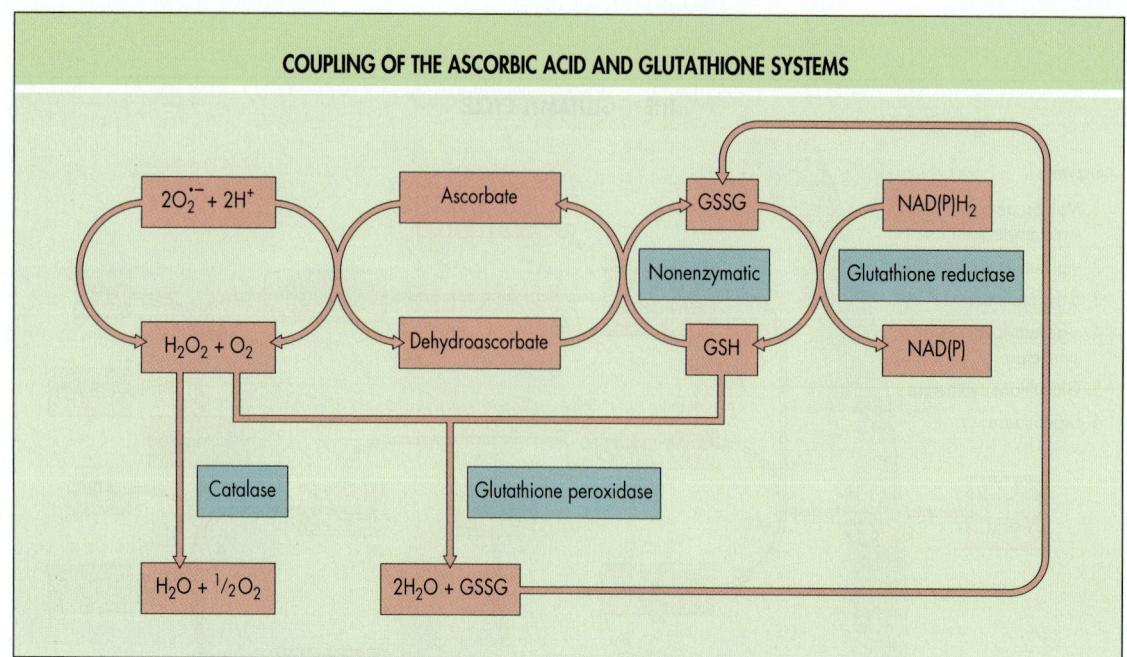

COUPLING OF THE ASCORBIC ACID AND GLUTATHIONE SYSTEMS

FIG. 31-3 ■ Coupling of the ascorbic acid and glutathione systems.

milieu (e.g., H_2O_2 is present at high levels in the aqueous humor [30 μmol/l in humans]).[3,10]

Highly reactive oxygen species have the capacity to damage the lens in several ways.[3,11]

- Peroxidizing membrane lipids results in the formation of malondialdehyde, which in turn can form cross-links between membrane lipids and proteins.
- Introducing damage into the bases of the DNA, such as base modifications (8-hydroxyguanosine), plana-lesions (cytosine glycols) and lesions leading to major helical distortions of the DNA (8'5 cyclopurine deoxyribonucleosides), initiates DNA repair mechanisms. However, 8-hydroxyguanosine can mispair with adenosine and so represents a mutagenic lesion.
- Polymerizing and cross-linking proteins result in crystallin aggregation and inactivation of many essential enzymes, including those with an antioxidant role (e.g., catalase and glutathione reductase).

Although these reactions would result rapidly in lens damage, the presence of a complex antioxidant system offers considerable protection. This system, however, is not 100% efficient and a low level of cumulative damage occurs throughout life.

Protection against damage induced by reactive oxygen species in the lens is achieved in a number of ways. The superoxide anion undergoes dismutation by superoxide dismutase or interaction with ascorbate (see below), which results in the formation of H_2O_2. This, along with the high levels of exogenous H_2O_2, is detoxified by the enzyme catalase or glutathione peroxidase or both (see Fig. 31-3).[12] Catalase is present in epithelial cells but is found at very low levels in fibers. Glutathione peroxidase, however, is found in significant amounts in both epithelial cells and fibers, although the highest levels are found in the epithelial cells. The glutathione system, therefore, is thought to provide the most protection against H_2O_2. A hydrogen atom is donated by GSH in a reaction, catalyzed by glutathione peroxidase, resulting in the formation of GSSG and water. Subsequently, GSSG is reduced by glutathione reductase and reenters the antioxidant system. In addition to neutralizing H_2O_2, the glutathione system provides important protection against the lipid free-radical chain reaction by the neutralization of lipid peroxides, although low levels of the antioxidants α-tocopherol and β-carotene also are present in the aqueous humor.[3,7,10,11]

Ascorbic acid (vitamin C) appears to play a major role in the antioxidant system in the lens, although this may be species dependent, because the human lens is rich in ascorbate (1.9 mg l/kg wet weight or 1.1 mmol/kg), while it is almost absent in the rat lens (0.08 mmol/kg). Ascorbate is present at high levels in the outer layers of the lens and virtually absent from the nucleus. It rapidly reacts with superoxide anions, peroxide radicals, and hydroxyl radicals to give dehydroascorbate. It also scavenges singlet oxygen, reduces thiol radicals, and is important in the prevention of lipid peroxidation. In the case of the superoxide anion, ascorbate acts by the donation of one electron to give dehydroascorbate and H_2O_2. The ascorbic acid and glutathione systems are coupled in that dehydroascorbate reacts with the reduced form of glutathione to generate ascorbate and GSSG (see Fig. 31-3).[4,10,13,14]

REFERENCES

1. Kador PF. Biochemistry of the lens: intermediary metabolism and sugar cataract formation. In: Albert DM, Jakobiec FA, eds. Principles and practice of ophthalmology. Basic sciences. Philadelphia: WB Saunders; 1994:146–67.
2. Harding JJ, Crabbe MJC. The lens: development, proteins, metabolism and cataract. In: Davson H, ed. The eye, ed 3. London: Academic Press; 1984:207–492.
3. Berman ER. Lens. In: Blakemore C, ed. Biochemistry of the eye. New York: Plenum Press; 1991:201–90.
4. Harding J. The normal lens. In: Harding J. Cataract: biochemistry, epidemiology and pharmacology. London: Chapman & Hall; 1991:1–70.
5. Bassnett S. The fate of the Golgi apparatus and the endoplasmic reticulum during lens fiber cell differentiation. Invest Ophthalmol Vis Sci. 1995;36:1793–803.
6. Lieska N, Krotzer K, Yang HY. A reassessment of protein synthesis by lens nuclear fiber cells. Exp Eye Res. 1992;54:807–11.
7. Reddy VN. Glutathione and its functions in the lens—an overview. Exp Eye Res. 1990;50:771–8.
8. Rathbun WB, Murray DL. Age-related cysteine uptake as rate-limiting step in glutathione synthesis and glutathione half-life in the cultured human lens. Exp Eye Res. 1991;53:205–12.
9. Kannan R, Yi JR, Zlokovic BV, Kaplowitz N. Molecular characterization of a reduced glutathione transporter in the lens. Invest Ophthalmol Vis Sci. 1995;36:1785–92.
10. Augusteyn RC. Protein modification in cataract. In: Duncan G, ed. Mechanisms of cataract formation in the human lens. London: Academic Press; 1981:72–115.
11. Lerman S. Free radical damage and defense mechanisms in the ocular lens. Lens Eye Toxic Res. 1992;9:9–24.
12. Costarides AP, Riley MV, Green K. Roles of catalase and the glutathione redox cycle in the regulation of anterior-chamber hydrogen peroxide. Ophthalmic Res. 1991;23:284–94.
13. Sasaki H, Giblin FJ, Winkler BS, et al. A protective role for glutathione-dependent reduction of dehydroascorbic acid in lens epithelium. Invest Ophthalmol Vis Sci. 1995;36:1804–17.
14. Varma SD, Richards RD. Ascorbic acid and the eye lens. Ophthalmic Res. 1988;20:164–73.

Evolution and Molecular Biology

MICHAEL BOULTON • LISA A. SAXBY

DEFINITION

- Crystallins represent the major protein of the lens and are derived from enzyme or stress protein genes which have been recruited to the lens during evolution.

KEY FEATURES

- The crystallins constitute 90% of the total protein content of the lens.
- Three groups of crystallins are predominant in all vertebrate species and can be divided in the α-, β-, and γ-crystallin families.
- α-Crystallin and β-crystallin occur as high–molecular-weight aggregates.
- α-Crystallin acts as a chaperone protein and protects the lens from damage.

CRYSTALLIN STRUCTURE

Up to 60% of the wet weight and most of the dry weight of the human lens is composed of proteins. These lens proteins can be divided on a laboratory basis into water-soluble (cytoplasmic proteins) and water-insoluble (cytoskeletal and plasma membrane) fractions. The water-soluble crystallins constitute approximately 90% of the total protein content of the lens.[1,2]

The three groups of crystallins found in all vertebrate species can be divided into the α-crystallin family and the β/γ-crystallin superfamily. The properties of these crystallins are summarized in Table 32-1. The α-crystallins have the largest molecular size of the crystallins. They form polymeric ellipsoid structures approximately 16nm in diameter, with a native molecular mass between 600kDa and 900kDa. These structures are composed of noncovalent aggregates of four major polypeptide subunits (αA, αA1, αB, and αB1) and up to nine minor subunits in most species. The thiol content of these subunits is low and the N-terminal amino acid is masked. Because each major subunit has a molecular weight of approximately 20kDa, α-crystallin normally contains between 30 and 45 subunits. α-Crystallins have a predominantly β–pleated sheet secondary structure with a small amount of helical structure (less than 10%).[1-5] Although the quaternary structure of α-crystallin is not known, experimental data support several different models, which include a three-layer structure, a micellar and layer model, a rhombic dodecahedron, and a pore-like structure (see Table 32-1).[6,7]

The β-crystallins are composed of light (βL) (c. 52kDa) and heavy (βH) (150–210kDa) fractions, which can be separated by gel chromatography. The light fraction can be further subdivided into two fractions, βL1 and βL2. The β-crystallins are aggregates of polypeptide subunits with a molecular mass between 23kDa and 32kDa. The light fraction, therefore, is composed of dimers and the heavy fraction of 7–38 subunits. Aggregates range in diameter from 5–15nm. Seven different β-crystallin polypeptides occur, which can be divided into three basic (βB1, βB2, and βB3

[26–32kDa]) and four acidic subunits (βA1, βA2, βA3, and βA4 [23–25kDa]). The thiol content of each subunit is high and the N-terminal amino acid masked. Each polypeptide subunit has a two-domain structure linked by a short connecting peptide (3–5 amino acids) and one or two terminal extensions, or "arms." Two "Greek key" motifs exist in each domain. Each motif has an antiparallel β–pleated sheet structure. The basic subunits have both N- and C-terminal extensions, whereas the acidic subunits only have the N-terminal extension. These extensions and some of the hydrophobic surface residues are required for aggregation.[1-5]

The smallest of the crystallins are the γ-crystallins. Six members of this family, known as γA–γF, have a molecular weight of 20kDa. They are monomers with a high net charge, high thiol content, and either glycine or alanine as the N-terminal amino acid. They have a two-domain structure with four Greek key motifs but, unlike the β-crystallins, no terminal extensions exist. The γ-crystallin domains, however, pair intramolecularly and therefore are unable to form polymers. There is also a seventh crystallin known as γs, a 24kDa polypeptide originally known as βs-crystallin. However, although several of its characteristics, such as molecular weight, amino acid composition, and blocked amino terminus, are characteristic of the β-crystallins, the nucleotide sequence is closer to that of the γ-crystallins so this protein was renamed γs in 1988 (Fig. 32-1).[1-5,8]

CRYSTALLIN GENE STRUCTURE AND SEQUENCE HOMOLOGY

The two major α-crystallin gene products are the αA and the αB subunits. Posttranslational modification of these peptides gives rise to all the other α-crystallin subunits. Subunits αA and αB are converted into αA1 and αB1 by the phosphorylation of serine residues via a cyclic adenosine monophosphate–dependent system. The vertebrate αA and αB sequences are approximately 57% homologous, which suggests that the genome originally contained one gene that must have duplicated itself as long as 750 million years ago. αA and αB are encoded by single-copy genes found on chromosomes 21 and 11, respectively. αA is composed of 173 amino acids and αB of 175 amino acids.[1-5]

The α-crystallin gene consists of three exons. In some mammalian species, such as mice and rats, a sequence composed of 69 base pairs, known as αA^{ins}, is inserted between exons 1 and 2. Although the remnants of this sequence still are found in the first intron of the human gene, no messenger RNA (mRNA) is produced from this pseudoexon. Exon 1, which codes the first 60 amino acids, comprises two homologous regions of 30 amino acids, which have arisen from an internal duplication. Exons 2 and 3 code for the remainder of the polypeptide.[1,9,10]

The β-crystallin gene family has six members that encode the seven subunits. Subunits βA1 and βA3 are encoded by the same gene but use different initiation sites. As a result βA3 has an extra 17 amino acids at the N-terminal end. βB1, βB2, βB3, and βB4 all are found on chromosome 22 in humans. βA1/βA3 has translocated to chromosome 17 and βA2 has not been located. The human genome has two copies of the βB2 gene, one of

TABLE 32-1

PROPERTIES OF DIFFERENT CRYSTALLINS

	α	β	γ	γs
Subunits	αA, αA1, αB, αB1, up to nine minor subunits	Basic: βB1, βB2, βB3 Acidic: βA1, βA2, βA3, βA4	γA–γF	γs
Subunit molecular weight	20kDa	Basic: 26–32kDa Acidic: 23–25kDa	20kDa	24kDa
Native molecular weight	600–900kDa	βH: 150–200kDa βL: c. 50kDa	20kDa	24kDa
Number of subunits	30–45	βH: 0–8 βL: 2	1	1
Thiol content	Low	High	High	High
N-Terminal amino acid	Masked	Masked	Glycine or alanine	Masked
Secondary structure	Predominantly β-pleated sheet	β-pleated sheet	β-pleated sheet	β-pleated sheet
Three-dimensional structure	Unknown	Two domains with four "Greek key" motifs	Two domains with four "Greek key" motifs	Two domains with four "Greek key" motifs
Chromosome	αA: 21 αB: 11	βB1–βB4: 22 βA1/ βA3: 17 βA2: ?	2	3

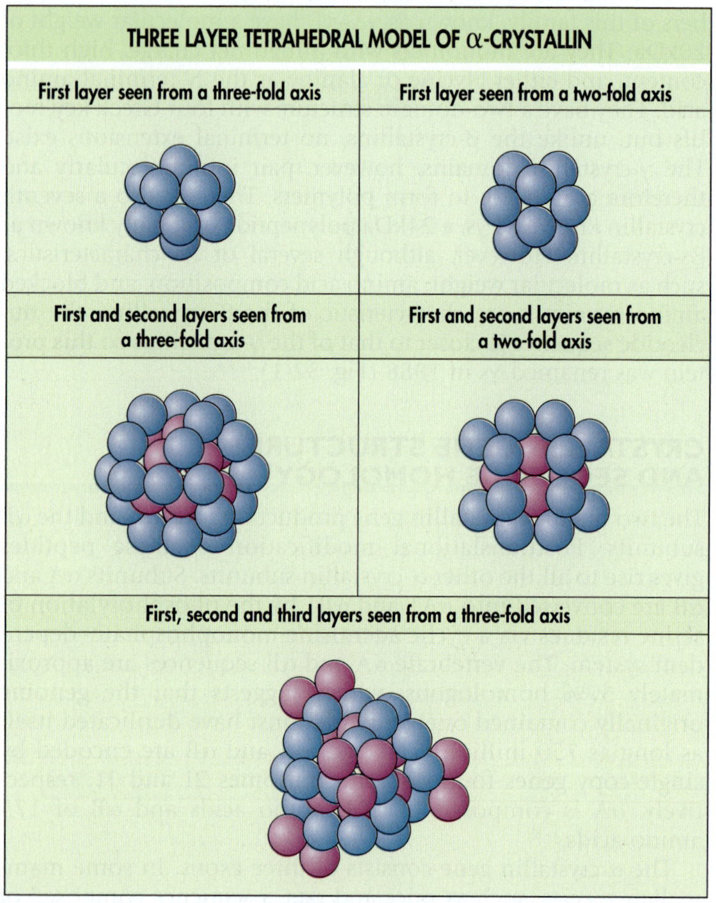

THREE LAYER TETRAHEDRAL MODEL OF α-CRYSTALLIN

First layer seen from a three-fold axis

First layer seen from a two-fold axis

First and second layers seen from a three-fold axis

First and second layers seen from a two-fold axis

First, second and third layers seen from a three-fold axis

FIG. 32-1 ■ Three-layer tetrahedral model of α-crystallin. In the lower part of the figure, only 12 equivalent sites are filled to yield a 48-subunit particle. Note that the subunits have been modeled as spheres. (From Tardieu A, Laporte D, Licinio P, et al. Calf lens α-crystallin quaternary structure. A three layer tetrahedral model. J Mol Biol. 1986;192:711–24.)

which is thought to be a pseudogene. The β-crystallin gene is composed of six exons. Exons 1 and 2 encode the amino acid terminal arm and the remaining four exons encode the motifs (100–150 nucleotides). Exons 3 and 5 are closely related, as are exons 4 and 6. Exon 6 also encodes the carboxyl terminal arm.[3,9] The β-crystallins have evolved from a single motif, which duplicated and then reduplicated to give a fourfold repeat of the ini-

tial structure. This structure then gave rise to both the βA and the βB subunits.[11] Sequence homology between the two domains is 45–60%. However, no homology exists between the N- and C-terminal extensions.[2] It is believed the β-crystallin gene family started to evolve at least 350 million years ago. The βA3/βA1 sequence is evolving the most slowly.[3,11]

The human genome contains two groups of γ-crystallin genes.
- γA–γF and a one-quarter gene fragment found on chromosome 2
- γs found on chromosome 3

Sequence comparisons between these two different branches suggest that they have not evolved recently. Although the β- and γ-crystallins have a similar tertiary structure, their gene structure is very different. The γ gene has three exons, the smallest of which (exon 1) contains three codons; exon 2 encodes both the first and the second motif, and the exon 3 encodes the third and fourth motif.[2,3,9] This gene arose from one gene that encoded a polypeptide with 40 amino acids, which duplicated itself, fused, and duplicated itself again to give one domain (two motifs) expressed in one exon. The two domains of γ-crystallin, therefore, show a high degree of homology. Homology between γA and γF is high, being at least 75% when comparing the amino acid sequences of rat, calf, and humans. Differences in the gene structure of the β- and γ-crystallins suggest that they must have separated after the duplication of the first motif. Comparisons among the members of the β/γ superfamily show that 30% sequence homology exists between the amino acid sequence of the globular domains of βB2 and γB in different species. Amino acids thought to be vital to maintain the structure of the β/γ-crystallins are particularly conserved.[1,11]

CRYSTALLIN EXPRESSION

Although αA-crystallin is expressed strongly in the lens, it also is found, but to a much lesser extent, in the spleen and the thymus. The αA gene promoter has four areas that are conserved significantly between the mouse, human, and chicken. These regions are called DE1, αA-CRYBP1, TATA/PE1, and PE2 in the mouse. Although these sequences are conserved, they have different functions in different species. For example, the αA-CRYBP1 site is needed for transcriptional activity in the mouse but not in the chicken. The DE1 sites are thought to bind different transcription factors and, although the mouse gene is expressed with only 111 base pairs upstream of the transcription start point, the chicken gene needs 162 base pairs for promoter activity. Other sequences, such as DE3, DE2A, DE2B, αCE1, αCE2, and αCE3, also have been identified in the chicken.[10,12,13]

αB-crystallin is expressed strongly in the lens also, is overexpressed in neurological and other degenerative diseases, and highly expressed in regions of high oxidative activity, such as the heart, bronchial epithelium, and skeletal muscle. The expression pattern of this gene, therefore, is far more complex. Most studies have been focused on the mouse gene and show that transcription is initiated 45 base pairs upstream of an ATG codon and 25 base pairs from the TATA box. Although the sequence −426/−164 of the promoter is needed for expression in heart and skeletal muscles, the region −164/+44 is needed for lens specificity. An enhancer is found between −426 and −257. Within the enhancer there are three regulatory sites: αBE-1, αBE-2, and αBE-3. A heat shock protein sequence is found between BE-1 and -2.[10,12,13]

Less research has been directed toward the β- and γ-crystallins. Sequences −434/+30 and −126/+30 of the βB1 chicken gene enable expression of a reporter gene in embryonic lens epithelial cells. Four functional elements, known as PL-1, PL-2, OL-1, and OL-2, also have been identified. The upstream region of the γ-crystallin genes contains a promoter that is lens specific. The γF gene also contains two enhancer-like elements. Although either the promoter or the enhancer is sufficient for expression during early lens development, both of these regulatory sequences are needed for expression in lens fibers.[13]

CRYSTALLIN GENE EXPRESSION DURING LENS GROWTH

The α-, β-, and γ-crystallins are synthesized in the human lens during gestation, and the absolute quantities of these three families increases during this developmental stage. The first crystallin to be synthesized is α-crystallin, which is found in all lens cells. The β- and γ-crystallins are first detected in the elongated cells that emerge from the posterior capsule to fill the center of the lens vesicle.[14] Throughout life the same pattern of synthesis is maintained, with the result that the α-crystallins are found in both lens epithelial cells and fibers, whereas the β- and γ-crystallins are found only in the lens fibers. α-Crystallin synthesis is far greater in the lens epithelium than in the fibers. The α-crystallins are found in both dividing and nondividing lens cells, whereas the β- and γ-crystallins are found only in nondividing lens cells. Differentiation of a lens epithelial cell into a fiber, therefore, may be one of the factors that triggers a decrease in translation of the α-crystallin gene and stimulates the synthesis of the β- and γ-crystallins.[15]

With increasing age there is an increase in both the complexity and the number of crystallin fractions found in the lens. The percentage of low–molecular-weight α-crystallin, as a proportion of the total lens crystallins, decreases. Significant increase occurs in the levels of high–molecular-weight aggregates, especially in the nucleus. This is predominantly thought to result from the polymerization of α-crystallin. β-Crystallin levels do not alter significantly and are found in roughly equal proportions in both the cortex and the nucleus throughout life. Because γA–γF crystallin synthesis ceases at a very young age, this family of crystallins is localized to the lens nucleus. Because γs is synthesized later in life, it is found to the greatest extent in the cortex.[16,17]

EVOLUTIONARY RELATIONSHIP BETWEEN CRYSTALLINS, ENZYMES, AND STRESS PROTEINS

Evolutionarily, crystallin genes are derived from enzymes or stress protein genes that have been recruited by the lens. Because the enzyme or protein acts as a refractive element in the lens but still has retained its original function elsewhere in the body, the gene is said to be *shared*. Some crystallins have arisen as the result of one or more gene duplications. These include the α-crystallins, which arose as the result of one duplication of the small heat shock protein (sHSP) gene, and

γs-crystallin, which arose as the result of many duplications of the glutathione-S-transferase gene. Other crystallins are derived from the same gene as the enzyme or stress protein, but the protein is expressed most strongly in the lens where it is post-translationally modified. An example is ε-crystallin/lactate dehydrogenase B.[9,11–13]

The α-crystallins are homologous to the sHSPs, a family of ubiquitous stress proteins expressed in all eukaryotes. Most of the 90–100 conserved amino acids are found at the C-terminal end in exons 2 and 3. Homology with the N-terminal domain has been found only with mammalian and chick sHSPs. Many similarities exist between these two families, including those that follow.

- Formation of large aggregates
- sHSPs and αB-crystallin contain heat shock elements (αA-crystallin has lost this element).
- β–Pleated sheet secondary structure is common to both.
- All act as molecular chaperones.
- α-Crystallin and mouse sHSP25 are expressed most strongly in the lens.

αA and αB crystallins are thought to have evolved as sHSPs before they were recruited to become crystallin subunits, which explains their different regulatory sequences and why their expression outside the lens is not the same.[3,10,13]

Although very little is known about the ancestral nonlens role of the β- and γ-crystallins, two nonlens members of the same superfamily are produced under osmotic stress, which suggests that these crystallins may have evolved from the osmotic stress proteins.[13]

CRYSTALLIN FUNCTIONS

The high concentration of crystallins and the gradient of refractive index are responsible for the refractive properties of the lens. The short-range order of these proteins ensures that the lens remains transparent (see Chapter 31). The crystallins also have other functions within the lens. The α- and βB1-crystallins are able to bind to cell membranes and the cytoskeleton. The importance of this binding is not clear, but is thought to be needed for the change in shape observed during the differentiation of an epithelial cell into a lens fiber. α-Crystallins also may be involved in the assembly and disassembly of the lens cytoskeleton. Similarities in structure between the sHSPs and αB-crystallin suggest that this crystallin family may provide the lens with stress-resistant properties.[2,3,13] α-Crystallins have chaperone-like functions that enable them to prevent the heat-denatured proteins from becoming insoluble and facilitate the renaturation of proteins that have been denatured chemically (Fig. 32-2).[18] They also act as chaperones under conditions of oxidative stress and, therefore, may help to maintain lens transparency.[19] It has been proposed that three regions (αA 32–37, αA 72–75, and αB 28–34) are the hydrophobic regions responsible for this activity.[20]

Although the function of the β-crystallins is unknown, their structural similarities with the osmotic stress proteins suggests that they also may act as stress proteins in the lens.[13] The γ-crystallins (with the exception of γs-crystallin) are found in the regions of low water content and high protein concentration, such as the lens nucleus. The presence of this family of crystallins correlates with the hardness of the lens. Concentrations are higher in those lenses that do not change shape during accommodation, as in fish, than in those that do, as in the human.[2] The exposed cysteine residues of γ-crystallins may be involved in electron transfer pathways and redox reactions.[5]

TAXON-SPECIFIC CRYSTALLINS

As already stated, α-, β-, and γ-crystallins are ubiquitous. However, some families of crystallin are restricted to certain species. δ-Crystallin is found in birds and reptiles, where it is the most predominant crystallin, composing up to 70% of the total

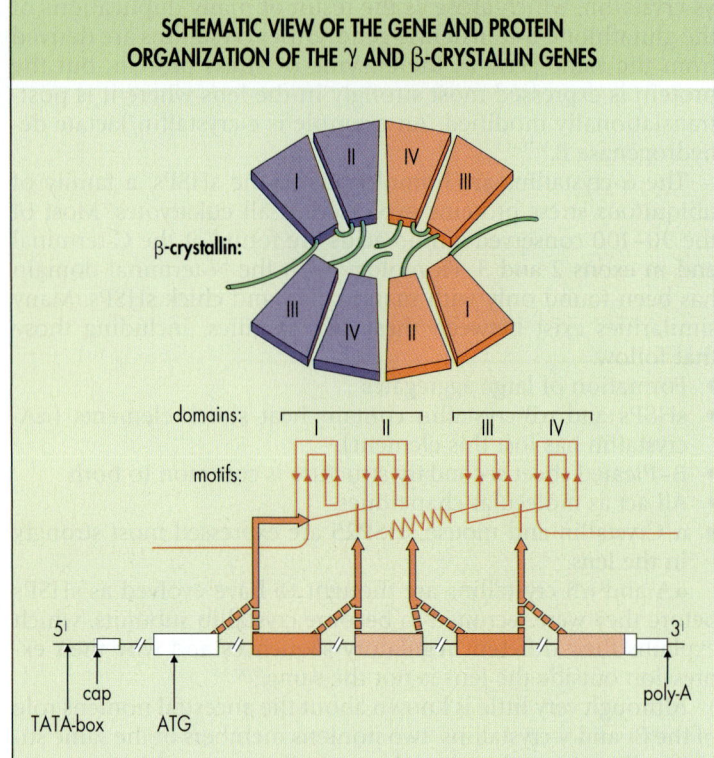

SCHEMATIC VIEW OF THE GENE AND PROTEIN ORGANIZATION OF THE γ AND β-CRYSTALLIN GENES

β-crystallin:

domains:

motifs:

5' TATA-box cap ATG poly-A 3'

FIG. 32-2 ■ Schematic view of the gene and protein organization of the γ- and β-crystallin genes. The bottom line represents the gene organization with the exons marked by boxes, where narrow boxes represent noncoding regions and the wider boxes the coding regions. The motif coding regions are shaded. The shading also indicates the internal homology within the coding sequence. The *Greek key motifs* are shown above their coding regions; the *arrows* show the sites of interruption of the coding regions by introns. The tertiary structure of the protein is shown schematically on top, and the roman numerals indicate the different motifs. One of the β-crystallin monomers has been shaded to emphasize the dimeric structure.

soluble protein. It is a tetramer of 200kDa, with a helical structure composed of subunits with a molecular weight of 48–50kDa. ε-Crystallin is found in birds and crocodiles. It is a tetramer composed of four subunits of 38kDa with a high helical content, and constitutes up to 23% of the protein of these species. ρ-Crystallin, a 200kDa polymer with subunits of 36kDa, is found in the frog, in which it constitutes up to 12% of the crystallin content. Many more taxon-specific crystallins exist

than the few mentioned here, such as η-, μ-, τ-, and λ-crystallins. For more details and a more extensive listing, see Harding,[1] Zigler,[2] and de Jong *et al.*[3] It should be emphasized that crystallins may also play an important role in maintaining corneal transparency because they have been identified in the cornea.[21]

REFERENCES

1. Harding J. The normal lens. In: Harding J. Cataract: biochemistry, epidemiology and pharmacology. London: Chapman & Hall; 1991:1–70.
2. Zigler JS. Lens proteins. In: Albert DM, Jakobiec FA, eds. Principles and practice of ophthalmology. Basic sciences. Philadelphia: WB Saunders; 1994:97–113.
3. de Jong WW, Lubsen NH, Kraft HJ. Molecular evolution of the eye lens. Prog Retina Eye Res. 1994;13:391–442.
4. Harding JJ, Crabbe MJC. The lens: development, proteins, metabolism and cataract. In: Davson H, ed. The eye, vol 1B, ed 3. London: Academic Press; 1984: 207–492.
5. Berman ER. Lens. In: Blakemore C, ed. Biochemistry of the eye. New York: Plenum Press; 1991:201–90.
6. Tardieu A, Laporte D, Licinio P, et al. Calf lens α-crystallin quaternary structure. A three layer tetrahedral model. J Mol Biol. 1986;192:711–24.
7. Groenen PJTA, Merck KB, de Jong WW, Bloemendal H. Structure and modifications of the junior chaperone α-crystallin. From lens transparency to molecular pathology. Eur J Biochem. 1994;225:1–19.
8. Smith JB, Yang Z, Lin P, et al. The complete sequence of human lens γs-crystallin. Biochem J. 1995;307:407–10.
9. Hejtmancik JF, Piatigorsky J. Molecular biology of the lens. In: Albert DM, Jakobiec FA, eds. Principles and practice of ophthalmology. Basic sciences. Philadelphia: WB Saunders; 1994:168–81.
10. Sax CM, Piatigorsky J. Expression of the α-crystallin/small heat-shock protein/molecular chaperone genes in the lens and other tissues. Adv Enzymol Relat Areas Mol Biol. 1994;69:155–201.
11. Lubsen NH, Aarts HJM, Schoenmakers JGG. The evolution of lenticular proteins: the β- and γ-crystallin super gene family. Prog Biophys Mol Biol. 1988;51:47–76.
12. Piatigorsky J, Kantorow M, Gopal-Srivastava R, Tomarev SI. Recruitment of enzymes and stress proteins as lens crystallins. EXS. 1994;71:241–50.
13. Wistow G, Richardson J, Jaworski C, et al. Crystallins: the over-expression of functional enzymes and stress proteins in the eye lens. Biotechnol Genet Eng Rev. 1994;12:1–38.
14. McAvoy JW. Cell division, cell elongation and the co-ordination of crystallin gene expression during lens morphogenesis in the rat. J Embryol Exp Morphol. 1978;45:271–81.
15. McAvoy JW. Cell division, cell elongation and the distribution of α-, β- and γ-crystallins in the rat lens. J Embryol Exp Morphol. 1978;44:149–65.
16. McFall-Ngai MJ, Ding LL, Takemoto LJ, Horwitz J. Spatial and temporal mapping of the age-related changes in human lens crystallins. Exp Eye Res. 1985; 41:745–58.
17. Pereira PC, Ramalho JS, Faro CJ, Mota MC. Age-related changes in normal and cataractous human lens crystallins, separated by fast-performance liquid chromatography. Ophthalmic Res. 1994;26:149–57.
18. Horwitz J. The function of α-crystallin. Invest Ophthalmol Vis Sci. 1993; 34:10–22.
19. Wang K, Spector A. α-Crystallin can act as a chaperone under conditions of oxidative stress. Invest Ophthalmol Vis Sci. 1995;36:311–21.
20. Smith JB, Liu Y, Smith DL. Identification of possible regions of chaperone activity in lens α-crystallin. Exp Eye Res. 1996;63:125–8.
21. Jester JV, Moller-Pedersen T, Huang J, et al. The cellular basis of corneal transparency: evidence for "corneal crystallins." J Cell Sci. 1999;112:613–22.

CHAPTER

33 Age Changes

MICHAEL BOULTON • LISA A. SAXBY

DEFINITION

- The lens exhibits age-related changes in structure, light transmission, metabolic capacity, and enzyme activity.

KEY FEATURES

- Overall light transmission decreases with age, partly through increased brunescence of the lens.
- The lens becomes less elastic, reducing its ability to accommodate and leading to presbyopia.
- The overall metabolic activity of the lens decreases with age.
- The reduction in antioxidant systems with age makes the lens more prone to oxidative damage.
- There are considerable changes in the crystallins; aggregation, degradation, and increased insolubility.
- Aging is associated with the appearance of lens opacities.

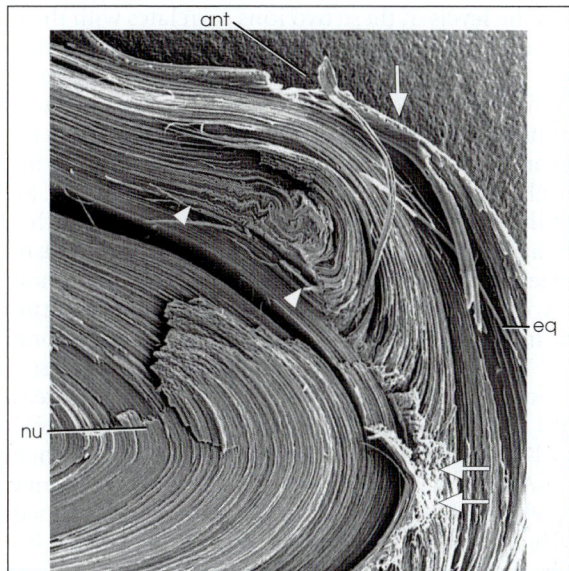

FIG. 33-1 ■ Survey scanning electron microscope of equatorial region of cortical fiber plasma membranes. Note the circular shade with the fracture of fibers in the deep equatorial cortex *(eq)* *(arrows)* and folding fibers in the anterior deep cortex *(ant)* *(arrowheads)*. *(nu, lens nucleus.)* (From Vrensen GFJM. Aging of the human eye lens—a morphological point of view. Comp Biochem Physiol A Physiol. 1995;111:519–32.)

MORPHOLOGY

Increases in both the mass and dimensions of the lens, which occur throughout life, are greatest during the first two decades (see Chapter 28). These increases result from the proliferation of lens epithelial cells and their differentiation into lens fibers. As a consequence of the unique pattern of growth of the lens, it contains cells of all ages. The oldest epithelial cells are found in the middle of the central zone under the anterior pole. Because cells are added to the periphery of this zone throughout life, the age of the cells decreases from the pole toward the outer units of this region so that the newest cells always are found near the pregerminative zone. Although the proliferative capacity of epithelial cells in the germinative zone is greater than in the pregerminative zone, both these populations of cells evolve constantly. Because newly formed fibers are internalized as more are added at the periphery of the lens, the oldest fibers are found in the center of the nucleus and the newest fibers in the outer cortex. Each growth shell, therefore, represents a layer of fibers that are younger than those in the shell immediately preceding.[1]

As the lens ages many morphological changes occur to the epithelial cells and fibers, and also to the capsule. Epithelial cells become flatter, flatten their nuclei, develop electron-dense bodies and vacuoles, and exhibit a dramatic increase in the density of their surface projections and cytoskeletal components. As a result of cellular flattening, the basal surface area of the cell increases; thus the number of cells needed to cover a region of the growing anterior capsule is less than that needed to cover a region of the same size in a younger lens. This, in combination with the decrease in proliferative capacity, means that epithelial cell density decreases as the lens ages.[1,2]

Lens fibers show a total loss or partial degradation of a number of plasma membrane and cytoskeletal proteins as the lens ages. The most significant degradation is that of major intrinsic protein 26 (MIP26) (see "Physiological Changes" section). Early in life, spectrin, vimentin, and actin are present in both the outer cortical fibers and the epithelial layer, however they are degraded as the fibers age and are further internalized. By 80 years of age expression of these cytoskeletal proteins is restricted to the epithelial cells. The cholesterol-to-phospholipid ratio of fiber cell plasma membranes increases throughout life, and consequently membrane fluidity decreases and structural order increases. These changes, which are known to occur from the second decade, are greatest in the nucleus and are therefore partially responsible for the increase in nuclear sclerosis (hardening).[3,4] Furthermore, it is thought that the changes in structure of the plasma membrane and the degradation of cytoskeletal components may contribute to the increase in the number of furrowed membranes and microvilli found on the fiber surface.[1] From the fourth decade onward, ruptures are found in the equatorial region of cortical fiber plasma membranes (Fig. 33-1). Reparation of these ruptures often prevents the formation of opacities. Any opacities that do develop become surrounded by deviated membranes and therefore isolated from the remainder of the lens. The deeper cortical fibers and nucleus are not prone to these ruptures, because the high cholesterol content of their membranes makes them more resistant to damage.[5]

The lens capsule thickens throughout life. It also increases in surface area as a result of the growth of the lens. Ultrastructural changes include the loss of laminations and an increase in the number of linear densities. Although the young lens capsule is known to contain collagen type IV and the aged capsule collagen types I, III, and IV, the presence of types I and III collagen in the young capsule has yet to be confirmed; however, their synthesis may be age related.[6]

PHYSIOLOGICAL CHANGES

Changes to the cellular junctions and alterations in cation permeability occur as the lens ages. The major gap junction protein MIP26 loses some of its amino acids to form new variants, which include polypeptides with molecular weights of 15, 20, and 22kDa.[3,4] The membrane potential of an isolated, perfused human lens may be –50mV at the age of 20 years, but only –20mV at the age of 80 years. Although potassium (K⁺) levels do not alter greatly, remaining at approximately 150mmol/l (150mEq/l), the sodium (Na⁺) content of the lens increases from 25mmol/l (25mEq/l) at the age of 20 years to 40mmol/l (40mEq/l) by the age of 70 years. Thus the Na⁺:K⁺ permeability ratio increases approximately sixfold, which results in a proportionately greater increase in the sodium content of the lens.[7] The change in the levels of these two ions correlates with the increase in optical density of the lens (Fig. 33-2).[8] This change in ion permeability with increasing fiber age is thought to occur due to a decrease in membrane fluidity as a result of the age-related increase in the cholesterol-to-phospholipid ratio. The lens, therefore, becomes more dependent on the Na⁺,K⁺-ATPase in the epithelial cells. Experiments on porcine lenses show that, although levels of the α_1 isoform of this ATPase do not alter with increasing lens age and membrane permeability, a new α_2 isoform is synthesized by the epithelial cells in an attempt to remove some of the excess Na⁺. It still is unclear why a new isoform is synthesized in preference to increasing the levels of the original α_1 isoform.[9] The decrease in membrane potential also results from changes in the free calcium (Ca⁺⁺) levels, which increase from 10μmol/l (0.04mg/dl) at the age of 20 years to approximately 15μmol/l (0.06mg/dl) by the age of 60 years. It is thought that the Ca⁺⁺-ATPase may be inhibited by the decrease in membrane fluidity, which decreases the rate that calcium is pumped out of the cell. It also is possible that the increase in Na⁺ and Ca⁺⁺ permeability may result from the increased activity of nonspecific cation channels.[7]

BIOPHYSICAL CHANGES

The absorption of both ultraviolet (UV) and visible light by the lens increases with age (see Chapter 30). Both free and bound aromatic amino acids (tryptophan, tyrosine, and phenylala-

nine), fluorophores, yellow pigments, and some endogenous compounds (such as riboflavin) are responsible for the absorption properties of the lens.[3] Tryptophan (which absorbs more than 95% of the photon energy absorbed by amino acids) is cleaved in the presence of sunlight and air to form N-formylkynurenine and a series of other metabolic products, which includes 3-hydroxykynurenine glucoside (3-HKG). Because more than 90% of the UV radiation that reaches the lens is UV-A (315–400nm), and 3-HKG absorbs light between 295–445nm whereas tryptophan only absorbs light between 295–340nm, this glucoside has a relative absorbance greater than that of tryptophan in the young human lens (95% compared with 5%) (Fig. 33-3).

As the lens ages it changes from colorless or pale yellow to darker yellow in adulthood, and brown or black in old age. These changes in coloration, which are limited to the nucleus, are thought to result from the attachment of 3-HKG and its metabolic derivatives to proteins to produce yellow-pigmented proteins that also absorb light. As the concentration of these pigments increases they compete with 3-HKG, but as the concentration of the kynurenines decreases further the yellow, aged proteins become the major absorbing species of the lens.[5,10] Because these yellow proteins are fluorescent species, the wavelength absorbed increases to approximately 500nm (see Fig. 33-3). A blue fluorophore, which absorbs between 330nm and 390nm and fluoresces between 440nm and 466nm, increases as the lens ages. The autofluorescent properties of the lens also change with age. A green fluorophore, which is excited between 441nm and 470nm and emits between 512nm and 528nm, then is formed by oxygen-dependent photolysis of the blue fluorophore.[11] This age-related shift in the spectral transmission of the lens explains the change in an artist's use of colors throughout a lifetime. The increased capacity of the lens to absorb visible light, in combination with the increased scattering properties of the lens (because of the aggregation of lens proteins and possibly the release of bound water), results in a decrease in transparency.[2] The increase in the total number of photons absorbed is accompanied by an age-related loss in antioxidant levels which, therefore, increases the amount of photo-oxidative stress.

Nonenzymatic glycation of proteins by the Maillard reaction results in the formation of advanced glycation end products,

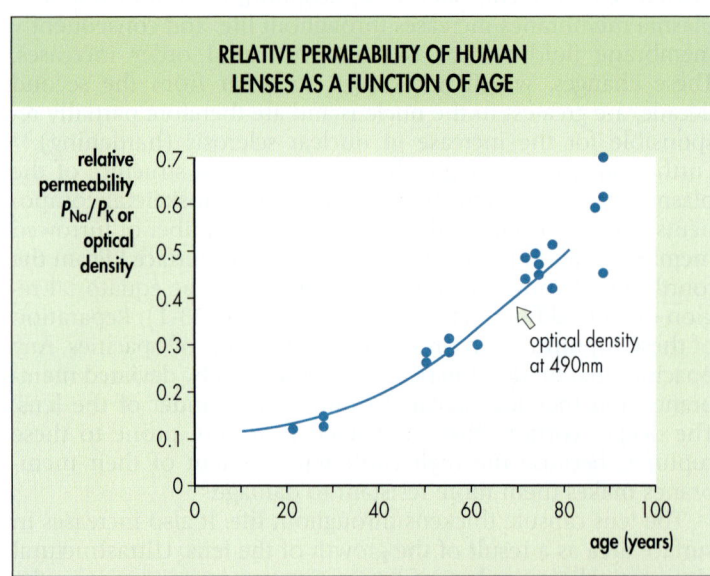

FIG. 33-2 ■ Relative permeability (P_{Na}/P_K) of human lenses as a function of age. The blue line shows the change with age of the mean optical density of the human lens measured at 490nm. Note that the scales for permeability ratio and optical density are the same. (From Duncan G, Hightower KR, Gandolfi SA, et al. Human lens membrane cation permeability increases with age. Invest Ophthalmol Vis Sci. 1989;30:1855–9.)

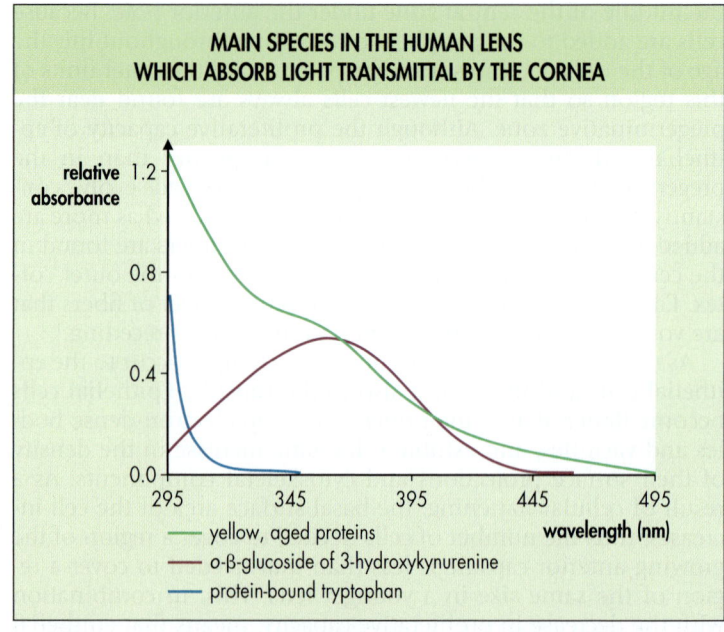

FIG. 33-3 ■ Main species in the human lens which absorb light transmitted by the cornea. (From Dillon J. The photophysics and photobiology of the eye. J Photochem Photobiol B. 1991;10:23–40.)

which also increase the yellowing of the lens. This reaction is initiated by the attachment of a sugar molecule (e.g., glucose) to an amino acid, normally valine or lysine. In young lenses, 1.3% of lysine residues of human crystallins (both soluble and insoluble) are glycated, but by the age of 50 years this increases to 2.7% and to approximately 4.2% in older lenses.[3] Yellow fluorescent photoproducts also are formed in the presence of ascorbic acid. Because ascorbic acid is found in the lens at much higher concentrations than glucose, and because the ascorbic acid reaction is faster, it probably plays a role in the formation of these yellow pigments.[12]

The amplitude of accommodation decreases throughout life from 13–14D at the age of 10 years to 6D at 40 years and almost 0D by the age of 60 years (Fig. 33-4). The older subject, therefore, is unable to focus clearly on near objects and is presbyopic. The change in accommodative power is attributable to a number of factors, including those listed.[13–15]

- Young's modulus of capsular elasticity decreases from $700N/cm^2$ at birth to $150N/cm^2$ by the age of 80 years.
- Stiffness of the lens substance increases, which renders the lens less deformable.
- Although the cortex increases in thickness throughout life, very little change occurs in the thickness of the nucleus. The effect of the rounding of the nucleus on the change in curvature of the anterior surface during accommodation, therefore, is reduced with age.
- Radius of curvature of the anterior capsule decreases, which renders the lens rounder. Contraction of the ciliary muscle, therefore, does not greatly alter the shape of the lens.
- Distance between the anterior surface of the lens and the cornea decreases.
- The internal apical region of the ciliary body moves forward and inward with age. The zonules, therefore, no longer put the lens under so much tension in the unaccommodated state.

The increases in curvature and thickness of the lens suggest that the refractive power should increase with age, resulting in myopia. This, however, does not happen because these changes are accompanied by small alterations to the gradient of refractive index. This gradient becomes flatter near the center of the lens and steeper near the surface and, therefore, the refractive power of the eye is lowered.[16]

BIOCHEMICAL CHANGES

The overall metabolic activity of the lens, as well as the activity of many glycolytic and oxidative enzymes, decreases with increasing age. This is attributed, in part, to decreasing activities in the cortex and nucleus. Loss of activity is not correlated always with a decrease in the formation of the protein, because in many cases posttranslational modifications are responsible for the alteration in catalytic properties of the enzyme. It is thought that for many of these enzymes the concentration of enzyme needs to be below a critical level before an enzyme's ability to carry out a particular function is compromised.[2]

The activity of many enzymes involved in the metabolism of glucose decrease with age. These include glyceraldehyde-3-phosphate dehydrogenase, glucose-6-phosphate dehydrogenase, aldolase, enolase, phosphoglycerate kinase, and phosphoglycerate mutase. Although overall metabolic activity decreases, the lens still maintains the capacity to synthesize proteins, fatty acids, and cholesterol at substantial rates. Decreased metabolic activity, therefore, does not serve as a significant limiting factor for the production of new lens fibers.[3,4]

A reduction in the activity or levels or both of many antioxidants occurs with increasing age. Because this decrease is greatest in the nucleus, fibers in this region of the lens are more susceptible to oxidative damage and lipid peroxidation. As a result they rely upon the overlying cortical fibers and epithelial layer to protect them. The activity of both catalase and superoxide dismutase decreases with age. A decrease also occurs in the levels of ascorbate and glutathione.[2] The reduced activity of both glutathione synthetase and γ-glutamylcysteine synthetase, accompanied by a decrease in the uptake of L-cysteine (an amino aid needed for glutathione synthesis), decreases the rate of synthesis of reduced glutathione (Fig. 33-5).[17] In the human lens a very slow decrease occurs in the total activity of glutathione reductase (converts oxidized glutathione into reduced glutathione). Glutathione peroxidase, which is involved in the breakdown of lipid peroxides and hydrogen peroxide, levels increase from birth until approximately 15 years of age and then slowly decrease throughout adulthood.[3,4] One study using human lenses ranging from newborn to 92 years showed that, with increasing age, protein-free reduced glutathione decreases 14-fold, protein-free oxidized glutathione increases 2.6-fold, cysteine uptake

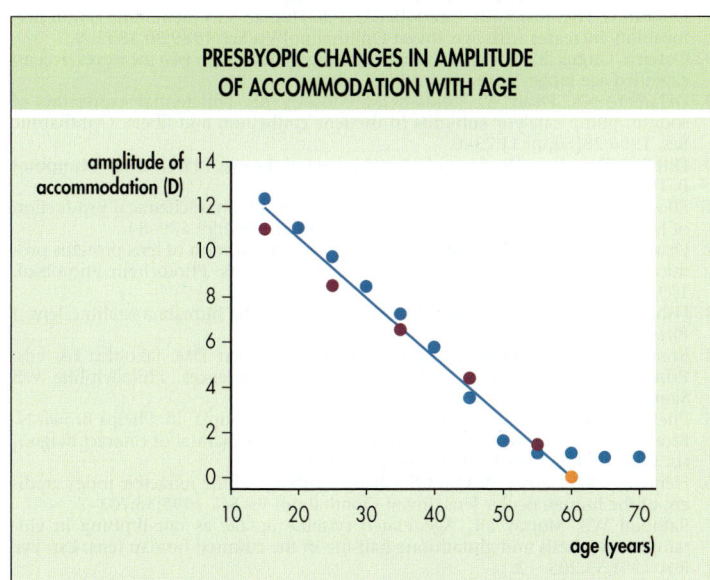

FIG. 33-4 ■ Presbyopic changes in the amplitude of accommodation with age. The different colored symbols represent the data obtained from different publications. (From Fisher RF. Presbyopia and the changes with age in human crystalline lens. J Physiol. 1973;223:765–79.)

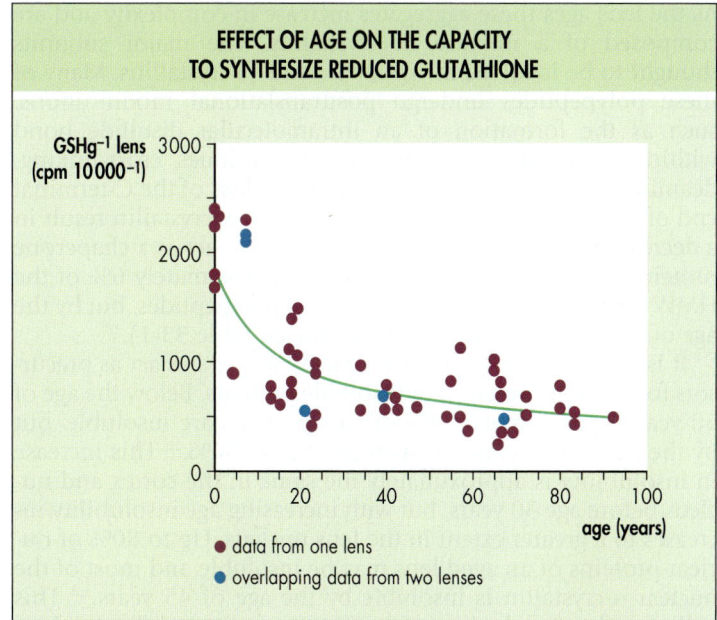

FIG. 33-5 ■ Effect of age on the capacity to synthesize reduced glutathione. (From Rathbun WB, Murray DL. Age-related cysteine uptake as rate-limiting in glutathione syntheses and glutathione half-life in the cultured human lens. Exp Eye Res. 1991;53:205–12.)

TABLE 33-I

LEVELS OF DEGRADED POLYPEPTIDES IN WATER-SOLUBLE HIGH–MOLECULAR-WEIGHT PROTEINS OF HUMAN LENSES

Donor's Age (years)	HMW Protein/Lens (mg)	HMW Protein-Associated Degraded Polypeptides/Lens (mg)	HMW Protein as Degraded Polypeptides (%)
16–19	0.16	0.009	5.6
38–39	0.93	0.17	18.2
49–51	2.17	0.255	11.75
55–56	2.2	0.42	19.1
60–80	2.3	0.62	26.9

(Adapted from Srivastava OP, Srivastava K, Silney C. Levels of crystallin fragments and identification of their origin in water soluble high molecular weight [HMW] proteins of human lenses. Curr Eye Res. 1996;15:511–20.)

reduces by 70%, synthesis of reduced glutathione decreases by 73%, and levels of total soluble oxidized glutathione increase from 2% to 18%.[17] This decreased antioxidant activity coupled with increased photon absorption with increasing age will advance photoxidative damage in the lens.

CRYSTALLINS

Many age-related changes develop in the crystallins.
- Accumulation of high–molecular-weight (HMW) aggregates
- Partial degradation of polypeptides
- Increased insolubility
- Photo-oxidation of tryptophan and the production of photosensitizers
- Loss of sulfhydryl groups
- Nonenzymatic glycation
- Deamidation of glutamine and asparagine residues
- Racemization of aspartic acid residues

These changes can alter the short-range spatial order of the crystallins and therefore decrease transparency.[2–5]

Levels of soluble HMW aggregates (greater than 15×10^3 kDa) increase from approximately 0.16 mg in the lenses of donors between the ages of 16 and 19 years to 2.3 mg by the age of 60 years (Table 33-1).[18] This increase occurs as the result of many factors, which include the inhibition of proteolytic enzymes that have the capacity to degrade these aggregates. Most of these aggregates are localized to the lens nucleus and are, in the majority of the young, principally composed of α-crystallin.[2] As the lens ages these aggregates increase in complexity and are composed of a mixture of crystallins. The major subunits thought to be involved are αA-, αB-, and γs-crystallins. Many of these polypeptides undergo posttranslational modifications, such as the formation of an intramolecular disulfide bond within αA-crystallin, glycation of lysine residues, cross-linking, deamidation of αA- and γs-crystallins and loss of the C-terminal end of αA-crystallin. Such modifications to α-crystallin result in a decrease in the capacity of this crystallin to act as a chaperone protein.[2,19] Below the age of 20 years, approximately 6% of the HMW protein is composed of degraded polypeptides, but by the age of 60 years this increases to 27% (see Table 33-1).[18]

It is thought that many of the HMW aggregates act as precursors for the accumulation of insoluble proteins. Below the age of 50 years, approximately 4% of lens proteins are insoluble, but by the age of 80 years this increases to 40–50%.[20] This increase in insolubility is approximately the same in the cortex and nucleus before age 30 years, but with increasing age insolubility increases to a greater extent in the lens nucleus. Up to 80% of nuclear proteins of an aged lens may be insoluble and most of the nuclear α-crystallin is insoluble by the age of 45 years.[3,4] This will contribute to the loss of lens transparency and the development of senile cataract.

Tryptophan residues in the crystallins are photo-oxidized to produce photosensitizers. This results in a decrease in tryptophan fluorescence and an increase in nontryptophan fluorescence throughout life (see "Biophysical Changes" section). The oxida-

tion of sulfhydryl groups results in the formation of disulfides, which may be one of the factors responsible for the age-related decrease in solubility of lens proteins. Because the γ-crystallins have sulfhydryl groups that are more exposed, they are more susceptible to this oxidation than are the α- and β-crystallins.[4] Increases in the glycation of crystallins in the presence of glucose or ascorbic acid results in protein cross-linking and the resultant formation of HMW proteins (see "Biophysical Changes" section). The α- and βH-crystallins rapidly cross-link; βL-crystallins are slower, but no γ-crystallin cross-linking occurs. One of the modifications that occurs most frequently to aging crystallins is deamidation of asparagine residues. This results in the formation of aspartic acid residues which can alter the structure, destabilize the protein, and increase its susceptibility to proteolytic degradation. Racemization of aspartyl residues, normally Asp-151, results in the conversion of the L-isomer (normal form) into the D-isomer, which increases in concentration throughout life at a rate of 0.14% per year.[2]

REFERENCES

1. Kuszak JR. The ultrastructure of epithelial and fiber cells in the crystalline lens. Int Rev Cytol. 1995;163:305–50.
2. Chylack LT. Aging changes in the crystalline lens and zonules. In: Albert DM, Jakobiec FA, eds. Principles and practice of ophthalmology. Basic sciences. Philadelphia: WB Saunders; 1994:702–10.
3. Berman ER. Lens. In: Blakemore C, ed. Biochemistry of the eye. New York: Plenum Press; 1991:201–90.
4. Harding J. The aging lens. In: Harding J. Cataract: biochemistry, epidemiology and pharmacology. London: Chapman & Hall; 1991:71–82.
5. Vrensen GFJM. Aging of the human eye lens—a morphological point of view. Comp Biochem Physiol. 1995;111A:519–32.
6. Marshall GE, Konstas AGP, Bechrakis NE, Lee WR. An immunoelectron microscope study of the aged human lens capsule. Exp Eye Res. 1992;54:393–401.
7. Duncan G, Hightower KR, Gandolfi SA, et al. Human lens membrane cation permeability increases with age. Invest Ophthalmol Vis Sci. 1989;30:1855–9.
8. Coren S, Girgus JS. Density of human lens pigmentation: in vivo measures over an extended age range. Vision Res. 1972;12:343–6.
9. Delamere NA, Dean WL, Stidam JM, Moseley AE. Differential expression of sodium pump catalytic subunits in the lens epithelium and fibers. Ophthalmic Res. 1996;28(Suppl 1):73–6.
10. Dillon J. The photophysics and photobiology of the eye. J Photochem Photobiol B. 1991;10:23–40.
11. Ellozy AR, Wang RH, Dillon J. Model studies on the photochemical production of lenticular fluorophores. Photochem Photobiol. 1994;59:479–84.
12. Ortwerth BJ, Linetsky M, Olesen PR. Ascorbic acid glycation of lens proteins produces UVA sensitizers similar to those in human lens. Photochem Photobiol. 1995;62:454–62.
13. Fisher RF. Presbyopia and the changes with age in the human crystalline lens. J Physiol. 1973;228:765–79.
14. Koretz JF. Accommodation and presbyopia. In: Albert DM, Jakobiec FA, eds. Principles and practice of ophthalmology. Basic sciences. Philadelphia: WB Saunders; 1994:270–82.
15. Phelps Brown N, Bron AJ. Accommodation and presbyopia. In: Phelps Brown N, Bron AJ, Phelps Brown NA. Lens disorders: a clinical manual of cataract diagnosis. Oxford: Butterworth–Heinemann; 1996:48–52.
16. Hemenger RP, Garner LF, Ooi CS. Change with age of the refractive index gradient of the human ocular lens. Invest Ophthalmol Vis Sci. 1995;36:703–7.
17. Rathbun WB, Murray DL. Age-related cysteine uptake as rate-limiting in glutathione synthesis and glutathione half-life in the cultured human lens. Exp Eye Res. 1991;53:205–12.
18. Srivastava OP, Srivastava K, Silney C. Levels of crystallin fragments and identification of their origin in water soluble high molecular weight (HMW) proteins of human lenses. Curr Eye Res. 1996;15:511–20.
19. Yang Z, Chamorro M, Smith DL, Smith JB. Identification of the major components of the high molecular weight crystallins from old human lenses. Curr Eye Res. 1994;13:415–21.
20. Lerman S. Composition and formation of the insoluble protein fraction in the ocular lens. Can J Ophthalmol. 1970;5:152–9.

34 Secondary Cataract

MICHAEL BOULTON • LISA A. SAXBY

DEFINITION

- Secondary cataract, predominantly posterior capsule opacification, occurs when remnant lens cells following cataract extraction cause opacification in the visual axis.

KEY FEATURES

- Capsular opacification can occur as fibrosis, Elschnig's pearls, or Soemmerring's ring.
- Fibrosis occurs when lens epithelial cells are deposited in a multilayer fashion on the posterior capsule and synthesize extracellular matrix.
- Elschnig's pearls represent the aberrant attempt of remnant epithelial cells to form lens fibers.
- Soemmerring's ring is the proliferation of cells and the synthesis of matrix within the space between the anterior and posterior capsule. It normally does not encroach on the visual axis.
- Posterior capsulectomy remains the preferred treatment, although new surgical, intraocular lens manufacturing, and pharmacological approaches are being evaluated.

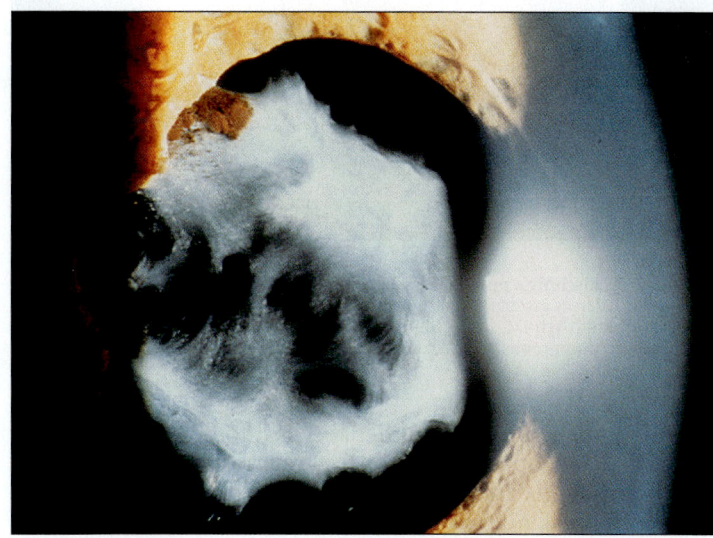

FIG. 34-1 ■ **Fibrosis of the posterior capsule.** This opacification developed in a 5-year-old child 20 days after extraction of a traumatic cataract (perforation with a knife). No intraocular lens was implanted. (From Rohrbach JM, Knorr M, Weidle EG, Steuhl KP. Nachstar: klinik, therapie, morphologic, and prophylaxe. Akt Augenheilkd. 1995;20:16–23.)

INTRODUCTION

Secondary cataract (also known as after cataract) is a significant late complication of extracapsular cataract extraction (ECCE). Posterior capsule opacification (PCO) is the most clinically significant type of secondary cataract and is the focus of this chapter. PCO develops in up to 50% of patients between 2 months and 5 years after the initial surgery. The frequency of PCO is age related; almost all children develop PCO after ECCE, but in adults the incidence is much lower. This is thought to be because of the higher proliferative capacity of lens epithelial cells in the young compared with the old.[1,2]

After ECCE the lens is composed of the remaining capsule and the residual epithelial cells and cortical fibers that were not removed at the time of surgery. The lens epithelial cells still possess the capacity to proliferate, differentiate, and undergo fibrous metaplasia. Migration of these cells toward the center of the previously acellular posterior capsule together with the synthesis of matrix components results in light being scattered, and the associated opacification reduces visual acuity. In the minority of cases, PCO results from the deposition of fibrin and other cell types onto the posterior capsule either at the time of surgery or postoperatively.[2]

MORPHOLOGICAL FORMS OF POSTERIOR CAPSULE OPACIFICATION

The two morphologically distinct types of PCO are fibrosis and Elschnig's pearls, which occur independently or in combination. In addition, ECCE procedures may result in the formation of a Soemmerring's ring (Figs. 34-1 to 34-4).[2,3]

Fibrosis-Type Posterior Capsule Opacification

Residual lens epithelial cells that are still attached to the anterior capsule after ECCE are thought to be the predominant cells involved in the formation of fibrous membranes. Although cases of fibrosis tend to appear within 2–6 months of ECCE, many are clinically insignificant.[2]

Remnant epithelial cells on the anterior capsule differentiate into spindle-shaped, fibroblast-like cells (myofibroblasts), which express α-smooth muscle actin (normally only expressed in smooth muscle cells) and become highly contractile. These fibroblastic cells proliferate and migrate onto the posterior capsule to form a cellular layer that secretes extracellular matrix components and a basal lamina-like material. Cellular contraction results in the formation of numerous fine folds and wrinkles in the posterior capsule. At this stage the capsule is only mildly opacified. No significant visual loss occurs until the cells migrate into the visual axis.[1,4]

More advanced stages of PCO result from further proliferation and multilayering of cells on the posterior capsule, and are associated with additional extracellular matrix production and the appearance of white fibrotic opacities. These cellular membranes increase the extent of capsular wrinkling which, in turn, further increases visual distortion. This capsular contraction can cause further complications, such as decentration of the intraocular lens (IOL). In some cases the cells partially or completely degrade and leave the extracellular matrix components.[1,4]

The majority of the extracellular matrix produced in the fibrosis-type of PCO is composed of types I and III fibrillar collagen with associated proteoglycans (dermatan sulfate and chondroitin sulfate).[5] The basal lamina-like material contains both collagen type IV and heparin sulfate proteoglycan.[5]

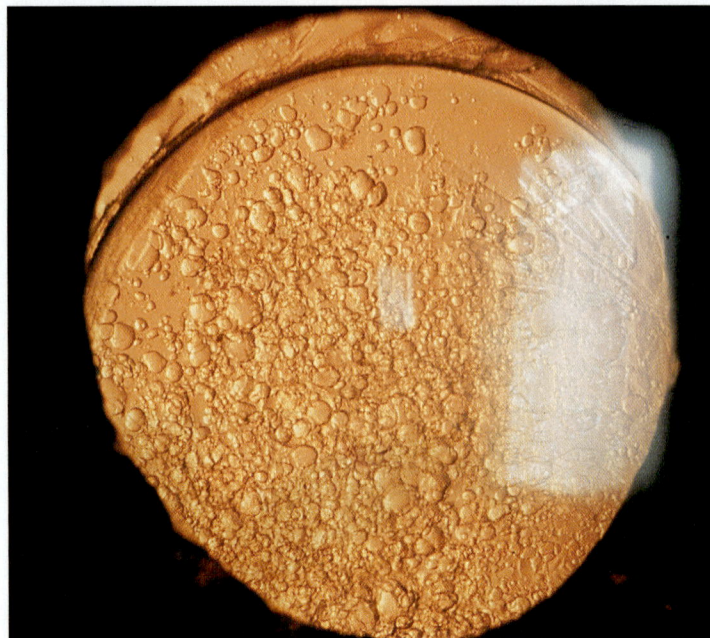

FIG. 34-2 ■ **Elschnig's pearls.** This opacification developed within 3 years of an extracapsular cataract extraction with implantation of a posterior chamber intraocular lens. (From Rohrbach JM, Knorr M, Weidle EG, Steuhl KP. Nachstar: klinik, therapie, morphologic, and prophylaxe. Akt Augenheilkd. 1995;20:16–23.)

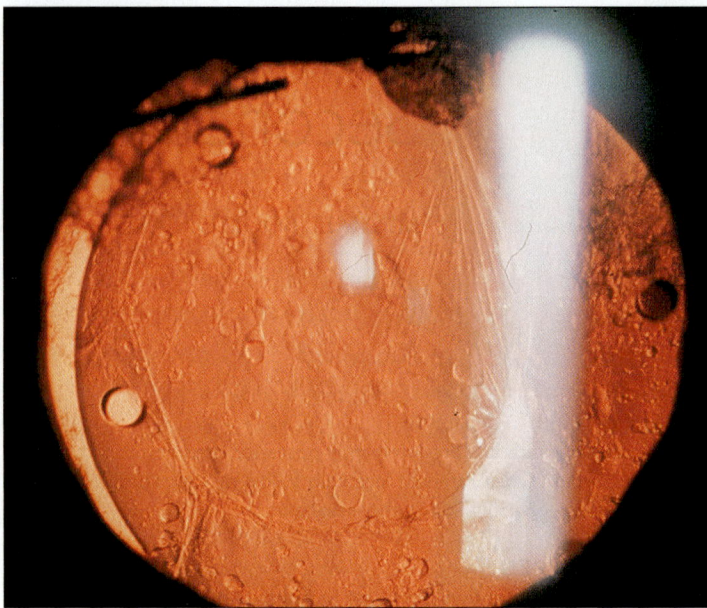

FIG. 34-3 ■ **Mixture of Elschnig's pearls and fibrosis on the posterior capsule.** This opacification developed in a 64-year-old woman 2 years after uncomplicated cataract surgery. Note the wrinkling of the posterior capsule. (Courtesy of M Knorr.)

Differentiation of lens epithelial cells into fibroblast-like cells also can cause opacification of the anterior capsule. Although technically this is another form of secondary cataract, it often is of no clinical significance because the opacification normally is away from the visual axis. In some cases of anterior capsular fibrosis the anterior capsule contracts centrifugally, which enlarges the capsular opening and may leave a sheet of cells attached to the IOL optic. Contraction of the anterior capsule, however, normally is centripetal, which shrinks the anterior capsular opening (capsule contraction syndrome). This reduction in size of the opening occurs more commonly in patients who have received a capsulorrhexis than in those who have undergone a "can-opener" capsulectomy. Vision is reduced only if the anterior capsular flap obscures the visual axis, but this can be corrected within a few weeks of the cataract surgery by making small radial incisions in the anterior capsule.[3]

In cases in which the cut edge of the anterior capsule rests on the IOL optic, residual anterior capsular cells may proliferate and extend from this cut edge onto the surface of the IOL, which results in the formation of a membranous outgrowth within approximately 1 week postoperatively.[6] Detailed studies using polymethylmethacrylate IOLs have shown that cells do not appear to cover the central part of the optic, and migration onto this optic decreases as the cells in the region of the anterior capsule in contact with the optic undergo fibrous metaplasia and begin to opacify. The cells on the IOL completely disappear within 3 months. It is also possible that cells may migrate around onto the posterior surface of the IOL implant and, therefore, contribute to the formation of PCO.

Growth factors present in both the aqueous and the vitreous humors have been implicated in the development of fibrosis-type PCO. These include acidic and basic fibroblast growth factors, insulin-like growth factor-I, epidermal growth factor, platelet-derived growth factor, hepatocyte growth factor, and transforming growth factor-β.

Pearl-Type Posterior Capsule Opacification

The pearls formed in this type of PCO are identical in appearance to Wedl (bladder) cells involved in the formation of posterior subcapsular cataracts. Because Wedl cells are known to originate from equatorial lens epithelial cells, it is believed that residual

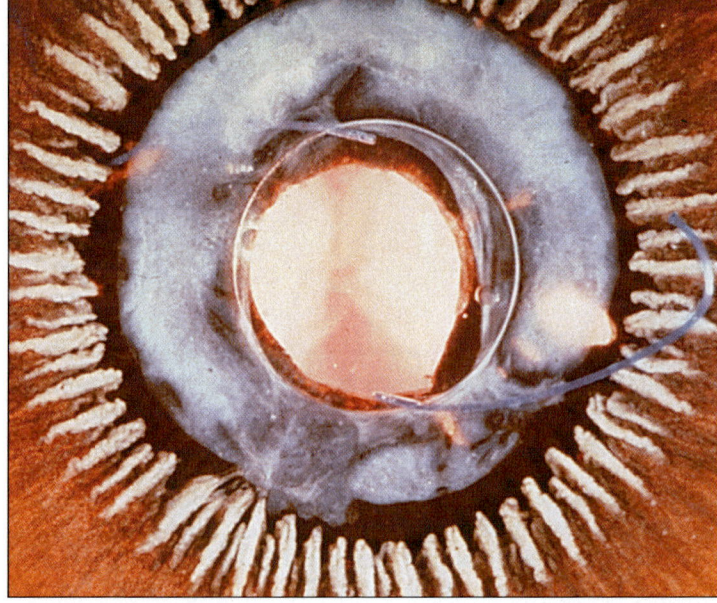

FIG. 34-4 ■ **Soemmerring's ring.** Taken from behind the lens of a human eye obtained postmortem. A three-piece, modified J, polypropylene loop posterior chamber intraocular lens is present. (From Apple DJ, Solomon KD, Tetz MR, *et al*. Posterior capsule opacification. Surv Ophthalmol. 1992;37:73–116.)

cells in this region of the capsule are the predominant cells involved in the formation of pearls. The possibility that the residual anterior capsular cells also are involved cannot be excluded completely. Clinically, cases of pearl formation occur somewhat later than those of fibrosis (up to 5 years postoperatively).[2]

Pearls were first observed by Hirschberg[7] in 1901 and then by Elschnig[8] in 1911; they now are referred to as Elschnig's pearls. After ECCE the fiber mass of the lens is no longer present and, as a result, no internal pressure exists. Newly formed lens fibers, therefore, are no longer forced in the anterior and posterior directions, which results in the formation of a mass of cells (normally large and globular, but sometimes spindle shaped), loosely connected and piled on top of each other. The diameters of these cells are in the range 5–120μm. Each pearl represents the aberrant attempt of one epithelial cell to differentiate into a new lens fiber, possessing characteristics of both epithelial cells and fibers, and may be embedded in an extracellular matrix. The fibrous granular cytoplasm and the possession of very few or no organelles are properties of lens fibers, but the pearls still have interdigitating processes and desmosomes between adjacent cells, which are traits of the original epithelial cells. Some pearls have a nucleus, which normally is lobulated but may be round or oval. Visual acuity is affected only if the pearls protrude into the center of the posterior capsule and therefore into pupillary space.[9-11]

Soemmerring's Ring

Soemmerring first noticed PCO in humans in 1828.[12] After ECCE, the cut edge of the remaining anterior capsular flap may attach itself to the posterior capsule within approximately 4 weeks postoperatively, through the production of fibrous tissue. Any residual cortical fibers and epithelial cells, therefore, are trapped within this sealed structure. The equatorial cells still retain the capacity to proliferate and differentiate into lens fibers. The increase in the volume of this lenticular material fills the space between the anterior and the posterior capsule, which results in the formation of a ring that often has the appearance of a string of sausages. Proliferating epithelial cells remain attached to the anterior capsule but also are found to a lesser extent on the posterior capsule, where they form small isolated groups. In some cases the epithelial cells escape from the ring and migrate onto the anterior surface of the anterior capsule. Although the newly formed peripheral fibers appear almost normal, those that are forced inward sometimes degenerate, containing clusters of recrystallized proteins embedded in an amorphous material. These proteins normally are rod-shaped structures, but they also may be spherical. In some cases, therefore, the ring remains clear and yellow, but in others opacities develop and the ring looks cataractous. Because the ring forms at the periphery of the lens, vision is not affected.[9,13,14]

At present, a considerable amount of disagreement exists as to whether the capsulorrhexis or capsulectomy diameter or both should be larger, smaller, or of the same size as that of the optic. The true seal needed for the formation of Soemmerring's ring occurs only if the cut edge of the anterior capsule comes into contact with the posterior capsule, because either the IOL optic is smaller than the opening or the capsule has retracted beyond the edge of the optic.[2] The ring has two important functions. First, the haptics of an implanted IOL, which extend to the equator of the capsular bag, are held in place, which prevents decentration. Second, the early fibrosis, which is known to seal the capsular surfaces, may help to contain the Elschnig's pearls by enhancing the seal between these two surfaces. The haptics of the IOL, however, are a region of loose adherence through which epithelial cells may escape; the cells have to migrate only a small distance before the center of the posterior capsule is reached. Some surgeons, therefore, believe that to keep the cut edge of the anterior capsular flap in front of the optic will ensure that the residual cells are kept further away from the center of the posterior capsule and thus reduce the incidence of PCO.[2,7,13]

Other Causes of Posterior Capsule Opacification

Cell types other than lens epithelial cells may be involved in PCO. ECCE is associated with the breakdown of the blood–aqueous barrier (normally greatest immediately after surgery), allowing inflammatory cells, erythrocytes, and many other components to be released from the blood into the aqueous humor. This elicits an inflammatory response, the severity of which is highly variable and may be increased by the implantation of an IOL. This foreign body reaction elicits a three-stage immune response that involves many different cell types, which include polymorphonuclear leukocytes, giant cells, and fibroblasts. As a result collagen is deposited onto the IOL and the capsule, which causes opacities, and fine wrinkles may form in the posterior capsule. In most cases, however, this inflammatory response is clinically insignificant.[2,9]

Bacteria and other organisms can enter the eye during surgery, find their way into the capsular bag, and cause postoperative localized endophthalmitis. These organisms, in conjunction with the inflammatory response they provoke, may form a white precipitate that opacifies the posterior capsule and mimics PCO. Iris melanocytes also have been shown to adhere to and migrate over the anterior surface of the posterior capsule.[2,9]

PREVENTION AND TREATMENT OF POSTERIOR CAPSULE OPACIFICATION

As yet there is no reliable treatment to prevent PCO. Experimental approaches being assessed include refinement of surgical technique, changes to the IOL design, and the development of pharmacological strategies either to kill the residual epithelial cells or to prevent their postoperative proliferation.

In an ideal world the best way to prevent PCO would be to remove all the lens epithelial cells and the cortical remnants at the time of the ECCE surgery. Many different approaches have been used, with variable success. Although insertion of the IOL probably knocks off a large number of cells, surgeons frequently concentrate on cleaning the posterior capsule rather than on removal of the residual epithelial cells. Polishing the posterior capsule, however, does not prevent the development of PCO.[15] Infusion of sterile saline under the capsule before the capsulectomy ruptures many, if not all, of residual epithelial cells. Corneal endothelial damage is prevented by filling the anterior chamber with a viscoelastic agent.[2] Anterior capsule cleaning with an ultrasonographic irrigating scratcher removes all fibers and reduces the number of residual epithelial cells.[1] Freezing of the posterior capsule with a cryoprobe results in the formation of intracellular ice crystals which destroy any remaining lens epithelial cells. The problem with this technique is the high risk of damage to the surrounding ocular tissues. Freezing of the vitreous humor may pull on the retina and cause additional complications.[16] The formation of PCO can be reduced also by minimizing the breakdown of the blood-aqueous barrier.[2]

An anterior capsulectomy is thought to provide a stimulus for lens epithelial cell proliferation. Originally the consensus was that to remove more of the anterior capsule would remove more lens epithelial cells and therefore reduce the risk of opacification. It is now thought that the wider the opening, the greater the number of epithelial cells released from contact inhibition, and therefore the greater the number of cells capable of proliferation and migration onto the posterior capsule. This is especially true of the can-opener technique.[1,17] Cases of PCO are less prevalent in patients who undergo a circular capsulorrhexis, because this technique enhances the efficiency of hydrodissection and subsequent cortical cleanup.[2] In patients who have a greater risk of developing PCO, such as children and those who have diabetes or uveitis, the center of the posterior capsule can be removed. Although it was thought that this posterior continuous circular capsulorrhexis would prevent the migration of cells into the center of the posterior capsule, a number of cases of partial or complete reclosure, either by fibrosis or the formation of pearls, have been observed.[18]

The implantation of a posterior chamber IOL into the capsular bag after ECCE is known to reduce the likelihood that a patient will develop PCO, because the IOL acts as a barrier to the migration of cells around and into the center of the posterior capsule. Posterior convex or biconvex optics sit in the capsular bag with their posterior surface firmly against the posterior capsule. As a result this capsular surface is stretched radially and flattened, so there should be no room for the cells to pass this mechanical barrier and migrate into the center of the posterior capsule. Barrier-ridge optics have a rim on the posterior surface of the IOL, which also should create a barrier to migrating cells.

Migration also has been shown to be dependent on the implant biomaterial. Trials have shown that the posterior capsules of patients who were given polyacrylic (AcrySof) implants were significantly clearer 2 years after implantation than the posterior capsules of those given polymethylmethacrylate or silicone implants. Lens epithelial cells also have been shown to regress in eyes implanted with polyacrylic IOLs.[19] Modifications of the surface of different types of IOL, by coating with heparin, indomethacin, or fibroblast growth factor conjugated with saporin, and surface passivation have been shown to reduce postoperative inflammation and PCO.[20]

Pharmacologic agents, antimetabolites, and other agents also have been used to try to reduce PCO. These compounds must be administered to the posterior chamber so that the highest concentrations occur in and around the remaining capsular bag to minimize damage to the surrounding tissues, but many of these agents still cause significant ocular toxicity. 5-Fluorouracil, methotrexate, colchicine, mitomycin C, and daunorubicin are antimitotic drugs that have been shown to reduce significantly the proliferative capacity of lens epithelial cells. 5-Fluorouracil experimentally used in combination with flurbiprofen also was found to reduce significantly the incidence of PCO.[2,21] LCM 1910, a synthetic peptide that recognizes the tripeptide arginine-glycine-aspartic acid (RGD sequence) found in moving extracellular matrix components, has been shown to decrease or totally inhibit lens cell migration by competing with capsule components for the integrin binding sites.[22] More directed approaches to lens epithelial cells include immunotargeting and gene therapy.[22] The potent protein synthesis inhibitor ricin has been conjugated to a human monoclonal antibody specific for lens epithelial cells and has been evaluated in cataract surgery. Although a significant inhibition of PCO was observed, postoperative flare and inflammation were a major complication. The transfer of suicide or growth-inhibiting genes into lens epithelial cells using viral vectors has been successful in animal models. However, this procedure will require considerable refinement before it can be used to inhibit PCO in patients.

Patients who have PCO who have significantly impaired vision need a posterior capsulectomy, which removes the central part of the posterior capsule and therefore instantly improves vision. Although this removal used to be achieved surgically, a neodymium yttrium-aluminum-garnet (Nd:YAG) laser is now used (Fig. 34-5). In a number of patients with posterior segment problems, however, massive proliferation of lens epithelial remnants has been observed within months of the capsulectomy. As a result of this proliferation, the size of the capsulectomy decreases, which may in turn reduce visual acuity. It has been postulated that this occurs because of "activation" of the cells, the release of growth factors from the vitreous humor, the direct stimulation of proliferation, or a combination of these factors.[23] Removal of the barrier between the posterior chamber and the vitreous cavity increases the risk of complications such as cystoid macular edema, retinal detachment, uveitis, and secondary glaucoma.[2]

REFERENCES

1. Green WR, McDonnell PJ. Opacification of the posterior capsule. Trans Ophthalmol Soc U K. 1985;104:727–39.
2. Apple DJ, Solomon KD, Tetz MR, et al. Posterior capsule opacification. Surv Ophthalmol. 1992;37:73–116.
3. Rohrbach JM, Knorr M, Weidle EG, Steuhl KP. Nachstar: klinik, therapie, morphologie und prophylaxe. Akt Augenheilkd. 1995;20:16–23.
4. McDonnell PJ, Stark WJ, Green WR. Posterior capsule opacification: a specular microscopic study. Ophthalmology. 1984;91:853–6.
5. Ishibashi T, Araki H, Sugai S, et al. Detection of proteoglycans in human posterior capsule opacification. Ophthalmic Res. 1995;27:208–13.
6. Pande MV, Spalton DJ, Marshall J. In vivo human lens epithelial cell proliferation on the anterior surface of PMMA intraocular lenses. Br J Ophthalmol. 1996;80:469–74.
7. Hirschberg J. Einführung in die Augenheilkunde. II. Hälkft I Abt. Leipzig: Themie; 1901:159.
8. Elschig A. Klinisch-anatomischer Beitrag zur Kenntnis des Nachstares. Klin Monatsbl Augenkeilkd. 1911;49:444–51.
9. Kappelhof JP, Vrensen GFJM. The pathology of after-cataract. Acta Ophthalmol. 1992;70(Suppl 205):13–24.
10. Sveinsson O. The ultrastructure of Elschnig's pearls in a pseudophakic eye. Acta Ophthalmol. 1993;71:95–8.
11. Kappelhof JP, Vrensen GFJM, de Jong PTVM, et al. An ultrastructural study of Elschnig's pearls in the pseudophakic eye. Am J Ophthalmol. 1986;101:58–69.
12. Soemmering DW. Beobachtungen von die organischen Veränderungen in Auge nach Staaroperationen. Frankfurt: Wesche; 1913.
13. Kappelhof JP, Vrensen GFJM, de Jong PTVM, et al. The ring of Soemmering in man: an ultrastructural study. Graefes Arch Klin Exp Ophthalmol. 1987; 225:77–83.
14. Jongebloed WL, Dijk F, Kruis J, Worst JGF. Soemmering's ring, an aspect of secondary cataract: a morphological description by SEM. Doc Ophthalmol. 1988; 70:165–74.
15. Meucci G, Esente S, Esente I. Anterior capsule cleaning with an ultrasound irrigating scratcher. J Cataract Refract Surg. 1991;17:75–9.
16. Zaturinsky B, Naveh N, Saks D, Solomon AS. Prevention of posterior capsular opacification by cryolysis and the use of heparinized irrigating solution during extracapsular lens extraction in rabbits. Ophthalmic Surg. 1990;21:431–4.
17. Green WT, Boase DL. How clean is your capsule? Eye. 1989;3:678–84.
18. Tassignon MJ, Smets RME, De Groot V, Vervecken F. Secondary closure of posterior continuous circular capsulorrhexis (PCCC) in diabetes and uveitis patients operated for cataract. Vision Res. 1995;36(Suppl):S112.
19. Pande M, Ursell PG, Spalton DJ. Lens epithelial cell regression on the posterior capsule with different intraocular lens materials. Br J Ophthalmol. 1998;82:1182–8.
20. Behar-Cohen FF, David T, D'Hermies F, et al. In vivo inhibition of lens regrowth by fibroblast growth factor 2-saporin. Invest Ophthalmol Vis Sci. 1995;36: 2434–48.
21. Ismali MM, Alio JL, Ruiz Moreno JM. Prevention of secondary cataract by antimitotic drugs: experimental study. Ophthalmic Res. 1996;28:64–9.
22. Bertelmann E, Kojetinsky C. Posterior capsule opacification and anterior capsule opacification. Curr Opin Ophthalmol. 2001;12:35–40.
23. Jones NP, McLeod D, Boulton ME. Massive proliferation of lens epithelial remnants after Nd-YAG laser capsulotomy. Br J Ophthalmol. 1995;79:261–3.

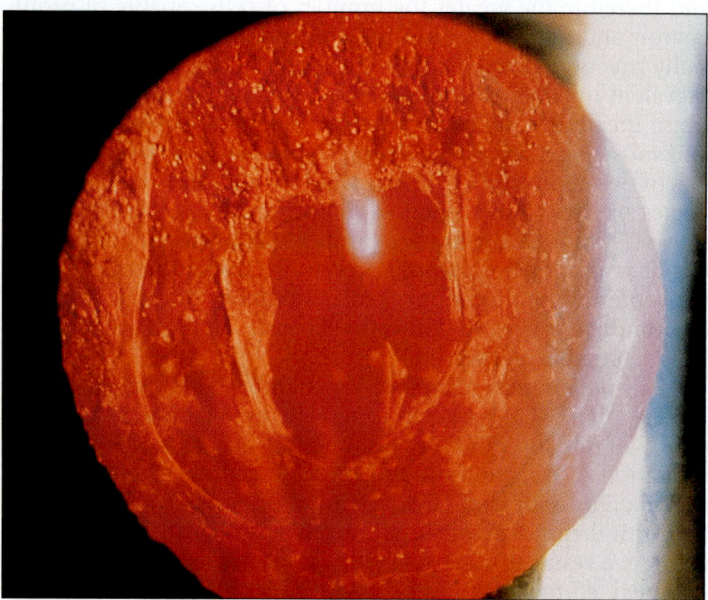

FIG. 34-5 ▓ Posterior capsule following a Nd:YAG laser posterior capsulectomy. (From Rohrbach JM, Knorr M, Weidle EG, Steuhl KP. Nachstar: klinik, therapie, morphologic, and prophylaxe. Akt Augenheilkd. 1995;20:16–23.)

CHAPTER 35

SECTION 2 CATARACT

Pathophysiology and Epidemiology of Cataract

DEEPAK K. CHITKARA • ANTHONY B. HALL • A. RALPH ROSENTHAL

INTRODUCTION

Lens abnormalities may be divided into two categories—abnormalities of lens size and shape, which are largely developmental, and abnormalities of lens clarity, or cataract. Cataract may be defined as any light scatter opacity in the lens, not necessarily with any demonstrable effect on vision. Cataract that is significant enough to impair vision is the leading cause of blindness worldwide.[1] In this chapter, lens abnormalities related to abnormal growth and the epidemiology and causal factors in cataract formation are discussed.

NORMAL LENS GROWTH

The human lens, unlike the lens in other species, continues to grow throughout life. In addition, the growth rate is not linear but has distinct phases. Growth is most rapid in the embryonic and prenatal phases. The lens induction precedes development of the optic vesicle. It is thought that a large area of head ectoderm acquires a "lens bias" in response to signals from the anterior end neural plate (Fig. 35-1). At the 2.6mm stage the optic vesicle develops from the forebrain. Signals from the optic vesicle cause the lens-biased tissue to differentiate further into the lens placode (or plate). As the placode grows, it forms the lens pit below its center. This lens pit is lined by flattened lens epithelial cells. As the pit enlarges into a lens vesicle, the epithelial cells within it break down and disappear by the 16mm stage. The enlarging pit forms a sac, which initially is open at the surface by the lens pore. This pore closes with further growth, which results in a spherical lens vesicle by the 8–9mm stage. The vesicle is approximately 0.2mm in diameter at this stage.

The cells of the posterior wall of the vesicle then elongate, which results in obliteration of the cavity of the vesicle. Meanwhile, the anterior cells become less crowded and assume a cuboidal shape—these cells will become the lens epithelium. Eventually, the cells of the posterior wall become separated from the epithelial cells anteriorly and the capsule posteriorly to form the embryonic nucleus. The lens capsule is secreted by the cells of the equator and those of the posterior wall by the 13mm stage. At the 17mm stage the lens diameter is about 350μm in the anteroposterior plane and 300μm in the equatorial diameter. Further growth takes place by the division of pre-equatorial epithelial cells, which become the germinative zone of the lens. New fibers are added here throughout life.

The lens at birth is almost spherical, with a slightly shorter sagittal than equatorial axis. After birth, lens growth slows down, but an important shape change occurs, such that most of the growth is equatorial in the first two decades.[2,3] The sagittal width may even decrease as a result of increased zonular tension and central compaction of lens fibers. As a result, the lens begins to take on the characteristic shape of the mature adult lens. Later, lens growth is in the sagittal axis with limited equatorial growth. This limitation leads to increased curvature of the lens, and the anterior chamber steadily shallows.

EMBRYONIC DEVELOPMENT OF THE LENS

— head ectoderm

optic vesicle —

— lens pit

lens placode —

— lens pore

cavity of primary optic vesicle —

— lens vesicle

cavity of primary optic vesicle —

cavity of secondary optic vesicle

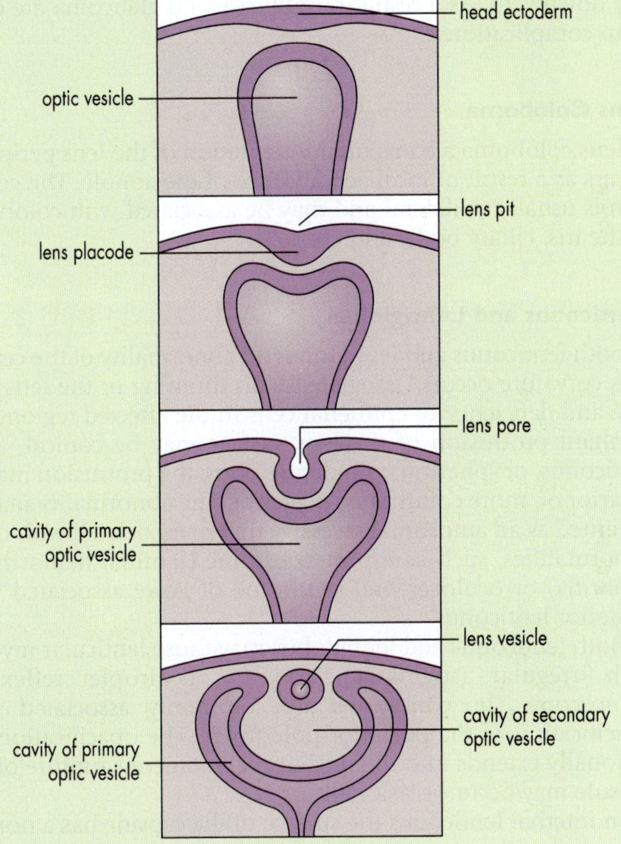

FIG. 35-1 ■ **Embryonic development of the lens.** The lens placode invaginates into the cavity of the secondary optic vesicle.

The suspensory ligaments of the lens develop as fibrils, which pass across the ciliary region of the neuroectoderm to the lens equator after the third month of intrauterine life at the 65mm stage. Their arrangement is regular by the 110mm stage.

ANOMALIES OF GROWTH

Aphakia

Aphakia may be primary or secondary. Primary aphakia is a rare condition associated with gross malformations such as microphthalmos, microcornea, and nystagmus.[4] It is proposed that a primary defect in surface ectoderm or in the formation of the optic cup is responsible.[5]

Secondary aphakia is distinguished from primary aphakia by the presence of some remnant of lens tissue or capsule. It may be associated with developmental abnormalities, such as micro-cornea, or it may occur as a result of partial or complete absorption of the lens in congenital cataract from rubella.[6]

Duplication of the Lens

A metaplastic change in surface ectoderm may prevent the invagination of lens placode and thereby the formation of a single vesicle, which may lead to a duplication of the lens. The condition is usually associated with corneal metaplasia and coloboma of the iris and choroid.

Microspherophakia

Microspherophakia is a bilateral condition in which a defect in the development of lens zonules leads to the formation of small, spherical lenses. The condition may be familial and occur as an isolated defect or it may be associated with other defects in the Weill-Marchesani syndrome and hyperlysinemia. The condition results in lenticular myopia and lens dislocation, which is usually downward. As a result, pupil block and glaucoma are common complications.

Lens Coloboma

In lens coloboma a congenital indentation of the lens periphery occurs as a result of localized absence of the zonule. The condition is usually unilateral and may be associated with coloboma of the iris, ciliary body, and choroid.

Lenticonus and Lentiglobus

In both lenticonus and lentiglobus an abnormality of the central lens curvature occurs, associated with thinning of the lens capsule and deficiency of epithelial cells in the affected region. The resultant protrusion of the lens surface may be conical, as in lenticonus, or spherical, as in lentiglobus; the protrusion may be anterior or, more commonly, posterior. The abnormality may be inherited as an autosomal recessive trait or associated with other abnormalities, such as Alport syndrome (familial hemorrhagic nephritis) or oculocerebral syndrome of Lowe associated with posterior lenticonus.

Both lenticonus and lentiglobus may cause lenticular myopia with irregular astigmatism and an oil droplet reflex on retinoscopy. The conditions are commonly associated with opacification of the posterior pole fibers. The opacification occasionally extends into the nucleus. Spontaneous rupture of the capsule may occur occasionally.

In internal lenticonus the surface of the capsule has a normal contour, but the nucleus within forms a cone anteriorly, posteriorly, or in both directions. This condition is very rare and may be a developmental defect in childhood or acquired in adult life.

Ectopia Lentis

A subluxation of the lens is described as a partial displacement, whereas a complete displacement is termed dislocation of the lens.

The causes of ectopia lentis may be familial or secondary to eye disease and trauma. Traumatic ectopia is by far the most common cause of ectopia lentis and is usually associated with signs of trauma to other ocular structures, such as angle recession. A history of ocular trauma, however, does not preclude other causes of ectopia lentis.

Ectopia may be secondary to a weakening of the zonule by uveitis or to its degeneration associated with hypermature cataracts, pseudoexfoliation of the lens capsule, and ciliary body tumors. Familial causes include an autosomal dominant form, which is usually bilateral and symmetrical and may be congenital or develop in youth.[7] A recessive form is also recognized, which is associated with other developmental abnormalities of

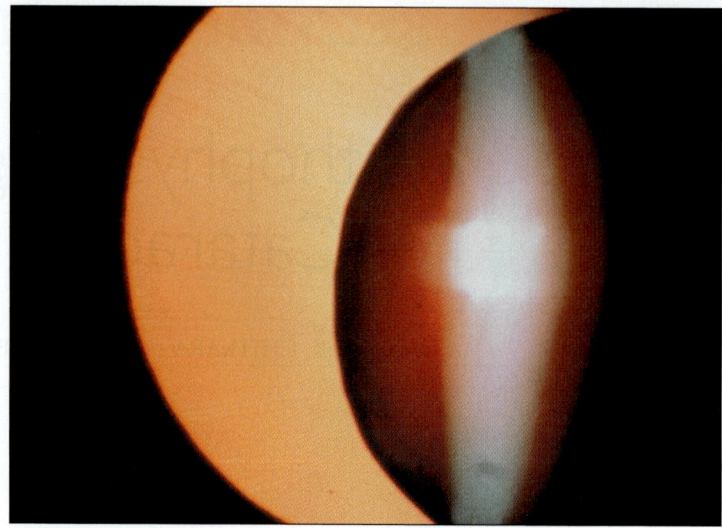

FIG. 35-2 ■ **Marfan syndrome.** A retroillumination slit-lamp photograph of ectopia lentis associated with Marfan syndrome.

the eyes such as iris coloboma, microspherophakia, aniridia, and ectopia pupillae congenita.[8]

Deficient development of the zonule causes ectopia lentis in association with other systemic conditions such as Marfan syndrome, Weill-Marchesani syndrome, homocystinuria, sulfite oxidase deficiency, and hyperlysinemia.

A subluxated lens causes a tremulous iris (iridodonesis), a fluctuating anterior chamber depth, and/or unstable lens movements (phacodonesis). The lens is commonly displaced vertically upward in Marfan syndrome and downward in Weill-Marchesani syndrome and homocystinuria (Fig. 35-2). Vitreous may herniate forward into the anterior chamber and pupil-block glaucoma may result from either vitreous or the lens, if it displaces anteriorly. Posterior displacement of the lens may cause lens-induced uveitis. The subluxated lens causes progressive-induced myopia and astigmatism, reduced amplitude of accommodation, and monocular diplopia.

INCIDENCE AND PREVALENCE OF CATARACT

The World Health Organization (WHO) estimated that in 1990 of the 38 million blind people in the world,[1] cataract accounted for 41.8%, nearly 16 million people. Blindness is defined in this context as a best-corrected visual acuity of less than 10/200 (3/60) in the better eye.[1]

Throughout the world the elderly population is increasing. For the period 1980–2020 the projected increase in the elderly population for the developed world is 186%, while in developing countries the projected increase is 356%. On this basis, the WHO estimated that there will be 54 million blind people aged 60 years or older by the year 2020.[1] Consequently, cataract surgery will continue to consume an increasing proportion of health care budgets in the developed nations. In the United States, current cataract-related expenditure is estimated to be over $3.4 billion annually.[9] In the developing world, the number of new cataract cases far outstrips the rate of surgical removal. In Africa alone, only about 10% of the 500,000 new cases of cataract blindness each year are likely to have their sight restored surgically.

RISK FACTORS

It is estimated that if onset of cataract could be delayed by 10 years the annual number of cataract operations performed would be reduced by 45%.[9,10] This requires identifying risk factors for cataract. Age-related cataract is a multifactorial disease in which genetic, environmental, socioeconomic, and biochemical factors may act synergistically. Epidemiological studies have identified a number of risk factors, which suggests that a substantial proportion of cataract blindness is avoidable.

Sunlight

The role of sunlight in the development of cataract is controversial.[9–12] Support for an association between cataract and ultraviolet B (UV-B) irradiation is provided by geographic correlation studies, which demonstrate an association between hours of sunshine or UV-B flux and the prevalence of cataract. The studies do show that areas with more hours of sunshine have a greater prevalence of cataract, which provides ecological evidence of an association between UV-B and cataract.[11]

Also, experimental studies reveal that artificial sources of UV-B produce lens opacities in animals, both *in vivo* and *in vitro*.[9,11,12] Although these lens opacities may have a different morphology from those found in human cataract, they do support the hypothesis that solar UV-B exposure may cause lens opacities in humans.[11] However, large-scale epidemiological studies in the United States do not show a consistent association with UV-B exposure.[11]

In summary, the epidemiological evidence supports an association between cortical cataract and UV-B exposure, but it is not strong enough to show a causal link.

Severe Diarrhea

Severe dehydration from diarrhea causes acidosis and increased plasma urea concentration. Two case-control studies from India indicate a three- to fourfold risk of cataract following remembered episodes of life-threatening diarrhea.[9,12] In England a weaker association was found.[12] Nevertheless, the frequency of dehydration in the developing world and the suggestion that up to 38% of cataract in India could be attributed to severe diarrhea warrant further study.[9,10,12]

Nutrition

Antioxidants, particularly the antioxidant vitamins A, C, and E, have the potential to protect the lens from oxidative damage. Evidence from case-control studies suggests a possible protective effect from a high intake of antioxidants and high serum antioxidant levels.[9,10,12,13] Population-based studies provide some support for this hypothesis. The Beaver Dam Eye Study found that high levels of serum β-carotene are protective against nuclear sclerosis in younger men.[14] However, high levels of some carotenoids and α-tocopherol are associated with nuclear sclerosis, particularly in women. Until the results of interventional trials are known, the recommendation of supplementation with vitamins to reduce the incidence of cataract cannot be justified.

A number of indicators of poor nutrition have been found to be associated with increased risk of cataract in India.[12,13] Patients with diarrhea are often malnourished. The confounding effect of these variables makes the risk attributable to each difficult to assess.

Diabetes

Many case-control studies demonstrate an association between diabetes and cataract. Two early prevalence studies confirmed an association between cortical cataract and diabetes in diabetics under the age of 65 years.[9] The Beaver Dam Eye Study found that diabetics are significantly more likely than nondiabetics to have cortical lens opacities or require cataract surgery.[15] Once again, the relationship is stronger in younger age groups. The apparent reduction in risk may arise because the effect of age on lens opacities becomes more important in both diabetics and nondiabetics. The difference may also be a result of higher mortality in older diabetics.

Smoking and Alcohol

Cross-sectional, longitudinal, and case-control studies show an increased risk of nuclear lens opacities in smokers.[9,10,12] Furthermore, the Beaver Dam study showed that previous heavy alcohol consumption is associated with an increased risk of all opacities.

Education

Data from case-control investigations in a variety of populations show a consistent association between low education and all types of cataract.[9,10] This effect persists after adjustment for various factors, such as diet, smoking, and UV-B exposure. No obvious biological link exists, and further research is needed.

Aspirin

Aspirin may protect the lens because it lowers plasma tryptophan, reduces the formation of sorbitol, and acetylates lens proteins.[12] Its protective role is supported by animal studies, but the epidemiological evidence is not consistent.[9,10] Some case-control studies show a protective effect for aspirin and aspirin-like analgesics.[12] However, a prospective study of aspirin use and cataract extraction in nurses failed to show a protective effect.[9] Similarly, a randomized, double-blind, placebo-controlled trial by U.S. physicians did not produce a significant reduction in cataract risk in those taking aspirin versus those taking placebo.

Corticosteroids

The association between corticosteroid use and posterior subcapsular cataract has been noted consistently since 1960.[9,10,12]

Gender

Population-based and case-control studies suggest a small, increased risk of cortical cataract in women. Evidence from the Beaver Dam Eye Study suggests that estrogen may have a protective effect against cataract.[16]

Glaucoma

Glaucoma has long been regarded as a risk factor for cataract. However, medical or surgical treatment of glaucoma may increase the risk of cancer. Sophisticated measurement of lens transmission and fluorescence indicated that untreated, primary, open-angle glaucoma or ocular hypertension does not seem to increase significantly the risk of developing cataract.[17]

Genetics

In the Beaver Dam Eye Study, segregation analysis was used to show that there may be recessive genes that predispose the population to both cortical and nuclear cataract.[18] Linkage analysis is required to identify these genes and locate them on the genome.

1. Thylefors B, Negrel A-D, Pararajasegaram R, Dadzie KY. Global data on blindness. Bull World Health Organ. 1995;73:115–21.
2. Manzitti E, *et al.* Eye length in congenital cataracts. In: Cotlier E, Lambert S, Taylor D, eds. Congenital cataracts. Austin: RG Landes; 1994:251–9.
3. Forbes JE, Holden R, Harris M, *et al.* Growth of the human crystalline lens in childhood. Proceedings of Xth ISER Meeting, Stresa, Italy (Abstract). Exp Eye Res. 1992;55:172.
4. Vogt A. Lehrbuch und Atlas der Spaltlampenmikroskopie des Lebenden Auges (Linse und Zonula), 2nd ed. Berlin: Springer-Verlag; 1931.
5. Mann I. Development abnormalities of the eye, 2nd ed. Philadelphia: Lippincott; 1957.
6. Smith GTH, Shun-Shin GA, Bron AJB. Spontaneous reabsorption of a rubella cataract. Br J Ophthalmol. 1990;74:564–5.
7. Jaureguy BM, Hall JG. Isolated congenital ectopia lentis with autosomal dominant inheritance. Clin Genet. 1979;15:97–109.
8. McKusick VA. Mendelian inheritance in man, 8th ed. Baltimore: Johns Hopkins University Press; 1988.

9. West SK, Valmadrid CT. Epidemiology of risk factors for age related cataract. Surv Ophthalmol. 1995;39:323–34.

10. Livingston PM, Carson CA, Taylor HR. The epidemiology of cataract: a review of the literature. Ophthalmic Epidemiol. 1995;2:151–64.

11. Dolin PJ. Ultraviolet radiation and cataract: a review of the epidemiological evidence. Br J Ophthalmol. 1994;78:478–82.

12. Harding JJ. Cataract: biochemistry, epidemiology and pharmacology. London: Chapman & Hall; 1991.

13. Sarma U, Brunner E, Evans J, Wormald R. Nutrition and the epidemiology of cataract and age-related maculopathy. Eur J Clin Nutr. 1994;48:1–8.

14. Mares-Perlman JA, Brady WE, Klein BEK, *et al.* Serum carotenoids and tocopherols and severity of nuclear and cortical opacities. Invest Ophthalmol Vis Sci. 1995;36:276–88.

15. Klein BEK, Klein R, Wang Q, Moss SE. Older onset diabetes and lens opacities. The Beaver Dam Eye Study. Ophthalmic Epidemiol. 1995;2:49–55.

16. Klein BEK, Klein R, Ritter LL. Is there evidence of an estrogen effect on age-related lens opacities? The Beaver Dam Eye Study. Arch Ophthalmol. 1994;112:85–91.

17. Kuppens EVM, van Best J, Sterk CC. Is glaucoma associated with an increased risk of cataract? Br J Ophthalmol. 1995;79:649–52.

18. Heiba IM, Elston RC, Klein BEK, Klein R. Evidence for a major gene for cortical cataract. Invest Ophthalmol Vis Sci. 1995;36:227–35.

CHAPTER
36

Cataract Formation Mechanisms

DEEPAK K. CHITKARA

INTRODUCTION

The main role of the lens is to focus objects onto the retina, thereby avoiding the need for excessive globe length. In addition, relaxation of the suspensory ligaments and elasticity of the lens enable near objects to be focused by accommodation. This is achieved only when the lens maintains its high transparency and refractive index. Any opacity in the lens that causes it to lose its transparency and/or scatter light is called a cataract.

NORMAL LENS TRANSPARENCY

The transparency of the lens is maintained by many interdependent factors that are responsible for its optic homogeneity. These factors include its microscopic structure and its chemical constituents. There is a regular arrangement of lens fibers that takes up minimal extracellular space—only 1.3% in total; only the superficial fibers are nucleated.

The major lens proteins are highly concentrated and are of small size,[1] which minimizes light scatter and maintains transparency of the cytoplasm. An increase in size of molecules or increased separation of the molecule via an excess of water causes light scatter; these processes may be responsible for the development of cataracts.[2,3]

The normal lens also absorbs electromagnetic radiation heavily in the 300–400nm band, which may be significant in cataract causation. In senile cataracts, increased absorption of light occurs through the development of nuclear brunescence of yellow-brown protein pigments.

The protective mechanisms of the lens operate at both the cellular and molecular levels. To protect the lens against oxidative damage, scavenger molecules, such as vitamin E, are present in the lens membranes. Reduced glutathione, a potent free-radical scavenger, is synthesized in the lens and is found in high concentration in the cortex and in the epithelium. It maintains lens protein thiols and ascorbate in a reduced state and scavenges for peroxides and radiation-induced free radicals.[4]

STRUCTURAL ALTERATIONS

The cellular and ultrastructural changes may affect any of the layers of the lens, either alone or in combination. In the epithelium, degenerative changes in the form of vacuolation occur in subcapsular cataracts. Ultrastructurally, the cytoplasmic density becomes variable with the presence of electron-dense bodies and convolution and distortion of the fiber membranes.

Anterior subcapsular cataracts appear to be caused by a metaplastic change in central lens epithelium. The cells become elongated, spindle shaped, and myofibroblast-like. They lie within a connective tissue plaque between the anterior capsule and the epithelium. The connective tissue contains types I, III, and IV collagen. This change is likely to result from direct trauma to the central epithelium such as is produced by ultraviolet (UV) radiation.[5]

Posterior subcapsular cataracts, however, appear to be caused by a dysplastic change in germinal epithelium. The differentiating

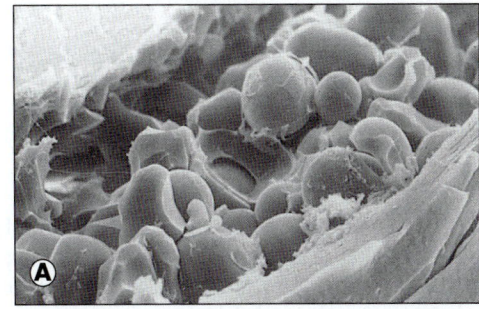
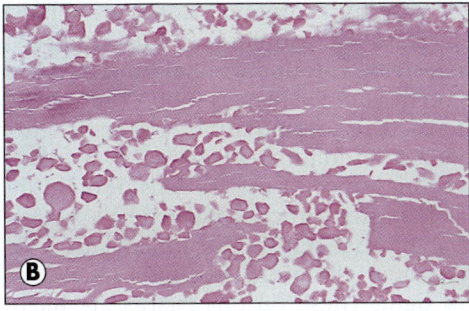

FIG. 36-1 ■ Cortical cataract. **A,** Scanning electron microscopic appearance of morgagnian globules in liquefied cortex. **B,** PAS-stained histological section shows morgagnian globules between fragmented lens "fibers" in cortex. (**A,** Courtesy of Dr RC Eagle Jr. **B,** From Yanoff M, Fine BS. Ocular pathology, ed 5. St. Louis: Mosby; 2002.)

cells are disorganized and imperfectly rotated and the dysplastic products migrate posteriorly, which gives rise to bladder cells of Wedl. The posteriorly migrating cells follow, preferentially, the suture lines. However, not all posterior subcapsular cataracts are associated with suture opacities.[6,7] Some cells may undergo fibrous metaplasia in association with retinal detachment.[8-10]

The cortical lens fibers may swell and the nuclei of the superficial fibers degenerate and disappear. The cytoplasm becomes reduced in density and vesicular, and the fiber membrane appears convoluted. Amorphous bodies and water clefts may form between the fibers. Eventually, the fiber breaks down and forms round Morgagnian globules (Fig. 36-1). When the entire anterior cortex undergoes Morgagnian globular degeneration, the lens appears white and is called a Morgagnian cataract (Fig. 36-2).

No major histological change appears to occur in the nucleus. The cataract seems to be the result of light scatter by accumulation of high-molecular-weight protein. The nucleus becomes yellow-brown and compacted (nuclear sclerosis).

As the cataract matures, cortical fiber breakdown proceeds further and massive water uptake occurs. As a result, the lens swells and the anterior chamber becomes shallower. If this progresses slowly, a shrunken lens with a wrinkled capsule and partially absorbed cortex, which contains calcium deposits, appears as a hypermature cataract. As the cortex liquefies, crystallin fragments may leak into the anterior chamber, which induces macrophage activity and phacolytic glaucoma.

273

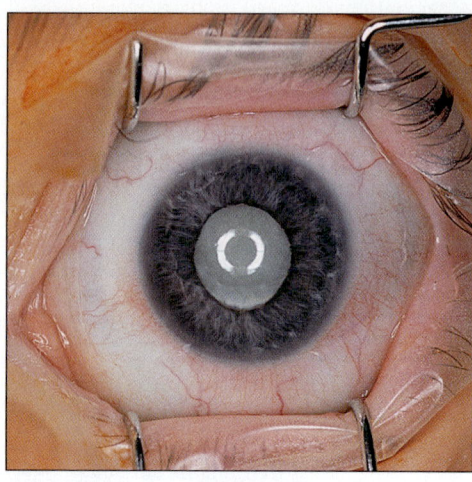

FIG. 36-2 ■ **Morgagnian cataract.** Liquefied, white cortex is present.

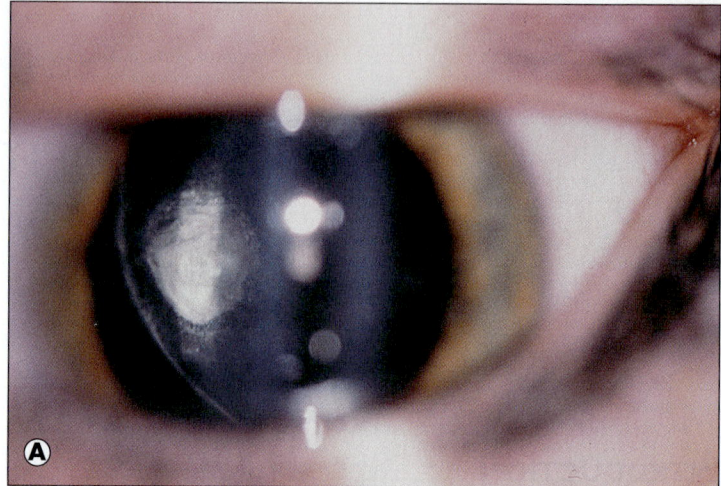

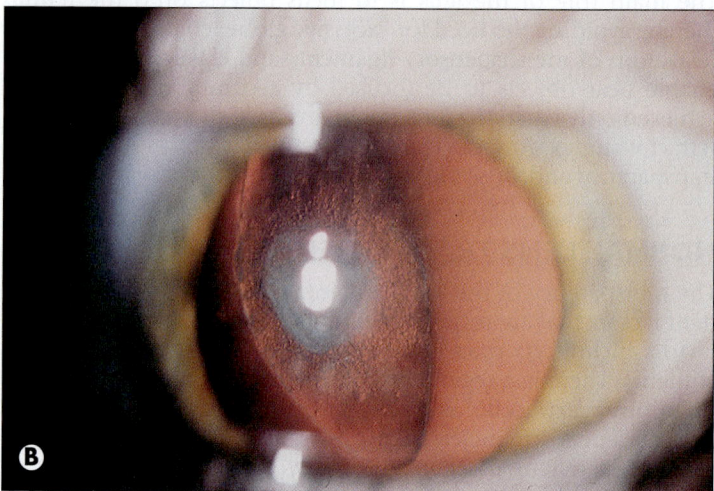

FIG. 36-3 ■ **Congenital cataract. A,** Opacification of nucleus and peripheral lamellae. **B,** Lamellar opacification seen with retroillumination.

BIOCHEMICAL ALTERATIONS

In a cataractous lens alterations occur in many of the biochemical processes that take place within the normal lens, such as changes in protein, water, vitamins, glutathione, and enzymes.

In cortical cataracts, the soluble protein content decreases. Although the insoluble protein content is relatively higher, overall a decrease in protein content results. In nuclear cataracts no decrease is found in total protein content, but the insoluble protein content increases and the water balance remains unaltered. The accumulation of specific chromophores, possibly from a combination of glucose or ascorbate with protein, causes brunescence of the nucleus. Protein denaturation may be caused by free radicals that oxidize, sugars that cause glycation, cyanate that results in carbamylation, or ascorbate that also may cause glycation. Free radicals may also be produced by UV light. These various factors are likely to have a combined effect, which causes a reduction of surface positive charges and, as a result, unfolding of the lens protein molecules. The unfolded proteins may form disulfide bonds that, under the appropriate conditions, form aggregates of larger molecules, which scatter light.

An accumulation of alcohol in the lens causes an osmotic hydration of lens in diseases of sugar metabolism, such as galactosemia and diabetes mellitus. The increased extracellular and intercellular water damages the lens fibers. This mechanism is responsible for the characteristic snowflake cortical cataract with subcapsular opacities, as seen in juvenile diabetics.

Enzymes, such as glutathione reductase and other respiratory enzymes, are depleted in cataracts,[4] while other proteolytic enzymes have enhanced activities during cataract maturation, as calcium concentration increases. This may cause the lens contents to liquefy as the proteins are broken down into their amino acid constituents.

The lens becomes increasingly susceptible to oxidative damage by free radicals because of a fall in glutathione levels and ascorbic acid concentration. Antioxidant vitamins, such as vitamins C and E, and β-carotene may be important in the prevention of cataracts.

FORMATION MECHANISMS

The lens has limited means of repair and regeneration and may lose its transparency in a number of basic ways. The most superficial fibers are most susceptible to mechanical and biochemical disturbances, such as trauma and hyperglycemia. Hence, many acquired cataracts are initially subcapsular. In a mature lens fiber, the opacity takes a limited form, depending on the anatomy of the lens fiber affected and its location. Thus, a lamellar cataract forms if the fibers within a particular fiber shell are affected. Similarly, if a group of fibers are affected, the appearance is that of a spoke. If the tips of the fibers are affected, the opacity appears in a branching pattern of the suture (e.g., traumatic or concussion cataract), where the suture line represents the base from which the petal-shaped cataract forms.

The newly formed fibers may be opaque at the outset. The lamellar cataract that may result is found only in congenital and developmental types of cataract (Fig. 36-3).

Fibrous metaplasia is associated with capsular trauma and with retinal detachment.[11,12] The epithelium may also opacify without a fibrous change; this may take the form of epithelial cell necrosis caused by trauma (e.g., chemical injury), an acute rise in intraocular pressure that causes glaukomflecken, and sometimes acute iritis. The epithelium may also calcify, as in hypermature and morgagnian cataract.

The normal human lens contains fluorescent compounds, the number of which increases with age—the more so in diabetic and cataractous lenses. With the development of senile brunescence, specific chromophores are produced and are associated with highly insoluble lens proteins, which are formed by glycation and by reaction of ascorbate with lens crystallins.

In a similar way, by-products of abnormal metabolism may accumulate in the lens in storage disorders, such as in Fabry's disease and mannosidosis. Drugs and their metabolites may also accumulate as fine granules, usually anteriorly in the capsule, or in the superficial cortex. Opaque granular material may be produced by damaged germinal epithelial cells. This process occurs in radiation cataracts and in posterior subcapsular cataracts.

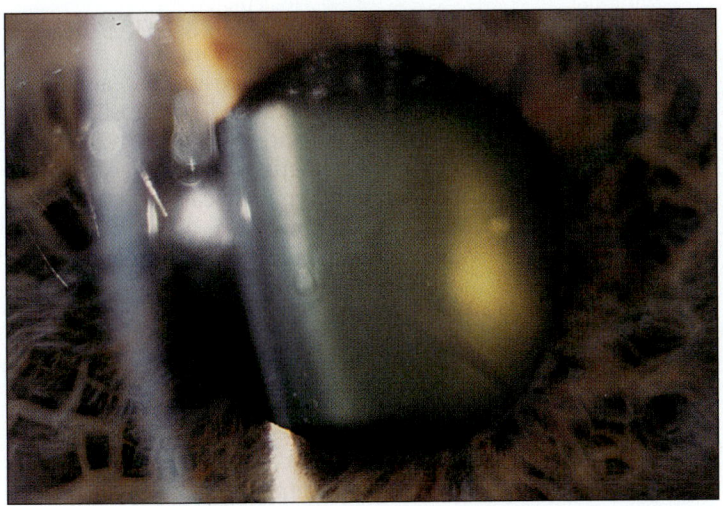

FIG. 36-4 ▪ Age-related cataract. Nuclear sclerosis and cortical lens opacities are present.

CAUSES OF CATARACTS

Numerous individual causes of cataracts exist and often multiple factors act together, with plenty of scope for overlap between the groups. Some causes predispose to a specific morphological variety of cataract, whereas other causes predispose to the common senile variety. Also, a given cause may produce many different morphological forms of cataracts.

Age-Related (Senile) Cataract

Senile cataract is the term used to describe any cataract that occurs after the age of 50 years and that has no evident cause. It is, however, more useful to use the term "age related" because age is the most important risk factor. Other influences, such as environmental, toxic, nutritional, and systemic factors, that affect an individual throughout life have a cumulative effect. It also is possible that genetic differences may influence an individual's susceptibility to these insults.

Age-related cataracts occur as cortical, nuclear, and subcapsular opacities, with cortical cataract the most and subcapsular the least frequent (see Fig. 36-4). This heterogeneity of cataract type may be related to unequal exposure of lens parts to a given cataractogenic influence. Thus, the pupillary area is exposed to aqueous humor, so topically applied drugs affect this region preferentially. Similarly, the pupillary zone of the lens is more exposed to UV light than other parts of the lens. It has been suggested that even more UV light reaches the lower and inferonasal quadrant of lens, which may be a factor responsible for the increased prevalence of cuneate cataract in the inferonasal quadrant of the lens.[13]

The lens equator is exposed to the highest concentration of blood-borne agents, such as glucose and drugs that can pass the blood-aqueous barrier. The posterior lens capsule, lens cortex, and posterior suture systems similarly are exposed to higher concentrations of toxic substances that arise from the posterior segment, such as occurs in degenerative retinal disorders and during retinal surgery. Conversely, all parts of the lens are susceptible to certain insults equally, such as ionizing radiation or physical trauma.

Just as various parts of the lens are exposed to different insults, the same insult on a different part of the lens may have different implications because the different lens parts have a variety of metabolic activity levels. Thus, the lens epithelium and superficial cortex possess organelles capable of aerobic and anaerobic metabolism, the pre-equatorial epithelium is the germinative zone of the lens, and the nucleus has little protein turnover—which renders the nucleus vulnerable to post-translational modification.

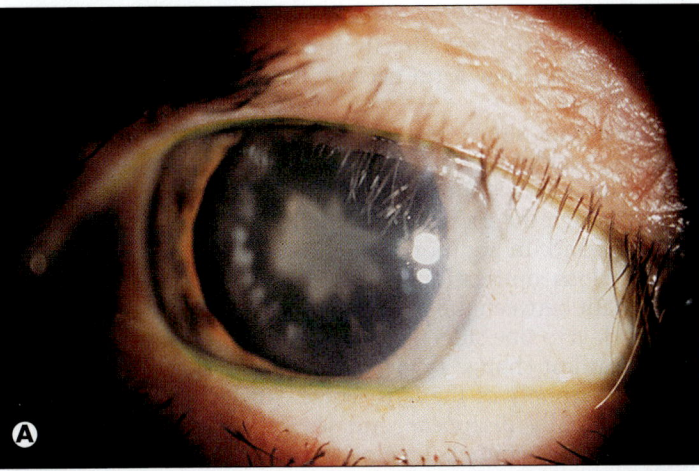

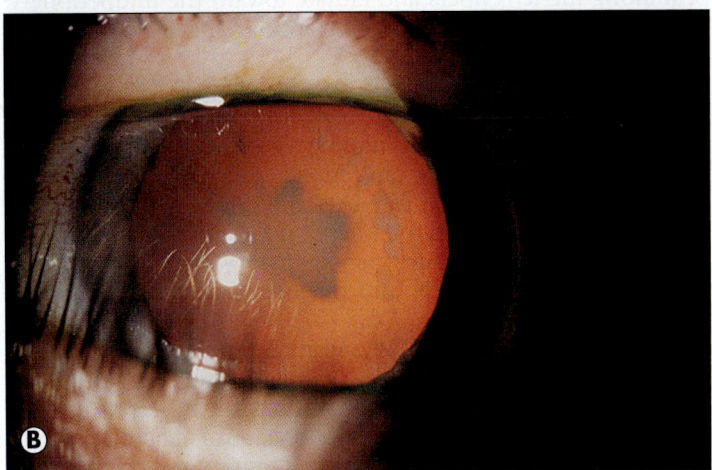

FIG. 36-5 ▪ Traumatic cataract. **A,** Typical flower-shaped pattern with coronary lens opacities. **B,** Seen in retroillumination in anterior subcapsular region.

Another feature of age-related cataract is the occurrence of specific cataract types within specific zones of the lens in a very predictable manner. Thus, a spoke-like senile lens opacity arises in the cortex, but never in the nucleus or perinucleus, and brunescent nuclear cataract does not affect the superficial cortex. This phenomenon is called zonal constraint.

Physical Factors

The lens may react in a number of ways to traumatic insults, be they concussion, sharp or "concussive" objects, a high-velocity foreign body, or electric shock.

In a concussion injury, the effect depends on whether the capsule is ruptured. If the capsule is not ruptured, a cataract may form. The earliest change is in the subcapsular region, both anteriorly and posteriorly. The fibers are thickened and edematous, and the anterior clear zone is lost. Later, the fibers become less swollen and whiten, and a characteristic flower-shaped pattern forms (Fig. 36-5). A Vossius ring may also be present. The flower-shaped pattern forms as a result of the spread of edema from the fiber tips because of the rupture of the processes that link one fiber tip to the next.

Alternatively, an amorphous anterior subcapsular opacity, which may be off axis, or a punctate subcapsular opacity that resembles glaukomflecken may form after trauma.

If the capsule is ruptured, usually posteriorly, water entry occurs rapidly and a mature cataract forms.

If the lens is ruptured by a penetrating object, the capsule may heal if the rupture is small, which results in a localized capsular and lens opacity. If the rupture is of significant size, the lens is overwhelmed by the entry of the water and rapidly progresses to a mature cataract. Surgical injury during peripheral iridectomy behaves similarly. During vitrectomy, even if the posterior capsule is not traumatized directly, a transient posterior subcapsular lens opacity may form because of overhydration of a group of lens fibers.

With electric shock, as a result of lightning or an industrial or domestic accident, cataracts may form with voltages as low as 220V. The current follows the path of least resistance from the head, through the eyes, into the brain, to the nerves, and finally to the ground. In addition to the cataract, the shock may cause memory loss, optic atrophy, and deafness. If the shock occurs equidistant between the two eyes, both eyes develop cataracts. If the shock is to one side, the cataract develops on that side.

The earliest change is formation of ring-shaped vacuoles in the midperiphery of the lens. These extracellular vacuoles coalesce, gradually disappear, and leave behind white, dust-like opacities in the epithelial region. Later, grayish white streaks appear along the lens fibers and radiate toward the midperiphery. Finally, these form an anterior subcapsular opacity.[14-16]

Radiation Cataract

All electromagnetic radiation and heavy, charged and uncharged particles, such as neutrons, can cause a radiation cataract of typical appearance. Radiation cataracts differ only in the energy required to cause them and the time of occurrence. The sources of ionizing radiation include cosmic rays, γ-rays, and artificial sources, such as industrial and diagnostic machines that produce X-rays.

Most of this radiation causes ionization of water and generation of free radicals, such as the hydroxyl and hydrogen radicals, and the hydrated electron. All these powerful reducing agents damage cell DNA, which results in transcriptional errors and altered protein synthesis. Such changes may inhibit mitosis and, therefore, affect cells that have a high mitotic rate, such as the lens equatorial fibers. Posterior subcapsular opacities, thus, are common.

Nonionizing radiation, such as infrared, is recognized as the cause of cataract in glassblowers and furnace workers, prior to availability of protective lenses. The mechanism here is a localized temperature rise of the iris pigment epithelium. The characteristic cataract is a posterior subcapsular cataract. A characteristic feature of infrared cataract is true exfoliation of the anterior lens capsule, which peels off from the periphery and coils up in the anterior chamber.

Ultraviolet radiation and perhaps blue light have also been implicated in cataract formation, possibly via the generation of free radicals. However, the cataract produced is reported to be nuclear, which would be expected to result from absorption of radiation by the yellowing, aging lens.

Poor nutrition is associated with a reduced antioxidant status, which can predispose to increased susceptibility to free-radical damage. Lack of antioxidant vitamins from a poor diet may explain, therefore, the increased incidence of cataract in those of low socioeconomic status.[17] Epidemiological studies have also shown an association of cataracts with chronic diarrhea, which may lead to dehydration.[18]

Systemic Disorders

GALACTOSEMIA. Absence of one of the three enzymes involved in the conversion of galactose into glucose may cause galactosemia, an autosomal recessive disorder. The cause of the cataract is an accumulation of galactitol (sugar alcohol of galactose) within the lens and an osmotic swelling of lens fibers. A deficiency of the enzyme galactose 1-phosphate uridyltransferase causes galactosemia in infancy and is associated with failure to thrive, mental retardation, hepatosplenomegaly, and cataract. The cataract is usually an anterior and posterior subcapsular opacity, which later becomes nuclear before it matures. The progression of cataract can be prevented if galactose is withheld from the diet.

Galactokinase deficiency is associated with galactosemia and cataract but without the systemic manifestations.[19]

DIABETES MELLITUS. Diabetics have lenses that are larger than normal for age and that have widened subcapsular clear zones. The lenses of an adult diabetic are said to be in the same condition as the lenses of a nondiabetic who is 15 years older. In diabetic adults, it has been shown that cataracts are more prevalent, are dependent on the duration of diabetes, and progress more rapidly. Morphologically, diabetic cataracts cannot be differentiated from nondiabetic, senile cataracts.[20-23] The mechanisms that result in excess cataracts in diabetic adults are unknown. All the mechanisms that cause post-translational protein modification, such as glycation, carbamylation of crystallins, and increased oxidative damage, may be responsible.

In uncontrolled young diabetics, younger than 30 years of age, a true diabetic cataract with characteristic morphology may occur. The onset of cataract may be preceded by myopia. The lens then becomes cataractous quickly, with dense, white, anterior and posterior subcapsular opacities in the cortex—"snowflake" cataract. Fine, needle-shaped polychromatic cortical opacities may also form. If appropriate treatment is given, the rapid progression to mature cataract may be arrested and a lamellar cataract may develop.

Infantile cataract, usually lamellar, may occur as a result of various forms of hypoglycemic insults during birth (e.g., idiopathic and ketotic). At the onset of hypoglycemic therapy, a reversible cataract may form.

FABRY'S DISEASE. This is an X-linked lysosomal storage disorder in which mild cataracts occur. A deficiency of the enzyme α-galactosidase occurs, which results in accumulation of glycolipid ceramide trihexoside. The patient suffers from episodic fever, pains, hypertension, renal disease, and a characteristic rash. In both the affected man and the carrier woman, a typical "spoke-like" cataract is found. The opacities are thought to result from incorporation of abnormal glycolipid into cell membranes.

LOWE'S OR OCULOCEREBRORENAL SYNDROME. This is a severe X-linked disorder that results in mental retardation, renal tubular acidosis, aminoaciduria, and renal rickets. Associated congenital glaucoma, congenital cataracts, and corneal keloids can all lead to blindness. The cataract is total, the lens being small and discoid. An early defect in embryogenesis results in poor demarcation between cortex and nucleus, and there is evidence of epithelial metaplasia. Female carriers may show focal dot opacities in the cortex.

ALPORT'S SYNDROME. The disorder may be inherited as a dominant, recessive, or X-linked trait and causes hemorrhagic nephropathy and sensorineural deafness. A generalized basement membrane abnormality occurs. Ocular features include congenital or postnatal cortical cataract, anterior or posterior lenticonus, and microspherophakia.

DYSTROPHIA MYOTONICA. Dystrophia myotonica is a dominantly inherited disorder and results in muscle wasting and tonic relaxation of skeletal muscles. Other features include premature baldness, gonadal atrophy, cardiac defects, and mental retardation. Cataract may be an early and prominent feature in 90% of patients. Other ocular features include hypotony, blepharitis, and pigmentary retinopathy. The cataracts may develop early, but most appear after 20 years of age and mature slowly. Early cataract consists of polychromatic dots and flakes in the superficial cortex. The dots are thought to result from the presence of multilamellar bodies, derived from fiber membranes. As the opacities mature, a characteristic stellate opacity appears at the posterior pole.

Dermatological Disorders

Both the skin and the lens share a common embryological origin, the ectoderm. It, therefore, is not surprising that many skin disorders are associated with cataract formation; many are inherited.

ATOPY. Atopic dermatitis and eczema may affect the cheeks, extensor aspects of limbs, flexure areas, face, hands, feet, or entire body. Cataract develops in about 10% of atopic adults, usually bilaterally; the "shield cataract" is characteristic. This is a dense, anterior subcapsular plaque that has radiating cortical riders, which cause wrinkling of the anterior capsule because of localized proliferation of lens epithelium. Posterior subcapsular opacity, similar to a complicated cataract, may also occur. Both these types of opacities progress rapidly. The mechanism of cataract formation in this condition is not known.

ICHTHYOSIS. Ichthyosis is an autosomal recessive disorder that features hypertrophic nails, atrophic sweat glands, cuneiform cataracts, and nuclear lens opacities.

ROTHMUND-THOMPSON SYNDROME. Rothmund-Thompson syndrome is an autosomal recessive disorder characterized by poikiloderma, hypogonadism, saddle-shaped nose, abnormal hair growth, and cataracts, which develop between the second and fourth decades of life and progress rapidly.

WERNER'S SYNDROME. Werner's syndrome is an autosomal recessive disorder with features that include premature senility, diabetes, hypogonadism, and arrested growth. Juvenile cataracts are common. The condition usually leads to death at about 40 years of age.

INCONTINENTIA PIGMENTI. Incontinentia pigmenti is an X-linked dominant disorder that affects skin, eyes, teeth, hair, nails, and the skeletal, cardiac, and central nervous systems. Skin lesions take the form of blisters soon after birth, followed by warty outgrowths. Ocular changes that cause blindness result from cataract, uveitis, chorioretinitis, pseudoglioma, or optic atrophy.

COCKAYNE'S SYNDROME. Cockayne's syndrome causes dwarfism, but with disproportionately long limbs with large hands and feet, deafness, and visual loss—the last results from pigmentary retinal degeneration, optic atrophy, and cataracts.

Central Nervous System Disorders

NEUROFIBROMATOSIS TYPE II. Neurofibromatosis type II is inherited dominantly; it is bilateral and associated with numerous intracranial and intraspinal tumors and acoustic neuromata. Ocular features include combined hamartoma of the retina and retinal pigment epithelium, epiretinal membranes, Lisch nodules, and cataracts that develop in the second or third decade of life. The cataracts are posterior cortical, posterior subcapsular, or peripheral, wedge-shaped cortical opacities.

ZELLWEGER SYNDROME. Zellweger syndrome is also known as hepatocerebrorenal syndrome. It is an autosomal recessive disorder, characterized by renal cysts, hepatosplenomegaly, and neurological abnormalities. Ocular features include corneal clouding, retinal degeneration, and cataracts.

NORRIE'S DISEASE. Norrie's disease is an X-linked recessive disorder that causes congenital infantile blindness and is associated with mental retardation and cochlear deafness. In the eye, vitreoretinal dysplasia, retinal detachment, vitreous hemorrhage, and formation of a white retrolental mass occur. Eventually, a cataract forms.

Local Ocular Disease

GLAUCOMA. Chronic open-angle glaucoma has no relationship with cataracts, but the use of miotics and other antiglaucoma drugs may result in cataract (see Toxic Causes later). An increased incidence of anterior subcapsular cataract occurs after glaucoma drainage surgery, which may be a complication of ocular hypotony and persistently shallow anterior chamber. Localized lens trauma during peripheral iridectomy may also result in cataract.

UVEITIS. Inflammation commonly results in posterior subcapsular or posterior cortical lens opacities. However, these may arise from corticosteroid treatment as well as the disease itself.[24] Uveitis is common in Fuchs' heterochromic iridocyclitis and juvenile rheumatoid arthritis.

RETINITIS PIGMENTOSA. All retinal pigment degenerations are associated with cataract formation. Most of these are poste-

rior subcapsular and are related to the onset of the disease—they occur at an earlier age in recessive and X-linked forms. The mechanism of cataract formation in retinitis pigmentosa is unclear. However, it is likely that damage results from toxic products released by degeneration of the retina or because of the absence of a factor synthesized by the retina that is important in normal lens growth. It is unlikely to be the result of a direct gene effect.

GYRATE ATROPHY. Gyrate atrophy (hyperornithemia) is an autosomal recessive disorder that causes night blindness, myopia, and peripheral chorioretinal atrophy. The disease is caused by deletion of the gene for the enzyme ornithine aminotransferase. Systemically, it causes abnormalities of muscle and hair and mental retardation. The cataracts are usually subcapsular with opacification of posterior sutures.

DEGENERATIVE MYOPIA. Degenerative myopia is associated with posterior cortical, subcapsular, and nuclear cataracts.

RETINAL DETACHMENT AND SURGERY. Retinal detachment and retinal surgery often cause a posterior subcapsular cataract, particularly in association with silicone oil injection and gas tamponade.[25] An anterior subcapsular form may develop because of metaplasia of the lens epithelium after vitreoretinal surgery.

A transient posterior subcapsular cataract appears within 24 hours of vitreoretinal surgery. It has the feathery appearance of a branching subcapsular sheet, which corresponds to the posterior suture system. The cataract gradually fades over about 2 weeks. The mechanism may involve transient overhydration of a group of lens fibers.

TUMORS. Ciliary body tumors may be associated with cortical or lamellar cataract in the affected quadrant.

ISCHEMIA. Anterior segment ischemia may cause a subcapsular or nuclear cataract, which progresses rapidly.

INFECTIVE CATARACT. Herpes zoster may cause cataract indirectly, as a result of uveitis. Occasionally, however, infective agents may gain access to the lens and cause abscess and cataract. In maternal rubella infection, the virus cannot traverse the lens capsule until the infant is about 6 weeks of age. Lens opacities, unilateral or bilateral, are usually present at birth but may develop several weeks or months later. The opacity is nuclear and has a dense, pearly appearance.

Toxic Causes

Many drugs and chemicals often cause characteristic cataracts.

CORTICOSTEROIDS. The association of posterior subcapsular cataract with prolonged corticosteroid therapy, either topical or systemic, is beyond dispute. However, the relationship between dose, duration of therapy, and development of cataract is unclear. It is believed generally that children are more susceptible to the cataractogenic effects of corticosteroids. Although a dose of prednisolone of 10mg/day or less for 1 year is usually regarded as a safe maintenance dose, the role of individual (genetic) susceptibility has been stressed. Therefore, it is suggested that the concept of a "safe" dose be abandoned in favor of reduction therapy to a minimum, consistent with control of the disease.[26,27]

Corticosteroid-induced cataracts show an axial, discoid posterior subcapsular opacity 2–3mm in diameter, which gradually increases in size. The borders of this discoid lesions are sharp, but they have a gray haze.

ANTICHOLINESTERASE AND MIOTIC DRUGS. Anticholinesterases were used for the treatment of chronic open-angle glaucoma and are an established cause of anterior subcapsular cataracts in the form of vacuoles. Cessation of treatment may stop, retard, or occasionally reverse cataract progression. The mechanism of cataract formation is unknown, but cholinesterases may be involved with ion transport in the lens.

PHENOTHIAZINES. Phenothiazines, such as chlorpromazine, may cause deposition of fine, yellow-brown granules under the

277

anterior capsule in the pupillary zone. These develop into large, stellate opacities and finally into anterior polar cataracts. A daily dose of 300mg up to a total dose of 500g appears to be the minimum required to produce ocular effects. Chlorpromazine absorbs energy because it is a photosensitizing agent, and this results in the formation of potent free radicals, which may be responsible for lens damage.

MITOTIC DRUGS. Antimitotic drugs, such as busulfan, used in the treatment of chronic myeloid leukemia, may cause posterior subcapsular cataract.

ANTIMALARIAL AGENTS. Chloroquine, but not hydroxychloroquine, may cause a white, flake-like posterior subcapsular lens opacity. Amiodarone is a drug used to treat cardiac arrhythmias. It may result in visually inconsequential anterior subcapsular opacities as well as corneal deposits.[28]

CHEMICALS. Toxic chemicals cause corneal burns that may result in anterior punctate lens opacities, which resemble glaukomflecken. Cigarette smoking is also a risk factor in cataract formation. The mechanism is thought to involve car-bamylation of lens proteins by the cyanide in cigarette smoke. The cataract is a nuclear type.

Some chemicals may have a protective effect against development of cataract, such as certain nonsteroidal anti-inflammatory agents, aspirin and ibuprofen, and acetaminophen (paracetamol).

CALCIUM. Hypocalcemia in hypoparathyroidism is a well-known cause of cataract. In children, the cataract is lamellar; in adults it produces an anterior or posterior punctate subcapsular opacity.

COPPER. Copper may be deposited in the eye from eyedrops that contain copper sulfate, from a copper-containing foreign body, or as part of Wilson's disease.

In Wilson's disease, an autosomal recessive disorder, defective copper metabolism develops as a result of a deficiency of the enzyme ceruloplasmin. A brown corneal ring, at the level of Descemet's membrane (Kayser-Fleischer ring), is characteristic, as is the development of a typical "sunflower" cataract. This is a disc-shaped polychromatic opacity in the pupil zone anteriorly, with petal-like spokes that extend toward the periphery. Metallic copper

---

BOX 36-1

Infantile Cataracts

ANTERIOR POLAR CATARACT
- Sharply defined opacities of the anterior capsule that affect the vision, usually dominantly inherited.
- The opacities may be caused by imperfect separation of lens from surface ectoderm, by epithelial damage, or by incomplete reabsorption of the vascular tunic of the lens.
- The opacity may have anterior or posterior conical projections; if it extends into the cortex in a rod shape, it is called a "fusiform" cataract.

SPEAR CATARACT
- A dominantly inherited polymorphic cataract with needle-like clusters of opacities in the axial region, which may not affect vision.

CORALLIFORM CATARACT
- A dominantly inherited cataract, which consists of round and oblong opacities, grouped toward the center of the lens; they resemble a coral.

FLORIFORM CATARACT
- A rare, ring-shaped, bluish white cataract in the axial region. It appears like a flower, often in the region of the fetal sutures.

LAMELLAR CATARACT
- A common form of infantile cataract, usually dominantly inherited, but it may have a metabolic or inflammatory cause.
- The cataracts are bilateral and symmetrical and appear as a round, gray shell of opacity that surrounds a clear nucleus. With time, the opacity is pushed deeper into the cortex as normal lens fibers are laid down around it.
- The opacity represents a generation or more of secondary lens fibers that have become opacified in response to a specific insult during their most active metabolic stage.

CATARACTA CENTRALIS PULVERULENTA
- A dominantly inherited, nonprogressive cataract within the embryonic or fetal nucleus.
- It is a biconvex or spheroid-shaped opacity and consists of fine, white, powdery dots (see Fig. 36-6).

CONGENITAL PUNCTATE CERULEAN CATARACT
- Consists of small, bluish dots scattered throughout the lens. They are bilateral, nonprogressive, and have little effect on vision.

CONGENITAL SUTURE (STELLATE) CATARACT
- Dominantly inherited and affects one or both fetal sutures, especially posteriorly.
- The opacity consists of bluish dots or a dense chalky band around the sutures and may interfere with vision (Fig. 36-7).

MITTENDORF'S DOT
- A small (about 1mm diameter), white condensation on the posterior pole of the lens capsule; it usually lies slightly inferonasally.
- It may be attached to a free-floating thread in the vitreous gel and represents the anterior part of the hyaloid artery remnant. It is nonprogressive.

CONGENITAL DISCIFORM CATARACT
- The central part of the lens is thinned and the peripheral part is of normal thickness—the lens, therefore, has a doughnut shape.
- It may arise from failure of development of the embryonic nucleus.

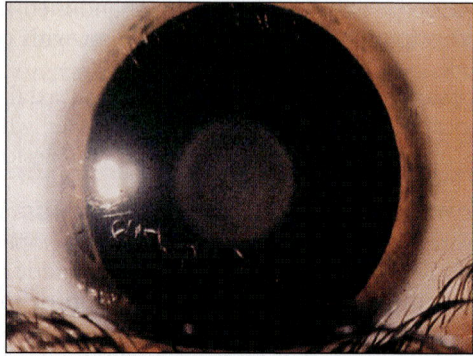

FIG. 36-6 ▓ Cataracta centralis pulverulenta. Opacification of fetal nucleus.

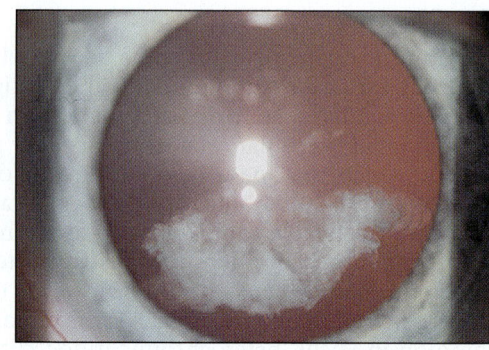

FIG. 36-7 ▓ Anterior sutural cataract in pigment dispersion syndrome.

is deposited in the lens capsule. The cataract is not visually disabling and may disappear on treatment of the disease with penicillamine.[29]

IRON. In siderosis that follows retention of a foreign body, iron deposits in the lens epithelium and iris, which results in a brown discoloration and iris heterochromia. A flower-shaped cataract may occur.

GOLD. Gold is deposited in the capsule and epithelium as fine, golden anterior capsular deposits.[30]

Hereditary Cataracts

Hereditary cataracts may present in infancy or later life and some are associated with other systemic syndromes, such as dystrophia myotonica. About one third of all congenital cataracts are hereditary and unassociated with any other metabolic or systemic disorders.[31]

Trisomy 21, or Down's syndrome, is the most common autosomal trisomy, with an incidence of 1 per 800 births. Systemic features include mental retardation, stunted growth, mongoloid facies, and congenital heart defects. Ocular features include visually disabling lens opacities in 15% of cases, narrow and slanted palpebral fissures, blepharitis, strabismus, nystagmus, light-colored and spotted irides (Brushfield spots), keratoconus, and myopia.[32]

Cataract is also associated with trisomy 13 (Patau's syndrome), trisomy 18 (Edwards' syndrome) and cri du chat syndrome (deletion of short arm of chromosome 5).

INFANTILE CATARACTS

Infantile cataracts, which include congenital and early postnatal cataracts, are of particular importance as a cause of amblyopia, strabismus, and nystagmus if bilateral. The incidence is about 0.4% of newborns, but the majority are not associated with poor vision. The visual problems (i.e., amblyopia) depend on the size, location, and density of the cataract. The causes of infantile cataracts are many and include maternal infections (such as rubella), systemic diseases, hereditary disorders, and local ocular disease. Several different types of infantile cataract occur (Box 36-1).

REFERENCES

1. Delaye M, Tardieu A. Short range order of crystallin proteins accounts for eye lens transparency. Nature. 1983;302:415–17.
2. Bendek GB. Theory of transparency of the eye. Appl Opt. 1971;10:459–73.
3. Philipson BT. Changes in lens, related to reduction in transparency. Exp Eye Res. 1973;16:29–39.
4. Pau H, Graf P, Sies H. Glutathione levels in human lens; regional distribution in different forms of cataract. Exp Eye Res. 1990;50:17–20.
5. Johnson G, Minassion D, Franken S. Alterations of the anterior lens capsule associated with climatic keratopathy. Br J Ophthalmol. 1989;73:229–34.
6. Kuszak JR, Deutsch TA. Anatomy of aged and senile cataractous lenses. In: Albert D, Jacobiec F, eds. Principles and practice of ophthalmology. Philadelphia: WB Saunders; 1991.
7. Eshagian J, Streeten BW. Human posterior sub-capsular cataract. An ultrastructural study of the posterior migrating cells. Arch Ophthalmol. 1980;98:134–43.
8. Yanoff M. Pathology of cataract. In: Bellows JG, ed. Cataract and abnormalities of the lens. New York: Grune & Stratton; 1975:155–90.
9. Scott JD. Lens changes in retinal detachment. Trans Ophthalmol Soc UK. 1979;99:241–3.
10. Scott JD. Lens epithelial proliferation in retinal detachment. Trans Ophthalmol Soc UK. 1982;102:385–9.
11. Scott JD. Lens changes in retinal detachment. Trans Ophthalmol Soc UK. 1979; 99:241–3.
12. Scott JD. Lens epithelial proliferation in retinal detachment. Trans Ophthalmol Soc UK. 1982;102:385–9.
13. Brown NP, Harris ML, Shun-Shin GA, et al. Is cortical spoke cataract due to lens fibre breaks? The relationship between fibre fold, fibre breaks, water clefts and spoke cataract. Eye. 1993;7:672–9.
14. Fraunfelder FT, Hanna C. Electric cataracts. I: Sequential changes, unusual and prognostic findings. Arch Ophthalmol. 1972;87:179–83.
15. Long JC. Electric cataract. Am J Ophthalmol. 1963;56:108–33.
16. Hanna C, Fraunfelder FT. Electric cataracts. II: Ultrastructural lens changes. Arch Ophthalmol. 1972;87:184–91.
17. Khan HA, Leibowitz HM, Ganley JP, et al. The Framingham eye study. I: Outline and major prevalence findings. Am J Ophthalmol. 1977;106:17–32.
18. Harding JJ, Van Heyningen R. Risk factors for cataracts. Br J Ophthalmol. 1989;73:579–80.
19. Elman MJ, Miller MT, Matalon R. Galactokinase activity in patients with idiopathic cataracts. Ophthalmology. 1986;93:210–15.
20. Harding JJ. Case control studies and risk factors for cataract: discussion paper. J R Soc Med. 1988;81:585–7.
21. Ederer F, Hiller R, Taylor HR. Senile lens changes and diabetes in two population studies. Am J Ophthalmol. 1981;91:381–95.
22. Hiller R, Sperduto RD, Ederer F. Epidemiological associations with cataract in the 1971–1972 National Health and Nutrition Examination Survey. Am J Ophthalmol. 1983;118:239–48.
23. Harding JJ. Pathophysiology of cataract. Curr Opin Ophthalmol 1993;4:14–21.
24. Fisher RF. The lens in uveitis. Trans Ophthalmol Soc UK. 1981;101:317–20.
25. Leaver PK, Grey RHB, Garner A. Silicone oil injection in the treatment of massive pre-retinal retraction. II: Late complications in 93 eyes. Br J Ophthalmol. 1979; 63:361–7.
26. Shalka HW, Prachal JT. Effect of corticosteroids on cataract formation. Arch Ophthalmol. 1980;98:1773–7.
27. Urban RC, Cotlier E. Corticosteroid-induced cataracts. Surv Ophthalmol. 1986; 31:102–10.
28. Flach AJ, Dolan BJ, Sudduth B, et al. Amiodarone induced lens opacities. Arch Ophthalmol. 1983;101:1554–6.
29. Walshe JM. The eye in Wilson's disease. Birth Defects Orig Artic Ser. 1976;3: 187–94.
30. McCormick SA, Di Bartolomeo AG, Raju VK, et al. Ocular chrysiasis. Ophthalmology. 1985;92:1432–5.
31. Maumenee IH. Classification of hereditary cataracts in children by linkage analysis. Ophthalmology. 1979;86:1554–9.
32. Shaprito MB, France TD. The ocular features of Down's syndrome. Am J Ophthalmol. 1985;99:659–63.

Morphology and Visual Effects of Lens Opacities of Cataract

DEEPAK K. CHITKARA • JOSEPH COLIN

INTRODUCTION

Age-related changes in the crystalline lens induce changes in visual function. The lens functions as an optical element and provides one third of the refractive power of the human eye. The eye's optical properties depend on the power of the lens, which in turn is determined by its physical dimensions (curvatures and thickness) and its refractive index as well as its transmissibility and the organization of its internal components. The progressive insolubilization of lens protein with age is believed to cause density fluctuations, which scatter light and impair vision.

The impact of a patient's cataract on the retinal image may be appreciated on funduscopic examination, which shows the blur of fine retinal vessels. The clinician is unable to resolve the retinal capillaries directly because of the scattering of light by opacities in the patient's lens. Light scattering also blurs the images of fine objects viewed by individuals with cataract.

DIAGNOSIS OF LENS OPACITIES

Slit-lamp biomicroscopy is the major method used to observe and assess cataracts. However, the image seen often fails to correlate with the patient's visual acuity or function. The relationship between alterations in the structural proteins, the increase in light scatter associated with conventional biomicroscopy, and the capacity of visual function is not a simple one. For all lens examinations, the pupil is dilated maximally.

CLASSIFICATION OF LENS OPACITIES

With age, the transparency of the lens decreases progressively and a wide variety of opacities may occur.[1] The morphological types of senile cataract fall into four basic categories: nuclear, cortical, posterior subcapsular cataracts, and advanced. These cataract types can be graded clinically and can be measured photographically.

Nuclear Opacities

Initially, an increase in optical density of the nucleus occurs (nuclear sclerosis). The fetal nucleus is first involved and then the whole adult nucleus. The increase in density is followed by an opacification (Fig. 37-1), which implies a change in color,

namely from an initial clear, to yellow, to a subsequent brown (brownish cataract).

In certain instances, crystals appear in the adult nucleus (or in the cortex) that, on slit-lamp examination, appear to be of different colors.

Cortical Opacities

The changes in transparency involve most of the cortex of the lens (Fig. 37-2). The changes evolve as follows:
- Hydration of the cortex with development of subcapsular vacuoles;
- Formation of ray-like spaces filled with liquid, which are at first transparent and later become opaque;
- Lamellar separation of the cortex with development of parallel linear opacities; and
- Formation of cuneiform opacities that originate at the periphery of the lens and spread toward the center.

Posterior Subcapsular Opacities

Posterior subcapsular opacities may develop as isolated entities or may be associated with other lens opacities. The opacity begins at the posterior polar region and then spreads toward the periphery. Often, granules and vacuoles are detectable in front of the posterior capsule.

Advanced Cataracts

The crystalline lens may swell and increase in volume because of cortical processes (intumescent cataract; Fig. 37-3). Complete opacification of the lens is called a mature (morgagnian) cataract.

If the liquefied cortical material is not, or is only partially, reabsorbed, the solid nucleus may "sink" to the bottom (Fig. 37-4). Reabsorption of the milky cortex causes a reduction in the lens volume, causing the capsule to form folds (hypermature cataract).

GRADING OF LENS OPACITIES

Gradations and classifications of cataracts are useful in cataract research, in studies to explore causation, and in trials of putative anticataract drugs. Devices designed to quantify lens opacifica-

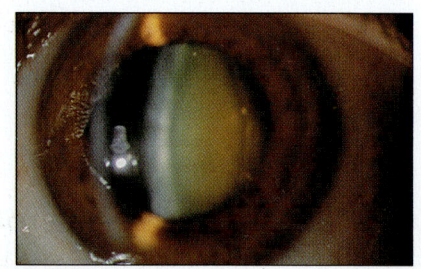

FIG. 37-1 ▪ Nuclear cataract. With continual generation of lens fibers in the equatorial periphery of the lens, the older material is continually compressed and eventually forms a nuclear cataract with changed optical density and altered transparency.

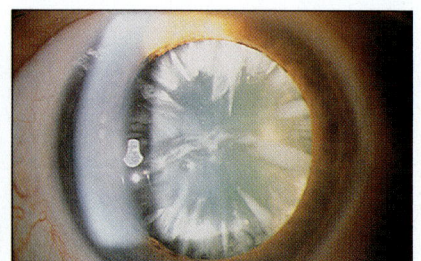

FIG. 37-2 ▪ Cortical cataract.

tion have been developed[2]—these instruments (such as the Kowa Early Cataract Detector and the Scheimpflug Photo slit lamp) appear to be more accurate when used to assess the formation of nuclear cataracts than that of cortical cataracts.

A rapid method for the gradation of cataract in epidemiological studies has been reported by Mehra and Minassian[3]—the area of lenticular opacity is assessed by direct ophthalmoscopy and graded on a scale from 0 to 5. Highly reproducible, validated systems (Lens Opacities Classification System II; see later) for cataract classification have been developed by Chylack *et al.*[4] to define the effects of specific cataract type and extent very accurately; these enable the effects of specific cataract types on specific visual functions to be quantified.

Lens Opacities Classification System II

For nuclear opalescence (NO), a slit beam is focused on the lens nucleus and the density of the lens is compared with a set of four standard photographs. If the density is equal to or less than that corresponding to the first photograph, NO is zero; NO is 1 if the density is equal to or less than that for the second photograph, and so on. The four standard photographs represent lens nuclei of increasing density, and the patient's cataract is graded accordingly. For cortical cataracts, a retroillumination view through the pupil is used to view the lens, focused first at the anterior capsule and then at the posterior capsule. The photographs are compared with standard photographs—each succeeding photograph shows the pupillary area covered by more cortical cataract. For posterior subcapsular cataract, a retroillumination view of the lens is used, focused at the posterior capsule. Again, the patient's cataract is graded according to standard photographs.

EFFECTS OF OPACITIES ON VISION

The nature of the effect of opacity on vision varies according to the degree of the cataract and the cataract morphology. No single test adequately describes the effects of cataract on a patient's visual status or functional ability.[5]

Visual Acuity Reduction

Measurement of visual acuity has been the standard tool by which to estimate the visual disability of patients and by which

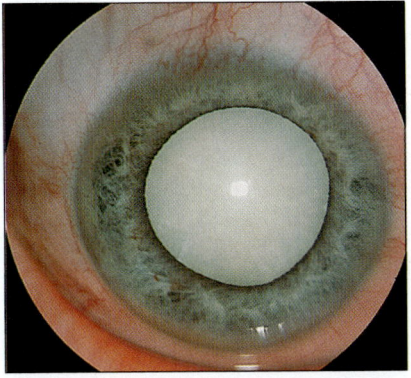

FIG. 37-3 ▓ Intumescent cataract. The crystalline lens increases in volume because of swelling processes that involve the cortex.

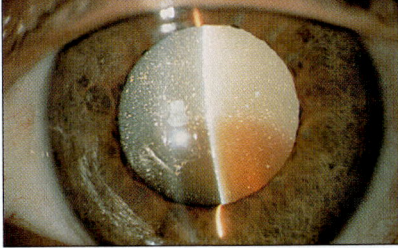

FIG. 37-4 ▓ Morgagnian cataract. The nucleus is seen as a "suntan" or a dark shadow in the inferior third of the pupil.

to detect changes in visual function induced by cataract over time.[6] However, it has been found clinically that visual acuity can remain high despite age-related lens opacities: the severity of the visual disability measured using high-contrast Snellen acuity charts is not sensitive to visual disability characterized by loss of contrast sensitivity.

Usually, visual acuity testing is conducted under ideal circumstances, which are not normally met in the real world, and so the results may not reflect visual disabilities that occur in less ideal conditions. Although not a definitive measurement of visual dysfunction, simple Snellen acuity is the most used index to determine whether cataract surgery should be performed. The Preferred Practice Pattern of the American Academy of Ophthalmology recommends Snellen acuity as the best general guide to the appropriateness of surgery but recognizes the need for flexibility with due regard to a patient's particular functional and visual needs, environment, and risks, which may vary widely.[7]

When the cataract is very dense and opaque, visual acuity may be reduced to light perception only (cataract is still the leading cause of blindness throughout the world).

Contrast Sensitivity Reduction

Cataract patients commonly complain of loss of the ability to see objects outdoors in bright sunlight and of being blinded easily by oncoming headlamps in nighttime driving.[8]

Typically, loss of contrast sensitivity in patients who have cataract has been reported to be greater at higher spatial frequencies. All cataracts lower contrast sensitivity—the posterior subcapsular opacities have been reported to be the most destructive.

Myopic Shift

The natural aging of the human lens produces a progressive hyperopic shift. Nuclear changes induce a modification of the refractive index of the lens and produce a myopic shift that may be of several diopters. It is possible to predict that an aging person who had emmetropia previously, but who can now read with no correction ("second sight"), is developing nuclear cataract.

If the lens structure becomes heterogeneous, with cortical spoke cataract for example, the change in refractive index may be uneven and may produce some degree of internal astigmatism.

Monocular Diplopia

Monocular diplopia is common in patients who have lens opacities, particularly cortical spoke cataract and in conjunction with water clefts that form radial wedge shapes and contain a fluid of lower refractive index than the surrounding lens. The patients, in some cases, may complain of polyopia.

Glare

Even minor degrees of lens opacity cause glare because of the forward scatter of light.[9] All forms of cataract can cause glare, especially cortical and posterior subcapsular. Such patients often see more poorly in daylight conditions and in the context of night driving. Unlike contrast sensitivity reduction, some glare may be produced by opacities that do not lie within the pupil diameter. The differences between measured visual acuity in a darkened room (and with a high-contrast chart) and acuity in ambient light that produces glare are interesting as subjective criteria for the justification of surgery.

Color Shift

The cataractous lens becomes more absorbent at the blue end of the spectrum, especially with nuclear opacities. Usually patients are not aware of this color visual defect, but it becomes obvious retrospectively after cataract surgery and visual rehabilitation.

Visual Field Loss

According to the morphology, the density, and the location of the opacities, the field of vision may be affected.

REFERENCES

1. Cardillo Piccolino F, Altieri G. Classification of cataract: In: Concepta Angellini, ed. Cataract. Roma: M Zingirian; 1985.
2. Harding JJ. Cataract epidemiology. Curr Opin Ophthalmol. 1990;1:10–15.
3. Mehra V, Minassian DC. A rapid method of grading cataract in epidemiological studies and eye surveys. Br J Ophthalmol. 1988;72:801–3.
4. Chylack LT, Leske MC, McCarthy D. Lens Opacities Classification System II (LOCS II). Arch Ophthalmol. 1989;107:991–7.
5. Phelps Brown NA. The morphology of cataract and visual performance. Eye. 1993;7:63–7.
6. Lasa MS, Datiles MB, Freidlin V. Potential vision tests in patients with cataracts. Ophthalmology. 1995;102:1007–11.
7. American Academy of Ophthalmology. Preferred Practice Pattern: Cataract in the otherwise healthy adult eye. San Francisco: American Academy of Ophthalmology; 1989.
8. Regan D, Giaschi DE, Fresco BB. Measurement of glare sensitivity in cataract patients using low-contrast letter chart. Ophthalmic Physiol Opt. 1993;13:115–23.
9. Lasa MS, Podgor MJ, Datiles MB, et al. Glare sensitivity in early cataracts. Br J Ophthalmol. 1993;77:489–91.

CHAPTER

38

Optics of Aphakia and Pseudophakia

JACK T. HOLLADAY

INTRODUCTION

The normal 72-year-old human eye has a total dioptric power of approximately 58D, with nearly 75% of the power from the cornea and 25% of the power from the crystalline lens (Fig. 38-1).[1] Removal of the crystalline lens leaves the eye extremely deficient in dioptric power, which must be replaced to restore vision. The replacement of the dioptric power can be in the form of spectacles, contact lenses, corneal onlays, corneal implants, or intraocular lenses. Although each modality can restore the patient's vision, the optical consequences are dramatically different and must be understood by the clinician to avoid unnecessary complications.

HISTORICAL REVIEW

The most common and successful method to replace crystalline lens power is to use an intraocular lens (IOL). The earliest documented IOL implant was performed by Harold Ridley in 1949.[2] Ridley's original IOL was made of polymethyl methacrylate (PMMA) and placed in the posterior chamber, in a manner very similar to that of the present method. Over the past 50 years, improvements in the purity of the PMMA, in the quality of lens manufacturing, and in the surgical techniques used have transformed this technique into one of the most successful surgical procedures performed today.

TREATMENT

Aphakia

Figure 38-2 shows the aphakic eye with a spectacle lens at a vertex of 14mm to correct the patient's vision. Replacement of the crystalline lens power with a spectacle lens causes the image that is formed on the patient's retina to be roughly 25% larger than the image formed with the crystalline lens. The actual magnification is determined by the exact power of the aphakic spectacles. There is approximately 2% of magnification for each diopter of power in the spectacles. The average aphakic spectacle is therefore 12.5D.

The magnification from aphakic spectacles causes other optical aberrations, such as a ring scotoma (Fig. 38-3), jack-in-the-box phenomenon (Fig. 38-4), and a pincushion distortion (Fig. 38-5). Because the image through the spectacles is magnified by 25%, the actual field of view through the spectacles is reduced by 25%, which makes it impossible to see the 25% of the peripheral

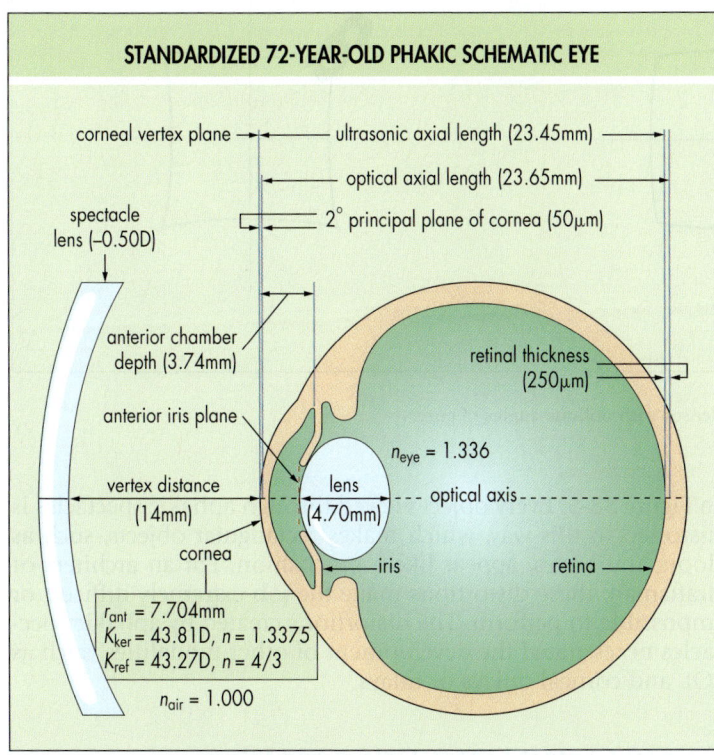

FIG. 38-1 ■ **Standardized 72-year-old phakic eye.** The values shown are the mean values for a phakic eye: keratometric power of the cornea (k_{ker}), net refractive power of the cornea (k_{ref}), and anterior radius of the cornea (r_{ant}). Indices of refraction (n) are 1.336 for the aqueous and vitreous (n_{eye}) and 1.000 for air (n_{air}).

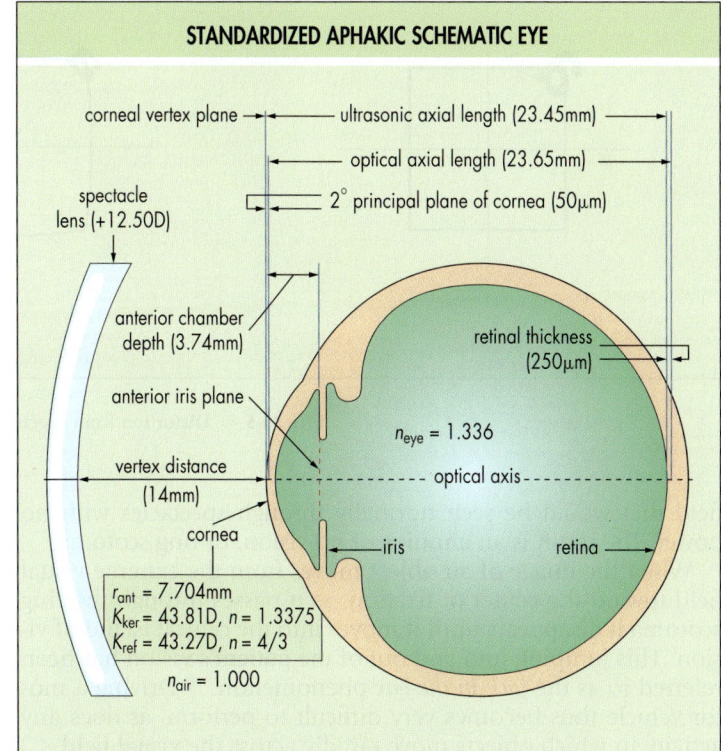

FIG. 38-2 ■ **Standardized 72-year-old aphakic eye.** The values shown are the mean values for a phakic eye: keratometric power of the cornea (k_{ker}), net refractive power of the cornea (k_{ref}), and anterior radius of the cornea (r_{ant}). Indices of refraction (n) are 1.336 for the aqueous and vitreous (n_{eye}) and 1.000 for air (n_{air}).

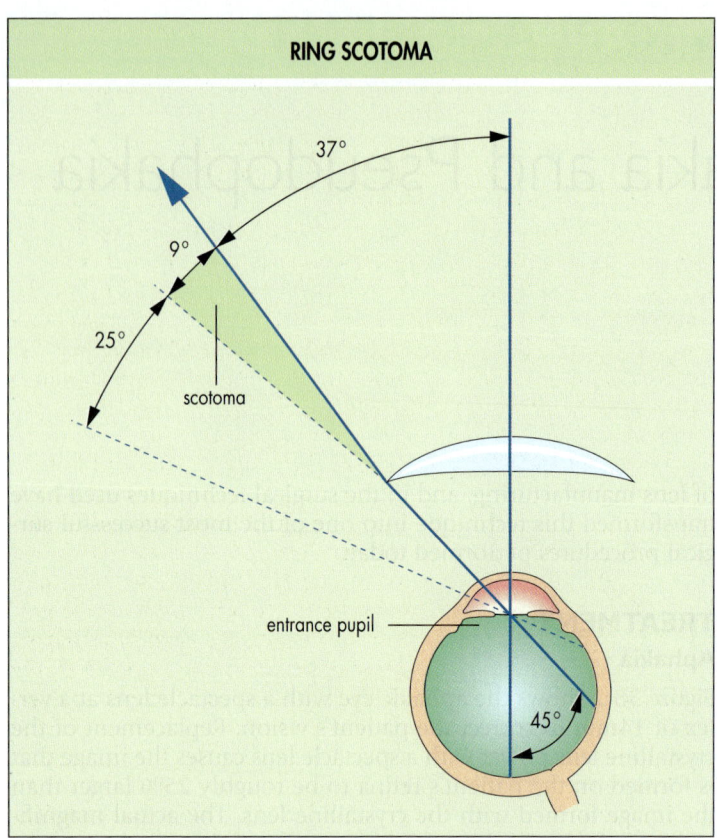

RING SCOTOMA

FIG. 38-3 ■ **Ring scotoma.** An area of about 9° of the field. The blind wedge extends around the circumference, hence the term ring scotoma.

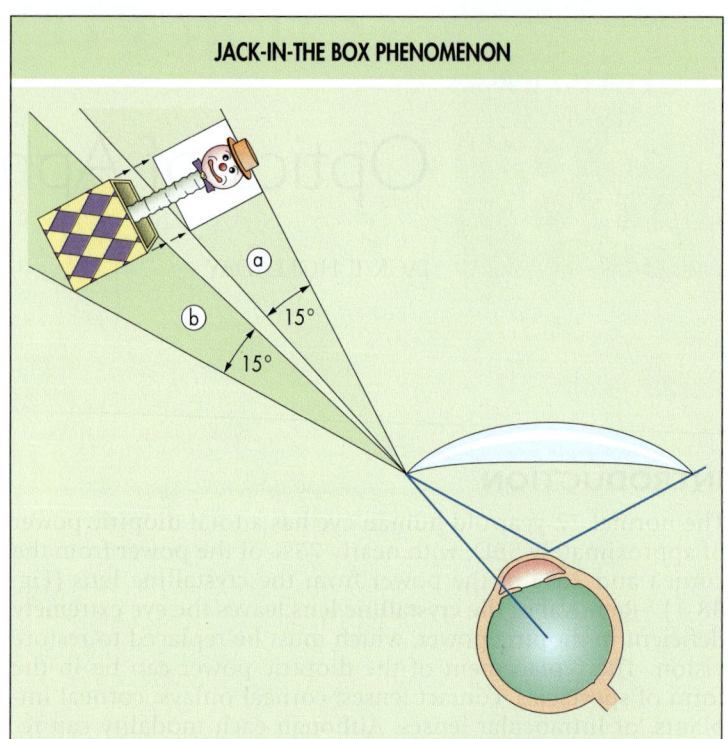

JACK-IN-THE BOX PHENOMENON

FIG. 38-4 ■ **The jack-in-the-box phenomenon. A,** Ring scotoma of an aphakic patient plotted by perimetry. The roving ring scotoma shifts centrally as the eye rotates peripherally. The result is the jack-in-the-box phenomenon, in which an object is seen with peripheral vision, the eye turns to look directly at the object, and the object disappears. Aphakic correction is by spectacle lenses. **B,** Perimeter of an aphakic eye that has a contact lens worn for correction of aphakia. Contact lenses remove the jack-in-the-box phenomenon entirely.

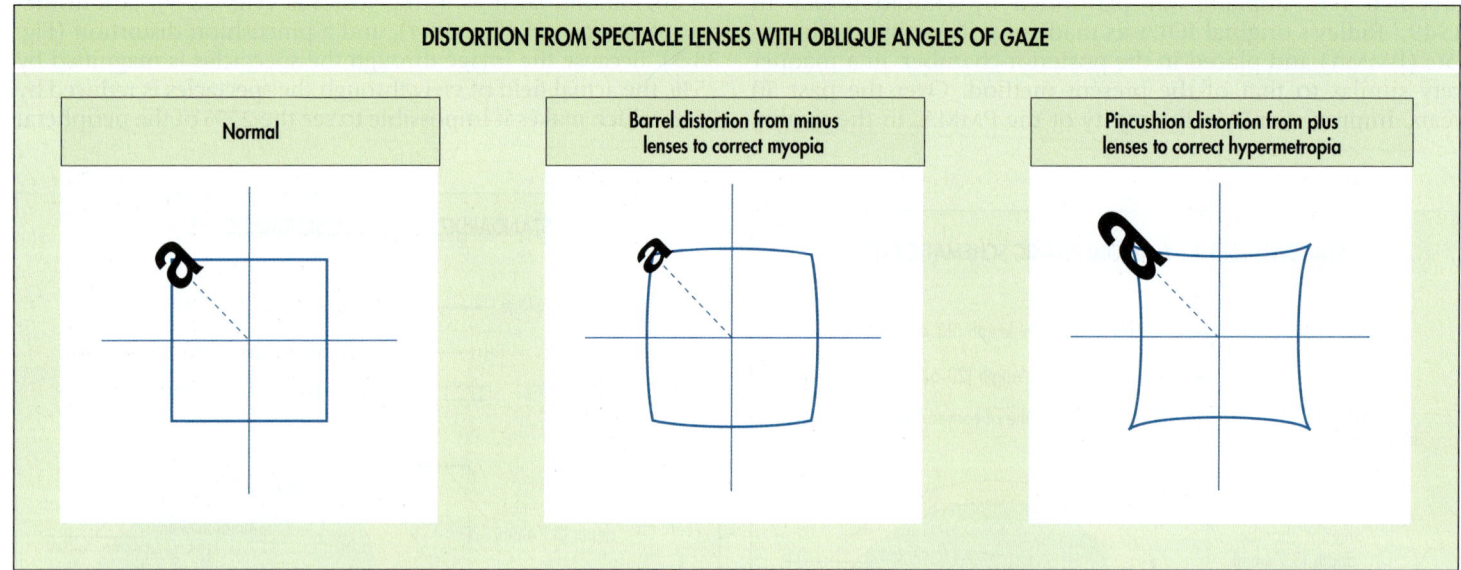

DISTORTION FROM SPECTACLE LENSES WITH OBLIQUE ANGLES OF GAZE

Normal

Barrel distortion from minus lenses to correct myopia

Pincushion distortion from plus lenses to correct hypermetropia

FIG. 38-5 ■ Distortion from spectacle lenses with oblique angles of gaze.

field that would be seen normally through spectacles with no power. The result is an annulus of no vision, or ring scotoma.

When the image of an object moves from the extreme visual field toward the center of fixation, as it passes through the ring scotoma it disappears until it moves into the central island of vision. This jumping into and out of the patient's vision has been referred to as the *jack-in-the-box* phenomenon.[3-5] Driving a motor vehicle thus becomes very difficult to perform, as does any activity in which objects move rapidly across the visual field.

Pincushion distortion is a property of all plus lenses and is proportional to their dioptric power. This distortion makes a square look like a pincushion—the corners of the square have a stretched-out appearance, and the sides are pushed in, as shown

in Figure 38-5. Every object viewed through aphakic spectacles is distorted in this way, which makes rectangular objects, such as doors and boxes, appear like a pincushion. For an architect or draftsman, these distortions make the job extremely difficult or impossible to perform. The distortions created by aphakic spectacles necessitated the development of other modalities, such as IOL and corneal onlays or inlays.

Corneal Contact Lenses, Onlays, and Inlays

To correct aphakia at the corneal plane involves the use of contact lenses or surgery that adds dioptric power to the cornea. As the position at which the optical correction is made moves

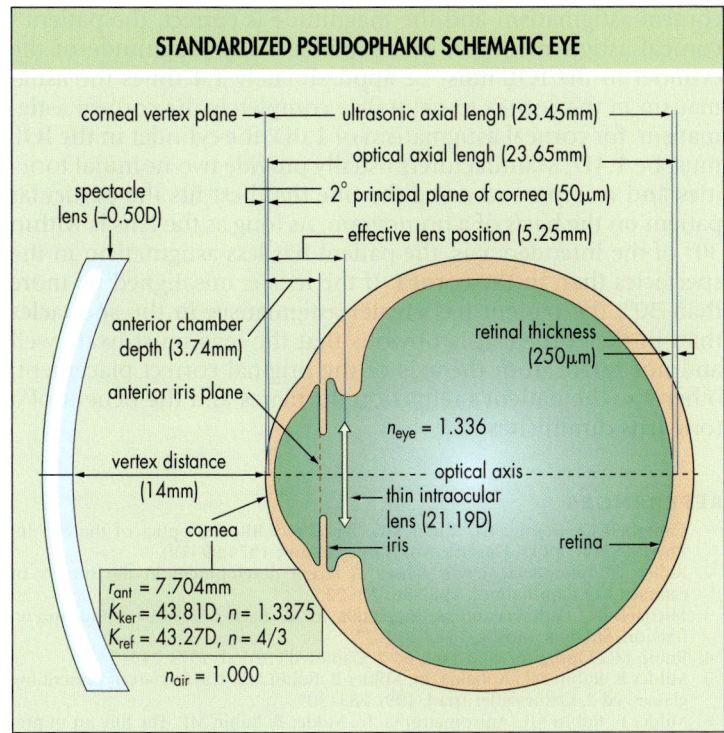

STANDARDIZED PSEUDOPHAKIC SCHEMATIC EYE

corneal vertex plane → ultrasonic axial lengh (23.45mm)

optical axial lengh (23.65mm)

spectacle lens (−0.50D)

2° principal plane of cornea (50μm)

effective lens position (5.25mm)

anterior chamber depth (3.74mm)

retinal thickness (250μm)

anterior iris plane

n_{eye} = 1.336

vertex distance (14mm)

optical axis

thin intraocular lens (21.19D)

cornea

iris

retina

r_{ant} = 7.704mm
K_{ker} = 43.81D, n = 1.3375
K_{ref} = 43.27D, n = 4/3

n_{air} = 1.000

FIG. 38-6 ■ Standardized 72-year-old pseudophakic eye (thin IOL). The values shown are the mean values for a pseudophakic eye: keratometric power of the cornea (k_{ker}), net refractive power of the cornea (k_{ref}), and anterior radius of the cornea (r_{ant}). Indices of refraction (n) are 1.336 for the aqueous and vitreous (n_{eye}) and 1.000 for air (n_{air}). Using these values, the required thin IOL power is 21.19D at an effective lens position (ELP) of 5.25mm.

closer to the retina, the necessary dioptric power increases but the subsequent magnification decreases. The power at the corneal plane that is equivalent to 12.5D at a vertex of 12mm is 14.7D; a patient who needs 12.5D in aphakic spectacles would need 14.7D in a soft or rigid contact lens. At the corneal plane the magnification is 6–8%. This value is near the limit of aniseikonia (image size disparity between the two eyes),[6,7] so most unilaterally aphakic patients can have binocular vision, with the aphakic eye corrected using a contact lens and the other eye phakic. Binocular vision is not possible with one aphakic spectacle and a normal phakic lens.

Corneal onlays, such as epikeratophakia, and inlays, such as the intracorneal lenticle, are still in the early phases of investigation and are not used commonly in clinical settings. The optical effects are no different from those of a contact lens, but onlays and inlays have the advantage that the patient need provide no maintenance. However, the excellent success of contact lenses and IOLs means that surgical techniques to correct aphakia at the cornea are not reasonable clinical alternatives at this time.

Pseudophakia

Figure 38-6 shows a posterior chamber lens in-the-bag following cataract extraction. Just as the average spectacle power for aphakia is 12.5D, the average power of an equiconvex IOL in-the-bag is approximately 21D. The average magnification of an IOL in this position is 1.5%, compared with the original crystalline lens. For an anterior chamber IOL the average power would be less, approximately 18D, and the magnification would be approximately 2.0%. Although some discerning patients can detect this disparity by alternately covering each eye, almost everyone can achieve binocular vision with one eye pseudophakic and the other phakic.[8]

PSEUDOPHAKIC LENS DESIGN. The IOLs currently available are either biconvex, convexoplano, or meniscus. As a result of clinical performance and optical analysis, the majority of lenses implanted today are biconvex.[9,10] The reasons for the

emergence of this design as the most superior are both optical and mechanical.

The quality of the optical design of an IOL is measured on the basis of its performance with respect to tilting, decentration, and spherical aberration. In terms of each of these, the positive meniscus lens performs miserably and rarely is used today. The original design concept was to create a "laser space," so that the posterior surface of the lens would not be in contact with the posterior capsule; this avoids pitting of the lens with yttrium–aluminum–garnet laser capsulotomy. When a meniscus lens is tilted or decentered, the induced astigmatism and power change are dramatic. A 10–15° tilt can induce enough regular and irregular astigmatism to make the spectacle correction intolerable and results in a best corrected vision of less than 20/20 (6/6), simply because of the poor optics.

Convexoplano IOLs (convex on the front surface and flat on the posterior surface) were the first to be designed. They are the simplest to manufacture, because one surface is flat and all the optical power lies in the other surface. These lenses have performed well over the years, but degradation of the retinal image with lens tilt or decentration is still greater than it is with biconvex lenses. Optical studies to determine the optimal lens design have shown that a biconvex design with a front surface much steeper than the back appears to minimize this aberration for most humans.[11] No clinical studies have demonstrated a difference in the spherical aberration of a convexoplano lens with respect to that of a biconvex lens that is steeper on the front surface.

The optimal optical and mechanical performance of an IOL in the human eye is that of biconvex lenses. In addition to minimizing the effects of tilt, decentration, and spherical aberrations, a convex posterior surface often reduces the migration of lens epithelial cells, a migration that may lead to opacification of the capsule; this is an additional mechanical advantage of biconvex over convexoplano lenses. The biconvex IOL has become the predominant lens style used today because of its superior optical and mechanical clinical performance.[9]

EDGE DESIGN. Reflections, shimmering peripheral lights, and flashes usually are related to the edge design of a lens. Flat edges from truncation (oval optics) or flat edges in round optics create unwanted external and internal reflections that the patient may see in low light levels.[12] Therefore, most lenses have rounded edges to avoid a coherent reflected image from the edge of a lens' flat surface. Oval (e.g., 5 × 6mm) optics flourished for a short time as a result of the desire to insert lenses through smaller and smaller incisions, until studies demonstrated an increased incidence of unwanted peripheral reflections from these lenses. It was shown that these unwanted reflections came from the flat, truncated edge of the lens.[12] Flat edges are no longer used in modern IOLs.

OPTICAL TRANSMISSION. The optical transmission through the human eye to the retina usually is considered to be in the range 400–700nm in wavelength. The cornea filters any wavelength shorter than 300nm, and the crystalline lens filters out any wavelength shorter than 400nm. When the crystalline lens is removed, wavelengths of 300–400nm reach the retina. PMMA that is not treated specially filters only light below 320nm, so in the late 1970s much discussion ensued as to whether the 320–400nm wavelengths that reached the pseudophakic retina could cause syneresis of the vitreous, macular degeneration, cystoid macular edema, and erythropsia.

Manufacturers began to modify PMMA to filter out wavelengths below 400nm (ultraviolet light [UV]), just as the crystalline lens does, to protect the retina. Clinical studies have found that this additional filter has no effect on any of these conditions except erythropsia (in which vision appears to be through a red transparency because blue cones have been bleached out by excessive UV). As a result, very few non–UV filtering IOLs are manufactured today.

MATERIAL. Commercially available IOLs are made of PMMA, silicone, or acrylic. Lenses made of hydroxyethyl methacrylate still are under investigation. The discussion here is limited to commercially available lenses. Silicone and acrylic lenses are foldable, so they can be implanted through small incisions (less than 3.5mm in length). The index of refraction for PMMA is 1.491, that for silicone is in the range 1.41–1.46, depending on the model and manufacturer, and for acrylic it is 1.55. The higher the index of refraction, the flatter the curvatures of the lens need to be to achieve the same refractive power. For a 20D biconvex IOL with 10D on each surface, the acrylic lens has the flattest curvatures and the silicone the steepest. As a consequence of the flatter curvatures, the acrylic lens is thinner than the PMMA lens which, in turn, is thinner than the silicone lens, provided all else is equal.

The velocity of ultrasound for these materials at eye temperature (35°C) is 2658m/sec for PMMA, 980–1090m/sec for silicones, and 2180m/sec for acrylic.[13] All three of these lens materials have performed well clinically, although the long-term results (over 10 years) are still awaited for silicone and acrylic lenses.

Specialty Intraocular Lenses

Two other special types of IOLs are manufactured currently—multifocal and toric. Multifocal IOLs have enjoyed a success similar to that of multifocal contact lenses. Multifocal IOLs produce two or more focal points, which create a focused and defocused image on the retina. The result is an image that is approximately 30% reduced in contrast with respect to monofocal lenses and unwanted optical images seen at night, such as halos or rings around headlights.[14] The reduced image quality must be weighed against the patient's desire to be less spectacle dependent. With (multifocal) contact lens failure, the problem is solved by returning to spectacles. A patient who is dissatisfied with a multifocal IOL is more difficult to deal with, and lens exchange occasionally is required. The success of these lenses is based almost entirely on appropriate patient selection.

Toric IOLs are simply spherocylindric lenses, just like spectacles. If the toric lens is aligned properly with the patient's corneal astigmatism and the magnitude is correct, the patient's corneal astigmatism can be neutralized. The magnitude of the cylinder in the IOL must be approximately 1.4 times the astigmatism in the cornea to neutralize completely the corneal astigmatism; for corneal astigmatism of 1.0D, the cylinder in the IOL must be 1.4D. Manufacturers usually provide two nominal toricities and recommend using the one that best fits the particular patient on the basis of a nomogram. As long as the lens is within 30° of the intended axis, the patient has less astigmatism in the spectacles than in the cornea. If the lens is misaligned by more than 30°, the patient has greater astigmatism in the spectacles than in the cornea. It is obvious that the lens must fixate well and not rotate from the axis of the original correct placement, otherwise the patient's refraction fluctuates and the benefit of a toric lens diminishes.

REFERENCES

1. Campbell CJ, Koester CJ, Rittler MC, Tackaberry RB. The optics of the eye. In: Physiological optics. Hagerstown: Harper & Row; 1974:99–110.
2. Ridley H. Intraocular acrylic lenses. A recent development in the surgery of cataract. Br J Ophthalmol. 1952;36:113–22.
3. Michaels DD. Aphakia and pseudophakia. In: Michaels DD. Visual optics and refraction. St Louis: Mosby; 1985:506–27.
4. Rubin ML. Optics for clinicians, ed 2. Gainesville: Triad; 1974:249–54.
5. Milder B, Rubin ML. Aphakia. In: Milder B, Rubin ML. The fine art of prescribing glasses, ed 2. Gainesville: Triad; 1991:283–309.
6. Milder B, Rubin ML. Anisometropia. In: Milder B, Rubin ML. The fine art of prescribing glasses, ed 2. Gainesville: Triad; 1991:217–53.
7. Burian HM, von Noorden GK. Visual acuity and aniseikonia. In: Binocular vision and ocular motility. St Louis: Mosby; 1974:130–41.
8. Holladay JT, Rubin ML. Avoiding refractive problems in cataract surgery. Surv Ophthalmol. 1988;32:357–60.
9. Holladay JT, Prager TC, Bishop JE, Blaker JW. The ideal intraocular lens. CLAO J. 1983;9:15–9.
10. Holladay JT. Evaluating the intraocular lens optic. Surv Ophthalmol. 1986;30:385–90.
11. Atchison DA. Optical design of intraocular lenses. I. On-axis performance. Optom Vision Sci. 1989;66:492–506.
12. Masket S, Geraghty E, Crandall AS, et al. Undesired light images associated with ovoid intraocular lenses. J Cataract Refract Surg. 1993;19:690–4.
13. Yang S, Lang A, Makker H, Azleski E. Effect of silicone sound speed and intraocular lens thickness on pseudophakic axial length corrections. J Cataract Refract Surg. 1995;21:442–6.
14. Holladay JT, Van Dijk H, Lang A, et al. Optical performance of multifocal intraocular lenses. J Cataract Refract Surg. 1990;16:413–22.

Measurements

JACK T. HOLLADAY

KEY FEATURES

- Several eye measurements help to determine the intraocular lens (IOL) power needed to achieve a desired refraction: central corneal refractive power (k readings), axial length (biometry), horizontal corneal diameter (horizontal white-to-white), anterior chamber depth, and lens thickness.
- The accuracy of prediction of the necessary power of an IOL is related directly to the accuracy of the measurements carried out.[1,2]

INTRODUCTION

Fedorov et al.[3] first estimated the optical power of an intraocular lens (IOL) using vergence formulas in 1967. Between 1972 and 1975, when accurate ultrasonic "A" scan units became available commercially, several investigators derived and published theoretical vergence formulas.[4-9] All of these formulas were identical, except for the form in which they were written and the choice of various constants, such as retinal thickness, optical plane of the cornea, and optical plane of the IOL.[10] The slightly different constants accounted for less than 0.50D in the predicted refraction. The use of different constants arose as a result of differences in lens styles, "A" scan units, keratometers, and surgical techniques used by the investigators.

IOL CALCULATIONS THAT REQUIRE AXIAL LENGTH

Theoretical Formulas

The theoretical formula for IOL power calculations has not changed since the original description by Fedorov et al.[3] in 1967. Although several investigators presented the theoretical formulas in different forms, the only differences were slight variations in the values of retinal thickness and corneal index of refraction. Six variables in the formula exist:

- Net corneal power (K)
- Axial length (AL)
- IOL power (IOLP)
- Effective lens position (ELP)
- Desired refraction (DPostRx)
- Vertex distance (V)

Normally, IOL power is chosen as the dependent variable and found by using the other five variables, where distances are given in millimeters and refractive powers are given in diopters, as in Equation 39-1.

Equation 39-1

$$IOLP = (1336/[AL - ELP]) - (1336/[1336/\{1000/([1000/DpostRx] - V) + K\} - ELP])$$

The only variable that cannot be chosen or measured preoperatively is ELP. The improvements in IOL power calculations

over the past 30 years are a result of improvements in the predictability of the variable ELP (see Fig. 38-6 for the physical locations of the variables).

The term effective lens position (ELP) was adopted by the U.S. Food and Drug Administration in 1995 to describe the position of the lens in the eye, because the often-used term anterior chamber depth (ACD) is not anatomically accurate for lenses in the posterior chamber and can lead to confusion for the clinician. The ELP used for IOLs before 1980 was a constant of 4mm for every lens in every patient (first-generation theoretical formula). This value actually worked well in most patients, because the majority of lenses implanted were of iris clip fixation type, in which the principal plane averages approximately 4mm posterior to the corneal vertex. In 1981, Binkhorst improved the prediction of ELP by using a single variable predictor, the axial length, as a scaling factor for ELP (second-generation theoretical formula).[11] If the patient's axial length was 10% greater than normal (normal being 23.45mm), the ELP used was increased by 10%. The average value of ELP used was increased to 4.5mm, because the preferred location of an implant was in the ciliary sulcus, approximately 0.5mm deeper than the iris plane. Also, most lenses were convex-plano, similar to the shape of the iris-supported lenses. By 1997 the average ELP used had increased to 5.25mm. This increased distance has occurred primarily for two reasons:

1. The majority of implanted IOLs are biconvex, which moves the principal plane of the lens even deeper into the eye.
2. The desired location for the lens is in the capsular bag, which is 0.25mm deeper than the ciliary sulcus.

In 1988, it was proved[2] that the use of a two-variable predictor (axial length and keratometry) could significantly improve the prediction of ELP, particularly in unusual eyes (third-generation theoretical formula). The original Holladay 1 formula was based on the geometric relationships of the anterior segment. Although several investigators have modified the original Holladay 1 formula, no comprehensive studies have shown any significant improvement using only these two variables.

In 1995, Olsen et al.[12] published a four-variable predictor that used keratometry and axial length, preoperative anterior chamber depth, and lens thickness. Their results showed an improvement over the two-variable prediction formulas, because the more information that is used to define the anterior segment value, the better the ELP can be predicted. (It is well known from prediction theory that the more variables that can be measured to describe an event, the more accurately the outcome can be predicted.)

In a recent study, Holladay et al.[13] discovered that the anterior segment and posterior segment of the human eye often are not proportional in size, which causes significant error in the prediction of the ELP in extremely short eyes (axial length <20mm). The authors found that even in eyes less than 20mm in axial length, the anterior segment was completely normal in the majority of cases. Because the axial lengths were so short, the two-variable prediction formulas severely underestimated ELP, which explains part of the large hyperopic prediction errors with the two-variable prediction formulas. Once this problem was

TABLE 39-1

CLINICAL CONDITIONS THAT DEMONSTRATE THE INDEPENDENCE OF THE ANTERIOR SEGMENT SIZE AND AXIAL LENGTH

Anterior Segment Size	Axial Length		
	Short	Normal	Long
Small	Small eye	Microcornea	Microcornea
	Nanophthalmos		Axial myopia
Normal	Axial hyperopia	Normal	Axial myopia
Large	Megalocornea	Megalocornea	Large eye
	Axial hyperopia		Buphthalmos
			Axial myopia

recognized, the authors began to take additional measurements on eyes that had extremely small or extremely large axial lengths, to determine whether the prediction of *ELP* could be improved by being able to describe the anterior segment more accurately. Table 39-1 shows the clinical conditions that illustrate the independence of the anterior segment size and the axial length.

For a year, data were gathered from 35 investigators around the world. Several additional measurements of the eye were taken, but only seven preoperative variables (axial length, corneal power, horizontal corneal diameter, anterior chamber depth, lens thickness, preoperative refraction, and age) were found to improve significantly the prediction of *ELP* in eyes of axial length in the range 15–35mm.

The improved accuracy of the prediction of *ELP* is not totally because of changes in the formula; it also is a function of the technical skills of surgeons who implant lenses in the capsular bag consistently. A 20D IOL that is displaced 0.5mm axially from the predicted *ELP* results in an error of approximately 1.00D in the stabilized postoperative refraction. However, when using piggy-back lenses that total 60D, the same axial displacement of 0.5mm causes a 3D refractive error; the error is directly proportional to the power of the implanted lens. This direct relationship is why the problem is much less evident in eyes of extremely large diameter, because the implanted IOL is either low plus or minus to achieve emmetropia following cataract extraction.

The Holladay 2 formula and the interim results of the 35 investigators were presented at the 1996 ASCRS meeting in Seattle. "A" scans and software programs that implement the new formula are now available. Once these additional measurements become routine among clinicians, a new flurry of prediction formulas using seven or more variables will emerge, similar to the activity that followed the first two-variable prediction formula in 1988.[2] The standard of care will reach a new level of prediction accuracy for extremely unusual eyes, just as it has for normal eyes. Predictions for patients who have eyes with axial lengths in the range 22–25mm and corneal powers in the range 42–46D will be accurate using current third-generation formulas (Holladay 1,[2] SRK/T,[14] and Hoffer Q[15]). In cases outside this range, the Holladay 2 formula should be used to ensure accuracy.

Normal Cornea with No Previous Keratorefractive Surgery

CLEAR LENSECTOMY FOR HIGH MYOPIA AND HYPEROPIA. The intraocular power calculations for clear lensectomy are the same as those for when a cataract is present. The patients usually are much younger, however, so the loss of accommodation should be discussed thoroughly. The actual desired postoperative refraction should be discussed, also, because a small degree of myopia (−0.50D) may be desirable to someone who has no accommodation so that the dependence on spectacles can be reduced.

This procedure usually is reserved for patients who are outside the range of other forms of refractive surgery. Consequently, the

values of axial length, keratometry, and other factors usually are quite different from those of the typical cataract patient because of the degree of refractive error. In most of the cases of high myopia, the axial lengths are extremely long (>26mm). In cases of high hyperopia, the axial lengths are very short (<21mm).

In patients who have myopia that exceeds 20D, removal of the clear lens often results in postoperative refractions near emmetropia with no implant. The exact result depends on the power of the cornea and the axial length. The recommended lens powers usually range from −10D to +10D, but the correct axial length measurement is very difficult to obtain in these cases because of the abnormal anatomy of the posterior pole. Staphylomas often are present in these eyes and the macula often is not at the location in the posterior pole where the "A" scan measures the axial length. In such cases, a "B" scan is recommended to locate the macula (fovea) and recheck the value determined using the "A" scan. Variations of 3–4D may occur because the macula is on the edge of the staphyloma, but the "A" scan measures to the deepest part of the staphyloma. Such a variation results in a hyperopic error, because the distance to the macula is much shorter than the distance to the center of the staphyloma. The third-generation theoretical formulas give excellent predictions if the axial length is stable and its measurements are accurate.

In patients who have hyperopia that exceeds +8D, axial lengths often are less than 21mm and require lens powers that exceed the normal range (>34D). In these cases piggy-back lenses are necessary to achieve emmetropia.[13] To date, the only formula available to use for these eyes is the Holladay 2. If the required lens power is less than or equal to 34D, then piggy-back lenses are not required and third-generation theoretical formulas may be used.

Piggy-Back IOLs to Achieve Powers Above 34D

For patients who have axial lengths shorter than 21mm the Holladay 2 formula should be used. In such cases, the size of the anterior segment has been shown to be unrelated to the axial length.[13] In many of these patients, the anterior segment size is normal; only the posterior segment is abnormally short. In a few cases, however, the anterior segment is proportionally small with respect to the axial length (nanophthalmos). The differences in the size of the anterior segment in these cases can cause an average of 5D hyperopic error when third-generation formulas are used, because they predict the depth of the anterior chamber to be very shallow. Use of the newer formula can reduce the prediction error in these eyes to less than 1D.

Accurate measurements of axial length and corneal power are especially important in these cases, because any error is magnified by the extreme dioptric powers of the IOLs. Placement of both lenses in the bag with the haptics aligned is essential. To place inadvertently one lens in the bag and the other in the sulcus can cause a 4D refractive surprise.

Patients with Previous Keratorefractive Surgery

BACKGROUND. The number of patients who have had keratorefractive surgery (radial keratotomy [RK], photorefractive keratectomy [PRK], or laser-assisted *in situ* keratomileusis [LASIK]) has increased steadily over the past 20 years. With the advent of the excimer laser, the number is predicted to increase dramatically. To determine corneal power accurately in such cases is difficult; usually it is the determining factor in the accuracy of the predicted refraction following cataract surgery. To provide this group of patients with the same accuracy of IOL power calculations as provided for standard cataract patients presents an especially difficult challenge to the clinician.

METHODS TO DETERMINE CORNEAL POWER. To determine accurately the central corneal refractive power is the most important and difficult part of the entire IOL calculation process.

> **BOX 39-1**
>
> **The Calculation Method**
>
> | | |
> |---|---|
> | Mean preoperative k | = 42.50 at 90° and 41.50 at 180° = 42.00D |
> | Preoperative refraction | = −10.00 + 1.00 × 90°, vertex = 14mm |
> | Postoperative refraction | = −0.25 + 1.00 × 90°, vertex = 14mm |
>
> **STEP 1**
>
> To calculate the spheroequivalent refraction for refractions at the corneal plane (SEQC) using the spheroequivalent refractions at the spectacle plane (SEQS) at a given vertex (V), use equations 39-2 and 39-3:
>
> SEQS = sphere + 0.5(cylinder) 39-2
> SEQC = 1000/[(1000/SEQS) − V] 39-3
>
> Using equations 39-2 and 39-3, we find the preoperative SEQS and SEQC are:
>
> PreOp SEQR = −10.00 + 0.5 × (1.00) = −9.50D
> PreOp SEQC = 1000/[(1000/−9.50) − 14] = −8.38D
>
> The postoperative spheroequivalent refraction at the corneal plane would be:
>
> PostOp SEQR = −0.25 + 0.5 × (1.00) = +0.25D
> PostOp SEQC = 1000/[(1000/0.25) − 14] = +0.25D
>
> **STEP 2**
>
> To calculate the change in refraction at the corneal plane, use equation 39-4,
>
> Change in refraction = preoperative SEQC − postoperative SEQC 39-4
> = −8.38 − (+0.25) = −8.63D
>
> **STEP 3**
>
> To calculate the postoperative corneal refractive power, use equation 39-5:
>
> $$\text{Mean postoperative } k = \left(\begin{array}{c}\text{mean}\\\text{preoperative}\\k\end{array}\right) - \left(\begin{array}{c}\text{change in}\\\text{refraction at}\\\text{corneal plane}\end{array}\right) \quad 39\text{-}5$$
>
> = 42.00 − 8.63 = 33.37D
>
> This value is the calculated central power of the cornea following the keratorefractive procedure. For IOL programs that require two k readings, this value is entered twice.

The explanation is quite simple—instruments used to measure corneal power make too many incorrect assumptions for corneas that have irregular astigmatism; the cornea can no longer be compared with a sphere centrally, the posterior radius of the cornea is no longer 1.2mm steeper than the anterior corneal radius, and so on. As a result of these limitations, the calculation method and the trial hard contact lens method are the most accurate, followed by corneal topography, automated keratometry and, finally, manual keratometry.

Calculation Method. For the calculation method, three parameters must be known—the *k* readings and refraction before the keratorefractive procedure, and the stabilized refraction after the keratorefractive procedure. It is important that the stabilized postoperative refraction be measured before any myopic shifts from nuclear sclerotic cataracts occur. Also, it is possible for posterior subcapsular cataracts to cause an apparent myopic shift, similar to capsular opacification, in which the patient wants more minus in the refraction to make the letters appear smaller and darker. The concept, described in 1989,[16] subtracts the change in refraction caused by the keratorefractive procedure at the corneal plane from the original *k* readings before the procedure, to arrive at a calculated postoperative *k* reading. This method usually is the most accurate because the preoperative *k* values and refraction usually are accurate to 0.25D. An example calculation is given in Box 39-1.

Trial Hard Contact Lens Method. The trial hard contact lens method requires a plano hard contact lens with a known base curve and a patient whose cataract does not prevent refraction to approximately ±0.50D. This tolerance usually requires a visual acuity of better than 20/80. The patient's spheroequivalent refraction is determined by normal refraction. The refraction then is repeated with the hard contact lens in place. If the spheroequivalent refraction does not change with the contact lens, then the power value for the patient's cornea must be the same as that for the base curve of the plano contact lens. If the patient has a myopic shift in the refraction with the contact lens, then the power value for the base curve of the contact lens is greater than that of the cornea by the amount of the shift. If there is a hyperopic shift in the refraction with the contact lens, then the power value for the base curve of the contact lens is less than that for the cornea by the amount of the shift.

For example, take a patient who has a current spheroequivalent refraction of +0.25D. With a plano hard contact lens of base curve 35.00D placed on the cornea, the spherical refraction changes to −2.00D. Because the patient experiences a myopic shift with the contact lens, the power value for the cornea must be lower than that for the base curve of the contact lens by 2.25D. Therefore, the cornea must be 32.75D (35.00–2.25D), which is slightly different from the value obtained by the calculation method (see Box 39-1). This method is compromised by the possible lack of accuracy of the refractions, which may be limited by the cataract.

Corneal Topography. Current corneal topography units measure more than 5000 points over the entire cornea and more than 1000 points within the central 3mm. This additional information provides greater accuracy in determining the power of corneas with irregular astigmatism compared with the data yielded by keratometry. The computer in topography units allows the measurement to account for the Stiles–Crawford effect, actual pupil size, and so on. These algorithms allow a very accurate determination of the anterior surface of the cornea. They provide no information, however, about the posterior surface of the cornea. In order to determine accurately the total power of the cornea, the power of both surfaces must be known.

In normal corneas that have not been subjected to keratorefractive surgery, the posterior radius of curvature of the cornea averages 1.2mm less than that of the anterior surface.[17] For a person who has an eye with an anterior corneal radius of 7.5mm and using the standardized keratometric index of refraction of 1.3375, the corneal power would be 45.00D. Several studies have shown that this power overestimates the total power of the cornea by approximately 0.56D. Hence, most IOL calculations today use a net index of refraction of 1.3333 (4/3) and the anterior radius of the cornea to calculate the net power of the cornea. Using this lower value, the total power of a cornea with an anterior radius of 7.5mm would be 44.44D. This index of refraction has provided excellent results in normal corneas for IOL calculations.

Following keratorefractive surgery, the assumptions that the central cornea can be approximated by a sphere (no significant irregular astigmatism or asphericity) and that the radius of curvature of the posterior cornea is 1.2mm less than that of the anterior cornea are no longer true. Corneal topography instruments can account for the changes in the anterior surface, but they are unable to account for any differences in the relationship to the posterior radius of curvature. In RK, the mechanism of having a peripheral bulge and central flattening apparently causes similar changes in both the anterior and posterior radii of curvature, with the result that using the net index of refraction for the cornea (4/3) usually gives fairly accurate results, particularly for optical zones larger than 4–5mm. In RKs with optical zones of 3mm or less, the accuracy of the predicted corneal power diminishes. Whether this inaccuracy occurs as a result of the additional central irregularity with small optical zones or of the difference in the relationship between the front and back radii of the cornea is unknown at this time. Studies in which the posterior radius of the cornea is measured are necessary to answer this question.

In PRK and LASIK, inaccuracies in the measurement of net corneal power are almost entirely due to the change in the relationship of the radii at the front and back of the cornea, because the irregular astigmatism in the central 3mm zone usually is minimal. In these two procedures, the anterior surface of the cornea is flattened, with little or no effect on the posterior radius. Using a net index of refraction (4/3) overestimates the power of the cornea by 14% of the change induced by the PRK or LASIK; if the patient had a 7D change in the refraction at the corneal plane from a PRK or LASIK with spherical preoperative *k* values of 44D, the actual power of the cornea is 37D, but the topography units give 38D. If a 14D change in the refraction occurs at the corneal plane, the topography units overestimate the power of the cornea by 2D.

In summary, corneal topography units do not provide accurate central corneal power following PRK, LASIK, or RKs with optical zones of 3mm or less. In RKs with larger optical zones the topography units become more reliable. The calculation method and hard contact lens trial always are more reliable.

Automated Keratometry. Automated keratometers usually are more accurate than manual keratometers for corneas of small optical zone (≤3mm) RKs, because they sample a smaller central area of the cornea (nominally 2.6mm). In addition, the automated instruments often have additional eccentric fixation targets that provide more information about the paracentral cornea. When a measurement error on an RK cornea occurs, the instrument almost always gives a central corneal power that is greater than the true refractive power of the cornea. This error occurs because the samples at 2.6mm are very close to the paracentral knee of the RK. The smaller the optical zone and the greater the number of the RK incisions, the greater the probability and magnitude of the error. Most automated instruments have reliability factors given for each measurement to help the clinician decide on the reliability of the measurement.

Automated keratometry measurements following LASIK or PRK yield accurate values of the front radius of the cornea, because the transition areas are far outside the 2.6mm zone that is measured. The measurements still are not accurate, however, because the assumed net index of refraction (4/3) is no longer appropriate for the new relationship of the front and back radius of the cornea after PRK or LASIK, just as with the topographic instruments. The change in central corneal power as measured by the keratometer used in PRK or LASIK must be increased by 14% to determine the actual refractive change at the plane of the cornea. Hence, the automated keratometer overestimates the power of the cornea proportionately to the amount of PRK or LASIK performed.

Manual Keratometry. Manual keratometers provide the least accurate measure of central corneal power following keratorefractive procedures, because the area that they measure usually is larger than 3.2mm in diameter. Therefore, measurements in this area are extremely unreliable for RK corneas that have optical zones less than or equal to 4mm. The one advantage of the manual keratometer is that the examiner actually is able to see the reflected mires and the amount of irregularity present. To see the mires does not help obtain a better measurement, but it does allow the observer to discount the measurement as unreliable.

The manual keratometer has the same problem with PRK and LASIK as topographers and automated keratometers and, therefore, is no less accurate. The manual keratometer overestimates the change in the central refractive power of the cornea by 14% following PRK and LASIK.

CHOOSING THE DESIRED POSTOPERATIVE REFRACTION TARGET. The procedure to determine the desired postoperative refractive target is no different from that used for other patients who have cataracts, in whom the refractive status and the presence of a cataract in the other eye are the major determining factors. A complete discussion as to how to avoid refractive problems with cataract surgery is beyond the scope of this text (for a thorough discussion see Holladay and Rubin[18]). A short discussion of the major factors follows.

If the patient has binocular cataracts, the decision is much easier because the refractive status of both eyes can be changed. The most important decision is whether the patient prefers to be my-

opic and read without glasses, or near emmetropic and drive without glasses. In some cases the surgeon and patient may choose the intermediate distance (-1.00D) for the best compromise. To target for monovision is certainly acceptable, provided the patient has used monovision successfully in the past. Monovision in a patient who has never experienced this condition may cause intolerable anisometropia and require further surgery.

Monocular cataracts restrict the choice of postoperative refraction, because the refractive status of the other eye is fixed. The general rule is that the operative eye must be within 2D of the nonoperative eye in order to avoid intolerable anisometropia. In most cases this means the other eye is matched or a target of up to 2D nearer emmetropia is set; if the nonoperative eye is -5.00D, then the target is -3.00D for the operative eye. If the patient successfully wears a contact in the unoperative eye or has demonstrated already the ability to accept monovision, an exception can be made to the general rule. It must be stressed, however, that should the patient not be able to continue wearing a contact lens, the necessary glasses for binocular correction may be intolerable and additional refractive surgery may be required.

SPECIAL LIMITATIONS OF IOL POWER CALCULATION FORMULAS. As discussed previously, the third-generation formulas (Holladay 1, Hoffer Q, and the SRK/T) and the new Holladay 2 are much more accurate than previous formulas the more unusual the eye. Older formulas, such as the SRK1, SRK2, and Binkhorst 1, should not be used in these cases. None of these formulas gives the desired result if the central corneal power is measured incorrectly. The resulting errors almost always are in the hyperopic direction following keratorefractive surgery, because the measured corneal powers usually are greater than the true refractive power of the cornea.

To further complicate matters, the newer formulas often use keratometry as one of the predictors to estimate *ELP* of the IOL. In patients who have had keratorefractive surgery, the corneal power is usually much flatter than normal and certainly flatter than before the keratorefractive procedure. In short, the *ELP* of a patient who has a 38D cornea with no keratorefractive surgery would not be expected to be similar to that of a patient who has a 38D cornea with keratorefractive surgery. New IOL calculation programs are being developed now to handle these situations and will improve predictions for these cases.

Intraoperative Evaluation

INTRAOPERATIVE VISUALIZATION AND CORNEAL PROTECTION. Intraoperative visualization is usually more difficult in patients who have had previous RK than in the normal cataract patient and is somewhat similar to the case with severe arcus senilis or other conditions that cause peripheral corneal haze. The surgeon should be prepared for this additional difficulty by ensuring that the patient is lined up such that the surgeon can visualize the cataract through the optical zone. This usually means aligning the microscope perpendicular to the center of the cornea, so that the surgeon looks directly through the optical zone at the center of the cataract. When the peripheral cortex is removed, the eye can be rotated so that visualization of the periphery is made through the central optical zone. It also is prudent to coat the endothelium with an ophthalmic visco-surgical device (OVD) to minimize any endothelial cell loss, because the keratorefractive procedure may have caused some prior loss.

INTRAOPERATIVE AUTOREFRACTOR AND RETINOSCOPY. Large refractive errors can be avoided by use of intraoperative retinoscopy or handheld autorefractors. These refractions should not be relied upon, however, when the IOL power is fine tuned, because many factors occur during surgery that may change during the postoperative period. Factors such as the pressure from the lid speculum, axial position of the IOL, intraocular pressure, and others may cause the intraoperative refraction to be different from the final stabilized postoperative refraction. If the intraoperative refraction is within 2D of the target refraction, no lens exchanges should be considered unless intraoperative keratometry also can be performed.

Postoperative Evaluation

REFRACTION ON THE FIRST POSTOPERATIVE DAY. On the first postoperative day following cataract surgery, patients who have had RK previously usually have a hyperopic shift, similar to that on the first postoperative day after their RK. This phenomenon occurs primarily because of the transient corneal edema that usually exaggerates the RK effect. These patients also exhibit the same daily fluctuations during the early postoperative period after their cataract surgery as exhibited after the RK. Usually this daily shift is in a myopic direction during the day, due to the regression of corneal edema after awakening in the morning.[19] Because the refractive changes are expected and vary significantly among patients, no lens exchange should be contemplated until after the first postoperative week or until after the refraction has stabilized, whichever is longer.

Very few results of cataract surgery following PRK and LASIK are available. In the few operations that have been performed, a much lower degree of hyperopic shift on the first day and less pronounced daily fluctuations occur. In most cases the stability of the cornea makes these cases no different than those of patients who have not had keratorefractive surgery.

LONG-TERM RESULTS. Long-term results of cataract surgery following RK are very good. The long-term hyperopic shifts and development of against-the-rule astigmatism over time following cataract surgery should be the same as in those that occur in long-term studies following RK. The problems with glare and starburst patterns usually are minimal, because the patients have had to adjust to these unwanted optical images following the initial RK. If a patient's primary complaint before cataract surgery is glare and starbursts, it should be made clear to the patient that only the glare due to the cataract will be removed by surgery—the symptoms caused by the RK will remain unchanged.

As yet, no long-term results exist following PRK and LASIK. Because no signs of hyperopic drift or development of against-the-rule astigmatism occur in the 5-year studies following PRK, such changes are not expected. However, the early studies following RK did not suggest any of these long-term changes, either. Only time will tell whether central haze, irregular astigmatism, and other effects will be problems that develop in the future.

IOL CALCULATIONS USING *K* VALUES AND PREOPERATIVE REFRACTION

Formula and Rationale for Using Preoperative Refraction Versus Axial Length

In a standard cataract removal with IOL implantation, the preoperative refraction is not very helpful for the calculation of the power of the implant, because as the crystalline lens is removed, so the dioptric power is being removed and then replaced. In cases in which power is not being reduced in the eye, such as secondary implant in aphakia, piggy-back IOL in pseudophakia, or a minus IOL in the anterior chamber of a phakic patient, the necessary IOL power for a desired postoperative refraction can be calculated from the corneal power and preoperative refraction—knowledge of the axial length is not necessary. The formula used to calculate the necessary IOL power is given in Equation 39-6,[20] where *ELP* is the expected lens position in millimeters (distance from corneal vertex to principal plane of IOL), *IOLP* is the IOL power in diopters, *k* is the net corneal power in diopters, *PreRx* is the preoperative refraction in diopters, *DPostRx* is the desired postoperative refraction in diopters, and *V* is the vertex distance in millimeters of refractions.

Equation 39-6

$$IOLP = (1336/[1336/\{(1000/[\{1000/PreRx\} - V])\} - k]) - ELP) -$$
$$(1336/[1336/\{1000/[1000/PostRx] - K\}]) - k\}]$$

Cases in Which to Use the Calculation from Preoperative Refraction

As mentioned above, the appropriate cases for which preoperative refraction and corneal power are used include the following:
- Secondary implant in aphakia
- Secondary piggy-back IOL in pseudophakia
- A minus anterior chamber IOL in a high myopic phakic patient

In each of these cases dioptric power is not being diminished in the eye, so the problem is simply to find the *IOLP* at a given distance behind the cornea *ELP* that is equivalent to the spectacle lens at a given vertex distance in front of the cornea. If emmetropia is not desired, then an additional term, the desired postoperative refraction (*DPostRx*), must be included. The formulas for calculating the predicted refraction and the back calculation of the *ELP* are given in Holladay.[20] Use of the formula for particular cases is outlined below.

Secondary Implant for Aphakia

The patient discussed here is 72 years old and is aphakic in the right eye and pseudophakic in the left eye. The right eye can no longer tolerate an aphakic contact lens. The capsule in the right eye is intact and a posterior chamber IOL is desired. The patient is −0.50D in the left eye and would like to be the same in the right eye. The mean keratometric *k* is 45.00D, aphakic refraction is +12.00 sphere at vertex of 14mm, manufacturer's anterior chamber depth (ACD) lens constant is 5.25mm, and the desired postoperative refraction is −0.50D.

Each of the values above can be substituted into Equation 39-6 except for the manufacturer's ACD and the measured *k* reading. The labeled values on IOL boxes are primarily for lenses implanted in the bag. Because this lens is intended for the sulcus, 0.25mm should be subtracted from 5.25mm to give the equivalent constant for the sulcus. The *ELP*, therefore, is 5.00mm. The *k* reading must be converted from the measured keratometric value ($n = 1.3375$) to the net *k* reading ($n = 4/3$), for the reasons described previously under corneal topography. The conversion is performed by multiplying the measured *k* reading by the fraction obtained in Equation 39-7 and inserting this into Equation 39-8.

Equation 39-7
$$\text{Conversion fraction} = ([4/3] - 1)/(1.3375 - 1) = (1/3)/0.3375 = 0.98765$$

Equation 39-8
$$\text{Mean refractive } k = \text{Mean keratometric } K \times \text{conversion fraction} = 45.00 \times 0.98765 = 44.44D$$

Using the mean refractive *K*, aphakic refraction, vertex distance, *ELP* for the sulcus, and the desired postoperative refraction in Equation 39-6, the patient needs a 22.90D IOL. A 23.00D IOL would yield a predicted refraction of −0.57D.[20]

Secondary Piggy-Back IOL for Pseudophakia

In patients who have a significant residual refractive error following the primary IOL implant, it often is easier surgically and more predictable optically to leave the primary implant in place and calculate the secondary piggy-back IOL power to achieve the desired refraction. This method does not require knowledge of the power of the primary implant or of the axial length; it is particularly important in cases in which the primary implant is thought to be mislabeled. The formula works for plus or minus lenses; however, negative lenses only now are becoming available.

The patient discussed here is a 55-year-old man who had a refractive surprise after the primary cataract surgery and was left with a +5.00D spherical refraction in the right eye. No cataract is present in the left eye, and the lens is plano. The surgeon and the patient both desire postoperative refraction of −0.50D, which was the target for the primary implant. The refractive surprise is felt to be caused by a mislabeled IOL, which is centered in the bag and very difficult to remove. The secondary piggy-back IOL will be placed in the sulcus. This is very important, because trying to place the second lens in the bag several weeks after primary surgery is very difficult. More importantly, it could displace the primary lens posteriorly, thus reducing its effective power and leaving the patient with a hyperopic error. To place the lens in the sulcus minimizes this posterior displacement. The mean keratometric k is 45.00D, pseudophakic refraction is +5.00 sphere at vertex of 14mm, manufacturer's ACD lens constant is 5.25mm, and the desired postoperative refraction is −0.50D.

Use of the same style lens and constant as in the case above and modifying the k reading to net power, Equation 39-6 yields a +8.64D IOL for a −0.50D target. The nearest available lens is +9.0D, which would result in −0.76D. In these cases extreme care should be taken to ensure that the two lenses are well centered with respect to one another. Decentration of either lens can result in poor image quality and can be the limiting factor in the patient's vision.

Primary Minus Anterior Chamber IOL in a High Myopic Phakic Patient

The calculation for a minus IOL in the anterior chamber is the same as for the aphakic calculation of an anterior chamber lens, with the exception that the power of the lens is negative. In the past, these lenses were reserved for high myopia that could not be corrected by radial keratotomy or photorefractive keratectomy. Because most of these lenses fixate in the anterior chamber angle, concerns of iritis and glaucoma have been raised. Nevertheless, several cases have been performed with good refractive results. Because successful laser-assisted *in situ* keratomileusis procedures have been performed in myopias up to −20.00D, these lenses may be reserved for myopia that exceeds this power. Interestingly, the power of the negative anterior chamber implant is very close to the spectacle refraction for normal vertex distances. Consider a case in which the mean keratometric k is 45.00D, phakic refraction is −20.00 sphere at vertex of 14mm, manufacturer's ACD

lens constant is 3.50mm, and the desired postoperative refraction is −0.50D. Using an *ELP* of 3.50 and modifying the k reading to net corneal power yields −18.49D for a desired refraction of −0.50D. If a −19.00D lens is used, the patient would have a predicted postoperative refraction of −0.10D.

REFERENCES

1. Holladay JT, Prager TC, Ruiz RS, Lewis JW. Improving the predictability of intraocular lens calculations. Arch Ophthalmol. 1986;104:539–41.
2. Holladay JT, Prager TC, Chandler TY, et al. A three-part system for refining intraocular lens power calculations. J Cataract Refract Surg. 1988;13:17–24.
3. Fedorov SN, Kolinko AI, Kolinko AI. Estimation of optical power of the intraocular lens. Vestn Oftalmol. 1967;80:27–31.
4. Fedorov SN, Galin MA, Linksz A. A calculation of the optical power of intraocular lenses. Invest Ophthalmol. 1975;14:625–8.
5. Binkhorst CD. Power of the prepupillary pseudophakos. Br J Ophthalmol. 1972;56:332–7.
6. Colenbrander MC. Calculation of the power of an iris clip lens for distant vision. Br J Ophthalmol. 1973;57:735–40.
7. Binkhorst RD. The optical design of intraocular lens implants. Ophthalmic Surg. 1975;6:17–31.
8. van der Heijde GL. The optical correction of unilateral aphakia. Trans Am Acad Ophthalmol Otolaryngol. 1976;81:80–8.
9. Thijssen JM. The emmetropic and the iseikonic implant lens: computer calculation of the refractive power and its accuracy. Ophthalmologica. 1975;171:467–86.
10. Fritz KJ. Intraocular lens power formulas. Am J Ophthalmol. 1981;91:414–5.
11. Binkhorst RD. Intraocular lens power calculation manual. A guide to the author's TI 58/59 IOL power module, ed 2. New York: Richard D Binkhorst; 1981.
12. Olsen T, Corydon L, Gimbel H. Intraocular lens power calculation with an improved anterior chamber depth prediction algorithm. J Cataract Refract Surg. 1995;21:313–9.
13. Holladay JT, Gills JP, Leidlein J, Cherchio M. Achieving emmetropia in extremely short eyes with two piggy-back posterior chamber intraocular lenses. Ophthalmology. 1996;103:1118–23.
14. Retzlaff JA, Sanders DR, Kraff MC. Development of the SRK/T intraocular lens implant power calculation formula. J Cataract Refract Surg. 1990;16:333–40.
15. Hoffer KJ. The Hoffer Q formula: a comparison of theoretic and regression formulas. J Cataract Refract Surg. 1993;19:700–12.
16. Holladay JT. IOL calculations following RK. J Refractive Corneal Surg. 1989;5:203.
17. Lowe RF, Clark BA. Posterior corneal curvature. Br J Ophthalmol. 1973;57:464–70.
18. Holladay JT, Rubin ML. Avoiding refractive problems in cataract surgery. Surv Ophthalmol. 1988;32:357–60.
19. Holladay JT. Management of hyperopic shift after RK. J Refract Corneal Surg. 1992;8:325.
20. Holladay JT. Refractive power calculations for intraocular lenses in the phakic eye. Am J Ophthalmol. 1993;116:63–6.

CHAPTER 40

Evolution of Intraocular Lens Implantation

LILIANA WERNER • ANDREA M. IZAK • ROBERT T. ISAACS • SURESH K. PANDEY • DAVID J. APPLE

INTRODUCTION

Cataract is the most prevalent ophthalmic disease. For 1998 the number of persons blind as a result of cataract was estimated to be about 20 million worldwide; this number was expected to double by early in the 20th century.[1,2] Although a pharmacological preventive or therapeutic treatment for this blinding disease is being sought actively, the solution still appears to be many years away. Therefore, surgical treatment for cataracts, which increasingly includes intraocular lens (IOL) implantation, remains the only viable alternative.

Treatment of cataracts has been practiced for centuries using various surgical and nonsurgical procedures. However, avoidance of complications and attainment of high-quality postoperative visual rehabilitation in the years before the introduction of modern IOLs were difficult problems. Because significant dioptric power resides in the crystalline lens, its removal results in marked visual disability.

Aphakic spectacle correction has been prescribed throughout history, but spectacles are less than satisfactory because of the visual distortions inherent in such high-power lenses.

It was not until the late 1940s that the tremendous optical advantages that an IOL could provide in visual rehabilitation were understood and acted upon by Harold Ridley.[3–7]

The implantation of IOLs is now a highly successful operation; the safety and efficacy of the procedure are now well established. For 1998 the number of IOL implants in the United States was estimated to be 1.6 million. Implantation data from other countries are scant, but the total number of implantations per year worldwide is increasing rapidly. Studies are still needed to determine which surgical technique(s) and which IOL design(s) are safest, most practical, and most economic for high-volume use in the less advantaged areas of the world. For general discussions that review the evolution and provide clinicopathologic overviews of IOLs, see Apple et al.[7–10] and Binkhorst.[11]

Posterior chamber IOLs, following a long period of disfavor after the Ridley lens was discontinued, were reintroduced in the mid-1970s and early 1980s. Jaffe and other authors compared posterior chamber lenses with iris-supported lenses and were impressed by the superior results achieved with the former type of lens using an extracapsular cataract extraction technique. The use of posterior chamber IOLs is now clearly the treatment of choice.

LENS DESIGN AND FIXATION

In 1967 Binkhorst[11] proposed a detailed classification of the various means of fixation for each IOL type. In a 1985 update of this classification, Binkhorst[12] listed four IOL types according to fixation sites:

- Anterior chamber angle-supported lenses;
- Iris-supported lenses;
- Capsule-supported lenses; and
- Posterior chamber angle (ciliary sulcus)-supported lenses.

TABLE 40-1

THE EVOLUTION OF INTRAOCULAR LENSES

Generation	Date	Description
I	1949–1954	Original Ridley posterior chamber lens
II	1952–1962	Early anterior chamber lenses
III	1953–1975	Iris-supported lenses
IV	1963–1990	Intermediate anterior chamber lenses
V	1975–1990	Improved posterior chamber lenses
VI	1990 to present	Modern capsular posterior chamber lenses and modern anterior chamber lenses

By common agreement, most surgeons today differentiate lens types as follows:

- Iris-supported lenses;
- Anterior chamber lenses; and
- Posterior chamber lenses.

From the time of Ridley's first lens implantation to the present day, the evolution of IOLs can be arbitrarily divided into six generations (Table 40-1).

Generation I (Original Ridley Posterior Chamber Lens)

A practical application of the concept of IOLs began with Harold Ridley,[3–7] and credit for the introduction of lens implants clearly belongs to him.

Ridley's first IOL operation was performed on a 49-year-old woman at St Thomas' Hospital in London on November 29, 1949. His original IOL was a biconvex polymethyl methacrylate (PMMA) disc designed to be implanted after nuclear expression extracapsular cataract extraction (BCCE) (Fig. 40-1).

Ridley's procedure was initially met with great hostility by several skeptical and critical ophthalmologists. However, good results were attained in enough cases to warrant further implantation of the Ridley IOL, although dislocation of the lens ultimately proved troublesome. It is gratifying to note that Ridley had lived to experience, finally, the acknowledgment, respect, and honor he so fully deserves for this innovation.

Generation II (Early Anterior Chamber Lenses)

As a consequence of the relatively high incidence of dislocations with the Ridley lens, a new implantation site was considered—the anterior chamber, with fixation of the lens in the angle recess.

The anterior chamber was chosen because less likelihood existed of dislocation within its narrow confines. In addition, anterior chamber lenses could be implanted after either an intracapsular cataract extraction (ICCE) or an ECCE. Also, anterior chamber placement of the pseudophakos was considered a simpler technical procedure than placement of the lens behind the iris.

293

Although many surgeons worked on the concept of this type of lens, Baron, in France, is generally credited as being the first designer and implanter of an anterior chamber lens (Fig. 40-2, A).[10] He first performed this procedure on May 13, 1952.

Late endothelial atrophy, corneal decompensation, and pseudophakic bullous keratopathy were observed with the original Baron lens and also developed with many subsequent anterior chamber lens designs. The entity now termed uveitis-glaucoma-hyphema (UGH) syndrome was described first when ocular tissue damage occurred that was clearly the result of poorly manufactured anterior chamber lenses.[13] It took many modifications of the haptic-loop configuration and the lens-vaulting characteristics (Fig. 40-2, B) to develop an anterior chamber lens that allowed a reasonable prediction of long-term success. This was achieved largely because of the advances in lens design by Dr. Peter Choyce of England and later by Dr. Charles Kelman of New York.

Generation III (Iris-Supported Lenses)

Relatively frequent dislocation of the Ridley lens and an unacceptably high rate of corneal decompensation associated with the anterior chamber lenses available in the early 1950s caused some surgeons to discontinue implantation of IOLs entirely.[14] However, iris-supported or iris-fixated IOLs were introduced subsequently in an attempt to overcome these problems.

Cornelius Binkhorst in The Netherlands was an early advocate of iris-supported IOLs.[11,12] His first lens was a four-loop, iris-clip IOL (Fig. 40-3, A) design. Although Binkhorst initially believed that IOL contact with the iris would not cause problems, he soon noted that iris chafing, pupillary abnormalities, and dislocation developed with the early iris-clip lens. Also, in an effort to circumvent dislocation, Binkhorst made the anterior loops of his four-loop lens longer, but this led to increased corneal decompensation from peripheral touch.

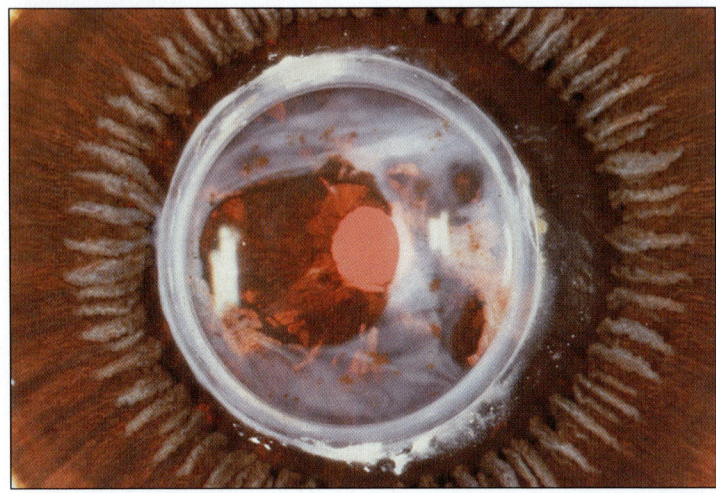

FIG. 40-1 ▪ Posterior view of an eye (obtained postmortem) showing the implantation site of a Ridley lens. To the time of death, almost 30 years after implantation, the patient's visual acuity remained 20/20 (6/6) in both eyes. Note the good centration and clarity of the all-polymethyl methacrylate optic in the central visual axis. The lens was implanted by Dr. W. Reese and Dr. T. Hammdi of Philadelphia.

FIG. 40-2 ▪ Sagittal section of the anterior segment of the eye. A, The original 1952 Baron anterior chamber lens, with fixation in the angle recess. Because this one-piece lens was rigid, sizing problems were unavoidable. Note the extremely steep anterior curvature of the lens. Such excessive anterior vaulting invariably caused corneal endothelial problems. B, Placement of a modern anterior chamber lens fixated in the angle recess. Note the more subtle anterior vaulting of the loops and lens optic.

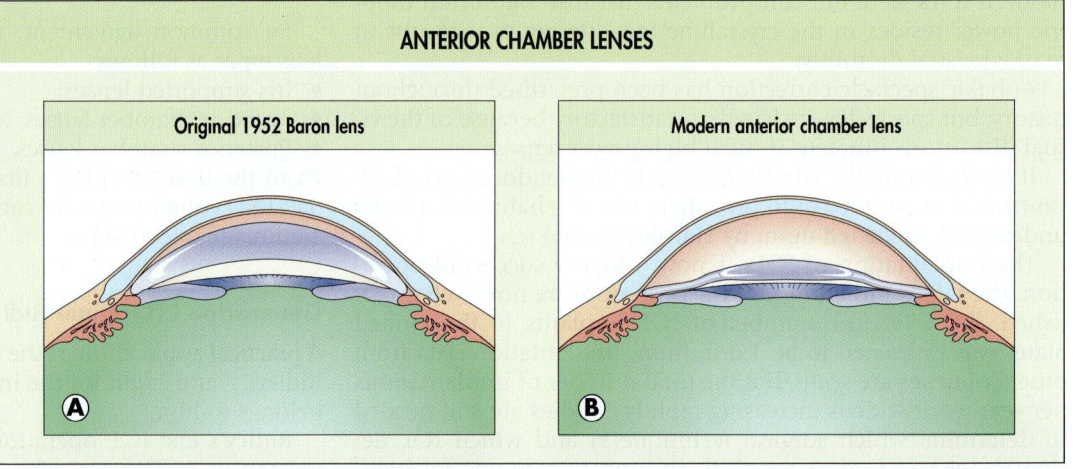

ANTERIOR CHAMBER LENSES

Original 1952 Baron lens

Modern anterior chamber lens

FIG. 40-3 ▪ Binkhorst iris-clip lenses. A, A correctly positioned Binkhorst four-loop, iris-clip lens, well centered in an eye that had good visual acuity. Moderate pupillary distortion and sphincter erosion occur. Note the iris-fixation suture superior to the site of the large iridectomy. B, Posterior view of an autopsy globe that contains a two-loop iridocapsular intraocular lens. Note the rod that helps to secure the lens to the iris through the iridectomy. An outer Soemmering ring is present, but the visual axis remains clear. The optic is well centered.

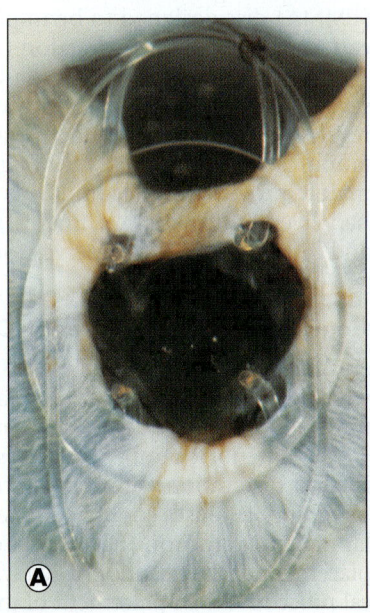

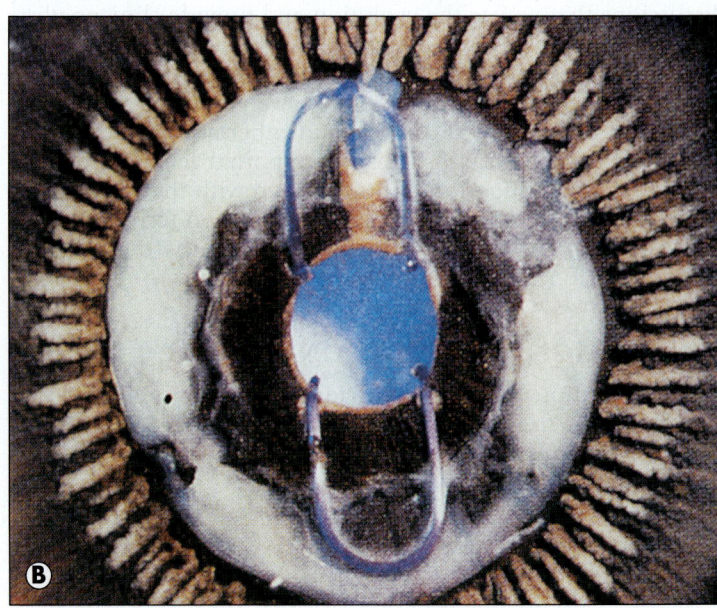

His initial implantations were done after ICCE, but occasionally he implanted his four-loop lens following ECCE. His positive experience with this procedure prompted him to modify his iris-clip lens design for implantation following ECCE. Binkhorst's change from ICCE to ECCE and the introduction of his two-loop iridocapsular IOL (Fig. 40-3, *B*) in 1965 were important advances in both IOL design and mode of fixation.[15] His and others' experiences with the two-loop lens style and its modifications were influential in the development of modern design concepts of IOLs, including capsular-bag fixated, posterior chamber IOLs. Binkhorst's innovative lens designs and his advocacy of ECCE came at a time when the entire future of IOL implantation was in jeopardy; they provided the major impetus that set the stage for modern posterior chamber lens implantations.

During the early years of iris-fixated IOLs, many clinical and subclinical problems emerged, such as dislocation, pupillary deformity and erosion, iris atrophy with transillumination defects, pigment dispersion, uveitis, hemorrhage, and opacification of the media. Many of these complications were the result of chronic rubbing or chafing of the iris by IOL loops or haptics. Problems were especially severe with metal loop IOLs and occurred frequently with multiple-looped lenses because uveal contact and chafing against the mobile iris tissues were unavoidable with these designs.

An increased incidence of corneal edema occurred in association with iris-supported lens designs. Corneal decompensation and pseudophakic bullous keratopathy became major indications for penetrating keratoplasty. The well-known coexistence of pseudophakic bullous keratopathy and cystoid macular edema (CME) has been termed corneal-retinal inflammatory syndrome by Obstbaum and Galin.[16] Binkhorst's return to ECCE, with the introduction of his two-loop iridocapsular lens in 1965 (see Fig. 40-3, *B*),[17] brought about an almost immediate reduction in the incidence of many of these complications.

Most iris-supported lenses were biplanar, with the optic placed in front of the pupil. In general, biplanar IOLs required a larger limbal wound opening for insertion. The change to capsular fixation after ECCE provided better stability for the pseudophakos. This important modification was a forerunner to capsular sac (in-the-bag) fixation of modern posterior chamber IOLs.

At the time when iris-supported lenses were in widespread use, and until the mid-1980s in many cases, manufacturing methods and surgical techniques were less sophisticated. It is now clear that most modern, high-quality anterior and posterior chamber IOLs provide better success than the IOLs that depend on the iris for support. At present, it is the consensus of surgeons that when a patient who has an iris-supported IOL develops late complications, such as inflammation or corneal decompensation that does not respond rapidly to conservative therapy, lens explantation and/or exchange is usually the best treatment.

Generation IV (Intermediate Anterior Chamber Lenses)

While iris-supported IOLs underwent major modifications in the early 1950s up to the beginning of the 1980s, several designs of anterior chamber IOLs were introduced.

The problems of tissue chafing and difficulties in correct sizing associated with rigid IOLs were addressed by the development of anterior chamber lenses with more flexible loops or haptics (Box 40-1). Unlike the ill-fated, nylon-looped lenses introduced by Dannheim in the early 1950s, the fixation elements of these anterior chamber IOLs were made from more stable polymers, usually PMMA and polypropylene. The best lenses were the various rigid[18] and flexible, open-loop, one-piece PMMA designs, such as the three- and four-point fixation Kelman IOLs.[19] Modifications of the latter have been in use since the late 1970s and are the styles most commonly implanted today (Fig. 40-4). These lenses now are well designed, correctly vaulted, and properly sized and can provide excellent long-term results. As with the early generation of anterior chamber IOLs,

---

BOX 40-1

Anterior Chamber Lenses

DISADVANTAGES OF CLOSED-LOOP ANTERIOR CHAMBER LENSES
Lenses may be difficult to size

Lenses may have inappropriate vault–compression ratios; when a lens is compressed, it may vault anteriorly or posteriorly—either type of response can cause deleterious effects

Small-diameter loops may cause a "cheese-cutter" effect, particularly if the lens is too large; subsequent erosion and chafing can cause uveitis, including cystoid macular edema and pseudophakic bullous keratopathy

Some lenses have a large contact zone over broad areas of the angle with the potential for secondary glaucoma

The poorly finished, sharp edges of some lens models can cause chafing, which leads to sequelae such as uveitis or the uveitis–glaucoma–hyphema syndrome

Synechiae formation around the small-diameter loops may make the lens difficult to remove when necessary; tearing of ocular tissues, hemorrhage, and iridocyclodialysis are possible complications of intraocular lens removal if correct procedures are not used

ADVANTAGES OF MODERN, OPEN-LOOP, ONE-PIECE, ALL-PMMA FLEXIBLE ANTERIOR CHAMBER LENSES
Most modern lenses have an excellent finish with highly polished smooth surfaces and rounded edges from tumble polishing; tissue contact with any component of these intraocular lenses is much less likely to result in chafing damage

Sizing is less critical with flexible, open-loop designs

In contrast to a closed-loop anterior chamber intraocular lens, the vault (a well-designed, open-loop lens) is maintained even under high compression—this minimizes intraocular lens touch against the cornea anteriorly, or against the iris posteriorly

Point fixation is possible, since the haptic may subtend only small areas of the angle outflow structures

Most open-loop intraocular lens designs are much easier to remove, when necessary, especially those with Choyce-like haptic or footplate fixation; the well polished surfaces of these lenses usually do not become completely surrounded by goniosynechiae or cocoon membranes, and, therefore, can usually be removed if necessary without undue difficulty or excessive tissue damage.

Disadvantages of the older, closed-loop anterior chamber lenses and advantages of the modern, open-loop, one-piece, all-polymethyl methacrylate (all-PMMA) flexible anterior chamber lenses.

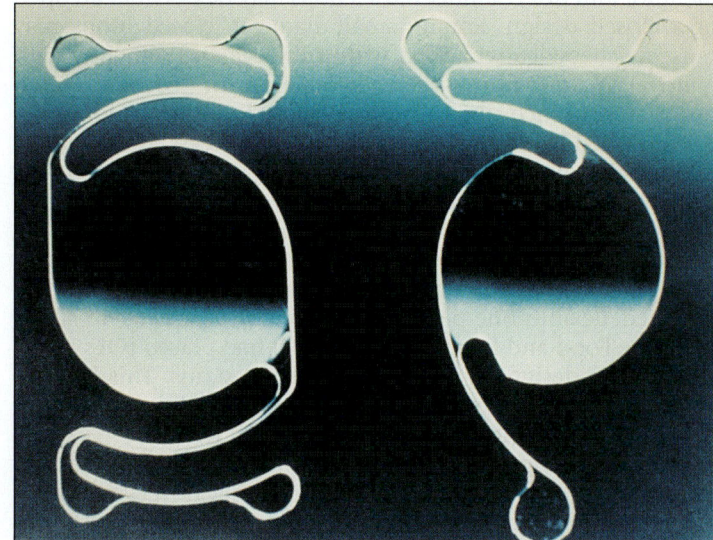

FIG. 40-4 ■ Modern one-piece, all-polymethyl methacrylate, Kelman-style anterior chamber lenses of four-point and three-point fixation designs. Note the excellent polishing and tissue-friendly Choyce-Kelman style footplates. These represent modern, state-of-the-art lenses that should be distinguished clearly from the earlier, unsatisfactory, closed-loop anterior chamber lenses.

new lens designs included both haptic (footplate) fixation lenses and small-diameter, round-looped IOLs.

Although in the 1950s implantations with early anterior chamber IOLs were often disappointing, some models of anterior chamber lenses provided good success, particularly when the lens was properly sized. Two important factors that led to an improved success rate with anterior chamber IOL use are:

- Improved lens designs; and
- Improved manufacturing techniques.

More appropriate lens flexibility has decreased the need for perfect sizing. Increased attention has been given to the anterior-posterior vaulting characteristics of IOLs, which has reduced the incidence of intermittent touch and uveal chafing problems. Design flaws in older lens styles have been identified and these lenses removed from the market in the United States. Tumble polishing of IOLs, particularly one-piece, all-PMMA lenses, produces excellent surfaces and edges. The elimination of sharp optic or haptic edges is critical in the production of anterior chamber IOLs. This is true even more so than for posterior chamber IOLs because anterior chamber IOLs are fixated in a confined space directly adjacent to delicate anterior segment tissues.

The two major disadvantages of an anterior chamber IOL, as compared with posterior chamber lens styles, are:

- The close proximity of the haptics or loops to delicate tissues such as the trabecular meshwork, corneal epithelium, angle recess, and anterior iris surface; and
- The difficulty often encountered in IOL sizing, particularly with rigid lens designs.

The close proximity of anterior chamber lens components to the corneal endothelium is an obvious disadvantage because of the potential for corneal decompensation and/or pseudophakic bullous keratopathy as a result of contact of the cornea with the IOL. In the past, the most common causes of pseudophakic bullous keratopathy were related to anterior chamber IOLs that were sized incorrectly, vaulted too steeply, or designed with an inappropriate amount of flexibility.[20]

Haptics or spatula-like footplates are one of the two types of fixation elements used for anterior chamber IOLs. Haptics or footplates, popularized by Peter Choyce, are often likened to the flattened portion of a spatula and were used originally with the more rigid IOL styles. They now are used with both rigid and flexible modern anterior chamber IOLs. When IOL removal is necessary for any reason, the footplate generally slides out of the eye much more easily than does a small-diameter loop and with minimal tissue damage.

Small-diameter lens loops are the second type of fixation element for anterior chamber IOLs. Loops may be of either an open or a closed design. Round, small-diameter, closed loops may cause a "cheese-cutter" effect within the eye and difficulty with removal. A 360° fibrouveal encapsulation, or "cocoon," often forms around such small-diameter, round loops as the loops become embedded in the tissues of the angle recess. If the correct explantation procedure is not used, these adhesions may result in tissue tears, hemorrhage, and iridocyclodialysis. These anterior chamber IOLs,[21-25] often generically classified together as "closed-loop lenses," do not provide the safety and efficacy achieved by other anterior chamber lens designs, such as finely polished, flexible, one-piece, all-PMMA lenses (see Fig. 40-4). By 1987 the Food and Drug Administration had placed IOLs of the closed-loop design on core investigational status. This had the effect of removing them from the market in the United States, although it did not prevent the export of such lenses.

The flexible, open-loop designs,[24-28] modifications of the original Kelman anterior chamber IOLs (with Choyce-style footplates), can be well finished using tumble polishing, which provides a rounded, "tissue-friendly" surface at points of haptic contact with delicate uveal tissues. One-piece IOLs, particularly those with a footplate design, are usually much easier to explant than IOLs with round, small-diameter loops, of either closed-loop or open-loop design.

Iris- or scleral-fixated, sutured posterior chamber IOLs may be used in cases formerly reserved for anterior chamber IOLs. Results are encouraging.[29,30] Uncertainty still exists as to whether a retropupillary lens is superior to a modern, well-manufactured, Kelman-style anterior chamber IOL for cases such as intraoperative capsular rupture or vitreous loss or as a secondary or exchange procedure. The technique is more difficult than insertion of a single anterior chamber lens and should, therefore, be carried out only by an experienced surgeon.

Generation V (Improved Posterior Chamber Lenses)

The return to Harold Ridley's[4-7] original concept of IOL implantation in the posterior chamber occurred after 1975. John Pearce[31] of England implanted the first uniplanar posterior chamber lens since Ridley.[32] It was a rigid tripod design with the two inferior feet implanted in the capsular bag and the superior foot implanted in front of the anterior capsule and sutured to the iris. Steven Shearing[33] of Las Vegas introduced a major lens design breakthrough in early 1977 with his posterior chamber lens. The design consisted of an optic with two flexible J-shaped loops. William Simcoe of Tulsa publicly introduced his C-looped posterior chamber lens shortly after Shearing's J-loop design appeared. Eric Arnott of London was an early advocate of

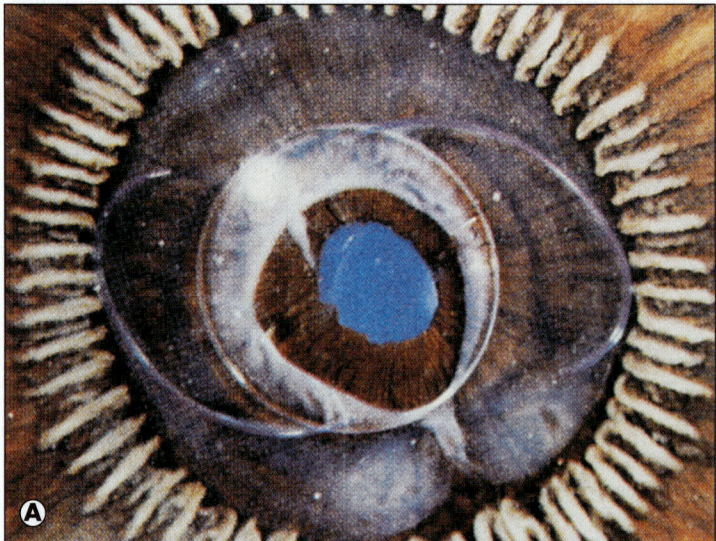

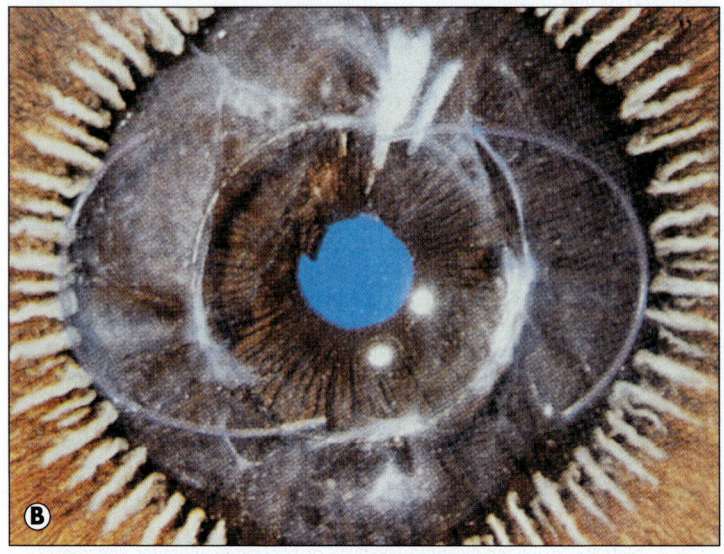

FIG. 40-5 ■ View from behind of an autopsy eye. **A,** A Sinskey-style, J-loop posterior chamber intraocular lens implanted within the lens capsular bag. The optic is well centered, the visual axis is clear, and there is only minimal regeneration of cortex in scattered areas. Moderate haziness or opacity occurs at the margins of the anterior capsulotomy, which does not encroach on the visual axis. **B,** The placement of the loop of this modified C-style intraocular lens in the capsular bag.

one-piece, all-PMMA posterior chamber IOLs. The flexible open-loop designs (J-loop, modified J-loop, C-loop, or modified C-loop) still account for the largest number of IOL styles available today (Fig. 40-5).

One obvious major theoretical advantage that a posterior chamber IOL has over an anterior chamber IOL is its position behind the iris, away from the delicate structures of the anterior segment.

As posterior chamber lens implantation evolved, the type of fixation achieved in the early years depended largely on chance or on the surgeon's individual preference. As Figure 40-6 illustrates, several loop-fixation sites are possible with modern, flexible-loop posterior chamber IOLs. In general, the loops were anchored in one of three ways:
- Both loops were placed in the ciliary region;
- Both loops were placed within the lens capsular sac; or
- One loop (usually the leading or inferior loop) was placed in the capsular sac and the other loop (usually the trailing or superior loop) in a variety of locations anterior to the anterior capsular flap.

These fixation sites have been confirmed histologically by analyses of postmortem globes implanted with posterior chamber IOLs.

The return to posterior chamber lenses coincided with the development of improved ECCE surgery. Shearing[33] identified four major milestones that have marked the evolution of ECCE surgery:
- Microscopic surgical techniques;
- Phacoemulsification;
- Iridocapsular fixation; and
- Flexible posterior chamber lenses.

Without microscopic surgery, modern IOL implantation would be far more difficult. Although phacoemulsification was promoted originally because it required only a small wound, it became clear that if an IOL were to be inserted, the wound would have to be enlarged after removal of the cataract, and thus nonultrasonic surgical methods were refined. By 1974, implan-

tation of IOLs again began to achieve significant acceptability. A natural marriage between phacoemulsification and implantation of IOLs occurred.

As noted previously, Cornelius Binkhorst[11,12,17] was one of the pioneers in the return to the ECCE procedure. Binkhorst recognized that an intact posterior capsule enhanced stability, and he also recognized the many advantages of IOL implantation within the capsular sac. Evidence continues to accumulate that CME and retinal detachment occur less frequently with ECCE than with ICCE.

The introduction of flexible posterior chamber lenses designed to be implanted following ECCE largely resolved the debate about ECCE versus ICCE clearly in favor of the extracapsular procedure.

Securing both loops in the lens capsular sac is the only type of fixation in which IOL contact with uveal tissues is avoided.[34] Placement of a lens with one or both loops outside the capsular bag is associated with various potential complications, including decentration and uveal erosion.[34,35] The consequences of uveal touch have been learned after experiences with the earlier iris-fixated IOLs. The excellent success rate now achieved with posterior chamber IOL implantation is associated with improved IOL designs and improved surgical techniques, including the meticulous placement of loops (Box 40-2).

Posterior capsular opacification (PCO); Elschnig pearls, secondary or after cataract) is a significant postoperative complication in IOL implantation. A well-designed posterior chamber lens in the lens capsular sac provides a gentle but taut radial stretch on the posterior capsule. Of the present open-loop flexible IOLs, the one-piece, all-PMMA posterior chamber designs with posterior convex or biconvex optics appear to be especially effective in providing a symmetrical stretch. Symmetrical stretch may help minimize PCO, as it reduces the folds in the capsular sac and holds the posterior capsule firmly against the posterior surface of the IOL optic. This is sometimes termed the "no space, no cells" concept.

The quality of surgery and the accuracy of loop placement are important factors that affect the outcome of the cataract operation. Two very helpful tools are available to surgeons that make precise loop or haptic placement possible:
- Ophthalmic visco-surgical devices (OVDs); and
- New methods to control the size, shape, and quality of the anterior capsulotomy.

The intercapsular (envelope) technique and its successor, circular continuous tear capsulorrhexis, greatly increase the ability to achieve accurate and permanent loop placement.

POSSIBLE PLACEMENT SITES OF POSTERIOR CHAMBER LENS LOOPS

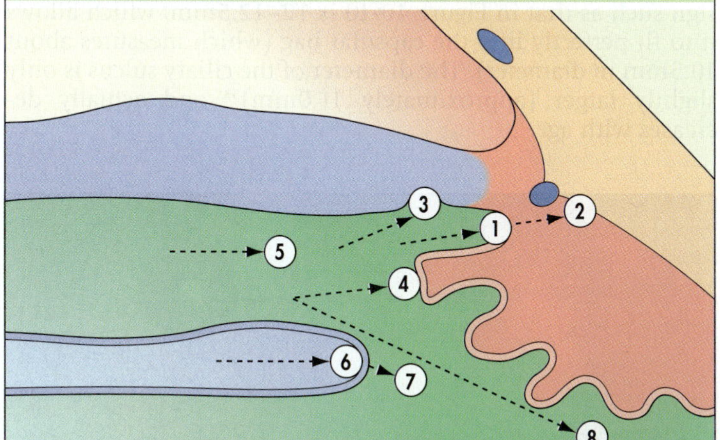

Site 1: loop in the ciliary sulcus.
Site 2: loop after erosion into the ciliary body stroma in the region of the major iris arterial circle.
Site 3: loop in contact with the iris root.
Site 4: loop attached to a ciliary process.
Site 5: loop in aqueous without tissue contact (can result in 'windshield wiper' syndrome because of inadequate fixation).
Site 6: loop in the lens capsular sac.
Site 7: loop ruptured through the lens capsular sac (a rare occurrence).
Site 8: loop in the zonular region between the ciliary sulcus and the lens capsular sac. The loop may penetrate the zonules (zonular fixation) or extend as far posteriorly as the pars plana (pars plana fixation).

FIG. 40-6 ▌▌ The possible placement sites of posterior chamber lens loops.

BOX 40-2

Advantages of Placing Both Loops in the Lens Capsular Sac

Intraocular lens is positioned in the proper anatomical site
Both loops can be placed symmetrically in the capsular sac as easily as in the ciliary sulcus
Intraoperative stretching or tearing of zonules by loop manipulations in front of the anterior capsular leaflet is avoided
Low incidence of lens decentration and dislocation
No evidence of spontaneous loop dislocation
Intraocular lens is positioned a maximal distance behind the cornea
Intraocular lens is positioned a maximal distance from the posterior iris pigment epithelium, iris root, and ciliary processes
Iris chafing (caused by postoperative pigment dispersion into the anterior chamber) is reduced
No direct contact by, or erosion of, intraocular lens loops or haptics into ciliary body tissues
Chronic uveal tissue chafing is avoided, and the probability of long-term blood–aqueous barrier breakdown is reduced
Surface alteration of loop material is less likely
Intraocular lens implantation is safer for children and young individuals
Posterior capsular opacification may be reduced
Intraocular lens may be easier to explant, if necessary

Generation VI (Modern Capsular Lenses—Rigid PMMA, Soft Foldable, and Modern Anterior Chamber)

By the end of the 1980s clinical laboratory studies demonstrated clearly that cataract surgical techniques and IOL design and manufacture had shown remarkable advances.[36–40] Surgical technique and IOL design and manufacture had advanced to a point at which the older techniques gave way to more modern ones that allowed consistent, secure, and permanent in-the-bag (capsular) fixation of the pseudophakos. A marriage between IOL design and improved surgical techniques has evolved into capsular surgery. The "capsular" IOLs are fabricated from both rigid and soft biomaterials.

The many changes in surgical techniques that occurred after 1980 and into the 1990s include the introduction of OVDs,[40–43] increased awareness of the advantages of in-the-bag fixation, the introduction of continuous curvilinear capsulorrhexis (CCC)[44–51] (Fig. 40-7), hydrodissection[52] (Fig. 40-8), and the increased use of phacoemulsification. This has allowed not only much safer surgery but also implantation through a smaller incision than was possible in the early days of extracapsular extraction.

The evolution from can opener toward capsulorrhexis (see Fig. 40-7) was initiated by Binkhorst, who developed a two-step (envelope) technique that eventually evolved into the single-step CCC. Two clear advantages of CCC exist over the early can-opener techniques. First, the formation of radial tears (Fig. 40-9) is reduced,[47] which minimizes radial tears of the anterior capsule; these reduce the stability of the capsular bag and may allow prolapse of haptics out of the capsular bag through the anterior capsular tear. Second, and less commonly recognized, capsulorrhexis provides a stable capsular bag that allows copious hydrodissection, which in turn is very helpful in cortical cleanup. With a frayed, emptier capsular edge, such as seen with the can-opener technique, hydrodissection is difficult without forming unwanted radial tears.

Hydrodissection (see Fig. 40-8) was a termed coined by Faust[52] in 1984. This technique, and the many variations thereof (e.g., cortical cleavage hydrodissection, hydrodelineation), makes the surgery much simpler in that mobilization and removal of cells and cortical material are rendered much easier. The long-term risk of PCO is, in turn, clearly minimized because of the more thorough removal of cells in cortical material, especially in the region of the equatorial fornix.

Modern phacoemulsification, pioneered by Charles Kelman, has now made possible the removal of lens material through small incisions and the implantation of IOLs through incisions down to 3mm in length, as opposed to incisions of 11–12mm length in the early days of ECCE. Many real advantages of small-incision cataract surgery exist, including safer healing (with fewer risks of complications such as inflammation), more rapid healing, and rapid recovery of visual rehabilitation (with less postoperative astigmatism).

In accompaniment with the developments of surgical techniques that allow secure in-the-bag implantation, IOLs have evolved that work well with these techniques—both rigid PMMA designs (Figs. 40-10 and 40-11) and foldable IOLs.[53] Figure 40-10 shows an example of a modern, state-of-the-art, one-piece, all-PMMA IOL that is designed for in-the-bag implantation. These can be inserted through incisions as small as 5.5–6mm in length and provide an excellent alternative for the surgeon who finds the almost 50-year history of PMMA as a lens biomaterial of comfort. Long-term results with these IOLs are excellent and, indeed, these lenses provide slightly better centration than do some of the more modern foldable lenses at the present time. The ideal diameter for a one-piece IOL design such as that in Figure 40-10 is 12–12.5mm, which allows it to fit perfectly into the capsular bag (which measures about 10.5mm in diameter). The diameter of the ciliary sulcus is only slightly larger (approximately 11.0mm)[53] and actually decreases with age.

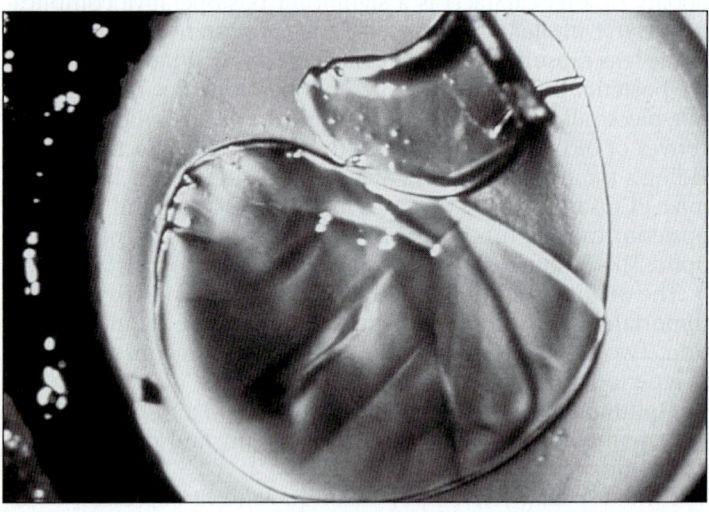

FIG. 40-7 ▓ Surgeon's view (cornea and iris removed) of a porcine eye showing the capsulorrhexis procedure. Notice the smooth edges of the anterior capsular tear, which is the key feature of this procedure.

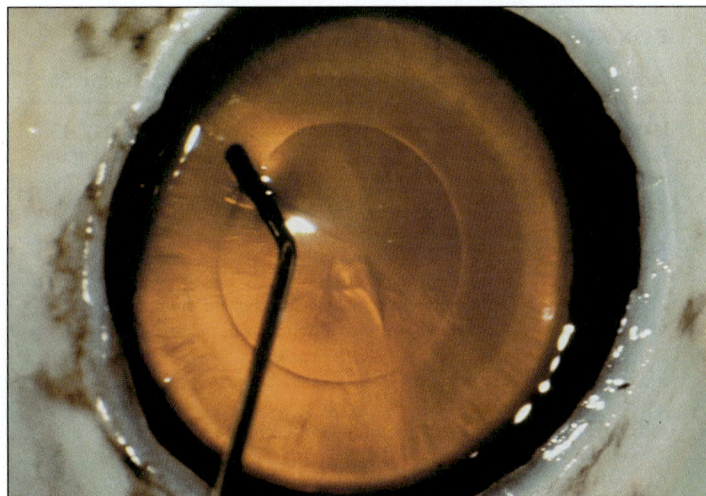

FIG. 40-8 ▓ Surgeon's view (cornea and iris removed) of a human eye (obtained postmortem) showing experimental hydrodissection. In this case the cannula is placed immediately under the anterior capsule (cortical cleavage hydrodissection). Hydrodissection is one of the most important maneuvers to help reduce the incidence of posterior capsular opacification.

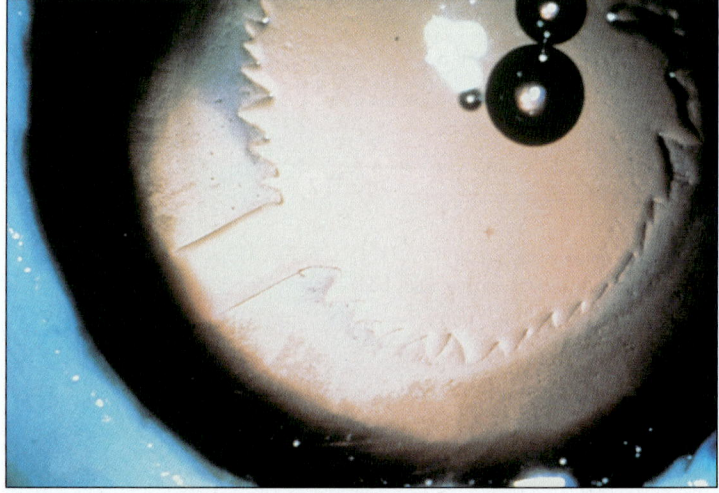

FIG. 40-9 ▓ Surgeon's view of an experimentally performed can-opener capsulectomy, with typical radial tears to the equator of the anterior capsule. The cornea and iris are removed from a human eye, obtained postmortem. Following clinical can-opener anterior capsulectomy, one to five radial tears invariably occur. (Reproduced with permission from Assia EI, Apple DJ, Tsai JC, Lim ES. The elastic properties of the lens capsule in capsulorrhexis. Am J Ophthalmol. 1991;111:628–32.)

These rigid PMMA IOL designs have been found to be very satisfactory in pediatric IOL implantation.[54,55] As 90% of the growth of the infantile globe occurs during the first 18 months to 2 years (Fig. 40-12), it is fair to assume that "adult" 12mm lenses can be safely implanted in children this age and older, with the achievement of good results (Figs. 40-12 and 40-13). The problem in the past with IOL implantation has been that of PCO. With present techniques, this is best prevented using primary posterior capsulectomy.

Improved small-incision surgical techniques and IOL designs have resulted in a natural evolution toward foldable lenses.[56-67] Most foldable lenses today are manufactured from silicone, hydrogel, or acrylic material (Figs. 40-14 to 40-16).

The earliest designs for which clinical usage was widespread were the plate lenses known as the "Mazzocco taco." In early years these were manufactured poorly and often not implanted properly into the capsular bag, so many complications ensued. In recent years manufacturing quality has become much better, and these lenses are now satisfactory for clinical usage (Figs. 40-17 and 40-18). The best plate lenses are those with large positioning holes that allow in-the-bag synechia formation, which enhances fixation and stability.[64]

The most commonly implanted designs at present are three-piece lenses that consist of silicone, acrylic, or hydrogel optics. Plate lenses continue to provide excellent results. These lenses can be implanted through incisions smaller than 5mm in length, and visual rehabilitation is now incredibly fast with various further modifications, such as clear corneal incisions and topical anesthesia. Such surgery is virtually analogous to arthroscopy of the eye.

Lens design and manufacture have improved to such an extent that perhaps the most important factor in the achievement of a successful result is not the IOL itself but the quality of surgery. These factors are very important now that there are high

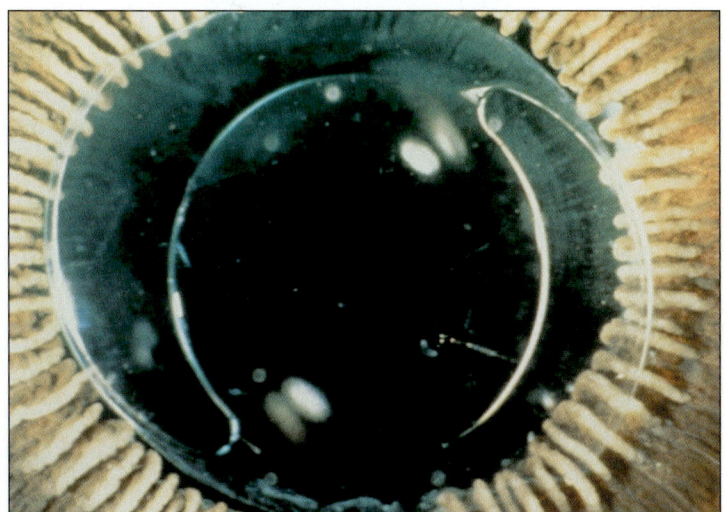

FIG. 40-10 ▥ A modern, one-piece, all-PMMA, capsular IOL implanted experimentally in a human eye: posterior view (Miyake technique) of the eye (obtained postmortem). Note the excellent centration and a perfect fit within the capsular bag.

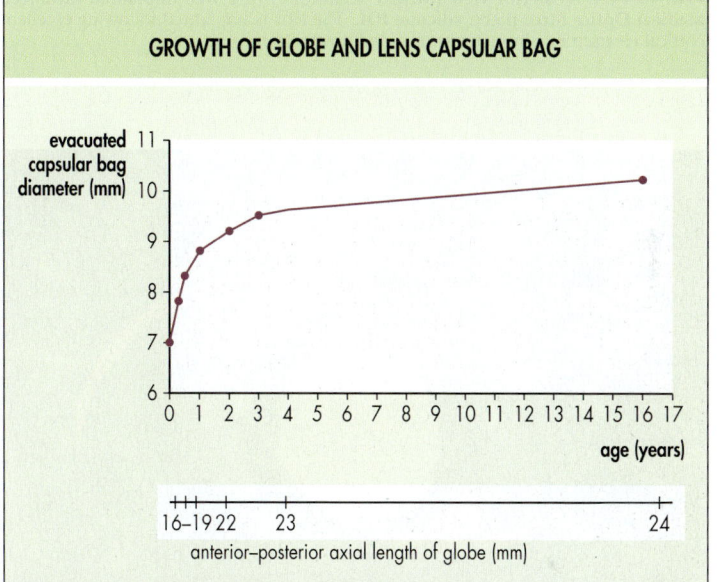

FIG. 40-12 ▥ **Growth of the globe and lens capsular bag.** These results are based on a study of 50 eyes obtained postmortem and demonstrate that the growth of the globe and lens capsular bag occurs relatively rapidly during the first 18 months to 2 years. (Reproduced with permission from Wilson ME, Apple DJ, Bluestein EC, Wang XH. Intraocular lenses for pediatric implantation: biomaterials, designs, and sizing. J Cataract Refract Surg. 1994;20:584–91.)

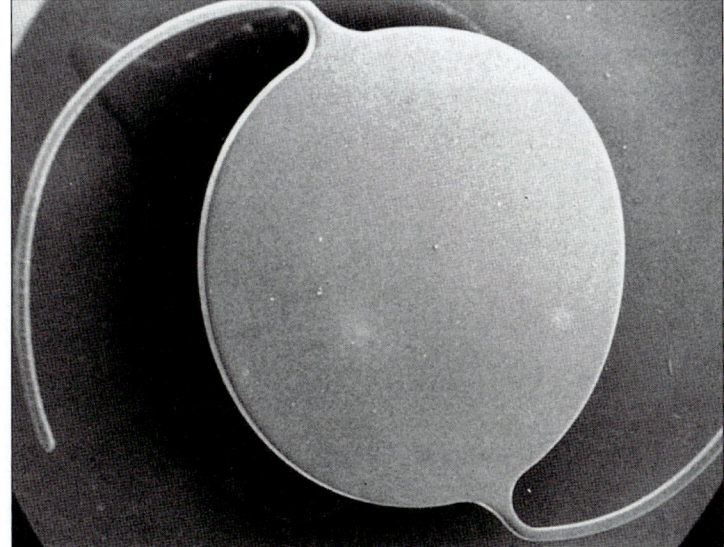

FIG. 40-11 ▥ Scanning electron micrograph of a well-designed, tumble-polished, modified C-loop, one-piece, all-PMMA posterior chamber IOL. The total length of this capsular IOL design is 12.0mm. Note the excellent, smooth finish of this well-polished IOL. (Original magnification ×10.)

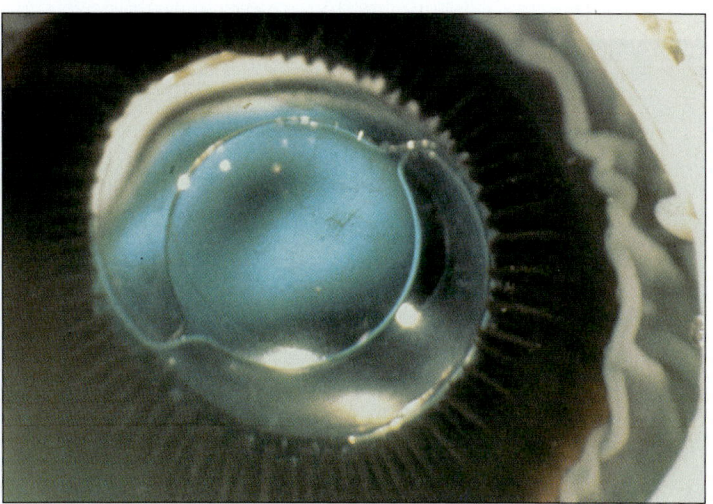

FIG. 40-13 ▥ Posterior view (Miyake technique) of an eye of a 2-year-old child (obtained postmortem). This was implanted experimentally with a 12mm, one-piece, all-PMMA IOL in the capsular bag. Note the excellent fit in the capsular bag. (Reproduced with permission from Wilson ME, Apple DJ, Bluestein EC, Wang XH. Intraocular lenses for pediatric implantation: biomaterials, designs, and sizing. J Cataract Refract Surg. 1994;20:584–91.)

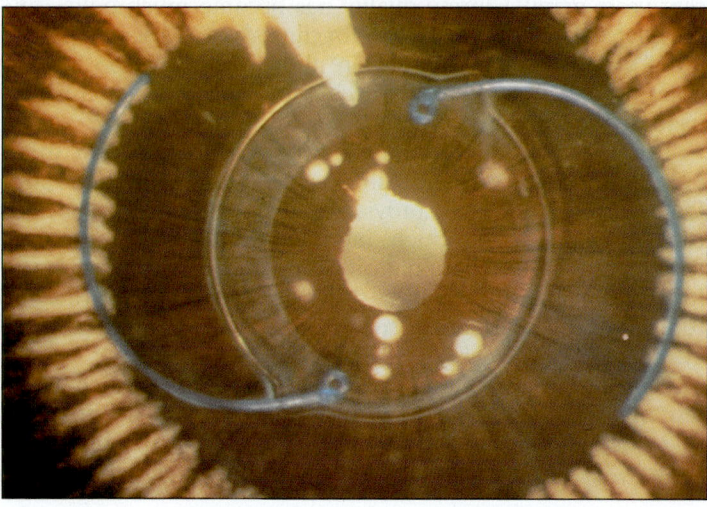

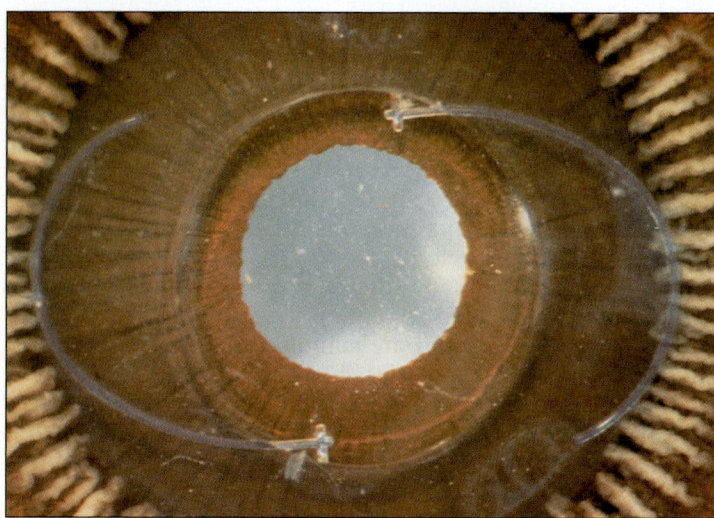

FIG. 40-14 ▮▮ Posterior view (Miyake technique) of a well-implanted Advanced Medical Optics three-piece, silicone IOL. The lens is implanted following excellent cortical cleanup in a human eye obtained postmortem.

FIG. 40-15 ▮▮ Posterior view (Miyake technique) of a well-implanted Alcon AcrySof acrylic IOL. The lens is well centered in the capsular bag after thorough cortical removal.

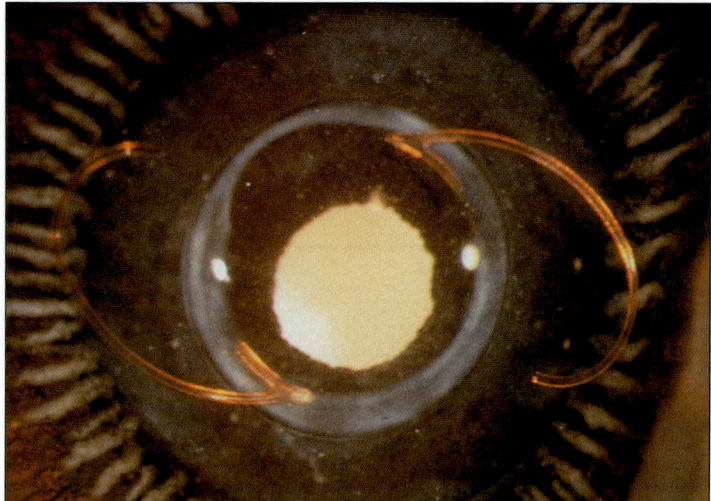

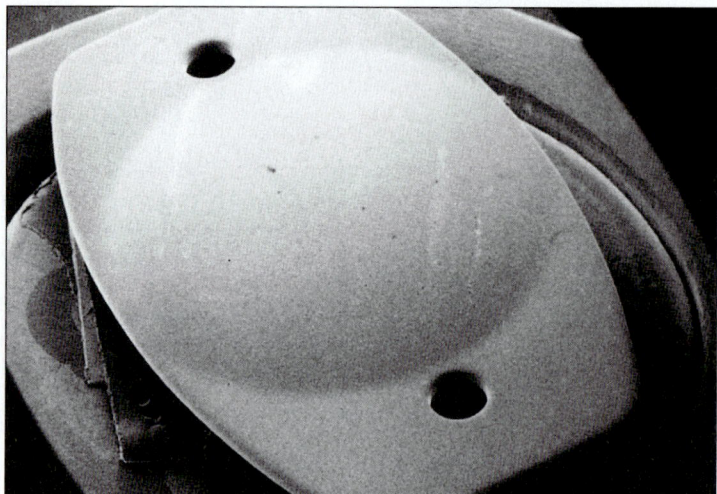

FIG. 40-16 ▮▮ A STAAR Surgical Corporation three-piece IOL with polyimide haptics: posterior view (Miyake technique) of an eye (obtained postmortem). The lens is well centered and positioned in a clean capsular bag.

FIG. 40-17 ▮▮ Scanning electron micrograph that shows the marked improvement in plate lens manufacture by the 1990s. Note the excellent overall design and manufacture finish. (Original magnification ×10.)

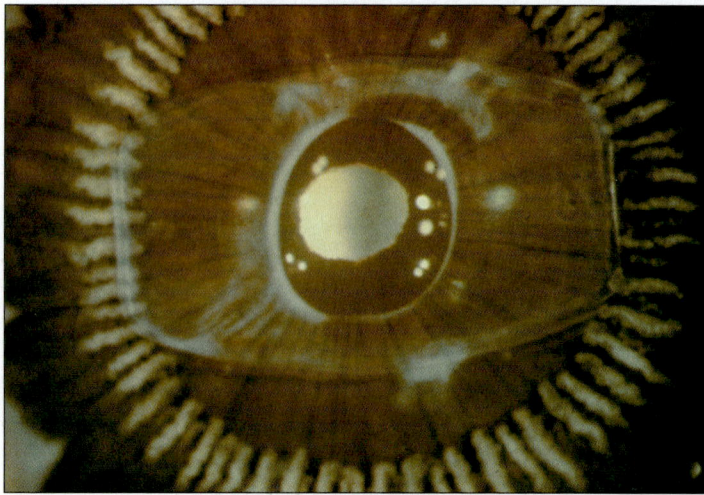

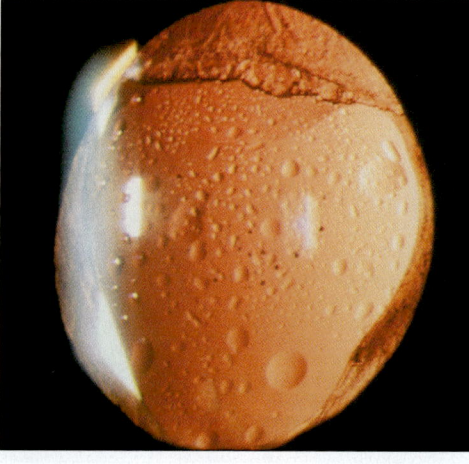

FIG. 40-19 ▮▮ View of a patient who has silicone IOL and who later required vitreoretinal surgery with silicone oil. Note the dense bubbles that cover the optic surface, which impair both vision and the surgeon's view into the eye.

FIG. 40-18 ▮▮ A well-implanted STAAR-Chiron style silicone plate IOL, with excellent cortical removal and centration. Posterior view (Miyake technique) of the eye (obtained postmortem).

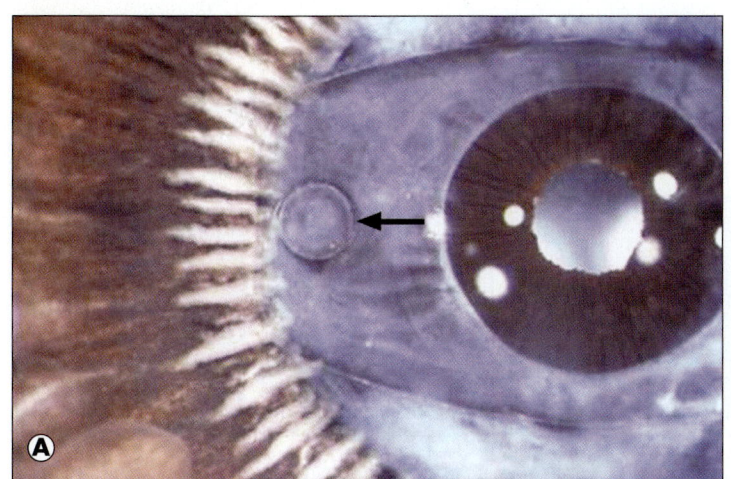

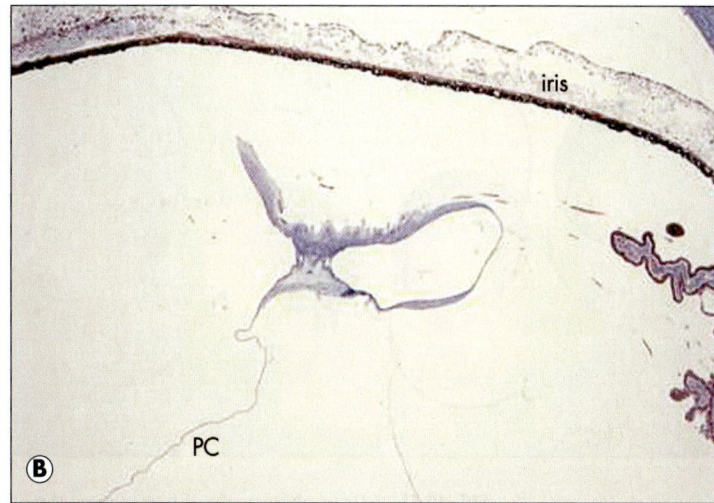

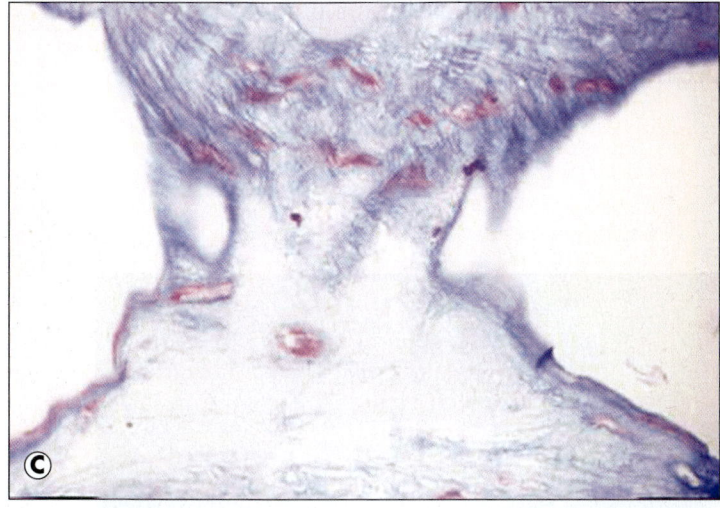

FIG. 40-20 ■ Gross and light microscopic photographs of a pseudophakic human eye obtained postmortem, implanted with a silicone plate lens, with large fenestrations. **A,** Miyake-Apple posterior photographic technique. The arrow indicates the fibrotic tissue growing through one of the large fenestrations. **B** and **C,** Fusion between anterior and posterior capsules promoted by the fibrocellular tissue growing through the fenestration (Masson's trichrome; original magnification ×100 and ×400, respectively). *PC,* Posterior capsule.

standards for results following IOL implantation, especially in this era when IOL implantation is considered not only a means of optical rehabilitation after cataract removal but also a bona fide refractive procedure. The development of bi- and multifocal IOL designs is one example of this evolutionary process. An increased interest in clear lens extraction for myopia and the use of phakic IOLs also exemplifies the evolution toward refractive IOLs. It is of utmost importance to achieve symmetrical capsular-bag fixation and good cortical cleanup to minimize the chance for complications, such as lens decentration and formation of a Soemmering ring.

The development of foldable lenses is one of fine tuning. For example, much effort is now being expended to develop ever more tissue-friendly optic biomaterials. Figure 40-19 reveals a complication that may occur occasionally in patients who have silicone lenses and who require subsequent vitreoretinal surgery using silicone oil.[68] Work is under way to address this complication by modifications of the biomaterial to change factors such as its surface characteristics.[69] Work is also in progress on the attachment of different styles of haptic materials to the optic to achieve better and more stable fixation of the haptics in the capsular bag.

Note that the various ultramodern designs of anterior chamber lenses developed for both aphakic and phakic implantations are considered to belong to generation VI. These include the various Kelman-Choyce designs and modifications by Baikoff and Clemente (see Fig. 40-4). These are categorized here to separate them from the myriad of generally inferior anterior chamber IOLs that were available in the earlier intermediate period between 1963 and 1990 (generation IV). The ultramodern designs are suitable for specific clinical indications and clearly should not be included in the generic concept that "all anterior chamber IOLs are bad."

RECENT ADVANCES

Our line of research at the Center for Research on Ocular Therapeutics and Biodevices, now transferred to the Moran Eye Center in Salt Lake City, Utah and renamed as the David J Apple MD Laboratories for Ophthalmic Devices Research, allows us to be in close contact not only with surgeons worldwide but also with virtually all companies manufacturing IOLs and related devices. One of the best means of discerning manufacturers' trends is to determine where they are investing energy and funds for the future. On the basis of our contacts and relationships with industry and after a close review of the available scientific literature, we have noted some general principles and tendencies with regard to the development of new foldable IOLs. Focusing on IOLs manufactured in the United States, we have identified seven selected innovative directions. Listed in appropriate chronological order of their introduction, they are as follows:

1. Large fixation holes or foramina have been incorporated in the haptic components of one-piece plate designs (Fig. 40-20, A). Fibrous adhesions often occur between the anterior and posterior capsules following ingrowth of fibrocellular tissue through the holes (Fig. 40-20, B and C). This helps enhance the fixation and stability of these designs within the capsular bag.[70-72] It is important to note that this fibrous growth requires at least 2 weeks and often much more to establish itself and help anchor the IOL. This design feature has been incorporated into lenses manufactured from silicone (including the Staar toric IOL), hydrogel (hydrophilic acrylic IOLs) and Collamer (Staar CC4203VF) materials.

2. For three-piece foldable designs, the preferred haptic materials are the relatively rigid materials with good material memory, such as PMMA, polyimide (Elastimide), or polyvinylidene fluoride (PVDF)[73,74] (Fig. 40-21). Examples of major

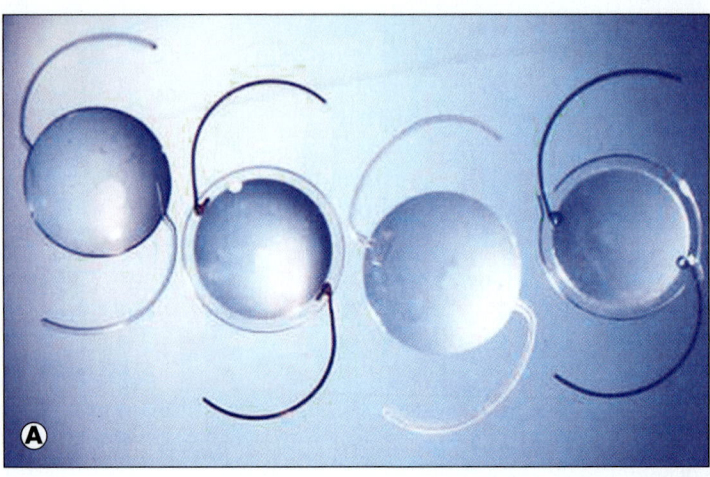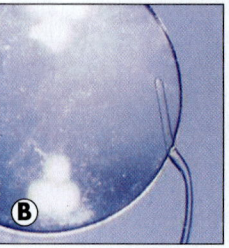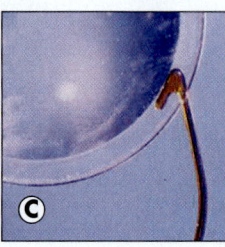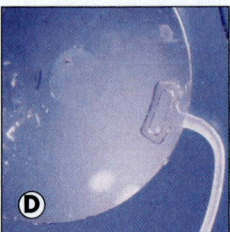

FIG. 40-21 ■ Gross photographs of four modern three-piece silicone lenses with different haptic materials. **A,** From left to right: PMMA (CeeOn 912, Pharmacia Inc., Peapack, NJ), Elastimide (AQ-2003, Staar Surgical, Inc., Monrovia, CA), polyvinylidene fluoride (PVDF) (CeeOn Edge 911, Pharmacia Inc.), and Prolene (SI-30 NB, AMO, Irvine, CA). **B–D,** Details of the optic-haptic junctions of the lenses having loops manufactured from relatively rigid materials (PMMA, Elastimide, and PVDF, respectively). (Reproduced from Izak AM, Werner L, Apple DJ, *et al.* Loop memory of different haptic materials used in the manufacture of posterior chamber intraocular lenses. J Cataract Refract Surg. 2002;28:1229–35.)

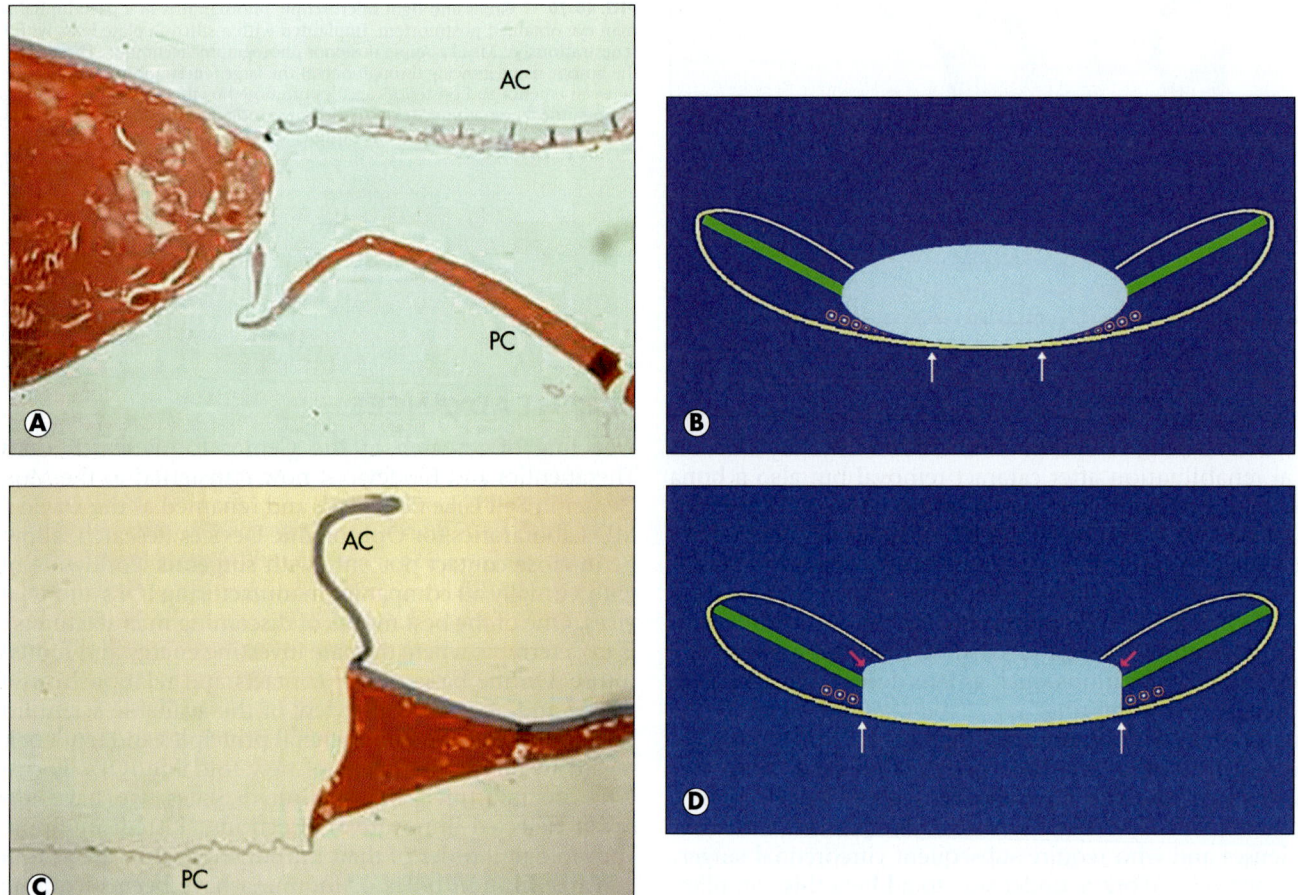

FIG. 40-22 ■ Light photomicrographs and schematic illustrations showing the subtle differences regarding the barrier effect of an IOL optic with a rounded edge versus a square truncated edge. **A,** Photomicrograph of the site of implantation of an IOL optic with a rounded edge. Note the large Soemmering ring on the left (red stain). Note also the migration of cortical material (red material) onto the posterior peripheral surface of the lens optic, a phenomenon that sometimes occurs with a rounded edge. Rarely does such growth extend onto the central visual axis (Masson's trichrome; original magnification ×100). **B,** Round edge: some cells may squeeze behind the posterior peripheral aspect of the optic, creating a paracentral rim of opacification *(arrows)* but usually sparing the visual axis. **C,** Photomicrograph of a case in which the Soemmering ring (red) remains totally confined to the right of the square optic edge, leaving the posterior capsule (lower left) cell-free (Masson's trichrome; original magnification ×50). **D,** Square truncated optic edge seems to provide an abrupt barrier *(arrows)*, leaving the entire optical zone free of cells. *AC,* Anterior capsule; *PC,* posterior capsule. (*A, B,* and *D,* Reproduced from Peng Q, Visessook N, Apple DJ, *et al.* Surgical prevention of posterior capsule opacification. Part III. Intraocular lens optic barrier effect as a second line of defense. J Cataract Refract Surg. 2000;26:198–213. *C,* Reproduced from Werner L, Apple DJ, Pandey SK. Postoperative proliferation on anterior and equatorial lens epithelial cells. In: Buratto L, Werner L, Zanini M, Apple DJ, eds. Phacoemulsification: principles and techniques. Thorofare, NJ: 2002, Slack; 603–23.)

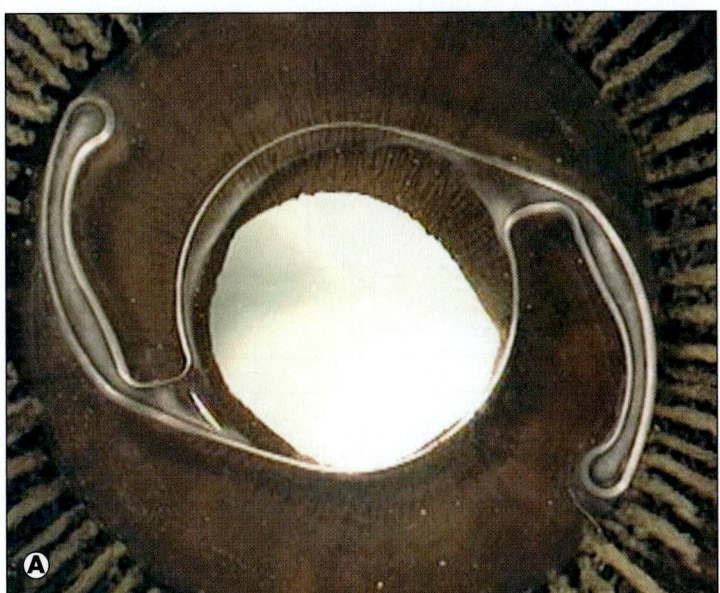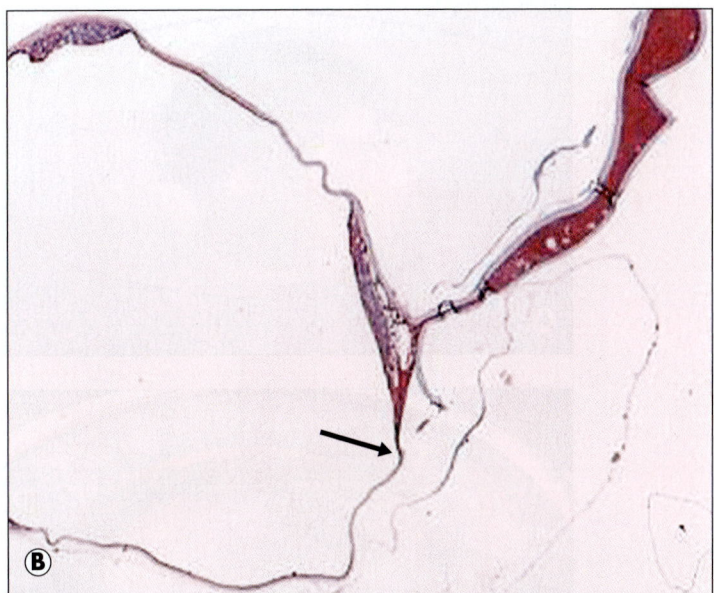

FIG. 40-23 ▮▮ Gross and light microscopy photographs of the first human eye obtained postmortem with a single-piece AcrySof lens (Alcon Laboratories, Forth Worth, TX) accessioned in our center. **A,** The lens is well centered and the capsular bag is clear. **B,** Light photomicrograph of a histological section from the same eye. The arrow indicates the imprint of the square edge of the lens optic on the capsular bag, causing a barrier effect that prevented retained/regenerative cortical material from the Soemmering ring to migrate onto the posterior capsule, opacifying the visual axis (Masson's trichrome; original magnification ×400). (Reproduced from Escobar-Gomez M, Apple DJ, Vargas LG, *et al.* Scanning electron microscopic and histologic evaluation of the AcrySof SA30AL acrylic intraocular lens. J Cataract Refract Surg. 2003;29[1]:164–69.)

designs of such lenses on the American market include the Advanced Medical Optics (AMO) SI40 NB with PMMA haptics, the Bausch & Lomb SoFlex C31UB and the Staar AQ-1016 with polyimide haptics, and the Pharmacia CeeOn Edge 911 with PVDF haptics. These haptics have appropriate memory characteristics that help enhance lens centration and stability and provide better resistance to postoperative contraction forces within the capsular bag.

3. One of the most important features that have been incorporated in new foldable lenses in terms of decreasing the incidence of PCO is the square, truncated optic edge. Various experimental animal studies by Nishi in Japan, analyses of human autopsy globes in our laboratory by Apple and associates, as well as several clinical studies with the three-piece AcrySof lens (MA30BA and MA60BM), the first design identified with this geometric characteristic, demonstrated an enhanced barrier effect against cell migration/proliferation on the posterior capsule toward the visual axis.[75-87] This IOL design feature has also been incorporated in other lenses such as the AMO Sensar IOL with the new OptiEdge optic configuration, a square posterior optic edge and a rounded anterior optic edge. Lenses manufactured from other materials, such as silicone (Pharmacia CeeOn Edge 911) and hydrophilic materials (Rayner Centerflex and the Ciba Vision MemoryLens), now present this design feature. The Bausch & Lomb Hydroview foldable hydrogel IOL does not yet have the truncated square optic edge technology, but the manufacturer is working to introduce it on updated models (Fig. 40-22).

4. Manufacturers have invested heavily and with great success in single-piece designs, all fabricated from the same material as the optic component. The Alcon (SA30AL and SA60AT) AcrySof IOL is a hydrophobic single-piece acrylic design that has provided excellent results (Fig. 40-23).

5. Manufacturers are also investing in the development of injector systems to be used with the new lens designs.

6. Perhaps the most energy and funding are being spent on new and complex IOLs that not only restore the refractive power of the eye after cataract surgery but also provide special features, including multifocality, toric corrections (Fig. 40-24, A), pseudoaccommodation (Fig. 40-24, B–C), postoperative adjustment of the IOL refractive power, and image magnifi-

cation (telescopic lenses) (Fig. 40-24, D).[88-91] Itemization of these IOL designs is not yet useful because proof of safety and efficacy is still in great flux.

With any IOL, the issue of "biocompatibility" must be assessed. Not only do surgeons today seem to be seeking IOLs that are easy to insert/inject through small incisions—perhaps the main factor influencing manufacturers' IOL development—but also more attention is being paid to the interaction of each IOL design within the surrounding capsular bag. Issues such as postoperative cell proliferation within the capsular bag, including PCO (Fig. 40-25), anterior capsule opacification (ACO) (Fig. 40-26), and interlenticular opacification (ILO) (Fig. 40-27) with piggyback IOLs, are used as one indication of lens biocompatibility.[92-99] This goes far beyond the normal postoperative inflammatory reaction observed after cataract surgery with IOL implantation. Different studies from our laboratory demonstrated that the choice of IOL design and material can largely influence the outcome of these complications, but the role of surgical techniques should not be underestimated. Last but not least, a "perfect" IOL would not be effective in preventing excess cell proliferation within the capsular bag after bad surgery.

7. The renewed interest in phakic IOLs, which we now realize can potentially correct any refractive error, is also progressing rapidly, and itemization of special IOL models as being those of choice is not yet possible. In our opinion, it is somewhat ironic that anterior chamber IOLs, previously relegated by many surgeons to a wastebasket of discarded devices, are now being resurrected and researched by both major and start-up manufacturers as a possible lens of choice for refractive correction.[100-102] Lenses designed for iris fixation and placement in the posterior chamber are also being studied, with good results to date. There is a trend for the use of foldable materials for these phakic lenses, designed to be inserted through small incisions (Figs. 40-28 and 40-29).

Although a large spectrum of lenses is available today, the IOL of choice still depends on a surgeon's personal preference based on multiple factors personalized to each individual, largely influenced by different features unique to each patient, such as the patient's history and clinical status, but also by the occurrence of intraoperative complications.

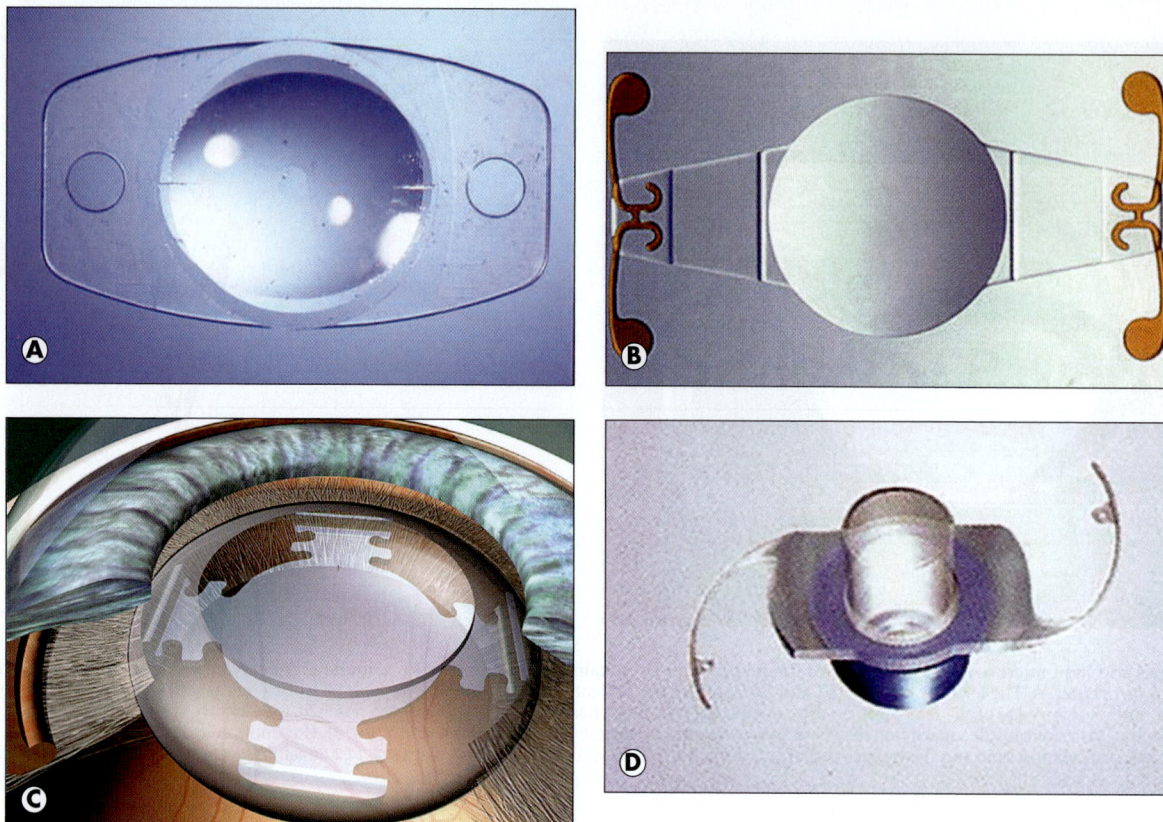

FIG. 40-24 ■ Special intraocular lenses. **A,** Gross photograph of a toric lens (AA-4203TF or AA-4203TL Staar Surgical, Inc.). This lens has basically the same design as single-piece, plate silicone posterior chamber lenses with large fenestrations but with an incorporated cylindrical correction. **B** and **C,** Schematic drawings representing two accommodative lenses, the AT-45 lens, manufactured by C&C Vision (Irvine, CA), and the AKKOMMODATIVE 1 CU, manufactured by HumanOptics (Erlangen, Germany), respectively. The first is essentially a plate haptic lens with Elastimide haptics. It is stated that redistribution of the ciliary body mass during effort for accommodation will result in increased vitreous pressure, which will move the optic of this lens anteriorly within the visual axis, creating a more plus powered lens. The second is a one-piece lens, manufactured from a hydrophilic acrylic material. It is stated that the special mechanical properties of this lens also enable it to change power during the contraction of the ciliary muscle. **D,** Schematic drawing representing the implantable miniaturized telescope (IMT) (VisionCare Ophthalmic Technologies Inc., Yehud, Israel). This is the only intraocular device available that is designed specifically to improve vision of patients suffering from age-related macular degeneration. The IMT is composed of two parts, an optical cylinder and a carrying device. The optic cylinder is made of pure glass. The carrying device is made of black PMMA. The latter has a general configuration of a posterior chamber intraocular lens, with two modified C-loops or haptics that hold the device in the capsular bag. Once in place, the anterior part of the optic extends anteriorly for approximately 1mm through the pupil. It is designed to be stabilized approximately 2mm posterior to the corneal endothelium. (**A–D,** Reproduced from Werner L, Apple DJ, Schmidbauer JM. Ideal IOL (PMMA and Foldable) for year 2002. In: Buratto L, Werner L, Zanini M, Apple DJ, eds. Phacoemulsification: principles and techniques. Thorofare, NJ: 2002, Slack; 435–52.)

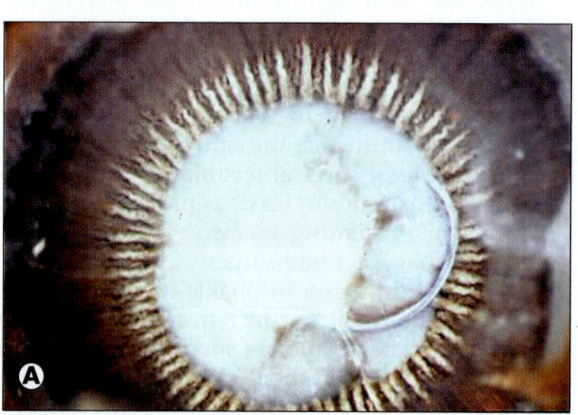

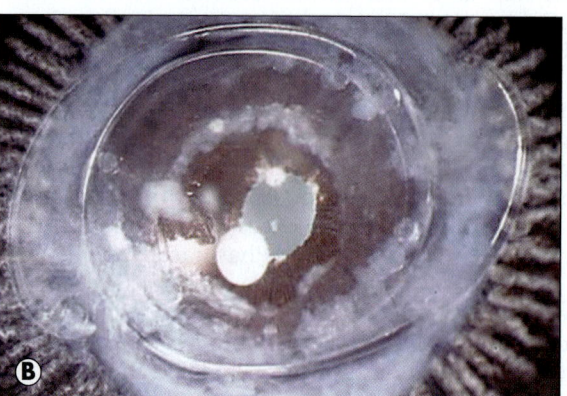

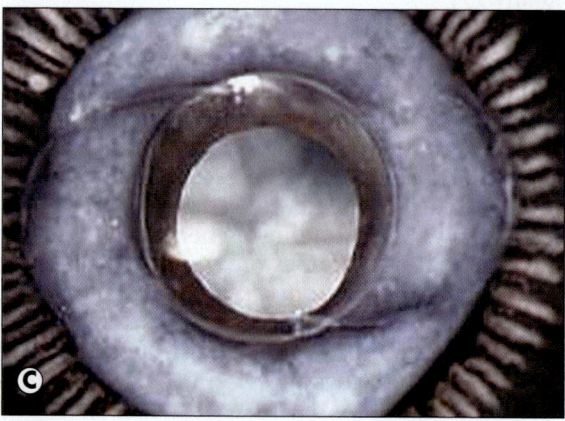

FIG. 40-25 ■ **Gross photographs from pseudophakic human eyes obtained postmortem showing different examples of posterior capsule opacification. A,** The eye was implanted with a rigid three-piece PMMA lens, which presents asymmetrical fixation (bag-sulcus). Massive opacification of the capsular bag can be observed. **B,** Eye implanted with a one-piece PMMA lens, presenting an important Soemmering ring formation and posterior capsule opacification, which required Nd:YAG laser posterior capsulotomy. Note the proliferation of Elschnig pearls around the orifice of the posterior capsulotomy. **C,** Eye implanted with a three-piece AcrySof lens. Although there is a significant Soemmering ring formation, the square edge of the lens prevented the retained/regenerative material from opacifying the visual axis. (**A,** Reproduced from Apple DJ, Solomon KD, Tetz MR, et al. Posterior capsule opacification. Surv Ophthalmol. 1992;37:73–116. **B,** Reproduced from Apple DJ. Influence of intraocular lens material and design on postoperative intracapsular cellular reactivity. Trans Am Ophthalmol Soc. 2000;98:257–83.)

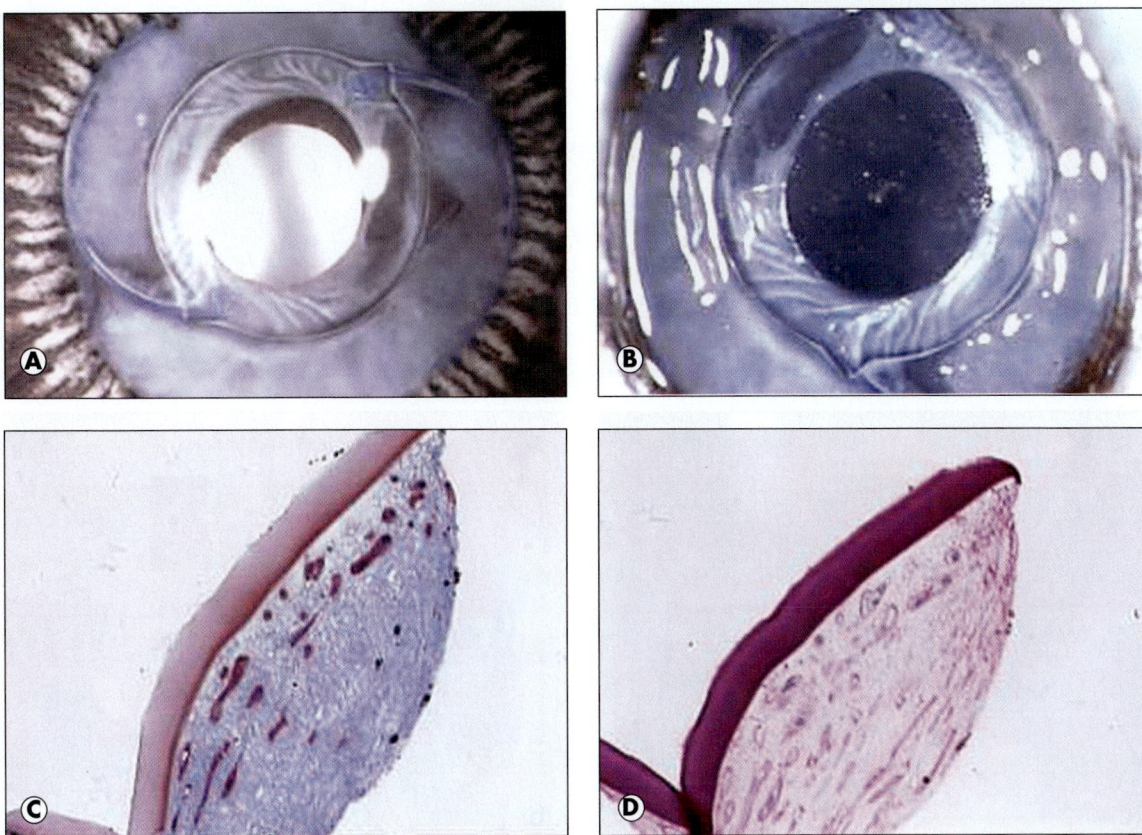

FIG. 40-26 ▮ **Gross and light microscopic photographs of a pseudophakic human eye obtained postmortem implanted with a three-piece silicone lens (SI-30 NB; AMO).** A and B, Opacification of the anterior capsule covering the lens optic from a posterior or Miyake-Apple view and from an anterior or surgeon's view, respectively. C and D, Histological sections from the same eye showing the fibrocellular tissue attached to the inner surface of the anterior capsule at the capsulorrhexis edge (Masson's trichrome and PAS stains, respectively; original magnification ×400). (A, Reproduced from Werner L, Apple DJ, Pandey SK. Postoperative proliferation of anterior and equatorial lens epithelial cells. In: Buratto L, Werner L, Zanini M, Apple DJ, eds. Phacoemulsification: principles and techniques. Thorofare, NJ: 2002, Slack; 603–23.)

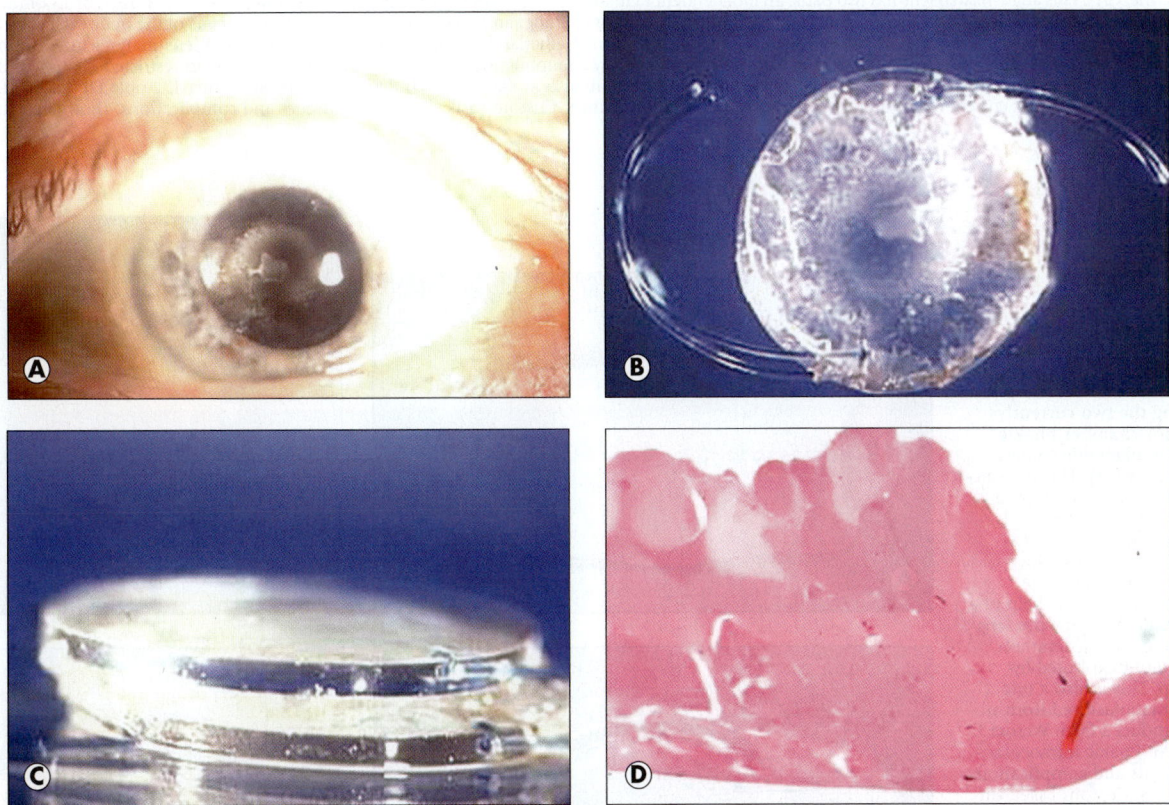

FIG. 40-27 ▮ **Clinical, gross and light microscopic photographs from a case of interlenticular opacification between two acrylic piggyback lenses implanted in a patient with high hyperopia** (case of Dr Johnny L. Gayton, Warner Robins, GA). The opacity observed (A) was caused by a membrane-like material sandwiched between the two lenses, which are practically fused together in the center (B and C). Histological examination demonstrated the presence of retained/regenerative cortical material and pearls (D), similar to what is observed in cases of posterior capsule opacification (hematoxylin and eosin stain; original magnification ×400). (A–D, Reproduced from Gayton JL, Apple DJ, Peng Q, et al. Interlenticular opacification: clinicopathological correlation of a complication of posterior chamber piggyback intraocular lenses. J Cataract Refract Surg. 2000;26:330–36.)

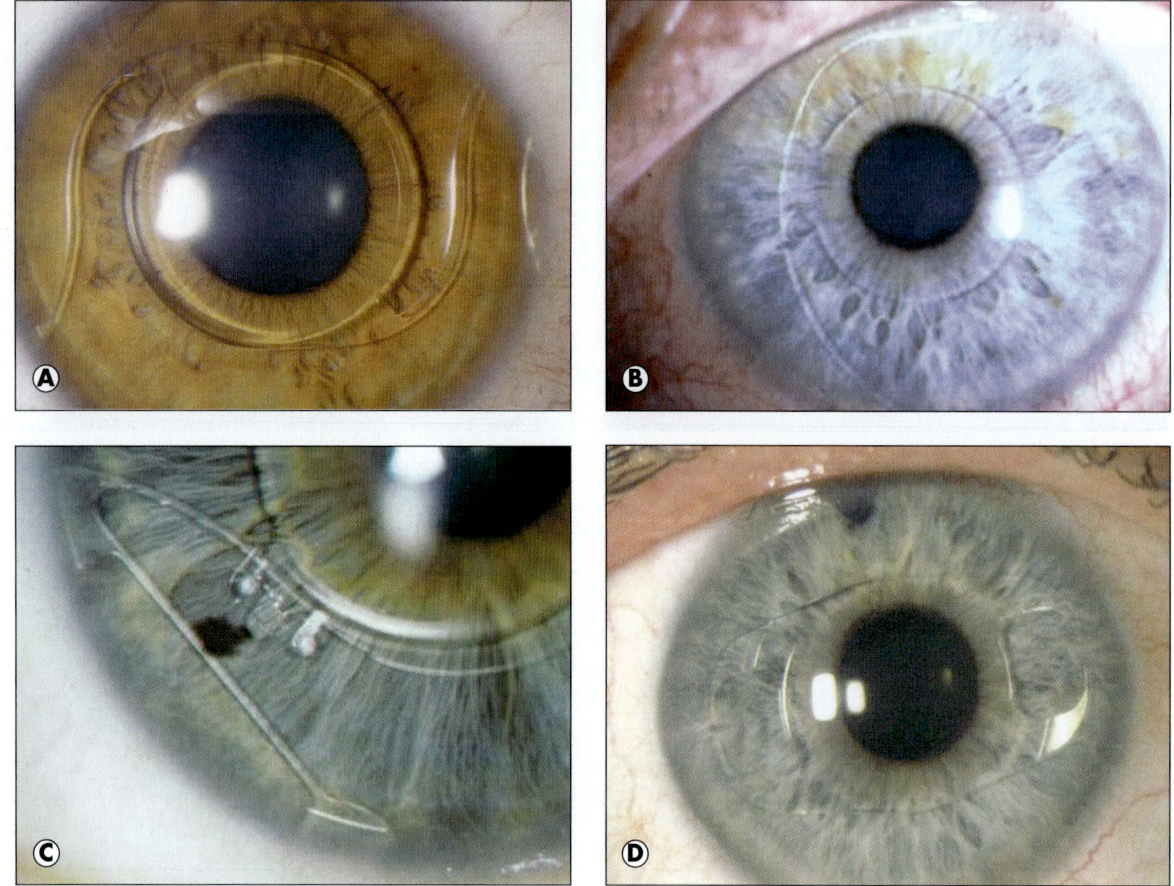

FIG. 40-28 ■ Clinical photographs of eyes implanted with different anterior chamber phakic intraocular lenses. **A,** ZSAL-4 (Morcher, Stuttgart, Germany). This is a one-piece PMMA angle-fixated lens, which has features similar to those of the ZB 5M model (Baïkoff's) concerning the haptic design and the angulation. Its optic is flat at the anterior surface and concave at the posterior surface. This allows more distance between the iris plane and the optic of the lens, also reducing the height of the optical edge, which leaves more space between it and the corneal endothelium. The lens is supplied in powers ranging from −10 to −23 diopters. It became available in Europe in January 1995. **B,** Vivarte lens, manufactured by IOLTECH (La Rochelle, France) and distributed by Ciba Vision Corp. (Duluth, GA). A manufacturing process termed selective polymerization allows the obtention of a one-piece IOL with flexible and rigid areas anywhere needed to optimize the mechanical properties of the lens. This angle-fixated lens thus has soft hydrophilic acrylic optic and footplates, while the haptics have rigidity similar to that of PMMA lenses. **C,** Kelman Duet lens, manufactured by TEKIA, Inc. (Irvine, CA). This angle-fixated lens has two parts: an independent Kelman tripod PMMA haptic, with an overall diameter of 12.0, 12.5, or 13.0mm, and a 5.5mm monofocal silicone optic. The latter is injected into the anterior chamber and then fixated to the haptic by means of the optic eyelets and haptic tabs using a Sinskey-type hook. **D,** Artisan lens (Ophtec, Groningen, Netherlands). This is a one-piece, iris-fixated lens manufactured from PMMA. Artisan haptics (fixation arms) attach to the midperipheral, virtually immobile iris stroma, thus allowing relatively unrestricted dilation and constriction of the pupil. Lenses with incorporated cylindrical correction are also available. (**A–D,** Reproduced from Werner L, Apple DJ, Izak AM. Phakic intraocular lenses: current trends and complications. In Buratto L, Brint S: Custom Lasik: surgical techniques and complications. Thorofare, NJ: 2002, Slack; 330–36.)

FIG. 40-29 ■ Gross and clinical photographs showing the two currently available posterior chamber phakic lenses. A and B, Implantable contact lens (ICL) (Staar Surgical). This is a one-piece plate lens manufactured from a proprietary hydrophilic collagen polymer know as Collamer. It can be inserted or injected into the anterior chamber, and then the haptics are placed behind the iris with the help of a spatula. C and D, Phakic refractive lens (PRL), manufactured by Medennium Inc. (Irvine, CA) and distributed by CIBA Vision Corp. This is also a one-piece plate lens, manufactured from silicone. (A–D, Reproduced from Werner L, Apple DJ, Izak AM. Phakic intraocular lenses: current trends and complications. In Buratto L, Brint S: Custom Lasik: surgical techniques and complications. Thorofare, NJ: 2002, Slack; 759–77.)

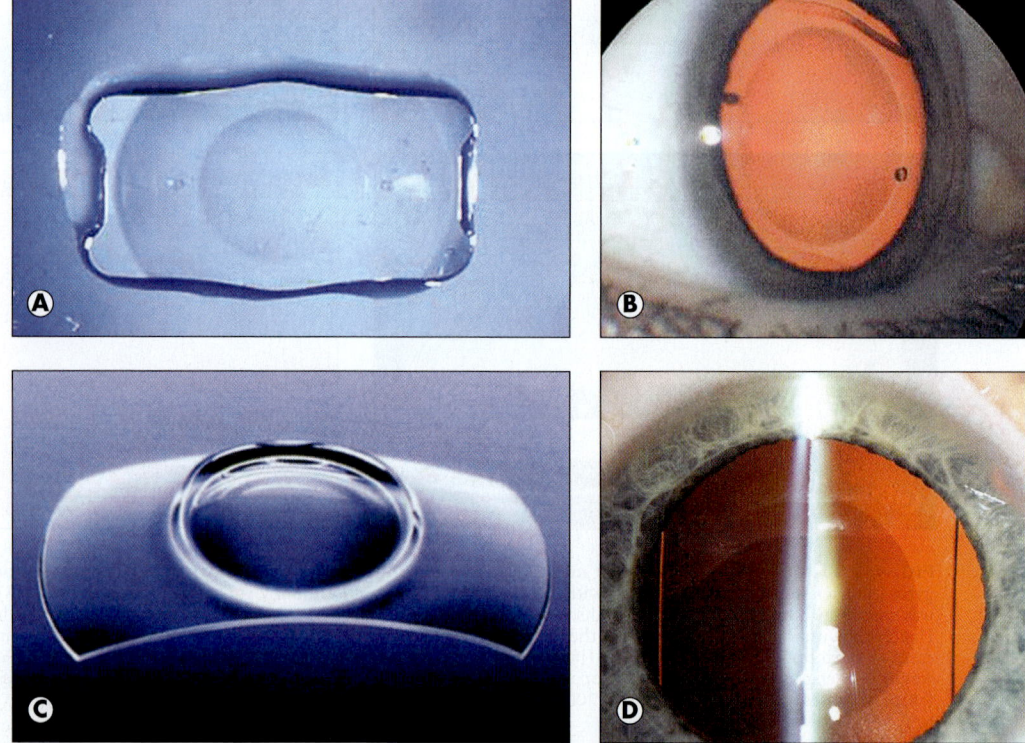

REFERENCES

1. Apple DJ, Ram J, Wang XH, Brown S. Cataract surgery in the developing world. Saudi J Ophthalmol. 1995;9(1):2–15.
2. Isaacs R, Ram J, Apple DJ. Cataract blindness in the developing world: is there a solution? J Agromed. 1996;3(4):7–21.
3. Kador PF. Overview of the current attempts toward the medical treatment of cataract. Ophthalmology. 1983;90:352–64.
4. Ridley H. Intra-ocular acrylic lenses. Trans Ophthalmol Soc UK. 1951;71:617–21.
5. Ridley H. Artificial intra-ocular lenses after cataract extraction. St Thomas Hosp Rep. 1952;7(2):12–14.
6. Apple DJ, Sims J. Harold Ridley and the invention of the intraocular lens. Surv Ophthalmol. 1995;40:279–92.
7. Apple DJ, Mamalis N, Loftfield K, et al. Complications of intraocular lenses: a historical and histopathological review. Surv Ophthalmol. 1984;29:1–54.
8. Apple DJ, Mamalis N, Brady SE, et al. Biocompatibility of implant materials: a review and scanning electron microscopic study. J Am Intraocul Implant Soc. 1984;10:53–66.
9. Apple DJ, Rabb MF. Ocular pathology: clinical applications and self-assessment, 5th ed. St Louis: CV Mosby; 1998.
10. Apple DJ, Kincaid MC, Mamalis N, Olson RJ. Intraocular lenses: evolution, designs, complications, and pathology. Baltimore: Williams & Wilkins; 1989.
11. Binkhorst CD. Lens implants (pseudophakoi) classified according to method of fixation. Br J Ophthalmol. 1967;51:772–4.
12. Binkhorst CD. About lens implantation. 2. Lens design and classification of lenses. Implant. 1985;3:11–4.
13. Ellingson FT. The uveitis-glaucoma-hyphema syndrome associated with the Mark VIII anterior chamber lens implant. J Am Intraocul Implant Soc. 1978;4:50–3.
14. Drews RC. The Barraquer experience with intraocular lenses: 20 years later. Ophthalmology. 1982;89:386–93.
15. Drews RC. Intracapsular versus extracapsular cataract extraction. In: Wilensky JT, ed. Intraocular lenses. Transactions of the University of Illinois Symposium on Intraocular Lenses. New York: Appleton-Century-Crofts; 1977.
16. Obstbaum SA, Galin MA. Cystoid macular edema and ocular inflammation: the corneo-retinal inflammatory syndrome. Trans Ophthalmol Soc UK. 1979;99:187–91.
17. Binkhorst CD. The iridocapsular (two-loop) lens and the iris-clip (four-loop) lens in pseudophakia. Trans Am Acad Ophthalmol Otolaryngol. 1973;77:589–617.
18. Choyce DP. The Mark VI, Mark VII and Mark VIII Choyce anterior chamber implants. Proc R Soc Med. 1965;58:729–31.
19. Kelman CD. Anterior chamber lens design concepts. In: Rosen ES, Haining WM, Arnott EJ, eds. Intraocular lens implantation. St Louis: CV Mosby; 1984.
20. Duffin RM, Olson RJ. Vaulting characteristics of flexible loop anterior chamber intraocular lenses. Arch Ophthalmol. 1983;101:1429–33.
21. Mamalis N, Apple DJ, Brady SE, et al. Pathological and scanning electron microscopic evaluation of the 91Z intraocular lens. J Am Intraocul Implant Soc. 1984;10:191–9.
22. Reidy JJ, Apple DJ, Googe JM, et al. An analysis of semiflexible, closed-loop anterior chamber intraocular lenses. J Am Intraocul Implant Soc. 1985;11:344–52.
23. Waring GO III. The 50-year epidemic of pseudophakic corneal edema. Arch Ophthalmol. 1989;107:657–9.
24. Apple DJ, Brems RN, Park RB, et al. Anterior chamber lenses. I. Complications and pathology and a review of designs. J Cataract Refract Surg. 1987;13:157–74.
25. Apple DJ, Hansen SO, Richards SC, et al. Anterior chamber lenses. II. A laboratory study. J Cataract Refract Surg. 1987;13:175–89.
26. Auffarth GU, Wesendahl TA, Apple DJ. Are there acceptable anterior chamber intraocular lenses for clinical use in the 1990s? An analysis of 4104 explanted anterior chamber intraocular lenses. Ophthalmology. 1994;101:1913–22.
27. Auffarth GU, Wesendahl TA, Brown SJ, Apple DJ. Update on complications of anterior chamber intraocular lenses. J Cataract Refract Surg, Special Issue: Best Papers of 1994 ASCRS Meeting. 1994:70–6.
28. Auffarth GU, Wesendahl TA, Brown SJ, Apple DJ. Update on complications of anterior chamber intraocular lenses. J Cataract Refract Surg. 1995;22:1–7.
29. Apple DJ, Price FW, Gwin T, et al. Sutured retropupillary posterior chamber intraocular lenses for exchange or secondary implantation (The Twelfth Annual Binkhorst Lecture, 1988). Ophthalmology. 1989;96:1241–7.
30. Duffey RJ, Holland EJ, Agapitos PJ, et al. Anatomic study of transsclerally sutured intraocular lens implantation. Am J Ophthalmol. 1989;108:300–9.
31. Pearce JL. Experience with 194 posterior chamber lenses in 20 months. Trans Ophthalmol Soc UK. 1977;97:258–64.
32. Drews RC. The Pearce tripod posterior chamber intraocular lens: an independent analysis of Pearce's results. J Am Intraocul Implant Soc. 1980;6:259–62.
33. Shearing SP. Evolution of the posterior chamber intraocular lenses. J Am Intraocul Implant Soc. 1984;10:343–6.
34. Apple DJ, Reidy JJ, Googe JM, et al. A comparison of ciliary sulcus and capsular bag fixation of posterior chamber intraocular lenses. J Am Intraocul Implant Soc. 1985;11:44–63.
35. Miyake K, Asakura M, Kobayashi H. Effect of intraocular lens fixation on the blood-aqueous barrier. Am J Ophthalmol. 1984;98:451–5.
36. Apple DJ, Lim ES, Morgan RC, et al. Preparation and study of human eyes obtained postmortem with the Miyake posterior photographic technique. Ophthalmology. 1990;97:810–6.
37. Assia EI, Castaneda VE, Legler UFC, et al. Studies on cataract surgery and intraocular lenses at the center for intraocular lens research. Ophthalmol Clin North Am. 1991;4:251–66.
38. Assia EI, Legler UFC, Apple DJ. The capsular bag after short- and long-term fixation of intraocular lenses. Ophthalmology. 1995;102:1151–7.
39. Apple DJ, Auffarth GU, Wesendahl TA. Pathophysiology of modern capsular surgery. In: Steinert RF, ed. Textbook of modern cataract surgery: technique, complication, and management. Philadelphia: WB Saunders; 1995.
40. Assia EI, Apple DJ, Lim ES, et al. Removal of viscoelastic materials after experimental cataract surgery in vitro. J Cataract Refract Surg. 1992;18:3–6.
41. Auffarth GU, Wesendahl TA, Solomon KD, et al. Evaluation of different removal techniques of a high viscosity viscoelastic (Healon GV). J Cataract Refract Surg, Special Issue: Best Papers of 1994 ASCRS Meeting. 1994:30–32.
42. Glasser DB, Katz HR, Boyd JE, et al. Protective effects of viscous solutions in phakoemulsification and traumatic lens implantation. Arch Ophthalmol. 1989;107:1047–51.
43. Madsen K, Stenevi U, Apple DJ, Harfstrand A. Histochemical and receptor binding studies of hyaluronic acid and hyaluronic acid binding sites on corneal endothelium. Ophthalmic Pract. 1989;7(3):1–8.
44. Neuhann T. Theorie und operationstechnik des kapsulorhexis. Klin Monatsbl Augenheilkd. 1987;190:542–5.
45. Gimbel H, Neuhann T. Development, advantages and methods of continuous circular capsulorrhexis techniques. J Cataract Refract Surg. 1990;16:31–7.
46. Assia EI, Apple DJ, Tsai JC, Lim ES. The elastic properties of the lens capsule in capsulorrhexis. Am J Ophthalmol. 1991;111:628–32.
47. Assia EI, Apple DJ, Tsai JC, et al. An experimental study comparing various anterior capsulectomy techniques. Arch Ophthalmol. 1991;109:642–7.
48. Assia EI, Apple DJ, Tsai JC, Morgan RC. Mechanism of radial tear formation and extension after anterior capsulectomy. Ophthalmology. 1991;98:432–7.
49. Wasserman D, Apple DJ, Castaneda VE, et al. Anterior capsular tears and loop fixation of posterior chamber intraocular lenses. Ophthalmology. 1991;98:425–31.
50. Assia EI, Legler UFC, Castaneda VE, et al. Clinicopathologic study of the effect of radial tears and loop fixation on intraocular lens decentration. Ophthalmology. 1993;100:153–8.
51. Auffarth GU, Wesendahl TA, Newland TJ, Apple DJ. Capsulorrhexis in the rabbit eye as a model for pediatric capsulectomy. J Cataract Refract Surg. 1994;20:188–91.
52. Faust KJ. Hydrodissection of soft nuclei. J Am Intraocul Implant Soc. 1984;10(1):75–7.
53. Ohmi S, Uenoyama K, Apple DJ. Implantation of IOLs with different diameters. Acta Soc Ophthalmol Jpn. 1992;96:1093–8.
54. Wilson ME, Apple DJ, Bluestein EC, Wang XH. Intraocular lenses for pediatric implantation: biomaterials, designs, and sizing. J Cataract Refract Surg. 1994;20:584–91.
55. Wilson ME, Wang XH, Bluestein EC, Apple DJ. Comparison of mechanized anterior capsulectomy and manual continuous capsulorrhexis in pediatric eyes. J Cataract Refract Surg. 1994;20:602–6.
56. Auffarth GU, Wilcox M, Sims JCR, et al. Analysis of 100 explanted one-piece and three-piece silicone intraocular lenses. Ophthalmology. 1995;102:1144–50.
57. Auffarth GU, Wilcox M, Sims JCR, et al. Complications of silicone intraocular lenses. J Cataract Refract Surg, Special Issue: Best Papers of 1995 ASCRS Meeting. 1995;38–41.
58. Auffarth GU, McCabe C, Wilcox M, et al. Centration and fixation of silicone intraocular lenses: an analysis of clinicopathological findings in human autopsy eyes. J Cataract Refract Surg. 1996;22:1281–5.
59. Buchen SY, Richards SC, Solomon KD, et al. Evaluation of the biocompatibility and fixation of a new silicone intraocular lens in the feline model. J Cataract Refract Surg. 1989;15:545–53.
60. Menapace R. Evaluation of 35 consecutive SI-30 phacoflex lenses with high-refractive silicone optic implanted in the capsulorrhexis bag. J Cataract Refract Surg. 1995;21:339–47.
61. Menapace R. English title: Current state of implantation of flexible intraocular lenses [in German]. Fortschr Ophthalmol. 1991;88:421–28.
62. Menapace R, Radax U, Amon M, Papapanos P. No-stitch, small incision cataract surgery with flexible intraocular lens implantation. J Cataract Refract Surg. 1994;20:534–42.
63. Tsai JC, Castaneda VE, Apple DJ, et al. Scanning electron microscopic study of modern silicone intraocular lenses. J Cataract Refract Surg. 1992;18:232–5.
64. Apple DJ, Kent DG, Peng Q, et al. Verbesserung der befestigung von silikon-schiffchenlinsen durch den gebrauch von positionierungslochern in der linsenhaptik. Proceedings of the 10th Annual Deutsche Gesellschaft fuer Intraokularlinsen Implantation Meeting, Budapest, Hungary, March 1996.
65. Percival SP, Pai V. Heparin-modified lenses for eyes at risk for breakdown of the blood-aqueous barrier during cataract surgery. J Cataract Refract Surg. 1993;19:760–5.
66. Apple DJ, Federman JL, Krolicki TJ, et al. Irreversible silicone oil adhesion to silicone intraocular lenses. A clinicopathologic analysis. Ophthalmology. 1996;103:1555–62.
67. Apple DJ, Park SB, Merkley KH, et al. Posterior chamber intraocular lenses in a series of 75 autopsy eyes. I. Loop location. J Cataract Refract Surg. 1986;12:358–62.
68. Apple DJ, Tetz M, Hunold W. Lokalisierte Endophthalmitis: Eine bisher nicht beschriebene Komplikation der extrakapsulären Kataraktextraktion. In: Jacobic KW, Schott K, Gloor B, eds. I. Kongress der Deutschen Gesellschaft für Intraokularlinsen Implantation (DGII). New York: Springer-Verlag; 1988.
69. Piest KL, Kincaid MC, Tetz MR, et al. Localized endophthalmitis: a newly described cause of the so-called toxic lens syndrome. J Cataract Refract Surg. 1987;13:498–510.
70. Kent DG, Peng Q, Isaacs RT, et al. Security of capsular fixation: small- versus large-hole plate-haptic lenses. J Cataract Refract Surg. 1997;23:1371–5.
71. Whiteside SB, Apple DJ, Peng Q, et al. Fixation elements on plate intraocular lens: large positioning holes to improve security of capsular fixation. Ophthalmology. 1998;105:837–42.
72. Kent DG, Peng Q, Isaacs RT, et al. Mini-haptics to improve capsular fixation of plate-haptic silicone intraocular lenses. J Cataract Refract Surg. 1998;24:666–71.
73. Assia EI, Legler UF, Castaneda VE, Apple DJ. Loop memory of posterior chamber intraocular lenses of various sizes, designs, and loop materials. J Cataract Refract Surg. 1992;18:541–6.
74. Izak AM, Werner L, Apple DJ, et al. Loop memory of different haptic materials used in the manufacture of posterior chamber intraocular lenses. J Cataract Refract Surg. 2002;28:1229–35.
75. Nishi O, Nishi K, Wickstrom K. Preventing lens epithelial cell migration using intraocular lenses with sharp rectangular edges. J Cataract Refract Surg. 2000;26:1543–9.
76. Apple DJ, Peng Q, Visessook N, et al. Surgical prevention of posterior capsule opacification. Part I. Progress in eliminating this complication of cataract surgery. J Cataract Refract Surg. 2000;26:180–7.
77. Peng Q, Apple DJ, Visessook N, et al. Surgical prevention of posterior capsule opacification. Part II. Enhancement of cortical clean up by focusing on hydrodissection. J Cataract Refract Surg. 2000;26:188–97.

78. Peng Q, Visessook N, Apple DJ, *et al.* Surgical prevention of posterior capsule opacification. Part III. Intraocular lens optic barrier effect as a second line of defense. J Cataract Refract Surg. 2000;26:198–213.

79. Werner L, Apple DJ, Pandey SK. Postoperative proliferation of anterior and equatorial lens epithelial cells. In: Buratto L, Osher RH, Masket S, eds. Cataract surgery in complicated cases. Thorofare, NJ: Slack; 2000:399–417.

80. Linnola RJ, Werner L, Pandey SK, *et al.* Adhesion of fibronectin, vitronectin, laminin and collagen type IV to intraocular lens materials in human autopsy eyes. Part I: histological sections. J Cataract Refract Surg. 2000;26:1792–1806.

81. Linnola RJ, Werner L, Pandey SK, *et al.* Adhesion of fibronectin, vitronectin, laminin and collagen type IV to intraocular lens materials in human autopsy eyes. Part II: explanted IOLs. J Cataract Refract Surg. 2000;26:1807–18.

82. Ram J, Pandey SK, Apple DJ, *et al.* Effect of in-the-bag intraocular lens fixation on the prevention of posterior capsule opacification. J Cataract Refract Surg. 2001;27:1039–46.

83. Apple DJ, Peng Q, Visessook N, *et al.* Eradication of posterior capsule opacification. Documentation of a marked decrease in Nd:YAG laser posterior capsulotomy rates noted in an analysis of 5416 pseudophakic human eyes obtained postmortem. Ophthalmology. 2001;108:505–18.

84. Schmidbauer JM, Vargas LG, Peng Q, *et al.* Posterior capsule opacification. Int Ophthalmol Clin. 2001;41:109–31.

85. Pandey SK, Wilson ME, Trivedi RH, *et al.* Pediatric cataract surgery and intraocular lens implantation: current techniques, complications and management. Int Ophthalmol Clin. 2001;41:175–96.

86. Pandey SK, Cochener B, Apple DJ, *et al.* Intracapsular ring sustained 5-fluorouracil delivery system for prevention of posterior capsule opacification in rabbits: a histological study. J Cataract Refract Surg. 2002;28:139–48.

87. Vargas L, Peng Q, Apple DJ, *et al.* An evaluation of three modern single-piece foldable intraocular lenses: a clinicopathological study in a rabbit model with special reference to posterior capsule opacification. J Cataract Refract Surg. 2002;28:1241–50.

88. Fine IH, Hoffman RS, Packer M. Clear-lens extraction with multifocal lens implantation. Int Ophthalmol Clin. 2001;41:113–21.

89. Avitablie T, Marano F. Multifocal intraocular lenses. Curr Opin Ophthalmol. 2001;12:12–6.

90. Kaskaloglu M, Uretmen O, Yagci A. Medium-term results of implantable miniaturized telescopes in eyes with age-related macular degeneration. J Cataract Refract Surg. 2001;27:1751–5.

91. Werner L, Kaskaloglu MM, Apple DJ, *et al.* Aqueous infiltration into an implantable miniaturized telescope. Ophthalmic Surg Lasers. 2002;33:343–8.

92. Werner L, Pandey SK, Escobar-Gomez M, *et al.* Anterior capsule opacification: a histopathological study comparing different IOL styles. Ophthalmology. 2000;107:463–71.

93. Werner L, Pandey SK, Apple DJ, *et al.* Anterior capsule opacification: correlation of pathologic findings with clinical sequelae. Ophthalmology. 2001;108:1675–81.

94. Apple DJ, Werner L. Complications of cataract and refractive surgery: a clinicopathological documentation. Trans Am Ophthalmol Soc. 2001;99:95–107; discussion 107–9.

95. Macky TA, Pandey SK, Werner L, *et al.* Anterior capsule opacification. Int Ophthalmol Clin. 2001;41:17–31.

96. Gayton JL, Apple DJ, Peng Q, *et al.* Interlenticular opacification: a clinicopathological correlation of a new complication of piggyback posterior chamber intraocular lenses. J Cataract Refract Surg. 2000;26:330–6.

97. Werner L, Shugar JK, Apple DJ, *et al.* Opacification of piggyback IOLs associated to an amorphous material attached to interlenticular surfaces. J Cataract Refract Surg. 2000;26:1612–9.

98. Trivedi RH, Izak A, Werner L, *et al.* Interlenticular opacification of piggyback intraocular lenses. Int Ophthalmol Clin. 2001;41:47–62.

99. Werner L, Apple DJ, Pandey SK, *et al.* Analysis of elements of interlenticular opacification. Am J Ophthalmol. 2002;133:320–6.

100. Visessook N, Peng Q, Apple DJ, *et al.* Pathological examination of an explanted phakic posterior chamber intraocular lens. J Cataract Refract Surg. 1999;25:216–22.

101. Werner L, Apple DJ, Izak A, *et al.* Phakic anterior chamber intraocular lenses. Int Ophthalmol Clin. 2001;41:133–52.

102. Werner L, Apple DJ, Pandey SK, *et al.* Phakic posterior chamber intraocular lenses. Int Ophthalmol Clin. 2001;41:153–74.

41 Corneal Topography in Cataract Surgery

MELANIE C. CORBETT • EMANUEL S. ROSEN

DEFINITION
- Topography is the description or representation in scientific detail of the features of a particular place: corneal topography refers to the assessment of corneal shape.

KEY FEATURES
- Knowledge and manipulation of the corneal shape during cataract extraction may improve the refractive and visual outcomes of surgery.
- Preoperative assessment of intraocular lens power and incision location is useful in patients who have corneal astigmatism.
- Intraoperative adjustment of suture tension is of limited value.
- Postoperative identification of sutures to be removed helps minimize astigmatism.

INTRODUCTION

Cataract surgery usually is performed to improve vision. Over the years, technological advances have enabled a greater and greater degree of improvement to be achieved. Originally, surgeons concentrated on removal of the opacified lens to enable light to enter the posterior portion of the globe. With the introduction of microsurgery and intraocular lenses (IOLs), patients could hope for a return of good best-corrected visual acuity. Since the most recent developments in cataract surgery, investigators now seek ways to ensure that light is brought to an optimal focus on the retina, providing patients with good uncorrected vision.

The lens contributes only one third of the total focusing power of the eye. The remaining two thirds arises from the convex shape of the anterior corneal surface, which has two important implications for cataract surgery. First, knowledge of the power contributed by the cornea is essential to calculate accurately the power of an IOL to be inserted. Second, very small changes in corneal shape may have a dramatic effect on the precision with which light rays are brought to a focus on the retina. Therefore, incisions made in the cornea or anterior sclera during cataract extraction may change the refraction of the eye. Assessments of corneal topography can be used to minimize the adverse results of these incisions, and even to use their effects to advantage.

HISTORICAL REVIEW

With the increasingly widespread use of spectacles at the beginning of the seventeenth century, interest developed in the shape of the cornea and the optical properties of the eye.[1] Early investigations of corneal topography were confined to gross estimates of corneal curvature by comparison with convex mirrors of known curvature (as performed by Scheiner in 1619). It became apparent that the corneal surface must be smooth to provide good vision, and this was assessed by viewing an image reflected from its surface (carried out by Cuignet in the 1820s). The target used for this purpose by Placido in 1882 was a disc that had black and white concentric rings, with an observation hole in the middle. This pattern still forms the basis of many of the topography systems used today.[2]

Keratometry

Corneal curvature was first quantified using a keratometer, by Helmholtz in 1845. This device measures the distance between two perpendicular pairs of points reflected from a 3mm annulus. It is calibrated in radius of corneal curvature (in millimeters), and the values are converted into corneal power (in diopters) using the standard keratometric index of 1.3375.

Keratometry measurements are accurate and reproducible for regular spherocylindrical surfaces, such as the paracentral area of the normal cornea. They are used routinely today in cataract surgery to calculate the power of IOLs and to identify tight sutures for removal. However, they are of only limited value for irregular corneas because the mire reflections may be distorted, and no information is provided about the corneal curvature other than at the four reference points.[3]

Photokeratoscopy

Attachment of a Placido-type disc to a keratometer increases the area of cornea that can be analyzed, as first shown by Javal in 1889. Photography of the rings rendered measurement of their sizes possible, as developed by Gullstrand in 1896, but manual analysis was very laborious and time consuming.

Videokeratoscopy

Since the recent developments in computer technology it has been possible to measure and analyze keratoscopic images rapidly, with great accuracy and detail. Curvature and power data are generated in less than a couple of minutes for over 6000 locations that cover 95% of the corneal surface.[1,2] However, because this equipment is more expensive than the keratometer, it is not yet available in all eye units.

New Topography Technology

Although clinically useful, keratometry and videokeratoscopy both have a number of limitations, because they use the principle of reflection to assess the corneal curvature. Newer techniques currently under development are based on the principle of projection (e.g., slit photography, raster stereography, moiré interference, and laser interferometry).[4] These systems measure the true corneal shape in terms of height above a reference plane, and have the additional benefit that measurements can be made from paralimbal areas and from irregular or nonreflective surfaces. In view of the currently limited availability of these systems, results of videokeratoscopy are presented in this chapter.

PURPOSE OF TOPOGRAPHY

The curvature of the anterior corneal surface determines the refractive power it provides. In a manner similar to keratoscope usage, videokeratoscopes are used to assess corneal curvature by measurement of the size of the images of a series of targets, or mires, reflected by the cornea.[1,2]

Hardware

The most commonly used mires are a Placido disc that contains 15–38 rings, which may be black and white, or colored (Fig. 41-1). The mires cover a corneal area in the range 0.3–11mm. The image of the mires reflected from the corneal surface is recorded by the charge-coupled device camera. A single video frame is captured and stored by the frame grabber. This image is digitized, the position of the rings identified, and the data analyzed by the computer software. Where the mires are small or close together, the cornea is steepest; and where they are wider apart, the cornea is flatter.

Software

The software establishes a reference point, such as the center of the innermost mire, from which the position of each point can be identified mathematically. Coordinates are given to each data point at which a semimeridian intersects a mire. Most commercial systems have 15–38 circular mires and 256–360 equally spaced semimeridians, which theoretically provides 6000–11,000 data points. The actual number of data points available for analysis may be reduced by mire distortion or shadows from the eyelids.

The position of the data points on the two-dimensional image is analyzed according to a mathematical formula (algorithm) to give the curvature of the corneal surface at the locations where they were reflected. The algorithms include a number of assumptions and estimations and, therefore, provide only an approximate reconstruction of the corneal surface. The accuracy and reproducibility of the measurements for the central cornea is 0.25D, which is below clinical significance. However, measurements are less accurate toward the corneal periphery and for unusually steep or flat corneas.

For optical lenses, measurements of radius of curvature (r) can be converted to power (P) using equation 41-1, where n1 is the refractive index of the first medium (in this case, air = 1), and n2 is the refractive index of the second medium (in this case, cornea = 1.376). The same formula also applies to the posterior corneal surface, but because the curvature of the posterior corneal surface is not easy to measure, the standard keratometric index (1.3375) is an approximation used in the conversion to take account of both surfaces of the cornea. Therefore, although it may be easier for the surgeon to use corneal power values when the patient's refraction is considered, these are less accurate than measurements of corneal curvature.

Equation 41-1 $$P = \frac{(n2 - n1)}{r}$$

Display

The corneal curvature or power is displayed most commonly in the form of a color-coded contour map (Fig. 41-2).[5] The warmer colors (red and yellow) represent the steeper areas, whereas the cooler colors (green and blue) mark the flatter ones. The curvature and dioptric scales beside each map must be studied first to determine the step interval used in a given map.

The radius of curvature (and therefore power) can be expressed in two ways—global (or axial or sagittal) radius of curvature was used initially, but recently local (or instantaneous or tangential) radius of curvature has been found to be more appropriate in some situations.[4] Global radius of curvature is a measure of the curvature of the cornea along each of the meridians with respect to the visual axis. In contrast, local radius of curvature is a measure of the curvature at each point with respect to its neighboring points along a tangent.

Quantitative descriptors of corneal contour provide numerical assessments of the regularity and asymmetry of the corneal surface as a whole. The change in corneal curvature or power that, for example, results from surgery, can be displayed by a

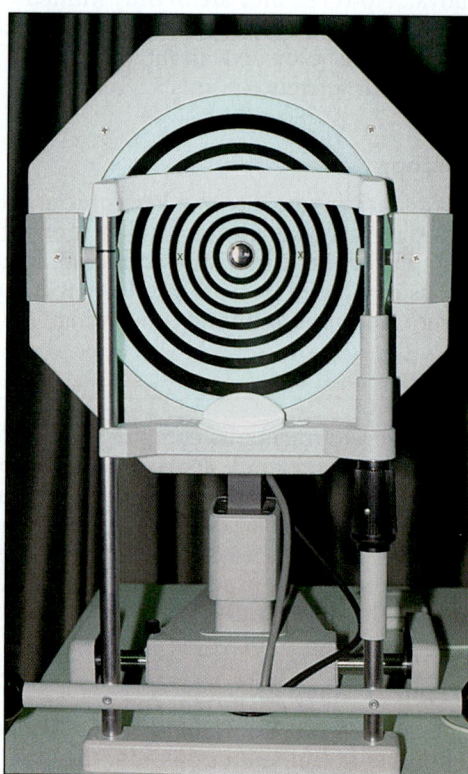

FIG. 41-1 ■ Cone of a videokeratoscope that carries Placido-type mires. The patient places his or her head against the chin and forehead supports. The cone is centered and focused in front of the eye to be tested. The image of the mires reflected from the corneal surface is recorded by the charge-coupled device video camera housed behind the central mire.

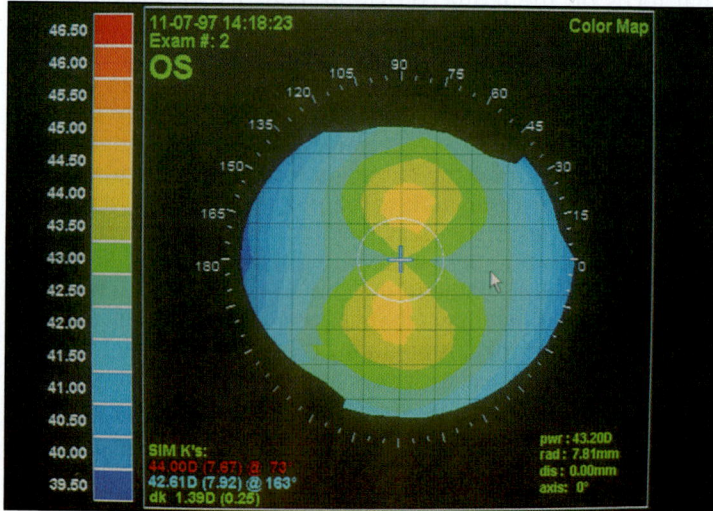

FIG. 41-2 ■ Topography of normal cornea. Note symmetry in vertical meridian of "with-the-rules," regular astigmatism, which respects either side of the horizontal meridian.

"change map." This is generated by the subtraction of the preoperative topography from the postoperative topography. Alternative representations of individual maps include keratographs, numerical maps, and three-dimensional wire nets.[1]

UTILITY OF TOPOGRAPHY

Over the years many different techniques for the construction and closure of incisions for cataract surgery have been proposed, each with its own claimed advantages. More recently, corneal topography has provided an objective means by which to compare the effects of various surgical parameters on optical outcome.

Nowadays the aim of cataract surgery is to return patients to good uncorrected vision. This requires that their final refraction be within 1D of emmetropia or a predetermined ametropic result, and that preexisting and surgically induced astigmatism be minimized.[6] To achieve this, the refractive element of each stage of surgery has to be optimized which, particularly in difficult cases, is facilitated by the use of corneal topography.

Preoperative Topography

The preoperative assessment of corneal topography has two roles in cataract surgery. First, as an alternative to keratometry, it can provide a representative measure of the corneal curvature or power necessary to calculate intraocular lens (IOL) power. Second, knowledge of the magnitude and location of preexisting astigmatism is important if it is to be reversed by appropriate placement and construction of the wound during surgery.

Calculation of Intraocular Lens Power

Prior to cataract surgery, the power of the IOL required to give the desired postoperative refraction is determined using measurements of corneal curvature and axial length in a mathematical formula. The final refractive result is dependent upon the accuracy of the biometric data and its appropriate use in the relevant calculations.

For these calculations, the corneal curvature commonly is measured by keratometry, and the mean of the two readings is used in the formula. For the majority of normal corneas, the small variability of the keratometry readings gives an accuracy of IOL power to within the 0.5D step interval of manufactured lenses. In this group, variability in the measurement of the axial length tends to be the main source of discrepancy in the IOL power prediction.

In contrast, this is not necessarily the case for patients who have corneal pathology or who have undergone previous corneal or refractive procedures.[7] When the cornea is irregular, a better prediction of the required IOL power can be obtained using corneal topography rather than keratometry to measure the corneal curvature.[3,8] As a result of the generation of many more data points, corneal topography has the advantage that it represents these corneas more accurately; but with it comes the difficulty of knowing which data points to use in the IOL power calculations. Moreover, different sets of data points may be more accurate with different formulas.[7] Examples of the data points which may be used include[8]:

- Keratometric equivalent at the 3mm zone (average of the steepest and flattest meridians)
- Average curvature of the 3mm ring
- Average curvature of the 4mm ring
- Mean central corneal power
- Centrally weighted mean corneal power

On the whole, measurements that use a greater number of data points that are nearer the central cornea are the most useful.

Planning the Incision

Corneal topography may be used to assess the magnitude, location, and regularity of preexisting corneal astigmatism. Vector analysis may be used to calculate the induced astigmatism that needs to be added to the existing astigmatism to produce the desired spherical end result. This may be achieved either by astigmatically neutral cataract surgery combined with a refractive corneal procedure, or by the appropriate modification of the cataract incision.[6,9] In the latter, the incision is centered on the steep meridian, and the wound construction–placement–closure combination that will produce the required astigmatic decay is carried out. The effect can be further titrated against the topography by selective suture removal.

INCISION LOCATION. Surgically induced change in corneal contour is less for the more peripheral (posterior) incisions in the sclera or limbus[7] than for those that involve the cornea. Some authors have claimed that for smaller incision surgery some incision sites (e.g., superotemporal) cause less astigmatism than others.[10]

INCISION LENGTH. A huge quantity of literature now exists to support the theory that smaller incisions are associated with less surgically induced change in corneal contour, a more stable refraction, earlier visual recovery, and a better uncorrected visual acuity, particularly early after surgery.[10–12] Since the introduction of IOLs that have flexible optics, it has been shown that an unsutured 3.2mm incision is associated with less than 0.5D against-the-rule shift in corneal astigmatism.

INCISION ARCHITECTURE. Multiplanar incisions commonly are used to aid vertical alignment and give the wound greater stability. As incisions have become smaller, tunnel constructions have been introduced to enable wounds to self-seal, and thereby avoid the need for sutures and the consequent suture-induced astigmatism.[7]

Intraoperative Topography

The majority of surgeons believe that intraoperative keratometry does not significantly reduce corneal astigmatism that is surgically induced.

Postoperative Topography

Postoperatively, corneal topography or keratometry can be used routinely to identify tight sutures that need to be removed (Fig. 41-3). Topography is valuable for patients who have an inadequate best-corrected visual acuity, and to determine whether corneal irregularities account for the poor level of vision. In patients who require surgical correction of a persistent refractive error or irregular astigmatism, corneal topography is essential.

Wound Closure

SUTURELESS INCISIONS. The use of well-constructed, self-sealing incisions avoids suture-related complications and is not usually associated with significant wound-related flattening (Fig. 41-4).[10,13]

SUTURED WOUNDS. If the wound requires sutures, monofilament nylon is used commonly. This is an inert, nonabsorbable suture that has a relatively high tensile strength and allows minimal natural decay of induced astigmatism (Figs. 41-5 and 41-6) until the suture is removed.[14,15]

To minimize surgically induced astigmatism, radial sutures must be relatively deep and of moderate length to prevent tissue compression or wound gape.[14,15] For tunnel incisions some studies suggest that horizontal, triangular, or mattress sutures are associated with less wound-related steepening than either radial or cross sutures (see Fig. 41-5).[6,7] Some surgeons advocate the use of a keratometer during the suturing of corneal wounds to reduce surgically induced astigmatism,[16] but many others are unconvinced of its value.

In wounds closed by nonabsorbable sutures, selective suture manipulation at 8–12 weeks postoperatively is an effective way to reduce wound-related corneal steepening.[17] For interrupted sutures, this involves removal of the tight suture(s) in the steep

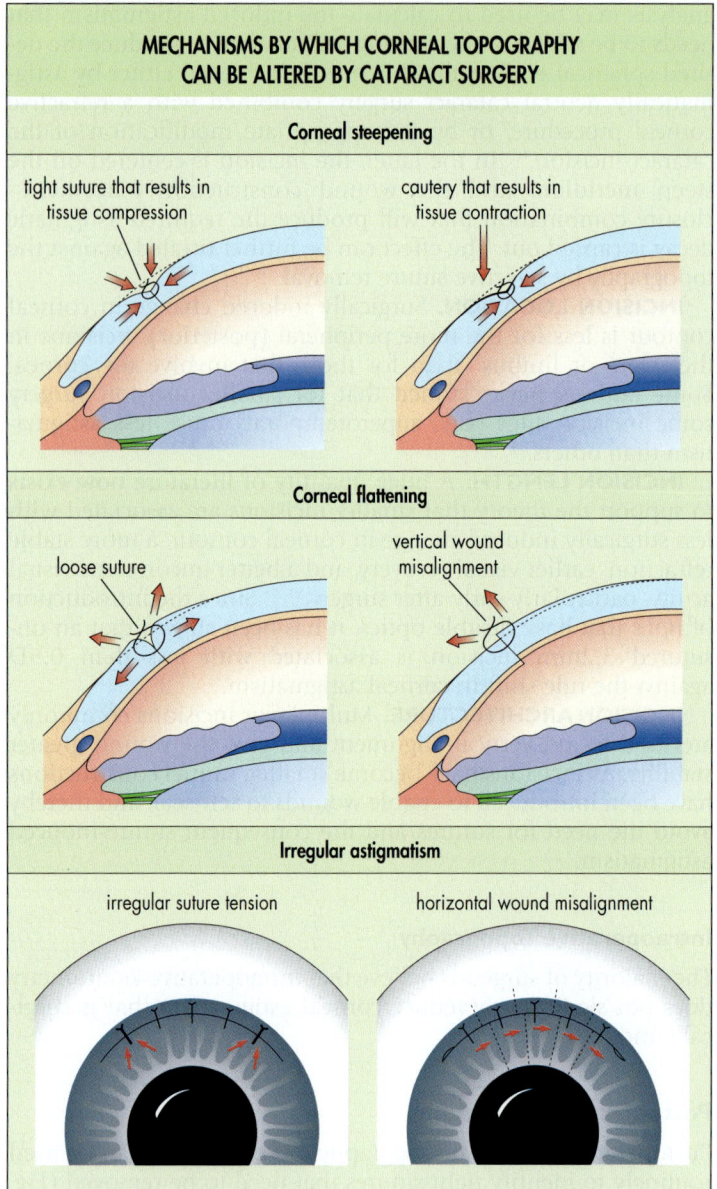

MECHANISMS BY WHICH CORNEAL TOPOGRAPHY CAN BE ALTERED BY CATARACT SURGERY

Corneal steepening

tight suture that results in tissue compression

cautery that results in tissue contraction

Corneal flattening

loose suture

vertical wound misalignment

Irregular astigmatism

irregular suture tension

horizontal wound misalignment

FIG. 41-3 ■ **Mechanisms by which corneal topography can be altered by cataract surgery.** Wound compression (corneal steepening), wound gape (corneal flattening), and wound misalignment (irregular astigmatism) are shown. The cornea is shown in section through the incision site, or from anteriorly; the *arrows* show the direction of the forces exerted; and the *dashed lines* show the original position of the corneal surface.

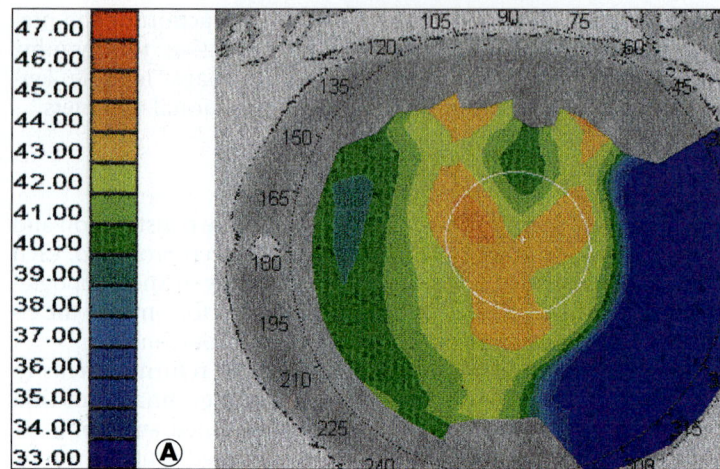

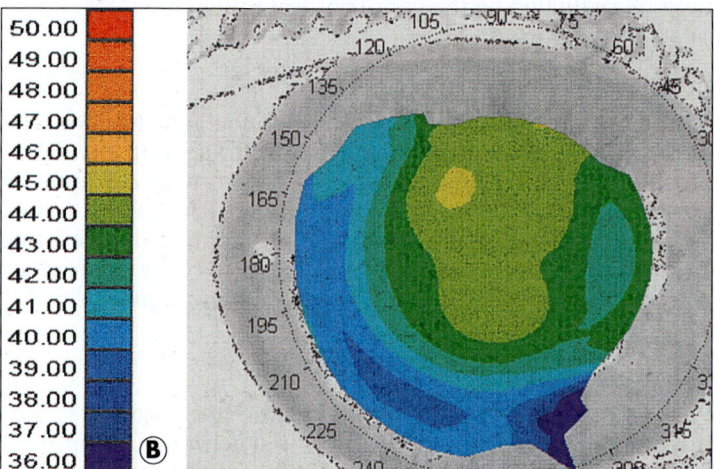

FIG. 41-4 ■ Corneal flattening after sutureless phacoemulsification. **A,** Immediately after phacoemulsification through a 3mm clear corneal tunnel, there was localized flattening superiorly that related to the site of the incision. **B,** After 1 year this had resolved spontaneously, and the corneal topography returned to its preoperative oval pattern.

axis or axes. Continuous sutures may be removed partly or entirely or, alternatively, the tension may be redistributed by easing the suture loop by loop from flat areas to steep areas.[18] Corneal topography is of greater benefit than keratometry for suture adjustment, because it enables the location of the tight sutures to be identified more accurately, particularly if more than one is tight (see Fig. 41-6).

Topographic Changes Induced by Cataract Surgery

The topographic changes induced by cataract surgery may be displayed on a change map or "difference" map, in which the preoperative measurements are subtracted from the postoperative measurements. Most of the primary changes relate to the incision site, but these may induce secondary changes in the perpendicular meridian as a result of "coupling."

Surgery may result in either steepening or flattening of one or more parts of the cornea, changes that can be classified according to their location relative to the wound and their magnitude[11,13]:

- Central: >1D, within the central 2 × 2mm
- Peripheral: >1D, away from the wound

- Wound-related—extending to within: +1D (central 7mm), +2D (central 5mm), or +3D (central 3mm)
- Astigmatic increase or decrease by >1D

CORNEAL STEEPENING. Wound-related corneal steepening (with-the-rule astigmatism for a superior incision) occurs secondary to compression of tissue at the wound site (see Figs. 41-3 and 41-5).[11] This is commonly a result of overly tight sutures or edema of the wound margin. It also may result from vertical wound malalignment, in which the central edge underrides the peripheral edge, or from cautery that causes tissue contraction.[7]

The compression of tissue at the limbus depresses the limbal cornea toward the center of the globe and, thereby, increases the curvature of the central cornea (i.e., causes a reduction in the radius of curvature).[15] A small area of flattening occurs immediately within the area of the suture and a secondary flattening in the meridian perpendicular to the suture as a result of coupling.

CORNEAL FLATTENING. Wound-related corneal flattening (against-the-rule astigmatism for a superior incision) occurs as a result of wound gape (see Figs. 41-3 and 41-4).[19] This sometimes is seen to a small extent in unsutured wounds, but more commonly if sutures are too loose either at the time of surgery or if subsequent cheese-wiring, knot slippage, suture-related inflammation, degradation, or removal occurs. Sutures that are placed too superficially may result in posterior wound gape, which has a similar topographic appearance. Vertical misalignment of the wound in which the central edge overrides the peripheral edge also produces wound-related corneal flattening. If the wound edges are in poor apposition and the gape area is filled by

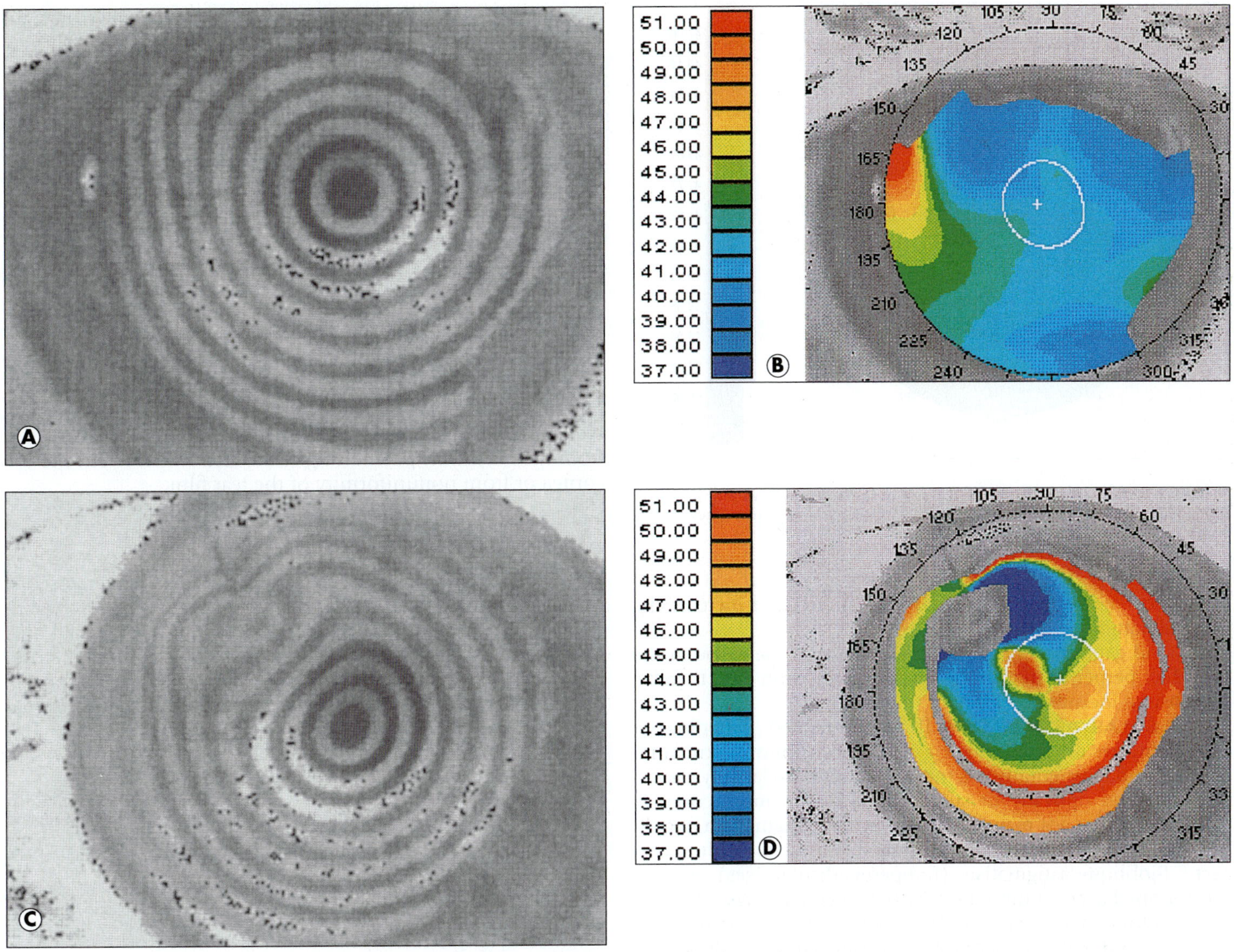

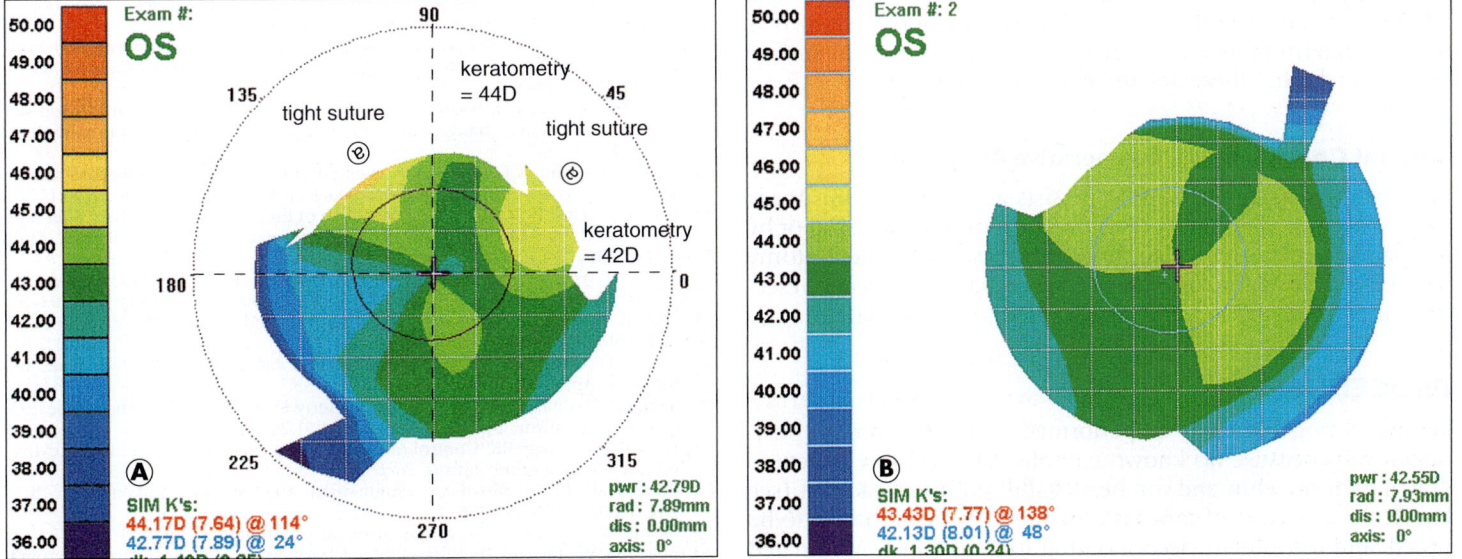

FIG. 41-5 ▮ **Corneal steepening that results from a tight suture. A,** The video image shows a tight suture at 80° after phacoemulsification and cataract extraction. **B,** The corneal topography shows this has resulted in a wound-related corneal steepening that extends into the central or 3mm zone. **C,** When the suture is removed there is a flattening of the cornea in the region of the incision, the degree of flattening depending upon the extent of the incision. **D,** The effect on the central cornea, though, is now relieved as shown in the topography where the central cornea is now spherical.

FIG. 41-6 ▮ **Corneal irregularity as a result of unequal suture tension. A,** After extracapsular cataract extraction, tight sutures caused steepening in the 30° and 320° meridians, which was obvious on videokeratoscopy. On keratometry the mires were distorted, and measurements taken from the positions shown by the circles gave readings of 44D at 90° and 42D at 0°. This demonstrates how the use of keratometry in irregular corneas can be misleading—in this case it would have resulted in the removal of the wrong sutures, and the astigmatism and corneal irregularity may have been made worse. **B,** Removal of the two tight sutures, at the locations demonstrated by videokeratoscopy, restored the cornea to a more normal spherocylindrical shape.

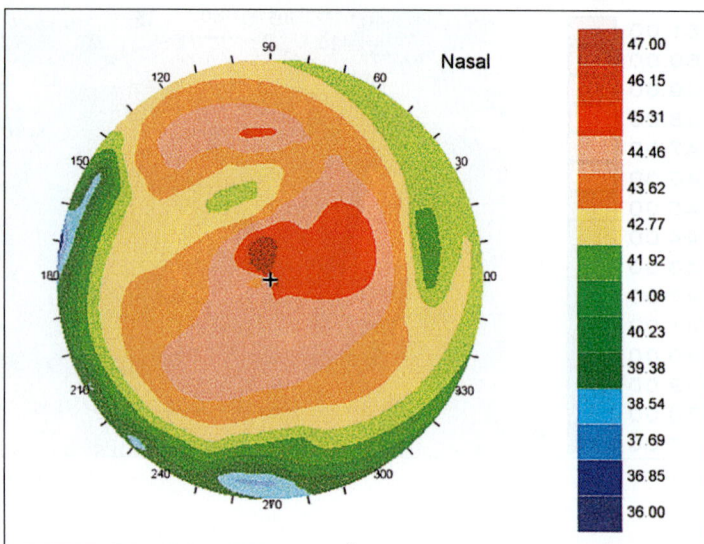

FIG. 41-7 ■ Corneal irregularity as a result of horizontal wound misalignment. Horizontal misalignment of the wound because of malposition of the sutures resulted in spiraling of the corneal topography.

fibrovascular scar tissue, this may later stretch and increase the corneal flattening.

Wound gape increases the circumference of the globe in the meridian perpendicular to the line of the incision and, thereby, flattens the incisional meridian.

IRREGULAR ASTIGMATISM. If wound-related flattening or steepening results from either a single or a uniform structural defect, regular astigmatism is most likely and is relatively easy to correct either optically or surgically. However, more complex anatomical changes may result in irregular astigmatism, which produces greater visual dysfunction and is more difficult to correct.[11] Bioblique astigmatism (nonperpendicular axes) may occur if nonadjacent sutures are over-tightened (see Figs. 41-3 and 41-6). A torsional effect results from a horizontal malalignment of the wound, whether because of a mismatch of its edges or of nonradial suture bites (see Figs. 41-3 and 41-7).

Investigation of Poor Outcome

Corneal topography is helpful after cataract surgery in cases in which the best-corrected visual acuity is not adequate, and where there are no other obvious causes for poor vision. It is used to determine whether irregularities of the corneal surface exist and whether these are amenable to correction.[3,11]

Surgical Correction of Postoperative Astigmatism

Postoperative astigmatism that persists after suture adjustment may be addressed either by revision of the original incision or by a separate corneal refractive procedure.[6] Astigmatic keratotomy may be performed across the steep meridian, and wedge resection or compressive sutures may be used to reverse flattening.

PROCEDURE

Corneal topography may be performed at any time pre- or post-operatively, because no known complications exist. A patient is seated with the chin and forehead stabilized by a head rest (see Fig. 41-1). The cone of mires is centered in front of the eye to be tested, and the patient views a central fixation target. Automated focusing devices ensure that the cone and charge-coupled device camera are positioned correctly relative to the cornea. The accuracy of the results is dependent upon proper alignment and patient fixation. At the touch of a button, the charge-coupled device camera records the image of the mires. The images are stored automatically and can be analyzed immediately or later.[1,2]

INTERPRETATION OF RESULTS

Once the mires have been analyzed, the operator determines how to display the data from a number of options.[1] The scale may be altered to emphasize aspects of the results, and grids, optical zones, astigmatic axes, and the pupil margin may be overlaid to assist interpretation.

Operators must be familiar with the range of appearances of the normal cornea and of artifacts before corneal pathology can be diagnosed or the effects of surgery assessed.[20] The appearance of the normal cornea has been classified as belonging to one of five patterns—round, oval, symmetrical bow-tie, asymmetrical bow-tie, or irregular. The bow-tie patterns tend to be associated more commonly with astigmatism. The two corneas of an individual are often mirror images of each other. Artifacts can arise from the inaccurate positioning of the instrument relative to the cornea or from nonuniformity of the tear film.

ALTERNATIVE TESTS

Keratometry is a widely available alternative to videokeratoscopy for the measurement of corneal curvature or power. However, as discussed above, it makes measurements over a very small area of cornea,[2] which is acceptable in most regular corneas the central portions of which are broadly either spherical or spherocylindrical. However, for more irregular corneas, the additional data provided by videokeratoscopy are preferred.

REFERENCES

1. Corbett MC, Rosen ES, O'Brart DPS. Corneal topography: principles and applications. London: BMJ Books; 1998.
2. Wilson SE, Klyce SD. Advances in the analysis of corneal topography. Surv Ophthalmol. 1991;35:269–77.
3. Sanders RD, Gills JP, Martin RG. When keratometric measurements do not accurately reflect corneal topography. J Cataract Refract Surg. 1993;19(suppl):131–5.
4. Corbett MC, Marshall J, O'Brart DPS, Rosen ES. New and future technology in corneal topography. Eur J Implant Refract Surg. 1995;7:372–86.
5. Wilson SE, Klyce SD, Husseini ZM. Standardised colour coded maps for corneal topography. Ophthalmology. 1993;100:1723–7.
6. Nordan LT, Lusby FW. Refractive aspects of cataract surgery. Curr Opin Ophthalmol. 1995;6:36–40.
7. Koch DD, Haft EA, Gay C. Computerized videokeratographic analysis of corneal topographic changes induced by sutured and unsutured 4mm scleral pocket incisions. J Cataract Refract Surg. 1993;19(suppl):166–9.
8. Cuaycong MJ, Gay CA, Emery J, et al. Comparison of the accuracy of computerized videokeratoscopy and keratometry for use in intraocular lens calculations. J Cataract Refract Surg. 1993;19(suppl):178–81.
9. Nielsen PJ. Prospective evaluation of surgically induced astigmatism and astigmatic keratotomy effects of various self-sealing small incisions. J Cataract Refract Surg. 1995;21:43–8.
10. Hayashi K, Hayashi H, Nakao F, Hayashi F. The correlation between incision size and corneal shape changes in sutureless cataract surgery. Ophthalmology. 1995;102:550–6.
11. Martin RG, Sanders DR, Miller JD, et al. Effect of cataract wound incision size on acute changes in corneal topography. J Cataract Refract Surg. 1993;19(suppl):170–7.
12. Kohnen T, Dick B, Jacobi KW. Comparison of the induced astigmatism after temporal clear corneal incisions of different sizes. J Cataract Refract Surg. 1995;21:417–24.
13. Oshika T, Tsuboi S, Yaguchi S, et al. Comparative study of intraocular lens implantation through 3.2 and 5.5mm incisions. Ophthalmology. 1994;101:1183–90.
14. Eve FR, Troutman RC. Placement of sutures used in corneal incisions. Am J Ophthalmol. 1976;82:786–9.
15. van Rij G, Waring GO III. Changes in corneal curvature induced by sutures and incisions. Am J Ophthalmol. 1984;98:773–83.
16. Samples JR, Binder PS. The value of the Terry Keratometer in predicting postoperative astigmatism. Ophthalmology. 1984;91:280–4.
17. Kronish JW, Forster RK. Control of corneal astigmatism following cataract extraction by selective suture cutting. Arch Ophthalmol. 1987;105:1650–5.
18. Roper-Hall MJ. Control of astigmatism after surgery and trauma. Br J Ophthalmol. 1982;66:556–9.
19. Swinger CA. Postoperative astigmatism. Surv Ophthalmol. 1987;31:219–48.
20. Bogan SJ, Waring GO, Ibrahim O, et al. Classification of normal corneal topography based on computer-assisted video keratography. Arch Ophthalmol. 1990;108:945–9.

SECTION 4 LENS SURGERY

CHAPTER

42

Indications for Lens Surgery and Different Techniques

HARRY B. GRABOW

KEY FEATURES
- Lens surgery is the most common eye operation.
- Technical indications for lens surgery are divided into two main categories: medical and optical.
- Socioeconomic conditions play a role in the indications for lens surgery.
- All lens surgery should be considered form of refractive surgery.
- Lens surgery may be divided into four major categories by technique:
  - Lens repositioning (couching)
  - Lens removal
  - Lens replacement
  - Lens enhancement

INTRODUCTION

The technical indications for lens surgery today may be classified into two main categories: medical, which might more properly be called surgical or pathological indications, and optical—currently known as refractive indications. Medical indications arise from pathological states of the lens of varying causes, usually related to lens clarity, lens position, or other lens-related conditions, such as inflammation or glaucoma. Non-lens-related conditions may also be an indication for lens surgery, such as aniridia. Surgical or pathological indications have existed for centuries, if not millennia, and are generally indisputable. Refractive indications for lens surgery, in contrast, include clear-lens ametropic refractive states. These are relatively new indications, only decades old, and they may or may not be considered pathological conditions. In some settings, surgery for such conditions is considered controversial, if not contraindicated. However, the ophthalmic subspecialty of refractive surgery gained a secure foothold in the late 1990s, and refractive lens surgery is rapidly becoming a common tool in the armamentarium of both cataract and refractive surgeons. The lens plays such a significant role in the visual refractive system of the eye that many, if not all, of the medical conditions of the lens also interfere with its optics. Similarly, surgical removal of the lens immediately and permanently alters the refractive state of the eye. Today, therefore, all lens surgery, for whatever indication, has properly come to be considered refractive surgery.

In addition to medical and optical indications, a third set of indications exists, particularly pertaining to cataract surgery, that relates not so much to the condition of the eye as it does to economic conditions in the various societies of the world. Thus, the socioeconomic conditions of a country may determine when lens removal is performed, how it is performed, and how available it is for a given population.

BOX 42-1

MEDICAL (PATHOLOGICAL) INDICATIONS FOR LENS SURGERY

I. Lenticular opacification (cataract)
II. Lenticular malposition
   A. Subluxation
   B. Dislocation
III. Lenticular malformation
   A. Coloboma
   B. Lenticonus
   C. Lentiglobus
   D. Spherophakia
IV. Uveal malformation
   A. Partial iris coloboma
   B. Total aniridia
V. Lens-induced inflammation
   A. Phacoanaphylactic endophthalmitis
VI. Lens-induced (phacolytic) glaucoma
VII. Postoperative retained lenticular material
   A. Capsule
   B. Cortex
   C. Nucleus
VIII. Postoperative complications
   A. Capsular ophthalmic visco-surgical device block
   B. Capsular hematoma
   C. Propioni endophthalmitis
IX. Postoperative capsular opacification
   A. Anterior
   B. Posterior
   C. Synechia
X. Lenticular tumor
   A. Epithelioma
   B. Epitheliocarcinoma

MEDICAL INDICATIONS FOR LENS SURGERY

Lenticular Opacification (Cataract)

The medical indications for lens surgery (Box 42-1) are true pathological states, some of which threaten the integrity of the whole organ (the eye). They also interfere with a major ocular function, focused vision. Lenticular opacification obstructs the pathway of light; reduces the available quantity of light; scatters light off axis; reduces contrast sensitivity; diminishes color intensity; reduces resolution acuity; may alter lens texture in such a way to contribute to a decrease in accommodation amplitude, particularly in the case of presenile nuclear sclerosis; and, in the case of progressive nuclear sclerosis, often results in a myopic alteration of a previously stable lifelong refractive state.

Lens opacification is by far the most common indication for lens surgery, and lens surgery is the most common eye operation, if not the most frequently performed of all human operations; yet cataract persists today as the most prevalent cause of

315

human blindness on earth. However, with the rapid acceptance, by both surgeons and patients, of corneal refractive surgery, particularly LASIK, and with the prevalence of ametropia far exceeding the prevalence of cataract in the world population, it may be only a few years before the number of cataract operations is exceeded by the number of refractive procedures.

Cataract, depending on severity, is a condition of the eye that, by interfering with vision, can simultaneously interfere with certain activities in life. It is generally agreed that surgical intervention is indicated when there is "functional" visual impairment. The levels of functional visual impairment necessitating surgical intervention, however, vary from culture to culture. In highly developed societies, the mere loss of the ability to follow a golf ball may qualify an eye for surgery; in third-world countries, leukocoria may precede nutritional deprivation, and lens surgery may be a matter of survival.

In highly structured societies, governments or third-party health insurance carriers pay for such surgical procedures, and these same institutions often set standards for lens surgery indications. Therefore, in developed societies where surgical technology is advanced, perceived economic conditions may be the factors that determine the prevalence and definition of "cataract blindness" for a population, and this changes as conditions change. In many underdeveloped nations, the prevalence of cataract blindness is determined by the availability of care.

In the United States, cataract surgeons often refer to measurable standards of visual performance as indications for cataract surgery. Visual acuity of 20/50 or worse as measured on a Snellen chart in dim ambient (mesopic) illumination with maximal refractive correction is an acceptable level of cataract to indicate surgery, according to the American Academy of Ophthalmology. Visual acuity of 20/50 or worse when tested with bright light imposition on the pupil, or glare testing, is considered a surgical level of cataract dysfunction in many states in the United States. Reduction of contrast sensitivity can be demonstrated and quantified, and the type and degree of lens opacification may be subjectively quantified by slit-lamp examination and categorized according to the Lens Opacification System III (LOCS-III) devised by Chylack et al.[1] The degree to which the opacification obstructs light can, additionally, be measured by laser interferometry.[2] Progressive changes in cataract density over time can be documented by Scheimpflug photography of nuclear cataracts[3] and by Neitz-Kawara retroillumination photography of posterior subcapsular cataracts.[4]

However, in structured economic societies, third-party payers and governmental regulatory agencies are not interested in the results of these sophisticated methods of analyzing loss of lens function; they are more interested in how the loss of lens function interferes with life functions. Loss of functional impairment due to visual impairment may range from minor impairment in luxury lifestyles, such as inability to follow a golf ball; to moderate impairment, such as inability to see well enough to drive an automobile; to severe impairment of life support functions, such as inability to see the units on an insulin syringe or the instructions on a bottle of cardiac medication—or even food on the table. Examples of such tests are the Visual Function Index (VF-14)[5-8] and the Activities of Daily Vision Scale (ADVS).[9,10]

CATARACT IN THE PRESENCE OF OTHER OCULAR DISORDERS. The decision to remove a cataract in an otherwise healthy eye usually depends on the cataract's impact on the visual function of the eye and the impact of that level of visual impairment on the person's life. In healthy eyes whose only disorder is cataract, the presumed outcome after uncomplicated surgery is better vision than before surgery. Indeed, in the most technologically advanced societies, patients are requesting emmetropia, and even restoration of accommodation. In such "healthy" eyes, cataract surgeons experience a rate of intraopera-

tive and postoperative complications of less than 2% or, conversely, an uncomplicated rate of 98%. Thus, when one applies a risk-benefit ratio with such a high degree of success, surgery is usually the mutually agreed on course.

However, such may not be the case when the cataract is associated with other disorders, especially if they are contributing factors to the loss of vision of an eye. Therefore, such conditions as amblyopia, corneal opacification, vitreous opacification, maculopathy, retinopathy, glaucoma, and optic neuropathy may alter or delay the decision to operate, based not so much on the expected risks but rather on the limited benefits. In some cases, lens surgery is indicated to preserve peripheral vision only for functional ambulation. In other cases, a progressive condition of the posterior segment is an indication for lens surgery, even when the expectation for visual improvement may be minimal.[11]

Systemic conditions may also play a role in deciding whether and when to remove a cataract. Is the patient's diabetes under control? Has there been a stroke with hemianopia? Is the patient on systemic anticoagulants? Is the patient terminally ill or immunologically suppressed? Does the patient have Alzheimer's disease or severe mental retardation?

Thus, the decision to remove a cataract may become a collaborative endeavor with participation by the patient, the patient's family, the patient's primary physician, the surgeon, a governmental agency, and a third-party payer. The decision, thus, is determined not only by technological findings and expectations but also by a "holistic" evaluation of the impact of such a decision on that person's life, as defined by that society.

Lenticular Malposition

Subluxation and dislocation of the lens are different degrees of the same phenomenon and result from dysfunction of the zonule. The zonule may be defective as a result of congenital malformation, total or partial agenesis, or a hereditary metabolic disorder, such as Marfan's syndrome. Chronic inflammation and pseudoexfoliation have been shown to be associated with a weakness in the zonular fibers or their attachments. Ocular trauma is an obvious cause.

Partial subluxation, in the absence of associated sequelae, may not be visually significant and may not be an indication for lensectomy. Similarly, complete dislocation of an intact lens into the inferior vitreous may be a quiescent event in the absence of inflammation and may simply produce a state of refractive aphakia, correctable nonsurgically with a spectacle or contact lens or surgically with intraocular lens (IOL) implantation. Partial subluxation to the extent that the equator of the lens is visible in the midsized pupil is usually visually significant, causing glare, fluctuating vision, and monocular diplopia. This symptom complex would qualify for lens surgery.

Lenticular Malformation

These conditions of abnormal lens development are congenital. They may be genetic, hereditary, or the result of intrauterine infection or trauma. These conditions include lens coloboma, lenticonus, lentiglobus, and spherophakia, as well as varieties of congenital cataract. Partial iris coloboma or total aniridia, whether congenital, traumatic, or surgical, may be an indication for lens surgery to improve visual function or for cosmesis. The availability of aniridia IOLs (Fig. 42-1) and opaque endocapsular rings (Figs. 42-2 and 42-3) offers great improvements for such patients.

The indications for surgery depend on the degree to which the specific malformation interferes with vision or the integrity of the involved eye. Such abnormalities may be associated with amblyopia. Early detection and surgical intervention should be incorporated with a plan for amblyopia therapy.

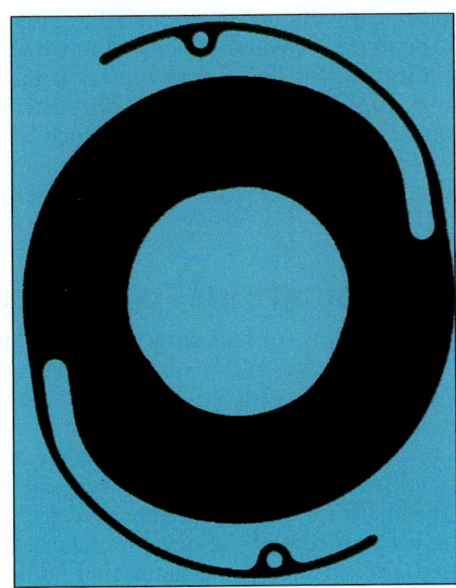

FIG. 42-1 ▓ Aniridia intraocular lens with opaque peripheral "pseudoiris." (Courtesy of Morcher, GMBh, Germany.)

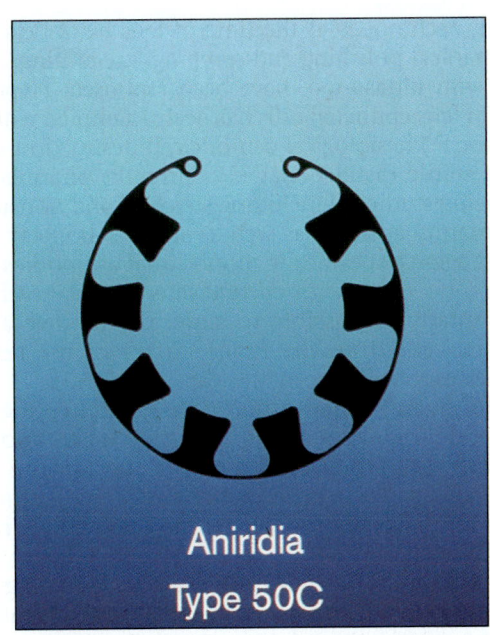

Aniridia
Type 50C

FIG. 42-2 ▓ Aniridia endocapsular ring. (Courtesy of Morcher, GMBh, Germany.)

Lens-Induced Ocular Inflammation

Certain specific prerequisites are necessary for phacoanaphylactic endophthalmitis to occur: the first is an immunologically mature and competent host; the second is a physical or chemical disruption of the lens capsule. Removal of the lens protein that is perceived to be foreign to the organism may be curative. This is one form of ocular inflammation for which surgery is the appropriate treatment.

Lens-Induced Glaucoma

Phacolytic glaucoma is not associated with a physical or chemical disruption of the lens capsule. Denatured lens protein leaks out through an intact capsule and is engulfed by macrophages. The macrophages then occlude an open angle. As with the lens-induced inflammatory syndromes, removal of the offending organelle, the lens, is usually curative, obviating the need for other forms of medical or surgical pressure management.

Postoperative Retained Lenticular Material

Retained remnants of nucleus following extracapsular surgery, particularly phacoemulsification, may cause ocular inflammation, ocular hypertension, cystoid macular edema, and corneal edema. Small remnants may inadvertently be left in the anterior chamber angle or posterior to the iris in the ciliary sulcus. A few days of observation and medical management with corticosteroids, cycloplegics, beta blockers and nonsteroidal anti-inflammatories may aid in controlling the inflammation and hypertension while phagocytosis occurs. However, significantly decreased visual acuity or elevated intraocular pressure may be an indication for surgical intervention.

Small fragments of nucleus in aqueous are usually hydrated after a few days and are easily aspirated with a cannula through a paracentesis incision. Larger fragments in the vitreous have been observed to cause either no reaction or significant vitritis. Those that cause no reaction may be completely embedded in, and surrounded by, formed vitreous and act as though they are insulated from uveal tissue. Others appear to be exposed to the uvea and incite an inflammatory reaction. These are also easily removed but usually require pars plana vitrectomy.

Retained remnants of cortex are a rare indication for surgical intervention, as small amounts of residual cortex appear to be

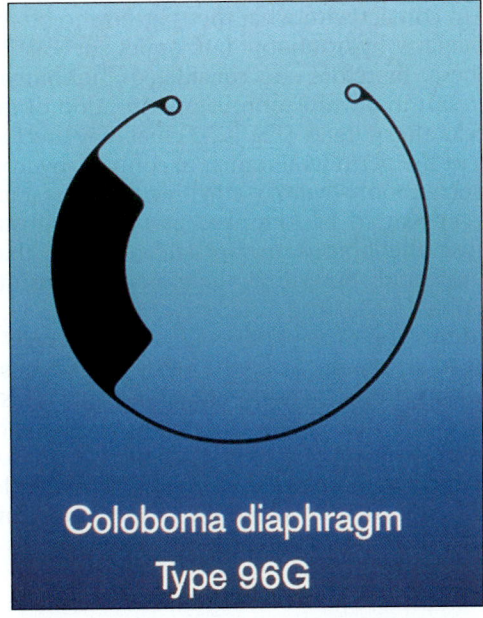

Coloboma diaphragm
Type 96G

FIG. 42-3 ▓ Iris coloboma endocapsular ring. (Courtesy of Morcher, GMBh, Germany.)

phagocytosed in a matter of weeks. Occasionally, however, a large wedge of adherent cortex may remain, either unintentionally or intentionally, and may cause excessive and prolonged postoperative inflammation, hypertension, and, if in the pupillary space, visual symptoms. These would be indications for surgical aspiration.

Some posterior subcapsular opacities are extremely adherent to the central posterior capsule and may be resistant to removal by vacuuming, polishing, curetting, or with forceps. The surgeon may then elect to perform primary posterior capsulorrhexis or to defer definitive primary treatment, for fear of disrupting the adjacent vitreous face, in favor of secondary postoperative yttrium-aluminum-garnet (YAG) laser posterior capsulectomy.

Postoperative Capsular Opacification

The prevention of capsular opacification following extracapsular extraction techniques is currently undergoing intense investigation. Primary techniques at the time of lens extraction, such as simple mechanical polishing and curetting, vacuuming, and even vacuuming with ultrasound, have been espoused. Hypothermic destruction of lens epithelial cells has been attempted with the use of a cryoprobe.[12] Physiological osmotic cell destruction was tried with simple sterile distilled water.[13] Currently, pharmacological agents are being studied,[14] including steroidal and nonsteroidal[15] anti-inflammatory agents,[16] as well as antimetabolites[17] and immunological agents, specifically monoclonal antibodies.[18]

It appears, however, with current lens removal technology, that it is virtually impossible to surgically remove all living lens epithelial cells from the inner surface of the remaining lens capsule, especially from the capsular fornix. It also appears that following extracapsular surgery, lens epithelial cells become mobile, diapedetic, and that they try to adopt three new functions: (1) repairing the rent created in the anterior capsule, (2) encapsulating the foreign body (IOL), and (3) replacing the removed natural crystalline lens with a new natural crystalline lens.

The first mission of the lens epithelial cells, repairing the rent in the anterior capsule, can result in the fibrotic phimotic contraction of the anterior capsular opening, in some cases resulting in successful complete closure (Fig. 42-4). This rare phenomenon, facilitated by a small initial surgical capsulectomy and by hydrophilic polymethyl methacrylate (PMMA) and silicone, results in obstruction of vision requiring correction with YAG laser. Fibrous metaplasia of the lens epithelial cells occurs when they come in contact with what they perceive to be foreign material, particularly hydrophobic IOL optics such as PMMA and silicone. These, therefore, are considered "nonbiocompatible" and often result in a white, fibrous opacification of the anterior capsule weeks after surgery (Fig. 42-5) that may preclude easy visualization of the peripheral retina. In contrast, hydrophilic IOL materials, such as poly-hydroxy-ethyl-methacrylate and collagen-copolymer, appear to be perceived as natural substances and do not cause the fibrous metaplastic response that the hydrophobic materials do. These, therefore, are considered more "biocompatible."

The third mission of remaining lens epithelial cells is to multiply rapidly in an attempt to fill the newly voided capsular space with a new, functional, natural crystalline lens. This rapid recrudescence of mitotic activity, lens epithelial cell hyperplasia, is engendered by the physical loss of contiguity of previously adjacent cells, which were removed at surgery, causing a loss of cellular contact inhibition. Without the proper embryonically created template, these now migratory lens epithelial cells can do no

better than to multiply in an uncontrollable and disorderly fashion and form optically disrupting epithelial "pearls" (Fig. 42-6). Symptomatic posterior capsular opacification by such a process may be an indication for either a secondary surgical posterior capsulectomy or capsulotomy or a YAG laser posterior capsulectomy. If surgical intervention is indicated, such as for IOL exchange or secondary "piggyback" IOL implementation, then simple vacuuming of the posterior capsule may remove soft epithelial pearls.

REFRACTIVE INDICATIONS FOR LENS SURGERY

The refractive indications for lens surgery include all the classic well-known refractive states of the "healthy" eye, which is why this new indication for lens surgery has been somewhat controversial. There may be no true histopathology to most of these eyes; however, some, such as those with extreme axial myopia, may be at risk for true pathology following surgical intervention. In addition, the historical development of spectacles and contact lenses, having long antedated the development of modern lens surgery, created a mind-set among many that "inborn errors of refraction" are not diseases and are therefore not conditions to be treated with medicine or surgery, especially if such treatment

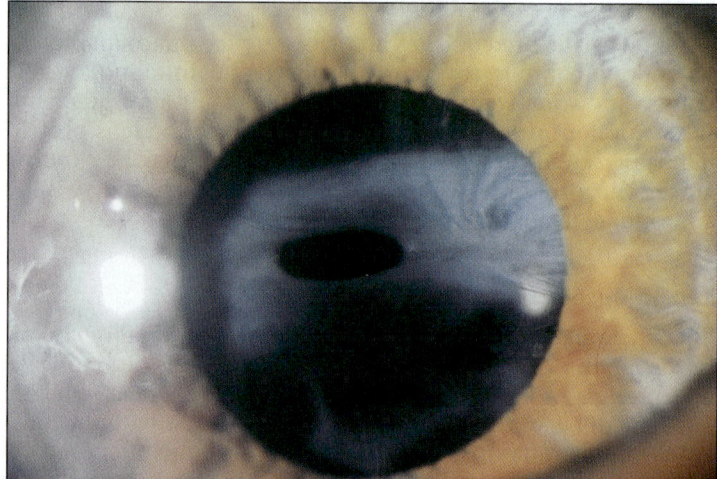

FIG. 42-5 ▉ **Fibrosis of the anterior capsule.** A "nonbiocompatible" reaction of lens epithelial cells (LECs) to hydrophobic intraocular lens materials.

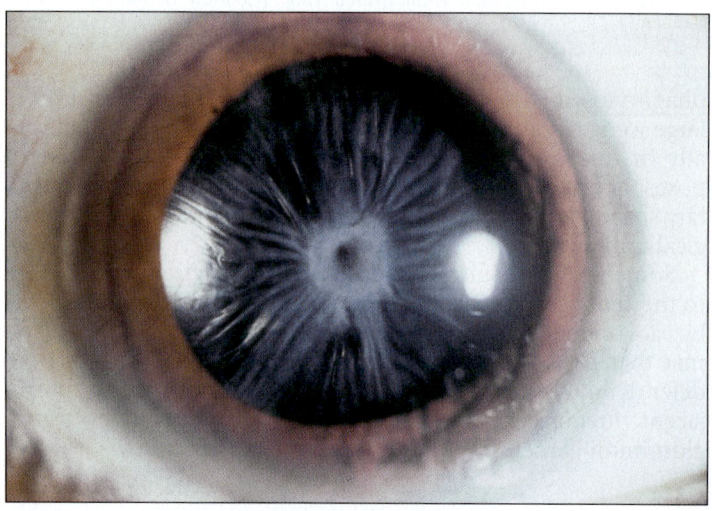

FIG. 42-4 ▉ Virtual complete closure of capsulorrhexis over a PMMA implant. (Courtesy of John Shepherd, M.D., Las Vegas, Nevada.)

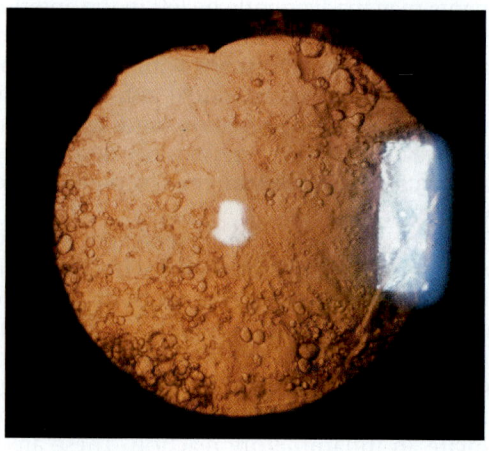

FIG. 42-6 ▉ Posterior capsular opacification by lens epithelial cell hyperplasia.

might unnecessarily endanger an eye or expose an otherwise "healthy" eye to undue risk. Although there may be merit to that argument, it is a concept that is rapidly losing popularity. Whether prudent or not, the global anterior segment ophthalmic surgical community has embarked on a new and enticing endeavor—rendering the human population emmetropic. The process began as an idea before its time in the 1950s, with the failed attempts of Sato at endothelial radial keratotomy and Barraquer and others at phakic anterior chamber IOL implantation.[18] The ophthalmic surgical "technolution" (technical revolution) that ensued over the following decades led to renewed interest in the surgical correction of refractive errors 30 years later in the 1980s, this time as an idea whose time had come. Refinements in ocular anesthesia, incision technology, lensectomy techniques, ophthalmic visco-surgical device (OVD) tissue protection, and IOL manufacturing and implantation allowed the successful return of the concept of intraocular correction of refractive errors, including both clear lensectomy and phakic implantation. All this, combined with the multitude of new keratorefractive procedures, has actually led to the development of a new, bona fide ophthalmic surgical subspecialty, that of refractive surgery.

As may be observed in Box 42-2, almost all the operable tissues and spaces of the eye have come under investigation as locations for refractive surgical modulation: corneal epithelial surface, corneal stroma, corneal endothelial surface, anterior chamber, iris, pupil, posterior chamber, lens, and sclera. The lens therefore assumes its role among the others as a popular location for surgical refractive modulation for those who prefer a familiar procedure that spares the cornea and saves the economic expense of an excimer laser. Those who decry the lenticular approach emphasize all the potential intraoperative and postoperative complications attendant with invasive intraocular procedures.

Despite the controversy, clear lens replacement stands as a viable procedure today for both myopia and hyperopia and has begun to be included in the surgical treatment of astigmatism and presbyopia. Toric IOLs are now available for the intraocular correction of astigmatism (Fig. 42-7). Multifocal IOLs represent some of the first attempts at the intraocular correction of presbyopia (Fig. 42-8). Other attempts at the development of a truly accommodative pseudophakos have included the intracapsular injection of liquid silicone[19-21] and the intracapsular placement of high-water-content poly-HEMA lenses, a liquid silicone-filled intracapsular balloon[22,23] (Fig. 42-9), multiple IOLs (polypseudophakia)[24,25] (Figs. 42-10 and 42-11), and flexible plate–haptic foldable accommodative IOLs.

BOX 42-2

REFRACTIVE SURGERY

I. Cornea
 A. Incisional keratotomy
  1. Radial (RK)
  2. Tangential astigmatic (AK)
 B. Laser thermal keratoplasty (LTK)
 C. Radiofrequency conductive keratoplasty (CK)
 D. Laser surface ablation (PRK)
 E. Subepithelial laser ablation (LASEK)
 F. Lamellar keratotomy/keratectomy
  1. Keratomileusis
  2. Keratophakia
  3. Automated lamellar keratectomy (ALK)
  4. Laser stromal ablation (LASIK)
 G. Intrastromal corneal inlays
  1. PMMA rings (Intacs)
  2. Hydrogel discs
  3. Gel injection
 H. Surface tissue onlays
  1. Epikeratophakia
  2. Epitheliokeratomileusis
II. Lens
 A. Clear lensectomy without IOL (aphakia)
 B. Clear lensectomy with monofocal or toric IOL (pseudophakia)
 C. Clear lensectomy with multiple monofocal IOLs (polypseudophakia)
 D. Clear lensectomy with multifocal IOL
 E. Clear lensectomy with accommodative IOL
III. Phakic IOL implantation
 A. Anterior chamber
  1. Angle fixation (Baikoff, Kelman)
  2. Iris fixation (Worst-Fechner, Singh)
  3. Scleral fixation (Maggi)
 B. Posterior chamber
  1. Pupillary fixation (Fyodorov)
  2. Zonular fixation (Fyodorov)
  3. Sulcus fixation (Fyodorov)
IV. Sclera
 A. Posterior homograft scleroplasty
 B. Scleral expansion/implantation (Schachar)
 C. Radial incisional sclerotomy (Thornton-Fukasaku)

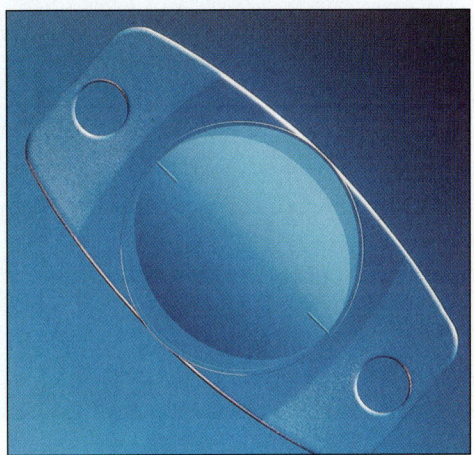
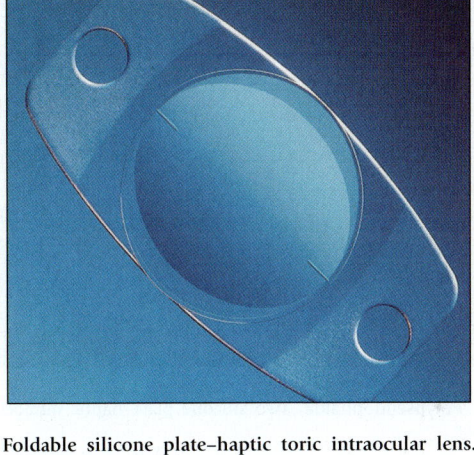

FIG.42-7 ▌ Foldable silicone plate–haptic toric intraocular lens. (Courtesy of STAAR Surgical, Monrovia, California.)

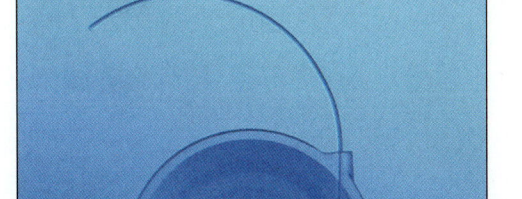

FIG. 42-8 ▌ Foldable silicone multifocal intraocular lens. (Courtesy of Advanced Medical Optics, Inc.)

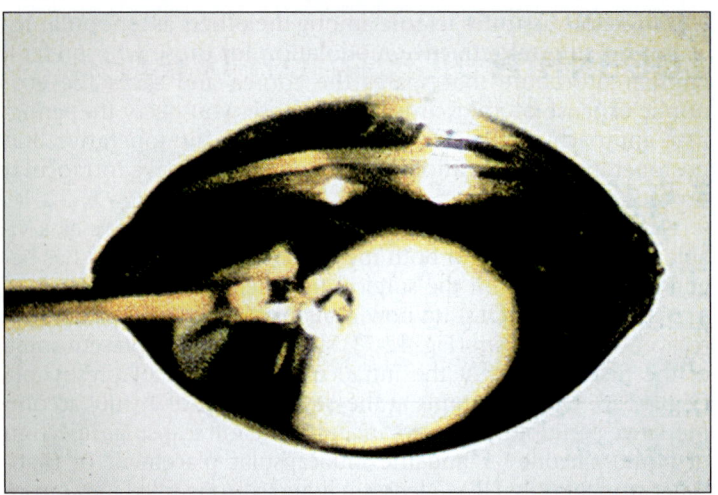

FIG. 42-9 ■ Accommodative inflatable silicone intracapsular balloon. (Courtesy O. Nishi, M.D., Osaka, Japan.)

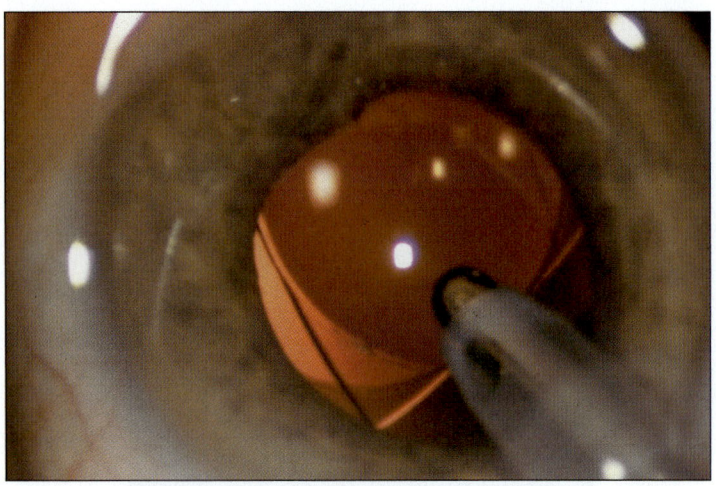

FIG. 42-10 ■ **Polypseudophakia.** Two silicone plate–haptic intraocular lenses in the capsular bag.

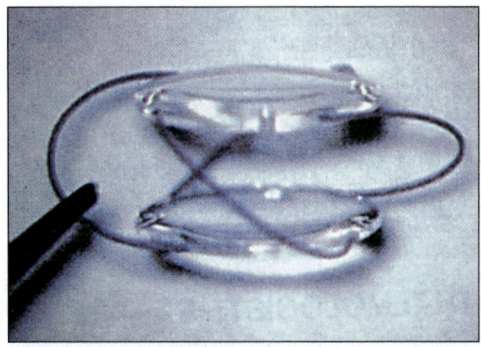

FIG. 42-11 ■ Accommodative PMMA polypseudophakic intraocular lens. (Courtesy of T. Hara.)

INDICATIONS FOR DIFFERENT LENS SURGERY TECHNIQUES

Surgery affecting the human lens can be organized historically by chronology of development (Table 42-1) or divided into four major categories by technique (Box 42-3):
• Lens repositioning
• Lens removal
• Lens replacement
• Lens enhancement

Lens repositioning, traditionally known as "couching," is perhaps the oldest form of lens surgery and is still in use in some

TABLE 42-1

HISTORY OF CATARACT SURGERY TECHNIQUES

Year	Technique	Place	Surgeon
800	Couching	India	Unknown
1015	Needle aspiration	Iraq	Unknown
1100	Needle aspiration	Syria	Unknown
1500	Couching	Europe	Unknown
1745	ECCE inferior incision	France	Daviel
1753	ICCE by thumb expression	England	Sharp
1860	ECCE superior incision	Germany	von Graefe
1880	ICCE by muscle-hook zonulysis and lens tumble	India	Smith
1900	ICCE by capsule forceps	Germany	Verhoeff Kalt
1940	ICCE by capsule suction erysiphake	Europe	Stoewer I. Barraquer
1949	ECCE with posterior chamber IOL and operating microscope	England	Ridley
1951	Anterior chamber IOLs	Italy Germany	Strampelli Dannheim
1957	ICCE by enzyme zonulysis	Spain	J. Barraquer
1961	ICCE by capsule cryoadhesion	Poland	Krawicz
1967	ECCE by phacoemulsification	United States	Kelman J. Shock
1975	Iris-pupil supported IOLs	Netherlands	Binkhorst Worst
1984	Foldable IOLs	United States South Africa	Mazzocco Epstein

ECCE, Extracapsular cataract extraction; *ICCE,* intracapsular cataract extraction; *IOL,* intraocular lens.

third-world countries today. In stark contrast, at the other end of the historical spectrum is the most recent category of lens surgery, that of lens functional enhancement. These new investigational techniques involve surgical procedures designed to enhance accommodation in the presbyopic eye.

The indications for a particular lens surgery technique may be determined by several factors (Box 42-4). Different medical conditions or pathological states of the eye and the lens may favor one technique over another. In some countries, the availability of equipment, as well as the level of training of the surgeon, may be factors that dictate technique. Certain countries have governmental agencies, professional organizations, academic institutions, insurance payers, or surgical facilities that regulate and control the types of surgical techniques surgeons may perform. For the purpose of this text, however, only specific medical or pathological conditions of the eye are discussed as factors determining the choice of surgical technique.

Couching

This is the oldest technique of lens surgery; it has been performed for more than 1000 years and is still in use today in some underdeveloped countries. The original method was an extracapsular technique that involved the placement of a sharp needle through the sclera at the pars plana, behind the iris, until the tip of the needle was visible in the pupil in front of the lens. The anterior capsule was then scratched open with the needle tip, and the nucleus was pushed inferiorly until the pupillary space appeared clear. This early extracapsular technique, which was being performed long before the development of topical anti-inflammatory medications, was associated with inflammation, secondary glaucoma, posterior synechiae, pupillary block, Soemmerring's rings, and capsular opacification, not to mention

BOX 42-3

LENS SURGERY TECHNIQUES

I. Lens repositioning ("couching")
  A. Extracapsular
  B. Intracapsular
    1. Physical (instrumental) zonulysis
    2. Pharmacological (enzymatic) zonulysis
II. Lens removal
  A. Total (intracapsular)
    1. Capsule forceps
    2. Suction erysiphake
    3. Cryoextraction
  B. Partial (extracapsular)
    1. Anterior capsulotomy/capsulectomy
      a. Discontinuous
      b. Continuous (capsulorrhexis)
      c. Linear
    2. Nucleus removal
      a. Assembled delivery (large incision)
        (1) Expression ("push")
        (2) Extraction ("pull")
      b. Disassembled extraction
        (1) Phacosection
        (2) Phacoemulsification-aspiration
          (a) Ultrasound
          (b) Laser
          (c) Water jet
          (d) Impeller
    3. Cortex removal
      a. Irrigation
      b. Aspiration
III. Lens replacement (intraocular lens implantation)
  A. Locations
    1. Anterior chamber
      a. Angle fixation
      b. Iris fixation
    2. Pupil
    3. Posterior chamber
      a. Iris fixation (sutured)
      b. Ciliary sulcus (sutured or unsutured)
    4. Lens capsule
      a. Anterior capsule
        (1) Haptic sulcus/optic bag
        (2) Optic posterior chamber/haptic bag
      b. Intracapsular ("bag-bag")
      c. Posterior capsule (haptic bag/optic Berger's space)
    5. Pars plana (sutured)
  B. Optic materials
    1. Hydrophobic
      a. PMMA
      b. Silicone
      c. Acrylic
    2. Hydrophilic
      a. Poly-HEMA
      b. Acrylic
      c. Collagen-copolymer
  C. Optic types
    1. Monofocal
      a. Spherical
        (1) Plus
        (2) Minus
      b. Toric
      c. Telescopic
      d. Prismatic
    2. Multifocal
    3. Accommodative
IV. Lens enhancement: reversal of presbyopia by scleral expansion
  A. Ciliary cerclage
  B. Radial anterior ciliary sclerotomy

BOX 42-4

LENS REMOVAL TECHNIQUES: OCULAR INDICATIONS

I. Intracapsular extraction
  A. Zonular absence/dialysis
  B. Lens subluxation
  C. Lens dislocation
II. Nuclear delivery
  A. Status of cornea
    1. Low endothelial cell count
    2. Guttate dystrophy
  B. Status of cataract
    1. Brunescent nuclear sclerosis
    2. Cataracta nigra
  C. Torn posterior capsule during phacoemulsification
  D. Zonulodialysis
III. Phacosection
  A. Same corneal, cataract, and capsular indications as nuclear delivery
  B. Astigmatism management
IV. Phacoemulsification
  A. Status of cornea
    1. Normal endothelial cell count
    2. No guttate dystrophy
  B. Status of cataract
    1. Immature nuclear sclerosis
    2. Cortical or subcapsular cataract
  C. Astigmatism management

couching can also be performed safely under an operating microscope in a matter of minutes following enzymatic zonulysis with α-chymotrypsin. Unlike the exposed nucleus and cortex in the extracapsular method, the intact, encapsulated, dislocated crystalline lens in the intracapsular method is immunologically inert. The low skill level required and the low cost of this simple, safe, fast, and effective procedure make it an attractive alternative for economically disadvantaged third-world countries, which harbor a large majority of the world's estimated 18 million cataract blind.

Intracapsular Extraction

The intracapsular method of lens removal has not been the procedure of choice in industrialized nations since the development of modern extracapsular techniques in the late 1970s, primarily because of lower rates of postoperative posterior segment complications such as hemorrhage, vitreous loss, retinal detachment, and cystoid macular edema. Current indications for planned intracapsular extraction, therefore, are related to intraocular conditions that preclude safe and successful extracapsular surgery. The absence or lysis of a significant number of zonular fibers, which may occur as an isolated congenital anomaly or as a result of Marfan's syndrome, pseudoexfoliation, trauma, or following pars plana surgery, may be an indication for intracapsular extraction. Significant subluxation or dislocation of the lens may leave no other option except for removal of the lens in its capsule.

Traditionally, intracapsular extraction involved removal of the complete intact lens through a large incision measuring 11–16mm. Later, implantation of a PMMA IOL, either primarily or secondarily, rendered these eyes pseudophakic, with both procedures requiring sutures. A more modern small incision intracapsular technique is one in which the capsule, cortex, and nucleus are all removed by phacoemulsification through a 3mm scleral incision, followed by PMMA anterior chamber IOL implantation through a 5–6mm scleral incision and no sutures. This rare technique may be of particular value in eyes that demonstrate no zonular support upon introduction of the phacoemulsification tip. In addition, a foldable silicone IOL can be implanted through the small incision and sutured to the posterior surface of the iris or to the sclera.

endophthalmitis. Considering current technology, there may be no indications for extracapsular couching today.

Intracapsular couching, however, is another matter. This procedure was (and still is) performed without anesthesia with the patient in the sitting position, sometimes outdoors. However,

Nuclear Delivery

This technique became popular in the 1980s as surgeons, who had been performing long incision intracapsular extraction and anterior chamber implantation, desired the benefits derived from an intact posterior capsule and posterior chamber implantation. The technique persists today and is performed in great numbers, particularly in Asian countries, where the more advanced small incision techniques of phacoemulsification and foldable lens implantation are not yet available. In Europe, Japan, and the United States, where phacoemulsification and foldable lens implantation are widely standard, the only ocular indication for planned nuclear delivery may be an advanced nucleus that is too hard to be emulsified safely. Corneas at risk for developing irreversible edema, such as those with low endothelial cell counts or guttate dystrophy, may be relative indications for nuclear delivery. However, small incision lens surgery in the presence of high-risk corneas remains a viable option, particularly when highly retentive dispersive ophthalmic visco-surgical devices are used in combination with endolenticular or intercapsular phacoemulsification.

Another indication for nuclear delivery is the occurrence of a tear in the posterior capsule during phacoemulsification. Although it may be possible to continue to emulsify the nucleus over ophthalmic visco-surgical device or over a lens glide (Michelson technique), a large capsular tear with presentation of vitreous may preclude safe emulsification, necessitating incision enlargement and nuclear delivery.

Phacosection

These techniques involve delivering the nucleus not as a single intact unit in one step through a large incision, but in parts through a small incision. The nucleus may be separated concentrically, delivering the smallest endonucleus separately from outer layers of epinucleus. This technique may be performed through a 7–8mm sutureless scleral incision using side-port irrigation through a chamber maintainer to hydroexpress the nuclear components, which delaminate as they pass through the incision. This has been called the "mini-nuc" technique.[26]

True intraocular phacosection involves bisecting or trisecting the nucleus by instrumentation, achieving geometrical nuclear division in the anterior chamber. The small sections may then be removed linearly with forceps through incisions as small as 3–4mm.[27]

The indications for phacosection techniques are the same as those for intact nuclear delivery, as a manual extracapsular technique, with the addition of astigmatism management. Unlike long incision, single-stage nuclear delivery, small incision phacosection may induce no change in astigmatism, particularly if a foldable lens is used and all is accomplished through a 3mm scleral incision.

Phacoemulsification

This technique of nucleus removal has been performed through incisions ranging from 3.2mm down to less than 1.0mm. Combined with foldable lens implantation, the major advantage of phacoemulsification is the small incision. Current techniques are using self-sealing, sutureless scleral and clear corneal incisions measuring 2.3–3.2mm. These incisions should be astigmatically neutral. Corneal incisions can be moved centrally from the limbus and can be grooved as two-plane, two-stage incisions, allowing the reduction of preexisting astigmatism, especially when used in combination with astigmatic keratotomy.[28] Therefore, the presence of corneal cylinder is an indication for phacoemulsification and foldable lens implantation, just as is the absence of corneal cylinder.

The status of both the nucleus and the cornea factors into the decision whether to perform phacoemulsification. It has been observed that with certain phacoemulsification techniques, the

longer the duration of ultrasound, the greater the loss of endothelial cells (Fig. 42-12). In addition, the closer the emulsification process is to the cornea, the more cells are lost (Table 42-2), and corneas with guttatae lose more cells than normal corneas do (Table 42-3). Therefore, the degree of nuclear sclerosis and the health of the cornea are indications for protective ophthalmic visco-surgical devices and for phacoemulsification as far away from the cornea as possible. When phacoemulsification was originally performed in the anterior chamber and in the iris plane, high-risk corneas and dense nuclei were considered contraindications, and nuclear delivery was recommended. However, long ultrasound times have been shown to be well tolerated when the ultrasonic energy is confined to the capsular bag. Newer emulsification techniques, such as phaco chop[29] and high vacuum, have also been shown to greatly reduce ultrasound times, providing further protection to the cornea (Box 42-5). Newer modalities of nuclear emulsification not involving ultrasound include sonic mode (Staar Wave), with axial movements of the tip reduced from 40,000 to 400 cycles per second; neodymium:YAG laser[30-34]; erbium:YAG laser[35-37]; pulsed water jet; "plasma blade" molecular bond disruption; impeller aspiration-emulsification; and others.

Lens Capsule Surgery

When capsulectomy was first conceived, it was performed in discontinuous fashion, either as multiple punctures ("can-opener") with a bent needle or cystotome or as triangular (Kelman) or square (Gills) capsulectomies facilitated with scissors (Fig. 42-13). Discontinuous openings, being weak, allow easy dislocation of the nucleus anteriorly for either delivery or emulsification. However, they are also prone to developing multiple radial anterior tears out to the equator, with possible extension around to the posterior capsule.[38] Postoperatively, they have a high rate of posterior synechia formation and anterior IOL loop dislocation.[39] Plate-haptic lenses are contraindicated in the presence of a discontinuous anterior capsular opening, as they have also been shown to dislocate anteriorly postoperatively. There is, therefore, rarely a current indication for a discontinuous capsulectomy, except possibly in the case of advanced nuclear sclerosis with absence of a red reflex and nonavailability of a biological capsule stain, such as trypan blue or indocyanine green.

Continuous curvilinear capsulectomy (CCC), also known as capsulorrhexis,[40] is much more desirable than previous discontinuous methods. The continuous anterior capsular opening is stronger and more resistant to radial tearing than are discontin-

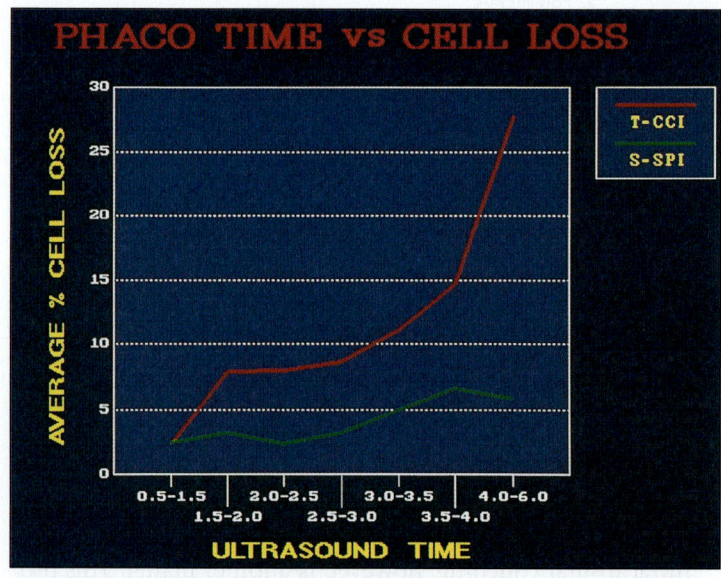

FIG. 42-12 ■ Endothelial cell loss in relation to (1) scleral versus corneal incision phacoemulsification and (2) duration of ultrasound.

uous openings.[41] The continuous anterior capsulectomy of the appropriate size and shape has also been shown to retain IOL haptics of all designs and materials within the capsular bag postoperatively virtually 100% of the time. A circular opening of 4–5mm also readily retains the nucleus for *in situ* or endolenticular emulsification techniques. Larger openings of 6–7mm allow nuclear prolapse for intact delivery, phacosection, or anterior chamber emulsification. Continuous openings that are too small may contract postoperatively due to fibrous metaplasia of LECs (see Figs. 42-4 and 42-5), obstructing not only the patient's vision but also the doctor's view, precluding examination and treatment of fundus disorders. YAG laser anterior capsulectomy would then be indicated, just as posterior capsulectomy is indicated for posterior capsular opacification. The ideal continuous anterior capsular opening is 1.0mm smaller than the diameter of the lens optic to be implanted.

The capsular contents may also be removed through a linear capsulotomy rather than a capsulectomy. Both discontinuous and continuous linear capsulotomy techniques have been employed for nuclear delivery[42] and emulsification.[43] The advantage of these intercapsular techniques, if the anterior capsule is left intact during surgery, is protection of the cornea. Leaving the anterior capsule in place also offers the postoperative possibility of total encapsulation of an accommodative pseudophakos. The implantation of a pliable refractive material into a complete, intact lens capsule may establish the potential for pseudophakic accommodation.

Animal experimental trials were begun in the early 1980s, first by Schanzlin's group, who evacuated the capsular contents through a 3mm linear capsulotomy and injected liquid silicone in rabbit eyes.[44] These procedures worked surgically; however, the resultant optical power of the liquid injectable material could not be controlled, the anterior capsules became opacified by white fibrosis in a few weeks, and accommodative function was not determined. In the late 1980s, Nishi *et al.*[23] developed a liquid silicone-filled intracapsular balloon and placed it in monkey eyes. The power of the IOL was now controllable, and Scheimpflug photography demonstrated 6D of apparent accommodation. Also in the late 1980s, the first potentially accommodating IOLs were placed in human eyes; they were 66% water, poly-HEMA "full-size" expandable IOLs.[45] Unfortunately, none of these first human subjects, approximately 46 in number, demonstrated accommodation. A more recent design is that of a flexible hinged plate–haptic silicone IOL.

Although there may be major surgical and clinical advantages to leaving most of the lens capsule in the eye, there are also disadvantages with present materials and techniques. The posterior capsule can opacify as a result of lens epithelial cell hyperplasia (see Fig. 42-6), and the anterior capsule can opacify as a result of lens epithelial cell fibrous metaplasia (see Fig. 42-5). In addition, excessive fibrosis can result in contraction of the entire capsule with deformation of the IOL haptics, decentration of the IOL optic, and zonular dialysis with capsular bag subluxation or dislocation. Efforts to prevent unwanted postoperative lens epithelial cell activity have included primary posterior capsulotomy, primary posterior capsulectomy,[46] and methods of mechanically cleaning the capsule, including vacuuming, vacuuming with ultrasound, curettage, and cryosurgery (Box 42-6).[47] Attempts at pharmacologically disabling the lens epithelial cell have included hypotonic hydrolavage, antiprostaglandins,[15,16] antimetabolites,[17] and immunosuppressors.[18] These techniques are currently under investigation. In addition, newer IOL materials that are hydrophilic, such as poly-HEMA, acrylic, and collagen-copolymer, appear to stimulate very low levels of lens epithelial hyperplasia and almost no fibrous metaplasia. The possibility of using hydrophilic IOLs as drug delivery systems is also very attractive. However, the most recent clinical advancement that has been demonstrated to reduce the incidence of posterior capsular opacification is the use of IOL optics with "square" posterior edges (Fig. 42-14). These are manufactured in acrylic (Alcon,

TABLE 42-2

ENDOTHELIAL CELL LOSS IN PHACOEMULSIFICATION

	Percent Cell Loss
Anterior chamber	20
Posterior chamber	14
Phaco-in-situ in the capsular bag	7
Intact anterior capsule (intercapsular phacoemulsification)	4

TABLE 42-3

ENDOTHELIAL CELL LOSS FOLLOWING PHACOEMULSIFICATION IN EYES WITH NORMAL CORNEAS VERSUS EYES WITH DISEASED CORNEAS

	Percent Cell Loss
Normal cornea	7
Guttatae	14

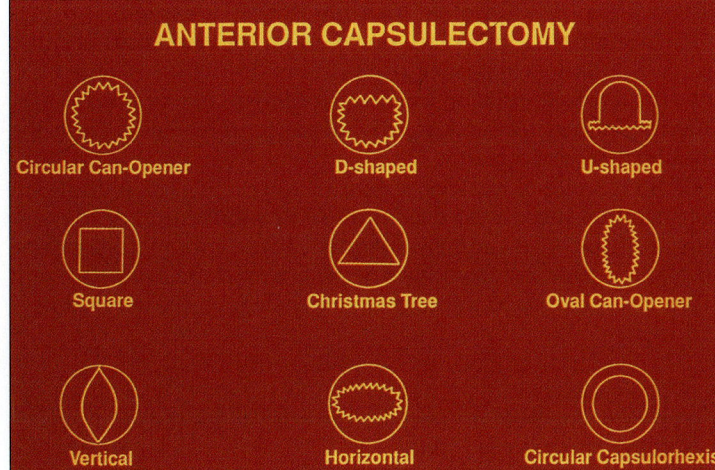

FIG. 42-13 ■ Anterior capsulectomy shapes used for extracapsular cataract surgery. (Courtesy of Adanced Medical Optics, Inc.)

BOX 42-5

PHACOEMULSIFICATION TECHNIQUES

I. Location
  A. Anterior chamber (Kelman, Brown)
  B. Iris plane (Kratz)
  C. Posterior chamber (supracapsular) (Maloney)
  D. Capsule (endolenticular, in situ)
    1. Anterior capsulectomy (Sinskey)
    2. Anterior capsulotomy (intercapsular) (Hara)
II. Techniques
  A. Carousel
  B. Chip-and-flip (Fine)
  C. Phacofracture
    1. Divide-and-conquer (Gimbel)
    2. Four-quadrant pregrooved (Shepherd)
    3. Nonstop chop (Nagahara)
    4. Stop-and-chop (Koch)
    5. Double chop (Kammann)

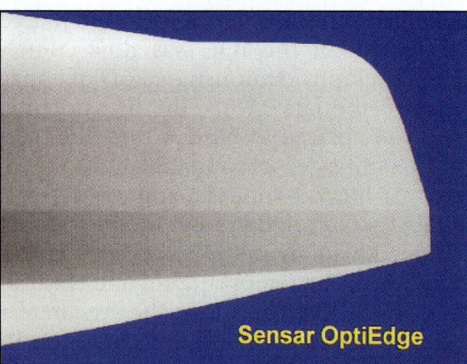

FIG. 42-14 ■ Acrylic intraocular lens optic, Sensar® AR40e, with rounded anterior edge and squared posterior edge. (Courtesy of AMO.)

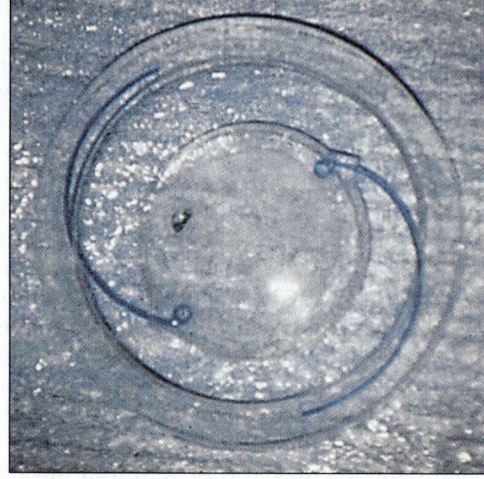

FIG. 42-15 ■ Complete closed, circular, foldable silicone endocapsular ring. (Courtesy of T. Hara.)

BOX 42-6

LENS EPITHELIAL CELL SURGERY

I. Primary procedures
  A. Mechanical
    1. Capsular polishing
    2. Capsular vacuuming
    3. Capsular vacuuming with ultrasound
    4. Capsular curettage
    5. Capsular cryo
  B. Pharmacological
    1. Hypotonic hydrolavage
    2. Antimetabolites
    3. Antiprostaglandins
  C. Immunological
    1. Monoclonal antibodies
  D. Prophylactic posterior capsulotomy/capsulectomy (CCC)
II. Secondary procedures
  A. Invasive
    1. Capsulotomy/capsulectomy (CCC)
    2. Curettage
    3. Vacuuming
  B. Noninvasive
    1. Nd:YAG laser capsulotomy/capsulectomy

AcrySof MA60AC and AMO, Sensar AR40e) and in silicone (AMO, ClariflexBand Pharmacia C911). The square edge has been shown to be a physical barrier to the central posterior migration of LECs.[23]

Zonular Surgery

The preceding discussion of the surgical management of the lens capsule concentrated on endocapsular techniques and management of the viable LECs on the interior surface of the lens capsule. The discussion would be incomplete if it did not address a significant, difficult, new area of capsular surgery that deals with an abnormality of the exterior capsule—management of the weak or partially absent zonule.

In most cases, the goal of this type of lens surgery is the same as that for eyes without a compromised zonule: to remove the contents of the capsular bag though a CCC and replace the contents with a foldable IOL. However, in these cases, the goal is extended to include performing the surgery without further compromising the zonule, without disrupting the vitreous, without jeopardizing the long-term integrity of the capsulozonular apparatus, and, if possible, to recircularize and recenter a subluxed capsule.

To accomplish these surgical goals and avoid a long incision, intracapsular extraction, vitrectomy, and anterior chamber IOL, several modifications to the standard procedure are planned for eyes with compromised zonules. In these eyes, there is some zonular support to the capsule (partial zonular absence), enough of a circumference of attached fibers to support CCC and implantation of an endocapsular ring. If only a small percentage of the zonule is attached, or if the zonule is completely absent, intracapsular extraction with anterior chamber IOL or sutured posterior chamber IOL may be the only technique available.

Endocapsular rings were originally conceived in Japan, not for the purpose of supporting the zonule, but for the purpose of placing pressure on the equatorial LECs to prevent posterior capsular opacification. Two models were manufactured in the early 1990s. A completely closed circular model, made of silicone for foldability and implantability through a 3mm incision, was designed by Hara (Fig. 42-15), and an open PMMA model was designed by Nagamoto. It was subsequently demonstrated in clinical trials and by phase-contrast videography of living LECs (Nagamoto and Bissen-Miyajima) that the presence of a ring in the capsular equator had no effect on the viability and migratory activity of LECs. Witchell *et al.* in Germany also designed an open PMMA ring for the purpose of supporting capsules with compromised zonules (Fig. 42-16), and Cionni (Cincinnati, Ohio) designed modifications to the PMMA capsule tension rings (CTRs) to allow them to be sutured to the eye wall,[48] thus creating a synthetic "pseudozonule" attached to an intracapsular skeletal supporting apparatus (Fig. 42-17). When surgery on such eyes is planned, if OVD is to be used for the CCC, care must be taken not to overinflate the eye, especially with a dispersive OVD, as this may stress or further tear zonular fibers. A CCC can usually be performed and should be large. This facilitates hydrodissection and allows for the possibility of nuclear hydro- or viscoexpression. Complete hydrodissection is essential so that nuclear manipulations place no stress on the remaining zonular fibers. Similarly, expressing the nucleus through the large CCC into the supracapsular space, the pupillary plane, or the anterior chamber allows for nuclear emulsification safely away from the zonulocapsular apparatus.

If the zonule is weak or absent in only a limited meridional arc such that there is no decentration or subluxation of the capsule, a simple CTR can be implanted. These simple rings can be implanted with forceps or by injection with a special instrument (Geuder) and can be implanted at any stage in the surgical procedure:

- After hydrodissection, before phacoemulsification
- During phacoemulsification
- After phacoemulsification, before cortical aspiration
- During cortical aspiration
- After cortical aspiration, before IOL implantation

If there is capsular subluxation, a Cionni CTR may be implanted; ideally, the ring is sutured to the sclera in the meridian that is the

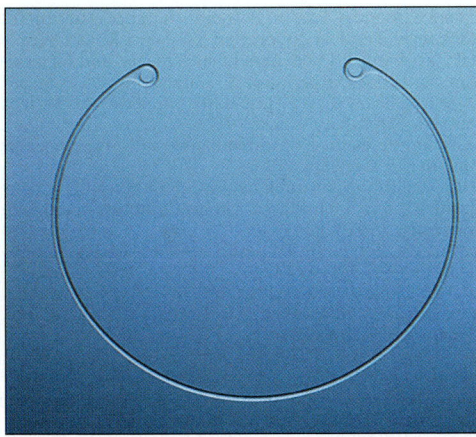

FIG. 42-16 ■ Open PMMA endocapsular ring. (Courtesy of Morcher, GMBh, Germany.)

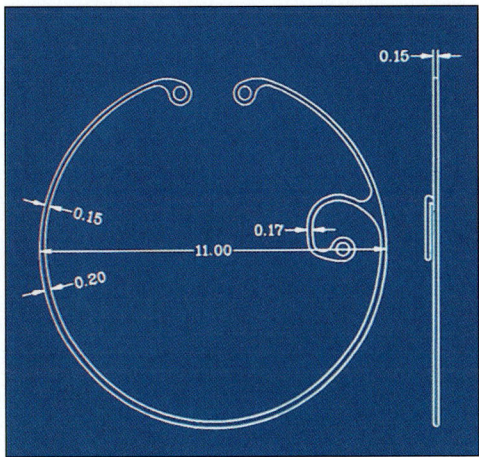

FIG. 42-17 ■ Cionni-modified endocapsular ring for suturing to sclera to create a pseudozonule. (Courtesy of Morcher, GMBh, Germany.)

center of the arc of zonular absence. The ring will recentralize the capsule, and the suture will recentralize the capsule and will re-elevate a posteriorly tilted capsule to the zonular plane.

Another modification to the routine technique is that of lowering the infusion bottle to a level that provides the slowest stream of irrigation beyond a drip, such that the phacotip is cooled and the chamber is maintained, but excessive volume with posterior displacement of the lens is avoided. The Cionni ring type of sutured skeletal support of the capsule is often strong enough to support careful endocapsular phacoemulsification techniques. Chopping performed with equicentripetal forces places no lateral stress on the zonule.

When choosing an IOL, it would be ideal to implant a material that induces no fibrous metaplasia of the LECs and a design that blocks the formation of central posterior capsular opacification. Therefore, PMMA and silicone are not ideal materials for these eyes. Among those currently available, the IOL of choice is one with an acrylic optic and a square posterior edge. Two such models are available, the Alcon AcrySof MA60AC and the AMO Sensar AR40e (see Fig. 42-14). Additionally, these hydrophobic acrylics unfold in a very slow, controlled fashion that produces zero stress on the capsule or zonule.

Surgery for Presbyopia

These new and experimental procedures are designed to enhance lens function; that is, they are performed to improve the amplitude of accommodation in a presbyopic eye. These proce-

dures are intended for purely presbyopic noncataractous eyes with no lenticular pathology other than the normal physiological middle-aged loss of accommodative function.

Although one could theoretically make a case for clear lens replacement with an accommodative pseudophakos, it has never been conclusively demonstrated that loss of elasticity of the lens is the sole or even the major cause of presbyopia—in fact, more to the contrary. Changes have been shown to occur in the area of insertion of the zonular fibers, as well as in the configuration of the ciliary muscle. With only this limited knowledge, the present procedures represent the first attempts at the surgical correction of presbyopia by altering the ciliary architecture. Scleral expansion over the ciliary muscle by implantation of four circumferential PMMA rods or by radial sclerotomy, restoring tension to the flaccid zonular fibers, has been shown in early clinical studies to have mixed success at restoring some accommodative power to the ciliary-zonule-lens mechanism.

REFERENCES

1. Chylack LT Jr, Wolfe JK, Singer DM, *et al.* The lens opacities classification system. Version III (LOCS-III). Arch Ophthalmol. 1993;111:831.
2. Lasa MSM, Datiles MB III, Freidlin V. Potential vision tests in patients with cataracts. Ophthalmology. 1995;102:1007–11.
3. Datiles MB III, Magno BV, Freidlin V. Study of nuclear cataract progression using the National Eye Institute Scheimpflug system. Br J Ophthalmol. 1995;79:527–34.
4. Lopez JLL, Freidlin V, Datiles MB III. Longitudinal study of posterior subcapsular opacities using the National Eye Institute computer planimetry system. Br J Ophthalmol. 1995;79:535–40.
5. Steinberg EP, Tielsch JM, Schein OD, *et al.* The VF-14: an index of functional impairment in patients with cataract. Arch Ophthalmol. 1994;112:630–8.
6. Steinberg EP, Tielsch JM, Schein OD, *et al.* National study of cataract surgery outcomes: variation in 4-month post-operative outcomes as reflected in multiple outcome measures. Ophthalmology. 1994;101:1131–41.
7. Schein OD, Steinberg EP, Cassard SD, *et al.* Predictors of outcome in patients who underwent cataract surgery. Ophthalmology. 1995;102:817–23.
8. Cassard SD, Patrick DL, Damiano AM, *et al.* Reproducibility and responsiveness of the VF-14: an index of functional impairment in patients with cataracts. Arch Ophthalmol. 1995;113:1508–13.
9. Mangione CM, Phillips RS, Lawrence MG, *et al.* Improved visual function and attenuation of declines in health-related quality of life after cataract extraction. Arch Ophthalmol. 1994;112:1419–25.
10. Mangione CM, Orav EJ, Lawrence MG, *et al.* Prediction of visual function after cataract surgery: a prospectively validated model. Arch Ophthalmol. 1995;113:1305–11.
11. Edwards MG, Schachat AP, Bressler SB, Bressler NM. Outcome of cataract operations performed to permit diagnosis, to determine eligibility for laser therapy, or to perform laser therapy of retinal disorders. Am J Ophthalmol. 1994;118:440–4.
12. Fukaya Y, Hara T, Hara T, Iwata S. Effect of freezing on lens epithelial cell growth. J Cataract Refract Surg. 1988;14:309–11.
13. McDonnell PJ, Krause W, Glaser BM. In vitro inhibition of lens epithelial cell proliferation and migration. Ophthalmic Surg. 1988;19:25–30.
14. Inan UU, Ozturk F, Kaynak S, *et al.* Prevention of posterior capsule opacification by intraoperative single-dose pharmacologic agents. J Cataract Refract Surg. 2001;27:1079–87.
15. Nishi O, Nishi K, Yamada Y, Mizumoto Y. Effect of indomethacin-coated posterior chamber intraocular lenses on post-operative inflammation and posterior capsular opacification, J Cataract Refract Surg. 1995;21:574–8.
16. Tetz M, Ries M, Lucas C, *et al.* Inhibition of posterior capsule opacification by an intraocular-lens-bound sustained drug delivery system: an experimental animal study and literature review. J Cataract Refract Surg. 1996;22:1070–8.
17. Power WJ, Neylav D, Collum LMT. Daunomycin as an inhibitor of human lens epithelial cell proliferation in culture. J Cataract Refract Surg. 1994;20:287–90.
18. Goins KM, Optiz JR, Fulcher SFA, *et al.* Inhibition of proliferating lens epithelium with antitransferrin receptor immunotoxin. J Cataract Refract Surg. 1994;20:513–5.
19. Gindi JJ, Wan WL, Schanzlin DJ. Endocapsular cataract surgery. I. Surgical technique. Cataract. 1985;2(5):6–10.
20. Haefliger E, Parel J-M, Fantes F, *et al.* Accommodation of an endocapsular silicone lens (Phaco-ersatz) in the non-human primate. Ophthalmology. 1987;94(5):471–7.
21. Haefliger E, Parel J-M. Accommodation of an endocapsular silicone lens (Phaco-ersatz) in the aging rhesus money. J Refract Corneal Surg. 1994;10:550.
22. Nishi O. Refilling the lens of the rabbit eye after endocapsular cataract surgery. Folia Ophthalmol Jpn. 1987;38:1615–8.
23. Nishi O, Hara T, Hayashi F, *et al.* Further development of experimental techniques for refilling the lens of animal eyes with a balloon. J Cataract Refract Surg. 1989;15:584–8.
24. Hara T, Hara T, Yasuda A, Yamada Y. Accommodative intraocular lens with spring action. Part 1. Design and placement in an excised animal eye. Ophthalmic Surg. 1990;21:128–33.
25. Hara T, Hara T, Yasuda A, *et al.* Accommodative intraocular lens with spring action. Part 2. Fixation in the living rabbit. Ophthalmic Surg. 1992;23:632–5.
26. Blumenthal M, Assia EI. Extracapsular cataract extraction. In: Nordan LT, Maxwell WA, Davison JA, eds. The surgical rehabilitation of vision. New York: Gower; 1992:ch 10.
27. McIntyre DJ. Cataract surgery: techniques, complications and management. In: Steinert RF, ed. Phacosection cataract surgery. Philadelphia: WB Saunders; 1995:119–22.

28. Kershner RM. Keratolenticuloplasty. In: Kersher RM, ed. Refractive keratotomy for cataract surgery and the correction of astigmatism. New Jersey: Slack; 1994:ch 3.

29. Koch PS, Katzen LE. Stop and chop phacoemulsification. J Cataract Refrac Surg. 1994;20:566–70.

30. Dodick JM, Christiansen J. Experimental studies on the development and propagation of shock waves created by the interaction of short Nd:YAG laser pulses with a titanium target. J Cataract Refract Surg. 1991;17:794–7.

31. Grabner G, Alzner E. Dodick laser phacolysis: thermal effects. J Cataract Refract Surg. 1999;25:800–3.

32. Kanellopoulos AJ, Dodick JM, Brauweiler P, Alzner E. Dodick photolysis for cataract surgery. Ophthalmology. 1999;106:2197–202.

33. Huetz WW, Eckhardt B. Photolysis using the Dodick-ARC laser system for cataract surgery. J Cataract Refract Surg. 2001;27:208–12.

34. Kanellopoulos AJ: Laser cataract surgery: a prospective clinical evaluation of 1000 consecutive laser cataract procedures using the Dodick photolysis Nd:YAG system. Ophthalmology. 2001;108:649–55.

35. Neubaur CC, Stevens S. Erbium:YAG laser cataract removal: role of fiber-optic delivery system. J Cataract Refract Surg. 1999;25:514–20.

36. Hoh H, Fischer E. Pilot study on erbium laser phacoemulsification. Ophthalmology. 2001;107:1053–62.

37. Duran SD, Zato M. Erbium:YAG laser emulsification of the cataractous lens. J Cataract Refract Surg. 2001;27:1025–32.

38. Assia E, Apple D, Barden O, et al. An experimental study comparing various anterior capsulectomy techniques. Arch Ophthalmol. 1991;109:642–7.

39. Apple D, Park S, Merkley K, et al. Posterior chamber intraocular lenses in a series of 75 autopsy eyes. Part I. Loop location. J Cataract Refract Surg. 1986;12:358–62.

40. Gimbel HV, Neuhann T. Development, advantages, and methods of the continuous circular capsulorrhexis technique. J Cataract Refract Surg. 1990;16:31–7.

41. Assia E, Apple D, Tsai J, Lim E. The elastic properties of the lens capsule in capsulorrhexis. Am J Ophthalmol. 1991;111:628–32.

42. Galand A. A simple method of implantation within the capsular bag. Am Intraocular Implant Soc J. 1983;9:330–2.

43. Hara T, Hara T. Intraocular implantation in an almost completely retained capsular bag with a 4.5 to 5.0 millimeter linear dumbbell opening in the human eye. Ophthalmic Surg. 1992;23:545–50.

44. Gindi JJ, Wan WL, Schanzlin DJ. Endocapsular cataract surgery. I. Surgical technique. Cataract. 1985;2(5):6–10.

45. Blumenthal M. Clinical evaluation of full-size hydrogel lens—concept and reality. Six years experience. Presented at Symposium on Cataract, IOL, and Refractive Surgery, Boston, April 9, 1991.

46. Galand A, Galand A, van Cauenberge F, Moosavi J. Posterior capsulorrhexis in adult eyes with intact and clear capsules. J Cataract Refract Surg. 1996;22:458–61.

47. Hara T, Hara T. Observations on lens epithelial cells and their removal in anterior capsule specimens. Arch Ophthalmol. 1988;106:1683–7.

48. Ahmed II, Crandall AS. Ab externo scleral fixation of the Cionni modified capsular tension ring. J Cataract Refract Surg. 2001;207:977–81.

43

Patient Work-up for Cataract Surgery

FRANK HOWES

KEY FEATURES

- Any patient undergoing cataract surgery, whether topical, local or general anesthesia is to be used, should have a general medical and an ophthalmological work-up.
- The general medical work-up should evaluate the patient for systemic disorders, particularly cardiac, bronchopulmonary, or cerebrovascular disease, as well as diabetes mellitus and systemic hypertension.
- A patient's social history may be important, particularly if there is a history of smoking or substance abuse.
- Specific preoperative ophthalmic tests include refraction and visual acuity, corneal topography, specular microscopy, biometry, and B-scan ultrasonography.

INTRODUCTION

Any patient who needs to undergo cataract surgery, whether topical, local or general anesthesia is used, has both a general medical and an ophthalmological work-up. Even if a topical anesthetic is used, surgery is stressful for a patient, especially if there is a coexistent medical disorder. Therefore, the patient's overall welfare is entrusted to a skilled physician, usually the anesthesiologist. The cataract surgeon concentrates on the eye and should not be distracted by the patient's systemic needs during surgery, even if the surgeon possesses the requisite skills. Although most cataract procedures are uneventful with regard to the patient's medical condition, any problem or crisis is potentially ruinous, especially if surgery becomes complicated or prolonged. It is therefore incumbent upon the surgical and anesthetic team to be aware of every patient's medical status.

Cataract management is a team affair. The family doctor provides the medical history and current therapeutic information. Nursing members of the team have more contact with the patient than does the surgeon, and they can address the patient's immediate needs as well as provide a confidence-boosting ambience. Technical and administrative personnel complete the team, along with the anesthesiologist and ophthalmic surgeon.

MEDICAL HISTORY AND CURRENT THERAPEUTIC REGIMEN

A history of cardiac, bronchopulmonary, or cerebrovascular incidents, especially if recent, influences the timing and management of surgery. Diabetes mellitus and systemic hypertension are common in the population predisposed to operable cataract formation, and these conditions may adversely influence both the surgery and the postoperative course of events.[1] Other medical conditions are noted, and although it is unusual for an ophthalmic team to perform a general examination, this is done if the history suggests that it may be worthwhile (to be forewarned is to be forearmed). Ram et al.,[2] in a study of more than 6000 patients who underwent cataract surgery, discovered multiple morbidities that arose from a

TABLE 43-1

MORBIDITY IN CATARACT SURGERY PATIENTS

Condition	Percentage
Significant medical history	84
Diabetes mellitus	16
Systemic hypertension	47
Ischemic heart disease	38
Hypothyroidism	18
Undiagnosed tumors	3

variety of conditions. The major causes included pulmonary disease, cardiovascular and hypertensive disorders, diabetes mellitus, and significant orodental problems that required intervention.

Ram et al.[2] also noted significant postoperative problems in 1.27% of their patients, nearly half of whom required hospitalization. Thus, they concluded that all patients for whom cataract surgery is planned should undergo evaluation for systemic disease to prevent morbidity, or even mortality, in the preoperative, intraoperative, and postoperative periods. It is not uncommon for thyroid disorders to be associated with cataract surgery; they may even be precipitated by the surgical intervention.[3] Fisher and Cunningham[4] noted an even higher morbidity in their cohort of patients who had cataract surgery (Table 43-1).

The presence of disorders that might make cooperation difficult during surgery must be determined so that the operating environment can be optimized. These include Parkinson's disease and other involuntary movement disorders involving the head, face, and lids; communication difficulty; and excessive fear or anxiety. These factors influence both the surgeon's and the anesthesiologist's decision about the form of anesthetic to use and the sedation required.

The patient's social history may provide useful information, especially with reference to smoking, because breathing difficulties during surgery and coughing after surgery could compromise the surgical outcome. Similarly, substance abuse may be linked to poor patient compliance during surgery, as well as having implications for postoperative medication and management. Good preoperative assessment and management can minimize the risks associated with operating on these patients.

Systemic disorders may provide clues to the existence of an association between the morphology and the corresponding lens opacities (Table 43-2). When a systemic disorder is present, ensuring a good understanding of the pharmacological and other therapeutic measures used in its management is an essential component of the preoperative work-up.

OPHTHALMIC HISTORY AND EXAMINATION

It is important to establish whether there are coexistent ophthalmic conditions that may influence the cataract surgery, postoperative recovery, or outcome. Both eyes are assessed fully by routine ophthalmological work-up, which includes tonometry,

TABLE 43-2

SYSTEMIC DISORDERS AND LENS OPACITIES

Systemic Disorder	Appearance in the Eye
Myotonic dystrophy	Blue dot cortical cataract and posterior subcapsular cataract
Wilson's disease	Green sunflower cataract (copper) anterior or posterior subcapsular
Atopic dermatitis	Blue dot cortical cataract and posterior subcapsular cataract
Hypocalcemia	Discrete white cortical opacities
Diabetes mellitus	Snowflake opacities located in anterior and posterior subcapsular cortex
Acute-onset diabetes	Cortical wedges caused by lens fiber swelling
Down syndrome	Snowflake opacities located in anterior and posterior subcapsular cortex

slit-lamp biomicroscope examination, and posterior segment observations under mydriasis. Care must be taken to determine the effective lens implant position and power (biometry qv) (see Chapters 38 and 39). Intercurrent ophthalmic disorders may prejudice the visual outcome; for example, uveitis may be exacerbated,[5] herpes zoster may have left an anesthetic cornea,[6] atopic disease may predispose the eye to infection,[7] and diabetes mellitus without retinopathy increases the prospects of postoperative macular edema.[1]

Patient counseling on the procedure and postoperative expectations is a vital part of the preoperative work-up. A written explanation of the background and process of cataract surgery is invaluable.

PREOPERATIVE TESTS AND THEIR RATIONALE

Refraction and Visual Acuity (Near and Distance), Corrected and Uncorrected

Snellen acuity is one test for visual performance, but it does not always relate to visual difficulties in environments of variable lighting conditions, in which glare and pupil constriction may reduce the effective visual acuity. Glare testing of acuity is therefore useful (see Chapter 11). Log mar charting provides a more accurate means of comparing postoperative and preoperative acuity, if required. Certain forms of cataract induce changes in color perception before loss of acuity occurs. Modern cataract surgery demands the coincidental adjustment of intrinsic refractive errors (and avoidance of induced errors). Preoperative knowledge of the spherical and astigmatic errors in each eye, therefore, contributes to the surgical planning process. Planning of the final refractive outcome needs to take into account the other eye and the patient's needs and desires in the context of his or her lifestyle when considering the usage of residual refractive error such as monovision.

Corneal Topography (Videokeratography, Corneal Mapping)

A number of structures in the visual axis of the eye can contribute to refractive error. The main refracting media nevertheless are the cornea and the lens. The refractive state of the lens can be variable, particularly with cataract development. Because the lens is removed at surgery, and because of the need to attain emmetropia following surgery, an awareness of corneal shape is important if shape alterations are required, since part of the surgical process is to adjust intrinsic refractive errors. Preoperative topographical tangential maps (to show the true corneal shape) also provide the basis for comparative postoperative maps, not only to judge the desired manipulation of corneal shape but also to enable the surgeon to understand the effects of an inci-

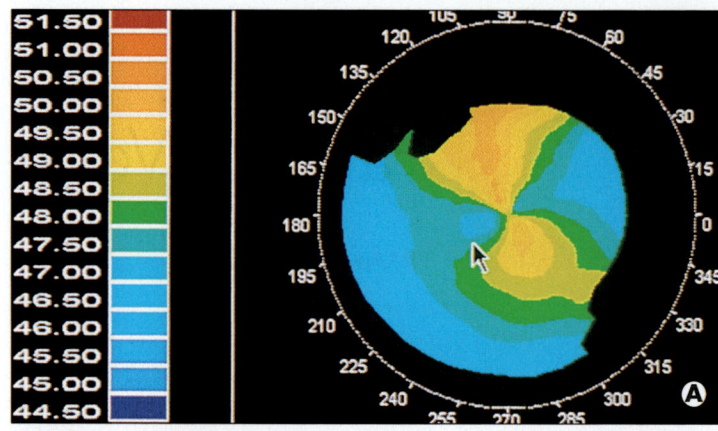

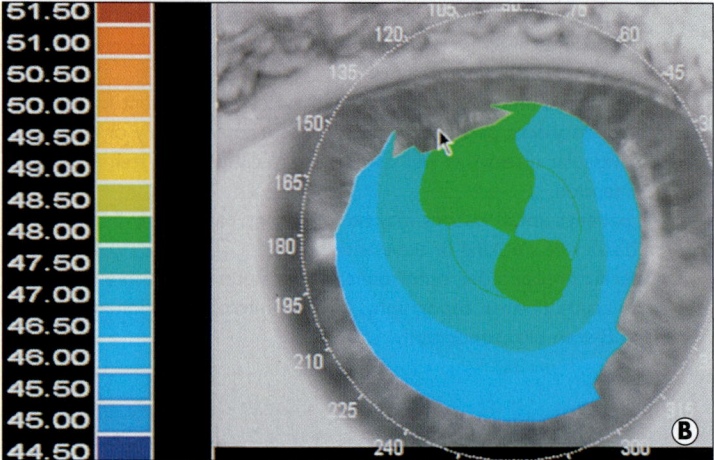

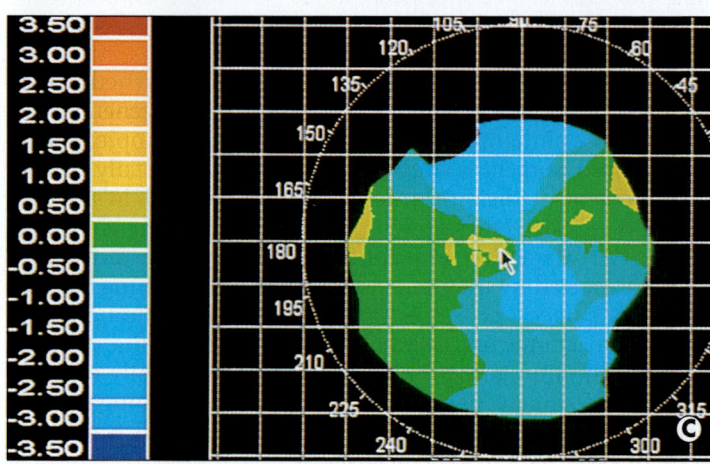

FIG. 43-1 ■ Topographical map of the cornea. **A,** Preoperative astigmatism before small incision cataract surgery. **B,** Postoperative minimal astigmatism after small incision cataract surgery. **C,** The difference map (incision on axis). The three-plane 3mm clear corneal incision was planned to be placed on the steep meridian of the cornea, because this form of incision induces 2D of corneal flattening in that meridian and results in a central cornea with an almost spherical refraction. The value of corneal topography in cataract surgery is illustrated by this one example.

sion in terms of both placement and form (Fig. 43-1; see also Chapter 41 on corneal topography).

Specular Microscopy

Because the corneal endothelium is vulnerable during the surgical process, it sometimes is useful to examine and record the status of the endothelium before surgery using specular microscopy (Fig. 43-2). Postoperative monitoring of the state of the corneal endothelial layer provides an indicator of the quality of the surgical intervention. The assessment also has a prognostic value for corneal survival. In the event that the cornea has a dystrophic or damaged endothelium before the opera-

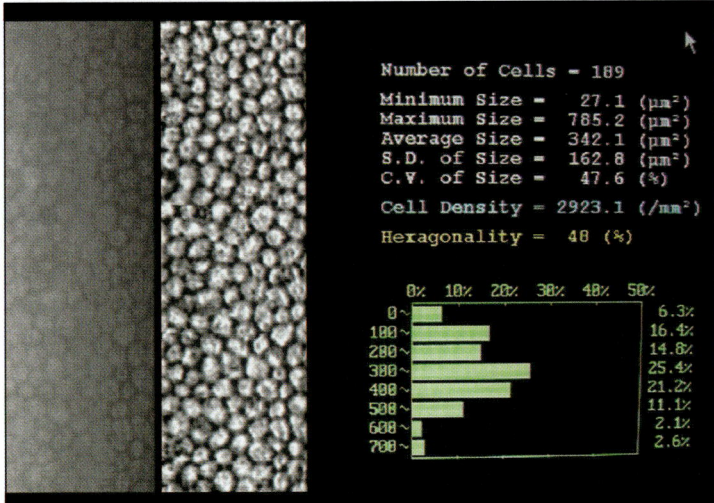

FIG. 43-2 ■ **Specular microscopy of the human cornea.** Shown is the endothelial cell analysis of a patient due to undergo intraocular surgery. The endothelium is healthy in this specular micrograph but should be recorded particularly if noted to be abnormal.

tion, the surgeon may document this to confirm that surgical misadventure was not the cause.

Biometry of the Eye

Biometry includes A-scan ultrasound measurement of the eye's axial length, anterior chamber depth, and crystalline lens thickness. Anterior segment dimensions include the white-to-white diameter of the cornea in its horizontal axis (for the implications of capsular bag size and ciliary sulcus diameter) and keratometry (manual or automated, with manual probably providing more accurate results). The A-scan ultrasound measurement can be performed by either contact or immersion methods. Immersion is considered to be more accurate.

Calculation of the power (dioptric value) of the intraocular lens (IOL) implant is essential. Adjustment of the preoperative refraction of an operated eye is required more often than not to obtain optimal focus and binocular balance. The importance of determining all the measurable parameters (e.g., axial length of the eye, anterior chamber depth, crystalline lens dimensions) is stressed in Chapter 39, as these enable the exact dioptric power of the replacement IOL to be calculated, taking into account the effective IOL location. Different IOL power calculation formulas are required for various axial lengths to ensure accurate IOL dioptric power (see Chapter 38).

B-Scan Ultrasonography

In eyes that have opaque cataracts, it is not always possible to perform a visual assessment of the posterior segment of the eye. In such eyes, a coincident pathology (e.g., detached retina, tumor) may be present and cause complications during cataract surgery. It may be clinically necessary to investigate the eye by B-scan ultrasonography to forewarn the surgeon of any additional pathology. This also enables the surgeon to advise the patient correctly as to the prospective surgical outcome.

INDICATIONS FOR SURGERY AND INFORMED CONSENT

The indications for surgery vary from patient to patient, especially with the current minimally invasive nature of cataract and lens implant surgery (compared with such surgery performed only a few years ago). The visual needs of patients vary according to their ages, occupations, and leisure interests. A clinical cataract may not be symptomatic. Visual symptoms and out-

come expectation affect the benefit-risk ratio. Although the risks of technically well performed small incision surgery are few in a healthy eye, patients require enough information on which to base the decision to proceed. Most patients are inclined to accept the professional judgment of the ophthalmic surgeon, but it is implicit that an adult of sound mind has the right to determine whether surgery should proceed. Therefore, in the context of cataract surgery, how much information is it necessary for an ophthalmologist to disclose to a patient? To what extent should an ophthalmologist shield a patient from the anxieties that can accompany a full explanation of diagnosis and treatment? An ophthalmologist must strike a balance between providing enough information to enable the patient to give informed consent with respect to treatment and engendering the confidence and trust that encompasses a joint decision to proceed. The surgeon shoulders the major responsibility for this, which should be accepted as a consequence of medical and specialist training.

In the application of professional judgment, the consideration of alternative management strategies, risks, and benefits allows a patient to make some sort of informed evaluation of the options. Statistical information based on published data may be confusing: Where does the patient fit into the statistics? What are the personal outcome statistics for the surgeon who offers advice? What guarantees are there that a particular surgeon will perform the surgery?

A problem arises if potential material risks and dangers are not disclosed to a patient before surgery and a complication occurs. The patient may claim that, with prior knowledge of such a risk, he or she would not have consented to the surgery. A risk is material when a rational patient considers the risk of undergoing a certain type of treatment to be significant.

Problems that arise from consent to perform surgical procedures can be minimized but not completely avoided, because every contingency cannot be reviewed completely. Taking the following steps will ensure that a thorough approach has been used.

First, appropriate patient education is required—the procedure is described in a manner that allows the patient to appreciate what will be done to treat the eye. Although the decision to proceed has to be the patient's, the surgeon must not pass all the responsibility on to the patient; rather, the surgeon should communicate the appropriate degree of confidence in the procedure's outcome. The surgeon has to assume much of the responsibility for treatment advice, because the patient cannot appreciate the intricacies of every surgical situation. Ultimately, the patient has to have faith in the ability of the surgeon not only to carry out the procedure but also to make the judgment that the benefits far outweigh the risks. An analogous situation might be that of a passenger contemplating a journey on a commercial airliner. If the passenger inquires of the pilot what the potential risks are, common sense suggests that the answer would be that they are high in number but low in expectation. A passenger who decides to make the trip has confidence in the airline and the aircrew to complete a successful journey. So it is with surgery: the patient must have confidence in the ability of the surgeon and the surgical team to carry out a successful procedure without knowing each and every pitfall that exists.

Alternative stratagems for the management of an ophthalmic condition are explained to the patient to enable patient participation in the final direction of treatment.

When uncertainties exist, the patient is advised of the predictability of the planned procedure, its stability, and its safety. Statistical information on outcome is of limited value when given in a general sense. Few surgeons are in a position to give specific statistical information about the outcome of their own practices or of certain procedures.

The patient must be given adequate time to decide. At the end of the consultation, a patient must have an opportunity to consider the treatment that has been advised or to reverse a decision to proceed. It is inappropriate to obtain a patient's signed con-

BOX 43-1

Issues to Discuss With a Patient Prior to Cataract Surgery

The purpose of surgery

The surgical procedure

The anesthetic requirements

Commonly experienced visual conditions after surgery, even if temporary

That temporary postsurgical visual conditions may become permanent under certain circumstances

The serious complications that may follow surgery

Potential pain or ocular discomfort

The refractive requirements after surgery (i.e., the need to wear and provision of glasses and/or contact lenses)

The potential need for additional procedures (planned staged procedures)

Alternative management of the condition

The patient should sign a consent form that states that the procedure has been explained fully in language that is comprehensible and that there has been sufficient opportunity to ask questions and reconsider consent prior to surgery. A written guide helps patients comprehend the nature of the planned surgery.

Any surgical intervention is essentially a matter of trust and confidence—the trust of the patient in the surgeon's ability and integrity, and the trust of the surgeon in the patient's ability to comprehend and follow the process and to comply with prescriptions for managing the condition before, during, and after surgery.

sent for a procedure and then proceed on very short notice (the same day) with that treatment. The delay between consent and treatment must be sufficient to allow the patient to consider the matter fully.

To ensure that a patient is fully informed with regard to consent for a surgical procedure, the issues listed in Box 43-1 should be covered.

REFERENCES

1. Wagner T, Knaflic D, Rauber M, Mester U. Influence of cataract surgery on the diabetic eye: a prospective study. Ger J Ophthalmol. 1996;5(2):79–83.
2. Ram J, Pandav SS, Ram B, Arora FC. Systemic disorders in age related cataract patients. Int Ophthalmol. 1994;18(3):121–5.
3. Hamed LM, Lingua DN. Thyroid disease presenting after cataract surgery. J Pediatr Ophthalmol Strabismus. 1990;27(1):10–5.
4. Fisher SJ, Cunningham RD. The medical profile of cataract patients. Geriatr Clin. 1985;1:339–44.
5. Jacquerie F, Comhaire-Poutchinian Y, Galand A. Cataract extraction in uveitis. Bull Soc Belge Ophthalmol. 1995;259:9–17.
6. Lightman S, Marsh RJ, Powell D. Herpes zoster ophthalmicus; a medical review. Br J Ophthalmol. 1981;65:539.
7. Hara T, Hoshi N, Hara T. Changes in bacterial strains before and after cataract surgery. Ophthalmology. 1996;103(11):1876–9.

44

The Pharmacotherapy of Cataract Surgery

STEVE A. ARSHINOFF • YVONNE A.V. OPALINSKI

KEY FEATURES

- Pharmacotherapeutic agents are used in the preoperative, intra-operative, and postoperative periods of cataract surgery.
- Preoperative medications are used as pupillary dilators, as prophylactic antibiotics, and as anesthetics.
- Intraoperative pharmacotherapeutic agents include irrigating solutions and additives to irrigating solutions, as well as ophthalmic viscosurgical devices.
- Postoperative medications include antibiotics, corticosteroids, and nonsteroidal anti-inflammatory drugs.

INTRODUCTION

With the recent rapid evolution of cataract surgical techniques, a corresponding change in the pharmacotherapeutic management of cataract patients has occurred. In this chapter, current pharmacotherapeutic practices in the pre-, intra-, and postoperative periods are reviewed.

PREOPERATIVE MEDICATIONS

Table 44-1 provides a summary of commonly used preoperative pharmacotherapeutic routines for cataract surgery.

Pupil Dilatation

Sympathomimetic mydriatic agents (such as phenylephrine 2.5%) and parasympatholytic cycloplegics (such as tropicamide or cyclopentolate 1.0%) usually are used together before extracapsular cataract extraction or phacoemulsification. If used in excess, sympathomimetics may increase the risk of a systemic hypertensive response and the associated systemic risks in the elderly.[1] For this reason, phenylephrine 10% is not recommended for routine use. To assist in adequate pupil dilatation, pilocarpine and other cholinergic miotics should be discontinued at least 12–24 hours before surgery.

Topical nonsteroidal anti-inflammatory drugs (NSAIDs) are commonly used in cataract surgery to prevent pupillary miosis, reduce surgically induced inflammation, and prevent postoperative cystoid macular edema.[2] Administration of NSAIDs decreases prostaglandin synthesis by the inhibition of cyclooxygenase, thus preventing the transformation of arachidonic acid into prostaglandins.[2,3] Prostaglandin E_2 (PGE_2) enhances the constrictor action of the iris sphincter through a mechanism that is not dependent on cholinergic receptors.[4,5] Topical flurbiprofen 0.03%, the first agent to be used for this indication, was demonstrated to be clinically superior to topical indomethacin 1%.[5] More recently, diclofenac 0.1% and ketorolac 0.5% have been used for the same indication.[6] No difference has been noted between diclofenac and flurbiprofen intraoperatively; both adequately maintain mydriasis during surgery.[7]

Anti-Infective Prophylaxis

Prophylactic antibiotic use in cataract surgery has been an accepted practice for decades. Preoperatively, the most important source of potential infectious organisms is the patient's own natural conjunctival and skin flora. Intraoperative cultures indicate that at least 5% of intraocular surgeries result in measurable anterior chamber contamination from indigenous flora; the vast majority of these patients develop no clinical adverse sequelae.[8] Cultures taken from the conjunctiva and anterior chamber of patients who subsequently developed endophthalmitis usually yielded the same bacterial strains. Staphylococci (*Staphylococcus epidermidis* and *S. aureus*), diphtheroids (*Corynebacterium*), streptococci (*Streptococcus viridans*), and gram-negative bacilli (anaerobic *Propionibacterium acnes* and others) are the infecting agents in decreasing order of occurrence.[9] Administered medications should adequately cover the bacteria most likely to cause potential endophthalmitis. Before cataract surgery, topical anti-infective regimens may include gramicidin–neomycin–polymyxin B sulfate, aminoglycosides such as gentamicin or tobramycin (which provide gram-negative and *Pseudomonas* coverage), and the fluoroquinolones—ciprofloxacin, norfloxacin, and ofloxacin in 0.3% concentrations. Of these, ciprofloxacin and ofloxacin appear to provide superior coverage and anterior chamber penetration.[7,10,11] Fluoroquinolones provide broad-spectrum coverage of gram-positive and gram-negative bacteria, including methicillin-resistant staphylococci; however, coverage of streptococci and anaerobes is suboptimal. The combination of trimethoprim and polymyxin B offers coverage of the common pathogens, except for *Pseudomonas*, anaerobes, and methicillin-resistant staphylococci. Based on existing data, tobramycin, a fluoroquinolone, and trimethoprim–polymyxin B are the most common choices for anti-infective prophylaxis in many types of ocular surgery.[3] However, complete conjunctival sterility through the elimination of such flora is not possible with the use of preoperative antibiotics alone.[7] The topical antiseptic povidone-iodine 5% instilled as a single drop before surgery is one of the most effective measures to decrease this bacterial flora[12] and is equal in efficacy to topical antibiotics.[13]

Anesthetics

Anesthetics are covered fully in Chapter 45. Periocular injection anesthesia is declining in popularity, and the use of intracameral lidocaine has gained popularity over the last few years, as has topical lidocaine gel. Lidocaine gel is claimed to provide increased corneal hydration and anesthesia equal to that of injections and drops[14,15] while minimizing patient discomfort.

TABLE 44-1

COMMONLY USED AGENTS IN THE ROUTINE PREOPERATIVE PHARMACOTHERAPY OF CATARACT SURGERY

	Class and Agent	Concentration	Dosage
Nonsteroidal anti-inflammatory drugs to prevent miosis	Diclofenac	0.10%	I drop 4 times over Ih preceding surgery
	Ketorolac	0.50%	
	Flurbiprofen	0.03%	
	Indomethacin	1%	
Cycloplegics	Tropicamide	1%	I drop 4 times over Ih preceding surgery
	Cyclopentolate	1%	
Mydriatics	Phenylephrine	2.50%	I drop twice over 0.5h preoperatively
Antibiotic prophylaxis	Gramicidin– neomycin– polymyxin B	0.025mg/ml 2.5mg/ml 10,000IU/ml	I drop 4 times over Ih preceding surgery
	Gentamicin	0.30%	
	Tobramycin	0.30%	
	Ciprofloxacin	0.30%	
	Ofloxacin	0.30%	
	Trimethoprim–polymyxin B	Img/ml (10,000IU/ml)	
Anesthetic: retrobulbar or parabulbar	Lidocaine	1–2%	3–9ml
	Mepivacaine	1–2%	
	Bupivacaine	0.25–0.75%	
Anesthetic: intracameral	Isotonic, nonpreserved lidocaine	1–2%	0.3–0.6ml
Anesthetic: topical	Proparacaine	1–2%	1–2 drops prior to surgery, and then every 10 minutes or as needed during surgery
	Tetracaine	0.50%	
	Benoxinate (oxybuprocaine)	0.40%	
	Lidocaine	4%	
	Bupivacaine	0.75%	

INTRAOPERATIVE MEDICATIONS

Additives to Irrigating Solutions

Table 44-2 gives a summary of commonly used intraoperative pharmacotherapeutic routines. In general, the addition of antibiotics, mydriatics, epinephrine (adrenaline), or lidocaine (lignocaine) is not recommended by the companies that produce irrigating solutions for cataract surgery, because any effect on stabilizers and preservatives in the solutions could alter their pH, chemical balance, or osmolarity and influence the potential toxicities of both irrigating solution and additive alike. Caution is therefore advised if any alteration to commercial irrigating solutions is considered.

The intraoperative use of antibiotics in irrigating solutions is a controversial issue in cataract surgery. It appears that surgical technique may play the most critical role in anterior chamber contamination, and the antibiotics administered in irrigating solutions may contribute minimally to reduce the risk of endophthalmitis.[8,16] A case of coagulase-negative staphylococcal endophthalmitis has been reported despite intraoperative vancomycin (1mg/0.1ml) injected intravitreally.[17] Furthermore, vancomycin remains the leading agent against methicillin-resistant S. aureus, and infectious disease epidemiologists regularly advise against the routine use of last-resort agents for fear that resistance will develop. Nevertheless, intraocular vancomycin (20µg/ml [0.02mg/ml]) in combination with gentamicin (8µg/ml [0.008mg/ml]) has been reported to eradicate gram-positive, coagulase-negative micrococci,[18] with minimal associated complications. Surgeons recognize that the postsurgical capsular bag is a sequestered avascular site that harbors a foreign body (the intraocular lens) and may act as the nidus for most cases of endophthalmitis. Therefore, vancomycin 1mg in 0.1ml BSS has also been injected directly into the capsular bag as the final step in the surgical procedure. This mode of delivery is considered superior to irrigated solution because it goes directly to where it is needed.[19] Gentamicin alone has been used intraoperatively in the dosage range of 8–80µg/ml, which appears sufficient to avoid retinal toxicity and at the same time decrease the intracameral bacterial load.[20] To prevent intraoperative miosis, nonpreserved epinephrine (1:1000) 0.5ml/500ml of irrigating solution is added frequently. This concentration appears not to be toxic to the corneal endothelium and allows normal endothelial function.[21]

Rapid miosis can be produced at the end of the surgical procedure using one of two available intraocular parasympathomimetics—acetylcholine chloride 1% or carbachol 0.01%.[22] Current preparations have shown no evidence of endothelial toxicity, and the choice of agent depends on the desired clinical features. Acetylcholine 1% has an onset time of less than 1 minute, has a relatively brief duration of action, and results in miosis for 10 minutes, whereas carbachol 0.01% takes 2 minutes to act and its effect has a duration of 2–24 hours. Both agents lower postoperative intraocular pressure spikes.[23]

Irrigating Solutions

In the early days of phacoemulsification, the only irrigating solutions available were normal saline, Plasma-Lyte, and lactated Ringer's solution. The main difficulty with these solutions was endothelial cell toxicity, which resulted in dysfunction and destruction. Irrigating solutions with calcium, glutathione, and bicarbonate form more physiologically balanced solutions (Table 44-3).[24] Several comparative studies have found BSS Plus to be superior to BSS and other irrigating solutions and protective of the corneal endothelium. Unlike BSS, BSS Plus is physiologically similar to human aqueous and vitreous, especially with regard to calcium concentration and the addition of glucose, glutathione, and bicarbonate. BSS Plus maintains endothelial cell function over periods ranging from 15 minutes to in excess of a few hours.[24] The buffer in BSS Plus is bicarbonate, which is an improvement over the sodium acetate and citrate buffers in BSS.

Corneal irrigation to maintain hydration and surgical clarity has traditionally been performed throughout intraocular procedures with BSS. The development of an elastoviscous hylan surgical shield 0.45%, which decreases the surgeon's dependence on manual corneal irrigation, has proved to be an improvement over BSS in maintaining corneal hydration and clarity intraoperatively.[25]

TABLE 44-2

COMMONLY USED AGENTS IN THE ROUTINE INTRAOPERATIVE PHARMACOTHERAPY OF CATARACT SURGERY

	Class and Agent	Concentration	Dosage
Agents added to irrigating solutions	Antibiotics		
	Vancomycin plus	20µg/ml	
	Gentamicin	8µg/ml	
	Gentamicin	8–80µg/ml	
	Sympathomimetics to prevent miosis		
	Nonpreserved epinephrine		0.5ml/500ml of 1:1000 nonpreserved epinephrine
Agents used at the end of the procedure	Antibiotics		0.1ml intracapsularly via sideport at end of procedure
	Vancomycin	1mg/0.1ml	
	Parasympathomimetics		0.5ml injected into anterior chamber via sideport to cause miosis
	Acetylcholine	1%	
	Carbachol	0.01%	

TABLE 44-3

CHEMICAL COMPOSITION OF HUMAN AQUEOUS HUMOR, VITREOUS HUMOR, BSS PLUS, AND BSS

Ingredient	Human Aqueous Humor	Human Vitreous Humor	BSS Plus	BSS
Sodium	162.9	144	160	155.7
Potassium	2.2–3.9	5.5	5	10.1
Calcium	1.8	1.6	1	3.3
Magnesium	1.1	1.3	1	1.5
Chloride	131.6	177	130	128.9
Bicarbonate	20.15	15	25	–
Phosphate	0.62	0.4	3	–
Lactate	2.5	7.8	–	–
Glucose	2.7–3.7	3.4	5	–
Ascorbate	1.06	2	–	–
Glutathione	0.0019	–	0.3	–
Citrate	–	–	–	5.8
Acetate	–	–	–	28.6
pH	7.38	–	7.4	7.6
Osmolality (mOsm)	304	–	305	298

(Adapted from Edelhauser HF. Intraocular irrigating solutions. In: Lamberts DW, Potter DE, eds. Clinical Ophthalmic Pharmacology. Boston: Little, Brown; 1987, pp. 431–44.) All concentrations are expressed in mmol/l or mEq/l of solution.

OPHTHALMIC VISCOSURGICAL DEVICES

The introduction of Healon in 1980 for use in ocular surgery ushered in the era of viscosurgery. Because all these ophthalmic viscosurgical devices (OVDs) tend to consist of solutions of long-chain biopolymers (almost always hyaluronic acid or hydroxypropyl methylcellulose) in low concentration, they are all pseudoplastic in their rheological behavior. Their physical properties tend to correlate (i.e., the most viscous solution is also the most elastic and the most cohesive) and are a function of the chain length distribution of the rheologically important constituent polymer and its concentration. This allows the classification of OVDs into viscoadaptives (extremely high zero-shear viscosity and cohesion), superviscous cohesives (very high zero-shear viscosity), viscous cohesives (high zero-shear viscosity), medium-viscosity dispersives (low zero-shear viscosity), and very-low-viscosity dispersives (Table 44-4). It is apparent that OVDs are not interchangeable and that many surgical maneuvers can be achieved more easily with one type of OVD than another. Before the advent of viscoadaptive OVDs, superviscous cohesive and viscous cohesive OVDs were recognized as the best for creating, stabilizing, and maintaining spaces (to deepen the anterior chamber in the presence of positive vitre-ous pressure, to stabilize the anterior chamber to facilitate capsulorrhexis, and to keep the capsular bag open and taut to facilitate foldable intraocular lens implantation). Conversely, lower-viscosity dispersive OVDs are excellent for the selective isolation of areas of the intraocular surgical field and for enabling fluid partition of the anterior chamber (to protect marginal corneas from the turbulence of phacoemulsification, or to keep a frayed piece of iris or bulging vitreous away from the phacoemulsifying or irrigation-aspiration tip).[26] Supercohesive and cohesive OVDs cannot be used to partition fluid-filled spaces. To achieve the benefits of both types of older OVDs and avoid having to deal with their disadvantages, the "soft shell technique" can be utilized.[27,28] Healon5 and Microvisc Phaco (iVisc Phaco, Hyvisc Phaco, BD Multivisc) are new viscoadaptive OVDs that exhibit either highly viscous cohesive or pseudodispersive properties, depending on fluid turbulence in the anterior chamber.[29] These characteristics allow their use for chamber partitioning and yield enhanced versatility over earlier OVDs during phacoemulsification.[30-34] The "ultimate soft shell technique" further enhances the scope of utility of viscoadaptive OVDs,[35,36] and enables the benefits of the soft shell technique to be attained using a single viscoadaptive OVD.

TABLE 44-4

OPHTHALMIC VISCOSURGICAL DEVICES—CONTENT, MOLECULAR WEIGHT, AND ZERO-SHEAR VISCOSITY

Class	Ophthalmic Viscosurgical Device (OVD)	Content (%)	Molecular Weight (Da)	Zero-Shear Viscosity (mPas)
HIGHER-VISCOSITY COHESIVE OVDs				
Viscoadaptives	MicroVisc Phaco (iVisc Phaco, Hyvisc Phaco, BD Multivisc)	NaHa (2.5)	7.9M	18.0M
	Healon5	NaHa (2.3)	4.0M	7.0M
Superviscous cohesives	MicroVisc Plus (iVisc Plus, Hyvisc Plus)	NaHa (1.4)	7.9M	4.8M
	Healon GV	NaHa (1.4)	5.0M	2.0M
Viscous cohesives	Microvisc (iVisc, Hyvisc)			
	Provisc	NaHa (1.0)	2.0M	280K
	Healon	NaHa (1.0)	4.0M	230K
	Biolon	NaHa (1.0)	3.0M	215K
	Amvisc	NaHa (1.2)	1.0M	100K
	Amvisc Plus	NaHa (1.6)	1.0M	100K
LOWER-VISCOSITY DISPERSIVE OVDs				
Medium-viscosity dispersives	Viscoat	NaHa (3.0)	500K	41K
		Chondroitin sulfate (4.0)	25K	
	Cellugel	Chemically modified HPMC (2.0)	100K	28K
	Vitrax	NaHa (3.0)	500K	25K
Very-low-viscosity dispersives	Occucoat	HPMC (2.0)	86K	4K
	Hymecel	HPMC (2.0)	86K	4K
	Adatocel	HPMC (2.0)	86K	4K
	Visilon	HPMC (2.0)	86K	4K
	Ocuvis	HPMC (2.0)	90K	4.3K

HPMC, Hydrooxypropylmethylcellulose; *K*, thousand; *M*, million; *mod*, chemically modified; *Mw(Da)*, molecular weight (daltons); *NaHa*, sodium hyaluronate; *V0(mPas)*, zero-shear viscosity (milliPascal seconds).

TABLE 44-5

COMMONLY USED AGENTS IN THE ROUTINE POSTOPERATIVE PHARMACOTHERAPY OF CATARACT SURGERY

	Class and Agent	Concentration	Dosage
Corticosteroids	Dexamethasone	0.10%	1 drop 4 times daily for 3–4 weeks postoperatively
	Prednisolone	1%	
	Betamethasone	0.10%	
Nonsteroidal anti-inflammatory drugs	Dicolfenac	0.10%	1 drop 4 times daily for 4 weeks postoperatively
	Ketorolac	0.50%	
Antibiotics	Gramicidin–neomycin–polymyxin B	0.025mg/ml 2.5mg/ml 10,000IU/ml	1 drop 4 times daily for 3–4 weeks postoperatively
	Gentamicin	0.30%	
	Tobramycin	0.30%	
	Ciprofloxacin	0.30%	
	Ofloxacin	0.30%	
	Trimethoprim–polymyxin B	1mg/ml (10,000IU/ml)	

POSTOPERATIVE MEDICATIONS

Postoperative drugs are listed in Table 44-5.

Antibiotics

Postoperative regimens of topical antibiotics vary but generally consist of one drop to the operated eye four times daily. The duration of treatment also varies from 5 days in uncomplicated surgery to weeks if prolonged inflammation or postoperative endophthalmitis occurs. Topical treatment is so efficacious that the use of injections and collagen shields is increasingly falling out of favor. Increasing resistance to antibiotics that have been used for decades and the lack of resistance to newer drugs (e.g., gentamicin versus ofloxacin) also influence the selection of postoperative anti-infective prophylaxis.

Subconjunctival injections of antibiotics deliver higher levels to the aqueous humor but have a greater risk associated with their administration, notably perforation of the eye, macular infarction, and retinal toxicity. Oral or parenteral antibiotics, such as the fluoroquinolones, may reach substantial levels in the anterior chamber but do not provide any advantages over topical routes of administration and are associated with increased side effects.[37,38]

Collagen shields, with a dissolution time of 12 hours, have been introduced to decrease the frequency of drop application and to increase the concentration and retention of the drug at the intended site of action. The shields, presoaked in an antibiotic and corticosteroid solution such as tobramycin and dexamethasone, or netilmicin and betamethasone, are placed on the eye immediately after surgery, and have been associated with minimal adverse effects.[39] A preoperative 60-minute application of a single-use collagen shield delivery system, presoaked in ofloxacin for 10 minutes, has also been proposed to achieve superior aqueous drug levels at the onset of surgery.[40] Postoperative application of collagen shields appears to be superior to subconjunctival injections of the same antibiotic-corticosteroid mix in terms of efficacy, toxicity, safety, and reduction of patient discomfort. The use of postoperative collagen shields has not been widely adopted because antibiotic concentrations in the shield may become toxic if they leach into the anterior chamber. Therefore, great caution should be exercised when using collagen shields in the absence of a well-sealed wound.[8] Furthermore, some combinations of antibiotic and corticosteroid have produced toxic precipitates.[31]

Corticosteroids and Nonsteroidal Anti-Inflammatory Drugs

Topical corticosteroids and NSAIDs are used after cataract surgery to reduce postoperative noninfectious inflammation. Corticosteroids and NSAIDs appear to be equally efficacious in decreasing inflammation,[6,41] and there is no difference between them in terms of astigmatic decay. The development of an intraocular biodegradable drug delivery system containing dexamethasone appears to be an effective alternative to topical drops,[42] and because a variety of drugs may be bound to the polymer matrix, it may play a role in the long-term prevention or treatment of cystoid macular edema. Topical NSAIDs have a specific advantage over corticosteroids if there are contraindications to corticosteroid use in a particular patient, such as corticosteroid-responsive elevations of intraocular pressure, recurrent herpes simplex infection,[43] or concern about delayed wound healing.[44] Ketorolac 0.5% has been shown to be equally effective as a single agent in antimiotic and anti-inflammatory activity when compared with an NSAID-prednisolone 1% combination.[45]

Pretreatment with an NSAID decreases the postoperative level of inflammation, provided the medication is administered over a period of 3 days.[46,47] Both corticosteroids and NSAIDs are used postoperatively, either interchangeably or together, although not as a single solution. The addition of an NSAID to an antibiotic-steroid postoperative regimen has been reported to decrease the incidence of noninfectious postoperative inflammatory conditions.[48] The corticosteroids dexamethasone 0.1%, prednisolone 1%, and betamethasone 0.1% are used most commonly. The most frequently used NSAIDs are diclofenac 0.1% and ketorolac 0.5%.[49,50] Corticosteroid and NSAID regimens are the same and consist of one drop to the affected eye four times daily for up to 4 weeks, usually used in conjunction with a topical antibiotic. Combination NSAID-antibiotic drops have been formulated to minimize the number of different bottles a patient must use postoperatively, without altering either drug's efficacy or penetration.[51]

LATE POSTOPERATIVE MEDICATIONS

Treatment of Endophthalmitis

Endophthalmitis has been treated with antibiotics systemically, intravitreally, and topically. See Chapter 169 for details.

Treatment of Cystoid Macular Edema

Cystoid macular edema (CME) usually manifests 1–3 months postoperatively as either decreased visual acuity or changes on fluorescein angiography that result from serous exudate leaking out of incompetent intraretinal capillaries into the outer plexiform layer of Henle.[52] Most patients spontaneously recover, with full restoration of visual acuity within 6 months; however, it may require 1–2 years for full spontaneous resolution to occur.[2] In approximately one third of patients, macular edema persists, accompanied by decreased visual acuity.

Prophylaxis and treatment have been suggested in the form of systemic and topical NSAIDs. Oral NSAIDs, with regimens of indomethacin 25mg three times daily 1 week before surgery and 3 weeks postoperatively,[2] or ibuprofen 200mg preoperatively and postoperatively, have received mixed reviews.[53] Literature supports the efficacy of topical NSAIDs,[54,55] such as flurbiprofen

0.03%, diclofenac 0.1%, and ketorolac 0.5%, used prophylactically and after surgery to reduce inflammation. Usually, preoperatively and postoperatively, one drop is administered four times daily for up to 3 weeks to prevent CME. Frequently, topical corticosteroids are used in conjunction with NSAIDs in the treatment of CME, and their combined effect in the acute postoperative period appears to be more beneficial than monotherapy with either agent.[56] In chronic cases, management continues until resolution.[2] It has been suggested that indefinite NSAID treatment may be required to maintain CME regression,[57] which increases interest in the utility of a long-term, intraocular drug delivery system.[46] Once established, CME has been treated with oral acetazolamide, topical corticosteroids with NSAIDs, or posterior sub-Tenon's injection of long-acting corticosteroids (see Chapter 131). CME unresponsive to oral or topical treatment has resolved in a small number of patients treated with high-dose methylprednisolone (1000mg for three days), with an improvement in visual acuity.[58] Antiglaucomatous prostaglandin analogs such as latanoprost may enhance disruption of the blood-aqueous barrier, increasing the incidence of CME after cataract surgery, but this appears to be a response to the drug's preservative, and not the drug itself. The concurrent application of NSAIDs decreases the incidence of CME secondary to these medications and does not adversely influence the antiglaucoma drug's effect on intraocular pressure.[59,60]

REFERENCES

1. Hoffman BB, Lefkowitz RJ. Catecholamines and sympathomimetic drugs. In: Hardman JG, Limberg LE, Goodman Gilman A, et al., eds. The pharmacological basis of therapeutics. Toronto: Pergamon Press; 1990:187–220.
2. Flach AJ. Cyclo-oxygenase inhibitors in ophthalmology. Surv Ophthalmol. 1992;36:259–84.
3. Arshinoff SA, Mills M, Haber S. Pharmacotherapy of photorefractive keratectomy. J Cataract Refract Surg. 1996;22:1037–44.
4. Keates R, McGowan K. Clinical trial of flurbiprofen to maintain pupillary dilation during cataract surgery. Ann Ophthalmol. 1984;16(10):919–21.
5. Miyake K. The significance of inflammatory reactions following cataract extraction and intraocular lens implantation. J Cataract Refract Surg. 1996;22(Suppl.):759–63.
6. Flach AJ, Kraff MC, Sanders DR, Tanenbaum L. The quantitative effect of 0.5% ketorolac tromethamine solution and 0.1% dexamethasone sodium phosphate solution on postsurgical blood-aqueous barrier. Arch Ophthalmol. 1988;106(4):480–3.
7. Roberts C. Comparison of diclofenac sodium and flurbiprofen for inhibition of surgically induced miosis. J Cataract Refract Surg. 1996;22(Suppl.):780–6.
8. Samad A, Solomon LD, Miller MA, Mendelson J. Anterior chamber contamination after uncomplicated phacoemulsification and intraocular lens implantation. Am J Ophthalmol. 1995;120:143–50.
9. Starr MB, Lally JM. Antimicrobial prophylaxis for ophthalmic surgery. Surv Ophthalmol. 1995;39(6):485–501.
10. Donnenfeld ED, Schrier A, Perry HD. Penetration of topically applied ciprofloxacin, norfloxacin and ofloxacin into the aqueous humor. Ophthalmology. 1994;101(5):902–5.
11. Leeming JP, Diamond JP, Trigg R. Ocular penetration of topical ciprofloxacin and norfloxacin drops and their effect upon eyelid flora. Br J Ophthalmol. 1994;78(7):546–8.
12. Dereklis DL, Bufidis TA, Tsiakiri EP, Palassopoulos SI. Preoperative ocular disinfection by the use of povidone-iodine 5%. Acta Ophthalmol. 1994;72(5):627–30.
13. Chaudhary U, Nagpal RC, Malik AK, Kumar A. Comparative evaluation of antimicrobial activity of polyvinylpyrrolidone (PVP)-iodine versus topical antibiotics in cataract surgery. J Indian Med Assoc. 1998;96(7):202–4.
14. Koch PS. Efficacy of lidocaine 2% jelly as a topical agent in cataract surgery. J Cataract Refract Surg. 1999;25:632–4.
15. Assia EI, Pras E, Yehezkel M, et al. Topical anesthesia using lidocaine gel for cataract surgery. J Cataract Refract Surg. 1999;25:635–9.
16. Parkkari M, Paivarinta H, Salminen L. The treatment of endophthalmitis after cataract surgery. J Ocular Pharmacol Ther. 1995;11(3):349–59.
17. Townsend-Pico WA, Meyers SM, Langston RH, Costin JA. Coagulase-negative staphylococcus endophthalmitis after cataract surgery with intraocular vancomycin. Am J Ophthalmol. 1996;121(3):318–9.
18. Han DP, Wisniewski SR, Wilson LA, et al. Spectrum and susceptibilities of microbiologic isolates in the Endophthalmitis Vitrectomy Study. Am J Ophthalmol. 1996;122(1):1–17.
19. Han DP, Wisniewski SR, Wilson LA, et al. Spectrum and susceptibilities of microbiologic isolates in the Endophthalmitis Vitrectomy Study. Am J Ophthalmol. 1996;122(1):1–17.
20. Dickey JB, Thompson KD, Jay WM. Intraocular gentamicin sulfate and post cataract anterior chamber aspirate cultures. J Cataract Refract Surg. 1994;20(4):373–7.
21. Glasser DB, Edelhauser HF. Toxicity of surgical solutions. Int Ophthalmol Clin. 1989;29(3):179–87.
22. Roberts CW. Intraocular miotics and postoperative inflammation. J Cataract Refract Surg. 1993;19(6):731–4.
23. Arshinoff SA, Calogero DX, Bilotta R, et al. The problems associated with OVD use in cataract surgery. Presented by S Senft at the annual meeting of the American Society of Cataract and Refractive Surgery, San Diego, California, April 16–22, 1998.

24. McDermott ML, Edelhauser HF, Hack HM, Langston RH. Ophthalmic irrigants: a current review and update. Ophthal Surg. 1988;19(10):724–33 (review).

25. Arshinoff SA, Khoury E. HsS versus a balanced salt solution as a corneal wetting agent during routine cataract extraction and lens implantation. J Cataract Refract Surg. 1997;23:1211–25.

26. Arshinoff SA. Dispersive and cohesive viscoelastics in phacoemulsification. Ophthalmic Pract. 1995;13(3):98–104.

27. Arshinoff SA. The viscoelastic soft shell technique for compromised corneas and anterior chamber compartmentalization. Presented at the American Society of Cataract and Refractive Surgery Symposium on Cataract, IOL, and Refractive Surgery, Seattle, Washington, 1996.

28. Arshinoff SA. "Soft shell" technique uses two types of viscoelastics. Reported by Harvey Black. Ocular Surg News, Int Ed. 1996;7(10):20.

29. Dick HB, Krummenauer F, Augustin AJ, et al. Healon5 viscoadaptive formulation: comparison to Healon and Healon GV. J Cataract Refract Surg. 2001;27:320–6.

30. Arshinoff SA, Hofman I. Prospective, randomized trial comparing MicroVisc Plus and Healon GV in routine phacoemulsification. J Cataract Refract Surg. 1998;24:814–20.

31. Miller KM, Colvard M. Randomized clinical comparison of Healon GV and Viscoat. J Cataract Refract Surg. 1999;25:1630–6.

32. Rainer G, Menapace R, Findl O, et al. Intraocular pressure after small incision cataract surgery with Healon5 and Viscoat. J Cataract Refract Surg. 2000;26:271–6.

33. Arshinoff SA. Why Healon5. The meaning of viscoadaptive. Ophthalmic Pract. 1999;17(6):332–4.

34. Arshinoff SA. Healon5. In: Buratto L, Giardini P, Bellucci R, eds. Viscoelastics in ophthalmic surgery. Thorofare, NJ: Slack; 2000.

35. Arshinoff S. The ultimate soft-shell technique. Ophthalmic Pract. 2000;18(6):289–90.

36. Arshinoff SA. Using BSS with viscoadaptives in "the ultimate soft shell technique." J Cataract Refract Surg. 2002;28:1509–14.

37. Bron AM, Pechinot AP, Garcher CP, et al. The ocular penetration of oral sparfloxacin in humans. Am J Ophthalmol. 1994;117(3):322–7.

38. Mounier M, Ploy MC, Chauvin M. Study of intraocular diffusion of ofloxacin in humans and rabbits. Pathol Biol. 1992;40(5):529–33.

39. Haaskjold E, Ohrstrom A, Uusitalo RJ, et al. Use of collagen shields in cataract surgery. J Cataract Refract Surg. 1994;20(2):150–3.

40. Taravella MJ, Balentine J, Young DA, et al. Collagen shield delivery of ofloxacin to the human eye. J Cataract Refract Surg. 1999;25:562–5.

41. Simone JN, Pendelton RA, Jenkins JE. Comparison of the efficacy and safety of ketorolac tromethamine 0.5% and prednisolone acetate 1% after cataract surgery. J Cataract Refract Surg. 1999;25:699–704.

42. Chang DF, Garcia IH, Hunkeler JD, et al. Phase II results of an intraocular steroid delivery system for cataract surgery. Ophthalmology. 1999;106:1172–7.

43. Masket M. Comparison of the effect of topical corticosteroids and nonsteroidals on postoperative corneal astigmatism. J Cataract Refract Surg. 1990;16(6):715–8.

44. Barba KR, Samy A, Lai C, et al. Effect of topical anti-inflammatory drugs on corneal and limbal wound healing. J Cataract Refract Surg. 2000;26:893–7.

45. Snyder RW, Siekert RW, Schwiegerling J, et al. Acular as a single agent for use as an antimiotic and anti-inflammatory in cataract surgery. J Cataract Refract Surg. 2000;26:1225–7.

46. Roberts CW. Pretreatment with topical diclofenac sodium to decrease postoperative inflammation. Ophthalmology. 1996;103:636–9.

47. El-Harazi SM, Ruiz RS, Feldman RM, et al. Efficacy of preoperative versus postoperative ketorolac tromethamine 0.5% in reducing inflammation after cataract surgery. J Cataract Refract Surg. 2000;26:1626–30.

48. Arshinoff SA, Strube YNJ, Yagev R. Simultaneous bilateral cataract surgery. J Cataract Refract Surg. 2003. In press.

49. Flach AJ, Lavelle CJ, Olander KW, et al. The effect of ketorolac tromethamine solution 0.5% in reducing postoperative inflammation after cataract extraction and intraocular lens implantation. Ophthalmology. 1988;95(9):1279–84.

50. Solomon KD, Cheetham JK, DeGryse R, et al. Topical ketorolac tromethamine 0.5% ophthalmic solution in ocular inflammation after cataract surgery. Ophthalmology. 2001;108:331–7.

51. Killer HE, Borruat FX, Blumer BK, et al. Corneal penetration of diclofenac from a fixed combination of diclofenac-gentamicin eye drops. J Cataract Refract Surg. 1998;24:1365–70.

52. Jaffe NS. Cataract surgery and its complications. St. Louis: Mosby; 1984:426–41.

53. Yanuzzi LA, Klein RM, Wallyn RH, et al. Ineffectiveness of indomethacin in the treatment of chronic cystoid macular edema. Am J Ophthalmol. 1977;84:517–9.

54. Rossetti L, Bujtar E, Castoldi D, et al. Effectiveness of diclofenac eye drops in reducing inflammation and the incidence of cystoid macular edema after cataract surgery. J Cataract Refract Surg. 1996;22(Suppl.):794–9.

55. Miyake K, Masuda K, Shirato S, et al. Comparison of diclofenac and fluorometholone in preventing cystoid macular edema after small incision cataract surgery: a multicentred prospective trial. Jpn J Ophthalmol. 2000;44:58–67.

56. Heier JS, Topping TM, Baumann W, et al. Ketorolac versus prednisolone versus combination therapy in the treatment of acute pseudophakic cystoid macular edema. Ophthalmology. 2000;107:2034–9.

57. Weisz JM, Bressler NM, Bressler SB, et al. Ketorolac treatment of pseudophakic cystoid macular edema identified more than 24 months after cataract extraction. Ophthalmology. 1999;106:1656–9.

58. Abe T, Hayasaka S, Nagaki Y, et al. Pseudophakic cystoid macular edema treated with high-dose intravenous methylprednisolone. J Cataract Refract Surg. 1999;25:1286–8.

59. Miyake K, Ota I, Mackubo K, et al. Latanoprost accelerates disruption of the blood-aqueous barrier and the incidence of angiographic cystoid macular edema in early postoperative pseudophakias. Arch Ophthalmol. 1999;117:34–40.

60. Miyake K, Ota I, Ibaraki N, et al. Enhanced disruption of the blood-aqueous barrier and the incidence of angiographic cystoid macular edema by topical timolol and its preservative in early postoperative pseudophakia. Arch Ophthalmol. 2001;119:387–94.

Anesthesia for Cataract Surgery

DONNA L. GREENHALGH

DEFINITION
- Adequate control of pain and eye movement to allow surgeon to achieve surgical goals.

KEY FEATURES
- Local anesthesia.
- General anesthesia.
- Topical anesthesia.

INTRODUCTION

As surgery has developed, and with the advent of small incision phacoemulsification, the requirements for anesthesia have changed. It is no longer essential to ensure complete akinesia, and as a consequence, peribulbar and topical anesthesia technique have been developed that feature variable or no akinesia. Moreover, self-sealing incisions with closed eye surgery mean that it is not essential to maintain very low intraocular pressures.

A team approach to ophthalmic surgery is important, with the surgeon concentrating on the operation and the anesthetist looking after the patient under either local or general anesthesia.

MEDICAL ASPECTS OF ANESTHESIA FOR CATARACT SURGERY

Cataract Type and Associated Conditions

Cataracts can be either congenital or acquired. Patients who have congenital cataracts often have associated syndromes and conditions, such as cerebral, ocular, facial, and skeletal syndrome, in which the patient has multiple facial and skeletal abnormalities and can be difficult to intubate. In those with Marfan syndrome, the underlying cardiac conditions may cause added problems. Patients who have acquired cataracts usually are elderly; the average age is 75. Medical conditions such as ischemic heart disease and chronic obstructive airway disease commonly coexist with cataracts. In one study 84% of patients had at least one concomitant serious medical disease.[1] The risk of cataract is increased in patients older than 49 years who use inhaled steroids.[2] Overall, cataract extraction is associated with a significant increase in overall mortality in those with the following conditions[3]:

- Hypertension (47%)
- Ischemic heart disease (38%)
- History of hypothyroidism (18%)
- Diabetes (16%)
- History of a new malignancy (3%)

Consequently, the Royal Colleges of Anaesthetists and Ophthalmologists recommend that patients undergoing local anesthesia for intraocular surgery be subject to a full preoperative history and examination, with appropriate investigations, to ensure that they are in the best possible condition to undergo surgery.[4]

Specific Conditions

ISCHEMIC HEART DISEASE. Stress may cause ischemia and can be provoked at the prospect of local or general anesthesia; neither of these should be given within 6 months of a myocardial infarction without appropriate medical consultation. Medication should be continued throughout the perioperative period. The application of phenylephrine drops for dilatation may result in a rise in blood pressure, and they should be administered with caution. The oxidative damage resulting in cataract formation is linked to free radical formation and atherosclerosis. A prospective study showed that patients undergoing cataract extraction have a higher risk of coronary artery heart disease, especially women with insulin-dependent diabetes.[3]

DIABETES MELLITUS. Local anesthesia causes the least disruption to diabetic management. However, in some cases, local anesthesia may not be possible, and general anesthesia may be necessary. Nowadays this need not disrupt diabetic therapy, as recovery from the new anesthetic agents is rapid.[5]

ANTICOAGULANTS. Most patients on oral anticoagulants, including aspirin, should not stop these before surgery. The risk of hemorrhage is less than the risk of cardiovascular complications. There are varying data, and until a large series of patients taking anticoagulants is studied, general anesthesia is the method of choice; sub-Tenon's block or peribulbar block is recommended if local anesthesia is indicated.[6] The prothrombin time should not be greater than twice the control level.

LOCAL ANESTHESIA

Local anesthesia can be classified into topical anesthesia, retrobulbar block, peribulbar block, and sub-Tenon's block.

General Considerations

The main advantage of local anesthesia is a conscious and alert patient. Sedation, even with midazolam, has variable effects and can result in a confused and uncooperative patient or one who suddenly "comes to" in the middle of the operation and tries to sit up. However, being awake may distress certain patients, or the stress of having a needle inserted around the eye may provoke an increase in blood pressure and possibly cause cardiac ischemia.

Many medical conditions common in the elderly population render patients unsuitable for local anesthesia, such as those who are unable to lie flat because of chronic obstructive airway disease or cardiovascular problems. However, evidence suggests that catecholamine release is reduced under local anesthesia; this improves cardiovascular stability, which may make local anesthesia a suitable technique for the elderly population.[7]

The fasting regimens for patients undergoing local anesthesia were recently surveyed among the members of the British Ophthalmic Anaesthesia Society.[8] The majority did not require fasting patients; 37% would give sedation and 27.8% analgesia without fasting. Almost two thirds gave sedation on some occasions, although some stopped if the patient became unmanageable and disoriented. In the United States, members of the American Society of Anesthesiologists do not differentiate between general anesthesia and regional anesthesia with or without sedation. They require patients to fast for 6 hours after eating food and for 2 hours after taking clear fluids before the administration of local anesthesia.

Minimal monitoring of the patient should include pulse oximetry, as many elderly patients become hypoxic when lying flat even with no sedation, and one third of patients have a saturation less than 95% when breathing air. Other monitoring includes an electrocardiogram, blood pressure measurements, and a trained observer, who must be an anesthetist if sedation is used, to maintain verbal contact with the patient. During the procedure, it is important to reduce the frequency of blood pressure measurements, as many patients find these uncomfortable and may move when the cuff tightens. Intravenous access always should be secured.

Supplemental oxygen is usually given to patients regardless of the use of sedation for the reasons stated earlier and to minimize the sensation of claustrophobia. Rebreathing can occur even at 6L/minute with oxygen just administered under the drapes. A Venturi system or oxygen at 2L/minute via nasal cannulae is a superior method.[9,10]

Inadvertent inhalation anesthesia has been reported when supplemental oxygen was given by the outlet on the anesthetic machine, a common practice. The recommendation is that the anesthetic machine be used only by an anesthetist.[11]

All operating room personnel must be trained in basic life support, and at least one member should have advanced training.[4]

It is recommended in the United Kingdom that an anesthetist (anesthesiologist) be present throughout the operation, whether local or general anesthesia is being used, to look after the patient's welfare.

Patients for whom local anesthesia may not be indicated are those:

- Who are unable to cooperate (e.g., with mental impairment)
- In whom communication is difficult (e.g., inability to speak the language or deafness)
- Who have involuntary movements (e.g., those with Parkinson's disease)
- Who are unable to lie flat or still
- Who have uncontrolled coughing or sneezing
- Who are severely anxious or claustrophobic
- Undergoing bilateral surgery
- For whom prolonged or difficult surgery is likely
- For whom general anesthesia is preferred, whether by the patient, the surgeon, or the anesthetist

The objectives of local anesthesia are as follows[12]:

- Ensure that the block procedure is painless
- Provide globe and conjunctival anesthesia
- Obtain a low pressure within the orbit and globe
- Avoid local and systemic complications

Sedative Agents Used in Local Anesthesia

Midazolam, a short-acting, water-soluble benzodiazepine with a half-life of 2 hours, is now the most frequently chosen sedative for its amnesic and anxiolytic properties, lack of venous sequelae, rapid patient recovery, and absence of hangover effects. It is administered intravenously in 1mg increments, and if it is given sufficient time to act in patients with a slow circulation, a total dose of 2–3mg usually is ample.

Diazepam (Diazemuls) has a longer half-life and a greater hangover effect and is less suitable than midazolam for sedation in cataract patients.

All the benzodiazepines can be reversed with flumazenil, a specific antagonist with a half-life of 1 hour. Therefore, resedation can be a problem.

Propofol, a short-acting phenol, is an intravenous induction agent suitable for infusion and sedation. It is characterized by a rapid and clear-headed recovery, with a low incidence of nausea

and vomiting. Respiratory depression is less than with thiopental sodium, but it can occur. Both these agents decrease the systolic and diastolic blood pressure.

Propofol and midazolam have been used for patient-controlled sedation, whereby patients self-administer a dose of either 3.3mg of propofol with no lockout (2.5mg for patients older than 60 years, with a lockout of 3 minutes) or 0.1mg of midazolam with no lockout. This has been shown to significantly reduce patients' level of anxiety, and they remain cooperative enough to press the button, eliminating the unpredictability of elderly patients' reaction to sedation. The heart rates were reduced in both groups; midazolam obtunded the rise in blood pressure during surgery but has a greater risk than propofol of stacking doses, resulting in oversedation.[13]

Fentanyl is a potent, short-acting narcotic analgesic with a duration of action of about 30 minutes. Given in doses of 25–50μg, it provides analgesia with minimal sedation. However, it has the side effects of all narcotic analgesics, including respiratory depression, nausea, and vomiting.

Remifentanil is an ultra-short-acting analgesic metabolized by esterases, resulting in an elimination half-life of 3–10 minutes. It produces intense analgesia, but it needs to be supplemented because it also wears off within 3–10 minutes when the infusion is stopped. It causes a fall in heart rate and blood pressure, though it is used in frail patients as a cardiac-stable anesthetic; it causes respiratory depression but less nausea and vomiting than morphine. Remifentanil is administered by infusion, given in conjunction with other induction agents. It is not recommended for use as a sole agent. The initial dose is a bolus of 1μg/kg over 30 seconds, followed by an infusion of 0.05–2μg/kg per minute.

Topical Anesthesia

The first modern use of topical anesthesia was by Koller in 1884 with cocaine. Since then, synthetic drugs have become available; cocaine is no longer used because of the potential risk of side effects and drug abuse. Benoxinate 0.4% (oxybuprocaine; 2-diethylaminoethyl-4-amino-3-butoxybenzoate), an ester anesthetic, is currently the most frequently used because of its high degree of safety. Other commonly used agents are tetracaine 0.5% or 1% amethocaine and proparacaine (proxymetacaine) 0.5%; both are short acting (20 minutes) and are the least toxic to the corneal epithelium. Lidocaine 4% (lignocaine) and bupivacaine 0.5% and 0.75% have a longer duration of action but an increased associated corneal toxicity.[14]

Relative contraindications to topical anesthesia are difficult or extended surgery, language barrier, deafness, and an uncooperative patient. Absolute contraindications are true allergy to local anesthesia and nystagmus.

The advantages and disadvantages of topical anesthesia are given in Box 45-1. Topical anesthesia may be combined with subconjunctival anesthesia. This allows subconjunctival and scleral manipulations to be carried out, with good toleration by patients.[15]

TECHNIQUE. The aim is to block the nerves that supply the superficial cornea and conjunctiva; namely, the long and short ciliary, nasociliary, and lacrimal nerves. The patient should be warned that application of the drops on the surface of the cornea stings (except for proxymetacaine). Drops are administered before the placement of the drapes.

Preparation of the unblocked eyelid requires the patient to keep the eye closed, but the eye is kept open when the plastic drape is applied in order to secure the lid and lashes. As visual perception is not lost, the patient is asked to focus on the source of the light, the intensity of which is reduced subsequently.[17] The subconjunctival injection of antibiotics can be painful, but this can be avoided by including these in the infusion bottle.

Thirty percent of all cataract operations in the United States were performed under topical anesthesia in 1998, though pain scores were higher than with other methods.

BOX 45-1

Advantages and Disadvantages of Topical Anesthesia

ADVANTAGES
- No risk associated at needle insertion
- No risk of periocular hemorrhage or hyphema with clear corneal incisions; systemic anticoagulation can be continued without any worry
- Functional vision is maintained; advantageous for uniocular patients
- No postoperative diplopia or ptosis
- Patients are fully alert

DISADVANTAGES
- An awake and talkative patient can be distracting for the surgeon
- No akinesia of the eye
- If difficulties or problems occur the anesthesia may not be adequate

ADVERSE EFFECTS OF TOPICAL OCULAR ANESTHETICS[16]
- Direct corneal effects—alteration of lacrimation and tear film stability
- Epithelial toxicity—healing has been shown to be delayed when an epithelial defect occurs (lidocaine does not appear to affect healing)
- Endothelial toxicity—this occurs when penetrating trauma is present and appears to be related to the preservative benzalkonium
- Systemic effects—lethal toxicity (this is only a problem with cocaine)
- Allergy and idiosyncratic reactions—contact dermatitis is the most common and occurs with proparacaine most frequently

SECONDARY ADVERSE EFFECTS
- Surface keratopathy

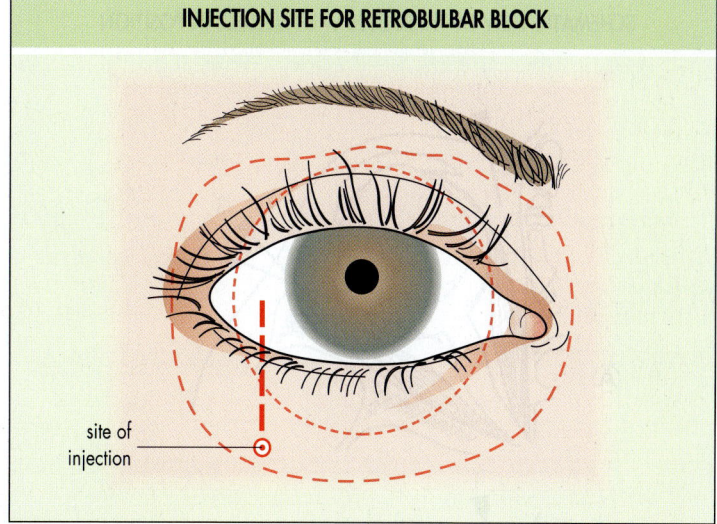

INJECTION SITE FOR RETROBULBAR BLOCK

site of injection

FIG. 45-1 ■ Injection site for retrobulbar block. The injection site through the lower lid lies halfway between the lateral canthus and the lateral limbus. (Adapted from Sanderson Grizzard W. Ophthalmic anaesthesia. Ann Ophthalmol. 1989;21:265–94.)

BOX 45-2

Risk Factors Predisposing to Perforation of the Eyeball[24]

Long eye, axial length >26mm; patients with axial myopia have a 30 times greater risk
Posterior staphyloma
Enophthalmos
Faulty technique
Uncooperative patient
Unnecessarily long needle
No appreciation of risk factors

INTRAOCULAR LIDOCAINE. Recently, intraocular lidocaine has been used to provide analgesia during surgery. The solution used is 1% isotonic, nonpreserved lidocaine 0.3ml administered intramurally.[15] At present, no side effects have been reported, except for possible transient retinal toxicity if lidocaine is injected posteriorly in the absence of a posterior capsule.[18] Its use obviates the need for intravenous and regional anesthetic supplementation in most patients. Adequate anesthesia is obtained in about 10 seconds.[19] As with all topical techniques, the ability of the patient to cooperate during surgery is desirable.

DEEP TOPICAL FORNIX NERVE BLOCK. In this technique, first described in 1995, local anesthetic (0.5% bupivacaine) is placed on sponges deep in the conjunctival fornices for 15 minutes. The agent diffuses across the conjunctiva into the peribulbar space to reach the scleral nerve behind the eye.

The advantage is a needle-free technique, useful for patients on anticoagulants or who will not accept injections. The disadvantage is that it causes patient discomfort that may not be tolerated. Reducing the size of the sponges helps.

Retrobulbar Block

Knapp described the first retrobulbar block in 1884 using 4% cocaine.[15] The anatomy of the orbit is described fully in Chapter 83.

The aim is to block the oculomotor nerves before they enter the four rectus muscles in the posterior intraconal space. Some activity may be retained in the superior oblique muscle because of its extraconal course.

POSITION OF THE EYE. The primary gaze is now the accepted position, as the optic nerve is directed away from the path of the needle toward the medial side of the midsagittal plane.[22]

SITE OF THE INJECTION. The injection site is immediately above the inferior orbital rim, between the temporal limbus and the lateral canthus; injection is subconjunctival either via the skin or by pulling the lower eyelid down. This is a relatively avascular area (Fig. 45-1).[23]

NEEDLES. A sharp 25- or 27-gauge needle is used, no more than 31mm in length to avoid piercing the optic nerve. Traditionally, a blunt, intermediate-gauge needle was thought to be safer, as it pushes the tissues aside, which causes less trauma

and makes it more difficult to penetrate the globe but causes more damage if penetration occurs (Box 45-2 lists the risk factor for penetration; see Fig. 45-2). Nowadays, a sharp cutting needle is used, as it results in less pain, less distortion, and less tissue damage. An increase in the gauge results in a reduced "feel" of the tissue planes as the needle passes through them.

LOCAL ANESTHETIC AGENT. The most common mixture used is bupivacaine 0.5% plus lidocaine 2% plus hyaluronidase 150u. Alternatively, bupivacaine 0.75% with lidocaine may be used. The mixture (2–4ml) is injected slowly to avoid patient discomfort. Aspiration prior to injection minimizes the risk of intravascular or subdural injection. Other agents used are mepivacaine 1–2%, lidocaine 1–2% solely, and bupivacaine 0.25–0.75% alone.

Epinephrine (adrenaline) 5μg/ml may be added to improve the onset time, quality, and duration of the block. However, it should be avoided in patients who have ischemic heart disease, tachycardia, and hypertension. Also, epinephrine has been implicated in optic artery thrombosis secondary to vasoconstriction. A 50% decrease in the pressure in the ophthalmic artery has been noted, so epinephrine is probably best avoided in patients who have generalized atherosclerosis.

Hyaluronidase breaks down C1-C4 bonds between glucosamine and glucuronic acid in connective tissue, which enables the local anesthetic to permeate the tissues more effectively; the required quantity of local anesthetic is therefore reduced, and the time to onset is decreased. It appears that 150IU decreases ocular movements more than 15IU does.[25] Hyaluronidase may help prevent damage to extraocular muscles, especially the inferior rectus muscle, and may prevent diplopia.[26]

SCHEMATIC VIEW OF THREE EYES WITH NEEDLES IN POSITION

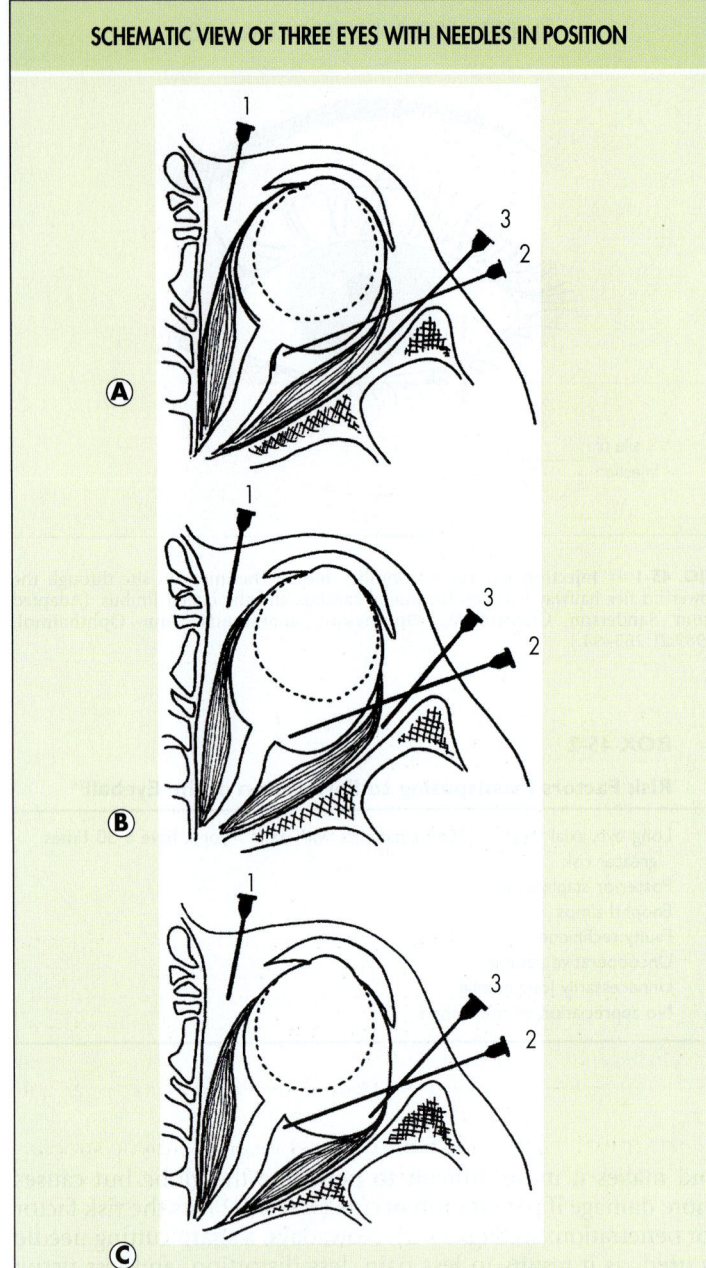

FIG. 45-2 ■ Schematic view of three eyes with needles in position. Dotted lines show outline of normal (non-myopic) eye. **A,** Severe myopia without staphyloma. **B,** Posterior staphyloma. **C,** Inferolateral staphyloma. Needles: *1,* medial canthus peribulbar block; *2,* retrobulbar block; *3,* inferolateral peribulbar block. Note that only the position of needle 1 does not risk perforation. (From Thind CS, Rubin AP. Editorial VI. Local anaesthesia for eye surgery—no room for complacency. Br J Anaesth. 2001;86:473–6.)

The use of "painless" local anesthetic to initially anesthetize the skin and subcutaneous tissues is becoming more popular. The solution is made by adding 1.5ml of lidocaine 2% to 15ml of balanced salt solution.

Amethocaine or EMLA cream applied to the skin at least 1 hour preoperatively removes the pain of injection if the needle will pass through the skin.[27]

TECHNIQUE OF INJECTION. With the globe in primary gaze, the needle is inserted at the lower temporal orbital margin, halfway between the lateral canthus and the lateral limbus, close to the bone. The needle is passed posteriorly parallel to the plane of the orbital floor at an angle of 10° to the horizontal until the tip passes the equator of the globe. This corresponds with the middle of the needle being in the plane of the iris. Then the needle is directed slightly upward and medially, avoiding the bony orbit and periosteum (which is painful if touched), so that it approaches but does not cross the midsagittal plane of the

ADVANCEMENT OF NEEDLE IN RETROBULBAR BLOCK

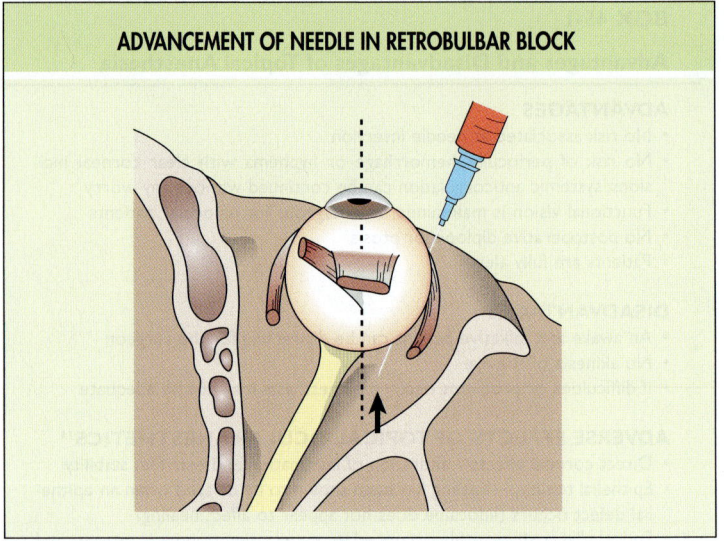

FIG. 45-3 ■ Advancement of needle in retrobulbar block. The needle is advanced beyond the equator of the globe and then directed toward an imaginary point behind the macula, with care taken not to cross the midsagittal plane of the eye. (Adapted from Sanderson Grizzard W. Ophthalmic anaesthesia. Ann Ophthalmol. 1989;21:265–94.)

globe, as though moving toward an imaginary point behind the macula. When the hub of the needle reaches the plane of the iris, the tip should be in the intraconal space, 4–5mm behind the globe if it is of normal axial length (Figs. 45-3 and 45-4).

After aspiration, the local anesthetic is injected slowly. Any movement of the globe is noted, as this is indicative of possible scleral puncture. Asking the patient to move the eye is dangerous, as movement increases the likelihood of vascular or optic nerve injury. A Honan balloon usually is used to spread the anesthetic and soften the eye.

Facial nerve blocks are not performed routinely, as adequate akinesia is generally obtained. They also are painful, cause a facial palsy that is disfiguring when working, and leave the cornea unprotected.[5]

It is imperative that proper training be given to either the ophthalmologist or anesthetist to decrease the risk of complications. Provided this occurs, there is no difference in the complication rate between the specialties.[28,29]

The advantages and disadvantages of retrobulbar block are given in Box 45-3. Complications associated with retrobulbar block include:

- Retrobulbar hemorrhage
- Ocular perforation (<0.1% incidence, but 1 in 140 injections in highly myopic eyes)[29]
- Subarachnoid or intradural injection, leading to brainstem anesthesia in 1 in 350–500 patients[6]
- Respiratory depression or arrest (0.29% incidence)
- Optic nerve contusion and atrophy
- Retinal vascular occlusion
- Grand mal seizure
- Decreased visual acuity
- Hypotony
- Contralateral amaurosis
- Muscle complications: ptosis from levator aponeurosis dehiscence, entropion and diplopia following extraocular muscle injection
- Pulmonary edema[31]
- Oculocardiac reflex, usually produced by pressure on the globe (vasovagal bradycardias are more common)

Overall, there is a 1–3% chance that complications will occur. However, even if only a minimal complication occurs, the operation is abandoned; the worst complications are life or sight threatening.[32] Hence, it is recommended that an anes-

RETROBULBAR BLOCK/INFEROTEMPORAL INTRACONAL BLOCK

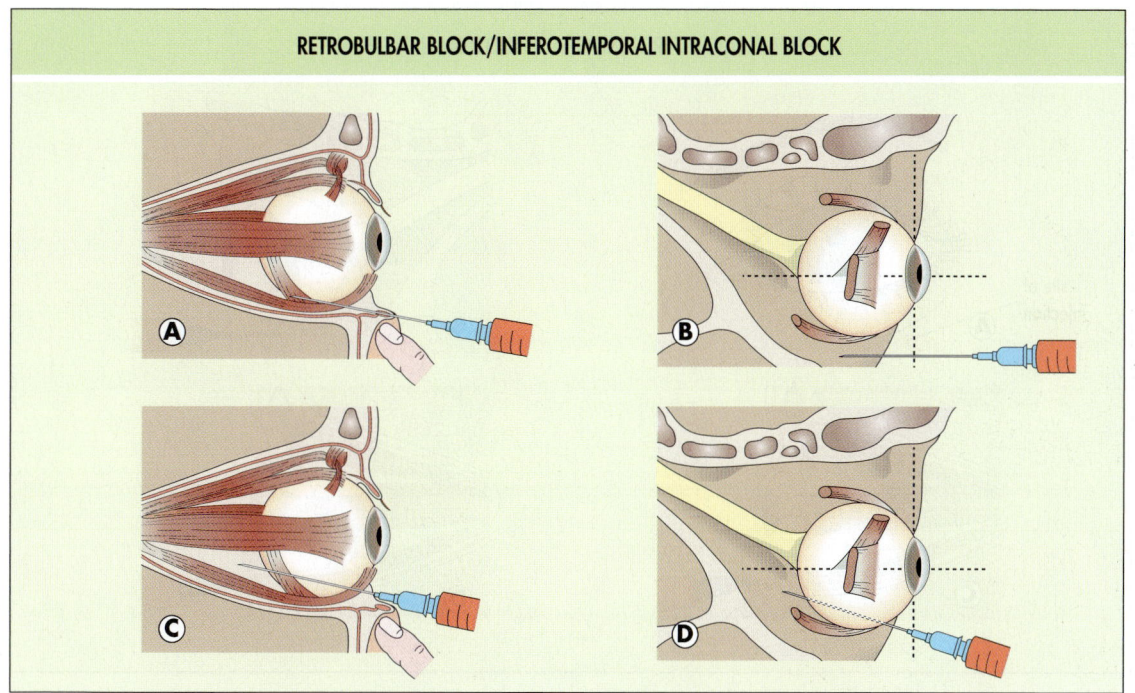

FIG. 45-4 ■ Inferotemporal intraconal block (retrobulbar block). **A,** The needle tip enters at the lower temporal orbital rim slightly up from the orbital floor and passes very close to the bone. **B,** At 10° elevation parallel to the orbital floor, the needle passes backward until its midshaft is at the iris. The tip is then at the equator of the globe. **C,** The needle is then directed at an imaginary point behind the globe on the axis formed by the pupil and macula. **D,** The needle does not pass the midsagittal plane of the globe. It enters the intraconal space after passing through the intermuscular septum. Any movement of the sclera is noted. After test aspiration, 4ml of anesthetic solution is injected. (Adapted from Hamilton RC. Techniques of orbital regional anaesthesia. Br J Anaesth. 2001;86:473–6.)

BOX 45-3

Advantages and Disadvantage of Retrobulbar Block

ADVANTAGES
- A retrobulbar block is reliable for producing excellent anesthesia and akinesia
- The onset of the block is quicker than with peribulbar; it usually occurs within 5 minutes
- Low volumes of anesthetic result in a lower intraorbital tension and less chemosis than with peribulbar blocks
- Loss of visual acuity occurs in a greater number of patients compared to peribulbar blocks, though this can be volume dependent[30]; some patients may be distressed by being able to see throughout the procedure

DISADVANTAGE
- The main disadvantage of retrobulbar blocks is that the complication rate is higher than for peribulbar blocks—the reason for the development of the peribulbar block

thetist be present to monitor and, if necessary, resuscitate the patient.

Peribulbar Block

The principle of this technique is to instill the local anesthetic outside the muscle cone and avoid proximity to the optic nerve. This utilizes high volumes of anesthetic and the application of a pressure device. The local anesthetic agents do not differ from those used in retrobulbar block, but typically shorter needles are used.

Prilocaine 3% has been used effectively for peribulbar blocks, with and without felypressin. The toxicity of prilocaine is less (although the volumes involved are well under the toxic range) and there are fewer cardiac side effects than with bupivacaine. When compared with lignocaine 2% and the mixture of lignocaine with bupivacaine, prilocaine produces a rapid onset, a dense block, and greater akinesia with reduced need for repeat

injections.[33] A single medial injection technique with prilocaine has good results and decreases the risk of problems by decreasing the number of injections.[34]

A single medial canthus injection of 7–9ml of 2% articaine has also been used to good effect.[35]

TECHNIQUE. The volume varies from 3–10ml; the usual volume is 5–7ml. Again, the eye is in primary gaze.

The initial injection is with painless local anesthetic subconjunctivally at the inferotemporal lower orbital margin, midway between the lateral canthus and the lateral limbus. The 27- or 25-gauge needle is then advanced parallel to the plane of the orbital floor and injected at a depth of about 2.5cm from the inferior orbital rim (in an eye of normal axial length). As with retrobulbar blocks, no resistance to injection should be felt, and aspiration should be performed (Figs. 45-5 and 45-6).

After 5 minutes, the amount of akinesia is assessed. Often, a second injection is required to block the superior oblique. A 25-gauge, 2.5cm needle is inserted between the medial canthus and the caruncle, which is another relatively avascular area; then the needle is directed immediately backward. The medial check ligament often is penetrated, and the medial rectus can be injected at this point. At a depth of 1.5cm, another 5ml of solution is injected to produce a more complete block, with akinesia of the orbicularis oculi and levator palpebrae superioris (see Fig. 45-6). This avoids the alternative option of injecting the superotemporal region and causing ecchymosis of the eyelid. A Honan balloon or pressure-lowering device is applied for 20–30 minutes. Four milliliters of local anesthetic can increase the intraocular pressure over 6.2mm Hg; ocular compression can decrease the intraocular pressure by 8.8mm Hg after 5 minutes and by 14.3mm Hg after 40 minutes. In compromised patients, ocular compression may be advantageous prior to insertion of the local anesthetic.[6]

A single medial canthus injection has been described at the junction of the caruncle and medial canthus, which is usually at the junction of the medial two thirds and lateral two thirds of the lower orbital rim. This is easily learned, and fewer injections decrease the complication rate.

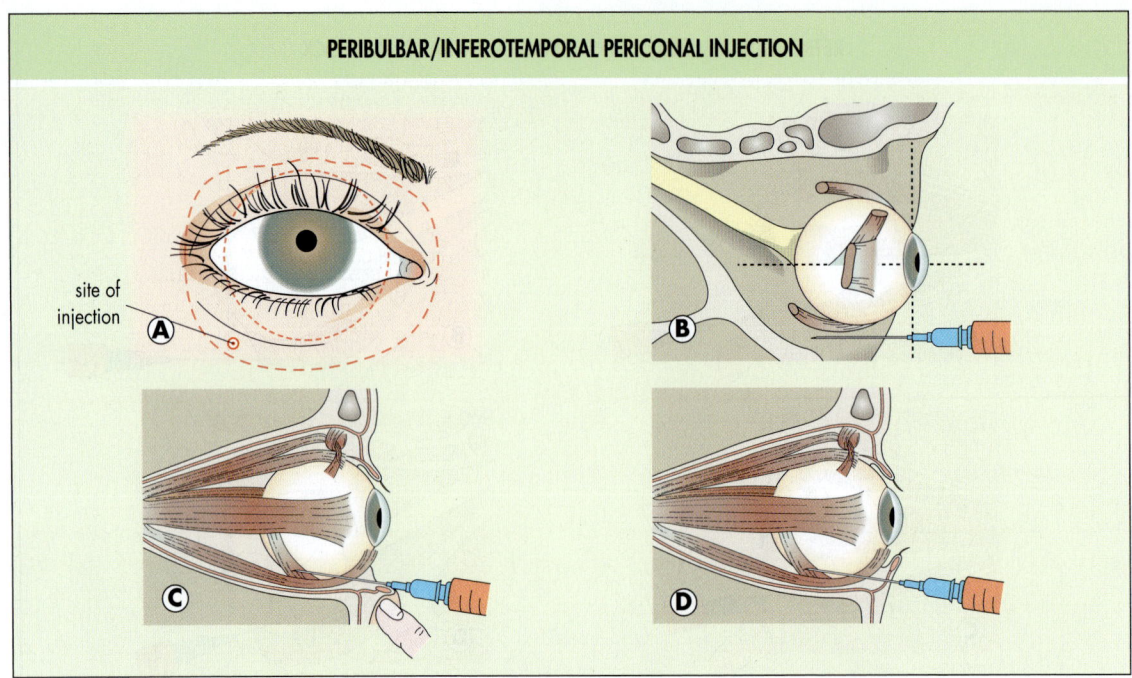

FIG. 45-5 ▓ **Inferotemporal periconal injection. A,** The needle enters the orbit at the junction of its floor with the lateral wall, very close to the bony rim. **B,** The needle passes backward in a sagittal plane parallel to the orbit floor. **C,** It passes the globe equator when the needle-hub junction reaches the plane of the iris. **D,** After test aspiration, up to 10ml anesthetic solution is injected. (Adapted from Hamilton RC. Techniques of orbital regional anaesthesia. Br J Anaesth. 2001;86:473–6.)

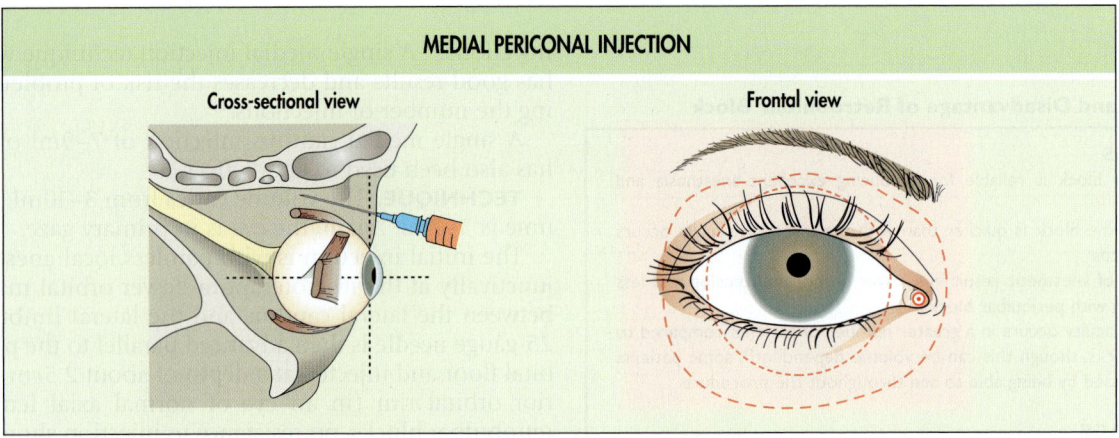

FIG. 45-6 ▓ **Medial periconal injection.** The globe is in the primary gaze. The needle enters transconjunctivally on the medial side of the caruncle at the extreme medial side of the palpebral fissure. With the bevel facing the orbit wall, it passes backward in the transverse plane, directed at a 5° angle away from the sagittal plane and toward the medial orbit wall. (Adapted from Hamilton RC. Techniques of orbital regional anaesthesia. Br J Anaesth. 2001;86:473–6.)

The advantages and disadvantages of peribulbar block are given in Box 45-4.

Sub-Tenon's Block

TECHNIQUE. The conjunctiva is anesthetized first using drops of local anesthetic, such as benzocaine. A bridle suture is placed around the superior rectus muscle. Then the capsule is incised under sterile conditions at a point 7–8mm from the corneal limbus, between the 1 o'clock and 2 o'clock positions. A specially designed needle is now available with the correct curved radius of 30mm and a flattened tip to ensure that it remains within the capsule and rigid (this enables feedback); it is 26mm long so that it passes beyond the equator. Some resistance is met at this point as the scleral Tenon bridging fibers are entered. Slow injection allows advancement of the needle and pushes the tissues away. A flexible needle, the Greenbaum cannula, has now

been designed, with excellent results.[36] Dissection is carried out down to bare sclera through the conjunctiva. The incision is small, so a few milliliters of local anesthetic are forced posteriorly. The mixture of 2.5–3.5ml of lidocaine 2% (5ml) plus bupivacaine 0.5% (5ml) plus 1500U hyaluronidase provides good anesthesia. Comparison with peribulbar anesthesia shows that it is a suitable alternative, with better akinesia, improved consistency, and a quicker onset.[22,37]

The advantages and disadvantages of sub-Tenon's block are given in Box 45-5.

GENERAL ANESTHESIA

General anesthesia is performed on those patients who are unsuitable candidates for local anesthesia, as described earlier. Anxious and nervous patients lead to anxious surgeons, which may impair surgical performance[39]—a strong indication for a

BOX 45-4

Advantages and Disadvantages of Peribulbar Block

ADVANTAGES
- The risk of complications associated with peribulbar block is low
- Peribulbar block has all the advantages of retrobulbar block

DISADVANTAGES
- Peribulbar blocks have all the disadvantages of retrobulbar blocks, but they occur less frequently
- The quality of akinesia and anesthesia may not be as good as with retrobulbar block
- Often more than one injection is required
- The block takes much longer to work—it can take up to 30 minutes
- The Honan balloon may be uncomfortable for the patient
- Chemosis occurs in 80% of cases, which makes operating conditions difficult
- In 5.8% of both retrobulbar and peribulbar blocks, ptosis can remain for up to 90 days
- One perforation for every 140 peribulbar blocks in eyes >26mm axial length

BOX 45-5

Advantages and Disadvantages of Sub-Tenon's Block

ADVANTAGES
- It is less painful than a retrobulbar block[38]
- No serious complications are associated with this technique
- No increase in intraocular pressure occurs with the administration of local anesthetic
- Surgery can begin almost immediately
- Lasts for 60 minutes and supplemental anesthetic agent can be given
- The globe can be voluntarily moved at the surgeon's instruction
- Low dose and low volume of anesthetic agent are used

DISADVANTAGES
- The local anesthetic agent must be injected into the capsule—double perforation of the conjunctiva results in anesthetic leaking out, which decreases the effectiveness of the block
- Although it is an advantage that the globe can be moved under instruction, it is important that the eye is not moved at other times—use of stabilizing sutures or forceps is advised
- Dissection of the capsule must be carried out under sterile conditions

BOX 45-6

Advantages and Disadvantages of General Anesthesia

ADVANTAGES
- Patient comfort
- Ideal operating conditions—a quiet, immobile patient and soft eye
- Allows for rapid alterations in intraocular pressure if required
- The method of choice for difficult cases
- Effective for more patients
- No risk of any of the complications associated with local anesthetic blocks
- No residual paralysis of the eye when the patient is awake
- Bilateral surgery can be performed, which is advantageous in the frail, elderly, and medically "unfit"
- Better conditions for teaching

DISADVANTAGES
- Slightly slower turnaround times, if only one anesthetist is available
- More expensive

general anesthetic. It is the method of choice for babies, children, and even some young adults.

The traditional method for administering a general anesthetic for cataract surgery was to intubate, paralyze, and ventilate the patient. Potential problems included an insufficiently paralyzed patient coughing when the eye was open or, conversely, a patient remaining paralyzed at completion, which delays the onset of spontaneous respiration and turnover. However, with the advent of phacoemulsification and small incision surgery, plus the introduction of propofol and the laryngeal mask, it is feasible to have the patient breathing spontaneously. Previously, it was necessary to intubate a spontaneously breathing patient because of the competition for space around the operative site. To enable the endotracheal tube to be tolerated, the patient had to be anesthetized deeply with volatile agents of high concentration. These all cause some degree of cardiac depression and, in the elderly, could result in severe hypotension, which is associated with increased morbidity and mortality. Consequently, not intubating the patient allows a lighter anesthetic to be given, which does not cause as much cardiovascular depression and has a faster recovery. Although a comparison of etomidate-vecuronium-isoflurane with propofol infusion resulted in faster recovery times in the former group, there was no difference at 2 hours when all patients were assessed as fit to go home.[40] However, in the over-80-year-old group, psychomotor testing showed that total intravenous anesthesia with propofol and remifentanil resulted in significantly faster recovery of cognitive function compared with etomidate-fentanyl-isoflurane.[41]

Technique

SPONTANEOUS RESPIRATION. A laryngeal mask is inserted and anesthesia is maintained with either a continuous propofol infusion or a volatile agent of choice. The propofol infusion is adjusted to the end-tidal carbon dioxide and blood pressure, as an inspired volatile agent would be altered. A starting infusion corresponds to a blood level of 6mg/ml dropping to 4mg/ml; a simpler procedure is to use half the induction dose in milligrams as ml/hr[42] (e.g., 150mg induction followed by 75ml/hr maintenance infusion rate). The introduction of target-controlled infusions may further simplify this technique. Propofol 4.5μg/ml bolus for induction followed by 3.25μg/ml maintenance target infusion levels are combined with either an alfentanil (target blood concentration 25ng/ml) or remifentanil (1–1.5ng/ml) infusion. The use of a laryngeal mask enables faster turnaround times and reduces the cough associated with extubation. It provides a stable, easily controlled anesthetic with rapid recovery and a low incidence of nausea and vomiting.[43]

VENTILATION. The traditional method involves endotracheal intubation. Suxamethonium is avoided, if possible, as a transient rise in intraocular pressure occurs with its use. Muscle pains also are a problem; they usually occur in ambulant younger patients and cause some debilitation. Short-acting nondepolarizers are used in preference, along with an induction agent; maintenance consists of using a volatile agent of choice or a propofol infusion. Although changeovers may be slower, especially if single handed, this technique also provides a stable, easily controlled anesthetic and is the method of choice for certain patients for whom spontaneous respiration is inappropriate (e.g., the obese and patients who cough despite adequate anesthetic).

CONCLUSION. Both spontaneous respiration and ventilation methods are suitable for day-case anesthesia.[44] They are both widely used in all other specialties. Topical local anesthesia can be used as an adjunct, as it reduces systemic anesthetic requirements. It also may allow opiates to be avoided, which results in a decrease in the incidence of postoperative nausea and vomiting. This is better for both the surgery and the well-being of the patient. Both propofol and the new volatile agents sevoflurane and desflurane provide a rapid and clear-headed recovery.

Hypotension needs to be aggressively treated with vasoconstrictors, such as ephedrine or metaraminol, to minimize morbidity.

The advantages and disadvantages of general anesthesia are given in Box 45-6.

POSTOPERATIVE CARE FOR BOTH LOCAL AND GENERAL ANESTHESIA

Cataract extraction by phacoemulsification is relatively pain free. In the majority of cases, simple analgesics are all that is required. Nonsteroidal anti-inflammatory drugs can be used with caution in the elderly to supplement analgesia, intravenously or orally. This can help reduce postoperative nausea and vomiting by avoiding opiates, though opiates are rarely needed for pain relief. Propofol also has antiemetic properties. The topical use of nonsteroidal anti-inflammatories has been shown to be equally effective in reducing the inflammatory response when compared with corticosteroids, and there are fewer side effects such as increased intraocular pressure, delayed wound healing, and infection. Corticosteroids can be reserved for the complicated cataract with more severe inflammation.[45]

REFERENCES

1. Fisher SJ, Cunningham RD. The medical profile of cataract patients. Geriatr Clin North Am. 1985;1:339–44.
2. Jick SS, Vasilakis-Scaramozza C, Maier WC. The risk of cataract among users of inhaled steroids. Epidemiology. 2001;12(2):229–34.
3. Hu FB, Hankinson SE, Stampfer MJ, et al. Prospective study of cataract extraction and the risk of coronary heart disease in women. Am J Epidemiol. 2001;153(9):875–81.
4. The Royal College of Anaesthetists & The Royal College of Ophthalmologists. Local anesthesia for intraocular surgery. July 2001.
5. Barker JP, Robinson PN, Vafidis GC, et al. Metabolic control of non-insulin-dependent diabetic patients undergoing cataract surgery: comparison of local and general anesthesia. Br J Anaesth. 1995;74:500–5.
6. Wong DHW. Review article: regional anaesthesia for intraocular surgery. Can J Anaesth. 1993;40(7):635–57.
7. Barker JP, Vafidis GC, Robinson PN, Hall GM. Plasma catecholamine response to cataract surgery. A comparison between general and local anesthesia. Anesthesia. 1991;46:642–5.
8. Steeds C, Mather SJ. Fasting regimes for regional ophthalmic anaesthesia. A survey of members of the British Ophthalmic Anaesthesia Society. Anaesthesia. 2001;56:638–42.
9. Risdall JE, Geraghty IF. Oxygenation of patients undergoing ophthalmic surgery under local anaesthesia. Anaesthesia. 1997;52:489–500.
10. Bosman YK, Krige SI, Edge KR, et al. Comfort and safety in eye surgery under local anaesthesia. Anaesth Intensive Care.1998;26:173–7.
11. Smith WQ. Inadvertent inhalation anaesthesia during surgery under retrobulbar eye block. Br J Anaesth. 1998;81:793–4.
12. Rubin AP. Local anesthesia for ophthalmic surgery: an anaesthetist's view. Eur J Implant Refract Surg. 1993;5:8–11.
13. Pac-Soo CK, Deacock S, Lockwood G, et al. Patient-controlled sedation for cataract surgery using peribulbar block. Br J Anaesth. 1996;77:370–4.
14. Davis DB, Mandeell MR. Anesthesia for cataract extraction. Int Ophthalmol Clin. 1993;33(4):13–32.
15. Anderson CI. Combined topical and subconjunctival anaesthesia in cataract surgery. Ophthalmic Surg. 1995;26(3):205–8.
16. Rosenwasser GOD. Complications of topical ocular anesthetics. Int Ophthalmol Clin. 1989;29(3):153–8.
17. Grabow HB. Topical anesthesia for cataract surgery. Eur J Implant Refract Surg. 1993;5:20–4.
18. Maloney WF. Intraocular lidocaine causes transient vision loss in small number of cases. Ocul Surg News. 1996;14(21):32.
19. Harvey B. Intraocular lidocaine eases pain after cataract surgery. Ocul Surg News. 1995;13(22):23.
20. Nicholson G, Mantovani C, Hall GM. Topical anaesthesia for cataract surgery. Br J Anaesth. 2001;86:900.
21. Aziz ES, Samura A. Prospective evaluation of deep topical fornix nerve block versus peribulbar block in patients undergoing cataract surgery using phacoemulsion. Br J Anaesth. 2000;85:314–6.
22. Hamilton RC. Techniques of orbital regional anesthesia. Br J Anaesth. 1995;75:88–92.
23. Sanderson Grizzard W. Ophthalmic anaesthesia. Ann Ophthalmol. 1989;21:265–94.
24. Thind CS, Rubin AP. Editorial VI. Local anaesthesia for eye surgery—no room for complacency. Br J Anaesth. 2001;86:473–6.
25. Mantovani C, Bryan AE, Nicholson G. Efficacy of varying concentrations of hyaluronidase in peribulbar anaesthesia. Br J Anaesth. 2001;86:876–8.
26. Brown SM, Brooks SE, Mazow ML, et al. Cluster of diplopia cases after periocular anesthesia without hyaluronidase. J Cataract Refract Surg. 1999;25:1245–9.
27. Joyce PW, Sunderraj P, Villada J, et al. A comparison of amethocaine cream with lignocaine-prilocaine cream (EMLA) for reducing pain during retrobulbar injection. Eye. 1994;8:465–6.
28. Kleinman B, Perlman J, Anderson C, et al. A collaborative regional ocular anesthesia training program: successes and failures. J Clin Anesth. 1999;11:301–4.
29. Edge R, Navon S. Scleral perforation during retrobulbar and peribulbar anesthesia: risk factors and outcome in 50,000 consecutive injections. J Cataract Refract Surg. 1999;25:1237–44.
30. Talks SJ, Chong NHV, Gibson JM, Francis IR. Visual acuity and pupillary reactions after peribulbar anesthesia. Br J Ophthalmol. 1994;78:41–3.
31. Kumar C, Lawler P. Case report. Pulmonary oedema after peribulbar block. Anaesthesia. 1999;82(5):777–9.
32. Rubin AP. Complications of local anesthesia for ophthalmic surgery. Br J Anaesth. 1995;75:93–6.
33. Bedi A, Carabine U. Peribulbar anaesthesia: a double-blind comparison of three local anaesthetic solutions. Anaesthesia. 1999;54:67–71.
34. Brahma K, Pemberton CJ, Ayeko M, Morgan LH. Single medial injection peribulbar anaesthesia using prilocaine. Anaesthesia. 1994;49:1003–5.
35. Allman KG, McFaden JG, Armstrong J, et al. Comparison of articaine and bupivacaine/lidocaine for single medial canthus peribulbar anaesthesia. Br J Anaesth. 2001;87:584–7.
36. Kumar CM. How to do a sub-Tenon's block. Cpd Anaesthesia. 2001;3(2):56–61.
37. Ripart J, Lefrant J-Y, Vivien B, et al. Ophthalmic regional anesthesia medial canthus episcleral (sub-Tenon) anesthesia is more efficient than peribulbar anesthesia. Anesthesiology. 2000;92(5):1278–85.
38. Tsuneoka H, Ohki K, Taniuchi O, Kitahara K. Tenon's capsule anesthesia for cataract surgery with IOL implantation. Eur J Implant Refract Surg. 1993;5:29–34.
39. Rosen E. Editorial review: anesthesia for cataract surgery. Eur J Implant Refract Surg. 1993;5:1–3.
40. Moffat A, Cullen PM. Comparison of two standard techniques of general anaesthesia for day-case cataract surgery. Br J Anaesth. 1995;74(2):145–8.
41. Kubitz J, Epple J, Bach A, et al. Psychomotor recovery in very old patients after total intravenous anaesthesia for cataract surgery. Br J Anaesth. 2001;86(2):203–8.
42. Jackson PW. In support of general anesthesia for cataract surgery. Eur J Implant Refract Surg. 1993;5:17–9.
43. Sutcliffe NP, Hyde R, Martay K. Use of "Diprifusor" in anaesthesia for ophthalmic surgery. Anaesthesia. 1998;53(suppl 1):49–52.
44. Moffat A, Cullen PM. Comparison of two standard techniques of general anesthesia for day-case cataract surgery. Br J Anaesth. 1995;74:145–8.
45. Simone J, Whitacre M. Effects of anti-inflammatory drugs following cataract extraction. Curr Opin Ophthalmol 2001;12:1263–7.

CHAPTER 46

The Mechanical and Hydrodynamic Aspects of Phacoemulsification

DAVID ALLEN

INTRODUCTION

As surgical techniques for the removal of cataract and drug modulation of the consequent biological responses have become more refined, the problems of postoperative infection and inflammation are less prominent in the thinking of lens surgeons. As a consequence, it has become possible to concentrate on the further refinement of the actual process of lens removal. Phacoemulsification (phaco) offers the surgeon the possibility to break the nucleus into smaller pieces and even into a fine emulsion of material, all of which can be removed through the probe used to achieve the breakup (Fig. 46-1). As a result, it is now possible to minimize trauma to the eye and to improve the stability of its shape after modern cataract surgery. To achieve this, however, requires the use of very powerful tools. Unfortunately, a good number of surgeons fail to understand the principles that underlie the machines they use. As a consequence of this relative ignorance, the surgery is sometimes performed less efficiently and possibly more dangerously than necessary.

HISTORICAL REVIEW

In February 1965 Charles Kelman suggested that the ultrasonic tool used at that time by some dentists to help descale teeth could also be used to fragment the nucleus of the crystalline lens and allow its removal without the need for a large incision. This liberated a powerful force, previously untried within the eye, but the equipment involved was large, inefficient, and extremely heavy. Nevertheless, he and others persevered.[1-4] Kelman's first operation using phaco on a human eye took 3 hours. At that time the patients were left aphakic or the incision needed considerable enlargement to allow insertion of the then relatively new, nonfoldable intraocular lenses (IOLs). Three developments—the technological progress of the 1970s and 1980s (particularly in solid-state electronic control mechanisms), new surgical techniques (particularly continuous curvilinear capsulorrhexis[5]), and the development of high-quality, foldable IOLs[6]—acted synergistically to enable the development of modern phaco surgery despite the considerable early resistance to this new technique.[7] Surgeons are now presented with increasingly sophisticated equipment that allows much more control of the surgical process. Understanding the basic principles of the equipment allows the surgeon to maximize this potential.

HANDPIECES AND TIPS

The phaco handpiece houses an ultrasonic transducer—a device that converts electrical energy into mechanical vibratory energy. Some crystals exhibit a relationship between mechanical stress and electricity—they are piezoelectric (electrostrictive). If an electric charge is applied to opposite faces of these crystals, a strain appears in the structure, which results in deformation. Similarly, magnetostrictive materials occur that are subject to strain when placed in a magnetic field; the transducer used in the first ophthalmic phaco handpieces was based on magnetostriction (Table

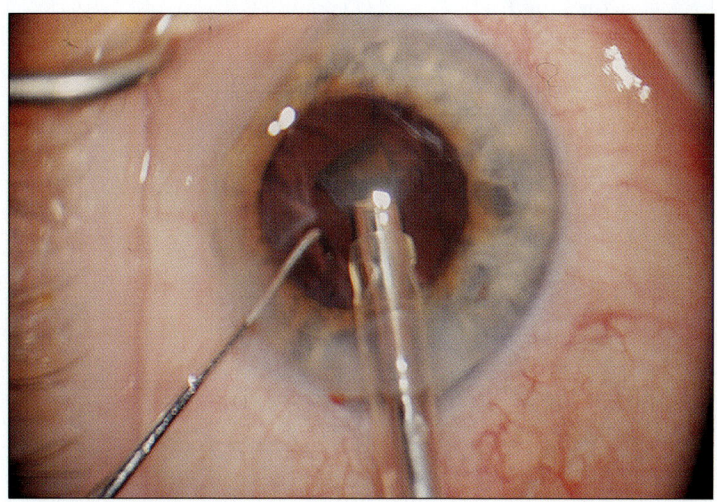

FIG. 46-1 ■ Phacoemulsification using the "Cobra tip."

TABLE 46-1

COMPARATIVE PROPERTIES OF THE TWO TYPES OF PHACO HANDPIECE

Property	Piezoelectric	Magnetostrictive
Power generation	More efficient	Less efficient
Power transfer	Less efficient	More efficient
Tip performance	No difference	No difference
Thermal stress	Vulnerable	Less vulnerable
Mechanical stress	Vulnerable	Less vulnerable
Purchase cost	Lower	Higher

46-1). The early magnetostrictive handpieces were inefficient and generated considerable heat, which required water cooling. Now efficient and powerful handpieces are available that use electrostrictive (piezoelectric) or magnetostrictive transducers.

The frequency at which a handpiece is set to work depends on the design and materials used. For each combination of mass and material a particular frequency exists at which the transducer works most efficiently. It now is possible to have the control unit continually "autotune" the handpiece (i.e., make small adjustments to compensate for the effects of changes in temperature, in the mass of the tip, etc.) so that the transducer always operates at the most efficient frequency. Adjustment of the power setting on the machine affects the stroke length (the distance traveled by the tip during one cycle) but not the frequency. It is clear that if the frequency remains constant but the distance traveled in each stroke increases, the acceleration of the tip and the maximum speed it reaches must be greater. This increases the effectiveness of the various processes at work that break up the nuclear material.

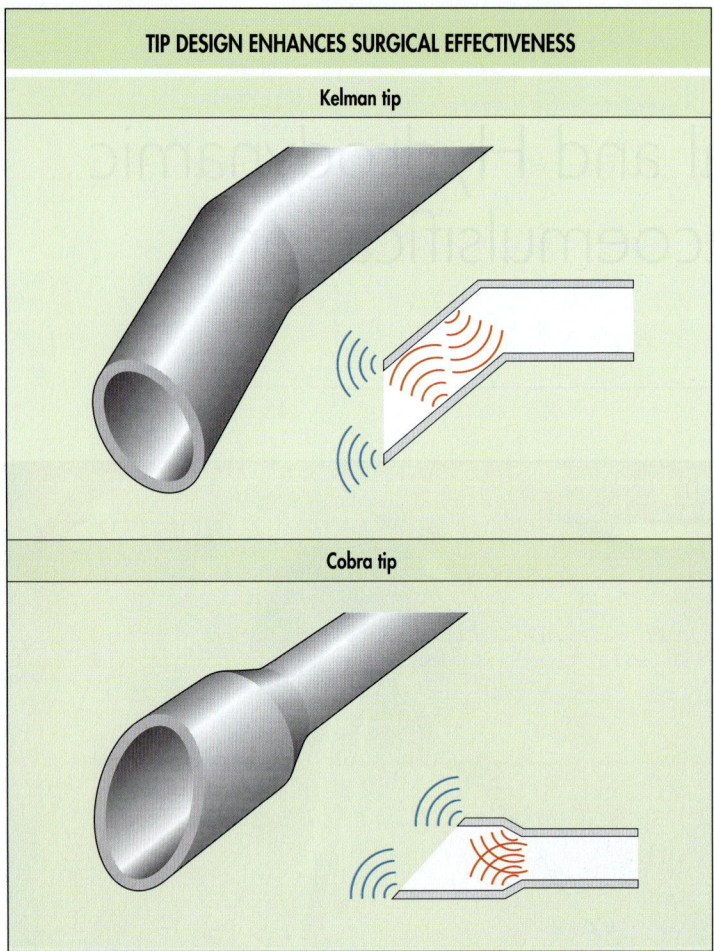

TIP DESIGN ENHANCES SURGICAL EFFECTIVENESS

Kelman tip

Cobra tip

FIG. 46-2 ■ **Tip design enhances surgical effectiveness.** In the Kelman tip and the Cobra tip, acoustic or shock waves (red) are generated within the tip and project forward, in addition to the conventional waves (blue) that are generated at the cutting edge of all tips.

The physical mechanisms that break up nuclear material when a phaco tip is used are complex, and the relative importance of the various factors is not yet entirely clear.[8,9] The direct, mechanical, hammer-like effect of the extremely hard titanium tip, although intuitively the most important, is probably not. A phaco tip operated at a frequency of 44kHz has a maximum speed of 66ft/sec (20m/sec) when operated at full power, and the acceleration of the tip is >168,300ft/sec^2 (>51,000m/sec^2). Under these conditions, direct impact of the tip breaks frictional forces within the nuclear material, but this may be relatively unimportant. This direct effect is reduced by the forward-propagating acoustic waves or fluid and particle waves generated by the tip, which tend to push away any piece of nucleus approached by an active tip. However, the acoustic shock waves themselves tend to weaken or break some of the bonds that hold nuclear material together.

Cavitation is being recognized increasingly as an extremely destructive process that occurs in a system with very rapid movement of metal objects in a fluid environment. The effect of a rapidly retreating phaco tip on the return part of its cycle is to create a void (and hence bubble) within the fluid, just in front of the retreating tip. As the tip retreats more, the size of the "bubble" increases until the forces generated within it cause it to implode. The mechanical and thermal forces that occur during such an implosion are surprisingly large and destructive and also tend to break down molecular bonds in the nucleus in the immediate vicinity.

The design of the tip plays an important part in determining the effectiveness of the acoustic and cavitational forces. One effect of the acoustic waves, and of the direct mechanical forces, is to push the nucleus away from the tip repeatedly. This needs to be countered by the aspiration through the tip (see later). Tips of

the same external diameter but with thicker walls have increased effective power because the surface area that emits acoustic and mechanical waves is greater. By reducing the lumen diameter of such a tip, the force available to hold the nucleus in contact with the tip is also reduced, which quite possibly may produce a less efficient tip overall. A fine balance needs to be struck by designers between these two forces in order to ensure that a given tip is efficient. Some tips, for example, have a bell-shaped end (e.g., Cobra Tip, Surgical Design) or a bend in the tip near the end (e.g., Kelman Tip, Alcon Laboratories). The effect of these design features is to make these particular tips very powerful by increasing the area from which the acoustic shock waves are generated as well as an increased cavitation effect (Fig. 46-2).

PUMPS AND FLUIDICS

The function of the phaco pump is to hold the nucleus onto the tip and remove debris created by the tip, but with modern techniques it is used increasingly to aspirate directly the softer parts of the nucleus. Traditionally, two pump principles have been used—peristaltic and a vacuum-driven system. A third type of pump—the scroll pump—is now available in the Concentrix module of the Bausch & Lomb Surgical (B&L) Millennium phaco machine.

Peristaltic Systems

Flow is generated by roller pumps that rotate against compressible tubing; this "milks" fluid along the lumen and creates a pressure gradient between pump and anterior chamber. Design changes in the rollers and sophisticated microprocessor controls have resulted in sophisticated, powerful, and well-controlled pump systems. Although the earlier peristaltic systems had a reputation for being unresponsive, modern systems are capable of producing a 500mmHg (66.5kPa) vacuum in about 1 second. The rate at which fluid is aspirated through the unoccluded phaco tip is set at the machine console in ml/min. To set a low value allows events within the anterior chamber to happen slowly; a high value speeds up events and generates more "pulling power." Fine adjustments of flow, by changing the speed at which the pump turns, allow for personal surgical style or different operating conditions. Some advanced systems sense when the tip is occluded partially and make fine adjustments to the pump to compensate for reduced aspiration.

The second pump parameter that can be adjusted is the vacuum level at which, once achieved, the pump stops. When the tip becomes occluded, the pump continues to turn, with reduction in the pressure in the lumen between tip and pump. Once the preset vacuum has been reached, the pump stops for as long as that vacuum level holds. The rate at which the maximum set vacuum level is reached is directly proportional to the flow rate, so that for a particular machine a level of 400mmHg (53.2kPa) is reached in 3.4 seconds when the flow rate is set at 8ml/min but in 1 second when it is set at 30ml/min.

Vacuum Based

These systems generate a vacuum level, which is adjustable, in a chamber in the machine using either a Venturi or a diaphragm pump. The rotary vane pump has a particular way of controlling the amount of vacuum generated. The pressure difference between this chamber and the tip generates flow. Once the tip is occluded, fluid continues to be removed from the tubing until the pressure within it equilibrates with that in the vacuum chamber (the vacuum in this chamber is the maximum achievable in the system). In this system, flow through the tip can be adjusted only indirectly because it is proportional to the vacuum level in the vacuum chamber. Thus, these two parameters cannot be modulated independently. It is possible, however, to introduce a damping effect into the system so that the equilibration of pressures does not take place instantaneously.

Scroll Pump

The scroll pump is a rigid pump with a very high compliance and in the Concentrix module of the B&L Millennium machine is coupled with sophisticated computer control with very sensitive, real-time flow and vacuum sensing. This allows the pump to be run either in a flow-dominant mode (simulating a peristaltic system) or in a vacuum-dominant mode that simulates a Venturi system.

ANTERIOR CHAMBER HYDRODYNAMICS

It is important to understand the correct meaning of various terms used to describe the physical aspects of phaco. Normally, "flow" is used to mean evacuation flow out of the eye. Fluid also flows out of the eye through the incisions at a variable rate[10]—a significant reduction of this incisional outflow is achieved by some sleeve designs (e.g., Microseal by B&L). To avoid confusion, if flow into the eye is being described, it is necessary to use the term "inflow." The rate of fluid inflow is determined by the height difference between the drip chamber of the fluid reservoir and the eye. Inflow is always passive; it is modulated by the resistance of the tubing and by any compression of the inflow sleeve around the phaco tip. "Vacuum" is taken to mean the preset maximum vacuum level indicated on the console. In neither peristaltic nor vacuum-based systems is the vacuum present in the anterior chamber. "Power" is expressed as a proportion of the maximum power available.

An active phaco tip (power applied) produces forces that push material away from it. This is countered by aspiration flow; a high flow rate holds material to the tip very well. It is essential that inflow potential at least equals, and if possible exceeds, the maximum outflow (combined incisional flow and machine-generated flow), otherwise anterior chamber collapse occurs. When working near the subincisional area a risk exists of partial occlusion of the infusion ports within the incision (particularly a corneal incision).

When a surgeon uses a technique that involves sculpting (e.g., "divide and conquer"[11] or "stop and chop"[12]), a relatively low flow (<10ml/min), with no tip occlusion, is required. The low flow allows sculpting near or even onto the capsule, without the risk of drawing the capsule into the port, and a tip slope of 30° or 45° allows the surgeon both to see the tip and to minimize occlusion potential. When using a technique that involves nucleus consumption (e.g., phaco chop), a high flow is required to help hold the nucleus against the tip and so increase the efficiency. Occlusion in these circumstances is enhanced by rotation of the tip so that the opening is aligned with the edge of nucleus being grasped. When using high flow and high vacuum settings, the surgeon must not approach the capsule with the tip, as high flow (particularly during postocclusion surge) may carry the capsule into the tip.[13,14]

The infusion ports in the infusion sleeve around the phaco tip are positioned close to the aspiration port and therefore can create turbulent flow that can disrupt the attractive force generated by aspiration. In addition, there is a certain amount of irrigation that enters the anterior chamber between the sleeve and the tip, particularly a soft silicone sleeve. Until recently these forces, which can be disruptive to the attractive aspiration force, have been unavoidable and therefore ignored. Recent developments, however (see later), may make it possible to dissociate in space the irrigation and aspiration ports.

POSTOCCLUSION SURGE

With any pump design, in the occluded state, vacuum is generated in the lumen of the tubing. In an unmodulated system, when the occlusion breaks, fluid rushes into the tubing to equilibrate the pressure difference between the anterior chamber and the lumen ("postocclusion surge"). During the period of occlusion, the walls of the tubing tend to collapse in proportion to the increase in vacuum (Fig. 46-3). With release of the occlusion the tubing reexpands and often rebounds, which results in a

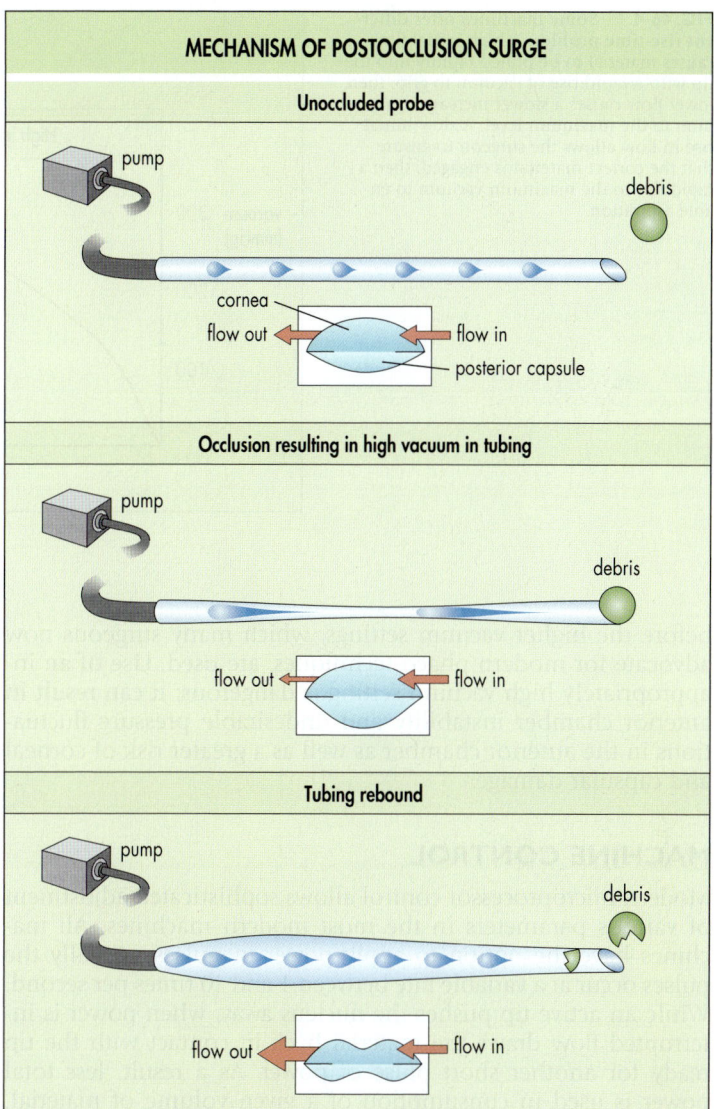

MECHANISM OF POSTOCCLUSION SURGE

FIG. 46-3 ■ The mechanism of postocclusion surge. (Top) Fluid flow through an unoccluded probe. (Middle) Occlusion that results in a high vacuum in the tubing (as a consequence of the blockage less fluid is extracted, so the eye swells). (Bottom) Tubing rebound with potential loss of the anterior chamber (as a result of an occlusion in the tubing the pump works harder and extracts more fluid than needed, so the eye may collapse).

larger postocclusion surge. In addition, if the foot pedal is still in position two (i.e., irrigation and aspiration), the pump immediately begins to turn. These factors may cause anterior chamber instability during removal of the nucleus.

Modern phaco machines incorporate various measures to reduce this instability, with varying success. One machine provides a pressure-sensing transducer in the vacuum line; at the first sign of rapid pressure fluctuation (i.e., when occlusion is just breaking), fluid is allowed directly into the vacuum line from a bottle higher than that which feeds the anterior chamber. The effect of this is to reverse the pressure difference immediately, which causes a slight reflux of fluid into the anterior chamber. Other systems have similar sensing devices that stop the pump for a brief period when an occlusion break is detected. This type of surge prevention or surge control has allowed surgeons to work with vacuum levels of 300–500mmHg (39.9–66.5kPa) or higher—the maximum safe level without such features is 120mmHg (15.96kPa) or less. A feature of all machines that operate at these enhanced vacuum levels is that they must be used in conjunction with specially adapted tubing that has a much reduced compliance to minimize the rebound effect mentioned before. It is vitally important that the surgeon is familiar with the properties of the particular machine being used and that the tubing is checked to ensure the correct type is in place

FIG. 46-4 ■ Some machines offer different rise-time profiles. A high initial flow causes material to be pulled rapidly into the tip with a rapid rise of vacuum to grip; then lower flow causes a slower increase in vacuum to the maximum level. A slow initial rise in flow allows the surgeon to ensure that the correct material is engaged, then a rapid rise to the maximum vacuum to enable aspiration.

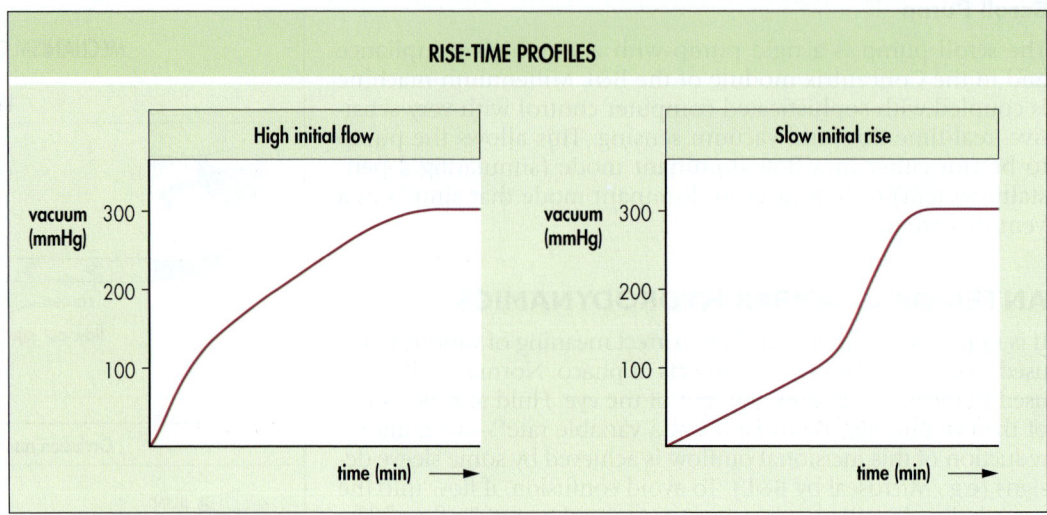

before the higher vacuum settings, which many surgeons now advocate for modern phaco techniques, are used. Use of an inappropriately high vacuum setting is dangerous; it can result in anterior chamber instability and undesirable pressure fluctuations in the anterior chamber as well as a greater risk of corneal and capsular damage.

MACHINE CONTROL

Modern microprocessor control allows sophisticated adjustment of various parameters in the most modern machines. All machines have the option to apply power in pulses—usually the pulses occur at a variable rate between 1 and 10 times per second. While an active tip pushes the nucleus away, when power is interrupted flow draws the material back in contact with the tip ready for another short pulse of power. As a result, less total power is used in consumption of a given volume of material. Increasingly machines have software that allows a "burst mode," which in its basic setting gives a 20 millisecond burst of power followed by a 1 or 2 second pause. Machines with burst mode usually offer the option of linear control of the burst frequency (with a fixed power level) in foot position three, with frequency increasing until continuous phaco is achieved with full depression of the pedal. A new development in 2001, "WhiteStar" software enhancement to the Sovereign machine (Allergan Inc.), uses ultrashort bursts with relatively long intervals. It is claimed that this allows the phaco tip to cool between bursts, removing the need for constant irrigation around the tip. Irrigation can be dissociated from the phaco tip, allowing cataract removal through 1mm incisions but also allowing more efficient anterior chamber hydrodynamics with enhanced aspiration efficiency without the turbulence normally associated with a coaxial irrigation sleeve.

Software enhancements now allow the setting of variations in machine parameters when occlusion is approaching (i.e., vacuum has reached 90% of preset level) or has been reached. Different flow rates, burst methods, and so forth can then be programmed to occur automatically (Fig. 46-4). The B&L Millennium machine has a sophisticated footpedal that allows simultaneous linear control of aspiration and control of phaco power. Both these technologies enable several different combinations of parameters to be used in the different phases of one operation and make it possible to deal with different types of cataract with slightly different techniques.

NEW DEVELOPMENTS

Phacoemulsification has allowed the development of small incision techniques. The use of small incisions is not, however, dependent on phacoemulsification and several new modalities have been introduced and are in the process of development. Staar Surgical has introduced a handpiece and control system that can operate at sonic (40–400Hz) frequencies. This is claimed to remove any incisional heating effects seen with standard ultrasonic handpieces. Alcon has introduced the Neosonix handpiece, which has the ability to oscillate the phaco tip 1° or 2° in the long axis of the tip, enhancing its action, particularly, they hope, with hard cataracts. The same company has a completely different modality in late stages of development—Aqualase—which uses rapid high-pressure pulses of warmed BSS as the destructive force. B&L have Avantix (previously known as Catarex)—an endocapsular vortex emulsification system, which has the potential to remove the contents of the lens through a 1mm capsulorrhexis, at a similar stage of development. Various companies have laser-phaco systems that are based on either an Nd:YAG or an erbium laser system, and these also have the potential advantage of allowing disassociated aspiration and irrigation, leading to 1mm maximum incision size. At the time of writing none of these new technologies, except Neosonics, has been sufficiently developed to allow removal of hard nuclei, but they show clear promise of being able to facilitate the development of foldable or injectable IOLs that can be delivered into the anterior chamber through a 1mm incision.

REFERENCES

1. Kelman C. Phaco-emulsification and aspiration. A new technique of cataract removal. A preliminary report. Am J Ophthalmol. 1967;64:23–35.
2. Kelman C. Cataract emulsification and aspiration. Trans Ophthalmol Soc UK. 1970;90:13–22.
3. Kraff MC, Sanders DR, Lieberman HL. Total cataract extraction through a 3-mm incision: a report of 650 cases. Ophthalmic Surg. 1979;10:46–54.
4. Cohen SW, Kara G, Rizzuti AB, et al. Automated phakotomy and aspiration of soft congenital and traumatic cataracts. Ophthalmic Surg. 1979;10:38–45.
5. Gimbel HV, Neuhann T. Development, advantages, and methods of the continuous circular capsulorrhexis technique. J Cataract Refract Surg. 1990;16:31–7.
6. Allarakia L, Knoll RL, Lindstrom RL. Soft intraocular lenses. J Cataract Refract Surg. 1987;13:607–20.
7. Illiff CE. Phacoemulsification—why? Trans Am Acad Ophthalmol Otolaryngol. 1977;83:213–15.
8. Pacifico RL. Ultrasonic energy in phacoemulsification: mechanical cutting and cavitation. J Cataract Refract Surg. 1994;20:338–41.
9. Davis PL. Mechanism of phacoemulsification. Letter to the editor. J Cataract Refract Surg. 1994;20:672–3.
10. Allen ED. Understanding phacoemulsification. I. Principles of the machinery. Eur J Implant Refract Surg. 1995;7:247–50.
11. Gimbel HV. Divide and conquer nucleofractis phacoemulsification: development and variations. J Cataract Refract Surg. 1991;17:281–91.
12. Koch PS, Katzen LE. Stop and chop phacoemulsification. J Cataract Refract Surg. 1994;20:566–70.
13. Allen ED. Understanding phacoemulsification. II. Principles applied to surgical practice. Eur J Implant Refract Surg. 1995;7:299–304.
14. Allen ED. Understanding phacoemulsification. III. Principles of nucleofractis techniques. Eur J Implant Refract Surg. 1995;7:347–53.

CHAPTER
47

Small Incision Cataract Surgery

I. HOWARD FINE • MARK PACKER • RICHARD S. HOFFMAN

INTRODUCTION

In the last decade marked improvements in phacoemulsification technology are correlated with continual improvements in phacosurgical techniques. Instruments with improved cutting capabilities are available widely. The development of fluid dynamic analysis allows much faster vacuum rise times and vacuum levels greater than those previously considered safe in the intraocular environment, yet with greater stability of the anterior chamber. Power modulations allow the application of phacoultrasound energy in a much more judicious manner, and the interrelationships between all the modalities are enhanced with microprocessor controls. These technological advances, increased user-friendliness, and the availability of small incision lenses result in the utilization of phacoemulsification as the preferred cataract surgical technique by approximately 88% of surgeons in the United States in 1997; other developed nations are following this trend. The availability of viscoelastic materials to provide space, cushion tissues, and protect the endothelium and posterior capsule has improved safety in the performance of both phacoemulsification of cataract and implantation of an intraocular lens (IOL).

GENERAL TECHNIQUES

Incisions

The scleral tunnel incision was introduced in the early 1980s in an attempt to provide better healing with less surgically induced astigmatism in wider incision nuclear expression cataract extraction[1]; this became the favored incision technique along with some modification for phacoemulsification. In 1990 the sutureless incision was developed, which utilized a longer scleral tunnel with linear grooves in the floor of the tunnel in the meridian of the incision. This incision could be stretched to admit a folded lens, and, when unsutured, still retains water-tight characteristics. The corneal entry was described as a one-way valve or corneal lip incision, which enabled the incision to self-seal. Subsequently, the temporal, sutureless, clear corneal incision for cataract surgery was described in 1992[2,3]; it has now become a favored technique for cataract surgery, in conjunction with foldable or small incision IOLs, for many surgeons internationally.

The temporal location is used because of the following:

- The vector forces of lid blink and gravity run parallel to the incision, in contradistinction to superiorly located incisions in which the same vector forces act perpendicular to the incision and contribute to postoperative against-the-rule drift in astigmatism.
- The temporal location at the periphery is farthest from the visual axis, with the result that any flattening of the incision site is less likely to be transmitted to the center.
- The need to work over the brow is eliminated.
- The eye does not have to be rotated down, and with the iris parallel to the floor the incident light from the microscope is perpendicular to the plane of the iris, which enhances the red reflex and allows better visualization of intraocular structures.
- The lateral canthal angle lies just beneath the incision, which facilitates drainage of the operative site.

The initial incision structure was based on the side-port incision or paracentesis in which a single plane incision is made through clear cornea. Later, a perpendicular groove of 300–400μm depth was added to the incision in order to give the superior lip of the incision more thickness, which resulted in less tendency for it to tear.[4] New technology blades have been developed that have helped to perfect incision architecture. The Fine Triamond Knife was developed in conjunction with Mastel Instruments so that the incision could be made with an extremely sharp, thin, and narrow knife without a necessity for dimpling down, which resulted in some tendency for tearing of tissue or scrolling of Descemet's membrane. Subsequently, in conjunction with Rhein Medical, the 3-D blade was developed, which had differential slope angles to the bevels on the anterior versus the posterior surface, resulting in an ability to just touch the eye at the location of the external incision and advance the blade in the plane of the cornea. The differential slopes on the anterior versus posterior aspects of the blade allowed the forces of tissue resistance to create an incision that was characterized by a linear external incision, a 2mm tunnel, and a linear internal incision without the need to dimple down or distort tissues to create the proper incision architecture. The trapezoidal 3-D blade also allowed enlargement of the incision to 3.5mm for IOL insertion without altering incision architecture.

Fixation via the Fine/Thornton fixation device or the side-port incision is important to stabilize the eye during incision construction.

Stromal hydration by injection of balanced salt solution into the cornea at the sides of the tunnel after completion of the surgical procedure results in thickening of the cornea at the site of the incision. This forces the floor and roof of the incision into contact with each other and enhances the effect of the corneal endothelial pump, which participates in early sealing of these incisions.

Incisions should be sized appropriately for the particular IOL implantation system. Unpublished data strongly suggest that the astigmatic neutrality of the incision is maintained more effectively when the incision is cut to the proper size. An undersized incision that stretches or tears to allow delivery of the IOL appears to have a greater impact on corneal astigmatism.

Continuous Curvilinear Capsulorrhexis

Capsulorrhexis, originally described by both Neuhann[5] (Germany) and Gimbel[6] (Canada), was originally performed with a bent needle or cystotome, but capsulorrhexis forceps provide added control; this has become the predominant technique used in an anterior chamber filled with viscoelastic material. A pinch-type forceps (e.g., Rhein Rhexis Forceps) helps to minimize the asymmetric force on the zonular apparatus during the initiation of the capsulorrhexis.

Hydrodissection and Hydrodelineation

Hydrodissection to mobilize the nucleus within the capsular bag ensures nucleus rotation for effective disassembly and removal. Cortical cleaving hydrodissection is a technique that not only mobilizes the lens in the capsule but also severs cortical capsular connections.[7] Cortical cleaving hydrodissection involves elevation of the anterior capsule leaf with a small (e.g., 26 gauge) cannula and slow, continuous injection of balanced salt solution from a 2ml syringe against the elevated capsular leaf. Fluid flows around the equator of the lens, peripheral to the cortex, into the posterior aspect of the lens capsule. As it continues forward, it finally reaches the dense adhesions between the capsule and the cortex at the equator, which prevent it from advancing circumferentially around the nucleus. As the volume of balanced salt solution posterior to the lens increases, the lens appears to move forward and the continuous curvilinear capsulorrhexis enlarges. At this point, prior to hydrodissecting the nucleus out of the capsule, injection of balanced salt solution is stopped and the nucleus depressed with the straight arm of the cannula toward the posterior pole of the eye. The trapped fluid is then forced circumferentially the rest of the way around the equator of the lens and ruptures cortical-capsular connections before flowing through the capsulorrhexis. The capsulorrhexis then assumes its earlier smaller diameter and radial striations are often noted, formed from cortical fibers washed toward the center of the capsulorrhexis.

Hydrodelineation is performed by injection of the fluid into the substance of the nucleus.[8,9] A tract is made midway between the center of the anterior surface of the nucleus and the equator. The cannula is advanced toward the central plane of the nucleus until the nucleus starts to move, which indicates abutment against the hard central portion of the nucleus. At that point, the direction of the needle is changed to horizontal and a tract is created at that depth in the nucleus by a to-and-fro motion of the cannula. The cannula is backed about halfway out of the tract, and fluid is injected continuously. Fluid flows along the path of least resistance, which is the junction between the soft epinucleus and the hard endonuclear mass; this results in the formation of a golden ring or dark circle at that junction. This completes the circumferential division of the nucleus, with the result that there is now a central endonucleus and a peripheral epinuclear shell with cortex attached. In about 70% of cases, the cortex is evacuated with the epinuclear removal. This is facilitated by trimming the roof and rim of the epinucleus.[10] Residual cortex, if present, may be viscodissected to the capsular fornix and evacuated along with residual viscoelastic material after IOL implantation. In this way, the posterior capsule is protected by the IOL from the aspiration port of the irrigation-aspiration (I/A) handpiece.

Nucleus Removal

In order to remove the nucleus through a small circular capsulorrhexis, it is necessary to disassemble the nucleus within the confines of the capsular bag. The divide-and-conquer technique utilizes sculpting and grooving with ultrasound energy prior to cracking to disassemble the nucleus. More recent chopping techniques rely instead on high vacuum and mechanical force for disassembly.

In the late 1980s, as phacoemulsification was increasing in popularity, the desire of most phacoemulsification surgeons was for increased power in order to address increasingly hard cataracts with the divide-and-conquer technique. In the 1990s increased power became available, as did other very important technical innovations such as high-vacuum tubing and cassettes, microprocessor controls integrated with central onboard computers, and downsized tips with better holding power and increased followability. These technological innovations permitted the use of higher vacuum and less ultrasound energy in the process of nuclear disassembly and extraction than had previously been thought possible.

In the late 1980s and early 1990s, two endolenticular phacoemulsification techniques were described, chip and flip and chop and flip phacoemulsification, in which pulse mode was

used for the removal of nuclear material. In doing so, decreased chattering and increased holding power of the nuclear material was obtainable. More recently, multiple modulations in the delivery of power are available that allow dramatic reductions in the total amount of ultrasound energy delivered into the eye. Today a technique relying almost entirely on chopping with high-vacuum extraction and ultrasound assistance with power modulation for cataract extraction is preferred. Only in cases of very soft nuclei or refractive lens exchange should the chip and flip technique previously described be employed.[10]

Intraocular Lens Implantation

Although IOLs, including foldable IOLs, can be implanted with an anterior chamber maintainer that continuously replenishes anterior chamber fluid, most surgeons prefer the safety of stable expansion of the capsular bag with a viscoelastic material. Multiple materials are now being utilized for foldable IOLs, including silicone, acrylic, collamer, and hydrogels.

If a foldable lens is not utilized, the incision has to be opened to 5–7mm in width. This may be accomplished with either a keratome or a knife. However, clear corneal incisions do not self-seal safely at widths greater than 4mm, and these larger incisions are not astigmatically neutral. There appears to be a distinct advantage to the use of foldable IOLs that can be inserted through an injector system in that the IOL is transferred directly from the sterile package into the capsular bag without touching any part of the surface of the eye or the surgical field, from which it may absorb bacterial contaminants.[9] Injectors enable IOL implantation through incisions considerably smaller than required for implantation with forceps.

Foldable plate haptic lenses and three-piece silicone lenses are being utilized routinely with incision widths in the range 2.5–3mm without enlargement, although some data indicate that these incisions, in fact, enlarge to an average width of about 3.1mm by stretching or tearing when the injector is inserted.[11,12] The potential for leakage certainly appears much greater with incisions that have been stretched. In general, foldable three-piece acrylic lenses require incision widths of 3.5–4mm.

Removal of Residual Viscoelastic Material and Residual Cortex

Removal of viscoelastic material is accomplished using the I/A handpiece. The various viscoelastic agents available differ in their degree of cohesiveness and in other properties, and this affects the ease with which they can be mobilized from the eye. Those that have bulk retention and low cohesiveness (e.g., Viscoat) tend to remain in the eye and must be flushed out by the irrigation flow as aspiration tip occlusion does not readily occur to facilitate vacuum evacuation. The viscoelastic materials, for example, Healon, that have high cohesiveness tend to be mobilized much more rapidly and can be evacuated readily.

Residual cortex can be mobilized and evacuated at the same time if cortical cleaving hydrodissection has been performed. This is accomplished by stripping the cortex in movements that run parallel to the plane of the pupil while at the same time depressing the IOL to expand the access to the capsular fornix. The I/A handpiece can also be slipped under the IOL, whether it is a looped haptic or plate haptic lens, to evacuate viscoelastic material behind the IOL. The aspiration port should be kept facing the IOL in these instances to avoid aspiration of the posterior capsule and its rupture.

For surgeons who wish to mobilize cortex as a separate step prior to IOL implantation, the options are either to increase the vacuum or increase the aspiration flow rate. Because occlusion of the tip and a rise in vacuum are almost always required to evacuate cortex, it seems more logical to utilize a fixed, relatively low aspiration flow rate with a programmable vacuum rise time. Subincisional cortex may be reached more easily with a bent tip or the use of separate handpieces, one for aspiration and one for irrigation, introduced through side-port incisions on opposite sides of the eye. Many surgeons prefer a continuous irrigation mode in cortical cleanup to prevent shallowing of the chamber, even with a tip occlusion; this again reduces the potential for capture of the posterior capsule and its possible tearing.

In capsular block syndrome with fluid expansion of the capsular bag, the anterior displacement of the IOL may result in induced myopia. Therefore it is important to ensure that all viscoelastic material is removed from the capsular bag.

CURRENT TECHNIQUE

Choo-Choo Chop and Flip Phacoemulsification[13]

A side-port incision is made to the left with a 1mm-trifaceted diamond knife, after which the anterior chamber is irrigated with $\frac{1}{2}$ ml preservative-free Xylocaine. Utilizing the soft-shell technique described by Arshinoff,[14] the physician places Viscoat (Alcon Surgical Inc.) into the anterior chamber angle distal to

the side port through the side-port incision. It fills the anterior chamber but allows the eye to remain relatively soft. Provisc is instilled on top of the center of the lens capsule under the Viscoat. Provisc (Alcon Surgical Inc.) forces the Viscoat up against the cornea, creating a soft shell, which helps stabilize the anterior chamber and protect the endothelium. In addition, Provisc, which is a cohesive viscoelastic, decreases any tendency for iris prolapse during the hydro steps. Following construction of a temporal 2.5mm × 2mm clear corneal incision, cortical cleaving hydrodissection is performed in the two distal quadrants followed by hydrodelineation. After the two hydro steps, the nucleus should rotate easily within the capsular bag. The Mackool/Kelman aspiration bypass micro flare tip on the Legacy is introduced bevel down to aspirate the epinucleus uncovered by the capsulorrhexis and is then turned bevel up. Alternatively on other systems, an MST chop series SP tip (Microsurgical Technology, Redmond, WA) or a 30° standard bevel-down tip is used throughout endonuclear removal (see Tables 47-1 through 47-6).

TABLE 47-1

ALCON LEGACY PHACOEMULSIFICATION SETTINGS: MICROTIP FLARED TIP ABS—MAX VAC

Memory	Chop Pulse Mem 1	Trim Bimodal Mem 1	Irrigation-Aspiration	Viscoat Removal
Power (%)	40	30		
Flow (ml/min)	32/35	42/33	38	60
Vacuum (mm Hg)	500	300	500	500
Mode	2 pulses/sec	Surg asp		
Bottle ht (in)	100	100	70	70

20 Ga tip.
ABS, Aspiration Bypass System; *Mem*, memory; *Surg asp*, surgeon aspiration.

TABLE 47-2

ALLERGAN DIPLOMAX

	High-Vacuum/Chop and Flip			Irrigation and Aspiration Control Surgical Vacuum Control	
	Chop phaco 1	Trim phaco 2	Flip phaco 3	Cortical Cleanup	Viscoat Removal
Power (%)	60	60	60		
Aspiration Cont Flow (ml/mm)	26/30	32/26	32/16	10	30
Vacuum (mm Hg)	50/250	40/90	70/150	500	500
Mode	Continuous burst Continuous irrigation	Continuous burst Continuous irrigation	Continuous burst Continuous irrigation	Continuous irrigation	Continuous irrigation
Bottle ht (in)	32	32	32	28	28

20 Ga tip.

TABLE 47-3

ALLERGAN SOVEREIGN

	Chop Phaco 1	Trim Phaco 2	Flip Phaco 3	Cortical Clean IA 1	Viscoat Removal IA 2
Power (%)	40/40	20/20	20/20		
Flow (ml/mm)	28/34	30/26	28/22	30	40 (linear)
Vacuum (mm Hg)	350/100	150/20	150/80	500 linear	500
Other	Continuous irrigation Linear vac	Continuous irrigation Linear vac	Continuous irrigation Linear vac	Continuous irrigation Linear vac	Continuous irrigation Linear asp
Mode	Long pulse 2 pps	Long pulse 2 pps	Long pulse 2 pps		
Bottle ht (in)	30	30	30	30	30

20 Ga tip.

TABLE 47-4

B & L/STORZ MILLENNIUM MICROFLOW

Phaco					IA/Viscoat
Mode	CHOP "Choo-choo chop Flow"	CHOP (Soft nucleus/small pupil) "Choo-choo chop vac"	TRIM "Linear Vac Trim"	FLIP "Linear Flow Flip"	I/A, "Irrigation-Aspiration"
Power (%)	20	20	10	10	N/A
Vacuum (mm Hg)	275-375	115-200	140-225	225	550
Flow (ml/min)	34	N/A	28	25-32	
Pulses	2	2	2	2	
Bottle ht (in)	95	90	90	90	80

20 Ga tip.

TABLE 47-5

MENTOR SIStem

Mode	Phaco 1 CHOP Pulsed Mem 1	Phaco 2 TRIM Pulsed Mem 2	Phaco 2 FLIP Fixed Phaco 2	IA Cortex Linear Vac	IA Viscoat Linear Asp
Power (%)	50	28	10		
Aspiration (ml/min)	22/28	20/18	26/20	26	40
Vacuum (mm Hg)	250	185	235	500	500
Bottle ht (in)	94	94	94	89	89
Pulse	2 pulses/sec Continuous irrigation	2 pulses/sec Continuous irrigation	2 pulses/sec Continuous irrigation		

20 Ga tip.
Asp, Aspiration; *Mem*, memory; *Vac*, vacuum.

TABLE 47-6

STAAR WAVE ULTRASONIC MODE

Memory	Chop Pulse Mem 1	Trim Pulse Mem 2	Flip Pulse Mem 3	Cortical IA Mem 3	Viscoat Rem Mem 4
Power (%)	30	20	20		
Aspiration (ml/min)	30	30	30	38	50
Vacuum (mm Hg)	350	250	180	Linear 550	Linear 550
Other	Continuous irrigation	Continuous irrigation	Continuous irrigation	Continuous irrigation	Continuous irrigation
Mode	Pulse 2	Pulse 2	Pulse 2		
Bottle ht (in)	46"	46"	46"		

20 Ga tip.
IA, Irrigation/aspiration; *Mem*, memory; *Rem*, removal.

The Fine/Nagahara chopper (Rhein Medical, Tampa, FL) is placed in the golden ring by touching the center of the epinucleus with the tip and pushing it peripherally so that it reflects the capsulorrhexis. The chopper is used to stabilize the nucleus by lifting and pulling toward the incision slightly (Fig. 47-1, *A*), after which the phaco tip "lollipops" the nucleus in either pulse mode at 2 pulses/sec or 80msec burst mode (Diplomax). Burst mode is a power modulation that utilizes a fixed percent power (panel control), a programmable burst width (duration of power), and a *linear interval* between bursts. As one enters foot position 3, the interval between bursts is 2sec; with increasing depressions of the foot pedal in foot position 3 the interval shortens until at the bottom of foot position 3 there is continuous phacoemulsification. In pulse mode, there is *linear power* (%) but a *fixed interval between pulses*, resulting in 2 pulses/sec in a 250msec pulse (linear power) followed by a 250msec pause in power followed by a 250msec pulse, and so forth. However, in both of these modulations with tip occlusion, vacuum is continuous throughout the pulse and pause intervals. With the energy delivered in this way, we minimize ultrasound energy into the eye and maximize our hold on the nucleus as the vacuum builds between pulses or bursts. Because of the decrease in cavitational energy around the tip at this low pulse rate or in burst mode, the tunnel in the nucleus in which the tip is embedded fits the needle very tightly and gives us an excellent hold on the nucleus, thus maximizing control of the nucleus as we score and chop it (Fig. 47-1, *B*) in foot position 2.

The Fine/Nagahara chop instrument is grooved on the horizontal arm close to the vertical "chop" element with the groove parallel to the direction of the sharp edge of the vertical element. In scoring the nucleus, the instrument is always moved in the direction the sharp edge of the wedge-shaped vertical element is facing (as indicated by the groove on the instrument), thus facilitating scoring. Bringing the chop instrument to the side of the phaco needle scores the nucleus. It is chopped in half by pulling the chopper to the left and slightly down while moving the phaco needle, still in foot position 2, to the right and slightly up. Then the nuclear complex is rotated. The chop instrument is again brought into the golden ring (Fig. 47-2, *A*), and the nucleus is again lollipopped, scored, and chopped with the resulting pie-shaped segment now lollipopped on the phaco tip (Fig. 47-2, *B*). The segment is then evacuated utilizing high vacuum

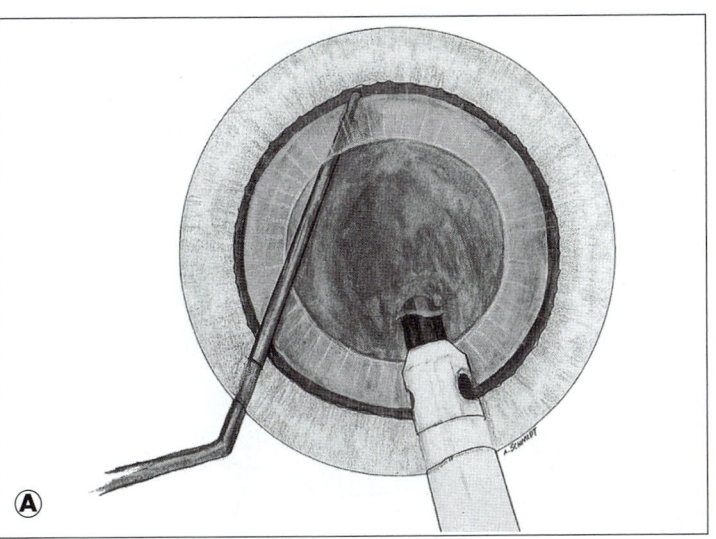
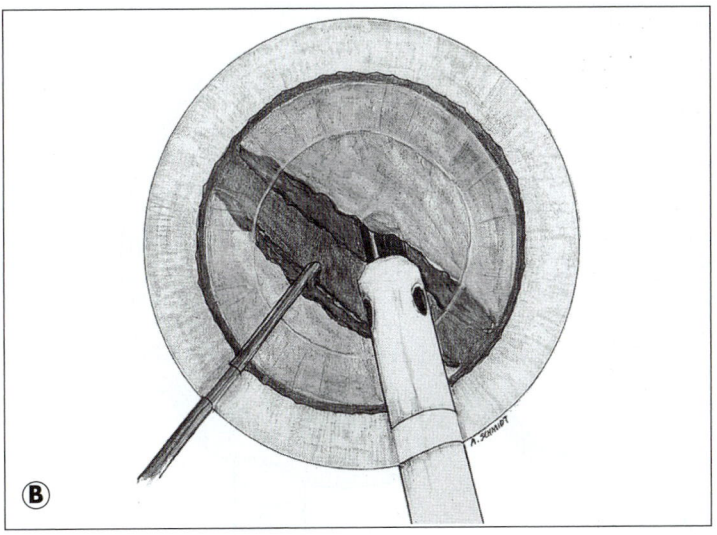

FIG. 47-1 ■ A, Stabilization of the nucleus during lollipopping for the initial chop. B, Completion of the initial chop. (Reproduced from Fine IH: Oper Tech Cataract Surg. 1998;1:61-5.)

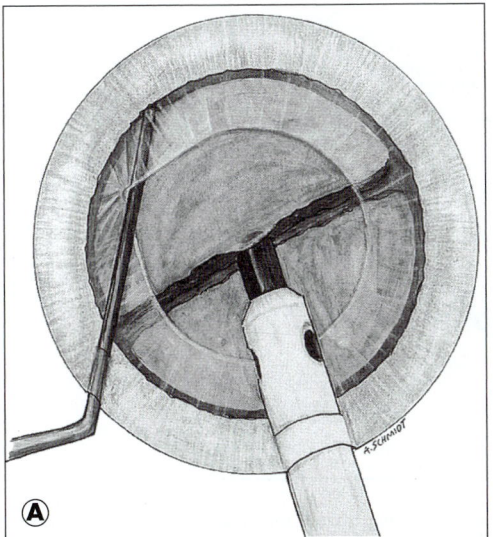
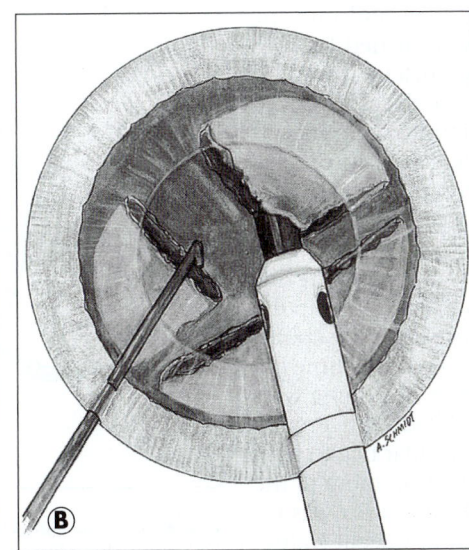
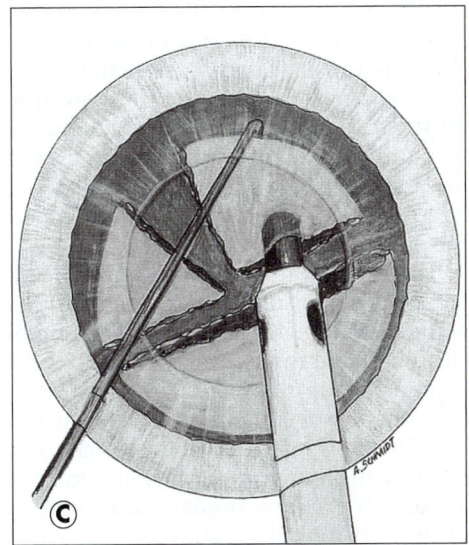

FIG. 47-2 ■ A, Stabilization of the nucleus prior to commencing the second chop. B, Pie-shaped segment adherent to the phaco tip following completion of the second chop. C, Mobilization of the first pie-shaped segment. (Reproduced from Fine IH: Oper Tech Cataract Surg. 1998;1:61-5.)

and short bursts or pulse mode phacoemulsification at 2 pulses/sec (Fig. 47-2, C). The nucleus is continually rotated so that pie-shaped segments can be scored, chopped, and removed essentially by the high vacuum assisted by short bursts or pulses of phacoemulsification. The short bursts or pulses of ultrasound energy continuously reshape the pie-shaped segments, which are kept at the tip, allowing occlusion and extraction by the vacuum. The size of the pie-shaped segments is customized to the density of the nucleus, with smaller segments for denser nuclei. Phacoemulsification in burst mode or at this low pulse rate sounds like "choo-choo-choo-choo," hence the name of this technique. With burst mode or the low pulse rate, the nuclear material tends to stay at the tip rather than chatter as vacuum holds between pulses. The chop instrument is utilized to stuff the segment into the tip or keep it down in the epinuclear shell.

After evacuation of the first heminucleus, the second heminucleus is rotated to the distal portion of the bag and the chop instrument stabilizes it while it is lollipopped. It is then scored (Fig. 47-3, A) and chopped. The pie-shaped segments can be chopped a second time to reduce their size (Fig. 47-3, B) if they appear too large to evacuate easily.

There is little tendency for nuclear material to come up into the anterior chamber with this technique. Usually it stays down within the epinuclear shell, but the chop instrument can control the position of the endonuclear material. The 30° bevel-down tip facilitates occlusion, as the angle of approach of the phaco tip to the endonucleus through a clear corneal incision is approximately 30°. This allows full vacuum to be reached quickly, which facilitates embedding the tip into the nucleus for chopping and allows mobilization of pie-shaped segments from above rather than having to go deeper into the endolenticular space as is necessary with a bevel-up tip. In addition, the cavitational energy is directed downward toward the nucleus rather than up toward the endothelium. Following evacuation of all endonuclear material (the 30° tip is turned bevel up) (Fig. 47-4), the epinuclear rim is trimmed in each of the three quadrants, mobilizing cortex as well in the following way. The distal rim and roof are purchased in foot position 2. Upon occlusion, the roof and rim are drawn central to the capsulorrhexis and then foot position 3 is entered. This results in mobilization of the roof and rim and clearance of occlusion. As each quadrant of the epinuclear rim is trimmed, the cortex in the adjacent cap-

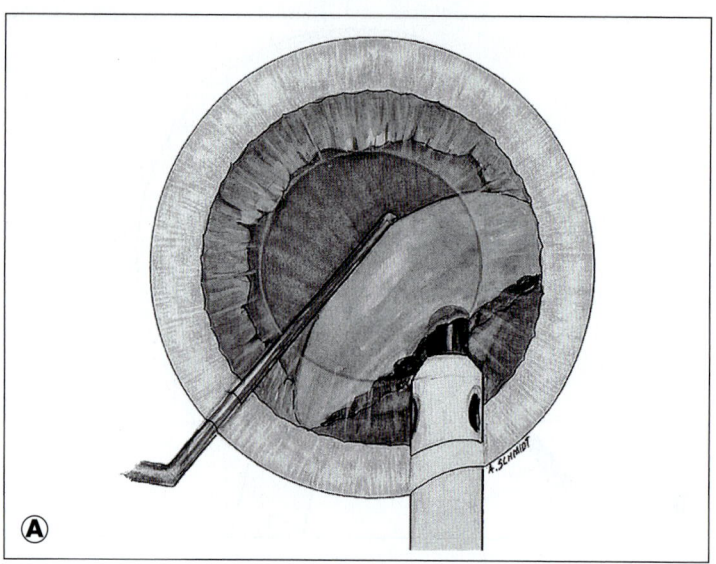 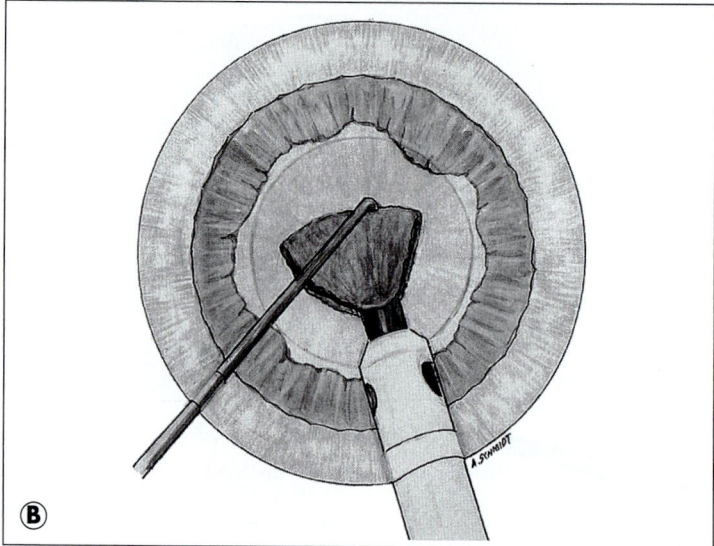

FIG. 47-3 ▦ **A,** Scoring of the second heminucleus. **B,** Mobilizing the final quadrant. (Reproduced from Fine IH: Oper Tech Cataract Surg. 1998;1:61-5.)

sular fornix flows over the floor of the epinucleus and into the phaco tip. Then the floor of the epinucleus is pushed back to keep the capsular bag on stretch and the epinucleus is rotated to bring a new quadrant of roof and rim to the distal position. This is repeated until three of the four quadrants of epinuclear rim and forniceal cortex have been evacuated. It is important not to allow the epinucleus to flip too early, thus avoiding a large amount of residual cortex remaining after evacuation of the epinucleus.

The epinuclear rim of the fourth quadrant is rotated to the distal position (i.e., nasally) and then utilized as a handle to flip the epinucleus (Fig. 47-5, *A*). As the remaining portion of the epinuclear floor and rim is evacuated from the eye, 70% of the time the entire cortex is evacuated with it (Fig. 47-5, *B*). Continuing with the soft-shell technique, the capsular bag is filled with Provisc and Viscoat is injected into the center of the capsular bag to help stabilize the anterior chamber and to blunt the movement of the foldable IOL as it is implanted into the eye. If the cortex was incompletely mobilized during epinuclear removal, Viscoat (rather than Provisc) is instilled first to viscodissect the cortex into the capsular fornix and drape some of it on top of the capsulorrhexis (Fig. 47-6, *A* and *B*). Provisc is then injected into the bottom of the bag, forcing the Viscoat anteriorly. The foldable IOL is then implanted. Residual cortex is evacuated with residual viscoelastic, the posterior capsule being protected by the optic of the IOL. Mobilization of Viscoat is greatly facilitated as it is encased within the much more highly cohesive Provisc and less time is necessary to evacuate residual viscoelastic.

The choo-choo chop and flip technique uses the same hydro forces to disassemble the nucleus but substitutes mechanical forces (chopping) for ultrasound energy (grooving) to further disassemble the nucleus. High vacuum is utilized as an extractive technique to remove nuclear material rather than using ultrasound energy to convert the nucleus to an emulsate that is evacuated by aspiration. This technique maximizes safety and control as well as efficiency in all cases and allows phacoemulsification of harder nuclei in the presence of a compromised endothelium. This technique facilitates the achievement of two goals: minimally invasive cataract surgery and maximally rapid visual rehabilitation.[15]

SPECIAL CASES
Pseudoexfoliation

A variety of special techniques are available to deal with pseudoexfoliation to minimize the likelihood of zonular ligament dehiscence or loss of nucleus. The use of an endocapsular ten-

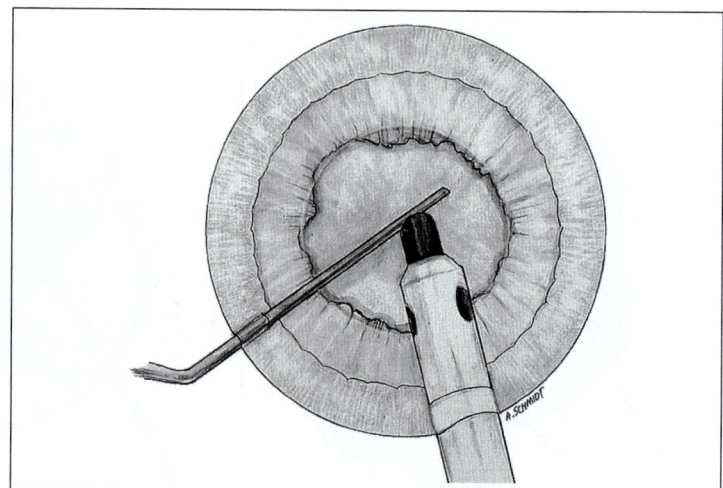

FIG. 47-4 ▦ **The epinuclear shell being rotated for trimming.** The bevel is shown here turned down because the epinucleus has not been removed. (Reproduced from Fine IH: Oper Tech Cataract Surg. 1998;1:61-5.)

sion ring[16] (Morcher, Stuttgart) to create a circumferential distribution of forces around the zonular apparatus is an aid to prevention of zonular dehiscence. Instead of adjacent zonular fibers being stressed by these forces, the capsular ring affects distribution of these forces to the entire zonular apparatus, which imparts greater safety to all the intracapsular manipulations that may be required. Postoperatively, the outward force of the endocapsular tension ring can prevent or reduce the tendency for capsulorrhexis phimosis to occur.

It is important to perform cortical cleaving hydrodissection very carefully, utilizing injections in several different quadrants and being quite delicate when depressing the nucleus to allow for rupture of cortical-capsular connections. The counterbalanced forces acting on the nucleus during horizontal chopping maneuvers limit stress on the zonular fibers and represent a real advantage over the unbalanced forces present during sculpting.

The greatest single threat in pseudoexfoliation cataract extraction is cortical cleanup, which can present an enormous challenge to the zonular fibers adjacent to the area of cortical stripping. For this reason, if an endocapsular ring has not been utilized, an IOL with polymethyl methacrylate haptics should be implanted prior to cortical aspiration so that the haptics can stabilize the bag. Postimplantation cortical cleanup takes

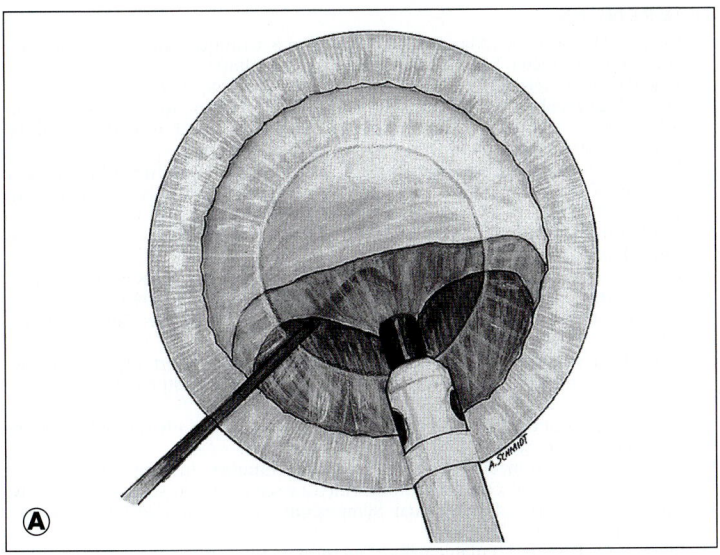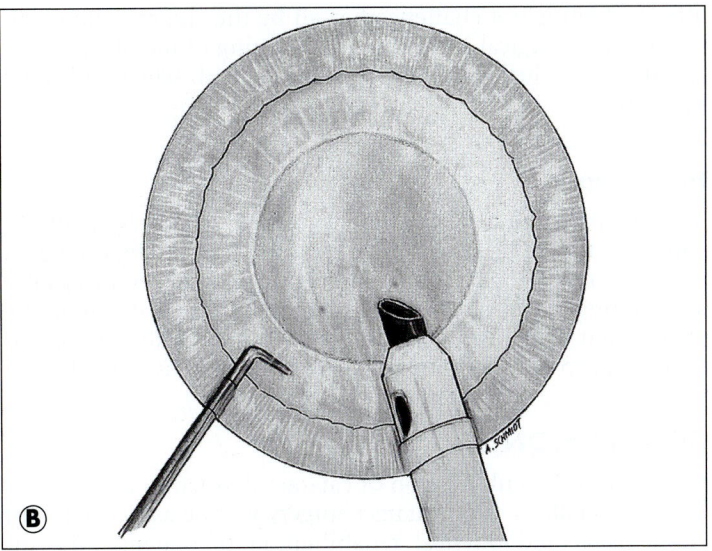

FIG. 47-5 ▮▮ **A,** Flipping of the epinucleus. **B,** Empty capsular bag following flipping of the epinucleus. (Reproduced from Fine IH: Oper Tech Cataract Surg. 1998;1:61-5.)

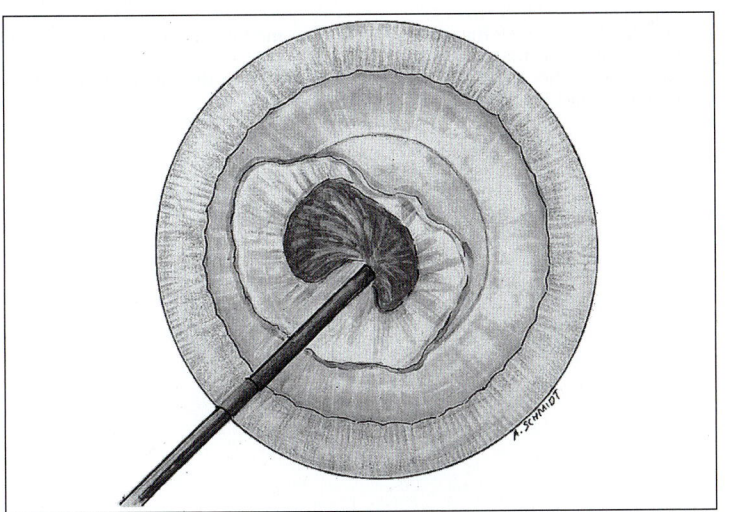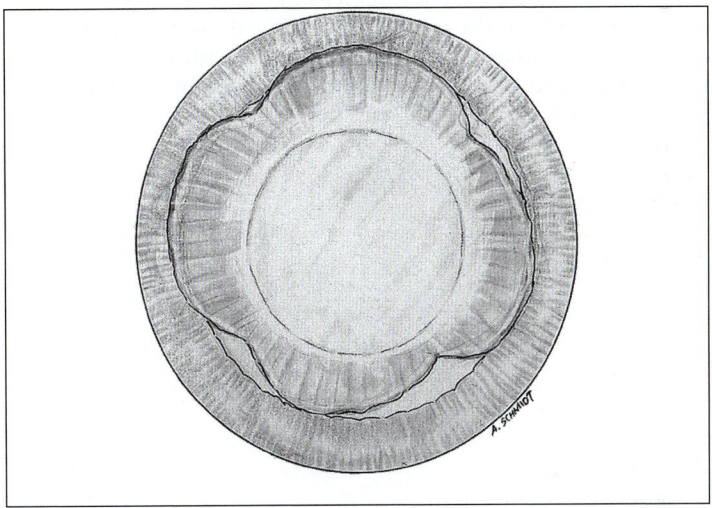

FIG. 47-6 ▮▮ Residual cortex draped over the capsulorrhexis rim following viscodissection. (Reproduced from Fine IH: Oper Tech Cataract Surg. 1998;1:61-5.)

longer but is safer, although not quite as safe as use of an endocapsular ring.

Posttrauma

Patients who have had previous eye trauma should be carefully examined for the possibility of zonular damage. However, on occasion zonular weakness or partial dialysis does not become evident until the time of surgery. This is another indication for the use of the endocapsular ring, which stabilizes the position of the lens capsule and allows surgery to proceed almost as though no compromise of the zonular apparatus existed.

Small Pupils

Small pupils used to be a relative contraindication for phacoemulsification. However, with the multitude of pupil-expanding techniques available, such as the use of iris retractors, expander rings, or the Beehler pupil expander (an elegant, atraumatic, simple instrument to operate), it is no longer reasonable to proceed to phacoemulsification with less than adequate visualization because of failure to address the small pupil. In a less than fully dilated pupil, it may be necessary to employ more manipulation than usual to bring the nuclear segments into view for

evacuation, but adequate visualization can almost always be achieved.

Hard Nuclei

A rock-hard nucleus was at one time a contraindication for phacoemulsification, but today this problem can be addressed with a variety of endolenticular phacoemulsification techniques. It is specifically in this area that the new modalities, with better cutting, higher vacuum, and power modulations, become so useful. Choo-choo chop and flip phacoemulsification chop is an ideal technique for hard nuclei; using this, it is easier to lollipop and easier to chop than to groove and crack. However, the epinucleus is very thin and hard and does not flip. Attempts to flip it uniformly result in a fracture of the epinuclear structure into three separate pie-shaped segments following the lines of the posterior Y suture. Each segment flips as it fractures, with the result that the maneuvers to remove the epinucleus in rock-hard nuclei are exactly the same as those for less hard nuclei.

Filtering Blebs

Postfiltration patients are especially suitable candidates for temporal, clear corneal phacoemulsification because the existing filtering bleb is not challenged at all by the surgery; the likelihood of postsurgical inflammation, scarring of the bleb, or surgical trauma injuring the bleb is less than with scleral or limbal incisions.

High Myopia

In these patients, a great tendency exists for the lens iris diaphragm to move posteriorly during surgery. High myopia therefore represents another indication for the endocapsular tension ring. Great care must be taken not to press down on the nucleus but to stabilize it, as in cases of pseudoexfoliation, and to try to keep it as high in the anterior segment as possible.

CONCLUSION

Modern phacoemulsification of cataracts has led to the expectation that small incision cataract surgery will be associated with rapid visual and physical rehabilitation of patients. The increased user-friendliness of the machines, along with the continuous improvements in phacoemulsification technology and the downsizing of phacoemulsification incisions and implantation devices, has enabled many incremental improvements to create safer and more rapid cataract surgical procedures. In many centers throughout the world, clear corneal cataract surgery under topical anesthesia is being performed with rapid visual rehabilitation and resumption of full activities by the patient in the immediate postoperative period.

REFERENCES

1. Colvard DM, Kratz RP, Mazzocco TR, Davidson B. Clinical evaluation of the Terry surgical keratometer. J Am Intraocul Implant Soc. 1980;6:249–51.
2. Fine IH. Uma incisao para a faco. Oftalmologia. 1992;9(30):1,12.
3. Fine IH. Corneal tunnel incision with a temporal approach. In: Fine IH, Fichman RA, Grabow HB, eds. Clear-corneal cataract surgery and topical anesthesia. Thorofare, NJ: Slack; 1993.
4. Williamson CH. Cataract keratotomy surgery. In: Fine IH, Fichman RA, Grabow HB, eds. Clear-corneal cataract surgery and topical anesthesia. Thorofare, NJ: Slack; 1993.
5. Neuhann T. Theoric und Operationstechnik der Kapsulorhexis. Klin Monatsbl Augenheilkd. 1987;190:542–45.
6. Gimbel HV, Neuhann T. Development, advantages and methods of the continuous circular capsulorrhexis technique. J Cataract Refract Surg. 1990;16:31–7.
7. Fine IH. Cortical cleaving hydrodissection. J Cataract Refract Surg. 1992;18;508–12.
8. Fine IH. Hydrodissection and hydrodelineation. In: Steinert RF, ed. Cataract surgery: technique, complications, and management. Philadelphia: WB Saunders; 1995.
9. Fine IH, Maloney WF, Dillman DM. Crack and flip phacoemulsification. J Cataract Refract Surg. 1993;19:797–802.
10. Fine IH. A spectrum of clear corneal phaco techniques. In: Long DA, ed. New Orleans Academy of Ophthalmology: Anterior segment and strabismus surgery. Proceedings of the 44th Annual Symposium. Amsterdam/New York: Kugler Publications; 1996.
11. Steinert RF, Deacon J. Enlargement of incision width during phacoemulsification and folded intraocular lens surgery. Ophthalmology. 1996;103:220–5.
12. Mackool RJ, Russell RS. Effect of foldable intraocular lens insertion on incision width. J Cataract Refract Surg. 1996;22:571–4.
13. Fine IH. The choo-choo chop and flip phacoemulsification technique. Oper Tech Cataract Refract Surg 1998;1:61–5.
14. Arshinoff SA. Dispersive-cohesive viscoelastic soft shell technique. J Cataract Refract Surg. 1999;25:167–73.
15. Fine IH, Packer M, Hoffman RS. Use of power modulations in phacoemulsification. J Cataract Refract Surg. 2001;27:188–97.
16. Cionni RJ, Osher RH. Endocapsular ring approach to the subluxed cataractous lens. J Cataract Refract Surg. 1995;21:245–9.

CHAPTER

48

Manual Cataract Extraction

FRANK HOWES

DEFINITION

- Removal of crystalline lens by nonautomated or manual techniques.

KEY FEATURES

- Major developments in cataract surgery over the past 20 years.
- Evolution of techniques with experience.
- Intracapsular cataract extraction or large incision full lens extraction.
- Extracapsular cataract extraction or large incision nuclear expression cataract surgery.
- "Mininuc" technique or manual nucleus expression lens surgery through a small incision.

INTRODUCTION

The technique of cataract surgery have changed substantially over the last 10 years. The mainstay of cataract surgery is now phacoemulsification through small corneal incisions, combined with the use of foldable intraocular lenses inserted through these small incisions to correct or minimize astigmatism. The techniques of large incision extracapsular surgery and intracapsular surgery are now used primarily as secondary procedures when faced with unusual intraoperative problems (e.g., nuclear sclerotic cataracts too dense for phacoemulsification or zonular loss disguised by posterior synechiae) or as primary procedures when certain conditions have been diagnosed preoperatively and are deemed inappropriate for phacoemulsification (e.g., dislocated lenses due to trauma, congenital conditions, or dystrophic conditions). The threshold for embarking on these procedures is dependent on the experience of the operating surgeon.

The decision about the choice of procedure, in the broader sense, is based on a spectrum of factors related primarily to socioeconomic environment (e.g., equipment) and competence (of the surgeon and the surgical team) on the one hand and to the ophthalmological condition of the patient on the other hand.

HISTORICAL ISSUES

Large incision nuclear expression cataract surgery, or extracapsular cataract extraction (ECCE), has been the mainstay of cataract surgery for the past three decades. The experiences gained from this form of surgery have in many ways contributed to the development of the smaller incision techniques. Much of the value of the large incision procedure is the lower cost and minimal instrumentation with which the surgery can be performed, a significant factor in third-world care. ECCE is also less demanding in terms of skill yet provides excellent rehabilitation of blindness caused by cataract at the expense of only recovery time and stability of refraction over the first year.[1]

Intracapsular cataract extraction (ICCE) still has a place in today's surgical environment, but that place is restricted mainly to eyes with dislocated or subluxed crystalline lenses in the first-world environment. Because cataract is a worldwide problem, particularly in the third world, advanced equipment should not reduce the capacity to treat multitudes of patients who require surgery. It is in conditions of destitution that ICCE remains necessary, and undoubtedly there are ways to improve that operation under such conditions.

Before World War II, both ECCE and ICCE were performed, but ECCE was predominant. In 1946 Stallard wrote, "The majority of conservative surgeons favour the extra-capsular method of extraction as being less dangerous from the point of view of vitreous loss."[2] However, the danger existed that lens cortex might remain in the eye after ECCE on an immature cataract, which sometimes excited devastating inflammation, including severe iritis, phacoanaphylaxis, the development of dense secondary membranes, and glaucoma. Then, as now, ECCE often required secondary capsulotomy, and in those days, this could be very traumatic. In skilled hands, ICCE gave better results.

Thus ICCE held favor until the ECCE method was improved with the introduction of microsurgery in the 1950s and automated infusion-aspiration and phacoemulsification in the 1970s, which enabled the complete removal of lens cortex by peeling from the equator. The improved stability of an intraocular lens (IOL) when placed in the capsular bag encouraged surgeons to return to ECCE.

With time, cataract removal became more successful, thanks to complete cortical removal and IOL stabilization against the capsular bag. This was followed by the desire to improve optical outcome by making smaller incisions with consequently less astigmatism and instability. The means of doing this slowly became available with the development of phacoemulsification, but the costs of equipment and the steepness of the learning curve created the need for techniques that reduced the requirement for sophisticated means of decreasing the nuclear size in order to remove fragments through smaller incisions. This led to the development of manual nuclear expression surgery through smaller incisions, or the so-called mininuc technique.[3]

The development of systems to provide continuous inflow of irrigating fluid while aspirating the lens remnant provided the cornerstones for all forms of extracapsular cataract surgery. These systems reached a high level of technological sophistication in the phacoemulsification techniques. In the mininuc systems, the need for high pressure and high flow for nuclear expression through a smaller incision led to the development of the wide-bore anterior chamber maintainer (ACM), which permitted such an intraocular environment. The independent infusion proved to be advantageous when used throughout the period of surgery because of the continuous flow and resultant positive pressure.[4–6]

As quoted by the inventor of the procedure[7]:

Small incision, machine-dependent phacoemulsification of the nucleus,[8] which is a common procedure in certain parts of the world, was designed to overcome the need to express the nucleus of the cataract out of the eye through a large incision. Reduction of the size of the nucleus ("mini-nuc") enables an alternative approach to nuclear expression that uses a manual technique.[4] This surgery is best achieved if the operation is performed throughout under positive intraocular pressure[9] (IOP), with the utilization of an anterior chamber maintenance system that provides continuous flow from the inside of the eye to the outside. The surgery is best performed through a sclerocorneal tunnel, the major portion of which is in the cornea. The nucleus is separated by hydrodissection and is manipulated manually in part or as a whole into the anterior chamber. Thereafter, nucleus expression is effected by the application of hydrostatic and external pressure, which enables lens implantation under the same conditions. A smaller incision than used in conventional nuclear expression can be made under topical anesthetic, and no sutures are required. Rehabilitation is rapid and the procedure is cost effective compared to phacoemulsification or any other manual nuclear expression extracapsular cataract extraction using viscoelastic material.

In summary, the objective of this procedure is to express the nucleus through an intact capsulorrhexis and thereafter through the smallest sclerocorneal[3] tunnel possible.

LARGER INCISION CATARACT SURGERY

Both intracapsular (ICCE) surgery and nuclear expression extracapsular (ECCE) surgery require large incisions, perhaps slightly larger in the ICCE group due to the increased size of the whole lens and the penalty of poor outcome should the capsule break on removal. In both techniques, however, attention to wound construction is vital if a good optical outcome is expected.

Incision

An incision of 8–10mm of arc length around the limbus (corneal, limbal, scleral, or a combination thereof) is required to manually express the nucleus from the capsular bag in ECCE, whereas an incision of 12–14mm around the limbus is required in ICCE. Variation in the incision position has a profound influence on the postoperative occurrence of cylindrical error[10]; this can be used to benefit the patient. The more corneal the section is placed, the stronger the influence on the cylindrical error. The more scleral the section is placed, the less the cylindrical induction, particularly if a three-plane (Fig. 48-1), valve-type incision is utilized. Combinations of both scleral and corneal sections can be used to correct preexisting cylindrical errors.[11] These sections can be rotated appropriately to reduce cylindrical error in any meridian.

When the incision is fashioned, the third plane of the incision (see Fig. 48-1) should be completed only when the anterior capsulectomy has been performed. This allows the anterior chamber to maintain depth, with or without viscoelastic material, while the anterior capsulectomy is undertaken. Once this is done, the internal incision may be completed.

Wound Closure

During closure of a wound cut in the three-plane format, the sutures must not be overtightened; the edges are merely opposed (incisional gape; see Fig. 48-1).[12] The valve effect of the incision seals the wound. In cases in which leakage is excessive, closure can be obtained by intracameral air.

A second chance to modify cylindrical effects arises when sutures are removed. This allows controlled dehiscence of the wound. Dehiscence induces negative cylindrical effect at the meridian of the suture removal (e.g., releasing a positive cylindrical effect induced by overly tight wound suturing). A rough guide to timing suture removal is as follows:
- After 1 month if major wound dehiscence is required to correct cylindrical error (3–6 diopters)
- After 2 months if minor dehiscence is required to correct cylindrical error (2–3 diopters)
- At 3–6 months to resume preoperative cylinder

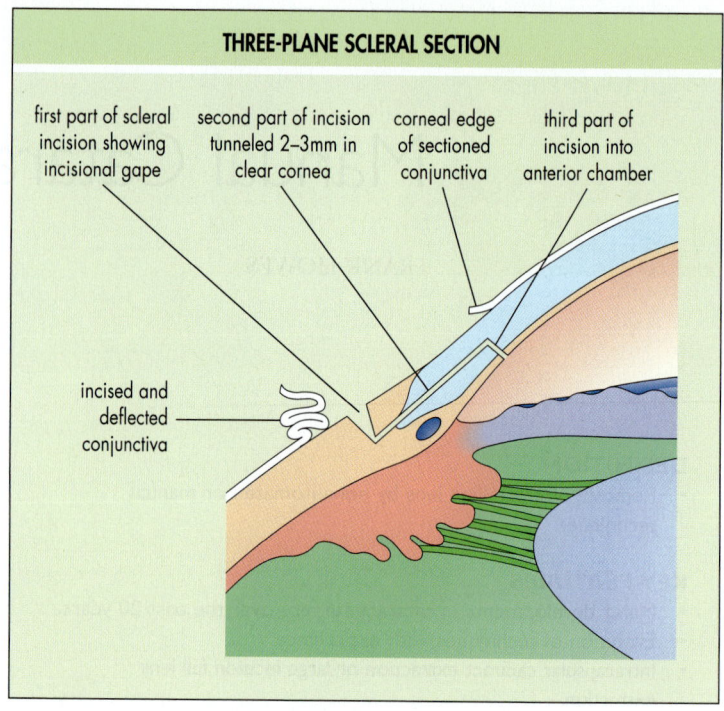

THREE-PLANE SCLERAL SECTION

first part of scleral incision showing incisional gape

second part of incision tunneled 2–3mm in clear cornea

corneal edge of sectioned conjunctiva

third part of incision into anterior chamber

incised and deflected conjunctiva

FIG. 48-1 ■ **Three-plane scleral section.** This incision is formed by the use of a sharp microsurgical knife for the initial vertical segment, followed by use of a curved dissecting blade to form the intralamellar section of the incision. The final vertical portion of the incision is best cut with corneal microscissors. Tissue elasticity produces the incisional gape.

- After 6 months to maintain surgically induced cylinder correction if appropriate

INTRACAPSULAR CATARACT EXTRACTION
General Technique[13]

After confirmation that the anesthetized eye is soft and akinetic, a speculum is inserted to retract the lids without pressure being applied to the globe. An incision is made large enough for lens delivery.

Endothelial touch must be avoided and a deep anterior chamber maintained during and after the procedure, with the lens removed in an intact capsule with minimal trauma and no disturbance of the vitreous face. Viscoelastic materials facilitate this process.

One or two iridectomies (Fig. 48-2) are necessary to prevent pupil block, which may result in iris adhesion, incarceration, or prolapse through the wound. Alpha-chymotrypsin is introduced through a cannula to pass behind the lower pupil border. Approximately 0.3ml of fluid is injected over the zonule to the sides and below it, as well as through an iridectomy over the zonule above it. The fluid serves to weaken the zonule, prove the patency of the iridotomy, and irrigate small amounts of blood or iris pigment from the anterior chamber. This enables removal of the lens without zonular traction on the peripheral retina.

The lens can be held by capsule forceps, by suction, or by freezing with a cryoprobe; the last is the most reliable. In the cryoprobe technique (Fig. 48-3), the cornea is lifted by the preplaced suture so that the iris can be retracted using a dry cellulose sponge swab to uncover the peripheral lens capsule. The swab also absorbs moisture from the lens surface before the cryoprobe is applied to the upper lens capsule. As the probe operates, an ice ball forms and is observed closely until it includes some of the lens substance. This allows traction to be applied with little risk of tearing the capsule. There should be no lines of tension showing on the anterior capsule. The lens is eased through the pupil by a combination of traction and expression. As the lens slides forward and upward, the full equatorial diameter engages and dilates the pupil. As soon as this point is

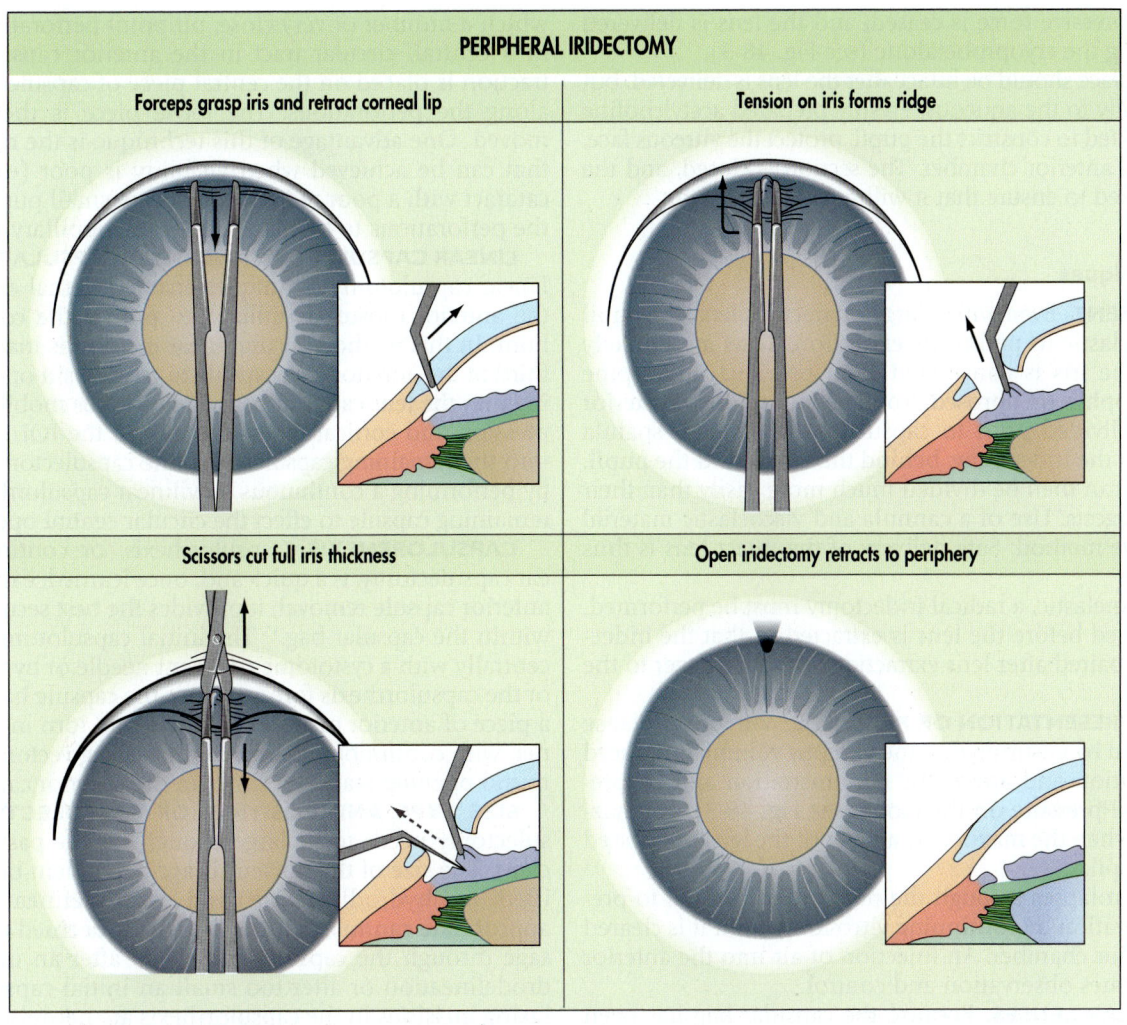

PERIPHERAL IRIDECTOMY

Forceps grasp iris and retract corneal lip	Tension on iris forms ridge
Scissors cut full iris thickness	Open iridectomy retracts to periphery

FIG. 48-2 ■ **The surgery of peripheral iridectomy.** The midzone iris stroma is grasped from below within the wound lips at the 12 o'clock position, and the iris is drawn out of the incision by about 1mm to tent its periphery. Curved or angled Vannas' scissors are introduced from above, with the blades across the tented iris. The blades are closed to cut through the iris. The resultant small iridectomy opens and retracts peripherally as the instruments are removed. Iris pigment should be observed from the excised piece of iris to ensure that the posterior portion of the iris has been cut, confirming patency. (Adapted from Roper-Hall MJ: Stallard's eye surgery, 7th ed. London: Wright; 1989.)

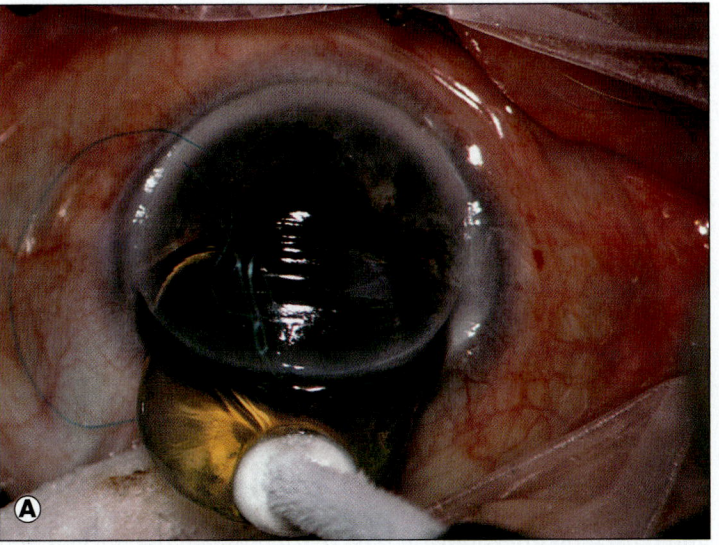
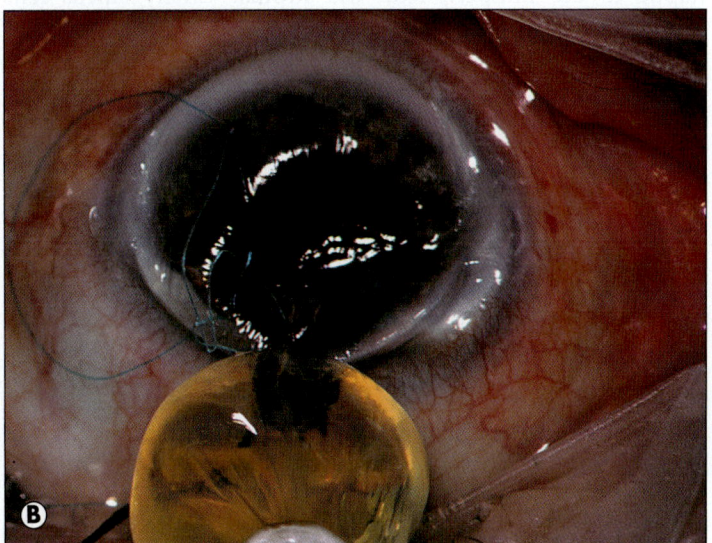

FIG. 48-3 ■ **Intracapsular delivery of the lens after it has been brought forward through the pupil with the cryoprobe. A,** The pupil constricts spontaneously as soon as the maximal diameter of the lens is through. In the lower left of the figure, the moist swab is shown as it and the lens are sliding. **B,** The cornea has a concave surface, showing that the eye is soft without forward pressure from the vitreous body. The anterior chamber is reformed with a physiological solution. (From Roper-Hall MJ: Stallard's eye surgery, 7th ed. London: Wright; 1989.)

reached, all expressive force is ceased, and the lens is delivered by sliding, using the cryoprobe alone (see Fig. 48-3).

The vitreous face should be intact after the lens is delivered, but it is exposed fully to the aqueous. Freshly prepared acetylcholine solution is injected to constrict the pupil, protect the vitreous face, and reform the anterior chamber. The section is closed, and the wound is checked to ensure that it will remain watertight.

Specific Techniques

IRIS MANAGEMENT. Even with a large cataractous lens, the pupil is sufficiently elastic to permit its extraction. Tears are unlikely except when the iris is constricted from previous pilocarpine therapy or atrophic or fibrosed from previous iritis. Posterior synechiae are divided prior to capsulating by using a spatula passed through the iridectomy, behind the iris toward the pupil. The adhesions can then be divided much more easily than their appearance suggests. Use of a cannula and viscoelastic material is an alternative method. Safe delivery of the intact lens is thus facilitated.

If the iris is inelastic, a radical iridectomy must be performed. A suture is placed before the lens is extracted so that the iridectomy can be repaired after lens extraction without danger to the vitreous face.

VITREOUS PRESENTATION OR PROLAPSE. Vitreous prolapse must be avoided by ensuring that the vitreous volume is reduced during preparation and anesthetic administration and by preventing external pressure on the globe (see Fig. 48-3). The hazard is greatest when the maximal diameter of the lens has passed through the pupil.

If vitreous prolapses through the pupil, it is essential to prevent its incarceration by continuing vitrectomy until it is cleared from the anterior chamber. An injection of air into the anterior chamber facilitates observation and control.

INTRAOCULAR LENSES. Because the capsular bag has been removed, the choice of IOL support is limited to the angle, the iris, or the ciliary sulcus support (fixated by suture).

The anterior chamber depth is maintained with viscoelastic material. An angle-supported lens must be fitted carefully to the individual chamber diameter so that it neither distorts nor moves. An iris-supported lens is stabler when placed in an oblique direction and prevented from rotating by suturing the haptic to the midperipheral iris stroma. Ciliary sulcus lens placement requires trans-scleral support by suture fixation and is useful when there is either iris damage (e.g., from trauma) or trabecular damage (e.g., associated with glaucoma). Adequate vitreous clearance is a prerequisite to all these placement sites, but particularly in ciliary sulcus placement.

EXTRACAPSULAR CATARACT EXTRACTION

Extracapsular surgery entails more steps than intracapsular surgery, in that the capsular bag is left in the eye, held in position by the zonules. The loss of the refracting power of the crystalline lens is replaced by a synthetic intraocular lens that can rest either in the capsular bag (preferentially) or in the ciliary sulcus. To initiate the process, a hole is made in the crystalline lens in a central position in the visual axis (anterior capsulectomy). The remainder of the process involves careful removal of the contents.

The important variables in this operation are the position and pattern of the incision, the position and method of the anterior capsulectomy, the method of nucleus expression, and the techniques of closure.

Anterior Capsulectomy

The techniques of anterior capsulectomy have changed over the past 20 years.[14]

"CAN-OPENER" CAPSULECTOMY. The simplest type of capsular opening or capsulectomy is the "can-opener" type, in which a number of very close, pinpoint perforations are created in a central, circular tract in the anterior capsule. Centripetal traction is placed on the central piece of capsule to create a tear along the perforations. The loose piece is then carefully removed. One advantage of this technique is the relative accuracy that can be achieved when visibility is poor (e.g., for a dense cataract with a poor red reflex or a very small pupil that requires the perforations to be made under the pupillary margin).

LINEAR CAPSULOTOMY AND INTERCAPSULAR TECHNIQUES. Linear capsulotomy techniques enable external expression while the anterior capsule is utilized to protect the corneal endothelium. In this method, a curvilinear incision is made in the upper third of the anterior lens capsule to create a slit or envelope opening into the lens capsular bag. After nucleus mobilization and expression and cortical material removal, the IOL can be inserted into the remaining capsular bag. The capsulectomy is completed by performing a continuous curvilinear capsulorrhexis across the remaining capsule to effect the circular central opening.

CAPSULORRHEXIS. Capsulorrhexis, or continuous curvilinear capsulectomy, is a quick and, once learned, easy technique for anterior capsule removal; it provides the best security for the IOL within the capsular bag.[15] The initial capsulotomy can be made centrally with a cystotome or a bent needle or by utilizing the tip of the capsulorrhexis forceps. Once the capsule has been opened, a piece of anterior capsule is grasped and torn in a circular manner, with continuous change of the tearing vectors to achieve the round opening (capsulectomy) in the anterior capsule.

SIZE, TYPE, AND POSITION OF CAPSULECTOMY. The capsulectomy needs to be large enough for the passage of the nucleus. The size of the nucleus is age dependent but can be modified by hydrodissection and hydrodelineation using an appropriate cannula.[16] If the nucleus is deemed too big for passage through the capsulectomy (e.g., after an unsuccessful hydrodelineation or after too small an initial capsulorrhexis), relaxing incisions in the capsulorrhexis are necessary to reduce the possibility of capsular dislocation and zonular damage during nucleus expression. During hydrodissection, if the anterior capsular opening is large enough, part of the equatorial rim of the nucleus can be expressed into the anterior chamber, then rotated into the anterior chamber and into the incision, and thus removed from the eye. Viscoelastic material between the corneal endothelial surface and the nuclear surface is necessary to prevent endothelial damage.

The size and shape of the capsulorrhexis can be varied by the surgeon. A large capsulectomy facilitates surgery, but when this exceeds approximately 6.5mm in diameter, the capsulorrhexis becomes difficult to control because of the presence of the insertion of the zonules.[17] When the anterior capsular ridge is crossed, the danger of a peripheral radial irretrievable split[18] is possible (particularly if the anterior chamber is not kept deep; a shallow anterior chamber creates tension on the anterior zonules). Peripheral splits are usually blocked by the zonules, but unwanted posterior capsular tears can occur by this mechanism.

NUCLEAR EXPRESSION. The scleral lip of the incision should be depressed to allow the leading pole of the nucleus to present into the incision. Gentle pressure at the 180° opposing limbus then expresses the nucleus. The appropriate pressure may be applied with a broad-based instrument, such as a vectis or squint hook.

Alternatively, internal expression using an irrigating vectis is effective, as long as the nucleus has undergone hydrodissection and partial hydroexpression. The space between the nucleus and the posterior capsule or cortex is opened with the irrigation function of the vectis. Viscoelastic material is also very useful in defining and holding these spaces and in preventing posterior capsular and endothelial damage.

CORTICAL WASHOUT. Removal of the remaining cortex using an irrigation-aspiration technique is not difficult, as long as the tip of the irrigation-aspiration cannula is kept in view to avoid unwanted capsular engagement. Difficulties can arise if the posterior globe pressure causes the anterior chamber to become shallow and causes closure of the fornix of the capsular bag. Partial closure of the wound and irrigation produce a deep and safe anterior chamber within which to work. Cleaning of the posterior capsule and removal of remaining resistant cortical remnants can be achieved by aspiration using a fine cannula with a polished tip.

INTRAOCULAR LENS INSERTION. Insertion of the IOL is performed under direct vision, with the second haptic inserted either by circular dialing of the IOL or by direct placement using fine forceps.[19] When the capsular bag is damaged by complication, the sites of intraocular placement become the same as those noted in the ICCE section. In some circumstances where there is still sufficient capsular support, in spite of capsular damage, posterior chamber implantation can be considered.

Mininuc Technique

ANTERIOR CHAMBER MAINTAINER. An oval ACM (Fig. 48-4) is inserted through clear cornea to the anterior chamber between the 4 o'clock and 8 o'clock positions, parallel to and near the limbus. The height of the infusion bottle determines the intraocular pressure (IOP). The continuous flow is responsible for the anterior chamber maintenance system.

CAPSULORRHEXIS. The IOP is increased to 40mmHg (5.3kPa). This pressure pushes the lens backward, which facilitates the formation of capsulorrhexis and prevents accidental radial capsule tear to the periphery.[18] A 5–6mm capsulorrhexis is preferred.

SCLEROCORNEAL POCKET TUNNEL. The scleral entrance incision to the sclerocorneal pocket tunnel is frown shaped and 5mm long and is placed 1mm behind the limbus (Fig. 48-5). At both ends of the incision, perpendicular backward continuation incisions 1mm long are cut. This extension helps accommodate the thickness of the nucleus as it passes through the tunnel. The tunnel is dissected anteriorly for 3–4mm (1mm in the sclera, 1mm in the limbus tissue, and 2mm in clear cornea). Also, the scleral dissection is enlarged on both sides of the tunnel beyond the 1mm backward scleral incision to make a pocket-like dissection (hence the term *pocket tunnel* rather than simply *tunnel*). The keratome internal incision is placed parallel to the curvature of the limbus and is 20% longer than the scleral outer incision. The pocket tunnel facilitates nucleus expression.

NUCLEUS MANIPULATION. Hydrodissection is performed in two separate, anatomically distinct parts of the lens: first, just under the capsule, and second, between the hard-core nucleus and the epinucleus.[20] Usually, the hydrodissection under the capsule partially moves the nucleus to the anterior chamber at the 12 o'clock position. If the nucleus does not move anteriorly, the hydrodissector cannula is lodged perpendicularly around the equator of the nucleus and then moved behind the nucleus. The positive IOP in the anterior segment pushes the posterior capsule away, which creates a counterforce to the anterior movement of the hydrodissector cannula while the hard-core small nucleus is being separated from the epinucleus and cortex. In this way, the smallest possible hard-core nucleus is isolated, to be delivered through the intact capsulorrhexis. At this stage, the nucleus is ready for expression.

NUCLEUS EXPRESSION. A plastic glide (4mm wide, 0.2mm thick) is introduced through the tunnel under the nucleus. Slight pressure is induced on the glide at the inner limbal area, which is used to guide the nucleus that is to be engaged in the sclerocorneal pocket tunnel. This pocket is made to accommodate the nucleus at this stage. When the nucleus is well lodged in the pocket, and no leakage of BSS is observed, slight scleral pressure is induced. The further the nucleus is expressed (Fig. 48-6), the more the location of the scleral pressure is moved backward. If the external pressure on the sclera is located near the internal incision throughout, an area of leakage is created rather than prevented, and nucleus expression cannot be completed. The IOP during nucleus expression is 40–45mmHg (5.3–6.0kPa), helping hydroexpression of the nucleus.

CORTEX REMOVAL AND INTRAOCULAR LENS IMPLANTATION. Cortex removal and IOL implantation are facilitated by the deep anterior chamber formation induced by the ACM system. The capsular bag is inflated during aspiration and during the IOL implantation. Insertion of the IOL is performed under direct vision, similar to ECCE, with the second haptic inserted either by circular

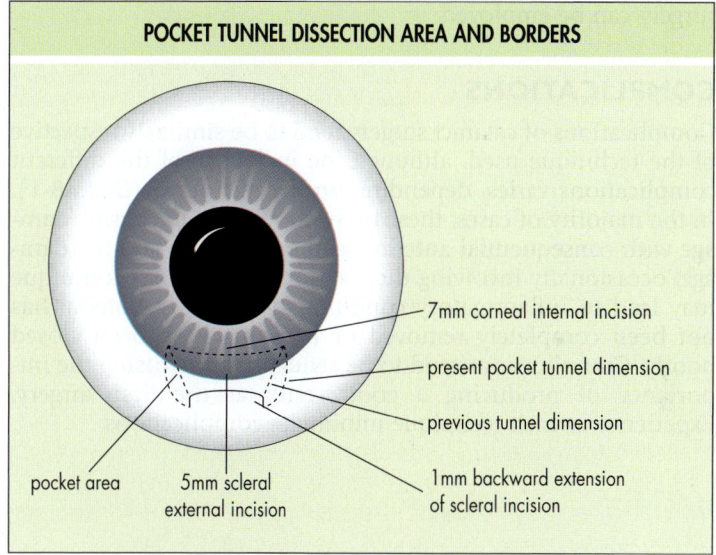

POCKET TUNNEL DISSECTION AREA AND BORDERS

- 7mm corneal internal incision
- present pocket tunnel dimension
- previous tunnel dimension
- 1mm backward extension of scleral incision
- pocket area
- 5mm scleral external incision

FIG. 48-5 ▐ Pocket tunnel dissection area and borders.

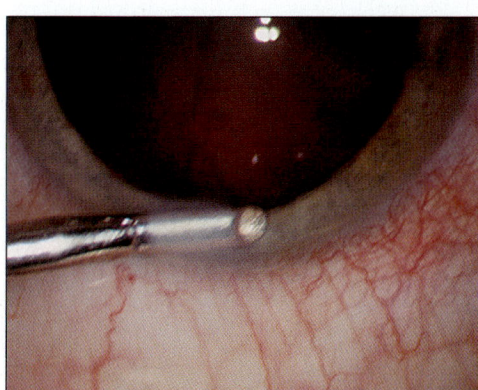

FIG. 48-4 ▐ Anterior chamber maintainer located at the 6 o'clock position, parallel and adjacent to the limbus, in clear cornea. The incision is made into the cornea with a stiletto 1.1mm wide and beveled 1.5–2mm.

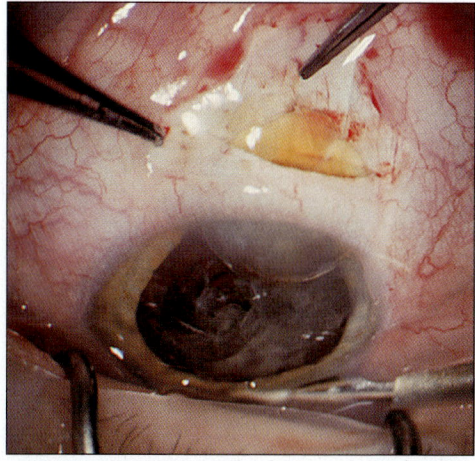

FIG. 48-6 ▐ The nucleus is lodged in the pocket tunnel and hydroexpressed out of the eye. The glide is located behind the nucleus. External expression is performed on the glide away from the external incision of the pocket tunnel.

BOX 48-1

Complications of Cataract Surgery

Optical power aberrations (sphere and cylinder)
Capsule rupture without vitreous loss
Capsule rupture with vitreous loss
Vitreous capture in incisional wound
Iris prolapse
Iris capture in incisional wound
Nuclear loss into the posterior segment
Intraocular lens loss into the posterior segment
Inability to primarily implant intraocular lens due to above
Glaucoma (aphakic, inflammatory, malignant, pupil block)
Chronic inflammatory disease
Cystoid macular edema
Retinal detachment
Hypotony
Choroidal edema and effusion
Choroidal hemorrhage
Infection

dialing of the IOL or by direct placement using fine forceps.[19] Once again, when the capsular bag is damaged by complication, the sites of intraocular placement become the same as those noted in the ICCE section.

With a smaller incision than both ECCE and ICCE, the techniques of foldable lens insertion per phacoemulsification surgery can be employed.

COMPLICATIONS

Complications of cataract surgery tend to be similar, irrespective of the technique used, although the incidence of the different complications varies, depending on the technique (Box 48-1). In the majority of cases, these occur in relation to capsule damage with consequential anterior segment vitreous and iris damage, occasionally involving the incision as well. Poor technique may lead to inflammatory conditions when lens material has not been completely removed or incisions have been closed poorly. Complications tend to be sequential, increasing the importance of producing a good result at the first surgery. Experience in each technique minimizes complications.

REFERENCES

1. Oshika T, Tsuboi S. Astigmatic and refractive stabilisation after cataract surgery. Ophthalmic Surg. 1995;26(4):309–15.
2. Stallard HB. Eye surgery, 1st ed. Bristol: Wright; 1946:263.
3. Blumenthal M. Manual ECCE, the present state of the art. Klin Monatsbl Augenheilkd. 1994;205:266–70.
4. Blumenthal M, Moisseiev J. Anterior chamber maintainer for extracapsular cataract extraction and intraocular lens implantation. J Cataract Refract Surg. 1987;13:204–6.
5. Blumenthal M, Cahane M, Ashkenazi I. Direct intraoperative continuous monitoring of intraocular pressure. Ophthalmic Surg. 1992;23(2):132–4.
6. Blumenthal M. Manual nucleus expression through a small incision. In: Yanoff M, Duker JS, eds. Ophthalmology, 1st ed. London: Mosby; 1999.
7. Obstbaum SA. Phacoemulsification, the favoured surgical technique. Editorial. J Cataract Refract Surg. 1991;17:267.
8. Blumenthal M, Assia E, Neuman D. Lens anatomical principles and their technical implication. J Cataract Refract Surg. 1991;17:211–7.
9. Blumenthal M, Assia E, Neuman D. The round capsulorrhexis capsulotomy and the rationale for 11mm diameter IOL. Eur Implant Refract Surg. 1990;2:15–9.
10. Storr-Paulsen A, Vangsted P, Perriard A. Long term natural and modified course of surgically induced astigmatism after extracapsular cataract extraction. Acta Ophthalmol (Copenh). 1994;72(5):617–21.
11. Howes G. Control of astigmatism in cataract surgery. Presentation at 1986 Annual Meeting of the Ophthalmological Society of South Africa (P.O. Box 339, Bloemfontein 9300, South Africa).
12. Koch P. Incisional gape. Mastering phacoemulsification, 4th ed. Thorofare: Slack; 1994:23–4.
13. Roper-Hall MJ. Intracapsular cataract extraction. In: Yanoff M, Duker JS, eds. Ophthalmology, 1st ed. London: Mosby, 1999.
14. Apple D, Legler VF, Assia EI. Comparison of various capsulectomy techniques in cataract surgery. An experimental study [in German]. Ophthalmologe. 1992;89(4):301–4.
15. Gimbel H, Neuhann T. Development, advantages, and methods of the continuous circular capsulorrhexis. J Cataract Refract Surg. 1990;16(1):31–7.
16. Blumenthal M. Manual ECCE, the present state of the art. Klin Monatsblad Augenheilkd. 1994;205(5):266–70.
17. Sakabe I, Lim SJ, Apple DJ. Anatomical evaluation of the anterior capsular zonular free zone in the human crystalline lens [in Japanese]. Nippon Ganka Gakkai Zasshi. 1995;99(10):1119–22.
18. Assia E, Apple D. Mechanism of radial tear formation and extension after anterior capsulectomy. Ophthalmology. 1991;98(4):432–7.
19. Assia EI, Leglar V, Merril JC, et al. Clinicopathologic study of the effect of radial tears and loop fixation on intraocular lens decentration. Ophthalmology. 1993;100(2):153–8.
20. Blumenthal M, Ashkenazi I, Assia E, Cahane M. Small incision manual extracapsular cataract extraction using selective hydrodissection. Ophthalmic Surg. 1992;23(10):699–701.

Combined Procedures

DAVID ALLEN

INTRODUCTION

Cataract develops mainly as a response to aging but also to chemical or biological insults to the eye. Frequently, these causative processes are associated with other conditions that may require surgical intervention. With the development of phacoemulsification and its attendant reduced inflammatory response and early ocular stability, it has become more common to combine this surgical approach with that used for the coexisting disease. The conditions commonly associated with cataract and that lend themselves to such a combined approach are glaucoma, corneal opacity, effects of penetrating trauma, and vitreoretinal disorders.

COMBINED PHACOTRABECULECTOMY

HISTORICAL REVIEW

Although surgeons have attempted to control intraocular pressure (IOP) at the time of cataract surgery for some time, it was with the development of trabeculectomy in the late 1960s and early 1970s that the combined procedure was recognized to have a legitimate role in the routine management of coexisting cataract and glaucoma. In 1976 Spaeth and Sivalingam[1] described the concept of modifying the shelved posterior lip of a (large) cataract incision to allow filtration interestingly. The concept when reborn in the mid-1990s with sutureless phacotrabeculectomy was regarded as new. The combined surgery concept was revisited in the 1990s because the inflammatory consequences of small-incision surgery have been shown to be much reduced in comparison with those of large-incision surgery.[2]

PREOPERATIVE EVALUATION AND DIAGNOSTIC APPROACH

Lens opacities often impair the accurate evaluation and monitoring of glaucoma, as they interfere with visualization of the optic disc or with visual field assessment. The proposition, therefore, is that the cataract requires removal to enable progress of the glaucoma to be monitored.

Other cases to be considered for combined surgery include those in which glaucoma is uncontrolled by medical treatment and some degree of cataract exists. Many surgeons also elect to remove early cataract in a combined procedure if trabeculectomy is otherwise indicated, in order to maximize the visual benefit for the patient, who can expect some worsening of cataract in the first 1–2 years following trabeculectomy.

The patient's expectation from combined procedures requires careful management. In this situation the use of some form of potential acuity assessment may be of help. The extent to which the pupil dilates also influences the surgical approach and enables the surgeon to assess the degree of increased risk of preoperative and early postoperative complications.

ANESTHESIA

The anesthetic techniques considered are no different from those considered for simple cataract surgery in the same patient.

When local anesthetic is injected, care must be taken, if ocular and/or orbital pressure is applied, not to cause further damage to a compromised and vulnerable optic disc.

SPECIFIC TECHNIQUES

Several studies have reported reduced complications from and increased efficacy of phacotrabeculectomy compared with manual extracapsular extraction combined with trabeculectomy.[3,4] Debate continues on whether a single-site or two-site approach is best. Several studies reported no significant difference in pressure-lowering effect. A single-site approach may be less time consuming, but a two-site approach allows the surgeon to use the familiar clear corneal approach with better visibility associated with avoidance of a superior scleral tunnel. There is similar controversy over fornix-based or limbus-based conjunctival flap. Randomized prospective studies have shown no difference in IOP control or visual improvement, but if the antimetabolite mitomycin C (MMC) is used there are increased complications with a limbus-based flap.[5]

In a single-site approach a standard 5mm wide trabeculectomy flap is fashioned, and phacoemulsification and implant insertion are performed through what would become the site of the sclerectomy. The sclerectomy is then completed with a blade or by using a punch (Fig. 49-1), followed by peripheral iridectomy. The scleral flap is then resutured in the normal way for a trabeculectomy (Chapter 240).

An alternative approach is to modify the standard self-sealing scleral tunnel phacoincision by removal of part of the posterior internal lip (see Fig. 49-2), which destroys its self-sealing properties but still allows a sutureless technique. In this technique, the surgeon creates a standard scleral tunnel incision that commences 2mm posterior to the limbus. After cataract removal and intraocular lens insertion, a scleral punch is used to remove part of the posterior internal lip (see Fig. 49-3). To facilitate this a relieving incision is often made, either at one end of the phacoemulsification tunnel or in the center to form a "T" incision (see Fig. 49-4). After sclerectomy and iridectomy a suture is used to secure the scleral flap (see Fig. 49-5), and the tightness of this

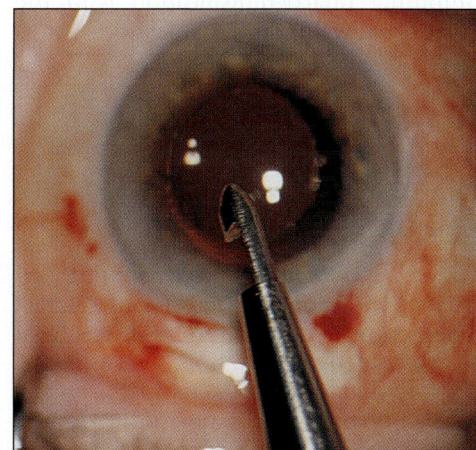

FIG. 49-1 Crozafon-deLaage punch. The guillotine-type cutter is visible clearly against the red reflex of the pseudophakic eye.

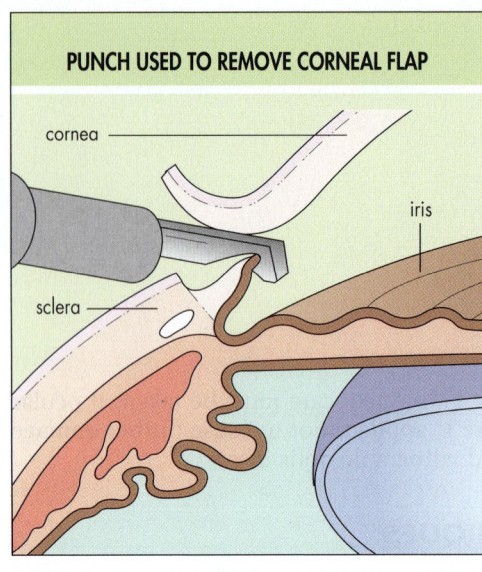

PUNCH USED TO REMOVE CORNEAL FLAP

cornea

iris

sclera

FIG. 49-2 ▌ Punch used to remove internal corneal lip. Note the position and effect of the punch.

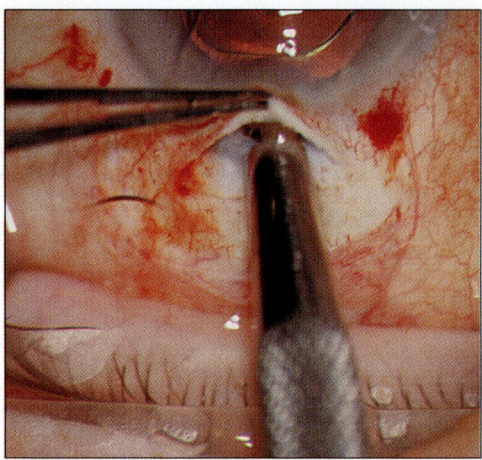

FIG. 49-3 ▌ Keratectomy performed using a punch.

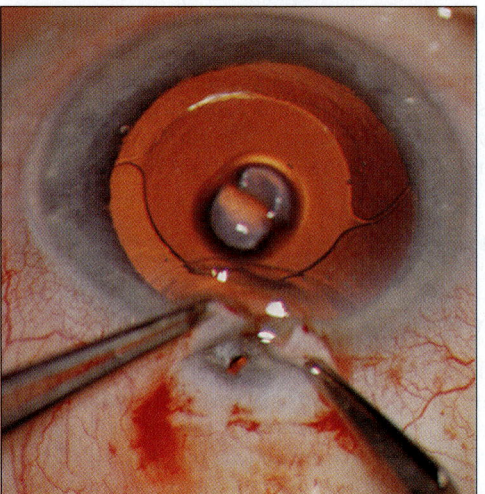

FIG. 49-4 ▌ "T" incision in the scleral flap. The anterior scleral flap has undergone a central relieving incision. The site of keratectomy excision is visible in the bed, and the two excised portions can be seen placed on the cornea. Note also that a peripheral iridectomy has been performed.

or the period before laser suture lysis can be titrated in the standard way, as for a trabeculectomy.

Nonpenetrating glaucoma surgery (deep sclerectomy or viscocanalostomy) has been combined with phacoemulsification. There are early reports that these new techniques are as effective as trabeculectomy when combined with phacoemulsification,[6,7] but more longer term studies are required before their true place in treatment of coexisting cataract and glaucoma can be determined.

COMPLICATIONS

The surgical approaches just described demand careful resuture of the conjunctival flap to minimize the possibility of a shallow and/or flat anterior chamber and to minimize the risk of intraocular infection. Postoperatively, a visible bleb is often thought to be a sign of successful drainage (Fig. 49-6), but in practice there seems to be little correlation between bleb presence and continued IOP control.[8] The incidence of inflammatory response in anterior chamber fibrinous uveitis and of other complications is reported to be higher with combined surgery than with single operations.[9]

OUTCOMES

Increasing evidence shows that trabeculectomy combined with phacoemulsification is more effective for the control of IOP than when combined with large-incision surgery.[3,4] The outcomes in terms of lowering IOP are good, and few additional complications occur.[10] The addition of MMC produces a greater IOP lowering but with added complications. The length of follow-up of surgery combining phacoemulsification with the newer nonpenetrating glaucoma techniques is still short.

LENS SURGERY COMBINED WITH KERATOPLASTY

HISTORICAL REVIEW

The underlying pathology in eyes that require penetrating keratoplasty is often associated with an increased risk of cataract (Fig. 49-7); this includes corneal perforation as a result of trauma or infection and age-related degeneration, such as Fuchs' corneal degeneration. Pseudophakic bullous keratopathy associated with the use of closed-loop anterior chamber or iris-fixated intraocular lenses (IOLs) became apparent during the 1980s and 1990s. These factors resulted in the development of a variety of

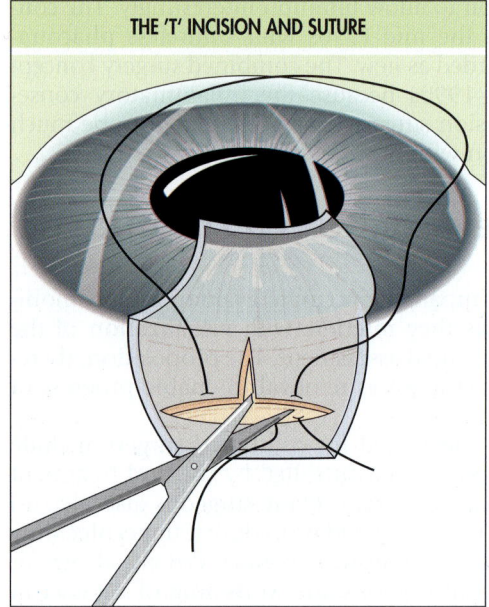

THE 'T' INCISION AND SUTURE

FIG. 49-5 ▌ "T" incision and suture.

techniques for combined primary cataract surgery and keratoplasty or IOL exchange combined with keratoplasty.

PREOPERATIVE EVALUATION, DIAGNOSTIC APPROACH, AND SURGICAL OPTIONS

The corneal evaluation of patients for penetrating keratoplasty is considered in Chapter 62. A retrospective analysis of eyes that underwent penetrating keratoplasty for Fuchs' endothelial dystrophy, with an average follow-up period of 6 years,[11] showed an

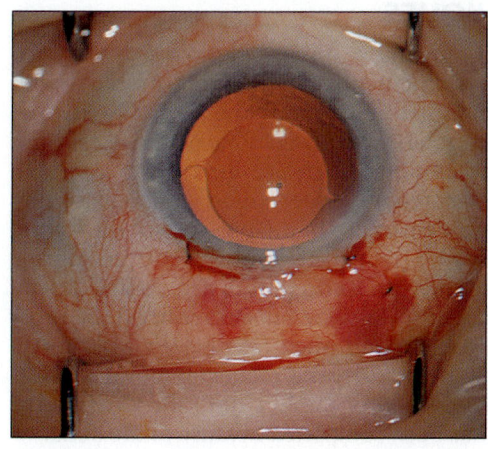

FIG. 49-6 ■ Diffuse subconjunctival bleb seen at the end of the phacotrabeculectomy procedure.

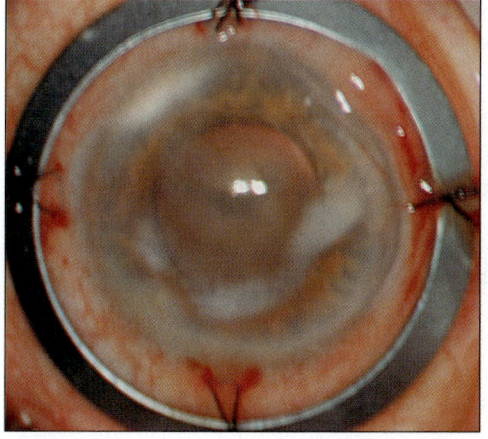

FIG. 49-7 ■ Patient with combined corneal and lens opacities. His degree of corneal opacity demands an open-sky approach to cataract removal.

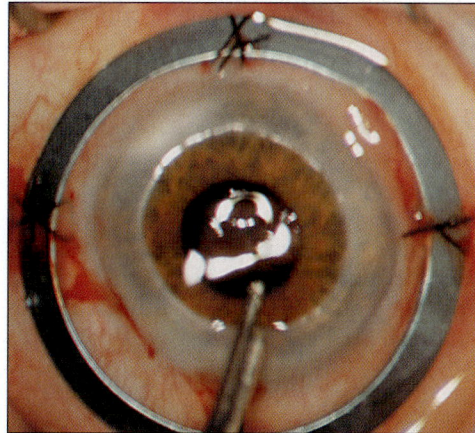

FIG. 49-8 ■ Abnormal reflexes make visualization of the posterior capsule difficult.

incidence of significant cataract in 75% of patients over 60 years of age. Of those who subsequently required lens surgery, 13% lost transplant clarity postoperatively. In addition, the eyes that had significant preexisting lens opacity had reduced visual benefit from keratoplasty if the lens remained unoperated. There are arguments, therefore, for simultaneous lens and corneal surgery.[11,12] Weighed against these are the problems associated with such a combined approach; the decision in individual cases depends on the balance of the risks and benefits that apply.

Choice of IOL depends on the individual circumstances. In the event that some form of extracapsular surgery is part of the primary procedure, a standard IOL can be placed in the capsular bag. If an IOL is already present and is considered either to be the cause of or to exacerbate the corneal decompensation, it should be replaced. If sufficient capsular and/or zonular fiber support exists, the best option is a sulcus-placed posterior chamber IOL. If adequate support is not available, the choice is either a modern open-loop, angle-supported lens or a transsclerally sutured IOL.[13]

If cataract surgery or IOL replacement is being considered, the preoperative evaluation must include some form of IOL power calculation. Keratoplasty unfortunately alters the axial length, keratometry, and anterior chamber depth, changes in all of which affect the calculation of IOL power for the required postoperative refraction. As a result, whereas most reported series of cataract extraction alone achieve refractive results within 2D in more than 90% of cases, reported results from combined cataract extraction and penetrating keratoplasty record a similar accuracy for between 26% and 67% of patients.[14] Strategies employed to overcome this deficiency included the use of fellow-eye keratometry readings in IOL regression formulas. Unfortunately, postoperative keratometry values bear more relation to the individual surgical technique (including donor and/or host size mismatch) than to the preexisting keratometry. Other strategies, therefore, are required, such as analysis of peripheral recipient corneal curvature.[14] Another approach is to analyze retrospectively a series of cases and make an assessment of the surgeon-specific, average

postkeratoplasty central corneal curvature and anterior chamber depth for use in regression formulas.[15]

After penetrating keratoplasty, the full visual rehabilitation routinely may be delayed for 12–18 months because of wound instability and the effects of healing and suture removal. In this context, another approach that some surgeons find acceptable is to remove the cataract at the time of keratoplasty but to insert the IOL as a secondary procedure some 12–18 months later, using the actual postkeratoplasty axial length and central keratometry to calculate the IOL power required. Although there are some reports of good outcomes using this approach, a comparative study showed no statistically significant difference in final refractive status with the technique.[12]

ANESTHESIA

Relatively prolonged periods with the ocular contents at atmospheric pressure make the use of topical anesthetic problematic. Most surgeons, therefore, prefer to use conventional injection of local anesthetic or general anesthesia. Safe local anesthesia is dependent on the use of agents that have an appropriate length of action to avoid the need for additional "top-up" injections during the procedure.

SPECIFIC TECHNIQUES

The techniques of keratoplasty are dealt with elsewhere. Technically, phacoemulsification surgery can be difficult when carried out as part of a combined approach because of the poor visibility in the anterior chamber as a result of the corneal disease. Selected cases may be suitable for a routine phacoemulsification procedure after a partial-thickness trephination of the cornea and removal of epithelium to aid anterior chamber and capsule visibility.[16] Such an approach is not always possible, and "open-sky" removal of the lens may be used. The altered anterior chamber and lens–iris diaphragm dynamics affect the ability to complete capsulorrhexis, but the open access allows the surgeon to employ capsule scissors more readily, if required. The use of phacoemulsification and irrigation-aspiration of the cortex is hampered by the abnormal light reflexes present in the open-sky situation (Fig. 49-8),[17] and control of anterior and posterior capsule is difficult; this results in an increased risk of capsule rupture or, alternatively, incomplete cortex removal.

For surgery on an aphakic or pseudophakic patient, complete clearance of any vitreous from the anterior chamber is mandatory. If a scleral-sutured IOL is to be fixed, clearance of vitreous from the posterior chamber and from the region of the pars plana–vitreous base is required. An open-sky approach to vitrectomy leads to problems of surgical visibility and of stability of the whole anterior segment, and use of a scleral support ring is helpful. The problems of an open chamber can be avoided by the use of a temporary corneal graft using material rejected by the eye bank, and this is replaced at the end of the lens surgery by a therapeutic graft.[18] Various methods of suture fixation of the IOL with scleral flaps, donor corneal buttons, or simple Tenon's capsule or conjunctival cover can be used; these are dealt with in more detail elsewhere.

COMPLICATIONS

Major complications of such combined procedures are the variability of refractive outcome and the delayed visual rehabilitation compared with straightforward cataract surgery. Apart from the possible inherent complications of keratoplasty, the combined procedure seems to offer an additional risk of cystoid macular edema. Weighed against this, however, is the additional risk of graft failure inherent in the alternative of a two-stage procedure.

OUTCOMES

The respective theoretical risks and benefits of a combined approach, a planned staged approach, and a keratoplasty wait-and-see approach have been discussed already. No definitive studies exist that provide hard evidence of the benefit of one approach over another.

COMBINED PHACOVITRECTOMY

HISTORICAL REVIEW

Planned vitrectomy through a pars plana was described first in 1972.[19] Since then, both technological support and surgical techniques have developed rapidly and surgical correction of severe vitreoretinal disorders is now possible. In two areas in particular a high incidence of significant associated problems with cataract exist—namely post-traumatic conditions (including retained intraocular foreign body) and proliferative diabetic retinopathy. The possibility of a simultaneous approach to the problems of the cataract and the retina in these conditions has become routinely available only with the widespread acceptance of small-incision (phaco) cataract surgery in the late 1980s and 1990s. The main advantage is that when the surgical approaches are combined, the vitreoretinal disease does not have time to progress significantly between procedures,[20] which increases the chances of a successful outcome in terms of retinal function.

PREOPERATIVE EVALUATION, DIAGNOSTIC APPROACH, AND SURGICAL OPTIONS

The presence of significant lens opacities in eyes that have suffered penetrating trauma involving the posterior segment or that have proliferative vitreoretinopathies makes definitive vitreoretinal surgery both more difficult and less likely to achieve the goals than when clear media are present. Assessment must be made, therefore, of whether the presence of lens opacities reduces the visibility of the posterior segment anatomy to a significant degree and also whether more minor opacities are likely to progress rapidly and require further intraocular surgery in the near future. When surgical options are considered for patients who have compromised general health, to perform a cataract removal and insert an IOL together would seem to add significant time to the procedure and thus increase the anesthetic risk. Weighed against this, however, is the possibility that vitreoretinal surgery can be accomplished more quickly in the presence of clear media, and so the final, total surgical time may be reduced significantly by a combined approach. Performance of posterior segment surgery can induce the rapid advancement of preexisting but mild lens opacities, and thus a second surgical episode with its attendant additional risks can possibly be avoided by combined primary surgery.

SPECIFIC TECHNIQUES

Although lensectomy remains a surgical option in combined cataract and posterior segment surgery, the main problem with this technique is that the anatomical barrier between anterior and posterior segments is inevitably destroyed. Phacoemulsification is now regarded as the technique of choice for cataract removal. Large-incision, nuclear expression surgery offers a particular problem with wound leak or dehiscence in the presence of the significantly higher than normal IOPs, which are often generated during posterior segment vitreoretinal procedures. Self-sealing scleral tunnel or corneal incisions for phacoemulsification, on the other hand, pose no such problem and often may be left without suture. Many surgeons choose to carry out cataract removal alone as a first stage and delay insertion of the IOL until the vitreoretinal part of the procedure has been completed because of the better visualization of the retinal periphery and vitreous base afforded by an aphakic rather than a pseudophakic eye. Once the posterior part of the surgery has been completed, the IOL can be placed in order to complete the procedure.

OUTCOMES

The technique described has been used for a relatively short period; the conditions to which it is applicable are difficult to standardize and subject to detailed stratified or randomized study. However, reports of small series of patients dealt with in this way indicate a favorable outcome.

REFERENCES

1. Spaeth GL, Sivalingam E. The partial punch: a new combined cataract-glaucoma operation. Ophthalmic Surg. 1976;7:53–7.
2. Lyle WA, Jin JC. Comparison of a 3 and 6 mm incision in combined phacoemulsification and trabeculectomy. Am J Ophthalmol. 1991;111:189–96.
3. Shingleton BJ, Jacobson LM, Kuperwaser MC. Comparison of combined cataract and glaucoma surgery using planned extracapsular and phacoemulsification techniques. Ophthalmic Surg Lasers. 1995;26:414–19.
4. Wishart PK, Austin MW. Combined cataract extraction and trabeculectomy: phacoemulsification compared with extracapsular technique. Ophthalmic Surg. 1993; 24:814–21.
5. Casson RJ, Salmon JF. Combined surgery in the treatment of patients with cataract and primary open-angle glaucoma. J Cataract Refract Surg. 2001;27:1854–63.
6. Gimbel HV, Anderson Penno EE, Ferensowicz M. Combined cataract surgery, intraocular lens implantation and viscocanalostomy. J Cataract Refract Surg. 1999; 25:1370–75.
7. Gianoli F, Scnyder CC, Bovey E, Mermoud A. Combined surgery for cataract and glaucoma: phacoemulsification and deep sclerectomy compared with phacoemulsification and trabeculectomy. J Cataract Refract Surg. 1999;25:340–46.
8. Simmons ST, Litoff D, Nichols DA, et al. Extracapsular cataract extraction and posterior chamber intraocular lens implantation combined with trabeculectomy in patients with glaucoma. Am J Ophthalmol. 1987;104:465–70.
9. Naveh N, Kottass R, Glovinsky J, et al. Long term effects on intraocular pressure of a procedure combining trabeculectomy and cataract surgery as compared with trabeculectomy alone. Ophthalmic Surg. 1990;21:339–45.
10. Jayamane DGR, Kostakis A, Phelan PS. The outcome of 2.3mm incision combined phacoemulsification, trabeculectomy and lens implantation of non-foldable intraocular lenses. Eye. 1997;11:91–4.
11. Payant JA, Gordon LW, VanderZwaag TO. Cataract formation following corneal transplantation in eyes with Fuchs' endothelial dystrophy. Cornea. 1990;9:286–9.
12. Pineros O, Cohen EJ, Rapuano CJ, Laibson PR. Long-term results after penetrating keratoplasty for Fuchs' endothelial dystrophy. Arch Ophthalmol. 1996; 114:15–18.
13. Hardten DR, Holland EJ, Doughman DJ, Nelson JD. Early postkeratoplasty astigmatism following placement of anterior chamber lenses and transsclerally sutured posterior chamber lenses. CLAO J. 1992;18:108–11.
14. Serdaravic ON, Renard GJ, Pouliquen Y. Videokeratoscopy of recipient peripheral corneas in combined penetrating keratoplasty, cataract extraction and lens implantation. Am J Ophthalmol. 1996;122:29–37.
15. Flowers CW, McLeod SD, McDonnell PJ, et al. Evaluation of intraocular lens power calculation formulas in the triple procedure. J Cataract Refract Surg. 1996;22:116–22.
16. Malbran ES, Malbran E, Buonsanti J, Adrogue E. Closed-system phacoemulsification and posterior chamber implant combined with penetrating keratoplasty. Ophthalmic Surg. 1993;24:403–6.
17. Groden LC. Continuous tear capsulotomy and phacoemulsification cataract extraction with penetrating keratoplasty. Refract Corneal Surg. 1990;6:458–9.
18. Nardi M, Giudice V, Marabotti A, et al. Temporary graft for closed-system cataract surgery during corneal triple procedures. J Cataract Refract Surg. 2001;27:1172–75.
19. Machemer R, Parel JM, Buettner H. A new concept for vitreous surgery: I. Instrumentation. Am J Ophthalmol. 1972;73:1–7.
20. Hurley C, Barry P. Combined endocapsular phacoemulsification, pars plana vitrectomy, and intraocular lens implantation. J Cataract Refract Surg. 1996; 22:462–6.

CHAPTER 50

Cataract Surgery in Complicated Eyes

GARY S. SCHWARTZ • STEPHEN S. LANE

INTRODUCTION

Following uncomplicated extracapsular cataract extraction, it is the standard of care that a posterior chamber intraocular lens implant (PCIOL) be placed within the capsular bag. Most surgeons agree that the intracapsular placement of a PCIOL minimizes not only the incidence of postoperative lens decentration but also the contact of the intraocular lens (IOL) with iris and ciliary body, thereby decreasing postoperative inflammation.

Occasionally, the surgeon must determine whether capsular bag placement is truly the preferred way to proceed after cataract extraction. Patients who have a previous history of trauma, pseudoexfoliation syndrome, or Marfan's syndrome may have areas of zonular dehiscence that preclude safe intracapsular IOL placement. Other patients may experience zonular dehiscence or posterior capsule rupture during cataract extraction, either of which forces the surgeon to rethink the decision of where to place the IOL. A host of factors, including a history of uveitis, the patient's age, status of the vitreous and capsule, and prior surgeries, may affect the decision concerning IOL placement after cataract extraction.

PREOPERATIVE EVALUATION AND DIAGNOSTIC APPROACH

When cataract surgery and IOL placement are planned, especially for a patient who has a prior history of ocular trauma, surgery, pseudoexfoliation syndrome, or crystalline lens subluxation (e.g., Marfan's syndrome), it is important to evaluate the status of the zonules. Whether or not the PCIOL is to be placed into the capsular bag or the ciliary sulcus, the zonules must hold the implant in place throughout the remainder of the life of that patient. Patients who do not have adequate zonular support may experience postoperative IOL decentration or dislocation.[1,2]

Zonular integrity should be evaluated preoperatively at the slit lamp by looking for the presence of phacodonesis or iridodonesis. If any question of loss of zonular integrity exists on the basis of slit-lamp evaluation, the zonules must be evaluated gonioscopically. If a patient has a history of ocular trauma, the eye should also be examined for iridodialysis and vitreous in the anterior chamber, either of which makes zonular dehiscence more likely.

The patient should also be evaluated for evidence of uveitis. Both uveitic inflammation and corticosteroids for treatment of uveitis can result in visually disabling cataract. The cause of the uveitis must be elucidated. Some forms of uveitis, such as pars planitis, Fuchs' heterochromic iridocyclitis, and human leukocyte antigen B27 (HLA-B27)–associated uveitis, heal well with IOL placement after cataract extraction.[3] In others, such as uveitis of Vogt-Koyanagi-Harada syndrome, sympathetic ophthalmia, and juvenile rheumatoid arthritis, the IOL may contribute to excessive intraocular inflammation, and, therefore, patients often do better if left aphakic.[4,5] However, at least one study discusses the successful implantation of PCIOLs in older patients who have cataract and a history of juvenile rheumatoid arthritis.[6]

In vitro and in vivo studies have demonstrated an advantage of heparin surface-modified polymethyl methacrylate (PMMA) lenses compared with regular PMMA lenses when looking at the adhesion of inflammatory cells.[7] For this reason, heparin surface-modified PMMA lenses probably have an advantage over regular PMMA lenses in patients with a history of uveitis. However, because of the necessity for a larger incision when using PMMA lenses, it remains to be seen whether heparin surface-modified lenses have an advantage over foldable silicone or acrylic IOLs when otherwise small-incision phacoemulsification is performed. If an IOL is to be placed in a patient who has a history of uveitis, an anterior chamber lens or a sulcus-supported posterior chamber lens should be avoided whenever possible, as increased contact with the iris and ciliary body may result in increased postoperative inflammation.

The presence of corneal astigmatism must also be established as part of the preoperative work-up, using either keratometry or videokeratography. If possible, placing the incision at the axis of the steep meridian of the corneal cylinder may be considered.[8]

OPTIONS TO SURGERY

Several options exist for IOL placement in combination with complicated cataract surgery (Table 50-1). Which is chosen depends upon many factors but mostly on the condition of the zonules and capsule and the experience of the surgeon.

Another option is to leave the patient aphakic. For such patients, visual rehabilitation may be achieved with the aid of aphakic spectacles or contact lenses. Epikeratophakia, although uncommon today, is another option for the aphakic patient.

GENERAL TECHNIQUES

Great care must be taken during the cataract extraction to preserve the integrity of the zonules, posterior capsule, and capsular fornices. The technique used for cataract extraction when the integrity of the zonules is in question depends upon the surgeon's experience and preference. Phacoemulsification can be performed with continuous-tear capsulorrhexis. Nuclear expression extracapsular cataract extraction is often done through either a can-opener capsulotomy or capsulorrhexis with relaxing incisions. The capsulorrhexis technique results in stronger capsular support during both nucleus and cortex removal.[9] In addition, because the nucleus is taken out in small pieces during phacoemulsification, its removal causes less stress on the capsule and zonules than does expression of the whole nucleus, as occurs in nuclear expression.

Phacoemulsification is usually the procedure of choice for patients who have a history of uveitis.[10] Phacoemulsification normally results in less trauma to the iris because of manipulation than does large-incision nuclear expression and, therefore, usually results in less postoperative inflammation. Larger incisions cause more postoperative inflammation and therefore should be avoided in uveitic patients whenever possible.

SPECIFIC TECHNIQUES

Zonular Dehiscence

Aside from a few specific precautions, cataract extraction in complicated eyes should be performed much as it is for uncomplicated ones. If the eye is compromised by loss of zonular support, as in cases of prior trauma, surgery, or pseudoexfoliation syndrome, care must be taken to preserve as much of the remaining supporting zonules as possible. A large capsulorrhexis (at least 5.5mm in diameter) is made to facilitate removal of nuclear fragments with minimal stress on the zonules. Careful and complete hydrodissection and hydrodelineation are carried out so that the nucleus rotates easily within the epinuclear bag, which decreases stress on the zonules during nuclear manipulation. The surgeon may choose to sublux the nucleus from the capsular bag and perform phacoemulsification within the anterior chamber. If phacoemulsification is to be carried out in the capsular bag, the phaco needle tip should be maneuvered to create troughs toward the area of the dehiscence whenever possible; this may necessitate the use of multiple incision sites. In this way the lens nucleus is always pushed toward the weakened area, which preserves the zonules, rather than pushed away from it (which may cause extension of the area of zonular dehiscence).

The surgeon may experience difficulty in performing capsulorrhexis in patients with significant zonular dehiscence because there are no zonules to offer resistance to the tearing forces applied by the surgeon's instrument.[11] A simple technique to stabilize the capsular bag and facilitate completion of the capsulorrhexis is the utilization of nylon iris fixation hooks. After starting the capsulorrhexis, the surgeon gently retracts the capsular edge with the iris hooks in the direction of the area of dehiscence. After the capsulorrhexis is completed, the nylon hooks can be left in place while hydrodissection and phacoemulsification are performed.

TABLE 50-1

OPTIONS FOR INTRAOCULAR LENS PLACEMENT AFTER CATARACT EXTRACTION

Procedure	Position of Optic	Position of Haptics	Haptic Fixation
Intracapsular posterior chamber intraocular lens implant	Capsular bag	Capsular bag	Capsular bag fornices
Foward-prolapsed optic	Posterior chamber	Capsular bag	Capsular bag fornices
Sulcus-supported posterior chamber intraocular lens implant	Posterior chamber	Ciliary sulcus	Ciliary sulcus
Optic bag–haptic sulcus	Capsular bag	Ciliary sulcus	Ciliary sulcus
Trans-sclerally sutured posterior chamber intraocular lens implant	Posterior chamber	Ciliary sulcus	Trans-scleral sutures
Iris-sutured posterior chamber intraocular lens implant	Posterior chamber	Ciliary sulcus	Iris sutures
Anterior chamber lens	Anterior chamber	Anterior chamber	Anterior chamber angle
Aphakia	None	None	None

The "forward-prolapsed optic" and "optic bag–haptic sulcus" techniques depend on an intact continuous curvilinear capsulorrhexis.

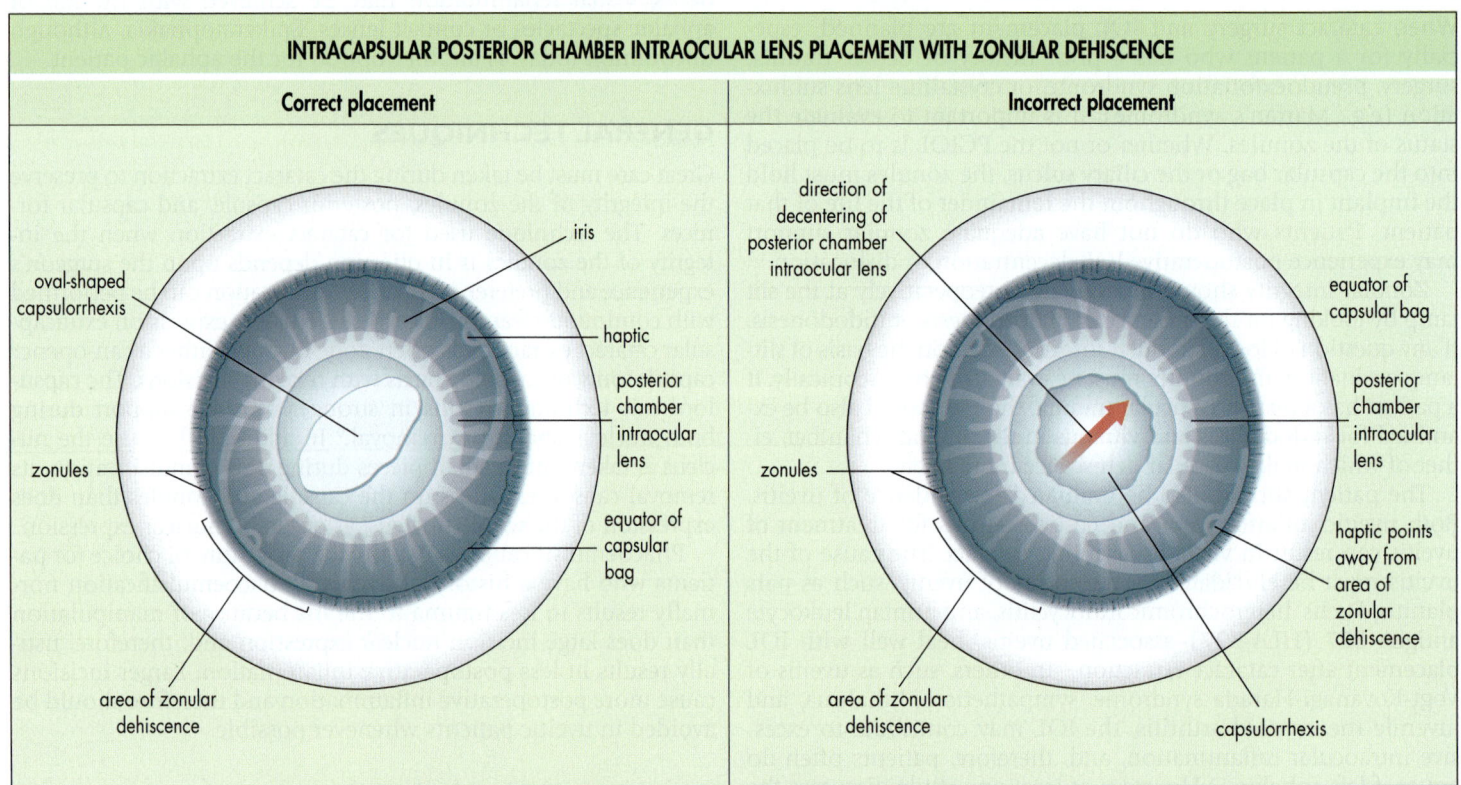

INTRACAPSULAR POSTERIOR CHAMBER INTRAOCULAR LENS PLACEMENT WITH ZONULAR DEHISCENCE

Correct placement	Incorrect placement

Correct placement labels: oval-shaped capsulorrhexis; iris; haptic; posterior chamber intraocular lens; zonules; equator of capsular bag; area of zonular dehiscence

Incorrect placement labels: direction of decentering of posterior chamber intraocular lens; equator of capsular bag; posterior chamber intraocular lens; zonules; haptic points away from area of zonular dehiscence; area of zonular dehiscence; capsulorrhexis

FIG. 50-1 ▪ Intracapsular posterior chamber intraocular lens implant placement with zonular dehiscence. The intraocular lens is first shown placed properly in the capsular bag with the haptics positioned toward the area of dehiscence. In this way, the bag is stretched toward the dehiscence and the optic does not decenter. Note that the capsulorrhexis is oval shaped because it has been pulled by the haptic in the direction of the dehiscence. The intraocular lens is then shown placed incorrectly in the bag with the haptics oriented 90° away from the dehiscence. A posterior chamber intraocular lens implant placed thus decenters away from the area of dehiscence in the direction of the arrow.

Once the nucleus and epinucleus have been removed, cortical cleanup should be performed both delicately and completely. With the nucleus removed, the capsular bag is floppier in nature, and the area of the dehiscence is drawn toward the aspiration tip. In such cases, it is often safer to separate the irrigation and aspiration ports and perform bimanual irrigation-aspiration. In this way, the irrigation tip can be used to hold back the capsular fornix of the area of dehiscence while the aspiration tip safely removes cortex.

After complete removal of the cataract, the IOL must be selected. Whenever possible, the IOL should be placed within the capsular bag for reasons described above. Intracapsular IOL placement is appropriate for patients who have up to 6 clock hours of zonular dehiscence. In such cases, the PCIOL is placed so that one of the haptics is in the meridian of the area of dehiscence, a position that spreads the bag out in that area (Fig. 50-1). If the haptics are rotated so that they are 90° away from the dehiscence, the optic will probably decenter in a direction away from the area of dehiscence.

Zonular dehiscence can also be managed by a PMMA capsular fixation ring during cataract extraction. Some fixation rings, such as the Cionni ring, have eyelets on them to allow fixation to the scleral wall with a Prolene suture.[12] These rings are left in place after surgery to help both expand and center the capsular bag postoperatively, thus keeping the lens implant from migrating away from areas of zonular dehiscence.

If the capsular support is felt to be inadequate for intracapsular lens placement, an alternative technique should be performed (see Table 50-1). A sulcus-supported PCIOL is placed so that the haptics are 90° away from the area of dehiscence (Fig. 50-2). This orientation prevents the haptic from slipping posteriorly into the vitreous chamber. If a continuous curvilinear capsulorrhexis has been performed, it may be advantageous to prolapse the optic into the capsular bag while the haptics are kept in the surgical sulcus. This technique often results in more stable optic centration in the presence of zonular dehiscence.

If not enough capsule is present to support both haptics, a PCIOL may be sutured to the iris or held in place with a trans-scleral suture. If no capsular support exists, both haptics may be sutured, either to the iris or trans-sclerally (Fig. 50-3).[13] Since transscleral and iris fixation procedures are technically more difficult to perform, the surgeon may opt for placement of an anterior chamber lens instead. Today's anterior chamber lenses, with their one-piece, PMMA, flexible, open-loop configuration, have proved to be a viable alternative.

Uveitis

Cataract extraction with IOL insertion in uveitic patients carries an increased complication rate due to small pupils, posterior synechiae, and postoperative inflammation. As a general rule, a patient should not be operated upon if the uveitis has recurred within the past year. Uveitic patients should receive oral prednisone 10mg/kg daily for up to 1 week prior to surgery, and many also benefit from intravenous methylprednisolone sodium succinate 125–250mg during the surgery. Oral prednisone may be tapered over 2–3 weeks after surgery.

In these patients, phacoemulsification is the procedure of choice because it allows the cataract to be removed with minimal manipulation of the sclera and uvea. Often, posterior synechialysis must be performed, which can be done with a cyclodialysis spatula or with viscodissection. The pupil may need to be enlarged by stretching it. The surgeon has the choice of stretching the pupil with two instruments usually found on the surgical tray (e.g., Beckert and chopper) or may use an instrument specifically designed for pupillary dilation (e.g., Beehler pupil dilator). If simple stretching does not provide the surgeon with an adequate pupil size to perform the surgery safely, self-retaining nylon iris hooks may be used. Once the pupil has been adequately dilated, cataract extraction then proceeds according to the surgeon's typical protocol.

After the cataract has been removed, the surgeon must address the question of which IOL to implant. As mentioned before, it is best to avoid anterior chamber lenses, iris-supported PCIOLs, and sulcus-supported PCIOLs as they have a tendency

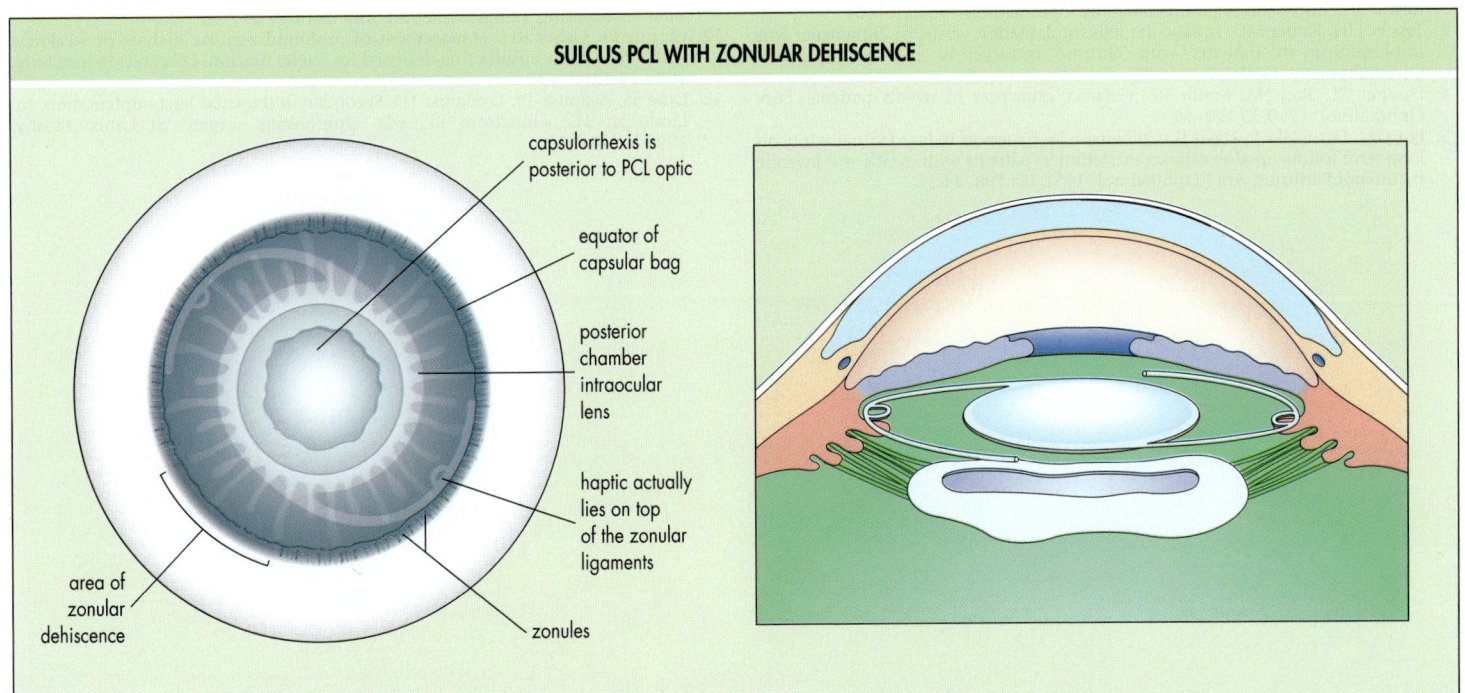

SULCUS PCL WITH ZONULAR DEHISCENCE

capsulorrhexis is posterior to PCL optic

equator of capsular bag

posterior chamber intraocular lens

haptic actually lies on top of the zonular ligaments

area of zonular dehiscence

zonules

FIG. 50-2 ▪ **Sulcus PCL with zonular dehiscence.** The IOL is properly placed in the ciliary sulcus. The haptics lie away from the area of the dehiscence and therefore are in the areas of greatest support. Placement here will decrease the likelihood that the haptics will prolapse backward into the vitreous cavity.

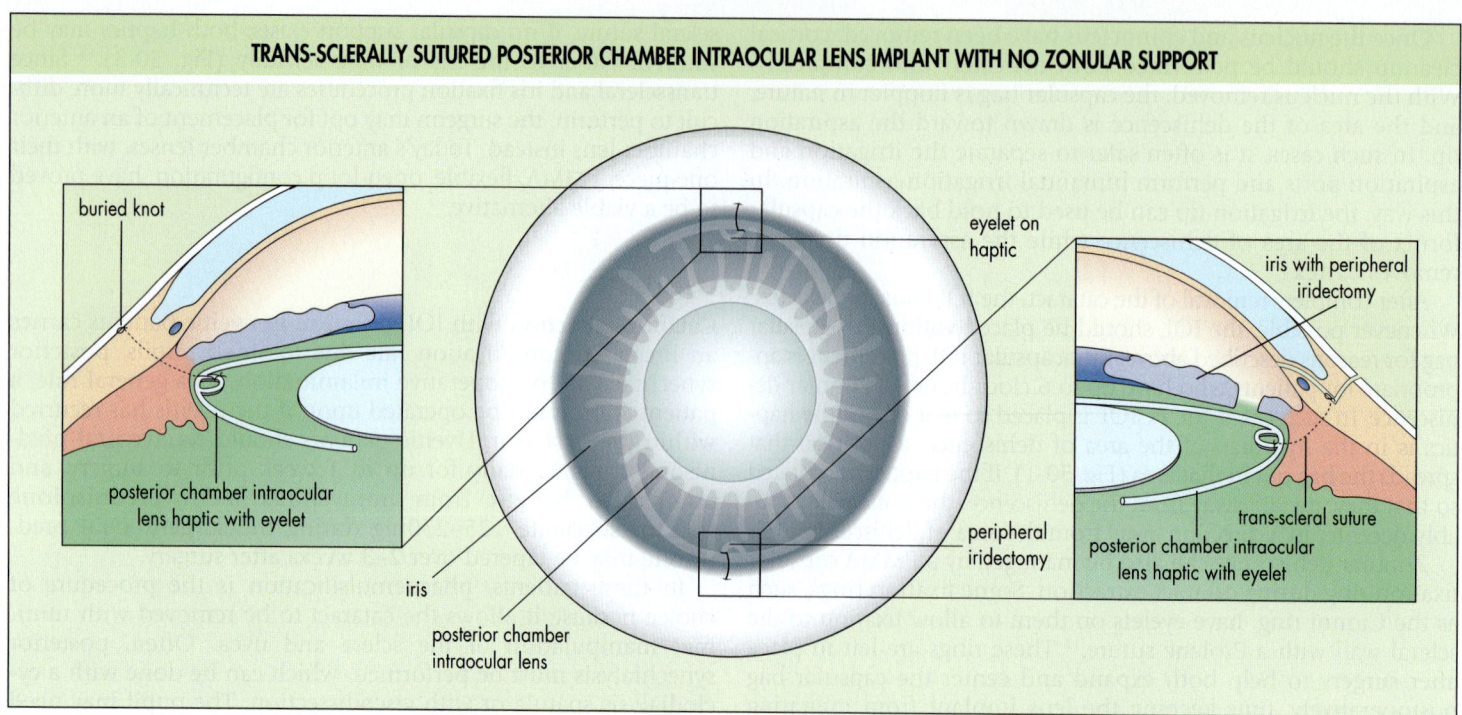

FIG. 50-3 ■ **Trans-sclerally sutured posterior chamber intraocular lens implant with no zonular support.** The intraocular lens has no natural support from the lens capsule and zonules. This implant is a one-piece, polymethyl methacrylate intraocular lens held in place by two trans-scleral 10-0 Prolene sutures tied to eyelets on the haptics. The knots are rotated to decrease the risk of long-term complications from knot erosion through the conjunctiva.

to cause postoperative inflammation as a result of contact with the iris and ciliary body. Whenever possible, a capsule-supported PCIOL is used. If capsular support is not present at the time of IOL implantation, a trans-sclerally sutured PCIOL may be used, or the patient may be left aphakic.

REFERENCES

1. Smith SG, Lindstrom RL. Report and management of the sunrise syndrome. J Am Intraocul Implant Soc. 1984;10:218–20.
2. Apple DJ, Mamalis N, Loftfield K, et al. Complications of intraocular lenses. A historical and histopathological review. Surv Ophthalmol. 1984;29:1–54.
3. Tessler HH, Farber MD. Intraocular lens implantation versus no intraocular lens implantation in patients with chronic iridocyclitis and pars planitis. Ophthalmology. 1993;110:1206–9.
4. Hooper PL, Rao NA, Smith RE. Cataract extraction in uveitis patients. Surv Ophthalmol. 1990;35:120–44.
5. Fox GM, Flynn HW Jr, Davis JL, Culbertson W. Causes of reduced visual acuity on long-term follow-up after cataract extraction in patients with uveitis and juvenile rheumatoid arthritis. Am J Ophthalmol. 1992;114:708–14.
6. Probst LE, Holland EJ. Intraocular lens implantation in patients with juvenile rheumatoid arthritis. Am J Ophthalmol. 1996;122:161–70.
7. Ygge J, Wenzel M, Philipson B, Fagerholm P. Cellular reactions on heparin surface-modified versus regular PMMA lenses during the first postoperative month. Ophthalmology 1990;97:1216–23.
8. Koch DD, Lindstrom RL. Controlling astigmatism in cataract surgery. Semin Ophthalmol. 1992;7:224–33.
9. Thim K, Krag S, Corydon L. Stretching capacity of capsulorrhexis and nucleus delivery. J Cataract Refract Surg. 1991;17:27–31.
10. Raizman MB. Cataract surgery in uveitis patients. In: Steinert RF, ed. Cataract surgery: technique, complications, and management. Philadelphia: WB Saunders; 1995:243–6.
11. Ahmed IIK, Crandall AS. Ab externo scleral fixation of the Cionni modified capsular tension ring. J Cataract Refract Surg. 2001;27:977–81.
12. Cionni RJ, Osher RH. Management of profound zonular dialysis or weakness with a new endocapsular ring designed for scleral fixation. J Cataract Refract Surg. 1998;24:1299–1306.
13. Lane SS, Agapitos PJ, Lindquist TD. Secondary intraocular lens implantation. In: Lindquist TD, Lindstrom RL, eds. Ophthalmic surgery. St Louis: Mosby; 1993:IG1–18.

51 Management of Eyes After Small Incision Phacoemulsification and Lens Implantation

FRANK HOWES

INTRODUCTION

Any intraocular surgery, including cataract surgery, can precipitate an inflammatory response initiated by a biochemical cascade of events.[1] The severity of this response varies from negligible to severe and depends on several factors (Box 51-1); it is not necessarily linked to the quality of the surgery. The management of these biochemical events is the same regardless of the type of surgery; the only major difference with cataract surgery is that incision size can be varied.

Cataract surgery may induce refractive errors, primarily through changes in corneal shape. If a corneal incision is greater than 3mm long, a change may be induced, especially if the wound has been sutured (Fig. 51-1). If a more posterior incision has been used, its form, width, and location determine its effect on the cornea.[2] Suture removal is considered more fully in Chapter 48.

BOX 51-1

Factors That Influence the Severity of Trauma in Cataract Surgery

SURGICAL
Form of surgery (i.e., large or small incision)
Duration of procedure (the longer, the more trauma)
Tissue manipulation (e.g., inadvertent corneal endothelial touch, uveal tissue damage, poor vitreous management)

INDIVIDUAL PATIENT
Individual response to trauma
Preexisting ocular disorders (e.g., active diabetic eye disease, uveitis, corneal endothelial disease)
Preexisting systemic disorders (e.g., collagen vascular disease, diabetes mellitus, atopic disease)

ENVIRONMENTAL
Surgical asepsis
Patient hygiene after operation

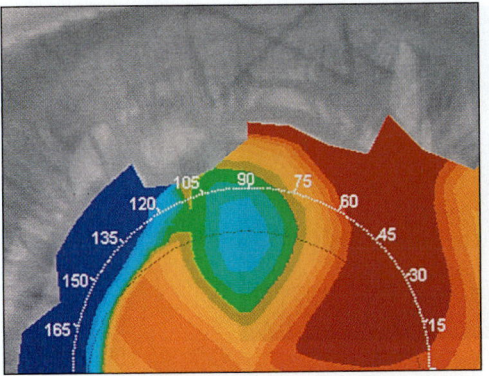

FIG. 51-1 ■
Peripheral corneal map illustrating irregular corneal shape. Uneven suture tension shows localized flattening where the limb of a suture is loose (blue area) and steepening where the limb of a suture is tight (red area). In this case, the peripheral effect is transmitted to the central optical portion of the cornea.

Postoperative management routines must be flexible enough to deal with unforeseen problems. A key aspect of postoperative management is patient cooperation—the patient must report adverse symptoms promptly. All patients must be made aware of the importance of visual symptoms, pain, redness, and discharge.

Cataract surgeons have their own individual regimens for postoperative management that vary according to each surgeon's technique and experience, but these regimens are based on a common theme. Some prefer intrusive management, while others prefer minimal management in recognition that patient compliance is variable and that uneventful surgery generally requires little aftercare.

IMMEDIATE POSTOPERATIVE PERIOD (DAYS 0–5)

Uneventful Surgery

If the surgery has been uneventful, topical antibiotics and corticosteroids are given three or four times a day for up to 1 month, often in diminishing doses. Antibiotics are given to treat potential pathogenic flora on the eyelids, lashes, and conjunctiva; these flora could contaminate the ocular surface and enter the eye by influx through an insecure wound, with possible milking of the globe by lid blinking in the immediate postoperative period. Corticosteroids are given to reduce the postoperative inflammation that is invariably present and quicken the rate of recovery.

The use of an eye pad after surgery is of questionable efficacy; a clear shield is probably adequate protection. An eye pad delays the return of vision to the eye (which should be immediate after either topical or general anesthetic), limits exposure of the ocular surface to atmospheric oxygen, and creates discomfort. Bandage contact lenses used after cataract surgery may entrap bacterial or fungal contaminants.[3,4]

Other topical medications are occasionally required. Mydriasis is indicated when surgery has been unusually traumatic and increased postoperative uveitis is expected. Ocular hypotensive agents (β-blockers, carbonic anhydrase inhibitors) are indicated when a sustained elevation of intraocular pressure (IOP) is anticipated or as a prophylactic measure against immediate postoperative ocular hypertension. This is especially important when viscoelastic materials have not been completely evacuated at the conclusion of surgery or in susceptible eyes with significant glaucomatous optic neuropathy.

Subconjunctival injections of corticosteroid, depot corticosteroid, antibiotics, or combinations of these are used routinely by some surgeons at the end of surgery, although their value has not been confirmed. It is accepted that such injections do no harm, apart from occasionally causing allergy and possible subconjunctival, periorbital, or even retrobulbar hemorrhage. Advocates argue that deposition of anti-inflammatory and antibiotic agents in the vicinity of the globe deters infection and inflammation.

Intra-cameral antibiotic (Cefuroxime 1mg/ml injecting 0.1mg in 0.1ml)[5] administered at the end of surgery has been advocated as a good prophylaxis against intraocular infection, thus avoiding the above-mentioned risks of hemorrhage.

Complicated Surgery

After complicated or prolonged surgery or in cases of an immediate heightened inflammatory response, topical dexamethasone is applied frequently with mydriasis until the inflammation subsides. If IOP is raised, topical β-blockers are given with, if necessary, oral acetazolamide 250mg two to four times per day, depending on the pressure. Rapid attention to severe postoperative inflammation is necessary if longer-term complications, such as the formation of synechiae between the pupil and lens capsule or intraocular lens (IOL) or secondary glaucoma (on a temporary basis), are to be prevented. This also applies to the formation of foreign body granulomata on the surface of certain intraocular lenses in association with inflammation (Fig. 51-2).[6] Medication is initially tailored to the severity of the inflammatory response and is then based on clinical judgment of the therapeutic response.

Surgery complicated by tissue or intraocular lens misplacement requires a return to the operating room at the earliest opportunity. Intensive postoperative medication as described earlier is usually necessary after such reconstruction.

EARLY POSTOPERATIVE PERIOD (DAYS 6–14)

After small incision cataract surgery using clear corneal incisions 3mm long (or limbal incisions of similar dimensions and certain scleral incisions), the refractive state of the eye is at or near its stable refraction.[2] Thus, following an uneventful surgery and postoperative course, refraction can be performed and a spectacle prescription given. Occasionally, however, capsular bag contracture can be asymmetrical, occurring predominantly anteriorly or posteriorly. This causes the IOL to shift either anteriorly (myopic shift) or posteriorly (hyperopic shift), requiring a change in spectacle correction. Medication is unnecessary unless there is persistent, mild uveitis, in which case topical corticosteroids are continued until the inflammation has resolved.

If surgery was uneventful but a mild fibrinous uveitis appears several days after the operation,[7] cycloplegia may be induced by the application of topical cycloplegic agents (the frequency depends on the severity of the inflammation). Systemic corticosteroids may supplement topical medication in more severe cases, and topical nonsteroidal anti-inflammatory drugs may be helpful when steroidal agents run the risk of causing complications (e.g., steroid-induced pressure rise or herpes simplex reactivation).

LATER POSTOPERATIVE PERIOD (WEEKS 3–6)

If there are no subjective or objective postoperative problems, the patient may be discharged from follow-up; no further medication is required. Most patients stabilize very rapidly after phacoemulsification cataract extraction and lens implantation through a small incision.

Visual Blurring and Image Distortion

If blurring of vision with image distortion occurs, the diagnosis may be transient postoperative cystoid macular edema. Subclinical inflammation is the usual cause of this condition, which requires anti-inflammatory medication (both steroidal and nonsteroidal), including oral acetazolamide 125mg twice daily for 1–2 weeks. In cases resistant to this treatment, posterior sub-Tenon administration of injectable steroid may be necessary. If surgery was traumatic, the risk of this complication increases, and appropriately vigorous treatment is required to pre-empt permanent damage. Any vitreous tags adherent to other tissues should be removed by neodymium:yttrium-aluminum-garnet (Nd:YAG) laser or by surgical intervention.[7]

Early Opacification of the Posterior Lens Capsule

The most common cause of this complication is poor cleaning of the posterior capsule at the time of surgery. Posterior capsular plaque and accumulation of inflammatory or infective debris (*Propionibacterium acnes*, *Staphylococcus epidermidis*) are less common causes. Posterior capsulotomy (usually performed using the Nd:YAG laser) should be delayed until approximately 3–6 months postoperatively to minimize the risk of retinal detachment, cystoid macular edema (see Chapter 131),[8,9] and endophthalmitis; infected material could be released into the vitreous following sequestration of the infected material in the lens capsular bag between the IOL and the posterior capsule.

LATE POSTOPERATIVE PERIOD (>3 MONTHS)

Foreign body giant cells may accumulate on the proteinaceous membrane on the surface of the IOL (Fig. 51-3). These may respond to intensive administration of topical corticosteroids. An alternative therapy is to release the membrane by low-dose Nd:YAG therapy to clear the light path if the cell membrane is dense. In severe cases, the IOL surface may need to be polished and the posterior synechiae broken to minimize recurrence.[6]

If poor uncorrected visual acuity develops because of induced astigmatism (through poor management of the cataract incision), the corneal shape may be corrected by selective suture removal (using corneal topography for guidance) or by arcuate keratotomy if the suture tension is not relevant or a sutureless technique was used.

Visual acuity deterioration and glare symptoms indicate posterior lens capsule opacification, which is treated by capsulotomy using the Nd:YAG laser to clear the visual axis and provide full transmission of light to the retina.[10,11] Potential complications of this treatment are immediate postlaser pressure spikes, cystoid macular edema, and subsequent retinal detachment (see Chapter 53).

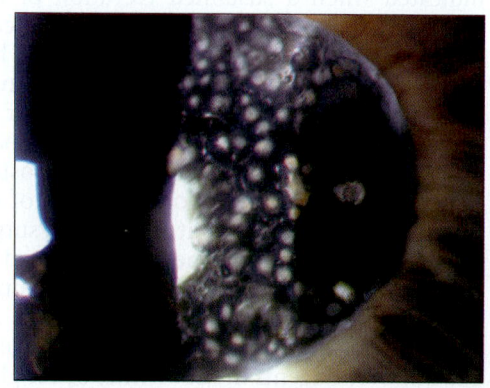

FIG. 51-2 ■ Slit-lamp photograph showing the clinical appearance of foreign body granulomata on the anterior surface of the intraocular lens.

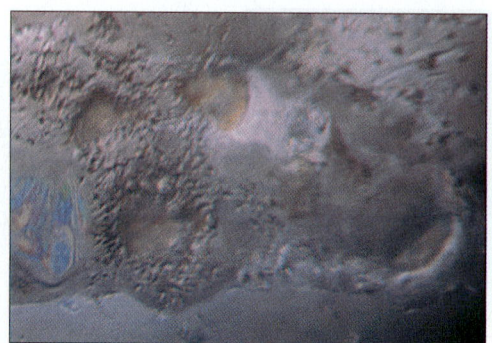

FIG. 51-3 ■ Specular microphotograph of an intraocular lens 3 months after implantation. Shown are foreign body giant cells adherent to the anterior surface.

POSTOPERATIVE EXAMINATION SEQUENCE

The postoperative examination sequence varies according to the logistics of the particular case. A few caveats in the planning of the postoperative sequence are important, however. An attempt must be made at the end of surgery to ensure that sutureless wound closure is sufficient to maintain a good anterior chamber depth. A poorly closed wound can create complications of hypotony and poses a risk of infection. The first check to ensure that the wound is closed and the anterior chamber depth is maintained should be within the first 48 hours. The patient should be instructed to report unusual symptoms such as pain and early visual loss. Intraocular infection usually manifests from the third day onward. If all is well at the end of the first week, serious complications are unlikely. A second visit between days 7 and 14 is valuable to exclude postoperative inflammation that is nonresponsive to routine medication and to ensure that the refractive state is within acceptable limits. The window of opportunity to make surgical adjustments in this respect is limited to the first 1–2 weeks. The final routine postoperative visit should be between 4 and 6 weeks. By this time, the eye should have settled completely, and the patient should be ready for final advice regarding future spectacle requirements. This is also the time to discuss the possibility of posterior capsule opacification and its symptoms. Medications have usually been discontinued by this time, and this examination should confirm the appropriateness of that.

COMPLICATIONS

Complications such as intraocular lens subluxation and dislocation, corneal decompensation, retinal detachment, glaucoma, endophthalmitis, and others are discussed in Chapter 53.

REFERENCES

1. Galin M. Causes of implant inflammation. In: Rosen ES, Haining W, Arnott EJ, eds. Intraocular lens implantation. St. Louis: Mosby; 1984:563–5.
2. Nielsen PJ. Prospective evaluation of surgically induced astigmatism and astigmatic effects of various self sealing small incisions. J Cataract Refract Surg. 1995;21:43–8.
3. Yee RW, Kosrirukvongs P, Meenakshi S, Tabbara K. Fungal keratitis. In: Tabarra KF, Hyndiuk RA, eds. Infections of the eye, 2nd ed. Boston: Little, Brown; 1996:350.
4. Faschinger C, Grasl M, Ganser K. Infectious corneal ulcers—once with endophthalmitis—after photorefractive keratotomy with disposable contact lens. Klin Monatsbl Augenheilkd. 1995;206:96–102.
5. Jenkins CDG, Tuft SJ, Sheraidah G, et al. Comparative intra-ocular penetration of topical and injected cefuroxime. Br J Ophthalmol. 1996;80(8):685–8.
6. Howes F, Chacko D. The management of foreign body granulomata on plate silicone intraocular lenses. OSUK; 2001.
7. Rose GE. Fibrinous uveitis and IOL implantation. Surface modification of polymethylmethacrylate during extracapsular cataract extraction. Ophthalmology. 1992;99:242–7.
8. Ruiz RS, Saatci OA. Visual outcome in pseudophakic eyes with cystoid macular edema. Ophthalmic Surg. 1991;22:190–3.
9. Piest KL, Kincaid MC, Tetz M, et al. Localized endophthalmitis: a new cause of the so called toxic lens syndrome. J Cataract Refract Surg. 1987;13:498–510.
10. Nasisse MP, Dykstra MJ, Cobo LM. Lens capsule opacification in aphakic and pseudophakic eyes. Graefes Arch Clin Exp Ophthalmol. 1995;233:67–70.
11. Altimara D, Guex C, Crosier Y, et al. Complications of posterior capsulotomy with the Nd:YAG laser. Klin Montasbl Augenheilk. 1994;204:286–7.

52 Pediatric Cataract Surgery

ELIE DAHAN

DEFINITION
- Cataracts occurring in the pediatric age group, arbitrarily birth to adolescence.

KEY FEATURES
- Two main approaches are used to remove cataracts in children: pars plana and limbal.
- Spectacles, contact lenses, and intraocular lenses are the most readily available means to correct aphakia in children.
- Posterior chamber intraocular lenses supplemented by spectacles are the best option for correction of aphakia in children because most of the correction is permanently situated inside of the eye.

Cataracts in childhood not only reduce vision but also interfere with normal visual development.[1-3] The management of pediatric cataracts is more complex, by far, than the management of cataracts in adults. The timing of surgery, the surgical technique, the choice of the aphakic correction, and the amblyopia management are of utmost importance to achieve good and long-lasting results in children.[4-10] Children's eyes are not only smaller than adults' eyes, but their tissues are much softer. The inflammatory response to surgical insult seems more pronounced in children, often because of iatrogenic damage to the iris.[11] During the past two decades, the refinements that have occurred in adult extracapsular cataract surgery have contributed to the development of pediatric cataract surgery.[2,4-8] Certain adaptations and modifications in surgical technique are required to achieve results similar to those achieved in adults.[2-8] Furthermore, postoperative amblyopia management forms an integral part of visual rehabilitation in children.[1-10]

HISTORICAL REVIEW

Discission of soft cataracts was first described by Aurelius Cornelius Celsius, a Roman physician who lived 2000 years ago. Because of its simplicity, discission remained the method of choice until the middle of the twentieth century. The technique consisted of lacerating the anterior capsule and exposing the lens material to the aqueous humor for resorption and/or secondary washout. Wolfe and Wolfe[12] in 1941 refined the technique by introducing the double-barreled aspirating-irrigating cannula, which allowed a one-step procedure. Repeated discissions were often required to manage the inevitable secondary cataracts.[2,11] Many early complications were associated with these early techniques; plastic iritis, glaucoma, and retinal detachments were the norms.[2,11] With the advent of vitrectomy machines and viscoelastic substances as well as the refinements in extracapsular cataract surgery, these complications have been reduced markedly over the past two decades.[2-10]

PREOPERATIVE EVALUATION AND DIAGNOSTIC APPROACH

A careful history demonstrates to the clinician the investigations required to determine the cause of cataracts in children.[2] Problems during pregnancy (e.g., infections, rashes or febrile illnesses, exposures to drugs, toxins or ionizing radiation) should be elicited. Family history of cataracts in childhood or other ocular abnormalities can be relevant. Both parents and all siblings should be examined with a slit lamp to determine any lens abnormalities. When family history is positive, consultation with a geneticist is recommended. A thorough examination by a pediatrician to assess the general health of the child and to elicit information as to other congenital abnormalities is mandatory.

Laboratory tests in children who have bilateral cataracts in nonhereditary cases are listed in Box 52-1. Most unilateral pediatric cataracts are idiopathic and do not warrant exhaustive laboratory tests.

The ophthalmologic part of the evaluation starts with a complete ocular examination, which includes an assessment of visual acuity, pupillary response, and ocular motility. Biomicroscopy follows and might necessitate sedation or even general anesthesia in very young patients. Fundus examination with dilated pupils is made unless the cataract is complete. A- and B-scan ultrasonography is carried out in both eyes to compare axial lengths and to discover any posterior segment abnormalities. Earlier photographs should be examined for the quality of the pupil's red reflexes. This might help to date the onset of the cataracts.

ALTERNATIVES TO SURGERY

The development of metabolic cataracts, such as those found in galactosemia, can be reversed if they are discovered in the early phases. With the elimination of galactose from the diet, the early changes in the lens, which resemble an oil droplet in the center of the lens, can be reversed.[13] Later on, lamellar or total cataracts develop, which require surgery.

When lens opacities are confined to the center of the anterior capsule or the anterior cortex, mild dilation of the pupils with homatropine 2% twice daily can improve vision and postpone the need for surgery. Photophobia and partial loss of accommodation are side effects of this measure. This temporary management should be implemented only in bilateral cataracts in which vision is equal in both eyes and better than 20/60 (6/18).

ANESTHESIA

General anesthesia is presently the only anesthetic option in pediatric cataract surgery. Neonates should be anesthetized by an anesthesiologist who is familiar with anesthesia of such young patients. It is extremely important to request deep anesthesia with paralysis and ventilation throughout the procedure.[5,7,8] The extraocular muscles are the last striated muscles to relax under drugs that cause paralysis. The sclera and cornea are very soft in childhood. Any tension on the extraocular muscles is

Laboratory Tests for Bilateral Nonhereditary Pediatric Cataracts

Full blood count
Random blood sugar
Plasma calcium and phosphorus
Urine assay for reducing substances after milk feeding
Red blood cell transferase and galactokinase levels
If Lowe's syndrome is suspected, screening for amino acids in urine
Toxoplasmosis titer
Rubella titer
Cytomegalovirus titer
Herpes simplex titer

transmitted to the sclera and results in increased intraocular pressure. A useful marker for anesthesia depth is the position of the eye during surgery. The cornea should be well centered without the help of any traction suture. If the cornea moves toward the superior rectus muscle, the anesthesia is too light and should be deepened. When this advice is followed, surgery is easier to perform and iatrogenic damage to the iris and cornea is diminished.

GENERAL TECHNIQUES

Unlike in adults, pediatric cataracts are soft. Their lens material can be aspirated through incisions that are 1–1.5mm long at the limbus or can be subjected to lensectomy through pars plana. When intraocular lens (IOL) implantation is intended, a larger wound is needed to introduce the IOL. This is best done through a scleral tunnel that is 5–6mm long. Unlike in adults, the tunnel should be securely sutured to prevent dehiscence of the wound with iris incarceration—a common complication in children.[11]

SPECIFIC TECHNIQUES

Two main approaches exist for the removal of cataracts in children: the pars plana approach and the limbal approach.

Both techniques have their advocates and opponents, and both have advantages and disadvantages. The pars plana approach was developed with the advent of vitrectomy machines in the late 1970s[14,15]; it was intended to deal mainly with very young infants in whom surgery is more difficult. With the continuing refinements in cataract and implant surgery in adults, the pars plana approach is gradually being abandoned in favor of the limbal approach, because the latter allows better preservation of the capsular bag for in-the-bag IOL placement.[2,5,7,8]

Pars Plana Approach

The pars plana approach is indicated mainly for neonates and infants under 2 years of age, particularly for those who have bilateral congenital cataracts for whom IOL implantation is not intended immediately.[2] The technique requires a guillotine-type vitrectome and balanced salt solution containing epinephrine (adrenaline) 1:500,000. The conjunctiva is opened at the 10 o'clock and 2 o'clock positions to expose the sclera at the level of the pars plana. The location of the pars plana in infants can be 2–3.5mm from the limbus. Two scleral perforations are made with a 20-gauge stiletto knife at the pars plana level; one for the vitrectomy probe and the second for the infusion cannula. A lensectomy–anterior vitrectomy is completed, sparing a 2–3mm peripheral rim of anterior and posterior capsule. These capsule remnants are used to create a shelf to support a posterior chamber IOL that may be implanted later on in life.[16] It is important to avoid vitreous incarceration in the wounds by turning off the infusion before withdrawing the vitrectome from the eye. This precaution reduces the chances of suffering

retinal traction and detachment later in life. The scleral incisions are sutured with 10-0 nylon, and the knots are buried to prevent irritation to the conjunctiva.

The pars plana approach can be performed relatively rapidly. It allows a permanently clear visual axis and spares the iris and the corneal endothelium. The postoperative course is normally less complicated than that after the limbal approach, because fewer maneuvers occur in the anterior chamber. Consequently, the iris and the corneal endothelium suffer less iatrogenic damage. In neonates who have bilateral cataracts, for whom the anesthetic risk is great, the two eyes can be operated on at the same sitting using different sets of instruments.[2,6] Simultaneous surgery also reduces the risk of relative amblyopia, which can occur when two operations are undertaken a few days apart.[2,6]

A possible disadvantage of the pars plana approach is the incarceration of vitreous in the scleral incisions. Subsequent vitreous traction may lead to retinal breaks and/or detachments.[2,17] Another hindrance with the pars plana approach arises when the pupil is dilated insufficiently; the lensectomy has to be performed under partially "blind" conditions, which means either leaving too much lens material in the periphery or too little peripheral capsular support for future posterior chamber IOL implantation.[16]

Limbal Approach

With the proper precautions, the limbal approach is the most versatile technique for pediatric cataract surgery.[2,4,5,7,8] Many surgeons have not yet recognized the importance of the anterior chamber maintainer (ACM) when operating on eyes in young patients. Although it is possible to use an aspiration-irrigation device or a vitrectome with an irrigation sleeve in order to remove a soft cataract, the use of an ACM makes the surgery safer (Figs. 52-1 and 52-2). Moreover, although viscoelastic materials maintain space, the ACM provides, in addition, a constant washout of blood, pigment, and prostaglandins that may be released during surgery to leave clear and "clean" media. The ACM also helps to keep the pupil well dilated throughout the procedure. It prevents collapse of the globe when the instruments are withdrawn from the eye and thus helps to reduce damage to the iris and corneal endothelium.

Two limbal incisions are made with a 20-gauge stiletto knife at the 10 o'clock and 2 o'clock positions; one for the ACM (connected to a balanced salt solution with epinephrine 1:500,000) and the other one for the aspiration cannula.

Various techniques have been described by which to open the anterior capsule.[2,4,14,15] Capsulorrhexis can be carried out with the help of high-viscosity ophthalmic visco-surgical devices (OVDs); however, the younger the child is, the more difficult it is to perform a capsulorrhexis. Infants have a very elastic anterior capsule, which easily tears toward the periphery. A practical alternative to manual capsulorrhexis is to use a vitrectomy probe to create a small central opening in the anterior capsule (Fig. 52-1). This initial hole can be enlarged gradually by "biting" into the anterior capsule with the vitrectome until the desired 4–5mm opening is achieved. The lens material can be aspirated manually or with an automatic aspiration device (Fig. 52-2).

Once the capsular bag is empty, the decision has to be made as to the management of the posterior capsule. Most authors agree that infants under 2 years of age should receive an elective posterior capsulectomy–anterior vitrectomy.[2,4-8,14,15] Posterior capsulorrhexis can be carried out either manually or with the vitrectome, as described for the anterior capsule.[2,4-8,14,15,18] The segment of capsulorrhexis tissue must be at least 4mm in diameter, and one third of the anterior vitreous must be removed to ensure a permanently clear visual axis (Fig. 52-3). Smaller posterior capsulectomies with shallow anterior vitrectomies tend to close down, especially in neonates.[19] Posterior capsulectomy, either alone or when combined with a shallow anterior vitrectomy, does not guarantee a permanently clear visual axis, because vitreous remnants serve as a scaffold for the lens epithelium to grow on, which results in the

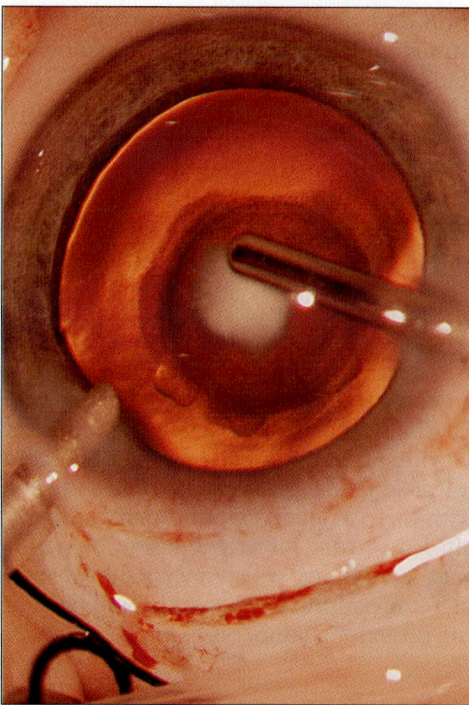

FIG. 52-1 ▦ **Anterior capsulectomy performed using a vitrectomy probe in a congenital cataract.** Note the use of the anterior chamber maintainer for a deep anterior chamber and a well-dilated pupil.

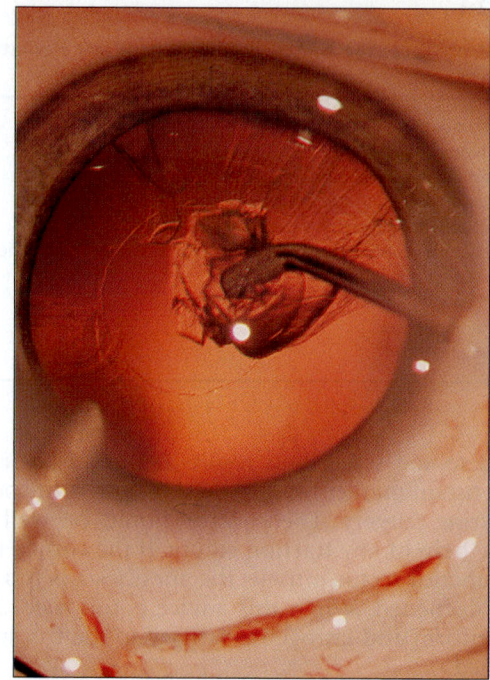

FIG. 52-2 ▦ **Completion of lens material aspiration within the capsular bag in a congenital cataract.** Note the use of the anterior chamber maintainer, which allows atraumatic maneuvers in a well-formed anterior chamber.

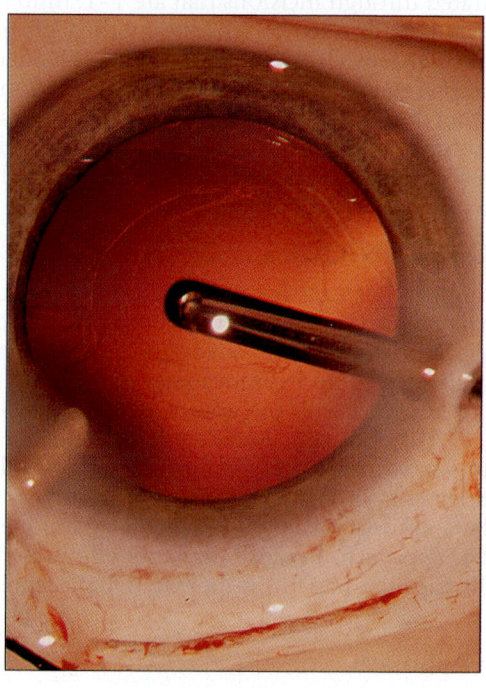

FIG. 52-3 ▦ **Elective posterior capsulectomy and a deep anterior vitrectomy.** This is performed using a vitrectomy probe, after all the lens material has been aspirated within the chamber bag.

formation of new opaque membranes. Furthermore, the immediate postoperative iritis seems markedly reduced when a generous anterior vitrectomy has been performed.[2,4,5,7,8,14] Management of the posterior capsule in children more than 2 years old remains controversial. Some authors prefer to leave it intact until opacification occurs; others perform an yttrium-aluminum-garnet (YAG) laser capsulectomy immediately after surgery. Experienced pediatric cataract surgeons choose to perform an elective posterior capsulectomy–anterior vitrectomy, routinely, in every child under 8 years of age in order to provide a one-stop treatment in this age group wherein amblyopia is still a risk. This alternative is logical when meticulous follow-up is uncertain.[4-10,14,15]

CHOICE OF APHAKIC CORRECTION IN CHILDREN

Spectacles, contact lenses, and IOLs are the most readily available means to correct aphakia in children. Epikeratophakia has been used in limited series, but this option has been abandoned by most surgeons because of complicated postoperative courses and lack of availability of the corneal lenticules.

Spectacles

Aphakic spectacles provide a satisfactory correction only in cases of bilateral aphakia in which anisometropia does not represent a problem.[2] Most of these patients develop good visual acuity with spectacles, provided the eyes are not excessively microphthalmic.[2] The disadvantages of spectacles are cosmetic blemish and the poor optical quality of high-plus lenses.

Contact Lenses

During the 1970s and 1980s contact lenses were described as the method of choice to correct unilateral and bilateral aphakia in childhood.[2,9,10] Contact lenses provide a better optical correction than spectacles, and their dioptric power can be adjusted throughout life. However, the management of contact lenses in children can be very difficult and costly. Frequent loss of lenses, recurrent infections, and inconsistent follow-up visits turn this theoretically ideal choice into the most impractical

option. Most ophthalmologists, therefore, now recommend the use of IOLs supplemented by spectacles in children rather than contact lenses.[2,4,5,7,8,10,14]

Intraocular Lenses

The IOL option was originally advocated in cases of unilateral pediatric cataracts because it facilitates amblyopia management by providing a more permanent correction.[2,4,5,7,8,10,14] Implanting an IOL in a growing eye is not an ideal solution, but it is currently the most practical one. The aim in the IOL option, unlike in the contact lens alternative, is to correct most, but not all, of

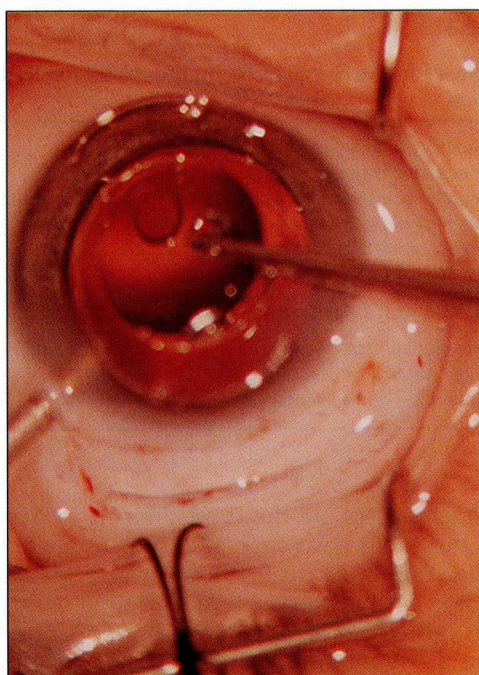

FIG. 52-4 ▪ One-piece polymethylmethacrylate posterior chamber pediatric intraocular lens, 11mm overall diameter, before its insertion in the capsular bag remnants. The insertion is made through a 6mm scleral tunnel that is prepared in advance at the start of surgery.

the aphakia; the residual refractive error has to be corrected using spectacles, which can be adjusted throughout life.

The implantation of anterior chamber IOLs in children was discontinued in the mid-1980s. Devastating complications, such as secondary glaucoma and corneal decompensation, were attributed to anterior chamber IOLs, especially in younger patients.[20] Posterior chamber IOL implantation represents, by far, the better method for the correction of aphakia in adults, and the same applies in children.

SELECTION OF INTRAOCULAR LENSES. The choice of which IOL of what dioptric power to implant in young children is the main difficulty that faces the ophthalmologist.[2] Pediatric IOLs are not yet readily available,[21,22] and the rapid growth of the eye during the first 2 years of life makes an effective choice difficult.[2,4,7,8,23-26] Nevertheless, in the 1990s increasingly positive reports were published on the use of posterior chamber IOLs in children and even in neonates.

The material from which the IOL is made must have a long track record of safety. Polymethylmethacrylate (PMMA) IOLs have been in use for more than 40 years; PMMA is currently the best material to be used for children, until a similar follow-up is obtained for other biomaterials.[21] The optimal size of the capsular bag and the ciliary sulcus in children has been ascertained by the work of Bluestein et al.[22] Posterior chamber IOLs, which were originally oversized, have been reduced from 13–14mm to 12–12.5mm in diameter in most modern models. In children it is even more important to implant an IOL of correct size.[22] Oversized IOLs act like loaded springs in the eye and can dislocate, especially when a child rubs his or her eyes, which can cause damage to intraocular structures. Pediatric IOLs should not exceed 12mm overall diameter because the average adult ciliary sulcus diameter rarely exceeds 11.5mm. Ideally, the pediatric IOL should be available in diameters of the range 10.5–12mm (Fig. 52-4).[22] The choice of the IOL size is determined mainly by the site of implantation (i.e., in-the-bag or ciliary sulcus).

Both the biometry and the age of the child determine the choice of the IOL dioptric power. Two main age groups exist in pediatric cataract surgery: patients younger than 2 years and patients between 2 and 8 years. In the first group the axial length and the keratometric (K) readings change rapidly, whereas in the second group the changes are slower and more moderate.[23-26] In order to minimize the need to exchange IOLs later in life, when a large myopic shift occurs, it is advisable to undercorrect children with IOLs so that they can grow into emmetropia or mild myopia in adult life.[23-26]

Those who are under 2 years of age should receive 80% of the power needed for emmetropia at the time of surgery. Since the K readings also change rapidly during the first 18 months of life, it is practical to rely on the axial length only when the IOL dioptric power is chosen for infants (Box 52-2). The postoperative residual refractive error is corrected by spectacles, which can be adjusted at will as the child grows. Infants and toddlers can tolerate up to 6D of anisometropia, which gradually disappears within 2–3 years.[25] Most of the infants who have unilateral pseudophakia need a patch over the sound eye for half their waking hours until 4–5 years of age. Patches alleviate the symptoms of anisometropia but at the same time affect the chances for good binocularity to develop.[27]

For the age range 2–8 years, the IOL dioptric power should be 90% of that needed for emmetropia at the time of surgery (Box 52-2). The induced anisometropia is moderate and lessens with the expected myopic shift that occurs in adolescence.[23-26]

The need for spectacles after IOL implantation in pediatric cataract surgery has some positive aspects:

- More dependency on the ophthalmologist is needed because spectacles have to be taken care of, adjusted, and repaired periodically; this increases the chances of good follow-up.
- The pseudophakic eye is protected from direct trauma by the spectacles.
- Spectacles can be used as an adjunct to amblyopia therapy by atropine penalization of the sound eye and alteration of the dioptric power of its lens.

IMPLANTATION IN CHILDREN UNDER 2 YEARS OF AGE. In unilateral cases, primary implantation is indicated as soon as the patient is fit for anesthesia, ideally between 2 and 3 months of age. The earlier the surgery is done, the better the chance that deep amblyopia can be overcome.

After the cataract has been aspirated, an elective posterior capsulectomy–anterior vitrectomy is performed. The posterior chamber IOL is inserted through a scleral tunnel, which is prepared in advance. The surgeon has to choose between ciliary sulcus and the bag according to the following criteria. Sulcus implantation is easier and also allows an easier explantation in cases where IOL exchange will be needed later in life.[25] This option is indicated in neonates and infants less than 1 year of age. The in-the-bag placement is more physiological, but more difficult technically. To facilitate in-the-bag insertion in pediatric cataract surgery, the following technique is used. The IOL haptics are compressed temporarily onto the optics with a suture, which reduces the overall IOL diameter. The compressed IOL is inserted into the bag fornices, and the suture is cut only after the correct position has been verified (Fig. 52-5).[28] An in-the-bag IOL is more difficult to explant; this option should be chosen for

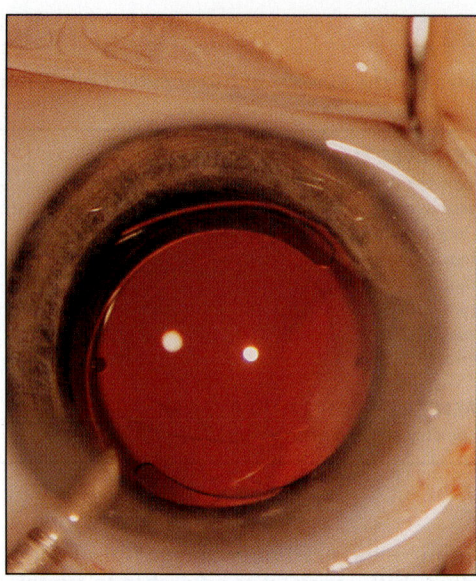

FIG. 52-5 ■ **Pediatric intraocular lens contained in the bag remnants.** Note both the anterior and posterior capsulectomies.

infants above 1 year of age because they are less likely to need an IOL exchange, provided they are undercorrected by 20%.

IMPLANTATION IN CHILDREN ABOVE 2 YEARS OF AGE. For children older than 2 years old, the IOL should be inserted in the bag because the eye has reached nearly the adult size, although its sclera is much softer. Gimbel[18] has described a special IOL implantation for this group of patients. The technique requires extreme dexterity as both anterior and posterior capsulorrhexises are performed. The IOL haptics are placed in the bag fornices, while the optic is protruded through both capsulorrhexises to be captured beneath the posterior capsule remnants.

POSTOPERATIVE TREATMENT. Topical medications are sufficient when surgery has not been excessively traumatic. A combination of antibiotic-corticosteroid drops (2) hourly with a mild mydriatic agent twice daily is given for the first week. Thereafter the medications are tapered off during the next 3 weeks. Some authors have used systemic corticosteroids to overcome the intense inflammatory response in young children's eyes.

COMPLICATIONS

A summary of the guidelines used to minimize complications in pediatric cataract surgery is given in Box 52-3.

Intraoperative complications usually are related to the surgeon's unfamiliarity with the child's soft ocular tissues. The anterior chamber tends to collapse, the iris can protrude through the surgical wounds, and the pupil constricts on injury to the iris. These events can be avoided by operating under deep anesthesia and by using an ACM.

Immediate postoperative complications include anterior plastic uveitis, high intraocular pressure, incarceration of iris tissue in the wound, and endophthalmitis. Atraumatic surgery, use of an ACM during surgery, thorough removal of OVDs at completion of surgery, and meticulous closure of the wound reduce the occurrence of these complications.

Late complications include dislocation of the IOL, chronic iritis, glaucoma, and retinal detachment. Close follow-up enables detection of these complications at an early stage. Their treatment is similar to that for the same occurrences in adults.

Amblyopia Management

The child's parents must understand that visual rehabilitation only starts with surgery and must be continued throughout childhood.

The unilateral cases are the most difficult to manage.[2,4,5,7-10] Amblyopia treatment starts soon after surgery, after clarification of the media. The initial treatment must be aggressive in order to boost vision in the deprived eye. Full-time occlusion of the sound eye is carried out for a few days—1 day per month of age. For example, a 3-month-old neonate should be subjected to occlusion for 3 consecutive days, a 4-month-old infant for 4 days, etc. Thereafter, occlusion is reduced to half the waking hours. The younger the infant, the easier it is to comply with the patch regimen. Autorefractometers, especially portable ones, help to determine the residual refractive error; retinoscopy is often difficult in pseudophakic children. Spectacles are prescribed from the age of 4 months onward. A bifocal lens with an add of +3.00 is prescribed in the pseudophakic eye from the age of 3 years, when the child becomes verbal. Unilateral pseudophakes should continue with half-day patches until 4–5 years of age. Thereafter, the patch time can be reduced gradually, but should not be abandoned until 10–12 years of age. After that age, amblyopia management is practically superfluous.

Cases of bilateral pseudophakia should be followed closely to detect and treat relative amblyopia.

Intraocular Lens Exchange and Alternative Options

Exchange of IOLs should be considered when a great myopic shift has occurred.[23-26] When the pseudophakic eye becomes 7D more myopic than the sound eye, the IOL should be exchanged, unless contact lens wear is a viable option. Refractive surgery in children is not yet an acceptable option. An experienced anterior segment surgeon who is familiar with IOL exchange should perform the procedure. An alternative to IOL exchange is to implant, preferably in the posterior chamber, an additional negative dioptric power IOL to correct the myopia. This procedure is easily performed when the primary IOL was inserted in the bag.

OUTCOME

The visual outcome depends largely on the type of cataract, the timing of intervention, the quality of surgery, and, above all, the amblyopia management. It is possible to achieve nearly normal vision even in unilateral congenital cataracts, provided amblyopia management is aggressive.[2-10,25] Binocularity is usually poor in these cases, but some gross stereopsis can be expected.[27] Aphakic and pseudophakic children certainly should be followed up throughout childhood and preferably throughout life.[29]

REFERENCES

1. Elston JS, Timms C. Clinical evidence for the onset of the sensitive period in infancy. Br J Ophthalmol. 1992;76:327–8.
2. Lambert SR, Drake AV. Infantile cataracts. Surv Ophthalmol. 1996;40:427–58.
3. Birch EE, Stager DR, Leffler J, Weakley D. Early treatment of congenital cataract minimizes unequal competition. Invest Ophthalmol Vis Sci. 1998;39:1560–66.
4. Ben-Ezra D, Paez JH. Congenital cataract and intraocular lenses. Am J Ophthalmol. 1983;96:311–14.

5. Dahan E. Lens implantation in microphthalmic eyes of infants. Eur J Implant Refract Surg. 1989;1:1–9.
6. Guo S, Nelson LB, Calhoun J, Levin A. Simultaneous surgery for bilateral congenital cataracts. J Pediatr Ophthalmol Strabismus. 1990;27:23–5.
7. Dahan E, Salmenson BD. Pseudophakia in children: precautions, techniques and feasibility. J Cataract Refract Surg. 1990;16:75–82.
8. Dahan E, Welsh NH, Salmenson BD. Posterior chamber implants in unilateral congenital and developmental cataracts. Eur J Implant Refract Surg. 1990; 2:295–302.
9. Neumman D, Weissman BA, Isenberg SJ, et al. The effectiveness of daily wear contact lenses for the correction of infantile aphakia. Arch Ophthalmol. 1993;111:927–30.
10. BenEzra D, Cohen E, Rose L. Traumatic cataract in children: correction of aphakia by contact lens or by intraocular lens. Am J Ophthalmol. 1997;123:773–82.
11. Hiles DA, Watson BA. Complications of implant surgery in children. Am Intraocul Soc J. 1979;5:24–32.
12. Wolfe OR, Wolfe RM. Removal of soft cataract by suction. New double-barreled aspirating needle. Arch Ophthalmol Chicago. 1941;26:127–8.
13. Burke JP, O'Keefe M, Bowell R, Naughten ER. Ophthalmic findings in classical galactosemia—a screened population. J Pediatr Ophthalmol Strabismus. 1989; 26:165–8.
14. Ahmadieh H, Javadi MA, Ahmadi M, et al. Primary capsulectomy, anterior vitrectomy, lensectomy, and posterior chamber lens implantation in children: limbal versus pars plana. J Cataract Refract Surg. 1999;25:768–75.
15. Koch DD, Kohnen T. Retrospective comparison of techniques to prevent secondary cataract formation after posterior chamber intraocular lens implantation in infants and children. J Cataract Refract Surg. 1997;23:657–63.
16. Dahan E, Salmenson BD, Levin J. Ciliary sulcus reconstruction for posterior implantation in the absence of an intact posterior capsule. Ophthalmic Surg. 1989;20:776–80.
17. McLeod D. Congenital cataract surgeries: a retinal surgeon's viewpoint. Aust NZ J Ophthalmol. 1986;14:79–84.
18. Gimbel HV, Debroff BM. Posterior capsulorrhexis with optic capture: maintaining a clear visual axis after pediatric cataract surgery. J Cataract Refractive Surg. 1994;20:658–64.
19. Morgan KS, Karcioglu ZA. Secondary cataracts in infants after lensectomies. J Pediatr Ophthalmol Strabismus. 1987;24:45–8.
20. Sawada T, Kimura W, Kimura T, et al. Long-term follow up of primary anterior chamber intraocular lens implantation J Cataract Refract Surg. 1998;24:1515–20.
21. Wilson ME, Apple DJ, Bluestein EC, Wang XH. Intraocular lenses for pediatric implantation: biomaterials, designs and sizing. J Cataract Refract Surg. 1994;20:584–91.
22. Bluestein EC, Wilson ME, Wang XH, et al. Dimensions of the pediatric crystalline lens: implications for intraocular lenses in children. J Pediatr Ophthalmol Strabismus. 1996;33:18–20.
23. Spierer A, Desatnik H, Blumenthal M. Refractive status in children after long-term follow-up of cataract surgery with intraocular lens implantation. J Pediatr Ophthalmol Strabismus. 1999;36:25–9.
24. Gordon RA, Donzis PB. Refractive development of the human eye. Arch Ophthalmol. 1985;103:785–9.
25. Dahan E, Drusedau MUH. Choice of lens and dioptric power in pediatric pseudophakia. J Cataract Refract Surg. 1997;23:1–6.
26. Flitcroft DI, Knight-Nanan D, Bowell R, et al. Intraocular lenses in children: changes in axial length, corneal curvature, and refraction. Br J Ophthalmol. 1999;83:265–9.
27. Tytla ME, Lewis TL, Maurer D, Brent HP. Stereopsis after congenital cataract. Invest Ophthalmol Vis Sci. 1993;34:1767–72.
28. Dahan E. Insertion of intraocular lenses in the capsular bag. Metab Pediatr Syst Ophthalmol. 1987;10:87–8.
29. Rabin J, Van Sluyters RC, Malach R. Emmetropization: a vision dependent phenomenon. Invest Ophthalmol Vis Sci. 1981;20:561–4.

SECTION 5 COMPLICATIONS AND OUTCOMES

CHAPTER

53 Complications of Cataract Surgery

THOMAS KOHNEN • LI WANG • NEIL J. FRIEDMAN • DOUGLAS D. KOCH

INTRODUCTION

Phacoemulsification; sutureless, self-sealing tunnel incisions; and foldable intraocular lenses (IOLs) have changed cataract surgery dramatically over the past two decades. Postoperative astigmatism and inflammation are typically minimal; visual recovery and patients' rehabilitation are accelerated. The published literature indicates that modern cataract surgery, though certainly not free of complications, is a remarkably safe procedure, regardless of which extraction technique is used.[1]

To put this into perspective, an overview of the visual outcomes and incidence of complications following cataract surgery is helpful. Using rigid criteria for scientific validity, Powe et al.[1] analyzed 90 studies published between 1979 and 1991 that addressed visual acuity ($n = 17,390$ eyes) or complications ($n = 68,316$ eyes) following standard nuclear expression cataract extraction with posterior chamber IOL implantation, phacoemulsification with posterior chamber IOL implantation, or intracapsular cataract extraction with anterior chamber IOL implantation. Strikingly, the percentage of eyes with postoperative visual acuity of 20/40 or better was 89.7% for all eyes and 95.5% for eyes with no preexisting ocular comorbidity. The incidence of sight-threatening complications was less than 2%.

In this chapter, the key elements in the prevention, recognition, and management of the major intraoperative and postoperative complications of cataract surgery are discussed.

INTRAOPERATIVE COMPLICATIONS

Cataract Incision

The cataract incision serves as more than just the port of access to the anterior segment; it is a critical step of the operation that affects ocular integrity and corneal stability. The traditional limbal or posterior limbal incision has been largely replaced by tunnel constructions, which can be located in the sclera, limbus, or cornea and are characterized by their greater radial length and an anterior entry into the anterior chamber to create the self-sealing internal corneal valve. Advantages of tunnel incisions are increased intraoperative safety, decreased postoperative inflammation and pain, increased postoperative watertightness, and reduced surgically induced astigmatism.[2]

Tunnel Perforation

Tearing of the roof of the tunnel predisposes to excessive intraoperative leakage that compromises anterior chamber stability, and to postoperative wound leakage. If the tear occurs at either edge of the roof, surgery usually can be completed using the initial incision, proceeding slowly and observing the wound carefully as instruments are introduced or manipulated in the eye. It usually is preferable to suture the incision at the conclusion of surgery, even if the wound is watertight, to restore a more normal architecture and prevent external wound gape.

If, however, the roof is perforated in the center of the flap and this is noted before the anterior chamber is entered, creation of a new incision should be considered. If the cut is extremely small (e.g., <0.5mm), sometimes the same procedure as for lateral roof tears (see above) can be used. Before IOL insertion, the opposite margin of the wound is enlarged, and to prevent further tearing, the incision is made larger than normal for IOL insertion. Suture closure usually is advisable to restore normal wound architecture.

If the floor of the tunnel is perforated, which can happen during scleral tunnel dissection, surgery usually can be performed through this wound; care must be taken to avoid trauma to any prolapsing uveal tissue. The perforation should be closed with sutures.

Descemet's Detachment

Detachment of Descemet's membrane can be a major postoperative complication; it results in persistent corneal edema and decreased visual acuity. To prevent Descemet's detachment, the surgeon should carefully observe the inner lip (cut edge of Descemet's membrane) at each phase of the procedure. To avoid blunt stripping of Descemet's membrane during enlargement of the wound, a sharp metal or diamond blade is recommended.

If detachment is caused by viscoelastic injection, the agent must be removed, such as by using a blunt cannula. Intraoperatively, repositioning of Descemet's membrane usually can be achieved by injecting balanced salt solution or occasionally air or an ophthalmic viscosurgical device (OVD) through the paracentesis site.

If a visually significant Descemet's detachment is present postoperatively, the authors prefer to intervene after 2–3 weeks; however, late spontaneous reattachment 2–3 months (in one case, 10 months) postoperatively has been reported.[3,4] To reattach Descemet's membrane, the patient is positioned at the slit lamp after several drops of anesthetic agent and antibiotics have been administered. A paracentesis incision is made inferotemporally. A 27- or 30-gauge cannula is attached to a syringe with a filter, and the syringe is filled with 0.5–1cm³ of air or, for eyes that have an unsuccessful injection of air alone, an expansive gas (e.g., sulfur hexafluoride SF6). Using the cannula, approximately 50% of the aqueous is drained, and the chamber is reformed with injection of the gas. Recently, a new technique for repairing Descemet's detachments using intracameral gas injection at the slit-lamp microscope was reported.[5] A 25-gauge needle on a 3ml syringe filled with the gas and another 25-gauge needle are advanced through the corneoscleral limbus at opposite clock hours with the bevel up and the needles oriented parallel to the iris plane. The plunger on the syringe is depressed to inject the gas and fill the anterior chamber while aqueous humor is allowed to egress from the opposing 25-gauge needle. More complicated cases may require direct suturing.[6]

Thermal Burns

Part of the energy produced by the phacoemulsification tip is dissipated as heat. This heat is conducted into the eye along the titanium tip and then cooled by the ongoing flow of the irrigation-

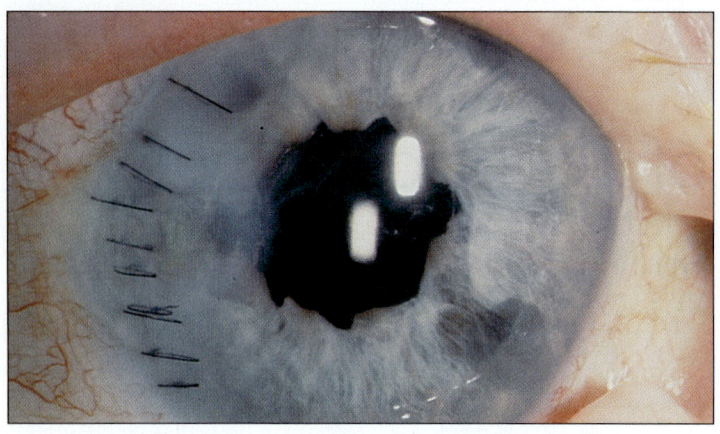

FIG. 53-1 ■ **Corneal burn following phacoemulsification.** In this patient who had an apparent filtering bleb, phacoemulsification was performed through a temporal, clear corneal incision. Posterior capsular rupture was suspected; the surgeon injected a highly retentive ophthalmic viscosurgical device beneath and in front of the nucleus to minimize the risk of posterior dislocation of the nucleus. Phacoemulsification was instituted with low flow and vacuum settings, and a severe corneal burn was immediately produced because of obstruction of the phacoemulsification tip by the viscoelastic material. The incision was closed with several interrupted sutures. Many of these pulled through the injured tissue, and as a result, additional suturing was required several days later. Postoperatively, the patient has 5D of surgically induced astigmatism that has persisted for more than 5 years.

aspiration fluid. If for any reason the flow is blocked, a corneal burn can occur within 1–3 seconds. The most common cause is inadequate flow through the phacoemulsification tip because it has been obstructed by a retentive OVD; this problem arises from using low flow and vacuum settings. The critical warning sign is the appearance of milky fluid that is produced around the tip as emulsification is begun.

To avoid corneal burns, phacoemulsification and irrigation-aspiration functions should always be tested before the eye is entered. Some of the viscoelastic material that overlies the nucleus can be aspirated before the start of emulsification to ensure that aspiration is adequate. To prevent constriction of the irrigating sleeve, an incision size that is appropriate for each particular phacoemulsification tip should be selected. If a burn does occur, meticulous suturing of the wound with multiple radial sutures (Fig. 53-1) is required. A bandage contact lens may assist with wound closure. Severe postoperative astigmatism can result.

Anterior Capsulectomy

PREVENTING RADIAL TEARS IN THE ANTERIOR CAPSULE. For phacoemulsification, the preferred method of anterior capsulectomy is capsulorrhexis. It is now recognized that radial tears in the anterior capsule can pose significant risks because of their tendency to tear into the equatorial region of the lens[7] and extend into the posterior capsule. This causes posterior capsular rupture, loss of lens material, and IOL decentration. The surgeon's goal, therefore, must be to retain an intact capsulorrhexis. A common cause of radial tears is irretrievable loss of the capsulorrhexis tear peripherally beneath the iris. To prevent this, the following steps should be considered:

- The anterior chamber should be reinflated with an OVD.
- The vector forces of the tear should be changed to redirect the tear in a more central direction.
- If the tear is lost beneath the iris, the capsulorrhexis should be restarted from its origin, proceeding in the opposite direction (if possible, this new capsulorrhexis should finish by incorporating the original tear in an outside-in direction; however, the original tear is often too peripheral to permit this, and a single radial tear is created).

An alternative approach to a "lost" capsulorrhexis is to convert to a can-opener capsulectomy. It may indeed be safer to have multiple tears rather than a single one, because forces that

extend these tears can be distributed to multiple sites, which reduces the likelihood of a tear extending equatorially.

EXCESSIVELY SMALL CAPSULORRHEXIS. If the diameter of the capsulorrhexis opening is excessively small, the tear should be directed more peripherally and continued beyond the original point of origin before completion of the capsulorrhexis; this procedure removes an annulus of capsule and enlarges the opening. If the capsulorrhexis has been terminated and the opening is too small, a new tear can be started by making an oblique cut with Vannas scissors. It usually is preferable to enlarge the capsulorrhexis after IOL implantation, to minimize the risk of radial tears during lens implantation.

MINIMIZING COMPLICATIONS WHEN RADIAL TEARS ARE PRESENT. If radial tears are present, several modifications in surgical technique should be considered to minimize the risk of tear extension into the posterior capsule:

- Hydrodissection or hydrodelineation is performed gently to minimize distension of the capsular bag.
- Cracks during emulsification are made gently away from the area(s) with radial tears. Alternatively, as much of the nucleus as possible is sculpted within the capsular bag, and the rest is removed at the iris plane. The height of the infusion bottle is kept low to prevent overinflation of the anterior chamber (which can cause the tear to extend peripherally).
- The IOL should be placed with the haptics 90° away from the tear. One-piece polymethyl methacrylate lenses tend to maintain better centration in these situations. Rotation of the IOL should be minimized. The OVD should be removed in small aliquots, while gentle infusion of balanced salt solution is performed through a side-port incision.
- It is important to avoid anterior chamber collapse at any phase of the operation when radial tears are present. Anterior bulging of the posterior capsule can place increased stress on a radial tear, which predisposes its extension into the equator and posterior capsule. To avoid this, the chamber is deepened each time the phacoemulsification or irrigation-aspiration tip is removed from the eye; this is done by injecting fluid, OVD, or perhaps air through the paracentesis incision with a syringe while the instrument is removed from the incision.

Nuclear Expression Cataract Extraction

Complications related to nuclear expression are covered in Chapters 47 and 48.

Complications During Phacoemulsification

HYDRODISSECTION. Hydrodissection was developed to permit easy rotation of the nucleus in the capsular bag and to facilitate removal of various layers of the lens by eliminating their adhesion to surrounding tissues. Two major complications of hydrodissection are inadequate hydrodissection and overinflation of the capsular bag. The former results in a nucleus that does not rotate, which predisposes to zonular dehiscence if excessive force is exerted on the nucleus. This can be avoided by making an additional hydrodissection, particularly in quadrants that have not been hydrodissected before. U-shaped cannulas are useful to hydrodissect subincisional regions of the lens not accessible with straight or angulated cannulas.

Overinflation of the capsular bag can predispose to nuclear prolapse into the anterior chamber, which might compromise the ease or safety of nucleus emulsification. A serious complication of overinflation is posterior capsular rupture with loss of the nucleus into the vitreous. This is more likely to occur in eyes with long axial lengths or with fragile posterior capsules, such as are found in patients who have congenital posterior polar cataracts.[8]

IRIS PROLAPSE OR DAMAGE. Iris prolapse usually is caused when the anterior chamber is entered too posteriorly, such as near the iris root. If this is noted early in the case and interferes with the easy introduction of instruments into the eye, it is advisable to suture the incision and move to another location.

A second and more ominous cause of iris prolapse is an acute increase of intraocular pressure (IOP) accompanied by choroidal effusion or hemorrhage. In this instance, the surgeon should attempt to identify the cause and lower the IOP. Sometimes digital massage on the eye, pressing directly on the incision, can successfully lower the pressure. It is useful to examine the fundus to ascertain whether a choroidal effusion or hemorrhage exists. With choroidal effusion, aspiration of vitreous can be helpful, as can the administration of intravenous mannitol. If a choroidal hemorrhage occurs or if the increased IOP from an effusion is resistant to treatment, it usually is best to terminate surgery. The wound is sutured carefully; intraocular miotics are administered, and a peripheral iridectomy may be performed to help reposition the iris. For effusions, surgery can be deferred until later in the day or the next day, when the fluid dynamics of the eye have returned to a more normal state. If a limited choroidal hemorrhage has occurred, it is best to wait 2–3 weeks before attempting further surgery.

Trauma to the iris from prolapse or emulsification with a phacoemulsification tip can produce an irregularly shaped pupil and iris atrophy and can predispose to posterior synechiae formation. If iris damage is produced inferiorly through contact with the phacoemulsification tip, loose strands of tissue should be cut to reduce the likelihood of these being aspirated into the phacoemulsification tip. Another option is to use a single iris hook to retract the inferior iris, holding it away from the phacoemulsification tip for the duration of the procedure.

TRAPPED NUCLEUS. In this situation, the nucleus seems to be trapped within the capsular bag; it resists rotation, elevation, or both. This usually indicates a nucleus that requires further hydrodissection, which should be repeated in regions not previously hydrodissected (e.g., laterally and inferiorly with angled or straight cannulas, superiorly with U-shaped cannulas; if these cannulas are not available, additional paracentesis sites can be created in strategic locations).[9] If this is unsuccessful in achieving adequate mobilization of the nucleus, viscodissection can be performed. An OVD is injected in the plane of the hydrodissection, which usually results in elevation of the nuclear remnant. When reentering the eye with the phacoemulsification tip, irrigation should not be used until a second instrument has been inserted through the stab incision and placed below the nucleus; when irrigation and aspiration begin and the OVD is removed, the second instrument prevents the nuclear piece from falling back into the posterior chamber.

If the capsulorrhexis is small and the nuclear circumference is intact, nuclear elevation through the capsulorrhexis may not be possible. Additional sculpting might be required to thin the nucleus centrally or to remove some of the peripheral nucleus. After the nucleus has been sufficiently thinned, an instrument such as a Sinskey hook or spatula can be teased posteriorly through the remaining nuclear tissue; this enables elevation of a portion of the nucleus and thereby facilitates access to the remainder.

SUBLUXATED LENS. The surgical approach for subluxated lenses (Fig. 53-2) is determined by lens stability, lens position, and nuclear density.[10] In a subluxated lens with adequate zonular support, phacoemulsification (or nuclear expression) can be performed. Viscoelastic material is injected as needed throughout the surgery to tamponade the vitreous in areas of zonular dehiscence. Extensive hydrodissection and viscodissection should be carried out. Depending on nuclear density, either phacoemulsification in the capsular bag or anterior chamber phacoemulsification under a retentive viscoelastic is performed. Any form of zonular stress should be minimized, particularly with nuclear rotation.

If phacodonesis is present but the lens has not fallen posteriorly, a soft nucleus sometimes can be removed by phacoemulsification-aspiration, whereas a hard nucleus should be extracted

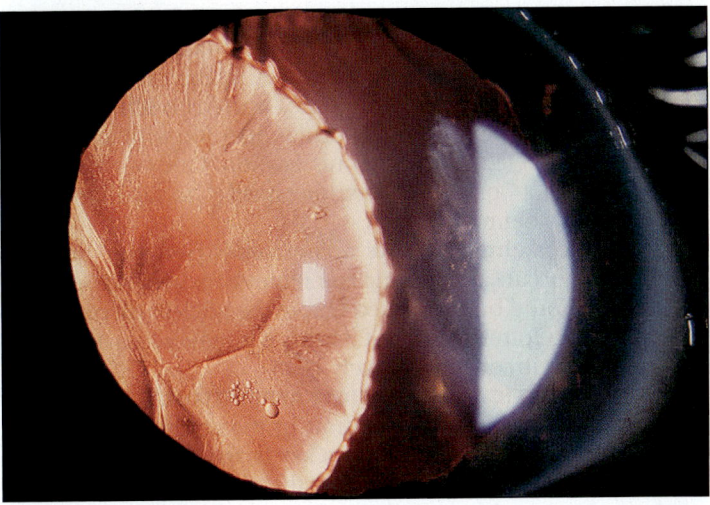

FIG. 53-2 ■ **Subluxated lens.** This patient had a subluxated lens caused by ocular trauma. The crystalline lens was removed using a pars plana approach, and a sulcus-sutured intraocular lens was implanted.

using an intracapsular approach. Pars plana vitrectomy is an excellent option for these cases as well; it certainly is preferred when the lens is subluxated posteriorly.

The location of the IOL placement depends on the status of the capsular bag after cataract removal. If zonular disruption is minimal (fewer than 3 clock hours), the IOL can be implanted into the capsular bag with the haptic orientated in the meridian of the zonular defect. If the zonular disruption is larger, options include:

- Ciliary sulcus implantation, possibly with scleral or iris fixation of one or both haptics.
- Insertion of one haptic into the capsular bag and suturing of the second haptic into the sulcus.
- Anterior chamber lens implantation.

An anterior chamber lens is acceptable if no anterior chamber angle pathology, glaucoma, or uveitis is present.

Recently, the use of an endocapsular polymethyl methacrylate ring has been introduced for zonular dialysis. This device allows expansion and stabilization of the capsular bag during phacoemulsification and following posterior chamber IOL implantation.[11,12]

Ruptured Posterior Capsule

Posterior capsule rupture is the most common serious intraoperative complication of cataract surgery[13]; however, proper management can result in minimal morbidity to the patient. A posterior capsular rent is more likely to occur in eyes with small pupils, hard nuclei, or pseudoexfoliation syndrome. Recent reports suggest that the visual prognosis of patients who have broken posterior capsules is excellent. The key factors are to minimize ocular trauma, meticulously clean prolapsed vitreous from the anterior segment, if present, and ensure secure fixation of the IOL.

BEFORE NUCLEUS REMOVAL. A capsular break noted before nucleus extraction is a potential disaster. The first objective is to prevent the nucleus from being dislodged into the vitreous cavity. An OVD can be injected posterior and anterior to the nucleus to prevent its posterior displacement and to cushion the corneal endothelium. Another alternative is to insert an instrument through a pars plana incision 3mm posterior to the limbus into the vitreous, which Kelman has described as "posterior assisted levitation" (Charles Kelman, personal communication). The nucleus is pushed gently anteriorly, so that it can be captured in front of the iris and safely removed from the eye. Once the nucleus or its remnants have been repositioned in the anterior chamber, the choice is to convert or to continue the emulsification. The latter course can be more hazardous and predisposes to enlarging the rent and possibly losing the nucleus into the vitreous. In most circumstances, the nucleus should be managed by sufficiently enlarging the wound to facilitate easy extraction of the nucleus on a lens loop. However, in the case of a small break or when only a small amount of nucleus is left, it may be possible to cover the posterior capsular opening with a retentive OVD and complete the phacoemulsification. One can also use a Sheets glide as a "pseudo–posterior capsule" to facilitate completion of phacoemulsification.

Vitreous loss almost always accompanies posterior capsular rupture that occurs before nucleus removal; whenever feasible, vitrectomy should be performed before the nuclear pieces are removed. Clearly, one should not do this if it makes loss of the nucleus into the vitreous more likely.

DURING CORTICAL IRRIGATION-ASPIRATION. When capsular rupture occurs during aspiration of the cortex (which is, in fact, the most common cause),[7,14] a key factor is the status of the vitreous. If no vitreous is present in the anterior segment, vitreous loss often can be averted. An OVD can be injected through the capsular opening to push the vitreous posteriorly. Cortical removal can be completed using low-flow irrigation. Options include using a manual system; a dry approach, aspirating with a cannula in the chamber filled with OVD; a bimanual approach through two paracentesis openings; and automated irrigation-aspiration with all settings reduced.[15] Cortex should be stripped first in the region farthest from the rent, and the direction of stripping should be toward the rent. Because it can be hazardous to remove cortex in the region of the rent, the cortex is sometimes better left in the eye, to avoid the possibility of enlarging the rent and precipitating vitreous loss. One option to prevent extension of the rent is to convert the tear into a small posterior capsulorrhexis, which eliminates any radially orientated tears that could extend with further surgical manipulation.

If vitreous is present in the anterior segment, vitrectomy should be performed first, with the necessary caution being taken to prevent extension of the rent. Depending on the type of capsular tear, the vitrectomy is performed through either the limbal incision or the pars plana. The former approach is used when the tear is located near the incision, which permits vitrectomy with minimal risk of enlargement of the tear. A pars plana approach is preferred when the tear is remote from the incision and therefore less accessible anteriorly. In either case, irrigation is provided with an infusion cannula in the paracentesis opening. After a thorough anterior vitrectomy, the remaining cortical material can be removed using one of the techniques described earlier or using the vitrector in the aspiration mode without cutting.

INTRAOCULAR LENS INSERTION. Careful inspection of the anatomy of the capsule and zonules is required to determine the appropriate site for IOL implantation. There are four choices: capsular bag, ciliary sulcus, sutured posterior chamber, and anterior chamber.

Capsular Bag. If the rent is small and relatively central, and if the anterior capsular margins are well defined, the posterior chamber IOL can be implanted into the capsular bag. If possible, conversion of posterior capsule tears to posterior continuous curvilinear capsulorrhexis (CCC) is recommended.[16] With the use of an OVD, posterior CCC is initiated by grasping the advancing tear in the posterior capsule with forceps, and then applying CCC principles. This technique is applied to avoid an anticipated extension of the inadvertent linear or triangular tear during maneuvers such as a required vitrectomy or lens placement. The surgeon should ensure that the haptics are orientated away from the rent (to avoid haptic placement or subsequent migration into the vitreous) and that the lens is inserted gently to avoid enlargement of the rent.

Ciliary Sulcus. If the rent exceeds 4–5mm in length or there is extensive zonular loss, the capsular bag probably is not adequate for IOL support. In such cases, the ciliary sulcus is opened with an OVD, and the iris is retracted in all quadrants to assess the status of the peripheral capsule and zonules. The IOL is inserted

with its haptics oriented away from the area of the rent and positioned in areas of intact zonules and capsule.

Another alternative, if the anterior capsulorrhexis is intact, is sulcus placement of the IOL, with capture of the optic through the capsulorrhexis. Finally, some surgeons advocate iris suture fixation of one or both haptics to prevent IOL decentration. After the IOL optic is captured through the pupil, McCannel sutures are used to secure the haptic(s) to the iris, and then the optic is repositioned through the pupil.

Sutured Posterior Chamber. If loss of more than 4–5 clock hours of capsule or zonules occurs, the ciliary sulcus may be inadequate for lens stability. The lens can be fixated to the sclera using single or dual 10–0 polypropylene sutures. If one region of solid peripheral capsule and zonules exists, one haptic can be inserted into the sulcus in this area, and the opposite haptic can be sutured to the sclera.

Anterior Chamber. A Kelman-type multiflex anterior chamber IOL design is a good option for patients who do not have glaucoma, peripheral anterior synechiae, or chronic uveitis. A peripheral iridectomy should be performed in these patients to prevent pupillary block.

Dropped Nucleus

Loss of nuclear material into the vitreous cavity (Fig. 53-3) is one of the most potentially sight-threatening complications of cataract surgery.[17] Clinical and cadaver eye studies implicate posterior extension of breaks in the capsulorrhexis as a common cause of this complication.[7,18] It therefore behooves the surgeon to use increased caution when phacoemulsification is performed with capsulorrhexis tears,[19] as noted earlier. Congenital posterior polar cataract, which predisposes to posterior capsular dehiscence, is another risk factor for dropped nucleus.[20]

Loss of the nucleus into the vitreous cavity can sometimes be avoided by recognizing the early signs of posterior capsular rupture. These include unusual deepening of the anterior chamber, decentration of the nucleus, or loss of efficiency of aspiration, which suggests occlusion of the tip with vitreous. If capsular rupture is noted, the steps outlined earlier should be taken to prevent nucleus loss.

Some controversy exists with regard to the appropriate management of loss of the nucleus into the vitreous. Most surgeons recommend completing the procedure with careful anterior vitrectomy and removal of remaining accessible lens material. In general, IOL implantation is permissible; one rare exception might be loss of an extremely hard, dense nucleus that would require removal through a limbal incision. If a significant amount

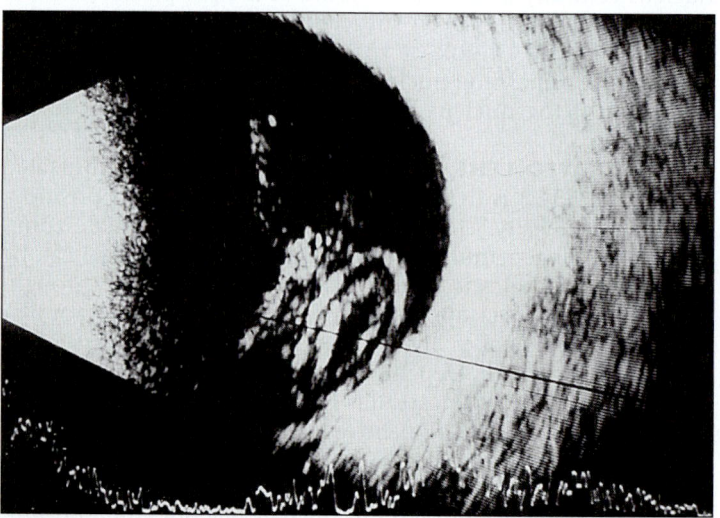

FIG. 53-3 ▓ **Dropped nucleus.** B-scan ultrasonography 1 day after dislocation of a lens nucleus into the vitreous cavity in a patient who has high myopia.

of nuclear material has been retained, the patient is referred to a vitreoretinal surgeon 1–2 days postoperatively. Patients whose eyes have small residual nuclear fragments may be observed and referred if increased IOP or uveitis refractory to medical treatment develops. Some surgeons advocate irrigating the vitreous with fluid in an attempt to float the nucleus back into position. An obvious concern is that this additional turbulence could increase vitreous traction on the retina and cause retinal tears.

Anterior Segment Hemorrhage

The presence of intraocular blood decreases the surgeon's view during the procedure, stimulates postoperative inflammation and synechia formation, and accelerates capsular opacification. To minimize the risk of bleeding, discontinuation of anticoagulant therapy before surgery can be considered if it does not pose a significant medical risk to the patient.[21] The sites of anterior segment hemorrhage are either the wound or the iris. Steps to minimize or eliminate bleeding from the wound include:

- Careful cautery of bleeding vessels in the vicinity of the incision.
- Creation of an adequate internal corneal valve to minimize the likelihood of scleral blood entering the anterior chamber.
- Performing a clear corneal incision.

Iris bleeding is caused by iris trauma. Intraocular bleeding can be stopped by:

- Temporarily elevating the IOP with a balanced salt solution or an OVD.
- Injecting a dilute solution of preservative-free epinephrine (adrenaline) 1:5000 (or a weaker solution).
- Direct cautery (if the bleeding vessel can be identified) with a needle-tipped cautery probe.

The most dire complication of cataract surgery is expulsive hemorrhage, which is actually a spectrum of conditions that ranges from suprachoroidal effusion to mild hemorrhage to severe hemorrhage with expulsion. A sign of any of these conditions is shallowing of the anterior chamber with posterior pressure that resists further deepening of the chamber, sometimes accompanied by a change in the red reflex. These conditions typically occur intraoperatively but also may occur postoperatively, usually when the IOP is below normal (Fig. 53-4). Choroidal effusion also may be a precursor to suprachoroidal hemorrhage, which presumably occurs from the rupture of a blood vessel that is placed under stretch. Risk factors for suprachoroidal hemorrhage include hypertension, glaucoma, nanophthalmos, high myopia, and chronic intraocular inflammation.[22]

If sudden shallowing of the anterior chamber occurs and the eye becomes firm, the retina is examined, if possible, to ascertain the cause. If a dark choroidal elevation is noted, a choroidal hemorrhage is likely, and the incision should be closed as

quickly as possible. The worst scenario is expulsion of intraocular contents through the wound. With tunnel incisions, the wound typically is self-sealing and resists expulsion of a significant amount of tissue. This self-sealing construction can save an eye from complete loss of intraocular contents. However, the surgeon can assist by using a finger tamponade on the wound while hyperosmotic solution is given intravenously. The wound should be closed and the anterior chamber deepened further, if possible, using a balanced salt solution or an OVD.

In the event of severe ongoing prolapse of tissue through the incision, a posterior sclerotomy should be performed; this must be done quickly. Time permitting, a conjunctival peritomy is made 3–4mm posterior to the limbus. A microsurgical steel knife is used to make a radial incision approximately 2mm in length, avoiding the horizontal plane, scratching through the sclera to the level of the suprachoroidal space. Usually, blood begins to ooze from this site. As this occurs, infusion of fluid and OVD into the anterior chamber is commenced in an attempt to restore normal anterior segment anatomy. This bleeding site can be left open, or it can be sutured once the rate of hemorrhage has diminished, the incision has been closed, and the normal anterior chamber depth has been restored. The goal in these cases is to preserve the eye; cataract surgery can always be completed at a later date, typically 2 or more weeks later.

POSTOPERATIVE COMPLICATIONS

Wound Dehiscence

With small-diameter tunnel incisions, wound dehiscence is relatively uncommon. The creation of an internal corneal valve typically prevents the major complications of wound leakage, inadvertent filtering bleb, and epithelial downgrowth. The wound healing process varies according to the site of the posterior entry. Scleral limbal incisions heal by the ingrowth of episcleral vascular tissue. New fibrovascular tissue is deposited with an orientation parallel to the edges of the incision and perpendicular to existing collagen bundles. Over the ensuing few years, collagen remodeling occurs so that the new collagen becomes oriented parallel to existing collagen bundles, which increases the strength of the healed area.[23] Ultimately, the strength of the healed area is approximately 70–80% that of the native tissue. For corneal incisions, closure of the external wound takes place by apposition or, in areas of wound gape, by epithelial ingrowth. A gradual process of remodeling then occurs; this consists of fibrocytic metaplasia of keratocytes with deposition of new collagen, again parallel to the incision, followed over a period of years by remodeling similar to that seen with scleral incisions. In the absence of vascular tissue, this process occurs much more slowly than in scleral or limbal tissue. Postoperative abnormalities in wound structure are produced by defects in the tunnel architecture or by defective wound healing because of systemic disorders, preexisting tissue abnormalities (e.g., excessively thin or weak tissue), or incarceration of material, such as lens, vitreous, or iris, in the wound, which inhibits the normal healing process.

Wound Leakage

A wound leak that occurs in the immediate postoperative period is usually the result of inadequate suture closure for a specific wound configuration. This entity is rare with tunnel constructions. Scleral pocket incisions have a longer tunnel and can readily be demonstrated to be watertight at the conclusion of surgery. Corneal incisions as small as 3.5mm in width seal remarkably well, even though intraoperative pinpoint posterior lip pressure in these eyes often can induce a wound leak. Some surgeons perform hydration of the corneal stroma to prevent a wound leak that can be elicited with posterior lip pressure; however, this hydration clears within a few minutes to hours, and it is uncertain whether it has any actual clinical value.

FIG. 53-4 ■ **Choroidal effusion.** This patient experienced deep ocular pain 1 day postoperatively. A choroidal hemorrhage was noted on close examination. This resolved over several months, leaving no permanent sequelae.

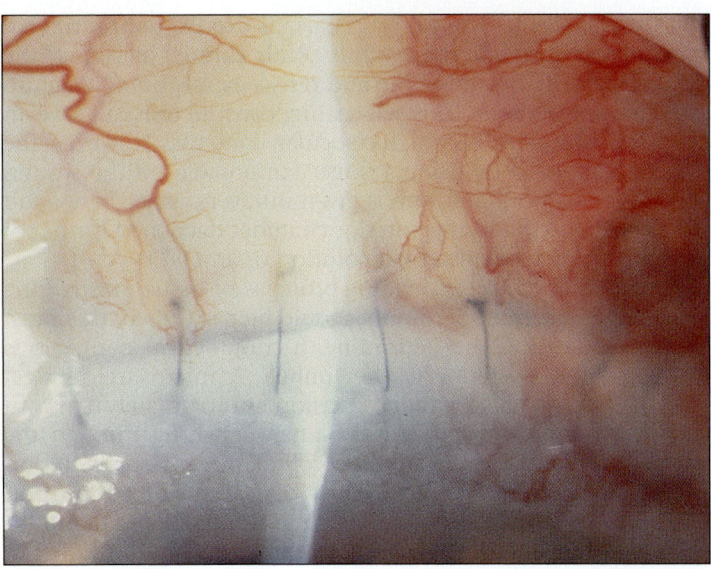

FIG. 53-5 ▓ **Wound dehiscence.** This patient had 5D of against-the-wound astigmatism following nuclear expression. The surgeon resutured the wound 4 weeks postoperatively, but the astigmatism immediately recurred. Note the thin, fragile sclera, sometimes characterized as scleral "melting."

Wound leaks in scleral incisions typically are covered by conjunctiva and usually resolve within a few days; occasionally, they lead to the formation of a filtering bleb. Medical management of scleral or corneal wound leaks may include the following:

- Decreasing or discontinuing corticosteroid therapy.
- Administration of prophylactic topical antibiotics.
- Pressure patching.
- Use of a collagen shield, bandage lens, or disposable contact lens.
- Administration of aqueous inhibitors.

It usually is necessary to suture a wound if the leak persists after 5–7 days or if there is a flat anterior chamber, iris prolapse, extensive external tissue gape, or excessive against-the-wound astigmatism (Fig. 53-5).

Inadvertent Filtering Bleb

Formation of a filtering bleb after cataract surgery occurs if the wound leaks under a sealed conjunctival flap. If early filtration is recognized, progression might be prevented by discontinuation of corticosteroid treatment. If the patient is asymptomatic, the physician can observe the bleb. Elimination of the bleb can be considered if it causes irritation, tearing, or infection. Blebs that tend to be more symptomatic are tall and cystic and encroach over the corneal surface. Options for late closure include cryotherapy, chemical cautery, neodymium:yttrium-aluminum-garnet (Nd:YAG) laser,[24] or surgical closure. The latter can be complex because of endothelialization of the fistula. The surgical approach requires excision of the conjunctival bleb, scraping or cryotherapy of the cells that line the fistula, and closure of the fistula, which sometimes requires a scleral patch graft.

Epithelial Ingrowth

Epithelial downgrowth is a rare but serious complication of intraocular surgery. It occurs most commonly after intracapsular cataract extraction and less often following nuclear expression; it is extremely rare after phacoemulsification. Surface epithelium that invades the intraocular structures, such as over the cornea, iris, ciliary body, lens capsule, and Bruch's membrane,[25] can cause corneal decompensation, chronic anterior uveitis, and intractable secondary angle-closure glaucoma. Conditions for the onset of this entity are highly variable, but it appears to be more common in patients who undergo multiple intraocular procedures or have postoperative wound dehiscence.

The presence of epithelial downgrowth may be confirmed by irradiation of the affected iris with an argon laser (epithelial tissue turns white with argon ablation, compared with the dark or brown appearance of normal iris) or diagnosed with specular micrography (noting a sheet of abnormal tissue that obliterates the normal endothelial mosaic); however, the definitive diagnosis is dependent on the histopathological confirmation of epithelial tissue in the eye. Treatment consists of complete destruction of all intraocular epithelial tissue using cryotherapy, iridocyclectomy, or pars plana vitrectomy. Unfortunately, the prognosis for this postoperative complication is poor, except for a well-defined cyst that can be excised en bloc.[26]

Postoperative Astigmatism

Complications related to postoperative astigmatism are covered in Chapters 41 and 54.

Corneal Edema and Bullous Keratopathy

Factors that predispose to corneal edema following cataract surgery include the following:

- Prior endothelial disease or cell loss.
- Intraoperative mechanical endothelial trauma.
- Excessive postoperative inflammation.
- Prolonged postoperative elevation of IOP.

Preoperatively, patients should be carefully examined for evidence of Fuchs' dystrophy or other conditions that produce a low endothelial cell count. Patients who have marginal corneal endothelial function may complain of poorer vision in the morning because of corneal edema produced by hypoxia overnight. Although most patients who have Fuchs' dystrophy have guttae that are readily visible with slit-lamp examination, in rare instances, patients can have low endothelial cell counts in the absence of guttae. It is often advisable to obtain an endothelial cell count in the fellow eye. Finally, corneal pachymetry can be helpful to assess such patients, because those with a corneal thickness in excess of approximately 0.63mm presumably have marginally compensated corneas and are at great risk of developing permanent postoperative corneal edema. If the corneal thickness is greater than 0.63mm but no corneal edema is evident, the authors generally perform cataract surgery alone and advise patients of the increased risk of developing postoperative corneal decompensation. If frank epithelial and stromal edema is present, a combined cataract extraction with penetrating keratoplasty may be advisable.

Several measures can be taken intra- and postoperatively to minimize the risk of corneal injury. For some surgeons, nuclear expression may be safer than phacoemulsification. Techniques to remove the nucleus in the posterior chamber seem to minimize endothelial cell loss,[27] and evidence exists that highly retentive OVDs are more protective when surgical removal of the nucleus near the endothelium is carried out. Postoperatively, inflammation should be aggressively treated with topical corticosteroids, and IOP should be controlled below 20mmHg. Mechanical factors, such as Descemet's detachment or retained nuclear fragments in the angle touching the endothelium, should be addressed. For symptomatic relief, hypertonic saline ointment is sometimes helpful as a temporary measure. Sequential corneal pachymetry is an excellent way to document the resolution of postoperative corneal edema, which may take up to 3 months; it is usually advisable to wait at least this long before recommending penetrating keratoplasty.

Hyphema

A postoperative hyphema is caused by bleeding from the wound or iris (Fig. 53-6). As the hyphema resolves, the IOP should be controlled. Surgical reintervention to remove a blood clot is indicated if severe, medically resistant pressure elevation exists for

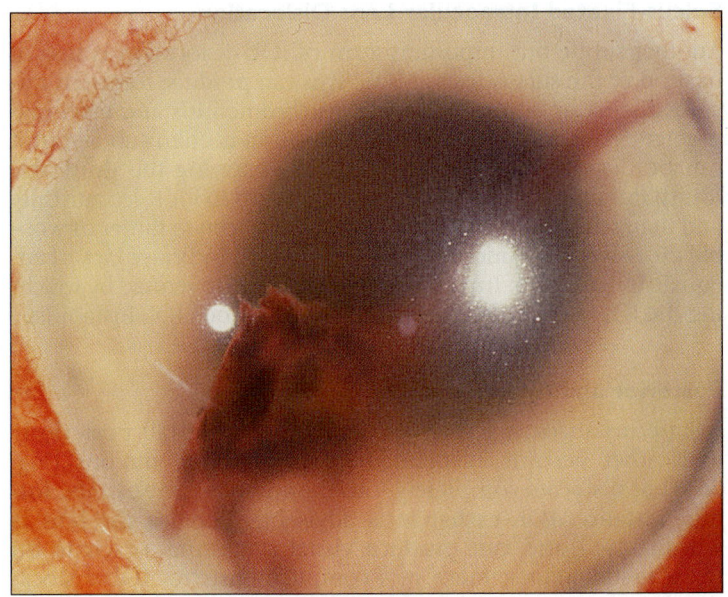

FIG. 53-6 ■ **Postoperative hyphema.** This hyphema was produced by hemorrhage from the scleral incision in a patient who had a small postoperative wound leak. The hyphema resolved once the incision closed, which led to cessation of ongoing bleeding and restoration of normal intraocular pressure.

several days. The duration of tolerated pressure elevation depends on the patient's age and the status of the optic nerve. The incidence of postoperative hyphema is reduced by making clear corneal incisions.

Late hyphema or microhyphema most often is caused by chafing of the IOL against the iris or ciliary body (uveitis-glaucoma-hyphema syndrome).[28] This most typically occurs because of loss of fixation of the sulcus-fixated posterior chamber IOL; micromovements of the lens cause chafing against a vessel, which produces the postoperative bleeding. Treatment consists of IOL exchange and ensuring that the new lens is well fixated; this might require suture fixation to the sclera or implantation of an anterior chamber lens. A rare cause of postoperative bleeding is hemorrhage from vascularization of the internal margin of the incision (Swan's syndrome)[29]; this can be diagnosed by noting neovascularization of the wound using gonioscopy, and it is treated by argon laser photocoagulation.

Endocapsular Hematoma

Endocapsular hematoma is the postoperative entrapment of blood between the posterior surface of the IOL and the posterior capsule.[30] It is a variant of hyphema, with the exception that the blood can become entrapped within the capsular bag for months or even permanently. Fortunately, in most instances the amount of blood is minimal and either does not significantly impair vision or is absorbed over a few weeks or months.[31] When the accumulation is extensive and persistent, Nd:YAG laser posterior capsulectomy is curative when used to enable the blood to flow immediately into the vitreous, where it can be resorbed.

Intraocular Pressure Elevation

Elevation of IOP following cataract surgery is a common occurrence. Fortunately, it usually is mild and self-limited and does not require prolonged antiglaucoma therapy. Causes of acute pressure elevation are retention of viscoelastic substances, obstruction of the trabecular meshwork with inflammatory debris, and pupillary or ciliary block. Patients who have preexisting glaucoma are at much greater risk of developing acute significant pressure elevation. Prevention of this problem includes careful removal of the OVD at the time of surgery, control of intraocular bleeding, and the use of intra- and postoperative antiglaucomatous agents. Intracameral injection of 0.01% carbachol at the

conclusion of surgery is effective, as is the postoperative administration of pilocarpine gel; topical beta blockers; apraclonidine; and topical, intravenous, or oral carbonic anhydrase inhibitors. If marked elevation of IOP is present on the first postoperative day, this can be immediately controlled by "venting" the anterior chamber. After topical anesthetic agents and antibiotics have been administered, a forceps or other fine instrument is used to depress the posterior lip of the paracentesis incision, which allows the egress of a small amount of OVD and aqueous.[32] This is repeated as necessary until the IOP is brought into the low-normal range. The patient can then be treated with topical antiglaucoma therapy and followed carefully to ensure that pressure is controlled.

Chronic IOP elevation can be caused by corticosteroid use, retained lens (particularly nuclear) material, chronic inflammation, peripheral anterior synechiae formation, endophthalmitis, and ciliary block. The correct diagnosis of the underlying cause is required to institute appropriate therapy.

Capsular Block Syndrome

Capsular block syndrome (CBS) is initially defined by the entrapment of an OVD in the capsular bag, because of apposition of the anterior rim of the capsulorrhexis with the anterior face of the IOL.[33,34] This may be more common with acrylic IOLs because of their slightly "stickier" surface. Postoperatively, the bag becomes more distended (perhaps through osmotic imbibition of aqueous), and the IOL is pushed anteriorly to create a myopic refractive shift. This can be prevented by meticulous removal of the OVD from the bag at the conclusion of surgery. To accomplish this, it is helpful to gently depress the IOL optic to displace the OVD trapped behind the IOL.[35] Treatment requires Nd:YAG laser puncture of the anterior capsule peripheral to the edge of the capsulorrhexis, which permits the OVD to escape into the anterior chamber. Alternatively, if the pupil is relatively small and the anterior capsule is not accessible to laser treatment, a small posterior capsulectomy can be performed, which permits the OVD to drain into the vitreous.

A new classification of CBS includes intraoperative CBS, early postoperative CBS, and late postoperative CBS.[36] Intraoperative CBS occurs during rapid hydrodissection using a large amount of BSS and has been discussed in the hydrodissection section. Early postoperative CBS represents the initial type of CBS, with accumulation of the OVD in the capsular bag, as discussed earlier. Late postoperative CBS refers to eyes with accumulation of a milky-white substance in the closed capsular bag.[37–39] Reduction of vision with this type of CBS is rare, and Nd:YAG laser capsulotomy can be performed, if necessary.

Intraocular Lens Miscalculation

Complications related to IOL miscalculation are covered in Chapters 38 and 39.

Intraocular Lens Decentration and Dislocation

Common causes of IOL dislocation are asymmetrical loop placement, sunset syndrome, loss of zonular support for a lens fixated in the capsular bag, and pupillary capture of the IOL optic.[40]

ASYMMETRICAL HAPTIC PLACEMENT. Pathological studies indicate that asymmetrical loop placement is an extremely common occurrence, particularly when can-opener capsulotomies are performed. The incidence of this complication has been greatly reduced with the advent of capsulorrhexis, which permits excellent visualization of the capsular edge and ensures that a lens placed in the capsular bag is retained there. An IOL with asymmetrical loop placement becomes symptomatic if the lens is decentered sufficiently relative to the pupil; symptoms include polyopia, glare, induced myopia (from looking through the peripheral portion of the IOL), and loss of best-corrected acuity. Depending on the severity of the symptoms, treatment includes IOL repositioning or IOL exchange. In some instances, topical miotics can be prescribed; however, few patients prefer this mode of management.

SUNSET SYNDROME. Sunset syndrome occurs when a sulcus-fixated posterior chamber IOL dislocates through a peripheral break in the zonules, typically inferiorly. Sunset syndrome is usually an acute, nonprogressive event. Treatment options again depend on the severity of the patient's symptoms. The authors have found that simple IOL repositioning is often unsuccessful and predisposes to recurrence. Therefore, several other options are recommended:

- Repositioning the lens, combined with iris fixation sutures.
- IOL exchange with a larger, more rigid lens.
- Scleral fixation of a posterior chamber lens.
- Replacement with an anterior chamber lens.

LENS-BAG DECENTRATION. In rare instances, a lens that is placed in the capsular bag can dislocate as a result of bag decentration caused by zonular rupture or dehiscence, especially in pseudoexfoliation syndrome. Treatment of this condition, if sufficiently severe, requires IOL exchange with some form of scleral fixation or implantation of an anterior chamber lens.

PUPILLARY CAPTURE. Pupillary capture of the IOL optic consists of the posterior migration of some portion of the iris beneath the IOL optic (Fig. 53-7). Predisposing factors are can-opener capsulectomy and sulcus implantation of the posterior chamber IOL, particularly in the absence of angulated haptics; however, in rare instances, pupillary capture can occur with capsular fixation of the lens after capsulorrhexis, especially when the capsulorrhexis is large.[41,42] Pupillary capture can produce acute and chronic iritis, posterior synechiae formation, visual loss from deposition of inflammatory cells on the IOL surface, and, if the lens is displaced sufficiently eccentrically and anteriorly, chronic endothelial trauma with corneal decompensation. Pupillary capture diagnosed within a few days of its occurrence can be treated pharmacologically or by manually repositioning the optic into the posterior chamber. Chronic pupillary capture may be more difficult to manage, because firm synechiae form between the iris and posterior capsule. In such situations, the IOL should be repositioned if there are visual symptoms, chronic uveitis, or corneal endothelial trauma. Chronic cellular precipitates on the IOL surface can often be managed by the administration of topical corticosteroids and occasional Nd:YAG laser "dusting" of the anterior IOL surface.[43]

Sulcus-Fixated Intraocular Lens Dislocation

Another subtle but important form of IOL dislocation is loss of fixation of the sulcus-fixated IOL. This can produce recurrent microhyphema or hyphema, as well as chronic iritis and even pigmentary glaucoma. The loss of lens fixation is often subtle, but it can be diagnosed at the slit lamp by observing the third and fourth Purkinje images. If the patient is asked to look eccentrically and then refix centrally, these images can be seen to flutter or wobble excessively (pseudophacodonesis), which indicates lack of adequate IOL fixation. Intraoperatively, this can be verified by touching the IOL with an instrument; there is obvious IOL instability.

Posterior and Anterior Dislocation

In rare instances, a posterior chamber lens can fall posteriorly and either become suspended in the anterior vitreous (Fig. 53-8) or dislocate completely into the vitreous cavity. In the former instance, IOL exchange is advisable, because the lens is within reach and can produce visual symptoms or chafe on uveal tissue. Management of a complete posterior IOL dislocation is more controversial. Although in some eyes this condition is well tolerated, in others, the lenses can become entrapped in the vitreous base and cause vitreous traction and retinal tears, or they can produce visual symptoms by intermittently moving into the visual axis. Consultation with a vitreoretinal surgeon is advised for the management of these patients.

Even more rarely, anterior luxation of a posterior chamber lens into the anterior chamber may occur.[44] This can be prevented with a small and continuous capsulorrhexis and in-the-bag implantation of the lens.

Intraocular Lens Exchange

Several principles of IOL exchange need to be emphasized. It is generally preferable to exchange lenses that have haptics that are poorly designed, too short, or deformed from lens malposition in the eye. Patients who have a marginal corneal endothelium status generally should be subjected to the least traumatic surgery possible, such as iris repositioning with iris fixation sutures rather than IOL exchange, particularly if the latter requires anterior vitrectomy. It is important to distinguish between IOL

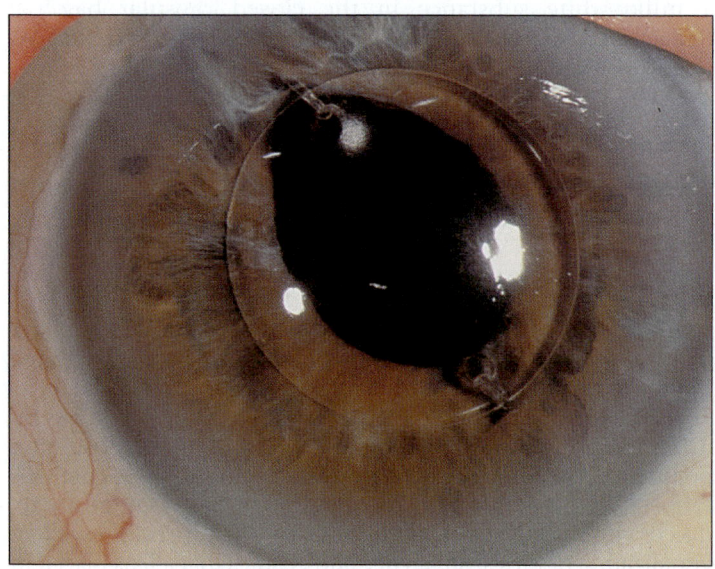

FIG. 53-7 ■ **Pupillary capture of the intraocular lens.** Predisposing factors in this patient included a can-opener capsulectomy, intraoperative iris trauma, and nonangulated haptics.

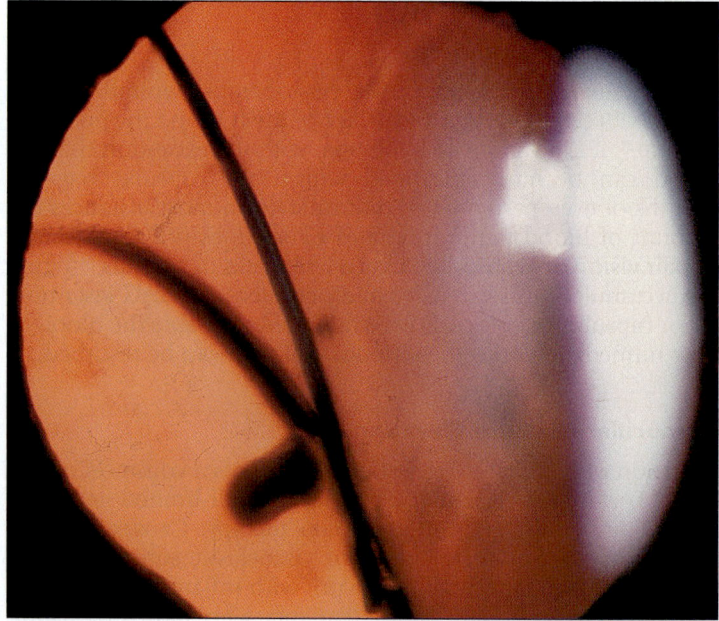

FIG. 53-8 ■ **Intraocular lens dislocation.** During surgery, a capsular rupture was noted. A lens was, however, implanted in the posterior chamber. On the morning following surgery, the lens was found to be dislocated posteriorly and inferiorly, and the patient was referred for treatment. At the time of lens exchange, it appeared that insufficient capsular support was present, and a new lens was sutured into the ciliary sulcus.

decentration and pupil displacement. In some instances, the patient's symptoms result from an eccentrically displaced pupil in the face of a relatively well-positioned IOL. Clearly, surgery, if indicated, should address the underlying problem by reconstructing the pupil. This can be done by suturing the pupil in the peripheral region and opening the pupil centrally with several small sphincterotomies. If certain complications are associated with the site of the dislocated IOL (e.g., recurrent microhyphema with a posterior chamber IOL or peripheral anterior synechiae with an anterior chamber IOL), it may be advisable to place the new lens in a new site. Finally, if sufficient intact posterior capsule exists, an attempt can be made to reopen the capsular flaps to permit fixation of the new lens within the capsular bag; this, clearly, is the most desirable location.

Cystoid Macular Edema

Cystoid macular edema (CME) is the most common cause of unexpected visual loss following cataract surgery. Fluorescein angiographic CME can occur in up to 50% of patients at 4–8 weeks postoperatively, but clinical CME occurs in less than 3% of patients. The typical time of onset of clinical CME is 3–4 weeks postoperatively. Predisposing factors are intraoperative complications (e.g., vitreous loss or severe iris trauma), vitreous traction at the wound, diabetic retinopathy,[45] and preexisting epiretinal membrane. In cases without predisposing factors, CME typically resolves over several weeks, although most surgeons prefer to treat this topically with nonsteroidal and corticosteroid drops. Other modes of treatment that have been employed include sub-Tenon's corticosteroid injection and administration of systemic nonsteroidal anti-inflammatory drugs with corticosteroids. In patients who have epiretinal membranes, CME may take months to resolve. When associated with diabetic retinopathy, CME often is resistant to medical therapy and can persist indefinitely; macular laser photocoagulation is sometimes helpful to document angiographically the leaking vessels and microaneurysms. Patients who have ongoing structural abnormalities, such as vitreous traction or extensive iris chafing, are less likely to experience spontaneous resolution of CME and may benefit from surgical correction of the precipitating factor.

Endophthalmitis

Endophthalmitis can occur in an acute or a chronic form. It is characterized by ciliary injection, conjunctival chemosis, hy-popyon, decreased visual acuity, and ocular pain. The acute form generally develops within 2–5 days of surgery and has a fulminant course (Fig. 53-9). Common causative organisms are gram-positive, coagulase-negative micrococci, *Staphylococcus aureus*, streptococcus species, and enterococcus species.[46,47]

Chronic endophthalmitis is caused by organisms of low pathogenicity, such as *Propionibacterium acnes* or *Staphylococcus epidermidis*. It typically is diagnosed several weeks or longer after surgery. Signs include decreased visual acuity, chronic uveitis with or without hypopyon formation, and, in some instances, plaque-like material on the posterior capsule. Histopathologically, this material consists of the offending microorganism embedded in residual lenticular tissue.

Treatment of endophthalmitis consists of culturing aqueous and vitreous aspirates, followed by administration of intravitreal,[48] topical, and subconjunctival antibiotics, as discussed elsewhere. In the Endophthalmitis Vitrectomy Study, no evidence was found of any benefit from the use of systemic antibiotics.[49] Pars plana vitrectomy helped increase the final visual outcome only of those patients who had an initial visual acuity of light perception or worse.[49] For further discussion of endophthalmitis, see Chapter 169.

Posterior Capsular Opacification

Secondary cataract formation is a major complication of IOL implantation after extracapsular cataract extraction (ECCE or phacoemulsification). The incidence is in the range of 18–50% in adults followed for as long as 5 years; in infants and juveniles, an opacification rate of 44% was found within 3 months of surgery after in-the-bag IOL implantation with an intact posterior capsule.[50] Posterior capsular opacification (PCO) is caused by proliferation and migration of residual lens epithelial cells. These can produce visual loss through two mechanisms:

- Formation of swollen, abnormally shaped lens cells called Elschnig's pearls, which migrate over the posterior capsule into the visual axis (Fig. 53-10).
- Transformation into fibroblasts, which may contain contractile elements (myofibroblasts) and cause the posterior capsule to wrinkle (see Fig. 53-8).

Standard treatment of PCO consists of opening the capsule with Nd:YAG laser. Complications of this treatment include

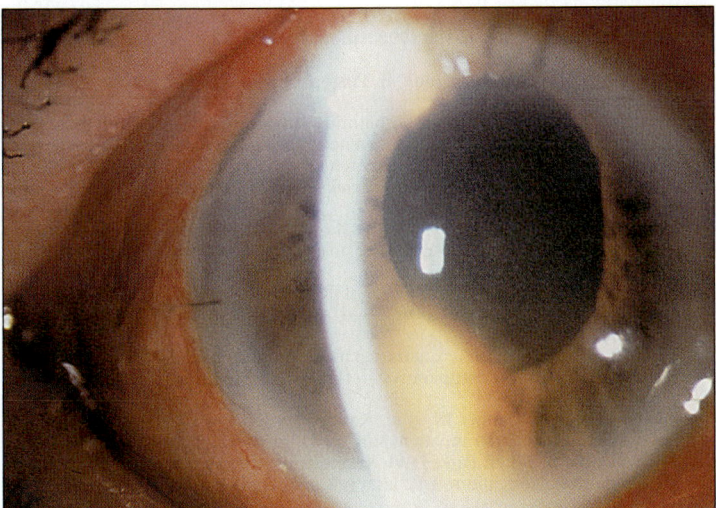

FIG. 53-9 ■ Postoperative endophthalmitis. This patient developed an acute postoperative endophthalmitis after clear cornea cataract surgery and implantation of a polymethyl methacrylate posterior chamber intraocular lens. During cataract surgery, a capsular break occurred, and an anterior vitrectomy was performed. The patient was treated successfully with vitrectomy and injection of intravitreal antibiotics combined with postoperative topical antibiotic therapy. Final visual acuity was 20/50 (6/15).

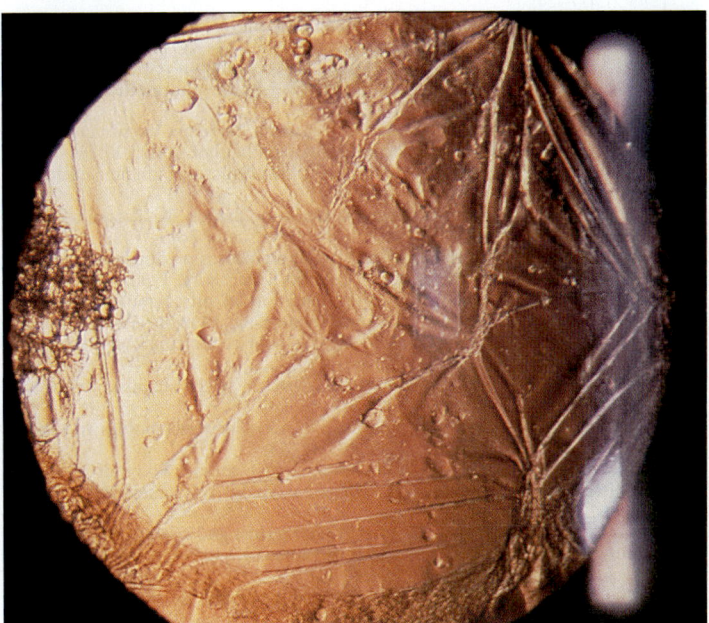

FIG. 53-10 ■ Posterior capsular opacification. Elschnig's pearl formation and capsular wrinkling causing a severe decrease of visual acuity.

acute and, in rare instances, chronic IOP elevation, pitting of the IOL, and retinal detachment. Factors that predispose to retinal attachment include an axial length greater than 24.5mm, male gender, and preexisting retinal pathology.[51–53]

A related and unusual abnormality is the formation of striae in the posterior capsule in the absence of abnormal proliferation of lens epithelial cells. In some patients, this produces a Maddox-rod effect; the typical symptoms are linear streaks that radiate from lights, and their orientation is 90° from the meridian of the striae. The cause is stretching of the capsular bag by the IOL, which produces the striae aligned with the axis of the lens haptics. Typically, this is present on the first postoperative day but may not be mentioned by the patient until later. In many eyes, the striae resolve in the first week or two after surgery as capsular contraction occurs, which counteracts the stretch forces of the IOL haptics. If the condition persists and is sufficiently symptomatic, it can be corrected readily with a laser posterior capsulectomy. For further discussion of PCO, see Chapter 34.

Retinal Detachment

Retinal detachment is a well-recognized complication of cataract surgery; it occurs in 0.2–3.6% of persons after extracapsular cataract surgery. The incidence of retinal detachment increases fivefold if an intracapsular procedure is performed.[54] Predisposing factors include Nd:YAG laser capsulectomy, axial length greater than 24.5mm, myopic refractive error, lattice degeneration, male gender, intraoperative vitreous loss, postoperative ocular trauma, posterior vitreous detachment, and history of retinal detachment in the fellow eye.[52,55,56] Steps to prevent retinal detachment include the following:

- A careful preoperative fundus examination.
- Preservation of the integrity of the posterior capsule at the time of surgery.
- Education of patients with regard to the symptoms of retinal tears and detachment.
- Regular postoperative dilated fundus examinations.

REFERENCES

1. Powe NR, Schein OD, Gieser SC, et al. Synthesis of the literature on visual acuity and complications following cataract extraction with intraocular lens implantation. Arch Ophthalmol. 1994;112:239–52.
2. Kohnen T, Dick B, Jacobi KW. Comparison of induced astigmatism after temporal clear corneal tunnel incisions of different sizes. J Cataract Refract Surg. 1995;21:417–24.
3. Assia EI, Levkovich-Verbin H, Blumenthal M. Management of Descemet's membrane detachment. J Cataract Refract Surg. 1995;21:714–7.
4. Iradier MT, Moreno E, Aranguez C, et al. Late spontaneous resolution of a massive detachment of Descemet's membrane after phacoemulsification. J Cataract Refract Surg. 2002;28:1071–3.
5. Kim T, Hasan SA. A new technique for repairing Descemet membrane detachments using intracameral gas injection. Arch Ophthalmol. 2002;120:181–3.
6. Amaral CE, Palay DA. Technique for repair of Descemet membrane detachment. Am J Ophthalmol. 1999;127:88–90.
7. Kohnen T. Kapsel und Zonularupturen als Komplikation der Kataraktchirurgie mit Phacoemulsifikation. MD dissertation, University of Bonn, 1989.
8. Osher RH, Yu BC-Y, Koch DD. Posterior polar cataracts: a predisposition to intraoperative posterior capsular rupture. J Cataract Refract Surg. 1990;16:157–62.
9. Koch DD, Liu JF. Multilamellar hydrodissection in phacoemulsification and planned extracapsular surgery. J Cataract Refract Surg. 1990;16:559–62.
10. Hakin KN, Jacobs M, Rosen P, et al. Management of the subluxated crystalline lens. Ophthalmology. 1992;99:542–5.
11. Cionni RJ, Osher RH. Endocapsular ring approach to the subluxed cataractous lens. J Cataract Refract Surg. 1995;21:245–9.
12. Gimbel HV, Sun R. Clinical applications of capsular tension rings in cataract surgery. Ophthalmic Surg Lasers. 2002;33:44–53.
13. Ng DT, Rowe NA, Francis IC, et al. Intraoperative complications of 1000 phacoemulsification procedures: a prospective study. J Cataract Refract Surg. 1998;24:1390–5.
14. Cruz OA, Wallace GW, Gay CA, et al. Visual results and complications of phacoemulsification with intraocular lens implantation performed by ophthalmology residents. Ophthalmology. 1992;99:448–52.
15. Brauweiler P. Bimanual irrigation/aspiration. J Cataract Refract Surg. 1996;22:1013–6.
16. Gimbel HV, Sun R, Ferensowicz M, et al. Intraoperative management of posterior capsule tears in phacoemulsification and intraocular lens implantation. Ophthalmology. 2001;108:2186–9.
17. Kim JE, Flynn HW Jr, Rubsamen PE, et al. Endophthalmitis in patients with retained lens fragments after phacoemulsification. Ophthalmology. 1996;103:575–8.
18. Assia EI, Apple DJ, Barden A, et al. An experimental study comparing various anterior capsulectomy techniques. Arch Ophthalmol. 1991;109:642–7.
19. Chern S, Yung C-W. Posterior lens dislocation during attempted phacoemulsification. Ophthalmic Surg. 1995;26:114–6.
20. Aasuri MK, Kompella VB, Majji AB. Risk factors for and management of dropped nucleus during phacoemulsification. J Cataract Refract Surg. 2001;27:1428–32.
21. Saitoh AK, Saitoh A, Taniguchi H, Amemiya T. Anticoagulation therapy and ocular surgery. Ophthalmic Surg Lasers. 1998;29:909–15.
22. Beatty S, Lotery A, Kent D, et al. Acute intraoperative suprachoroidal haemorrhage in ocular surgery. Eye. 1998;12(Pt 5):815–20.
23. Koch DD, Smith SH, Whiteside SB. Limbal and scleral wound healing. In: Beuerman RW, Crosson CE, Kaufman HE, eds. Healing processes in the cornea. Houston: Gulf Publishing; 1989:165–82.
24. Geyer O. Management of large, leaking, and inadvertent filtering blebs with the neodymium:YAG laser. Ophthalmology. 1998;105:983–7.
25. Küchle M, Green W. Epithelial ingrowth: a study of 207 histopathologically proved cases. Ger J Ophthalmol. 1996;5:211–23.
26. Knauf HP, Rowsey JJ, Margo CE. Cystic epithelial downgrowth following clear-corneal cataract extraction. Arch Ophthalmol. 1997;115:668–9.
27. Koch DD, Liu JF, Glasser DB, et al. A comparison of corneal endothelial changes after use of Healon or Viscoat during phacoemulsification. Am J Ophthalmol. 1993;115:188–201.
28. Johnson SH, Kratz RP, Olson PF. Iris transillumination and microhyphema syndrome. J Am Intraocul Implant Soc. 1984;10:425–8.
29. Swan KC. Hyphema due to wound vascularization after cataract extraction. Arch Ophthalmol. 1973;89:87–90.
30. Hagan JC III, Menapace R, Radax U. Clinical syndrome of endocapsular hematoma: presentation of a collected series and review of the literature. J Cataract Refract Surg. 1996;22:379–84.
31. Hater MA, Yung CW. Spontaneous resolution of an endocapsular hematoma. Am J Ophthalmol. 1997;123:844–6.
32. Laube T, Koch HR, Çubuk H, Kohnen T. Druckentlastung nach Staroperation (abstract). Klin Monatsbl Augenheilkd. 1995;206:59.
33. Davison JA. Capsular bag distension after endophacoemulsification and posterior chamber intraocular lens implantation. J Cataract Refract Surg. 1990;16:312–4.
34. Masket S. Postoperative complications of capsulorrhexis. J Cataract Refract Surg. 1993;19:721–4.
35. Kohnen T, von Ehr M, Schütte E, Koch DD. Evaluation of intraocular pressure with Healon and Healon GV in sutureless cataract surgery with foldable lens implantation. J Cataract Refract Surg. 1996;22:227–37.
36. Miyake K, Ota I, Ichihashi S, et al. New classification of capsular block syndrome. J Cataract Refract Surg. 1998;24:1230–4.
37. Eifrig DE. Capsulorrhexis-related lacteocrumenasia. J Cataract Refract Surg. 1997;23:450–4.
38. Miyake K, Ota I, Miyake S, Horiguchi M. Liquefied aftercataract: a complication of continuous curvilinear capsulorrhexis and intraocular lens implantation in the lens capsule. Am J Ophthalmol. 1998;125:429–35.
39. Namba H, Namba R, Sugiura T, Miyauchi S. Accumulation of milky fluid: a late complication of cataract surgery. J Cataract Refract Surg. 1999;25:1019–23.
40. Tappin MJ, Larkin DF. Factors leading to lens implant decentration and exchange. Eye. 2000;14(Pt 5):773–6.
41. Nagamoto S, Kohzuka T, Nagamoto T. Pupillary block after pupillary capture of an AcrySof intraocular lens. J Cataract Refract Surg. 1998;24:1271–4.
42. Khokhar S, Sethi HS, Sony P, et al. Pseudophakic pupillary block caused by pupillary capture after phacoemulsification and in-the-bag AcrySof lens implantation. J Cataract Refract Surg. 2002;28:1291–2.
43. Brauweiler P, Ohrloff C. Das Polieren eiweibeschlagener Intraokularlinsen mit dem Nd:YAG-Laser. Fortsch Ophthalmol. 1990;87:78–9.
44. Faucher A, Rootman DS. Dislocation of a plate-haptic silicone intraocular lens into the anterior chamber. J Cataract Refract Surg. 2001;27:169–71.
45. Schatz H, Atienza D, McDonald HR, Johnson RN. Severer diabetic retinopathy after cataract surgery. Am J Ophthalmol. 1994;117:314–21.
46. Han DP, Wisniewski SR, Wilson LA, et al. Spectrum and susceptibilities of microbiologic isolates in the Endophthalmitis Vitrectomy Study. Am J Ophthalmol. 1996;122:1–17.
47. Montan P, Lundstrom M, Stenevi U, Thorburn W. Endophthalmitis following cataract surgery in Sweden. The 1998 national prospective survey. Acta Ophthalmol Scand. 2002;80:258–61.
48. Mamalis N, Kearsley L, Brinton E. Postoperative endophthalmitis. Curr Opin Ophthalmol. 2002;13:14–8.
49. Group EVS. Results of the Endophthalmitis Vitrectomy Study. A randomized trial of immediate vitrectomy and of intravenous antibiotics for the treatment of postoperative bacterial endophthalmitis. Arch Ophthalmol. 1995;113:1479–96.
50. Apple DJ, Solomon KD, Tetz RM, et al. Posterior capsule opacification. Surv Ophthalmol. 1992;37:73–116.
51. Koch DD, Liu JF, Fill EP, Parke DWI. Axial myopia increases the risk of retina complications after neodymium–YAG laser posterior capsulotomy. Arch Ophthalmol. 1989;107:986–90.
52. Tielsch JM, Legro MW, Cassard SD, et al. Risk factors for retinal detachment after cataract surgery. A population-based case-control study. Ophthalmology. 1996;103:1537–45.
53. Ninn-Pedersen K, Bauer B. Cataract patients in a defined Swedish population, 1986 to 1990. V. Postoperative retinal detachments. Arch Ophthalmol. 1996;114:382–6.
54. Javitt JC, Vitale S, Canner JK, et al. National outcomes of cataract extraction. I. Retinal detachment after inpatient surgery. Ophthalmology. 1991;98:895–902.
55. Koch DD, Liu JF, Fill EP, Parke DWI. Axial myopia increases the risk of retina complications after neodymium–YAG laser posterior capsulectomy. Arch Ophthalmol. 1989;107:986–90.
56. Haddad WM, Monin C, Morel C, et al. Retinal detachment after phacoemulsification: a study of 114 cases. Am J Ophthalmol. 2002;133:630–8.

54 Outcomes of Cataract Surgery

JACK T. HOLLADAY

KEY FEATURES

- Outcomes of cataract surgery can be classified according to subjective and objective findings.
- Subjective findings are evaluated best with interviews or questionnaires. Several questionnaires to help assess a patient's change in functional vision following cataract surgery are available. These surveys are especially helpful in the evaluation of patient satisfaction.[1]
- Objective measures of functional vision include much more than best-corrected visual acuity. Parameters such as uncorrected visual acuity, contrast sensitivity, glare disability, visual field, and color vision are also important.

INTRODUCTION

For many years, the only measure used to assess the outcome of cataract surgery was the patient's best-corrected visual acuity. This may be the most important measure, as it is often used to determine whether a person is eligible to operate a motor vehicle, qualify for a job as a pilot, and so forth. As a result of the transition from intracapsular cataract surgery (with 7 days of bed rest and use of aphakic glasses) to small incision surgery (with no rehabilitation period and a reduced dependence on spectacles), expectations of cataract surgery have increased dramatically. Over this same period, the functional assessment of vision also has improved. This chapter delineates the parameters a clinician should measure to assess the objective outcome of cataract surgery.

EVALUATION OF OUTCOMES

Functional vision assessment implies the ability to characterize parameters of vision and translate them into how well daily activities are performed with respect to vision. To do this objectively, the parameters that characterize vision must first be determined. In both clinical practice and research, these parameters can be allocated to five major areas:
- Limiting resolution (high-contrast visual acuity).
- Contrast performance (contrast sensitivity and threshold).
- Performance at various background illuminations (glare disability).
- Field of view (visual field).
- Color performance (color vision).

If these characteristics are known in a camera, an ophthalmic instrument, or, most importantly, a patient, their performance in any situation can be predicted and evaluated objectively. Instruments currently developed for the military, such as night-vision scopes, virtual-reality displays in aircraft, and remote interactive missile-guidance equipment, already employ such objective parameters to describe the optical performance of the systems subserved. Just as with a device, the visual system of an individual must be characterized using these same five parameters to describe accurately and completely the performance of the system.

Translating a patient's visual performance or functional vision into the ability to perform a specific activity necessitates knowledge of the visual requirements needed to carry out the activity being evaluated. In most cases, the use of these parameters to characterize the visual requirements for even the simplest activities, such as reading, has begun only recently.[2] For more complex activities, such as driving, the primitive requirements for visual acuity and visual field date back to the early 1950s and are known not to correlate with driving performance and safety.[3] For example, the U.S. Food and Drug Administration currently requires manufacturers to evaluate the effect of multifocal intraocular lenses (IOLs) compared with monofocal lenses on a person's ability to drive in daylight and at night. The differences in the five parameters using these IOLs have been delineated very accurately and objectively over the past 10 years for these two types of lenses.[4-6] The impact on vision can be demonstrated both numerically and photographically, but translating these parameters into a determination of whether a person is a safe driver is much more difficult, because many nonvisual activities, such as reaction time, hearing ability, cognitive skills, emotional state, and personality, may have a greater impact on driving safety than vision alone.

The difficulty of determining the visual requirements of various activities and the variation in daily activities from one individual to another result in difficulty correlating significant improvement in visual performance in the five areas with improvement in the patient's quality of life.[7-9] The ability to demonstrate changes in the quality of life lies not in objectively and accurately describing the patient's visual system but in determining the visual requirements for performing daily activities at an acceptable level.

Fully evaluating the visual system using these five parameters in a patient who has a cataract is important. In many cases, the patient does not present to the clinician with the diagnosis of cataract. The patient usually presents with complaints of decreased vision, and it is the clinician's role to evaluate the patient's history and examine the patient to determine the cause of the reduced vision. After the diagnosis of a cataract—or any other diagnosis—has been made, some of the five parameters that describe visual performance may become less important. Not fully evaluating a patient's vision in these five areas may be harmful in two major ways: it can result in unnecessary therapy being rendered or necessary therapy being withheld.

A common example is a 75-year-old patient who has a cataract and pigment mottling in the macula and a visual acuity of 20/80 (6/24). Is the poor acuity the result of cataract or of age-related macular degeneration? No clinician can accurately assess the impact of a cataract on the visual system using the biomicroscope, direct ophthalmoscope, retinoscope, or indirect ophthalmoscope. Although estimates can be made of the reduction in visual acuity resulting from a cataract, the optics are far too complex to be exact. An objective measurement of the retinal acuity can be made with a laser interference pattern[10,11] or projected retinal acuity chart.[8,12–14] Several comparisons of these two modalities have been made, with good results for both.[9,15–17] Finding a good retinal acuity of 20/20 (6/6) and recommending cataract surgery to the patient is just as important as finding a poor retinal acuity of 20/80 (6/24) from macular degeneration and not recommending cataract surgery.

Cataracts have a unique effect on functional vision with respect to the five areas considered here. At the outset, it should be clear that none of these parameters on its own is sufficient to determine the exact cause of reduced vision, even in the presence of a cataract. When they are considered collectively, however, the diagnosis of most ocular diseases is very specific.

FIVE PARAMETERS THAT DESCRIBE VISUAL FUNCTION

Visual Acuity

STANDARDIZED VISUAL ACUITY TESTING. Standardized visual acuity tests measure the patient's ability to recognize standardized optotypes (usually Snellen acuity letters) at a specified visual angle, illumination, and contrast. In the 1980s, the International Council of Ophthalmology adopted the standard that the elements of the 10 Snellen letters should subtend an angle of 1 minute of arc, to make the entire letter 5 minutes in angular height.[18] A minimum of five letters should be on a line, and the lines should increase or decrease in size by 0.1 log units (25%) between lines. These standards were incorporated into a standardized chart by Bailey and Lovie.[19] The letters should be greater than 85% contrast (black letters on a white background) with a background illumination of 85cd/m². Under these conditions, the "normal" individual can recognize letters with elements 1 minute in angular magnitude. The visual acuity can be recorded in various notations, for which normal vision would be Snellen units (20/20 or 6/6), decimal (1.0), or LogMAR (0.0).

BEST-CORRECTED VISUAL ACUITY. Best-corrected visual acuity implies that the patient has been corrected optically to achieve the best visual acuity possible. In most cases, this value is obtained with the best spherocylindrical spectacle refraction. In cases of irregular corneal astigmatism, the best-corrected visual acuity may be attained with a rigid contact lens, not with spectacles. In recent studies in which preoperative pathology was excluded (best-case analysis),[5,6,20] more than 95% of the patients who had received cataract surgery achieved 20/40 (6/12) best spectacle-corrected visual acuity or better.

UNCORRECTED VISUAL ACUITY. Uncorrected visual acuity refers to the patient's vision in standard conditions with no extraocular optical correction. Unlike best-corrected visual acuity, there are several additional factors (such as pupil size, degree of refractive error, amount of regular astigmatism) that influence the measured visual acuity.[5,6,20] With best-corrected visual acuity, if the regular astigmatism is corrected completely, the amount of astigmatism and pupil size should not influence the measured visual acuity.

Uncorrected visual acuity is most useful in the evaluation of specialty lenses, such as multifocal and toric IOLs. The goal when using these lenses is to reduce or eliminate the patient's dependence on glasses. Unfortunately, the performance of such specialty lenses is related directly to the extent of postoperative corneal astigmatism, which in turn is related to the degree of preexisting astigmatism and the amount of surgically induced astigmatism. In patients who have less than 1.5D of postoperative astigmatism, the multifocal lenses substantially reduce the need for spectacles for reading compared with monofocal lenses, with a commensurate decrease in the contrast of the retinal image.[5,6,21]

TARGET REFRACTION PREDICTION ERROR. Another factor in the determination of uncorrected visual acuity is the ability to achieve the target postoperative refraction. Most surgeons target the majority of their patients for postoperative refractions in the range 0.0–0.5D. With newer IOL formulas, personalization of lens constants, and improvements in surgical technique, at least 50% of patients should have a spheroequivalent refraction within ±0.5D of the intended target, 90% of patients within 1D, and 99.9% within ±2D.[22,23] For compulsive surgeons whose staffs are dedicated to quality and attention to detail, 90% of patients are within ±0.5D. This performance is well above the prevailing standard of care and is a level to which all should aspire.

POTENTIAL RETINAL ACUITY TESTING. A special type of acuity test used in cataract patients is the assessment of potential retinal acuity. This test is essential for patients who have pigment mottling in the macula and reduced vision, particularly in the presence of a cataract or other optical aberrations of the eye. In the cataract age group, the incidence of macular degeneration is at least 10% and may exceed 15%, depending on the age of the patient. This test probably helps avoid unnecessary cataract surgery.

It is important that both the surgeon and the patient have realistic expectations about the quality of postsurgery vision, which helps both to assess the risk-benefit ratio. Studies showing the accuracy of this test are documented in the literature referenced earlier. Although there are different modalities, such as laser interferometry, super pinholes, entoptic phenomenon, and projected retinal acuity charts, all have been shown to be helpful in various situations. In dense, mature cataracts, the entoptic phenomenon is the only modality expected to function, because the others require some small optical window or windows for the transmission of coherent light. It is often difficult to show an exact correlation with final postoperative acuity because of changes that might occur as a result of the surgery (such as cystoid macular edema and optical irregularities in the cornea) that would not be expected to agree with the preoperative estimate.[15,17,24]

Removal of a significant cataract should always be considered, even in the presence of an abnormal macula or if the predicted acuity is low. Cataracts are progressive, they affect contrast sensitivity and glare, and even if the patient does not gain an improvement in acuity after cataract removal, a subjective improvement may occur, along with protection from vision degradation through progression of the cataract. Cataract surgery today encourages the surgeon to render the eye in the best optical condition, while advising the patient that preexisting disease will limit visual potential.

Contrast Sensitivity Testing

Contrast sensitivity testing assesses both sensory disease and media opacities. Contrast sensitivity has been documented as undergoing specific changes in many disorders, such as media opacities, generalized retinal disorders (e.g., diabetes), localized retinal disorders (e.g., macular degeneration and cystoid macular edema), and optic neuropathies (ranging from multiple sclerosis to ischemic optic neuropathy).[25–27]

With media opacities, such as cataracts, there is a general depression of contrast sensitivity at all points, with a slightly greater effect in the depression at the lower contrasts. The changes occurring with the sensory disorders mentioned earlier are much more specific, and when the contrast sensitivity curve is not depressed evenly, the clinician should be suspicious that the cataract is not the only reason for the reduced vision and visual complaints.

This is an area of active research in which types of stimuli (letter targets, sinusoidal and square-wave gratings), number of sample points, and methods of reporting are being standardized. However, there is no question of its value to the clinician. Figures 54-1 and 54-2 show the normal curves for contrast sensitivity tests using Snellen acuity letters and sinusoidal gratings. Cataracts uniformly reduce the contrast sensitivity for various object sizes, so the shape of the curve remains the same, with the curve being depressed (lowered) uniformly. Because the shape of the curve does not change when a cataract is the only pathology, the effect at lower contrast levels can often be predicted by

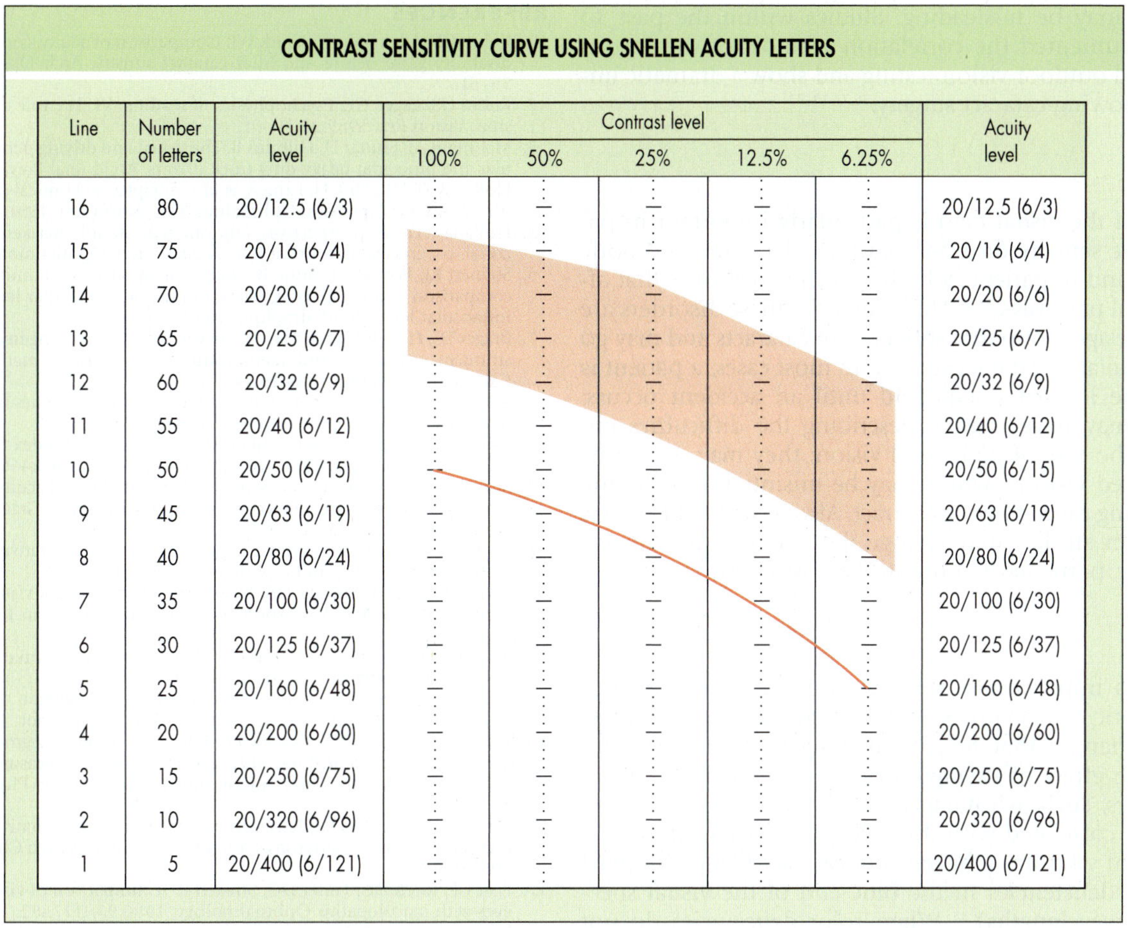

CONTRAST SENSITIVITY CURVE USING SNELLEN ACUITY LETTERS

Line	Number of letters	Acuity level	Contrast level					Acuity level
			100%	50%	25%	12.5%	6.25%	
16	80	20/12.5 (6/3)						20/12.5 (6/3)
15	75	20/16 (6/4)						20/16 (6/4)
14	70	20/20 (6/6)						20/20 (6/6)
13	65	20/25 (6/7)						20/25 (6/7)
12	60	20/32 (6/9)						20/32 (6/9)
11	55	20/40 (6/12)						20/40 (6/12)
10	50	20/50 (6/15)						20/50 (6/15)
9	45	20/63 (6/19)						20/63 (6/19)
8	40	20/80 (6/24)						20/80 (6/24)
7	35	20/100 (6/30)						20/100 (6/30)
6	30	20/125 (6/37)						20/125 (6/37)
5	25	20/160 (6/48)						20/160 (6/48)
4	20	20/200 (6/60)						20/200 (6/60)
3	15	20/250 (6/75)						20/250 (6/75)
2	10	20/320 (6/96)						20/320 (6/96)
1	5	20/400 (6/121)						20/400 (6/121)

FIG. 54-1 ■ **Contrast sensitivity curve using Snellen letters.** The shaded area represents the normal letter contrast sensitivity for all ages. Contrast sensitivities of younger individuals lie nearer the top of the shaded area, and those of older individuals are usually nearer the bottom. The single line corresponds to a 65-year-old patient with 20/50 (6/15) standard Snellen acuity.

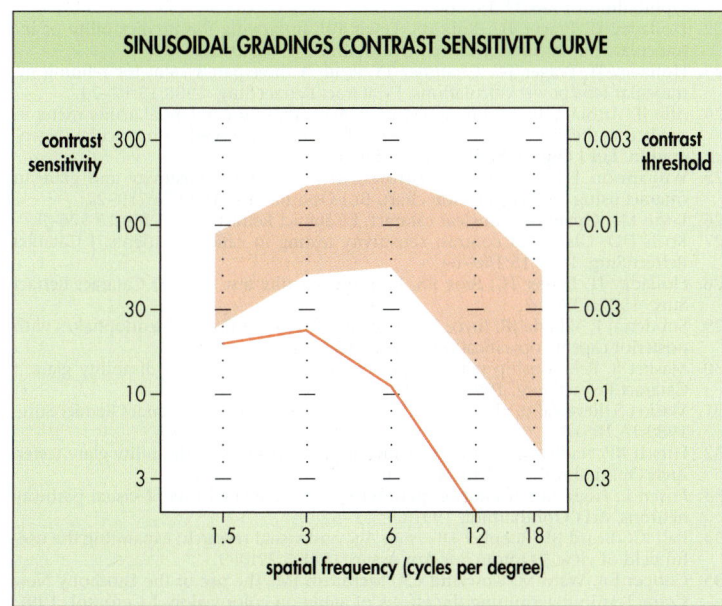

SINUSOIDAL GRADINGS CONTRAST SENSITIVITY CURVE

FIG. 54-2 ■ **Sinusoidal gradings contrast sensitivity curve.** The shaded area represents the normal sinusoidal gradings contrast sensitivity for all ages. Contrast sensitivities of younger individuals lie nearer the top of the shaded area, and those of older individuals are usually nearer the bottom. The single line corresponds to a 65-year-old patient with 20/30 (6/9) standard Snellen acuity.

Glare Testing

Glare testing is important in the assessment of media opacities such as cataracts. The effect is negligible in sensory disorders, except for the few macular disorders such as cystoid macular edema, where intraocular light scatter occurs in the superficial layers of the retina.[15,24] Even with this disorder, the changes in glare disability are minimal. Glare testing can be very sensitive and specific to media opacities, but more important, it gives visual acuity values or equivalents that relate to a person's vision in daylight, not in a dark room with high-contrast letters. Researchers and instrument developers have tried to simulate the patient's vision in daylight conditions (overcast days, clear days, etc.) without having to move the patient outside for testing. Although the design and specific characteristics of each of these instruments vary, the central theme is to simulate vision outside in daylight, in contrast to the dark examining room.[28]

Glare and contrast sensitivity testing have not yet been standardized completely and remain an area of active research and development. This has led the American Association of Ophthalmologists to develop associated modules. The value of glare testing to the clinician both to evaluate a patient's vision (as part of the diagnostic assessment) and to demonstrate improvement following cataract surgery is considerable.

It is important to realize that a patient's history of glare symptoms is difficult to interpret, because the meaning of the word "glare" is ambiguous to most patients. A patient often uses "glare" to describe unwanted images on spectacles or a windshield or originating from the sidewalk surface, which have nothing to do with the patient's visual symptoms, much less a cataract. The value of both glare testing and contrast sensitivity testing is to provide the clinician with objective data, to corroborate both examination and history. Without these tests, the pa-

the reduction in standard visual acuity. However, if routine preoperative tests reveal greater reduction in contrast sensitivity at lower contrasts, the clinician should be suspicious of a sensory defect. Following cataract surgery, in the absence of other ocular disease, the contrast sensitivity returns to normal.

tient's history may be misleading. Studies within the past 10 years have documented the correlation of most of the instruments used and outdoor vision testing and show a dramatic improvement following cataract surgery.[26,27,29–32]

Visual Fields

The integrity of the visual field is particularly important in patients who have sensory disorders, such as glaucoma and optic neuropathies, and in patients who have suffered strokes that affected the visual pathways.[33,34] Unfortunately, these disorders are common in the age group that suffers from cataracts and may go undetected until after cataract surgery. In most cases, a patient is unaware of the loss of visual field until an accident occurs. Patients also may have trouble describing the difficulties encountered by the loss of peripheral vision; they may use terms such as "reduced vision," which may be misinterpreted by the clinician as being caused by the cataract. Also, visual field defects that result from strokes may change the risk-benefit ratio for cataract surgery, particularly if the stroke was recent.

Color Vision

Color vision is important in sensory diseases such as retinopathies and optic neuropathies, which often show characteristic color vision changes that help in making the diagnosis and monitoring the effect of therapy. In patients who have ocular media disorders, such as cataracts, the changes in color vision can usually be correlated with the color of the cataract; for example, a patient who has a brunescent cataract (yellow-brown) has significant deficiencies in the blue end of the visual spectrum (shorter wavelengths).[35] When color deficiencies do not correlate, sensory disorders should be suspected.

Following cataract surgery in patients who have blue color deficiencies caused by the cataract, the return to normal color vision is important to some patients but unnoticed by others. The artist, the decorator, and the individual who appreciates the blue sky on a clear day all find such an improvement remarkable; some attribute the ability to continue in a chosen profession or avocation to the restoration of good-quality vision. Although color vision testing is very sensitive in disorders such as central serous maculopathy and cystoid macular edema, because of the "bleaching" or reduction of apparent brightness, other parameters such as visual acuity, visual field, and contrast sensitivity are also affected, which makes routine color testing unnecessary. In a patient who has a cataract and unusual color vision complaints, the results of color vision testing can be very helpful in diagnosing and treating the concomitant disease. Color vision returns to normal in the absence of other ocular disease.

SUMMARY

It is extremely important that the outcome of cataract surgery with respect to quality of life be evaluated, particularly because of the significant costs of this procedure. Any clinician realizes that a good history, thorough examination, and quantification of the five areas that describe functional vision are all important in determining the indications for surgery and its outcome.

REFERENCES

1. Rubin GS, Adamsons IA, Stark WJ. Comparison of acuity, contrast sensitivity, and disability glare before and after cataract surgery. Arch Ophthalmol. 1993;111: 56–61.
2. Rubin GS, Legge GE. Psychophysics of reading. VI. The role of contrast in low vision. Vision Res. 1989;29:79–91.
3. McKnight AJ, Shinar D, Hilburn B. The visual and driving performance of monocular and binocular heavy-duty truck drivers. Accid Anal Prev. 1991;23:225–37.
4. Holladay JT, Van Dijk H, Lang A, et al. Principles and optical performance of multifocal intraocular lenses. Ophthalmol Clin North Am. 1991;4:295–311.
5. Holladay JT. A prospective, randomized, double-masked comparison of a zonal–progressive multifocal IOL. A discussion. Ophthalmology. 1992;99:860.
6. Steinert RF, Post CT Jr, Brint SF, et al. A prospective, randomized, double-masked comparison of a zonal–progressive multifocal intraocular lens and a monofocal intraocular lens. Ophthalmology. 1992;99:853–60.
7. Prager TC, Urso RG, Holladay JT, Stewart RH. Glare testing in cataract patients: instrument evaluation and identification of sources of methodological error. J Cataract Refract Surg. 1989;15:149–57.
8. Miller ST, Graney MJ, Elam JT, et al. Predictions of outcomes from cataract surgery in elderly persons. Ophthalmology. 1988;95:1125–9.
9. Graney MJ, Applegate WB, Miller ST, et al. A clinical index for predicting visual acuity after cataract surgery. Am J Ophthalmol. 1988;105:460–5.
10. Strong N. Interferometer assessment of potential visual acuity before YAG capsulotomy: relative performance of three instruments. Graefes Arch Clin Exp Ophthalmol. 1992;230:42–6.
11. Faulkner W. Laser interferometric prediction of postoperative visual acuity in patients with cataracts. Am J Ophthalmol. 1983;95:626–36.
12. Tetz MR, Klein U, Volcker HE. Measurement of potential visual acuity in 343 patients with cataracts. A prospective clinical study. German J Ophthalmol. 1992; 1:403–8.
13. Severin TD, Severin SL. A clinical evaluation of the potential acuity meter in 210 cases. Ann Ophthalmol. 1988;20:373–5.
14. Sherman J, Davis E, Schnider C, et al. Presurgical prediction of postsurgical visual acuity in patients with media opacities. J Am Optom Assoc. 1988;59:481–8.
15. Barrett BT, Davison PA, Eustace PE. Effects of posterior segment disorders on oscillatory displacement thresholds, and on acuities as measured using the potential acuity meter and laser interferometer. Ophthalmic Physiol Opt. 1994;14: 132–8.
16. Datiles MB, Edwards PA, Kaiser-Kupfer MI, et al. A comparative study between the PAM and the laser interferometer in cataracts. Graefes Arch Clin Exp Ophthalmol. 1987;225:457–60.
17. Fish GE, Birch DG, Fuller DG, Straach R. A comparison of visual function tests in eyes with maculopathy. Ophthalmology. 1986;93:1177–82.
18. National Research Council Committee on Vision. Recommended standards for the clinical measurement and specification of visual acuity. Adv Ophthalmol. 1980;41:103–48.
19. Bailey IL, Lovie JE. New design principles for visual acuity letter charts. Am J Optom Physiol Opt. 1976;53:740–5.
20. Lindstrom RL. Food and Drug Administration update. One-year results from 671 patients with the 3M multifocal intraocular lens. Ophthalmology. 1993;100:91–7.
21. Holladay JT, Rubin ML. Avoiding refractive problems in cataract surgery. Surv Ophthalmol. 1988;32:357–60.
22. Holladay JT, Prager TC, Ruiz RS, Lewis JW. Improving the predictability of intraocular lens calculations. Arch Ophthalmol. 1986;104:539–41.
23. Holladay JT, Prager TC, Chandler TY, et al. A three-part system for refining intraocular lens power calculations. J Cataract Refract Surg. 1988;13:17–24.
24. Alio JL, Artola A, Ruiz-Moreno JM, et al. Accuracy of the potential acuity meter in predicting the visual outcome in cases of cataract associated with macular degeneration. Eur J Ophthalmol. 1993;3:189–92.
25. Williamson TH, Strong NP, Sparrow J, et al. Contrast sensitivity and glare in cataract using the Pelli-Robson chart. Br J Ophthalmol. 1992;76:719–22.
26. Levin ML. Opalescent nuclear cataract. J Cataract Refract Surg. 1989;15:576–9.
27. Koch DD. Glare and contrast sensitivity testing in cataract patients. J Cataract Refract Surg. 1989;15:158–64.
28. Holladay JT, Prager TC, Ruiz RS. Brightness acuity test (BAT). J Cataract Refract Surg. 1987;13:67–9.
29. Sunderraj P, Villada JR, Joyce PW, Watson A. Glare testing in pseudophakes with posterior capsule opacification. Eye. 1992;6:411–3.
30. Masket S. Relationship between postoperative pupil size and disability glare. J Cataract Refract Surg. 1992;18:506–7.
31. Masket S. Reversal of glare disability after cataract surgery. J Cataract Refract Surg. 1989;15:165–8.
32. Hirsch RP, Nadler MP, Miller D. Clinical performance of a disability glare tester. Arch Ophthalmol. 1984;102:1633–6.
33. Frisen L. High-pass resolution perimetry and age-related loss of visual pathway neurons. Acta Ophthalmol. 1991;69:511–5.
34. Ball KK, Beard BL, Roenker DL, et al. Age and visual research: expanding the useful field of view. J Optom Soc Am Assoc. 1988;5:2210–9.
35. Cooper BA, Ward M, Gowland CA, McIntosh JM. The use of the Lanthony New Color Test in determining the effects of aging on color vision. J Gerontol. 1991; 46:320–4.

CORNEA AND EXTERNAL DISEASE

Joel Sugar

CHAPTER 55

Disorders of the Conjunctiva and Limbus

JONATHAN B. RUBENSTEIN • SHARON L. JICK

CONGENITAL ANOMALIES

Choristomas

Choristomas are common congenital lesions that possess little growth potential. They contain both dermal and epithelial elements that are not normally found in the conjunctiva. Three types of conjunctival choristomas are found—the solid limbal dermoid, the more diffuse dermolipoma, and the complex choristoma.

Solid limbal dermoids are compact, pale yellow growths that typically occur unilaterally at the inferotemporal limbus (Fig. 55-1).[1] Most limbal dermoids are superficial and only minimally involve the cornea and sclera. However, some tumors can penetrate deeply into the cornea, sclera, and conjunctiva. Surgical excision usually involves shaving the lesion off the cornea and sclera; however, complete excision of the dermoid may require reconstruction with lamellar or penetrating keratoplasty.[2] Histological examination reveals a thick, collagenous lesion that may contain hair, sweat glands, fat, sebaceous glands, or teeth (Fig. 55-2). Eyelid colobomas may occur in association with limbal dermoids, which suggests the postulate that both anomalies may result from incomplete fusion of the lids with displacement of skin elements into the dermoid tumor.[1]

Dermolipomas are less dense than solid dermoids and contain more adipose tissue. These are true choristomas, because fatty tissue is usually not found anterior to the orbital septum. They are typically found on the superior temporal bulbar conjunctiva.[3] These masses can extend from the limbus anteriorly to the posterior aspect of the globe and orbit between the superior and lateral rectus. Care must be taken during surgical removal not to damage the extraocular muscles, levator, or lacrimal gland.[4] Usually, surgery is restricted to partial resection of the anterior portion of the tumor.

Bilateral limbal dermoids or dermolipomas are found in children who have Goldenhar's syndrome (oculoauriculovertebral dysplasia).[5,6] Unilateral colobomas of the upper lid may also be seen, along with iris colobomas and aniridia. Other systemic features of this first branchial arch syndrome include preauricular skin tags, blind-ended preauricular fistulas, hypoplasia of the facial bones, and other vertebral anomalies.

Complex choristomas consist of variable combinations of ectopic tissues such as cartilage, adipose tissue, smooth muscle, and acinar glands. Clinically, these lesions resemble dermoids and lipodermoids.[4] When acinar elements compose the majority of the tumor, complex choristomas may assume a fleshier, vascularized appearance with raised translucent nodules. These raised nodules have been referred to as ectopic lacrimal glands.[5] Although mild growth may occur, especially during puberty, malignant transformation is rare. As these tumors also tend to invade deeply into the globe, excision is usually avoided.

Epibulbar Osseous Choristomas

Osseous choristomas are solitary nodules that resemble dermoids. However, they can be differentiated from dermoids clinically because of their location 5–10mm posterior to the limbus[4] and their more discrete borders. They are composed of mature, compact bone along with other typical choristomatous elements such as pilosebaceous units and hair follicles. Usually, excision is performed for cosmetic reasons only.[7,8]

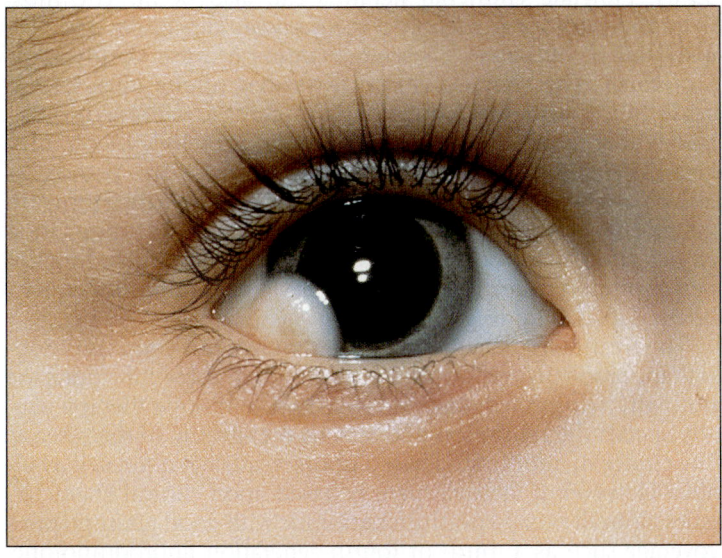

FIG. 55-1 ▌ **Limbal dermoid in a 5-year-old child.** This is typically located at the inferotemporal limbus.

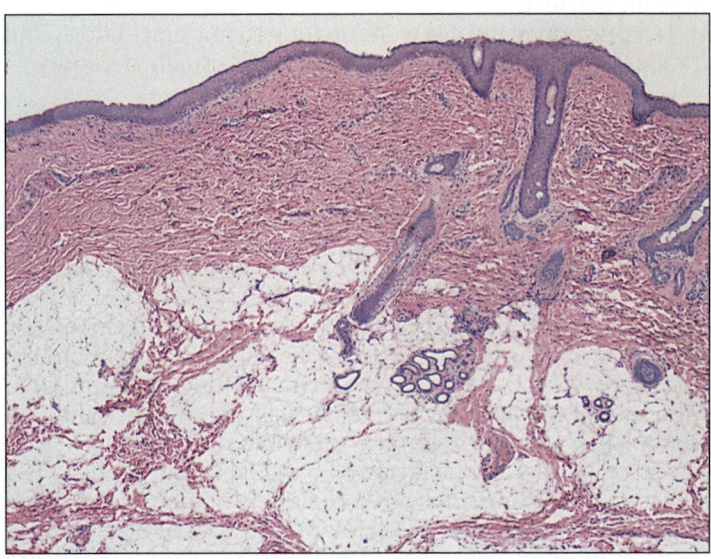

FIG. 55-2 ▌ **Corneal dermoid.** Histological section shows epidermis, dermis, epidermal appendages, and adipose tissue.

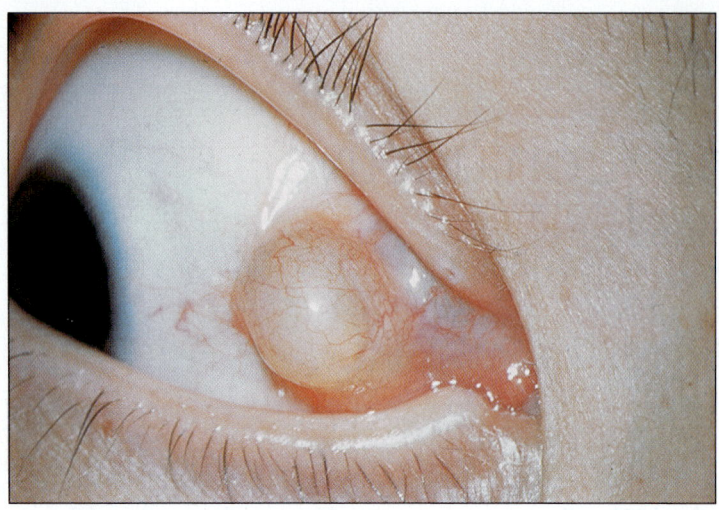

FIG. 55-3 ■ **Epithelial inclusion cyst.** This cyst occurred at the site of a conjunctival incision that accompanied muscle surgery.

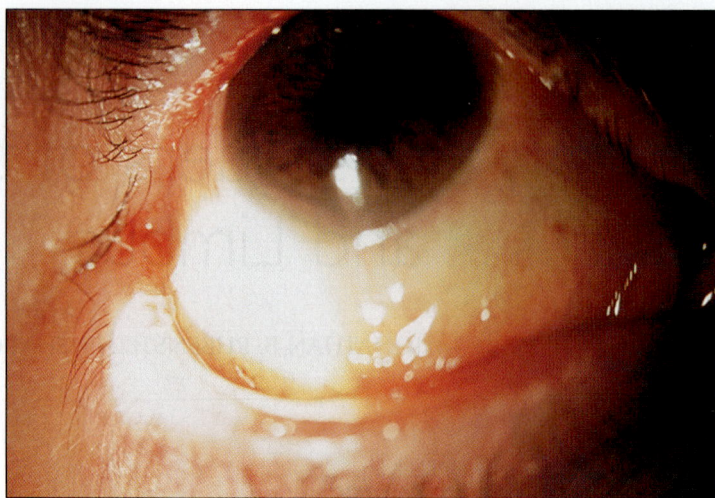

FIG. 55-4 ■ **Conjunctival amyloidosis.** Associated with primary systemic amyloidosis.

Epithelial Cysts

Epithelial inclusion cysts can be found in both the bulbar and palpebral conjunctiva. They are filled with clear fluid and lined with nonkeratinized, stratified squamous epithelium (Fig. 55-3). They remain symptom free and present only a cosmetic concern. Treatment, if desired, consists of simple excision; however, these cysts can recur.

AMYLOIDOSIS

Amyloid, an avascular, noncollagenous protein, may be deposited in the conjunctiva, cornea, adnexal tissues, vitreous, retina, choroid, ciliary body, and orbit. Ocular involvement is most common in primary systemic or localized amyloidosis but may also occur as secondary localized amyloidosis associated with trichiasis, trachoma, chronic keratitis, keratoconus, and stromal corneal dystrophies.[1] Conjunctival amyloidosis is usually asymptomatic. It presents as a discrete, nontender, nonulcerative, waxy, yellow-white, firm subconjunctival mass. It is most often found in the inferior fornix but can also occur anywhere on the bulbar conjunctiva or at the limbus (Fig. 55-4).[3]

Usually, the diagnosis is suspected on clinical grounds; however, definite diagnosis is made on the basis of biopsy. The histochemical reactions include birefringence and dichroism with Congo red, metachromasia with crystal violet, and fluorescence with thioflavin-T.

Treatment may involve work-up for systemic amyloidosis, but local excision of conjunctival masses is not usually necessary.

INFECTIONS
Bacterial Infections

Bacterial conjunctivitis, which is uncommon, is characterized by a rapid onset of unilateral conjunctival hyperemia, lid edema, and mucopurulent discharge. The second eye typically becomes involved 1–2 days later.

The pathogenesis of bacterial conjunctivitis usually involves a disruption of the host defense mechanisms. Examples are abnormalities of the ocular surface secondary to eyelid abnormalities, surface trauma, tear film abnormalities, or a preceding infection such as herpes simplex.[9] Systemic immunosuppression may also increase the incidence of bacterial conjunctivitis.[9,10]

Bacterial conjunctivitis can be classified into three clinical types—acute, hyperacute, and chronic (Table 55-1). The most common conjunctival pathogens include *Staphylococcus, Streptococcus pneumoniae, Haemophilus* species, *Moraxella, Corynebacterium diphtheriae, Neisseria* species, and enteric gram-negative rods.[9]

TABLE 55-1

PATHOGENS THAT CAUSE BACTERIAL CONJUNCTIVITIS

Acute	Hyperacute	Chronic
Staphylococcus aureus	*Neisseria gonorrhoeae*	*Staphylococcus aureus*
Streptococcus pneumoniae	*Neisseria meningitidis*	*Moraxella lacunata*
Haemophilus influenzae		Enteric bacteria

Conjunctival membranes and pseudomembranes are among the findings associated with bacterial conjunctivitis and may be produced in association with *Neisseria gonorrhoeae*, β-hemolytic streptococci, and *C. diphtheriae*, among others. Pseudomembranes are a combination of inflammatory cells and an exudate that contains mucus and proteins (Fig. 55-5). They are loosely adherent to the underlying conjunctival epithelium and can be peeled away with no bleeding or damage to the epithelium. True membranes occur with more intense inflammation. The conjunctival epithelium becomes necrotic, and firmer adhesions are formed between the necrotic cells and the overlying coagulum. When the membrane is peeled, the epithelium tears to leave a raw, bleeding surface.

ACUTE BACTERIAL CONJUNCTIVITIS. Acute bacterial conjunctivitis usually begins unilaterally with hyperemia, irritation, tearing, mucopurulent discharge, and mattering of the lids (Fig. 55-6). Punctate epithelial keratitis can also occur. The most common pathogens include *Staphylococcus aureus*, *Str. pneumoniae*, and *H. influenzae*.[9] The most common cause worldwide is *Str. aureus*. The characteristic disease that results ranges from acute mucopurulent conjunctivitis to chronic, smoldering disease. Other common ocular manifestations include blepharitis, keratitis, marginal ulcers, and phlyctenulosis.[11] The pathogens *Str. pneumoniae* and *H. influenzae* occur more commonly in young children and may occur in institutional epidemics. Often *H. influenzae* is associated with systemic infection, including upper respiratory infection and fever. Systemic antibiotics should be used if such findings are present.

The treatment of acute bacterial conjunctivitis consists of topical antibiotic drops or ointments. Although these infections are normally self-limited, lasting 7–10 days, antibiotic therapy usually speeds the resolution and lessens the severity of the disease. The choice of antibiotic is based upon results of cultures, if available. However, if the treatment is based upon clinical characteristics alone, a broad-spectrum antibiotic with good gram-positive coverage such as a third- or fourth-generation fluoroquinolone, 10% sodium sulfacetamide, or trimethoprim-polymyxin may be used for 7–10 days.

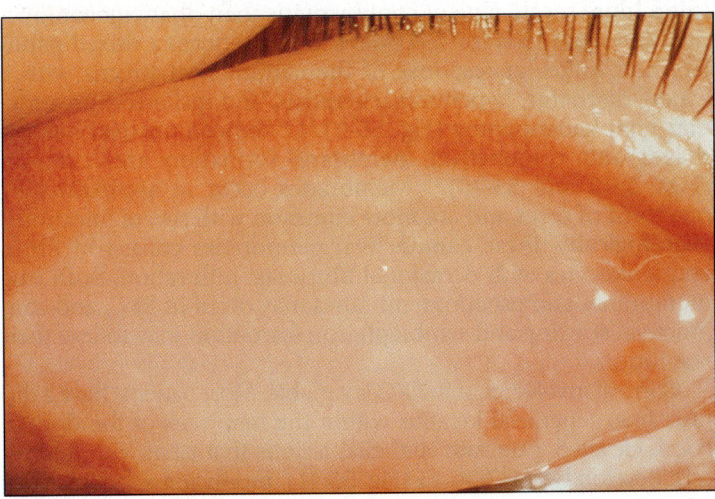

FIG. 55-5 ▌ **Pseudomembrane.** A combination of inflammatory cells, mucus, and protein exudate covers the superior tarsal conjunctiva.

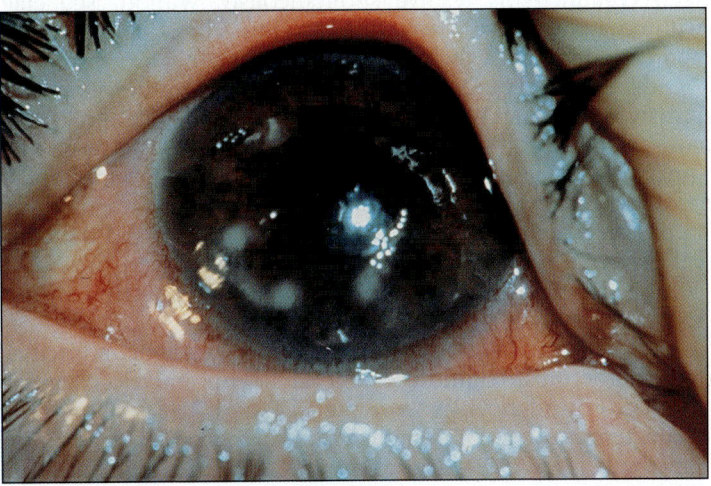

FIG. 55-7 ▌ **Staphylococcal marginal keratitis.** Note the inferior marginal corneal ulcers and the blepharoconjunctivitis.

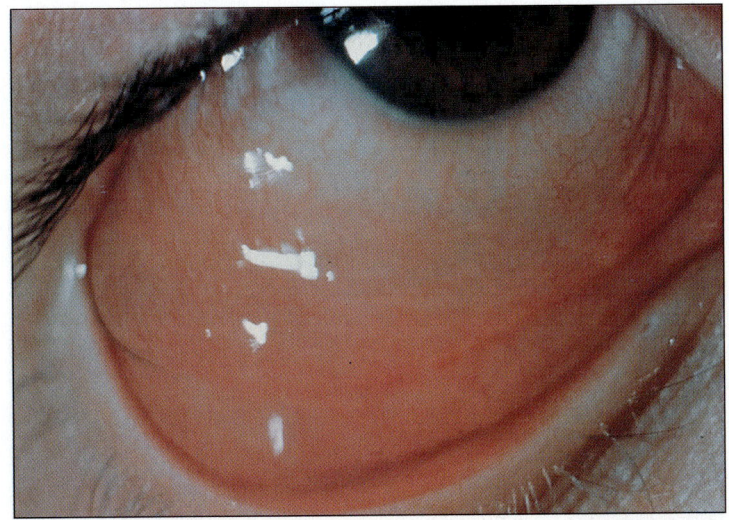

FIG. 55-6 ▌ **Acute bacterial conjunctivitis.** This patient was culture positive for pneumococcus.

HYPERACUTE BACTERIAL CONJUNCTIVITIS. The most common cause of hyperacute bacterial conjunctivitis is *N. gonorrhoeae*.[9] This oculogenital disease is seen primarily in neonates and sexually active young adults. A careful history helps to identify contacts that may be in need of antibiotic treatment. Signs include profuse, thick, yellow-green purulent discharge, painful hyperemia, chemosis of the conjunctiva, and tender preauricular nodes. Untreated cases may lead to peripheral corneal ulceration and eventual perforation with possible endophthalmitis. A similar, but somewhat milder, form of conjunctival and corneal disease is caused by *N. meningitidis*.[12]

The treatment of hyperacute bacterial conjunctivitis is directed at the specific pathogen. Conjunctival scraping for Gram stain and culture on blood and chocolate agar are strongly suggested. If gram-negative diplococci are seen, suspect gonococcus. Gonococcal conjunctivitis is treated with both topical and systemic antibiotics. An effective regimen includes 1g of intramuscular ceftriaxone followed by a 2- to 3-week course of oral tetracycline or erythromycin. Topical medications may include penicillin (333,000U/ml) or bacitracin or erythromycin ointment every 2 hours. As large amounts of tenacious discharge occur, frequent irrigation of the ocular surface is helpful. Patients need to be seen daily in case of corneal involvement.

CHRONIC BACTERIAL CONJUNCTIVITIS. Chronic bacterial conjunctivitis, which is defined by a duration of longer than 3 weeks, may result from a number of organisms. The most common of these are *S. aureus* and *Mo. lacunata;* other causative organisms include the enteric bacteria *Proteus mirabilis, Escherichia coli, Klebsiella pneumoniae,* and *Serratia marcescens* and *Branhamella catarrhalis* from the upper respiratory tract.[9] The most common causative agent in chronic bacterial blepharoconjunctivitis is *S. aureus,* which colonizes the eyelid margin, from which it causes direct infection of the conjunctiva or conjunctival inflammation through its elaboration of exotoxins.[13] Chronic angular blepharoconjunctivitis of the inner and outer canthal angles most commonly results from *Mo. lacunata.* A chronic follicular conjunctivitis may accompany both chronic angular blepharoconjunctivitis and chronic staphylococcal conjunctivitis.

The clinical signs of chronic staphylococcal conjunctivitis include diffuse conjunctival hyperemia with either papillae or follicles, minimal mucopurulent discharge, and conjunctival thickening. Eyelid involvement may comprise redness, telangiectasis, lash loss, collarettes, recurrent hordeolae, and ulcerations at the base of the cilia. Chronic staphylococcal blepharoconjunctivitis may lead to marginal corneal ulcers (Fig. 55-7), which usually occur along the inferior limbus and probably result from an immune-mediated reaction to staphylococcal toxins. Maceration and crusting of the lateral canthal angle are seen in chronic angular blepharitis caused by *Moraxella* species. Corneal findings include an inferior punctate epithelial keratitis.

The treatment of chronic bacterial conjunctivitis combines proper antimicrobial therapy and good lid hygiene, which includes hot compresses and eyelid scrubs. Scrubs may be performed using a commercial product or a dilute, gentle shampoo applied with a washcloth, followed by complete rinsing with lukewarm water. Erythromycin and bacitracin ointments are effective adjunct topical antibiotics. When severe inflammation exists, antibiotic and corticosteroid combination drops or ointments can be rubbed into the lid margins after the eye scrubs. Oral therapy with tetracycline 250mg four times a day or doxycycline 100mg twice a day may be needed for more severe infections.

Viral Infections

Viral conjunctivitis is extremely common and is one of the most frequent reasons for visits to an emergency room or doctor's office. The diagnosis can usually be made clinically, so viral culture and laboratory investigation are rarely undertaken.[13] Viral conjunctivitis usually has an acute onset, unilateral at first, with involvement of the second eye within 1 week. It is manifested by a watery discharge and conjunctival hyperemia and is usually accompanied by preauricular lymphadenopathy on the affected side. Most cases of viral conjunctivitis resolve spontaneously, without sequelae, within days to weeks. Many different viruses cause conjunctivitis, and each produces a slightly different disease.

Adenoviruses produce two of the most common viral conjunctivitides, pharyngoconjunctival fever and epidemic keratoconjunctivitis. Of the 41 adenovirus serotypes, 19 can cause conjunctivitis.[14] These infections are spread via respiratory droplets or direct contact from fingers to the lids and conjunctival surface. The incubation period is usually 5–12 days, and the clinical illness is present for 5–15 days.[15] After recovery, immunocompetent hosts are protected from further infection by the specific serotype that caused the infection.

PHARYNGOCONJUNCTIVAL FEVER. Pharyngoconjunctival fever is the most common ocular adenoviral infection[16] and is produced by adenovirus serotypes 3, 4, and 7. It is a condition characterized by a combination of pharyngitis, fever, and conjunctivitis (Fig. 55-8). The conjunctivitis is predominantly follicular with a scant watery discharge, hyperemia, and mild chemosis. The cornea may be involved with a fine punctate epitheliopathy, and preauricular lymph nodes are enlarged in about 90% of cases. As the disease resolves spontaneously within 2 weeks, treatment is usually supportive with cold compresses, artificial tears, and vasoconstrictor eyedrops.

EPIDEMIC KERATOCONJUNCTIVITIS. Another common form of viral conjunctivitis is epidemic keratoconjunctivitis (EKC), usually produced by adenovirus serotypes 8, 19, and 37.

It is a more severe type of conjunctivitis than pharyngoconjunctival fever and lasts for 7–21 days. EKC produces a mixed papillary and follicular response of the conjunctival stroma with a watery discharge, hyperemia, chemosis, and ipsilateral preauricular lymphadenopathy (Fig. 55-9).[13,17] Subconjunctival hemorrhages and conjunctival membrane formation are common (Figs. 55-9 and 55-10).[18] Membranes occur in approximately one third of cases and are more common with severe infections. Histologically, these conjunctival membranes consist of fibrin and leukocytes with occasional fibroblast infiltration. Both true membranes and pseudomembranes may occur in EKC, and conjunctival scarring and symblepharon formation may follow their resolution.

Corneal involvement in EKC is variable. Most patients have a diffuse, fine, superficial keratitis within the first week of the disease. Focal, elevated, punctate epithelial lesions that stain with fluorescein develop by day 6 to 13 (Fig. 55-11), producing a foreign body sensation. By day 14, subepithelial opacities develop under the focal epithelial lesions in 20–50% of cases (Fig. 55-12). Often, these opacities are visually disabling and may persist for months to years, but eventually they resolve with no scarring or vascularization.[19]

Treatment of EKC consists of amelioration of symptoms and minimization of transmission of this highly contagious disease. Patients may be infectious for up to 14 days after onset,[18,20,21] and outbreaks are especially common in ophthalmology offices and clinics. Transmission usually occurs from eye to fingers to eye,

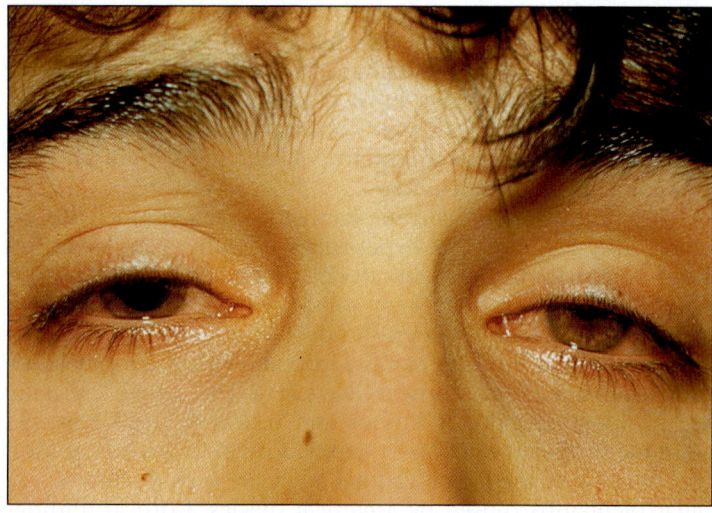

FIG. 55-8 ■ **Acute bilateral viral conjunctivitis.** This 22-year-old man has pharyngoconjunctival fever, and the conjunctivitis was preceded by a viral upper respiratory tract infection.

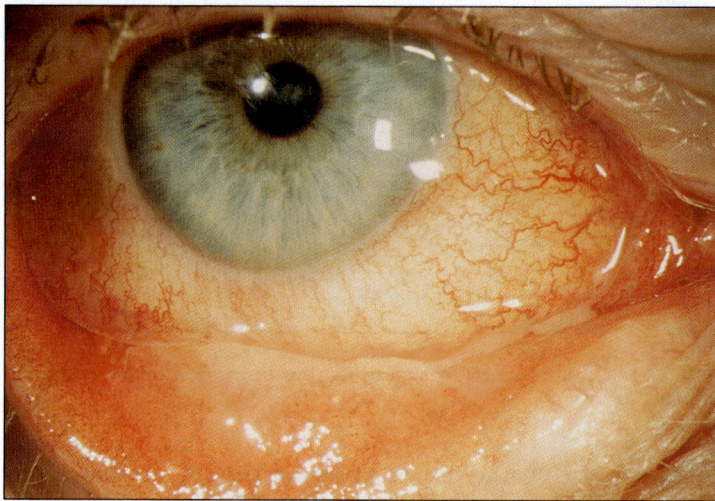

FIG. 55-10 ■ **Pseudomembrane in epidemic keratoconjunctivitis.** An early pseudomembrane is forming in the inferior fornix.

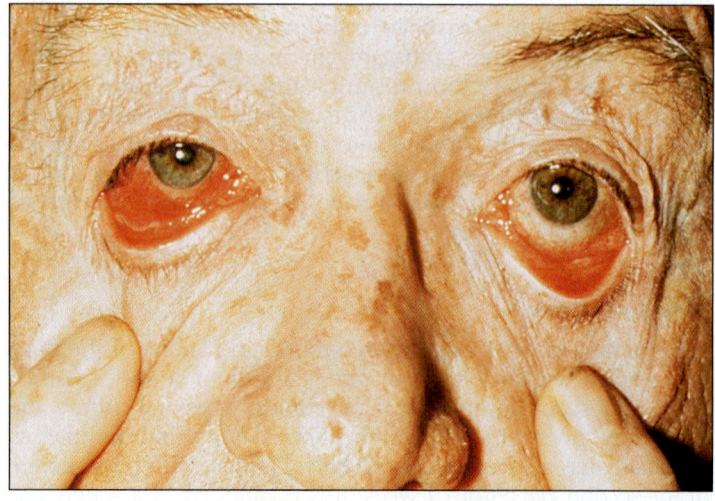

FIG. 55-9 ■ **Epidemic keratoconjunctivitis.** Early pseudomembrane formation may be seen in the inferior fornix.

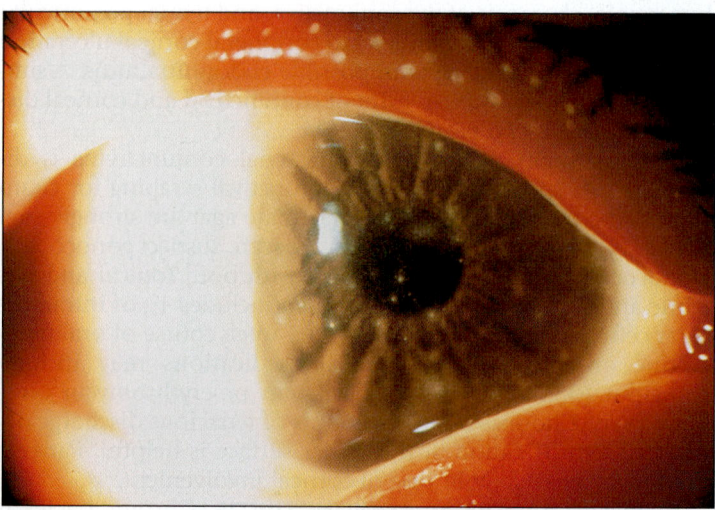

FIG. 55-11 ■ **Epidemic keratoconjunctivitis subepithelial infiltrates.** These infiltrates develop 2 weeks after the onset of the disease and persist for months to years.

but tonometers, contact lenses, and eyedrops are other routes of transmission. Preventive measures include frequent hand washing, relative isolation of infected individuals in an office setting, and disinfection of ophthalmic instruments.[22,23] During the stage of acute conjunctivitis, treatment is usually supportive and includes cold compresses and decongestant eyedrops. An antihistamine drop may be considered in cases of severe itching. When patients have decreased visual acuity or disabling photophobia from subepithelial opacities, topical corticosteroid therapy may be beneficial. High-dose topical corticosteroids, such as 1% prednisolone acetate three to four times a day, eliminate the subepithelial infiltrates.[24] Cidofovir, an antiviral agent, has been investigated in the treatment of EKC.[25,26] Although the application of cidofovir drops may prevent the formation of corneal opacities, use has been limited by local toxicity, and a commercial product is not yet available.

ACUTE HEMORRHAGIC CONJUNCTIVITIS. Acute hemorrhagic conjunctivitis, also known as Apollo disease, was first described in Ghana during the time of the lunar landing mission of 1969.[27] Two picornaviruses, enterovirus 70 and coxsackievirus A24, are the usual causative agents.[3,28] The signs of the disease include rapid onset of severe, painful papillary conjunctivitis with chemosis, tearing, and the development of tiny subconjunctival hemorrhages. The hemorrhages are petechial at first and then coalesce. The cornea may be involved with a fine punctate keratopathy but rarely with subepithelial opacities. The conjunctivitis resolves within 4–6 days, but the hemorrhages clear more slowly. The disease tends to occur in epidemics, especially in developing countries, with more than 50% of the local population affected in some cases.

HERPES SIMPLEX CONJUNCTIVITIS. Primary herpes simplex conjunctivitis usually occurs in children under 5 years of age. Most cases go undiscovered and undocumented because of their nonspecific nature. Typical signs include ocular irritation, watery discharge, follicular conjunctivitis, and preauricular lymphadenopathy. Epidermal vesicular eruptions of the eyelids and lid margins may accompany the conjunctivitis (Fig. 55-13), and the cornea may be involved. Corneal involvement may include a coarse, punctate epithelial keratitis, marginal infiltrates, or a dendritic ulcer (see Chapter 62). Although herpetic blepharoconjunctivitis is associated mainly with the primary disease, it may occur as a manifestation of recurrent disease with or without typical herpetic keratitis.[15] Most ocular herpetic infections result from herpes simplex virus type 1. Infections that result from the type 2 serotype may be seen in newborns or adults who have a history of orogenital contact.[29,30]

The conjunctivitis usually resolves spontaneously without treatment, although some physicians administer topical antiviral drops to patients with corneal involvement or to patients with lid vesicles with the goal of preventing corneal involvement. Care should be taken to avoid the cavalier use of corticosteroids in the treatment of patients who have acute follicular conjunctivitis, as some of these patients may have herpetic disease and corticosteroids may enhance the severity of herpetic epithelial keratitis.

OTHER CAUSES. Other causes of viral conjunctivitis include the rubella, rubeola, varicella-zoster, Epstein-Barr, and Newcastle disease viruses.[3] Rubella virus produces a nondescript, catarrhal conjunctivitis associated with the systemic disease, and a follicular reaction may occur. Rubeola produces a catarrhal, papillary conjunctivitis with tearing, pain, and photophobia. Pale, discrete, avascular spots, which resemble Koplik's spots seen in the mouth, may appear on the conjunctiva. Varicella-zoster virus produces pustules and phlyctenule-like lesions on the conjunctiva, and a follicular conjunctivitis may occur with the recurrent skin disease. The follicular conjunctivitis associated with the Epstein-Barr virus occurs in association with infectious mononucleosis.[31] Newcastle disease viral conjunctivitis occurs in poultry workers and veterinarians in whom direct conjunctival inoculation of the virus has occurred while infected birds are handled.[32] The disease is self-limited, lasts 7–10 days, and leaves no ocular sequelae.

Chronic Follicular Conjunctivitis

A follicular conjunctivitis that lasts for more than 16 days is considered to be a chronic follicular conjunctivitis (Box 55-1).[13] *Chlamydia trachomatis* is the most common cause of chronic follicular conjunctivitis; the organism causes three clinical syndromes—trachoma, adult inclusion conjunctivitis, and neonatal conjunctivitis.

TRACHOMA. Trachoma results from *C. trachomatis* serotypes A–C, is endemic in many parts of the world, and is especially prevalent in areas of close human contact and poor hygiene. Blinding trachoma still occurs in parts of Africa, the Middle East, India, and Southeast Asia. Trachoma begins as a follicular con-

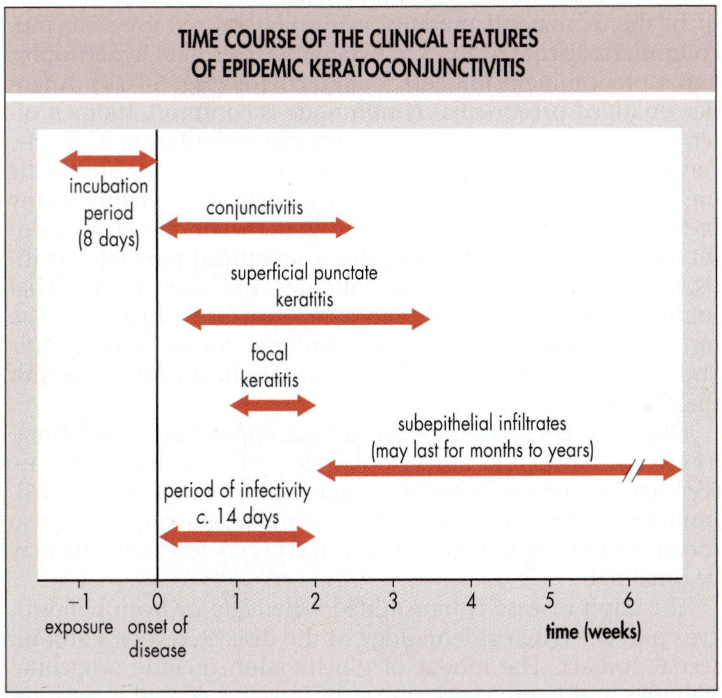

TIME COURSE OF THE CLINICAL FEATURES OF EPIDEMIC KERATOCONJUNCTIVITIS

incubation period (8 days)

conjunctivitis

superficial punctate keratitis

focal keratitis

subepithelial infiltrates (may last for months to years)

period of infectivity c. 14 days

−1 exposure, 0 onset of disease, 1, 2, 3, 4, 5, 6 time (weeks)

FIG. 55-12 ▌ Time course of the clinical features of epidemic keratoconjunctivitis.

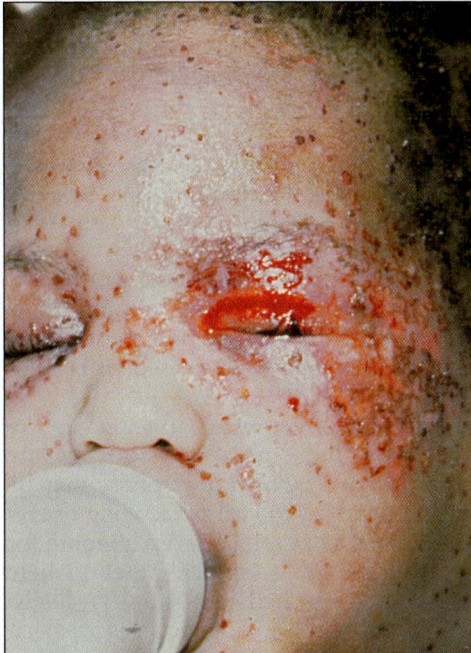

FIG. 55-13 ▌ Primary herpes simplex blepharoconjunctivitis. Note the bilateral vesicular eruptions in this child who has a primary herpes simplex infection.

BOX 55-1

Causes of Chronic Follicular Conjunctivitis

Chlamydial
- trachoma
- adult inclusion conjunctivitis

Molluscum contagiosum
Drug-induced or toxic
Bacterial
Axenfeld's chronic follicular conjunctivitis
Merrill–Thygeson type follicular conjunctivitis
Parinaud's oculoglandular syndrome
Folliculosis of childhood

TABLE 55-2

MACCALLAN CLASSIFICATION OF TRACHOMA

Stage	Description
I	Early lymphoid hyperplasia with immature follicle formation on the superior tarsal conjunctiva, diffuse punctate keratitis, and early pannus
IIA	Mature follicles on the superior tarsus
IIB	Florid inflammation with increases in pretarsal and limbal follicular and papillary hypertrophy and increasing pannus
III	Resolution of papillary hypertrophy, continued tarsal follicles, and early conjunctival cicatrization
IV	No active inflammation; replacement of papillae and follicles with scar and resolution of pannus

Stages of the disease based upon conjunctival findings.

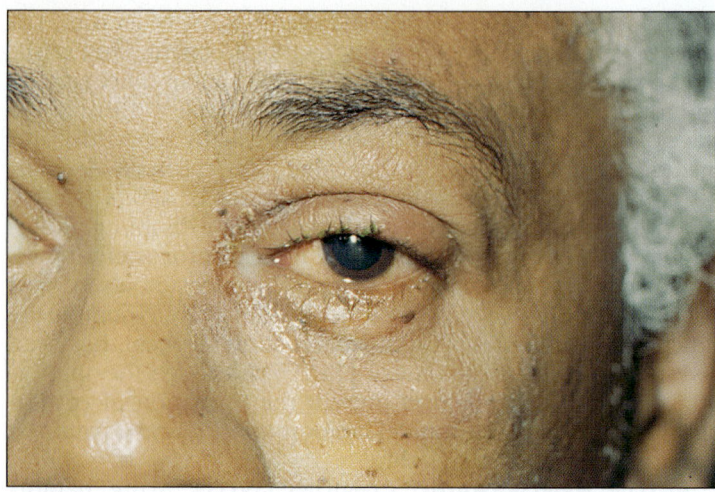

FIG. 55-14 ■ **Adult inclusion conjunctivitis.** This 50-year-old man had prominent follicular conjunctivitis with a large and tender preauricular lymph node.

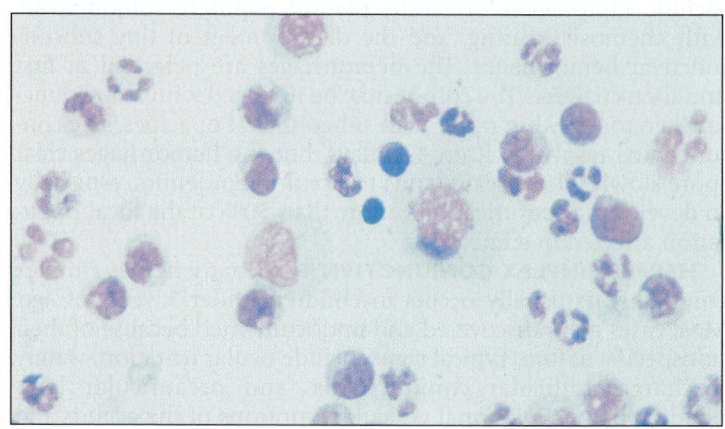

FIG. 55-15 ■ **Giemsa stain of a conjunctival scraping.** The epithelial cells show basophilic cytoplasmic inclusions typical of a chlamydial infection.

junctivitis of the upper palpebral conjunctiva with associated limbal follicles. Other early findings include conjunctival papillary hypertrophy, a mucopurulent discharge, a superiorly based superficial corneal pannus, and a fine epithelial keratitis. Eventually, the inflammation leads to scarring and cicatrization of the cornea, conjunctiva, and eyelids. In 1908, MacCallan divided the disease into four stages based on the conjunctival findings (Table 55-2). The World Health Organization has also developed a grading system for trachoma, structured around the presence or absence of follicular conjunctivitis, diffuse inflammation, tarsal scarring, trichiasis, and corneal opacification.[33]

The complications of trachoma that cause blindness occur as a result of corneal ulceration and scarring secondary to severe conjunctival scarring and eyelid deformities.[34] Proliferation of connective tissue in the conjunctiva results in cicatrization. Arlt's line (a horizontal line that results from conjunctival scarring at the junction of the anterior one third and posterior two thirds of the conjunctiva) is a characteristic finding on the superior pretarsal conjunctiva. Herbert's pits are a unique sequel of trachoma[35]; these sharply delineated depressions occur after cicatrization of the limbal follicles, and the resultant clear space is filled with epithelium. A diffuse haze of the superior cornea can result after regression of the superior pannus.

Eyelid deformities such as trichiasis, distichiasis, entropion, and ectropion may all occur. Resulting corneal complications include scarring, vascularization, ulceration, and perforation. The resultant poor ocular surface leads to decreased visual acuity and possible blindness.

Treatment of trachoma usually consists of a 3- to 4-week course of oral tetracycline (tetracycline 1g/day or doxycycline 100mg/day) or oral erythromycin. The clinical response may be slow and take 9–18 weeks. Therefore, topical tetracycline or erythromycin ointment is used twice a day for 5 days each month for 6 months.[14] Repeated topical therapy is especially useful where the disease is endemic and repeated exposure is likely. Widespread use of systemic antibiotics in endemic areas has been tried in an attempt to eradicate the disease. Oral azithromycin has shown promise in this regard.[36,37]

ADULT INCLUSION CONJUNCTIVITIS. Adult inclusion conjunctivitis results from *C. trachomatis* serotypes D–K, which cause a chronic follicular conjunctivitis that can occur in adults or in the neonate. It presents as a unilateral red eye with mucopurulent discharge, marked hyperemia, papillary hypertrophy, and a predominant follicular conjunctivitis (Fig. 55-14). A tender, enlarged preauricular lymph node is common. Women often have a concomitant vaginal discharge secondary to a chronic cervicitis, and men may have symptomatic or nonsymptomatic urethritis. The conjunctivitis is often chronic, lasting many months. Keratitis may develop during the second week after onset. Corneal involvement includes a superficial punctate keratitis, small marginal or central infiltrates, EKC-like subepithelial infiltrates, limbal swelling, and a superior limbal pannus. The untreated disease has a chronic, remittent course, and keratitis and possible iritis occur more commonly in the later stages of the disease.

Diagnosis is based upon the clinical appearance plus laboratory tests. Basophilic intracytoplasmic epithelial inclusions are seen with Giemsa staining of conjunctival scrapings (Fig. 55-15). Immunofluorescent staining of the conjunctival scrapings is also useful. Serum immunoglobulin G (IgG) titers to chlamydia may be obtained.

The adult disease is transmitted venereally or from hand-to-eye contact.[38] The epidemiology of the disease revolves around sexual contact. The modes of transmission include orogenital activities and hand-to-eye spread of infective genital secretions. The incubation period is 4–12 days. It is estimated that 1 in 300 patients who have genital chlamydial disease develops adult inclusion conjunctivitis.[39] It is important to treat all sexual part-

TABLE 55-3

CAUSES OF NEONATAL CONJUNCTIVITIS

Causes	Time of Onset (Postpartum)
Chemical (silver nitrate)	1–36 hours
Chlamydia	5–14 days
Neisseria gonorrhoeae	24–48 hours
Bacteria (*Staphylococcus, Streptococcus, Haemophilus*)	2–5 days
Virus (herpes simplex virus types 1 and 2)	3–15 days

The cause of the conjunctivitis is established by the clinical picture, time course, and laboratory confirmation.

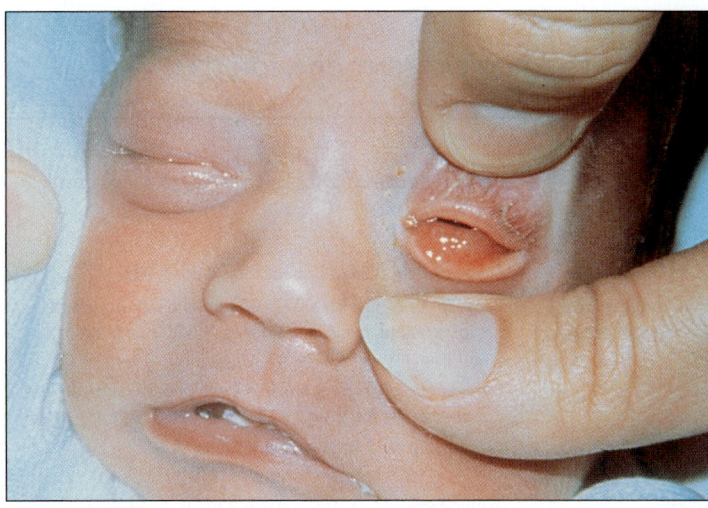

FIG. 55-16 ▌ **A 10-day-old infant who has unilateral conjunctivitis.** The mother had an untreated chlamydial infection of the birth canal.

ners simultaneously to prevent reinfection. It also is prudent to examine all sexual partners for other venereal diseases, such as gonorrhea and syphilis. Treatment consists of systemic antibiotics, as topical antibiotics are relatively ineffective in the treatment of the eye disease. Recommended treatment, which is given for 3 weeks, includes either oral tetracycline 500mg four times a day, oral doxycycline 100mg twice a day, or oral erythromycin stearate 500mg four times a day. Tetracycline should be avoided in children younger than 7 years of age and in pregnant or lactating women.

NEONATAL CONJUNCTIVITIS (OPHTHALMIA NEONATORUM). Conjunctivitis of the newborn is defined as any conjunctivitis that occurs within the first 4 weeks of life (Table 55-3).[40] It may be caused by a bacterial, viral, or chlamydial infection or by a toxic response to topically applied chemicals. Because the infectious agent may produce a severe localized infection of the eye plus a potentially serious systemic infection, precise identification of the cause is essential.

A number of factors contribute to neonatal conjunctivitis, including the following:

- Organisms harbored in the mother's birth canal,
- Maternal infections during pregnancy,
- Exposure of the infant to infectious organisms,
- Inadequacy of ocular prophylaxis immediately after birth,
- Susceptibility of the infant's eye to infection, and
- Ocular trauma during delivery

All infants are exposed to infectious agents in the birth canal; the duration of the exposure is an important factor in the development of disease.

CHEMICAL CONJUNCTIVITIS. Chemical conjunctivitis classically results from the instillation of silver nitrate drops used for infection prophylaxis. Credé[41] introduced this practice in 1881 to protect against gonococcal infection. The chemical conjunctivitis begins a few hours after delivery and lasts for 24–36 hours. Approximately 90% of infants who receive silver nitrate develop mild, transient conjunctival injection with tearing.[42] The severity of these symptoms has been lessened since the development of single-use 1% buffered silver nitrate ampules. Before this, silver nitrate was kept in large, multiuse bottles, which often resulted in more concentrated doses of the chemical being obtained when an aliquot was drawn from the bottom of the bottle. Although effective against *N. gonorrhoeae*, silver nitrate has a relatively limited spectrum of activity against bacteria and is ineffective against chlamydial or viral infections.[43] Silver nitrate may injure epithelial cells and thus render them more susceptible to invasion by other infectious agents. Although this method is still used in the majority of countries as the primary means of infection prophylaxis, many hospitals are changing to the use of erythromycin or tetracycline ointments.

CHLAMYDIAL INFECTIONS. The most frequent cause of neonatal conjunctivitis in the United States is *C. trachomatis*. The Centers for Disease Control and Prevention estimates that 3 million new cases of chlamydial infection occur annually.[44] Chlamydial infections occur in 4–10% of pregnant women in the United States.[45] Infants whose mothers have untreated

chlamydial infections have a 30–40% chance of developing conjunctivitis and a 10–20% chance of developing pneumonia.[46] Symptoms typically develop 5–14 days after delivery and may be unilateral or bilateral. Initially, infants have a watery discharge that may progressively turn mucopurulent. Signs include lid edema, a papillary conjunctival response, and pseudomembrane formation (Fig. 55-16). Usually, the infection is mild and self-limited; however, severe cases may occur and result in conjunctival scarring and a peripheral corneal pannus with corneal scarring. If either erythromycin or tetracycline ointment is applied within 1 hour of delivery, the chance of developing chlamydial conjunctivitis is essentially eliminated.[47]

Laboratory data are very helpful in the diagnosis of chlamydia. Originally, the two most common techniques for the identification of inclusion bodies involved the use of a Giemsa stain of a conjunctival scraping and a McCoy cell culture. Unfortunately, the Giemsa test is only 50–90% sensitive, and a well-trained technician must read the slides. The cell culture is expensive, and it takes 2–3 days to obtain results. Fortunately, other laboratory tests are now available for the diagnosis of chlamydia. An enzyme-linked immunoassay test is nearly 90% sensitive, over 95% specific, and provides results within several hours. A direct immunofluorescent monoclonal antibody stain of conjunctival smears is probably the most useful serological test as it has over 95% sensitivity and 77–90% specificity for chlamydia, depending on the prevalence of the disease. It may show infections missed by the other assays and can be read immediately. DNA detection techniques including polymerase chain reaction and ligase chain reaction are also available and are approximately 90% sensitive and 100% specific.[48]

The objectives of the treatment of infants who have chlamydial conjunctivitis include the resolution of infectious conjunctivitis and the eradication of respiratory colonization. Topical therapy alone is not sufficient to treat chlamydial conjunctivitis. The recommended treatment is oral erythromycin syrup 50mg/kg/day in four divided doses for 14 days (see Table 55-4). If a complete response does not occur, a second course of the same therapy may be given. The mother and sexual partners are treated with either oral tetracycline 500mg four times a day or oral erythromycin 500mg four times a day for 7 days[49] (pregnant or breast-feeding women are given erythromycin). Prevention still remains the best treatment as good prenatal care and treatment of chlamydial, gonococcal, or herpetic infections during pregnancy significantly lower the incidence of neonatal conjunctivitis. Proper eye cleaning using sterile cotton followed by the instillation of an antibiotic ointment immediately after birth provides the necessary prophylaxis to prevent neonatal ocular infection.

403

TABLE 55-4

GUIDELINES FOR TREATMENT OF NEONATAL CONJUNCTIVITIS

Infection	Treatment
Chlamydia	Oral erythromycin 50mg/kg/day in four divided doses for 14 days
Bacteria	
Gram-positive	Erythromycin 0.5% ointment four times a day
Gram-negative, gonococcal	Penicillin G drops 10,000–20,000 units every hour and intravenous penicillin G drops 100,000 units/kg/day in four divided doses for 7 days
	Intravenous or intramuscular ceftriaxone 25–50mg/kg/day once a day for 7 days
Gram-negative, others	Gentamicin or tobramycin ointments
Viral	Trifluorothymidine drops every 2 hours for 7 days

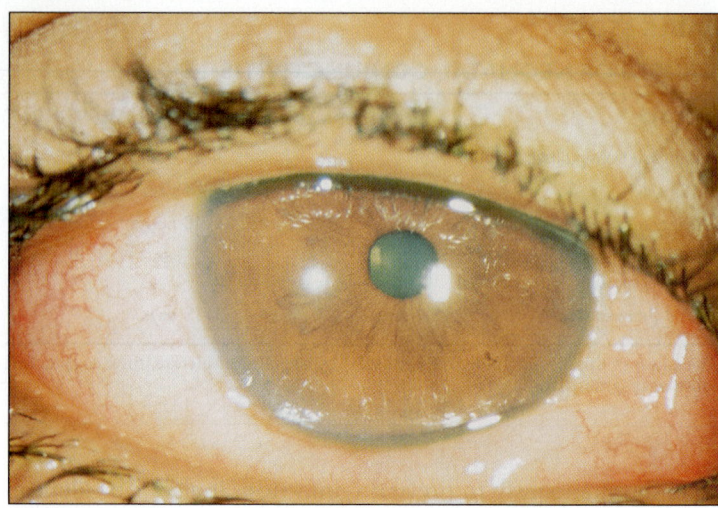

FIG. 55-17 ■ **Acute atopic conjunctivitis.** A man with itching, mucoid discharge, chemosis, and a papillary conjunctival reaction.

NEISSERIAL INFECTIONS. Neonatal conjunctivitis caused by *N. gonorrhoeae*, a gram-negative diplococcus that can penetrate an intact epithelium, has decreased significantly since the advent of prophylaxis. The clinical picture of gonococcal conjunctivitis consists of the development of a hyperacute conjunctivitis 24–48 hours after birth characterized by marked eyelid edema, profound chemosis, and excessive purulent discharge. The discharge is often so copious that it reaccumulates immediately after the eye has been wiped clean. Conjunctival membrane formation may occur. Because the organism may penetrate an intact epithelium, corneal ulceration with possible perforation can also occur if the conjunctivitis is not treated adequately.[40]

Diagnosis is made by identification of gram-negative intracellular diplococci on smears from the conjunctiva. The organism is best cultured on chocolate agar or Thayer-Martin agar incubated at 37°C in 10% carbon dioxide, and sensitivities are obtained after culture. Prompt diagnosis by examination of an immediate Gram stain is essential to timely and effective therapy.

Local treatment consists of aqueous penicillin G 10,000–20,000 units. Drops are given every hour with a loading dose of one drop every 5 minutes for 30 minutes. Systemic therapy should also be instituted with either intravenous aqueous penicillin G 100,000 units/kg/day in four divided doses or penicillin G benzathine 50,000 units/kg/day for 7 days. Intravenous or intramuscular ceftriaxone 25–50mg/kg once a day for 7 days is also effective if there is suspicion of a penicillinase-producing strain (see Table 55-4).

OTHER BACTERIAL INFECTIONS. Many different organisms can cause bacterial neonatal conjunctivitis. Bacteria are probably transmitted through the air to the infant shortly after birth, and there may be an association with obstruction of the nasolacrimal duct. Usually, these infections are caused by gram-positive bacteria such as *S. aureus, Str. pneumoniae, Str. viridans,* and *S. epidermidis*. Gram-negative organisms that have been implicated include *Haemophilus* species, *E. coli, Proteus* species, *K. pneumoniae, Enterobacter* species, and *Ser. marcescens.*[50] A rare cause, *Pseudomonas* sp., deserves particular mention in that infection with this organism can result in corneal ulceration and perforation.[51]

Typically, these infections arise 2–5 days after birth but may occur at any time within the postpartum period. Signs include lid edema, chemosis, and conjunctival injection with discharge. The work-up includes conjunctival scrapings for Gram stain and cultures, the results of which direct the choice of therapy. For gram-positive organisms, erythromycin 0.5% ointment four times a day is administered. Gentamicin, tobramycin, or fluoroquinolone drops or ointment four times a day can be used for gram-negative organisms (see Table 55-4).

VIRAL INFECTIONS. Viral conjunctivitis of the newborn is rare but can be associated with significant morbidity and mortality. Both herpes simplex virus type 1 and herpes simplex type 2 can be associated with conjunctivitis, but type 2 infection is more common.[52] Type 1 may be transmitted by a kiss from an adult who has an active "cold sore," and type 2 is more commonly transmitted through the birth canal. Onset is usually within the first 2 weeks of life and may be associated with vesicular skin lesions of the lid or lid margin (see Fig. 55-13). The conjunctivitis may be followed by herpetic keratitis or keratouveitis. The keratitis consists of microdendrites or small geographical ulcers. Vitritis, retinitis, retinal detachment, optic neuritis, and cataract have all been reported in association with neonatal ocular herpes. The diagnosis may be confirmed by the presence of eosinophilic intranuclear inclusions on smears, positive viral cultures, or positive monoclonal antibody immunoassays.

Treatment consists of trifluorothymidine 1% drops every 2 hours for 7 days or acyclovir ointment five times a day (see Table 55-4). Herpes simplex type 2 may be more resistant to treatment. In cases of systemic disease associated with pneumonitis, septicemia, and meningitis, systemic acyclovir should be used. Good prenatal care and frequent culture and treatment of mothers who have known herpes genital infections decrease the incidence of herpetic neonatal conjunctivitis.

Guidelines for Work-up

Prompt examination, work-up, and therapy are essential for proper resolution of neonatal conjunctivitis. A detailed maternal history is obtained with attention to a background of venereal disease or exposure during pregnancy. The results of any vaginal or cervical cultures are checked. A history of the labor, including duration and any premature rupture of membranes, is noted.

A conjunctival scraping with a spatula or moistened Ca^{2+} alginate swab is obtained. Gram and Giemsa stains are performed. Cultures are sent to the laboratory on blood agar, chocolate agar, and Thayer-Martin agar plates. Viral and chlamydial cultures are requested. The laboratory is informed about the organisms that are suspected and the importance of a rapid and accurate diagnosis.

Results of the laboratory tests are checked early and often. Treatment is based on the results of conjunctival scrapings and cultures, not on the clinical findings of severity of disease and time of onset, because these are nonspecific and may be misleading.

INFLAMMATIONS

Allergic Conjunctivitis

ACUTE ATOPIC CONJUNCTIVITIS. Acute atopic conjunctivitis is an immediate type (type 1) allergic response mediated by IgE. This response is stimulated by airborne allergens such as dust,

TABLE 55-5

MEDICATIONS USED IN THE TREATMENT OF ALLERGIC CONJUNCTIVITIS

Category	Examples	Comments
H₁ receptor agonists	Levocabastine, emedastine difumarate	Use for isolated, acute allergic attacks. Use alone or in combination with mast cell stabilizers and nonsteroidal anti-inflammatory drug (NSAID) medication
Mast cell stabilizers	Cromolyn sodium, lodoxamide, pemirolast, nedocromil sodium	Most useful for chronic allergies. May take 1–2 weeks to be effective. Pemirolast and nedocromil have antihistamine effects as well. Nedocromil also reduces eosinophil and neutrophil chemotaxis
Antihistamines with mast cell–stabilizing activity	Olopatadine, ketotifen fumarate, azelastine	These medications combine the immediate effect of selective antihistamines with the long-term effects of mast cell stabilization. They have convenient twice-a-day-dosing. Ketotifen and azelastine have anti-inflammatory properties as well.
Topical NSAIDs	Ketorolac	Can reduce itching but stings when applied
Vasoconstrictors	Naphazoline/pheniramine, naphazoline/antazoline	Available over the counter; instruction must be given to patients to avoid chronic use and rebound redness.
Topical steroids	Loteprednol, fluorometholone, rimexolone	May be useful in serious cases or until control is achieved with other agents. Side effects limit chronic use.
Oral antihistamines	Fexofenadine, loratadine, cetirizine	Useful when systemic allergic symptoms are present but may cause dry eyes.

molds, pollens, spores, and animal dander. Symptoms consist of the sudden onset of itching, burning, hyperemia, and conjunctival edema, followed by the development of a glassy chemosis and a watery or mucoid discharge (Fig. 55-17).[53] The reaction may be limited to the eye, or it may be part of a generalized allergic reaction with nasal and respiratory symptoms. Often, a family history of atopy is present, and cytological examination of conjunctival scrapings shows eosinophils. Unfortunately, avoidance of the offending antigens is usually impossible. Many new medications have become available for the treatment of allergic conjunctivitis (see Table 55-5). Histamine (H₁ receptor specific) agonists such as levocabastine and emedastine difumarate are used for intermittent, acute allergic reactions from a limited exposure to the antigen. Mast cell stabilizers such as cromolyn sodium, lodoxamide, pemirolast, and nedocromil sodium are used for chronic allergies. Combination medications that act as both mast cell stabilizers and H₁-specific antihistamines such as olopatadine, ketotifen fumarate, and azelastine are effective for acute and chronic antigen exposure. Some of these medications have additional inhibitory effects on late phase leukocyte recruitment. Vasoconstrictors with nonspecific antihistamines can still be used symptomatically with mild allergic reactions. Topical steroids and nonsteroidal anti-inflammatory agents can be used to reduce the acute inflammatory response until the mast cell stabilizers and antihistamines take effect. Therapy should be tailored to the individual's clinical picture, keeping in mind that some medications may not be effective for up to 2 weeks. Evaluation by an allergist is often useful in severe cases.

CHRONIC ATOPIC CONJUNCTIVITIS. Chronic atopic conjunctivitis is characterized by the same symptoms as in the acute condition, but there is a longer duration of the signs of inflammation. The conjunctiva exhibits a pale edema with papillary hypertrophy and a mild, mucopurulent discharge. Giant cobblestone papillae may occur (Fig. 55-18). Conjunctival scrapings reveal numerous eosinophils. As this chronic condition also occurs in atopic individuals who have a compromised immune system, secondary infections must also be ruled out in these patients.[54]

ALLERGIC DERMATOCONJUNCTIVITIS. Contact allergy of the eyelids and conjunctiva represents the most common form of allergic reaction seen by the ophthalmologist. It represents a delayed, cell-mediated (type IV) hypersensitivity reaction. Previous sensitization can have occurred as little as 5 days or as long as years previously. The most common stimuli for this reaction are eyedrops, cosmetics, clothing, jewelry, plastics, animal or vegetable products, and industrial chemicals.[3] The ocular drugs commonly associated with this reaction include neomycin, gentamicin, idoxuridine, atropine, thimerosal, and

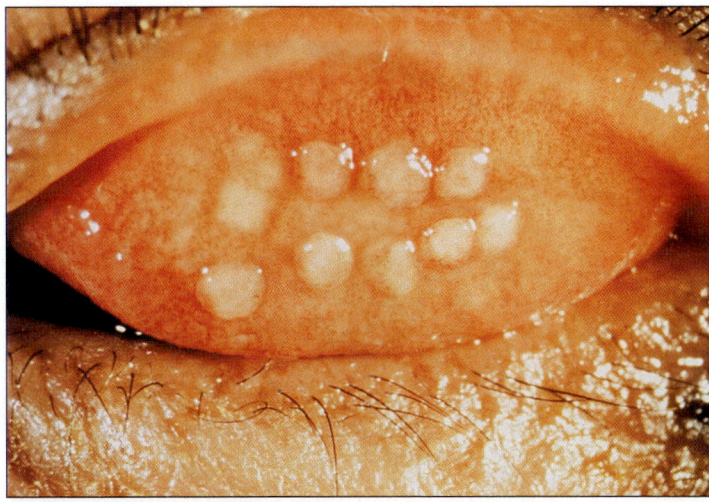

FIG. 55-18 ▓ **Chronic atopic conjunctivitis.** Mild conjunctival injection with numerous giant cobblestone papillae.

penicillin.[55] Other preservatives may stimulate allergy as well. The allergic reaction usually begins with severe itching and a papillary conjunctivitis that is worse on the inferior palpebral conjunctiva. A mucoid or mucopurulent discharge is seen. The adjacent skin of the lower lids and lateral canthi become involved in a typical eczematous dermatitis (Fig. 55-19). Chronic use of the allergen can lead to keratinization of the lid with eventual punctal edema and stenosis. The cornea may show punctate epithelial keratitis and erosions. Conjunctival scrapings show monocytes, polymorphonuclear neutrophil leukocytes, mucus, and eosinophils. Treatment consists of eliminating the antigenic stimulus and quieting the eye with topical corticosteroids.

MICROBIALLERGIC CONJUNCTIVITIS. Microbiallergic conjunctivitis is a type IV hypersensitivity response to the toxic protein breakdown products of bacterial disintegration. In the eyes, the most common cause of this reaction is chronic staphylococcal blepharoconjunctivitis. This common infection results in the formation of breakdown products of the bacteria, which cause an allergic response in the conjunctiva and cornea.[56] Usually, there is no history of allergy. Culture of the conjunctiva is negative for staphylococci. Marginal infiltrates of the cornea can be associated with this condition (Fig. 55-20).[3]

Phlyctenular keratoconjunctivitis is another manifestation of microbiallergic conjunctivitis. In the past, this condition was commonly associated with tuberculosis. Today, it is most frequently seen with chronic staphylococcal blepharoconjunctivi-

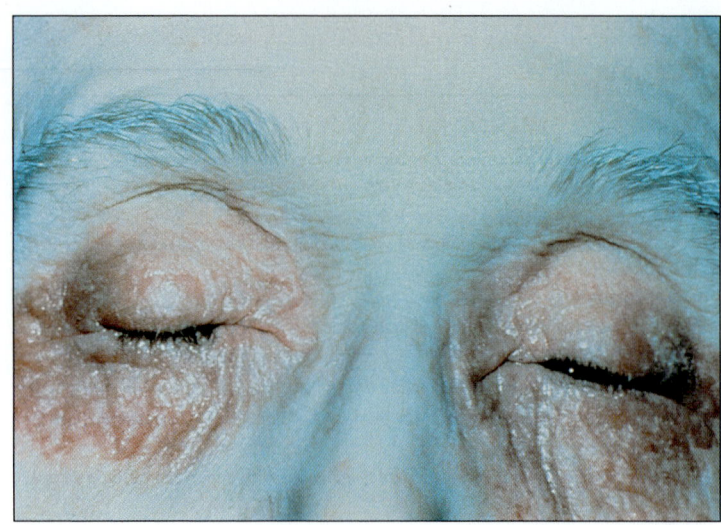

FIG. 55-19 ▮ **Allergic dermatoconjunctivitis.** Contact allergy of the eyelids after exposure to neomycin eyedrops. The skin shows a typical eczematous dermatitis.

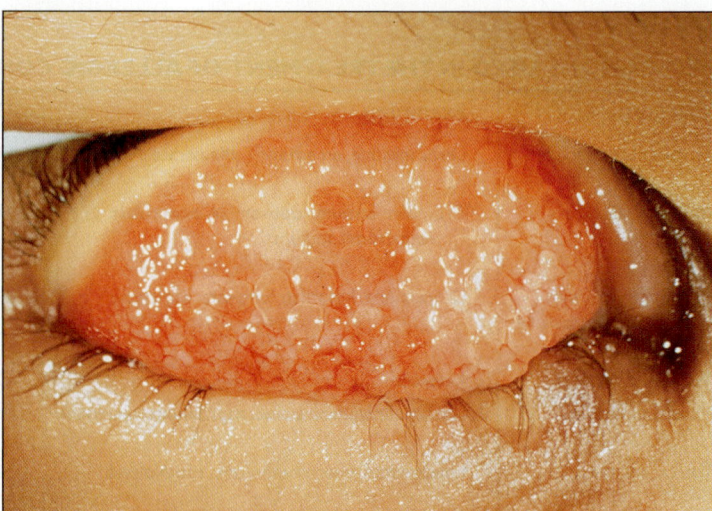

FIG. 55-21 ▮ **Vernal conjunctivitis.** Cobblestone papillae cover the superior tarsal conjunctiva.

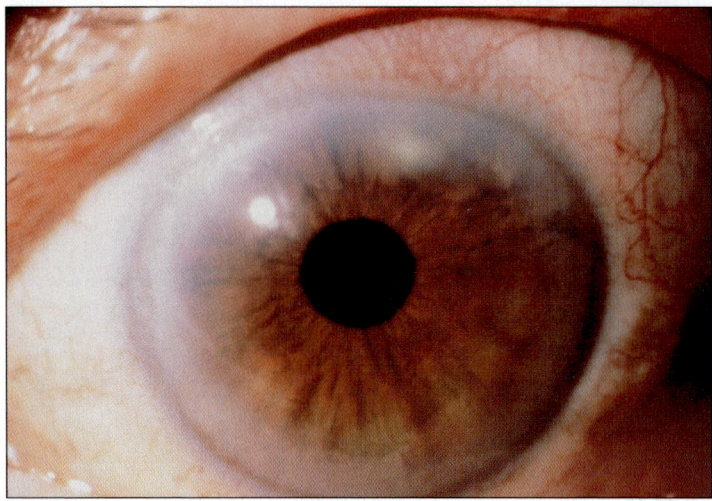

FIG. 55-20 ▮ **Microbiallergic keratoconjunctivitis associated with staphylococci.** A staphylococcal marginal infiltrate is seen in the superior cornea.

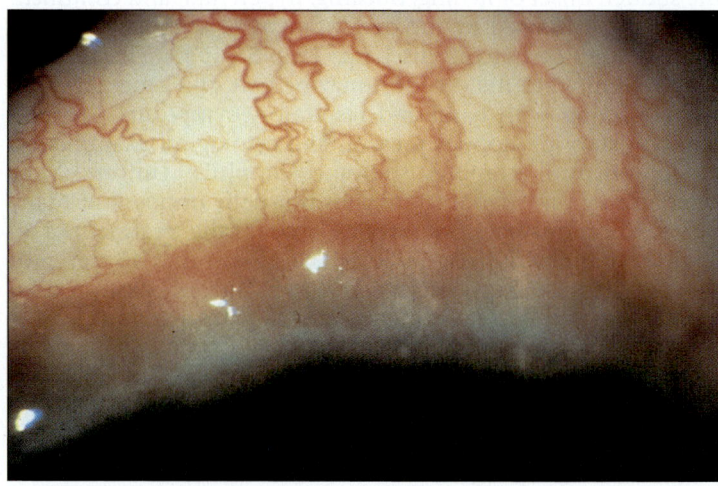

FIG. 55-22 ▮ **Vernal catarrh.** Clinical appearance of the less commonly seen limbal reaction. (Courtesy of Dr. IM Raber.)

tis. Other possible sources include *Candida albicans, Coccidioides immitis, Chlamydia,* parasites, and lymphogranuloma venereum. Phlyctenular disease presents as slightly raised, small, pinkish white or yellow nodules surrounded by dilated vessels. After a few days, the superficial part of the raised nodule becomes gray and soft; then the center of the lesion ulcerates, sloughs, and clears without scarring. Phlyctenules may occur both on the conjunctiva near the limbus and on the peripheral cornea. Classically, there is no clear zone between the limbus and the lesion. Involvement is usually bilateral and seasonal (occurring more in spring and summer), and the condition occurs most frequently in children and young adults.

Treatment of these microbiallergic conjunctivitides requires an attempt to identify the inciting organism and eradicate it. In chronic staphylococcal disease, elimination of the inciting bacteria can be difficult. Twice-daily lid scrubs (mechanical débridement of the lid margins with dilute baby shampoo or commercially prepared lid scrub pads) can usually achieve symptomatic improvement. Topical antibiotic or antibiotic-corticosteroid combination ointments or drops rubbed into the lid margins may also reduce the number of bacterial colonies. Corticosteroids are reserved for chronic recalcitrant blepharoconjunctivitis and are beneficial early in the treatment of phlyctenular disease. Tuberculosis should be ruled out in children or young adults as well as any adult who has had a recently converted purified protein derivative skin test. Systemic antibiotics, such as oral tetra-

cycline 250mg four times a day or oral doxycycline 100mg twice a day, can help in cases of nontuberculous phlyctenular disease or persistent staphylococcal blepharoconjunctivitis.

VERNAL CONJUNCTIVITIS. Vernal conjunctivitis is a bilateral, recurrent inflammation of the conjunctiva that tends to occur in children. Its onset is most common in the spring and summer (hence the name vernal, which refers to spring), and the inflammation often goes into remission during the cooler months.[57] The highest incidence of the disease is in the warm, temperate Middle East–Mediterranean region and Mexico. The condition occurs mainly in children and young adults in the age range 5–20 years, with peak incidence between 11 and 13 years. Boys are affected twice as frequently as girls, but the male-to-female ratio evens out when the disease affects adults.[58] A family history of atopy is common. The disease is self-limited in children, with an average duration of 4–10 years. In adults, a more severe form of the disease may recur indefinitely. The prominent symptom is itching. Other complaints include photophobia, burning, tearing, mild ptosis, and a thick, ropy, yellow, mucoid discharge.

The three forms of the vernal conjunctivitis are palpebral, limbal, and mixed.[59] The palpebral form is marked by cobblestone papillae on the superior tarsal conjunctiva (Fig. 55-21) while the lower lid is minimally affected. The initial change is papillary hypertrophy, after which the connective tissue of the substantia propria undergoes hyperplasia and proliferation to form giant papillae. Then the pressure of the cornea flattens the tops of the giant

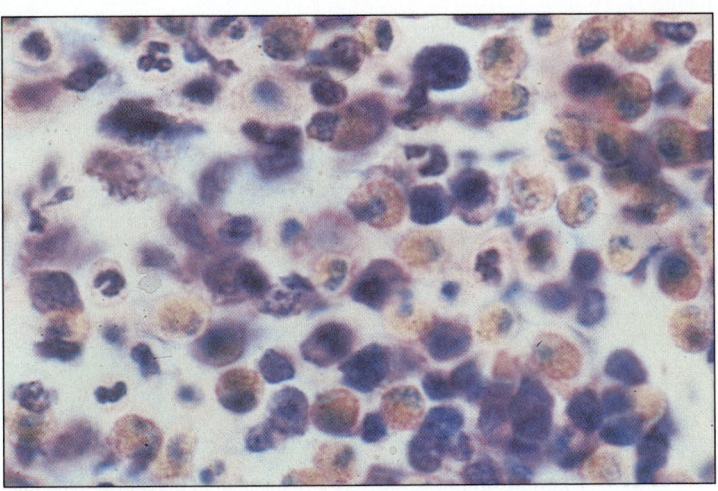

FIG. 55-23 ▮ **Vernal catarrh.** Histological examination of a conjunctival smear shows the presence of many eosinophils. (Courtesy of Dr. IM Raber.)

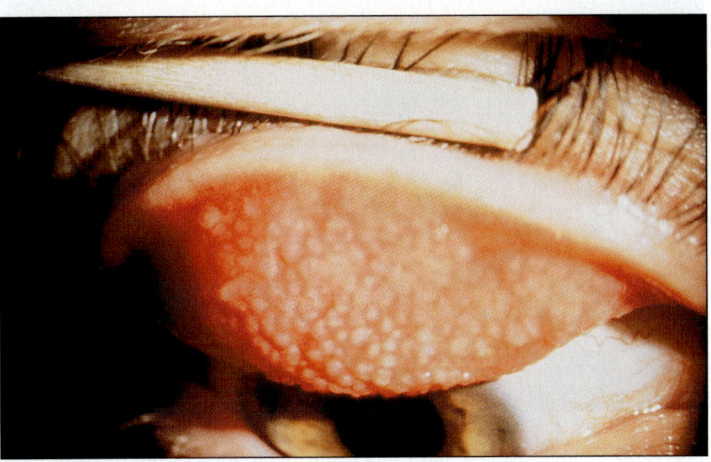

FIG. 55-24 ▮ **Giant papillary conjunctivitis.** Giant papillae cover this patient's superior tarsal conjunctiva after chronic exposure to soft contact lenses.

papillae to produce a pattern that resembles cobblestones. Tiny twigs of vessels are found in the centers of the papillae, which helps to differentiate these from large follicles such as may be seen in trachoma. When wiped with a cotton-tipped applicator, a milky veil that overlies the cobblestones pulls off in a stringy fashion. The limbal form is marked by a broad, thickened, gelatinous opacification of the superior limbus that can override the cornea (Fig. 55-22). Again, tiny, twig-like vessels arise in the centers of these rounded lumps, whereas in limbal follicles the vessels appear around the sides of the elevations only. Histologically, the tissue is infiltrated with lymphocytes, plasma cells, macrophages, basophils, and many eosinophils (Fig. 55-23). A characteristic manifestation of limbal vernal conjunctivitis is the presence of Horner-Trantas dots, which are white, chalk-like dots composed of eosinophils and epithelial debris.

The cornea can be involved in up to 50% of cases. Corneal manifestations include a superficial pannus and a punctate epithelial keratitis. Small, gray patches of necrotizing epithelium may involve the upper one third to two thirds of the cornea—in severe cases, the cornea appears to be dusted with flour.[59] The affected area stains with fluorescein. A vernal ulcer is a horizontally oval, shallow, nonvascularized, indolent ulcer of the superior cornea (see Fig. 55-23). The edges are composed of shaggy, gray, dead epithelial cells, and there is infiltration of the underlying superficial stroma. After the ulcer heals, a mild corneal opacity may persist at the level of Bowman's layer.

The chronic nature of the disease must be considered when the treatment is decided. Topical corticosteroids certainly provide the patient with significant relief from symptoms. However, the chronic use of corticosteroids carries the risks of glaucoma, cataract, and, possibly, infectious keratitis. It may be difficult to persuade the patient to limit the use of corticosteroids because they provide such potent symptomatic relief. Cromolyn sodium 4% works well as long-term treatment.[60] This drug works by preventing mast cell degranulation. A good strategy by which to control the acute exacerbation of symptoms is to start with frequent topical corticosteroids combined with topical cromolyn. The corticosteroids are then tapered off over a 2- to 3-week period as the therapeutic effects of the cromolyn take hold. Severe cases respond well to topical cyclosporin 2%. Cold compresses provide some relief as well. Finally, a move to a colder climate decreases the likelihood of disease recurrence.

Giant Papillary Conjunctivitis

Giant papillary conjunctivitis (GPC) is a syndrome of inflammation of the upper palpebral conjunctiva associated with con-

tact lens wear, ocular prostheses, and protruding ocular sutures.[61,62] Primarily, this is a syndrome linked to contact lens wear and is seen 10 times more frequently in soft lens wearers than in rigid lens wearers.[62] The average time for the development of symptoms is 8 months for soft lens wearers and 8 years for hard lens wearers. Estimates of the prevalence vary from 1–5% of soft lens users to 1% of rigid lens users.

The symptoms of GPC appear before the signs of superior tarsal involvement. Patients complain of mild itching after removal of the contact lenses and increased mucus on the lenses and in the nasal canthus upon awaking. They also complain of increased lens awareness, blurring of vision after hours of lens wear, excessive lens movement, and eventual contact lens intolerance. Signs of GPC initially include a generalized thickening and hyperemia of the superior pretarsal conjunctiva. The normally small papillae become elevated. The conjunctiva becomes more translucent and eventually becomes opaque secondary to cellular infiltration. Macropapillae (0.3–1.0mm) and giant papillae (1.0–2.0mm) then form (Fig. 55-24). Trantas dots and gelatinous nodules may develop at the limbus.[63] Inspection of the contact lenses almost always reveals whitish deposits.

The histology of GPC shows irregular thickening of the conjunctival epithelium over the papillae, with epithelial downgrowth into the stroma. The epithelium and stroma show infiltration of lymphocytes, plasma cells, polymorphonuclear neutrophil leukocytes, eosinophils, basophils, and macrophages along with fibroblast proliferation. The number of eosinophils and basophils is considerably lower than that seen in vernal conjunctivitis.

The cause of GPC is probably multifactorial. Patients are likely to have environmental antigens adhere to the mucus and proteins that normally coat the surface of all contact lenses.[64] These antigens, which persist as deposits on the contact lenses, are forced into repeated contact with the superior tarsal conjunctiva with blinking. Mechanical trauma is also an important factor in the pathogenesis of GPC that develops in patients who have ocular prostheses and exposed suture ends. This repeated exposure to antigen combined with the trauma to the upper tarsal conjunctiva from contact lens wear may result in stimulation of a type IV basophil hypersensitivity of the conjunctiva, which resembles cutaneous basophil hypersensitivity. A type I IgE-mediated immediate hypersensitivity reaction occurs as well. Conditions that favor the development of GPC in lens wearers include increased lens deposits, increased wearing time, extended number of years the lenses have been worn, larger diameter lenses, and soft lenses.

Treatment of the condition initially requires discontinuation of lens wear until the inflammation subsides. Lens wear may resume

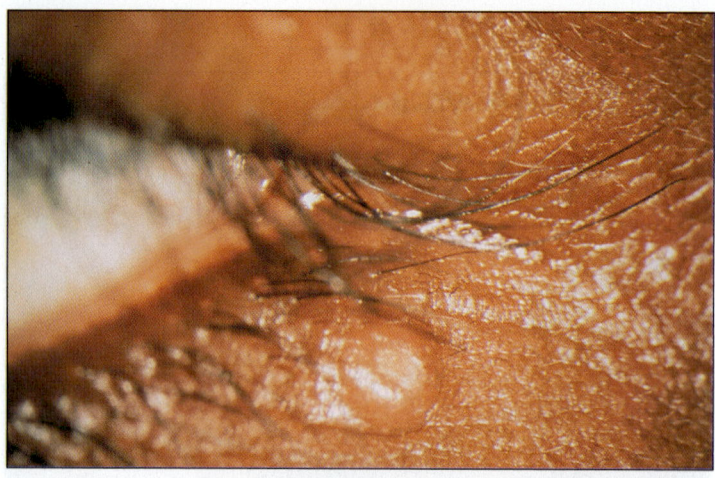

FIG. 55-25 ■ Molluscum contagiosum lesion on the lower eyelid. This patient had an accompanying chronic follicular conjunctivitis secondary to the toxic effect of viral proteins from this lesion.

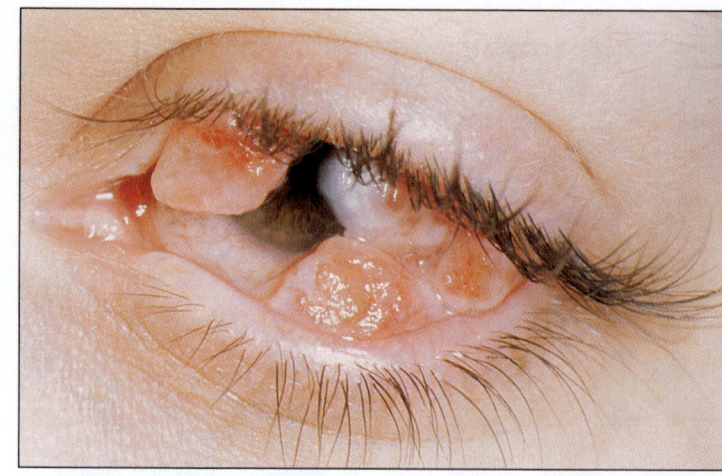

FIG. 55-26 ■ Ligneous conjunctivitis. Woody induration of the superior and inferior tarsal conjunctiva.

---

when the eye quiets down, but good care is essential. Patients must be instructed to clean their contacts thoroughly each night, and an attempt should be made to remove preservatives from the lens care system. Hydrogen peroxide disinfection is used. Patients should also clean their lenses enzymatically at least once a week and as often as each night with a papain enzymatic cleaner. Initially, a new lens of the same design may be used, but if this is not tolerated, a different lens design should be substituted. A silicone-containing lens such as the CSI lens or frequent replacement soft lenses may be successful. If soft lenses do not work, a rigid gas-permeable lens often does. When used in the early stages of GPC, cromolyn sodium 4% can be effective in the resolution of symptoms such as mucus production and itching. A short course of topical corticosteroids can lessen the symptoms in severe cases.

Toxic Follicular Conjunctivitis

Toxic follicular conjunctivitis follows chronic exposure of the conjunctiva to a variety of foreign substances, including molluscum contagiosum of the lid margin, infection of the lashes by *Phthirus pubis*, use of eye cosmetics, and prolonged use of various eye medications. Molluscum contagiosum infections are caused by a poxvirus and are common in the setting of human immunodeficiency virus infection. They are characterized by elevated, round, pearly white, waxy, noninflammatory lesions with umbilicated centers (Fig. 55-25). When these lesions occur on or near the eyelid margin, the viral proteins spill into the conjunctiva to cause a chronic follicular conjunctivitis.[65] The virus itself does not grow in the conjunctiva; rather the conjunctivitis is a toxic reaction to its proteins. Removal of the lesion or curettage until it bleeds internally eliminates this condition.

Most commonly, toxic follicular conjunctivitis occurs in association with eye medications, such as neomycin, gentamicin, idoxuridine, and other topical antivirals, as well as many glaucoma medications including brimonidine, pilocarpine, and other miotics (Box 55-2). These drugs incite a type IV delayed hypersensitivity reaction with periocular erythema and a follicular conjunctivitis. The process is sometimes called "pseudotrachoma," with follicles on the superior tarsus, papillary hypertrophy, conjunctival scarring, keratitis, and pannus. Herbert's pits do not occur, however. A marked follicular response can also accompany the use of eye cosmetics such as mascara and eyeliner. A common finding is dark granules from the cosmetic incorporated in the follicles. If symptomatic, patients usually respond well to discontinuation of the cosmetic and substitution of smaller amounts of hypoallergenic preparations.

Ligneous Conjunctivitis

Ligneous conjunctivitis is a rare chronic conjunctivitis that has an acute onset. It is characterized by a woody induration of the tarsal conjunctiva associated with a membrane or pseudomembranes (Fig. 55-26). Plasminogen deficiency, both homozygous and heterozygous, has been identified as a cause of ligneous conjunctivitis.[66,67] The condition is often associated with an acute infection or trauma of the upper respiratory tract, urinary tract, middle ear, sinuses, cervix, or vagina.[68] Therefore, fever and other constitutional symptoms may accompany the conjunctivitis. Chronic, recurrent inflammation of the upper pretarsal conjunctiva becomes compacted and granulated to produce the woody membrane. The cornea may become involved secondarily with scarring and vascularization.

The pathophysiology of this disease involves increased vascular permeability of the conjunctival blood vessels. Widened spaces between endothelial cells are found. The membrane produced is composed of fibrin, albumin, IgG, new blood vessels, plasma cells, and activated T and B lymphocytes.[3]

Many different therapies have been tried. Surgical excision of the membranes is technically difficult and usually results in a recurrence. Cryotherapy has been reported to have mixed results but overall is probably not helpful. Chymotrypsin, hyaluronidase, various antibiotics, topical corticosteroids alone, antiviral agents, cautery, and beta and X-ray irradiation all have been tried with little success. The most promising treatment to date is a combination of cyclosporin 2% and topical corticosteroids.[69] It is thought that cyclosporin interferes with T-cell recruitment and activation because it decreases the production of or response to interleukin-2. Treatment with intravenous plasminogen has been shown to be beneficial in case studies.[70]

Cicatricial Pemphigoid

Cicatricial pemphigoid is a rare disorder characterized by recurrent blisters or bullae of the skin and mucous membranes that

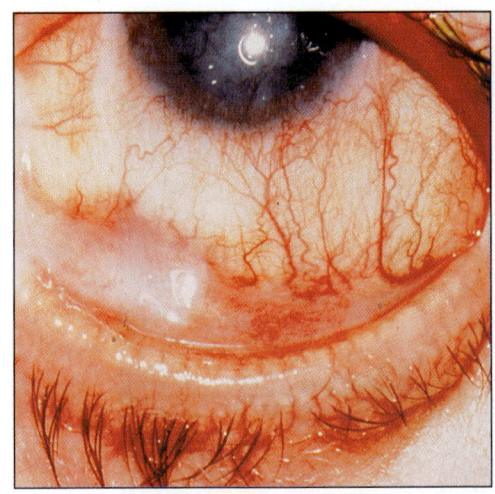

FIG. 55-27 Cicatricial pemphigoid. Marked subepithelial fibrosis has resulted in shrinkage of the inferior conjunctival fornix, with overlying keratinization of the conjunctiva.

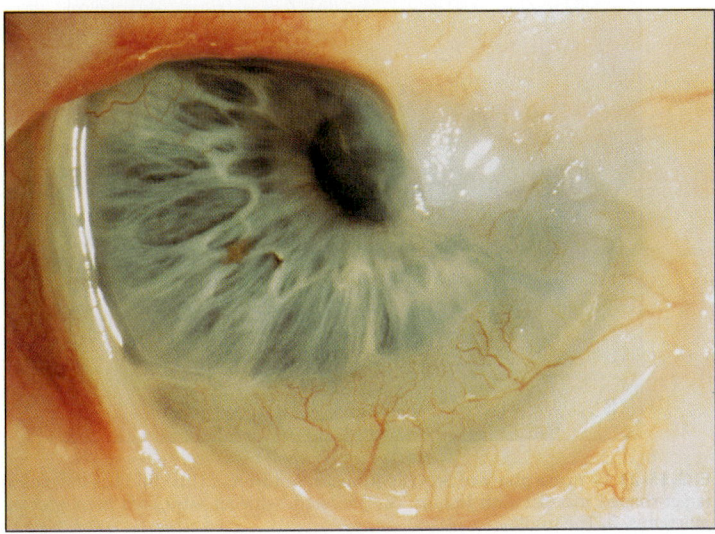

FIG. 55-28 Symblepharon formation. Lower and upper lids to the cornea in cicatricial pemphigoid.

result in scar formation.[71] It is a disease of older people (mean age of 70 years) and affects women more frequently than men. Oral and ocular involvements are common. In ophthalmic studies, 15–50% of patients show oral involvement and 100% show ocular involvement.[72,73] Skin may be involved in up to 25% of cases, with either a recurrent vesiculobullous, nonscarring eruption of the inguinal area or extremities or a localized erythematous plaque with overlying bullae and vesicles on the face near the involved mucous membranes; this can result in smooth atrophic scars. Mucous membrane involvement may include the conjunctiva, nose, mouth, pharynx, larynx, esophagus, anus, vagina, or urethra.

The course of ocular involvement is usually slow but unremittingly progressive. Often, asymmetrical bilateral involvement is seen. The initial symptoms are chronic conjunctival irritation, burning, and tearing, sometimes with a mucopurulent discharge. Secondary bacterial conjunctivitis is common, especially with coagulase-positive staphylococci. Conjunctival inflammation progresses to subepithelial fibrosis, which is the hallmark of the disease.[72] Symblepharon, fibrotic bands, and blunting of the fornices occur next and most frequently involve the inferior fornix (Fig. 55-27). Eventual obliteration of the fornices, ankyloblepharon, and a keratinized ocular surface epithelium occur at the end stage (Fig. 55-28). Cicatricial pemphigoid is associated with dry eye because fibrosis beneath the conjunctival epithelium can cause occlusion of the ducts of the lacrimal

and accessory lacrimal glands and result in an aqueous deficiency. Progressive conjunctival scarring results in loss of goblet cells and a mucin deficiency.[74] Chronic associated staphylococcal blepharitis may produce meibomian gland dysfunction and a resultant lipid tear film abnormality. Therefore, all the components of the tear film are altered along with the decrease in the volume of tears. Entropion, trichiasis, and lagophthalmos occur. As a result of the severe dry eye and the mechanical irritation from the disturbed eyelid architecture, the cornea may develop recurring epithelial erosions, keratinization, neovascularization, ulcer formation, possible perforation, and secondary bacterial infection.[75] In one study, 21% with treated ocular cicatricial pemphigoid progressed to legal blindness.[76]

The pathogenesis of the disease is thought to involve an autoimmune attack of immunoglobulins (mostly IgG) on the basement membrane of the conjunctiva, which suggests a type II reaction.[72,73] The target autoantigen has been identified as the β4 subunit of the α6β4 integrin dimer.[77] Both the classical and alternative complement pathways are stimulated, which results in an inflammatory response.[78] Conjunctival biopsies demonstrate immunoglobulins and complement bound to the basement membrane.[79] In the acute stages, subepithelial bullae with a separation between basal cells and the basement membrane occur. An infiltration of lymphocytes (mostly helper T cells), plasma cells, occasional eosinophils, and few neutrophils is seen. Later stages show pronounced fibrosis with hyperproliferation of conjunctival fibroblasts.

The differential diagnosis involves all other conditions that produce conjunctival scarring[80] including radiation, thermal, or severe chemical burns. Sjögren's syndrome, severe atopic keratoconjunctivitis, scleroderma, and sarcoidosis also produce conjunctival scarring and symblepharon. Postsurgical scarring and conjunctival carcinoma must also be considered. In addition, infections such as trachoma, adenoviral EKC, primary herpes simplex, diphtheria, and β-hemolytic streptococcus result in conjunctival scarring. Medications such as systemic practolol, topical epinephrine (adrenaline), idoxuridine, echothiophate iodide, pilocarpine, timolol, demecarium, and dipivefrin may cause a drug-induced ocular cicatricial pemphigoid.[81] This condition can be self-limited or progressive and essentially cannot be differentiated from true cicatricial pemphigoid. Erythema multiforme major may produce a clinical picture similar to that of cicatricial pemphigoid. Other bullous diseases, such as bullous pemphigoid and pemphigus, usually do not cause conjunctival scarring. The former is primarily a skin disease and the latter causes intraepithelial bullae.

Treatment can be difficult. Nonpreserved artificial tears are the mainstay of treatment of the dry eye. Although artificial tears can increase comfort and temporarily improve the ocular surface, they do not halt the progression of the disease. Punctal occlusion can be performed if the puncta do not scar closed. A therapeutic soft contact lens with frequent artificial tears can be tried in some patients who suffer continual corneal damage from trichiasis or lid abnormalities. Caution is needed, however, because of the increased risk of infection. The chronic staphylococcus blepharitis may be controlled with regular lid scrubs followed by an antibiotic ointment, such as bacitracin or erythromycin, rubbed into the lid margins. Oral tetracycline or doxycycline also helps to control the posterior aspect of blepharitis. Trichiasis can be treated with electrolysis for sporadic lashes or cryotherapy to eradicate large areas of trichiatic lashes. With advanced scarring, oculoplastic procedures to restore normal lid position and architecture can be tried but may activate the inflammatory process.[82] Mucous membrane grafts can be used to replace scarred conjunctiva. However, the usual sources for mucous membranes (contralateral eye, oral mucosa) may be damaged by the disease. Amniotic membrane grafts can be used as a replacement for conjunctival basement membrane.

Long-term systemic immunosuppressive therapy can control the disease,[83,84] an approach that works best in the earlier stages.

Many different modalities are available. Dapsone is a good choice for patients who have only mild to moderate inflammation. Methotrexate, azathioprine, or cyclophosphamide may be the best choice for highly active cases; adjunctive oral prednisone (1mg/kg/day) may be beneficial. Patients often need to have systemic immunosuppression for at least 12 months, and use of more than one medication is often necessary.[76] Preliminary studies indicate that disease that is refractory to conventional treatment may respond to intravenous immunoglobulin or subconjunctival mitomycin C.[84,85] Corneal transplant surgery, even with preoperative stem cell transplants, is associated with a very poor prognosis. Some surgeons have found success with a keratoprosthesis.

Caution must be exercised when any surgical procedure is carried out on an eye that has cicatricial pemphigoid.[72,86] Cataract, glaucoma, or oculoplastic surgery may activate the conjunctival inflammatory process unless the patient's disease is controlled adequately by systemic immunosuppressive therapy. If cataract surgery is needed, a clear corneal temporal incision, without conjunctival manipulation, is preferred.

Erythema Multiforme Major (Stevens-Johnson Syndrome)

Erythema multiforme, unlike cicatricial pemphigoid, is an acute, generally self-limited, nonprogressive inflammatory disorder of the skin and mucous membranes; it is classified into minor and major forms. The minor form primarily involves the skin and lasts 2–3 weeks in its acute phase. Erythema multiforme major, also known as Stevens-Johnson syndrome, is the more serious variant, characterized by skin lesions and erosive involvement of mucous membranes that lasts up to 6 weeks.[79] There are signs of systemic toxicity, which include malaise, fever, headache, and fluid imbalance. Toxic epidermal necrolysis is a severe variant of erythema multiforme major that is characterized by massive denudation of the epidermis.[87] Erythema multiforme major classically occurs in previously healthy young people, men more than women, in their first three decades of life.[87] There may be a genetic predisposition for the development of Stevens-Johnson syndrome with ocular involvement, as seen in the association of human leukocyte antigens HLA-Bw44 and HLA-B12.[88] The disease can be fatal in 2–25% of patients, with death often secondary to sepsis. Twenty percent of those who have erythema multiforme suffer a recurrence over their lifetime.

The exact cause of erythema multiforme is unknown, although the disease seems to be precipitated by numerous antigens including bacteria (e.g., *Mycoplasma pneumoniae*), viruses, fungi, and drugs. Herpes simplex virus and *Mycoplasma* have a particularly strong association. Drugs implicated in the development of erythema multiforme include the sulfonamides, penicillin, barbiturates, salicylates, mercurial agents, arsenic, phenylbutazone, and phenytoin.[89] Also, erythema multiforme has been reported following the use of topical ophthalmic scopolamine (hyoscine), tropicamide, and proparacaine. In addition, the onset of the disease has been related to neoplasms, radiation therapy, collagen vascular diseases, and vaccinations.[87]

Erythema multiforme often begins with the symptoms of malaise, fever, and headache as well as symptoms of an upper respiratory tract infection. Next, skin lesions develop symmetrically on the extremities, but the trunk is often spared (Fig. 55-29). Crops of skin lesions can reoccur every 2 weeks or so over a period of 6 weeks. The primary cutaneous lesion is a round, erythematous macule that develops into a papule and then a vesicle or bulla. Eventually, large bullae can rupture, which results in epidermal necrosis. The characteristic skin finding is a target lesion characterized by a red center surrounded by a pale zone and then an outer red ring. If extensive skin necrosis occurs, the condition is labeled toxic epidermal necrolysis (Fig. 55-30). The extent of mucous membrane involvement usually parallels the extent of skin involvement. Any mucous membrane may be involved, but the mouth and eyes are affected most frequently and most se-

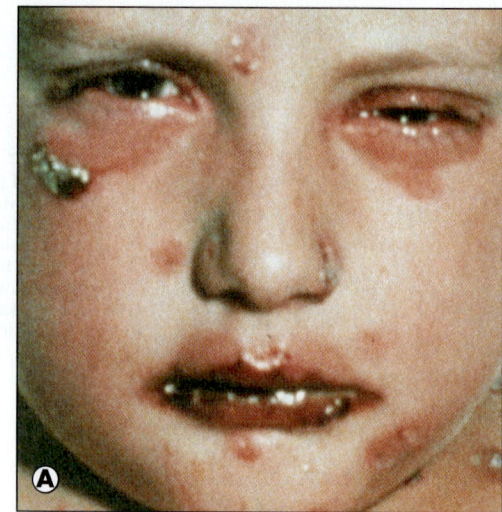

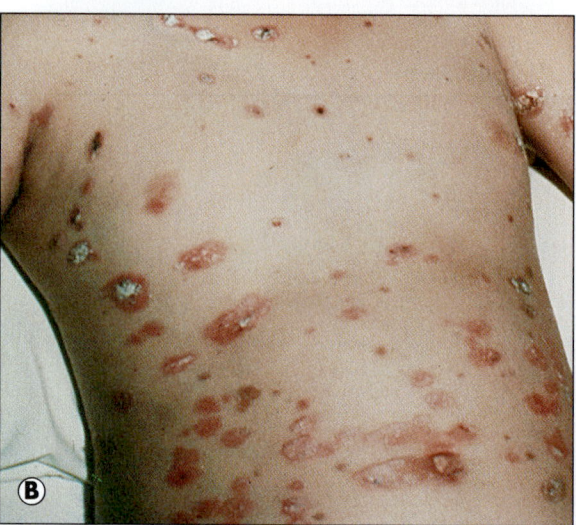

FIG. 55-29 ■ **Acute phase of Stevens-Johnson syndrome.** This child has the typical target-shaped macular skin lesions. **A,** The head, with an associated blepharoconjunctivitis. **B,** The trunk.

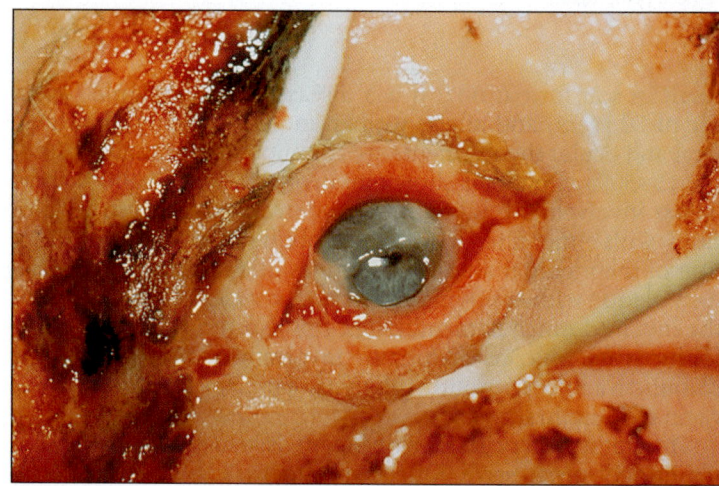

FIG. 55-30 ■ **Severe skin and conjunctival necrosis.** The patient has toxic epidermal necrolysis.

verely. In one study, 100% of patients had stomatitis and 63% had conjunctivitis.[90]

The acute phase of ocular involvement lasts 2–3 weeks.[91] The lids become swollen, ulcerated, and crusted. Patients develop an acute bilateral mucopurulent conjunctivitis, and those affected more severely develop chemosis, vesicles and bullae, pseudomembranes or membranes, and eventual ulceration. A

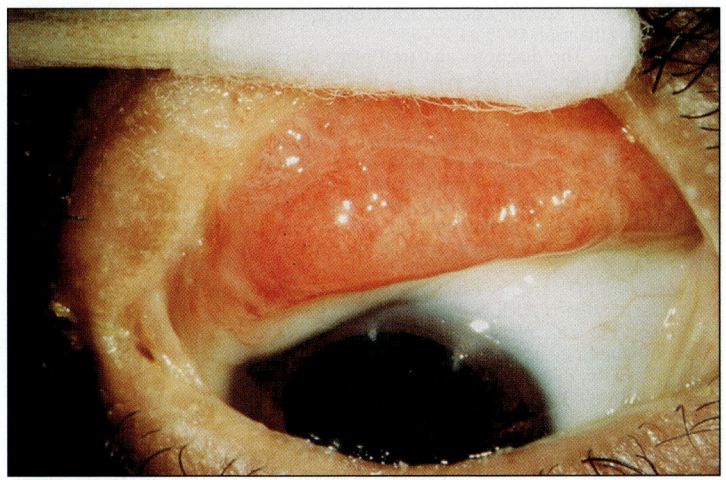

FIG. 55-31 ■ **Stevens-Johnson syndrome.** Residual conjunctival scarring is evident over the superior tarsal plate. Symblepharon formation and fibrous bands are present at the canthal angles.

TABLE 55-6

CLINICAL FORMS OF EPIDERMOLYSIS BULLOSA

Type	Inheritance	Ophthalmic Involvement
Simple	Dominant	Bilateral small cysts at epithelial basal cell layer
Junctional	Recessive	Severe conjunctival scarring—resembles pemphigoid
		Corneal clouding
Dystrophic	Dominant	Little conjunctival involvement—can have scarring
		Primarily corneal—with clouding, recurrent erosions, ulcers, and opacification
	Recessive	None

more purulent conjunctivitis may develop as a result of bacterial secondary infection.[89] The major ocular problems occur from the cicatricial stage, after the acute toxic episode subsides. Conjunctival scarring and symblepharon may occur despite all supportive measures (Fig. 55-31). Destruction of the conjunctival goblet cells, lacrimal gland, and accessory lacrimal gland tissue results in a severe dry eye, just as in cicatricial pemphigoid. Entropion, trichiasis, and lagophthalmos combined with the dry eye can produce severe corneal problems such as ulceration, vascularization, opacification, and eventual perforation.[91] Although the acute phase of erythema multiforme may leave extensive conjunctival scarring in its wake, progressive scarring does not occur when the acute disease has subsided, unlike the situation in cicatricial pemphigoid. Fortunately, recurrences of erythema multiforme rarely involve the conjunctiva.

The histological changes in erythema multiforme suggest an underlying vasculitis or perivasculitis.[79] Mononuclear cells, eosinophils, and polymorphonuclear neutrophil leukocytes accumulate around the vessels or within the vessel wall and induce fibrinoid necrosis of the wall. Subepithelial bullae are seen in the acute phase, and pseudomembranes and true membranes are found. Conjunctival goblet cell densities are reduced. Circulating immune complexes have been demonstrated in the sera of these patients. Also, immunoglobulins and complement are deposited at the dermal-epidermal junction.

Treatment often varies with the severity of the condition. Patients who have a more severe initial presentation suffer the worst late ocular complications. In the acute phase, local treatment involves lubrication of the ocular surface. Frequent lysis of developing symblepharon may have no effect on the eventual structure. Unfortunately, local treatment of the acute condition seems to have little influence on the severity of the eventual cicatricial complications. However, systemic corticosteroids (prednisone 60–80mg/day for 3–4 weeks) may help control the acute disease.[92] Secondary bacterial conjunctivitis should be suspected and treated if present, although care must be taken not to use an antibiotic that could stimulate another toxic reaction. The cicatricial stage is treated with frequent nonpreserved artificial tears and/or ointments. If not already scarred, the puncta may be closed to help the dry eye. Surgery to correct lid keratinization, entropion, and trichiasis should be considered. Unlike that in cicatricial pemphigoid, eyelid or conjunctival surgery does not stimulate further scarring. Conjunctival or buccal mucous membrane grafts may be considered in order to restore the ocular surface. Amniotic membrane grafts may also be used to repair areas of conjunctival destruction. Stem cell transplantation through the use of living-related or cadaveric conjunctival and limbal allografts holds promise for the treatment of corneal surface disease,[93] and trials incorporating cultivated corneal epithelial stem cells using denuded amniotic membrane as a carrier have had encouraging results.[94]

Epidermolysis Bullosa

Epidermolysis bullosa comprises a group of skin and mucous membrane diseases that are characterized by the tendency to form blisters after minor trauma.[95] Symptoms occur shortly after birth or in early childhood and have a tendency to recur throughout the patient's life. Men and women are affected equally, and both hereditary and acquired autoimmune forms exist.[96] The hereditary forms of epidermolysis bullosa may be classified as simple (autosomal dominant), junctional (autosomal recessive), and dystrophic (autosomal dominant or recessive) (Table 55-6).

Ocular problems have been described with all three types of epidermolysis bullosa; however, they are most common with the dystrophic form, which is also the most common form of the disease. Such patients may have marked conjunctival scarring, which includes symblepharon formation. A granular epithelial clouding of the cornea can occur, as can ulcers and opacification secondary to conjunctival scarring similar to that seen in cicatricial pemphigoid or erythema multiforme. Patients who have the junctional form, a rare type, have more primary corneal problems, such as recurrent erosions, and little conjunctival involvement. The acquired, autoimmune form may have both primary corneal subepithelial vesicles and secondary corneal involvement associated with conjunctival scarring and symblepharon.

REFERENCES

1. Spencer WH. Ophthalmic pathology: an atlas and textbook, Vol 1, 3rd ed. Philadelphia: WB Saunders; 1985:176–7.
2. Grove AS. Dermoid. In: Fraunfelder FT, Roy FH, eds. Current ocular therapy, 3. Philadelphia: WB Saunders; 1995:233–4.
3. Rheinstrom SD. The conjunctiva. In: Chandler JW, Sugar J, Edelhauser HF, eds. Textbook of ophthalmology, Vol 8: External diseases. London: Mosby; 1994:2.8–9.
4. Conlon MR, Alfonso EC, Starck T, et al. Tumors of the cornea and conjunctiva. In: Albert DM, Jakobiec FA, eds. Principles and practice of ophthalmology. Clinical practice. Philadelphia: WB Saunders; 1994:276–91.
5. Goldenhar M. Associations malformatives de l'oeil et de l'oreille en particulier le syndrome dermoide épibulbaire–appendices auriculaires–fistula auris congénita et ses relations avec la dysostose mandibulo-faciale. J Genet Hum. 1952;1:243–82.
6. Sugar HS. The oculoauriculovertebral dysplasia syndrome of Goldenhar. Am J Ophthalmol. 1966;62:678–82.
7. Hayasaka S, Sekimoto M, Setogawa T. Epibulbar complex choristoma involving the bulbar conjunctiva and cornea. J Pediatr Ophthalmol Strabismus. 1989;26:251–3.
8. Pokorny KS, Hyman BM, Jakobiec FA, et al. Epibulbar choristomas containing lacrimal tissue. Clinical distinction from dermoids and histologic evidence of an origin from the palpebral lobe. Ophthalmology. 1987;94:1249–57.
9. Mannis MJ. Bacterial conjunctivitis. In: Tasman W, Jaeger EA, eds. Duane's clinical ophthalmology, Vol 4. Philadelphia: JB Lippincott; 1990:5.3–7.
10. Friedlander MH. Immunology of ocular infections. In: Friedlander MH, ed. Allergy and immunology of the eye. Philadelphia: Harper & Row; 1979:10–20.
11. Allansmith MR. The eye and immunology. St Louis: CV Mosby; 1982:75–81.
12. Brook I, Bateman JB, Pettit TH. Meningococcal conjunctivitis. Arch Ophthalmol. 1979;97:890–1.

13. Thygeson P, Kimura S. Chronic conjunctivitis. Trans Am Acad Ophthalmol Otolaryngol. 1963;67:494–517.
14. Dawson CR, Sheppard JD. Follicular conjunctivitis. In: Tasman W, Jaeger EA, eds. Duane's clinical ophthalmology, Vol 4. Philadelphia: JB Lippincott; 1990:7.2–20.
15. Thygeson P, Dawson CR. Trachoma and follicular conjunctivitis in children. Arch Ophthalmol. 1966;75:3–12.
16. Schmitz HR, Wigand R, Heinrich W. Worldwide epidemiology of human adenovirus infection. Am J Epidemiol. 1983;117:455–66.
17. Bell JA, Rowe WP, Engler JI, *et al.* Pharyngoconjunctival fever. Epidemiological studies of a recently recognized disease entity. JAMA. 1955;157:1083–5.
18. Hogan MJ, Crawford JW. Epidemic keratoconjunctivitis with a review of the literature and a report of 125 cases. Am J Ophthalmol. 1942;25:1059–78.
19. Dawson C, Hanna L, Wood TR, *et al.* Adenovirus type 8 in the United States. III. Epidemiologic, clinical and microbiologic features. Am J Ophthalmol. 1970;69:473–80.
20. Dawson CR, Hanna L, Togni B. Adenovirus infections in the United States. IV. Observations on the pathogenesis of lesions in severe eye disease. Arch Ophthalmol. 1972;87:258–68.
21. Dawson CR, Darrell R, Hanna L, *et al.* Infections due to adenovirus type 8 in the United States. II. Community-wide infection with adenovirus type 8. N Engl J Med. 1963;268:1034–7.
22. Dawson CR, Darrell R. Infections due to adenovirus type 8 in the United States. I. An outbreak of epidemic keratoconjunctivitis originating in a physician's office. N Engl J Med. 1963;268:1031–3.
23. Vastine DW, West C, Yamashiroya H, *et al.* Simultaneous nosocomial and community outbreak of epidemic keratoconjunctivitis with types 8 and 19 adenovirus. Trans Am Acad Ophthalmol Otolaryngol. 1976;81:826–40.
24. Laibson PR, Ortolan G, Dhiri S, *et al.* The treatment of epidemic keratoconjunctivitis (adenovirus type 8) by corticosteroid therapy. XXI Concilium Ophthalmologicum, Mexico. Amsterdam: Excerpta Medica; 1970:1246–50.
25. Hillenkamp J, Reinhard T, Ross RS, *et al.* Topical treatment of acute adenoviral keratoconjunctivitis with 0.2% cidofovir and 1% cyclosporin A. Arch Ophthalmol. 2001;119:1487–91.
26. Hillenkamp J, Reinhard T, Ross RS, *et al.* The effects of cidofovir 1% with and without cyclosporin A 1% as a topical treatment of acute adenoviral keratoconjunctivitis. Ophthalmology. 2002;109:845–50.
27. Chatterjee S, Quarcoopome CO, Apenteng A. An epidemic of acute conjunctivitis in Ghana. Ghana Med J. 1970;9:9–11.
28. Yin-Murphy M. Viruses of acute hemorrhagic conjunctivitis. Lancet. 1973;1: 545–6.
29. Oh JO. Ocular infections of herpes simplex virus type II in adults. In: Darrell RW, ed. Viral diseases of the eye. Philadelphia: Lea & Febiger; 1985:59–62.
30. Sumers KD, Sugar J, Levine R. Endogenous dissemination of genital *Herpesvirus hominis* type II to the eye. Br J Ophthalmol. 1980;64:770–2.
31. Garau J, Kabins S, DeNosaquo S, *et al.* Spontaneous cytomegalovirus mononucleosis with conjunctivitis. Arch Intern Med. 1977;137:1631–2.
32. Trott DG, Pilsworth R. Outbreaks of conjunctivitis due to Newcastle disease virus in chicken broiler factory workers. Br J Med. 1965;3377:1514–17.
33. Thylefors B, Dawson CR, Jones BR, *et al.* A simple system for the assessment of trachoma and its complications. Bull World Health Organ. 1987;65:477–83.
34. Dawson CR, Jones BR, Tarizzo M. Guide to trachoma control. Geneva: World Health Organization; 1981:56.
35. Dawson CR, Juster R, Marx R, *et al.* Limbal disease in trachoma and other ocular chlamydial infections: risk factors for corneal vascularization. Eye. 1989;3:204–9.
36. Fraser-Hunt N, Bailey RL, Cousens S, *et al.* Efficacy of oral azithromycin versus topical tetracycline in mass treatment of endemic trachoma. Bull World Health Organ. 2001;79:632–40.
37. Schacher J, West SK, Mabey D, *et al.* Azithromycin in control of trachoma. Lancet. 1999;354:630–5.
38. Dawson CR, Schachter J. TRIC agent infections of the eye and genital tract. Am J Ophthalmol. 1967;63:1288–98.
39. Tullo AB, Richmond SJ, Esty PL. The presentation and incidence of paratrachoma in adults. J Hyg. 1981;87:63–9.
40. Chandler JW. Neonatal conjunctivitis. In: Tasman W, Jaeger EA, eds. Duane's clinical ophthalmology, Vol 4. Philadelphia: JB Lippincott; 1995:6.2–6.
41. Credé CSF. Die Verhutung der augenentzundung der neugeborenen. Arch Gynaekol. 1881;17:50–5.
42. Nishida H, Risemberg HM. Silver nitrate ophthalmic solution and chemical conjunctivitis. Pediatrics. 1975;56:368–73.
43. Laga M, Plummer FA, Piot P, *et al.* Prophylaxis of gonococcal and chlamydial ophthalmia neonatorum: a comparison of silver nitrate and tetracycline. N Engl J Med. 1988;318:653–7.
44. *Chlamydia trachomatis* infections: policy guidelines for prevention and control. MMWR Morb Mortal Wkly Rep. 1985;34(Suppl 3):53S–74S.
45. Holmes KK. The chlamydia epidemic. JAMA. 1981;245:1718–23.
46. Harrison JR, English MG. *Chlamydia trachomatis* infant pneumonitis. N Engl J Med. 1978;298:702–8.
47. Rapoza PA, Chandler JW. Neonatal conjunctivitis: diagnosis and treatment. In: Focal Points 1988: clinical modules for ophthalmologists. San Francisco: American Academy of Ophthalmology; 1988:5–6.
48. Goroll AH, Mulley AG, May LA, eds. Primary care medicine: office evaluation and management of the adult patient, 4th ed. Philadelphia: Lippincott, Williams & Wilkins; 2000:742.
49. Sanders LL, Harrison HR, Washington AE. Treatment of sexually transmitted chlamydial infections. JAMA. 1986;255:1750–6.
50. Prentice MJ, Hutchinson JR, Taylor-Robinson D. A microbiological study of neonatal conjunctivae and conjunctivitis. Br J Ophthalmol. 1977;61:601–7.
51. Burns RP, Rhodes DH Jr. Pseudomonas eye infection as a cause of death in premature infants. Arch Ophthalmol. 1961;65:517–25.
52. Whitley RJ, Nahmias AJ, Visintine AM, *et al.* The natural history of herpes virus infection of mother and newborn. Pediatrics. 1980;66:489–94.
53. Tuft SJ, Kemeny DM, Dart JK, *et al.* Clinical features of atopic keratoconjunctivitis. Ophthalmology. 1991;98:150–8.
54. Seamone CD, Jackson WB. Immunology of the external eye. In: Tasman W, Jaeger EA, eds. Duane's clinical ophthalmology, Vol 4. Philadelphia: JB Lippincott; 1995:2.29–32.
55. Wilson FM II. Adverse external ocular effects of topical ophthalmic medications. Surv Ophthalmol. 1979;24:57–88.
56. Woods AC. The diagnosis and treatment of ocular allergy. Am J Ophthalmol. 1949;32:1457–78.
57. Beigelman MN. Vernal conjunctivitis. Los Angeles: University of Southern California Press; 1950.
58. Neumann E, Gutmann MJ, Blumenkrantz N, *et al.* A review of four hundred cases of vernal conjunctivitis. Am J Ophthalmol. 1959;47:166–72.
59. Stock EL, Meisler DM. Vernal conjunctivitis. In: Tasman W, Jaeger EA, eds. Duane's clinical ophthalmology, Vol 4. Philadelphia: JB Lippincott; 1995:9.1–5.
60. Foster CS, Duncan J. Randomized clinical trial of topically administered cromolyn sodium for vernal keratoconjunctivitis. Am J Ophthalmol. 1980;90: 175–81.
61. Srinivasan BD, Jacobiec FA, Iwamoto T, *et al.* Giant papillary conjunctivitis with ocular prosthesis. Arch Ophthalmol. 1979;97:892–5.
62. Binder PS. The physiologic effects of extended wear soft contact lenses. Ophthalmology. 1980;87:745–9.
63. Meisler DM, Zaret CR, Stock EL. Trantas' dots and limbal inflammation associated with soft contact lens wear. Am J Ophthalmol. 1980;89:66–9.
64. Fowler SA, Allansmith MR. Evolution of soft contact lens coatings. Arch Ophthalmol. 1980;98:95–9.
65. Jones BR. Immunological specificity of follicles in conjunctivitis due to molluscum contagiosum, adenovirus and cat scratch disease. In: Nichols R, ed. Trachoma and related disorders. Princeton: Excerpta Medica; 1971:243–5.
66. Schuster V, Seidenspinner S, Zeitler P, *et al.* Compound heterozygous mutations in the plasminogen gene predispose to the development of ligneous conjunctivitis. Blood. 1999;93:3457–60.
67. Chen S, Wishart M, Hiscott P. Ligneous conjunctivitis: a local manifestation of a systemic disorder? J AAPOS. 2000;4:313–5.
68. Hidayat AA, Riddle PJ. Ligneous conjunctivitis: a clinicopathologic study of 17 cases. Ophthalmology. 1987;94:949–59.
69. Kraft J, Lieb W, Zeitler P, *et al.* Ligneous conjunctivitis in a girl with severe type I plasminogen deficiency. Graefes Arch Clin Exp Ophthalmol. 2000;238:797–800.
70. Holland EJ, Chan CC, Kuwabara T, *et al.* Immunohistologic findings and results of treatment with cyclosporine in ligneous conjunctivitis. Am J Ophthalmol. 1989;107:160–6.
71. Mondino BJ. Cicatricial pemphigoid and erythema multiforme. Ophthalmology. 1990;97:939–52.
72. Mondino BJ, Brown SI. Ocular cicatricial pemphigoid. Ophthalmology. 1981; 88:95–100.
73. Foster CS. Cicatricial pemphigoid. Trans Am Ophthalmol Soc. 1986;84:527–663.
74. Ralph RA. Conjunctival goblet cell density in normal subjects and dry eye syndromes. Invest Ophthalmol. 1975;14:299–302.
75. Ormerod LD, Fong LP, Foster CS. Corneal infection in mucosal scarring disorders and Sjögren's syndrome. Am J Ophthalmol. 1988;105:512–18.
76. Miserocchi E, Baltatzis S, Roque MR, *et al.* The effect of treatment and its related side effects in patients with severe ocular cicatricial pemphigoid. Ophthalmology. 2002;109:111–8.
77. Chan RY, Bhol K, Natarajan K, *et al.* The role of antibody to human β4 integrin in conjunctival basement membrane separation: possible in vitro model for ocular cicatricial pemphigoid. Invest Ophthalmol Vis Sci. 1999;40:2283–90.
78. Rogers RS, Perry HO, Bean SF, *et al.* Immunopathology of cicatricial pemphigoid: studies of complement deposition. J Invest Dermatol. 1977;68:39–43.
79. Leonard JN, Hobday CM, Haffenden GP, *et al.* Immunofluorescent studies in ocular cicatricial pemphigoid. Br J Dermatol. 1988;118:209–17.
80. Mondino BJ. Bullous diseases of the skin and mucous membranes. In: Tasman W, Jaeger EA, eds. Duane's clinical ophthalmology, Vol 4. Philadelphia: JB Lippincott; 1991:12.11–17.
81. Fiore PM, Jacobs IH, Goldberg DB. Drug induced pemphigoid. Arch Ophthalmol. 1987;105:1660–3.
82. Mondino BJ, Brown SI. Immunosuppressive therapy in ocular cicatricial pemphigoid. Am J Ophthalmol. 1983;96:453–9.
83. Foster CS, Wilson LA, Ekins MB. Immunosuppressive therapy for progressive ocular cicatricial pemphigoid. Ophthalmology. 1982;89:340–53.
84. Foster CS, Ahmed AR. Intravenous immunoglobulin therapy for ocular cicatricial pemphigoid: a preliminary study. Ophthalmology. 1999;106:2136–43.
85. Donnenfeld ED, Perry HD, Wallerstein A, *et al.* Subconjunctival mitomycin C for the treatment of ocular cicatricial pemphigoid. Ophthalmology 1999;106:72–8.
86. Mondino BJ, Brown SI, Lempert S, *et al.* The acute manifestations of ocular cicatricial pemphigoid: diagnosis and treatment. Ophthalmology. 1979;86:543–55.
87. Huff JC, Weston WL, Tonnesen MG. Erythema multiforme: a critical review of characteristics, diagnostic criteria and causes. J Am Acad Dermatol. 1983;8:763–75.
88. Mondino BJ, Brown SI, Biglan AW. HLA antigens in Stevens-Johnson syndrome with ocular involvement. Arch Ophthalmol. 1982;100:1453–4.
89. Dohlman CH, Doughman DJ. The Stevens-Johnson syndrome. In: Castroviejo R, ed. Symposium on the cornea. Transactions of the New Orleans Academy of Ophthalmology. St Louis: CV Mosby; 1972:236–52.
90. Yetiv JZ, Bianchine JR, Owen JA. Etiologic factors of the Stevens-Johnson syndrome. South Med J. 1980;73:599–602.
91. Arstikaitis MJ. Ocular aftermath of Stevens-Johnson syndrome. Arch Ophthalmol. 1973;90:376–9.
92. Tonnesen MG, Soter NA. Erythema multiforme. J Am Acad Dermatol. 1979;1: 357–64.
93. Tsubota K, Shimmura S, Shinozaki N, *et al.* Clinical application of living-related conjunctival-limbal allograft. Am J Ophthalmol. 2002;133:134–5.
94. Koizumi N, Inatomi T, Suzuki T, *et al.* Cultivated corneal epithelial stem cell transplantation in ocular surface disorders. Ophthalmology. 2001;180:1569–74.
95. Fine JD. Epidermolysis bullosa: clinical aspects, pathology and recent advances in research. Int J Dermatol. 1986;25:143–57.
96. Boothe WA, Mondino BJ, Donzis PB. Epidermolysis bullosa. In: Gold DH, Weingeist TA, eds. The eye in systemic disease. Philadelphia: JB Lippincott; 1990: 634–6.

CHAPTER 56 Corneal Epithelium

AYAD A. FARJO • H. KAZ SOONG

DEFINITION
- The anterior-most cellular layer of the cornea.

KEY FEATURES
- Together with the tear film, it is the major refractive surface of the eye.
- Tight junctions provide barrier function.
- Limbal basal epithelium contains the reservoir of stem cells.
- Corneal epithelial dystrophies: map-dot-fingerprint, Meesmann.

ASSOCIATED FEATURES
- Recurrent erosions and persistent epithelial defects.
- Epithelial neoplasia and dysplasia.

INTRODUCTION

A healthy corneal epithelium is necessary to provide a proper anterior refractive surface and to protect the eye against infection and structural damage to the deeper components of the eye.

ANATOMY AND PHYSIOLOGY

Embryologically, the corneal epithelium is derived from surface ectoderm at approximately 5–6 weeks of gestation. It is composed of nonkeratinized, nonsecretory, stratified squamous epithelium (Fig. 56-1), which is 4–6 cell layers thick (40–50μm). The epithelium is covered with a tear film of 7μm thickness, which is optically important in smoothing out microirregularities of the anterior epithelial surface. Without this film, degradation of visual images would result. The tear–air interface, together with the underlying cornea, provides roughly two thirds of the total refractive power of the eye. The mucinous portion of tears, which forms the undercoat of the tear film and is produced by the conjunctival goblet cells, interacts closely with the corneal epithelial cell glycocalyx to allow hydrophilic spreading of the tear film with each eyelid blink. Recent studies have shown that part of this mucinous layer may be secreted by the corneal epithelial cells.[1,2] Loss of the glycocalyx from injury or disease results in loss of stability of the tear film. The tear film also helps protect the corneal surface from microbial invasion, as well as from chemical, toxic, or foreign body damage. Thus the ocular surface tear film and the corneal epithelium share an intimate mutual relationship, both anatomically and physiologically.

Corneal epithelial cells undergo orderly involution, apoptosis (programmed cell death), and desquamation. Complete turnover of corneal epithelial cells occurs in about 7–10 days,[3] with the deeper cells eventually replacing the desquamating superficial cells in an orderly, apically directed fashion. The most superficial cells of the corneal epithelium form an average of two to three layers of flat, polygonal cells. Extensive apical microvilli and microplicae characterize the cell membranes of the superficial cells, which in turn are covered by a fine, closely apposed, charged glycocalyceal layer. The apical membrane projections increase the surface area of contact and adherence between the tear film's mucinous undercoat and the cell membrane. Laterally adjacent superficial cells are joined by barrier tight-junctional complexes, which restrict entry of tears into the intercellular spaces. Thus a healthy epithelial surface repels dyes such as fluorescein and rose bengal. This is consistent with the high resistance ($12–16k\Omega cm^2$) and low ionic conductance of the apical tight junctions.[4] Superficial cells contain relatively sparse intracytoplasmic organelles.

Beneath the superficial cell layer are the suprabasal or wing cells, so named for their cross-sectional alar shapes. This layer is about 2–3 cells deep and consists of cells that are less flat than the overlying superficial cells, but possess similar tight, lateral, intercellular junctions. Beneath the wing cells are the basal cells, which comprise the deepest cellular layer of the corneal epithelium. The basal cell layer is composed of a single-cell layer of columnar epithelium approximately 20μm tall. Besides the stem cells and transient amplifying cells (*vide infra* in the "Epithelial Regeneration" section), basal cells are the only corneal epithelial cells capable of mitosis.[5,6] Thus they possess relatively large numbers of intracytoplasmic organelles, mitochondria, filaments (intermediate filaments, microfilaments [e.g., actin], and microtubules), and glycogen granules. Basal cells, which are the source of both wing and superficial cells, possess lateral intercellular junctions characterized by gap junctions and zonulae adherens. The basal cells are attached to the underlying basement membrane by an extensive basal hemidesmosomal system. This attachment is of pivotal importance in preventing the detachment of the multilayer epithelial sheet from the cornea. Abnormalities in this bonding system may result clinically in either recurrent corneal erosion syndromes or in persistent, nonhealing epithelial defects.

The basement membrane is composed of an extracellular matrix material secreted by the basal cells. Following destruction of the basement membrane, about 6 weeks is required for it to reconstitute and heal. The epithelial bond to the underlying, newly laid basement membrane tends to be unstable and weak during this period. The epithelium also adheres relatively poorly to bare stroma or Bowman's layer. Under ordinary conditions, type IV collagen and laminin are the major components of the basement membrane; however, fibronectin production increases to high levels during acute epithelial injury. The basement membrane, approximately 0.05μm in thickness, adheres to the underlying Bowman's membrane through a poorly understood mechanism that involves anchoring fibrils and plaques.[7]

The central cornea is normally devoid of antigen processing and presenting cells. Under certain conditions (e.g., corneal graft rejection, *herpesvirus* infection, or injury), immunologically active dendritic macrophages (Langerhans' cells) migrate rapidly from the limbal periphery. These cells are derived from the bone marrow and express major histocompatibility complex class II molecules that, upon interacting with CD4-positive T-lymphocytes, release immunomodulatory cytokines.

413

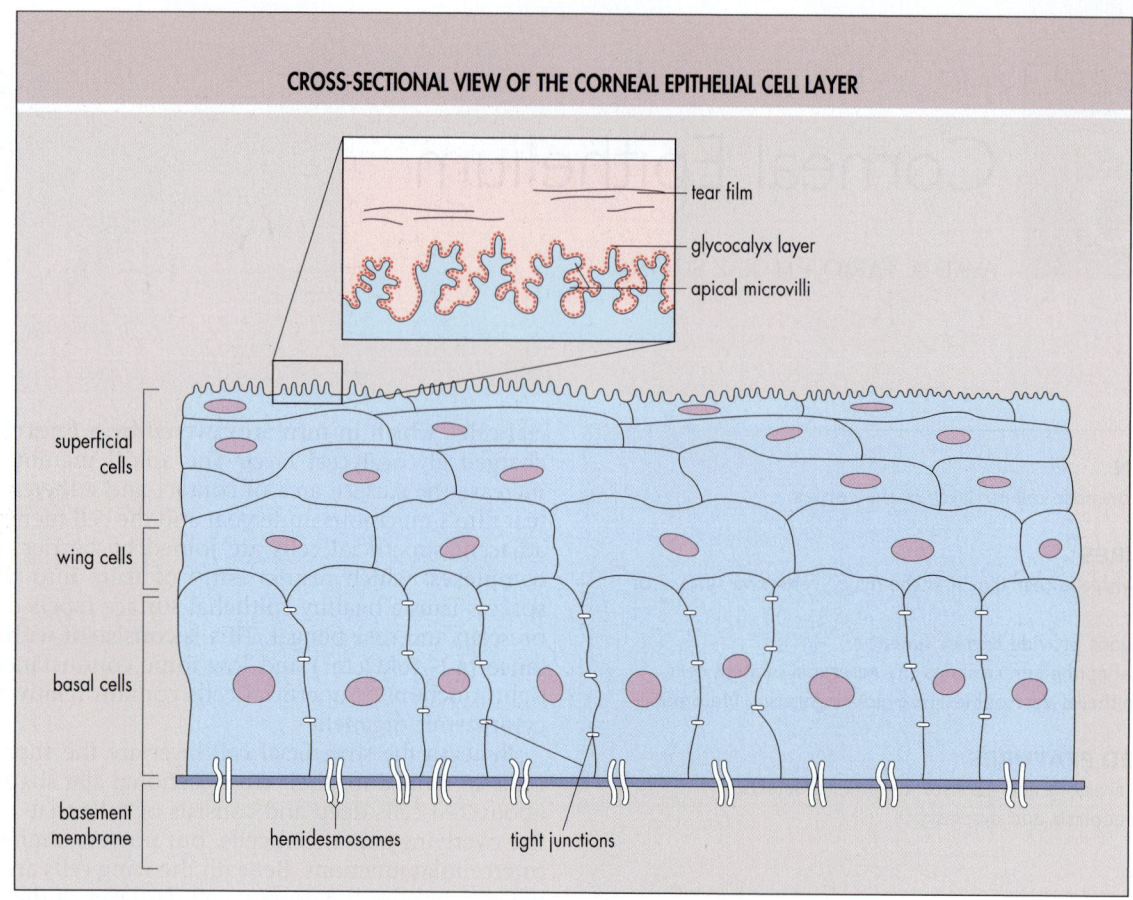

CROSS-SECTIONAL VIEW OF THE CORNEAL EPITHELIAL CELL LAYER

tear film
glycocalyx layer
apical microvilli

superficial cells

wing cells

basal cells

basement membrane

hemidesmosomes

tight junctions

FIG. 56-1 ▪ Cross-sectional view of the corneal epithelial cell layer.

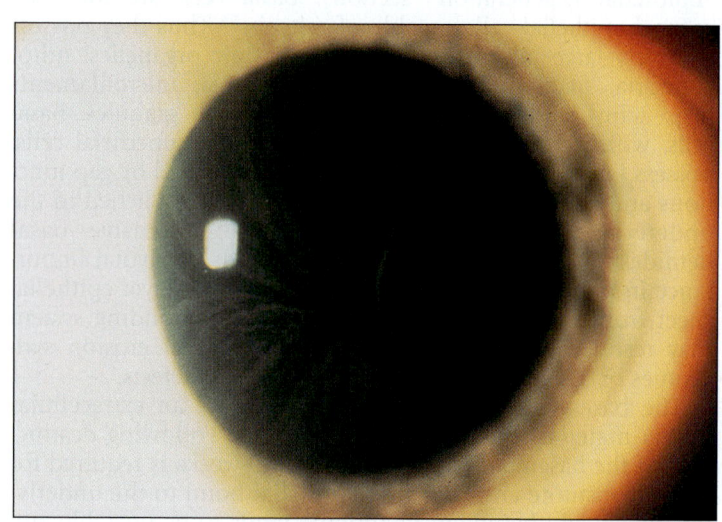

FIG. 56-2 ▪ Whorl-like deposition keratopathy in corneal epithelium seen in Fabry's disease.

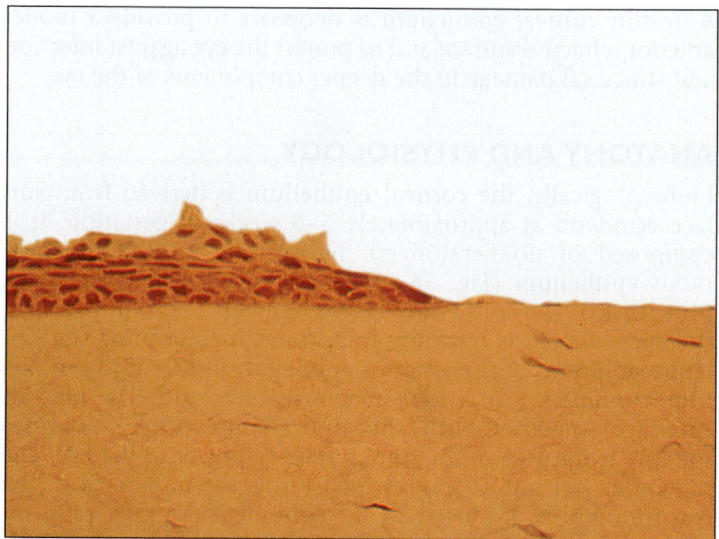

FIG. 56-3 ▪ Light micrograph that shows the leading edge of migrating rat corneal epithelium as it tapers to a layer of one-cell thickness. As the epithelial defect is rapidly covered by migrating cells, it is initially coated with a thin, rarefied cell population prior to onset of mitotic activity (hematoxylin & eosin).

Epithelial Regeneration

Epithelial stem cells—undifferentiated pluripotent cells that serve as an important source of new corneal epithelium—have been localized to the limbal basal epithelium. As the cells migrate to the central cornea, they differentiate into transient amplifying cells (cells capable of multiple, but limited cellular division) and basal cells. The corneal epithelial cell layer mass appears to be the complex resultant of three phenomena. According to the "X, Y, Z hypothesis," X is the proliferation of basal epithelial cells, Y is the centripetal mass movement of peripheral epithelial cells, and Z is the cell loss resulting from

death and desquamation.[8] These three phenomena probably are not totally independent of each other, but rather are controlled by a complex interactive feedback mechanism that maintains the status quo, vis-à-vis cell density, cell distribution and polarity, and cell layer thickness. These cytodynamics are likely to be responsible for the striking verticillate (vortex or whorl-like) biochemical deposition patterns seen in Fabry's disease (Fig. 56-2) and drug deposition keratopathies (e.g., from chloroquine and amiodarone). Newly formed limbal cells are thought to migrate toward the central cornea in such an arcuate, whorl-like pattern.

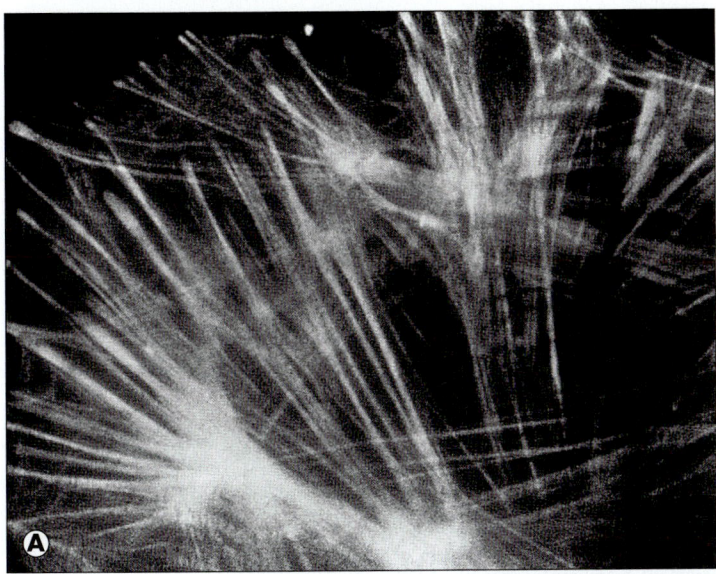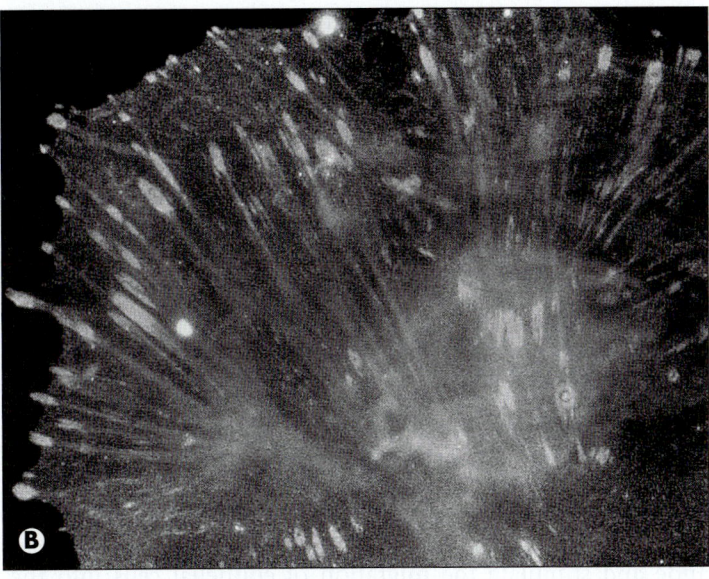

FIG. 56-4 ■ Double-fluorescent labeling at the leading edge of a migrating corneal epithelial cell in tissue culture. This is for, **A**, actin and, **B**, vinculin. Vinculin-rich adhesion foci are abundant in cell membrane protrusions and at the front edge of the cell. Actin fibers terminate into these foci and are oriented in the direction of cell migration.

WOUND HEALING

Within minutes after a small corneal epithelial injury, cells at the edge of the abrasion begin to cover the defect as rapidly as possible by a combination of cell migration and cell spreading. A longer delay of up to 4–5 hours is seen in larger defects. This lag phase is necessary for the preparatory cellular changes of an anatomical, physiological, and biochemical nature to occur before rapid cell movement. Various cell membrane extensions, such as lamellipodia, filopodia, and ruffles, develop at the leading edge of the wound. Anchoring hemidesmosomes disappear from the basal cells. This early nonmitotic wound coverage phase is remarkable for its speed; the cells have been measured to migrate at a rate of 60–80μm/h (Fig. 56-3).[9] The migrating sheet of epithelial cells is attached most firmly to the underlying substrate at the leading margin.[10] The relatively firmer adhesion at the leading margin suggests that the epithelial sheet movement may have "front-wheel drive," with the less well-anchored cells behind the leading margin being pulled forward, possibly by intracellular contractile mechanisms that involve actin.[11] Vinculin, a 130kD cytoplasmic protein found specifically in focal adhesion plaques on the cytoplasmic side of the cell membrane, may be involved in the linkage of intracytoplasmic actin stress fibers to the cell membrane at these focal junctions. Vinculin links actin fibers to the cell membrane protein, talin, which in turn is linked to integrin, a major cell-to-substrate adhesion protein.[12] These adhesion protein complexes are most numerous at the leading edge of the migrating cells, which enables the cells to adhere to the basement membrane in the absence of hemidesmosomes. The contraction of actin fibers ostensibly pulls the soma (cell body) forward in the direction of the leading edge (Fig. 56-4). Fibronectin, a ubiquitous extracellular matrix protein present in plasma and in fresh wounds, is thought to be a key element in the mediation of cell-to-substrate adhesion and cell migration. Present on the extracellular side of adhesion plaques, it is thought to mediate the linkage between the vinculin–talin–integrin complex and the substrate during epithelial migration after a wound has occurred (Fig. 56-5). Laminin, a less ubiquitous extracellular matrix protein, is thought to serve a similar function.

At 24–30 hours after medium-sized epithelial injuries, mitosis or cell proliferation begins and restores the rarefied epithelial cell population. After large epithelial injuries, significant increases in cellular division occur as late as 96 hours.[13] Only the basal cells, transient amplifying cells, and the limbal stem cells partake in this reconstitutive mitosis.[5,6]

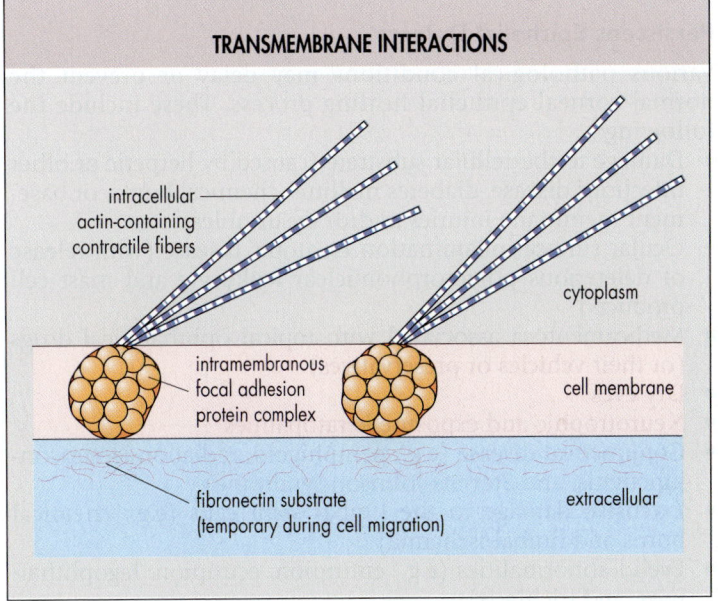

TRANSMEMBRANE INTERACTIONS

intracellular actin-containing contractile fibers

cytoplasm

intramembranous focal adhesion protein complex

cell membrane

fibronectin substrate (temporary during cell migration)

extracellular

FIG. 56-5 ■ Transmembrane interactions. The transmembrane interactions between the intracellular (intracytoplasmic) actin-containing contractile fibers, the focal intramembranous adhesion protein complexes, and the extracellular substrate of fibronectin during epithelial migration in wound healing are shown. After wound healing, more permanent and firmly rooted hemidesmosomal attachments become established.

In laboratory and clinical trials, various agents known to influence epithelial migration, mitosis, apoptosis, adhesion, and differentiation have been studied as possible therapeutic agents to enhance corneal epithelial healing. These include growth factors, fibronectin, and retinoids (see Soong[14] for review). Although primarily mitogenic agents, growth factors also stimulate production of extracellular matrix components to enhance cell-to-substrate adhesion. Whether growth factors enhance cellular migration and spread remains in dispute. Topical fibronectin eyedrops effectively accelerate corneal epithelial healing in persistent epithelial defects associated with several conditions; these include herpes simplex keratitis, cataract surgery, and trophic keratitis.[15] On the other hand, fibronectin eyedrops show no significant efficacy in the treatment of epithelial defects that follow corneal alkali injury or that occur in dry eye conditions.[16] Furthermore, exogenous fibronectin by itself did not enhance epithelial wound closure rates in an *in vitro* study of scraped corneal epithelial wounds, nor did it enhance the concomitant effects of growth factor.[17] The lack of efficacy of exogenously applied fibronectin in these studies may be caused by the presence of endogenously produced fibronectin at the wound site, in response to the injury.[17] Topical tretinoin (all-*trans*-retinoic acid), a vitamin A analog, promotes differentiation of epithelial cells and enhances corneal epithelial wound closure rates in rabbits.[18,19] It may also indirectly promote the healing of corneal epithelium by maintaining the proper anatomy, differentiation, and function of the conjunctival and stem cells.[18]

Several extrinsic factors are involved in the control of directed cell movements during cell migration. These include contact inhibition, chemotaxis, haptotaxis (cell migration guided by signals within the extracellular matrix substrate), and contact guidance. Corneal epithelial cells also have been shown to generate electrical fields during wound healing (injury currents). Interestingly, the movement of the cells appears to be influenced by these biological, self-generated fields. Such fields may serve to guide and stimulate the migration of epithelial cells into the area of the defect (galvanotropism and galvanotaxis).[20] It is attractive to hypothesize that these biologically generated electrical fields may constitute an alternative form of nonhumoral intercellular communication.[20]

Persistent Epithelial Defects

Various pathological conditions may delay or prevent the normal corneal epithelial healing process. These include the following:

- Damage to the cellular substrate (caused by herpetic or other infectious disease, diabetes mellitus, chemical burns, or basement membrane injuries and/or dystrophies)
- Ocular surface inflammation or atopic disease (with release of deleterious polymorphonuclear leukocyte and mast cell products)
- Medicamentosa associated with topical ophthalmical drugs (or their vehicles or preservatives)
- Dry eyes
- Neurotrophic and exposure keratopathies
- Conjunctival disease (e.g., pemphigoid, radiation keratoconjunctivitis, and Stevens-Johnson syndrome)
- Extensive damage to the limbal stem cells (e.g., chemical burns and limbal ischemia)
- Eyelid abnormalities (e.g., entropion, ectropion, lagophthalmos, and trichiasis)

The epithelial healing problems of postinfectious (metaherpetic) ulceration, seen after acute herpetic keratitis, are believed to be caused by damage to the basement membrane from antiviral drug toxicity or from overzealous iatrogenic scraping of the corneal surface using either mechanical or chemical means.[21] In neurotrophic corneas it is possible that interruption of corneal innervation results in depletion of substance P, a neurogenic chemical known to regulate corneal physiological functions. Diabetic corneas may manifest abnormally thickened and easily delaminated basement membranes (Fig. 56-6), perhaps akin to basement membrane abnormalities elsewhere, as in the renal glomeruli.[22] Persistent epithelial defects associated with topical anesthetic abuse may be caused by a combination of pharmacological interruption of corneal nerve function and damage to the epithelial cells and substrate.[23,24] Limbal stem cell deficiency is an increasingly recognized cause of nonhealing epithelial defects.

Treatment is directed toward the underlying condition in a stepwise fashion. Unless absolutely needed, all topical medications should be discontinued with the use of only preservative-free lubricants. Punctal occlusion should be performed in the presence of dry eyes with treatment of concomitant ocular surface inflammation as needed. Autologous serum eyedrops, bandage soft contact lenses, and amniotic membrane transplanta-

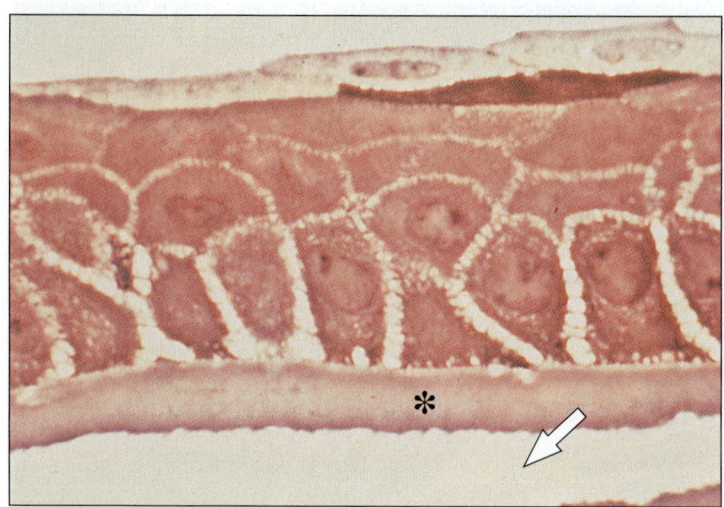

FIG. 56-6 ■ Recurrent erosion in a diabetic cornea. Note the abnormally thick basement membrane *(asterisk)* and the intralamellar split within *(arrow)* (hematoxylin & eosin).

tion can be used. Ultimately, tarsorrhaphy appears to remain the best means of healing persistent epithelial defects.

RECURRENT CORNEAL EROSIONS

Although most corneal epithelial defects heal quickly and permanently, some may be characterized by recurrent breakdowns of the epithelium as late as several years after the initial episode. The majority of corneas that have recurrent epithelial erosions often show abnormalities in the underlying basement membrane microstructure. Microscopic derangement in the epithelial basement membrane either may occur as sequelae of trauma or may be a result of dystrophy or disease. Recurrent corneal erosions are a relatively common problem. The majority of cases occur after corneal trauma, frequently following superficial epithelial abrasions from fingernails, paper, or mascara brushes. Although less commonly encountered, chemical and thermal burns also may lead to recurrent epithelial breakdown.

Post-Traumatic Erosions Without Primary Basement Membrane Abnormalities

Posttraumatic, nondystrophic, recurrent corneal erosion is clinically the most common form of repetitive corneal epithelial breakdown. After corneal surface injury, basement membrane thickening, discontinuities, and duplications are typically seen for 8-12 weeks; the overlying epithelium is vulnerable to detachment during this period.[25-27] These changes occasionally may persist for a prolonged period, in which case the cornea is susceptible to repetitive breakdown even years after the original injury. Slit-lamp findings similar to those in epithelial basement membrane dystrophy may be seen in some patients, whereas in others the cornea may clinically look disarmingly normal between erosive episodes.

Erosions Associated with Corneal Dystrophy

Epithelial basement membrane dystrophy (Cogan's microcystic dystrophy; map–dot–fingerprint dystrophy) is frequently seen in general ophthalmic practice and is the most common form of anterior corneal dystrophy. Intraepithelial lesions that resemble geographic map-like gray patches, dots or microcysts, and fingerprint or whorl-like patterns (Figs. 56-7 and 56-8) characterize this dystrophy. No known systemic associations occur. Slit-lamp examination under direct illumination may not be sufficient to elicit the often subtle and small intraepithelial lesions. Retroillumination through a dilated pupil in a dark examining room best highlights fingerprint lines and microcystic dots. Rapid

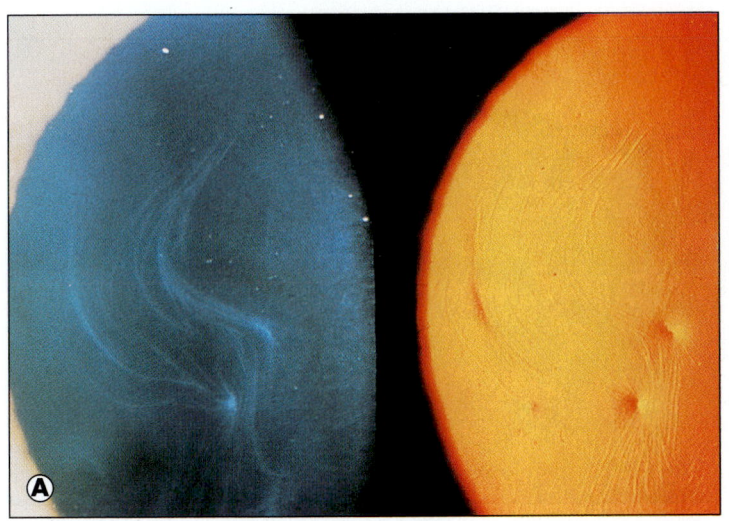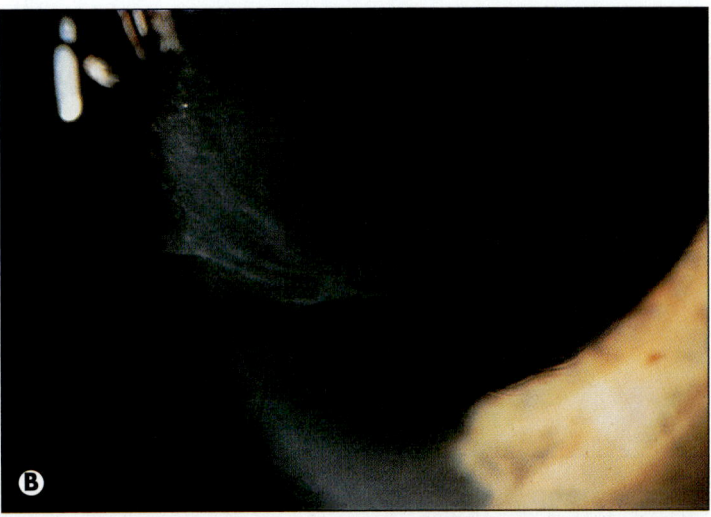

FIG. 56-7 ▮ **Epithelial basement membrane dystrophy. A,** Slit-lamp view of fingerprint lines and microcysts under direct illumination *(left)* and retroillumination *(right)*. **B,** Map lesion under direct illumination.

tear-film breakup resulting from subtle surface contour irregularities also occurs over these lesions, especially the maplike patches.

Clinicopathologically, epithelial basement membrane dystrophy is associated with three basic elemental findings[28]:

- Thickening of the basement membrane with fingerlike or lamellar extensions into the overlying epithelial layer
- Intraepithelial microcysts formed by trapped, degenerating epithelial cells
- Fibrillar material between the basement membrane and the underlying Bowman's layer (as viewed by electron microscopy)

This dystrophy of the epithelial basement membrane is associated with recurrent corneal erosions in up to 10% of cases. From a converse perspective, 50% of individuals with recurrent corneal erosions may show clinical findings compatible with this disorder.[29] Most cases of epithelial basement membrane dystrophy are bilateral and remain asymptomatic. Although they probably are autosomal dominant in inheritance,[28] many show no apparent familial pattern. Other studies have observed similar corneal findings incidentally during routine examination in a large proportion of the general population.[30] Irregular astigmatism from these superficial lesions sometimes can lead to decreased visual acuity. Irregular astigmatism may be readily diagnosed by keratometry, keratoscopy, or computed topography.

Painful, recurrent corneal erosions are more common after the third decade of life and usually are self limited, with spontaneous resolution after several years. Permanent deficits in visual acuity are extremely rare. The recurrent erosions may occur either in association with a history of previous trauma or spontaneously without any obvious antecedent precipitating incidents. Histopathologically, erosions result from poor epithelial adhesion to the abnormal basement membrane or from lamellar splitting and/or shearing of the abnormally fragile membrane. Large, single sheets of loose epithelium may often be peeled off the cornea during therapeutic debridement. Recurrent erosions may occur in other anterior corneal dystrophies, such as Reis-Bücklers' and Meesmann's dystrophies.

Meesmann's epithelial dystrophy is an autosomal dominant, inherited, bilateral disorder usually seen as early as the first year of life as multiple tiny intraepithelial vesicles (Fig. 56-9, *A-B*).[28] No systemic associations occur. The patient remains asymptomatic until middle age, at which time the diffusely distributed intraepithelial vesicles break through the anterior epithelial surface and cause punctal staining (Fig. 56-9, *C*), intermittent irritation, and irregular astigmatism.

Histopathologically, the epithelial layer is thickened and contains intraepithelial cysts mostly in its anterior aspect (Fig. 56-10). These correspond to vesicles seen clinically and may

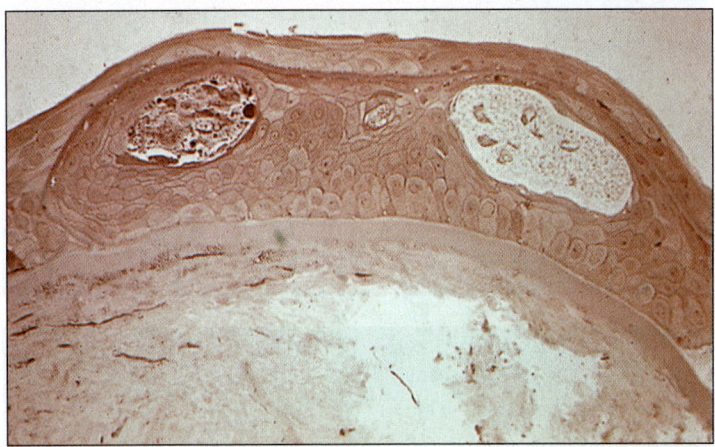

FIG. 56-8 ▮ **Cogan's microcystic dystrophy.** The dot pattern is caused by cysts that contain desquamating surface epithelial cells. (From Yanoff M, Fine BS. Ocular pathology, ed 5. St Louis, Mosby; 2002.)

stain with fluorescein and rose bengal stains. The basement membrane may show multilaminar thickening with occasional projections into the overlying epithelial layer. These basement membrane changes may be responsible for disordered epithelial adhesion to the substrate. Ultrastructurally, an intracytoplasmic fibrillogranular "peculiar substance" is seen consistently in Meesmann's dystrophy.[28]

Anterior involvement in lattice, macular, and granular stromal dystrophies may be associated with epithelial erosions. Recurrent epithelial breakdown in Fuchs' dystrophy is due to an edematous process, rather than to abnormalities in the substrate.

Erosions Associated with Diabetes Mellitus

Recurrent corneal erosions are not uncommon in severe diabetics and may further compromise vision already made tenuous by concomitant retinopathy. These erosions usually are post-traumatic following apparently mild injuries; however, epithelial breakdown may also occur after ophthalmic surgery, such as cataract extraction and vitrectomy procedures. In some instances the surgeon may elect to scrape off the epithelium intraoperatively to improve visualization of the intraocular structures. As mentioned earlier, a thickened and fragile basement membrane (Fig. 56-6), reduced penetration of the basal anchoring fibrils into Bowman's layer, and effete duplication of anchoring fibrils in diabetic corneas have been described.[31] Unlike the case with nondiabetic erosions, these diabetic corneas not only are prone to recurrent erosions, but also tend to have persistent nonheal-

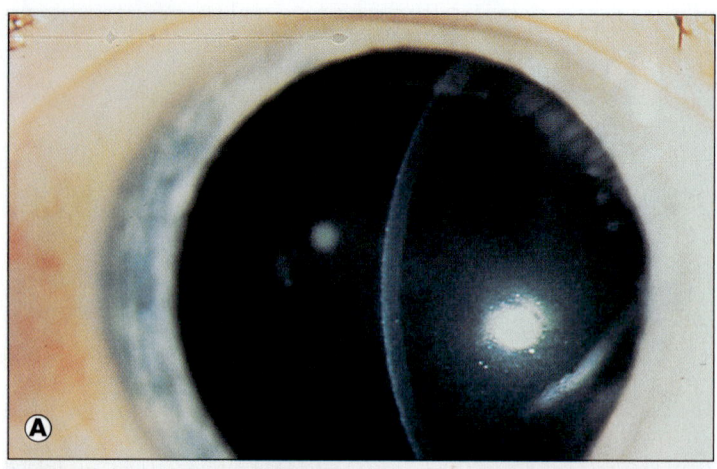

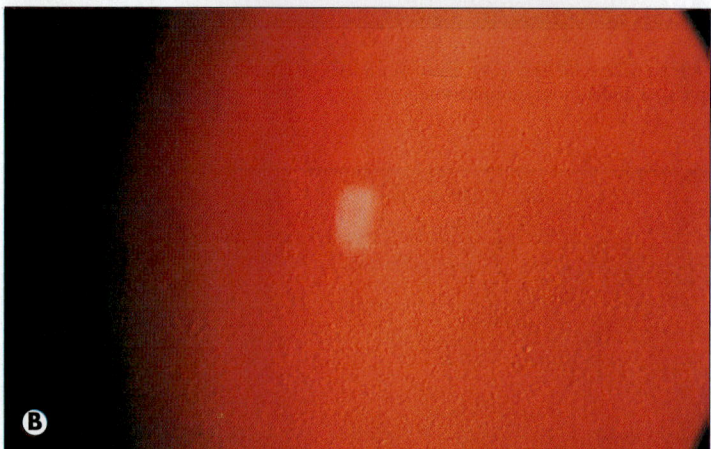

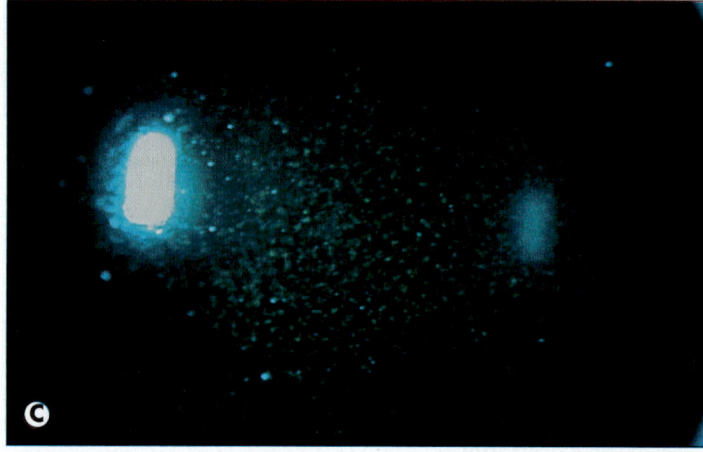

FIG. 56-9 ▓ Meesmann's epithelial dystrophy with intraepithelial vesicles. A, Direct illumination. B, Retroillumination. C, Punctate staining of Meesmann's corneal epithelium with fluorescein.

ing epithelial defects. This may be caused by additional factors such as neurotrophic disease and limbal vasculopathy.

Clinical Symptoms and Signs of Recurrent Erosion

Typically, the onset of corneal erosion is upon awakening in the morning, although it may occur at any time. This propensity may be caused by relative anoxia, hypercapnia, or edema of the corneal epithelium when the eyelids are closed during sleep. Also, the sudden opening of the eyelids upon awakening may easily rub off the vulnerable epithelium. The patient frequently experiences pain, blurring, photophobia, foreign-body sensation, blepharospasm, and tearing. The symptoms may vary among individuals and with the extent of the surface breakdown. Depending on the severity, the erosion may spontaneously resolve within minutes to weeks, or alternatively may be

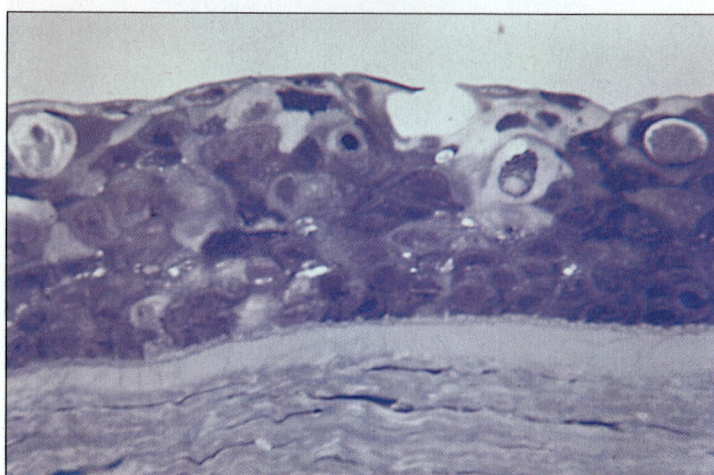

FIG. 56-10 ▓ Meesmann's dystrophy. In this thin, plastic-embedded section, numerous tiny cysts of uniform size and one surface pit are present within the epithelium. One cyst to the right of center resembles a cell. (From Yanoff M, Fine BS. Ocular pathology, ed 5. St Louis, Mosby; 2002.)

subject to multiple brief, repetitive breakdown episodes before finally subsiding.

Slit-lamp examination may show a frank epithelial defect, often with an entire loose sheet of epithelium hanging tenuously from the corneal surface. Filamentary keratitis, intraepithelial microcysts, fingerprint lines, bullae, epithelial irregularity, subepithelial haze, and epithelial edema may also be present. Between erosive episodes, the basement membrane changes may be difficult to see on direct illumination; however, retroillumination against the background of a dilated pupil may bring out subtle epithelial and subepithelial lesions (Fig. 56-7, A).

Treatment of Recurrent Corneal Erosion

For mild erosions, the use of ocular surface lubricants (artificial tears and/or ointments) or pressure patches may be enough to improve patient comfort and perhaps reduce the deleterious frictional effects of each eyelid blink. The efficacy of pressure patching a corneal abrasion is currently debatable. Hypertonic sodium chloride eyedrops and ointments may have an additional yet poorly understood (and disputed) beneficial effect. Typically, hypertonic eyedrops are used 3–4 times during waking hours, and the ointment form is used at bedtime for at least 3 months. Although the ointment form has superior lubrication effects and pharmacologic contact time, it does significantly compromise visual acuity. Antimicrobial prophylaxis and cycloplegics are given at the discretion of the physician. For beneficial long-term behavior modification, patients should learn to open their eyes slowly, cautiously, and with deliberation when awakening from sleep.

In cases of more extensive erosion accompanied by large, loose sheets of epithelium and devitalized cells, scraping and debridement of the affected area with a cellulose spear (Weck-cel) or a smooth-edged, nonincisional instrument, such as the Kimura spatula, may help provide a smoother and more hospitable epithelial substrate. Sharp instruments or chemicals should not be used, since they may cause excessive damage to the substrate. Surrounding areas also should be checked for the presence of loosely adherent epithelial sheets by gently probing suspicious-looking regions with a cellulose spear or a cotton-tipped applicator. Lifting with fine surgical forceps may facilitate removal of these poorly adherent epithelial sheets.

Extended-wear bandage soft contact lenses may provide comfort and support the healing process, with minimal compromise of vision. They have the additional benefit of protecting and isolating the fragile, healing epithelium from the windshield-wiper effects of blinking eyelids. These lenses should remain on the cornea for at least 6–8 weeks to allow the basement membrane

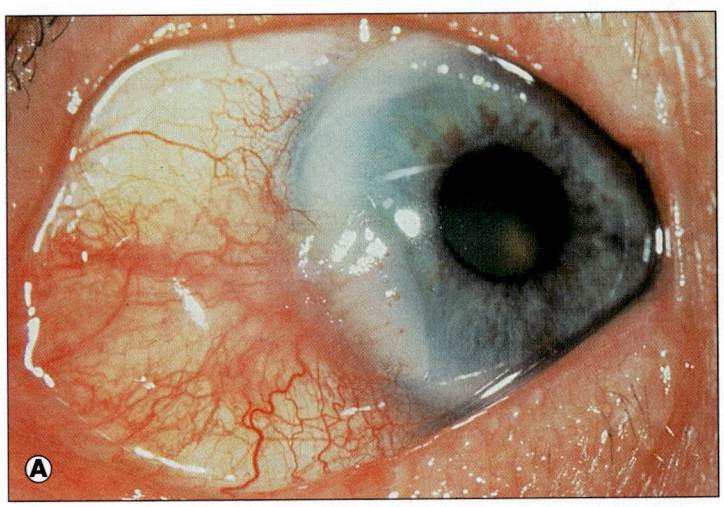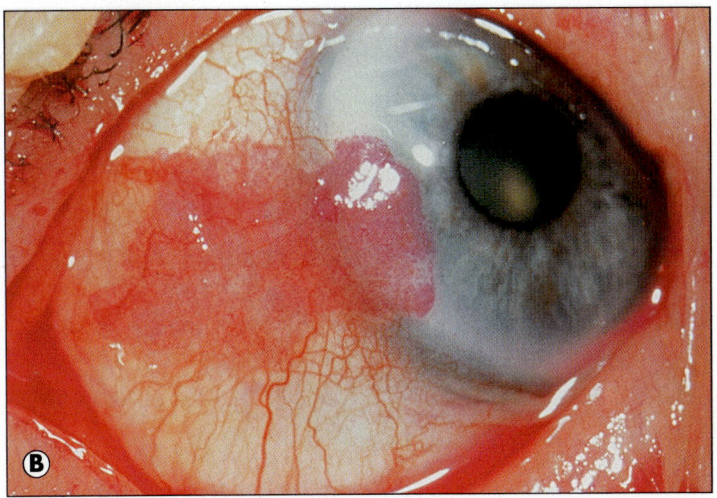

FIG. 56-11 ■ Carcinoma in situ of the conjunctiva, limbus, and cornea. A, Slit-lamp appearance. B, The dysplastic conjunctival and corneal epithelia stained with rose bengal.

and hemidesmosomes time to reorganize. The patient should be warned of the slight risk of microbial infection associated with the use of extended-wear lenses. The authors remove the bandage lens once at 4 weeks and insert either a new lens or reinsert the original one after sterilization; concomitant antibiotic prophylaxis generally is not used. In the acute phase of erosion marked by inflammation, bandage lenses should be checked within 24 hours after insertion for any evidence of the tight-lens syndrome. If the lens is tolerated poorly, it either should be replaced with a smaller diameter, flatter lens or should be removed and not replaced. Cautious and judicious use of topical corticosteroids and cycloplegics may reduce inflammation and enhance patient comfort. Hypertonic sodium chloride preparations should not be used in conjunction with these high water content lenses. An alternative for short-term relief and epithelial support is a collagen shield.

If the erosions are severe or frequent, anterior stromal micropuncture or superficial keratectomy are the therapeutic options. Superficial stromal micropuncture for recurrent corneal erosions, first described by McLean et al.,[32] is highly efficacious in the stabilization of susceptible epithelium and very effective in the provision of a long-term cure for erosions. The mechanism of action is unclear, but epithelial plugs remain in the puncture sites as anchors for months after therapy.[33] The action is analogous to tacking down a loose carpet with nails. The procedure is performed at the slit lamp, using a 25- or 27-gauge sterile hypodermic needle. Some clinicians prefer to use a larger (20-gauge) needle, which covers more area and perhaps reduces the likelihood of corneal perforation; however, these larger needles cause more scarring because of the sheer size of the micropuncture wound they create. The needle may be attached to a 1cm³ tuberculin syringe for surgeon comfort and ease of application. A 60–90° bend is made in the direction of the bevel, being careful not to blunt the tip in the process. The bend enhances the surgeon's ergonomic comfort and provides a mechanical stop to reduce the chance of corneal perforation. Since only the superficial stroma needs be punctured, there is little reason to push excessively hard with the needle into the cornea. Multiple punctures are applied to include the surrounding normal cornea and to ensure that the erosion does not spread centrifugally. Some clinicians do treat the central visual axis lightly in severe cases and apparently encounter little or no significant visual sequelae, but others prefer to leave at least a 3.0mm clear central optical zone. If necessary, the anterior stromal micropuncture procedure may be repeated later, with either extension of the treatment beyond the original zone or additional filling in of the area previously treated. The use of argon or YAG laser, surface cauterization, or diathermy to perform this procedure does not offer any advantages over the needle technique and may cause more scarring and corneal topographic changes than does the micropuncture technique.

Superficial keratectomy is an effective treatment for recurrent corneal erosions. It removes the diseased basement membrane down to the Bowman's layer and superficial stroma. A scarifier blade or blunt lamellar dissection blade may be used to peel and dissect off gently the abnormal superficial tissue. Sharp blades may cause excessive damage to the stroma and should be avoided. The fine-grade diamond polishing drill (Ugo-Fisch) is a very simple and effective instrument with which to remove superficial corneal tissue. Compared with dissectional methods, the polishing procedure is less technically demanding and creates a very smooth corneal surface.[34] Alternatively, excimer laser phototherapeutic keratectomy may be used to achieve the same ends. Induced hyperopia with excimer laser keratectomy for recurrent corneal erosions is usually minimal because of the superficial nature of the treatment.

CORNEAL EPITHELIAL DYSPLASIA AND NEOPLASIA

Dysplastic disturbances of squamous cells constitute the most common true neoplastic processes of the corneal epithelium. Owing to the intimate anatomical, functional, and cytological relationships between corneal and conjunctival epithelia, such tumors appear to be inseparable from those that affect the conjunctiva. The majority of dysplastic corneal epithelial lesions, consequently, have a portion of the lesion in direct contiguity with the highly mitotic stem cells at the limbus (Fig. 56-11). Dysplastic cells manifest increased nuclear:cytoplasmic ratio, atypical size and shape, and disturbed polarity and maturation. Most such lesions occur in the exposed interpalpebral regions in fair-skinned, older men, which suggests the causal role of actinic transformation. Dysplastic corneal epithelium appears translucent or gelatinous, in contrast to clear, normal epithelium. Occasionally, keratinization from squamous metaplasia may impart a whitish, leukoplakic appearance to the lesion. Another useful way to distinguish dysplastic epithelium from normal epithelium is to apply fluorescein or rose bengal stain (Fig. 56-11). Normal epithelium does not stain, whereas dysplastic epithelium shows diffuse, punctate staining.

Squamous dysplasia and carcinoma in situ are histopathologically distinguished by the degree of anaplastic involvement (loss of differentiation, increased mitotic figures, and dysmaturation). In squamous dysplasia, atypical cells replace only a portion of the corneal epithelium, whereas in carcinoma in situ these cells occupy the entire epithelial layer from basement

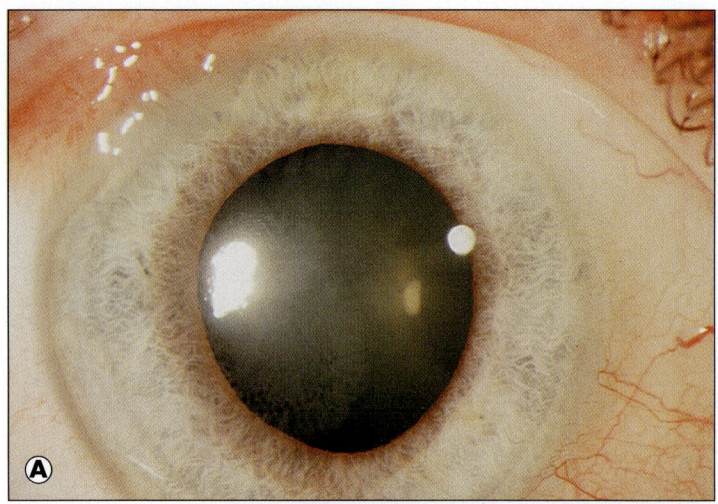

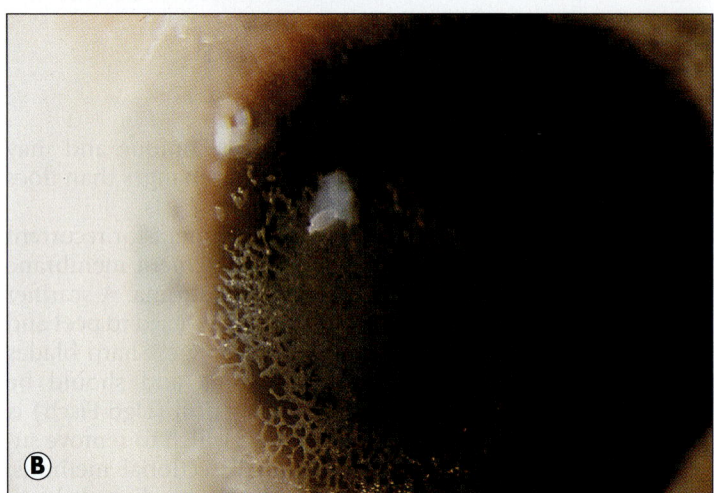

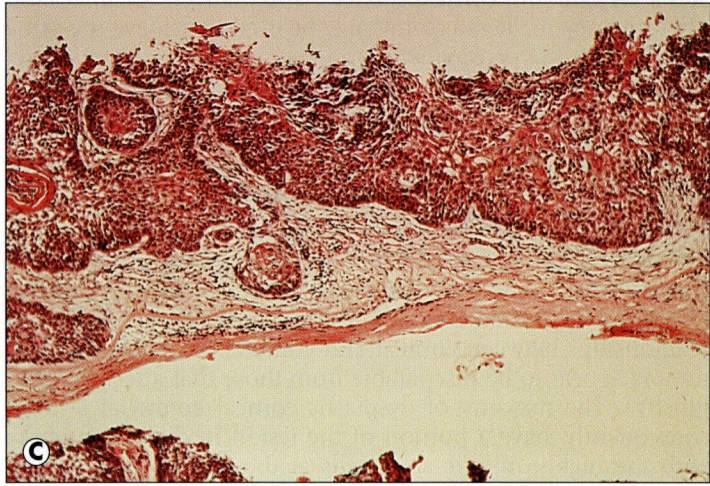

FIG. 56-12 ▪ Corneal and limbal conjunctival squamous cell carcinoma in situ. **A**, Clinical appearances. **B**, Close-up view of the corneal epithelial lesion with fimbriated edges. **C**, Histopathology of the limbal conjunctiva showing dysplasia of the entire epithelial layer (hematoxylin & eosin).

membrane to the superficial cells. In both cases the basement membrane is intact. The practicality of this distinction is questionable, and some now prefer to use the term "intraepithelial neoplasia" to encompass both entities (Fig. 56-12).

Squamous dysplasia and carcinoma in situ are treated by scraping off the affected corneal epithelium, preferably with a blunt instrument such as a Kimura or Paton spatula, which reduces damage to the basement membrane. Occasionally, an adherent fibrovascular pannus may be present and must be dissected from Bowman's layer using sharp dissection. Some surgeons recommend additional chemical devitalization of the limbus with absolute alcohol. Contiguous limbal and conjunc-

tival lesions are excised down to bare sclera, and additional lateral margins (1–2mm) of apparently normal conjunctiva are removed. The limbus, peripheral cornea, base, and conjunctiva are treated with a cryoprobe in a rapid double- or triple-freeze fashion. Extensive, prolonged, or deep treatment is not recommended, however, because of the superficiality and ready accessibility of these lesions. In these noninvasive lesions, it is unnecessary to risk deep structural freeze damage to the cornea, trabecular meshwork, ciliary body, and retina. The eye should be regularly examined for evidence of recurrent disease. Although recurrent lesions generally are treated in the same way as primary lesions, the margins of excision and the degree of cryotherapy need to be increased because of the small but not negligible potential for the development of invasive carcinoma. Early evidence suggests that application of topical mitomycin-C, adjunctively in cases of recurrence or primarily in instances in which surgical excision cannot be performed, may be a safe and effective treatment modality.[35]

Primary corneal epithelial dysplasia is a relatively rare condition that predominantly involves the corneal epithelium, with disproportionately little or absent lesional involvement of the limbus. The involved corneal epithelium appears frosted or opalescent, with either fimbriated, serpiginous, scalloped, geographic, or smooth edges, and usually without a fibrovascular pannus. The corneal lesions may be single or multiple and abut the limbus or form islands away from the limbus. These lesions may show extensive waxing and waning alterations in shape and size over months to years.[36] Cytologically, the involved epithelium shows signs of atypia and dysmaturation. Treatment consists of simple scraping of the corneal epithelium, taking special care not to damage the basement membrane protective barrier. Any associated limbal mass or lesion should be excised, leaving wide margins, with the option for additional cryotherapy left to the discretion of the surgeon. Recurrences are common.

Invasive squamous cell carcinoma can arise from squamous dysplasia or carcinoma in situ if the underlying basement membrane barrier is broken. The underlying Bowman's layer and corneal stroma, or the subepithelial conjunctival tissues, may be invaded. Treatment consists of wide excision of the lesion with inclusion of the involved corneal stroma and sclera by lamellar dissection. Extensive cryotherapy of the lateral and deep margins is indicated, more aggressively than for the noninvasive situations. Cryotherapy reduces the recurrence rate of these lesions from 40% to under 10%.[37] Scleral, intraocular, or orbital invasion also may occur. Involvement of the uvea or trabecular meshwork may afford the neoplastic cells access to the systemic circulation. Fortunately, regional metastasis is rare[38] and widespread systemic metastasis is even rarer. Deaths from this type of tumor are extremely uncommon. Enucleation is indicated for intraocular invasion, and exenteration is indicated in orbital extension.

REFERENCES

1. Ubels JL, McCartney MD, Lantz WK, et al. Effects of preservative-free artificial tear solutions on corneal epithelial structure and function. Arch Ophthalmol. 1995;113:371–8.
2. Gipson IK, Yankaukas M, Spurr-Michaud SJ, et al. Characteristics of a glycoprotein in the ocular surface glycocalyx. Invest Ophthalmol Vis Sci. 1992;33:218–27.
3. Hanna C, Bicknell DS, O'Brien JE. Cell turnover in the adult human eye. Arch Ophthalmol. 1961;65:695–8.
4. Klyce SD, Crosson CE. Transport processes across the rabbit corneal epithelium: a review. Curr Eye Res. 1985;4:323–31.
5. Gipson IK, Friend J, Spurr-Michaud SJ. Transplant of corneal epithelium to rabbit corneal wounds in vitro. Invest Ophthalmol Vis Sci. 1985;26:425–33.
6. Wiley L, SunderRaj N, Sun TT, Thoft RA. Regional heterogeneity in human corneal and limbal epithelia: an immunohistochemical evaluation. Invest Ophthalmol Vis Sci. 1991;32:594–602.
7. Hogan MJ, Alvarado JA, Weddell E. Histology of the human eye. Philadelphia: WB Saunders; 1971:55–111.
8. Thoft RA, Friend J. The X, Y, Z hypothesis of corneal epithelial maintenance. Invest Ophthalmol Vis Sci. 1983;24:1442–3.
9. Matsuda M, Ubels JL, Edelhauser HF. A larger corneal epithelial wound closes at a faster rate. Invest Ophthalmol Vis Sci. 1985;26:897–900.
10. DiPasquale A. Locomotory activity of epithelial cells in culture. Exp Cell Res. 1975;94:191–215.

11. Soong HK. Vinculin in focal cell-to-substrate attachments of spreading corneal epithelial cells. Arch Ophthalmol. 1987;105:1129–32.
12. Zieske JD, Bukusoglu G, Gipson IK. Enhancement of vinculin synthesis by migrating stratified squamous epithelium. J Cell Biol. 1989;109:571–6.
13. Arey LB, Cavode WM. The method of repair in epithelial wounds of the cornea. Anat Rec. 1943;86:75–82.
14. Soong HK. Penetrating keratoplasty for ocular surface disease. In: Krachmer JH, Mannis MJ, Holland EJ, eds. Cornea, Vol. 3. St. Louis: Mosby Yearbook; 1996:1781–8.
15. Nishida T, Nakagawa S, Awata T, et al. Fibronectin promotes epithelial migration of cultured rabbit cornea in situ. J Cell Biol. 1983;97:1653–7.
16. Fujikawa LS, Foster CS, Harrist TJ, et al. Fibronectin in healing rabbit corneal wounds. Lab Invest. 1981;45:120–9.
17. Soong HK, Hassan T, Varani J, et al. Fibronectin does not enhance epidermal growth factor-mediated acceleration of corneal epithelial wound closure. Arch Ophthalmol. 1989;107:1052–4.
18. Tseng SCG, Maumenee AE, Stark WJ, et al. Topical retinoid therapy for various dry-eye disorders. Ophthalmology. 1985;92:717–27.
19. Ubels JL, Edelhauser HF, Austin KH. Healing of experimental corneal wounds treated with topically applied retinoids. Am J Ophthalmol. 1985;95:353–8.
20. Soong HK, Parkinson WC, Bafna S, et al. Movements of cultured corneal epithelial cells and stromal fibroblasts in electric fields. Invest Ophthalmol Vis Sci. 1990;31:2278–82.
21. Kaufman HE. Epithelial erosion syndrome: metaherpetic keratitis. Am J Ophthalmol. 1964;57:983–7.
22. Taylor HR, Kimsey RA. Corneal epithelial basement membrane changes in diabetics. Invest Ophthalmol Vis Sci. 1981;20:548–53.
23. Bisla K, Tanelian DL. Concentration-dependent effects of lidocaine on corneal epithelial wound healing. Invest Ophthalmol Vis Sci. 1992;33:3029–33.
24. Dass B, Soong HK, Lee B. Effects of proparacaine on actin cytoskeleton of corneal epithelium. J Ocul Pharmacol. 1988;4:187–94.
25. Goldman JN, Dohlman CH, Kravitt BA. The basement membrane of the human cornea in recurrent epithelial erosion syndrome. Trans Am Acad Ophthalmol Otolaryngol. 1969;73:471–81.
26. Khodadoust AA, Silverstein AM, Kenyon KR, Dowling JE. Adhesion of regenerating corneal epithelium: the role of the basement membrane. Am J Ophthalmol. 1968;65:339–48.
27. Kenyon KR, Fogle JA, Stone DL, Stark WJ. Regeneration of corneal epithelial basement membrane following thermal cauterization. Invest Ophthalmol Vis Sci. 1977;16:292–301.
28. Brown NA, Bron AJ. Recurrent erosion of the cornea. Br J Ophthalmol. 1976;60:84–96.
29. Waring GO III, Rodrigues MM, Laibson PR. Corneal dystrophies. I. Dystrophies of the epithelium, Bowman's layer and stroma. Surv Ophthalmol. 1978;23:71–122.
30. Werblin TP, Hirst LW, Stark WJ, et al. Prevalence of map–dot–fingerprint change in the cornea. Br J Ophthalmol. 1981;65:401–9.
31. Kenyon KR. Recurrent corneal erosion: pathogenesis and therapy. Int Ophthalmol Clin. 1979;19:169–75.
32. McLean EN, MacRae SM, Rich LF. Recurrent erosion. Treatment by anterior stromal puncture. Ophthalmology. 1986;93:784–8.
33. Judge D, Payant J, Frase S, Wood TO. Anterior stromal micropuncture: electron microscopic changes in the rabbit cornea. Cornea. 1990;9:152–60.
34. Soong HK, Farjo QA, Meyer RF, Sugar A. Diamond burr superficial keratectomy for recurrent corneal erosions. Br J Ophthalmol. 2002;86:296–8.
35. Frucht-Pery J, Sugar J, Baum J, et al. Mitomycin C treatment for conjunctival-corneal intraepithelial neoplasia: a multicenter experience. Ophthalmology, 1997;104:2085–93.
36. Waring GO, Ross AM, Ekins MB. Clinical and pathological description of 17 cases of corneal intraepithelial neoplasia. Am J Ophthalmol. 1984;97:547–59.
37. Fraunfelder FT, Wingfield D. Management of intraepithelial conjunctival tumors and squamous cell carcinomas. Am J Ophthalmol. 1983;95:359–63.
38. Zimmerman LE. The cancerous, precancerous, and pseudocancerous lesions of the cornea and conjunctiva. Corneoplastic surgery. In: Rycroft PV, ed. Proceedings 2nd Annual International Corneoplastic Conference. London: Pergamon Press; 1969:547–55.

Corneal Endothelium

MARK L. MCDERMOTT • HARVINDER K. S. ATLURI

DEFINITION
- Hexagonal nonreplicating monolayer of neural crest–derived tissue that regulates the hydration state of corneal stroma.

KEY FEATURE
- A tissue containing large quantities of membrane-bound Na$^+$, K$^+$-ATPase with specialized intercellular junctions that establish a pump–leak process in the maintenance of corneal deturgescence.

ASSOCIATED FEATURE
- A delicate tissue subject to alteration from age, trauma, systemic or ocular disease, contact lens wear, surgery, intraocular solutions, and unique dystrophic conditions. This chapter discusses normal corneal endothelial anatomy and physiology, the effects of extrinsic and intrinsic stressors on edothelial structure and function, and the endothelial dystrophies.
- Endothelial abnormalities: Fuchs' dystrophy, congenital hereditary endothelial dystrophy, posterior polymorphous dystrophy, and endothelial trauma are discussed.

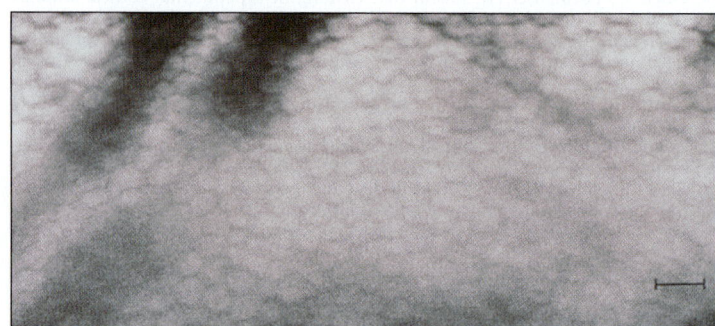

FIG. 57-1 ▮ **Specular photomicrograph of normal endothelium.** Note the dark, well-defined cell borders, the regular hexagonal array, and the uniform cell size. (Bar = 50μm.)

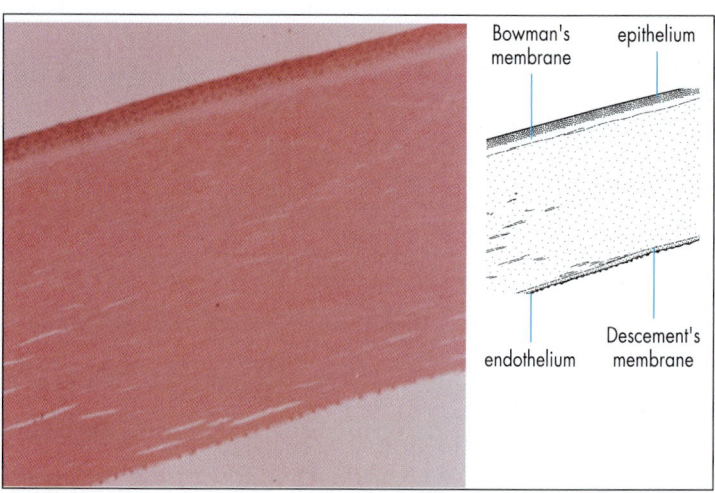

FIG. 57-2 ▮ **Light micrograph of normal endothelium (×100).** Note the single-cell endothelial layer with a Descemet's membrane of uniform thickness (epithelial surface at top of figure). (Courtesy of Dr. David Barsky.)

INTRODUCTION

The effects of external trauma and of ophthalmic and systemic disease on human corneal endothelium are best understood by reviewing the anatomy and physiology of the adult human endothelium.

ANATOMY

Embryology

In early embryogenesis, the posterior cornea is lined with a neural crest–derived[1] monolayer of orderly arranged cuboidal cells.[2] By the 78mm stage, the cells become flattened and abut one another. At this stage, immediately anterior to the flattened layer is a discontinuous, homogeneous acellular layer that in time becomes Descemet's membrane.[2] By the 120mm and 165mm stages of development, the endothelial monolayer is uniform in thickness, spans the entire posterior corneal surface, and fuses with the cells of the trabecular meshwork.[2] Similarly, Descemet's membrane becomes continuous and uniform and fuses with the trabecular beams.[2] The fusion site, known as Schwalbe's line, is a gonioscopic landmark that defines the end of Descemet's membrane and the start of the trabecular meshwork. At birth, the endothelium is approximately 10μm thick.[3]

Morphology and Development

The intact human endothelium is a monolayer that appears as a honeycomb-like mosaic when viewed from the aqueous side (Fig. 57-1). The individual cells flatten as the person ages; they stabilize at about 4μm in height in adulthood (Fig. 57-2).[3] The surface of the endothelium on the aqueous side is devoid of sur-

face villi, except in certain pathological conditions, when it may develop epithelial characteristics. Adjacent cells share extensive lateral interdigitations and possess gap and tight junctions spread along their lateral cell borders. The lateral membranes contain a high density of Na$^+$, K$^+$-adenosinetriphosphatase (ATPase) pump sites.[4] The basal side of the endothelial membrane contains numerous hemidesmosomes that promote adhesion to Descemet's membrane. Endothelial cells contain numerous mitochondria and a prominent Golgi apparatus (Fig. 57-3).

Endothelium continuously secretes Descemet's membrane throughout life, beginning *in utero* at the 8-week stage. The anterior portion of Descemet's membrane formed *in utero* has a distinctive banded appearance when viewed by electron microscopy and is approximately 3μm thick. Descemet's membrane thickens with age, reaching up to 10μm, but any Descemet's membrane produced after birth is not banded and has an amorphous texture when viewed by electron microscopy.

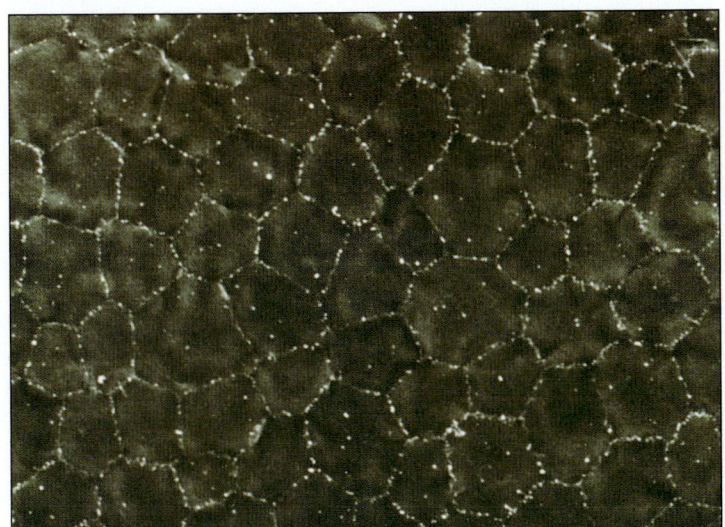

FIG. 57-3 ▌ Scanning electron micrograph of normal endothelium (×500). Note the hexagonal cellular array and surface topography.

Throughout life, endothelial cell density and topography change. From the second to eighth decades, endothelial cell density declines from approximately 3000–4000 cells/mm² to around 2600 cells/mm², and the percentage of hexagonal cells declines from about 75% to around 60%.[5]

Physiology

The anatomy of the endothelium is ideally suited to its primary physiological role of fluid regulation. Thermodynamically, the hexagonal arrangement of individual cells is the most favorable one for cells to cover a surface without gaps, thereby facilitating barrier function.[6–8] This geometrical arrangement also minimizes individual circumferential cell area, thereby allowing a maximal number of cells per unit area and maximizing pump site density.

The primary site of fluid regulation through the endothelium's activity is the corneal stroma. As a result of this endothelial activity, the stroma is maintained in a relatively deturgesced state (78% water content), which allows an orderly lattice of collagen fibrils to enmesh in glycosaminoglycans and create a transparent tissue.[9] One hypothesis is that this endothelial activity is mediated by a pump–leak process; net fluid egress from the corneal stroma follows movement down an osmotic gradient from a relatively hypo-osmotic stroma toward a relatively hypertonic aqueous humor. This bulk fluid movement requires no energy. The energy-requiring processes are the intracellular and membrane-bound ion transport systems, which generate the osmotic gradient. The two most important ion transport systems are the membrane-bound Na^+, K^+-ATPase sites and the intracellular carbonic anhydrase pathway.[10] Activity in both these pathways produces a net flux from stroma to aqueous humor.

The barrier portion of the endothelium is unique, in that it is permeable to some degree, permitting the ion flux necessary to establish the osmotic gradient.[11,12] This permeability can be modulated, depending on ambient calcium ion. Exposure of endothelium to calcium-free media results in large reductions in barrier function.

Assessment of Endothelial Function

In vivo assessment of endothelial function relies on measurements of corneal thickness or observation of the endothelial monolayer using specular microscopy. Measurement of the corneal thickness (pachymetry) indirectly reflects endothelial function, because corneal thickness reflects the state of corneal deturgescence. The average central corneal thickness is around 0.5mm, which gradually increases toward the periphery to around 0.7mm. Pachymetry may be carried out ultrasonically or optically. Both methods are reproducible, but they are not always directly comparable. Moreover, pachymetry as an indicator of corneal function is time dependent. A normal patient has slightly thicker corneas immediately upon awaking than he or she does later in the day. This increased thickness is the result of the loss of the open-eye desiccating effect on the cornea, as well as reduced metabolic activity of the endothelium under nocturnal lid closure. Such nocturnal swelling is exaggerated in dysfunctional endothelium and is often noticed by patients as a morning blur in vision that improves during the day.

Direct observation using specular microscopy[13] also is used to evaluate endothelial status. By using a wide-field specular microscope, a photomicrograph can be obtained and subsequently digitalized and analyzed.[5] In cases in which corneal edema may not allow adequate visualization of the endothelium by specular microscopy, confocal microscopy may be of value. Confocal microscopy allows real-time *in vivo* assessment of different layers of the cornea. Although not precluded by corneal edema, it is technically more difficult to perform than specular microscopy.[14,15] Analysis of images from these techniques provides data that reflect endothelial cell density and morphology. At birth, the normal cornea is lined by about 3500–4000 cells/mm². Central endothelial cell density decreases at an average rate of 0.6% per year in normal corneas.[16] Little, if any, mitotic potential exists within the endothelium. The exact number of cells/mm² required to maintain corneal deturgescence is not known, but corneas with cell counts below 1000 cells/mm² in multiple areas may be at risk for the later development of corneal edema. This prediction is difficult to verify, because nonuniform cell loss results in regional variation in cell density, which leads to sampling errors during specular microscopy. Besides actual cell density, endothelial cell morphology (size and shape) can affect function. Endothelial monolayers with increased variation in cell size (polymegathism) and increased variation in cell shape (pleomorphism) are less effective in achieving deturgescence in a cornea swollen by hypoxic stress than in a cornea with normal morphology.[17,18]

Endothelial Function Research Techniques

In vivo assessment of global endothelial function can be carried out by examining the curve obtained by plotting corneal thickness over time after induction of corneal edema by hypoxia.[19] This technique permits the comparison of eyes with morphometric or cell density alterations to the eyes of age-matched controls. Barrier function can be evaluated using fluorophotometry.[20] In this technique, the change in concentration of the fluorescein molecule in the corneal and aqueous compartments is determined over time and used to calculate transfer coefficients that reflect the relative permeability of the barrier between the two compartments. This technique generally is used in research studies rather than clinical practice because of the duration of the experiment and the requirement for multiple fluorescence measurements.

Endothelial Responses to Stress

The endothelium has a rather restricted response to stress. Mild stress may result in morphometric changes, and greater stresses may result in cell loss as well as morphometric changes. Morphometric changes are believed to result from alterations in the endothelial cytoskeleton.[21] Sources of stress may be metabolic (from hypoxia or hyperglycemia) or toxic (from drugs or preservatives); stress may also be caused by alterations in pH, ionization, or osmolarity or by trauma from surgery.

A common hypoxic stress is that generated by contact lens wear. All contact lenses present a hypoxic stress to the endothelium to varying degrees.[22] Over time, this results in alteration of the morphometry of the endothelium.[23] With contact lens wear, the coefficient of variation for cell size increases, and the percentage of hexagons decreases.[24] The severity of this change is re-

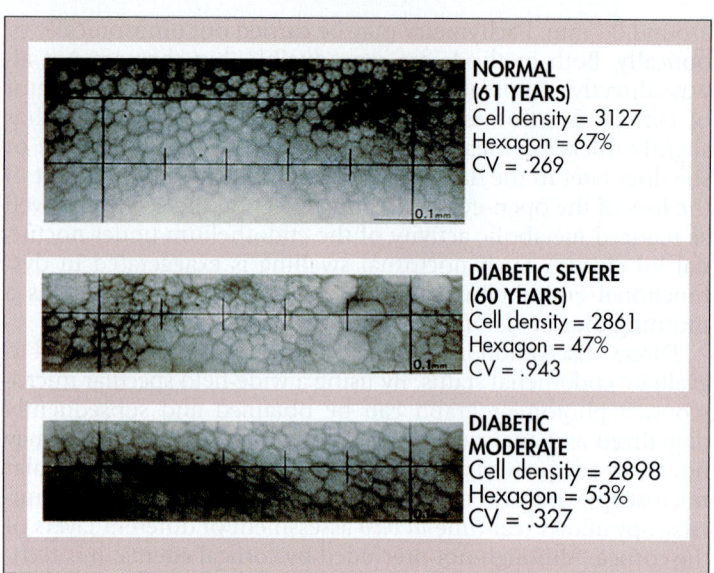

NORMAL
(61 YEARS)
Cell density = 3127
Hexagon = 67%
CV = .269

DIABETIC SEVERE
(60 YEARS)
Cell density = 2861
Hexagon = 47%
CV = .943

DIABETIC
MODERATE
Cell density = 2898
Hexagon = 53%
CV = .327

FIG. 57-4 ■ **Age-matched comparison of diabetic and normal endothelia.** Note the reduction in the percentage of hexagons and the increase in the coefficient of variation of cell size in both severe and moderate diabetics compared with the age-matched controls. (Courtesy of Dr. Henry Edelhauser.)

lated to contact lens composition, duration of use, and type of lens wear. The greatest changes in morphometry are seen in patients who have worn polymethyl methacrylate lenses for multiple decades.[25,26] Less severe changes are seen in other forms and types of contact lens use.[27] Although earlier studies found no difference in endothelial cell density among contact lens wearers, recent studies demonstrate a significant reduction in endothelial cell density with increased duration of contact lens wear.[28] This decrease in cell count is preceded by pleomorphism and polymegathism and may be a late indicator of altered corneal endothelium in long-term contact lens users.[28] The morphometric changes induced by contact lens wear do not regress upon cessation of wear.[29] A physiological correlate to the altered morphometry induced by contact lens wear is the *in vivo* observation that the corneal deswelling (deturgescence) response after induction of edema by hypoxia is significantly less in long-term contact lens wearers compared with age-matched controls.[30]

Another metabolic stress is hyperglycemia. The corneal endothelium in type I and type II diabetics, when compared with that of age-matched controls, has morphometric and morphological alterations manifested as lower mean cell density and greater pleomorphism and polymegathism.[31] These changes are more pronounced in type I diabetics.[31] There are conflicting results regarding functional abnormalities associated with these morphological alterations, but it is recognized that the diabetic cornea has a higher susceptibility to mechanical or surgical stress or additional metabolic stress[31] (Fig. 57-4).

Besides adverse systemic conditions, the endothelium can be damaged by the introduction of intraocular agents during surgery. The potential for damage to the endothelium and other tissues is related to chemical composition, pH, and osmolality.[32,33]

Intraocular surgery commonly results in endothelial damage. During cataract surgery, contact of the endothelium with jets of irrigation fluid, nucleus particles, instruments, or intraocular lenses causes focal endothelial cell death. Repair of these areas takes place via the process of cell slide from adjacent undamaged areas. A permanent reduction in cell density occurs, and individual cell size is increased.[34] Often the mosaic suggests the area of injury by elongation of cells or the production of giant cells with 10 or more sides. Ophthalmic viscoelastic devices (composed of hydroxypropyl methylcellulose, chondroitin sulfate, or sodium hyaluronate) are now widely used in cataract surgery and provide significant protection against trauma to the endothelium.[35]

Glaucoma has also been associated with endothelial cell loss. A recent study found significantly lower endothelial cell counts in patients who have glaucoma and ocular hypertension compared with age-matched controls.[36] Cell counts were inversely proportional to the mean intraocular pressure in the glaucoma and ocular hypertension groups. Mechanisms of cell loss may include direct damage from intraocular pressure, congenital alterations of endothelium in glaucoma, and medication toxicity.[36]

FUCHS' DYSTROPHY

INTRODUCTION

Fuchs' dystrophy (combined dystrophy) is defined as bilateral, noninflammatory, progressive loss of endothelium that results in reduction of vision. The key features are guttae, folds in Descemet's membrane, stromal edema, and microcystic epithelial edema. Corneal endothelial degeneration is the primary defect; corneal edema is secondary. Associated features are prominent corneal nerves, stromal opacification, recurrent corneal erosions, open-angle glaucoma, female gender, and familial predisposition.

EPIDEMIOLOGY AND PATHOGENESIS

Fuchs' dystrophy is perhaps the most common corneal dystrophy to require keratoplasty, accounting for approximately 15% of all penetrating keratoplasties in the United States in 2000.[37] Pedigree analysis is complex but suggests that Fuchs' dystrophy is an inherited dystrophy with an autosomal dominant inheritance pattern.[38] A significant variation occurs in expressivity between males and females, with a 4:1 female-male ratio at the time of keratoplasty.[39] It is equally common among whites and African Americans who undergo keratoplasty, but in Asians it is a relatively rare cause for keratoplasty.[40]

Development of guttae and the onset of symptoms are more common in middle age.[38] Fuchs' dystrophy patients are believed to have an increased incidence of open-angle glaucoma.[41] Short axial length, shallow anterior chamber, and angle-closure glaucoma also have been seen in conjunction with Fuchs' dystrophy,[42] but only rarely has it been associated with keratoconus.[43,44] Fuchs' dystrophy is characterized by progressive loss of endothelial function that is primary in nature rather than secondary to any alteration in aqueous humor flow rate[45] or constituency.[46] Endothelial dysfunction is primarily a result of a reduction in Na^+,K^+-ATPase pump activity,[47] which leads to a reduction in ion flux across the endothelium but the relative maintenance of barrier function throughout the course of the disease.[45]

Mutations in the gene that codes for the α_2 chain of type VIII collagen have been reported in patients who have Fuchs' endothelial dystrophy, as well as in families with posterior polymorphous corneal dystrophy. A defect in type VIII collagen may play a role in these disorders.[48]

OCULAR MANIFESTATIONS

The earliest slit-lamp finding in Fuchs' dystrophy is the presence of excrescences of Descemet's membrane, called guttae (cornea guttata), in the central corneal endothelium (Fig. 57-5). Guttae are not pathognomonic for Fuchs' dystrophy; they may be seen in asymptomatic patients and in the setting of uveitis and nonspecific superficial keratopathies. Up to 11% of eyes in patients older than 50 years have guttae.[49] Identical lesions that present in peripheral Descemet's membrane are known as Hassall-Henle warts and are part of the normal aging process (see Chapter 60). The guttae initially appear on specular reflection as scattered, discrete, isolated dark structures, smaller than an individual endothelial cell.[50] An associated fine pigment dusting occurs

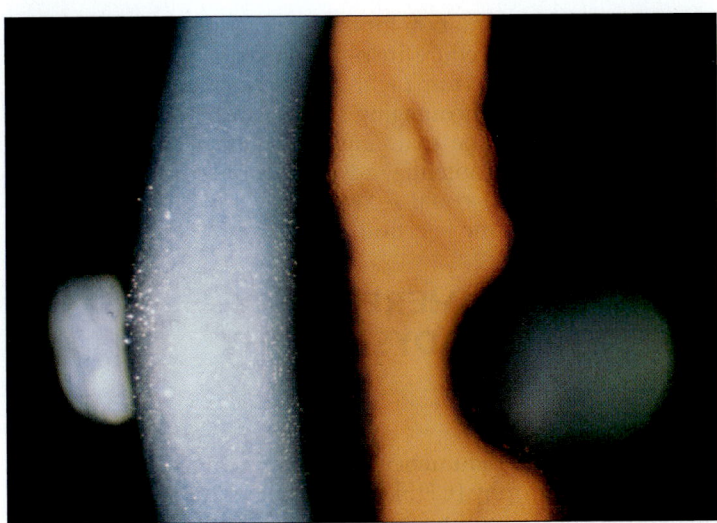

FIG. 57-5 ■ **Slit-lamp view of Fuchs' dystrophy.** Note the guttae on the specularly reflected image of the endothelium.

FIG. 57-6 ■ **Specular photomicrograph of Fuchs' dystrophy.** Note dark areas that represent guttae adjacent to areas of enlarged endothelial cells. (Spacing of grid 0.1mm.)

within the central endothelium. At this stage, referred to as stage 1, the patient's vision is normal, and the stroma and epithelium are uninvolved.[49] Over time, these individual excrescences increase in number, enlarge, and may fuse with adjacent guttae to disrupt the normal endothelial monolayer's specular reflection.[50] This produces a roughened surface with a specular reflection similar to beaten metal in appearance. Eventually, this process expands from the center of the cornea to involve the corneal periphery as well. As the disorder progresses, the endothelial monolayer becomes attenuated in thickness, with an increase in average cell size, a decrease in the percentage of hexagons, and an increase in the coefficient of variation in cell size. In the last stages of the dystrophy, effacement of the endothelium results in overlying stromal edema. The endothelium becomes unobservable using conventional specular microscopy but still may be seen using confocal microscopy techniques.[14]

As endothelial function progressively declines, the fluid accumulated in the stroma during nighttime lid closure is removed at a reduced rate, which results in significant stromal edema upon awakening.[51] This heralds the onset of stage 2.[49] Patients note blurred vision, glare, and colored haloes around lights. It is not uncommon for there to be asymmetry between involved eyes. Initially, the stromal edema is localized in front of Descemet's and behind Bowman's membranes.[52] Eventually the entire stroma swells, taking on a ground-glass appearance. With the increase in corneal thickness, the posterior stroma and Descemet's membrane are thrown into folds. Vision at this time is variable but may be only mildly reduced in the afternoon hours due to posterior irregular astigmatism produced from the folds in Descemet's membrane. With progressive endothelial dysfunction, bulk fluid flow across the cornea results in microcystic and bullous epithelial edema. With involvement of the epithelial layer, the optical quality of the tear–air interface is severely degraded, which produces a profound reduction in vision.

With the onset of epithelial edema, basal adhesion complexes become disrupted to produce recurrent corneal erosions. As a slit-lamp marker of recurrent epithelial slough, duplication of basement layers occurs, which creates fingerprint and map changes. If erosions are prominent, a vascular pannus between epithelium and Bowman's membrane may be induced; this accelerates the deposition of a subepithelial fibrotic layer and results in an anterior stromal haze, with further reduction in vision. This development represents stage 3 of the disease.[49] However, this fibrotic layer often reduces or eliminates the painful recurrent epithelial erosions experienced by the patient. With the progressive increase in stromal water content, gly-

cosaminoglycans elute from the stroma,[53] causing disorganization of the collagen fibrils, which contributes to additional stromal opacification.

DIAGNOSIS AND ANCILLARY TESTING

The earliest observable change suggestive of Fuchs' dystrophy is the presence of guttae on slit-lamp examination (see Fig. 57-5). Using specular microscopy, a photographic record can be obtained and is a useful educational aid for the patient (Fig. 57-6). Cell counts are readily determined from the micrograph. Subtle stromal edema can be observed using sclerotic scatter techniques. As the disease progresses, corneal pachymetry can be used to document increased corneal thickness over the normal thickness of 0.5mm centrally. Later, more obvious signs include folds in Descemet's membrane, stromal haze, microcystic and bullous epithelial edema, subepithelial fibrosis, and pannus formation. When corneal opacification precludes specular microscopy, confocal microscopy can be used to image the endothelium. Pathological changes in Fuchs' dystrophy can be demonstrated in all corneal layers, and reliable endothelial cell counts can be obtained by confocal microscopy.[14,15]

DIFFERENTIAL DIAGNOSIS

Differential diagnosis includes posterior polymorphous dystrophy, congenital hereditary endothelial dystrophy, aphakic or pseudophakic bullous keratopathy, and Hassall-Henle bodies. No associated systemic diseases exist.[49]

PATHOLOGY

Light microscopy of keratoplasty buttons from patients with Fuchs' dystrophy shows a thickened Descemet's membrane, which may be laminated in appearance with buried guttae, guttae on the surface, or devoid of guttae but thickened (Fig. 57-7).[39] The endothelial layer is attenuated but present. Descemet's membrane, however, has been shown to be abnormal before the onset of clinically observable guttae. Transmission electron micrographs of Descemet's membrane in buttons obtained at the time of keratoplasty in Fuchs' dystrophy patients demonstrate an abnormal posterior banded layer and a fibrillar layer, both of which result in gross thickening of Descemet's membrane. The production of this morphologically abnormal Descemet's membrane serves as a marker for a dysfunctional endothelium.[54] Recent molecular biological studies of corneal buttons from patients who have Fuchs' dystrophy, using nucleus la-

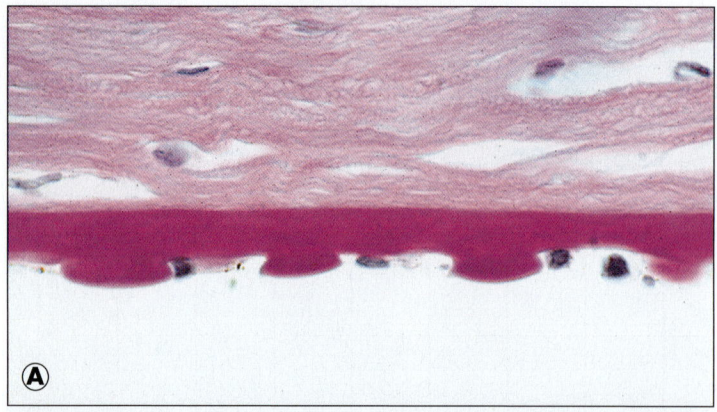

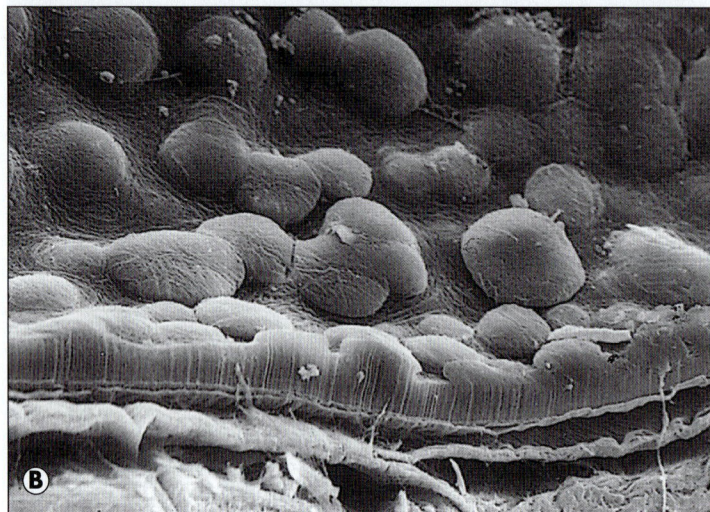

FIG. 57-7 ▮ **Characteristic wart-like bumps present within Descemet's membrane. A,** Periodic acid–Schiff stain. **B,** Scanning electron microscopy shows this better. (**A,** From Yanoff M, Fine BS. Ocular pathology, ed 5. Philadelphia: WB Saunders; 2002. **B,** Courtesy of Dr. R. C. Eagle, Jr. In Yanoff M, Fine BS. Ocular pathology, ed 4. London; Mosby, 1996.)

beling and electron microscopy techniques, suggest that apoptosis (programmed cell death) may play an important role in endothelial cell degeneration in this disorder.[55] It is unclear whether this is a primary process or secondary to modification of the composition of Descemet's membrane or loss of contact between endothelial cells and the basement membrane. If further study confirms the role of apoptosis in endothelial cell loss, pharmacological inhibition of apoptosis may be possible.[55]

TREATMENT

Treatment is usually supportive and temporizing until keratoplasty. Medical management includes the use of hypertonic solutions or ointments and a hair dryer to decrease ambient humidity and increase tear evaporation. If intraocular pressure (IOP) is above 20mmHg (2.67kPa), attempts to lower it may reduce the force that drives fluid into the stroma. Treatment measures for painful erosions include hypertonics, bandage contact lenses, anterior stromal puncture, and conjunctival flaps.

COURSE AND OUTCOME

With progressive corneal edema, the cornea becomes refractory to supportive measures, so keratoplasty is usually offered. Long-term results show that graft clarity is close to 90%, and approximately 60% of patients have 20/40 (6/12) or better visual acuity following keratoplasty.[56] If the patient is older than 60 years and shows early lens changes, keratoplasty should be combined with cataract extraction.[57] Recently, posterior lamellar keratoplasty (also known as endokeratoplasty or deep lamellar keratoplasty) has been presented as an alternative to conventional full-thick-

ness corneal transplantation for the treatment of endothelial disorders.[58-60] This procedure involves replacing the diseased endothelium and deep stroma with a posterior lamellar disc of tissue and has shown encouraging results in early clinical trials. If interface clarity can be maintained, posterior lamellar keratoplasty may offer the potential advantages of reduced postoperative astigmatism and visual recovery time and a possible reduction in risk of immune rejection.

CONGENITAL HEREDITARY ENDOTHELIAL DYSTROPHY

INTRODUCTION

First described by Maumenee[61] in 1960, congenital hereditary endothelial dystrophy (CHED) is but one of the many causes of bilateral corneal clouding in full-term infants that usually requires keratoplasty. Key features of this autosomal dominant or recessive condition are a corneal thickness two to three times normal, normal IOP, and normal corneal diameter. Associated features are corneal pannus, nystagmus, and esotropia.

EPIDEMIOLOGY AND PATHOGENESIS

Prevalence, incidence, and sex distribution for this disorder are unknown. The onset is usually at birth in a term infant; corneal clouding may be maximal at birth or progress over a period of years. Family pedigree studies support autosomal dominant and recessive forms, as well as sporadic occurrence. Autosomal recessive inheritance is associated with the presence at birth of bilateral corneal edema without photophobia but with nystagmus.[62] Autosomal dominant inheritance is associated with the progressive onset of corneal edema 1–2 years postpartum with associated photophobia but without nystagmus.[62] Autosomal dominant CHED has been linked to the pericentric region of chromosome 20 within the genetic interval containing the posterior polymorphous dystrophy locus.[63] Genetic studies in autosomal recessive pedigrees indicate that the locus for autosomal recessive CHED is distinct from this region of chromosome 20, but it has not yet been identified.[63]

CHED is believed to result from abnormal neural crest cell terminal induction during the late term to perinatal period. At this time, failure to complete final differentiation of the endothelial monolayer occurs, which results in a dysfunctional endothelium.[64] This dysfunctional endothelium is believed to have faulty growth regulation mechanisms that lead to accumulation of a functionally abnormal and structurally exaggerated form of posterior nonbanded Descemet's membrane.[65]

OCULAR MANIFESTATIONS

The usual presentation is in an otherwise healthy term infant who is found to have bilateral symmetrically edematous, cloudy corneas.[62] Examination under anesthesia reveals the corneas to have a diffuse gray-blue ground-glass coloring.[62] Corneal thickness is two to three times normal and often greater than 1mm centrally. Both IOP and horizontal corneal diameter are normal. Rarely, CHED is associated with glaucoma and should be considered if corneal opacification fails to resolve after normalization of IOP.[66]

Closer examination reveals the texture of the epithelial surface to be irregular, with a diffuse pigskin-like roughness.[62] Despite the epithelial surface irregularity, recurrent epithelial erosions are uncommon. The stromal opacification is ground glass in consistency but may vary in optical density from one area of the cornea to another. Within a given area, however, the density is uniform from anterior to posterior. Occasionally, discrete white dots also may be seen in the stroma. In areas where stromal opacification is less dense, Descemet's membrane appears gray and on specular reflection may have a *peau d'orange* texture.[62] The endothelial layer may or may not be visualized. A fine corneal pannus may be seen, as well as low-grade inflammation.

DIAGNOSIS

A tentative diagnosis is usually possible when examination under anesthesia demonstrates the typical bilateral stromal opacification, gross corneal thickening, normal horizontal diameter, normal IOP, and absence of breaks in Descemet's membrane.

DIFFERENTIAL DIAGNOSIS

Differential diagnosis is glaucoma without buphthalmos, posterior polymorphous dystrophy, macular stromal dystrophy, mucopolysaccharidosis, intrauterine infection, and birth trauma from forceps. One family has an association with sensory neural deafness.[67]

PATHOLOGY

Light microscopy of the keratoplasty buttons shows epithelial atrophy with basal cell hydrops, subepithelial calcification or fibrosis, patchy loss of Bowman's membrane, and variable vascularization or spheroidal degeneration of the stroma.[65] Descemet's membrane is thickened, often with discrete laminations, and the endothelial layer is attenuated.[65] Electron microscopy of Descemet's membrane shows the anterior banded zone to be normal and the posterior nonbanded layer to be grossly abnormal. These abnormalities include the deposition of a basement membrane–like material, a long-spaced collagen region, and a posterior collagenous layer of a fibrillary nature.[65]

TREATMENT

If the edema is stationary and mild, use of hypertonics and desiccating measures may be employed. Usually, however, these patients require keratoplasty due to the bilateral nature of the corneal edema. Keratoplasty in infants and children is a high-risk procedure and is technically difficult, and the long-term prognosis for graft clarity is worse than for adults. No definitive clinical guidelines have emerged regarding the timing of surgical intervention due to significant heterogeneity in disease severity, follow-up periods, and ages at diagnosis and surgery among the few published studies.[68]

The decision regarding surgery may be difficult, because despite significant corneal haze and absence of a red reflex, patients often seem to see much better than expected.[69] If patients maintain good fixation with normal alignment, surgery may be delayed; loss of fixation or development of nystagmus should lead to prompt intervention.[69]

COURSE AND OUTCOME

In one large study, 38% of patients younger than 12 years of age who underwent keratoplasty had haze or opaque grafts at the most recent office visit. In the same study, the 5-year graft survival rate was about 50%.[70] First graft survival rates range from 25% at 3 months in earlier studies to 62–90% at 2–3 years in more recent series.[68,69] Visual acuity is always limited by degrees of amblyopia.

POSTERIOR POLYMORPHOUS DYSTROPHY

INTRODUCTION

First described in 1916 by Koeppe, this rare dystrophy has a clinical spectrum that ranges from congenital corneal edema to late-onset corneal edema in middle age. Many cases are subclinical—the majority of patients have good vision and only subtle slit-lamp and specular micrographic abnormalities. Posterior polymorphous dystrophy (PPMD) is a bilateral autosomal dominant disorder characterized by polymorphic posterior corneal surface irregularities with variable degrees of corneal decompensation. Key features are:

- Vesicular, curvilinear, and placoid irregularities found on slit-lamp examination
- Rounded dark areas with central cell detail that produce a doughnut-like pattern on specular microscopy
- Epithelial-like transformation of endothelium on histological examination
- Reduced vision from the corneal edema

Associated features are iridocorneal adhesions, peripheral anterior synechiae, glaucoma, and a tendency to recur in graft patients. Some of these features overlap with iridocorneal endothelial (ICE) syndrome, Peters' anomaly, and Axenfeld-Rieger syndrome, suggesting that PPMD may be part of a broader spectrum of disorders united by abnormalities of terminal neural crest cell differentiation.[71,72] PPMD associated with posterior amyloid degeneration of the cornea, keratoconus, and Alport's syndrome has been reported.[71,73,74]

EPIDEMIOLOGY AND PATHOGENESIS

This disorder is a rare reason for corneal transplantation. Its prevalence in the general population is unknown. It is believed to be mainly autosomal dominant with variable penetrance, but cases of autosomal recessive inheritance are seen.[75] The autosomal dominant form has been linked to the long arm of chromosome 20.[63] The pathogenesis is thought to be due to focal metaplasia of endothelial cells into a population of aberrant keratinized epithelial-like cells.[71,74] Immunohistochemical analyses of these transformed cells show that they contain antigens and cytokeratins that are usually associated with epithelial cells.[76] The transformation of a single-cell layer of endothelium into a multilayered epithelium-like tissue is believed to be responsible for the loss of stromal deturgescence, the observed specular microscopic patterns, and the tendency toward synechiae formation. These concepts, however, are based on analysis of keratoplasty buttons from patients who have severe disease; it is unknown whether the proposed mechanisms of pathogenesis can be extrapolated to the more common asymptomatic patient who has a few scattered vesicular lesions on the corneal endothelium.

As in Fuchs' dystrophy, a different defect in the gene that codes for the α_2 chain of type VIII collagen has been found.[48]

OCULAR MANIFESTATIONS

PPMD has a spectrum of slit-lamp findings. The most common finding is isolated vesicles bilaterally, which appear as circular or oval transparent cysts with a gray halo at the level of Descemet's membrane, best viewed by retroillumination with a widely dilated pupil (Fig. 57-8).[77] The vesicular or doughnut-like lesions have diameters in the range of 0.2–1mm.[78] They may be few or many, widely separated or clustered close together to create confluent geographic patches. Less common are band-shaped or "snail track" areas, which typically have scalloped edges and are about 1mm across (Fig. 57-9).[77] Their length can range from 2 to 10mm.[78] In both vesicular and band presentations, the overlying stroma and epithelium are uninvolved, and vision is normal. The least common slit-lamp finding is placoid or diffuse involvement of the endothelium.[77] Patients who have placoid-type PPMD often present with reduced vision. Specular microscopy of the presenting lesions shows them to be sharply demarcated from uninvolved endothelium. In this presentation, Descemet's membrane and the posterior stroma are hazy, and usually areas of corneal edema and iridocorneal adhesions occur.[78]

On specular microscopy the vesicles appear as circular dark rings around a lighter, though mottled, center in which some

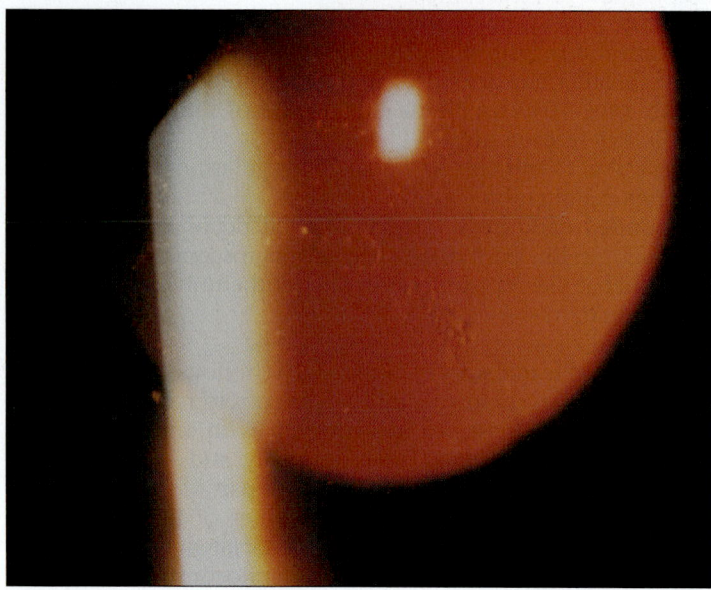

FIG. 57-8 ■ Slit-lamp appearance of vesicles in posterior polymorphous dystrophy. Note the small vesicular lesions on retroillumination. (Courtesy of Dr. Richard Yee.)

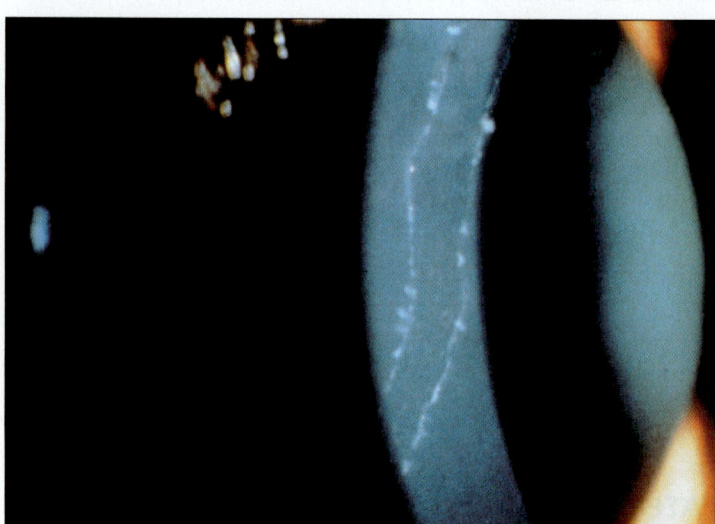

FIG. 57-9 ■ Slit-lamp appearance of the band form of posterior polymorphous dystrophy. Note the vertical serpentine band. (Courtesy of Dr. Richard Yee.)

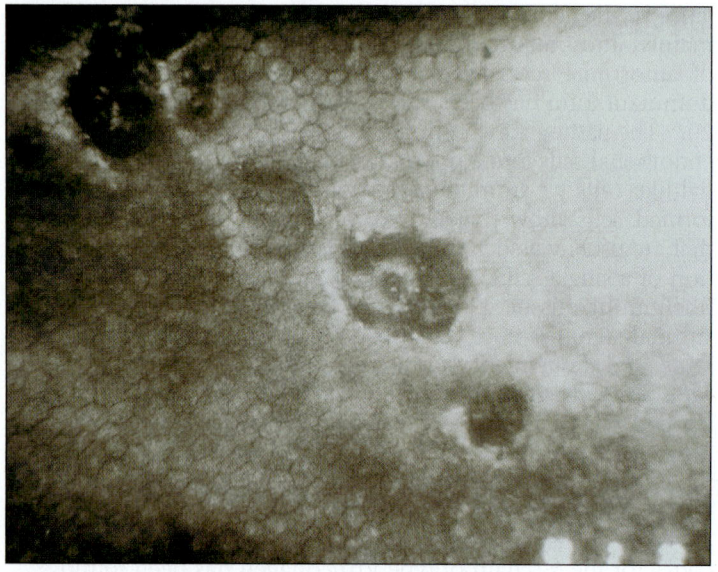

FIG. 57-10 ■ Specular photomicrograph of vesicles in posterior polymorphous dystrophy. Note the doughnut-like appearance of the vesicles. (Courtesy of Dr. Richard Yee.)

cellular detail is evident.[77-79] These vesicles represent steep-sided, shallow depressions in the endothelium[77]; the steep sides correspond to the peripheral dark ring seen on specular reflection, and the depressed center corresponds to the lighter, mottled central portion (Fig. 57-10). Specular microscopy of the band-shaped areas shows them to be composed of a chain of overlapping vesicles, which create a shallow trench with scalloped borders that represent the edges of individual vesicles that have fused.[77] Rarely, patients who have the typical corneal endothelial changes of PPMD exhibit broad-based iridocorneal adhesions and peripheral anterior synechiae. These are most often seen in corneas with placoid areas of involvement.[78] Elevation of IOP refractory to medical measures is common in this group of patients. All patients who have PPMD have reduced endothelial cell counts compared with age-matched controls.[77,79]

DIAGNOSIS

The majority of patients are diagnosed using the slit lamp by observing vesicular, band-like, or placoid areas on the posterior corneal surface. The diagnosis of PPMD in patients with corneal edema of unknown cause is based on light and electron microscopy of the excised buttons obtained during keratoplasty.

DIFFERENTIAL DIAGNOSIS

Differential diagnosis includes tears in Descemet's membrane, interstitial keratitis, Fuchs' dystrophy, and ICE syndrome. ICE syndrome is a group of disorders resulting from an underlying corneal endothelial abnormality with features overlapping those of PPMD. ICE syndrome is discussed in detail in Chapter 230, Glaucoma Associated with Abnormalities of Cornea and Iris, Tumors, and Retinal Disease. As in PPMD, endothelial cells in ICE syndrome may show epithelial characteristics, leading to speculation that they represent a spectrum of the same disease.[72] However, unlike PPMD, ICE syndrome is unilateral, occurs sporadically, is more common in women, and is typically progressive and symptomatic. Glaucoma and iris changes can be found in PPMD but are much more prominent features of ICE syndrome. No systemic associations exist except for rare reports of PPMD associated with Alport's syndrome.

PATHOLOGY

Light microscopy of keratoplasty buttons shows pits in the posterior corneal surface, which correspond to the vesicles seen on slit-lamp examination. Descemet's membrane in these areas is attenuated, and the endothelium may be multilayered (Fig. 57-11).[80,81] In other areas, Descemet's membrane appears multilayered, of variable thickness, and with attenuation or loss of endothelium. Discontinuities in Descemet's membrane with anterior migration of cells to form slit-like structures or clefts in pre-Descemet's stroma have been described.[73] Scanning electron microscopy of keratoplasty buttons may show a striking juxtaposition of normal-appearing endothelial cells adjacent to epithelial cell–like areas that show myriad surface microvilli.[80,81] Transmission electron microscopy of these layers shows the cells to be multilayered and to contain numerous desmosomes and intracytoplasmic filaments.[80,81] Cell culture studies of these cells demonstrate features similar to cultured epithelial cell lines.[81]

TREATMENT

The majority of patients require no treatment, but those who have corneal opacification are offered keratoplasty.

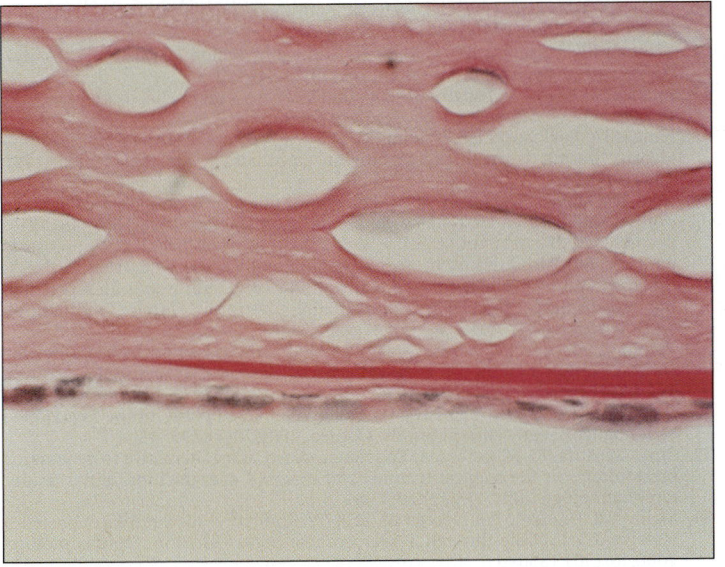

FIG. 57-11 ■ Light micrograph of keratoplasty button from posterior polymorphous dystrophy (hematoxylin & eosin). Note the multilayered epithelial-like endothelium and variably attenuated Descemet's membrane. (Courtesy of Dr. Richard Yee.)

COURSE AND OUTCOME

It is unknown whether the majority of patients who have PPMD progress. It is believed, however, to be a nonprogressive type of dystrophy, usually without vision impairment. Those patients who require keratoplasty appear to be at risk for recurrence of this dystrophy in the grafted cornea,[82,83] as well as for the development of a difficult-to-manage glaucoma.[81] It is thought that the genesis of this behavior is due to the epithelial-like transformation and subsequent migration of host endothelium to encroach on donor corneal tissue and host angle structures.[81]

ENDOTHELIAL TRAUMA

INTRODUCTION

As mentioned in the section on endothelial responses to stress, endothelial trauma can be a significant cause of corneal edema, because endothelial cells that are destroyed cannot be replaced by the production of new cells.

EPIDEMIOLOGY AND PATHOGENESIS

Although superficial trauma is common, endothelial trauma is fortunately less so. Direct puncture injuries to the anterior cornea, such as those that occur when the cornea is struck by high-velocity small particles, may cause annular buckling stress on the endothelium. Buckling of the cornea also can arise as a result of surgical trauma in large incision surgeries. Lens fragments striking the endothelium also can cause trauma during cataract surgery. All these injuries represent focal destruction of endothelial cells. Sliding in of surrounding healthy endothelial cells leads to rapid replacement of the damaged cells, and clinically the changes are no longer evident 1–3 days after injury. In addition to focal endothelial trauma, more severe trauma may rupture Descemet's membrane. This can occur as a result of severe indentation injuries to the cornea, forceps delivery, or corneal stretching (as with buphthalmos or keratoconus). As in keratoconus, Descemet's membrane curls in toward the stroma. Surrounding endothelial cells slide in to cover the defect and produce new Descemet's membrane. The corneal edema resolves as the endothelial cells fill the defect, which leads to deturgescence of the cornea.

OCULAR MANIFESTATIONS

Buckling stress on the endothelium leads to the clinical appearance of a grayish ring on the posterior cornea. Buckling of the cornea may lead to "snail tracks" due to grayish swelling of endothelial cells. Endothelial swelling as a result of trauma appears as dark spots at the level of the endothelium. This also may be seen in eyes with inflammation in the presence of keratic precipitates and in eye bank corneas stored in refrigerated media. The appearance may resemble the guttae in Fuchs' dystrophy, but it is reversible, more regular in size, and not associated with the presence of pigment. More severe trauma may lead to acute, massive corneal swelling or hydrops. As described elsewhere (see Chapter 59, Stromal Corneal Dystrophies and Ectasias), Descemet's membrane curls in toward the stroma. Surrounding endothelial cells slide in to cover the defect and produce new Descemet's membrane. The corneal edema resolves as the endothelial cells, which have filled the defect, deturgesce the cornea.

DIAGNOSIS

Diagnosis is based on history and clinical appearance.

DIFFERENTIAL DIAGNOSIS

Differential diagnosis includes guttae from Fuchs' dystrophy and the presence of endothelial keratic precipitates.

PATHOLOGY

Specular microscopy shows the endothelial disruption as dark spots. Histopathology is not usually obtained, but with massive trauma leading to keratoplasty, the acute absence of endothelial cells in the area of trauma is seen.

TREATMENT

Usually no treatment is necessary, as the surrounding endothelial cells enlarge and slide in to fill the defect. When inflammation is the source of the trauma, anti-inflammatory treatment is appropriate. In acute hydrops, hypertonic saline may be of benefit, and in the presence of persistent edema, keratoplasty may be indicated.

COURSE AND OUTCOME

Recovery is usually rapid. However, if a sufficient number of endothelial cells is lost, persistent edema may result. Also, if recovery of corneal compensation occurs, the combination of the acute loss of endothelial cells from trauma and the normal attrition over time may lead to late corneal decompensation.

REFERENCES

1. Beebe DC, Coats JM. The lens organizes the anterior segment: specification of neural crest cell differentiation in the avian eye. Dev Biol. 2000;220(2):424–31.
2. Sevel D, Isaacs R. A reevaluation of corneal development. Trans Am Ophthalmol Soc. 1988;136:178–207.
3. Nuijts RMMA. Ocular toxicity of intraoperatively used drugs and solutions. New Amsterdam: Kugler Publications; 1995.
4. Stiemke MM, Edelhauser HF, Geroski DH. The developing corneal endothelium: correlation of morphology, hydration and Na/K ATPase pump site density. Curr Eye Res. 1991;10(2):145–56.
5. Yee RW, Matsuda M, Schultz RO, Edelhauser HF. Changes in the normal corneal endothelial cellular pattern as a function of age. Curr Eye Res. 1985;4(6):671–7.
6. Thompson DW. The forms of tissues on cell-aggregates. In: Bonner JT, ed. On growth and form. Cambridge: University Press; 1969:88–119.
7. Rao GN, Lohman LE, Aquavella JV. Cell-size–shape relationships in corneal endothelium. Invest Ophthalmol Vis Sci. 1982;22:271.
8. Honda H. Geometrical models for cells in tissues. Int Rev Cytol. 1983;81:191–248.
9. Geroski DH, Matsuda M, Yee RW, Edelhauser HF. Pump function of the human corneal endothelium, effects of age and corneal guttata. Ophthalmology. 1985;92(6):759–63.
10. Riley M. Transport of ions and metabolites across the corneal endothelium. In: McDevitt D, ed. Cell biology of the eye. New York: Academic Press; 1982:53–95.
11. Watsky MA, McDermott ML, Edelhauser HF. In vitro corneal endothelial permeability in rabbit and human: the effects of age, cataract surgery and diabetes. Exp Eye Res. 1989;49:751–67.

12. Watsky MA, McCartney MD, McLaughlin BJ, Edelhauser HF. Corneal endothelial junctions and the effect of ouabain. Invest Ophthalmol Vis Sci. 1990;31(5): 933–41.
13. Doughty MJ, Muller A, Zaman ML. Assessment of the reliability of human corneal endothelial cell-density estimates using a noncontact specular microscope. Cornea. 2000;19(2):148–58.
14. Chiou AG, Kaufman SC, Beuerman RW, et al. Confocal microscopy in cornea guttata and Fuchs' endothelial dystrophy. B J Ophthalmol. 1999;83(2):185–9.
15. Mustonen RK, McDonald MB, Srivannaboon S, et al. In vivo confocal microscopy of Fuchs' endothelial dystrophy. Cornea. 1998;17(5):493–503.
16. Bourne WM, Nelson LR, Hodge DO. Central corneal endothelial cell changes over a ten year period. Invest Ophthalmol Vis Sci. 1997;38(3):779–82.
17. Polse KA, Brand RJ, Cohen SR, Guillon M. Hypoxic effects on corneal morphology and function. Invest Ophthalmol Vis Sci. 1990;31:1542–54.
18. McMahon T, Polse K, McNamara N. Long-term PMMA contact lens wear reduces corneal function. ARVO abstracts. Invest Ophthalmol Vis Sci. 1993;34:1008.
19. Polse KA, Brand R, Mandell R, et al. Age differences in corneal hydration control. Invest Ophthalmol Vis Sci. 1989;30(3):392–9.
20. McLaren JW, Brubaker RF. A two-dimensional scanning ocular fluorophotometer. Invest Ophthalmol Vis Sci. 1985;26:144–52.
21. Kim EK, Geroski DH, Holly GP, et al. Corneal endothelial cytoskeletal changes in F-actin with aging, diabetes, and after cytochalasin exposure. Am J Ophthalmol. 1992;114:329–35.
22. Klyce SD, Beuerman RW. The effects of contact lenses on the normal physiology and anatomy of the cornea: symposium summary. Curr Eye Res. 1985;4(6): 719–44.
23. Polse KA, Brand RJ, Cohen SR, Guillon M. Hypoxic effects on corneal morphology and function. Invest Ophthalmol Vis Sci. 1990;31(8):1542–54.
24. MacRae SM, Matsuda M, Shellans S, Rich LF. The effects of hard and soft contact lenses on the corneal endothelium. Am J Ophthalmol. 1986;102:50–7.
25. MacRae SM, Matsuda M, Yee R. The effect of long-term hard contact lens wear on the corneal endothelium. CLAO J. 1985;11:322–6.
26. Schoessler JP. The corneal endothelium following 20 years of PMMA contact lens wear. CLAO J. 1987;13:157–60.
27. Orsborn GN, Schoessler JP. Corneal endothelial polymegathism after extended wear of rigid gas-permeable contact lenses. Am J Optom Physiol Opt. 1988; 65:84–90.
28. Lee JS, Park WS, Lee SH, et al. A comparative study of corneal endothelial changes induced by different durations of soft contact lens wear. Graefes Arch Clin Exp Ophthalmol. 2001;239(1):1–4.
29. Sibug ME, Datiles MB, Kashima K, et al. Specular microscopy studies on the corneal endothelium after cessation of contact lens wear. Cornea. 1991;10(5): 395–401.
30. Nieuwendaal CP, Odenthal MTP, Kok JHC, et al. Morphology and function of the corneal endothelium after long-term contact lens wear. Invest Ophthalmol Vis Sci. 1994;35(7):3071–7.
31. Roszkowska AM, Tringali CG, Colosi P, et al. Corneal endothelium evaluation in type I and type II diabetes mellitus. Ophthalmologica. 1999;213(4):258–61.
32. Hyndiuk RA, Schultz RO. Overview of the corneal toxicity of surgical solutions and drugs: and clinical concepts in corneal edema. Lens Eye Toxic Res. 1992;9(3–4):331–50.
33. McDermott ML, Edelhauser HF, Hack HM, Langston RHS. Ophthalmic irrigants: a current review and update. Ophthalmic Surg. 1988;19(10):724–33.
34. Schultz RO, Glasser DB, Matsuda M, et al. Response of the corneal endothelium to cataract surgery. Arch Ophthalmol. 1986;104:1164–9.
35. Holzer MP, Tetz MR, Auffarth GU, et al. Effect of Healon5 and 4 other viscoelastic substances on intraocular pressure and endothelium after cataract surgery. J Cataract Refract Surg. 2001;27(2):213–8.
36. Gagnon MM, Boisjoly HM, Brunette I, et al. Corneal endothelial cell density in glaucoma. Cornea. 1997;16(3):314–8.
37. 2000 Eye banking statistical report. Washington, DC: Eye Bank Association of America; 2000.
38. Wilson SE, Bourne WM. Fuchs' dystrophy. Cornea. 1988;7(1):2–18.
39. Lang GK, Naumann GOH. The frequency of corneal dystrophies requiring keratoplasty in Europe and the USA. Cornea. 1987;6(3):209–11.
40. Santo RM, Yamaguchi T, Kanai A, et al. Clinical and histopathologic features of corneal dystrophies in Japan. Ophthalmology. 1995;102(4):557–67.
41. Kolker AE, Hetherington J Jr. Becker-Shaffer's diagnosis and therapy of the glaucomas, 5th ed. St Louis: CV Mosby; 1983:275.
42. Pitts JF, Jay JL. The association of Fuchs' corneal endothelial dystrophy with axial hypermetropia, shallow anterior chamber, and angle closure glaucoma. Br J Ophthalmol. 1990;74:601–4.
43. Lipman RM, Rubenstein JB, Torczynski E. Keratoconus and Fuchs' corneal endothelial dystrophy in a patient and her family. Arch Ophthalmol. 1990;108: 993–4.
44. Orlin SE, Raber IM, Eagle RC Jr, Scheie HG. Keratoconus associated with corneal endothelial dystrophy. Cornea. 1990;9(4):299–304.
45. Wilson SE, Bourne WM, O'Brien PC, Brubaker FR. Endothelial function and aqueous humor flow rate in patients with Fuchs' dystrophy. Am J Ophthalmol. 1988;106:270–8.
46. Wilson SE, Bourne WM, Maguire LJ, et al. Aqueous humor composition in Fuchs' dystrophy. Invest Ophthalmol Vis Sci. 1989;30(3):449–53.
47. McCartney MD, Wood TO, McLaughlin BJ. Moderate Fuchs' endothelial dystrophy ATPase pump site density. Invest Ophthalmol Vis Sci. 1989;30(7):1560–4.
48. Biswas S, Munier FL, Yardley J, et al. Missense mutations in COL8A2, the gene encoding the alpha2 chain of type VIII collagen, cause two forms of corneal endothelial dystrophy. Hum Mol Genet. 2001;21:2415–23.
49. Wilson SE, Bourne WM. Fuchs' dystrophy. Cornea. 1988;7(1):2–18.
50. Laing RA, Leibowitz HM, Oak SS, et al. Endothelial mosaic in Fuchs' dystrophy. Arch Ophthalmol. 1981;99:80–3.
51. Mandell RB, Polse KA, Brand RJ, et al. Corneal hydration control in Fuchs' dystrophy. Invest Ophthalmol Vis Sci. 1989;30(5):845–52.
52. Adamis AP, Filatov V, Tripathi BJ, Tripathi RC. Fuchs' endothelial dystrophy of the cornea. Surv Ophthalmol. 1993;38(2):149–68.
53. Kangas TA, Edelhauser HF, Twining SS, O'Brien WJ. Loss of stromal glycosaminoglycans during corneal edema. Invest Ophthalmol Vis Sci. 1990;31(10): 1994–2002.
54. Levy SG, Moss J, Sawada H, et al. The composition of wide-spaced collagen in normal and diseased Descemet's membrane. Curr Eye Res. 1996;15(1):45–52.
55. Borderie VM, Baudrimont M, Vallee A, et al. Corneal endothelial cell apoptosis in patients with Fuchs' dystrophy. Invest Ophthalmol Vis Sci. 2000;41(9):2501–5.
56. Pineros O, Cohen EJ, Rapuano CJ, Laibson PR. Long-term results after penetrating keratoplasty for Fuchs' endothelial dystrophy. Arch Ophthalmol. 1996;114:15–18.
57. Payant JA, Gordon LW, VanderZwaag R, Wood TO. Cataract formation following corneal transplantation in eyes with Fuchs' endothelial dystrophy. Cornea. 1990;9(4):286–9.
58. Terry MA, Ousley PJ. Deep lamellar endothelial keratoplasty in the first United States patients: early clinical results. Cornea. 2001;20(3):239–43.
59. Busin M, Arffa RC, Sebastiani A. Endokeratoplasty as an alternative to penetrating keratoplasty for the surgical treatment of diseased endothelium: initial results. Ophthalmology. 2000;107(11):2077–82.
60. Melles GR, Lander F, van Dooren BT, et al. Preliminary clinical results of posterior lamellar keratoplasty through a sclerocorneal pocket incision. Ophthalmology. 2000;107(10):1850–6.
61. Maumenee AE. Congenital hereditary corneal dystrophy. Am J Ophthalmol. 1960;50(6):1114–24.
62. Waring GO III, Rodrigues MM, Laibson PR. Corneal dystrophies. II. Endothelial dystrophies. Surv Ophthalmol. 1978;23(2):147–67.
63. Kanis AB, Al-Rajhi AA, Taylor CM, et al. Exclusion of AR-CHED from the chromosome 20 region containing the PPMD and AD-CHED loci. Ophthalmic Genet. 1999;20(4):243–9.
64. Bahn CF, Falls HF, Varley GA, et al. Classification of corneal endothelial disorders based on neural crest origin. Ophthalmology. 1984;91(6):558–63.
65. Kirkness CM, McCartney A, Rice SC, et al. Congenital hereditary corneal oedema of Maumenee: its clinical features, management, and pathology. Br J Ophthalmol. 1987;71:140–4.
66. Mullaney PB, Risco JM, Teichmann K, Millar L. Congenital hereditary endothelial dystrophy associated with glaucoma. Ophthalmology. 1995;102(2):186–92.
67. Harboyan G, Mamo J, Der Kaloustian V, Karam F. Congenital corneal dystrophy: progressive sensorineural deafness in a family. Arch Ophthalmol. 1981;85:27–32.
68. Schaumberg DA, Moyes AL, Gomes JA, et al. Congenital hereditary endothelial dystrophy. Multicenter Pediatric Keratoplasty Study. Am J Ophthalmol. 1999;127(4):373–8.
69. Sajjadi H, Javadi MA, Hemmati R, et al. Results of penetrating keratoplasty in CHED: congenital hereditary endothelial dystrophy. Cornea. 1995;14(1):18–25.
70. Dana M-R, Moyes AL, Gomes JAP, et al. The indications for and outcome in pediatric keratoplasty. Ophthalmology. 1995;102(4):1129–38.
71. Molia LM, Lanier JD, Font RL. Posterior polymorphous dystrophy associated with posterior amyloid degeneration of the cornea. Am J Ophthalmol. 1999;127(1): 86–8.
72. Anderson NJ, Badawi DY, Grossniklaus HE, et al. Posterior polymorphous membranous dystrophy with overlapping features of iridocorneal endothelial syndrome. Arch Ophthalmol. 2001;119(4):624–5.
73. Feil SH, Barraquer J, Howell DN, et al. Extrusion of abnormal endothelium into the posterior corneal stroma in a patient with posterior polymorphous dystrophy. Cornea. 1997;16(4):439–46.
74. Ross JR, Foulks GN, Sanfilippo FP, et al. Immunohistochemical analysis of the pathogenesis of posterior polymorphous dystrophy. Arch Ophthalmol. 1995;113(3):340–5.
75. Cibis GW, Krachmer JA, Phelps CD, Weingeist TA. The clinical spectrum of posterior polymorphous dystrophy. Arch Ophthalmol. 1977;95:1529–37.
76. Ross JR, Foulks GN, Sanfilippo FP, Howell DN. Immunohistochemical analysis of the pathogenesis of posterior polymorphous dystrophy. Arch Ophthalmol. 1995; 113:340–5.
77. Laganowski HC, Sherrard ES, Kerr Muir MG. The posterior corneal surface in posterior polymorphous dystrophy: a specular microscopical study. Cornea. 1991;10(3):224–32.
78. Hirst LW, Waring GO III. Clinical specular microscopy of posterior polymorphous endothelial dystrophy. Am J Ophthalmol. 1983;95:143–55.
79. Brooks AMV, Gillies WE. Differentiation of posterior polymorphous dystrophy from other posterior corneal opacities by specular microscopy. Ophthalmology. 1989;96(11):1639–45.
80. Henriquez AS, Kenyon KR, Dohlman KH, et al. Morphologic characteristics of posterior polymorphous dystrophy: a study of nine corneas and review of the literature. Surv Ophthalmol. 1984;29(2):139–47.
81. Krachmer JH. Posterior polymorphous corneal dystrophy: a disease characterized by epithelial-like endothelial cells which influence management and prognosis. Trans Am Ophthalmol Soc. 1985;83:413–75.
82. Boruchoff SA, Weiner MJ, Albert DM. Recurrence of posterior polymorphous corneal dystrophy after penetrating keratoplasty. Am J Ophthalmol. 1990;109: 323–8.
83. Sekundo W, Lee WR, Aitken DA, Kirkness CM. Multirecurrence of corneal posterior polymorphous dystrophy. Cornea. 1994;13(6):509–15.

CHAPTER 58

Congenital Corneal Anomalies

JOEL SUGAR

DEFINITION
- Developmental abnormalities of the cornea present at birth.

KEY FEATURES
- Present at birth.
- Generally involve defects in the migration of mesenchyme in the anterior segment of the eye.
- Often associated with iris and lens anomalies.

INTRODUCTION

A number of corneal anomalies may be present at birth. The cause can be genetic, the result of a teratogen, or idiopathic. An awareness of the basic embryology of the anterior segment enables the possible developmental anomalies to be understood. At the fifth week of gestation, the lens vesicle separates from the surface ectoderm. Mesenchymal neural crest cells migrate between the surface ectoderm and the optic cup in what will become the anterior chamber.[1] The first wave of mesenchyme becomes the corneal endothelium and trabecular meshwork, the second becomes the corneal stromal keratocytes, and the third becomes the anterior iris stroma. Separation of these forms the anterior chamber. Alterations in this process result in the anomalies of corneal size, shape, and clarity described here. Many other congenital corneal disorders are described in other chapters of this book.

SIZE AND SHAPE ANOMALIES

MICROCORNEA

The cornea's horizontal diameter is normally 9.5–10mm at birth and 10–12.5mm in adulthood. The horizontal diameter of the cornea normally exceeds the vertical because of the broader limbus inferiorly and superiorly. An adult cornea less than 10mm in horizontal diameter is called microcornea. Microcornea may occur as part of microphthalmos. Microphthalmos is a diffusely small eye and may be associated with other anomalies, such as coloboma of the iris, retina, choroid, and even the optic nerve (Fig. 58-1).

Epidemiology, Pathogenesis, and Ocular Manifestations

Most cases are sporadic, although autosomal recessive and autosomal dominant pedigrees are reported.[2] Microphthalmos in association with dermal aplasia and sclerocornea is known as MIDAS syndrome. This has been found to be due to a deletion in Xp22.[3] In microcornea, the adult corneal diameter is less than 10mm, while the remainder of the eye is normal in size. This disparity may result in angle-closure glaucoma as the lens enlarges.

Again, most cases are sporadic, although an autosomal dominant variant associated with cataract and other anterior segment anomalies has been described.[4] Microcornea has been associated with numerous other anomalies, including the "micro" syndrome of microcornea, congenital cataract, mental retardation, retinal dystrophy, optic atrophy, hypogenitalism, and microcephaly.[5]

MEGALOCORNEA

Epidemiology, Pathogenesis, and Ocular Manifestations

Megalocornea is characterized by bilateral anterior segment enlargement with a corneal horizontal diameter of 12mm or greater at birth and 13mm or greater after 2 years of age (Fig. 58-2). It is distinct from buphthalmos, which manifests as elevated intraocular pressure and an enlarged globe as well as an enlarged cornea. The cause appears to be related to defective growth of the optic cup, which leaves a larger space for development of the cornea. In utero, elevated intraocular pressure, which spontaneously arrests, may result in similar changes, but presumably the endothelial cell density decreases, and the entire globe enlarges.

A number of variants of this disorder have been described. Autosomal dominant megalocornea without other ocular abnormalities is the least common. X-linked recessive megalocornea is reported more frequently and is associated with iris transillumination, pigment dispersion, lens subluxation, arcus, and central crocodile shagreen.[6,7] Endothelial cell density is normal, which confirms that the enlargement does not arise from corneal stretching,[8] and corneal clarity and thickness are usually normal. The genetic locus for X-linked megalocornea appears to be in the region Xq21–q22.6. Megalocornea has been reported in association with congenital miosis,[9] ectopia lentis and ectopia pupillae, and mental retardation.[10] Megalophthalmos, an enlarged cornea in an overall enlarged eye that does not have glaucoma, is most likely autosomal recessive and gives findings similar to X-linked megalocornea, with, in addition, an increased axial length (often >30mm), juvenile cataract, and high myopia.[6]

Treatment

Treatment is not necessary except for spectacle correction of myopic refractive error, which commonly occurs.

CORNEAL ABSENCE

Isolated absence of the cornea cannot occur. Concomitant, usually severe developmental anomalies of the entire anterior segment or the entire eye are seen because of the intimate relationship between the ocular structures in the development of the cornea. Anophthalmos is the extreme; absence of the cornea as well as other describable ocular structures may occur as part of more extreme genetic developmental disorders. Cryptophthalmos, with partial or complete failure of development of the eyelids, may be associated with a skin-like cornea, an incompletely developed anterior segment, or a rudimentary cyst-like globe with an absent an-

431

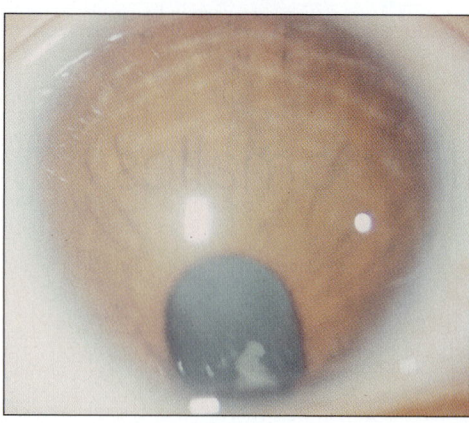

FIG. 58-1 ▌▌ **Colobomatous microphthalmos.** Right eye; note the small cornea and typical coloboma.

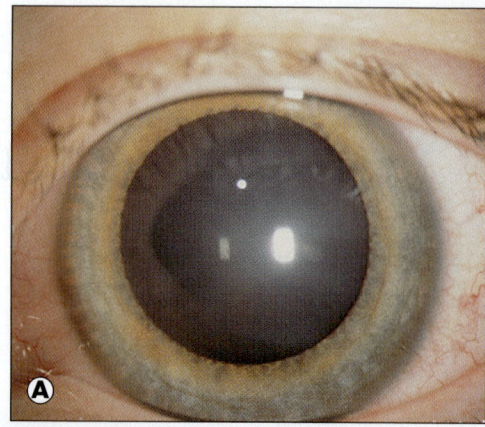

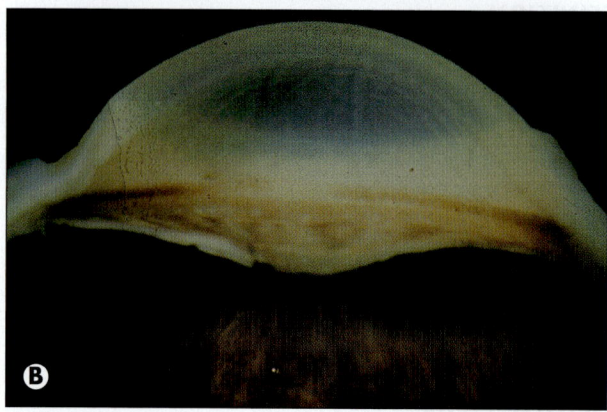

FIG. 58-2 ▌▌ **Megalocornea. A,** This patient has corneal diameters of 14mm bilaterally. **B,** Gross examination shows an enlarged cornea and a very deep anterior chamber. (From Yanoff M, Fine BS, eds. Ocular pathology, ed 5. Philadelphia, 2002; WB Saunders.)

terior segment. Cryptophthalmos also may be associated with systemic anomalies, which include syndactyly and genitourinary anomalies; this cryptophthalmos syndrome is inherited as an autosomal recessive trait. Pseudocryptophthalmos occurs when the lids fail to separate and the underlying globe is intact.

CONGENITAL CORNEAL ECTASIA

Keratoglobus (discussed in Chapter 59) is not congenital, but corneal ectasia may be present at birth as part of congenital anterior staphyloma, which is often part of Peters' anomaly. With congenital corneal ectasia, more marked corneal thinning and bulging occur than in Peters' anomaly alone (see Fig. 58-6), presumably as a consequence of the same developmental abnormalities in the migration of mesenchyme. This anomaly is usually unilateral and is often associated with iris developmental defects. Anterior staphyloma also may occur, presumably as a result of inflammatory or infectious corneal thinning *in utero*.

ANOMALIES OF CORNEAL CLARITY

Anomalies of neural crest mesenchyme migration may result in anomalies of the anterior segment and alterations in corneal clarity. Disordered events in the first wave of mesenchyme result in anomalies of the corneal endothelium and anterior chamber angle, while those in the second wave lead to corneal stromal alterations, and those in the third wave to iris abnormalities. Often the factors that result in maldevelopment act at more than one phase of this process to produce anomalies that involve more than one tissue derived from neural crest.

ANTERIOR EMBRYOTOXON

Anterior embryotoxon has been used to refer to a congenital broad limbus superiorly with an otherwise normal anterior segment, representing merely a broad transition from sclera to cornea. The term also is used to describe an appearance similar to arcus senilis (arcus juvenilis) present at birth. Though it is often sporadic, autosomal dominant and autosomal recessive pedigrees have been described.

POSTERIOR EMBRYOTOXON

Posterior embryotoxon is probably the most frequently seen anomaly, occurring in as many as 24% of a random population.[11] It consists of thickening and anterior displacement of Schwalbe's line, which is seen most readily at the slit lamp in the temporal cornea (Fig. 58-3). The term *toxon* is derived from the Greek word for "bow," in reference to the crescent of Schwalbe's line; when present alone, this has no functional significance.

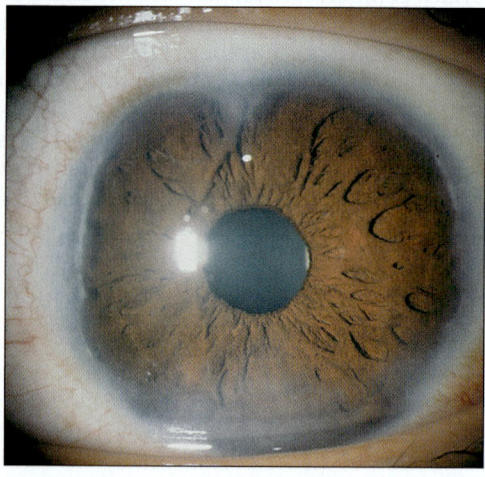

FIG. 58-3 ▌▌ **Posterior embryotoxon.** Schwalbe's line is evident nasally, superiorly, and temporally in the eye of this patient.

CORNEAL KELOIDS

Keloids are white, glistening, protuberant lesions that involve all or part of the cornea. Although usually resulting from trauma or ocular inflammation, they may be present at birth. Histopathologically, they represent hypertrophic scar with irregularly arrayed collagen bundles, fibroblasts, and capillaries arising in the corneal stroma. They may be progressive and have been associated with disorders that involve oculodigital manipulation, as in Lowe's syndrome. For bilateral lesions in otherwise healthy eyes, a rare occurrence, keratoplasty is appropriate.[12] For lesions in which progressive growth results in discomfort, dissection of the lesion from the cornea followed by covering with a conjunctival flap may halt progression.

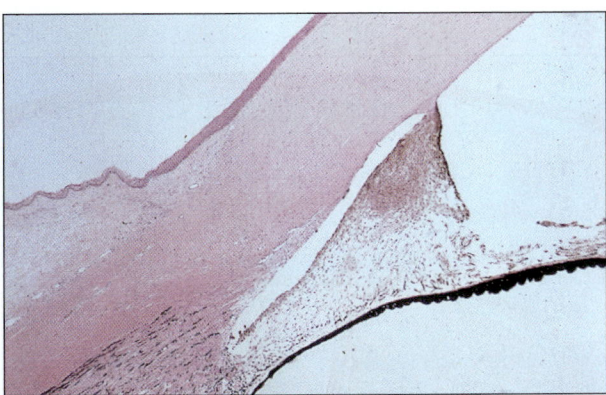

FIG. 58-4 ■ **Axenfeld's anomaly (posterior embryotoxon).** Histological section shows an iris process attached to the anteriorly displaced Schwalbe's ring. (Courtesy of Dr. R. Y. Foos. and Yanoff M, Fine BS, eds. Ocular pathology, ed 5. Philadelphia, 2002; WB Saunders.)

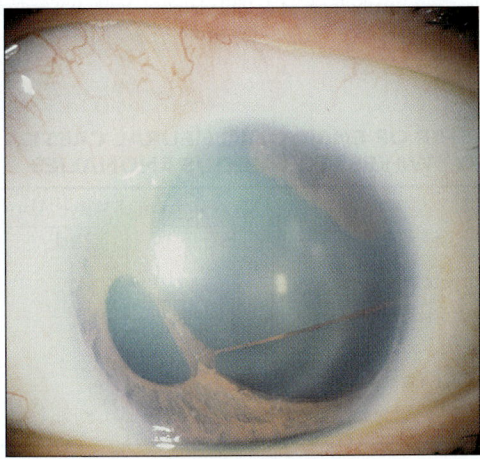

FIG. 58-5 ■ **Axenfeld-Rieger syndrome.** This patient has bilateral glaucoma as well as dental and facial anomalies.

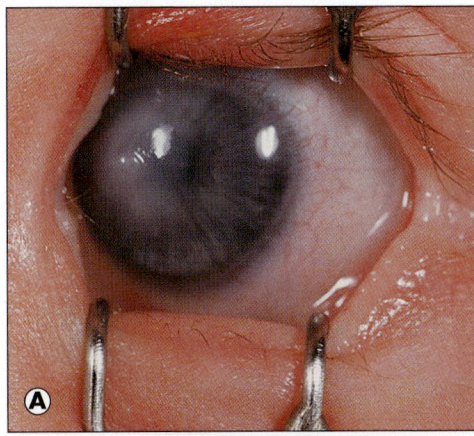

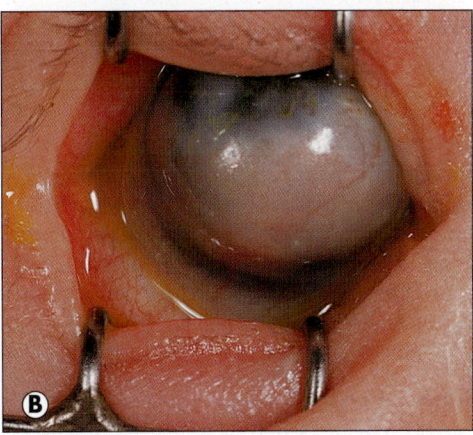

FIG. 58-6 ■ **Peters' anomaly in a neonate.** A, Typical Peters' anomaly type I. B, Severe Peters' involvement with corneal thinning and ectasia. This is called a congenital anterior staphyloma.

DERMOIDS

As discussed in Chapter 55, dermoids (choristomas, or growths of tissue not normally present) may be found on the cornea, usually at the inferotemporal limbus. At times they may involve larger areas of the cornea, the entire limbus, the entire cornea, or the interior of the eye. They usually are round, domed, and pink to white to yellow in color. They may have hair, or in the lipodermoid variant, fat globules are evident on slit-lamp examination. Induced astigmatism may be present and even amblyopia. Limbal dermoids may be associated with other malformations. The most common of these is Goldenhar's syndrome, which involves lid colobomas, hemifacial microsomia, preauricular skin tags, and other ear anomalies. Limbal dermoids also may be associated with mandibular and other facial anomalies.

Histopathology confirms the presence of skin-like collagen with skin adnexal appendages, which include hair follicles, sweat and sebaceous glands, and fat. Treatment consists of simple excision, since a plane can be developed between the lesion and normal sclera, limbus, and cornea, and the dermoid can be readily removed. Infrequently the lesion is of sufficient depth to warrant concurrent lamellar keratoplasty to fill the defect.[13] The depth can be ascertained by ultrasound biomicroscopy.[14]

AXENFELD'S ANOMALY AND RIEGER'S SYNDROME

Axenfeld's anomaly consists of bilateral posterior embryotoxon with iris strands adherent to Schwalbe's line (Fig. 58-4). Rieger's syndrome includes the changes of Axenfeld's anomaly along with iris atrophy, corectopia, and polycoria. Dental anomalies and a flattened midface and nasal bridge are associated with the

Axenfeld-Rieger syndrome (Fig. 58-5). The term *anomaly* refers to the localized anatomical changes seen, while the term *syndrome* refers to the more widespread ocular and systemic findings. Glaucoma occurs in about half of the patients who have Axenfeld-Rieger syndrome. It appears that Axenfeld's anomaly and Rieger's syndrome arise from retention of neural crest remnants and primordial endothelium on the iris and chamber angle.[15] Defects in the PITX 2 gene on chromosome 4q25 and in the FKHL7 gene on 6p25, as well as other defects, have been found in different families with the Axenfeld-Rieger phenotype.[16] Differential diagnosis includes the iridocorneal endothelial syndrome, which is acquired and usually unilateral; posterior polymorphous dystrophy with iridocorneal adhesions; and the iridogoniodysgenesis syndrome.[17]

PETERS' ANOMALY
Ocular Manifestations

Among the spectrum of malformations that occur with alterations in the mesenchymal formation of anterior chamber components, Peters' anomaly includes a variety of possible findings. Most cases are sporadic. The pathogenesis is alteration of the migration of waves of neural crest. Type I consists of a central or paracentral corneal opacity with iris strands that arise from the collarette and attach to the periphery of the opacity. Initially, a defect in corneal endothelium and Descemet's membrane is present, often with marked corneal edema, which may extend well beyond the defect (Fig. 58-6). Over time the surrounding endothelium covers the defect and produces new basement membrane, and the edema regresses to leave the corneal opacity only.[18] Posterior keratoconus and posterior ulcer of von Hippel may be thought of as Peters' anomaly that does not have iris adhesions. Peters' anomaly type II has lens involvement as well lens adherence to the posterior cornea, failure of complete sep-

433

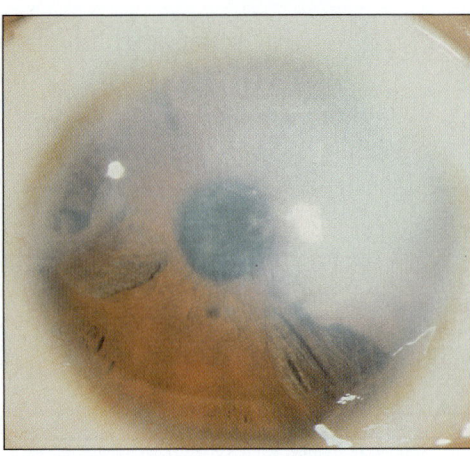

FIG. 58-7 ■ **Severe Peters' anomaly.** This infant has bilateral glaucoma, Peters' anomaly type II, and features of sclerocornea.

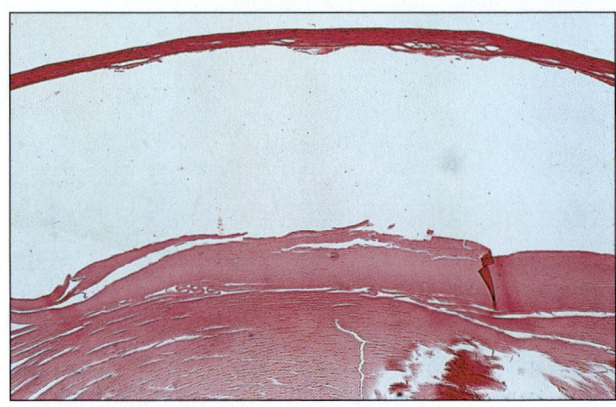

FIG. 58-8 ■ **Peters' anomaly.** Histologic section shows considerable corneal thinning centrally. The space between the cornea and the lens material is artifactitious and secondary to shrinkage of the lens cortex during processing of the eye. (From Yanoff M, Fine BS, eds. Ocular pathology, ed 5. Philadelphia, 2002; WB Saunders.)

aration of the lens from the cornea, and/or cataract. Type I most often is unilateral, while type II most frequently is bilateral. Peters' anomaly may be associated with other ocular anomalies (Fig. 58-7), including chorioretinal coloboma, iris coloboma, persistence and hyperplasia of the primary vitreous, microphthalmos, and optic nerve hypoplasia.

Systemic Associations

The systemic association of Peters' anomaly with short stature, facial dysmorphism, developmental delay, and delayed skeletal maturation is known as the Krause-Kivlin syndrome, which is autosomal recessive in inheritance. The Peters'-plus syndrome, consisting of Peters' anomaly with syndactyly, genitourinary anomalies, brachycephaly, central nervous system anomalies, cardiac disease, or deafness, is of uncertain inheritance pattern.[19,20] Peters' anomaly also has been reported as part of the fetal alcohol syndrome.[21] Most interesting is the finding of mutations at the PAX 6 locus on chromosome 11p13 in some Peters' anomaly patients.[22] The PAX 6 gene appears to play a regulatory role in embryogenesis and also has been found to be abnormal in aniridia and autosomal dominant keratitis.[23] PAX 6 is normal, however, in most patients with Peters' anomaly.[24] A defect in the same gene as Axenfeld-Rieger, 4q25, has also been found in Peters'.[25]

Pathology

Pathology of Peters' anomaly shows absence of Descemet's membrane and endothelium in the area of opacity initially (Fig. 58-8). As mentioned earlier, over time, the endothelial and Descemet's membrane defects are repaired by surrounding cells. Except for residual fibrosis in the posterior stroma, the remainder of the cornea, except for a usually absent central Bowman's membrane, is normal.

Treatment and Outcome

Treatment of Peters' anomaly includes treatment of the associated glaucoma. When corneal opacification is bilateral, penetrating keratoplasty should be considered. Although visual outcomes often are not ideal, the establishment of some formed vision is worthwhile.[26]

SCLEROCORNEA

Sclerocornea refers to scleral-like clouding of the cornea, which may be peripheral or diffuse. It results from a disordered second wave of mesenchyme migration and may be associated with corneal flattening or cornea plana because of the partici-

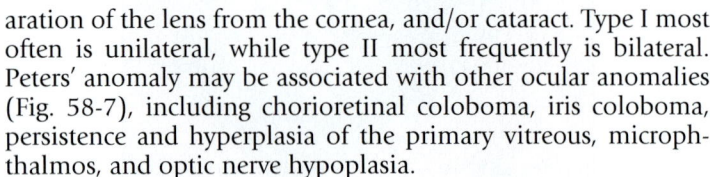

TABLE 58-1

RELATIONSHIP OF EMBRYONIC NEURAL CREST MIGRATORY "WAVES" TO VARIOUS ANOMALIES

Anomaly	Mesenchymal Wave Abnormality		
	1st	2nd	3rd
Posterior embryotoxon	X		
Axenfeld-Rieger syndrome	X		X
Peters' anomaly	X		X
Posterior keratoconus	X		
Sclerocornea		X	

pation of this wave in the formation of the limbus. Peripheral forms need to be differentiated from a congenital broad limbus or anterior embryotoxon. Sclerocornea may be associated with other anomalies of anterior segment development, such as Peters' anomaly; indeed, all the anterior segment developmental abnormalities discussed here may be considered part of a spectrum and often have many overlapping findings. Glaucoma is common. Associations with systemic anomalies and other ocular anomalies may occur, as in the MIDAS syndrome noted earlier, which results from a defect at Xp22. Inheritance may be autosomal dominant or recessive. Most cases, however, are sporadic and usually bilateral. Treatment consists of keratoplasty once the glaucoma has been controlled. Outcomes are poor, usually because of the difficulty in maintaining glaucoma control.

A review of the relationship of the embryonic neural crest migratory waves to the anomalies discussed is given in Table 58-1.

REFERENCES

1. Cook CS. Experimental models of anterior segment dysgenesis. Ophthalmic Pediatr Genet. 1989;10:33–46.
2. Vingolo EM, Steindl K, Forte R, et al. Autosomal dominant simple microphthalmos. J Med Genet. 1994;31:721–5.
3. Zvulunov A, Kachko L, Manor E, et al. Reticulolinear aplasia cutis congenita of the face and neck: a distinctive cutaneous manifestation in several syndromes linked to Xp22. Br J Dermatol. 1998;138:104–52.
4. Salmon JF, Wallis CE, Murray ADN. Variable expressivity of autosomal dominant microcornea with cataract. Arch Ophthalmol. 1988;106:505–10.
5. Warburg M, Sjo O, Fledelius HC, Pedersen SA. Autosomal recessive microcephaly, microcornea, congenital cataract, mental retardation, optic atrophy and hypogenitalism. Am J Dis Child. 1993;147:1309–12.
6. Meire FM. Megalocornea, clinical and genetic aspects. Doc Ophthalmol. 1994;87:1–121.
7. Pletz C, Hentsch R. Hereditary anterior megalophthalmos—a genealogical study of 12 patients in 4 generations. Klin Monatsbl Augenheilkd. 2000;217:284–8.
8. Skuta GL, Sugar J, Ericson ES. Corneal endothelial cell measurements in megalocornea. Arch Ophthalmol. 1983;101:51–3.
9. Meire FM, Delleman JW. Autosomal dominant congenital miosis with megalocornea. Ophthalmic Paediatr Genet. 1992;13:123–9.

10. Antinolo G, Rufo M, Borrego S, Morales C. Megalocornea–mental retardation syndrome: an additional case. Am J Med Genet. 1994;52:196–7.
11. Özeki H, Shirai S, Majima A, et al. Clinical evaluation of posterior embryotoxon in one institution. Jpn J Ophthalmol 1997;41:422–5.
12. Mejia LF, Acosta C, Santamaria JP. Clinical, surgical, and histopathologic characteristics of corneal keloid. Cornea. 2001;20:421–4.
13. Mader TH, Stulting D. Technique for the removal of limbal dermoids. Cornea. 1998;17:66–7.
14. Lanzl M, Augsburger JJ, Hertle RW, et al. The role of ultrasound biomicroscopy in surgical planning for limbal dermoids. Cornea. 1998;17:604–6.
15. Shields MB, Buckley E, Klintworth GK, Thresher R. Axenfeld-Rieger syndrome: a spectrum of developmental disorders. Surv Ophthalmol. 1985;29:387–409.
16. Alward WL. Axenfeld-Rieger syndrome in the age of molecular genetics. Am J Ophthalmol. 2000;130:107–15.
17. Walter MA, Mirzayans F, Means AJ, et al. Autosomal-dominant iridogoniodysgenesis and Axenfeld-Rieger syndrome are genetically distinct. Ophthalmology. 1996;103:1907–15.
18. Townsend WM, Font RL, Zimmerman LE. Congenital corneal leukomas II. Histopathologic findings in 19 eyes with central defect in Descemet's membrane. Am J Ophthalmol. 1974;77:192–206.
19. Heon E, Barsoum-Homsy M, Cevrette L, et al. Peters' anomaly, the spectrum of associated ocular malformations. Ophthalmic Pediatr Genet. 1992;13:137–43.
20. Mayer UM. Peters' anomaly and combination with other malformations. Ophthalmic Pediatr Genet. 1992;13:131–5.
21. Miller MT, Epstein RJ, Sugar J, et al. Anterior segment anomalies associated with the fetal alcohol syndrome. J Pediatr Ophthalmol Strabismus. 1984;21:8–18.
22. Hanson IM, Fletcher JM, Jordan T, et al. Mutations at the PAX 6 locus are found in heterogeneous anterior segment malformations including Peters' anomaly. Nat Genet. 1994;6:168–73.
23. Mirzayans F, Pearce WG, MacDonald IM, Walter MA. Mutation of the PAX 6 gene in patients with autosomal dominant keratitis. Am J Hum Genet. 1995;57:539–48.
24. Churchill AJ, Booth AP, Anwar R, Markham AF. PAX 6 is normal in most cases of Peters' anomaly. Eye. 1998;12:299–303.
25. Doward W, Periseen R, Lloyd GC. A mutation in the RIEG 1 gene associated with Peters' anomaly. J Med Genet. 1999;36:152–5.
26. Dana MR, Schaumberg DA, Moyes AL, Gomes JA. Corneal transplantation in children with Peters anomaly and mesenchymal dysgenesis. Multicenter Pediatric Keratoplasty Study. Ophthalmology. 1997;104:1580–6.

59 Stromal Corneal Dystrophies and Ectasias

JOEL SUGAR

DEFINITION
- A disorder in which an abnormal substance accumulates in the cornea.

KEY FEATURES
- Characteristically bilateral
- Progressive
- Isolated to the cornea

ASSOCIATED FEATURES
- Usually autosomal dominant
- Not associated with systemic disease

INTRODUCTION

A corneal dystrophy is a disorder that is typically bilateral, progressive, and isolated to the cornea; usually it presents in the central cornea. Most disorders are inherited, characteristically in a dominant fashion, and often appear clinically to involve only one layer of the cornea. With the present and ongoing identification of the genes involved in many of these entities, much hope exists that a better pathophysiological understanding. Ultimately this should lead to better treatment for these diseases. The epithelial and endothelial dystrophies are discussed in the chapters on the corneal epithelium (Chapter 56) and corneal endothelium (Chapter 57), respectively.

ANTERIOR MEMBRANE DYSTROPHIES

The anterior membrane dystrophies involve Bowman's membrane and appear to involve the epithelium as well. The category *anterior membrane* is somewhat arbitrary, since many of the so-called stromal dystrophies also involve Bowman's layer and epithelium. The recent genetic understanding of many of these disorders makes this classification even less appropriate, and many of these conditions will ultimately be better classified and named by their specific biochemical defects (Table 59-1).

REIS-BÜCKLERS' DYSTROPHY

"True" Reis-Bücklers' dystrophy, also known as corneal dystrophy of Bowman's I (CDB I) or granular dystrophy type III, is discussed here. Grayson-Willbrandt and Stocker-Holt dystrophies appear to be variants of Reis-Bücklers' dystrophy.

Epidemiology and Pathogenesis

The cause of Reis-Bücklers' dystrophy is unknown (see the "Avellino Dystrophy" section). It is autosomal dominant in in-

heritance and recently has been linked to a specific defect in the keratoepithelin gene on chromosome 5q. An arginine replaced by a glycine at codon 555 has been found in most families with this disorder, although other defects have been found in other families.[1,2] No systemic associations are known. The diagnosis is made on the basis of clinical appearance, although differentiation from honeycomb dystrophy is often difficult.

Ocular Manifestations

Reis-Bücklers' dystrophy is characterized by recurrent painful corneal epithelial erosions that typically begin in the first 1–2 years of life. Minimal corneal changes are seen at first, but then ring-like and map-like opacities appear at the level of Bowman's membrane; these become denser and more irregular over time (Fig. 59-1). By the second or third decade of life the painful erosions diminish as corneal sensitivity decreases, but the increasing fibrosis results in visual dysfunction.

Pathology

Pathology shows eosinophilic and fibrotic material beneath the corneal epithelium and in the anterior stroma, with destruction of Bowman's membrane. The material is somewhat granular in appearance. Electron microscopy shows rod-shaped bodies that replace Bowman's layer and lie between epithelial cells. These pathological findings are the same as those seen in superficial granular dystrophy.

Treatment

Treatment of Reis-Bücklers' dystrophy is symptomatic for the recurrent erosions. Superficial keratectomy, either by mechanical stripping or by excimer laser ablation, is the appropriate treatment for the visual disturbance. Recurrence may be relatively rapid, and after multiple treatments, penetrating keratoplasty may become necessary.

HONEYCOMB DYSTROPHY

Also known as Thiel-Behnke dystrophy, Waardenburg and Jonkers dystrophy, or corneal dystrophy of Bowman's membrane II (CDB II), honeycomb dystrophy is often confused in the literature with Reis-Bücklers' dystrophy. Patients have recurrent erosions, although less severe than those associated with Reis-Bücklers' dystrophy, and develop a reticular array of anterior stromal opacities that elevate the corneal epithelium in a "sawtooth" pattern. The disorder is inherited as an autosomal dominant. A defect has been found in the keratoepithelin gene.[3] In other families a defect has been found on chromosome 10. No known associated systemic abnormality exists. Histopathology shows wavy, subepithelial fibrosis with disruption of Bowman's membrane and of epithelial basement membrane. Electron mi-

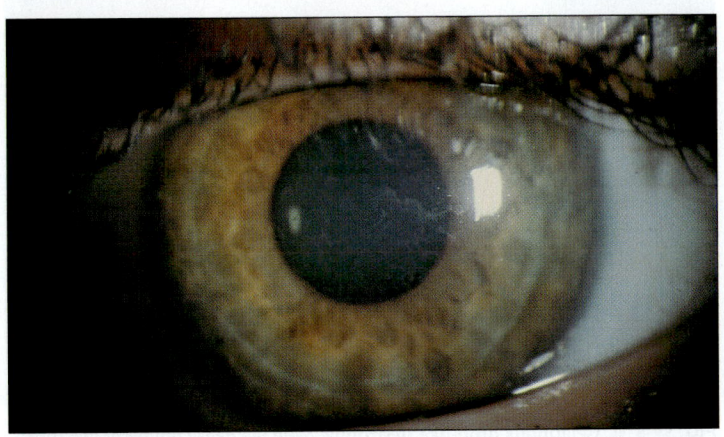

FIG. 59-1 ■ Reis-Bücklers' corneal dystrophy. Note the irregular opacities at the level of Bowman's layer.

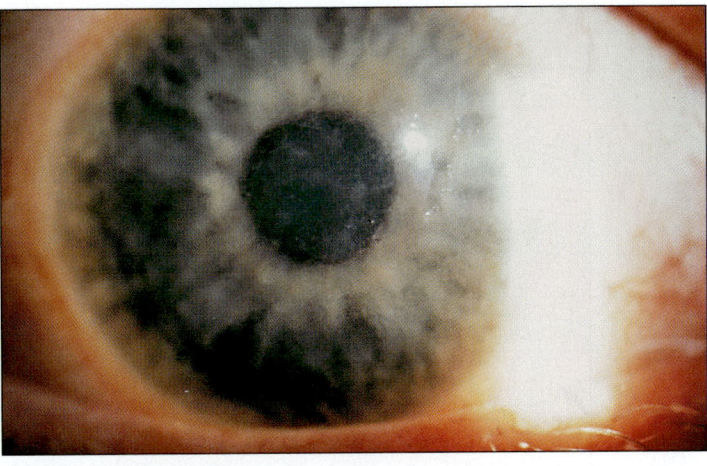

FIG. 59-2 ■ Lattice dystrophy Type I. This patient has very fine, rod-like opacities in the anterior stroma.

TABLE 59-1

CORNEAL DYSTROPHIES DUE TO KERATOEPITHELIN GENE DEFECTS

Dystrophy	Defect
Reis-Bücklers'	Arg555Gly, Arg124Leu, Arg555Gln
Thiel-Behnke	Arg124Leu (other families chromosome 10)
Lattice I	Arg124Lys
Lattice IIIA	Arg124Thr, Pro501Thr
Lattice IV	Leu527Arg
Granular I	Arg555Trp, Arg124Ser
Granular II (Avellino)	Arg124His

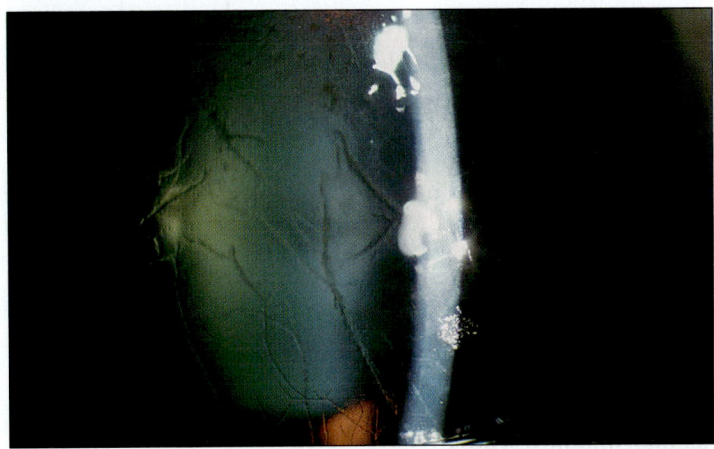

FIG. 59-3 ■ Lattice dystrophy Type I. Denser, ropier opacities than those shown in Figure 59-2.

croscopy reveals that curly collagen filaments replace Bowman's layer.[4] Treatment is the same as for Reis-Bücklers' dystrophy, namely superficial keratectomy or excimer ablation. Keratoplasty may become necessary after multiple recurrences.

SUPERFICIAL GRANULAR DYSTROPHY

Superficial granular dystrophy is likely a variant of Reis-Bücklers' and has been referred to as granular dystrophy Type III. It occurs less frequently with recurrent erosions but may occur early in life with photophobia and decreased vision. Histopathology and electron microscopy findings are the same as those for Reis-Bücklers' dystrophy. Some family members of patients who have this entity have a more typical stromal granular dystrophy. Treatment consists of excimer ablation or lamellar keratoplasty.

STROMAL DYSTROPHIES

The stromal dystrophies are classified as such because their clinical manifestation is the accumulation of material predominantly in the stroma. Nonetheless, like anterior membrane dystrophies, strong evidence exists that in at least some of these disorders the epithelium plays a significant role.

Lattice dystrophy is a term given to a subgroup of stromal dystrophies. All the lattice dystrophies have amyloid accumulation in the stroma, arranged in a branching pattern.

LATTICE DYSTROPHY TYPE I

Ocular Manifestations

The most frequently found lattice dystrophy is Type I, which has been referred to as Biber-Haab-Dimmer corneal dystrophy. Generally, rod-like glassy opacities appear in the anterior stroma

in the first or second decade of life, which become denser over time; linear, often branching, opacities are seen (Figs. 59-2 and 59-3). Recurrent erosions often occur and over time central anterior stromal haze may develop. The opacities usually are densest anteriorly and centrally in the cornea with a clear zone in the corneal periphery. The lines are relatively fine, as opposed to the ropier opacities seen in lattice dystrophy Type III. While the disorder is bilateral, asymmetry is found and occasional unilateral involvement may occur.

Diagnosis

Diagnosis of lattice dystrophy Type I is based on clinical appearance. Inheritance is autosomal dominant, and the disorder has been demonstrated to be due to defects at various codons on the BIGH3 gene. The most frequent defect is at codon 124 where the amino acid arginine is replaced by cysteine.[5]

Pathology

Histopathologically, dense deposits are seen in the stroma, which stain with Congo red, periodic acid–Schiff, and Masson's trichrome (Fig. 59-4). Dichroism and birefringence are seen with polarized light and fluorescence is seen with thioflavin-T. All of these findings are characteristic for amyloid, a β-pleated protein structure. The amyloid appears to be distinct from that seen in Type II lattice dystrophy.[6] Some granular deposits, typical of those seen in granular dystrophy, have been described in histopathologic evaluations of specimens of patients who have lattice dystrophy Type I.[7]

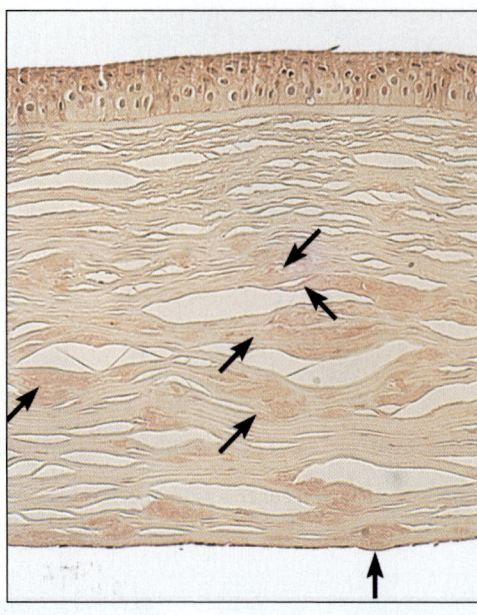

FIG. 59-4 ◼ **Lattice dystrophy Type 1.** Histopathology using Congo red stain shows the amyloid accumulations throughout the stroma *(arrows)*.

Treatment

Treatment consists of patching and soft contact lenses for episodes of corneal epithelial erosion. When acuity decreases significantly, penetrating keratoplasty is the treatment of choice. Recurrence is common and may respond to phototherapeutic keratectomy using the excimer laser. This same modality is of benefit in some early cases as an alternative to keratoplasty.

LATTICE DYSTROPHY TYPE II

Ocular Manifestations

Lattice dystrophy Type II is part of the systemic disorder familial amyloid polyneuropathy Type IV (Finnish type), also known as Meretoja's syndrome. In this disorder, fine lattice lines extend to the limbus. The lattice lines are not related to corneal nerves although the subbasal nerve density is reduced.[8] Recurrent erosions are less frequent and visual disturbance is less.

Systemic Associations

The frequency of glaucoma is increased with lattice dystrophy Type II. In addition, these patients have cranial neuropathy with facial weakness and systemic amyloid deposition. Lattice dystrophy Type II results from a single amino acid substitution in the plasma protein gelsolin, the consequence of a single nucleotide guanine to adenine change in the gene for gelsolin on chromosome 9q 32–34, leading to replacement of aspartic acid by asparagine or tyrosine at amino acid 187.[6]

Pathology

The pathology is similar to lattice dystrophy Type I.

Treatment

Treatment, if necessary, is the same as for lattice dystrophy Type I, although additional consideration must be given to the risk of corneal exposure from the facial neuropathy present in these patients.

LATTICE DYSTROPHY TYPE III

Lattice dystrophy Type III is a disorder characterized by the presence of thick, ropy lattice lines in the cornea without corneal erosions. This appears to be autosomal recessive and occurs later

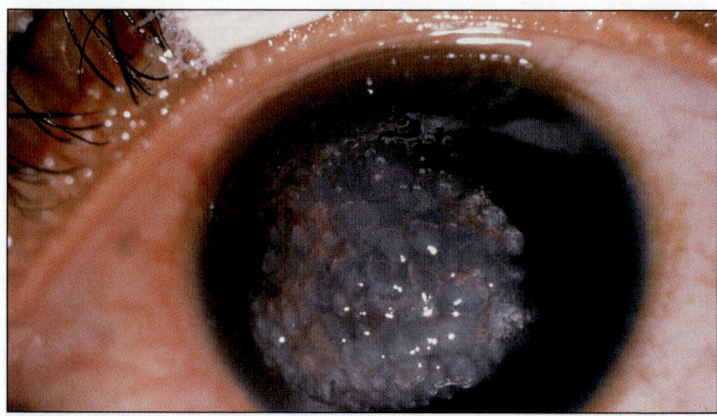

FIG. 59-5 ◼ **Gelatinous drop-like dystrophy.** Note the dense mulberry-like subepithelial accumulation. (Courtesy Deepak Edward, MD.)

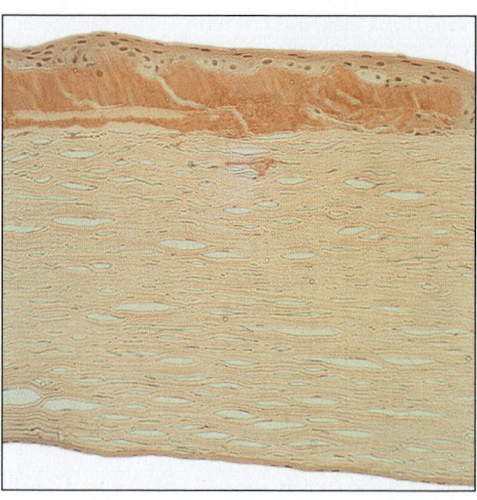

FIG. 59-6 ◼ **Gelatinous drop-like dystrophy.** Histopathology using Congo red stain shows the subepithelial accumulation of amyloid. (Courtesy Deepak Edward, MD.)

than lattice dystrophy Type I, often after 40 years of age. Histopathology shows amyloid deposition in the mid stroma, as well as in the superficial stroma beneath Bowman's membrane.[9] A lattice dystrophy Type IIIA that has identical corneal changes, but also the presence of recurrent erosions and a dominant inheritance pattern, has been described.[10] This disorder is due to a defect in the keratoepithelin gene, demonstrated at various codons (see Table 59-1).[11] A late-onset lattice dystrophy, Type IV, with deep stromal opacities has also been reported.[12]

GELATINOUS DROP-LIKE DYSTROPHY

Gelatinous drop-like dystrophy, also known as familial subepithelial amyloidosis of the cornea, appears to be an autosomal recessive disorder. The majority of reported cases have been from Japan, although some families have been reported in the United States as well as in Europe, Africa, and India. The disorder presents with severe photophobia, tearing, and decreased vision. Gray to white to yellow subepithelial nodules appear in the central cornea in the first or second decade of life. Over time these become confluent and give a nubbly, mulberry surface to the cornea (Fig. 59-5). Late in the progress of the disorder, superficial vascularization and deeper corneal deposition of amyloid occur. Histopathology shows subepithelial and anterior stromal accumulation of amyloid (Fig. 59-6).[13] The gene responsible appears to be the M1S1 gene on chromosome 1p with a Q118X mutation.[14] Treatment consists of superficial keratectomy, which needs to be repeated approximately every 2 years. Keratoplasty is followed by early recurrences.

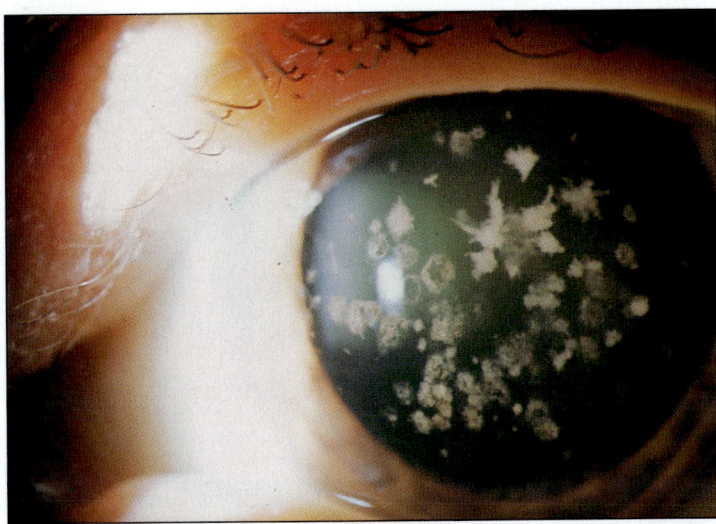

FIG. 59-7 ▮ **Granular dystrophy.** Note the crumb-like opacities in this patient who has sufficient clear cornea to have normal acuity.

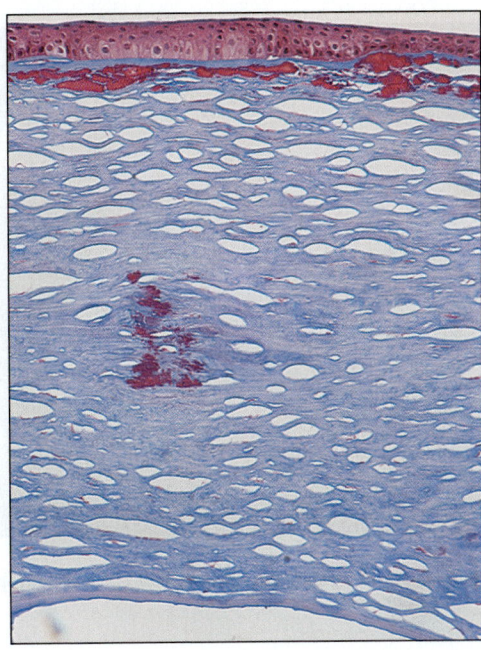

FIG. 59-8 ▮ **Granular corneal dystrophy.** Masson trichrome stain shows accumulation of hyaline material in the corneal stroma and beneath the epithelium.

Other forms of corneal amyloid deposition are seen, including secondary amyloidosis. Degenerative amyloid also occurs and can anatomically resemble lattice dystrophy in polymorphic amyloid corneal degeneration (see Chapter 60).

GRANULAR CORNEAL DYSTROPHY (GROENOUW TYPE I)

Ocular Manifestation

Granular corneal dystrophy is characterized by the presence of discrete opacities in the corneal stroma, with the stroma between opacities being clear. The opacities have irregular crumb-like or flake-like shapes and are whitish or slightly glassy in appearance (Fig. 59-7). The pattern within a given family appears to be consistent.

Diagnosis

In many patients no symptoms occur, whereas occasionally patients develop recurrent erosions. In the fifth decade or later some patients develop sufficient visual difficulties to require keratoplasty. The disorder is autosomal dominant and maps to chromosome 5q as do lattice Type I, Reis-Bücklers', and Avellino dystrophies. The most common defect is Arg555Trp on the BIGH3 (keratoepithelin) gene although other defects including those at codon 124 have been found.[20] No systemic associations are known.

Pathology

Histopathologic findings show red staining (Fig. 59-8) with Masson trichrome[21] without Congo red staining, although Congo red staining has been noted around the hyaline granules in some patients.[9] Electron microscopy shows electron-dense, rod-like deposits and microfibrils, which are present in keratocytes as well as epithelial cells.[22] The material is thought to be phospholipid.

Treatment

Patients who require keratoplasty do well, although the granules recur superficially in the graft, at times in a swirling pattern that suggests the epithelium is the source of the deposits.[18] Superficial recurrences may respond to keratectomy or excimer ablation.

AVELLINO DYSTROPHY

A dystrophy that combines features of both granular and lattice dystrophies has been described, with the majority of patients from the Avellino region of Italy. This is also referred to as *granular dystrophy Type II*. These patients have granular deposits in the anterior stroma as well as the presence of lattice-like lines deeper within the stroma. Gray subepithelial haze may develop centrally in the cornea, and corneal erosions and significant visual decline may occur. The disorder is autosomal dominant in inheritance and also is due to defects in the gene for keratoepithelin (BIGH3) with arginine replaced by histidine at residue 124.[19] Histopathology shows superficial, discrete, red granular deposits with Masson trichrome stain, as well as mid-to-deep stromal fusiform deposits with the typical Congo red and other stains (which are characteristic of lattice dystrophy Type I).[20] Treatment is the same as for granular and lattice dystrophies.

MACULAR CORNEAL DYSTROPHY

Ocular Manifestations

Macular corneal dystrophy is autosomal recessive. Faint anterior stromal white opacities are seen early in life, often in the first decade. The opacities become denser over time and a grainy, ground-glass haze becomes evident between the opacities, and then throughout the stroma (Fig. 59-9).

Diagnosis

Decreased vision and photophobia become evident in the second and third decades, and keratoplasty for decreased vision is often necessary in the fourth decade. This disorder appears to be the result of a metabolic abnormality in keratan sulfate.

Macular corneal dystrophy is autosomal recessive, and two types have been defined. In Type I, typical sulfated keratan sulfate is not present in the cornea or in the serum. The material accumulated in the cornea is an abnormal keratan sulfate, which results in altered corneal transparency and hydration. In macular corneal dystrophy Type II, antigenic keratan sulfate is present in both the cornea and the serum. In a Type I patient characteristic antigenic keratan sulfate is absent in the cartilage as well.[21] Clinically and histopathologically, Types I and II are indistinguishable.[22] Heterozygote carriers of macular corneal dystrophy Type I have normal serum antigenic keratan sulfate levels.[23] Mutations in the carbohydrate sulfotransferase 6 gene (CHST6) on chromosome 16q have been found to cause both types of macular corneal dystrophies.[24]

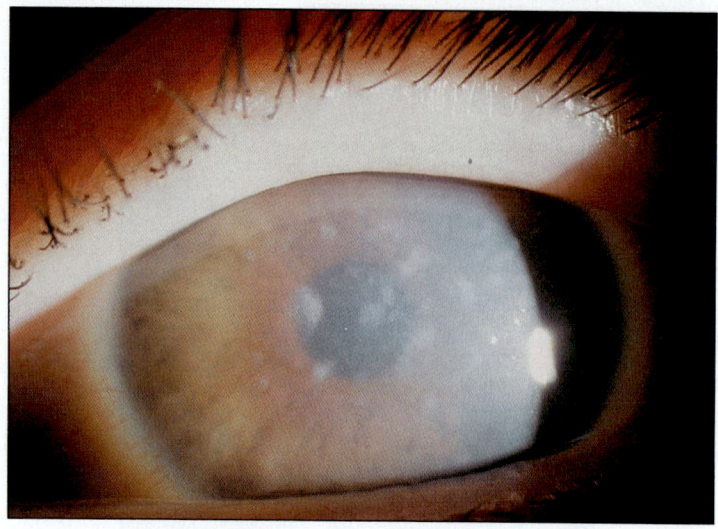

FIG. 59-9 ■ Forty-year-old woman who has macular corneal dystrophy. Note the stromal haze between the denser macular opacities.

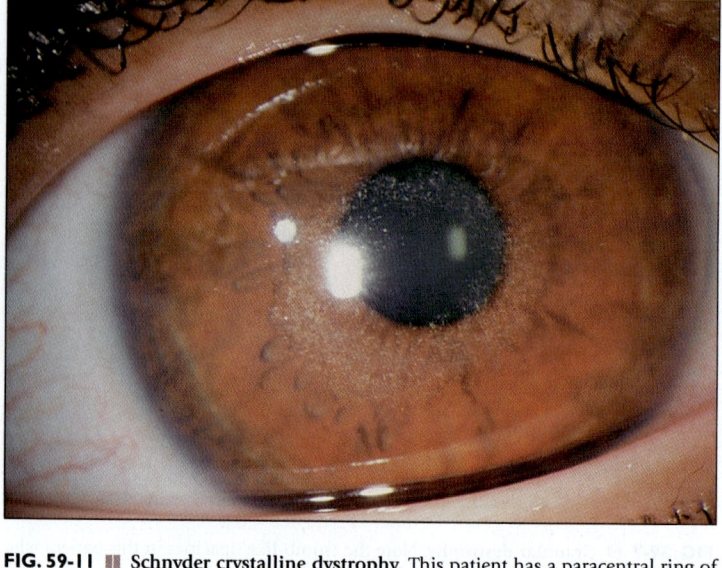

FIG. 59-11 ■ Schnyder crystalline dystrophy. This patient has a paracentral ring of crystals. (Courtesy Frederick Brightbill, MD.)

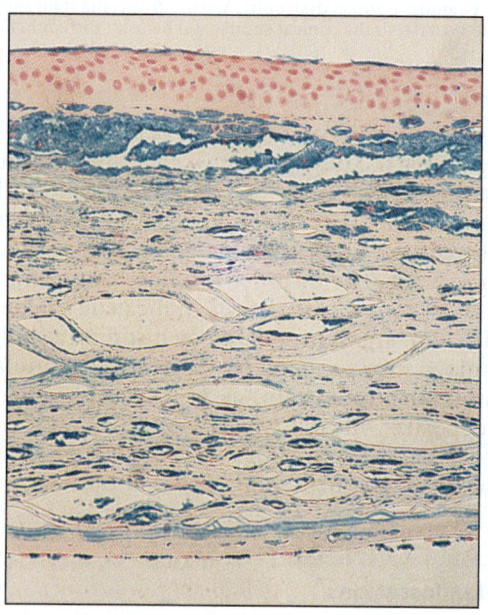

FIG. 59-10 ■ Macular corneal dystrophy. Colloidal iron shows accumulation of glycosaminoglycan (blue) at all levels of the cornea.

Systemic Associations

Although abnormalities in keratan sulfate in the blood and in cartilage have been reported, no systemic clinical abnormalities have been found in patients who have macular corneal dystrophy.

Pathology

Pathology shows glycosaminoglycan accumulation within and outside stromal keratocytes, beneath the corneal epithelium, and within corneal endothelial cells. This is evident with alcian blue, colloidal iron (Fig. 59-10), and periodic acid-Schiff stains. Electron microscopy shows intracytoplasmic vacuoles that contain glycosaminoglycans.

Treatment

Treatment consists of penetrating keratoplasty and has good outcomes. Recurrence in grafts has been reported, although infrequently.

SCHNYDER CRYSTALLINE DYSTROPHY
Ocular Manifestations

Schnyder crystalline dystrophy is an autosomal dominant disorder with variable phenotypic expression; it begins with central subepithelial corneal crystals, often in a ring pattern (Fig. 59-11). The crystals usually are evident in the first decade of life. With advancing age, arcus lipoides and more diffuse stromal haze may become evident. In other patients, however, even in those from the same families, such crystals may not be evident, but there is a central corneal haze that becomes more diffuse and denser with advancing age. This has been called Schnyder crystalline dystrophy *sine* crystals by Weiss.[25] Corneal sensitivity diminishes and acuity decreases from the fourth decade of life. The gene has been localized to chromosome 1p.[26]

Systemic Associations

Systemic hypercholesterolemia is frequent both in affected and unaffected family members. Genu valgum (knock knees) is associated infrequently.

Pathology

Histopathology shows oil-red O-positive lipid material throughout the stroma, which is more prominent peripherally, in Bowman's membrane, and just anterior to Descemet's membrane. Electron microscopy shows membrane-bound intracellular and extracellular vacuoles that contain electron-dense material throughout the stroma,[27] and cholesterol clefts may be seen in the anterior stroma. The accumulated material appears to be phospholipid and esterified and unesterified cholesterol.

Treatment

Treatment consists of corneal graft when the acuity declines sufficiently, although phototherapeutic keratectomy may be beneficial in some patients.[28] Crystals have been reported to diminish after corneal erosions.[29]

CENTRAL CLOUDY DYSTROPHY

Central cloudy dystrophy, also known as central cloudy dystrophy of Francois, has the same clinical appearance as Vogt's posterior crocodile shagreen, the difference being that central cloudy dystrophy appears to be dominantly inherited whereas posterior crocodile shagreen appears to be sporadic. These disorders have central corneal haze in a mosaic pattern like crocodile skin that involves the posterior stroma (Fig. 59-12). Patients typically are asymptomatic, and histopathology shows a "sawtooth" disarray of the corneal stromal lamellae.[30]

FLECK DYSTROPHY

Fleck dystrophy, also referred to as speckle or Francois-Neeten's dystrophy or cornea en mouchetee, is autosomal dominant. Patients have discrete, small, white-to-gray opacities, which may be solid in appearance or have clear centers, scattered throughout the stroma. The corneal epithelium and endothelium are uninvolved. Most patients are asymptomatic, although the occasional patient may be photophobic. Pathology shows distention of some keratocytes with membrane-bound vacuoles filled with electron-dense material. Electron microscopy shows staining with oil-red O consistent with the presence of lipid and acid mucopolysaccharide.[31] The epithelium and endothelium are normal. No treatment is necessary.

POSTERIOR AMORPHOUS CORNEAL DYSTROPHY

Posterior amorphous corneal dystrophy is a rare disorder, dominantly inherited, and defined by the presence of central and peripheral, deep corneal, gray, broad sheets of opacification.[32] Some patients have only peripheral changes (which extend to the limbus); corneal flattening and thinning are associated, and iridocorneal adhesions have been reported. The disorder appears to be nonprogressive, which prompts the suggestion that this entity be considered a dysgenesis rather than a dystrophy.[33] Pathologic evaluation has shown irregular disorganization of the corneal lamellae anterior to Descemet's membrane, with lipid deposition in the cytoplasm of some keratocytes.[34] A case has also been reported in which subepithelial deposits and a thick collagenous layer posterior to Descemet's membrane were found.[35] Usually, vision is affected only minimally, so treatment is unnecessary. The pathology reports come from two cases that had sufficient visual decrease to warrant keratoplasty.

CONGENITAL HEREDITARY STROMAL DYSTROPHY

Epidemiology and Pathogenesis

Congenital hereditary stromal dystrophy is present at birth and nonprogressive, so it better fits the category of congenital anomalies. Nonetheless, since it is named a dystrophy and resembles many of the dystrophies, it is discussed here.

Ocular Manifestations

Congenital hereditary stromal dystrophy is a very rare autosomal dominant disorder that is characterized by the presence of bilateral feathery or flaky, white, diffuse stromal clouding, most prominent centrally in the cornea. The corneal epithelium is normal. No corneal edema occurs. The opacification is present at birth and is nonprogressive. Without treatment visual acuity is reduced significantly and nystagmus may ensue.

Differential Diagnosis

The differential diagnosis includes congenital corneal edema (as a result of congenital hereditary endothelial dystrophy), congenital glaucoma, and posterior polymorphous dystrophy. The absence of epithelial edema and the presence of normal corneal thickness and intraocular pressure, however, exclude these. Corneal haze from metabolic disorders usually is less evident at birth, increases over time, and is associated with systemic find-

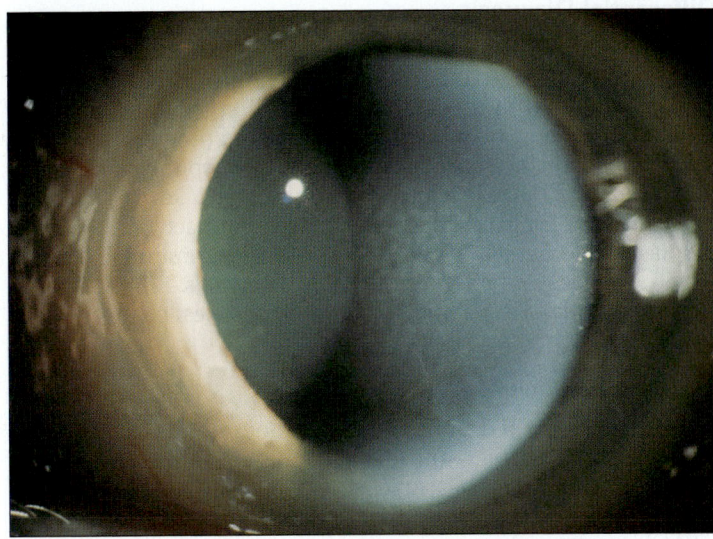

FIG. 59-12 ■ Findings typical of central cloudy dystrophy (posterior crocodile shagreen) are shown. Such patients are almost always asymptomatic.

ings. In congenital hereditary stromal dystrophy, no known systemic abnormalities occur.

Pathology

Pathologic evaluation of corneas removed at keratoplasty reveals normal epithelium and Bowman's layer, whereas the stroma shows separation of lamellae with layers of normal fibrillar arrangement separated by loosely packed layers of irregularly arrayed collagen. The collagen fibrils are about half the normal diameter. The normally banded anterior portion of Descemet's membrane lacks bandings, but the posterior portion of Descemet's membrane and the endothelium are normal.[36]

Treatment

Treatment consists of penetrating keratoplasty, usually with good outcomes.

CORNEA FARINATA

Cornea farinata is probably more a degeneration than a dystrophy. It is characterized by the presence of numerous, small, dustlike particles anterior to Descemet's membrane. This disorder is of no functional significance.

AUTOSOMAL DOMINANT KERATITIS

Epidemiology and Pathogenesis

Autosomal dominant keratitis is a rare autosomal dominant disorder. The cause is unknown, but similarities between this disorder and the corneal findings of aniridia suggest that it may be a variant of aniridia with the genetic defect at the PAX6 gene locus.[37]

Ocular Manifestations

Clinically, patients with this disorder have recurrent episodes of ocular erythema and photophobia. Over time, progressive, pannus-like fibrovascular tissue grows circumferentially onto the cornea, and central anterior stromal haze may develop. Iris abnormalities may be present with ectropion uveae, stromal atrophy, and an irregular pupil shape. Mild macular hypoplasia is common in some series. Other series of patients, however, show neither iris abnormalities nor fovea hypoplasia and may represent a different entity.[38]

Differential Diagnosis

The differential diagnosis of autosomal dominant keratitis includes aniridia and ectodermal dysplasia. Aniridia has associated corneal pannus with irregular subepithelial fibrosis and vascularization, which may be present early in life and progress over time. Studies show the presence of conjunctival-like epithelial cells and the absence of limbal stem cells in aniridia.[39] Likewise, ectodermal dysplasia, such as that seen in the ectrodactyl–ectodermal dysplasia–clefting syndrome, is associated with similar corneal surface changes and absence of limbal stem cells. KID syndrome (keratitis, ichthyosis, deafness) has similar corneal changes.

Systemic Anomalies

Whereas autosomal dominant keratitis does not have associated systemic abnormalities, aniridia, which is so similar as to possibly be a variant of the same entity, may be associated with Wilms' tumor, genitourinary anomalies, and mental retardation (WAGR syndrome).

Pathology

Pathology shows epithelial thinning, replacement of Bowman's membrane with fibrovascular tissue, and vessels and inflammatory cells in the anterior corneal stroma.

Treatment

Patients who have significant corneal clouding that results from autosomal dominant keratitis and progresses over time may undergo keratoplasty with variable outcomes—some have pannus and vascularization recur in the graft.

PRIMARY BAND KERATOPATHY

Epidemiology, Pathogenesis, and Ocular Manifestations

Rarely, patients have been reported to have an autosomal recessive form of band keratopathy. This disorder appears in early childhood, with whitish deposition of calcium in the interpalpebral zone of the cornea that begins at the limbus, nasally and temporally, and progresses centrally. Clear spaces are often seen in the opacity. Central involvement may reduce vision, fragmentation of the calcium may disrupt the corneal epithelium and cause pain, and corneal scarring and vascularization may ensue.[40] An adult form that appears later in life with similar findings has also been reported.

Differential Diagnosis

The differential diagnosis includes secondary causes of band keratopathy, such as ocular inflammatory disease, trauma, hypercalcemia, hypophosphatasia, and renal failure.

Pathology

Pathologic evaluation shows calcium deposition at the level of Bowman's membrane, in the epithelial basement membrane, and often in the anterior stroma.

Treatment

If vision is reduced or painful erosions occur, after epithelial removal the involved area is soaked with disodium ethylenediaminetetraacetic acid and the calcium débrided. Recurrence may take place.

CORNEAL ECTASIAS

Corneal ectasias, a group of disorders of corneal shape, include keratoconus, pellucid marginal corneal degeneration, and keratoglobus. Although keratoglobus and the related brittle cornea syndrome are congenital anomalies, they are discussed here. Posterior keratoconus, unrelated to the above disorders except by name, is also discussed here.

Keratoconus

Keratoconus is a disorder characterized by progressive corneal steepening, most typically inferior to the center of the cornea, with eventual corneal thinning, induced myopia, and both regular and irregular astigmatism.

EPIDEMIOLOGY AND PATHOGENESIS. The cause of keratoconus is unknown and, indeed, evidence exists that keratoconus may not be a single disorder, but rather a phenotypic expression of perhaps many causes. Recent studies suggest that enzyme abnormalities in the corneal epithelium, such as increased expression of lysosomal enzymes and decreased levels of inhibitors of proteolytic enzymes, may play a role in corneal stromal degradation. Gelatinolytic activity in the stroma has also been described, which perhaps occurs because of decreased function of enzyme inhibitors. Promoters of the genes involved in these enzyme activities may be abnormal as well.[41] Regulatory proteins that may play a role in controlling the numerous enzymes involved are being studied. Other investigators have suggested that abnormalities in corneal collagen and its cross-linking may be the cause of keratoconus.[42] Eye rubbing[43] and other factors such as contact lens wear may play a role.[44] The cytokine interleukin-1 has been suggested as a mediator of eye rubbing and stromal degradation.[45]

The prevalence of keratoconus in the general population appears to be relatively high, although the definition of cases varies in different series. A long-term study of a well-evaluated population in Minnesota found a prevalence of 54.5 cases per 100,000.[46] As new techniques of assessment of corneal topography become more widespread, the prevalence may well be found to be much greater. In a series of patients who sought refractive surgery for myopia, changes suggestive of keratoconus were found in 5 of 91 patients (5.5%) when computerized videokeratography was used to make the evaluation.[47]

OCULAR MANIFESTATIONS. The ocular manifestations of keratoconus are limited to the cornea. They include steepening of the cornea, especially inferiorly (Fig. 59-13), thinning of the corneal apex, clearing zones in the region of Bowman's layer, scarring at the level of Bowman's layer, and deep stromal stress lines that clear when the lids are pressed upon during slit-lamp examination. A ring of iron deposition (Fig. 59-14) accumulates in the epithelium at the base of the cone (Fleischer ring). The steepening of the cornea leads to clinical signs, which include protrusion of the lower eyelid on downgaze (Munson's sign), focusing of a light beam shown from temporally across the cornea in an arrowhead pattern at the nasal limbus (Rizutti's sign), and a dark reflex in the area of the cone on observation of the cornea with the pupil dilated using a direct ophthalmoscope set on plano (Charleaux's sign). Other signs have been described, such as pulsation of the mires on applanation tonometry and pulsation of the reflected images on standard keratometry because the thinned cornea readily transmits the ocular pulse. In some patients who have keratoconus, acute rupture of Descemet's membrane (acute hydrops) may occur and result in acute overhydration of the cornea and accumulation of lakes of fluid within the corneal stroma. The overlying corneal epithelium may become edematous, and fluid may leak through the corneal epithelium. The ruptured Descemet's membrane curls in on itself, and over time endothelial cells spread over the posterior stromal defect to lay down a new Descemet's membrane and recompensate the cornea. Subsequent to this, the corneal steepness may reduce.

DIAGNOSIS. More recently, computerized videokeratography has been used to confirm the diagnosis of keratoconus and in some cases to even make the diagnosis (Fig. 59-15). Rabinowitz[48] has suggested that the diagnosis of keratoconus can be made on the basis of observation of the presence of ker-

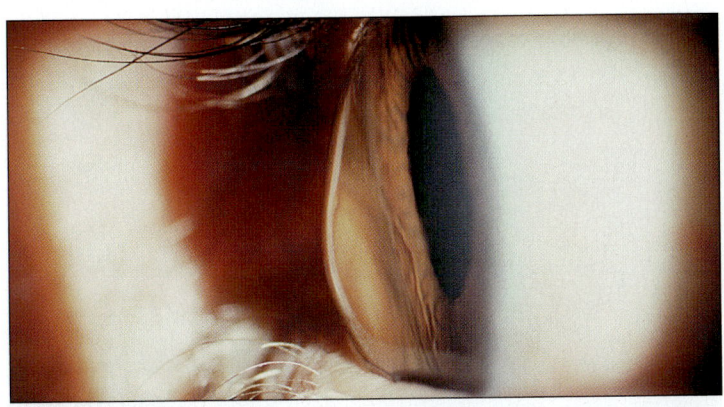

FIG. 59-13 ■ Lateral view of the inferior displacement of the cone apex in keratoconus.

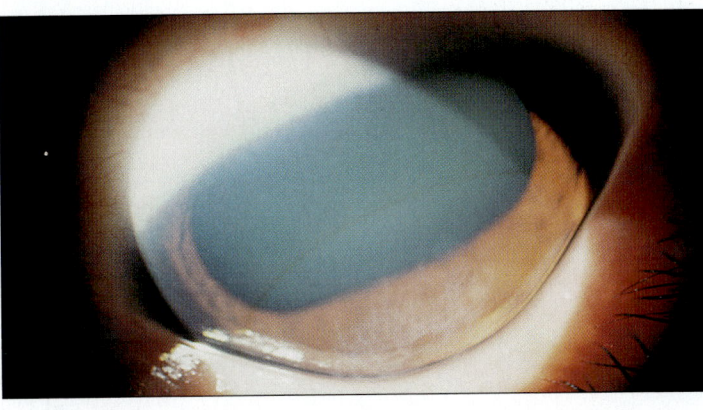

FIG. 59-14 ■ Keratoconus with the surrounding Fleischer ring.

atometry >47.20D, steepening of the inferior cornea compared with the superior cornea of >1.2D, and skewing of the radial axis of astigmatism by greater than 21°. These findings have a sensitivity of 98% and a specificity of 99.5% for the diagnosis of keratoconus. Such analyses have been used to demonstrate that keratoconus is almost always a bilateral disease, even when not evident at the slit lamp in one eye. The inheritance pattern of keratoconus is defined incompletely still. In the past it was believed that more than 90% of cases were sporadic. With the advent of videokeratography to assess family members, however, pedigrees have been analyzed. These studies show corneal changes consistent with keratoconus in some family members, which suggests an autosomal dominant pattern of inheritance.[49]

DIFFERENTIAL DIAGNOSIS. The differential diagnosis of keratoconus includes the other corneal ectasia disorders listed here. Posttraumatic corneal ectasia or protrusion of the cornea subsequent to corneal thinning from ulceration is also included in the differential diagnosis. The symptoms of keratoconus, which include decreased acuity, polyopia, and decreased contrast sensitivity, may be seen in other disorders, especially early nuclear sclerotic cataract.

SYSTEMIC ASSOCIATIONS. A number of systemic and ocular disorders have been described in association with keratoconus. Atopy commonly is associated and is seen in as many as 35% of patients,[50] vernal keratoconjunctivitis is not infrequent, and the eye rubbing seen in systemic atopy may play a role in the development of the cone.[43] Down's syndrome patients have been reported to show keratoconus in 5.5% of cases.[51] Among these patients the frequency of acute hydrops is higher, perhaps because of eye rubbing and/or because these patients are treated infrequently with keratoplasty and their disease is allowed to progress longer. Other systemic associations include Ehlers-Danlos, Marfan's, Cruzon's, Apert's, and other syndromes. Ocular-associated disorders include Leber's congenital amaurosis, retinitis pigmentosa, and retinopathy of prematurity. Fuchs' dystrophy and posterior polymorphous dystrophy have been reported as well. Given the relatively high prevalence of keratoconus in the general population, some of these associations may be coincidental.

PATHOLOGY. Examination of pathologic specimens from keratoconus shows central stromal thinning, irregular epithelium, breaks in Bowman's layer, and fibrosis filling in the breaks that extends beneath the epithelium (Fig. 59-16). With hydrops, breaks at the layer of Descemet's membrane are seen, with inward curling of Descemet's membrane, which is otherwise normal. Electron microscopy shows decreased thickness of the cornea with fewer lamellae. The collagen fibrils in the lamellae are thickened mildly and the space between fibrils is increased.[52]

TREATMENT. Treatment consists of spectacles for astigmatism and myopia initially, and rigid contact lenses once spectacle-corrected acuity becomes inadequate. When contact lenses no

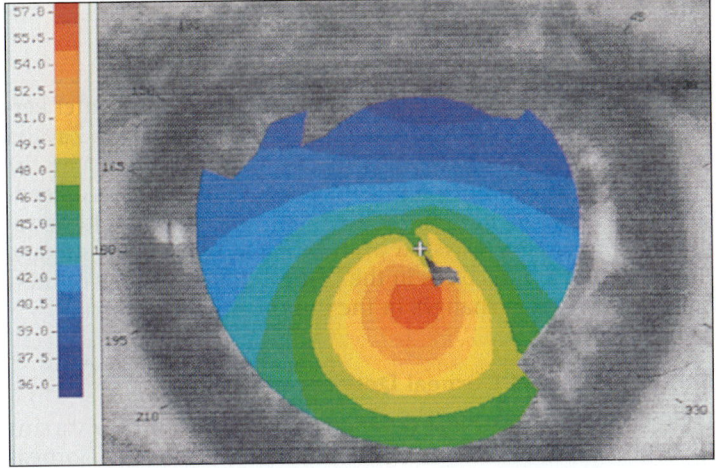

FIG. 59-15 ■ Computerized videokeratography. The inferior steeping of the cornea in keratoconus is shown.

longer provide adequate acuity, contact lens comfort becomes inadequate, or the steepness of the cornea is such that lenses cannot be maintained in position, surgical treatment is indicated. Also, if thinning progresses toward the limbus such that keratoplasty becomes more difficult and riskier, many surgeons proceed with keratoplasty. In one series, the most frequent reason for contact lens failure that resulted in the need for keratoplasty was inadequate acuity (43%), followed by inadequate lens tolerance (32%), frequent lens displacement (13%), and peripheral thinning (12%).[53]

Standard surgical treatment consists of keratoplasty; lamellar keratoplasty is effective, but most surgeons prefer not to use this because of the technical difficulties involved and the slightly reduced visual outcome.[54] Epikeratoplasty has successes as well, but largely has been abandoned because of the suboptimal visual outcome. By far the most frequent procedure is penetrating keratoplasty, which accounted for over 14.5% of all penetrating keratoplasties carried out in the United States in 2000.[55] At the time of keratoplasty, decreasing the donor/recipient size disparity reduces postkeratoplasty myopia.[56] Intracorneal ring segments have achieved some success in patients without corneal scarring in reducing the myopia and astigmatism and improving spectacle corrected visual acuity.[57]

COURSE AND OUTCOMES. Outcomes in terms of graft clarity and improved vision are excellent, although residual astigmatism and myopia remain problematic. Despite the proven outcome with keratoplasty, it is still the author's belief that contact lens use should be the treatment of choice for most patients who have keratoconus. A recent publication suggested that keratoplasty should be carried out once keratoconus patients do not see well with spectacles, although this approach is contro-

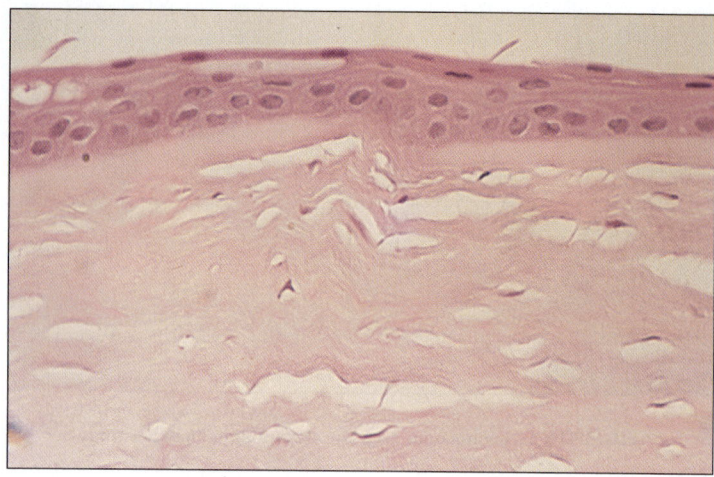

FIG. 59-16 ▮ Keratoconus. Breaks in Bowman's layer, with fibrosis that extends beneath the epithelium, can be seen. The stroma shows scarring.

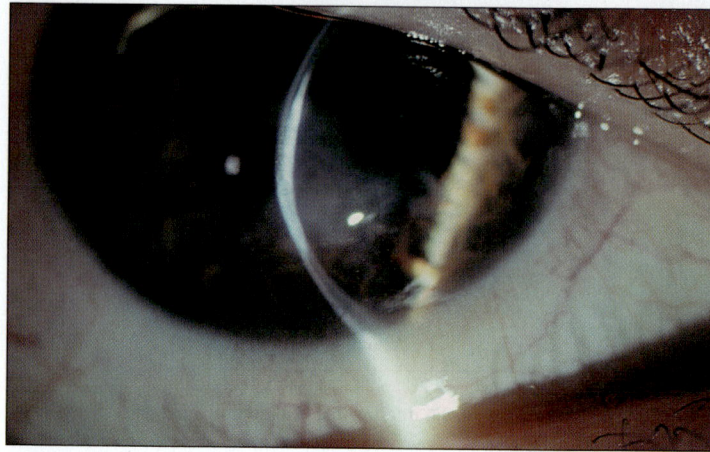

FIG. 59-17 ▮ Typical inferior thinning of pellucid marginal corneal degeneration. Note the subepithelial fibrosis from keratoconus (which is also present more centrally).

versial.[58] The complication of a fixed and dilated pupil after keratoplasty for keratoconus has been described (Urrets-Zavalia syndrome), but it is rare and appears to be related to iris ischemia.[59] Recurrence of keratoconus after keratoplasty is exceedingly rare. Authors have postulated that recurrence could be related to incomplete excision of the cone at the time of surgery, unrecognized keratoconus in the corneal donor, or host cellular activity that causes changes in the donor corneal material.[60]

Pellucid Marginal Corneal Degeneration

Pellucid marginal corneal degeneration appears to be a variant of keratoconus, with some different clinical features. Corneal thinning and protrusion are seen in the inferior peripheral cornea; the thinning begins 1–2mm inside the inferior limbus in a horizontal oval band approximately 2mm in radial extent and 6–8mm in horizontal extent (Fig. 59-17). The involved area is clear, and usually no iron line occurs central to it. Hydrops may occur. The central cornea is regular, but usually with marked against-the-rule astigmatism. Some patients who have pellucid may have more typical central corneal changes of keratoconus, as may family members, although the inheritance of pellucid is not clear. Pathology appears to be the same as in keratoconus. Treatment, as for keratoconus, consists of spectacles or contact lenses. When these are insufficient, in the author's experience results are best with large, eccentric penetrating keratoplasty. Lamellar keratoplasty, thermokeratoplasty, and corneal imbrication have all been reported as treatments that have limited success.

Keratoglobus

EPIDEMIOLOGY AND PATHOGENESIS. At least two forms of keratoglobus appear to exist: a congenital or juvenile form and an acquired adult form. The acquired form may be an end-stage form of keratoconus—patients have been described with initial keratoconus followed by later keratoglobus—or acquired keratoglobus may be seen with no known prior keratoconus. This form of keratoglobus has been seen in association with vernal keratoconjunctivitis, blepharitis, and orbital diseases that cause proptosis.[61] The congenital form appears to be part of at least two different autosomal recessive syndromes. One is Ehlers-Danlos syndrome Type VI. Another clinically similar syndrome, but with normal lysyl hydroxylase activity, is brittle corneal syndrome with associated blue sclera and red hair, which mimics Ehlers-Danlos syndrome Type VI.[62]

OCULAR MANIFESTATIONS. Keratoglobus is a disorder characterized by the presence of limbus-to-limbus corneal thinning with globular corneal protrusion. Usually the thinning is greatest in the corneal periphery or midperiphery. Hydrops occurs not infrequently, and perforations may occur with relatively minor trauma. In Ehlers-Danlos syndrome Type VI, patients have diffuse corneal thinning with corneal rupture spontaneously or after minor trauma, and corneal hydrops also is common. Blue sclera is present and is most apparent over the ciliary body; it creates a "blue halo" around the limbus. These patients may have systemic connective tissue abnormalities as well, with hyperextensible joints, bony anomalies, and hearing loss.[63] A defect in lysyl hydroxylase activity is present.

PATHOLOGY. Pathology of acquired keratoglobus is similar to that of keratoconus, whereas congenital keratoglobus shows an absence of Bowman's membrane, stromal disorganization, and thickening of Descemet's membrane with breaks.[64]

TREATMENT. Treatment includes protection from trauma. Lamellar epikeratoplasty has been used successfully to reinforce thin corneas and, in some cases, to improve vision.[65] For acquired keratoglobus, large penetrating keratoplasty may be successful.

Posterior Keratoconus

Posterior keratoconus refers to a congenital corneal anomaly in which the posterior corneal surface protrudes into the stroma, which usually occurs in a localized area, but may be more diffuse. This disorder usually is sporadic and unilateral and is nonprogressive. Bilateral and familial cases do occur but are less frequent. Often, the anterior corneal contour is affected minimally, although anterior protrusion and even a surrounding iron line have been described. Frequently, scarring occurs in the stroma anterior to the Descemet's bulge. On pathologic examination, scarring at the level of Bowman's membrane is seen and thinning of Descemet's membrane with excrescences has been reported variably.[66] The Descemet's membrane changes and congenital nature of this disorder suggest that it is a variant of corneal mesenchymal dysgenesis. Treatment usually is not necessary, although occasionally keratoplasty is indicated.

REFERENCES

1. Mullahy JE, Afshari MA, Steinert RF, et al. Survey of patients with granular, lattice, Avellino, and Reis-Bückler's corneal dystrophies for mutations in the BIGH3 and gelsolin genes. Arch Ophthalmol. 2001;119:16–22.
2. Takahashi K, Murakami A, Okisaka S. Keratoepithelin mutation (R555Q) in a case of Reis-Bückler's corneal dystrophy. Jpn J Ophthalmol. 2001;44:191.
3. Yee RW, Sullivan LS, Lai HT, et al. Linkage mapping of Thiel-Behnke corneal dystrophy (CDB2) to chromosome 10q 23-q24. Genomics. 1997;46:152–4.
4. Kuchle M, Green WR, Volcker AG, Barraquer J. Reevaluation of corneal dystrophies of Bowman's layer and the anterior stroma (Reis-Bücklers' and Thiel-Behnke types): a light and electron microscopy study of eight corneas and a review of the literature. Cornea. 1995;14:333–54.
5. Korvatska E, Munier FL, Djemai A, et al. Mutation hot spots in 5q31–linked corneal dystrophies. Am J Hum Genet. 1998;62:320–4.

6. deLaChapelle A, Tolvanen R, Boysen G, et al. Gelsolin-derived familial amyloidosis caused by asparagine or tyrosine substitution for aspartic acid at residue 187. Nat Genet. 1992;2:157–60.

7. Folberg R, Stone EM, Sheffield VC, Mathers WD. The relationship between granular, lattice type I and Avellino corneal dystrophies. A histopathologic study. Arch Ophthalmol. 1994;112:1080–5.

8. Rosenberg ME, Tervo TMT, Gullen J, et al. Corneal morphology and sensitivity in lattice dystrophy type II (familial amyloidosis, Finnish type). Invest Ophthalmol Vis Sci. 2001;42:634–41.

9. Hida T, Proia AD, Kigasawa K, et al. Histopathologic and immunological features of lattice corneal dystrophy Type III. Am J Ophthalmol. 1987;104:249–54.

10. Stock EL, Feder RS, O'Grady RB, et al. Lattice corneal dystrophy type III A: clinical and histopathologic correlations. Arch Ophthalmol. 1991;109:354–8.

11. Kawasaki S, Nishida K, Quantock AJ, et al. Amyloid and Pro 501 Thr-mutated Big-h3 gene product colocalize in lattice corneal dystrophy type IIIA. Am J Ophthalmol. 1999;127:456–8.

12. Fujiki K, Hotta Y, Nakayasu K, et al. A new L527 mutation of the BIGH3 gene in patients with lattice corneal dystrophy with deep stromal opacities. Hum Genet. 1998:103:286–9.

13. Li S, Edward DP, Ratnakar KS, et al. Clinicohistopathological findings of gelatinous droplike corneal dystrophy among Asians. Cornea. 1996;15:355–62.

14. Tsujikawa M, Kurahashi H, Tanaka T, et al. Identification of the gene responsible for gelatinous drop-like corneal dystrophy. Nat Genet. 1999;21:420–3.

15. Dighiero P, Niel F, Ellies P, et al. Histologic phenotype—genotype correlation of corneal dystrophies associated with eight distinct mutations in the TGFB1 gene. Ophthalmology. 2001;108:818–23.

16. Jones ST, Zimmerman LE. Histopathologic differentiation of granular, macular and lattice dystrophies of the cornea. Am J Ophthalmol. 1961;51:394–410.

17. Rodrigues MM, Streeten BW, Krachmer JA, et al. Microfibrillar protein and phospholipid in granular corneal dystrophy. Arch Ophthalmol. 1983;101:802–10.

18. Lyons CJ, McCartney AC, Kirkness CM, et al. Granular corneal dystrophy: visual results and pattern of recurrence after lamellar or penetrating keratoplasty. Ophthalmology. 1994;101:1812–7.

19. Kanishi M, Yamada M, Nakamura Y, Mashima Y. Immunohistology of keratoepithelin in corneal stromal dystrophies associated with R124 mutations of the BIGH3 gene. Curr Eye Res. 2000;21:891–96.

20. Holland EJ, Daya SM, Stone EM, et al. Avellino corneal dystrophy, clinical manifestations and natural history. Ophthalmology. 1992;99:1564–8.

21. Edward DP, Thonar EJ-MA, Srinivasan M, et al. Macular dystrophy of the cornea, a systemic disorder of keratan sulfate metabolism. Ophthalmology. 1990; 97:1194–200.

22. Edward DP, Yue BYJT, Sugar J, et al. Heterogeneity in macular cornea dystrophy. Arch Ophthalmol. 1988;106:1579–83.

23. Jonasson F, Oshima E, Thonar EJ-MA, et al. Macular corneal dystrophy in Iceland: a clinical, genealogic, and immunohistochemical study of 28 patients. Ophthalmology. 1996;103:1111–17.

24. Akama TO, Nishida K, Nakayama J, et al. Macular corneal dystrophy type I and type II are caused by distinct mutations in a new sulfotransferase gene. Nat Genet. 2000;26:237–41.

25. Weiss JS. Schnyder crystalline dystrophy sine crystals; recommendation for a revision of nomenclature. Ophthalmology. 1996;103:465–73.

26. Shearman AM, Hudson TJ, Andresen JM, et al. The gene for Schnyder's crystalline corneal dystrophy maps to human chromosome 1p 34.1-p36. Hum Mol Genet. 1996;5:1667–72.

27. McCarthy M, Innis S, Dubord P, White V. Panstromal Schnyder corneal dystrophy: a clinical pathologic report with quantitative analysis of corneal lipid composition. Ophthalmology. 1994;101:895–901.

28. Paparo LG, Rapuano CJ, Raber IM, et al. Phototherapeutic keratectomy for Schnyder's crystalline corneal dystrophy. Cornea. 2000;19:343–7.

29. Chern KC, Meisler DM. Disappearance of crystals in Schnyder's crystalline corneal dystrophy after epithelial erosion. Am J Ophthalmol. 1995;120:802–3.

30. Meyer JC, Quantock AJ, Thonar EJ-MA, et al. Characterization of a central corneal cloudiness showing features of posterior crocodile shagreen and central cloudy dystrophy of Francois. Cornea. 1996;15:347–54.

31. Nicholson DH, Green WR, Cross HT, et al. A clinical and histopathologic study of Francois-Neetens speckled corneal dystrophy. Am J Ophthalmol. 1977;83: 544–60.

32. Carpel EF, Sigelman RJ, Doughman DJ. Posterior amorphous corneal dystrophy. Am J Ophthalmol. 1977;83:629–32.

33. Grimm BB, Waring GO, Grimm SB. Posterior amorphous corneal dysgenesis. Am J Ophthalmol. 1995;120:448–55.

34. Johnson AT, Folberg R, Vrabec MP, et al. The pathology of posterior amorphous corneal dystrophy. Ophthalmology. 1990;97:104–9.

35. Roth SI, Mittelman D, Stock EL. Posterior amorphous corneal dystrophy: an ultrastructural study of a variant with histopathologic features of an endothelial dystrophy. Cornea. 1992;11:165–72.

36. Witschel H, Fine BS, Grutzner P, McTigue JW. Congenital hereditary stromal dystrophy of the cornea. Arch Ophthalmol. 1978;96:1043–51.

37. Pearce WG, Mielke BW, Hassard DTR, et al. Autosomal dominant keratitis: a possible aniridia variant. Can J Ophthalmol. 1995;30:131–7.

38. Kivlin JD, Apple DJ, Olson JR, Mantley R. Dominantly inherited keratitis. Arch Ophthalmol. 1986;104:1621–3.

39. Nishida K, Kinoshita S, Ohashi Y, et al. Ocular surface abnormalities in aniridia. Am J Ophthalmol. 1995;120:368–75.

40. Ticho U, Lhav M, Ivry M. Familial band-shaped keratopathy. J Pediatr Ophthalmol Strabismus. 1979;16:183–5.

41. Maruyama Y, Wang X, Li Y, et al. Involvement of sp1 elements in the promoter activity of genes affected in keratoconus. Invest Ophthalmol Vis Sci. 2001;42:1980–5.

42. Bron AJ. Keratoconus. Cornea. 1988;7:163–9.

43. Karseras AG, Ruben M. Aetiology of keratoconus. Br J Ophthalmol. 1976;60:522–5.

44. Macsai MS, Varley GA, Krachmer JH. Development of keratoconus after contact lens wear: patient characteristics. Arch Ophthalmol. 1990;108:534–8.

45. Wilson SE, Yu Guang HE, Weng J, et al. Epithelial injury induces keratocyte apoptosis: hypothesized role for the interleukin-1 system in the modulation of corneal tissue organization and wound healing. Exp Eye Res. 1996;62:325–37.

46. Kennedy RH, Bourne WM, Dyer JA. A 48-year clinical and epidemiologic study of keratoconus. Am J Ophthalmol. 1986;101:267–73.

47. Nesburn AB, Bahri S, Salz J, et al. Keratoconus detected by videokeratography in candidates for photorefractive keratectomy. J Refractive Surg. 1995;11:194–201.

48. Rabinowitz YS. Videokeratographic indices to aid in screening for keratoconus. J Refractive Surg. 1995;11:371–9.

49. Gonzalez V, McDonnell PJ. Computer-assisted corneal topography in parents of patients with keratoconus. Arch Ophthalmol. 1992;110:1412–4.

50. Rahi A, Davies P, Ruben M, et al. Keratoconus and coexisting atopic disease. Br J Ophthalmol. 1977;61:761–4.

51. Cullen JF, Butler HG. Mongolism (Down's syndrome) and keratoconus. Br J Ophthalmol. 1963;47:321–30.

52. Pouliquen Y. Doyne lecture: keratoconus. Eye. 1987;1:1–14.

53. Dana MR, Putz JS, Viana MAG, et al. Contact lens failure in keratoconus management. Ophthalmology. 1992;99:1187–92.

54. Waller SG, Steinert RF, Wagoner MD. Long-term results of epikeratoplasty for keratoconus. Cornea. 1995;14:84–8.

55. Eye Bank Association of America. 2000 statistical report. Washington: Eye Bank Association of America; 2001.

56. Wilson SE, Bourne WM. Effect of recipient–donor trephine size disparity on refractive error in keratoconus. Ophthalmology. 1989;96:299–305.

57. Colin J, Cochenee B, Savary G, et al. Intacs inserts for treating keratoconus: one-year results. Ophthalmology. 2001;108:1409–14.

58. Buzard KA, Fundisland BR. Corneal transplant for keratoconus: results in early and late disease. J Cataract Refractive Surg. 1997;23:398–406.

59. Tuft SJ, Buckley RJ. Iris ischaemia following penetrating keratoplasty for keratoconus (Urrets-Zavalia syndrome). Cornea. 1995;14:618–22.

60. Bechrakis N, Blom ML, Stark WJ, Green WR. Recurrent keratoconus. Cornea. 1994;13:73–7.

61. Cameron JA. Keratoglobus. Cornea. 1993;12:124–30.

62. Royce PM, Steinmann B, Vogel A, et al. Brittle cornea syndrome: an heritable connective tissue disorder distinct from Ehlers-Danlos syndrome type VI and fragilitas oculi, with spontaneous perforations of the eye, blue sclerae, red hair, and normal collagen lysyl hydroxylation. Eur J Pediatr. 1990;149:465–9.

63. Cameron JA. Corneal abnormalities in Ehlers-Danlos syndrome type VI. Cornea. 1993;12:54–9.

64. Pouliquen Y, Dhermy P, Espinasse MA, et al. Keratoglobus. J Fr Ophthalmol. 1985;8:43–54.

65. Cameron JA, Cotter JB, Risco JM, Alvarez H. Epikeratoplasty for keratoglobus associated with blue sclera. Ophthalmology. 1991;98:446–52.

66. Al-Hazzaa SAF, Specht CS, McLean IW, Harris DJ. Posterior keratoconus: case report with scanning electron microscopy. Cornea. 1995;14:316–20.

CHAPTER

60 Conjunctival and Corneal Degenerations

QAIS A. FARJO • ALAN SUGAR

DEFINITION
- Secondary deterioration or deposition in the cornea and/or conjunctiva, distinct from the dystrophies.

KEY FEATURES
- Common.
- Bilateral usually.
- Typically does not affect vision.

ASSOCIATED FEATURES
- Increased prevalence with age.
- Often associated with chronic light exposure.
- May follow past inflammation.
- Not inherited.

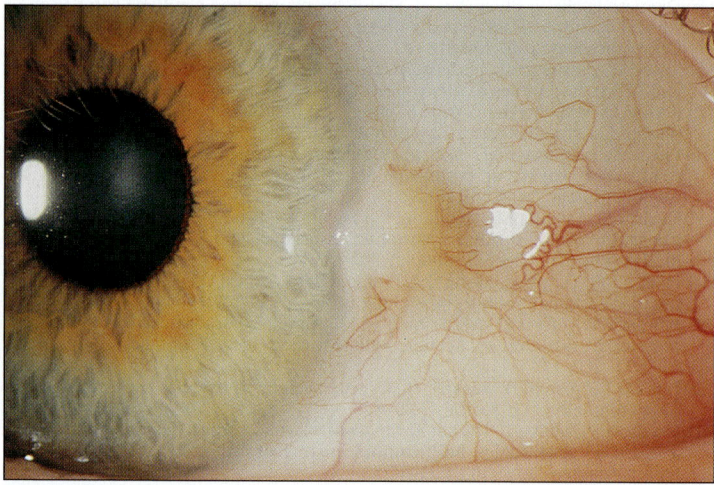

FIG. 60-1 ▮ Nasal pinguecula. Elevated conjunctival lesion encroaches on nasal limbus.

INTRODUCTION

Degenerations of the cornea and conjunctiva are common conditions that have, in most cases, relatively little effect on ocular function and vision. These conditions increase in prevalence with increasing age—as a result of past inflammation, of long-term toxic effects of environmental exposure, or of aging itself. Unlike corneal dystrophies, corneal degenerations are not inherited, may be unilateral or bilateral, and are often associated with corneal vascularization. Degenerations tend to involve the peripheral cornea and may overlap the limbus and conjunctiva. Conjunctival degenerations are discussed first, followed by those that involve the cornea.

CONJUNCTIVAL DEGENERATIONS

Pinguecula

Pingueculae are areas of bulbar conjunctival thickening that adjoin the limbus in the palpebral fissure area (Fig. 60-1). They are elevated, white to yellow in color, and horizontally oriented. Also, they are less transparent than normal conjunctiva, often have a fatty appearance, are usually bilateral, and are located nasally more often than temporally. When a pinguecula crosses the limbus onto the cornea, it is called a pterygium. Current information, however, suggests that pinguecula does not progress to pterygium and that the two are distinct disorders.

The causes of pingueculae are not known with certainty. Good evidence exists, however, of an association with increasing age and ultraviolet light exposure. Pingueculae are seen in most eyes by 70 years of age and in almost all by 80 years of age.[1,2] Chronic sunlight exposure has been found to be a factor by association with outdoor work and equatorial residence. In some studies, the strength of this association is less than that for pterygium.[3] The association with light exposure has also been found

in welders, for whom a higher rate of pingueculae occurs than for nonwelders as well as an increasing rate with increasing welding exposure.[4] It is thought that the predominantly nasal location is related to reflection of light from the nose onto the nasal conjunctiva. The effect of ultraviolet light may be mediated by mutations in the *p53* gene.[5]

Pingueculae are associated only rarely with any symptoms other than a minimal cosmetic defect. They may become red with surface keratinization. When inflamed, the diagnosis of pingueculitis may be given.

Distinguishing pingueculae from other lesions is usually not a problem because of the typical appearance. Conjunctival intraepithelial neoplasia may be difficult to differentiate from keratinization of a pinguecula. Gaucher's disease type I is said to be associated with tan pingueculae, but this is probably not a specific finding.[6]

The histopathology of pingueculae is characterized by elastotic degeneration with hyalinization of the conjunctival stroma, collection of basophilic elastotic fibers, and granular deposits.[7]

Pingueculitis responds to a brief course of topical corticosteroids or nonsteroidal anti-inflammatory agents.[8] Chronically inflamed or cosmetically unsatisfactory pingueculae rarely warrant simple excision.

Pterygium

Pterygium is a growth onto the cornea, usually nasally, of fibrovascular tissue that is continuous with the conjunctiva. It occurs in the palpebral fissure area, more often nasally than temporally, although either or both ("double" pterygium) occur (Fig. 60-2). Like pinguecula, it is a degenerative lesion, although it

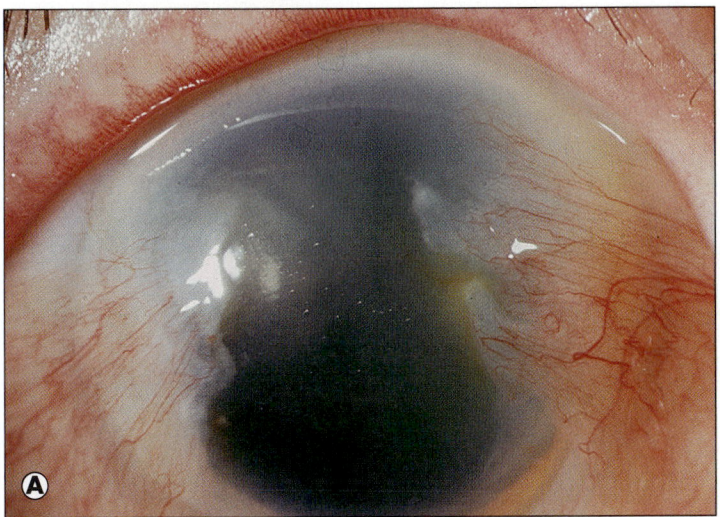

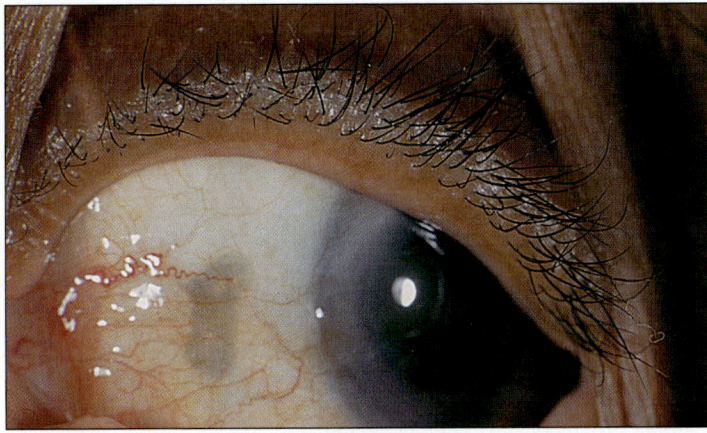

FIG. 60-3 ▮ **Senile scleral plaque.** Calcium deposition appears as a gray scleral plaque under the medial rectus muscle insertion.

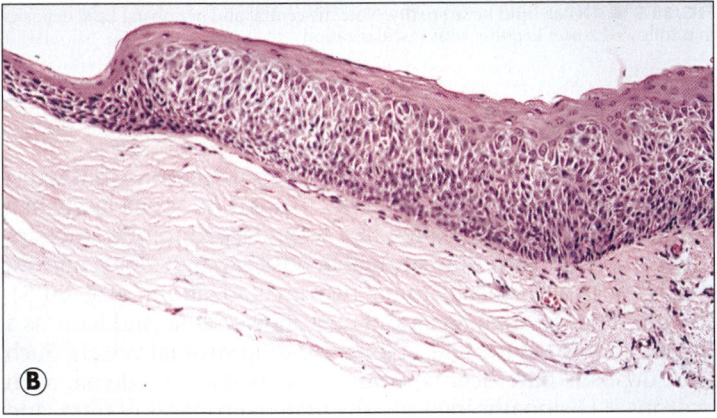

FIG. 60-2 ▮ **Double pterygium. A,** Note both nasal and temporal pterygia in a 57-year-old farmer. **B,** It is the invasion of the cornea that distinguishes a pterygium from a pinguecula.

may appear similar to pseudopterygium, which is a conjunctival adhesion to the cornea secondary to previous trauma or inflammation such as peripheral corneal ulceration. A pseudopterygium often has an atypical position and is not adherent at all points, so a probe can be passed beneath it peripherally.

Like pinguecula, pterygium is associated with ultraviolet light exposure. It occurs at highest prevalence and most severely in tropical areas near the equator and to a lesser and milder degree in cooler climates.[9,10] Both blue and ultraviolet light have been implicated in its causation, as demonstrated in watermen.[9] Outdoor work in situations with high light reflectivity, including from sand and water, enhances pterygium development, and the use of hats and sunglasses is protective.[10] In the past, the pathogenesis of pterygium was thought to be related to disturbance of the tear film spread central to a pinguecula. New theories include the possibility of damage to limbal stem cells by ultraviolet light and by activation of matrix metalloproteinases.[11,12] The histopathology of pterygium is similar to that of pinguecula except that Bowman's membrane is destroyed within the corneal component.[13]

Pterygia warrant treatment when they encroach upon the visual axis, induce significant regular or irregular astigmatism, or become cosmetically bothersome. A variety of surgical techniques have been developed. Most methods for small primary pterygia involve simple excision of the pterygium on the cornea and sclera. For larger and recurrent pterygia, the goal of treatment has been prevention of recurrence. The recurrence rates after older techniques have been very high: 50% reoccur within 4 months of excision and nearly all within 1 year.[14] Beta radiation applied postoperatively to the pterygium base was popular for many years and is moderately effective. It is now used less be-

cause of reports of late scleral necrosis.[15] Currently, the most widely used techniques are conjunctival autografting and mitomycin C application. These methods are equally effective.[16] Topical mitomycin C applied at the time of surgery appears to be relatively safe[17] and to decrease the potential toxicity of postoperative applications, although scleral and corneal melting may still occur.[18] Human amniotic membrane grafts have also been shown to be effective.[19]

Senile Scleral Plaques

Senile scleral plaques occur in the sclera rather than the cornea or conjunctiva, but they are frequently misinterpreted as a melting process similar to that of corneal degenerations or as conjunctival depositions. These lesions appear as yellow, gray, or black vertical bands just anterior to the insertion of the medial and lateral rectus muscles in elderly patients (Fig. 60-3). They become more common after the age of 60 years and, like pinguecula and pterygium, may be related to ultraviolet light exposure.[20] Histologically, calcium deposits along with decreased cellularity and hyalinization are seen. These lesions do not need therapy.

Amyloid

See later under Corneal Degenerations.

CORNEAL DEGENERATIONS

No adequate system exists by which to categorize logically all corneal degenerations, as this is a diverse group of conditions. The conditions that occur in the corneal periphery are discussed first, followed by the conditions that occur more centrally. This is an arbitrary division as many conditions, such as spheroidal degeneration or band keratopathy, can be found in either or both locations.

Corneal Arcus (Arcus Senilis)

Corneal arcus is the deposition in the corneal periphery of a gray to white or occasionally yellow band of opacity. It comprises fine dots and has a clear zone between it and the limbus, about 0.3mm wide, known as the clear interval of Vogt. Arcus usually has a diffuse central border and a sharper peripheral border (Fig. 60-4). It begins superiorly and inferiorly, possibly because of increased corneal temperature in unexposed areas, and gradually spreads to involve the entire corneal periphery but becomes densest and widest above. The deposits occur in the deep stroma initially and later in superficial stroma, with less density in the midstroma. The central extent may show crossing lines of dark-

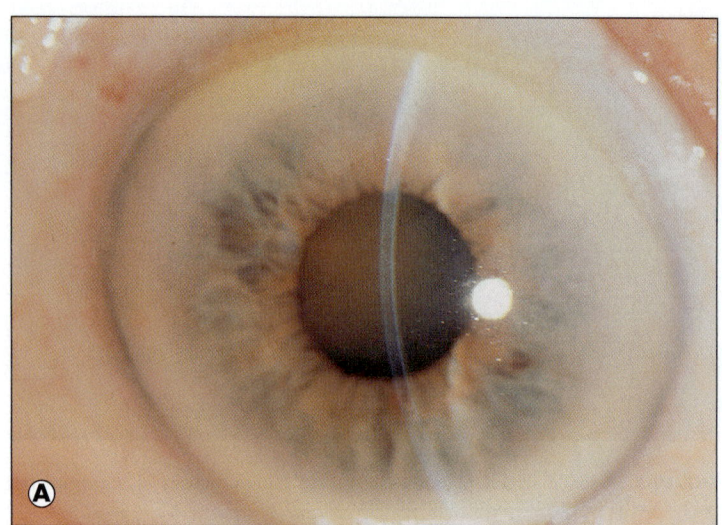

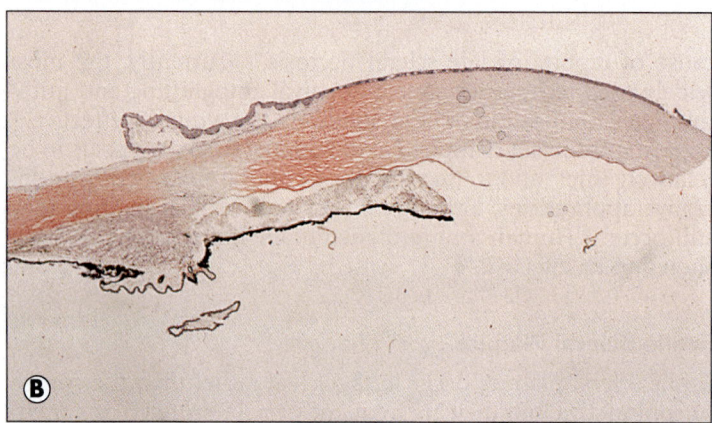

FIG. 60-4 ▮ **Arcus senilis. A,** Corneal arcus in an elderly man. **B,** Histologic section shows that the lipid is concentrated in the anterior and posterior stroma as two red triangles, apex to apex, with the bases being Bowman's and Descemet's membranes, both of which are infiltrated heavily by fat (red staining), as is the sclera. (From Yanoff M, Fine BS. Ocular pathology, ed 5. St. Louis: Mosby, 2002.)

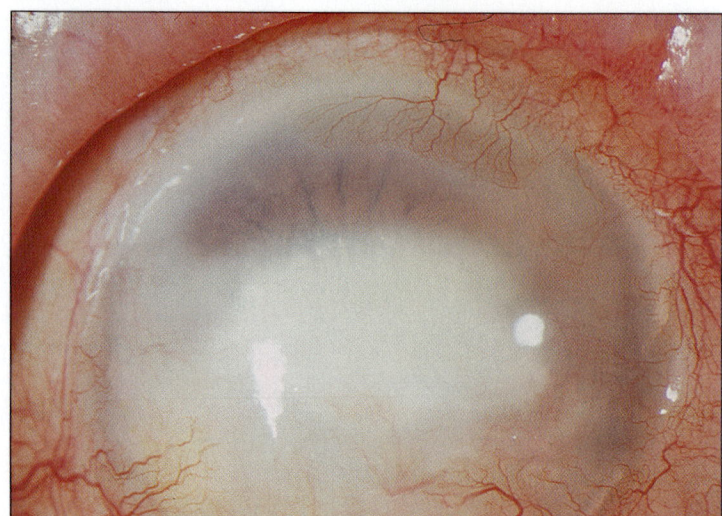

FIG. 60-5 ▮ **Dense lipid keratopathy.** Note the central and peripheral lipid deposits that followed zoster keratitis with vascularization.

Lipid Keratopathy

Lipid keratopathy may be peripheral, central, or diffuse but is discussed here because of its similarity to arcus. It occurs rarely in a primary form and more often in a secondary form; the latter appears as a white or yellow stromal deposit separated by a narrow, clear zone from corneal stromal neovascularization[27] (Fig. 60-5). It is often denser than arcus and may appear rather suddenly as a circular deposit at the end of long-standing stromal vessels. Such lipid deposits have been known to follow corneal edema, as in hydrops.[28] Histopathologically, the material consists of intra- and extracellular lipids, similar to those of arcus.[29]

Primary lipid keratopathy has features of a corneal dystrophy. It is usually bilateral and occurs in a previously normal cornea. Central lipid, often with cholesterol crystals, may severely decrease vision and warrant penetrating keratoplasty.[30]

Vogt's White Limbal Girdle

Vogt[31] described many of the corneal degenerations in his classic atlas of 1930. He was the first to describe two types of limbal girdle—white, arc-like opacities in the cornea central to the limbus in the 3 and 9 o'clock positions. What Vogt described as type I is probably a mild, early form of calcific band keratopathy with a peripheral clear zone and scattered clear holes. The much more common type II lacks a peripheral clear zone between the arc and the limbus and consists of fine, white radial lines, located nasally more often than temporally (Fig. 60-6). As with most degenerations, this condition increases in prevalence with age. It is present in normal eyes in 50% of those who are 40–60 years of age and increases to essentially 100% in those older than 80 years.[32]

Histologically, Vogt's limbal girdle type II is made up of hyperelastotic and hyaline deposits peripheral to Bowman's membrane. These findings are similar to those seen in pinguecula and pterygium.

Senile Corneal Furrow Degeneration

A peripheral corneal furrow that occurs between corneal arcus and the limbus in the elderly is found, but rarely.[31] The lucid interval peripheral to arcus may appear to be furrowed because of the clarity of the superficial cornea, but it was considered to be falsely thinned by Vogt.[31] Rarely, true thinning with no inflammation, vascularization, or induced corneal astigmatism can occur in this region, usually in the very elderly. It requires no therapy, but it should be considered when cataract incisions are made in these patients.

ness or lessened deposition, similar to the patches seen in the central cornea in crocodile shagreen, discussed later. The roughly circular path of the arcus may deviate centrally in areas of corneal vascularization. The arcus is almost always bilateral. It may be asymmetric when carotid vascular disease on one side is associated with decreased arcus or when arcus is increased in eyes with chronic hypotony.[21]

The frequent designation of corneal arcus as arcus senilis recognizes its association with aging. Arcus is the most common of the corneal degenerations. In men, it occurs with increasing frequency from the ages of 40–80 years, in 90% of normal men between 70 and 80 years of age, and in essentially all those older than 80 years. In women a similar pattern is seen, but with a delay of about 10 years.[21]

The deposits of arcus are made up of extracellular steroid esters of lipoproteins, most of a low density. Lipid material leaks from limbal capillaries, but its central flow is limited by a functional barrier to the flow of large molecules in the cornea, which keeps the deposits in their peripheral location.[22,23]

The most important systemic association of corneal arcus is with aging. Also, good evidence exists for an association with increased plasma cholesterol and low-density lipoprotein cholesterol, particularly in men younger than 50 years (arcus juvenilis). Young patients who have arcus also have an increased risk for type IIa dyslipoproteinemia but a decreased risk for type IV.[24] Men with arcus juvenilis have a fourfold increased relative risk of mortality from coronary heart disease and cardiovascular disease. Arcus in young men therefore is a useful clinical indication for the need for lipid and cardiovascular evaluation.[25] In older patients, including diabetics, arcus does not correlate with mortality.[26]

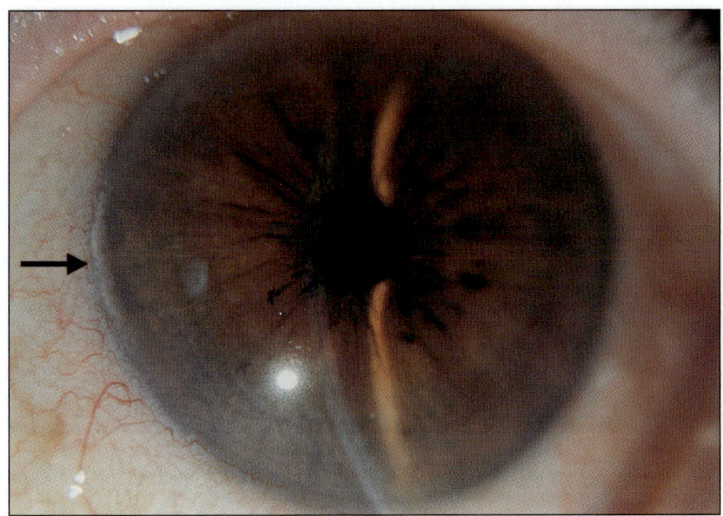

FIG. 60-6 ▌ **Vogt's limbal girdle.** The fimbriated peripheral corneal opacity is visible in the 9 o'clock position *(arrow).*

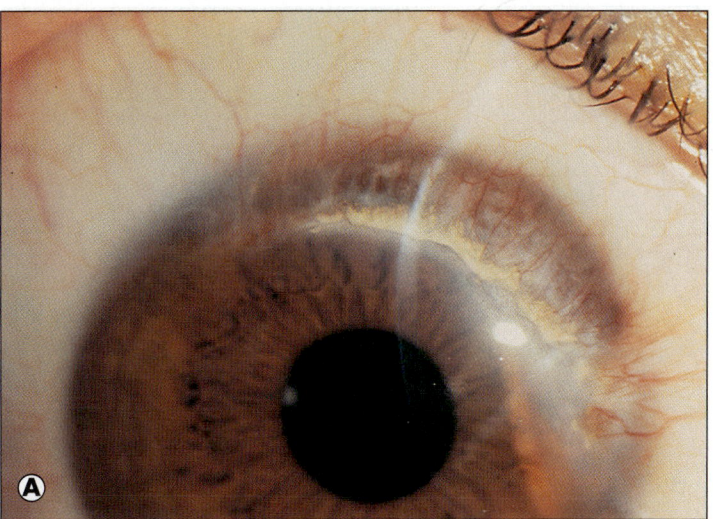

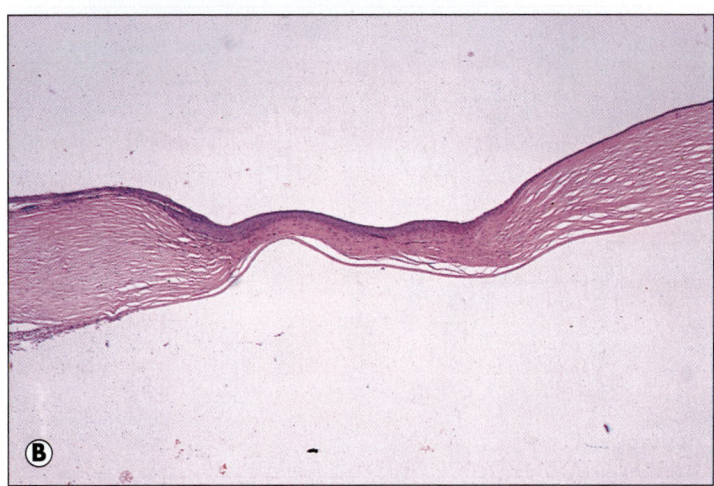

FIG. 60-7 ▌ **Terrien's marginal corneal degeneration. A,** Note the lipid deposit along the central edge. **B,** Histologic section shows limbus on the left (iris not present) and central cornea to the right. Note marked stromal thinning. (From Yanoff M, Fine BS. Ocular pathology, ed 5. St. Louis: Mosby, 2002.)

Terrien's Marginal Corneal Degeneration

Terrien's degeneration is a condition with marginal corneal ectasia and was described originally as a dystrophy. It occurs at any age, from children to the elderly, although it is said to occur most frequently in middle-aged to elderly men. Most cases are bilateral, although the timing of development on each side may be different.[33]

Terrien's degeneration initially arises with peripheral corneal haze, usually superiorly. This gradually vascularizes superficially and is followed by corneal thinning, typically with a sloping central edge and a fairly steep peripheral edge to the resultant furrow. A lipid deposit is present along the central edge (Fig. 60-7). Slowly, this progresses around the limbus and somewhat centrally—the progression may occur over many years or decades. Astigmatism develops from the associated corneal flattening, which may be irregular, and the resulting visual deterioration is more likely than other symptoms to lead to presentation. Usually no pain or inflammation occurs, although some patients have periodic episodes of redness and discomfort that respond to topical corticosteroid treatment.[34] A pseudopterygium, often in an axis other than that of a typical pterygium, occurs in many patients. Corneal thinning may progress, despite intact epithelium, to the point at which a deep corneal break leads to hydrops or even to frank perforation.[35] In such cases, corneal inlay lamellar grafting or excision of the ectatic tissue with direct resuturing may be indicated. Fuchs' superficial marginal keratitis has similar findings but more conjunctival involvement and is more localized (see Chapter 61).

Although the cause of Terrien's disease is unknown, it is likely to be different from the causes of most degenerations that occur with age. Histopathologically, the chief findings are those of stromal thinning, fibrosis and vascularization. Phagocytosis of corneal stromal collagen may be seen.[36]

Pellucid marginal corneal degeneration is another condition with peripheral corneal thinning. It is not a true degeneration but rather a variant of keratoconus (see Chapter 59).

Peripheral Corneal Guttae

The corneal endothelium undergoes degeneration with age, as manifested by a decreasing endothelial cell density[37] and thickening of the posterior, nonbanded layer of Descemet's membrane.[38] Degenerating endothelial cells produce localized nodular thickenings of Descemet's membrane, known as guttae. The incidence of central guttae increases with age.[38] The relationship of central guttae to Fuchs' corneal endothelial dystrophy is discussed elsewhere with the corneal dystrophies. Peripheral guttae, known as Hassall-Henle warts, are visible in normal adult

corneas and are thought to be truly degenerative and unrelated to Fuchs' dystrophy (see Chapter 57). They are not associated with functional corneal changes.

Calcific Band Keratopathy

Band keratopathy is a common corneal degeneration that can occur at any age and can occur peripherally or centrally. Whereas primary idiopathic forms rarely occur, it most commonly occurs in eyes with chronic disease, particularly uveitis, glaucoma, keratitis, or trauma. It also occurs with elevated serum calcium or phosphate. A toxic form resulting from mercurial preservatives in pilocarpine has been described. Associated systemic diseases include sarcoidosis, hyperparathyroidism, vitamin D toxicity, and extensive metastatic neoplasm to bone, all of which are associated with elevated serum calcium. In children, band keratopathy may be the presenting sign of chronic uveitis as a result of juvenile rheumatoid arthritis. It may also occur in patients with chronic renal failure from secondary hyperparathyroidism. Local corneal damage has occurred as a result of intraocular silicone oil, viscoelastics manufactured in the past with high phosphate levels, and phosphate forms of corticosteroids.[39-41]

The mechanism of calcium deposition in the cornea is unknown, but it is associated with corneal exposure, as deposition occurs primarily in the exposed area. It may result from precipitation left as tears evaporate or because of a lower pH in this region.[42]

As the name implies, calcium is deposited in the cornea as a horizontal band that begins near the corneal periphery and ap-

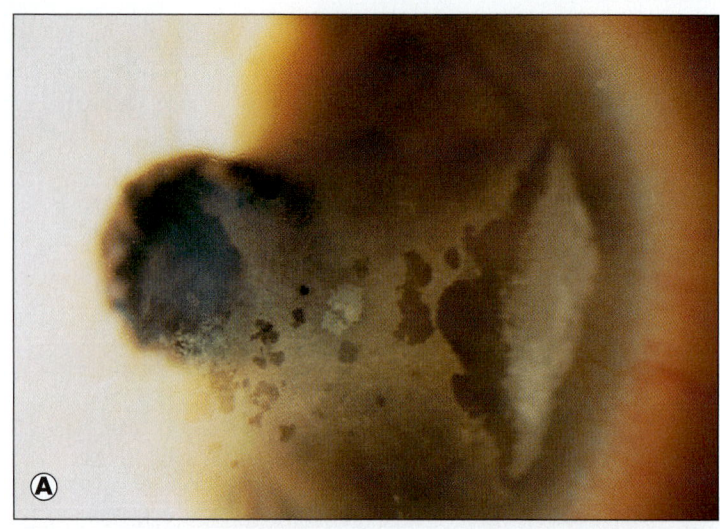

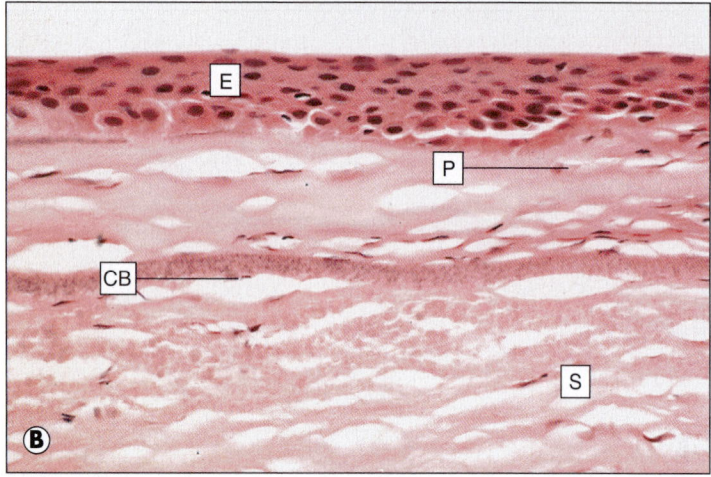

FIG. 60-8 ■ **Band keratopathy. A,** Calcium deposits in the cornea of a 13-year-old with juvenile rheumatoid arthritis. **B,** A fibrous pannus *(P)* is present between the epithelium *(E)* and a calcified Bowman's membrane *(CB)*. Some deposit is also present in the anterior corneal stroma *(S)*. (From Yanoff M, Fine BS. Ocular pathology, ed 5. St. Louis: Mosby, 2002.)

pears as a hazy deposit in the peripheral stroma separated from the limbus by a clear zone (Fig. 60-8). The more central areas have clear circles where Bowman's membrane is traversed by nerve endings. Gradually, the deposits move centrally, although the central areas may occasionally occur first. The most severely affected area is centered on the junction of the middle and inferior thirds of the cornea, the area of greatest exposure to the atmosphere. The deposits begin as a gray haze but can become densely white with a rough, pebbly surface that elevates the epithelium and results in pain, foreign body sensation, recurrent corneal erosions, and decreased vision. The rate of development is variable; it may take many years, although it may occur rapidly in very dry eyes.[43]

Histopathologically, calcium is deposited as the hydroxyapatite salt in the epithelial basement membrane, basal epithelium, and Bowman's membrane.[42] The deposits are usually extracellular, although hypercalcemia may cause intracellular epithelial accumulation.

Band keratopathy usually does not decrease vision and requires no treatment or only treatment of the underlying condition. If persistent discomfort or decreased vision occurs, the central deposits may be removed. Traditionally, this is done by removal of the epithelium over the deposits and the application of 0.05mol/l disodium ethylenediaminetetraacetic acid as a chelator of calcium. After several minutes the surface is rubbed with a sponge or blade. This process is repeated until the central cornea becomes clear. Coverage of the resulting corneal defect by transplanted amniotic membrane may help to restore the surface.[44] A diamond burr may be used to help remove dense de-

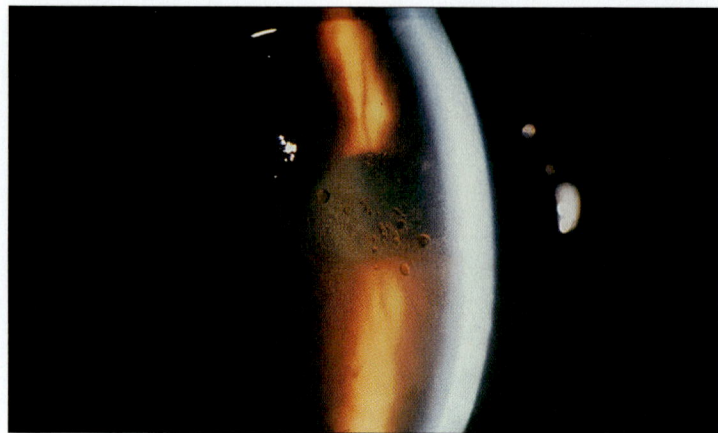

FIG. 60-9 ■ **Spheroidal degeneration.** Central spheroidal droplets in the cornea of an eye that is blind from glaucoma.

posits. Excimer laser phototherapeutic keratectomy may also be used to remove band keratopathy, although visual improvement is often limited by the underlying disease.[45]

Spheroidal Degeneration

Spheroidal degeneration may have a distribution in the cornea similar to that of band keratopathy, and it also occurs in the conjunctiva. It has been given a variety of names, of which the most commonly used are climatic droplet keratopathy, hyaline degeneration, and local designations such as Labrador keratopathy.[46] Spheroidal degeneration occurs as a primary corneal form, a secondary corneal form in eyes with prior keratitis or trauma, and a conjunctival form. Its frequency varies with geographic location and increases with age. It occurs most often in areas that have high sunlight exposure and sunlight reflection off snow or sand, in combination with wind-driven corneal damage by snow and sand. It is twice as prevalent in men as in women. Prevalence varies from 6% in England to over 60% in males in Labrador. It is thought to be a result of ultraviolet light exposure and may also be associated with blue-light exposure.[4,9] Drying of the cornea and repeated corneal trauma are thought to be risk factors. An association exists with conjunctival pinguecula, which is thought to have a similar cause. The secondary forms occur with corneal scars after keratitis or trauma, lattice corneal dystrophy, and glaucoma.

Typically, spheroidal degeneration is characterized by the presence of fine droplets, yellow or golden in color, beneath the conjunctival or corneal epithelium (Fig. 60-9). The droplets appear oily, although they are not of lipid origin. They may be clear but often become cloudy or opaque over time. In the cornea they may occur along the edge of scars. In the primary form, they begin peripherally and advance toward the center in the palpebral fissure area. As the condition advances, the droplets become larger and more nodular and lift the central corneal epithelium. Three stages of the primary form have been described:

- Grade I—fine shiny droplets are present only peripherally without symptoms.
- Grade II—the central cornea is involved and vision may be as low as 20/100 (6/30).
- Grade III—there are large corneal nodules and vision is no better than 20/200 (6/60).

These forms are always bilateral. Stage III disease may be rapidly progressive followed by ulceration of involved areas of cornea, with secondary bacterial infection.[47]

In histologic sections the deposits of spheroidal degeneration appear as extracellular amorphous globules, which may coalesce to form larger masses in Bowman's membrane. These globules are made up of a protein material with elastotic features, as in pinguecula. The source of the protein is unknown, but it has

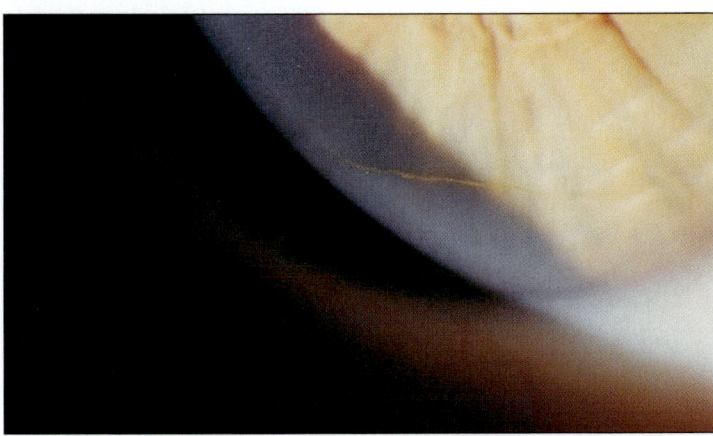

FIG. 60-10 ■ Hudson–Stähli line. Thin horizontal brown line in inferior cornea of a healthy 57-year-old male. (Courtesy of the photography department, WK Kellogg Eye Center, University of Michigan.)

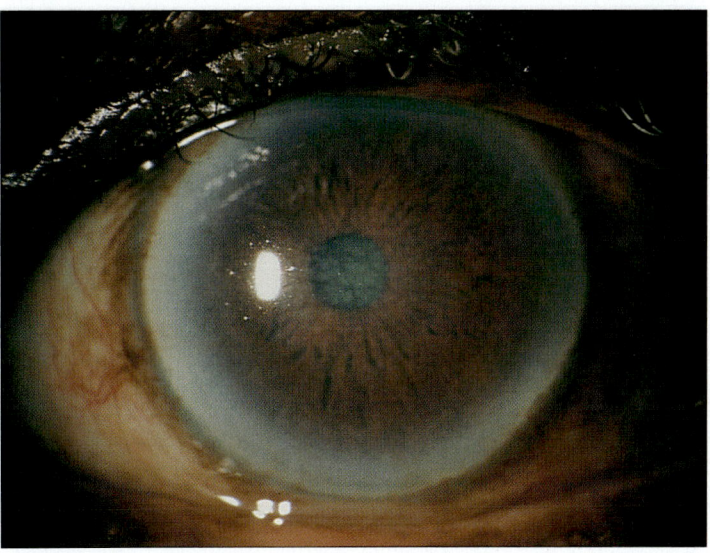

FIG. 60-11 ■ Posterior crocodile shagreen. A mottled, gray pattern is visible in the central cornea.

been postulated to result from the action of ultraviolet light on proteins that diffuse into the stroma from limbal vessels.[46,48]

The majority of cases of spheroidal degeneration are asymptomatic. In those who have visual loss from central corneal lesions, as occurs frequently in the developing tropical areas, superficial keratectomy and lamellar or penetrating keratoplasty have been used. Reports of excimer laser phototherapeutic keratectomy in the climatic form have shown encouraging results.[49]

Iron Deposition

Iron deposition occurs in the deep corneal epithelium in several clinical situations in which the smooth spreading of the tear film is disturbed. The prototype is the Hudson–Stähli line, which is located at the junction of the middle and lower thirds of the cornea (Fig. 60-10). It is yellow-brown in color and curves downward at its center. It is usually about 0.5mm wide and 1–2mm long. It is seen most clearly in blue light as a black line. Hudson–Stähli lines occur in most patients over the age of 50 years and decrease in density and frequency after the age of 70 years.[50] Similar iron deposition occurs at the base of the cone in keratoconus (Fleischer ring), around filtering blebs (Ferry line), central to pterygium (Stocker line), and around Salzmann's nodules. Iron lines occur within the margin of corneal grafts, between radial keratotomy scars, and following laser *in situ* keratomileusis (LASIK).[51] It is postulated that altered tear flow secondary to distorted corneal shape is a factor in the formation of these lines and that epithelial migration patterns affect the shape of the Hudson-Stähli line. The source of the iron is unknown, but it most likely comes from the tear film.

Histologically, the iron associated with these conditions is deposited intracellularly in the corneal epithelial cells as a ferritin-like material, possibly hemosiderin.[52] The Hudson-Stähli lines do not affect vision or cause any symptoms and thus require no treatment.

Coats' white ring is an iron deposition that occurs just deep to the corneal epithelium in the anterior portion of Bowman's membrane. It appears as a tiny ring of white dots, most often inferiorly. It is thought to result from previous iron deposition by a corneal foreign body and occurs long after resolution of the corneal iron ring. It has no symptoms.[53]

Crocodile Shagreen

Anterior or posterior polygonal opacities in the corneal stroma occur as a consequence of aging. Crocodile shagreen was first described by Vogt[31] in an elderly woman who had a gray opacity of the central cornea, with opacities separated by darker clear zones. The pattern resembles that of crocodile skin and is thought to be related to the oblique insertion of the collagen lamellae that constitute the corneal stroma.[54] The same pattern is transmitted to the normal corneal epithelium and may be seen after fluorescein is applied to the cornea and pressure applied through the closed lid, in hypotony of the globe, and in contact lens wearers with keratoconus. No information is available on the incidence of this degeneration, but it is a very common, although frequently subtle, finding in older patients. The anterior form is thought to be more common than the posterior, but posterior crocodile shagreen is similar, although it occurs in the deep central stroma (Fig. 60-11). The opacities in posterior crocodile shagreen may occur peripherally, in which case they may be indistinguishable from the central extension of corneal arcus.

Histology is rarely available as surgical treatment is almost never indicated. Postmortem histology shows a serrated configuration of collagen lamellae in the stroma with widely spaced collagen fibers rather than any abnormal deposition of material.[55]

Familial forms of posterior crocodile shagreen have been described in a dominant juvenile form and in a form associated with X-linked megalocornea. Central cloudy dystrophy of François appears to be similar, but it is a true dystrophy that is inherited dominantly. This dystrophic form rarely interferes with vision (see Chapter 59).

Cornea Farinata

Like many of the other degenerations, this common but subtle finding was described by Vogt.[31] It occurs in the corneas of older patients and is always an incidental finding as it causes no symptoms. The corneal opacities in this condition are very fine, dust-like dots of white or gray color in the deep central stroma, just anterior to Descemet's membrane. The name farinata, meaning "like wheat flour," refers to the appearance of the dots. The bilateral deposits are very difficult to visualize at the slit lamp, except by retroillumination. The cause of the condition is unknown. The histology of similar conditions suggests that the deposits may be composed of lipofuscin in stromal keratocytes.[56,57]

Salzmann's Corneal Degeneration

This degenerative condition was described originally as a dystrophy. It may occur at any age but is primarily a condition of the elderly. It develops in corneas with previous keratitis but often several decades later. It has been associated particularly with past phlyctenular keratitis but may also follow interstitial keratitis, vernal keratitis, trachoma, or Thygeson's superficial punctate

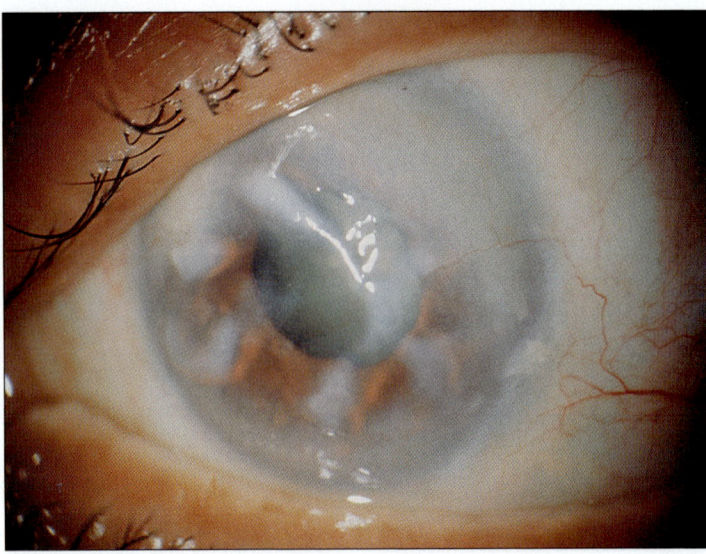

FIG. 60-12 ■ Salzmann's nodular degeneration. Severe corneal involvement in an elderly woman.

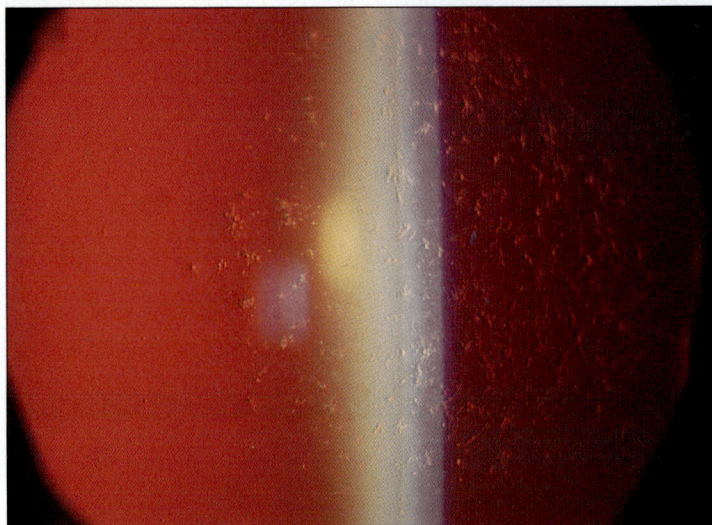

FIG. 60-13 ■ Polymorphic amyloid degeneration. Glassy, fine deep corneal deposits in the central cornea of an elderly woman.

keratitis, or it may occur with no history of prior corneal disease. It may be unilateral or bilateral and occurs more often in women than in men.

Salzmann's degeneration is characterized by the presence of white to gray or light blue nodules that elevate the epithelium in the superficial corneal stroma (Fig. 60-12). They may be single or occur as clusters in a circular array, often at the edge of old corneal scars. Each nodule is about 0.5–2mm in diameter, not vascularized, and separated from other nodules by clear cornea. An epithelial iron line may outline the base of the lesion. The onset of the lesions is gradual, over many years, during which time they increase in both size and number. They may decrease vision as they encroach upon the central cornea or, more often, as they alter the corneal shape and may be associated with recurrent corneal erosions.[58]

Histologic examination of excised nodules shows thinned epithelium that overlies hyalinized avascular collagen. Bowman's membrane is damaged or focally absent and replaced by material that is similar to basement membrane.[59] Usually, evidence is seen of old keratitis in the surrounding stroma.

Many elderly patients who have peripheral Salzmann's nodules are asymptomatic and require no treatment. If vision is altered or if recurrent erosions are frequent, the nodules may be removed. Often, they may be peeled from the underlying stroma. Excimer laser phototherapeutic keratectomy has been used to remove these lesions, with success in improving vision.[45] In the past, lamellar or penetrating keratoplasty has been used. Recurrences have been found after all forms of treatment.[60]

Corneal Amyloid Degeneration

Amyloid is a group of hyaline proteins deposited in tissues in a variety of systemic and localized conditions. These conditions may be primary or secondary, localized or systemic, and familial or nonfamilial. The deposits of proteins may be derived from immunoglobulin light chains as in primary systemic amyloidosis, from amyloid A protein in secondary amyloid, from some forms of albumin in familial amyloidosis, and as a protein known as AP. Primary systemic amyloidosis causes heart failure, neuropathies, and other disorders. Secondary systemic amyloid follows long-standing inflammatory diseases such as tuberculosis or syphilis. Nonfamilial localized amyloidosis of a primary form can present with conjunctival or lid nodules. Familial localized amyloidosis is seen in the cornea as lattice, Avellino, and gelatinous drop-like corneal dystrophies discussed in Chapter 59.

The degenerative forms of amyloid seen in the cornea and conjunctiva are secondary, localized, and nonfamilial. These occur as nonspecific corneal deposits that follow corneal trauma or keratitis. They may also follow chronic intraocular inflammation. Usually, they are not diagnosed clinically as amyloid deposits but are seen histopathologically, often in nonspecific corneal opacities.[61] Histologic diagnosis can be made with Congo red staining of extracellular hyaline deposits or with immunofluorescence staining for specific amyloid proteins.

A more specific form of corneal amyloid degeneration has been described as polymorphic amyloid degeneration.[62] Usually, this condition is an incidental finding in the elderly. It is characterized by the presence of glass-like deposits in the deep central corneal stroma, which often indent Descemet's membrane. The deposits are punctate or rod-like and may appear identical to the deposits of lattice dystrophy, although they are usually much less dense (Fig. 60-13). They are bilateral, generally occur after the age of 50 years, and do not affect vision. Histologically, they appear similar to lattice dystrophy deposits and are composed of amyloid. The cause is unknown and the condition requires no treatment.

Another stromal deposition with features of both spheroidal degeneration and amyloid deposition has been called climatic proteoglycan stromal keratopathy.[63] This has been described in Saudi Arabian patients, and the risk factors are similar to those of spheroidal degeneration. The patients have bilateral, horizontal, oval, central anterior stromal, ground glass haze. Some have refractile stromal lines. Both proteoglycan and amyloid have been found histopathologically. This condition does not usually affect vision.[63]

REFERENCES

1. Hinnen E. Die Altersveranderungen des vorderen bulbusabschnittes. Z Augenheilkd. 1921;45:129–34.
2. Panchapakesan J, Hourihan F, Mitchell P. Prevalence of pterygium and pinguecula: the Blue Mountains Eye Study. Aust NZ J Ophthalmol. 1998;26(suppl 1):s2–5.
3. Taylor HR, West SK, Rosenthal FS, et al. Corneal changes associated with chronic UV irradiation. Arch Ophthalmol. 1989;107:1481–4.
4. Norn M, Franck C. Long-term changes in the outer part of the eye in welders. Acta Ophthalmol. 1991;69:382–6.
5. Dushku N, Hatcher SL, Albert DM, Reid TW. P53 expression and relation to human papillomavirus infection in pingueculae, pterygia and limbal tumors. Arch Ophthalmol. 1999;117:1593–9.
6. Chu FU, Rodriguez MM, Cogan DG, Barranger JD. The pathology of pingueculae in Gaucher's disease. Ophthalmol Paediatr Genet. 1984;4:7–11.
7. Austin P, Jakobiec FA, Iwamoto T. Elastodysplasia and elastodystrophy as pathologic bases of ocular pterygium and pinguecula. Ophthalmology. 1983;90:96–109.
8. Frucht-Pery J, Siganos CS, Solomon A, et al. Topical indomethacin solution versus dexamethasone solution for treatment of inflamed pterygium and pinguecula: a prospective randomized clinical study. Am J Ophthalmol. 1999;127:148–52.

9. Taylor HR, West S, Munoz B, *et al.* The long-term effects of visible light on the eye. Arch Ophthalmol. 1992;110:99–104.

10. Mackenzie FB, Hirst LW, Battistutta D, Green A. Risk analysis in the development of pterygia. Ophthalmology. 1992;99:1056–61.

11. Kwok LS, Coroneo MT. A model for pterygium formation. Cornea. 1994;13:219–24.

12. Di Girolamo N, Coroneo MT, Wakefield D. Active matrilysin (MMP-7) in human pterygia: potential role in angiogenesis. Invest Ophthalmol Vis Sci. 2001;42:1963–8.

13. Dushku N, Reid TW. Immunohistochemical evidence that human pterygia originate from an invasion of vimentin-expressing altered limbal epithelial basal cells. Curr Eye Res. 1994;13:473–81.

14. Hirst LW, Sebban A, Chant D. Pterygium recurrence time. Ophthalmology. 1994;101:755–8.

15. Moriarty AP, Crawford GJ, McAllister IL, Constable IJ. Severe corneoscleral infection. A complication of beta irradiation scleral necrosis following pterygium excision. Arch Ophthalmol. 1993;111:947–51.

16. Chen PP, Ariyasu RG, Kaza V, *et al.* A randomized trial comparing mitomycin C and conjunctival autograft after excision of primary pterygium. Am J Ophthalmol. 1995;120:151–60.

17. Frucht-Pery J, Siganos CS, Ilsar M. Intraoperative application of topical mitomycin C for pterygium surgery. Ophthalmology. 1996;103:674–7.

18. Rubinfeld RS, Pfister RR, Stein RR, *et al.* Serious complications of topical mitomycin-C after pterygium surgery. Ophthalmology. 1992;99:1647–54.

19. Ma DH, See LC, Liau SB, Tsai RJ. Amniotic membrane graft for primary pterygium: comparison with conjunctival autograft and topical mitomycin C treatment. Br J Ophthalmol 2000;84:973–8.

20. Scroggs MW, Klintworth GK. Senile scleral plaques: a histopathologic study using energy-dispersive X-ray microanalysis. Hum Pathol. 1991;22:557–62.

21. Barchiesi BJ, Eckel RH, Ellis PP. The cornea and disorders of lipid metabolism. Surv Ophthalmol. 1991;36:1–22.

22. Cogan DG, Kuwabara T. Arcus senilis, its pathology and histochemistry. Arch Ophthalmol. 1959;61:553–60.

23. Green K, DeBarge LR, Cheeks L, Phillips CI. Centripetal movement of fluorescein dextrans in the cornea: relevance to arcus. Acta Ophthalmol (Copenh). 1987;65:538–44.

24. Segal P, Insull W, Chambless LE, *et al.* The association of dyslipoproteinemia with corneal arcus and xanthelasma. The Lipid Research Clinics Program Prevalence Study. Circulation. 1986;73:108–18.

25. Chambless LE, Fuchs FD, Linn S, *et al.* The association of corneal arcus with coronary heart disease and cardiovascular disease in the lipid research clinics mortality follow-up study. Am J Public Health. 1990;80:1200–4.

26. Moss SE, Klein R, Klein BE. Arcus senilis and mortality in a population with diabetes. Am J Ophthalmol. 2000;129:676–8.

27. Cogan DG, Kuwabara T. Lipid keratopathy and atheromas. Circulation. 1958;18:519–25.

28. Shapiro LA, Farkas TG. Lipid keratopathy following corneal hydrops. Arch Ophthalmol. 1977;95:456–8.

29. Croxatto JO, Dodds CM, Dodds R. Bilateral and massive lipoidal infiltrates of the cornea (secondary lipoidal degeneration). Ophthalmology. 1985;92:1686–90.

30. Duran JA, Rodriguez-Ares MT. Idiopathic lipid corneal degeneration. Cornea. 1991;10:166–9.

31. Vogt A. Textbook and atlas of slit lamp microscopy of the living eye. Bonn: Wayenborgh Editions; 1981.

32. Sugar HS, Kobernick S. The white limbus girdle of Vogt. Am J Ophthalmol. 1960;50:101–7.

33. Beauchamp GR. Terrien's marginal corneal degeneration. Ophthalmology. 1990;97:1188–93.

34. Austin P, Brown SI. Inflammatory Terrien's marginal corneal disease. Am J Ophthalmol. 1981;92:189–92.

35. Soong HK, Fitzgerald J, Boruchoff A, *et al.* Corneal hydrops in Terrien's marginal degeneration. Ophthalmology. 1986;93:340–3.

36. Iwamoto T, DeVoe AG, Farris RL. Electron microscopy in cases of marginal degeneration of the cornea. Invest Ophthalmol. 1972;11:241–57.

37. Carlson KH, Bourne WM, McLaren JV, Brubaker R. Variations in human corneal endothelial cell morphology and permeability to fluorescein with age. Exp Eye Res. 1988;47:27–41.

38. Lorenzetti DW, Uotila MH, Parikh N, *et al.* Central cornea guttata, incidence in the general population. Am J Ophthalmol. 1967;64:1155–8.

39. Azen SP, Scott IU, Flynn HW, *et al.* Silicone oil in the repair of complex retinal detachments. A prospective observational multicenter study. Ophthalmology. 1998;105:1587–97.

40. Nevyas AS, Raber IM, Eagle RC, *et al.* Acute band keratopathy from intracameral Viscoat. Arch Ophthalmol. 1987;105:958–64.

41. Taravella MJ, Stulting RD, Mader TH, *et al.* Calcific band keratopathy associated with the use of topical steroid-phosphate preparations. Arch Ophthalmol. 1994;112:608–13.

42. O'Connor GR. Calcific band keratopathy. Trans Am Ophthalmol Soc. 1972;70:58–85.

43. Lemp MA, Ralph RA. Rapid development of band keratopathy in dry eye. Am J Ophthalmol. 1977;83:657–9.

44. Anderson DF, Prabhasawat P, Alfonso E, Tseng SC. Amniotic membrane transplantation after primary surgical management of band keratopathy. Cornea. 2001;20:354–61.

45. Maloney RK, Thompson V, Ghiselli G, *et al.* A prospective multicenter trial of excimer laser phototherapeutic keratectomy for corneal vision loss. Am J Ophthalmol. 1996;122:144–60.

46. Gray RH, Johnson GJ, Freedman A. Climatic droplet keratopathy. Surv Ophthalmol. 1992;36:241–53.

47. Ormerod LD, Dahan E, Hagele JE, *et al.* Serious occurrences in the natural history of advanced climatic keratopathy. Ophthalmology. 1994;101:448–53.

48. Johnson GJ, Overall M. Histology of spheroidal degeneration of the cornea in Labrador. Br J Ophthalmol. 1978;62:53–61.

49. Badr IA, Al-Rajhi A, Wagoner MD. Phototherapeutic keratectomy for climatic droplet keratopathy. J Refract Surg. 1996;12:112–22.

50. Norn MS. Hudson-Stähli's line of cornea I. Incidence and morphology. Acta Ophthalmol (Copenh). 1968;46:106–18.

51. Probst LE, Almassawy MA, Bell J. Pseudo-Fleischer ring after hyperopic laser in situ keratomileusis. J Cataract Refract Surg. 1999;25:868–70.

52. Gass JDM. The iron lines of the superficial cornea. Arch Ophthalmol. 1964;71:348–58.

53. Nevins RC, Davis WH, Elliott JH. Coats' white ring of the cornea—unsettled metal fettle. Arch Ophthalmol. 1968;80:145–6.

54. Tripathi RL, Bron AJ. Secondary anterior crocodile shagreen of Vogt. Br J Ophthalmol. 1975;59:59–63.

55. Krachmer JH, Dubord PJ, Rodriguez MM, *et al.* Corneal posterior crocodile shagreen and polymorphic amyloid degeneration. Arch Ophthalmol. 1983;101:54–9.

56. Curran RE, Kenyon KR, Green WR. Pre-Descemet's membrane corneal dystrophy. Am J Ophthalmol. 1974;77:711–16.

57. Durand L, Bouvier R, Burillon C, *et al.* Cornea farinata à propos d'un cas: etude clinique, histologique et ultrastructurale. J Fr Ophtalmol. 1990;13:449–55.

58. Wood TO. Salzmann's nodular degeneration. Cornea. 1990;9:17–22.

59. Vannas A, Hogan MJ, Wood I. Salzmann's nodular degeneration of the cornea. Am J Ophthalmol. 1975;79:211–19.

60. Severin M, Kirchof B. Recurrent Salzmann's corneal degeneration. Graefes Arch Clin Exp Ophthalmol. 1990;222:101–4.

61. Dutt S, Elner VM, Soong HK, *et al.* Secondary localized amyloidosis in interstitial keratitis (IK): clinicopathologic findings. Ophthalmology. 1992;99:817–23.

62. Mannis MJ, Krachmer JH, Rodriguez MM, *et al.* Polymorphic amyloid degeneration of the cornea. Arch Ophthalmol. 1981;99:1217–23.

63. Waring GO, Malaty A, Grossniklaus H, *et al.* Climatic proteoglycan stromal keratopathy, a new corneal degeneration. Am J Ophthalmol. 1995;120:330–41.

CHARLES S. BOUCHARD

DEFINITION
• Corneal inflammation with no known infectious cause.

KEY FEATURE
• Diverse group of diseases with corneal inflammation as the common feature.

ASSOCIATED FEATURE
• Systemic inflammatory disease.

INTRODUCTION

In this chapter well-characterized clinical entities that to date have no known infectious cause are presented. A complete list of noninfectious corneal inflammatory diseases is given in Box 61-1.[1]

Noninfectious keratitis is typically characterized by persistent corneal epithelial defects, stromal inflammation, and enzymatic degradation of the corneal collagen.[1] This results in part from the proximity of the peripheral cornea to the afferent and efferent cellular pathways of the limbal vasculature. Clinical symptoms associated with noninfectious keratitis include photophobia, pain, redness, and decreased visual acuity. Visual loss may result from an irregular surface, corneal opacity, or altered topography from corneal thinning. General therapeutic principles include determination of the specific cause; promotion of epithelial healing; limitation of ulceration and stromal loss; and support of repair.[1] Both local and systemic routes of therapy may be necessary for effective management.

THYGESON'S SUPERFICIAL PUNCTATE KERATOPATHY

EPIDEMIOLOGY AND PATHOGENESIS

Thygeson's superficial punctate keratopathy (TSPK) is a bilateral, epithelial keratitis of unknown cause first described by Phillips Thygeson in 1950.[2] It is characterized by an insidious onset of corneal inflammation with a long duration of exacerbations and remissions. The disease has been known to *last* from 1 month to 24 years, with an average duration of 3.5 years. The *onset* of TSPK is most common in the second and third decades (mean age, 29 years), with a range of 2.5–70 years. No clear sex predilection exists, although a female preponderance has been suggested.

No established cause for this disease is known, nor are there any clear trigger mechanisms or associated systemic illnesses. However, allergic, viral, and dyskeratotic mechanisms have been proposed. The clinical manifestations of TSPK resemble those of a viral keratitis. Although viral isolation from TSPK lesions has been reported,[3] this has not been confirmed.

The characteristic exacerbations and remissions of the disease may be caused by an altered immune response to an unknown exogenous or endogenous antigen. A genetic predisposition to develop TSPK may also be present. In some TSPK patients there is an increase in HLA-Dw3 and HLA-DR3 expression, both of which are HLA loci associated with immune response genes.[4]

OCULAR MANIFESTATIONS

The lesions of TSPK typically appear in the central cornea as small, round or oval, discrete, granular, white-gray, fine, intraepithelial dot-like opacities. The number of lesions ranges between 3 and 40, and occasionally the lesions appear stellate (Fig. 61-1). Corneal edema and associated cellular infiltration are generally absent (Fig. 61-2). Subepithelial opacities occur in 44% of patients. TSPK is bilateral in 96% of patients. Characteristically, no conjunctival inflammation is associated with the keratitis.

Active lesions are resistant to mechanical removal and appear elevated following fluorescein staining. During remissions, the epithelium is flat and without stain over the previous area of keratitis. Recurrences may occur in different areas. Most lesions are central; however, peripheral lesions do occur and may be associated with delicate, peripheral vascularization in chronic cases. Fine filaments also may be associated with the keratitis.

Symptoms include tearing, foreign body sensation, photophobia, and burning. Visual acuity may be decreased by the subepithelial opacities, but generally it returns to normal following resolution of the keratitis. Corneal sensation usually is normal, but mild hypesthesia may occur rarely.

DIAGNOSIS

Thygeson[2] outlined five characteristic features of TSPK:
• Chronic, bilateral punctate inflammation
• Long duration, with remissions and exacerbations
• Healing without significant scarring
• Absent clinical response to topical antibiotics
• Striking symptomatic response to topical corticosteroids

The diagnosis of TSPK generally can be made from the clinical history, the slit-lamp examination, and the unusually rapid response to topical corticosteroids. No specific systemic associations have been reported for this disease.

DIFFERENTIAL DIAGNOSIS

One of the most characteristic features of TSPK is its lack of associated conjunctival inflammation. All the other disease entities in Box 61-2 have either obvious associated features or signs of local or diffuse conjunctival inflammation.

Noninfectious Keratitis

Dermatologic	Mucous membrane pemphigoid
	Erythema multiforme
	Rosacea
Mechanical	Ectropion/entropion
	Lid defects
	Trichiasis
	Lagophthalmos
	Exophthalmos
	Dellen
Immunologic/allergic	Collagen vascular disease
	Mooren's ulcer
	Staphylococcal marginal infiltrate
	Phlyctenular keratoconjunctivitis
	Vernal keratoconjunctivitis
	Graft versus host disease
	Atopic keratoconjunctivitis
Lacrimal	Keratoconjunctivitis sicca (primary, secondary)
Neurologic	Neurotrophic keratitis (cranial nerve V, diabetes)
	Neuroparalytic keratitis (cranial nerve VII)
Nutritional	Keratomalacia
Postinfectious	Viral
	Bacterial
	Fungal
Postsurgical	Delayed epithelial healing (diabetes mellitus)
	Homograft reaction
	Diffuse lamellar keratitis (DLK)
Traumatic	Chemical injury (alkali, acid)
	Thermal injury
	Radiation
Other	Thygeson's superficial punctate keratitis
	Acute leukemia
	Pyoderma gangrenosum
	Cutaneous porphyria
	Terrien's marginal degeneration

Adapted from Kenyon KR: Decision-making in the therapy of external eye disease. Noninfected corneal ulcers. Ophthalmology. 89:44–51, 1982.

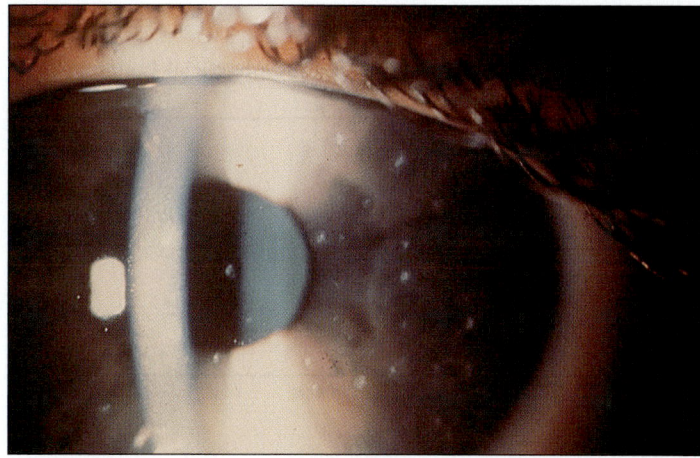

FIG. 61-1 ▌ Corneal punctate lesions characteristic of Thygeson's superficial punctate keratopathy. These typically occur in a noninflamed eye. (Courtesy of Joel Sugar, MD.)

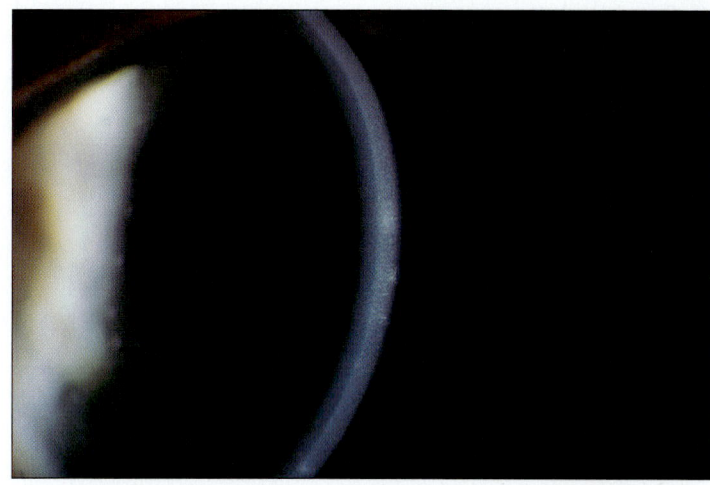

FIG. 61-2 ▌ A patient who has Thygeson's superficial punctate keratopathy. Slit-lamp appearance of the fine subepithelial haze and relative lack of corneal inflammation between lesions are shown.

PATHOLOGY

Corneal scrapings of the lesions demonstrate nonspecific findings, which include atypical and degenerated epithelial cells and a mild mononuclear and polymorphonuclear cell infiltrate. Focal cell destruction without the cell-to-cell pattern typical of herpes keratitis has been reported. However, the presence of specific viral particles has not been documented. Confocal microscopy of two cases of TSPK demonstrated fine deposits of highly reflected material below the basal lamina.[5]

TREATMENT

Topical corticosteroids clearly decrease the signs and symptoms of TSPK and probably are most effective during acute exacerbations. A rapid taper of the dose to maintain control of the symptoms is recommended. The course of the disease may be prolonged with the chronic use of corticosteroids. Topical 2% cyclosporine has been effective in the management of TSPK, with few side effects.[6] Therapeutic bandage contact lenses may be used to improve visual acuity, as well as to reduce the irritative symptoms in more symptomatic patients. The use of antiviral agents has been evaluated, but no convincing evidence exists that they are effective.[7] Idoxuridine may actually increase the risk of subepithelial scarring. Scraping of the lesions is not effective and may stimulate scarring. Photorefractive keratectomy may reduce the recurrences in the central ablated cornea, suggesting that some unknown inflammatory signal may reside in the superficial corneal stroma.[8]

COURSE AND OUTCOME

Most patients who have TSPK recover completely with no loss of visual acuity, although up to 44% may be left with faint subep-

ithelial opacities. Proper counseling about the exacerbations and remissions that occur with this disease helps patients deal with this frustrating and bothersome clinical entity.

SUPERIOR LIMBIC KERATOCONJUNCTIVITIS OF THEODORE

EPIDEMIOLOGY AND PATHOGENESIS

Superior limbic keratoconjunctivitis (SLK) is a chronic, focal, ocular surface disease characterized by episodes of recurrent inflammation of the superior cornea and limbus, as well as of the superior tarsal and bulbar conjunctiva.[9] It occurs primarily in adults between 30 and 55 years of age and is more common in women (3:1). It is typically bilateral, but unilateral disease may occur.

Although the pathophysiology is unclear, mechanical trauma from tight upper lids or loose redundant conjunctiva could lead to the known disruption of normal epithelial development.[10] This mechanical hypothesis is supported by the increased lid apposition of exophthalmic thyroid patients, who are known to have an increased incidence of SLK,[11] as well as increased lubrication as an effective treatment modality.[12]

BOX 61-2

Differential Diagnosis of Thygeson's Superficial Punctate Keratitis

Herpes simplex keratitis
Other viral keratitis (adenovirus)
Molluscum contagiosum
Exposure keratitis
Blepharokeratitis
Neurotrophic keratopathy
Staphylococcal keratitis
Traumatic keratopathy
Dry eye (see Chapter 62)

BOX 61-3

Differential Diagnosis of Superior Limbic Keratoconjunctivitis of Theodore

KERATOCONJUNCTIVITIS WITH FILAMENTS
Ptosis/lid occlusion
Keratoconjunctivitis sicca
Neurotrophic keratitis
Herpes simplex epithelial keratitis
Recurrent corneal erosion
Trauma
Bullous keratopathy
Medicamentosa

KERATOCONJUNCTIVITIS WITHOUT FILAMENTS
Keratoconjunctivitis induced by contact lens
Limbal vernal keratoconjunctivitis
Phlyctenulosis
Thygeson's superficial punctate keratitis

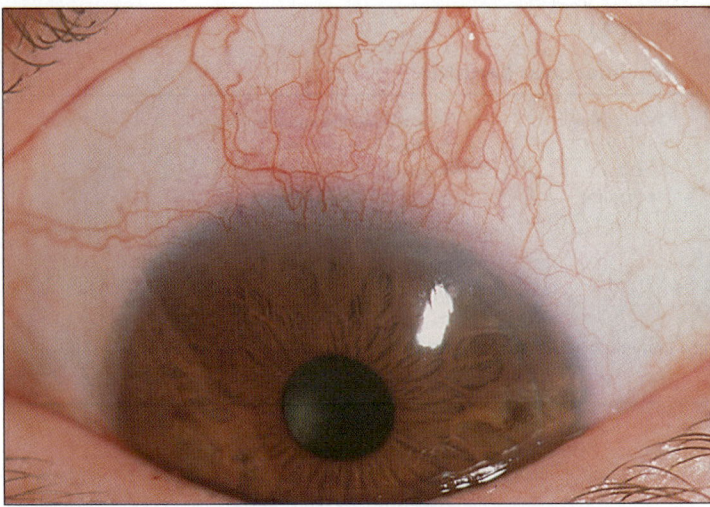

FIG. 61-3 ■ Superior limbic keratoconjunctivitis. Slit-lamp appearance of focal superior bulbar conjunctival injection is shown with rose bengal staining.

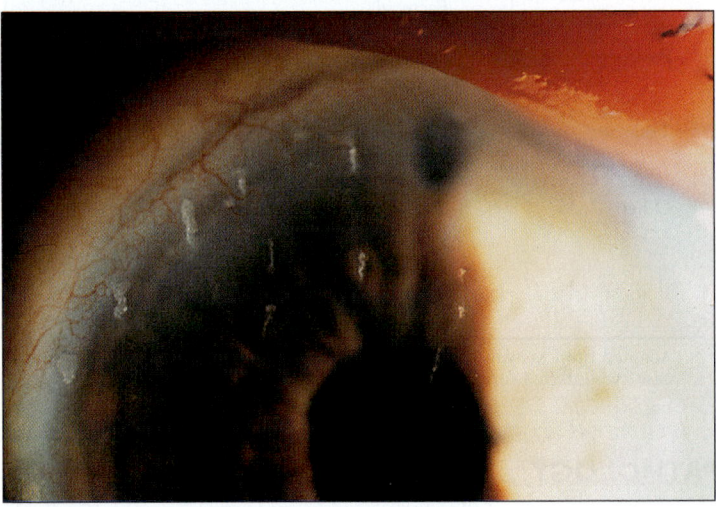

FIG. 61-4 ■ Superior limbic keratoconjunctivitis. Slit-lamp appearance of superior filamentary keratitis is shown.

OCULAR MANIFESTATIONS

The classic sign of SLK is bilateral local hyperemia of the superior bulbar conjunctiva (Fig. 61-3), which also appears keratinized, thickened, and redundant. The opposing superior palpebral conjunctiva demonstrates a delicate papillary reaction with associated hyperemia. Fine fluorescein or rose bengal punctate staining is usually evident. Keratoconjunctivitis sicca occurs in 25–50% of patients and must be evaluated in all patients who have SLK.[11] A fine filamentary keratitis of the superior cornea and limbus may also be present (Fig. 61-4). A delicate superior corneal pannus suggests more long-standing disease. Corneal hypesthesia is not uncommon.

Characteristic symptoms include a gradual onset of burning, tearing, foreign body sensation, mild photophobia, and sometimes mucous discharge. Patients may notice pain and a decrease in vision if the filamentary component is severe or occurs within the visual axis. Pseudoptosis and blepharospasm also may develop with severe or chronic disease.

DIAGNOSIS

The diagnosis of SLK is made from the history of irritation and photophobia and the specific pattern of superior corneal and conjunctival inflammation and staining. Localized superior filamentary keratitis reinforces the diagnosis.

DIFFERENTIAL DIAGNOSIS

The differential diagnosis is shown in Box 61-3. Other common causes of chronic, bilateral papillary conjunctivitis include keratoconjunctivitis sicca, blepharokeratoconjunctivitis, toxic keratoconjunctivitis, and floppy eyelid syndrome. Filamentary keratitis may occur in up to 40% of SLK patients. The distribution of fila-

ments on the upper cornea and limbus may help differentiate SLK from dry eye syndrome, in which filaments occur more typically in the lower half of the cornea. Isolated TSPK and limbal vernal and phlyctenular disease rarely demonstrate filaments. Typically no corneal infiltration is associated with the limbal inflammation, which distinguishes SLK from marginal ulcers.

An inflammatory condition associated with soft contact lens wear may resemble SLK. Although many signs and symptoms of this contact lens–related SLK are similar to those of SLK of Theodore, filaments are usually absent, vision may be decreased (unusual in SLK), and there is no female predilection or associated thyroid dysfunction. More importantly, symptoms generally improve with discontinuation of contact lens wear. Contact lens–induced keratoconjunctivitis may be a more appropriate term for this entity, with SLK reserved for the specific condition described by Theodore.[9]

SYSTEMIC ASSOCIATIONS

Systemic associations are thyroid disease and collagen vascular disease. Sixty-five percent of patients in a referral university setting who had SLK also had thyroid dysfunction.[11] Of the patients who had SLK and thyroid disease, 90% had ophthalmopathy and 49% had severe thyroid disease that required orbital decompression. SLK is a strong negative prognostic factor for patients who have thyroid disease.[11]

PATHOLOGY

The superior bulbar conjunctiva demonstrates keratinization of the epithelium with intracellular accumulation of glycogen and abnormal chromatin. A predominantly polymorphonuclear infiltrate exists. Acanthosis, squamous metaplasia, dyskeratosis, balloon degeneration of nuclei, and decreased goblet cell density also occur, as well as conjunctival stromal edema. Up-regulation of transforming growth factor-beta2 and tenascin support an increase in mechanical stress.[12] Altered expression of cytokeratins also suggests an abnormality of epithelial differentiation.[13]

Changes in the superior palpebral conjunctiva are somewhat different, with an increase in polymorphonuclear neutrophil leukocytes, lymphocytes, and plasma cells. The overlying epithelium contains hypertrophic goblet cells.

TREATMENT

Several surgical and nonsurgical modes of treatment have been used, with variable long-term results. Since a large proportion (25–50%) of patients who have SLK also have dry eyes, care must be taken to treat any concurrent aqueous tear deficiency with unpreserved teardrops and, if indicated, punctal occlusion.[14] Associated blepharitis also must be managed aggressively if it is severe. Any lid surgery, especially ptosis repair, should be evaluated carefully, since possible exacerbation of SLK may arise from the resultant lid tightening and possible secondary exposure.

Silver nitrate ($AgNO_3$) 0.5% solution had been used with some success for the initial treatment of SLK, but the solution is no longer available. Sticks of $AgNO_3$ or washings from the sticks are contraindicated, since the $AgNO_3$ concentration is too high and may result in a severe keratitis.

Surgical approaches to treatment involve the destruction or resection of the presumed abnormal conjunctival epithelium. Simple resection or recession of the conjunctiva with Tenon's capsule can be very effective. Cryotherapy and thermocautery have been reported, with symptom improvement in 75% of patients treated using the latter.[15]

Bandage contact lenses and pressure patching have been used to manage severe symptoms of photophobia, ocular discomfort, and associated filamentary keratitis. The SLK often recurs, however, after lens wear has been discontinued.

Topical hypertonic saline solutions may help reduce the excessive mucus production and associated filaments. N-acetylcysteine (Mucomyst), in a 10–20% solution, may offer relief in severe cases. Topical cromolyn or lodoxamide also may offer symptomatic relief of itching.[16]

Corticosteroids offer little help for this recurrent condition, and chronic use should be discouraged. Antibiotic and antiviral agents are not effective either. Topical vitamin A eyedrops have been reported to be variably effective during inflammatory periods.[17]

COURSE AND OUTCOME

Many of the proposed therapies have been effective, and the overall prognosis is excellent, since the visual axis usually is not affected. Counseling patients about the recurrent nature of the disease is important.

MOOREN'S ULCER

EPIDEMIOLOGY AND PATHOGENESIS

Mooren's ulcer is a rare, chronic, painful, peripheral ulcerative keratitis (PUK) that was first described in detail as a clinical entity by Mooren in 1867.[18] Two clinical types of primary Mooren's ulcers have been described.[19] The limited type is typically unilateral, occurs in older patients (fourth decade and older), and is more responsive to local surgical and medical therapy. The second type, which is more resistant to systemic immunosuppression, involves a bilateral, painful, relentless, progressive destruction of the cornea, usually in younger individuals (third decade), many of whom are of African descent.

The pathogenesis of Mooren's ulcer is unknown but appears to involve an autoimmune reaction against a specific target molecule in the corneal stroma, which may occur in genetically susceptible individuals.[20] Both cellular and humoral mechanisms are postulated. Tissue-specific autoantigens may stimulate the host immune response, which results in complement activation, cellular infiltration, and collagenolytic destruction of corneal stroma. Gottsch et al.[20,21] identified a corneal stromal protein (CO-Ag) produced by corneal keratocytes whose cDNA sequence is identical to that of human neutrophil calgranulin C (CaGC), a neutrophil protein found on the surface of filarial nematodes. Lymphocytes and plasma cells are present in the conjunctiva of patients who have Mooren's ulcer, which supports an immune-mediated mechanism.[22] Antigen–antibody interaction could activate the classic complement pathway in the peripheral cornea, where the concentration of complement C1 is much higher than in the central cornea. The presence of circulating antibodies to corneal antigens and circulating immune complexes supports the involvement of an antibody-mediated mechanism.[22]

T-cell abnormalities also have been reported, including a decrease in suppressor T cells and an altered ratio of T helper/suppressor T cells.[23] A depressed number of suppressor T cells may permit production of autoantibodies responsible for the corneal inflammation. HLA expression is also up-regulated in Mooren's ulcer, and in one series, HLA-DR17 and HLA-DQ were positive in 83% of patients.[24]

Interestingly, there have been several reported cases of Mooren's ulcer in patients who have concurrent hepatitis C and whose corneal inflammation responded to systemic interferon α.[25] These cases suggest a common antigenic source.[26]

OCULAR MANIFESTATIONS

Mooren's ulcer is characterized by a progressive, crescentic, peripheral corneal ulceration that is slightly central to the corneoscleral limbus. It is associated with a characteristic extensive, undermined, "overhanging" edge (Fig. 61-5). It typically progresses with an anterior, stromal, yellow-white infiltrate at the advancing margin. An overlying epithelial defect then develops. Progressive stromal melting follows, which affects first the deeper and subsequently the anterior stroma. The ulcer progresses circumferentially and centrally. A re-epithelialized, conjunctivalized, thinned cornea remains. Patients in whom Descemet's membrane has a minimal overlying stroma may be predisposed to perforation either spontaneously or following minor trauma.

In the more aggressive form of Mooren's ulcer, the inflammation may affect the entire cornea and perilimbal tissue. Perforation is not uncommon in this form, occurring in about one third of patients. Associated cataract, secondary glaucoma, and uveitis also may be seen.

Chronic Mooren's ulcer ultimately results in a central island of hazy stromal tissue with severe peripheral thinning (Fig. 61-6). Topography demonstrates severe irregular astigmatism and peripheral steepening (Fig. 61-7). No scleral involvement occurs, although associated conjunctival and episcleral inflammation may be seen. No clear zone exists between the ulcer and the limbus, which distinguishes Mooren's ulcer from other forms of PUK. Visual loss as a result of severe, irregular corneal astigmatism and scarring is common.

DIAGNOSIS

Mooren's ulcer is, by definition, not associated with any systemic abnormality, except for the occasional association with hepatitis C.

457

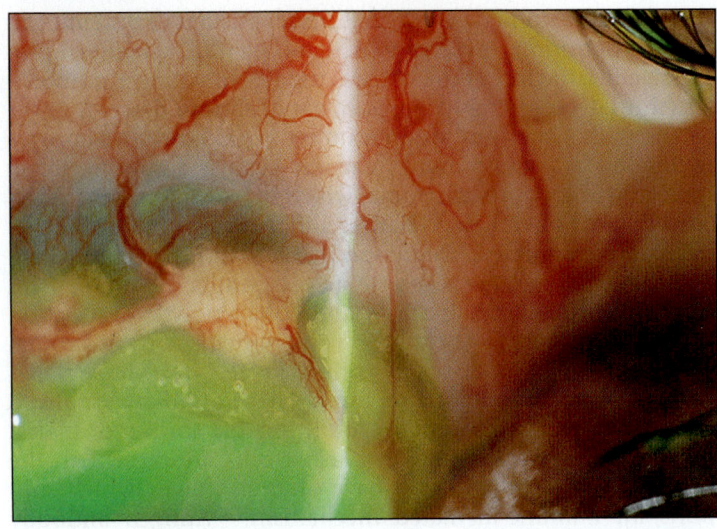

FIG. 61-5 ▌ Acute Mooren's ulcer. Peripheral thinning and an overlying epithelial defect are present in an inflamed eye. (Courtesy of Joel Sugar, MD.)

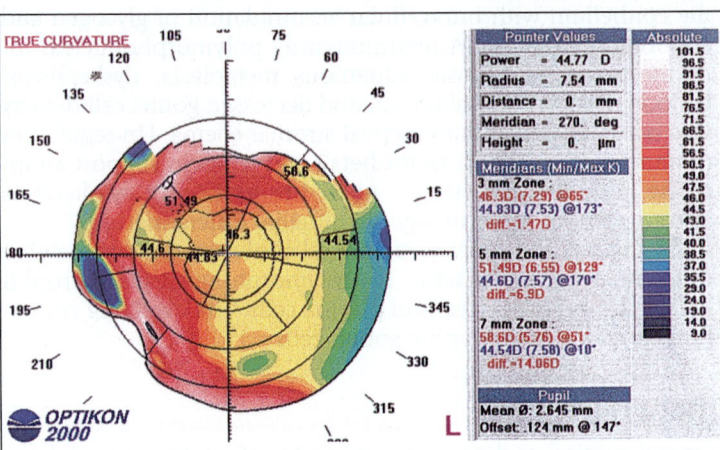

FIG. 61-7 ▌ Topographic image showing peripheral steepening. This is the same patient shown in Figure 61-1.

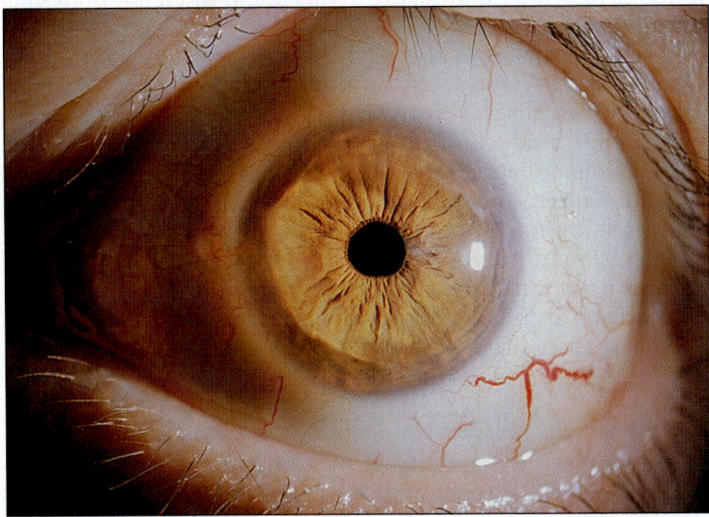

FIG. 61-6 ▌ Mooren's ulcer. Peripheral thinning is present in a quiet eye in this patient who had a history of Mooren's ulcer, now in remission.

It is not associated with scleritis. This distinguishes it from other, more common types of PUK associated with collagen vascular disease, which must be excluded. Patients should also be tested for hepatitis C virus.[26] Patients who have other systemic diseases, including leukemia, pyoderma gangrenosum, and syphilis, may also develop PUK.[27]

A secondary Mooren's ulcer–like PUK may occur following other types of corneal inflammations, including trauma, cataract surgery,[28] herpes simplex keratitis, alkali injury, and herpes zoster. Although these are not diagnostic of true Mooren's ulcer, they do support the involvement of an altered autoantigen pathogenic mechanism. In addition, these cases seem to respond better to treatment.

Patients complain of severe ocular pain, photophobia, and tearing. The overlying epithelium in other degenerative corneal lesions remains intact. This includes Terrien's, pellucid, and involutional marginal degenerations.

DIFFERENTIAL DIAGNOSIS

Although there are many other causes of PUK (Box 61-4), Mooren's ulcer is an unusual and severe inflammatory disease without known associated systemic disease. In Terrien's marginal degeneration, the epithelium is present, and there is not the severe, debilitating pain associated with Mooren's. An addi-

---

BOX 61-4

Differential Diagnosis of Mooren's Ulcer

COLLAGEN VASCULAR DISEASE
Rheumatoid arthritis
Juvenile rheumatoid arthritis
Systemic lupus erythematosus
Wegener's granulomatosis
Progressive systemic sclerosis
Relapsing polychondritis
Polyarteritis nodosa
Cogan's syndrome

OCULODERMATOLOGIC CONDITIONS
Stevens-Johnson syndrome
Rosacea
Psoriasis
Benign mucous membrane pemphigoid
Ichthyosis
Pyoderma gangrenosum

CORNEAL DEGENERATIONS
Terrien's marginal degeneration
Pellucid marginal degeneration
Involutional marginal degeneration

OTHER
Staphylococcal marginal infiltrate

---

tional characteristic feature of Mooren's is the overhanging edge of the cornea, which is absent in Terrien's.

PATHOLOGY

Three zones of corneal involvement have been described in Mooren's ulcer. The superficial stroma contains lymphocytes, plasma cells, polymorphonuclear neutrophil leukocytes, disrupted collagen lamellae, and neovascular elements. The midstroma demonstrates an increase in the number of fibroblasts, and the deep stroma is infiltrated primarily by macrophages. The epithelial basement membrane is disrupted at the leading edge, and the characteristic infiltrate contains primarily neutrophils.

Conjunctival resections from patients who have Mooren's ulcer demonstrate a mononuclear infiltrate in the substantia propria, which contains plasma cells, histiocytes, and eosinophils.[29] The presence of tissue-fixed autoantibodies and complement also has been reported in the epithelial basement membrane of the cornea and conjunctiva.

TREATMENT

The stepladder approach used to manage this aggressive disease includes local, systemic, and surgical therapy.[29] Initial treatment should be with topical corticosteroids, followed by conjunctival resection if the inflammation is not controlled. Topical cyclosporine drops also have been effective in some cases.[22] In addition, bandage contact lenses may reduce discomfort and promote epithelial healing. Subconjunctival heparin injections and topical collagenase inhibitors have also been used.

Systemic immunosuppression with cyclophosphamide followed by azathioprine may be initiated if treatment with conjunctival resection fails. Systemic immunosuppressive treatment of the more aggressive bilateral disease has included the use of corticosteroids, cyclosporine, and methotrexate.[23,29] Plasma exchange also has been tried, but with no clear efficacy. Systemic interferon α-2b has been effective in the treatment of patients positive for the hepatitis C virus who have Mooren's ulcer.[25]

Systemic work-up for vasculitis or collagen vascular disease is mandatory for patients who are suspected of having Mooren's ulcer. The primary goal of therapy is to slow the severe progression of the corneal loss, although 50% of cases may be unresponsive to all medical therapy.[29]

Other surgical interventions have included lamellar keratoplasty, epikeratoplasty, delimiting keratotomy, conjunctival flap, and patch grafts of periosteum, fascia lata,[30] or Gore-Tex, although poor results with the last were reported.[31] Some investigators advocate removal of the presumed antigenic corneal source (central lamellar keratectomy) in an attempt to mediate a more rapid resolution of the inflammation.[29]

Small perforations can be managed with cyanoacrylate adhesive; large perforations may require lamellar keratoplasty.

Surgical management for visual rehabilitation is a challenge; penetrating keratoplasty is usually associated with disease recurrence and graft rejection and melting. Successful cataract surgery has been reported in a patient with Mooren's ulcer who was systemically immunosuppressed with cyclophosphamide for 14 months.[32]

COURSE AND OUTCOME

Most patients who have unilateral disease respond fairly well to topical corticosteroids and conjunctival resection. For more severe bilateral cases, the prognosis is poor, and the primary goal is to reduce the likelihood of perforation and preserve the structure of the eye.

NONSYPHILITIC INTERSTITIAL KERATITIS (COGAN'S SYNDROME)

EPIDEMIOLOGY AND PATHOGENESIS

Cogan's syndrome is a rare inflammatory multisystem disease that affects the eye (deep nonsyphilitic interstitial keratitis) and ear (vestibuloauditory dysfunction).[33] It is also associated with life-threatening vasculitis in 10% of patients. It typically affects younger individuals.

The cause is unknown, but it is presumed to be an autoimmune reaction to a common autoantigen in the cornea and middle ear. Majoor et al.[34] reported the presence of circulating antibodies to corneal epithelium, which decreased with systemic corticosteroid therapy. Serum antibodies to various infectious agents (Lyme disease, *Chlamydia*, type 1 poliovirus) reportedly have been associated with Cogan's syndrome.

OCULAR MANIFESTATIONS

The most common eye finding in Cogan's syndrome is a chronic, bilateral interstitial keratitis. The keratitis begins with an acute

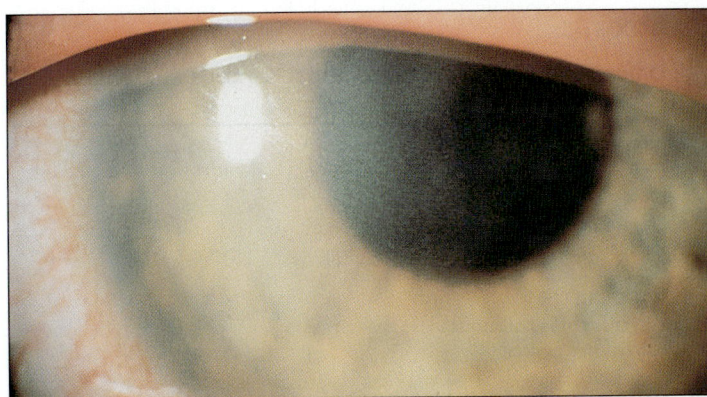

FIG. 61-8 ■ Cogan's syndrome (interstitial keratitis). Slit-lamp appearance of anterior stromal keratitis. (Courtesy of Gary N. Foulks, MD.)

onset of paralimbal injection associated with diffuse or sectoral anterior stromal, subepithelial infiltrates 0.5–1mm in diameter (Fig. 61-8). Topical corticosteroid treatment at this point may reduce the viral-like infiltrates and inhibit the development of the classic late interstitial keratitis. This nummular anterior stromal keratitis may be misdiagnosed as a viral keratitis. Bullae may form within the edematous epithelium. Symptoms of acute keratitis include redness, irritation, photophobia, tearing, and decreased vision; blepharospasm may occur.

The process usually regresses over a period of months, with clearing of the peripheral infiltration. It then may remain peripheral or progress centrally. Late corneal findings include vascularization, scarring, and associated irregular corneal astigmatism. Vascular flow gradually decreases to leave characteristic ghost vessels.

Mild conjunctivitis and anterior uveitis with fine keratic precipitates also may develop in association with the keratitis; 10% of cases may present with episcleritis, scleritis, or other noninterstitial keratitis anterior segment inflammatory disease, which has been termed *atypical Cogan's syndrome.*

Posterior signs may include vitritis, choroiditis, pars planitis, or cotton-wool spots.

DIAGNOSIS

The diagnosis of Cogan's syndrome is made with the identification of the acute onset of vestibuloauditory findings concomitant with the ocular disease.[35] The former may include fluctuating sensory hearing impairment, tinnitus, vertigo, and a reduced vestibular response. Atypical Cogan's syndrome may include posterior scleritis, episcleritis, or uveitis associated with vertigo, tinnitus, and deafness. Immediate diagnosis and medical intervention may provide optimal auditory recovery and preservation.

DIFFERENTIAL DIAGNOSIS

The differential diagnosis of interstitial keratitis is given in Box 61-5. Luetic interstitial keratitis is probably the most common infectious cause of interstitial keratitis. It differs from Cogan's syndrome in that the inflammation is typically bilateral and more progressive and severe in its course. The corneal inflammation in Cogan's is also more anterior, whereas luetic disease is more posterior. Finally, positive serology and other systemic clinical manifestations of congenital syphilis are present.

SYSTEMIC ASSOCIATIONS

The most common systemic findings associated with Cogan's syndrome include abnormalities of the skin, auditory, and cardiovascular systems.[35] Vasculitis does not appear to be the cause of the cochlear disease.

The most common ear findings include an acute onset of Meniere-like syndrome with tinnitus, nausea, vomiting, and vertigo. Common vestibuloauditory findings include nystagmus, oscillopsia, and hearing loss. Immediate diagnosis and systemic immunosuppressive therapy are necessary to prevent hearing loss. Most patients (60–80%) become deaf if the syndrome is not treated.[36]

The major systemic complication is vasculitis and the associated life-threatening aortitis, which develops in 10% of patients. Nonspecific weight loss, fever, headache, arthralgias, and myalgias also may occur.

PATHOLOGY

The cornea demonstrates a lymphocytic infiltrate with old, deep stromal vascularization and a thickened corneal epithelium.

Immunoglobulins A and G (IgA and IgG) have been identified against *Chlamydia trachomatis* without direct evidence of the organism in aortic adventitial biopsy specimens and urogenital smears.[37] Increases in HLA-B17, HLA-A9, HLA-Bw35, and HLA-Cw4 have been reported, which suggests a genetic predilection for the disease.[34] Leukocytosis is common, and elevation in erythrocyte sedimentation rate and C-reactive protein also may be found.

Calcific bony and soft tissue obliteration of the intralabyrinth fluid spaces in patients who have Cogan's syndrome may be demonstrated. Cochlear hydrops also may occur.

TREATMENT

A multidisciplinary approach to the management of patients who have Cogan's syndrome should be implemented; the ophthalmologist and otolaryngologist should be involved, as well as an internal medicine physician to evaluate and manage the vestibular and cardiovascular problems. Audiological assessment and erythrocyte sedimentation rate and C-reactive protein levels may be used to monitor disease activity.[38]

Most patients require oral corticosteroids for 2–6 months to manage the vestibuloauditory signs, typically with a good prognosis.[39] High-dose combination therapy with cyclophosphamide and cyclosporine may be required for more severe ocular or systemic inflammatory disease, including large vessel aortitis. Aortic valve replacement may be required for severe insufficiency, which develops in 10% of patients. Corticosteroids used late in the course of the disease may exacerbate the hearing loss if cochlear hydrops is present.

COURSE AND OUTCOME

The acute stage typically lasts months to years, and the chronic phase lasts indefinitely.

NEUROTROPHIC KERATITIS

EPIDEMIOLOGY AND PATHOGENESIS

Lesions of the fifth cranial nerve from the trigeminal nucleus to the cornea may lead to interruption of the normal sensation and trophic stimulation of the cornea and result in neurotrophic ulceration. The trophic ulceration results from abnormal repair of corneal epithelium secondary to abnormal epithelial cell turnover and reduced reflex tearing. Normally, a bidirectional interaction occurs between epithelial cells and nerve endings. Adrenergic stimulation leads to increased cyclic adenosine monophosphate, which inhibits mitosis.[40] Cholinergic stimulation leads to increased cyclic guanosine monophosphate, which increases cell turnover.[40] Substance P may play a role in normal and abnormal epithelial cell turnover.[41,42] Disruption of the sensory and sympathetic pathways is thought to lead to decreased cell division.[40] Cells therefore fail to resist the effects of trauma (microtrauma) and desiccation, which normally lead to reflex tearing.[43,44]

Varicella-zoster (8% of patients) and herpes simplex keratitis are the most common causes of neurotrophic keratitis. Traumatic nerve damage to the ophthalmic branch of the fifth cranial nerve may result after various surgical procedures. Stroke, irradiation to eye or adnexa, aneurysm, multiple sclerosis, toxic chemical reactions, and brainstem hemorrhages may also lead to trigeminal dysfunction and corneal ulceration.

OCULAR MANIFESTATIONS

Mackie[45] characterized three stages of neurotrophic keratitis. Stage one includes an often subtle irregular corneal surface, which later develops into an easily recognized punctate keratitis. Stage two is characterized by a frank epithelial defect, which typically is associated with mild anterior stromal inflammation (Fig. 61-9). Folds in Descemet's membrane often develop. The epithelium at the edges of the defect tends to be characteristically "heaped up" with grayish, swollen epithelium. The ulcer is typically found in the lower, exposed, paracentral cornea and is generally oval in shape (Fig. 61-10). Stage three involves stromal melting and occasionally perforation. Other characteristic symptoms include red eye, mild foreign body sensation, blurred vision, and lid edema.

DIAGNOSIS

A history of surgery, irradiation, stroke, or decreased hearing should be established, in addition to a previous history of red eye. Decreased corneal sensation typically is evident with or without a decrease in conjunctival sensation. Decreased sensation in either cornea or conjunctiva suggests a viral (herpetic) cause. Excess mucus also is common and results from increased conjunctival epithelial turnover. Decreased aqueous tear production may also be associated with neurotrophic keratopathy.[44]

DIFFERENTIAL DIAGNOSIS

The differential diagnosis of decreased corneal sensation is given in Box 61-6. Herpes simplex and herpes zoster are the most common causes, and each has a characteristic clinical presentation. The role of topical medications and contact lens wear may be difficult to establish but may contribute to corneal hypesthesia. Finally, diabetes is a well-described cause of neurotrophic keratitis and may result in epithelial healing problems.

SYSTEMIC ASSOCIATIONS

Diabetic peripheral neuropathy may result in decreased corneal sensation.

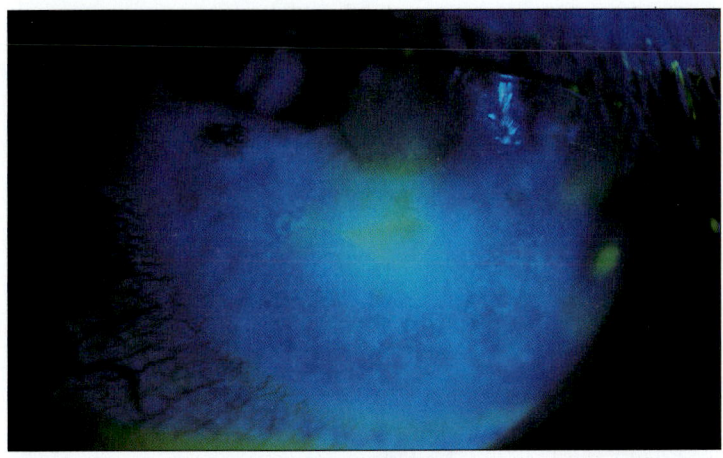

FIG. 61-9 ■ Neurotrophic keratitis. Slit-lamp appearance in a patient who developed a paracentral epithelial defect with minimal subepithelial inflammation.

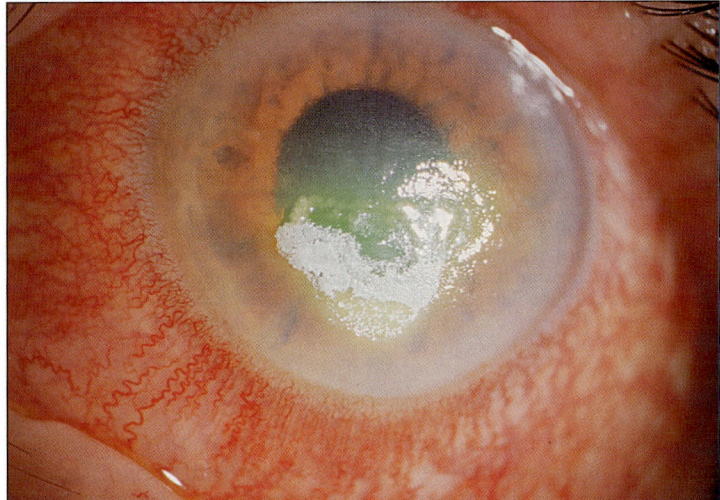

FIG. 61-10 ■ Neurotrophic keratitis. Slit-lamp appearance in a patient who has a partial seventh nerve palsy. He was treated with ciprofloxacin and developed deposits of the antibiotic on the cornea.

PATHOLOGY

Histological changes include acanthotic, hyperplastic epithelium with rete peg formation, stromal scarring, destruction or disruption of Bowman's membrane, and corneal vascularization. Intracellular edema, irregularity and loss of the epithelial microvilli, and loss of the superficial epithelial cell layer of the cornea may be seen.[40] Epithelial cell attachment is also abnormal.

TREATMENT

For mild punctate keratitis, lubrication with unpreserved artificial teardrops and ointment may be effective. Aqueous tear deficiency should be documented and punctal occlusion performed; if tear deficiency is severe, and especially with associated epithelial defects, frequent unpreserved artificial tear therapy is required.

For small epithelial defects, topical ointment with patching may aid in healing. Mild topical corticosteroids may reduce the associated anterior stromal scarring but should be used cautiously, as they may lead to stromal lysis.

For persistent epithelial defects and stromal lysis, patching or soft contact lens wear may be tried, but patients usually respond best to lateral or medial tarsorrhaphy (temporary or permanent). More recently, Bonini et al.[46] demonstrated improved corneal sensation and promotion of epithelial healing following treatment with topical nerve growth factor in 45 eyes of patients with neurotrophic keratitis. Autologous serum may also be effective.

Conjunctival flaps may be necessary in severe cases. Corneal perforation can be managed with tissue glue and lamellar or penetrating keratoplasty. Amniotic membrane has also been used as an effective multilayer patch graft in the management of deep corneal neurotrophic ulcers refractory to conventional treatment.[47] Management of any eyelid abnormality, including blepharitis, entropion, ectropion, and seventh nerve palsy, must be aggressive.

COURSE AND OUTCOME

Patients who have superficial punctate staining should be maintained on regular lubrication. Persistent defects respond best to tarsorrhaphy. Signs of infection must be followed closely. Patients should be advised that neurotrophic ulcers tend to recur and are difficult to heal. More severe, progressive, sterile, or infectious ulcers may progress to descemetocele or perforation.

TERRIEN'S MARGINAL DEGENERATION

EPIDEMIOLOGY AND PATHOGENESIS

Terrien's marginal degeneration is a slowly progressive, bilateral, peripheral corneal thinning disorder associated with corneal neovascularization, opacification, lipid deposition, and thinning. There may be high degrees of astigmatism. Up to one third of patients may have episcleral or scleral inflammation. Patients are typically 20–40 years of age, although it may present in childhood. It is found more commonly in men than in women (3:1).[48]

The cause is unknown, although inflammatory, degenerative, and immune mechanisms have been proposed. Two types have been documented. One type occurs primarily in the older population. It is usually asymptomatic and slowly progressive. The other, more inflammatory type characteristically occurs in younger patients and may be associated with episcleritis or scleritis.[49] It has also been reported in patients who have posterior polymorphous dystrophy,[50] anterior basement membrane dystrophy,[51] and erythema elevatum diutinum.[52]

OCULAR MANIFESTATIONS

Terrien's degeneration usually starts superiorly with mild, punctate, subepithelial and/or anterior stromal opacities. A clear area exists between the opacities and the limbus. This opacification is followed by the development of a peripheral, superficial, fine vascular pannus, which progresses over years to include subepithelial opacity at the advancing edge. The thinning slowly be-

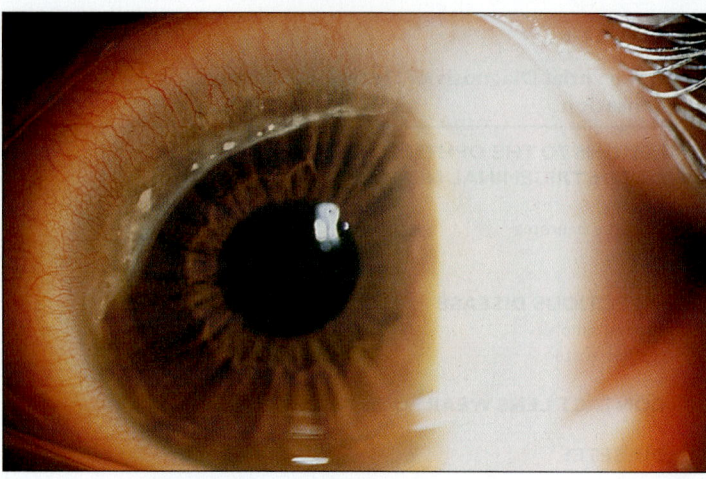

FIG. 61-11 ▮ **Terrien's marginal degeneration.** Advancing lipid deposits and superficial vascular pannus are present. (Courtesy of Joel Sugar, MD.)

BOX 61-7

Differential Diagnosis of Terrien's Marginal Degeneration

Marginal furrow degeneration
Dellen
Collagen vascular disease
Pellucid marginal degeneration
Sclerokeratitis
Keratoconjunctivitis sicca
Staphylococcal marginal keratitis
Infectious corneal ulcer

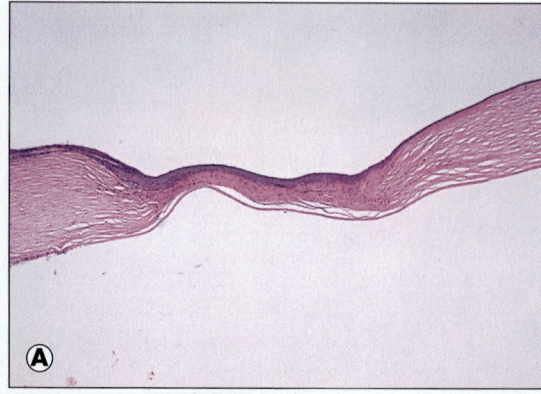
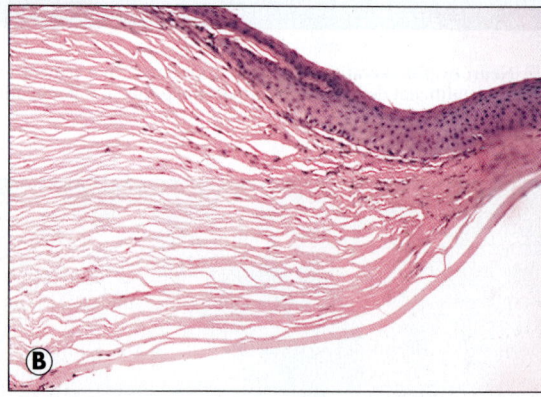

FIG. 61-12 ▮ **Terrien's degeneration. A,** Histological section shows limbus on the left (iris not present) and central cornea to the right. **B,** Note the marked stromal thinning, thickened epithelium, and loss of Bowman's membrane on the limbal side. (Courtesy Yanoff M, Fine BS. Ocular pathology, ed. 5, St Louis: Mosby; 2002.)

---

gins between the limbus and the line of lipid deposition. Characteristically, a steeper sloping of the cornea occurs at the advancing edge (Fig. 61-11), without the overlying edge characteristic of Mooren's ulcer. The thinning progresses circumferentially, but the overlying epithelium typically remains intact. Perforation is rare but may occur. Corneal hydrops also has been reported, which may present as a clear intracorneal pocket of aqueous rather than stromal clouding.[53]

Irregular corneal astigmatism from progressive flattening of the vertical meridian and high against-the-rule astigmatism is characteristic. Initial conservative management includes the use of rigid gas-permeable contact lenses. Rarely, Terrien's degeneration may present as a pseudopterygium with a broad, flat, leading edge that arises in an oblique axis. This variant may be the same as Fuchs' superficial marginal keratitis. Underlying corneal thinning should be monitored carefully. Intraocular lenses have been placed successfully through the furrow.

DIAGNOSIS

Terrien's marginal degeneration is distinguished from other peripheral corneal thinning disorders by the lack of inflammation, presence of superficial vascularization, advancing linear deposition of lipid, lack of epithelial defect, and slow progressive course. Occasionally, Terrien's may present with recurrent painful episodes of inflammation. Collagen vascular disease should be ruled out. No known systemic associations occur with Terrien's.

DIFFERENTIAL DIAGNOSIS

The differential diagnosis of Terrien's marginal degeneration is outlined in Box 61-7. Terrien's is generally easy to distinguish from Mooren's, since there is usually no pain or inflammation. The epithelium is intact, and there is no overhanging edge. Inflammatory staphylococcal lesions usually have a lucid inter-

val between the limbus and infiltrate. There is only rarely stromal thinning, and there is typically more local inflammation. Marginal furrow degeneration is bilateral and avascular, with only minimal, if any, thinning.

PATHOLOGY

The epithelium may be normal, thickened, or thinned. Bowman's membrane is typically absent or has degenerated (Fig. 61-12). Thinning and occasional breaks in Descemet's membrane may be seen. Subepithelial fibrillar collagen degeneration has been demonstrated by light microscopy, and an unknown stromal material in phagocytic cells has been demonstrated by electron microscopy.[49] Degeneration of the peripheral corneal stroma with lipid accumulation unaccompanied by significant inflammatory cells is characteristic. Lamellar specimens demonstrated less than 25% HLA-DR+ cells and a 1:1 ratio of CD4 to CD8 T lymphocytes. This differed from Mooren's ulcer, which had 75% HLA-DR+ cells and a 24:1 CD4-to-CD8 ratio.[54]

TREATMENT

Usually no treatment is required, unless perforation or impending perforation occurs. Severe astigmatism may be managed with spectacles or rigid contact lenses. More severe thinning may require crescentic, full-thickness, or lamellar keratoplasty.[55] Eccentric, full-thickness grafts have been performed, with an increase in graft rejection.

COURSE AND OUTCOME

Most patients who have Terrien's degeneration do not progress to corneal perforation and can be managed successfully with glasses or rigid contact lenses. Because Terrien's degeneration typically lacks an associated epithelial defect, the risk of infectious keratitis and acute corneal thinning is low, but these patients must be monitored regularly.

RHEUMATOID-ASSOCIATED CORNEAL ULCERATION

EPIDEMIOLOGY AND PATHOGENESIS

Many collagen vascular diseases can result in unilateral or bilateral noninfectious peripheral corneal inflammation. However, it is beyond the scope of this chapter to discuss all of them. Rheumatoid arthritis (RA) and secondary Sjögren's syndrome are probably the most common and serve here as models for this complex group of systemic diseases. In this section the focus is on RA, since it is the most common collagen vascular disease; it affects 3–5% of the adult population,[56] women more than men. The average age of onset is 35–40 years.

The etiology of RA is not understood completely, although autoimmune (increased T helper/T suppressor cell ratio, elevated serum rheumatoid factor), genetic (increased frequency of HLA-DR4 and HLA-DR1), and hormonal influences probably contribute.[56]

There are two types of rheumatoid-mediated ulcerative keratitis: peripheral and paracentral. The paracentral ulcers (keratolysis) typically present without significant conjunctival inflammation, usually in patients who have severe dry eye.[57] The mechanism is postulated to involve an altered epithelial barrier, which results in inflammatory mediators that enter the stroma, where they effect a sterile keratolysis.

The pathophysiology of peripheral corneal thinning results from an obliterative microangiitis at the level of the limbal vascular arcades, the episcleral meshwork, or the deeper vascular networks.[58] Inappropriate peripheral deposition of immune complexes in the limbal vasculature results in an immune microangiopathy and leakage of inflammatory cells and proteins, especially in the setting of scleral inflammation. The area of tissue loss corresponds to the degree of vascular occlusion. Collagenases and proteases, released by infiltrating polymorphonuclear neutrophil leukocytes and activated stromal keratocytes, degrade stromal collagen. The classic complement pathway also may be activated.

OCULAR MANIFESTATIONS

RA can affect almost all ocular structures, including the posterior segment (involving the retina, choroid, optic nerve), extraocular muscles, and anterior segment (keratoconjunctivitis sicca, punctate keratopathy, keratitis, scleritis, and episcleritis).[59] It may affect the sclera alone (scleritis), both sclera and cornea (sclerosing keratitis), or only the cornea (keratitis). In this section the focus is on the corneal manifestations of RA.

Patients who have RA and noninfectious corneal inflammation may present with complaints of foreign body sensation, dryness, photophobia, and blurred vision—signs and symptoms commonly associated with dry eye. These patients should be examined carefully for the presence of corneal inflammation. Many types of keratitis have been described that may be associated with scleral inflammation, including[60]:

- Peripheral limbal furrow or gutter
- Peripheral corneal thinning
- Keratolysis
- Acute stromal keratitis
- Sclerosing keratitis

Limbal (Marginal) Furrow

Patients who have RA may develop peripheral corneal thinning without infiltration or overlying epithelial defect. This usually occurs in a relatively quiet eye, with minimal infiltration and associated neovascularization. The marginal furrow is a benign condition that results from a slowly progressive resorption of peripheral corneal tissue.

Peripheral Ulcerative Keratitis and Keratolysis

Peripheral corneal thinning (Fig. 61-13) and keratolysis (Fig. 61-14) were described earlier in the epidemiology and pathogenesis subsection.

Acute Stromal Keratitis

Acute onset of stromal infiltration or opacity associated with stromal edema may occur with or without an overlying epithelial defect. The opacity gradually resolves to leave an area of superficial vascularization and stromal thinning, if severe.

Sclerosing Keratitis

Patients who have scleritis contiguous with the limbus often develop fibrotic lesions that appear as a deep stromal haze in the same area. This process is referred to as sclerosing keratitis.

DIAGNOSIS

The diagnosis of RA depends on a set of criteria established by the American Rheumatism Association: (1) morning stiffness; (2) arthritis in three or more joints; (3) arthritis of the proximal interphalangeal, metacarpophalangeal, or wrist joint; (4) rheumatoid nodules; (5) positive rheumatoid factor; (6) radiographic erosions; and/or (7) periarticular osteopenia in the hand or wrist joints. These confirm the associated systemic disease.[56,59]

DIFFERENTIAL DIAGNOSIS

The differential diagnosis of peripheral corneal thinning is large and includes a variety of collagen vascular diseases as well as in-

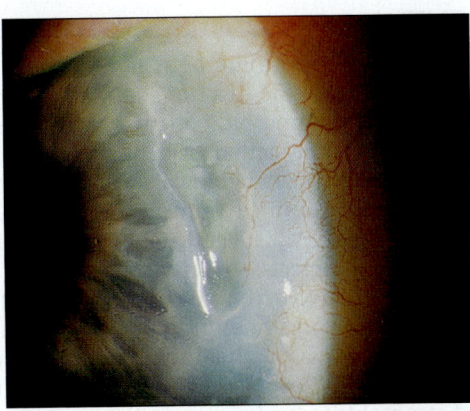

FIG. 61-13 ■ Peripheral corneal thinning in a patient who has rheumatoid arthritis.

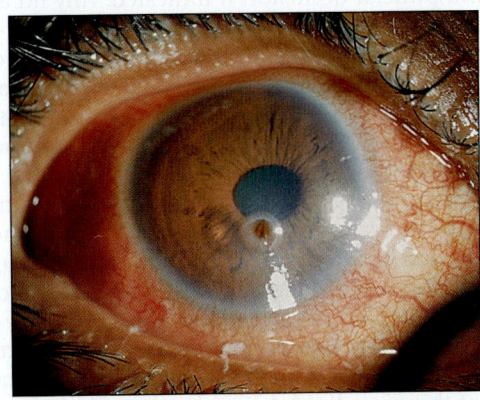

FIG. 61-14 ■ Paracentral corneal thinning in a patient who has severe dry eye.

fectious and inflammatory processes, most notably herpes simplex keratitis, which may result in severe stromal inflammation and thinning. Wegener's granulomatosis, a potentially life-threatening disease, may present with peripheral corneal thinning and should be carefully ruled out by history, examination, and serological screening (antineutrophil cytoplasmic antibodies).[60] There are also many dermatological conditions, most commonly rosacea, that can cause peripheral corneal ulceration. Other systemic clinical features help differentiate these entities (see Box 61-1).

PATHOLOGY

The pathology of paracentral rheumatoid ulceration involves infiltration by monocytes, macrophages, and T cells, as well as immunoglobulin deposition in the epithelium. The infiltration is also associated with strong HLA-DR expression by stromal keratocytes and epithelium, which results from interferon gamma released by TH2 lymphocytes.[56]

Interleukin-1 and tumor necrosis factor-α are the predominant local cytokines that induce the production of collagenase and protease in synovial fibroblasts of rheumatoid patients; they also may play a role in corneal ulceration.[57]

Conjunctival biopsies in patients who have peripheral corneal thinning secondary to collagen vascular disease have demonstrated inflammation that is more accurately a microangiopathy than a microvasculitis, since the vessels lack a tunica media. Polymorphonuclear neutrophil leukocyte invasion of the vessels, fibrinoid necrosis, and deposits of IgA, IgG, IgM, C3, and C4 may be found.[59] Adjacent episcleritis or scleritis is common in rheumatoid-associated keratitis.

Immunohistochemistry of corneas with paracentral corneal melts associated with rheumatoid keratitis demonstrate HLA-DR expression on stromal keratocytes and epithelial cells and immunoglobulin deposition in the corneal epithelium.[57] CD11c macrophages also are seen in the epithelium and subepithelium of the edge of the ulcer.

TREATMENT

Although peripheral corneal thinning is not always a manifestation of systemic autoimmune disorders, the onset of peripheral corneal thinning in a rheumatoid patient may indicate the presence of a severe, potentially lethal vasculitis requiring aggressive systemic immunosuppressive therapy. Elevated levels of rheumatoid factor, circulating immune complexes, low complement levels, and cryoglobulinemia all suggest severe systemic disease.[59]

Persistent epithelial defects, stromal inflammation, and enzymatic degradation are involved in the pathogenesis of noninfectious corneal ulceration.[1] As in all noninfectious corneal ulceration, general principles of therapy include promotion of epithelial healing, reduction of inflammation, limitation of ulceration and stromal loss, and support of repair.[1]

The promotion of epithelial healing includes the administration of mucolytic agents, the frequent use of unpreserved artificial tears, and punctal occlusion if indicated. Any lid abnormalities should be corrected.

Many therapeutic approaches to the management of peripheral corneal thinning secondary to collagen vascular disease have been advocated. These include topical and systemic immunosuppression with or without cytotoxic immunosuppressive agents.[56,61] Methotrexate has been recommended as a first-line drug for the management of peripheral corneal thinning in RA patients, with cyclophosphamide as a second-line drug in cases of drug intolerance or treatment failure.[59] Nonsteroidal anti-inflammatory agents also are important for the control of inflammation.

Photographs of the lesions may help assess progression, as the lesions often recur and progress over years. Systematic documentation of thinning, lipid deposition, vascularization, and intensity of blood flow may help evaluate responses to therapy.

Concurrent surgical approaches include conjunctival recession or resection, tarsorrhaphy, cyanoacrylate adhesive use, lamellar keratoplasty, and scleral grafting.[59] Such approaches must always be accompanied by immunosuppressive therapy and are inadequate as isolated treatment modalities.

For the paracentral ulcers, conjunctival resection may not be effective, because conjunctival microangiopathy may not be the cause of the ulceration. Topical 2% cyclosporine has been used with some success, as it may enable epithelial healing while reducing cell-mediated immune reactions in the cornea.[57] Topical metalloproteinase inhibitors also may help reduce stromal lysis.

For peripheral corneal infiltrates without thinning, a short course of topical corticosteroids may be helpful. For marginal corneal furrows without infiltration and a clear zone between the limbus and the furrow, topical corticosteroids should not be used because of the risk of further keratolysis and perforation. Corneal thinning with infiltration that begins at the limbus and extends centrally and circumferentially may respond to short courses of topical corticosteroids. Caution must be exercised, because an increased incidence of corneal perforation in these ulcers has been reported.

Perforations or impending perforations may require the application of cyanoacrylate adhesive, lamellar grafting, or the creation of a conjunctival flap, in addition to punctal occlusion, tarsorrhaphy, and the use of copious quantities of nonpreserved artificial tears.

Paracentral keratolysis may develop in RA patients after cataract surgery and should be monitored carefully. Patients who have high preoperative rheumatoid factor levels and circulating immune complex levels may benefit from preoperative immunosuppression. Measures to maintain epithelial integrity should be taken postoperatively.

Concurrent treatment of dry eye and lid margin disease should be aggressive. This may include frequent use of unpreserved teardrops, punctal occlusion, ointment at bedtime, topical cyclosporine, topical tretinoin (vitamin A), or autologous sera.

Penetrating keratoplasty usually has a poor visual prognosis in severe cases, although structural integrity of the globe may be achieved.[59]

COURSE AND OUTCOME

Patients who have mild disease usually can be managed effectively with local therapy. Systemic immunosuppression is necessary in most cases of severe peripheral corneal thinning and should be managed in consultation with a rheumatologist or oncologist. Elevated rheumatoid factor may correlate with a worse prognosis. Initial treatment failures usually occur when local therapy is pursued without management of the systemic autoimmune process.

Paracentral keratolysis may be more difficult to manage. The use of topical cyclosporine drops may play a role in its management.

REFERENCES

1. Kenyon KR. Decision-making in the therapy of external eye disease. Noninfected corneal ulcers. Ophthalmology. 1982;89:44–51.
2. Thygeson P. Superficial punctate keratitis. JAMA. 1950;144:1544–9.
3. Lemp MA, Chambers RW, Lundy J. Viral isolate in superficial punctate keratitis. Arch Ophthalmol. 1974;91:8–10.
4. Darrell RW. Thygeson's superficial punctate keratitis: natural history and association with HLA-DR3. Trans Am Ophthalmol Soc. 1981;74:486–516.
5. Dighiens P, Mayer F, Hernandez-Quintela E, et al. Confocal microscopy of 2 cases with HLA-DR3. Trans Am Ophthalmol Soc. 1981;74:486–516.
6. Del Castillo JM, Del Castillo JB, Garcia-Sanchez J. Effect of topical cyclosporine A on Thygeson's superficial punctate keratitis. Doc Ophthalmol. 1996;93:193–8.
7. Nesburn AB, Lowe GH, Lepoff NJ, Maguen E. Effect of topical trifluridine on Thygeson's superficial punctate keratitis. Ophthalmology. 1984;91:1188–92.
8. Fite SW, Chodosh J. Photorefractive keratectomy for myopia in the setting of Thygeson's superficial punctate keratitis. Cornea. 2001;20:425–6.
9. Theodore FH. Superior limbic keratoconjunctivitis. Eye, Ear, Nose Throat Monthly. 1963;42:25–8.
10. Cher I. Superior limbic keratoconjunctivitis: multifactorial mechanical pathogenesis. Clin Exp Ophthalmol. 2000;28:181–4.

11. Kadramas EF, Bartley GB. Superior limbic keratoconjunctivitis. A prognostic sign for severe Graves' ophthalmopathy. Ophthalmology. 1995;102:1472–5.

12. Matsuda A, Tagawa Y, Matsududa H. TGF-beta2, tenascin, and integrin beta1 expression in superior limbic keratoconjunctivitis. Jpn J Ophthalmol. 1999;43:251–6.

13. Matsuda A, Tagawa Y, Matsuda H. Cytokeratin and proliferative cell nuclear antigen expression in superior limbic keratoconjunctivitis. Curr Eye Res. 1996;15:1033–8.

14. Yang HY, Fujishima H, Toda I, et al. Lacrimal punctal occlusion for the treatment of superior limbic keratoconjunctivitis. Am J Ophthalmol. 1997;124:80–7.

15. Udell IJ, Kenyon KR, Sawa M. Treatment of superior limbic keratoconjunctivitis by thermocauterization of the superior bulbar conjunctiva. Ophthalmology. 1986;93:162–6.

16. Grutzmacher RD, Foster RS, Feiler LS. Lodoxamide tromethamine treatment for superior limbic keratoconjunctivitis. Am J Ophthalmol. 1995;120:400–1.

17. Ohashi Y, Watanabe H, Kinoshita S, et al. Vitamin A eyedrops for superior limbic keratoconjunctivitis. Am J Ophthalmol. 1988;105:523–7.

18. Mooren A. Ophthalmiatrische Beobachtungen. Berlin: A Hirschwald; 1867:107–10.

19. Wood TO, Kaufman HE. Mooren's ulcer. Am J Ophthalmol. 1971;71:417–22.

20. Gottsch JD, Li Q, Ashraf F, et al. Cytokine-induced calgranulin C expression in keratocytes. Clin Immunol. 1999;91:34–40.

21. Gottsch JD, Liu SH. Cloning and expression of human corneal calgranulin C (CO-Ag). Curr Eye Res. 1998;17:870–4.

22. Zhao JC, Jin XY. Immunological analysis and treatment of Mooren's ulcer with cyclosporin A applied topically. Cornea. 1993;12:481–8.

23. Foster CS. Systemic immunosuppressive therapy for progressive bilateral Mooren's ulcer. Ophthalmology. 1985;92:1436–9.

24. Taylor CJ, Smith SI, Morgan CH, et al. HLA and Mooren's ulceration. Br J Ophthalmol. 2000;84:72–5.

25. Mozami G, Auran JD, Florakis GJ, et al. Interferon treatment of Mooren's ulcers associated with hepatitis C. Am J Ophthalmol. 1995;119:365–6.

26. Wilson SE, Lee WM, Murakami C, et al. Mooren-type hepatitis C virus associated corneal ulceration. Ophthalmology. 1994;101:736–45.

27. Bouchard CS, Meyer M, McDonnell JF. Peripheral ulcerative keratitis in a leukemic patient with pyoderma gangrenosum. Cornea. 1997;16:480–2.

28. David T, Morel X, Bigorgne C, et al. Mooren's ulcer following combined extracapsular crystalline lens extraction and trabeculectomy. J Fr Ophthalmol. 1997;20:619–23.

29. Brown SI, Mondino BJ. Therapy of Mooren's ulcer. Am J Ophthalmol. 1984;98:1–6.

30. Kinoshita S, Ohashi Y, Ohji M, Manabe R. Long-term results of keratoepithelioplasty in Mooren's ulcer. Ophthalmology. 1991;89:438–45.

31. Huang WJ, Hu FR, Chang SW. Clinicopathological study of Gore-Tex patch graft in corneoscleral surgery. Cornea. 1994;13:82–6.

32. Akova YA, Aslan BS, Duman S. Phacoemulsification and intraocular lens implant in a patient with Mooren's ulcer. Ophthalmic Surg Lasers. 1997;28:769–71.

33. Cogan DS. Syndrome of nonsyphilitic interstitial keratitis and vestibuloauditory symptoms. Arch Ophthalmol. 1945;33:144–9.

34. Majoor MH, Albers FW, van der Gaag R, et al. Corneal autoimmunity in Cogan's syndrome? A report of two cases. Ann Otol Rhinol Laryngol. 1992;101:679–84.

35. McCallum RM, Allen NB, Cobo LM, et al. Cogan's syndrome: clinical features and outcomes. Arthritis Rheum. 1992;35(suppl. 9):S51.

36. Haynes BF, Kaiser-Kupfer MI, Mason P, Fauci AJ. Cogan's syndrome: studies in thirteen patients, long term follow up, and a review of the literature. Medicine. 1980;59:426–40.

37. Hammer M, Witte T, Mugge A, et al. Complicated Cogan's syndrome with aortic insufficiency and coronary stenosis. J Rheumatol. 1994;21(3):552–5.

38. Allen NB, Cox CC, Cobo M, et al. Use of immunosuppressive agents in the treatment of severe ocular and vascular manifestations of Cogan's syndrome. Am J Med. 1990;88(3):296–301.

39. Cote DN, Molony TB, Waxman J, Parsa D. Cogan's syndrome manifesting as sudden bilateral deafness: diagnosis and management. South Med J. 1993;86(9):1056–60.

40. Cavanagh HD, Colley AM. The molecular basis of neurotrophic keratitis. Acta Ophthalmol Suppl. 1989;192:115.

41. Reid TW, Murphy CJ, Iwahashi CK, et al. Stimulation of epithelial cell growth by the neuropeptide substance P. J Cell Biochem. 1993;52:476–85.

42. Araki-Sasaki K, Aizawa S, Hiramoto M, et al. Substance P induced cadherin expression and its signal transduction in a cloned human corneal epithelial cell line. J Cell Physiol. 2000;182:189–95.

43. Gilbard JP, Rossi SR. Tear film and ocular surface changes in a rabbit model of neurotrophic keratitis. Ophthalmology. 1990;97:308–12.

44. Heigle TJ, Pflugfelder SC. Aqueous tear production in patients with neurotrophic keratitis. Cornea. 1996;15:135–8.

45. Mackie IA. Role of the corneal nerves in destructive disease of the cornea. Trans Ophthalmol Soc UK. 1978;98:343–7.

46. Bonini S, Lambiase A, Rama P, et al. Topical treatment with nerve growth factor for neurotrophic keratitis. Ophthalmology. 2000;107:1347–51.

47. Kruse FE, Rohrschneidwer K, Volcker HE. Multilayer amniotic membrane transplantation for reconstruction of deep corneal ulcers. Ophthalmology. 1999;106:1504–10.

48. Austin P, Brown SI. Inflammatory Terrien's marginal corneal disease. Am J Ophthalmol. 1981;92:189–92.

49. Iwamoto T, DeVoe AG, Farris RL. Electron microscopy in cases of marginal degeneration of the cornea. Invest Ophthalmol Vis Sci. 1972;11:241–57.

50. Wagoner MD, Teichman KD. Terrien's marginal degeneration associated with posterior polymorphous dystrophy. Cornea. 1999;18:612–5.

51. Donshik PC, Tedesco J, Carlton R, Telfer A. Terrien's marginal degeneration associated with central anterior basement membrane–like dystrophic like changes. Cornea. 1987;6:246–9.

52. Shimizaki J, Yang HY, Shimmura S, Tsubota K. Terrien's marginal degeneration associated with erythema elevatum diutinum. Cornea. 1998;17:342–4.

53. Ashenhuurst M, Slomovic A. Corneal hydrops in Terrien's marginal degeneration: an unusual complication. Can J Ophthalmol. 1987;22:328–30.

54. Lopez JS, Price FW, Whitcup SM, et al. Immunohistochemistry of Terrien's and Mooren's corneal degeneration. Arch Ophthalmol. 1991;109:988–92.

55. Hahn TW, Kim JH. Two step annular tectonic lamellar keratoplasty in severe Terrien's marginal degeneration. Ophthalmic Surg. 1993;24:831–4.

56. Harris ED Jr. Rheumatoid arthritis: pathophysiology and implications for therapy. N Engl J Med. 1990;322:1277–89.

57. Kervick GN, Pflugfelder SC, Haimovici R, et al. Paracentral rheumatoid corneal ulceration: clinical features and cyclosporine therapy. Ophthalmology. 1992;99:80–8.

58. Watson PG. Vascular changes in peripheral corneal destructive disease. Eye. 1990;4:65–73.

59. Messmer EM, Foster CS. Destructive corneal and scleral disease associated with rheumatoid arthritis. Cornea. 1995;14:408–17.

60. Soukiasian SH, Foster CS, Niles JL, Raizman MB. Diagnostic value of anti-neutrophil cytoplasmic antibodies in scleritis associated with Wegener's granulomatosis. Ophthalmology. 1992;99:125–32.

61. Liegner JT, Yee RW, Wild JH. Topical cyclosporine therapy for ulcerative keratitis associated with rheumatoid arthritis. Am J Ophthalmol. 1990;109:610–12.

DEFINITION
• Corneal disease caused by bacterial, viral, fungal, or protozoal organisms.

KEY FEATURES
• Cellular infiltration of the corneal epithelium or stroma, corneal inflammation, and necrosis.

ASSOCIATED FEATURES
• Lid edema.
• Conjunctival inflammation.
• Discharge.
• Anterior chamber reaction.
• Hypopyon.

INTRODUCTION

Infectious keratitis is one of the leading causes of blindness in the world. Because, in most cases, these infections represent preventable or treatable ophthalmic disease, a thorough understanding of the epidemiology, diagnosis, and treatment of the various forms of infectious keratitis is essential for eye care practitioners and public health officials.

BACTERIAL KERATITIS

EPIDEMIOLOGY AND PATHOGENESIS

Bacterial keratitis is considered a leading cause of monocular blindness in the developing world.[1] In this environment, corneal infections often follow trauma, but they also contribute significantly to corneal blindness associated with trachoma and xerophthalmia.

Although no reliable surveys exist, an estimated 30,000 cases occur annually in the United States. Given the potential blinding complications of severe bacterial keratitis, these infections are a significant public health issue.[2] The increasing popularity of contact lens wear has contributed to a rising incidence of bacterial keratitis in the developed world. Current estimates are that 10–30 persons per 100,000 who wear contact lenses develop ulcerative keratitis annually in the United States.[3,4] A host of bacterial organisms can cause infectious keratitis. These organisms are commonly grouped by their staining pattern with Gram's iodine and their response to oxygen, that is, gram positive versus gram negative, and aerobic versus anaerobic. The incidence of infection by specific organisms varies by region, and practitioners should be aware of the local epidemiological patterns of corneal infection. Whereas staphylococcal species are most commonly seen in

Canada and the eastern and northeastern United States, *Pseudomonas* infection is more common in the southern United States. Indeed, *Streptococcus pneumoniae* was once the most common pathogen isolated from bacterial corneal ulcers, but as contact lens wear and related infectious keratitis have increased, the relative incidence of pseudomonad and staphylococcal infection has increased. These two organisms account for the majority of infections associated with contact lens wear, followed by *Serratia marcescens.*[5] Corneal infections that occur in patients with systemic debilitating diseases such as alcohol abuse, malnutrition, or diabetes are often associated with *Moraxella.* In the developing world, streptococcal corneal infection remains the most common, followed by staphylococcal and pseudomonad keratitis.

The corneal surface is normally well protected by a variety of mechanisms. The eyelids form a physical barrier to foreign material, and blinking regularly sweeps away debris trapped in the mucin layer of the tears. The corneal and conjunctival epithelial cells are tightly bound together, providing another barrier to microbial invasion, and epithelial cells themselves can phagocytize and transport microbes.

Tears also contain immunoactive substances such as lactoferrin, lysozyme, beta lysin, tear-specific albumin, and immunoglobulin A (IgA). Lactoferrin is a major protein constituent of human tears and is secreted by the lacrimal gland. It appears to affect certain bacterial strains directly, helps regulate the production of granulocyte- and macrophage-derived colony-stimulating factors, and inhibits complement activation, thus decreasing inflammation.[6] Lysozyme is active against certain gram-positive organisms, promotes microbial aggregation, and enhances IgA-mediated lysis of bacterial cell membranes.[7] Beta lysin also causes bacteriolysis. Secretory IgA causes bacterial agglutination and inhibits bacterial adherence to the corneal and conjunctival surface.

A number of immune mediators operate to protect the corneal surface. Most are provided by the conjunctiva. The conjunctiva contains mast cells that, when activated, induce vascular dilatation and increased vascular permeability, which results in the production of an antimicrobial transudate. The conjunctiva also contains conjunctiva-associated lymphoid tissue (CALT), which consists of nodules of small and medium-sized lymphocytes responsible for local antigen processing. Plasma cells, macrophages, and a variety of T cells are also present, as well as IgG, IgA, and IgM, which are brought in by the conjunctival vasculature.

The natural microbial environment of the ocular surface consists of both sessile and free-floating bacteria. This population is kept in check by the antimicrobial features of the tear film, as well as by the products of resident microbes; these products, called bacteriocins, are high-molecular-weight proteins that inhibit the growth of pathogens such as pneumococci and gram-negative bacilli.

In the majority of cases in which bacterial keratitis develops, at least one risk factor that represents a compromise of one or more of these defense mechanisms can be identified. Lid abnormalities

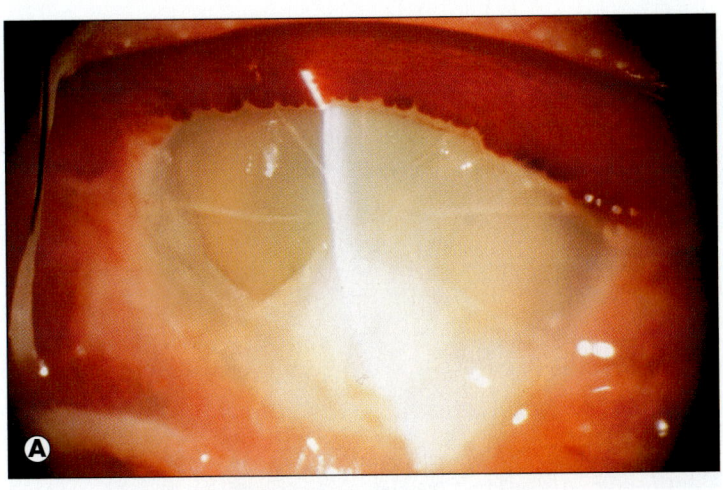
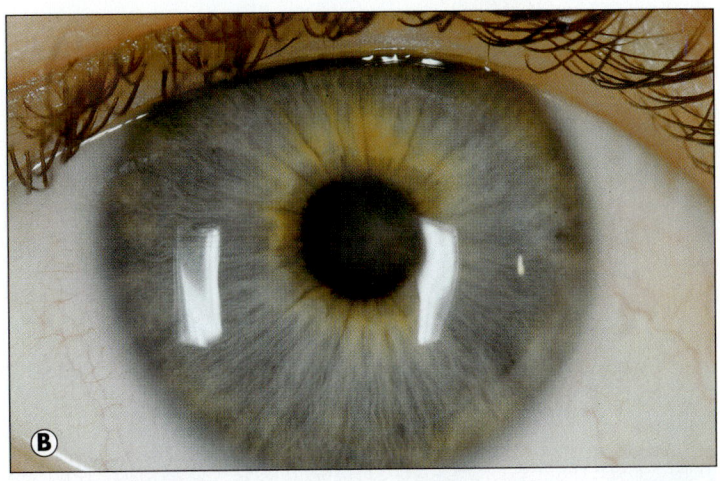

FIG. 62-1 ■ **Keratitis.** **A,** Severe *Pseudomonas* keratitis following radial keratotomy. **B,** Scarring at the interface of a LASIK flap and bed following *Aspergillus* keratitis.

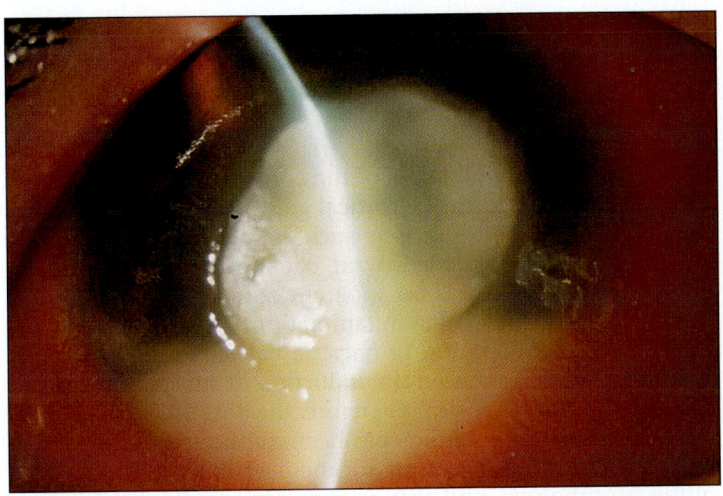

FIG. 62-2 ■ Epithelial defect, stromal infiltrate, and hypopyon associated with crack cocaine use. Candidal, streptococcal, and *Haemophilus* species were recovered from scrapings of the infiltrate.

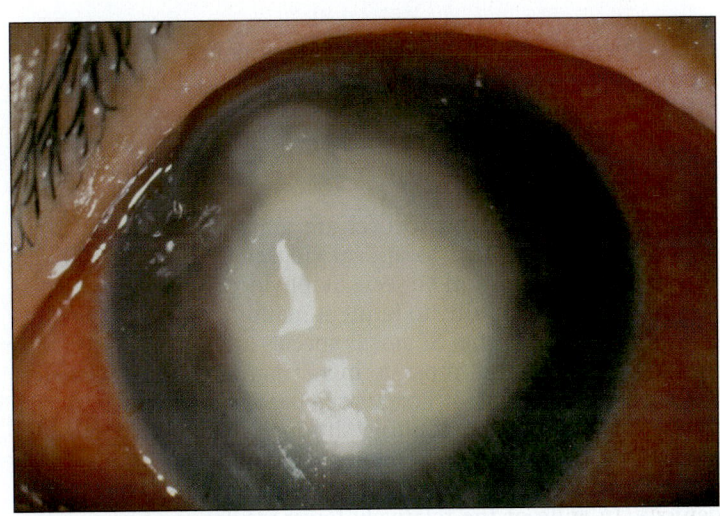

FIG. 62-3 ■ Bacterial corneal infection with dense central necrotic ulcer and infiltrate.

such as entropion or ectropion, exposure of the corneal surface, or trichiasis can cause breakdown of the protective corneal epithelium. Poor tear production can lead to a reduction of antimicrobial tear components and epithelial desiccation and damage. Epithelial problems such as bullous keratopathy, medication toxicity, prior herpetic infection, and trauma associated with contact lens use can allow microbial adherence and invasion.

With the increasing popularity of laser *in situ* keratomileusis (LASIK) and other keratorefractive procedures that involve epithelial disruption and stromal incision, a wide variety of postsurgical corneal infections have been reported. Organisms can be introduced directly into the stroma at the time of keratorefractive incisional surgery or can gain admission later via abnormal epithelium that overlies the incisions[8] (Fig. 62-1).

The use of smokable drugs such as cocaine and methamphetamine has been associated with microbial keratitis, probably due to a direct toxic effect, exposure keratopathy, neurotrophic changes, or mechanical trauma[9,10] (Fig. 62-2). Local or systemic immune compromise can lead to impairment of local immune defenses. This is most commonly caused by the use of topical corticosteroids, but it can also be caused by immunosuppression, malignancy, malnutrition, or extensive burns. It is worth noting that at present it does not appear that acquired immunodeficiency syndrome (AIDS) is an independent risk for the development of infectious keratitis, but infectious keratitis in AIDS patients might follow a more aggressive course.

Although disruption of the continuity of the epithelium is the most common event that allows the establishment of a corneal infection, a few organisms such as *Corynebacterium diphtheriae*, *Haemophilus aegyptius*, *Neisseria gonorrhoeae* and *N. meningitidis*, and *Shigella* and *Listeria* species can penetrate an intact epithelium. Occasionally, keratitis can be established via the corneoscleral limbus by hematogenous spread.

CLINICAL FEATURES

The clinical signs and symptoms of bacterial keratitis depend greatly on the virulence of the organism and the duration of infection. Other influential factors include the previous status of the cornea and the use of corticosteroids. Patients may describe decreased vision, pain, and photophobia. The cardinal corneal sign is a localized or diffuse infiltration of the epithelium or stroma (Fig. 62-3). Commonly, there is epithelial absence over a gray-white necrotic stromal infiltrate. Alternatively, a stromal abscess can appear beneath an intact epithelium. Infiltration and edema of the cornea can appear distant to the primary site of infection. Occasionally, bacterial keratitis can present with predominantly multifocal epithelial infiltration, especially in the setting of hydrophilic contact lens wear.

Other ocular structures usually demonstrate associated inflammation. There is often some degree of lid erythema and edema, conjunctival injection and chemosis, tearing, and discharge. A nonspecific conjunctival papillary response might be seen. Anterior chamber inflammation is often present, with cells and flare. The inflammatory response might be so severe as to produce a hypopyon, but in the absence of a full-thickness

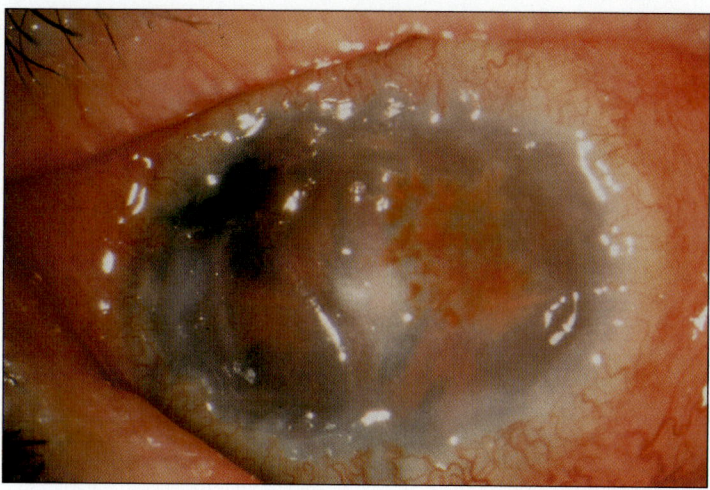

FIG. 62-4 ■ Streptococcal bacterial keratitis with infiltration of the central cornea. (Courtesy of Alan Sugar, MD.)

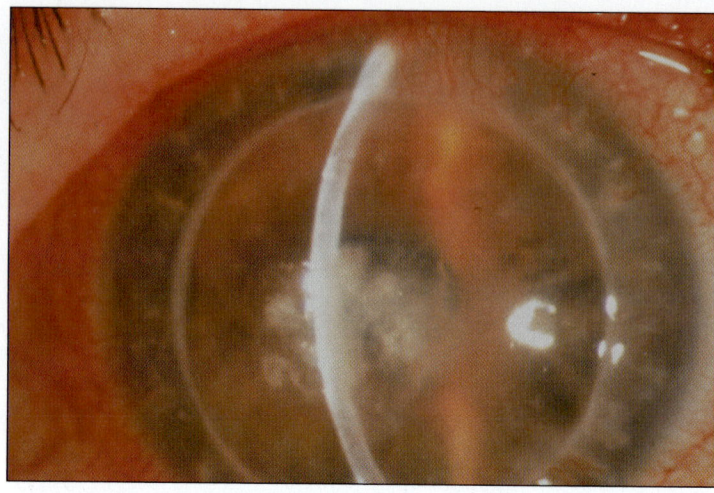

FIG. 62-5 ■ Infectious crystalline keratopathy caused by *Streptococcus viridans*.

corneal perforation, this most often represents a sterile accumulation. The aqueous might become dense and fibrinoid, and fibrinous endothelial plaques might develop.

Gram-Positive Cocci

STAPHYLOCOCCI. Staphylococci are gram-positive cocci that, on stained smears, tend to appear singly or in pairs, although clusters of organisms can be seen. Staphylococcal species are distinguished by their ability to ferment mannitol and by their ability to coagulate plasma. *S. aureus* species are, by definition, coagulase positive, and most ferment mannitol. *S. epidermidis* belongs to the group of coagulase-negative staphylococci and tends not to ferment mannitol. Although *S. aureus* is generally considered to be more pathogenic than non-*aureus* strains, mannitol fermentation is not a reliable indicator of a lack of pathogenicity. In spite of the relatively lower virulence of non-*aureus* strains, antibiotic resistance tends to be more common, and aggressive keratitis occasionally occurs.

Staphylococci are commonly found on the skin, lids, and conjunctiva and are considered opportunistic pathogens. Infection tends to occur in compromised corneas, such as those with bullous keratopathy, herpetic disease, and persistent epithelial defect. There is usually a well-defined, cream-colored or gray-white stromal infiltrate with an overlying epithelial defect. Sometimes multiple foci of abscesses can develop that resemble fungal satellite lesions. *S. aureus* tends to cause more severe infiltration and necrosis than *S. epidermidis*. Over time, the former can extend deep into the stroma, and necrosis of this abscess can lead to perforation. A hypopyon and endothelial plaque can be seen.

STREPTOCOCCI. Streptococci are gram-positive cocci. On stained smears, most species tend to appear in chains, but they can also be arranged singly, in pairs, or in loose clusters. Pneumococci are lancet-shaped diplococci arranged with the flattened ends together. Streptococcal species are distinguished by their ability to hemolyze red blood cells. *S. viridans* and *S. pneumoniae* do so partially (alpha hemolysis), *S. pyogenes* completely (beta hemolysis), and gamma-hemolytic species do not hemolyze red blood cells at all.

Pneumococci do not readily invade an intact corneal epithelium, and pneumococcal conjunctivitis rarely leads to keratitis. However, corneal infection can follow trauma, and infiltration that begins at the site of injury can readily spread (often toward the center of the cornea), producing a deep stromal abscess, fibrin deposition, plaque formation, severe anterior chamber reaction, hypopyon, and iris synechiae (Fig. 62-4). The advancing necrosis often produces an undermined leading edge with overhanging tissue. Inadequately treated keratitis often leads to perforation. *S. pyogenes* infection occurs less frequently but has a

similar, severe presentation and course. *S. viridans* tends to cause less aggressive disease and is associated with a more indolent course, as is seen in infectious crystalline keratopathy.

Infectious crystalline keratopathy describes a particular pattern of corneal infiltration characterized by needle-like opacities that can be found at all levels of the corneal stroma (Fig. 62-5). It most frequently occurs in corneal grafts but has also been associated with other conditions such as incisional keratotomy, epikeratophakia, contact lens wear, chemical burns, and topical anesthetic abuse. There is no apparent cellular infiltrate and little or no attendant ocular inflammation. This pattern is produced by the proliferation of bacteria between the lamellae of the corneal stroma without the induction of substantial corneal inflammation or necrosis.[11] Therefore, the anti-inflammatory effect of topical corticosteroids has been implicated in the lack of corneal suppuration necessary for the development of this crystalline morphology, and this pattern can also be seen in immunocompromised patients. The appearance of these crystalline opacities can range from fine, feathery, and white to thick, brown, arborizing aggregations. Some bacteria responsible for this pattern of infection can produce agents that suppress an inflammatory host response. Although the *viridans* group of streptococci accounts for most cases, other organisms associated with infectious crystalline keratopathy include *S. pneumoniae*, *Haemophilus aphrophilus*, *Peptostreptococcus*, *Pseudomonas aeruginosa*, and a number of other bacteria, as well as *Candida* and *Alternaria* fungal species.

Gram-Positive Bacilli

BACILLUS. *B. cereus* is an aerobic, spore-forming, typically gram-positive rod, although considerable variability in staining characteristics has been noted. They are ubiquitous and are found in water, in soil, and on vegetation. Corneal infection can therefore be seen after penetrating injury, especially when there is soil contamination. Bacillus infection has also been reported in contact lens–related keratitis. Post-traumatic infection characteristically develops within 24 hours of injury and is associated with chemosis, profound lid edema, and proptosis. There is often diffuse or a peripheral ring of microcystic edema, followed by a circumferential corneal abscess. This is an extremely virulent organism, and perforation of the cornea can develop within hours.

CORYNEBACTERIA. The corynebacteria, which include *C. diphtheriae*, are gram-positive, club-shaped or pleomorphic rods arranged in the so-called Chinese-letter formation, Y's, or palisades. They infrequently cause corneal disease, but diphtheria infection might be associated with pseudomembranous conjunctivitis and preauricular lymphadenopathy. The keratitis characteristically begins with diffuse epithelial haze, followed by stromal necrosis and melting. Other corynebacteria species tend to be associated with less virulent keratitis.

LISTERIA. *L. monocytogenes* is a gram-positive, short, rod-shaped facultative anaerobe. Infection usually occurs in animal handlers. It can colonize persistent epithelial defects and lead to a necrotizing keratitis. Typically, there is a ring ulcer and an exuberant anterior chamber reaction with fibrinous exudate and a hypopyon.

CLOSTRIDIUM. Clostridia are anaerobic, spore-forming, gram-positive bacilli. Infrequently, clostridial conjunctivitis can be associated with the development of a marginal keratitis. Direct corneal infection is associated with marked edema and a frothy, bullous keratitis caused by trapped intraepithelial, subepithelial, and intrastromal gas produced by the organism. Gas might also be seen in the anterior chamber.[12]

PROPIONIBACTERIUM ACNES. *P. acnes* is an anaerobic, non-spore-forming, gram-positive rod. It forms part of the normal flora of the eyelid and conjunctiva. Keratitis can be established in the event of corneal disease, trauma, surgery, contact lens wear, or chronic topical corticosteroid use.[13] Although *P. acnes* keratitis can assume the appearance of typical infectious keratitis, the infection can be indolent, with a stromal abscess covered by an intact epithelium.

Filamentous Bacteria

ACTINOMYCES AND NOCARDIA. *Actinomyces* and *Nocardia* are gram-positive, filamentous bacteria. *Actinomyces* is obligatorily anaerobic and non-acid-fast, whereas *Nocardia* is obligatorily aerobic and variably acid-fast. On Gram's stain, the filaments of these organisms are branching and intertwined; some might display terminal clubs, and the filaments often fragment into bacillary and coccoid forms.

Actinomycotic keratitis is typically part of a mixed infection with other organisms that might have different antibiotic sensitivities. Infection is rare and usually follows trauma. Typically, the ulcer bed appears dry and necrotic and is surrounded by a yellow demarcating gutter.[14] The ulcers tend to progress slowly, but ultimately, necrosis can lead to descemetocele formation, followed rapidly by perforation. Alternatively, ring abscesses have been described. Inflammation can be severe, with iritis and a hypopyon.

Nocardia infections also tend to follow trauma, especially if there is soil contamination. The ulcer is typically superficial, with irregular gray-white infiltrates and an undermined necrotic edge. The base might assume a cracked windshield appearance. *Nocardia* keratitis often resembles fungal infection, with a filamentous-appearing border and satellite lesions. Infection appears to be indolent, and the anterior chamber reaction is often minimal. However, more severe anterior chamber reaction and hypopyon can rarely be seen.

Gram-Negative Rods

PSEUDOMONAS. *P. aeruginosa* is the most common gram-negative organism isolated from corneal ulcers and is a frequent cause of contact lens–associated keratitis. These aerobic bacilli are found in moist environments and frequently contaminate inadequately chlorinated swimming pools and hot tubs, ventilators, nebulizer and vaporizer solutions, and ophthalmic solution bottles. The last have occasionally been implicated in corneal infection. The organism readily adheres to damaged epithelium, and stromal invasion is rapid.

Pseudomonas keratitis tends to progress rapidly if inadequately treated. Most commonly, the organism produces destructive enzymes such as protease, lipase, elastase, and exotoxin, which results in necrotic, soupy ulceration. The organism's surface glycocalyx protects it against phagocytosis and complement attack. The ulcer often extends peripherally and deeply within hours and can rapidly involve the entire cornea (Fig. 62-6). Ring ulcers

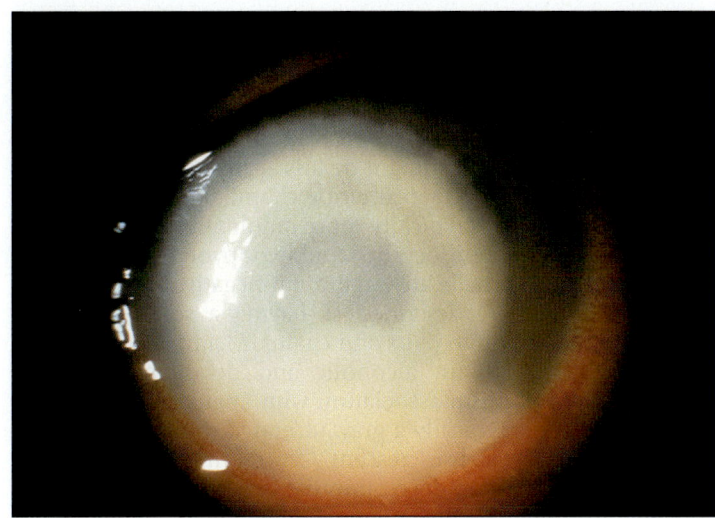

FIG. 62-6 ‖ *Pseudomonas* infection of the cornea, with liquefying necrosis, advanced central thinning, and hypopyon formation.

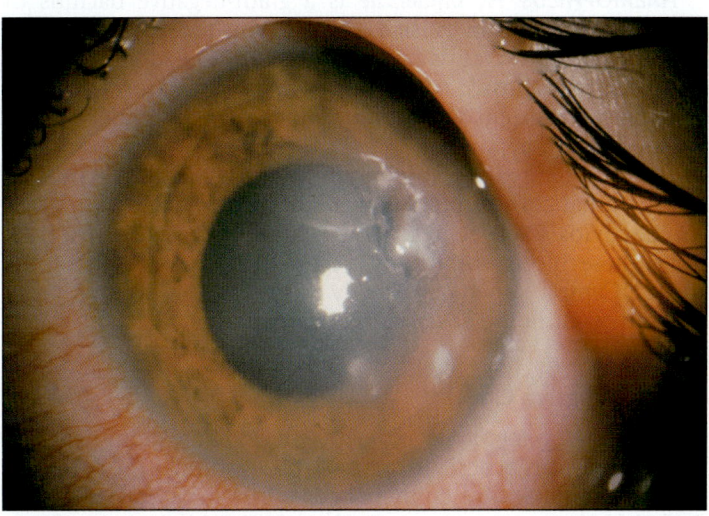

FIG. 62-7 ‖ Intraepithelial infiltration of the cornea by *Pseudomonas* organisms in a hydrophilic contact lens wearer.

can develop, and the corneal epithelium peripheral to the primary ulcer typically develops a diffuse gray, ground-glass appearance. The corneal stroma appears to dissolve into a greenish yellow mucous discharge that fluoresces under ultraviolet (but not under cobalt blue) light. The suppurative ulcer frequently thins to a descemetocele that perforates. The ulcer is often associated with a marked anterior chamber reaction and hypopyon formation. Extensive keratitis can extend to the limbus and produce an infectious scleritis.

Less virulent strains produce less aggressive corneal necrosis and follow a more indolent course. Multifocal epithelial infection can also be seen, with multiple intraepithelial gray-white nodules accompanied by a granular-appearing stromal infiltrate and anterior chamber inflammation (Fig. 62-7). Diffuse epithelial disease is most commonly seen in association with hydrophilic contact lens wear.

SERRATIA. These gram-negative rods are found in soil, water, food, and the gastrointestinal tract. Keratitis often occurs in association with hydrophilic contact lens wear. The infection may begin as a superficial central or paracentral ulcer that invades the deeper layers of the cornea, producing a deep, ring-shaped keratitis. Exotoxins and protease can produce aggressive ulceration and perforation. Contact lens–associated disease can also present with multiple gray intraepithelial nodules that assume a branching linear pattern, accompanied by a granular-appearing stromal infiltrate and anterior chamber inflammation.

ESCHERICHIA, KLEBSIELLA, AND PROTEUS. Infection by this group of gram-negative rods is associated with contact lens wear and diseased eyes. The features of corneal infection can be similar to those seen in a virulent pseudomonad infection, with aggressive necrosis, ring ulcer formation, and perforation. Alternatively, the keratitis might be less aggressive with indolent ulceration and a moderate anterior chamber reaction. *E. coli* suppurative keratitis is typically more indolent but is usually accompanied by severe iridocyclitis and hypopyon formation.

MORAXELLA. *Moraxella* are large, gram-negative (or gram-variable) bacilli that are described as having a square "boxcar" shape. They are found in pairs and chains. *Moraxella* keratitis occurs most frequently in alcoholic and debilitated patients. Marginal ulcers occur in association with angular blepharoconjunctivitis; there is typically a gray, ulcerated infiltrate separated from the limbus by a clear crescent. Central indolent ulcers also occur. These most often develop in the lower half of the cornea as a gray infiltrate that eventually forms an oval-shaped ulcer. The infection tends to extend deeply rather than peripherally and does so slowly, although the anterior chamber reaction can be vigorous. Perforation can occur but is uncommon.

HAEMOPHILUS. *H. influenzae* is a gram-negative bacillus or coccobacillus that can cause a conjunctivitis that leads to keratitis. Infrequently, keratitis has also been associated with contact lens wear and chronic corneal disease. The infection is usually superficial but extensive; it can be suppurative and might be associated with a hypopyon.

H. aegyptius are long, thin, gram-negative bacilli. The superficial marginal corneal ulcer that might be associated with acute conjunctivitis likely represents a type III hypersensitivity reaction. These ulcers commonly occur in the lower half of the cornea. Central, superficial, slowly progressive or suppurative ulcers can occur in the absence of conjunctivitis.

Gram-Negative Cocci

NEISSERIA. *N. gonorrhoeae* and *N. meningitidis* are gram-negative, intracellular diplococci. In corneal and conjunctival scrapings they are found within epithelial cells. In a newborn with ophthalmia neonatorum, gonorrheal conjunctivitis is a significant concern, because the organism can invade through an intact epithelium. Corneal infection is often peripheral and can progress to perforation and endophthalmitis. In adults, ocular gonorrhea is accompanied by a copious weeping, hyperpurulent discharge. Keratitis most commonly occurs after prolonged conjunctivitis. The transient, usually peripheral subepithelial infiltrates that might be seen likely represent a type III hypersensitivity reaction. Keratitis is characterized by diffuse edema or a ring ulcer with hypopyon, and there is a significant risk of corneal necrosis and perforation.

Meningococcal conjunctivitis can also be complicated by keratitis, although this is less common than with gonococcal conjunctivitis. Typically, the keratitis is multifocal, and a peripheral infiltrate progresses to ulceration.

BRANHAMELLA CATARRHALIS. *B. catarrhalis* is a gram-negative diplococcus that resembles *N. gonorrhoeae*. However, on smears of the conjunctiva, it is not found within epithelial cells. It can be a constituent of the normal flora of the conjunctiva and is an opportunistic pathogen. Although it can be associated with both neonatal and adult conjunctivitis, it is an infrequent cause of keratitis.

Mycobacteria

NONTUBERCULOUS MYCOBACTERIA. Of this group of organisms, *Mycobacterium fortuitum* and *M. chelonae* are most commonly associated with ocular disease, although *M. avium-intracellulare* and *M. gordonae*[15,16] have also been reported to cause infectious keratitis. These long rods are acid-fast; that is, they retain red basic fuchsin dye with Ziehl-Neelsen staining. Nontuberculous my-

cobacteria can grow in disinfectant and are found free in the environment, including soil. Keratitis most commonly follows trauma or surgery and has been associated with penetrating keratoplasty and lamellar refractive surgery. These corneal ulcers tend to be indolent and have been confused with mycotic keratitis. The infiltrated base of this typically nonsuppurative ulcer characteristically assumes a "cracked windshield" appearance, with multiple radiating lines. Satellite lesions, immune ring, and endothelial plaque formation might develop as the infection progresses.

TUBERCULOSIS. Corneal manifestations of *M. tuberculosis* include phlyctenulosis, sectoral interstitial keratitis, sclerosing keratitis, and, in association with ulcerative granuloma of the conjunctiva, tuberculous pannus. Tuberculous conjunctivitis or scleritis can also progress to produce an indolent corneal ulcer. These ulcers are associated with neovascularization and can go on to perforate. Systemic treatment is required.

MYCOBACTERIUM LEPRAE. It is estimated that 10–12 million people worldwide are affected with leprosy (Hansen's disease) due to systemic infection by *M. leprae*.[17] Ocular involvement is frequent, with estimates ranging from 6–100%.[18] The systemic and ocular manifestations of leprosy depend on the severity of disease, which is largely dictated by the host response to the organism. The clinical manifestations range from lepromatous through borderline to tuberculoid. Lepromatous disease is characterized by extensive clinical manifestations, including numerous macules, papules, plaques, and nodules over cooler areas of the body, and is associated with a weak immune response. There are numerous poorly defined skin lesions with elevated centers. The facial skin, especially over the forehead, thickens, leading to the classic leonine appearance; the ears become pendulous; and loss of the outer third of the eyebrows is common. Nasal symptoms and obstructed breathing can be early symptoms, and septal perforation and nasal collapse lead to saddlenose.

At the other extreme, tuberculoid disease is characterized by more limited clinical manifestations, relatively few lesions, and a more robust granulomatous inflammatory response. Although peripheral nerve involvement occurs in all forms of leprosy, damage to the major nerve trunks is most pronounced in the tuberculoid forms of the disease. Early skin lesions are typically hypoesthetic, hypopigmented macules with sharply demarcated borders. Peripheral neuropathy occurs early and leads to muscular atrophy and contractures. As the disease progresses, hypoesthesia of the extremities can lead to repeated trauma, ulceration, and infection, which ultimately results in resorption of the digits and severe deformity.

Involvement of the external eye and adnexa is common in all forms of leprosy. Neuropathy of the seventh nerve can lead to ectropion and lagophthalmos, resulting in exposure keratopathy. Conjunctival nodules and episcleritis can be seen in lepromatous

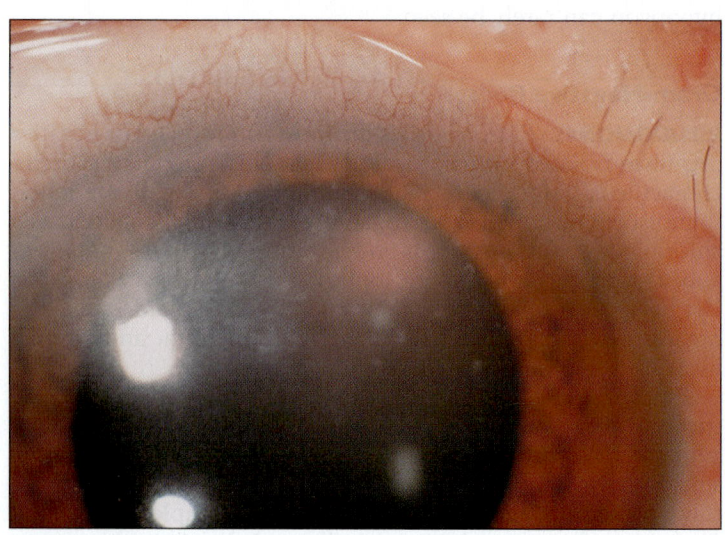

FIG. 62-8 ■ Focal avascular keratitis seen in leprosy.

disease. A number of corneal changes can be observed. Corneal nerve beading is due to aggregates of organisms and the accompanying granulomatous response typical of lepromatous disease. Lepromas consisting of *M. leprae* organisms, macrophages, and lymphocytes[19] can accumulate in the anterior stroma (although they might occasionally appear in deeper layers of the cornea), producing discrete, chalky-appearing opacities. These lesions can progress and coalesce, leading to a diffuse anterior corneal haze that, late in the course of disease, might become vascularized to produce lepromatous pannus (Fig. 62-8).

Other ocular findings include acute iritis or, more commonly, chronic iritis; iris pearls (considered pathognomonic for leprosy) that consist of white to yellow clusters of bacilli within mononuclear cells, devoid of surrounding inflammatory reaction; iris atrophy; cataract; and glaucoma. Posterior segment inflammation is uncommon, except as a consequence of scleritis.

DIAGNOSIS

The presumptive diagnosis of infectious keratitis is based primarily on the clinical history and physical examination, but confirmation of infectious (as opposed to sterile) infiltration and definitive identification of the offending organism can be achieved only by examining stained smears of corneal scrapings and laboratory cultures of these scrapings. In practice, specific identification of the offending organism and antibiotic sensitivity data are necessary only insofar as they advise modification of antibiotic treatment if the initial antibiotic regimen fails. Since approximately 95% of suspected bacterial ulcers respond favorably to a well-chosen initial antibiotic regimen,[20,21] treatment modification is rarely necessary. Many practitioners therefore defer diagnostic stains and cultures for selected cases of suspected bacterial keratitis, although the advisability of this practice, and the specific types of cases for which it is appropriate, have yet to be determined in a prospective fashion. There is some evidence, however, that small infiltrates that are not associated with advanced suppuration or severe intraocular inflammation respond favorably to this approach.[21] There is no debate that scrapings are mandatory if the infection is advanced or central or if the patient's history or the appearance of the infection is at all suggestive of filamentous bacterial, nontuberculous mycobacterial, gonococcal, mycotic, or protozoal infection.

When scrapings of corneal ulcers are obtained, material should be taken from the most active regions. The eye is anesthetized with topical anesthetic, and a heat-sterilized platinum spatula or blade is used to firmly scrape the leading edges of the ulcer. Multiple areas of a large ulcer should be sampled. If significant corneal thinning is evident, care must be exercised not to precipitate perforation. Some investigators have reported ac-

ceptable organism recovery rates with scrapings performed with a calcium alginate swab moistened with soy broth.[22] Scrapings should be placed on a slide for staining and directly applied to culture media, such as plates and broth, to maximize the chance of recovery. The commonly used culture media are described in Table 62-1. Multiple C streaks should be used on agar plates, because it is often difficult to identify an organism recovered in culture as the offending pathogen, and growth outside of the C streak might indicate contamination.

The most commonly applied stains are Gram's and Giemsa stains (Table 62-2). Gram's stain is useful to identify bacteria and yeasts, and Giemsa stain is useful for cytology and to identify bacteria (all stain blue), fungi, and chlamydia inclusions. If filamentous bacterial or nontuberculous mycobacterial infection is suspected, a Ziehl-Neelsen stain should be performed.

Corneal biopsy is indicated when an apparent infection fails to resolve in spite of antimicrobial treatment, the identity of the organism is in doubt, and conventional scrapings have failed to demonstrate a reasonably culpable organism.[23] Corneal stromal biopsy is sometimes necessary to identify protozoan, mycobacterial, or mycotic organisms. As with corneal scrapings, the corneal biopsy specimen should incorporate the active edge and base of the ulcer. If the infiltrate is sequestered within the stroma, a lamellar technique is required. Tissue obtained by biopsy should be sectioned, with a portion submitted to the pathologist for microscopic examination, and a portion used for direct inoculation of plates and broth for microbial culture and antibiotic sensitivity studies.

DIFFERENTIAL DIAGNOSIS

See Box 62-1.

SYSTEMIC ASSOCIATIONS

Mechanisms that protect the cornea from infection involve both mechanical and immunological strategies. Systemic conditions that affect the mechanical protective function of the lids due to lagophthalmos or reduced blinking include chronic alcoholism, dementia, parkinsonism, general anesthesia, and coma. Bullous conditions that affect both skin and eye, such as erythema multiforme and ocular cicatricial pemphigoid, are associated with an

TABLE 62-1

COMMON CULTURE MEDIA

Medium	Organism	Comment
Blood agar	Aerobic bacteria Saprophytic fungi	37° C for bacteria Room temperature for fungi
Chocolate agar	*Haemophilus, Neisseria, Moraxella*	5–10% CO_2
Brain-heart infusion (BHI)	Bacteria Fungi	
Sabouraud dextrose agar	Fungi	Room temperature
Enriched thioglycollate broth	Aerobic and anaerobic bacteria	Good for small inocula
Löwenstein-Jensen agar	Nontuberculous mycobacteria	
E. coli plated non-nutrient agar	*Acanthamoeba*	Transport sample to plate in Page saline

TABLE 62-2

STAINS FOR SMEARS AND CORNEAL SCRAPINGS

Stain	Organism	Comment
Gram's	Bacteria, fungi, *Acanthamoeba*, microsporidia	Stains walls of fungi
Giemsa	Bacteria, fungi, chlamydial inclusions, *Acanthamoeba*, microsporidia	All stain blue; does not demonstrate intranuclear inclusions; stains fungal cytoplasm
Gomori's methenamine silver	Fungi	Difficult technique
Ink–potassium hydroxide	Fungi	Displays fungal walls
Periodic acid–Schiff (PAS)	Fungi	
Acridine orange	Bacteria, fungi, *Acanthamoeba*	Requires fluorescent microscope
Calcofluor white	Fungi, *Acanthamoeba*	Requires fluorescent microscope
Weber	Microsporidia	
Ziehl-Neelsen	Mycobacteria, *Nocardia*, Actinomyces	

BOX 62-1

Differential Diagnosis of Corneal Infiltration and Ulceration

INFECTIOUS	NONINFECTIOUS
Bacteria	Chronic epithelial defect
Fungi	Autoimmune disease
Parasites	Rheumatoid arthritis
Acanthamoeba	Mooren's ulcer
Microsporidiosis	Terrien's marginal degeneration
Onchocerciasis	Staphylococcal marginal disease
Viruses	Phlyctenulosis
Herpes simplex virus	Contact lens-related infiltration
Varicella-zoster virus	Vernal keratoconjunctivitis (shield ulcer)
Epstein-Barr virus	Smokable drug-induced
Measles	Anesthetic abuse
Mumps	Xerophthalmia, keratomalacia
Spirochetes	
Syphilis	
Lyme disease	

increased risk of infectious keratitis due not only to lagophthalmos but also to inflammatory cicatricial conjunctival changes.

As mentioned earlier, local or systemic immune compromise might lead to impairment of local immune defenses, increasing the risk or severity of infectious keratitis. Although it is not clear that patients with systemic immune disorders such as AIDS have an increased risk of developing infectious keratitis, they sometimes follow a more fulminant or protracted course.[24] Malnutrition and conditions due to vitamin deficiency, such as xerophthalmia and scurvy, appear to increase the risk of post-traumatic infection.

PATHOLOGY

For a bacterial keratitis to become established, microbial adhesins must bind to host cell receptors. Certain adhesins not only aid in fixing bacteria to the host cells but also are toxins. Adhesion is facilitated by surface pili or a glycocalyx coat that also serves a protective function. Most commonly, bacterial adherence to the cornea requires a defect in the continuity of the corneal epithelium. Although bacteria bind to exposed corneal stroma, they appear to demonstrate increased attachment to the edges of epithelial wounds.[25]

Once attachment has occurred, the destructive processes of inflammation, necrosis, and angiogenesis can ensue. Certain bacteria produce toxins that inhibit protein synthesis and proteases, such as alkaline protease and elastase, that stimulate necrosis. They also interfere with host defense by degrading complement, immunoglobulins, interferon, interleukin-1, interleukin-2, and tumor necrosis factor.[26,27] Host lysozymal enzymes and oxidative products of neutrophils, keratocytes, and epithelial cells might also contribute significantly to stromal necrosis.[28]

Corneal infection stimulates the immigration of polymorphonuclear leukocytes (PMNs) that arrive initially via the tear film and later via proliferating limbal blood vessels. These PMNs phagocytize bacteria and necrotic stroma. Complement component C3 also appears to play a role in corneal defense.[29] If the bacterial population overwhelms the cornea's protective mechanisms, or necrosis progresses unchecked, corneal perforation and possibly endophthalmitis will result. Alternatively, if the infection is brought under control, the infiltrate will decrease in size and the epithelium will heal over the ulcer. Scar tissue is produced by activated keratocytes and transformed histiocytes. Angiogenesis might be stimulated by the inflammation, but these vessels usually regress with time.

TREATMENT

Because progression of disease with disastrous consequences can be rapid, infectious keratitis should be considered an ocular emergency. Treatment is directed toward halting the proliferation of bacteria, minimizing destructive inflammation and pain,

and encouraging corneal healing. Antibiotic therapy must be initiated promptly. Topical administration is the route of choice, because it provides rapid, high levels of drug in the cornea and anterior chamber (Table 62-3). Subconjunctival injection is associated with increased pain and inflammation, patient apprehension, and risk of globe perforation, while failing to provide enhanced corneal levels of antibiotic compared with topical drops.[30] Oral or parenteral administration establishes a relatively low level of antibiotic in the cornea and does not appear to contribute significantly to the effect of topically applied drugs.[31] Systemic antibiotics are therefore advised only when keratitis is complicated by scleritis or there is a risk of perforation or endophthalmitis. Antibiotic-soaked collagen shields can also be used to enhance topical delivery. Desiccated collagen shields are rehydrated with antibiotic and placed over the cornea. Drops are intermittently placed over the shield, which acts as a drug reservoir. Although animal models demonstrate enhanced corneal drug levels, the clinical usefulness of this method has not been established.

Significantly higher corneal levels of drug can be established with more frequent application of drops. Various schedules can be employed to rapidly achieve and maintain therapeutic levels. One such strategy is to apply a drop of antibiotic every 5 minutes for five doses, followed by a drop every 15 minutes for the next 6–12 hours. If a combination of two antibiotics is prescribed, the drops are given in an alternating fashion, so that initially a drop is applied every 5 minutes, but each antibiotic is given every 10 minutes for five doses of each. Thereafter, each antibiotic is applied every 30 minutes, but alternated so that a drop is instilled every 15 minutes, for 6–12 hours. The frequency of application is later reduced to each drop every hour. Sometimes the frequency is further reduced for a few hours during the night to allow for longer periods of sleep. Subsequent reductions are dictated by the response of the infection.

Empirical therapy must be initiated before the results of any scrapings for culture and antibiotic sensitivity testing are available to advise antibiotic choice. Although controversial, it is the opinion of many authorities that Gram's stain cannot be relied on for modification of the initial regimen, because such results do not consistently correlate with cultures, especially if the observer is inexperienced or if no organisms or multiple organisms are seen.[32] Since the effectiveness of the initial regimen is predictive of ultimate treatment success, and the consequences of not effectively treating a causative organism are dire, many authorities recommend that therapy be initiated with a broad-spectrum regimen.[33] Arguably, the advantages of this approach outweigh the disadvantages of an increased risk of antibiotic side effects and antagonism.

Broad-spectrum coverage can be achieved with a fluoroquinolone antibiotic alone or combined with another agent, or with the combination of an aminoglycoside and a cephalosporin or vancomycin (see Table 62-3). Because of concerns about emerging vancomycin resistance, initial empirical use of this antibiotic is not encouraged. Studies have reported that an initial regimen of a fluoroquinolone, or an aminoglycoside combined with a cephalosporin, is effective in approximately 95% of cases of bacterial keratitis[20,34] and have suggested that these regimens are equivalently effective in a majority of cases.

The fluoroquinolones commercially available for topical ophthalmic use are ciprofloxacin, ofloxacin, levofloxacin, gatifloxacin, and moxifloxacin. Ciprofloxacin, ofloxacin, and levofloxacin demonstrate excellent activity against gram-negative organisms, with good to excellent activity against gram-positive organisms but variable activity against anaerobes and *S. pneumoniae*.[35] Levofloxacin may offer enhanced gram-positive coverage compared with ofloxacin and ciprofloxacin,[36] but mutations that confer resistance to ciprofloxacin have been noted to confer cross-resistance to levofloxacin.[37] Ocular *S. aureus* and *P. aeruginosa* isolates that are resistant to ciprofloxacin and ofloxacin have also shown resistance to levofloxacin.[38] Gatifloxacin and moxifloxacin represent the most recently introduced generation

TABLE 62-3

COMMONLY USED ANTIBIOTICS FOR THE TREATMENT OF BACTERIAL KERATITIS

Antibiotic	Concentration	Route	Activity
Aminoglycosides			Gram-negatives, staphylococci, some streptococci (not pneumococcus)
Amikacin	6.7mg/ml	Topical	Also active against nontuberculous mycobacteria
	50mg/ml	Subconjunctival	
Gentamicin	14mg/ml	Topical	
	40mg/ml	Subconjunctival	
Tobramycin	14mg/ml	Topical	
	40mg/ml	Subconjunctival	
Cephalosporins			Active against non-penicillinase-producing gram-positive organisms, some gram-negative bacilli
Cefazolin	75–100mg/ml	Topical	
	200mg/ml	Subconjunctival	
Fluoroquinolones			Active against gram-negatives, fair to good against gram-positives, variable against anaerobes and pneumococcus
Ciprofloxacin	3mg/ml	Topical	
Ofloxacin	3mg/ml	Topical	
Levofloxacin	3mg/ml	Topical	
Gatifloxacin	3mg/ml	Topical	Improved gram-positive activity, as well as activity against nontuberculous mycobacteria
Moxifloxacin	5mg/ml	Topical	Improved gram-positive activity, as well as activity against nontuberculous mycobacteria
Penicillins			
Penicillin G	100,000U/ml	Topical	Active against non-penicillinase-producing gram-positive organisms
	1,000,000U/ml	Subconjunctival	
Methicillin	50mg/ml	Topical	Active against penicillinase-producing gram-positive organisms
	200mg/ml	Subconjunctival	
Piperacillin	7mg/ml	Topical	Active against gram-positives and some gram-negatives, including *Pseudomonas*
	200mg/ml	Subconjunctival	
Vancomycin	33mg/ml	Topical	Active against gram-positive organisms, including methicillin-resistant staphylococci
	100mg/ml	Subconjunctival	

of fluoroquinolones that demonstrate improved activity against gram-positive pathogens, including *S. epidemidis, S. aureus,* and *S. pneumoniae,* as well as excellent activity against atypical pathogens such as non-tuberculous mycobacteria *Mycoplasma, Legionella, Chlamydia* species and the anaerobic *Propionibacterium acnes.*

Because of the broad gram-positive and gram-negative coverage provided by fluoroquinolones, their ready commercial availability, and the minimal discomfort on instillation, topical ophthalmic fluoroquinolone use has rapidly increased in the community over the last few years. Parenteral use of fluoroquinolones has also greatly increased, leading to the emergence of more widespread resistance in numerous strains of *S. aureus,*[39,40] *E. coli,*[41] and *N. gonorrhoeae*[42] among others. Surveys of resistance patterns seen in ocular isolates have demonstrated increasing earlier generation fluoroquinolone resistance to common causes of infectious keratitis, such as *P. aeruginosa*[43,44] and staphylococcal,[40,45,46] and streptococcal species.[40,45,46]

Based on the observed emergence of resistance to ocular isolates, fluoroquinolone monotherapy should be applied with great caution and with careful observation for a clinical response particularly with regards to the earlier generation compounds. Patients considered for fluoroquinolone monotherapy should be limited to those at lowest risk for infection with potentially resistant gram-positive organisms (e.g., contact lens–related infiltrates) and at low risk for rapid advancement with visual compromise (small size; minimal infiltration and necrosis; peripheral; no history or appearance suggestive of filamentous bacterial, non-tuberculous mycobacterial, gonococcal, mycotic, or protozoal infection). Later generation fluoroquinolone (moxifloxacin and gatifloxacin) should be considered for cases likely to be caused by gram-positive organisms.

The aminoglycosides most commonly used for the treatment of infectious keratitis are gentamicin and tobramycin. Both are prepared at a "fortified" concentration of 10–20mg/ml. These antibiotics provide excellent gram-negative coverage and are also active against staphylococci and some streptococci but not against pneumococcus. Whereas gentamicin appears to be effective against

a greater number of streptococci,[32] tobramycin appears to be more active *in vivo* against *P. aeruginosa.*[47] Both tend to inhibit epithelial wound healing and can cause a punctate epitheliopathy.

The cephalosporin most commonly used for the treatment of infectious keratitis is cefazolin. These compounds are effective against non-penicillinase-producing gram-positive organisms, as well as some gram-negative bacilli such as *E. coli, Klebsiella,* and *P. mirabilis.* Cefazolin is relatively nontoxic to the corneal epithelium.

The penicillins are effective against many gram-positive organisms such as streptococcal and staphylococcal species, as well as gonococcal and some anaerobic species. However, many staphylococcal strains produce beta-lactamase, which inactivates penicillin. There is also a 10% rate of allergic reaction to penicillins. The semisynthetic penicillins such as dicloxacillin, methicillin, and nafcillin are useful against penicillinase-producing staphylococci but will incite an allergic reaction in patients sensitive to penicillin. The extended-spectrum penicillins such as amoxicillin, ampicillin, piperacillin, and ticarcillin have broad-spectrum activity against gram-positive and gram-negative organisms such as pseudomonad species, but they are ineffective as independent agents against penicillinase-producing staphylococci. The penicillin and penicillin-derived antibiotics can be administered both topically and subconjunctivally.

Vancomycin is a useful agent against staphylococcal organisms when cephalosporins or penicillin and penicillin-related compounds are ineffective or poorly tolerated. To minimize the development of resistance, empirical therapy is not encouraged.[48] Subconjunctival injections are not recommended, since sloughing can result.

Amikacin is a semisynthetic aminoglycoside that is useful in the treatment of infection due to gram-negative organisms resistant to gentamicin and tobramycin. It is also active against nontuberculous mycobacterial organisms.

Although empirical therapy with a fluoroquinolone or a first-generation cephalosporin and aminoglycoside is effective and equivalent in a majority of cases, microbiological investigation may reveal an organism that requires a modification of therapy for effective treatment. For example, fluoroquinolone treatment is significantly more effective in the treatment of Neisseria infection than is an aminoglycoside combined with a cephalosporin. *N. gonorrhoeae* should be treated systemically with 125–250mg of intramuscular ceftriaxone. Alternatively, 1g intravenous penicillin G can be given four times daily for 5–10 days. The conjunctival sac should be irrigated frequently with normal saline, followed by topical administration of a fluoroquinolone antibiotic solution. Meningococcal infections should be treated with 6 million units of intravenous penicillin G every 6 hours for 7–10 days, along with a topical fluoroquinolone.

Actinomyces infections are treated with topical sulfacetamide or penicillin. Penicillin can also be administered subconjunctivally, along with systemic iodides. Nocardia infection is also responsive to treatment with sulfonamides. A combination of trimethoprim and sulfamethoxazole should be administered both topically and systemically. In cases of filamentous bacterial infection, lamellar or penetrating keratoplasty may reduce the load of the infected tissue and promote healing.

Nontuberculous mycobacterial keratitis has been successfully treated with fluoroquinolone antibiotics, and some infections respond well to topically applied amikacin. The fourth-generation fluoroquinolone gatifloxacin and moxifloxacin have been shown to be particularly effective against these organisms. Combination therapy of amikacin and a fourth-generation fluoroquinolone should be considered. Prolonged therapy of these recalcitrant infections is often necessary, and in certain cases, lamellar or penetrating keratoplasty might be necessary. The treatment of leprosy requires a broad multidisciplinary approach and prolonged systemic antimicrobial therapy. Standard practice in the United States is to treat paucibacillary disease with a combination of dapsone and rifampin, and multibacillary disease with a combination of dapsone, rifampin, and clofazimine or ethionamide.

Modification of treatment is required if the infection fails to improve. The strongest argument in favor of pretreatment scrapings is that if organisms are recovered, laboratory data might be available to advise any necessary changes in the antibiotic regimen. Whether or not pretreatment scrapings were obtained, samples for smears and culture and sensitivity studies must be obtained from corneal ulcers that fail to improve. In the case of indolent infections, antibiotic treatment might be interrupted for 24–48 hours to decrease the inhibitory effect of antibiotic treatment and therefore increase the probability of recovering the organism. If antibiotic sensitivity studies are available, these data can be used as a relative guide in choosing antibiotics that might have a higher probability of eradicating the offending microbe.

It is important to recognize that these data serve only as a guide. Antibiotic sensitivities are measured by disc diffusion or, more commonly, by serial dilution methods, and they report minimum inhibitory concentration (MIC) and minimum lethal concentration (MLC). Whether a particular organism is described as "sensitive" to a particular antibiotic is, for most laboratories, based not on the expected corneal concentration of the antibiotic but on the expected serum concentration. With frequent application of a fortified preparation, relatively high corneal concentrations of many antibiotics can be established; therefore, organisms cultured from a corneal infiltrate may be reported as "resistant" to a particular antibiotic but respond to treatment because of the effect of high local concentration.[49]

If no organism is recovered in bacterial culture and the disease worsens, noninfectious and nonbacterial causes of ulcerative keratitis must be considered (see Box 62-1). Appropriate cultures for nontuberculous mycobacteria, fungi, and protozoal organisms should be obtained, and corneal biopsy might be necessary. Corneal stromal necrosis might progress in spite of effective antimicrobial treatment because of the lytic activity of immigrant leukocytes. Immunological ring infiltrates can appear many days after the initiation of effective antimicrobial treatment and might be erroneously interpreted to indicate worsening of the infection.

The initial sign of effective treatment is failure of the infiltrate to worsen; however, it is not uncommon for ulcers to initially worsen before stabilizing, even with an effective initial antibiotic regimen. The early signs of a resolving infection include stabilization of the area and depth of the infiltrate and reduced activity at the infiltrate's margins. Signs of continuing improvement include progressive healing of the epithelial defect, clearing of the infiltrate, reduced corneal edema adjacent to the infiltrate, and decreasing inflammation and anterior chamber reaction.

If a single antibiotic is chosen initially and is effective in treating the infection, there is seldom a reason to change medicines. If a combination of antibiotics is initially effective, administration of the less effective (by sensitivity studies) of the two can often be halted after a few days. Fortified preparations can be replaced by commercial preparations, and the frequency of application can be gradually tapered. Treatment should be continued at least until the epithelium has completely healed. *P. aeruginosa* can reappear after apparent resolution if treatment is halted early, and antibiotic administration should be maintained for at least a week after epithelial healing.

Aside from antimicrobial therapy, adjunctive treatments have been employed in an effort to minimize the adverse sequelae of corneal infection such as perforation, vascularization, and scarring. Corticosteroids can be used to suppress the inflammatory response that leads to these adverse sequelae. However, the precise role that corticosteroids should play in the treatment of bacterial corneal infections is poorly defined. In this setting, corticosteroids have been associated with inhibition of wound healing, and if antibiotic therapy is inadequate, corticosteroids have been found to promote bacterial replication. Corticosteroids should therefore not be used if there is doubt about the efficacy of the antimicrobial regimen. It is safest to add these agents after there is initial evidence of successful antibiotic treatment. Nonsteroidal anti-inflammatory agents might also help reduce the adverse sequelae of infectious inflammation, but again, they should be used only in the presence of effective antimicrobial treatment.[50]

Cycloplegic agents can be useful in reducing discomfort due to ciliary body spasm, and they can be used periodically to decrease synechiae formation. Collagenase inhibitors such as acetylcysteine and heparin have not proved to be clinically useful in reducing stromal necrosis.

If necrosis progresses to perforation, surgical intervention is warranted. Small perforations that do not exist within an extensive bed of necrotic material can be treated by the application of cyanoacrylate glue (Fig. 62-9). If the perforation is large or necrosis is extensive, penetrating keratoplasty might be necessary. There is evidence that favorable surgical results might be achieved in this setting,[51] although the procedure can be complicated by the difficulties involved in operating on a perforated globe, concurrent infection, and inflammation that threatens graft success.

Conjunctival flaps can be used to treat infections that fail to improve with medical therapy, and they might be especially useful in peripheral infectious ulceration. The vascularized conjunctival tissue helps admit blood vessels that aid in healing and scarring. Conjunctival flaps should not be placed over a corneal perforation.

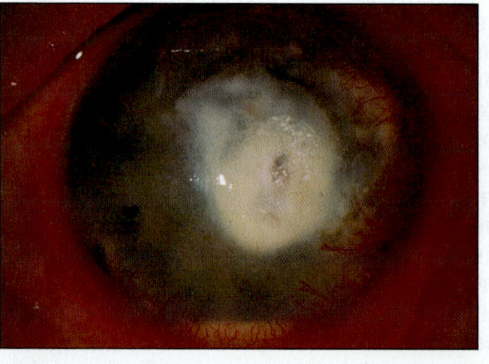

FIG. 62-9 ▮ Bacterial infection leading to central necrosis, thinning, and perforation, sealed with cyanoacrylate tissue adhesive.

OUTCOME

The visual outcomes of bacterial keratitis vary greatly. Relatively small infiltrates that do not involve the entrance pupil might leave stromal scarring that is only faintly discerned on slit-lamp examination and has no visual consequence; more extensive ulceration and infiltration can result in significant scarring and irregular astigmatism. Although it tends to fade over time, residual scarring can be visually debilitating. Persistent anterior stromal scars can sometimes be removed by excimer laser phototherapeutic keratectomy, but deeper scars require lamellar or penetrating keratoplasty. In the absence of significant opacification, irregular astigmatism is best treated with a rigid contact lens.

Corneal inflammation can lead to neovascularization; these vessels may regress with time, and regression might be aided by corticosteroid therapy. Ocular inflammation can also lead to synechiae formation, elevated intraocular pressure, and cataract.

VIRAL KERATITIS

INTRODUCTION

Viruses are obligate intracellular parasites that contain only one type of nucleic acid within the infectious unit and are unable to replicate by binary fission. Viruses that cause corneal disease with significant ocular morbidity include herpes simplex (HSV), varicella-zoster (VZV), Epstein-Barr (EBV), and adenovirus. Cytomegalovirus (CMV) can also cause keratitis and may become more a common entity in association with AIDS.

HERPES SIMPLEX VIRAL KERATITIS

Epidemiology and Pathogenesis

HSV, VZV, EBV, and CMV are all members of the family Herpesviridae. These are DNA viruses whose central core is surrounded by a protein capsid, all enclosed within an envelope of glycoprotein, lipid, and carbohydrate. There are two types of HSV; HSV-1 is more commonly associated with labial and ocular infection, and HSV-2 with genital infection. Formerly, it was presumed that this pattern was explained by a preference for HSV-1 to inhabit the trigeminal ganglion and HSV-2 to inhabit the sacral, but recent evidence has suggested that HSV-1 and HSV-2 are found equally in each site. Therefore, it is more likely that local host factors are responsible for different patterns of recurrence.[52]

Ocular herpes simplex infection is a leading cause of corneal blindness in the developing world. Although difficult to accurately assess, the estimated prevalence is approximately 150 per 100,000 population.[53] Experimental infection can be induced in other animals, but humans are the exclusive natural hosts of HSV, and infection is ubiquitous. HSV can be identified in the cadaveric trigeminal ganglia of 18% of people younger than 21 years and nearly 100% of those older than 60 years.[54] The virus is transmitted by direct contact and has an incubation period of 1–28 days. Although the initial infection is subclinical in 94–99% of cases, all infected individuals continue to carry the virus. Saliva droplet transmission commonly leads to oral infection, which can then be transmitted to the eye via the trigeminal nerve. Ocular HSV-2 infection is likely spread directly by oculogenital contact or via contaminated fingers. Infection of newborns might occur via the placenta but is far more commonly a consequence of vaginal infection, either ascending to infect the fetus or infecting it as it passes through the birth canal. Ocular infection occurs in about 20% of cases of neonatal HSV infection.[55]

Corneal scarring and decreased visual acuity due to ocular HSV infection are usually due to recurrent disease. Approximately 15% of patients suffer significant decreased visual acuity due to recurrent infections experienced over 3–15 years.[56] Recurrence rates are estimated to be 10–20% within 1 year, 20–30% within 2 years, 40% within 5 years, and 60% at 20 years.[53,57] The time between recurrences can be very variable and ranges from weeks to decades, although the disease course in some individuals appears to be characterized by short intervals between repeated attacks.[57] A multitude of potential risk factors for the recurrence of ocular HSV disease has been identified, including stress, trauma, surgery, and menstrual period. Since ultraviolet radiation appears to be associated with increased recurrence, excimer laser photoablation is also considered a risk. Malnourishment and measles infection, which might accompany vitamin A deficiency in the developing world, have also been associated with severe and bilateral ulcerative herpes keratitis.[58] States of immunocompromise such as inherited immune disorder, chemotherapy, and severe burns have been associated with bilateral and severe recurrent disease.[59] It is not clear that the immunocompromise seen in AIDS leads to a greater incidence of ocular HSV infection, but when contracted, the disease appears to follow a more prolonged course with more frequent recurrences.[60,61]

Fortunately, ocular HSV tends to be a unilateral disease, with only one eye affected by primary disease in approximately 80–90% of cases.[62] Atopy appears to be a significant risk factor for bilateral disease, which has also been associated with diseases such as gastric cancer, lumbar zoster, malaria, and pulmonary tuberculosis.[57]

Clinical Features

The clinical manifestations of HSV disease can be categorized by congenital and neonatal infection, primary infection, and recurrent disease.

NEONATAL INFECTION. Because of its association with maternal genital herpetic infection, about 80% of neonatal HSV infection is by the type 2 virus.[63] The disease can remain localized to the eye, can specifically affect the central nervous system, or can be widely disseminated, involving multiple organs including the eye. Because of the potential seriousness of systemic herpetic infection, neonates must be treated promptly with systemic acyclovir.

At presentation, neonatal ocular HSV can include conjunctivitis, epithelial or stromal keratitis, cataract, iridocyclitis, iris atrophy and synechiae, chorioretinitis, and optic neuritis.[64] The visual prognosis is best for disease restricted to the anterior segment, since immune-mediated destruction is limited in neonates. Late sequelae of neonatal ocular HSV infection include strabismus, chorioretinal scarring, optic atrophy, and cortical blindness.

PRIMARY INFECTION. Neonates are usually protected by maternal antibodies against HSV infection throughout the first 6 months of life. Thereafter, primary infection by HSV-1 usually occurs within the first few years of life. Transmission is most commonly via contaminated adult saliva, with an incubation period of 3–12 days. It is much more common for primary disease to involve the oral mucosa than the eye, and the disease is often subclinical or mild.

Primary ocular and periocular disease in all age groups is less common. Periocular disease is characterized by a vesicular or ulcerative blepharitis, and ocular disease by a unilateral acute follicular conjunctivitis that can become pseudomembranous or demonstrate dendrites (Fig. 62-10). Both ocular and periocular

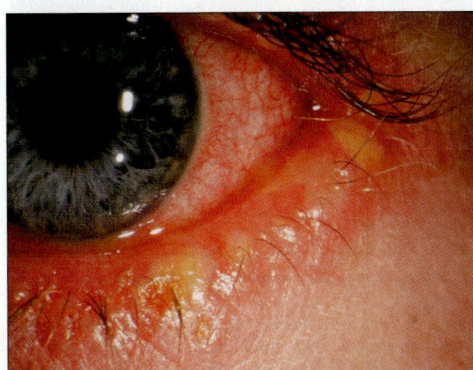

FIG. 62-10 ■ Vesicles of the eyelid caused by herpes simplex virus primary infection.

disease might be accompanied by fever, malaise, and local lymphadenopathy. Keratitis, which is seen in a third to a half of cases, tends to lag conjunctivitis and lid disease by 1–2 weeks. Corneal signs are usually confined to the epithelium and are diffuse but variable in morphology. There can be diffuse punctate epitheliopathy, evolving microdendrites, typical dendrites, or geographical ulcers. Infrequently, stromal keratitis or iridocyclitis can occur in primary disease. Whereas the vesicular lid lesions and conjunctivitis tend to resolve over 2 weeks, corneal disease can be more persistent.

RECURRENT INFECTION. Recurrent disease most often affects the cornea, but lid and conjunctival disease can occur in the form of a follicular conjunctivitis, lid vesicles, and blepharitis. Recurrent corneal disease can affect any or all layers of the cornea. The characteristic epithelial lesions are dendrites: thin, meandering, arborizing epithelial ulcerations, sometimes with terminal bulbs at the ends of fine branches (Fig. 62-11). This morphology probably represents a pattern of cell-to-cell viral spread. The central ulcerated area stains with fluorescein dye, whereas the peripheral cells that contain live virus stain with rose bengal. These dendrites might be observed to evolve from fine, opaque epithelial lesions that coalesce and enlarge. Dendrites can be multiple, and recurrent lesions tend to occur in the same area. Herpetic dendrites might resolve spontaneously or with treatment over 1–2 weeks, or they can develop into geographical ulcers, which are larger serpiginous areas of ulceration with heaped edges and various degrees of underlying stromal opacity. These lesions can be very slow to heal, and epithelial defects can persist after live virus has been eradicated. Decreased corneal sensation accompanies corneal lesions. During earlier episodes, the decreased sensation tends to be localized to the area of the lesion, but with repeated recurrences, the hypoesthesia becomes more diffuse.

Epithelial defects might also recur after live virus disappears, assuming a round, oval, or dendritic form. These postinfectious or "metaherpetic" ulcers have heaped edges of epithelial cells that fail to migrate over the ulcer bed, as opposed to the flatter edges of actively infected ulcers. These metaherpetic ulcers can also be distinguished from infected ulcers, in that the base of the former stains with both rose bengal and fluorescein, whereas the bed of the latter stains only with fluorescein. Poor healing is probably due to basement membrane damage, stromal denervation, tear film instability, and persistent inflammation.[65] Over time, these ulcers can lead to corneal perforation.

Recurrent keratitis can also involve the corneal stroma. Stromal disease might be immune related or infectious, or it may invoke combined mechanisms. The commonly described patterns of stromal herpetic disease include disciform edema, necrotizing stromal keratitis, and immune ring formation. In disciform edema, the dominant feature is disc-shaped stromal edema without neovascularization or necrosis; it can be focal in milder disease, but is extensive and diffuse in more severe disease. Folds in Descemet's membrane might accompany the corneal thickening, and keratic precipitates accumulate under the area of edema, with or without a mild anterior chamber reaction.

In necrotizing stromal keratitis, there is inflammatory necrosis with infiltration of the cornea by PMNs, macrophages, lymphocytes, and plasma cells.[66] This cellular infiltration produces stromal edema and necrosis (Fig. 62-12). The necrotizing focus can be located at any level of the corneal stroma, with or without epithelial ulceration. Ring infiltrates that resemble those seen in fungal and Acanthamoeba keratitis might develop. In some cases, diffuse patches of infiltration appear beneath an intact epithelium, followed by local neovascularization, the so-called interstitial keratitis pattern. Lipid deposition, stromal melting, descemetocele formation, and perforation are all potential complications of advanced necrotizing stromal keratitis. If the peripheral cornea is involved, inflammation and necrosis can spread to the sclera, producing a sclerokeratitis.

Sometimes the corneal endothelium appears to be primarily affected. Typically, a line of endothelial precipitates resembling a corneal rejection line develops that demarcates an overlying zone of stromal edema. Endotheliitis is sometimes accompanied by trabeculitis, which often results in elevated intraocular pressure. In some cases of ocular HSV, a recurrent, nongranulomatous iridocyclitis is the dominant feature. In some cases, live virus has been recovered from the aqueous.[67] Herpetic uveitis can be accompanied by a fibrinoid reaction, hypopyon, and synechiae formation.

Diagnosis

The diagnosis of neonatal, primary, and recurrent ocular HSV disease is based on a constellation of history, physical examination, examination of smears, and viral culture. More recently, the polymerase chain reaction (PCR) has provided an effective means of identifying minute quantities of HSV viral DNA in tissue samples and pathological specimens, aqueous, and tears.

The history should include questions concerning past episodes of conjunctivitis or keratitis. Physical examination should include an assessment of corneal sensation, and the epithelium's staining characteristics should be evaluated with fluorescein and rose bengal dye. Giemsa-stained smears of corneal scrapings might reveal mononuclear cells, PMNs, multinucleated giant epithelial cells, and eosinophilic Lipschütz inclusion bodies in cell nuclei. The last are best seen with Papanicolaou's stain.

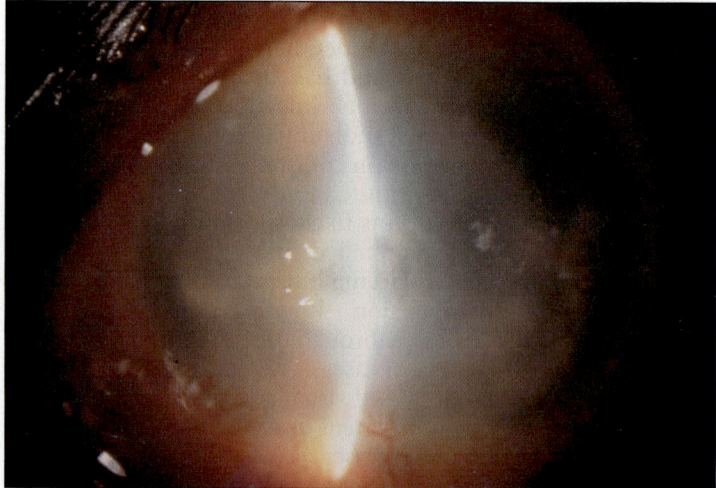

FIG. 62-11 ■ Dendritic lesions of recurrent herpes simplex epithelial disease. *Left,* unstained. *Right,* stained with fluorescein and rose bengal.

FIG. 62-12 ■ Active necrotizing stromal disease of recurrent herpes simplex infection. Note the central corneal infiltration and thinning, inflammation, and hypopyon formation.

A definitive diagnosis might be made with viral culture if active virus is present. If viral cultures are contemplated, rose bengal stain should be deferred until cultures are obtained, since this dye has antiviral properties. Enzyme-linked immunosorbent assay (ELISA) tests are available that identify viral antigens, whether or not live virus is present. HSV antigen can also be identified by direct immunofluorescence, but this technique is less sensitive than ELISA or tissue culture. PCR techniques can be applied to a wide range of tissue sources, and recent reports have described techniques for the detection of HSV in tear samples.[68]

Recurrent as opposed to primary disease can be distinguished on the basis of serum assays of HSV titers separated by 4–6 weeks. Because of fluctuations in titers, comparative assays are not useful in identifying specific episodes of recurrent disease.

Differential Diagnosis

The differential diagnosis of corneal ulceration is described in Box 62-1, and the distinguishing features of HSV and VZV epithelial disease are listed in Table 62-4. Since the stromal inflammation of VZV is intrinsically indistinguishable from that of HSV, other clinical elements such as history, recurrence patterns, and associated skin lesion should be considered in distinguishing the two conditions. Other causes of disciform and necrotizing stromal keratitis include EBV, mumps, and syphilis.

HSV disease should be suspected in a child with a follicular or pseudomembranous conjunctivitis, but this might also represent adenoviral or chlamydial disease. Lid vesicles that might signify HSV disease can also be seen in vaccinia, zoster, and chickenpox. Of note, it is important that fungal or Acanthamoeba keratitis be considered along with HSV disease in the differential diagnosis of disciform keratitis or a ring infiltrate. It might be difficult to distinguish recurrent herpetic disease in a corneal graft from endothelial rejection, but keratic precipitates in the latter are more likely to be confined to the graft.

Systemic Associations

Neonatal ocular herpes can be associated with disseminated systemic disease or central nervous system disease, as noted earlier. Lesions can involve the eyes, mucosa, or skin, and skin lesions can resemble the dermatomal clusters of herpes zoster. Hepatosplenomegaly might develop, and the lungs and adrenal glands can also be involved. Central nervous system infection produces meningeal signs, as well as convulsions, stupor, and coma. This infection can be fatal within a week. Due to the potential severity of neonatal HSV disease, systemic antiviral treatment in cooperation with neonatal specialists is mandatory.

Although the majority of primary infections are subclinical, they can be associated with fever, malaise, myalgia, and regional lymphadenopathy. Recurrent disease can also cause these symptoms, but they tend to be less acute and severe. Skin lesions can occur anywhere on the body. They tend not to scar, so long as secondary infection does not develop.

TABLE 62-4

DISTINGUISHING FEATURES OF DENDRITES ASSOCIATED WITH HERPES SIMPLEX VIRUS (HSV) VERSUS VARICELLA-ZOSTER VIRUS (VZV)

Feature	HSV	VZV
Overall appearance	Fine, lacy	Thick, ropy
Epithelium	Linear defect with bared stroma, surrounded by edematous epithelial cells	Elevated, painted-on appearance
Staining	Base stains with fluorescein, diseased border epithelial cells stain with rose bengal	Minimal fluorescein staining
Terminal bulbs	Frequent	None

Generalized herpetic infections can occur in atopic and immunosuppressed patients. Skin lesions are often atypical, and oral lesions can be persistent. Visceral organs can be affected, including hepatitis without jaundice and tender splenomegaly. Meningoencephalitis is unrelated to the patient's immune status and can be fatal. Infection is characterized by headache, meningeal signs, confusion, and coma.

Pathology

HSV disease is established on initial infection. The initial replication of the virus occurs at the peripheral site of infection (skin, mucosa, conjunctiva), but thereafter, the virus spreads by way of sensory nerves to neuronal cell bodies of ganglia, such as the trigeminal, ciliary, or sympathetic, or to the mesocephalic nucleus of the brainstem, where a latent infection is established. When reactivation is stimulated, the neuron begins to shed live virus, which is transported to the periphery. Further viral replication can occur there.

Epithelial disease marked by dendrite formation results from lysis of infected cells and cell-to-cell transfer of released virus. Whereas epithelial disease is dominated by live virus damage, stromal and endothelial disease involves both live virus activity and the immune reaction to viral antigen. In disciform edema, it has been proposed that live virus infection might lead to endothelial cell lysis and subsequent endothelial dysfunction and stromal edema.[69,70] However, at this time, viral particles have not yet been definitively identified in human endothelium obtained from corneas with disciform disease. Experimental evidence provides stronger support for the theory that stromal edema might be attributed to a delayed-type hypersensitivity reaction against HSV antigens in the corneal stroma or endothelium.[66,70]

Live virus has been isolated from some corneas demonstrating stromal disease, which implies that along with viral antigen, active infection might play a role in the immunopathology of necrotizing and interstitial keratitis.[66] However, the relative importance of these factors is not known. In necrotizing disease, the cellular infiltrate consists of PMNs, macrophages, lymphocytes, and plasma cells. The precise mechanism of immunopathology mediated by these cells is unknown, but both delayed-type hypersensitivity and cytotoxic T cell mechanisms have been implicated. Studies of the role of cytokines, including interleukin-1 and tumor necrosis factor-α, suggest that these inflammatory cytokines are upregulated in corneas experiencing recurrent HSV and might be expected to promote destructive inflammation through chemotaxis and activation of inflammatory and antigen-presenting cells, upregulation of adhesion molecules, enhancement of neovascularization, and function as a cofactor in lymphocyte activation.[71]

The diverse manifestations of ocular HSV disease may be caused by immune features of the host as well as by the varying characteristics of different HSV strains. Isolates associated with epithelial as opposed to stromal disease have been distinguished on the basis of the identity and quantity of soluble glycoprotein released in vitro.

Treatment

Antiviral agents commonly used in the treatment of ocular HSV are listed in Table 62-5. In the United States, trifluridine is the first drug of choice for topical treatment, since it has far greater solubility (and thus ocular penetration) than idoxuridine (IDU). It also appears to induce less epithelial toxicity than IDU and can be effective in the treatment of vidarabine (ara-A)– and IDU-resistant cases, since resistance to trifluridine is rare. In Europe, topical acyclovir is popularly used, since it has excellent transepithelial corneal penetration and antiviral activity and demonstrates less epithelial toxicity than trifluridine, ara-A, and IDU. At present, it is available in the United States for investigational use only.

TABLE 62-5

ANTIVIRAL MEDICINES USED IN THE TREATMENT OF HERPES SIMPLEX VIRUS OCULAR DISEASE

Antiviral	Route	Form	Frequency	Action
Idoxuridine (IDU)	Topical	0.1% solution	Hourly while awake	Inhibits viral thymidine kinase, thymidylate kinase, and DNA polymerase
Vidarabine (ara-A)	Topical	3% ointment	5 times daily	Inhibits viral DNA polymerase
Trifluridine	Topical	1% solution	Every 2 hours while awake	Inhibits viral thymidylate synthetase
Acyclovir	Topical Oral	3% ointment	5 times daily 400mg 5 times daily	Activated by viral thymidine kinase to inhibit DNA polymerase

Topical antiviral treatment is associated with significant toxicity, and oral antiviral therapy provides an effective alternative. Oral acyclovir administered at a dose of 400mg five times a day has been shown to establish excellent trough levels in the tear film and to provide effective therapy for corneal herpetic disease.[72] Other antimicrobials such as valacyclovir or penciclovir that are known to be effective against herpesviruses are also presumed to be effective. Famciclovir, the oral pro-drug of penciclovir, has been demonstrated to be effective in a rabbit model of HSV corneal disease.[73]

In order to better define, among other issues, the role of oral antiviral agents and topical corticosteroids in the treatment and prevention of recurrent HSV ocular disease, a prospective, placebo-controlled, masked study termed the Herpetic Eye Disease Study (HEDS) was conducted at multiple sites around the United States. The results of this study have greatly influenced the treatment rationale for herpetic eye disease and are discussed in the following paragraphs whenever applicable.

BLEPHARITIS AND CONJUNCTIVITIS. Although it generally resolves without scarring, herpes blepharitis is treated by some practitioners with topical antiviral agents to minimize the risk of corneal infection. Although follicular conjunctivitis is often not treated with antiviral agents, they are sometimes used if conjunctival dendrites appear, and the drugs are continued until their resolution.

DENDRITIC EPITHELIAL DISEASE WITHOUT STROMAL INVOLVEMENT. Infected epithelial cells should be débrided by rolling a cotton-tipped applicator over the lesion, followed by application of a topical antiviral agent or initiation of an oral agent (see Table 62-5). The agent should be used until the epithelial ulcer has healed and then continued for 3 more days. Topical antiviral agents exert a considerable toxic effect on the epithelium that can contribute to poor epithelial healing or the development of a punctate keratopathy. This should be considered, especially in cases of prolonged treatment, and oral antiviral treatment can be a useful and effective alternative. A cycloplegic agent can provide some measure of relief from mild iridocyclitis. Corticosteroids are generally not administered for epithelial disease without significant stromal involvement.

The HEDS evaluated the effect of a 3-week course of oral acyclovir administered prophylactically against subsequent HSV stromal keratitis or iritis in patients concurrently treated with topical trifluridine.[74] No apparent benefit was observed.

STROMAL KERATITIS. The use of corticosteroids in the treatment of stromal keratitis has been the subject of active debate. Although corticosteroids can be useful in reducing destructive corneal inflammation, they have been implicated in prolonging the duration of infection and increasing the risk of secondary complications. In a study of the effect of topical corticosteroids for herpes simplex stromal keratitis, the HEDS investigators concluded that along with topical antiviral therapy, corticosteroid application reduced the persistence or progression of stromal inflammation and shortened the duration of stromal keratitis.[75] Because inflammation tends to flare as the corticosteroid drops are tapered, a high initial concentration and frequent application should be followed by a careful and gradual taper of corticosteroids.

The HEDS investigation of the role of oral acyclovir along with topical corticosteroids and topical antivirals did not find oral acyclovir to be of benefit in addition to topical Viroptic,[76] but it is expected to be at least as effective as Viroptic as a single agent.

POSTINFECTIOUS ULCERS. In the event of persistent epithelial defect or progressive thinning, active viral infection or secondary bacterial infection should be ruled out. If the ulcer is truly metaherpetic, an antiviral agent serves no purpose and most likely will only inhibit epithelial regeneration. Treatment is directed toward encouraging epithelial healing. Initially, the eye should be generously lubricated. If unsuccessful, a pressure patch with prophylactic antibiotic can be placed. Alternatively or subsequently, a therapeutic soft contact lens can be placed. If these measures are unsuccessful, a tarsorrhaphy should be performed. Amniotic membrane grafts have reportedly improved HSV-1 necrotizing keratitis in a murine model, but human data are lacking.[77] If thinning ensues, cyanoacrylate glue can be applied, and a bandage contact lens placed over the glue. A conjunctival flap might be necessary to maintain the integrity of the eye. If a perforation develops, it might be sealed with cyanoacrylate glue to delay penetrating keratoplasty, but a transplant may be unavoidable.

TRABECULITIS AND IRIDOCYCLITIS. Patients with trabeculitis and iridocyclitis should be treated with a combination of topical corticosteroid and topical antiviral agents. Corticosteroid should be administered quite frequently to begin with, followed by a careful taper. The HEDS investigation of oral acyclovir for iridocyclitis caused by HSV suggested a benefit of oral acyclovir, so concurrent administration of an oral antiviral agent is recommended.[78]

RECURRENT OCULAR DISEASE AND SYSTEMIC ANTIVIRAL PROPHYLAXIS. To examine the question of whether long-term treatment with antiviral agents prevents recurrences of ocular HSV disease, the HEDS group randomized patients to treatment with 400mg acyclovir or placebo twice daily for 12 months, followed by 6 months of observation. After the resolution of ocular HSV disease, prophylactic treatment reduced the rate of recurrent ocular HSV disease significantly. The cumulative probability of recurrent stromal disease was reduced to 14% in the acyclovir group, compared with 28% in the placebo group; the cumulative probability of nonocular HSV was reduced to 19% in the acyclovir group, compared with 36% in the placebo group.[79] No rebound in the rate of HSV disease was noted in the 6 months after discontinuation of acyclovir treatment. Based on these observations, long-term prophylactic treatment should be considered in patients at risk for visual loss due to a pattern of repeated HSV stromal keratitis.

Outcome

The visual prognosis of most cases of ocular HSV is quite good. Two thirds of individuals are expected to maintain a visual acuity of 20/30 or better; however, if vision falls permanently to 20/40, a high proportion of these patients can be expected to go on to suffer significant vision loss[56] (Fig. 62-13).

Significant scarring and opacity can be successfully treated by penetrating keratoplasty, which has a markedly better prognosis

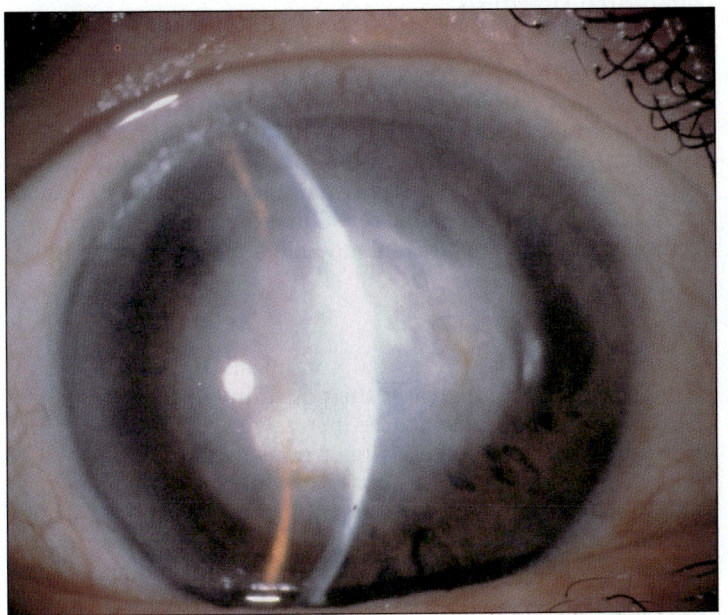

FIG. 62-13 ▮ Significant central corneal scarring following necrotizing stromal disease caused by recurrent herpes simplex virus infection.

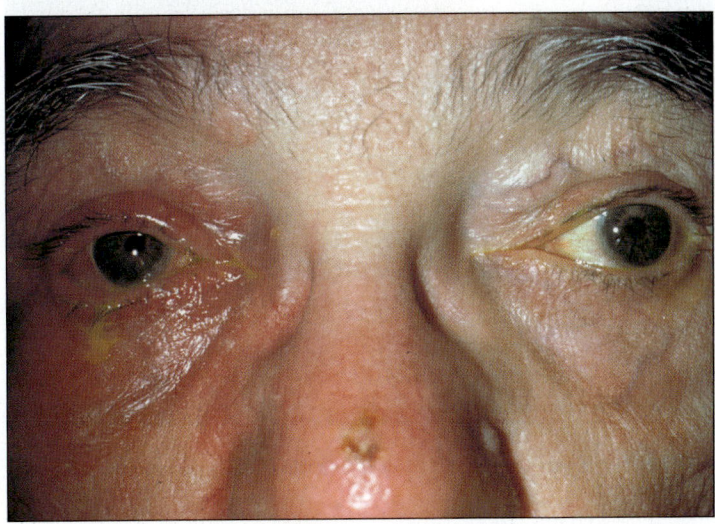

FIG. 62-14 ▮ Herpes zoster ophthalmicus demonstrating inflammation of the right brow, periorbital skin, conjunctiva, and tip of the nose (Huchinson's sign). These areas are all served by fibers from the frontal and nasociliary branches of the first division of the trigeminal nerve.

than transplantation performed in the event of acute perforation. Overall long-term graft survival in elective cases can be as high as 80%.[80] Epithelial herpetic disease has been noted to recur in corneal grafts. To maximize the probability of graft success, loose sutures should be removed promptly, and any sign of herpes recurrence or rejection should be treated promptly and aggressively. Since long-term antiviral treatment can significantly reduce recurrence rates, sustained antiviral prophylaxis should be considered.

VARICELLA-ZOSTER VIRUS KERATITIS

Epidemiology and Pathogenesis

VZV is a herpesvirus that causes varicella (chickenpox) on initial infection and shingles, or zoster, on recurrence. By age 60 years, 90% of the population will be seropositive for VZV,[81] but far fewer (approximately 20%) will have suffered a reactivation that represents zoster.[82] Whereas the vast majority of initial varicella infections occur in childhood, there is an increased incidence of zoster with age and an overall incidence of 2–4% per annum.[83] This is probably due to a decreasing cellular immune response with age. However, second recurrences are rare and develop in only 2% of the nonimmunosuppressed population.[83] In general, immunosuppressed patients, such as organ transplant recipients or those suffering from AIDS, neoplasm, or blood dyscrasia, are at an increased risk of developing recurrent disease. Recurrent disease can occur through reactivation of latent ganglionic virus or, less commonly, after exposure to persons with active varicella or zoster disease.[84]

Herpes zoster ophthalmicus (HZO) is a consequence of trigeminal nerve infection, which is second in frequency as a site of recurrence after the thoracic region. Involvement of the first (ophthalmic) division occurs far more commonly than involvement of the second or third divisions of the trigeminal nerve, and of the first division, the frontal nerve is the most commonly involved branch. Virus resides in a latent state in the dorsal root ganglion or trigeminal ganglion and, when reactivated, spreads from the ganglion along the sensory nerve to the skin, eye, and adnexae.

Clinical Features

The primary disease varicella can present in the form of congenital varicella syndrome or as disseminated varicella. The former results from infection *in utero*, usually during the first or second trimester,

and is characterized systemically by dermatomally distributed cicatricial skin lesions and delayed development, and by ocular findings of congenital cataract, chorioretinitis, and optic nerve atrophy. The latter is the well-recognized chickenpox, characterized by a disseminated maculopapulovesicular rash that appears in successive crops, accompanied by fever and malaise. Vesicular lesions can appear on the lids and conjunctiva, most commonly at the limbus. Although these lesions can develop into red, inflamed punched-out lesions, they most often resolve without sequelae. A punctate keratopathy or coarse dendritiform corneal lesions can develop. Features that aid in distinguishing these lesions from those of herpes simplex keratitis are listed in Table 62-4. In rare cases, iridocyclitis and subsequent cataract might develop.

HZO that represents recurrent disease can involve virtually all ocular and adnexal tissues (Fig. 62-14). Reactivation is often preceded by headache, malaise, and fever, followed by neuralgia that is later replaced by redness, pain, and swelling in the periorbital skin. A few days later, vesicles begin to erupt in successive crops as older lesions rupture and crust over. The upper eyelid is involved as a consequence of frontal nerve infection. Edema and vesicles can appear, which usually resolve without sequelae, but if there is scarring, lid retraction and exposure can develop. Conjunctivitis can be follicular or necrotizing. Occasionally, conjunctival vesicles appear, which can lead to scarring. Episcleritis and scleritis (which is frequently recurrent) can occur, leading to staphyloma formation on resolution.

Corneal involvement, which appears in approximately two thirds of cases of HZO,[85] can accompany the acute event or follow it by months to years. Protean manifestations of HZO keratitis include, in decreasing order of frequency, punctate keratopathy, pseudodendrites, anterior stromal infiltrates, keratouveitis-endotheliitis, neurotrophic keratitis, delayed mucous plaques, exposure keratitis, disciform keratitis, peripheral ulcerative keratitis, and sclerokeratitis.[85] The punctate keratopathy represents coarse, elevated patches of epithelium that contain live virus and stain with rose bengal. These can resolve spontaneously or progress, either developing anterior stromal infiltrates or coalescing to form elevated dendritiform lesions. These lesions differ from the dendrites of HSV in a number of characteristics (see Table 62-4), but like those associated with HSV, they contain live virus. They appear most often during the acute event but can occur many weeks after, and they typically resolve spontaneously over a few weeks. These should be distinguished from mucous plaques, which are gray, elevated, linear or branching lesions that stain with rose

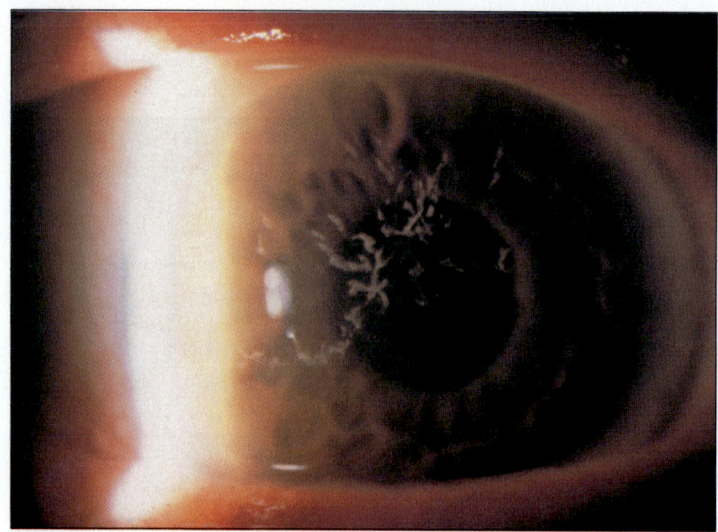

FIG. 62-15 ▓ Epithelial mucous plaques following herpes zoster corneal disease.

bengal and are loosely adherent to underlying degenerating epithelium and inflamed stroma (Fig. 62-15). These plaques usually appear 3–4 months after the acute event and vary in appearance from day to day.

Chronic dendritiform lesions have been observed in patients with AIDS up to 6 years after an episode of cutaneous zoster. In many such patients, VZV was detected on immunofluorescence, by culture, or by PCR. Such lesions stain vividly with rose bengal and might be accompanied by significant discomfort.[86]

Neurotrophic keratitis is considered a consequence of corneal nerve damage that manifests as decreased corneal sensation. Corneal hypoesthesia tends to be more severe than that seen in HSV disease and can be accompanied by a persistent epithelial defect that precedes stromal necrosis and perforation.

Stromal keratitis resembling the disciform or necrotizing keratitis of HSV disease usually occurs 3–4 months following the acute event but can occur many years later. The immune mechanisms involved in HZO-related stromal keratitis are thought to be similar to those involved in HSV-related disease.

HZO *sine herpete* is a long-recognized but uncommon manifestation of HZO. PCR analysis and VZV serology have confirmed the role of VZV—not preceded by an episode of shingles—in producing disciform keratitis, recurrent iritis, and acute iridoplegic iridocyclitis.[87]

Postherpetic neuralgia refers to the spontaneous pain associated with minor stimuli and the altered sensation that follow herpes zoster infection long after the skin lesions have healed. It is found with increased incidence in patients with HZO. It is probably due to injury to the peripheral nerves and altered central nervous system signal processing. Symptoms resolve or persist unpredictably, but in the long term, they tend to decrease over time.

Diagnosis

The diagnosis of herpes zoster disease is usually evident clinically, based on the appearance of the characteristic dermatomal rash. However, the diagnosis can be confirmed in the laboratory by examination of smears prepared with Giemsa or Papanicolaou's stain. These reveal multinucleated giant epithelial cells and intranuclear eosinophilic inclusion bodies. Viral particles can be identified by electron microscopy, and immunological tests such as immunofluorescence microscopy, radioimmunoassay, and ELISA can also aid in making the diagnosis. If exudate from lesions up to 7 days old is introduced to human tissue culture, virus can often be recovered.

Serology for VZV IgG and IgM may prove helpful in confirming the diagnosis, and PCR has become increasingly useful in the analysis of corneal tissue or vitreous specimens, as well as those from corneal scrapings or tears.[68]

Differential Diagnosis

The dendritiform epithelial lesions of VZV should be distinguished from those of HSV (see Table 62-4), as should the stromal inflammation. Whereas the dendritiform lesions are themselves clinically distinct, the stromal inflammation of VZV is intrinsically indistinguishable from that of HSV, and other clinical elements such as history, recurrence patterns, and associated skin lesions should be considered. Other causes of disciform and necrotizing stromal keratitis include EBV, mumps, and syphilis.

Systemic Associations

Varicella infection is a potential complication of immunosuppression, which also increases the possibility of recurrent zoster disease. Such conditions include increasing age, malignancy, immunosuppression following organ transplantation, and AIDS. Zoster can appear at a focal locus of immunosuppression, such as at an irradiation site[88]; conversely, it can develop into widely disseminated disease when arising in severely immunocompromised individuals. Since zoster in patients younger than 50 years old is uncommon, human immunodeficiency virus (HIV) infection must be considered in this age group. In such patients, there is an increased risk for second recurrences of disease and for a complicated, protracted disease course.

Pathology

During primary infection, the varicella virus infects the skin and then migrates via sensory nerves to the ganglia, where latent infection is established. Reactivation is associated with decreased cell-mediated immunity, which allows replicating virus to produce local ganglionic inflammation and destruction, after which the activated virus migrates down the peripheral nerve to the skin dermatome or eye, where peripheral inflammation develops. There is a prominent vasculitis, with granulomatous or lymphocytic infiltration, which suggests that tissue damage caused by zoster infection is due both to inflammation and to vasculitis-induced ischemia.

The disciform keratitis of corneal zoster is considered to be due to a delayed-type hypersensitivity reaction,[85,89] although a granulomatous inflammation of Descemet's membrane has been observed.[90]

Treatment

Disseminated varicella disease in children older than 2 years should be treated with oral acyclovir, 800mg four times daily for 5 days. There are no established conventions regarding limited ocular disease. However, lid and conjunctival lesions are sometimes treated with topical antiviral agents such as vidarabine ointment four times daily for 10–14 days. Disciform keratitis should be treated with topical corticosteroids, which are then tapered slowly over a number of weeks.

HZO should be treated with systemic antiviral agents. The mainstay is oral acyclovir, 800mg five times daily for 7–10 days, ideally initiated within 72 hours of the onset of symptoms. Oral acyclovir has been demonstrated to accelerate the resolution of skin rash and the healing of skin lesions, reduce the period of lesion formation and viral shedding, and reduce the incidence of episcleritis, keratitis, and iritis. Oral acyclovir also appears to reduce acute zoster-associated pain, but the effect on postherpetic neuralgia is unclear.[91]

Newer antiviral agents are currently available for the treatment of herpes zoster. The nucleoside analog famciclovir has *in vitro* activity against VZV that is similar to the activity of acyclovir, but it is more bioavailable on oral administration, and its active metabolite, pencyclovir triphosphate, has an intracellular half-life nearly 10 times that of acyclovir. The recommended dose is 500mg/day for 7 days. Valacyclovir is a pro-drug of acyclovir that is highly available when administered orally. It reaches plasma acyclovir concentrations almost three times greater than those achievable with oral acyclovir, which is comparable to those achieved with intravenous acyclovir.[92] It is administered at a dose of 1000mg three times daily for 7–10 days. Both famciclovir and valacyclovir appear to be superior to acyclovir in reducing the duration of zoster-associated pain.[91]

Systemic corticosteroids used in combination with systemic antiviral medication appear to reduce acute zoster-associated pain and significantly improve patient function during the acute event, but they do not consistently affect long-term postherpetic neuralgia.[91] There is an increased risk of disseminated viral infection associated with systemic corticosteroid use, although this risk is reduced by the presence of systemic antiviral agents. This is of particular concern in immunocompromised HIV-positive individuals with unrecognized disease. Therefore, the use of systemic corticosteroids along with a systemic antiviral agent is best limited to patients 50 years of age or older with moderate to severe pain who appear to have age-normal immunocompetence and in whom corticosteroids are not otherwise contraindicated.[91] Systemic corticosteroids should also be considered in the treatment of the inflammatory complications of HZO, such as severe scleritis and uveitis or orbital inflammation.

Established postherpetic neuralgia is difficult to treat. As an initial approach, topical lidocaine-prilocaine cream or 5% lidocaine gel should be applied. If ineffective, tricyclic antidepressant medication such as amitriptyline or desipramine at a low dose of 12.5–25mg at bedtime can be added to the regimen and increased slowly. Substantial relief may not occur for several weeks. Many authorities are skeptical about the efficacy of topical capsaicin, which causes a burning sensation when applied, followed by anesthesia. The burning is intolerable for up to one third of patients and renders masked studies impossible. Given the risks of sedation and dependence, narcotics are probably best administered by a pain-management specialist who might also employ other nonpharmacological techniques. Neurosurgical procedures such as dorsal root electrocoagulation remain treatments of last resort and carry a substantial risk of postoperative motor and sensory deficit.[91]

Local ocular treatment of HZO is directed toward reducing the damage associated with inflammation. Although topical antiviral agents are not commonly employed in the treatment of HZO keratitis, certain cases of delayed pseudodendritic keratitis have been reported to respond to topical antiviral treatment.[93] Topical corticosteroids are useful for reducing corneal and scleral inflammation and iridocyclitis and, unlike their effect on the dendritic disease of HSV infection, do not appear to exacerbate keratitis. They should be tapered carefully over a few weeks. Topical antibiotics should be administered if there is an epithelial defect to minimize the risk of bacterial infection.

Neurotrophic ulceration is a major complication of HZO; persistent epithelial defect and corneal ulceration can be complicated by vascularization, superinfection, and perforation. Persistent neurotrophic epithelial defect might be successfully treated with bandage contact lens wear or lateral or complete tarsorrhaphy. Cyanoacrylate glue or a conjunctival flap can be used in an attempt to arrest severe thinning that threatens corneal integrity. Severe necrotizing keratitis or postherpetic neurotrophic ulceration might lead to severe scarring or corneal perforation that requires corneal transplantation. If the eye has been quiet for a number of months prior to surgery, penetrating keratoplasty has a reasonably good chance of success.[94] If the disease is active at the time of surgery, a tarsorrhaphy over the graft might be useful in preserving the corneal surface.[95]

Outcome

In immunocompromised states, there is an increased risk of recurrent HZO with attendant inflammatory damage that is related to the degree of immunocompromise. In nonimmunocompromised individuals, the chance of a second episode of recurrent HZO disease is extremely low. However, inflammation during any event of HZO can lead to lid scarring and exposure, corneal scarring, neurotrophic keratitis, and postherpetic neuralgia, all of which may require therapy long after the acute event.

EPSTEIN-BARR VIRUS KERATITIS
Epidemiology and Pathogenesis

EBV is a DNA virus that infects more than 90% of the adult population.[96] Persons of lower socioeconomic groups acquire the virus at a younger age. The most common route of transmission is by saliva, although infection after transfusion has been reported. Following infection, EBV enters B-lymphocytes and establishes a latent phase from whence reactivation can occur.

Clinical Features

EBV ocular disease can affect virtually all the tissues of the eye. Conjunctival manifestations include follicular conjunctivitis,[97] conjunctival mass, and Parinaud's oculoglandular syndrome.[98] Corneal findings include multifocal epithelial dendritic keratitis; subepithelial infiltrates; multifocal, well-demarcated granular anterior stromal opacities; multifocal, coin-shaped peripheral translucent lesions at all levels of the cornea; multifocal nonsuppurative stromal keratitis; and peripheral, deep infiltrative keratitis often associated with vascularization.[99] Iritis and panuveitis can occur, sometimes months after the acute event.

Diagnosis

The diagnosis of EBV infection is made on the basis of detecting heterophile antibodies that, as predominantly IgM antibodies, are indicative of acute infection. However, these antibodies, which are targeted by the popular monospot agglutination test, are undetectable in 10–20% of individuals with acute infection.[100] Alternatively, serological tests can be performed for EBV capsid antigen and EBV nuclear antigen. The former are found in patients with acute disease, and the latter appear several weeks to months after the acute infection. Antibodies persist throughout life.

Differential Diagnosis

Anterior stromal and subepithelial EBV keratitis can be distinguished from the lesions associated with adenovirus, in that the former are more pleomorphic and tend to appear at deeper levels of the stroma. Other causes of nummular keratitis that should be considered include HSV and VZV, sarcoid, syphilis, tuberculosis, leprosy, and onchocerciasis.

Systemic Associations

Systemic primary EBV infection (infectious mononucleosis) is characterized by the triad of fever, sore throat, and lymphadenopathy. These manifestations are often preceded by a prodrome of chills, malaise, headache, myalgia, and arthralgia. A fraction of patients subsequently develops neurological symptoms that include optic nerve edema and optic neuritis, abducens nerve palsy, and ophthalmoplegia.[101]

Treatment

Systemic disease is usually managed with supportive care only, since there is little evidence that systemic antiviral therapy affects systemic symptoms. Both EBV iritis and stromal keratitis respond well to topical corticosteroid therapy, which can be administered initially every 2 hours and subsequently tapered, based on response. Some practitioners prescribe oral antiviral therapy such as acyclovir, 800mg five times daily, but there is little support for this practice in the literature.

Outcome

Keratitis usually responds well to therapy, with resolution of epithelial disease and clearing of the infiltrates. Patients with posterior inflammation such as panuveitis, choroiditis, and papillitis may suffer a protracted disease course that might be improved with systemic acyclovir and corticosteroid treatment.

CYTOMEGALOVIRUS KERATITIS
Epidemiology and Pathogenesis

CMV disease of the external eye is extremely uncommon, and few reports exist in the literature. CMV infection of the conjunctiva has been reported in association with HIV infection,[102] and cases of keratitis have been reported in association with cardiac transplantation,[103] penetrating keratoplasty,[104] and AIDS.[105] CMV is not usually present in the corneal or conjunctival epithelium of AIDS patients,[106] but systemic CMV infection likely leads to lacrimal gland and conjunctival infection, which in turn might lead to corneal infection. It is unclear why infection of the cornea and conjunctiva is so rare in immunosuppressed patients compared with retinal infection.

Clinical Features

CMV epithelial keratitis resembles the epithelial disease of HZO and is characterized by dendritic epithelial lesions with edematous epithelial cells and adherent mucus. The case of stromal CMV keratitis described by Wehrly et al.[104] occurred in a corneal graft and demonstrated a noninfiltrated epithelial defect, endothelial plaque, and hypopyon. Too few cases of epithelial or stromal disease have been reported to confidently characterize the presentation of this rare manifestation of CMV infection.

Diagnosis

Corneal scrapings of CMV epithelial lesions demonstrate numerous multinucleated syncytial giant cells and intranuclear inclusions.[105] Scrapings can be submitted for viral culture, from which CMV might be recovered. However, care must be taken in procuring the corneal specimen, as positive cultures might be attributable to infection of the tear film rather than of conjunctival or corneal tissue. If tissue is obtained by biopsy, immunostaining using anti-CMV antibodies can identify cytoplasmic and intranuclear inclusions as due to CMV. Routine electron microscopy is not useful, because CMV and herpes simplex or zoster virions are indistinguishable by this technique.

Differential Diagnosis

The dendritic appearance of CMV epithelial disease must be distinguished from that of HSV and VZV.

Systemic Associations

CMV keratitis has been reported in both the immunocompetent and the immunosuppressed; however, because immunosuppression is considered a risk for disseminated CMV infection, it should be considered a risk for CMV keratitis.

Pathology

Histopathological examination of CMV-infected conjunctiva has demonstrated cytomegalic cells with prominent intranuclear inclusions associated with dilated conjunctival vessels. Electron microscopy of these cells revealed intranuclear and intracytoplasmic viral particles and intracytoplasmic membrane-bound dense bodies characteristic of CMV.[102] Histopathological examination of CMV stromal keratitis has demonstrated basophilic intranuclear inclusion in keratocytes.[104]

Treatment

CMV keratitis has reportedly responded to simple superficial débridement.[103] However, recurrent keratitis unresponsive to antiviral chemotherapy with oral acyclovir, oral famciclovir, topical foscarnet, topical trifluridine, and topical acyclovir has been observed, probably due to systemic infection with repeated local reinfection.[105] Therefore, the optimal treatment of this uncommon disorder is unknown.

Outcome

As described earlier, CMV keratitis may respond completely to treatment, or it may recur persistently. Further experience is necessary to better characterize this disease.

FUNGAL KERATITIS

INTRODUCTION

Fungal infections of the cornea are relatively infrequent in the developed world but constitute a larger proportion of keratitis cases in many parts of the developing world.[107] Although these infections can cause devastating damage if allowed to progress unchecked, advances in antimicrobial therapy and surgical technique have improved their prognosis. Therefore, recognition and prompt, aggressive therapy of fungal infections are extremely important.

EPIDEMIOLOGY AND PATHOGENESIS

Fungi are ubiquitous organisms that are recognized more frequently as ocular pathogens in agrarian, tropical countries than in the developed world. The incidence of fungal keratitis in the United States is estimated to be on the order of 1500 cases per year,[108] with the majority of cases arising in the warmer southern and southwestern states. In these areas (and around the world), septate filamentous fungi, most notably Fusarium and Aspergillus, are the most common causative organisms, whereas in the northern states, Candida is the most commonly isolated fungal organism.

In the warmer states and in the tropics, corneal trauma, which might be trivial, frequently precedes infection. Concurrent contamination with plant material presents an increased risk for fungal keratitis. However, in colder climates, where Candida infections predominate, corneal disease and local immunosuppression caused by chronic corticosteroid use and systemic disease states that lower host resistance are associated with these infections.

For clinical purposes, fungi can be classified on a morphological basis into filamentous, yeast, and diphasic forms. Filamentous organisms are multicellular with branched hyphae. Some, the so-called septate organisms such as Fusarium, Cephalosporium, Aspergillus, Curvularia, and Alternaria species, have hyphae that are divided by cell walls, whereas other filamentous fungi such as Mucor and Rhizopus are nonseptate. Yeasts, such as Candida and Cryptococcus, are unicellular fungi that reproduce by budding, but in tissue, they might develop elongated buds (pseudohyphae) or real hyphae. Dimorphic fungi such as Histoplasma, Coccidioides, and Blastomyces demonstrate both a yeast phase that occurs in tissues and a mycelial phase that appears on culture media and saprophytic surfaces.

CLINICAL FEATURES

As described earlier, fungal infection tends to arise in traumatized, diseased, and immunocompromised corneas. The kerati-

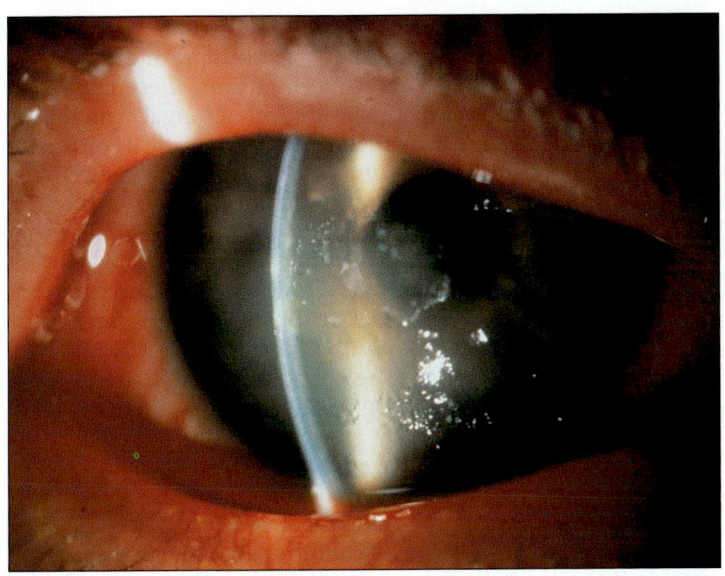

FIG. 62-16 ▪ Feathery stromal infiltrates typical of fungal keratitis.

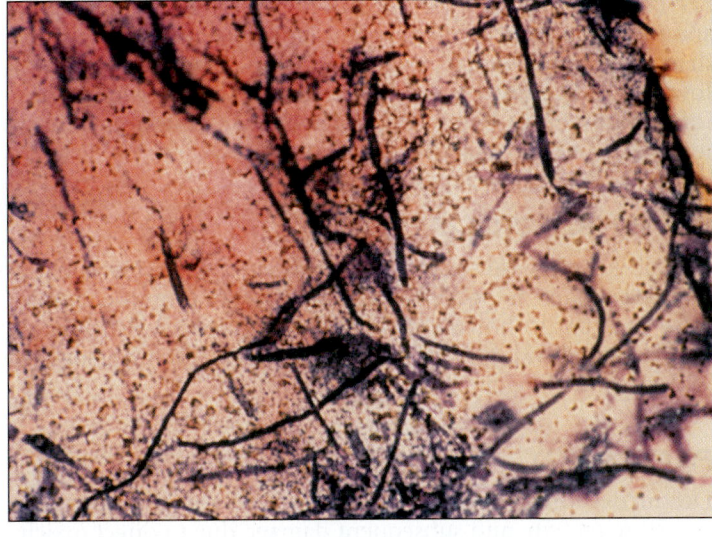

FIG. 62-18 ▪ Gram's stain of scraping from *Fusarium* corneal ulcer demonstrating branching fungal hyphae.

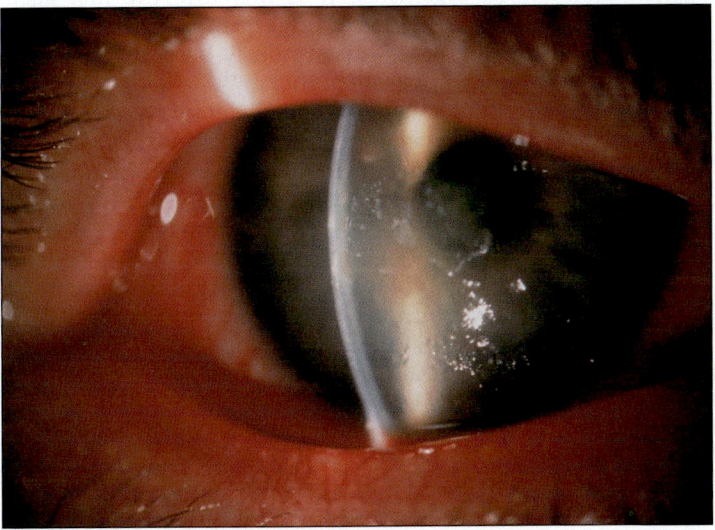

FIG. 62-17 ▪ *Fusarium* fungal keratitis.

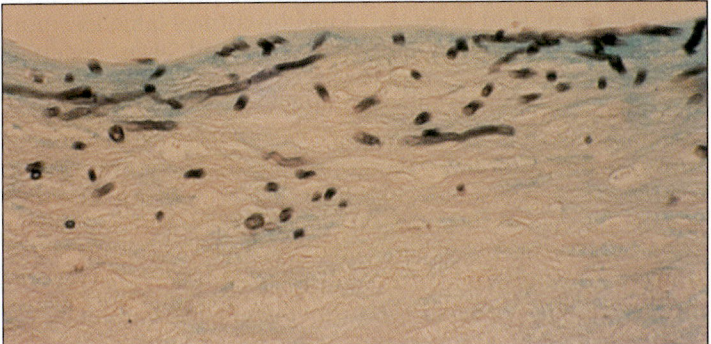

FIG. 62-19 ▪ A keratoplasty specimen demonstrates fungal infiltration of the anterior stroma and inflammatory cells.

tis tends to be slowly progressive and insidious, but a fairly rapid infiltrate development does not rule out fungal infection. In some cases, the epithelium might heal over an intrastromal infiltrate that produces little inflammation and minimal discomfort. Conversely, inflammation might be so severe as to result in hypopyon formation. The ulcer and infiltrate itself can assume protean appearances and might be indistinguishable from a bacterial ulcer. However, certain features suggest a fungal infection, including feathery edges or a dry, gray, elevated infiltrate and satellite lesions (Fig. 62-16). Although a ring infiltrate and endothelial plaque are frequently suggested as indicators of fungal keratitis, many cases do not demonstrate these features, which merely reflect corneal and anterior chamber inflammation.

DIAGNOSIS

A high level of suspicion for nonbacterial keratitis must be maintained at all times, especially in those areas where the incidence of fungal keratitis is relatively high (Fig. 62-17). Important historical elements include preexisting corneal disease, chronic corticosteroid use, or trauma, with attention to the possibility of vegetable matter contamination. With increasing frequency, numerous cases of fungal infection at the lamellar interface have been described following LASIK.[109,110]

Definite diagnosis requires laboratory confirmation, and treatment for fungal keratitis should not be initiated until such evidence has been acquired. Scrapings for stains and culture should be obtained as described for bacterial keratitis. If fungal infection is suspected following LASIK, the flap must be elevated to obtain samples. Gram's stain demonstrates darkened fungal walls, and Giemsa stain demonstrates the walls in contrast to highlighted cytoplasm (Fig. 62-18). A useful adjunctive stain is ink–potassium hydroxide, which demonstrates the dark outline of fungal walls. Gomori's methenamine silver stain is generally considered the stain that best demonstrates fungal organisms, but it is time-consuming and difficult to perform. Although not widely available, confocal microscopy might be useful in the identification of fungal hyphae *in vivo* within the cornea.[111]

Culture media should include blood agar (upon which *Fusarium* grows well at room temperature) and either Sabouraud medium or brain-heart infusion broth. Cycloheximide should not be included in the medium, since it inhibits fungal growth. Most ocular fungal isolates demonstrate growth within 2–3 days, although it is prudent to wait 2 weeks before confirmation of no growth. Although identification of the causative fungal organism is critical for the decision to initiate antifungal therapy, it is not helpful to use specific antimicrobial sensitivity studies to advise antifungal choice, since test criteria are poorly standardized.

Since some cases of keratitis may develop deep in the stroma with intact overlying corneal tissue, a deep corneal biopsy might be necessary to obtain tissue for laboratory studies (Fig. 62-19).

DIFFERENTIAL DIAGNOSIS

See Box 62-1. Owing to indolent progression and failure to respond to antibacterial medication, fungal keratitis is often misdiagnosed as herpetic or amoebic disease. Fungal infection following LASIK must be differentiated from the sterile interface infiltration of post-LASIK diffuse lamellar keratitis and from infection due to bacterial species.

SYSTEMIC ASSOCIATIONS

Fungal keratitis caused by less virulent organisms such as *Candida* is often associated with conditions of immunocompromise such as alcoholism, diabetes, and vitamin A deficiency.[112] Unlike fungal endophthalmitis, fungal keratitis is not associated with systemic fungemia.

PATHOLOGY

Destructive fungal infection is advanced by organism adherence, invasion, growth, and subsequent damage due to direct toxicity and host response. Adherence is facilitated by a number of surface molecule adhesins, some of which also appear to inhibit neutrophil attachment, thus protecting the invading organism within the corneal stroma.[113] Whereas the mycelia of filamentous organisms tend to extend along the corneal lamellae, more virulent organisms can cross lamellae and even penetrate Descemet's membrane, leading to intracameral infection.[114,115] The inflammatory host response is similar to that described in bacterial infection, and damage is augmented by mycotoxins and proteolytic enzymes. Fungi produce a variety of proteases specific for the substrates on which they grow, some of which may be directed against corneal collagen.[116,117] Moreover, in the presence of viable fungal elements, invading neutrophils elaborate a number of proteolytic enzymes, including corneal matrix metalloproteinases, leading to further tissue degradation.[117]

TREATMENT

The efficacy of currently available antifungal agents is limited, and there is a relatively high medical treatment failure rate. These agents fall into three main groups: the polyenes, the azoles, and the fluorinated pyrimidines (Table 62-6). The polyenes, such as amphotericin B, natamycin, and nystatin, bind to fungal cell wall ergosterol, thus disrupting the cell. Imidazoles, such as miconazole, clotrimazole, and ketoconazole, and triazoles, such as fluconazole and itraconazole, appear to have two mechanisms of action. At low concentrations, these agents inhibit ergosterol synthesis by the inhibition of fungal cytochrome P-450–dependent 14-α demethylase, which is critical for the incorporation of ergosterol into the fungal cell membrane. Ergosterol precursors subsequently accumulate within the fungal membrane, inhibiting fungal growth. At higher concentrations, the triazoles appear to cause direct damage to cell walls independent of ergosterol synthesis. However, the concentrations required for the latter fungicidal action are higher than can be achieved in the cornea, so only the former mechanism is considered practically effective. The pyrimidine flucytosine is converted into a thymidine analog within fungal cells that blocks fungal thymidine synthesis.

The polyenes are effective against both filamentous and yeast forms. Amphotericin B is particularly effective against yeasts but less effective against filamentous organisms; it is therefore the first agent of choice against yeasts. Although penetration is comparable if the epithelium has been débrided, the penetration of topically applied amphotericin B is less than that of topically applied natamycin through an intact epithelium.[118] Natamycin is effective against yeasts and has a broad spectrum of activity against filamentous organisms. It is therefore the first agent of choice against filamentous fungi. Amphotericin B and natamycin can be alternated on an hourly basis for infections that fail to respond to single-agent therapy.

The azoles and flucytosine are generally employed as alternative agents when the fungal ulcer is particularly advanced or fails to improve with polyene treatment. Because experimental models have suggested antagonism between amphotericin B and the imidazoles,[119] some authorities do not recommend that they be used in combination, although in some cases, clinical evidence has been contradictory. Azoles should be included in the initial management of *Paecilomyces*, which frequently exhibits resistance against the polyenes.[120] Topically applied, the imidazoles have relatively poor corneal penetration, so they are more effective in treating superficial infections. Miconazole can be applied topically, subconjunctivally, or systemically and is particularly useful in the treatment of poorly responsive Aspergillus infection. Ketoconazole administered topically, subconjunctivally, and systemically achieves effective corneal levels and is effective against both yeast and filamentous organisms, including *Aspergillus, Candida, Curvularia,* and *Fusarium*.[121] The triazole fluconazole demonstrates ready corneal penetration when applied topically or subconjunctivally. Oral absorption is also excellent, and therapeutic corneal levels can be achieved by this route. It is effective against candidal infections and is also useful against *Aspergillus.* Although its clinical role has yet to be precisely defined, given its systemic absorption characteristics, oral fluconazole should be considered in the management of deep fungal keratitis that threatens intracameral infection. A number of new triazole derivatives (voriconazole, posaconazole, and ravuconazole) demonstrate potent, broad-spectrum antifungal activity. Along with novel agents such as the echinocandin antifungals, the sodarin derivatives, and the nikkomycins, these antimicrobials might substantially improve the treatment of fungal keratitis.[122]

Flucytosine is well absorbed when administered orally, and it can also be applied as a topical solution. It is very effective against *Candida,* but resistance develops rapidly. Therefore, flucytosine should always be administered in combination with an azole or amphotericin B.

Once the diagnosis has been made, fungal keratitis should be treated with frequently applied topical antifungal medication. Initially, drops can be administered every 5 minutes for five doses, followed by hourly application during the day and every 2 hours at night. If an azole is added to the regimen, a subconjunctival injection can be administered, and oral supplements should be considered for deep stromal infection. As stability is achieved, the frequency of nighttime application can be reduced,

TABLE 62-6

ANTIFUNGAL ANTIBIOTICS

Agent	Route	Dosage/Concentration
Polyenes		
Amphotericin B	Topical	0.15%
	Subconjunctival	0.5–1mg
	Intracameral	7.5–10mg in 0.1ml
Natamycin	Topical suspension	5%
Imidazoles		
Clotrimazole	Topical	1%
Ketoconazole	Topical	5%
	Oral	300mg/day
Miconazole	Topical suspension	1%
	Topical cream	2%
	Subconjunctival	5–10mg
Triazoles		
Fluconazole	Topical	0.2%
	Oral	200mg/day
Itraconazole	Topical	1%
	Oral	100–200mg BID
Pyrimidines		
Flucytosine	Topical	2%
	Oral	50–150mg/kg/day divided BID

followed by a reduction in the daytime frequency. As a method of circumventing the poor intraocular penetration of topically applied antifungals, intracameral injection of amphotericin B (7.5–10µg in 0.1ml) has reportedly been successful in controlling cases resistant to topical and oral antifungal preparations.[123]

Since these infections can be so tenacious, and host suppression of infection is so important, corticosteroid use is generally not recommended in the management of fungal keratitis. Corticosteroids should be employed with the greatest caution and exclusively when it appears that excessive inflammation is the cause of progressive damage and effective antifungal medicine has eliminated viable organisms. The propensity for corticosteroids to enhance microbial viability can present a particular dilemma for the treatment of fungal infection in a corneal graft. In vitro studies have suggested that topical cyclosporine A might possess antifungal properties,[124] and this agent has been used as an alternative for reducing inflammation and the subsequent risk of graft failure in the setting of fungal graft infection.[125]

The course of treatment is typically protracted, and antifungal treatment is usually maintained over 12 weeks, with strict vigilance as medicines are tapered. If fungal keratitis fails to respond to medical therapy, surgical intervention should be considered. Because of the propensity for fungal elements to invade deeply and, in some cases, penetrate Descemet's membrane, advanced cases require penetrating keratoplasty to ensure complete removal of the invading fungus. In general, penetrating keratoplasty should be performed sooner rather than later to maximize the probability of a graft margin free of infection and to minimize the risk of endophthalmitis or infectious scleritis. As generous a clear margin as possible should be included in the excised cornea.[126] Less advanced cases might be amenable to lamellar keratoplasty, but the surgeon must be confident that the entire infection has been encompassed by the lamellar dissection. If there is any question about the depth of infection, the procedure should be converted to a full-thickness penetrating excision.[127]

OUTCOME

Patients with deep stromal infection and those treated with corticosteroids appear to respond particularly poorly to medical therapy.[120] Forster and Rebell[128] reported a medical failure rate of approximately 20%. Although penetrating keratoplasty can successfully eliminate the organism and restore the integrity of the eye, a delay in surgery or advanced disease might allow catastrophic extension of infection to the anterior chamber and sclera.

PARASITIC KERATITIS

INTRODUCTION

Parasitic infections of the cornea are a significant cause of ocular morbidity. Although Onchocerca infection is commonly encountered in some parts of the developing world, Acanthamoeba keratitis is increasingly recognized in the developed world as a potentially disastrous complication of contact lens wear, and one that requires early, aggressive treatment.

ACANTHAMOEBA

Epidemiology and Pathogenesis

Numerous free-living phagotrophic amebae cause opportunistic infection in humans. Since 1973, Acanthamoeba has been recognized to cause a severe, blinding keratitis. Only six cases were reported up to 1981, after which the number of cases recognized increased steadily throughout the 1980s. Use of the confocal microscope as a diagnostic tool may have contributed to the increased recognition of Acanthamoeba infection.[129] To date, eight species of Acanthamoeba are known to cause keratitis. The most common of these pathogens is A. castellani.[130] Other amebic genera, such as Vahlkampfia and Hartmannella, have also been found to cause a keratitis with similar clinical features.[131]

Acanthamoeba thrives in soil and water environments such as ponds, swimming pools, hot tubs, and contact lens saline solutions. In almost all cases, a history of exposure to contaminated water or corneal trauma can be elicited. Whereas some studies suggest associated contact lens use or exposure to contaminated water in as many as 93% of cases,[132] other authors suggest that recall bias may spuriously affect these data with a more accurate figure being 40%.[130] Of interest, cases reported from India are infrequently associated with contact lens use.[133] A particular risk exists for persons who prepare saline for contact lens use with salt tablets and distilled water. Furthermore, co-contamination with bacteria appears to be an important risk for the adherence of Acanthamoeba to hydrogel lenses.[134] Once contact lenses and supplies are contaminated, the risk of infection is established, since the organism can adhere to and penetrate an intact epithelium.

Clinical Features

Acanthamoeba keratitis is often confused with other causes of infectious keratitis, particularly fungal and herpetic keratitis (Fig. 62-20). Since a delay in treatment has been shown to adversely affect visual outcome, clinicians must be aware of the sometimes subtle indications of early Acanthamoeba infection.[135] Early infection can be confined to the epithelium, which demonstrates irregularity and infiltration, pseudodendrites, or elevated epithelial ridges (Fig. 62-21). Infiltrates might be seen around corneal nerves. Nonspecific stromal infiltration or a characteristic ring infiltrate that resembles stromal herpetic disease often develops, along with uveitis. Conjunctival injection and chemosis are often associated with infection (Fig. 62-22). Satellite lesions can appear, and corneal neovascularization is uncommon. When present, fluctuating, nongranulomatous anterior chamber inflammation may contribute to the formation of cataract or elevated intraocular pressure.[136] In the most severe cases, hypopyon, diffuse or nodular anterior scleritis, or posterior scleritis (sometimes associated with optic neuritis) can occur.

It has been reported frequently that patients experience severe pain far out of proportion to clinical findings, but this is an unreliable diagnostic sign, as is the oft-quoted radial perineuritis, which in many cases does not appear (Fig. 62-23).

Diagnosis

Although not widely available, the confocal microscope can be helpful in establishing the diagnosis of Acanthamoeba keratitis,

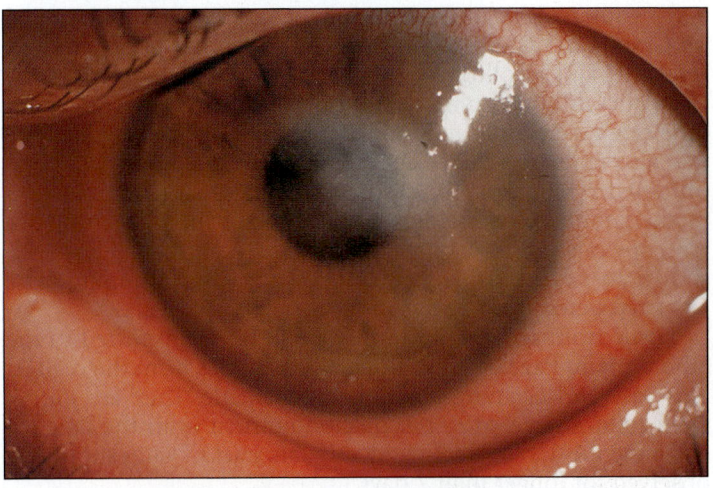

FIG. 62-20 ▪ Nonspecific infiltration of the corneal stroma caused by *Acanthamoeba* infection. (Courtesy of Joel Sugar, MD.)

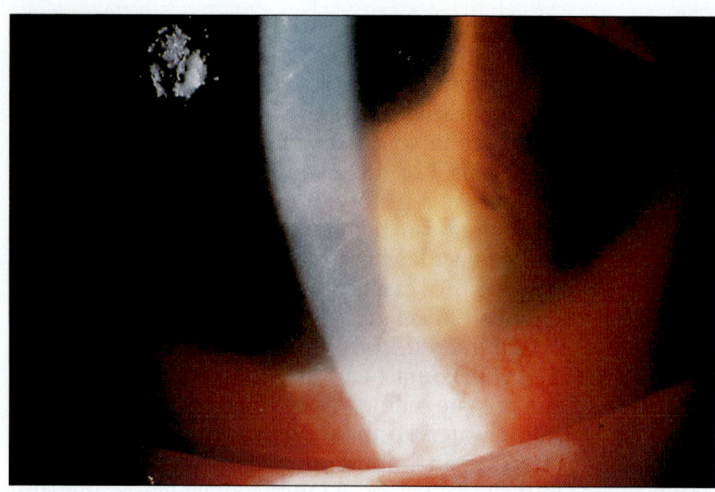

FIG. 62-21 ■ Epithelial ridges seen in *Acanthamoeba* keratitis. (Courtesy of Joel Sugar, MD.)

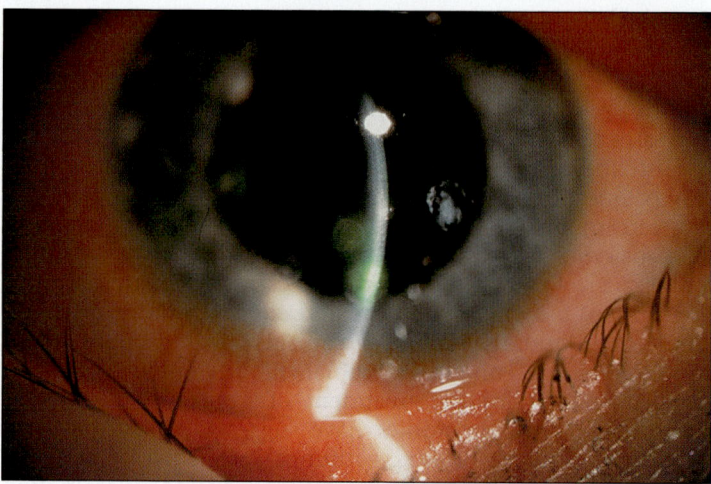

FIG. 62-23 ■ Perineuritis seen in *Acanthamoeba* keratitis. (Courtesy of Joel Sugar, MD.)

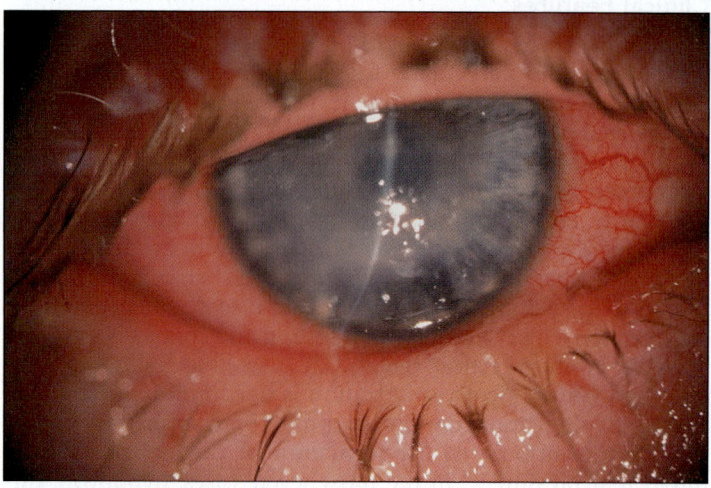

FIG. 62-22 ■ Disciform keratitis seen in *Acanthamoeba* corneal infection. (Courtesy of Joel Sugar, MD.)

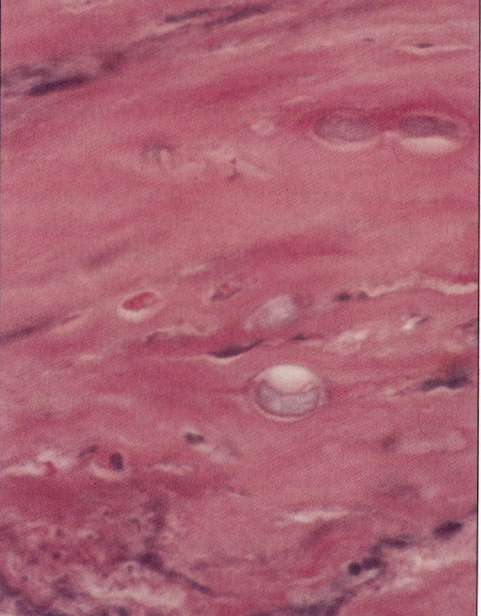

FIG. 62-24 ■ Light microscopic view of a corneal section demonstrating *Acanthamoeba* cysts. (Courtesy of Joel Sugar, MD.)

based on the visualization of pear-shaped cysts (measuring 11–15μm) and irregular trophozoites.[129,137] Otherwise, laboratory diagnosis is essential, since the patient must be committed to a protracted treatment course. Corneal epithelial scrapings should be procured for stains and cultures of epithelial or subepithelial lesions. If there is little epithelial disease but a predominant stromal infection, biopsy should be considered. Phase-contrast microscopy of a wet mount can be employed to identify motile trophozoites, which possess a large karyosome and a contractile vacuole. Acanthamoeba cysts can be identified on Gram's and Giemsa stains of scrapings or biopsy specimens (Fig. 62-24). Calcofluor white stain effectively demonstrates the walls of cysts but requires a fluorescent microscope, as does acridine orange. An immunofluorescent antibody stain is available that also requires a fluorescent microscope. If a biopsy has been obtained, hematoxylin-eosin, periodic acid–Schiff, and methenamine silver stains should be performed. Electron microscopy can also reveal organisms. More recently, PCR has been shown to be a sensitive method of detecting Acanthamoeba DNA recovered from ocular surface scrapings or tears.[130]

Tissue from scraping or biopsy should be transported to the laboratory in Page's saline, along with samples from the contact lens case and cleaning solutions, if available. They are inoculated onto a lawn of *E. coli* on non-nutrient agar; the amebae consume the *E. coli*, creating identifiable tracks. Plates should be observed for longer than 7 days.

Buffered charcoal-yeast extract agar is an alternative medium that is more readily available in many laboratories. However, it offers lower recovery rates (72%) compared with non-nutrient agar with live bacterial overlay.[138]

Differential Diagnosis

See Box 62-1. The pseudodendrites of early disease and the ring infiltrate of more advanced disease are often mistakenly identified as representing herpetic keratitis. In those cases that are refractory to treatment, herpetic keratitis and bacterial superinfection should be considered.[136]

Pathology

Acanthamoebae exist in both dormant cystic and active trophozoite forms. Trophozoites bind to the corneal epithelium and establish infection. This is followed by thinning and necrosis of the epithelium, which allows the organism to enter the stroma, where it may enter progressively deeper layers of the stroma and eventually penetrate the anterior chamber. The organism can become encysted in the corneal stroma, and recrudescence after partially successful treatment is considered to be due to an inflammatory response to the necrotic cysts and may not be related to the presence of viable and active amebae, as previously thought.[139]

TABLE 62-7

ANTIAMEBIC MEDICATIONS

Agent	Trade Name	Manufacturer	Dosage Form	Concentration for Ocular Use	Availability	Comment
Cationic antiseptics						
Chlorhexidine			Solution	0.02%	As 20% concentrate	Used as disinfectant
Polyhexamethylene biguanide (PHMB)	Baquacil	Zeneca	Solution	0.02%	As 20% pool disinfectant	Used also as a preservative, contact lens solutions
Aromatic diamidines						
Propamidine isethionate	Brolene	Mays & Baker	Solution	0.1%w/v 10ml	Over-the-counter in UK	
Aminoglycosides						
Neomycin	Neosporin	Burroughs Wellcome/ generic	Solution Ointment	10,000U/ml 10,000U/g 10ml/3.5g	As Neosporin, combined with polymyxin B and either bacitracin (ointment) or gramicidin (drops)	Not available as only neomycin
Azoles						
Clotrimazole	Lotrimin	Schering	Suspension	1%	As powder from manufacturer to make	Poor suspension; difficult
Fluconazole	Diflucan	Roerig	Solution	0.2%	As 2mg/ml solution	Withdraw from vial with filter needle
Ketoconazole	Nizoral	Janssen	Oil solution	5%	As 200mg tablet	In mortar, dissolve 2.5 200mg tablets in 10ml of peanut oil
Miconazole	Monistat	Janssen	Solution	1%	As 10mg/ml solution	Simple 1:1 solution or directly from vial via filter

(Courtesy of Richard G. Fiscella, RPh, MPH.)

Treatment

Although numerous effective antiamebic antimicrobials exist, the preferred treatment of Acanthamoeba keratitis has not yet been established, and a combination of agents is commonly recommended.[140,141] Suggested antimicrobials include cationic antiseptics (chlorhexidine and polyhexamethylene biguanide [PHMB]), which inhibit membrane function; aromatic diamidines (hexamidine, pentamidine, and propamidine), which inhibit DNA synthesis; aminoglycosides (neomycin and paromomycin), which disrupt the plasmalemma of the organism and facilitate the entry of effective drugs into the cornea; and imidazoles (clotrimazole, fluconazole, ketoconazole, and miconazole), which destabilize cell walls (Table 62-7).[142] Dimethyl sulfoxide (DMSO) has also been used in conjunction with propamidine to increase corneal penetration.[142]

Rational combination therapy takes advantage of antimicrobial agents with different and additive or synergistic mechanisms. Many authors suggest using propamidine or PHMB, both of which are active against trophozoites, along with a diamidine, which is active against trophozoites and cysts.[143] Other authors espouse simple débridement or cryosurgery along with topical therapy.[144,145] As an initial approach in our institution, we recommend either chlorhexidine or PHMB in combination with an imidazole or propamidine. Once the diagnosis has been made, drops are usually administered on the hour for 48 hours; then the frequency of nighttime administration is gradually reduced while maintaining hourly daytime administration. As the infection and inflammation subside, the frequency can be reduced over a number of weeks to four times a day, a level that is then maintained for several months. It has recently been suggested that the persistent corneal and scleral inflammation characteristic of acanthamoebic keratitis may be due to necrotic protozoa and amebic cyst walls rather than active trophozoites; therefore, excessively prolonged and aggressive antiamebic therapy may merely increase the morbidity of the disease.[139] The role of

corticosteroids in the treatment of Acanthamoeba infection has not been established. Corticosteroids prevent the encystment of trophozoites in vitro and may therefore enhance the effectiveness of topical treatment.[143] Topical corticosteroids have been shown to prolong effective treatment time but have not necessarily been correlated with increased treatment failure rates.[135] Corticosteroid application should probably be limited to specific indications such as limbitis, scleritis, and uveitis.[146]

Outcome

With timely diagnosis, in a majority of cases, Acanthamoeba organisms can be eradicated from the cornea by medical therapy. However, due to severe inflammation and necrosis, substantial scarring that impairs vision can result, necessitating penetrating keratoplasty for visual rehabilitation. If the infection is controlled, penetrating keratoplasty carries a good prognosis. If penetrating keratoplasty is performed to eradicate an infection that has failed medical therapy and the infected region of the cornea is not included entirely within the donor button, the infection can recur (often at the graft-host interface), with catastrophic consequences.

MICROSPORIDIOSIS

Epidemiology and Pathogenesis

Microsporidia are ubiquitous organisms that exist as obligate intracellular protozoal parasites. Three species of Encephalitozoon (E. hellem, E. cuniculi, and E. intestinalis) have been associated with human ocular infection in HIV-positive patients. Species reported to have caused stromal keratitis after ocular trauma in immunocompetent patients include the following: Vittaforma corneae, Nosema ocularum, Brachiola algerae, Trachiplestophora hominis, Microsporidium africanum, and M. ceylonensis.[147,148] Microsporidial keratitis was first described in 1973 in an immunocompetent boy.[149] Since then, a handful of cases have been reported that developed in immunocompetent patients, but many more have occurred in individuals who were HIV positive.

Clinical Features

In immunocompetent individuals, microsporidiosis infection appears to produce a stromal keratitis, sometimes associated with iritis, whereas immunocompromised patients typically develop conjunctivitis and an epithelial keratitis accompanied by pain, photophobia, blurred vision, and foreign body sensation. The epitheliopathy is characterized by multiple coarse, white to gray epithelial opacities (the more superficial of which stain with fluorescein), decreased corneal luster, and a fusiform swelling in the inferior fornix from which microsporidia might be recovered.[150] These infections rarely lead to corneal ulcers.[151]

Diagnosis

Microsporidia are difficult to recover in culture, and the diagnosis is usually made by direct observation of the organism or by immunofluorescent antibody studies. Serological assays have been established to detect IgG and IgM; however, they are unable to distinguish between acute or latent infections and previous contact with the pathogen. PCR, used in combination with light microscopy, offers an excellent diagnostic approach, with the added advantage of species differentiation of microsporidiosis.[148] On Gram's stain, microsporidia appear as gram-positive, ovoid, intracytoplasmic inclusions. Variable staining characteristics are observed with Giemsa, Gomori's methenamine silver, and Ziehl-Neelsen staining. Periodic acid–Schiff stain reveals a typical body at one end of the organism. An improved hot Gram-chromotrope technique has shortened the previously time-consuming process to 5 minutes. This chromotrope-based stain involves a trichrome stain that effectively demonstrates dense concentrations of individual intracellular spores.[152,153] The confocal microscope can reveal intraepithelial microsporidia, but these organisms (which measure 1 by 2 μm) approach the resolution limits of this instrument.[154] Electron microscopy performed on body fluids is considered the gold standard for diagnosis of microsporidial infection.

Differential Diagnosis

See Box 62-1.

Systemic Associations

Microsporidial infection can involve nearly every organ system in severely immunocompromised HIV-infected patients (usually CD4 cell counts <100/μl). The gastrointestinal system is most commonly involved, representing a major cause of malabsorption and diarrhea in AIDS patients. Ocular infections are second in frequency and may result from nasopharyngeal infection or from urine-to-finger-to-eye contamination. When ocular microsporidial infections are diagnosed, the patient must be fully examined for other areas of involvement. Other common infections include sinusitis, hepatitis, peritonitis, cholangitis, myositis, bronchiolitis, pneumonia, encephalitis, cystitis, and nephritis. Rare manifestations include urethritis, prostatic abscess, tongue ulcer, and skeletal and cutaneous involvement.[147]

Treatment

Treatment regimens for ocular microsporidiosis have included oral itraconazole, oral albendazole, topical propamidine, and topical fumagillin (Fumadil B).[155,156] Fumagillin appears to be most effective in reducing the symptoms of keratoconjunctivitis. A 10mg/ml suspension can be applied hourly for 24 hours and then tapered. Complete resolution of symptoms has been reported in

as short a period as 3 days.[157] Combination antiretroviral therapy, which includes protease inhibitors, can restore immunity to microsporidiosis and has been shown to improve symptoms.[158]

Outcome

Topical treatment of microsporidiosis keratoconjunctivitis with fumagillin has resulted in elimination of the organism from the cornea.[159] However, in some cases, symptoms have returned upon the discontinuation of treatment; in such an event, a low maintenance dose of one drop a day might be sufficient to control the keratoconjunctivitis. Alternatively, albendazole, a broad-spectrum anthelmintic, has been used when ocular microsporidiosis was refractory to topical therapy.[156] Others have administered itraconazole, a broad-spectrum oral antifungal, after albendazole treatment failure.[160] Disease involving the corneal stroma is difficult to treat, and recrudescence is common. Some authors advocate full-thickness keratoplasty in these cases, as lamellar keratoplasty does not preclude recurrence.[161]

ONCHOCERCIASIS
Epidemiology and Pathogenesis

Onchocerciasis, also known as river blindness, is a major cause of blindness worldwide; approximately 18 million people are infected with the parasite *Onchocerca volvulus*, of whom 270,000 are rendered blind or visually impaired.[162] Ninety-nine percent of these cases occur in the 30 countries in Africa where the disease is still endemic.[163,164] The causative organism is a filarial nematode that is transmitted by the Simulium black fly, which breeds in the fast-flowing rivers and streams of Africa, Brazil, Mexico, the Middle East, and parts of Central America. The fly feeds on the skin of infected humans and becomes infected with microfilariae. These microfilariae become infective within the fly after a week and are transmitted back to humans by the feeding fly. The larvae mature within the skin and then migrate around the body, either directly or along blood vessels and nerve sheaths and via the bloodstream. The worms can survive for up to 15 years, with males achieving a length of about 4cm and females up to 50cm.

Although most cases are transmitted by the black fly, transplacental infection can occur. Children are commonly infected, and infection in males occurs more frequently, appears at a younger age, and follows a more severe course. Eye disease is related to the inflammatory response generated by the nematodes, which can be found in the conjunctival epithelium, corneal stroma, iris, ciliary body, sclera, extraocular muscles, and optic nerve sheath.

Clinical Features

Early infection with the Onchocerca worm is marked by mild and intermittent to intense and constant pruritus, which can lead to infected excoriation due to scratching. Hyperpigmented patches and variably distributed papules develop on the skin; the latter represent intraepithelial abscesses laden with microfilariae. As the infection progresses, the skin develops patches of depigmentation and becomes generally dry and atrophic. Subcutaneous nodules that contain adult worms develop; typically, they occur above the waist in Central America (particularly on the head), about the pelvis in Africa, and below the waist in the Middle East. They can be deep and nonpalpable or more superficially located. If more superficial, they appear as nontender, freely movable nodules, usually grouped in lobulated masses about 0.5–1cm in diameter, with occasional satellite masses.

Ocular findings tend to develop more than a year after skin symptoms, and the severity of these findings depends not only on the duration and severity of infection but also on the strain of microfilariae. The savanna strain from the savanna regions of West Africa is known to induce a more severe inflammatory response and a sclerosing keratitis, which is typically absent in infections caused by the rain forest strain.[165-167] Symptoms and signs can involve virtually all ocular tissues. Lid nodules and edema, chronic conjunctivitis with injection, chemosis, and phlyctenule-like conjunctival masses can develop. Corneal involvement is marked by a fine interpalpebral, epithelial punctate keratitis that overlies white subepithelial flake-like opacities and discrete nummular scars, and stromal edema caused by an intrastromal worm. These worms can be visualized at the slit lamp on retroillumination at all corneal levels as S- or C-shaped fine, motile filaments. Conjunctival pigment can migrate onto the cornea. Sclerosing keratitis represents more severe, blinding corneal disease. It tends to appear as an anterior stromal haze centered at the 3 and 9 o'clock positions separated from the limbus by a clear zone. Both infiltration and neovascularization progress and can encroach on the visual axis as the entire cornea becomes involved. Calcific band keratopathy and uveitis can develop, as well as a scleritis.

Microfilariae might be observed in the anterior chamber, especially in the inferior angle on gonioscopy, or on the anterior lens capsule. In some cases, the accompanying uveitis can be severe, leading to corectopia, synechiae, occluded pupil, and secondary glaucoma. Chorioretinal lesions are associated with iridocyclitis and tend to appear as asymmetrical lesions peripheral to the macula or around the optic nerve head. Peripapillary chorioretinitis with optic nerve edema can result in optic atrophy, another significant cause of visual impairment.

Diagnosis

Diagnosis is based on observation and identification of the worm. It can be recovered from the skin, by taking a bloodless skin snip from the scapula, iliac crest, or lower calf, or from an excised nodule. The worm count in skin snips is correlated with the intensity of infection. More recently, Onchocerca-specific antigens have been detected by enzyme-labeled antibodies. They include the dipstick immunobinding assay for ocular microfilariae (DSIA), which is employed on tear samples; the transblot immunobinding assay for the detection of skin microfilariae (TADA); and the dot-blot immunobinding assay for detecting urinary microfilariae and their antigens (DIA). These dipstick tests are cost-effective yet offer high sensitivity and specificity rates.[168] Diagnosis can also be made by the Mazzotti test: oral diethylcarbamazepine, which induces widespread onchocercal death with antigen release and resultant eosinophilia, is administered under close supervision. Within 30 minutes, but possibly up to 24 hours later, the patient develops pruritus, erythema, and flu-like symptoms, which might be severe. After the first few hours of drug administration, microfilariae can be recovered from the blood and urine.

Differential Diagnosis

Similar skin lesions can be seen in association with *Mansonella perstans* microfilarial infection. Skin nodules and uveitis can also be seen with sarcoidosis.

Systemic Associations

Besides being present in the skin lesions, the microfilariae can be identified in blood vessels, visceral organs, the central nervous system, urine, and sputum. Superficial lymph nodes draining areas with cutaneous concentrations of the worms can become painlessly enlarged.

Pathology

The destructive inflammation caused by Onchocerca infection is stimulated by antigens released by dead and dying organisms. This process initiates a Th2 response in the lymphoid tissue, including interleukin-4 production, which stimulates B cell anti-body production, and interleukin-5, which stimulates eosinophil production and activation. When microfilariae begin to die in the cornea, parasite antigens are recognized, triggering a cascade that results in secretion of chemokines and expression of vascular endothelium adhesion molecules. Eosinophils and neutrophils migrate into the corneal stroma in response to these signals. Surface-bound immunoglobulin molecules on these cells cross-link with parasite antigen, causing the inflammatory cells to degranulate. These eosinophil and neutrophil granule proteins are cytotoxic and disrupt the normal functioning of the corneal cells responsible for maintaining clarity, resulting in corneal opacification. The pathways leading to corneal neovascularization and fibrosis have yet to be elicited.[162]

In the skin, subcutaneous nodules are found that consist of adult worms surrounded by granulation tissue composed of fibrin, lymphocytes, macrophages, eosinophils, PMNs, and giant cells.

Treatment

The mainstay of treatment is oral ivermectin given as a single dose (150μg/kg), and repeated yearly.[169] Ivermectin slowly eliminates the microfilariae over 6 months, minimizing the destructive inflammatory response for up to 18 months.[169] Oral ivermectin reverses even advanced sclerosing keratitis and iridocyclitis and has been reported to improve the appearance of optic atrophy in some cases. However, improvement in chorioretinal lesions has not been observed. Iridocyclitis should be treated with corticosteroids and cycloplegia.

Outcome

Although anterior segment inflammation and lesions respond well to treatment, severe visual impairment can result from chorioretinitis that, in advanced cases, often continues to progress in spite of treatment. Health programs are aimed at blindness prevention through treatment, prevention, and vector control; eradication of the parasite in highly endemic areas is estimated to require nearly three decades of annual treatment.[170]

REFERENCES

1. Whitcher JP. Corneal ulceration. Int Ophthalmol Clin. 1990;30:30–2.
2. Pepose JS, Wilhelmus KR. Divergent approaches to the management of corneal ulcers (editorial). Am J Ophthalmol. 1992;114:630–2.
3. MacRae S, Herman C, Stulting RD, et al. Corneal ulcer and adverse reaction rates in premarket contact lens studies. Am J Ophthalmol. 1991;111:457–65.
4. Poggio EC, Glynn RJ, Schein OD, et al. The incidence of ulcerative keratitis among users of daily-wear and extended-wear soft contact lenses. N Engl J Med. 1989;321:779–83.
5. Bowden FW III, Cohen EJ. Corneal ulcerations with contact lenses. Ophthalmol Clin North Am. 1998;2:267–73.
6. Arnold RR, Cole MF, McGhee JR. A bacterial effect for human lactoferrin. Science. 1977;197:263–5.
7. Rotkis WM. Lysozyme: its significance in external ocular disease. In: O'Connor GR, ed. Immunologic diseases of the mucous membranes: pathology, diagnosis and treatment. New York: Masson; 1980:27–31.
8. McLeod SD, Flowers CW, Lopez PF, et al. Endophthalmitis and orbital cellulitis after radial keratotomy. Ophthalmology. 1995;102:1902–7.
9. Sachs R, Zagelbaum BM, Hersh PS. Corneal complications associated with the use of crack cocaine. Ophthalmology. 1993;100:187–91.
10. Chuck RS, Williams JM, Goldstein MA, Lubniewski AJ. Recurrent corneal ulcerations associated with smokeable methamphetamine abuse. Am J Ophthalmol. 1996;121:571–2.
11. Butler TK, Dua HS, Edwards R, Lowe JS. In vitro model of infectious crystalline keratopathy: tissue architecture determines pattern of microbial spread. Invest Ophthalmol Vis Sci. 2001;42:1243–6.
12. Ostler HB, Ostler MW. Diseases of the cornea. In: Diseases of the external eye and adnexa: a text and atlas. Baltimore: Williams & Wilkins; 1993:137–251.
13. Zaidman GW. *Propionibacterium acnes* keratitis. Am J Ophthalmol. 1992;113:596–8.
14. McLean JM. Oculomycosis. Trans Am Acad Ophthalmol Otolaryngol. 1963;67:149–63.
15. Knapp A, Stern GA, Hood CI. *Mycobacterium avium-intracellulare* corneal ulcer. Cornea. 1987;6:175–80.
16. Moore MB, Newton C, Kaufman HE. Chronic keratitis caused by *Mycobacterium gordonae*. Am J Ophthalmol. 1986;102:516–21.
17. Binford H, Meyers WM, Walsh GP. Leprosy. JAMA 1982;247:2283–92.
18. Sugar J, Hill C. Leprosy. In: Eye and skin diseases. Philadelphia: Lippincott-Raven; 1996:543–50.
19. Allen JH, Byers JL. The pathology of ocular leprosy. I. Cornea. Arch Ophthalmol. 1960;64:216–20.

20. O'Brien TP, Maguire MG, Fink NE, *et al.* Efficacy of ofloxacin vs cefazolin and tobramycin in the therapy for bacterial keratitis: report from the bacterial keratitis study research group. Arch Ophthalmol. 1995;113:1257–65.
21. McLeod SD, Kolahdouz-Isfahani A, Rostamian K, *et al.* The role of routine smears, cultures and antibiotic sensitivity testing in the management of suspected infectious keratitis. Ophthalmology. 1996;103:23–8.
22. Benson WH, Lanier JD. Comparison of techniques for culturing corneal ulcers. Ophthalmology. 1992;99:800–4.
23. Alexandrakis G, Haimovici R, Miller D, Alfonso EC. Corneal biopsy in the management of progressive microbial keratitis. Am J Ophthalmol. 2000;129:571–6.
24. Nanda M, Pflugfelder SC, Holland S. Fulminant pseudomonal keratitis and scleritis in human immunodeficiency virus–infected patients. Arch Ophthalmol. 1991;109:503–5.
25. Stern GA, Weitzenkorn D, Valenti J. Adherence of *Pseudomonas aeruginosa* to the mouse cornea. Epithelial vs stomal adherence. Arch Ophthalmol. 1982;100:1956–8.
26. Kharazmi A. Mechanisms involved in the evasion of the host defence by *Pseudomonas aeruginosa.* Immunol Lett. 1991;30:201–5.
27. Hazlett LD, Rudner IL, Mclellan SA, *et al.* Role of IL-12 and IFN-gamma in *Pseudomonas aeruginosa* corneal infection. Invest Ophthalmol Vis Sci. 2002;43:419–24.
28. Steuhl KP, Doring G, Henni A, *et al.* Relevance of host-derived and bacterial factors in *Pseudomonas aeruginosa* corneal infections. Invest Ophthalmol Vis Sci. 1987;28:1559–68.
29. Cleveland RP, Hazlett LD, Leon MA, Berk RS. Role of complement in murine corneal infection caused by *Pseudomonas aeruginosa.* Invest Ophthalmol Vis Sci. 1983;24:237–42.
30. Baum J, Barza M. Topical vs subconjunctival treatment of bacterial corneal ulcers. Ophthalmology. 1983;90:162–8.
31. Davis SD, Sarff LD, Hyndiuk RA. Comparison of therapeutic routes in experimental *Pseudomonas* keratitis. Am J Ophthalmol. 1979;87:710–6.
32. Arffa RC. Infectious ulcerative keratitis: bacterial. In: Grayson's diseases of the cornea, 3rd ed. St. Louis: Mosby Year Book; 1991:163–98.
33. McLeod SD, LaBree LD, Tayyanipour R, *et al.* The importance of initial management in the treatment of severe infectious corneal ulcers. Ophthalmology. 1995;102:1943–8.
34. Panda A, Ahuja R, Sastry SS. Comparison of topical 0.3% ofloxacin with fortified tobramycin plus cefazolin in the treatment of bacterial keratitis. Eye. 1999;13:744–77.
35. Anonymous. Ciprofloxacin. Med Lett Drugs Ther. 1988;30:11–3.
36. Esposito S, Noviello S, Ianniello F. Comparative in vitro activity of older and newer fluoroquinolones against respiratory tract pathogens. Chemotherapy. 2000;46:309–14.
37. Varon E, Gutmann L. Mechanisms and spread of fluoroquinolone resistance in *Streptococcus pneumoniae.* Res Microbiol. 2000;151:471–3.
38. Kowalski RP, Pandya AN, Karenchak LM, *et al.* An in vitro resistance study of levofloxacin, ciprofloxacin, and ofloxacin using keratitis isolates of *Staphylococcus aureus* and *Pseudomonas aeruginosa.* Ophthalmology. 2001;108:1826–9.
39. Lister PD. Emerging resistance problems among respiratory tract pathogens. Am J Manag Care. 2000;6:S409–18.
40. Alexndrakis G, Alfonso EC, Miller D. Shifting trends in bacterial keratitis in south Florida and emerging resistance to fluoroquinolones. Ophthalmololgy. 2000;107:1497–502.
41. Goettsch W, van Pelt W, Nagelkerke N, *et al.* Increasing resistance to fluoroquinolones in *Escherichia coli* from urinary tract infections in the Netherlands. J Antimicrob Chemother. 2000;46:223–8.
42. Anonymous. Fluoroquinolone-resistance in *Neisseria gonorrhoeae,* Hawaii 1999, and decreased susceptibility to azithromycin in *N. gonorrhoeae,* Missouri, 1999. MMWR Morb Mortal Wkly Rep. 2000;49:833–7.
43. Garg P, Sharma S, Rao GN. Ciprofloxacin-resistant *Pseudomonas* keratitis. Ophthalmology. 1999;106:1319–23.
44. Kunimoto DY, Sharma S, Garg P, Rao GN. In vitro susceptibility of bacterial keratitis pathogens to ciprofloxacin. Emerging resistance. Ophthalmology. 1999;106:80–5.
45. Knauf HP, Silvany R, Southern PM Jr, *et al.* Susceptibility of corneal and conjunctival pathogens to ciprofloxacin. Cornea. 1996;15:66–71.
46. Goldstein MH, Kowalski RP, Gordon YJ. Emerging fluoroquinolone resistance in bacterial keratitis: a 5 year review. Ophthalmology. 1999;106:1313–8.
47. Neu HC. Tobramycin: an overview. J Infect Dis. 1976;134(suppl):S3–19.
48. Fiscella RG. Vancomycin use in ophthalmology. Arch Ophthalmol. 1995;133:1353–4.
49. Ormerod LD, Heseltine PNR, Alfonso E, *et al.* Gentamicin-resistant pseudomonal infection: rationale for a redefinition of ophthalmic antimicrobial sensitivities. Cornea. 1989;8:195–9.
50. Gritz DC, Lee TY, Kwitko S, McDonnell PJ. Topical anti-inflammatory agents in an animal model of microbial keratitis. Arch Ophthalmol. 1990;108:1001–5.
51. Hill JC. Use of penetrating keratoplasty in acute bacterial keratitis. Br J Ophthalmol. 1986;70:502–6.
52. Obara Y, Furuta Y, Takasu T, *et al.* Distribution of herpes simplex virus types 1 and 2 genomes in human spinal ganglia studied by PCR and in situ hybridization. J Med Virol. 1997;52:136–42.
53. Liesegang TJ, Melton LJ III, Daly PJ, Ilstrup DM. Epidemiology of ocular herpes simplex: incidence in Rochester, Minn, 1950 through 1982. Arch Ophthalmol. 1989;107:1155–9.
54. Liedtke W, Opalka B, Zimmermann CW, Lignitz E. Age distribution of latent herpes simplex virus 1 and varicella-zoster virus genome in human nervous tissue. J Neurol Sci. 1993;116:6–11.
55. Liesegang TJ. Herpes simplex virus epidemiology and ocular importance. Cornea. 2001;20:(1):1–13.
56. Claoue CMP, Menage MJ, Easty DL. Severe herpetic keratitis. I. Prevalence of visual impairment in a clinic population. Br J Ophthalmol. 1988;72:530–3.
57. Shuster JJ, Kaufman HE, Nesburn AB. Statistical analysis of the rate of recurrence of herpesvirus ocular epithelial disease. Am J Ophthalmol. 1981;91:328–31.
58. Foster A, Sommer A. Corneal ulceration, measles, and childhood blindness in Tanzania. Br J Ophthalmol. 1987;71:331–43.
59. Pepose JS. External ocular herpesvirus infections in immunodeficiency. Curr Eye Res. 1991;10(suppl):587–95.
60. Shuler JD, Engstrom RE Jr, Holland GN. External ocular disease and anterior segment disorders associated with AIDS. Int Ophthalmol Clin. 1989;29:98–104.
61. Hodge WG, Seiff SR, Margolis TP. Ocular opportunistic infection incidences among patients who are HIV positive compared to patients who are HIV negative. Ophthalmology. 1998;105:895–900.
62. Wilhelmus KR, Falcon MG, Jones BR. Bilateral herpetic keratitis. Br J Ophthalmol. 1981;65:385–7.
63. Nahmias AJ, Alford CA, Korones SB. Infection of the newborn with *Herpesvirus hominis.* Adv Pediatr. 1970;17:185–226.
64. Nahmias AJ, Visintine AM, Caldwell DR, Wilson LA. Eye infections with herpes simplex viruses in neonates. Surv Ophthalmol. 1976;21:100–5.
65. Kaufman HE. Epithelial erosion syndrome: metaherpetic keratitis. Am J Ophthalmol. 1964;57:983–7.
66. Pepose JS. Herpes simplex keratitis: role of viral infection versus immune response. Surv Ophthalmol. 1991;35:345–52.
67. Kaufman HE, Kanai A, Ellison ED. Herpetic iritis: demonstration of virus in the anterior chamber by fluorescent antibody techniques and electron microscopy. Am J Ophthalmol. 1971;71:465–9.
68. Robert PY, Traccard I, Adenis JP, *et al.* Multiplex detection of herpesviruses in tear fluid using the "stair primers" PCR method: prospective study of 93 patients. J Med Virol. 2002;66:506–11.
69. Sundmacher R, Neumann-Haefelin D. Herpes simplex virus–positive and negative keratouveitis. In: Silverstein AM, O'Connor GR, eds. Immunology and immunopathology of the eye. New York: Masson; 1979:225–9.
70. Nagy RM, McFall RC, Sery TW, *et al.* Scanning electron microscope study of herpes simplex virus experimental keratitis. Br J Ophthalmol. 1978;52:838–42.
71. Keadle TL, Usui N, Laycock KA, *et al.* IL-1 and TNF-alpha are important factors in the pathogenesis of murine recurrent herpetic stomal keratitis. Invest Ophthalmol Vis Sci. 2000;41(1):96–102.
72. Collum LM, McGettrick P, Akhtar J, *et al.* Oral acyclovir (Zovirax) in herpes simplex dendritic corneal ulceration. Br J Ophthalmol. 1986;70(6):435–8.
73. Loutsch JM, Sainz B Jr, Marquart ME, *et al.* Effects of famciclovir on herpes simplex virus type 1 corneal disease and establishment of latency in rabbits. Antimicrob Agents Chemother. 2001;45(7):2044–53.
74. The Herpetic Eye Disease Study Group. A controlled trial of oral acyclovir for the prevention of stomal keratitis or iritis in patients with herpes simplex virus epithelial keratitis. The epithelial keratitis trial. Ophthalmology. 1997;115(6):703–12.
75. Wilhelmus KR, Gee L, Hauck WW, *et al.* Herpetic eye disease study: a controlled trial of topical corticosteroids for herpes simplex stromal keratitis. Ophthalmology. 1994;101:1883–96.
76. Barron BA, Gee L, Hauck WW, *et al.* Herpetic eye disease study: a controlled trial of oral acyclovir for herpes simplex stromal keratitis. Ophthalmology. 1994;101:1871–82.
77. Heiligenhaus A, Bauer D, Meller D, *et al.* Improvement of HSV-1 necrotizing keratitis with amniotic membrane transplantation. Invest Ophthalmol Vis Sci. 2001;42(9):1969–74.
78. The Herpetic Eye Disease Study Group. A controlled trial of oral acyclovir for iridocyclitis caused by herpes simpex virus. Arch Ophthalmol. 1996;114:1065–72.
79. The Herpetic Eye Disease Study Group. Acyclovir for the prevention of recurrent herpes simplex virus eye disease. N Engl J Med. 1998;339:300–6.
80. Cohen EJ, Laibson PR, Arentsen JJ. Corneal transplantation for herpes simplex keratitis. Am J Ophthalmol. 1983;95:645–50.
81. Gershon AA, Steinberg SP. Antibody responses to varicella-zoster virus and the role of antibody in host defense. Am J Med Sci. 1981;282:12–7.
82. Liesegang TJ. Diagnosis and therapy of herpes zoster ophthalmicus. Ophthalmology. 1991;98:1216–29.
83. Ragozzino MW, Melton LJ III, Kurland LT, *et al.* Population-based study of herpes zoster and its sequelae. Medicine. 1982;61:310–6.
84. Weller TH. Varicella and herpes zoster. Pt 1. N Engl J Med. 1983;309:1362–8.
85. Liesegang TJ. Corneal complications from herpes zoster ophthalmicus. Ophthalmology. 1985;92:316–24.
86. Chern KC, Conrad D, Holland GN, *et al.* Chronic varicella-zoster virus epithelial keratitis in patients with acquired immunodeficiency syndrome. Arch Ophthalmol. 1998;116:1011–7.
87. Chern KC, Margolis TP. Varicella zoster virus ocular disease. Int Ophthalmol Clin. 1998;38:149–60.
88. Arvin AM, Pollard RB, Rasmussen LE, Merigan TC. Cellular and humoral immunity in the pathogenesis of recurrent herpes viral infections in patients with lymphoma. J Clin Invest. 1980;65:869–78.
89. McGill J. The enigma of herpes stromal disease. Br J Ophthalmol. 1987;71:118–25.
90. Green WR, Zimmerman L. Granulomatous reaction of Descemet's membrane. Am J Ophthalmol. 1967;64:555–8.
91. Kost RG, Straus SE. Postherpetic neuralgia—pathogenesis, treatment, and prevention. N Engl J Med. 1996;335:32–42.
92. Beutner KR. Valacyclovir: a review of its antiviral activity, pharmacokinetic properties, and clinical efficacy. Antiviral Res. 1995;28:281–90.
93. Pavan-Langston D, Yamamoto S, Dunkel EC. Delayed herpes zoster pseudodendrites. Polymerase chain reaction detection of viral DNA and a role for antiviral therapy. Arch Ophthalmol. 1995;113:1381–5.
94. Soong HK, Schwartz AE, Meyer RF, Sugar A. Penetrating keratoplasty for corneal scarring due to herpes zoster ophthalmicus. Br J Ophthalmol. 1989;73:19–21.
95. Reed JW, Joyner SJ, Knauer WJ III. Penetrating keratoplasty for herpes zoster keratopathy. Am J Ophthalmol. 1989;107:257–61.
96. Fleisher GR, Bolognese R. Seroepidemiology of Epstein-Barr virus in pregnant women. J Infect Dis. 1982;145:537–41.
97. Jones BR, Howie JB, Wilson RP. Ocular aspects of an epidemic of infectious mononucleosis. Proc Univ Otago Med Sch. 1952;30:1–4.
98. Meisler DM, Bosworth DE, Krachmer JH. Ocular infectious mononucleosis manifested as Parinaud's oculoglandular syndrome. Am J Ophthalmol. 1981;92:722–6.
99. Matoba AY, Wilhelmus KR, Jones DB. Epstein-Barr viral stromal keratitis. Ophthalmology. 1986;93:746–51.

100. Erlich KS. Laboratory diagnosis of herpesvirus infections. Clin Lab Med. 1987;7:759–76.

101. Silverstein A, Steinberg G, Nathanson M. Nervous system involvement in infectious mononucleosis: the heralding and-or major manifestations. Arch Neurol. 1972;26:353–8.

102. Brown HH, Glasgow BJ, Holland GN, Foos RY. Cytomegalovirus infection of the conjunctiva in AIDS. Am J Ophthalmol. 1988;106:102–4.

103. Yee RW, Sigler SC, Lawton AW, et al. Apparent cytomegalovirus epithelial keratitis in a cardiac transplant recipient. Transplantation. 1991;51:1040–3.

104. Wehrly SR, Manning FJ, Proia AD, et al. Cytomegalovirus keratitis after penetrating keratoplasty. Cornea. 1995;14:623–33.

105. Wilhelmus KR, Font RL, Lehmann RP, Cernoch PL. Cytomegalovirus keratitis in acquired immunodeficiency syndrome. Arch Ophthalmol. 1996;114:869–72.

106. Pastor SA, Shuster AR, Miller MM, Lam K-W. Use of impression cytology to demonstrate a retrovirus in AIDS patients with cytomegalovirus retinitis. Cornea. 1991;10:511–5.

107. Houang E, Lam D, Fan D, Seal D. Microbial keratitis in Hong Kong: relationship to climate, environment and contact-lens disinfection. Trans R Soc Trop Med Hyg. 2001;95:361–7.

108. O'Day DM. Fungal keratitis. In: Pepose JS, Holland GN, Wilhelmus KR, eds. Ocular infection and immunity. St. Louis: Mosby Year Book; 1996:1048–61.

109. Kuo IC, Margolis TP, Cevallos V, Kwang DG. Aspergillus fumigatus keratitis after laser in situ keratomileusis. Cornea. 2001;20:342–4.

110. Sridhar MS, Garg P, Bansal AK, Sharma S. Fungal keratitis after laser in situ keratomileusis. J Cataract Refract Surg. 2000;26(4):613–5.

111. Winchester K, Mathers WD, Sutphin JE. Diagnosis of Aspergillus keratitis in vivo with confocal microscopy. Cornea. 1997;16:27–31.

112. Arffa RC. Infectious keratitis: fungal and parasitic. In: Grayson's diseases of the cornea, 3rd ed. St. Louis: Mosby Year Book; 1991:199–223.

113. Nelson RD, Shibata N, Podzorski RP, Herron MJ. Candida mannan: chemistry, suppression of cell-mediated immunity, and possible mechanisms of action. Clin Microbiol Rev. 1991;4:1–19.

114. Naumann G, Green WR, Zimmerman LE. Mycotic keratitis: the histopathologic study of 73 cases. Am J Ophthalmol. 1967;64:668–82.

115. Ishida N, Brown AC, Rao GN, et al. Recurrent Fusarium keratomycosis: a light and electron microscopic study. Ann Ophthalmol. 1984;16:354–66.

116. Zhu WS, Wojdyla K, Donlon K, et al. Extracellular proteases of Aspergillus flavus. Diagn Microbiol Infect Dis. 1990;13:491–7.

117. Gopinathan U, Ramakrishna T, Willcox M, et al. Enzymatic, clinical and histologic evaluation of corneal tissues in experimental fungal keratitis in rabbits. Exp Eye Res. 2001;72:433–42.

118. O'Day DM, Head WS, Robinson RD, Clanton JA. Corneal penetration of topical amphotericin B and natamycin. Curr Eye Res. 1986;5:877–82.

119. Brajtburg J, Kobayashi D, Medoff G, Kobayashi GS. Antifungal action of amphotericin B in combination with other polyene or imidazole antibiotics. J Infect Dis. 1982;146:138–46.

120. Forster RK. Fungal keratitis and conjunctivitis: clinical disease. In: Smolin G, Thoft RA, eds. The cornea. Scientific foundations and clinical practice, 3rd ed. Boston: Little, Brown; 1994:239–52.

121. Thienpont D, Van Cutsem J, Van Gerven F, et al. Ketoconazole: a new broad spectrum orally active antimycotic. Experientia. 1979;35:606–9.

122. Ernst EJ. Investigational antifungal agents. Pharmacotherapy. 2001;21(8 pt 2):165S–74S.

123. Kaushik S, Ram J, Brar GS, et al. Intracameral amphotericn B: initial experience in severe keratomycosis. Cornea. 2001;20:715–9.

124. Bell NP, Karp CL, Alfonso EC, et al. Effects of methylprednisolone and cyclosporine A on fungal growth in vitro. Cornea. 1999;18:306–13.

125. Perry HD, Doshi SJ, Donnenfeld ED, Bai GS. Topical cyclosporin A in the management of therapeutic keratoplasty for mycotic keratitis. Cornea. 2002;21:161–3.

126. Xie L, Dong X, Shi W. Treatment of fungal keratitis by penetrating keratoplasty. Br J Ophthalmol. 2001;85:1070–4.

127. Xie L, Shi W, Liu Z, Li S. Lamellar keratoplasty for the treatment of fungal keratitis. Cornea. 2002;21:33–7.

128. Forster RK, Rebell G. Therapeutic surgery in failures of medical treatment for fungal keratitis. Br J Ophthalmol. 1975;59:366–71.

129. Mathers WD, Sutphin JE, Folberg R, et al. Outbreak of keratitis presumed to be caused by Acanthamoeba. Am J Ophthalmol. 1996;121:129–42.

130. Mathers WD, Nelson SE, Lane J. Confirmation of confocal microscopy diagnosis of Acanthamoeba keratitis using polymerase chain reaction analysis. Arch Ophthalmol. 2000;118:178–83.

131. Aitken D, Hay J, Kinnear FB, et al. Amebic keratitis in a wearer of disposable contact lenses due to a mixed Vahlkampfia and Hartmannella infection. Ophthalmology. 1996;103:485–94.

132. Radford CF, Lehmamm OJ, Dart JK. Acanthamoeba keratitis: multicentre survey in England 1992–6. Br J Ophthalmol. 1998;82:1387–92.

133. Sharma S, Prashant G, Gullapalli R. Patient characteristics, diagnosis, and treatment of non–contact lens related Acanthamoeba keratitis. Br J Ophthalmol. 2000;84:1103–8.

134. Gorlin AI, Gabriel MM, Wilson LA, Ahearn DG. Effect of adhered bacteria on the binding of Acanthamoeba to hydrogel lenses. Arch Ophthalmol. 1996;114:576–80.

135. Park DH, Palay DA, Daya SM. The role of topical corticosteroids in the management of Acanthamoeba keratitis. Cornea. 1997;16(3):277–83.

136. Lindquist TD. Treatment of Acanthamoeba keratitis. Cornea. 1998;17(1):11–6.

137. Pfister DR, Cameron JD, Krachmer JH, Holland EJ. Confocal microscopy findings of Acanthamoeba keratitis. Am J Ophthalmol. 1996;121:119–28.

138. Penland RL, Wilhelmus KR. Laboratory diagnosis of Acanthamoeba keratitis using buffered charcoal-yeast extract agar. Am J Ophthalmol. 1998;126(4):590–2.

139. Yang YF, Matheson M, Dart JK. Persistence of Acanthamoeba antigen following Acanthamoeba keratitis. Br J Ophthalmol. 2001;85:277–80.

140. Hay J, Kirkness CM, Seal DV, Wright P. Drug resistance and Acanthamoeba keratitis: the quest for alternative antiprotozoal chemotherapy. Eye. 1994;8:555–63.

141. D'Aversa G, Stern GA, Driebe WT Jr. Diagnosis and successful medical treatment of Acanthamoeba keratitis. Arch Ophthalmol. 1995;113:1120–3.

142. Wysenbeek YS, Blank-Porat D, Harizman N. The reculture technique: individualizing the treatment of Acanthamoeba keratitis. Cornea. 2000;19(4):464–7.

143. O'Day DM, Head WS. Advances in the management of keratomycosis and Acanthamoeba keratitis. Cornea. 2000;19(5):681–7.

144. Brooks JG, Coster DJ, Badenoch PR. Acanthamoeba keratitis. Resolution after epithelial débridement. Cornea. 1994;13:186–9.

145. Amoils SP, Heney C. Acanthamoeba keratitis with live isolates treated with cryosurgery and fluconazole. Am J Ophthalmol. 1999;127(6):718–9.

146. Bacon AS, Frazer DG, Dart JKG. A review of 72 consecutive cases of Acanthamoeba keratitis. Eye. 1993;7:719–25.

147. Franzen C, Muller A. Molecular techniques for detection, species differentiation, and phylogenetic analysis of microsporidia. Clin Microbiol Rev. 1999;12(2):243–85.

148. Franzen C, Muller A. Current focus: microsporidia, intracellular parasites causing emerging diseases. Microsporidiosis: human diseases and diagnosis. Microbes Infect. 2001;3(5):389–400.

149. Ashton N, Wirasinha PA. Encephalitozoonosis (nosematosis) of the cornea. Br J Ophthalmol. 1973;57:669–74.

150. Friedberg DN, Stenson SM, Orenstein JM, et al. Microsporidial keratoconjunctivitis in acquired immunodeficiency syndrome. Arch Ophthalmol. 1990;108:504–8.

151. Reboucas Martins SA, Muccioli C, Belfors R. Resolution of microsporidial keratoconjunctivitis in an AIDS patient treated with highly active antiretroviral therapy. Am J Ophthalmol. 2001;131(3):378–9.

152. Weber R, Schwartz DA, Deplazes P. Laboratory diagnosis of microsporidiosis. Microsporidia Microsporidiosis. 1999;315–62.

153. Weber R, Bryan RT, Owen RL, et al. Improved light-microscopical detection of microsporidia spores in stool and duodenal aspirates. N Engl J Med. 1992;326:161–6.

154. Shah GK, Pfister D, Probst LE, et al. Diagnosis of microsporidial keratitis by confocal microscopy and the chromatrope stain. Am J Ophthalmol. 1996;121:89–91.

155. Theng J, Chan C, Ling ML. Microsporidial keratoconjunctivitis in a healthy contact lens wearer without human immunodeficiency virus infection. Ophthalmology. 2001;108(5):976–8.

156. Gritz DC, Holsclaw DS, Neger RE. Ocular and sinus microsporidial infection cured with systemic albendazole. Am J Ophthalmol. 1997;124(2):241–3.

157. Wilkins JH, Joshi N, Margolis TP, et al. Microsporidial keratoconjunctivitis treated successfully with a short course of fumagillin. Eye. 1994;8:703–4.

158. Carr A, Marriott A, Field E. Treatment of HIV-1–associated microsporidiosis and cryptosporidiosis with combination antiretroviral therapy. Lancet. 1998;351:256–61.

159. Rosberger DF, Sedarevic ON, Erlandson RA, et al. Successful treatment of microsporidial keratoconjunctivitis with topical fumagillin in a patient with AIDS. Cornea. 1993;12:261–5.

160. Rossi P, Urbani C, Donelli G. Resolution of microsporidial sinusitis and keratoconjunctivitis by itraconazole treatment. Am J Ophthalmol. 1999;127:210–2.

161. Font RL, Samaha A, Keener MJ. Corneal microsporidiosis: report of case, including electron microscopic observations. Ophthalmology. 2000;107(9):1769–75.

162. Hall LR, Pearlman E. Pathogenesis of onchocercal keratitis (river blindness). Clin Microbiol Rev. 1999;12(3):445–53.

163. Lewallen S, Courtright P. Blindness in Africa: present situation and future needs. Br J Ophthalmol. 2001;85(8):897–903.

164. World Health Organization. WHO expert committee on onchocerciasis, third report. WHO Tech Rep Ser. 1987;752:1–167.

165. Dadzie K, Remme J, Baker A. Ocular onchocerciasis and intensity of infection in the community. III. West African rainforest foci of the vector Simulium sanctipauli. Trop Med Parasitol. 1990;41:376–82.

166. Dadzie K, Remme A, Thylefors B. Ocular onchocerciasis and intensity of infection in the community. II. West African rainforest foci of the vector Simulium yahense. Trop Med Parasitol. 1989;40:348–52.

167. Pearlman E, Diaconu E, Hazlett FE. Identification of an epitope of a recombinant Onchocerca volvulus protein that induces corneal pathology. Mol Biochem Parasitol. 1997;89:123–35.

168. Ngu JL, Nkenfou C, Capuli E. Novel, sensitive and low-cost diagnostic tests for "river blindness"—detection of specific antigens in tears and dermal fluid. Trop Med Int Health. 1998;3(5):339–48.

169. Mabey D, Whitworth JA, Eckstein M. The effects of multiple doses of ivermectin on ocular onchocerciasis. A six-year follow-up. Ophthalmology. 1996;103(7):1001–8.

170. Plaisier AP, van Oortmarssen GJ, Remme J, et al. The risk and dynamics of onchocerciasis recrudescence after cessation of vector control. Bull World Health Organ. 1991;69:169–78.

CHAPTER

63

Corneal and Conjunctival Surgery

MING X. WANG • CAROL L. KARP • ROBERT P. SELKIN • DIMITRI T. AZAR

KERATOPLASTY

INTRODUCTION

Recent years have seen remarkable progress in the technologies involved in keratoplasty. The successful outcomes enjoyed by patients who undergo modern penetrating keratoplasty and lamellar keratoplasty are the result of advances in operating microscope design, suture technology, surgical techniques, and corneal topography and of the availability of carefully preserved corneal tissue along with a better understanding of corneal and ocular surface physiology.

HISTORICAL REVIEW

Corneal grafting techniques date back to the latter part of the 19th century and earlier part of the 20th century,[1] as exemplified by pioneer ophthalmologists such as Reisinger,[2] von Hippel,[3] and Elschnig.[4] Today, penetrating keratoplasty is the most common and successful human transplantation procedure. Over 40,000 corneal transplantations are performed in the United States each year. Optical results have improved greatly as a result of advances in tissue selection and preservation, trephines, and management of postoperative astigmatism. Corneal grafts are generally performed for two reasons—to restore globe integrity and to restore vision.

Lamellar corneal grafts date back to 1886, when von Hippel[3] successfully performed the first lamellar graft in a human. Developments in lamellar grafting techniques, surgical instrumentation, anesthetic agents, and donor tissue preservation have contributed to the success of this surgical technique. However, in the past few decades, lamellar keratoplasty has become less popular because of the remarkable success of the penetrating corneal graft technique.

ANESTHESIA

Corneal transplant surgeries may be performed using local or general anesthetic. Local anesthetic is used for adult and cooperative patients. Typically, local anesthetic consists of peribulbar or retrobulbar injection of lidocaine (lignocaine) 2%, bupivacaine 0.75%, and hyaluronidase. Peribulbar anesthetic may be preferred over retrobulbar injection to avoid globe penetration. To prevent squeezing during surgery, a lid block may be employed. General anesthetic is reserved for the pediatric age group and uncooperative adults or for use in open globes.

SPECIFIC TECHNIQUES

Lamellar Keratoplasty

Lamellar keratoplasty is a procedure in which a partial-thickness graft of donor tissue is used to provide tectonic stability and/or optical improvement. A partial-thickness section of donor stroma or sclera is used. There are generally two types of lamellar keratoplasty: anterior lamellar keratoplasty and posterior lamellar keratoplasty.

In an anterior lamellar keratoplasty procedure, the transplanted tissue does not include corneal endothelium, and thus donor tissue is obtained more easily from older eyes and this procedure avoids endothelial rejection. Indications for anterior lamellar keratoplasty mainly include anterior corneal pathology in which the posterior cornea is unaffected.

In recent years deep lamellar keratoplasty and posterior lamellar keratoplasty techniques have been developed in which the main objective is to replace diseased corneal endothelium while keeping the anterior corneal surface intact, thus reducing refractive error and irregular astigmatism.

PREOPERATIVE EVALUATION AND DIAGNOSTIC APPROACH. Two major indications exist for anterior lamellar keratoplasty[5,6]—tectonic graft for structural support and/or cosmesis and optical grafts. For posterior lamellar keratoplasty, the aim is to replace the diseased endothelium.

A tectonic graft is the most common type of anterior lamellar keratoplasty performed. It is used to reinforce areas of thinned cornea to prevent melting and perforation or to restore ocular surface integrity, such as after pterygium surgery.

Optical grafts are used to replace diseased anterior cornea to improve visual function and require that the posterior stroma of the recipient is healthy. Lamellar optical grafts are seldom used today because of the increased use of phototherapeutic keratectomy and the excellent outcomes with penetrating keratoplasty.

Regarding posterior lamellar keratoplasty, the main advantage is the preservation of the anterior corneal tissue and thus maintenance of the refractive character of the cornea.

The rationale for a lamellar keratoplasty must be examined carefully and the various surgical options thoroughly discussed with patients. Compared with penetrating keratoplasty, anterior lamellar keratoplasty eliminates the chance of endothelial rejection, is an extraocular procedure, and carries a lower risk of endophthalmitis. In addition, the healing period after lamellar keratoplasty is shorter than that after penetrating keratoplasty. The disadvantages of anterior lamellar keratoplasty include the technical difficulty of the surgery and the possible opacification and vascularization of the donor-recipient interface. Penetrating keratoplasty offers a significantly better visual prognosis[5] but requires careful screening of donor endothelium and carries risks of rejection and infection (see later sections on penetrating keratoplasty). With regard to posterior lamellar keratoplasty, the risk of the intraocular procedure and the increased surgical difficulty in performing posterior lamellar grafts need to be carefully considered and weighed against the risk and benefit of penetrating keratoplasty.

SURGICAL TECHNIQUES

Anterior Lamellar Dissection of the Host Tissue. If necessary, the globe is stabilized with bridle sutures passed beneath both superior and inferior rectus muscles. A trephine is used gently to mark the extent of graft needed. After the position of the graft has been confirmed, a partial-thickness trephination is performed until the desired depth of dissection is reached (see Fig. 63-1). A blade or a microkeratome is then used to extend the dissection plane along the entire host corneal tissue until the

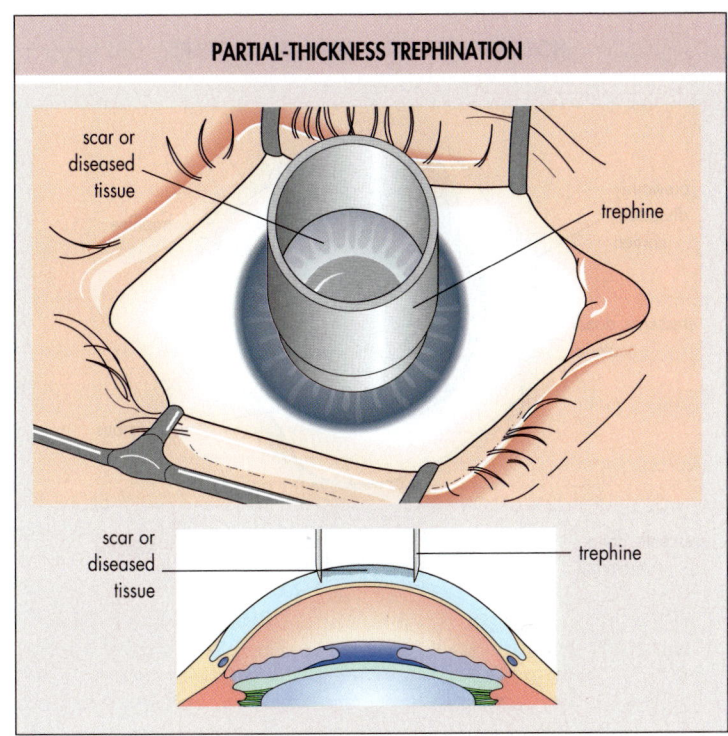

FIG. 63-1 ■ **Partial-thickness trephination.** This is performed on the host in the desired location and to the desired depth. Care must be taken not to perforate the cornea.

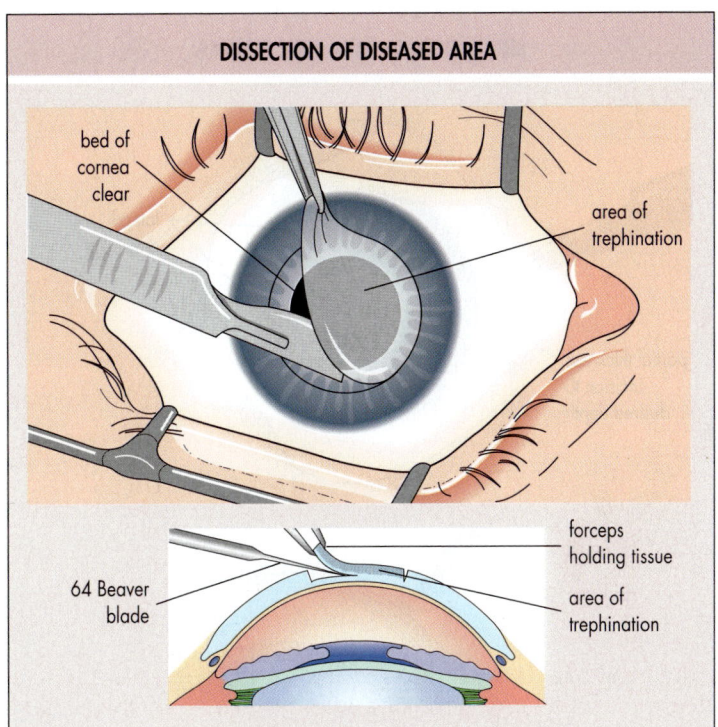

FIG. 63-2 ■ **Dissection of diseased area.** The diseased area in the host cornea is dissected gently to create a uniplanar, disease-free bed.

dissection of the host tissue is completed. The goal is to create a smooth, uniplanar recipient bed (see Fig. 63-2). If globe perforation occurs, the procedure is converted into a penetrating keratoplasty. This is also generally why dissection of the host tissue is performed prior to preparation of the donor cornea when a lamellar keratoplasty is performed. In recent years, another technique has been developed for deep anterior lamellar dissection.[7,8] In this new technique, aqueous fluid is first exchanged with air, creating an air-endothelium interface for visualization. A deep stromal pocket is then created using viscoelastic material followed by trephination of the anterior lamellar disc.

In posterior lamellar keratoplasty, there are mainly two techniques: microkeratome-assisted posterior lamellar keratoplasty[9-13] and posterior lamellar keratoplasty using a deep stromal pocket approach.[14-17] In the first technique, a corneal flap is created using a microkeratome similar to that used in a LASIK procedure. Posterior stroma tissue is then excised by trephination and replaced by a donor disc. The anterior lamellar flap is then repositioned to its original place and sutured. In the second approach to posterior lamellar keratoplasty, a deep stromal pocket is created across the cornea through a superior scleral incision. A posterior lamellar disc is then excised using a custom-made flat trephine placed into the deep stromal pocket.

Donor Preparation. In general, the criteria that donor tissue for anterior lamellar keratoplasty must meet are less stringent than those for donor tissue used in penetrating keratoplasty because the donor endothelium is not used; the tissue does not need to be as fresh as that used in penetrating keratoplasty. The corneal stroma may be used up to 7 days postmortem.[18] In contrast, posterior lamellar keratoplasty requires the same stringency of donor tissue as in penetrating keratoplasty because the endothelium is to be transplanted. A fresh or frozen whole donor eye should be used to fashion the anterior lamellar donor tissue.[19] In anterior lamellar keratoplasty, using a scalpel, an incision is made just inside the limbus of the donor cornea to reach the depth of the desired dissection (see Fig. 63-3). A Martinez dissector or a cyclodialysis spatula is used to extend the dissection plane within the corneal stroma and harvest the donor tissue (see Fig. 63-4). The tissue harvested may be circular, annular, or any other shape, depending on the needs of the

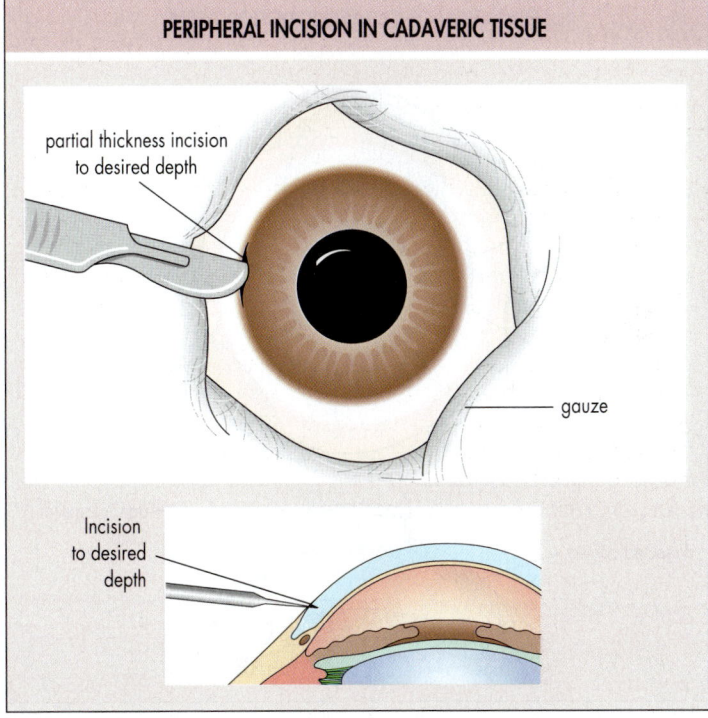

FIG. 63-3 ■ **Peripheral incision in donor cadaveric tissue.** The incision is made to the desired depth at the limbus using a scalpel.

patient (Figs. 63-5 and 63-6). Both cornea and sclera may be used. Usually, donor tissue is slightly oversized (0.25–0.5mm) compared with the recipient bed. As described previously, donor tissue suitable for penetrating keratoplasty is made available in case perforation occurs in the lamellar dissection of the host tissue. Newer microkeratomes may allow future anterior donor dissection. In posterior lamellar keratoplasty, either an inflated whole globe should be used or an artificial chamber can be used to anchor the scleral rim when only anterior corneal-sclera donor tissue is available. Donor tissue is fashioned in a manner similar to that of the recipient counterpart.

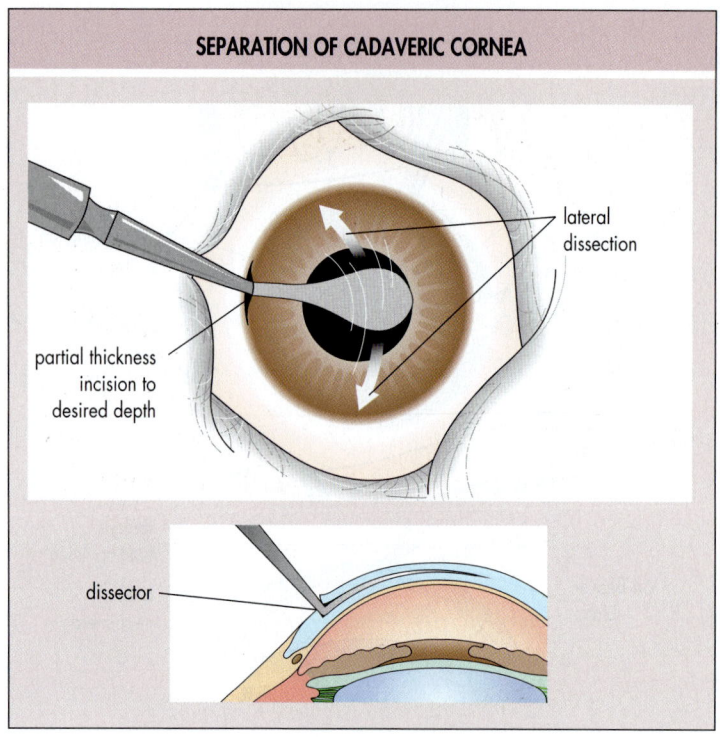

FIG. 63-4 ▌ **Separation of cadaveric cornea.** A dissector, such as the Martinez dissector or a cyclodialysis spatula, is used to separate gently the cornea along the lamellar cleavage plane through the entire cornea.

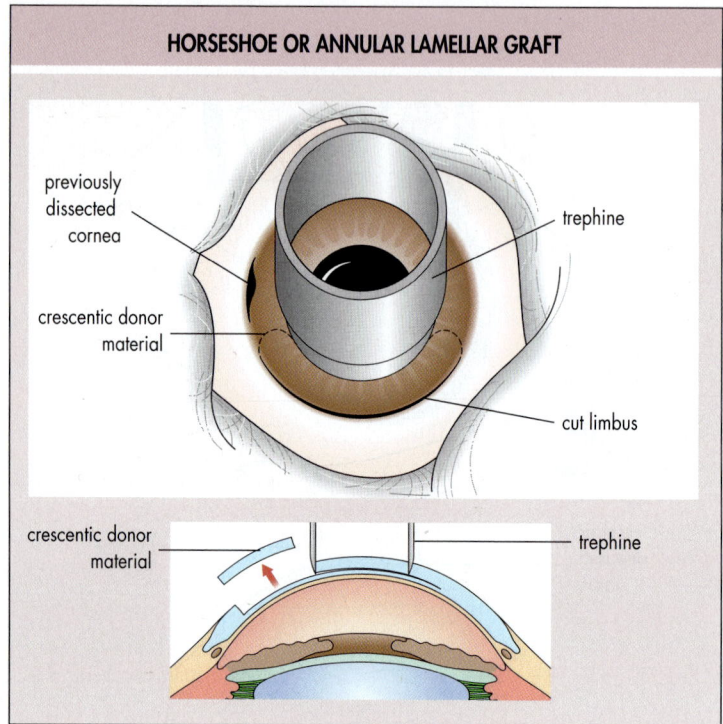

FIG. 63-6 ▌ **Horseshoe or annular lamellar graft.** A combination of corneal and scleral tissue may be harvested to give a different tissue shape.

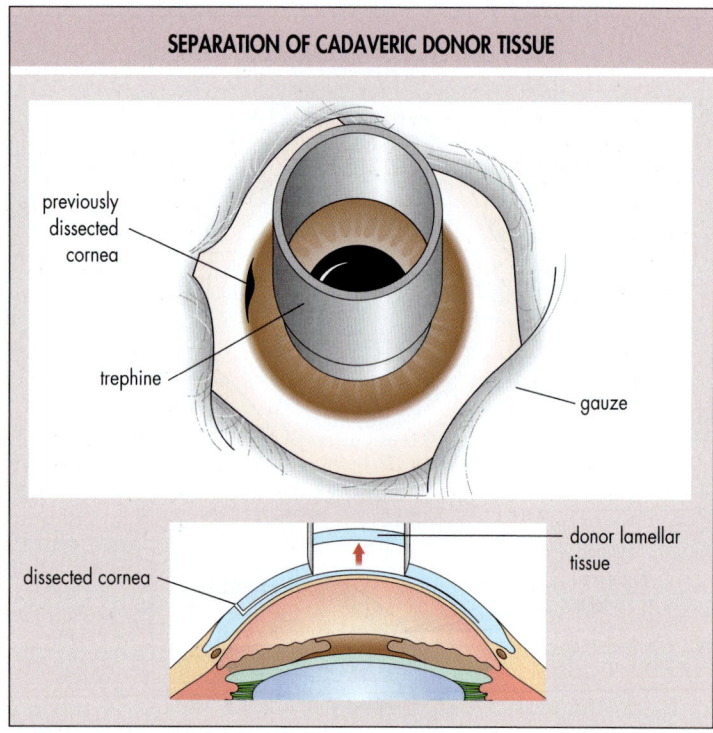

FIG. 63-5 ▌ **Donor tissue is harvested.** A trephine is placed on the cadaveric globe in the size and the shape desired. A circular lamellar graft is being harvested here.

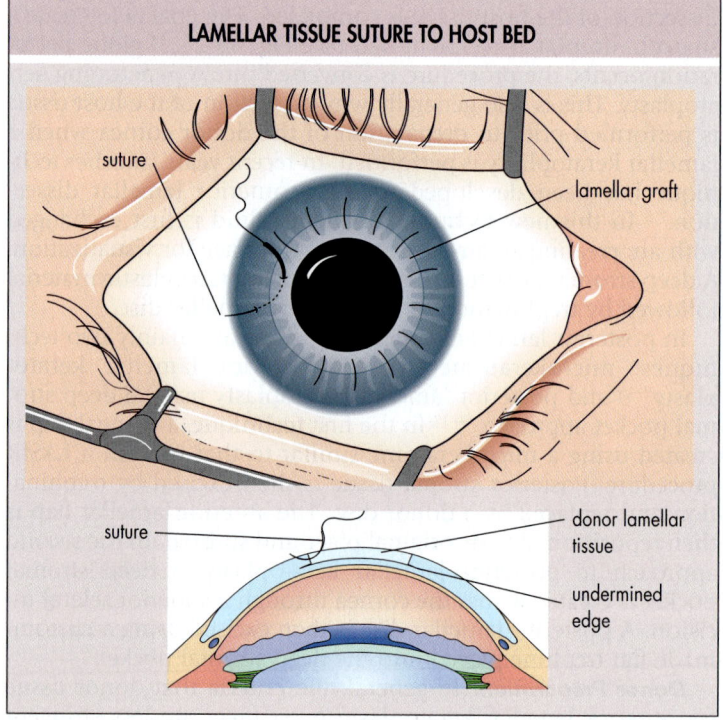

FIG. 63-7 ▌ **The lamellar tissue is sutured to the host bed.** Suture placement is facilitated if the edge of the host bed is undermined. Traditionally, the graft is sutured with 10-0 nylon.

Suture of the Donor Lamellae to Host Bed. In anterior lamellar keratoplasty, to improve the apposition of the graft-host junction, the edge of the host bed should be undermined to create a horizontal groove using a Paufique knife.[19] The donor lamella is placed on the recipient bed and secured with interrupted 10-0 nylon sutures (Fig. 63-7). The depth of the suture is about 90% of the corneal stroma's depth. Particular attention must be paid where the sutures are placed to avoid penetration of the globe. The donor tissue margins should not ride anterior to the rim of the recipient bed. At times, an anterior chamber paracentesis may become necessary before lamellar sutures are placed.

In microkeratome-assisted posterior lamellar keratoplasty, the posterior lamellar disc is sutured onto the recipient posterior stromal rim using 10-0 or 11-0 nylon. The knots are rotated and buried. The anterior stromal flap is then reflected back and repositioned in its original position and sutured. With the deep stromal pocket approach to posterior lamellar keratoplasty, the donor posterior lamellar disc is placed within the recipient rim via the anterior chamber but not sutured.

COMPLICATIONS AND POSTOPERATIVE MANAGEMENT. In general, an anterior lamellar graft can be extremely successful (Figs. 63-8 and 63-9). The complications are less frequent or se-

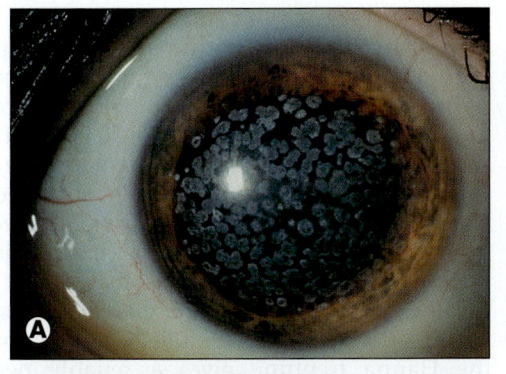

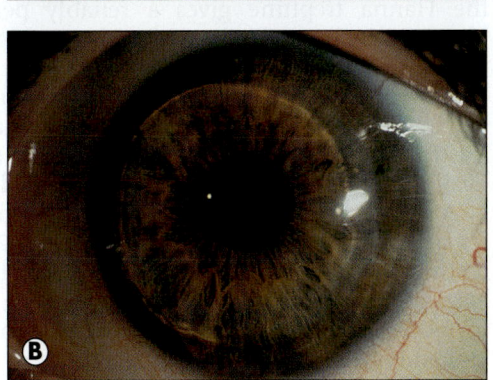

FIG. 63-8 ■ Lamellar keratoplasty for granular dystrophy. **A,** Preoperative appearance of a patient who had granular dystrophy limited to the anterior cornea. **B,** Postoperative appearance following lamellar keratoplasty. (Courtesy of Dr WW Culbertson.)

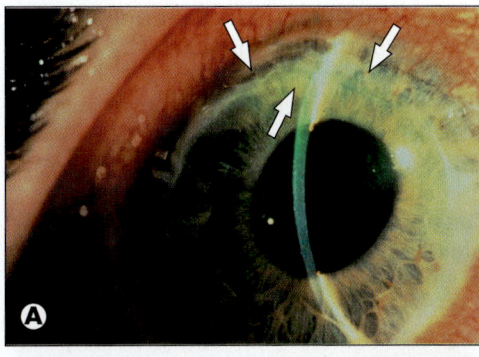

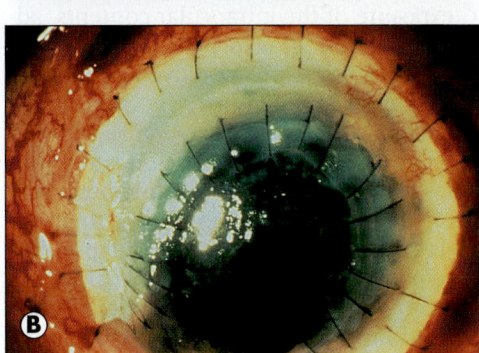

FIG. 63-9 ■ Lamellar keratoplasty for peripheral corneal melt and perforation. **A,** Preoperative appearance of a patient who had a peripheral corneal melt and perforation (*see arrows*). **B,** Postoperative appearance after the placement of a horseshoe corneal scleral lamellar graft. (Courtesy of Dr WW Culbertson.)

rious in nature than those of penetrating keratoplasty. Possible complications of lamellar graft include perforation of the recipient cornea, interface scarring and vascularization, persistent epithelial defect, inflammatory necrosis of the graft and graft melting, infection, astigmatism, and allograft rejection. Careful irrigation and cleaning of the host bed may reduce the incidence of such complications. With regard to allograft rejection, lamellar keratoplasty has a significantly reduced incidence as there is no transplantation of foreign endothelium. Posterior lamellar keratoplasty carries the same risk of graft rejection as in penetrating keratoplasty. In addition, both the posterior and anterior lamellar tissues need to be sealed adequately so wound leak resulting from poor tissue apposition may occur.

Penetrating Keratoplasty

Penetrating keratoplasty refers to the full-thickness replacement of diseased corneal tissue with a healthy donor. Penetrating keratoplasty has become the most frequently performed transplant of human tissues, thanks to advances in microsurgery techniques, suture material, donor tissue handling and storage, and postoperative management.

PREOPERATIVE EVALUATION AND DIAGNOSTIC APPROACH. Penetrating keratoplasty may be used to provide tectonic support, such as in corneal thinning and perforation, and improvement of visual outcome, such as in the replacement of a scarred cornea. Indications for penetrating keratoplasty include keratoconus, pseudophakic or aphakic bullous keratopathy, graft failure, Fuchs' endothelial dystrophy, graft rejection, corneal scars, chemical burns, corneal ulcers (bacterial, fungal, parasitic, or viral), corneal dystrophies and degenerations, herpetic keratitis, trauma, or any other causes of corneal decompensation. The rate of success of penetrating keratoplasty for the first four indications listed is excellent, but the chance of graft rejection increases significantly in instances of active or recurrent infection, inflammation, corneal vascularization, or previous graft rejection.

Because penetrating keratoplasty involves a significant amount of postoperative care, it is important to perform a careful preoperative evaluation and thoroughly discuss with patients the surgery, visual expectation, possible complications, and, in particular, the long process of postoperative care. The recipient must be prepared for lifelong management of the eye. In general, important considerations for preoperative evaluation for penetrating keratoplasty are as follows:

- Evaluation of visual potential—a careful ocular history, which includes strabismus, amblyopia, glaucoma, and retinal and optic nerve abnormalities, is important to assess the best potential visual outcome of the surgery.
- Ocular surface abnormality—a variety of ocular surface diseases must be recognized and treated prior to penetrating keratoplasty. These include rosacea, dry eyes, blepharitis, trichiasis, exposure keratopathy, ectropion, and entropion.
- Intraocular pressure (IOP) must be controlled adequately prior to penetrating keratoplasty to ensure a successful surgical outcome.
- Ocular inflammation—both intraocular and ocular surface inflammation may compromise graft success. Inflammatory conditions such as uveitis must be recognized and treated, as these conditions markedly increase the chance of elevated IOP, macular edema, graft rejection, and failure. Patients who suffer from active infectious processes with an inflamed "hot" eye also have an increased risk of graft rejection or failure.
- Prior corneal diseases and vascularization—a history of herpetic keratitis significantly reduces the chance of graft success as a result of several factors, which include recurrent disease in the graft, vascularization, trabeculitis with increased IOP, and persistent inflammation that causes rejection.
- Peripheral corneal melting—corneal thinning and melting, such as that associated with rheumatoid arthritis, may significantly affect the surgical outcome of penetrating keratoplasty and thus must be treated adequately prior to the surgery. Corneal surgery in these eyes can be technically difficult. Surgical complications include irregular astigmatism because of peripheral ectasia and recurrent corneal thinning.

Donor Selection. The Eye Bank Association of America has developed a set of criteria for donor corneas.[20] Contraindications for the use of donor tissue for penetrating keratoplasty include:

- Death of unknown cause;
- Central nervous system diseases, such as Creutzfeldt-Jakob disease, subacute sclerosing panencephalitis, rubella, Reye's syndrome, rabies, and infectious encephalitis;
- Infections such as human immunodeficiency virus, hepatitis, septicemia, syphilis, and endocarditis;

- Eye diseases such as retinoblastoma, malignant tumor of anterior segment, and active ocular inflammation (e.g., uveitis, scleritis, retinitis, and choroiditis);
- Prior ocular surgery (although pseudophakic eyes may be used with good cell densities);
- Congenital or acquired anterior segment abnormalities such as keratoconus and Fuchs' endothelial dystrophy.

Prior to penetrating keratoplasty, donor blood must be evaluated for communicable disease and donor tissues inspected by the surgeon under the slit lamp. A new factor will be donors with previous corneal refractive surgery.

SURGICAL TECHNIQUES. Because penetrating keratoplasty involves an "open sky" exposure of the intraocular contents, adequate decompression of the globe prior to penetrating keratoplasty is an important step as excessive preoperative IOP may increase the risk of expulsive choroidal hemorrhage. Intravenous mannitol or mechanical ocular decompression, such as with the Honan balloon, may be considered. Patients who undergo a simple penetrating keratoplasty have miotics placed preoperatively to protect the lens during surgery. Scleral supporting rings are used when the surgeon is concerned about ocular collapse during the procedure—principally in aphakic eyes. These rings are sutured to the sclera with 6-0 silk or Vicryl suture, with care taken to balance the suture positions and tensions. Inadvertent misalignment of the rings may result in an irregular trephination.

Using a caliper, the horizontal and vertical diameters of the recipient cornea are measured and the size of the graft is determined based on pathology and clinical judgment. Traditionally, a size disparity in which the donor tissue is 0.25mm larger in diameter than that of the recipient is used. In certain circumstances, a larger (0.5mm) donor, such as in a hyperopic eye, or a same size or smaller (0.25mm) donor button, such as in a recipient with keratoconus, may be chosen judiciously. The center of the recipient cornea is marked with a marking pen. A radial keratotomy marker stained with ink may be used to mark the peripheral cornea. A paracentesis port is made with a No. 75 Beaver blade, followed by injection of viscoelastic material into the anterior chamber. If a sclerally sutured intraocular lens (IOL) is planned, the scleral flaps are made prior to trephination, and the IOL is prepared. Alternatively, the surgeon may choose not to use scleral flaps but instead simply to rotate the Prolene suture knot into the sclera.

Attention is directed to the donor tissue, and a donor corneal button is punched. Several systems are available for donor trephination, which include a handheld trephine, the universal punch, and the Katena trephine blade attached to a gravity corneal punch (Fig. 63-10). These devices all cut the donor from endothelium to epithelium. In some of these systems, the epithelium may be marked prior to trephination to help with tissue distribution. The donor may also be cut from epithelium to endothelium with a system such as the Hanna artificial anterior chamber. This has the theoretical advantage that both the donor and recipient are cut in the same fashion with the same blade, which reduces donor-recipient disparity and potentially reduces astigmatism.

The recipient cornea may be cut using a variety of trephines, such as the Hessburg-Barron suction trephine, Hanna trephine (Fig. 63-11), Castroviejo trephine, and a number of other designs, such as the Lieberman single-point corneal trephine and the Grieshaber contact lens corneal cutter. The Hessburg-Barron suction trephine consists of a circular blade assembly that has a vacuum chamber attached to a spring-loaded syringe. The Hanna trephine has a unique, funnel-shaped design with a vacuum chamber created around a circular disposable blade. The Castroviejo trephine is made of a circular blade in a handle. Ideally, to achieve optimal graft-host tissue apposition, the trephination cut lies perpendicular to the corneal surface. Use of the Hanna trephine gives a reliably perpendicular profile. However, in instances in which the recipient ocular surface is not sufficiently large to accommodate the size of the Hanna trephine, the Hessburg-Barron trephine is used—it requires less surface area to achieve an adequate vacuum. The handheld Castroviejo trephine may be used for decentered grafts in which flexibility of orientation of the trephine is desired.

A partial-thickness trephination followed by a controlled entry into the anterior chamber using a No. 75 Beaver blade or a continued trephination that is stopped as soon as aqueous egress shows the anterior chamber has been entered may be performed. Suction is released the moment entry is noted. The recipient button is then excised using forceps and corneal scissors (Fig. 63-12). Alternatively, the button is removed using a blade such as a No. 75 Beaver, with care taken not to traumatize the iris inadvertently. The edge of the recipient bed is made perpendicular for optimal graft-host apposition. The anterior chamber may be reformed using a small amount of viscoelastic.

Depending on the case, the patient may need cataract extraction, IOL explantation, anterior vitrectomy, or the placement of a new IOL (Figs. 63-13 and 63-14). The donor button is placed over the recipient bed and sutured in place with four cardinal sutures (see Fig. 63-15). The depth of suture is typically 90% of the corneal thickness. Proper tissue distribution is paramount. It is beneficial to avoid a full-thickness pass, which may increase the chance of subsequent infection or epithelial downgrowth. After

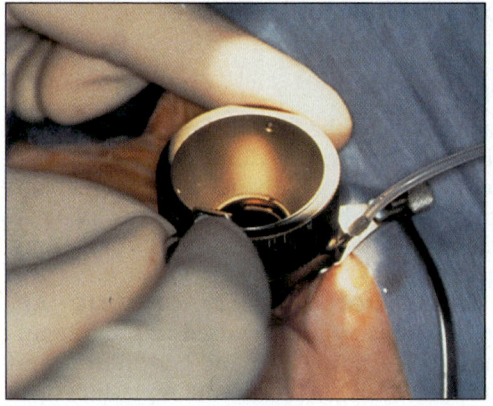

FIG. 63-11 ■ Hanna suction trephine. The anterior chamber of the patient may be filled with viscoelastic material and trephination then performed. (Courtesy of Dr WW Culbertson.)

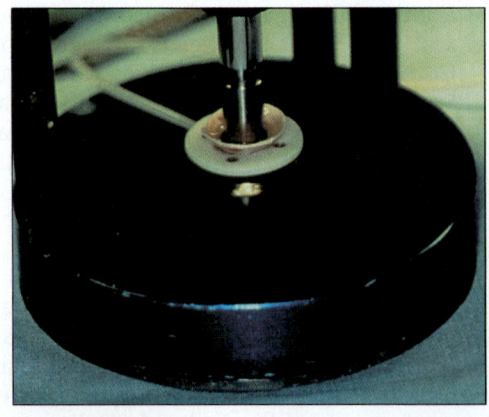

FIG. 63-10 ■ The corneal button is cut. A Katena blade mounted on a gravity punch may be used to cut the button from the endothelial side. (Courtesy of Dr WW Culbertson.)

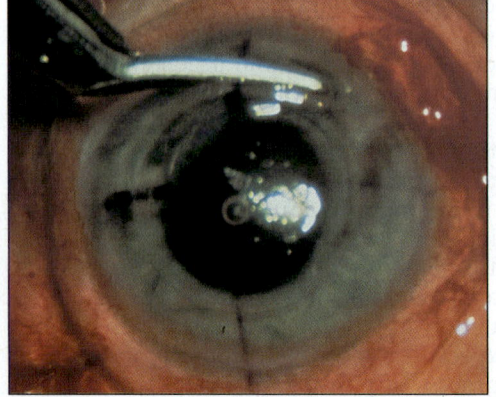

FIG. 63-12 ■ Excision of corneal button. The corneal button is removed completely using corneal scissors. (Courtesy of Dr WW Culbertson.)

placement of the 12 o'clock suture, particular attention is paid to the 6 o'clock suture such that these two sutures follow a vertical line and bisect the entire donor button. The 3 and 9 o'clock sutures are similarly placed. The marks on the recipient sclera and donor tissue may serve as guides, but the surgeon must decide the best suture placement.

The rest of the sutures are a combination of interrupted and running sutures (Fig. 63-16) or solely interrupted sutures. Interrupted sutures are suited for vascularized or thinned cornea as subsequent selective removal may be necessary to prevent the advancement of vessels or to control astigmatism. Running sutures, on the other hand, have the advantage of speedy placement intraoperatively and better tension distribution and healing. Prior to the completion of all sutures, the viscoelastic material in the anterior chamber is removed. The running sutures may be adjusted intraoperatively by using a keratoscope, such as the Hyde astigmatic ruler, to project a circular image onto the donor cornea. If the ring image is oval rather than circular, excessive tightness is indicated in one meridian and the running suture adjusted accordingly. When the graft sutures are completed, the security of the wound is tested by the injection of balanced salt solution into the anterior chamber; any fluid leak through the graft-host junction is sought. If a scleral-sutured IOL is used, the surgeon must ensure that the knots are either rotated and buried or covered by a partial-thickness scleral flap.

COMPLICATIONS AND POSTOPERATIVE MANAGEMENT. Most of the intraoperative complications can be avoided by using adequate surgical planning and techniques. Possible intraoperative complications include poor graft centration, excessive bleeding, damage to ocular structures (such as donor endothelium, iris, lens, or posterior capsule), or expulsive hemorrhage. During the process of excision of the recipient button, it is imperative to monitor continuously the depth of the anterior chamber and the red reflex. A sudden shallowing of the anterior chamber or disappearance of the red reflex may signify an impending expulsive choroidal hemorrhage. Having Cobo prosthesis available, which can be placed quickly on the recipient bed to seal the globe in the event of expulsive choroidal hemorrhage, is recommended.

The success of penetrating keratoplasty depends significantly on adequate postoperative care and management. The surgeon must be able to recognize and manage a variety of possible complications, such as wound leak and infection, glaucoma, and graft rejection or failure. The common postoperative complications and their management are discussed in the following subsections.

Wound Leak. A shallow anterior chamber in a soft globe the day after penetrating keratoplasty may indicate a wound leak. Measures that can be taken to manage wound leak include patching, aqueous suppressant, lubrication, or bandage contact lenses. Significant wound leak that arises from either a broken suture or poor wound apposition may require the wound to be resutured.

Flat Anterior Chamber with Increased Intraocular Pressure. Flat anterior chamber with increased IOP may result from pupillary block, anterior rotation of the lens-iris diaphragm (such as is found in choroidal hemorrhage), choroidal effusion, or malignant glaucoma. The cause must be identified and treated.

Endophthalmitis. Postoperative endophthalmitis may result from a variety of factors, such as contamination of donor or host tissue or postoperative infection. It is a devastating complication that requires aggressive management, which includes aqueous and vitreous cultures, intraocular antibiotics, and possibly vitrectomy (Fig. 63-17).

Persistent Epithelial Defect. Typically, an epithelial defect after penetrating keratoplasty heals within 1 week postoperatively. Persistent epithelial defects occur in eyes that have ocular surface disorders, such as dry eye, blepharitis, exposure keratopathy, and

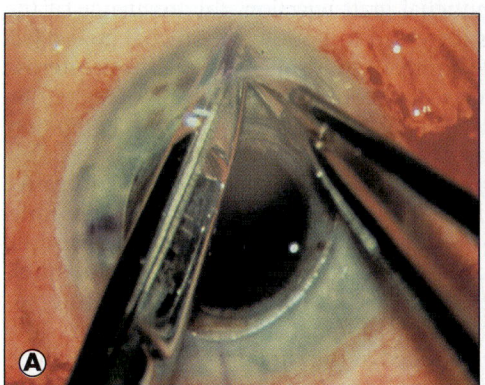
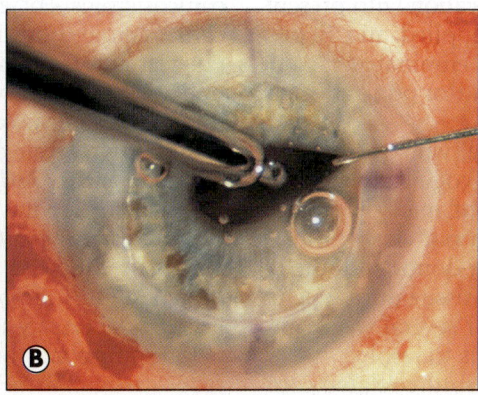
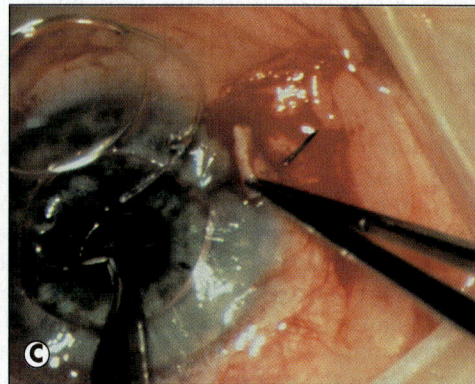

FIG. 63-13 ■ Removal of anterior chamber intraocular lens. **A,** Care is taken when the anterior chamber haptics are removed, as they may become encysted in the peripheral iris and bleeding may occur on removal. **B,** An anterior vitrectomy is performed—an iris hook may be used to improve visualization. **C,** A 10-0 Prolene suture is passed beneath the iris and through the scleral sulcus and out through the previously prepared scleral flap. This is performed on both sides. (Courtesy of Dr WW Culbertson.)

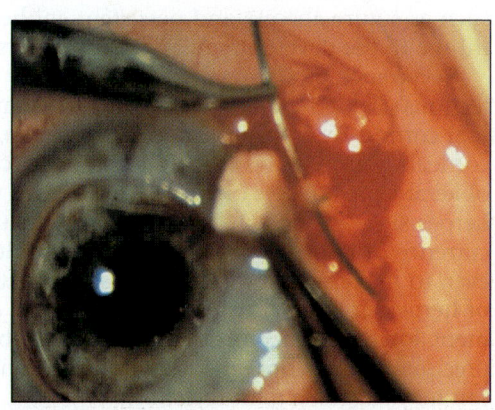

FIG. 63-14 ■ Prolene suture passed through the sclera and tied under the flap. This is carried out after the suture supported lens has been placed in the sulcus. The Prolene suture is tied to itself beneath the scleral flap. Alternatively, the knot may be rotated beneath the sclera. (Courtesy of Dr WW Culbertson.)

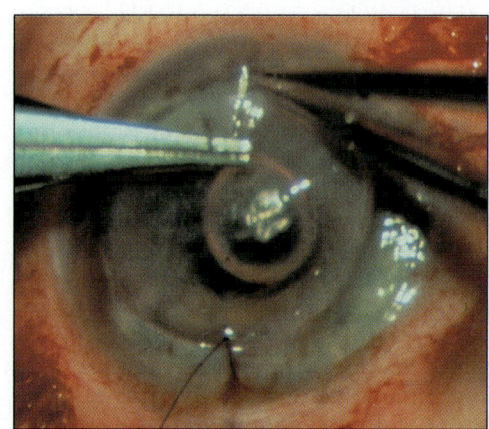

FIG. 63-15 ■ The corneal button is placed. Care is taken in the placement of cardinal sutures to ensure adequate tissue distribution. (Courtesy of Dr WW Culbertson.)

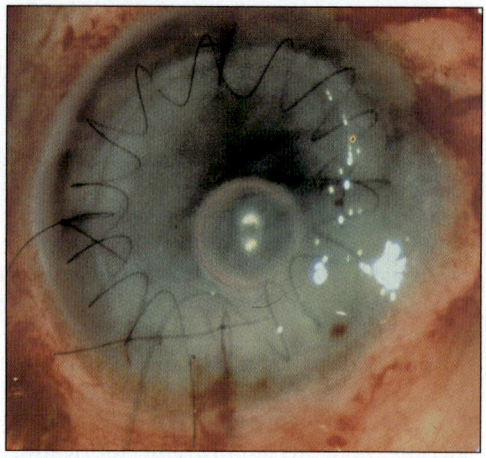

FIG. 63-16 ▮ Place-ment of a 10-0 run-ning suture. (Courtesy of Dr WW Culbertson.)

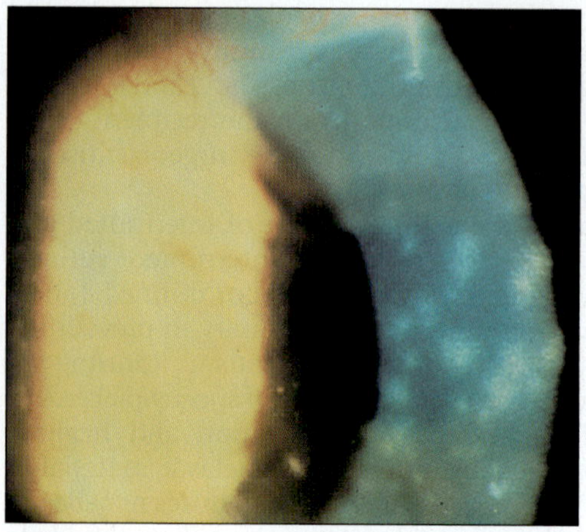

FIG. 63-18 ▮ Subepithelial infil-trates secondary to subepithelial graft re-jection. (Courtesy of Dr WW Culbertson.)

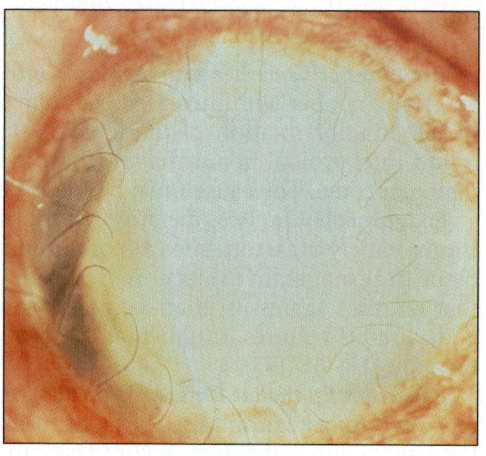

FIG. 63-17 ▮ Endophthalmitis. This was caused by *Proteus* infection 5 weeks fol-lowing penetrating ker-atoplasty. (Courtesy of Dr RK Forster.)

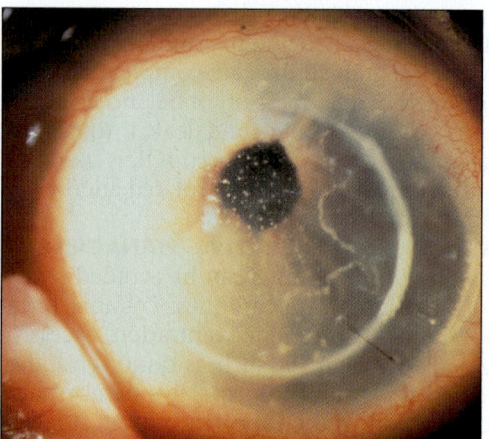

FIG. 63-19 ▮ Graft rejection. Note the in-flammatory precipi-tates and Khodadoust line secondary to en-dothelial rejection. (Courtesy of Dr EC Alfonso.)

rosacea, or in patients who have systemic diseases, such as dia-betes or rheumatoid arthritis. Frequent lubrication with preserv-ative-free drops and lubricating ointment is applied, and all pos-sible causes of topical toxicity must be eliminated. If the problem does not resolve, a tarsorrhaphy and/or punctal occlu-sion may be necessary.

Primary Graft Failure. Primary graft failure (which is different from graft rejection—see the following) is recognized when sig-nificant edema of the donor tissue in a noninflamed eye is pres-ent on the first postoperative day and does not clear. Primary graft failure may be attributed to either poor donor endothelial function or iatrogenic damage to the donor tissue during pene-trating keratoplasty. The graft is observed for several weeks and a regraft considered if the corneal edema fails to resolve.

Problems Related to Sutures. A variety of suture-related com-plications may occur after penetrating keratoplasty. If found, a loose or broken suture must be removed because it may result in vascularization or abscesses.

Graft Rejection. Graft rejection remains the most common cause of graft failure. Alldredge and Krachmer[21] reported an over-all incidence of endothelial graft rejection of 21%. Symptoms of endothelial graft rejection include pain, photophobia, redness, and decreased vision. Patients must be educated carefully with regard to these symptoms, and must seek medical attention im-mediately should they occur.

Graft rejection may be divided anatomically into three categories:
• Epithelial rejection—may be recognized by observation of an epithelial line, which represents the replacement of the donor epithelium by that of the recipient;
• Subepithelial rejection—multiple subepithelial infiltrates limited to the corneal graft may be observed (Fig. 63-18);
• Endothelial rejection (the most severe type characterized by keratic precipitates, iritis, and corneal edema)—a Khodadoust line may be seen, which represents the advanc-ing front of the host immunological and inflammatory cells against a receding front of donor endothelium (Fig. 63-19).

The treatment of graft rejection consists primarily of topical corticosteroids. For epithelial graft rejection, the frequency of the corticosteroid drops is increased to hourly; endothelial graft rejec-tion warrants frequent (hourly or more often) topical corticosteroid until the process is reversed. Subconjunctival injection of corticoste-roid may also be used. Systemic steroids (oral or intravenous) may be utilized in severe cases but are usually not necessary.

Treatment for Astigmatism. Adequate control of postoperative astigmatism is vital to achieve the best visual acuity possible. Typically starting at 6–8 weeks after penetrating keratoplasty, the patient is followed using serial corneal topography and inter-rupted sutures are removed selectively or a running suture ad-justed as necessary to reduce astigmatism. The continuous 10-0 nylon sutures may be adjusted at the slit lamp postoperatively to reduce astigmatism.[22] Early removal of sutures may have a more significant effect on astigmatism, although care is required with regard to wound stability if sutures are removed too early. Astigmatic keratotomy may be performed late if a significant amount of residual astigmatism remains after all the sutures have been removed and the patient is intolerant of contact lenses.

Corneal Ulcers. Patients who have undergone penetrating keratoplasty are more susceptible to infectious keratitis. Factors such as suture abscess and persistent epithelial defect may con-tribute to the development of corneal ulcers.

Recurrence of Diseases. Various corneal dystrophies and in-fections (Fig. 63-20) may recur in grafts. Among the three stro-mal corneal dystrophies (macular, granular, and lattice), lattice corneal dystrophy has the highest recurrence rate. In the setting of keratic precipitates on a graft in a patient who has a history of herpes simplex virus, it is sometimes difficult to distinguish re-currence of a disease from graft rejection. It is important, how-ever, to make such a distinction as the treatment for recurrence of herpes simplex virus (antiviral agent) is different from treat-ment for rejection (corticosteroid). The observation of keratic precipitates and corneal edema confined only to the donor but-ton may suggest a graft rejection.

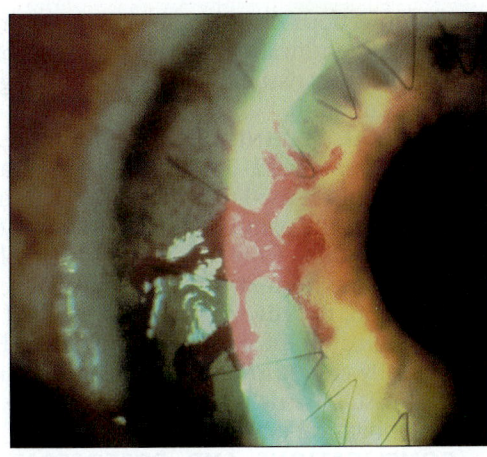

FIG. 63-20 ▮▮ **Herpetic keratitis recurrence in graft.** Note positive staining with rose bengal. (Courtesy of Dr EC Alfonso.)

Triple Procedure (Combined Procedure)

PREOPERATIVE EVALUATION AND DIAGNOSTIC APPROACH. A combined procedure or triple procedure refers to penetrating keratoplasty, cataract extraction, and IOL implantation. The procedure is indicated for patients who have visually significant cataract and who require penetrating keratoplasty for visual rehabilitation. The leading indication for a triple procedure is Fuchs' endothelial dystrophy, which accounts for up to 77% of eyes that require a triple procedure.[23-26] Other indications for triple procedures include corneal leukoma, keratoconus, herpes simplex infection, and interstitial keratitis.

Compared with penetrating keratoplasty, a combined procedure requires the additional, appropriate calculation of the power of the IOL required to achieve the optimal refractive result. The authors use the Sanders-Retzlaff-Kraff formula (Equation 1),[27] in which A is the constant for an IOL, AL is the axial length, and K is the keratometric measurement. The determination of K varies from surgeon to surgeon. The authors normally advocate one of two alternative approaches. Either the average of the past postoperative keratometric readings associated with the surgical technique or the K reading from the contralateral eye is used for IOL calculation. In the instances in which an over- or undersized graft is required, 1-2D is subtracted from the IOL power for a 0.5mm oversized graft or 1-2D is added to the IOL power for 0.5mm undersizing.[19]

Equation 1 $$IOL\ power = A - 2.5\ AL - 0.9\ K$$

SURGICAL TECHNIQUES. The detailed surgical technique for penetrating keratoplasty is as described previously. The additional components of the surgery related to cataract extraction and IOL implantation are described here. After the recipient button has been excised, a can-opener type of anterior capsulectomy, a continuous curvilinear capsulorrhexis, or a square capsulectomy using Vannas scissors may be performed. The capsulectomy must be sufficiently large to allow subsequent expression of the lens nucleus. Care is taken during the capsulorrhexis because the lens-iris diaphragm is rotated anteriorly with an open-sky eye. No counterpressure is used on the anterior chamber to keep the anterior capsule flat, and thus the capsulectomy tends to extend peripherally if excessive IOP or insufficient use of preoperative mannitol occurs.

After hydrodissection using balanced salt solution and mobilization of the lens nucleus, the lens is expressed gently using pressure at the 6 o'clock position to tilt the superior or inferior edge of the lens anteriorly above the plane of the anterior capsular opening. The lens is rotated out using a No. 25 gauge needle or a lens loop. The remaining cortical material is removed using a manual irrigation and aspiration device, which must be carried out carefully because the anterior and posterior capsules tend to collapse together. The posterior chamber is then inflated with viscoelastic material and the appropriate posterior IOL is inserted using a lens forceps. In the event that a posterior capsular tear and anterior extension of vitreous occur, a limited anterior vitrectomy

is performed and the IOL either inserted in the bag or sulcus or sutured to the sclera, depending on the available capsular support (see Figs. 63-13 and 63-14). An open-loop anterior chamber IOL may also be used. The remainder of the procedure for penetrating keratoplasty is the same as that described in the appropriate sections earlier. Phacoemulsification is often difficult to perform because it requires a clear view through the cornea, which is rarely the case in patients undergoing a triple procedure.

COMPLICATIONS AND POSTOPERATIVE MANAGEMENT. Intraoperative complications of a triple procedure include capsular rupture with vitreous loss and suprachoroidal hemorrhage. Postoperatively, the complications associated with penetrating keratoplasty (as described earlier) are possible, which include failure and graft rejection, postoperative glaucoma, endothelial cell loss, cystoid macular edema, retinal detachment, and endophthalmitis.[23,26,28-30] In addition, posterior capsular opacification in combined procedures can occur with an incidence similar to that in routine extracapsular cataract extraction alone.[31]

OUTCOMES

Corneal grafting techniques, such as penetrating keratoplasty, lamellar keratoplasty, and triple procedures, have become reliable and popular surgical techniques. Patients who undergo these types of surgery achieve significantly improved vision in the majority of cases. Careful attention to preoperative evaluation, surgical techniques, and postoperative management will improve surgical outcome and patients' satisfaction.

SUPERFICIAL CORNEAL PROCEDURES

HISTORICAL REVIEW

Superficial corneal procedures include corneal glue application, superficial keratectomy for anterior corneal degenerations and dystrophies, treatment of band keratopathy using ethylenediaminetetraacetic acid (EDTA), and corneal biopsy. Corneal glue consists of cyanoacrylate polymer. Webster *et al.*[32] reported in 1968 the first use of cyanoacrylate to seal corneal perforations. In the past 30 years, the application of tissue adhesive has been shown to restore globe integrity effectively and to delay penetrating keratoplasty; thus, complications related to corneal graft in an acute setting are reduced.[33-36] With regard to superficial keratectomy for corneal dystrophies and other anterior pathologies, the advent of excimer laser phototherapeutic keratectomy has offered an effective alternative (discussed later).

ANESTHESIA

Superficial corneal procedures are performed mostly using topical anesthetic. Proparacaine hydrochloride eyedrops are used frequently.

SPECIFIC TECHNIQUES

Superficial Keratectomy

PREOPERATIVE EVALUATION AND DIAGNOSTIC APPROACH. Superficial keratectomy may be carried out either mechanically or by using excimer lasers (see later). Mechanical keratectomy consists of removal of pathological epithelial or subepithelial tissues. The procedure is indicated in patients who have[19]:
- Anterior corneal dystrophies;
- B-band keratopathy;
- Superficial pannus or scar;
- Corneal dermoid, pterygium, or Salzmann's nodules; and
- Excision of retained foreign bodies.

In addition, superficial keratectomy is used to obtain corneal tissue for microbiological or histological examination in the setting of infection.

SURGICAL TECHNIQUES. After the epithelium has been removed, the plane between abnormal tissue and the underlying normal tissue is identified. The lesion is dissected in a lamellar fashion using a sharp or blunt blade. The corneal bed is left as smooth as possible to facilitate epithelialization. If possible, injuries to the limbal epithelium are avoided as limbal stem cells are important for the subsequent reepithelialization. Bandage contact lenses or antibiotic ointment with a patch can be administered after keratectomy.

COMPLICATIONS AND POSTOPERATIVE MANAGEMENT. Bandage soft lenses, an eye patch, antibiotic drops, or aggressive lubrication is continued until the corneal epithelium has healed. Complications after superficial keratectomy include persistent epithelial defect, infection, and corneal scarring. Occasionally, a limbal stem cell transplant is necessary to provide a source for reepithelialization.

Treatment of Band Keratopathy Using Ethylenediaminetetraacetic Acid

PREOPERATIVE EVALUATION AND DIAGNOSTIC APPROACH. Band keratopathy has a variety of causes, which include chronic uveitis (such as juvenile rheumatoid arthritis), interstitial keratitis, corneal edema, phthisis bulbi, and long-standing glaucoma. Less commonly, band keratopathy may result from a hypercalcemic state (caused by hyperparathyroidism, sarcoidosis, vitamin D intoxication, or Paget's disease), gout, renal failure, or chronic exposure to irritants.

SURGICAL TECHNIQUES. A solution of disodium EDTA 1.5–3.0% is used. An aliquot (2ml) of EDTA (150mg/ml) is added to sterile saline (8ml) to make up the 3% solution. After application of topical anesthetic, débridement of corneal epithelium is performed. A cellulose sponge soaked in the EDTA solution is then wiped over the lesion repeatedly until the calcium is removed. Repeated saturation of the sponge in the EDTA solution may be necessary and the entire process may take as long as several minutes. Alternatively, the patient is placed in a supine position and a well placed over the eye into which the EDTA solution is poured. The cornea is soaked for several minutes and then débrided to remove the calcium.

COMPLICATIONS AND POSTOPERATIVE MANAGEMENT. Postoperatively, either a bandage contact lens or antibiotic ointment is applied. Repeated treatment may be necessary to remove recurrent calcium. The patient must be observed carefully during the process of reepithelialization to ensure that complications of infection are avoided.

Corneal Biopsy

PREOPERATIVE EVALUATION AND DIAGNOSTIC APPROACH. Corneal biopsy is indicated in a patient who has an unresponsive and culture-negative corneal ulcer.[37] Infections that arise from atypical mycobacteria, fungus, and *Acanthamoeba* and crystalline keratopathy as a result of *Streptococcus viridans* are examples of infectious disorders that may require corneal biopsy for definitive identification of the causative organisms. A corneal biopsy provides tissue for both microbiological and histopathological evaluation.

SURGICAL TECHNIQUES. After topical anesthetic, a sterile, handheld trephine (2–3mm diameter dermatological punch) under a slit lamp is used to achieve a partial-thickness trephination that contains the pathological specimen. The size of the trephine depends on that of the lesion, and the trephine is positioned to straddle some normal corneal tissue. After the partial-thickness trephination, the edge of the lesion is lifted using a 0.12 forceps and dissected off the cornea using a blade (Figs. 63-21 to 63-23). It is usually easiest to begin the dissection in the area of normal corneal tissue. Tissue is divided and sent for microbiological and histopathological evaluation.

COMPLICATIONS AND POSTOPERATIVE MANAGEMENT. Intraoperatively, it is important to gauge the depth of the trephination appropriately to avoid perforation. This is especially important in the setting of microbial infection with corneal thinning. Continual broad-spectrum antibiotic therapy is maintained until positive identification of the causative organism is achieved.

Corneal Glue Application

PREOPERATIVE EVALUATION AND DIAGNOSTIC APPROACH. Application of cyanoacrylate tissue adhesive is indicated when a small corneal perforation is present because of microbial infection, sterile thinning, or trauma. This is usually successful in perforations <1.5mm in diameter and is probably contraindicated in cases with vitreous or iris prolapse.

SURGICAL TECHNIQUES. After the application of topical anesthetic, the corneal epithelium and necrotic tissue are débrided and the area is dried with sponges. The glue may be applied using either the "disc" or "drip" technique. The authors prefer the disc technique, in which a round punch of a sterile plastic drape (2–3mm diameter) is made using a dermatological trephine—the size used depends on extent of the perforation (Fig. 63-24). A small amount of ophthalmic oint-

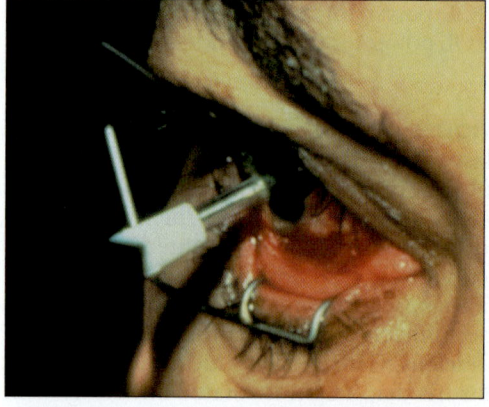

FIG. 63-22 ■ Partial trephination of the cornea. A 3mm dermatological trephine is used to trephinate the cornea partially—both infected and noninfected cornea are straddled. (With permission from Karp CL, Forster RK. The corneal ulcer. In: Krachmer JH, Mannis MJ, Holland EJ, eds. Cornea. St Louis: Mosby; 1997:403–8.)

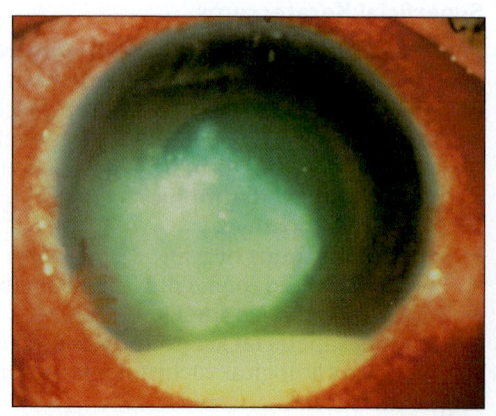

FIG. 63-21 ■ Nonresolving culture-negative corneal ulcer. (With permission from Karp CL, Forster RK. The corneal ulcer. In: Krachmer JH, Mannis MJ, Holland EJ, eds. Cornea. St Louis: Mosby; 1997:403–8.)

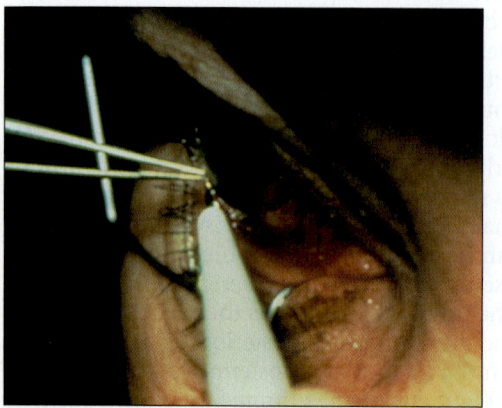

FIG. 63-23 ■ A blade is used gently to dissect the corneal tissue. (With permission from Karp CL, Forster RK. The corneal ulcer. In: Krachmer JH, Mannis MJ, Holland EJ, eds. Cornea. St Louis: Mosby; 1997:403–8.)

ment is placed on the flat end of a sterile cotton applicator and the plastic disc is placed on the ointment (Fig. 63-25). A small amount of tissue glue is placed on the disc (Fig. 63-26)—it is important to use the least amount of glue possible. The patient, with a lid speculum in place, is either in the supine position or sitting at the slit lamp. The glue and disc are placed gently on the prepared, dry perforation site (Fig. 63-27), and the disc becomes an integral part of the glue. A bandage contact

lens is placed (Fig. 63-28). For the drip technique, the same preparation of the donor is carried out, and the patient is placed in the supine position. A tiny drop of glue is placed on the cornea using a 30-gauge needle. The drip technique is also very effective, but the disc technique may provide better control of the quantity of glue applied and provides the extra reinforcement of a fine plastic disc.

COMPLICATIONS AND POSTOPERATIVE MANAGEMENT. The patient is examined regularly to monitor the status of the glue, the anterior chamber depth, and infection if present. As the cornea heals, the epithelium grows under the glue and eventually dislodges it when the healing process has been completed.

OUTCOMES

Eyes that undergo superficial corneal procedures, such as superficial keratectomy, EDTA scrub, corneal biopsy and adhesive application, in general heal well. The success of these techniques depends on the rate of reepithelialization and the underlying ocular surface pathology.

CONJUNCTIVAL SURGERY

HISTORICAL REVIEW

Conjunctival procedures include conjunctival flap preparation, pterygium surgery, and limbal cell transplantation. In a conjunctival flap procedure, a hinged flap of conjunctiva is created to cover an unstable or painful corneal surface. Originally described by Gundersen,[38] conjunctival flaps have remained an effective procedure for the treatment of unresponsive corneal ulcers in which visual expectation is poor. The conjunctival flap provides a source of blood vessels and cellular nutrients, and the goal is to reduce ocular surface inflammation. Corneal procedures for visual rehabilitation may be performed at a later date.

Pterygium surgery dates back to 1855, when Desmarres[39] first performed a transposition of the pterygium head. Arlt in 1872 recognized the importance of covering the epibulbar defect after pterygium excision and described the first conjunctival graft.[40] With respect to limbal transplantation, Kenyon and Tseng[41] described the technique of limbal autograft transplantation for ocular surface disorders. The recognition of limbal stem cell function has enhanced greatly the surgeon's ability to treat patients who have ocular surface diseases secondary to limbal deficiency. The techniques of limbal cell transplantation have allowed patients to enjoy improved ocular surfaces, and enhanced success of corneal transplantation has occurred in these cases.

ANESTHESIA

Conjunctival surgeries may be performed using either local or general anesthetic. Local anesthetic is indicated for adult and co-

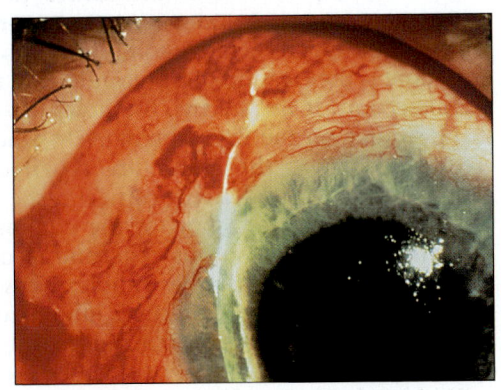

FIG. 63-24 ▓ Corneal perforation. Preoperative appearance of a patient who has a small, 1.5mm corneal perforation at the 10 o'clock limbus. (Courtesy of Dr RK Forster.)

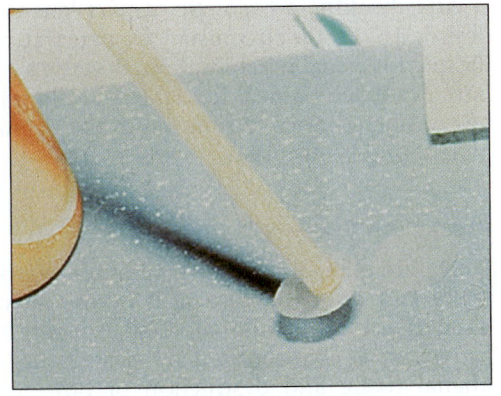

FIG. 63-25 ▓ Plastic sterile disc. A 2–3mm plastic sterile disc is placed on the end of a cotton tip applicator. (Courtesy of Dr RK Forster.)

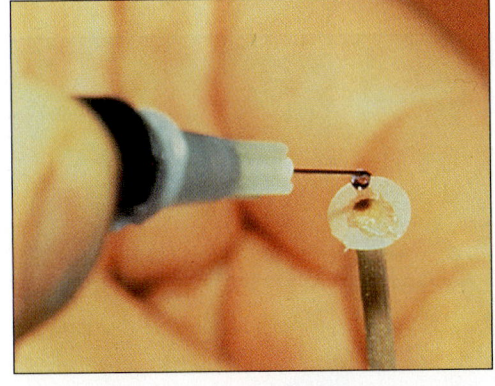

FIG. 63-26 ▓ Cyanoacrylate glue. A small amount of cyanoacrylate glue is placed on top of the plastic disc. (Courtesy of Dr RK Forster.)

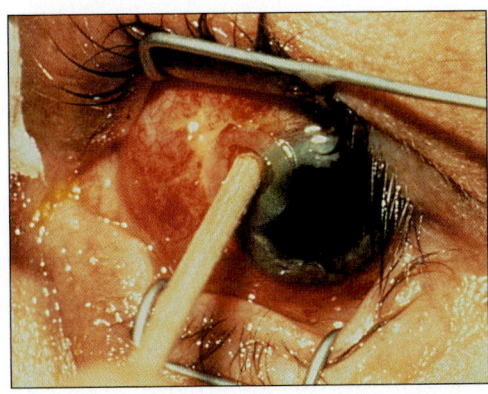

FIG. 63-27 ▓ Placement of corneal glue and plastic disc to the area of perforation. (Courtesy of Dr RK Forster.)

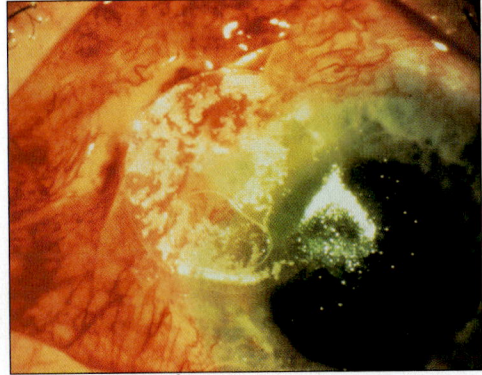

FIG. 63-28 ▓ Immediate postoperative appearance. The soft contact lens is in place. (Courtesy of Dr RK Forster.)

operative patients and consists of peribulbar or retrobulbar injection of lidocaine (2%), bupivacaine (0.75%), and hyaluronidase. Peribulbar anesthetic may be preferred over retrobulbar injection to avoid globe penetration. Sometimes, when a conjunctival flap procedure is carried out, a reinforcement injection over the superior fornix is indicated. To prevent squeezing during surgery, a lid block is sometimes employed. General anesthetic is reserved for pediatric patients and uncooperative adults.

SPECIFIC TECHNIQUES

Conjunctival Flap

PREOPERATIVE EVALUATION AND DIAGNOSTIC APPROACH.
Common indications for conjunctival flap include:

- Nonhealing sterile corneal ulcerations secondary to chemical or thermal injuries, herpetic infections, exposure keratopathies, and neurotrophic diseases;
- Painful bullous keratopathy in eyes that have low visual potential in which penetrating keratoplasty is not indicated and in which simpler management techniques, such as soft contact lenses or anterior stromal puncture, have failed;
- Blind eyes in need of surface preparation for prosthetic shells or contact lenses.

Contraindications for conjunctival flap include active bacterial or fungal keratitis and corneal perforation. An active infection should be treated first before the application of a conjunctival flap, as the flap may reduce the access of antibiotics to the infection site beneath it. A perforated cornea should be sealed before the use of a conjunctival flap is considered because a perforated cornea may continue to leak under the conjunctival flap. As a result of advances in antimicrobial therapy, bandage lenses, tarsorrhaphy, and penetrating keratoplasty, conjunctival flaps are used less frequently today.

SURGICAL TECHNIQUES.
The availability of mobile conjunctiva is evaluated. If superior conjunctival scarring precludes mobilization, a conjunctival flap may be fashioned from the inferior bulbar conjunctiva, although often less tissue is available. When superior conjunctiva is available, the globe is rotated inferiorly using a traction suture placed at the 12 o'clock limbus. A semicircular incision, parallel to the superior corneal limbus, is made as posterior as possible using Westcott scissors. Using a smooth forceps, the dissection of a thin conjunctival flap is carried inferiorly until the superior corneal limbus is reached. Adequate dissection and undermining of this flap laterally is important for the subsequent downward mobilization of the flap over the cornea and to prevent traction. It is imperative in the dissection process that particular care is taken not to create buttonholes in the conjunctival flap.

The conjunctival flap is freed completely of its underlying Tenon's capsule to enable adequate movement of the flap. With the use of a No. 64 Beaver blade, the corneal epithelium is removed completely. Application of lidocaine 4% or absolute alcohol may help loosen the corneal epithelium. A 360° limbal peritomy is performed using Westcott scissors or a blade (Fig. 63-29). The well-mobilized conjunctival flap is stretched to cover the desired area (Fig. 63-30). The superior and inferior aspects of the flap are secured on the sclera using interrupted or running 10-0 nylon sutures. The inferior edges of the conjunctiva may also be reapposed with 8-0 Vicryl suture in a running fashion (Fig. 63-31).

A partial Gundersen flap is used in certain circumstances, such as for focal nonhealing corneal ulcers. The procedure also includes scraping of the corneal epithelium, mobilization of the conjunctiva in the appropriate quadrant, and suturing of the conjunctival flap over a localized corneal defect.

COMPLICATIONS AND POSTOPERATIVE MANAGEMENT. The most common perioperative complication of a conjunctival flap procedure is the creation of a buttonhole on the conjunctiva during dissection. If this occurs, the holes are closed using purse-string sutures on the flap. Alternatively, when the flap has covered the cornea, the holes are repaired by suturing the conjunctiva to the underlying corneal tissue. Postoperative complications include retraction of the conjunctival flap, hemorrhage and epithelial mucous cysts, and recurrence of infection, such as that caused by herpes simplex virus.[42] Adequate undermining during the flap dissection minimizes the likelihood of subsequent flap retraction. To avoid the subsequent creation of epithelial cysts, it is important that when the conjunctival flap is secured on the corneal limbus, only the edge of the conjunctival tissue is used.

After healing, a cosmetic contact lens is fitted if the patient desires. In certain circumstances, penetrating keratoplasty is indicated for visual rehabilitation. Because a conjunctival flap may have destroyed corneal limbal stem cells, a limbal allograft may be considered prior to removal of the conjunctival flap and the penetrating keratoplasty.

Pterygium Surgery

Pterygium refers to conjunctival or fibrovascular growth over the sclera and onto the cornea; it occurs most commonly in the nasal aspect of the interpalpebral exposure zone. Pathologically, pterygium is characterized by elastoid degeneration of subepithelial tissue and destruction of Bowman's membrane. The cause of pterygium is believed to be related to ultraviolet and

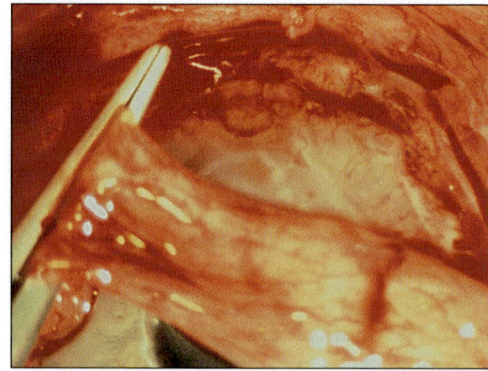

FIG. 63-30 ■ Mobilization of the conjunctival flap to the desired area of the cornea. (Courtesy of Dr RK Forster.)

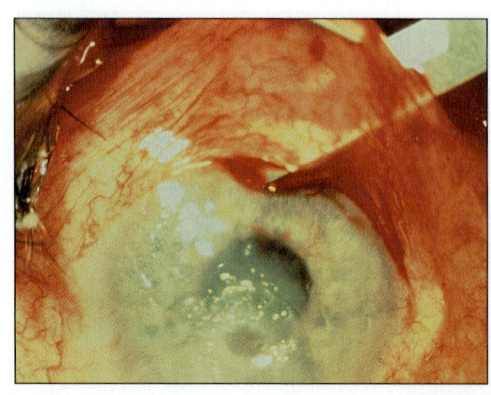

FIG. 63-29 ■ 360° peritomy. Westcott scissors is used. The dissection is carried out toward the corneal limbus with care not to buttonhole the conjunctiva. (Courtesy of Dr RK Forster.)

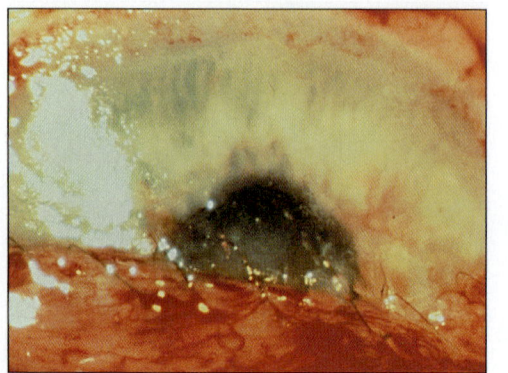

FIG. 63-31 ■ Here, the conjunctival flap covers the area of sterile ulceration. The flap is sutured into position with 10-0 nylon sutures superiorly and 7-0 Vicryl sutures through the inferior limbal episclera. (Courtesy of Dr RK Forster.)

dust exposure. Clinically, a characteristic iron line (Stocker's line) may be seen at the advancing front of a pterygium.

PREOPERATIVE EVALUATION AND DIAGNOSTIC APPROACH.

Surgical indications for a pterygium excision include:

- Growth of pterygium such that it has impinged on the visual axis;
- Reduced vision as a result of astigmatism induced by the pterygium;
- Severe irritation not relieved by medical therapy;
- Surgery for cosmesis; and
- Reduced motility secondary to pterygium.

Recurrence after surgical excision is a risk, and recurred lesions grow more aggressively than the primary lesions. It is therefore imperative that patients are made fully aware of these possibilities as well as of the other complications discussed later.

SURGICAL TECHNIQUES.

Several techniques are available for the excision of pterygium, which include the bare sclera technique, autograft, antimetabolites, radiation, and the recently developed techniques using amniotic membranes.

Bare Sclera Technique. The bare sclera technique is technically simple, although it is associated with a recurrence rate as high as 40%.[43] Surgically, the lesion may be outlined using spot cautery. To facilitate the dissection, the eye is rotated laterally using traction sutures (6-0 Vicryl or silk) placed at the corneal limbus at the 6 and 12 o'clock positions. The dissection may be initiated at the corneal side of the pterygium. Using forceps, the head of pterygium is lifted and dissected off the cornea in a lamellar fashion using a No. 64 or No. 69 Beaver blade (Fig. 63-32). The scleral portion of the pterygium is excised using Westcott scissors (see Fig. 63-33). Care is taken to identify the rectus muscle, especially in surgery for recurrent pterygium in which fibrous tissue may be adherent to the underlying muscle. The dissected area near the limbus is polished using a diamond burr (see Fig. 63-34). Alternative techniques include removal of the scleral portion first, followed by blunt dissection or avulsion of the corneal portion.

Autograft. A conjunctival autograft after pterygium excision has been shown to decrease significantly the chance of recurrence to 5%.[43] After excision of the pterygium, as already described, the size of the bare sclera defect is measured. Commonly, the supero-

temporal conjunctiva is used as donor if the pterygium is located nasally. The tractional sutures may be used to rotate the eye downward. The donor conjunctiva is outlined using spot cautery and a conjunctival flap is dissected with smooth forceps and Westcott scissors (Fig. 63-35). It is important to handle the conjunctiva carefully to avoid the creation of buttonholes. The orientation of the conjunctival flap is maintained when it is transferred to the recipient bed to ensure the proper positioning of limbal stem cells, although the presence of limbal cells may not be necessary. Alternatively, the conjunctival flap may be rotated on a pedicle. The authors use a 10-0 nylon suture at the limbus to secure the graft and several interrupted 8-0 Vicryl sutures elsewhere (Fig. 63-36). The nylon sutures are removed 2 weeks postoperatively and the Vicryl sutures are left to be reabsorbed. In general, the donor conjunctival defect is left unsutured.

Antimetabolites and Radiation. Mitomycin has been used both intraoperatively and postoperatively and appears to reduce significantly the recurrence rate. In addition, beta radiation using strontium-90 has been employed and has decreased recurrence successfully. However, radiation treatment may cause significant complications such as scleral necrosis, cataract, and persistent epithelial defect. As a result, beta radiation and mitomycin treatment after pterygium surgery have been supplanted largely by conjunctival transplantation.

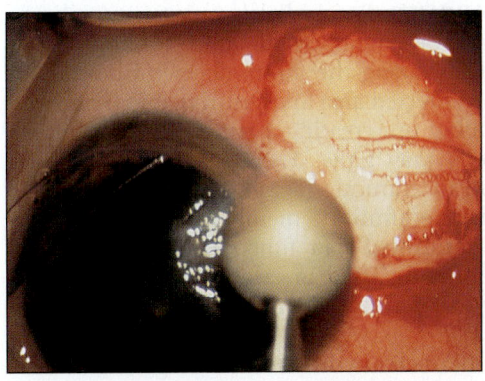

FIG. 63-34 ▮ A diamond burr is used to smooth the corneal tissue.

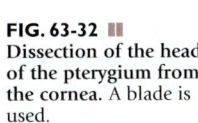
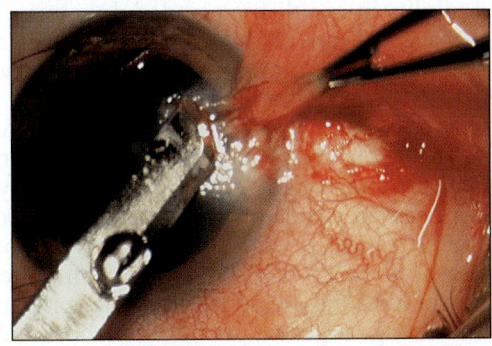

FIG. 63-32 ▮ Dissection of the head of the pterygium from the cornea. A blade is used.

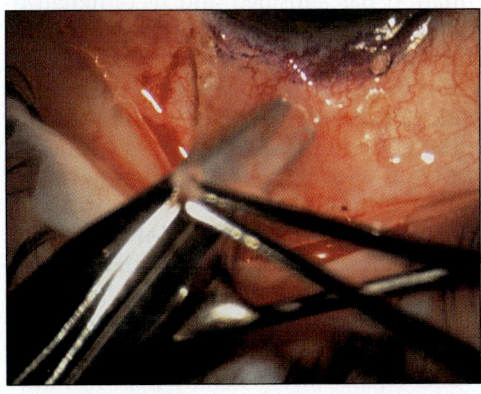

FIG. 63-35 ▮ Dissection of the conjunctiva. The limbus is marked and the healthy conjunctiva is harvested. The conjunctiva is dissected gently with care not to buttonhole the donor tissue.

FIG. 63-33 ▮ Removal of the body of the pterygium. Westcott scissors are used with care to avoid damage to the underlying rectus muscle.

FIG. 63-36 ▮ Conjunctival autograft in position over the previously excised pterygium. Two 10-0 nylon sutures are placed at the limbus and 8-0 Vicryl sutures are used along the conjunctiva in an interrupted fashion. Care is taken to maintain the limbus-to-limbus position of the graft.

Amniotic Membrane Transplantation (AMT)

PREOPERATIVE EVALUATION AND DIAGNOSTIC APPROACH.
Amniotic membrane has been increasingly used for various clinical indications for ocular surface reconstruction.[44,45] Amniotic membrane provides two main favorable clinical effects: the promotion of epithelialization and the inhibition of inflammation and fibrosis. In the promotion of epithelialization, amnion basement membrane facilitates the migration of epithelial cells,[46] reinforces basal epithelial adhesion,[47,48] prevents cellular apoptosis,[49,50] and promotes cellular differentiation.[51-54] In addition, clinical studies indicate that amniotic membrane possesses anti-inflammatory properties[55,56] that decrease neovascularization and fibrosis. Rabbit studies have shown that AMT suppresses corneal stromal inflammatory cells after alkali injury[57] and after excimer laser ablation.[58-61]

To date, amniotic membrane has been used to treat an ever-widening range of disorders, including persistent epithelial defects and sterile ulceration.[55,56,62-67] AMT has also been used to treat descemetocele formation and corneal perforation[66] as well as scleral perforation.[66,68] It has also been used as an adjunct to limbal stem cell transplantation.[69,70] AMT has also been used to treat the ocular surface in the acute[71,72] and chronic[63,64,66,69,73-75] phase of chemical or thermal burn. In the conjunctiva, AMT has been used to cover the defects created after excision of conjunctival intraepithelial neoplasia and tumors,[76,77] symblephara,[64,67,76-78] and conjunctivochalasis[77,78] as well as covering on top of scleral grafts[76] and in pterygium surgery.[67,76,79-82]

SURGICAL TECHNIQUES. Surgically, amniotic membrane can be applied in three ways: inlay, overlay, and "filling." The inlay technique[62] involves sizing the amniotic membrane to be slightly larger than the affected area and suturing it in place with the epithelial side facing up, creating a surface on which new corneal epithelial cells may grow. The overlay technique, in which the orientation of amniotic membrane is not as important, involves placing the amniotic membrane over the entire cornea, limbus, and perilimbal area, functioning like a biological contact lens.[63,64] Filling is used in cases of deep stromal ulceration: multiple layers of amniotic membrane may be used to fill the ulcer cavity

After AMT, a large-diameter hydrophilic bandage contact lens is often applied, and topical antibiotic and steroid medications are used until inflammation has subsided and reepithelialization is complete. Systemic immunosuppression is in general not necessary. Amniotic membrane is not completely transparent but does allow navigational vision. When used in the overlay fashion, amniotic membrane usually dissolves within weeks or months, whereas the inlayed amniotic membrane is frequently preserved for a longer period of time.[55,56,65] It is often necessary to apply amniotic membrane multiple times.[63]

COMPLICATIONS AND POSTOPERATIVE MANAGEMENT.
Amniotic membrane dehiscence, postoperative irritation, and pain are the most common complications seen after AMT. Ocular surface health and lubrication are critical for maintenance of amniotic membrane on the eye for the appropriate period of time to achieve its effect. AMT generally does not have the mechanical strength to serve as a tectonic graft, and hence wound leak can been seen when it is used in that setting.

Limbal Cell Transplant

The corneal limbus is believed to contain stem cells capable of regeneration and is the source of new corneal epithelium. The limbal stem cells also serve as the junctional barrier between corneal and conjunctival epithelium. Limbal deficiency or dysfunctional limbal stem cells may result in poor corneal epithelialization with persistent defects or erosions, corneal vascularization, corneal scarring, and conjunctivalization of the cornea. True limbal deficiency is confirmed pathologically by the detection of goblet cells on the corneal surface—this may be done using impression cytology.[83]

PREOPERATIVE EVALUATION AND DIAGNOSTIC APPROACH.
Limbal stem cell transplantation is indicated in the setting of limbal cell deficiency. Limbal deficiency may be secondary to chemical or thermal injuries, Stevens-Johnson syndrome, multiple surgery or cryotherapy to the limbal area, contact lens injury, aniridia, multiple endocrine deficiency, or idiopathic causes. Limbal cell transplantation refers to the transplantation of a ring or a sectorial portion of corneal limbal tissue from a healthy donor eye. The donor may be the contralateral eye from the same patient (autograft) or from a corneal donor (allograft). Autograft carries a lower chance of rejection than allograft, but allograft is used in cases of bilateral limbal deficiency or when either the surgeon or the patient prefers to leave the contralateral eye undisturbed.[84]

With regard to allograft, a major limitation of success of the surgery is the lack of a robust and consistently effective drug regimen for systemic immunosuppression that provides a prolonged period of survival of these grafts. The limbal tissue is highly antigenic because it is vascularized and has more Langerhans' cells than the rest of the cornea. The existing systemic immunosuppression regimens consist mostly of cyclosporin (CsA) or prednisone as single drugs or in combination.[85-92] The efficacy of most of these existing drug regimens is limited, and the 5-year survival rate of limbal stem cell allograft (LSA) is still quite low with the majority of the grafts rejected.[92] Most of the acute rejection episodes occurred within the first 6 months postoperatively, suggesting that early and sufficient immunosuppression is of utmost importance. However, intensive systemic immunosuppression for any prolonged period of time significantly increases the likelihood of dose-related and cumulative drug toxicity.

In an attempt to find more efficacious and safer immunosuppressive drugs, the authors[93] identified a triple drug regimen to help overcome the shortcomings with current regimens. This regimen is analogous to those used in renal transplantation[94,95] with the addition of mycophenolate mofetil (MMF, Cellcept) to CsA and prednisone. We reasoned that an ideal drug regimen for LSA should be one that has the flexibility of providing not only a short-term intense drug treatment in the early postoperative period when the acute rejection rate is high but also a sustained and prolonged period of drug coverage to address the critical issue of long-term graft survival. Hence, a single drug regimen may not be the best choice, whereas in a multidrug regimen, one has more flexibility in establishing graded drug treatment intensity as well as staggered time durations. Furthermore, compared with single drug treatment, a multidrug approach may involve lower drug toxicity because the dose of each drug can be reduced, particularly if the toxicity target organ is different for each drug.

This triple drug regimen for allograft consists of three drugs: CsA, prednisone, and MMF. MMF selectively inhibits T cells and has been an effective immunosuppressive drug in recent years. These three drugs work synergistically and have different toxicity target organs. MMF is started at 1 month preoperatively and CsA and prednisone are added at 3 days prior to the surgery. These three drugs together provide the short-term intense immunosuppression needed to curb the high rejection rate in the immediate postoperative period (the first 6 months). CsA doses are kept relatively low, as in the treatment for rheumatoid arthritis, to limit its dose-related toxicity. Duration of use for CsA and prednisone is also shortened to reduce cumulative toxicities. Beyond 6 months, only MMF is maintained, which provides more sustained drug coverage to prolong graft survival in the late postoperative period. Our preliminary result using the triple drug therapy shows promising improvement over the existing regimen.

A new promising alternative to limbal stem cell auto- or allografting involves the *ex vivo* expansion of limbal tissue.[96] In this method, cell culture techniques are used to cultivate a sheet of epithelial cells from a harvested limbus biopsy from a patient's contralateral eye[96,97] or the eye of a living relative.[98]

The advantage is that a smaller amount of tissue is harvested, limiting the risk to the donor eye. Investigators have learned that sheets of cultured epithelial cells are fragile and difficult to manipulate and have subsequently used amniotic membrane as the substrate onto which the limbal epithelial cells are expanded.[99-101] Amniotic membrane provides advantages over other extracellular matrices: it has been shown to promote epithelialization and decrease inflammation, it contains components similar to those of conjunctival basement membranes, and it is readily available. Success has been shown in treating patients with ocular surface disorders using limbal epithelium expanded on amniotic membrane.[97] In these cases, epithelial cells that were cultured on amniotic membrane were transplanted along with the amniotic membrane onto the ocular surface of damaged eyes.

Limbal cell transplantation may be carried out in conjunction with pterygium surgery or in anticipation of a future penetrating keratoplasty. Limbal deficiency may be focal or diffuse. Appropriate surgical approaches need to be selected depending on the requirements of the patient.

SURGICAL TECHNIQUES. After peribulbar or retrobulbar anesthetic and insertion of a lid speculum, a peritomy is performed in the appropriate quadrant(s). The peritomy extends 2–3mm posterior to the limbus. A lamellar keratectomy may be performed, depending on the degree of scarring. Pannus tissue, if present, is stripped off the corneal surface. The graft is prepared from the donor site of the fellow eye or from a donor cadaveric eye. The surgeon removes sectorial annular grafts of limbal tissue, which extend approximately 0.5mm onto the clear cornea and approximately 4mm onto the bulbar conjunctiva peripherally. The length and quantity of transplanted tissue depend on the needs of the recipient eye. If the graft is taken from the patient's other eye, the minimal amount of limbal tissue is removed to ensure no iatrogenic limbal deficiency. The donor sites are left unsutured. When a cadaveric eye is used, every effort is made to use the freshest possible tissue (i.e., within 24 hours). The authors prefer to use an annular graft, either sectorial or a complete ring. Other authors have performed keratoepithelioplasty by cutting lenticules from the donor cadaveric limbus and suturing these to the recipient so that the peripheral limbus is oriented centrally.[102,103] In the setting of using *ex vivo* expanded limbal stem cells, a sheet of amniotic membrane containing corneal epithelial cells grown on its surface in a laboratory is used.

The autografts are secured to their corresponding positions using 10-0 nylon sutures; 8-0 Vicryl sutures are used to secure the conjunctival margins. A bandage contact lens or a tarsorrhaphy may be used to help with the resurfacing. Studies are under way to investigate the use of amniotic membrane as a potential adjunct to this surgery.[43]

COMPLICATIONS AND POSTOPERATIVE MANAGEMENT. Graft rejection is the most common complication seen after limbal cell transplantation. In additional to topical corticosteroids, systemic immunosuppression is critical and the patients need to be monitored regularly to identify drug-related side effects. With our triple-drug therapy,[93] all three systemic medications are kept on board for the first 6 months, followed by slow tapering of steroid and cyclosporin with Cellcept being kept on beyond that point. Patients are monitored weekly to monthly and the tapering regimen adjusted according clinical examination. Sub-Tenon's capsule injection of corticosteroid may also be necessary.

OUTCOMES

Conjunctival procedures, such as conjunctival flap, pterygium surgery, and limbal cell transplantation, are important surgical techniques for corneal surgeons. The success of these procedures depends on the appropriate consideration of surgical indications and judicious selection of the optimal surgical approach.

EXCIMER LASER TREATMENT OF CORNEAL PATHOLOGY

INTRODUCTION

The use of high-energy ultraviolet radiation of wavelength 193nm to treat corneal pathology and smooth corneal surface irregularities has generated great interest in the field of ophthalmology. Laser energy emitted by the argon-fluoride (ArF) excimer laser for these purposes is termed phototherapeutic keratectomy (PTK). The concept was first suggested by Trokel in 1983, and investigational protocols using PTK in clinical trials have been under way since 1988; these culminated in United States Food and Drug Administration approval of PTK in 1995. Advantages of excimer laser technology in the treatment of corneal pathology include:

- Corneal tissue can be ablated with precision and minimal thermal damage to nonablated tissue;
- The depth and diameter of treatment can be controlled carefully (which enables precise removal of epithelium, Bowman's membrane, and anterior stromal tissue); and
- A smooth template is provided for reepithelialization.

Enormous potential lies in the ability of the ArF excimer laser to treat anterior corneal pathology and thereby postpone or eliminate the need for lamellar or penetrating keratoplasty.[104]

Despite the precision of the excimer laser in the treatment of anterior corneal pathology, PTK should be viewed as an adjunct to more conservative measures, and its limitations must be understood. Optimal results occur with pathology in the superficial 100μm of the cornea, and treatment must always allow the cornea to have at least 350μm thickness after the procedure.[105]

PREOPERATIVE EVALUATION AND DIAGNOSTIC APPROACH

Preoperative evaluation includes uncorrected visual acuity, best corrected visual acuity by manifest refraction, hard contact lens fitting, pupil size measurements in room light and in near-dark lighting, slit-lamp biomicroscopy, dilated fundus examination, keratometry, corneal topography, and wavefront analysis. The type of pathology and the depth estimated by optical pachymetry are documented, as well as the proximity of the pathology to the pupillary center. To plan the most effective procedure, determination of the type of pathology and its ablation characteristics is also important.

Indications for PTK include anterior basement membrane dystrophy, Bowman's membrane dystrophies (Reis-Bückler), and stromal dystrophies, such as lattice, Schnyder's, and granular. Additional indications include superficial corneal scars (traumatic, surgical, or infectious), Salzmann's nodules, and fibroblastic nodules in keratoconus patients. Band keratopathy may be treated using the excimer laser, but a highly irregular base is often left because of the nonuniformity of the calcium density in the band across the cornea.[106-108] Chelation with EDTA is attempted first. Irregular corneal surfaces that result from pterygium removal and climatic droplet keratopathy are further possibilities for treatment.[109,110]

Contraindications to PTK include severe keratoconjunctivitis sicca, uncontrolled uveitis, severe blepharitis, lagophthalmos, and systemic immunosuppression. Also, PTK should be avoided in patients who have neurotrophic corneas (including previous herpes simplex or zoster or trigeminal nerve injury), exposure keratitis, collagen vascular disease, and diabetes because of potential problems with wound healing. Because it is possible that microorganisms may be spread during treatment, PTK should not be used for deep corneal scars and microbial keratitis, including infectious crystalline keratopathy.[111,112] Significant corneal thinning is a further contraindication. Hyperopia is a relative contraindication because removal of corneal lesions centrally causes significant central flattening and further hyperopia.

The surgeon should anticipate the hyperopic shift, and this includes hyperopic PRK as a component of the treatment.

SURGICAL TECHNIQUES
Corneal Dystrophies, Scars, and Elevated Opacities

The goal of treatment of anterior stromal dystrophies is to ablate the confluent opacities in the visual axis and remove the least amount of tissue possible to achieve the optimal visual outcome. Typically, anterior stromal dystrophies have the bulk of lesions anteriorly (see Fig. 63-37).[113] The middle and deep stroma often have fewer lesions with intervening clear stroma. In the course of treatment, deeper lesions are not ablated. In corneas that have smooth epithelium, it is typically best to remove the epithelium using the excimer laser rather than manually. This may have added benefit because lesions often extend from the stroma into the epithelium. The epithelium, therefore, serves as a natural masking agent by filling in the irregularities. A large-diameter (6–7mm) ablation zone is centered over the entrance pupil. Once the epithelium has been ablated and an irregular lesion encountered, the treatment is halted and masking fluid applied as needed to provide for a smoother ablation.[106,114]

Masking fluids fill in depressions and expose elevations of an irregular corneal surface; they also absorb laser energy and thus shield depressions and expose tissue peaks. Numerous masking fluids are available. The most important principle is to use just enough masking fluid to cover the "valleys." Carboxymethyl-cellulose 0.5% is of medium viscosity and efficiently covers the valleys and exposes the elevated areas. Methylcellulose 1–2% is a high-viscosity fluid that may cover peaks, whereas hydroxypropylmethylcellulose 0.1% with dextran is of low viscosity and may leave valleys as well as peaks partly exposed. It is often best to use more than one agent depending on the particular corneal surface. It is essential that, even with a preoperative determination of the depth of the lesion, the surgeon always errs on the side of undertreatment and then examines the patient at the slit lamp. The patient may be brought back to the laser to receive further treatment.

Corneal dystrophies may recur after PTK in much the same way that dystrophies recur after penetrating keratoplasty. Recurrences are usually more superficial and may be retreated with PTK or, in a corneal graft, treated with PTK for the first time.

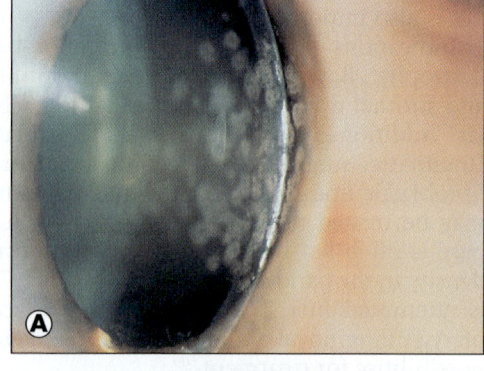

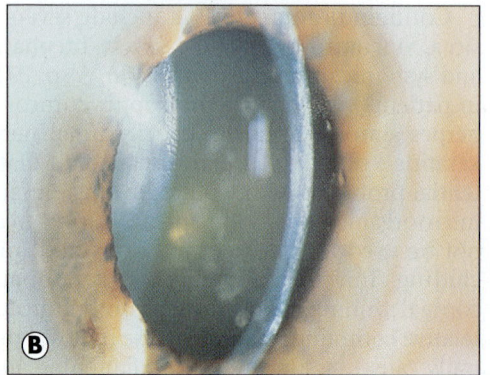

FIG. 63-37 ▌
Granular dystrophy. **A,** Preoperative anterior appearance of the opacities in a patient who has granular dystrophy. **B,** The same eye 3 months after phototherapeutic keratectomy. (With permission from Salz JJ, McDonnell PJ, McDonald MB, eds. Corneal laser surgery. St Louis: Mosby; 1995.)

The success rate for recurrent granular or lattice dystrophy is extremely high and comparable to the high success rate for primary Reis-Bückler dystrophy, in which the deposits occur at Bowman's layer.[104] Macular and Aellino dystrophies have deeper lesions, and macular has intervening confluence; both are usually not amenable to PTK.

Postinfectious, post-traumatic, trachomatous, climatic droplet keratopathy and pterygium-related scars have been treated with success using PTK. Superficial corneal scars, such as those following pterygium surgery, often have better rates of successful treatment than deeper, postinfectious, and post-traumatic scars. Superficial herpetic scars have also been treated successfully, but numerous studies document recurrence of herpetic disease after PTK.[104,107,115,116] Corneal scars often ablate at a different rate than the normal stroma, which may result in an irregular treatment surface. Corneal surface abnormalities often cause irregular astigmatism, and seemingly minor focal abnormalities may give rise to visually significant problems. The use of hyperopic PRK as part of the treatment is important to reduce the degree of surgically induced hyperopia.

Elevated corneal opacities represent a major challenge to the PTK surgeon. This type of pathology is often amenable to manual keratectomy using a blade, which is efficacious when a suitable plane is found to leave a smooth surface on the cornea; this is especially valuable in vascularized pannus. When a plane cannot be found, it is possible to "debulk" the elevation and smooth the remaining area using the excimer laser. Alternatively, the epithelium may be removed from the area over the elevated lesion and photoablation performed upon the pathology.[106] The surrounding epithelium is left in place to serve as a masking agent, to avoid the ablation of normal tissue around the lesion. After removal of the nodule, the entire area is smoothed with additional use of masking agents, such as hydroxypropyl-methylcellulose 0.1% with dextran. In this way, Salzmann's nodular degeneration and keratoconus nodules have been treated successfully.[117]

Phototherapeutic Keratectomy in the Treatment of Photorefractive Keratectomy Complications

Photorefractive keratectomy (PRK) complications include subepithelial scarring, astigmatism, decentration, and central islands. Central islands are topographical changes after PRK that result from insufficient flattening of the central cornea compared with the edge of the treated area. They cause blurred vision, glare, and halos (see Chapter 18). PTK has shown promise in the treatment of subepithelial collagen plaques after PRK. Although haze after PRK often clears over a period of 3–6 months, confluent, dense haze may cause a qualitative difference in vision as well as myopia and night glare. During treatment, the epithelium is ablated using the excimer laser and the collagen plaque treated with an optical zone at least as large as the PRK optical zone. Masking fluids may also help to achieve a smooth postoperative surface. Collagen plaques are often 20–40mm thick.[118] The shoot and check technique, in which the patient is checked at the slit lamp and taken back to the laser, if necessary, is used. The plaque is ablated partially, as total removal to leave a clear cornea may induce unwanted hyperopia. Residual haze, on the other hand, can be treated with mitomycin C and typically leaves the patient with an improved quality of vision and less refractive change after the procedure.[118]

Irregular astigmatism is one potential undesirable outcome after PRK. Gibralter and Trokel[119] described a method for the treatment of irregular astigmatism using the excimer laser in a corneal graft. They used small-diameter ablations to neutralize the irregular astigmatism by treating steep areas of the cornea identified topographically.[119] The diameter and steepness of the irregular areas were estimated preoperatively. Residual myopia was corrected using PRK parameters.[119] This approach has been replaced by wavefront–guided laser treatment.

Decentered ablations and central islands are other possible complications of PRK. Glare and halos may be troublesome to the patient. It is important to differentiate between treatment displacement and intraoperative drift.[120] Tangential topography is valuable in the differentiation of these forms of decentration. Patients who have pure, tangential displacement may not require additional treatment unless the displacement is excessive or is associated with undercorrection. Patients who suffer treatment drift may be better candidates for retreatment because their symptoms may be secondary to irregularities in the ablation bed, which can be remedied using the appropriate surgical technique.[120,121] Talamo et al.[122] reported successful treatment of a nasally decentered PRK with grade 2.0 haze at the temporal part of the ablation. The epithelium was removed using the excimer laser temporally, and not nasally, to achieve a more temporal stromal ablation. Carboxymethylcellulose 1% was applied nasally as a masking agent, and additional pulses were applied to remove haze and flatten the temporal area further. Azar et al.[123] reported using corneal topography to plan the treatment sequences of epithelial PTK and PRK, guided by the epithelial fluorescence over the intended area of correction. A 6.0–6.5mm PTK is performed in a transepithelial fashion until a crescent of stromal ablation is observed (manifest as an arc of "loss of epithelial fluorescence"). Treatment of the residual refractive error using PRK is performed when the crescent of stromal PTK ablation reaches the center of the entrance pupil. This technique applies to the treatment of decentrations and of central islands. Topographic systems that display maps of actual corneal elevations rather than reflected ring images may help identify focal irregularities to improve PTK in the future. The smooth surface after wavefront–guided treatment using scanning slit or flying spot lasers also appears promising.[123–127]

POSTOPERATIVE CARE. Immediately postoperatively, a bandage soft contact lens is applied and the patient is instructed to use topical antibiotics, often a broad-spectrum antibiotic such as a fluoroquinolone. Alternatively, bacitracin or erythromycin ophthalmic antibiotic ointment is applied along with a cycloplegic drop (homatropine), and a pressure patch is placed. Topical corticosteroid such as prednisolone acetate 1%, dexamethasone phosphate 0.1%, or fluorometholone 0.1%, four times a day, is used. The corticosteroid is tapered to once daily within 1 month. In many compromised corneas that undergo PTK, the benefits of continued corticosteroid drops may be outweighed by the potential side effects of a rise in IOP, cataract, risk of microbial infection, or recurrent herpetic disease. Topical nonsteroidal anti-inflammatory drops given for 1 day may help control pain, which may be severe.[104,128–130]

Patients are examined every 24–72 hours until epithelialization is complete, which generally occurs within 1 week. Eye examinations are performed at 1 month, 3 months, 12 months, and annually thereafter.[115]

COMPLICATIONS
Hyperopia

The most common side effect of PTK is induced hyperopia, which results from flattening of the central cornea and may require postoperative contact lenses. A number of possible reasons may explain the hyperopic shift. The excimer laser beam is focused centrally and is delivered to the central cornea at a 90° angle, whereas the periphery receives an angled beam that ablates less tissue than the perpendicular central beam.[124] More important, epithelial and stromal hyperplasia and a flatter tear meniscus peripherally may result in greater central flattening, and the periphery may be shielded by ablation products. Nevertheless, strategies to decrease induced hyperopia have been used with variable success. Sher's buff and polish technique[131] is performed by moving the patient's head in a circular manner under a laser beam of varying aperture size. Sher et al.[131] also performed hyperopic ablations in a number of other cases immediately after

PTK. Stark et al.[104] and Chamon et al.[108] used a modified taper technique to treat the ablation margins with a 20mm deep, 2.0mm diameter annulus. The authors' preferred method is to include 1D of hyperopic correction for every 25m of PTK tissue ablation. The depth of the ablation correlates with the amount of induced hyperopia. Therefore, the judicious use of masking agents and avoidance of ablation of deeper lesions help to prevent a case that appears to be an anatomical success to the surgeon (because of the clarity of the cornea after ablation of pathology) from being a visual failure to the patient.

Myopia/Myopic Astigmatism

Myopia and myopic astigmatism may be induced when the periphery or paracentral cornea undergoes a deeper ablation than the central cornea, which may occur in the treatment of paracentral opacities. Sher et al.[131] observed myopic shift in 3% of PTK-treated patients, and Campos et al. found a rate of 16.6%.[107]

Irregular Astigmatism and Decentration

Irregular astigmatism is an undesirable potential outcome that may be minimized by using masking agents to help achieve a smooth corneal contour postoperatively. Decentration may also lead to irregular astigmatism. When extensive pathology needs ablation, the ablation zone must be large and centered about the entrance pupil. Proper patient fixation is critical, and treatment is interrupted if fixation is lost. Alignment of the laser beam and microscope is also of great importance to avoid decentered ablations. Preoperative use of miotics may cause superonasal displacement of the pupil, which may result in a decentered ablation if the beam is centered at the entrance pupil.

Pain

Pain may be severe after excimer laser photoablation. Judicious use of topical nonsteroidal anti-inflammatory agents, which include diclofenac sodium, ketorolac tromethamine (ketorolac trometamol), and flurbiprofen sodium, has helped in pain control after excimer laser treatment.

Delayed Epithelialization

Epithelial healing is usually complete within the first week. It is desirable to avoid prolonged epithelial healing because without an intact epithelium, a port of entry into the subepithelial tissue exists for microorganisms, visual acuity is reduced, and pain may be severe. Persistent epithelial defects or recurrent erosions are possible complications that may result and seem to be more common in patients who have preoperative epitheliopathy. The damage to Bowman's layer from PTK, postoperative iatrogenic toxicity from drops, or active inflammation may result in epithelial healing difficulties. Systemic disorders, such as collagen vascular diseases or diabetes, may also be involved. Chamon et al.[108] noted a history of heavy alcohol intake in one patient whose epithelium took 3–4 weeks to heal after PTK. Active inflammation is treated aggressively. Bandage contact lenses and lubrication are typically very helpful in the promotion of epithelial healing.[104] Punctal plugs are often helpful in patients who have dry eye signs or symptoms, and tarsorrhaphy may be considered in recalcitrant cases. Preoperative epitheliopathy must be treated and medications carefully reviewed.

Bacterial Keratitis

Bacterial keratitis is a feared postoperative complication because of the existence of an epithelial defect and the placement of a contact lens on what may be an already compromised cornea. Al-Rajhi et al.[132] reported three cases of bacterial keratitis, all of which had a preoperative diagnosis of climatic droplet keratopathy, out of 258 eyes that underwent PTK. All three had gram-positive keratitis. However, the authors maintain that the risk of infection after PTK is lower than the risk associated with the natural history of the disease. Most PTK surgeons believe the ability of bandage contact lenses to decrease pain and help epithelial wound healing outweighs the risk of bacterial keratitis. Prophylactic antibiotic drops are used postoperatively. In addition, stromal infiltrates are managed similarly to those in patients who have not had PTK. Nonsteroidal anti-inflammatory agents, contact lenses, and infectious keratitis may also produce infiltrates.

Viral Keratitis

Herpes simplex virus may be reactivated after PTK. Pepose *et al.*[133] demonstrated reactivation in latently infected mice, possibly related to irritation of the corneal nerve plexus by excimer keratectomy. In a study of 166 eyes, Fagerholm *et al.*[134] reported one patient who had three recurrences of herpes simplex. Vrabec *et al.*[116] described two cases of recurrence of herpetic dendritic keratitis in which PTK was performed to ablate stromal scars secondary to recurrent herpes simplex. McDonnell *et al.*[135] reported recurrence of herpes epithelial keratitis after excimer astigmatic photokeratectomy in a corneal graft. Whenever possible, treatment of patients who have a history of herpes is avoided. In cases that are treated, regimens of preoperative and postoperative acyclovir are given. Campos *et al.*[107] described a successful outcome in a patient using oral acyclovir 200mg four times a day preoperatively and continued for 10 days postoperatively. Topical antiviral agents should be considered, and corticosteroids are used sparingly.

Recurrence and Haze

Corneal dystrophies treated with PTK may recur, as they do in corneal grafts. Retreatment may be undertaken, although the possibility of the inducement of further hyperopia and possibly anisometropia must be considered. Best corrected visual acuity may be improved by PTK retreatment, but anisometropia and contact lens intolerance may be problematic. Alternative options, which include mechanical keratectomy, should be considered. Furthermore, haze often results after PTK and may be confluent and visually significant. Haze often decreases over time, and a period of 12 months is allowed to elapse before the haze is treated.[124]

Graft Rejection

Corneal graft rejection in PTK-treated patients has been reported, as in patients treated by Hersh *et al.*[136] for recurrent lattice dystrophy and Epstein and Robin[137] for postoperative astigmatism. Medical treatment of the rejection episodes was successful in both instances.

OUTCOMES

Corneal Light Scattering and Wound Healing after Phototherapeutic Keratectomy

The transparency and minimal degree of light scatter of the cornea largely result from the tight packing and small diameter of stromal collagen fibrils. Fibrils within lamellae scatter light inefficiently, and each lamella scatters light. The light scattered by the different lamellae undergoes mutually destructive interference.[138] Further, the cornea is a thin structure, which also helps to decrease light scatter. A functional endothelium is necessary for corneal transparency because corneal edema increases the packing distance between fibrils.[139]

After ablation of the anterior cornea using the ArF excimer laser, reepithelialization occurs within the first week.[104,128–130] One hypothesis is that photoablation leads to the formation of a "pseudomembrane," which serves as a template for migrating hyperplastic epithelial cells, as well as a water barrier, and thus helps prevent corneal edema after photoablation.[140,141] The use of mitomycin C (during PTK) to treat corneal scarring after PRK has reduced the likelihood of recurrences of haze and scarring and improved visual outcomes.[142–144]

Anchorage of the epithelium to the stroma occurs approximately 1–3 months after photoablation through the reformation of three different structural groups that participate in the bonds between the epithelium and stroma—hemidesmosomes, anchoring fibrils containing type VII collagen, and basal laminae. These groups are restored over a period of many months, but abnormalities may still persist after a year and perhaps become a permanent feature.[145] Although such abnormalities are noted after PTK, the technique has been used successfully to treat disorders of the cornea that involve faulty epithelial adhesion, such as recalcitrant recurrent erosion syndrome.[109]

Stromal wound healing occurs simultaneously with reformation of the anchoring complexes. Activated keratocytes repopulate the area and actually increase in number by the third week after photoablation. Histologically, the activity of the cells is evident by a large increase in rough endoplasmic reticulum. New collagen, predominantly type III, and proteoglycan matrix, believed to be primarily keratan sulfate, are produced.[146,147]

The activated keratocytes and their products (newly formed collagen and proteoglycans in an irregular network) result in the haze that contributes to light scatter.[105,147,148] Morphological studies of animal and human endothelium have failed to show evidence of endothelial cell loss in ablations at least 40mm anterior to Descemet's membrane.[105,149,150]

SUMMARY

In conclusion, the 193nm ArF excimer laser has great potential for the treatment of anterior corneal pathology and surface irregularities. The expenses and risks of penetrating keratoplasty, including the risks of intraocular surgery and anesthesia, may be avoided. The use of PTK in the treatment of complications of PRK will continue to evolve and will be coupled with wavefront–guided laser ablation with or without mitomycin C. However, the limits of PTK must be accepted. Deep corneal pathology must not be treated. During PTK, the use of masking fluids helps to achieve a smooth corneal surface. Treatment must be individualized depending on the type of pathology and its ablation characteristics and depth. Clinical studies have demonstrated the success of PTK for anterior corneal pathology.[151,152] Its use is an exciting addition to the treatment options available to corneal surgeons.

REFERENCES

1. Boruchoff SA, Thoft RA. Keratoplasty: lamellar and penetrating. In: Smolin G, Thoft RA, eds. The cornea. Boston: Little, Brown; 1994:645–65.
2. Reisinger F. De Keratoplastic, ein Versuch zur Erweiterring dev Augenhelkunde. Baiersche Ann Abhandl. 1824;1:207.
3. von Hippel A. On transplantation of the cornea. Berichte Ophthalmol Gesellschaft Herdelberg. 1886;18:54.
4. Elschnig A. On keratoplasty. Prag Med Wochenschr. 1914;39:30.
5. Paton D. Lamellar keratoplasty. In: Symposium on medical and surgical disease of the cornea. Transactions of the New Orleans Academy of Ophthalmology. St Louis: Mosby–Year Book; 1980:406–27.
6. Arentsen JJ. Lamellar keratoplasty. In: Brightbill FS, ed. Corneal surgery, theory, technique and tissue. St Louis: Mosby–Year Book; 1993:360–8.
7. Melles GR, Remeijer L, Geerardes AJ, Beekhuis WH. A quick surgical technique for deep, anterior lamellar keratoplasty using visco-dissection. Cornea. 2000;19:427–32.
8. Melles GR, Lander F, Rietveld FJ, et al. A new surgical technique for deep stromal, anterior lamellar keratoplasty. Br J Ophthalmol. 1999;83:327–33.
9. Azar DT, Jain S. Microkeratome-assisted posterior keratoplasty. J Cataract Refract Surg. 2002;28:732–3.
10. Yeung EF, Chi CC, Li J, et al. Microkeratome-assisted posterior lamellar keratoplasty. J Cataract Refract Surg. 2001;27:1903–4.
11. Jain S, Azar DT. New lamellar keratoplasty techniques: posterior keratoplasty and deep lamellar keratoplasty. Curr Opin Ophthalmol. 2001;12:262–8.
12. Azar DT, Jain S, Sambursky R, Strauss L. Microkeratome-assisted posterior keratoplasty. J Cataract Refract Surg. 2001;27:353–6.
13. Ehlers N, Ehlers H, Hjortdal J, Moller-Pedersen T. Grating of the posterior cornea. Description of a new technique with 12-month clinical results. Acta Ophthalmol Scand. 2000;78:543–6.

14. Melles GR, Lander F, Nieuwendaal C. Sutureless, posterior lamellar keratoplasty: a case report of a modified technique. Cornea. 2002;21:325–7.
15. Terry MA, Ousley PJ. Endothelial replacement without surface corneal incisions or sutures. Cornea. 2001;20:14–18.
16. Melles GR, Lander F, van Dooren BT, *et al.* Preliminary clinical results of posterior lamellar keratoplasty through a sclerocorneal pocket incision. Ophthalmology. 2000;107:1850–6.
17. Melles GR, Lander F, Beekhuis WH, *et al.* Posterior lamellar keratoplasty for a case of pseudophakic bullous keratopathy. Am J Ophthalmol. 1999;127:340–1.
18. Steele ADM, Kirkness CM. Manual of systematic corneal surgery. New York: Churchill Livingstone; 1992:57.
19. Hersh PS. Ophthalmic surgical procedures. Boston: Little, Brown; 1988:213.
20. O'Day DM. Donor selection. In: Brightbill FS, ed. Corneal surgery, theory, technique and tissue. St Louis: Mosby–Year Book; 1993:549–62.
21. Alldredge OC, Krachmer JH. Clinical types of corneal transplant rejection. Arch Ophthalmol. 1981;99:599–604.
22. McNeill JL, Wessels IF. Adjustment of single continuous suture to control astigmatism after penetrating keratoplasty. Refract Corneal Surg. 1989;5:216–23.
23. Pamel GJ, Taylor DM. Combined procedures. In: Brightbill FS, ed. Corneal surgery, theory, technique and tissue. St Louis: Mosby–Year Book; 1993:177–92.
24. Binder PS. Refractive errors encountered with the triple procedure. In: Cornea, refractive surgery, and contact lens. Transactions of the New Orleans Academy of Ophthalmology. New York: Raven Press; 1987:111–20.
25. Meyer RF, Musch DC. Assessment of success and complications of triple procedure surgery. Trans Am Ophthalmol Soc. 1987;85:350–67.
26. Taylor DM, Stern AL, McDonald P. The triple procedure: 2–10 year follow-up. Trans Am Ophthalmol Soc. 1986;84:221–49.
27. Retzlaff J. Posterior chamber implant power calculation: regressive formula. J Am Intraocular Implant Soc. 1980;6:268–73.
28. Katz HR, Forster RK. Intraocular lens calculation in combined penetrating keratoplasty, cataract extraction and intraocular lens implantation. Ophthalmology. 1985;92:1203–7.
29. Mattax JB, McCulley JP. The effect of standardized keratoplasty technique on IOL power calculation of the triple procedure. Acta Ophthalmol. 1989;67:24–9.
30. Skorpik C, Menapace R, Gnad HD, Grasl M. The triple procedure—results in cataract patients with corneal opacity. Ophthalmologica. 1988;196:1–6.
31. Jaffe NS, Jaffe MS, Jaffe GF. Cataract surgery and its complications. Philadelphia: Lippincott; 1990.
32. Webster RG Jr, Slansky HH, Refojo MF, *et al.* The use of adhesive for the closure of corneal perforations. Arch Ophthalmol. 1968;80:705–9.
33. Hirst LW, Smiddy WE, Stark WJ. Corneal perforations: changing methods of treatment, 1960–1980. Ophthalmology. 1982;89:630–4.
34. Kenyon KR. Corneal perforations: discussion. Ophthalmology. 1982;89:634–5.
35. Hirst LW, Smiddy WE, DeJuan E. Tissue adhesive therapy for corneal perforation. Aust J Ophthalmol. 1983;11:113–18.
36. Nobe JR, Moura BT, Robin JB, Smith RE. Results of penetrating keratoplasty for the treatment of corneal perforations. Arch Ophthalmol. 1990;108:939–41.
37. Karp CL, Forster RK. The corneal ulcer. In: Krachmer JH, Mannis MJ, Holland EJ, eds. Cornea. St Louis: Mosby; 1997:403–8.
38. Gundersen T. Conjunctival flaps in the treatment of corneal disease with reference to a new technique of application. Arch Ophthalmol. 1958;60:880.
39. Desmarres LA. Traité théorique et practique des maladies des yeux, Vol. 2. Paris: G Bailliere; 1855.
40. Rosenthal JW. Chronology of pterygium therapy. Am J Ophthalmol. 1953;36: 1601.
41. Kenyon KR, Tseng SCG. Limbal autograft transplantation for ocular surface disorders. Ophthalmology. 1989;96:709–22.
42. Rosenfeld SI, Alfonso EC, Gollamudi S. Recurrent *Herpes simplex* infection in a conjunctival flap. Am J Ophthalmol. 1993;116:242–4.
43. Jaros PA, deLuise VP. Pingueculum and pterygium. Surv Ophthalmol. 1988;33:41–9.
44. Kim JC, Tseng SCG. Transplantation of preserved human amniotic membrane for surface reconstruction in severely damaged rabbit corneas. Cornea. 1995;14:473–84.
45. Trelford JD, Trelford-Sauder M. The amnion in surgery, past and present. Am J Obstet Gynecol. 1979;134:833–45.
46. Terranova VP, Lyall RM. Chemotaxis of human gingival epithelial cells to laminin. A mechanism for epithelial cell apical migration. J Periodontol. 1986; 57:311–17.
47. Sonnenberg A, Calafat J, Janssen H, *et al.* Integrin alpha 6/beta 4 complex is located in hemidesmosomes, suggesting a major role in epidermal cell-basement membrane adhesion. J Cell Biol. 1991;113:907–17.
48. Khodadoust AA, Silverstein AM, Kenyon DR, *et al.* Adhesion of regenerating corneal epithelium. The role of basement membrane. Am J Ophthalmol. 1968;65:339–48.
49. Boudreau N, Synpson CJ, Werb Z, *et al.* Suppression of ICE and apoptosis in mammary epithelial cells by extracellular matrix. Science. 1995;267:891–3.
50. Boudreau N, Werb Z, Bissell MJ. Suppression of apoptosis by basement membrane requires three-dimensional tissue organization and withdrawal from the cell cycle. Proc Natl Acad Sci U S A 1996;93:3509–13.
51. Barcellos-Hoff MH, Aggeler J, Ram TG, *et al.* Functional differentiation and alveolar morphogenesis of primary mammary cultures on reconstituted basement membrane. Development. 1989;105:223–35.
52. Guo M, Grinnell F. Basement membrane and human epidermal differentiation in vitro. J Invest Dermatol. 1989;93:372–8.
53. Streuli CH, Bailey N, Bissell MJ. Control of mammary epithelial differentiation: basement membrane induces tissue-specific gene expression in the absence of cell-cell interaction and morphological polarity. J Cell Biol. 1991;115:1383–95.
54. Meller D, Tseng SC. Conjunctival epithelial cell differentiation on amniotic membrane. Invest Ophthalmol Vis Sci. 1999;40:878–86.
55. Kruse FE, Rohrschneider K, Volcker HE. Multilayer amniotic membrane transplantation for reconstruction of deep corneal ulcers. Ophthalmology. 1999;106:1504–11.
56. Chen HJ, Pires RT, Tseng SC. Amniotic membrane transplantation for severe neurotrophic corneal ulcers. Br J Ophthalmol. 2000;84:826–33.
57. Kim JS, Kim JC, Na BK, *et al.* Amniotic membrane patching promotes healing and inhibits proteinase activity on wound healing following acute corneal alkali burn. Exp Eye Res. 2000;70:329–37.
58. Park WC, Tseng SC. Modulation of acute inflammation and keratocyte death by suturing, blood, and amniotic membrane in PRK. Invest Ophthalmol Vis Sci. 2000;41:2906–14.
59. Wang MX, Gray TB, Park WC, *et al.* Reduction in corneal haze and apoptosis by amniotic membrane matrix in excimer laser photoablation in rabbits. J Cataract Refract Surg. 2001;27:310–19.
60. Choi YS, Kim JY, Wee WR, *et al.* Effect of the application of human amniotic membrane on rabbit corneal wound healing after excimer laser photorefractive keratectomy. Cornea. 1998;17:389–95.
61. Woo HM, Kim MS, Kweon OK, *et al.* Effects of amniotic membrane on epithelial wound healing and stromal remodeling after excimer laser keratectomy in rabbit cornea. Br J Ophthalmol. 2001;85:345–9.
62. Lee SH, Tseng SC. Amniotic membrane transplantation for persistent epithelial defects with ulceration. Am J Ophthalmol. 1997;123:303–12.
63. Letko E, Stechschulte SU, Kenyon KR, *et al.* Amniotic membrane inlay and overlay grafting for corneal epithelial defects and stromal ulcers. Arch Ophthalmol. 2001;119:659–63.
64. Azuara-Blanco A, Pillai CT, Dua HS. Amniotic membrane transplantation for ocular surface reconstruction. Br J Ophthalmol. 1999;83:399–402.
65. Shiroma H, Shimmnura S, Shimazaki J, *et al.* Histopathological study of amniotic membrane after transplantation. Invest Ophthalmol Vis Sci. 2001;42:S270.
66. Hanada K, Shimazaki J, Shimmura S, *et al.* Multilayered amniotic membrane transplantation for severe ulceration of the cornea and sclera. Am J Ophthalmol. 2000;131:324–31.
67. Gabric N, Mravicic I, Dekaris I, *et al.* Human amniotic membrane in the reconstruction of the ocular surface. Doc Ophthalmol. 1999;98:273–83.
68. Rodriguez-Ares MT, Tourino R, Capeans C, *et al.* Repair of scleral perforation with preserved scleral and amniotic membrane in Marfan's syndrome. Ophthalmic Surg Lasers. 1999;30:485–7.
69. Tseng SC, Prabhasawat P, Barton K, *et al.* Amniotic membrane transplantation with or without limbal deficiency. Arch Ophthalmol. 1998;116:431–41.
70. Pires RT, Chokshi A, Tseng SC. Amniotic membrane transplantation or conjunctival limbal autograft for limbal stem cell deficiency induced by 5-fluorouracil in glaucoma surgeries. Cornea. 2000;19:284–7.
71. Meller D, Pires RT, Mack RJ, *et al.* Amniotic membrane transplantation for acute chemical or thermal burns. Ophthalmology. 2000;107:980–90.
72. Sridhar MS, Bansal AK, Sangwan VS, *et al.* Amniotic membrane transplantation in acute chemical and thermal injury. Am J Ophthalmol. 2000;130:134–7.
73. Shimazaki J, Yang HY, Tsubota K. Amniotic membrane transplantation for ocular surface reconstruction in patients with chemical and thermal burns. Ophthalmology. 1997;104:2068–76.
74. Morgan S, Murray A. Limbal autotransplantation in the acute and chronic phases of severe chemical injuries. Eye. 1996;10:349–54.
75. Dos Santos MS, Fairbanks D, Donato WBC, *et al.* Amniotic membrane transplantation for ocular surface reconstruction in chemical burn. Invest Ophthalmol Vis Sci. 2001;42:S267.
76. Tesavibul N, Prabhasawat P. Amniotic membrane transplantation in conjunctival surface reconstruction: a prospective study. Invest Ophthalmol Vis Sci. 2001; 42:S270.
77. Tseng SC, Prabhasawat P, Lee SH. Amniotic membrane transplantation for conjunctival surface reconstruction. Am J Ophthalmol. 1997;124:765–74.
78. Meller D, Maskin SL, Pires RT, *et al.* Amniotic membrane transplantation for symptomatic conjunctivochalasis refractory to medical treatments. Cornea. 2000;19:796–803.
79. Ma DH, See LC, Liau SB, *et al.* Amniotic membrane graft for primary pterygium: comparison with conjunctival autograft and topical mitomycin C treatment. Br J Ophthalmol. 2000;84:973–8.
80. Prabhasawat P, Barton K, Burkett G, *et al.* Comparison of conjunctival autografts, amniotic membrane grafts, and primary closure for pterygium excision. Ophthalmology. 1997;104:974–85.
81. Solomon A, Pires RT, Tseng SC. Amniotic membrane transplantation after extensive removal of primary and recurrent pterygia. Ophthalmology. 2001;108: 449–60.
82. Shimazaki J, Shinozaki N, Tsubota K. Transplantation of amniotic membrane and limbal autograft for patients with recurrent pterygium associated with symblepharon. Br J Ophthalmol. 1998;82:235–40.
83. Tseng SCG. Staging of conjunctival squamous metaplasia by impression cytology. Ophthalmology. 1985;92:728–33.
84. Holland EJ, Schwarte GS. The evolution of epithelium transplantation for severe ocular surface disease and a proposed classification system. Cornea. 1996;15: 549–56.
85. Tsai RJ, Tseng SC. Human allograft limbal transplantation for corneal surface reconstruction. Cornea. 1994;13:389–400.
86. Tsubota K, Toda I, Saito H, *et al.* Reconstruction of the corneal epithelium by limbal allograft transplantation for severe ocular surface disorders. Ophthalmology. 1995;102:1486–96.
87. Tsubota K, Satake Y, Ohyama M, *et al.* Surgical reconstruction of the ocular surface in advanced ocular cicatrical pemphigoid and Stevens-Johnson syndrome. Am J Ophthalmol. 1996;122:38–52.
88. Tsubota K, Satake Y, Kaido M, *et al.* Treatment of severe ocular-surface disorders with corneal epithelial stem-cell transplantation. N Engl J Med. 1999;340: 1697–703.
89. Holland EJ. Epithelial transplantation for the management of severe ocular surface disease. Trans Am Ophthalmol Soc. 1996;94:677–743.
90. Holland EJ, Schwartz GS. The evolution of epithelial transplantation for severe ocular surface disease and a proposed classification system. Cornea. 1996;15: 549–56.
91. Tan DTH, Ficker LA, Buckley RJ. Limbal transplantation. Ophthalmology. 1996; 103:29–36.
92. Tseng SCG, Prabhasawat P, Barton K, *et al.* Amniotic membrane transplantation with or without limbal allografts for corneal surface reconstruction in patients with limbal stem cell deficiency. Arch Ophthalmol. 1998;116:431–41.

93. Ge Q, Fuchs H, Wang MX. A new triple-drug regimen for systemic immunosuppression for limbal stem cell allograft. Invest Ophthalmol Vis Sci. 2002;46:B208.

94. Tricontinental Mycophenolate Mofetil Renal Transplantation Study Group. A blinded randomized clinical trial of mycophenolate mofetil for the prevention of acute rejection in cadaveric renal transplantation. Transplantation. 1996;61:1029–37.

95. European Mycophenolate Mofetil Cooperative Study Group. Mycophenolate mofetil in renal transplantation: 3-year results from the placebo-controlled trial. Transplantation. 1999;68:391–6.

96. Pellegrini G, Traverso CE, Franzi AT, et al. Long-term restoration of damaged corneal surfaces with autologous cultivated corneal epithelium. Lancet. 1997;349:990–3.

97. Tsai RJ, Li LM, Chen JK. Reconstruction of damaged corneas by transplantation of autologous limbal epithelial cells. N Engl J Med. 2000;343:86–93.

98. Schwab IR, Reyes M, Isseroff RR. Successful transplantation of bioengineered tissue replacements in patients with ocular surface disease. Cornea. 2000;19:421–6.

99. Koizumi N, Fullwood NJ, Bairaktaris G, et al. Cultivation of corneal epithelial cells on intact and denuded human amniotic membrane. Invest Ophthalmol Vis Sci. 2000;41:2506–13.

100. Meller D, Pires RTF, Tseng SCG. Ex vivo preservation and expansion of human limbal epithelial progenitor cells by amniotic membrane. Invest Ophthalmol Vis Sci. 1999;40:S329.

101. Koizumi N, Inatomi T, Quantock AJ, et al. Amniotic membrane as a substrate for cultivating limbal corneal epithelial cells for autologous transplantation in rabbits. Cornea. 2000;19:65–71.

102. Thoft RA. Keratoplasty. Am J Ophthalmol. 1984;97:1–6.

103. Turgeon PW, Nauhem RC, Roat MI. Indication for keratoepithelioplasty. Arch Ophthalmol. 1990;108:233–6.

104. Stark WJ, Chamon W, Kamp MT, et al. Clinical follow-up of 193nm ArF excimer laser photokeratectomy. Ophthalmology. 1992;99:805–11.

105. Marshall J, Trokel S, Rothery S, Krueger RR. Photoablative reprofiling of the cornea using an excimer laser: photorefractive keratectomy. Lasers Ophthalmol. 1986;1:23–44.

106. Rapuano CJ. Excimer laser phototherapeutic keratectomy. Int Ophthalmol Clin. 1996;36:127–36.

107. Campos M, Nielson S, Szerenyi K, et al. Clinical follow-up of phototherapeutic keratectomy for treatment of corneal opacities. Am J Ophthalmol. 1993;115:433–40.

108. Chamon W, Azar DT, Stark WJ, et al. Phototherapeutic keratectomy. Ophthalmol Clin North Am. 1993;6:399–413.

109. Ohman L, Fagerholm P, Tengroth B. Treatment of recurrent corneal erosions with the excimer laser. Acta Ophthalmol. 1994;72:461–3.

110. Hersh PS, Spinak A, Garrana R, Mayers M. Phototherapeutic keratectomy: strategies and results in 12 eyes. Refract Corneal Surg. 1993;9(2 Suppl):90–5.

111. Gottsch JD, Gilbert ML, Goodman DF, et al. Excimer laser ablative treatment of microbial keratitis. Ophthalmology. 1991;98:146–9.

112. Eiferman RA, Forgey DR, Cook YD. Excimer laser ablation of infectious crystalline keratopathy. Arch Ophthalmol. 1992;110:18.

113. Salz JJ, McDonnell PJ, McDonald MB, eds. Corneal laser surgery. St Louis: Mosby; 1995.

114. Thompson V, Durrie DS, Cavanaugh TB. Philosophy and technique for excimer laser phototherapeutic keratectomy. Review. Refract Corneal Surg. 1993;9(2 Suppl):81–5.

115. Azar DT, Jain S, Woods R, et al. Phototherapeutic keratectomy: the VISX experience. In: Salz JJ, McDonnell PJ, McDonald MB, eds. Corneal laser surgery. St Louis: Mosby; 1995:213–26.

116. Vrabec MP, Anderson JA, Rock ME, et al. Electron microscopic findings in a cornea with recurrence of herpes simplex keratitis after excimer laser phototherapeutic keratectomy. CLAO J. 1994;20:41–4.

117. Azar DT, Jain S, Stark W. Phototherapeutic keratectomy. In: Azar DT (ed). Refractive surgery. Stamford, CT: Appleton & Lange; 1996:503–4.

118. Machat JJ. PRK retreatment techniques and results. In: Machat JJ. Excimer laser refractive surgery: practice and principles. Thorofare, NJ: Slack; 1996:215–33.

119. Gibralter R, Trokel SL. Correction of irregular astigmatism with the excimer laser. Ophthalmology. 1994;101:1310–15.

120. Azar DT, Yeh PC. Corneal topographic evaluation of decentration in photorefractive keratectomy: treatment displacement vs. intraoperative drift. Am J Ophthalmol. 1997;124:312–20.

121. Azar DT, Jain S, Stark W. Phototherapeutic keratectomy. In: Azar DT. Refractive surgery. Stamford, Conn: Appleton & Lange; 1997:501–17.

122. Talamo JH, Wagoner MD, Lee SL. Management of ablation decentration following excimer photorefractive keratectomy. Arch Ophthalmol. 1995;113:706–7.

123. Azar DT, Stark WJ, Steinert RF. Surgical management of PRK complications. In: Azar DT, Steinert RF, Stark WJ, eds. Excimer laser phototherapeutic keratectomy. Baltimore: William & Wilkins; 1997:169–72.

124. Azar DT, Talamo JH, Helena MC, et al. PTK: Indications, surgical techniques, postoperative care, and complications management. In: Talamo JH, Krueger RR, eds. The excimer manual: a clinician's guide to excimer laser surgery. Boston: Little, Brown; 1997:173–98.

125. McRae SM, Krueger RR, Applegate RA. Customized corneal ablation. The quest for supervision. Wavefront standards. Optical Society of America. Thorofare, NJ: Slack; 2000:347–62.

126. Roberts C, Dupps WJ. Corneal biomechanics and their role in corneal ablative procedures. In: McRae SM, Krueger RR, Applegate RA. Customized corneal ablation. The quest for supervision. Wavefront standards. Optical Society of America. Thorofare, NJ: Slack; 2000:347–62.

127. Gatinel D, Hoang-Xuan T, Azar DT. Determination of corneal asphericity after myopic surgery with the excimer laser: a mathematical model. Invest Ophthalmol Vis Sci. 2001;42:1736–42.

128. Salz JJ, Maguen E, Macy JI, et al. One-year results of excimer laser photorefractive keratectomy for myopia. Refract Corneal Surg. 1992;8:270–3.

129. Gaster RN, Binder PS, Coalwell K, et al. Corneal surface ablation by 193 nm excimer laser and wound healing in rabbits. Invest Ophthalmol Vis Sci. 1989;30:90–7.

130. Sanders D. Clinical evaluation of phototherapeutic keratectomy—VISX Twenty/Twenty excimer laser. Submitted to the FDA; 1994. Written Communication 2/7/94.

131. Sher NA, Bowers RA, Zabel RW, et al. Clinical use of 193-nm excimer laser in the treatment of corneal scars. Arch Ophthalmol. 1991;109:491–8.

132. Al-Rajhi AA, Wagoner MD, Badr IA, et al. Bacterial keratitis following phototherapeutic keratectomy. J Refract Surg. 1996;12:123–7.

133. Pepose JS, Laycock KA, Miller JK, et al. Reactivation of latent Herpes simplex virus by excimer laser photokeratectomy. Am J Ophthalmol. 1992;114:45–50.

134. Fagerholm P, Fitzsimmons TD, Orndahl M, et al. Phototherapeutic keratectomy: long-term results in 166 eyes. Refract Corneal Surg. 1993;9(2 Suppl):76–81.

135. McDonnell PJ, Moreira H, Clapham TN, et al. Photorefractive keratectomy for astigmatism. Arch Ophthalmol. 1991;109:1370–3.

136. Hersh PS, Jordan AJ, Mayers M. Corneal graft rejection episode after excimer laser phototherapeutic keratectomy. Arch Ophthalmol. 1993;111:735–6.

137. Epstein RJ, Robin JB. Corneal graft rejection episode after excimer laser phototherapeutic keratectomy. Arch Ophthalmol. 1994;112:157.

138. Farrell RA. Corneal transparency. In: Albert DM, Jakobiec FA, eds. Principles and practice of ophthalmology: basic sciences. Philadelphia: WB Saunders; 1994:64–81.

139. Olsen BR, McCarthy MT. Molecular structure of the sclera, cornea, and vitreous body. In: Albert DM, Jakobiec FA, eds. Principles and practice of ophthalmology: basic sciences. Philadelphia: WB Saunders; 1994:47–8.

140. Gordon M, Brint SF, Durrie DS, et al. Photorefractive keratectomy at 193 nm using an erodible mask. In: Parel JM, ed. Ophthalmic technologies II. Bellingham, WA: SPIE; 1992.

141. Campos M, Wang X, Hertzog LL, et al. Ablation rates and surface ultrastructure of 193 nm excimer laser keratectomies. Invest Ophthalmol Vis Sci. 1993;34:2493–500.

142. Majmudar PA, Forstot SL, Dennis RF, et al. Topical mitomycin C for subepithelial fibrosis after refractive corneal surgery. Ophthalmology. 2000;107:89–94.

143. Azar DT, Jain S. Topical MMC for subepithelial fibrosis after refractive corneal surgery. Ophthalmology. 2001;108:239–40.

144. Jain S, McCally RL, Connolly PJ, Azar DT. Mitomycin C reduces corneal light scattering after excimer keratectomy. Cornea. 2001;20:45–9.

145. Fountain TR, De la Cruz Z, Green WR, et al. Reassembly of corneal epithelial adhesion structures after excimer laser keratectomy in humans. Arch Ophthalmol. 1994;112:967–72.

146. Fantes FE, Hanna KD, Waring GO, et al. Wound healing after excimer laser keratomileusis (photorefractive keratectomy) in monkeys. Arch Ophthalmol. 1990;108:665–75.

147. Tuft SJ, Zabel RW, Marshall J. Corneal repair following keratectomy. Invest Ophthalmol Vis Sci. 1989;30:1769–77.

148. Courant D, Fritsch P, Azema A, et al. Corneal wound healing after photo-keratomileusis treatment on the primate eye. Lasers Light Ophthalmol. 1990;3:189–95.

149. Bende T, Seiler T, Wollensak J. Side effects in excimer corneal surgery: corneal thermal gradients. Graefes Arch Clin Exp Ophthalmol. 1988;226:277–80.

150. Ozler SA, Liaw LL, Neev J, et al. Acute ultrastructural changes of cornea after excimer laser ablation. Invest Ophthalmol Vis Sci. 1992;33:540–6.

151. Ashraf F, Azar D, Odrich M. Clinical results of PTK using the VISX excimer laser. In: Azar DT, Steinert RF, Stark WJ, eds. Excimer laser phototherapeutic keratectomy. Baltimore: William & Wilkins; 1997:169–72.

152. Steinert RF. Clinical results with the Summit Technology excimer laser. In: Azar DT, Steinert RF, Stark WJ, eds. Excimer laser phototherapeutic keratectomy. Baltimore: William & Wilkins; 1997:155–66.

CHAPTER

64

Episcleritis, Scleritis, and Other Scleral Disorders

DEBRA A. GOLDSTEIN • HOWARD H. TESSLER

Episcleritis

DEFINITION
• Inflammation of the connective tissue between the sclera and conjunctiva.

KEY FEATURES
• Self-limited condition.
• Less pain than with scleritis.
• Blanches with topical neosynephrine.

ASSOCIATED FEATURES
• Underlying blepharitis.
• Systemic association in about a third of patients.

Scleritis

DEFINITION
• A rare disorder of inflammation and necrosis centered within the sclera.

KEY FEATURES
• Focal or diffuse redness or violaceous discoloration.
• Scleral thickening.
• Nodules.
• Necrosis.
• Pain.

ASSOCIATED FEATURES
• Keratitis and iritis.
• Glaucoma.
• Exudative retinal detachment.
• Systemic association in about half the patients.

INTRODUCTION

The sclera is a dense, poorly vascularized connective tissue structure composed of types I, III, IV, V, VI, and VIII collagen, as well as elastin, proteoglycans, and glycoproteins. It is embryologically derived from neural crest and mesoderm.

The sclera may be affected by a number of inflammatory and noninflammatory processes. In this chapter some scleral anomalies are outlined, but the focus is on the more frequently seen and clinically important inflammatory conditions—episcleritis and scleritis.

INFLAMMATORY DISEASES

EPISCLERITIS

Epidemiology and Pathogenesis

Episcleritis refers to inflammation of the loose connective tissue between the sclera and the conjunctiva; it is a much more benign condition than scleritis. Patients with episcleritis may complain of discomfort or irritation rather than true pain, which is commonly present in scleritis. Slit-lamp examination usually localizes any edema to the area that overlies the sclera. The sclera itself is not thickened. An accompanying uveitis is very rare.

In contrast to scleritis, episcleritis is a self-limited condition. Untreated, it generally runs its course in a few days. Although recurrence is common, structural damage of the eye does not occur.

Diagnosis and Ocular Manifestations

Episcleritis can be described as simple, in which all or part of the episclera is diffusely inflamed, or nodular, in which inflammation is confined to a localized area with the presence of a well-defined red nodule. The nodule can be differentiated from a conjunctival nodule, such as a phlyctenule, because the nodule of episcleritis is not mobile with the conjunctiva. Nodular episcleritis is often associated with more discomfort and a more prolonged course than is simple episcleritis. Typically, topical phenylephrine blanches overlying conjunctival vessels and inflamed episcleral vessels.

Differential Diagnosis

The differential diagnosis includes conjunctivitis, which is more superficial, and scleritis, which is deeper.

Systemic Associations

An underlying cause for episcleritis is found in one third of cases. In one large series of 94 patients who had episcleritis, 68% were found to have no associated disease, 13% had a connective tissue or vasculitic disease, 7% had rosacea, and 7% had atopy. Herpes zoster, herpes simplex, chemical injury, and gout were believed to be responsible in one case each.[1]

Treatment

Episcleritis does not always require treatment. However, certain patients may require treatment for cosmesis or for the alleviation of discomfort. Many physicians elect to treat with topical corticosteroids, as these were demonstrated in a randomized double-blind trial to be superior to placebo for the treatment of episcleritis.[2] It also has been suggested, however, that the use of topical corticosteroids may be detrimental, with significant rebound inflammation when corticosteroids are tapered.[1] Some patients with episcleritis respond well to topical nonsteroidal anti-inflammatory drugs (NSAIDs). Systemic NSAIDs also may be used for the treatment of severe or recurrent episcleritis, although significant side effects may be associated with their use (see the section on scleritis). Treatment of underlying blepharitis is important.

SCLERITIS

Epidemiology and Pathogenesis

Scleritis is a rare condition—most ophthalmologists see only one or two new patients with this condition each year. Scleritis is associated with different systemic diseases than is uveitis, so the evaluation and treatment of these patients differ. Most scleral inflammation is noninfectious. However, scleral infection by bacterial or fungal organisms, such as *Pseudomonas* or *Aspergillus*, may cause a severe scleritis that is difficult to treat. On rare occasions, tuberculosis may be the cause of scleral nodules.[3]

Histopathology may show granulomatous or nongranulomatous inflammation, vasculitis, and scleral necrosis.[1] Antigen-antibody complexes appear to play a role in many cases of scleritis, although T cells have been implicated in some cases of posterior scleritis.[4-6] Of patients who have scleritis, 50% appear to

have no underlying systemic disease. In the other 50%, an underlying systemic disorder, usually a connective tissue disease, is present.

Ocular Manifestations

Scleritis may be unilateral, simultaneously bilateral, or alternate from eye to eye. The duration of inflammation is variable—active inflammation may last only a few months or persist for years.

In cases of scleritis, the eye is often red, but because the inflammation is in deeper tissues, the discoloration may appear violaceous (Fig. 64-1). The whole eye may be involved, or the inflammation may be limited to one or more quadrants. The eye is usually tender to palpation in the involved area, although pain may occur even in seemingly uninvolved areas. The pain typically is deep and boring in nature and often wakes the patient from sleep. It is important to assess the whole eye by turning on the examination room lights and lifting the eyelids. This provides a global view of the eyes, which can be missed in a darkened room at the slit lamp.

On slit-lamp examination, the overlying conjunctival vessels are usually found to be engorged. The episclera may also be edematous and inflamed. Episcleral vessels are often domed up by thickened sclera. At times, the secondary inflammation in the conjunctiva and episclera makes it difficult to determine whether there is underlying scleral inflammation. Topical phenylephrine 2.5% or 10% blanches the overlying conjunctiva and, to a much lesser extent, the episclera. This may permit better delineation of the depth of inflammation. The red-free (green) light on the slit lamp may also be used to clear overlying haze and better determine the level of inflammation.

Anterior scleritis is usually classified as diffuse or nodular. It also may be necrotizing or non-necrotizing. Necrotizing scleritis usually is extremely painful and presents with areas of avascularity in the sclera. Avascular areas may slough to leave scleral thinning, which can progress to staphyloma formation and exposure of bare uvea (Fig. 64-2).

Scleromalacia perforans is a type of painless necrotizing scleritis that typically occurs in women with a long-standing history of rheumatoid arthritis. In these cases, yellow scleral nodules develop without much redness or pain. These nodules, which are histopathologically very similar to rheumatoid nodules, may necrose and slough to leave defects in the sclera[7] (Fig. 64-3).

The term *posterior scleritis* refers to inflammation behind the equator of the globe. If anterior scleritis is also present, the di-

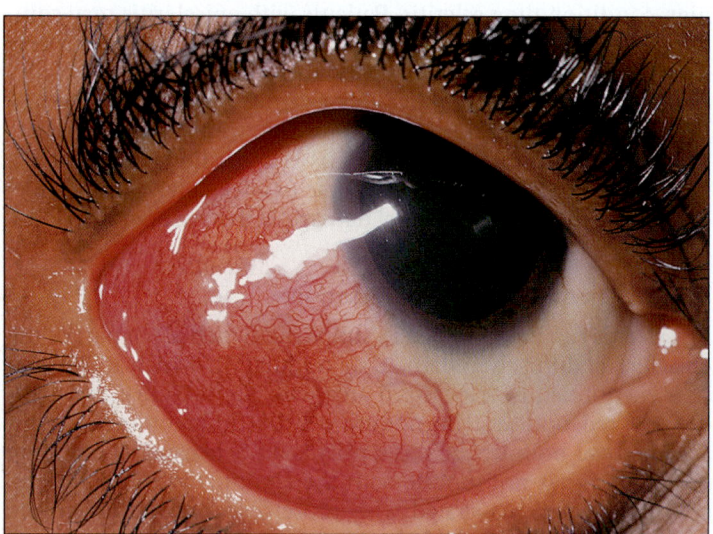

FIG. 64-1 ■ Diffuse scleritis with a violaceous hue due to deep inflammation. Vessels do not blanch with topical phenylephrine.

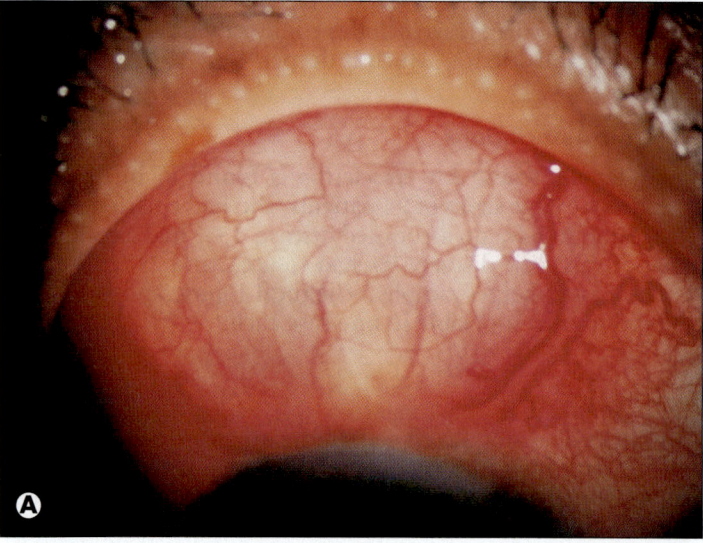
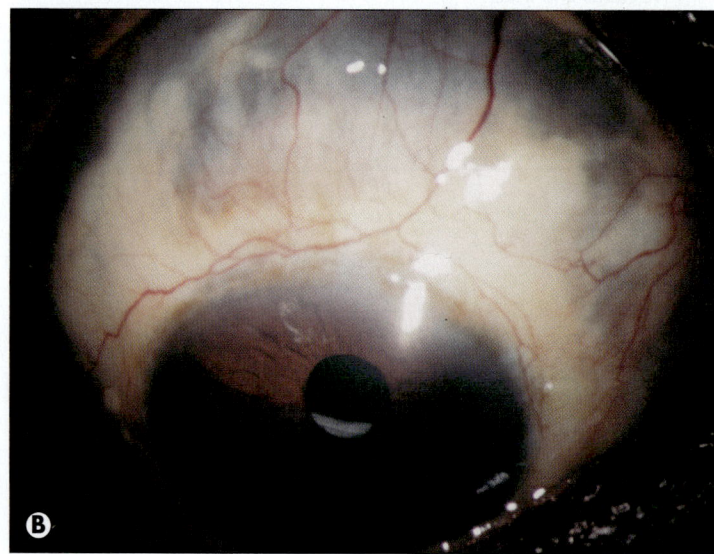

FIG. 64-2 ■ **Large scleral nodule. A,** Seventy-year-old woman with large scleral nodule of undetermined etiology; note the yellow area, which probably represents scleral necrosis. **B,** Same patient 6 months later after completing a 3-month course of chlorambucil; note the lack of activity, coupled with marked scleral thinning and transparency, which allows dark uvea to show through.

agnosis is not difficult. However, in the case of purely posterior scleritis with a quiet anterior segment, the diagnosis is often missed. Symptoms of posterior scleritis may include pain, blurred vision, and photophobia, although the patient also may be fairly asymptomatic. Some patients who have posterior scleritis develop proptosis, shallowing of the anterior chamber, exudative retinal detachments, choroidal detachments, disc swelling, and chorioretinal changes. Chorioretinal changes may consist of subretinal exudates and hemorrhages, as well as a stippled appearance to the retinal pigment epithelium in long-standing disease (Fig. 64-4).

Scleritis frequently is associated with a secondary uveitis—either iritis or choroiditis. The ophthalmologist must therefore carry out a thorough examination of the sclera in any patient who has anterior segment inflammation to avoid misdiagnosing a case of scleritis as endogenous anterior uveitis. Patients who have sclerouveitis may develop keratic precipitates, posterior synechiae, and, if posterior scleritis is present, exudative retinal changes, hemorrhage, and retinal pigmentary changes.

Scleral inflammation may cause structural damage to the eye. Scleral translucency and thinning regularly occur (see Fig. 64-2).

Scleritis adjacent to the cornea may be associated with a focal or diffuse keratitis. Focal keratitis may manifest as a ring infiltrate at the limbus, without the peripheral clear zone that is seen with staphylococcal marginal infiltrates (Fig. 64-5). Sclerokeratitis also may present with crystalline deposits that have the appearance of spun sugar or cotton candy in the deep cornea. This variant is known as sclerosing keratitis[7] (Fig. 64-6).

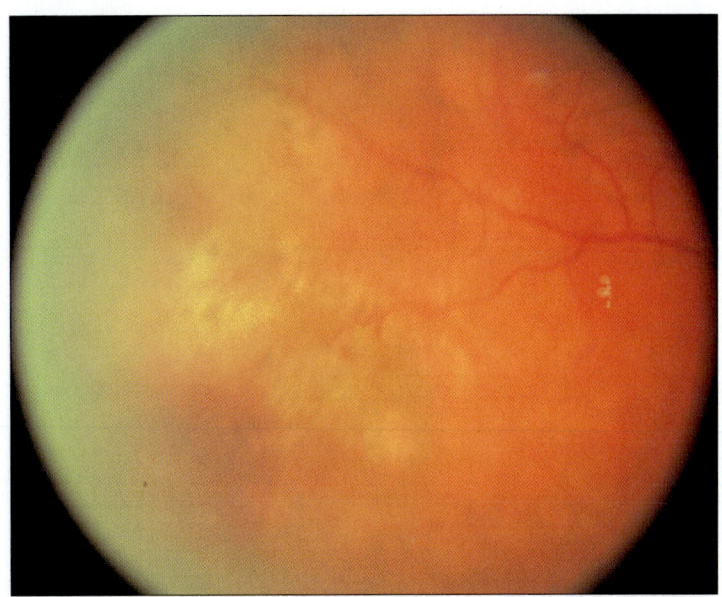

FIG. 64-4 ▮ Subretinal hemorrhage and exudate in a patient who has necrotizing scleritis.

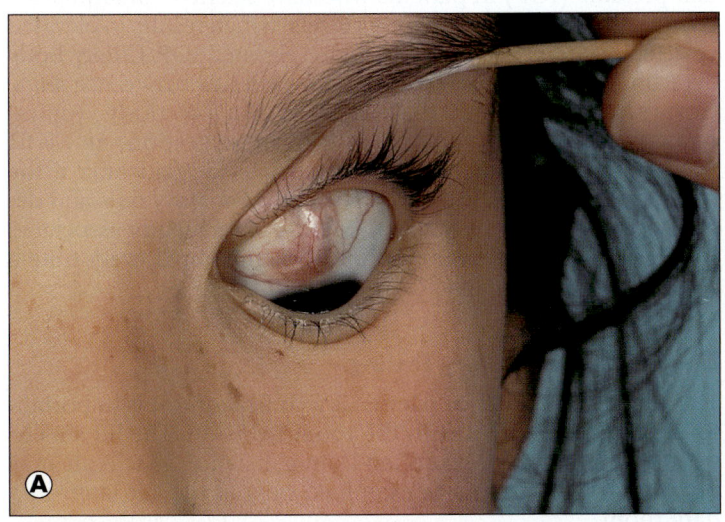

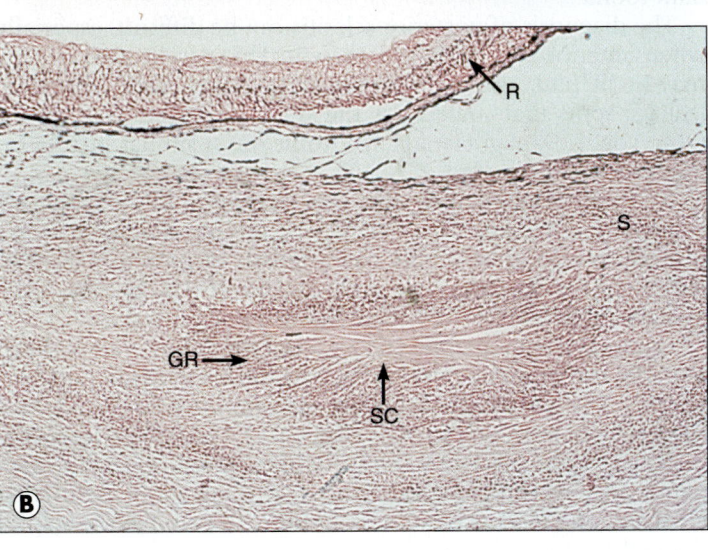

FIG. 64-3 ▮ Nodular scleritis. A, Twelve-year-old girl with nodular scleritis of undetermined cause. B, Histological section of another case shows a zonal granulomatous reaction (GR) around necrotic scleral collagen (SC). R, Retina; S, sclera. (Presented by Dr. I. W. McLean to the AFIP Alumni, 1973.)

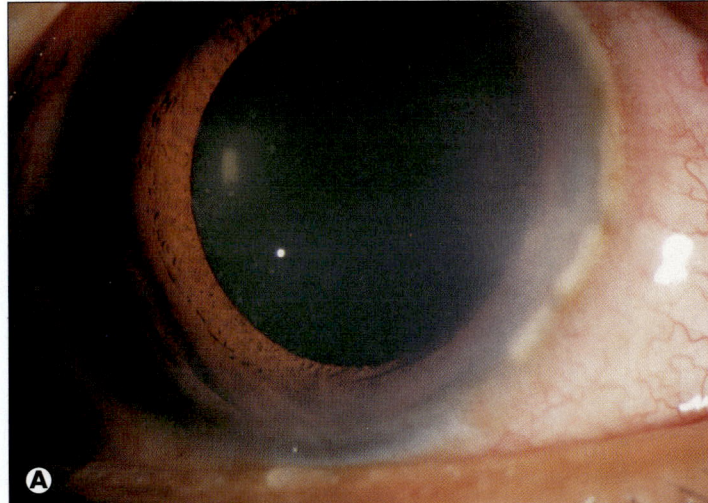

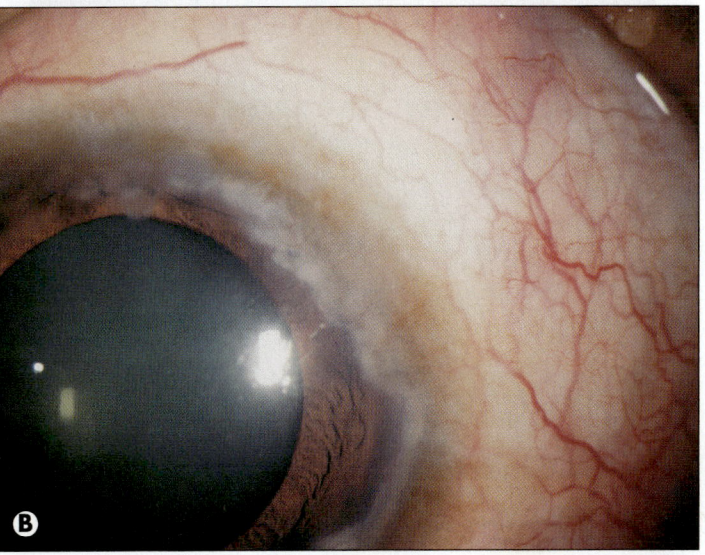

FIG. 64-5 ▮ Ring corneal ulcer in a patient with rheumatoid arthritis and scleritis. A, Note the white, creamy infiltrate in the cornea, indicating active inflammation, and the lack of a lucid interval from the limbus to the ulcer. B, Other eye of the same patient. Note the scarring and vascularization from a previous active ring ulcer.

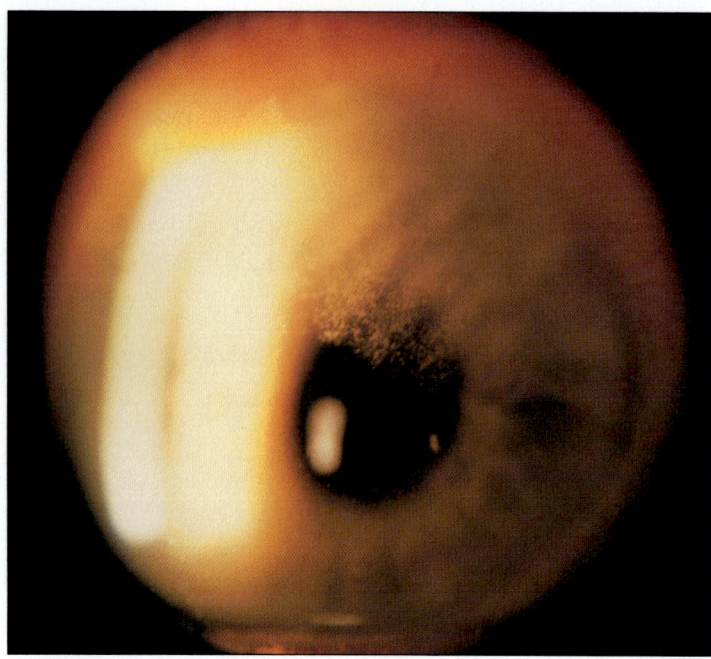

FIG. 64-6 ▮ Inactive sclerokeratitis in a patient who has ulcerative colitis. White dotlike lesions in the pre-Descemet's stroma are crystalline in appearance, resembling spun sugar. They may represent immunoglobulin deposits.

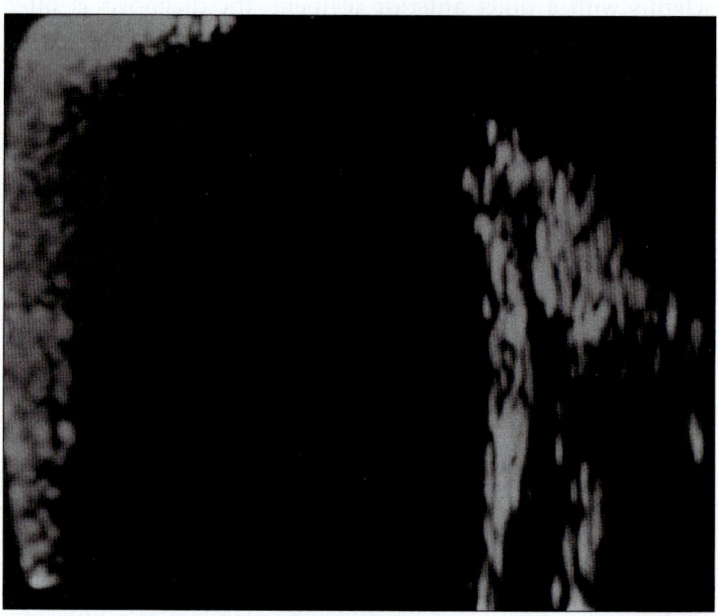

FIG. 64-8 ▮ B-scan ultrasonography showing the dark area behind Tenon's capsule. This forms the "T-sign" with the dark optic nerve pattern, which is believed to be due to fluid in Tenon's capsule and is very characteristic of posterior scleritis, but it is not always present.

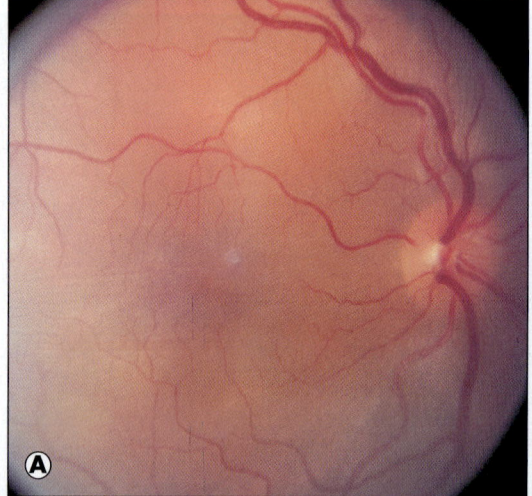

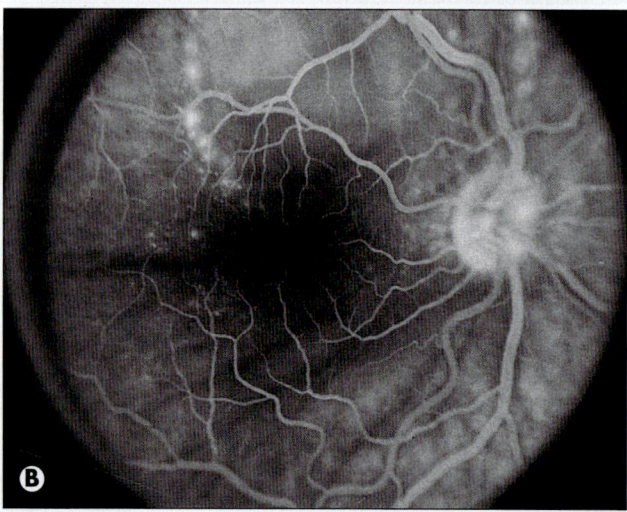

FIG. 64-7 ▮ Fluorescein angiography. A, Exudative retinal detachment and choroidal folds in posterior scleritis. B, The same eye shows choroidal folds and areas of subretinal leakage, which increase in intensity in the late phases of the angiogram. Only Vogt-Koyanagi-Harada syndrome and posterior scleritis exhibit this subretinal leakage pattern. Many patients with posterior scleritis do not have this leakage pattern, however.

A number of mechanisms may result in elevation of intraocular pressure (IOP) in patients who have scleritis. Inflammatory cells may block scleral emissary vessels, which results in elevated episcleral venous pressure and hence elevated IOP. Ciliary body detachment adjacent to areas of active scleritis may cause angle closure as the lens–iris diaphragm rotates anteriorly. Topical corticosteroids also may induce an elevation in IOP. Accompanying uveitis may be responsible for glaucoma if the trabecular meshwork is clogged with inflammatory cells and debris. Whatever the mechanism, scleritis is frequently associated with secondary glaucoma. IOP must be measured every time a scleritis patient is evaluated.

Diagnosis and Ancillary Testing

The diagnosis of anterior scleritis is a clinical one. It is important to examine the patient with the room lights on. The lid should be lifted and the eyes examined from a distance, as scleritis may be missed if the patient is examined only at the slit lamp in a dark room.

The diagnosis of posterior scleritis can be difficult, especially when anterior scleritis is not present. Fluorescein angiography may be helpful, as it may demonstrate characteristic subretinal leakage spots that coalesce as the study progresses (Fig. 64-7). Only Vogt-Koyanagi-Harada syndrome has a similar picture on fluorescein angiogram.[8]

B-scan ultrasonography also may be helpful in the diagnosis of posterior scleritis. The T-sign, representing fluid in Tenon's capsule, is said to be highly characteristic of posterior scleritis, although it is not always present (Fig. 64-8). Thickening of the posterior sclera can usually be demonstrated on B-scan.[9]

Computed tomography (CT) scan of the orbits with contrast material can be very helpful in making the diagnosis of posterior scleritis. The so-called ring sign of enhancement of the sclera is suggestive of posterior scleritis (Fig. 64-9). However, scleritis patients can have negative CT scans with contrast. Magnetic resonance imaging (MRI) has not proved to be any more useful than CT scans, and evidence exists that MRI may even be less helpful than CT.[10]

The work-up of a patient with active scleritis includes an evaluation for evidence of vasculitis, connective tissue disease, and infection. Much of this information can be gained from a detailed

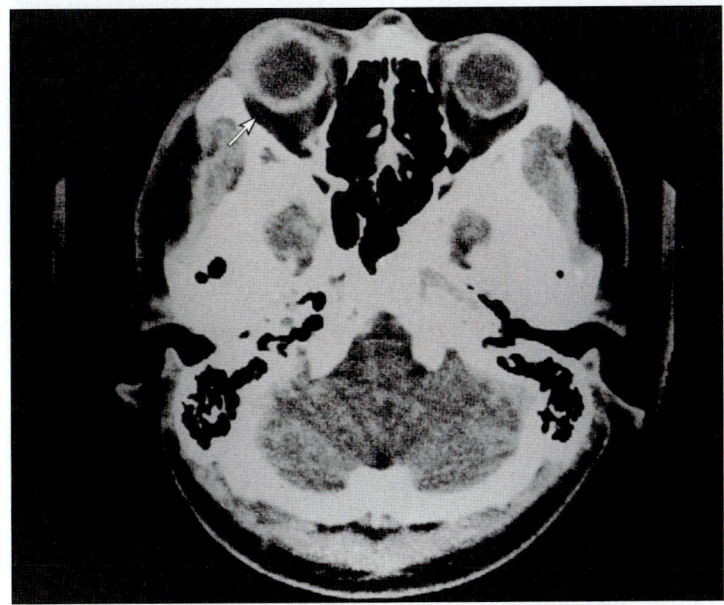

FIG. 64-9 ■ Computed tomography scan of orbits with infusion in a patient with posterior scleritis. On the right *(arrow),* the ring sign, due to the concentration of contrast material in the sclera, is present.

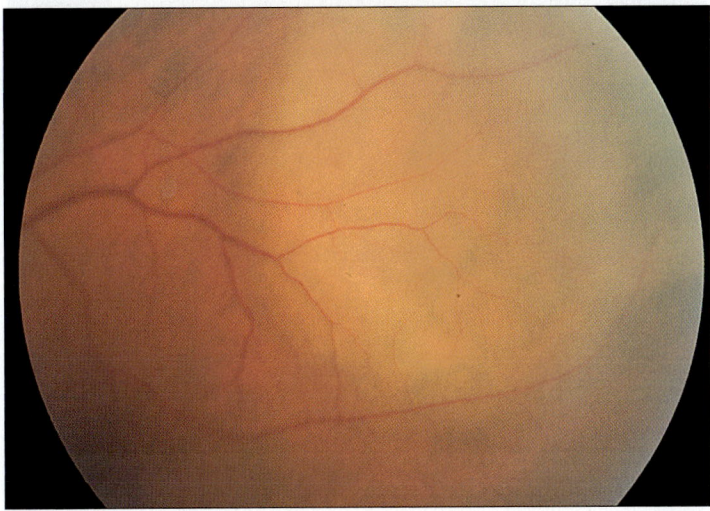

FIG. 64-10 ■ Subretinal mass mimicking an amelanotic melanoma in a patient who has scleritis. In this patient, the mass disappeared with cyclophosphamide therapy.

history. Appropriate laboratory tests might include erythrocyte sedimentation rate, rheumatoid factor, and antinuclear antibody to look for evidence of systemic connective tissue disease. A fluorescent treponemal antibody absorption (FTA-ABS) test, MHA-TP (microhemagglutination test for *Treponema pallidum*), or other specific serological test for syphilis should be done on all patients to rule out latent syphilis. A complete blood count and urinalysis may be considered. A chest radiograph may be obtained to look for evidence of tuberculosis, sarcoid, or Wegener's granulomatosis. An antineutrophil cytoplasmic antibody (ANCA) test should be carried out for all patients suspected of having vasculitic disease. It is often positive in cases of Wegener's granulomatosis, microscopic polyarteritis, and other related vasculitides.[11] Two different patterns of immunofluorescence staining have been identified. Classic ANCA (C-ANCA) produces a coarsely granular, centrally attenuated immunofluorescence, and perinuclear ANCA (P-ANCA) produces a perinuclear staining pattern. Of these, C-ANCA is more specific for Wegener's granulomatosis and other closely related vasculitides and is rarely positive in other patients, whereas P-ANCA is less specific and may be positive in patients who have inflammation of nonvasculitic cause. The positivity of this test may depend, in part, on disease activity; in some patients, the tests become negative with a decrease in disease activity.[12]

Differential Diagnosis

Other causes of red eyes must be considered in the differential diagnosis of scleritis. Conjunctivitis usually can be differentiated from scleritis by the presence of discharge, superficial inflammation that clears with topical phenylephrine, and the lack of severe aching or pain.

Episcleritis is the most challenging differential diagnosis in patients who have scleritis; differentiating features were discussed earlier.

The ciliary flush that accompanies acute iritis may be confused with scleritis. However, the ciliary flush usually is restricted to the area adjacent to the limbus, and iritis appears to be the predominant finding.

Solid-appearing subretinal masses that mimic melanomas can occur in patients who have scleritis (Fig. 64-10).[13,14] CT scanning may be helpful in making the diagnosis of scleritis in these cases, demonstrating a contrast-enhancing mass that is uniformly iso-

dense with sclera. A-scan ultrasonography usually demonstrates high internal reflectivity in scleritis (as opposed to low internal reflectivity in melanoma). A B-scan may demonstrate thickened sclera.

Systemic Associations

Underlying systemic disease is present in approximately 50% of patients with scleritis.[15] Rheumatoid arthritis is the most frequently associated condition.[16] Other connective tissue diseases that can present with scleritis include Wegener's granulomatosis, polyarteritis nodosa, systemic lupus erythematosus, and relapsing polychondritis (Fig. 64-11).

Psoriatic arthritis and ankylosing spondylitis, although usually associated with acute iritis, can at times be associated with scleritis.[16]

Inflammatory bowel disease, especially Crohn's disease, can be associated with scleritis[17] (Fig. 64-12). Patients who have inflammatory bowel disease, especially those that are HLA-B27 positive, also may develop both acute and chronic iridocyclitis. Scleritis is more often associated with inflammatory bowel disease when large joint peripheral arthritis occurs. Iritis is more often associated with inflammatory bowel disease when the patient also has ankylosing spondylitis.[17] Pyoderma gangrenosum and Cogan's syndrome also can be associated with scleritis.[18] Sarcoidosis can cause scleral granulomas.

Infectious conditions such as tuberculosis, syphilis, and leprosy have been reported to cause granulomas in the sclera. Herpes zoster and herpes simplex may also cause scleritis (Fig. 64-13). When herpesviruses cause scleritis, it is usually in the late recovery phase of the disease rather than during the acute infection.[15]

Necrotizing scleritis can be triggered by ocular surgery (Fig. 64-14); it has been reported weeks to months after cataract surgery, penetrating keratoplasty, muscle surgery, glaucoma surgery, and even pterygium surgery.[19–21] Evidence exists of underlying connective tissue disease in some of these patients, but in others, no causative factor can be found.

Pathology

The histopathology of scleritis appears to be similar whether or not a systemic autoimmune disease is present. Inflammatory cells are seen in the sclera. Nongranulomatous inflammation is

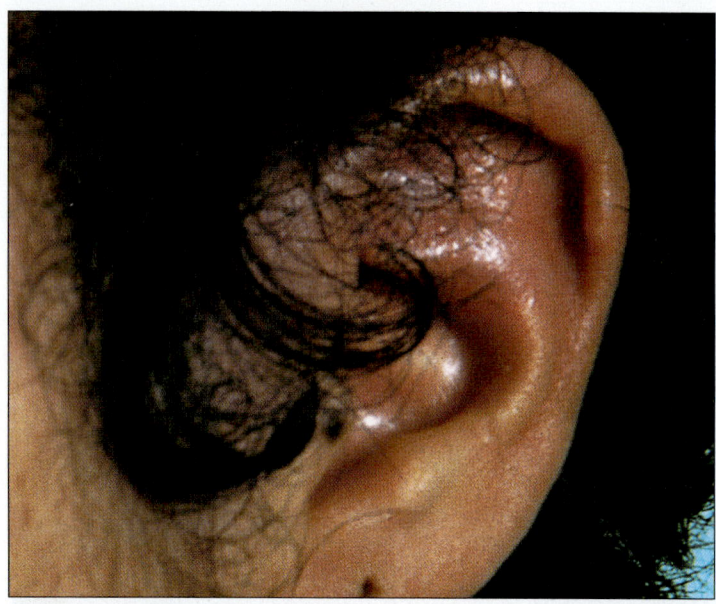

FIG. 64-11 ■ Patients with relapsing polychondritis. Note inflammation of the superior half of the pinna.

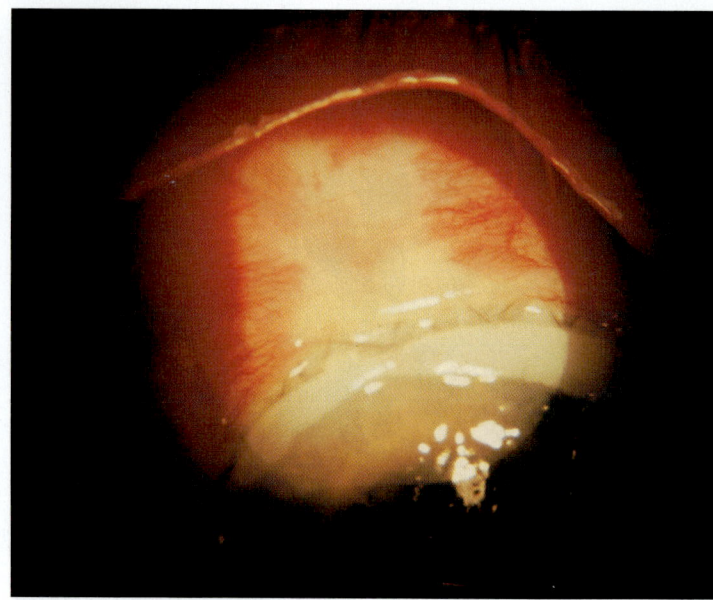

FIG. 64-13 ■ Necrotizing anterior scleritis secondary to herpes zoster. The patient underwent extracapsular cataract extraction 2 weeks earlier, which precipitated ophthalmic zoster and led to anterior segment necrosis.

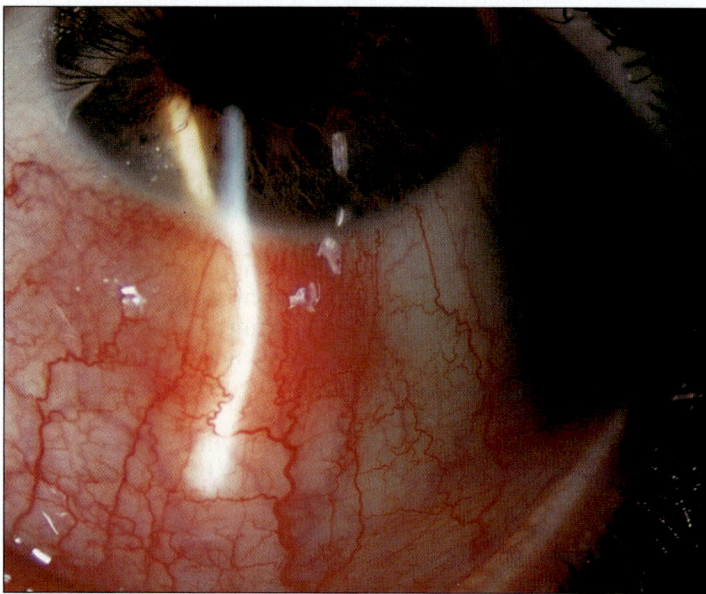

FIG. 64-12 ■ Nodular scleritis in patient who has Crohn's disease.

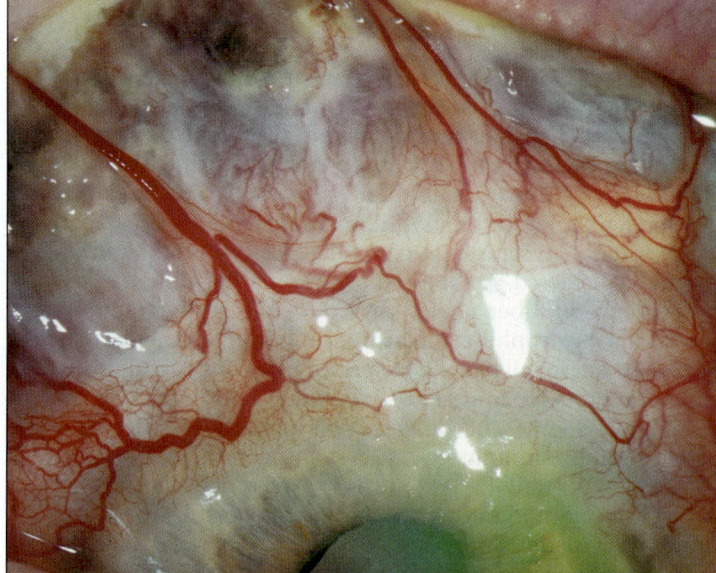

FIG. 64-14 ■ Necrotizing scleritis induced by trabeculectomy surgery. Note the large conjunctival vessels seen in this 75-year-old woman; these are frequently seen after severe scleritis.

composed primarily of mononuclear cells, including lymphocytes, plasma cells, and macrophages. Granulomatous inflammation is characterized by the presence of epithelioid cells, which may coalesce to form multinucleated giant cells. In necrotizing scleritis, one sees eosinophilic fibrinoid material, often in the center of a granuloma.

Scleral biopsy should be done only in exceptional circumstances. The surgeon should be prepared to either place a scleral reinforcement graft or use some other tissue, such as periosteum, to replace the sclera that is biopsied, as severe thinning of the sclera can result in an unexpected encounter with intraocular contents.

Treatment

MEDICAL TREATMENT. Most patients who have active scleritis require therapy. Some controversy exists in the literature as to what constitutes active disease that requires treatment. Certainly,

patients who have pain and marked redness require therapy to alleviate the pain and prevent structural damage to the eye. Some physicians recommend that treatment be continued until all redness is gone from the eye. However, if there is no pain and no evidence of any damage to the eye, the side effects of the therapy may outweigh the benefits. Patients who have mild redness, no active secondary uveitis or keratitis, and no visual problems may not require therapy.

Topical nonsteroidal agents may be of some benefit in patients who have mild episcleritis, but they are of minimal or no benefit in true scleritis. Topical corticosteroids seldom have any marked beneficial anti-inflammatory effect in cases of true scleritis, although they may be helpful in controlling secondary uveitis.

Oral NSAIDs should be considered the first line of treatment in patients who have mild and moderately severe scleritis. Indomethacin 50mg three times a day or, in the sustained-release form, 75mg twice a day can be very effective. Another nonsteroidal agent that appears to work well is piroxicam 20mg daily. Ibuprofen, naproxen, tolmetin, sulindac, and others may be of benefit.

All these nonsteroidal agents carry the risk of significant side effects. Allergic reactions, gastrointestinal problems, and kidney damage from long-term therapy can all occur. Patients who take NSAIDs may require other medications to prevent or treat gastrointestinal side effects. Options include histamine H_2 receptor antagonists (e.g., ranitidine, famotidine, cimetidine), agents that coat the ulcer site (e.g., sucralfate), gastric acid secretion inhibitors (e.g., the synthetic prostaglandin E_1 analog misoprostol), and proton pump inhibitors (e.g., omeprazole). The NSAIDs that are selective COX-2 inhibitors, such as refecoxib and celecoxib, may have fewer gastrointestinal side effects but appear to be less potent anti-inflammatory agents.

Corticosteroids are usually required for patients who have moderately severe to severe scleritis. The usual starting dose is 1mg/kg/day of prednisone, but in severe cases, doses up to 1.5mg/kg/day may be required. The prednisone is then slowly tapered to a best-tolerated dose. Some patients require daily prednisone for 6 months to a year or longer. Adrenal suppression can be reduced with an every-other-day dosing regimen. Occasionally, patients who take their full dose of oral prednisone in the morning experience pain at night. If the dose is divided and taken twice a day, this night pain may be relieved without increasing the total dose.

Pulse intravenous methylprednisolone at 0.5–1g may be required in some patients who have severe scleritis. This high dose may be used once a day for 3 days or once every other day for 3 days and then reduced to once a week. Oral prednisone is usually required to supplement the pulses.[22]

All systemic corticosteroids may result in adrenal suppression, weight gain, mood changes, blood pressure elevation, blood sugar elevation, osteoporosis, and aseptic necrosis of the femoral head. Any patient who is on oral prednisone for longer than 1 year, even on an every-other-day schedule, should have a bone density evaluation.

Subconjunctival injection has been proposed as a method of corticosteroid delivery in cases of non-necrotizing anterior scleritis.[23] Although this treatment has been found to be safe and effective in selected cases, it must not be performed if there is any suggestion of scleral thinning or in lieu of systemic therapy in sight- or life-threatening disease. Its use, as the study authors suggest, should probably be limited to adjunctive therapy in select cases of non-necrotizing localized disease.

Immunosuppressive drugs can be vision saving and even life-saving in patients who have scleritis who are unresponsive to or intolerant of prednisone (Fig. 64-15). The morbidity and mortality of patients who have severe rheumatoid arthritis and Wegener's granulomatosis are reduced with the use of immunosuppressive agents.[24] Many patients who have necrotizing scleritis require immunosuppressive therapy to preserve vision. Immunosuppressives also may be required in patients who develop corticosteroid toxicity or who have been on prednisone for more than 3–6 months. Evidence exists that many immunosuppressives may have less long-term toxicity than high- or moderate-dose prednisone.[25]

Low-dose methotrexate (7.5–15mg weekly) has been reported to be of benefit in reducing or eliminating the need for prednisone.[26] Azathioprine at a dose of 1.5–2mg/kg/day also may reduce or eliminate the need for corticosteroids.[3] However, both these agents can result in hepatic and hematological toxicity. These drugs may be used alone but are more often used in combination with corticosteroids. Mycophenolate mofetil is in the same family as azathioprine but may have lower toxicity and higher efficacy. There are few or no data on its use in scleritis. Alkylating agents, such as chlorambucil and cyclophosphamide, also may be of benefit[27] and usually enable oral prednisone to be tapered or discontinued. In many cases, a 3–6-month course of chlorambucil, with reduction of the white blood cell count to

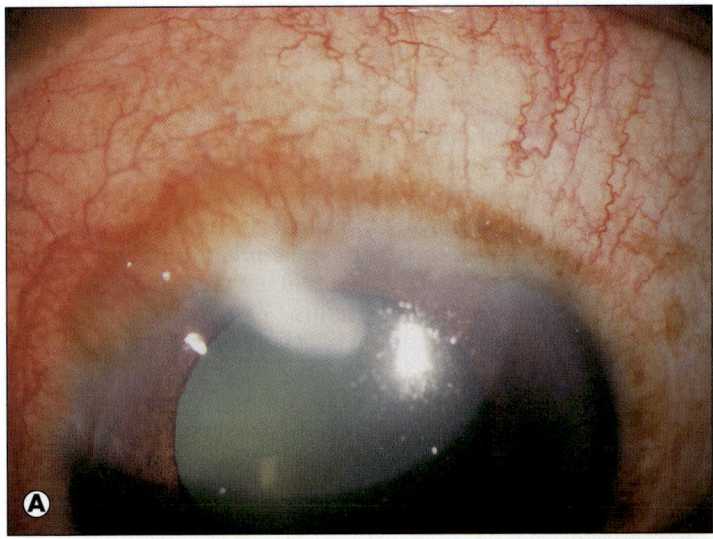
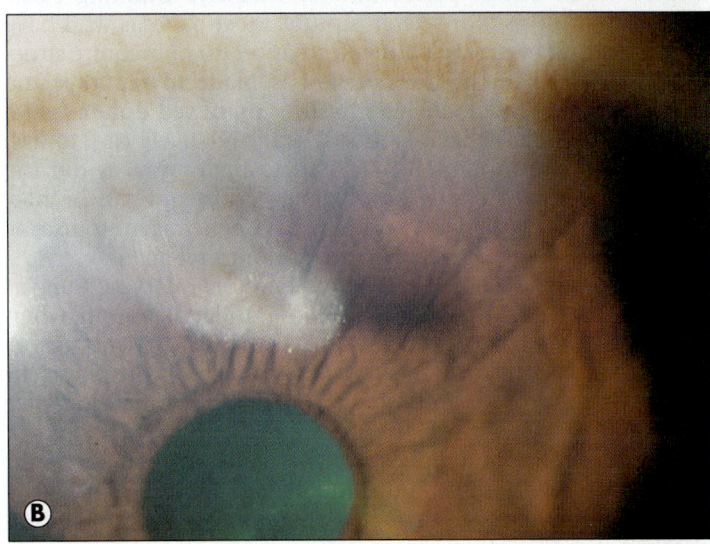

FIG. 64-15 ■ Necrotizing sclerokeratitis secondary to rheumatoid arthritis. **A**, Sixty-year-old man with necrotizing sclerokeratitis secondary to rheumatoid arthritis. **B**, Same patient 6 months later while on cyclophosphamide. Note the scar in the cornea but the lack of scleral inflammation and corneal infiltration. The patient still required cyclophosphamide to keep inflammation in check 1 year after these photographs were taken.

2400–3500, causes prolonged remission of ocular inflammatory disease.[28,29] Alkylating agents do not cause hepatic problems but do have hematological toxicity. Blood counts must be monitored frequently. Cyclophosphamide has the added risk of hemorrhagic cystitis, so adequate hydration is imperative. Cyclophosphamide works more rapidly (frequently within a few days to a week) than does chlorambucil, which has a slower onset. Cyclophosphamide given once a week or once a month may be less toxic than daily oral cyclophosphamide, although it may be less effective. Pulse intravenous cyclophosphamide also has been used in severe sight- or life-threatening disease. Because prolonged use may increase the risk of late malignancy and sterility, informed consent should be obtained before starting therapy with an immunosuppressive agent. Women must be advised that pregnancy must be avoided, as these agents may be teratogenic.

Cyclosporine, which acts, at least in part, by interfering with interleukin-2, has been used with some success in the treatment of scleritis.[30] At doses of 10mg/kg/day it is nephrotoxic, so it is almost always used at lower doses, such as 5mg/kg/day as an initial dose, and 3–5mg/kg/day as a maintenance dose. However, at these doses it may be impossible to discontinue the use of corticosteroids, so the main use has been as adjunctive therapy, permitting the use of lower doses of systemic corticosteroids.[30,31] Systemic hypertension, renal failure, hirsutism, and gingival hyperplasia all may occur with cyclosporine. Because cyclosporine is not associated with the development of sterility, it may be an attractive agent to use in young patients. Again, the risk of developing late malignancy is much lower with cyclosporine than with other immunosuppressive agents. Tacrolimus (FK-506) has a different structure than cyclosporine but similar intracellular actions. There are no data on its efficacy in scleritis, but it has been shown to be useful in the treatment of a number of types of uveitis. Tumor necrosis factor inhibitors such as etanercept and infliximab are used to treat diseases associated with scleritis, such as rheumatoid arthritis and Crohn's disease. There are no current data, but these drugs may be of benefit in the long-term control of scleritis.

Anecdotal reports suggest that plasmapheresis may be of benefit in patients who have scleritis. However, it is immune stimulating, so the concomitant use of an immunosuppressive agent is required. Radiation therapy may be used in a subset of patients who have posterior scleritis that represents a form of orbital pseudotumor.

SURGICAL TREATMENT. Surgery for scleritis may be performed when scleral perforation or extensive thinning exists with significant risk for scleral rupture. Most patients who have thin sclera and even staphyloma formation do not require structural reinforcement. If the decision is made to reinforce the sclera, available agents include fresh or preserved donor sclera, periosteum, or fascia lata. Donor sclera is relatively easy to use, but after several months it may start to melt away, as did the originally diseased tissue. Autologous periosteum can be harvested from the tibial crest and may be a better agent to use, as it may be less likely to necrose than is donor sclera.[32]

Many patients who have scleritis develop cataracts. Surgery for cataracts in such patients should be undertaken only when the disease has been in remission for at least 2–3 months. A small incision clear corneal extraction is preferred. The physician should be alert for a recrudescence of scleral inflammation after surgery.

Again, it must be emphasized that glaucoma can occur in scleritis patients, both from the underlying disease and from the corticosteroids used to treat it. Patients must have their IOP checked at each visit, and any pressure rises must be handled appropriately. Often a decrease in the frequency or potency of corticosteroid drops is enough to reduce the pressure. If this is unsuccessful and the IOP remains high or evidence exists of glaucomatous damage, the IOP must be controlled with pharmacological agents or, rarely, surgery.

Course and Outcome

Most patients who have mild or moderate scleritis maintain excellent vision. The length of time during which scleritis is active varies from patient to patient. In a minority of patients, the disease is active for only a few months and then goes into long-term remission. In other patients, the disease is active for several years. In some patients, the disease seems to move from eye to eye or to move from one area of sclera to another.

Necrotizing scleritis portends a worse prognosis than does non-necrotizing disease. Patients who have necrotizing scleritis have a high incidence of visual loss[33] and a 21% 8-year mortality.[15] Immunosuppressive therapy appears to lessen these risks.

NONINFLAMMATORY DISEASES

Noninflammatory processes that affect the sclera are rarely encountered by the general ophthalmologist. They may be congenital or acquired and may reflect an underlying systemic disease. Noninflammatory processes that involve the sclera may be considered in two broad categories—those that thicken the sclera, and those that thin it. The former may do so via thickening of otherwise normal sclera, as in nanophthalmos; via deposits within the sclera, as in cystinosis or alkaptonuria; or via the formation of scleral masses, such as dermoid choristomas or squamous cell carcinomas. The sclera may be thinned in congenital disease, such as osteogenesis imperfecta, or in acquired disease, such as iron deficiency anemia.[1]

OSTEOGENESIS IMPERFECTA

Osteogenesis imperfecta is an inherited condition that involves the skeleton, ear, joints, teeth, skin, and eyes. Van der Hoeve in 1918 described the three main signs of osteogenesis imperfecta: blue sclera, deafness, and bone fractures.[34] Four clinical types occur, summarized in Table 64-1. The old terms *congenita* and *tarda* have been replaced.

The characteristic blue sclera is caused by thinness and transparency of the collagen fibers of the sclera that allow visualization of the underlying uvea. In types III and IV, the blue sclera fades with age, with the result that the sclera may have normal color by adolescence or adulthood.[35] Blue sclera can be an inherited trait in some families without evidence of bone fragility. Central corneal thickness has been found to be reduced in osteogenesis imperfecta. Keratoconus, megalocornea, and anterior embryotoxon also have been reported.

Other ocular manifestations sporadically reported include congenital glaucoma, zonular cataract, dislocated lens, choroidal sclerosis, and retinal and subhyaloid hemorrhage. Optic neuropathy and atrophy are due to compression by deformities and skull bone fractures.[36] The disease is due to abnormalities of the type I collagen gene.

NANOPHTHALMOS

Nanophthalmos refers to a bilateral inherited condition consisting of short axial length, normal-sized crystalline lens, and thick sclera. Nanophthalmos is usually autosomal recessive, but dominant cases have been reported.[37]

The axial length in nanophthalmos measures 14–20mm. Frequently, the visual acuity is good in youth, but the patients are very hyperopic (+10–+20D) and have been described as phakic patients who wear cataract glasses.[37] The abnormally thick sclera contains large collagen bundles and increased glycosaminoglycans.[38,39] Nanophthalmos has been reported in association with the mucopolysaccharidoses, fetal alcohol syndrome, myotonic dystrophy, and achondroplasia.[37,40]

Aging nanophthalmic sclera becomes less elastic and may result in increased resistance to venous outflow through the vortex veins and via trans-scleral fluid passage. This aging change can lead to choroidal congestion, choroidal thickening, and eventu-

TABLE 64-1

FOUR CLINICAL TYPES OF OSTEOGENESIS IMPERFECTA

Type	Inheritance	Dental Abnormalities	Deafness	Other	Blue Sclera
Type I	Autosomal dominant	±	Otosclerosis	–	+
Type II	Recessive or sporadic, dominant	+	Severe	Very severe, uniformly lethal	Dark blue, ++
Type III	Heterogeneous	Variable	Variable	Normal at birth	Variable
Type IV	Heterogeneous	Less severe	Less common	Less severe	Less common

ally choroidal effusion. Choroidal effusion may occur spontaneously or after sudden decompression of the eye at the time of intraocular surgery for cataract and glaucoma. Scleral resection (window) surgery or sclerotomy to drain suprachoroidal fluid can be effective therapy in these cases.[37] Because choroidal effusions can occur at the time of intraocular surgery, some authors recommend prophylactic sclerotomy before anterior segment surgery.[41]

Angle-closure glaucoma regularly occurs in nanophthalmic eyes because of the large lens in the small eye. Laser iridectomy and gonioplasty may be used to treat the angle closure.

CHORISTOMAS

Choristomas represent heterotopic rests of tissue and are present congenitally. They may involve episclera and, more rarely, sclera.

Epibulbar limbal dermoids are choristomas most frequently found in the inferotemporal quadrant near the limbus. Histopathologically, dermoids contain epidermal and mesodermal elements, often with keratin, hair follicles, and sebaceous glands. Clinically, they are usually yellowish white solid or cystic nodules that may be firm, rubbery, or soft in consistency and are usually mobile with conjunctival and subconjunctival tissue. Limbal dermoids may be associated with systemic abnormalities in up to 30% of cases, most commonly Goldenhar's syndrome.[42] Excision of limbal dermoids may be undertaken for relief of cosmetic deformity, ocular irritation, or decreased vision because of encroachment on the visual axis or the presence of significant regular or irregular astigmatism. One series of 10 epibulbar dermoids that were surgically removed showed a two-line improvement in visual acuity in 2 patients, with no significant change in acuity in 8 patients. All 10 patients had improvement in cosmesis, with no visually significant adverse effects.[43]

Episcleral osseous choristomas are usually located in the superotemporal quadrant and contain mature, compact bone with no epidermoid structures. In contrast to epibulbar dermoids, these lesions may be densely adherent to sclera and do not tend to be associated with systemic abnormalities.[44]

REFERENCES

1. Foster CS, Sainz de la Maza M. The sclera. New York: Springer-Verlag; 1994.
2. Lyons CJ, Hakin KN, Watson, PG. Topical flurbiprofen: an effective treatment for episcleritis? Eye. 1990;4:521–5.
3. Nanda M, Pflugfelder SC, Holland S. *Mycobacterium tuberculosis* scleritis. Am J Ophthalmol. 1989;108:736–7.
4. Rao NA, Marak GE, Hidayat AA. Necrotizing scleritis: a clinicopathologic study of 41 cases. Ophthalmology. 1985;92:1542–9.
5. Fong LP, Sainz de la Maza M, Rice BA, et al. Immunopathology of scleritis. Ophthalmology. 1991;98:472–9.
6. Bernauer W, Buchi ER, Daicker B. Immunopathological findings in posterior scleritis. Int Ophthalmol. 1995;18:229–31.
7. Watson PG, Hazleman BL. The sclera and systemic disorders. Philadelphia: WB Saunders; 1976.
8. Rabb MF, Jennings T. Fluorescein angiography and uveitis. In: Tasman W, Jaeger AE, eds. Duane's clinical ophthalmology, vol. 4. Philadelphia: Lippincott; 1995:4–5.
9. Benson WE. Posterior scleritis. Surv Ophthalmol. 1988;32(5):297–316.
10. Chaques VJ, Lam S, Tessler HH, Mafee MF. Computed tomography and magnetic resonance imaging in the diagnosis of posterior scleritis. Ann Ophthalmol. 1993;25(3):89–94.
11. Pulido JS, Gueken JA, Nerad JA, et al. Ocular manifestations of patients with circulating antineutrophil cytoplasmic antibodies. Arch Ophthalmol. 1990;108:845–50.
12. Young DW. The antineutrophil antibody in uveitis. Br J Ophthalmol. 1991;75:208–11.
13. Calthorpe CM, Watson PG, McCarthy ACE. Posterior scleritis: a clinical and histological survey. Eye. 1988;2:267–77.
14. Finger PT, Perry HD, Packer S, et al. Posterior scleritis as an intraocular tumor. Br J Ophthalmol. 1990;74:121–2.
15. Watson PG, Hayreh SS. Scleritis and episcleritis. Br J Ophthalmol. 1976;60:163–91.
16. Sainz de la Maza M, Foster CS, Jabbur NS. Scleritis associated with systemic vasculitic disease. Ophthalmology. 1995;102(4):687–92.
17. Soukiasian SH, Foster CS, Raizman MB. Treatment strategies for scleritis and uveitis associated with inflammatory bowel disease. Am J Ophthalmol. 1994;118:604–11.
18. Shah P, Luqmani RA, Murray PI, et al. Posterior scleritis—an unusual manifestation of Cogan's syndrome. Br J Rheumatol. 1994;33:774–5.
19. Sainz de la Maza M, Foster CS. Necrotizing scleritis after ocular surgery: a clinicopathologic study. Ophthalmology. 1991;98:1720–6.
20. O'Donoghue E, Lightman S, Tuft S, Watson P. Surgically induced necrotizing scleritis (SINS): precipitating factors and response to treatment. Br J Ophthalmol. 1992;76:17–21.
21. Galanopoulos A, Snibson G, O'Day J. Necrotizing anterior scleritis after pterygium surgery. Aust N Z J Ophthalmol. 1994;22(3):167–73.
22. Wakefield D, McCluskey P, Penny R. Intravenous pulse methylprednisolone therapy in severe inflammatory eye disease. Arch Ophthalmol. 1986;104:847–51.
23. Tu EY, Culbertson WW, Pflugfelder SC, et al. Therapy of nonnecrotizing anterior scleritis with subconjunctival corticosteroid injection. Ophthalmology. 1995;102(5):718–24.
24. Foster CS, Forstot SL, Wilson LA. Mortality rate in rheumatoid arthritis patients developing necrotizing scleritis or peripheral ulcerative keratitis: effects of systemic immunosuppression. Ophthalmology. 1984;91(10):1253–63.
25. Tamesis RR, Rodriguez A, Christen WG, et al. Systemic drug toxicity trends in immunosuppressive therapy of immune and inflammatory ocular disease. Ophthalmology. 1996;103:768–75.
26. Schall SS, Louder Cy, Schmitt MA, et al. Low dose methotrexate therapy for ocular inflammatory disease. Ophthalmology. 1992;99:1419–23.
27. Jampol LM, West C, Goldberg M. Therapy of scleritis with cytotoxic agents. Am J Ophthalmol. 1978;86:266–71.
28. Tessler HH, Jennings T. High-dose short-term chlorambucil for intractable sympathetic ophthalmia and Behçet's disease. Br J Ophthalmol. 1990;74:353–7.
29. Goldstein DA, Fontanilla FA, Kaul S, et al. Long-term follow-up of patients treated with short-term high-dose chlorambucil for sight-threatening ocular inflammation. Ophthalmology. 2002;109:370–7.
30. Wakefield D, McCluskey P. Cyclosporin therapy for severe scleritis. Br J Ophthalmol. 1989;73:743–6.
31. Hakin KN, Ham J, Lightman SL. Use of cyclosporin in the management of steroid dependent non-necrotizing scleritis. Br J Ophthalmol. 1991;75:340–1.
32. Koenig SB, Sanitato JJ, Kaufman HE. Long-term follow-up study of scleroplasty using autogenous periosteum. Cornea. 1990;9(2):139–43.
33. Tuft SJ, Watson PG. Progression of scleral disease. Ophthalmology. 1991;98:467–71.
34. Khalil M. Osteogenesis imperfecta. In: Gold DH, Weingeist TA, eds. The eye and systemic disease. Philadelphia: Lippincott; 1990:549–50.
35. Sillence D, Butler B, Latham M, et al. Natural history of blue sclerae in osteogenesis imperfecta. Am J Med Genet. 1993;45:183–6.
36. Khalil M. Subhyaloid hemorrhage in osteogenesis imperfecta tarda. Can J Ophthalmol. 1983;18:251–2.
37. Brockhurst RJ. Nanophthalmos. In: Fraunfelder FT, Roy FH, eds. Current ocular therapy. Philadelphia: WB Saunders; 1995:611–2.
38. Tagami N, Uyama M, Yamada K, et al. Histological observations on the sclera in uveal effusion. Acta Soc Ophthalmol Jpn. 1993;97:268–74.
39. Stewart DH, Strecten BW, Brokhurst RJ, et al. Abnormal scleral collagen in nanophthalmos. Arch Ophthalmol. 1991;109:1017–25.
40. Weiss A, Kousseff BG, Ross EA. Simple microphthalmos. Arch Ophthalmol. 1989;107:1625–30.
41. Singh OS, Sofinski SJ. Nanophthalmos: guidelines for diagnosis and therapy. In: Albert DM, Jakobiec FA, eds. Principles and practice of ophthalmology. Philadelphia: WB Saunders; 1994:1528–40.
42. Mansour AM, Barber JC, Reinecke RD, Wang FM. Ocular choristomas. Surv Ophthalmol. 1989;33(5):339–58.
43. Panton RW, Sugar J. Excision of limbal dermoids. Ophthalmic Surg. 1991;22(2):85–9.
44. Gonnering RS, Fuerste FH, Lemke BN, Sonneland PR. Epibulbar osseous choristomas with scleral involvement. Ophthalmic Plast Reconstr Surg. 1988;4(1):63–6.

CHAPTER

65

Dry Eye

ELMER Y. TU • STEPHEN RHEINSTROM

DEFINITION
- Dry eye syndrome is a clinical condition characterized by deficient tear production or excessive tear evaporation resulting in ocular discomfort.

KEY FEATURES
- Ocular irritation.
- Conjunctival injection.
- Ocular surface disruption.

ASSOCIATED FEATURES
- Possible autoimmune disease.
- Possible conjunctival or lid abnormalities.
- Systemic and topical medications.
- Blurred or unstable vision.

INTRODUCTION

Dry eye syndrome (DES) is characterized by ocular irritation resulting from an alteration of the tear film. The effects of DES can vary from minor inconvenience for most sufferers to rare sight-threatening complications in severe cases. Although the diagnosis of DES has traditionally focused on inadequate secretion, or aqueous tear deficiency, the tear film is a complex and delicately balanced unit dependent on the normal function of several distinct components.[1,2] Both systemic and local conditions can affect these individual components, and these conditions can be identified through a detailed history and examination.

Current treatment is heavily weighted toward supplementation, stimulation, or preservation of aqueous tears, which is satisfactory for most patients. DES, however, often involves multiple deficiency states that, when disregarded, can result in treatment failure and frustration for both the patient and the physician. A more thorough understanding of DES and its interaction with the ocular surface is leading to promising and more complete approaches to treatment.

EPIDEMIOLOGY AND PATHOGENESIS
Normal Physiology

The tear film is composed of mucin, aqueous, and lipid components stratified into distinct layers in the resting tear film. The mucin layer consists of high–molecular-weight glycoproteins that adhere to surface epithelium and its secreted glycocalyx. This mucinous coating of the hydrophobic epithelial cell surface provides a level, hydrophilic surface,[3] permitting smooth distribution of the overlying aqueous layer. Although recent studies have demonstrated mucin secretion by squamous epithelial cells of the cornea and conjunctiva,[4] its primary source is conjunctival goblet cells. The aqueous layer is approximately $70\mu m$ thick and constitutes the largest volume of the tear film. In an undisturbed state, it rests above the mucin but deep to the lipid layer.

The aqueous is secreted by the main lacrimal gland and accessory glands of Krause and Wolfring, with a small contribution from conjunctival vessels and the cornea. As the name implies, the aqueous layer consists primarily of water but also contains electrolytes (Na, K, Cl) and myriad proteins, including epidermal growth factor, immunoglobulins (IgA, IgG, IgM), lactoferrin, lysozyme, and other cytokines.[5,6] The precise role of these proteins is unknown, but they likely play both a protective and a homeostatic role for the ocular surface. Last, meibomian glands secrete the lipid layer, which contains chiefly sterol esters and wax monoesters.[7,8] Although only $0.1\mu m$ thick, the lipid layer serves to stabilize the tear film by increasing surface tension and retarding evaporation.

The tear layer has a variety of different functions, including maintenance of a smooth surface for optical clarity, lubrication to facilitate eyelid blink, and protection against ocular infection.[1] Average tear flow is about $1.2\mu m/min$.[9] Blinking serves to periodically distribute tears evenly over the ocular surface and promotes the constant turnover of tears by encouraging both secretion and mechanical drainage of tears through the lacrimal drainage system. Regulation of secretion is not completely understood, but it appears to involve both neuronal and hormonal pathways. Direct innervation of the lacrimal gland, meibomian glands, and goblet cells has been demonstrated, with M3 class cholinergic receptors predominating in the lacrimal gland.[10] The effect of hormonal triggers is less clear, but androgens appear to have a positive effect on the secretion of both aqueous and lipid tears.[11,12]

The tear film and ocular surface form a highly interdependent complex. Deficiencies of the tear film lead to either hyperosmolar toxicity or direct exposure of the cornea and conjunctiva; persistent DES leads to reactive structural and cellular changes of the ocular surface.[13] Squamous metaplasia of the conjunctiva and cornea, corneal epitheliopathy, and filamentary keratitis can all be associated with chronic low tear volume.

Classification of Dry Eye

The National Eye Institute/Industry Workshop adopted the following definition of dry eye[14]: Dry eye is a disorder of the tear film due to tear deficiency or excessive tear evaporation which causes damage to the interpalpebral ocular surface and is associated with symptoms of ocular discomfort. This definition encompasses all the clinical entities associated with systemic disease, as well as idiopathic dry eye disease. As a result of these workshops, a classification system algorithm for dry eye was produced (Fig. 65-1).

TEAR-DEFICIENT DRY EYE. Defective lacrimal function as a cause of dry eye subdivides into two categories: non–Sjögren's tear deficiency (NSTD), and Sjögren's syndrome tear deficiency (SSTD). NSTD has no association with systemic autoimmune disease, which is a cardinal feature of SSTD. The description of keratoconjunctivitis sicca (KCS) that Sjögren[15] gave in his 1933 article has become associated with his name. The term *KCS–Sjögren's syndrome* is used in much of the world literature for the ocular surface disease that occurs in Sjögren's syndrome,

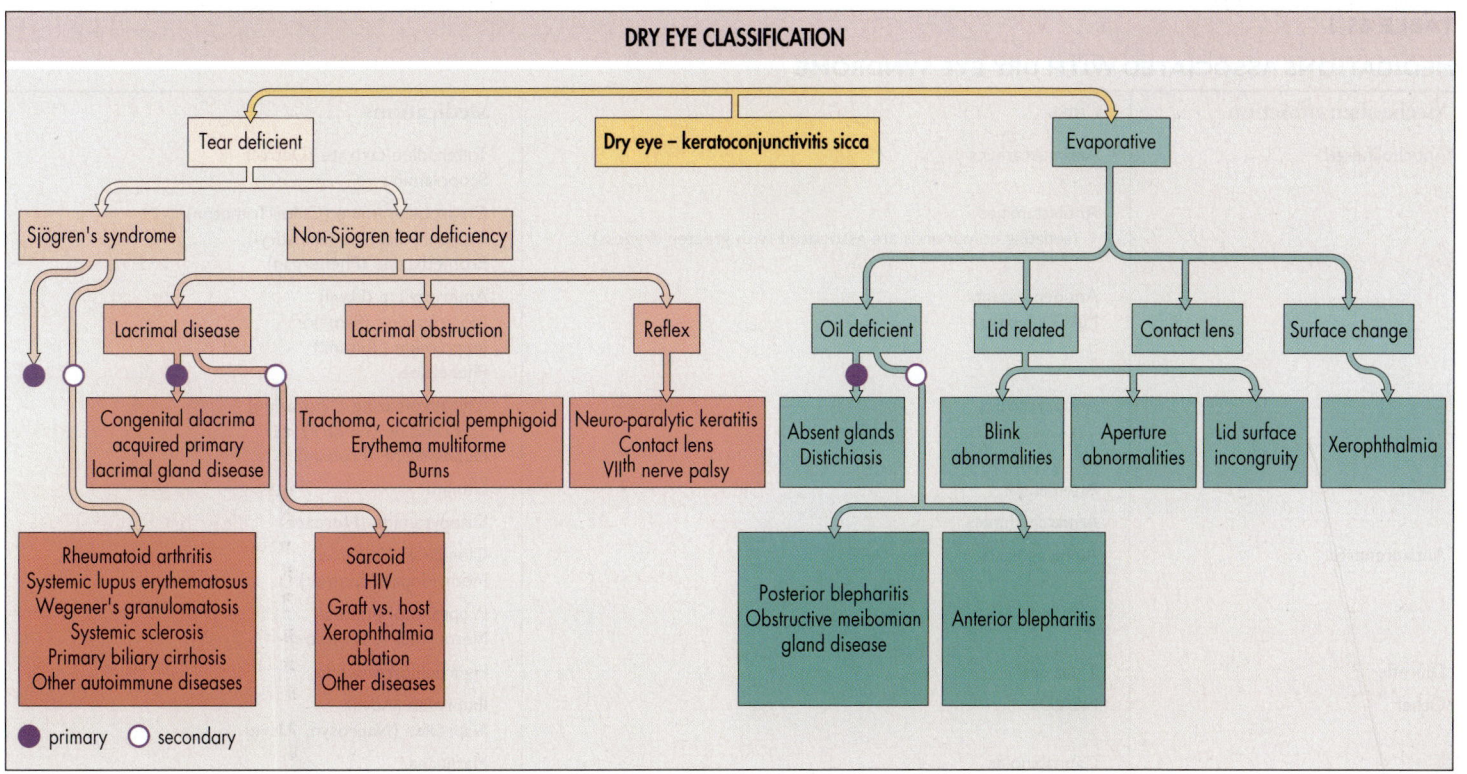

FIG. 65-1 ■ Dry eye classification. (With permission from Lemp MA. The 1998 Castroviejo lecture. New strategies in the treatment of dry-eye states. Cornea. 1999;18[6]:625–32.)

whereas the term *non–Sjögren's syndrome KCS* is used for primary, age-related tear deficiency.

Non–Sjögren's Tear Deficiency. NSTD can occur from impaired glandular production, impaired afferent or efferent stimulation, or local ocular surface disease. Primary lacrimal deficiency may result from congenital alacrima, a rare condition of children born with absent or hypoplastic lacrimal glands. Another inborn disease, Riley-Day syndrome, features aberrant parasympathetic innervation in a functional lacrimal gland with intact reflex tearing. The large majority of patients who have DES, however, are categorized as having acquired lacrimal gland deficiency, primary lacrimal deficiency, or idiopathic KCS syndrome. The pathogenesis is unknown, but DES may result from either age-related changes in the lacrimal gland[16] or an immune mechanism evidenced by round cell infiltration of the lacrimal gland and ductal tissue.[17]

Secondary lacrimal deficiency can result from infiltration of the lacrimal gland. Lymphoma, sarcoidosis, hemochromatosis, amyloidosis, human immunodeficiency virus infection, and graft-versus-host disease all can result in dry eye from this process.[18,19] Similarly, surgical or radiation-induced destruction of lacrimal tissue can result in severe dry eye.

Systemic medications are a common source for the inhibition of efferent lacrimal gland stimulation. Numerous medications are associated with DES (Table 65-1), many of which reduce lacrimation through either anticholinergic inhibition of the lacrimal gland or systemic dehydration.[20] Mechanical trauma to efferent secretomotor fibers to the lacrimal gland also may result in dry eye.[18]

DES has been reported in association with menopause.[21] Although most systemic symptoms of menopause are related to decreasing levels of estrogen, supplementation studies have not shown a beneficial effect in DES.[22] The cause of postmenopausal DES, therefore, is hypothesized to be due to alterations in other hormones, especially androgens, which are also reduced during menopause.

Interruption of the afferent stimulus of tear production, or sensory loss (denervation), results in decreased tear secretion and reduced blink rate. Tear flow decreases by 60–75%, and blink rate decreases by 30% after topical instillation of anesthetic.[23,24] Damage to afferent sensory fibers resulting in dry eye has been reported after incisional surgery of the cornea (penetrating keratoplasty, radial keratotomy, and limbal cataract incision) and after damage to the first division of the trigeminal ganglion from trauma, tumor, herpes simplex, or zoster. Physiologically, denervation also results in corneal epithelial atrophy, compounding the risk of corneal ulceration.

LASIK and photorefractive keratectomy are increasingly recognized as precipitating causes of dry eye.[25] Postsurgical findings of decreased corneal sensation, tear production, and blink rate lasting 6–18 months or more are evidence of neurotrophic DES.[26–28] The incidence may be higher in LASIK because the incision involves 270° of the corneal circumference, severing penetrating branches of the long ciliary nerves.[25] Donnenfeld et al.[29] reported significantly greater dry eye in patients with superior hinge placement, suggesting that nasal hinge placement may preserve a greater number of these nerve branches. The resultant contour of the corneal surface may also prevent proper tear distribution. Avoidance of surgery, especially LASIK, in patients at risk for corneal neuropathy (i.e., those with advanced diabetes or preexisting severe dry eye) is strongly recommended.

Sjögren's Syndrome Tear Deficiency. Sjögren's syndrome is a clinical condition of aqueous tear deficiency combined with dry mouth. The syndrome is classified as primary—patients without a *defined* connective tissue disease—and secondary—patients who have a confirmed connective tissue disease, most often rheumatoid arthritis. Secondary SSTD is also associated with systemic lupus erythematosus, polyarteritis, Wegener's granulomatosis, scleroderma, polymyositis, dermatomyositis, and primary biliary cirrhosis. All feature progressive lymphocytic infiltration of the lacrimal and salivary glands and can be associated with severe and painful ocular and oral discomfort. The pathogenesis of the tear deficit in SSTD is infiltration of the lacrimal gland by B and CD4 lymphocytes (with some CD8 lymphocytes) and by plasma cells, with subsequent fibrosis. Fox[19] laid out criteria to establish the diagnosis of Sjögren's syndrome:
• Abnormally low Schirmer's test result.
• Objectively decreased salivary gland flow.

TABLE 65-1

MEDICATIONS ASSOCIATED WITH DRY EYE SYNDROME

Mechanism of Action	Class	Medications
Anticholinergic	Antimuscarinics	Tolterodine tartrate (Detrol) Scopolamine
	Antihistamines (sedating compounds are associated with greater dryness)	Chlorpheniramine (Chlor-Trimeton) Diphenhydramine (Benadryl) Promethazine (Phenergan)
	Antidepressants MAO inhibitors	Amitriptyline (Elavil) Nortriptyline (Pamelor) Imipramine (Tofranil) Phenelzine
	Antipsychotics	Chlorpromazine (Thorazine) Thioridazine (Mellaril) Fluphenazine (Prolixin)
	Antimanics	Lithium
	Antiarrhythmics	Disopyramide (Norpace)
Antiadrenergic	Alpha agonists	Clonidine (Catapres) Methyldopa (Aldomet)
	Beta blockers	Propranolol (Inderal) Metoprolol (Lopressor)
Diuretic	Thiazides	Hydrochlorothiazide
Other	NSAIDs	Ibuprofen (Advil) Naproxen (Naprosyn, Aleve)
	Cannabinoids	Marijuana

- Biopsy-proved infiltration of the labial salivary glands.
- Serum autoantibodies (antinuclear antibody, rheumatoid factor, or the specific antibodies anti-Ro [SS-A] and anti-La [SS-B]).

When all four factors are present, a definite diagnosis of Sjögren's syndrome is made; if three of the four are met, a provisional diagnosis can be made.

EVAPORATIVE DRY EYE. Excessive evaporation that occurs in specific periocular disorders can cause dry eye disease with or without concurrent aqueous tear deficiency. Evaporation leads to both loss of tear volume and a disproportionate loss of water, resulting in hyperosmolarity. Environmental conditions such as high altitude, dryness, or extreme heat accelerate tear loss even in normal individuals.

Meibomian Gland Disease and Blepharitis. Meibomian gland dysfunction (MGD) leads to both decreased secretion and abnormal composition of the tear film lipid layer. The meibomian gland secretions (meibum) are altered in MGD, leading to meibomian gland blockage as well as reducing its effectiveness in the tear film. The abnormal lipids cause both ocular surface and eyelid inflammation, perpetuating a cycle of inflammation, scarring, hyperkeratosis, stenosis, and further MGD. The resultant lipid layer is unable to maintain stability of the tear film and retard evaporation.

MGD is associated with abnormal bacterial colonization, acne rosacea, and seborrheic dermatitis. Abnormal bacterial colonization may act directly by altering secreted lipids or indirectly by causing inflammation. Acne rosacea is a dermatological disorder resulting in vascular dilatation, telangiectasias, and plugging of sebaceous glands of both facial and eyelid skin.

Exposure. Excessive exposure of the ocular surface leads to increased evaporative loss of tears; thus, any disorder that results in increased ocular exposure can cause evaporative dry eye. Trauma to the eyelid, whether mechanical or neurological, that results in impaired or reduced blinking, lagophthalmos, or an increased palpebral fissure width can result in an evaporative dry eye. Evaporative dry eye can be seen in thyroid eye disease secondary to proptosis or lid retraction. Comatose patients and some psychiatric patients may have central nervous system–induced exposure from an impaired blink reflex.

Mucin Deficiency. Local ocular surface disorders such as cicatrizing diseases of the conjunctiva or surgical trauma may result in aqueous tear deficiency by scarring of the tear ducts. More im-

portant, these processes destroy mucin-producing goblet cells and cause anatomical abnormalities of the conjunctiva, preventing proper tear distribution. Although uncommon in incidence, trachoma, mucous membrane pemphigoid, Stevens-Johnson syndrome, and chemical and thermal burns can result in severe DES not amenable to aqueous tear replacement therapy. Vitamin A deficiency similarly can result in extensive goblet cell loss and squamous metaplasia.[30]

OCULAR MANIFESTATIONS

Most forms of dry eye have symptoms, interpalpebral surface damage, tear instability, and tear hyperosmolarity. Many symptoms of DES are the same, regardless of cause. Typical complaints include burning, itching, foreign body sensation, stinging, dryness, photophobia, ocular fatigue, and redness. Although symptoms are usually nonspecific, careful attention to a patient's complaints will help refine the diagnosis.

Patients commonly describe a diurnal pattern. Aqueous tear deficiency typically presents with worsening symptoms over the day and decompensation in particular environmental conditions. Low humidity in airline cabins and in modern office buildings with climate control can be exacerbating factors for the development of symptomatic DES.[31] Video display terminals have been associated with both decreased blink rate and increased tear evaporation, which can contribute to dry eye.[32] Conversely, nighttime exposure, floppy eyelid syndrome, and inflammatory conditions often present with discomfort on awakening and improvement over the day.

Patients with an unstable tear film report intermittent visual blurring and discomfort. A gritty or sandy sensation is common in meibomian gland disease. It is important to recognize that diabetic patients and patients with other corneal neuropathies may exhibit signs of DES with or without discomfort. Recognition of corneal neurosensory loss is critical in determining the course of therapy and observation, since these patients are at high risk for keratolysis.

Common signs of DES include conjunctival injection, decreased tear meniscus, photophobia, increased tear debris, and loss of corneal sheen. Findings are more common in the exposed interpalpebral fissure. DES patients may experience excess

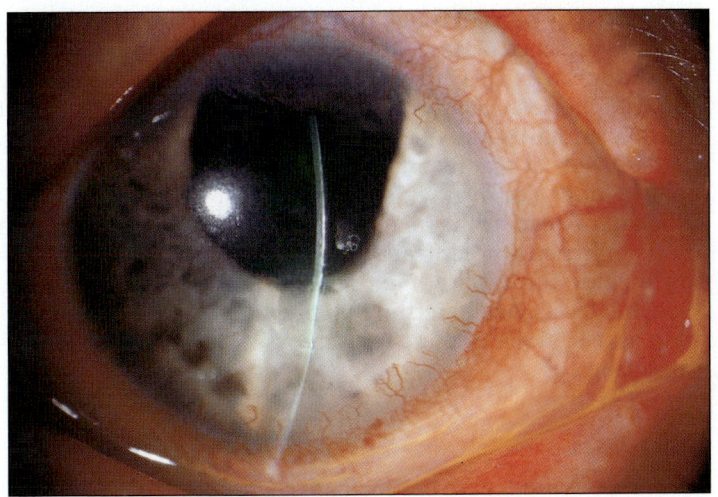

FIG. 65-2 ■ Seventy-three-year-old patient with rheumatoid arthritis and secondary Sjögren's syndrome.

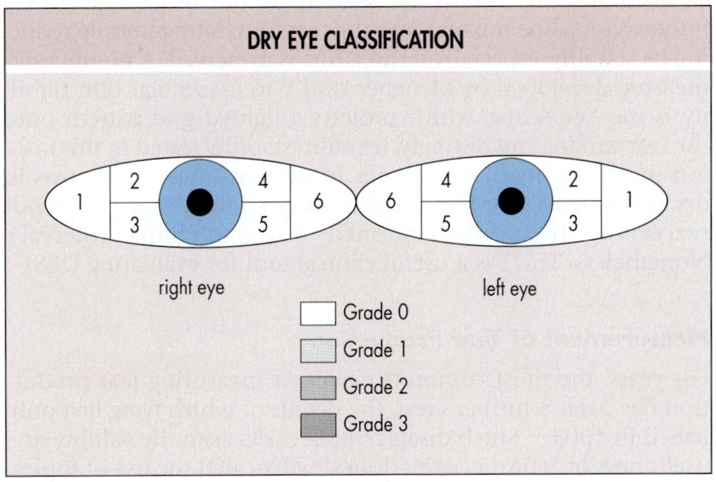

DRY EYE CLASSIFICATION

right eye   left eye

☐ Grade 0
☐ Grade 1
☐ Grade 2
☐ Grade 3

FIG. 65-3 ■ Modified van Bijsterveld conjunctival rose bengal grading map. The density of rose bengal staining is recorded on a scale of 0–3 for each of six areas of the conjunctiva, and then summed for each eye. (With permission from Lemp MA. The 1998 Castroviejo lecture. New strategies in the treatment of dry-eye states. Cornea. 1999;18[6]:625–32.)

tearing or even epiphora as a result of reflex tearing. DES patients are also at greater risk for external infections secondary to decreased tear turnover and desiccation of the surface epithelium. Instability of the surface epithelium and disordered mucin production may lead to painful and recurrent filamentary keratitis. Keratinization may occur in chronic DES, but vitamin A deficiency should also be suspected. Meibomian gland inspissation, telangiectasias, glandular dropout (seen on transillumination of the tarsus), chalazions, and eyelash debris are found in meibomian gland disease and blepharitis.

Patients who have SSTD tend to have more severe symptoms and more serious findings than do NSTD patients. Sterile ulceration may be seen in SSTD. Ulceration of the cornea can be peripheral or paracentral; both thinning and perforation of these ulcers can occur. Figure 65-2 shows a patient with paracentral ulceration secondary to SSTD. Acute lacrimal enlargement may be seen in SSTD but should be differentiated from Mikulicz's disease, which results from infiltration of the gland without surface findings.[33]

The result of DES is hyperosmolar toxicity and exposure of the underlying ocular surface. Chronically present, this leads to a loss of conjunctival goblet cells, epithelial cell dysfunction, and, in advanced cases, metaplasia and keratinization. These changes manifest as "dry" patches and keratinization of the conjunctiva. Disruption of the normal epithelial barrier promotes release of the pro-inflammatory cytokines interleukin-1, interleukin-6, interleukin-8, and tumor necrosis factor, among others, leading to further epithelial damage. The cornea exhibits similar changes, with disruption of tight junctions and abnormal epithelial-mucin interaction.

DIAGNOSIS AND ANCILLARY TESTING
Diagnostic Dye Evaluation

Fluorescein is a large molecule that is normally unable to traverse the tight junctions of an intact epithelium. These tight junctions in advanced DES are disrupted, producing characteristic diffuse subepithelial or punctate staining. Rose bengal, a derivative of fluorescein, is used to detect ocular surface damage by staining devitalized epithelial cells. Feenstra and Tseng[34] showed that rose bengal stains healthy epithelial cells if a normal amount of mucin does not overlie the cell surface. Since 1% rose bengal solution is no longer commercially available, impregnated strips wetted with artificial tears may be used. Proparacaine should be avoided because it dilutes rose bengal poorly and may desiccate the ocular surface, creating spurious results.

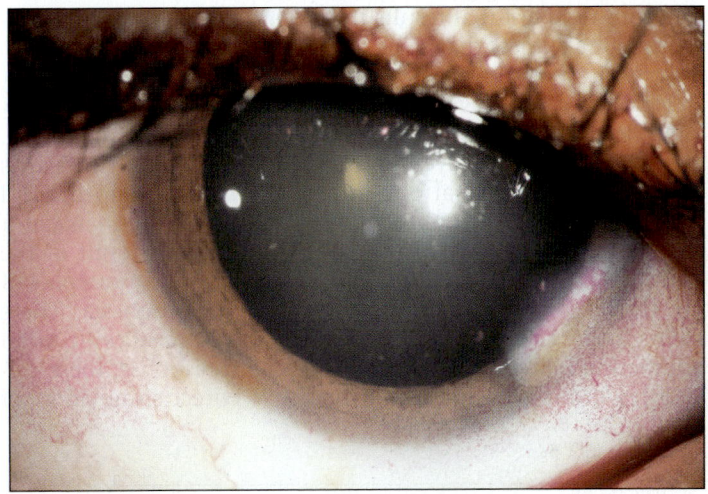

FIG. 65-4 ■ Dry eye syndrome with rose bengal staining.

Van Bijsterveld[35] created a grading scale for rose bengal dye that divides the ocular surface into three zones: nasal bulbar conjunctiva, cornea, and temporal bulbar conjunctiva. Each zone is evaluated for density of stain in the range 0–3 (0, none; 3, confluent staining). An additive zone stain total of 3.5 or more in the eye constitutes a positive test for dry eye. Typically, the conjunctiva stains to a greater extent than the cornea, and the nasal conjunctiva shows more stain than the temporal.[16] Lemp and the National Eye Institute/Industry Workshop group[14] suggest that the conjunctiva be divided into six areas and graded in a similar manner (Fig. 65-3). Figure 65-4 is a clinical example of an eye with KCS stained with rose bengal. Also widely available, lissamine green does not irritate the eye and stains for cell death or degeneration, as well as cell-to-cell junction disruption.[36]

Tear Film Stability

Tear film instability may be a result of either tear deficiency or evaporative DES. One of the common objective tests used to help make a diagnosis of dry eye is tear breakup time (TBUT), described by Norn and revised by Lemp and Holly.[37] Tears are stained with fluorescein dye, and the time interval is measured between a complete blink to the first appearance of a dry spot in the precorneal tear film. Theoretically, TBUTs shorter than the blink interval of 5 seconds could result in surface damage, and very short TBUTs (less than 2 seconds) indicate KCS.

Unfortunately, results are skewed by the introduction of a fluorescein-saline mixture into the tear film, iatrogenically reducing its stability, especially if the saline is preserved. A noninvasive measure developed by Mengher et al.[38] to assess tear film stability is the Xeroscope, which projects a lighted grid pattern onto the tear surface. Interestingly, tear film stability tested in this fashion measured about 40 seconds in normal subjects, whereas in dry eye patients, tear film stability survived for about 12 seconds (exceeding the aforementioned 5-second blink interval). Nonetheless, TBUT is a useful clinical tool for evaluating DES.

Measurement of Tear Production

For years, the most common means of measuring tear production has been Schirmer's test, the details of which were first published in 1903.[39] Much disagreement exists as to the validity and usefulness of Schirmer's test. Jones[40] advocated the use of topical anesthesia combined with a Schirmer's test strip for 5 minutes to reduce the effect of the presence of the filter paper strip; this has become the "basal" test. False-negative and false-positive results cloud the usefulness of each test. The application of Schirmer's test is fraught with inconsistencies that limit its repeatability in DES,[41] but it still enjoys widespread use. With these caveats in mind, the following general guidelines are recommended:

- A 5-minute test that results in less than 5mm of wetting confirms the clinical diagnosis of DES.
- A result of 6–10mm of wetting suggests a dry eye problem.

Hamano et al.[42] developed the phenol red thread test in an attempt to overcome some of the disadvantages of Schirmer's test. In this test, 3mm of dye-impregnated 75mm cotton thread is placed under the lateral one fifth of the inferior palpebral lid margin; it is allowed to absorb tears for 15 seconds—its color changes to bright orange from tear contact (as a result of the slightly alkaline pH of tears). The patient has little awareness of the thread, which eliminates the need for anesthesia. There seems to be a racially biased variation of response, with Asian populations showing a lessened wet-length response; these differences diminish with advancing age.[43] Direct stimulation of the nasociliary nerve through irritation of the nasopharynx confirms the presence or absence of reflex tearing.

Although it is clear that tears in dry-eye patients generally have a higher osmolarity than normal and that measurement of tear osmolarity provides a sensitive test, it is not specific, standardized, or readily attainable. Also, the degree of tear osmolarity does not distinguish between tear-deficient and tear-sufficient dry eye, as the increased evaporation in the latter also results in hyperosmolar tears. Other tests for reduced tear function include fluorophotometry for decreased protein content, lysozyme levels, ocular ferning, impression cytology, and lactoferrin assays. None of these tests enjoys widespread use in clinical settings.

Other Tests

Corneal sensation may be qualitatively assessed with a cotton wisp, but quantification requires an instrument such as the Cochet-Bonnet aesthesiometer, a subjective test using a thin standardized wisp of varying length. More predictive than Schirmer's test, the tear clearance test measures tear turnover with serial tear collection after instillation of a standardized volume of dye.[41,44] Serological tests, including antinuclear, anti-Ro, and anti-La antibodies, should be performed in patients suspected of having autoimmune DES. A definitive diagnosis of Sjögren's syndrome requires, however, minor salivary or, rarely, lacrimal gland biopsy.

Diagnosis

Neither clinical presentation nor individual ancillary tests alone are sufficient for an accurate diagnosis of DES. Because of the therapeutic importance of appropriate categorization of patients, Pflugfelder et al.[45] combined standard subjective examination with ancillary tests in the evaluation of SSTD, NSTD, inflammatory MGD, and atrophic MGD patients. Clinically important results were identified and compiled into an algorithm that helps differentiate DES patients with available tests (Fig. 65-5).

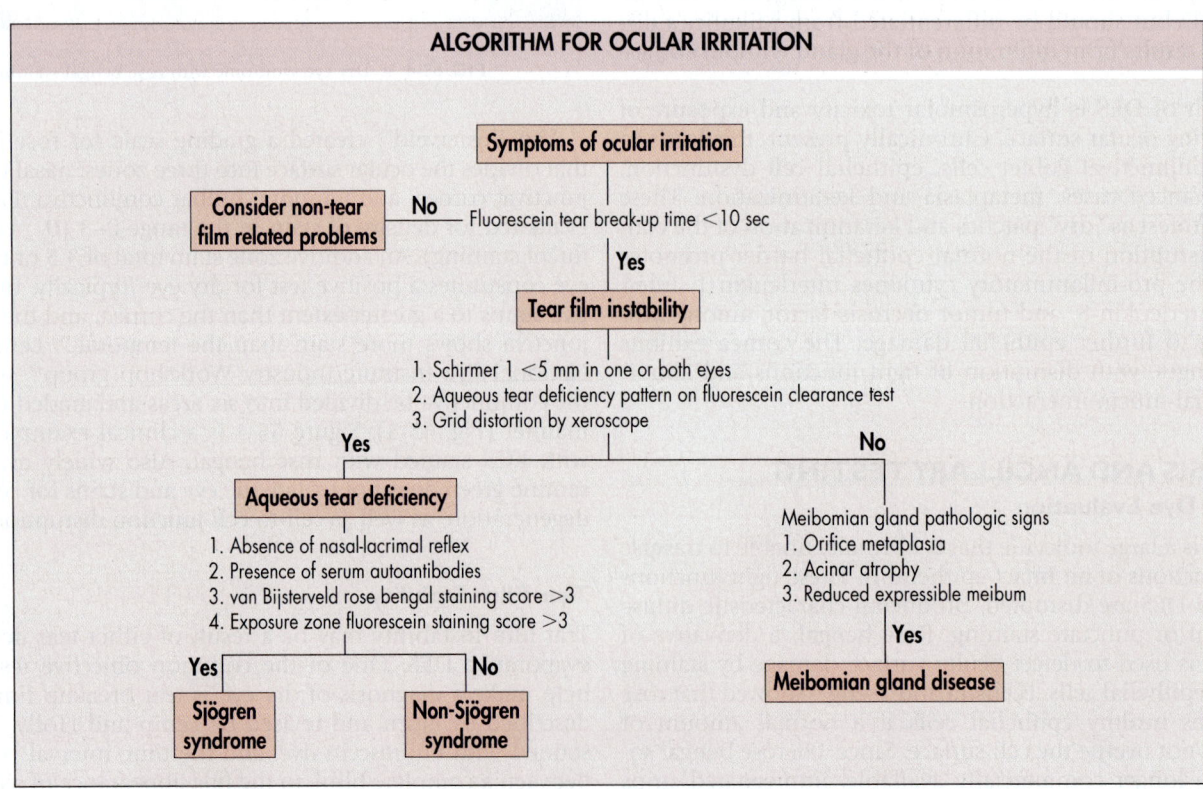

FIG. 65-5 ▮ **Diagnostic algorithm for ocular irritation.** (With permission from Pflugfelder SC, Tseng SC, Sanabria O, et al. Evaluation of subjective assessments and objective diagnostic tests for diagnosing tear-film disorders known to cause ocular irritation. Cornea. 1998;17[1]:38–56.)

TREATMENT

Significant advances have been made in treating the many facets of dry eye, but it remains a disorder of long-term maintenance rather than permanent cure. Current therapy focuses on tear supplementation to allow resident healing mechanisms to restore a normal ocular surface. Chronic DES, however, induces aberrant inflammatory and cellular changes that impede healing. Evolving therapeutic approaches are directed toward modulation of these aberrant processes as well as promotion of normal tear secretion. Since the tear film is a highly integrated unit, optimizing each layer, regardless of how minor the abnormality, is central to the successful treatment of DES.

Aqueous Tear Deficiency

As the first line of treatment, artificial tears both increase available tears and lower tear osmolarity through dilutional effects. A large number of artificial tears are available commercially, differing in electrolyte composition and preservative. The addition of "thickening" agents such as methylcellulose, hydroxypropyl methylcellulose, and polyvinyl alcohol can prolong retention of the tears on the ocular surface. Physiological buffering and hypotonicity may be beneficial to the ocular surface and decrease hyperosmolarity further. The compatibility of a tear preparation is highly dependent on an individual patient's preferences, which may involve such disparate concerns as cost, comfort, visual blurring, and ease of delivery. It is clear, however, that the use of traditionally preserved tears in moderate or severe dry eye is poorly tolerated and harmful. For patients with significant dry eye, single-dose, nonpreserved tear preparations are the mainstay of therapy. Because of the cost, inconvenience, and difficulty in handling the vials, bottled tear products utilizing sodium perborate or a stabilized oxychloro complex are a reasonable alternative. These preservatives have good antimicrobial activity but are converted to harmless compounds when in contact with the ocular surface. Artificial tear ointments can be effective for longer-lasting control of symptoms, but visual blurring limits their usefulness for many patients. They are most effective in balancing decreased tear production and exposure in the nighttime hours.

Secretagogues are agents that stimulate lacrimal gland secretion and increase available tears, requiring functional glandular tissue. Oral pilocarpine (Salagen) and cevimeline (Evoxac) are two M3 cholinergic agonists approved for use in dry mouth that also stimulate tear secretion.[10,46] The effect tends to be greater in oral dryness than in dry eye, and systemic cholinergic side effects may limit their use. Buccal salivary gland transplantation and parotid duct transposition have been largely abandoned but may have utility in specific cases.[47] Various nutritional supplements are also touted for DES but without scientific confirmation of their safety or efficacy. Punctal occlusion retards tear drainage, thereby increasing tear volume on the ocular surface and lowering tear osmolarity. Occlusion may be achieved irreversibly by cauterization or reversibly with the use of various silicone plugs. YAG laser occlusion is characterized by a high incidence of recanalization. The use of collagen or 5-0 chromic gut for temporary occlusion can help identify those borderline patients at risk for epiphora prior to permanent occlusion. It should be noted that epiphora in the presence of one functional punctum in patients with little or no tear production is uncommon.

Evaporative Dry Eye

Primary treatment of tear evaporation involves stabilizing the lipid tear layer. Since lipid tear substitutes are investigational and not widely available, treatment is focused on improving the quality and quantity of native meibomian gland secretions. Lid hygiene, in the form of warm compresses and lid massage, is effective in improving meibomian gland secretion. Lid scrubs with dilute detergents can decrease seborrheic or bacterial load, help-ing to break the pro-inflammatory cycle of MGD. The addition of a systemic tetracycline has also been shown to decrease local inflammation and improve meibomian gland function, resulting in improved patient comfort. Treatment must continue for several weeks to see an effect.

Correction of eyelid abnormalities that increase exposure of the ocular surface, such as lower lid ptosis and lagophthalmos, can stabilize a decompensated ocular surface. In severe cases, a partial or complete tarsorrhaphy or a conjunctival flap may be necessary to prevent complete decompensation of the cornea. The use of humidifiers, moist chambers, glasses, or goggles decreases evaporative pressure. New high-Dk, high-water-content contact lenses and new polymer lenses, accompanied by proper tear supplementation and hygiene, are effective in treating DES patients with poor corneal wetting.

Ocular Surface Inflammation

Treating the secondary inflammatory response and consequential cellular changes of dry eye is more controversial. DES-induced ocular surface inflammation disrupts the epithelial and mucin layers, further exacerbating tear film breakdown. Persistent inflammation can prevent effective treatment of either aqueous or lipid tear deficiency. Immune modulators such as corticosteroids, cyclosporine A, and tetracyclines have all been used with some success in reversing the destructive effects of KCS.[47-49] Control of these reactive epithelial changes has been shown to restore normal cell morphology, cell-to-cell interactions, and critical mucin production and clearly has a role in the treatment at all forms of DES. A better understanding of surface inflammation and the development of specific agents are needed to prevent and reverse the structural changes induced by dry eye.

REFERENCES

1. Rolando M, Zierhut M. The ocular surface and tear film and their dysfunction in dry eye disease. Surv Ophthalmol. 2001;45(Suppl 2):S203–10.
2. Tseng SC, Tsubota K. Important concepts for treating ocular surface and tear disorders. Am J Ophthalmol. 1997;124(6):825–35.
3. Argueso P, Gipson IK. Epithelial mucins of the ocular surface: structure, biosynthesis and function. Exp Eye Res. 2001;73(3):281–9.
4. Watanabe H, Fabricant M, Tisdale AS, et al. Human corneal and conjunctival epithelia produce a mucin-like glycoprotein for the apical surface. Invest Ophthalmol Vis Sci. 1995;36(2):337–44.
5. Barton K, Nava A, Monroy DC, Pflugfelder SC. Cytokines and tear function in ocular surface disease. Adv Exp Med Biol. 1998;438:461–9.
6. Solomon A, Dursun D, Liu Z, et al. Pro- and anti-inflammatory forms of interleukin-1 in the tear fluid and conjunctiva of patients with dry-eye disease. Invest Ophthalmol Vis Sci. 2001;42(10):2283–92.
7. Driver PJ, Lemp MA. Meibomian gland dysfunction. Surv Ophthalmol. 1996;40(5):343–67.
8. Bron AJ, Tiffany JM. The meibomian glands and tear film lipids. Structure, function, and control. Adv Exp Med Biol. 1998;438:281–95.
9. Mishima S, Gasset A, Klyce SD Jr, Baum JL. Determination of tear volume and tear flow. Invest Ophthalmol. 1966;5(3):264–76.
10. Fox RI, Michelson P. Approaches to the treatment of Sjogren's syndrome. J Rheumatol Suppl. 2000;61:15–21.
11. Krenzer KL, Dana MR, Ullman MD, et al. Effect of androgen deficiency on the human meibomian gland and ocular surface. J Clin Endocrinol Metab. 2000;85(12):4874–82.
12. Lemp MA. The 1998 Castroviejo lecture. New strategies in the treatment of dry-eye states. Cornea. 1999;18(6):625–32.
13. Stern ME, Beuerman RW, Fox RI, et al. The pathology of dry eye: the interaction between the ocular surface and lacrimal glands. Cornea. 1998;17(6):584–9.
14. Lemp MA. Report of the National Eye Institute/Industry Workshop on Clinical Trials in Dry Eyes. CLAO J. 1995;21(4):221–32.
15. Sjögren H. Zur kenntnis der keratoconjunctivitis sicca (Keratitis filiformis bei hypofunktion der tranendrusen). Acta Ophthalmol (Copenh). 1933;2:1–151.
16. Obata H, Yamamoto S, Horiuchi H, Machinami R. Histopathologic study of human lacrimal gland. Statistical analysis with special reference to aging. Ophthalmology. 1995;102(4):678–86.
17. Nasu M, Matsubara O, Yamamoto H. Post-mortem prevalence of lymphocytic infiltration of the lacrimal gland: a comparative study in autoimmune and non-autoimmune diseases. J Pathol. 1984;143(1):11–5.
18. Gilbard J, ed. Dry eye disorders. In: Albert JF, ed. Principles and practice of ophthalmology. Philadelphia: WB Saunders; 1994:257–76.
19. Fox RI. Systemic diseases associated with dry eye. Int Ophthalmol Clin. 1994; 34(1):71–87.
20. Fraunfelder F, Fraunfelder FW. Drug-induced ocular side effects, 5th ed. Boston: Butterworth-Heinemann; 2001.
21. Mathers WD, Stovall D, Lane JA, et al. Menopause and tear function: the influence of prolactin and sex hormones on human tear production. Cornea. 1998;17(4):353–8.

22. Schaumberg DA, Buring JE, Sullivan DA, Dana MR. Hormone replacement therapy and dry eye syndrome. JAMA. 2001;286(17):2114–9.

23. Jordan A, Baum J. Basic tear flow. Does it exist? Ophthalmology. 1980;87(9):920–30.

24. Collins M, Seeto R, Campbell L, Ross M. Blinking and corneal sensitivity. Acta Ophthalmol. 1989;67(5):525–31.

25. Ang RT, Dartt DA, Tsubota K. Dry eye after refractive surgery. Curr Opin Ophthalmol. 2001;12(4):318–22.

26. Battat L, Macri A, Dursun D, Pflugfelder SC. Effects of laser in situ keratomileusis on tear production, clearance, and the ocular surface. Ophthalmology. 2001;108(7):1230–5.

27. Wilson SE. Laser in situ keratomileusis–induced (presumed) neurotrophic epitheliopathy. Ophthalmology. 2001;108(6):1082–7.

28. Benitez-del-Castillo JM, del Rio T, Iradier T, et al. Decrease in tear secretion and corneal sensitivity after laser in situ keratomileusis. Cornea. 2001;20(1):30–2.

29. Donnenfeld ED, Perry HD, Ehrenhaus M, et al. The effect of hinge position on corneal sensation and dry eye signs and symptoms. New Orleans: 2001, American Academy of Ophthalmology.

30. Smith J, Steinemann TL. Vitamin A deficiency and the eye. Int Ophthalmol Clin. 2000;40(4):83–91.

31. Sommer HJ, Johnen J, Schongen P, Stolze HH. Adaptation of the tear film to work in air-conditioned rooms (office-eye syndrome). German J Ophthalmol. 1994;3(6):406–8.

32. Tsubota K, Nakamori K. Dry eyes and video display terminals. N Engl J Med. 1993;328(8):584.

33. Tsubota K, Fujita H, Tsuzaka K, Takeuchi T. Mikulicz's disease and Sjogren's syndrome. Invest Ophthalmol Vis Sci. 2000;41(7):1666–73.

34. Feenstra RP, Tseng SC. Comparison of fluorescein and rose bengal staining. Ophthalmology. 1992;99(4):605–17.

35. van Bijsterveld OP. Diagnostic tests in the sicca syndrome. Arch Ophthal. 1969;82(1):10–4.

36. Norn MS. Lissamine green. Vital staining of cornea and conjunctiva. Acta Ophthalmol. 1973;51(4):483–91.

37. Lemp MA, Holly FJ. Recent advances in ocular surface chemistry. Am J Optom Arch Am Acad Optom. 1970;47(9):669–72.

38. Mengher LS, Bron AJ, Tonge SR, Gilbert DJ. A non-invasive instrument for clinical assessment of the pre-corneal tear film stability. Curr Eye Res. 1985;4(1):1–7.

39. Schirmer O. Studien zur Physiologie und Pathologie der Tranenabsonderung und Tranenabfuhr. Albrecht von Graefes Arch Ophthalmol. 1903;56:197–291.

40. Jones LT. The lacrimal secretory system and its treatment. J All India Ophthalmol Soc. 1966;14(5):191–6.

41. Afonso AA, Monroy D, Stern ME, et al. Correlation of tear fluorescein clearance and Schirmer test scores with ocular irritation symptoms. Ophthalmology. 1999;106(4):803–10.

42. Hamano T, Mitsunaga S, Kotani S, et al. Tear volume in relation to contact lens wear and age. CLAO J. 1990;16(1):57–61.

43. Sakamoto R, Bennett ES, Henry VA, et al. The phenol red thread tear test: a cross-cultural study. Invest Ophthalmol Vis Sci. 1993;34(13):3510–4.

44. Macri A, Pflugfelder S. Correlation of the Schirmer 1 and fluorescein clearance tests with the severity of corneal epithelial and eyelid disease. Arch Ophthalmol. 2000;118(12):1632–8.

45. Pflugfelder SC, Tseng SC, Sanabria O, et al. Evaluation of subjective assessments and objective diagnostic tests for diagnosing tear-film disorders known to cause ocular irritation. Cornea. 1998;17(1):38–56.

46. Vivino FB, Al-Hashimi I, Khan Z, et al. Pilocarpine tablets for the treatment of dry mouth and dry eye symptoms in patients with Sjogren syndrome: a randomized, placebo-controlled, fixed-dose, multicenter trial. P92-01 Study Group. Arch Intern Med. 1999;159(2):174–81.

47. Sieg P, Geerling G, Kosmehl H, et al. Microvascular submandibular gland transfer for severe cases of keratoconjunctivitis sicca. Plast Reconstr Surg. 2000;106(3):554–60; discussion 561–2.

48. Marsh P, Pflugfelder SC. Topical nonpreserved methylprednisolone therapy for keratoconjunctivitis sicca in Sjogren syndrome. Ophthalmology. 1999;106(4):811–6.

49. Kunert KS, Tisdale AS, Stern ME, et al. Analysis of topical cyclosporine treatment of patients with dry eye syndrome: effect on conjunctival lymphocytes. Arch Ophthalmol. 2000;118(11):1489–96.

CHAPTER

66

Corneal and External Eye Manifestations of Systemic Disease

ANNA C. NEWLIN • JOEL SUGAR

DEFINITION
• Disorders with cornea and external eye manifestations as part of systemic syndromes.

KEY FEATURE
• Anterior segment anomalies as well as systemic abnormalities.

ASSOCIATED FEATURE
• Usually genetic defect with multisystem clinical findings.

INTRODUCTION

As seen in many sections throughout this book, the eye commonly exhibits manifestations of more widespread systemic disorders. Although these disorders are too numerous to discuss at length, this chapter presents in tabular form some of the conditions that involve the cornea and external eye. The grouping of these presentations is in some cases obvious and in others more arbitrary. In many, if not most, cases, the listings are incomplete, because the intention is to present only disorders that have corneal and external ocular findings. Many other disorders are discussed elsewhere in this book. Where it is appropriate and information is available, genetic localizations are provided.

CONGENITAL DISORDERS

Congenital disorders are nonmetabolic disorders present at birth that have generalized systemic findings as well as ocular abnormalities of the anterior portion of the eye. These groupings are arbitrary and may change as genetic information allows more specific categorizations. Some of the craniofacial malformation syndromes with associated corneal and external disease findings are given in Table 66-1. These disorders usually are readily recognizable. Their management requires a multidisci-

plinary approach with involvement of ophthalmologists, facial plastic surgeons, neurosurgeons, and others.

CHROMOSOMAL DISORDERS

The chromosomal disorders are defined by the location of the abnormality in the genetic material (Table 66-2). In the future, a more thorough understanding of the regulatory or other gene mechanisms involved will allow better interpretation of the widespread, multisystemic findings in these disorders (see Chapter 2). It is often striking how different chromosomal defects may lead to similar phenotypic abnormalities.

INHERITED CONNECTIVE TISSUE DISORDERS

Some of the inherited connective tissue disorders are given in Table 66-3. More detailed discussions of these disorders are found elsewhere in this text (see Chapter 59).

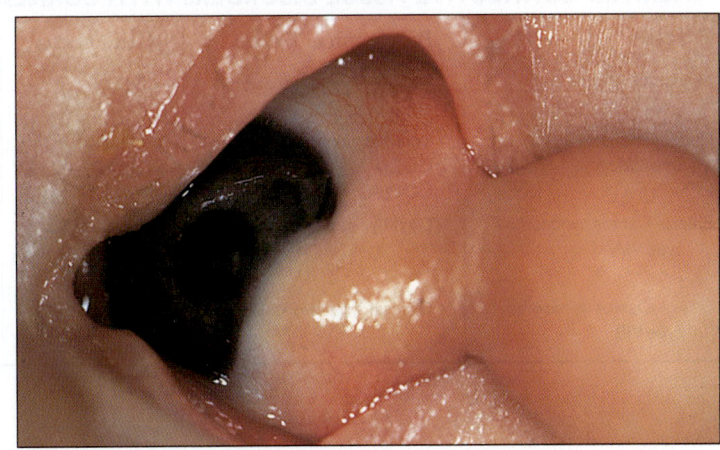

FIG. 66-1 ■ **Goldenhar's syndrome.** Pedunculated temporal limbal dermoid present in a patient who had Goldenhar's syndrome. (With permission from Ziavras E, Farber MG, Diamond G. A pedunculated lipodermoid in oculoauriculovertebral dysplasia. Arch Ophthalmol. 1990;108:1032–3.)

TABLE 66-1

CRANIOFACIAL MALFORMATION SYNDROMES WITH CORNEAL INVOLVEMENT

Syndrome	Ocular Manifestations	Systemic Manifestations	Gene Locus
Crouzon and Apert	Shallow orbits, decreased motility, secondary corneal exposure	Craniofacial malformation and syndactyly (Apert)	10q26[1]
Meyer-Schwickerath (oculodentodigital dysplasia)	Microphthalmos and microcornea	Syndactyly, dysplastic tooth enamel	6q22–q24[2]
Goldenhar (oculoauriculovertebral dysplasia)	Limbal dermoids, microphthalmos, anophthalmos, lid notching, blepharophimosis (Fig. 66-1[3])	Facial asymmetry, vertebral anomalies, ear deformities	
Hallermann–Streiff	Microphthalmos, spontaneously resorbing cataracts, macular pigment changes, Coats' disease	Facial malformation, hypoplastic mandible, short stature, skin atrophy	

TABLE 66-2

CHROMOSOMAL DISORDERS WITH CORNEAL MANIFESTATIONS

Genetic Findings	Ocular Manifestations	Systemic Manifestations
13q deletion	Hypertelorism, ptosis, epicanthal folds, microphthalmos, retinoblastoma	Microcephaly, facial malformation, absent thumbs
18p deletion	Ptosis, epicanthal folds, hypertelorism, corneal opacity, keratoconus, microphthalmos	Brachycephaly, growth retardation, mental retardation
18q deletion	Hypertelorism, epicanthal folds, nystagmus, corneal opacity, microphthalmos, corneal staphyloma, microcornea	Growth retardation, mental retardation, facial malformation, microcephaly
18r	Same as 18p deletion, 18q deletion	Growth retardation, mental retardation, facial malformation, microcephaly
4p deletion (Wolf–Hirschhorn syndrome)	Hypertelorism, ptosis, microphthalmos, strabismus, cataract	Growth retardation, microcephaly, micrognathia, hypotonia seizures
Ring D chromosome	Ptosis, epicanthal folds, microphthalmos, strabismus, nystagmus	Mental retardation, microcephaly, facial malformation
Turner syndrome (45 × 0)[4]	Ptosis, epicanthal folds, strabismus, rarely microcornea, blue sclera, corneal opacity	Female, short stature, webbed neck
Trisomy 13 (Patau syndrome)	Microphthalmos, corneal opacity, Peters' anomaly, cataract, retinal dysplasia (Fig. 66-2)	Microcephaly, cleft lip and palate, low set ears
Trisomy 18 (Edwards syndrome)	Corneal opacity, ptosis, epicanthal folds, microphthalmos, colobomas, cataract, retinal dysplasia	Low birth weight; failure to thrive; brain hypoplasia; cardiac, gastrointestinal, renal, and musculoskeletal anomalies
Trisomy 21 (Down syndrome)	Shortened, slanted palpebral fissure, neonatal ectropion, later trichiasis and entropion, keratoconus, cataract	Cardiac defects, mental retardation, short stature, characteristic facies
Partial trisomy 22 (cat's eye syndrome)	Microphthalmos, hypertelorism, colobomas	Mental retardation, microcephaly, cardiac anomalies, ear anomalies, anal atresia

TABLE 66-3

INHERITED CONNECTIVE TISSUE DISORDERS WITH CORNEAL MANIFESTATIONS

Disease	Biochemical Defect	Gene Locus	Ocular Manifestations	Systemic Manifestations
Marfan syndrome[5]	Fibrillin-1 gene mutations	15q21.1	Megalocornea, lens subluxation, high myopia, retinal detachment	Long extremities, lax joints, aortic/mitral dilatation, aortic dissection
Osteogenesis imperfecta[6]	Type I procollagen COL1A1 COL1A2	17q21.31–q22 7q22.1	Blue sclera, keratoconus, megalocornea, optic nerve compression	Bone deformities, otosclerosis, dental anomalies
Ehlers–Danlos syndrome type VIA[7]	Lysyl hydroxylase	1p36.3–p36.2	Blue sclera, keratoconus, keratoglobus, lens subluxation, myopia, ocular fragility to trauma	Skin stretching, scarring joint hypermobility, scoliosis
Ehlers–Danlos syndrome type VIB[7]	Normal lysyl hydroxylase	Unknown	Same as VIA	Same as VIA

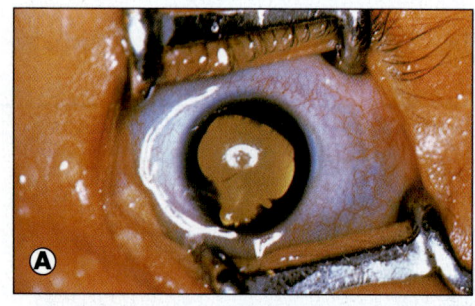 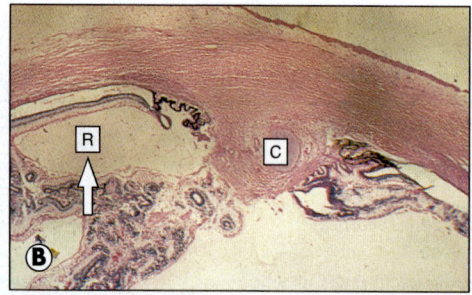 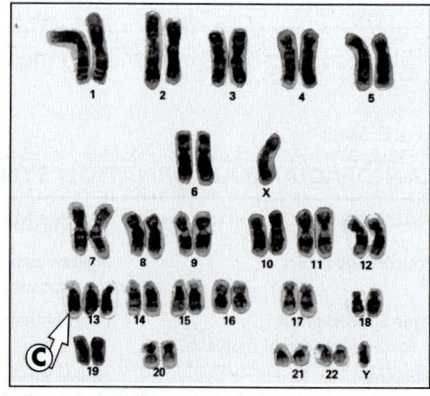

FIG. 66-2 ■ **Trisomy 13. A,** An inferior nasal iris coloboma and leukokoria are present. **B,** A coloboma of the ciliary body is filled with mesenchymal tissue that contains cartilage *(C)*; note the retinal dysplasia *(R)*. Generally, in trisomy 13, cartilage is present in eyes less than 10mm in size. **C,** A karyotype shows an extra chromosome in group 13 *(arrow).* (**A,** Courtesy of Shaffer DB. In: Yanoff M, Fine BS. Ocular pathology, 4th ed. London: Mosby; 1996. **C,** Courtesy of Drs. B.S. Emanuel and W.J. Mellman. In: Yanoff M, Fine BS. Ocular pathology, ed 4. London: Mosby; 1996.)

TABLE 66-4

DISORDERS OF PROTEIN AND AMINO ACID METABOLISM

Disorder	Enzyme Deficiency	Gene Locus	Metabolite Accumulated	Mode of Inheritance	Ocular Manifestations	Systemic Manifestations
Cystinosis[8]	Probable defect of lysosomal cysteine transport protein	17p13	Cystine	Autosomal recessive	All forms—conjunctival and corneal cystine crystal deposition (needle-shaped, refractile, polychromatic crystals in full thickness of peripheral corneal and anterior central stroma), band keratopathy, photophobia. Infantile and adolescent forms—patchy retinal abnormalities, occasional macular changes (Fig. 66-3)	Infantile form, renal failure, death. Adolescent form, renal failure. Adult form, no renal failure
Tyrosinemia[9] type II (tyrosinosis, Richner–Hanhart syndrome)	Tyrosine transaminase deficiency	16q22.1–22.3	Tyrosine	Autosomal recessive	Dendritiform corneal epithelial changes (branches or snowflake opacities), red eye, photophobia	Palmar–plantar hyperkeratosis, mental retardation, growth retardation
Alkaptonuria[10]	Homogentisate-1, 2-dioxygenase	3q21–q23	Homogentisic acid	Autosomal recessive	Triangular patches of intrascleral pigmentation near insertion of horizontal rectus muscles, "oil-droplet" opacities in limbal corneal epithelium and Bowman's layer, pigmented pingueculae, irregular pigmented granules in episclera, no functional changes	Joint pain and stiffness
Wilson disease[11]	Defective excretion of copper from hepatic lysosomes	13q14.3–q21.1	Copper	Autosomal recessive	Kayser–Fleischer ring, "sunflower" cataract (Fig. 66-4)[12]	Liver dysfunction, spasticity, behavior disturbance, nephrotic syndrome
Lattice dystrophy type II (Meretoja syndrome)[13]	Gelsolin gene defect	9q34	Amyloid	Autosomal dominant	Lattice dystrophy, ptosis, glaucoma	Progressive cranial neuropathy, cardiac disease

METABOLIC DISORDERS

A number of systemic metabolic disorders of genetic origin affect the anterior portion of the eye. These disorders usually are autosomal recessive, and a single enzyme deficiency accounts for the clinical manifestations. In many of these disorders, the specific gene locus has been determined, as has the biochemical defect. Unlike the corneal changes in many of the corneal dystrophies, the corneal changes in metabolic disorders may involve more than one layer of the cornea, affect the peripheral as well as the central cornea, and progress over time. The disorders are subdivided according to the biochemical group in which the abnormality is found.

Protein and Amino Acid Metabolic Defects

Protein and amino acid metabolic defects are listed in Table 66-4. These disorders are quite diverse, both clinically and biochemically.

Mucopolysaccharidoses

The mucopolysaccharidoses (Table 66-5) are a group of related disorders in which mucopolysaccharides or glycosaminoglycans are progressively accumulated in lysosomes. Glycosaminoglycans are carbohydrates made up of chains of uronic acids and amino and neutral sugars. These chains are joined to protein and form proteoglycans, the ground substance be-

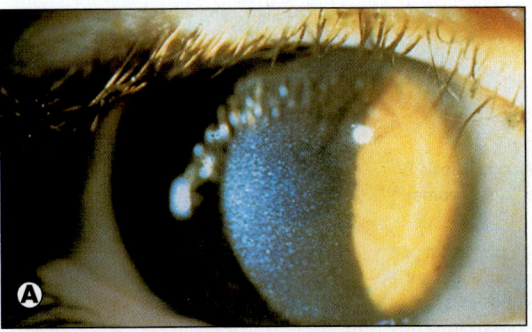

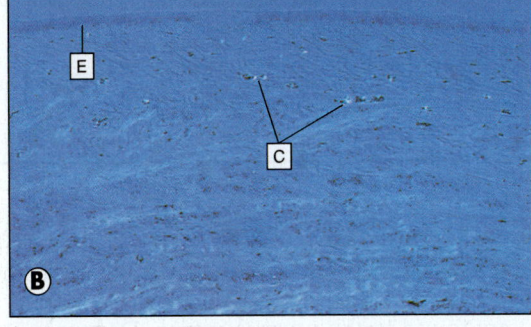

FIG. 66-3 ■ Cystinosis. **A**, Myriad tiny opacities give the cornea a cloudy appearance. **B**, Polarization of an unstained histological section of the cornea shows birefringent cystine crystals *(C)*. *E*, Epithelium. (**A**, Courtesy of Shaffer DB. In: Yanoff M, Fine BS. Ocular pathology, ed 4. London: Mosby; 1996.)

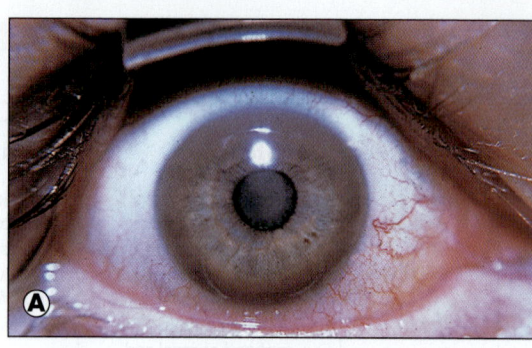
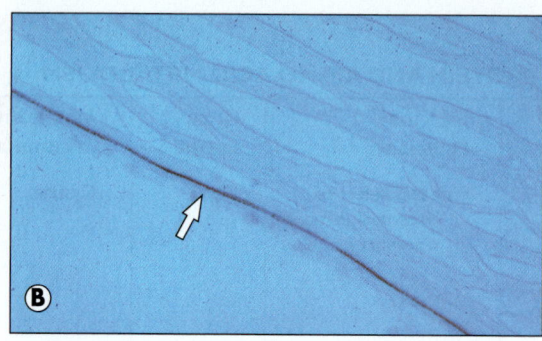

FIG. 66-4 ■ **Wilson's disease, Kayser-Fleischer ring. A,** The deposition of copper in the periphery of Descemet's membrane, seen as a brown color, partially obstructs the view of the underlying iris, especially superiorly. A "sunflower" (disciform) cataract is present in the lens of this patient who has Wilson's disease. **B,** An unstained section shows copper deposition *(arrow)* in the inner portion of peripheral Descemet's membrane. (Modified from Tso MOM, Fine BS, Thorpe HE. Kayser-Fleischer ring and associated cataract in Wilson's disease. Am J Ophthalmol. 1975;79:479–88.)

TABLE 66-5

THE MUCOPOLYSACCHARIDOSES

Disorder	Enzyme Deficiency	Metabolite Accumulated	Mode of Inheritance	Gene Locus	Ocular Manifestations	Systemic Manifestations
Mucopolysaccharidosis I-H (Hurler syndrome)[14]	α-L-Iduronidase	Heparan sulfate Dermatan sulfate	Autosomal recessive	4p16.3	Corneal clouding, pigmentary retinopathy, optic atrophy, trabecular involvement	Gargoyle facies, mental retardation, dwarfism, skeletal dysplasia
Mucopolysaccharidosis I-S (Scheie syndrome)	α-L-Iduronidase	Heparan sulfate Dermatan sulfate	Autosomal recessive	4p16.3	Corneal clouding, pigmentary retinopathy, optic atrophy, glaucoma	Coarse facies, claw-like hands, aortic valve disease
Mucopolysaccharidosis I-H/S (Hurler–Scheie syndrome; Fig. 66-5)	α-L-Iduronidase	Heparan sulfate Dermatan sulfate	Autosomal recessive	4p16.3	Corneal clouding, pigmentary retinopathy, optic atrophy (Fig. 66-5)	More severe than I-S, less severe than I-H
Mucopolysaccharidosis II (Hunter syndrome)[15]	Iduronate sulfate sulfatase (iduronate sulfatase)	Heparan sulfate Dermatan sulfate	X-Linked recessive	Xq28	Rare corneal clouding, pigmentary retinopathy, optic atrophy	Similar to I-H with less bony deformity
Mucopolysaccharidosis III (Sanfilippo syndrome)[16,17]	A: heparan-S-sulfaminidase (heparan sulfate N-sulfatase) B: α-N-acteyl-glucosaminidase (N-acetyl D-glucosaminidase) C: acetyl-CoA-glucosaminidase-N, N-acetyltransferase D: N-acetylglucosamine-6-sulfate sulfatase	Heparan sulfate	Autosomal recessive	17q25.3 17q21.1 12q14 Chr #14	All forms: clinically clear cornea, occasional slit-lamp corneal opacities (mucopolysaccharide accumulation in intracytoplasmic vacuoles in keratocytes, endothelium and epithelium), pigmentary retinopathy, optic atrophy	All forms: mild dysmorphism, progressive dementia
Mucopolysaccharidosis IV (Morquio syndrome)[18,19]	A: galactose-6-sulfatase B: β-galactosidase	Keratan sulfate	Autosomal recessive Autosomal recessive	16q24.3 3p21.33	Corneal clouding, optic atrophy	Severe bony deformity, aortic valve disease, normal intelligence
Mucopolysaccharidosis V (reclassified as mucopolysaccharidosis I-S)						
Mucopolysaccharidosis VI (Maroteaux–Lamy syndrome)	N-acetylgalactosamine-4-sulfatase	Dermatan sulfate	Autosomal recessive	5q11–q13	Corneal clouding, optic atrophy	Similar to I-H, but normal intellect
Mucopolysaccharidosis VII (Sly syndrome)	β-Glucuronidase	Dermatan sulfate Heparan sulfate	Autosomal recessive	7q21.1	Corneal clouding	Similar to I-H

tween the collagen fibrils in the corneal stroma. Keratan sulfate (lumican) and chondroitin sulfate or dermatan sulfate (decorin) are found in the normal cornea. Dermatan sulfate is also found in corneal scars. In the mucopolysaccharidoses, deficiency in a catabolic enzyme results in accumulation of glycosaminoglycan. The excess of dermatan sulfate and keratan sulfate in the cornea produces corneal clouding, while excess heparan sulfate results in retinal and central nervous system dysfunction.

Sphingolipidoses

The sphingolipidoses also arise from dysfunction of catabolic enzymes that results in accumulation of sphingolipids (Table

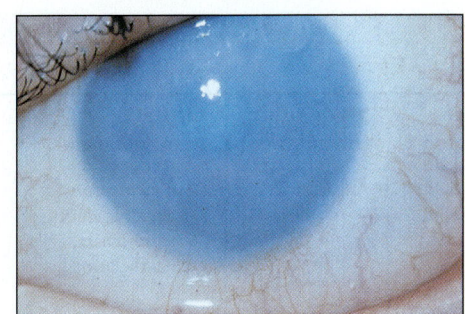

FIG. 66-5 ■ The mucopolysaccharidoses. The cornea is clouded diffusely in this case of Hurler-Scheie syndrome. (Courtesy of Shaffer DB. In: Yanoff M, Fine BS. Ocular pathology, ed 4. London: Mosby; 1996.)

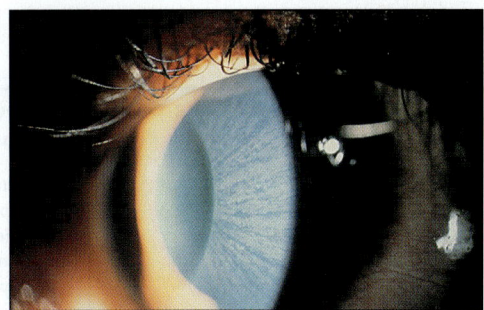

FIG. 66-6 ■ Fabry's disease. Verticillate changes in the cornea of a carrier.

TABLE 66-6

THE SPHINGOLIPIDOSES

Disorder	Enzyme Deficiency	Gene Locus	Metabolite Accumulated	Mode of Inheritance	Ocular Manifestations	Systemic Manifestations
GM₂ gangliosidosis II (Sandhoff disease)	Hexosaminidase B, HEX B chain	5q13	Ganglioside GM₂	Autosomal recessive	Membrane-bound vacuoles within corneal keratocytes, cherry-red macula	Psychomotor retardation, hepatosplenomegaly
Metachromatic leukodystrophy (Austin's juvenile form)[20,21]	Arylsulfatase A isozymes	22q13.31-qter	Sulfatide	Autosomal recessive	Corneal clouding	Mental retardation, seizures
Fabry disease[22]	α-Galactosidase	Xq22	Ceramide trihexoside	X-Linked recessive	Conjunctival and retinal vascular tortuosity, white granular anterior subcapsular lens opacities, oculomotor abnormalities, whorl-like corneal epithelial changes (cornea verticillata; Fig. 66-6)	Renal failure, peripheral neuropathy

TABLE 66-7

THE DYSLIPOPROTEINEMIAS[23]

Disorder	Deficiency	Gene Locus	Metabolite Accumulated	Mode of Inheritance	Ocular Manifestations	Systemic Manifestations
Lecithin–cholesterol acyltransferase deficiency[24]	Lecithin–cholesterol acyltransferase	16q22.1	Free cholesterol	Autosomal recessive	Dense peripheral arcus, diffuse grayish dots in central stroma, no visual changes	Atherosclerosis, renal insufficiency
Fish eye disease (high-density lipoprotein lecthin–cholesterol acyltransferase)[25]	α-Lecithin–cholesterol acyltransferase	16q22.1	Triglycerides, very low density lipoproteins; low-density lipoproteins	Autosomal dominant	Progressive gray–white–yellow dot corneal clouding, increased corneal thickness	None
Tangier disease (analphalipoproteinemia)	High-density lipoprotein	9q22–q31	Triglycerides (low high-density lipoproteins, cholesterol and phospholipids)	Autosomal recessive	Fine dot corneal clouding, severe visual loss, incomplete eyelid closure, ectropion, no arcus	Lymphadenopathy hepatosplenomegaly, coronary artery disease
Hyperlipoproteinemia I (hyperchylomicronemia)[26]	Lipoprotein lipase	8p22	Triglycerides, chylomicrons	Autosomal recessive	Lipemia retinalis, palpebral eruptive xanthomata	Xanthomas

Continued

66-6). A number of sphingolipidoses in which corneal abnormalities do not occur have been described but are not included in this discussion.

Dyslipoproteinemias

The dyslipoproteinemias (Table 66-7) are an often vague group of disorders because of the large number of lipid metabolic processes that exist. They are characterized by accumulation of lipid in the cornea, in retinal blood vessels, or in the eyelid skin. Greater understanding of these disorders has led to the subdivision of some categories and more specific nomenclature based on the pathophysiological processes involved.

Mucolipidoses

The mucolipidoses are characterized by the presence of abnormalities in the carbohydrate moiety of both glycoprotein and glycolipid. Oligosaccharides accumulate, which results in changes similar to those seen in the mucopolysaccharidoses and the sphingolipidoses (Table 66-8).

OCULAR ANATOMICAL DISORDERS

Although such a classification of disorders is not biochemically rational, it does provide a framework within which potential associations between disorders that involve both nonocular organs and the eye may be considered. The corneorenal syndromes are

TABLE 66-7

THE DYSLIPOPROTEINEMIAS[23]—cont'd

Disorder	Deficiency	Gene Locus	Metabolite Accumulated	Mode of Inheritance	Ocular Manifestations	Systemic Manifestations
Hyperlipoproteinemia II hyper-β-lipoproteinemia IIa hyper-β-lipoproteinemia IIb	Thought to be defective or absent low-density lipoprotein receptors		Low-density lipoproteins, cholesterol Low-density lipoproteins, very low density lipoproteins, cholesterol, triglycerides, hypertriglyceridemia	Autosomal dominant	Both forms; corneal arcus, conjunctival xanthomata, xanthelasma	Coronary artery disease
Hyperlipoproteinemia III (dys-β-lipoproteinemia; broad β-disease)	Defective remnant metabolism in the liver caused by an abnormality in apolipoprotein E	19q13.2	Very low density lipoprotein remnants, cholesterol, triglycerides	Autosomal recessive with pseudo dominance	Arcus, xanthelasma, lipemia retinalis	Peripheral vascular disease, diabetes mellitus
Hyperlipoproteinemia IV (hyperpre-β-lipoproteinemia)	Unknown		Triglycerides, very low density lipoproteins, cholesterol usually normal	Autosomal dominant	Arcus, xanthelasma, lipemia, retinalis	Vascular disease, diabetes mellitus
Hyperlipoproteinemia V (hyperprelipoproteinemia and hyperchylomicronemia)	Unknown		Very low density lipoproteins, chylomicrons	Unknown	Lipemia retinalis, no arcus	Xanthomas, hepatosplenomegaly

TABLE 66-8

THE MUCOLIPIDOSES

Disorder	Enzyme Deficiency	Gene Locus	Metabolite Accumulated	Mode of Inheritance	Ocular Manifestations	Systemic Manifestations
Mucolipidosis I (dysmorphic sialidosis, Spranger syndrome)[27]	Glycoprotein sialidase (neuraminidase I)	6p21.3	Unknown	Autosomal recessive	Macular cherry-red spot, tortuous retinal and conjunctival vessels, spoke-like lens opacities, progressive corneal clouding	Coarse facies, hearing loss, normal IQ
Mucolipidosis II (I-cell disease)[28]	GluNac-1-phosphotransferase	4q21–q23	Increased plasma lysosomal hydrolases	Autosomal recessive	Small orbits, hypoplastic supraorbital ridges and prominent eyes, glaucoma, megalocornea, corneal clouding	Hurler-like facies, mental retardation
Mucolipidosis III (pseudo-Hurler polydystrophy)[29]	GluNac-1-phosphotransferase	4q21–q23	Increased plasma lysosomal hydrolases	Autosomal recessive	Corneal clouding	Milder growth and mental retardation
Mucolipidosis IV (Berman syndrome)	Possible ganglioside sialidase	19p13.3–p13.2	Sialogangliosides	Autosomal recessive	Corneal clouding, retinal degeneration	Slowed psychomotor development
Goldberg syndrome (galactosialidosis)	β-Galactosidase Neuraminidase	20q13.1	Unknown	Autosomal recessive	Macular cherry-red spot, diffuse mild corneal clouding, conjunctival telangiectases	Seizures, mental retardation, hearing loss, hemangiomas
Mannosidosis[30]	α-D-Mannosidase	19cen–21q	Unknown	Autosomal recessive	No corneal abnormalities or mild corneal clouding, lens opacities	Coarse facies, mental retardation, hearing loss
Fucosidosis	α-L-Fucosidase	1p34	Unknown	Autosomal recessive		Coarse facies, mental retardation, angiokeratoma

TABLE 66-9

CORNEORENAL SYNDROMES

Syndrome	Gene Locus	Ocular Manifestations	Systemic Manifestations
Alport mainly X-linked dominant	Xq22.3 COL4A5	Posterior polymorphous corneal dystrophy, juvenile arcus, pigment dispersion, lenticonus, retinal pigmentary changes	Renal failure, hearing loss
Also X-linked recessive and autosomal recessive	2q36–q37 COL4A3-COL4A4		
Cystinosis	17p13	See Figure 66-3	Infantile form: renal failure, death Intermediate form: renal failure Adult form: no renal failure
Fabry disease	Xq22	See Figure 66-6	Renal failure, peripheral neuropathy
Lowe syndrome (oculocerebrorenal)	Xq26.1	Corneal keloids, glaucoma, cataracts	Mental retardation, amino acid urea, renal tubular acidosis, angiokeratomas
Wegener granulomatosis	Nongenetic	Marginal keratitis, scleritis, episcleritis	Granulomatous vasculitis of lungs, kidneys, nasopharynx
WAGR	11p13	Superficial corneal opacity and vascularization, aniridia, glaucoma, foveal hypoplasia, optic nerve hypoplasia	Wilms' tumor, mental retardation, craniofacial anomalies, growth retardation
Zellweger	2p15(PEX13) 1q22 12p13.3(PEX5) 7q21–q22(PEX1) 6q23–q24	Axenfeld's anomaly, corneal clouding, glaucoma, retinal degeneration	Craniofacial anomalies, hypotonia seizures, retardation, hepatic degeneration, cystic kidneys, cardiac defects, early death

WAGR, Wilms' tumor, aniridia, genital anomalies, and mental retardation.

TABLE 66-10

HEPATOCORNEAL SYNDROMES

Syndrome	Gene Locus	Ocular Manifestations	Systemic Manifestations
Gaucher disease	1q21	Prominent pingueculae, white deposits in corneal epithelium, vitreous opacities, paramacular gray ring	Hepatosplenomegaly, bone pain, accumulation of glucocerebroside
Wilson disease	13q14.3–q21.1	Kayser–Fleisher ring (see Fig. 66-4)	Liver dysfunction; neurological dysfunction with dysarthria, spasticity, behavior disturbances
Zellweger syndrome	7q21–q22	See Table 66-9	See Table 66-9
Alagille syndrome[31]	20p11.2–p12	Posterior embryotoxon, anterior chamber anomalies, eccentric or ectopic pupils, chorioretinal atrophy, retinal pigment clumping	Cholestatic liver disease, structural heart defects

a disparate group of disorders in which corneal abnormalities combine with renal disease (Table 66-9). The hepatocorneal syndromes are less common (Table 66-10). The cutaneous disorders with anterior segment ocular findings are numerous, and only a few are listed here (see Table 66-11). This tabular review serves to emphasize the frequent associations between systemic disorders and the cornea and external eye. Numerous other disorders exist but are not included in this summary.

CONCLUSION

This brief overview of systemic diseases with corneal involvement, even though incomplete, emphasizes the importance of taking into account the whole patient, not just the cornea or the eye. As our understanding of the basic mechanisms involved in the disorders discussed increases, these conditions will be important areas for new therapeutic interventions.

TABLE 66-11

CUTANEOUS DISORDERS

Syndrome	Gene Locus	Ocular Manifestations	Cutaneous/Systemic Manifestations
Basal cell nevus syndrome	9q22.3, 9q31, 1p32	Multiple basal cell carcinomas of the eyelid, hypertelorism	Multiple basal cell carcinomas, jaw cysts, bony anomalies
Xeroderma pigmentosum	3p25	Lid neoplasms, conjunctival and corneal neoplasia, corneal exposure, drying	Basal cell carcinoma, squamous cell carcinomas, and malignant melanomas develop in sun-exposed areas
Ichthyosis (multiple types)	1q21, 12q11-q13, 14q11.2, X922.32, 19p12-q12	Eyelid and lash scaling (all types), ectropion with corneal exposure (lamellar ichthyosis)	Scaly skin
Keratitis–ichthyosis–deafness syndrome		Keratoconjunctivitis with corneal pannus formation	Ichthyosis, deafness
Epidermolysis bullosa (numerous types)	1q32, 1q25–q31, 10q24.3	Corneal epithelial cysts, blebs, corneal erosions, corneal scarring, conjunctival bullae, eyelid deformities	Skin blistering, contractures in severe dystrophic type
Ectrodactyly–ectodermal dysplasia–clefting	7p11.2–q21.3	Dysplasia of meibomian glands, blepharitis, corneal pannus formation, corneal scarring	Lobster-claw deformity of hands and feet, ectodermal dysplasia, cleft lip and palate
Porphyria (numerous types)		Corneal conjunctival and eyelid scarring, scleral necrosis	Photosensitivity of skin
Richner–Hanhart syndrome (tyrosinemia type II)	16q22.1–q22.3	See Table 66-4	See Table 66-4

REFERENCES

1. Wilkie AO, Slaney SF, Oldridge M, et al. Apert syndrome results from localized mutations of FGFR2 and is allelic with Crouzon syndrome. Nat Genet. 1995;9:165–72.
2. Gladwin A, Donnai D, Metcalfe K, et al. Localization of a gene for oculodentodigital syndrome to human chromosome 6q22-q24. Hum Mol Genet. 1997; 6:123–7.
3. Ziavras E, Farber MG, Diamond G. A pedunculated lipodermoid in oculoauriculovertebral dysplasia. Arch Ophthalmol. 1990;108:1032–33.
4. Chrousos GA, Ross JL, Chrousos G, et al. Ocular findings in Turner syndrome. Ophthalmology. 1984;91:926–8.
5. Ramirez F. Fibrillin mutations in Marfan syndrome and related phenotypes. Curr Opin Genet Dev. 1996;6:309–15.
6. Willing MC, Pruchno CJ, Byers PH. Molecular heterogeneity in osteogenesis imperfecta type I. Am J Med Genet. 1993;45:223–7.
7. Hautala T, Byers MG, Eddy RL, et al. Cloning of human lysyl hydroxylase: complete cDNA-derived amino acid sequence and assignment of the gene (PLOD) to chromosome 1p36.3-p36.2. Genomics. 1992;13:62–9.
8. Jean G, Fuchshuber A, Town MM, et al. High-resolution mapping of the gene for cystinosis, using combined biochemical and linkage analysis. Am J Hum Genet. 1996;58:535–43.
9. Natt E, Kida K, Odievre M, et al. Point mutations in the tyrosine aminotransferase gene in tyrosinemia type II. Proc Natl Acad Sci U S A. 1992;89:9297–301.
10. Fernandez-Canon JM, Granadino B, Beltran-Valero de Bernabe D, et al. The molecular basis of alkaptonuria. Nat Genet. 1996;14:19–24.
11. Thomas GR, Roberts EA, Walshe JM, Cox DW. Haplotypes and mutations in Wilson disease. Am J Hum Genet. 1995;56:1315–9.
12. Tso MOM, Fine BS, Thorpe HE. Kayser-Fleischer ring and associated cataract in Wilson's disease. Am J Ophthalmol. 1975;79:479–88.
13. Haltia M, Levy E, Meretoja J, et al. Gelsolin gene mutation—at codon 187—in familial amyloidosis, Finnish: DNA-diagnostic assay. Am J Med Genet. 1992;42:357–9.
14. Scott HS, Ashton LJ, Eyre HY, et al. Chromosomal localization of the human alpha-L-iduronidase gene (IDUA) to 4p16.3. Am J Hum Genet. 1990;47:802–7.
15. Wilson JP, Meaney CA, Hopwood JJ, Morris CP. Sequence of the human iduronate 2-sulfatase (IDS) gene. Genomics. 1993;17:773–5.
16. Zhao HG, Li HH, Bach G, et al. The molecular basis of Sanfilippo syndrome type B. Proc Natl Acad Sci U S A. 1996;93:6101–5.
17. Zaremba J, Kleijer WJ, Huijmans JG, et al. Chromosomes 14 and 21 as possible candidates for mapping the gene for Sanfilippo disease type IIIC. J Med Genet. 1992;29:514.
18. Tomatsu S, Fukuda S, Yamagishi A, et al. Mucopolysaccharidosis IV A: four new exotic mutations in patients with N-acetylgalactosamine-6-sulfate deficiency. Am J Hum Genet. 1996;58:950–62.
19. Takano T, Yamanouchi Y, et al. Assignment of human beta-galactosidase-A gene to 3p21.33 by fluorescence in situ hybridization. Hum Genet. 1993;92:403–4.
20. Stein C, Gieselmann V, Kreysing J, et al. Cloning and expression of human arylsulfatase A. J Biol Chem. 1989;264:1252–9.
21. Gieselmann V, Zlotogora J, Harris A, et al. Molecular genetics of metachromatic leukodystrophy. Hum Mutat. 1994;4:233–42.
22. Bishop DF, Calhoun DH, Bernstein HS, et al. Human alpha galactosidase A; nucleotide sequence of a cDNA clone encoding the mature enzyme. Proc Natl Acad Sci U S A. 1986;83:4859–63.
23. Barchiesi BJ, Eckel RH, Ellis PP. The cornea and disorders of lipid metabolism. Surv Ophthalmol. 1991;36:1–22.
24. McLain J, Fielding C, Drayna D, et al. Cloning and expression of human lecithin–cholesterol acyltransferase cDNA. Proc Natl Acad Sci U S A. 1986;83:2335–9.
25. Funke H, von Eckardstein A, Pritchard PH, et al. A molecular defect causing fish eye disease: an amino acid exchange in lecithin–cholesterol acyltransferase (LCAT) leads to the selective loss of alpha-LCAT activity. Proc Natl Acad Sci U S A. 1991;88:4855–9.
26. Ma Y, Henderson HE, Venmurthy MR, et al. A mutation in the human lipoprotein lipase gene as the most common cause of familial chylomicronemia in French Canadians. N Engl J Med. 1991;324:1761–6.
27. Bonton E, van der Spoel A, Fornerod M, et al. Characterization of human lysosomal neuraminidase defines the molecular basis of the metabolic storage disorder sialidosis. Genes Dev. 1996;10:3156–69.
28. Mueller OT, Honey NK, Little LE, et al. Mucolipidosis II and III: the genetic relationships between two disorders of lysosomal enzyme biosynthesis. J Clin Invest. 1983;72:1016–23.
29. Mueller OT, Wasmuth JJ, Murray JC, et al. Chromosomal assignment of N-acetylglucosaminylophosphotransferase, the lysosomal hydrolase targeting enzyme deficient in mucolipidosis II and III. Cell Genet. 1987;46:664.
30. Nebes VL, Schmidt MC. Human lysosomal alpha-mannosidase: isolation and nucleotide sequence of the full-length cDNA. Biochem Biophys Res Commun. 1994;200:239–45.
31. Hol FA, Hamel BCJ, Geurds MPA, et al. Localization of Alagille syndrome to 20p11.2–p12 by linkage analysis of a three-generation family. Hum Genet. 1995; 95:687–90.

CHAPTER
67

Tumors of Conjunctiva and Cornea

JAMES J. AUGSBURGER • SUSAN SCHNEIDER

DEFINITION
- Malignant and benign neoplasms, choristomas, and hamartomas arising from or within tissues of the anterior ocular walls and its coverings

KEY FEATURES
- Solid mass or discrete lesion of cornea, conjunctiva, or both
- Principal categories include the following:
  1. Tumors of stratified squamous epithelium
  2. Melanocytic tumors
  3. Lymphoid tumors
  4. Choristomatous tumors
  5. Miscellaneous other tumors

TUMORS OF STRATIFIED SQUAMOUS EPITHELIUM

Tumors of the stratified squamous epithelium of the conjunctiva and cornea encompass a wide spectrum of lesions, ranging from benign disturbances of epithelial maturation (actinic keratosis, pseudoepitheliomatous hyperplasia) to frankly malignant neoplasms (squamous cell carcinoma and its variants). Although advanced malignant lesions frequently exhibit clearly invasive features, less advanced malignant lesions typically resemble their benign counterparts quite closely. Consequently, lesions of the conjunctiva and cornea suspected of being neoplasms of the stratified squamous epithelium should be excised (if possible) or a biopsy done to establish their histopathological nature and provide a sound basis for subsequent management.

EPIDEMIOLOGY AND PATHOGENESIS

Tumors of the stratified squamous epithelium of the conjunctiva and cornea are almost certainly the most common type of primary ocular neoplasm encountered in clinical practice around the world. The average annual incidence of squamous cell carcinoma of the conjunctiva across all age groups has been estimated to be approximately 17 to 20 cases per million persons per year.[1] For a population with an average life expectancy of 70 years, this average annual incidence translates to a cumulative lifetime incidence of approximately 1 case per 700 to 850 persons. By and large, they are tumors of older adults. They affect all racial groups and both sexes. Risk factors for occurrence of such tumors[2–4] include a history of repeated intense sunlight exposure, male sex, outdoor occupations, advanced age, cigarette smoking, a history of squamous cell carcinoma of the skin of the head and neck, blonde hair, light complexion, xeroderma pigmentosum, acquired immunodeficiency syndrome (AIDS), and conjunctival infection by human papilloma viruses 16 and 18.

The pathogenesis of tumors of the stratified squamous epithelium appears to be disordered maturation of the epithelium induced by various irritants. Cytogenetic studies of conjunctival squamous cell carcinomas have not revealed any consistent chromosomal or gene changes in tumor cells. Xeroderma pigmentosum, a rare autosomal recessive disorder, conveys a substantially increased risk of developing one or more neoplasms of the stratified squamous epithelium of the conjunctiva or cornea following sunlight exposure.[5] These tumors tend to develop much earlier in life than do typical squamous cell carcinomas of the conjunctiva and their variants. Persons with AIDS also tend to develop tumors of the stratified squamous epithelium of the conjunctiva and cornea at a younger age than do individuals without this disorder.[6] Their tumors also tend to be substantially more aggressive on average than the typical squamous cell carcinomas of the conjunctiva.

OCULAR MANIFESTATIONS

Tumors of the stratified squamous epithelium of the conjunctiva and cornea appear most frequently as focal epibulbar lesions at the corneoscleral limbus temporally or nasally. Three morphological patterns are most common. The *leukoplakic lesion* (Fig. 67-1) appears as a focal thickening of the stratified squamous cell epithelium with a superficial plaque of opaque white hyperkeratosis. The *papillomatous lesion* (Fig. 67-2) appears as a highly vascularized soft tissue mass. The *gelatinous lesion* (Fig. 67-3) appears as an ill-defined translucent thickening that is not usually as prominent as the papillomatous or leukoplakic lesions. When the disordered epithelial maturation involves the corneal epithelium, it frequently appears as a zone of translucent corneal epithelial clouding (Fig. 67-4) visible by slit-lamp biomicroscopy. The affected individual may or may not recognize the lesion. If symptomatic, the patient typically complains of mild foreign body sensation and visual blurring attributable to the lesion. Development of a neoplasm of the stratified squamous cell epithelium within the palpebral conjunctiva or in the superior or inferior fornix is extremely uncommon.

The larger the lesion, the greater the likelihood of its malignant histology. Other features indicative of probable malignant histology include prominent epibulbar vasculature of the lesion, corneoscleral or intraocular invasion, anterior orbital invasion, spontaneous bleeding, umbilication, and strong broad-based adhesion to the globe away from the limbus.[2,7–10]

DIAGNOSIS AND ANCILLARY TESTING

Clinical diagnosis of a probable or possible squamous cell carcinoma of the conjunctiva or cornea is based upon detection of a lesion having some or all of the findings mentioned in the preceding paragraph. Any discrete thickening of the conjunctiva associated with prominent conjunctival vasculature should probably be excised or sampled for biopsy without undue delay.

BASELINE EVALUATION

Patients with a suspected neoplasm of the stratified squamous epithelium of the conjunctiva or cornea require a comprehensive ophthalmologic evaluation, with mapping of the lesion at

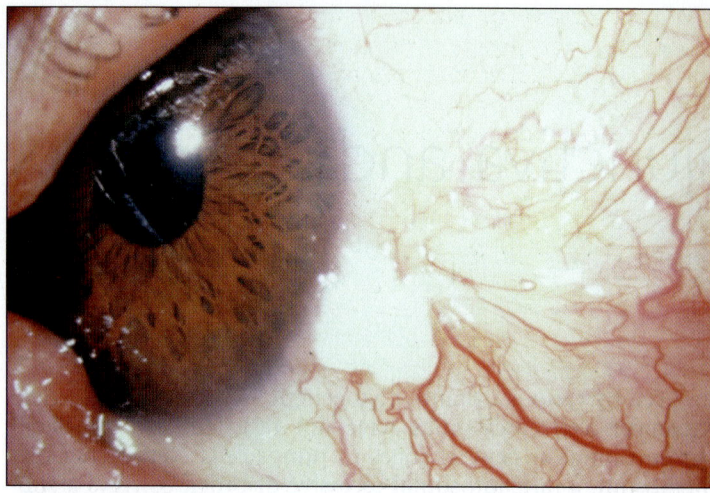

FIG. 67-1 ■ **Leukoplakic squamous cell carcinoma of conjunctiva.** Discrete white hyperkeratotic limbal plaque is associated with prominent conjunctival blood vessels.

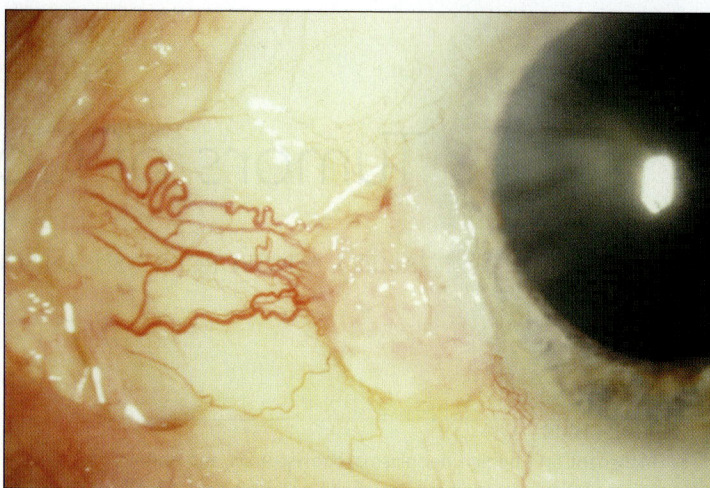

FIG. 67-3 ■ **Gelatinous squamous cell carcinoma of conjunctiva.** Translucent limbal mass is associated with dilated afferent and efferent conjunctival blood vessels.

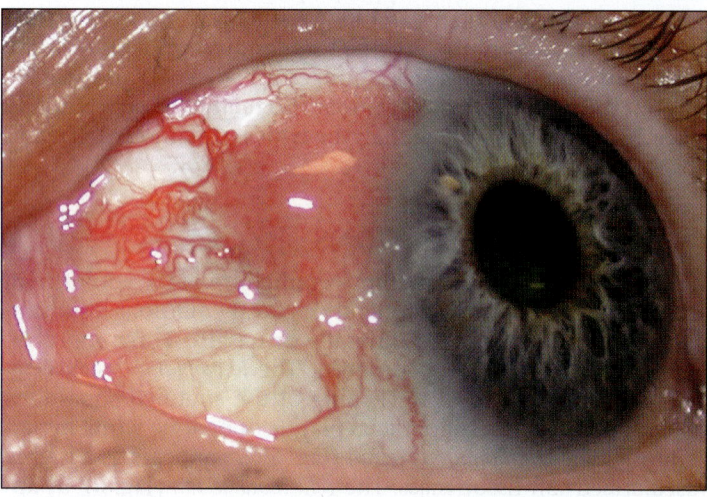

FIG. 67-2 ■ **Papillomatous squamous cell carcinoma of conjunctiva.** Pink limbal tumor contains multiple fine intralesional corkscrew blood vessels and is associated with dilated afferent and efferent conjunctival blood vessels.

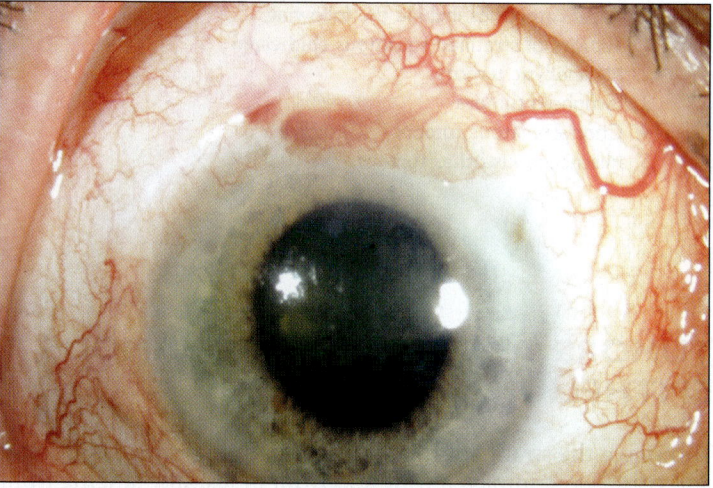

FIG. 67-4 ■ **Corneal intraepithelial neoplasia.** Lesion appears as faint gray clouding of corneal epithelium.

the slit lamp and identification of invasive features, if present. Ultrasonographic biomicroscopy may be helpful if corneal or scleral invasion is suspected.

PATHOLOGY

Tumors of the stratified squamous epithelium of the conjunctiva are regarded as malignant when they exhibit anaplasia, invasion of the substantia propria of the conjunctiva, or invasion of the underlying sclera, cornea, or both. The following are the most common types of tumors of the stratified squamous epithelium of the conjunctiva and cornea that appear on pathology reports:

- Hyperplasia: benign thickening of the stratified squamous epithelium with disordered transition from basal to superficial layers, but no cells with nuclear features suggestive of malignancy[11]
- Dysplasia: abnormal epithelial maturation from basal to superficial layers of stratified squamous epithelium, accompanied by partial thickness replacement of epithelium by atypical but not frankly malignant cells[12]; intermediate lesion between benign hyperplasia and intraepithelial neoplasia: the more numerous and more atypical the abnormal cells, the greater the concern about neoplasia
- Intraepithelial neoplasia (carcinoma *in situ*): abnormal malignant-appearing (anaplastic) epithelial cells replacing the conjunctival stratified squamous epithelium[13]; may involve partial thickness or full thickness of epithelium

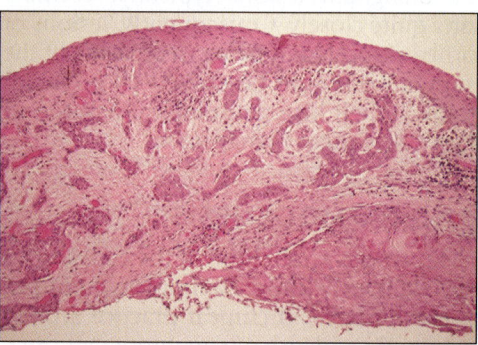

FIG. 67-5 ■ **Pathology of squamous cell carcinoma of conjunctiva.** Tumor consists of neoplastic squamous epithelial cells thickening epithelium and extending deeply into substantia propria.

- Squamous cell carcinoma: mass composed of malignant-appearing stratified squamous epithelial cells with invasion into substantia propria (Fig. 67-5) and possibly into corneal or scleral stroma[13]
- Mucoepidermoid carcinoma: similar to squamous cell carcinoma, but with nests of cells that elaborate mucin; tends to be highly invasive[14]

TREATMENT

Treatment options for squamous cell carcinoma of the conjunctiva range from simple excision to exenteration. A number of factors influence the method of treatment recommended for individual patients. These factors include the size of the lesion

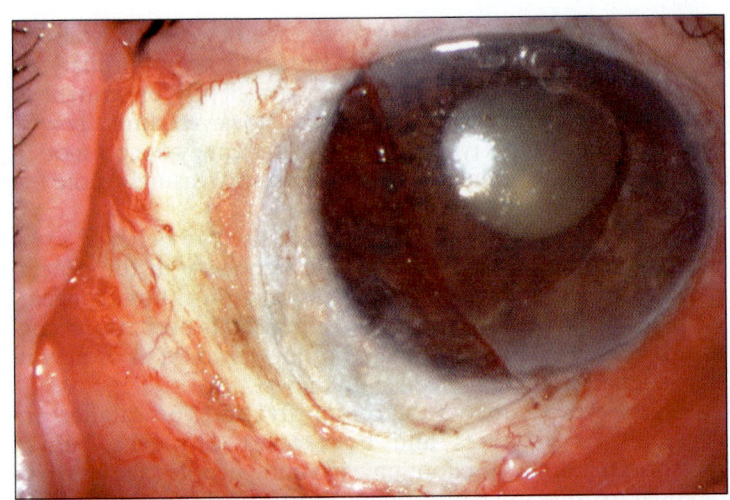

FIG. 67-6 ◼ Excision of squamous cell carcinoma of conjunctiva with lamellar keratosclerectomy. Superficial D-shaped area of excised inner scleral and corneal lamellae straddling limbus.

(basal area and thickness), location of the lesion, clinical invasiveness of the lesion, the status of the fellow eye, and the age and general health of the patient. If the lesion in question is a discrete nodular limbal mass, it frequently can be removed completely by simple excision.[15] To maximize the likelihood of complete lesion excision, the margins of the lesion can be marked with a sterile methylene blue pen prior to making the first conjunctival incision. The bulbar conjunctiva is incised around the lesion about 2mm from its marked margins. The incision is carried down to bare sclera. The conjunctiva containing the limbal lesion is separated from the underlying sclera up to the limbus using blunt or sharp dissection, and the conjunctival specimen is excised as a single piece. Depending on the size of the conjunctival defect created by the excision, the defect can either be left to granulate in or closed surgically with or without a conjunctival transposition flap or mucous membrane graft.

If the lesion is strongly adherent to the sclera at the limbus, superficial lamellar keratosclerectomy can be performed to increase the chance of complete removal of the tumor (Fig. 67-6). A surgical blade is used to create a partial thickness scleral incision around the area of strong adhesion. A thin lamellar scleral flap is dissected under the lesion and into the peripheral clear cornea. The conjunctiva and adherent limbal corneoscleral flap are then excised as a single piece with Westcott or Vannas scissors. Immediately following excision of the specimen, a cotton-tipped applicator stick soaked in absolute alcohol is applied briefly to the peripheral cornea adjacent to the now bare bulbar sclera to loosen the epithelium. Using a surgical blade, the loosened peripheral corneal epithelium is then removed. Some authors have also suggested a microscopically controlled excision approach similar to the Mohs' micrographic technique used for skin cancers to increase the likelihood of complete tumor excision.[16] This method of excision is not used widely.

A word about handling the excised specimen to maximize the likelihood of satisfactory histopathological assessment of completeness of lesion excision is appropriate. The ophthalmic surgeon who excises a conjunctival specimen should flatten the specimen on either a segment of a sterile tongue blade or a heavyweight paper (e.g., the paper in suture packets), unrolling all of the edges as he or she does so, allowing it to air dry momentarily, and then immersing it in formaldehyde or paraformaldehyde for delivery to and processing by the ophthalmic pathologist. If the specimen is allowed to roll up, it will be virtually impossible for the pathologist to determine completeness of excision reliably.

Cryotherapy to the bulbar conjunctiva adjacent to the incision around the lesion and to the sclera underlying the site of the excised limbal lesion frequently is performed immediately

following excision to reduce the likelihood of local tumor recurrence.[17] It can also be performed as a separate procedure following early postoperative healing if histopathological study reveals tumor extension to the margins of the resected specimen. To avoid performing inadvertent cyclocryotherapy, the surgeon should inject anesthetic into the substantia propria of the conjunctiva to elevate the stratified squamous epithelium from the sclera before freezing the conjunctiva. The elevated epithelium typically is frozen for about 10–30 seconds, allowed to thaw, and then refrozen for another 10–30 seconds. Cryotherapy typically causes pronounced local tissue swelling that may take several weeks to subside. It can also cause symblepharon, restricted ocular motility, and scleral melting.

During the past decade, quite a few patients with extensive conjunctival or corneal intraepithelial neoplasia (CIN), incompletely excised intraepithelial neoplasia of the bulbar conjunctiva by histopathological criteria, and recurrent intraepithelial neoplasia following prior excision have been treated by topical chemotherapy using mitomycin C (0.02–0.04% solution) or 5-fluorouracil (1% solution) drops.[18–21] Such usage of mitomycin C and 5-fluorouracil is not approved by the U.S. Food and Drug Administration. Treatment with topical chemotherapeutic drops is most often considered for eyes with extensive CIN of the cornea, diffuse or multifocal residual or recurrent intraepithelial neoplasia of the bulbar conjunctiva after prior excision, or both. Because application of mitomycin C and 5-fluorouracil to bare sclera and de-epithelialized cornea following pterygium surgery has been associated with occasional corneoscleral melting, the bulbar conjunctiva and corneal epithelium should be allowed to heal prior to initiation of such therapy. Typical regimens call for administration of one drop to the surface of the affected eye 4 times daily for 2 weeks, a 2-week period during which the drops are not given, and a second 2-week course of treatment if there appears to be any clinically apparent residual intraepithelial disease. Most intraepithelial tumors of the stratified squamous epithelium respond favorably to this therapy. Topical chemotherapy is not considered appropriate for deeply invasive epithelial neoplasms of the stratified squamous epithelium of the conjunctiva and cornea.

An alternative to topical chemotherapy that has been used in selected patients with CIN and residual intraepithelial conjunctival neoplasia of the bulbar conjunctiva is topical immunotherapy with interferon alfa-2b.[22] This therapy appears to provide results similar to topical chemotherapy but may be less toxic to the normal epithelium or the cornea and conjunctiva.

Contact radiation therapy with high–dose rate strontium-90 applicators or moderate-to-low–dose rate temporary ruthenium-106 or iodine-125 plaques is used occasionally to treat both incompletely excised and recurrent invasive carcinomas of the stratified squamous epithelium of the conjunctiva.[23,24] It is an effective therapy when tumor extends deeply into the lamellar cornea or sclera at the limbus and is incompletely excised. Treatment generally targets the eye wall to receive approximately 60Gy at 1mm depth. The selected applicator or plaque must cover the entire area to be treated. Consequently, contact radiation therapy is not usually employed to treat diffuse or multifocal conjunctival intraepithelial disease. One potential complication of contact radiation therapy is corneoscleral breakdown at the treatment site due to disintegration of an extensive tumor infiltrate that has replaced the eye wall tissue, tissue necrosis induced by the radiation, tissue breakdown attributable to collagenases and other factors acting on the bare sclera following loss of conjunctiva, or some combination of these factors.

Enucleation usually is advised when a malignant neoplasm of the stratified squamous epithelium of the conjunctiva and cornea has invaded through the cornea or sclera into the eye. Although a few patients with intraocular invasion have undergone successful eye wall resection with placement of a scleral or corneoscleral patch graft,[25] most such procedures have not been successful long term. Exenteration usually is recommended when an epibulbar neoplasm of the conjunctival stratified squamous epithelium has invaded the anterior orbit.[26] Such surgery can eliminate residual or recurrent tumor, but local failures frequently occur even following this aggressive intervention.

COURSE AND OUTCOMES

Patients whose tumors of the stratified squamous epithelium of the conjunctiva and cornea are excised completely by histopathological criteria are usually cured.[7-9] In contrast, patients whose tumors are excised incompletely have a substantial risk of local tumor recurrence. Because of this, virtually all patients with incompletely excised malignant neoplasms of the stratified squamous epithelium of the conjunctiva and cornea are advised to undergo supplemental treatment (e.g., wider excision, cryotherapy, contact radiation therapy, topical chemotherapy). Patients who experience a local relapse of their epibulbar neoplasia of stratified squamous epithelium are much less likely to be cured by local treatment than are patients who do not.

As mentioned above, aggressive malignant neoplasms of the conjunctiva and cornea occasionally invade the eye or the orbit. These advanced forms of the disease typically require enucleation or exenteration for cancer eradication. Mucoepidermoid carcinoma is a form of neoplasia of the stratified squamous epithelium of the conjunctiva that is particularly aggressive and most frequently requires enucleation or exenteration.[14]

Although metastasis of malignant neoplasms of the conjunctiva and cornea occurs infrequently, it is observed in occasional advanced cases due to patient neglect and in persons with extremely aggressive tumors.[27] Patients with concurrent AIDS are particularly likely to exhibit rapidly progressive malignant neoplasms of the conjunctival and corneal stratified squamous epithelium and metastasis of those neoplasms.[6] Tumors arising from the temporal limbal area most frequently metastasize initially to preauricular lymph nodes, while those arising from the medial limbal area most frequently metastasize initially to anterior cervical lymph nodes.

MELANOCYTIC TUMORS

Melanocytic tumors of the conjunctiva and cornea comprise a spectrum of lesions ranging from benign nevi and primary acquired melanosis (PAM) to invasive malignant melanoma. Although most melanocytic tumors appear darkly melanotic, some are predominantly or completely amelanotic. These hypomelanotic and amelanotic lesions are particularly likely to be mistaken for tumors of the stratified squamous epithelium of the cornea or conjunctiva or some other lesion. Because of potentially fatal outcome in patients with conjunctival melanoma, prompt excision or other definitive treatment of any tumor strongly suspected of being a malignant melanoma of the conjunctiva or cornea is advised strongly.

EPIDEMIOLOGY AND PATHOGENESIS

Conjunctival melanoma is substantially less common than squamous cell carcinoma of the conjunctiva and cornea.[28] Its annual incidence in the white race is only about 2 to 4 new cases per 10 million persons per year, and its cumulative lifetime incidence in the white race is approximately 1 in 50,000 to 75,000 persons. The frequency of conjunctival melanoma in blacks is approximately 8 times lower.[29]

In contrast to conjunctival melanoma, primary acquired melanosis of the conjunctiva is extremely common. In one study of white persons without known non-European ancestry (a group selected to avoid cases of racial melanosis), over one third of patients were found to have at least one patch of conjunctival

melanosis in one eye.[30] Most of these patches were limited in extent and not worrisome clinically. The frequency of primary acquired melanosis of the conjunctiva sufficiently prominent to warrant biopsy or excision is unknown. However, clinically worrisome lesions of this type appear to be extremely uncommon in persons under 20 years of age and become increasingly more frequent in persons of older age groups.

Melanocytic nevi of the conjunctiva also are believed to be relatively common, but their precise frequency in the general population and in racial subgroups is unknown. Both congenital and acquired melanocytic conjunctival nevi are recognized.[31,32] The relative frequencies of these two types of nevi in the general population are also unknown.

Melanocytic tumors of the conjunctiva and cornea affect individuals of all races and both sexes. However, benign melanocytic tumors predominate in young people (age less than or equal to 20 years) while pre-malignant (PAM) and malignant lesions (melanomas) predominate in older individuals. Recognized risk factors for pre-malignant and malignant melanocytic conjunctival tumors include white race, older age (over 20 years), and history of repeated intense sunlight exposures. Some nevi are believed to undergo malignant transformation, but this phenomenon appears to be uncommon.[31-34] In contrast, malignant transformation of clinically significant PAM is relatively common.[35] The presence of atypical melanocytic hyperplasia within PAM is an important prognostic factor for malignant transformation (see Pathology section below).

OCULAR MANIFESTATIONS

The typical melanocytic conjunctival nevus (Fig. 67-7) appears as a dark brown elevated lesion of the limbal or perilimbal conjunctiva nasally or temporally in the interpalpebral fissure. Less common sites of such lesions are in the extralimbal bulbar conjunctiva in the interpalpebral fissure, semilunar fold, and caruncle (Fig. 67-8). Melanocytic nevi involving the superior or inferior limbal or bulbar conjunctiva, the palpebral conjunctiva, and the superior or inferior forniceal conjunctiva are all extremely uncommon.[36] Many conjunctival nevi have a stippled reddish brown appearance on slit-lamp biomicroscopy, while others appear homogeneously dark brown and well defined. Occasional nevi are predominantly or completely amelanotic and appear tan to pink (Fig. 67-9). Many conjunctival nevi contain intralesional microcysts visible on slit-lamp biomicroscopy. They usually have few, if any, associated prominent conjunctival or episcleral blood vessels.

Primary acquired melanosis typically appears as a flat patch of brown conjunctiva in the interpalpebral fissure, most frequently

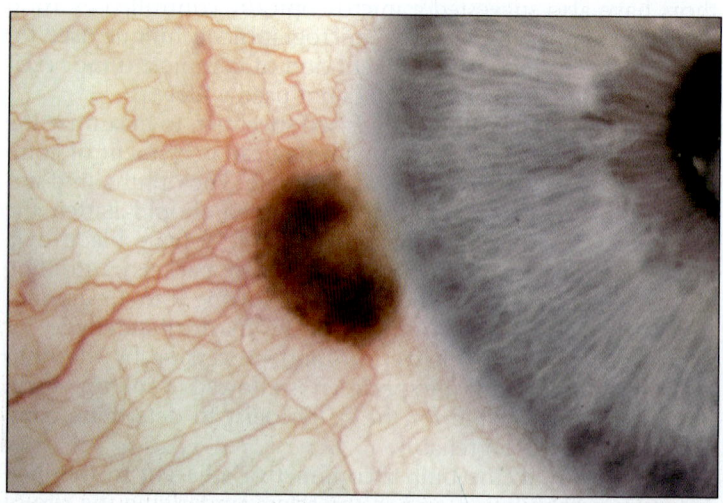

FIG. 67-7 ■ Melanotic melanocytic nevus of bulbar conjunctiva adjacent to limbus.

adjacent to the limbus (Fig. 67-10). Amelanotic PAM has been reported but appears to be uncommon.[37] Unlike the scleral melanocytic pigmentation that occurs in ocular melanocytosis, PAM clearly involves the conjunctiva and can, therefore, be moved over the underlying sclera. Slit-lamp biomicroscopy frequently shows faint conjunctival melanotic stippling beyond the margins of the grossly visible lesion. More than one patch may be present in the same eye. The melanotic pigmentation occasionally extends to the conjunctival fornices and onto the palpebral conjunctiva or into the corneal epithelium (Fig. 67-11). In the cornea, PAM typically appears as a poorly defined zone of melanotic epithelial stippling extending from a focus of limbal melanotic conjunctival pigmentation.[35] Focal thickenings within melanotic PAM generally appear darker brown than thinner portions of the lesion. Such foci are highly suspicious for malignant transformation. Although there are no established clinical criteria for distinguishing benign conjunctival melanosis from clinically significant premalignant PAM, lesions that are large, multifocal, darkly melanotic, or progressive during short-term observation, and those involving unusual locations (i.e., fornix, semilunar fold, caruncle, palpebral conjunctiva, extralimbal bulbar conjunctiva) should certainly be regarded as clinically significant and be sampled for biopsy or excised.[29]

Malignant melanoma of the conjunctiva that arises *de novo* typically appears as a focal nodular melanotic epibulbar mass, with multiple prominent epibulbar blood vessels extending to and from the lesion and involving the mass (Fig. 67-12). Although most conjunctival melanomas are darkly melanotic,[34] some are hypomelanotic or amelanotic (Fig. 67-13).[37] The most commonly recognized site of such lesions is at the limbus in the interpalpebral fissure. Conjunctival melanomas

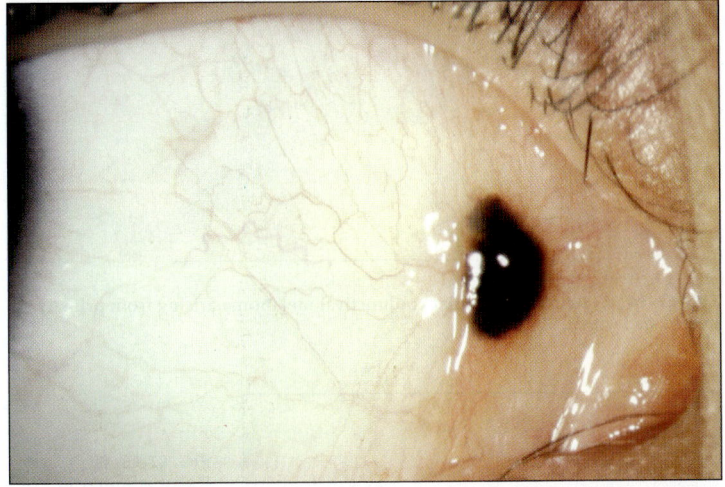

FIG. 67-8 ▪ Melanotic melanocytic nevus of conjunctiva of semilunar fold.

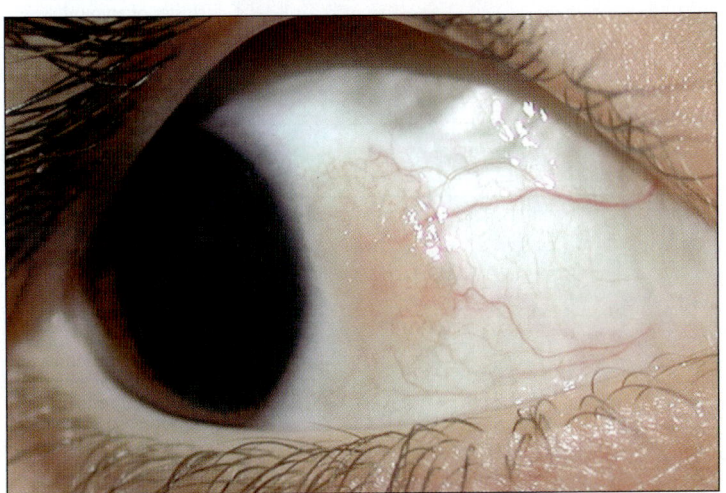

FIG. 67-9 ▪ Amelanotic melanocytic nevus of bulbar conjunctiva. Note absence of dilated conjunctival blood vessels associated with lesion.

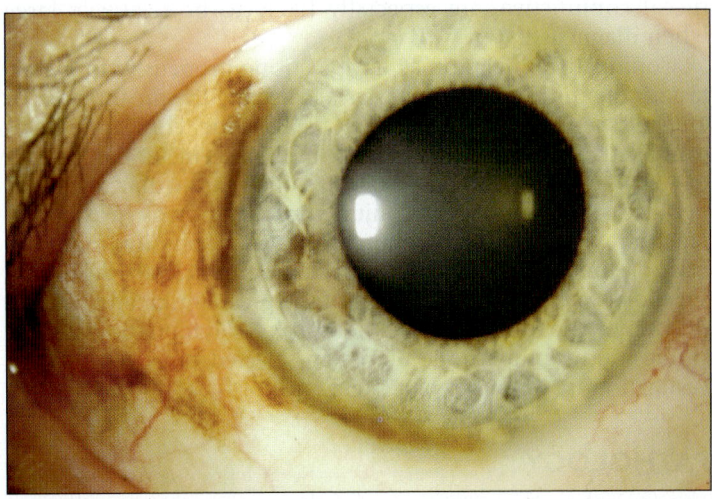

FIG. 67-11 ▪ Primary acquired melanosis of conjunctiva and cornea. Note darkly melanotic conjunctival pigmentation along limbus inferiorly and temporally and extension of melanotic cells into adjacent corneal epithelium.

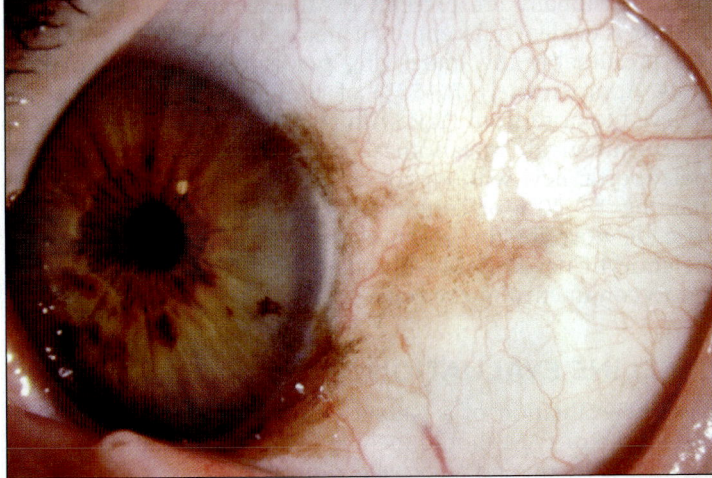

FIG. 67-10 ▪ Primary acquired melanosis of bulbar conjunctiva. Melanotic flat conjunctival lesion involves bulbar conjunctiva adjacent to limbus. Note nonuniform pigment density and absence of dilated conjunctival blood vessels associated with lesion.

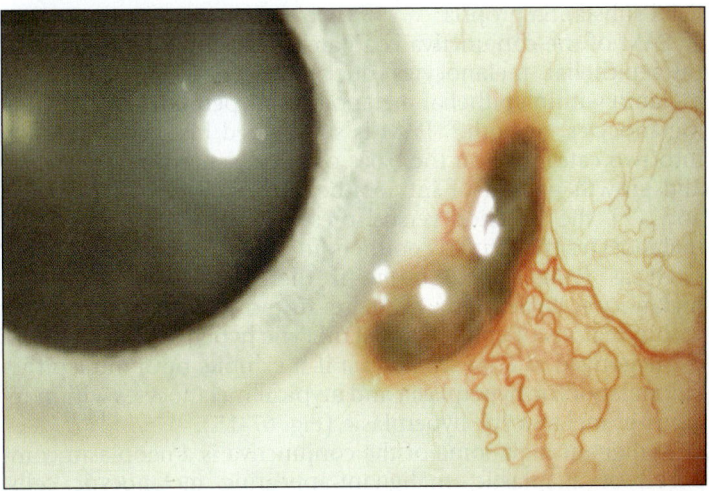

FIG. 67-12 ▪ Nodular melanotic conjunctival melanoma at limbus. Note dilated afferent and efferent conjunctival blood vessels associated with the lesion.

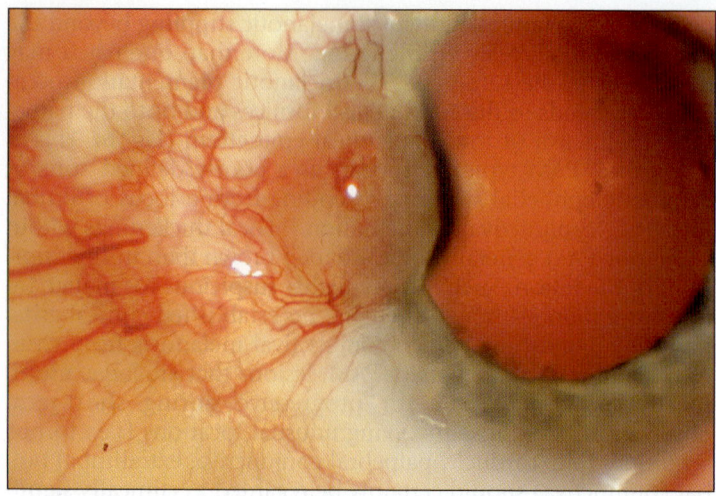

FIG. 67-13 ▌ Amelanotic nodular conjunctival melanoma at limbus. Note prominent afferent and efferent conjunctival blood vessels associated with the lesion.

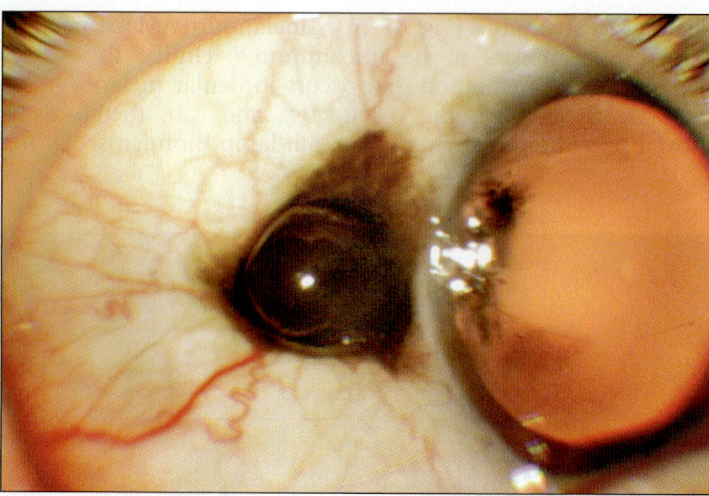

FIG. 67-14 ▌ Melanotic nodular conjunctival melanoma arising from primary acquired melanosis.

that arise from PAM (Fig. 67-14) develop from any portion of the lesion, including the superior or inferior fornix and palpebral conjunctiva, and may also develop on the cornea.[38] A nodular melanoma can be small (less than 3mm in diameter, less than 1mm thick) to quite large (greater than 10mm in diameter, greater than 3mm thick) when noted initially. Tumors arising in hidden locations, such as the superior bulbar or forniceal conjunctiva, are especially likely to be relatively large when diagnosed.

Conjunctival melanomas have a strong propensity to metastasize. The initial site of metastasis is usually the preauricular or anterior cervical lymph nodes.[39–41] Baseline clinical features prognostic of regional lymph node metastasis include larger size of the tumor, forniceal location, and caruncular location. Because of the tendency of conjunctival melanomas to extend to regional lymph nodes, baseline pretreatment physical examination of the patient with a suspected conjunctival melanoma should always include palpation of the preauricular and cervical regions of the head and neck. The role of lymphatic drainage studies and sentinel node biopsy in selected cases is under investigation in a number of centers.

PATHOLOGY

The typical melanocytic nevus of the conjunctiva is a discrete mass composed of nests of benign-appearing melanocytes within the superficial substantia propria and epithelium of the conjunctiva.[31] These nests of melanocytic cells frequently are associated with epithelial microcysts and inclusions in the superficial substantia propria.

PAM of the conjunctiva is a patch of abnormally prominent intraepithelial melanocytes due to excessive production of melanin within epithelial melanocytes, hyperplasia of epithelial melanocytes, or both.[35] PAM is subdivided histopathologically into two categories on the basis of (1) absence versus presence and growth pattern of intraepithelial melanocytic hyperplasia and (2) the absence versus presence of atypical epithelial melanocytes (particularly epithelioid cells). The lesion is categorized as *PAM without atypia* if there is no intraepithelial melanocytic hyperplasia or there are no atypical melanocytes within regions of epithelial melanocytic hyperplasia. The lesion is categorized as *PAM with atypia* if it exhibits both intraepithelial melanocytic hyperplasia and atypical melanocytes within regions of melanocytic hyperplasia (Fig. 67-15).

Malignant melanoma of the conjunctiva is a neoplasm composed of anaplastic, malignant-appearing melanocytic cells, some of which involve the substantia propria of the conjunctiva (Fig. 67-16).[34,39,40] Tumor cells may invade blood vessels, lym-

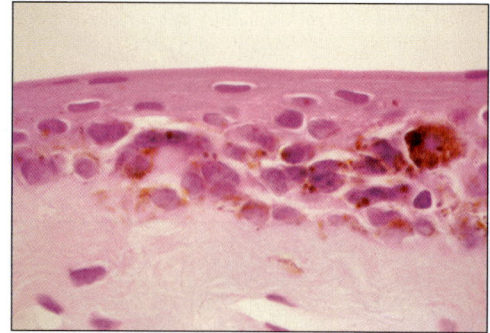

FIG. 67-15 ▌ Histopathology of primary acquired melanosis of conjunctiva with atypical melanocytic hyperplasia. Note prominent cluster of atypical melanocytes in basal epithelium of conjunctiva.

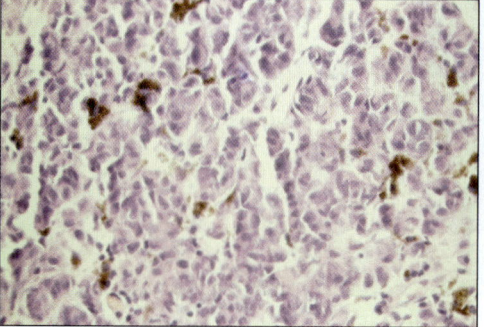

FIG. 67-16 ▌ Histopathology of conjunctival melanoma. Densely packed cords of malignant melanocytic cells, some of which contain prominent intracytoplasmic melanin granules.

phatic vessels, cornea, or sclera. The tumor frequently contains numerous prominent blood vessels. Scattered inflammatory cells occasionally are present. PAM with atypia or nevus frequently is evident adjacent to an area of invasive melanoma and was presumably the underlying predisposing lesion in these cases. Approximately 70–75% of conjunctival melanomas are believed to arise from PAM with atypia.[34,35] Only about 5–10% of conjunctival melanomas are believed to arise from melanocytic nevi without coexistent PAM with atypia. The remaining 15–20% of conjunctival melanomas are believed to arise de novo in the absence of either PAM with atypia or melanocytic nevus. PAM without atypia does not appear to give rise to conjunctival melanoma.

BASELINE EVALUATION

Baseline evaluation of a patient with a suspected conjunctival melanoma or PAM should include detailed clinical mapping of the visible lesion and associated clinical features and palpation of the head and neck to identify preauricular or cervical lymphadenopathy that might be present. Worrisome conjunctival lesions should be excised completely (if possible) or a biopsy taken for pathology evaluation.

TREATMENT

The principles of treatment of conjunctival melanocytic tumors are similar to those for tumors of the stratified squamous epithelium of the conjunctiva and cornea, with only a few exceptions. Factors influencing the method of treatment recommended include the size of the tumor, the location of the tumor, the presence or absence of regional lymphadenopathy and distant metastasis, the presence or absence of associated PAM, the completeness of initial excision, the age of the patient, the general health of the patient, and biases of the patient and physician.[41]

Conjunctival nevi that are congenital or juvenile in onset frequently are excised in childhood. However, most of these tumors probably could be left alone because of their extraordinarily low rate of malignant transformation.[31,32] Although these lesions can enlarge and become darker over time, they are very unlikely to transform into malignant melanomas. Conjunctival nevi that appear initially in adolescents have a somewhat higher rate of malignant transformation, and excision probably is warranted because of this risk. But conjunctival nevi with the highest risk of malignant transformation are those that arise in adults.[34] A melanocytic conjunctival tumor that appears in adulthood should usually be excised without undue delay.

PAM of the conjunctiva, which almost always shows up initially in adults, usually is managed by simple observation if it is limited in extent and not rapidly progressive. In contrast, prominent or progressive PAM lesions usually are excised (if small) or a biopsy taken (if too large to excise). If pathological study shows PAM without atypia, then the residual conjunctival lesion (assuming that the entire lesion was not excised) usually is left untreated. A biopsy may have to be repeated at some later time if the lesion exhibits any worrisome changes (e.g., darkening, thickening). In contrast, if pathological study reveals PAM with atypia, then the ophthalmologist must either excise the residual lesion completely (if possible) or arrange for alternative definitive therapy (e.g., cryotherapy,[42] topical chemotherapy,[43] contact radiation therapy[44]) for that residual disease. (See treatment section of preceding text on tumors of the stratified squamous epithelium for details on these treatment methods.) If pathological study shows both PAM and invasive melanoma, one must be even more aggressive with attempts to excise the residual melanoma and PAM or treat the residual lesion by cryotherapy, topical chemotherapy, or contact radiation therapy.

For nodular conjunctival melanoma arising *de novo* or from a preexisting conjunctival nevus, the ophthalmologist must either excise the entire lesion or perform an incisional biopsy. If biopsy confirms invasive melanoma, complete excision coupled with cryotherapy to the normal-appearing conjunctiva surrounding the lesion usually is performed. If complete excision is impossible because of the extent of the lesion, then supplemental treatment of the residual lesion with cryotherapy or contact radiation therapy is indicated. Alternatively, some small nodular conjunctival melanomas can be treated effectively by contact radiation therapy after the biopsy.

If physical examination reveals preauricular or cervical lymphadenopathy, a comprehensive staging evaluation is indicated to identify any clinically apparent distant metastasis. If that evaluation fails to detect metastasis, then a head and neck surgeon should be called upon to perform excision of the suspicious regional lymph nodes.

Enucleation is indicated rarely in patients with conjunctival melanoma; however, this surgical method may be appropriate for the rare cases with intraocular invasion by tumor. Exenteration is employed much more frequently than enucleation for conjunctival melanoma. This aggressive surgical method is indicated for patients with massive unresectable tumor or frank orbital invasion by tumor but no evidence of metastatic disease.[45]

COURSE AND OUTCOMES

The natural history of untreated patients with conjunctival melanoma is virtually unknown. Almost all patients with worrisome clinical lesions are treated promptly following detection of the lesion. Several relatively large retrospective studies have shown actuarial rates of death from metastatic disease following initial diagnosis and treatment of primary conjunctival melanoma to be about 15–20% after 5 years, 25–30% after 10 years, and 30–35% after 15 years. Prognostic factors associated with increased risk of metastasis of conjunctival melanoma include larger tumor size, tumor location in unfavorable sites (fornix, semilunar fold, caruncle, and tarsal conjunctiva), epithelioid melanoma cells on histopathological study of the primary tumor, orbital invasion by tumor, recurrent tumor following initial treatment, and older patient age.[39,41] Prognostic factors associated with local tumor recurrence following initial treatment include larger tumor size, incomplete tumor excision by histopathological criteria, unfavorable tumor location, orbital invasion by tumor, origin of the tumor from PAM with atypia, and aggressiveness of initial treatment.[39,41] Because local recurrence of conjunctival melanoma is an unfavorable prognostic factor for metastasis and survival, one must make every reasonable effort to eradicate all tumor with initial treatment.

LYMPHOID TUMORS

Lymphoid tumors of conjunctiva comprise a spectrum of benign to malignant infiltrative masses that involve the substantia propria and lymphatic tissue of the conjunctiva.[46] The tumors range from benign reactive lymphoid hyperplasia through lymphoid neoplasms of indeterminate malignant potential (atypical lymphoid hyperplasia) to frankly malignant lymphomas. Many, if not most, such tumors originate within the lymphoid follicles and lymphatic vessels of the conjunctiva, but some develop as metastatic masses in patients with systemic lymphoma. Conjunctival lymphoid tumors do not tend to impair vision or destroy the eye, and local treatments tend to be highly effective for local tumor control or eradication.

EPIDEMIOLOGY AND PATHOGENESIS

Lymphoid tumors of the conjunctiva and cornea are quite rare. However, figures for annual and cumulative lifetime incidence of lymphoid tumors of the conjunctiva as an entire group and for conjunctival lymphomas as a subgroup are not available.[47] Malignant lymphoid tumors of the conjunctiva tend to be tumors of middle-aged to elderly adults, while benign lymphoid tumors of the conjunctiva are more frequent in older children and younger adults.[46] Recognized risk factors for occurrence of conjunctival lymphoma include older patient age, history of systemic (visceral) lymphoma, and systemic immunosuppression (medically induced or from AIDS).[46,48,49]

CLINICAL MANIFESTATIONS

The typical conjunctival lymphoid tumor appears as a pink, smoothly elevated subepithelial mass of the bulbar or forniceal conjunctiva (Fig. 67-17). The inferior fornix appears to be the most common location of such lesions.[49] The lesions tend to be compressible when indented. The conjunctival blood vessels associated with the mass tend to be slightly more prominent than normal but usually are not grossly enlarged. In some patients, the lesion is multifocal. The patient may be asymptomatic or complain of mild foreign body sensation or a visible epibulbar mass.

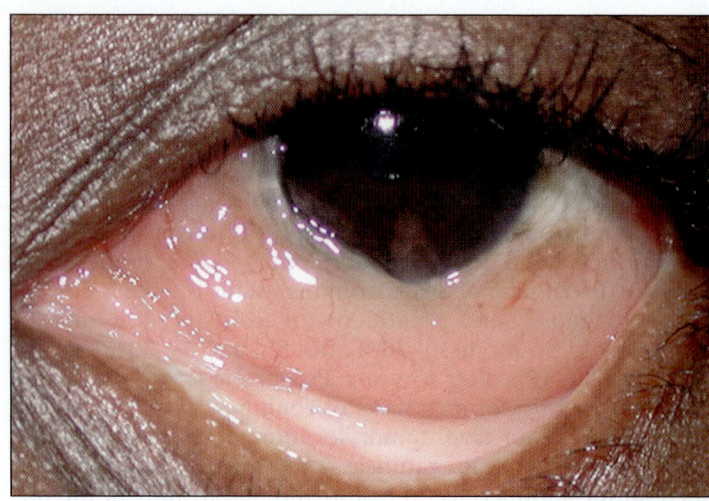

FIG. 67-17 ◼ Lymphoid tumor (malignant lymphoma) of bulbar conjunctiva. Tumor involves inferior bulbar and forniceal conjunctiva.

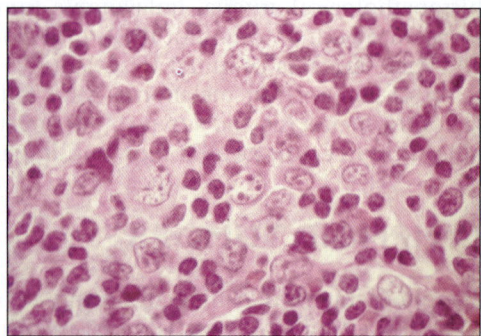

FIG. 67-18 ◼ Histopathology of conjunctival lymphoma. Tumor consists of a dense collection of neoplastic lymphoid cells.

Occasional patients with diffuse benign reactive lymphoid hyperplasia of the conjunctiva have had concurrent diffuse choroidal lymphoid thickening.[49] However, most patients with a conjunctival lymphoid tumor do not have a concurrent choroidal lymphoid mass. Bilateral but asynchronous or asymmetrical involvement is relatively common. At least 20% of patients in most series exhibit bilateral ocular lesions.[46,48,49]

In certain forms of lymphoma (e.g., Burkitt's lymphoma and AIDS-associated lymphoma), the lymphoid masses tend to develop suddenly and enlarge rapidly.[50] In most other forms of conjunctival lymphoid neoplasia, the conjunctival masses tend to develop rather slowly and exhibit an indolent course.

PATHOLOGY

As the term *lymphoid tumor* implies, masses in this category are composed of stimulated (reactive) or neoplastic lymphocytic cells. As such, they tend to appear as small, round, blue cells on conventional hematoxylin and eosin–stained microslides (Fig. 67-18).[46] Benign reactive tumors tend to be composed of polyclonal lymphoid cells and frequently exhibit abortive or well-developed germinal centers.[51] In contrast, lymphomas of the conjunctiva tend to be monoclonal or pauciclonal by morphological criteria and do not exhibit germinal centers.[46,48]

An important part of the pathological evaluation of suspected lymphoid tumors of the conjunctiva is processing fresh tumor specimens by flow cytometry and gene rearrangement studies. Flow cytometry helps to identify the monoclonal, pauciclonal, or polyclonal nature of the tumor cells, identify the origin of these cells as B cells or T cells, and detect DNA content abnormalities of those cells. Gene rearrangement studies are performed frequently to confirm the clonality of the tumor cells. Immunohistochemical stains typically are used to further refine the identity of the lymphoid cells.

Most conjunctival lymphomas encountered in the United States are B cell–derived tumors.[46,48] Special subcategories that may be helpful for prognostication of systemic associations include MALT lymphoma (marginal B-cell lymphoma) and mantle cell lymphoma.[52]

BASELINE EVALUATION

Any patient with a suspected lymphoid tumor of the conjunctiva deserves a comprehensive review of the medical-surgical history, a complete physical examination, a complete blood count with differential, and probably imaging studies (e.g., computed tomography scans, magnetic resonance imaging) of the chest, abdomen, and pelvis to identify any associated systemic lymphoma. The conjunctival lesion or lesions should be mapped completely and documented photographically. A biopsy of the suspected conjunctival lymphoid tumor should be taken to confirm its pathological nature and direct subsequent evaluation and treatment.

TREATMENT

If systemic evaluation reveals no evidence of extra-ophthalmic lymphoma, conventional treatment for conjunctival lymphoid tumors is governed by the pathological findings of the conjunctival lesion. If the lymphoid tumor is categorized as benign reactive lymphoid hyperplasia, one may either observe the lesion without treatment or try a course of oral or topical corticosteroids for several weeks. Many benign lymphoid tumors regress spontaneously. Those that do not usually respond promptly to corticosteroid therapy. If the lesion fails to respond to this treatment, or if pathological study reveals a low-grade lymphoid neoplasia, then conventional current therapy is low-dose fractionated external beam radiation therapy to the affected eye or eyes.[53] The target dose of radiation in such cases is usually 30–35Gy. The cornea and lens are shielded during this treatment. In contrast, if pathological study reveals frank lymphoma (especially if it is of an aggressive subtype), the target dose of radiation typically is increased to 40–45Gy. Most conjunctival lymphomas regress quickly and completely following such therapy.

If systemic evaluation shows extra-ophthalmic lymphoma, the conventional initial treatment is an appropriate regimen of intravenous chemotherapy for that systemic lymphoma. The precise regimen employed should be based on the pathological findings and available information about the expected effectiveness of various regimens in patients with the identified form of lymphoma. External beam radiation therapy can be used to treat ocular or extraocular foci of lymphoma that fail to regress or respond incompletely to chemotherapy.

Cryotherapy can be performed as an alternative to external beam radiation therapy for localized extranodal lymphoma confined to the conjunctiva.[54] This therapy usually induces complete local regression of the treated tumors but may have to be repeated several times. Lesions that do not respond to cryotherapy usually are managed with radiation therapy.

COURSE AND OUTCOMES

Most patients with a localized conjunctival lymphoid tumor without prior or concurrent evidence of systemic lymphoma have a favorable course. The conjunctival tumors tend to respond well to the local therapies mentioned above, and only about 20–30% of patients subsequently develop extra-ophthalmic lymphoma.[46,48] In one relatively large series of patients with conjunctival lymphoid tumors,[49] 14% of them had a history of systemic lymphoma and 17% developed systemic lymphoma subsequent to detection of the conjunctival tumor. The actuarial probabilities of developing systemic lymphoma among patients with a conjunctival lymphoid tumor but no systemic disease at evaluation were 7% after 1 year, 12% after 2 years, 15% after 5 years, and 28% after 10 years. When one restricts attention to patients in that series who had pathologically confirmed malignant lymphoma of the conjunctiva (i.e., excluding cases of benign reactive lymphoid hyperplasia and atypical lymphoid hyperplasia) but no systemic disease at evaluation, the actuarial probabilities of developing systemic lymphoma increased to 12% after 1 year, 30% after 2 years, 38% after 5 years, and 79% after 10 years. Fortunately, most patients who developed systemic lymphoma responded favorably to treatment. Only one patient in that series died of lymphoma. Recognized prognostic factors for development of systemic lymphoma in patients with a conjunctival lymphoid tumor include bilateral involvement, malignant histopathological features of the conjunctival tumor, and lymphoma subtype established by pathological study.[49,52] The survival prognosis of patients who develop systemic lymphoma is a function of the pathological subtype of lymphoma determined by comprehensive pathological studies, the stage of the lymphoma, the aggressiveness of the particular form of lymphoma, and its responsiveness to chemotherapy. Regardless of the initial pathological findings, patients with a lymphoid tumor of the conjunctiva should be reevaluated periodically to look for local tumor relapse or new conjunctival or systemic lymphoid tumors.

MISCELLANEOUS OTHER TUMORS

A variety of other tumors occur within the conjunctiva and cornea. Choristomatous tumors of the conjunctiva and cornea are described elsewhere in this text. Degenerative tumors (pinguecula and pterygium) are common acquired non-neoplastic lesions well known to ophthalmologists. These lesions deserve no further mention here. Similarly, a number of inflammatory tumors, including inflammatory papillomas (viral and nonviral), pyogenic granulomas, and sarcoid granulomas, are also well known to ophthalmologists and require no comments in this chapter. However, one specific vascular tumor of the conjunctiva, Kaposi's sarcoma, and three other categories of lesions, the secondary and metastatic tumors and leukemic infiltrates, merit at least passing mention.

KAPOSI'S SARCOMA OF THE CONJUNCTIVA

Kaposi's sarcoma of the conjunctiva is a rapidly growing acquired neoplasm composed of malignant stromal cells densely vascularized by blood vessels of capillary size.[55] The typical lesion appears as an expanding, bright red subepithelial mass that projects through and replaces the overlying conjunctival epithelium (Fig. 67-19). Spontaneous bleeding leading to bloody tears or a subconjunctival hematoma is relatively common. Kaposi's sarcoma occurs in two clinical settings, one being as a rare subtype of soft tissue sarcoma in otherwise healthy individuals and the other being a relatively common occurrence in patients with AIDS.[55] During the early years of the AIDS epidemic in the United States, Kaposi's sarcoma ultimately developed in approximately 80% of patients with AIDS. Between 5–10% of those patients developed conjunctival Kaposi's sarcoma. Since that time, the frequency of Kaposi's sarcoma in patients with AIDS has decreased steadily, reflecting the development of effective drug therapy for this condition. The incidence of Kaposi's sarcoma in patients with AIDS is currently less than 1%. However, the proportion of patients with AIDS and Kaposi's sarcoma who ultimately develop conjunctival tumors appears to be about the same. Pathologically, the typical Kaposi's sarcoma consists of a delicate matrix of capillaries surrounding a matrix of malignant stromal cells of uncertain origin. There are no morphological differences between lesions of this type that occur sporadically and those associated with AIDS. Conjunctival Kaposi's sarcoma can be treated by excision, cryotherapy, radiation therapy (exter-

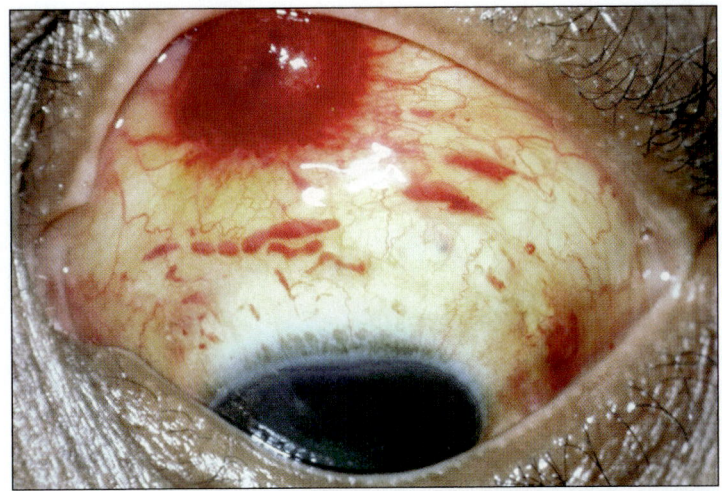

FIG. 67-19 ■ **Kaposi's sarcoma of bulbar conjunctiva.** Note intensely red color of mass and associated subconjunctival blood. This patient had underlying acquired immunodeficiency syndrome.

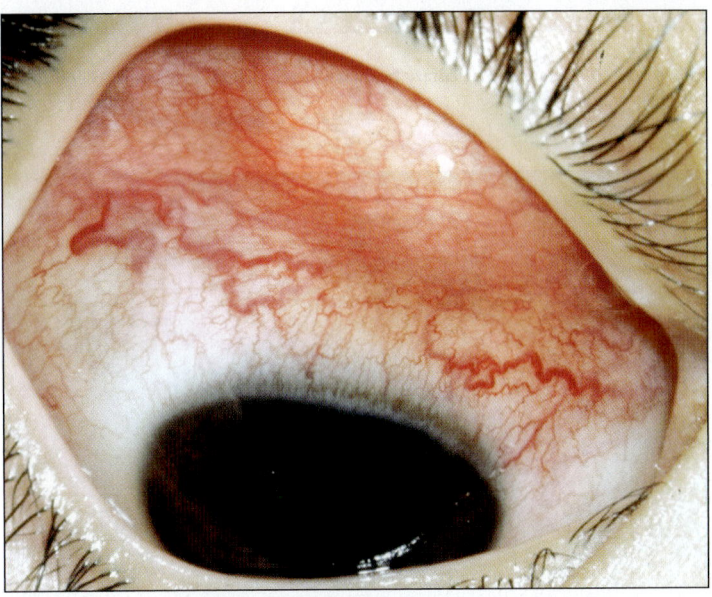

FIG. 67-20 ■ **Rhabdomyosarcoma of conjunctiva and orbit manifesting as epibulbar mass.** Tumor appears as pink mass arising from superior fornix.

nal beam or contact therapy), chemotherapy, or topical or intralesional interferon-α.[56–58]

SECONDARY TUMORS OF THE CONJUNCTIVA

Secondary tumors of the conjunctiva are malignant neoplasms of the eye, orbit, or eyelids that involve the conjunctiva by direct extension. Probably the most important orbital tumor that occasionally appears as a conjunctival mass is the rhabdomyosarcoma of the orbit (Fig. 67-20).[59] The reader is referred to the chapter on orbital tumors for additional information about this neoplasm. Several intraocular tumors occasionally appear as episcleral masses attributable to trans-scleral extension along neural or vascular foramina in the sclera. In adults, the most common intraocular tumor that exhibits extension to the exterior of the globe anteriorly is the ciliary body melanoma (Fig. 67-21). In children, both retinoblastoma and medulloepithelioma occasionally develop anterior episcleral extension. Squamous cell carcinomas and sebaceous carcinomas of the eyelid, as well as a few other malignant skin tumors, occasionally extend into the palpebral and forniceal conjunctiva and invade the orbit or globe.

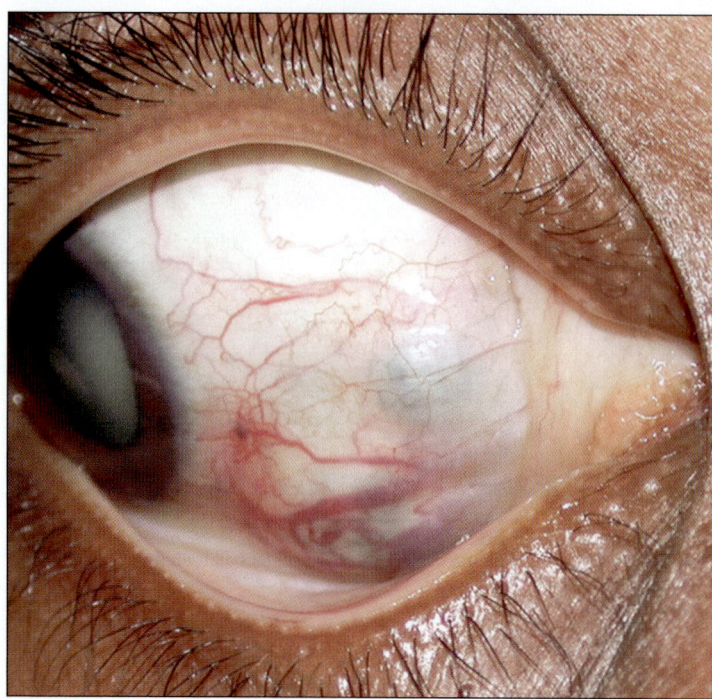

FIG. 67-21 Melanoma of ciliary body with transscleral extension to epibulbar surface.

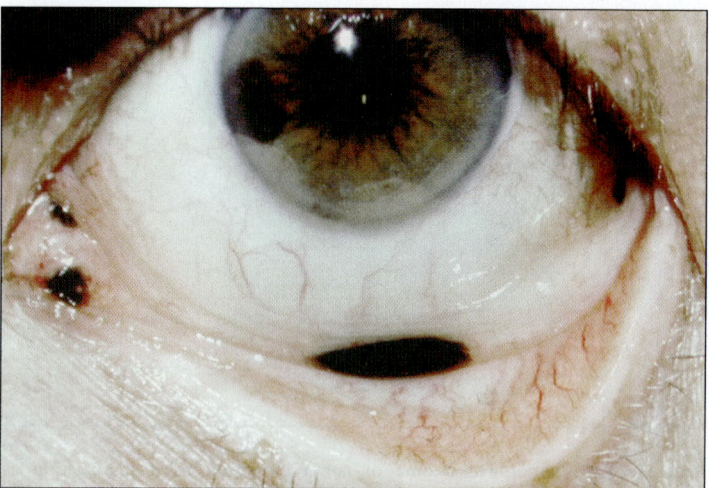

FIG. 67-22 Metastatic cutaneous melanoma to conjunctiva. Note melanotic conjunctival lesions in inferior fornix and caruncle and associated iris metastasis.

METASTATIC CARCINOMAS TO THE CONJUNCTIVA

Metastatic carcinomas to the conjunctiva are conjunctival deposits of malignant cells derived from a distant extra-ophthalmic primary cancer.[60] They are subepithelial masses that appear suddenly and typically enlarge progressively in the absence of effective local or systemic treatment. Most are unifocal, unilateral lesions, but bilateral and multifocal conjunctival metastatic tumors (Fig. 67-22) occur occasionally. Most patients with a metastatic conjunctival tumor have a well-documented history of the cancer that gave rise to the conjunctival lesion. They frequently are associated with concurrent ipsilateral intraocular or orbital metastatic tumors and usually are associated with concurrent metastatic tumors in other organs or tissues. Metastatic conjunctival tumors are extremely rare.

LEUKEMIC INFILTRATES OF THE CONJUNCTIVA

Leukemic infiltrates of the conjunctiva tend to be rapidly enlarging pale to pink subepithelial masses (Fig. 67-23). They are

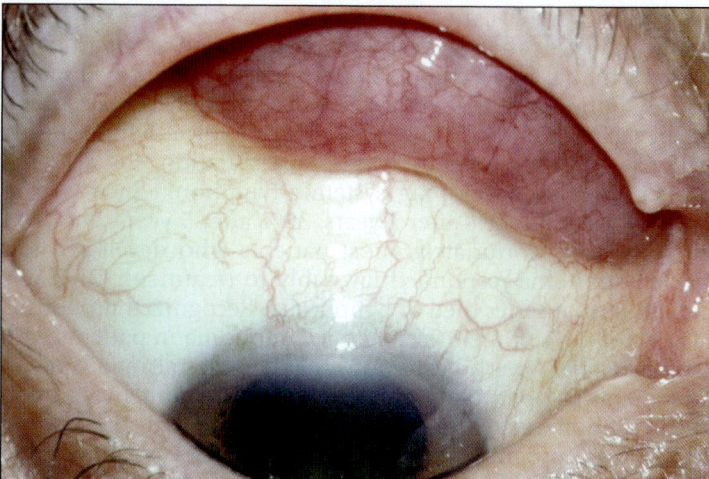

FIG. 67-23 Leukemic conjunctival tumor. Tumor appears as reddish pink mass involving superior fornix.

usually unilateral and localized, but bilateral and diffuse lesions sometimes are encountered.[61] In most cases, the patient has a well-documented history of leukemia prior to development of the conjunctival tumor. However, a conjunctival tumor is occasionally the first recognized manifestation of underlying leukemia. Conjunctival involvement appears to be more common in patients with acute lymphocytic and lymphoblastic leukemia than in those with other forms of the disease. Patients with conjunctival leukemic infiltrates must undergo a comprehensive staging examination, after which they usually are treated with a chemotherapeutic regimen appropriate to the type and stage of their leukemia. Conjunctival tumors that fail to regress with chemotherapy typically are managed with radiation therapy.

REFERENCES

1. Lee GA, Hirst LW. Incidence of ocular surface epithelial dysplasia in metropolitan Brisbane. A 10-year survey. Arch Ophthalmol. 1992;110:525–7.
2. Sun EC, Fears TR, Goedert JJ. Epidemiology of squamous cell conjunctival cancer. Cancer Epidemiol Biomarkers Prev. 1997;6:73–7.
3. Lee GA, Hirst LW. Ocular surface squamous neoplasia. Surv Ophthalmol. 1995; 39:429–50.
4. Lee GA, Williams G, Hirst LW, Green AC. Risk factors in the development of ocular surface epithelial dysplasia. Ophthalmology. 1994;101:360–4.
5. Kraemer KH, Lee MM, Scotto J. Xeroderma pigmentosum. Cutaneous, ocular, and neurologic abnormalities in 830 published cases. Arch Dermatol. 1987;123:241–50.
6. Kaimbo Wa Kaimbo D, Parys-Van Ginderdeuren R, Missotten L. Conjunctival squamous cell carcinoma and intraepithelial neoplasia in AIDS patients in Congo Kinshasa. Bull Soc Belge Ophtalmol. 1998;268:135–41.
7. Seitz B, Fischer M, Holbach LM, Naumann GO. Differential diagnosis and prognosis of 112 excised epithelial tumors. Klin Monatsbl Augenheilkd. 1995; 207:239–46.
8. McKelvie PA, Daniell M, McNab A, et al. Squamous cell carcinoma of the conjunctiva: a series of 26 cases. Br J Ophthalmol. 2002;86:168–73.
9. Tunc M, Char DH, Crawford B, Miller T. Intraepithelial and invasive squamous cell carcinoma of the conjunctiva: analysis of 60 cases. Br J Ophthalmol. 1999; 83:98–103.
10. Shields JA, Shields CL, Gunduz K, Eagle RC. Intraocular invasion of conjunctival squamous cell carcinoma in five patients. Ophthal Plast Reconstr Surg. 1999;15: 153–60.
11. Margo CE, Grossniklaus HE. Pseudoadenomatous hyperplasia of the conjunctiva. Ophthalmology. 2001;108:135–8.
12. Mauriello JA, Napolitano J, McLean I. Actinic keratosis and dysplasia of the conjunctiva: a clinicopathological study of 45 cases. Can J Ophthalmol. 1995; 30:312–6.
13. Erie JC, Campbell RJ, Liesegang TJ. Conjunctival and corneal intraepithelial and invasive neoplasia. Ophthalmology. 1986;93:176–83.
14. Hwang IP, Jordan DR, Brownstein S, et al. Mucoepidermoid carcinoma of the conjunctiva. A series of three cases. Ophthalmology. 2000;107:801–5.
15. Shields JA, Shields CL, De Potter P. Surgical management of conjunctival tumors. Arch Ophthalmol. 1997;115:808–15.
16. Buuns DR, Tse DT, Folberg R. Microscopically controlled excision of conjunctival squamous cell carcinoma. Am J Ophthalmol. 1994;117:97–102.
17. Peksayar G, Soyturk MK, Demiryünt M. Long-term results of cryotherapy on malignant epithelial tumors of the conjunctiva. Am J Ophthalmol. 1989;107:337–49.
18. Yeatts RP, Engelbrecht NE, Curry CD, et al. 5-Fluorouracil for the treatment of intraepithelial neoplasia of the conjunctiva and cornea. Ophthalmology. 2000;107:2190–5.
19. Wilson MW, Hungerford JL, George SM, Madreperla SA. Topical mitomycin C for the treatment of conjunctival and corneal epithelial dysplasia and neoplasia. Am J Ophthalmol. 1997;124:303–11.

20. Frucht-Pery J, Rozenman Y, Pe'er J. Topical mitomycin-C for partially excised conjunctival squamous cell carcinoma. Ophthalmology. 2002;109:548–52.

21. Shields CL, Naseripour M, Shields JA. Topical mitomycin C for extensive, recurrent conjunctival-corneal squamous cell carcinoma. Am J Ophthalmol. 2002; 133:601–6.

22. Karp CL, Moore JK, Rosa RH. Treatment of conjunctival and corneal intraepithelial neoplasia with topical interferon α-2b. Ophthalmology. 2001;108:1093–8.

23. Kearsley JH, Fitchew RS, Taylor RGS. Adjunctive radiotherapy with strontium-90 in the treatment of conjunctival squamous cell carcinoma. Int J Radiat Oncol Biol Phys. 1988;14:435–43.

24. Zehetmayer M, Manapace R, Kulnig W. Combined local excision and brachytherapy with ruthenium-106 in the treatment of epibulbar malignancies. Ophthalmologica. 1993;207:133–9.

25. Char DH. The management of lid and conjunctival malignancies. Surv Ophthalmol. 1980;24:679–89.

26. Levin PS, Dutton JJ. A series of orbital exenteration. Am J Ophthalmol. 1991;112: 496–501.

27. Bhattacharyya N, Wenokur RK, Rubin PAD. Metastasis of squamous cell carcinoma of the conjunctiva: case report and review of the literature. Am J Otolaryngol. 1997;18:217–9.

28. Seregard S, Kick E. Conjunctival malignant melanoma in Sweden 1969–91. Acta Ophthalmol. 1992;70:289–96.

29. Singh AD, Campos OE, Rhatigan RM, et al. Conjunctival melanoma in the black population. Surv Ophthalmol. 1998;43:127–33.

30. Gloor P, Alexandrakis G. Clinical characterization of primary acquired melanosis. Invest Ophthalmol Vis Sci. 1995;36:1721–9.

31. Folberg R, Jakobiec FA, Bernardino VB, Iwamoto T. Benign conjunctival melanocytic lesions. Clinicopathologic features. Ophthalmology. 1989;96: 436–61.

32. McDonnell JM, Carpenter JD, Jacobs P, et al. Conjunctival melanocytic lesions in children. Ophthalmology. 1989;96:986–93.

33. Gerner Nf, Morregaard JC, Jensen OA, Prause JU. Conjunctival naevi in Denmark 1960–1980. A 21-year follow-up study. Acta Ophthalmol Scand. 1996;74:334–7.

34. Jakobiec FA, Folberg R, Iwamoto T. Clinicopathologic characteristics of premalignant and malignant melanocytic lesions of the conjunctiva. Ophthalmology. 1989;96:147–66.

35. Folberg R, McLean IW, Zimmerman LE. Primary acquired melanosis of the conjunctiva. Hum Pathol. 1985;16:129–35f.

36. Buckman G, Jakobiec FA, Folberg R, McNally LM. Melanocytic nevi of the palpebral conjunctiva. An extremely rare location usually signifying melanoma. Ophthalmology. 1988;95:1053–7.

37. Paridaens ADA, McCartney ACE, Hungerford JL. Multifocal amelanotic conjunctival melanoma and acquired melanosis sine pigmento. Br J Ophthalmol. 1992; 76:163–5.

38. Tuomaala S, Afine E, Saari KM, Kivelä T. Corneally displaced malignant conjunctival melanomas. Ophthalmology. 2002;109:914–9.

39. Paridaens ADA, Minassian DC, McCartney ACE, Hungerford JL. Prognostic factors in primary malignant melanoma of the conjunctiva: a clinicopathological study of 256 cases. Br J Ophthalmol. 1994;78:252–9.

40. Anastassiou G, Heiligenhaus A, Bechrakis N, et al. Prognostic value of clinical and histopathological parameters in conjunctival melanomas: a retrospective study. Br J Ophthalmol. 2002;86:163–7.

41. Shields CL, Shields JA, Gunduz K, et al. Conjunctival melanoma. Risk factors for recurrence, exenteration, metastasis, and death in 150 consecutive patients. Arch Ophthalmol. 2000;118:1497–507.

42. Jakobiec FA, Rini FJ, Fraunfelder FT, Brownstein S. Cryotherapy for conjunctival primary acquired melanosis and malignant melanoma. Experienced with 62 cases. Ophthalmology. 1988;95:1058–70.

43. Demirci H, McCormick SA, Finger PT. Topical mitomycin chemotherapy for conjunctival malignant melanoma and primary acquired melanosis with atypia. Clinical experience with histopathologic observations. Arch Ophthalmol. 2000;118:885–91.

44. Lommatzsch PK, Lommatzsch RE, Kirsch I, Fuhrmann P. Therapeutic outcome of patients suffering from malignant melanomas of the conjunctiva. Br J Ophthalmol. 1990;74:615–9.

45. Paridaens AD, McCartney AC, Minassian DC, Hungerford JL. Orbital exenteration in 95 cases of primary conjunctival malignant melanoma. Br J Ophthalmol. 1994;78:520–8.

46. Knowles DM, Jakobiec FA, McNally L, Burke JS. Lymphoid hyperplasia and malignant lymphoma occurring in the ocular adnexa (orbit, conjunctiva, and eyelids): a prospective multiparametric analysis of 108 cases during 1977 to 1987. Hum Pathol. 1990;21:959–73.

47. Freeman C, Berg JW, Cutler SJ. Occurrence and prognosis of extranodal lymphomas. Cancer. 1972;29:252–60.

48. Coupland SE, Krause L, Delecluse HJ, et al. Lymphoproliferative lesions of the ocular adnexa. Analysis of 112 cases. Ophthalmology. 1998;105:1430–41.

49. Shields CL, Shields JA, Carvalho C, et al. Conjunctival lymphoid tumors. Clinical analysis of 117 cases and relationship to systemic lymphoma. Ophthalmology. 2001;108:979–84.

50. Weisenthal RW, Streeten BW, Dubansky AS, et al. Burkitt lymphoma presenting as conjunctival mass. Ophthalmology. 1995;102:129–34.

51. McLeod SD, Edward DP. Benign lymphoid hyperplasia of the conjunctiva in children. Arch Ophthalmol. 1999;117:832–5.

52. Hardman-Lea S, Kerr-Muir M, Wotherspoon AC, et al. Mucosal-associated lymphoid tissue lymphoma of the conjunctiva. Arch Ophthalmol. 1994;112: 1207–12.

53. Dunbar SF, Linggood RM, Doppke KP, et al. Conjunctival lymphoma: results and treatment with a single anterior electron field. A lens sparing approach. Int J Radiat Oncol Biol Phys. 1990;19:249–57.

54. Eichler MD, Fraunfelder FT. Cryotherapy for conjunctival lymphoid tumors. Am J Ophthalmol. 1994;118:463–7.

55. Shuler JD, Holland GN, Miles SA, et al. Kaposi's sarcoma of the conjunctiva and eyelids associated with the acquired immunodeficiency syndrome. Arch Ophthalmol. 1989;107:858–62.

56. Dugel PU, Gill PS, Frangieh GT, Rao NA. Treatment of ocular adnexal Kaposi's sarcoma in acquired immune deficiency syndrome. Ophthalmology. 1992;99: 1127–32.

57. Ghabrial R, Quivey JM, Dunn JP, Char DH. Radiation therapy of acquired immunodeficiency syndrome-related Kaposi's sarcoma of the eyelids and conjunctiva. Arch Ophthalmol. 1992;110:1423–6.

58. Hummer J, Gass JD, Huang AJ. Conjunctival Kaposi's sarcoma treated with interferon α-2a. Am J Ophthalmol. 1993;116:502–3.

59. Shields CL, Shields JA, Honavar SG, Demirci H. Primary ophthalmic rhabdomyosarcoma in 33 patients. Trans Am Ophthalmol Soc. 2001;99:133–42.

60. Kiratli H, Shields CL, Shields JA, DePotter P. Metastatic tumours to the conjunctiva: report of 10 cases. Br J Ophthalmol. 1996;80:5–8.

61. Kincaid MC, Green WR. Ocular and orbital involvement in leukemia. Surv Ophthalmol. 1983;27:211–32.

STRABISMUS

Gary R. Diamond

CHAPTER

68

Anatomy and Physiology of the Extraocular Muscles and Surrounding Tissues

BRIAN N. CAMPOLATTARO • FREDERICK M. WANG

EMBRYOLOGY

The extraocular muscles are of mesodermal origin, development beginning at 3–4 weeks' gestation.[1] The muscles originate from three separate foci of primordial cells, one for the muscles innervated by the oculomotor nerve, one for the superior oblique muscle, and one for the lateral rectus muscle. All of the extraocular muscles develop *in situ*; they do not begin development at their origins and sprout toward their respective insertions. The extraocular muscles receive input from their respective cranial nerves as early as 1 month of gestation.[2]

The tissues that surround the extraocular muscles also develop early in gestation. Formation of the trochlea begins at 6 weeks' gestation, and early fascial coverings can be detected around the extraocular muscles by 3 months' gestation.[3] Tissues destined to become intermuscular septa and orbital fat differentiate in the fourth and fifth months of gestation, respectively. All of the extraocular muscle and their surrounding tissues are present and in their final anatomical positions by 6 months' gestation, merely enlarging throughout the remainder of gestation.

GROSS ANATOMY OF THE EXTRAOCULAR MUSCLES

The alignment of the eye is determined by the extraocular muscles and their surrounding tissues. Primary position is defined as the position when the eye and head are both directed straight ahead. The primary position of the eye is approximately 23° nasal to the position of the orbits (the medial orbital walls are approximately parallel to each other); this relationship explains and determines both the cardinal positions of gaze and the fact that all vertical extraocular muscles have vertical, rotational, and horizontal (i.e., primary, secondary, and tertiary) actions on the globe when the globe is in primary position (Fig. 68-1). (Remember, the horizontal rectus muscles do have vertical actions on the globe, but not in primary position, where the primary, secondary, and tertiary actions of the extraocular muscles are defined.)

Origin of the Extraocular Muscles

Five of the six extraocular muscles (the inferior oblique excepted) originate at the orbital apex. The superior, inferior, medial, and lateral rectus muscles arise from the annulus of Zinn, an oval, fibrous ring at the orbital apex. The superior oblique muscle arises just above the annulus of Zinn. The following structures pass through the annulus of Zinn (Fig. 68-2):
• The superior and inferior divisions
• The oculomotor nerve
• The abducens nerve
• The optic nerve

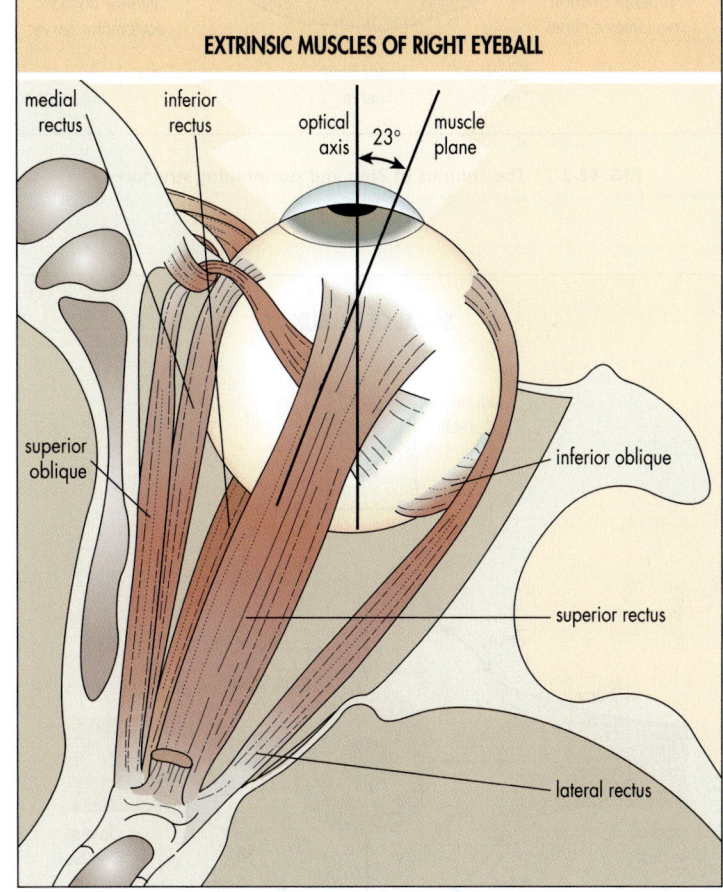

EXTRINSIC MUSCLES OF RIGHT EYEBALL

medial rectus — inferior rectus — optical axis — 23° — muscle plane — inferior oblique — superior oblique — superior rectus — lateral rectus

FIG. 68-1 ■ The extrinsic muscles of the right eyeball in the primary position, seen from above. The muscles are shown partially transparent.

• The nasociliary nerve
• The ophthalmic artery

The sixth extraocular muscle, the inferior oblique, originates from the maxillary bone, adjacent to the lacrimal fossa, posterior to the orbital rim.

Insertion of the Extraocular Muscles

The rectus muscles insert into the sclera via their tendons anterior to the equator of the globe. Although the rectus insertions may vary slightly, the spatial formation created by connecting their insertion is called the spiral of Tillaux (Fig. 68-3).[4] Note that the *medial rectus tendon* inserts closest to the limbus, followed by the inferior, lateral, and superior recti in that order.

THE ANNULUS OF ZINN AND SURROUNDING STRUCTURES

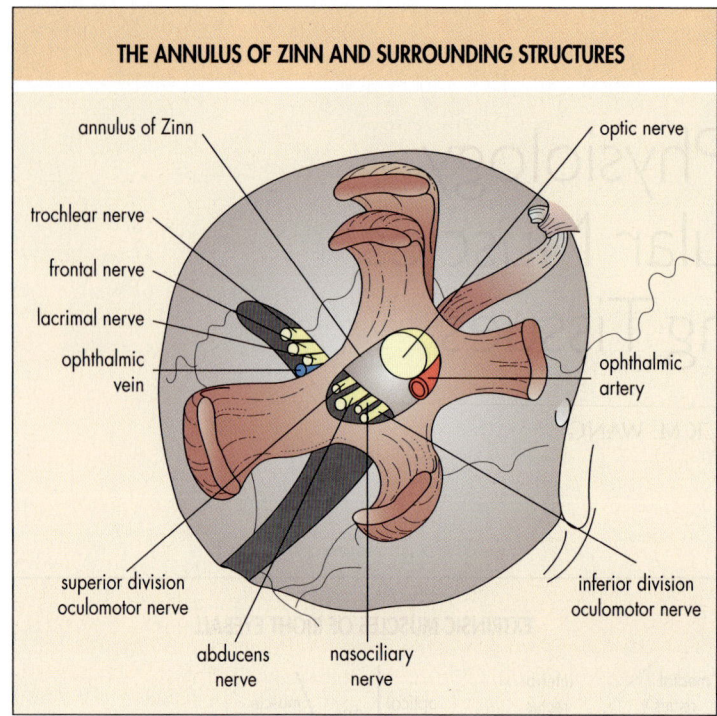

FIG. 68-2 ■ The annulus of Zinn and surrounding structures.

SPIRAL OF TILLAUX

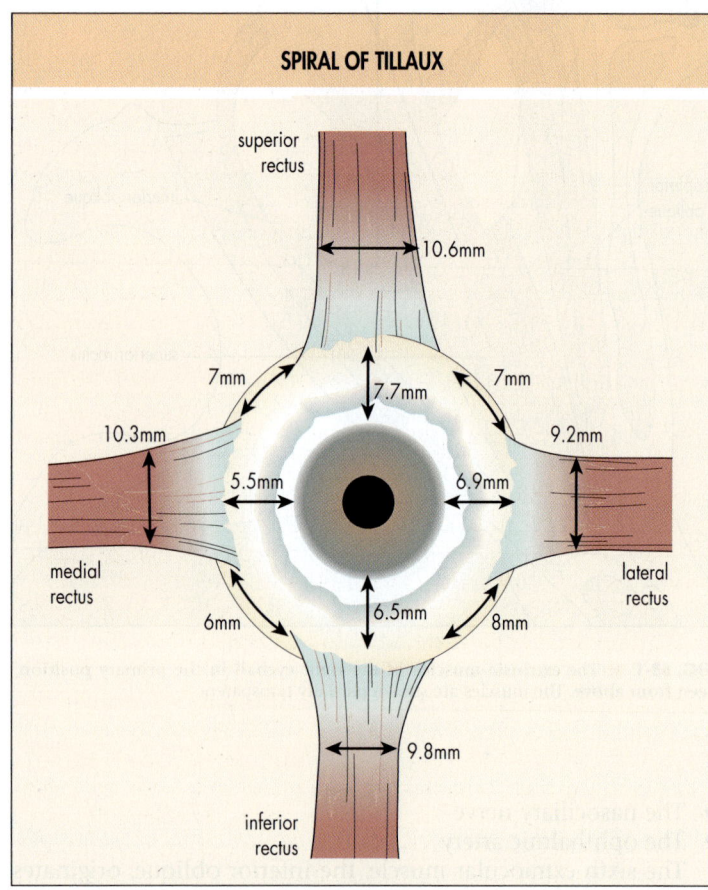

FIG. 68-3 ■ Spiral of Tillaux. The structure of the rectus muscle insertions.

Also note that the tendinous insertion line of the superior and inferior recti migrates posteriorly from the nasal to the temporal edge of the tendon. The sclera is thinnest (approximately 0.3mm thick) just posterior to the tendinous rectus insertions. Because the distance between the rectus insertions is less than the width of each rectus insertion, a thorough knowledge of the

POSTERIOR VIEW OF RIGHT EYE WITH TENON'S CAPSULE REMOVED

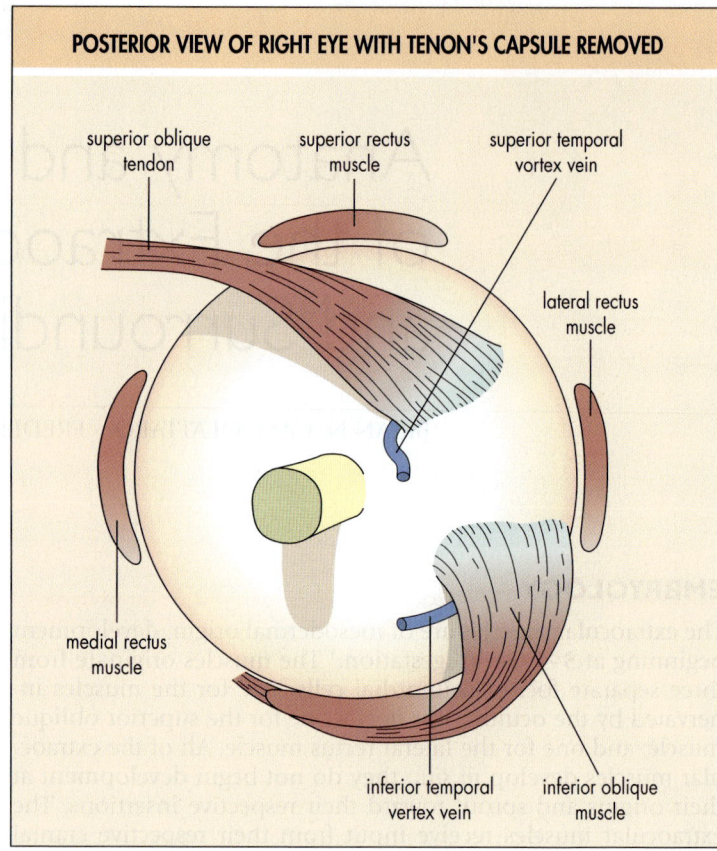

FIG. 68-4 ■ Posterior view of the eye with Tenon's capsule removed. (Adapted with permission from Parks MM. Extraocular muscles. In: Duane TD. Clinical ophthalmology. Philadelphia: Harper & Row; 1982:1–12.)

anatomy of the region is essential to ensure proper surgery on the correct muscles during strabismus surgery.

The oblique muscles insert into the sclera posterior to the equator of the globe (Fig. 68-4). The *superior oblique tendon* inserts into the posterior, superolateral sclera in a broad, fan-shaped fashion under the superior rectus muscle. The tendon insertion extends from the temporal pole of the superior rectus muscle to near the optic nerve. The insertion may be up to 18mm wide and extend near the superotemporal vortex vein. The tendon insertion is functionally separated into two parts, the anterior one third and the posterior two thirds. The anterior one third of the tendon functions almost exclusively to incyclo-tort the globe. The posterior two thirds of the tendon functions to depress and abduct the globe. This distinction allows surgical treatment of cyclovertical strabismus through manipulation of the anterior tendon fibers, such as by the Harada-Ito procedure.[5]

The *inferior oblique muscle*, which has almost no tendon at its insertion, inserts into the posterior, inferolateral sclera. The insertion lies in close proximity to both the macula and the infer-otemporal vortex vein. In general, the point of insertion of the oblique muscles is more variable than that of the rectus muscles.[6]

Course of the Extraocular Muscles

The extraocular muscles are belt-shaped structures with their thickest section residing posterior to the globe. The path of the extraocular muscles from their origin to their insertion determines their effects on eye movement, and a thorough knowledge of the relationship of the muscles with each other as they course to their insertions is requisite for successful orbital and strabismus surgery.

The *medial rectus muscle* leaves the nasal edge of the annulus of Zinn and courses anteriorly along the medial wall of the orbit to insert on the nasal anterior sclera. The proximity of the muscle to the medial orbital wall means that the medial rectus

ACTIONS OF THE RIGHT SUPERIOR RECTUS MUSCLE

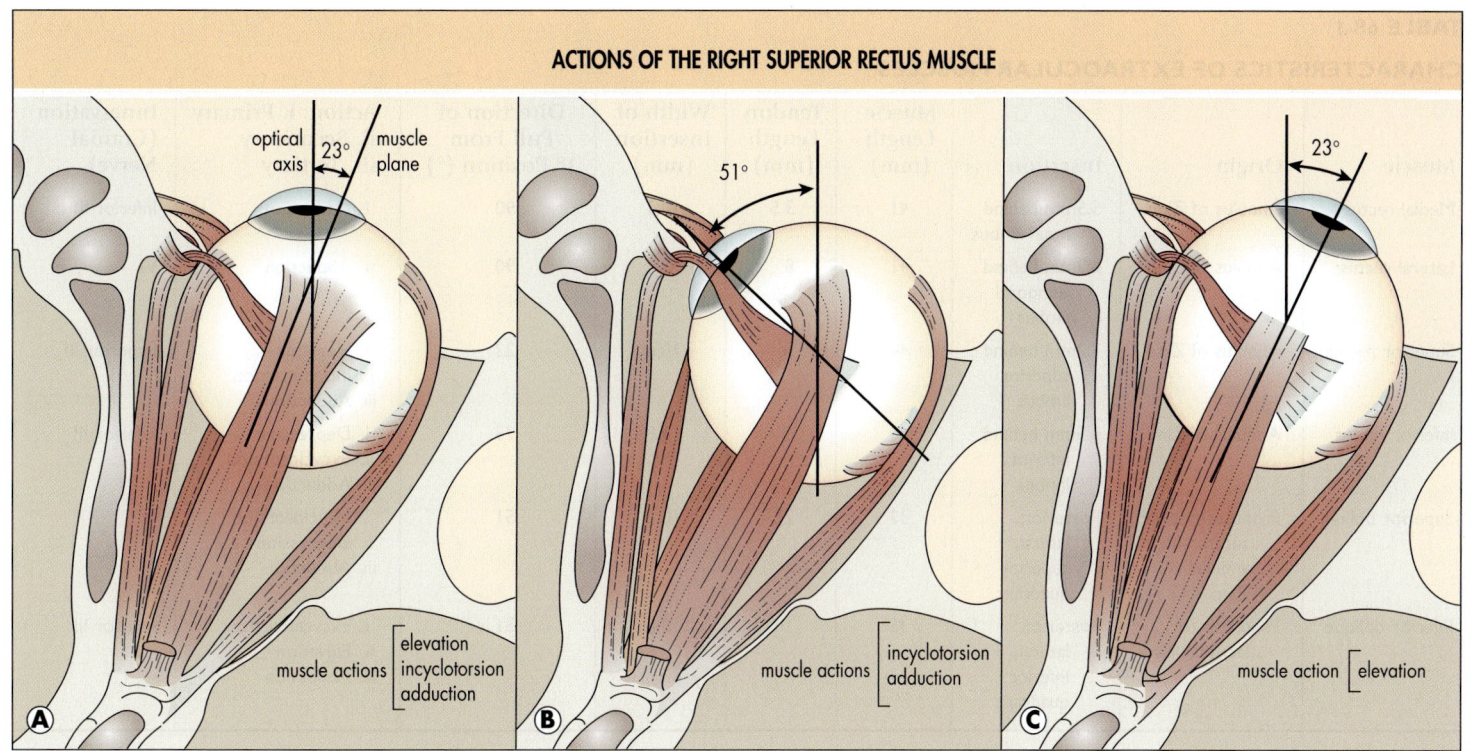

FIG. 68-5 ■ The actions of the right superior rectus muscle. **A,** Primary position. **B,** Adduction. **C,** Abduction.

can sustain inadvertent damage during standard or endoscopic ethmoid sinus surgery. The medial rectus is the only rectus muscle that does not have a fascial attachment to an oblique muscle; thus, the medial rectus muscle is at greatest risk for slippage or loss during orbital or strabismus surgery.

The *lateral rectus muscle* leaves the temporal edge of the annulus of Zinn and courses anteriorly in the lateral orbit to insert on the temporal anterior sclera. The inferior border of the lateral rectus passes just superior to the insertion of the inferior oblique muscle, and fascial connections between the two muscles here (8–9mm from the insertion of the lateral rectus) allow the surgeon to retrieve the lateral rectus at this location if inadvertent muscle detachment occurs.[7]

The *superior rectus muscle* leaves the superior edge of the annulus of Zinn and courses anteriorly, laterally, and superiorly in the superior orbit to insert on the anterior globe. In the primary position, the muscle forms an angle of 23° with the visual axis (Fig. 68-1). This angle determines the secondary and tertiary actions of the superior rectus muscle in the primary position. In primary position, the superior rectus functions to elevate, incyclotort, and adduct the globe. If the globe is abducted 23°, the visual axis and the muscle axis align and the sole action (in theory) of the superior rectus is elevation of the globe.

The cardinal positions of gaze refer to positions of the globe that minimize the angle between the axis of the extraocular muscle being evaluated and the visual axis. Minimizing this angle minimizes the secondary and tertiary actions of the muscle on the globe.

Nomenclature defines secondary and tertiary actions of the extraocular muscles in the primary position. In reality, if the globe is abducted more than 23°, the actions of the superior rectus muscle on the globe are elevation, abduction, and excyclotorsion (Fig. 68-5).

The *superior rectus muscle* courses between the tendon of the superior oblique muscle and the levator palpebrae muscle prior to its insertion, and fascial attachments from the superior rectus extend to both muscles. Failure to remove these connections to the levator muscle during superior rectus muscle recession or resection may lead to subsequent eyelid-fissure widening or narrowing, respectively.

The *inferior rectus muscle* leaves the inferior edge of the annulus of Zinn and courses anteriorly, laterally, and downward along the orbital floor to insert on the anterior globe. In the primary position, the muscle forms an angle of 23° with the visual axis. In primary position, the inferior rectus muscle functions to depress, excyclotort, and adduct the globe. If the globe is abducted 23°, the only action of the inferior rectus is depression of the globe.

The inferior rectus muscle courses between the globe and the inferior oblique muscle prior to its insertion, and fascial attachments exist between the inferior rectus, the inferior oblique, and the lower lid retractors. Failure to dissect these connections during inferior rectus recession or resection may lead to eyelid-fissure widening or narrowing, respectively. Some clinicians suggest that late overcorrections after inferior rectus recession may be caused by reattachment of these connections postoperatively even if dissection is performed.[8] If inadvertent disinsertion of the inferior rectus muscle occurs, this fascial network may allow retrieval of the muscle in the region of Lockwood's ligament.[9] These fascial relationships are described in detail later in this chapter.

The *superior oblique muscle* leaves the orbital apex at its anatomical origin above the annulus of Zinn and courses anteriorly along the superomedial wall of the orbit. The superior oblique muscle becomes tendinous as it passes through the trochlea, where its direction is altered. Connective tissue attachments exist between the trochlea and the superior oblique tendon.[10] The trochlea becomes the functional origin of the superior oblique tendon, and the tendon exits the trochlea inferiorly, posteriorly, and laterally to insert on the posterior globe. In the primary position, the superior oblique tendon forms an angle of 51° with the visual axis. In primary position, the superior oblique muscle functions to incyclotort, depress, and abduct the globe. If the globe is abducted 39°, the major action of the superior oblique muscle is incyclotorsion of the globe. If the globe is adducted 51°, the major action of the superior oblique muscle is depression of the globe. (The globe can move up to 50° in each direction from the primary position, but head movement usually occurs after it moves 15–20° from the primary position.)

The *superior oblique tendon* courses between the globe and the superior rectus muscle prior to its insertion, and fascial attachments exist between the tendon and the superior rectus muscle.

TABLE 68-1

CHARACTERISTICS OF EXTRAOCULAR MUSCLES

Muscle	Origin	Insertion	Muscle Length (mm)	Tendon Length (mm)	Width of Insertion (mm)	Direction of Pull From 1° Position (°)	Action: i. Primary ii. Secondary iii. Tertiary	Innervation (Cranial Nerve)
Medial rectus	Annulus of Zinn	5.5mm behind nasal limbus	41	3.5	10.3	90	i. Adduction	Inferior III
Lateral rectus	Annulus of Zinn	6.9mm behind temporal limbus	41	8	9.2	90	i. Abduction	VI
Superior rectus	Annulus of Zinn	7.7mm behind superior limbus	42	5	10.6	23	i. Elevation ii. Incyclotorsion iii. Adduction	Superior III
Inferior rectus	Annulus of Zinn	6.5mm behind inferior limbus	40	6	9.8	23	i. Depression ii. Excyclotorsion iii. Adduction	Inferior III
Superior oblique	Frontoethmoidal suture above annulus of Zinn	Posterior, lateral, superior quadrant	32	26	10.8	51	i. Incyclotorsion ii. Depression iii. Abduction	IV
Inferior oblique	Posterior to lacrimal fossa	Posterior, lateral, inferior quadrant	35	1	9.6	51	i. Excyclotorsion ii. Elevation iii. Abduction	Inferior III

The *inferior oblique muscle* leaves the lacrimal fossa and courses posteriorly, laterally, and temporally; it passes beneath the inferior rectus muscle to its insertion, which is adjacent to the inferior border of the lateral rectus. Fascial attachments exist between the inferior oblique muscle and the inferior and lateral rectus muscles. In the primary position, the inferior oblique muscle forms an angle of 51° with the visual axis. In primary position, the inferior oblique functions to excyclotort, elevate, and abduct the globe. If the globe is abducted 39°, the major action of the inferior oblique muscle is excyclotorsion of the globe. If the globe is adducted 51°, the major action of the muscle is elevation of the globe.

Other pertinent information about the extraocular muscles is listed in Table 68-1.

Innervation

The *third cranial (oculomotor) nerve* innervates multiple extraocular muscles after separating near the orbital apex into a superior and an inferior division. The superior division innervates the levator palpebrae and superior rectus muscles, and the inferior division innervates the medial rectus, inferior rectus, and inferior oblique muscles. The *fourth cranial (trochlear) nerve* innervates the superior oblique muscle. The *sixth cranial (abducens) nerve* innervates the lateral rectus muscle.

All rectus muscles are innervated from the intraconal surface of the muscle belly at approximately the junction of the middle and posterior third of each muscle. The inferior oblique muscle receives its innervation just lateral to the inferior rectus muscle. Inadvertent trauma to the nerve at this location may cause ipsilateral mydriasis because the parasympathetic fibers responsible for pupillary constriction also travel with the nerve to the inferior oblique muscle. The superior oblique muscle is innervated from its orbital surface, in several branches, near the middle of the muscle. Because the fibers of the fourth cranial nerve pass outside the muscle cone, the superior oblique muscle is not usually affected by retrobulbar anesthesia.

Blood Supply

The *ophthalmic artery* sends muscular branches to most of the extraocular muscles. The medial muscular branch supplies the medial rectus, inferior rectus, and inferior oblique muscles. The lateral muscular branch supplies the superior rectus, lateral rectus, and superior oblique muscles as well as the levator palpebrae muscle. Also, the *lacrimal artery* supplies the lateral rectus muscle and the infraorbital artery supplies the inferior rectus and inferior oblique muscles. The blood vessels that supply the oblique muscles do not carry any circulation to the anterior segment. The blood vessels that supply the rectus muscles are termed *anterior ciliary arteries*; these anterior ciliary arteries also supply the anterior segment of the eye. Usually, each rectus muscle contains two anterior ciliary arteries, with the exception of the lateral rectus muscle, which contains one such artery, but variations have been reported. These branches travel on the anterior surface of the rectus muscles and then pierce the sclera just anterior to the tendinous rectus insertions. They anastomose with conjunctival vessels at the limbus before connecting with the major arterial circle of the iris. The long *posterior ciliary arteries* also supply the anterior segment of the eye with blood via the major arterial circle of the iris. These long posterior ciliary arteries allow collateral blood flow after rectus muscle surgery.

Surgical manipulation of the rectus muscles permanently disrupts the anterior ciliary arteries. If surgery is performed on multiple rectus muscles simultaneously, anterior segment ischemia may result.[11] Usually, anterior segment circulation is most dependent on arteries from vertical rectus muscles and least dependent on arteries from the lateral rectus muscle, although exceptions have been reported.[12] Other risk factors for the development of anterior segment ischemia include sickle cell anemia, lupus erythematosus, hyperviscosity syndromes, arteriosclerosis, and advanced age. Anterior segment ischemia can lead to pain, uveitis, or even phthisis bulbi. Dissection of the anterior ciliary arteries from the rectus muscles prior to muscle surgery allows sparing of these vessels, minimizing the risk of anterior segment ischemia.[13]

The *superior and inferior orbital veins* supply venous drainage for the extraocular muscles.

Microscopic Anatomy

Extraocular muscle is unique because of its combination of different forms of muscle cells. Although five types have been reported, these can be represented by two main groups of muscle cells.

Fibrillenstruktur fibers are similar to the muscle fibers of skeletal muscle—they are singly innervated with large myelinated axons, motor end plates that resemble *en plaque* nerve endings, and many glycolytic enzymes that allow anaerobic metabolism. Their firing rate is proportional to conducted action potentials.[14] These characteristics allow a rapid, all-or-none response to a single nerve stimulus, which is necessary for rapid eye movements such as saccades. Within each extraocular muscle, these relatively large fibers reside on the global side.

The second group of muscle cells form *Felderstruktur* fibers. These fibers are unique to extraocular muscle—they are multiply innervated via small axons and multiple *en grappe* nerve endings and have a high concentration of mitochondria for aerobic metabolism. Their firing rate is proportional to the nerve impulse rate, not to conducted action potentials.[15] These characteristics allow a graded response to repetitive nerve stimuli, which is necessary for slow, precise eye movements, such as smooth pursuit, or for a tonic response necessary for gaze fixation. Within each extraocular muscle, these relatively small fibers reside on the orbital side. Because these fibers with high mitochondrial content are more physiologically "active" and consume more oxygen than *Fibrillenstruktur* fibers, capillaries are most prevalent on the orbital surface of the muscle.

Both groups demonstrate a high ratio of nerve fibers to eye muscle fibers compared with true skeletal muscle (approximately 1:50 to 1:100 in true skeletal muscle), especially *Felderstruktur* fibers (1:4).[16]

Unlike the situation in skeletal muscle, individual muscle cells, both *Fibrillenstruktur* and *Felderstruktur* types, are surrounded by connective tissue. This complex of mucopolysaccharide, collagen, and elastin harbors blood supply and nerve input to the muscle.[17]

Muscle spindles that detect length changes of extraocular muscles (proprioception) do exist, although they are less well developed than muscle spindles in skeletal muscle. They are most prevalent at the muscle-tendon interface.[18] Their importance in eye position and extraocular muscle activity, however, is unclear.

THE ORBITAL INFRASTRUCTURE AND ANATOMY

Within the orbit, there exists a delicate fibrous infrastructure that suspends the globe, compartmentalizes the cushioning fat pads, and directs the traversing muscles, nerves, and vessels (Fig. 68-6).[19–21] Tenon's capsule is a fibroelastic membrane that begins 1mm from the limbus, where it is fused with the conjunctiva; it then caps the globe posteriorly to the optic nerve.[19] Its inner surface is smooth, which allows free gliding of the adjacent structures within it. Its equatorial region is penetrated by the extraocular muscles. The rectus muscles penetrate Tenon's capsule just posterior to the equator (approximately 10mm posterior to the extraocular muscle insertions), and the oblique muscles penetrate Tenon's capsule just anterior to the equator. Tenon's capsule is arbitrarily divided into anterior and posterior segments at the sites of rectus penetration.

Tenon's capsule thickens in the equatorial region, where it is penetrated by the extraocular muscles.[20] At the site of penetration, a sleeve is formed around the penetrating extraocular muscle with increasing cross-linked collagen and elastin. This sleeve has significant fibroelastic attachments to the periorbita and adjacent sleeves (Figs. 68-7 and 68-8, *A*). These sleeves create compliant pulleys that redirect the extraocular muscles and act as functional origins.[20,22,23] The sleeve-like pulleys are centered at and just posterior to the equator of the globe with total anteroposterior extents of 13–19mm, although it is likely that only the middle 5–8mm of this extent is mechanically stiff. The pulley sleeves contain collagen, elastin, and innervated smooth muscle. Whether or not the smooth muscle dynamically changes pulley function is not known at present.[22] The sleeves extend both

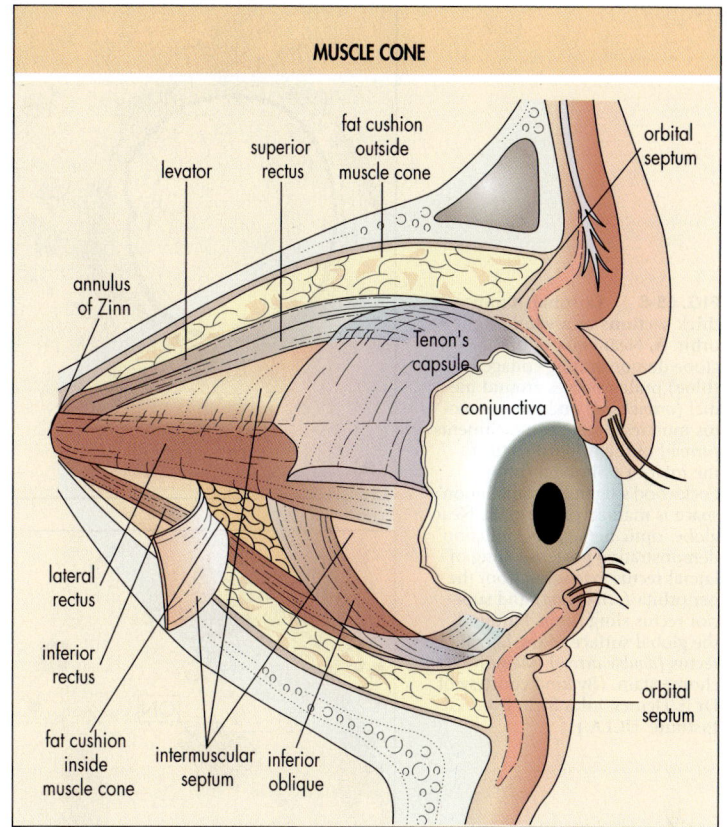

FIG. 68-6 ■ **Muscle cone.** (Adapted with permission from Parks MM. Extraocular muscles. In: Duane TD, ed. Clinical ophthalmology. Philadelphia: Harper & Row; 1982:1–12.)

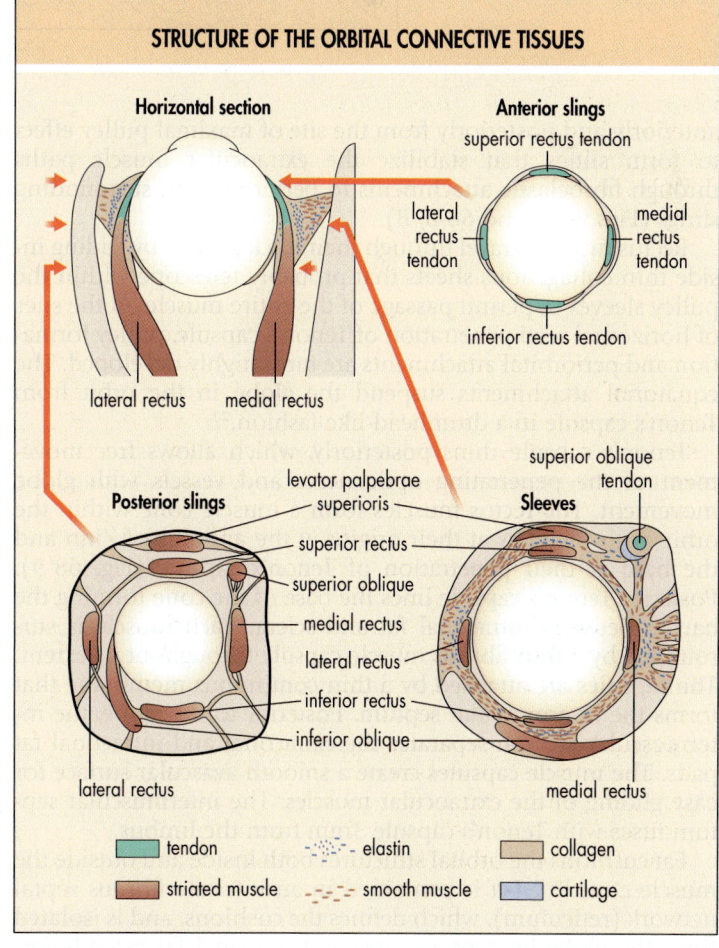

FIG. 68-7 ■ **The structure of the orbital connective tissues.** (Adapted with permission from Slack Incorporated. Demer JL, Miller JM, Poukens V, *et al.* Evidence for fibromuscular pulleys of the recti extraocular muscles. Invest Ophthalmol Vis Sci. 1995;36:1125–36.)

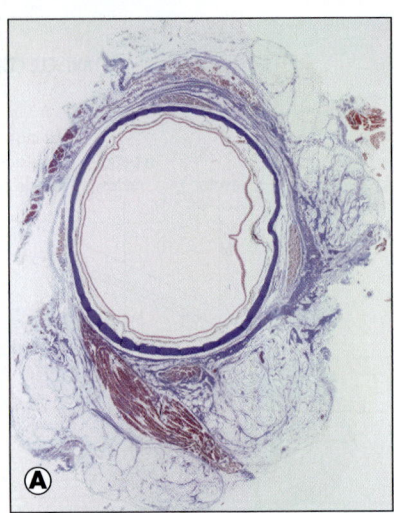

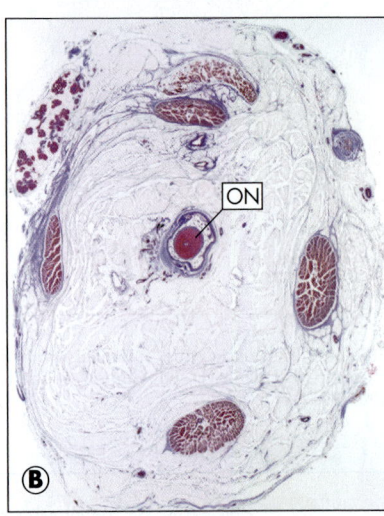

FIG. 68-8 ■ Coronal 10mm thick sections of a whole right orbit. **A,** Near equator of the globe demonstrating collagen (blue) pulley sleeves around medial *(arrowhead)* and inferior rectus muscles. Note the attachments *(arrow)* of the inferior rectus to the inferior oblique forming Lockwood's ligament. Sub-Tenon's space is marked *(asterisk)*. **B,** Near globe–optic nerve *(ON)* junction demonstrating posterior sling of lateral rectus extending from the periorbita *(arrowhead)* and superior rectus sling *(arrow)* around the global surface of the lateral rectus *(double arrow)*. Masson's trichome stain. (By kind courtesy of Dr JL Demer, Jules Stein Eye Institute, UCLA.)

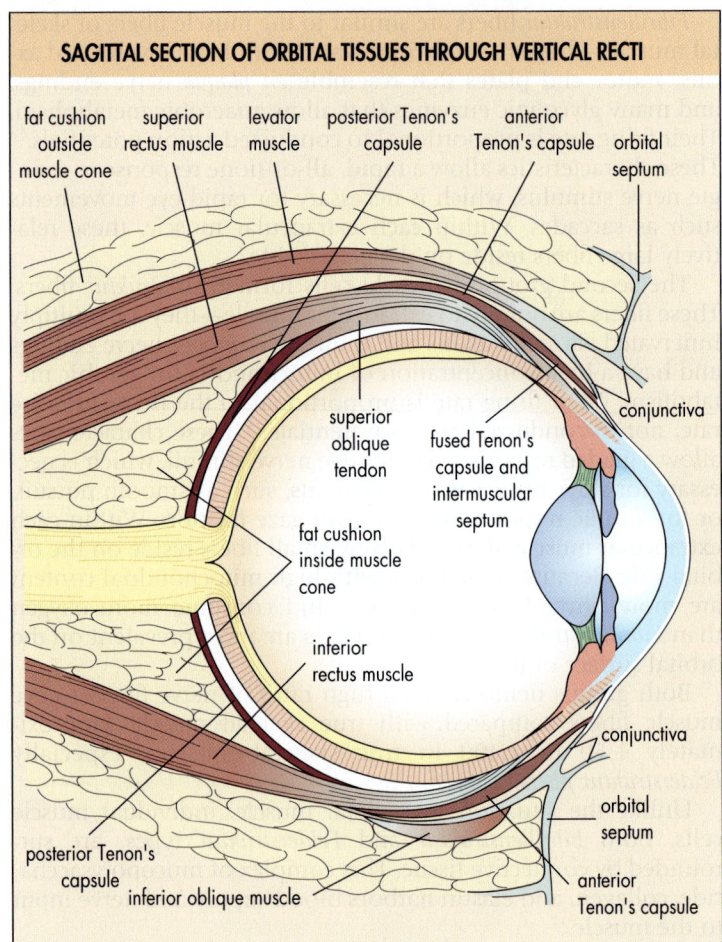

SAGITTAL SECTION OF ORBITAL TISSUES THROUGH VERTICAL RECTI

FIG. 68-9 ■ Sagittal section of orbital tissues through the vertical recti. (Adapted with permission from Parks MM. Extraocular muscles. In: Duane TD, ed. Clinical ophthalmology. Philadelphia: Harper & Row; 1982:1–12.)

anteriorly and posteriorly from the site of maximal pulley effect to form slings that stabilize the extraocular muscle paths through fibroelastic attachments to periorbita and surrounding slings (Figs. 68-7 and 68-8, *B*).

Rectus muscles travel through their thick pulleys by sliding inside thin collagenous sheets that probably telescope within the pulley sleeves to permit passage of the entire muscle. At the sites of horizontal recti penetration of Tenon's capsule, pulley formation and periorbital attachments are most highly developed. The equatorial attachments suspend the globe in the orbit from Tenon's capsule in a drumhead-like fashion.[20]

Tenon's capsule thins posteriorly, which allows free movement of the penetrating optic nerve and vessels with globe movement. The rectus muscles form a muscle cone within the orbit, with the apex at their origins at the annulus of Zinn and the base at their penetration of Tenon's capsule (Fig. 68-9). Posterior Tenon's capsule lines the base of the cone forming the barrier between intraconal fat and sclera. Each muscle is surrounded by a thin fibrous muscle capsule throughout its extent. The capsules are attached by a thin continuous membrane that forms the intermuscular septum. Posterior to the globe, the intermuscular septum separates the extraconal and intraconal fat pads. The muscle capsules create a smooth avascular surface for easy gliding of the extraocular muscles. The intermuscular septum fuses with Tenon's capsule 3mm from the limbus.

Fat cushions the orbital structures both inside and outside the muscle cone.[19–21] Fat is contained in an intricate fibrous septal network (reticulum), which defines the cushions, and is isolated from the globe by Tenon's capsule. Extraconal fat extends forward 10mm from the limbus, being limited in its anterior extent by the close apposition and fine areolar connections between Tenon's capsule and conjunctiva.

The trochlea is a cartilaginous saddle attached to periorbita of the frontal bone in the superior nasal orbit (Fig. 68-10).[24] The superior oblique tendon passes through the trochlea, changing direction in the fashion of a simple pulley. This cartilaginous saddle is 5.5mm long, 4mm wide, and 4mm deep with a 2mm groove along its long axis. Within the cartilaginous saddle and separated from it by a bursa-like space is a fibrillovascular sheath. The tendon of the superior oblique runs within this sheath. Movement of the tendon through the trochlea occurs by telescoping of the tendon fibers, the more internal fibers moving farther than the peripheral ones (Fig. 68-11). The tendon penetrates Tenon's capsule 2mm nasally and 5mm posteriorly to the nasal insertion of the superior rectus, where its capsule becomes continuous with the anterior intermuscular septum to the superior rectus. The superior oblique tendon has no special "sheath." This concept arose because the technique for capturing the superior oblique tendon frequently resulted in its being enveloped with a combination of Tenon's and intermuscular septum, which gave the appearance of a sheath.

The inferior oblique arises from the orbital plate of the maxilla, traveling through the extraconal fat cushion until it penetrates Tenon's capsule at the nasal border of the inferior rectus. It crosses beneath the inferior rectus, at which point extensions from the muscle capsules of the two muscles become continuous to form the "suspensory ligament of Lockwood."[25] This particular structure may have no unique suspensory or ligamentous function.[26] It is instead one part of the continuous fibrous infrastructure. After crossing beneath the inferior rectus, the posterior lateral surface of the inferior oblique abuts Tenon's capsule near the muscle's insertion. The surface capsule of the inferior oblique is continuous with the intermuscular septum of the lateral rectus.

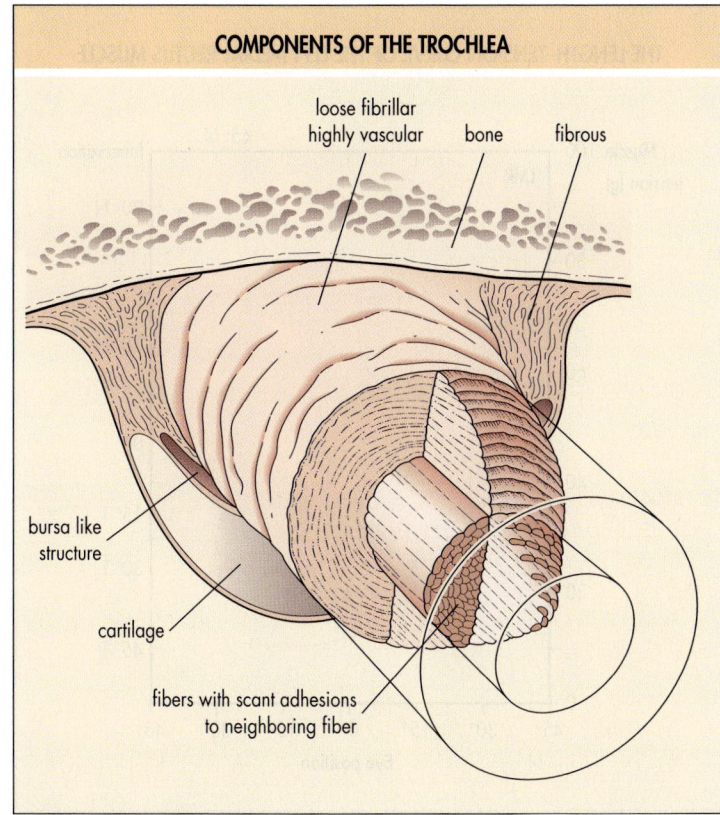

FIG. 68-10 ▮▮ **Components of the trochlea.** (Adapted with permission from Helveston EM, Merriam WW, Ellis RD, *et al*. The trochlea: a study of the anatomy and physiology. Ophthalmology. 1989;89:124–33.)

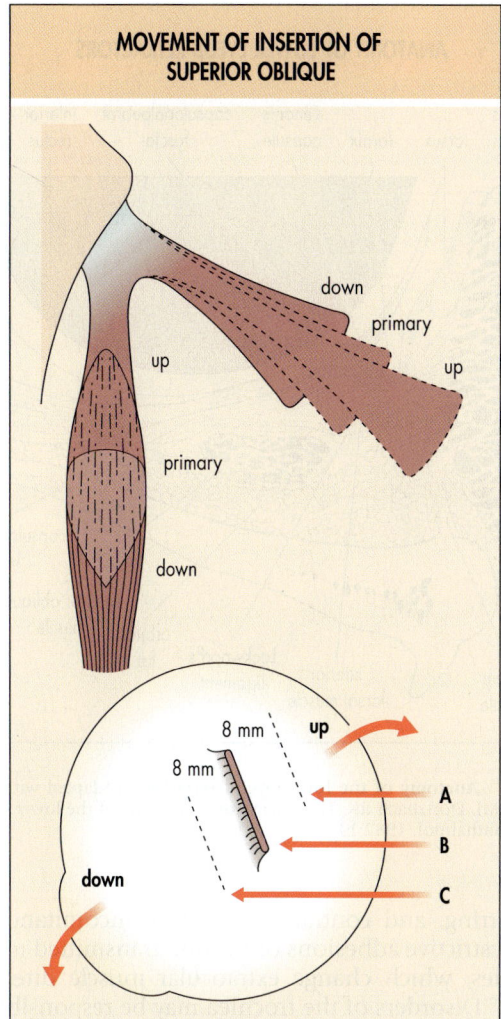

FIG. 68-11 ▮▮ **Movement of the insertion of the superior oblique.** The eye is shown in 50° adduction. From elevation A to primary position B is 8mm and from primary position B to downgaze C is 8mm. (Adapted with permission from Helveston EM, Merriam WW, Ellis RD, *et al*. The trochlea: a study of the anatomy and physiology. Ophthalmology. 1989;89:124–33.)

Fibrous septa arise from the orbital surface of the capsule of the inferior rectus 15mm from the limbus and extend forward to form the capsulopalpebral head of the inferior rectus (Fig. 68-12).[25,27] The fibroelastic tissue of the capsulopalpebral head divides above and below the inferior oblique while fusing with its capsule. Anterior to the inferior oblique, the fibers of the two portions of the capsulopalpebral head come together to form Lockwood's ligament. The capsulopalpebral head divides, sending fibers inferiorly through orbital fat to attach to the orbital septum; the bulk of the fibers continue anteriorly. This anterior extension proceeds forward as the capsulopalpebral fascia, being joined by smooth muscle fibers, the "inferior tarsal muscle." This fibromuscular band extends forward and attaches in slips to the tarsus on its anterior, basal, and posterior surfaces. Some fibers also extend through the preseptal orbicularis oculi muscle toward the skin, probably contributing to the lower eyelid crease.

CLINICAL CORRELATES

A thorough knowledge of and careful respect for the orbital infrastructure are the keys to successful strabismus and orbital surgery. Violating Tenon's capsule disrupts the globe's free movement by allowing adherence of fat to the globe, which restricts excursions.[28] Tenon's capsule is most often violated during strabismus surgery by either of the following:

- Making fornix incisions more than 9mm posterior to the limbus that expose the extraconal fat cushion, or
- Penetrating posterior Tenon's capsule to expose the intraconal fat cushion while working on the segment of the inferior oblique that is apposed to Tenon's capsule.

The muscle pulleys redirect the rectus muscles and limit the effect of transposition surgery.[23] The system of sleeves and slings limits the sideslip of the muscles that occurs during transposition procedures, thereby lessening the effective change in pulling direction that would occur if such structures were not

present. Whether or not there are entities of pulley dysfunction that produce incomitant strabismus remains to be elucidated.

Maintaining the integrity of the muscle capsules during surgery eliminates bleeding and preserves free-sliding upper surfaces. The intermuscular septal connections, especially between the obliques and their adjacent recti, help prevent surgical "loss" of the muscles through their pulleys at the sites of penetration of Tenon's capsule. Once the muscle slips through Tenon's pulley, it is difficult to find it within the orbital fat; the process of finding it may violate various tissue planes with attendant complications. The intermuscular septal connections and check ligaments attached to Tenon's capsule should be carefully severed when resecting or transposing muscles. This prevents the relocation of adjacent muscles and fat compartments. For example, if the attachments between the lateral rectus and inferior oblique are not severed, the inferior oblique is moved anteriorly during a resection of the lateral rectus. Severing of the intermuscular septal connections is not necessary for rectus recessions.[29]

Recession of the inferior rectus results in a posterior displacement of the capsulopalpebral head, which causes lowering of the lower lid. The capsulopalpebral septa, therefore, should be carefully severed during inferior rectus recession surgery. With moderate or large recessions of the inferior rectus, it is best to replace these septa at their normal distance from the limbus in order to minimize the lowering of the lower lid.[27]

Disruption of the reticulum of the fat cushions may result from various surgical procedures but most commonly occurs with orbital floor fracture. Resultant incarceration of orbital

555

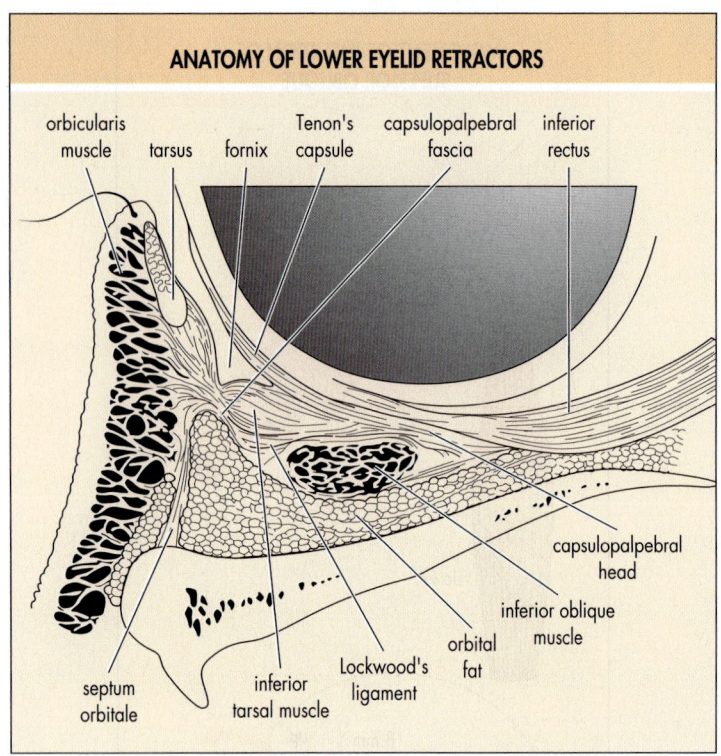

FIG. 68-12 ■ **Anatomy of the lower eyelid retractors.** (Adapted with permission from Hawes MJ, Dortzbach RK. The microscopic anatomy of the lower eyelid retractors. Arch Ophthalmol. 1982;100:1313–18.)

septa, scarring, and contracture produce incomitance of gaze through restrictive adhesions or traction transmitted to the muscle capsules, which change extraocular muscle direction and function.[30] Disorders of the trochlea may be responsible for certain inflammatory and traumatic Brown syndromes.[24]

EXTRAOCULAR MUSCLE PHYSIOLOGY

For globe movement, extraocular muscles must generate a force that overcomes the stiffness of passive tissues and the resting tension of the antagonist extraocular muscles. The contractile force produced by an eye muscle depends on its innervation and its length.

Length-tension curves summarize these forces for each extraocular muscle (Fig. 68-13).[31] For example, in primary position the medial rectus muscle has a resting tension of approximately 15g. This resting tension balances the tension of the lateral rectus muscle and the resistance of the surrounding tissues. With medial rectus contraction, tension of the muscle increases and the muscle shortens. However, the continued force available for muscle contraction decreases as a muscle shortens (due partly to changes in sarcomere length), with the result that continued contraction leads to higher tension but smaller force within the medial rectus muscle for further contraction. At the same time, the lateral rectus muscle is being stretched. Although, first, innervation to the lateral rectus is decreased during this adduction and, second, initial stretching places the lateral rectus muscle at its lowest resting tension, further stretching increases the tension in the lateral rectus muscle. Continued stretching leads to continued increases in the tension of the lateral rectus muscle and decreases in the force of contraction remaining in the medial rectus muscle until the opposing forces balance and a new eye position and resting tension are achieved. The resting tension of the medial rectus at this new eye position is less than the maximal tension within the muscle during the saccade to the new eye position. These forces are affected by paralysis, scar formation, abnormal innervation, and muscle contracture.

In the past, the length-tension curve provided the sole explanation for globe movement and for the resultant eye position af-

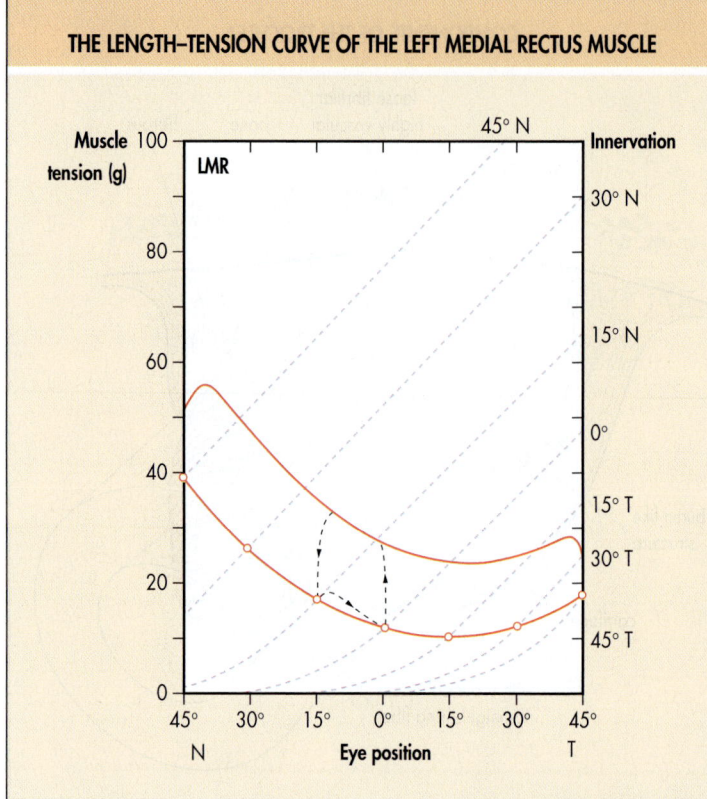

FIG. 68-13 ■ **The length-tension curve of the left medial rectus muscle.** (From Collins C, O'Mear DM, Scott AB. Muscle tension during unrestrained human eye movement. J Physiol. 1975;245:351–69.)

ter strabismus surgery. More recent evidence demonstrates that sarcomere reorganization occurs after extraocular muscle recession, resection, or paralysis, and these changes may be partly responsible for the resultant eye position after strabismus surgery.[32]

In normal, tonically innervated muscle, sarcomeres are of a precise length to maximize their contractility. Recession of extraocular muscle causes temporary "slack" of each sarcomere in that muscle. An analogy to decreasing the length of each sarcomere during muscle recession is to push the two sides of an accordion together, with each fold representing one sarcomere (Fig. 68-14). In time (8–12 weeks), each sarcomere reorganizes to its original length for maximal contractility. Now, however, the total number of sarcomeres in the muscle is decreased from preoperative levels. Similarly, muscle resection creates a temporary "stretch" of each sarcomere in that muscle (because tendon has been removed in the resection process and the remaining muscle must now reach from origin to insertion), and sarcomeric reorganization to its original length causes an increase in the total number of sarcomeres in the resected muscle.[33] How an increase or decrease in the number of sarcomeres per muscle ultimately affects extraocular muscle function, however, remains to be elucidated.

Principles and Terms

For convenience, it is assumed that the eye rotates about a fixed point 13.5mm behind the cornea, the center of rotation, on the visual axis. The three axes that pass through this fixed point can describe all globe rotations and are termed the *axes of Fick*.[34] These axes are the *x*-axis, which is horizontally orientated for vertical globe movement, the *z*-axis, which is vertically orientated for horizontal globe movement, and the *y*-axis, which is orientated on the visual axis for rotational globe movement. Listing's equatorial plane also passes through the center of rotation and includes the *x*- and *z*-axes (Fig. 68-15).[35]

Donder's law states that the orientation of the eye is determined solely by the horizontal and vertical coordinates plotted

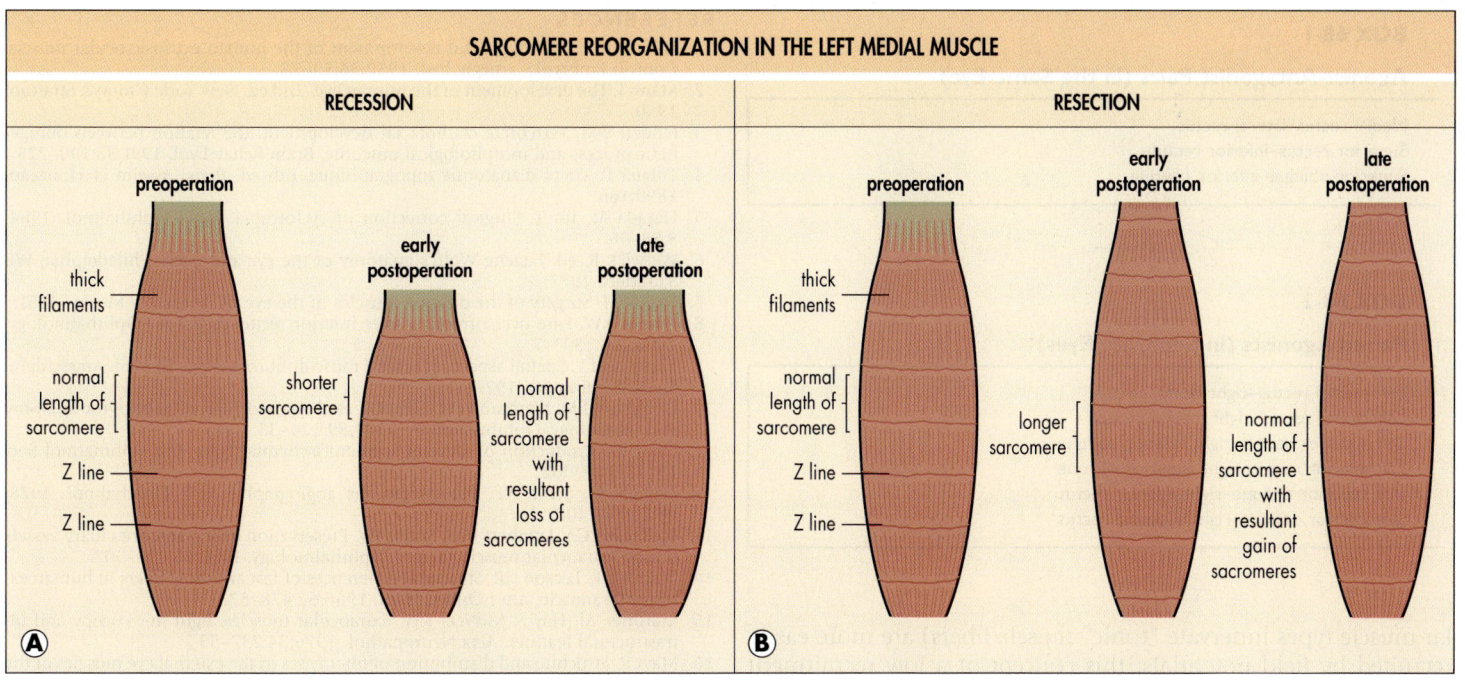

SARCOMERE REORGANIZATION IN THE LEFT MEDIAL MUSCLE

FIG. 68-14 ▌ Sarcomere reorganization of the left medial rectus muscle. (A, Recession. B, Resection.)

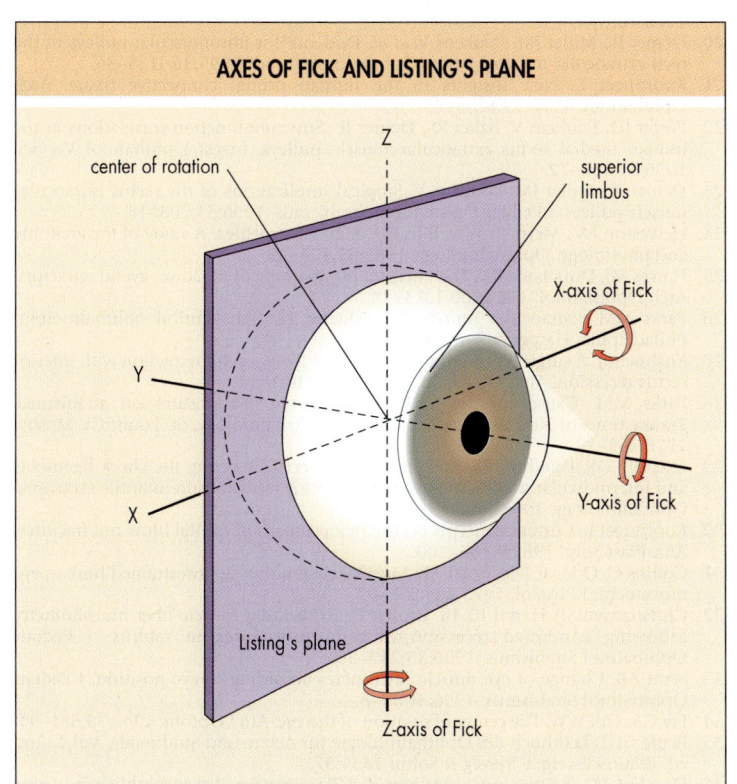

FIG. 68-15 ▌ The axes of Fick and Listing's plane.

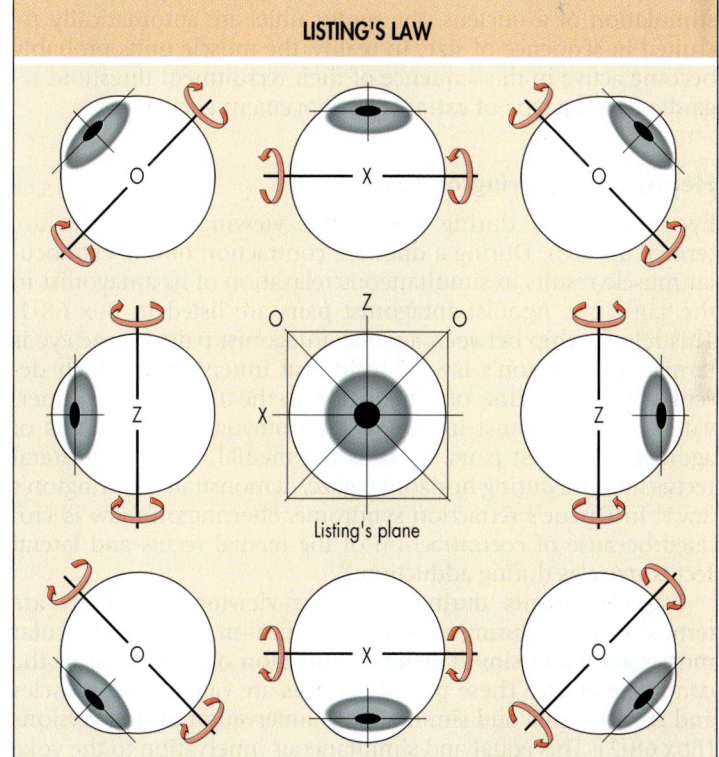

FIG. 68-16 ▌ **Demonstration of Listing's law.** All positions of gaze can be achieved by rotations around axes that lie on Listing's plane. Note pseudotorsion of the cornea during rotation around the oblique axes.

on the axes of Fick; preceding eye movements have no effect on subsequent orientation.[36] This law does not apply to smooth pursuit movements or eye movements in the presence of head tilt.

Listing's law specifies the orientation of the globe as a function of gaze direction and states that all positions of gaze can be achieved by rotations around axes that lie on Listing's plane. On Listing's plane, an oblique (O-) axis is present between the z- and x-axes of Fick, which allows oblique eye rotation. Listing's law does not apply in the presence of head tilt because countertorsion is elicited (Fig. 68-16).

Central Innervational Patterns

Individual muscle fibers fire at a rate dependent on both eye position and velocity of movement regardless of the type of eye movement.[37] Each extraocular muscle fiber, classified simply as a "fast-saccadic" type or "slow-tonic" type, is innervated by a neuron with a particular electric threshold at which it becomes active. In the spinal cord, a "size order of nerve recruitment" exists for motor neurons; the concept seems to apply to extraocular muscle innervation as well.[38] This means that smaller neurons with smaller axons (which in the simplified concept of extraocu-

---

BOX 68-1

Agonist-Antagonist Pairs (in the Same Eye)

Medial rectus–lateral rectus
Superior rectus–inferior rectus
Superior oblique–inferior oblique

BOX 68-2

Paired Agonists (in Separate Eyes)

Left medial rectus–right lateral rectus
Left lateral rectus–right medial rectus
Left superior rectus–right inferior oblique
Left inferior rectus–right superior oblique
Left superior oblique–right inferior rectus
Left inferior oblique–right superior rectus

---

lar muscle types innervate "tonic" muscle fibers) are more easily recruited by field potentials; this concept of a low recruitment threshold for neurons that innervate tonic muscle fibers provides an efficient method of stimulating continuous extraocular muscle activity for pursuit or gaze fixation.[39] For saccades, a larger field potential is required to recruit the larger neurons with larger axons (which innervate fast muscle fibers). Thus, with increasing stimulation of a nucleus, the motor units are automatically recruited in sequence of size. In reality, the muscle units probably become active in the sequence of their recruitment threshold regardless of the type of extraocular movement elicited.

Hering and Sherrington Laws

Eye movements during monocular viewing conditions are termed *ductions*. During a duction, contraction of one extraocular muscle results in simultaneous relaxation of its antagonist in the same eye. Agonist-antagonist pairs are listed in Box 68-1. This relationship between agonist-antagonist pairs in one eye is termed Sherrington's law of reciprocal innervation, which describes the inhibition of innervation to the antagonist as innervation to the agonist increases. Electromyogram recordings of agonist-antagonist pairs, such as the medial rectus and lateral rectus muscles during horizontal gaze, demonstrate Sherrington's law.[40] In Duane's retraction syndrome, Sherrington's law is violated because of cocontraction of the medial rectus and lateral rectus muscles during adduction.[41]

Eye movements during binocular viewing conditions are termed *versions*. During a version, contraction of one extraocular muscle results in simultaneous contraction of an agonist in the contralateral eye. These paired agonists are called yoke muscles and receive equal and simultaneous innervation during versions (Box 68-2). This equal and simultaneous innervation to the yoke muscles during versions is called Hering's law of motor correspondence.[42] Hering's law is often violated during saccadic eye movements, when dynamic overshoot and slightly different innervational signals to the yoke muscles may occur.[43] Hering's law explains the findings of primary and secondary deviations in the setting of paralytic strabismus. Innervation to the yoke muscles is always determined by the fixing eye. When the normal eye fixates, the resultant strabismus is termed the primary deviation. When the paretic eye fixates, the resultant strabismus is termed the secondary deviation and is often the larger of the two deviations.

REFERENCES

1. Gilbert PW. The origin and development of the human extrinsic ocular muscle. Contrib Embryol Carnegie Inst. 1957;36:59–78.
2. Mann I. The development of the human eye, 2nd ed. New York: Grune & Stratton; 1950.
3. Noden DM. Vertebrate craniofacial development: the relation between ontogenetic process and morphological outcome. Brain Behav Evol. 1991;38:190–225.
4. Tillaux P. Traité d'anatomie topographique, 6th ed. Paris: Asselin et Houzeau; 1890:166.
5. Harada M, Ito Y. Surgical correction of cyclotropia. Jpn J Ophthalmol. 1964; 8:88–96.
6. Warwick R, ed. Eugene Wolff's anatomy of the eye and orbit. Philadelphia: WB Saunders; 1977.
7. Fink WH. Surgery of the oblique muscles of the eye. St. Louis: CV Mosby; 1951.
8. Wright KW. Late overcorrection after inferior rectus recession. Ophthalmology. 1996;103:1503–7.
9. Koornneef L. Spatial aspects of orbital musculofibrous tissue in man. Amsterdam: Swets & Zeitlinger; 1977.
10. Helveston EM, Merriam WW, Ellis RD, et al. The trochlea: a study of the anatomy and physiology. Ophthalmology. 1989;89:124–33.
11. Hiatt RL. Production of anterior segment ischemia. Trans Am Ophthalmol Soc. 1977;75:87–102.
12. Hayreh SS, Scott WE. Fluorescein iris angiography. Arch Ophthalmol. 1978; 96:1390–1400.
13. McKeown CA, Lambert HM, Shore JW. Preservation of the anterior ciliary vessels during extraocular muscle surgery. Ophthalmology. 1989;96:498–507.
14. Brandt DE, Leeson CR. Structural differences of fast and slow fibers in human extraocular muscle. Am J Ophthalmol. 1966;62:478–87.
15. Martinez AJ, Hay S, McNeer KW. Extraocular muscles, light microscopy and ultrastructural features. Acta Neuropathol. 1976;34:237–53.
16. Mayr R. Structure and distribution of fiber types in the external eye muscles of the rat. Tissue Cell. 1971;3:433–62.
17. Ringel SP, Wilson WB, Barden MT, Kaiser KK. Histochemistry of human extraocular muscle. Arch Ophthalmol. 1978;96:1067–72.
18. Cooper S, Daniel PM. Muscle spindles in human extrinsic eye muscles. Brain. 1949;72:1–24.
19. Parks MM. The role of the fascia in muscle surgery. J Int Ophthalmol Clin. 1976;16(3):17–37.
20. Demer JL, Miller JM, Poukens V, et al. Evidence for fibromuscular pulleys of the recti extraocular muscles. Invest Ophthalmol Vis Sci. 1995;36:1125–36.
21. Koornneef L. New insights in the human orbital connective tissue. Arch Ophthalmol. 1977;95:1269–73.
22. Porter JD, Poukens V, Baker RS, Demer JL. Structure-function correlations in the human medial rectus extraocular muscle pulleys. Invest Ophthalmol Vis Sci. 1996;37:468–72.
23. Demer JL, Miller JM, Poukens V. Surgical implications of the rectus extraocular muscle pulleys. J Pediatr Ophthalmol Strabismus. 1996;33:208–18.
24. Helveston EM, Merriam WW, Ellis FD, et al. The trochlea. A study of the anatomy and physiology. Ophthalmology. 1982;89:124–33.
25. Hawes MJ, Dortzbach RK. The microscopic anatomy of the lower eyelid retractors. Arch Ophthalmol. 1982;100:1313–18.
26. Parks MM. Extraocular muscles. In: Duane TD, ed. Clinical ophthalmology. Philadelphia: Harper & Row; 1982:1–12.
27. Kushner BJ. A surgical procedure to minimize lower-eyelid retraction with inferior rectus recession. Arch Ophthalmol. 1992;110:1011–14.
28. Parks MM. Causes of the adhesive syndrome. Symposium on strabismus. Transactions of New Orleans Academy of Ophthalmology. St. Louis: CV Mosby; 1978:269–79.
29. Friendly DS, Parelhoff ES, McKeown CA. Effect of severing the check ligaments and intermuscular membranes on medial rectus recessions in infantile esotropia. Ophthalmology. 1993;100:945–8.
30. Koornneef L. Current concepts on the management of orbital blow-out fractures. Ann Plast Surg. 1982;9:185–200.
31. Collins C, O'Mear DM, Scott AB. Muscle tension during unrestrained human eye movement. J Physiol. 1975;245:351–69.
32. Christiansen SP, Harral RL III, Brown H. Extraocular muscle fiber morphometry following combined recession-resection procedures in rabbits. J Pediatr Ophthalmol Strabismus. 1996;33:247–50.
33. Scott AB. Change of eye muscle sarcomeres according to eye position. J Pediatr Ophthalmol Strabismus. 1996;31:85–8.
34. Fry GA, Hill WW. The center of rotation of the eye. Am J Optom. 1962;39:581–95.
35. Reute CGT. Lehrbuch der Ophthalmologie fur Aerzte und Studirende, Vol 1, 2nd ed. Braunschweig: F Vieveg & Sohn; 1855:37.
36. Donders FC. Beitrag zur Lehre von den Bewegungen des menschlichen. Auges Holl Beitr Anat Physiol Wiss. 1846;1:105–45.
37. Robinson DA. Oculomotor unit behavior in the monkey. J Neurophysiol. 1970; 33:393–404.
38. Henneman E, Somjen G, Carpenter DO. Functional significance of cell size in spinal motoneurons. J Neurophysiol. 1965;28:560–80.
39. Henneman E, Somjen G, Carpenter DO. Excitability and inhibitability of motoneurons of different sizes. J Neurophysiol. 1965;28:560–80.
40. Sherrington CS. Experimental note on two movements of the eye. J Physiol. 1894; 17:27–9.
41. Strachan IM, Brown BH. Electromyography of extraocular muscles in Duane's syndrome. Br J Ophthalmol. 1972;56:594–9.
42. Bridgeman B, Stark L. The theory of binocular vision. New York: Plenum; 1977.
43. Bahill AT, Cuiffreda KJ, Kenyon R, Stark L. Dynamic and static violations of Hering's law of equal innervation. Am J Optom Physiol Opt. 1976;53:786–96.

CHAPTER

69

Evaluating Vision in Preverbal and Preliterate Infants and Children

GARY R. DIAMOND

DEFINITION

- Visual acuity, in preverbal infants, is defined as a motor or sensory response to a threshold stimulus of known size at known testing distance. In preliterate but verbal children, visual acuity is defined as the smallest target of known size at known testing distance correctly verbally identified by a child.

KEY FEATURES

- In preverbal children, visual acuity may be quantified by a motor response (opticokinetic nystagmus testing, forced choice preferential looking) as well as by a sensory response (visual evoked responses).
- In preliterate but verbal children, visual acuity may be quantified by verbal or motor identification of graded non-Snellen optotypes (Landolt rings, HOTV test, tumbling E game, Sheridan-Gardner method.)

INTRODUCTION

Specialized techniques for visual acuity quantitation are necessary when evaluating children younger than about 5 years of age. These techniques include observation, the use of fixation targets, opticokinetic nystagmus, visual evoked potentials, forced choice preferential looking, and specially constructed graded optotypes. Each of these techniques is described in this chapter.

HISTORICAL AND OBSERVATIONAL TECHNIQUES

Much can be learned from the historical descriptions of a young child's visual behavior with family members and at playtime. Parents or caretakers are asked routinely whether the child responds to a silent smile, enjoys silent mobiles, and follows objects around the environment. Pertinent observations include strabismus, nystagmus, persistent staring, and inattention to objects. A younger sibling's visual behavior may be compared with that of an older child.

The pupillary light response is not equivalent to visual ability, but its presence indicates intact afferent visual neurologic pathways to the level of the brachium of the superior colliculus and efferent pathways to the iris sphincter. This reflex is present in premature babies over 29–31 weeks of gestational age.[1] Visualization in very young children sometimes requires a magnifying glass, as their pupils are smaller than those of older children (because of decreased sympathetic tone) and the light responses are of small amplitude. Dilatation to direct illumination has been described in Leber's congenital amaurosis, optic nerve hypoplasia, congenital cone dystrophy, and congenital stationary night blindness.[2] Nystagmus is absent in cortical blindness[3] and is not found often in association with unilateral visual defects.

The blink to a bright light is a behavior learned by 30 weeks of gestational age and occasionally is present in decorticate infants. The blink to a threatening gesture is another learned reflex, usually present by 5 months; when testing, care must be taken not to brush air against the child's corneas and elicit a blink by that mechanism.

FIXATION TARGETS

Visual fixational abilities may be demonstrated in term newborns if the appropriate target, such as a human face, is utilized. A flashlight is a poor target as it has no edges; stripes, dots, or checkerboards are preferred because they have edges. Term infants younger than 3 months of age follow by means of hypometric saccades when the target is small[4]; term infants may generate smooth pursuit movements to a large target such as an opticokinetic drum. Because saccadic palsies are common in young children who have central nervous system damage, spinning an upright child demonstrates the presence of saccades as the rapid recovery phase of the spin-induced nystagmus. If no rapid phase can be stimulated, the child's vision cannot be evaluated by its ability to "follow" a small target, as neither a saccadic nor a smooth pursuit system is available. In addition, a child who has normal fixational behavior should dampen spin-induced nystagmus in 3–5sec; a blind or poorly sighted child cannot use fixational dampening and beats for 15–30sec until mechanical dampening occurs.

In somewhat older children, small, colorful, nonthreatening familiar toys generate the best, albeit often momentary, interest. Small coins and breakfast cereals have been used to quantify roughly visual acuity, often with success, but the rule remains: "one toy earns one look."

OPTICOKINETIC NYSTAGMUS

Evaluation of the presence or absence of opticokinetic nystagmus was the first "technologic" approach to acuity measurement in preverbal children; square-wave gratings (alternating black and white stripes with sharp, distinct interfaces) placed on arcs were moved across an infant's visual field.[5] Standardized drums that contain stripes that subtend small fractions of the infant's visual field are available (Fig. 69-1) but often do not hold interest, are frequently spun at varying and uncalibrated rates, and are bathed in variable illumination. More disturbing is the realization that normal responses[6] may occur in the occasional decorticate infant, which indicate that subcortical areas of the occipital cortex may generate opticokinetic responses. When determination is performed binocularly, term infants have approximately 20/400 (6/120) acuity at birth and reach 20/20 (6/6) by 26–30 months. This method measures acuity by means of a motor response technique (eye movement), but using this can result in underestimation of the acuity in some children who have

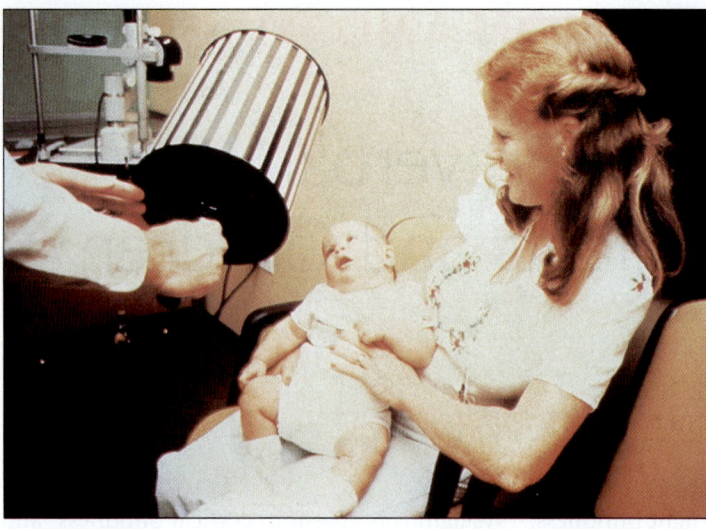

FIG. 69-1 ■ The infant responds to the optokinetic drum.

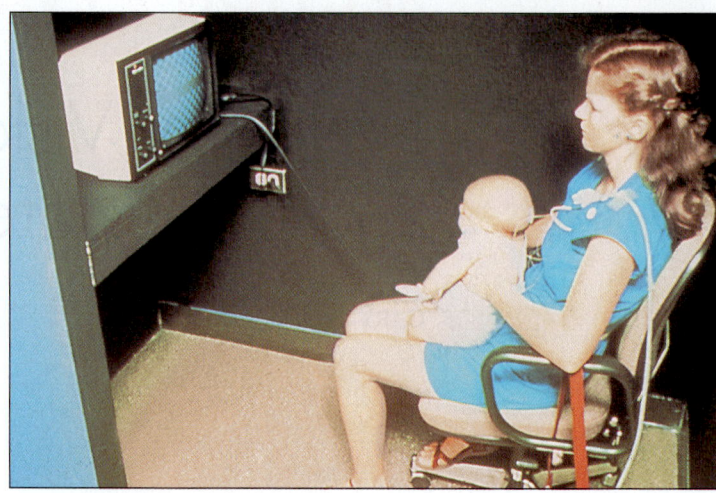

FIG. 69-3 ■ Checkerboard pattern for evoked potential test.

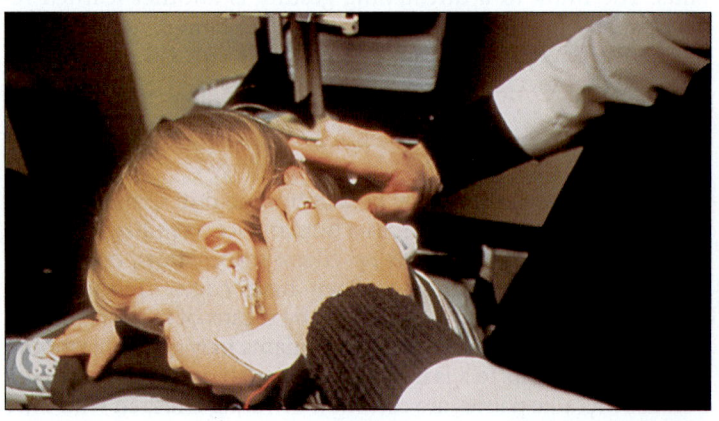

FIG. 69-2 ■ Evoked potential test. The occipital electrodes are placed in position.

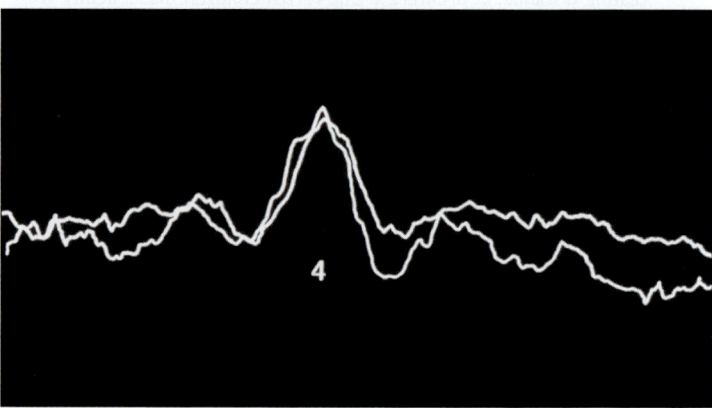

FIG. 69-4 ■ Waveform of typical visual evoked potential. The amplitude of the major positive wave and elapsed time from stimulus onset to this wave are the most important features of the visual evoked potential.

disturbed oculomotor systems. Whereas the horizontal saccadic system is present at term birth, the vertical saccadic system does not develop until 4–6 weeks later; thus, vertical responses are not present until that time.

As the testing drums are reasonably priced, portable, and rarely break, this technique remains in use as a quick and easy method with which to evaluate infant acuity.

VISUAL EVOKED POTENTIALS

On the basis of the observation that visual stimuli yield a measurable electroencephalographic pattern received by occipital scalp electrodes, various methods, which include the use of bright-flash stimuli, square-wave gratings, and phase-alternating checkerboards, have been employed to evaluate acuity. Only the last two targets can be calibrated. Many investigators using visual evoked potentials have found 20/200 (6/60) acuity in term newborns.[7] Acuity of 20/20 (6/6) may be demonstrated by 6–12 months, considerably before the age indicated by opticokinetic nystagmus testing, which perhaps reflects that this electrophysiologic test evaluates acuity by direct recording of sensory afferents, the only test to do so.

Visual evoked potential testing can be used to evaluate acuity in aphakic,[8] amblyopic,[9] and strabismic children and in those who have large refractive errors. Although the test directly evaluates vision by means of a sensory process, a waveform of normal appearance has been recorded in the occasional decorticate infant who later behaves as if blind, which implies a subcortical

contribution; the exact origin of the response remains unknown.[10] As the response waveform changes markedly between 1 and 6 months, care must be taken to compare waveforms with those of age-matched controls.

Difficulties with this test include reliance upon expensive, delicate equipment (and the subsequent need for technical assistance) and lack of standardization of equipment. Intense interest in this technique continues, as do technologic improvement and miniaturization (Figs. 69-2 to 69-4).

FORCED CHOICE PREFERENTIAL LOOKING

This behavioral technique is based on the observation that infants prefer to view a pattern stimulus rather than a homogeneous field.[11] Using flat, calibrated, square-wave gratings, this tendency may be observed by a trained individual.[12] As with the opticokinetic nystagmus test results, a term newborn differentially responds to 20/400 (6/120) gratings; the response to 20/20 (6/6) gratings occurs at 18–24 months.[13,14] A smaller and simpler apparatus, with the target presenter unmasked, has been devised; this is more suitable for clinical applications (Figs. 69-5 and 69-6).[15]

The child must be alert and able to generate neck and eye movements, which disqualifies many whose hypotonia and inattention prevent such purposeful movement—a significant limitation in the evaluation of developmentally delayed infants. Thus, as with the opticokinetic nystagmus technique, vision is evaluated by means of a motor response. In addition, this test presents a resolution acuity task, not a recognition acuity task, and thus

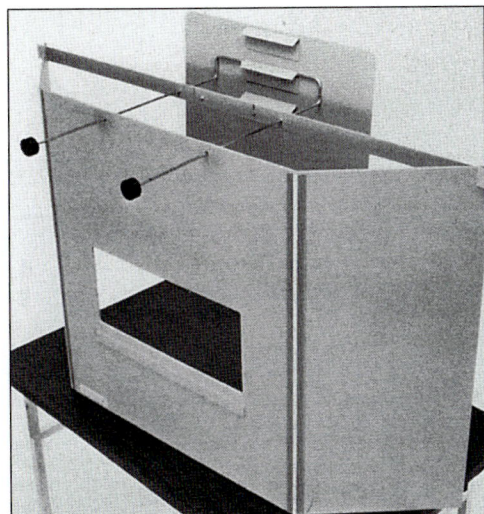

FIG. 69-5 ▌▌ Forced choice preferential looking device. (Courtesy of Visitech Consultants, Inc.)

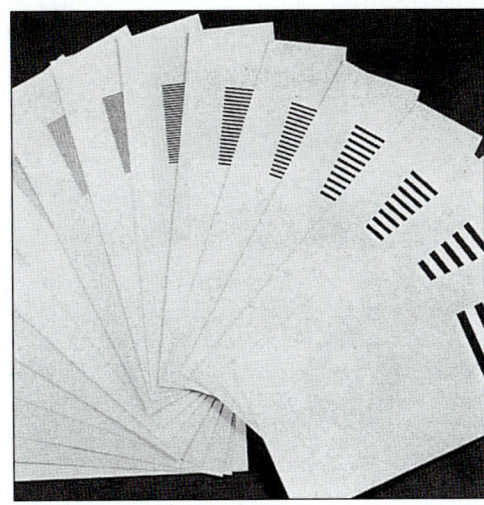

FIG. 69-6 ▌▌ Teller acuity cards.

may be less ideal for the detection of amblyopia than the visual evoked response test.[16,17] However, the testing cards are simple, portable, and cannot lose calibration; in a typical child, the testing of both eyes often takes less than 20 minutes. Evidence exists of experiential effects, and as the cards can be presented with the stripes in one orientation (vertical) only, the acuities of some optically uncorrected astigmatic children may be estimated erroneously using this technique.[18] Children who have nystagmus may be unable to fixate on the targets accurately, and those who have visual field defects may have difficulty finding the targets.

GRADED OPTOTYPES

Rarely, children as young as 18 months can respond to Snellen optotypes, but it is uncommon for children under 4.5 years to read a standardized Snellen acuity chart dependably. Tests useful in the age range 2.5–4.5 years include Allen picture cards, Landolt rings, the HOTV test, the Tumbling E test, and the Sheridan-Gardner test.

Allen picture cards are quite useful (the near test card is slightly easier for the younger child) but have certain disadvantages:

- Pictures are not constructed according to the Snellen formula (each element in the target subtends 1min of visual angle);
- Some (the telephone) may not be familiar to modern children because of their antiquated form;
- Targets are variably larger than the corresponding Snellen letter target; and
- Smallest target size is labeled 20/30 (6/9).

Despite these difficulties, most children respond readily to this familiar and easily obtainable test (Fig. 69-7).

The HOTV test requires pattern recognition and matching of progressively smaller optotypes with those on a hand-held card. These letters are chosen to be of average recognition difficulty and have a vertical axis of symmetry, which obviates the issue of right-left confusion so common in this age group. An advantage is the exact correspondence of the target to the graded Snellen optotypes (Fig. 69-8).

Landolt rings are discontinuous circles; the child points to a similar ring on a hand-held card. The test often confuses the younger child and perhaps is more useful for illiterate adults; it does have the advantage of corresponding directly to the Snellen chart. The familiar Tumbling E test requires matching orientation of the letter E with a figure or the child's fingers; unfortunately, right-left disorientation is common in this age range and limits the usefulness of the test. Its major advantage is the direct correspondence to graded Snellen optotypes.

The Sheridan-Gardner method requires children to match familiar object patterns viewed at distance with those on a

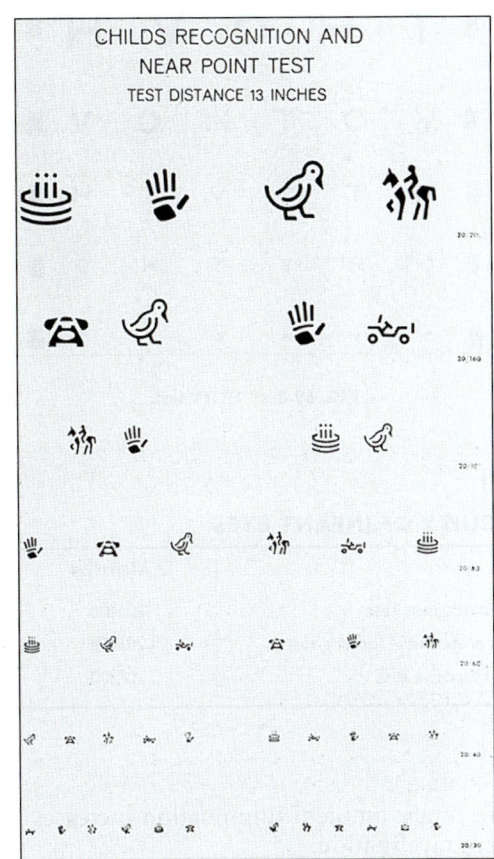

FIG. 69-7 ▌▌ Allen picture card.

near card. Some children respond to isolated Snellen optotypes, or graded numerical optotypes, before linear Snellen presentations.

MATURATION OF VISUAL ACUITY

Although the central cones function by term birth, acuity as measured by the preceding techniques does not approach 20/20 (6/6) until from 6 to 30 months (depending upon the examination technique used; see Fig. 69-9). Reasons for this delay include the incomplete development and specialization of photoreceptors, maturation of synapses in the inner retinal layers, and myelination of the upper visual pathways. Foveal cones do not attain adult appearance until 4 months after term birth.[19] Visual pathway myelination continues until 2 years of

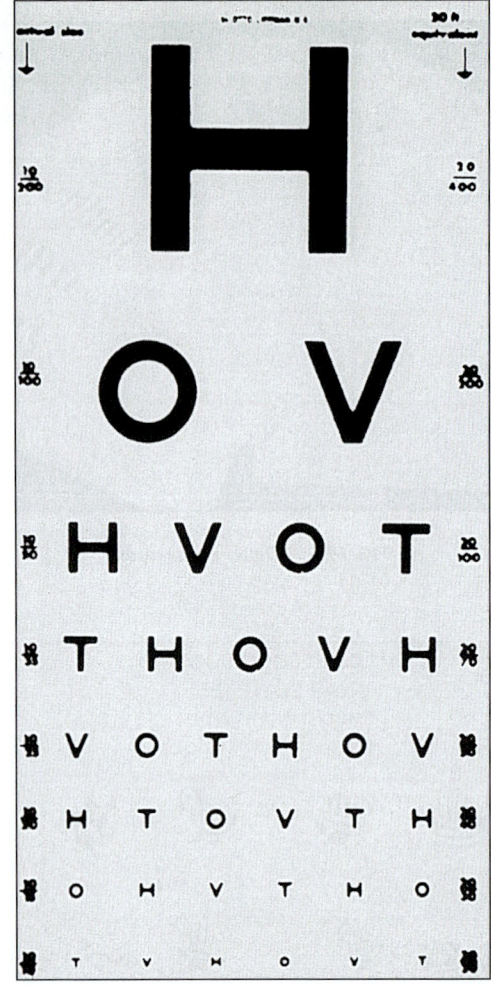

FIG. 69-8 ▉ HOTV test.

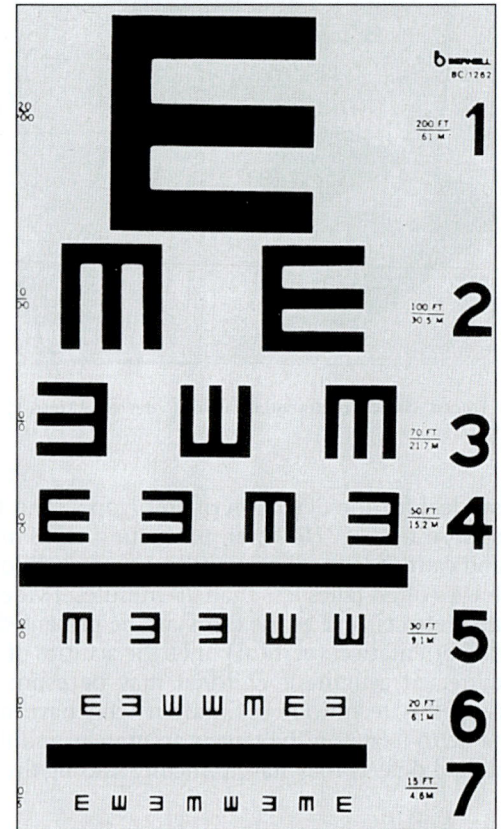

FIG. 69-9 ▉ Tumbling E test.

TABLE 69-1

VISUAL ACUITY OF INFANT EYES

Test	2 Months	4 Months	6 Months	1 Year	Attainment (months)
Opticokinetic nystagmus test	20/400	20/400	20/200	20/80	24–30
Forced choice preferential looking test	20/400	20/200	20/200	20/50	18–24
Visual evoked response test	20/200	20/80	20/60–20/20	20/40–20/20	6–12

age.[20] Interestingly, ambient illumination increases the rate of visual system myelination.[21]

Occasionally, infants fail to develop visual fixational abilities up to 6–12 months of age but at that later age develop normal visual behavior. These challenging children, often small for gestational age or developmentally delayed, have a normal or sluggish pupillary response, no nystagmus, and normal globe structure. The electroretinogram is completely normal; the visual evoked response has been reported variously as normal,[22] reduced in amplitude, or absent.[21] These children are postulated to have a cortical synaptic developmental delay. No clear explanation exists for children who have normal visual evoked response tests but present with visual inattention and other aspects of this syndrome. The parents are reassured and the child examined frequently during this time period until visual attention becomes as expected.

Interest among researchers in the potential precocity of visual development in premature infants has resulted in the following finding—no precocity in expected acuity, as measured by the opticokinetic nystagmus and forced choice preferential looking techniques, has been found, but initial precocity of attained acuity as measured by visually evoked potentials has been demon-

strated (Table 69-1). Premature infants tested by the latter lead similarly aged term infants for roughly 6 months, but acuity development then slows to match the acuity of the term infants (see Chapter 68).

REFERENCES

1. Robinson RJ. Assessment of gestational age by neurologic examination. Arch Dis Child. 1966;41:437–43.
2. Goldhammer Y. Paradoxical pupillary light reaction. In: Smith JL, ed. Neuroophthalmology update. New York: Masson; 1977:39–42.
3. Yee RD, Balon RW, Hanrubia Y. Study of congenital nystagmus. Br J Ophthalmol. 1980;64:926–30.
4. Albin RV, Salpatek P. Saccadic localization of peripheral targets by the very young human infant. Percept Psychophysiol. 1975;17:293–7.
5. Gorman JJ, Cogan DG, Gellis SS. An apparatus for grading the visual acuity of infants on the basis of opticokinetic nystagmus. Pediatrics. 1957;9:1088–91.
6. Berlyne DE. The influence of the albedo and complexity of stimulus on visual fixation in the human infant. Br J Psychol. 1958;49:315–18.
7. Marg E, Freeman DN, Pelzman P, Goldstein PJ. Visual acuity development in human infants: evoked potential measurements. Invest Ophthalmol Vis Sci. 1976;15:150–4.
8. Beller R, Hoyt CS, Marg E, Odom JV. Good visual fixation after neonatal surgery for congenital monocular cataracts. Am J Ophthalmol. 1981;91:559–64.
9. Lombrosco CT, Duffy FH, Ross RM. Selective suppression of cerebral evoked potentials to patterned light in amblyopia exanopsia. Electroencephalogr Clin Neurophysiol. 1969;27:238–43.

10. Spelmann R, Gross RA, Ho SU, *et al.* Visual evoked potentials and postmortem findings in a case of cortical blindness. Ann Neurol. 1977;2:531–4.
11. Fantz RL. Pattern vision in young infants. Psychol Res. 1958;8:43–50.
12. Atkinson J, Bradick O, Moar K. Development of contrast sensitivity in the first three months of life in the human infant. Vision Res. 1977;17:1057–60.
13. Dobson V, Mayer DL, Lee CP. Visual acuity screening of preterm infants. Invest Ophthalmol Vis Sci. 1980;19:1498–503.
14. Mayer DL, Beiser AS, Werner AF, *et al.* Monocular acuity norms for the Teller acuity cards between ages 1 month and 4 years. Invest Ophthalmol Vis Sci. 1995; 36:671–85.
15. Teller D, McDonald M, Preston K, *et al.* Assessment of visual acuity in infants and children: the acuity card procedure. Dev Med Clin Neurol. 1986;28:779–84.
16. Kushner BJ, Lucchese NH, Morton GV. Grating visual acuity with Teller cards compared with Snellen visual acuity in literate patients. Arch Ophthalmol. 1995;113:485–93.
17. Hainline L, Evelyn L, Abramov I. Acuity cards: what do they measure? ARVO abstracts. Invest Ophthalmol Vis Sci. 1989;30:310.
18. Raye K, Pratt E, Rodier D, *et al.* Acuity and card grating orientation: acuity of normals and patients with nystagmus. ARVO abstracts. Invest Ophthalmol Vis Sci. 1991;3:96.
19. Hollenberg MJ, Spira AW. Human retinal development: ultrastructure of the retina. Am J Anat. 1973;137:357–69.
20. Magoon EH, Robb RM. Development of myelin in human optic nerve and tract. A light and electron microscopic study. Arch Ophthalmol. 1981;99:655–64.
21. Mellor DH, Fielder AR. Dissociated visual development: electrodiagnostic studies in infants who are 'slow to see'. Dev Med Clin Neurol. 1980;22:307–14.
22. Lambert SR, Kriss A, Taylor D. Delayed visual development. Ophthalmology. 1989;96:524–9.

70 Examination of Ocular Alignment and Eye Movements

GARY R. DIAMOND

DEFINITIONS
- Phoria: a latent visual axis deviation held in check by fusion.
- Tropia: a manifest visual axis deviation.
- Intermittent tropia: an intermittent visual axis deviation that may exist only in certain gaze positions or target distances.
- Ductions: monocular movements into various gaze positions; each eye views in the same direction.
- Vergences: binocular eye movements into opposite gaze directions.

KEY FEATURES
- Alignment of the visual axes can be evaluated by objective and subjective clinical methods.
- Evaluation of eye movements can be accomplished by objective and subjective techniques.
- Patients who have mechanical limitations of eye movements, if cooperative, can be evaluated in an outpatient setting using forced duction testing and active force generation testing.

EVALUATION OF OCULAR ALIGNMENT

INTRODUCTION

The clinician who undertakes evaluation of ocular alignment must first decide the information that is required—the eye alignment during everyday binocular viewing, or the maximal deviation of the visual axes under conditions of disrupted binocular vision, or both of these. Subjective methods are useful for cooperative, communicative older patients, but objective methods must be used in younger patients or those less cooperative. Finally, some testing methods are useful only under research laboratory conditions.

LABORATORY METHODS

Most laboratory tests are objective. The absolute position of the eye in space may be determined by measurement of the quantity of light reflected by the sclera from a deviated eye. The electro-oculogram (EOG) generated by alterations in direct current between the front and back of the eye changes as the eye rotates; this voltage change is detected by suitably placed electrodes. Finally, insulated wire placed in a silicone rubber limbal annulus (eye coil) generates a current in response to a magnetic field; this very precise technique is limited by irritation from the device but may be used to detect horizontal, vertical, and torsional changes in eye position.

CLINICAL METHODS

The clinician should accompany a new patient from the waiting room to the examination chair and carefully note the position of the patient's head when it is mobilized in free space. Atypical head positions may indicate restrictive or paralytic strabismus, the presence of a null point in a patient who has nystagmus, or alphabet pattern strabismus. Usually, a patient places the head in a position that provides comfortable single binocular vision for the straightened view, but occasionally the head is placed to separate diplopic images maximally. The examiner must differentiate between head turns, tilts, and vertical head positions and attempt to quantitate these to within 5°.

Once the patient is seated in the examination chair, the patient's lid position is noted; in patients who have vertical strabismus, lid asymmetry is usually found. If hypotropia is present and the nonfixing eye is lower than the fixing eye, the lid position is lower in the nonfixing eye; this is termed *pseudoptosis* if the lid regains normal position when the previously hypotropic eye fixes in primary position. Other soft tissue and bone structures that surround the eye may confound the family and the examiner. Epicanthal skin folds that extend over the nasal sclera in a small child may simulate esotropia. Vertical displacement of an orbit may simulate vertical strabismus, and hypertelorism may simulate exotropia. The examiner can declare a patient to be strabismic only after the appropriate alignment testing has been performed.

The optic axis can be determined accurately only by alignment of the Purkinje images with a coaxial light through a telescope; this light intersects the retina between the disc and fovea.[1] For clinical purposes, the optic axis may be assumed to strike the fovea. An observer considers the eye to view along its pupillary axis, a line through the pupillary center perpendicular to the cornea. The visual axis outside the eye is usually nasal to the pupillary axis ("positive angle κ") at an average angle of 5° in emmetropic eyes, 7.5° in hyperopic eyes, and 2° in myopic eyes (Fig. 70-1).[2] In some myopic eyes the visual axis is temporal to the pupillary axis, which gives a "negative angle κ." In some children who have cicatricial retinopathy of prematurity, the fovea is dragged temporally, which results in large positive angle κ and pseudoexotropia.

OBJECTIVE CLINICAL METHODS

Objective clinical methods to determine and measure deviations of the visual axes include corneal light reflex tests, cover tests, and haploscopic tests. These tests do not require any response by the patient and thus are independent of the patient's ability to interpret the testing environment.

Corneal Light Reflex Tests

Corneal light reflex tests, the oldest testing methods, are suitable for all patients. They do not take into account the angle κ and do not require both eyes to discern a fixation target or be able to move into a given position to take up fixation of the target. The Hirschberg method relies on a pupil size of 4mm and assumes

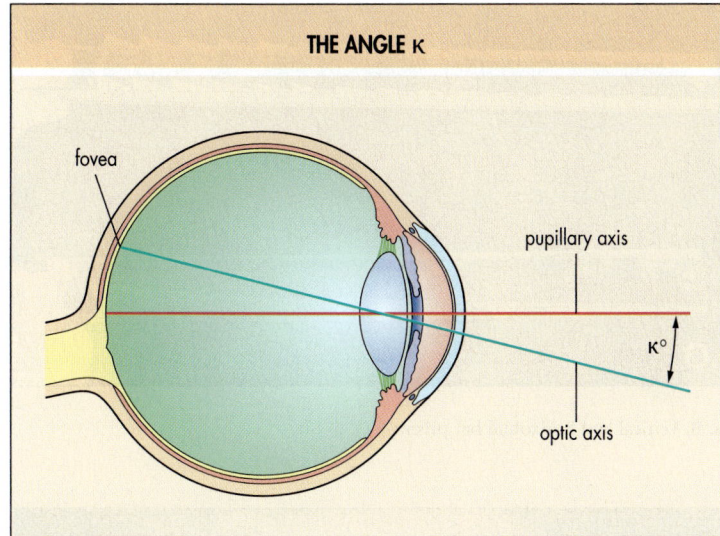

FIG. 70-1 ■ **The angle κ.** This is the displacement in degrees of the pupillary axis from the optic axis. The positive angle κ provides the illusion of exotropia in this left eye.

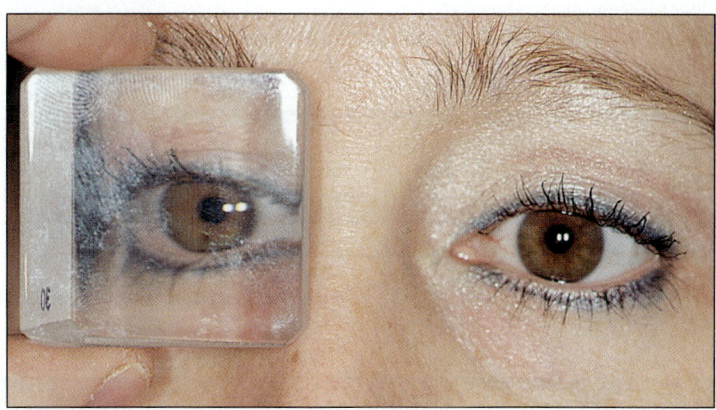

FIG. 70-3 ■ **Krimsky light reflex method (same patient as in Fig. 70-2).** The strength of a base-out prism over the fixing right eye sufficient to center the pupillary light reflex in the esotropic left eye is defined as the amount of left esotropia.

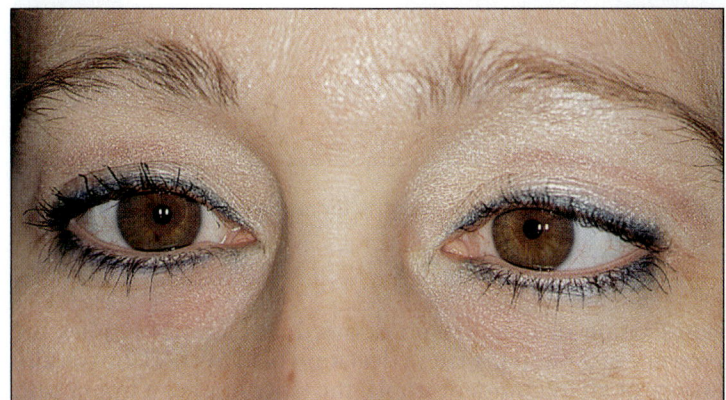

FIG. 70-2 ■ **Hirschberg light reflex method.** The patient has a left esotropia. Note the corneal light reflex at the temporal pupillary border of the left eye while the reflex is centered in the pupil of the right eye.

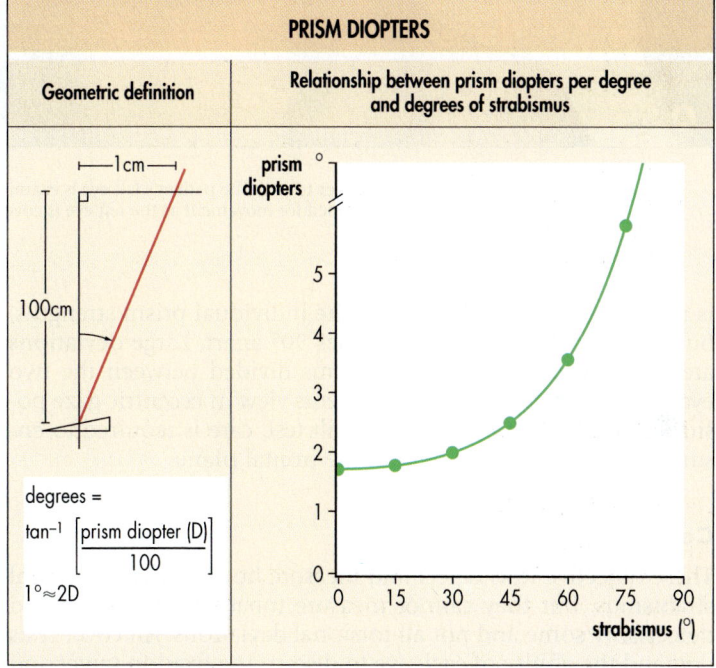

FIG. 70-4 ■ **Prism diopters.** Geometric definition of the prism diopter, a tangent function. The relationship between prism diopters per degree and degrees of strabismus is nonlinear (90° represents an infinite number of prism diopters).

each millimeter of light displacement across the cornea is equivalent to 7° of decentration or 15Δ. A light reflection at the pupillary border signifies a 15° or 30Δ deviation (see Fig. 70-2), at the midiris a deviation of 30° or 60Δ, and at the limbus a deviation of 45° or 90Δ. Studies indicate that 1mm of light displacement is equal to 18° of strabismus, 21° if referred to the frontal plane by photographic techniques.[3] The test should be performed with the light centered in each eye's pupil to detect the presence of secondary deviations (see later). The disadvantages of this test are the estimations necessary to measure the eye deviation and the inability to control accommodation when testing at near fixation, as the measuring light serves as the fixation target. Distance testing is difficult because of the dimness of the target light reflected in the corneas.

The Krimsky test quantifies the light reflex displacement using appropriately held prisms. The original description suggested placing the prism before the aligned eye (Fig. 70-3), but most users today find it easier to hold the prism before the deviating eye.[4] The results are identical unless a secondary deviation (measurement taken with the paretic or mechanically restricted eye fixing) exists. An arc perimeter may be used to measure larger deviations by alignment of a light in the deviated eye, with the deviation read in degrees from the arc perimeter scale. The Maddox tangent scale at 3.3ft (1m) or 16.5ft (5m) testing distance may be used in a manner similar to that with the arc perimeter. Using the

major amblyoscope, a light may be projected on each cornea and the tubes moved to center the light reflexes.

Prisms must be appropriately handled to yield accurate measurement of strabismus.[5] They deflect light toward their base, but the patient views the light as deflected toward the prism apex. The prism diopter is defined as the strength of prism necessary to deflect a light beam 0.4in (1cm) at 3.3ft (1m) distance (Fig. 70-4). As a tangent function, the prism diopter is not linear and increases in size as the deviation increases, but for small deviations 1° approximates 1.7Δ. Glass prisms are manufactured rarely today but are calibrated to be held in the Prentice position with the back surface perpendicular to the visual axes. Plastic prisms, whether loose or in bar form (Fig. 70-5), must be held with the rear surface in the frontal plane to approximate closely the position of minimal deviation of light through the prism. Prisms cannot be stacked base to base as the sum prism strength

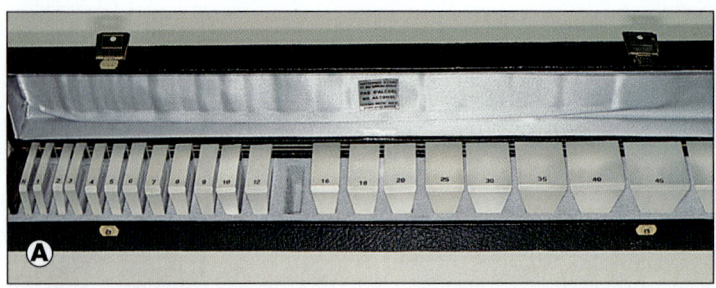
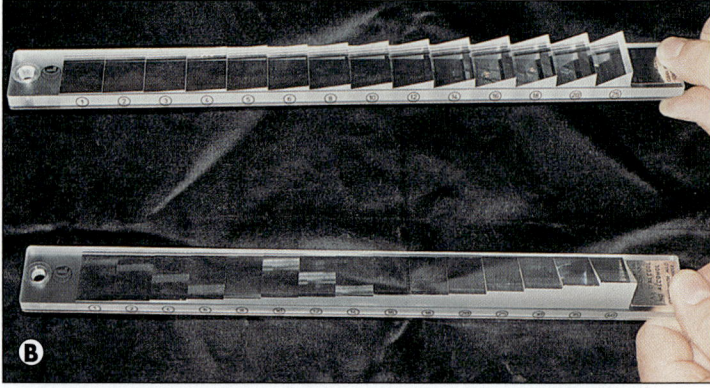

FIG. 70-5 ■ Prisms. A, Loose plastic prisms. B, Vertical and horizontal bar prisms.

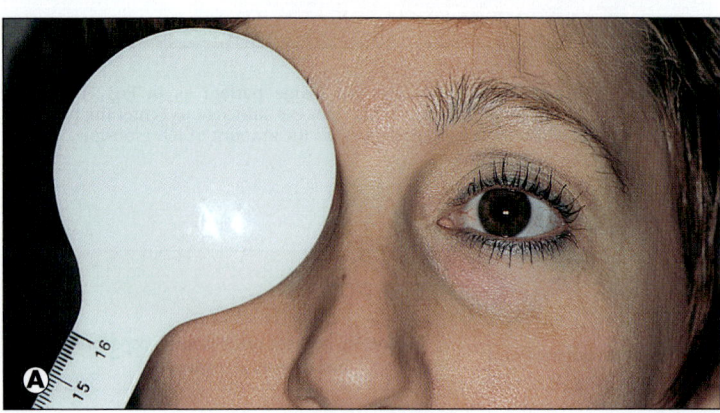
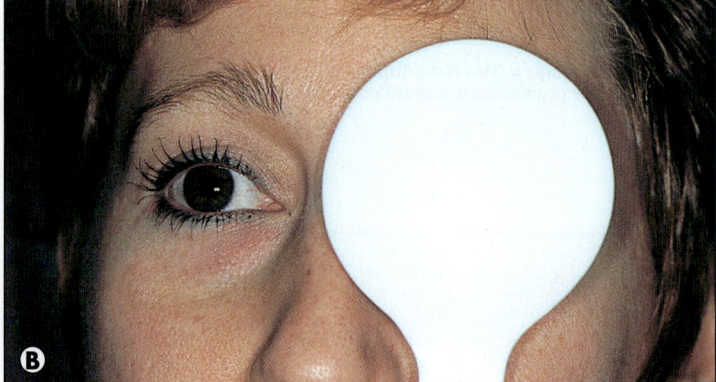

FIG. 70-6 ■ Cover test. A, The patient's left eye is examined for movement as the right eye is covered. B, The patient's right eye is examined for movement as the left eye is covered.

is much greater than the sum of the individual prism strengths, but they may be stacked with bases 90° apart. Large deviations are best neutralized with the prisms divided between the two eyes. For measurements when patients view in eccentric gaze positions and for those in the head tilt test, care is required to ensure that the prisms are held in the frontal plane.

Cover Tests

These objective tests detect and measure horizontal and vertical strabismus, but they cannot measure torsional deviations and detect only some and not all torsional deviations. All cover tests demand the ability of each eye to discern the fixation target and to move to take up fixation upon that target.

The cover test detects tropias—constant visual axis deviations. The examiner observes the uncovered eye for movement as its fellow is covered with a paddle, thumb, or remote occluder (Fig. 70-6).[6] A nasal movement implies exotropia (Fig. 70-7, A), temporal movement esotropia (Fig. 70-7, B), upward movement hypotropia, and downward movement hypertropia (Fig. 70-7, C) of the uncovered eye.[7] Each eye is covered in turn. An accommodation-controlling fixation target of about 20/40 (6/12) size is presented to the patient, who ideally describes the target. Small toys are suitable for young children, but bright white lights are avoided as the patient cannot accommodate on the contours of a light. Tropias established by the cover test may be measured using the simultaneous prism and cover test; a prism of appropriate strength held in the appropriate direction is introduced before one eye as its fellow is covered (Fig. 70-8). Prism strength is increased until eye movement ceases; this prism strength corresponds to the size of the strabismus. The test is then repeated with the prism before the other eye.

The uncover test requires observation of the covered eye as the cover is removed. If that eye deviated under cover, it may re-

gain fixation or may remain deviated. The former implies the presence of a phoria, a latent deviation held in check by sensory fusion, or an intermittent tropia; the latter implies a tropia with fixation preference for the fellow eye.

Phorias may be detected more directly using the alternate cover test, in which each eye is occluded alternately to dissociate the visual axes maximally. Care must be taken to permit time for each eye to reside behind the cover (the cover must not be "fanned" before the eyes). Appropriately held prisms enable quantitation of the phoria (Fig. 70-9). Some patients have poorly defined end points and a range over which eye movements shift from one direction to the opposite as prism strength is increased; the strabismus measurement may be estimated as the midpoint between clearly defined movements in each direction. For most clinical purposes, measurements within 2D are sufficiently accurate. Cover test measurements are influenced by the presence of eccentric fixation; its presence must be investigated in patients who have severe amblyopia.

The eye behind the prism is the "fixing" eye. If the cause of strabismus is paralytic or restrictive, patients may have greater cover test measurements when the paretic or restricted eye fixes in a given gaze position (secondary deviation) than when the sound eye fixes (primary deviation). This phenomenon arises from Hering's law, which demands equal innervation to yoke muscles; thus, the yoke of a paralyzed or restricted muscle receives excess innervation when the pathologic eye is fixing.

Strabismus should be detected and measured in primary position at distance and near fixation and in gaze up, down, right, and left 30° from primary position. The nine "diagnostic gaze positions" include the above plus up and right, up and left, down and right, and down and left; these are useful to measure cyclovertical muscle palsies. For patients who have oblique muscle dysfunction, measurements are taken with the head tilted 30° right and left at distance fixation.

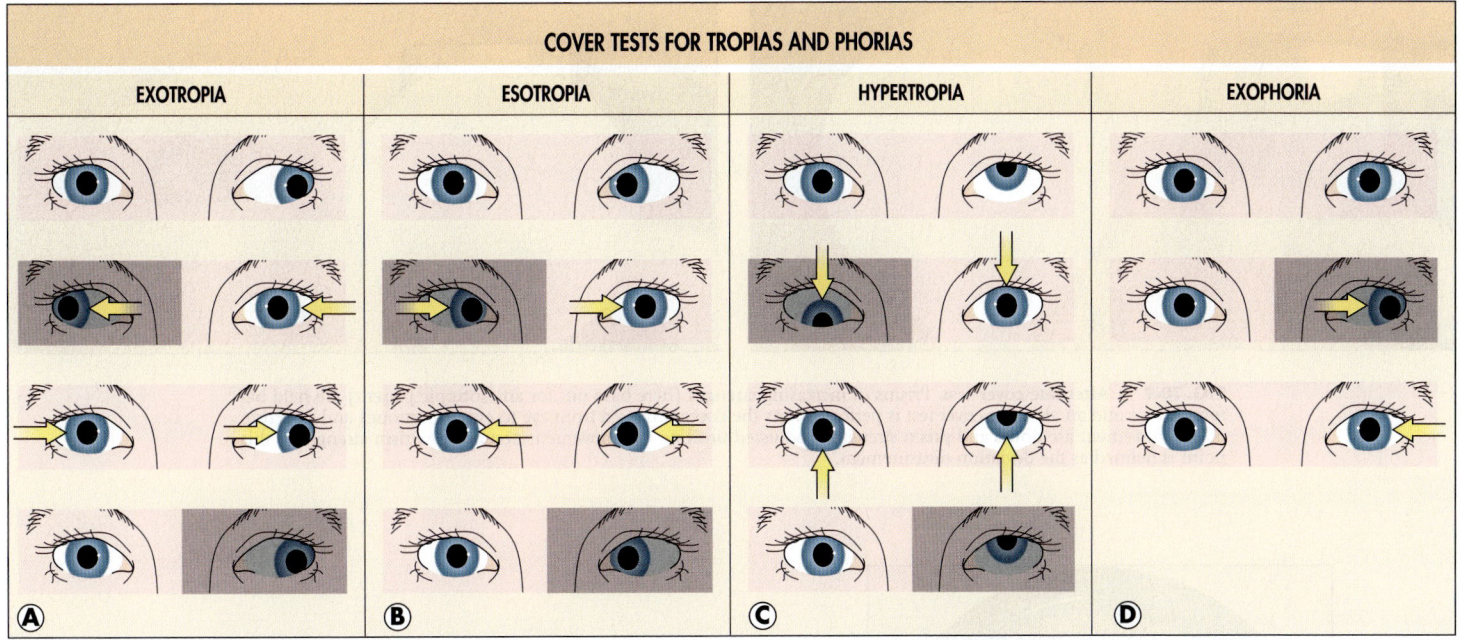

COVER TESTS FOR TROPIAS AND PHORIAS

EXOTROPIA	ESOTROPIA	HYPERTROPIA	EXOPHORIA

A   B   C   D

FIG. 70-7 ▪ Cover test for tropias. A, For exotropia, covering the right eye drives inward movement of the left eye to take up fixation; uncovering the right eye shows recovery of fixation by the right eye and leftward movement of both eyes; covering the left eye discloses no shift of the preferred right eye. B, For esotropia, covering the right eye drives outward movement of the left eye to take up fixation; uncovering the right eye shows recovery of fixation by the right eye and rightward movement of both eyes; covering the left eye discloses no shift of the preferred right eye. C, For hypertropia, covering the right eye drives downward movement of the left eye to take up fixation; uncovering the right eye shows recovery of fixation by the right eye and upward movement of both eyes; covering the left eye shows no shift of the preferred right eye. D, For exophoria, the left eye deviates outward behind a cover and returns to primary position when the cover is removed. An immediate inward movement denotes a phoria, a delayed inward movement denotes an intermittent exotropia. (Redrawn with permission from Diamond G, Eggers H. Strabismus and pediatric ophthalmology. London: Mosby; 1993.)

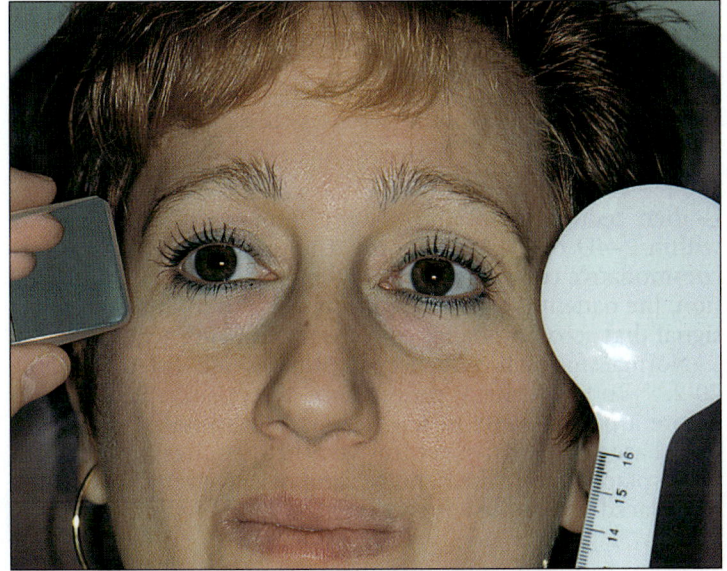

FIG. 70-8 ▪ Simultaneous prism and cover test with right eye fixing. The prism is moved before the fixing right eye simultaneously with the cover held before the left eye.

Subjective Clinical Methods

Subjective clinical methods include diplopia tests and haploscopic tests, which require cooperation, intelligence, and the ability of the patient to communicate the sensory percept to the examiner.

The red glass test requires the patient to alert the examiner when the red light viewed behind a red filter before the right eye and a white light viewed with the left eye are superimposed or displaced one from the other. Fusion is disrupted by the red glass and thus horizontal and vertical phorias are uncovered and measured; torsional deviations are not detected by this method.

The gaze position of maximal image separation is a clue to the identity of paretic or restricted muscles. This is a useful bedside test, but accommodation is not controlled.

The Maddox rod consists of closely aligned, powerful glass or plastic cylinders. When illuminated, these cylinders project a line upon the patient's retina perpendicular to the groove orientation. The line is aligned horizontally to detect and measure horizontal phorias (accommodation cannot be controlled with this test). Torsion may be detected and quantitated; the Maddox rod is placed in a trial frame scaled in degrees (Fig. 70-10). It is common to place two Maddox rods of different colors in each trial frame cell and permit the patient to rotate each to his or her perception of the horizontal. The torsional position of each eye may be read directly in degrees from the angular scale used for cylinder axes. Figure 70-11 exhibits a red Maddox rod before the right eye of a patient who has 10° of excyclotorsion, as read directly from the trial frame.

Haploscopic devices, such as the major amblyoscope, present each eye with a target significantly different from that presented to its fellow eye. These devices measure horizontal, vertical, and torsional deviations by alternately illuminating the fixation targets presented to each eye; the tubes are positioned appropriately until no eye movements occur.

Diplopia tests also present different images to the two eyes. These images may be identified by red-green (anaglyph) glasses or by mirrors. The Lancaster red-green test uses a screen marked in 2° increments viewed from a distance of 6.6ft (2m). The examiner projects a red or green line on the screen; the patient views through the anaglyph glasses and projects the appropriate colored line upon the examiner's projected line. The results are recorded and the glasses reversed or the projecting wands switched. Torsion may be evaluated.

The Hess screen contains illuminated red lights at fixed distances on a black screen; the patient places a green pointer light on the red lights while wearing anaglyph glasses. The glasses are reversed to test the other eye. Torsion cannot be detected.

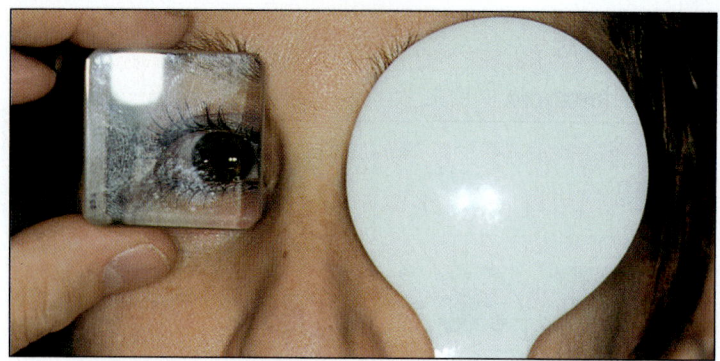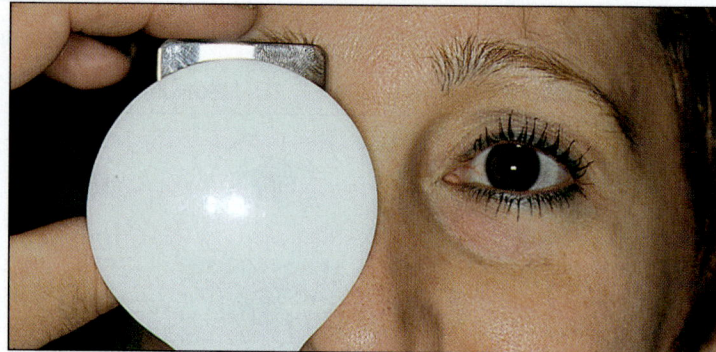

FIG. 70-9 ■ **Alternate cover test.** Prisms of increasing strength (here base out for an esotropic patient) are held before the eye and an alternate cover test is performed. As the cover is moved from eye to eye, the amount and direction of eye movement are noted and prism strength is adjusted until no eye movement occurs. The prism strength at this point is defined as the deviation measurement.

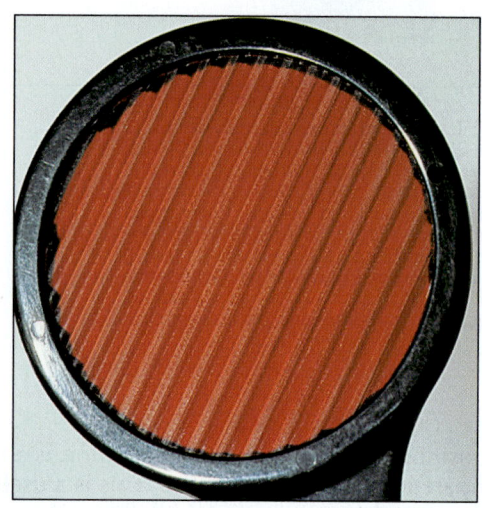

FIG. 70-10 ■ **Maddox rod.** A series of aligned strong cylinders, here placed in a paddle handle.

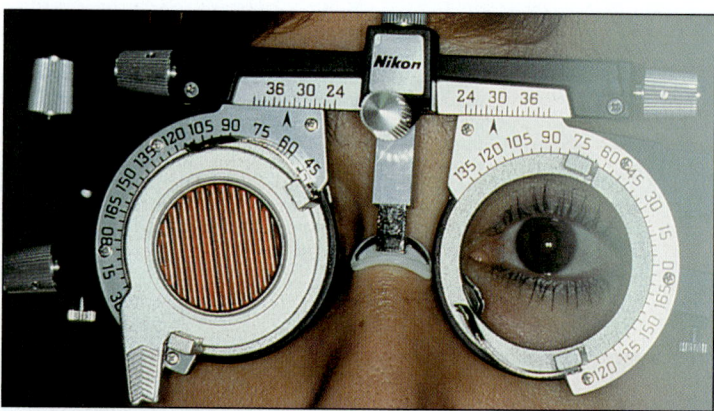

FIG. 70-11 ■ **Red Maddox rod.** A red Maddox rod in a trial frame may be used to evaluate subjective ocular torsion. The grooves must be aligned with the mark on the rim, as they tend to rotate within.

EYE MOVEMENT EXAMINATIONS

Evaluation of ductions, versions, and vergences is essential to understand a patient's eye movement system completely. A commonly accepted terminology system is given in Table 70-1. *Ductions* are monocular eye movements, generally evaluated with the fellow eye occluded. Extreme gaze positions are investigated. In full and normal abduction, the temporal limbus touches the lateral canthus. Full adduction brings the junction of the nasal and middle corneal thirds to a position above the inferior tear punctum.[8] Each eye elevates 10mm and depresses 5–7mm. Tertiary gaze positions are also evaluated and compared with those in the fellow eye.

Measurements of eye movements may be performed by estimation or quantification using the arc perimeter, Goldmann perimeter, or tangent screen. Rotations of 50° in all directions are considered normal.

Versions are binocular movements in which the eyes view in the same direction. Vergences are binocular movements in which the eyes gaze in opposite gaze directions; these are slow movements made as part of the near synkinesis or to achieve better alignment to facilitate sensory fusion. Fusional vergence amplitudes (convergence amplitudes to correct an exodeviation, divergence amplitudes an esodeviation, etc.) may be measured by the introduction of increasingly strong prisms before one eye of a patient who views an accommodation-controlling target. The patient reports when the image doubles or the examiner notes the sudden appearance of strabismus. The power of prism necessary to reach this "break" point is the vergence amplitude at a given testing distance in a given direction. The prism power

is then reduced until the patient "remakes" fusion, usually within 2–4D of the break point. The patient may generate accommodative convergence to aid fusion, especially at near fixation; the patient is asked to report target blur to the examiner, a signal that accommodative convergence is being generated.

Normal fusional vergence amplitudes are listed in Table 70-2.[9,10] To test fusional convergence, the prism is held base in before a patient's eye; to test fusional divergence, the prism is held base out. Positive vertical vergence requires a base-down prism placed before the right eye, and negative vertical vergence, one placed before the left eye.

MECHANICAL TESTS OF EYE MOVEMENT LIMITATION

Patients who have duction limitations may suffer from paralysis or paresis, or mechanical restriction of full duction movement, or both. Forced duction testing and active force generation testing may help to differentiate these. In cooperative patients these tests may be performed in the office, but in young or uncooperative patients these tests are reserved for the operating room, when the patient is under local or general anesthesia.

Forced Duction Test

The forced duction test is an attempt by the examiner to move a patient's eye farther in a given direction than the patient can move it. Topical anesthetic is placed on the appropriate limbal location (generally 180° away from the duction limitation) with a small cotton swab and the limbal conjunctiva is grasped

TABLE 70-1

EYE MOVEMENT TERMINOLOGY

	Terminology	Movement
Ductions:	Adduction	Nasal rotation
	Abduction	Temporal rotation
	Depression	Downward rotation
	Elevation	Upward rotation
	Intorsion	Upper corneal pole rotates inward
	Extorsion	Upper corneal pole rotates outward
	Dextrocycloduction	Upper corneal pole rotates rightward
	Levocycloduction	Upper corneal pole rotates leftward
Versions:	Dextroversion	Both eyes rotate to patient's right
	Levoversion	Both eyes rotate to patient's left
	Supraversion	Both eyes rotate upward
	Infraversion	Both eyes rotate downward
	Dextrocycloversion	Upper corneal poles of both eyes rotate to patient's right
	Levocycloversion	Upper corneal poles of both eyes rotate to patient's left
Vergences:	Convergence	Both eyes rotate nasally
	Divergence	Both eyes rotate temporally
	Positive vertical vergence	Right eye rotates higher than left
	Negative vertical vergence	Left eye rotates higher than right
	Incyclovergence	Upper corneal poles of both eyes rotate inward
	Excyclovergence	Upper corneal poles of both eyes rotate outward

TABLE 70-2

NORMAL FUSION VERGENCE AMPLITUDES

Testing Distance (m)	Convergence (D)	Divergence (D)	Vertical Vergence (D)
6	14	6	2.5
0.025	38	16	2.5

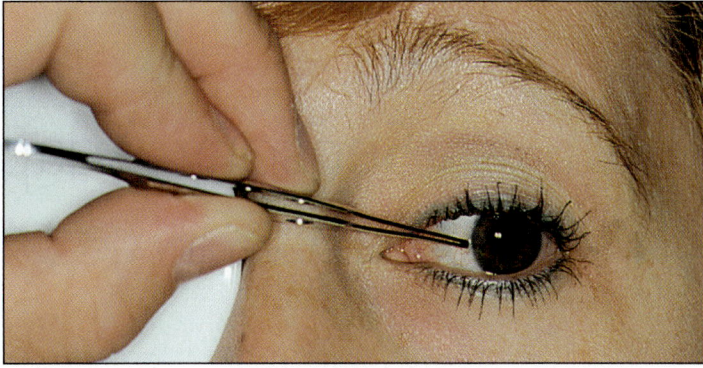

FIG. 70-12 ▮▮ **Forced duction testing.** The patient has left esotropia and limited abduction. The patient is abducting her left eye from a position of maximal adduction and the examiner is attempting to abduct the eye farther than the patient can.

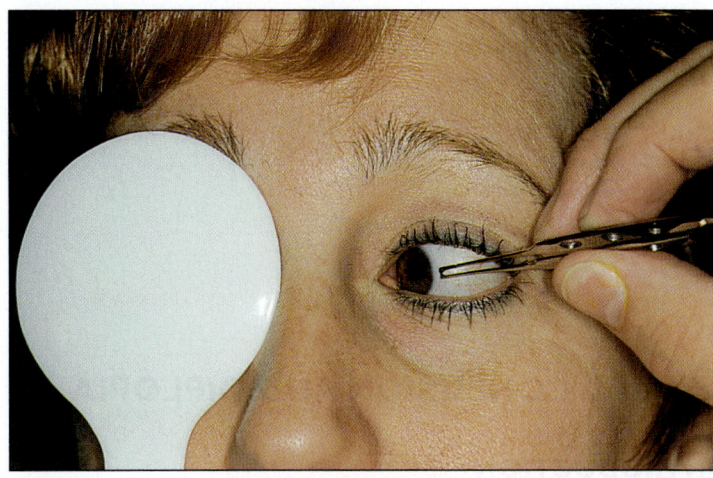

FIG. 70-13 ▮▮ **Active force generation test.** The patient has left esotropia and limited abduction. The patient abducts her left eye from a position of maximal adduction and the examiner estimates the force of abduction through the forceps.

firmly with a toothed forceps. The patient is asked to rotate the eye fully in the direction of the limited duction. An attempt is then made by the examiner to rotate the eye beyond the position attained by the patient while avoiding globe retraction (Fig. 70-12). Care must be taken not to abrade the cornea. Patients who have pure nerve palsy exhibit no restriction to full movement by the examiner; patients who have pure restriction (dysthyroid orbitopathy, entrapment of ocular contents after blowout fracture) exhibit restricted movements (sometimes termed a positive forced duction test). Some patients initially have a pure nerve palsy, but contracture of the antagonist muscle results in secondary mechanical restriction of movement. Suction cup devices have been developed for examiners who are wary of using toothed instruments at the limbus; a cotton swab may be a sufficient tool in some patients.

Forced duction testing of oblique muscles may be performed, but two forceps are used and the globe is depressed forcibly into the orbit. To test tension in the superior oblique tendon, the globe is grasped in the limbal meridian of the tendon (the 2:30 position in the right eye, the 10:30 position in the left) and 180° away. The globe is rocked clockwise and counterclockwise over the taut tendon and the tendon tension is evaluated; experience with normal tendons is essential to obtain an accurate evaluation. To test tension in the inferior oblique muscle, the globe is grasped at the 4:30 position limbus and 180° away in the right eye, at the 7:30 position limbus and 180° away in the left eye; the globe is rocked similarly and the muscle tension evaluated.

Active Force Generation Test

Active force generation testing may be used to evaluate the ability of a muscle to move the eye against a resisting force. The forceps is placed at the limbus of the anesthetized globe in the meridian of the muscle whose duction is limited and the patient requested to rotate the eye in the direction of the limited duction; the examiner judges through the forceps the relative amount of force generated. Strain gauges have been devised that enable quantitation of this force. In Figure 70-13 a patient has abduction maximum in the left eye. The examiner can gauge the relative abduction strength as the patient attempts to move her eye to the left.

REFERENCES

1. Tscherning H. Optique physiologique. Paris: Georges Carre et C. Naud; 1898.
2. Donders FC. On the anomalies of accommodation and refraction of the eye. London: The New Sydenham Society; 1864.
3. Brodie SE. Photographic calibration of the Hirschberg test. Invest Ophthalmol Vis Sci. 1987;28:736–42.
4. Krimsky E. The binocular examination of the young child. Am J Ophthalmol. 1943;26:624–5.
5. Thompson JT, Guyton DL. Ophthalmic prisms: measurement errors and how to minimize them. Ophthalmology. 1983;90:204–10.
6. Guyton DL. Remote optical systems for ophthalmic examinations. Trans Am Ophthalmol Soc. 1986;84:869–919.
7. Diamond G, Eggers H. Strabismus and pediatric ophthalmology. London: Mosby; 1993.
8. Kestenbaum A. Clinical methods of neuro-ophthalmic examination, 2nd ed. New York: Grune & Stratton; 1961.
9. Ellerbrock VJ. Experimental investigations of vertical fusional movements. Am J Optom. 1949;26:327–33.
10. Hofmann FB, Bielschowsky A. Die Verwertung der Kopfneigung zur Diagnose der Augen muskellahmungen. Graefes Arch Ophthalmol. 1900;51:174–85.

Sensory Adaptations in Strabismus

GARY R. DIAMOND

DEFINITION
- Physiologic adaptations to strabismus in order to avoid visual confusion or diplopia.

KEY FEATURES
- Suppression.
- Monofixation syndrome.
- Anomalous retinal correspondence.

VISUAL CONFUSION AND DIPLOPIA

INTRODUCTION

If binocularity is established early in an infant's life, it is maintained unless sight is lost in either eye. When an individual develops strabismus, the corresponding retinal elements in the two eyes are no longer directed toward identical objects. This puts the individual at risk for development of two specific visual phenomena, both potentially quite uncomfortable—visual confusion and diplopia. These terms have specific meanings. Visual confusion is the simultaneous perception of dissimilar objects that project upon corresponding retinal elements (the two foveas, for example). Diplopia is the perception of one object that projects upon two different (noncorresponding) retinal areas (Fig. 71-1). If the retina is considered to be divided into a central, rod-free area that roughly corresponds to the fovea (central 2.5°) and a peripheral area, it is clear that the newly strabismic patient who has binocularity is confronted by four separate potential problems—central confusion, central diplopia, peripheral confusion, and peripheral diplopia.

OCULAR MANIFESTATIONS

Central confusion is immediately obviated in individuals of any age as the rod-free retinal areas cannot simultaneously perceive disparate targets. The fovea in the strabismic eye is immediately enveloped in a scotoma of roughly 2.5° diameter.[1] This can be demonstrated in oneself by manual displacement of one eye with a finger; there is an immediate decrease of visual acuity in that eye.

TREATMENT, COURSE, AND OUTCOME

The onset of a new strabismus in children older than 7–9 years of age and in all adults causes peripheral confusion, central diplopia, and peripheral diplopia unless it is controlled successfully by the fusional vergence system or by the occlusion of one eye or severely decreased visual acuity is present in one eye. Even patients who have acuity as low as 2/200 (0.6/60) may experience severe symptoms from visual confusion and diplopia.

SUPPRESSION AND ANOMALOUS RETINAL CORRESPONDENCE

INTRODUCTION

Children younger than 7–9 years are usually able to achieve the sensory adaptations of suppression and anomalous retinal correspondence (ARC).[2] These adaptations may develop rapidly or slowly after the appearance of strabismus and usually occur together.

OCULAR MANIFESTATIONS

Suppression scotomas obviate central diplopia because they encompass the retinal area on which the foveally viewed image in the aligned eye projects within a facultative, absolute scotoma (facultative in that the scotoma is present only when that eye is strabismic and absolute in that no image can be visualized within). When the strabismic eye fixes, the scotoma immediately disappears, only to reappear when the eye is again misaligned.

Interestingly, the shape and size of the suppression scotoma are different in an esotrope compared with an exotrope.[3] An esotrope usually exhibits a small, round scotoma that envelops only the nasal retinal area within which the foveally viewed image in the aligned eye projects, although occasionally a somewhat larger, suppressed retinal area is demonstrated. An exotropic patient's suppression scotoma is much larger and encompasses the temporal retinal area on which the foveally viewed image in the aligned eye projects and, in addition, the entire area that extends to a vertical line that bisects the fovea (Fig. 71-2). Postulated explanations for this difference include developmental and teleologic differences between the nasal and temporal hemiretinas, the intermittent nature of many exodeviations, the constant nature of many esodeviations, and others, but no explanation is entirely convincing. Suppression scotomas can be demonstrated in patients who have strabismus by using the testing techniques described in Chapter 72.

DIAGNOSIS AND ANCILLARY TESTING

As described in Chapter 72, different sensory tests may demonstrate persistence of normal retinal correspondence in certain patients who have known ARC and, conversely, persistence of ARC in patients who have realigned visual axes; thus, the limitations of the various sensory tests commonly used to diagnose ARC must be understood. As ARC is infinitely flexible, fusional vergence is not required for visual comfort and, in fact, is demonstrated rarely. Stereoptic appreciation, as shown by read-

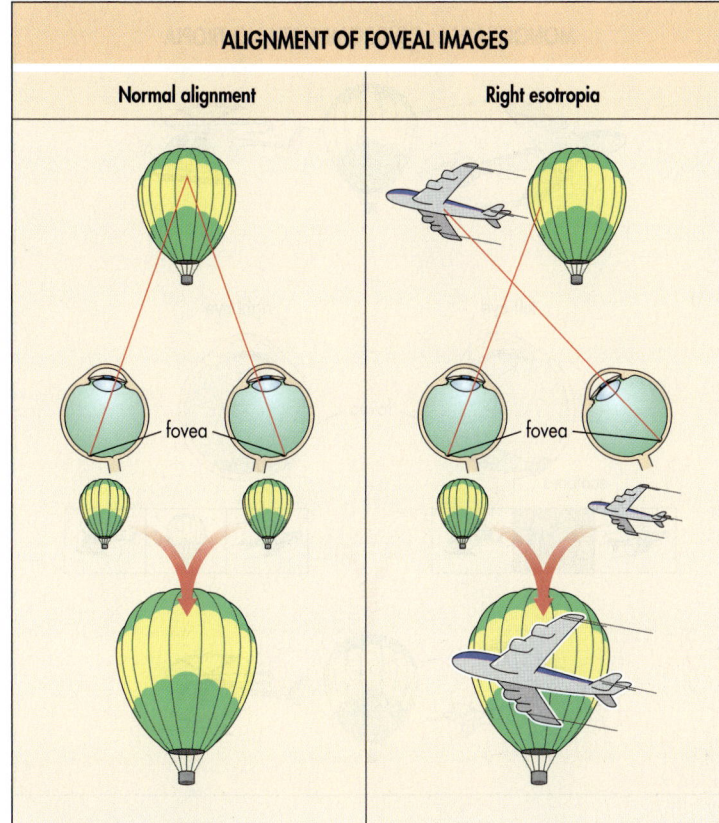

FIG. 71-1 ◼ **Alignment of foveal images.** Normal alignment of a typical patient who has straight eyes fuses foveal targets. Right esotropia in a binocular patient results in visual confusion of foveal targets. This does not exist clinically, as the fovea in the turned eye cannot accept an image disparate from that seen by the fovea in the straight, fixing eye.

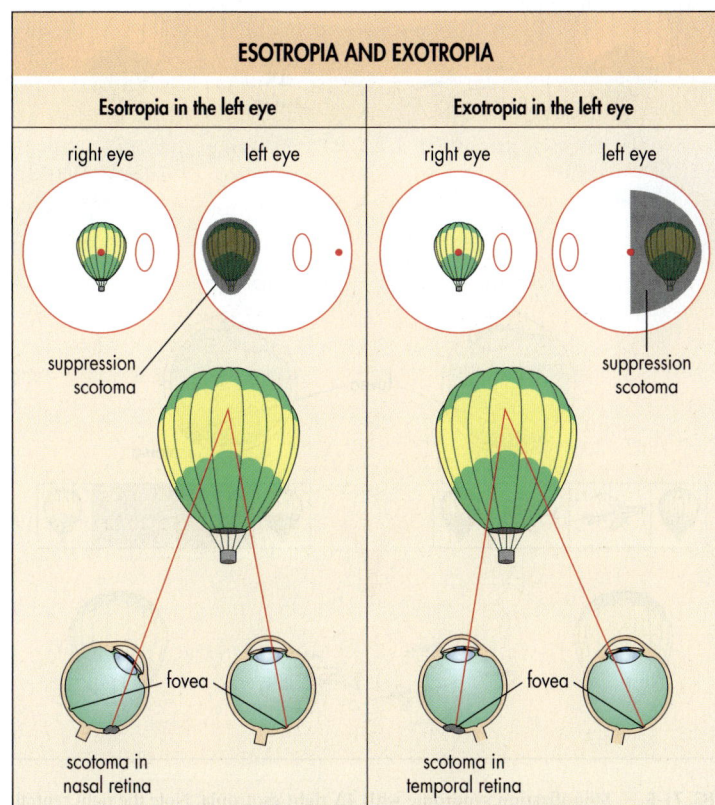

FIG. 71-2 ◼ **Esotropia and exotropia.** Esotropia in the left eye—a nasal retinal suppression scotoma obviates central diplopia. Exotropia in the left eye—a temporal retinal suppression scotoma obviates central diplopia.

ily available clinical tests, is also not found in patients who have ARC, although specialized testing may demonstrate primitive stereoptic appreciation in some patients.[4]

TREATMENT, COURSE, AND OUTCOME

Peripheral visual confusion and peripheral diplopia are obviated in the newly strabismic child by both the development of ARC and the reassignment of cortical directional values to "impose" comfortable, simultaneous perception on dissimilar retinal elements—essentially, a "superimposition" of such dissimilar elements (Fig. 71-3). This reassignment of cortical directional values is flexible and enables patients who have incomitant and intermittent forms of strabismus to maintain visual comfort despite various deviation angles in different gaze positions.

MONOFIXATION SYNDROME

INTRODUCTION

Many binocular patients who have a small or absent tropia (up to 8Δ esotropic or exotropic and 2Δ vertically up or down) and possible superimposed phoria exhibit monofixation syndrome (MFS), a sensory state that comprises features of both normal retinal correspondence and ARC (Box 71-1). Initially known by many terms, each of which explains one sensory or motor component of the complete syndrome (Box 71-2), the generally ac-

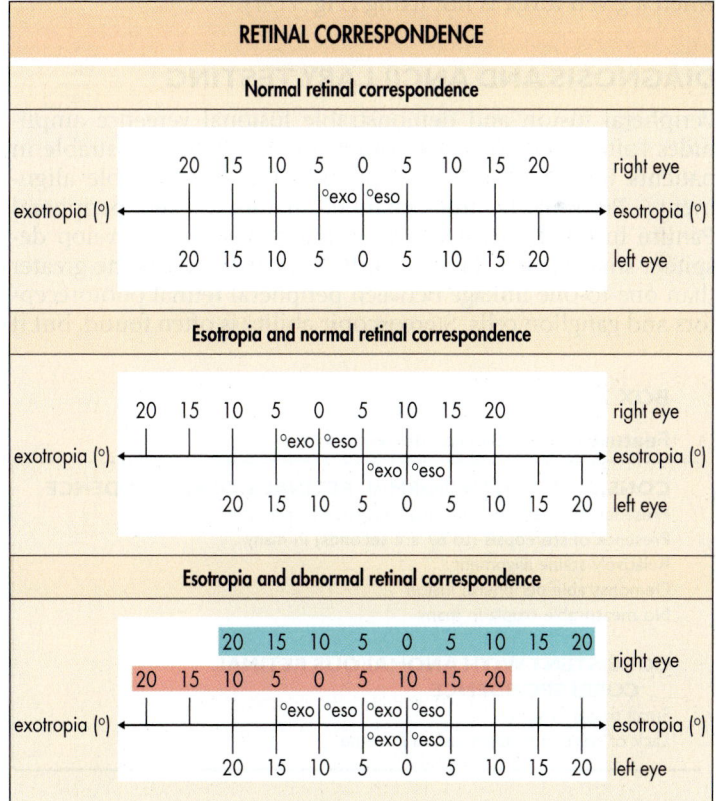

FIG. 71-3 ◼ **Retinal correspondence.** Normal retinal correspondence in aligned eyes, in which the visual cortex interprets the location of objects eccentric to fixation in each eye as coming from the same direction in space (noted as degrees from fixation). Right esotropia and normal retinal correspondence, in which the visual cortex receives images of two objects for each direction in space; the result is peripheral confusion. Also, each object in space stimulates noncorresponding retinal elements in the eyes, which results in peripheral diplopia. Right esotropia and abnormal retinal correspondence, in which the visual cortex reassigns directional values to objects viewed with the deviating eye to correspond with those values in the aligned eye. These subjective directional values (shown in blue) permit a form of comfortable, single, binocular vision by obviating peripheral confusion and peripheral diplopia. The objective alignment of the right eye appears 10° esotropic to the examiner (red values).

cepted name MFS emphasizes the essential feature of this syndrome, the presence of peripheral fusion without central fusion.[5] This means that only one rod-free retinal area (fovea) views at a given time.

The syndrome may develop spontaneously by unknown means, may be caused by anisometropia, is the best-expected sensory state in almost all patients who have "congenital" strabismus after successful surgical alignment, and is found in patients who have acquired unilateral organic foveal lesions (such as toxoplasmosis), although in the last instance the scotoma is usually larger.

Central fusion (bifoveal viewing with the possibility for superb stereoptic appreciation) may occur in the presence of very minimal deviation of the visual axes, less than that detectable by cover testing, and is termed *fixation disparity*; it measures roughly 14min of arc (perhaps 0.5Δ) and is present in most individuals.[6] It should not be confused with MFS.

Precise terminology restricts the term *suppression scotoma* to apply to that which arises to obviate central diplopia. Because many patients who have MFS have no tropia, central diplopia presumably does not occur consistently. If the viewing foveas alternate freely in a young child, amblyopia does not occur; if one fovea is preferred, amblyopia may occur even in patients who do not have a demonstrably strabismic appearance, which emphasizes the need for amblyopia screening in the young.

OCULAR MANIFESTATIONS

Patients who have MFS demonstrate an absolute, facultative, central scotoma that usually measures 2.5–3° in diameter, and, like a suppression scotoma seen in binocular patients who have childhood-onset strabismus and larger tropias, it is present only when a given fovea is not fixing (Fig. 71-4).

DIAGNOSIS AND ANCILLARY TESTING

Peripheral fusion and demonstrable fusional vergence amplitudes (often of a normal amount) are usually demonstrable in patients who have MFS and provide a generally stable alignment.[7] Presumably, the expanded nature of the peripheral Panum fusional area permits peripheral fusion to develop despite a small tropia (Fig. 71-5). Perhaps this reflects the greater than one-to-one linkage between peripheral retinal photoreceptors and ganglion cells. Stereoscopic ability is often found, but it

> ### BOX 71-1
>
> **Features of Monofixation Syndrome**
>
> **CONSISTENT WITH NORMAL RETINAL CORRESPONDENCE**
> Presence of measurable fusional vergence amplitudes
> Presence of stereopsis (to 67 arc seconds) in many
> Relatively stable alignment
> Demonstrable peripheral fusion
> No measurable tropia in many
>
> **CONSISTENT WITH ANOMALOUS RETINAL CORRESPONDENCE**
> Small tropia in some
> Lack of stereoptic appreciation in some

> ### BOX 71-2
>
> **Older Terms for Monofixation Syndrome**
>
> Monofixational phoria
> Microtropia
> Microstrabismus
> Esotropic flick strabismus
> Small angle strabismus

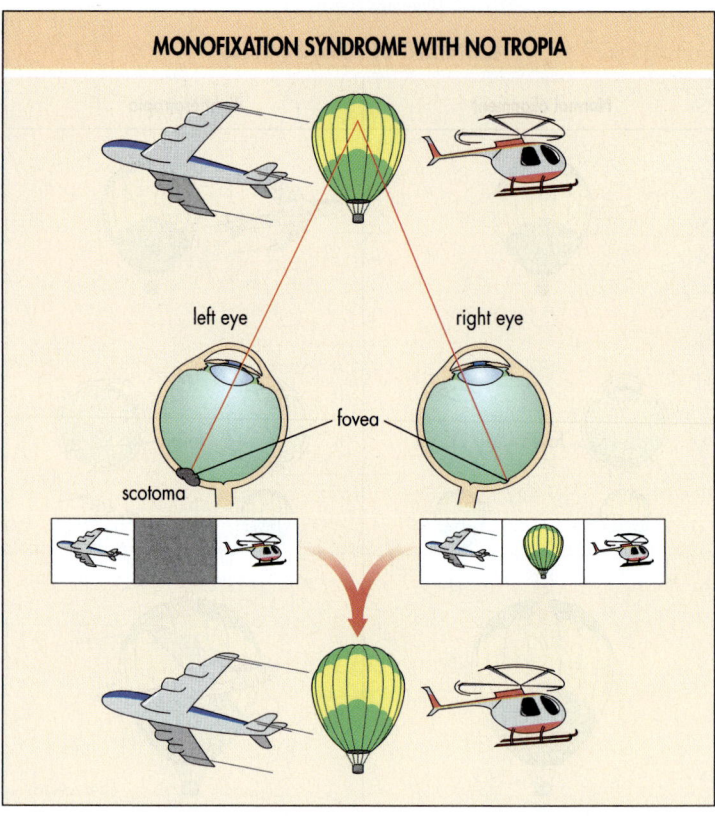

FIG. 71-4 ▌▌ **Monofixation syndrome with no tropia.** Note the central scotoma that envelops the area seen by the left fovea and fusion of peripheral information.

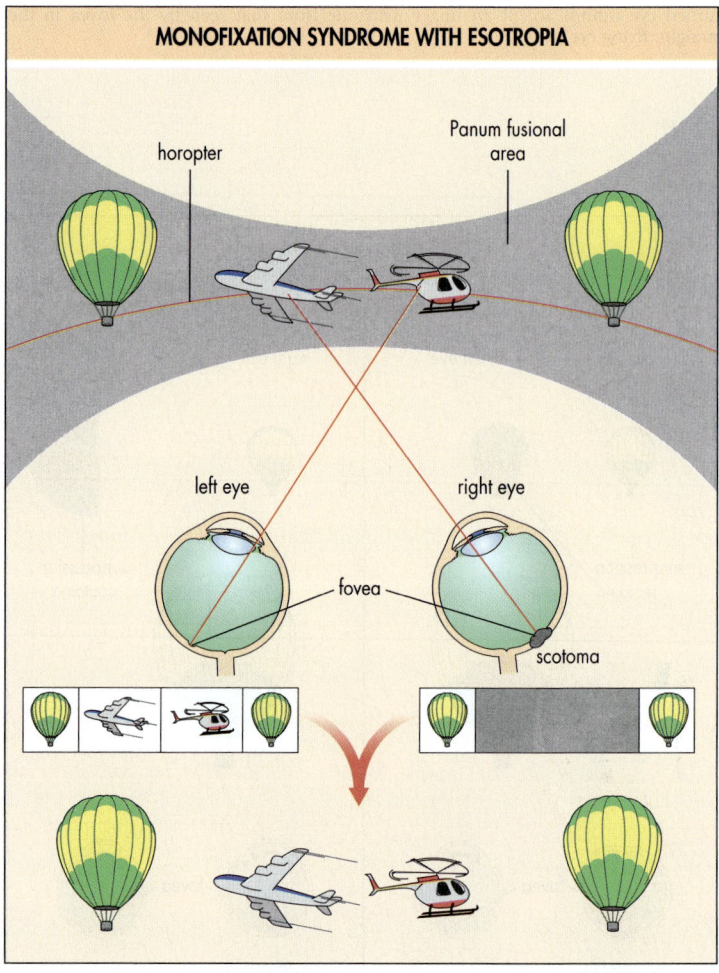

FIG. 71-5 ▌▌ **Monofixation syndrome with 4Δ right esotropia.** Note the right central scotoma that prevents perception of the plane and helicopter under binocular viewing conditions and fusion of peripheral information (balloons). The horopter is an infinitely thin surface in space that contains all the object points that project to corresponding retinal points. It is surrounded by the Panum fusional area, within which objects in space can be fused even though they project onto noncorresponding retinal points.

is rarely better than 67 arc seconds, as only one fovea is used in binocular viewing.[8] Note that the sensory status of patients who have MFS is the same whether or not a small tropia exists, although those who have large, superimposed phorias may sometimes have asthenopic symptoms.

Sensory testing shows peripheral without central fusion, possible stereoscopic appreciation (although never to normal limits), and generally normal fusional vergence amplitudes. If the patient has a phoria superimposed on a small tropia, alternate cover testing demonstrates larger strabismus than does cover-uncover or simultaneous prism-and-cover testing.[9]

Patients who have MFS exhibit sensory characteristics closer to normal retinal correspondence than ARC, that is, the presence of fusional vergence amplitudes and possible gross stereoptic appreciation, although those who have a small tropia do not have precise alignment of corresponding retinal elements. Cover testing shows roughly 22% without phoria or tropia, 34% with phoria only, and 44% with tropia and superimposed phoria, occasionally up to 20Δ. Only MFS permits the existence of a measurable tropia and superimposed phoria.

COURSE AND OUTCOMES

The absence of simultaneous foveal viewing means that young patients are at risk for development of amblyopia, and approximately two thirds do become amblyopic—90% if they also have a tropia. In the absence of anisometropia, three fourths of MFS patients are amblyopic. Of successfully aligned congenital esotropes who have MFS, one third are amblyopic. The amblyopia is treated as described elsewhere, but once lost, central fusion (bifoveality) cannot be reestablished (see Chapter 79).

REFERENCES

1. Adler FH. Physiology of the eye. St. Louis: CV Mosby; 1959.
2. Burian HM. The sensorial retinal relationships in comitant strabismus. Arch Ophthalmol. 1947;37:336–40.
3. Jampolsky A. Characteristics of suppression in strabismus. Arch Ophthalmol. 1955;54:683–9.
4. Hansell R. Stereopsis and ARC. Am Orthopt J. 1991;41:122–7.
5. Parks MM. The monofixation syndrome. In: Dabezies O, ed. Strabismus. Transactions New Orleans Academy of Ophthalmology. St. Louis: CV Mosby; 1971.
6. Ogle KN. Fixation disparity. Am Orthopt J. 1954;4:35–40.
7. Asrch BW, Smith JT, Scott WE. Long term stability of alignment in the monofixation syndrome. J Pediatr Ophthalmol Strabismus. 1989;26:244–9.
8. Parks MM. Stereoacuity as an indicator of bifixation. In: Knapp P, ed. Strabismus symposium. New York: Karger; 1968.
9. Parks MM. Small angle esotropia/monofixation: avoid the traps. Am Orthopt J. 1991;41:34–5.

CHAPTER

72

Sensory Status in Strabismus

GARY R. DIAMOND

DEFINITION

- Fusion: cortical integration of slightly dissimilar images perceived by the two eyes into a unified percept.
- Horopter: the locus in space representing the intersection of all points that stimulate corresponding retinal points.
- Panum fusional area: area in space surrounding the horopter in which objects can be fused.
- Stereopsis: a form of depth perception that demands binocular vision and usually sensory fusion.
- Monofixation syndrome: a form of binocular vision found in many patients who have small amounts of strabismus that permits peripheral fusion, stereopsis, and alignment stability.

KEY FEATURES

- Subjective tests for binocular vision and retinal correspondence are an important part of every patient's examination.
- Monofixation syndrome can be diagnosed reliably only by sensory testing.

INTRODUCTION

Binocular patients who develop strabismus before the age of 7–9 years usually develop the sensory adaptations of suppression and anomalous retinal correspondence to obviate diplopia and visual confusion (see Chapter 71). Older patients who develop strabismus for the first time suffer from diplopia and visual confusion as long as vision remains in both eyes, until the eyes are aligned or the patient learns to ignore one image. Nonbinocular patients (or those who perceive with one eye at a time) are not troubled by symptoms of double vision if their eyes become strabismic.

Clinical testing of sensory status in strabismic patients is easier to understand after the basic physiology of sensory fusion and stereopsis has been mastered.

SENSORY FUSION

Sensory fusion is the cerebral cortical integration of the slightly dissimilar images perceived by the two eyes into a unified percept. If images are sufficiently dissimilar, they cannot be fused; examples are red and green variants of the same object or lines seen vertically by one eye and horizontally by the other. Binocular rivalry usually occurs under these conditions, and a varying percept is obtained. Motor fusion with vergence amplitudes, and even stereopsis, may be produced by rivalrous stimuli in the absence of sensory fusion. Such stimuli are fortunately uncommon in daily life.

A retinal element is a small retinal patch that has an associated directional value. The fovea's directional value is defined subjectively as straight ahead; peripheral retinal elements possess directional values in other orientations. Corresponding retinal points are a pair of retinal elements, one in each eye, that have the same directional value. Comfortable single binocular vision occurs when objects in the binocular field stimulate corresponding retinal points and the higher cortical function—termed *sensory fusion*—occurs.

The locus in space that represents the intersection of all points in space that stimulate corresponding retinal points is termed the *horopter*. Interestingly, sensory fusion still occurs if the object that projects upon a retinal element in one eye projects upon a range of elements that surrounds the corresponding retinal element in the second eye. The area in space that projects from this range of elements in the second eye that intersects with the projection from the retinal element in the first eye is termed the *Panum fusional area* (Fig. 72-1). This Panum fusional area surrounds the horopter anteriorly and posteriorly; it permits fusion to take place when exact retinal correspondence does not occur. The binocularly perceived object imaged on noncorresponding retinal loci, but fused within the Panum fusional area, is perceived to have one subjective visual direction. The foveal Panum area is circular, of diameter about 14min of arc; thus, an object projected upon the fovea of one eye may be displaced by this amount and the patient still maintains bifoveal vision. The size of the Panum fusional area increases toward the retinal periphery (see Fig. 71-5), but the ultimate size and shape depend upon the temporal and spatial frequency of the patient's alignment drift when fixing upon a stationary target.[1]

Objects in front of or behind the Panum fusional area stimulate physiologic diplopia, which is not usually noted but may in turn stimulate fusional vergence eye movements. The horopter shape may be defined in a pair of perfectly spherical eyes that have refractive seats at the nodal points of each eye as the locus of points of zero vertical disparity relative to the fixation point. In a horizontal plane, the horopter, which includes the fovea, is the Vieth-Müller circle (Fig. 72-2).[1,2] In a living animal visual system the horopter is flatter (the Hering-Hellebrand horopter deviation). The vertical horopter tilts away from the observer, who stands on the horopter; the inclination is a function of fixation distance.[3]

DEPTH PERCEPTION AND STEREOPSIS

Depth perception may occur without binocular vision and depends on both monocular (Box 72-1) and binocular clues. Stereopsis is a form of depth perception that demands binocular vision and usually sensory fusion but under certain conditions may be stimulated by rivalrous objects whose images cannot be fused. Stereopsis is the perception of depth stimulated by objects that possess horizontal disparity, with one object also usually located before or behind the fixation point. Horizontal disparity alone is sufficient to stimulate the stereoptic percept. Visual contours are not necessary, and disparity may be stimu-

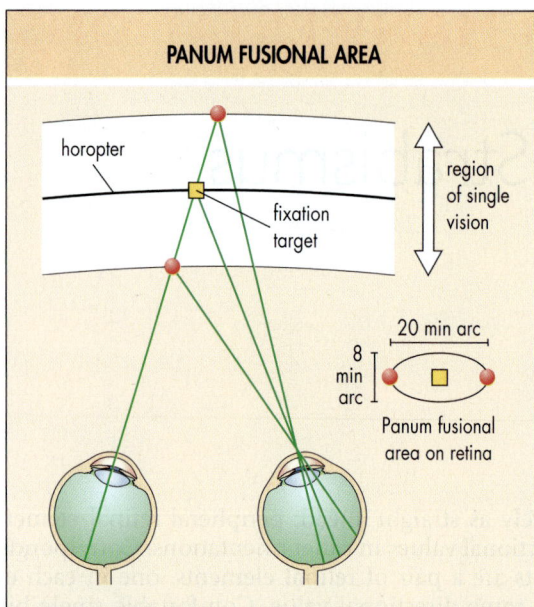

FIG. 72-1 ▮ **Panum fusional area.** The left eye fixates a square target, and a search object visible only to the right eye is moved before and behind this target. The ellipse of retinal area, for which typical dimensions are given for the parafoveal area, is the projection of the Panum fusional area. Diplopia is not perceived for two targets within this area.

FIG. 72-2 ▮ **Vieth–Müller circle.** If the eyes are assumed to be spherical with rotational centers at the nodal points, all points in space that have a zero disparity fall on this circle. Angle a_1 = angle a_2; thus, equal retinal distances map into equal angles in space in this idealized system.

lated by random dots.[4,5] Stereoacuity, the disparity threshold at which a depth difference may just be appreciated, is best at the fovea and depends on the level of visual acuity in each eye. Stereoacuity dissipates rapidly into the peripheral visual field and with increasing object distance[6] and is proportional to interpupillary distance. Under ideal conditions, foveal stereoacuity is 10sec of arc.[7]

CLINICAL TESTING

The clinician must determine the sensory status of each patient, specifically whether the patient is binocular and if so whether the patient has normal retinal correspondence (NRC) or abnormal retinal correspondence (ARC) and suppression (see Chapter 71). Binocular patients who have constant tropias measurable on cover testing may exhibit NRC with diplopia and visual confusion, ARC and suppression, or monofixation syndrome. The last possesses features of both NRC and ARC but is considered closer to the former.

Asymptomatic patients who have tropias >8Δ horizontally or 4Δ vertically usually have ARC and suppression, although these may be difficult to demonstrate. Asymptomatic binocular patients who have smaller tropias, or a smaller tropia with superimposed phoria, usually have monofixation syndrome.

Many sensory tests are available to the busy clinician, but access to and understanding of just a few enable evaluation of the patient's sensory status. It is important to perform sensory testing at the beginning of the examination; prolonged monocular occlusion to evaluate visual acuity may dissociate the eyes and confound determination of the patient's ambient sensory status.

Testing for Binocularity (Simultaneous Perception)

Many tests require simple tools to demonstrate binocularity. Holding a red lens before one eye and presenting a white light detects perception of two lights, red and white, in patients who have NRC and diplopia. Prisms may be used to project one light beyond the bounds of a suppression scotoma in patients who have ARC and suppression or NRC-monofixation syndrome. Commercially available Polaroid projection slides, when viewed through polarized lenses, present one half of an optotype line to each eye; binocular patients view the entire line, whereas nonbinocular patients

---

BOX 72-1

Monocular Clues to Depth Perception

Apparent size of objects of known size
Superimposition of near object on more distant object
Loss of contrast of distant object
Movement parallax (shift in relative position of two objects as subject moves head)
Light and shape effects
Linear perspective (such as convergent railroad tracks)
Fading of texture with distance

Binocular vision is not always necessary to determine the relative position of objects in space.

---

view the half perceived by the foveating eye only. Prismatically, overcorrection of a strabismic patient elicits diplopic symptoms, which proves the presence of binocular vision.

The Worth four-dot test uses a fixed wall target for distance fixation (Fig. 72-3) and a handheld wand for testing at variable near-fixation distances (Fig. 72-4). The stimulus is an array of four round targets ("dots"), usually presented with the red dot above two green dots that in turn are above one white dot. The diameter of the target array subtends 6° at 20ft (6m) and 1.25° at 1ft (33cm). The targets are viewed through red-green (anaglyph) glasses, and the patient describes the percept to the examiner or simply counts the lights viewed. Binocular patients perceive red and green lights simultaneously, but the near wand must be held very close to a patient with a large strabismic deviation to project the target beyond the bounds of a suppression scotoma (Fig. 72-5). Nonbinocular patients see two red or three green lights at all testing distances (Fig. 72-6).

Bagolini lenses are finely ruled plano lenses that give a streak appearance to a point light source perpendicular to the ruled direction. The lenses are placed in orthogonal orientation (traditionally at 135° right eye and 45° left eye; Fig. 72-7) in a trial frame and the patient views a light at distance fixation. Binocular patients perceive an "X" figure or, if a suppression scotoma exists, one complete line and the peripheral elements of the second. Nonbinocular patients see only one entire line.

Haploscopes, for example, the major amblyoscope, may present slightly different but fusible images to each eye; if por-

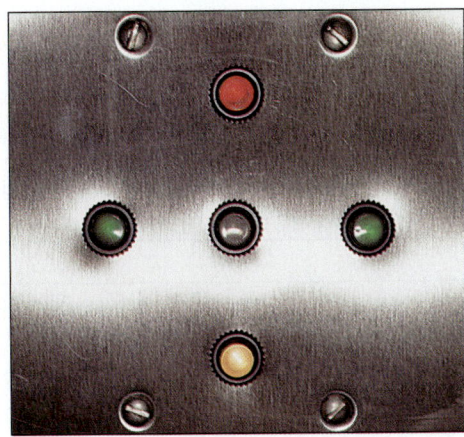

FIG. 72-3 ▌▌ **Distant Worth four-dot target.** This is fixed to a wall, traditionally with the red dot placed at the top.

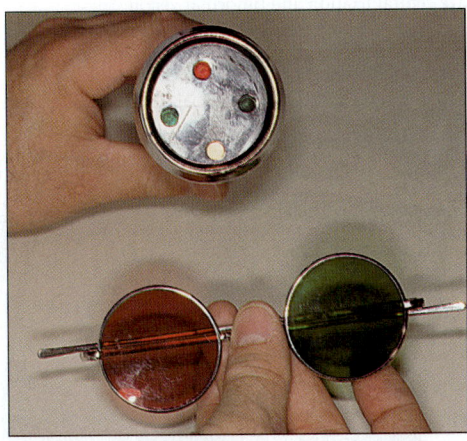

FIG. 72-4 ▌▌ **Near Worth four-dot target and anaglyph glasses.** The near target is brought to the face to elicit a binocular response in patients who have strabismus and large scotomas.

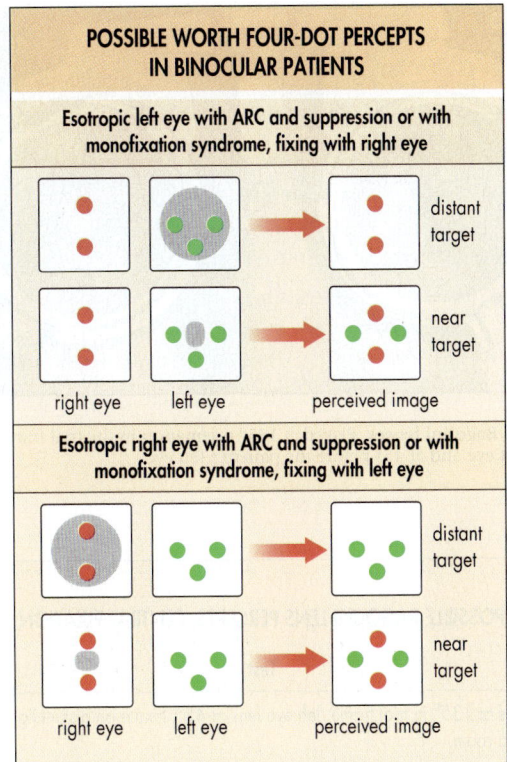

FIG. 72-5 ▌▌ **Possible Worth four-dot percepts in binocular patients.** Note the similar distant responses in patients who have esotropia with abnormal retinal correspondence (ARC) and suppression and in those who have monofixation syndrome. Patients who have exotropia with ARC and suppression give the same responses, but the suppression scotoma is larger and shaped somewhat differently (see Fig. 71-2). The red lens is over the right eye and the green lens over the left eye.

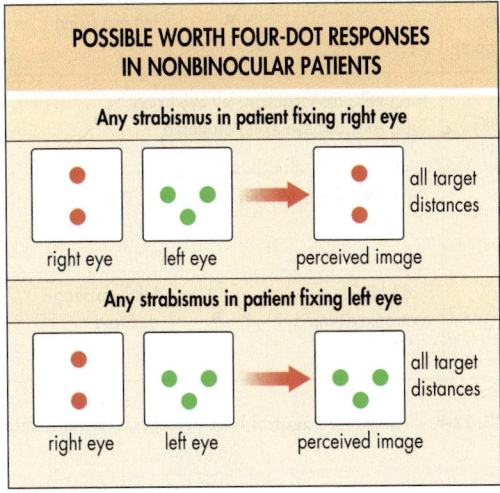

FIG. 72-6 ▌▌ **Possible Worth four-dot responses in patients who do not have binocularity.** The red lens is over the right eye and the green lens over the left eye.

tions of each image are perceived, the patient is binocular. The viewing tubes may be displaced to the strabismic angle if such exists, or the tubes may be kept in the straight position and targets used that are large enough to project beyond the suppression scotoma.

Tests of Retinal Correspondence

Many of the preceding tests may be used in binocular patients to diagnose ARC and suppression, NRC bifoveality, or NRC-monofixation syndrome at a given testing distance at a given moment. As ARC exists only under binocular testing conditions, some tests may yield an ARC response at a given moment whereas other tests yield an NRC response, depending on the room illumination and the length of time ARC has been present. Tests that confound correctable single binocular vision and that poorly reproduce ordinary binocular viewing conditions demonstrate ARC later than tests that closely simulate typical binocular viewing conditions. Retinal correspondence tests are listed by depth of abnormal correspondence in Box 72-2.

The Worth four-dot test demonstrates suppression of one eye when presented with a distant viewing target and fusion of lights of the near viewing target in patients who have ARC and suppression and NRC-monofixation syndrome (Fig. 72-5); thus, it cannot be used to differentiate ARC from NRC easily.[8]

The Bagolini lens test most closely simulates ordinary viewing and is the least dissociating of all retinal correspondence tests.[9] Central (foveal) fixation must be assumed and the alignment of the eyes known; possible outcomes are given in Figure 72-8.

The afterimage test is most removed from ordinary binocular viewing and the most dissociating of all commonly performed retinal correspondence tests; an ARC response on this test declares the ARC to be deep seated. An afterimage (positive in dim illumination, negative in bright) is imprinted on each retina in turn with a photographic flash device. The fellow eye is covered during the flash. Usually a vertical flash is presented to one eye and a horizontal flash to the other. The fovea is protected by a central mask with fixation target and thus "labeled" as the center of an afterimage line. An NRC response yields a cross pattern (see Fig. 72-9) as the fovea in each eye retains the straight-ahead directional value. A crossed heteronymous localization occurs in ARC with esotropia, as the straight-ahead directional value lies in

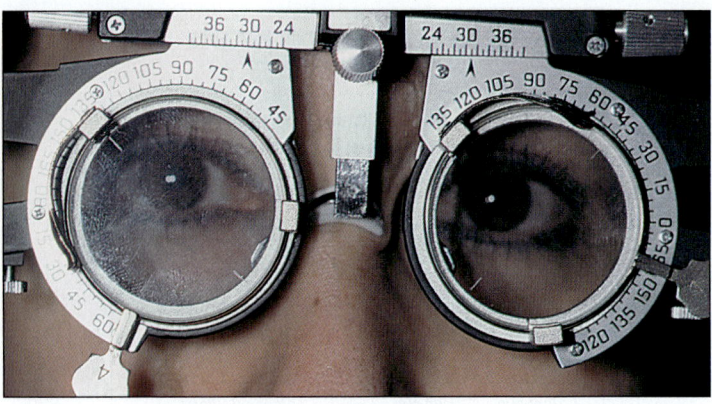

FIG. 72-7 ▌ **Bagolini lenses.** Placed at 135° orientation in the trial frame before the patient's right eye and at 45° before the patient's left eye.

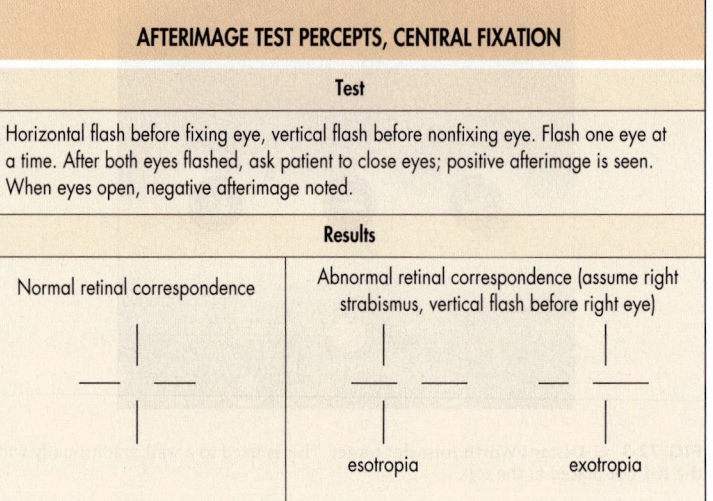

AFTERIMAGE TEST PERCEPTS, CENTRAL FIXATION

Test
Horizontal flash before fixing eye, vertical flash before nonfixing eye. Flash one eye at a time. After both eyes flashed, ask patient to close eyes; positive afterimage is seen. When eyes open, negative afterimage noted.

Results	
Normal retinal correspondence	Abnormal retinal correspondence (assume right strabismus, vertical flash before right eye)
	esotropia exotropia

FIG. 72-9 ▌ **Afterimage test percepts, central fixation.** Shown are those possible in patients who have central fixation and binocular vision.

POSSIBLE BAGOLINI LENS PERCEPTS, CENTRAL FIXATION

Test
Right eye lens at 135° in trial frame, left eye lens at 45°. Fixate on distant light in semidarkened room.
Closest sensory test to normal viewing, first to exhibit abnormal retinal correspondence (ARC) strabismus, first to revert to normal retinal correspondence (NRC) when eyes aligned.

Results		
Cover–uncover test irrelevant	No binocularity, right eye fixing	No binocularity, left eye fixing
No shift on cover–uncover testing (no tropia)	NRC bifoveal	NRC monofixation, left eye fixing
Shift on cover–uncover testing (tropia)	≤8Δ NRC monofixation, left eye fixing >8Δ ARC, left eye fixing esotropia	
	>8Δ ARC, left eye fixing exotropia	
	>8Δ NRC, esotropic diplopia	NRC, exotropic diplopia

FIG. 72-8 ▌ Possible Bagolini lens percepts, central fixation.

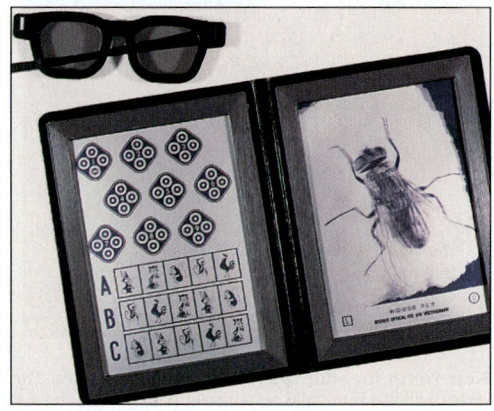

FIG. 72-10 ▌ **Titmus stereotest with Polaroid glasses.**

BOX 72-2

Retinal Correspondence Testing

Bagolini striated lenses; Aulhorn phase-difference haploscope
Synoptophore (major amblyoscope)
Red glass test
Worth four-dot test; Polaroid lens and mirror test
Afterimage test
Dazzle test

The lower the listing of an abnormal retinal correspondence response, the more the depth of the abnormal correspondence. After successful treatment, a normal retinal correspondence response develops with time, initially shown by the bottom tests and then through to the top. Not all listed tests are described in the text.

the nasal retina of the strabismic eye; the fovea has a temporal directional value.[10] In patients who have ARC and exotropia, the afterimage percept is an uncrossed homonymous localization.

Clinicians who have access to a major amblyoscope may set the tubes at the objective angle of strabismus; if the targets are superimposed, NRC exists. Crossed diplopia occurs in patients who have ARC and esotropia and uncrossed diplopia in patients who have ARC and exotropia. An "angle of anomaly" is defined when the patient moves the tubes until the targets are superimposed; this subjective angle equals the objective angle in "harmonious" ARC and is less or greater in "unharmonious" ARC.

Stereopsis Tests

Clinically useful stereopsis tests provide slightly different views of the same target to each eye; each unique view is maintained by either Polaroid filters (Titmus, Wirt, Randot, Lang) or anaglyph glasses (TNO).

The Titmus stereotest (Fig. 72-10) provides disparity in the range 3000sec of arc at 40cm testing distance (fly wings above background) to 40sec of arc (ninth circle). Younger children may respond to the depth illusion of three sets of five animals, one of which appears to float above the background (400, 200, 100sec of arc). The older Wirt stereotest provided circles with disparity as fine as 14sec of arc. The first few circles may be identified accurately by nonstereoptic patients because the circles possess monocular clues[11]; the Randot test (Fig. 72-11) avoids this problem because it provides similar targets as random dots with no monocular clues.

TABLE 72-1

SYNOPSIS OF SENSORY TESTING IN STRABISMUS

Test	NRC–Bifoveal	NRC–Monofixation	Abnormal Retinal Correspondence	Diplopia	No Binocularity
Worth four-dot, distance (6m)	4	2 or 3	2 or 3	5	2 or 3
Worth four-dot, near (40cm)	4	4	4	5	2 or 3
Stereo	None to 14sec arc	None to 67sec arc	None	None	None

The Worth four-dot test and Titmus stereotest are used to define a patient's sensory status. Appreciation of four distant lights demands normal retinal correspondence (*NRC*) and bifoveality, as does recognition of seven or more circles on the stereotest. Any level of stereoptic appreciation on this test signifies NRC at that moment at that testing distance. Appreciation of four lights on the Worth test at any testing distance signifies binocular vision.

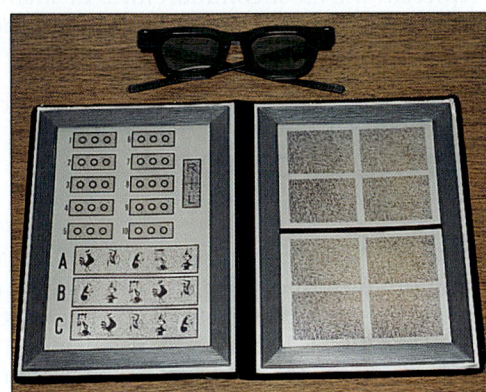

FIG. 72-11 ■ Randot stereotest with Polaroid glasses.

Children who reject the Polaroid glasses may be tested using the similarly targeted Lang test,[12] in which random-dot stereograms are presented through a cylinder grating that overlies the target. The TNO stereotest uses random-dot stereograms viewed through anaglyph glasses and contains disparities in the range 480 down to 15sec of arc.

Test for Monofixation Syndrome

One feature of this syndrome (see Chapter 71) is a small, round scotoma that surrounds the fovea of one eye under binocular viewing conditions. As the patient views a distant target, a 4Δ prism, usually held base out, is introduced before one eye. If held before the fixing eye, it will saccade to the new target position toward the prism's apex, as does the fellow eye. A slower fusional vergence movement in the fellow eye in the opposite direction follows. When the prism is held before a nonfixing eye there is no saccade, as the image displacement falls within a scotoma and is therefore not perceived. The test must be performed with the prism before each eye. Some patients switch fixation to the fellow eye when a prism is introduced before either and no saccadic shift is generated.

The busy clinician may determine the sensory status of most patients by using two straightforward and easily available tests—the Worth four-dot test and the Titmus stereotest. A summary of sensory testing interpretation using these commonly available testing devices is given in Table 72-1.

REFERENCES

1. Schor LE, Tyler CW. Spatio-temporal properties of Panum's fusional area. Vision Res. 1981;21:683–92.
2. Hillebrand F. Lehre von der Gesichtsempfindungen. Vienna: Springer; 1929.
3. Amigo G. A vertical horopter. Optica Acta. 1974;21:277–92.
4. Julesz B. Binocular depth perception of computer-generated patterns. Bell Syst Technol J. 1967;46:1203–21.
5. Julesz B. Foundations of cyclopean perception. Chicago: University of Chicago Press; 1971.
6. Blakemore C. The range and scope of binocular depth discrimination in man. J Physiol (Lond). 1970;211:599–622.
7. Richards W. Stereopsis and stereoblindness. Exp Brain Res. 1970;10:380–8.
8. Roundtable discussion. In: Gregerson E, ed. Transactions of the European Strabismological Association. Copenhagen: Jencodan Tryk; 1984:215–24.
9. Bagolini B. Anomalous correspondence: definition and diagnostic methods. Doc Ophthalmol. 1967;23:638–51.
10. Bielschowsky A. Application of the after image test in the investigation of squint. Am J Ophthalmol. 1937;20:408–13.
11. Kohler L, Stigmar G. Vision screening in four-year-old children. Acta Paediatr Scand. 1973;63:17–25.
12. Lang J. A new stereotest. J Pediatr Ophthalmol Strabismus. 1983;20:72–4.

CHAPTER

73 Esotropia

GARY R. DIAMOND

CONGENITAL ESOTROPIA

DEFINITION

- Inward deviation of the visual axes, with an onset before 6 months of age.

KEY FEATURES

- Esotropia greater than 30Δ.
- Cross-fixation.
- No binocular vision.
- Typical refractive error (between +1.50 and +3.00).
- Initially, similar deviation at distance and near fixation.

ASSOCIATED FEATURES

- Inferior oblique overaction.
- Dissociated vertical deviation.
- Latent horizontal and manifest rotary nystagmus.
- Amblyopia in about one third of patients.

ACCOMMODATIVE ESOTROPIA

DEFINITION

- Inward deviation of the visual axes caused by high hyperopia or a high accommodative convergence–to–accommodation ratio, or both.

KEY FEATURES

- Initially intermittent acquired esotropia.
- Esotropia larger at near than distance fixation.

ASSOCIATED FEATURES

- Patients who have a high accommodative convergence–to–accommodation ratio may have any refractive error.
- Age of onset usually between 18 months and 3 years.

DUANE'S SYNDROME

DEFINITION

- Congenital miswiring of the medial or lateral rectus muscles, or both, often associated with strabismus.

KEY FEATURE

- Retraction of the affected globe(s) on attempted adduction.

ASSOCIATED FEATURES

- Ptosis on attempted adduction.
- Elevation or depression of the globe on attempted adduction.
- Limitation of abduction, adduction, or both.
- Esotropia or exotropia in some patients, usually acquired and rarely larger than 30°.

INTRODUCTION

Esotropias represent the most common form of strabismus and include congenital, accommodative, cyclic, and nonaccommodative forms. They also are seen in some patients who have Duane's and Möbius' syndromes.

CONGENITAL ESOTROPIA

INTRODUCTION

The most common form of esotropia is "congenital" esotropia, somewhat arbitrarily defined as esotropia that presents before 6 months of age (Fig. 73-1). Recent work has demonstrated that many infants begin life with a moderate exodeviation that disappears between 2 and 4 months of age; prospective studies have determined that this is the age at which congenital esotropia is first noted. For younger children, it cannot be predicted which ones will develop congenital esotropia by age 2–4 months.[1] These important observations suggest that the causes of congenital strabismus are neither purely motor nor purely sensory in most cases; rather, there is a difficulty in coupling the two systems.

EPIDEMIOLOGY AND PATHOGENESIS

The incidence of congenital esotropia is roughly 1% in most series and may be more common in children who have neurological disorders.[2] The term *congenital esotropia* is so widely used that it should be retained despite evidence that few, if any, children are truly esotropic from birth. Sex and racial distributions are equal. Concordance in one series was 81% in monozygous twins and 9% in dizygous twins.[3] It is common to find accommodative esotropia or other cases of congenital esotropia in other members of the proband's family.

OCULAR MANIFESTATIONS

Amblyopia occurs in 25–40% of patients, but the majority "cross-fixate"—use the right eye to fix across the nose to view objects to the left of the patient, and vice versa[4] (Fig. 73-2). A child who does not have amblyopia switches fixation at the midline as an object is brought from one side to the other and does not maintain fixation and adopt a progressive head turn. As a rule, the deviation is >35Δ and comitant, measuring roughly the same in all gaze positions, distance and near.

Inferior oblique overaction is noted in up to 75% of patients, with an onset most frequently during the second year of life; it may be unilateral or bilateral (Fig. 73-3).[5] Early surgical correction of the esotropia does not prevent the later development of inferior oblique overaction. This must be differentiated from dissociated vertical deviation (DVD), which also occurs in roughly 75% of these patients and has similar onset patterns (Fig. 73-4)[6]; DVD may be manifest or latent, is very asymmetrical, and may present as any combination of elevation, abduction, and excyclotorsion (Box 73-1). Although its

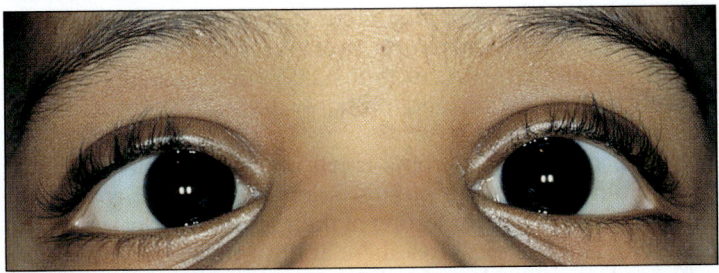

FIG. 73-1 ▮ **Congenital esotropia.** The child is fixing with her left eye; note the decentered light reflex in the right eye.

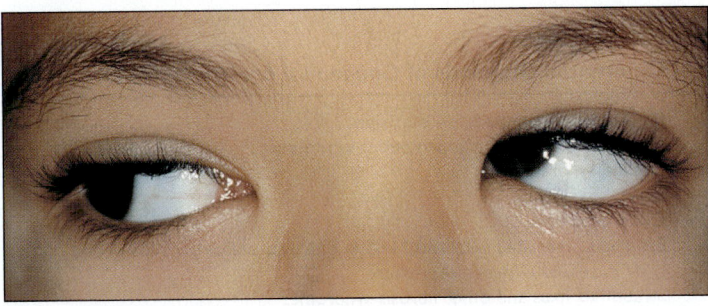

FIG. 73-3 ▮ **Overelevation in adduction of the left eye.** This arose from inferior oblique overaction and must be differentiated from dissociated vertical deviation, which also may cause overelevation in adduction.

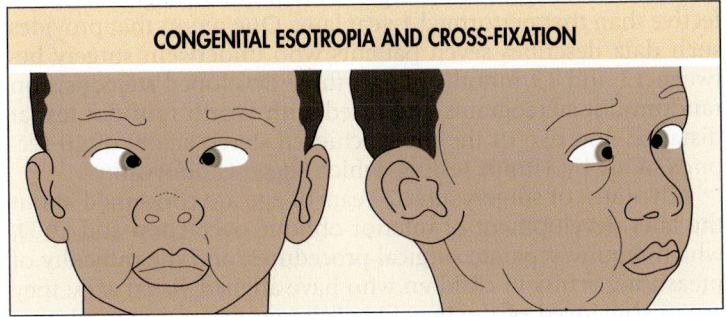

FIG. 73-2 ▮ **Congenital esotropia and cross-fixation.** The infant uses the right eye to view left, and vice versa. Doll's head maneuver shows full abduction.

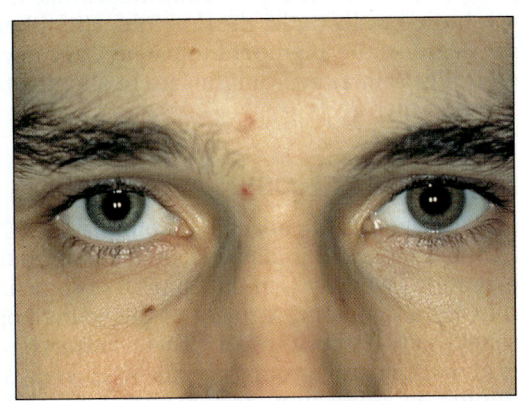

FIG. 73-4 ▮ **Dissociated vertical deviation in the right eye.** If the patient fixes with the right eye, no hypodeviation is seen in the left. Therefore, dissociated vertical deviation does not obey the Hering law. (Reproduced with permission from Cheng KP, Biglan AW, Hiles DA. Pediatric ophthalmology. In: Zitelli BJ, Davis HW, eds. Atlas of pediatric physical diagnosis, 2nd ed. New York: Gower Medical Publishing; 1992:19.1.)

BOX 73-1

Dissociated Vertical Deviation Compared With Inferior Oblique Overaction

DISSOCIATED VERTICAL DEVIATION	INFERIOR OBLIQUE OVERACTION
Present in all gaze positions	Present in adduction only
Does not obey the Hering law	Obeys the Hering law
Slow floating abduction, elevation, excyclotorsion movement	Rapid elevation, abduction movement
Not associated with A or V pattern	Often associated with V pattern
Proportional to ambient illumination in fixing eye	Not proportional to illumination in fixing eye
No objective fundus torsion	Objective fundus excyclotorsion

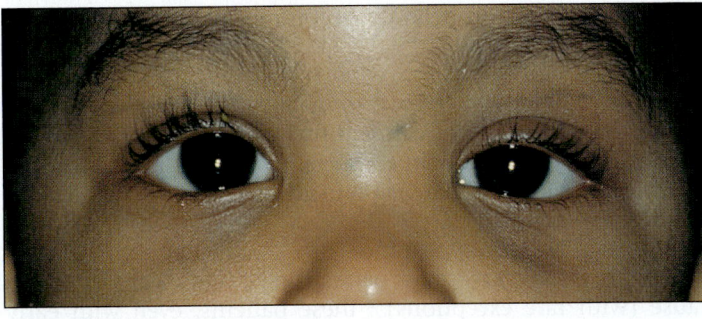

FIG. 73-5 ▮ **Pseudostrabismus.** This results from a flat nasal bridge, wide epicanthal folds, and small interpupillary distance. (Reproduced with permission from Cheng KP, Biglan AW, Hiles DA. Pediatric ophthalmology. In: Zitelli BJ, Davis HW, eds. Atlas of pediatric physical diagnosis, 2nd ed. New York: Gower Medical Publishing; 1992:19.1.)

---

cause is unknown, DVD may represent a primitive eye movement pattern uncovered by deficient fusion. Brodsky[7] concluded that DVD is a dorsal light reflex in which asymmetrical input evokes a vertical divergence, serving in lower lateral-eyed animals as a righting response by equalizing visual input to each eye. Nystagmus may be present in both manifest rotary and latent horizontal forms. The former is uncommon and tends to diminish during the first decade of life. Latent nystagmus with fast phase toward the unoccluded eye is found in approximately 50% of patients.

Asymmetrical monocular pursuit is a feature of congenital esotropia, as measured by opticokinetic nystagmus (OKN). Temporal-to-nasal pursuit is favored; patients who have congenital esotropia show poor nasal-to-temporal OKN regardless of the degree of stereopsis or the timing of surgery.[8]

Roughly half of young children sent to ophthalmologists by pediatricians for esotropia have pseudostrabismus, an illusion caused by a wide and flat nasal bridge, wide epicanthal folds, and the ability of young children to converge accommodatively to very close distances (Fig. 73-5).[9]

DIAGNOSIS

Cover test measurements to detect amblyopia may be difficult in very young children, and a variation of the light reflex test in which the deviation is neutralized by prisms held apex-to-apex before both eyes may be required. The deviation tends to be constant but may vary; rarely, spontaneous resolution may occur during a 3–4-year period. Refractive errors tend to be similar to those of normal children of the same age.

Nystagmus may confound attempts at monocular acuity measurement; fogging one eye with plus lenses or the use of anaglyph (red–green) lenses may provide a more accurate acuity measurement in the face of latent nystagmus.

Side gaze observations by nonophthalmologists may be particularly deceptive in the case of pseudostrabismus, as the adducted eye is buried easily under the skin fold. Hirschberg's light reflexes may demonstrate alignment to parents, as can elevation of the nasal bridge skin away from the face to alter the facial appearance temporarily.

DIFFERENTIAL DIAGNOSIS

The differential diagnosis of congenital esotropia (Box 73-2) includes the entities discussed in detail later. The nystagmus blockage (compensation) syndrome, in the opinion of some investigators, accounts for a significant segment of the young population with large-angle, early-onset esotropia.[10] These patients have a large esotropia and nystagmus at a young age; the nystagmus is of minimal amplitude in adduction and maximal in abduction.[11] Therefore, the patient makes a continuous effort to maintain both eyes in adduction through the use of convergence, and it may be impossible to neutralize the esodeviation using prisms held before one or both eyes. Although nystagmus may occur in patients who have the common form of congenital esotropia, it is present in equal degrees in all gaze positions. Various series imply that nystagmus blockage syndrome affects 10–12% of esotropic patients, but many investigators believe that it is much less common.

TREATMENT

The theoretical goals of treatment include:
- Excellent visual acuity in each eye;
- Perfect single binocular vision in all gaze positions at distance and near; and
- A normal esthetic appearance.

All are obtainable except for perfect single binocular vision, because (with rare exceptions)[12] these patients, even with early treatment, do not view with both foveae simultaneously. However, as discussed later, most obtain peripheral fusion and the monofixation syndrome and generally stable alignment. Other reported benefits of successful surgical alignment include improvement in fine motor skills, heightened bonding of parents and child, and enlarged binocular visual field.

Amblyopia traditionally is treated preoperatively, because compliance is usually better, acuity may be evaluated more easily (the eye moves to take up fixation in the presence of a large strabismus), and amblyopia responds more quickly in a younger child. A common approach is to occlude the better-sighted eye for all waking hours and evaluate the child at intervals related to age. For example, a 1-year-old child is evaluated 1 week after the onset of occlusion, a 2-year-old at 2 weeks, and a 6-month-old at 3 days. After acuity has equalized, the duration of patching may be decreased to approximately 2 hours per day, with good assurance that amblyopia will not return; in compliant children, patching may be discontinued, with a 50% or better assurance that amblyopia will not return. Some investigators have induced cycloplegia in the better-sighted eye, if hyperopic, using atropine or via occlusion with an opaque contact lens, with success.

The impact of treatment of refractive errors of less than +2.00D usually is variable and minimal. Larger refractive errors are corrected, and the deviation is remeasured, because postoperative exotropia may occur if surgery is performed on uncorrected, highly hyperopic eyes. An occasional patient responds to miotic treatment, but such patients usually have an intermittent deviation and probably have an early-onset accommodative esotropia.

When congenital esotropia is left untreated, patients do not display binocular vision of any variety when they become old enough to cooperate for testing of their visual sensory status; the primary goal of surgical treatment at this age is to align the eyes sufficiently to stimulate the development of binocularity. This binocularity usually fulfills the criteria for monofixation syndrome as defined by Parks[13] and is generally a stable alignment.

The mainstay of therapy for this form of strabismus is surgery. Ing[14] found that surgical alignment before the age of 24 months resulted in peripheral fusion in 93% of patients; surgery after 24 months resulted in similar results in only 31% of patients. Few available data suggest that surgery at 6 months of age is more effective than that performed 1 year later. One report that provides such data describes seven patients who underwent surgery between 13 and 19 months of age; three developed stereopsis on random dot stereograms and fused with Worth four-dot test at distance, and two of the three achieved stereo acuity of 40 seconds of arc by Titmus testing, which suggests bifoveality.

Advocates of surgery after 2 years of age are concerned about the later development of inferior oblique overaction and DVD, which require separate surgical procedures, and the difficulty of measuring acuity in children who have aligned visual axes; they are unconvinced of the benefits of the monofixation syndrome (peripheral fusion without central fusion). Given reproducible strabismus measurements, informed and supportive parents, the availability of safe pediatric anesthetic, and the absence of amblyopia, most strabismus surgeons in the United States opt for attainment of horizontal alignment by age 2 years.

The two major surgical options for correction are symmetrical medial rectus recessions on both eyes (possibly adding a monocular or binocular lateral rectus resection) and a recession of one medial rectus combined with resection of the opponent lateral rectus on the same eye. Some surgeons prefer a limbal incision because of the ease of access and orientation, as well as the ability to recede contracted conjunctiva and thus augment the effect of the medial rectus recession. Many prefer the fornix approach popularized by Parks because it often does not require suture closure and avoids proximity to the cornea, which enables rapid patient mobilization.

A novel approach to congenital esotropia is the use of botulinum toxin, originally popularized by Scott and studied further by Magoon.[15] He injected one medial rectus in 15 children and obtained excellent results, stable for at least 1 year. Most children required ketamine sedation, and many required more than one injection.

Because patients with DVD usually exhibit no binocularity when DVD is present, they are asymptomatic. The major reason for treatment of DVD is esthetic. If DVD is monocular or highly asymmetrical, optical means may enable fixation to be switched to the eye that has DVD and thus render it entirely latent. Usually, however, surgical treatment is necessary. This can be symmetrical or asymmetrical and may involve significant recessions of the superior rectus muscles or resection of the inferior rectus muscles. Some surgeons combine the former with a posterior fixation suture, which alone is ineffective. It is crucial to dissect the intermuscular septum from the vertical recti so that lid position is not affected.

Treatment of inferior oblique overaction is often undertaken primarily for esthetic reasons, but the condition may interfere with binocular function if elevation of the adducted eye occurs close to fixation and if it is bilateral. Because of the frequency of increased overaction in an unoperated, overactive oblique muscle after the other is weakened, unilateral surgery is reserved for those cases that are clearly unilateral. Traditional weakening

TABLE 73-1

SURGERY FOR CONGENITAL ESOTROPIA

Deviation (Δ)	Symmetric	Asymmetric (one eye)	
	Recede Medial Rectus, Both Eyes (mm)	Resect Lateral Rectus (mm)	Recede Medial Rectus (mm)
35	5.0	5.0	8.0
40 or 45	5.5	5.5	9.0
50 or 55	6.0	6.0	10.0
60 or 65	6.5	6.5	10.0
≥70	7.0	7.0	10.0

procedures include disinsertion, myectomy, denervation and extirpation, and measured recession. Anteriorization of the oblique insertion to the margin of the inferior rectus significantly weakens the muscle and may be effective treatment for simultaneous DVD. Clear separation between DVD and inferior oblique overaction is necessary, however, because weakening of a normally functioning inferior oblique muscle may cause limitation of elevation in adduction, compensatory head postures, and all the signs and symptoms of cyclovertical muscle palsy.

COURSE AND OUTCOME

Whatever the approach, a recent tendency toward larger medial rectus recessions has improved the surgical success rates significantly. Recent series quote rates as high as 90% for alignment to within 10Δ of perfect alignment. Some surgeons prefer to perform recessions measured from the limbus rather than the original muscle insertion, because of increased uniformity and better results. A common protocol for surgical treatment is given in Table 73-1.

As a result of the instability of postoperative alignment, children who have surgery for congenital esotropia require long-term follow-up. Residual esotropia of >10Δ found 4–6 weeks after initial surgery may respond to antiaccommodative measures if the patient is significantly hyperopic, but it probably requires a second surgical procedure. This might consist of bilateral lateral rectus resection for those who initially underwent bilateral medial rectus recessions, and a recess-resect procedure on the unoperated eye for those who underwent a unilateral procedure. A significant fraction of patients who initially achieve alignment later develop accommodative esotropia and require treatment with glasses or miotics.[16] Asymmetrical monocular pursuit as measured by OKN testing persists indefinitely and may be a perpetual marker for congenital esotropia.

ACCOMMODATIVE ESOTROPIA

INTRODUCTION

Accommodative esotropia is characterized by two mechanisms that may occur in variable proportions in the same individual. The first cause is high hyperopia, with an an average of +4.50D, and the second is a larger eso tendency at near fixation than can be controlled comfortably by fusional divergence. A third cause may be anisometropia greater than or equal to 1D, especially in patients who have lower overall hyperopia (less than +3.00D).[17]

EPIDEMIOLOGY AND PATHOGENESIS

The typical history is of intermittent esotropia that appears between 6 months and 7 years of age (average 30 months) toward the end of the day or when the child is very tired, ill, or daydreaming (especially at near fixation distances, such as across the dinner table). At onset, the child may experience asthenopia as fusional divergence amplitudes are stressed and may rub the

BOX 73-3

Accommodative Convergence–to–Accommodation Ratio Calculations

HETEROPHORIA METHOD

Determine phoria by prism and alternate cover test at optical infinity and 0.33m distances. Control accommodation and correct acuity to 20/30 (6/9) using least plus lens.

$$AC/A = IPD(cm) + \frac{(\Delta_2 - \Delta_1)}{F}$$

where

AC/A = accommodative convergence to accommodation

IPD = interpupillary distance

Δ_1 = distance phoria

Δ_2 = near phoria (eso is +, exo is −)

F = near fixation distance in diopters of vergence

Example:

IPD = 60mm or 6cm

Δ_1 = 4 eso

Δ_2 = 30 eso

F = 1/33cm = 3D

$$AC/A = 6 + \frac{30 - 4}{3}$$

= about 15/1

GRADIENT METHOD

Determine phoria by prism and alternate cover test at a fixed distance, generally 0.33m. Control accommodation and correct acuity to 20/30 (6/9) with least plus lens. Vary lens power held before eyes and remeasure alignment.

$$AC/A = \frac{(\Delta_2 - \Delta_1)}{D}$$

Δ_1 = original phoria in diopters

Δ_2 = new phoria with new lens

D = power of lens

Example:

Δ_2 = 2 eso

Δ_1 = 6 eso

D = +1.00

$$AC/A = \frac{6 - 2}{1}$$

= 4/1

eyes or squint; an older child may complain of headaches or diplopia. As the esotropia becomes more frequent, abnormal retinal correspondence and suppression, when extant, relieve asthenopic symptoms at the possible expense of fusional divergence amplitudes. Some children maintain intermittent esotropia for long periods, whereas others progress quickly to constant esotropia, especially at near fixation.

OCULAR MANIFESTATIONS

Patients who have high hyperopia must generate large, accommodative input to see clearly at near fixation and thus stress fusional divergence amplitudes. They may choose blurred vision and maintain comfortable single binocular vision, or they may choose clear vision and risk asthenopia or esotropia. Those patients who have high hyperopia but do not develop esotropia, yet who maintain excellent acuity, often have low ratios of accommodative convergence to accommodation (AC/A).

Patients who have typical hyperopia (average +2.25D) or myopia and who develop an esodeviation greater at distance than near have an overactive convergence response to a given accommodation requirement—a high AC/A ratio. This ratio can be calculated by two methods, the heterophoria method and the gradient method, as described in Box 73-3. Some patients have mildly high hyperopia and mildly high AC/A ratios and therefore have a mixed mechanism of accommodative esotropia. In all cases, however, the patient's fusional divergence amplitudes are insufficient to control the eso tendency.

DIAGNOSIS AND ANCILLARY TESTING

The ophthalmologist must be alert to historical clues, evaluate the AC/A ratio, and, if possible, measure fusional divergence amplitudes at distance and near fixation. Historically, atropine has been considered essential to obtain the maximal hyperopic refractive error; however, its use requires a return visit, and its cycloplegic effect is prolonged. The outpatient use of cyclopentolate and tropicamide permits immediate treatment and, in most patients, provides results within +0.50D of the refractive error obtained using atropine, although a few patients have greater uncovered hyperopia.

It is important to recognize that most individuals without strabismus have flexible AC/A ratios that adjust to changes in refractive error over the person's lifetime; however, patients who have accommodative esotropia often have rigid AC/A ratios that respond inflexibly to changes in refractive correction. This fact may be used to the patient's benefit through the prescription of a hyperopic correction.

In older patients, the fusional divergence amplitudes may be measured and prove to be deficient. As successful treatment proceeds, normal fusional measurements are obtained.

If the esodeviation cannot be found on initial attempts, occlusion of one eye for 45 minutes to 3 hours may be carried out, or cycloplegia can be induced and cover testing performed using suitably large targets. An esodeviation after cycloplegia provides strong confirmation of parental observations and may be sufficient to warrant initiation of treatment.

DIFFERENTIAL DIAGNOSIS

Differential diagnosis includes variable esotropia accompanied by normal AC/A ratios and refractive errors; these (uncommon) patients exhibit fusional divergence amplitudes equally deficient at distance and near. Some of these patients respond to antiaccommodative measures, and others do not. Another group of patients has a V-pattern esotropia with greater deviation in downgaze. It is important to measure near deviations in primary position to avoid confusion with V-pattern esotropes.

TREATMENT, COURSE, AND OUTCOME

Treatment consists of antiaccommodative measures, primarily the prescription of much or all of the patient's hyperopic refractive error (to do the focusing for the child, so as not to stimulate accommodation and thus convergence). In very young children or myopes, the uncoupling of accommodation from convergence using miotics may be considered.

Glasses are a problem in children younger than approximately 1 year of age because of their weight, flat nasal bridge, lack of cooperation, and small face, which makes fitting difficult. Treatment of accommodative esotropia in this group is often better initiated with miotics such as ecothiopate iodide 0.125% used every evening for 2 weeks. If this is successful, less frequent administration may be attempted. To decrease the risk of pupillary margin cysts, phenylephrine 2.5% may be added 2 weeks after miotic initiation to maintain pupillary dilation. Because ecothiopate is a true cholinesterase inhibitor with a potential systemic effect, parents must be warned to alert all physicians to the child's use of this drug, especially if general anesthesia is indicated; nondepolarizing agents may be used to avoid prolonged anesthesia reversal. Despite years of experience using this drug in the treatment of accommodative esotropia, when it is used at this frequency and strength in children, no cases of cataract or retinal

detachment have been described. Older children may complain of brow ache and miotic spasm, so an attempt is made to switch patients to glasses at age 1 year when possible; however, many parents prefer to continue using the miotic because it has no esthetic disadvantages, works consistently well, and does not demand the child's cooperation. At present, ecothiopate iodide is difficult to obtain in the United States.

In children 1–4 years of age, the full cycloplegic refraction is given, and the child is re-evaluated after a month's full-time wear of the prescription. If the distance and near esodeviations are reduced to within the monofixational range ($\leq 8\Delta$ of esotropia) and the child has a comfortably controlled phoria and no asthenopic signs or symptoms, the treatment is considered initially successful and the patient is re-evaluated 3–6 months later, depending on age. At every visit, assessment of visual acuity at distance and near, assessment of alignment at distance and near, and sensory testing are performed. Cycloplegic refractions are repeated every 6 months. If the distance tropia is greater than the above limit, the cycloplegic refraction is repeated; if it is still so with the new refraction or no change has occurred in the refraction, the patient becomes a candidate for surgery. If the distance deviation is controlled but an esotropia greater than the above limit is present at near fixation, or if a symptomatic phoria at near fixation persists, the patient is given bifocal glasses (Fig. 73-6). Parents must be warned that a newly fitted child exhibits larger and more frequent esodeviations when glasses are removed.

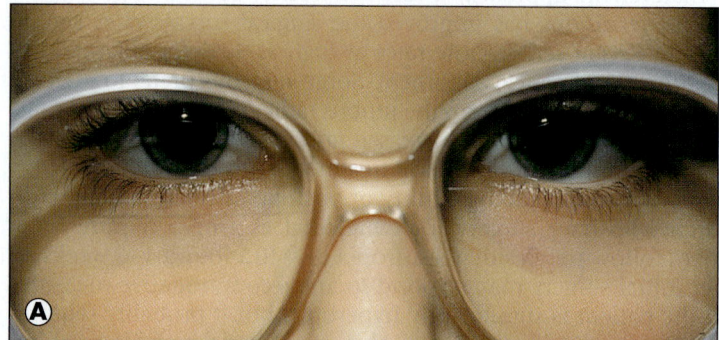

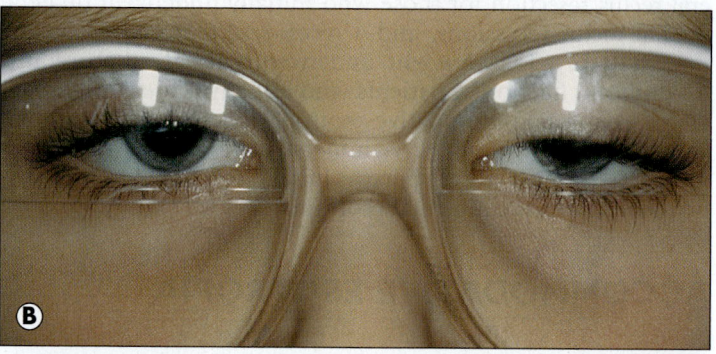

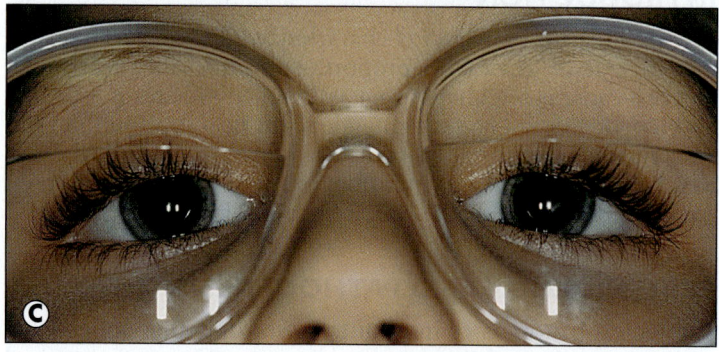

FIG. 73-6 ▌ **Hyperopic child with right esotropia. A,** Esotropia controlled at distance fixation through distance (top) segment of bifocals. **B,** Esotropia near fixation through distance segment of bifocals. **C,** Aligned eyes at near fixation through near (bottom) segment of bifocals.

The bifocals are prescribed high enough to split the pupil in primary position; strengths above +1.00D may be prescribed as executive style, but lower strengths often can be ground only as a large flat-top style. The initial bifocal strength may be estimated from measurement of the near esodeviation using various strengths of trial frame lenses or arbitrarily given as +2.50–+3.00D. The patient is asked to wear the bifocals for 1 month and then return for re-evaluation; rarely, except for V-pattern esotropia, does the near deviation not respond to bifocal prescription if the distance deviation is controlled using full cycloplegic refraction. Patients who have V-pattern accommodative esotropia may require miotics alone or in addition to single-vision glasses, as bifocals require downgaze fixation and the deviation is largest in downgaze in such patients.

As a rule, glasses and miotics are equally effective treatments, and it is rare for a patient to respond to one but not the other; conversely, use of both together rarely salvages a patient who does not respond to one or the other. An intellectual preference exists for refractive treatment for the highly hyperopic "refractive" accommodative esotrope and miotic treatment for the patient who has a high AC/A ratio.

When the successfully treated child is about 5 years of age, the parents note less esodeviation without glasses; at about 6 years of age, the glasses may be weakened progressively, roughly 0.50–0.75D every 6 months, beginning with the bifocals. A common practice is to place the weaker correction in a trial frame and perform cover testing; occasionally, a patient appears aligned during this office evaluation but develops a significant esodeviation, asthenopic symptoms, or both when the weaker correction is worn. In such cases, the patient must return to the previous stronger prescription. It is often possible to rid children of their bifocals by 8 or 9 years of age and of their mild to moderate hyperopic correction by the early teens. Patients who have high hyperopia, significant astigmatism, or anisometropia may require optical correction for acuity purposes after their accommodative esotropia has resolved; for some, treatment may consist of wearing contact lenses.

Patients whose treatment is initiated at 4–8 years of age may not accept their full hyperopic correction without a period of cycloplegia. Ideally, the minimal correction necessary to provide and maintain comfortable single binocular vision and (in the case of high hyperopia) good visual acuity is prescribed. After 6 years of age the AC/A ratio tends to normalize, but the hyperopia may increase. Initiation of treatment in children older than 9 years of age is difficult but is similar to that described earlier; some of these older patients may respond to miotics.

At any time after a period of successful antiaccommodative treatment, a patient may develop an esotropia that is not controlled with glasses or miotics.[18] Repeat refraction is carried out, and if greater hyperopia is found, it is prescribed. It is difficult to predict the effect of even as little as +0.50D additional correction on a decompensated accommodative esotrope. If no effect is obtained after a few weeks' trial, the patient should undergo strabismus surgery. The contribution of high hyperopia, a high AC/A ratio, progressively increasing hyperopia, undercorrection of hyperopia, and overactive inferior oblique muscles to decompensation of accommodative esotropia is still somewhat unclear. The clinical experience of this author is that significant inferior oblique overaction implies less likelihood that weaning from glasses can be achieved and a greater incidence of decompensation; the same is true of increased interpupillary distance.

Strabismus surgery classically is directed toward only the nonaccommodative component of the distance esodeviation, with an arbitrary addition (1mm additional recession per medial rectus) for a high AC/A ratio. Some investigators believe that posterior fixation sutures combined with medial rectus recessions benefit patients with high AC/A ratios.[19] Some surgeons favor directing surgery toward the near esodeviation; others operate for the average deviation between distance and near fixation. Parents must be warned of the continual need for antiaccommodative treatment even after strabismus surgery.

A difficult group of patients consists of teenagers who are well controlled in bifocals or high hyperopic correction but who have esthetic concerns. A switch to contact lenses places less accommodative demand on the patient and may enable comfortable single binocular vision at near fixation without the need for separate reading glasses. Bifocal contact lenses may be tolerable to some patients; few are satisfied with "monovision" fitting of one lens for distance needs and another for near. Blended bifocals may be tolerated by some teenagers and permit persistent bifocal treatment without the dysesthetic impact of a bifocal line. Some teenagers accept miotics in addition to single-vision glasses to avoid bifocal lenses. Finally, cautious single medial rectus recession, or small bimedial rectus recession, may be performed in those patients who fuse at distance when wearing single-vision lenses and who wish to be rid of their bifocals.

The effective management of accommodative esotropia demands a long period of cooperation among patient, physician, and parents and is as much art as science. Nowhere else in strabismus management are communication skills so important.

CYCLIC ESOTROPIA

First reported by Burian[20] in 1958, this curious condition most commonly presents as alternating 24-hour periods of perfect alignment followed by constant, usually large-angled (30–40Δ) esotropia. The age of onset is generally 3–4 years. Other cycles of alternation, often 12 or 36 hours, have been described.[21] When the eyes are aligned, excellent fusional abilities and stereopsis are found; when esotropia is present, patients exhibit abnormal retinal correspondence and suppression. Some patients who have cyclic esotropia display irritability and emotional withdrawal during the periods of strabismus. The incidence has been estimated as 1 in 5000 cases of strabismus (roughly 150 cases appear in the literature). Aids to diagnosis include a strong suspicion and a log of the strabismus periods kept by the parents. This condition differs from intermittent esotropia because, during the aligned periods, little or no strabismus may be elicited despite prolonged occlusion.

The cause is unknown but may be related to the "biological clock" phenomenon popularized by Richter.[22] Some patients develop a cyclic esotropia after head trauma, neurosurgical procedure, strabismus surgery, or infection. The course is usually stable, but some patients decompensate to a persistent strabismus.

Antiaccommodative measures usually have little effect during the periods of strabismus and are not needed during the aligned periods. Surgical treatment is typically successful in 75–90% of cases in attaining alignment with one operation, whether performed during aligned or strabismic periods.

MÖBIUS' SYNDROME

Möbius' syndrome, in its full presentation, consists of bilateral abduction limitation with or without esotropia, upper motor neuron seventh nerve palsies, and twelfth nerve palsy with atrophy of the tongue.[23] Some patients have difficulty suckling as young infants, as well as abnormal phonation. Close inspection of the tongue reveals atrophy of its terminal third. The upper motor neuron seventh nerve palsies cause smooth facies, absent nasolabial folds, round mouth, and decreased facial emotional responses. Lid closure is variable. Patients who have esotropia (38%) generally have tight medial recti on forced duction testing[24]; those who have gaze palsy and straight eyes do not. Esotropia, when present, is quite large, and the patients cross-fixate in a manner similar to congenital esotropes; as a rule, however, abduction to the midline cannot be performed.

The syndrome is not defined strictly; some patients are included who also have vertical gaze palsies and lower motor neuron seventh nerve palsies. The cause of the esotropia may include both involvement of the sixth nerve fascicles and nuclei and aberrant medial rectus insertion, as some patients have medial recti that insert quite close to the limbus. No treatment is necessary or successful in patients who have gaze palsies alone; those who are esotropic and unable to abduct to the midline require medial rectus recessions. These recessions may be technically quite challenging because the muscles are very tight and difficult to hook, suture, and safely detach from the globe; double-overlapping marginal myotomies may be safer in some situations. Resections of the nonfunctioning lateral recti are avoided, as they are fruitless.

Systemic associations include mental retardation, polydactyly, syndactyly, brachydactyly, clubbed feet, peroneal mus-

cular atrophy, and a peculiar gait.[25] Brainstem auditory evoked responses often are abnormal.

DUANE'S SYNDROME

EPIDEMIOLOGY AND PATHOGENESIS

Duane's syndrome, which accounts for 1% of all strabismus, is a congenital miswiring of the medial and lateral rectus muscles, such that globe retraction on attempted adduction occurs, as well as limitation of adduction, abduction, or both. Its most common variant (type I; 85% of cases) presents in the left eye (60%) (Fig. 73-7),[26] predominantly in girls (60%), as severely limited or absent abduction (Fig. 73-8).

OCULAR MANIFESTATIONS

Neuropathologically, this disorder has been shown to be caused by an absent sixth nerve nucleus and nerve and innervation of the lateral rectus by a branch from the inferior division of the third nerve.[27] Thus, classic electromyographical findings of absent lateral rectus firing upon attempted abduction, and firing of both horizontal recti upon attempted adduction, are explained.[28] No mechanism exists to improve the abduction limitation. About 40% of patients who develop esotropia and tight medial rectus muscles adopt a head turn toward the affected eye to maintain single binocular vision, or they maintain a straight head but accept esotropia, abnormal retinal correspondence, and suppression, if extant.

Duane's syndrome is bilateral in roughly 20% of cases; the sex and eye predominance pertain only to type I. Less common forms include type II (14%), with limitation of adduction and a tendency toward exotropia, and type III (1%), with limitation of both abduction and adduction and any form of horizontal strabismus. Often associated is a "tether" phenomenon, which con-

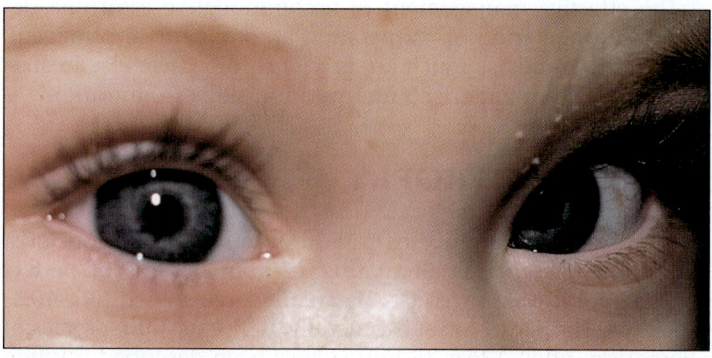

FIG. 73-7 ■ Head posture in left Duane's syndrome type I. This child shows a face turn to the left to compensate for deficient abduction in the left eye. (Reproduced with permission from Fells P, Lee JP. Strabismus. In: Spalton DJ, Hitchings RA, Hunter PA, eds. Atlas of clinical ophthalmology. London, New York: Gower Medical Publishing; 1984:6.7.)

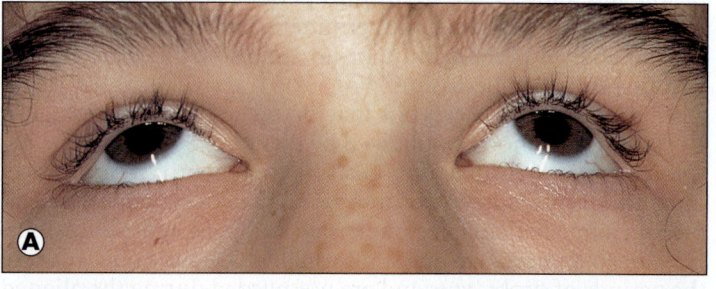

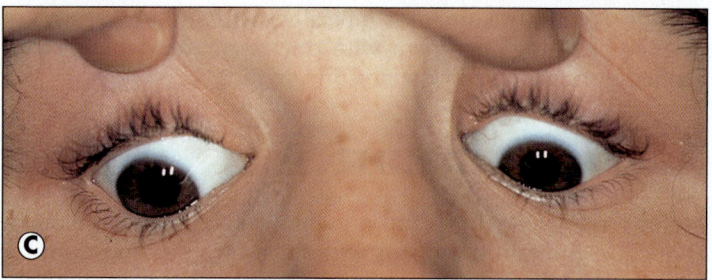

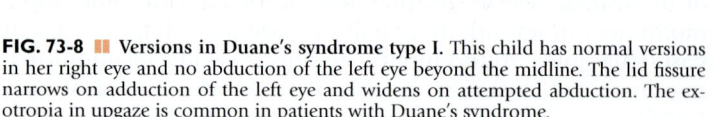

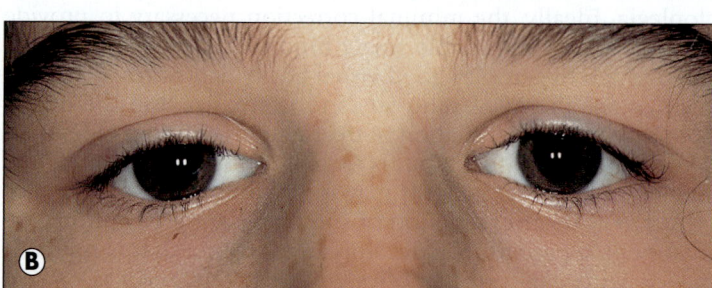

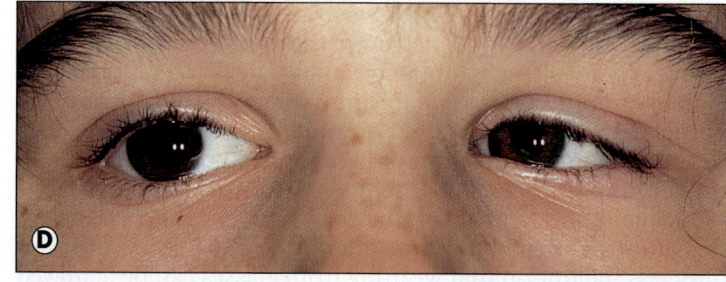

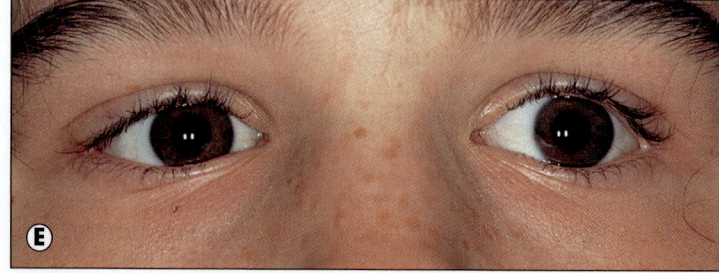

FIG. 73-8 ■ Versions in Duane's syndrome type I. This child has normal versions in her right eye and no abduction of the left eye beyond the midline. The lid fissure narrows on adduction of the left eye and widens on attempted abduction. The exotropia in upgaze is common in patients with Duane's syndrome.

sists of overelevation, overdepression, or both in adduction as the retracted globe escapes from its horizontal rectus restrictions.

TREATMENT

The amount of esotropia in monocular Duane's syndrome type I is rarely greater than 30Δ. Recession of the medial rectus muscle in the involved eye aligns the eye but does not improve abduction beyond primary position. Rarely, very large weakening procedures on the medial rectus result in consecutive exotropia, but the mechanisms are unclear. A small medial rectus recession in the opposite eye helps stabilize the pathologic eye in primary position by application of the Hering law[29,30]; resection of the lateral rectus generally is avoided, as it increases retraction and may not improve abduction. However, Morad et al.[31] showed improved abduction with no worsening of globe retraction after modest unilateral medial rectus recession and lateral rectus resection in carefully selected patients with mild globe retraction and good preoperative adduction. Lateral transposition of the vertical rectus muscles has been shown to improve abduction of the affected eye, but almost half the patients required additional medial rectus recession, and 15% developed vertical strabismus.[32]

The tether phenomenon may be improved surgically using horizontal rectus posterior fixation sutures or by horizontal splitting of the lateral rectus into a "Y" structure, with resuturing of the muscle above and below the axis of the lateral rectus. If extreme retraction with pseudoptosis is dysesthetic, both horizontal recti may be receded to relieve the retraction.

SYSTEMATIC ASSOCIATIONS

Systemic associations in 30% of cases include Goldenhar's syndrome; Klippel-Feil syndrome; a rare autosomal dominant form; and the Wildervanck association of Duane's syndrome, Klippel-Feil syndrome, and congenital labyrinthine deafness. Pairs of identical twins who have mirror-image Duane's syndrome have been described. Brainstem auditory evoked responses occasionally are abnormal, which suggests widespread neurological abnormalities.

STRABISMUS FIXUS

This rare, congenital, stationary, very large-angle esotropia of unknown cause may represent a form of congenital fibrosis of the medial rectus muscles. Usually, no abduction is possible, and strabismus surgery on these very tight muscles is often of little benefit.

ESOTROPIA IN THE NEUROLOGICALLY IMPAIRED

The incidence of strabismus is higher in the population of neurologically impaired children than in the general population. In addition to the previously mentioned categories, children with neurological impairment may have a variable intermittent esotropia that is unresponsive to antiaccommodative measures; it may be stable, worsen to a constant tropia, or disappear with maturity. Surgery is avoided unless measurements of the deviation are reproducible; the patient is intellectually capable of benefiting from improved binocular function; and the effects of any neurotropic medications, especially sedatives, are considered. Surgical outcome may be less successful in these patients, but antiaccommodative measures may be helpful.[33] In addition, a patient under significant emotional stress occasionally presents with a temporary esotropia, sometimes related to accommodative spasm.

ESOTROPIA ASSOCIATED WITH VISUAL DEFICIT

Children who have impaired vision in one or both eyes are at risk for the development of strabismus. Esotropia develops in a high proportion of infants younger than 2 years of age who have decreased acuity secondary to congenital cataract, corneal opacity, retinal pathology, or other devastating media-clarity impairment. The prognosis for the development of stable single binocular vision with early treatment of the media pathology and surgical alignment is poor; therefore, in most cases, surgical treatment is performed primarily for esthetic improvement.

REFERENCES

1. Archer SM, Sondhy N, Helveston EM. Strabismus in infancy. Ophthalmology. 1989;96:133–8.
2. Ing MR. Early surgical alignment for congenital esotropia. Trans Am Ophthalmol Soc. 1981;79:625–33.
3. Waardenburg PJ. Squint and heredity. Doc Ophthalmol. 1954;7:422–94.
4. Costenbader F. Infantile esotropia. Trans Ophthalmol Soc UK. 1970;59:397–429.
5. Hiles DA, Watson A, Biglan AW. Characteristics of infantile esotropia following early bimedial rectus recession. Arch Ophthalmol. 1980;98:697–703.
6. Helveston EM. Dissociated vertical deviation, a clinical and laboratory study. Trans Am Ophthalmol Soc. 1981;78:734–79.
7. Brodsky MC. Dissociated vertical divergence: a righting reflex gone wrong. Arch Ophthalmol 1999;117:1216–22.
8. Aiello A, Wright KW, Borchert M. Independence of optikokinetic nystagmus asymmetry and binocularity in infantile esotropia. Arch Ophthalmol 1994;112:1580–3.
9. Cheng KP, Biglan AW, Hiles DA. Pediatric ophthalmology. In: Zitelli BJ, Davis HW, eds. Atlas of pediatric physical diagnosis, 2nd ed. New York: Gower Medical Publishing; 1992:19.1.
10. Van Noorden GK. The nystagmus blockage syndrome. Trans Am Ophthalmol Soc. 1976;74:220–36.
11. Ciancia AO. On infantile esotropia with nystagmus in abduction. J Pediatr Ophthalmol Strabismus. 1995;32:280–8.
12. Wright KW, Edelman PM, McVey JH, et al. High-grade stereo acuity after early surgery for congenital esotropia. Arch Ophthalmol. 1994;112:913–9.
13. Parks MM. The monofixation syndrome. In: Dabezies O, ed. Strabismus. Transactions New Orleans Academy of Ophthalmology. St Louis: CV Mosby; 1971.
14. Ing MR. Early surgical alignment for congenital esotropia. Trans Am Ophthalmol Soc. 1981;79:625–63.
15. Magoon EH. Infantile esotropes treated under age one with botulinum chemodenervation routinely show motor fusion. Invest Ophthalmol Vis Sci. 1984;25:74–8.
16. Szymd SM, Nelson LB, Calhoun JC, Spratt C. Large bimedial rectus recessions in congenital esotropia. Br J Ophthalmol. 1985;69:271–4.
17. Weakley DR, Birch E, Kip K. The role of anisometropia in the development of accommodative esotropia. J AAPOS. 2001;5:153–7.
18. Baker JD, Parks MM. Early-onset accommodative esotropia. Am J Ophthalmol. 1980;90:11–8.
19. Elsas FJ, Mays A. Augmenting surgery for sensory esotropia with near/distance disparity with a medial rectus posterior fixation suture. J Pediatr Ophthalmol Strabismus. 1996;3:28–30.
20. Burian M. Cyclic esotropia. In: Allen H, ed. Strabismus ophthalmic symposium II. St Louis: CV Mosby; 1958.
21. Costenbader F, Manuel D. Cyclic esotropia. Arch Ophthalmol. 1964;71:150–4.
22. Richter C. Biologic clocks in medicine and psychiatry. Springfield: CC Thomas; 1965.
23. Henderson JC. The congenital facial diplegia syndrome: clinical features, pathology and aetiology. A review of 61 cases. Brain. 1939;62:381–403.
24. Parks MM. Ophthalmoplegic syndromes and trauma. In: Duane TD, Jaeger E, eds. Clinical ophthalmology. Philadelphia: JB Lippincott; 1985.
25. Gadoth N, Bioedner B, Torde G. Möbius' syndrome and Poland anomaly: case report and review of the literature. J Pediatr Ophthalmol Strabismus. 1978;16:374–6.
26. Fells P, Lee JP. Strabismus. In: Spalton DJ, Hitchings RA, Hunter PA, eds. Atlas of clinical ophthalmology. London, New York: Gower Medical Publishing; 1984:6.7.
27. Hotchkiss MG, Miller NR, Clark AW, et al. Bilateral Duane's retraction. A clinical-pathologic report. Arch Ophthalmol. 1980;98:870–4.
28. Huber A. Electrophysiology of the retraction syndrome. Br J Ophthalmol. 1974;58:293–300.
29. Pressman SH, Scott WE. Surgical treatment of Duane's syndrome. Ophthalmology. 1986;93:29–38.
30. Saunders RA, Wilson MF, Bluestein EC, Sinatra RB. Surgery on the normal eye in Duane's retraction syndrome. J Pediatr Ophthalmol Strabismus. 1994;31:162–9.
31. Morad Y, Kraft SP, Mims JL. Unilateral recession and resection in Duane syndrome. J AAPOS. 2001;5:158–63.
32. Molarte AB, Rosenbaum AL. Vertical rectus muscle transposition surgery for Duane's syndrome. J Pediatr Ophthalmol Strabismus. 1990;27:171–7.
33. Pickering JB, Simon JW, Ratliff CD, et al. Alignment success following medial rectus recessions in normal and delayed children. J Pediatr Ophthalmol Strabismus. 1995;32:225–7.

DEFINITION
- An acquired or, rarely, congenital, outward deviation of the visual axis of one or both eyes, which may be constant, intermittent, or latent.

KEY FEATURE
- An intermittent exotropia that measures greater at distance than at near fixation.

ASSOCIATED FEATURES
- History of squinting one eye in bright sunlight.
- Amblyopia, if present, is usually mild unless exotropia is constant.
- Common inferior or superior oblique muscle overaction.
- Common A, V, or other "alphabet" patterns.

INTRODUCTION

Exotropia is a manifest outward deviation of the visual axes of one or both eyes and may be either constantly or intermittently present. The term is also used loosely to describe a latent outward deviation that, more accurately, is termed *exophoria*. Patients who have intermittent exotropia compose a spectrum that extends from those who are easy to dissociate to those who are very difficult to dissociate; thus, there is a continuum of patients who have a form of exodeviation, as portrayed in Figure 74-1.

Intermittent exotropia (Fig. 74-2) is by far the most frequent cause of exodeviation and is often a progressive disease; an exophoria decompensates to an intermittent exotropia and finally to a constant exotropia. The angle of deviation usually does not increase until secondary contracture of the lateral recti ensues, but the deviation at near often increases to approach that at distance. Von Noorden[1] reported that 75% of 51 patients progressed, 9% did not, and 16% improved with time. Women represent 60–70% of patients who have intermittent exotropia in most series; refractive errors tend to follow a normal distribution.

EPIDEMIOLOGY AND PATHOGENESIS

Exotropia is about one third as common as esotropia and may be more prevalent in the Middle East, Asia, and Africa; Nepal appears to have the highest incidence of exotropia compared with esotropia, at 76%.[2]

Some patients who have exotropia also have orbital anomalies (craniosynostosis syndromes), mechanical restrictions (Duane's syndrome type II), or neurological pathologies (third nerve palsy) that account for the strabismus; some develop exotropia after strabismus surgery for esotropia. These causative disorders are not present in most patients; the majority are believed to have a primary deficiency of fusional convergence. Evidence exists that when an exotropia starts to manifest, neurons of the lateral rectus muscle of the deviating eye begin to fire, which suggests an active divergence contribution to the final deviation; secondary

contracture also may intervene.[3] A tendency toward exotropia may be inherited; Knapp[4] reported a family history in 28% of cases of exotropia, and Burian and Spivey[5] in 21.5%. Knapp suggested that the actual figure may be higher, as the disorder remains undetected in many family members because of the infrequent manifestation of an intermittent exotropia.

Chavasse[6] noted that the visual axes migrate from a lateral to a frontal position as phylogeny progresses, while oculomotor control migrates from the midbrain to the cerebral cortex. He speculated that exotropia represents an atavistic loss of cortical control. Exotropia provides an enlarged visual field and may have had a protective function at one time; aligned eyes provide better binocular vision, with heightened stereopsis, and are more suited to effective hunting and manipulation for tool making. Patients who have intermittent exotropia tend to have excellent alignment at near with superb stereopsis; at distance, where stereopsis is less effective, they have the benefit of an enlarged visual field. These patients, according to this theory, have developed an alignment strategy that provides an ideal system for those who are sometimes hunters and sometimes hunted, albeit with cosmetic and functional consequences.

OCULAR MANIFESTATIONS

Ocular manifestations, in addition to the outward deviation of the eye, are squinting in bright sunlight, contracture of lateral recti in long-standing cases, true overaction of oblique muscles, lateral gaze incomitance, alphabet patterns, and accommodative spasm. Most patients who have intermittent exotropia possess normal retinal correspondence when their eyes are aligned and anomalous retinal correspondence when deviated.[7]

Many patients who have intermittent exotropia squint the deviated eye in bright sunlight for reasons that are unclear; some speculations include glare avoidance and obviation of diplopia and visual confusion in circumstances in which the sensory adaptations are less effective. This feature is much less common in patients who have esotropia and, if historical, strongly confirms the accuracy of the parents' observations.

Contracture of the lateral recti may occur in patients who have long-standing intermittent exotropia and those who have constant exotropia. Adduction may be limited, and the tight lateral recti may act as tethering cords; on attempted elevation and depression in adduction, the globe may overelevate or overdepress, and oblique muscle dysfunction may be erroneously diagnosed. Confusingly, both the inferior oblique and superior oblique muscles may become truly overactive in patients with intermittent exotropia. Forced duction testing of the oblique muscles differentiates those with true oblique muscle overaction from those with merely tight lateral recti. Another interesting cause of pseudo-oblique overaction in patients with large-angle exotropia is the horizontally oriented, oval form of the maximal duction rotation of the eye in the orbit; a patient who fixes with the maximally abducted exotropic eye can elevate and depress the adducted eye more than the abducted eye, which is at the "point" of the oval.[8]

Some patients who have intermittent exotropia have less misalignment on side gaze than in the primary position and histor-

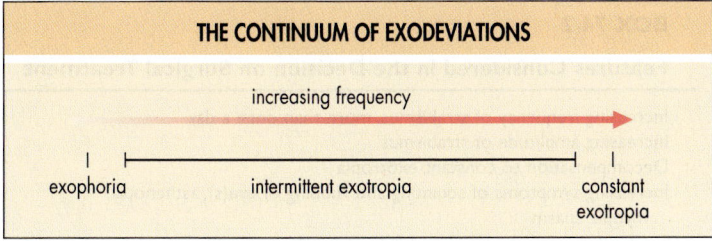

THE CONTINUUM OF EXODEVIATIONS

increasing frequency

exophoria   intermittent exotropia   constant exotropia

FIG. 74-1 ■ The continuum of exodeviations.

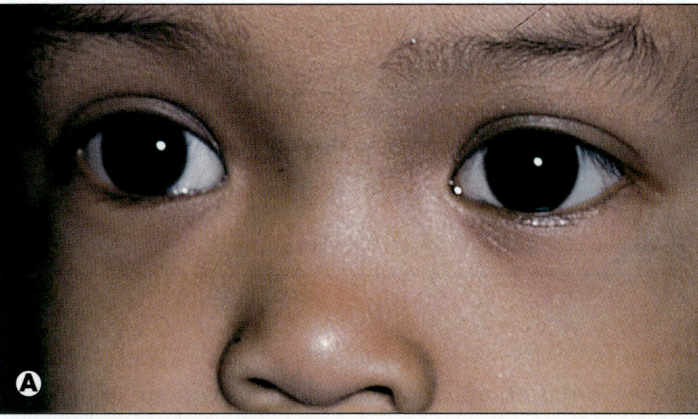

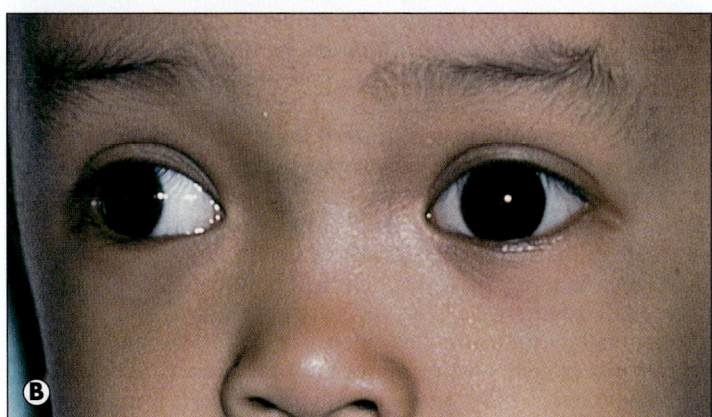

FIG. 74-2 ■ Intermittent exotropia. **A,** Eyes straight. **B,** A few moments later, the exotropia has become manifest. (Courtesy of Howard Eggers.)

ically have been considered at greater risk for surgical overcorrection.[9] This phenomenon was challenged as the result of an artifact of faulty prism technique when deviations are measured with the head turned to the side.[10] Many patients have greater deviations in upgaze or downgaze, or both, than in primary position; some have oblique overactions, which may explain the incomitance. All so-called alphabet patterns may be found, from the common A (greatest deviation in downgaze) and V (greatest deviation in upgaze) patterns to the X, Y, and lambda patterns.

Some patients who have greater intermittent exotropia at near fixation than at distance fixation recruit accommodative convergence to compensate for the deficiency in fusional convergence and thus maintain alignment at near fixation; prolonged accommodative convergence may lead to spasm and pseudomyopia with distance fixation.

DIAGNOSIS AND ANCILLARY TESTING

Intermittent exotropia typically presents between the ages of 18 months and 4 years with a gradual, but more frequently noted, exodeviation when the child fixes on a distant target. Squinting of the deviating eye and eye rubbing in bright sunlight are noted so frequently as to be volunteered by parents and may be the presenting complaint. A family history of strabismus should be sought, as well as an estimation of age of onset, progression in frequency and severity, and recognition by family, friends, and teachers. At about age 4 years, cosmetic issues become relevant as other children begin to notice the misalignment of the visual axes and squinting. Previous treatment for this or other strabismus should be noted.

The ophthalmologist should study the alignment of the eyes as the child enters the room and during the medical history to gain insight into the alignment under ordinary viewing conditions. Cover testing is the initial diagnostic test during the examination, using an accommodation-controlling target in primary position at distance (ideally 20ft [6m]) and near (1ft [0.3m]) fixation and in gazes right, left, up, and down at distance fixation. Near measurements used to calculate the accommodative convergence–to–accommodation (AC/A) ratio should be made after 1 hour of monocular occlusion to eliminate those who have pseudo-high AC/A ratios. Those rare patients who have intermittent exotropia and true high AC/A ratios often have an esophoria at 6in (0.15m) or 3in (0.07m) testing distance.[11] Ductions and versions are then evaluated to search for oblique muscle dysfunction or contracture of the lateral recti with adduction limitation. Evaluation of alignment at far distance fixation (horizon seen through a window or at the end of a long hallway) is attempted, because accommodative convergence may be generated even in an examination lane 20ft (6m) long, and the deviation decreased accordingly. Many also add tests at near fixation with the patient wearing +3.00D lenses before each eye to relax accommodative convergence. Sensory tests in a cooperative child for the presence of anomalous retinal correspondence, suppression, and stereopsis are performed and evaluated, as discussed in Chapters 71 and 72.

Frequently, the parents note strabismus at home, but the physician cannot detect misalignment with typical cover tests.

Occlusion of one eye to disrupt fusion may be performed for periods from 30 minutes to 2 hours, and the eye uncovered at the moment of alternate cover testing. Occasionally, the diagnosis must be deferred and the child scheduled for re-examination at a later time.

DIFFERENTIAL DIAGNOSIS

Only rarely is intermittent exotropia confused with another form of strabismus; should it decompensate to constant exotropia, it must be differentiated from congenital exotropia and exotropia associated with Duane's syndrome (see Chapter 73), convergence paralysis, third nerve palsy (see Chapter 77), and orbital anomalies (Box 74-1). Constant, large-angle exotropia can occur before 1 year of age ("infantile" or "congenital" exotropia) and is about 3% as common as infantile or congenital esotropia. Inferior oblique muscle overaction and dissociated vertical deviation are common, but latent nystagmus is rare. Sometimes spontaneous alignment occurs by 1 year of age; surgical correction by 2 years of age provides alignment with monofixation syndrome in most cases.[12]

TREATMENT
Nonsurgical Treatment

Successful treatment of intermittent exotropia is enhanced by correction of significant refractive errors and amblyopia. Undercorrected myopia is corrected fully not only to improve visual acuity at distance but also to stimulate accommodative convergence at near fixation. Significant amounts of uncorrected hyperopia (greater than +3.00D) are corrected as well, because uncorrected high hyperopia may be associated with hypoaccommodation.[13] Correction of amblyopia alone rarely improves alignment, but treatment compliance is often better before surgery, and it is easier to follow visual acuity levels in each eye in nonverbal children before the eyes are aligned.

589

Active orthoptic training is based on the concept of deficient motor fusion and has been performed in some fashion for more than 80 years. Fusional vergence amplitudes are enhanced, when deficient, by using a major amblyoscope or fusional training exercises in free space. Other techniques utilize monocular targets that are progressively more difficult to fuse, beginning with large, detailed stereoscopic targets at near. Eventually, simple targets at distance are presented. Results vary depending on the success criteria, but most practitioners agree that intermittent, comitant deviations that measure less than 25Δ have a better prognosis than large, incomitant, constant exotropias. Diplopia recognition is used less frequently because of the fear of intractable diplopia after sensory adaptations have been dissipated.

Monocular occlusion has been used by some authors, initially continuously and more recently for specific periods (3–8 hours per day).[14] A decrease in frequency of exotropic alignment and improvement from intermittent exotropia to exophoria have been noted; speculated reasons for the improvement include disruption of suppression development and subsequent improvement in fusional amplitudes.[15] Those for whom monocular occlusion therapy failed and who subsequently underwent surgery showed postoperative alignment equal to that of those who had not undergone occlusion.

Overcorrecting minus lenses (-2.00 to $-4.00D$ over the habitual distance prescription) have been prescribed to stimulate accommodative convergence, with some success. After improved alignment, the patients were weaned slowly from the overcorrected lenses. The treatment did not stimulate further development of myopia in these patients.[16]

Use of therapeutic (base-in) prisms has been attempted in some patients who have intermittent exotropia, with questionable long-term efficacy; typically, about 50% of the maximal distance deviation is corrected with prisms. Most younger patients relax fusional convergence in response to the prism ("eat" the prism), and the physician may have to increase the prism strength progressively; older patients who have more constant exotropia and limited fusional amplitudes may respond more positively. Intermittent exotropia may become more constant when the prism glasses are removed.[17] Prisms greater than 5D are difficult to incorporate into lenses; thus, Fresnel membrane prisms are more useful for larger deviations, but they also have disadvantages (see Chapter 80).

Auditory biofeedback has been attempted by a few investigators, with an infrared eye movement monitor linked to a variably pitched tone. Patients who had intermittent exotropia greater at distance than at near fixation responded well, but patients who had equivalent measurements did not.[18]

Surgical Treatment

Surgical treatment of strabismus is appropriate only after non-surgical approaches have been attempted and the results found to be unsatisfactory to the patient or physician. Patients who have intermittent exotropia become reasonable surgical candidates when many of the features listed in Box 74-2 are present. Usually, tropias under 10Δ are associated with the monofixation syndrome and do not require, nor is the patient's sensory status

benefited by, surgery unless a symptomatic, superimposed phoria is present. Some investigators believe that surgery deferred until after 4 years of age provides improved results, while others do not.

The surgeon must then decide between symmetrical surgery (recession of both lateral recti or resection of both medial recti) and asymmetrical surgery (recession of one lateral rectus combined with resection of its antagonist medial rectus). The historical approach was to reserve recession of both lateral recti for patients with "true divergence excess" intermittent exotropia, in whom the deviation remained larger at distance fixation than at near fixation after a trial of $+3.00D$ lenses at near. Patients with a greater intermittent exotropia at near fixation than at distance fixation ("convergence insufficiency") received resection of both medial recti, and all others received asymmetrical surgery. Some reports suggest that, except for those with convergence insufficiency, all patients may be given bilateral lateral rectus recessions, because the results are equivalent to those obtained with asymmetrical procedures. One prospective study found that patients with "basic-type" intermittent exotropia (near deviation equal to distance deviation) had better outcomes after unilateral recess-resect procedures.[19] The advantages and disadvantages of symmetrical and asymmetrical surgery are listed in Table 74-1.

Most published series show that symmetrical and asymmetrical surgery give equivalent results. Patients who receive the former are often esotropic for a few weeks after surgery. Patients who undergo asymmetrical surgery are less likely to be esotropic in the immediate postoperative period, and final alignment is often recorded after 1 week.

The amounts of recession and resection for intermittent exotropia or exotropia for given deviations are suggested in Table 74-2; these figures provide a roughly 5% ultimate overcorrection rate and a 15% ultimate undercorrection rate. These amounts are modified from data of Dr. Marshall M. Parks and require the suture to be placed 1.0–1.5mm from the lateral rectus insertion. If symmetrical surgery is chosen, each muscle is receded by the amount shown in the appropriate column. If asymmetrical surgery is chosen, the appropriate amount of surgery shown is performed on each muscle. Most surgeons operate for the maximal deviation uncovered at far distance fixation, except in patients with convergence insufficiency; in those patients, surgeons operate for the maximal deviation at near fixation distance. Those who have lateral gaze incomitance of more than 10Δ less than the primary position measurement should have 1.0mm less lateral rectus recession performed on the eye on the side of the lesser deviation. All patients who have binocular vision should be warned of the possibility of postoperative diplopia in the event of postoperative esotropia.

COURSE AND OUTCOME

Published surgical results vary, depending on criteria for success and length of follow-up. Cosmetic success is often defined as an esotropia or exotropia of less than 15Δ, and functional success is often defined as a small asymptomatic phoria or constant tropia less than 10Δ with peripheral fusion, or small residual intermittent exotropia, which rarely occurs. Typical published suc-

TABLE 74-1

ADVANTAGES AND DISADVANTAGES OF SYMMETRICAL AND ASYMMETRICAL SURGERY

	Advantages	Disadvantages
Symmetrical surgery (recession of both lateral recti or resection of both medial recti)	Recessions technically easier than resections Does not create lid fissure anomalies on side gaze Recessions do not sacrifice muscle tissue Does not alter refractive error	Bilateral surgery may be difficult to explain to patients who note monocular strabismus Monocular surgery lends itself more readily to local anesthetic techniques
Asymmetrical surgery (recession of one lateral rectus and resection of one medial rectus)	Preferred if one eye deeply amblyopic Preferred if patient demands surgery on one eye Monocular surgery lends itself more easily to local anesthetic techniques	Resections involve disposal of muscle tissue Induces plus cylinder axis 90° for 6 weeks postoperatively Often leads to subtle lid tissue anomalies on side gaze (wider in abduction than adduction)

TABLE 74-2

SUGGESTED EXTENT OF SURGERY FOR PATIENTS WITH EXOTROPIA

Deviation (Δ)	Recede Lateral Rectus by (mm)	Resect Medial Rectus by (mm)
12	3.5	2.5
15	4.0	3.0
20	5.0	4.0
25	6.0	5.0
30	7.0	6.0
35	7.5	7.0
40	8.0	8.0
45	8.5	9.0
50	9.0	10.0
60	10.0	
70	11.0	

Adapted from data from Marshall M. Parks, MD.

cess rates after one operation are in the range 60–90% for functional success and 70–95% for cosmetic success. Patients should be warned of the smaller lateral visual field expanse that occurs after successful surgery; some miss the panoramic visual field inherent in intermittent exotropia.

REFERENCES
1. Von Noorden GK. Some aspects of exotropia. In: Binocular vision and ocular motility. Theory and management of strabismus. St Louis: CV Mosby; 1990;236.
2. Jenkins R. Demographic geographic variations in the prevention and management of exotropia. Am Orthoptic J. 1992;421:82–7.
3. Blodi FC, Van Allen M. Electromyography in intermittent exotropia; recordings before, during, and after corrective operation. Doc Ophthalmol. 1962;26:21–34.
4. Knapp P. Intermittent exotropia: evaluation and therapy. Am Orthoptic J. 1953;3:27–33.
5. Burian HM, Spivey BE. The surgical management of exodeviations. Am J Ophthalmol. 1965;59:603–20.
6. Chavasse BF. Worth's squint or the binocular reflex and the treatment of strabismus, 7th ed. Philadelphia: Blakiston & Son; 1939:ch 2–3; 107–8.
7. Jampolsky A. Physiology of intermittent exotropia. Symposium: intermittent exotropia. Am Orthoptic J. 1952;2:5–14.
8. Capo H, Mallotte R, Guyton D. Overacting obliques in exotropia: a mechanical explanation. Presented at the American Association for Pediatric Ophthalmology and Strabismus Meeting; 1988.
9. Moore S. The prognostic value of lateral gaze incomitance in intermittent exotropia. Am Orthoptic J. 1969;19:69–74.
10. Repka MX, Arnoldi KA. Lateral incomitance in exotropia: fact or artifact. J Pediatr Ophthalmol Strabismus. 1991;28:125–30.
11. Kushner B. Diagnosis and treatment of exotropia with a high accommodation convergence–accommodation ratio. Arch Ophthalmol. 1999;117:221–4.
12. Biglan AW, Davis JS, Cheng KP, Pettapiece MC. Infantile exotropia. J Pediatr Ophthalmol Strabismus. 1996;33:79–84.
13. Iacobucci I, Archer S, Giles C. Children with exotropia respond to spectacle correction of hyperopia. Am J Ophthalmol. 1993;116:79–83.
14. Calhoun JT, McKinney S, Rosenhouse M. Management of intermittent exotropia. In: Moore S, Mein J, Stockbridge L, eds. Orthoptics: past, present, and future. New York: Stratten International; 1976:563–8.
15. Iacobucci I, Henderson SW. Occlusion in the preoperative management of exotropia. Am Orthoptic J. 1965;15:42–7.
16. Cattrider N, Jampolsky A. Overcorrecting minus lens therapy for treatment of intermittent exotropia. Ophthalmology. 1983;96:1160–5.
17. Veronneau-Troutman S, Shippman S, Clahane AC. Prisms as an orthoptic tool in the management of primary intermittent exotropia. In: Moore S, Mein J, Stockbridge L, eds. Orthoptics: past, present, and future. New York: Stratten International; 1976:653–8.
18. Goldrich SG. Oculomotor biofeedback therapy for exotropia. Am J Optom Physiol Opt. 1982;59:306.
19. Kushner B. Selective surgery for intermittent exotropia based on distance/near differences. Arch Ophthalmol. 1998;116:324–8.

Oblique Muscle Dysfunctions

GARY R. DIAMOND

DEFINITION
- Dysfunction of inferior or superior oblique muscle enough to cause measurable deviation.

KEY FEATURES
- Hyperdeviation.
- A- and V-pattern deviations.

ASSOCIATED FEATURES
- Primary inferior oblique overaction.
- Secondary inferior oblique overaction.
- Inferior oblique underaction.
- Primary superior oblique overaction.
- Secondary superior oblique overaction.
- Superior oblique underaction.

INTRODUCTION

Overactions and underactions of both oblique muscles are well recognized. Often, the term "primary" is used to indicate ignorance of the cause of the dysfunction, and "secondary" is appended when the dysfunction is caused by known pathology of another cyclovertical muscle. Gobin[1] suggested that many oblique dysfunctions are caused by a mismatch between the course of the inferior oblique muscle and that of the superior oblique tendon. If the trochlea is positioned anterior to the bony origin of the inferior oblique when viewed coronally, a mechanical advantage accrues to the superior oblique; conversely, if the trochlea is positioned behind the inferior oblique origin, the inferior oblique obtains a mechanical advantage (Fig. 75-1). The former situation occurs in some patients who have midface retrusion or hydrocephalus (Fig. 75-2), and the latter occurs in some patients who have orbital roof retrusion. However, many patients with oblique muscle dysfunction have normal orbital anatomy and unknown reasons for the dysfunction.

PRIMARY INFERIOR OBLIQUE OVERACTION

EPIDEMIOLOGY AND PATHOGENESIS

Overelevation in adduction caused by inferior oblique overaction develops in about 72% of congenital esotropes, 34% of accommodative esotropes, and 32% of intermittent exotropes who are followed for longer than 5 years.[2] In a study by Wilson and Parks,[2] the incidence of inferior oblique overaction in patients with congenital esotropia was not related to age at strabismus onset, time from onset to surgery for the esotropia, age at first surgery, or decompensation of horizontal alignment; it was,

however, related to the number of surgeries necessary to align the eyes horizontally. The mean age of onset was 3.6 years. The presence of fundus excyclotorsion in children with congenital esotropia may predict the later development of inferior oblique overaction.

Primary inferior oblique overaction is usually asymmetrical and may be unilateral at onset (23%). Frequently, the second eye becomes involved soon after unilateral surgery for inferior oblique weakening.

OCULAR MANIFESTATIONS

The hyperdeviation in the affected eye may present a few degrees in adduction, in full adduction only, or only in the field of action of the inferior oblique (Fig. 75-3). Several grading systems have been devised for this overaction, but none is ideal (Table 75-1). If extreme bilateral overaction is present, the patient has only a narrow range of comfortable, single binocular vision to either side of primary position.

A V-pattern strabismus is often associated with inferior oblique overaction and yields greater exodeviation in upgaze than in downgaze. This is explained easily by the tertiary abduction ability of the inferior oblique muscles in upgaze, but it is unclear why all patients with inferior oblique overaction do not develop a V-pattern strabismus. Vertical strabismus in primary position is quite uncommon, despite asymmetry of overaction.

DIAGNOSIS

Patients who have primary inferior oblique overaction exhibit no subjective symptoms of ocular torsion, but they do have objective evidence of excyclotorsion of the involved globes. The Parks-Bielschowsky three-step test (see Chapter 77) is negative, and no torsion is admitted by the patient on Maddox rod, Bagolini lens, or Lancaster red–green testing. However, examination of the fundus by camera shows the fovea to be positioned below its normal position of 0.3 disc diameters below a horizontal line that extends from the center of the disc (inverted, of course, by indirect ophthalmoscopy). Forced duction testing shows the inferior oblique muscles to be tighter than normal.[3] Presumably, for patients with primary inferior oblique overaction, sensory adaptations are available to reconcile globe excyclotorsion and thus maintain comfortable single binocular vision.

DIFFERENTIAL DIAGNOSIS

The differential diagnosis of primary inferior oblique overaction is listed in Box 75-1. Dissociated vertical deviation often coexists with inferior oblique overaction, especially in patients who have congenital esotropia. Capo et al.[4] presented a form of pseudo–inferior oblique overaction that may explain normalization of function after exotropia surgery. Semantically, the situation is clouded between primary and secondary inferior oblique overaction in some patients who have long-standing exotropia, in whom all obliques contract and overact.

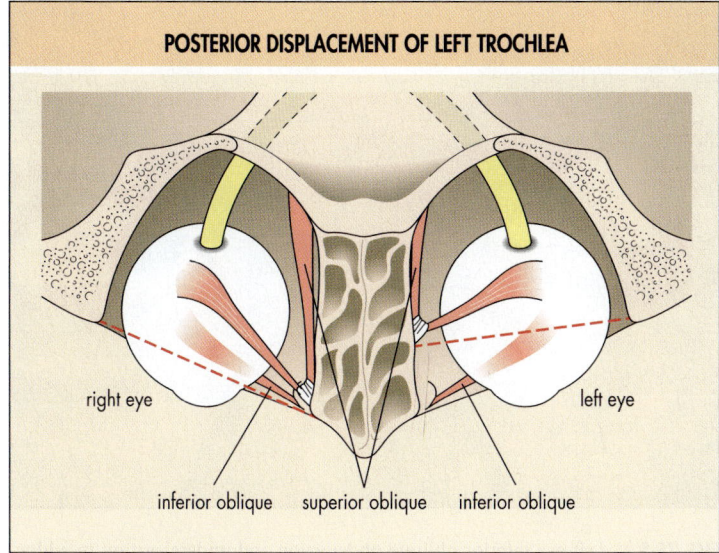

FIG. 75-1 ▮ **Posterior displacement of the left trochlea.** This may give mechanical advantage to the left inferior oblique muscle.

right eye   left eye

inferior oblique   superior oblique   inferior oblique

POSTERIOR DISPLACEMENT OF LEFT TROCHLEA

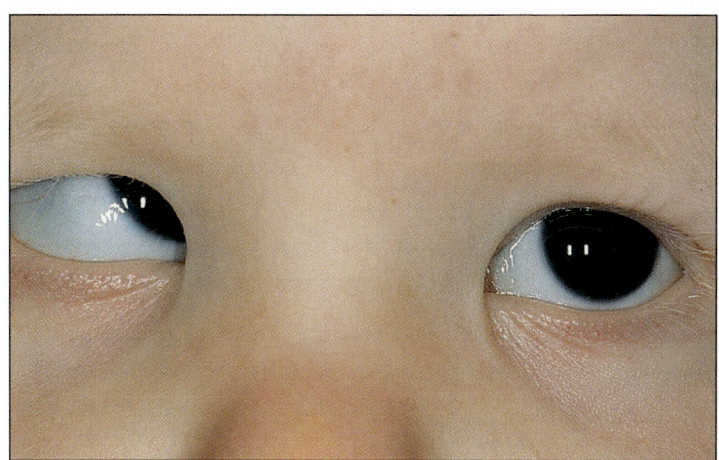

FIG. 75-3 ▮ **Right eye inferior oblique overaction and overelevation in adduction.**

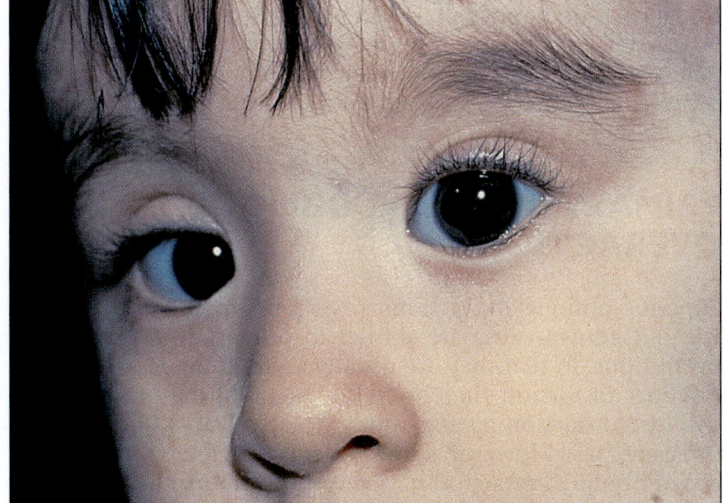

FIG. 75-2 ▮ **Hydrocephalus and frontal bossing.** As the frontal floor advances, it pulls the trochlea forward. This trochlear advance is postulated to give mechanical advantage to the superior oblique muscles, with resultant overdepression in adduction and an A-pattern strabismus.

TABLE 75-1

GRADING OF HYPERDEVIATION

Grade	Elevation or Depression in Adduction (D)
Trace	5
1+	10
2+	20
3+	30
4+	45

BOX 75-1

Differential Diagnosis of Overelevation in Adduction

Inferior oblique overaction
Dissociated vertical deviation
Aberrant regeneration of cranial nerve III
Rectus rotation in patients who have craniosynostosis
Tether effect in patients who have Duane's syndrome
Tight lateral rectus muscle syndrome

TREATMENT

Although treatment of primary inferior oblique overaction is usually performed for esthetic purposes, it often provides a functional benefit as well, because duction normalization permits a wider range of single binocular vision. The only effective treatment is surgery on the overacting muscle. Care must be taken to include the entire muscle in the procedure; in addition, direct visualization of the muscle should prevent rupture of a vortex vein or violation of Tenon's capsule. The latter may lead to fibrofatty proliferation of orbital fat on the sclera or contracture of radial fibrous tissue orbital septa, which results in an "adherence syndrome" of progressive hypotropia, excyclotropia, and elevation limitation. Excessive traction on the inferior oblique muscle may traumatize parasympathetic fibers of the ciliary ganglion and result in a (usually) transient pupillary dilatation and decreased accommodative tone. Postoperatively, patients with primary inferior oblique overaction do not usually complain of torsional diplopia, and primary position horizontal or vertical alignment is not affected.

Patients who have trace or 1+ overaction usually do not require treatment unless the inferior oblique muscle in the other eye is being weakened. In such cases, a 10mm recession is performed (Fig. 75-4), which requires that the muscle be disinserted and reattached to a point 3mm posterior and 2mm temporal to the temporal border of the inferior rectus insertion. Patients who have 2+ overaction usually receive a 10mm recession.

Patients who have 3+ or more overaction may be offered a number of powerful weakening procedures. The 14mm recession places the new muscle insertion on the sclera that straddles the inferotemporal vortex vein ampulla. The irreversible myectomy removes as much inferior oblique muscle as the surgeon can harness, extending from Tenon's capsule to the muscle's insertion; this may be combined with denervation.[5] Anteriorization places the insertion at or anterior to the temporal border of the lateral rectus insertion and cripples the elevating action of the muscle, transforming it into a supplementary depressor[6,7]; unilateral procedures are restricted to placement of the insertion at the level of the inferior rectus so as not to create a postoperative hypotropia.

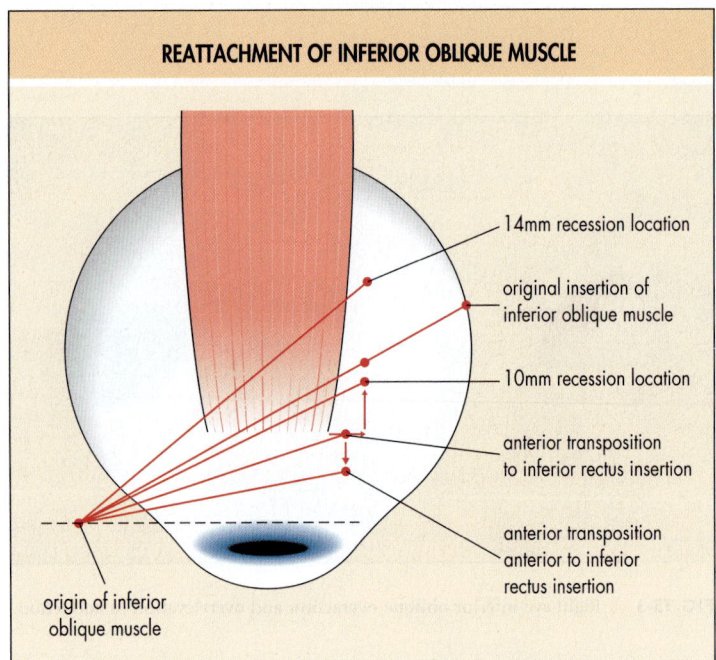

FIG. 75-4 ▍ Reattachment of inferior oblique muscle after disinsertion.

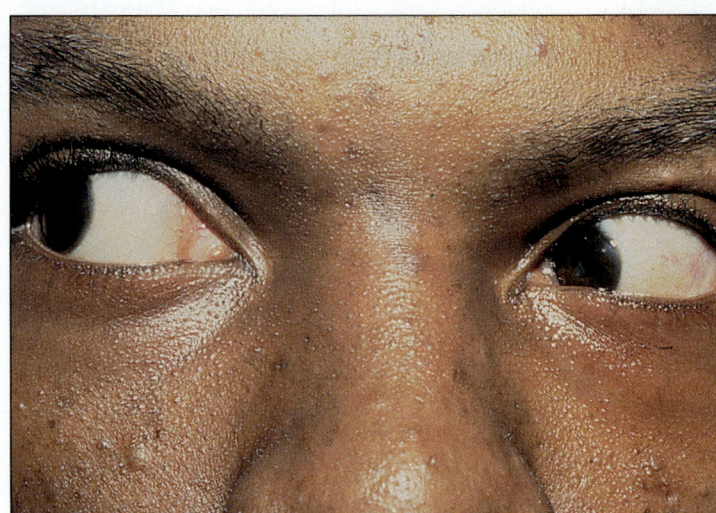

FIG. 75-5 ▍ Left eye inferior oblique underaction and underelevation in adduction. This must be differentiated from the more common Brown's syndrome.

SECONDARY INFERIOR OBLIQUE OVERACTION

Secondary inferior oblique overaction is usually caused by paresis of the antagonist superior oblique muscle with contracture, but occasionally it may be associated with superior rectus palsy in the opposite eye. Patients who have secondary overaction often have a vertical strabismus in primary position. Adult patients with a recent onset of palsy may complain of vertical and torsional diplopia and may also have a positive Parks-Bielschowsky three-step test. Of course, these patients also have the objective signs of oblique dysfunction mentioned earlier—excyclotorsion of the fovea around the optic nerve and positive forced duction testing. Head tilts and turns to avoid diplopia are common in this group.

Therapy is indicated not only for esthetic reasons and to increase the range of comfortable single binocular vision but also to obviate the need for changes in head posture to avoid visual confusion and diplopia. Some patients respond positively to vertical prisms, but many require surgery. Older patients must be warned of the possibility of temporary postoperative diplopia.

INFERIOR OBLIQUE UNDERACTION

Many patients who have limitation of elevation in adduction have Brown's syndrome, associated with V-pattern exotropia in upgaze, duction and version limitations of elevation of similar degree (worse in adduction than abduction), and tight forced duction testing. A few have true inferior oblique palsy, a difficult entity to reconcile neuroanatomically, but one that is analogous to superior oblique palsy.[8-10] These patients may have a hypodeviation in primary position if fixing with the nonparetic eye (Fig. 75-5), secondary overaction of the antagonist superior oblique muscle, and an A-pattern exotropia with better elevation in abduction than adduction. Elevation is better on duction than version testing, and forced duction testing is unrestricted unless the superior oblique is contracted. Some patients respond well to vertical prisms, but many require surgery; recession of the contralateral superior rectus or weakening of the ipsilateral superior oblique is the usual procedure.[11]

Secondary inferior oblique underaction caused by inhibitional palsy of the yoke of the antagonist to a paretic inferior rectus is seen occasionally. If the patient chooses to fixate with the paretic eye, a hypodeviation in the other eye in primary position is present.

PRIMARY SUPERIOR OBLIQUE OVERACTION

Superior oblique overactions (overdepression in adduction) without known cause are similar to primary inferior oblique overactions, in that they are usually asymptomatic and exhibit evidence of torsion (here incyclotorsion) of the fundus, positive forced duction testing, and a negative Parks-Bielschowsky three-step test. However, some patients affected by primary superior oblique overaction have a vertical strabismus in primary position. As a result of the tertiary abduction effect of the superior oblique in downgaze, some have an A-pattern strabismus as well (see Fig. 75-6). Superior oblique overactions may be seen in esotropia and exotropia and occasionally without any horizontal strabismus. Antagonist inferior oblique function often is normal, but occasional underactions may be demonstrated.

Prism therapy for a vertical strabismus benefits some patients. If the condition is esthetically significant, the superior oblique may be weakened by tenotomy, tenectomy, graded recession, or lengthening with biological plastic (Silastic) bands. If the tenotomy spares the intermuscular septum, contractile force is transmitted around the tenotomy to the distal tendon and thus prevents superior oblique palsy; some investigators advocate simultaneous inferior oblique weakening to delay or prevent the onset of superior oblique palsy.

Tenectomy is more associated with palsy than is tenotomy.[12] Measured recessions, although more technically challenging, offer reproducibility and less likelihood of palsy.[13,14] Lengthening by the interposition of Silastic material appears to be a promising method of superior oblique weakening.[15] Many are cautious about weakening overacting superior obliques in patients who show fusion in the primary position and choose to treat A-pattern strabismus with horizontal or vertical rectus translations. Reports describe little if any eso shift in primary position after bilateral superior oblique weakening procedures.[16]

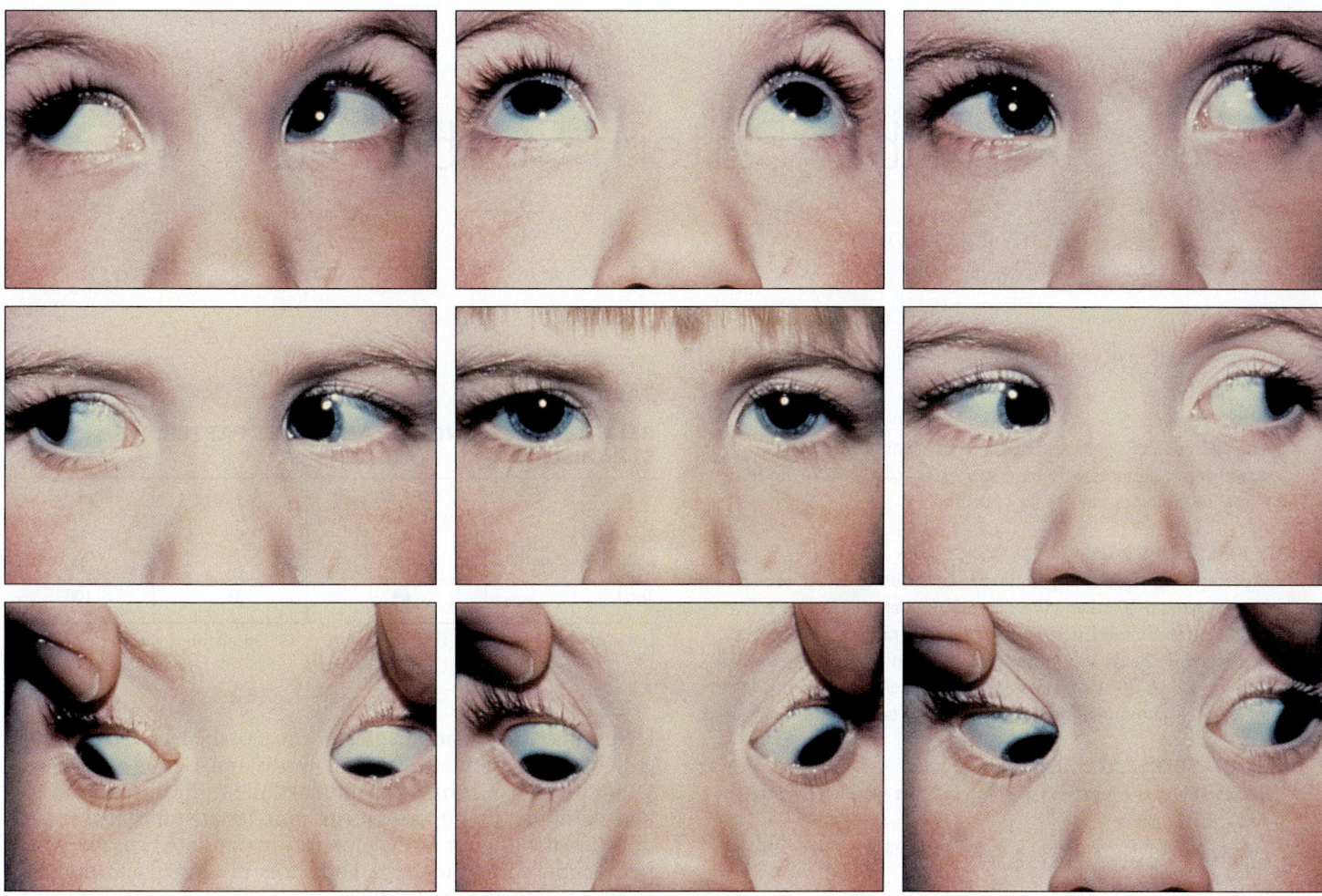

FIG. 75-6 ▐▐ Child who has bilateral superior oblique overaction, overdepression in adduction, and an A-pattern exotropia.

SECONDARY SUPERIOR OBLIQUE OVERACTION

Secondary superior oblique overactions are usually caused by ipsilateral inferior oblique palsy or contralateral inferior rectus palsy (if the patient fixes with the paretic eye). In the latter case, the patient may exhibit a hypodeviation in the nonparetic eye. Patients who have secondary superior oblique overaction may have a vertical deviation in primary position and a compensatory head posture, and they are expected to show a positive Parks-Bielschowsky three-step test. They also have objective evidence of globe torsion, as mentioned earlier. Some patients can be treated using vertical prisms, but many require strabismus surgery.

SUPERIOR OBLIQUE UNDERACTION

Superior oblique palsy is the most common form of cyclovertical muscle weakness. Its diagnosis and treatment are described in Chapter 77. Before spread of comitance to other cyclovertical muscles, underdepression in adduction, excyclotorsion of the fundus of the paretic eye, and a compensatory head posture occur. The Parks-Bielschowsky three-step test is positive. Adults with recent-onset superior oblique palsy show torsion on Maddox rod, Bagolini lens, or Lancaster red–green testing; children or adults with chronic palsy often do not. Some patients respond well to vertical prisms, but many require surgery.

Occasionally, a patient with superior rectus palsy in the contralateral eye presents with a secondary superior oblique underaction if he or she chooses to fix with the paretic eye.

REFERENCES

1. Gobin MH. Sagittallization of the oblique muscles as a possible cause for the "A," "V," and "X" phenomena. Br J Ophthalmol. 1968;52:13–21.
2. Wilson ME, Parks MM. Primary inferior oblique overaction in congenital esotropia, accommodative esotropia, and intermittent exotropia. Ophthalmology. 1989;96:7–11.
3. Guyton DL. Exaggerated traction test for the oblique muscles. Ophthalmology. 1981;88:1035–40.
4. Capo H, Mallette RA, Guyton DL. Overacting oblique muscles in exotropia: a mechanical explanation. J Pediatr Ophthalmol Strabismus. 1988;25:281–5.
5. Del Monte AA, Parks MM. Denervation and extirpation of the inferior oblique. Ophthalmology. 1983;90:1178–83.
6. Mims JL, Wood RC. Bilateral anterior transposition of the inferior oblique muscle. Arch Ophthalmol. 1989;107:41–4.
7. Elliot RL, Nankin SJ. Anterior transposition of the inferior oblique. J Pediatr Ophthalmol Strabismus. 1981;18:35–41.
8. Scott WE, Nankin SJ. Isolated inferior oblique paresis. Arch Ophthalmol. 1977; 95:1586–93.
9. Pollard ZF. Diagnosis and treatment of inferior oblique palsy. J Pediatr Ophthalmol Strabismus. 1993;30:936–9.
10. Hunter DG, Lam GC, Guyton DL. Inferior oblique muscle injury from local anesthesia for cataract surgery. Ophthalmology. 102;3:501–9.
11. Kutschke PJ, Scott WE. Postoperative results in inferior oblique palsy. J Pediatr Ophthalmol Strabismus. 1996;33:72–8.
12. Olivier P, von Noorden GK. Results of superior oblique tendon tenectomy for inferior oblique palsy and Brown's syndrome. Arch Ophthalmol. 1982;100:581–4.
13. Romano P, Roholt P. Measured graduated recession of the superior oblique muscle. J Pediatr Ophthalmol Strabismus. 1983;20:134–40.
14. Caldeira JAF. Graduated recession of the superior oblique muscle. Br J Ophthalmol. 1975;59:513–59.
15. Wright KW. Superior oblique silicone expander for Brown syndrome and superior oblique overaction. J Pediatr Ophthalmol Strabismus. 1991;28:101–7.
16. Diamond GR, Parks MM. The effect of superior oblique weakening procedures on primary position horizontal alignment. J Pediatr Ophthalmol Strabismus. 1981;18:1–3.

Alphabet Pattern Strabismus

GARY R. DIAMOND

DEFINITION
- The presence of significant incomitance from upgaze to downgaze in patients who have esotropia, exotropia, or no horizontal misalignment in primary position.

KEY FEATURES
- V pattern—at least 15D greater exodeviation or lesser esodeviation in gaze up 30° than gaze down 30° when the patient is fixing on an accommodation-control distance target.
- A pattern—at least 10D lesser exodeviation or greater esodeviation in gaze up 30° than gaze down 30° when the patient is fixing on an accommodation-control distance target.

ASSOCIATED FEATURES
- Inferior oblique overaction in some patients who have V patterns and Y patterns.
- Superior oblique overaction in some patients who have A patterns and lambda patterns.
- Both superior and inferior oblique overactions in some patients who have X patterns.

INTRODUCTION

This diverse group of ocular misalignments has incomitance from upgaze to downgaze as its unifying theme. It should be suspected in any patient who has a history or presentation of chin-up or chin-down posture, and it can be associated with eso-, exo-, or no deviation in primary position. Every patient must be evaluated for alphabet pattern strabismus using prism and alternate-cover test measurements at distance fixation with the chin elevated 30°, depressed 30°, and in primary position. The relative incidence of alphabet pattern strabismus is given in Table 76-1.

Every muscle group has been incriminated as causative in these patients. Patients who do not have oblique overaction have been postulated to have anatomical alterations in their rectus positions on the globe. Those who have A-pattern esotropia tend to have lateral canthi higher than medial ("mongoloid" facies), and those who have V-pattern esotropia tend to have lateral canthi lower than medial ("antimongoloid" facies), but no predilection can be determined for exotropes.[2,3] Demer *et al.*[4] demonstrated that compliant pulleys of collagen and elastin surround each rectus muscle at the eye's equator and serve as the functional origin of the muscles; pulley ectopia could cause alphabet pattern strabismus in some cases.

V-PATTERN ESOTROPIA

INTRODUCTION

The cause of the V pattern is obscure in patients who have normally functioning oblique muscles. Some authorities have postulated the existence of anatomical variations in the horizontal

TABLE 76-1

RELATIVE INCIDENCE OF ALPHABET PATTERN STRABISMUS

	V (%)	A (%)	Total (%)
Esotropia	41	25	66
Exotropia	23	11	34
Total	64	36	100

Data from Costenbader FD. Trans Am Acad Ophthalmol Otolaryngol. 1964; 68:354–5.

rectus muscles that permit greater effect of the lateral rectus muscles in upgaze and the medial rectus muscles in downgaze.[5] Other investigators have incriminated the vertical rectus muscles and claim that the superior rectus muscles are translated temporally and the inferior rectus muscles are translated nasally, which permits the former to act as abductors in upgaze and the latter to act as adductors in downgaze.

OCULAR MANIFESTATIONS

This common pattern presents with esotropia greatest in downgaze and often with a chin-down posture to maintain comfortable single binocular vision. The cause of the V pattern in some patients is inferior oblique overaction, as the abductive effect of the inferior obliques in upgaze produces an exo shift in horizontal alignment. The ultimate deviation in upgaze represents a sum of the underlying esodeviation and the abductive pull of the inferior obliques in upgaze (Fig. 76-1).

DIAGNOSIS

A three-step head tilt test is performed in all patients with V-pattern esotropia to investigate the presence of bilateral superior oblique palsy, which may accompany this picture. A left hyperdeviation on left head tilt and a right hyperdeviation on right head tilt with bilateral fundus extorsion confirm the diagnosis.

TREATMENT

Mild amounts of incomitance (less than 15Δ difference from upgaze to downgaze) may be ignored unless a compensatory chin posture results. Antiaccommodative measures (plus lenses or miotics) are effective for some patients, but the progressively increasing esotropia in downgaze confounds the use of bifocals in most patients who have V-pattern esotropia and a high accommodative convergence–to–accommodation ratio. If surgery is indicated, inferior oblique overaction is reduced, together with the horizontal misalignment; inferior oblique weakening procedures do not affect horizontal ocular alignment in the primary position. If the oblique muscles function normally, the lateral recti may be translated upward and the medial recti downward to a variable degree, up to perhaps one half the tendon width. Likewise, the superior rectus muscles may be trans-

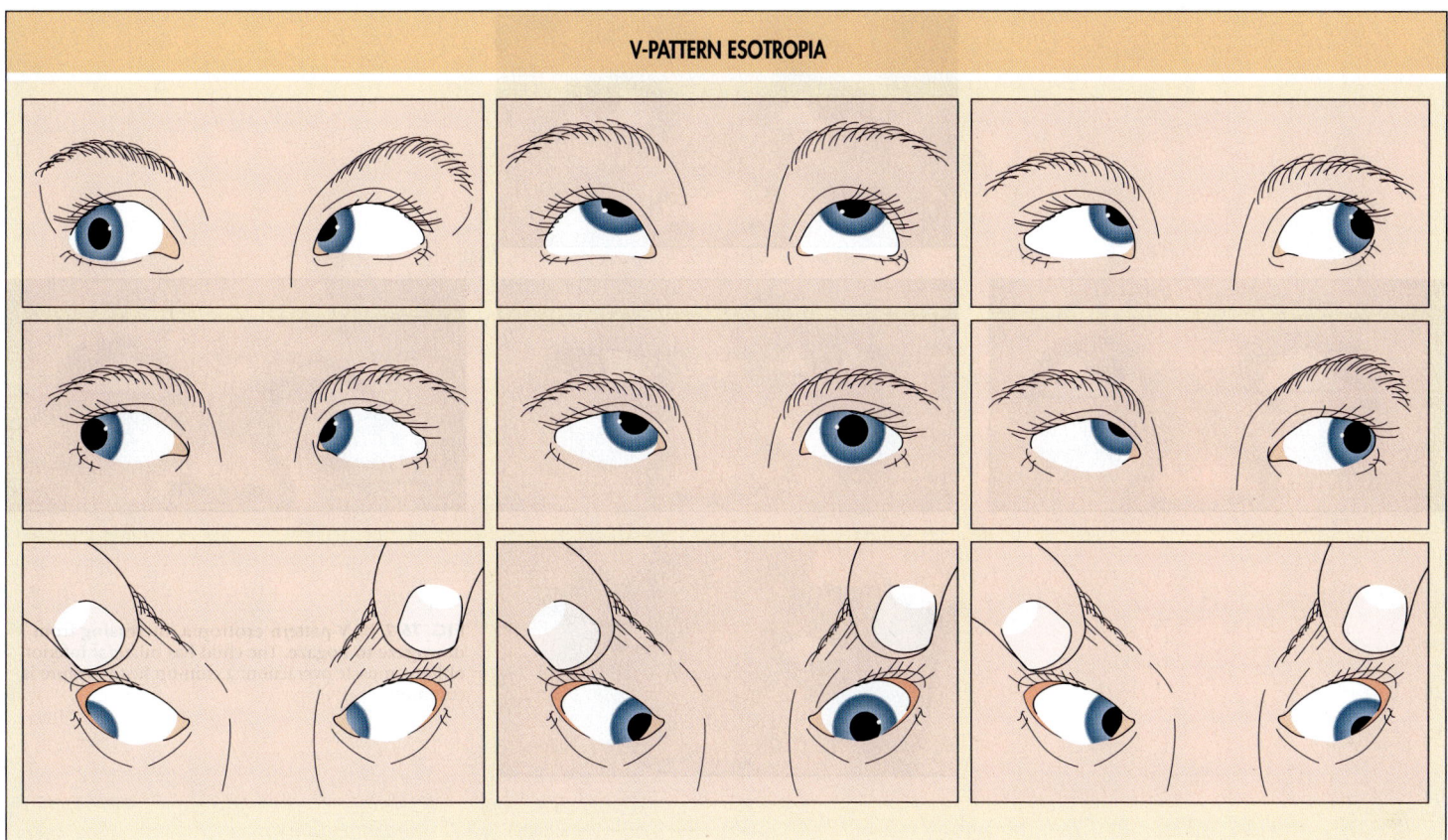

V-PATTERN ESOTROPIA

FIG. 76-1 ■ **V-pattern esotropia, increasing from upgaze to downgaze.** The eyes of a child who has bilateral inferior oblique muscle overaction; a chin-down head posture is common.

lated nasally and the inferior rectus muscles temporally to a similar degree. Translations larger than one half the tendon width tend to be unpredictable. In children, the resultant globe torsion is well tolerated; adults may complain postoperatively of torsional diplopia. To avoid overcorrection in patients who have great incomitance between upgaze and primary position, horizontal surgery for the least esodeviation (upgaze) is performed when combined with horizontal tendon translations.

V-PATTERN EXOTROPIA

OCULAR MANIFESTATIONS

Patients who have V-pattern exotropia commonly present with a chin-up head posture to place the eyes in a position of least horizontal strabismus (Fig. 76-2). Mild incomitance (less than 15Δ difference from upgaze to downgaze) may be ignored unless it results in a compensatory chin posture.

TREATMENT

Evidence of overaction of the inferior oblique muscles must be sought, and if surgery is undertaken, the inferior oblique muscles should be weakened. If the oblique muscles function normally, the lateral rectus muscles may be translated upward and the medial recti downward, as discussed earlier. To avoid overcorrection in patients who have great incomitance between downgaze and primary position, horizontal surgery for the least exodeviation (downgaze) is performed in combination with horizontal tendon translations.

The occasional patient with a Y-pattern strabismus that consists only of exotropia in upgaze can be treated with inferior oblique weakening alone if the oblique muscles overact, or with a pure upward translation of the lateral rectus muscles if the oblique muscles do not overact.

A-PATTERN ESOTROPIA

OCULAR MANIFESTATIONS

This common pattern is suspected in patients who maintain a chin-up posture and have esotropia in upgaze. Some patients have overaction of the superior oblique muscles and harness the abduction effect of the superior obliques in downgaze to overcome the esotropia partially or totally. Other patients have oblique muscles that act normally, and in these cases, the reason for the A pattern is less clear (Fig. 76-3). Mild amounts of incomitance (less than 10Δ difference from upgaze to downgaze) may be ignored unless a compensatory chin posture results.

TREATMENT

Traditionally, caution was recommended when superior oblique weakening procedures were considered for patients in whom fusion in primary position occurred, because postoperative primary position hyperdeviations and excyclotorsional diplopia were feared. Modern, graded superior oblique recession procedures and silicone tendon expander techniques[6] have become available and provide symmetrical superior oblique weakening in such patients with less risk than in previous techniques. Superior oblique weakening procedures do not affect primary position horizontal alignment. Those patients whose superior oblique muscles act normally benefit from downward translation of the lateral rectus muscles, upward translation of the medial rectus muscles,[6] or both, combined with the necessary surgery to reduce horizontal strabismus. To avoid overcorrection in patients who have great incomitance between downgaze and primary position, horizontal surgery for the least esodeviation (downgaze) is performed, along with horizontal tendon translation. An approach for patients who have little horizontal misalignment is temporal translation of the superior rectus muscles, nasal translation of the inferior rectus muscles, or both.

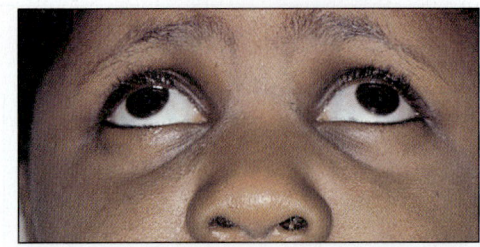

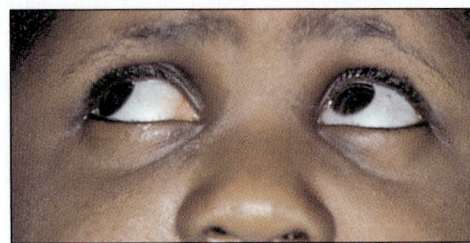
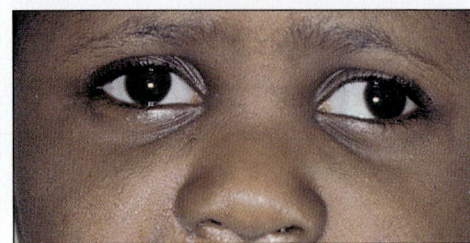

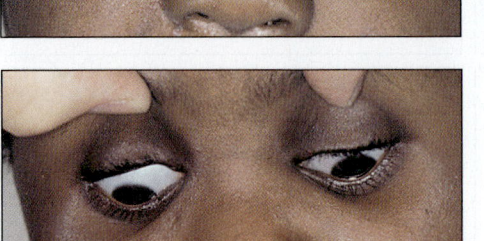

FIG. 76-2 ■ V-pattern exotropia, increasing from downgaze to upgaze. The child has bilateral inferior oblique muscle overaction; a chin-up head posture is common.

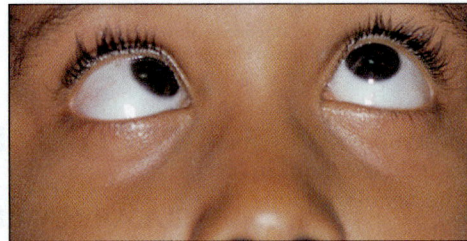

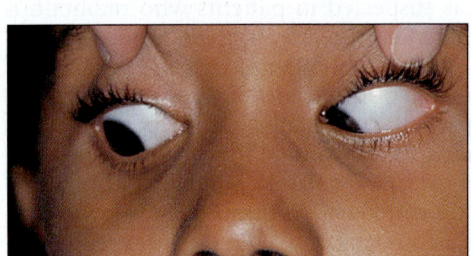
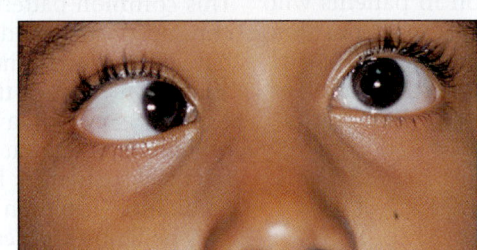
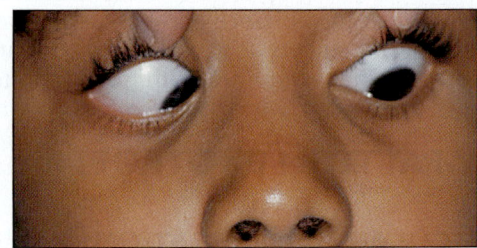

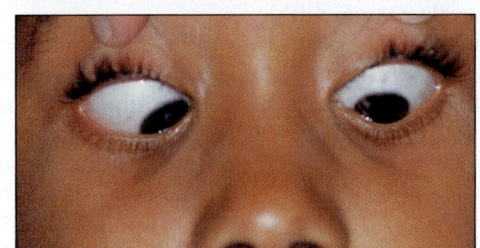

FIG. 76-3 ■ A-pattern esotropia, increasing from downgaze to upgaze. The child has bilateral superior oblique muscle overaction; a chin-up head posture is common.

X-PATTERN STRABISMUS

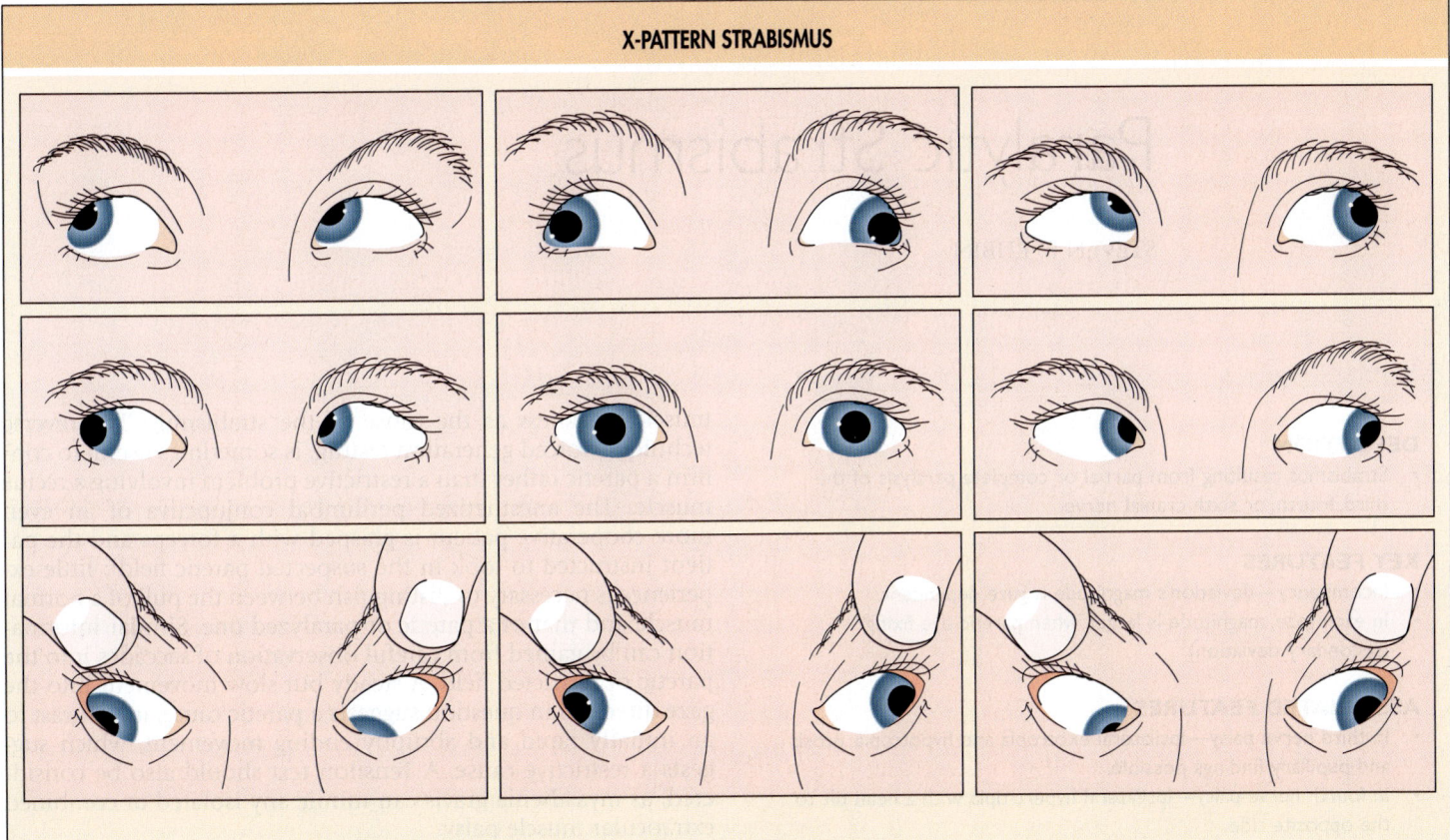

FIG. 76-4 ▮ **X-pattern strabismus with straight eyes in primary position.** Both overelevation and overdepression in adduction in each eye.

A-PATTERN EXOTROPIA

OCULAR MANIFESTATIONS

Patients who have this pattern have a chin-down posture to move the eyes away from the position of maximal exotropia (see Fig. 75-6). Mild amounts of incomitance (less than 10D from upgaze to downgaze) may be ignored unless a compensatory chin position results.

TREATMENT

Patients who do not have superior oblique overaction should undergo translation of the lateral rectus muscles downward, translation of the medial rectus muscles upward, or both, together with surgery for the exotropia. To avoid overcorrection in patients who have great incomitance between upgaze and primary position, horizontal surgery for the least exodeviation (upgaze) is performed in combination with horizontal tendon translations. Graded recessions of the superior oblique muscles[7] or silicone tendon expander techniques,[8] if the muscles are overactive, prevent asymmetrical weakening by tenotomy or tenectomy[9] and creation of a vertical strabismus and excyclodiplopia in primary position. Patients who have little exodeviation in primary position (lambda, or λ, pattern) may benefit from pure translation of the lateral rectus muscles downward or the inferior rectus muscles nasally.

X-PATTERN STRABISMUS

Patients who have long-standing exotropia may develop secondary contracture of all four oblique muscles and an X-pattern strabismus (Fig. 76-4). Alternatively, the lateral rectus muscles

may contract, which results in a "tether" effect on upgaze and downgaze and creates an X pattern. Because each of these visual axis deviations is approached by a different surgical technique, evidence of true oblique overaction must be sought by forced duction testing and observation of fundus torsion in upgaze and downgaze, and staged surgery should be considered. Lateral rectus recessions alone alleviate the X pattern if it is caused by a tether effect alone.

REFERENCES

1. Costenbader FD. Introduction on symposium: the "A" and "V" patterns in strabismus. Trans Am Acad Ophthalmol Otolaryngol. 1964;68:354–5.
2. Urrets-Zavalia A, Solares-Zamora J, Olmos H. Anthropological studies on the nature of cyclovertical squint. Br J Ophthalmol. 1961;45:578–96.
3. Helveston E. Atlas of strabismus surgery. St Louis: CV Mosby; 1977:4.
4. Demer JL, Miller JM, Poukens V. Surgical implications of the rectus extraocular muscle pulleys. J Pediatr Ophthalmol Strabismus. 1996;33:208–18.
5. Knapp P. Vertically incomitant horizontal strabismus: the so-called "A" and "V" syndromes. Trans Am Ophthalmol Soc. 1969;67:304–10.
6. Ribeiro G de B, Brooks SE, Archer SM, Del Monte MA. Vertical shift of the medial rectus muscles in the treatment of A-pattern esotropia: analysis of outcome. J Pediatr Ophthalmol Strabismus. 1995;32:167–71.
7. Romano P, Roholt P. Measured graduated recessions of the superior oblique muscles. J Pediatr Ophthalmol Strabismus. 1983;20:134–9.
8. Wright KW. Superior oblique silicone expander for Brown syndrome and superior oblique overaction. J Pediatr Ophthalmol Strabismus. 1991;28:101–7.
9. Shin GS, Elliott RL, Rosenbaum AL. Posterior superior oblique tenectomy at the scleral insertion for collapse of A-pattern strabismus. J Pediatr Ophthalmol Strabismus. 1996;33:211–8.

Paralytic Strabismus

STEVEN E. RUBIN

DEFINITION
- Strabismus resulting from partial or complete paralysis of the third, fourth, or sixth cranial nerve.

KEY FEATURES
- Incomitancy—deviation's magnitude is gaze dependent.
- In each gaze, magnitude is larger when paretic eye fixing (secondary deviation).

ASSOCIATED FEATURES
- In third nerve palsy—ipsilateral exotropia and hypotropia; ptosis and pupillary findings possible.
- In fourth nerve palsy—ipsilateral hypertropia with a head tilt to the opposite side.
- In sixth nerve palsy—ipsilateral esotropia with head turn to the affected side.

INTRODUCTION

The most common type of strabismus, by far, is the comitant variety—the angle of deviation varies little with gaze direction. Less commonly, muscle overactions or underactions cause a vertical gaze-dependent variation in a regular fashion to give an "alphabet pattern" strabismus, discussed in Chapter 76. Least common are the disorders that result from deficient innervation of one or more extraocular muscles. In this chapter, the comitant variety is not at issue because paralytic strabismus causes the incomitant variety.

In contrast to the straightforward evaluation of nonparetic and nonrestrictive strabismus, an expanded array of diagnostic techniques must be employed in patients who have paralytic strabismus. Accurate classification of a strabismus requires measurement in the cardinal fields (as discussed in Chapter 70) to detect the characteristic incomitance, or variability, of paretic or restrictive disorders. In general, the measured deviation is greatest in the field of action of the offending muscle(s). In some cases, the measured deviation may be "infinite" if the affected muscle is completely unable to move the affected eye into the field of gaze that is being measured.

With nonrestrictive and nonparetic strabismus syndromes, prism measurements are independent of the fixing eye, even in patients who have a fixation preference for one eye (suggesting amblyopia). If the measurements change when the fellow eye takes up fixation, a paretic or restrictive cause is usually the reason. The deviation is larger when the affected eye is used for fixation, termed *secondary deviation*.

A restrictive cause can be confirmed by the use of forced duction testing, whereby the anesthetized perilimbal conjunctiva of the affected eye of a very cooperative patient is grasped with a forceps and manually "forced" into the suspected paretic field; significant resistance indicates mechanical restriction rather than

muscle weakness as the cause of the strabismus. The reverse technique, forced generation testing, is sometimes useful to confirm a paretic rather than a restrictive problem involving a rectus muscle. The anesthetized perilimbal conjunctiva of an even more cooperative patient is grasped with a forceps and the patient instructed to look in the suspected paretic field[1]; little experience is necessary to distinguish between the pull of a normal muscle and that of a paretic or paralyzed one. Similar information can be gained from careful observation of saccades into the paretic or restricted field. A steady but slow movement into the gaze direction in question suggests a paretic cause, in contrast to an initially rapid and abruptly ending movement, which suggests a restrictive cause. A Tensilon test should also be considered, as myasthenia gravis can mimic any isolated or combined extraocular muscle palsy.

In acquired palsies that affect adults and cooperative children, the resulting diplopia can be assessed with binocular visual fields. A slight modification can incorporate the effect of torsion. This technique utilizes a standard Goldmann perimeter to identify and quantify the extent of the diplopic and nondiplopic areas of gaze.

Patients who have extraocular muscle palsies also require consideration for more extensive evaluation. Whereas comitant strabismus is only rarely secondary to a neurological or other systemic disease, paralytic forms of strabismus are often secondary to other causes, many of which are amenable to treatment, sometimes lifesaving. For children and adults, the lists of possible causes of a muscle palsy differ; this is discussed with individual disorders subsequently. Although congenital palsies are the main cause in children, they can also be the cause of fourth nerve palsies in adults, who can keep their deviation latent for many years or even decades.

Management of paralytic strabismus follows the same general guidelines as for any difficult condition—less invasive and risky remedies are tried or considered before those that involve greater risk. Hence, patients with a small or slowly improving paresis can be offered occlusion or prism therapy before surgery is considered. Because almost any focus of management for these conditions is a treatment and not a cure, the precise goals must be made exceedingly clear to the patient and family. Ocular alignment in primary position and downgaze (for reading) has priority over achieving alignment in all fields; the latter is almost always unattainable in these incomitant deviations.

Appropriate informed consent for surgery, if indicated, requires discussion of all the alternative treatments, including the option of no treatment. If and when surgery is planned, the muscle(s) at work in the field(s) of greatest deviation must be targeted. Details of surgical strategies are discussed in the following sections with the individual muscle palsies.

THIRD NERVE PALSY

Because the third nerve innervates the inferior oblique, inferior rectus, and medial rectus muscles (by the inferior division) and the superior rectus and levator muscles (by the superior divi-

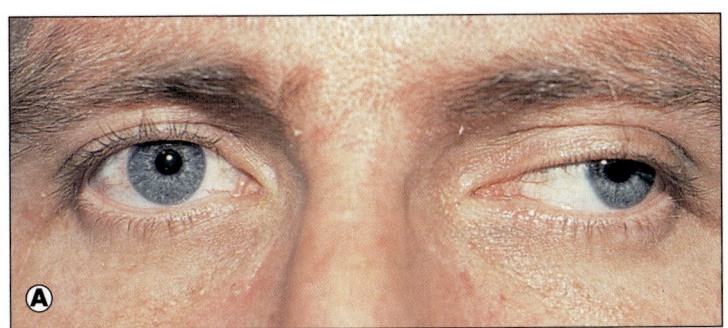

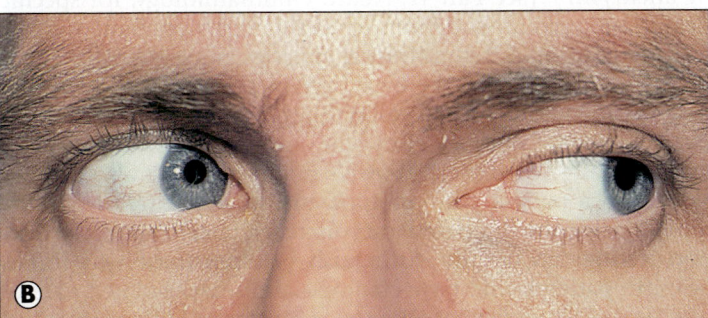

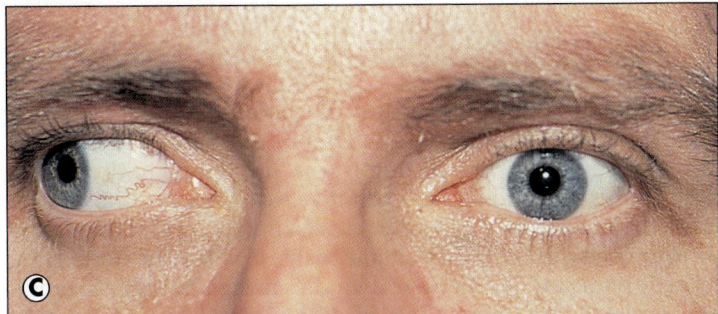

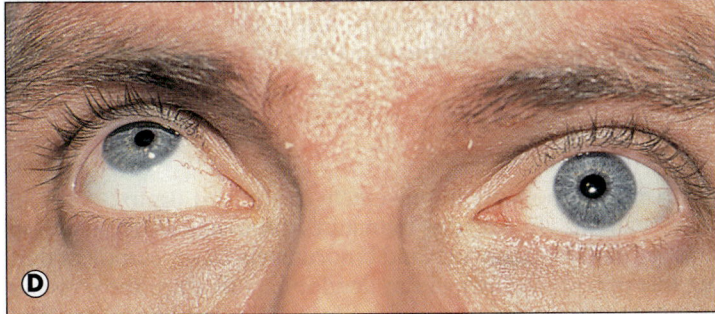

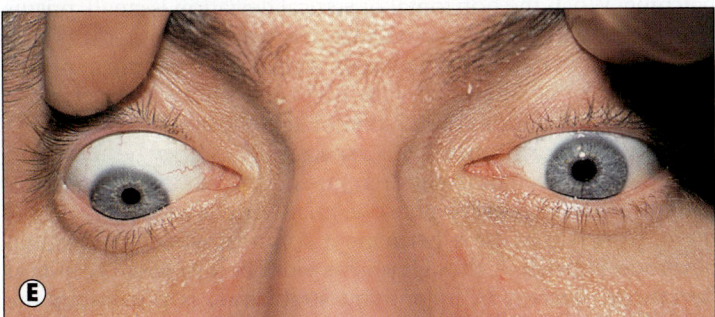

FIG. 77-1 ■ **Adult who has a partial left third nerve palsy. A,** Primary gaze showing slightly larger pupil, mild ptosis, left exotropia, and left hypotropia. **B,** Normal left gaze. **C,** No adduction of the left eye on right gaze. **D,** Poor elevation. **E,** Poor depression.

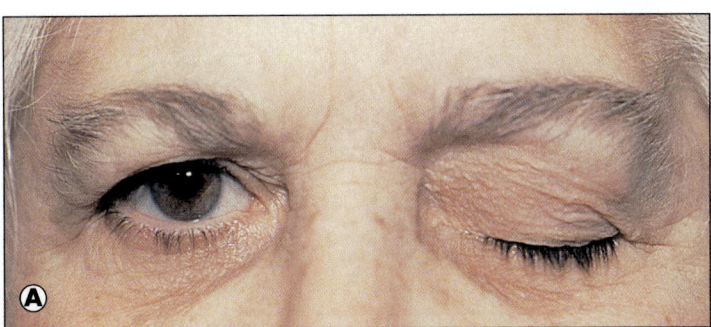

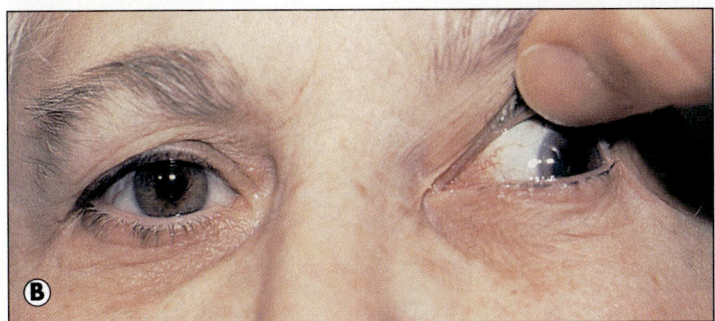

FIG. 77-2 ■ **Elderly woman who has complete left third nerve palsy. A,** Complete ptosis, left eye. **B,** Left exotropia and (small) left hypotropia.

cumulative with an already calamitous effect on their immature, developing visual system.

OCULAR MANIFESTATIONS

Third nerve palsies can be congenital or acquired; each can be partial, affecting one or more muscles (Fig. 77-1), or complete (Fig. 77-2). Possible causes, manifestation, associated features, and treatment vary according to the type of palsy. Cyclic palsies have also been reported.[2]

Among conditions that affect ocular motility, aberrant regeneration is a phenomenon peculiar to third nerve palsies, hence the alternative term *oculomotor synkinesis*. After injury or other compromise of function, the extramedullary axons can heal and regenerate, but not necessarily to their original locations.[3] Hence, action potentials that resulted in adduction prior to injury may produce, instead of or in addition to adduction, depression, retraction from simultaneous vertical rectus muscle contraction, globe elevation, lid elevation, or pupillary constriction. The two most common manifestations are lid elevation (pseudo-Graefe sign) and pupillary constriction, each of which occurs on adduction, downgaze, or both.

Congenital Third Nerve Palsies

Congenital third nerve palsies (generally idiopathic) are quite rare—most reports consist of only a handful of cases, yet they span decades and are from large institutions (Fig. 77-3). Affected children most often have unilateral involvement and no other neurological abnormalities.[3] Some of the latter have been reported[4] but are thought to represent concurrent injury rather than cause. These cases cannot be considered traumatic in origin as excessive birth trauma is not found in all cases.

Most often, all of the extraocular muscles innervated by the third nerve are affected in some way, resulting in exotropia (from unaffected lateral rectus muscle function), hypotropia (from the small depressor effect of the functioning superior oblique muscle, now unopposed by the paretic superior rectus and inferior oblique muscles), and ptosis (due to levator involvement) of varying amounts. The measured deviation is largest in the field of action of the affected muscle(s). Pupillary involvement in congenital palsies can result from either a primary manifestation of

sion), palsies and paresis of this nerve can have a comprehensive effect upon ocular motility; this nerve innervates extraocular muscles responsible for motility in all three planes (horizontal, vertical, and torsional) and is also the major determinant of levator muscle function. In the case of affected young children who develop a significant ptosis, the visual axis obstruction is

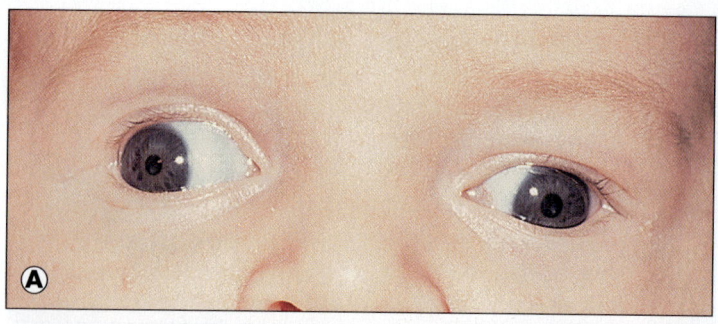

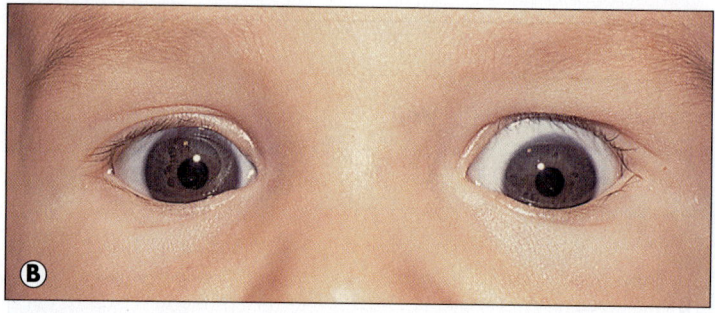

FIG. 77-3 ▮ Congenital left third nerve palsy in an otherwise healthy boy. **A,** At 6 weeks of age, large left exotropia. **B,** At 4 months of age, after spontaneous improvement, left exotropia is 16D.

TABLE 77-1

CAUSES OF ACQUIRED THIRD NERVE PALSY BY AGE GROUP

Cause	Children (%)	Adults (%)
Trauma	40	14
Neoplasm	14	11
Aneurysm	0	12
Vascular/diabetic	0	23
Other	29	16
Undetermined	17	24

Reproduced with permission from Kodsi SR, Younge BR. Acquired oculomotor, trochlear, and abducent cranial nerve palsies in pediatric patients. Am J Ophthalmol. 1992;114:568–74.

the palsy (a larger pupil from deficient sphincter innervation) or aberrant regeneration (pupillary constriction with adduction or downgaze). Pupillary sparing is not a reliable indicator of congenital origin as its presence in congenital cases is inconsistent.[3,5] When ptosis is either absent or incomplete, to optimize their binocularity affected children may develop an abnormal head posture (torticollis) consisting of chin elevation or a contralateral face turn to neutralize the hypotropia, ptosis, or exotropia. Most such children suffer loss of binocular function from ptosis or constant exotropia in addition to amblyopia.

Neurological evaluation of affected children is generally indicated for several reasons. Any associated (noncausative) neuropathology, alluded to earlier, must be sought. In addition, significant central nervous system pathology that may be the cause of the palsy, however infrequent, should be ruled out (see Part 11, Neuro-Ophthalmology, for more detailed recommendations for evaluation).

Acquired Third Nerve Palsies

Acquired third nerve palsies, although more common than their congenital counterpart, are still unusual, so any incidence data are imprecise. They also are rarely bilateral. Possible causes are age dependent (Table 77-1).

Acquired palsies of the oculomotor nerve produce findings similar to those of a congenital palsy. Exotropia, hypotropia, and ptosis are manifest commensurate with involvement of the

respective divisions or subnuclei, along with the characteristic incomitant deviation largest in the field of action of the affected muscle(s). In addition, visually mature adults report diplopia and visual confusion unless they also have significant ptosis. Torticollis (contralateral face turn or chin-up posture) also develops if the posture neutralizes the diplopia.

Patients who have an acquired third nerve palsy require further neurological evaluation as the palsy is often an ominous sign, especially in younger patients,[6] although exceptions occur.[7] Once thought indicative of benign and non–life-threatening vascular disease, pupillary sparing can occur even in cases caused by aneurysm[8,9] (see Part 11, Neuro-Ophthalmology, for specific details and recommendations for evaluating these patients).

Isolated pareses of individual muscles innervated by either branch of the third nerve have been described[10] and generally defy neuroanatomic localization. They are almost never indicative of serious pathology elsewhere, and manifestations depend upon the affected muscle. Brown's syndrome must also be considered in a patient with an apparent isolated inferior oblique muscle palsy; the three-step test (discussed later) and forced duction testing can usually distinguish between these two conditions. In patients who have craniofacial disease, isolated pareses may be due to congenital absence of a rectus or oblique muscle.[11]

TREATMENT

Third nerve palsy is among the most difficult and challenging of the paralytic strabismus syndromes because of the relatively large number of muscles and different motility planes involved and the significant risk of amblyopia in young children from both strabismus and ptosis. Definitive treatment is almost never immediately required as many cases exhibit at least some degree of improvement, either spontaneously or when an underlying cause is removed or otherwise dwindles in significance. The therapeutic goals are elimination of diplopia and optimization of binocularity in as many gaze positions as possible. Restoration of normal motility is generally not attainable except in the mildest of cases, so realistic goals should be made clear to the patient and family in the early stages of treatment.

Nonsurgical Treatment

The period of possible improvement can extend up to 3 years in some patients. In visually immature children, careful attention must be paid to monocular and binocular visual development during this period. Amblyopia can develop rapidly from the constant exotropia-hypotropia or occlusion by the lid, requiring aggressive patching. When the horizontal or vertical deviation is small, prisms may be beneficial to keep binocular development on track.

In visually mature individuals without a complete ptosis, diplopia may be alleviated with occlusion during the period of expectant observation. Even incomplete occlusion, accomplished by applying translucent tape to a spectacle lens, may be sufficient.

In visually immature children, in addition to their temporary use during the recovery phase to maintain binocular development, prisms may be a permanent solution when the residual deviation is small. Although prisms work best in small comitant deviations, success in incomitant strabismus is possible if the prism's magnitude is chosen to match the functionally important primary position and downgaze.

Botulinum toxin therapy can be a useful adjunct to treatment in the acute phase. Injecting the antagonist muscle(s), either by direct surgical visualization or transconjunctivally under audible electromyographic control, can prevent permanent contracture, which would otherwise interfere with recovery or complicate subsequent surgical treatment, or both.[12,13]

Surgical Treatment

Surgical treatment should be undertaken when little if any expectation of additional subsequent recovery exists. When some medial rectus muscle function is present, a large recess-resect procedure may produce acceptable results for the horizontal deviation[14]; this has been advocated in some patients with complete paralysis if combined with a traction suture.[15] Generally, in a complete palsy or when no demonstrable medial rectus function exists, some other method to generate adducting force is necessary in addition to functional crippling of the lateral rectus muscle; the latter requires recession at least 16mm from the original insertion.[16] This can be accomplished by transposition of the superior oblique tendon insertion to a position adjacent to the medial rectus insertion, either with[17] or without[18] its removal from the trochlea. Resections of completely nonfunctional muscles have little long-term effect as the nonfunctioning muscle stretches with time.

Although advocated by some for routine use in all cooperative strabismus surgical patients, adjustable sutures have an even greater indication in surgery for paralytic strabismus. The great variability in the degree of weakness of affected muscles makes published tables of graded recessions and resections somewhat less reliable in third, fourth, and sixth nerve palsies. This suggests a greater potential role for an adjustable suture technique.

An accompanying ptosis is generally addressed after ocular alignment has been optimized. If done in reverse order, raising the lid of a hypotropic eye unable to utilize Bell's phenomenon to protect the cornea may produce significant exposure keratitis. However, this strategy may have to be followed in visually immature children to prevent the development or worsening of amblyopia.

With isolated muscle palsies, the prognosis for an acceptable outcome is much greater because only one muscle is affected, producing a deviation in only one direction and without lid involvement. Such pareses are generally treated by weakening the antagonist muscle along with strengthening (resection) of the affected muscle, provided some of its function remains. In the case of isolated inferior oblique muscle paresis, antagonist weakening (of the superior oblique muscle) must be done with caution because of the resulting effects on ocular torsion. In such cases, vertical rectus muscle weakening can also be effective.[19]

Whenever multiple rectus muscles on the same eye are operated upon, anterior segment ischemia (ASI) is a possible complication. This condition may result when perfusion of the anterior segment is abruptly compromised by sudden loss of the contribution made from the anterior ciliary arteries that normally accompany the rectus muscles and penetrate the sclera at the muscle insertions. The contribution from the vertical rectus muscles is generally greater than that from the horizontal rectus muscles. With time, lost contribution to the anterior segment can be replaced, at least in part, by augmented circulation from another source (the posterior ciliary circulation). Although this lends support to the strategy of staging surgery by waiting several months to operate on additional muscles when multiple rectus muscles need to be operated upon, ASI can occur many years after the initial extraocular surgery.[20] Acute manifestations of ASI include pain, corneal edema, Descemet's membrane folds, and anterior chamber inflammation. Late effects include iris atrophy, an eccentric pupil, and infrequent visual loss.[21] Although ASI usually arises only with surgery on three or four rectus muscles, circumstances such as circulatory disorders or advanced age can increase the risk with surgery on fewer muscles. Preservation of the anterior ciliary circulation during rectus muscle surgery, either with[22] or without[23] use of the operating microscope, has been proposed to reduce if not eliminate the risk of this complication.

FOURTH NERVE PALSY

Unlike third nerve palsies with their protean manifestations, fourth (and sixth) nerve palsies generally have less complicated clinical pictures because these two cranial nerves each innervate only one extraocular muscle. The fourth (trochlear) nerve controls the superior oblique muscle, and the sixth (abducens) nerve innervates the lateral rectus muscle. As the superior oblique muscle acts as a depressor and is the major intorter of the eye, manifestations of its weakness or paralysis are more complicated than those of the sixth nerve, which has no torsional or vertical effects.

Although incidence data are age dependent, large series generally indicate that palsies of the fourth nerve occur somewhat less often than those of the third cranial nerve.[14,24-26] Data from a practice based on strabismus surgery, however, might indicate that they are the most common palsy.[10] The much greater ability of patients to keep a fourth nerve palsy latent (with the development of large vertical fusional vergence amplitudes) may influence the reported statistics.

EPIDEMIOLOGY AND PATHOGENESIS

The cause of an isolated fourth nerve palsy, congenital or acquired, is usually less of a concern than it is for third or sixth nerve palsies, as fourth nerve palsies rarely have a sinister cause. When a history of recent major trauma is lacking, a neurological work-up may be considered but is usually unproductive. Most cases are congenital (idiopathic) or post-traumatically acquired in origin.[3,27] The fourth cranial nerve is uniquely susceptible to trauma[28] as it is the only one with a ventral exit from the brainstem, which results in the longest intracranial course. A patient who has a "unilateral" palsy, especially in traumatic cases, should be very carefully and meticulously examined for evidence of bilateral involvement, which may not become evident until after surgery.[10]

Congenital fourth nerve palsy is almost always sporadic; there are only rare reports of familial occurrence.[29,30] Although the diagnosis in many patients is not made in childhood or youth, inspection of old photographs often reveals a consistent characteristic head tilt. The patients also commonly exhibit the facial asymmetry discussed earlier. Amblyopia is almost never a complication in congenital or early acquired cases.[31] In rare cases, a fourth nerve "palsy" is due to congenital absence of the superior oblique tendon or muscle,[32] especially in patients who have craniofacial disorders.[11] This can be suspected preoperatively on finding an associated horizontal deviation, amblyopia, a large primary-position hypertropia, spread of comitance, and/or pseudo-overaction of the contralateral superior oblique muscle.[33]

OCULAR MANIFESTATIONS

Weakness of the superior oblique muscle allows unopposed action of its direct antagonist, which results in an ipsilateral hypertropia and excyclotorsion. Vertical diplopia or vague reports of "eyestrain" or other difficulty reading in downgaze are the most common complaints vocalized in fourth nerve palsy. Some of the more observant and articulate patients also report excyclotorsion; affected engineers even draw the equivalent of Lancaster screen findings, including the effect on torsion.

The classical sign of a unilateral fourth nerve palsy is a preferred head position consisting of a contralateral head tilt (an "ocular" torticollis). It is exhibited by most patients and is usually the sole presenting sign in children. In this tilted position, reflex compensatory ocular countertorsion (to counteract the head tilt in direction but not degree for degree in magnitude) of the affected eye recruits the inferior oblique and inferior rectus muscles to produce compensatory excyclotorsion of the affected eye and avoids stimulation of the paretic superior oblique. When those normally acting cyclovertical muscles produce this reflex countertorsion, their opposite vertical effects are mutually neutralized and no vertical deviation results, allowing the patient to maintain fusion. However, with a tilt to the ipsilateral side (the side of the paretic eye), the countertorsion of the affected eye recruits the incyclotorters, the superior rectus and paretic superior oblique muscles. The vertical effect of the normal superior rectus muscle, which produces elevation, is unopposed or insufficiently neutralized by the weakened superior oblique muscle, resulting in an ipsilateral hypertropia[34] (Fig. 77-4). Paradoxically, some patients maintain a head tilt to the ipsilateral side, presumably to increase the vertical separation

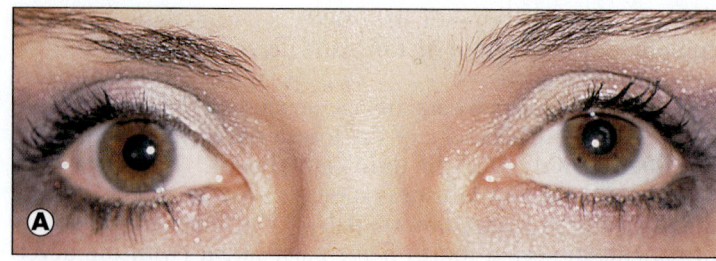

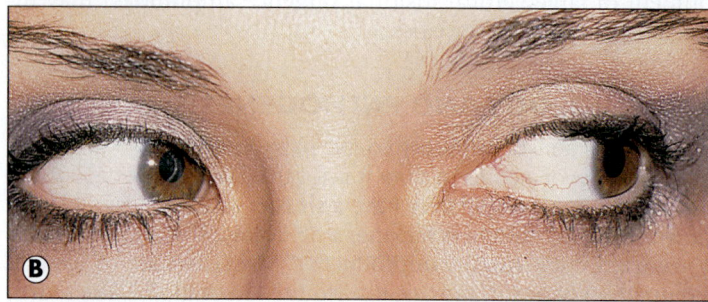

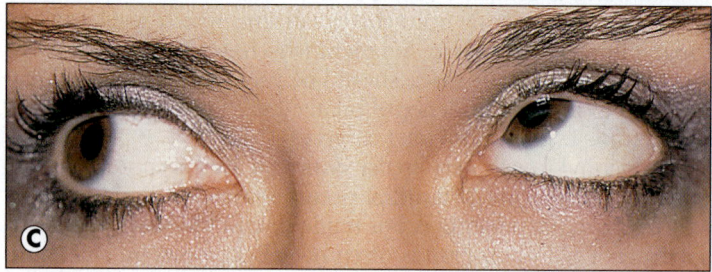

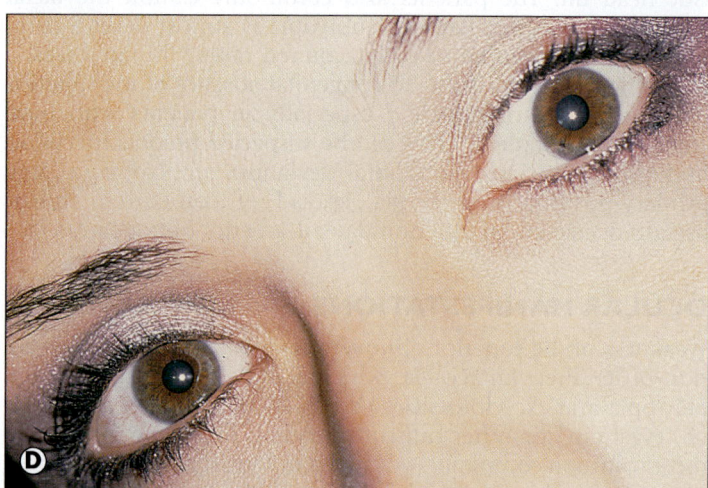

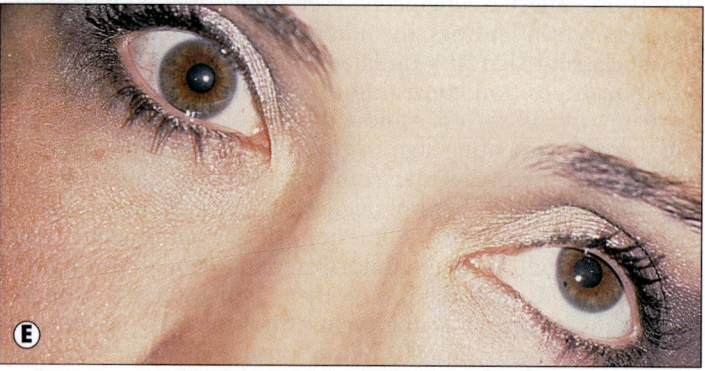

FIG. 77-4 ■ **Young woman who has idiopathic (presumed congenital) left fourth nerve palsy. A,** Primary position left hypertropia from loss of the depressor effect of the paretic left superior oblique muscle. **B,** Normal motility in left gaze, away from the fields of action of the paretic left superior oblique muscle. **C,** Compensatory overaction of the antagonist left inferior oblique muscle in its field of action in right gaze. **D,** No vertical deviation on contralateral head tilt, when reflex excyclotorsion of the affected left eye is accomplished by the unaffected inferior rectus and inferior oblique muscles. **E,** Large left hypertropia on ipsilateral head tilt, when reflex incyclotorsion recruits the superior rectus muscle and the paretic superior oblique muscle, and the vertical effect of the unaffected superior rectus muscle cannot be neutralized by the paretic superior oblique muscle.

between the images and make it easier simply to ignore one of them.[35] A contralateral face turn may also occur to put the affected eye farther away from the adducted position in which the superior oblique muscle has its greatest action.

The Bielschowsky head-tilt test[36] can be used to confirm the presence of a fourth nerve palsy or of any isolated cyclovertical muscle palsy if vision in each eye is adequate for fixation and there are no restrictions on either globe. It must be performed while the patient is erect or else the vestibular input, upon which this test is heavily dependent, will be eliminated. The test was modified by Parks[37]; it is now often termed the *three-step test* and is summarized in Table 77-2. Each of the three steps consists of an alternate cover test measurement of the deviation in the indicated gaze position(s): primary position for step one, right and left gaze for step two, and head tilt (of about 45°) to each side for step three. Table 77-3 summarizes the eight possible outcomes of the *three-step test* as well as which of the eight cyclovertical muscles is the culprit in each condition. It is important to remember that a positive three-step test does not prove the existence of a cyclocervical muscle paresis—it may be positive due to other causes such as Brown's syndrome.

Patients who have a bilateral palsy often have bilateral "reversing" hypertropias (e.g., a right hypertropia on left gaze and a left hypertropia on right gaze) and a bilaterally positive third step of the three-step test (right hypertropia on right head tilt and left hypertropia on left head tilt). A bilateral palsy often causes a chin-down head position in response to a V-pattern esotropia, resulting from the loss of the superior oblique muscle's tertiary abductive action in downgaze and large degrees of cyclotorsion, as discussed subsequently.

Although symptoms of cyclotropia should be evident in any acquired fourth nerve palsy, it is often not a significant problem except in acquired bilateral cases, which typically result from closed head trauma. In congenital or very early acquired cases, sensory reorientation of the retinal meridians develops to eliminate subjective cyclotropia.[38,39] When both superior oblique muscles are weak or completely paralyzed, their opposing hyper-

TABLE 77-2

THE THREE-STEP TEST FOR DIAGNOSIS OF AN ISOLATED SINGLE CYCLOVERTICAL MUSCLE PALSY

Step	Test
1	Determine whether there is a right or left hypertropia in or near primary gaze.
2	Determine the lateral gaze direction that worsens the hypertropia.
3	Determine the side to which tilting the head increases the hypertropia.

TABLE 77-3

CHARACTERISTIC THREE-STEP TEST PATTERNS AND THEIR INTERPRETATION

Test Outcome (Step 1–Step 2–Step 3)	Affected Cyclovertical Muscle
R–L–R	Right superior oblique muscle
L–R–L	Left superior oblique muscle
L–L–L	Right inferior oblique muscle
R–R–R	Left inferior oblique muscle
L–L–R	Left inferior rectus muscle
R–R–L	Right inferior rectus muscle
L–R–R	Right superior rectus muscle
R–L–L	Left superior rectus muscle

This test requires each eye to have vision sufficient for fixation and no restrictions. The test is not helpful in patients who have more than one weak cyclovertical muscle in each eye and may be positive in patients with Brown's syndrome, muscle entrapment, or other causes of restricted eye movement.

tropias can nullify each other, but their cyclodeviations are additive; the paresis on each side produces an ipsilateral excyclotropia that worsens the effect of the excyclotropia of the fellow eye. This effect is maximized in downgaze, the field of greatest action of both superior oblique muscles. When the excyclotorsion (as measured by double Maddox rod) exceeds 10°[40] or 15°,[41,42] a bilateral fourth nerve palsy is strongly suggested, although smaller amounts of torsion do not rule out a bilateral palsy.[27] Such affected patients, having no hypertropia to cause them to develop a compensatory head tilt, may still prefer a chin-down head position to keep their eyes in the upgaze position. In this gaze position, the paretic superior oblique muscles contribute least to ocular alignment, thus minimizing the cyclotropia and V-pattern esotropia. Assessment of the relative positions of the disc and fovea with indirect ophthalmoscopy can be used to assess torsion in preverbal children or otherwise uncooperative patients.[43,44]

Congenital or long-standing fourth nerve paresis can cause physiological and anatomic changes that may be helpful in suggesting the time of onset. These patients are constantly challenged to maintain fusion despite a slowly increasing vertical deviation, allowing very large vertical vergence amplitudes to develop; 15–20 prism diopters are not unusual in these patients, a normal value being 3–4 prism diopters.[45] In addition, the constant head tilt is strongly associated with facial asymmetry; the ipsilateral side is vertically shortened and hypoplastic. In such patients, a line drawn through both pupils and another line drawn through the corners of the mouth intersect near the face on the side of the tilt instead of running parallel as in patients who have symmetrical facies. The asymmetry was once thought to be due to ipsilateral carotid artery compression, but more recent work suggests that it is due to deformational molding from monotonous ipsilateral positioning during sleep.[46] Early surgery in congenital cases is thought to prevent this asymmetry.[46,47]

TREATMENT

General principles of treatment apply in fourth nerve palsies—small, asymptomatic deviations can usually be ignored until they produce a bothersome head tilt or other discomfort. In children, a persistent head tilt can, in some cases, induce scoliosis.[48]

Small, symptomatic deviations may, in some cases, be successfully treated using prisms. Even though incomitant deviations such as fourth nerve palsies are not ideal indications for prism treatment, some palsies exhibit spread of comitance (a "smoothing out" of the deviation) that makes these palsies more amenable to prism therapy. In cases without spread of comitance, prisms may still be successfully used by addressing primary position and downgaze deviations and by taking advantage of the patient's large vertical vergence amplitudes. As with third nerve palsies, acquired fourth nerve palsies, usually traumatic, should initially be nonsurgically treated during a period of observation lasting at least 6 months; improvement or even complete resolution frequently occurs. However, unlike their third nerve counterparts, congenital fourth nerve palsies almost always progress to the point at which surgery is required.

Surgical Treatment

Surgical treatment of fourth nerve palsies follows the general principles of treatment for any incomitant deviation in that the muscle(s) selected for manipulation must be the one(s) active in the field of largest deviation, especially when primary position and downgaze (reading position) are concerned. One approach is to assume that the antagonist inferior oblique muscle always overacts to some degree and that weakening the inferior oblique muscle with recession, myectomy, or other procedures resolves up to approximately 15Δ of primary position hypertropia. Patients who have larger primary position hypertropias require additional muscle surgery to address the additional deviation, usually with recession of the contralateral inferior rectus muscle

(the yoke of the paretic superior oblique muscle) with or without an adjustable suture technique.

A comprehensive surgical management plan for this difficult problem was codified by Knapp[49] in 1974 and is summarized in Box 77-1; it accounts for the observed spread of comitance and follows the general principles already outlined.

In class 1 and 2, where only one gaze field has a large deviation, the muscle whose field of greatest action lies within that gaze field is operated on. The overacting inferior oblique muscle is weakened in class 1 cases, and the paretic superior oblique muscle is strengthened with a tendon tuck or plication in class 2 cases. A small Brown's syndrome (inability to elevate the eye in adduction) is a desirable result following this surgery for class 2 cases.

In class 3, where all contralateral fields are affected, inferior oblique weakening (or superior oblique strengthening, as originally recommended) can be performed alone for vertical deviations below 20Δ; larger deviations require a graded recession of the contralateral inferior rectus muscle. Class 4 cases evolve from class 3 cases—the deviation extends from the lateral gaze positions to affect all three downgaze positions as well. Knapp[49] recommended the same treatment as in class 3 cases, then to wait for the downgaze deviation to resolve after the lateral gaze deviation had been treated, presuming that it is due to temporary underaction of the ipsilateral inferior rectus muscle. If it did not resolve, he advocated resection of the inferior rectus muscle. More recent analysis attributes this development to contracture of the ipsilateral superior rectus muscle from constant hypertropia[27]; this muscle may be receded for treatment if it is thought that oblique surgery alone will be insufficient.

Class 5 pareses have maximum deviations in the downgaze fields and are unusual. Although Knapp's original recommendation was to tuck the affected superior oblique muscle in combination with tenotomy of the contralateral superior oblique muscle, this strategy may convert a unilateral palsy into a bilateral one.

Bilateral superior oblique palsies constitute Knapp's class 6; he recommended a bilateral tuck of the superior oblique tendon. Successful treatment has been accomplished more recently by the Fells modification[40,50]—bilateral transposition of the anterior half of the superior oblique tendon as originally described by Harada and Ito.[51]

Combined paresis and restriction of the superior oblique muscle constitute class 7 cases; these are usually due to trauma, especially dog bites,[49] directly to the trochlear region. Surgery on the frontal sinus can also be responsible.[10] Knapp offered no solution for this difficult situation; initial alleviation of the restriction with subsequent treatment of the paretic component has since been recommended.

The vast majority of congenital cases have a demonstrable laxity or other abnormality of the tendon, which is infrequently found in acquired cases.[52] When present, this finding strongly suggests treat-

---

BOX 77-1

Knapp Classification of Superior Oblique Paresis

CLASS

1. Greatest deviation is with the affected eye elevated in adduction, the field of the ipsilateral (antagonist) inferior oblique muscle.
2. Greatest deviation is with the affected eye depressed in adduction, the field of the affected paretic superior oblique muscle.
3. Greatest deviation is in all contralateral gazes (down, level, and up).
4. Greatest deviations are in all contralateral gaze and in all downgaze positions (contralateral, straight, and ipsilateral).
5. Greatest deviations are in all downgaze positions.
6. V-Pattern esotropia, cyclotropia, and bilaterally positive three-step test indicates a bilateral palsy.
7. Poor elevation and depression in adduction of the affected eye, resulting from direct injury to the superior oblique muscle, causing its restriction and paresis.

Adapted from Knapp P. Classification and treatment of superior oblique palsy. Am Orthopt J. 1974;24:18–22.

ment with a tendon-strengthening procedure, perhaps combined with weakening of the antagonist inferior oblique muscle.[53]

SIXTH NERVE PALSY

Palsies or paralyses of the sixth cranial nerve have presentations that are much less complex than those of the third or fourth nerves. Because only the lateral rectus muscle is affected, a deviation in the horizontal plane alone is produced, no torsional effects exist, and the lid is uninvolved, thus reducing the amblyogenic causes in susceptible children. Sixth nerve palsies are far more common than either third or fourth nerve palsies in all age groups.[14,24–26]

EPIDEMIOLOGY AND PATHOGENESIS

Truly congenital sixth nerve palsy is unusual and in many cases resolves rapidly[54] (Fig. 77-5). If improvement is not forthcoming after frequent observation, a neurological evaluation should be strongly considered. More often, an esotropia with poor abduction of one or both eyes dating from birth represents another condition (Box 77-2), most commonly congenital esotropia. These children, who have a large, constant esotropia, often exhibit cross-fixation, looking to the right with their left eye and vice versa, thus never having to abduct either eye. A sixth nerve palsy can be ruled out by provoking abduction, either by unilateral occlusion for a few days (risking an occlusion amblyopia in a young infant) or preferably by utilizing the vestibulo-ocular reflex. The examiner holds the baby in front of his or her face at a close distance while they both spin, first to one side and then the other. An examination chair that swivels facilitates this maneuver; caution should be observed when using this procedure on a postprandial baby! If the reflex saccades in the opposite direction are brisk and abduction full, a sixth nerve palsy can be discounted. Möbius' syndrome[55] should be considered, although children with this disorder have other obvious problems (mask-like facies, poor feeding, hypoglossal atrophy, skeletal abnormalities) related to the other elements of this syndrome, which include palsies of the 7th and 12th nerves in addition to the 6th. Also, Duane's syndrome should be considered in the differential diagnosis of a congenital sixth nerve palsy, and congenital gaze palsy has been reported[56] as a cause of an abduction deficit.

As it has a long intracranial course similar to that of the fourth nerve and the longest subarachnoid course of any cranial nerve, the sixth nerve is prone to both injury from trauma and an extensive array of nontraumatic diseases of contiguous and nearby structures, summarized in Box 77-2. A benign ipsilateral recurrent palsy that follows a viral illness or immunization can affect children[57,58]; the adult counterpart has no known cause.[59] Studies indicate that in children trauma is a more common cause of an acquired sixth nerve palsy than neoplasm.[14,24] Earlier studies indicated the reverse, perhaps because of the delayed diagnosis of tumors prior to the advent of computed tomography and magnetic resonance imaging, a delay that allowed a paralytic strabismus to develop.[24] Acquired, bilateral palsies are more ominous than their unilateral counterpart.

Despite the lengthy list of possible causes, acquired unilateral sixth nerve weakness (Fig. 77-6) is often benign. However, careful examination must be performed to make sure the palsy is truly isolated and not accompanied by any other neurological findings that may suggest a serious cause. Patients who have a truly isolated paresis may be observed with serial examination for up to 6 months before any further investigation is indicated.[60] Prompt, spontaneous resolution of a sixth nerve palsy, however, does not rule out neoplasm as a cause in children or adults.[61] The appearance of new indicative findings or progression of the paresis demands immediate investigation. Although rare since the advent of antibiotics, children should be evaluated for otitis media as the cause; Gradenigo's syndrome occurs if contiguous inflammation of the petroclinoid

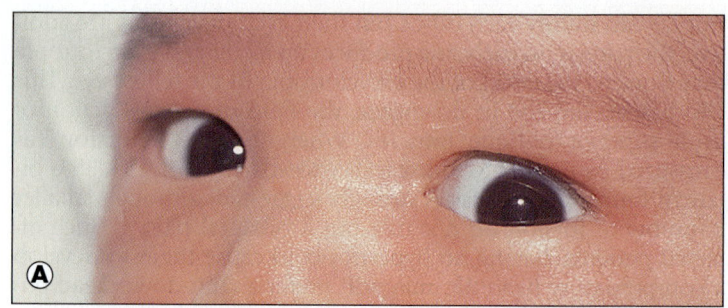
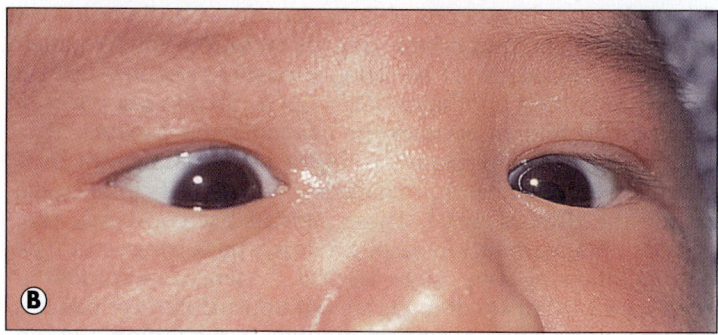

FIG. 77-5 ■ A 1-month-old infant who has congenital right sixth nerve palsy. **A,** Little or no deviation in contralateral (left) gaze. **B,** Large esotropia in ipsilateral (right) gaze.

BOX 77-2

Possible Causes of Abduction Deficits

CONGENITAL	ACQUIRED
Congenital esotropia	Trauma
Möbius' syndrome[58]	Neoplasm
Duane's syndrome	Meningitis
Congenital horizontal gaze palsy	Hydrocephalus
	Benign recurrent sixth nerve palsy[60–62]
	Pseudotumor cerebri
	Gradenigo's syndrome
	Demyelinating disease
	Vascular disease
	Aneurysm
	Postmyelography
	Postimmunization
	Postviral

---

ligament affects the adjacent sixth nerve as it passes through Dorello's canal.[62]

OCULAR MANIFESTATIONS

With its solitary innervation of the lateral rectus muscle, the only result of a sixth nerve palsy is an esotropia, which almost always affects the primary position. In congenital palsies that result from Möbius' syndrome an esotropia may be lacking, which raises the question of whether this syndrome (discussed later) produces a true sixth nerve palsy or, more accurately, a gaze palsy because the horizontal gaze center is very close to or even coincides with the sixth nerve nucleus.[63,64] When present, the esotropia of a sixth nerve palsy initially exhibits the typical findings of a paralytic strabismus; the deviation is maximized in ipsilateral horizontal gaze and smallest in gaze to the opposite side (incomitancy). In addition, in a given gaze position the deviation is larger when the paretic eye is fixing (secondary deviation). However, contracture of its antagonist and yoke muscles (the ipsilateral medial rectus and the contralateral medial rectus muscles, respectively) can rapidly convert the deviation into a comitant esotropia.[65] In unilateral cases that have not yet devel-

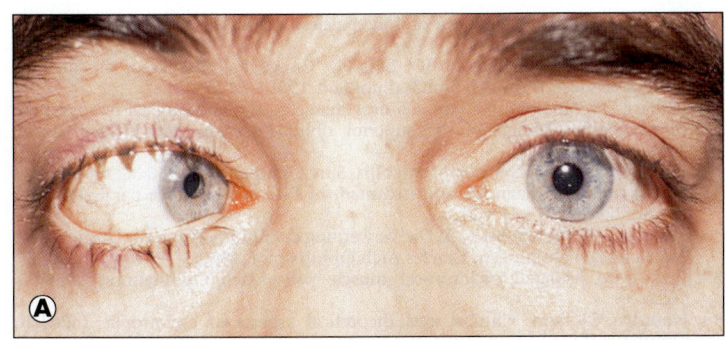

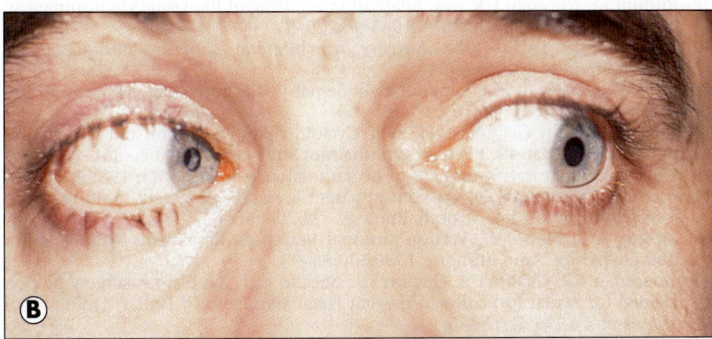

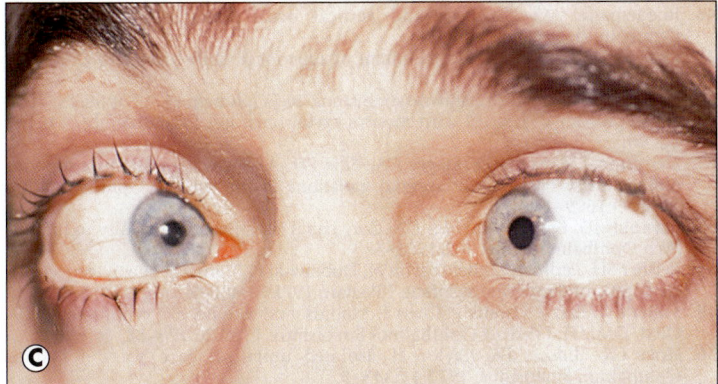

FIG. 77-6 ■ A 33-year-old man who has a right sixth nerve palsy. **A,** Right esotropia in primary position. **B,** No deviation in contralateral (left) gaze. **C,** Large esotropia in ipsilateral (right) gaze—the affected right eye cannot even get to midline position.

oped comitancy, an ipsilateral face turn may be adopted to maintain binocularity.

TREATMENT

As with palsies of the third and fourth cranial nerves, surgical treatment of sixth nerve palsy should be deferred whenever a chance for improvement exists and at least for the first 6 months after onset.

Nonsurgical Treatment

During this period of expectant observation, young children who do not adopt the characteristic ipsilateral face turn to maintain binocularity should undergo alternate occlusion to minimize the possibility of developing amblyopia. They should also be given spectacles with their full hypermetropic correction to minimize accommodation, which can worsen their esotropia. Adults may also appreciate unilateral occlusion to eliminate their uncrossed diplopia.

Small deviations may be amenable to treatment using prisms, especially because the originally incomitant deviation can rapidly become comitant due to contracture of both medial rectus muscles, as discussed earlier. To nurture continued improvement, the minimum amount of horizontal prism that allows fusion should be prescribed, with attempts to decrease prism strength further on subsequent evaluation.

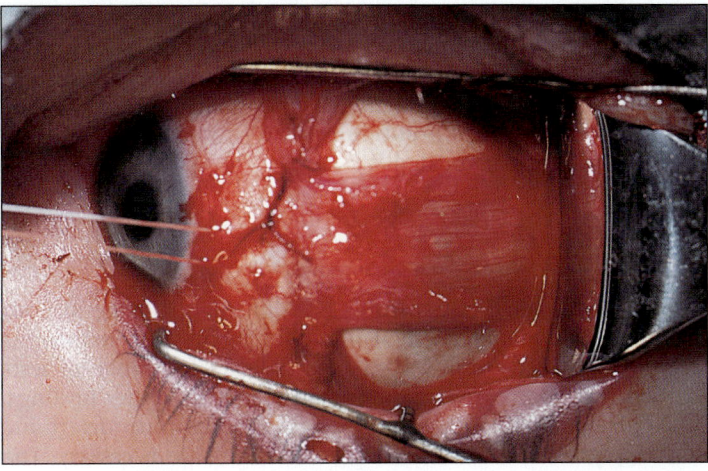

FIG. 77-7 ■ Full-tendon "transposition" of the superior and inferior rectus muscles to the insertion of the left lateral rectus muscle. (Courtesy of R. Scott Foster, MD.)

Chemodenervation with botulinum toxin can be used during the acute phase of a sixth nerve palsy to prevent contracture of the antagonist medial rectus muscle while the lateral rectus muscle recovers function.[12,13,66] Despite its frequent lack of lasting benefit as a sole remedy for chronic palsy,[12,13,66] some patients may require or even prefer its repeated use as their treatment.[67] It is very useful as an adjunct to surgical management and sometimes essential to prevent or minimize the risk of postoperative anterior segment ischemia.

Surgical Treatment

Surgical treatment should be considered when more than 6 months have passed after onset, serial examinations are stable (which indicates that subsequent improvement is unlikely), and the deviation is too large for use of prisms to be considered reasonable. The goals of treatment are primary position alignment and expansion of the diplopia-free field, which may be found only prior to treatment with face turn. The surgical plan is largely determined by the depth of the palsy and the quantity of medial rectus muscle contracture. Remaining lateral rectus muscle function can be assessed directly by a forced generation test,[1] discussed earlier. Careful observation of ipsilateral saccades and modified electro-oculography can provide similar information.[68] Traditional forced duction testing estimates the degree of medial rectus contracture.

When the preceding tests reveal that at least some lateral rectus muscle function remains (usually with an esotropia of less than 30Δ), a graded recess-resect procedure based on published tables often succeeds. Effective treatment when little or no abducting force remains generally requires a new source of abducting force provided by a muscle transposition procedure, together with weakening the usually contracted antagonist medial rectus muscle.

Abducting force can be supplied by moving the adjacent vertical rectus muscles to the lateral rectus muscle insertion or by nonsurgical union of the adjacent halves of the lateral and vertical rectus muscles. The many variations of these techniques are reviewed elsewhere.[69]

The original Hummelsheim procedure[70] involves longitudinally splitting the superior and inferior rectus muscles and transposing each lateral half to the insertion of the paretic lateral rectus muscle. Full-tendon "transpositions," more accurately termed "translations" (Fig. 77-7), can transfer more force and are equally effective; a proposed modification utilizes a posterior fixation suture to better direct the transferred force as horizontally as possible.[71] The Jensen procedure[72] entails longitudinal splitting of the lateral rectus and the vertical rectus muscles. The adjacent halves are then joined with an unabsorbable suture, usually in conjunction with medial rectus recession. Because only one rectus muscle is actually severed from the globe, interrupting its anterior ciliary artery circulation, it was originally thought that this procedure would eliminate the risk of ASI, a theory that has since been disproved.[73] To minimize this risk and at the same time preserve the effectiveness of full-tendon transposition, adjunctive chemodenervation of the medial rectus muscle with botulinum toxin (instead of surgical recession) has been advocated.[74]

SUMMARY

In summary, paralytic strabismus is a difficult challenge in both diagnosis and management. Patterns of incomitant strabismus must be analyzed using the strabismologist's full range of tests and maneuvers to arrive at the correct diagnosis. Other findings, both historical and physical, must be sought to determine whether systemic evaluation or consultations are necessary. The management of paralytic strabismus, especially with surgery, challenges us to maximize alignment and motility with fewer normally functioning muscles than in the original complex design.

REFERENCES

1. Scott AB. Active force tests in lateral rectus paralysis. Arch Ophthalmol. 1971;85:397–404.
2. Bateman DE, Saunders M. Cyclic oculomotor palsy: description of a case and hypothesis of the mechanism. J Neurol Neurosurg Psychiatry. 1983;46:451–3.
3. Miller NR. Walsh and Hoyt's clinical neuro-ophthalmology, 4th ed, Vol 2, Ch 35. Baltimore: Williams & Wilkins; 1985:652–784.
4. Balkan R, Hoyt CS. Associated neurologic abnormalities in congenital third nerve palsies. Am J Ophthalmol. 1984;97:315–19.
5. Ing EB, Sullivan TJ, Clarke MP, Buncic JR. Oculomotor nerve palsies in children. J Pediatr Ophthalmol Strabismus. 1992;29:331–6.
6. Abdul-Rahim AS, Savino PJ, Zimmerman RA, et al. Cryptogenic oculomotor nerve palsy: the need for repeated neuroimaging studies. Arch Ophthalmol. 1987; 107:387–90.
7. Mizen TR, Burde RM, Klingele TG. Cryptogenic oculomotor nerve palsies in children. Am J Ophthalmol. 1985;100:65–7.
8. Trobe JD. Third nerve palsy and the pupil: footnotes to the rule. Arch Ophthalmol. 1988;106:601–2.
9. Lustbader JM, Miller NR. Painless, pupil-sparing but otherwise complete oculomotor nerve paresis caused by basilar artery aneurysm. Arch Ophthalmol. 1988; 106:583–4.
10. Noorden GK von. Binocular vision and ocular motility, Ch 18. St Louis: Mosby–Year Book; 1996:392–429.
11. Diamond GR, Katowitz JA, Whitaker LA, et al. Variations in extraocular muscle number and structure in craniofacial dysostosis. Am J Ophthalmol. 1980; 90:416–18.
12. Ad Hoc Committee on Ophthalmic Procedures Assessment of the American Academy of Ophthalmology. Botulinum toxin therapy of eye muscle disorders. Ophthalmology. 1989;96(suppl):37–41.
13. Metz HS, Mazow M. Botulinum treatment of acute sixth and third nerve palsy. Graefes Arch Clin Exp Ophthalmol. 1988;226:141–4.
14. Harley RD. Paralytic strabismus in children. Etiologic incidence and management of the third, fourth, and sixth nerve palsies. Ophthalmology. 1980;87:24–43.
15. Helveston EM. Surgical management of strabismus, 4th ed. St Louis: Mosby–Year Book; 1993:302.
16. Nelson LB. Strabismus disorders. In: Nelson LB, Calhoun JH, Harley RB, eds. Pediatric ophthalmology, 3rd ed, Ch 7. Philadelphia: WB Saunders; 1991: 128–75.
17. Reinecke RD. Surgical management of third and sixth cranial nerve palsies. In: Nelson LB, Wagner RS, eds. Strabismus surgery. International ophthalmology clinics. Boston: Little, Brown; 1985:139–48.
18. Scott AB. Transposition of the superior oblique. Am Orthopt J. 1977;27:11–14.
19. Pollard ZF. Diagnosis and treatment of inferior oblique palsy. J Pediatr Ophthalmol Strabismus. 1993;30:15–18.
20. Saunders RA, Sandall GS. Anterior segment ischemia syndrome following rectus muscle transposition. Am J Ophthalmol. 1982;93:34–8.
21. France TD, Simon JW. Anterior segment ischemia syndrome following muscle surgery: the AAPO&S experience. J Pediatr Ophthalmol Strabismus. 1986;23: 87–91.
22. McKeown CA, Lambert HM, Shore JW. Preservation of the anterior ciliary vessels during extraocular muscle surgery. Ophthalmology. 1989;96:498–507.
23. Freedman HL, Waltman DD, Patterson JH. Preservation of anterior ciliary vessels during strabismus surgery: a nonmicroscopic technique. J Pediatr Ophthalmol Strabismus. 1992;29:38–43.
24. Kodsi SR, Younge BR. Acquired oculomotor, trochlear, and abducent cranial nerve palsies in pediatric patients. Am J Ophthalmol. 1992;114:568–74.
25. Rucker CW. Paralysis of the third, fourth and sixth cranial nerves. Am J Ophthalmol. 1958;46:787–94.
26. Rucker CW. The causes of paralysis of the third, fourth, and sixth cranial nerves. Am J Ophthalmol. 1966;61:1293–8.
27. Noorden GK von, Murray E, Wong SY. Superior oblique paralysis. A review of 270 cases. Arch Ophthalmol. 1986;104:1771–6.
28. Mansour AM, Reinecke RD. Central trochlear palsy. Surv Ophthalmol. 1986;30: 279–97.
29. Astle WF, Rosenbaum AL. Familial congenital fourth nerve palsy. Arch Ophthalmol. 1985;103:532–5.
30. Harris DJ Jr, Memmen JE, Katz NNK, Parks MM. Familial congenital superior oblique palsy. Ophthalmology. 1986;93:88–90.
31. Robb RM. Idiopathic superior oblique palsies in children. J Pediatr Ophthalmol Strabismus. 1990;27:66–9.
32. Helveston EM, Giangiacomo JD, Ellis FD. Congenital absence of the superior oblique tendon. Trans Am Ophthalmol Soc. 1981;79:123–35.
33. Wallace DK, Noorden GK von. Clinical characteristics and surgical management of congenital absence of the superior oblique tendon. Am J Ophthalmol. 1994;118:63–9.
34. Rubin SE, Wagner RS. Ocular torticollis. Surv Ophthalmol. 1986;30:366–76.
35. Gobin MH. The diagnosis and treatment of IVth cranial nerve paralysis. Ophthalmologica. 1976;173:292–5.
36. Hofmann FB, Bielschowsky A. Die Verwertung der Knipfneigung zur Diagnose der Augenmuskellahmungen. Graefes Arch Ophthalmol. 1900;51:174.
37. Parks MM. Isolated cyclovertical muscle palsy. Arch Ophthalmol. 1958;60: 1027–35.
38. Noorden GK von. Clinical and theoretical aspects of cyclotropia. J Pediatr Ophthalmol Strabismus. 1984;21:126–32.
39. Ruttum M, Noorden GK von. Adaptation to tilting of the visual environment in cyclotropia. Am J Ophthalmol. 1983;96:229–37.
40. Mitchell PR, Parks, MM. Surgery for bilateral superior oblique palsy. Ophthalmology. 1982;89:484–8.
41. Ellis FD, Helveston EM. Superior oblique palsy: diagnosis and classification. Int Ophthalmol Clin. 1976;16:127–35.
42. Kraft SP, O'Reilly C, Quigley PL, et al. Cyclotorsion in unilateral and bilateral superior oblique paresis. J Pediatr Ophthalmol Strabismus. 1993;30:361–7.
43. Guyton DL. Clinical assessment of ocular torsion. Am Orthopt J. 1983;33:7–15.
44. Bixenman WW, Noorden GK von. Apparent foveal displacement in normal subjects and in cyclotropia. Ophthalmology. 1982;89:58–62.
45. Mottier ME, Mets MB. Vertical fusional vergences in patients with superior oblique palsies. Am Orthopt J. 1990;100:88–93.
46. Goodman CR, Chabner E, Guyton DL. Should early strabismus surgery be performed for ocular torticollis to prevent facial asymmetry? J Pediatr Ophthalmol Strabismus. 1995;32:162–6.
47. Wilson ME, Hoxie J. Facial asymmetry in superior oblique muscle palsy. J Pediatr Ophthalmol Strabismus. 1993;30:315–18.
48. Ruedemann AD. Scoliosis and vertical ocular muscle imbalance. Arch Ophthalmol. 1956;56:389–414.
49. Knapp P. Classification and treatment of superior oblique palsy. Am Orthopt J. 1974;24:18–22.
50. Fells P. Management of paralytic strabismus. Br J Ophthalmol. 1974;58:255–65.
51. Harada M, Ito Y. Surgical correction of cyclotropia. Jpn J Ophthalmol. 1964;8: 88–96.
52. Helveston EM, Krach D, Plager DA, Ellis FD. A new classification of superior oblique palsy based on congenital variations in the tendon. Ophthalmology. 1992;99:1609–15.
53. Reynolds JD, Biglan AW, Hiles DA. Congenital superior oblique palsy in infants. Arch Ophthalmol. 1984;102:1503–5.
54. Reisner SH, Perlman M, Ben-Tovim N, Dubrawski C. Transient lateral rectus muscle paresis in the newborn infant. J Pediatr. 1971;78:461–5.
55. Miller MT, Ray V, Owens P, Chen F. Möbius' and Möbius-like syndromes (TTV-OFM, OMLH). J Pediatr Ophthalmol Strabismus. 1989;26:176–88.
56. Hoyt CS, Billson FA, Taylor H. Isolated unilateral gaze palsy. J Pediatr Ophthalmol Strabismus. 1977;14:343–5.
57. Bixenman WW, Noorden GK von. Benign recurrent VI nerve palsy in childhood. J Pediatr Ophthalmol Strabismus. 1981;18:29–34.
58. Werner DB, Savino PJ, Schatz NJ. Benign recurrent sixth nerve palsies in childhood. Secondary to immunization or viral illness. Arch Ophthalmol. 1983;101:607–8.
59. Hamilton SR, Lessell S. Recurrent idiopathic lateral rectus muscle palsy in adults. Am J Ophthalmol. 1991;112:540–2.
60. Savino PJ, Hilliker JK, Cassell GH, Schatz NJ. Chronic sixth nerve palsies. Are they really harbingers of serious intracranial disease? Arch Ophthalmol. 1982;100:1442–4.
61. Volpe NJ, Lessell S. Remitting sixth nerve palsy in skull base tumors. Arch Ophthalmol. 1993;111:1391–5.
62. Gradenigo G. A special syndrome of endocranial otitic complications (paralysis of the motor oculi externus of otitic origin). Ann Otol Rhinol Laryngol. 1904;13:637.
63. Brodsky MC, Baker RS, Hamed LM. Pediatric neuro-ophthalmology, Ch 6. New York: Springer-Verlag; 1996:201–50.
64. Glaser JS. Infranuclear disorders of eye movement. In: Tasman W, Jaeger EA, eds. Duane's clinical ophthalmology, Vol 2, Ch 12. Philadelphia: Lippincott-Raven; 1995:1–56.
65. Parks MM, Mitchell PR. Cranial nerve palsies. In: Tasman W, Jaeger EA, eds. Duane's clinical ophthalmology, Vol 1, Ch 19. Philadelphia: Lippincott-Raven; 1995:1–12.
66. Scott AB, Kraft SP. Botulinum toxin injection in the management of lateral rectus paresis. Ophthalmology. 1985;92:676–83.
67. Lee J. Modern management of sixth nerve palsy. Aust NZ J Ophthalmol. 1992;20:41–6.
68. Metz HS, Scott AB, O'Meara D, Stewart HL. Ocular saccades in lateral rectus palsy. Arch Ophthalmol. 1970;84:453–60.
69. Helveston EM. Surgical management of strabismus, 4th ed. St Louis: Mosby–Year Book; 1993:292–3.
70. Hummelsheim E. Weitere Erfahrungen mit partieller Sehnenuberpflanzung an den Augenmuskeln. Arch Augenheilkd. 1908–1909;62:71–4.
71. Foster RS. Vertical muscle transposition augmented with lateral fixation. J Am Assoc Pediatr Ophthalmol Strabismus. 1997;1:20–30.
72. Jensen CDF. Rectus muscle union: a new operation for paralysis of the rectus muscles. Trans Pacific Coast Ophthalmol Soc. 1964;45:359–87.
73. Noorden GK von. Anterior segment ischemia following the Jensen procedure. Arch Ophthalmol. 1976;94:845–7.
74. Rosenbaum AL, Kushner BJ, Kirschen D. Vertical rectus muscle transposition and botulinum toxin (Oculinum) to medial rectus for abducens palsy. Arch Ophthalmol. 1989;107:820–3.

78 Other Vertical Strabismus Forms

HOWARD M. EGGERS

DEFINITION
- Vertical strabismus not paretic in origin.

KEY FEATURES
- Incomitance.
- Supranuclear or mechanical causation.

INTRODUCTION

The various findings in nonparetic vertical strabismus group into several clinical entities. All share incomitance as a feature. The cause is frequently unknown, although the phenomenology of the deviation is descriptively either supranuclear, a mechanical restriction to rotation, or a local orbital cause of poor muscle contraction.

DISSOCIATED VERTICAL DIVERGENCE

INTRODUCTION

Dissociated vertical divergence (or dissociated vertical deviation; DVD) is characterized by a spontaneous upward deviation of either eye (dissociation) while the other eye fixates a target (Fig. 78-1).[1] The deviation is variable within an episode and from one dissociated episode to another. After a period of usually no more than a few tens of seconds or on a shift of gaze, the eye returns down and may even become mildly hypotropic. The amplitude of the deviation and the frequency of spontaneous dissociation are usually not equal in the two eyes. The spontaneous deviation may occur with or without daydreaming or fatigue, although these states make the deviation worse or the spontaneous dissociation more common.

EPIDEMIOLOGY AND PATHOGENESIS

Although DVD is most common with congenital esotropia, it can occur with any strabismus that develops early in life. While usually associated with a strabismus, DVD may occur as an isolated defect. Elevation in adduction, which produces an apparent inferior oblique overaction, is a common initial presentation. Latent or manifest nystagmus commonly occurs with DVD in congenital esotropia. Seldom present at birth, DVD is frequently a new finding after the age of 2–3 years. In isolated cases of DVD that appear to develop later in life, seldom has it been positively and totally ruled out as a preexisting condition.

OCULAR MANIFESTATIONS

In cover testing, updrift occurs behind the occluder, and the eye returns downward when the occluder is removed and vision restored. Although vision thus plays a role in stabilization of the

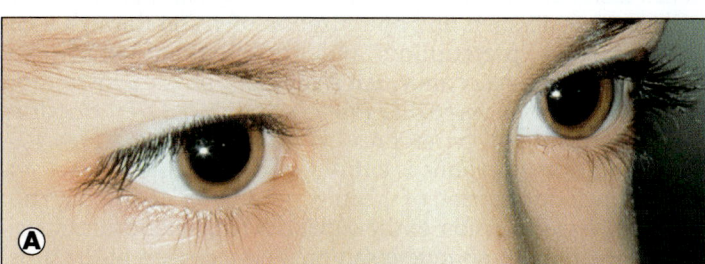
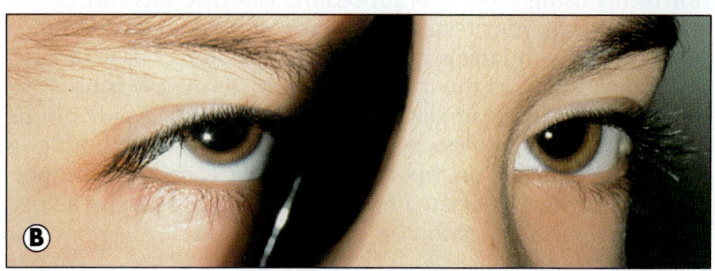

FIG. 78-1 ■ **Dissociated vertical divergence. A,** The eyes are approximately straight in primary position. **B,** Occlusion of an eye leads to an upward drift of the covered eye. Dissociated vertical divergence is usually bilateral, although it may show asymmetrical amounts of drift. On cover testing, each eye drifts up when under cover. A measure of a simultaneous vertical deviation is the prism power that equalizes the amplitude of the vertical drift in the two eyes.

eye position, the deviated eye is suppressed, so visual symptoms seldom occur.[2] Rarely, the suppression is not deep enough and vertical diplopia occurs. Occasionally, a patient may find it physically uncomfortable for the eye to turn upward. The spontaneous deviation may disturb psychosocial function.

Because each eye drifts upward under cover and moves downward on removal of the cover, it is not possible to measure accurately a vertical deviation in the presence of DVD, but the prism power that makes the residual vertical drift symmetrical can be used as an estimate of the deviation. The upward movement is typically accompanied by extorsion of the eye and sometimes a horizontal movement in the exotropic direction. Occasionally, the drift movement is chiefly horizontal and the term dissociated horizontal deviation is used[3]; if it is chiefly torsional, the term dissociated torsional deviation is used.

DIFFERENTIAL DIAGNOSIS

The characteristic findings in DVD eliminate the need for any differential diagnosis except in cases that have minimal involvement, concurrent vertical deviation, or difficulty in examination because of young age. Overaction of the inferior oblique (primary or secondary) and superior oblique paresis must be ruled out. In cases of vertical strabismus, a coexisting DVD may be difficult to diagnose.

DIAGNOSIS

The cause of DVD is the subject of much speculation. The normal versions and ductions imply a defect in supranuclear control of eye position. Eye movement studies implicate an abnormal vertical vergence system.[4] The Bielschowsky phenomenon is a curious characteristic of DVD that must be related to the abnormal supranuclear control of vertical eye position. It is demonstrated by occlusion of one eye to make it deviate upward. Then, a neutral density wedge is placed before the opposite, unoccluded eye. The eye behind the cover makes a gradual downward movement in proportion to the attenuation of light that reaches the open eye.

TREATMENT

Although binocular sensory and motor fusions are poor in DVD, the aim of nonsurgical therapy for DVD is to strengthen the patient's fusional mechanisms. This is done by elimination of any concurrent strabismus and optimization of vision through accurate refractive prescription and treatment of amblyopia. Indications for surgery are visual symptoms, physical discomfort from a large deviation, or disfigurement produced by the updrift. A variety of surgical procedures have been advocated for DVD, which indicates that none is entirely satisfactory. Advocated procedures include resection of the inferior recti, tuck of the superior obliques, large recession of the superior recti, anterior transposition of the inferior oblique insertion, and recession of the superior rectus using the Faden procedure. Good results can be obtained with superior rectus recession combined with the Faden procedure,[5,6] with large superior rectus recessions,[7] or with anterior transposition of the inferior oblique.[8] If one eye is used habitually for fixation, surgery needs to be performed only on the opposite eye. If either eye is used at times for fixation, both eyes need to be operated on, but asymmetrically, each eye in proportion to its drift. Dissociated horizontal deviation can be helped by a lateral rectus recession on the involved side.

STRABISMUS SURSOADDUCTORIUS

EPIDEMIOLOGY AND PATHOGENESIS

Strabismus sursoadductorius may be the result of primary overaction of the inferior obliques (i.e., the cause for the overaction is unknown). Although neurological factors are difficult to rule out, it seems more likely that anatomical variations play a role in its cause. A difference in the plane of action of the superior and inferior obliques, referred to as desagittalization, may leave the inferior oblique with a stronger vertical action in adduction than the superior oblique.[9] Excycloduction of the globe or orbit may raise the insertion of the medial rectus above the horizontal midline to give it a vertical action that assists elevation in adduction and simulates inferior oblique overaction.

OCULAR MANIFESTATIONS

Strabismus sursoadductorius refers to a marked elevation of an eye when in the adducted position under binocular viewing conditions. It is commonly ascribed to overaction of the inferior oblique (Fig. 78-2). No vertical deviation occurs in primary position, and a right hypertropia is seen in left gaze and a left hypertropia in right gaze. The elevation in adduction may be bilaterally symmetrical or asymmetrical. The head-tilt test result is negative. The patient may have esotropia, exotropia, or a V pattern.

DIFFERENTIAL DIAGNOSIS

The differential diagnosis includes secondary inferior oblique overaction (from a paretic ipsilateral superior oblique or contralateral superior rectus), Duane's syndrome, and DVD. Overaction secondary to superior oblique paresis shows a positive head-tilt test. The differentiation of DVD from inferior oblique overaction is important because different surgical procedures are used, depending on the diagnosis.

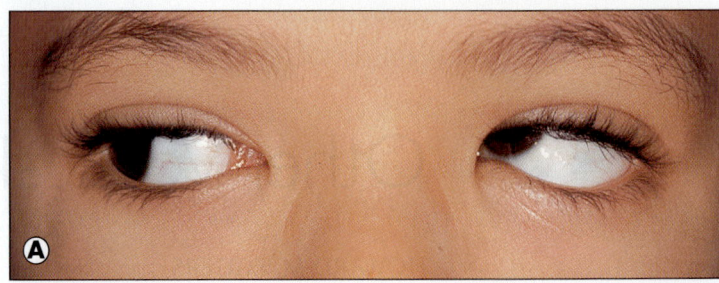
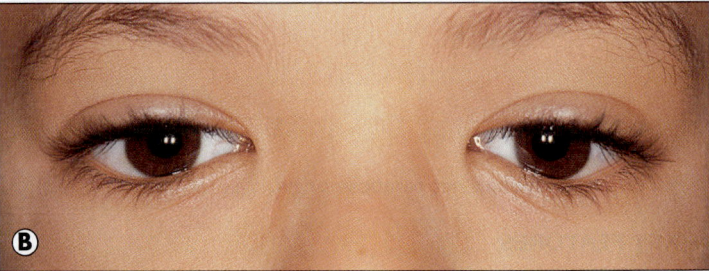
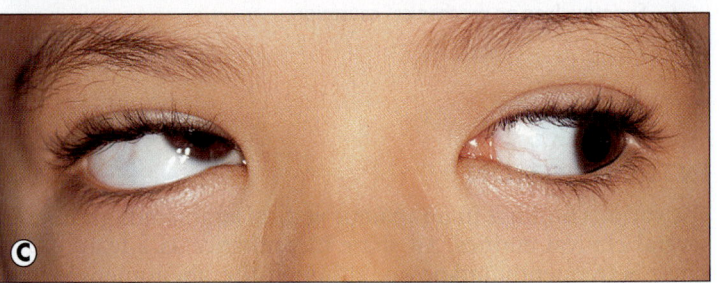

FIG. 78-2 ■ Elevation in adduction. The apparent overaction of the inferior oblique must be confirmed with cover testing. A dissociated vertical divergence frequently gives the same appearance on testing versions. True inferior oblique overaction gives a measurable deviation in lateral gaze and may produce a V pattern. In dissociated vertical divergence, the abducted eye may circumduct under occlusion. **A,** Right gaze. **B,** Gaze in primary position. **C,** Left gaze. Note elevation of adducted eye in lateral gaze to either side.

Strabismus sursoadductorius commonly occurs in congenital esotropia and is frequently confused with DVD. Genuine inferior oblique overaction should produce a V pattern and show measurable vertical deviations in lateral gaze. The abducted eye becomes lower as the high, adducted eye takes up fixation. The deviation is the same regardless of which eye fixates. The vertical fixation shift with alternation of the cover is fast and occurs at saccadic velocities.

In DVD, dissociation of the eyes occurs by occlusion of much of the visual field of the adducted eye by the nose and eyebrow, which results in elevation of the occluded eye. If the adducted eye is the fixating eye, much less or no elevation occurs in adduction. Occlusion of the abducted eye may make that eye elevate and thus reverse the hypertropia findings. The deviation in lateral gaze is not subject to routine prism and cover measurements because each eye moves downward on shift of the occluder to the opposite eye. The updrift and recovery movements are slower than in true tropia of inferior oblique overaction and are frequently accompanied by torsional movements, extorsion as the eye rises, and intorsion during recovery.

TREATMENT

When elevation in adduction genuinely results from inferior oblique overaction, a weakening procedure is required for these muscles.[10] If, in fact, a DVD is responsible for the elevation in adduction, weakening the muscles has little effect, and a procedure for DVD is required. Unilateral, inferior oblique weakening may result in overaction of the opposite inferior oblique after surgery. With the assumption that no mechanical restriction results from inferior oblique surgery, this indicates that a DVD was probably initially the cause. Apparent overaction of the inferior obliques may also disappear after surgery for esotropia.

DOUBLE ELEVATOR PALSY

INTRODUCTION

The apparent paralysis of both elevators (superior rectus and inferior oblique) of one eye that results in a rather large hypotropia on the affected side is uncommon. The levator palpebrae may or may not be involved, and Bell's phenomenon may be present but is usually absent; if it is present, a supranuclear lesion is implied. The pupil is normal, as are horizontal rotations.

EPIDEMIOLOGY AND PATHOGENESIS

Double elevator palsy may be congenital or acquired. The cause of the congenital forms is not known. The anatomical improbability that both the superior rectus and inferior oblique are weakened by a single lesion suggests that a long-standing superior rectus palsy may be the underlying cause. The acquired cases have all been adults who have small lesions in the pretectum[11]; this series of cases that have central nervous system lesions suggests that neuroimaging be carried out in all acquired cases.

DIFFERENTIAL DIAGNOSIS

The differential diagnosis includes mechanical restriction of elevation (orbital floor fracture, Graves' disease, congenital fibrosis of the inferior rectus) and Brown's syndrome (which can sometimes affect primary position).

TREATMENT, COURSE, AND OUTCOMES

A traction test must be carried out to confirm any mechanical restriction of movement. Surgical treatment consists of transferring the entire tendon of both the medial and lateral rectus muscles to the ends of the superior rectus insertion (Knapp's procedure).[12,13] In the absence of inferior rectus restriction, the result may be good. Horizontal rotations are impaired only slightly, and vertical rotations are improved remarkably. If the inferior rectus is restricted, it has to be recessed, either before or after the muscle transposition. Because four anterior ciliary arteries are sacrificed for the transposition, it is best to allow 6 months for adaptation of the blood supply before operation on a third rectus muscle. Alternatively, dissection and preservation of the anterior ciliary arteries from the muscle may enable the third muscle to be included at the initial operation. If the lid height does not improve with the raising of eye position, lid surgery may also be required.

A similar entity of double depressor paralysis occurs only in a congenital form. The inverse surgical procedure is effective.

BROWN'S SYNDROME

INTRODUCTION

The motility features of the superior oblique tendon sheath syndrome are the result of a short anterior sheath of the superior oblique tendon (Fig. 78-3).[14] Brown[14] differentiated true from simulated sheath syndrome on the basis of whether the causative defect was a short anterior sheath or some other anomaly. This differentiation cannot be based on clinical features but can be made only at the time of surgery.

EPIDEMIOLOGY AND PATHOGENESIS

In Brown's original series there was a 3:2 predominance of women to men and nearly twice as many cases involved the

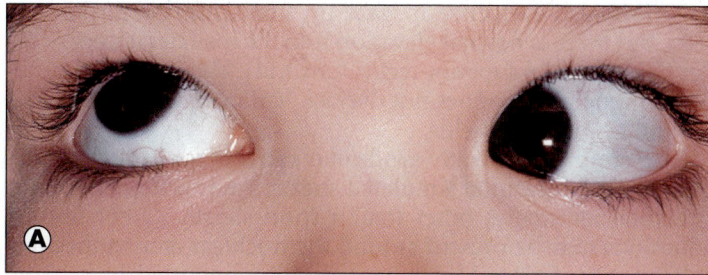
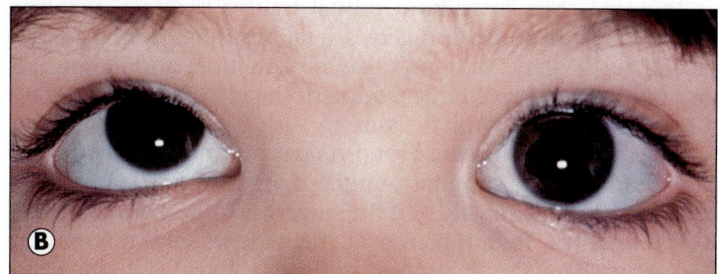
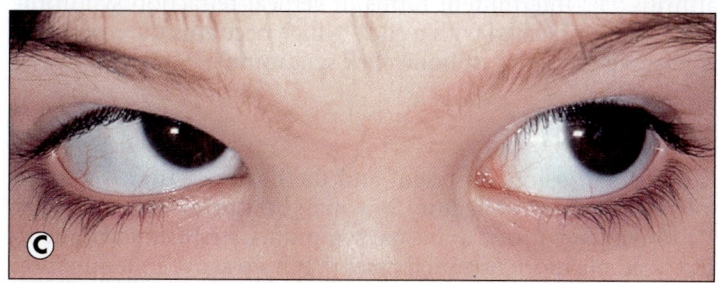
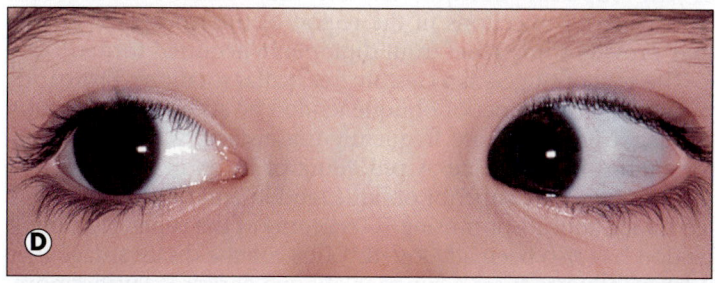
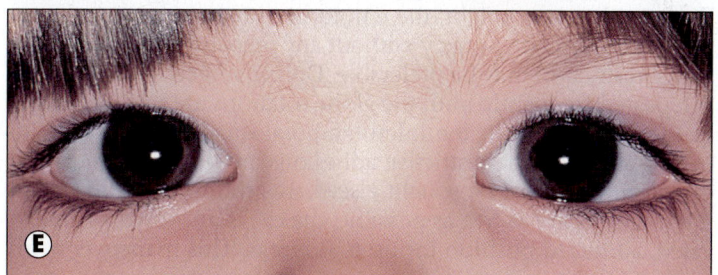

FIG. 78-3 ▌ **Brown's syndrome.** Elevation of the left eye is impaired most in right gaze. The differential diagnosis is one of inferior rectus paresis. Brown's syndrome is characterized by a positive traction test for elevation in adduction, but muscle paresis is not. **A,** Gaze to right and up. Note limitation of elevation of adducted left eye. **B,** Gazing upward shows mild limitation of elevation of left eye. **C,** Gazing left and up shows no restrictions. **D,** Gazing to the right shows no vertical deviation in this case, but one may be present. **E,** Primary position shows no deviation.

right eye as the left; 10% of cases showed bilaterality. Familial occurrence of Brown's syndrome has been reported.[15]

OCULAR MANIFESTATIONS

The most striking clinical feature is restriction of elevation in adduction, which is limited to the horizontal plane. The lid fissure may widen when the eye is adducted. Because the limitation arises from mechanical factors, it is the same on version, duction, and traction tests. The maximal elevation possible increases as the eye moves from adduction to abduction, in which it is normal. Divergence in gaze up from primary position is seen, but there is normal elevation into the ipsilateral upper corner field (normal superior rectus function). The ipsilateral superior oblique usually does not overact. Variable features are head tilt and tropia in all fields.

The simulated sheath syndrome can be congenital or acquired. The congenital simulated sheath syndrome results from structural anomalies other than a short sheath. Other fibrous adhesions may be present around the trochlear area. Adhesions around the inferior oblique have also been reported.

Acquired cases arise from orbital trauma,[16] direct trochlear trauma, orbit or muscle surgery, scleral buckling, frontal sinusitis or sinus surgery, Molteno valve implantation, and inflammation of the superior oblique tendon or sheath. Orbital floor fractures may trap the orbital tissue in such a way as to simulate Brown's syndrome. Brown's syndrome is produced easily during surgery to tuck the superior oblique if the tendon sheath is not stripped away adequately or if the surgery is carried out too close to the trochlea. Inflammation of the superior oblique tendon has occurred in rheumatoid arthritis and juvenile rheumatoid arthritis.[17-19] Intermittent forms of vertical retraction syndrome have been associated with a click, which occurs as the restriction is released (superior oblique click syndrome).[20,21]

TREATMENT

If binocular vision is present and the head position is correct, treatment is not obligatory but may be carried out electively. Treatment is required for visual symptoms, strabismus, or incorrect head position. Acquired cases that have active inflammation of the superior oblique tendon may benefit from local corticosteroid injections in the region of the trochlea.[17] Prisms may provide some relief from diplopia in acquired forms.

The goal of surgery is to restore free ocular rotations. Brown advocated that the superior oblique tendon be stripped. The results of such a procedure are frequently unsatisfactory because of reformation of scar tissue. A procedure of luxation of the whole trochlea, with the superior oblique tendon and orbital structures left intact, appears promising.[22] Tenotomy of the superior oblique tendon has also been advocated.[23] This has the disadvantage that it frequently produces a superior oblique paresis.[24] Furthermore, if the tendon is not tight, the tenotomy may not improve the restricted movement. Surgery without any preconception about the site of restriction may be preferable. During surgery, a traction test is repeated frequently until the globe rotations are free. Recession of the conjunctiva in the inferotemporal quadrant may help to free rotations. If the restrictive adhesions are not found near the trochlea, they must be sought elsewhere around the globe. After the rotations are as free as possible, the eye is anchored in an elevated, adducted position for up to 2 weeks. This maneuver is intended to prevent the reformation of scar tissue in the same places. In healing, the eye position shifts for several months after surgery, and a second procedure is frequently required. If a vertical strabismus is present, satisfactory mechanical freeing needs to be followed by treatment of the strabismus.

CONGENITAL FIBROSIS

A rare and usually familial form of vertical strabismus is congenital fibrosis.[25-27] The inheritance pattern is often autosomal dominant. One or both eyes are typically tethered in a downward position by a fibrotic inferior rectus. Blepharoptosis and a compensatory elevated chin position occur. Attempts at upward eye movements may result in convergence. Many of the extraocular muscles are fibrotic, not just the inferior recti. Histology shows replacement of muscle fibers with fibrotic tissue. The differential diagnosis includes Graves' disease, Brown's syndrome, orbital floor fracture, double elevator palsy, and chronic progressive external ophthalmoplegia.

Surgical treatment can relieve only the extreme downward tethering of the eyes. The head position improves as a result. The lids may need to be raised, but caution is necessary because the upward rotation of the eyes is limited and the normal Bell's phenomenon does not occur with blinking. It is, therefore, easy to produce corneal exposure. It is best to use a removable material to raise the lids in case exposure occurs and they need to be lowered again.

FRACTURES OF THE ORBITAL FLOOR

OCULAR MANIFESTATIONS

Ocular motility may be impaired in orbital floor fractures as a result of proptosis and edema from the original trauma, muscle contusion, intraorbital hemorrhage, herniation of the orbital fascia, and muscle entrapment.[28] Eye movements in general, but particularly elevation and depression, may be limited. The inferior rectus is the muscle most commonly affected.

DIAGNOSIS

The diagnosis of inferior rectus entrapment is made on the basis of the presence of limited elevation on the affected side, which results in hypotropia, and a positive traction test. Mild cases show hypotropia only in upgaze. Depression may also be limited by entrapment or by damage to the nerve to the inferior rectus. Diplopia may persist after the inferior rectus has been freed.

The pathophysiology of any resultant strabismus is the herniation of the orbital contents—fat, connective tissue septa, and muscle—into the fracture and consequent tethering of the eye. If the entrapment is old, the muscle can become permanently fibrotic and inelastic, which results in a reduced range of rotation. A paresis of the inferior rectus may also occur, which presumably arises from trauma to the nerve that supplies the inferior rectus. On occasion, the inferior rectus may be devitalized by compromise of its blood supply. The muscle is then found to be quite friable at the time of surgery.

TREATMENT

A floor fracture does not require repair if no disturbance of motility exists.[29] The initial treatment of the restricted motility consists of waiting for up to 2 weeks for regression of the edema, which may result in significantly improved motility. Surgery is carried out for the hypotropia that remains with restricted elevation on forced duction testing. The lid is incised just below the lash line and the periosteum at the orbital edge. A silicone plate is placed under the periosteum of the orbital floor to extend as far back as the fracture site and hold in the herniated orbital contents. This procedure may still not free the inferior rectus adequately, as determined by traction testing, and the muscle may need direct freeing from scarring and adhesions within the orbit. Implantation of a Supramid sleeve around the muscle blocks the reformation of adhesions. Frequently, a second procedure is required to deal with inferior rectus paresis.

GRAVES' OPHTHALMOPATHY (DYSTHYROID ORBITOPATHY)

INTRODUCTION

Graves' ophthalmopathy is an autoimmune inflammatory condition that involves the orbital tissues, primarily the muscles and fat.[30] The muscles are affected by a myositis, which shows histological features of interstitial edema and round cell infiltration. The muscles enlarge and become fibrotic and inelastic. Other findings are lid edema, proptosis, lid retraction, and optic neuropathy. Proptosis results from edema and enlargement of the muscles and fat spaces.

OCULAR MANIFESTATIONS

The usual motility findings are caused by the inelasticity of the muscles. In addition to muscle stiffness, orbital inflammation can result in diffuse adhesions of Tenon's capsule and orbital tissues to the globe. All the muscles become stretched and the range of rotation is limited by the lack of relaxation of antagonists because of the fibrotic changes. The inferior rectus is the muscle most commonly affected, which results in a limitation of elevation. When the condition is more severe, the eye may be tethered down by the inferior rectus to produce a hypotropia in primary position. The medial rectus is the next most commonly involved muscle, followed by the superior and lateral recti. The inferior oblique may also be involved. The restriction of rotation is away from the field of action of the stiff muscle (e.g., in abduction for a stiff medial rectus). Involvement is frequently asymmetrical between the two eyes.

DIAGNOSIS

The diagnosis is largely clinical. The patient may have any level of thyroid activity and still have thyroid ophthalmopathy. Thyroid ophthalmopathy may recur after many quiescent years. Orbital computed tomography, magnetic resonance imaging, or B-scan ultrasonography shows enlargement of the muscles. The traction test (forced duction test) demonstrates that the muscles are restricted. Intraocular pressure becomes elevated as the eye attempts to rotate against a restriction. Measurement of the intraocular pressure in upgaze, primary position, and downgaze may provide information similar to that obtained from a traction test.[31] Usually, at least some of the eye findings of Graves' disease are present in addition to any motility disturbance.

TREATMENT

General treatment of Graves' ophthalmopathy is not discussed here, as any abnormality of the thyroid state is corrected by an endocrinologist. The patient must be observed until the deviation has stopped changing and the orbital inflammation has subsided for 6 months. Although some improvement in motility may occur as a result of subsidence of orbital edema, the fibrotic changes in the muscles prevent resolution of the portion of the deviation that arises from restrictive muscle changes. Surgery performed too soon after the period of inflammation may lead to reactivation of the inflammation during the postoperative period.

The goal of surgery is single vision in primary position and downgaze. The strabismus may be difficult to treat because of the limitations in eye movements. Fresnel prisms may provide some relief of diplopia until the deviation has stabilized. Because more than one muscle is usually involved, both horizontal and vertical deviations are present and oblique prismation is the norm. Botulinum toxin appears to have little role because of the mechanical nature of the motility defect, although evidence for active muscle contraction in recent-onset Graves' disease provides a rationale for this treatment to be tried in the earliest stages.[32]

A further goal of surgery is to reduce the incomitance and the deviation. Tight muscles are recessed to enable better movement. Resection of normally elastic muscles may be carried out without detriment; however, resection of an inelastic muscle limits rotations even more. Recession of a normal muscle produces the largest effect in the field of action of the muscle. Recession of an inelastic muscle may produce the greatest effect in the field of action of the direct antagonist. The recessed muscle then also underacts in its field of action. The result is that the range of single vision may be reduced significantly compared with normal. Diffuse ad-

hesions to the sclera must be dissected free. Reformation is blocked through implantation of a Supramid sleeve.

A tight inferior rectus is recessed sufficiently to allow fusion in primary position. Upgaze is the least useful of the gaze positions, and diplopia may be allowed to exist if it allows better alignment in the more useful positions of primary gaze and downgaze. It may not be possible to achieve vertical alignment with the eyes lowered for reading. The reading material then must be held higher, or the head lowered for reading, or prism reading glasses prescribed. Recession of the medial rectus may be necessary for single vision in lateral gaze but tends to produce a convergence insufficiency. Convergence is also compromised by recession of the inferior recti, which then have less secondary convergence action in lowered gaze for reading. Recession of both superior and inferior recti may be indicated. Recession of the superior rectus may improve downgaze through release of restriction. Frequently, a prism is required to achieve single vision after surgery. Many times the extreme preoperative incomitance precludes satisfactory single vision with a prism.

HEAVY EYE SYNDROME

Heavy eye syndrome is an association of anisometropia, usually with high myopia, and hyperphoria or hypertropia. The more myopic eye is hypotropic. This disorder was called heavy eye syndrome on the basis of the fanciful idea that the larger, more myopic eye is in a relatively low position, as though it were too heavy. Of course, gravity has no discernible role in the causation, which appears to be an abnormally low muscle path of the lateral rectus in the involved eye(s).[33]

In the usual clinical situation, anisomyopia or unilateral high myopia exists, in the range 2–20D. The vertical deviation ranges from 2 to 25D, although there is no association between the amount of anisometropia and the amount of hypotropia. Elevation of the low eye may be limited. Frequently, the head tilts to the side of the hypotropic eye, which may be compensatory to achieve single vision by the creation of a base-up prism effect before the hypotropic eye. The heavy eye syndrome was first described by Hugonnier, but the most accessible description in English is by Ward.[34]

ADHERENCE SYNDROME

Adhesions, as a developmental anomaly between the sheaths of the superior rectus and superior oblique or between the lateral rectus and inferior oblique, are rare.[35] The clinical presentation is that of superior rectus or lateral rectus paresis. The traction test shows restriction and may help to differentiate this entity from true paralysis.

Adherence of fibrofatty scar tissue to the globe in the inferotemporal quadrant may follow surgery on the inferior oblique. A hypotropia of the affected eye in primary position and restricted elevation occur, which are shown by the traction test.

Treatment involves freeing of the adhesions and prevention of their reformation, as effected by the implantation of a Supramid sleeve or cap, a nonabsorbable plastic sheet.

REFERENCES

1. Bielschowsky A. Die einseitigen und gegensinnigen ('dissoziierten') Vertikalbewegungen der Augen. Graefes Arch Ophthalmol. 1930;25:493–553.
2. MacDonald AI, Pratt-Johnson A. The suppression patterns and sensory adaptations to dissociated vertical divergent strabismus. Can J Ophthalmol. 1974;9:113–19.
3. Wilson ME, McClatchey SK. Dissociated horizontal deviation. J Pediatr Ophthalmol Strabismus. 1991;28:90–5.
4. Zubcov AA, Goldstein HP, Reinecke RD. Dissociated vertical deviation (DVD). The saccadic eye movements. Strabismus. 1994;2:1–11.
5. Sprague JB, Moore S, Eggers HM, Knapp P. Dissociated vertical deviation. Treatment with the Faden operation of Cüppers. Arch Ophthalmol. 1980;98:465–8.
6. von Noorden GK. Indication of the posterior fixation suture. Ophthalmology. 1978;85:512–20.

7. Magoon E, Cruciger M, Jampolsky A. Dissociated vertical deviation: an asymmetric condition treated with large bilateral superior rectus recession. J Pediatr Ophthalmol Strabismus. 1982;19:152–6.

8. Burke JP, Scott WE, Kutschke PJ. Anterior transposition of the inferior oblique muscle for dissociated vertical deviation. Ophthalmology. 1993;100:245–50.

9. Fink W. The role of developmental anomalies in vertical muscle deficits. Am J Ophthalmol. 1955;40:529–52.

10. Parks MM. The weakening surgical procedures for eliminating overaction of the inferior oblique muscle. Am J Ophthalmol. 1972;73:102–22.

11. Jampel RS, Fells P. Monocular elevation paresis caused by a central nervous system lesion. Arch Ophthalmol. 1968;80:45–55.

12. Knapp P. The surgical treatment of double elevator paralysis. Trans Am Ophthalmol Soc. 1969;67:304–23.

13. Burke JP, Ruben JB, Scott WE. Vertical transposition of the horizontal recti (Knapp procedure) for the treatment of double elevator palsy: effectiveness and long term stability. Br J Ophthalmol. 1992;76:734–7.

14. Brown HW. True and simulated superior oblique tendon sheath syndromes. Doc Ophthalmol. 1973;34:123–36.

15. Moore AT, Walker J, Taylor D. Familial Brown's syndrome. J Pediatr Ophthalmol Strabismus. 1988;25:202–4.

16. Zipf RF, Trokel SL. Simulated superior oblique tendon sheath syndrome following orbital floor fracture. Am J Ophthalmol. 1973;75:700–5.

17. Hermann JS. Acquired Brown's syndrome of inflammatory origin. Arch Ophthalmol. 1978;96:1228–32.

18. Killian PJ, McClain B, Lawless OJ. Brown's syndrome. An unusual manifestation of rheumatoid arthritis. Arthritis Rheum. 1977;20:1080–4.

19. Wang FM, Wertenbaker C, Behrens MM, Jacobs JJ. Acquired Brown's syndrome in children with juvenile rheumatoid arthritis. Ophthalmology. 1984;91:23–6.

20. Roper Hall MJ. The superior oblique click syndrome. In: Mein J, Bierlaagh JJM, Brummel Kamp–Dons TE, eds. Orthoptics, Proceedings of the Second International Orthoptic Congress. Amsterdam: Excerpta Medica Foundation; 1972.

21. Girard LJ. Pseudoparalysis of the inferior oblique muscle. South Med J. 1956;49:342–6.

22. Mombaerts I, Koornneef L, Everhard-Halm YS, et al. Superior oblique luxation and trochlear luxation as new concepts in superior oblique muscle weakening surgery. Am J Ophthalmol. 1995;120:83–91.

23. Crawford JS, Orton R, Labow-Daily L. Late results of superior oblique muscle tenotomy in true Brown's syndrome. Am J Ophthalmol. 1980;89:824–9.

24. Eustis HS, O'Reilly C, Crawford JS. Management of superior oblique palsy after surgery for true Brown's syndrome. J Pediatr Ophthalmol Strabismus. 1987; 24: 10–16.

25. Brown HW. Congenital structural muscle anomalies. In: Allen JH, ed. Strabismus ophthalmic symposium. St. Louis: CV Mosby; 1950:205–36.

26. Harley RD, Rodrigues MM, Crawford JS. Congenital fibrosis of the extraocular muscles. Trans Am Ophthalmol Soc. 1978;76:197–226.

27. Hansen E. Congenital general fibrosis of the extraocular muscles. Acta Ophthalmol. 1968;46:469–76.

28. Hötte HHA. Orbital fractures. Springfield: CC Thomas; 1970.

29. Emery JM, von Noorden GK, Schlernitzauer DA. Orbital floor fractures: long-term follow-up of cases with and without surgical repair. Am J Ophthalmol. 1972;74:299–306.

30. Dunnington JH, Berke RN. Exophthalmos due to chronic orbital myositis. Arch Ophthalmol. 1943;30:446–66.

31. Manor RS, Kurz O, Lewitus Z. Intraocular pressure in endocrinologic patients with exophthalmos. Ophthalmologica. 1974;168:241–52.

32. Simonsz HJ, Kommerell G. Increased muscle tension and reduced elasticity of affected muscles in recent-onset Graves' disease caused primarily by active muscle contraction. Doc Ophthalmol. 1989;72:215–24.

33. Krzizok TH, Kaufmann H, Traupe H. Elucidation of restrictive motility in high myopia by magnetic resonance imaging. Arch Ophthalmol. 1997;115:1019–27.

34. Ward DM. The heavy eye phenomenon. Trans Ophthalmol Soc UK. 1967;87:717–26.

35. Johnson LV. Adherence syndrome: pseudoparalysis of the lateral or superior rectus muscle. Arch Ophthalmol. 1950;44:870–8.

Amblyopia

GARY R. DIAMOND

DEFINITION
- Amblyopia is a developmental defect of spatial visual processing that occurs in the central visual pathways of the eye.

KEY FEATURES
- Decreased recognition and vernier and grating acuity.
- Decreased contrast sensitivity and spatial localization.

ASSOCIATED FEATURES
- Accentuation of the "crowding" phenomenon.
- Stable acuity behind neutral density filters.
- Mild afferent pupillary defect in severely amblyopic eyes.
- Decreased saccadic amplitudes and impaired pursuit movements.

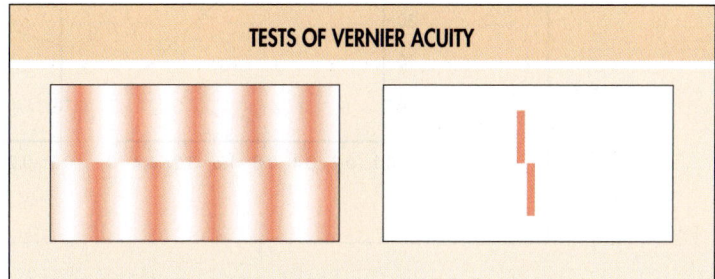

TESTS OF VERNIER ACUITY

FIG. 79-1 ■ Tests of vernier acuity. The vernier resolution task is to detect the offset in the grating (*left*) or line (*right*). The smallest detectable offset (threshold) is expressed as an angle at the viewing distance used. Under optimal conditions, vernier acuity may be as good as 3–6 arc seconds.

INTRODUCTION

Amblyopia is a "developmental defect of spatial visual processing that occurs in the central visual pathways of the brain."[1] It presents most dramatically as loss of visual acuity in one or, rarely, both eyes, but amblyopia is more than this; certain forms of amblyopia also present with diminished contrast sensitivity, vernier acuity, grating acuity, and spatial localization of objects. These defects may be explained by the mechanism of lack of use of an eye because of media opacity or extreme refractive errors that cause a chronically blurred image to form on the fovea of that eye; however, the cause of amblyopia in an eye that has strabismus is not as easily determined and is the result of abnormal binocular interaction.

Anisometropic Amblyopia

Patients who have anisometropia and decreased visual acuity in the more ametropic eye and who possess the sensory characteristics of monofixation syndrome (Chapter 71) are almost always amblyopic; the decreased acuity does not improve totally with corrective lenses alone. These patients have decreased acuity, as measured using graded optotypes (Chapter 68), gratings, and vernier testing (Fig. 79-1) in the same proportion. This acuity loss extends to the peripheral visual field equally nasally and temporally, which implies uniform degradation of the visual system by an amount proportional to the anisometropia.[2] As monocular visual function in the far temporal periphery of the visual field is spared, the acuity defect found in the more central field must result from, in some part, binocular interaction.[3]

The contrast sensitivity curve shows substantial losses at high spatial frequencies only (Fig. 79-2).[3] Spatial localization as measured by Hess and Holliday[4] is decreased in proportion to contrast sensitivity loss (see Fig. 79-3).

Stimulus-Deprivation Amblyopia

Amblyopia that results from a media opacity of early onset in one or both eyes may be devastating visually and sometimes irreversible. Common causes include congenital or early-onset cataract, corneal opacity from glaucoma or dystrophy, lid masses (Fig. 79-4), and persistent hyperplastic primary vitreous.

Strabismic Amblyopia

Amblyopia in patients who have strabismus occurs only if one eye is preferred for fixation; free alternation of fixation between the eyes is incompatible with the development of strabismic amblyopia. The fovea of the eye that is used less loses acuity in proportion to the amount of fixational preference shown to the other eye and the age of the child at onset of the preference.

EPIDEMIOLOGY AND PATHOGENESIS
Anisometropic Amblyopia

The initial development of amblyopia from any cause rarely occurs in children older than about 5.5 years, but once it has developed and been reversed by therapy, it may reappear until about 9 or 10 years of age. Anisometropic amblyopia rarely occurs unless the anisometropia has been present for more than 2 years.[5] Children at birth frequently have modest amounts of astigmatism equal in each eye, which disappears without permanent effect by the age of 6 months. The critical period for the development of anisometropic amblyopia in humans is not known more precisely (see later in this chapter).

Stimulus-Deprivation Amblyopia

Constant monocular occlusion of the visual axis for more than 1 week per year of life places a child at significant risk for the development of stimulus-deprivation amblyopia until about 5.5 years of age. Significant monocular congenital lens opacities

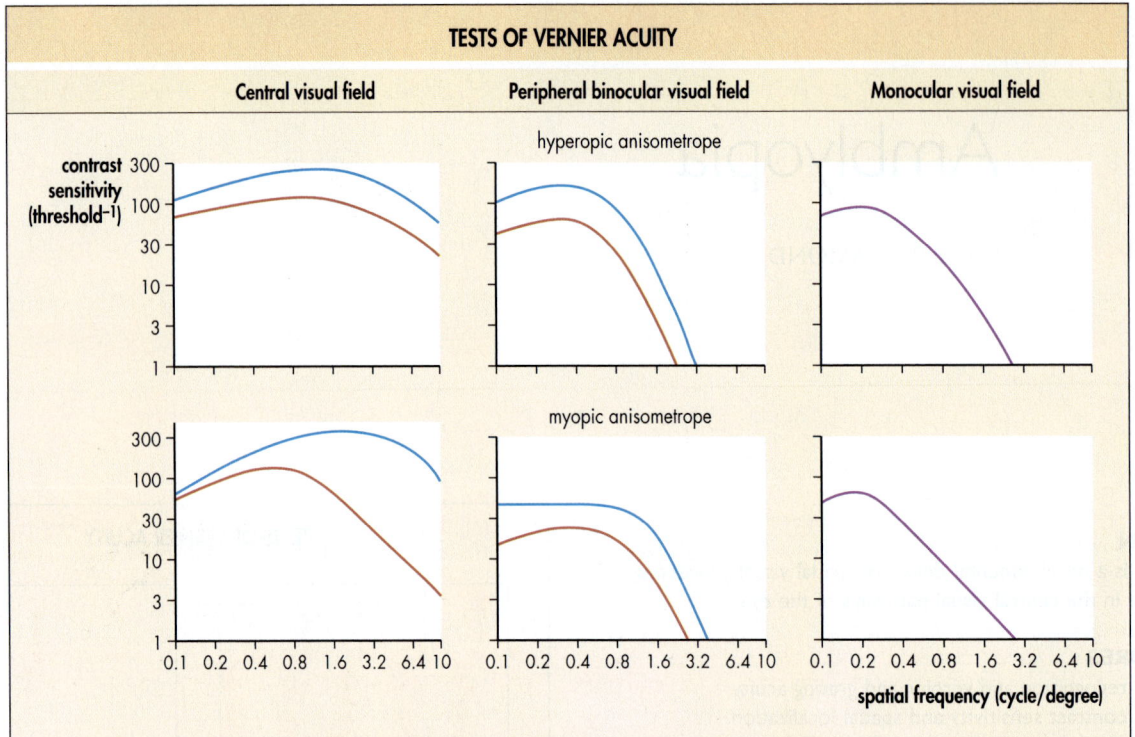

FIG. 79-2 ▌ **Contrast sensitivity for hyperopic and myopic anisometropes in binocular and monocular visual field.** Red lines represent the amblyopic eye, blue lines the sound eye, and mauve the monocular visual field. (Data from Hess RF, Pointer JS. Differences in the neural basis of human amblyopia: the distribution of the anomaly across the visual field. Vision Res. 1985;25:1577–94.)

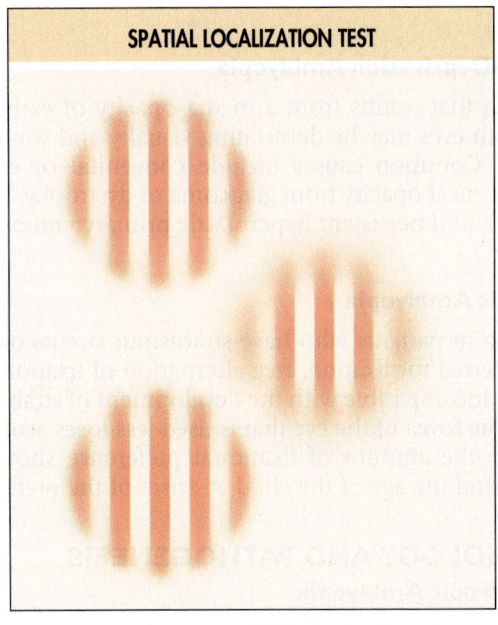

FIG. 79-3 ▌ **Spatial localization test.** The goal of this test is to align the middle grating between the upper and lower gratings.

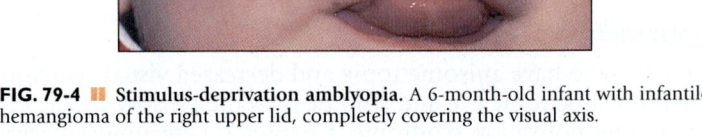

FIG. 79-4 ▌ **Stimulus-deprivation amblyopia.** A 6-month-old infant with infantile hemangioma of the right upper lid, completely covering the visual axis.

(axial diameter = 3.0mm) must be removed and the eye optically corrected at as young an age as feasible, certainly during the first few weeks of life; binocular similarly significant opacities must be removed before about 6 weeks of age.

Strabismic Amblyopia

Strabismic amblyopia may occur initially from birth to about 5.5 years of age, but even if successfully treated it may recur until about 9 or 10 years of age. The peak age for development of fixation preference in strabismic children is about 1 year of age (range 9 months to 2 years),[6] but fixation preference can occur until about 8–9 years of age. Numerous publications describe

successful improvement of visual acuity in strabismic or anisometropic amblyopia in older teenagers[7]; the loss of the better-sighted eye has led to spontaneous improvement in visual acuity in the remaining amblyopic eye of middle-aged adults! Perhaps the critical period for reversal of strabismic and anisometropic amblyopia really has no end.

OCULAR MANIFESTATIONS

Anisometropic Amblyopia

The two most common forms of anisometropic amblyopia occur in anisometropic hyperopes and unilaterally high myopes. Patients who have anisometropic hyperopia exert sufficient ac-

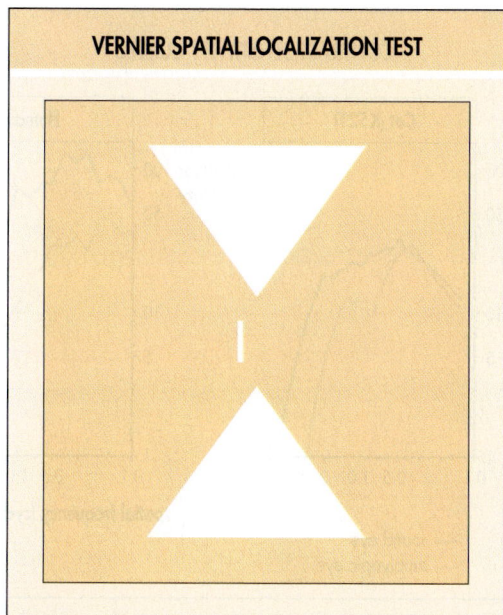

FIG. 79-5 ▮ **Vernier spatial localization test.** The goal of this test is to align the small vertical line between the triangle points.

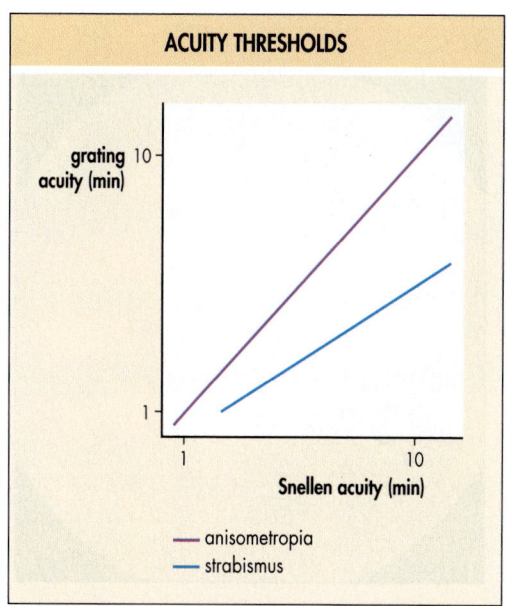

FIG. 79-6 ▮ **Grating acuity thresholds versus crowded Snellen acuity thresholds.** Snellen acuity is affected much more than grating acuity in strabismic amblyopia.

commodation to provide clear visual acuity in the less hyperopic eye and leave the other blurred; these patients may have better distance than near acuity in the amblyopic eye. Patients who have unilaterally high myopia often have better near than distance visual acuity. Anisometropic amblyopia may occur in patients who have monocular astigmatism alone but may be confined to a meridian in which maximal unfocusing occurs; detection of this type of "meridional" amblyopia often requires special testing.

Stimulus-Deprivation Amblyopia

All forms of visual acuity (optotype, vernier, grating) are affected equally, as are spatial localization (Fig. 79-5) and contrast sensitivity.

Strabismic Amblyopia

Optotype visual acuity is usually worse than grating acuity,[8] probably because the gratings are larger than the area suppressed under binocular viewing conditions, and distortion renders optotypes (letters, numbers, pictures) more difficult to identify than grating orientations (Fig. 79-6). Vernier acuity, about six times more precise than grating or optotype acuity in normal individuals and patients who have anisometropic amblyopia, is less precise in patients who have strabismic amblyopia.[9] This degradation of vernier acuity occurs at both fine and coarse levels. Contrast sensitivity in strabismic amblyopes may be normal or abnormal at high spatial frequencies.[4]

DIAGNOSIS AND ANCILLARY TESTING

Amblyopia should be suspected in any strabismic child who has a preference for fixation with one eye, but it is important to recognize that many patients who have amblyopia have aligned eyes (monofixation syndrome with amblyopia). Amblyopia should also be suspected as a contributor to decreased visual acuity when the hyperopic refractive errors between the two eyes differ by more than about 2.00D, when the myopic refractive errors differ by more than about 4.00D, and when astigmatic errors differ by more than about 1.25D.[10] A deeply amblyopic eye (<20/400 [<6/120]) may have a mild afferent pupillary defect, but a moderate or marked defect implies an organic cause for decreased acuity. Color vision is generally normal in amblyopic

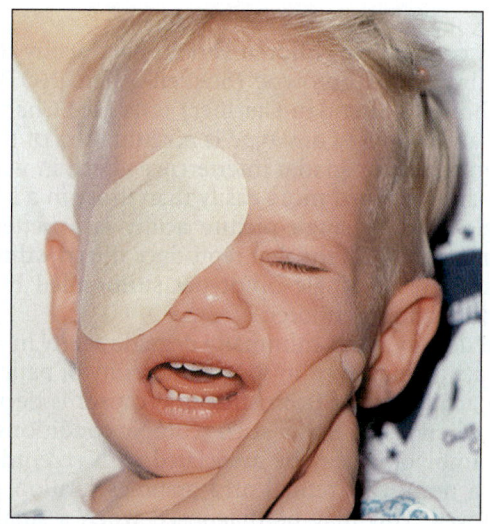

FIG. 79-7 ▮ **Application of a patch to the sound eye of a child.** This reduces vision in proportion to the degree of amblyopia. It frequently results in crying or efforts to remove the patch, which may be used to diagnose poor vision in one eye.

eyes if the eye can discern the target. Accommodation is deficient in many amblyopic eyes.[11]

For children who do not respond to graded optotype acuity testing, acuity may be evaluated by behavior with monocular occlusion. A child who rejects occlusion of only one eye by moving away from the cover or by crying is presumed to have decreased acuity in that eye (Fig. 79-7). Fixation preference in children who have aligned eyes may be evaluated by the creation of a vertical misalignment of the visual axes with a 10D prism held vertically before one eye. Alternating fixation implies equal acuity in each eye; progressively deeper amblyopia permits fixation to be held through a blink, to a blink, for a few seconds only, or momentarily, until it shifts to the better-sighted eye.

The ability to fix and follow a small target with each eye can be evaluated and a quantitative acuity measurement calculated from trigonometric principles. Acuity quantitation may be performed with optikokinetic nystagmus testing, visually evoked response testing, and forced-choice preferential-looking (Teller acuity card) testing; as noted earlier, strabismic amblyopes have acuity in the amblyopic eye that is overestimated by grating (opticokinetic nystagmus and Teller acuity card) techniques.

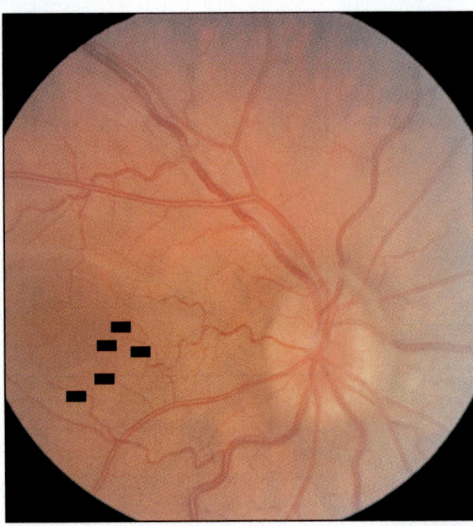

FIG. 79-8 ■ **Diagnosis of eccentric fixation.** A target is projected onto the retina using a special ophthalmoscope. The observer examines where the fixation target falls on the retina relative to the fovea. The marks indicate the locations of successive fixations in a case of eccentric fixation. In general, the poorer the vision, the greater the scatter and the greater the distance from the fovea.

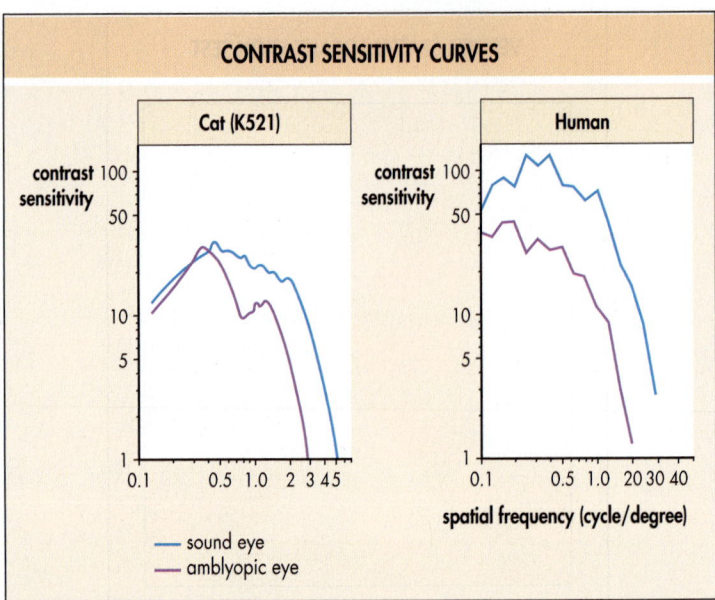

FIG. 79-9 ■ **Contrast sensitivity curves.** Cat (K521) curve is from visual cortex cells recorded in a cat reared with a −12.00D lens over the right eye. Human curve is from an anisometropic. Red lines represent the amblyopic eye and blue lines the sound eye. (Data from Eggers HM, Blakemore C. Physiological basis of anisometropic amblyopia. Science. 1978;201:264–6.)

Literate, cooperative children should have acuity in each eye measured by graded optotype (Snellen, Allen, HOTV, Landolt ring, tumbling E, Sheridan-Gardner) tests (see Chapter 68). A feature of amblyopia of any type is accentuation of the "crowding" phenomenon or spatial interference effect, in which single optotypes are discerned more easily than those in a larger array; thus, single-letter or single-picture acuity is a better measure than linear acuity.[12] Charts that reproduce the crowding effect of a linear array using single optotypes surrounded by lines are available for younger children.

Neutral density filters minimally degrade acuity in amblyopic eyes, and acuity may even improve; the acuity of patients whose decreased acuity results from structural causes is decreased significantly when tested under such scotopic conditions.[13]

Severe amblyopia may be associated with eccentric fixation, in which a nonfoveal retinal area assumes fixation preference over the fovea. This may be diagnosed when a small target is projected through a direct retinoscope onto the posterior retina and the patient asked to fixate upon it; those who have eccentric fixation fixate upon an extrafoveal area in preference to the fovea (Fig. 79-8). Esotropes and exotropes may fixate on either side of the fovea; eccentric fixation is correlated (but loosely) with anomalous retinal correspondence.

Eye movements in both eyes of an amblyopic patient may be affected. The better-sighted eye may show unsteady fixation and asymmetry of smooth tracking. Saccadic amplitudes are smaller in the amblyopic eye, more so in the temporal direction; pursuit movements are also impaired in the temporal direction, with a decrease in velocity and saccadic correction to the final end point.[14]

Experimental Anatomical and Physiological Changes in Amblyopia

ANISOMETROPIC AMBLYOPIA. An eye may be defocused and anisometropia created by rearing animals with a powerful lens (concave or convex) placed over one eye or atropine instilled to obviate accommodation. In primates given atropine, cells in the visual cortex driven by the eye that has had atropine instilled have reduced contrast sensitivity (Fig. 79-9)[15]; this is noted most prominently in layers of the striate cortex outside layer IV, is not seen in the lateral geniculate nucleus, and is present in moderate degree in cells of the striate cortex layer IV.[16] Also, a reduction

occurs in the fraction of binocularly driven cortical neurons and a small shift in dominance toward the normal eye occurs. Anatomical changes in the lateral geniculate nucleus are seen only in the parvicellular layers that subserve high spatial frequency and consist of diminution of cell size.[17]

STIMULUS-DEPRIVATION AMBLYOPIA. Monocular deprivation of images by lid closure in a cat or monkey for 3 months results in severe amblyopia. If the eye is opened and visual cortical cells are recorded, very few are found to be activated by the deprived eye.[18] The retina in the sutured eye is normal, as are the physiological properties of cells in the lateral geniculate nucleus driven by that eye. However, arbors of fine-detail cells (X cells) in the geniculate are larger than normal, and arbors of movement cells (Y cells) are smaller than normal[19]; thus, fewer Y cells are recorded and the spatial contrast sensitivity of X cells is reduced.

Projections from the lateral geniculate nucleus to the visual cortex are similarly affected. Cortical stripes from the affected eye are narrower than normal and stripes from the sound eye wider than normal.[20] The effects of monocular deprivation reflect competition from the open eye as well as loss of connections with the deprived eye (Fig. 79-10).[21] Binocular deprivation permits up to one third of cortical cells to be driven by one or both eyes, and these have normal receptive fields; thus, binocular deprivation is not physiologically or anatomically equivalent to monocular deprivation of both eyes.[22]

STRABISMIC AMBLYOPIA. Strabismus may be created in experimental animals by disinsertion of an extraocular muscle tendon, recession of a muscle, injection of botulinum toxin in a muscle belly to paralyze it temporarily, or rearing the animal with prisms placed before its eyes. Strabismus also occurs naturally in some cats and monkeys.

Loss of binocular function and depth perception is related to reduction in the number of cells in the visual cortex that can be activated by both eyes.[22] A reduction in the number of cells driven by the deviating eye may also occur (see Fig. 79-11). A reduction in acuity and contrast sensitivity is found in animals that have both natural and experimental esotropia.[23,24]

Critical Periods

During visual development, a period of time (known as the critical period) exists in which the anatomy and physiology of the

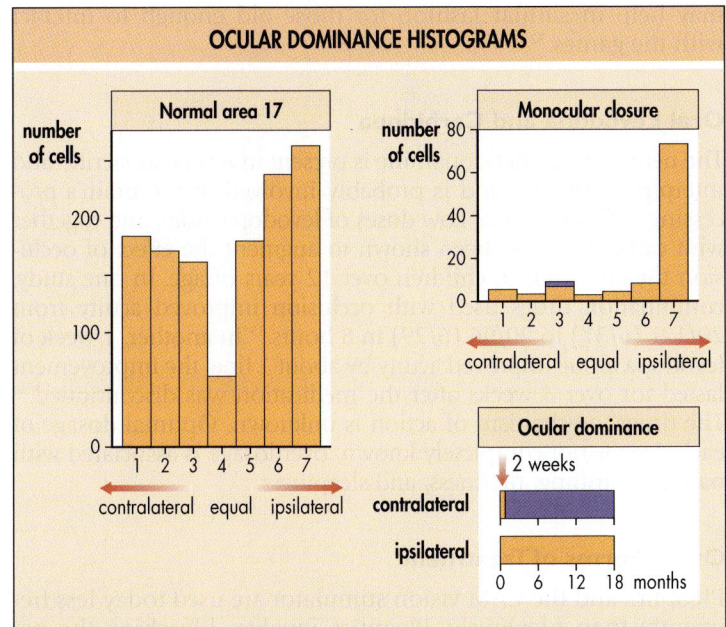

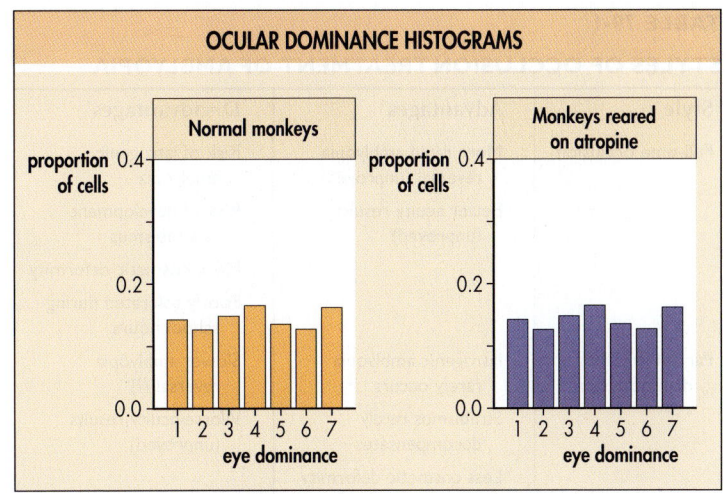

FIG. 79-10 ■ **Ocular dominance histograms.** Normal area 17 depicts a normal monkey and is derived from 1256 recordings of visual cortex cells in monkeys of all ages. Monocular closure is from a monocularly deprived monkey (the right eye was occluded from 2 weeks to 18 months of age; recordings were taken from the left hemisphere). Each cell is driven solely by the ipsilateral eye (group 7), contralateral eye (group 1), both eyes (group 4), or somewhere in between (groups 2, 3, 5, and 6). (Data from Hubel DH, Weisel TN, LeVay S. Functional architecture of area 17 in normal and monocularly deprived macaque monkeys. Cold Spring Harbor Symp Quant Biol. 1975;40:581–9.)

FIG. 79-11 ■ **Ocular dominance histograms.** Normal monkeys' histogram represents pooled data from four normal control monkeys (384 cells). Monkey reared on *atropine* had chronic atropinization of the right eye and provides a model of anisometropic amblyopia (316 cells). Cells dominated by the eye given *atropine* are in groups 1–3, cells dominated by the untreated eye are in groups 5–7. Group 4 responds equally well to receptive field stimulation in either eye. Adjacent groups are progressively unequal in responses until groups 1 and 7 respond to only one eye. The monkey given atropine shows a mild loss of binocular cells and more cells that respond to the untreated eye. The reduction in number of cells that respond through the amblyopic eye is not amblyopia per se but a corollary finding. The quality of cell function is not addressed by the ocular dominance histogram. (Data from Movshon JA, Eggers HM, Gizzi MS, *et al.* Effects of early unilateral blur on the macaque's visual system. III. Physiological observations. J Neurosci. 1987;7:1341–51.)

visual system are malleable; once this period is past, visual deprivation and reversal of deprivation occur only partially or not at all.

Animal experiments provide useful insights into the physiological and anatomical processes that occur in humans. Monocular deprivation (brought on by lid closure) in cats is most devastating between 4 and 6 weeks of age, during which time 3 days of monocular closure results in most cortical cells being driven by the open eye. Susceptibility decreases from 6 weeks to 3 months of age; some susceptibility persists until 9 months of age.[25] Alterations in cortical cell dominance that arise from strabismus follow a similar time course.[26] The visual system seems to maintain plasticity for a longer time period at the higher processing levels; thus, visual association areas are more plastic at a given age than primary visual cortical areas, and the latter are more plastic than the lateral geniculate nucleus. Connections for movement tend to mature earlier than those for fine visual acuity.

The critical period in the macaque monkey begins at about 4 weeks of age and ends a little after 1 year of age.[27]

No studies have been performed in experimental animals that have induced anisometropia. In naturally strabismic monkeys, acuity develops more slowly than in normal monkeys and final acuity in the strabismic eye is worse than normal. Monkeys seem susceptible to the development of strabismic amblyopia if strabismus begins between birth and 10 weeks of age, but the end of the critical period for strabismic amblyopia is not known.[28]

DIFFERENTIAL DIAGNOSIS

The differential diagnosis of amblyopia includes optic nerve, geniculate, optic tract, and visual cortex pathology. Subtle and overlooked causes of monocular visual acuity loss in children include keratoconus, posterior lenticonus or other lenticular opacity, and macular lesions such as those caused by toxoplasmosis and toxocariasis. Rarer but more ominous causes of monocular visual acuity loss in children include hypothalamic gliomas and craniopharyngiomas.

TREATMENT

Although patients who have amblyopia usually have no detectable structural lesions in the eye, the converse is not true; some patients who have structural lesions have a superimposed amblyopia. Many patients who have structural eye lesions benefit from a trial of amblyopia therapy.[29] Correction of significant refractive errors is an essential preparation for active amblyopia treatment. Accommodative balance between the eyes needs to be maintained, and prescription of a portion of a hyperopic amblyopic patient's refractive error should occur, as many amblyopes have deficient accommodation.

Occlusion

A patch over the better-sighted eye remains the mainstay of active treatment of amblyopia, even in patients who have eccentric fixation. Naturally, all media opacities are cleared if possible before the initiation of occlusion. Many styles of occlusion are possible and effective; some involve patches over the sound eye for all waking hours; others, patches for 5 hours a day for amblyopia reversal and then 1–2 hours a day for maintenance until the age of 9 years. The advantages and disadvantages of each style are listed in Table 79-1. Yet another style is to patch the sound eye for 2–7 days and the amblyopic eye for 1 day, with the cycle repeated as necessary. Patients who undergo full-time occlusion are reevaluated at intervals of a week per year of life; thus, a 6-month-old child returns in 3 days. Half of children for whom patches are discontinued when younger than 9 years of age again lose acuity; this is usually reversible with reinstitution of occlusion.

Many commercial brands of orthoptic patch are available. Elastoplast patches are thicker and may better block incoming images; Opticlude Eye Occlusors are thinner but less allergenic. Fair-complected children may develop irritation with removal of the patch; skin preparation with baby oil or powder and trimming of one half to two thirds of the mucilage may help prevent skin irritation.

Initiation of occlusion in a child who has severe amblyopia may be difficult. The parent must be encouraged to stimulate

TABLE 79-1

STYLES OF OCCLUSION TREATMENT OF AMBLYOPIA

Style	Advantages	Disadvantages
Full-time occlusion	More rapid amblyopia reversal (unproved)	Risk of iatrogenic amblyopia
	Better acuity results (unproved)	Risk of development of strabismus
		More cosmetic deformity
		Poorly tolerated during school hours
Part-time (5 hour/day) occlusion	Iatrogenic amblyopia rarely occurs	Slower amblyopia reversal (?)
	Strabismus rarely decompensates	Worse acuity results (unproved)
	Less cosmetic deformity	
	Can occlude outside of school hours	

constantly the patched child with games and activities and the child encouraged not to remove or loosen the patch over the nasal bridge. Occasionally, elbow restraints such as commercial cleft palate restraints or homemade restraints from juice cans are indicated. Patches held by elastic around the head are better tolerated by some children, especially if decorated by the child. Older children tend to reject occlusion in warm weather—an offer to speak personally over the phone to the child often improves compliance. As acuity improves, patch tolerance also improves. Children with acuity better than about 20/50 (6/15) tolerate a patch placed on a spectacle lens and do not peek around the patch.

Forms of occlusion other than opaque patches include fixation of a neutral density filter or clear nail polish on a spectacle lens. Benefits include better cosmesis and less disruption to peripheral fusion, but most amblyopes peek around the lenses. Neonates may tolerate extended-wear, large-diameter fogging or opaque contact lenses.

Iatrogenic amblyopia of the initially sound eye may occur with full-time occlusion before the acuity in the amblyopic eye reaches 20/20 (6/6) and tends to occur in younger children; it is rare in patients who are patched for 5 hours a day. Parents are instructed to call the physician if the child's fixation preference changes. Iatrogenic amblyopia does not always respond to occlusion of the initially amblyopic eye, and the child may conclude youth with two eyes that are visually compromised.[30]

Occlusion, whether full-time or 5 hours per day, continues until at least 6 months have passed with good compliance and no further improvement in visual acuity at distance or near fixation. Unilaterally high myopes experience increased near visual acuity before distance acuity improves substantially. The goal of all amblyopia treatment is equal and normal near and distance linear acuity in each eye.

Penalization

Atropine treatment of the sound eye with distance correction may encourage use of the amblyopic eye for near tasks; alternatively, the sound eye may be corrected for near fixation and the amblyopic eye for distance.[31] Best results are obtained in high hyperopes who have acuity better than 20/50 (6/15) in the amblyopic eye.

Game Therapy

Active visual involvement of the amblyopic eye is commonly encouraged; such tasks as to color within lines and to connect dots are useful if the targets are of the appropriate size. Video games may help in similar fashion for those old enough to interact with the games.[32]

Oral Levodopa and Carbidopa

The neurotransmitter dopamine is present in retinal amacrine and interplexiform cells and is probably involved in the brain's processing of information. Low doses of levodopa alone and together with carbidopa have been shown to augment the effect of occlusion therapy, even in children over 12 years of age. In one study, combination drugs used with occlusion improved acuity from 20/121 (6/37) to 20/96 (6/29) in 8 hours.[33] In another, 1 week of levodopa alone improved acuity by about 1 line; the improvement lasted for over 3 weeks after the medication was discontinued.[34] The drugs' mechanism of action is unknown. Optimal dosage of each drug is not completely known; overdosage is associated with nausea, vomiting, tiredness, and sleepiness.

Other Forms of Treatment

Pleoptics and the CAM vision stimulator are used today less frequently than previously. Pleoptics involves bleaching the peripheral retina via a powerful modified direct ophthalmoscope and stimulation of the fovea. Controlled studies showed occlusion to be as effective as pleoptics.[35] The CAM vision stimulator is a disc imprinted with bar gratings; discs of varying spatial frequencies are rotated slowly before the amblyopic eye, with the sound eye occluded. Weekly treatments of 7 minutes each were reported to be highly successful initially, but the results could not be reproduced. Daily treatments were found to be no more successful than patches.[36]

COURSE AND OUTCOMES

Why treat amblyopia? Direct benefits include potentially improved stereoptic appreciation and the occasional realignment of strabismic eyes with attainment of improved visual acuity. For most patients, the creation of a better-sighted "spare tire" should trauma or disease claim the sound eye is all that can be promised logically. Of interest is a study that showed a threefold greater risk of loss of the sound eye if the other is amblyopic.[37]

Strabismus surgery is traditionally deferred until after amblyopia has been treated successfully—the assumption is that surgical results are improved thereby. This assumption has not been proved by prospective, matched, controlled studies; a retrospective study suggested that surgical results are not dependent upon amblyopia reversal.[38] However, treatment of amblyopia before surgery probably enjoys better parental compliance, and evaluation of visual acuity by fixational ability of each eye as it moves to take up fixation is easier if the eyes are strabismic. Also, if amblyopia is reversed before surgery, postoperative occlusion is limited to 1–2 hours a day for maintenance of acuity and thus is less likely to disrupt peripheral fusion.

REFERENCES

1. Eggers HM. Amblyopia. In: Diamond GR, Eggers HM, eds. Strabismus and pediatric ophthalmology, Vol 5 in Podos SM, Yanoff M, eds. Textbook of ophthalmology. London: Mosby; 1993:13.1–17.
2. Sireteanu R, Fronius M. Naso-temporal asymmetries in human amblyopia: consequence of long-term interocular suppression. Vision Res. 1881;21:1055–63.
3. Hess RF, Pointer JS. Differences in the neural basis of human amblyopia: the distribution of the anomaly across the visual field. Vision Res. 1985;25:1577–94.
4. Hess RF, Holliday IE. The spatial localization defect in amblyopia. Vision Res. 1992;32:1319–39.
5. Abrahamsson M, Fabian G, Sjostrand J. A longitudinal study of a population based sample of astigmatic children. II. The changeability of anisometropia. Acta Ophthalmol. 1990;68:435–40.
6. Birch EE, Stager DE. Monocular acuity and stereopsis in infantile esotropia. Invest Ophthalmol Vis Sci. 1985;26:1624–30.
7. Birnbaum MH, Koslowe K, Sarret R. Success in amblyopia therapy as a function of age: a literature survey. Arch Ophthalmol. 1953;54:269–75.
8. Gstalder RJ, Green DG. Laser interferometric acuity in amblyopia. J Pediatr Ophthalmol Strabismus. 1971;8:251–6.
9. Flom ML, Bedell HE. Identifying amblyopia using associated conditions, acuity, and nonacuity features. Am J Optom Physiol Opt. 1985;62:153–60.

10. Kutschke PJ, Scott WE, Keech RV. Anisometropic amblyopia. Ophthalmology. 1991;98:258–63.
11. Abraham SV. Accommodation in the amblyopic eye. Am J Ophthalmol. 1961;52:197–200.
12. Stuart JA, Burian HM. A study of separation difficulty. Am J Ophthalmol. 1963;53:471–7.
13. von Noorden GK, Burian HM. Visual acuity in normal and amblyopic patients under reduced illumination. I. Behavior of visual acuity with and without neutral density filters. Arch Ophthalmol. 1959;61:533–5.
14. Schor C. A directional impairment of eye movement control in strabismic amblyopia. Invest Ophthalmol Vis Sci. 1975;14:692–7.
15. Eggers HM, Blakemore C. Physiological basis of anisometropic amblyopia. Science. 1978;201:264–6.
16. Movshon JA, Eggers HM, Gizzi MS, et al. Effects of early unilateral blur on the macaque's visual system. III. Physiological observations. J Neurosci. 1987;7: 1341–51.
17. Hendrickson AE, Movshon JA, Eggers HM. Effects of early unilateral blur on the macaque's visual system. II. Anatomical observations. J Neurosci. 1987;7: 1327–39.
18. Wiesel TN, Hubel DH. Single cell responses in striate cortex of kittens deprived of vision in one eye. J Neurophysiol. 1963;26:1003–17.
19. Sur M, Humphrey AH, Sherman SM. Monocular deprivation affects X- and Y-cell terminations in cats. Nature. 1982;300:183–5.
20. Hubel DH, Wiesel TN, LeVay S. Functional architecture of area 17 in normal and monocularly deprived macaque monkeys. Cold Spring Harbor Symp Quant Biol. 1975;40:581–9.
21. Hubel DH, Wiesel TN, LeVay S. Plasticity of ocular dominance columns in monkey striate cortex. Philos Trans R Soc Lond Ser B. 1977;278:377–409.
22. Wiesel TN, Hubel DH. Comparison of the effects of unilateral and bilateral closure on cortical unit responses in kittens. J Neurophysiol. 1965;28:1029–40.
23. Kiorper L, Boothe RG. Naturally occurring strabismus in monkeys (Macaca nemistrima). Invest Ophthalmol Vis Sci. 1981;20:257–63.
24. von Norden GK, Dowling JE, Ferguson DC. Experimental amblyopia in monkeys. Arch Ophthalmol. 1970;84:206–14.
25. Daw NH, Fox K, Sato H, Czepita D. Critical period for monocular deprivation in the cat visual cortex. J Neurophysiol. 1992;67:197–202.
26. Levitt FB, Van Sluyters RC. The sensitive period for strabismus in the kitten. Dev Brain Res. 1982;3:323–7.
27. LeVay S, Wiesel TN, Hubel DH. The development of ocular dominance columns in normal and visually deprived monkeys. J Comp Neurol. 1980;191:1–51.
28. Kirpes L, Carlson MR, Alfi D. Development of visual acuity in experimentally strabismic monkeys. Am Vision Sci. 1989;4:95–106.
29. Bradford GM, Kutschke PJ, Scott WE. Results of amblyopia therapy in eyes with unilateral structural abnormalities. Ophthalmology. 1992;99:1616–21.
30. Hardesty HH. Occlusion amblyopia. Report of a case. Arch Ophthalmol. 1959;62:314–16.
31. Haase W. Optische penalization als therapeutisches Hilfsmittel beim Fruhkindlichen strabismus. Adv Ophthalmol. 1978;35:26–44.
32. Friden SJ, Kuperwaser MC, Stromberg AE, Goldman SG. Stripe therapy for amblyopia with a modified television game. Arch Ophthalmol. 1981;99:1596–9.
33. Laguire LE, Regan GL, Bremer DL, et al. Levodopa/carbidopa for childhood amblyopia. Invest Ophthalmol Vis Sci. 1995;34:3090–5.
34. Gottlob I, Charlier J, Reinecke RD. Visual acuities and scotoma after one week levodopa administration in human amblyopia. Invest Ophthalmol Vis Sci. 1992;33:2722–8.
35. Fletcher MK, Abbott W, Girard LJ, et al. Results of the biostatistical study of the management of suppression amblyopia by intensive pleoptics versus conventional patching. Am Orthopt J. 1969;19:8–30.
36. Mehdorn E, Matthews W, Schuppe A, et al. Treatment for amblyopia with rotating gratings and subsequent occlusion: a controlled study. Int Ophthalmol. 1981;3:161–6.
37. Tommilla V, Tarkkanen A. Incidence of loss of vision in the healthy eye in amblyopia. Br J Ophthalmol. 1981;65:575–7.
38. Lam GC, Repka MX, Guyton DL. Timing of amblyopia therapy relative to strabismus surgery. Ophthalmology. 1993;100:1751–6.

CHAPTER

80

Forms of Nonsurgical Strabismus Management

GARY R. DIAMOND

DEFINITIONS
- Sector occlusion: occlusion of a portion of a spectacle lens with translucent adhesive paper to treat strabismus or amblyopia.
- Orthoptics: a wide range of techniques used to expand fusional vergence amplitudes and permit improved single binocular vision.

KEY FEATURES
- Numerous techniques other than glasses are available to treat strabismus and should be considered before strabismus surgery is performed.

SECTOR OCCLUSION

A popular form of strabismus management in Europe, not well known in the United States, involves the use of partial lens occlusion, termed "sector occlusion." A sector is a piece of translucent adhesive paper applied to the posterior surface of a lens or lenses to obstruct vision of an eye in a particular direction (Fig. 80-1). This method, unlike prisms or optical penalization, does not alter the shape, size, or localization of a viewed object.

Sector occluders are devised to obstruct the areas responsible for diplopia and visual confusion. A large frame is provided to enable exact placement of the sector occluders.

In one study, in 384 children who had constant horizontal strabismus, orthophoria was obtained in 169 (44%). Orthophoria was obtained in 85% of those who had a deviation less than 30Δ, in 25% of those who had a deviation in the range 30–50Δ, and in only 3% of those who had a deviation greater than 50Δ. An additional 57 (15%) achieved a final deviation less than 15Δ, and the remaining 157 children (41%) required surgery.[1]

Sector occluders of different shapes are used for the treatment of amblyopia (Fig. 80-2).

ORTHOPTICS

The treatment of strabismus by means of orthoptics (literally, "straight eyes") has a long history, although perhaps this technique is used more extensively in Europe than in the United States. Its basic principle is the gradual expansion of fusional vergence amplitudes by exercises, either in open space or using targets viewed through devices intended to isolate the eyes—haploscopic devices, such as the major amblyoscope. Fusional vergence amplitudes are expanded through the use of gradually stronger prisms held in the appropriate direction before one or both eyes or through the use of spherical lenses to utilize the accommodation-convergence relationship to change ocular alignment.

Historically, the success of orthoptic training was greatest in cooperative patients who had phorias or intermittent strabismus

of comitant nature. The patients who suffered alphabet pattern strabismus, torsional symptoms, or highly incomitant strabismus and who gave little cooperation fared less well. Patients affected by long-standing constant tropias were less likely to regain fusional vergence amplitudes despite orthoptic training.

Today, the most common indications for orthoptic expansion of fusional vergences include convergence insufficiency, intermittent exotropia of relatively small amplitude, and decompensating accommodative esotropia. Published series of successfully treated patients followed for long terms are difficult to find, and it is unclear whether orthoptic training must be continued throughout life to be effective. It also is unclear whether preoperative fusional expansion improves long-term surgical results.

Diplopia recognition training for patients who have anomalous retinal correspondence and suppression is performed rarely today because of the risk of intractable diplopia.

PRISMS

Prisms may be very useful in the treatment of certain patients who have a small degree of horizontal and vertical strabismus.[2,3]

Patients who have superior oblique palsy and a vertical deviation in primary position may benefit from a vertical prism before the paretic eye. The usefulness of this technique is confounded by the simultaneous excyclotorsion associated with this palsy; some patients, however, cyclofuse successfully if the vertical deviation is collapsed with a prism. The minimal amount of prismatic correction necessary to provide comfortable single binocular vision is prescribed after an office and home trial with Fresnel membrane prisms, as described subsequently. Because many patients who suffer this palsy have incomitant deviations when viewing from right to left, the field of single binocular vision is likely to be limited. In addition, vertical fusional vergence amplitudes are likely to wither under prism correction, and the patient becomes more strabismic when the prism is removed.

Some patients who have sixth nerve palsies and esotropia in primary position benefit from a base-out prism over the paretic eye; this may obviate the need for a face turn to view in the forward position. Some patients who have congenital nystagmus and a compensating face posture may benefit from prisms before one or both eyes to position the null point of least nystagmus and best acuity in the forward position, with the head straight. In the case of a horizontal face position, the bases of the prisms are placed in the direction of the face turn. Because the amount of prismatic correction is quite large, this approach is usually impractical.

The use of prisms to treat patients who have typical intermittent horizontal and vertical strabismus is often contraindicated because they place fusional vergence amplitudes at rest and consign the patient to permanent, often increasing, prismatic correction. However, certain elderly or debilitated patients may benefit from prismatic correction when surgery is not indicated or when the deviation is small and symptomatic.

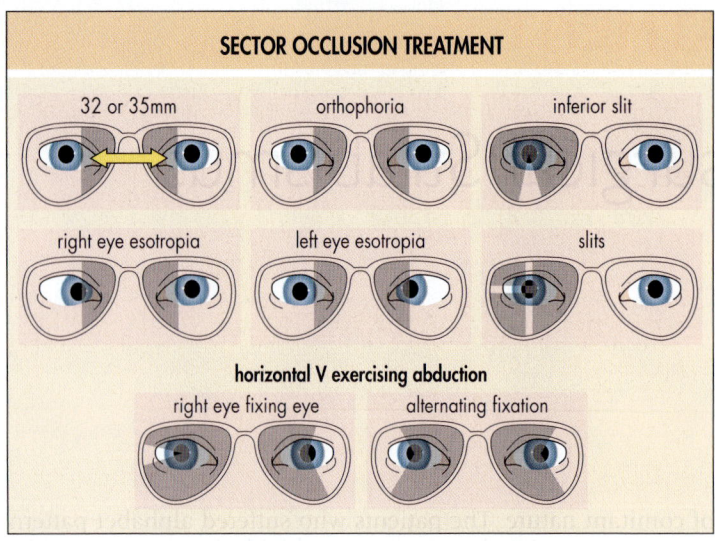

SECTOR OCCLUSION TREATMENT

32 or 35mm

orthophoria

inferior slit

right eye esotropia

left eye esotropia

slits

horizontal V exercising abduction

right eye fixing eye

alternating fixation

FIG. 80-1 ■ Sector occlusion treatment. Various forms for strabismus, diplopia, and visual confusion.

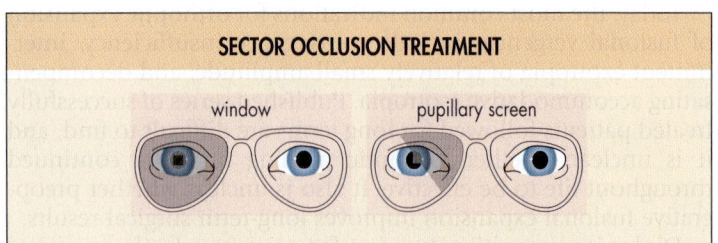

SECTOR OCCLUSION TREATMENT

window

pupillary screen

FIG. 80-2 ■ Sector occluder shapes for amblyopia.

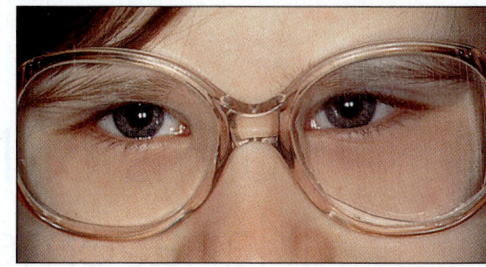

FIG. 80-3 ■ Prism adaptation test. A child with esotropia is wearing a Fresnel membrane prism over the left eye, of sufficient strength to neutralize the esotropia.

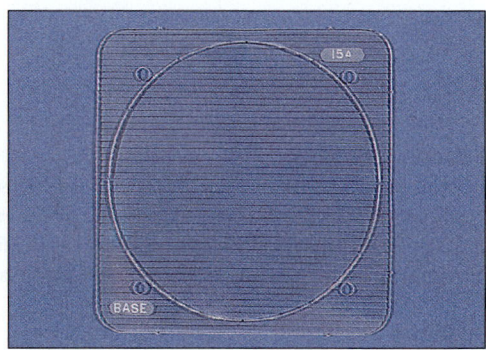

FIG. 80-4 ■ A Fresnel membrane prism. The prisms are prepunched in circular format and the base is clearly marked.

The prism adaptation test involves the preoperative use of prisms to neutralize a deviation with prisms for a given period of time, followed by surgery for the amount of strabismus fully neutralized by the prisms. Thus, the prism neutralization may be used to predict the outcome of surgery for a given deviation, to determine the maximum deviation, and to estimate fusion potential at that deviation (see Fig. 80-3). In addition, some patients exhibit a different deviation with the prism adaptation test than with cover testing. It remains to be shown whether the former deviation provides better surgical results than the latter. In a controlled, randomized study of patients who had acquired esotropia, 60% underwent prism adaptation and 40% did not; of those who responded to prisms with motor stability and sensory fusion, half underwent conventional surgery and half underwent augmented surgery based on the prism-adapted deviation.[4] Success rates were highest (89%) in the prism adaptation responders who underwent augmented surgery, 79% in those who underwent traditional amounts of surgery, and lowest (72%) in those who did not undergo prism adaptation.

The amount of prism to give a patient for comfortable single binocular vision may be assumed arbitrarily to be one third to one half of the maximal phoria obtained on cover testing, or it may be titrated to the subjective response of the patient.[5] Fresnel membrane prisms are obtained easily, are relatively inexpensive, and are easy to adjust in strength (Fig. 80-4). They are somewhat dysesthetic, yellow, peel after about 3 months in place, and do degrade acuity (about one line per 5Δ). Available in the range 1–30Δ, they may be confined to one or both lenses (plano carriers in the case of patients who are not wearing a correction); trimmed to fit a bifocal segment, distance correction, or part of the field of a lens; or prescribed to an oblique axis orientation for those who have both horizontal and vertical deviations. Patients are given a trial of Fresnel prism wear. If it is agreeable and the deviation is relatively small (under about 10Δ), the prism may be ground permanently into spectacles. Some prefer to continue to wear the Fresnel membrane prism and simply change it after 3 months or so.

BOTULINUM TOXIN

The use of type A *Clostridium botulinum* toxin (oculinum) to paralyze temporarily human extraocular muscles by chemodenervation and thus permit the antagonist to contract and effect a permanent alignment change is credited to Alan B. Scott[6] and colleagues at the Smith-Kettlewell Eye Research Foundation. The toxin interferes with acetylcholine release from nerve endings by antagonization of serotonin-mediated calcium ion release. The toxin is usually injected in the conscious patient, with the syringe needle connected to an auditory electromyogram device that amplifies the muscle action potentials; upon successful injection, the muscle immediately becomes silent as the action potential disappears. Within 3 days, the injected muscle becomes paralyzed and an overcorrection is noted. Alternatively, the muscle may be injected under direct visualization and a general anesthetic.

Oculinum is provided as a freeze-dried lyophil in vials that contain 50ng of toxin prepared under supervision of the U.S. Food and Drug Administration. The toxin is stable for up to 4 years at freezer temperature but degrades within 1 hour if thawed to room temperature. Immediately before use it is reconstituted with normal saline. Each vial contains less than 1/40 of the lethal dose for 50% of humans; the nanogram dose injected is too small to stimulate antibody formation.

Oculinum is predicted to be most useful in cooperative adults but has been injected successfully in children as young as 9 years. Younger children may be sedated in the operating room using ketamine and then injected with oculinum. The protocol suggests titrated dosages proportional to the deviation, with children's dosages also proportional to body weight. Injections are preceded by administration of topical anesthetic drops.

Many series of patients have been reported. In a series reported by Biglan *et al.*,[7] best results were found in patients who had surgical overcorrections (87.5% controlled with oculinum) and mild sixth nerve palsy (43.7% controlled) and worst results in patients who had comitant exotropia (13.3% controlled) and infantile esotropia (33.3% controlled). Significant complications included blepharoptosis, hypertropia, globe perforation, and subconjunctival hemorrhage. Complications reported by others include transient pupillary dilatation, retrobulbar hemorrhage, spread of paralysis to noninjected muscles, missed injection site, patient disorientation, diplopia, and corneal irritation.[8]

Oculinum appears to be most useful in patients who are not medically fit for surgery (because of illness or a history of malignant hyperthermia), who refuse surgery, who have had multiple strabismus operations, or who have acute sixth nerve palsies and mild esotropia in primary position. Oculinum is contraindicated in patients who have a history of myasthenia gravis and is unlikely to be effective in patients who have mechanical restriction of eye movement caused by scar tissue or entrapment of tissue.

REFERENCES

1. Sarniguet-Badoche J. Early medical treatment of strabismus. In: Reinecke R, ed. Strabismus II. Orlando: Grune & Stratton; 1984:83–9.
2. Kutschke PJ. Use of prisms: are they really helpful? Am Orthopt J. 1996;46:61–4.
3. Sinelli JM, Repka MX. Prism treatment of incomitant horizontal deviations. Am Orthopt J. 1996;41:123–6.
4. Prism Adaptation Study Research Group. Efficacy of prism adaptation in the surgical management of acquired esotropia. Arch Ophthalmol. 1990;108:1248–56.
5. Berard P. Prisms: their therapeutic use in strabismus. In: Knapp P, ed. International Strabismus Symposium: an evaluation of present status of orthoptics, pleoptics, and related diagnosis and treatment regimes. New York: Karger; 1968:339–44.
6. Scott A. Botulinum toxin injection of eye muscles to correct strabismus. Trans Am Ophthalmol Soc. 1981;79:734–70.
7. Biglan A, Burnstine R, Rogers G, Saunders R. Management of strabismus with botulinum A toxin. Ophthalmology. 1989;96:935–43.
8. Lingua R. Sequelae of botulinum toxin injection. Am J Ophthalmol. 1985; 100:305–7.

81

Techniques of Strabismus Surgery

ROBERT W. LINGUA • GARY R. DIAMOND

KEY FEATURES
- The ideal strabismus surgery should be pain free during and after surgery, performed under sterile conditions, be nontraumatic to ocular tissue, heal without scarring, and yield perfect alignment in all gaze positions and testing distances in a single operation without causing anesthetic morbidity.

INTRODUCTION

Strabismus surgery becomes the appropriate therapeutic approach when all nonsurgical methods to reduce visual axis deviations have failed. Many of these nonsurgical methods are discussed in Chapters 73–78 and 80. It is important that the surgeon defer to surgery until reproducible measurements are obtained, the patient is sufficiently systemically stable to be able to tolerate the procedure and attendant anesthetic, and the patient (or parent) understands the goals and limitations of the planned surgery.

Except in unusual cases, the following are goals of all strabismus surgery:
- Attainment of peripheral fusion with fusional vergence amplitudes sufficient to maintain alignment of the eyes
- Comfortable single binocular vision to enable the patient to perform visual tasks without asthenopia
- Improved esthetic appearance

In the uncommon case of an older patient (over 4 years of age) who has no preoperative binocular vision, surgery provides at best a temporary esthetic improvement with little hope of stable postoperative alignment; naturally, the patient or parent must be warned of this.

HISTORICAL REVIEW

The first eye muscle procedure (horizontal rectus muscle tenotomy) was probably performed in the middle of the eighteenth century by Chevalier John Taylor.[1] The first successful operation for strabismus using horizontal rectus tenotomy was performed on a living patient (a 7-year-old boy with esotropia) in 1839 by Johann Dieffenbach.[2] Von Graefe[3] performed partial tenotomy in 1851 and advancement of a rectus muscle in 1857. By the late 19th century sutures were being used to shorten a muscle, and measured resections and recessions followed soon afterward. More recent contributions include the use of adjustable sutures and techniques for operation on the oblique and vertical rectus muscles.

Over the past 20 years, major advances have occurred in magnification techniques, improved overhead lighting, instrument technology, and suture development. Modern sutures for stra-

bismus surgery are usually absorbable and swaged to needles with cutting edges directed away from the center of the globe.

PREOPERATIVE EVALUATION AND DIAGNOSTIC APPROACH

Ideal preoperative evaluation of the strabismus surgical patient includes quantitation of the misalignment in primary positions at distance and at near as well as in the nine diagnostic gaze positions (Box 81-1). In most patients, the maximal deviation under conditions of complete dissociation of the visual axes is the deviation for which surgery is to be designed. As indicated, measurements are taken both with and without the appropriate optical correction. Finally, duction and version testing and, when appropriate, forced duction and force-generation testing are performed. These topics are discussed in greater detail in Chapters 70–78.

ANESTHETIC

The choice of anesthetic technique is individualized and depends upon the circumstances of the procedure chosen, age, ability of the patient to tolerate discomfort, and patient's choice. Strabismus surgery on children younger than about 16 years usually requires general anesthetic; some older patients request general anesthetic for psychological reasons. Newer anesthetic agents may decrease postoperative nausea and vomiting; preoperative discussion with the anesthesiologist concerning availability may reduce the incidence of these events. The benefit of general anesthetic is an immobile, insensate patient; the disadvantages include the attendant risks of general anesthetic, increased recovery time, and delay of postoperative suture adjustment of final eye position.

Retrobulbar injection provides sufficient akinesia and anesthetic for sufficiently cooperative older teenagers and adults to be able to tolerate the injection. Preinjection intravenous dissociative agents or narcotics are often helpful, and lid block is usually not required. The benefits of retrobulbar injection include obviation of general anesthetic risks, briefer recovery room time, and more rapid return to normal routine. Disadvantages include risks of globe or nerve perforation,[4] rare cases of presumed brainstem anesthetic with respiratory suppression,[5] inability to immobilize the superior oblique muscle, inability to operate on both eyes in one session unless another technique is used for the second eye, and injection into a muscle belly with resultant contracture. Particular caution must be exercised in those who have large globes (e.g., myopia, buphthalmos) or encumbered orbits (patients who have dysthyroid orbitopathy and enlarged extraocular muscles) because of the increased risk of globe perforation or vascular compromise.

Many cooperative older patients can tolerate epibulbar injection of anesthetic agent around the appropriate muscle(s); generally, the patient who tolerates forced duction testing in the office is a candidate for epibulbar injection or even topical anesthetic. The advantages of epibulbar injection are similar to those of retrobulbar injection; disadvantages include somewhat greater discomfort (especially when the muscle is hooked) and rare cases of globe perforation. Some patients may have muscle adjustment performed at the time of surgery when they fixate upon a target.

GENERAL TECHNIQUES

Strabismus surgery demands meticulous planning. Barring unusual circumstances or unusual anatomy, the surgical plan is prepared before anesthetic is given. It is helpful to keep a description of the surgical plan for ready reference before and during surgery.

The exact location and number of conjunctival incisions depend upon the muscles to be operated, preexisting scarring, and the patient's previous surgical history. Limbal incisions more easily permit accurate surgery without a trained assistant, may expedite surgery in patients who have experienced multiple procedures upon a given muscle, may minimize conjunctival shredding in older patients who have limited Tenon's capsule and inelastic conjunctiva, and permit conjunctival recessions if the tissue is contracted.[6] However, patients experience increased discomfort because of corneal proximity, the incisions may compromise the conjunctival contribution to the anterior segment circulation, and the incision heals slightly more slowly than when other options are used.

Fornix incisions permit rapid access to the muscles, stimulate less discomfort than limbal incisions, preserve conjunctival vascular supply, and may not require suture or diathermic closure.[7] However, they do require the presence of a more skilled assistant, a better knowledge of muscle anatomy to avoid surgery on the wrong muscle, and relatively elastic conjunctiva. It is important not to incise conjunctiva more than 8mm posterior to the limbus so as not to invade orbital fat.

Incisions at the anterior border of the muscle tendon (Swan's approach)[8] have fallen from favor because of the tendency for significant postoperative subconjunctival scarring between the limbus and muscle insertion. However, certain patients who undergo reoperation may benefit from such an approach.

Absorbable sutures are generally utilized when vascular healing of tissues occurs, such as in typical recession and resection techniques. These sutures usually absorb within 7–10 days if covered with conjunctiva, slightly longer if exposed. Permanent sutures are utilized if avascular tissue such as the superior oblique tendon is harnessed, as in the superior oblique tuck or silicone (Silastic) band-lengthening procedure.

SPECIFIC TECHNIQUES

Recession of a Rectus Muscle

MEDIAL RECTUS. To perform a medial rectus recession, the assistant grasps the eye at the conjunctiva–Tenon's capsule junction with a 0.3mm forceps and rotates the eye into elevation and abduction (Fig. 81-1). The surgeon then elevates the conjunctiva at the base of the fornix and incises the conjunctiva 8mm from the limbus (Fig. 81-2). At this point, all visible conjunctival vessels are cauterized lightly to ensure good visibility during localization of the tendon. The assistant and surgeon grasp the fascia within the conjunctival incision with gentle pressure against the sclera and elevate it from the globe (Fig. 81-3). The scissors are then used to incise Tenon's capsule at this point and expose bare sclera (Fig. 81-4). Visualization of the bare sclera is maintained using the posterior forceps.

The Greene self-retaining muscle hook is then passed behind the medial rectus muscle with no posterior movement of the hook farther than the site of the incision itself (Fig. 81-5). When the medial rectus is on the hook, the surgeon confirms that the entire tendon is engaged. The posterior arm of the 0.3mm forceps may be used as a probe to locate the superior pole of the muscle (Fig. 81-6). The pole is secured using the forceps, and the muscle hook is withdrawn to the inferior aspect of the tendon (Fig. 81-7)—ensure

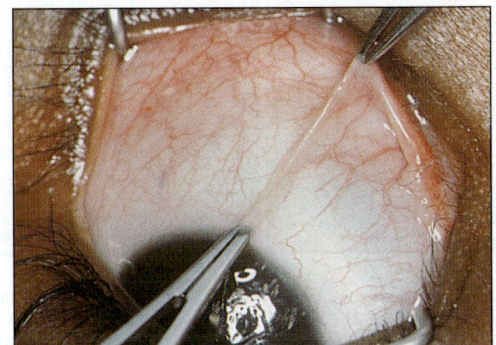

FIG. 81-1 Recession of medial rectus muscle. Figures 81-1 through 81-29 demonstrate recession of the left medial rectus as seen from the surgeon's 12 o'clock position. A 0.3mm forceps is placed at the 7:30 position and the conjunctiva and Tenon's capsule are grasped at the limbus. The eye is elevated and abducted. A second 0.3mm forceps is used to elevate the conjunctiva about 8mm posterior to the limbus.

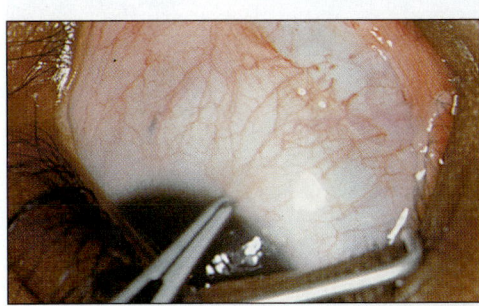

FIG. 81-2 The conjunctiva is incised (fornix incision) using Westcott scissors.

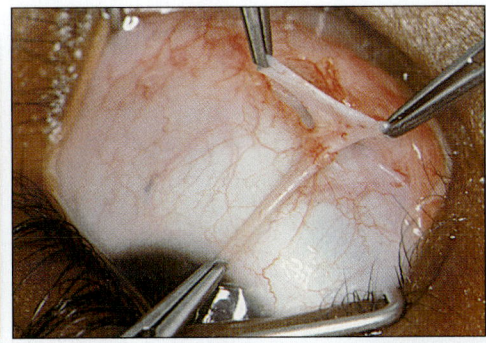

FIG. 81-3 Both surgeon and assistant elevate Tenon's capsule out of the plane of the conjunctival incision.

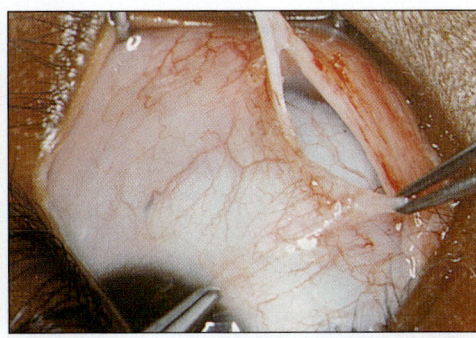

FIG. 81-4 Tenon's capsule is incised, which exposes sclera.

that the hook is released from entrapment in the insertion. Then the hook is passed beyond the superior pole held by the forceps (Fig. 81-8). In this way, it is certain that the full length of the tendon is secured completely. A large Jameson muscle hook, or the Greene hook, is useful in the following dissection.

The small tenotomy hook is introduced between the insertion of the tendon and Tenon's capsule anterior to it (Fig. 81-9) and used to dissect bluntly the fascia from the surface of the tendon as it is moved posteriorly along its long axis (Fig. 81-10). At this point, it is important to overcome any resistance to blunt dissection if the tendon is to be visualized adequately during the remainder of the procedure. When the conjunctiva and Tenon's capsule have been reflected satisfactorily over the tip of the large muscle hook (Fig. 81-11), the scissors are used to incise the superior aspect of Tenon's fascia (Fig. 81-12). Visualization of bare sclera superiorly is accomplished by the introduction of the

closed scissor blades into the fascial incision and rotation of these over the tip of the hook (Figs. 81-13 and 81-14). Two small tenotomy hooks are passed posteriorly along the tendon, against bare sclera, and elevated to expose the intermuscular fascia (Figs. 81-15 and 81-16) for dissection. The 0.5mm Castroviejo locking forceps are then applied to the distal aspect of the tendon superiorly (Fig. 81-17) and inferiorly. These forceps serve as globe handles throughout the procedure, which obviates the need for traction sutures at the limbus. Also, the superior forceps maintains full exposure of the insertion and keep the retracted conjunctiva and fascia securely above the superior pole when the inferonasal fornix incision is used.

Gentle traction by the assistant, away from the operated muscle, allows the surgeon to control the hook beneath the tendon and accomplish suture passage at the insertion (Fig. 81-18). The surgeon may then control the forceps during the scleral

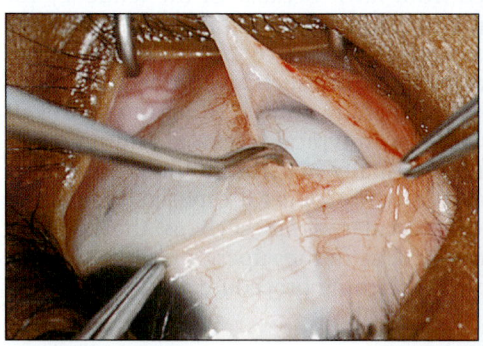 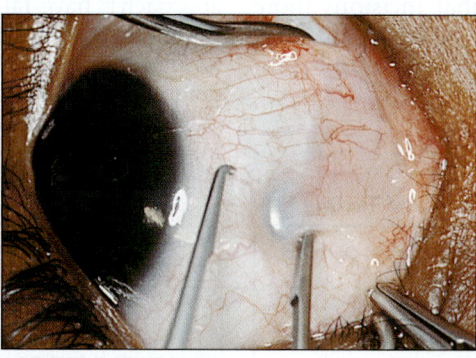 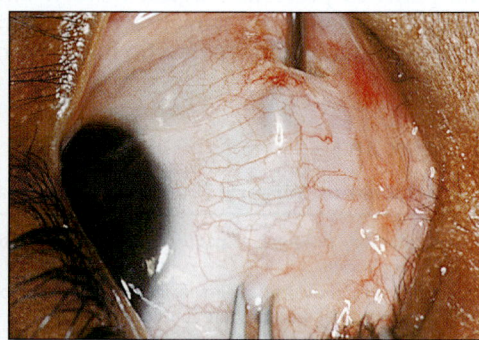

FIG. 81-5 ▌ The Greene or Jameson muscle hook is inserted under the tendon of the medial rectus muscle. The toe of the hook is kept flat against the sclera at all times.

FIG. 81-6 ▌ The surgeon grasps the superior pole of the muscle through the conjunctiva. This ensures that the entire tendon is on the muscle hook.

FIG. 81-7 ▌ The superior pole of the rectus muscle is held by the forceps. The muscle hook is partially withdrawn.

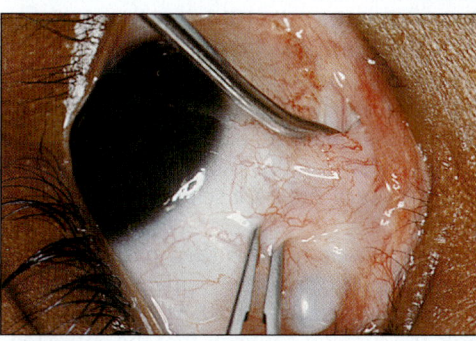 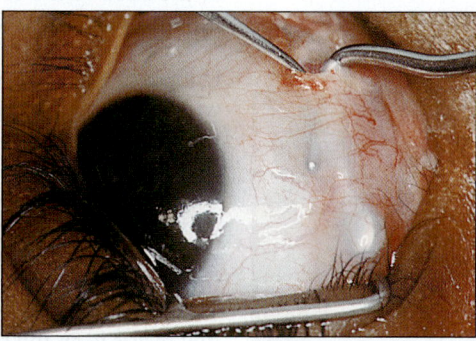 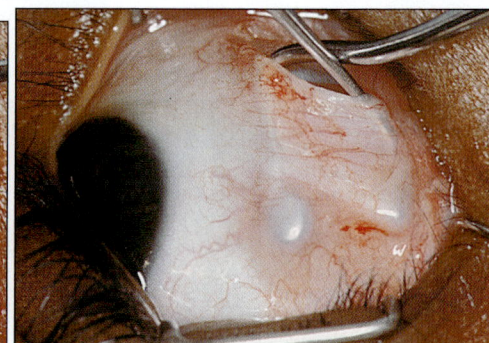

FIG. 81-8 ▌ The muscle hook has been replaced to clear the forceps and capture the entire tendon.

FIG. 81-9 ▌ A small Stevens muscle hook is placed under the conjunctiva on the limbal side of the rectus muscle tendon.

FIG. 81-10 ▌ The small Stevens hook is moved forward and backward over the tendon and under the conjunctiva. This separates conjunctiva from the underlying Tenon's capsule and tendon.

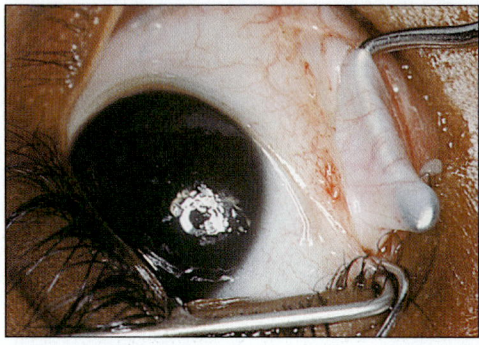 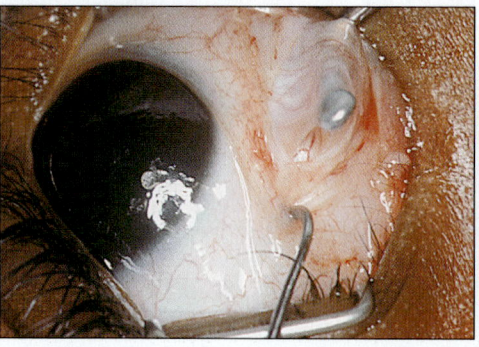 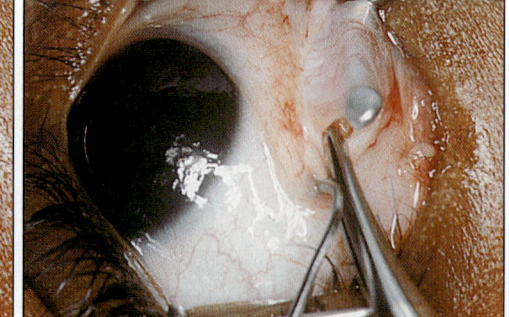

FIG. 81-11 ▌ The small muscle hook is placed perpendicular to the globe at the superior tendon border. This exposes intermuscular septum and Tenon's capsule.

FIG. 81-12 ▌ A small opening is created at the tip of the muscle hook through intermuscular septum and Tenon's capsule.

FIG 81-13 ▌ The closed scissors may be used to dissect bluntly the superior pole of the tendon.

passes to position optimally and control the globe. The needle is passed from the middle to the superior edge of the tendon, 1.0–1.5mm posterior to the tendon insertion, where it is positioned for regrasping. A second "through-and-through" lock to the edge of the tendon (Figs. 81-19 to 81-21) is performed. The Westcott scissors suffice for removal of the tendon (Fig. 81-22). Visualization of the tendon may be preserved if a dry cotton pledget is passed between the tendon and globe (Fig. 81-23). The anterior pole of the caliper is positioned at the crotch of the original insertion (Fig. 81-24). The ideal scleral pass imparts an opaque translucency to the needle (Fig. 81-25). The needle is laid flat on the sclera before the tip engages scleral tissue.

Because the spatula or inverted lancet needle is a side-cutting needle, it is important to avoid the tract of the previously passed suture and not cut it inadvertently. Likewise, it is important to position the exits of the sutures not so far apart as to create a buckling effect when the knot is tied; ideally, the needle paths overlap in sclera by 1mm (Fig. 81-26). The sutures are then drawn in the direction in which they were passed (Fig. 81-27) to avoid breaking the sutures out of the sclera. The receded muscle is demonstrated where an attempt is made to preserve the original orientation of the tendon to the globe at its normal width (Fig. 81-28). After the tendon has been secured to the globe, the tenotomy hook is introduced above the superior pole of the earlier insertion and the fascia is rotated inferiorly (Figs. 81-29 and 81-30) over the operative site. The incision is closed with a single 6-0 plain suture in a "bury-the-knot" fashion to minimize foreign body sensation (Fig. 81-31). In the young, the conjunctiva is routinely closed because the complication of Tenon's capsule prolapse may require additional anesthetic for management.

LATERAL RECTUS AND VERTICAL RECTI. The principles of recession are the same as described previously for the medial

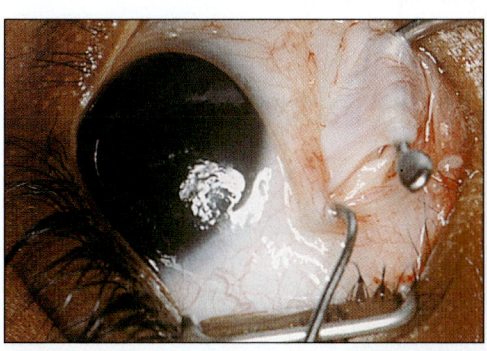

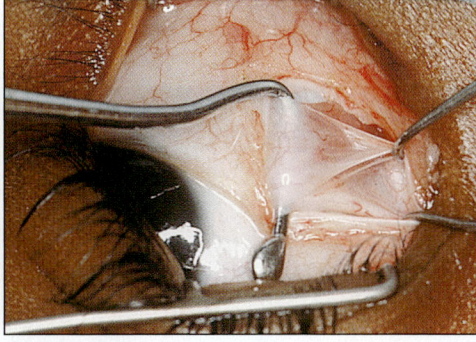

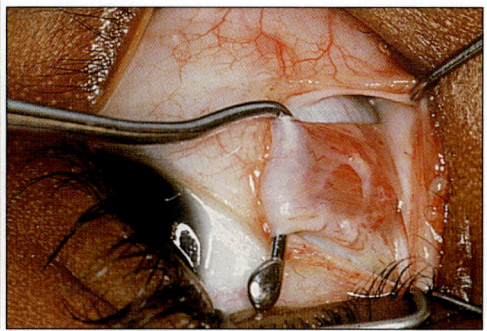

FIG. 81-14 ■ A Stevens muscle hook is placed perpendicular to the sclera through the incision. It is swept around the superior pole of the tendon to ensure that the entire tendon is captured on the muscle hook.

FIG. 81-15 ■ Two Stevens muscle hooks retract the conjunctiva and Tenon's capsule to expose the length of muscle.

FIG. 81-16 ■ The muscle is exposed as far posteriorly as desired.

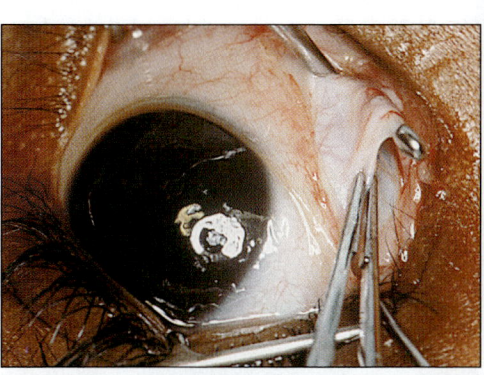

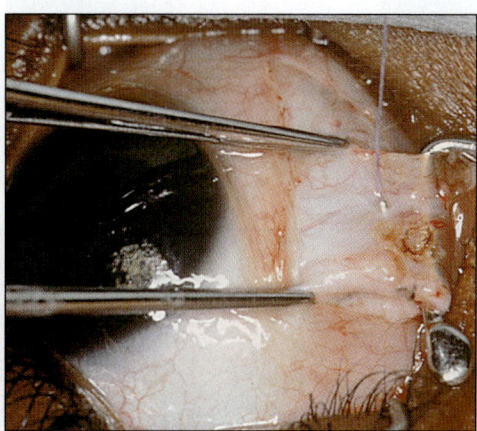

FIG. 81-17 ■ The locking forceps are applied to both the superior and inferior poles of the tendon insertion. This is to control the exposure as well as the position of the globe.

FIG. 81-18 ■ The surgeon holds the muscle hook and the assistant the locking forceps.

FIG. 81-19 ■ The position of the eye is controlled using the muscle hook. Simultaneously, the surgeon places the suture from the middle of the tendon to the margin, parallel to the insertion.

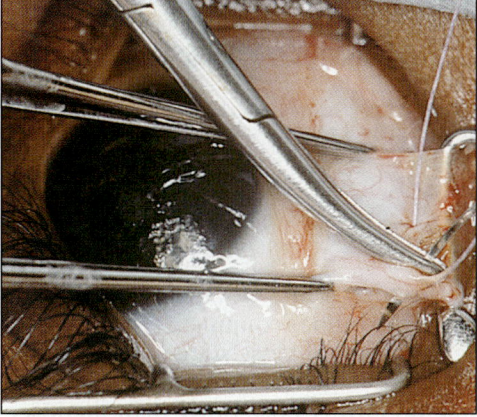

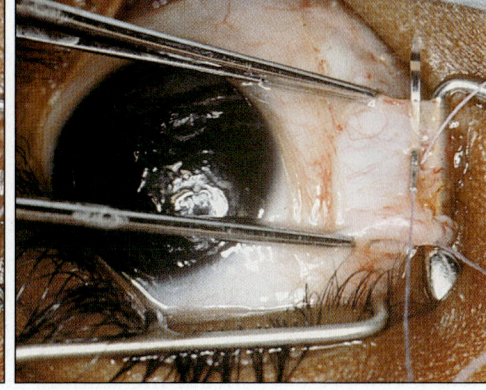

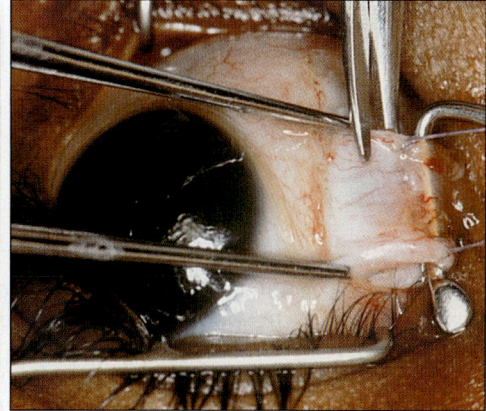

FIG. 81-20 ■ A lock bite is performed at the margin of the muscle.

FIG. 81-21 ■ A similar maneuver is performed. The second arm of the double-armed suture is placed through the remaining half of the tendon.

FIG. 81-22 ■ The tendon is disinserted from the globe.

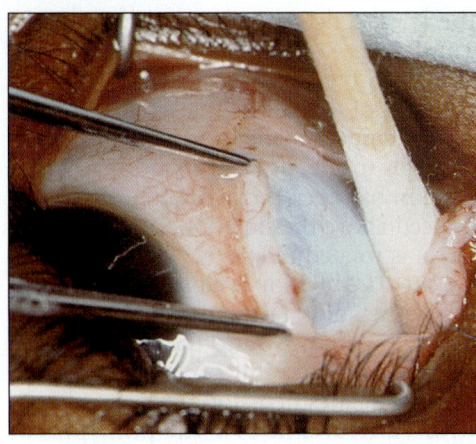

FIG. 81-23 ▌ Note the thin sclera posterior to the muscle insertion. Any hemorrhage from the cut tendon can be controlled with cotton swabs.

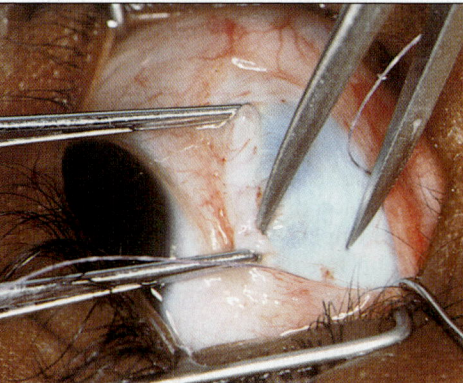

FIG. 81-24 ▌ The appropriate position for muscle reattachment is measured from the original insertion.

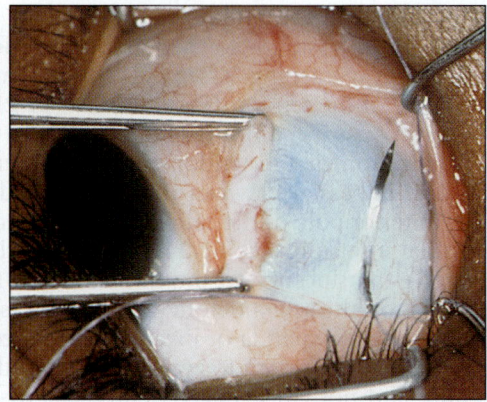

FIG. 81-25 ▌ The first arm of the double-armed suture is placed through the sclera. This placement is parallel to the original insertion.

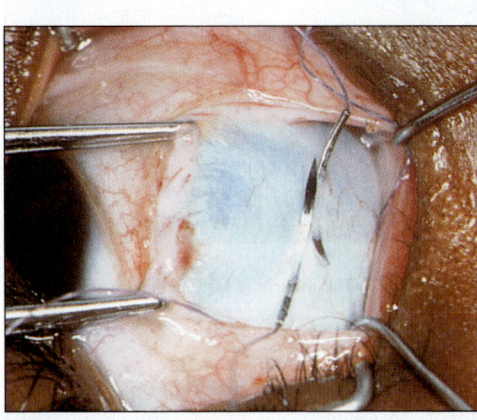

FIG. 81-26 ▌ The second needle of the double-armed suture is placed in similar fashion to the first. Ensure a slight overlap of exit sites.

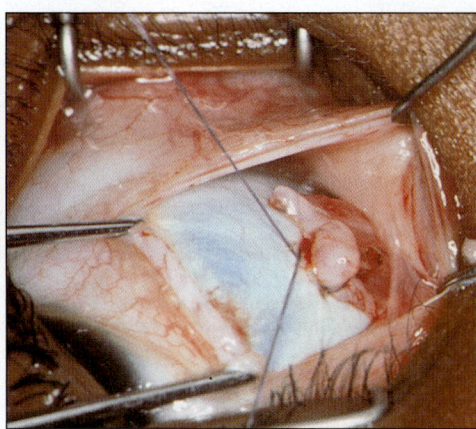

FIG. 81-27 ▌ The muscle is pulled fully to the desired recession site.

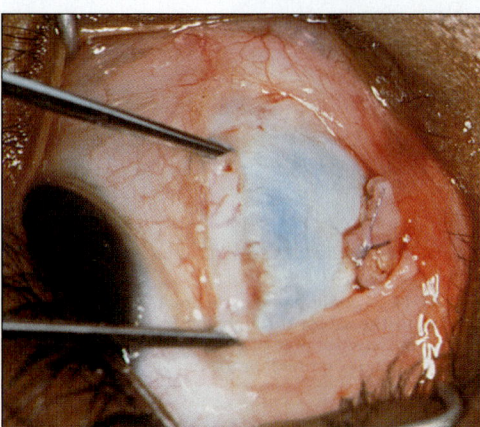

FIG. 81-28 ▌ The sutures are tightened, tied, and cut.

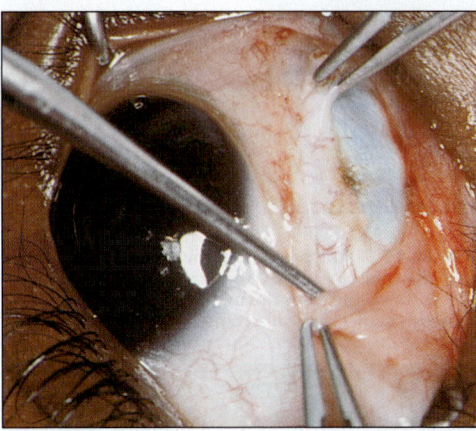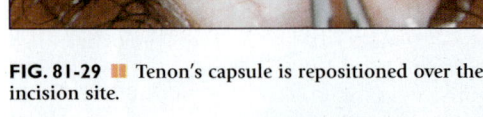

FIG. 81-29 ▌ Tenon's capsule is repositioned over the incision site.

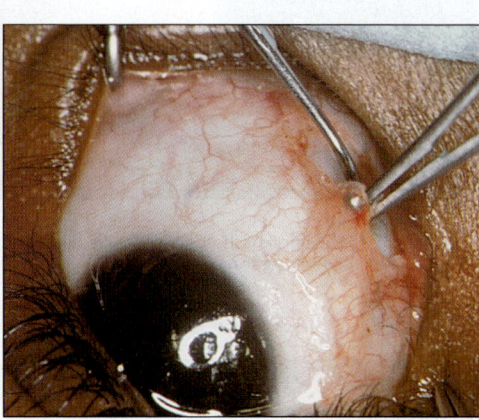

FIG. 81-30 ▌ The conjunctiva is smoothed over the incision site.

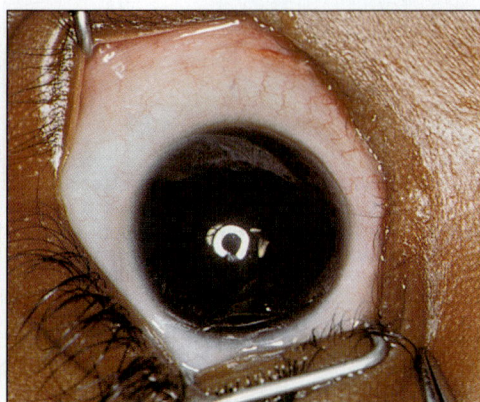

FIG. 81-31 ▌ The incision may be closed with a single buried knot suture.

rectus. However, recession of the lateral rectus and vertical recti includes visualization and preservation of the neighboring oblique muscles before the procedure is performed. The frenulum between the superior rectus and superior oblique is visualized and incised; the common fascial attachments between the lateral or inferior rectus and inferior oblique are likewise removed to avoid undesired effects on oblique muscle functions.

Resection of a Rectus Muscle

MEDIAL RECTUS. The semilunar fold is elevated (Fig. 81-32) to visualize its junction with the bulbar conjunctiva, which is incised (Fig. 81-33). The conjunctival vessels are cauterized and Tenon's fascia is entered. The large muscle hook is passed beneath the tendon, going no farther posteriorly than the insertion itself (Figs. 81-34 and 81-35). The Tenon's capsule beneath the olive tip of the large muscle hook is incised (Fig. 81-36) in

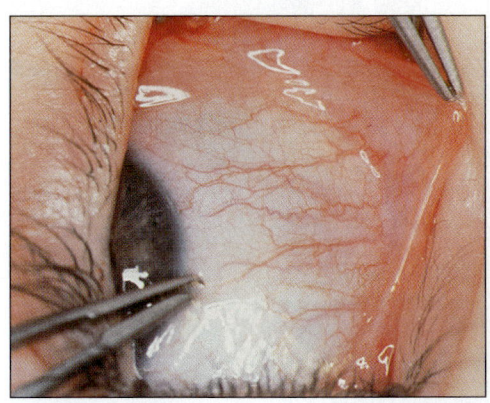

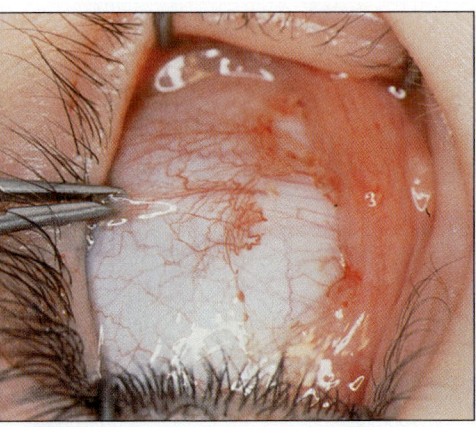

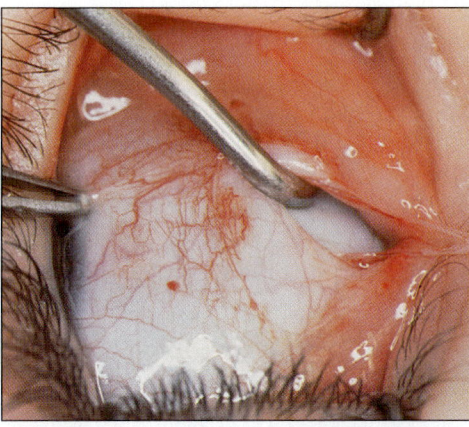

FIG. 81-32 ■ Resection of a rectus muscle. Figures 81-32 through 81-47 demonstrate a resection of the left medial rectus as viewed from the surgeon's 12 o'clock position. The surgeon has chosen a superonasal incision site, so the eye is grasped with 0.3mm forceps at the 10:30 limbus and held inferotemporally.

FIG. 81-33 ■ The conjunctiva and Tenon's capsule are incised in layers.

FIG. 81-34 ■ A large muscle hook is placed under the insertion of the rectus muscle.

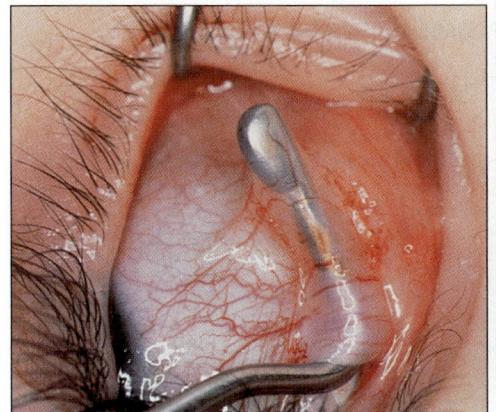

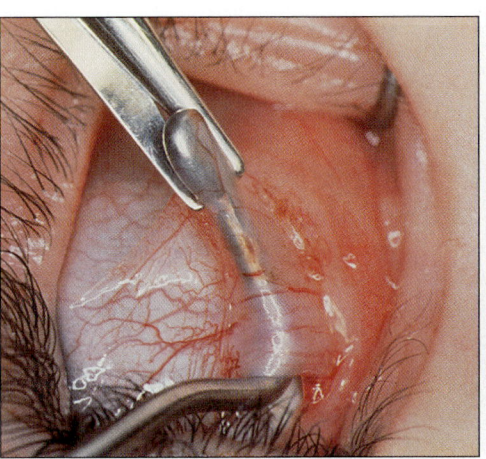

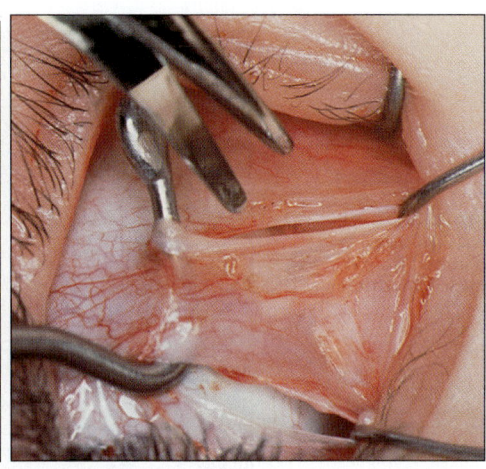

FIG. 81-35 ■ Appearance of the tendon after the conjunctiva has been displaced from the muscle belly.

FIG. 81-36 ■ A small incision is made in the inferior pole of the tendon through Tenon's capsule and intermuscular septum.

FIG. 81-37 ■ Two small Stevens muscle hooks are used to lift Tenon's capsule and intermuscular septum from the muscle belly for incision.

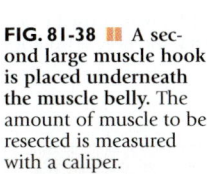

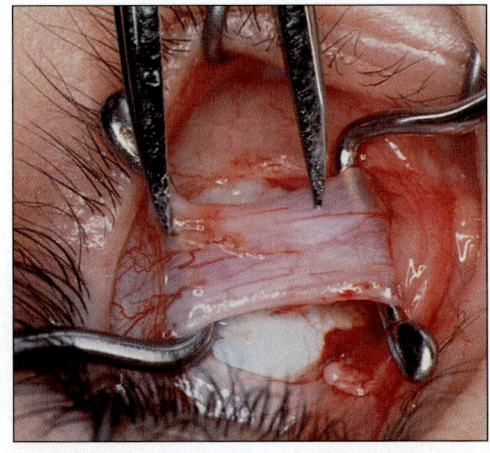

FIG. 81-38 ■ A second large muscle hook is placed underneath the muscle belly. The amount of muscle to be resected is measured with a caliper.

order to visualize bare sclera at both poles of the tendon. Two small tenotomy hooks are passed along the long axis of the tendon so that the perimuscular fascia can be exposed for incision (Fig. 81-37). A second large muscle hook is passed beneath the tendon, and traction is applied between the two muscle hooks with the insertion and both hook tips kept parallel. The anterior arm of the caliper is placed on the midportion of the anterior hook, and the posterior portion delineates the site for needle passage (Fig. 81-38). A marking pen or the cautery may be used if it is not desirable to remeasure during suture passage.

The same technique of suture passage is employed as described earlier for recession. The needle is passed tangentially to the tendon and globe and woven through the tendon from its midportion to the superior pole and then locked upon itself. The needle at the opposite end of the suture is then passed from the midportion to the inferior pole and once again locked, and the tendon is secured at the point of desired resection (Fig. 81-39). A "mosquito" hemostat is placed across the tendon just ahead of the suture (Fig. 81-40). The tendon is cut ahead of the clamp (Fig. 81-41), and the resection of tendon is completed at the original insertion (Fig. 81-42). The hemostat can remain on the tendon until all scleral passes have been performed, which permits a clean operating field.

Passage of the needles through the original insertion takes advantage of the differential scleral width at this location. Scleral thickness is at its minimum just posterior to the insertion; a differential step of 0.5–0.7mm exists from just behind to just in front of the insertion. Orientation of each needle tangentially to the globe just posterior to the insertion allows a forward movement of the needle through the step of sclera, which enables a secure attachment without the need to direct the tip of the needle toward the globe (Fig. 81-43). The passage of the needles through the insertion may be made in a diagonal fashion so that the normal width of the tendon is maintained at the posterior insertion and yet the needles' exit points still approximate one another to facilitate tying (Fig. 81-44).

Once the surgeon is satisfied with the location and depth of the scleral pass, the first suture throw is placed before the muscle is drawn forward and knotted (Figs. 81-45 and 81-46). The

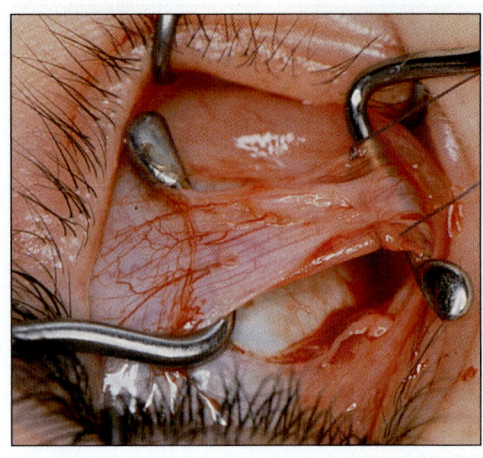

FIG. 81-39 ▪ A double-armed suture is placed in the measured position for the resection procedure.

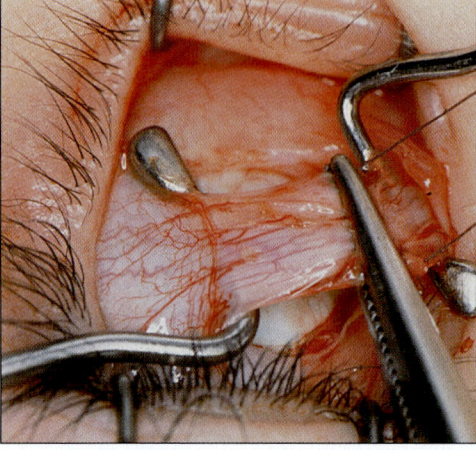

FIG. 81-40 ▪ A small hemostat is placed just anterior to the suture in the muscle belly.

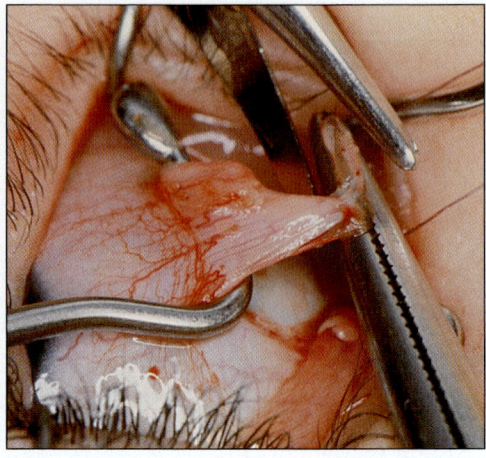

FIG. 81-41 ▪ The tendon is cut just anterior to the hemostat.

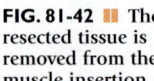 FIG. 81-42 ▪ The resected tissue is removed from the muscle insertion.

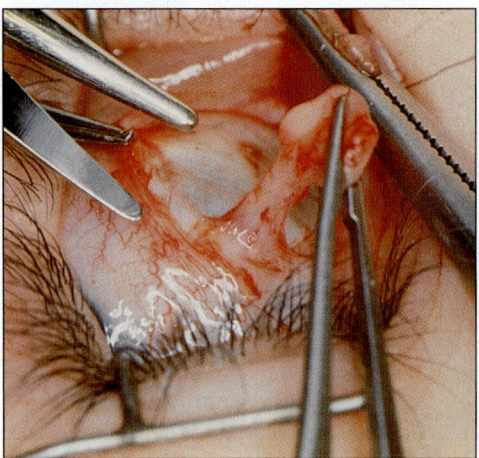

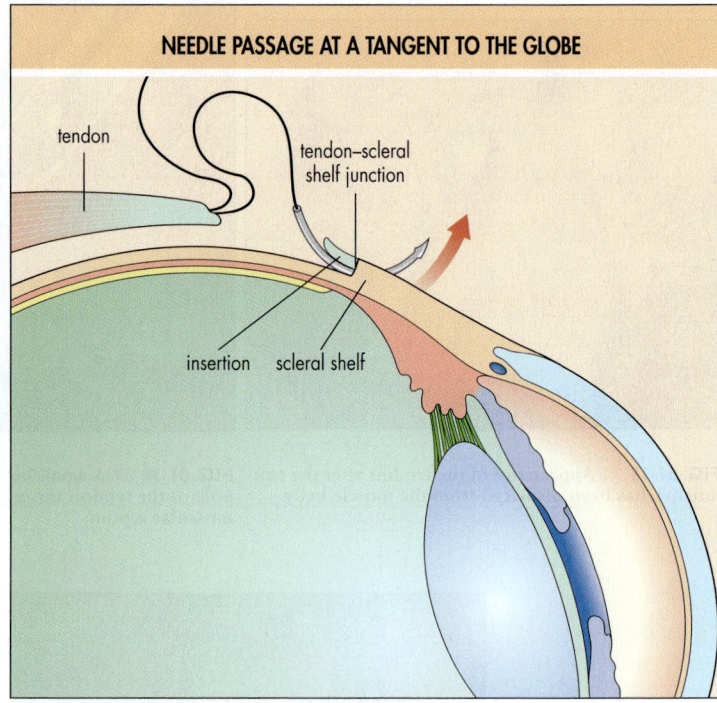

NEEDLE PASSAGE AT A TANGENT TO THE GLOBE

tendon

tendon–scleral shelf junction

insertion   scleral shelf

FIG. 81-43 ▪ Needle passage at a tangent to the globe. If this angle is used when the needle is returned through the insertional step of the sclera, the needle tip does not have to be directed toward the globe.

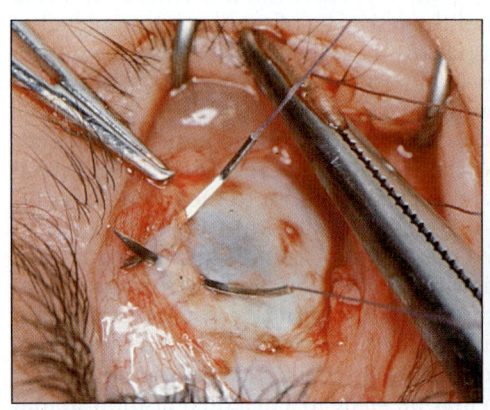

FIG. 81-44 ▪ The needles can be returned in diagonal fashion. This maintains normal tendon width.

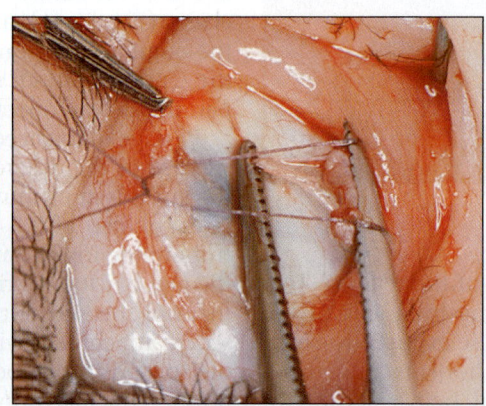

FIG. 81-45 ▪ The hemostat is released. The distal muscle is brought to the original insertion.

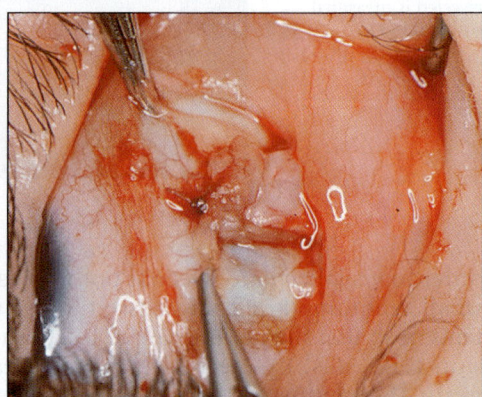

FIG. 81-46 ▪ The resected muscle has been returned to the original insertion.

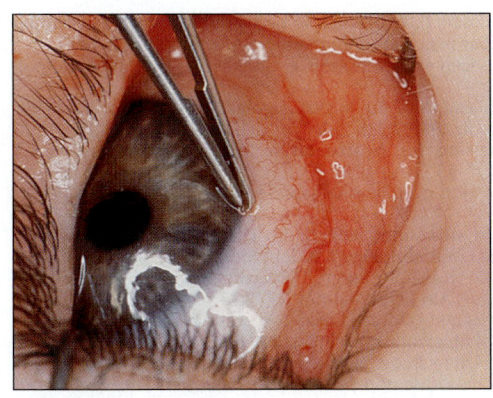

FIG. 81-47 ■ Tenon's capsule and conjunctiva are replaced in their original position. The incision is closed.

assistant may adduct the globe slightly at this time to minimize the suture tension required to complete the knot. The conjunctiva can be closed with two interrupted 6-0 plain sutures in a bury-the-knot fashion (Fig. 81-47). The conjunctiva from the limbus to the insertion is left undisturbed.

LATERAL RECTUS AND VERTICAL RECTI. The principles of resection are the same as described previously for the medial rectus. However, resections of the lateral rectus and vertical recti include visualization and preservation of the neighboring oblique muscles before the procedure is performed. The frenulum between the superior rectus and superior oblique should be visualized and incised and the common fascial attachments between the lateral rectus and inferior oblique likewise removed to avoid undesired effects on oblique muscle functions.

Other Surgical Techniques

Readers interested in surgical approaches to the superior oblique tendon and inferior oblique muscle, adjustable suture technique, and technique for posterior fixation suture are referred to Lingua,[9] Parks,[10] Romano and Roholt,[11] Fierson et al.,[12] and Guyton.[13]

COMPLICATIONS

Meticulous hemostasis is required at each step in the procedure, whichever conjunctival approach to the muscle is used. Attention to the corneal surface prevents inadvertent drying or instrument-derived abrasion. Particular caution is required with patients who have thin sclera (such as myopes), have a history of scleritis, or have undergone previous scleral procedures, especially when tenotomy is performed or the muscle is reattached to the globe. The surgeon must be aware of the location of contiguous vortex veins, especially during oblique muscle surgery.

Violation of the Posterior Tenon's Capsule

Violation of the posterior Tenon's capsule permits release of orbital fat into the space contiguous to the globe, with fibrofatty proliferations that involve sclera and nearby extraocular muscles.[14] This usually occurs after surgery on the inferior oblique muscle but may occur after surgery on any muscle; the best prevention is to perform all incisions under direct visualization. If a Tenon's capsule perforation is recognized, an attempt can be made to repair the defect with absorbable sutures. In the case of inferior oblique surgery, the patient often presents with a progressive hypotropia, esotropia, and excyclotropia in the involved eye because of tightening of the tissues around the inferior rectus muscle. Surgical treatment in these cases is difficult and unpredictable.

Anterior Segment Ischemia

Anterior segment ischemia with uveitis, hypotony, or cataract, a rare complication, appears to occur after strabismus surgery in older patients who have systemic vascular disease.[15] Surgery tra-

ditionally avoids removal of more than three rectus muscles in one eye at one time or within 6 months of previous rectus muscle detachment. However, anterior segment ischemia has been described in rare cases when less surgery was performed or rectus muscles were not detached from the globe but rather were split and joined to others (Jensen's procedure); it is thus difficult to provide exact guidelines. Most surgeons recommend caution in operations on patients who have systemic vascular disease, especially if vertical rectus muscle surgery is planned, as these muscles appear to contribute more significantly to anterior segment circulation. Evidence also exists that the avoidance of limbal conjunctival incisions preserves the conjunctivally transmitted oxygen contribution. Most patients who have postoperative anterior segment ischemia escape permanent visual sequelae if treated with topical or systemic corticosteroids.

Epithelial Cysts

Epithelial inclusion cysts may form if the conjunctiva folds under itself at any incision site. It is helpful to reappose the edges of a conjunctival incision carefully at the procedure's end. Older patients tolerate office removal of cysts with topical anesthetic.

Globe Perforation

The most ominous adverse occurrence during strabismus surgery is globe perforation. If the needle passes in the suprachoroidal space, no treatment is necessary. If the retina is perforated, vitreous may appear at the needle entrance or exit site. This should be trimmed and the retina examined; any retinal detachment must be addressed promptly. Usually, the retina appears attached and the perforation site is surrounded by retinal hemorrhage. Appropriate immediate treatment in these cases is controversial; some investigators suggest immediate cryotherapy, others frequent observation only. Most strabismus surgery is performed on children who have formed vitreous, and retinal detachment after perforation is rare; when retinal detachment occurs, however, the prognosis is guarded because of a typical delay in treatment.[16]

Undercorrection or Overcorrection

The most common "complication" after strabismus surgery is under- or overcorrection. After a suitable period of observation—depending on the individual clinical situation—and a trial of nonsurgical treatment, reoperation may be necessary. When possible and appropriate, nonoperated muscles are approached.

Lost or Slipped Muscles

Only the medial rectus muscle lacks a fascial connection to an oblique muscle, and thus it is the one most at risk of being "lost" should its sutural attachment to the globe slip. The medial rectus retracts within the posterior Tenon's capsule against the medial orbital wall. Excellent illumination, scleral retraction sutures to hold the globe in maximal abduction, and meticulous technique may enable the surgeon to reacquire the muscle. Particular care must be devoted to preservation of Tenon's capsule and prevention of adherence syndrome. Immediate reoperation is required as soon as the condition is suspected, but if some time has elapsed, the rectus contracts. The reattachment site is determined after consideration of the amount of strabismus and the amount of contracture. If the muscle cannot be identified, a translation procedure using the adjacent rectus muscle must be performed and the antagonist muscle crippled. The striated muscle may "slip" within its capsule, which results in underaction but not paresis of the muscle[17]; careful examination of the site demonstrates capsule alone attached to sclera. The muscle itself is advanced to its intended position.

OUTCOMES

Patients who undergo recession-resection procedures on one eye usually attain their final alignment within 2–3 days of surgery; patients who undergo recession of the same horizontal rectus muscle in each eye usually do not attain final alignment until 10–14 days have passed. Adults who undergo cyclovertical muscle surgery may not attain final motor and sensory stability until 4–6 weeks after surgery.

Surgical success rates are dependent upon many variables, some of which are unique to a given clinical situation. Large series (especially prospective series) with long follow-up are uncommon. Surgical results are described in the chapters that address the various forms of strabismus.

REFERENCES

1. Taylor J. A dissertation on the art of restoring the healthful position of the eye. Milan; 1756.
2. Dieffenbach JF. Über das Schielen und die Heilung desselben durch eine Operation. Berlin: A Foerstner; 1842.
3. von Graefe A. Symptomeniehre des Augensmuskellaehmungen. Berlin: H. Peters; 1867.
4. Hay A, Flynn HW, Hoffman JI, et al. Needle perforation of the globe during retrobulbar and peribulbar injections. Ophthalmology. 1991;98:1017–24.
5. Feibel RM. Current concepts in retrobulbar anesthetic. Surv Ophthalmol. 1985;30:102–10.
6. von Noorden GK. Modification of the limbal approach to surgery of the rectus muscles. Arch Ophthalmol. 1969;2:349–50.
7. Parks MM. Fornix incision for horizontal rectus muscle surgery. Am J Ophthalmol. 1968;65:907–15.
8. Swan CK, Talber T. Recession over Tenon's capsule. Arch Ophthalmol. 1954;51:32–41.
9. Lingua R. Techniques in strabismus surgery. In: Diamond G, Eggers H, eds. Strabismus and pediatric ophthalmology. London: Mosby; 1993:15.10–15.18.
10. Parks MM. A study of the weakening surgical procedure for eliminating overaction of the inferior oblique. Am J Ophthalmol. 1972;73:107–22.
11. Romano P, Roholt P. Measured graduated recession of the superior oblique muscle. J Pediatr Ophthalmol Strabismus. 1983;20:134–40.
12. Fierson WM, Boger WP, Dioro PC, et al. The effect of bilateral superior oblique tenotomy on horizontal deviation of A-pattern strabismus. J Pediatr Ophthalmol Strabismus. 1980;17:363–71.
13. Guyton DL. The posterior fixation procedure: mechanism and indications. Int Ophthalmol Clin. 1985;25:79–88.
14. Parks MM. The overacting inferior oblique. The XXXVI DeSchweinitz lecture. Am J Ophthalmol. 1974;77:787–97.
15. von Noorden GK. Anterior segment ischemia following the Jensen procedure. Arch Ophthalmol. 1976;94:845–7.
16. Basmadjian G, Labelle P, Dumas J. Retinal detachment after strabismus surgery. Am J Ophthalmol. 1975;79:305–9.
17. Bloom JN, Parks MM. The etiology, treatment and prevention of the "slipped muscle." J Pediatr Ophthalmol Strabismus. 1981;18:6–11.

ORBIT AND OCULOPLASTICS

Jonathan J. Dutton

SECTION I ORBITAL ANATOMY AND IMAGING

CHAPTER

82

Clinical Anatomy of the Eyelids

JONATHAN J. DUTTON

DEFINITION
- The eyelids are mobile, flexible, multilamellar structures that cover the globe anteriorly.

KEY FEATURES
- The eyelids provide protection from desiccation and airborne foreign matter.
- The eyelids anatomically contain both superficial musculocutaneous elements anteriorly and orbital components posteriorly.

INTRODUCTION

The eyelids serve a vital function by protecting the globe. They provide important elements of the precorneal tear film and help distribute the tear film evenly over the surface of the eye. The eyelids collect tears and propel them to the medial canthus, where they enter the lacrimal drainage system. The eyelashes sweep airborne particles from the front of the eye, and the constant voluntary and reflex movements of the eyelids protect the cornea from injury and glare.

ANATOMY OF THE EYELIDS

In young adults the interpalpebral fissure measures 10–11mm vertically. With advancing age this decreases to only about 8–10mm.[1] The horizontal length of the fissure is 30–31mm. The upper and lower eyelids meet at an angle of approximately 60° medially and laterally. In primary position the upper eyelid margin lies at the superior corneal limbus in children and 1.5–2mm below it in adults. The lower eyelid margin rests at the inferior corneal limbus.

The margin is covered by cutaneous epithelium through which the eyelashes emerge anteriorly; posteriorly it is interrupted by meibomian gland orifices. The cutaneous epithelium is continuous with the conjunctival epithelium at the posterior border of the lid margin.

Orbicularis Muscle

The orbicularis oculi is a complex striated muscle sheet that lies just below the skin. It is divided anatomically into three contiguous parts (Fig. 82-1): orbital, preseptal, and pretarsal.

The orbital portion overlies the bony orbital rims. It arises from insertions on the frontal process of the maxillary bone, the orbital process of the frontal bone, and the common medial canthal tendon. Its fibers pass around the orbital rim to form a continuous ellipse without interruption at the lateral palpebral commissure.

The palpebral portion of the orbicularis muscle overlies the mobile eyelid from the orbital rims to the eyelid margins. The muscle fibers sweep circumferentially around each eyelid as a

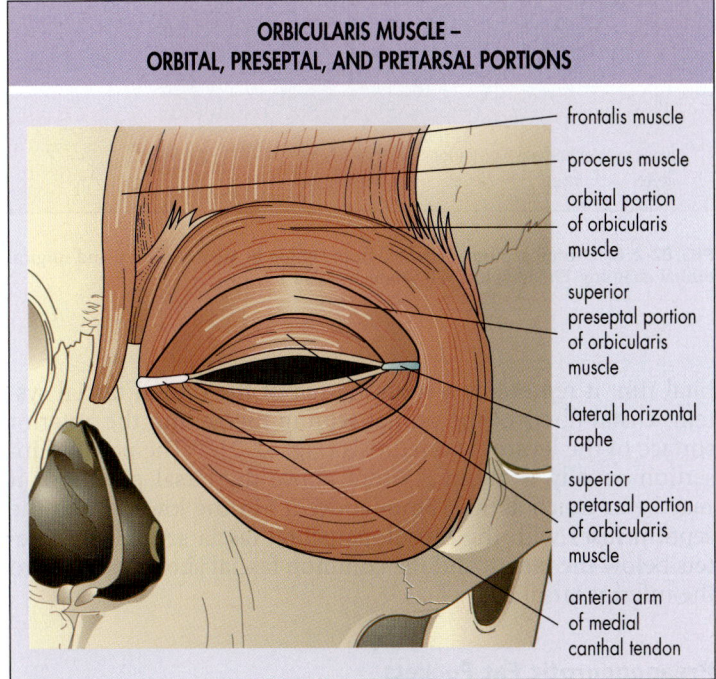

ORBICULARIS MUSCLE – ORBITAL, PRESEPTAL, AND PRETARSAL PORTIONS

frontalis muscle
procerus muscle
orbital portion of orbicularis muscle
superior preseptal portion of orbicularis muscle
lateral horizontal raphe
superior pretarsal portion of orbicularis muscle
anterior arm of medial canthal tendon

FIG. 82-1 ■ Orbicularis and frontalis muscles. (Adapted from Dutton JJ: Atlas of clinical and surgical orbital anatomy. Philadelphia: WB Saunders; 1994.)

half ellipse, fixed medially and laterally at the canthal tendons. It is further divided topographically into two parts, the preseptal and pretarsal orbicularis.

The preseptal portion of the muscle is positioned over the orbital septum in both upper and lower eyelids, and its fibers originate perpendicularly along the upper and lower borders of the medial canthal tendon. Fibers arc around the eyelids and insert along the lateral horizontal raphe. The pretarsal portion of the muscle overlies the tarsal plates. Its fibers originate from the medial canthal tendon via separate superficial and deep heads, arc around the lids, and insert onto the lateral canthal tendon and raphe. Contraction of these fibers aids in the lacrimal pump mechanism.[2] Medially, the deep heads of the pretarsal fibers fuse to form a prominent bundle of fibers, Horner's muscle, that runs just behind the posterior limb of the canthal tendon. It inserts onto the posterior lacrimal crest. Horner's muscle helps maintain the posterior position of the canthal angle, tightens the eyelids against the globe during eyelid closure, and may aid in the lacrimal pump mechanism.[3]

Orbital Septum

The orbital septum is a thin, fibrous, multilayered membrane that begins anatomically at the arcus marginalis along the or-

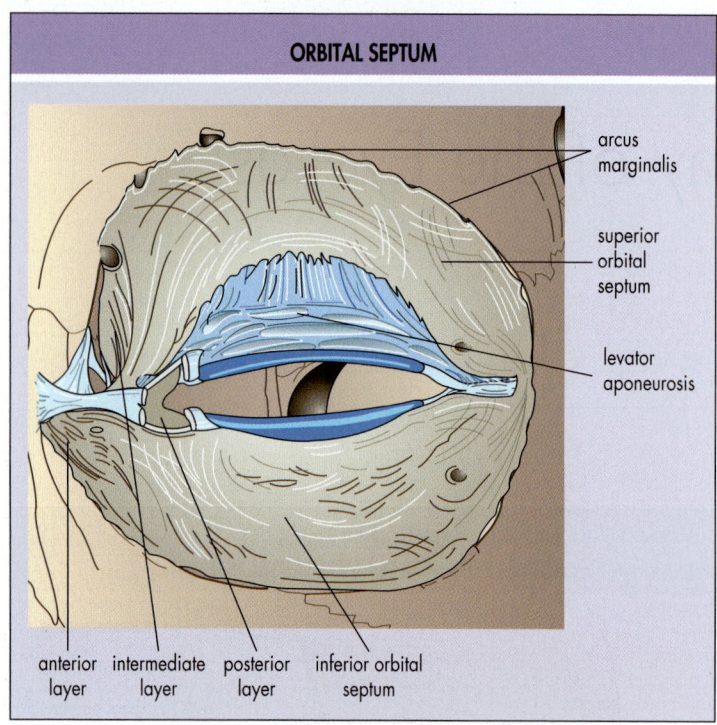

ORBITAL SEPTUM	

arcus marginalis

superior orbital septum

levator aponeurosis

anterior layer   intermediate layer   posterior layer   inferior orbital septum

FIG. 82-2 ■ **Orbital septum.** (Adapted from Dutton JJ: Atlas of clinical and surgical orbital anatomy. Philadelphia: WB Saunders; 1994.)

LEVATOR APONEUROSIS	

Whitnall's ligament

levator palpebrae superioris muscle

levator aponeurosis

lateral horn

lateral canthal tendon

medial canthal tendon   medial horn   fascial slips to orbicularis muscle   capsulopalpebral fascia

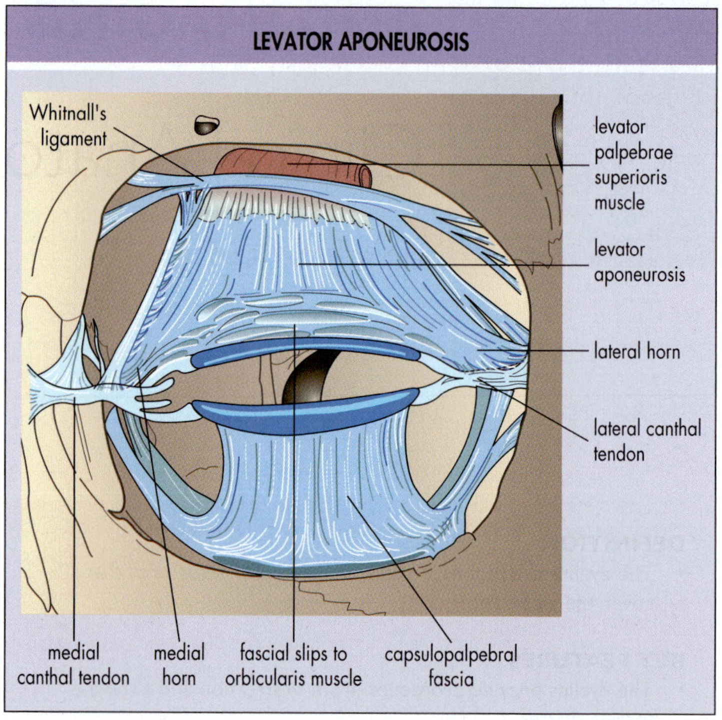

FIG. 82-3 ■ **Levator aponeurosis and medial and lateral canthal tendons.** (Adapted from Dutton JJ: Atlas of clinical and surgical orbital anatomy. Philadelphia: WB Saunders; 1994.)

bital rim; it represents a continuation of the orbital fascial system. Distal fibers of the orbital septum merge into the anterior surface of the levator aponeurosis (Fig. 82-2).[4,5] The point of insertion usually is about 3–5mm above the tarsal plate, but it may be as much as 10–15mm above it.[6] In the lower eyelid the septum fuses with the capsulopalpebral fascia several millimeters below the tarsus, and the common fascial sheet inserts onto the inferior tarsal edge.[7,8]

Preaponeurotic Fat Pockets

The preaponeurotic fat pockets in the upper eyelid and the precapsulopalpebral fat pockets in the lower eyelid are anterior extensions of extraconal orbital fat. These eyelid fat pockets are surgically important landmarks and help identify a plane immediately behind the orbital septum and anterior to the major eyelid retractors. In the upper eyelid, two fat pockets typically occur—a medial pocket and a central one. Laterally, the lacrimal gland may be mistaken for a third fat pocket. In the lower eyelid, three pockets occur—medial, central, and lateral.

Major Eyelid Retractors

The retractors of the upper eyelid consist of the levator palpebrae and Müller's muscles. The levator palpebrae superioris arises from the lesser sphenoid wing and runs forward just above the superior rectus muscle. Near the superior orbital rim, a condensation is seen along the muscle sheath,[9] which attaches medially and laterally to the orbital walls and soft tissues. This is the superior transverse orbital ligament of Whitnall. It appears to provide some support for the fascial system that maintains spatial relationships between a variety of anatomical structures in the superior orbit.

From Whitnall's ligament the muscle passes into its aponeurosis (Fig. 82-3). This sheet continues downward 14–20mm to its insertion near the marginal tarsal border. The aponeurotic fibers are most firmly attached at about 3–4mm above the eyelid margin.[10,11] Beginning near the upper edge of the tarsus, the aponeurosis also sends numerous delicate interconnecting slips forward and downward to insert onto the interfascicular septa of the pretarsal orbicularis muscle and subcutaneous tissue. These

multilayered slips maintain the close approximation of the skin, muscle, aponeurosis, and tarsal lamellae, and thus integrate the distal eyelid as a single functional unit. This relationship defines the upper eyelid crease of the Caucasian and black eyelid. In the Asian eyelid the crease is lower and less well defined.

As the levator aponeurosis passes into the eyelid from Whitnall's ligament, it broadens to form the medial and lateral "horns." The lateral horn forms a prominent fibrous sheet that indents the posterior aspect of the lacrimal gland, and so defines its orbital and palpebral lobes. The medial horn is not as well developed. It blends with the intermediate layer of the orbital septum and inserts onto the posterior crus of the medial canthal tendon and the posterior lacrimal crest. Together, the two horns serve to distribute the forces of the levator muscle along the aponeurosis and the tarsal plate.

In the lower eyelid, the capsulopalpebral fascia is a fibrous sheet that arises from Lockwood's ligament and the sheaths around the inferior rectus and inferior oblique muscles. It passes upward and generally fuses with fibers of the orbital septum about 4–5mm below the tarsal plate. From this junction, a common fascial sheet continues upward and inserts onto the lower border of the tarsus.

Sympathetic Accessory Retractors

Smooth muscles innervated by the sympathetic nervous system are present in both the upper and lower eyelids and serve as accessory retractors.[12] In the upper eyelid, the supratarsal muscle of Müller originates abruptly from the undersurface of the levator muscle just anterior to Whitnall's ligament.[13] It runs downward, posterior to the levator aponeurosis, to which it is adherent, and inserts onto the anterior edge of the superior tarsal border. In the lower eyelid, the sympathetic muscle is not as well defined. Fibers run behind the capsulopalpebral fascia to insert 2–5mm below the tarsus.[14]

Disruption of sympathetic innervation to these muscles results in Horner's syndrome. This is characterized by the classic triad of ptosis, miosis, and ipsilateral anhidrosis of the face. Specific clinical findings vary according to the location of the lesion along the polysynaptic pathway.

Tarsal Plates

The tarsal plates consist of dense, fibrous tissue 1–1.5mm thick that imparts structural integrity to the eyelids. Each plate measures about 25mm horizontally and is curved gently to conform to the contour of the anterior globe; the central height of the tarsal plates is 8–12mm in the upper eyelid and 3.5–4mm in the lower. Medially and laterally they taper to 2mm in height as they pass into the canthal tendons. Within each tarsus are the meibomian glands, numbering about 25 in the upper lid and 20 in the lower lid. These are holocrine-secreting sebaceous glands that are not associated with lash follicles. They produce the lipid layer of the precorneal tear film.

Canthal Tendons

Medially, the tarsal plates pass into fibrous bands that form the crura of the medial canthal tendon. These lie between the orbicularis muscle anteriorly and the conjunctiva posteriorly. The superior and inferior crura fuse to form a stout common tendon that inserts via three limbs (see Fig. 82-3).[2] The anterior limb inserts onto the orbital process of the maxillary bone in front of and above the anterior lacrimal crest. It provides the major support for the medial canthal angle. The posterior limb arises from the common tendon near the junction of the superior and inferior crura and passes between the canaliculi. It inserts onto the posterior lacrimal crest just in front of Horner's muscle. The posterior limb directs the vector forces of the canthal angle backward to maintain close approximation with the globe. The superior limb of the medial canthal tendon arises as a broad arc of fibers from both the anterior and posterior limbs. It passes upward to insert onto the orbital process of the frontal bone. The posterior head of the preseptal orbicularis muscle inserts onto this limb, and the unit forms the soft tissue roof of the lacrimal sac fossa. This tendinous extension may provide vertical support to the canthal angle,[15] but it also appears to play a significant role in the lacrimal pump mechanism.

Laterally, the tarsal plates pass into not very well developed fibrous strands that become the crura of the lateral canthal tendon. The lateral canthal tendon is a distinct entity separate from the orbicularis muscle; it measures about 1mm in thickness, 3mm in width, and approximately 5–7mm in length.[16] The insertion of these fibrous strands extends posteriorly along the lateral orbital wall, where it blends with strands of the lateral check ligament from the sheath of the lateral rectus muscle.

Conjunctiva

The conjunctiva is a mucous membrane that covers the posterior surface of the eyelids and the anterior pericorneal surface of the globe. The palpebral portion is applied closely to the posterior surface of the tarsal plate and the sympathetic tarsal muscle of Müller. It is continuous around the fornices above and below, where it joins the bulbar conjunctiva. Small accessory lacrimal glands are located within the submucosal connective tissue.

A small mound of tissue, the caruncle, is at the medial canthal angle. The caruncle consists of modified skin that contains fine hairs, sebaceous glands, and sweat glands. Just lateral to the caruncle is a vertical fold of conjunctiva, the plica semilunaris.

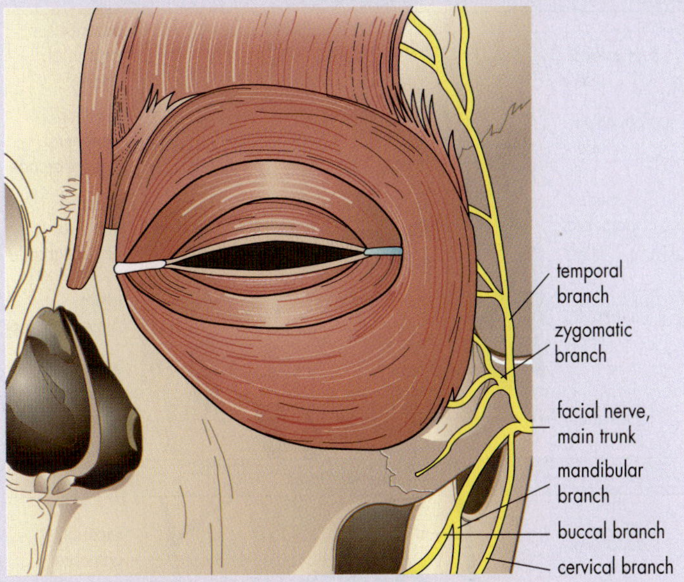

NERVES TO THE EYELIDS

The motor nerves to the orbicularis oculi muscle derive from the facial nerve (seventh cranial nerve) through its temporal and zygomatic branches (Fig. 82-4). The facial nerve separates into two divisions, the upper temporofacial and the lower cervicofacial.[17] The upper division further subdivides into the temporal and zygomatic branches, which innervate the frontalis and orbicularis muscles, respectively. The lower cervicofacial division gives rise to the buccal, mandibular, and cervical branches, which innervate muscles of the lower face and neck.

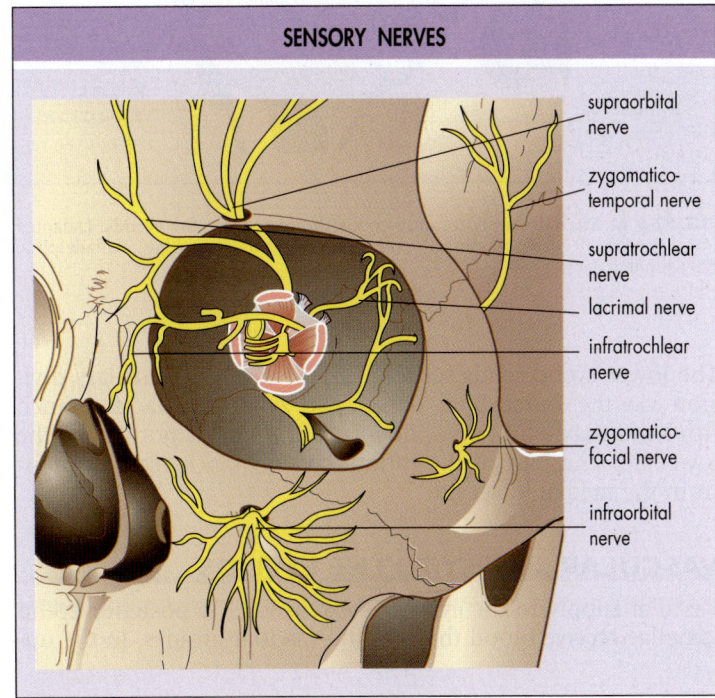

MOTOR NERVES

temporal branch
zygomatic branch
facial nerve, main trunk
mandibular branch
buccal branch
cervical branch

FIG. 82-4 ▪ Motor nerve supply to the eyelids; the facial nerve. (Adapted from Dutton JJ: Atlas of clinical and surgical orbital anatomy. Philadelphia: WB Saunders; 1994.)

SENSORY NERVES

supraorbital nerve
zygomatico-temporal nerve
supratrochlear nerve
lacrimal nerve
infratrochlear nerve
zygomatico-facial nerve
infraorbital nerve

FIG. 82-5 ▪ Sensory nerve supply from the eyelids. (Adapted from Dutton JJ: Atlas of clinical and surgical orbital anatomy. Philadelphia: WB Saunders; 1994.)

The sensory nerves to the eyelids derive from the ophthalmic and maxillary divisions of the trigeminal nerve (Fig. 82-5). Sensory input from the upper lid passes to the ophthalmic division primarily through its main terminal branches, the supraorbital, supratrochlear, and lacrimal nerves. The infratrochlear nerve receives sensory information from the extreme medial portion of both upper and lower eyelids. The zygomaticotemporal branch of the maxillary nerve innervates the lateral portion of the upper eyelid and temple. These branches also innervate portions of the adjacent brow, forehead, and nasal bridge.

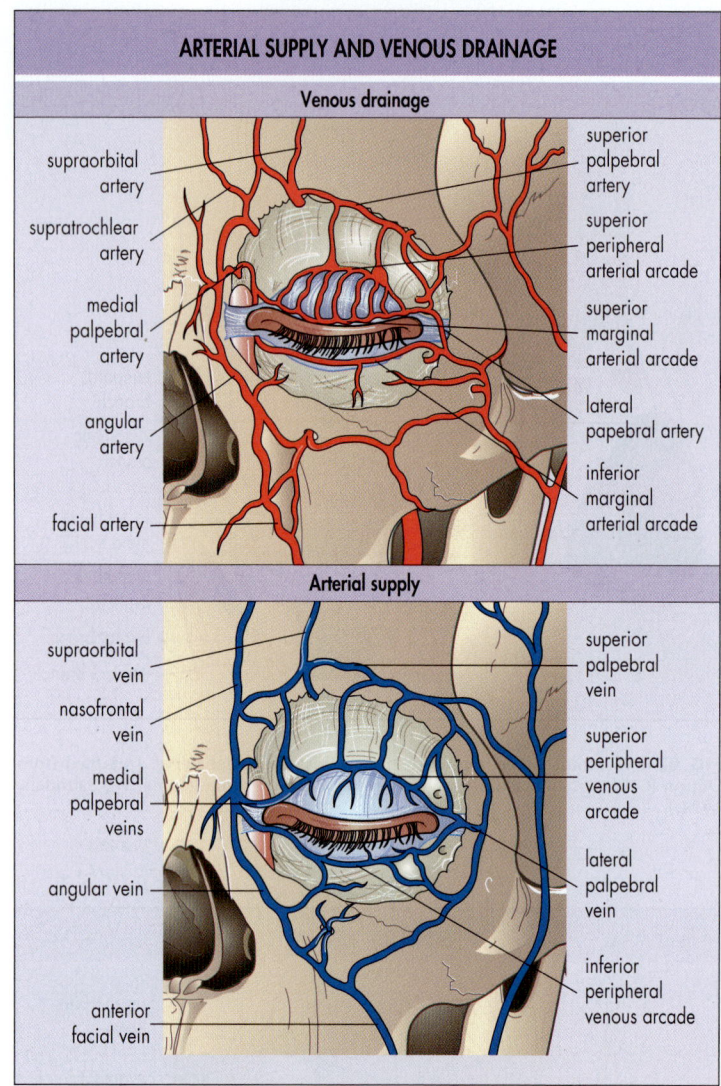

ARTERIAL SUPPLY AND VENOUS DRAINAGE

Venous drainage

- supraorbital artery
- supratrochlear artery
- medial palpebral artery
- angular artery
- facial artery

- superior palpebral artery
- superior peripheral arterial arcade
- superior marginal arterial arcade
- lateral papebral artery
- inferior marginal arterial arcade

Arterial supply

- supraorbital vein
- nasofrontal vein
- medial palpebral veins
- angular vein
- anterior facial vein

- superior palpebral vein
- superior peripheral venous arcade
- lateral palpebral vein
- inferior peripheral venous arcade

FIG. 82-6 ■ **Arterial supply to and venous drainage from the eyelids.** (Adapted from Dutton JJ: Atlas of clinical and surgical orbital anatomy. Philadelphia: WB Saunders; 1994.)

The lower eyelid sends sensory impulses to the maxillary division via the infraorbital nerve. The zygomaticofacial branch from the maxillary nerve innervates the lateral portion of the lower lid, and part of the infratrochlear branch receives input from the medial lower lid.

VASCULAR SUPPLY TO THE EYELIDS

Vascular supply to the eyelids is extensive. The posterior eyelid lamellae receive blood through the vascular arcades. In the up-

per eyelid, a marginal arcade runs about 2mm from the eyelid margin, and a peripheral arcade extends along the upper border of the tarsus between the levator aponeurosis and Müller's muscle (Fig. 82-6). These arcades are supplied medially by the superior medial palpebral vessel from the terminal ophthalmic artery and laterally by the superior lateral palpebral vessel from the lacrimal artery. The lower lid arcade receives blood from the medial and lateral inferior palpebral vessels.

The venous drainage system is not as well defined as the arterial system. Drainage is mainly into several large vessels of the facial system (see Fig. 82-6). Lymphatic drainage from the eyelids is restricted to the region anterior to the orbital septum. Drainage from the lateral two thirds of the upper eyelid and the lateral one third of the lower eyelid proceeds inferiorly and laterally into the deep and superficial parotid and submandibular nodes. Drainage from the medial one third of the upper eyelid and the medial two thirds of the lower eyelid occurs medially and inferiorly into the anterior cervical nodes.

REFERENCES

1. Hrecko T, Farkas LG, Katic M. Clinical significance of age-related changes in the palpebral fissure between ages 2 and 18 in healthy Caucasians. Acta Chir Plast. 1968;32:194–204.
2. Dutton JJ. Atlas of clinical and surgical orbital anatomy. Philadelphia: WB Saunders; 1994.
3. Ahl NC, Hill JC. Horner's muscle and the lacrimal system. Arch Ophthalmol. 1982;100:488–93.
4. Barker DE. Dye injection studies of orbital fat compartments. Plast Reconstr Surg. 1977;59:82–5.
5. Putterman AM, Urist MJ. Surgical anatomy of the orbital septum. Ann Ophthalmol. 1974;6:290–4.
6. Anderson RL, Dixon RS. The role of Whitnall's ligament in ptosis surgery. Arch Ophthalmol. 1979;97:705–10.
7. Harvey JT, Anderson RL. The aponeurotic approach to eyelid retraction. Ophthalmology. 1981;88:513–24.
8. Meyer DR, Linberg JV, Wobig JL, McCormick S. Anatomy of the orbital septum and associated eyelid connective tissue. Ophthal Plast Reconstr Surg. 1991;7:104–13.
9. Lemke BN, Stasior OG, Rosenberg PN. The surgical relations of the levator palpebrae superioris muscle. Ophthal Plast Reconstr Surg. 1988;4:25–30.
10. Anderson RL, Beard C. The levator aponeurosis. Attachments and their clinical significance. Arch Ophthalmol. 1977;95:1437–41.
11. Collin JRO, Beard C, Wood I. Experimental and clinical data on the insertion of the levator palpebrae superioris muscle. Am J Ophthalmol. 1987;85:792–801.
12. Manson PN, Lazarus RB, Magar R, Iliff N. Pathways of sympathetic innervation to the superior and inferior (Müller's) tarsal muscles. Plast Reconstr Surg. 1986;78:33–40.
13. Kuwabara T, Cogan DG, Johnson CC. Structure of the muscles of the upper eyelid. Arch Ophthalmol. 1975;93:1189–97.
14. Hawes MJ, Dortzbach RK. The microscopic anatomy of the lower eyelid retractors. Arch Ophthalmol. 1982;100:1313–8.
15. Anderson RL. The medial canthal tendon branches out. Arch Ophthalmol. 1977;95:2951–61.
16. Gioia VM, Linberg JV, McCormick SA. The anatomy of the lateral canthal tendon. Arch Ophthalmol. 1987;105:529–32.
17. Malone B, Maisel RH. Anatomy of the facial nerve. Am J Otolaryngol. 1988;9:494–504.

CHAPTER
83
Clinical Anatomy of the Orbit

JONATHAN J. DUTTON

DEFINITION
- The orbit is the anatomical space bounded by the orbital bones and enclosed within the multilamellar periorbita.

KEY FEATURES
- Anteriorly the orbit is limited by the orbital septum, which represents the anteriormost layer of the orbital septal system and separates the orbit from the eyelid.
- The orbit contains the eye and extraocular muscles, along with the nerves, vascular elements, and connective tissue support systems that subserve the visual system.

INTRODUCTION

An understanding of orbital disease demands a clear concept of normal orbital anatomy and physiological function. Only with this foundation can the clinician identify and characterize pathological states. The development of better surgical techniques requires, in addition, a comprehensive knowledge of the structural relationships among the numerous anatomical systems that are crowded into the small space available.

GENERAL ORGANIZATION

The human orbit is a small cavity that has the approximate shape of a pear with the stem directed posteriorly. Within this defined space are juxtaposed a complex array of closely packed structures, most of which subserve visual function.[1,2] Lobules of orbital fat surrounded by connective tissue fascia completely fill the spaces between the muscles, nerves, and vascular elements. These fat lobules provide a cushion to protect these delicate structures from injury during ocular movement. The entire anatomical region is bound together in a functional unit, the complexity and precision of which are unmatched elsewhere in the vertebrate body.

OSTEOLOGY OF THE ORBIT

The bony orbit develops from mesenchyme, which encircles the optic vesicle from as early as the sixth week of the embryonic stage. The individual orbital bones arise from a complex series of primary or secondary ossifications around the evolving optic cup and stalk. Initially, the optic vesicles are positioned 170–180° apart, on opposite sides of the forebrain. Later, these begin to rotate anteriorly as the primordial orbital bones are laid down around them.[3]

In adults the bony orbit encloses a volume of about 30cm³. It is composed of seven bones, simplified from a complex of der-

---

BOX 83-1

Bones of the Orbit

Ethmoid bone	Palatine bone
Frontal bone	Sphenoid bone
Lacrimal bone	Zygomatic bone
Maxillary bone	

---

mal and endochondral elements that evolved from earlier vertebrates (Box 83-1). Except for a series of canals, fissures, and foramina that communicate with extraorbital compartments, the orbit is a closed compartment with a broad opening anteriorly (Fig. 83-1).

Orbital Roof

The orbital roof is composed of the orbital plate of the frontal bone, with a small contribution from the lesser wing of the sphenoid bone at the apex. This bone is a thin lamina that separates the orbit from the frontal sinus anteriorly and from the anterior cranial fossa posteriorly. The roof slopes backward and downward from the orbital rim toward the apex, where it ends at the optic canal and superior orbital fissure. The optic canal measures 5–6mm in diameter and 8–12mm in length; it is oriented posteromedially about 35° to the midsagittal plane and upward about 38° to the horizontal plane.[4]

Lateral Orbital Wall

The lateral wall is formed by the greater wing of the sphenoid bone posteriorly and by the zygomatic process of the frontal bone and the orbital process of the zygomatic bone anteriorly. It lies at a nearly 45° angle to the midsagittal plane. The lateral wall is bounded below by the inferior orbital fissure, and medially by the superior orbital fissure. Behind the thick lateral orbital rim, the wall becomes quite thin where the zygomatic bone joins the greater sphenoid wing at a vertical suture line. The convoluted frontozygomatic suture line runs approximately horizontally and crosses the superotemporal rim near the lacrimal gland fossa. At 5–15mm above this line, the frontal bone widens as it passes around the front end of the anterior cranial fossa. About halfway along the anteroposterior depth of the lateral wall, in the sphenoid wing near the frontosphenoid suture, is a small canal that carries an anastomotic branch between the lacrimal and meningeal arteries. Elevation of the periorbita during lateral orbital dissection may result in brisk bleeding from this vessel. Just behind the zygomaticosphenoid suture line, the greater wing widens as it passes around the anterior tip of the middle cranial fossa. As the greater wing is removed during lateral orbitotomy procedures, the appearance of cancellous bone warns of the imminence of reaching the dura.

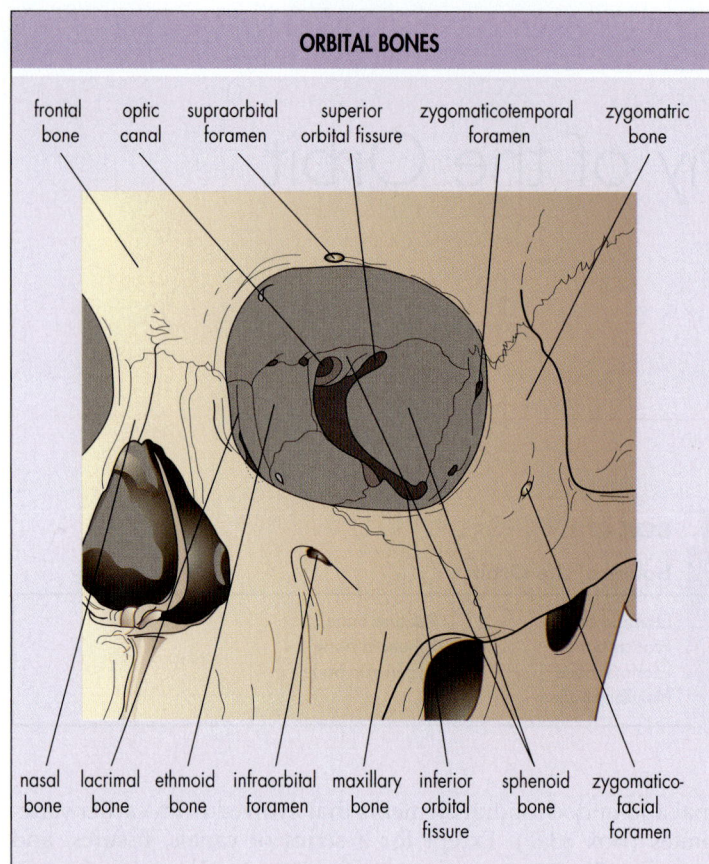

ORBITAL BONES

frontal bone · optic canal · supraorbital foramen · superior orbital fissure · zygomaticotemporal foramen · zygomatric bone

nasal bone · lacrimal bone · ethmoid bone · infraorbital foramen · maxillary bone · inferior orbital fissure · sphenoid bone · zygomatico-facial foramen

FIG. 83-1 ■ Bony anatomy of the orbit in frontal view. (Redrawn with permission from Dutton JJ. Atlas of clinical and surgical orbital anatomy. Philadelphia: WB Saunders; 1994.)

Orbital Floor

The floor is the shortest of the orbital walls; it extends back only 35–40mm from the inferior rim. The orbital floor is composed primarily of the maxillary bone; the zygomatic bone forms the anterolateral portion, and the palatine bone lies at the posterior extent of the floor. The surface of the orbital floor forms a triangular segment that extends from the maxillary–ethmoid buttress horizontally to the inferior orbital fissure, and from the orbital rim back to the posterior wall of the maxillary sinus. The orbital floor is thinnest just medial to the infraorbital canal, which is the most common site for blowout fractures. Despite its thinness, the floor is strengthened by one or more trabeculae in the roof of the maxillary sinus. The orbital floor shows the greatest degree of deformation when external force is applied,[5] which explains the high rate of floor fractures associated with even minor degrees of blunt trauma.

The infraorbital groove begins at the inferior orbital fissure and runs forward in the maxillary bone. About 15mm from the orbital rim, this groove is usually bridged over with a thin lamina of bone to form the infraorbital canal. Within this canal runs the maxillary division of the trigeminal nerve and the maxillary artery. These exit just below the central orbital rim at the infraorbital foramen.

The floor is separated from the lateral orbital wall by the inferior orbital fissure, which is approximately 20mm in length and runs in an anterolateral to posteromedial direction. At the orbital apex just below the optic canal, the inferior fissure joins the superior orbital fissure. The inferior fissure transmits structures into the orbit from the pterygopalatine fossa posteriorly and from the infratemporal fossa anteriorly. Multiple branches from the inferior ophthalmic vein pass through this opening to communicate with the pterygoid venous plexus. The inferior fissure also transmits the maxillary division of the trigeminal nerve from the foramen rotundum to the infraorbital sulcus.

Orbital Bones Contributing to Each Wall

ROOF
Frontal bone
Lesser wing of the sphenoid bone

MEDIAL WALL
Frontal process of the maxillary bone
Lacrimal bone
Ethmoid bone
Body of the sphenoid bone

FLOOR
Maxillary bone
Zygomatic bone
Palatine bone

LATERAL WALL
Zygomatic bone
Greater wing of the sphenoid bone

Postganglionic parasympathetic secretory and vasomotor neural branches from the pterygopalatine ganglion enter the orbit through the inferior orbital fissure, where they join with the maxillary nerve for a short distance before they pass to the lacrimal gland.

Medial Orbital Wall

The medial walls of the orbits are approximately parallel to each other and to the midsagittal plane. The medial wall is composed largely of the thin lamina papyracea of the ethmoid bone. This plate is exceptionally fragile, measuring only 0.2–0.4mm in thickness, and separates the orbit from air cells of the ethmoid sinus labyrinth. It is a frequent site of fracture in orbital trauma and is breached easily during transnasal ethmoid sinus surgery. The lamina papyracea offers little resistance to expanding ethmoid sinus mucoceles and commonly transmits inflammatory and infectious processes from sinusitis into the orbit.

Posterior to the ethmoid bone, the body of the sphenoid bone completes the medial wall to the apex. This portion of the wall is quite thick and is only rarely involved in orbital trauma or sinus pathology. The medial wall ends at the optic foramen, where the sphenoid forms the medial wall of the optic canal.

Anterior to the ethmoid is the lacrimal bone, a thin plate that contains the posterior lacrimal crest and forms the posterior half of the lacrimal sac fossa. In the midportion of the fossa the lacrimal bone joins the orbital process of the maxillary bone. The latter is a thick bone that forms the medial orbital rim. During lacrimal bypass surgery, entrance into the nose can be achieved most easily with a hemostat by applying gentle pressure on the lacrimal portion of the fossa.

Within the frontoethmoid suture line in the superomedial orbit are two openings, the anterior and posterior ethmoidal foramina. The former usually lies 20–25mm behind the anterior lacrimal crest, and the latter about 32–35mm behind the anterior crest and 5–10mm anterior to the optic canal.[6,7] These foramina transmit branches of the ophthalmic artery and nasociliary nerve into the ethmoid sinus and nose. These vessels frequently are injured in orbital trauma and are the major sources of subperiosteal hematomas. These openings mark the approximate level of the roof of the ethmoid labyrinth and the floor of the anterior cranial fossa. The cribriform plate may lie up to 10mm below this level, just medial to the root of the middle turbinate, and can be fractured during medial wall surgery.

A summary of the orbital bones is given in Box 83-2.

CONNECTIVE TISSUE SYSTEM

In the human, an extensive system of connective tissue forms a framework for compartmentalization and support of all orbital structures. It is essential to maintain the appropriate anatomical relationships between structural components and to allow precise and coordinated ocular movements.[8–12] Some connective tissue septa are aligned with directions of force that resist displacement of extraocular muscles during contraction. Others suspend and support delicate orbital vascular and neural elements. The essential components of this system include the periorbita, the orbital septal systems, and Tenon's capsule.[13,14]

Periorbita

The orbit is lined with periosteum that is loosely adherent to the underlying orbital bones. Applied to the inner surface of the periosteum are multiple layers of orbital connective tissue that are continuous with the transorbital septal systems. Together, this complex layer is known as the periorbita. It is attached firmly at the arcus marginalis along the orbital rim, at the lateral orbital tubercle, adjacent to the trochlea, around the optic foramen, and along the inferior and superior orbital fissures. Where the periorbita joins the margins of the optic canal and superior orbital fissure, it is fused to dura, so trauma or surgery in these areas may be complicated by cerebrospinal fluid leakage.

Within the orbit the periorbita serves to support the extensive septal systems and to stabilize anatomical structures. It forms the boundaries of the entire orbital compartment. At the orbital rim, the periorbita separates into its component layers. Periosteum continues over the rims and remains in contact with the outer table of the cranial bones. The inner layers of the connective tissue system separate from periosteum at the arcus marginalis and extend into the eyelids as the orbital septum. Thus the septum represents the anteriormost boundary of the orbital compartment.

Orbital Septal System

Suspended from the periorbita to form a complex radial and circumferential web of interconnecting slings are connective tissue septa.[8–11] These septa form fine capsules around the intraconal and extraconal fat lobules; they also surround the extraocular muscles, optic nerve, and neurovascular elements and suspend these structures from the adjacent orbital walls. The fascial slings provide support and maintain constant spatial relationships between these structures during ocular movements. These septa are responsible for the transmission of restrictive forces from incarcerated or hemorrhagic orbital fat to extraocular muscles after trauma, even in the absence of true muscle entrapment. Septa that encircle the optic nerve may confine hemorrhage or air, which may result in compressive optic neuropathy after trauma.

The anterior fascial system of the orbit primarily supports the globe, anterior orbital structures (such as the lacrimal gland and superior oblique tendon), and the eyelids. It consists of a number of well-developed condensations and ligaments, as well as a more diffuse system of fibrous septa. These structures include Lockwood's inferior ligament, Whitnall's superior suspensory ligament, the lacrimal ligaments, and the intermuscular septum. They coordinate movements between the globe and eyelids and suspend the globe so that gaze movements occur around stable axes of rotation (Fig. 83-2).

The connective tissue system is best developed in the midorbit. Here it forms well-defined fascial slings and suspensory complexes associated with each of the extraocular muscles. The fascial layers involved serve to maintain constant muscle alignment, minimize vector shifts during eye movement, and reduce sideslip over the rotating globe (Fig. 83-3).

In the posterior half of the orbit, the connective tissue septal system is not as well developed as in the anterior orbit. The in-

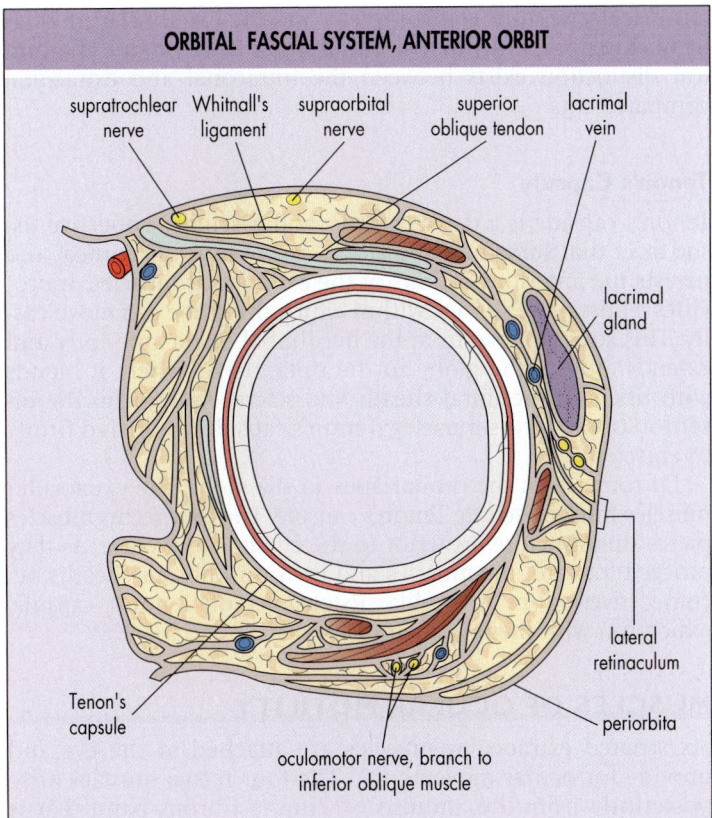

ORBITAL FASCIAL SYSTEM, ANTERIOR ORBIT

supratrochlear nerve — Whitnall's ligament — supraorbital nerve — superior oblique tendon — lacrimal vein — lacrimal gland — lateral retinaculum — periorbita — oculomotor nerve, branch to inferior oblique muscle — Tenon's capsule

FIG. 83-2 ■ The connective tissue system in cross-sectional frontal view through the anterior orbit at the level of Whitnall's ligament. (Adapted with permission from Dutton JJ. Atlas of clinical and surgical orbital anatomy. Philadelphia: WB Saunders; 1994.)

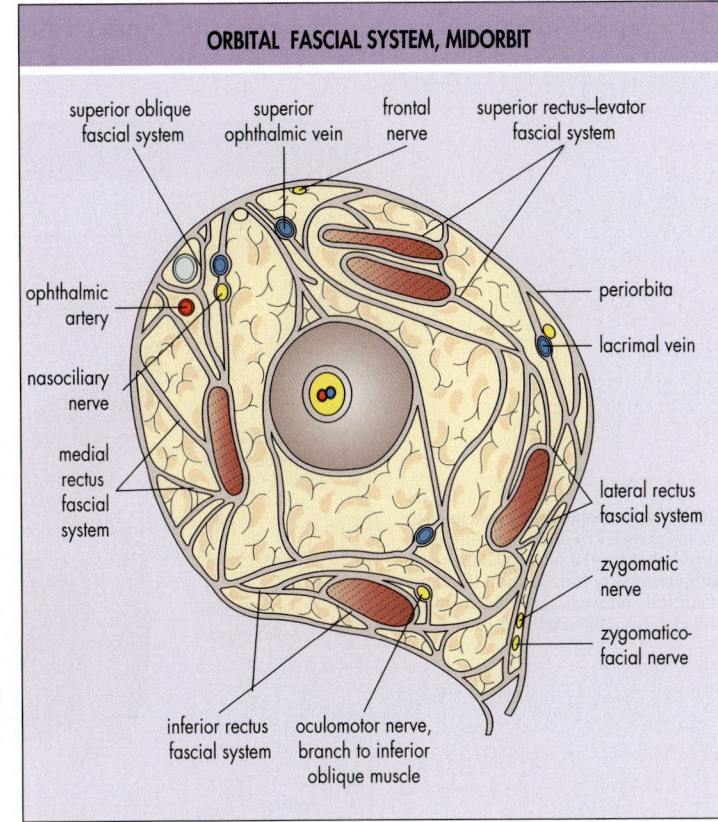

ORBITAL FASCIAL SYSTEM, MIDORBIT

superior oblique fascial system — superior ophthalmic vein — frontal nerve — superior rectus–levator fascial system — ophthalmic artery — nasociliary nerve — medial rectus fascial system — periorbita — lacrimal vein — lateral rectus fascial system — zygomatic nerve — zygomatico-facial nerve — inferior rectus fascial system — oculomotor nerve, branch to inferior oblique muscle

FIG. 83-3 ■ The connective tissue system in cross-sectional frontal view through the midorbit. (Adapted with permission from Dutton JJ. Atlas of clinical and surgical orbital anatomy. Philadelphia: WB Saunders; 1994.)

termuscular septum is incomplete, and the extraocular muscles lie in closer proximity to the orbital walls. Thus, no true anatomical distinction exists between the intraconal and extraconal compartments.

Tenon's Capsule

Tenon's capsule is a dense, elastic, and vascular connective tissue layer that surrounds the globe, except over the cornea, and invests the anterior portions of the extraocular muscles. It provides a bursa-like surface within which the globe can move easily. This structure begins at the perilimbal sclera anteriorly and extends around the globe to the optic nerve, where it blends with fibers of the dural sheath and sclera. Anterior to the insertion of the rectus muscles, Tenon's capsule is adhered firmly to episclera.

En route from the orbital apex to the globe, the extraocular muscles must penetrate Tenon's capsule. The four rectus muscles pierce this structure posterior to the equator of the eye. As they proceed forward, the muscles and their thin fibrous sheaths become invested by sleevelike extensions of Tenon's capsule, which run with them to their insertions.

MUSCLES OF OCULAR MOTILITY

Six striated extraocular muscles are attached to the eye and provide for ocular movement.[15] The four rectus muscles arise posteriorly from the annulus of Zinn, a fibrous band that is continuous with the periorbita and dura at the optic foramen.[16,17] The muscles run forward from the annulus of Zinn, and only a thin layer of extraconal fat separates them from the periorbita along the orbital walls. Each is surrounded by a sheath continuous with the orbital fascial systems. It is through these connective tissue septa that the muscles are held in position relative to the orbital walls. These fascial systems help keep the muscles in proper alignment and minimize the vector shifts that would otherwise be associated with ocular movement (Fig. 83-4).[18,19]

The superior oblique muscle arises above the annulus of Zinn, just superior and medial to the optic foramen. It runs forward along the superomedial orbital wall to the cartilaginous trochlea, through which its tendon slides before it turns sharply laterally to insert on the superoposterior aspect of the globe.[20]

The inferior oblique muscle arises anteriorly from a small depression just below and lateral to the lacrimal sac fossa. It passes laterally and slightly backward to insert on the inferoposterior surface of the globe near the macula. Along its course, the sheath of the inferior oblique muscle joins that of the inferior rectus muscle and Tenon's capsule just behind the orbital rim to form Lockwood's inferior suspensory ligament. The capsulopalpebral fascia extends anteriorly from this ligament to the inferior tarsal plate. During surgery in the inferior orbit, care must be taken when the orbital septum is opened, since the inferior oblique muscle and Lockwood's ligament lie immediately behind the orbital rim.

The levator palpebrae superioris muscle originates from the annulus of Zinn and lesser sphenoid wing. It runs forward along the orbital roof in close approximation to the superior rectus muscle. Fine check ligaments interconnect the levator to the superior rectus, as well as to periosteum of the frontal bone. Near the orbital rim, fine suspensory ligaments extend from the levator sheath to the superior conjunctival fornix. Also, at about this point, a horizontal condensation is seen within the muscle sheath to form the prominent transverse ligament of Whitnall.[21] The latter fuses to the orbital wall near the trochlea and around the lacrimal gland. Whitnall's ligament is an important suspensory structure for the superior orbit and eyelid and should not be cut. Anterior to Whitnall's ligament, the levator muscle passes into a thin, fibrous aponeurosis that turns inferiorly and fans out into the eyelid. It inserts onto the inferior two thirds of the anterior tarsal face.

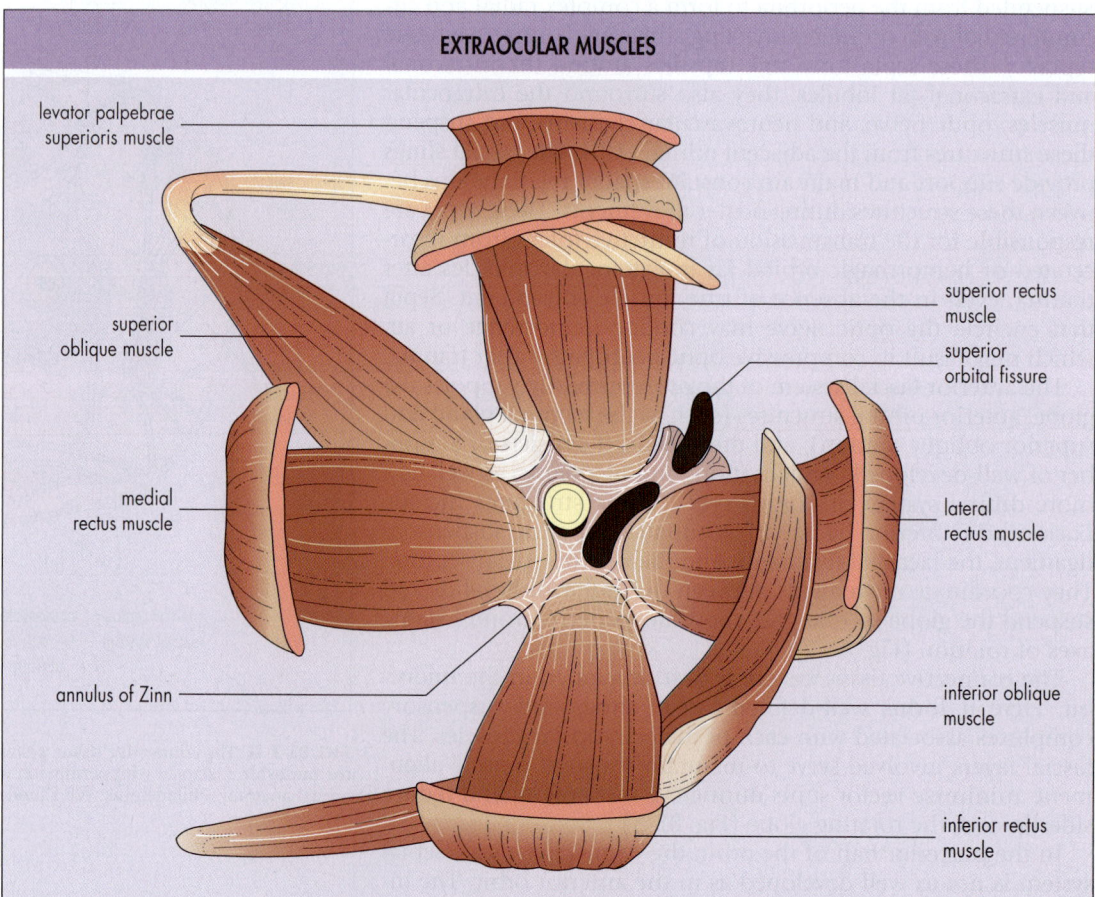

EXTRAOCULAR MUSCLES

levator palpebrae superioris muscle

superior oblique muscle

superior rectus muscle

superior orbital fissure

medial rectus muscle

lateral rectus muscle

annulus of Zinn

inferior oblique muscle

inferior rectus muscle

FIG. 83-4 ▌ **Extraocular muscles.** Orbital muscles of ocular motility as seen in the coronal plane. (Adapted with permission from Dutton JJ. Atlas of clinical and surgical orbital anatomy. Philadelphia: WB Saunders; 1994.)

MOTOR NERVES OF THE ORBIT

The extraocular muscles are innervated by the third, fourth, and sixth cranial nerves.[22] The oculomotor nerve (cranial nerve III) arises from the oculomotor nuclear complex in the midbrain and exits at the medial border of the cerebral peduncle. It passes forward in the lateral cavernous sinus, where it divides into superior and inferior divisions just before these enter the intraconal space through the superior orbital fissure. The superior branch innervates the superior rectus and levator muscles. The inferior branch sends fibers to the inferior rectus, medial rectus, and inferior oblique muscles. These branches are applied to the inner surface of the muscles, where they are cushioned and protected by the fibrous muscle sheaths. With the inferior division of the oculomotor nerve run parasympathetic fibers that arise from the Edinger-Westphal subnucleus. These synapse in the ciliary ganglion, just lateral and inferior to the optic nerve at 1.5–2cm behind the globe.[23] They progress via the short ciliary nerves to the ciliary body and iris sphincter.[24] Little redundancy occurs to these nerves, so they may be injured easily during orbital dissection. This results in disturbances of pupillary function and accommodation.

The trochlear nerve (cranial nerve IV) arises in the midbrain, exits below the inferior colliculus, and passes forward in the lateral cavernous sinus. It enters the extraconal space of the superior orbit through the superior orbital fissure above the annulus of Zinn. Here it crosses over the superior rectus and levator muscle complex and runs along the external surface of the superior oblique muscle before penetrating its substance in the posterior third of the orbit. In this position against the orbital roof, the trochlear nerve is damaged easily during blunt trauma.

The abducent nerve (cranial nerve VI) arises in the pons and passes forward in the cavernous sinus below the trochlear nerve. It enters the intraconal space of the orbit through the superior orbital fissure and annulus of Zinn. The nerve runs laterally to supply the lateral rectus muscle.

Sympathetic nerves enter the orbit via a number of different pathways to innervate the vascular muscular walls, the iris, and the accessory eyelid retractor muscles of Müller (Fig. 83-5).[25]

SENSORY NERVES OF THE ORBIT

The optic nerve is technically not a sensory nerve but a central nervous system tract that arises from the retinal ganglion cells. Nasal fibers decussate in the optic chiasm. Fibers in the optic tracts continue backward and synapse in the lateral geniculate nuclei, from which they radiate to the occipital cortex. The orbital portion of the nerve is somewhat redundant, to allow for ocular movement. It measures about 3cm in length and takes a sinusoidal path from the globe to the optic canal. In close approximation to the nerve are the ophthalmic artery, near the orbital apex, and the superior ophthalmic vein, in the midorbit. Both these vessels lie superior to the nerve in most individuals. The central retinal artery runs along the inferolateral side of the nerve to enter the dura about 1cm behind the globe. The short and long posterior ciliary arteries lie close to the nerve for much of its length and are highly convoluted and redundant near the globe.

Sensory innervation to the orbit is primarily from the ophthalmic division of the trigeminal nerve (cranial nerve V) (Fig. 83-6). The maxillary division supplies portions of the inferior orbit. The ophthalmic division divides into branches in the cavernous sinus just as it passes into the superior orbital fissure.[26] The lacrimal nerve enters above the annulus of Zinn and proceeds in the extraconal space just inside the periorbita along the superolateral orbit to the lacrimal gland and upper eyelid. The frontal nerve runs forward between the levator muscle and the superior periorbita and exits the orbit at the supraorbital notch. At about the level of the posterior globe, it gives rise to the supratrochlear nerve, which exits the orbit at the superomedial rim.

The nasociliary nerve is a branch of the ophthalmic division that enters the orbit through the superior orbital fissure and

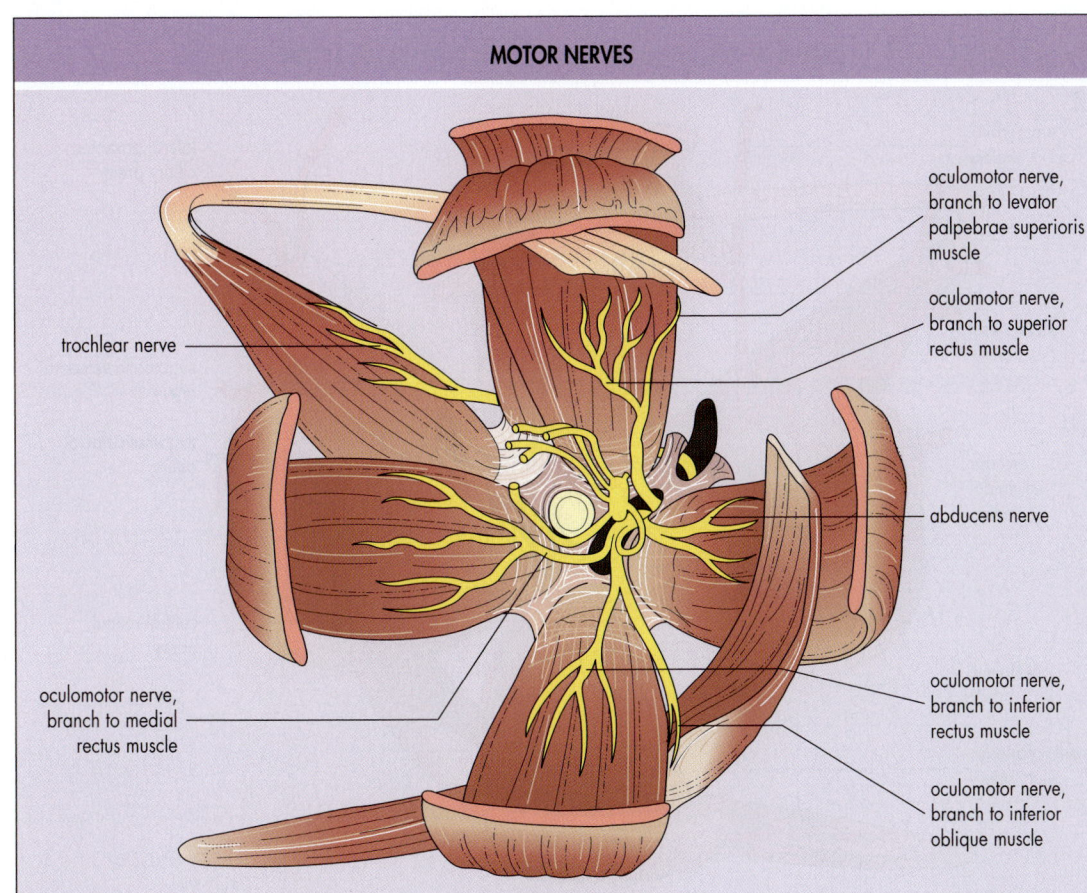

MOTOR NERVES

- trochlear nerve
- oculomotor nerve, branch to levator palpebrae superioris muscle
- oculomotor nerve, branch to superior rectus muscle
- abducens nerve
- oculomotor nerve, branch to medial rectus muscle
- oculomotor nerve, branch to inferior rectus muscle
- oculomotor nerve, branch to inferior oblique muscle

FIG. 83-5 ■ Motor nerves of the orbit that serve the muscles of ocular motility, in coronal view. (Adapted with permission from Dutton JJ. Atlas of clinical and surgical orbital anatomy. Philadelphia: WB Saunders; 1994.)

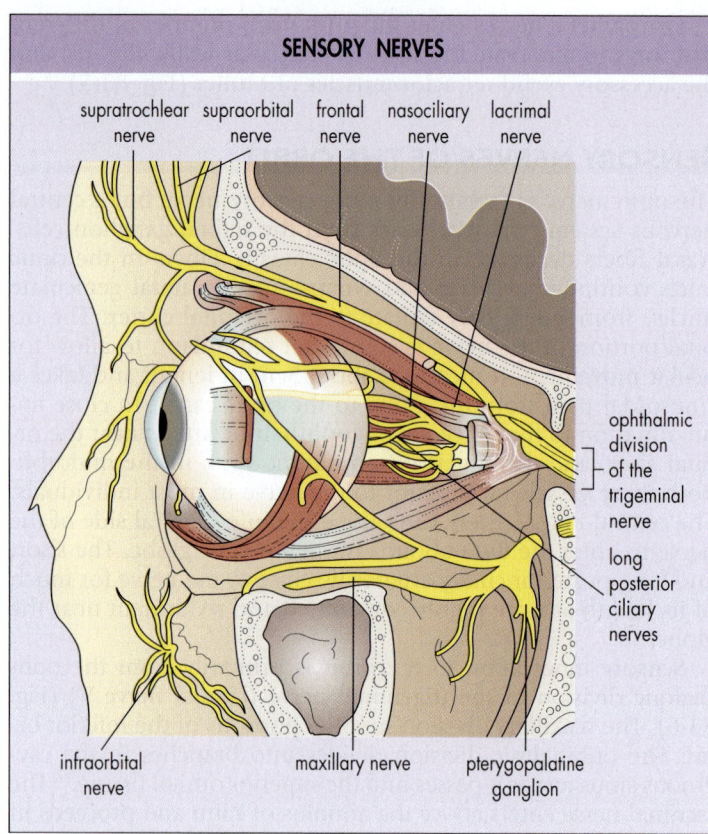

SENSORY NERVES

supratrochlear nerve · supraorbital nerve · frontal nerve · nasociliary nerve · lacrimal nerve

ophthalmic division of the trigeminal nerve

long posterior ciliary nerves

infraorbital nerve · maxillary nerve · pterygopalatine ganglion

FIG. 83-6 ■ **Sensory nerves of the orbit, in lateral view.** (Adapted with permission from Dutton JJ. Atlas of clinical and surgical orbital anatomy. Philadelphia: WB Saunders; 1994.)

annulus of Zinn. It crosses from lateral to medial over the optic nerve, after sending small sensory branches that pass through the ciliary ganglion without synapse and continue to the globe with the short ciliary nerves. As it passes to the lateral side of the optic nerve, the nasociliary nerve gives off the long posterior ciliary nerves, which extend to the posterior globe. The nasociliary nerve continues forward in the medial orbit, where it gives rise to the posterior and anterior ethmoidal nerves. It exits the anterior orbit at the superomedial rim as the infratrochlear nerve.

ARTERIAL SUPPLY TO THE ORBIT

The arterial supply to the orbit arises from the internal carotid system through the ophthalmic artery, with anastomotic connections anteriorly from the external carotid system through the superficial facial vessels.[26] The ophthalmic artery enters the orbit through the optic canal inferotemporal to the optic nerve (Fig. 83-7). In about 83% of individuals the vessel crosses over the nerve to the medial side of the orbit; in the remaining 17% it crosses below the nerve.[27,28] Shortly after it enters the orbit, the ophthalmic artery gives off a number of branches, with some variability in the sequence between individuals. The central retinal artery is usually the first branch. It runs along the inferior aspect of the optic nerve to penetrate the dura anywhere from 8 to 15mm behind the globe. The lacrimal artery generally arises next and courses upward and forward, pierces the intermuscular septum, and runs extraconally to the lacrimal gland just above the lateral rectus muscle. It gives rise to the zygomaticotemporal artery, which penetrates the lateral wall at about the midorbit, and to the zygomaticofacial artery, which runs inferolaterally to exit through a small foramen in the zygomatic bone. Through the latter two vessels the lacrimal artery anastomoses with the external carotid system via the transverse facial and superficial temporal arteries. The lacrimal artery terminates in the lids as the lateral inferior and superior palpebral arteries.

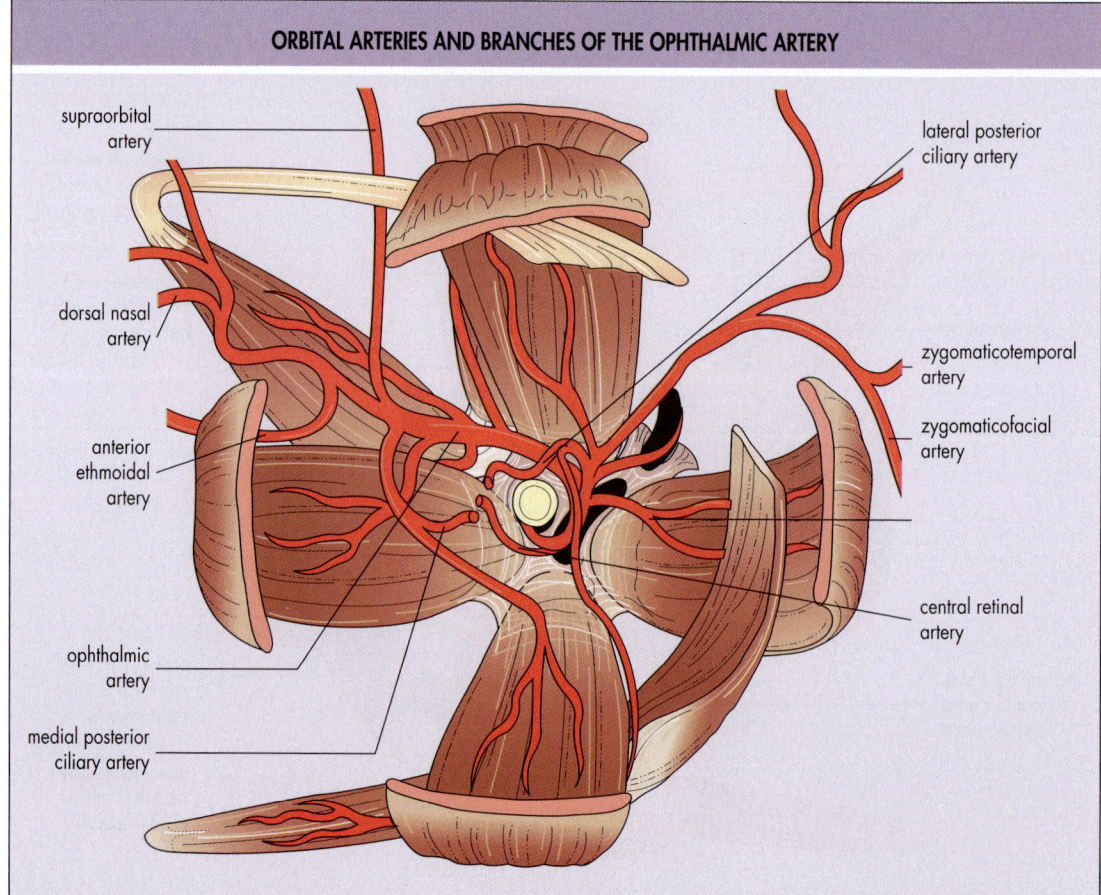

ORBITAL ARTERIES AND BRANCHES OF THE OPHTHALMIC ARTERY

supraorbital artery

dorsal nasal artery

anterior ethmoidal artery

ophthalmic artery

medial posterior ciliary artery

lateral posterior ciliary artery

zygomaticotemporal artery

zygomaticofacial artery

central retinal artery

FIG. 83-7 ■ **Arterial supply to the orbit, in coronal view.** (Adapted with permission from Dutton JJ. Atlas of clinical and surgical orbital anatomy. Philadelphia: WB Saunders; 1994.)

As the ophthalmic artery passes toward the medial orbit, the supraorbital branch is given off. This passes through the intermuscular septum medial to the levator muscle and runs forward with the frontal nerve to the supraorbital notch. In the medial orbit, the ophthalmic artery gives rise to the posterior and anterior ethmoidal arteries, which enter the ethmoidal foramina. The ophthalmic artery then continues forward as the nasofrontal artery to exit just above the medial canthus. Here, it gives off the inferior and superior medial palpebral arteries to the eyelids and terminates as the supratrochlear and dorsal nasal arteries, with anastomotic connections to the angular vessels. Branches to the extraocular muscles are given off along the course of the ophthalmic artery. The branching order is summarized in Box 83-3.

BOX 83-3

Most Common Branching Order of the Ophthalmic Artery

1. Central retinal artery
2. Lateral posterior ciliary artery
3. Lacrimal artery
4. Muscular branch to superior rectus and levator muscles
5. Posterior ethmoidal and supraorbital arteries
6. Medial posterior ciliary artery
7. Muscular branch to medial rectus muscle
8. Muscular branch to superior oblique muscle
9. Branch to connective tissue
10. Anterior ethmoidal artery
11. Inferior medial palpebral artery
12. Superior medial palpebral artery
T1. Dorsal nasal artery
T2. Supratrochlear artery

VENOUS DRAINAGE FROM THE ORBIT

Venous drainage from the orbit is primarily through the superior and inferior ophthalmic veins (Fig. 83-8).[29-31] The superior ophthalmic vein originates at the superomedial orbital rim from branches of the angular, supratrochlear, and supraorbital veins.[32,33] As it passes backward along the medial orbit, it is joined by branches draining the medial and superior rectus muscles and the levator muscle, and by the superior vortex veins, the anterior ethmoidal vein, and collateral branches from the inferior ophthalmic vein. At about the midorbit it crosses to the lateral orbit, just below the superior rectus muscle. Here it is joined by the lacrimal vein and continues posteriorly to enter the cavernous sinus through the superior orbital fissure.[34]

The inferior ophthalmic vein has an indistinct origin in a plexus of small vessels in the inferior orbit. It passes backward along the inferior rectus muscle and is joined by branches draining the inferior rectus and inferior oblique muscles, the inferior vortex veins, and the lateral rectus muscle. A branch exits through the inferior orbital fissure to join the pterygoid plexus before the vessel terminates at the superior ophthalmic vein, just before it enters the cavernous sinus.

REFERENCES

1. Doxanas MT, Anderson RL. Clinical orbital anatomy. Baltimore: Williams & Wilkins; 1984.
2. Dutton JJ. Atlas of clinical and surgical orbital anatomy. Philadelphia: WB Saunders; 1994.
3. De Haan AB, Willekins BL. Embryology of the orbital walls. Mod Probl Ophthalmol. 1975;14:57–64.
4. Goalwin HA. One thousand optic canals. Clinical, anatomic and roentgenologic study. JAMA. 1922;89:1745–8.
5. Jo A, Rizen V, Nikolic V, Banovic B. The role of orbital wall morphological properties and their supporting structures in the etiology of "blow-out" fractures. Surg Radiol Anat. 1989;11:241–8.
6. Ducasse A, Delattre JF, Segal A, et al. Anatomical basis of the surgical approach to the medial wall of the orbit. Anat Clin. 1985;7:15–21.
7. Kirchner JA, Gisawae Y, Crelin ES. Surgical anatomy of the ethmoidal arteries. A laboratory study of 150 orbits. Arch Otolaryngol. 1961;74:382–6.
8. Koornneef L. A new anatomical approach to the human orbit. Mod Probl Ophthalmol. 1975;14:49–56.

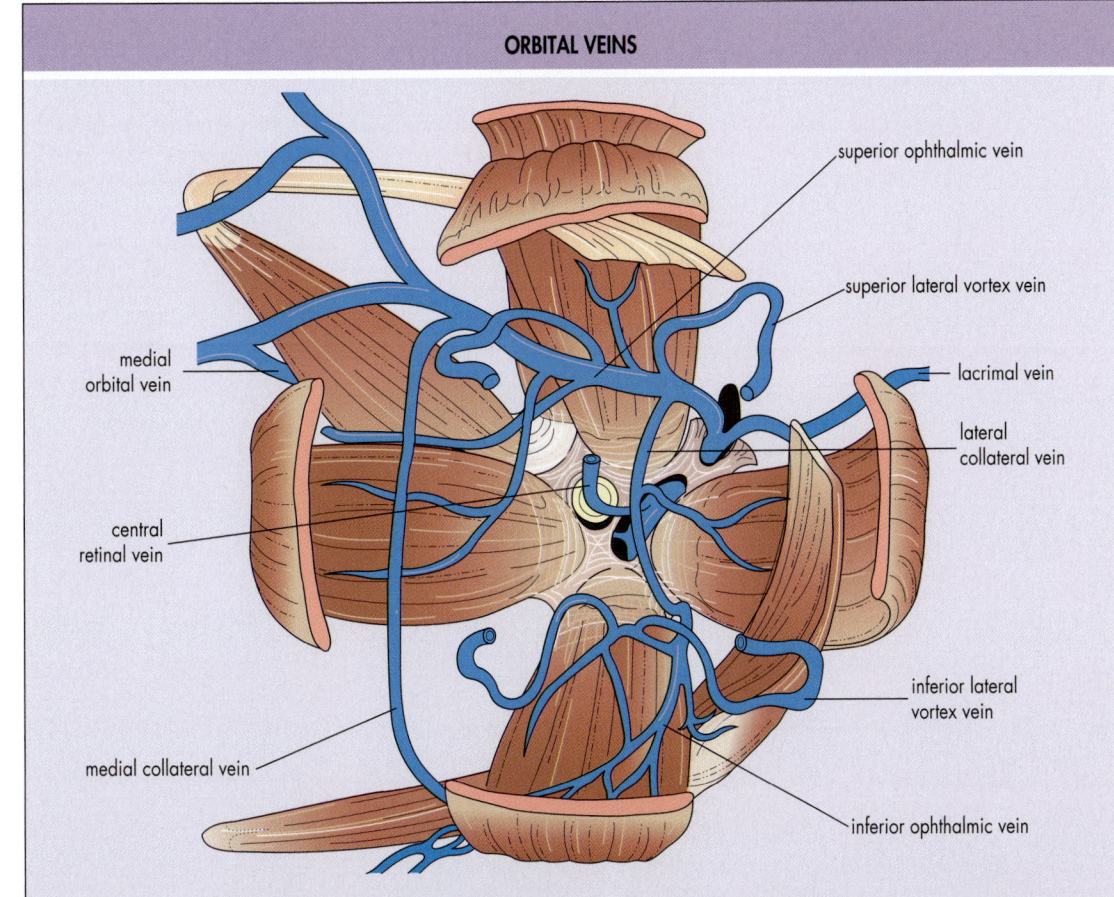

ORBITAL VEINS

superior ophthalmic vein

superior lateral vortex vein

lacrimal vein

lateral collateral vein

medial orbital vein

central retinal vein

medial collateral vein

inferior lateral vortex vein

inferior ophthalmic vein

FIG. 83-8 ▌ **Orbital veins.** Venous drainage from the orbit, in coronal view. (Adapted with permission from Dutton JJ. Atlas of clinical and surgical orbital anatomy. Philadelphia: WB Saunders; 1994.)

9. Koornneef L. The architecture of the musculo-fibrous apparatus in the human orbit. Acta Morphol Neerl Scand. 1977;15:35–64.

10. Koornneef L. New insights into the human orbit connective tissue. Arch Ophthalmol. 1977;95:1269–73.

11. Koornneef L. Orbital septa: anatomy and function. Ophthalmology. 1979;86: 876–80.

12. Manson PN, Clifford CM, Su CT, et al. Mechanisms of global support and post-traumatic enophthalmos. I. The anatomy of the ligament sling and its relation to intramuscular cone orbital fat. Plast Reconstr Surg. 1986;77:193–202.

13. Koornneef L. Eyelid and orbital fascial attachments and their clinical significance. Eye. 1988;2:130–4.

14. Koornneef L. Spatial aspects of the orbital musculofibrous tissue in man. Amsterdam: Lisse, Swets & Zeitlinger; 1977:890.

15. Sevel D. The origins and insertions of the extraocular muscles: development, histologic features, and clinical significance. Trans Am Ophthalmol Soc. 1986;84:488–526.

16. Eggers HM. Functional anatomy of the extraocular muscles. In: Jakobiec FA, ed. Ocular anatomy, embryology, and teratology. Philadelphia: Harper & Row; 1982:827.

17. Gilbert PW. The origin and development of the human extrinsic ocular muscles. Contrib Embryol Carnegie. 1957;36:59–78.

18. Miller JM. Functional anatomy of normal human rectus muscles. Vision Res. 1989;29:223–40.

19. Demer JL. The orbital pulley system: a revolution in concepts of orbital anatomy. Ann N Y Acad Sci. 2002;956:17–32.

20. Helveston EM, Merriam WW, Ellis FD, et al. The trochlea: a study of the anatomy and physiology. Ophthalmology. 1982;89:124–33.

21. Whitnall SE. Anatomy of the human orbit and accessory organs of vision, 2nd ed. London: Oxford Medical Publishers; 1932.

22. Sacks JG. Peripheral innervation of the extraocular muscles. Am J Ophthalmol. 1983;95:520–6.

23. Sinnreich Z, Nathan H. The ciliary ganglion in man (anatomic observations). Anat Anz. 1981;150:287–97.

24. Grimes P, von Sallmann L. Comparative anatomy of the ciliary nerves. Arch Ophthalmol. 1960;64:81–91.

25. Manson PN, Lazarus RB, Morgan R, Iliff N. Pathways of sympathetic innervation to the superior and inferior (Müller's) tarsal muscles. Plast Reconstr Surg. 1986;78:33–40.

26. Shankland WE. The trigeminal nerve. Part II: the ophthalmic division. Cranio. 2001;19:8–12.

27. Lang J, Kageyama I. The ophthalmic artery and its branches, measurements and clinical importance. Surg Radiol Anat. 1990;12:83–90.

28. Hayreh SS. The ophthalmic artery, III. Branches. Br J Ophthalmol. 1962;46: 212–47.

29. Hayreh SS, Dass R. The ophthalmic artery, II. Intra-orbital course. Br J Ophthalmol. 1962;46:165–85.

30. Bergin MP. A spatial reconstruction of the orbital vascular pattern in relation to the connective tissue system. Acta Morphol Neerl Scand. 1982;20:117–37.

31. Spektor S, Piontek E, Umansky F. Orbital venous drainage into the cavernous sinus space: microanatomic relationships. Neurosurgery. 1997;40:532–9.

32. Bergin MP. Relationships between the arteries and veins and the connective tissue system in the human orbit. I. The retrobulbar part of the orbit: apical region. Acta Morphol Neerl Scand. 1982;20:1–42.

33. Brismar J. Orbital phlebography. II. Anatomy of the superior ophthalmic vein and its tributaries. Acta Radiol Diagn (Stockh). 1974;15:481–96.

34. Brismar J. Orbital phlebography. III. Topography of the orbital veins. Acta Radiol Diagn (Stockh). 1974;15:577–94.

CHAPTER
84 Orbital Imaging Techniques

JONATHAN J. DUTTON

DEFINITIONS

- Computed tomography: An imaging technique where contrast differences are based on tissue density based on the passage of X-rays through tissues.
- Magnetic resonance imaging: An imaging technique where density differences are based on tissue proton density and their resonance characteristics based on biochemical relationships within the atomic lattice.
- Orbital echography: An imaging system where density differences are based on tissue characteristics reflecting the passage, reflection, and refraction of sound waves through the tissue.

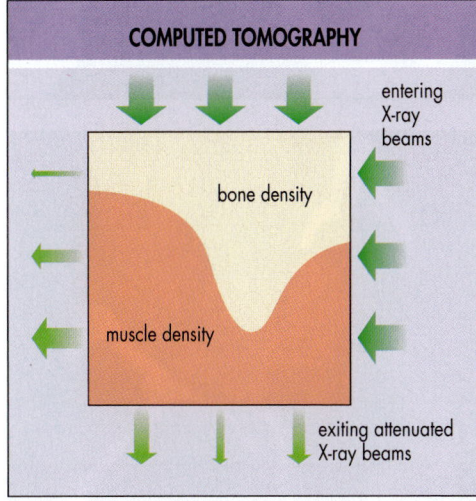

COMPUTED TOMOGRAPHY

entering X-ray beams

bone density

muscle density

exiting attenuated X-ray beams

FIG. 84-1 Computed tomography. Intersecting matrix of collimated X-ray beams passes through tissue and is attenuated according to differences in tissue density.

INTRODUCTION

Radiographic examination is an essential step in the evaluation of all patients who have suspected orbital disease. This routine frequently contributes to a specific diagnosis and also may help the physician plan the most appropriate medical therapy or surgical approach.[1] Computed tomography and magnetic resonance imaging have largely replaced older techniques. Orbital echography is another valuable tool that can provide information not obtained easily with other techniques.

COMPUTED TOMOGRAPHY

In computed tomography (CT), thin, collimated X-ray beams pass through tissue along the rows and columns of an intersecting matrix. The area defined by any two intersecting beams is referred to as a pixel and is analogous to a single dot in a newspaper photograph. Since the X-ray beam has a certain thickness, the area of the beam intersection actually defines a volumetric space, referred to as the voxel. As X-ray beams traverse the body, they are weakened or attenuated according to the density of the tissues through which they pass (Fig. 84-1). The degree of attenuation of any two intersecting beams that emerge from a volume of tissue allows the calculation of the mean attenuation value for all the tissues included within the area of intersection of the beams, or voxel. The smaller the pixel and the thinner the tissue slice, the smaller the volume of the voxel and the higher the resolution of the final image.

Each voxel is assigned an average attenuation value by the computer based on the mean attenuation of the X-rays that pass through the voxel. These values are designated in Hounsfield units, a 2000-unit scale from −1000 to +1000. By arbitrary convention, the density of air is assigned a value of −1000, the density of water is 0, and the density of bone is +1000. For visualization by the human eye, this scale is reduced to 32–64 gray levels between black and white on the radiographic film. Thus, air appears black on the film, and bone appears white. A density greater than that of bone, such as that of a metallic foreign body, also appears white.

For specific anatomical detail, the image is manipulated by setting "windows." The window level refers to the Hounsfield unit on which a narrow range of units is to be centered. The window range is the inclusive number of Hounsfield units above and below this level that are to be expanded into the black-to-white scale for imaging. In the examination of a soft tissue lesion such as a hemangioma, for example, the window level may be set to +50, the density of muscle, and the window range to plus and minus 200 units. With these window settings, −150 on the scale appears black, and +250 appears white. All attenuation values below −150 also appear black, so there is no detail visible in the orbital fat. Also, all those values above +250 appear white, so there is no detail seen in bone. Similarly, bone windows are centered on about +800 for visualization of bone details (Fig. 84-2).

Orbital CT routinely should include scans in both the axial and the coronal planes. Contrast enhancement is generally less useful than for brain studies because of the lack of a blood-orbit barrier, but it may provide valuable information about the nature of particular types of lesions. Unless contraindicated, contrast studies should be included in all orbital scans. Surface coil technology and fat-suppression algorithms may significantly increase resolution and contrast.[2-5]

MAGNETIC RESONANCE IMAGING

The technique of magnetic resonance imaging (MRI) offers several advantages over CT.[6-8] Because low-resonance signal is generated by bone, soft tissue visualization in the region of the orbital apex, optic canal, and cavernous sinus is not as degraded as in CT scans.[9-11] Manipulation of resonance signals provides contrast variability and tissue differentiation unobtainable with any X-ray technique. Surface coil technology, improvements in signal-to-noise ratios, and techniques to suppress the high fat signal on T1-weighted images have improved visualization of orbital lesions.[5,12-15] For intracranial lesions in the vicinity of the optic chiasm and suprasellar cistern, MRI has proved especially valuable and has all but replaced older techniques.[16]

The generation of a magnetic resonance signal depends on the presence of magnetic isotopes of common elements in biological

649

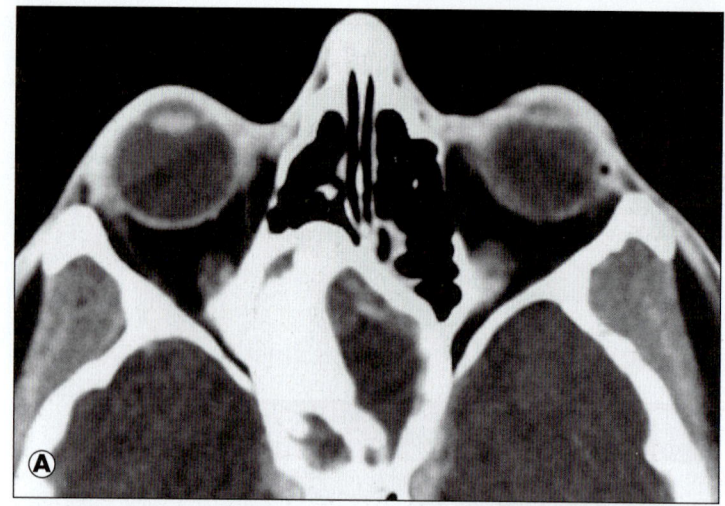

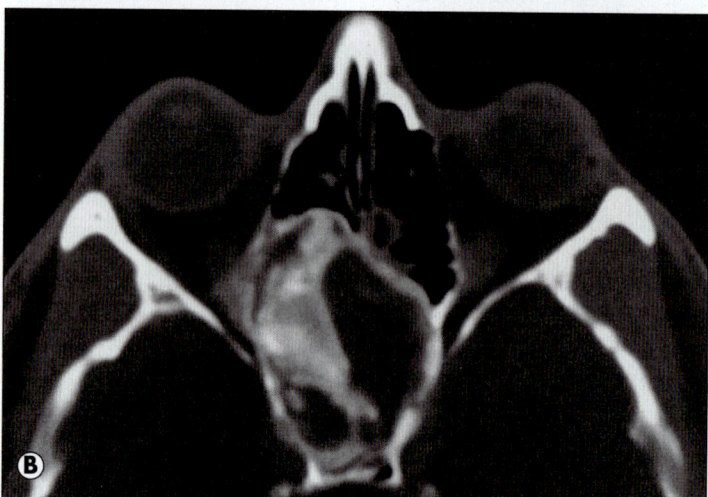

FIG. 84-2 ■ Axial computed tomography of the orbits. A, Tissue density window. B, Bone density window.

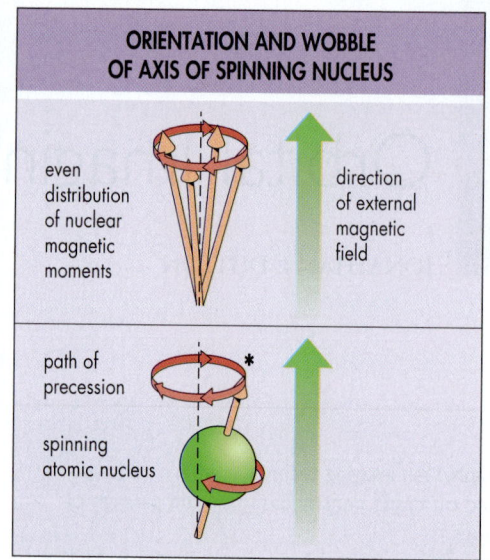

ORIENTATION AND WOBBLE OF AXIS OF SPINNING NUCLEUS

even distribution of nuclear magnetic moments

direction of external magnetic field

path of precession

*

spinning atomic nucleus

FIG. 84-4 ■ **Orientation of spinning nuclei.** In the top diagram, all spinning nuclei are distributed evenly around the magnetic moment. In the bottom diagram, each spinning nucleus exhibits a wobble of its axis with one end (*) precessing around the direction of the mean magnetic moment.

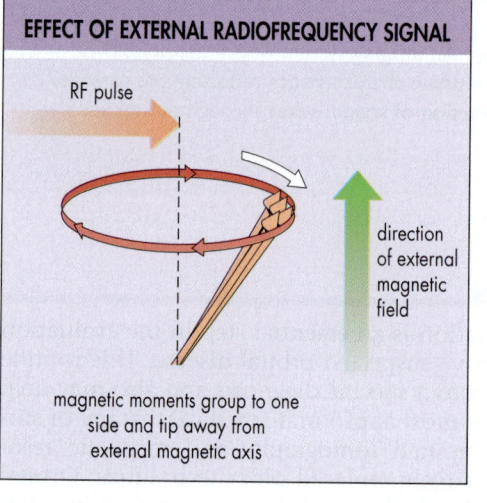

EFFECT OF EXTERNAL RADIOFREQUENCY SIGNAL

RF pulse

direction of external magnetic field

magnetic moments group to one side and tip away from external magnetic axis

FIG. 84-5 ■ **Radiofrequency signal.** With exposure to an external radiofrequency (RF) signal at the Larmor frequency, the spinning nuclear axes tip away from the direction of the magnetic field and group to one side.

SPINNING PROTON NUCLEI

Normal tissue: no net magnetic moment	External magnetic field: parallel magnetic moment

direction of external magnetic field

FIG. 84-3 ■ **Spinning proton nuclei.** The left diagram depicts random orientation found in normal tissues with no set magnetic field. The right diagram depicts orientation with a net magnetic moment aligned with an external magnetic field.

tissues.[17] The isotope most frequently imaged is the ubiquitous hydrogen nucleus or proton.[18,19] This proton is normally in a state of axial spin. This spinning charged particle generates a magnetic field, with north and south poles, analogous to a bar magnet. Under normal conditions, all the nuclei in a given volume of tissue are oriented randomly, with no net magnetic vector. When placed within a strong external magnetic field, the in-

dividual protons align with the direction of the external magnetic field, either parallel or antiparallel (Fig. 84-3). Because a slight preponderance of alignments is parallel to the direction of the magnetic field, the tissue assumes a mean magnetic moment in the same orientation.[20] Most of the axes of individual protons are not aligned perfectly with the direction of the magnetic field, but lie at various small angles to the mean magnetic moment. They are distributed equally through the 360° around the magnetic moment like spinning tops, and these inclined axes wobble, with one pole remaining stationary and the other revolving, or "precessing," around the direction of the mean magnetic moment (Fig. 84-4). The rotating axes, therefore, describe a conical surface. The angular velocity of precession is determined by the strength of the external magnetic field and by an intrinsic property of the particular atomic nucleus. This is called the gyromagnetic ratio, which is proportional to the magnetic moment.[21] The relationship between these parameters is defined by the Larmor equation, and the resultant angular velocity is the resonant or Larmor frequency.

When this system is exposed to an external radiofrequency (RF) pulse at the Larmor frequency, energy is absorbed by the atomic nuclei. As the spinning nuclei move to higher energy levels, the angular orientation of their axes to the direction of the external magnetic field increases. Also, an induced magnetic field perpendicular to the RF pulse direction realigns the individual atomic axes to one side of the direction of the external magnetic field (Fig. 84-5). When the RF signal is turned off, the spinning nuclei return to equilibrium by giving up energy to the environment, again at the Larmor frequency. Return to equilibrium occurs by two simultaneous decay, or relaxation, processes—T1 and T2.

During T1 relaxation, the individual nuclear axes realign parallel to the direction of the external magnetic field. In the process, they give up their absorbed energy. The time required for this process is the T1, or spin-lattice, relaxation time. It is influenced by the interaction of the proton with other atoms within the molecular lattice, by temperature, and by viscosity of the tissue. A high T1 relaxation time yields maximal energy release per unit time and, therefore, a higher resonance signal and brighter image.

During the RF pulse signal, while the atomic nuclei are still grouped on one side of the mean magnetic axis, they generate a resonant signal. This results from the tipped net magnetic vector of the spinning protons constantly cutting across the lines of force of the external magnetic field, thus generating a small alternating-current voltage. After the RF pulse is stopped, the atomic nuclei redistribute themselves evenly 360° around the direction of the external magnetic field; as they do so, the strength of this signal decreases because of canceling vectors. The time for complete decay of this resonant signal is the T2, or spin–spin relaxation time. It is influenced by the induced magnetic fields generated around adjacent spinning nuclei. As with the T1 times, biochemical differences between tissues confer slightly different T2 relaxation times to the protons in the tissue. Since the T1 and T2 signal strengths determine the contrast intensity, these biochemical differences result in contrast differentiation on the final image. Since small differences in T1 and T2 relaxation can be detected easily, contrast differentiation between adjacent tissues on MRI is considerably better than that with CT.

The T1 and T2 signals are measured by RF detectors. They detect in mass fashion all similar signals at the Larmor frequency, regardless of their specific location within the tissue. Spatial encoding of resonant signals from particular small blocks of tissue is necessary to create a visually meaningful two-dimensional image. This is achieved by deformation of the external magnetic field using gradient coils, such that the protons in every small volume of examined tissue (voxel) have a unique magnetic field strength and, therefore, a unique Larmor frequency. The detected Larmor frequency identifies the precise location of the signal, and thereby a topographical image can be created. The introduction of surface receiver coils placed close to the region of study has improved detection efficiency and the signal-to-noise ratio, thus decreasing the influence of surrounding magnetic aberrations.

Normal Orbital Anatomy in the Axial Plane

AXIAL SECTION THROUGH THE LOWERMOST ORBIT. The orbital floor appears as a thin, oblique density that runs from anteromedial to posterolateral, separating the orbit from the maxillary sinus.[22,23] Since the floor gradually slopes backward and upward, successively higher cross sections are cut in axial scan sequences. The orbital cavity is bounded medially by the anterior lacrimal crest and laterally by the lateral rim of the zygomatic bone. Posterior to the orbit is the cranial base.[24] A thin line arches across the orbital opening from the medial to the lateral bony rims; this represents the lower eyelid and orbital septum.[1]

Depending on the level of the cut, the orbital cavity may appear empty (because it contains only orbital fat), or it may contain a rounded density that represents the sclera cut tangentially. Occasionally, the inferior oblique muscle is seen as an oblique band of medium-density tissue, and in slightly higher sections, the inferior rectus muscle may appear as a density adjacent to the globe posteriorly.

AXIAL SECTION THROUGH THE INFERIOR ORBIT. In low axial sections through the inferior orbit, the floor again appears as a thin density that separates the orbital cavity from the maxillary sinus. In the posterolateral corner of the orbit, where the floor approaches the lateral wall, a channel separates the body of the sphenoid bone from the greater wing. This is the inferior orbital fissure. Posteriorly, behind the inferior rectus muscle, this fissure

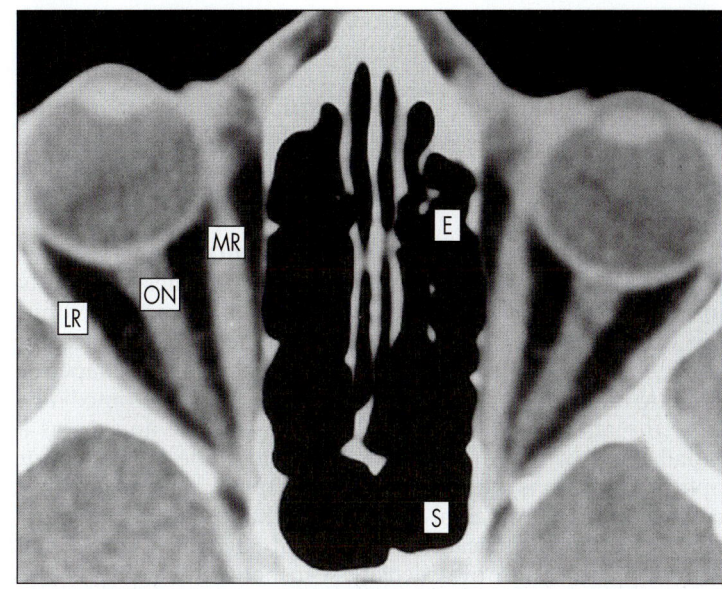

FIG. 84-6 Axial CT scan through the midorbit. The globe and optic nerve are seen in the axial plane, along with the medial and lateral rectus muscles. *E,* Ethmoid sinus; *LR,* lateral rectus; *MR,* medial rectus; *ON,* optic nerve; *S,* sphenoid sinus.

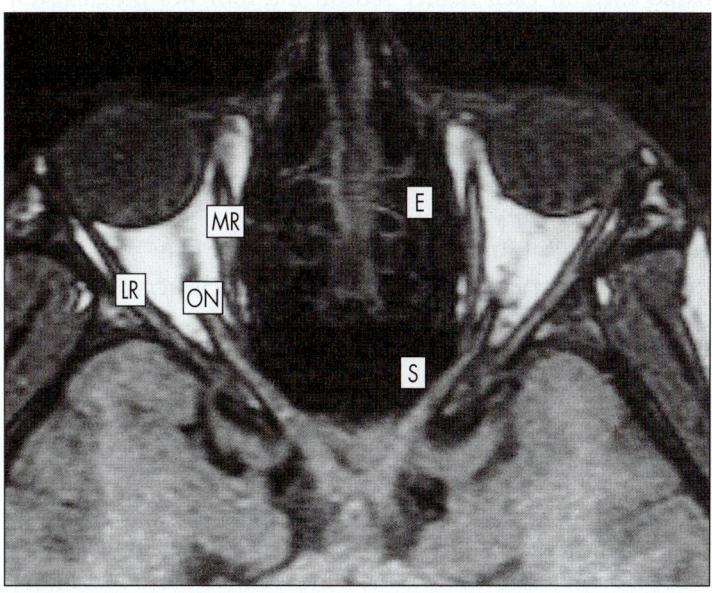

FIG. 84-7 Axial MRI scan through the midorbit. The section is slightly higher than in Figure 84-6. The optic nerves are seen passing back to the optic chiasm. *E,* Ethmoid sinus; *LR,* lateral rectus; *MR,* medial rectus; *ON,* optic nerve; *S,* sphenoid sinus.

communicates between the orbital space and the pterygopalatine fossa. In the anteromedial corner of the orbit, the lacrimal sac fossa is seen as a depression in the orbital process of the maxillary bone.

Within the orbital space, a central rounded density represents the globe. Since the vitreous is primarily aqueous, it appears empty (black) on CT. However, on MRI scans, the vitreous appears dark on T1-weighted sequences and bright on T2-weighted sequences. Just posterior to the globe is a rounded density that lies on the midportion of the orbital floor and is discontinuous with the globe. This is the inferior rectus muscle cut in cross section.

AXIAL SECTION THROUGH THE MIDORBIT. On axial scans through the midorbit, the globe is seen in equatorial section (Figs. 84-6 and 84-7). Anteriorly, the lens is seen as an oval density. On MRI sections, the ciliary body can be distinguished on either side of the lens.[1] Behind the globe, the optic nerve is seen to emerge from the posterior sclera and run toward the orbital apex.[25]

In the midorbit, a gently curved enhancing line crosses the orbit from lateral to medial. This is the superior ophthalmic vein.[26] Near the orbital apex, a small enhancing vessel is seen to cross over the optic nerve from lateral to medial. This is the second portion of the ophthalmic artery. Along the orbital walls are the lateral and medial rectus muscles. At slightly higher levels, both the medial rectus and superior oblique muscles are often seen together. On either side of the midline are the ethmoid sinuses, with the thin lamina papyracea that forms the medial orbital wall. Just medial to the laminae are the ethmoid air cells.

AXIAL SECTION THROUGH THE SUPERIOR ORBIT. At this level, the orbital contour is narrower and terminates posteriorly in a rounded angle above the level of the optic canals. Within the orbital outline, the globe is represented in cross section above the level of the lens. Along the medial wall is the superior oblique muscle that passes through the trochlea anteromedially. Near the orbital apex, the superior rectus muscle appears as a broad band of tissue directed toward the globe. The superior ophthalmic vein is seen as a curvilinear enhancing structure that crosses from anteromedial to posterolateral just below the muscle. Anterolaterally, near the lateral orbital rim, the lacrimal gland appears as an oval density seen between the zygomatic bone and the globe.

AXIAL SECTION THROUGH THE ORBITAL ROOF. In axial sections above the level of the globe, the orbit appears as a rounded contour posteriorly. Since the roof lies in a plane oblique to the tissue slice, in each higher section the roof lies progressively more anteriorly as it approaches the orbital rim. The levator muscle is seen as a broad band that extends from the superior orbital rim backward along the roof. Anteromedially, the trochlea is seen clearly, and at appropriate levels the superior oblique tendon can be visualized as it fans out over the superior globe below the superior rectus muscle insertion.

Normal Orbital Anatomy in the Coronal Plane

CORONAL SECTION THROUGH THE ANTERIORMOST ORBIT. In coronal sections through the anteriormost orbit, the globe is cut through the level of the eyelids. In the midline of the orbital roof, below the frontal lobes of the brain, is the frontal sinus. The anterior segment of the globe may appear as several concentric densities that represent the cornea, lens, and anterior sclera. In the superior medial corner of the orbit are the trochlea and tendon of the superior oblique muscle. Inferiorly, the inferior oblique muscle can be seen as a linear shadow that runs from the inferomedial orbital wall toward the lateral orbit.

CORONAL SECTION THROUGH THE ANTERIOR ORBIT. Sections cut through the anterior midorbit pass through the globe near its equator. At this level, the orbital roof is seen as a thin, curved plate of bone with an upper surface that undulates against the overlying frontal lobes. In the midline is the crista galli, and on either side are the cribriform plate and roof of the ethmoid sinus.

The orbital floor is a thin plate of bone that extends from the lowermost extent of the lamina papyracea and slopes downward and laterally to the inferolateral orbital wall. Immediately below the floor is the triangular maxillary sinus.

Centrally, the globe is seen to fill most of the orbital space (Figs. 84-8 and 84-9). Superiorly, the thin superior rectus muscle lies adjacent to the globe, and above it is the levator muscle. Medially, the flattened medial rectus muscle lies within the orbital fat between the lamina papyracea and the globe. Just below the eye is the inferior rectus muscle, and laterally is the lateral rectus muscle. In the superomedial corner, a small, round shadow is the superior oblique muscle. At the medial edge of the superior rectus–levator muscle complex is a round enhancing structure, the superior ophthalmic vein.

CORONAL SECTION THROUGH THE CENTRAL ORBIT. In coronal sections behind the globe, the orbital walls appear as in more anterior sections. Within the central space of the orbit lies the round optic nerve cut in cross section (Figs. 84-10 and 84-11).

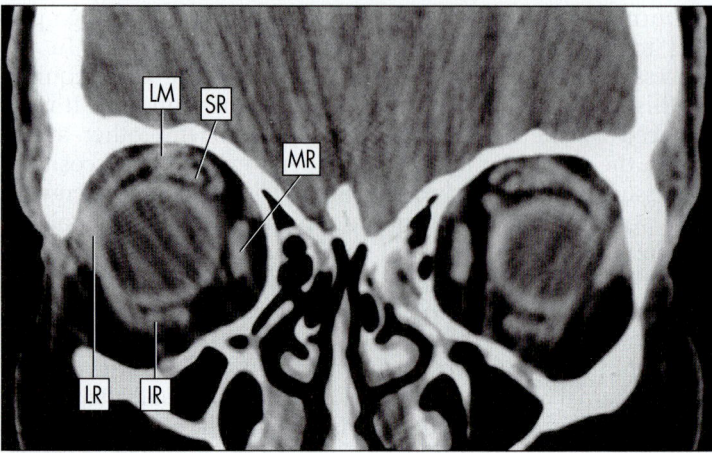

FIG. 84-8 ■ Coronal CT scan through the anterior portion of the orbit. The globes are cut in cross section, and the rectus muscles are seen as flattened densities near the sclera. *IR,* Inferior rectus; *LM,* levator muscle; *LR,* lateral rectus; *MR,* medial rectus; *SR,* superior rectus.

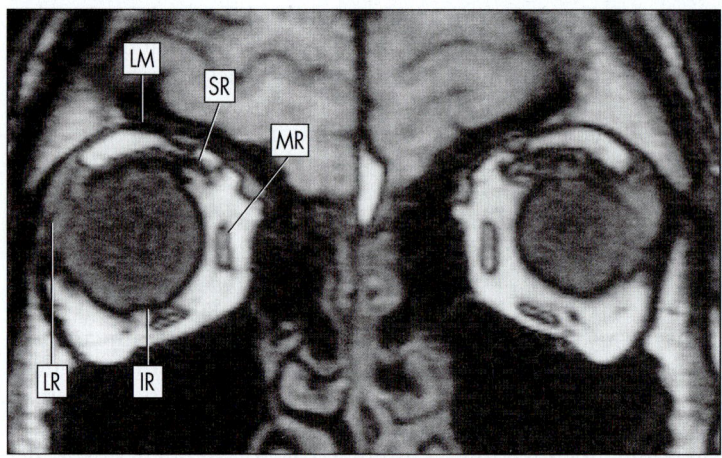

FIG. 84-9 ■ Coronal MRI scan through the anterior portion of the orbit. The cut is similar to that seen in Figure 84-8. *IR,* Inferior rectus; *LM,* levator muscle; *LR,* lateral rectus; *MR,* medial rectus; *SR,* superior rectus.

On MRI scans, the central nerve can easily be distinguished from the nerve sheaths; the two are separated by the clear subarachnoid space. The four rectus muscles are seen against their respective orbital walls cut across their midbellies. The levator muscle appears as a separate thin strap just above and medial to the superior rectus. Above the medial rectus muscle, along the superomedial corner or the orbit, is the superior oblique muscle. The superior ophthalmic vein is a small enhancing circular density between the optic nerve and the superior rectus muscle, en route to the lateral orbit.

CORONAL SECTION THROUGH THE ANTERIOR ORBITAL APEX. Toward the apex, the bony orbit narrows to a triangular section. Inferolaterally, the contour opens into the inferior orbital fissure that communicates with the infratemporal fossa. Within the orbit, the optic nerve, the superior oblique muscle, and all four rectus muscles can still be identified as separate structures. The superior ophthalmic vein is found more laterally, to the lateral edge of the superior rectus muscle. The ophthalmic artery is seen just above the optic nerve as it crosses over the nerve from lateral to medial.

CORONAL SECTION THROUGH THE POSTERIOR ORBITAL APEX. At this level, the orbit is reduced to a small rounded space, open inferiorly to the pterygopalatine fossa. It is bounded laterally by the greater wing of the sphenoid and medially by the body of the sphenoid adjacent to the sphenoid sinus. Superolaterally, the orbit opens into the middle cranial fossa through the superior orbital fissure.

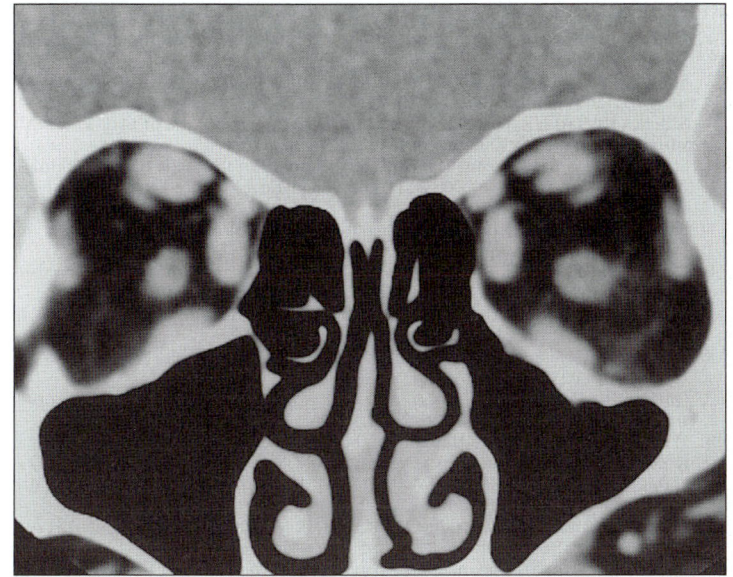

FIG. 84-10 ■ **Coronal CT scan through the midorbit.** The optic nerve lies centrally, surrounded by the rectus muscles. Just below the lateral edge of the superior rectus is the superior ophthalmic vein.

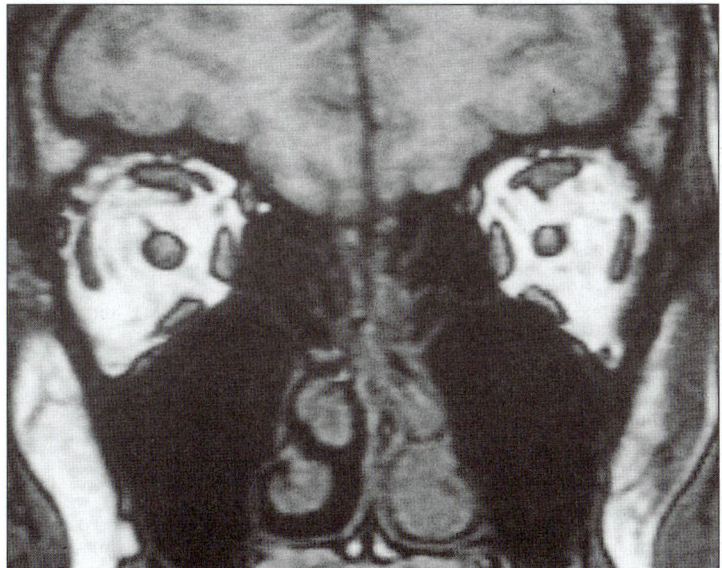

FIG. 84-11 ■ **Coronal MRI scan through the midorbit.** Structures are similar to those observed in Figure 84-10.

ORBITAL ECHOGRAPHY

Echography, or ultrasonography, is a technique that utilizes high-frequency sound waves to image tissue.[27] Sound waves are generated by a piezoelectric crystal and are directed through the tissues of interest. Here they behave as light does—they demonstrate density-dependent velocity, as well as reflection, refraction, and scatter. Tissue characteristics such as cell compaction and reflective surfaces determine the specific echographic pattern.

Sound waves in the range of 8–10mHz pass through orbital tissues from the probe tip. As the waves encounter tissues of different density and reflectivity, some are deflected and refracted, but others are reflected back to the probe, where they are detected and displayed on an oscilloscope. The amount of energy returned and detected by the probe determines the height (A-scan) or intensity (B-scan) of the resultant image. Thus, echography produces an image in which contrast reflects differences in the reflectivity of sound waves. The more reflective the interfaces within a tissue, the greater the amount of sound energy returned to the probe (Fig. 84-12).

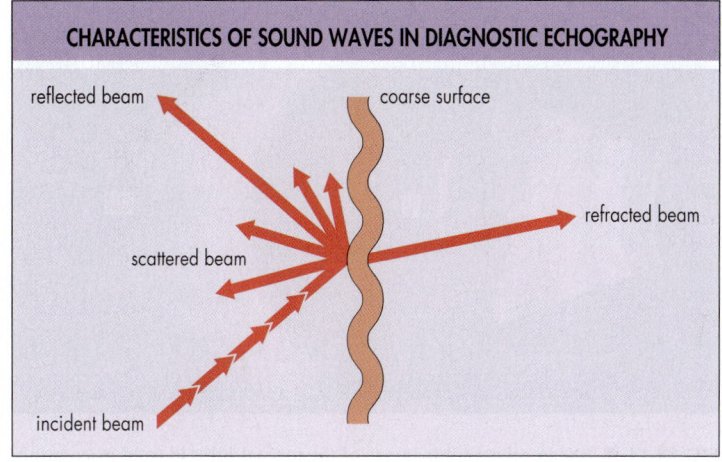

CHARACTERISTICS OF SOUND WAVES IN DIAGNOSTIC ECHOGRAPHY

FIG. 84-12 ■ Physical characteristics of sound waves in diagnostic echography.

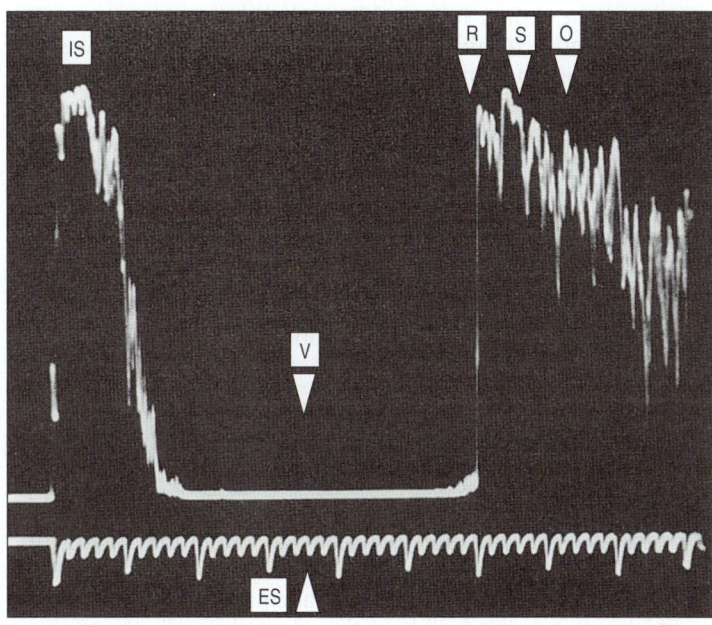

FIG. 84-13 ■ A-scan echographic image of the normal orbit. *ES,* Time scale in microseconds; *IS,* initial spike; *O,* orbital fat; *R,* retina; *S,* sclera; *V,* vitreous cavity.

Echography has the advantages of ease of use, no ionizing radiation, excellent tissue differentiation, and cost effectiveness. However, sound waves at 8–10mHz do not penetrate beyond the midorbit. Also, echography cannot image both orbits simultaneously and is difficult for a nonspecialist to interpret.

A-Scan Echography

The A-scan echographic image shows a one-dimensional array of spikes displayed along a baseline (Fig. 84-13). The height of the spikes represents the signal strength or amplitude of the reflected echo, whereas the horizontal spacing between the spikes is dependent on the time required for the sound to reach its target and return to the receiver. This distance is proportional to the distance from the probe to the tissue target.

For orbital examinations, a standardized tissue sensitivity is used.[28] Lesions are identified by their patterns, which are distinct from normal orbital echographic patterns. This technique is best for detecting tissue differentiation, surface characteristics, reflectivity, and vascularity.

On the normal orbital A-scan, the initial spike (see Fig. 84-13, far left) represents echoes generated in the probe tip. The vitreous cavity is typically echolucent at baseline. The posterior pole

653

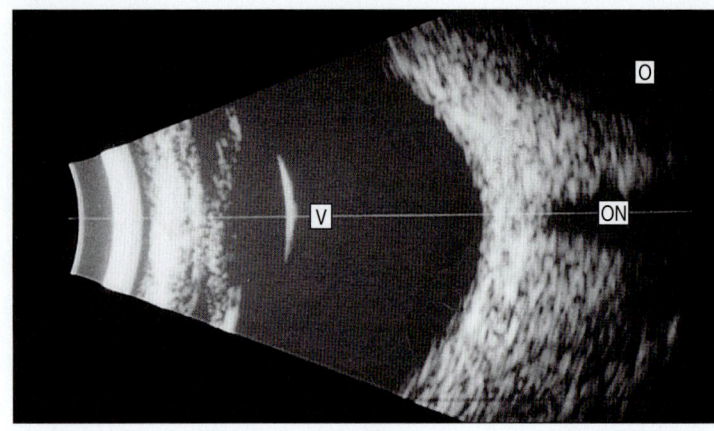

FIG. 84-14 ▌ B-scan echographic image of the normal orbit in axial orientation. *O*, Orbital fat; *ON*, optic nerve; *V*, vitreous cavity.

complex is seen as a sharply rising perpendicular spike that represents the retina, followed by a slightly lower narrow zone (choroid) and a double-peaked maximally elevated spike that represents the inner and outer walls of the sclera. The orbital fat is seen as a descending chain of high irregular spikes, with rapid attenuation. Orbital lesions may appear as a zone of different reflectivity within the fat signals.

B-Scan Echography

The B-scan echographic image shows a two-dimensional array that represents a "slice" through the tissue (Fig. 84-14). The intensity or brightness of echoes is proportional to the strength of the sound waves returned to the detector. As with the A-scan, the spacing between echoes from left to right on the screen represents time or, more importantly, distance from the probe tip to the target tissue.

The basic B-scan examination requires scans in the transverse, longitudinal, and axial orientations, with visualization along all the orbital walls and the meridians of the globe. For orbital scans, the sound waves are usually directed through the eye. For some anteriorly placed lesions, a paraocular approach—with the sound beam passing beside, rather than through, the globe—may be more useful to demonstrate a lesion in relation to the eye. The B-scan is best used for the evaluation of topography, localization, and general contour.

The normal orbital B-scan image shows a cross section of the targeted area with a lucent (black) circular region that represents the globe (see Fig. 84-14). Behind this is a zone of brightly reflective echoes from the fat and interlobular septa. Several areas of lucency may represent the optic nerve or extraocular muscles.

REFERENCES

1. Dutton JJ. Atlas of clinical and surgical orbital anatomy. Philadelphia: WB Saunders; 1994:201–40.
2. Sullivan JA, Harms SE. Characterization of orbital lesions by surface coil MR imaging. Radiographics. 1987;7:19–27.
3. Schenck JF, Hart HR, Foster TH, et al. Improved imaging of the orbit at 1.5T with surface coils. AJR Am J Roentgenol. 1985;144:1033–6.
4. Schenck JF, Hart HR, Foster TH, et al. High resolution magnetic resonance imaging using surface coils. In: Kressel HY, ed. Magnetic resonance annual 1986. New York: Raven; 1986:123–60.
5. Simon J, Szumowski J, Totterman S, et al. Fat-suppression MR imaging of the orbit. AJNR Am J Neuroradiol. 1988;9:261–8.
6. Dortzbach RK, Kronish JW, Gentry LR. Magnetic resonance imaging of the orbit. Part II. Clinical applications. Ophthal Plast Reconstr Surg. 1989;5:160–70.
7. DePotter P, Flanders AE, Shields CL, Shields JA. Magnetic resonance imaging of orbital tumors. Int Ophthalmol Clin. 1993;33:163–73.
8. DePotter P, Shields JA, Shields CL. MRI of the eye and orbit. Philadelphia: JB Lippincott; 1995:3–17.
9. Daniels DL, Pech P, Mark L, et al. Magnetic resonance imaging of the cavernous sinus. AJR Am J Roentgenol. 1985;145:1145–6.
10. Daniels DL, Yu S, Pech P, Haughton VM. Computed tomography and magnetic resonance imaging of the orbital apex. Radiol Clin North Am. 1987;25:803–17.
11. Hammerschlag SB, O'Reilly GVA, Naheedy MH. Computed tomography of the optic canals. AJNR Am J Neuroradiol. 1981;2:593–4.
12. Atlas SW, Grossman RI, Hackney HI, et al. STIR MR imaging of the orbit. AJR Am J Roentgenol. 1988;151:1025–30.
13. Atlas SW, Galetta SL. The orbit and visual system. In: Atlas SW, ed. Magnetic resonance imaging of the brain and spine. New York: Raven Press; 1991:709–22.
14. Harms SE. The orbit. In: Edelman RR, Hesselink JR, eds. Clinical magnetic resonance imaging. Philadelphia: WB Saunders; 1990:598–603.
15. Tien RD, Chu PK, Hesselink JR, Szumowski J. Intra- and paraorbital lesions: value of fat-suppression MR imaging with paramagnetic contrast enhancement. AJNR Am J Neuroradiol. 1991;12:245–53.
16. Dutton JJ, Klingele TG, Burde RM, Gado M. Evaluation of the suprasellar cistern by computed tomography. Ophthalmology. 1982;89:1220–5.
17. DeMarco JK, Bilaniuk LT. Magnetic resonance imaging: technical aspects. In: Newton TH, Bilaniuk LT, eds. Modern neuroradiology, vol 4, Radiology of the eye and orbit. New York: Raven Press; 1990:1–14.
18. Dortzbach RK, Kronish JW, Gentry LR. Magnetic resonance imaging of the orbit. Part I. Physical principles. Ophthal Plast Reconstr Surg. 1985;5:151–9.
19. Gore JC, Emery EW, Orr JS, Doyle FH. Medical nuclear magnetic resonance imaging: I. Physical principles. Invest Radiol. 1981;16:269–74.
20. Horowitz AL. MRI physics for radiologists, 2nd ed. New York: Springer-Verlag; 1992:4–54.
21. Sassani JW, Osbakken MD. Anatomic features of the eye disclosed with nuclear magnetic resonance imaging. Arch Ophthalmol. 1984;102:541–6.
22. Zonneveld FW, Koornneef L, Hillen B, de Slegte RGM. Normal direct multiplanar CT anatomy of the orbit with correlative anatomic cryosections. Radiol Clin North Am. 1987;25:381–407.
23. Dutton JJ. Radiographic evaluation of the orbit. In: Doxanas MT, Anderson RL, eds. Clinical orbital anatomy. Baltimore: Williams & Wilkins; 1984:35–56.
24. Beyer-Enke SA, Tiedemann K, Görich J, Gamroth A. Dünnschichtecomputertomographie der Schädelbasis. Radiologe. 1987;27:483–8.
25. Langer BG, Mafee MF, Pollock S, et al. MRI of the normal orbit and optic pathway. Radiol Clin North Am. 1987;25:429–46.
26. Artmann H, Grau A, Lösche CC. Aussagefähigkeit der Computertomograpgie der Ophthalmologischen Diagnostik. Radiol Diagn. 1989;30:621–8.
27. Byrne SF, Green RL. Ultrasound of the eye and orbit. St. Louis: Mosby–Year Book; 1992:1–51.
28. Byrne SF. Standardized echography. Part I: A-scan examination procedures. Int Ophthalmol Clin. 1979;19:267–75.

SECTION 2 EYELIDS

CHAPTER

85

Eyelid Retraction

GENE R. HOWARD

DEFINITION
- Deviation from the normal position of the upper or lower eyelid margin with respect to the limbus of the eye.

KEY FEATURES
- Upper eyelid margin above superior corneal limbus.
- Lower eyelid margin below inferior corneal limbus.

ASSOCIATED FEATURES
- Secondary epiphora.
- Corneal exposure.
- Dry eye symptoms.

INTRODUCTION

At first glance, eyelid retraction may appear to be an uncomplicated anatomic variant of eyelid position. The differential diagnosis, however, is extensive and encompasses congenital abnormalities, systemic infectious and inflammatory processes, degenerative disease, involutional changes, and traumatic or postoperative repercussions.

Management options for eyelid retraction may be as varied and complex. Medical treatment may return the eyelids to their normal position. Other cases require surgical repositioning to restore normal eyelid anatomy.

PREOPERATIVE EVALUATION AND DIAGNOSTIC APPROACH

The Ophthalmic History

Eyelid retraction is defined as a deviation from the normal position of the upper or lower eyelid margin with respect to the limbus of the eye. Simple observation of most normal individuals confirms that the upper eyelid margin usually rests 1–2mm below the superior limbal border. The lower eyelid margin rests at the level of the inferior limbus. Elevation of the superior eyelid margin above this level or depression of the lower eyelid margin below this level is a variation from the vast majority of the population. Furthermore, retraction may be unilateral or bilateral. In most cases, this retraction manifests itself as a visible zone of sclera above or below the limbal margin.

Mild retraction of the lower eyelids may occur as a variant of eyelid position in otherwise normal individuals. Individuals with axial myopia, familial congenital shallow orbits, or maxillary hypoplasia often have modest (1–2mm) lower eyelid retraction. Involutional changes with laxity of the tarsal canthal tendons also presents with lowering of the inferior eyelid margin.

During the initial evaluation, a careful history of the presentation of retraction should be taken. The distinction between an acute and a chronic process as perceived by patients is not always helpful because it is common for them to remain unaware of long-term subtle changes in eyelid position. An extensive medical history helps to establish any further tests required to confirm a diagnosis. Particular attention should be directed to symptoms of thyroid disease. Several other rare causes are discussed in this chapter to widen the differential diagnosis for the practicing physician.

The Ophthalmic Examination

A complete periocular examination is essential to form a diagnosis. It is important to measure and document the position of the upper and lower eyelids with respect to the limbus. Other helpful measurements should include the palpebral fissure heights, the degree of lagophthalmos or lid lag on downgaze, levator muscle function, and the distances from eyelid margin to central corneal reflex; exophthalmometry can also be used. Further examination of the eyelid position should be completed in all fields of gaze and with movement of the mouth to uncover possible traumatic rectus muscle entrapment, Graves' disease, cranial nerve regeneration, jaw-winking ptosis, and Duane's syndrome. Traction on the eyelids may uncover fibrosis and scarring. Forced duction testing is helpful to diagnose the existence of fibrotic or incarcerated rectus muscles. Palpation of the globe in conjunction with exophthalmometry may be used to assess axial myopia or reveal the presence of orbital tumors. Palpation and observation of the orbital rims may expose old bone trauma or maxillary hypoplasia. Traction on the lower eyelid tissue is helpful in diagnosing involutional laxity and cicatricial changes in the anterior and posterior eyelid lamellae.

Pseudoretraction may be seen in cases of contralateral eyelid blepharoptosis with a Hering effect. In the presence of unilateral ptosis, equal central nuclear outputs to both levator muscles may result in elevation and retraction of the previously normal opposite eyelid. Pseudoretraction of the elevated eyelid is suggested when digital elevation of the more ptotic lid results in lowering of the retracted lid. Similarly, digital closure of the retracted lid results in elevation of the opposite ptotic eyelid. Examination of ocular and orbital structures may detect several other causes of the aberrant eyelid position. Buphthalmos, intraocular tumors, enlargement of the rectus muscles, or orbital tumors may present with unilateral or bilateral proptosis and eyelid retraction. Orbital apex crowding, from either a mass lesion or enlarged infiltrated rectus muscles, may result in increased intraocular pressure and abnormal visual fields. This phenomenon may also yield abnormal results for optic nerve function and optic nerve head edema or pallor on ophthalmoscopy.

Ancillary Tests

Orbital examination may be augmented by ultrasound or radiological studies such as computed tomography or magnetic resonance imaging (MRI). The latter studies are particularly helpful in the diagnosis of Graves' disease, orbital trauma, and orbital tumors. Classically, there is enlargement of the belly of the rectus muscle in Graves' disease. Enlargements of the inferior rectus muscle and medial rectus muscle are most common, although enlargement or infiltration of all rectus muscles may occur unilaterally or bilaterally. Thyroid function tests are commonly ordered in cases of upper eyelid retraction. They may not clearly rule out thyroid disease because Graves' disease can be present in euthyroid patients. Initial tests should include serum thyroxine, triiodothyronine (T_3), thyroid-stimulating hormone levels, and resin T_3 uptake. Euthyroid patients who have suspected Graves' disease may warrant further testing with antithyroglobulin and antimicrosomal antibodies. Elevated thyroid antibody titers may confirm a thyroid-related rectus muscle infiltrative process, even in the presence of normal thyroid hormone levels. If all of these tests remain normal, a thyrotropin-releasing factor test may further refine the diagnosis, although in some cases of euthyroid Graves' disease all chemical diagnostic tests are normal.

DIFFERENTIAL DIAGNOSIS

The most definitive work on the differential diagnosis and classification of eyelid retraction has been published by Bartley.[1] A schema of three main classes has been proposed, which includes neurogenic, myogenic, and mechanistic causes. As with all such classification schemata, there are limitations to accommodating so many diverse disease processes in only three or four groups.

Neurogenic Retraction

Neurogenic eyelid retraction (Box 85-1) encompasses a diverse group of diseases within which are several well-known causes, such as dorsal midbrain syndrome resulting in Collier's sign.[2–4] Other more common neurogenic causes include aberrant regeneration or innervation of the oculomotor nerve[5] and Marcus Gunn (jaw-winking) syndrome.[6–11] Orbital floor fractures may fall into both the neurogenic and mechanistic classes. In the first case, retraction is associated with increased innervation to the

superior rectus and levator muscles in an attempt to overcome mechanical restriction.[12] In the second case, retraction is caused by traction on the connective tissue sheath or a postoperative complication in the lower eyelid after repair of a blowout fracture.[13] Bartley[1] lists 39 separate causes for neurogenically induced retraction of the eyelids.

One important subgroup in this neurogenic category is the phenomenon of pseudoretraction associated with ptosis of the contralateral upper eyelid. This subgroup is significant because pseudoretraction may be seen in 66.7% of ptosis patients.[14] In these cases, Hering's law, or effect, induces an artificial elevation of the contralateral upper eyelid, often misdiagnosed in much the same manner that unilateral enophthalmos is mistaken for contralateral proptosis. Surgical correction of the ptotic eyelid frequently unmasks ptosis in the previously retracted eyelid. Pseudoretraction has also been noted in association with thyroid orbitopathy,[15] although many of these cases may be caused by levator aponeurogenic ptosis.

Myogenic Retraction

The myogenic eyelid retraction (Box 85-2) class is the smallest in the Bartley classification,[1] although it includes Graves' disease, which is undoubtedly the most common cause of true upper eyelid retraction (see Box 85-3). Controversy remains over the cause of upper eyelid retraction associated with Graves' disease. Proposed mechanisms for retraction include orbital proptosis secondary to enlargement of the rectus muscles, levator and Müller's muscle infiltration with fibrosis, excessive sympathetic innervation, abnormal adhesions between the levator and adjacent tissues, and fixation duress.[16] The last and less well-known cause occurs when fixating with an eye that has inferior rectus muscle restriction. The result is excessive stimulation of the ipsilateral superior rectus levator complex.[17,18] Thickening of the levator muscle seen on T1-weighted sagittal MRI in patients with Graves' disease is closely associated with upper eyelid retraction, which has also been suggested as a causative factor for retraction.[19]

Other important entrants in the myogenic subgroup are myasthenia gravis, botulinum toxin injection, and postsurgical complications of vertical rectus muscle recessions, ptosis overcorrection, and defects following enucleation. Myasthenia gravis is known more as a cause of myogenic ptosis than of eyelid retraction; however, one study showed that 4 of 150 patients with

---

BOX 85-1

Neurogenic Causes of Eyelid Retraction

- Benign transient conjugate downward gaze in preterm infants
- "Eye-popping" reflex in infants
- Dorsal midbrain; Parinaud's syndrome; sylvian aqueduct syndrome (Koerber-Salus-Elschnig syndrome)
- Pinealoma
- Hydrocephalus
- Subthalamic or midbrain arteriovenous malformations
- Basilar artery disease
- Thalamic–mesencephalic infarction
- Unilateral lesion of nucleus of posterior commissure
- Disseminated sclerosis
- Bulbar poliomyelitis
- Encephalitis
- Tertiary syphilis
- Closed head injury
- Impending tentorial herniation
- Guillain-Barré syndrome
- Epilepsy
- Oculogyric crisis
- Palatal myoclonus
- Eyelid nystagmus
- Lateral medullary syndrome

- Cerebellar disease
- Postencephalitic parkinsonism
- Progressive supranuclear palsy
- Lesion of nondominant cerebral hemisphere
- "Levator spasticity" or failure of inhibition during coma ("coma vigil")
- Marcus Gunn (jaw-winking) syndrome (trigemino-oculomotor synkinesis)
- Seesaw jaw-winking
- Horizontal gaze palsy (congenital or acquired)
- Aberrant innervation or regeneration of the oculomotor nerve (congenital or acquired)
- Cyclic oculomotor paralysis
- Partial palsy of superior rectus muscle
- Esotropia, dissociated vertical deviation, latent nystagmus
- Sympathetic irritation (Horner-Bernard syndrome)
- Pseudoretraction associated with contralateral blepharoptosis
- Weakness of orbicularis oculi (e.g., facial nerve paralysis)
- Orbital floor ("blowout") fracture (globe hypertropia; increased innervation to superior rectus and levator muscles)
- Sympathomimetic eyedrops (phenylephrine, apraclonidine)
- Volitional

From Conway ST. Lid retraction following blow-out fracture of the orbit. *Ophthalmic Surg.* 1988;19:279–81.

this disease had eyelid retraction.[20] This phenomenon may be truly pseudoretraction rather than an intrinsic problem associated with myasthenia gravis. Botulinum toxin injection is most likely to result in lower eyelid retraction secondary to loss of orbicularis oculi muscle tone. The postsurgical complications in general have obvious causes, with correction by partial reversal of the initial surgery.

Mechanistic Retraction

The last major classification, referred to as mechanistic (Box 85-3), comprises a vast array of causes primarily related to architectural changes in the eyelid structure. This is also probably the major cause of Graves' eyelid retraction. These changes may be congenital, cicatricial, traumatic, neoplastic, or postoperative. In theory, diagnosis in this category is simpler than in the categories of neurogenic and myogenic causes. Most diagnoses are straightforward and based on obvious morphological changes in the patient, such as craniosynostosis. Consequently, repair of the anatomic defect should in many cases correct the eyelid malposition.

Miscellaneous Causes of Retraction

A miscellaneous category (Box 85-4) has also been developed for cases in which eyelid retraction is reported but no clear explanation of cause and effect can be determined.

BOX 85-2

Myogenic Causes of Eyelid Retraction

- Congenital upper or lower eyelid retraction
- Congenital hyperthyroidism
- Congenital, paradoxical lower eyelid retraction on upgaze
- Congenital myotonia; myotonic dystrophy
- Graves' ophthalmopathy
- Hypokalemic/hyperkalemic familial periodic paralysis
- Myasthenia gravis
- Botulinum toxin injection
- Postsurgical: inferior rectus recession (lower eyelid); superior rectus recession (upper eyelid); blepharoptosis repair; enucleation

From Conway ST. Lid retraction following blow-out fracture of the orbit. Ophthalmic Surg. 1988;19:279–81.

BOX 85-3

Mechanistic Causes of Eyelid Retraction

- Congenital horizontal tarsal kink
- Severe myopia
- Buphthalmos
- Proptosis; orbital; mass idiopathic
- Graves' ophthalmopathy
- Cherubism
- Craniosynostosis
- Paget's disease of bone
- Eyelid neoplasms
- Herpes zoster ophthalmicus
- Smallpox
- Atopic dermatitis
- Scleroderma
- Burns: thermal, chemical
- Orbital floor ("blowout") fracture (upper lid retracted from traction on connective tissue sheath)
- Lax socket syndrome
- Contact lens wearer
- Embedded hard contact lens in upper eyelid

- Hemangioma of orbit (ascribed to fibrosis of levator)
- Silent sinus syndrome
- After irradiation of orbit or sinus
- Postoperative:
  - scleral buckle
  - osteoplastic frontal sinusotomy
  - blepharoplasty
  - orbicularis myectomy
  - glaucoma filtering operation with prominent bleb
  - extracapsular cataract extraction
  - orbital floor ("blowout") fracture repair or orbitotomy (lower eyelid)
  - maxillectomy cheek flap

From Conway ST. Lid retraction following blow-out fracture of the orbit. Ophthalmic Surg. 1988;19:279–81.

ALTERNATIVES TO SURGERY

Eyelid retraction may be related to systemic disease, such as Guillain-Barré syndrome or myasthenia gravis, in which case it should be treated using systemic medication if appropriate. Other cases may respond to topical treatments, such as corticosteroid ointment for atopic dermatitis. Discontinuation of topical drops, such as apraclonidine, may also resolve drug-induced retraction. Eyelid retraction associated with Graves' disease may show some improvement following high-dose oral corticosteroids or radiotherapy used in the treatment of compressive optic neuropathy or severe orbital congestion.

ANESTHESIA

As with all surgery involving alterations in upper eyelid position, it is best to perform corrections of eyelid retraction under local anesthesia whenever possible. This allows more precise adjustment of eyelid height. The use of epinephrine (adrenaline) in the local anesthetic mixture stimulates Müller's sympathetic muscle; if this muscle is left intact, some compensation should be allowed for the loss of Müller's tone following the procedure.

SURGICAL TECHNIQUES

Surgical management of eyelid retraction can be separated into direct and indirect approaches. The direct method specifically addresses abnormalities of eyelid tissue. This approach can be further divided into treatment of upper eyelid and that of lower eyelid retraction. The indirect approach addresses a fundamental architectural abnormality of the orbit responsible for the retraction, such as seen in Paget's disease of bone or in craniosynostosis. Other indirect surgical treatment may involve excision of orbital neoplastic processes responsible for proptosis and subsequent eyelid retraction.

Levator Aponeurosis Recession with Excision of Müller's Muscle

The aponeurotic approach to this surgery begins with marking the appropriate eyelid crease. The skin beneath the crease is infiltrated with a small amount of local anesthetic, such as 2% lidocaine (lignocaine) with epinephrine 1:100,000. After adequate anesthesia is achieved, the crease is incised and dissection continues through the orbicularis oculi muscle to the septum. The septum is identified and incised 1–2mm above its insertion into the aponeurosis. Orbital fat can be gently pushed superiorly with cotton-tipped applicators. The inferior attachments of the aponeurosis are freed from the superior border of the tarsus. Dissection under the aponeurosis and above Müller's muscle is continued up to Whitnall's ligament. A small amount of local anesthetic can be injected into Müller's muscle at this time. Müller's muscle is excised from the superior border of the tarsus up to the level of Whitnall's ligament.

The patient's corneal shield is removed, and the patient is elevated to a sitting position. The position of the eyelid relative to

---

BOX 85-4

Miscellaneous Causes of Eyelid Retraction

- Optic nerve hypoplasia
- Microphthalmos
- Down syndrome
- Essential hypertension
- Hepatic cirrhosis
- Meningitis
- Sphenoid wing meningioma
- Lymphoma in superior cul-de-sac

From Conway ST. Lid retraction following blowout fracture of the orbit. Ophthalmic Surg. 1988;19:279–81.

the superior limbus is evaluated. The lid should be ptotic, and the procedure now becomes a ptosis repair. The aponeurosis may be advanced to tarsus or sutured directly to conjunctiva so that the eyelid margin lies at the appropriate height. In the case of conjunctival sutures, there is a risk of corneal abrasion. Attention is directed toward correcting any medial or lateral flare by severing attachments of the medial and lateral horns of the levator. Tightening the attachment of the superior lateral canthal tendon also improves lateral scleral flare or exposure. Placement of a Frost suture at the completion of the procedure may assist in prevention of short-term recurrence of retraction.

Placement of spacers to lengthen the upper eyelid has been recommended, most commonly contralateral tarsus and autologous sclera.[21,22] However, this has not met with the same success as their use to raise the lower eyelid position. The primary problem associated with spacers in the upper eyelid is the obvious increased risk of corneal irritation and abrasion. Mourits and Koornneef[22] reported a series of 62 consecutive patients in whom sclera was used as a spacer. In this series only 50% of patients had an acceptable result after one operation. The main complications were persistent temporal retraction and nasal overcorrection. Mourits and Koornneef[22] concluded that no distinct advantages could be found in the use of sclera as an upper eyelid spacer over other standard lengthening techniques.

Lower Eyelid Recession with Spacer Graft

In some cases of involutional or cicatricial lower eyelid retraction, repair of canthal tendon laxity and anterior lamellar contraction needs to be addressed. Lateral canthal tendon support can be augmented by several surgical procedures, including the lateral tarsal strip or sling.[23,24] Anterior lamellar augmentation is performed with split- and full-thickness skin grafts as well as orbicularis oculi muscle transposition. However, in the presence of proptosis, the primary emphasis in treating lower lid retraction is to place a spacer in the posterior lamella to lengthen the retractors and give eyelid support. Numerous materials have been utilized for this purpose, including auricular cartilage,[25–28] nasal septal cartilage,[29] autologous sclera,[30–32] costochondral cartilage,[32] fascia lata,[33–35] autogenous tarsus,[36] and hard palate.[36]

There are advantages and disadvantages to the harvesting and usage of each of these tissues. Cartilage, whether from the ear or the nasal septum, is relatively easy to harvest. The most significant limitation to cartilage in lower eyelid reconstruction is its lack of pliability, which can produce disfiguring contour abnormalities. Sclera is readily available through the eye bank, but unpredictable rates of shrinkage limit its value as a lower eyelid spacer. Reoperation for recurrent eyelid retraction is consequently higher when sclera is used. Costochondral cartilage is more difficult to obtain than other grafts. Fascia lata is available as autologous tissue but lacks the rigidity necessary for lower eyelid support. Autologous tarsus is an excellent spacer but is available in rather limited quantities because excessive harvest of upper eyelid tarsus may distort the position of the donor eyelid. Hard palate mucosa provides one of the optimal spacers for several reasons. The tissue is easily harvested and is available in adequate quantities for most cases of lower eyelid retraction. This tissue is rigid enough to support elevation of the inferior tarsus and pliable enough to avoid contour abnormalities.

Hard palate mucosal grafts are harvested by first infiltrating local anesthetic into the hard palate in the posterior region of the transverse palatine folds and adjacent to the palatine raphe. Excision of the graft, which includes mucosa, submucosa, and a small amount of fat, is completed with straight and angled surgical blades. A No. 66 Beaver blade is very helpful in this excision. Gentle cautery is used in the graft bed. The surgeon should be careful to avoid injury to the anterior palatine artery as continued postoperative bleeding can occur. The mucosal graft can vary in height and width with an average graft size of about 5mm by 20mm. The graft bed may be left to heal without treat-

ment or packed and covered with a custom-molded dental plate. The latter apparatus adds time and cost to the procedure and may not completely resolve the postoperative pain associated with surgery on the palate.

More recently, a high-density porous polyethylene graft has become available for lower eyelid retraction. It is easily inserted through a small lateral eyelid incision and placed into a pocket between the orbiculans muscle and orbital septum. Although long-term results are not yet available, early indications suggest that this may be a useful procedure.

Placement of the graft requires an incision into the lower eyelid just below the tarsal border. The graft is trimmed to the appropriate thickness, removing excess fat or submucosa. Suturing the graft is completed by running a dissolvable suture, such as plain gut, and burying the knots. Frequently, this surgery is done in conjunction with a lateral canthal tightening procedure.

COMPLICATIONS

The most common complications of surgery for eyelid retraction are undercorrection and overcorrection. The postoperative eyelid position can be highly variable despite a surgeon's best efforts and careful preoperative and intraoperative assessments. Continued flare of the lateral upper eyelid may not be so much a complication as an incomplete treatment of this problem. However, both the patient and the surgeon may see this as a less than optimal result. Lower lid elevation can be limited by the height of the spacer, and in most cases only a finite amount of spacer is available from any one source. Postoperative shrinkage of a spacer such as sclera is well known and unpredictable, potentially resulting in recurrence of the retraction. Also, some spacers such as nasal or auricular cartilage are difficult to contour and can lead to a bulky lower lid appearance. Spacers in either the upper or lower eyelid can cause epithelial erosion of the corneal surface.

OUTCOMES

In the majority of cases, the eyelid can be restored to a normal position and results in better protection of the cornea. In patients with Graves' disease, recession can also mask some degree of proptosis.

REFERENCES

1. Bartley GB. The differential diagnosis and classification of eyelid retraction. Ophthalmology. 1996;103:168–76.
2. Collier J. Nuclear ophthalmoplegia, with especial reference to retraction of lids and ptosis and to lesions of posterior commissure. Brain. 1927;5:488–98.
3. Francois MJ. L'hypertonie unilatérale du releveur de la paupiere supérieur dans le syndrome de Basedow. Bull Soc Belge Ophthalmol. 1951;97:138–60.
4. Burde RM, Savino PJ, Trobe JD. Clinical decisions in neuro-ophthalmology. St. Louis: Mosby; 1985:257–9.
5. Stout AU, Borchert M. Etiology of eyelid retraction in children: a retrospective study. J Pediatr Ophthalmol Strabismus. 1993;30:96–9.
6. Gunn RM. Congenital ptosis with peculiar associated movements of the affected lid. Trans Ophthalmol Soc UK. 1883:3:283–7.
7. Parry R. An unusual case of the Marcus Gunn syndrome. Trans Ophthalmol Soc UK. 1957;77:181–5.
8. Sano K. Trigemino-oculomotor synkineses. Neurologia. 1959;1:29–51.
9. Kirkham TH. Familial Marcus Gunn phenomenon. Br J Ophthalmol. 1969; 53:282–3.
10. Kirkham TH. Paradoxical elevation of eyelid on smiling. Am J Ophthalmol. 1971; 72:207–8.
11. Pratt SG, Beyer CK, Johnson CC. The Marcus Gunn phenomenon. A review of 71 cases. Ophthalmology. 1984;91:27–30.
12. Putterman AM, Urist MJ. Upper eyelid retraction after blowout fractures. Arch Ophthalmol. 1976;94:112–16.
13. Conway ST. Lid retraction following blow-out fracture of the orbit. Ophthalmic Surg. 1988;19:279–81.
14. Kratky V, Harvey JT. Tests for contralateral pseudoretraction in blepharoptosis. Ophthalm Reconstr Surg. 1992;8:22–5.
15. Gonnering RS. Pseudoretraction of the eyelid in thyroid-associated orbitopathy. Arch Ophthalmol. 1988;106:1078–80.
16. Hamed LM, Lessner AM. Fixation duress in the pathogenesis of upper eyelid retraction in thyroid orbitopathy. A prospective study. Ophthalmology. 1994; 101:608–11.
17. Wesley RE, Bond JB. Upper eyelid retraction from inferior rectus restriction in dysthyroid orbit disease. Ann Ophthalmol. 1987;19:34–6.

18. Ohnishi T, Noguchi 5, Murakami N, *et al.* Levator palpebrae superioris muscle: MR evaluation of enlargement as a cause of upper eyelid retraction in Graves' disease. Radiology. 1993;188:115–18.

19. Kansu T, Subutay N. Lid retraction in myasthenia gravis. J Clin Neuroophthalmol. 1987;7:145–8.

20. Stout AU, Borchert M. Etiology of eyelid retraction in children: a retrospective study. J Pediatr Ophthalmol Strabismus. 1993;30:96–9.

21. Crawford JS, Easterbrook M. The use of bank sclera to correct lid retraction. Can J Ophthalmol. 1976;11:309–22.

22. Mourits MP, Koornneef L. Lid lengthening by sclera interposition for eyelid retraction in Graves' ophthalmopathy. Br J Ophthalmol. 1991;75:344–7.

23. Anderson RL, Gordy DD. The tarsal strip procedure. Arch Ophthalmol. 1979;97:2192–6.

24. Tenzel RR, Buffam FV, Miller GR. The use of the 'lateral canthal sling' in ectropion repair. Can J Ophthalmol. 1977;12:199–202.

25. Baylis HI, Rosen N, Neuhaus RW. Obtaining auricular cartilage for reconstructive surgery. Am J Ophthalmol. 1982;93:709–12.

26. Marks MW, Argenta LC, Friedman RJ, Hall JD. Conchal cartilage and composite grafts for correction of lower lid retraction. Plast Reconstr Surg. 1989;33:629–35.

27. Jackson IT, Dubin B, Harris J. Use of contoured and stabilized conchal cartilage grafts for lower eyelid support: a preliminary report. Plast Reconstr Surg. 1989;83:636–40.

28. Mustarde JC. Problems in eyelid reconstruction. Ann Ophthalmol. 1972;4:883–901.

29. Flanagan JC. Eye bank sclera in oculoplastic surgery. Ophthalmic Surg. 1974;5:45–53.

30. Waller RR. Lower eyelid retraction: management. Ophthalmic Surg. 1978;9:41–7.

31. Hurwitz JJ, Archer KF, Gruss JS. Treatment of severe lower eyelid retraction with scleral and free skin grafts and bipedicle orbicularis flap. Ophthalmic Surg. 1991;2:167–72.

32. Mehrota ON. Repairing defects of the lower eyelid with a free chondromucosal graft. Plast Reconstr Surg. 1977;59:689–93.

33. Beyer CK, Albert DM. The use and fate of fascia lata and sclera in ophthalmic plastic and reconstructive surgery. Ophthalmology. 1981;88:869–86.

34. Flanagan JC, Campbell CB. The use of autogenous fascia lata to correct lid and orbital deformities. Trans Am Ophthalmol Soc. 1981;79:227–42.

35. Gardner TA, Kennerdell JS, Buerger GF. Treatment of dysthyroid lower lid retraction with autogenous tarsus transplants. Ophthalmol Plast Reconstr Surg. 1992;8:26–31.

36. Patipa M, Patek BCK, McLeish W, Anderson RL. Use of hard palate grafts for treatment of postsurgical lower eyelid retraction: a technical overview. J Craniomaxillofac Traumatol. 1996;2:18–28.

CHAPTER

86 Blepharoptosis

PHILIP L. CUSTER

DEFINITION
- An abnormally low position of the upper eyelid margin, determined while the eye is looking in primary gaze.

KEY FEATURES
- Blepharoptosis (ptosis) may result from trauma, masses, and congenital or acquired abnormalities of the levator or Müller neuromuscular complexes.
- May present with various symptoms, including visual field obstruction, headache, and fatigue.
- Surgery is considered in patients who are symptomatic or displeased with the appearance of their eyelid.
- The goal of ptosis repair is to elevate the eyelid without causing excessive lagophthalmos or ocular exposure.

INTRODUCTION

Blepharoptosis was initially repaired by excising upper eyelid skin, essentially suspending the eyelid from the brow. The frontalis suspension was popularized in the 19th century, when a variety of subcutaneous implants were used to create a direct connection between the eyelid and forehead. Motais[1] and Parinaud[2] introduced the superior rectus suspension in 1897. A portion of the superior rectus muscle was transposed and attached to the eyelid. Enthusiasm for this procedure declined as patients developed late complications from the resultant lagophthalmos.

Bowman (1857) first described shortening of the levator–Müller's muscle complex through a conjunctival incision.[3] Anterior levator resection was subsequently reported in 1883 by Eversbusch and Snellen.[4,5] In 1975, Jones et al.[6] published the successful repair of acquired ptosis by levator aponeurotic reattachment or resection.

Modern physicians use a variety of procedures, depending upon the levator muscle function. Patients with poor levator function usually require frontalis suspension. Anterior levator aponeurotic resection or posterior müllerectomy is often used in patients who have good levator activity.

PREOPERATIVE EVALUATION AND DIAGNOSTIC APPROACH

The Ocular and Medical History

The initial evaluation is directed toward determining the cause of the ptosis. The history should ascertain the onset, duration, severity, and variability of the condition. Reviewing old photographs is helpful in documenting the progression of the disorder. There may be a positive family history in some forms of hereditary ptosis. Prior ocular trauma, surgery, or disease can contribute to the development of ptosis or alter the treatment plan. Ptosis repair is considered with caution in patients who have symptoms of ocular irritation, dryness, photophobia, or diplopia. True eyelid pto-

sis must be differentiated from the various causes of pseudoptosis including dermatochalasis, contralateral eyelid retraction, enophthalmos, and hypotropia.

Concomitant ocular signs are helpful in making a diagnosis. Ipsilateral miosis is suggestive of Horner's syndrome, and mydriasis is found in cases of oculomotor paralysis. Patients who have surgically or traumatically enlarged pupils often experience photophobia, a symptom that can be exacerbated by ptosis surgery. Ocular inflammation or dryness may cause reactive ptosis. These conditions must be corrected before considering ptosis repair. A basic tear secretory rate is obtained in adult patients. Surgery is often limited or avoided in patients with dry eyes.

Preoperative photographs document the severity of ptosis. Visual fields with and without elevation of the drooping eyelids determine the degree of visual obstruction. Additional diagnostic studies, such as orbital imaging or neuromuscular testing, are indicated when clinical examination fails to determine the cause of the ptosis.

Hering's Law

The levator muscles obey Hering's law of equal innervation.[7] These muscles are innervated from a single midline nucleus, resulting in equal central neural output. In cases of bilateral asymmetrical ptosis, the less affected eyelid may maintain a normal level of elevation due to excessive innervational stimulation determined by the more ptotic eyelid. This condition can be detected prior to surgery by manually elevating the ptotic eyelid. An immediate fall of the contralateral eyelid confirms the presence of bilateral, asymmetrical ptosis masked by levator "overaction."[8]

Levator Muscle Function

Levator function is indirectly measured by determining the excursion of the eyelid margin as the patient looks from downgaze to upgaze. The eyebrow is manually fixed against the supraorbital rim during this measurement, preventing the frontalis muscle from contributing to eyelid movement. Many patients subconsciously raise their eyebrow in a compensatory effort to elevate the drooping lid, a beneficial finding in individuals requiring frontalis suspension. Normal adults typically demonstrate 13–16mm of levator function.[9] Lesser measurements may indicate the presence of a developmental or acquired myopathy.

Other Measurements

The upper eyelid margin is normally positioned 1–2mm below the superior limbus. The location of the lid margin is measured with the patient looking in primary gaze. This may be recorded as the position (in millimeters) of the eyelid margin with respect to the pupillary light reflex (margin-to-reflex distance or MRD).

The amount of redundant skin (dermatochalasis) and the position of the upper eyelid creases are recorded. Ocular motility is assessed. Coexisting strabismus may be present in cases of congenital ptosis, acquired neurological or myopathic disease, and

Differential Diagnosis of Upper Eyelid Blepharoptosis

CONGENITAL PTOSIS
Myopathic ptosis
Blepharophimosis syndrome
Marcus Gunn's jaw-winking syndrome

ACQUIRED PTOSIS
Third nerve palsy
Horner's syndrome
Myasthenia gravis
Chronic progressive external ophthalmoplegia
Aponeurotic ptosis
Mechanical ptosis

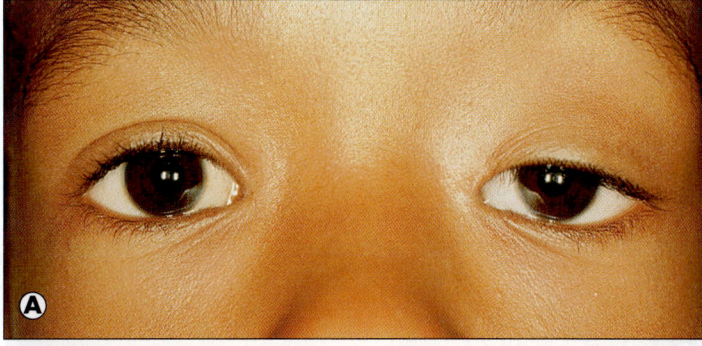

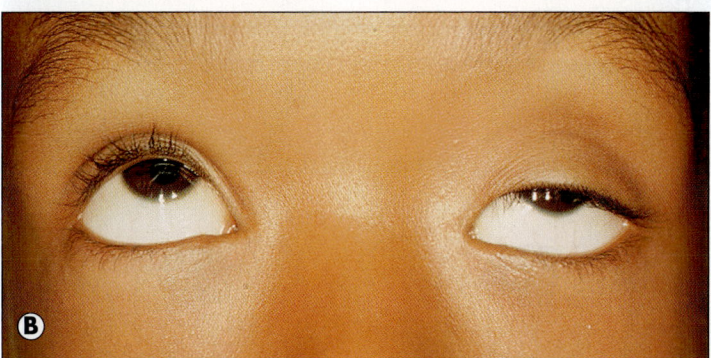

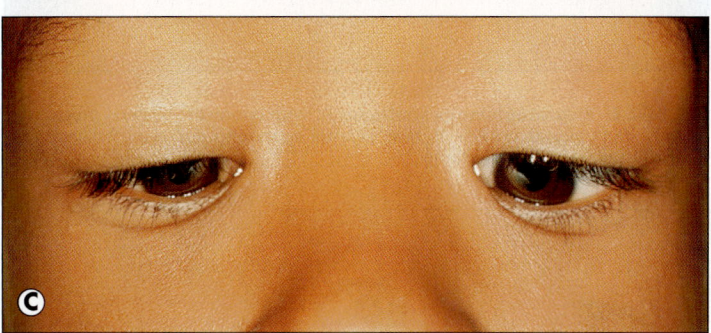

orbital masses. Ptosis patients who have hypotropia typically have a component of pseudoptosis. In patients who have reduced or absent Bell's phenomenon, ptosis repair should be conservative to avoid postoperative exposure.

DIFFERENTIAL DIAGNOSIS

Blepharoptosis may be categorized by age of onset (congenital vs. acquired), severity, and physiological etiology. The differential diagnosis of blepharoptosis is shown in Box 86-1.

Congenital Ptosis

SIMPLE CONGENITAL (MYOPATHIC) PTOSIS. The majority of children with congenital ptosis have a *developmental myopathy of the levator muscle.* The ptosis is present at birth and remains stable throughout life. Levator function is decreased in proportion to the severity of the ptosis. The fibrotic levator muscle limits inferior mobility of the eyelid, causing less ptosis in downgaze (Fig. 86-1). The upper eyelid crease is usually indistinct or absent. Compensatory elevation of the eyebrows or a chin-elevated head position is often present.

Simple congenital ptosis is unilateral in 69% of cases.[10] Bilateral involvement may be symmetrical or asymmetrical in appearance. Coexisting strabismus is present in approximately 30% of children.[11-13] Hypotropia is common, a possible manifestation of developmental failure affecting both the superior rectus and levator muscles.[14] Anisometropia is present in 12% of patients with simple congenital ptosis.[15,16] Strabismus and anisometropia may lead to amblyopia, which is found in 20% of patients who have simple congenital ptosis.[17] Occlusion amblyopia is less common and should be considered a diagnosis of exclusion. Early surgery is indicated in cases with obstruction of the visual axis. Treatment is otherwise delayed until the late preschool years.

Children who have good levator function are effectively repaired with anterior levator aponeurotic-muscle resection, whereas children with severe ptosis and poor function often require frontalis suspension. Treatment of severe unilateral congenital ptosis is challenging. Unilateral frontalis suspension may be considered in children who have compensatory elevation of the eyebrow. Maximal levator resection can also be used, although this procedure can be complicated by postoperative lagophthalmos. Bilateral frontalis suspension combined with ablation of the uninvolved levator muscle provides symmetrical eyelid appearance and function. However, many parents are hesitant to consider surgery on the normal eyelid.

BLEPHAROPHIMOSIS SYNDROME. Approximately 6% of children with congenital ptosis demonstrate the typical findings of blepharophimosis syndrome.[10] There is severe bilateral ptosis with poor levator function. The palpebral fissures are horizontally shortened (blepharophimosis) with resultant telecanthus (Fig. 86-2). True hypertelorism is occasionally present.[18]

FIG. 86-1 ■ Simple congenital ptosis. **A,** Decreased levator muscle function occurs along with an indistinct upper eyelid crease. **B,** The ptosis is exaggerated in upgaze due to the poor function of the levator muscle. **C,** In downgaze, the ptosis is reduced or absent because the fibrotic levator muscle cannot stretch.

Epicanthus inversus is another common finding. Mild ectropion of the temporal lower eyelids is seen in severe cases. The inferior puncta often are displaced laterally and the eyebrows may be abnormally wide. Some patients demonstrate low-set, "lop" ears.

Blepharophimosis is a dominantly inherited condition, although the severity of findings varies among affected family members.[19] Sporadic cases also occur. Blepharophimosis is associated with primary amenorrhea in some family lines.[20]

Treatment of blepharophimosis usually requires a staged approach. The telecanthus and epicanthal folds are initially repaired with medial canthal tendon plication and local skin flaps.[18,21] Bilateral frontalis suspension is subsequently performed. Skin grafting may be necessary to relieve coexisting lower eyelid ectropion.

MARCUS GUNN'S JAW-WINKING SYNDROME. The jaw-winking syndrome was initially described by Marcus Gunn in 1883.[22] This form of synkinetic ptosis is typically unilateral and not hereditary. There is intermittent elevation of the ptotic eyelid, coinciding with contraction of the muscles of mastication, resulting in a "winking" movement during eating or chewing (Fig. 86-3). The synkinesis commonly involves the ipsilateral external pterygoid muscle, which moves the jaw toward the opposite side. The severity of the ptosis and the amplitude of the wink are proportionally related. Measurable levator function is variable or decreased. The upper eyelid crease is usually intact. Hypotropia and other forms of strabismus may be seen in the jaw-winking syndrome.[23]

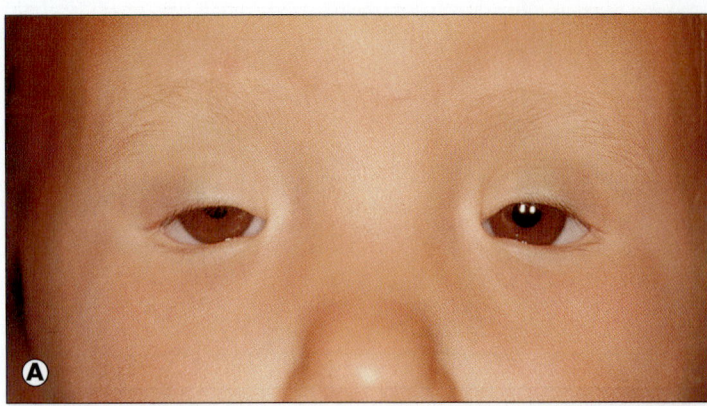

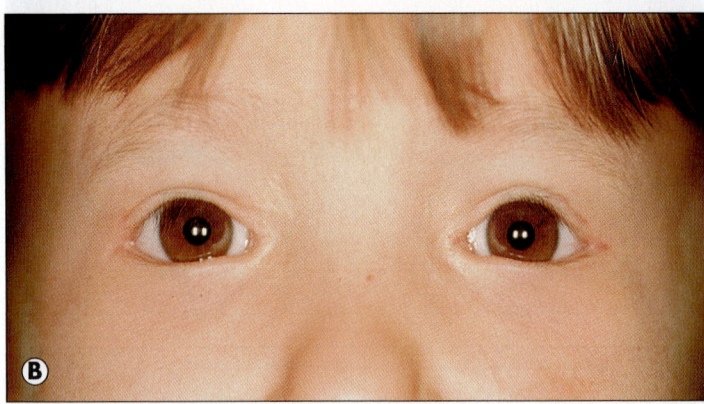

FIG. 86-2 ▮▮ **Blepharophimosis syndrome. A,** With symmetric bilateral ptosis, tele-canthus, and epicanthal folds. **B,** Postoperative appearance following bilateral can-thoplasty and frontalis suspension.

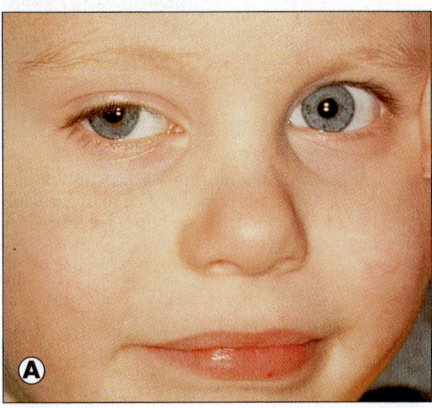

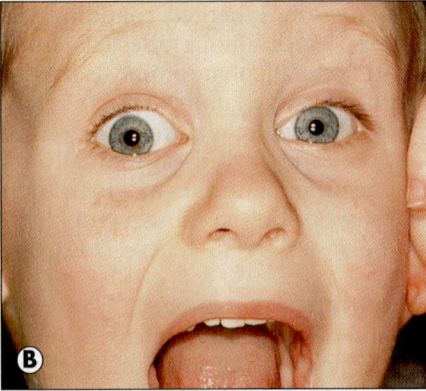

FIG. 86-3 ▮▮ **Marcus Gunn's jaw-winking syndrome. A,** In primary gaze with the mouth closed, there is right upper eyelid ptosis. **B,** With the jaw opened the right upper eyelid elevates due to synkinesis.

The cause of this condition is unknown, although there appears to be misdirection of either the efferent motor innervation or afferent proprioceptive fibers of the third and fifth cranial nerves.[24,25] The wink often becomes less noticeable with age, as patients learn to limit oral movements that stimulate the synkinesis.[26] Mild cases can be treated with levator aponeurotic-muscle resection. Patients with large-amplitude winking may require ablation of the levator, followed by frontalis suspension.[27]

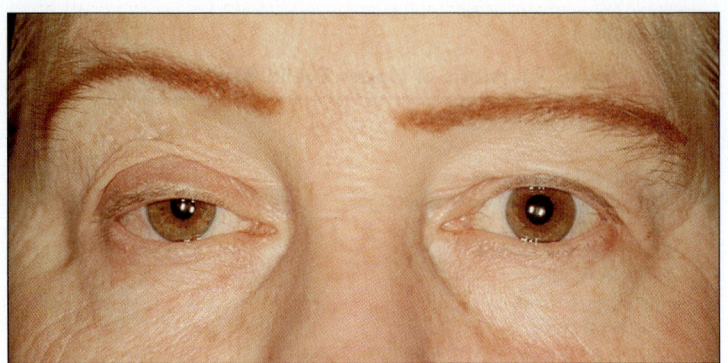

FIG. 86-4 ▮▮ Horner's syndrome with ipsilateral right upper eyelid ptosis and pupillary miosis.

Acquired Ptosis

THIRD CRANIAL NERVE PALSY. The levator muscle is innervated by the superior division of the third cranial nerve. The levator subnucleus is central and unpaired. Intranuclear lesions thus result in symmetrical, bilateral ptosis. Peripheral third nerve deficits are much more common and are often caused by trauma, ischemia (microvascular disease), inflammation, neoplasm, and aneurysms. Ptosis with decreased or absent levator function, mydriasis, and strabismus typically are present. Spontaneous recovery may occur, although a partial deficit often remains. Aberrant regeneration is frequent and occasionally results in gaze-directed eyelid retraction.

Repair of paralytic ptosis usually requires frontalis suspension. Surgery is delayed until it is certain that spontaneous recovery will not occur (6–12 months).[28] Coexisting strabismus is corrected prior to ptosis repair; otherwise eyelid elevation may result in intractable diplopia.

HORNER'S SYNDROME. Müller's muscle is sympathetically innervated and provides several millimeters of eyelid elevation. Sympathetic denervation (Horner's syndrome) results in moderate ptosis with preserved levator function (see Fig. 86-4). Weakness of the inferior tarsal muscle elevates the lower eyelid, contributing to a narrowed palpebral fissure. Ipsilateral miosis is uniformly present. Many patients also experience hemifacial anhidrosis. Heterochromia can be seen in patients who have congenital Horner's syndrome.[29] The ipsilateral iris is lighter in color.

Pharmacological (cocaine) testing confirms the diagnosis of this condition. The neurological deficit may result from ischemia, trauma, neoplasm, or iatrogenic insults. A medical evaluation is indicated in patients who have newly diagnosed Horner's syndrome of unknown causes. Surgical correction is indicated in patients who have significant, persistent ptosis. External levator aponeurotic-muscle resection and posterior müllerectomy are effective methods of repair.

MYASTHENIA GRAVIS. Ptosis and diplopia are presenting symptoms in about one half of patients who have myasthenia and subsequently appear in 96% of individuals with this condition.[30] The ptosis may be unilateral, bilateral, or alternating. Levator function is either decreased or variable. There is rapid fatigability of the affected levator muscle. The eyelid twitches or slowly falls with prolonged upgaze.[31] This finding is distinct from the increased ptosis associated with systemic fatigue, suffered by all ptosis patients, irrespective of cause. A minority of myasthenic patients have a purely ocular form of the disease; the majority develop systemic involvement.[32,33]

This autoimmunological condition affects the neuromuscular junction and has a predilection for muscles innervated by the cranial nerves. Antibodies to acetylcholine receptor protein are present in most patients with systemic disease.[32] The history and clinical findings usually lead the clinician to the diagnosis, which is confirmed by Tensilon testing, electrophysiological studies, or acetylcholine receptor antibody levels (Fig. 86-5). Myasthenia is treated medically. Selected patients may benefit

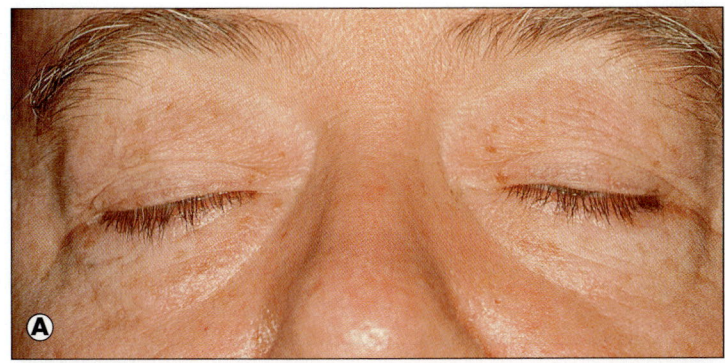

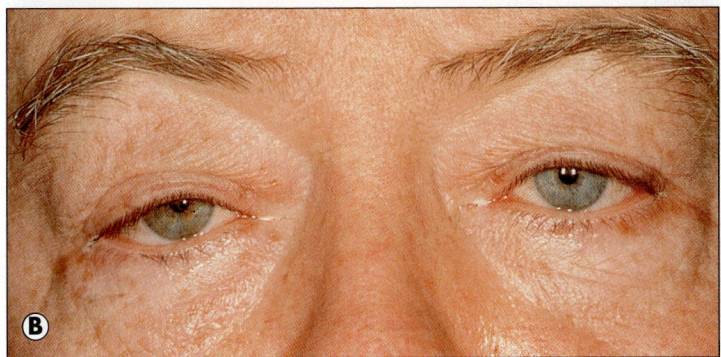

FIG. 86-5 ■ Myasthenia gravis with severe bilateral ptosis. A, Before treatment. B, The same patient after administration of intravenous Tensilon.

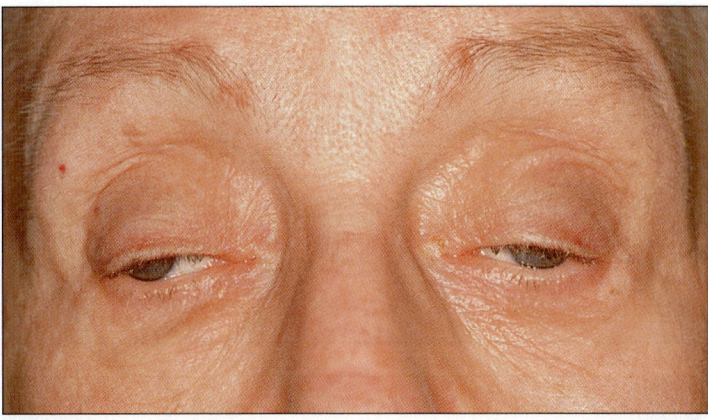

FIG. 86-6 ■ Chronic progressive external ophthalmoplegia (CPEO) with bilateral ptosis and ocular motility abnormality.

from thymectomy.[33] Ptosis repair is reserved for individuals with refractory, visually debilitating disease. Limited frontalis suspension is usually performed. Myasthenia patients are at increased risk for developing postoperative ocular exposure from coexisting orbicularis muscle weakness or a poor Bell's phenomenon.

CHRONIC PROGRESSIVE EXTERNAL OPHTHALMOPLEGIA. Chronic progressive external ophthalmoplegia (CPEO) includes a group of conditions that are either hereditary or sporadic in nature. Most patients present with symmetrical, bilateral ptosis in early adulthood (Fig. 86-6). The mitochondrial myopathy results in decreased levator function. Extraocular muscles are affected later, resulting in diffuse ophthalmoplegia. Associated systemic findings are present in some forms of this disease, including cardiac conduction defects (Kearns-Sayre syndrome) and dysphagia (oculopharyngeal dystrophy).[34-36]

Muscle biopsy may be necessary to confirm the diagnosis of CPEO. Ptosis repair is delayed until the patient is visually debilitated. Limited frontalis suspension is often the procedure of choice, avoiding postoperative lagophthalmos and resultant ocular exposure.

APONEUROTIC REDUNDANCY OR DEHISCENCE. Most patients who have acquired ptosis develop the condition secondary to involutional changes in the levator aponeurosis. Gradual stretching or dehiscence of this structure causes slowly progressive ptosis. Chronic contact lens wearers may also develop ptosis on this basis. Aponeurotic dehiscence may occur following ocular surgery or trauma. Ptosis develops in approximately 6% of patients following cataract surgery.[37]

Levator function is not reduced in this form of ptosis. Loss of the aponeurotic attachment results in an abnormally high or indistinct upper eyelid crease (Fig. 86-7). The superior sulcus deepens and the upper eyelid may appear to be unusually thin, occasionally allowing visualization of the iris through the eyelid tissue. Surgical repair of the aponeurosis through an anterior approach corrects the ptosis.

MECHANICAL PTOSIS. Mechanical ptosis develops from cicatricial processes, tumors, or enophthalmos. Scarring involving any of the anatomic layers of the upper eyelid or symblepharon between the lid and globe may limit eyelid mobility and cause ptosis. Encapsulated orbital lesions may alter levator function

secondary to a mass effect, and infiltrative conditions restrict muscle activity. The relative severity of mechanical ptosis often varies in different gaze positions. Effective treatment of mechanical ptosis requires correction of the underlying abnormality.

PTOSIS REPAIR

Ptosis repair is an elective procedure. Surgery should be avoided or limited in individuals who have preexisting ocular irritation or photophobia. Patients who have poor tear production can develop symptomatic dryness following eyelid elevation. Ptosis repair in a patient who has an enlarged pupil or sector iridectomy may cause intractable light sensitivity. Individuals who have poor Bell's phenomena are at an increased risk for exposure keratitis should there be postoperative lagophthalmos. Limited surgery can be performed should these patients develop visually debilitating ptosis. Nonsurgical elevation of the eyelid with a ptosis crutch attached to the spectacle frame is occasionally helpful, although these devices often limit blinking, resulting in ocular irritation.

ANESTHESIA

Ideally, ptosis repair is performed with local anesthesia. An alert patient facilitates the intraoperative adjustment of the eyelid. Subcutaneous injection of a mixture of 2% lidocaine (lignocaine) with 1:200,000 epinephrine (adrenaline) and 0.75% bupivacaine provides adequate analgesia. A minimal volume (1–2cm³ per eyelid) of anesthetic is required. Larger volumes or deeper orbital injections may alter levator function, compromising muscle adjustment. General anesthesia is necessary for young children, for apprehensive adults, and when harvesting fascia lata.

GENERAL TECHNIQUES

The type of ptosis and amount of levator function are considered when choosing the best procedure for an individual patient. Anterior levator aponeurotic-muscle reattachment or resection is effective in patients who have moderate to good levator function. Maximal levator resection can be used in cases with poor levator activity, although postoperative lagophthalmos is more common. Some surgeons perform a posterior resection of Müller's muscle in patients who demonstrate adequate elevation of the eyelid following instillation of topical phenylephrine.[38,39]

Frontalis suspension is performed in patients who have severe ptosis, poor levator activity, and intact frontalis muscle function. Autologous fascia lata is the preferred implant material in pediatric cases. Donor fascia may also be used, although recurrent ptosis may occur secondary to implant absorption.[40] Alloplastic implants such as silicone rods are placed in patients in whom it is impractical to harvest fascia lata. These implants are occasionally complicated by extrusion, infection, or breakage.

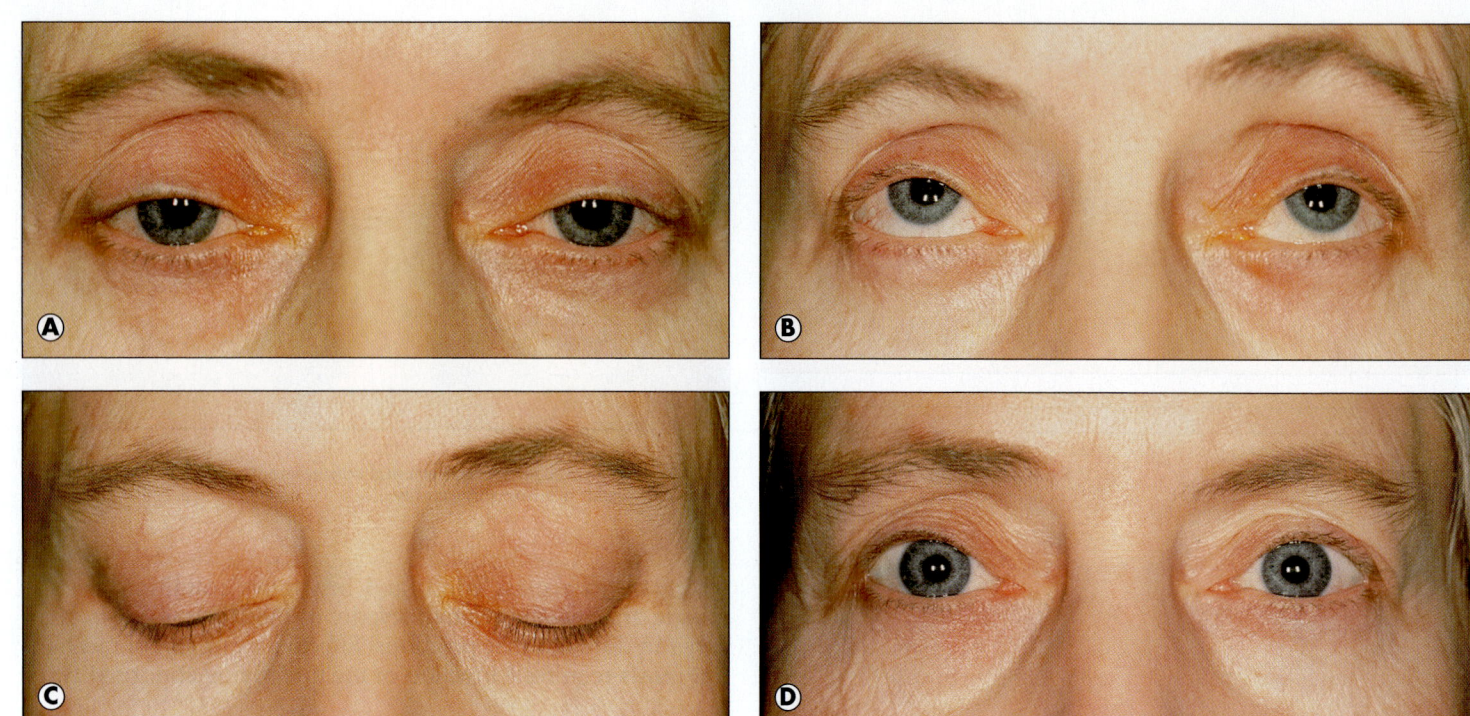

FIG. 86-7 ▪ Levator function. **A,** Bilateral ptosis from levator aponeurosis dehiscence demonstrating a high indistinct lid crease. **B,** In upgaze, levator muscle function is of normal amplitude. **C,** The indistinct eyelid crease and ptosis remain in downgaze. **D,** Normal lid height following levator aponeurosis advancement.

The quality of Bell's phenomenon, lacrimal production, and orbicularis activity are considered when determining the amount of eyelid elevation to perform. Selected patients tolerate mild lagophthalmos, which may be necessary to achieve an acceptable cosmetic result. Marked lagophthalmos should generally be avoided due to the risks of corneal exposure.

The skin incision is placed in the location of the desired eyelid crease. The position of the contralateral crease is matched in cases of unilateral ptosis. Eyelid creases are absent or indistinct in many cases of bilateral disease, in which case the incisions are marked about one third of the distance from the eyelashes to the lower edge of the brow.[41] The central incision is approximately 9–10mm above the lashes in adult women. The adult male crease is usually placed 1–2mm lower. Combined blepharoplasty and ptosis repair can be performed in patients undergoing bilateral surgery.

Early surgical intervention may be indicated in infants who have occlusion amblyopia. Ptosis repair in young children is otherwise deferred until 3 to 5 years of age, facilitating both preoperative measurements and postoperative care. It is difficult to obtain sufficient fascia lata in children younger than 3 years.

SPECIFIC TECHNIQUES

Anterior Levator Aponeurosis Advancement

The patient is examined both sitting and supine. Any change in eyelid position is noted because surgery is performed with the patient recumbent. A standard full-face surgical wash is performed. The desired position of the upper eyelid crease incision is marked, and subcutaneous infiltrative anesthesia is administered.

After creating the skin incision (Fig. 86-8, *A*), the orbicularis muscle is divided parallel to its muscle fibers. The septum is divided and the preaponeurotic fat pads are retracted upward to expose the underlying levator muscle (Fig. 86-8, *B*). Hemostasis is maintained throughout the procedure.

The opaque levator aponeurosis may be thin or completely dehisced from the tarsus. Any remaining attachments of the aponeurosis are divided, exposing the tarsus. The aponeurosis is separated from underlying Müller muscle with blunt and sharp dissection (Fig. 86-8, *C*). In severe congenital ptosis, the com-

bined aponeurosis–Müller muscle complex may have to be advanced to achieve adequate lid elevation. The dissection in these cases is performed between Müller's muscle and conjunctiva. The awake patient is asked to look in primary gaze, allowing the surgeon to determine whether the dissection has altered the preoperative eyelid level.

Two partial-thickness 6-0 polyester (Mersilene) sutures are placed in the central third of the tarsus. The posterior surface of the lid is examined to ensure that the sutures are not exposed. These sutures are used to reattach or advance the aponeurosis (Fig. 86-8, *D*). Any change in the lid position noted from supine to upright positioning or resulting from surgical dissection is considered when determining the amount of lid elevation to perform. The eyelid is adjusted empirically in patients under general anesthesia, considering the preoperative levator function and amount of ptosis. Redundant aponeurotic tissue is excised. The eyelid crease is reformed by suturing the cut edge of the pretarsal orbicularis muscle or subcutaneous tissue to the aponeurosis (7-0 polyglactin sutures) (Fig. 86-8, *E*). The skin incision is closed with a running 7-0 polypropylene suture (Fig. 86-8, *F*).

Patients are observed after surgery to detect early postoperative hemorrhage or other complications. Cold compresses are used during the first 48 hours to minimize edema and ecchymosis. Subsequent wet and warm compresses assist in wound hygiene. A topical antibiotic ointment is placed on the incision several times daily. Suture removal is performed 5–7 days following surgery. There may be transient lagophthalmos and poor blink after surgery, attributable to orbicularis underaction. These findings usually improve several weeks after surgery. A variable period of time is required for complete resolution of the postoperative edema and stabilization of the eyelid level.

Frontalis Suspension

Incision location and pattern of the implanted material are determined by brow contour. A pentagonally shaped sling is used in patients who have diffuse brow elevation. Medial and lateral incisions are marked at the superior border of the brow, just outside the medial and lateral corneal limbus (Fig. 86-9, *A*). A central forehead incision is placed approximately 10mm above the

LEVATOR APONEUROSIS ADVANCEMENT

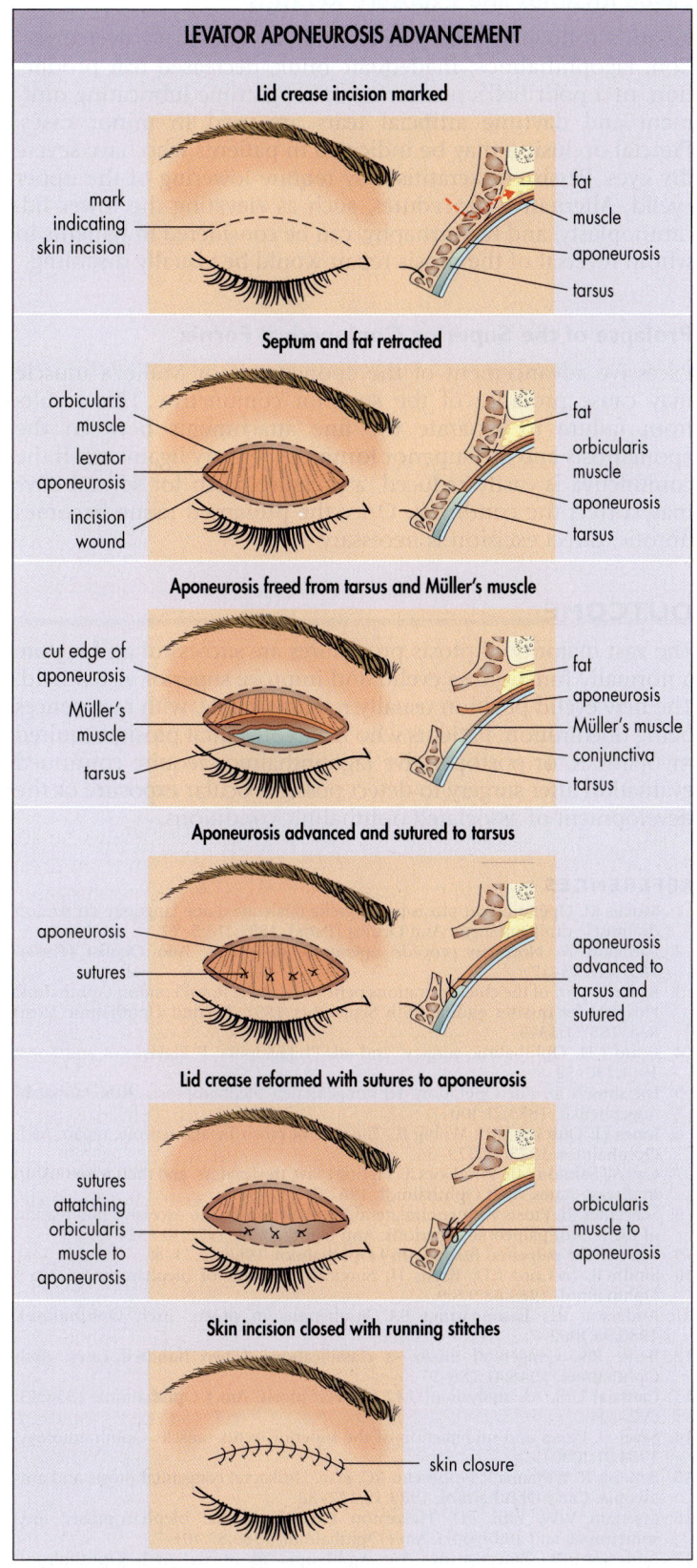

Lid crease incision marked

mark indicating skin incision

fat
muscle
aponeurosis
tarsus

Septum and fat retracted

orbicularis muscle
levator aponeurosis
incision wound

fat
orbicularis muscle
aponeurosis
tarsus

Aponeurosis freed from tarsus and Müller's muscle

cut edge of aponeurosis
Müller's muscle
tarsus

fat
aponeurosis
Müller's muscle
conjunctiva
tarsus

Aponeurosis advanced and sutured to tarsus

aponeurosis
sutures

aponeurosis advanced to tarsus and sutured

Lid crease reformed with sutures to aponeurosis

sutures attatching orbicularis muscle to aponeurosis

orbicularis muscle to aponeurosis

Skin incision closed with running stitches

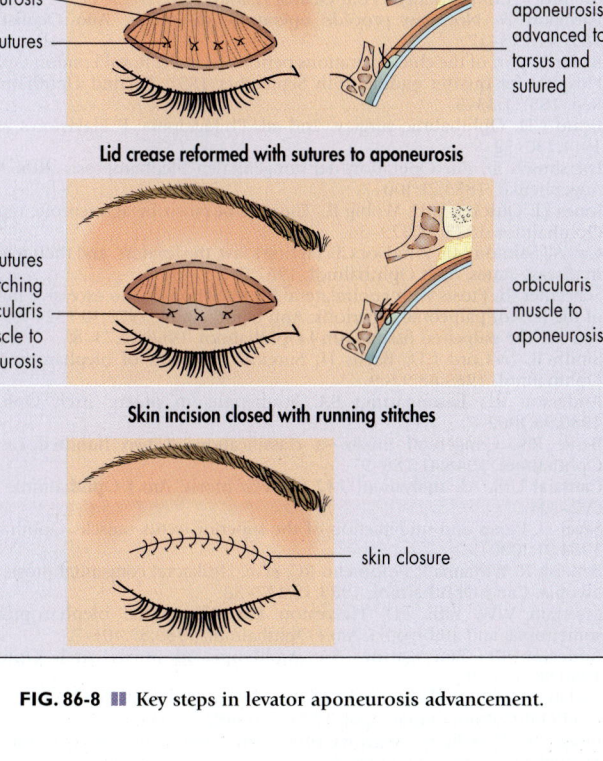

skin closure

FIG. 86-8 ▮ Key steps in levator aponeurosis advancement.

FRONTALIS SUSPENSION

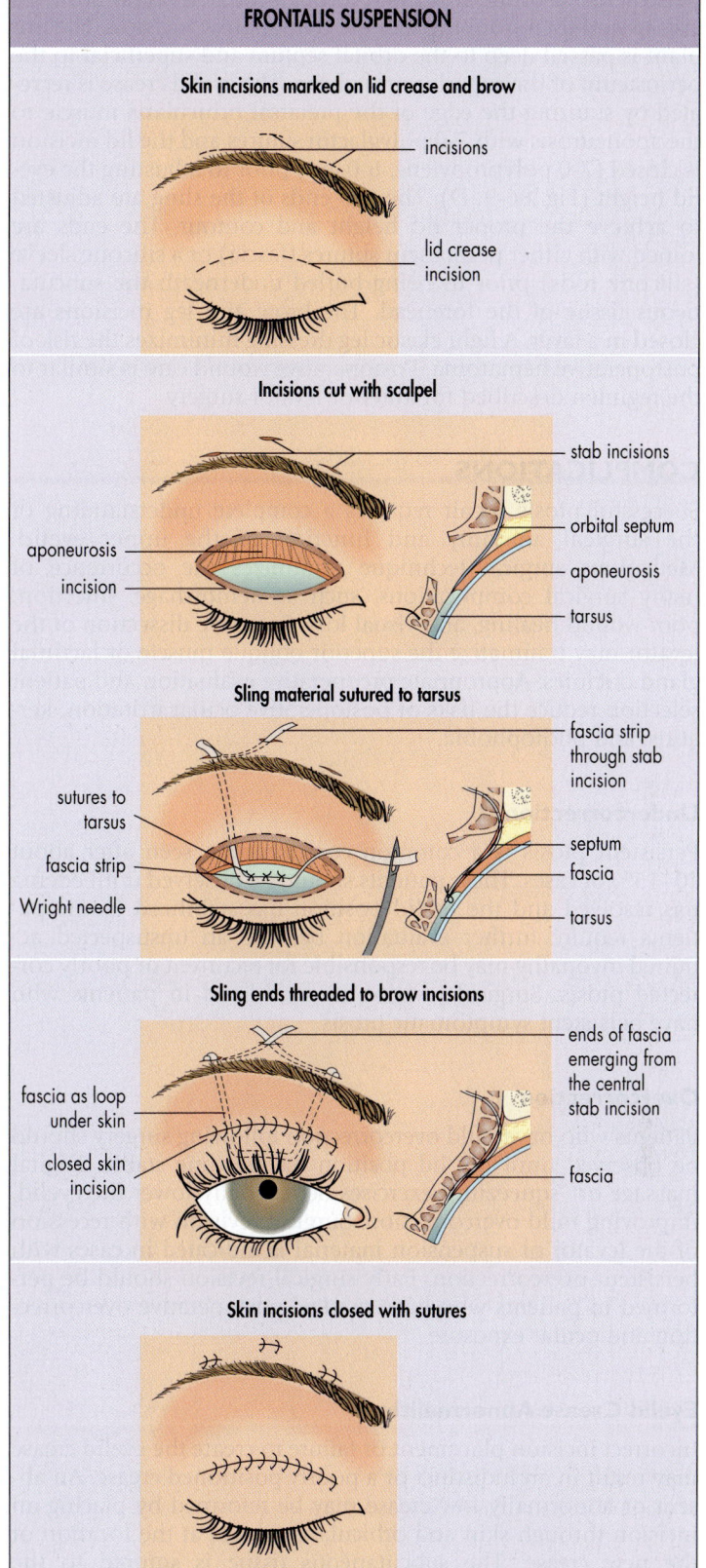

Skin incisions marked on lid crease and brow

incisions

lid crease incision

Incisions cut with scalpel

aponeurosis
incision

stab incisions
orbital septum
aponeurosis
tarsus

Sling material sutured to tarsus

sutures to tarsus
fascia strip
Wright needle

fascia strip through stab incision
septum
fascia
tarsus

Sling ends threaded to brow incisions

fascia as loop under skin
closed skin incision

ends of fascia emerging from the central stab incision
fascia

Skin incisions closed with sutures

FIG. 86-9 ▮ Key steps in frontalis suspension.

brow, between the other two incisions. Triangular slings are more ideal in individuals who have segmental brow elevation. They utilize a single incision above the portion of the brow exhibiting maximal movement.

The brow incisions are created through skin and subcutaneous tissue, exposing the frontalis muscle. A crease incision is used to expose the tarsus (Fig. 86-9, *B*). Fascia lata must be harvested in patients who undergo autologous grafting. A 3cm incision is made on the lower thigh, just above the lateral condyle of the femur. The white, glistening fascia lata is visible underneath the subcutaneous fat. Blunt dissection is performed on the anterior surface of the fascia, up the lateral aspect of the leg for about 15–20cm. A strip of fascia 6–8mm wide and 15–20cm long is harvested using a fascial stripper and cutter. The fascia is cleaned of adherent subcutaneous fat and divided into strips 2–3mm wide.

The implant material is sutured to the upper anterior surface of the central tarsus with several partial-thickness 6-0 polyester sutures (Fig. 86-9, *C*). Eyelid contour is adjusted by altering the width of this attachment. A Wright fascial needle is then used to pass each end of the sling, first through the peripheral brow incisions and then from these to the central brow incision. The implant is passed deep to the orbital septum and superficial to the periosteum of the superior orbital rim. The eyelid crease is recreated by suturing the edge of the pretarsal orbicularis muscle to the aponeurosis with 7-0 polyglactin sutures and the lid incision is closed (7-0 polypropylene, 6-0 gut) prior to adjusting the eyelid height (Fig. 86-9, *D*). The two ends of the sling are adjusted to achieve the proper lid height and contour. The ends are joined with either permanent sutures (fascia) or a silicone sleeve (silicone rods) prior to being buried underneath the subcutaneous tissue of the forehead. The brow and leg incisions are closed in a layer. A light elastic leg dressing minimizes the risk of postoperative hematoma. Postoperative wound care is similar to the regimen described for anterior levator surgery.

COMPLICATIONS

Successful ptosis repair requires a complete understanding of the surgical anatomy and function of the upper eyelid. Meticulous surgical technique minimizes the occurrence of many surgical complications, such as hemorrhage, infection, poor wound healing, and visual loss. Excessive dissection of the levator may traumatize the superior oblique muscle or lacrimal gland ductules. Appropriate preoperative evaluation and patient selection reduce the risks of postoperative ocular irritation, keratitis, and photophobia.

Undercorrection

Persistent ptosis is a common complication, seen after about 10–15% of cases. These patients should be observed until edema has resolved and the eyelid position has stabilized. Some patients require further evaluation because an unsuspected acquired myopathy may be responsible for recurrent or poorly corrected ptosis. Surgical revision is considered in patients who have persistent symptomatic ptosis.

Overcorrection

Patients who have mild overcorrection following surgery should be observed until the lid position has become stable. Digital massage or "squeezing" exercises occasionally lower the eyelid, improving mild overcorrection. Surgical revision with recession of the levator or suspension material is indicated in cases with persistent overcorrection. Early surgical revision should be performed in patients who have marked postoperative overcorrection and ocular exposure.

Eyelid Crease Abnormalities

Incorrect incision placement or failure to create the eyelid crease may result in an indistinct or a poorly positioned crease. An absent or abnormally low crease may be reformed by placing an incision through skin and orbicularis muscle at the location of the new crease. The subcutaneous tissue is sutured to the aponeurosis prior to skin closure.

It is difficult to lower an abnormally high crease. The attachment between the skin–orbicularis muscle and the aponeurosis must be separated. Soft tissue, such as orbital fat, should then be mobilized between these layers in an effort to minimize the establishment of a new adhesion in the same location. The new crease is then established at a lower level.

Abnormalities of Eyelid Margin Contour

Distortions of the eyelid margin contour result from uneven advancement of the aponeurosis. Surgical revision is often required. The lid contour is adjusted by tightening or loosening individual aponeurotic sutures.

Lagophthalmos and Exposure Keratitis

Keratitis following ptosis repair may be related to overcorrection, lagophthalmos, inadequate blink, decreased tear production, or a poor Bell's phenomenon. Nighttime lubricating ointment and daytime artificial tears are used in minor cases. Punctal occlusion may be indicated in patients who have severe dry eyes. Persistent keratitis may require lowering of the upper eyelid. Alternative procedures, such as elevating the lower lid, canthoplasty, and tarsorrhaphy, can be considered in patients in whom reversal of the ptosis repair would be visually disabling.

Prolapse of the Superior Conjunctival Fornix

Excessive advancement of the aponeurosis or Müller's muscle may cause prolapse of the superior conjunctiva. This results from failure to separate the fine attachments between the aponeurosis and the superior fornix suspensory ligaments. If the conjunctiva is easily reduced, a pressure patch for several days may correct the condition. Once the prolapsed tissue becomes fibrotic, direct excision is necessary.

OUTCOME

The vast majority of ptosis procedures are successful and restore a normally functioning eyelid and improve superior visual field. The new eyelid position usually remains stable, with recurrences being uncommon. Patients who have congenital ptosis, acquired myopathies, or postoperative lagophthalmos require continued evaluation after surgery to detect possible ocular exposure or the development of associated ophthalmic conditions.

REFERENCES

1. Motais M. Opération du ptosis par la greffe tarsienne d'une languette du tendon du muscle droit supérieur. Ann Oculist (Paris). 1897;118:5–12.
2. Parinaud H. Nouveau procédé opératoire du ptosis. Ann Oculist (Paris). 1897;118:13–17.
3. Bader. Report of the chief operations performed at the Royal London Ophthalmic Hospital for quarter ending 25th September 1857. R Lond Ophthalmic Hosp Rep. 1857;1:33–5.
4. Beard CH. Ophthalmic surgery, 2nd ed. Philadelphia: P Blakiston's and Sons; 1914:230–52.
5. Eversbusch O. Zur Operation der congenitalen Blepharoptosis. Klin Monatsbl Augenheilkd. 1883;21:100–7.
6. Jones LT, Quickert MH, Wobig JL. The cure of ptosis by aponeurotic repair. Arch Ophthalmol. 1975;93:629–34.
7. Gay AJ, Salmon ML, Windsor CE. Hering's law, the levators, and their relationship in disease states. Arch Ophthalmol. 1967;77:157–60.
8. Schechter RJ. Ptosis with contralateral lid retraction due to excessive innervation of the levator palpebrae superioris. Ann Ophthalmol. 1978;10:1324–8.
9. Fox SA. The palpebral fissure. Am J Ophthalmol. 1966;62:73–8.
10. Smith B, McCord CD, Baylis H. Surgical treatment of blepharoptosis. Am J Ophthalmol. 1969;68:92–9.
11. Anderson RL, Baumgartner SA. Strabismus in ptosis. Arch Ophthalmol. 1980;98:1062–7.
12. Berke RN. Congenital ptosis—a classification of two hundred cases. Arch Ophthalmol. 1948;41:188–97.
13. Carbajal UM. An analysis of 142 cases of ptosis. Am J Ophthalmol. 1958;45:692–704.
14. Sevel D. Ptosis and underaction of the superior rectus muscle. Ophthalmology. 1984;91:1080–5.
15. Beneish R, Williams F, Polomeno RC, et al. Unilateral congenital ptosis and amblyopia. Can J Ophthalmol. 1983;18:127–30.
16. Merriam WW, Ellis FD, Helveston EM. Congenital blepharoptosis, anisometropia, and amblyopia. Am J Ophthalmol. 1980;89:401–7.
17. Anderson RL, Baumgartner SA. Amblyopia in ptosis. Arch Ophthalmol. 1980;98:1068–9.
18. Callahan A. Surgical correction of the blepharophimosis syndromes. Trans Am Acad Ophthalmol Otolaryngol. 1973;77:op687–op695.
19. Briggs HH. Hereditary congenital ptosis with report of 64 cases conforming to the Mendelian rule of dominance. Am J Ophthalmol. 1919;2:408–17.
20. Townes PL, Muechler EK. Blepharophimosis, ptosis, epicanthus inversus, and primary amenorrhea—a dominant trait. Arch Ophthalmol. 1979;97:1664–6.
21. Mustarde JC. Experiences in ptosis correction. Trans Am Acad Ophthalmol Otolaryngol. 1968;72:173–85.
22. Gunn RM. Congenital ptosis with peculiar associated movements of the affected lid. Trans Ophthalmol Soc UK. 1883;3:283–5.
23. Oesterle CS, Faulkner WJ, Clay R, et al. Eye bobbing associated with jaw movement. Ophthalmology. 1982;89:63–7.
24. Lewy FH, Groff RA, Grant FC. Autonomic innervation of the eyelids and the Marcus Gunn phenomenon. Arch Neurol Psychiatry. 1937;37:1289–97.
25. Spaeth EB. The Marcus Gunn phenomenon. Am J Ophthalmol. 1947;30:143–158.
26. Pratt SG, Beyer CK, Johnson CC. The Marcus Gunn phenomenon (a review of 71 cases). Ophthalmology. 1984;91:27–30.

27. Bullock JD. Marcus Gunn jaw-winking ptosis: classification and surgical management. J Pediatr Ophthalmol Strabismus. 1980;17:375–9.

28. Krohel GB. Blepharoptosis after traumatic third-nerve palsies. Am J Ophthalmol. 1979;88:598–601.

29. Weinstein JM, Zweifel TJ, Thompson HS. Congenital Horner's syndrome. Arch Ophthalmol. 1980;98:1074–8.

30. Mattis RD. Ocular manifestations in myasthenia gravis. Arch Ophthalmol. 1941;26:969–82.

31. Cogan DG. Myasthenia gravis. Arch Ophthalmol. 1965;74:217–21.

32. Oasterhuis HJ. The ocular signs and symptoms of myasthenia gravis. Doc Ophthalmol. 1982;52:363–78.

33. Seybold ME. Myasthenia gravis. A clinical and basic science review. JAMA. 1983; 250:2516–21.

34. Duranceau AC, Beauchamp G, Jamiewon GG, et al. Oropharyngeal dysphagia and oculopharyngeal muscular dystrophy. Surg Clin North Am. 1983;63:825–32.

35. Johnson CC, Kuwabara T. Oculopharyngeal muscular dystrophy. Am J Ophthalmol. 1974;77:872–9.

36. Bastiaensen LA, Frenken CW, TerLaak HJ, et al. Kearns syndrome: a heterogeneous group of disorders with CPEO, or a nosological entity? Doc Ophthalmol. 1982;52:207–25.

37. Feibel RM, Custer PL, Gordon MO. Postcataract ptosis—a randomized, double-masked comparison of peribulbar and retrobulbar anesthesia. Ophthalmology. 1993;100:660-5.

38. Putterman AM. Müller muscle—conjunctiva resection—technique for treatment of blepharoptosis. Arch Ophthalmol. 1975;93:619–23.

39. Weinstein GS, Buerger GF. Modifications of the Müller's muscle–conjunctival resection operation for blepharoptosis. Am J Ophthalmol. 1982;93:647–51.

40. Crawford JS. Recent trends in ptosis surgery. Ann Ophthalmol. 1975;7:1263–7.

41. Zamora RL, Becker WL, Custer PL. Normal eyelid crease position in children. Ophthalmic Surg. 1993;25:42–7.

87 Entropion

JAMES W. GIGANTELLI

DEFINITION

- Entropion: an inward rotation of the tarsus and eyelid margin (Fig. 87-1).

KEY FEATURES

- Foreign body sensation.
- Secondary blepharospasm.
- Ocular discharge.
- Epiphora.
- Conjunctival metaplasia.
- Superficial keratopathy.
- Corneal scarring.

ASSOCIATED FEATURES

- It is progressive.
- Numerous corrective techniques for this anomaly are reported.
- Multiple pathogenic factors, including tarsotendinous instability, capsulopalpebral fascia dysfunction, and preseptal orbicularis muscle override.
- Surgical goals are to normalize eyelid function and appearance.

INTRODUCTION

There are over 400 publications in the medical literature that address entropion and its treatment. Early procedures can be categorized as vertically shortening the anterior lamella (skin and orbicularis muscle), vertically lengthening the posterior lamella (tarsus and conjunctiva), and/or controlling lamellar rotation. The ancient Egyptians and Arabians are credited with the earliest entropion treatment—everting the lower eyelid through skin and orbicularis muscle cautery. Celsus and others described procedures directed at foreshortening the anterior lamella or stabilizing its position. Procedures involving horizontal eyelid tightening were popularized by Fox, Bick, and others.[1] Wies[2] described a procedure that utilized full-thickness blepharotomy and eyelid margin rotation. Despite the nonphysiological basis of this procedure, it gained wide acceptance because of its technical ease and nonreliance upon a knowledge of eyelid anatomy.

The mid-twentieth century heralded an anatomic approach to entropion repair. In 1963, DeRoetth[3] and Jones et al.[4] separately identified the lower eyelid retractor system as pivotal in acquired entropion development. Jones et al.[5] also described a surgical correction via lower eyelid retractor repair. Lower eyelid retractor microanatomy and physiology were further refined by Hawes and Dortzbach,[6] Goldberg et al.,[7] and others.[8,9] Orbicularis muscle functions in acquired and congenital entropion were clarified by Dalgleish and Smith[8] and Tse et al.,[10] and tarsal plate and canthal tendon physiologies were advanced by Benger and Musch,[9] Shore,[11] and Liu and Stasior.[12] Finally, the importance of autologous tarsoconjunctival support in entropion was contributed by Shorr et al.[13] and Baylis and Hamako[14] and led to improved posterior lamellar substitutes and grafting technique by Silver[15] and others.[16]

PREOPERATIVE EVALUATION AND DIAGNOSTIC APPROACH

A complete ocular history, including all prior eyelid procedures, and physical examination are essential. A general medical history and physical examination may be critical in uncovering systemic manifestations predisposing to entropion development or altering the selection of treatment options.

The Capsulopalpebral Fascia

Capsulopalpebral fascia dysfunction is central to the evaluation of both congenital and acquired entropion (see Box 87-1 and Chapter 82). Although many authors suggest that entropion results from disinsertion or dehiscence of the fascia from the inferior tarsus, histological observations disclose only an attenuation of the conjoint capsulopalpebral fascia and orbital septum complex.[6] Clinical observations that identify possible lower lid retractor dysfunction include a higher eyelid resting position in primary gaze, an increased passive vertical distraction, and a reduced vertical eyelid excursion. Benger and Musch,[9] however, could not demonstrate a loss of lower lid excursion in patients who have entropion. They noted that normal lower lid excursion, in the presence of capsulopalpebral fascia disinsertion or attenuation, parallels the normal upper eyelid excursion in patients with aponeurogenic blepharoptosis.

Schwab et al.[17] determined the normal depth of the central inferior fornix to be 11mm. In cases of retractor dysfunction, the fornix depth often increases. In some cases, a white band, representing the disinserted edge of the capsulopalpebral fascia, can be observed beneath the palpebral conjunctiva.

The Tarsus and Canthal Tendons

The appositional pressure between the eyelid and globe is a factor in entropion development. Bick[1] demonstrated that entropion could be temporarily corrected by the intraconal injection of 2–4ml of saline. Although an age-related lengthening of the lower eyelid or tarsus remains unproved, some studies suggest that age-related horizontal lower lid laxity occurs, especially in patients who have chronic entropion.[12] This laxity often results from stretching of the lateral canthal tendon. The horizontal eyelid distraction test remains the best way to judge horizontal eyelid laxity. The central eyelid is passively pulled from the ocular surface while the eye is in the primary gaze position. Measurements of greater than 6mm between the eyelid margin and corneal surface are considered abnormal.

Enophthalmos

Another determinant of the appositional pressure between globe and eyelid is the relative position of the globe. Although widely discussed in the literature, involutional enophthalmos has not been verified. Kersten et al.[18] demonstrated no association between "involutional" entropion and globe position as measured by Hertel's exophthalmometry. Lower eyelid medial entropion has been reported following enophthalmos induced by orbital

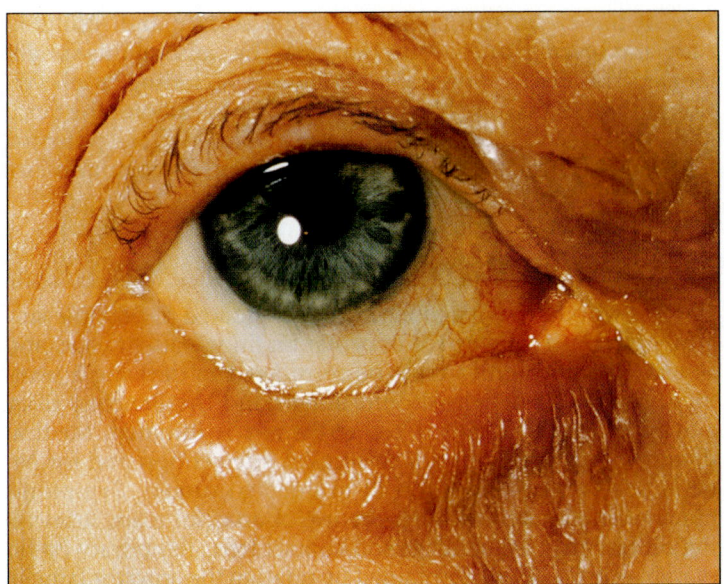

FIG. 87-1 ▪ **Right lower eyelid entropion.** Note the inward rotation of the tarsal plate about the horizontal axis and the resultant contact between the mucocutaneous junction and ocular surface. This patient may have multiple anatomic defects contributing to the eyelid presentation.

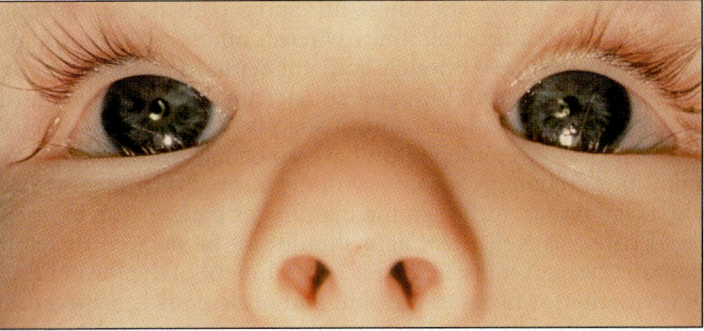

FIG. 87-2 ▪ **Epiblepharon.** Note the bilaterality, loss of the lower eyelid skin crease, and overriding skin fold. The normal orientation of the tarsal plate distinguishes this condition from entropion.

BOX 87-1

Preoperative Assessment of Entropion

ASSESSMENT OF CAPSULOPALPEBRAL FASCIA LAXITY
- Higher eyelid resting position in primary gaze
- Increased passive vertical eyelid distraction
- Increased depth of inferior conjunctival fornix
- Presence of a white infratarsal band

ASSESSMENT OF HORIZONTAL EYELID LAXITY
- Passive horizontal eyelid distraction

ASSESSMENT OF RELATIVE ENOPHTHALMOS
- Exophthalmometry

ASSESSMENT OF PRESEPTAL ORBICULARIS MUSCLE OVERRIDE

ASSESSMENT OF POSTERIOR LAMELLAR SUPPORT
- Height of tarsal plate
- Presence of cicatrizing conjunctival disease

ASSESSMENT OF MARKED ORBITAL FAT PROLAPSE

---

decompression in Graves' orbitopathy.[19] Enophthalmos alone may be insufficient to cause entropion.

Orbicularis Muscle

The historical subclassification of a spastic entropion variant implied a cause-and-effect relationship with increased orbicularis muscle tone. Dalgleish and Smith[8] demonstrated a superior migration of the preseptal orbicularis subunit toward, but not beyond, the inferior tarsal border in lower lid entropion. It is unclear whether this muscular bunching is a primary phenomenon or epiphenomenon. Clinical evaluation for preseptal orbicularis override is subjective and should be carried out with the eye in primary gaze position, after a spontaneous blink, and following forceful eyelid closure. Eyelids with preseptal override are often described as having a thickened appearance. In contrast to observations in eyelids with isolated capsulopalpebral fascia dysfunction, the inferior tarsal border is not easily visualized in orbicularis override.

The Posterior Lamella

Reduced posterior lamellar support in entropion may be more widespread than appreciated. Its vertical contracture in cicatrizing conjunctival disease has been distinctly categorized (cicatricial entropion). Several studies, however, imply a role for tarso-conjunctival loss even in noncicatrizing disease. An age-related decrease in the vertical dimension of the tarsal plate and a reduced tarsal height associated with involutional entropion have been documented.[8,20]

In the setting of posterior lamellar foreshortening, knowledge of the underlying disease process is paramount in deciding the timing and type of surgery. The majority of these cases involves trachoma, Stevens-Johnson syndrome, ocular cicatricial pemphigoid, chronic meibomian gland inflammation, chemical and radiation injury, and postoperative fibrosis. Additional diagnostic considerations include topical medication toxicity, sarcoidosis, atopic keratoconjunctivitis, ocular rosacea, toxic epidermal necrolysis, membranous conjunctivitis, herpes zoster ophthalmicus, progressive systemic sclerosis, dysthyroidism, and neoplasm. Patients who have progressive processes need preoperative and perioperative immunomodulation to stabilize their disease.[21,22] When the primary process is uncertain, a diagnostic conjunctival biopsy is indicated. Kemp and Collin[23] offered a grading system for cicatricial change. This system focuses on the position of the meibomian gland orifices, conjunctivalization of the eyelid margin, the position and orientation of the cilia, assessment of tarsal plate structure, keratinization of the palpebral conjunctiva, assessment of posterior lamellar scarring, and symblepharon formation.

Other Factors

Case reports suggest profoundly prolapsed orbital fat as a risk factor for lower eyelid entropion. Both Raina and Foster[24] and Bartley et al.[25] reported entropion in pediatric patients who have either morbid obesity or facial dysmorphism. Carter et al.[26] reported excessive orbital fat prolapse associated with lower eyelid entropion in the Asian population.

DIFFERENTIAL DIAGNOSIS

Other clinical entities may be confused with entropion and must be eliminated from the differential diagnosis. Epiblepharon, distichiasis, trichiasis, and eyelid retraction arise from different pathophysiologies, follow a different clinical course, and necessitate different therapies.

Epiblepharon

In epiblepharon, a horizontal fold of redundant pretarsal skin and orbicularis muscle extends beyond the eyelid margin and compresses the eyelashes against the globe (Fig. 87-2). The condition is usually bilateral, prevalent in Asian populations, and commonly involves the lower lid. Some patients demonstrate the clinical findings at all times, whereas others are symptomatic only in downgaze. Although both epiblepharon and congenital entropion result from lower eyelid retractor defects, their clinical presentation and course contrast sharply.[27] Nearly 80% of children who show epiblepharon have no ocular complaints.[28] The condition frequently resolves with the normal vertical growth of the facial bones. Although the majority of patients can be managed conservatively, treatment should not be delayed in symptomatic cases. A transcutaneous reattachment of the lower lid retractor anterior fibers to the skin and orbicularis is achieved by reforming the lower eyelid crease through the removal of a horizontal skin and orbicularis muscle strip and deep fixational suture closure.[27,29]

Distichiasis

Distichiasis refers to an accessory row of cilia arising from the meibomian gland orifices. It may occur in an autosomal dominant inheritance pattern. The tarsal plate in distichiasis manifests a normal position and orientation. It is the eyelash follicles that emerge from an abnormal position, the result of metadifferentiation of the primary epithelial germ cells originally intent upon meibomian gland development. The lashes are directed posteriorly toward the ocular surface and may not become symptomatic until about 5 years of age. Treatment modalities include mechanical epilation, electrolysis, radiofrequency ablation, laser photoablation, and cryotherapy to the posterior eyelid lamella.

Trichiasis

Trichiasis is an acquired condition in which cilia arising from their normal anterior lamellar position are misdirected toward the ocular surface. This usually results from inflammatory disruption and scarring of the eyelash follicles. The underlying inflammation may involve both eyelid lamellae and produce a coexistent entropion. Treatment is usually based upon the number, distribution, and severity of the misdirected cilia. Treatment modalities include epilation, electrolysis, radiofrequency ablation, laser photoablation, cryotherapy to the posterior eyelid lamella, anterior eyelid lamellar recession, and surgical excision of the eyelash bulbs.

Eyelid Retraction

Eyelid retraction may be clinically confused with entropion. The retracted eyelid is pulled toward the orbital rim with the eyelashes obscured by the resulting fold of eyelid skin (pseudodermatochalasis), resembling entropion. Some underlying disease conditions can result in the coexistence of entropion and lid retraction. The key in differentiating eyelid retraction from entropion remains the orientation of the tarsal plate. In isolated lid retraction, the tarsal plate maintains its normal orientation relative to the globe surface, and the eyelid margin is in a normal but vertically displaced position.

Congenital Entropion

Fewer than 50 cases of true congenital lower eyelid entropion have been reported in the medical literature, and the hypothesized pathophysiology is derived mostly from intraoperative observation.[25,27,29] Current belief is that in congenital lower eyelid entropion both the anterior and posterior attachments of the capsulopalpebral fascia are dysfunctional. This accounts for the poorly formed lower lid skin crease in addition to the inward tarsal rotation in affected children. Unlike epiblepharon, congenital entropion does not resolve spontaneously and requires prompt surgical intervention.

A rare form of congenital upper eyelid entropion is known as the horizontal tarsal kink syndrome. In this condition, a fixed right-angled inward rotation of the tarsal margin causes apposi-

tion of the eyelid margin to the ocular surface and results in early and severe corneal complications. The cause of this variant remains speculative. Surgical interventions, including tarsal eversion sutures, transverse blepharotomy, and resection of the tarsal kink with eversion sutures, have been advocated.[30] The potential for severe corneal complications requires early recognition and prompt therapy.

ALTERNATIVES TO SURGERY

Patients who have entropion must be evaluated as possible surgical candidates. The extent of ocular findings, patient's age, and systemic comorbidities must be considered in devising a treatment plan. The patient should understand the benefits, risks, and treatment alternatives before therapy is initiated. Medical therapy is appropriate prior to surgical intervention and for patients who refuse or are too ill to undergo surgery. Symptoms may be ameliorated through the use of artificial tears, lubricating ointments, or a bandage soft contact lens. Temporary eyelid margin eversion can be obtained by rotating the anterior lamella away from the globe with tape.

Quickert-Rathbun Sutures

Eyelid margin rotation and lamellar migration can be corrected by placing several well-spaced and tightly tied full-thickness sutures.[31] Chromic gut, nylon, and silk sutures are equivalent for scar induction, but silk and nylon sutures unfortunately incite epithelial ingrowth along the suture tract.[32] Despite Quickert and Rathbun's[33] reported 0% recurrence with up to 5 years of follow-up, the consensus is that suture entropion repair leads to late recurrence.[31] This shortcoming may be acceptable in patients who are poor surgical risks or for whom a temporary repair is adequate.

Botulinum Toxin

Chemodenervation of the orbicularis muscle with botulinum toxin may provide temporary entropion correction when the patient demonstrates significant preseptal muscle override.[34] Subcutaneous or intramuscular injection into the nasal and temporal lower eyelid can be performed in the office setting. Chemodenervation is noted within 3–5 days following administration and may last up to 6 months (see also Chapter 91). Injections in the medial lower eyelid may be complicated by temporary medial ectropion, punctal eversion, or inferior oblique muscle paresis.

ANESTHESIA

Entropion surgery is an outpatient procedure usually performed in the physician's office or in an ambulatory surgical center under local anesthesia. Pediatric patients require general inhalational anesthesia, although local subcutaneous infiltration is often utilized for additional hemostasis.

A 1:1 dilution of lidocaine 2% with 1:100,000 epinephrine (adrenaline) and bupivacaine 0.75% combined with hyaluronidase (150 units per 10ml of injectable anesthetic) provides excellent anesthesia. Hyaluronidase enhances anesthetic solution diffusion within connective tissues, reduces tissue distortion, and better preserves normal tissue anatomy. When coadministered with epinephrine, it does not reduce the anesthetic duration of action.

For many patients, the pain elicited during the local anesthetic injection is the most distressing aspect of the surgery. Sodium bicarbonate (1ml of 1mEq/ml [1mmol/ml] solution per 10ml of injectable anesthetic) can be added to local anesthetic solutions to decrease pain upon injection.[35] Sodium bicarbonate, however, decreases the pharmaceutical half-life of the anesthetic agent and admixed epinephrine. Thus, buffered anesthetic-epinephrine mixtures should be utilized within 1 week of preparation.[36] A nonpharmacological method of reducing injection discomfort is to provide the patient with adequate verbal support and to infiltrate the tissues slowly. Tissue infiltration or a regional nerve block is best performed with a 27- or 30-gauge hypodermic needle on a control syringe. The onset of epinephrine-induced vasoconstriction requires up to 10 minutes, so tissue infiltration should be performed prior to the surgical skin preparation and patient draping.

Monitored anesthesia care combines intravenous sedation with local analgesia. Its principal advantage is the sedative-induced amnesia. Propofol is an intravenous sedative that is neither a benzodiazepine nor a sedative-hypnotic. Its onset of action is equal to that of thiopental and it has a rapid recovery of less than 5 minutes.[37] It is excellent for the induction and maintenance of monitored anesthesia care sedation. It can produce undesirable cardiorespiratory depression, including systemic hypotension, peripheral vasodilatation, and respiratory depression. The use of intravenous sedatives necessitates appropriate preoperative evaluation and intraoperative monitoring of systemic blood pressure, cardiac rhythm, respiratory rate, and oxygen saturation.

GENERAL TECHNIQUE

The advances and improved surgical success in entropion management occurred through the appreciation of its pathophysiology and anatomic basis.[38] The preoperative assessment mandates the determination of all contributing defects. The planned surgical procedure is a sequential correction of each underlying defect. In most cases, entropion is multifactorial in origin and requires the correction of a combination of defects. Several authors have demonstrated that a single entropion procedure used for all cases is insufficient in providing adequate short- and long-term results.[39,40] In broad terms, entropion surgery includes:

- The correction of capsulopalpebral fascia dysfunction
- The reduction of horizontal lower eyelid laxity
- The debulking of significant lower lid fat
- The prevention of preseptal orbicularis muscle shifting
- The reconstruction of posterior eyelid lamellar foreshortening

In cases of capsulopalpebral fascia dysfunction, the fascia must be advanced or reattached to the inferior tarsal border. Transcutaneous and transconjunctival approaches are described for this repair.[39,41] Both approaches can be combined with techniques to correct horizontal laxity, prolapsed orbital fat, and preseptal orbicularis muscle override. The transconjunctival approach readily lends itself to the synchronous placement of a posterior lamellar graft. Some eyelid surgeons better appreciate the anatomic exposure as viewed through the transcutaneous approach. A recent study suggests a higher surgical success rate with the transcutaneous approach.[42]

The capsulopalpebral fascia can be advanced to the inferior tarsal border with or without its separation from the orbital septum. Separation of the septum from the fascia allows broader fascial exposure and a reduced likelihood of entrapping orbital septum in the advancement.

Surgical approaches to horizontal eyelid laxity address foreshortening by resection of the tarsal plate or plication-resection of the lateral canthal tendon. Evidence suggests that the dysfunction resides in the canthal tendon and its attachments rather than in the tarsal plate itself.[11] A surgical approach directed toward resection and reconstruction of the lateral canthal tendon is therefore preferred over purely tarsal resections performed in the central eyelid. This removes the dysfunctional canthal tendon, preserves the integrity of the healthy tarsus, places the incision within the cosmetically forgiving lateral laugh lines, and reduces the probability of a marginal notch, contour abnormality, or trichiasis.

Orbicularis muscle dysfunction is corrected by creating a fibrous barrier between the skin and deeper eyelid structures at the junction of the pretarsal and preseptal subunits. This can be achieved through a cutaneous incision placed at this level, the stimulation of fibrosis through the use of sutures, or the extirpation of a preseptal muscular subunit.[39]

Knowledge of the underlying disease process is essential in the treatment of posterior lamellar foreshortening. The timing of surgery and selection of the procedure are directly linked to the underlying process and its level of activity at the time of intervention. Progressive processes, such as ocular cicatricial pemphigoid, scleroderma, and sarcoidosis, are likely to require local and/or systemic immunomodulators to stabilize the disease course prior to surgical intervention.[22,43] In certain disease states, a local inflammatory exacerbation may follow posterior lamellar manipulation.[44] In this instance, deviation from direct correction of the pathophysiological defect may be appropriate. A modest advance of the capsulopalpebral fascia may suffice to correct mild to moderate "cicatricial" entropion and obviate the need for potentially dangerous physical manipulation of the tarsus and conjunctiva.[43]

In most cases of tarsoconjunctival foreshortening, once the process is identified and optimal immunosuppression achieved, a posterior lamellar technique is performed. This usually takes the form of a tarsal out-fracture with marginal rotation or placement of a posterior lamellar graft. The transverse tarsotomy is physiological in that it directly addresses the eyelid structures affected by the underlying disease process.[45,46] By limiting dissection to these layers, the risks of avascular necrosis of the lid, cutaneous scarring, and levator aponeurosis damage are minimized. The tarsotomy incision location is determined by the eyelid microvasculature and the degree of marginal eversion needed.

When posterior lamellar support or buttressing is needed, the selection of appropriate donor material is essential. Functionally, the posterior eyelid lamella is composed of a semirigid support material (tarsus) and a mucosal lining (conjunctiva). Although an autologous tarsoconjunctival composite flap or graft provides the most exact reconstruction, this tissue may be in short supply, especially if the primary disease process is bilateral. When replacement tissue is selected, an autologous, epithelium-covered, semirigid composite graft is favored. Materials utilized for tarsoconjunctival reconstruction or replacement have included tarsoconjunctival flaps and grafts, hard palate mucosa, nasal chondromucosa, and nasal mucoperiosteum. The hard palate mucosa and nasal mucoperiosteum are the current donor tissues of choice.[16] They are autologous, plentiful, easy to harvest, minimally resorptive, structurally similar to tarsus, and can be harvested repeatedly if necessary. Graft materials that may be used to lengthen the tarsus only include amniotic membrane, periosteum, temporalis fascia, banked sclera, irradiated homologous aorta, porous polyethylene, and polytef.[13,14,47–49]

SPECIFIC TECHNIQUES

Retractor Reattachment

In patients who do not demonstrate posterior lamellar foreshortening, the author advocates a transcutaneous surgical approach to lower eyelid entropion repair. A 4-0 silk traction suture is passed horizontally through the central lower eyelid margin and clamped to the drape above the brow (Fig. 87-3). The lid is put on mild vertical traction and a subciliary incision is made 4mm inferior to the eyelid margin (or 2.5mm inferior to the lower lid lashes). This is extended from just lateral to the lacrimal punctum to beyond the lateral canthal angle. As vertical traction is increased on the intramarginal suture, the multiple tissue layers of the eyelid are separated and assume a planar orientation. The orbicularis muscle is buttonholed at the junction of the pretarsal and preseptal subunits (see Chapter 82) and separated for the full skin incision length (Fig. 87-4). A myocutaneous flap is developed to the inferior orbital rim using blunt and sharp dissection posterior to the orbicularis plane.

The "free edge" of the capsulopalpebral fascia is often visualized several millimeters inferior to the tarsal border. The orbital septum is buttonholed 1mm inferior to its fusion with the capsulopalpebral fascia and opened the horizontal length of the anterior lamellar incision. The point of fusion between septum and capsulopalpebral fascia may vary within the lid, especially in cases of lower eyelid retractor dysfunction. An important surgical landmark

671

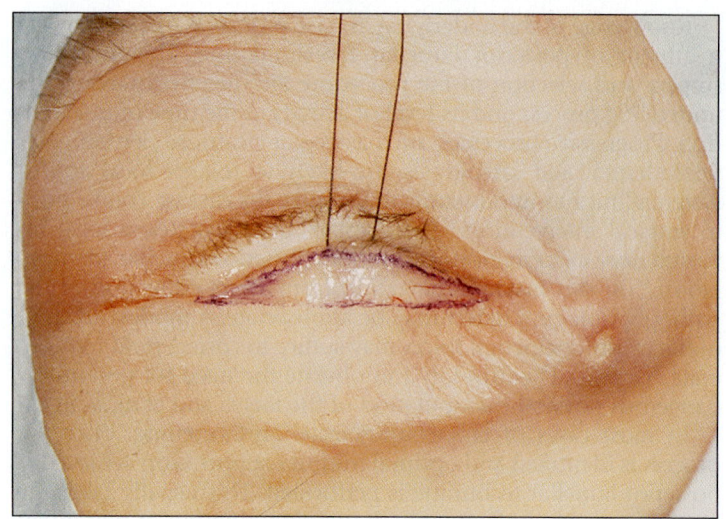

FIG. 87-3 ▪ A subciliary incision has been made following the placement of an intramarginal 4-0 silk traction suture.

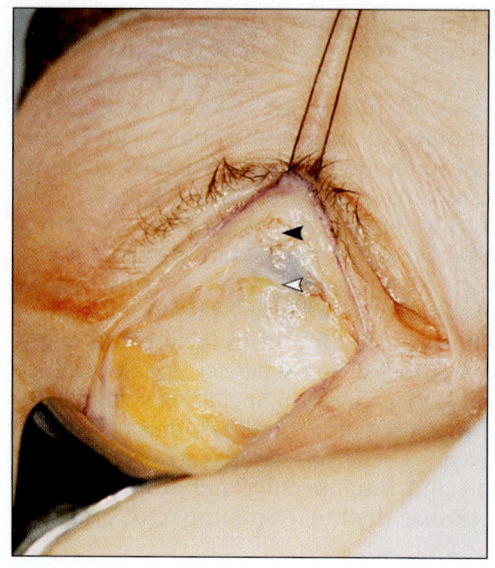

FIG. 87-5 ▪ Following opening of the orbital septum, the lower eyelid fat is retracted inferiorly. The capsulopalpebral fascia (open arrow) appears disinserted from the inferior tarsus (closed arrow).

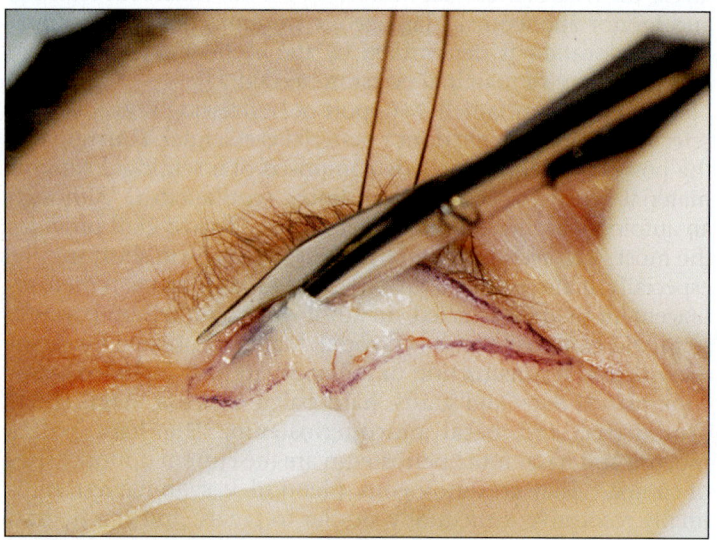

FIG. 87-4 ▪ Westcott scissors divide the pretarsal and preseptal subunits of the orbicularis muscle.

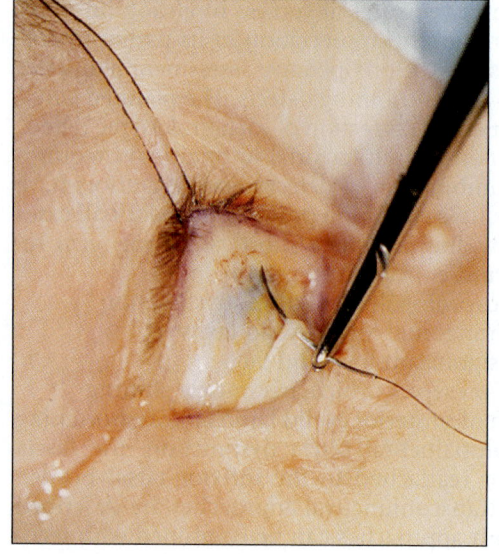

FIG. 87-6 ▪ The free edge of the capsulopalpebral fascia can be elevated easily from the underlying conjunctiva. In cases in which horizontal eyelid laxity is also present, the fascial advancement is performed following the lateral tarsal strip procedure.

is the lower eyelid fat, which anatomically rests between the septum and fascia. The three lower lid fat pads are gently dissected from the anterior surface of the capsulopalpebral fascia (Fig. 87-5).

In patients who have marked lower lid fat prolapse, fat debulking should be done at this time. This is performed using a standard lower eyelid blepharoplasty technique. Care is taken to ensure complete hemostasis and to preserve the inferior oblique muscle, which courses between the nasal and central fat pads (see Chapter 89).

The capsulopalpebral fascia is then advanced upward and reattached to the inferior tarsal border (Figs. 87-6 through 87-8). Grasping the tissue in toothed forceps and having the patient gaze inferiorly can confirm fascial identification. When an apparent disinsertion or dehiscence is present, the fascia is advanced to the inferior tarsal border. In cases in which the fascia is attenuated but not disinserted, the fascia is surgically disinserted by the surgeon, a narrow horizontal strip excised, and the fascia reattached to the inferior tarsal border. Reattachment to the tarsus is performed with several interrupted 6-0 Prolene sutures. Care is taken to ensure that a sufficient purchase of the tarsal plate is incorporated in the suture and that the fascia is not excessively advanced superiorly along the anterior tarsal surface.

In patients demonstrating preoperative preseptal orbicularis muscle override, the extirpation of a preseptal muscle strip is performed. Dissection and hemostasis are facilitated through dif-

fuse infiltration of the myocutaneous flap with an epinephrine-containing local anesthetic solution. A 6–10mm wide horizontal strip of muscle is dissected en bloc from the eyelid (Fig. 87-9). The subciliary skin incision can be closed with a running 6-0 mild chromic or nylon suture. Topical antibiotic ointment is sufficient for postoperative infection prophylaxis.

Lateral Tarsal Strip Procedure

A horizontal tightening of the lower lid may be combined with reattachment of the retractors or be done as a separate procedure (see Chapter 88). The tightening is best performed using a standard lateral tarsal strip technique. A lateral canthotomy and inferior cantholysis of the canthal tendon are performed. Within the temporal eyelid, the anterior and posterior lamellae must be separated from one another at the gray line and the lid margin de-epithelialized. The palpebral conjunctiva is disinserted from the inferior tarsal border to complete the tarsal strip. The redundant tissues of the strip are determined by gently drawing the strip to the lateral orbital tubercle. The excess tissue is excised and the new lateral border of tarsus is attached to periosteum at the lateral orbital tubercle with either two interrupted sutures or a single horizontal mattress suture. The small-radius, half-circle (P-2, S-2, or D-2) needle facilitates the periosteal anchor at the lateral orbital tubercle.

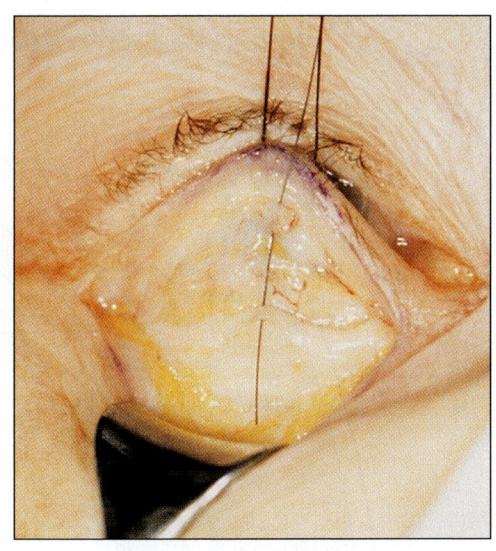

FIG. 87-7 ■ The capsulopalpebral fascia is advanced and sutured to the inferior border of the tarsal plate. Care must be taken to obtain a solid purchase of the inferior tarsus and to avoid advancing the fascia superiorly along the tarsal anterior surface.

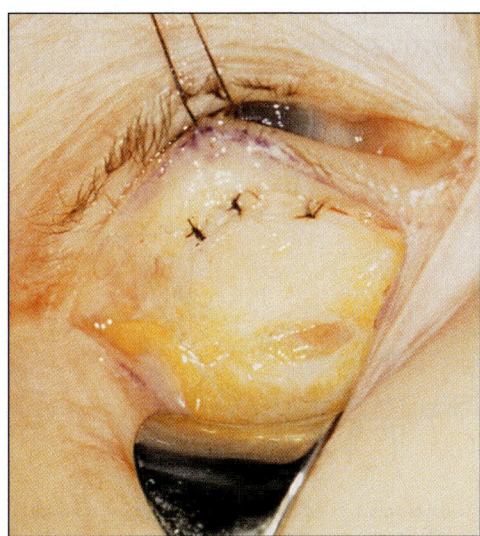

FIG. 87-8 ■ The completed lower eyelid retractor advancement. Multiple point fixation with nonabsorbable suture ensures permanence.

Absolute hemostasis should be established prior to closure. An absorbable 6-0 horizontal mattress canthopexy suture creates an acute canthal angulation and prevents imbrication of the upper lid over the temporal lower lid. To enhance esthetics, a small Burow triangle may be excised from the inferior skin wound margin lateral to the canthal angle. The lateral canthotomy is closed in a layered fashion.

Transverse Tarsotomy

In moderate cicatricial entropion, a posterior transverse tarsotomy with eyelid margin rotation is the procedure of choice. A 4-0 silk traction suture is placed horizontally through the central eyelid margin and the lid everted over a Desmarres retractor. A complete transverse tarsotomy is performed through the palpebral conjunctiva using a scalpel blade. The tarsotomy should be made equal to or greater than 3mm from the eyelid margin to avoid the marginal vascular arcade (Fig. 87-10). The marginal rotation is accomplished using double-armed 6-0 nonabsorbable sutures at multiple sites along the eyelid. The suture is first passed in a horizontal mattress fashion through the anterior edge of the nonmarginal tarsal plate. Each arm of the suture is then passed between the planes of the marginal tarsus and orbicularis muscle exiting the eyelid immediately anterior to the ciliary line. By tying under appropriate tension, the eyelid margin is everted. The immediate postoperative appearance should reveal a mild overcorrection of rotation.

Hard Palate Mucosal Graft

In cases of severe cicatricial entropion, the posterior eyelid lamella often requires buttressing. After everting the nonmarginal tarsal plate over a Desmarres retractor and performing the transverse tarsotomy, a limited dissection is performed in the plane between the tarsus and orbicularis muscle. This releases traction exerted by the eyelid retractors, septum, and conjunctiva. The posterior eyelid lamellar defect is measured and a template fashioned for graft harvesting. The graft should be mildly oversized to allow postoperative contraction.

A hard palate graft may be harvested using a local anesthetic block of the greater palatine and nasopalatine nerves followed by diffuse submucosal infiltration. The palatal mucosa is dried with suction and the graft template applied between the median raphe and alveolar process. The mucosa is outlined with a marking pen, the template removed, and the palate incised with a scalpel blade. The graft is undermined with the scalpel or a sharp periosteal elevator. Avoiding the areas of the greater palatine foramen and palatine vessels minimizes excessive bleeding. The palatal defect is not closed but may be covered with an acrylic retainer or the patient's upper dentures, if available.

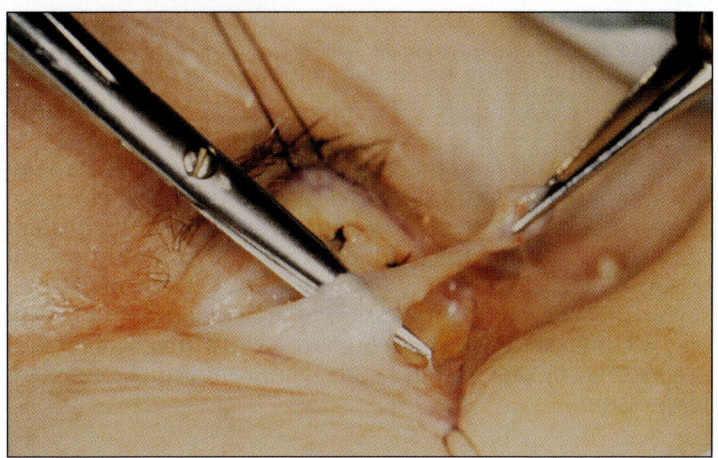

FIG. 87-9 ■ A strip of preseptal orbicularis muscle is extirpated using Westcott scissors. Muscle manipulation predisposes to hemorrhage; thus, thorough wound evaluation and complete hemostasis are essential.

The graft is thinned of fatty tissue on its submucosal surface and secured in the posterior eyelid lamellar defect with 6-0 absorbable sutures along its nonmarginal and lateral borders (Fig. 87-11). The rotated marginal strip of the eyelid is then secured to the anterior surface of the graft with three double-armed sutures, as previously described for the transverse tarsotomy procedure. In severe entropion, rotational overcorrection is desired. To achieve a more pronounced eversion, the tarsotomy can be placed a greater distance from the eyelid margin or the double-armed rotational sutures can be made to exit the skin more anteriorly than the lash line.

The treatment of upper lid entropion with tarsoconjunctival foreshortening differs slightly from that of the lower eyelid. For mild to moderate entropion, the transverse tarsotomy with marginal rotation is the procedure of choice. For severe cicatricial entropion, a posterior lamellar buttressing procedure is recommended. Postoperative application of a prophylactic topical antibiotic ointment is sufficient, although some authors utilize oral antibiotics following graft placement. When a posterior lamellar graft is placed in either the upper or lower eyelid, a Frost traction suture and pressure dressing are used for 5–7 days to immobilize the lid in a stretched position. When hard palate grafts are placed in the upper lid, corneal protection by copious surface lubrication or a bandage contact lens is frequently necessary.

COMPLICATIONS

Most postoperative complications can be avoided through meticulous preoperative planning and intraoperative tech-

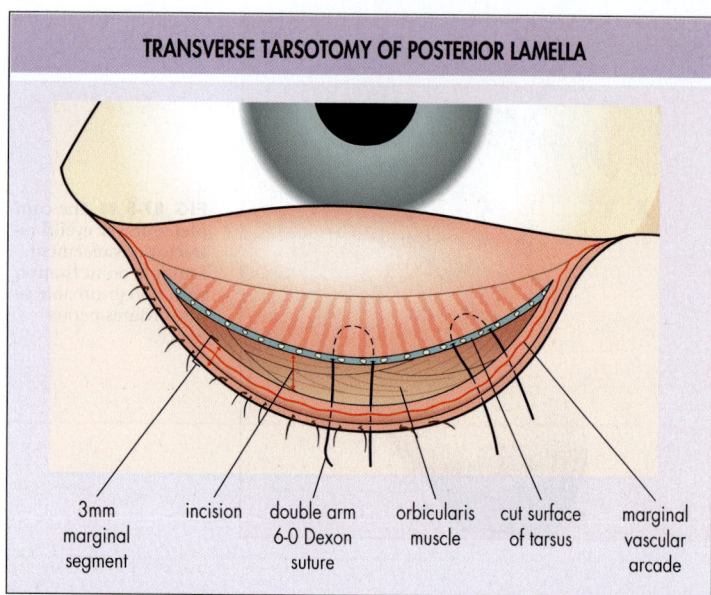

TRANSVERSE TARSOTOMY OF POSTERIOR LAMELLA

3mm marginal segment | incision | double arm 6-0 Dexon suture | orbicularis muscle | cut surface of tarsus | marginal vascular arcade

FIG. 87-10 ■ The transverse tarsotomy of the posterior lamella allows rotation of the marginal eyelid segment. Incision placement preserves the integrity of the marginal vascular arcade.

nique. The best way to prevent recurrent entropion is through the appropriate selection of surgical procedures. When entropion recurs during the early postoperative period, the patient must be reevaluated for overlooked or undercorrected predisposing factors. Recurrences that present a year or more after surgery may be due to progression of underlying pathophysiology. Recurrences in patients who have a cicatrizing conjunctival process may be due to graft failure, graft contracture, or disease progression.

Overcorrection

Overcorrection of eyelid margin position, or consecutive ectropion, is desired only in patients who have undergone transverse tarsotomy and marginal rotation procedures. When an unintended consecutive ectropion is present, the patient should be evaluated for excessive advancement of the capsulopalpebral fascia, attachment of the fascia too high on the anterior tarsal surface, uncorrected horizontal eyelid laxity, and incorporation of the orbital septum in the advancement or surgical closure. Postoperative ectropion can also occur following unintended extirpation of the pretarsal orbicularis subunit, excessive skin resection, or skin contracture after orbicularis extirpation. In such instances, if the degree of ectropion is mild and tolerated by the patient, conservative management with time, warm compresses, and massage may suffice. When it is severe, full-thickness skin grafting or the transposition of a preseptal orbicularis strip closer to the eyelid margin may be necessary.

Hematoma

The risk of hematoma can be reduced by appropriately discontinuing medications that impair platelet function and the clotting cascade. Intraoperative hemostasis can be achieved by meticulous cautery. Special attention must be given to the lateral branches of the palpebral arcades following lateral cantholysis. Extirpation of the preseptal orbicularis subunit increases the risk of hematoma. When eyelid hematomas occur, they are usually self-limiting and resolve with conservative management. In the setting of brisk bleeding or neuro-ophthalmic signs, reexploration of the surgical field with evacuation of the hematoma and cautery of vessels is indicated. Hemorrhage that occurs at a hard palate donor site usually originates from the greater palatine or nasopalatine artery. It can be controlled with digital pressure, submucosal epinephrine injection, conservative electrocautery,

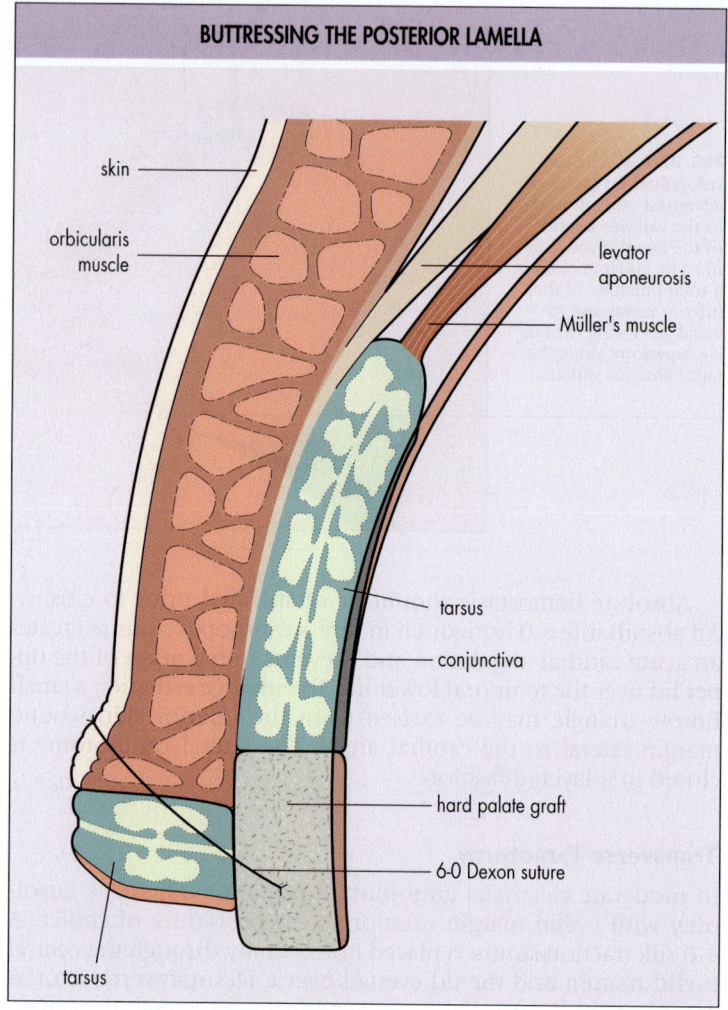

BUTTRESSING THE POSTERIOR LAMELLA

skin | orbicularis muscle | levator aponeurosis | Müller's muscle | tarsus | conjunctiva | hard palate graft | 6-0 Dexon suture | tarsus

FIG. 87-11 ■ Posterior lamella buttressing is accomplished through a hard palate graft. Graft bed preparation and marginal segment rotation are performed similarly to those for posterior tarsotomy.

chemical cautery, cellulose sponge, collagen sponge, periodontal putty, or a palatal stent.[50]

Eyelid Retraction

Postoperative eyelid retraction is usually the result of excessive horizontal tightening of the tarsus or excessive vertical advancement of the capsulopalpebral fascia. It is also important to ensure reattachment of the lateral tarsus to Whitnall's lateral orbital tubercle rather than the lateral raphe of the orbicularis complex. An excessively shortened tarsal strip should be resuspended from either the superior crus of the lateral canthal tendon or a periosteal strip elevated from the lateral orbital wall. When it is performed in the same surgical repair, the capsulopalpebral fascia should be advanced and reattached to the inferior tarsal border following the correction of horizontal laxity.

Exposure Keratopathy

Corneal epithelial damage can develop from exposed conjunctival sutures, lagophthalmos, and keratinized hard palate grafts. This risk is higher following upper lid entropion repair. Treatment includes ocular surface lubricants, collagen shields, bandage soft contact lens, early suture removal, and dermabrasion of the keratinized graft.

Postoperative mechanical lagophthalmos most commonly results from incorporation of the orbital septum into the capsulopalpebral advancement or skin closure—appreciation of the anatomic layers is necessary during wound closure. Treatment ranges from conservative observation to surgical exploration and release of the septum.

Granuloma Formation

Conjunctival granulomas may develop following manipulation or incision of the posterior lamella. Exuberant granulation tissue often develops as a result of chronic inflammation initiated by suture material or another surgical foreign body. Granulomas may resolve spontaneously but frequently necessitate treatment using topical or intralesional corticosteroids, cautery, excision, or removal of the inciting foreign body.

Symblepharon

Symblepharon results from tissue manipulation that allows apposition of two or more abraded epithelial surfaces. The conjunctiva is at risk for symblepharon development if not handled with care intraoperatively. Its occurrence can be reduced through the use of symblepharon rings, fornix reformation sutures, or topical and systemic immunomodulators.

Ptosis

Aponeurogenic ptosis can complicate the repair of cicatricial upper lid entropion. The posterior fibers of the levator aponeurosis attach to the inferior one third of the tarsal plate anterior surface. These fibers can be inadvertently disrupted during posterior tarsotomy with a resultant postoperative aponeurogenic ptosis.

Other Complications

Eyelash loss and eyelid necrosis can occur after entropion surgery and are most often due to vascular insufficiency of the marginal arcade. Patients who undergo transverse blepharotomy or repeated surgery are at particular risk. Tissue necrosis and atrophy are often segmental. The damaged segment can be excised and the defect closed directly or reconstructed using typical eyelid reconstructive techniques (see Chapter 94).

OUTCOMES

Appropriate patient evaluation and surgical procedure selection should result in the immediate correction of the eyelid malposition. Most patients report symptomatic relief as early as their first postoperative day. Except in cases of posterior lamellar foreshortening, the appropriate surgical management of entropion has a success rate of 97% or greater.[41] When tarsoconjunctival contraction is present, surgical success still exceeds 90%. An exception occurs in ocular cicatricial pemphigoid, where lower success is predicted.[23,45] Advances in the understanding of entropion have provided surgeons with improved, more reproducible, and longer lasting treatment options. A systematic approach to the evaluation and treatment of this condition ensures that patients will benefit from these therapeutic outcomes.

REFERENCES

1. Bick MW. Surgical management of orbital tarsal disparity. Arch Ophthalmol. 1966;75:386–9.
2. Wies FA. Spastic entropion. Trans Am Acad Ophthalmol Otolaryngol. 1955;59:503–5.
3. DeRoetth A. Mechanism of senile entropion. Trans Pacific Otoophthalmol Soc. 1963;44:173–7.
4. Jones LT, Reeh MJ, Tsujimura JK. Senile entropion. Am J Ophthalmol. 1963;55:463–9.
5. Jones LT, Reeh MJ, Wobig JL. Senile entropion: a new concept for correction. Am J Ophthalmol. 1972;74:327–9.
6. Hawes MJ, Dortzbach RK. The microscopic anatomy of the lower eyelid retractors. Arch Ophthalmol. 1982;100:1313–18.
7. Goldberg RA, Lufkin R, Farahani K, et al. Physiology of the lower eyelid retractors: tight linkage of the anterior capsulopalpebral fascia demonstrated using dynamic ultrafine surface coil MRI. Ophthalmol Plast Reconstr Surg. 1994;10:87–91.
8. Dalgleish R, Smith JLS. Mechanics and histology of senile entropion. Br J Ophthalmol. 1966;50:79–91.
9. Benger RS, Musch DC. A comparative study of eyelid parameters in involutional entropion. Ophthalmic Plast Reconstr Surg. 1989;5:281–7.
10. Tse DT, Anderson RL, Fratkin JD. Aponeurosis disinsertion in congenital entropion. Arch Ophthalmol. 1983;101:436–40.
11. Shore JW. Changes in lower eyelid resting position, movement, and tone with age. Am J Ophthalmol. 1985;99:415–23.
12. Liu D, Stasior OG. Lower eyelid laxity and ocular symptoms. Am J Ophthalmol. 1983;95:545–51.
13. Shorr N, Christenbury JD, Goldberg RA. Tarsoconjunctival grafts for upper eyelid cicatricial entropion. Ophthalmic Surg. 1988;19:316–20.
14. Baylis HI, Hamako C. Tarsal grafting for correction of cicatricial entropion. Ophthalmic Surg. 1979;10:42–8.
15. Silver B. The use of mucous membrane from the hard palate in the treatment of trichiasis and cicatricial entropion. Ophthalmic Plast Reconstr Surg. 1986;2:129–31.
16. Bartley GB, Kay PP. Posterior lamellar eyelid reconstruction with a hard palate mucosal graft. Am J Ophthalmol. 1989;107:609–12.
17. Schwab IR, Linberg JV, Gioia VM, et al. Foreshortening of the inferior conjunctival fornix associated with chronic glaucoma medications. Ophthalmology. 1992;99:197–202.
18. Kersten RC, Hammer BJ, Kulwin DR. The role of enophthalmos in involutional entropion. Ophthalmic Plast Reconstr Surg. 1997;13:195–8.
19. Goldberg RA, Christenbury JD, Shorr N. Medial entropion following orbital decompression for dysthyroid orbitopathy. Ophthalmic Plast Reconstr Surg. 1988;4:81–5.
20. Bashour M, Harvey J. Causes of involutional ectropion and entropion—age-related tarsal changes are the key. Ophthalmic Plast Reconstr Surg. 2000;16:126–30.
21. Tauber T, de la Maza MS, Foster CS. Systemic chemotherapy for ocular cicatricial pemphigoid. Cornea. 1991;10:185–95.
22. Shore JW, Foster CS, Westfall CT, Rubin PA. Results of buccal mucosal grafting for patients with medically controlled ocular cicatricial pemphigoid. Ophthalmology. 1992;99:383–5.
23. Kemp EG, Collin JRO. Surgical management of upper lid entropion. Br J Ophthalmol. 1986;70:575–9.
24. Raina J, Foster JA. Obesity as a cause of mechanical entropion. Am J Ophthalmol. 1996;122:123–5.
25. Bartley GB, Nerad JA, Kersten RC, Maquire LJ. Congenital entropion with intact lower eyelid retractor insertion. Am J Ophthalmol. 1991;112:437–41.
26. Carter SR, Chang J, Aguilar GL, et al. Involutional entropion and ectropion of the Asian lower eyelid. Ophthalmic Plast Reconstr Surg. 2000;16:45–9
27. Jordan R. The lower lid retractors in congenital entropion and epiblepharon. Ophthalmic Surg. 1993;24:494–6.
28. Noda S, Hayasaka S, Setogawa T. Epiblepharon with inverted eyelashes in Japanese children. I: Incidence and symptoms. Br J Ophthalmol. 1989;73:126–7.
29. Millman AL, Mannor GE, Putterman AM. Lid crease and capsulopalpebral fascia repair in congenital entropion and epiblepharon. Ophthalmic Surg. 1994;25:162–5.
30. Sires BS. Congenital horizontal tarsal kink: clinical characteristics from a large series. Ophthalmic Plast Reconstr Surg. 1999;15:355–9.
31. Wright M, Bell D, Scott C, Leatherbarrow B. Everting suture correction of lower lid involutional entropion. Br J Ophthalmol. 1999;83:1060–3.
32. Seiff SR, Kim M, Howes EL Jr. Histopathological evaluation of rotation sutures for involutional entropion. Br J Ophthalmol. 1989;73:628–32.
33. Quickert MH, Rathbun E. Suture repair of entropion. Arch Ophthalmol. 1971;85:304–5.
34. Steel DH, Hoh HB, Harrad RA, Collins CR. Botulinum toxin for the temporary treatment of involutional lower lid entropion: a clinical and morphological study. Eye. 1997;11:472–5.
35. McKay W, Morris R, Mushlin P. Sodium bicarbonate attenuates pain on skin infiltration with lidocaine, with or without epinephrine. Anesth Analg. 1987;66:572–4.
36. Stewart JH, Cole GW, Klein JA. Neutralized lidocaine with epinephrine for local anesthesia. J Dermatol Surg Oncol. 1989;10:1081–83.
37. Marshall BE, Longnecker DE. General anesthetics. In: Gilman AG, Rall TW, Nies AS, Taylor P, eds. Goodman and Gilman's pharmacological basis of therapeutics, 8th ed. New York: Pergamon Press; 1990:285–310.
38. Boboridis K, Bunce C, Rose GE. A comparative study of two procedures for repair of involutional lower lid entropion. Ophthalmology. 2000;107:959–61.
39. Nowinski TS. Orbicularis oculi muscle extirpation in a combined procedure for involutional entropion. Ophthalmology. 1991;98:1250–6.
40. Jordan DR. Ectropion following entropion surgery; an unhappy patient and physician. Ophthalmic Plast Reconstr Surg. 1992;8:41–6.
41. Dresner SC, Karesh JW. Transconjunctival entropion repair. Arch Ophthalmol. 1993;111:1144–8.
42. Cook T, Lucarelli MJ, Lemke BN, Dortzbach RK. Primary and secondary transconjunctival involutional entropion repair. Ophthalmology. 2001;108:989–93.
43. Elder MJ, Dart JK, Collin R. Inferior retractor plication surgery for lower lid entropion with trichiasis in ocular cicatricial pemphigoid. Br J Ophthalmol. 1995;79:1003–6.
44. Mauriello JA, Lopresti-Solis AE, DeRose DA, et al. Conjunctival scarring after eyelid surgery as first sign of ocular cicatricial pemphigoid. Ophthalmic Plast Reconstr Surg. 1994;10:142–5.
45. Kersten RC, Kleiner FP, Kulwin DR. Tarsotomy for the treatment of cicatricial entropion with trichiasis. Arch Ophthalmol. 1992;110:714–17.
46. Al-Rajhi AA, Hidayat A, Nasr A, al-Faran M. The histopathology and the mechanism of entropion in patients with trachoma. Ophthalmology. 1993;100:1293–6.
47. Jordan DR, McDonald H, Anderson RL. Irradiated homologous aorta in eyelid reconstruction. Part II: Human data. Ophthalmic Plast Reconstr Surg. 1994;10:227–33.
48. Levin PS, Dutton JJ. Polytef (polytetrafluoroethylene) alloplastic grafts as a substitute for mucous membrane. Arch Ophthalmol. 1990;108:282–5.
49. Matsuo K, Hirose T. The use of conchal cartilage graft in involutional entropion. Plast Reconstr Surg. 1990;86:968–70.
50. Mauriello JA, Wasserman B, Allee S, Robinson L. Molded acrylic mouthguard to control bleeding at the hard palate graft site after eyelid reconstruction. Am J Ophthalmol. 1992;113:342–4.

CHAPTER 88

Ectropion

FIONA O. ROBINSON • J. RICHARD O. COLLIN

DEFINITION
- Ectropion is an abnormal eversion of the eyelid margin away from the eye.

KEY FEATURES
- The eyelid margin and lash drive are turned away from the cornea.
- The conjunctival surface is exposed, sometimes resulting in keratinization of the epithelium.
- Corneal exposure results in foreign body sensation, corneal dryness, and occasionally ulceration.

ASSOCIATED FEATURES
- Photophobia
- Epiphora
- Conjunctival infection
- Decreased vision
- Ocular surface pain

INTRODUCTION

Ectropion, or eversion of the eyelid, is a common lid malposition frequently seen in clinical practice. It has various causes and may be broadly classified as follows:
- Congenital ectropion—congenital ectropion is rare and is due to a shortage of skin in the eyelids. It most commonly is seen in Down's syndrome, in which it may affect all four lids. It is also seen in blepharophimosis syndrome and can be idiopathic. If corneal exposure is mild, treatment with topical lubricants may be adequate. In more severe cases, skin grafting is necessary to avoid permanent corneal scarring and amblyopia. It is often a temptation to treat the corneal exposure with a simple lateral tarsorrhaphy, but this causes an inflammatory reaction, does not control the exposure, and so should not be attempted. If a shortage of skin exists, it must be replaced. However, skin grafting should be avoided in very young children, if possible, as postoperative scars are unattractive when they develop at an early age.
- Acquired ectropion—involutional, cicatricial, mechanical, paralytic; by far the most common
  — Involutional ectropion, in which aging changes result in a generalized laxity of lower lid structures. Treatment depends on the anatomical defect that predominates and on the region of the lid that shows maximum laxity. The first sign of lower lid ectropion is often punctal eversion, which prevents tears from reaching the inferior canaliculus and may cause epiphora. As the ectropion progresses exposure causes secondary inflammatory changes in the conjunctiva and thickening of the tarsus, which further worsens the ectropion. Marked ectropion may result in lagophthalmos with resultant corneal exposure and, in extreme cases, corneal ulceration. Treatment of the ectropion in the early stages should avoid such late complications.
  — Cicatricial ectropion is caused by a vertical shortening of the anterior lamella of the lower lid. The onset may be gradual, as seen with many skin diseases, or sudden when due to surgery, trauma, or acute allergic skin reactions. It often is associated with horizontal lid laxity. If the cicatricial changes are mild, correction of the horizontal component alone may suffice. If both elements are significant, the cicatricial changes should be corrected first. Whenever possible, the original cause (e.g., cicatricial skin diseases) should be treated medically. When the scarring is permanent and the cicatricial element is generalized, a full-thickness skin graft or pedicle transposition flap is necessary to correct the deformity. A Z-plasty corrects any localized scar.
  — Mechanical ectropion results from mass lesions that displace the lid margin away from the globe. Causes include tumors, scars, conjunctival cysts, and edema. Treatment should be directed at the primary cause—it should include surgery only if residual ectropion remains following the initial treatment.
  — Paralytic ectropion occurs in facial palsy. It results from loss of muscle tone and weakening of orbicularis muscle contraction. If the paresis is temporary, surgical treatment is usually not indicated. Topical lubrication of the eye is all that is needed until recovery is complete. If the palsy is permanent, surgery is usually necessary. In younger patients who have better elasticity and lid tone, loss of orbicularis function may result in only mild ectropion. Older patients who already have some lower lid laxity prior to the facial palsy may develop a marked ectropion. The ectropion is usually most severe in the region of the medial canthal tendon, which is the tendon of insertion of the orbicularis muscle. The choice of surgical procedure to correct paralytic ectropion depends not only on the extent and area of lid affected but also on the presence of other ocular sequelae, including corneal exposure, epiphora, and poor cosmesis. Procedures should be carefully individualized depending on the degree of anatomical deformity and lid dysfunction. With good lid elasticity, medial and/or lateral canthal support may be sufficient. If lid laxity is also present, a horizontal tightening procedure should be performed, but care must be taken not to overtighten the lid, which can increase lower lid retraction.

HISTORICAL REVIEW

In 1812 Sir William Adams[1] described a new operation for the cure of ectropion, which consisted of a V-shaped shortening at the lateral canthus, closed with one suture. In 1831 Von Ammon[2] excised a wedge of tissue from the center of the lid to cure the defect, later moving the excision toward the lateral canthus. The classical Kuhnt[3] (1883) and Symanowski[4] (1870) procedure has remained popular since its conception, albeit with various alterations over the years. In the past century, many modifications and new techniques were developed for the treatment of ectropion.

More recently, the importance of aiming the surgical correction at the major underlying anatomical defect or defects has been realized. The choice of operation depends on the findings at preoperative evaluation.[5]

PREOPERATIVE EVALUATION AND DIAGNOSTIC APPROACH

Ectropion may be caused or exacerbated by one or more anatomical defects of the eyelid structures. A thorough preoperative evaluation of these separate elements is essential because treatment needs to be directed at the predominant defect(s). Hence, more than one surgical procedure may be necessary to correct fully the malpositioned lid.

A full ocular history should be taken prior to examination of the malpositioned lid. The surgeon should ask specifically about a history of facial palsy, lid trauma, and previous lid surgery. Specific examination procedures should include tests for horizontal and vertical lid laxity, integrity of the canthal tendons, orbicularis muscle tone, and changes in the overlying lid skin.

Eyelid Laxity

To test for eyelid laxity the lower lid is pulled away from the globe. A distance of more than 10mm between the lower lid and globe is abnormal and confirms horizontal laxity. Alternatively, the lid is gently pulled downward, away from the globe, and upon release of the lid the speed of return back to its original position is observed. In the normal lid, the lid snaps back snugly into position almost immediately. If laxity exists, the lid recoils slowly or only with the help of a few blinks. The position of maximum lid laxity (i.e., medial, lateral, or generalized) should be noted. Once laxity is established, the specific anatomical cause, that is, lax canthal tendon(s) or generalized tarsal redundancy, must be determined.

Medial Canthal Tendon Laxity

The lid is pulled laterally and the lateral excursion of the inferior punctum measured. Normally, the punctum should lie just lateral to the caruncle at rest and should not be displaced more than 1–2mm with lateral lid traction. If lid laxity is severe, the punctum may move to lie below the pupil. It is unusual to find medial canthal tendon laxity without also finding horizontal lid laxity. If medial canthal tendon laxity and horizontal lid laxity exist together, the medial canthal tendon is tightened first and the horizontal element should be reassessed subsequently.

Lateral Canthal Tendon Laxity

A history of watering that occurs mainly from the lateral aspect of the lower lid suggests lateral lid laxity. The lateral canthal angle should first be evaluated with the lid at rest. It should have an acute angular contour and lie 1–2mm medial to the lateral orbital rim (palpate with your finger). If the canthus has a rounded appearance, marked laxity is present. The lateral part of the lid is then pulled medially and the movement of the lateral canthal angle assessed. In normal lids the canthal angle should move no more than 1–2mm.

Position of the Lacrimal Puncta

The inferior lacrimal punctum should lie just lateral to the caruncle at rest and directly below the superior punctum (see Chapter 82). In a normal lid, the inferior punctum is directed posteriorly against the globe and should not be visible without pulling the lid downward. In this position, the punctum dips into the lacus lacrimalis (tear lake). Direction of the punctum away from the globe is often the earliest sign of medial lid ectropion. Relative punctal stenosis or even frank occlusion may

be seen with long-standing ectropion. Note that even in patients who have ectropion, a complaint of epiphora demands evaluation of the lacrimal drainage system to rule out concomitant nasolacrimal system obstruction (see Chapter 98).

Cicatricial Skin Changes

Vertical shortening of the skin of the lower lid may lead to eversion of the lid margin. A localized vertical contraction from scarring is usually immediately obvious. More subtle causes of skin shortening are more difficult to demonstrate. Vertical skin shortage is evaluated by gently pushing the lid back into its correct position. This is impossible to accomplish if skin deficiency is severe. In milder cases one simply sees vertical tension lines in the eyelid skin. Manual elevation of the cheek skin typically corrects the ectropion, as tension on the lid is reduced. Alternatively, ask the patient to look up and at the same time to open his or her mouth widely. If a shortage of skin exists, the lower lid immediately moves downward and everts further as the skin is pulled more tightly.

Cicatricial changes are often accompanied by horizontal lid laxity, and both may require correction. In such cases, the cicatricial restriction should always be freed by dissection first, then the other elements(s) corrected. The cicatricial element is then repaired as discussed in the following.

Orbicularis Muscle Weakness

This is usually due to a complete or partial facial nerve palsy. Orbicularis muscle weakness is evaluated during forced eyelid closure. Lagophthalmos and reduced force of contraction demonstrate muscle weakness. Other signs of facial nerve palsy, such as brow ptosis, loss of forehead wrinkles, and a mouth droop, should also be noted. Remember that facial palsy may be bilateral.

Lid Masses

Mass lesions on the lid, such as tumors or cysts, may result in a mechanical ectropion, where the lid margin is physically displaced away from the globe. Such lesions are usually evident on initial inspection. The conjunctival surface and deep fornices should be examined in all cases of ectropion.

Inferior Lid Retractor Laxity

A mild degree of lower lid retractor laxity is commonly associated with horizontal lid laxity and rarely occurs alone. It can present as a tarsal or marginal ectropion.[6] In this condition the lid is completely everted with the tarsal plate turned upside down. It often becomes manifest only when other elements have been corrected.

The inferior movement of the lower lid in downgaze is reduced and the inferior fornix is deeper than usual due to laxity or loss of retractor attachment in this area. The resting lower lid position may be raised, and a horizontal infratarsal red band may appear on the conjunctival surface that corresponds to the defect in the retractors. This condition is said to be due to the orbicularis muscle now being directly visible through the conjunctiva. The edge of the retractors may be seen directly below this band.

Treatment requires reinsertion of the lower lid retractors into the inferior edge of the tarsal plate (Box 88-1).[7]

ALTERNATIVES TO SURGERY

No completely satisfactory nonsurgical approaches exist in the management of symptomatic ectropion. When the condition is mild, the patient may experience only mild irritation from conjunctival exposure, usually associated with epiphora and perhaps a foreign body sensation from corneal drying. Artificial tears during the day and ointments at night usually ameliorate

Preoperative Evaluation of Ectropion

Full ocular history
General ocular examination
Examination of specific eyelid changes:
- Lid laxity: horizontal lid laxity
                     medial canthal tendon laxity
                     lateral canthal tendon laxity
- Position of punctum
- Cicatricial skin changes
- Orbicularis weakness
- Lid masses
- Inferior lid retractor laxity or disinsertion

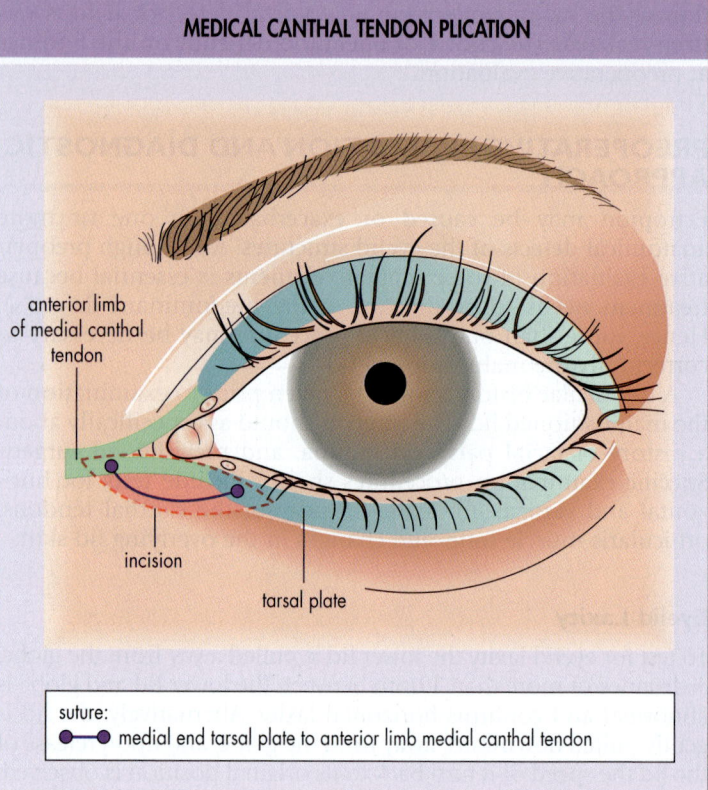

MEDICAL CANTHAL TENDON PLICATION

anterior limb
of medial canthal
tendon

incision

tarsal plate

suture:
medial end tarsal plate to anterior limb medial canthal tendon

FIG. 88-1 ■ Plication of the anterior limb of the medial canthal tendon.

the symptoms. When the lid malposition is so severe that corneal breakdown results, even aggressive medical management may not be adequate.

ANESTHESIA

Local infiltrative anesthesia may be used in almost all types of ectropion correction. It is often preferable to give a general anesthetic if a postauricular skin graft is to be harvested or if the patient is a child. For transcutaneous approaches, a subcutaneous injection of local anesthetic is adequate. However, for any surgery that involves the posterior lamella, a subconjunctival injection may be needed.

GENERAL TECHNIQUES

Correction of lower lid ectropion is directed toward the anatomical cause. When the primary defect is horizontal laxity, lid shortening (either tarsal or canthal tendon) should be the treatment of choice. When vertical laxity is responsible, shortening or reattachment of the lower lid retractor is necessary. In many cases, some degree of each condition is present and multiple procedures are required.

In cases of cicatricial ectropion, disparity exists in the lengths of the anterior and posterior lamellae; specifically, a shortage of skin occurs. When the condition is mild, simple horizontal lid tightening may prove beneficial. But with more significant cicatricial changes, lengthening of the anterior lamella must be achieved by tissue rearrangement, local flaps, or skin grafts.

SPECIFIC TECHNIQUES

Plication of the Anterior Limb of the Medial Canthal Tendon

This procedure is most often performed in patients who have involutional ectropion and in those with facial palsy. It is indicated for mild medial canthal tendon laxity (see tendon evaluation earlier), without displacement of the canthal angle at rest. This operation is rarely performed alone, usually being done in conjunction with a lateral horizontal lid-shortening procedure. The aim of surgery is to give support to the medial canthal tendon.

A wire probe is placed into the inferior canaliculus to mark its precise location. This should remain in place throughout the procedure. A horizontal skin incision is made below the canaliculus, starting at the medial canthus and extending to below the inferior punctum (Fig. 88-1). The inferior border of the medial canthal tendon and the medial end of the tarsus are exposed beneath the orbicularis muscle. A 5-0 nonabsorbable suture is passed through the medial edge of the tarsal plate and then through the anterior limb of the medial canthal tendon.

The suture is tightened sufficiently to stabilize the canthal angle in its normal position. It should not be overtightened, as this results in anterior displacement of the lid margin as well as wrin-

kling of the skin and underlying canaliculus. The skin incision is closed with 6-0 silk sutures, which are removed after 5 days.

Medial Canthal Resection

This is the procedure of choice when marked medial canthal tendon laxity is present that results in dystopia of the medial canthal angle at rest.[8] This may be associated with many forms of ectropion but is seen most commonly with involutional changes.

The procedure involves resection of the medial canthal structures combined with horizontal lid shortening. The posterior limb of the medial canthal tendon is reconstructed with a permanent suture, and the cut inferior canaliculus is marsupialized into the conjunctival sac of the lower fornix.[9] This gives good long-term results with relief of epiphora in the majority of patients.

A vertical full-thickness cut is made through the lower lid just lateral to the caruncle to include the canthal tendon and canaliculus (Fig. 88-2). The canaliculus is preserved by placing a probe into it prior to the cut and moving the scissors laterally after the initial vertical incision is made. The conjunctival incision is continued onto the bulbar surface, posterior to the plica. It may be necessary to resect the lateral half of the caruncle if it is especially prominent. This plane is followed back along the medial orbital wall with blunt-ended scissors until the posterior lacrimal crest is encountered. The exposure is improved by the use of two small malleable retractors. Each half-circle needle of a double-armed 5-0 nonabsorbable suture is passed through the periosteum of the posterior lacrimal crest, one at the level of the medial canthal tendon and one 2mm higher on the medial orbital wall. The cut lateral part of the lid is pulled toward the posterior lacrimal crest and an appropriate amount of lid is resected. The two ends of the fixation suture are passed through the cut edge of the tarsal plate. Before tying, the exposed segment of canaliculus on the medial side of the lid incision is cut longitudinally to form anterior and posterior flaps, and the anterior flap is sutured to the posterior edge of the tarsus with one or two 8-0 absorbable sutures. The fixation suture is tied to re-

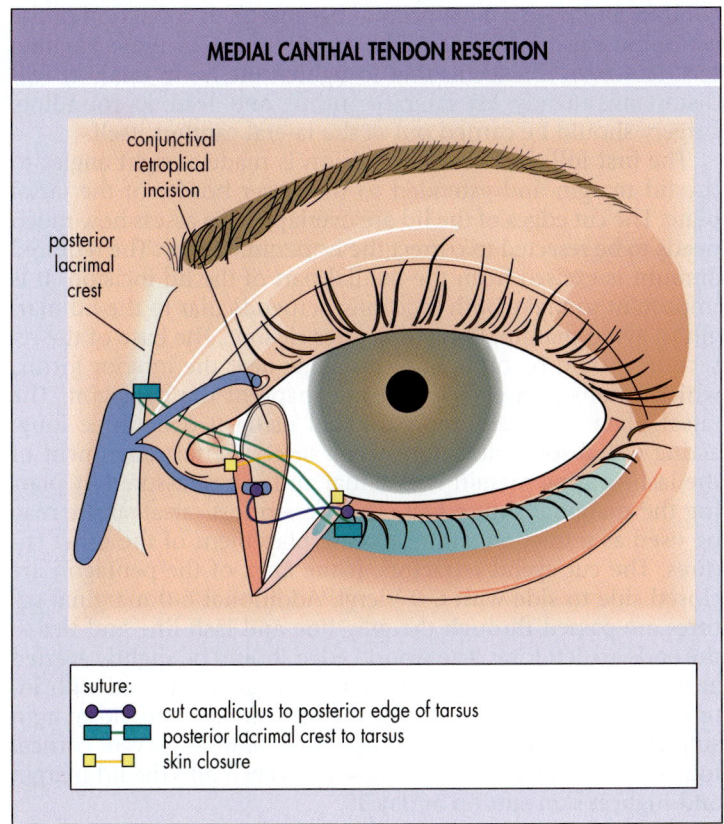

MEDIAL CANTHAL TENDON RESECTION

conjunctival
retroplical
incision

posterior
lacrimal
crest

suture:
● — cut canaliculus to posterior edge of tarsus
■ — posterior lacrimal crest to tarsus
□ — skin closure

FIG. 88-2 ▐▌ Medial canthal tendon resection, with posterior fixation and canalicular repair.

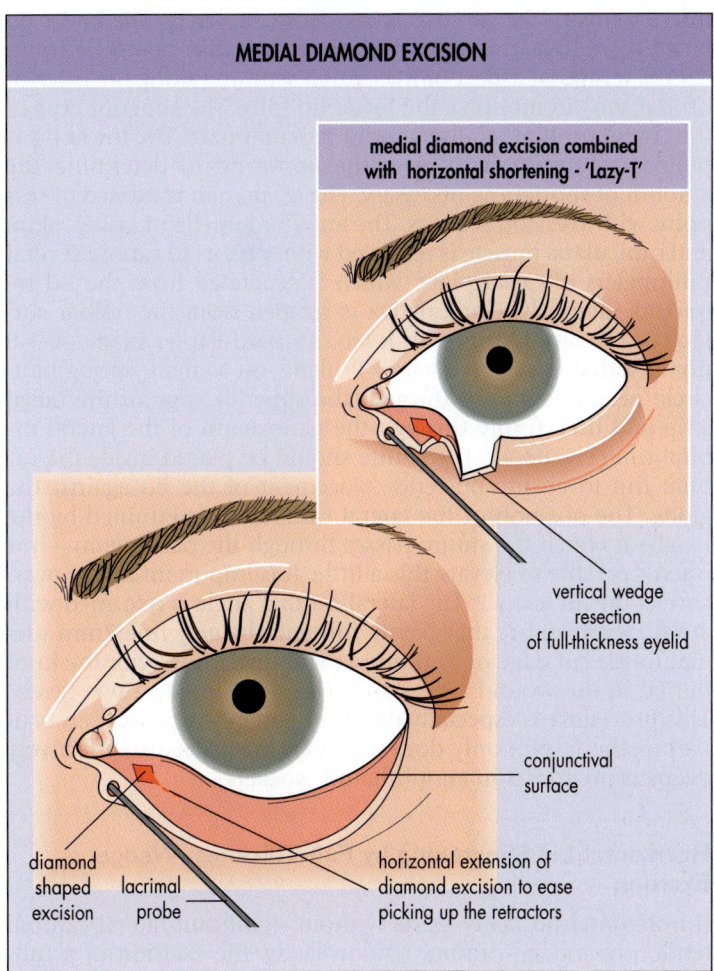

MEDIAL DIAMOND EXCISION

medial diamond excision combined
with horizontal shortening - 'Lazy-T'

vertical wedge
resection
of full-thickness eyelid

conjunctival
surface

diamond
shaped
excision

lacrimal
probe

horizontal extension of
diamond excision to ease
picking up the retractors

FIG. 88-3 ▐▌ **Medial diamond excision.** Inset shows the same procedure combined with a horizontal lid shortening procedure—the lazy-T procedure.

form the medial canthal angle. The lid margin and skin are reapproximated with 6-0 silk.

Excision of a Diamond of Tarsoconjunctiva

If punctal eversion is present but no significant horizontal lid laxity exists and the medial canthal tendon is normal, a vertical shortening of the posterior lamella corrects localized medial lid ectropion. This procedure also includes shortening of the medial lid retractors and can be used in cases of mild involutional ectropion or with mild cicatricial changes.[10]

A canalicular probe is passed into the inferior canaliculus. A diamond-shaped segment of tarsus and conjunctiva is resected directly below the punctum (Fig. 88-3). Care should be taken to place the edge of the diamond at least 2mm below the lid margin to avoid entering the canalicular ampulla when the inverting suture is placed. One arm of a double-armed 6-0 absorbable suture is passed through the superior apex of the diamond from the conjunctival surface to emerge within the wound. The other end of the suture is passed through the conjunctiva and lower lid retractors at the inferior apex of the diamond and again emerges within the wound. As the suture is tied, the medial lid margin and punctum are rotated inward. The punctal inversion should be overdone at the time of surgery as the lid will relax outward postoperatively. If the inversion is not sufficient, an inverting suture can be placed. For this, a double-armed 4-0 catgut mattress suture is passed from the conjunctiva immediately below the closed wound, anteriorly and somewhat downward through orbicularis and skin, and tied over a bolster. This suture advances the anterior lamella upward and thus enhances the correction.

Medial Diamond Excision Plus Horizontal Lid Shortening ("Lazy-T")

This procedure was first described by Byron Smith[11] and remains the treatment of choice for medial ectropion with punctal eversion associated with predominantly medial horizontal lid laxity.

A full-thickness incision is made through the lid margin 4mm lateral to the punctum. The cut is extended inferiorly to below the inferior tarsal edge. The amount of redundant lid to be resected is assessed by overlapping the cut edges, and this amount is excised as a full-thickness pentagon lateral to the first incision (Fig. 88-3). In most cases, a resection of 5mm or less is sufficient. As described previously for medial diamond excision, a diamond of tarsus and conjunctiva is excised, but the closing suture is not tied. The vertical lid defect is repaired first as described for horizontal lid shortening subsequently. Finally, the diamond is closed by tying the preplaced suture.

Lateral Tarsal Strip Procedure

The lateral canthal sling was first described by Tenzel[12] in 1969. Various modifications have been made since then, the most well known being the lateral tarsal strip procedure.[13] This procedure can be used to correct both lateral canthal tendon laxity and generalized horizontal lid laxity.

The lid is tightened at the lateral canthus and is shortened by the amount necessary to produce snug apposition of lid and globe. In addition to tightening, the canthal angle can be elevated, which may be necessary to aid tear drainage. This is very effective in the correction of ectropion from many causes and is cosmetically useful in the restoration of a normal canthal configuration.

The area of the lateral canthus is infiltrated with local anesthetic down to the orbital rim and along the periorbita just inside the rim. A lateral canthotomy is performed by dividing the lateral canthal tendon horizontally from the canthal angle to the lateral orbital rim. A blunt dissection is carried through the orbicularis to expose periosteum of the orbital rim. The lower lid is pulled upward and medially to place it under tension, and the inferior crus of the canthus is divided completely. The lower lid is felt to yield as the tendon is released. It may be necessary to cut the temporal aspect of the orbital septum (along the inferior orbital rim) to mobilize the lower lid fully. The superior crus of the lateral canthal tendon should remain intact. The lower lid is pulled up and laterally over the upper lid to determine the amount of shortening necessary. The lid margin is excised to this point with Westcott scissors. The anterior lamella of lashes, skin, and orbicularis muscle is removed with scissors to expose several millimeters of tarsal plate, which is separated from the lid retractors inferiorly. Conjunctiva is scraped from the bulbar surface of the tarsal strip with a No. 15 Bard-Parker blade. A 5-0 nonabsorbable suture, such as Prolene, on a small, strong half-circle needle is passed through the superior edge of the tarsal strip and then firmly through the periosteum of the lateral orbital rim (Fig. 88-4). The suture should be placed inside the orbital rim to ensure posterior placement of the lid against the globe. The position of the lateral canthus is determined by the height at which the suture passes through the periosteum—it is often desirable to elevate this a little. It is important not to overcorrect the lid laxity.[14] The lateral canthal angle is reformed with a 6-0 Dexon suture that passes through the gray line 2mm medial to the cut edge of both upper and lower lids, with the knot buried in the wound. The skin incision is closed in two layers. This procedure is especially useful in patients who wear an ocular prosthesis. Not only does it tighten the lid, it also effectively deepens the fornix in anophthalmic sockets.

Horizontal Lid Shortening by Full-Thickness Wedge Excision

If horizontal lid laxity exists without significant lateral canthal tendon or medial canthal tendon laxity, the excision of a full-thickness pentagon of lid often corrects the ectropion completely. It is a simple procedure that can be performed at any point on the lower lid, although the preferred site is usually in the lateral third. It is especially useful if the lateral canthal angle

contour and position are normal because then correction of the ectropion can be achieved with no alteration of these parameters. However, if it seems that to tighten the lid in this way will distort an already lax lateral canthus and lead to rounding, surgery should be carried out at the lateral canthus itself.

The first full-thickness lid incision is made at right angles to the lid margin and extended to the lower border of the tarsal plate. The cut edges of the lid are overlapped to assess how much needs to be resected to correct the horizontal laxity. The required amount is excised from the medial part of the lid incision. It is important to make both incisions perpendicular to the lid margin to avoid marginal notching after closure. The base of the resection should be brought to an angle near the inferior fornix, which results in a defect with the shape of the pentagon. The tarsal plate edges are approximated using two or three long-acting 6-0 absorbable sutures (Fig. 88-5). Perfect alignment of the lash-bearing margin is essential and is best assured by placing the marginal suture first. This uppermost tarsal suture may be used as a traction suture to ease placement of the other sutures. The cut eyelid retractors at the apex of the pentagon are closed side to side with 6-0 Vicryl. Additional 6-0 marginal sutures are passed through the gray line and lash line and tied—the ends are left long. The wound edge should be slightly everted at this stage to avoid notching later. The skin is closed with interrupted 6-0 silk sutures, with the long ends of the lid margin sutures incorporated into the uppermost knot to prevent corneal touch. The skin sutures are removed at day 5 and the lid margin and highest skin sutures at day 10.

Horizontal Lid Shortening Plus Blepharoplasty (Kuhnt-Symanowski Procedure)

This procedure is useful when there is an excess of lower lid skin in addition to generalized horizontal lid laxity. It is used primarily in cases of involutional ectropion.

A subciliary incision is cut through skin 2mm below the lashes, from the punctum to the lateral canthal angle. At the lat-

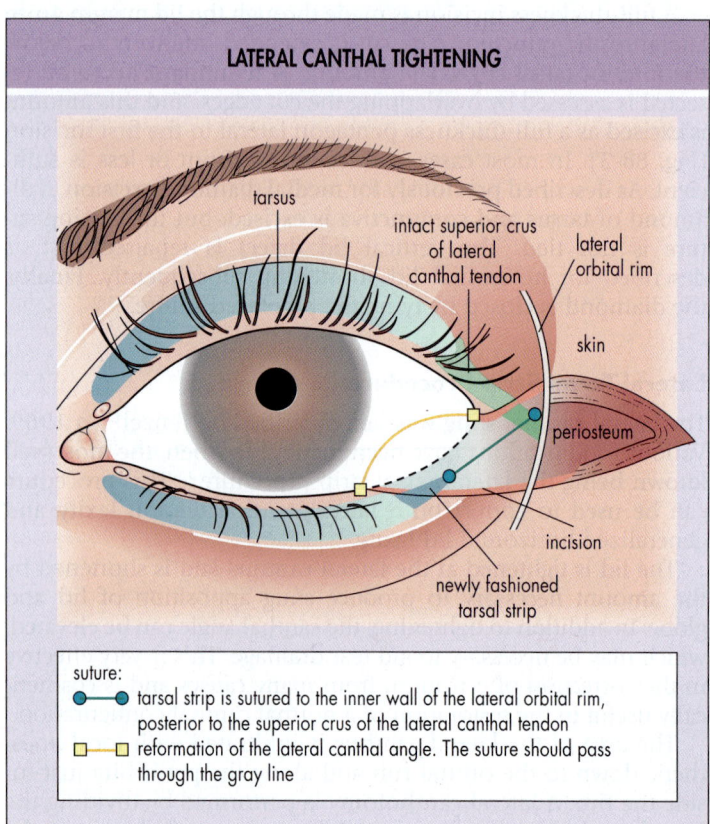

FIG. 88-4 ▮ Tightening of the lateral canthal tendon using the lateral tarsal strip procedure.

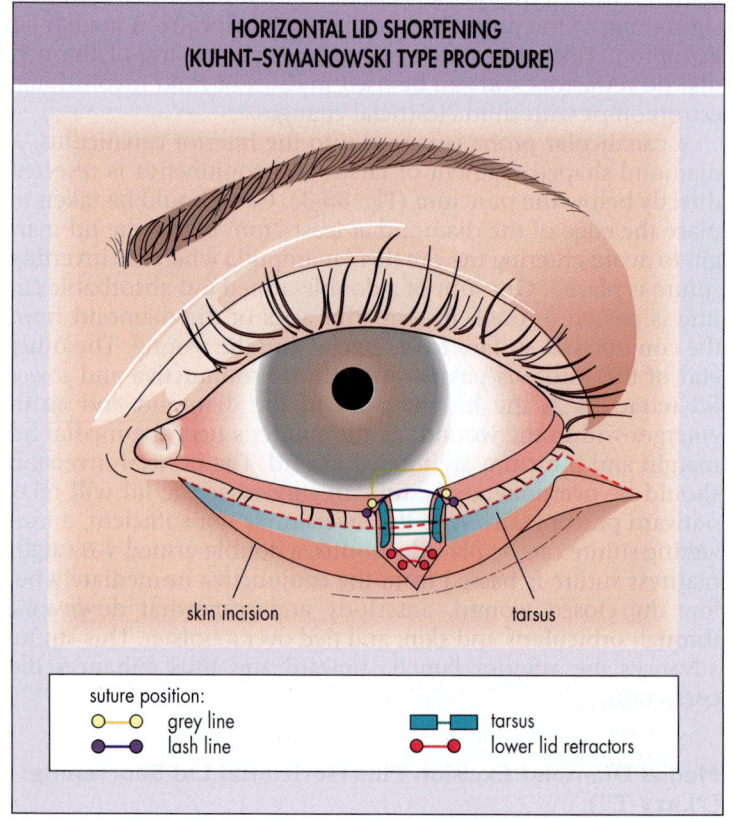

FIG. 88-5 ▮ Horizontal lid shortening with a full-thickness wedge resection combined with a blepharoplasty excision of redundant skin. (Modified Kuhnt-Symanowski procedure.)

eral canthus the incision is continued obliquely downward in a natural skin crease for a distance of 10mm (Fig. 88-5), and the skin flap is undermined to the level of the orbital rim. A full-thickness pentagonal wedge excision is cut from posterior lamella at the lateral portion of the lid and repaired as described previously. The redundant skin flap is pulled laterally and the excess is cut as a triangle, as for a standard lower lid blepharoplasty (see Chapter 89). The subciliary skin incision is closed with a continuous 6-0 nylon suture and the lateral extension with interrupted 6-0 sutures.

Z-Plasty

A Z-plasty is a flap rearrangement procedure used to correct skin shortening due to a focal linear scar. The transposition of two flaps of skin cut in a defined configuration increases the length of the scar line at the expense of shortening skin at right angles to it. The Z-plasty may have to be combined with other procedures to correct ectropion effectively.[15]

The edges of the scar are marked, but if the lid margin is involved and notched it should be excised using a pentagonal full-thickness resection before the Z-plasty is performed. A 4-0 nylon traction suture is placed across the lid margin in the line of the scar. The planned Z-shaped incision is fashioned by drawing a line from each end of the scar line to form a 60° angle with it (see Fig. 88-6). Each of these lines should be equal in length to the scar line itself. If the scar is especially long, two or more Zs may be marked in tandem along its length. The skin flaps are cut and extensively undermined beneath the surrounding tissue. Any obvious scar tissue should be excised. The triangular skin flaps are transposed and closed with 6-0 sutures. Upward traction should be maintained on the lid for 48 hours using the marginal suture placed previously.

Pedicle Transposition Flap

If cicatricial changes in the lid are mild, the transposition of a pedicle of skin from the upper lid to the lower lid corrects the ectropion. This may be performed using the medial or lateral can-

thus (or both) as the flap base, depending on the position of greatest skin shortage. The pedicle transposition flap provides additional skin as well as support for the lower lid. A moderate excess of skin must be present in the upper lid to allow the transposition.

The skin pedicle is marked on the upper lid and a subciliary incision of equal length is marked along the lower lid area into which the flap is to be transposed (Fig. 88-7). In the upper lid the flap should straddle the skin crease if the crease is to remain in the same position postoperatively. The lower border of the flap base should join the subciliary incision just above the lateral canthal angle, and the upper border should lie above and lateral to this. If the base of the flap lies below the lateral canthal angle, it will not support the lower lid. The flap should be a little wider than the vertical deficit to be corrected. The lower lid incision is cut, the skin dissected, and scar tissue excised until the ectropion is fully corrected. The transposition flap is cut and freed from the upper lid and rotated into the lower lid defect. The flap is shortened as necessary to give adequate support to the canthal angle. All skin incisions are closed with 6-0 sutures. Owing to the length of the flap and its narrow width, the distal part should be treated as a free graft and a pressure dressing should be applied for 24 hours. All sutures are removed at day 5.

Skin Graft

If a cicatricial ectropion is caused by diffuse skin shortage, the skin area must be increased. For the lower lid, a full-thickness skin graft is taken from the postauricular area (most commonly), upper lid, supraclavicular fossa, or inner arm.

The lower lid host site is prepared by placing two 4-0 nylon traction sutures through the lid margin. A horizontal incision is cut 2–3mm below the lashes, along the area of skin shortage. It is best to extend the incision beyond the limits of the scarred area and above the canthi to allow for postoperative graft shrinkage (the theory is that if postoperative contraction occurs, it will tend to pull the lower lid up due to support at the canthal areas). The skin is undermined and scar tissue is resected to whatever depth is necessary to relieve the ectropion completely

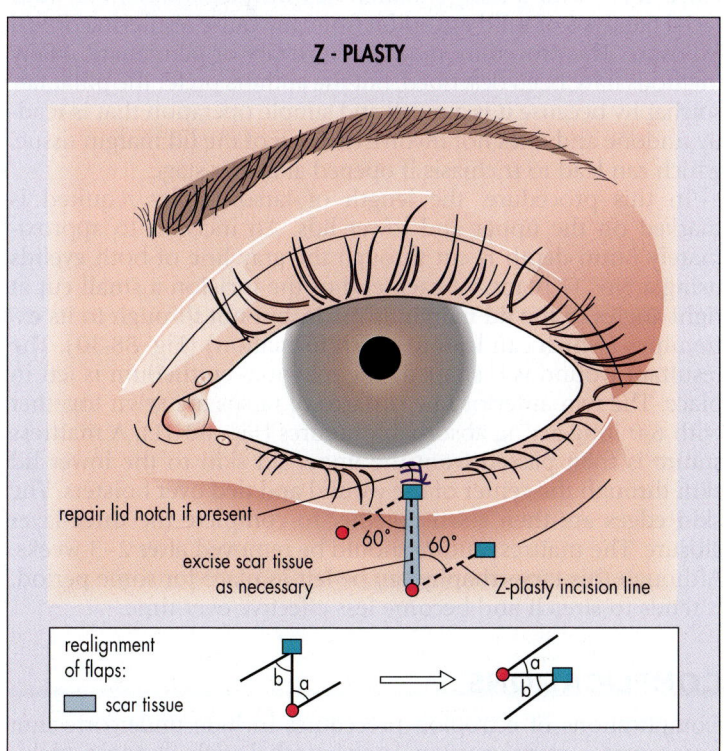

FIG. 88-6 ▐▌ Z-plasty procedure for lengthening focal cicatricial scarring. Flaps *a* and *b* are transposed to lengthen the scar line.

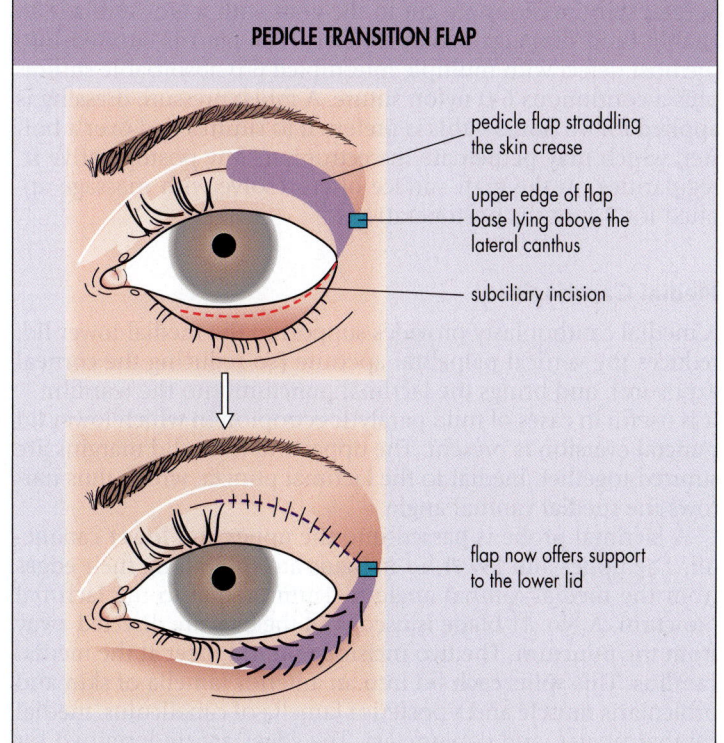

FIG. 88-7 ▐▌ Pedicle transposition flap of skin and muscle from upper lid to lower lid for cicatricial ectropion.

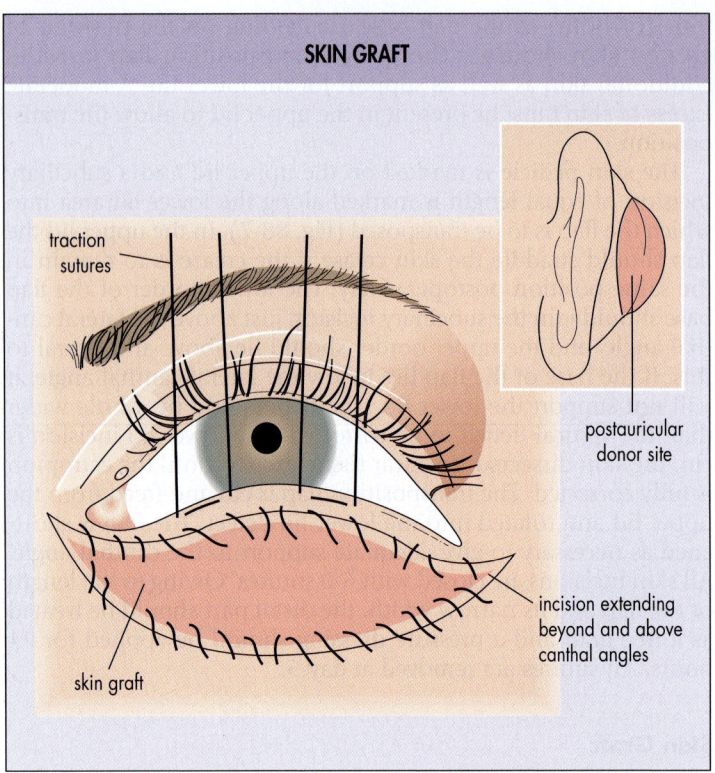

FIG. 88-8 ■ Full-thickness skin graft for lower lid cicatricial ectropion. Inset shows the retroauricular donor site.

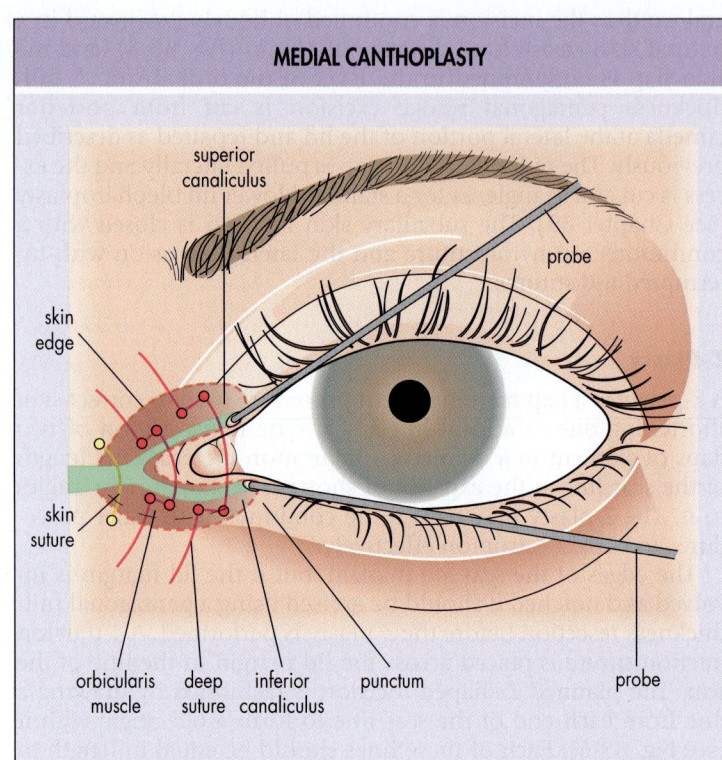

FIG. 88-9 ■ Medial canthoplasty shortens the palpebral fissure.

and return the eyelid to its normal position. Adequate hemostasis is essential to avoid hematoma formation under the graft. The traction sutures exaggerate the defect. A template of the lower lid defect is used to mark the donor site. The donor graft should be marked slightly larger than the defect to allow for shrinkage. If the retroauricular area is used as the donor site, equal amounts of skin are removed from either side of the postauricular crease (Fig. 88-8). The donor defect is repaired with a continuous 4-0 nylon suture and covered with a light dressing for 24 hours. The sutures are removed at day 10. Subcutaneous tissue is dissected from the donor skin graft. Several stab incisions are cut in the graft with a No. 11 blade to enable fluid drainage postoperatively. The graft is sutured into the host defect with multiple interrupted 6-0 absorbable sutures plus a continuous 6-0 nylon suture. A moist pressure dressing is applied for 48 hours—this is preferred to sutures tied over a bolster, which may perpetuate the ectropion. Any postoperative irregularities on the graft surface often resolve with massage applied for 3 months postoperatively.

Medial Canthoplasty

A medial canthoplasty provides support to the medial lower lid, reduces the vertical palpebral aperture (so reducing the corneal exposure), and brings the lacrimal punctum into the tear film.[16] It is useful in cases of mild paralytic ectropion in which lower lid punctal eversion is present. The upper and lower lid margins are sutured together, medial to the lacrimal puncta, which thus narrows the medial canthal angle.

A lacrimal probe is passed into the upper and lower canaliculi. The upper and lower lid margins are split along their edges from the medial canthal angle to 1mm medial to the lacrimal punctum. A No. 11 blade is used, and the cuts are directed away from the punctum. The two incisions should meet at the medial canthus. This splits each lid into an anterior lamella of skin and orbicularis muscle and a posterior lamella of canaliculus, medial canthal tissues, and conjunctiva. The edges are undermined for 5mm using sharp-pointed scissors.

The orbicularis muscles just anterior to the inferior canaliculus and just above the superior canaliculus are approximated

with two 6-0 long-acting absorbable sutures (Fig. 88-9). On tying the sutures, the two canaliculi are brought together and rotated inward so that the puncta become inverted. The skin edges are closed after any excess of skin has been excised. Sutures are removed at day 5.

Lateral Tarsorrhaphy

Lateral tarsorrhaphy is a procedure used to shorten the palpebral fissure horizontally by fusing the lid margins over a variable distance. It is useful for any situation in which lagophthalmos from facial paralysis or mild ectropion from any cause results in corneal exposure. The procedure may be temporary or permanent. Many methods have been described, but the authors prefer the pillar tarsorrhaphy because it is a quick and simple operation that is readily undone and does not involve excision of the lid margin tissue, which can lead to trichiasis if opened at a later stage.

In this procedure, the length of tarsorrhaphy required is marked on the upper and lower lids. An incision to approximately 3mm depth is cut through the gray line of both eyelids using a No. 11 blade. At each end of the incision a small cut at right angles to the lid margin is made, but not through to its extremities (which can lead to notch formation) (Fig. 88-10). The resultant wound is H shaped. The marginal epithelium is left in place. The two anterior raw surfaces of tarsus are sewn together with 6-0 long-acting absorbable sutures (Fig. 88-11). A mattress suture is then passed from the upper lid skin to the lower lid skin through the center of the wound and tied over bolsters. The skin edges are then sewn together to complete the three-layer closure. The mattress suture should be removed after 2–3 weeks. Although this tarsorrhaphy can be left in place for some period, it tends to stretch and become less effective over time.

COMPLICATIONS

Complications of ectropion procedures include undercorrection or recurrence, overcorrection, lateral canthal angle dystopia, trichiasis, canalicular injury, corneal abrasion, and eyelid notching.

Undercorrection results from shrinkage of graft materials, lack of support for the canthal angles, inadequate horizontal

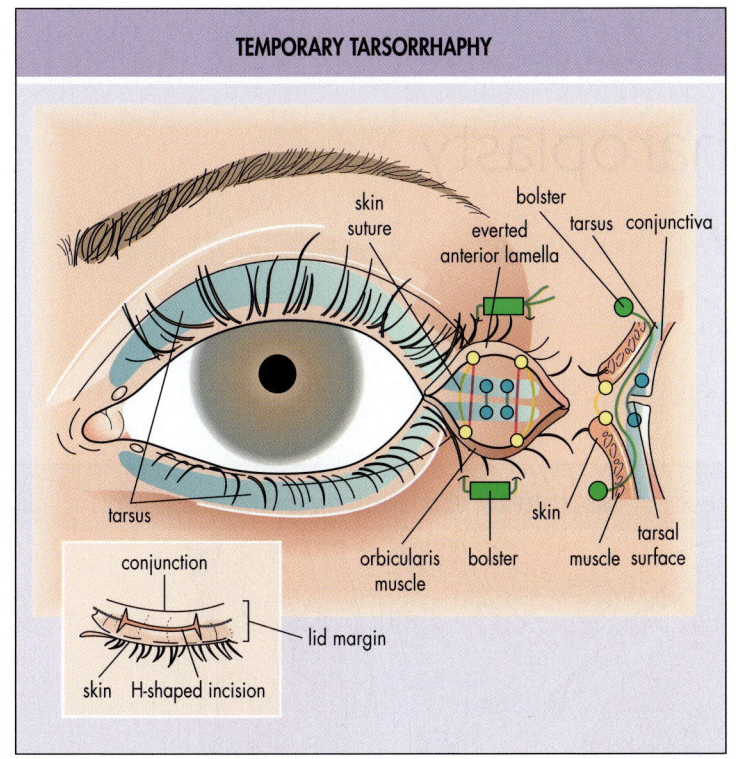

FIG. 88-10 ■ **Temporary tarsorrhaphy procedure.** Inset shows the lid margin incision.

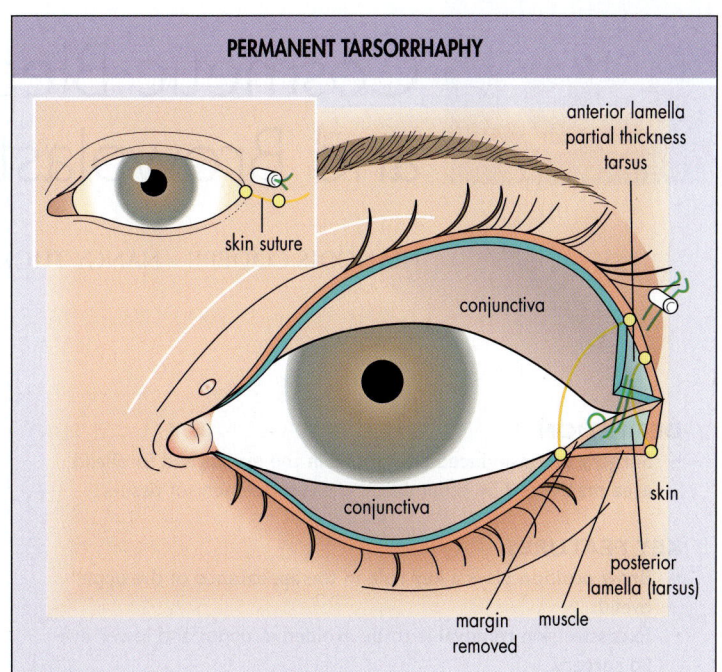

FIG. 88-11 ■ **Permanent tarsorrhaphy procedure.** Inset shows appearance of end result.

shortening of the lid, or loss of suture fixation. It can be avoided by careful preoperative planning, selection of the appropriate procedure for the pathology, and meticulous technique. Allowance must be made for the expected shrinkage of skin grafts and for the effects of gravity when the patient is supine. In most cases, reoperation is needed for undercorrection.

Overcorrection is related to aggressive tightening of inverting sutures when the posterior lamella is shortened or to excessive lid shortening so that retraction of the lid margin results. This usually stretches over time, which can be hastened with massage. In some cases surgical intervention may be necessary; occasionally a periosteal or fascial graft is required to lengthen the canthal tendons.

Poor alignment of the lid margin following full-thickness excisions may result in a lid notch, irregular marginal surface, and trichiasis with resultant corneal complications. The trichitic lashes can be removed with cryosurgery or electrohyphrecation. In most cases it is preferable to repair the lid margin with excision and repair of the notched area.

Injury to the canaliculi is a potential complication of any surgery carried out in the area of the medial canthus. The location of the canaliculi must be delimited with an indwelling probe whenever the surgical site is nearby, and the dissection must be meticulous. If any question of potential injury arises during the procedure, it is best to place a silicone stent in the canaliculus for several weeks or months.

OUTCOME

The surgical treatment of ectropion aims to restore the lower lid margin and punctum to their normal positions with respect to the globe. When the ectropion is mild and primarily of cos-

metic concern, simple procedures usually correct the problem completely. In more advanced cases associated with involutional changes, tightening of redundant tissues restores both functional and esthetic deficits. When ectropion is severe, especially when it results from facial paralysis, cicatricial changes, or significant scarring, the results are less predictable and full correction may require multiple procedures over a period of time.

REFERENCES

1. Adams W. Practical observations on ectropion. London: J Callow; 1812.
2. Von Ammon FA. Zeitschrift für die Ophthalmologie im Verlag der Walterschen hof und Buchhandlung. Dresden; 1831.
3. Kuhnt H. Beitrage zur Operationen augenheikunder. Jena: G Fischer; 1883:44–55.
4. Symanowski J. Handbuch der Operationen chirurgie. Berlin: Braunschweig; 1870:243.
5. Frueh BR, Schoengarth LD. Evaluation and treatment of the patient with ectropion. Ophthalmology. 1982;89:1049–54.
6. Fox SA. Marginal (tarsal) ectropion. Arch Ophthalmol. 1960;63:660–2.
7. Tse DT, Kronish JW, Delyse BUUS. Surgical correction of lower eyelid tarsal ectropion by reinsertion of the retractors. Arch Ophthalmol. 1991;109:427–31.
8. Collin JRO. A manual of systematic eyelid surgery. Edinburgh: Churchill Livingstone; 1989.
9. Crawford GJ, Collin JRO, Moriarty PAJ. The correction of paralytic medial ectropion. Br J Ophthalmol. 1984;68:639–41.
10. Nowinski TS, Anderson RL. The medial spindle procedure for involutional medial ectropion. Arch Ophthalmol. 1985;103:1750–53.
11. Smith B. The lazy-T correction of ectropion of the lower punctum. Arch Ophthalmol. 1976;94:1149–50.
12. Tenzel RR. Treatment of lagophthalmos of the lower eyelid. Arch Ophthalmol. 1969;81:366–8.
13. Anderson RL, Gordy DD. The tarsal strip procedure. Arch Ophthalmol. 1979;97:2192–6.
14. Jordan DR, Anderson RL. The lateral tarsal strip revisited. Arch Ophthalmol. 1989;107:604–6.
15. Tyers AG, Collin JRO. Colour atlas of ophthalmic plastic surgery. Edinburgh: Churchill Livingstone; 1995.
16. Lee OS. An operation for the correction of everted lacrimal puncta. Am J Ophthalmol. 1951;34:575–8.

CHAPTER

89

Cosmetic Blepharoplasty and Browplasty

FRANÇOIS CODÈRE • NANCY TUCKER

DEFINITION
• Surgery of age-induced alterations in the eyelids and forehead area manifested by redundancy and displacement of tissues.

KEY FEATURES
• Brow position plays a key role in the appearance of the upper eyelid.
• Excessive skin removal is to be avoided in upper and lower eyelid surgery.
• Position of the fat pad determines the position of the lid crease.
• In the lower eyelid, repositioning the lid should precede any removal of skin.
• Eventual forehead surgery is considered when planning upper blepharoplasty.

INTRODUCTION

Aging changes in the eyelids and the face are related to loss of tone in the various layers underlying the skin. Changes that occur in the upper eyelid skin are usually due to passive stretching, loss of support, or redundancy of skin secondary to lowering of the brows.

Most patients do not appreciate the extent to which brow malposition contributes to the overall appearance of the aging periorbital area. This needs to be pointed out specifically to help the patient understand why a blepharoplasty alone often will not fully correct the problem. If a manual lift of the brow to the desired position significantly improves the patient's appearance, a browplasty, either alone or combined with blepharoplasty, should be considered. If a blepharoplasty is performed without recognizing any associated brow ptosis, the lateral eyebrow can appear pulled down, which produces an undesirable, sad appearance.

ANATOMICAL CONSIDERATIONS
Eyelids

Key anatomical features that cause excess upper eyelid skin include brow ptosis from the loss of forehead deep tissue support, loss of the deep invagination of the eyelid skin in the principal lid crease as a result of anterior displacement of the suborbicularis fat pads, and stretching of attachments between the levator aponeurosis and the skin. To understand the anatomy, the lid may be arbitrarily divided into two distinct portions (Fig. 89-1).

UPPER EYELID. In the upper eyelid the first segment spans the zone between the lid margin and the lid crease. From anterior to posterior, it consists of skin, orbicularis muscle, levator aponeurosis, tarsus or Müller's muscle higher up, and, finally, conjunctiva (see Chapter 82). These layers are held tightly together by

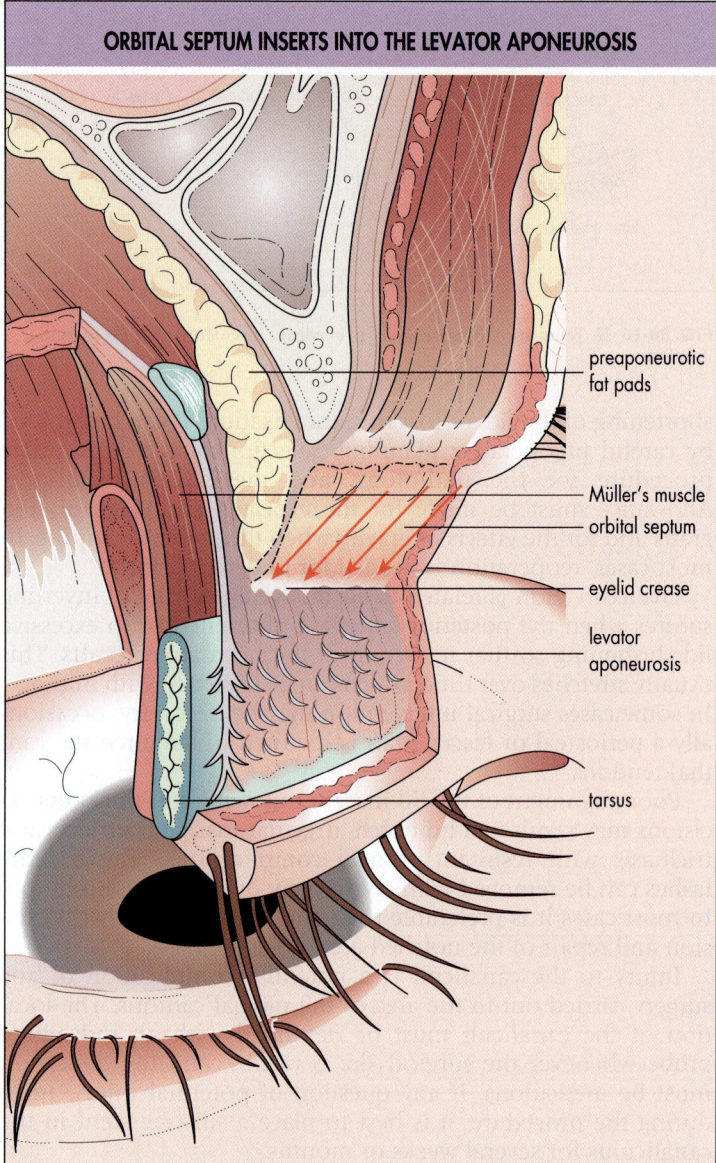

ORBITAL SEPTUM INSERTS INTO THE LEVATOR APONEUROSIS

preaponeurotic fat pads

Müller's muscle
orbital septum

eyelid crease

levator aponeurosis

tarsus

FIG. 89-1 ■ **The orbital septum inserts into the levator aponeurosis (arrows).** The preaponeurotic fat pads are located posterior to the septum. In downgaze the lid crease becomes attenuated (weakened), and in a normal young eyelid the fold is absent. (Adapted with permission from Zide BM, Jelks GW. Surgical anatomy of the orbit, Ch 4. New York: Raven Press; 1985:23.)

fibers of the levator aponeurosis that cross the orbicularis and insert into the dermis.[1] The second segment of the lid begins at the crease and extends to the superior orbital rim. Its layers consist of skin and orbicularis muscle, the orbital septum, the preaponeurotic fat pads, the levator aponeurosis, Müller's muscle, and conjunctiva. The eyelid crease is formed by upper limit of septal

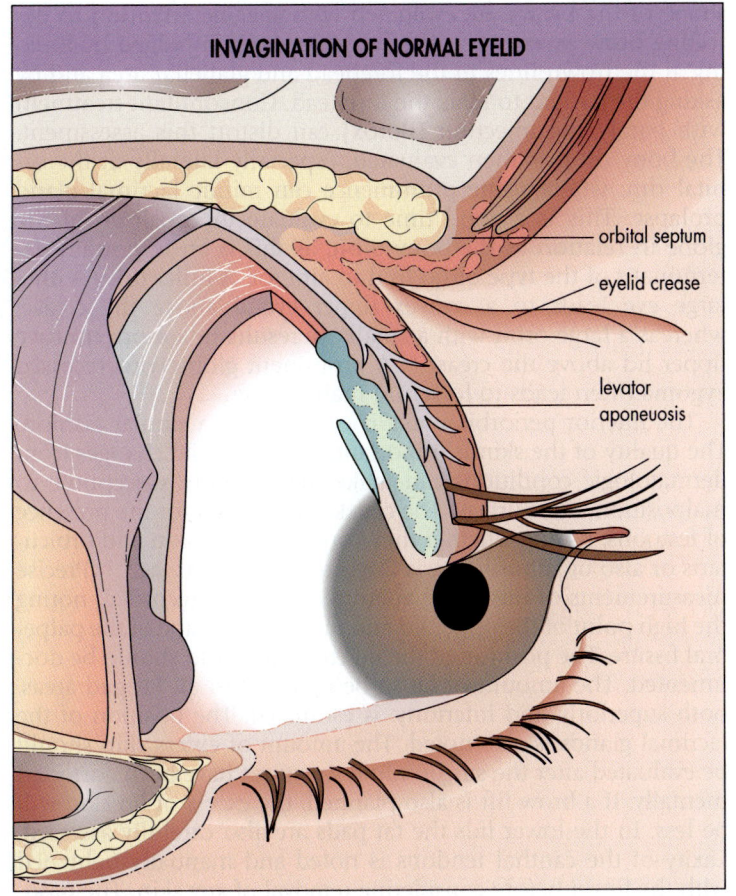

INVAGINATION OF NORMAL EYELID

orbital septum

eyelid crease

levator aponeuosis

FIG. 89-2 ▮▮ The invagination of the normal eyelid crease is created by the posterior pull on the septal insertion by the elevating levator aponeurosis. The preaponeurotic fat is also retracted by the septum. The flat portion of the lid under the crease slips inside the upper preseptal portion. (Adapted with permission from Zide BM, Jelks GW. Surgical anatomy of the orbit, Ch 4. New York: Raven Press; 1985:23.)

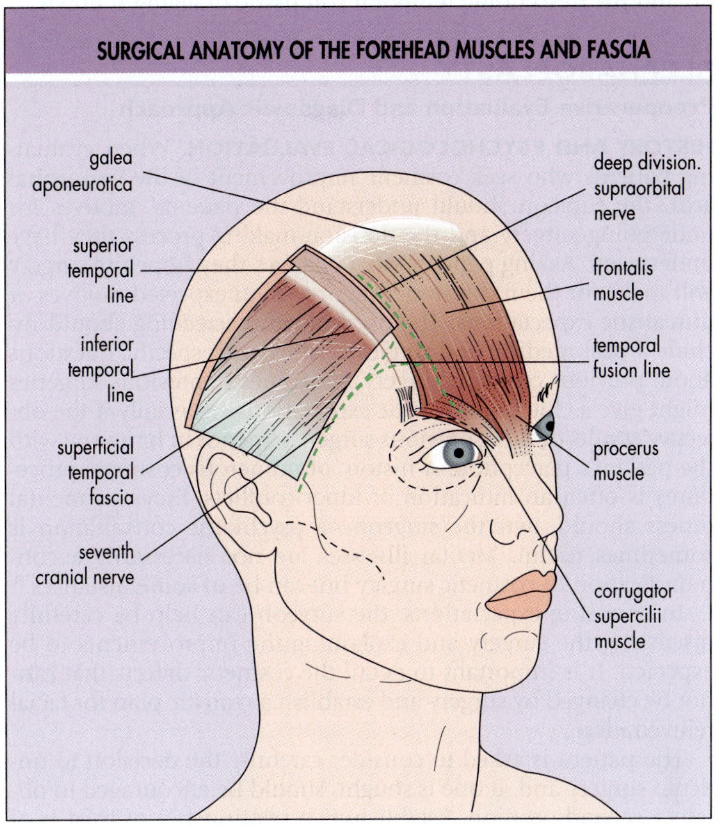

SURGICAL ANATOMY OF THE FOREHEAD MUSCLES AND FASCIA

galea aponeurotica

superior temporal line

inferior temporal line

superficial temporal fascia

seventh cranial nerve

deep division. supraorbital nerve

frontalis muscle

temporal fusion line

procerus muscle

corrugator supercilii muscle

FIG. 89-3 ▮▮ Surgical anatomy of the forehead muscles and fascia.

fibers from the aponeurosis inserting onto the orbicularis intermuscular septa and the skin. It marks the position where the septum inserts into the aponeurosis, which is also the lowest extent of the preaponeurotic fat pads.[2] If the fat recedes, the crease appears higher. When the levator aponeurosis becomes stretched or disinserted from the tarsus, it retracts upward, pulling up the septal insertion. In Asiatic eyelids, the crease (if present) is lower because of the low insertion of the septum into the aponeurosis and thus the lower extension of fat.[3]

When the eyelid opens, the lid crease skin is pulled upward and backward by the aponeurosis as it retracts under the fat pad (see Fig. 89-2).[4] The portion of the lid above the crease bulges slightly as this fat pushes the skin forward. During downgaze, tension in the aponeurosis becomes lax, resulting in a weakened or absent lid crease. These anatomical relations are also influenced by the size and position of the eye within the orbit.[5]

LOWER EYELID. The lower eyelid has a similar, but simpler, anatomy. The capsulopalpebral fascia, equivalent to the levator aponeurosis, fuses with the orbital septum at or only a few millimeters below the lower border of the tarsus. Integrity of the medial and lateral canthal tendons (see Chapter 82) is very important to maintain a proper lid position with aging, but the bony configuration of the midface also plays a key role. Movement of the lower lid is of small amplitude. The crease, if present, is faint and lies close to the lid border.

Brows

A thorough understanding of the forehead anatomy is essential to evaluate brow ptosis (Fig. 89-3). The layers in the midforehead are skin, dermis, superficial galea, frontalis muscle, deep galea, and periosteum. The forehead skin is much thicker than

the eyelid skin. The dermis and subcutaneous fat are connected to the underlying frontalis muscle by multiple fibrous septa. The paired frontalis muscles originate just anterior to the coronal suture line. A smooth fibrous sheath, the galea aponeurotica, envelops the frontalis to form both superficial and deep galeal layers. The periosteum lies beneath the deep galeal layer.

Laterally, the frontalis muscle ends or becomes markedly attenuated along the temporal fusion line of the skull. Here, the superficial galea, the superficial temporalis fascia, and the periosteum of the frontal bone fuse. The confluence of these tissue planes is called the "zone of fixation." The eyebrow fat pad (subgaleal fad pad) is a transverse band of fibroadipose tissue 2–2.5cm above the orbital rim. It allows movement of the frontalis muscle in the lower forehead. The eyebrow fat pad is continuous inferiorly with the suborbicularis space in the eyelid.

Centrally, the procerus muscle is continuous with the medial portion of the frontalis muscle and inserts into the nasal bone glabellar subcutaneous tissue. It causes horizontal wrinkles of the glabella. The corrugator supercilii muscle is obliquely oriented, passing from the subcutaneous brow to the frontal bone medially. It causes vertical glabellar furrows.[6,7]

Several important neurovascular structures occur in the forehead. The frontal branch of the facial nerve lies within the superficial temporal fascia before entering the frontalis muscle. At the superior rim there are the lacrimal nerve laterally, the supraorbital nerve with its deep and superficial division, and the supratrochlear nerve more nasally.

Several factors contribute to the appearance of the aging forehead and brow. These include changes in the quality of the skin, loss of tissue support, and forehead and glabellar furrows related to action of the underlying facial muscles.[8–10] The lateral eyebrow segment is more prone to become ptotic because of less structural support in this area.. The final brow position depends on the dynamics between the frontalis muscle pulling the brow up and the descending temporal soft tissue dragging it down.[7]

BLEPHAROPLASTY

Preoperative Evaluation and Diagnostic Approach

HISTORY AND PSYCHOLOGICAL EVALUATION. When evaluating patients who seek cosmetic improvement of the periorbital area, the surgeon should understand the patients' motives for undergoing surgery and the decision-making process they have undertaken. Asking patients what changes they hope the surgery will make for them can sometimes reveal unexpected motives or unrealistic expectations. The psychological screening should include a past medical and surgical history with specific questions about previous cosmetic surgery. Outcomes of previous surgeries might give a clue to unrealistic expectations, especially if the objective results of these previous surgeries are not in harmony with the patient's perception. A history of numerous cosmetic procedures is often an indication of inner conflicts. Previous mental illness should alert the surgeon—a psychiatric consultation is sometimes useful. Mental illnesses are not necessarily a contraindication to cosmetic surgery but can be in some instances.[11]

In assessing expectations, the surgeon can help by carefully discussing the surgery and explaining the improvements to be expected. It is important to detail the cosmetic defects that cannot be changed by surgery and establish a realistic plan for facial rejuvenation.

The patient is asked to consider carefully the decision to undergo surgery and, if one is sought, should be encouraged to obtain a second opinion. Establishing a relationship of trust is of paramount importance. If in any doubt, even for unclear objective reasons, a conservative attitude is recommended.

PHYSICAL EXAMINATION. The position and shape of the different periorbital structures are evaluated along with the quality of the skin. In the forehead area, the level and shape of the hairline, the quality of skin of the forehead, and the position and

shape of the brows are evaluated with specific attention to detecting brow asymmetry. The muscular layer is judged by looking at the frown lines in the forehead and glabellar area and by asking the patient to relax the forehead. Concomitant treatment with paralyzing injection (Botox) can distort this assessment. The bony orbit is then evaluated, especially laterally at the orbital rim, where some prominence can mimic lacrimal gland prolapse. This is a good time to evaluate the position of the globe in relation to the bony orbit, as this is an important determinant of the type of lid fold to aim for. A fuller orbit with a large eye leads to a convex upper eyelid above the crease, whereas a large orbit with a small eye results in a more concave upper lid above the crease.[12] A prominent globe with recessed zygoma often leads to lower lid malposition.

The inferior periorbital area is evaluated in a similar fashion. The quality of the skin is important, and cicatricial changes from dermatologic conditions can make the lid more susceptible to malposition after surgery. The cheek is examined for the presence of festoons, noting whether they consist of only skin and orbicularis or also of suborbicularis fascia and/or orbital fat.[13,14] Precise measurements of the eyelid aperture should be recorded, noting the high point of the upper lid and the general shape of the palpebral fissure. The position of the lid crease and fold should be documented. The amount of fat to be removed in all fat pad areas, both superiorly and inferiorly, is estimated. The position of the lacrimal glands is also noted. The amount of excess skin should be evaluated after the surrounding structures have been corrected mentally. If a brow lift is also planned, the excess of lid skin will be less. In the lower lids the fat pads are also carefully assessed. Laxity of the canthal tendons is noted and manually tightened with the finger before considering removal of any skin. The nasojugal area should be examined to detect tear trough deformities, which may need correction instead of fat pad removal.[15]

The use of a flow sheet to outline systematically the physical findings is an excellent way to plan present and future surgery (Fig. 89-4).[16] Surgery planning must take into account the patient's desires, what he or she is willing to undergo, and what the

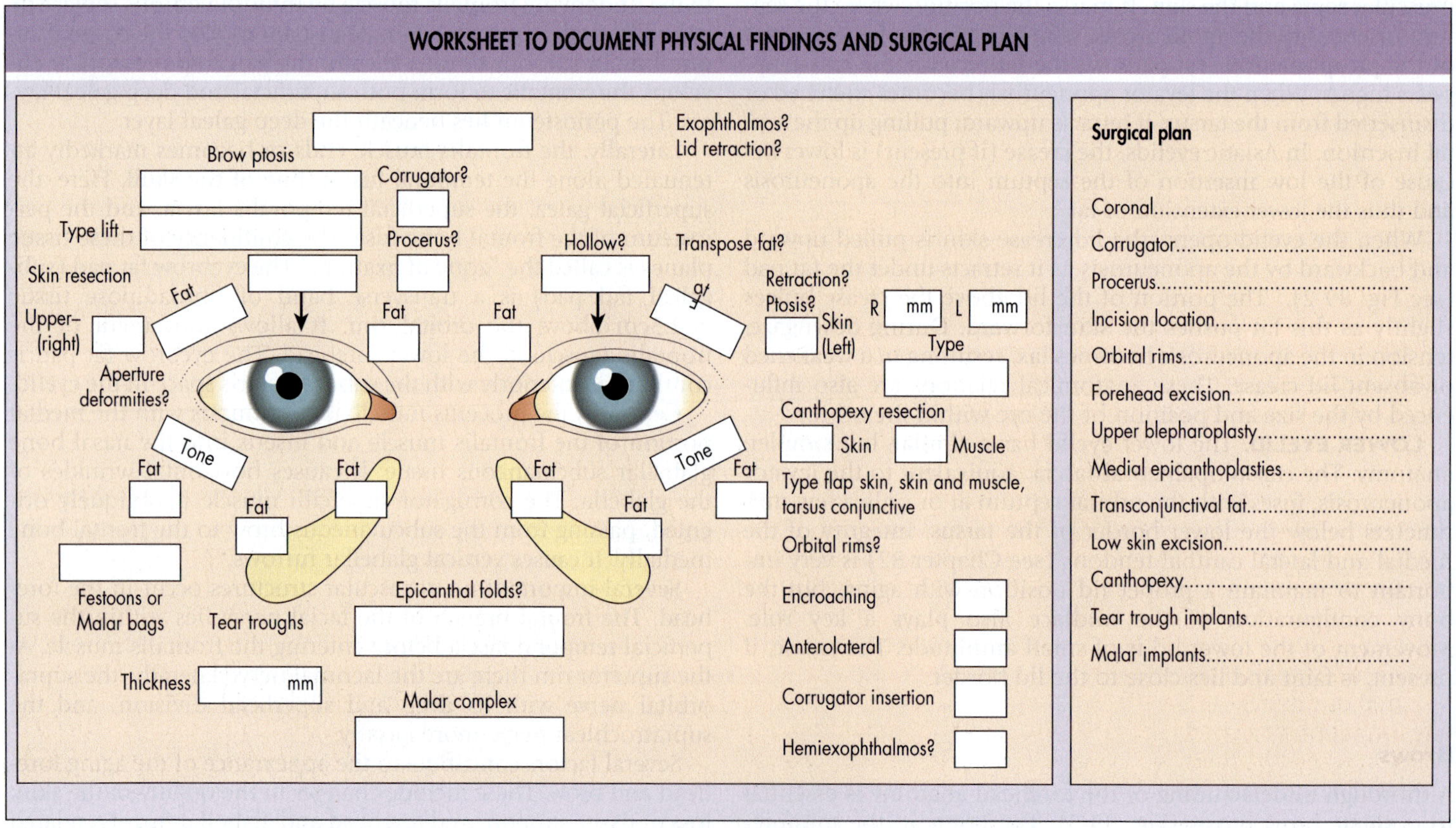

WORKSHEET TO DOCUMENT PHYSICAL FINDINGS AND SURGICAL PLAN

FIG. 89-4 ▪ A sample worksheet to document the physical findings and surgical plan. (Adapted with permission from Flowers RS, Flowers SS. Precision planning in blepharoplasty. Clin Plast Surg. 1993;20:303–10.)

surgeon thinks is reasonable and safe. Figure 89-4 gives an overview of the evaluation of the patient consulting for blepharoplasty and brow malposition. A good set of photographs should carefully document the changes noted and be kept as part of the patient's chart.

Anesthesia

Local infiltrative anesthesia containing epinephrine for hemostasis is adequate for all blepharoplasty procedures.

General Techniques

The patient should avoid using makeup on the day of surgery. Draping should be done carefully to avoid distortion of the brow and lateral canthi[17] and to allow the patient to sit up, if necessary, during the operation. The amount of skin to be removed is marked before infiltration. In the upper eyelid, excessive removal of thin lid skin and dragging down of thick brow skin are a nonesthetic shortcut and should not be substituted for adequate repositioning of the brows. In the lower lids the same principle applies: the lid should be repositioned and the scleral show corrected before any skin is removed. The ideal brow position is determined with the patient supine. Then, by letting the brow drop to its natural state, the amount of brow elevation required can be determined.

Specific Techniques

UPPER LID BLEPHAROPLASTY. The lid crease is first marked at 8–10mm above the lash line, taking into account the racial background of the patient. The crease marking usually goes from a point above the superior punctum to, but not beyond, the lateral orbital rim. Skin excess should be evaluated so that in downgaze the crease is attenuated without lid retraction, and a gentle fold reforms over it in primary position. Proper crease reformation and adequate excision of prolapsed fat allow the skin fold to be pulled into the orbit in upgaze. In general, 20–24mm of skin should be left between the brows and the lid margin.[18] Even if associated brow ptosis is not to be corrected at the same time, excessive skin removal should be avoided. The long-taught rule that the eyes should not close on the operating table has certainly become obsolete. Excessive skin removal medially may result in hood formation. If disproportionate tissue is still present in this region after surgery, a glabellar lift should be considered. An optional small triangular flap of skin can be added to the usual skin pattern medially to minimize folding of the skin at the time of closure in patients with an unusual excess of skin medially (Fig. 89-5).

The lid is placed under traction. A Bard-Parker No. 15 blade is used to incise the skin to the level of the dermis. The skin flap is then removed with a blade or scissors, leaving the orbicularis intact at this stage.

Gentle pressure on the globe prolapses the orbital fat and helps identify the orbital septum. The fat is exposed by making a small buttonhole centrally through the orbicularis and the septum above its insertion on the aponeurosis. The septum is opened laterally and medially from this buttonhole (Fig. 89-6). Each fat pad capsule is opened. The fat is gently prolapsed and sectioned. The section line can be cauterized with a bipolar cautery (Fig. 89-6). The paler nasal fat pad should be specifically exposed and resected to ensure a clean medial canthal area.

The orbicularis muscle is thinned down. The aponeurosis is bared of orbicularis just above the tarsal border to encourage the formation of a good adherence between the aponeurosis and the skin where the lid crease is to be formed. Invagination of the skin by fixing the skin edge to the aponeurosis at the time of closure ensures a good position of the crease in fuller lids but is not always necessary. The orbicularis can be tacked down to the aponeurosis immediately under the upper skin edge using two

or three 6-0 plain sutures. This defines the position of the eyelid crease and controls the position of the fat pad in the lid (Fig. 89-7). These techniques minimize the risks of ptosis and allow better attenuation of the lid crease in downgaze than firmer skin fixation.

The lid is closed with 6-0 nylon. The area beyond the lateral canthal angle is closed with interrupted sutures to obtain an edge-to-edge closure without folds. The rest of the lid is usually closed with a simple nonlocking continuous running suture (Fig. 89-8).

LOWER LID BLEPHAROPLASTY. Two specific techniques are popular for lower lid blepharoplasty. The skin approach allows modification of the interaction between the muscle and the skin planes and makes lid tightening or canthal repositioning easier. When only fat prolapse is present, the transconjunctival approach allows surgical access without visible scar and avoids the risk of lid malposition.

Skin Approach. In the skin approach, the skin is marked 3mm below the lash line from the inferior punctum to the lateral canthal angle. If excess skin is to be removed or if the orbicularis muscle is to be tightened, the incision is extended laterally and downward toward the earlobe for a short distance. Local anesthetic can be injected through the conjunctiva.

The skin is incised with a no. 15 blade and scissor dissection exposes the suborbicularis plane and the anterior surface of the orbital septum. The septum is easily identified by pushing gently on the globe to prolapse the fat and opened with scissors. The temporal and central fat pads are one continuous pad separated by a vertical band of fascial connections between the capsulopalpebral fascia and the orbital septum.[3] The capsule of each of the fat pads is opened. Care is taken to tease the fat out of the respective pockets without undue traction in order to avoid deep bleeding in the orbit. In the medial lid the fat capsule is opened separately, and care must be taken to protect the inferior oblique at the time of excision. The fat is carefully examined for bleeders before it is allowed to retract into the orbit

A canthopexy can be used to lift a sagging lateral angle by placing a suture through the lateral canthus and attaching it to periosteum.[19] If horizontal lid laxity is present, a tarsal strip procedure can be performed (see Chapter 88). A small triangle of skin and orbicularis muscle may be excised laterally. Closure of the orbicularis as a sliding flap often helps to rejuvenate an older lid. Hemostasis is attained carefully before the skin is closed with a continuous suture of 6-0 nylon.

Transconjunctival Approach. With the transconjunctival approach, the lid is everted over a medium-size Desmarres retractor. The lateral fat pad is often the most difficult to expose—a buttonhole through the conjunctiva laterally about 4mm from

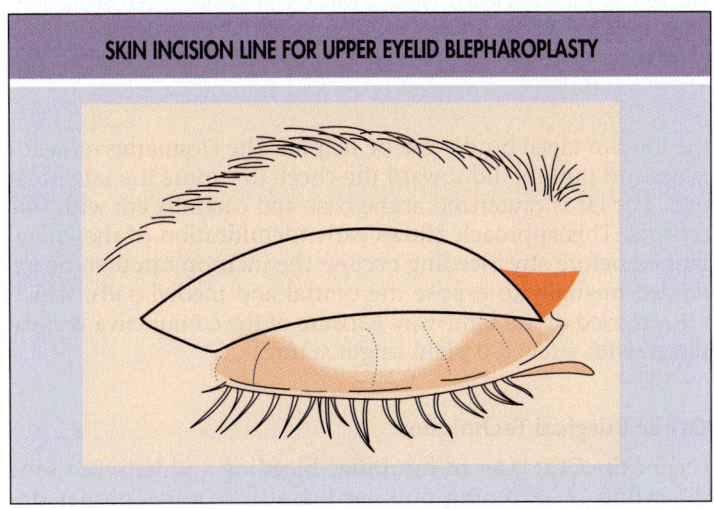

SKIN INCISION LINE FOR UPPER EYELID BLEPHAROPLASTY

FIG. 89-5 ■ Typical skin incision line used for upper eyelid blepharoplasty. A small additional medial flap is added (shaded area) if a dog-ear or fold develops because of excessive skin nasally.

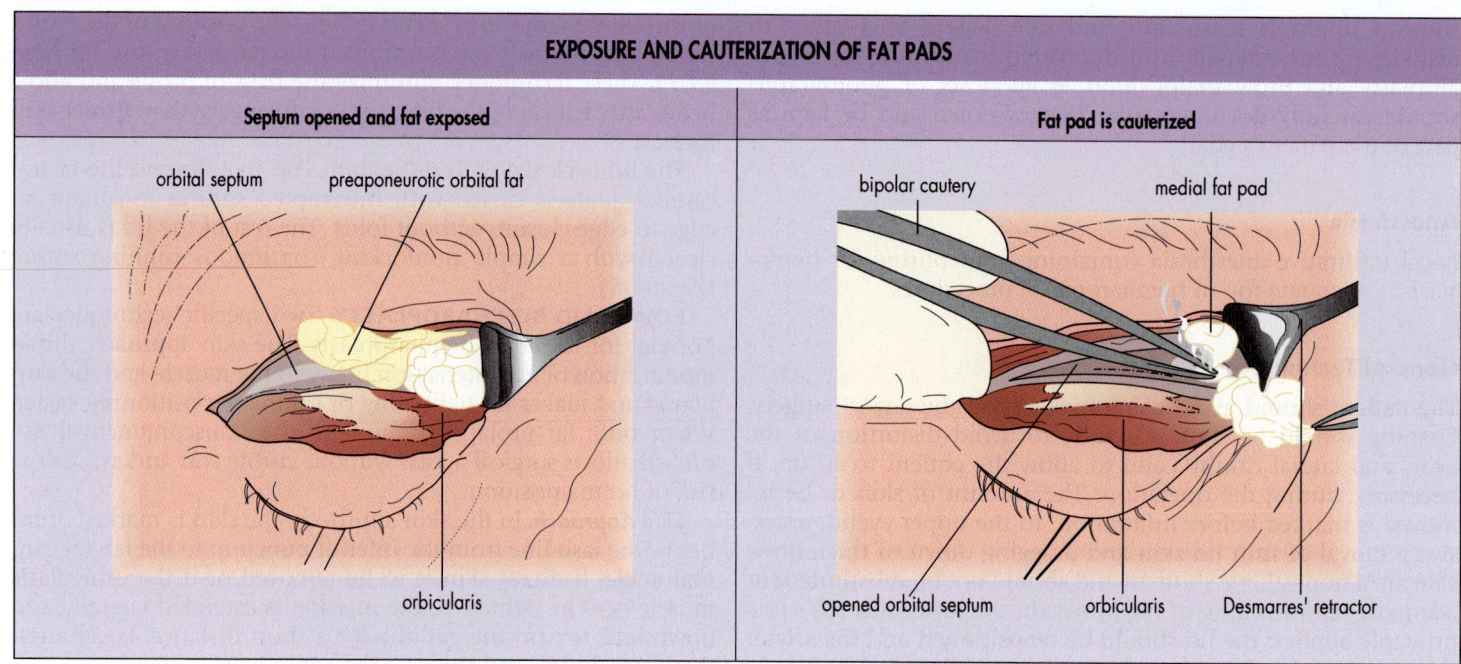

FIG. 89-6 ■ **Exposure and cauterization of fat pads.** Preaponeurotic fat pads are a key landmark just anterior to the aponeurosis. The orbital septum is opened to expose the fat, and each pad is carefully cauterized along its base before being cut with scissors.

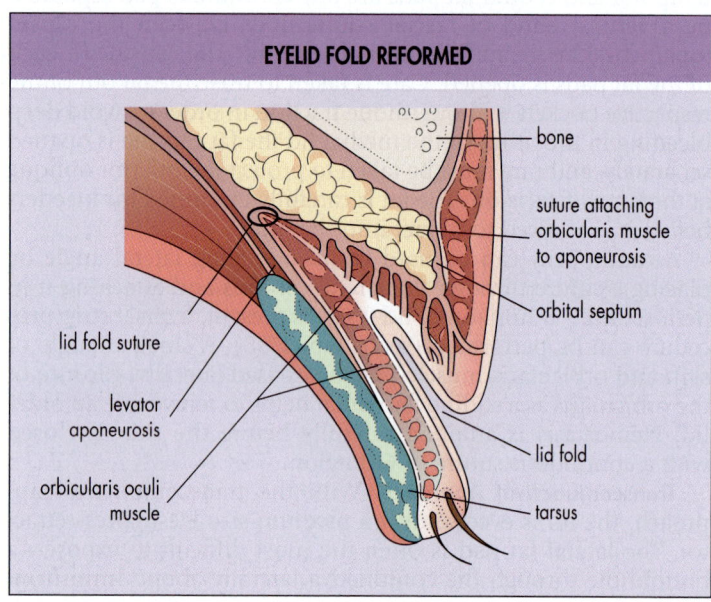

FIG. 89-7 ■ The eyelid fold or crease is reformed by passing several sutures from the orbicularis muscle to the aponeurosis at the appropriate height.

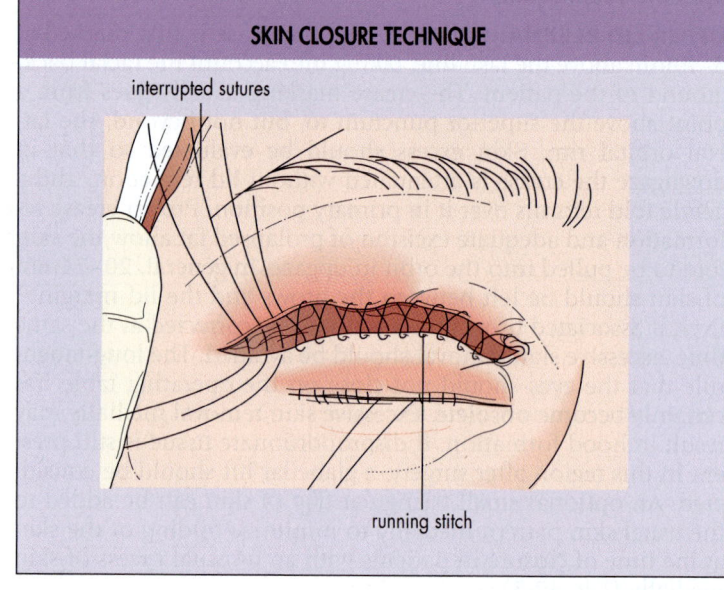

FIG. 89-8 ■ The skin is closed with two to three interrupted sutures laterally, where the skin is thicker, and with a running suture along the remainder of the wound.

the inferior tarsal border can be helpful. The Desmarres retractor is used to pull the lid toward the cheek to expose the lateral fat pad. The fat is cauterized at the base and carefully cut with fine scissors. This approach allows early identification of the lateral fat pad before any bleeding occurs. The incision can then be extended medially to expose the central and medial pads, which are removed in the same way. Closure of the conjunctiva is completed with a few 6-0 plain catgut sutures.

Other Surgical Techniques

Use of the CO_2 laser to minimize bleeding and help in tissue dissection is becoming popular but still requires proper understanding of lid anatomy and the general surgical principles of blepharoplasty. Resurfacing of the skin with the ultrapulse CO_2 laser or chemical peeling solutions offers new opportuni-

ties to correct persistent wrinkles and lax skin that remain after blepharoplasty.[20,21]

Specific techniques should be used when operating on Asian eyelids—the goals determine the technique to be used. In general, the skin incision is made lower toward the lid margin, depending upon the desired position of the resulting crease. Some preaponeurotic fat should be left to act as a barrier between the levator and the skin if the Asian-type lid is to be preserved.

Postoperative Care

A medium-pressure bandage is applied to the lids with an appropriate antibiotic ointment. The patient can remove the patches rapidly after surgery and start applying cold packs to the surgical site for 10 minutes each hour during the first evening and then four or five times the next day. Light analgesia for blepharoplasty is usually sufficient. Severe pain is not expected and warrants immediate examination to rule out orbital hemorrhage or corneal abrasion. The sutures on the skin can be removed 5–7 days postoperatively if nylon 6-0 is used.

Complications

Complications of blepharoplasty are of two orders. One group of complications can occur from events unrelated to the technique used; a second group can occur following improper surgery for a particular deformation. For example, infection, despite the best surgical techniques, will occur in a small number of patients; the same is true of milia formation along a scar line. Lower lid ectropion or canthal angle rounding in the lower eyelid is usually the result of improper surgical planning or techniques. In the first group, careful follow-up and good patient teaching prevent most major problems. In the latter group, prevention is always better than secondary correction.

ORBITAL HEMORRHAGE AND BLINDNESS. Orbital hemorrhage following blepharoplasty is an emergency. It has been associated with permanent loss of vision in some cases, especially if the lower eyelid is involved.[18,22] Prevention involves careful preoperative screening for use of anticoagulants, including aspirin. Meticulous hemostasis, gentle manipulation of fat during surgery, and good control of blood pressure postoperatively are important. Early removal of patches and application of cold packs minimize swelling. Strenuous activities should be avoided for the first 3–4 days. Anticoagulants should not be administered for at least 5–6 days after surgery. The surgeon and medical staff should be alerted by unusual pain, swelling under tension, or double or blurred vision. If in doubt, the patient must be seen immediately for an assessment of visual acuity and pupillary response. In the presence of a deep hematoma the patient should be admitted for close monitoring of optic nerve function. If optic nerve dysfunction appears, the wounds are opened and the blood is evacuated. The use of concomitant hyperosmotic agents (e.g., mannitol) has been advocated.[18] A lateral cantholysis helps decompress the soft tissues of the orbit, but with a deep hemorrhage an orbital exploration may be required. If all else fails, an orbital decompression, as done for compressive neuropathy in Graves' disease, may become necessary (see Chapter 96).

INFECTIONS. Fortunately, the eyelids are well vascularized so that infections after blepharoplasty are rare. Patients should be aware that an increase in swelling with redness and pain may be the first sign of infection. If it is confirmed by examination, appropriate cultures and sensitivities should be obtained and the patient started immediately on wide-spectrum systemic antibiotics. Close follow-up to rule out abscess formation in the orbit is necessary in severe cases and proper orbital imaging should be obtained. Blindness is a rare complication of infection, but it has occurred following blepharoplasty.[23]

TELANGIECTASIAS, CHEMOSIS, MILIA, AND SUTURE TRACTS. Telangiectasias can form or previously present rosacea can become more evident in the lids after surgery, especially in the zone between the lid border and the incision in the upper eyelid. With time, these usually fade. Minimal dissection in this area prevents this annoying complication. In some cases, ecchymoses may stain the skin for up to a year. Careful suturing and early removal of sutures minimize the risks of inclusion cysts, milia, and suture tracts.

PTOSIS. Ptosis may be present but unrecognized on initial preoperative examination in patients with severe skin excess. Palpebral fissures should be evaluated along with the levator action as if all patients were consulting for ptosis (see Chapter 86). If present, ptosis should be corrected by advancing the levator aponeurosis on the tarsal surface. Otherwise, at the time of blepharoplasty care should be taken not to damage the aponeurosis. If impending ptosis is present and the lid crease is reconstructed by supratarsal fixation, a slight tightening of the aponeurosis may be wise. When ptosis appears after surgery,

conservative observation for 6 months is recommended. If it persists, surgical correction may be necessary.

LAGOPHTHALMOS, LOWER LID RETRACTION, ECTROPION, AND LATERAL CANTHAL DEFORMITIES. If excessive skin has been removed in the upper lid, resulting in lagophthalmos, time is often of help; the brows continue their downward drift and the lagophthalmos often progressively decreases. Massage and ocular lubricants in the first few months after surgery may bring the patient out of this difficult phase. But if keratitis ensues and threatens the integrity of the eye, surgical correction should be done. In the lower lid, gravity works against spontaneous improvement. Frank ectropion might resolve with massage but almost invariably leaves lower scleral show. Using the transconjunctival approach when minimal or no skin excess is present, tightening the lateral canthal tendon if necessary, and avoiding excessive skin removal are the best ways to prevent this complication.[24,25] Revision using a lateral tarsal strip procedure combined with a disinsertion of the lower eyelid retractors can give satisfactory results in mild cases. A midfacial lift or a skin graft may become necessary with more severe deformities.[26–28]

OTHER COMPLICATIONS. Tearing after blepharoplasty can be a complex problem, especially if lagophthalmos is present. Investigation of this complication should include a full lacrimal work-up with assessment of the reflex component if keratitis is present. The integrity of the canaliculi and the position of the lid margin and puncta are all evaluated before planning correction (see Chapter 98). Injury to the extraocular muscles can occur, especially in the lower lid, where the inferior oblique and inferior rectus are prone to damage with exploration of the medial fat pad.[29] The superior oblique tendon can also be damaged in upper lid surgery.[30] In these instances, a follow-up of at least 6 months is necessary prior to considering surgical interventions, as spontaneous resolution is fortunately the rule.

Outcome

Most patients who seek cosmetic eyelid or brow surgery expect some improvement in their appearance and in their self-image and are usually happy with the result. Some, in whom the anatomical deformity interferes with visual function, as in severe overhanging dermatochalasis, can also notice improvement in their visual field. The patients who enter into surgery with unrealistic goals, either physical or social, are more at risk of not being satisfied with the results.

BROW MALPOSITION
Preoperative Evaluation and Diagnostic Approach

The ideal brow position and shape are subjective, but in general the brow is straighter and at the superior orbital rim in a man and more curved and slightly above the rim in a woman. An evaluation of the most cosmetically pleasing brows in women suggests that the medial eyebrow should be positioned at or below the supraorbital rim, with the eyebrow shape having an apex lateral slant.[31,32]

The clinical evaluation should include brow position (estimated by the difference between the actual resting brow position and the desired position), the amount of excess forehead skin and degree of furrowing, the hairline position, and the length of the forehead. The length of the forehead can be determined by passing imaginary horizontal lines through the hairline, the upper border of the eyebrows, and directly below the nose. These lines divide the balanced face into three equal portions. An increase or reduction of the upper segment is an important factor when selecting the incision site using the coronal approach.[33] The extent to which the procerus and corrugator muscles contribute to furrowing of the forehead should be determined. A family history of male pattern baldness should be sought. It is important to determine how extensive a surgery the patient is willing to undergo to achieve the best results; often the

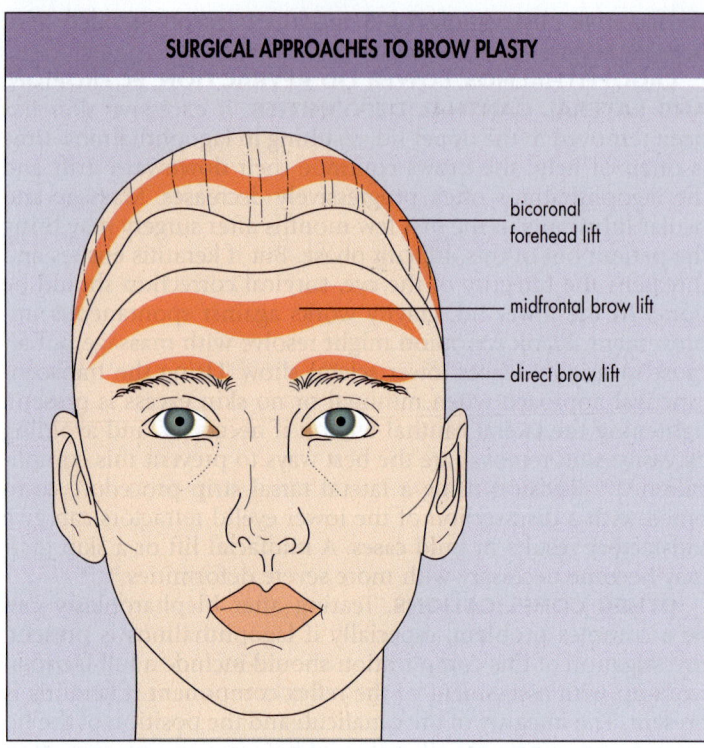

SURGICAL APPROACHES TO BROW PLASTY

bicoronal
forehead lift

midfrontal brow lift

direct brow lift

FIG. 89-9 ▌▌ Surgical incision sites for correction of brow ptosis.

final surgical choice is a compromise between the most effective technique and the least invasive procedure.

Anesthesia

Anesthesia is provided by supraorbital and supratrochlear regional blocks along with direct local infiltration, depending on the extent of anesthesia desired for each of the various techniques. In selected patients, general anesthesia may be considered. Gentle but constant pressure minimizes the formation of hematomas that can distort anatomy.

General Techniques

Surgical approaches to the correction of brow ptosis include direct, midfrontal, and bicoronal brow lifts (see Fig. 89-9). More recently, endoscopic and small incision browplasties have been described. Minimal brow elevation can also be approached through an eyelid crease incision at the time of blepharoplasty.[34] The choice of technique depends on the amount of correction required and on the patient's expectations.

Specific Techniques

THE BICORONAL FOREHEAD LIFT. The bicoronal forehead lift allows the maximal effect of brow elevation with a well-camouflaged incision site.[35] It is ideally suited for patients with significant brow ptosis, without frontal baldness, and with a normal to low hairline.

The incision is hidden posterior to the hairline (post-trichion). Alternatively, in patients who have a high forehead, the incision can be placed at the hairline (pretrichion) to avoid further elevating the hairline. There are two major choices for the surgical dissection plane: subcutaneous and subgaleal.[33] Factors that influence the choice of dissection plane include the quality and elasticity of the skin, the amount of skin wrinkling, and the depth of the furrows, but surgeon preference is likely to be the most significant factor.[8,33] A combined coronal brow lift and blepharoplasty can be used in patients with excessive eyelid fat and brow ptosis but little or no dermatochalasis.[36] The major disadvantages of the bicoronal technique include its invasive

surgical approach, which can be intimidating to the patient, and the increased risk of hematoma and nerve injury.

THE MIDFRONTAL BROW LIFT. The midfrontal approach provides less brow lift effect than does the bicoronal but more than the direct brow lift approach. Advantages include less risk of hematoma (because only moderate undermining is required and it is performed above the frontalis muscle) and less risk of nerve damage. The corrugator supercilii and procerus may be resected directly through this approach. It is ideally suited for patients who have deep horizontal furrows in the forehead (usually men), especially when frontal baldness prevents the use of a bicoronal incision. Some surgeons use this as their procedure of choice for brow ptosis in men and women.[32] There are various types of incisions that can be used for the following:

- Along a furrow line the entire length of the forehead.
- Along a furrow line staggered centrally.
- Two separate fusiform excisions, each extending from the medial to lateral end of the brow.

The major disadvantage of this technique is the resultant scar line.

THE DIRECT BROW LIFT. The direct brow lift is the oldest and simplest surgical approach. Its advantages include a less invasive surgical dissection with less risk of damage to the facial nerve and minimal risk of hematoma. It is ideally suited for patients with bushy brows and mild brow ptosis. It can also be used in patients who have unilateral brow ptosis, which most commonly occurs following peripheral facial nerve palsy. It does not fully correct the medial brow ptosis, and it results in a visible scar even when placed directly above the eyebrow with often an unnaturally sharp border due to loss of the fine upper brow hairs. In patients who have large bushy brows, the incision tends to be less apparent. Modifications include a more temporal skin excision to correct isolated temporal brow ptosis.

ENDOSCOPIC BROW LIFT. Recently, less invasive techniques have emerged in an attempt to reduce complications and achieve faster recovery. These techniques include endoscopic procedures, which involve small incisions placed temporally and/or centrally on the scalp, posterior to the hairline. A subperiosteal or subgaleal dissection is carried down to the level of the brow. The procerus and corrugator muscles are usually cut and excised, and the periosteum is transected at the superior orbital rim. The forehead is pulled upward and the periosteum fixed into position.

TRANSBLEPHAROPLASTY BROW FIXATION. For minimal brow ptosis, the brow can be elevated through a blepharoplasty incision by suturing the sub-brow dermis higher on to the frontalis muscle. This approach can help correct mild brow ptosis or small asymmetries.[34]

Complications

Complications of browplasty depend on the technique used. There are two major groups of complications, those related to the incision site and those related to the extent of dissection. Complications related to the incision site are visible scar and alopecia.

EXCESSIVE CUTANEOUS SCAR AND ALOPECIA. The forehead skin is thicker and less vascular than the eyelid skin, so incisions in the forehead often heal with a visible scar. Meticulous closure with adequate subdermal tension-bearing sutures and careful approximation of the wound edges is important. However, placement of the incision is the main determinant of scar visibility. It is generally preferable to locate the incision site at or above the hairline. Alopecia can be secondary to tension of wound, ischemia, or superficial dissection.

PARESTHESIA AND HEMATOMA. Related to the extent of dissection are the potential associated nerve injuries, which can result in frontal paresis, numbness, and an increased risk of hematoma formation. Temporary paresthesia following browplasty is common but usually resolves within 6 months. Hematomas can occur after bicoronal brow lift. They can be prevented at the end of surgery by placement of suction drains under the flaps. Small hematomas often resolve spontaneously, but larger ones should be evacuated to avoid flap necrosis, especially with a subcutaneous dissection where necrosis is more likely.

OVERCORRECTION AND UNDERCORRECTION. Overcorrection of brow position or loss of movement of the brow can result in a "look of perpetual surprise," particularly if the brow has been fixed to the underlying periosteum in an overzealous direct brow lift. Undercorrection occurs when insufficient elevation is achieved; it is more common with the endoscopic technique and with posterior fixation of the brow through a blepharoplasty incision.

Outcome

Following brow elevation procedures, the patient should experience an improvement in appearance and a restoration of superior visual field. In order to achieve these results, the brow repair may have to be combined with a blepharoplasty.

REFERENCES

1. Anderson RL, Beard C. The levator aponeurosis. Attachments and their clinical significance. Arch Ophthalmol. 1977;95:1437–41.
2. Flowers RS. Upper blepharoplasty by eyelid invagination. Clin Plast Surg. 1993;20:193–207.
3. Doxanas MT, Anderson RL. Eyebrows, eyelids and anterior orbit, Ch 4. In: Doxanas MT, Anderson RL, eds. Clinical orbital anatomy. Baltimore: Williams & Wilkins; 1984:57–88.
4. Zide BW, Jelks BW. Surgical anatomy of the orbit, Ch 4. New York: Raven Press; 1985:23.
5. Jelks GW, Jelks EL. Preoperative evaluation of the blepharoplasty patient. Bypassing the pitfalls. Clin Plast Surg. 1993;20:213–24.
6. Knize DM. Limited-incision forehead lift for eyebrow elevation to enhance upper blepharoplasty. Plast Reconstr Surg. 1996;97:1334–42.
7. Knize DM. An anatomically based study of the mechanism of eyebrow ptosis. Plast Reconstr Surg. 1996;97:1321–33.
8. Ortiz-Monasterio F, Barrera G, Olmedo A. The coronal incision in rhytidectomy—the brow lift. Clin Plast Surg. 1978;5:167–79.
9. Connell BF. Eyebrow, face and neck lifts for males. Clin Plast Surg. 1978;5:15–23.
10. Katzen LB. The history of cosmetic oculoplastic surgery. In: Putterman A, ed. Cosmetic oculoplastic surgery, 2nd ed. Philadelphia: WB Saunders; 1993:2–10.
11. Shulman BH. Psychiatric issues in cosmetic blepharoplasty. In: Putterman AM, ed. Cosmetic eyelid surgery. Philadelphia: WB Saunders; 1993:44–9.
12. Flowers RS. The art of eyelid and orbital aesthetics: multiracial surgical considerations. Clin Plast Surg. 1987;14:703–21.
13. Furnas DW. Festoons, mounds, and bags of the eyelids and cheeks. Clin Plast Surg. 1993;20:367–85.
14. Furnas DW. Festoons of orbicularis muscle as a cause of baggy eyelids. Plast Reconstr Surg. 1978;61:540–6.
15. Flowers RS. Tear trough implants for correction of tear trough deformities. Clin Plast Surg. 1993;20:403–15.
16. Flowers RS, Flowers SS. Precision planning in blepharoplasty. Clin Plast Surg. 1993;20:303–10.
17. Bosniak SL. Cosmetic blepharoplasty. New York: Raven Press; 1990:37–58.
18. Kulwin DR, Kersten RC. Blepharoplasty and brow elevation. In: Dortzbach RK, ed. Ophthalmic plastic surgery: prevention and management of complications. New York: Raven Press; 1994:91–111.
19. Flowers RS. Canthopexy as a routine blepharoplasty component. Clin Plast Surg. 1993;20:351–65.
20. Baker TM, Stuzin JM, Baker JB, Gordon HL. What's new in aesthetic surgery? Clin Plast Surg. 1996;23:3–16.
21. Rosenberg GJ, Gregory RO. Lasers in aesthetic surgery. Clin Plast Surg. 1996; 23:29–48.
22. McCord CD, Shore JW. Avoidance of complications in lower lid blepharoplasty. Ophthalmology. 1983;90:1039–46.
23. Morgan SC. Orbital cellulitis and blindness following a blepharoplasty. Plast Reconstr Surg. 1979;64:823–6.
24. Zarem HA, Resnick JI. Minimizing deformities in lower blepharoplasty. Clin Plast Surg. 1993;20:317–21.
25. Tomlinson FB, Hovey LM. Transconjunctival lower lid blepharoplasty for removal of fat. Plast Reconstr Surg. 1975;56:314–8.
26. Anderson RL, Gordy DD. The tarsal strip procedure. Arch Ophthalmol. 1979; 97:2192–7.
27. Lisman RD, Hyde K, Smith B. Complications of blepharoplasty. Clin Plast Surg. 1988;15:309–35.
28. Tenzel RR. Complications of blepharoplasties. Clin Plast Surg. 1981;8:797–802.
29. Harley RD, Nelson LB, Flannagan JC, Callahan JH. Ocular motility disturbances following cosmetic blepharoplasty. Ophthalmology. 1980;89:517–21.
30. Wesley RE, Pollard ZF, McCord CD Jr. Superior oblique paresis after blepharoplasty. Plast Reconstr Surg. 1980;66:283–7.
31. Freund RM, Nolan WB. Correlation between brow lift outcomes and aesthetic ideals for eyebrow height and shape in females. Plast Reconstr Surg. 1996; 97:1343–8.
32. Cook TA, Browwrigg PJ, Wang TD, Quatela VC. The versatile midforehead browlift. Arch Otolaryngol Head Neck Surg. 1989;115:163–8.
33. Guyuron B. Subcutaneous approach to forehead, brow, and modified temple incision. Clin Plast Surg. 1992;19:461–76.
34. Knize DM. Transpalpebral approach to the corrugator supercilii and procerus muscles. Plast Reconstr Surg. 1995;95:52–60.
35. Dingman DL. Transcoronal blepharoplasty. Plast Reconstr Surg. 1992;90:815–19.
36. Ellenbogen R. Transcoronal eyebrow lift with concomitant upper blepharoplasty. Plast Reconstr Surg. 1983;71:490–9.

CHAPTER 90

Esthetic Laser Skin Treatments

MARC S. COHEN • NANCY G. SWARTZ

INTRODUCTION

The medical and surgical treatment of skin appearance has changed dramatically over the past several years.[1] Botulinum neurotoxin (Botox), topical agents, minimally invasive procedures (glycolic peels, intense pulsed light, microdermabrasion), and laser skin resurfacing have captured the imagination of the public and have improved substantially our therapeutic options. The number of treatments to improve the appearance of skin far exceeds that of any other cosmetic procedure. This chapter will focus on the use of the CO_2 laser to improve skin texture.

Skin responds to age and sun damage in characteristic ways.[2] With aging, the skin produces less collagen, elastin, and glycosaminoglycans and is less able to respond to injury.[3] Ultraviolet radiation from the sun injures dermal collagen and elastin. The epithelium loses its normal polarity, atypia develops, and pigment abnormalities occur. The result is thin, dry, sallow, fragile, and wrinkled skin which has poor elasticity, uneven pigmentation, and malignancies. There are many treatment options, and the cosmetic surgeon must be familiar with each of these to determine what is best suited to each patient's needs.[2] Botulinum neurotoxin is best suited to treat dynamic wrinkles such as crow's-feet. A sallow complexion and hyperpigmentation often is treated successfully with topical agents such as tretinoin, bleaching agents, microdermabrasion, and light peels. Deeper pigmentation and increased vascularity can be improved with intense pulsed light. It is our belief that the best treatment of moderately deep static rhytids (such as most lower eyelid wrinkles) is laser resurfacing with the CO_2 laser.

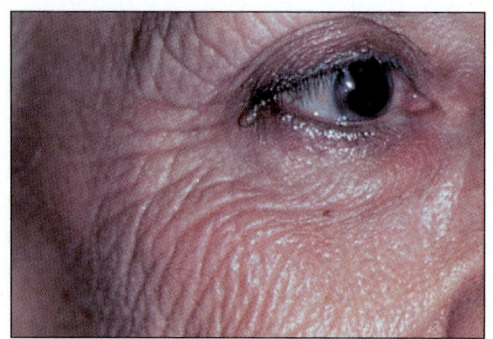

FIG. 90-1 ▮▮
Preoperative view of a patient awaiting full-face laser resurfacing.

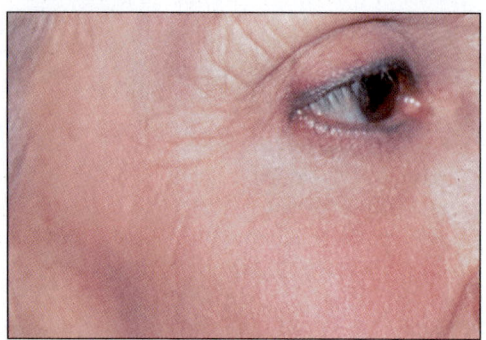

FIG. 90-2 ▮▮
Postoperative appearance of the patient shown in Figure 90-1, 6 months after full-face CO_2 laser resurfacing.

Skin rejuvenation may be achieved when the top layers of aged and environmentally damaged skin are removed and replaced by healthier skin. The advantage of CO_2 laser resurfacing lies in the laser's ability to deliver extremely short pulses of high energy to a precisely controlled depth.[4] The energy is absorbed by water in the cells, which results in cellular vaporization with minimal thermal damage to adjacent tissues.[5–7] This removes the superficial, damaged layers of skin and irritates the underlying skin just enough to stimulate new collagen development. The result is healthier, younger looking skin that has a smoother texture and more even pigmentation (Figs. 90-1 and 90-2).

PREOPERATIVE EVALUATION AND PATIENT PREPARATION

The best candidates for laser skin resurfacing are patients with a fair complexion. The more pigmented the skin, the greater is the risk of development of postinflammatory hyperpigmentation. Patients who have Fitzpatrick skin types I–III (Table 90-1) are at relatively low risk, while those who have Fitzpatrick skin types IV–VI are considered at high risk for hyperpigmentation.[8] Patients who have a history of hypertrophic scar or keloid formation are at greater risk for scarring. Patients who have a history of herpes simplex virus infections are at risk for recurrent infection with scarring. Recent use of isotretinoin, recent laser resurfacing, recent chemical peeling, or radiation therapy within the past 6 months should be considered contraindications to this procedure.

Realistic patient expectations are the hallmark of success. Wrinkles and skin imperfections can be reduced, but not eliminated, with this procedure. Patients must be educated about skin care and postoperative expectations. The healing period usually is longer than implied by the lay press. Patients must understand that a significant disruption of their routine will occur for about 1 week and that they will not be able to wear cover-up makeup until epithelium has healed completely (approximately 10 days). It is essential that patients avoid sun exposure during healing, because this induces hyperpigmentation.

Skin should be treated with tretinoin and bleaching agents prior to resurfacing,[9] which enables a more rapid re-epithelialization and reduces the risk of postoperative pigment abnor-

TABLE 90-1

FITZPATRICK SKIN CLASSIFICATION SYSTEM

Skin Type	Skin Color	Characteristics
I	White	Always burns, never tans
II	White	Usually burns, tans less than average
III	White	Sometimes mild burn, tans about average
IV	White	Rarely burns, tans more than average
V	Brown	Rarely burns, tans profusely
VI	Black	Never burns, deeply pigmented

malities. Ideally, such treatments should begin at least 3 to 4 weeks prior to resurfacing. Hydroquinone, the most commonly used bleaching agent, inhibits tyrosinase and thereby prevents melanin production.

Successful results rely on uncomplicated healing after the procedure. Bacterial, fungal, and viral infections can occur postoperatively and may lead to scarring. Laser resurfacing can activate herpes simplex but, because many patients are unaware that they have herpes, all are treated with antibiotics and antiviral agents prophylactically.

PROCEDURE

The skin is divided into esthetic units—the periocular region, perioral region (within the nasolabial folds and the chin), forehead, nose, and cheeks. Some surgeons always treat the entire face; others treat specific esthetic units only, as determined preoperatively.

On the morning of the procedure, the patient is instructed to cleanse the skin with a mild cleanser only. The skin is prepared with antiseptic solution, which must be allowed to dry fully, because moisture on the skin interferes with the laser absorption. The patient's head is draped in a saline-soaked cloth or crumpled aluminum foil to cover areas that are not to be treated, and metallic scleral shields are used to protect the patient's eyes. All others in the treatment room must wear protective glasses. The procedure is performed under local anesthesia, with or without sedation. Oxygen must be turned off and the tubes removed from the field prior to treatment.

Achieving the appropriate depth of ablation can be learned only through experience, because no simple formula exists by which to determine laser settings or depth of treatment. Each brand of laser has different settings, and different settings are required for different skin types and the same skin type in different locations on the body.

Each laser pulse vaporizes a small spot of the skin, which leaves visible debris. The surgeon treats the entire esthetic unit with confluent spots. Many lasers can be used to treat a relatively large area more quickly by using a computer-generated pattern of many individual spots that are ablated on a single pass. Sterile, saline-soaked gauze or a cotton-tipped applicator is then used to wipe away the debris gently (Fig. 90-3).

The skin then is examined to determine the depth of the treatment. A pink color indicates epithelial ablation (Fig. 90-4), a gray color is seen in the papillary dermis, and a chamois yellow color denotes treatment to the upper reticular dermis. The skin is treated with repeated passes, as needed, but treatment should not be deeper than the upper reticular dermis. While gaining experience, it is far better to undertreat and plan on "touch-up" treatments, if necessary. If the entire face is not treated, feathering the edges by applying less total energy provides a smooth transition into untreated skin.

Laser resurfacing is very effective for the treatment of lower eyelid rhytids and crow's-feet.[5] The upper eyelids usually are not treated or are treated only lightly, and upper eyelid pretarsal skin is not treated. The procedure can be performed in conjunction with upper eyelid or transconjunctival lower eyelid blepharoplasty. In the treatment of lower eyelid rhytids and textural skin problems, it is important to apply laser to the lower eyelid pretarsal skin lightly to prevent ectropion. Lower eyelid laxity must be corrected prior to treatment using a lid-shortening procedure (see Chapters 88 and 89). Laser resurfacing should not be combined with a transcutaneous lower eyelid blepharoplasty, because the skin flap created results in decreased blood flow to the eyelid skin. This impedes skin healing and could result in scarring.

POSTOPERATIVE CARE

Until re-epithelialization is complete, skin must be kept moist and protected from physical stress. This can be accomplished with occlusive dressings (e.g., Flexzan), water-soluble hydrogel dressings (e.g., Vigilon, Second Skin), or topical preparations (e.g., Crisco shortening). The authors prefer occlusive dressings for the first 5 days, which are associated with more rapid wound healing and less discomfort, and which require less patient care. During this time, the dressing is changed carefully by the physician or appropriately trained staff and the skin is inspected. After 5 days, the patient is instructed to use a bland moisturizer until the epithelium has healed completely. Crusting may form and should be rinsed or soaked with warm water. It must be emphasized to the patient that to pick at the crusts can result in dermal injury and permanent scarring. As noted above, oral antibiotics and antiviral agents are used prophylactically. Discomfort is minimal and usually can be controlled well with acetaminophen (paracetamol).

After 10 days, the patient may wear makeup. Protection with sunscreen is essential. Bleaching agents are restarted prophylactically 2 weeks postoperatively to prevent excessive melanin formation. Most patients resume their normal skin care routine after 3–4 weeks. Skin health maintenance with stimulators, such as tretinoin or α-hydroxyl acids, may be resumed 1 month postoperatively.

COMPLICATIONS

Complications of skin laser resurfacing are uncommon when patients have been selected carefully, prepared, treated properly, and given appropriate treatment postoperatively.[10] However, even with ideal selection and care, complications can occur. Hyperpigmentation and hypopigmentation, persistent erythema, hypertrophic scarring, lower eyelid retraction and ectropion, and infections (bacterial, viral, and fungal) all have been reported. With early detection and intervention, permanent problems usually can be prevented.

CONCLUSION

Cosmetic skin treatments are the most commonly performed cosmetic procedures. Skin care has evolved dramatically over the past few years. CO_2 laser skin resurfacing remains the treatment of choice for most lower eyelid rhytids. Although technology continues to provide new avenues for skin rejuvenation, the basic principles of skin care and wound healing remain unchanged.

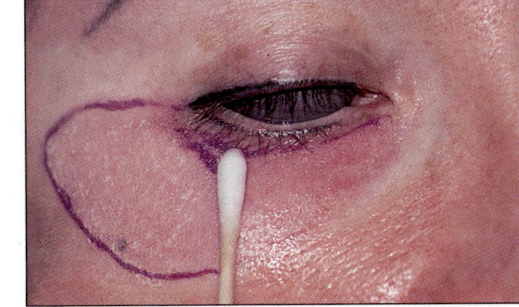

FIG. 90-3 ■ Periocular CO_2 laser–ablated skin, with the medial aspect débrided.

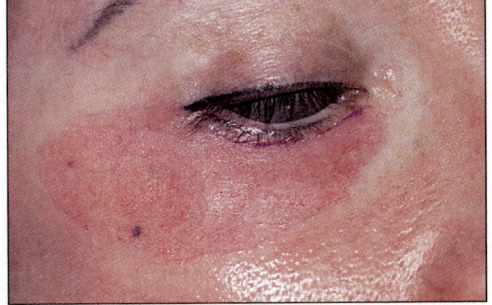

FIG. 90-4 ■ Periocular CO_2 laser–treated skin, with epithelium ablated.

REFERENCES

1. http://surgery.org/statistics.html, accessed February 25, 2003.
2. http://www.asds-net.org/index.html, accessed February 25, 2003.
3. RoTenigk HH Jr. Treatment of the aging face. In: Pinski JB, Pinski KS, eds. Cosmetic dermatology. Dermatol Clin. 1995;3(Suppl I):245–61.
4. Fitzpatrick RE, Goldman MP. Advances in carbon dioxide laser surgery. Clin Dermatol. 1995;13:35–47.
5. Green HA, Burd E, Nishioka NS, et al. Mid-dermal wound healing. Arch Dermatol. 1992;128:639–45.
6. Reid R. Physical and surgical principles governing carbon dioxide laser surgery on the skin. Dermatol Clin. 1991;9:297–316.
7. McKenzie AL. How far does thermal damage extend beneath the surface of CO_2 laser incisions? Phys Med Biol. 1983;28:905–12.
8. Ho C, Nguyen Q, Lowe NJ, et al. Laser resurfacing in pigmented skin. Dermatol Surg. 1995;21:1035–7.
9. Vagotis FL, Brundage SR. Histologic study of dermabrasion and chemical peel in an animal model after pretreatment with Retin-A. Aesthetic Plast Surg. 1995;19:243–6.
10. Weinstein C. Ultrapulse carbon dioxide laser removal of periocular wrinkles in association with laser blepharoplasty. J Clin Laser Med Surg. 1994;12:205–9.

CHAPTER 91

Essential Blepharospasm

DONALD C. FAUCETT

DEFINITION

- Essential blepharospasm is a variable, progressive bilateral focal dystonia characterized by contraction of the orbicularis oculi muscles, which causes spasmodic involuntary eyelid closure in the absence of any other ocular or adnexal cause.

KEY FEATURES

- Bilateral involuntary spasmodic closure of the eyelids.
- Symptoms exacerbated by stress, fatigue, bright lights, interpersonal interactions.
- Fluctuation of symptoms marked by transient remissions and exacerbations.
- Spasms absent when asleep.
- Spasms improve with relaxation.

ASSOCIATED FEATURES

- Decrease in tear production.
- Dystonic activity of facial muscles (Meige's syndrome).
- Dystonic activity of the neck muscles (cranial–cervical dystonia).
- Dystonic activity of the vocal cords (spastic dysphonia).
- Dysphagia, blepharoptosis, eyebrow ptosis, entropion, canthal tendon abnormalities.

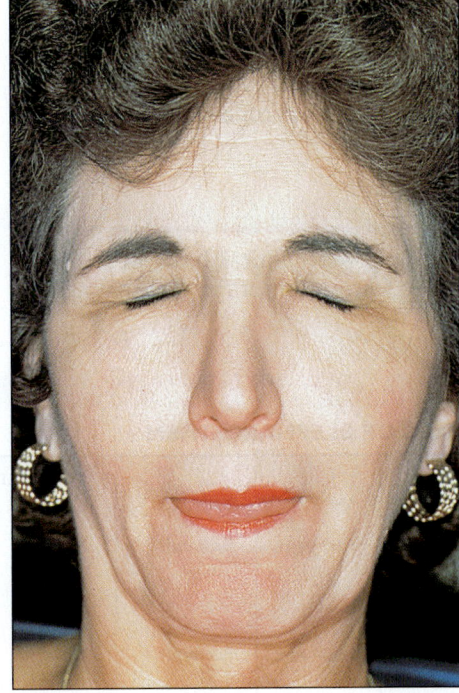

FIG. 91-1 ▌ Involuntary spasms of the orbicularis and procerus muscles in essential blepharospasm. These spasms are associated with oromandibular dystonia involving the middle and lower face.

INTRODUCTION

Blepharospasm refers to a tonic spasm of the orbicularis oculi muscle that produces intermittent and often complete closure of the eyelids.[1] Benign essential blepharospasm (BEB) is bilateral focal dystonia of idiopathic origin; in its most severe form, it results in functional blindness, depression, and social isolation.[2,3] Additionally, it is often misdiagnosed as a psychiatric disorder, which typically delays definitive treatment. Secondary blepharospasm is the result of adnexal or ocular disease. It is not uncommon to see both benign essential and secondary blepharospasm concurrently in a patient.[4] Other disease entities, such as hemifacial spasm and tardive dyskinesia, may manifest similar clinical characteristics.

OCULAR MANIFESTATIONS

In the earliest stages of essential blepharospasm, patients frequently complain of photophobia and ocular surface disorders, especially dry eye symptoms. Associated with these symptoms is an increase in the frequency of blinking.[2,4] The blinking progresses over a variable period of 2–7 years to become more frequent, forceful, and sustained, and often results in intermittent functional blindness due to the inability to control these spasms (Fig. 91-1).[1,4] The factors which seem to exacerbate the disease include stressful situations such as are found at the work place or in social gatherings. As with other dystonias, patients are often able to employ sensory "tricks" to arrest the spasms temporarily. These include whistling, singing, and application of pressure to points on the face.[1,4]

On clinical examination the spasms may be variable, ranging from absent to intense. For this reason, it is most important to question patients as to the subjective severity of their symptoms outside of the clinical environment. Spasms may spread to involve the midface over a variable period. This extension of essential blepharospasm to include adjacent focal oromandibular dystonia usually is referred to as *Meige's syndrome*. As the disease progresses to involve the face, patients frequently complain of difficulty in talking, eating, or swallowing. In severe cases, pronounced bruxism occurs, often resulting in problems with dentition and, subsequently, nutritional deficiency.

Other associated features may include decreased tear production,[5] adjacent dystonias (such as spastic dysphonia and torticollis), and anatomical changes (such as eyelid and brow ptosis, dermatochalasis, entropion, and canthal tendon abnormalities).[6]

DIAGNOSIS

The diagnosis of essential blepharospasm is one of exclusion. For this reason, a careful examination must be conducted to rule out the various causes of secondary blepharospasm. The more common causes of secondary blepharospasm include blepharitis, trichiasis, dry eye syndrome, corneal and external disease, glaucoma, and uveitis.[1] The diagnosis of this disease is rather straightforward from historical and clinical evidence alone. In atypical cases, however, in which dystonic activity may be associated with muscular weakness, associated signs and symptoms may alert the clinician to an alternative primary diagnosis. In such instances, a complete neurological evaluation and neuroimaging are mandatory to rule out other neurological diseases.[7]

Numerous rating scales are useful in the development of new treatment modalities. The most widely used scale was developed by Jankovic[8] with a severity rating as follows:

- 0 = No spasms
- 1 = Minimal spasms with increased blinking only with external stimuli (e.g., bright light, wind, reading, driving)
- 2 = Mild, noticeable eyelid fluttering without functional disability
- 3 = Moderate, very noticeable spasms involving the eyelids only and causing some visual disability
- 4 = Severe, incapacitating spasms, often involving other facial muscles and causing functional blindness

DIFFERENTIAL DIAGNOSIS

A number of disorders are associated with dystonic movements of the orbicularis muscles and, therefore, can simulate blepharospasm (Table 91-1). A careful evaluation usually helps to differentiate these disorders.

PATHOLOGY

The anatomical origin and the biochemical basis of essential blepharospasm are unknown.[9] Most authorities feel that abnor-malities in the basal ganglia or midbrain are responsible. Abnormal auditory brainstem response potentials have been noted in patients who have BEB and Meige's syndrome, which implicates involvement of the brainstem.[10] Additionally, abnormal levels of neurotransmitters have been demonstrated in the midbrain and brainstem nuclei of patients with Meige's syndrome.[1,10] Animal studies have demonstrated similar activity with stimuli near the facial, parabrachial, red, and interstitial nuclei.[11] Postmortem studies and neuroimaging findings have been normal.[4]

TREATMENT

The goal in the treatment of essential blepharospasm is to minimize or eliminate the disabling spasms. Pharmacological measures have variable success. Selective peripheral facial nerve avulsion, along with other surgical measures, has been tried, but complications such as facial paralysis, ectropion, and high recurrence rates have decreased its popularity.[6,9]

Myectomy

Myectomy is the major surgical treatment for BEB, in which the orbicularis, procerus, and corrugator muscles are extirpated.[12] A modified or limited myectomy has been introduced more re-

TABLE 91-1

DIFFERENTIAL DIAGNOSIS OF BLEPHAROSPASM

Differential Diagnosis	Sex	Age	Side	Voluntary Control	Present in Sleep	Clinical Characteristics	Diagnostic Etiology	Tests
Essential blepharospasm	F > M, 2–3:1	>50 years	Bilateral	No	No	Isolated spasms of the orbicularis oculi	1. Uncertain 2. Basal group ganglia 3. Brainstem	None in typical cases
Meige's syndrome	F > M, 2–3:1	>50 years	Bilateral	No	No	Blepharospasm plus midfacial spasm	Same as for BEB	Same as for BEB
Hemifacial spasm	F > M, 3:2	>45 years	Unilateral, L > R	No	Yes	Tonic–clonic spasms in the distribution of the 7th cranial nerve	Usually a vascular compression of the 7th cranial nerve root	CT or MRI; must rule out a posterior fossa tumor
Apraxia of eyelid opening; involuntary levator inhibition	—	—	—	No	—	1. Passive involuntary closure of eyelids; raised eyebrows; relaxed eyelids 2. Occasionally seen with essential blepharospasm	Unknown; seen in extrapyramidal disease such as Parkinson's, Huntington's, Wilson's disease, or with supranuclear palsy, and Shy–Drager syndrome	Orbicularis oculi muscle EMG inactive; total inhibition of levator muscle
Facial myokymia	F = M	Any	Unilateral	No	Yes	Rapid undulating flicking muscles	1. Uncertain 2. Multiple sclerosis, intramedullary tumor 3. Caffeine, stress	EMG
Facial tic	F = M	Childhood	Unilateral or bilateral	Yes	Yes	Stereotypic movements, brief repetitive, suppressible	Tourette syndrome	None
Facial seizure	F = M	Any age	Unilateral	No	—	Movements occurring with head; questionable eye deviation	Focal cortical lesion	CT, MRI
Facial synkinesis	Equally affected	Any	Unilateral	No	Yes	1. Unilateral contracture with weakness 2. Gustatory lacrimation	Prior history of facial paralysis	EMG evidence of synkinesis, fibrillation potential, reduced motor units

cently, in which only the orbicularis muscle in the upper lid is removed. The limited myectomy offers a quicker recovery and most of the benefits of the radical myectomy with less morbidity.

Chemomyectomy is another type of myectomy under investigation. Local injections of doxorubicin produce permanent orbicularis oculi weakness. In one study, over 50% of patients required no further treatment. However, high concentrations of drug can result in skin ulceration, but a modified technique may be less deleterious. Although doxorubicin is known to be carried in a retrograde fashion to the brain and is a known neurotoxin, animal studies have failed to demonstrate a measurable loss of facial neurons.[13,14]

Pharmacological Agents

Oral pharmacological agents have been used with variable results. Benzodiazepines, such as lorazepam 0.5–2.0mg 2 to 3 times a day, clonazepam 0.5–5mg 3 times a day, or oxazepam 10–30mg 3 to 4 times daily, have been somewhat effective.

Chemodenervation

The treatment of choice for the initial treatment of BEB is botulinum toxin type A.[3,9] This is one of seven antigenic-specific neurotoxins (A, B, C1, D, E, F, and G) produced by the bacterium *Clostridium botulinum*.[15] Botulinum neurotoxin blocks neuromuscular transmission by acting on peripheral cholinergic nerve endings to prevent acetylcholine release from presynaptic terminals.[16]

The onset of effect is within 24–72 hours, with a plateau usually at 3–5 days but, occasionally, onset may be delayed as long as 2–4 weeks.[9,15,17] The duration of denervation averages 3 months for BEB and slightly longer for hemifacial spasm.[9,15] For BEB, the usual injection sites are as shown in Figure 91-2. Frequently, the procerus and corrugator muscles also are involved and so require injection. Other periorbital or facial sites may require treatment, as determined on an individual basis. In the upper eyelid, the injections should be subcutaneous only in order to prevent migration of the toxin below the orbital septum, which otherwise results in paralysis of the levator muscle.[15] Frequently, injections in the lower lid alone have a pronounced effect on spasms in the lower face, thus eliminating or decreasing the dosage required in the lower face for Meige's syndrome and hemifacial spasm. The recommended starting dosage for botulinum toxin type A is 1.25–5 units per injection site. If a suboptimal response occurs, the dosage should be doubled. Less toxin usually is required with dystonic activity with paresis.

Recovery of function following toxin injection results from axonal sprouting and formation of new neuromuscular junctions.[16,18]

The reported response rate to botulinum toxin is 95–98%.[16] Antibody formation to previous or current toxin exposure may be responsible for the 2–5% failure rate with this modality and has been reported most often when high doses of toxin are used at frequent intervals.[15] It, therefore, is recommended that toxin should not be given more frequently than every 3 months, and the dosage should not exceed 200 units in a 30-day period. In cases in which antibodies are demonstrated and no response occurs to botulinum toxin type A, other antigenically distinct serotypes, such as type F, may be of help.

The major adverse reactions to botulinum toxin include ptosis, epiphora, keratitis, dry eyes, and diplopia.[16] These effects are usually transient and resolve long before the beneficial effects of the drug are exhausted. A flu-like syndrome has been reported following botulinum toxin injections for blepharospasm, most common with higher doses. Studies also suggest the possibility of a transient increase in intraocular pressure and an abnormal emptying of the gallbladder, with secondary biliary colic as additional side effects.

COURSE AND OUTCOMES

As noted above, botulinum toxin currently is the initial treatment of choice for BEB. Oral pharmacological agents often are helpful for milder cases of BEB or as adjunctive therapy, especially for dampening dystonic activity in the lower face in Meige's syndrome and hemifacial spasm. Myectomy usually is reserved for those individuals who respond poorly to more conservative therapy or for those patients who have anatomical problems, such as ptosis, which need correction. Application of these various treatment modalities based on an individual assessment and the response characteristics of each patient usually results in a favorable prognosis for the vast majority of patients.

In hemifacial spasm, in which the pathology is an abnormal compression of the seventh cranial nerve root by a blood vessel, botulinum toxin is the initial treatment of choice. However, in the proper hands, neurosurgical decompression of the seventh nerve has a high success rate.[19]

REFERENCES

1. Holds JB, White GL Jr, Thiese SM, Anderson RL. Facial dystonia, essential blepharospasm and hemifacial spasm. Am Fam Physician. 1991;43(6):2113–20.
2. Jankovic J, Orman J. Blepharospasm: demographic and clinical survey of 250 patients. Ann Ophthalmol. 1984;16:371–6.
3. Patrinely JR, Anderson RL. Essential blepharospasm: a review. Geriatr Ophthalmol. Jul/Aug 1986:27–33.
4. Jankovic J, Hallett M. Therapy with botulinum toxin. New York, Hong Kong: Marcel Dekker; 1994:191–7.
5. Price J, O'Day J. A comparative study of tear secretion in blepharospasm and hemifacial spasm patients treated with botulinum toxin. J Clin Neuroophthalmol. 1993;13:67–71.
6. Bodker FS, Olson JJ, Putterman AM. Acquired blepharoptosis secondary to essential blepharospasm. Ophthalmic Surg. 1993;24:546–9.
7. Paulson GW, Gill W. Oral and facial movements of blepharospasm. Arch Neurol. 1993;25:380–2.
8. Allergan, Inc. Clinical investigator's brochure. Botox (botulinum toxin type A). Irvine: Allergan, Inc; 1995:10.
9. Dutton JJ, Buckley EG. Botulinum toxin in the management of blepharospasm. Arch Neurol. 1986;43:380–2.
10. Creel DJ, Holds JB, Anderson RL. Auditory brain-stem responses in blepharospasm. Electroencephalogr Clin Neurophysiol. 1993;86:138–40.
11. Klemm WR, Bratton GR, Hudson LC, et al. A possible feline model for human blepharospasm. Neurol Res. 1993;15(1):41–5.
12. Hurwitz JJ, Kazdan M, Codere F, Pashby RC. The orbicularis stripping operation for intractable blepharospasm: surgical results in eighteen patients. Can J Ophthalmol. 1986;21:167–9.
13. Wirtschafter JD. Chemomyectomy of the orbicularis oculi muscle for the treatment of localized hemifacial spasm. J Neuroophthalmol. 1994;14(4):199–204.
14. McLoon LK, Kirsch JD, Cameron S, Wirtschafter JD. Injection of doxorubicin in to rabbit eyelid does not result in loss of facial motor neurons. Brain Res. 1994;641(1):105–10.
15. Gonnering RS. Pharmacology of botulinum toxin. Int Ophthalmol Clin. 1993:33(4):203–27.
16. Dutton JJ. Acute and chronic, local and distant effects of botulinum toxin. Surv Ophthalmol. 1996;40:51–65.
17. Physician's Desk Reference 50th Edition. Montvale, NJ: Medical Economics Company; 1996:477–8.
18. Holds JB, Anderson, RL, Fogg SG, Anderson RL. Motor nerve sprouting in human orbicularis muscle after botulinum A injection. Invest Ophthalmol Vis Sci. 1990; 31:964–7.
19. Wilkins RH. Hemifacial spasm: a review. Surg Neurol. 1991;36:251–77.

INJECTION SITES FOR BLEPHAROSPASM

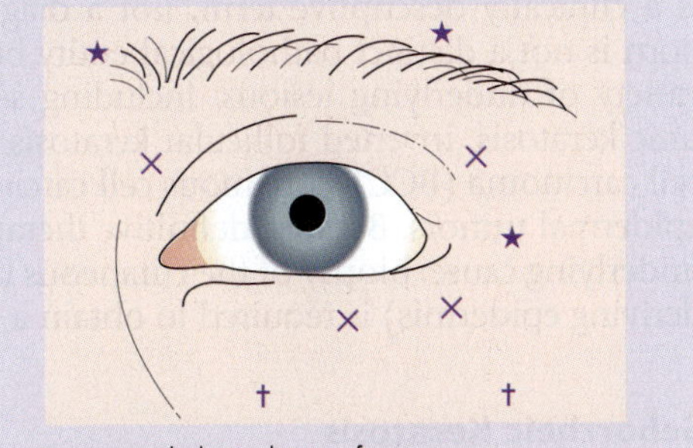

FIG. 91-2 ■ Sites of injection for botulinum toxin in the treatment of benign essential blepharospasm (BEB).

✕ Recommended initial sites of injection;

★ other sites frequently used in essential blepharospasm;

† sites used for Meige's syndrome and hemifacial spasm in addition to the usual sites for BEB

CHAPTER 92 Benign Eyelid Lesions

ANN G. NEFF • KEITH D. CARTER

INTRODUCTION

The eyelids may be affected by a wide spectrum of benign and malignant lesions. In a study that analyzed all eyelid lesions submitted for histopathological examination over a 38-year period, benign lesions were 3 times more frequent than malignant neoplasms.[1] Many lesions which affect the eyelids may occur on any skin surface, but some occur exclusively or more frequently on the eyelids.

The more common benign eyelid lesions are presented here, classified by origin, with each discussion highlighting the important clinical features, differential diagnosis, pertinent systemic associations, histopathology, and treatment.

EPITHELIAL TUMORS

Epithelial cells of the epidermis are arranged in four layers, from deep to superficial:

- The stratum germinativum, known as the *basal layer*
- The stratum spinosum, referred to as the *squamous* or *prickle cell layer*
- The stratum granulosum, called the *granular layer*
- The stratum corneum, also known as the *horny* or *keratin layer*

A variety of histopathological changes that affect these layers of the epidermis may be observed within lesions affecting the eyelids. Such changes may be helpful to distinguish the vast variety of lesions that may be found on the eyelids. Hyperkeratosis, or thickening of the keratin layer, is seen clinically as an adherent scale. Parakeratosis is a form of hyperkeratosis characterized by incomplete keratinization, with retention of nuclei within the keratin layer. Dyskeratosis is abnormal keratinization of cells within the squamous layer. Acanthosis, or thickening of the squamous layer, is seen commonly in proliferative epithelial lesions. Acantholysis refers to separation of epithelial cells.

Each type of epithelial tumor may exhibit some variability in its clinical picture and morphological features. In addition, different types of tumors may share similar clinical and morphological features, which results in clinical diagnostic confusion. A definitive diagnosis of these various lesions depends upon histopathological examination.

Squamous Papilloma

The most common benign lesion of the eyelid is the squamous papilloma, also known as a *fibroepithelial polyp, acrochordon,* or *skin tag.* These lesions may be single or multiple and commonly involve the eyelid margin. Squamous papillomas characteristically are flesh colored and may be sessile or pedunculated (Fig. 92-1). Diagnosis is made by the typical clinical appearance and histological characteristics. The differential diagnosis includes seborrheic keratosis, verruca vulgaris, and intradermal nevus. Microscopically, the lesion has finger-like projections with a fibrovascular core, and the overlying epidermis demonstrates acanthosis and hyperkeratosis. Treatment is simple excision at the base of the lesion.

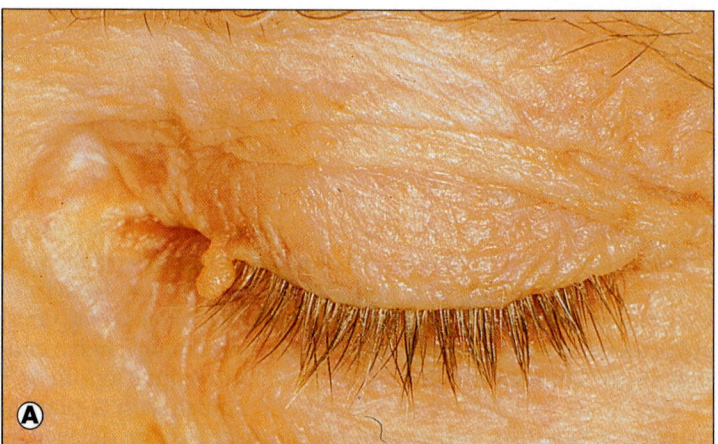

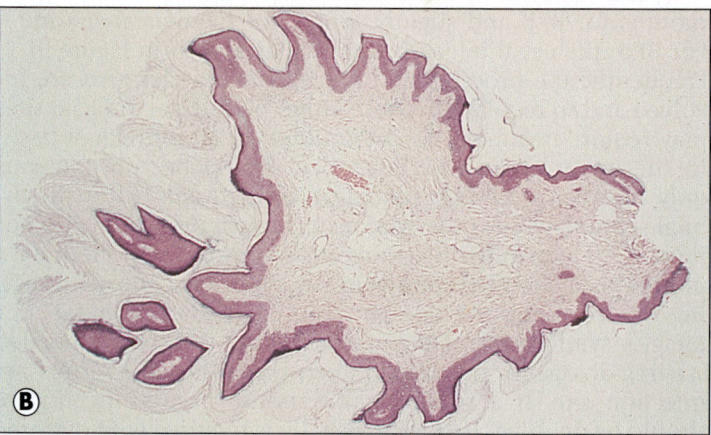

FIG. 92-1 ■ Squamous papilloma. **A,** Typical flesh-colored, pedunculated skin tag involving the left upper eyelid. **B,** Fibroepithelial papilloma consists of a narrow-based (to the right) papilloma with fibrovascular core and finger-like projections covered by acanthotic, hyperkeratotic epithelium. (**B,** From Yanoff M, Fine BS. Ocular pathology, ed 5. St. Louis: Mosby; 2002.)

Cutaneous Horn

A cutaneous horn is a projection of packed keratin (Fig. 92-2). This is a clinically descriptive term, not a diagnostic one. Cutaneous horn is not a distinct pathological entity but may develop from a variety of underlying lesions, including seborrheic keratosis, actinic keratosis, inverted follicular keratosis, verruca vulgaris, basal cell carcinoma (BCC), squamous cell carcinoma (SCC), and other epidermal tumors. Because definitive therapy is dependent on the underlying cause, biopsy of the cutaneous horn (including the underlying epidermis) is required to obtain a histological diagnosis.[2]

Seborrheic Keratosis

Seborrheic keratosis, also known as *senile verruca,* is a common benign epithelial neoplasm which may occur on the face, trunk, and extremities. These lesions usually affect middle-aged and older adults, occurring as single or multiple, greasy, stuck-on plaques (Fig. 92-3). Eyelid lesions are often pedunculated. Color

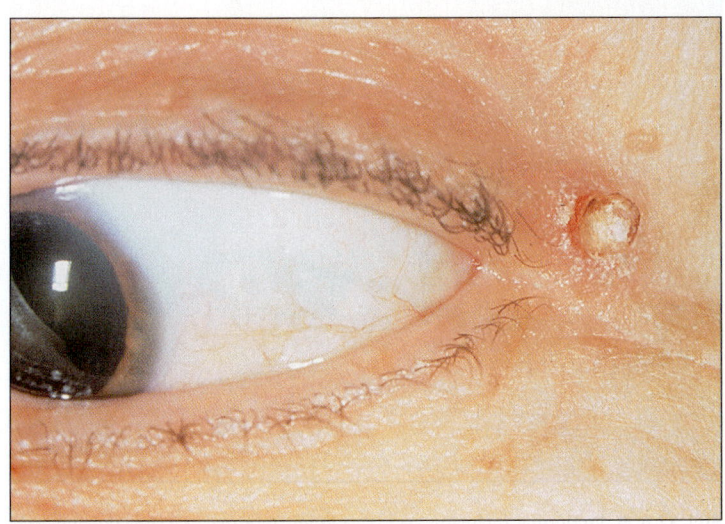

FIG. 92-2 ▮▮ Cutaneous horn. Note the projection of packed keratin that arises from the skin in the region of the left lateral canthus.

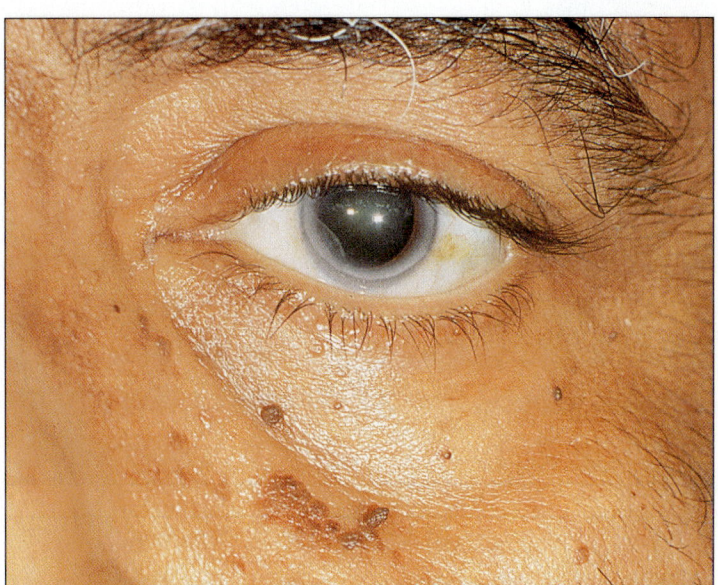

FIG. 92-4 ▮▮ Dermatosis papulosa nigra. Multiple pigmented papules involving the malar region.

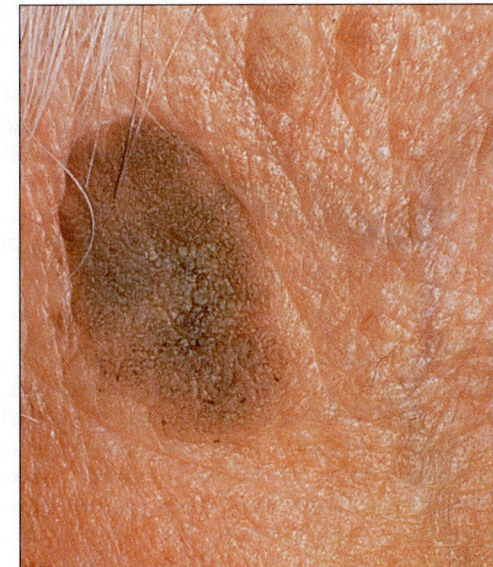

FIG. 92-3 ▮▮ Seborrheic keratosis. Brown, stuck-on plaque, typical of seborrheic keratosis.

varies from tan to brown, and the surface is frequently papillomatous. The differential diagnosis includes skin tag, nevus, verruca vulgaris, actinic keratosis, and pigmented BCC. Seborrheic keratoses are not considered premalignant lesions. A systemic association, however, known as the *sign of Leser–Trélat*, denotes a rapid increase in the size and number of seborrheic keratoses which may occur in patients with occult malignancy.[3]

A variant of seborrheic keratosis, which shares a similar histopathological appearance, is dermatosis papulosa nigra, which occurs primarily in dark-skinned individuals. These lesions usually appear on the cheeks and periorbital region as multiple pigmented papules (Fig. 92-4).

Although different histopathological types of seborrheic keratoses exist, all lesions share features of hyperkeratosis, acanthosis, and papillomatosis.[4] Most lesions contain horn cysts, which are keratin-filled inclusions within the acanthotic epidermis, and pseudohorn cysts, which represent invaginations of surface keratin.[5] Simple excision may be performed for biopsy or cosmesis, or to prevent irritation.

Inverted Follicular Keratosis

Inverted follicular keratosis, also known as *basosquamous cell acanthoma*, usually appears as a small, solitary, papillomatous lesion on the face. It is a well-demarcated, keratotic mass, which may appear as a cutaneous horn. The lesion may resemble verruca vulgaris and seborrheic keratosis—many consider it an irritated seborrheic keratosis.[6] Histopathology reveals hyperkeratosis and lobular acanthosis. Proliferation of basaloid cells occurs with areas of acantholysis and zones of squamous cells, often arranged in whorls called *squamous eddies*. Treatment is complete excision, because recurrence is common after incomplete removal.

Pseudoepitheliomatous Hyperplasia

Pseudoepitheliomatous, or pseudocarcinomatous, hyperplasia is a benign epithelial proliferation which often develops rapidly over several weeks. It appears elevated, with an irregular surface which may be hyperkeratotic or ulcerated. This lesion represents an epidermal response to an underlying disorder, often inflammatory in nature. Associated conditions include mycotic infections, burns, ulcers, surgical wounds, radiation therapy, and insect bites. It also may occur adjacent to malignant neoplasms such as basal and squamous cell carcinomas. Histopathology reveals acanthotic squamous epithelium irregularly invading the dermis, with an inflammatory reaction, often involving the overlying epidermis. Although the squamous cells usually lack atypical changes, differentiation from low-grade SCC may be difficult. Biopsy is necessary for diagnosis, with treatment directed at the underlying condition.

Keratoacanthoma

Keratoacanthoma most commonly appears as a solitary, rapidly growing nodule on sun-exposed areas of middle-aged and older individuals. The nodule is usually umbilicated, with a distinctive central crater filled with a keratin plug (Fig. 92-5). The lesion develops over weeks and typically undergoes spontaneous involution within 6 months to leave an atrophic scar. Lesions which occur on the eyelids may produce mechanical abnormalities, such as ectropion or ptosis, and occasionally may cause destructive changes.[7] The differential diagnosis includes SCC, BCC, verruca vulgaris, and molluscum contagiosum (MC). Patients with Muir–Torre syndrome may develop, in association with internal malignancy, multiple keratoacanthomas and sebaceous neoplasms.

Microscopically, there is cup-shaped elevation of acanthotic squamous epithelium which surrounds a central mass of keratin. Microabscesses which contain necrotic keratinocytes and neutrophils may be found within the proliferative epithelium. The base is usually noninfiltrating and often demarcated from

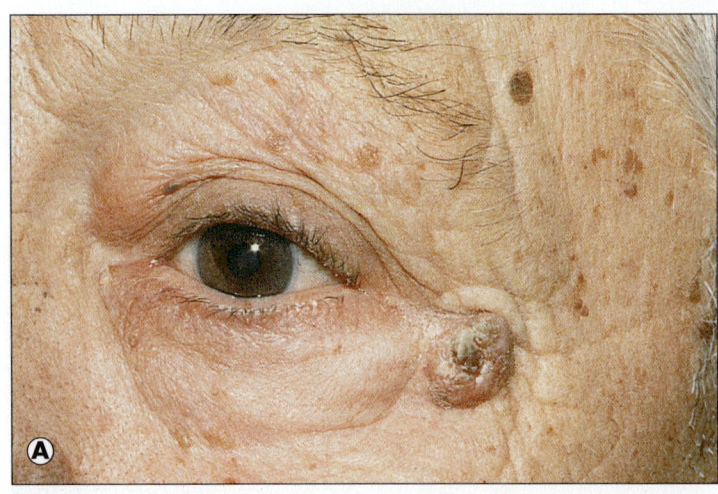

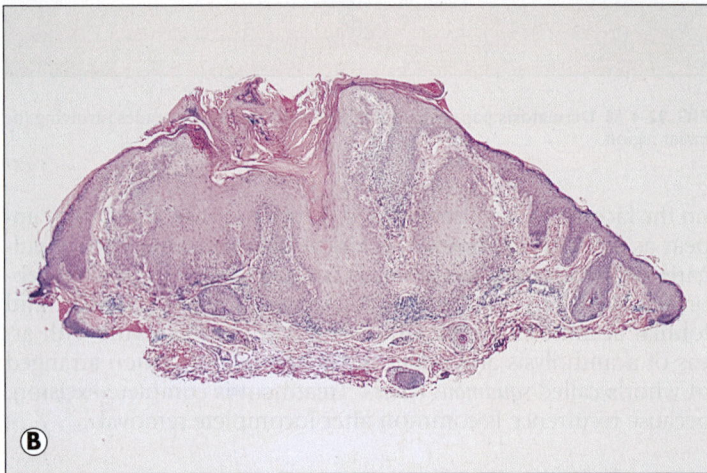

FIG. 92-5 ■ Keratoacanthoma. A, Lesion shows typical clinical appearance; history was also typical. **B,** The lesion that can be seen above the surface epithelium has a cup-shaped configuration, and a central keratin core. The base of the acanthotic epithelium is blunted (rather than invasive) at the junction of the dermis.

the underlying dermis by an inflammatory reaction. Cellular atypia may be present, making differentiation from SCC difficult. Many pathologists consider keratoacanthoma a type of low-grade SCC.[8] Treatment may speed recovery, limit scarring, and confirm the diagnosis. Complete excision is recommended because an invasive variant exists, with the potential for perineural and intramuscular spread.[8] Both radiotherapy and intralesional fluorouracil have been advocated.[9,10]

Actinic Keratosis

Actinic keratosis, also known as *solar* or *senile keratosis,* is not truly a benign condition, being the most common premalignant skin lesion. The lesions develop on sun-exposed areas and commonly affect the face, hands, and scalp and, less commonly, the eyelid. They usually appear as multiple, flat-topped papules with an adherent white scale. The development of SCC in untreated lesions reportedly ranges as high as 20% (see Chapter 93).[11] Microscopically, actinic keratoses display hyperkeratosis, parakeratosis, and dyskeratosis. Epidermal atrophy, or thinning, often is present. Atypical keratinocytes in the deep epidermal layers often form buds which extend into the papillary dermis. The underlying dermis usually contains chronic inflammation. Management is surgical excision or cryotherapy (following biopsy).

Epidermal Inclusion Cyst

Epidermal inclusion cysts appear as slow-growing, round, firm lesions of the dermis or subcutaneous tissue. Eyelid lesions are usually solitary, mobile, and less than 1cm in diameter. These

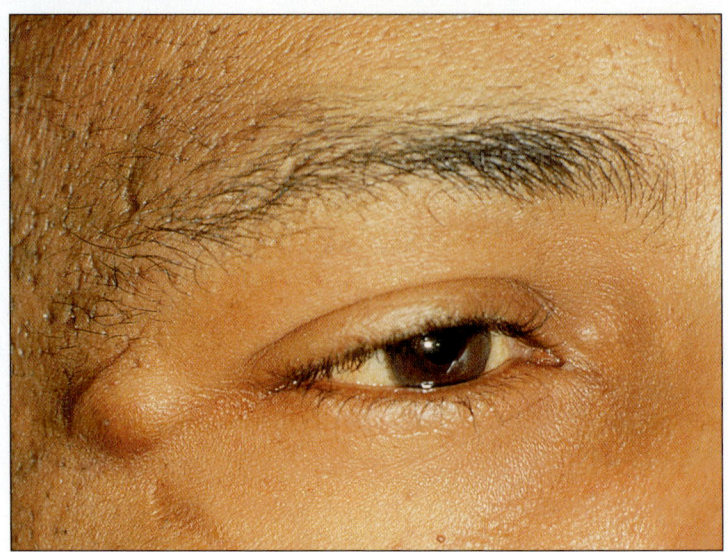

FIG. 92-6 ■ Epidermal inclusion cyst. This lesion appeared as a slow-growing, cystic lesion in a region of previous penetrating trauma.

cysts may be congenital in origin or may arise from traumatic implantation of surface epidermis (Fig. 92-6). Cysts may become infected or may rupture, producing a surrounding foreign body granulomatous reaction.

Diagnosis is based on the clinical appearance and histopathology. Differential diagnosis includes dermoid cyst, pilar cyst, and neurofibroma. Microscopically, the cyst is filled with keratin and is lined by a keratinizing, stratified squamous epithelium. Adnexal structures are not present in the cyst wall.[12] Treatment is complete excision, preferably of the entire cyst wall, to prevent recurrence.

Pilar Cyst

Pilar cysts, formerly known as *sebaceous cysts,* are smooth, round, movable dermal or subcutaneous masses, clinically identical to epidermal inclusion cysts. The differentiation within these cysts is thought to be toward hair keratin.[13] These cysts tend to occur in areas with large numbers of hair follicles and are found most commonly on the scalp. They may occur occasionally in the periocular region, particularly in the brow or along the eyelid margin. Histopathology reveals an epithelium-lined cyst, with palisading of the basal layer. The lining lacks a granular layer, unlike that of epidermal cysts. Eosinophilic material within the cyst comprises desquamated cells and keratin, and commonly calcifies. Cyst rupture may occur and incite a foreign body granulomatous response. Treatment is complete surgical excision—incomplete excision may result in recurrence.

Epidermoid and Dermoid Cysts

Although generally considered in discussions of orbital lesions (see Chapter 94), epidermoid and dermoid cysts are included here because they may appear as an eyelid mass. These cysts can occur as superficial, subcutaneous, or deep orbital lesions. Both are choristomas that are firm, slowly enlarging, nontender masses, most commonly in the lateral upper eyelid and brow region (Fig. 92-7). Superficial lesions usually are recognized during early childhood.[14] These cysts presumably occur secondary to entrapment of skin along embryonic closure lines. Attachment to underlying bony sutures often is present, most commonly the frontozygomatic suture (see Chapter 82). Lesions may extend posteriorly into the orbit. Diagnosis is suspected clinically, confirmed after excision with histopathological examination.

Microscopically, both dermoid and epidermoid cysts are lined by a stratified squamous keratinizing epithelium. Dermoid cysts also contain adnexal elements in the cyst wall, including hair fol-

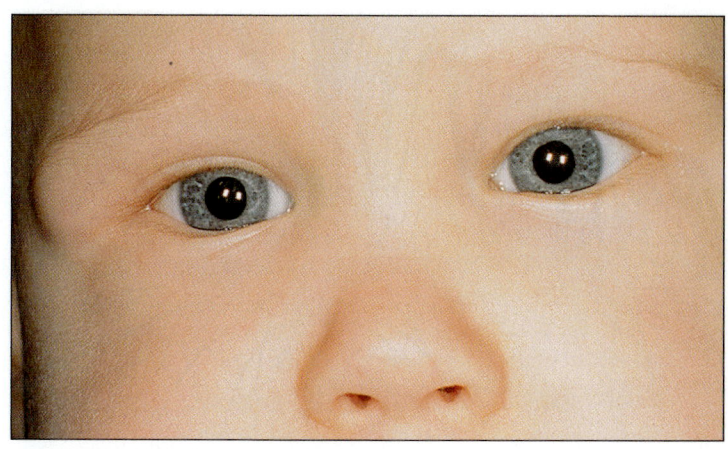

FIG. 92-7 ■ **Dermoid cyst.** Cystic, subcutaneous lesion in the right upper lid and brow region, attached to the underlying frontozygomatic suture.

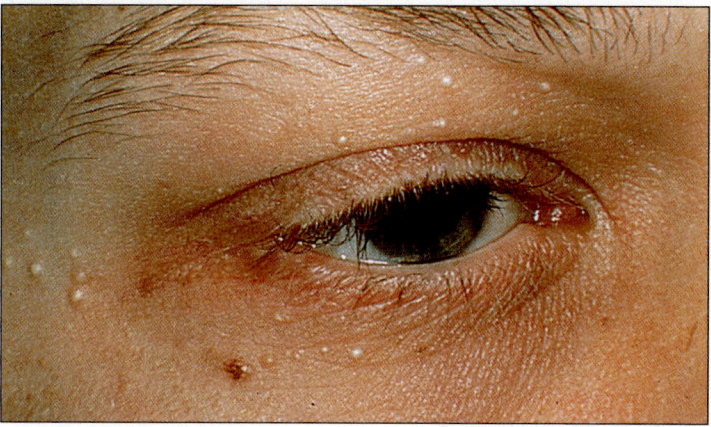

FIG. 92-8 ■ **Milia.** Multiple, small, white lesions that affect the upper and lower eyelids.

licles and sebaceous and eccrine glands; these elements are lacking in epidermoid cysts. Treatment is complete surgical excision. Preoperative orbital imaging is indicated if the entire cyst cannot be palpated or if orbital extension is suspected. Complete excision eliminates the potential for cyst rupture, which can produce secondary foreign body granulomatous inflammation.

Nevus Verruca

Nevus verruca, or linear epidermal nevus, is a flesh-colored lesion composed of a linear series of hyperkeratotic papules. This localized form usually appears at birth or early in life. A generalized, widespread form of nevus verruca also exists, which may be associated with skeletal and central nervous system abnormalities.[15] Diagnosis is based on the typical clinical appearance and biopsy findings. Histopathology reveals papillomatosis, hyperkeratosis, and acanthosis of the epidermis, with no dermal involvement. Treatment modalities include surgical excision, cryotherapy, electrodesiccation, and dermabrasion.

Nevus Sebaceus of Jadassohn

The nevus sebaceus of Jadassohn may be confused clinically with linear epidermal nevus. The nevus sebaceus typically is found on the face during early childhood and appears as a well-defined, yellow, papillomatous lesion, which typically enlarges during adolescence. Initially it is characterized by epithelial hyperplasia, but subsequent hyperplasia of the adnexal structures occurs. Secondary tumor formation often develops during adulthood. Syringocystadenoma papilliferum, a benign tumor of apocrine origin, may appear.[16] BCC and SCC have been associated rarely with nevus sebaceus.

ADNEXAL TUMORS

Lesions of adnexal origin arise from the epidermal appendages, which include the sebaceous glands of Zeis, meibomian glands, pilosebaceous units (consisting of hair follicles and associated sebaceous glands), eccrine sweat glands, and apocrine sweat glands of Moll.

Benign Lesions of Sebaceous Origin

Sebaceous lesions of the eyelid may arise from several sources: the glands of Zeis, found in association with the eyelashes; the meibomian glands, located within the fibrous tarsal plates; and sebaceous glands, associated with hair follicles of the eyebrows and on the cutaneous surfaces of the eyelids. The sebaceous glands create their secretions by a holocrine mechanism, in which the central cells undergo disintegration and subsequent extrusion into a common excretory duct.

MILIA. Milia form as multiple, firm, white lesions which range from 1–4mm in diameter. They usually appear on the face and commonly affect the eyelids, nose, and malar region (Fig. 92-8). Lesions may occur spontaneously or secondarily due to trauma, radiotherapy, skin infection, or bullous diseases. Occlusion of pilosebaceous units with retention of keratin is thought to be the causative mechanism. Histopathology reveals a dilated, keratin-filled hair follicle, with compression and atrophy of the adjacent sebaceous glands.[17] Treatment includes simple incision, electrodesiccation of the surface, or puncture and expression of the contents.

ACQUIRED SEBACEOUS GLAND HYPERPLASIA. This lesion occurs predominantly in elderly patients, usually on the skin of the face and scalp. Skin lesions appear as multiple, small, yellow, slightly umbilicated papules. Individual lesions may resemble BCC. The meibomian glands may also be affected, to produce nodular thickening of the lids. Sebaceous carcinoma must be considered (see Chapter 93). Microscopically, numerous sebaceous gland lobules are grouped around a central dilated duct. Multiple management options exist, including excision, cryotherapy, and carbon dioxide laser.

SEBACEOUS ADENOMA. This uncommon lesion usually appears in the elderly as a solitary, yellow papule, with a predilection for the eyelid and brow. The importance of this and other benign sebaceous neoplasms is the association with internal malignancy, known as the Muir–Torre syndrome. Even a single cutaneous sebaceous neoplasm may be significant, so patients should be evaluated accordingly.[18] Patients with this syndrome also may develop multiple keratoacanthomas. Microscopically, the sebaceous adenoma is a well-circumscribed lesion, with lobules containing an outer layer of basal germinal cells, which become lipidized centrally. Treatment is complete surgical excision, because incompletely excised lesions commonly recur.

Benign Lesions of Eccrine Origin

The eccrine sweat glands are found throughout the cutaneous surface of the eyelids. They are composed of three segments, including an intradermal secretory coil, an intradermal duct, and an intraepidermal duct.

ECCRINE HIDROCYSTOMA. Eccrine hidrocystomas, also known as *sudoriferous* or *sweat gland cysts*, appear as solitary or multiple, small nodules on the eyelids. The overlying skin is shiny and smooth, and the cyst usually is translucent and fluid filled (Fig. 92-9). Eccrine hidrocystomas are thought to be ductal retention cysts, which tend to increase in size in hot, humid weather. The differential diagnosis includes apocrine hidrocystoma and epidermal inclusion cyst. Histopathology reveals a dermal cyst lined by a double-layered cuboidal epithelium without papillary infoldings. Treatment is complete excision.

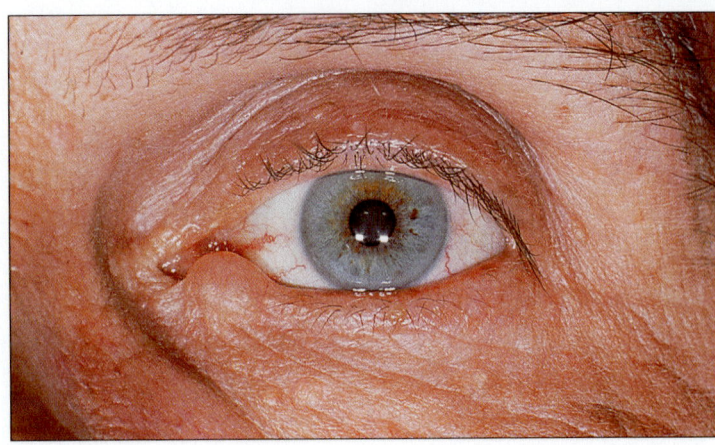

FIG. 92-9 ■ **Eccrine hidrocystoma.** Cystic lesion involving the left lower eyelid margin. The lesion was filled with translucent fluid.

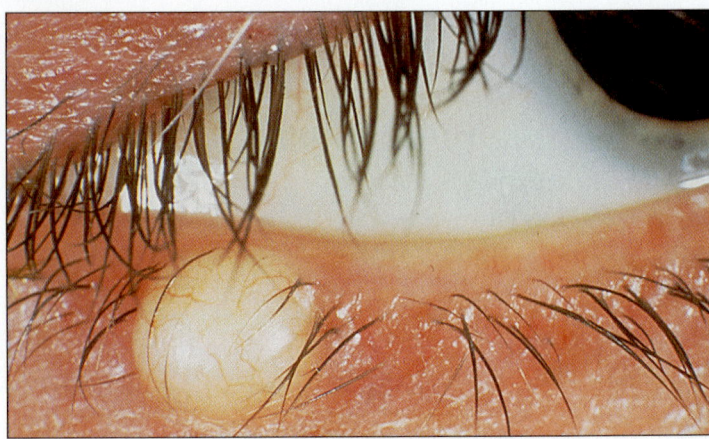

FIG. 92-10 ■ **Apocrine hidrocystoma.** Cystic lesion, filled with milky fluid, involving the right lower eyelid margin.

SYRINGOMA. The syringoma is a common adnexal tumor arising from adenomatous proliferation of the intraepidermal duct of eccrine glands. They occur primarily in young females, occurring as multiple, small (1–3mm diameter), skin-color to yellowish papules distributed symmetrically on the lower eyelids and cheeks. Microscopically, syringomas contain ducts lined by double-layered cuboidal epithelium, embedded in a dense fibrous stroma. The ducts may taper to a solid core of cells, to produce a comma-shaped or "tadpole" configuration.[19] Treatment modalities include surgical excision, electrodesiccation, and carbon dioxide laser.[20]

CHONDROID SYRINGOMA. Chondroid syringoma, also known as *pleomorphic adenoma* or *mixed tumor of the skin*, most commonly occurs in the head and neck region and, rarely, may involve the eyelid.[21] It appears as a 0.5–3cm in diameter, asymptomatic, dermal nodule. The lesions are thought to arise from eccrine sweat glands and owe their name to the mixture of sweat gland and cartilaginous elements. Differential diagnosis includes epidermal inclusion cyst, pilar cyst, neurofibroma, and pilomatrixoma. Microscopically, it is identical to pleomorphic adenoma of the lacrimal gland. Ducts lined with an inner secretory layer and an outer myoepithelial layer are embedded in a stroma with areas of chondroid metaplasia. Treatment is surgical excision. Malignant variants have been reported.

ACROSPIROMA. Acrospiroma, also known as *clear-cell hidradenoma*, appears as a solid or cystic subcutaneous nodule, with flesh-colored or erythematous overlying skin which may ulcerate.[22] Acrospiroma occurs in young adults and may appear at any cutaneous site, occasionally on the eyelid. Lesions may resemble keratoacanthoma. Pain may be elicited in approximately 20% of cases on applying pressure to the lesion. Histopathology reveals a well-demarcated dermal mass with ductal and secretory elements. Large, glycogen-rich clear cells and polyhedral cells with eosinophilic cytoplasm are present in the solid portions of the tumor.[23] Treatment is surgical excision. Malignant variants are reported to exist.

Benign Lesions of Apocrine Origin

The apocrine glands of Moll are found along the eyelid margin in association with the eyelash follicles. They are modified sweat glands which contain a secretory coil, an intradermal duct, and an intraepithelial duct. Their secretions are produced by decapitation of the secretory cells.

APOCRINE HIDROCYSTOMA. Apocrine hidrocystoma, also known as *cystadenoma*, usually appears as a solitary, translucent cyst on the face, sometimes at the eyelid margin. The cyst is usually small (less than 1cm in diameter) and filled with clear or milky fluid, with shiny, smooth overlying skin (Fig. 92-10). Lesions may display a bluish coloration, attributed to the Tyndall effect. Unlike the eccrine variety, these lesions are thought to be proliferative in origin and do not increase in size in hot weather.

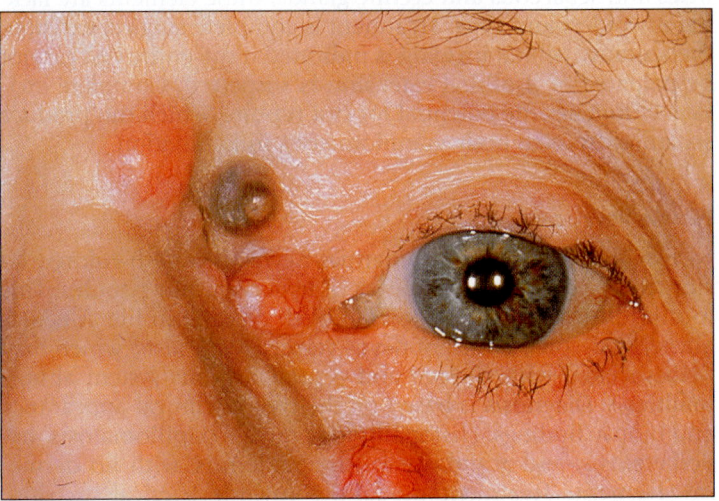

FIG. 92-11 ■ **Cylindroma.** Multiple, pinkish-red dermal nodules involving the eyelids, forehead, nose, and malar region.

The differential diagnosis includes eccrine hidrocystoma and cystic BCC. An association has been reported, thought to represent an ectodermal dysplasia, in which patients display multiple apocrine hidrocystomas, hypodontia, palmar–plantar hyperkeratosis, and onychodystrophy.[24]

Histopathology reveals a dermal cyst with papillary infoldings, lined by an inner secretory layer with eosinophilic columnar cells and an outer myoepithelial layer. Treatment is complete excision.

CYLINDROMA. Cylindroma, presumably of apocrine origin, may occur on the eyelid or brow. It usually appears as a dome-shaped, skin-colored, or pinkish-red, dermal nodule (Fig. 92-11). Solitary lesions usually occur in adulthood in the head and neck region and may appear similar to a pilar or epidermal inclusion cyst. Multiple lesions are inherited in an autosomal dominant fashion and usually appear on the scalp, where extensive involvement is referred to as a *turban tumor*. Multiple lesions have been associated with trichoepitheliomas. Microscopically, the cylindroma consists of islands with large, pale-staining cells centrally and small, cuboidal cells peripherally, surrounded by an eosinophilic basement membrane. Treatment is surgical excision.

Benign Lesions of Hair Follicle Origin

Benign lesions of hair follicle origin are rather rare tumors, often confused clinically with BCC, the most common malignant eyelid lesion. Confirmation of diagnosis by incisional biopsy is helpful for suspicious-looking lesions, which allows less extensive resection of lesions confirmed as benign.[25]

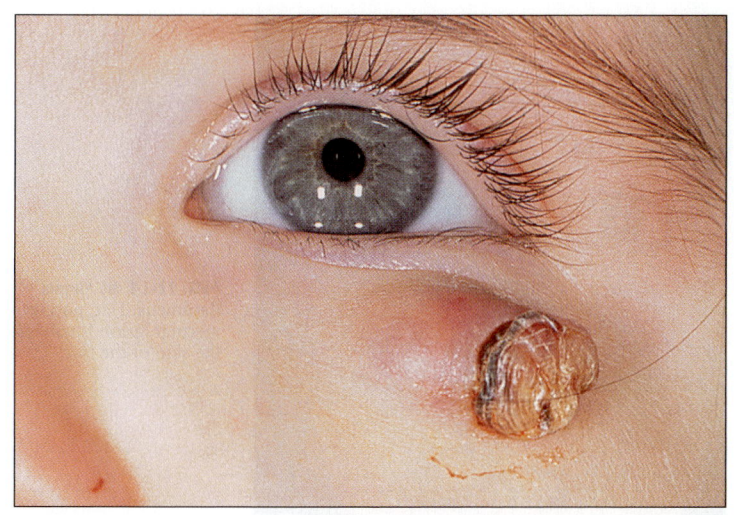

FIG. 92-12 ■ Pilomatrixoma. Reddish nodule arising from the left lower eyelid.

TRICHOEPITHELIOMA. Trichoepithelioma is a tumor of hair follicle origin with a predilection for the face, including the eyelids and forehead. The solitary lesion tends to occur in older individuals as an asymptomatic, flesh-colored to yellowish, firm papule that rarely ulcerates. Clinical differentiation from BCC and other adnexal tumors may be difficult to make.

Multiple lesions, also known as *multiple benign cystic epithelioma* or *Brooke's tumor*, are inherited in an autosomal dominant pattern with variable penetrance. Lesions appear during adolescence as multiple firm nodules involving the face, and also the scalp, neck, and trunk. They may increase in size and number but rarely ulcerate. Diagnosis is made by the clinical appearance, family history, and histopathology. Differential diagnosis includes basal cell nevus syndrome, in which lesions tend to ulcerate more frequently (see Chapter 93).

Histopathology reveals multiple, keratin-filled horn cysts surrounded by islands of basaloid cells which display peripheral palisading. The abundant fibrous stroma is well demarcated from the surrounding dermis. Lesions may histologically resemble BCC, and rare reports of transformation to BCC exist.[26] Treatment includes surgical excision of solitary lesions and cryosurgery or laser for multiple lesions.

TRICHOFOLLICULOMA. Trichofolliculoma is a fairly well-differentiated hamartomatous lesion, usually appearing as an asymptomatic, solitary, flesh-colored nodule during adulthood on the face or scalp. A central umbilication usually is present, which is the opening of a keratin-filled follicle. Small white hairs may protrude from the central pore and are suggestive of the diagnosis. The lesion may be confused clinically with a pilar cyst, nevus, or BCC.[17] Histopathology reveals a dilated follicle, filled with keratin and hair shafts, and lined by stratified squamous epithelium continuous with the epidermis. Surgical excision is curative.

TRICHILEMMOMA. Trichilemmoma is a tumor which arises from the outer hair sheath. A solitary lesion generally appears during adulthood as an asymptomatic, flesh-colored, nodular, or papillomatous lesion. The nose is the most common site of occurrence, followed by the eyelid and the brow.[27] The lesion may appear as a cutaneous horn or may resemble verruca vulgaris or BCC.

Multiple trichilemmomas are a marker for Cowden's disease, or multiple hamartoma syndrome, a rare genodermatosis inherited in an autosomal dominant fashion. In addition to the facial trichilemmomas, patients may develop acral keratoses and oral papillomas. Patients are at increased risk of developing breast and thyroid carcinoma, as well as multiple hamartomas. The mucocutaneous lesions usually precede the onset of malignancy.[28]

Microscopically, glycogen-rich cells with clear cytoplasm proliferate in lobules, with peripheral palisading and a distinct basement membrane. Hair follicles may be present. Treatment is surgical excision, cryosurgery, or laser.

PILOMATRIXOMA. The pilomatrixoma, also known as the *calcifying epithelioma of Malherbe*, is a benign tumor of hair matrix origin.[29] The lesion tends to occur in children and young adults on the head and upper extremities. Lesions may occur in the periorbital region, particularly the upper eyelid and brow.[30] Usually a solitary lesion, it appears as a solid or cystic, mobile, subcutaneous nodule with normal overlying skin. It is firm, irregular, often reddish blue, and may contain chalky white nodules (Fig. 92-12). Histopathology reveals islands of basophilic epithelial cells, which transform into shadow cells located more centrally. Most tumors contain masses of calcified shadow cells, which may incite a giant cell granulomatous response. Rare cases of malignant transformation have been reported. Treatment is surgical excision.

VASCULAR TUMORS
Capillary Hemangioma

The capillary hemangioma, also known as a *benign hemangioendothelioma*, is a common vascular lesion of childhood, which occurs in 1–2% of infants and is the most common orbital tumor found in children. Girls are more commonly affected than boys, with a 3:2 ratio. A periorbital hemangioma may appear as a superficial cutaneous lesion, subcutaneous lesion, deep orbital tumor, or combination of these types. Approximately one third of lesions are visible at birth, with the remainder manifest by 6 months of age. There is typically an initial rapid growth phase within 6 months of diagnosis, followed by a period of stabilization and subsequent involution over several years. It is estimated that approximately 75% regress to some extent by the time the child reaches 7 years of age.

The classic superficial lesion, the strawberry nevus, appears as a red, raised, nodular mass which blanches with pressure (Fig. 92-13). It may first be seen as a flat lesion with telangiectatic surface vessels. A subcutaneous lesion appears as a bluish-purple, spongy mass. Deep orbital lesions may cause proptosis and globe displacement, with no associated cutaneous findings.

The most common ocular complication is amblyopia, which may result from occlusion of the visual axis due to eyelid involvement, or from anisometropia due to induced astigmatism. Strabismus may occur secondary to the amblyopia or be caused by orbital involvement with restriction of ocular motility.[31]

Lesions that involve the eyelid and anterior orbit usually can be diagnosed by clinical findings. Cutaneous lesions may be confused with nevus flammeus, which is usually flatter, darker, and does not blanch with pressure. The differential diagnosis of orbital lesions includes rhabdomyosarcoma, neuroblastoma, encephalocele, lymphangioma, and inflammatory masses (see Chapter 95). Ultrasonography, computed tomography, and magnetic resonance imaging may aid in diagnosis and in determining the extent of involvement (see Chapter 84). Biopsy may be needed for patients who have a rapidly expanding orbital mass or for those in whom noninvasive methods are not diagnostic.

Systemic complications are rare in isolated periorbital lesions. However, patients who have extensive visceral hemangiomas may develop thrombocytopenia related to entrapment of platelets within the lesion, with resulting hemorrhagic diathesis, known as the *Kasabach–Merritt syndrome*. Patients with orbital hemangiomas have a predilection for noncontiguous hemangiomas in the head and neck region.

Microscopically, the early proliferative phase of the lesion contains lobules of plump endothelial cells separated by fibrous septa, with frequent mitotic figures and small, irregular vascular lumina. Mature lesions contain more prominent vascular structures and flatter endothelial cells diminished in number. As regression takes place, progressive fibrosis occurs, with thickening of the fibrous septa and replacement of endothelial lobules by adipose tissue. Atrophy of the vascular component of the lesion eventuates.

Because most capillary hemangiomas undergo spontaneous regression to some extent, treatment generally is reserved for patients who have specific ocular, dermatologic, or systemic in-

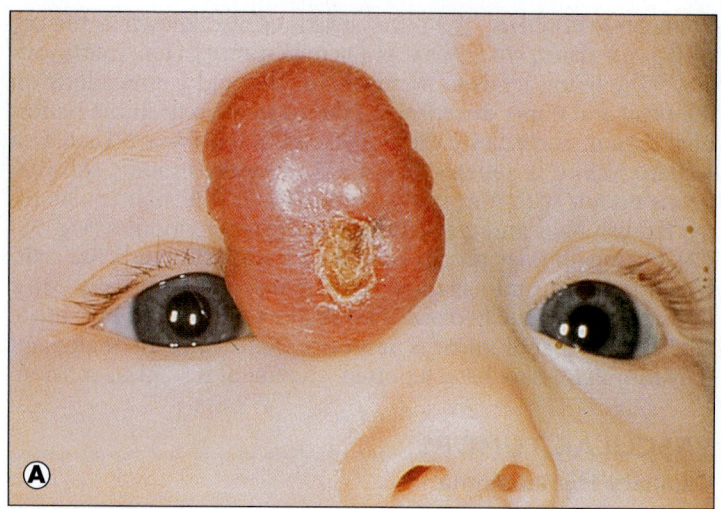

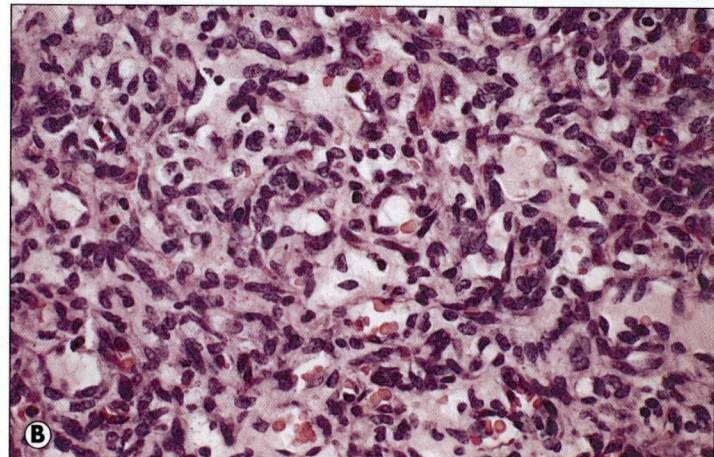

FIG. 92-13 ■ **Capillary hemangioma. A,** Superficial, raised, red mass involving the right upper eyelid and medial canthal region. **B,** High magnification of endothelial cells. (**B,** From Yanoff M, Fine BS. Ocular pathology, ed 5. St. Louis: Mosby; 2002.)

dications for intervention. Various management modalities have been advocated, each with potential significant risks which are beyond the scope of this discussion. Ocular indications include amblyopia, compressive optic neuropathy, and proptosis with globe exposure. Treatment modalities include intralesional corticosteroid injection,[32,33] systemic corticosteroids, radiotherapy, laser therapy, systemic interferon, and surgery. Intralesional corticosteroid injection is the favored management, especially for cutaneous hemangiomas. Surgery should be considered for localized, noninfiltrative lesions, or for those which fail to respond to corticosteroids.[34] Amblyopia should be treated with appropriate patching and spectacle correction, as indicated.

Cavernous Hemangioma

Cavernous hemangioma is the most common benign orbital tumor of adults (only occasionally occurring as a primary eyelid lesion); the lesions usually appear during adulthood and normally do not undergo spontaneous regression. Superficial skin lesions are dark blue, compressible and, unlike the orbital variety, not encapsulated. The differential diagnosis includes lymphangioma, with associated hemorrhage, and varices, which are formed by dilatation of preexisting vascular channels. A rare syndrome exists, termed the *blue rubber bleb nevus syndrome,* which is characterized by multiple cutaneous lesions consistent with cavernous hemangiomas, associated with gastrointestinal hemangiomas which often bleed.[35] Histologically, cavernous hemangiomas contain dilated, endothelium-lined vascular spaces, often with thrombosis and phlebolith formation. Treatment is surgical excision.

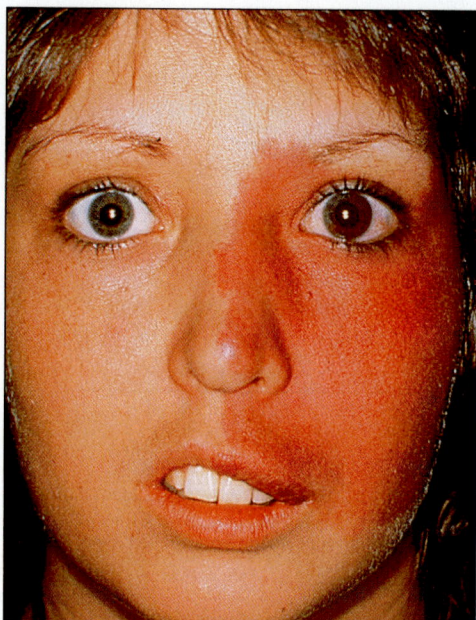

FIG. 92-14 ■ **Nevus flammeus.** Flat, purple, vascular lesion involving the skin of the face.

Lymphangioma

Lymphangiomas may involve the eyelid, conjunctiva, or orbit.[36] Lesions often appear at birth or early in childhood, and only occasionally in adulthood. They often are poorly circumscribed, with an infiltrative growth pattern. Eyelid involvement may occur as a superficial lesion with multiple cyst-like excrescences, or as a complex of channels that cause lid thickening and distortion. Hemorrhage into the lesion may occur, to produce a hematoma when the eyelid is involved or proptosis when orbital lesions are present (see Chapter 95). Biopsy may be needed for definitive diagnosis. Microscopically, dilated, thin-walled vascular spaces lined by endothelial cells are present. Lymphoid aggregates may be present which, in the context of orbital lesions, may undergo proliferation associated with upper respiratory infections and cause worsening proptosis. Surgical excision is indicated for optic nerve compromise in orbital lesions, cosmesis, or eyelid malposition. Large lesions may be difficult to manage due to extensive infiltration. Carbon dioxide laser is a useful modality when excision is required.

Nevus Flammeus

Nevus flammeus, also known as a *port-wine stain,* presents as a flat, purple, vascular lesion, usually unilateral and in the distribution of a branch of the trigeminal nerve (Fig. 92-14). It is congenital and does not undergo spontaneous regression. If associated with ocular and leptomeningeal vascular hamartomas, it represents the Sturge–Weber syndrome. Ocular manifestations of this syndrome include diffuse choroidal hemangioma, ipsilateral glaucoma, and serous retinal detachment. Histopathology of the skin lesion reveals dilated, telangiectatic capillaries within the dermis. Management is primarily with cosmetics. Tunable dye laser therapy also may be used to improve the appearance of the lesion.[37]

Pyogenic Granuloma

Pyogenic granuloma is the most common acquired vascular lesion to involve the eyelids.[17] It usually occurs after trauma or surgery as a fast-growing, fleshy, red-to-pink mass, which readily bleeds with minor contact (Fig. 92-15). Lesions also may develop in association with inflammatory processes, including chalazia. The differential diagnosis includes Kaposi's sarcoma and intravascular papillary endothelial hyperplasia, a rare endothelial proliferation. Microscopically, there is granulation tissue consisting of fibroblasts and blood vessels, with acute and

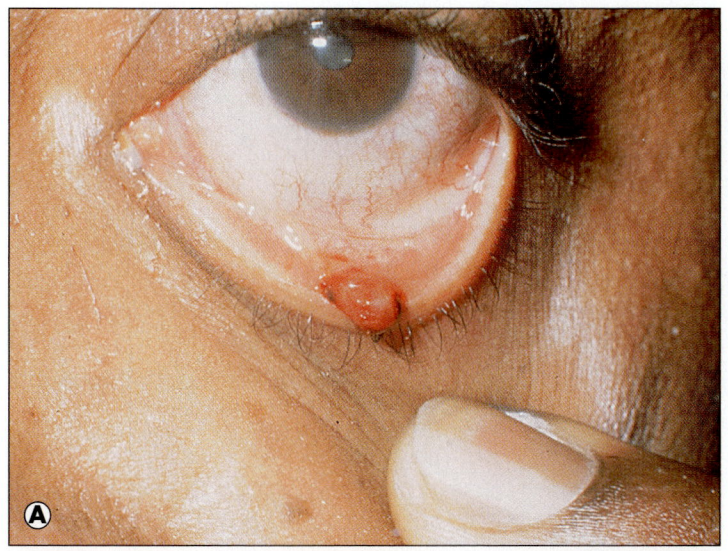

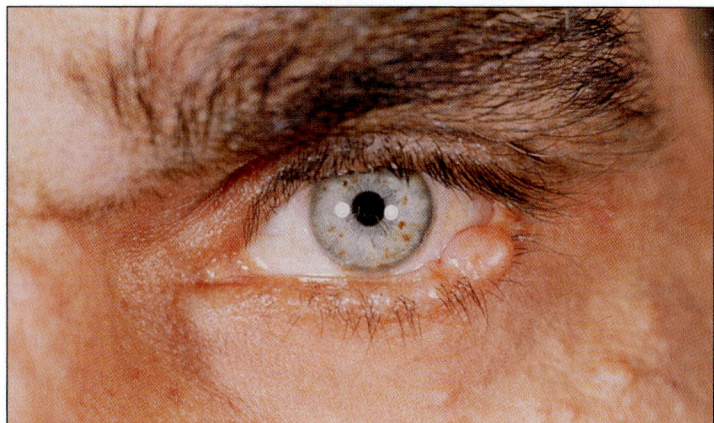

FIG. 92-16 ▮▮ **Neurofibroma.** Note the fleshy mass on the eyelid of this patient with disseminated cutaneous neurofibromas.

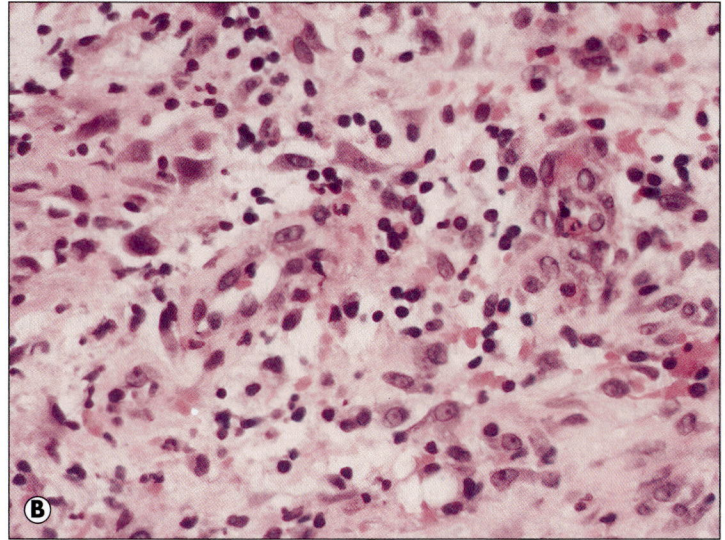

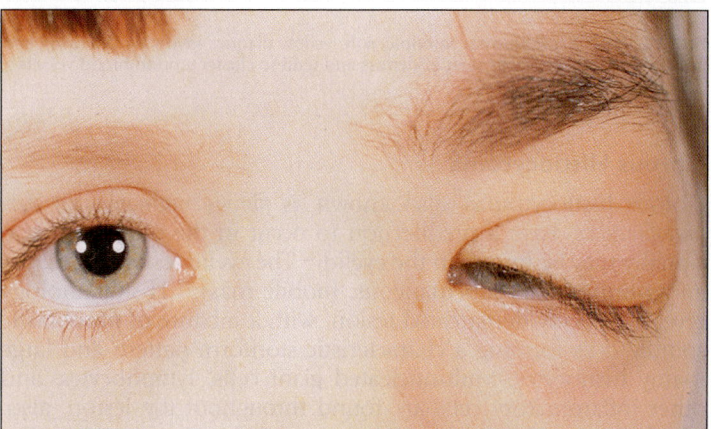

FIG. 92-17 ▮▮ **Plexiform neurofibroma.** Note the ptosis and typical S-shaped curvature of the upper lid.

FIG. 92-15 ▮▮ **Pyogenic granuloma. A,** Red mass arising from the palpebral conjunctiva and protruding over the eyelid margin. This lesion developed in association with a chalazion. **B,** Vascularized tissue (granulation tissue) that consists of inflammatory cells (polymorphonuclear lymphocytes and fibroblasts) and the endothelial cells of budding capillaries.

chronic nongranulomatous inflammatory cells. Notably, the lesion is neither pyogenic nor granulomatous. Treatment is by surgical excision at the base of the lesion.

TUMORS OF NEURAL ORIGIN

Neurofibroma

Neurofibromas most commonly are considered in the context of neurofibromatosis, in which patients often develop multiple cutaneous lesions in association with other stigmata of the disease, usually apparent by adolescence.[38] The neurofibromas may occur on any cutaneous surface, including the eyelid, and typically enlarge slowly over many years. They appear as soft, fleshy, often pedunculated masses (Fig. 92-16). Isolated cutaneous neurofibromas, often resembling intradermal nevi, also may occur in individuals with no other associated abnormality.

The plexiform neurofibroma, characteristic of type 1 neurofibromatosis, often occurs as a diffuse infiltration of the eyelid and orbit. The upper eyelid is usually ptotic, with an S-shaped curvature (Fig. 92-17). On palpation, the lesion feels like a "bag of worms." Histopathology reveals units of proliferating axons, Schwann cells, and fibroblasts, with each unit surrounded by a perineural sheath.

Management depends on the site and extent of disease. Isolated cutaneous lesions, unrelated to neurofibromatosis, may

be excised surgically. Surgical debulking may be performed for plexiform neurofibromas which produce mechanical ptosis or cosmetic deformity. However, due to the infiltrative nature of these lesions, complete excision is usually impossible and recurrence is common.

XANTHOMATOUS LESIONS

Xanthomatous lesions are characterized by the presence of histiocytes which have accumulated lipid, resulting in a foamy appearance of the cytoplasm histologically.

Xanthelasma

Xanthelasma palpebrarum is the most common cutaneous xanthoma, typically occurring in middle-aged and older adults as soft, yellow plaques on the medial aspect of the eyelids (Fig. 92-18). The diagnosis often can be made clinically. Hyperlipidemia is reported to occur in approximately 50% of patients with xanthelasma,[39,40] therefore screening is recommended.[41] Type IIa is the most commonly associated hyperlipidemia. The differential diagnosis of atypical lesions includes Erdheim–Chester disease, a systemic xanthogranulomatous disorder which has lesions that typically appear more indurated.

Microscopically, xanthelasmas are composed of foamy, lipid-laden histiocytes (xanthoma cells) clustered around blood vessels and adnexal structures within the superficial dermis. Surrounding fibrosis and inflammation may be observed. Treatment modalities include surgical excision, carbon dioxide laser ablation, and topical trichloroacetic acid. Recurrence is common.

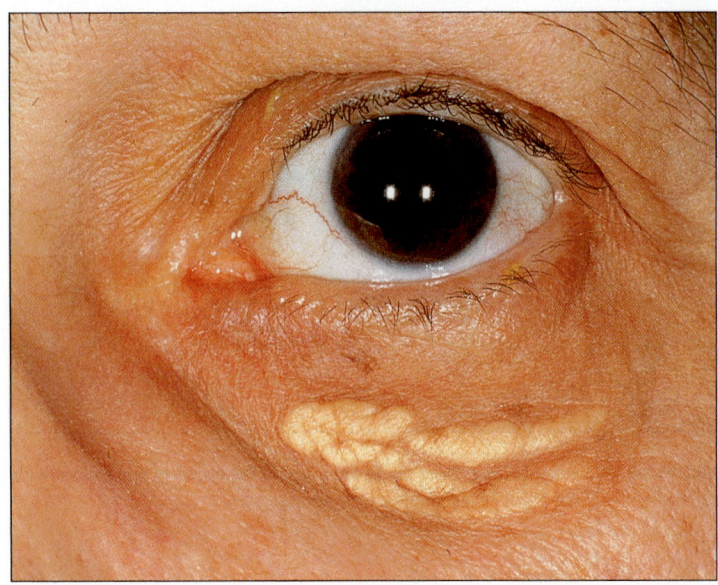

FIG. 92-18 ■ **Xanthelasma.** Multiple, soft, yellow plaques involving the lower eyelid. Lipid-laden foam cells seen in dermis and tend to cluster around blood vessels.

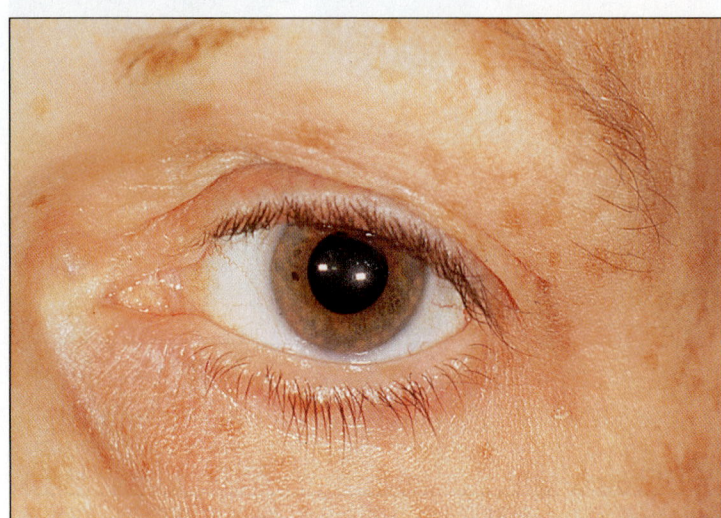

FIG. 92-19 ■ **Freckles.** Multiple, tan–brown, small macules, involving the skin of sun-exposed areas.

Fibrous Histiocytoma

Fibrous histiocytomas, also known as *fibrous xanthomas* or *dermatofibromas,* have a predilection to occur in the orbit but occasionally may be found on the eyelid.[42] The eyelid lesion appears as an asymptomatic, subcutaneous, mobile mass.[43] Histopathology reveals a poorly demarcated lesion, with a mixture of fibroblastic spindle cells forming a characteristic storiform pattern and large foamy histiocytes. Multinucleated giant cells, lymphocytes, and other inflammatory cells are found throughout the lesion, also. Complete surgical excision is recommended.

Juvenile Xanthogranuloma

Juvenile xanthogranuloma (JXG), also known as *nevoxanthoendothelioma,* is a benign histiocytic proliferation which most commonly affects the skin. It occurs mainly in children less than 2 years of age and usually appears within the first year of life. The skin lesions most commonly appear in the head and neck region as elevated orange, red, or brown nodules, which are generally self-limited. They typically increase in size and number initially but subsequently regress spontaneously into an atrophic scar over months to years. Lesions which appear in adulthood are more likely to persist and often require treatment to induce regression.

The most common site of extracutaneous involvement is the eye, with a predilection for the iris.[44] The iris may contain localized vascular nodules or diffuse infiltration of tumor. Complications include hyphema, uveitis, and glaucoma, with resulting visual loss and phthisis. Treatment, which includes topical and subconjunctival corticosteroids, is recommended for intraocular lesions,[45] because they rarely regress spontaneously and complications are common.

Biopsy of skin lesions helps to confirm the clinical diagnosis in patients who have cutaneous disease alone and in patients who have suspicious eye findings associated with skin lesions. Microscopically, lesions contain an infiltrate of lipid-laden histiocytes, lymphocytes, eosinophils, and Touton giant cells. Fibrosis appears in older lesions. Skin lesions may be treated by excision or, if necessary, corticosteroid injection.

PIGMENTED LESIONS OF MELANOCYTIC ORIGIN

Skin lesions of melanocytic origin arise from one of three cell types:
- Epidermal, or dendritic, melanocytes which lie between the basal cells of the epidermis

- Nevus cells, or nevocytes, which usually form nests of cells within the epidermis
- Dermal, or fusiform, melanocytes which lie in the subepithelial tissues

Melanocytes are derived from neural crest cells. Epidermal melanocytes produce melanin, which is transferred to surrounding epidermal cells, with tanning and racial pigmentation resulting from this process.

Freckles

Freckles, also known as *ephelides,* arise from epidermal melanocytes. They appear as small (1–3mm diameter), tan-to-brown macules in sun-exposed areas, including the eyelids (Fig. 92-19). Freckles occur more commonly in light-complected individuals and darken with sun exposure. These lesions reflect melanocytic overactivity, not proliferation. Microscopically, hyperpigmentation occurs within the basal layer of the epidermis. No treatment is necessary, but sunscreen may help prevent further darkening of lesions.

Lentigo Simplex

Lentigo simplex is another epidermal melanocytic lesion which may appear on skin and mucous membranes as small, brown macules. They usually appear during childhood and are unaffected by sun exposure. Lesions may be solitary and have an appearance similar to that of junctional nevi. Multiple lesions may be a manifestation of a systemic syndrome, such as Peutz–Jeghers syndrome. Patients who have this syndrome develop multiple lesions, often periocular and perioral in distribution, in association with gastrointestinal polyps,[46] which may undergo malignant transformation. Multiple lesions may resemble freckles but do not change in pigmentation with sun exposure as freckles often do. Microscopically, lentigo simplex has hyperpigmentation along the basal layer of the epidermis, with an increased number of melanocytes. Elongation of the rete ridges occurs along with mild lymphocytic infiltration of the superficial dermis. Intervention is not required, because these lesions are thought to have no malignant potential.

Solar Lentigo

Lesions of solar lentigo, also of epidermal melanocytic origin, are tan-to-brown macules found commonly in sun-exposed areas of older individuals. They also are known as *senile lentigines* but may occur in younger individuals after prolonged sun exposure. These lesions also are found commonly in patients who have xeroderma pigmentosum, often appearing during the first decade of life. Lesions usually have slightly irregular borders but are evenly pigmented. Initially, lesions are a few millimeters in diameter but slowly increase in size. They may resemble junctional nevi and seborrheic keratoses. Lesions should be differentiated from lentigo maligna, a premalignant condition, which usually has variable pigmentation and more prominent border irregularity and notching. Biopsy should be performed on suspicious-looking lesions.

Histologically, solar lentigo lesions display hyperpigmentation of the basal layer of the epidermis, with proliferation of melanocytes. More extensive elongation of the rete ridges is found in comparison with lentigo simplex. Treatment is not required, unless desired for cosmetic reasons.

Melanocytic Nevi

Melanocytic nevi, also known as *nevocellular nevi*, are derived from nevocytes. They are extremely common lesions, especially in fair-complected individuals.[47] These lesions frequently occur on the eyelid skin and eyelid margin. The clinical appearance often is predictive of the histological type, which may be junctional, compound, or intradermal.

Lesions typically occur during childhood as small, flat, tan macules which gradually increase in size radially. Nests of nevus cells are found within the epidermis, at the dermal–epidermal junction, representing a junctional nevus. As the lesion ceases to increase in diameter in older children and young adults, nests of cells "drop off" into the dermis, forming a compound nevus. Clinically, compound nevi are slightly elevated and pigmented. Lesions further evolve as the remaining epidermal nests migrate into the dermis, to produce an intradermal nevus. This lesion, most common in adults, may be dome-shaped, pedunculated, or papillomatous, and usually is less pigmented or amelanotic (Fig. 92-20). Later in life, as the nevus cells induce fibroplasia within the dermis, the cells decrease in number and are replaced by normal dermal tissue.

Diagnosis usually is based on the typical clinical appearance. Malignant transformation may occur rarely, generally in the junctional or compound stages. Thus, suspicious-looking lesions that demonstrate irregular growth or appearance should be excised. Otherwise, removal of common nevi is not required, unless desired for cosmesis or relief of mechanical irritation.

Congenital Melanocytic Nevus

These lesions are derived from nevocytes and occur in approximately 1% of newborns. Lesions may be single or multiple, and usually are deeply pigmented. The border often is irregular and the surface may be covered with hair. Congenital nevi that appear in a symmetrical fashion on adjacent portions of the upper and lower eyelids are referred to as *kissing nevi* and are formed as a result of melanocytic migration to the lids prior to separation of the embryonic eyelids (Fig. 92-21).

The size of congenital nevi is critical in management, because large lesions are associated with a higher risk of malignant transformation. Controversy exists regarding the definition of "large" and "small" congenital nevi. Large lesions in the head and neck region commonly are defined as those greater than or equal to the area of the patient's palm. The risk of malignant transformation is estimated at 5%.[48]

Histologically, congenital nevi display a variety of patterns. Many lesions contain features of compound nevi, with nevus cells in the dermis and the dermal–epidermal junction. Nevus cells often extend into the deep dermis and subcutaneous tissue. Malignant melanoma usually develops within the deep dermis, which makes early diagnosis difficult. Thus, any suspicious-

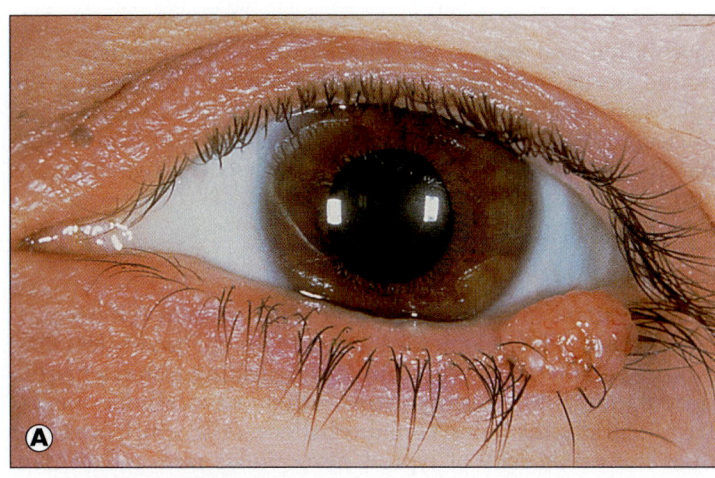
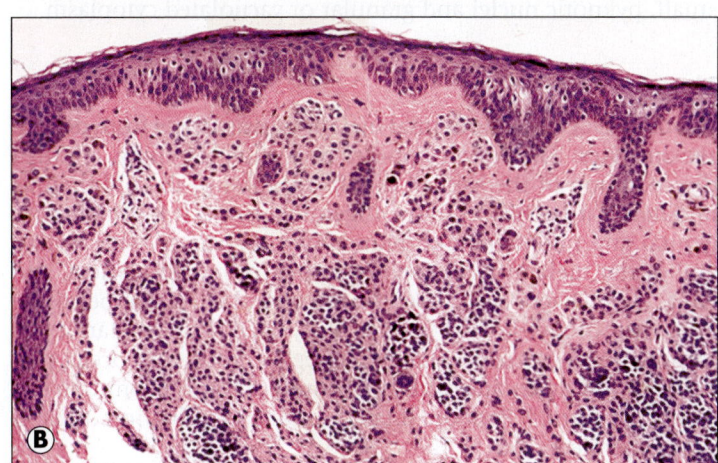

FIG. 92-20 ■ **Intradermal nevus. A,** Elevated, papillomatous lesion, amelanotic in color, involving the eyelid margin. **B,** Nests of nevus cells fill the dermis except for a narrow area just under the epithelium. The nuclei of the nevus cells become smaller, thinner or spindle-shaped, and darker as they go deeper into the dermis (i.e., they show normal polarity). (**B,** From Yanoff M, Fine BS. Ocular pathology, ed 5. St. Louis: Mosby; 2002.)

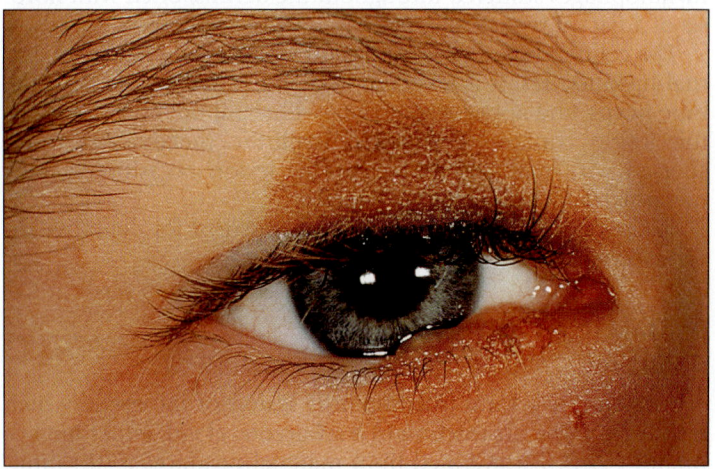

FIG. 92-21 ■ **Kissing nevus.** Congenital melanocytic nevus in a symmetrical fashion on adjacent portions of the upper and lower eyelids.

looking lesion should be sampled for biopsy. Large lesions should be excised, but complete excision is impossible in some patients due to the size and extent of the lesion. The management of small lesions is controversial—some advocate excision of all congenital nevi.[49]

Spindle–Epithelioid Cell Nevus

Another variant of nevocellular nevi, the spindle–epithelioid cell nevus, also has been termed *benign juvenile melanoma* and

707

Spitz nevus. It appears as a pink-to-orange, dome-shaped nodule in children and young adults. Microscopically, this is a compound nevus, with spindle or epithelioid cells throughout the epidermis and dermis. Lesions may contain mitotic figures and nuclear atypia, making histological differentiation from malignant melanoma difficult. Excision provides definitive diagnosis and treatment.

Balloon Cell Nevus

A third variant of nevocellular nevi is the balloon cell nevus. It appears as a lightly pigmented, elevated lesion, usually less than 5mm in diameter. No clinically distinguishing features help to differentiate this lesion from other nevocellular nevi.[13] Histologically, the lesion contains balloon cells, which are larger than the nevus cells of typical nevocellular nevi and contain small, pyknotic nuclei and granular or vacuolated cytoplasm.

Nevus of Ota

Nevus of Ota, or oculodermal melanocytosis, arises from dermal melanocytes. The lesion appears as a blue-to-purple, mottled discoloration of the skin in the distribution of the ophthalmic and maxillary divisions of the trigeminal nerve. It is usually congenital and unilateral and frequently is associated with ipsilateral ocular melanocytosis involving the conjunctiva, sclera, and uveal tract. Diagnosis is based on the typical clinical appearance. Histopathology reveals pigmented, dendritic melanocytes throughout the dermis. Malignant degeneration may occur, particularly in Caucasians, with the choroid the most common site of involvement.[50] Periodic dilated fundus examination, thus, is recommended.

Blue Nevus

The blue nevus appears as a solitary blue nodule, usually less than 1cm in diameter. The differential diagnosis includes melanoma, pigmented BCC, and vascular lesions. Microscopically, the lesion is composed of pigmented dendritic melanocytes and melanophages scattered throughout the dermis, often with fibrosis of adjacent tissue.

The cellular blue nevus is a lesion which also arises from dermal melanocytes. It is less common and usually larger than the blue nevus, and appears as a solitary blue papule. Histologically, the lesion contains pigmented dendritic melanocytes interspersed with pale spindle cells. This lesion occasionally may metastasize to regional lymph nodes.

Excision of these lesions may be performed for definitive diagnosis or cosmesis.

INFLAMMATORY LESIONS

Chalazion

A chalazion is a focal inflammatory lesion of the eyelid which results from the obstruction of a sebaceous gland, either meibomian or Zeis. Extravasated lipid material produces a surrounding chronic lipogranulomatous inflammation. A chalazion may occur acutely with eyelid edema and erythema and evolve into a nodule, which may point anteriorly to the skin surface or, more commonly, through the posterior surface of the lid. The lesion may drain spontaneously or persist as a chronic nodule, usually a few millimeters from the eyelid margin. Lesions also may appear insidiously as firm, painless nodules (Fig. 92-22). Large lesions on the upper lid may even induce astigmatism. Chalazia often occur in patients with blepharitis and rosacea.

Diagnosis is based on the typical clinical features. Acute lesions appear similar to hordeola in appearance—differentiation is nearly impossible to make clinically. In recurrent lesions, a sebaceous gland carcinoma needs to be excluded; thus, histopathological examination is important. Histopathology reveals

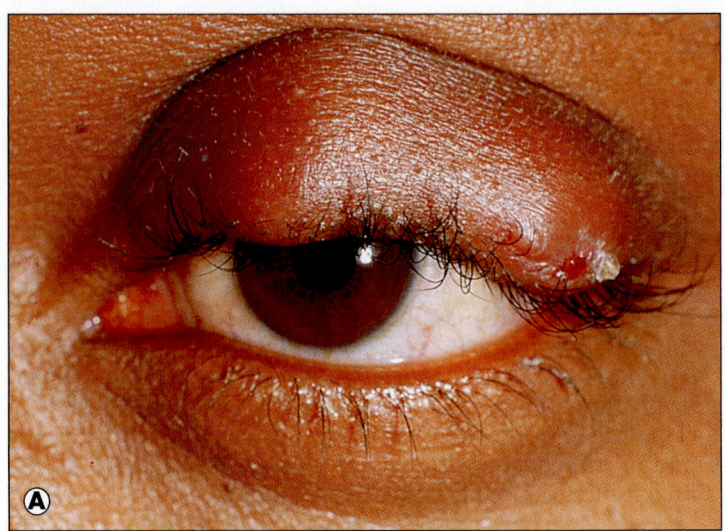

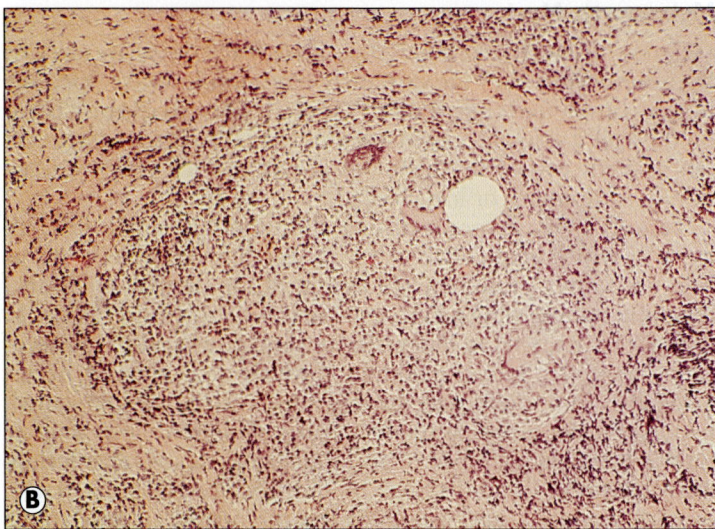

FIG. 92-22 ■ Chalazion and external hordeolum. **A,** The medial lesion of the upper eyelid appeared as a firm, painless nodule, consistent with a chalazion. The lateral lesion caused pain and eyelid erythema, subsequently becoming more localized, with drainage of purulent material through the skin surface. **B,** A clear circular area surrounded by epithelioid cells and multinucleated giant cells can be seen. In processing the tissue, lipid is dissolved out, leaving a clear space.

lipogranulomatous inflammation, with clear spaces corresponding to lipid, surrounded by foreign body giant cells, epithelioid cells, neutrophils, lymphocytes, plasma cells, and eosinophils. A fibrous pseudocapsule may form around a lesion.

Treatment varies according to the stage of a lesion. Acute lesions are treated with hot compresses to encourage localization and drainage. Chronic chalazia may be treated using intralesional corticosteroid injection or surgical drainage. Vertical transconjunctival incisions allow adequate exposure of lesions and limit damage to surrounding meibomian glands.[51] Small chalazia, which may resolve spontaneously, can be removed with incision and curettage.

Hordeolum

A hordeolum is an acute purulent inflammation of the eyelid. An external hordeolum, or stye, results from infection of the follicle of a cilium and the adjacent glands of Zeis or Moll. The lesion typically causes pain, edema, and erythema of the eyelid, which becomes localized and often drains anteriorly through the skin near the lash line (see Fig. 92-22). An internal hordeolum occurs due to obstruction and infection of a meibomian gland. Initially, a painful edema and erythema localizes as an inflammatory abscess on the posterior conjunctival surface of the tarsus. In both external and internal lesions, cellulitis of the surrounding soft tissue may develop. Diagnosis is based on the clinical appearance and culture, with *Staphylococcus aureus* most frequently isolated. Hordeola frequently occur in association with blepharitis. Histopathology reveals an abscess or a focal collection of polymorphonuclear leukocytes and necrotic tissue.

Although the inflammatory process usually is self-limited, with drainage and resolution occurring within 5–7 days, hot compresses and topical antibiotics help confine the spread of the lesion. Rarely, incision and drainage are necessary. Systemic antibiotics are used only if significant cellulitis exists. Treatment of accompanying blepharitis is helpful to prevent the formation of new lesions.

INFECTIOUS LESIONS

Molluscum Contagiosum

A common viral skin disease, MC is caused by a large DNA pox virus. Infection usually arises from direct contact or fomites in children and by a sexually transmitted route in adults. The typical lesion appears as a raised, shiny, white-to-pink nodule with a central umbilication filled with cheesy material. Lesions may be single or multiple, but usually fewer than 20 are present. Eyelid margin lesions may produce a follicular conjunctival reaction. Other ocular manifestations include epithelial keratitis, pannus formation, conjunctival scarring, and punctal occlusion. Primary conjunctival or limbal lesions occur rarely.

Diagnosis of MC usually is based on the clinical appearance of the lesion. Biopsy rarely is required in an otherwise healthy individual. The differential diagnosis includes keratoacanthoma, verruca vulgaris, squamous papilloma, milia, and SCC or BCC (see Chapter 93).

Patients who have acquired immunodeficiency syndrome (AIDS) often have an atypical clinical picture of MC. Disseminated disease may be present and lesions often are more confluent. Patients may have 30–40 lesions on each eyelid, or a confluent mass (Fig. 92-23). Secondary keratoconjunctivitis develops less frequently.

Histopathology of MC shows invasive acanthosis, with lobules of epithelial hyperplasia invaginating into the dermis. The epithelium at the surface degenerates and sloughs into a central cavity, which opens through a pore to the epidermal surface. Intracytoplasmic inclusions containing virions, referred to as *molluscum bodies*, are round and eosinophilic in the lower layers of the epidermis. These inclusions increase in size and are more basophilic in the granular and horny layers.

Usually, MC spontaneously resolves within 3–12 months but the patient may be treated to prevent corneal complications, reduce transmission, and speed recovery. Various treatment options exist, including simple incision or excision, incision and curettage, cryosurgery, and electrodesiccation. Management is more difficult in patients with AIDS because of extensive involvement and recurrences. Hyperfocal cryotherapy has been effective in these patients.[52]

Verruca Vulgaris

Verruca vulgaris, or the common cutaneous wart, is caused by epidermal infection with the human papillomavirus, which is spread by direct contact and fomites. Verruca vulgaris is more common in children and young adults and may occur anywhere on the skin, occasionally on the eyelid. Lesions appear elevated with an irregular, hyperkeratotic, papillomatous surface (Fig. 92-24). Lesions along the lid margin may induce a mild papillary conjunctivitis due to shedding of virus particles into the tear film. Patients also may develop a superficial punctate keratitis and may have pannus formation. Primary conjunctival lesions also may occur.[53]

Diagnosis is based on the typical appearance and is confirmed by biopsy. Histologically, papillomatosis is present, with hyperkeratosis, acanthosis, and parakeratosis. Large, vacuolated ker-

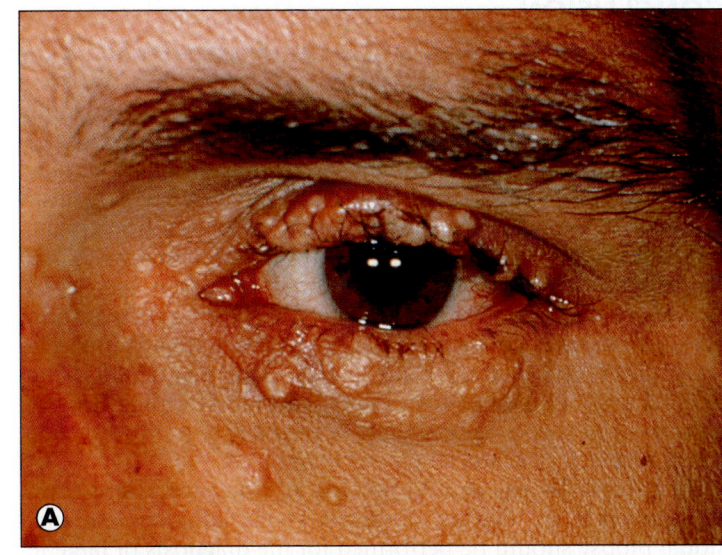

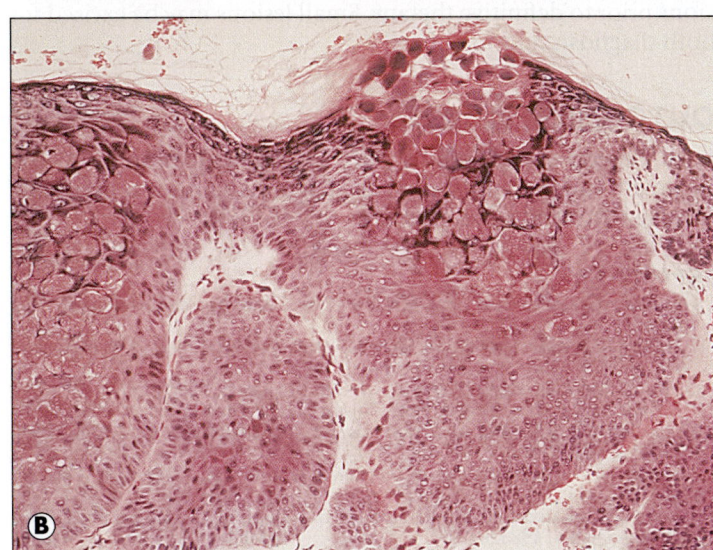

FIG. 92-23 ▌▌ Molluscum contagiosum. **A,** Multiple raised nodules, with areas of confluent lesions, affecting the eyelids of a patient with AIDS. **B,** Intracytoplasmic, small, eosinophilic molluscum bodies occur in the deep layers of epidermis. The bodies become enormous and basophilic near the surface. The bodies may be shed into the tear film where they cause a secondary, irritative, follicular conjunctivitis. (**B,** From Yanoff M, Fine BS. Ocular pathology, ed 5. St. Louis: Mosby; 2002.)

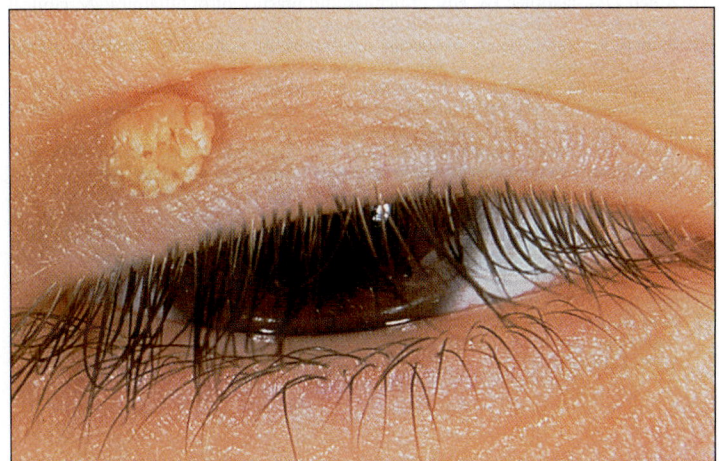

FIG. 92-24 ▌▌ Verruca vulgaris. Skin-colored, irregular lesion with a papillomatous surface appearing on the upper eyelid.

atinocytes are seen, with deeply basophilic nuclei surrounded by a clear halo. Observation is recommended if no ocular complications occur, because most lesions are self-limiting. Treatment, if necessary, is either cryotherapy or complete surgical excision. Incomplete excision may cause multiple recurrences.

CONCLUSION

The eyelids may be affected by a variety of benign lesions, some indicative of local pathology, others associated with or resulting from systemic pathology. Some lesions may be identified readily by the clinical appearance and behavior. However, many pose a diagnostic challenge, because different lesions may appear similar. Also, individual types of lesions may occur in a variety of forms.

Most important is the differentiation of benign from malignant lesions, because management often differs. Biopsy with ocular pathology consultation is, thus, warranted for any suspicious-looking lesion. Epithelial lesions which display painless growth, irregular or pearly borders, ulceration, induration, or telangiectasis should raise concern for malignancy. Signs that herald malignant change in pigmented lesions include irregular borders, asymmetrical shape, color change or presence of multiple colors, recent changes, or diameter greater than 5mm.

In general, biopsy should precede all extensive tumor resections, even if the clinical diagnosis seems apparent. An incisional biopsy should be performed for the diagnosis of large lesions prior to definitive therapy. Small lesions may be excised for both diagnosis and treatment.

OUTCOMES

Most benign eyelid lesions have an excellent prognosis. The treatment varies according to site, diagnosis, concurrent systemic involvement, and other factors.

REFERENCES

1. Aurora AL, Blodi FC. Lesions of the eyelids: a clinicopathological study. Surv Ophthalmol. 1970;15:94–104.
2. Folberg R. Eyelids: terminology of eyelid pathology. In: Folberg, R. Pathology of the eye [CD-ROM]. St Louis: Mosby–Year Book; 1996.
3. Ellis DL, Yates RA. Sign of Leser-Trélat. Clin Dermatol. 1993;11:141–8.
4. Kobalter AS, Roth A. Benign epithelial neoplasms. In: Mannis MJ, Macsai MS, Huntley AC, eds. Eye and skin disease. Philadelphia: Lippincott–Raven; 1996:345–55.
5. Sanderson KV. The structure of seborrheic keratosis. Br J Dermatol. 1968;80:588–93.
6. Lever WF. Inverted follicular keratosis is an irritated seborrheic keratosis. Am J Dermatopathol. 1983;5:474.
7. Boynton JR, Searl SS, Caldwell EH. Large periocular keratoacanthoma: the case for definitive treatment. Ophthalmic Surg. 1986;17:565–9.
8. Grossniklaus HE, Wojno TH, Yanoff M, Font RL. Invasive keratoacanthoma of the eyelid and ocular adnexa. Ophthalmology. 1996;103:937–41.
9. Farina AT, Leider M, Newall J, Carella R. Radiotherapy for aggressive and destructive keratoacanthomas. J Dermatol Surg Oncol. 1977;3:177–80.
10. Eubanks SW, Gentry RH, Patteson JW, et al. Treatment of multiple keratoacanthomas with intralesional fluorouracil. J Am Acad Dermatol. 1982;7:126–9.
11. Scott KR, Kronish JW. Premalignant lesions and squamous cell carcinoma. In: Albert DM, Jakobiec FA, eds. Principles and practice of ophthalmology: clinical practice, vol 3. Philadelphia: WB Saunders; 1994:1733–44.
12. Folberg R. Eyelids: study of specific conditions. In: Folberg, R. Pathology of the eye [CD-ROM]. St Louis: Mosby–Year Book; 1996.
13. Campbell RJ. Tumors of the eyelids, conjunctiva, and cornea. In: Garner A, Klintworth GK, eds. Pathobiology of ocular disease: a dynamic approach, part B, ed 2. New York: Marcel Dekker; 1994:1367–403.
14. Weiss RA. Orbital disease. In: McCord CD, Tanenbaum M, Nunery WR, eds. Oculoplastic surgery, ed 3. New York: Raven Press; 1995:417–76.
15. Ectodermal tumors of the eyelid. In: Griffith DG, Salasche SJ, Clemons DE, eds. Cutaneous abnormalities of the eyelid and face: an atlas with histopathology. New York: McGraw-Hill; 1987:195–254.
16. Rodgers IR, Jakobiec FA, Hidayat AA. Eyelid tumors of apocrine, eccrine, and pilar origins. In: Albert DM, Jakobiec FA, eds. Principles and practice of ophthalmology: clinical practice, vol. 3. Philadelphia: WB Saunders; 1994:1770–96.
17. Font RL. Eyelids and lacrimal drainage system. In: Spencer WH, ed. Ophthalmic pathology: an atlas and textbook, vol. 4, ed 4. Philadelphia: WB Saunders; 1996:2218–437.
18. Jakobiec FA, Zimmerman LE, La Piana F, et al. Unusual eyelid tumors with sebaceous differentiation in the Muir–Torre syndrome. Ophthalmology. 1988;95:1543–8.
19. Ni C, Dryja TP, Albert DM. Sweat gland tumors in the eyelids: a clinicopathological analysis of 55 cases. Int Ophthalmol Clin. 1982;22:1–22.
20. Nerad JA, Anderson RL. CO_2 laser treatment of eyelid syringomas. Ophthalmic Plast Reconstr Surg. 1988;4:91–4.
21. Jordan DR, Nerad JA, Patrinely JR. Chondroid syringoma of the eyelid. Can J Ophthalmol. 1989;24:24–7.
22. Ferry AP, Hadad HM. Eccrine acrospiroma (porosynringoma) of the eyelid. Arch Ophthalmol. 1970;83:591–3.
23. Grossniklaus HE, Knight SH. Eccrine acrospiroma (clear cell hidradenoma) of the eyelid: immunohistochemical and ultrastructural features. Ophthalmology. 1991;98:347–52.
24. Font RL, Stone MS, Schanzer MC, Lewis RA. Apocrine hidrocystomas of the lids, hypodontia, palmar–plantar hyperkeratosis, and onychodystrophy: a new variant of ectodermal dysplasia. Arch Ophthalmol. 1986;104:1811–3.
25. Simpson W, Garner A, Collin JRO. Benign hair-follicle derived tumours in the differential diagnosis of basal-cell carcinoma of the eyelids: a clinicopathological comparison. Br J Ophthalmol. 1989;73:347–53.
26. Sternberg I, Buckman G, Levine MR, Sterin W. Trichoepithelioma. Ophthalmology. 1986;93:531–3.
27. Hidayat AA, Font RL. Trichilemmoma of eyelid and eyebrow: a clinicopathologic study of 31 cases. Arch Ophthalmol. 1980;98:844–7.
28. Bardenstein DS, McLean IW, Nerney J, Boatwright RS. Cowden's disease. Ophthalmology. 1988;95:1038–41.
29. O'Grady RB, Spoerl G. Pilomatrixoma (benign calcifying epithelioma of Malherbe). Ophthalmology. 1981;88:1196–7.
30. Orlando RG, Rogers GL, Bremer DL. Pilomatrixoma in a pediatric hospital. Arch Ophthalmol. 1983;101:1209–10.
31. Haik BG, Karcioglu ZA, Gordon RA, Pechous BP. Capillary hemangioma (infantile periocular hemangioma). Surv Ophthalmol. 1994;38:399–426.
32. Kushner B. Intralesional corticosteroid injection for infantile adnexal hemangioma. Am J Ophthalmol. 1982;93:496–506.
33. Glatt HJ, Putterman AM, Van Aalst JJ, et al. Adrenal suppression and growth retardation after injection of periocular capillary hemangioma with corticosteroids. Ophthalmic Surg. 1991;22:95–7.
34. Walker RS, Custer PL, Nerad JA. Surgical excision of periorbital capillary hemangiomas. Ophthalmology. 1994;101:1333–40.
35. McCannel CA, Hoenig J, Umlas J, et al. Orbital lesions in the blue rubber bleb nevus syndrome. Ophthalmology. 1996;103:933–6.
36. Pang P, Jakobiec FA, Iwamoto T, Hornblass A. Small lymphangiomas of the eyelids. Ophthalmology. 1984;91:1278–84.
37. Tan OT, Gilchrest BA. Laser therapy for selected cutaneous vascular lesions in the pediatric population: a review. Pediatrics. 1988;82:652–62.
38. Woog JJ, Albert DM, Solt LC, et al. Neurofibromatosis of the eyelid and orbit. Int Ophthalmol Clin. 1982;22:157–87.
39. Bergman R. The pathogenesis and clinical significance of xanthelasma palpebrarum. J Am Acad Dermatol. 1994;30:236–42.
40. Vinger P, Sach B. Ocular manifestations of hyperlipidemia. Am J Ophthalmol. 1970;70:563–73.
41. Ribera M, Pintó X, Argimon JM, et al. Lipid metabolism and apolipoprotein E phenotypes in patients with xanthelasma. Am J Med. 1995;99:485–90.
42. John T, Yanoff M, Scheie HG. Eyelid fibrous histiocytoma. Ophthalmology. 1981;88:1193–5.
43. Jordan DR, Anderson RL. Fibrous histiocytoma. An uncommon eyelid lesion. Arch Ophthalmol. 1989;107:1530–1.
44. Zimmerman LE. Ocular lesions of JXG (nevoxanthoendothelioma). Trans Am Acad Ophthalmol Otolaryngol. 1965;69:412–39.
45. Casteels I, Olver J, Malone M, Taylor D. Early treatment of juvenile xanthogranuloma of the iris with subconjunctival steroids. Br J Ophthalmol. 1993;77:57–60.
46. Traboulsi EI, Maumenee IH. Periocular pigmentation in the Peutz-Jeghers syndrome. Am J Ophthalmol. 1986;102:126–7.
47. Sigg C, Pelloni F. Frequency of acquired melanonevocytic nevi and their relationship to skin complexion in 939 schoolchildren. Dermatologica. 1989;179:123–8.
48. Margo CE, Habal MB. Large congenital melanocytic nevus: light and electron microscopic findings. Ophthalmology. 1987;94:960–5.
49. Solomon LM. The management of congenital melanocytic nevi. Arch Dermatol. 1980;116:1017.
50. Dutton JJ, Anderson RL, Schelper RL, et al. Orbital malignant melanoma and oculodermal melanocytosis: report of two cases and review of the literature. Ophthalmology. 1984;91:497–507.
51. Goldberg RA, Shorr N. 'Vertical slat' chalazion excision. Ophthalmic Surg. 1992;23:120–2.
52. Bardenstein DS, Elmets C. Hyperfocal cryotherapy of multiple molluscum contagiosum lesions in patients with the acquired immune deficiency syndrome. Ophthalmology. 1995;102:1031–4.
53. Scharf BH. Viral eyelid infections. In: Krachmer JH, Mannis MJ, Holland EJ, eds. Cornea. Vol II: cornea and external disease: clinical diagnosis and management. St Louis: Mosby–Year Book; 1997:641–51.

93 Eyelid Malignancies

GREGORY J. VAUGHN • RICHARD K. DORTZBACH • GREGG S. GAYRE

DEFINITION

- Cutaneous cancers that arise from the epidermis, dermis, or adnexal structures of the eyelid. Rarely they may be metastatic from distant sites. They include a number of histologically distinct tumors from diverse skin cell types.

KEY FEATURES

- Flat, eroded, or elevated lesion on the eyelid margin, eyelid skin, or brow.
- Nodular and well circumscribed or irregular with indistinct borders.
- Ulcerated with a central crater or benign in appearance with some telangiectatic vessels.
- Slow, generally painless, growth.

ASSOCIATED FEATURES

- Dilated blood vessels.
- Ectropion from skin contracture.
- Firm induration.
- Loss of eyelashes.
- Palpable preauricular nodes.
- Proptosis.
- Ptosis.
- Restricted ocular motility.
- Thickened eyelid margin.

Malignant lesions are common around the eyes, partly because many are induced by sun exposure or develop from sun-related benign lesions. Most of these are small and grow slowly, which results in minimal concern for the patient and a low index of suspicion for the physician. Although most eyelid malignancies rarely metastasize, they can be very destructive locally. Any periocular lesion that shows some growth, especially when associated with chronic irritation or bleeding, should undergo biopsy for diagnosis. Confirmation of histopathology is also mandatory before committing the patient to a major resection or reconstructive procedure.

BASAL CELL CARCINOMA

INTRODUCTION

Basal cell carcinoma (BCC) is a malignant tumor derived from cells of the basal layer of the epidermis. The etiology of BCC is linked to excessive ultraviolet light exposure in fair-skinned individuals. Other predisposing factors include ionizing radiation,

arsenic exposure, and scars. Although metastases are rare, local invasion is common and can be very destructive.

EPIDEMIOLOGY AND PATHOGENESIS

BCC is the most common malignant tumor of the eyelids and constitutes 85–90% of all malignant epithelial eyelid tumors at this site.[1] Over 99% of BCCs occur in whites; about 95% of these lesions occur between the ages of 40 and 79 years, with an average age at diagnosis of 60 years.[2] BCC arises from a pleuripotential stem cell in the epidermis that proliferates, amplifies, and eventually terminally differentiates.[3,4] Ultraviolet light exposure is one of the most important risk factors, especially in light-skinned individuals. Proposed mechanisms for BCC invasion include enhanced tumor cell motility and collagenase content.[1] Having had one BCC is a prognostic factor for the development of additional lesions.

OCULAR MANIFESTATIONS

Up to 50–60% of BCCs affect the lower eyelid. The medial canthus is involved 25–30% of the time. The upper eyelid is involved nearly 15% of the time and the lateral canthus is only rarely involved (5%).[5] On the basis of their histopathological presentation, BCCs may be classified into five basic types:
- Nodular-ulcerative
- Pigmented
- Morphea or sclerosing
- Superficial
- Fibroepithelioma

Two additional, although very rare, types are the linear basal cell nevus and generalized follicular basal cell nevus.[6]

The nodular type of BCC, the most common lesion, has the classical appearance of a pink or pearly papule or nodule with overlying telangiectatic vessels. As the nodule grows in size, central ulceration may occur surrounded by a rolled border (Fig. 93-1). This appearance is often described as a "rodent ulcer."

The pigmented BCC is similar to the noduloulcerative type in morphology but with brown or black pigmentation. These lesions represent the most common pigmented malignancy on the eyelids and may resemble malignant melanoma.

The morphea or sclerosing type of BCC appears as a flat, indurated, yellow-pink plaque with ill-defined borders. It may simulate a blepharitis or dermatitis. As it has a flat appearance, it may not be as clinically noticeable as others. However, this form of BCC is aggressive and may invade the dermis deeply. It characteristically occurs in the medial canthal region and may invade into the paranasal sinuses and orbit.

Superficial BCC appears as an erythematous, scaling patch with a raised pearly border. Fibroepithelioma BCC presents as a pedunculated or sessile smooth, pink nodule. Both the superficial and fibroepithelioma types typically arise on the trunk rather than the eyelid.[7]

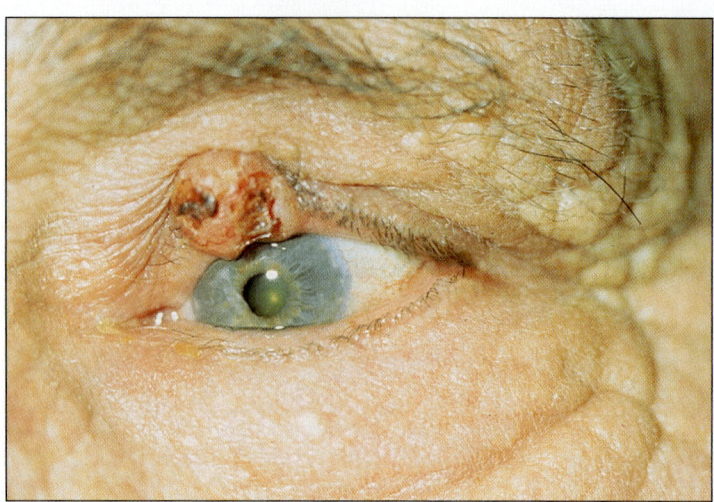

FIG. 93-1 ▌▌ **Nodular basal cell carcinoma of the eyelid.** A firm, pink-colored left upper eyelid BCC is seen with raised border, superficial telangiectatic vessels, and characteristic central ulceration. These lesions are more commonly seen on the lower eyelid. (Courtesy of Dr Morton Smith.)

DIAGNOSIS

The diagnosis of BCC is initially made from its clinical appearance, especially with the noduloulcerative type with its raised pearly borders and central ulcerated crater. Definitive diagnosis, however, can be made only on histopathological examination of biopsy specimens.

DIFFERENTIAL DIAGNOSIS

The differential diagnosis of BCC and of other periocular malignant lesions may be divided into several categories: other malignant lesions, premalignant lesions, benign adnexal tumors and cysts, and inflammatory and infectious conditions (Table 93-1; see Chapter 92).[8] In many cases the diagnosis depends upon histopathology.

SYSTEMIC ASSOCIATIONS

Basal cell nevus syndrome (Gorlin-Goltz syndrome) is inherited as an autosomal dominant disorder with high penetrance and variable expressivity. Basal cell nevus syndrome is rare, occurring in less than 1% of individuals with BCC.[9] The group of clinical findings described in 1960 as a syndrome by Gorlin and Goltz[10] includes:

- Multiple BCCs affecting the face, trunk, and extremities
- Cysts of the jaw (odontogenic keratocysts)
- Skeletal abnormalities (e.g., bifid ribs)
- Neurological abnormalities (e.g., mental retardation, ectopic calcification, cerebellar medulloblastoma)
- Endocrine disorders (e.g., ovarian cysts and testicular disorders)[7]

Palmar and plantar pits also develop in young adulthood. The BCCs in this syndrome typically develop at puberty and have a predilection for the periorbital region and face.[2] Multiple lesions occur with a high rate of recurrence. Other rare BCC syndromes include Bazex's syndrome, linear unilateral basal cell nevus, and Rombo syndrome.

Also, BCC may be associated with albinism, xeroderma pigmentosum, and nevus sebaceus.

PATHOLOGY

The BCCs may be grouped as either undifferentiated or differentiated by their histopathological appearance.[6] The typical histopathology of an undifferentiated BCC consists of nests, lobules, and cords of tumor cells with peripheral palisading of cells and stromal retraction (Fig. 93-2). Undifferentiated BCCs include the solid noduloulcerative, morphea or sclerosing, pig-

TABLE 93-1

DIFFERENTIAL DIAGNOSIS OF PERIOCULAR MALIGNANCIES

Simulating Lesion	BCC	SCC	SGC	MM	KS	MCT
OTHER MALIGNANT LESIONS						
Amelanotic melanoma						X
Basal cell carcinoma		X	X			
Glomus tumor						X
Lymphoma					X	X
Malignant melanoma	X				X	
Metastatic oat cell carcinoma						X
Sebaceous cell carcinoma	X	X				X
Squamous cell carcinoma	X		X			
Squamous cell carcinoma *in situ*	X	X				
PREMALIGNANT LESIONS						
Actinic keratosis	X	X				
Radiation dermatitis	X					
Keratoacanthoma	X	X				
ADNEXAL TUMORS AND CYSTS						
Cavernous hemangioma				X		
Cutaneous horns	X					
Dermoid and sebaceous cysts	X					
Eccrine and apocrine cysts	X					
Inverted follicular keratosis		X				
Nevus cell and nevocellular nevi, pigmented lesions of epidermal and dermal melanocyte origin				X		
Papillomatous lesions	X	X	X			
Pseudoepitheliomatous hyperplasia		X				
Seborrheic keratosis nevus	X	X				
Trichilemomma		X				
INFLAMMATORY/INFECTIOUS CONDITIONS						
Blepharitis	X		X			
Chalazion	X		X		X	
Eczema	X					
Foreign body granuloma					X	
Fungal infections		X				X
Hordeolum	X					
Psoriasis	X					
Pyogenic granuloma					X	
Seborrheic dermatitis	X					
Superior limbic keratoconjunctivitis			X			
Verruca vulgaris		X				
OTHER						
Conjunctival hemorrhage				X	X	

BCC, Basal cell carcinoma; *SCC,* squamous cell carcinoma; *SGC,* sebaceous gland carcinoma; *MM,* malignant melanoma; *KS,* Kaposi's sarcoma; *MCT,* Merkel cell tumor.

mented, superficial, and fibroepithelioma forms. The morphea or sclerosing form is characterized by strands of proliferating, malignant basal cells in a fibrous stroma (Fig. 93-3).

The adenoid and metatypical or basosquamous are the most common differentiated forms. These tumors differentiate to-

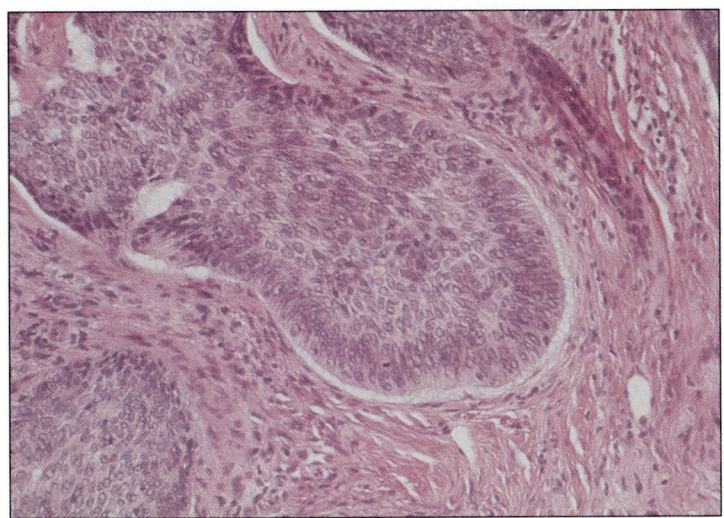

FIG. 93-2 ▮▮ Nodular basal cell carcinoma of the eyelid. Basophilic nests of proliferating epithelial tumor cells are shown with characteristic peripheral, palisading nuclei and stromal reaction. (Courtesy of Dr Morton Smith.)

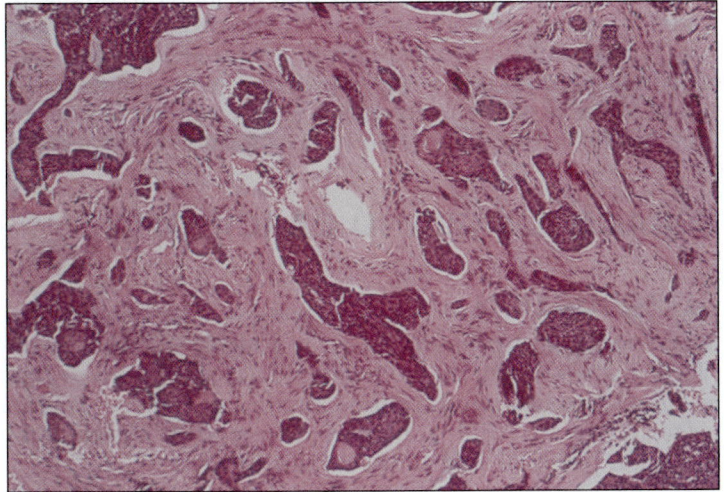

FIG. 93-3 ▮▮ Morphea or sclerosing type of basal cell carcinoma of the eyelid. Strands and islands of basaloid cells are shown within a dense connective tissue matrix. (Courtesy of Dr Morton Smith.)

ward glandular structures with mucinous stroma. They exhibit morphological features between those of basal cell and squamous cell carcinoma. The metatypical BCCs are more aggressive and invasive with a higher recurrence rate and potential for metastasis.[11]

TREATMENT

The goal of therapy is the complete removal of tumor cells with preservation of unaffected eyelid and periorbital tissues. Although nonsurgical treatments such as cryotherapy, electrodesiccation, and laser ablation are advocated by some, surgical therapy is generally accepted as the treatment of choice for removal of BCCs. Some BCCs, especially the morphea and multicentric types, may extend far beyond the area that is apparent clinically. Therefore, histological monitoring of tumor margins is essential. Mohs' micrographic surgery and excisional biopsy with frozen section control are the two basic techniques available. An incisional biopsy may be performed prior to definitive treatment to confirm the clinical suspicion of BCC.[12]

Surgery

Mohs' micrographic surgery provides the highest cure rate with the most effective preservation of normal tissue. Tissue is excised

in layers that provide a three-dimensional mapping of the excised tumor. These layers are processed as frozen sections and viewed under the microscope. Any areas of residual tumor are identified, and the map is used to direct additional tumor excision.[13,14] This technique is particularly useful for morphea and multicentric-type BCCs in the medial canthal region, which may exhibit subclinical extension to orbital bone or sinuses. Mohs' micrographic surgery technique is somewhat limited if the tumor has extended to the plane of orbital fat. In addition, it requires the collaboration of a trained Mohs' surgeon and dermatopathologist.

Excisional biopsy with frozen section control is also an effective way to remove BCCs and can be performed by the ophthalmologist. Several studies have reported no recurrences after excision of BCCs with frozen section monitoring.[5,15,16] However, following simple excisional biopsy without frozen section control, recurrence rates up to 50% have been reported.[17]

Eyelid reconstruction should be performed within 2–3 days after tumor excision. Various reconstructive surgical techniques may be used depending upon the location and size of the residual defect (see Chapter 94).

Radiation Therapy

Radiation therapy is generally not recommended in the initial treatment of periocular BCCs. However, it may be useful in the treatment of advanced or recurrent lesions in the medial canthal region or elsewhere. Doses are in the range 4000–7000cGy.[18] Radiation therapy is less effective in treating morphea BCCs, with the likelihood of BCC recurrence following radiotherapy being higher than that for previously described surgical techniques.[19] A recurrence rate of 12% was noted in one series following radiation therapy.[20] Surgical management is very difficult after radiation treatment of an affected area. Radiotherapy complications include skin atrophy and necrosis, madarosis, cicatricial entropion and ectropion, dry eye syndrome, cataract, and corneal ulceration.[21] Radiation therapy is contraindicated in basal cell nevus syndrome and is associated with significant complications in patients who have scleroderma or acquired immunodeficiency syndrome (AIDS).[22]

Cryotherapy

Cryotherapy is often used to treat BCCs outside the periorbital area. Around the eyelids it may be used to treat eyelid notching and malpositions, symblepharon formation with fornix foreshortening, and pigmentary changes. It is associated with a higher recurrence rate than the surgical approaches. Cryotherapy is contraindicated in lesions greater than 1cm in diameter, medial canthal lesions, morphea-like lesions, and recurrent BCC.[23]

Chemotherapy and Photodynamic Therapy

Topical, intralesional, and systemic chemotherapeutic agents, including 5-fluorouracil, cisplatinum, doxorubicin, bleomycin, and interferon, have been used to treat BCCs. However, these agents are generally not recommended for tumors in the periorbital region.[2]

Photodynamic therapy may be considered as an alternative treatment for large numbers of cutaneous BCCs (e.g., basal cell nevus syndrome). However, long-term follow-up of patients treated with this modality is not yet available.[24]

COURSE AND OUTCOME

Complete surgical excision of BCC is almost always curative because these lesions rarely metastasize. The incidence of metastasis ranges from 0.028–0.55%.[7] Tumor-related death is exceedingly rare, but when it does occur, it is usually caused by direct orbital and intracranial extension.

SQUAMOUS CELL CARCINOMA

INTRODUCTION

Squamous cell carcinoma (SCC) is a malignant tumor of the squamous layer of cells of the epidermis. It is much less common than BCC on the eyelids and carries a greater potential for metastatic spread.

EPIDEMIOLOGY AND PATHOGENESIS

Typically, SCC affects elderly, fair-skinned individuals. In the region of the eye it is usually found on the lower eyelid. Although SCC is 40 times less common than BCC of the eyelid, it is more common than BCC on the upper eyelid and lateral canthus.[25,26]

The exact mechanism of the pathogenesis of SCC is not known. However, environmental and intrinsic stimuli initiate a process in which cell growth and regulation are lost. Most periorbital SCCs arise from actinic lesions, but they may also arise *de novo*. Environmental factors may contribute to the development of SCC, including cumulative ultraviolet radiation (sun exposure), ionizing radiation, arsenic ingestion, psoralen plus ultraviolet A (PUVA) therapy for psoriasis, and the human papilloma virus.[27]

Intrinsic factors that contribute to the development of SCC include the autosomal recessive conditions xeroderma pigmentosum and oculocutaneous albinism. Chronic skin dermatoses, ulceration, and scarring are also associated with the development of this tumor. In fact, scarring of the skin is the most common intrinsic factor leading to SCC in black patients.[28]

OCULAR MANIFESTATIONS

Typically, SCC presents as an erythematous, indurated, hyperkeratotic plaque or nodule with irregular margins. These lesions have a high tendency toward ulceration and tend to affect the eyelid margin and medial canthus. Lymphatic spread and perineural invasion are possible.

DIAGNOSIS

The diagnosis of SCC is often suspected from the clinical appearance. However, because so many other malignant and benign processes can be confused with SCC, the diagnosis requires biopsy for histological confirmation.

DIFFERENTIAL DIAGNOSIS

A number of lesions can be mistaken for SCC (see Table 93-1). These include both other malignant tumors and benign lesions.[27]

PATHOLOGY

Well-differentiated SCC exhibits polygonal cells with abundant eosinophilic cytoplasm and hyperchromatic nuclei (Fig. 93-4). Dyskeratosis, keratin pearls, intercellular bridges, and abnormal mitotic figures are prominent. Poorly differentiated lesions show little keratinization and fewer intercellular bridges.[7]

TREATMENT

Before planning any therapy, the clinical diagnosis of SCC should be confirmed by incisional biopsy. Compared with BCC, SCC is a more aggressive and invasive tumor, but early SCC lesions of the eyelid rarely metastasize. Surgery, irradiation, and cryotherapy management options are similar to those described previously for BCC.

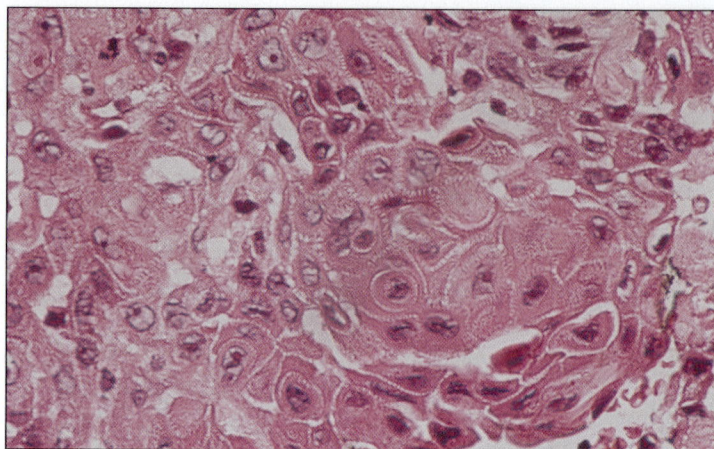

FIG. 93-4 ■ **Squamous cell carcinoma of the eyelid.** Anaplastic squamous cells with hyperchromatic nuclei, abundant eosinophilic cytoplasm, and intercellular bridges. (Courtesy of Dr Morton Smith.)

COURSE AND OUTCOME

Wide local surgical excision, either with the Mohs' technique or under frozen section control, is usually curative. Advanced cases may be associated with metastasis to the preauricular and submandibular lymph nodes, which heralds a more guarded prognosis. Invasion of the deep orbital tissues may sometimes be seen and frequently requires orbital exenteration for cure.

SEBACEOUS GLAND CARCINOMA

INTRODUCTION

Sebaceous gland carcinoma (SGC) is a highly malignant neoplasm that arises from the meibomian glands, the glands of Zeis, and the sebaceous glands of the caruncle and eyebrow. It is an aggressive tumor with a high recurrence rate, a significant metastatic potential, and a notable mortality rate.

EPIDEMIOLOGY AND PATHOGENESIS

Although it is relatively rare, SGC is the third most common eyelid malignancy, accounting for 1–5.5% of all eyelid cancers. It affects all races, occurs in women more often than men, and usually presents in the sixth to seventh decades, but cases in younger patients have been reported.[29-31]

The cause of SGC is unclear. However, there are reported associations that link SGC with prior radiation therapy[32] and with the production of nitrosamines and photosensitization from prior diuretic use.[33]

OCULAR MANIFESTATIONS

The upper eyelid is the site of origin in about two thirds of all cases, but SGC may arise from any of the periocular structures previously mentioned[7] and may have a variety of clinical appearances. It often presents as a firm, yellow nodule that resembles a chalazion. It may present as a plaque-like thickening of the tarsal plate with destruction of meibomian gland orifices and tumor invasion of eyelash follicles leading to madarosis, or loss of lashes (Fig. 93-5). Also, SGC may mimic a chronic blepharoconjunctivitis, meibomianitis, or chalazion that does not respond to standard therapies, thus the term "masquerade syndrome."

SGC tends to invade overlying epithelium, which may form nests of malignant cells (pagetoid spread), or it may result in diffuse spread that replaces the entire thickness of the conjunctiva (intraepithelial carcinoma). The carcinoma may exhibit multi-

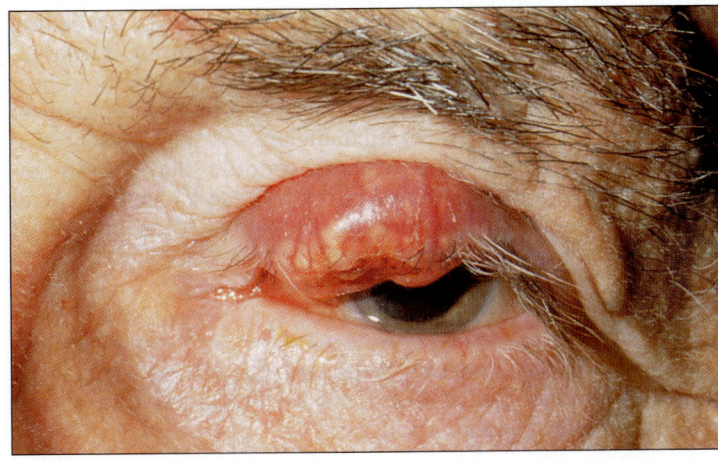

FIG. 93-5 ■ Sebaceous cell carcinoma of the eyelid. A large, firm, irregular nodule with yellowish coloration of the left upper eyelid is shown. Associated inflammation, telangiectatic vessels, and loss of cilia are observed. (Courtesy of Dr Morton Smith.)

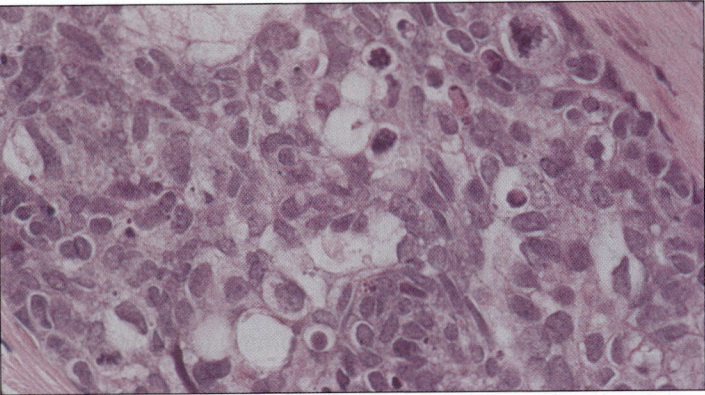

FIG. 93-6 ■ Sebaceous cell carcinoma of the eyelid. Large, hyperchromatic neoplastic cells with vacuolated (frothy), basophilic cytoplasm are observed. (Courtesy of Dr Morton Smith.)

centric spread to the other eyelid, conjunctiva, or corneal epithelium.[7] This neoplasm may spread through the canaliculus to the lacrimal excretory system and even to the nasal cavity.[33]

DIAGNOSIS

The clinical appearance of SGC must be confirmed by a full-thickness wedge biopsy of the affected eyelid. Because of potential multicentric spread, multiple biopsy specimens should also be taken from the adjacent bulbar and palpebral conjunctiva and the other ipsilateral eyelid. The pathologist should be alerted to the clinical suspicion of SGC, and fresh tissue should be submitted to pathology so that special lipid stains may be performed on the specimen to confirm the diagnosis.

DIFFERENTIAL DIAGNOSIS

Unfortunately, SGC is frequently confused with a large number of other lesions, especially benign inflammatory and infectious diseases (see Table 93-1). As this tumor is so rare, it is usually not considered by the physician, but its potential consequences demand a high index of suspicion. This is especially true for any benign-appearing lesion that does not respond to the usual medical management.

PATHOLOGY

Dysplasia and anaplasia of the sebaceous lobules in the meibomian glands are exhibited by SGC, with associated destruction of tarsal and adnexal tissues. Intraepithelial (pagetoid) spread to conjunctiva distant from the primary tumor may be observed. The intraepithelial spread may resemble SCC *in situ.*

Typically, SGC shows highly pleomorphic cells arranged in lobules or nests with hyperchromatic nuclei and vacuolated (foamy or frothy) cytoplasm due to a high lipid content (Fig. 93-6). Histologically, SGC may resemble the appearance of SCC. However, the cytoplasm in SGC tends to be more basophilic compared with the eosinophilic appearance of SCC. Also, SCC cells tend not to exhibit a regular, lobular arrangement. Four histological patterns have been described: lobular, comedocarcinoma, papillary, and mixed. Special stains for lipid (e.g., oil red O) on fresh tissue may assist in the histopathological diagnosis of SGC (Fig. 93-7).[7,34]

TREATMENT

Successful treatment of SGC depends largely upon heightened clinical suspicion and awareness of the possible masquerade

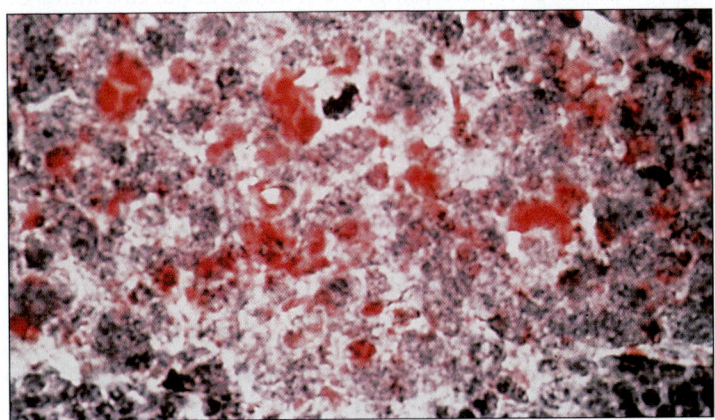

FIG. 93-7 ■ Lipid stain (oil red O) of sebaceous gland carcinoma. Tumor cells stain strongly positive (red) for lipid. (Courtesy of Dr Morton Smith.)

syndrome followed by early confirmatory biopsy. Wide surgical excision with microscopic monitoring of the margins is the procedure of choice. Mohs' micrographic surgical excision may be used, but it may not be as successful as in BCC or SCC because of the possibility of multicentric and pagetoid spread. If the tumor is very large or recurrent with demonstrated spread to bulbar conjunctiva, to the other eyelid, or to orbital tissues, a subtotal or complete exenteration may be necessary.[2,30,31,33,35] If evidence of spread to regional lymph nodes is present, the patient should be referred to a head and neck surgeon for possible lymph node or radical neck dissection.[34]

Radiation therapy may be considered as an adjunct to local surgery. However, primary treatment of the tumor with irradiation alone is inadequate. Recurrence of tumor usually occurs within 3 years following radiotherapy alone.[36]

COURSE AND OUTCOME

An invasive, potentially lethal tumor, SGC may cause extensive local destruction of eyelid tissues. It carries a risk of metastasis to preauricular and submandibular lymph nodes or may spread hematogenously to distant sites. It may invade locally into the globe, the orbit, the sinuses, or the brain. Early reports demonstrated a high (30%) tumor-related mortality rate.[32] More recent reviews show a much lower mortality rate, attributed to heightened clinical suspicion and early diagnosis of the tumor.[30] Nonmetastatic disease has a 0–15% mortality rate. However, the presence of distant metastases carries a very poor prognosis with a 50–67% 5-year mortality.[29,32]

MALIGNANT MELANOMA

INTRODUCTION

Cutaneous malignant melanoma is an invasive proliferation of malignant melanocytes. Melanoma may also arise from the conjunctiva, where it constitutes a distinct entity (see Chapter 56). Cutaneous malignant melanoma may be classified into four different types[7]:

- Lentigo maligna melanoma (5%)
- Superficial spreading melanoma (70%)
- Nodular melanoma (16%)
- "Other," including acral lentiginous melanoma (9%)

Nodular melanoma is the most common type to affect the eyelids.[37]

EPIDEMIOLOGY AND PATHOGENESIS

Cutaneous malignant melanoma of the eyelid accounts for about 1% of all eyelid malignancies. The incidence of malignant melanoma has been increasing, and it causes about two thirds of all tumor-related deaths from cutaneous cancers. The incidence increases with age but remains relatively stable from the fifth to the seventh decades.[38]

Risk factors for the development of malignant melanoma include congenital and dysplastic nevi, changing cutaneous moles, excessive sun exposure and sun sensitivity, family history (genetic factors), age greater than 20 years, and Caucasian race. Malignant melanoma is 12 times more common in whites than in blacks and 7 times more common in whites than in Hispanics.[39] In contrast to BCC, a history of severe sunburns rather than cumulative actinic exposure is thought to be a major risk factor for developing malignant melanoma.[38]

Cutaneous malignant melanoma arises from the neoplastic transformation of intraepidermal melanocytes derived from the neural crest. Initially, a noninvasive horizontal growth phase occurs, which is followed by an invasive vertical growth phase.

OCULAR MANIFESTATIONS

Lentigo maligna melanoma and its precursor, lentigo maligna (melanotic freckle of Hutchinson), present as a flat macule with irregular borders and variable pigmentation. It may have a long *in situ* (horizontal growth) phase, in which the pigmentation extends for up to several centimeters in diameter and lasts many years. This phase is associated with variable growth and spontaneous regression of the lesion with alteration in pigmentation. It typically occurs in sun-exposed areas and commonly involves

the lower eyelid and canthi (Fig. 93-8). Superficial spreading melanoma is typically a smaller pigmented lesion with mild elevation and irregular borders. It tends to have a more rapid progression to the invasive phase, characterized by development of nodules and induration. Nodular melanoma may present as a markedly pigmented or amelanotic nodule that rapidly increases in size with associated ulceration and bleeding. Acral lentiginous melanoma occurs on the palms, soles, and distal phalanges as well as on the mucous membranes.[7,38]

DIAGNOSIS

The diagnosis of cutaneous malignant melanoma is made by clinical suspicion and confirmed with excisional biopsy and histopathological examination.

DIFFERENTIAL DIAGNOSIS

The differential diagnosis of malignant melanoma of the eyelid primarily comprises nonmalignant pigmented nevi that affect the eyelids (see Table 93-1).[7]

SYSTEMIC ASSOCIATIONS

The dysplastic nevus syndrome (also known as B-K mole syndrome) is an autosomal dominantly inherited condition characterized by multiple, large, atypical cutaneous nevi. The moles appear in childhood and continue to grow through adulthood. Patients with this syndrome have a high risk of developing malignant melanoma.[40]

PATHOLOGY

Lentigo maligna is hyperpigmentation in the epidermis characterized by a diffuse hyperplasia of atypical melanocytes throughout the basal cell layer. The entity is regarded as lentigo malignant melanoma when dermal invasion occurs during the transition to the vertical growth phase (Fig. 93-9). Superficial spreading melanoma is typified by atypical melanocytes that occur in nests or singly throughout all levels of the epidermis. Pagetoid spread into the epidermis is characteristic. A mixture of epithelioid, spindle, and nevus-like cells may be present. In nodular melanoma dermal invasion is always present; it exhibits large, anaplastic epithelioid cells.

TREATMENT

Wide surgical excision, with 1cm of skin margins (when possible) confirmed by histological monitoring, is the procedure of choice for treatment of cutaneous malignant melanoma of the

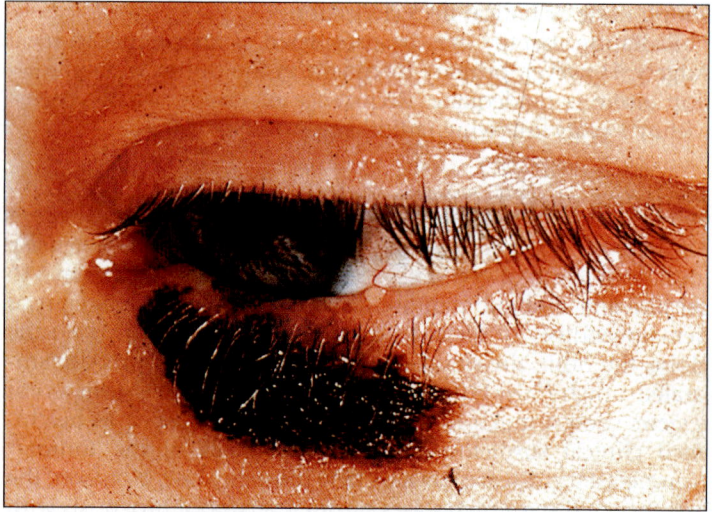

FIG. 93-8 ▐▐ **Lentigo maligna melanoma (Hutchinson freckle).** Clinical appearance of acquired pigmented lesion of the left lower lid.

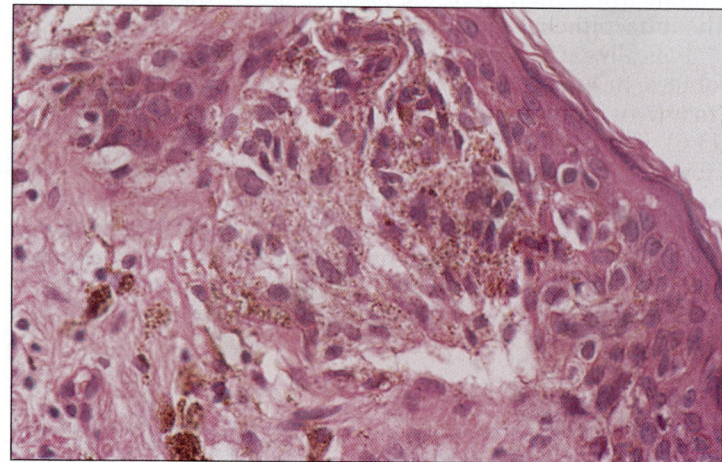

FIG. 93-9 ▐▐ **Malignant melanoma.** Subepithelial pigmented, spindle-shaped melanoma cells invade the dermis. (Courtesy of Dr Morton Smith.)

eyelid. Regional lymph node dissection should be performed for tumors greater than 1.5mm in depth and/or for tumors that show evidence of vascular or lymphatic spread. A metastatic evaluation is also recommended for patients who have such tumors. Cryotherapy may be useful in treating some conjunctival malignant melanomas, but it is not an effective treatment option for cutaneous malignant melanoma of the eyelid.[37]

COURSE AND OUTCOME

Prognosis and metastatic potential are linked to the depth of invasion and thickness of the tumor. Clark and associates[41] correlated prognosis with depth of invasion, characterized at five levels:

- Level 1: tumor confined to the epidermis with an intact basement membrane.
- Level 2: tumor extension beyond the basement membrane with early invasion of the papillary dermis.
- Level 3: tumor fills the papillary dermis and reaches the interface between the papillary and reticular dermis.
- Level 4: tumor penetrates the reticular dermis.
- Level 5: tumor invasion of the subcutaneous tissues.

For lentigo maligna melanoma in levels 1 and 2 there is a 100% survival rate after therapy, whereas for nodular melanoma extending to level 4 there is a 65% survival rate following treatment. The survival drops dramatically to only 15% with extension of any type to level 5.[42]

Breslow[43] related prognosis to tumor thickness—malignant melanomas less than 0.76mm thick are associated with a 100% 5-year survival rate after excision; tumors greater than 1.5mm in thickness are associated with a less than 50% 5-year survival rate. Therefore, nodular melanoma has the worst prognosis and lentigo maligna melanoma has the most favorable prognosis of all tumor types. The Clark and Breslow systems may be used in conjunction to predict the prognosis for patients with malignant melanoma.

In a review by Tahery et al.,[44] malignant melanoma involving the eyelid margin was found to have a poorer prognosis than eyelid malignant melanoma that did not affect the margin. This worse prognosis was attributed to conjunctival involvement in the eyelid margin tumors.

KAPOSI'S SARCOMA

INTRODUCTION

Kaposi's sarcoma is a rare neoplasm that may affect the cutaneous or mucosal surfaces of the eyelids. Prior to the advent of AIDS, this tumor was exceedingly rare, but it is now seen more commonly in those with AIDS.

EPIDEMIOLOGY AND PATHOGENESIS

Ophthalmic involvement with Kaposi's sarcoma occurs in 24–30% of AIDS patients. Generally, Kaposi's sarcoma is associated with slowly progressive disease, but the condition may resolve spontaneously.[45] A rare form of systemic Kaposi's sarcoma is seen in elderly men of southern Mediterranean origin. Studies suggest that the endothelial cells characteristic of this tumor may be of lymphatic or viral origin.[46,47]

OCULAR MANIFESTATIONS

Usually Kaposi's sarcoma presents as highly vascular, purple or red nodules on the cutaneous aspect of the eyelids and caruncle or on the conjunctiva (Fig. 93-10), but it may also involve the lacrimal sac and, rarely, the orbit. Intraocular involvement has not been described.[48,49]

DIFFERENTIAL DIAGNOSIS

A number of lesions can be confused with Kaposi's sarcoma (see Table 93-1),[50] but in the setting of an immunocompromised host the diagnosis is usually not difficult to make.

SYSTEMIC ASSOCIATION

The most important systemic association is AIDS.

PATHOLOGY

Kaposi's sarcoma is composed of slit-like vascular channels lined by endothelial cells and surrounded by spindle-shaped mesenchymal cells and collagen (Fig. 93-11).

TREATMENT, COURSE, AND OUTCOME

The goal of therapy is to relieve ocular irritation, mass effect, and disfigurement. Cryotherapy, irradiation, surgical excision, and intralesional chemotherapy have been described.[49,50] Therapy may reduce or clear the visible lesions, but it is not curative.

MERKEL CELL TUMOR (CUTANEOUS NEUROENDOCRINE CARCINOMA)

INTRODUCTION

Merkel cell tumor is a rare neoplasm composed of nondendritic and nonkeratinocytic epithelial clear cells of neural crest origin.[51] It is characterized by frequent local recurrences following excision and by lymphatic spread.[52]

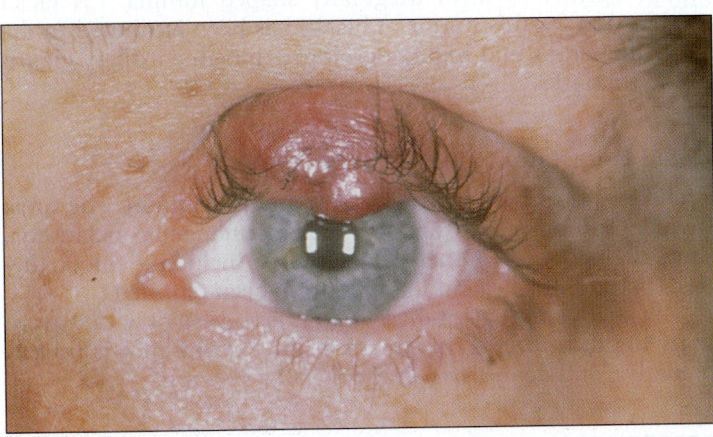

FIG. 93-10 ■ **Kaposi's sarcoma of the eyelid margin.** A solitary, vascular reddish purple nodule of the left upper eyelid. (Courtesy of Dr Morton Smith.)

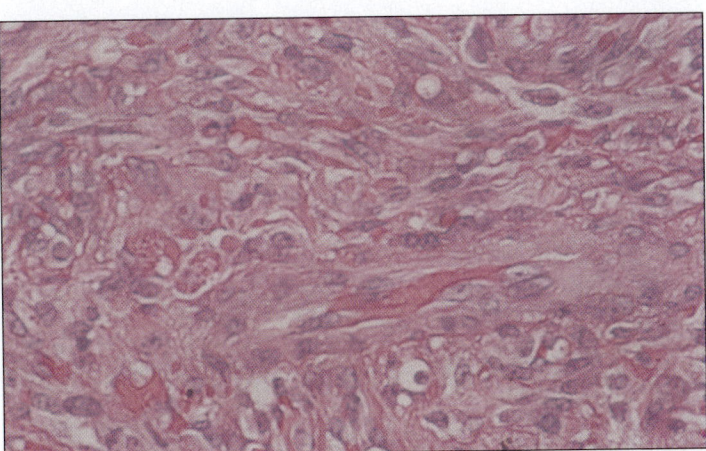

FIG. 93-11 ■ **Kaposi's sarcoma.** A network of plump endothelial cells line slit-like vascular channels. (Courtesy of Dr Morton Smith.)

EPIDEMIOLOGY AND PATHOGENESIS

Nearly equal incidences of Merkel cell tumors are seen in men and women, primarily in the elderly, and the tumors have a predilection for the head and neck region. The upper eyelid tends to be involved more than other periocular sites. No tumors have been reported in blacks.[7]

The Merkel cell as the origin for cutaneous neuroendocrine carcinoma was described after electron microscopic ultrastructural analysis demonstrated neurosecretory granules.[53]

OCULAR MANIFESTATIONS

Clinically, Merkel cell tumors of the eyelid present as solitary, vascularized, nontender, red or violaceous nodules (Fig. 93-12). Tumors of the upper eyelid may cause a mechanical blepharoptosis.

DIFFERENTIAL DIAGNOSIS

The most common lesions in the differential diagnosis are given in Table 93-1.

PATHOLOGY

Light microscopy demonstrates tumor cells with uniformly sized nuclei, scant cytoplasm, and numerous mitotic figures. Tumor cells invade the dermis and are arranged in sheets or in a trabecular pattern (Fig. 93-13). Hair follicles may be involved, but the epidermis is usually spared. Ultrastructural examination reveals secretory granules, microfilaments, desmosomes, and intranuclear rodlets.[7]

TREATMENT

Wide surgical excision with frozen section control of the margins is the treatment of choice. Patients should be evaluated for evidence of metastasis. The possible roles of chemotherapy and radiotherapy are unclear.

COURSE AND OUTCOME

A high incidence of local, multiple recurrences occurs with Merkel cell tumors, with recurrent disease being more common in men. Tumor-related death is usually attributed to distant metastatic disease. The mean survival period after diagnosis of distant metastasis is 16 months in men and 23 months in women.[54]

OTHER RARE TUMORS OF THE EYELIDS

INTRODUCTION, PATHOLOGY, AND TREATMENT

Mucinous Sweat Gland Adenocarcinoma

Mucinous sweat gland adenocarcinoma is a rare malignancy of the eccrine sweat glands that may present in the skin of the eyelid and typically affects male, middle-aged adults. These tumors occur more frequently in blacks. Although it usually presents as a skin-colored, firm, indurated nodule or lobulated mass, it may occasionally have a red-blue, cystic appearance. The clinical differential diagnosis includes benign cysts, keratoacanthomas, and BCC.[55]

Histopathologically, the tumor exhibits cords and lobules of epithelial cells in a pool of mucin, separated by thin fibrovascular septa. The tumor cells are cuboidal or polygonal in shape with nuclear pleomorphism. The tumor is composed of both light and dark cell populations—the dark cells are generally located closer to the periphery and produce mucin and the light cells are located more centrally. Light cells have a paucity of intracellular organelles.[7]

Wide surgical excision with frozen section control of the margins is the treatment of choice for mucinous adenocarcinomas. As these have a propensity for local recurrence, long-term follow-up is required. However, they have low metastatic potential and a better prognosis than other sweat gland carcinomas.

Adenocarcinoma of the Gland of Moll

Adenocarcinoma of the gland of Moll is an exceedingly rare tumor that arises from apocrine sweat glands. It is characterized by a glandular arrangement of large cells that have eosinophilic cytoplasm with evidence of decapitation secretion. The cells may group together to form irregularly shaped lumina.[56] A racial predilection for this tumor in blacks has been attributed to the more numerous and highly developed apocrine axillary glands found in blacks.[57]

Eyelid Metastases

Eyelid metastases from distant sites are uncommon. The most frequent primary sites are the breast, cutaneous melanoma, lung, and stomach. Other primary sites, including colon, thyroid, parotid, trachea, and kidney, have been reported.[7]

The histopathology of these lesions is consistent with the primary tumor of origin. Treatment of the eyelid tumor is usually palliative, and definitive therapy must be systemic.

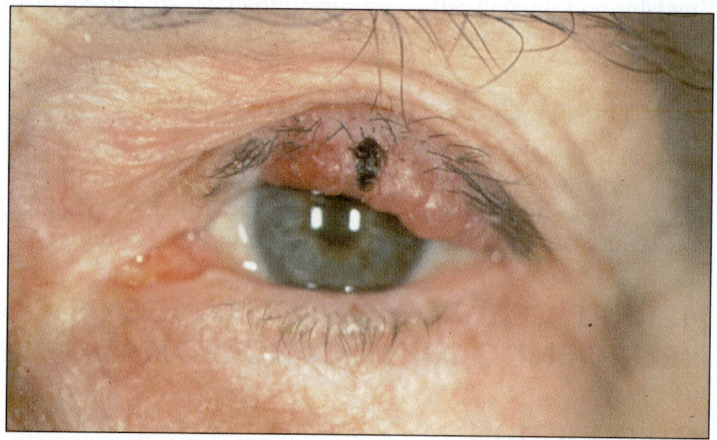

FIG. 93-12 ■ **Merkel cell tumor of the eyelid.** A large, firm, reddish nodule that resembles an angiomatous lesion of the left upper eyelid. Telangiectatic vessels appear on the surface of the nodule. These lesions are typically more violaceous in coloration. (Courtesy of Dr Morton Smith.)

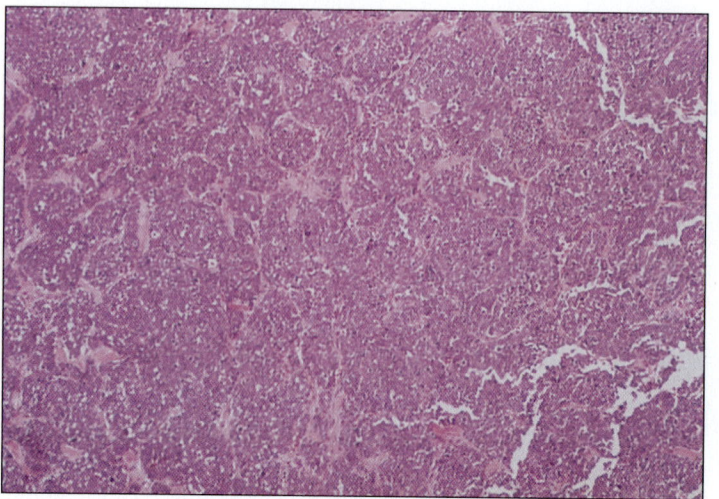

FIG. 93-13 ■ **Merkel cell tumor.** Sheets of densely packed basophilic, round, and ovoid tumor cells with scant cytoplasm are observed. (Courtesy of Dr Morton Smith.)

REFERENCES

1. Margo CE, Waltz K. Basal cell carcinoma of the eyelid and periocular skin. Surv Ophthalmol. 1993;38:169–92.

2. Haas AF, Kielty DW. Basal cell carcinoma. In: Mannis MJ, Macsai MS, Huntley AC, eds. Eye and skin disease. Philadelphia: Lippincott-Raven; 1996:395–403.

3. Cotsarelis G, Cheng S, Dong D. Existence of slow cycling limbal epithelial basal cells that can be preferentially stimulated to proliferate: implications on epithelial stem cells. Cell. 1989;57:201–9.

4. Lavker RM, San T. Heterogeneity in epidermal basal keratinocytes: morphological and functional correlations. Science. 1982;215:1239–41.

5. Doxanas MT, Green WR. Factors in successful surgical management of basal cell carcinoma of the eyelids. Am J Ophthalmol. 1981;91:726–36.

6. Lever WF, Schaumburg-Lever G. Tumors of the epidermal appendages. In: Histopathology of the skin, 7th ed. Philadelphia: JB Lippincott; 1990:578–650.

7. Font RL. Eyelids and lacrimal drainage system. In: Spencer WH, ed. Ophthalmic pathology: an atlas and textbook, 4th ed, Vol 4. Philadelphia: WB Saunders; 1996:2218–433.

8. Yanoff M, Fine BS. Skin and lacrimal drainage system. In: Yanoff M, Fine BS, eds. Ocular pathology. Hagerstown: Harper & Row; 1975:177–232.

9. Kahn LB, Gordon W. Nevoid basal cell carcinoma syndrome. S Afr Med J. 1967;41:832–5.

10. Gorlin RJ, Goltz RW. Multiple nevoid basal cell epithelioma, jaw cysts and bifid rib, a syndrome. N Engl J Med. 1960;262:908–12.

11. Borel DM. Cutaneous basosquamous carcinoma. Review of the literature and report of 35 cases. Arch Pathol. 1973;95:293–7.

12. Warren RC, Nerad JA, Carter KD. Punch biopsy technique for the ophthalmologist. Arch Ophthalmol. 1990;108:778–9.

13. Waltz K, Margo CE. Mohs' micrographic surgery. Ophthalmol Clin North Am. 1991;4:153–63.

14. Mohs FE. Micrographic surgery for microscopically controlled excision of eyelid tumors. Arch Ophthalmol. 1986;104:901–9.

15. Glatt HJ, Olson JJ, Putterman AM. Conventional frozen sections in periocular basal cell carcinoma: a review of 236 cases. Ophthalmic Surg. 1992;23:6–9.

16. Frank HJ. Frozen section control of excision of eyelid basal cell carcinoma: 8½ years' experience. Br J Ophthalmol. 1989;73:328–32.

17. Einaugler RB, Henkind P. Basal cell epithelioma of the eyelid: apparent incomplete removal. Am J Ophthalmol. 1969;67:413–17.

18. Westgate SJ. Radiation therapy for skin tumors. Otolaryngol Clin. 1993;26:265–76.

19. Wiggs EO. Morphea-form basal cell carcinomas of the canthi. Trans Am Acad Ophthalmol Otolaryngol. 1975;79:649–53.

20. Payne JW, Duke JR, Buther R, Eifrig DE. Basal cell carcinoma of the eyelids. A long-term follow-up study. Arch Ophthalmol. 1969;81:553–8.

21. Rodrequez-Sains RS, Robbins P, Smith B, Bosniak S. Radiotherapy of periocular basal cell carcinoma: recurrence rates and treatment with special attention to the medial canthus. Br J Ophthalmol. 1988;72:693–7.

22. Anscher M, Montana G. Radiotherapy. Surv Ophthalmol. 1993;38:193–212.

23. Fraunfelder FT, Zacarian SA, Wingfield DL, et al. Results of cryotherapy for eyelid malignancies. Am J Ophthalmol. 1985;97:184–8.

24. Wilson BD, Mang TS, Stoll H, et al. Photodynamic therapy for the treatment of basal cell carcinoma. Arch Dermatol. 1992;128:1597–601.

25. Kwitko ML, Boniuk M, Zimmerman LE. Eyelid tumors with reference to lesions confused with squamous cell carcinoma. I. Incidence and errors in diagnosis. Arch Ophthalmol. 1963;69:693–7.

26. Lederman M. Discussion of carcinomas of conjunctiva and eyelid. In: Boniuk M, ed. Ocular and adnexal tumors. St Louis: CV Mosby; 1964:104–9.

27. Haas AF, Tucker SM. Squamous cell carcinoma. In: Mannis MJ, Macsai MS, Huntley AC, eds. Eye and skin disease. Philadelphia: Lippincott-Raven; 1996:405–11.

28. Mora RG, Perniliaro C. Cancer of the skin in blacks. I. A review of 163 black patients with cutaneous squamous cell carcinoma. J Am Acad Dermatol. 1981;5:535–43.

29. Rao NA, Hidayat AA, McLean IW, et al. Sebaceous gland carcinomas of the ocular adnexa: a clinicopathologic study of 104 cases, with five-year follow-up data. Hum Pathol. 1982;13:113–22.

30. Doxanas MT, Green WR. Sebaceous gland carcinoma. Arch Ophthalmol. 1984;102:245–9.

31. Kass LG, Hornblass A. Sebaceous carcinoma of the ocular adnexa. Surv Ophthalmol. 1989;33:477–90.

32. Boniuk M, Zimmerman LE, Sebaceous carcinoma of the eyelid, eyebrow, caruncle, and orbit. Trans Am Acad Ophthalmol Otolaryngol. 1968;72:619–41.

33. Khan JA, Grove AS, Joseph MP, et al. Sebaceous gland carcinoma: diuretic use, lacrimal system spread, and surgical margins. Ophthalmic Plast Reconstr Surg. 1989;5:227–34.

34. Kostick DA, Linberg JV, McCormick SA. Sebaceous gland carcinoma. In: Mannis MJ, Macsai MS, Huntley AC, eds. Eye and skin disease. Philadelphia: Lippincott-Raven; 1996:413–17.

35. Harvey JT, Anderson RL. The management of meibomian gland carcinoma. Ophthalmic Surg. 1982;13:56–60.

36. Nunery WR, Welsh MG, McCord CD Jr. Recurrence of sebaceous carcinoma of the eyelid after radiation therapy. Am J Ophthalmol. 1983;96:10–15.

37. Garner A, Koornneef L, Levene A, et al. Malignant melanoma of the eyelid skin: histopathology and behavior. Br J Ophthalmol. 1985;69:180–6.

38. McCormick SA, DeLuca RL. Tumors of melanocytic origin. In: Mannis MJ, Macsai MS, Huntley AC, eds. Eye and skin disease. Philadelphia: Lippincott-Raven; 1996:381–93.

39. Rhodes AR, Weinstock MA, Fitzpatrick TB, et al. Risk factors for cutaneous melanoma: a practical method of recognizing predisposed individuals. JAMA. 1987;258:3146–54.

40. Clark WH Jr, Reimer RR, Greene MH, et al. Origin of familial malignant melanoma from heritable melanocytic lesions. The B-K mole syndrome. Arch Dermatol. 1978;114:732–8.

41. Clark WH Jr, Ainsworth AM, Bernardino EA, et al. Developmental biology of primary human malignant melanomas. Semin Oncol. 1975;2:83–103.

42. Kopf AW, Bart RS, Rodriguez-Sain RS, et al. Malignant melanoma. New York: Masson; 1979.

43. Breslow A. Thickness, cross-sectional areas and depths of invasion in the prognosis of cutaneous melanoma. Ann Surg. 1970;172:902–8.

44. Tahery DP, Goldberg R, Moy RL. Malignant melanoma of the eyelid: a report of eight cases and a review of the literature. J Am Acad Dermatol. 1992;27:17–21.

45. Friedman-Kien AE, Saltzman BR. Clinical manifestations of classical, endemic African and epidemic AIDS-associated Kaposi's sarcoma. J Am Acad Dermatol. 1990;22:1237–50.

46. Bookstead JH, Wood GS, Fletcher V. Evidence for the origin of Kaposi's sarcoma from lymphatic endothelium. Am J Pathol. 1985;119:292–300.

47. Cesarman E, Knowles DM. Kaposi's sarcoma–associated herpes virus. Semin Diagn Pathol. 1997;14:54–66.

48. Dugel PU, Gill PS, Frangieh GT, et al. Ocular adnexal Kaposi's sarcoma in acquired immunodeficiency syndrome. Am J Ophthalmol. 1990;110:500–3.

49. Shuler JD, Holland GN, Miles SA, et al. Kaposi sarcoma of the conjunctiva and eyelids associated with the acquired immunodeficiency syndrome. Arch Ophthalmol. 1989;107:858–62.

50. Dugel PU, Gill PS, Frangieh GT, et al. Treatment of ocular adnexal Kaposi's sarcoma in acquired immune deficiency syndrome. Ophthalmology. 1992;99:1127–32.

51. Yanoff M, Fine BS, eds. Skin. In: Ocular pathology: a text and atlas, 3rd ed. Philadelphia: JB Lippincott; 1989:164–213.

52. Kivela T, Tarkkanen A. The Merkel cell and associated neoplasms in the eyelids and periocular regions. Surv Ophthalmol. 1990;35:171–87.

53. Wick MR, Millns JL, Sibley RK, et al. Secondary neuroendocrine carcinomas of the skin: an immunohistochemical comparison with primary neuroendocrine carcinoma of the skin ('Merkel cell' carcinoma). J Am Acad Dermatol. 1985;13:134–42.

54. Pitale M, Session RB, Husain S. An analysis of prognostic factors in cutaneous neuroendocrine carcinoma. Laryngoscope. 1992;102:244–9.

55. Wright JD, Font RL. Mucinous sweat gland adenocarcinoma of the eyelid: a clinicopathologic study of 21 cases with histochemical and electron microscopic observations. Cancer. 1979;44:1757–68.

56. Rodgers IR, Jakobiec FA, Hidayat AA. Eyelid tumors of apocrine, eccrine, and pilar origins. In: Albert DM, Jakobiec FA, eds. Principles and practice of ophthalmology, Vol 3. Philadelphia: WB Saunders; 1994:1771–96.

57. Warkel RL, Helwig EB. Apocrine gland adenoma and adenocarcinoma of the axilla. Arch Dermatol. 1978;114:198–204.

CHAPTER 94

Eyelid Trauma and Reconstruction Techniques

JEFFREY P. GREEN • GEORGE C. CHARONIS • ROBERT ALAN GOLDBERG

DEFINITION
• Injuries varying from simple skin abrasions to more complex cases with extensive tissue loss and underlying fractures of the facial skeleton.

KEY FEATURES
• Caused by blunt or penetrating facial trauma.
• Partial-thickness eyelid injury.
• Eyelid margin lacerations.
• Eyelid injuries with tissue loss.
• Full-thickness eyelid injury.

INTRODUCTION

Injuries that involve the eyelids and periorbital area are common after blunt or penetrating facial trauma. Such injuries can vary from simple skin abrasions to more complex cases that have extensive tissue loss and underlying fractures of the facial skeleton. A complete assessment of the trauma patient is critical to determine the extent of the underlying systemic damage, but stabilization of vital systems should be the first priority in the management of these patients. After successful stabilization of the patient's systemic condition has been achieved, attention can be directed toward the specific ocular adnexal injuries. Restoration of structure and function along with adherence to basic esthetic principles should be the primary concern of the reconstructive surgeon involved in the management of such injuries.

In this chapter, general principles for the evaluation and management of eyelid trauma are discussed. The most common types of adnexal injuries are presented in a systematic approach. Ocular adnexal trauma can be very challenging and often tests the ingenuity of the reconstructive surgeon. Several management principles and surgical techniques that can minimize postoperative complications and improve esthetic results and function are explained. This can often have a dramatic impact on the patient's life, as secondary defects can be very difficult or even impossible to correct in later surgery.

PREOPERATIVE EVALUATION AND DIAGNOSTIC APPROACH

Systemic Stabilization

The evaluation of periorbital injuries begins after the traumatized patient has been stabilized and life-threatening injuries addressed. The role of the ophthalmologist in the evaluation and management is very important—good communication must exist between the trauma team and the ophthalmologist. The presence of subjective symptoms related to the visual system or physical evidence of periorbital injuries demands the immediate attention of the ophthalmologist. The incidence of ocular injuries in craniofacial trauma is high, ranging between 15 and 60% in various studies.[1]

Medical History

A complete history is obtained to determine the time course and circumstances of the injury. For children, consideration must be given to the possibility of child abuse as the cause of ocular and periorbital injury. A history consistent with injuries from high-speed projectile particles may require the appropriate imaging studies to determine the presence of intraocular or intraorbital foreign bodies. Animal and human bites deserve particular attention and are managed accordingly with the administration of appropriate antibiotics. The site of injury is inspected carefully for any missing tissue, and any amputated tissue found at the site of injury is preserved and placed on ice as soon as possible. In most cases this tissue can be sutured back to the proper anatomic location.

Ophthalmologic Examination

Assessment of visual acuity is mandatory and made prior to any reconstructive efforts. The pupils are checked and, if a relative afferent pupillary defect is found, the potential of poor visual outcome is discussed with the patient prior to surgical repair. The extraocular muscles are evaluated and any diplopia documented prior to surgery. The external examination includes a complete bone assessment of the facial skeleton, with particular emphasis on the periorbital region. A palpable step-off, crepitus, or unstable bone requires radiological evaluation. The baseline measurement of globe projection is documented with Hertel exophthalmometry because enophthalmos is a common late sequela of orbital trauma. Eyelid position, orbicularis muscle function, and any evidence of lagophthalmos are documented thoroughly. Measurement of the intercanthal distance and evaluation of the integrity of the canthal tendons are also performed because traumatic tendon dehiscence and telecanthus are frequently associated with periorbital injuries. The integrity of the lacrimal system is checked, with a high index of suspicion for canalicular lacerations (see Chapter 98).

Medicolegal Documentation

All injuries are documented precisely and completely. This can be done with detailed drawings on the patient's charts or, even better, with photographic documentation. Bullets and other projectiles must be retained and marked so that no break occurs in the chain of evidence. The medicolegal implications can be significant, so every effort must be made to complete the preoperative documentation of every injury.

TABLE 94-1

GUIDELINES FOR TETANUS PROPHYLAXIS IN WOUND TREATMENT

Immunization History	Clean, Minor Wound	Other Type of Wound
Uncertain history	Tetanus and diphtheria toxoids*	Tetanus and diphtheria toxoids + tetanus immune globulin
None or one previous dose	Tetanus and diphtheria toxoids*	Tetanus and diphtheria toxoids + tetanus immune globulin
Two previous doses	Tetanus and diphtheria toxoids*	Tetanus and diphtheria toxoids†
More than three previous doses	None unless the last dose is more than 10 years previously	None unless the last dose is more than 10 years previously

Adapted from Mustarde JC. Eyelid reconstruction. Orbit. 1983;1:33–43.
*Adult type; for children less than 7 years of age, DTP (diphtheria, tetanus, pertusis).
† For wounds more than 24 hours old, add tetanus immune globulin.

Laboratory and Radiographic Evaluation

Usually, an appropriate laboratory evaluation is performed by the emergency room team. A complete blood count and serum chemistry analysis are often needed for anesthetic purposes. Coagulative studies may be helpful in selected cases, and blood chemistry studies for alcohol and other toxic substances are necessary in others. When the clinical suspicion of orbital fractures is high, appropriate orbital imaging studies, mainly computed tomography, should be ordered (see Chapter 84). Ultrasonic examination of the globe contents, extraocular muscles, optic nerve, and orbit sometimes can be an important adjunctive study.

Infection Prophylaxis

Prevention of infection is a primary concern. A complete tetanus immunization history is obtained and the appropriate management followed if the patient is not up to date with immunizations (see Table 94-1).[2] If an animal bite is known or suspected, all information about the site of injury, the owner of the animal, and any abnormal animal behavior must be obtained and the local animal care department notified. The standard rabies protocol is followed. A section on dog bites is presented later and contains more detailed information on the evaluation and management of such injuries.

Cat bites, and even wounds caused by cat claws, carry a high risk for infection, mainly with *Pasteurella multocida* (see the later section on dog bites). Appropriate prophylaxis includes penicillin VK (phenoxymethylpenicillin) 500mg a day for 5–7 days. In allergic patients tetracycline may be given.[3]

Human bite injuries require the administration of appropriate antibiotics, such as penicillin, Augmentin (amoxicillin and clavulanic acid), erythromycin, or dicloxacillin, as the potential exists to inoculate a large number of bacteria.[3] Additional consideration should be given to human immunodeficiency virus and hepatitis and the appropriate testing administered.

Following any type of bite injury, copious irrigation of all injured tissues and removal of superficial foreign bodies lodged in the conjunctival fornices are performed. Vigorous irrigation and removal of foreign bodies are generally sufficient to prevent wound infection in most bites.

Timing of Repair

The timing of the repair is governed by several factors. Every effort must be made to reconstruct the injured tissues as soon as possible after the patient has been thoroughly evaluated and appropriate ancillary studies have been obtained. However, waiting for 24–48 hours to assemble the most efficient and experienced reconstructive team is a viable alternative unless amputated tissue needs to be replaced. It must be emphasized here that the best chances for restoration of structure and function and for successful cosmesis exist in the initial surgery. To try to address complications or a poor outcome in secondary procedures can be difficult. Should a slight delay in treatment be deemed necessary, the wound should be kept moist with continuous application of soaked saline gauze pads to prevent wound drying and desiccation. Adequate eye protection with copious lubrication must be given or even a temporary tarsorrhaphy performed if a significant threat of exposure keratopathy exists.

ANESTHESIA

The choice of anesthetic for the repair of adnexal injuries depends on several factors. Obviously, the patient's age is critical because almost all children require general anesthetic for the best reconstructive results to be achieved. Large injuries with extensive soft tissue and osseous involvement are best managed in a similar setting. However, even with general anesthetic, local infiltration of epinephrine (adrenaline) is essential for hemostasis. The majority of adult injuries can be repaired with local infiltrative or regional anesthetic of 1–2% lidocaine (lignocaine) with 1:100,000 epinephrine. Infiltrative anesthetic can cause significant tissue distortion; this can be minimized with the use of hyaluronic acid (hyaluronidase), which facilitates spreading of the anesthetic solution. Regional anesthesia of the infraorbital, supraorbital, infratrochlear, and supratrochlear nerves can be a very effective adjunct and causes no associated tissue distortion.

GENERAL TECHNIQUES

The techniques of eyelid and orbital reconstruction after trauma are numerous and varied; which is used largely depends upon the extent of the injury and the specific adnexal structures involved. The general approach is to address each anatomic structure independently and to respect appropriate priorities—eye protection first, then function, and finally cosmesis. In many cases, a number of reconstructive techniques are combined to achieve an acceptable result.

SPECIFIC TECHNIQUES
Partial-Thickness Eyelid Injuries

Small, superficial eyelid lacerations that do not involve the lid margin and that are parallel to the relaxed skin tension lines can be stabilized with skin tape. Larger lacerations and those that are perpendicular to the relaxed skin tension lines require careful approximation and eversion of the skin edge. This can be accomplished with simple interrupted 6-0 or 7-0 absorbable or nonabsorbable sutures. If the full thickness of the orbicularis muscle is involved, it should be repaired separately. Penetration of the orbital septum (see Chapter 82) with resultant levator aponeurosis injury must be ruled out in upper eyelid injuries; if present, such injuries must be repaired.

Eyelid Margin Lacerations

This type of adnexal trauma requires the most meticulous eyelid approximation, which must be precise to avoid eyelid notching and margin malposition. A good esthetic result depends heavily upon wound preparation. All tarsal irregularities at the wound edges are trimmed to allow good tarsal-to-tarsal approximation of the repaired edges. This is done along the entire vertical height of the tarsus to prevent tarsal buckling, even though the primary laceration may involve only the marginal tarsus.[4] The repair begins with the placement of a 6-0 suture in the plane of the meibomian glands at the lid margin, approximately 2mm from the wound edges and 2mm deep (Fig. 94-1, *A*). Historically, the margin sutures used are nonabsorbable. However, the authors have routinely used absorbable sutures (such as 6-0 Dexon that comes with a convenient half-circle D1 needle; Davis & Geck) and have not experienced complications from premature suture absorption. This option is particularly useful in children.

The traction suture is pulled to determine whether a satisfactory approximation of the margin edges has occurred. A good margin eversion should be the goal. This suture is left long and untied, and traction is applied to facilitate repair of the remaining lid segments. The tarsus is next closed with fine, interrupted, partial-thickness sutures, such as 6-0 or 7-0 Dexon, polyglactin (Vicryl), or 7-0 silk. The knots are tied on the anterior tarsal surface to avoid corneal irritation (Fig. 94-1, *B*). Additional margin sutures are then placed, usually in the eyelash line and in the gray line. These sutures are tied and left long. The anterior lamella of the eyelid is closed next, with fine interrupted sutures. The long margin sutures are tied through these skin sutures to prevent the suture ends from abrading the cornea (Fig. 94-1, *C*). When nonabsorbable sutures are used, they are removed after approximately 2 weeks.

Eyelid Injuries with Tissue Loss

Injuries of the eyelid that result in tissue loss provide a difficult reconstructive challenge. It is incumbent on the surgeon, when the patient with eyelid trauma is evaluated, to define not only whether and how much of the eyelid is missing but also which layers of the eyelid are absent. In the evaluation of these patients, it is very useful to consider the eyelid as a structure that has anterior and posterior lamellae, the skin and orbicularis being the anterior lamella and the tarsus and conjunctiva the posterior lamella (see Chapter 82). If a full-thickness loss of eyelid tissue leads to lagophthalmos and corneal exposure, aggressive lubrication with antibiotic ointments is instituted or a temporary tarsorrhaphy placed until definitive repair can be accomplished.

Tissue loss that involves only the anterior lamella may be repaired, if the tissue loss is small and the defect lies anterior to the septum, by allowing the defect to granulate. This method may obviate the need for skin grafts and myocutaneous flaps; however, the wound must be monitored carefully for infection and late contracture. The result of allowing the eyelid to granulate spontaneously can be equal to, or even surpass, the outcome of primary repair.[5]

If the loss of anterior lamella is more extensive, with exposure of the underlying fat and posterior lamellar tissue, local advancement flaps and skin grafts are required. Acute skin grafting may produce an excellent cosmetic result; also, it may reduce the possibility of a shrinkage phase, which can result in lagophthalmos, lid retraction, and the corneal exposure that is likely to occur if the eyelid is left to granulate spontaneously. Caution must be observed in the employment of grafts and large flaps, as their use in the acute setting is associated with an increased incidence of infection and failure. Whether the surgeon chooses to employ acute skin grafting or other means of repair, it must be recognized that immediate repair is directed at protection of the integrity of the globe, with the recognition that further reconstructive surgery may be necessary to achieve the maximal functional and cosmetic result.[6]

Full-Thickness Eyelid Lacerations

Full-thickness lacerations that do not involve the eyelid margin may be associated with significant internal disarrangement of lid structures and perforation of the globe. These injuries require adequate layer-by-layer inspection of the wound to assess the integrity of the orbital septum, levator muscle and levator aponeurosis, conjunctiva, rectus muscles, and the globe. Meticulous layered closure is required, with the septum left unsutured.

If the posterior lamella of the eyelid is involved in a full-thickness eyelid injury but can be reapproximated without undue tension, it is repaired directly. Tarsal alignment is achieved best through interrupted buried sutures. The authors prefer to use 6-0 or 7-0 polyglactin (Vicryl) sutures; however, Dexon, silk, and chromic sutures are all adequate for tarsal closure. In the upper eyelid these sutures must be passed through the tarsus but remain subconjunctival because full-thickness sutures may result in corneal contact and irritation.

When an injury is severe enough to result in full-thickness tissue loss that involves both the anterior and posterior lamellae of the eyelid, the technique of repair depends on the amount and location of tissue loss. Many of the repair techniques for such injuries are used in lid reconstructions implemented after eyelid skin cancer resections.

The amount of tissue loss usually can be ascertained only after careful reapproximation of the wound. Fortunately, tissue

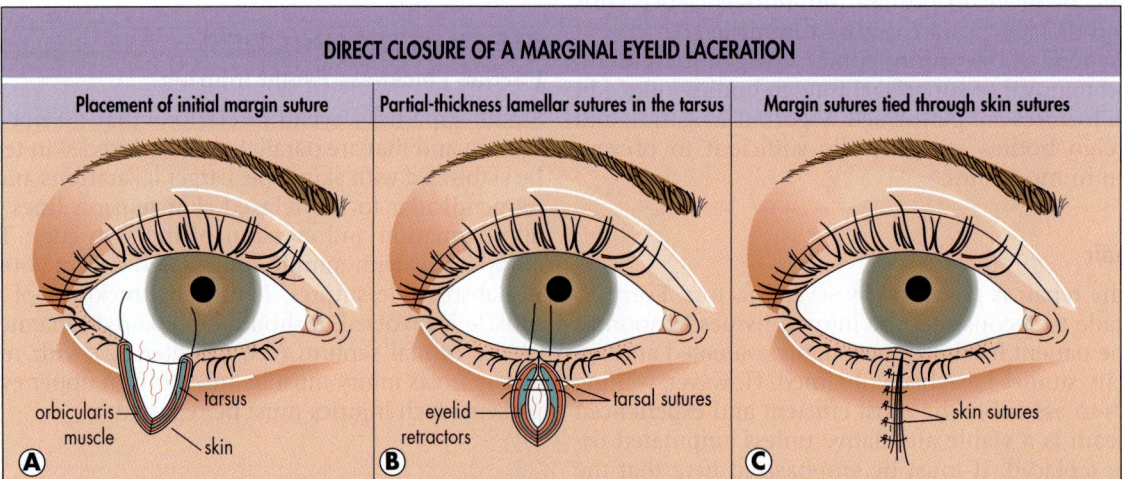

DIRECT CLOSURE OF A MARGINAL EYELID LACERATION

Placement of initial margin suture	Partial-thickness lamellar sutures in the tarsus	Margin sutures tied through skin sutures

FIG. 94-1 ■ **Direct closure of a marginal eyelid laceration. A,** The suture is placed precisely in the plane of the meibomian glands at the eyelid margin, approximately 2mm from the wound edges and 2mm deep. This placement should provide adequate margin eversion. **B,** Partial-thickness lamellar sutures are placed across the tarsus and tied anteriorly. **C,** The anterior skin and muscle lamella is closed with fine sutures, and these are tied over the long marginal sutures to prevent corneal touch.

loss is usually less significant than the initial presentation may suggest, as retraction of the tissue gives the appearance of greater tissue loss than actually has occurred. Every effort is made to preserve all tissue. The generous adnexal vascular supply usually preserves even narrow pedicles, and even largely avulsed tissue can be reattached with significant survival rates. If large defects persist, standard methods of eyelid reconstruction are employed to complete the anatomic repair.[7]

Upper and Lower Full-Thickness Eyelid Injuries

TISSUE LOSS OF 0–25%. If either the upper or lower eyelid has sustained a full-thickness injury that results in less than 25% loss of tissue (including the eyelid margin), the repair can generally be closed primarily. However, it is often necessary to "freshen up" the eyelid margins prior to reconstruction. This not only removes any necrotic, nonviable tissue but also allows the surgeon to create two perpendicular, tarsal-to-tarsal wound edges to prevent any postoperative abnormalities of the lid contour. Other than this minimal débridement required to square off the tarsal edges, no other eyelid tissue should be discarded. Closure of the resultant defect can be accomplished with the same technique as used for full-thickness marginal lid lacerations. In older patients, because of increased eyelid laxity, primary closure of both the upper and lower eyelid may be accomplished for injuries that have up to 40% tissue loss.[8] Injuries with greater than 25% full-thickness tissue loss (40% in the elderly) require borrowing or advancing adjacent tissue for closure.

TISSUE LOSS OF 25–60%. Primary closure of upper or lower eyelid injuries with full-thickness tissue loss that includes the margin can be accomplished by release and advancement of lateral tissues. Some injuries that are at the upper limit of primary closure may have their closure facilitated by a lateral canthotomy, followed by cantholysis of the lateral canthal tendon of the involved upper or lower eyelid.

If more tissue is required to reconstruct an upper or lower eyelid defect, the lateral canthotomy can be made in a semicircular fashion. The entire semicircular skin-muscle flap can be rotated into the lid defect area as described by Tenzel and Stewart[9] (see Fig. 94-2). A periosteal flap can be used to supplement the lateral posterior lamella when either the upper or lower eyelid is reconstructed[2] (see Fig. 94-3). Also, the lateral posterior lamella can be supplemented with hard palate or ear cartilage grafts.[10] Initially, the eyelid may appear tense, but it gradually relaxes over time.

Another technique for upper lid defects with tissue loss between 25 and 60% is the Mustarde lid-switch technique. This technique is useful in patients who have broad, shallow defects of the upper eyelid. It is a two-stage procedure in which the first stage involves the transfer of a pedicle flap from the lower eyelid to the upper eyelid (Fig. 94-4, A). An advantage of this flap is that lashes are transferred to the upper eyelid. The amount of tissue that can be transferred without the need to reconstruct the lower eyelid with an advancement flap is 6mm. The width of the flap is 7–8mm, and it contains the marginal artery. As the middle portion of the lower eyelid has the longest eyelashes and is away from the canthal regions, it is often the best donor site. The second stage, in which the pedicle flap is separated, should be performed 2–3 weeks after the first stage (Fig. 94-4, B).

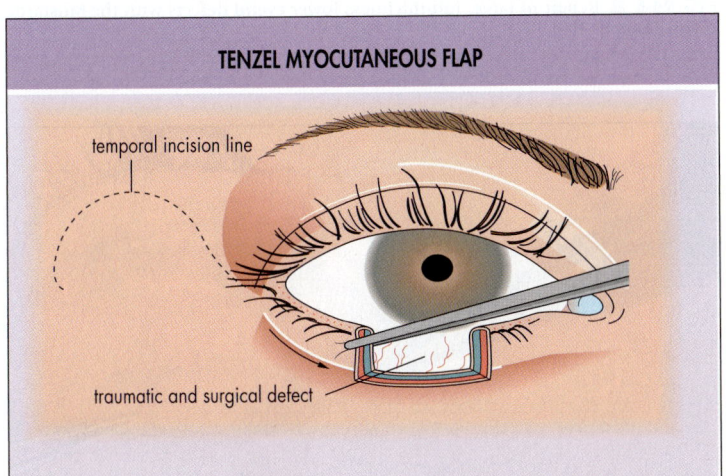

FIG. 94-2 ▐▌ Repair of a lower eyelid defect with the Tenzel myocutaneous flap.

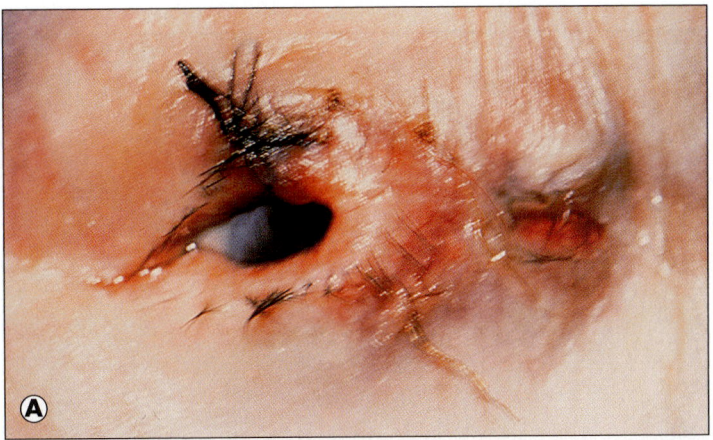

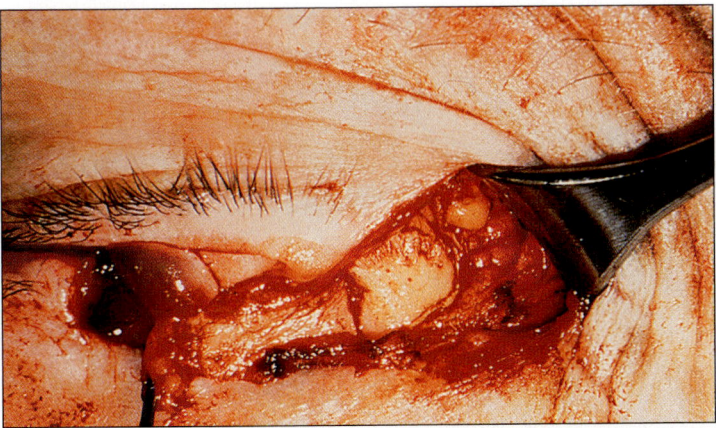

FIG. 94-3 ▐▌ A periosteal flap can be rotated to supplement the lateral posterior lamella in eyelid reconstruction. (Courtesy of Regents of the University of California, 1997, reprinted with permission.)

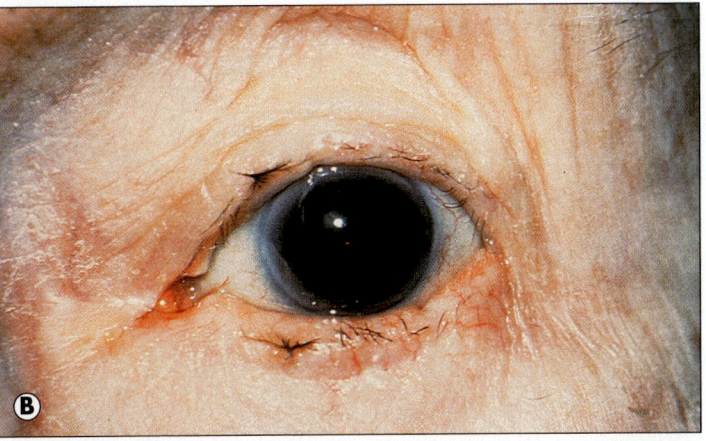

FIG. 94-4 ▐▌ The Mustarde eyelid switch is a very helpful technique in patients who have broad, shallow defects of the upper eyelid. **A,** A pedicle flap of marginal eyelid is cut from the central lower lid and rotated into the upper eyelid defect. **B,** After 2–3 weeks the flap is separated and repaired to restore satisfactory upper and lower eyelid contours, with preservation of lashes. (Courtesy of Regents of the University of California, 1997, reprinted with permission.)

Full-Thickness Eyelid Injuries with Greater Than 60% Tissue Loss

LOWER EYELID. The repair of large tissue defects of the lower lid requires supplemental tissue from adjacent regions. The Hughes tarsoconjunctival flap is a two-stage procedure best suited to large, centrally located, lower eyelid full-thickness defects that spare the eyelid margins medially and laterally[11] (Fig. 94-5).

Shallow, full-thickness, lateral lower eyelid defects may be addressed with the transposition tarsoconjunctival flap described by Hewes *et al.*[12] This is a one-stage procedure in which the superolateral portion of the upper lid tarsus is used as a flap based at the lateral canthus. The flap is rotated down and sutured to the tarsus and conjunctiva in the lower lid, with the tarsal margin in the downmost position. This transposed tarsoconjunctival flap is then covered with a full-thickness skin graft from a suitable donor site.[12]

The Mustarde flap is a large, rotational, skin-muscle cheek flap that, if necessary can, be relied on to cover virtually any lower lid defect[13] (Fig. 94-6). It may be considered a progression in size from the smaller Tenzel semicircular rotational flap. This flap is most useful for vertical, deep, medial, full-thickness lower lid defects. The advantage of this procedure is that it is a one-stage, complete lower lid reconstruction. The disadvantages of this procedure are the excessively long scar on the face and the adynamic nature of the reconstructed lower lid. A graft of either hard palate or ear cartilage is needed for posterior lamellar support.

The authors have used an advancement of suborbital ocularis oculi fascia in lower lid defects that cannot be closed primarily. This myocutaneous advancement flap allows reconstruction of the lower lid posterior and anterior lamellar structures in a vertical direction, by directing cheek tissue superiorly.[14] In conjunction with lifted suborbital ocularis oculi fascia, posterior lamel-lar and anterior lamellar grafts can be used as needed to complete the lower eyelid reconstruction.

UPPER EYELID. When large, upper eyelid defects are reconstructed, the surgeon must appreciate the effects of both horizontal and vertical tension on the final result. Excessive horizontal tension on the upper lid causes tether ptosis, and excessive vertical tension causes lagophthalmos. Care must be taken to avoid these postoperative complications. Multiple surgical modalities exist to address full-thickness tissue loss greater than 60%, all of which share the principles of replacement of both posterior and anterior lamellar structures.

A large, horizontal advancement of an upper eyelid tarsoconjunctival flap is useful for full-thickness defects of up to two

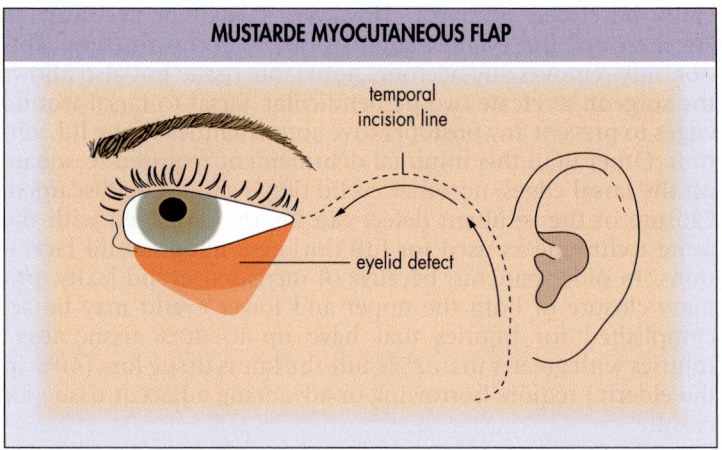

MUSTARDE MYOCUTANEOUS FLAP

temporal incision line

eyelid defect

FIG. 94-6 ■ Repair of large, full-thickness lower eyelid defects with the Mustarde myocutaneous flap.

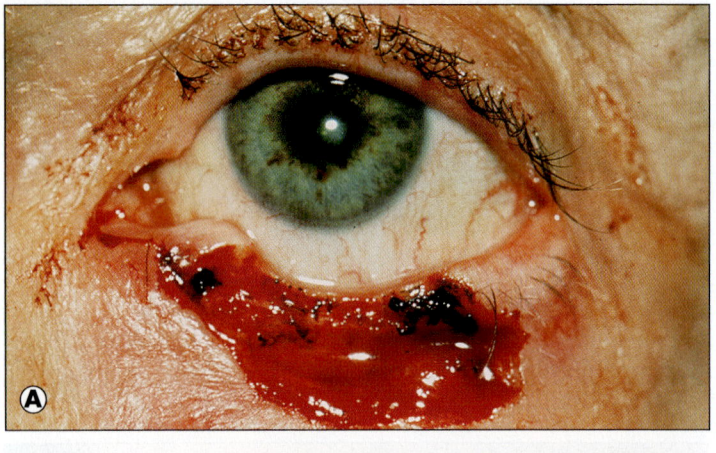

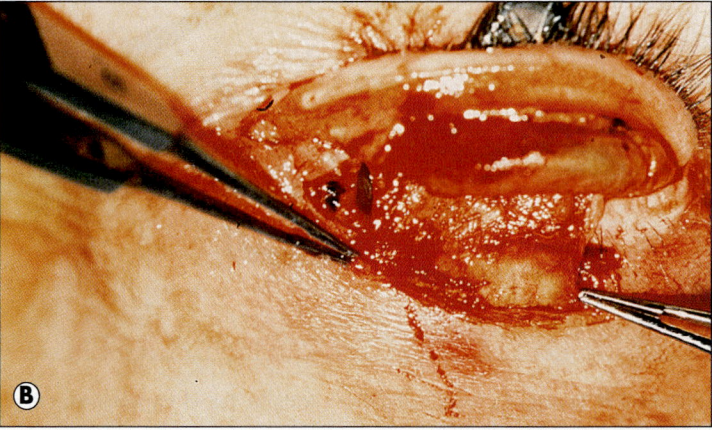

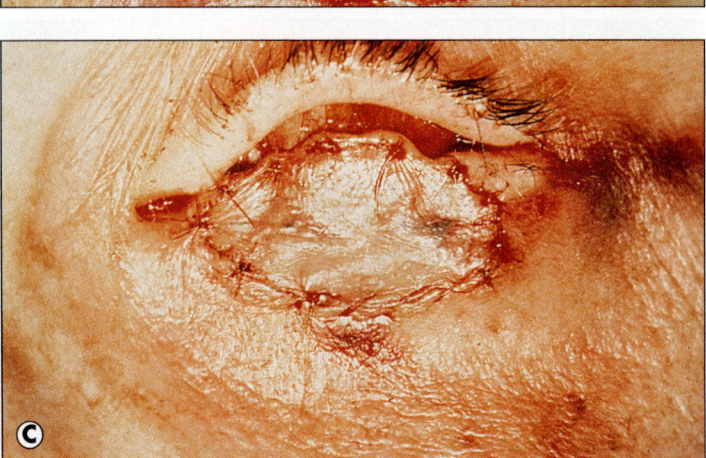

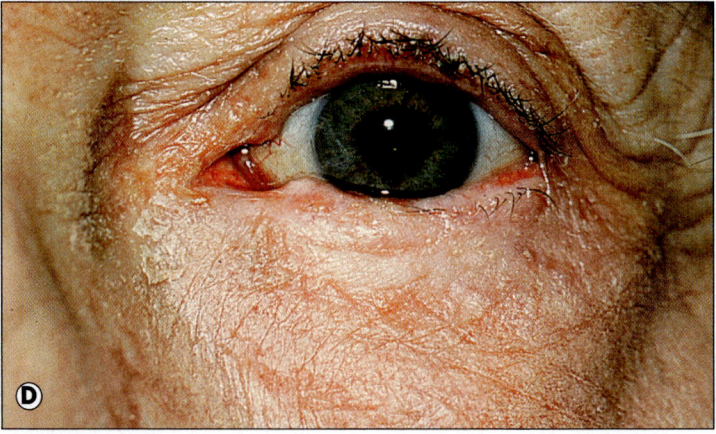

FIG. 94-5 ■ The Hughes tarsoconjunctival flap procedure. **A,** The lower eyelid defect is examined to estimate the width of the flap. **B,** The flap is dissected from the posterior lamella of the upper eyelid. At least 4mm of tarsus must remain along the upper eyelid margin to enable stabilization. **C,** A skin graft can provide adequate anterior lamella of the lower eyelid. **D,** After 4–6 weeks the flap is divided to restore the eyelid margins. (Courtesy of Regents of the University of California, 1997, reprinted with permission.)

thirds the length of the upper lid margin. The anterior lamella can be replaced with a full-thickness skin graft.

A Cutler-Beard bridge flap reconstruction is useful for upper eyelid defects covering up to 100% of the eyelid margin (Fig. 94-7).[15] This technique, a two-stage procedure, takes tissue from the lower eyelid to reconstruct the upper eyelid. First, skin, muscle, and conjunctiva are advanced from the lower eyelid to replace the defect in the upper eyelid; the second stage can usually be performed 3–4 weeks after the initial reconstruction. This procedure does not replace lost eyelashes of the upper eyelid and is also fraught with the need for secondary corrective procedures.

Postoperative Care

For the first 2 days after any reconstructive surgery on the eye, the patient should be instructed to use ice compresses on the wound and to keep the head of the bed elevated. These steps help to reduce postoperative edema. If there is concern that the patient may rub the wound, a Fox shield can be applied. The authors prefer not to bandage the patient's eye unless skin grafts have been used. Antibiotic ointment placed on the wound two to three times a day not only helps to prevent infection but also assists in lubrication of the wound. This helps to débride the wound and prevent the sutures from becoming crusted. The antibiotic ointment also helps to hasten re-epithelialization of portions of the wound that may be left to granulate spontaneously. The authors generally remove skin sutures at 5–7 days and lid margin sutures at 10–14 days.

Patients are instructed to stay out of direct sunlight and to use sun block on the maturing scar for at least 6 months postoperatively. This helps to avoid abnormal pigmentation of the scar. When the cicatricial phase of wound healing commences, at 3–4 weeks, the patient is instructed to massage the wound. It is hoped that this lessens late contracture of the wound, and it prevents cicatricial changes such as ectropion, entropion, or lagophthalmos and the resultant exposure keratopathy.

Late Repair of Eyelid Injuries

It is not uncommon for the patient who has undergone extensive traumatic eyelid repair to require secondary surgery. Skin grafts on the upper eyelid for lagophthalmos and on the lower eyelid for lower eyelid cicatricial ectropion are often necessary in the late postoperative period (Fig. 94-8). To improve the postoperative esthetic result, donor sites for skin grafts should be matched to the area of skin loss. The contralateral upper eyelid,

pre- or postauricular areas, and supraclavicular areas have been used with excellent results for skin grafts on eyelids and the periocular region. When skin grafts are used in either the acute setting of trauma or the late postoperative period, the involved upper or lower eyelid should be kept on stretch using a traction suture (Frost or reverse Frost suture). Alternatively, a vertical scar in the lower eyelid that causes vertical shortening can be corrected with Z-plasty techniques. If the patient has shortening of the posterior lamella in the late postoperative period, hard palate or mucous membrane grafts can be implemented to treat cicatricial entropion.

Dog Bites

Of the 44,000 facial dog bites that present to emergency rooms in the United States each year, orbital and periorbital injuries occur in 4–8% of cases.[16,17] In a recent series in the ophthalmic literature, over half of these bites occurred in children younger than 5 years and two thirds in children younger than 10 years.

It is essential to ascertain information about the dog's health and rabies vaccination status. Immunocompromised patients, those who have undergone prior splenectomy, patients who suffer from chronic obstructive pulmonary disease or alcoholism, and even healthy infants are at particular risk for the development of fulminant septicemia 24–48 hours after the bite. *Pasteurella multocida* is identified in up to 50% of dog bite injury infections[18]; *Pa. multocida* infections commonly occur within 48 hours of inoculation and are characterized by prominent wound inflammation and drainage. The organism is a small gram-negative coccobacillus that grows in both aerobic and anaerobic environments.[18]

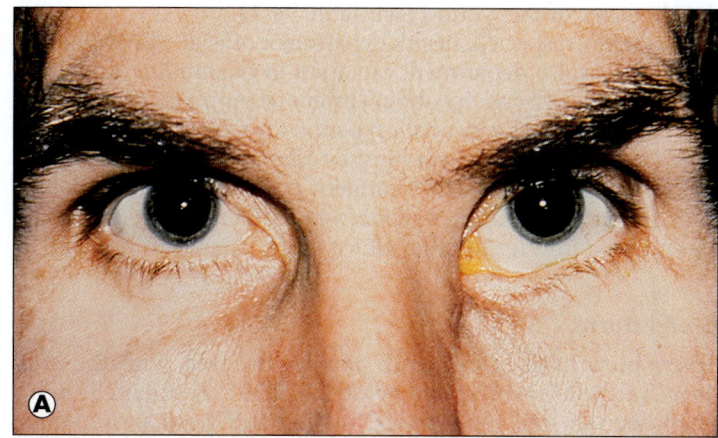

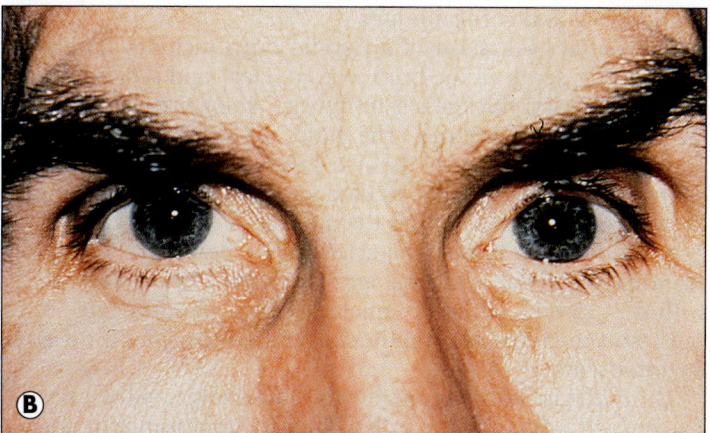

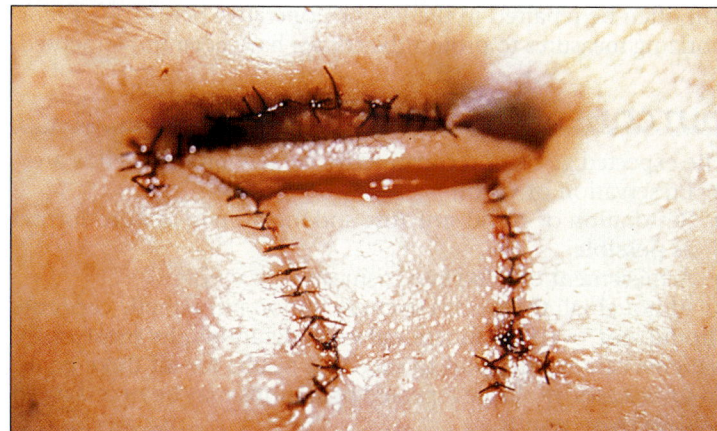

FIG. 94-7 ▮ **The Cutler-Beard bridge flap.** A full-thickness flap of lower eyelid tissue is advanced beneath a marginal bridge into the upper eyelid defect. After 3–4 weeks the flap is cut at the appropriate level and the lower lid is repaired. (Courtesy of Regents of the University of California, 1997, reprinted with permission.)

FIG. 94-8 ▮ **A patient had an obvious cicatricial left medial canthal dystopia as a result of trauma. A,** Primary repair did not address the reconstruction of the critical deep portion of the medial canthal tendon. **B,** The same patient as in A after left medial canthoplasty and anterior lamella reconstruction with a skin graft. It is imperative to reconstruct all elements of the medial canthal complex to achieve satisfactory eyelid apposition to the globe. (Courtesy of Regents of the University of California, 1997, reprinted with permission.)

Septicemia, meningitis, and, in rare cases, death have been reported as a result of infection by a gram-negative, non–spore-forming rod, *Capnocytophaga canimorsus*. The organism was previously referred to as CDC group DF-2 (Centers for Disease Control and Prevention group Dysgonic Fermenter-2) and can be cultured from the mouths of healthy dogs.[18–24]

Gonnering,[25] in a study of periorbital dog bites, found no penetration injuries of the globe and no tissue loss. Disruption of the lacrimal system was present in 14 of the 16 cases. All dog bite wounds are presumed to be contaminated and, therefore, must be decontaminated prior to surgical repair to limit infection. Forceful irrigation with at least 200ml of normal saline using a 35ml syringe and 18-gauge irrigating cannula is recommended, while the cornea is protected with a scleral contact lens.[26]

Surgical repair is carried out as for any other eyelid reconstruction, with restoration of normal anatomic structure and function. Care should be taken to evaluate and repair medial canthal tendon avulsions as well as lacrimal system injuries.

Adjunct medical therapy includes tetanus prophylaxis and rabies prophylaxis if the rabies status of the dog is unknown or positive. The need for prophylactic antibiotics in dog bites is controversial. Adequate wound decontamination is probably the single most important modality that prevents infection. Various studies have isolated many different pathogens as the cause of infections after dog bites. No single antimicrobial agent is optimal against these various pathogens, which may include *Staphylococcus aureus*, *S. epidermidis*, *Pseudomonas aeruginosa*, and anaerobes in addition to *Pa. multocida* and *C. canimorsus*. Recommended choices of antibiotic prophylaxis include penicillin, Augmentin (amoxicillin and clavulanic acid), cefuroxime, and cephalexin.[25] Alternatives for the penicillin-allergic patient include erythromycin and tetracycline. Decisions about tetanus prophylaxis depend on the patient's immunization history and the character of the wound (see Table 94-1).

If rabies is suspected, health department officials should be notified. The health department can assist in quarantine of the animal as well as offer advice about current recommendations for rabies prophylaxis. The incubation period for rabies averages 30–50 days. Prophylactic treatment must be administered before the onset of clinical disease. The treatment consists of inactive rabies virus human diploid cell vaccine, which offers active immunity, and rabies immune globulin, which offers passive immunity.[18]

Eyelid Burns

Severe burn injuries frequently involve the face, with the incidence of eyelid involvement being 20–30%.[27] Fortunately, Bell's phenomenon, the blink reflex, rapid reflex head movements, and shielding of the eyes with arms and hands often prevent conjunctival and corneal injury.

The initial evaluation of an eyelid burn includes an assessment of the depth of the burn wound. First- and second-degree burns are partial-thickness skin injuries, and third-degree burns are full-thickness injuries. The mild swelling, erythema, and pain of first-degree burns (which involve only the epidermis) generally resolve within 5–10 days with no compromise of eyelid function and structure, as the damage is quite superficial.

Second-degree burns, characterized by erythema, bulla formation, considerable edema, and pain, often heal uneventfully within 7–14 days without sequelae. A deep second-degree burn can result in cicatricial eyelid deformities, especially if superinfection occurs.

Third-degree burns represent the most severe burn injuries. The burned lids may have a dark, leathery appearance or appear translucent or waxy white. These burns are not very painful because the terminal nerve endings have been destroyed. A thick black eschar forms and then separates within 2–3 weeks. Granulation tissue then forms and the myofibroblasts produce contracture, with ensuing eyelid retraction, cicatricial ectropion, and lagophthalmos.

Acute treatment of all eyelid burns requires frequent lubrication with artificial tear drops and lubricating ointment at bedtime. If associated corneal and conjunctival injuries exist, appropriate topical antibiotic ointment is used as well. The topical antibiotic is continued until the cornea has re-epithelialized. Topical burn medications are placed on the periorbital skin in coordination with the burn-team care.

In the intermediate phase (1–4 weeks) of eyelid burn healing, first-degree burns generally do not undergo significant cicatricial changes and often heal without sequelae. Second- and third-degree burns are accompanied by cicatrization and shortage of skin surface area. This results in lagophthalmos secondary to lower eyelid ectropion and upper eyelid retraction. Corneal exposure may lead to epithelial compromise, and it may be followed by sterile or infectious corneal ulcers. In this intermediate period, prior to full cicatrization before the wounds are ready for skin grafts, it is best to perform temporizing measures. If heavy ocular lubrication is not sufficient, surgical scar release using Frost suture eyelid closure or non–margin-injuring tarsorrhaphy can be performed.[28]

When burn wounds are healed completely and the cicatricial phase of healing is over, definitive eyelid reconstruction may be undertaken. Usually, full-thickness skin grafts are used for eyelid reconstruction. Optimal donor sites for a full-thickness graft are the non–hair-bearing retroauricular, contralateral eyelid, and supraclavicular skin. In a severely burned patient, any available donor site may be used for full-thickness tissue, and split-thickness skin grafts may be used if necessary.

The technique used for skin grafts in the burn patient is similar for both the upper and lower eyelid. The only exception is that the lower eyelid may require a horizontal eyelid-shortening procedure in addition to the skin graft. The eyelid that is to receive the graft is placed on stretch. In the upper lid, the scar tissue is released with a lid crease incision, and a subciliary incision is employed to release scar tissue in the lower eyelid. After all the scar tissue has been released, the eyelid remains on stretch, and the skin graft is harvested and placed in the recipient bed. The graft is sutured into position with numerous interrupted 6-0 sutures, with one arm of each suture left long. A stent or bolster is placed over the graft, and the sutures are tied over this graft so that they press the graft down onto the host site. A pressure dressing is applied over the bolster with mild pressure, and after 5–6 days the dressing and bolster are removed.[29]

The late phase of eyelid-burn healing may also lead to scar formation (webbing) of the lateral and medial canthi. Skin grafts and Z-plasty techniques can be employed to address this canthal webbing.[30]

In the treatment of the eyelid-burn patient, emphasis is placed on protection of the cornea and conjunctiva. Skin deformities can often be repaired in the late postoperative period, after temporizing measures to protect the cornea have been implemented.

OUTCOMES

The expected goals of reconstructive surgery on the eyelids are:
- Preservation of vision
- Restoration of eyelid structure and function to as near normal as possible
- Achievement of adequate cosmesis

Although all three objectives are important, esthetic concerns should not override functional considerations. In most cases, patients can expect good to excellent results for all three goals. In some cases, multiple repeated operations may be necessary to achieve these results.

REFERENCES

1. Gossman MD, Roberts DM, Barr CC. Ophthalmic aspects of orbital injury: a comprehensive diagnostic and management approach. Clin Plast Surg. 1992;19:71–85.
2. Mustarde JC. Eyelid reconstruction. Orbit. 1983;1:33–43.

3. Walton RL, Matory WE Jr. Wound care. In: Ho MT, Saunders CE, eds. Current emergency diagnosis and treatment, 3rd ed. Norwalk, CT: Appleton & Lange; 1990:756–80.

4. Gossman MD, Berlin AJ. Management of acute adnexal trauma. In: Stewart WB, ed. Surgery of the eyelid, orbit and lacrimal system, Vol 1. San Francisco: American Academy of Ophthalmology; 1993:170–85.

5. Mehta HK. Spontaneous reformation of upper eyelid. Br J Ophthalmol. 1988;72:856–62.

6. Rubin PAD, Shore JW. Penetrating eyelid and orbital trauma. In: Albert DM, Jakobiec FA, eds. Principles and practices of ophthalmology: clinical practice. Philadelphia: WB Saunders; 1994:3426–40.

7. McNab AA, Collin JRO. Eyelid and canthal lacerations. In: Linberg JV, ed. Oculoplastic and orbital emergencies. Norwalk, CT: Appleton & Lange; 1990:1–13.

8. McCord CD Jr. System of repair of full-thickness lid defects. In: McCord CD Jr, Tanenebaum M, Nunery WR, eds. Oculoplastic surgery, 3rd ed. New York: Raven Press; 1995:85–97.

9. Tenzel RR, Stewart WB. Eyelid reconstruction by semi-circular flap technique. Trans Am Soc Ophthalmol Otolaryngol. 1978;85:1164–9.

10. Hughes WL. Reconstruction of the lids. Am J Ophthalmol. 1945;28:1203–11.

11. Hughes WL. Total lower lid reconstruction: technical details. Trans Am Ophthalmol Soc. 1976;74:321–9.

12. Hewes EH, Sullivan JH, Beard C. Lower eyelid reconstruction by tarsal transposition. Am J Ophthalmol. 1976;81:512–14.

13. Mustarde JC. Major reconstruction of the eyelids—functional and aesthetic considerations. Clin Plast Surg. 1988;15:255–62.

14. Shorr N, Goldberg RA, Green JP. The SOOF lift in aesthetic and reconstructive surgery. Presented at the American Society of Ophthalmic Plastic and Reconstructive Surgery Fall Symposium; Chicago; 1996.

15. Cutler NL, Beard C. A method for partial and total upper lid reconstruction. Am J Ophthalmol. 1955;39:1–7.

16. Karlson TA. The incidence of facial injuries from dog bites. JAMA. 1984;251:3265–7.

17. Palmer J, Rees M. Dog bites of the face; a 15 year review. Br J Plast Surg. 1983;36:315–18.

18. Herman DC, Bartley GB, Walker RC. The treatment of animal bite injuries of the eye and ocular adnexa. Ophthal Plast Reconstr Surg. 1987;3(4):237–41.

19. Findling JW, Pohlmanss GP, Rose HD. Fulminant gram-negative bacillemia (DF-2) following a dog bite in an asplenic woman. Am J Med. 1980;68:154–6.

20. Hicklin H, Verghese A, Alvarez S. Dysgonic fermenter 2 septicemia. Rev Infect Dis. 1987;9:884–90.

21. Perez RE. Dysgonic fermenter-2 infections. West J Med. 1988;148:90–2.

22. Dankner WM, Davis CE, Thompson MA. DF-2 bacteremia following a dog bite in a 4 month old child. J Pediatr Infect Dis. 1987;6:695–6.

23. Bailie WE, Stowe EC, Schmitt AM. Aerobic bacterial flora of oral and nasal fluids of canines with reference to bacteria associated with bites. J Clin Microbiol. 1978;7:223–31.

24. Brenner DJ, Hollis DG, Fanning GR, et al. Capnocytophaga canimorsus sp. Nov. (formerly CDC Group DF-2), a cause of septicemia following dog bite, and C. cynodegnmi sp. Nov., a cause of localized wound infection following dog bite. J Clin Microbiol. 1989;27:231–5.

25. Gonnering RS. Ocular adnexal injury and complications in orbital dog bites. Ophthalmic Plast Reconstr Surg. 1987;3:231–5.

26. Stevenson TR, Thacker JG, Rodenheaver GT, et al. Cleansing the traumatic wound by high pressure syringe irrigation. J Am Coll Emerg Physicians. 1976;5:17–21.

27. Glover AT. Eyelid burns. In: Shingleton BJ, Hersh PS, Kenyon KR, eds. Eye trauma. St Louis: Mosby–Year Book; 1991:315–22.

28. Kulwin DR, Kersten RC. Management of eyelid burns. Focal points; clinical modules for ophthalmologists. American Academy of Ophthalmology San Francisco; 1990:8.

29. Hartford CE. Methods of reducing burn scar formation. In: Stark RB, ed. Plastic surgery of the head and neck, Vol 1. New York: Churchill Livingstone; 1987:282–5.

30. Waltman SR, Keates RH, Hoyt CS, et al. Surgery of the eye. New York: Churchill Livingstone; 1988.

SECTION 3 ORBIT AND LACRIMAL GLAND

CHAPTER

95

Orbital Diseases

JONATHAN J. DUTTON

DEFINITION

- The orbit is the bony cavity that contains the eye, eye muscles, lacrimal gland, and neural and vascular structures that serve eye function. Numerous diseases occur in the orbit that can affect visual function.

KEY FEATURES

- A mass lesion of the orbit may cause proptosis or displacement of the eye.
- Orbital lesions may be the presenting sign of systemic diseases, such as metastatic cancer.
- Demographics such as age, sex, and location within the orbit may be helpful in making a specific diagnosis.
- Treatment of orbital lesions may be medical, such as the use of steroids or radiotherapy for inflammatory disease, and does not always require surgery.

TABLE 95-1

FREQUENCY OF ORBITAL LESIONS BY MAJOR DIAGNOSTIC GROUP

Diagnostic Group	Frequency (%)
Thyroid orbitopathy	50
Cystic lesions	10
Inflammatory lesions	11
Vascular neoplasms	4
Vascular, structural	1
Lacrimal gland lesions	2
Lymphoproliferative lesions	5
Secondary tumors	4
Mesenchymal lesions	4
Metastatic tumors	2
Optic nerve tumors	3
Other and unclassified	5

(Data from Dutton JJ, Frazier Byrne S, Proia A. Diagnostic atlas of orbital diseases. Philadelphia: WB Saunders; 2000:1–5.)

INTRODUCTION

During the past few decades, advances in diagnostic instrumentation and surgical technique have helped elevate the orbit to an anatomical area of great clinical interest. Computed tomography, magnetic resonance imaging (MRI), and orbital echography have dramatically improved diagnostic accuracy and allow more careful therapeutic planning. Orbital surgery has become safer and more precise, and treatment results are significantly enhanced. The operating microscope, specialized orbital instruments, fiberoptic illumination, endoscopy, and hypotensive anesthesia have allowed orbital surgeons to perform complex, deep dissections more easily and with fewer complications.

CLINICAL EVALUATION

The initial step in the evaluation of orbital disease is a complete ophthalmic examination.[1] A careful medical and ophthalmic history, including time course of the disease, past trauma, ocular surgery, and systemic illnesses, must be obtained. A complete clinical examination includes assessment of visual acuity and visual fields, anterior and posterior segment evaluation, and external and periorbital inspection. The use of modern imaging techniques is almost always indicated—the choice depends on the disease processes suspected.

In this chapter, the most common orbital lesions are categorized by diagnostic criteria, to enable the reader to evaluate patients more easily and establish a meaningful differential diagnosis (Tables 95-1–95-3).[1,2] In addition, the key points and diagnostic criteria for each lesion are given.

METASTATIC TUMORS

Metastatic tumors represent 2–3% of all orbital tumors. In 30–60% of patients, orbital metastases develop before the diagnosis of the primary tumor (Table 95-4). Metastases reach the orbit via hematogenous spread and occur less commonly than do uveal metastases. In adults, most metastases are carcinomas. In children, metastases are more likely to be sarcomas and embryonal tumors of neural origin. Only 4% of orbital metastases are bilateral. Clinical symptoms include proptosis, axial displacement of the globe, ptosis, diplopia, pain, and chemosis.

Metastatic Carcinoma

KEY POINTS. The most common primary sites of metastatic carcinoma to the orbit are the breast, lung, prostate, gastrointestinal tract, and kidney.[3-5] Key features are:

- For breast carcinoma, the interval from primary diagnosis to orbital metastasis is 3–5 years.
- In scirrhous cell breast carcinoma and gastric carcinoma, enophthalmos may result from orbital fibrosis.
- Metastatic lung cancer is seen most commonly in smoking males aged 45–60 years.
- Prostatic metastases occur most common in elderly men, and pain is more common because of bony involvement.

Metastases are characterized by a rapid onset of orbital symptoms, which include exophthalmos and globe displacement.

TABLE 95-2

AGE DISTRIBUTION OF COMMON ORBITAL DISEASES

Diagnostic Group	Frequency (%)		
	Childhood and Adolescence (0–20 years)	Middle Age (21–60 years)	Later Adult Life (61+ years)
Adenoid cystic carcinoma of lacrimal gland	18	73	9
Capillary hemangioma	100	0	0
Cavernous hemangioma	10	75	15
Cystic lesions	77	3	4
Fibrous histiocytoma	25	50	25
Infectious processes	35	3	3
Inflammatory lesions	12	5	9
Lymphangiomas	6	1	0
Lymphoproliferative diseases	1	3	12
Optic nerve glioma	5	1	1
Optic nerve meningioma	4	88	8
Pleomorphic adenoma of lacrimal gland	0	89	11
Rhabdomyosarcoma	98	2	0
Secondary and metastatic malignancies	1	2	9
Thyroid orbitopathy	4	59	40
Trauma	7	4	2

(Modified from Dutton JJ, Frazier Byrne S, Proia A. Diagnostic atlas of orbital diseases. Philadelphia: WB Saunders; 2000:1–5.)
Data rounded to the nearest percentage point.

TABLE 95-3

TEMPORAL ONSET OF COMMON ORBITAL DISEASES

Hours	Days	Weeks	Months	Years
Traumatic	Inflammatory	Inflammatory	Neoplastic	Neoplastic
Hemorrhagic	Infectious	Neoplastic	Lymphoid	Degenerative
Infectious	Traumatic	Traumatic	Vascular	Lymphoid
	Hemorrhagic	Lymphoid	Inflammatory	Vascular
	Vascular	Vascular	Degenerative	Inflammatory

(Modified from Dutton JJ, Frazier Byrne S, Proia A. Diagnostic atlas of orbital diseases. Philadelphia: WB Saunders; 2000:1–5.)

TABLE 95-4

PRIMARY ORIGINS OF METASTATIC TUMORS OF THE ORBIT

Origin	Percent
Breast	53
Prostate	11
Gastrointestinal	11
Lung	4
Sarcomas and other	21

(Modified from Dutton JJ, Frazier Byrne S, Proia A. Diagnostic atlas of orbital diseases. Philadelphia: WB Saunders; 2000:1–5.)

ORBITAL IMAGING. Metastatic carcinomas usually are poorly defined, nonencapsulated, diffuse masses that are somewhat infiltrative. Extraocular muscles often are involved. Osteoblastic changes may be seen with prostatic carcinoma. On MRI, the T1-weighted image is usually isointense and the T2-weighted image hyperintense to muscle.

BOX 95-1

Causes of Abaxial Globe Displacement

DOWNWARD DISPLACEMENT
Fibrous dysplasia
Frontal mucocele
Lymphoma
Neuroblastoma
Neurofibroma
Schwannoma
Subperiosteal hematoma
Thyroid orbitopathy

UPWARD DISPLACEMENT
Lacrimal sac tumors
Lymphoma
Maxillary sinus tumor
Metastatic tumors

LATERAL DISPLACEMENT
Ethmoid mucocele
Lacrimal sac tumors
Lethal midline granuloma
Metastatic tumors
Nasopharyngeal tumors
Rhabdomyosarcoma

MEDIAL DISPLACEMENT
Lacrimal fossa tumors
Sphenoid wing meningioma

The direction of ocular displacement may be helpful in narrowing the differential diagnosis.

ECHOGRAPHY. A metastatic carcinoma has an irregular shape with a surface that can be poorly to well defined. The carcinoma often is diffuse, with a medium to high internal reflectivity, but low reflectivity is seen with small cell carcinoma of the lung. Vascularity is minimal to absent.

TREATMENT AND PROGNOSIS. Treatment requires chemotherapy combined with local radiotherapy. Orchiectomy may be indicated for prostate carcinoma, and hormonal therapy for breast carcinoma.

Orbital metastases from carcinoma reflect more widespread systemic disease, so the prognosis for survival is generally poor.

LACRIMAL GLAND LESIONS

Lesions of the lacrimal gland include infiltrative processes (such as inflammatory diseases and lymphoma), structural disorders (such as cysts), and epithelial neoplasms.[6–10] Epithelial tumors represent 20–25% of all lacrimal gland lesions. The appropriate management of lacrimal fossa lesions requires a thorough evaluation and determination of the cause. Almost all lacrimal gland lesions result in a mass effect, with swelling of the lateral eyelid and often with a downward and medial displacement of the globe (Box 95-1). Inflammatory processes are more commonly associated with pain, eyelid edema, and conjunctival chemosis and injection.

Pleomorphic Adenoma (Benign Mixed Cell Tumor)

KEY POINTS. Pleomorphic adenomas occur mainly in the orbital lobe and rarely in the palpebral lobe of the lacrimal gland.[11–16] They are composed of epithelial and mesenchymal elements (thus the term benign "mixed" cell tumor), but both elements are derived from epithelium. Key features are:
- They represent 3–5% of all orbital tumors, 25% of lacrimal mass lesions, and 50% of epithelial lacrimal gland tumors.
- Most commonly they occur in the second to fifth decades of life (mean age, 39 years).
- The male-female ratio is 1.5:1.

Orbital symptoms are painless exophthalmos, axial downward displacement of the globe, diplopia, retinal striae, fullness

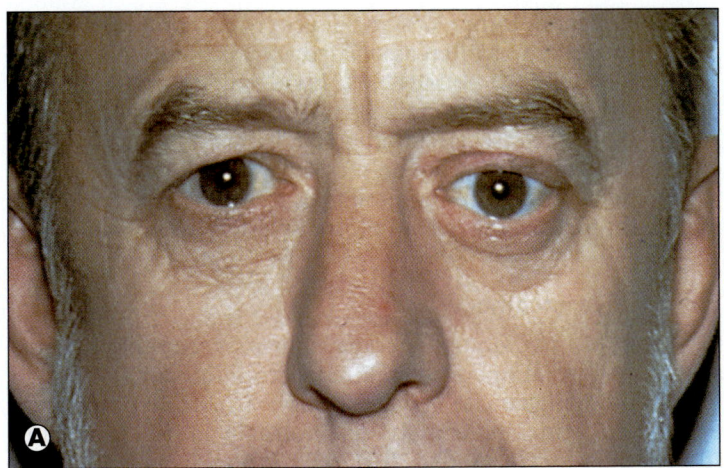

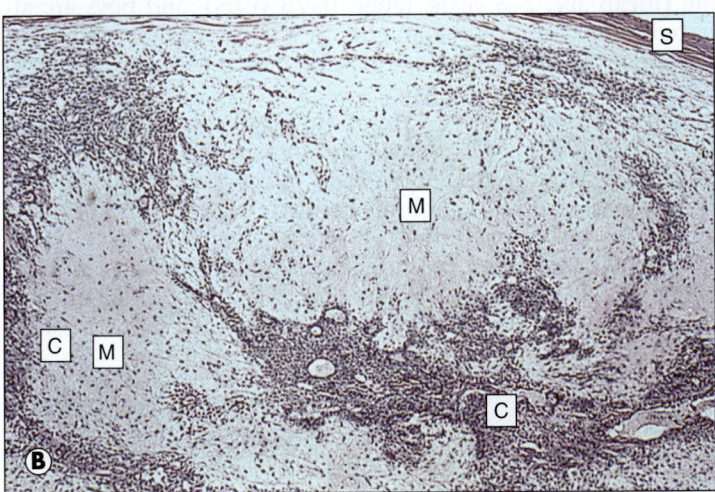

FIG. 95-1 ■ **Benign mixed tumor. A,** The patient had proptosis of the left eye for quite some time. It had gradually increased in severity. **B,** The characteristic diphasic pattern is shown. It consists of a pale background that has a myxomatous stroma and a relatively amorphous appearance, contiguous with quite cellular areas that contain mainly epithelial cells. *C,* Cellular epithelial areas; *M,* myxomatous stroma; *S,* surface of tumor. (From Yanoff M, Fine BS. Ocular pathology, ed 5. St. Louis: Mosby, 2002.)

of the upper eyelid, and a palpable eyelid mass. These tumors are slowly progressive over 12 or more months.

ORBITAL IMAGING. Well-circumscribed, round to oval, encapsulated lesions are typical. Remolding of the bone may be seen with long-standing tumors, but no bone destruction occurs. The tumors may be cystic and may contain areas of calcification. On MRI the T1-weighted image is hypointense and the T2-weighted image hyperintense to muscle.

ECHOGRAPHY. Round to oval shapes with well-defined surface spikes are seen, with medium to high reflectivity, a regular acoustic structure, and moderate sound attenuation. Cystic cavities may occur.

PATHOLOGY. Pleomorphic adenomas are encapsulated tumors that demonstrate ducts, cords, and squamous pearls, with myxoid and chondroid tissue (Fig. 95-1).

TREATMENT AND PROGNOSIS. These adenomas must be excised completely with an intact capsule; biopsy may result in recurrence associated with infiltration. Malignant degeneration occurs at a rate of 10% in 10 years.

The prognosis is generally very good, despite the possibility of malignant transformation.

Adenoid Cystic Carcinoma

KEY POINTS. Adenoid cystic carcinoma accounts for 23% of all epithelial tumors of the lacrimal gland and is the most common epithelial malignancy of the lacrimal gland (Table 95-5).[17] Key features are:

- It occurs most commonly in the fourth decade of life but may be seen at any age.

TABLE 95-5

FREQUENCY OF LACRIMAL FOSSA LESIONS

Lesion	Frequency (%)
Dacryoadenitis	51
Pleomorphic adenoma	18
Reactive lymphoid hyperplasia	9
Adenoid cystic carcinoma	7
Dacryops (epithelial cyst)	5
Lymphoma	4
Mucoepidermoid carcinoma	3
Pleomorphic adenocarcinoma	2
Plasmacytoid lesions	1

(Modified from Rootman JL. Diseases of the orbit. A multidisciplinary approach. Philadelphia: JB Lippincott; 1988:119–39; and Shields JA, ed. Diagnosis and management of orbital tumors. Philadelphia: WB Saunders; 1989:291–315.)

- It is slightly more common in women.
- The duration of symptoms is generally short—often less than 6 months, and usually less than 12 months.

Orbital symptoms include exophthalmos, downward globe displacement, ptosis, and diplopia. Orbital pain as a result of perineural spread of tumor is common, seen in 10–40% of cases.

ORBITAL IMAGING. Computed tomography and MRI usually show a poorly demarcated, irregular lesion that may extend along the lateral wall to the orbital apex. Bone destruction is common, and foci of calcification are seen frequently. On MRI the T1- and T2-weighted images are hyperintense to muscle, and the signal is heterogeneous.

ECHOGRAPHY. Adenoid cystic carcinoma usually appears as a diffuse, infiltrative lesion with indistinct borders (although it may be well defined), with medium to high internal reflectivity and an irregular internal structure. Sound attenuation is moderate to strong.

PATHOLOGY. Solid cords of malignant epithelial cells are seen, with cystic spaces ("Swiss cheese" appearance) or hyalinization of cylinders of connective tissue (Fig. 95-2).

TREATMENT AND PROGNOSIS. Treatment consists of radical *en bloc* excision or exenteration, with wide margins including bone. Adjunctive radiotherapy for incompletely excised lesions may be necessary. The prognosis is dismal, with relentless recurrences. The mortality rate is high.

MESENCHYMAL TUMORS

Nonosseous mesenchymal tumors arise from fibroblasts, myoblasts, and lipoblasts. Classification of such lesions is difficult, as their features overlap, so the terminology is confusing. Together, these orbital lesions form an important group that accounts for about 8% of all orbital lesions.[18-31]

Fibrous Histiocytoma

KEY POINTS. Fibrous histiocytoma is a benign or malignant mesenchymal tumor that arises from fascia, muscle, or other soft tissues.[32,33] In children, it may result from early orbital radiotherapy. In adults, it is the most common mesenchymal orbital tumor, usually seen in middle-aged patients (40–60 years).

The upper nasal quadrant is the most common orbital site. Symptoms are exophthalmos, decreased vision, diplopia, ptosis, motility restriction, and epiphora. The lesions may be circumscribed or infiltrative and can be locally aggressive.

ORBITAL IMAGING. Usually a well-defined, rounded mass is seen, as in other benign lesions, but the tumor may be more infiltrative. On MRI the signal is heterogeneous, with isointense T1 and variable T2 signals with respect to muscle. Enhancement with gadolinium is moderate.

ECHOGRAPHY. The lesion is well outlined, with a regular internal structure of low to medium reflectivity and moderate sound attenuation. Vascularity is variable.

PATHOLOGY. The tumor is a mixture of spindle-shaped fibroblasts and histiocytes arranged in a storiform pattern, twisted about a central focus (Fig. 95-3). The benign form (63% incidence) is a well-circumscribed, slow-growing lesion with a fine capsule. A small potential exists for malignant degeneration.

The malignant form (37% incidence) is more infiltrative and rapidly growing; it is often associated with pain and necrosis.

TREATMENT AND PROGNOSIS. Local surgical excision or orbital exenteration is required, with recurrences being common (in up to 30% of cases). Radiotherapy offers no benefit, and the effects of chemotherapy are unknown.

For the benign form, the prognosis for life is excellent. With malignant tumors, the overall mortality rate is more than 40%.

Rhabdomyosarcoma

KEY POINTS. Rhabdomyosarcoma is the most common soft tissue mesenchymal tumor in children, accounting for 3.4% of all childhood malignancies.[34–37] The tumors arise from pluripotential mesenchymal precursors that normally differentiate into striated muscle cells. About 70% occur during the first decade of life (mean age, 7–8 years; range, 0–78 years), and boys are affected more commonly than girls, at a ratio of 5:3. In the orbit, the most common histological variant is the embryonal type, followed by the alveolar type.

Symptoms may be acute to subacute, with rapidly progressive exophthalmos, eyelid edema, and ptosis. This rapidity may cause diagnostic confusion with an infectious process. The tumor is located in the retrobulbar muscle cone in 50% of cases, and in the superior orbit in 25% of cases.

ORBITAL IMAGING. Typically, the tumor presents as an irregular but well-defined soft tissue mass (Fig. 95-4). Bony erosion may be seen but is uncommon. On MRI the T1 signal is isoin-

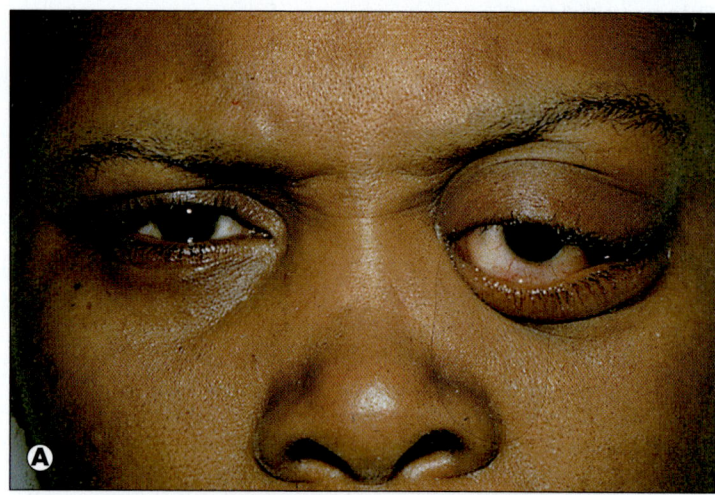

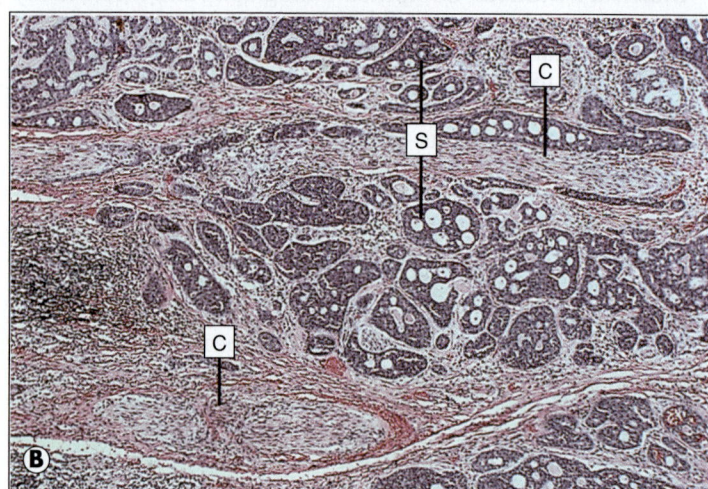

FIG. 95-2 ▪ **Adenoid cystic carcinoma. A,** The patient had a rapidly progressing proptosis of the left eye. **B,** The characteristic "Swiss cheese" pattern (*S*) of adenoid cystic carcinoma is shown. The "Swiss cheese" tumor is also present in the perineural sheath around the ciliary nerve (*C*). Adenoid cystic carcinoma is noted for its rapid invasion of ciliary nerves. (From Yanoff M, Fine BS. Ocular pathology, ed 5. St. Louis: Mosby, 2002.)

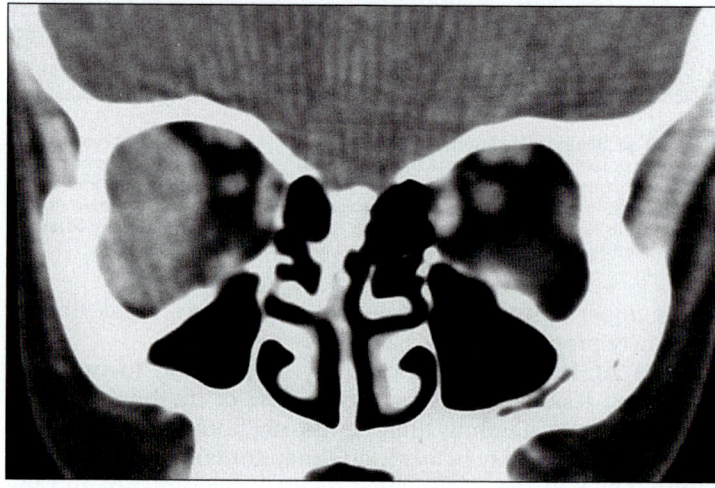

FIG. 95-4 ▪ Rhabdomyosarcoma of the lateral orbital wall in a 7-year-old girl.

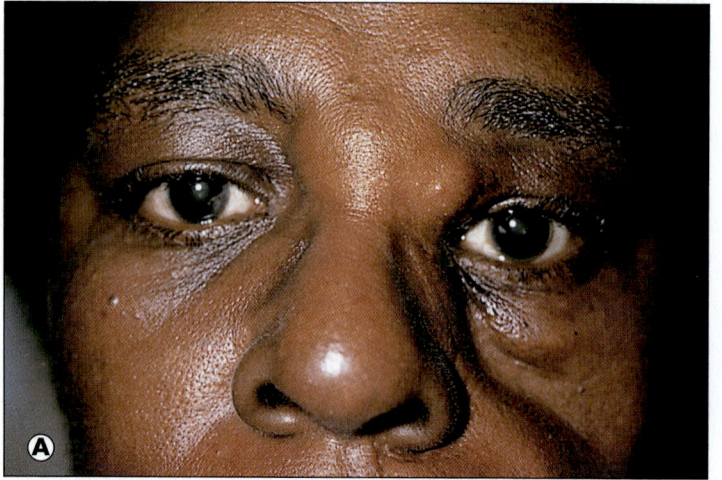

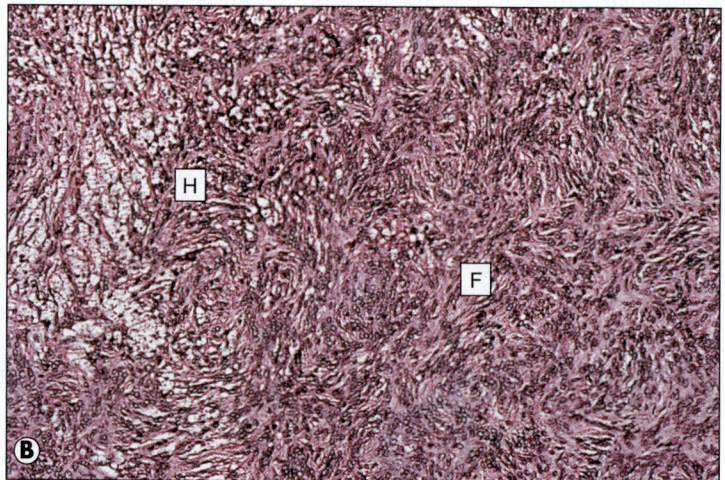

FIG. 95-3 ▪ **Fibrous histiocytoma. A,** This is the fourth recurrence of an orbital tumor that was first excised 10 years previously. The histology of the primary lesion and of the four recurrences appear identical. **B,** A histological section shows the diphasic pattern consisting of a histiocytic component (*H*), mainly on the far left, and a fibrous component (*F*). (Case reported by Jones WD III, Yanoff M, Katowitz JA. Recurrent facial fibrous histiocytoma. Br J Plast Surg. 1979; 32:46–51.)

tense to hyperintense, and the T2 signal is hyperintense with respect to muscle.

ECHOCARDIOGRAPHY. The lesion has variable borders (but they are usually well circumscribed; occasionally there are bony defects), low to medium reflectivity, moderate sound attenuation, and a somewhat irregular structure. Vascularity is variable.

PATHOLOGY. Cross-striations may be seen in 50–60% of embryonal-type tumors and in 30% of the alveolar type (Fig. 95-5). Myoglobulin is a specific immunohistochemical marker. Electron microscopy shows actin myofilaments and myosin filaments.

DIFFERENTIAL DIAGNOSIS. The differential diagnosis includes inflammatory processes, orbital cellulitis, metastatic neuroblastoma, chloroma, lymphangioma, and ruptured dermoid cyst.

STAGING. There are four stages:
I. Localized tumor, completely resected
II. Regional spread, positive nodes, grossly resected
III. Gross residual tumor remaining after incomplete resection
IV. Distant metastases

TREATMENT AND DIAGNOSIS. An immediate biopsy is required to confirm the diagnosis. Surgical excision is carried out only if the lesion is well circumscribed. The excision can be performed easily without excessive tissue damage. Local radiotherapy doses are 4000cGy for stage II and 5000cGy for stages III and IV. Adjuvant chemotherapy is given, using vincristine, actinomycin D, and cyclophosphamide. (Some centers prefer only surgery and chemotherapy, to avoid the potential for radiation-induced orbital malignancies in children.)

The 5-year survival rate is 95%; there is a more favorable prognosis for orbital tumors because of the near absence of orbital lymphatics. For local treatment failures, orbital exenteration may be necessary.

NEUROGENIC TUMORS

Peripheral nerves in the orbit are subject to tumors that arise from various cellular components such as Schwann cells, axons, endoneural fibroblasts, and nerve sheaths (Table 95-6). In contrast, the optic nerve, which represents a white-matter tract of the central nervous system (CNS), may give rise to CNS tumors such as astrocytomas and meningiomas.

Plexiform Neurofibroma

KEY POINTS. Plexiform neurofibroma is the most common benign peripheral nerve tumor in the eyelid and orbit and is considered characteristic of neurofibromatosis type 1.[38–41] The tumor grows along the nerve, is invasive, and is not encapsulated. Key features are:
- A propensity for sensory nerves, but also may involve motor, parasympathetic, and sympathetic nerves.
- Children in the first decade of life are affected most commonly.
- 31% of plexiform neurofibromas occur in the eyelids.

Clinically, this tumor has been described as a palpable "bag of worms," with thickened overlying skin and an S-shaped eyelid (Fig. 95-6).

It may be associated with uveal neurofibromas (50%), iris (Lisch) nodules (77%), prominent corneal nerves (25%), optic nerve gliomas (15%), and pulsatile proptosis from an absence of the greater sphenoid wing.

ORBITAL IMAGING. A diffuse, irregular mass is seen with variable contrast enhancement. It may involve extraocular muscles, orbital fat, and the cavernous sinus. On MRI the T1 is hypointense and the T2 hyperintense to muscle.

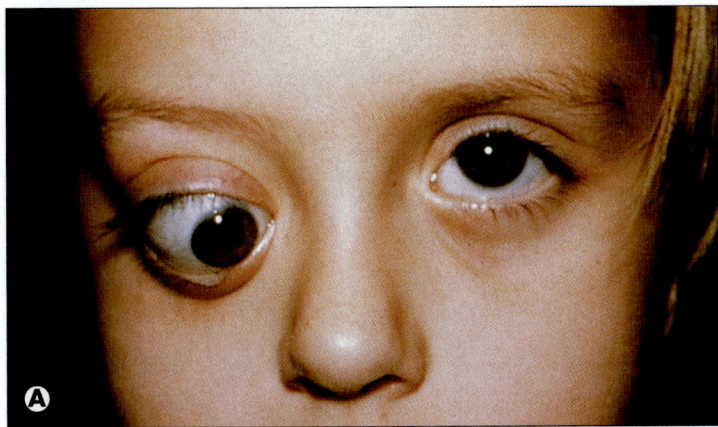

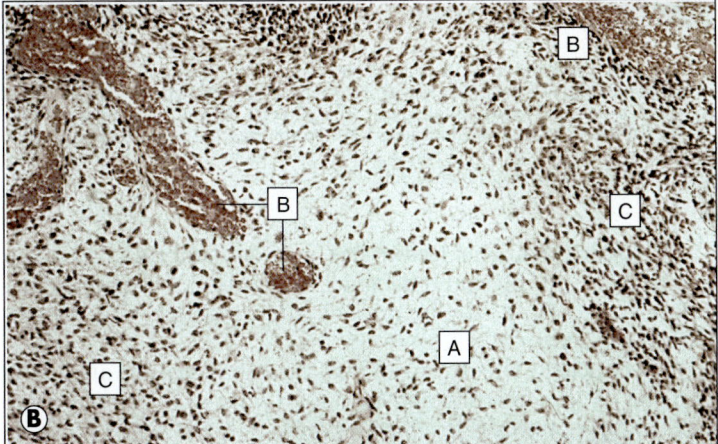

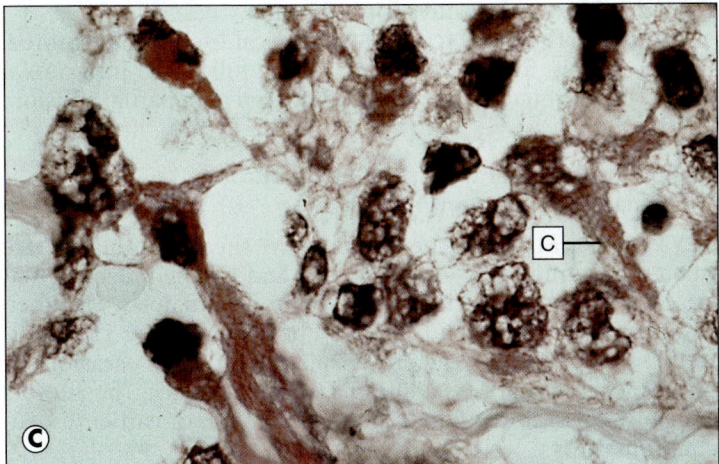

FIG. 95-5 ▮ Embryonal rhabdomyosarcoma. A, The patient has a unilateral right ocular proptosis of very recent onset. Often, rhabdomyosarcoma presents rapidly, causes lid redness, and is mistaken for orbital inflammation. **B,** A marked embryonic cellular pattern is shown, hence the term *embryonal rhabdomyosarcoma* (*A,* relatively acellular area; *B,* blood vessels; *C,* relatively cellular area). **C,** A trichrome stain shows characteristic cross-striations in the cytoplasm of some of the rhabdomyoblasts. Cross-striations (*C*), although not abundant in embryonal rhabdomyosarcoma, can be seen in sections stained with hematoxylin and eosin but are easier to see with special stains. (**A–C,** From Yanoff M, Fine BS. Ocular pathology, ed 5. St. Louis: Mosby, 2002.)

TABLE 95-6

FREQUENCY OF THE MOST COMMON NEUROGENIC ORBITAL LESIONS

Lesion	Frequency (%)
Sphenoid wing meningioma	30
Optic nerve glioma	22
Neurofibroma	19
Schwannoma	14
Optic sheath meningioma	11
Other	4

(Data from Rootman JL. Diseases of the orbit. A multidisciplinary approach. Philadelphia: JB Lippincott; 1988:119–39; Shields JA, ed. Diagnosis and management of orbital tumors. Philadelphia: WB Saunders; 1989:291–315; and the author's personal data.)

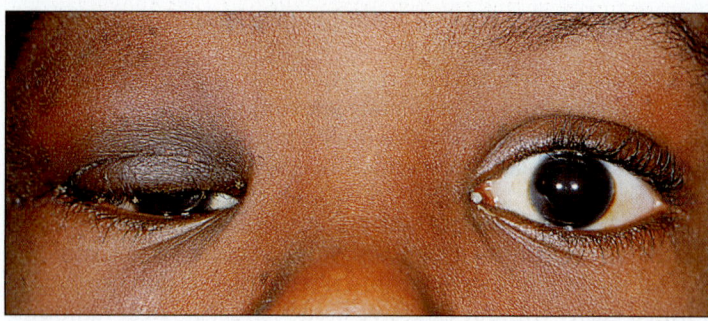

FIG. 95-6 ■ Plexiform neurofibroma of the right eyelid in a child with neurofibromatosis.

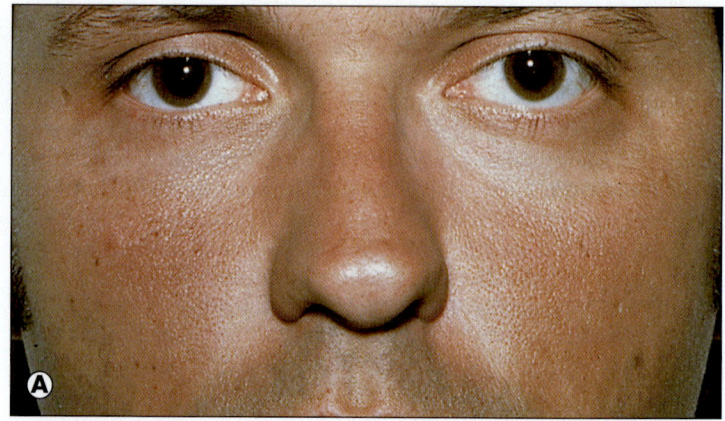

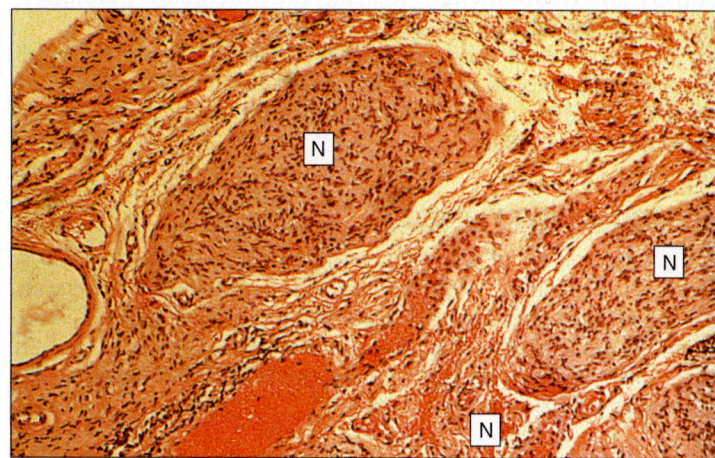

FIG. 95-7 ■ Plexiform neurofibroma. Diffuse proliferation of Schwann cells within the nerve sheath enlarges the nerve. *N,* Thickened abnormal nerves. (From Yanoff M, Fine BS. Ocular pathology, ed 5. St. Louis: Mosby, 2002.)

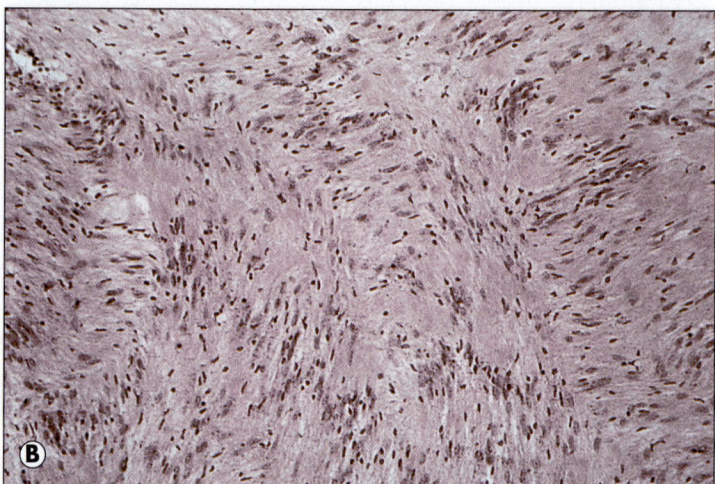

FIG. 95-8 ■ Neurilemmoma. **A,** Proptosis of the patient's left eye had been present for many months and was increasing in size. An orbital tumor was removed. **B,** Ribbons of spindle Schwann cell nuclei can be seen. This shows a tendency toward palisading. Areas of relative acellularity, mimicking tactile corpuscles, are called Verocay bodies. This pattern is called the Antoni type A pattern. (**A-B,** From Yanoff M, Fine BS. Ocular pathology, ed 5. St. Louis: Mosby, 2002.)

ECHOCARDIOGRAPHY. The lesion has a poorly outlined, irregular contour, with high internal reflectivity, minimal attenuation, and an irregular internal structure.

PATHOLOGY. Interwoven bundles of axons, Schwann cells, and endoneural fibroblasts are seen in a mucoid matrix (Fig. 95-7). A characteristic cellular perineural sheath defines the tumor cords. Immunohistochemistry is positive for S100 stain.

TREATMENT AND PROGNOSIS. Surgical excision is generally difficult and frustrating, with excessive bleeding and a poor cosmetic result. Repeated debulking may be necessary for severe symptoms, and orbital exenteration for extensive cases. Radiotherapy offers no benefit.

There is a small risk of malignant transformation. These tumors may occasionally erode into the anterior cranial fossa, which results in death.

Schwannoma (Neurilemmoma)

KEY POINTS. Schwannoma is a Schwann cell tumor that arises as an outpouching from peripheral or cranial nerves (e.g., acoustic neuroma); it has a neural crest origin.[42,43] Schwannomas represent 1% of all orbital tumors and 35% of peripheral nerve tumors; they are mostly benign but rarely may undergo malignant transformation in patients with neurofibromatosis.

Schwannoma is seen most commonly in young adults to middle-aged individuals (20–50 years). It presents as a slow-growing, painless, well-defined solitary mass, usually in the superior orbit, and is frequently cystic. Orbital symptoms may include exophthalmos, diplopia, and visual loss from optic nerve compression.

ORBITAL IMAGING. The tumor is typically an extraconal, fusiform, well-defined, sometimes cystic mass that is aligned anteroposteriorly along the involved nerve. On MRI the signal is homogeneous to heterogeneous; T1 is hypointense and T2 isointense to muscle.

ECHOGRAPHY. The lesion has well-defined surface spikes, low to medium internal reflectivity, and a regular acoustic structure. Cystic cavities may be present, and moderate sound attenuation may occur.

PATHOLOGY. The encapsulated mass has yellow areas and patterns of cells described as Antoni A (whorls) or Antoni B (no palisading) patterns (Fig. 95-8). Spindle cells are seen with vesiculated nuclei in a palisading configuration. The cells are negative for alcian blue and positive for S100 stain.

TREATMENT AND PROGNOSIS. Surgical excision is required. The prognosis for life is good, except following intracranial spread. Late orbital recurrences may be seen after partial excision.

Malignant Peripheral Nerve Sheath Tumor (Malignant Schwannoma)

KEY POINTS. Malignant peripheral nerve sheath tumors are rare malignant tumors of Schwann cells and perineural cells that arise *de novo* or in association with neurofibromatosis.[44,45] When associated with neurofibromatosis, the onset is slow, characterized by exophthalmos, globe displacement, and occasionally pain, ptosis, visual loss, diplopia, and chemosis. The tumors generally occur in patients 20–50 years of age, or earlier in neurofibromatosis.

The clinical course is characterized by relentless invasion along tissue planes to the middle cranial fossa. Metastases to the lungs are common.

ORBITAL IMAGING. A poorly defined, irregular mass is seen. Bone destruction may occur when the lesion is large.

ECHOGRAPHY. The lesion appears as an irregular mass with low internal reflectivity.

PATHOLOGY. The tumor has plexiform, swollen nerve bundles and spindle-shaped cells in whorls of interlacing fascicles.

TREATMENT AND PROGNOSIS. Wide surgical resection is required. Ancillary chemotherapy and radiotherapy may be palliative only. Prognosis is very poor, with death from metastases or intracranial spread.

Neuroblastoma

KEY POINTS. Neuroblastoma is an undifferentiated malignant tumor of primitive neuroblasts, which may be metastatic to the orbit.[46,47] It represents the second most common orbital tumor in children, after rhabdomyosarcoma. It arises from the sympathetic system and ganglia and represents the peripheral nervous system counterpart of retinoblastoma. Rarely, neuroblastomas may represent primary lesions in the orbit, where they may arise from the ciliary ganglion. Key features are:

- 60% of the primary tumors occur in the abdomen.
- 10–40% of systemic neuroblastomas result in orbital metastases, on average 3 months after diagnosis.
- 90% of orbital lesions originate from the abdomen.
- Only 8% of cases first present with an orbital lesion; in 92% of cases the presence of an extraorbital primary tumor is already known.
- 40% of orbital lesions are bilateral.
- The mean age at presentation is 2 years old.
- 75% of cases occur before the age of 4 years.

Symptoms include rapid progression of exophthalmos over several weeks, lid ecchymosis from necrosis and hemorrhage, eyelid edema, ptosis, Horner's syndrome (from mediastinal tumors), papilledema, retinal striae, and decreased vision. Systemic symptoms may involve fever, weakness, and an abdominal or thoracic mass.

ORBITAL IMAGING. An irregular, poorly circumscribed mass is seen, frequently associated with bone destruction and separation of sutures, especially at the zygoma. Metastases to the skull bones occur in 74% of cases.

PATHOLOGY. The lesion is a soft, friable, bluish mass; small round cells that resemble lymphocytes with specks of calcium and areas of necrosis are seen. Electron microscopy reveals neurosecretory tubules.

TREATMENT AND PROGNOSIS. If no systemic primary disease exists, the orbital tumor can be excised. With systemic primary disease, chemotherapy yields resolution in 60–70% of cases in 4–6 months. Radiotherapy (1500cGy in children and 4000cGy in patients older than 10 years old) may be used for local orbital disease.

Recurrences may be seen in 90% of cases over 1–2 years, and a 50–60% mortality rate occurs after 2 years. Bony and orbital metastases are associated with a poorer prognosis.

Optic Nerve Glioma (Pilocytic Astrocytoma of Childhood)

KEY POINTS. Optic nerve glioma is a neoplasm of astrocytes[48] that affects primarily children (mean age, 8 years). No sex predilection exists. The optic nerve alone is affected in 28% of cases; 72% involve the optic chiasm, and of these, 43% involve the chiasm and midbrain. In neurofibromatosis, the lesion may be bilateral. In 29% there is an association with type 1 neurofibromatosis.

Symptoms include slow loss of vision, optic atrophy or edema, and exophthalmos. After an initial decrease, vision remains stable in 80% of patients. Hypothalamic signs may be seen in 22% of cases. Rapid enlargement of the lesion occurs from mucoid degeneration and arachnoid hyperplasia.

ORBITAL IMAGING. Typically, the lesion appears as an intraconal, fusiform enlargement of the optic nerve, with or without a chiasmal mass. The nerve may appear kinked with cystic spaces. On MRI the T1 signal is hypotense to isointense, and the T2 signal shows variable intensity compared to muscle (Fig. 95-9). Enhancement with gadolinium is variable.

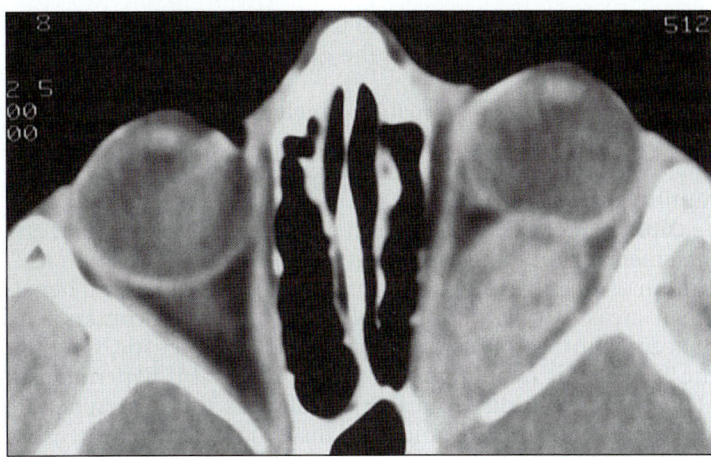

FIG. 95-9 ▌▌ Optic nerve glioma in a child with neurofibromatosis type 1.

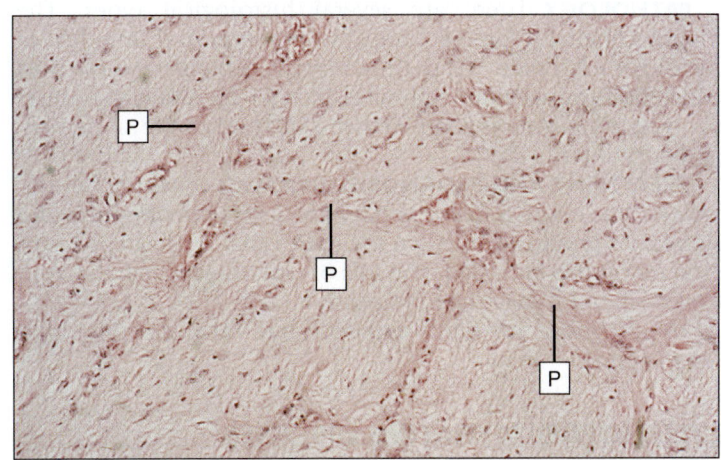

FIG. 95-10 ▌▌ Optic nerve "glioma." Well-differentiated astrocytes spread out the pial septa *(P)*. (From Yanoff M, Fine BS. Ocular pathology, ed 5. St. Louis: Mosby, 2002.)

ECHOGRAPHY. Echography demonstrates a smooth, fusiform enlargement of the optic nerve with low to medium and regular internal reflectivity. The 30° test for increased subarachnoid fluid is usually negative.

PATHOLOGY. Juvenile pilocytic astrocytomas demonstrate cystic spaces that contain a mucoid material and pial septae that are separated by well-differentiated astrocytes (Fig. 95-10). Eosinophilic Rosenthal fibers may represent degenerated astrocytic processes. Immunohistochemistry is positive for neuron-specific enolase.

TREATMENT AND PROGNOSIS. Treatment consists of observation if the vision is good. The patient should be followed with serial MRI scans. Surgical excision is offered if a tumor approaches the chiasm. Surgery also is indicated for pain or disfiguring proptosis. The role of radiotherapy remains controversial; it may be associated with CNS complications. More recently, chemotherapy has shown promising results.[49]

Prognosis for vision is poor. For lesions confined initially to the optic nerve, prognosis for life is good, with a mortality of 10%. For those lesions that involve the chiasm, mortality approaches 20%. Once the midbrain and hypothalamus are involved, the overall prognosis is poor, with mortality exceeding 55%.

Optic Nerve Sheath Meningioma

KEY POINTS. Optic nerve sheath meningioma is a benign neoplasm of meningothelial cells of arachnoid tissue[50] that affects primarily middle-aged adults (20–60 years). Women are involved slightly more commonly than men, at a ratio of 3:2. In 4–9% of cases there is an association with type 1 neurofibromatosis, and in 6% of cases the lesion may be bilateral; 5% of meningiomas are confined to the optic canal, which makes diagnosis difficult.

Symptoms and signs include slowly progressive exophthalmos over several years, visual loss, optic disc edema, optic atrophy, development of opticociliary shunt vessels, and ocular motility restriction.

ORBITAL IMAGING. The lesion usually is seen as a tubular enlargement of the optic nerve with a characteristic "tram-track" pattern of an enhancing nerve sheath with a lucent central nerve. Small areas of calcification may be seen. Marked contrast enhancement on computed tomography is characteristic. On MRI the T1 signal is hypointense, and the T2 signal is hyperintense. Heterogeneity results from low signal areas that represent calcium. Areas of subarachnoid fluid distention are hyperintense.

ECHOGRAPHY. Enlargement of the optic nerve is seen, with medium to high internal reflectivity, and calcification may be apparent. The 30° test may be positive anterior to the tumor, indicating increased subarachnoid fluid.

PATHOLOGY. There are several histological types. The meningothelial type of lesion shows syncytial lobules of meningothelial cells. The psammous type demonstrates calcified concretions or psammoma bodies (Box 95-2). A rare angioblastic type contains vascular elements that resemble a hemangiopericytoma.

TREATMENT AND PROGNOSIS. Treatment consists of observation if the vision remains good. In patients with blindness and significant proptosis, or when the optic canal is threatened, surgical excision is indicated. The role of radiotherapy remains controversial, but it may slow progression.

The prognosis for life is excellent, but visual outcome typically is poor.

LYMPHOPROLIFERATIVE DISEASES

Lymphoid lesions are uncommon in the orbit and account for 6% of all orbital mass lesions (Table 95-7). This group includes lymphocytic, plasmacytic, and leukemic lesions. Among the lymphoid infiltrates, lesions are divided into three categories: idiopathic inflammations (pseudotumors), lymphoproliferative reactive and atypical diseases, and lymphomas. The relationships between the last two groups and their relationship to systemic disease are not always clear, and some confusion still surrounds the diagnosis and prognosis of each.

Benign Reactive Lymphoid Hyperplasia

KEY POINTS. This disease constitutes a benign proliferation of lymphoid follicles that contain polymorphic lymphocytes that are immunohistochemically polyclonal.[51,52] Benign reactive lymphoid hyperplasia (BRLH) occurs most commonly in the anterior superior orbit, with a predilection for the lacrimal gland (15%). The clinical course is indolent, with painless exophthalmos, globe displacement, and typically normal vision. A firm, rubbery mass is often palpable beneath the orbital rim, and there may be a pink subconjunctival "salmon-patch" infiltrate.

ORBITAL IMAGING. An infiltrative mass is seen in the eyelids or anterior orbit. It typically molds to the globe and other adjacent structures and may extend along the rectus muscles. On MRI the T1 signal is hypointense and the T2 signal hyperintense to muscle.

BOX 95-2

Calcified Orbital Lesions

Phlebolith
Orbital varix
Lymphangioma
Thrombosed atrioventricular shunt
Chronic inflammation
Malignant lacrimal gland tumors
Optic nerve sheath meningioma
Dermoid cyst
Mucocele walls
Fibro-osseous tumors

TABLE 95-7

FREQUENCY OF LYMPHOPROLIFERATIVE DISEASES OF THE ORBIT

Disease	Frequency (%)
Lymphoma	51
Reactive and atypical lymphoid hyperplasia	36
Plasma cell dyscrasias	7
Leukemia	2
Histiocytoses	4

(Modified from Dutton JJ, Frazier Byrne S, Proia A. Diagnostic atlas of orbital diseases. Philadelphia: WB Saunders; 2000:1–5.)

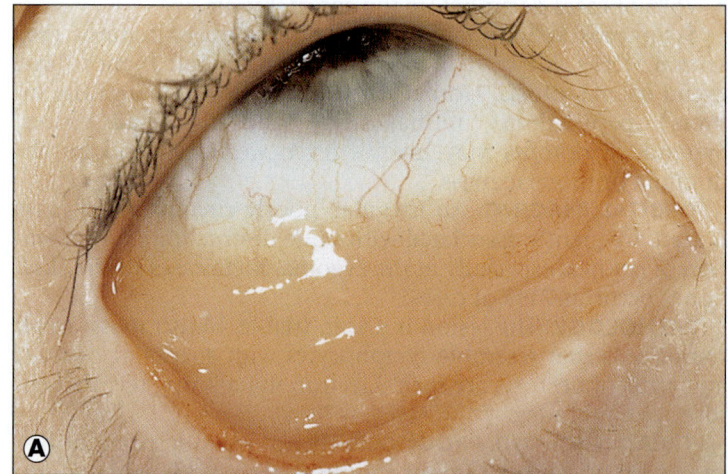
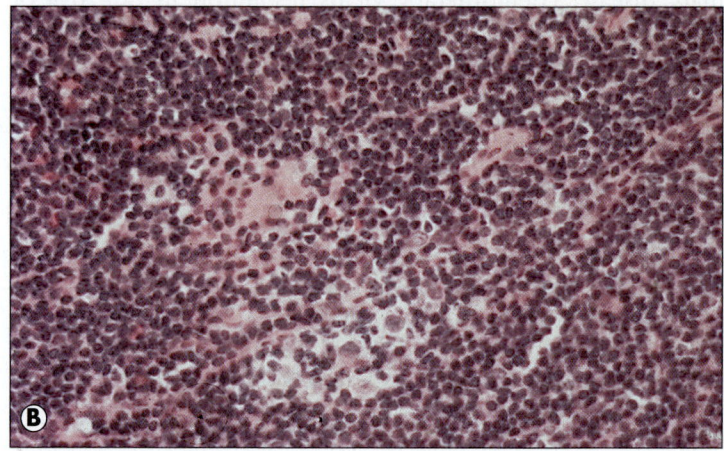

FIG. 95-11 ▪ **Reactive lymphoid hyperplasia. A,** The patient noted a fullness of the lower right lid. Large, thickened, redundant folds of conjunctiva in the inferior cul-de-sac are seen. The characteristic "fish flesh" appearance of the lesion suggests the clinical differential diagnosis of a lymphoid or leukemic infiltrate or amyloidosis. **B,** Lymphocytes are mature, quite small, and uniform; occasional plasma cells are large monocytoid lymphocytes. The uniformity of the lymphocytes makes it difficult to differentiate this benign lesion from a well-differentiated lymphosarcoma. The very mature appearance of the cells and the absence of atypical cells, along with the presence of plasma cells, suggests the diagnosis of a benign lesion. In such cases, testing using monoclonal antibodies may be quite helpful. If the population is of mixed B and T cells, the chances are that the tumor is benign. If it is predominantly of one cell type or the other, usually B cells, it is probably malignant and may represent mucosal-associated lymphoid tissue of the conjunctiva. (**A-B,** From Yanoff M, Fine BS. Ocular pathology, ed 5. St. Louis: Mosby, 2002.)

ECHOGRAPHY. The lesion has a variable shape and borders. A-scan shows a regular acoustic structure with low to medium reflectivity.

PATHOLOGY. Typically, the tumor is a polymorphous array of small lymphocytes and plasma cells, with mitotically active germinal centers (Fig. 95-11). Immunohistochemistry is positive for polyclonal T- and B-cell markers.

TREATMENT AND PROGNOSIS. Treatment involves systemic corticosteroids or local radiotherapy at 1500–2000cGy. Some lesions may require cytotoxic agents (chlorambucil) for control. There is a 15–25% chance of developing systemic lymphoma within 5 years.

Atypical Lymphoid Hyperplasia

KEY POINTS. Atypical lymphoid hyperplasia (ALH) represents an intermediate between BRLH and malignant lymphoma and may be unilateral or bilateral.[53] Presentation is as for BRLH, but ALH may involve other systemic organs and more frequently does not respond to corticosteroids. There is a 15% incidence of extraorbital involvement, and systemic lymphoma may develop.

ORBITAL IMAGING AND ECHOGRAPHY. Computed tomography and MRI scans are similar to those for BRLH.

PATHOLOGY. Monomorphous sheets of lymphocytes that have larger nuclei than those of BRLH are seen. Some abortive follicles may be present.

TREATMENT AND PROGNOSIS. If no systemic involvement exists, radiotherapy at 2500–3000cGy is appropriate. There is a 40% chance of systemic lymphoma developing within 5 years.

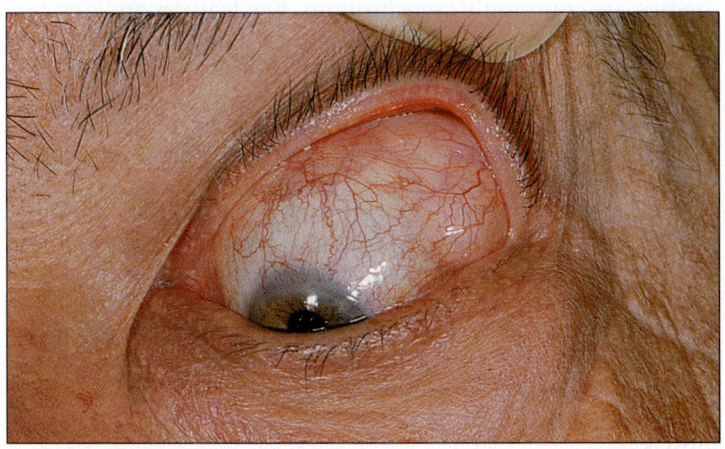

FIG. 95-12 ■ Subconjunctival anterior orbital lymphoma.

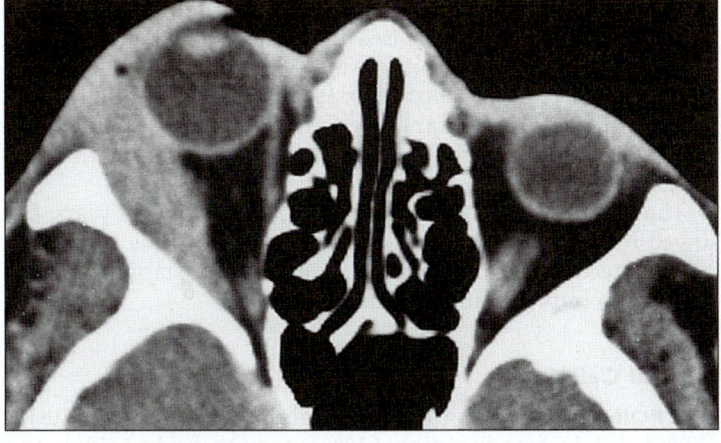

FIG. 95-13 ■ Lymphoma infiltrating along the lateral orbital wall.

Malignant Orbital Lymphoma (Lymphosarcoma)

KEY POINTS. Malignant orbital lymphoma is a low-grade malignancy characterized by a proliferation of monoclonal B cells (non-Hodgkin's), which arise in lymph nodes or in an extranodal site such as the orbit.[54,55] Most commonly affected is the older age group (50–70 years). Clinically, a palpable mass may be present in the anterior orbit. Symptoms include exophthalmos, occasional diplopia, lid edema, and ptosis (Fig. 95-12).

In 75% of cases the process is unilateral, and in 25% it is bilateral; 40% of cases are associated with systemic disease at the time of diagnosis.

ORBITAL IMAGING. A well-defined mass is seen that molds to encompass adjacent structures. Most lesions are located in the anterior, superior, and lateral orbit and frequently involve the lacrimal gland (Fig. 95-13).

ECHOGRAPHY. The lesion has a variable shape and borders, with a regular acoustic structure and low to medium reflectivity.

PATHOLOGY. Infiltrative, anaplastic lymphocytes with large cleaved nuclei and frequent nucleoli are seen. Follicles are absent. Immunohistochemistry reveals a monoclonal proliferation of B cells.

TREATMENT AND PROGNOSIS. If no systemic involvement occurs, observation is warranted for low-grade differentiated lesions. For less well-differentiated types, chemotherapy or radiotherapy at 2500–3000cGy is recommended.

When the disease is confined to the orbit, the visual prognosis is excellent, but the overall prognosis for life is variable. A 60% chance exists of developing systemic lymphoma within 5 years.

HISTIOCYTIC TUMORS

Histiocytic tumors are rare proliferative disorders of histiocytes that range from solitary benign lesions to those that exhibit a more malignant course. A typical feature of all these lesions is the presence of Langerhans' cells, a type of histiocyte normally found in the epidermis.

Eosinophilic Granuloma (Histiocytosis X)

KEY POINTS. Eosinophilic granuloma is the most common and benign form of the histiocytosis X group.[56] The disease affects primarily children and teenagers (from birth to 20 years of age). It consists of a unifocal, granulomatous proliferation in the bone. Orbital involvement occurs in up to 20% of cases, most commonly in the superotemporal orbit.

Clinically, a rapid onset of abaxial displacement of the globe occurs, and painful superolateral swelling. Erythema and inflammatory signs are seen in the overlying skin.

ORBITAL IMAGING. Typically, an osteolytic lesion is seen near the superotemporal bony rim. Usually an irregular contour is noted, with marginal hyperostosis. Occasionally, the lesion may extend into the cranial fossa.

ECHOGRAPHY. A well-circumscribed mass with low internal reflectivity occurs in the superotemporal orbit. It typically is associated with a bony defect.

PATHOLOGY. This is a soft, friable, tan–yellow tumor with sheets of binuclear histiocytes, eosinophils, and giant cells (Fig. 95-14). Characteristic Langerhans' granules are seen in the cytoplasm.

TREATMENT AND PROGNOSIS. Surgical curettage generally is curative, but radiotherapy at 900–1500cGy also may be used. The prognosis is very good.

INFLAMMATIONS AND INFECTIONS

Inflammatory diseases are common orbital lesions that may simulate neoplasms. They include a variety of acute and subacute idiopathic processes, chronic inflammations, and specific inflammations of uncertain etiology. Most notable among these

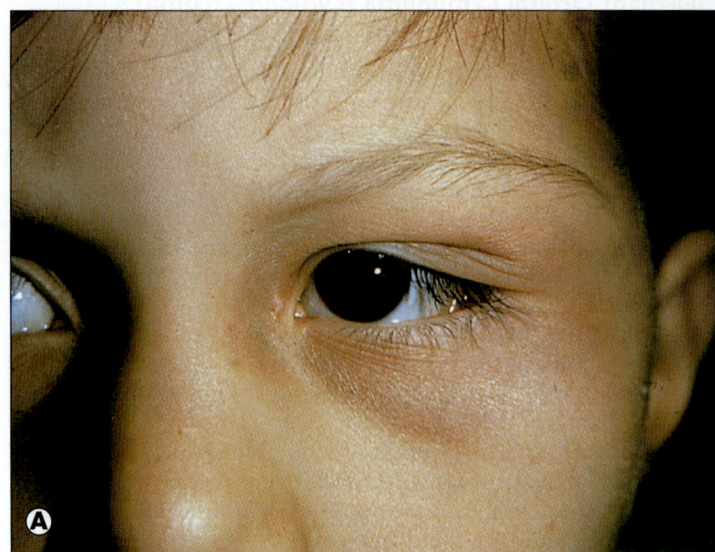

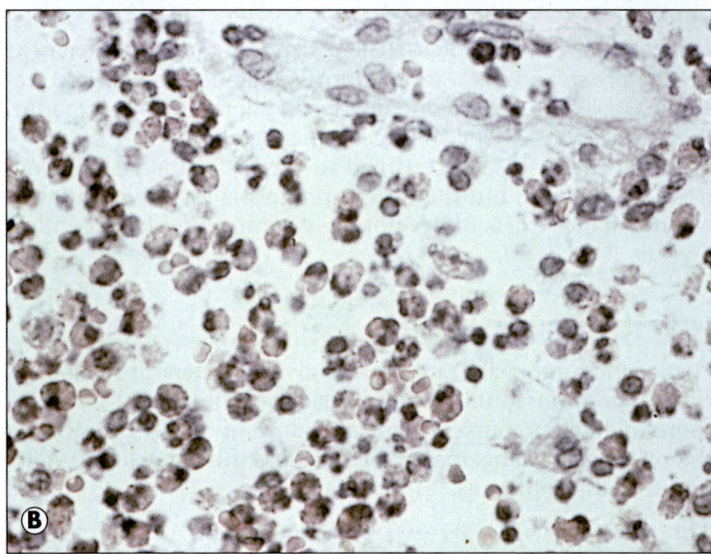

FIG. 95-14 ■ Eosinophilic granuloma. A, A 4-year-old boy presented clinically with rapid onset of erythema and swelling over the lateral edge of the left orbit. Osteomyelitis versus rhabdomyosarcoma was diagnosed clinically; the area was explored surgically. **B,** Histological section shows large histiocytes (abnormal Langerhans' cells) and numerous eosinophils characteristic of a solitary eosinophilic granuloma. (**A,** Courtesy of Dr. D.B. Schaffer. In: Yanoff M, Fine BS. Ocular pathology, ed 5. St. Louis: Mosby, 2002. **B,** From Yanoff M, Fine BS. Ocular pathology, ed 5. St. Louis: Mosby, 2002.)

lesions is Graves' orbitopathy, which accounts for more than half of all such cases.

Diffuse Idiopathic Orbital Inflammation (Pseudotumor)

KEY POINTS. Diffuse orbital pseudotumor is a nongranulomatous acute to subacute inflammatory disease with no systemic manifestations that may affect teenagers to the elderly.[57] Most commonly it occurs in the anterior or mid orbit, and it frequently involves the lacrimal gland. It is typically unilateral but rarely may be bilateral. Uveitis and retinal detachment may be associated with scleritis.

Symptoms include abrupt pain, conjunctival injection, chemosis, lid edema, exophthalmos, and motility restriction. A palpable mass is detected in 50% of cases.

ORBITAL IMAGING. Posterior Tenon's capsule shows thickening and enhancement. A shaggy orbital infiltrate or discrete mass is present, which may mold to the globe or optic nerve sheath. The lacrimal gland may be enlarged. On MRI the T1 signal is hypointense and the T2 signal is hyperintense to muscle. Moderate enhancement occurs with gadolinium.

ECHOGRAPHY. The lesion has a variable shape and borders, with low to medium reflectivity, a regular acoustic structure, and weak sound attenuation. Edema in Tenon's capsule may appear as an area of lucency behind the globe.

PATHOLOGY. The pseudotumor is a gray rubbery mass composed of a polymorphic infiltrate of lymphocytes, eosinophils, plasma cells, and polymorphonuclear leukocytes. In the sclerosing type, the dominant feature is scarification and collagen deposition.

TREATMENT AND PROGNOSIS. Systemic corticosteroids typically result in a dramatic improvement. Rarely, some lesions may require cytotoxic agents. The sclerosing type shows little or no response to treatment.

Prognosis generally is excellent, with complete resolution of disease.

Myositis

KEY POINTS. An acute to subacute idiopathic inflammation of the extraocular muscles, myositis may affect teenagers to the elderly.[58] Typically, the disease is unilateral and involves only one muscle, most commonly the superior or lateral rectus.

Symptoms include pain, motility restriction, exophthalmos, and displacement of the globe.

ORBITAL IMAGING. Enlargement of an extraocular muscle is seen, with involvement of the entire muscle from origin to insertion.

ECHOGRAPHY. Echography shows a thickened muscle with low internal reflectivity and a regular acoustic structure.

TREATMENT AND PROGNOSIS. Systemic corticosteroids generally result in prompt resolution. The prognosis is excellent.

Thyroid Orbitopathy (Graves' Disease)

KEY POINTS. Thyroid orbitopathy is an immunological disorder that affects the orbital muscles and fat.[59] Hyperthyroidism is seen with orbitopathy at some point in most patients, although the two are commonly asynchronous. Key features are:

- Middle-aged adults (30–50 years) are affected most frequently.
- The disease is seen in women more commonly than in men, in a ratio of 3–4:1.
- It is always a bilateral process but is often asymmetrical.
- Multiple muscles are involved simultaneously, most commonly the inferior and medial rectus.

Symptoms and signs include dry eyes, conjunctival injection, lid retraction, exophthalmos, diplopia, corneal exposure, and rarely optic nerve compression. Graves' disease usually runs a progressive course for 3–5 years and then stabilizes.

ORBITAL IMAGING. Increased fat lucency is seen, as well as extraocular muscle enlargement confined to the bellies, but with sparing of the insertions and origins. On MRI the T1 is isointense and the T2 isointense to slightly hyperintense to muscle.

ECHOGRAPHY. Thickened muscles with medium to high internal reflectivity and an irregular acoustic structure are seen on echography.

PATHOLOGY. The enlarged, rubbery muscles show variable amounts of edema and infiltration with inflammatory round cells (Fig. 95-15). An increased amount of acid mucopolysaccharides infiltrates the orbital tissue.

TREATMENT AND PROGNOSIS. Symptomatic therapy is given until the disease stabilizes. Systemic corticosteroids or radiotherapy may be indicated for acute orbital inflammation and congestion.

The orbital disease is usually progressive over 1–5 years, followed by stabilization. Eyelid recession, strabismus surgery, or orbital decompression may be offered after stabilization, as needed, to improve function and cosmesis.

Orbital Cellulitis

KEY POINTS. The major causes of orbital cellulitis are sinusitis (58%), lid or face infection (28%), foreign body (11%), and hematogenous (4%).[60] *Staphylococcus* and *Streptococcus* are the most common causative organisms in adults, *Haemophilus in-*

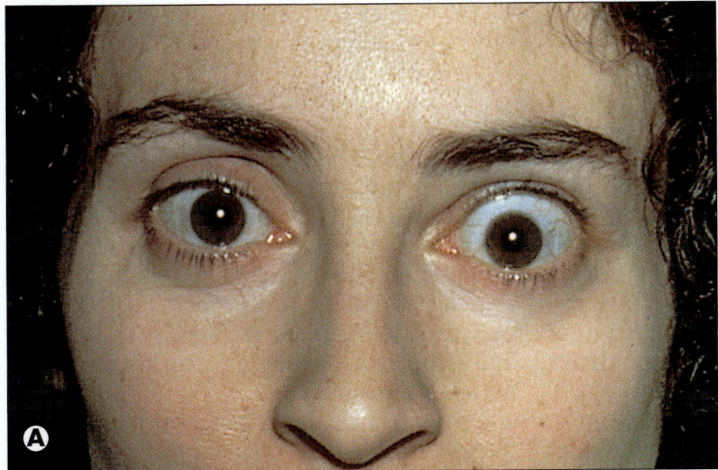

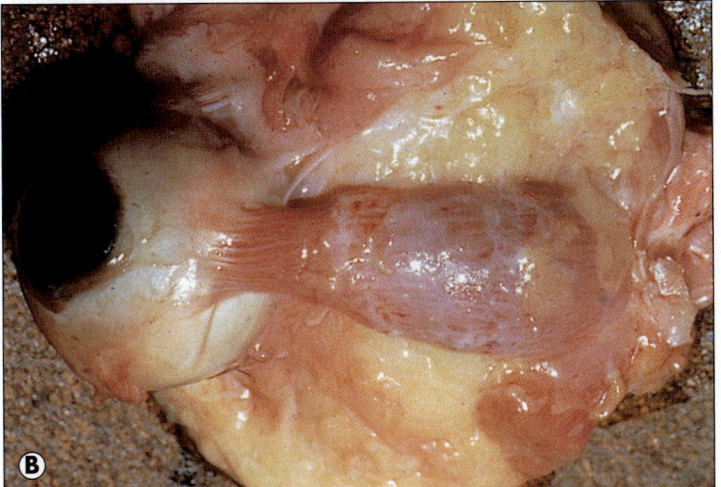

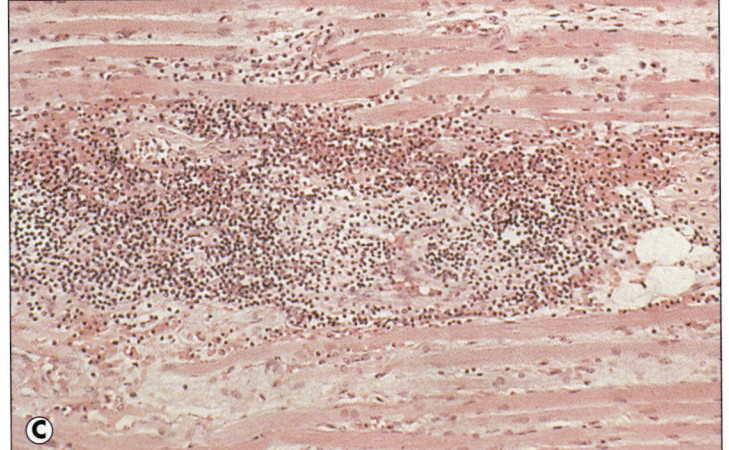

FIG. 95-15 ■ Graves' disease. **A,** In Graves' disease, exophthalmos often looks more pronounced than it actually is because of the extreme lid retraction that may occur. This patient, for instance, had minimal proptosis of the left eye but marked lid retraction. **B,** The orbital contents obtained post mortem from a patient with Graves' disease. Note the enormously thickened extraocular muscle. **C,** Both fluid and inflammatory cells separating the muscle bundle may be seen. The inflammatory cells are predominantly lymphocytes, plus plasma cells. (**A,** Courtesy Dr. HG Scheie. In: Yanoff M, Fine BS. Ocular pathology, ed 5. St. Louis: Mosby, 2002. **B–C,** Courtesy Dr. RC Eagle Jr. In: Hufnagle TJ, *et al.* Opthalmology. 1984; 91:1411.)

fluenzae in children. Less common organisms are *Pseudomonas* and *Escherichia coli.*

Orbital symptoms are pain, lid edema and erythema, chemosis, and axial proptosis if diffuse disease occurs or abaxial displacement if an abscess forms. Decreased ocular motility is common, and intraocular pressure may be elevated. A rapid loss of vision from optic nerve compression, optic neuritis, or vasculitis may ensue. With posterior extension, cavernous sinus thrombosis, subdural empyema, and intracranial abscess may develop.

Systemic symptoms may include malaise and fever. If the cavernous sinus is involved, headache, nausea, vomiting, and decreased consciousness may supervene.

The warning signs of orbital cellulitis are a dilated pupil, marked ophthalmoplegia, loss of vision, afferent pupillary defect, papilledema, perivasculitis, and violaceous lids.

ORBITAL IMAGING. Diffuse orbital infiltrate is seen, often with opacification of adjacent sinuses.

TREATMENT AND PROGNOSIS. In children, treatment is with systemic antibiotics; sinus drainage is needed in only 50% of cases. In adults, the drainage of sinuses and abscesses may be needed in 90% of cases.

The prognosis is very good with prompt antibiotic therapy and surgical drainage when indicated.

Wegener's Granulomatosis

KEY POINTS. Wegener's granulomatosis is a necrotizing granulomatosis of the upper respiratory tract, characterized by vasculitic pneumonitis, glomerulonephritis, sinusitis, and mucosal ulcerations of the nasopharynx.[61] A limited form does not involve the kidney. The cause is T-cell immune complex formation secondary to inhaled antigens. Key features are:

* Peak incidence is in adults 40–50 years of age.
* Men are more commonly affected than women, in a ratio of 2:1.
* Classic antineutrophil cytoplasmic antibody is positive in 80% of cases.
* 40–50% of patients may have ocular involvement (mostly contiguous from the sinus or pharynx, but it may be isolated).
* 18–22% of patients demonstrate orbital involvement, usually bilateral.

Symptoms are chemosis, exophthalmos, motility restriction, papilledema, and decreased vision. Ocular tissue involvement may include scleritis and episcleritis (20–38%), uveitis (10–20%), peripheral corneal guttering (14–28%), and retinal vasculitis (7–18%).

ORBITAL IMAGING. A diffuse orbital mass may be bilateral and may involve the adjacent nasopharynx.

PATHOLOGY. The pathology is necrotizing granulomatous vasculitis with giant cells.

TREATMENT AND PROGNOSIS. Treatment consists of administration of systemic corticosteroids plus cyclophosphamide or azathioprine. Radiotherapy is of doubtful value. Improvement with systemic therapy is usual, with up to 90% remission.

Patients who have the more limited form of the disease have a better prognosis.

STRUCTURAL LESIONS

Structural lesions of the orbit include choristomatous lesions such as dermoid cysts, which arise from errors in embryogenesis, and anatomical abnormalities such as mucoceles, which result from local disease processes (Box 95-3).

Dermoid Cyst

KEY POINTS. A dermoid cyst is a developmental choristoma, lined with epithelium and filled with keratinized material.[62] The majority of such cysts are located in the eyelids and orbit (Fig. 95-16). These cysts represent 24% of all orbital and lid masses, 6–8% of deep orbital masses, and 80% of cystic orbital lesions. Dermoid cysts may lie latent for many years before growth and may be located superficially in the eyelid and anterior orbit or deep in the orbit.

SUPERFICIAL LESIONS. Superficial lesions arise from a sequestration of epithelium during embryogenesis along bony suture lines. They are present in early infancy, typically in the superotemporal or superonasal quadrants. Clinically, they present as a slowly enlarging, unilateral, painless, firm mass; they may be mobile or fixed to underlying structures and are free from overlying skin.

ORBITAL IMAGING. The round, well-defined lesions have an enhancing rim that may contain calcium, and a lucent center. They may be associated with a well-corticated bone defect.

ECHOGRAPHY. The lesion is well defined, with medium to high internal reflectivity and a somewhat irregular acoustic structure; it usually shows some compressibility.

PATHOLOGY. The cyst usually has a thin, fibrous capsule and a central lumen lined with keratinized stratified squamous epithelium. If derived from conjunctiva, the lining may be cuboidal with goblet cells. The cyst wall contains hair follicles and sweat and sebaceous glands. The cyst contains keratin debris, hair shafts, and oily material. About 38% of cysts are associated with chronic granulomatous inflammation.

TREATMENT AND PROGNOSIS. Complete surgical excision in one piece is required. The prognosis is excellent, but recurrences with infiltration may follow incomplete excision or rupture of the capsule.

DEEP LESIONS. Deep lesions are seen in both children and adults. They are associated with any bony suture in the orbit and may extend across bones into the frontal sinus, temporal fossa, or cranium.

Symptoms from the slow-growing mass include proptosis, occasionally motility restriction, and decreased vision. Spontaneous rupture produces marked orbital inflammation.

ORBITAL IMAGING. The well-defined lesion has an enhancing rim that may contain areas of calcification. The central lumen is nonenhancing and of variable density, depending on its contents; it may show a fluid-fat interface. A bone defect may be seen.

ECHOGRAPHY. A cystic mass with low to absent internal reflectivity is seen, but higher echoes occur when the cyst is filled with keratin debris and fat.

PATHOLOGY. A smooth, thin rim of keratinized squamous epithelium, which may have goblet cells if derived from conjunctiva, lines the cyst. The cyst wall contains hair shafts, and sweat and sebaceous glands are characteristic.

TREATMENT AND PROGNOSIS. Treatment consists of total excision without rupture of the capsule. The prognosis is excellent.

Mucocele

KEY POINTS. Mucoceles arise from a primary obstruction of a paranasal sinus following trauma, sinusitis, or, rarely, a tumor.[63] Frequently, they expand into the orbit by expansion of a bony wall. Mucoceles consist of a cystic mass filled with mucus and may be bounded by an eggshell layer of bone (when they become infected, mucoceles are referred to as pyoceles). The majority of mucoceles (70%) occur in adults (aged 40–70 years), and the frontal and ethmoid sinuses are most commonly involved—rarely the sphenoid sinus.

Symptoms include headache, exophthalmos, and a palpable fluctuant mass in the medial or superomedial orbit.

ORBITAL IMAGING. An opacified frontal or ethmoid sinus, loss of ethmoid septae, and a bony dehiscence (Fig. 95-17) are observed. The cystic content shows variable density and is nonenhancing.

ECHOGRAPHY. Echography reveals a very well-defined mass with sharp surface spikes and low internal reflectivity. Mucocele is associated with a large bony defect adjacent to a paranasal sinus.

PATHOLOGY. The lining is composed of pseudostratified, ciliated columnar epithelium with goblet cells. The cyst content is mucoid with chronic inflammatory debris.

TREATMENT AND DIAGNOSIS. Treatment consists of surgical excision with restoration of sinus drainage. Obliteration of the sinus with fat or muscle may be necessary to treat recurrences.

The prognosis is very good, but there is a significant rate of recurrence.

VASCULAR NEOPLASTIC LESIONS

Neoplastic lesions that arise from the vascular system include both benign and malignant tumors (Table 95-8). Unlike nonneoplastic vascular lesions, which usually reflect the hemodynamic functions of the underlying vascular structures, neoplastic lesions typically manifest only a mass effect, occasionally modified by some hemodynamic characteristics. They may be well circumscribed or infiltrative.

Capillary Hemangioma (Hemangioendothelioma)

KEY POINTS. Capillary hemangioma is a congenital hamartoma of tightly packed capillaries that typically presents during the first 6 months of life.[2,54,64] It is generally unilateral and usually visible on the surface, but it may lie deep in the orbit (Fig. 95-18). More common in the superonasal quadrant of the up-

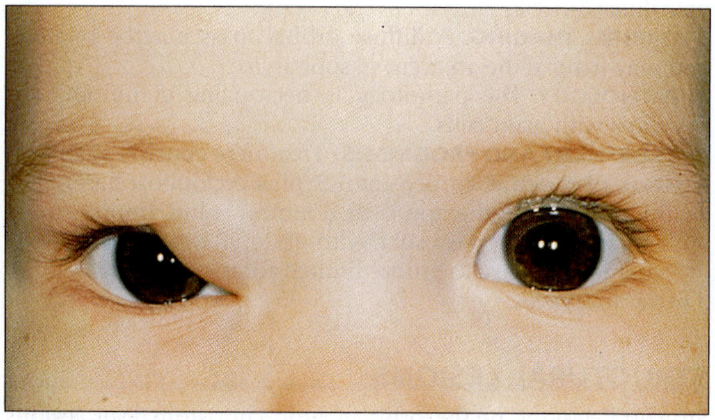

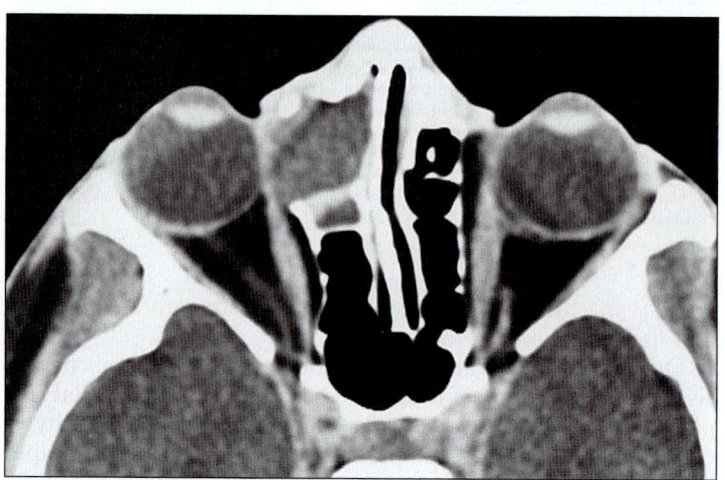

FIG. 95-16 ▮ Right superomedial superficial orbital dermoid cyst in a young child.

FIG. 95-17 ▮ Anterior ethmoid sinus mucocele eroding into the orbit.

per lid, capillary hemangioma appears as a fluctuant mass that may involve the overlying skin as a reddish lesion. Capillary hemangiomas show rapid growth over weeks to months, followed by slow spontaneous involution over months to years.

SUPERFICIAL LESIONS. Also known as the "strawberry nevus," capillary hemangioma is confined to the dermis. It may be single or multiple and is generally elevated.

Symptoms include ptosis, sometimes associated with astigmatism and amblyopia.

TREATMENT AND PROGNOSIS. Observation is warranted in most cases, since involution usually occurs. For severe cosmetic deformity or deprivation amblyopia, intralesional (40mg/ml triamcinolone plus 6mg/ml betamethasone) or systemic corticosteroids (1–2mg/kg/day prednisone) may be used. Radiotherapy, yellow dye laser, and, more recently, topical corticosteroids also have been advocated. Surgery is useful for small, circumscribed lesions, but for larger ones, this may result in cosmetic compromise.

The prognosis is good; 30% of cases involute by 3 years of age, 60% by 4 years, and 75% by 7 years of age. Large lesions may not completely disappear.

DEEP LESIONS. Deep lesions occur most frequently in the lids or posterior to orbital septum and are more common in the superonasal quadrant.

Symptoms are proptosis, displacement of the globe, subtle pulsations as a result of high vascular flow, and increasing size with Valsalva's maneuver or crying. Secondary amblyopia may result from distortion of the globe. Large lesions may sequester platelets.

ORBITAL IMAGING. A well-defined to infiltrating intraconal or extraconal lesion is observed, with moderate to intense enhancement. On MRI the signals are homogeneous to heterogeneous, being hypointense on T1 and hyperintense on T2 images.

TABLE 95-8

FREQUENCY OF THE MOST COMMON VASCULAR ORBITAL LESIONS

Lesion	Frequency (%)
Cavernous hemangioma	50
Capillary hemangioma	18
Hemangiopericytoma	13
Lymphangioma	10
Orbital varices	5
Other	5

(Modified from Shields JA, ed. Diagnosis and management of orbital tumors. Philadelphia: WB Saunders; 1989:291–315.)

Flow voids appear as hypointense regions. Moderate enhancement is seen with gadolinium.

ECHOGRAPHY. The lesion is poorly outlined, with an irregular shape, high internal reflectivity, and an irregular acoustic structure. Sound attenuation is variable.

PATHOLOGY. A florid proliferation of capillary endothelial cells and small capillaries is seen, with few spaces (Fig. 95-19). Mitoses are common, but this is not a malignant tumor.

TREATMENT AND PROGNOSIS. Treatment consists of observation, since many lesions will involute, although few orbital lesions completely disappear. If the lesion is large or amblyopia is present, local radiotherapy (500cGy) or corticosteroids (systemic or local) may be indicated. If the lesion is small and well defined, surgery may be attempted.

The prognosis is excellent for vision and for life.

Cavernous Hemangioma

KEY POINTS. Cavernous hemangioma is a benign, noninfiltrative, slowly progressive tumor of large endothelial-lined channels.[1,2] Although it is congenital, it typically becomes symptomatic in adults (aged 20–40 years). Cavernous hemangioma is usually found in an intraconal location, more commonly in the temporal quadrant. Rarely, it may be intraosseous.

Symptoms relate to its mass effect, which produces proptosis and late motility restriction. When cavernous hemangiomas are very large, choroidal folds and decreased vision may result. The lesions may enlarge during pregnancy.

ORBITAL IMAGING. A well-defined, oval to round, typically intraconal mass is seen with minimal enhancement. With large, long-standing lesions, molding of bone and internal calcification may occur. On MRI the lesion is isointense on T1 and hyperintense on T2 with respect to muscle. Signal voids represent calcific phleboliths. Enhancement with gadolinium is moderate.

ECHOGRAPHY. The lesions are well circumscribed and round to oval, with high internal reflectivity and a regular acoustic structure. Vascular flow is poor.

PATHOLOGY. The encapsulated nodular mass is dilated, with vascular spaces lined by flattened endothelial cells (Fig. 95-20). Septae may contain smooth muscles cells.

TREATMENT AND PROGNOSIS. Surgical excision is required if the lesion is symptomatic—typically, there is little or no bleeding. There is no role for radiotherapy. The prognosis is excellent for vision and life.

Lymphangioma

KEY POINTS. Lymphangioma is a rare vascular hamartoma of lymphatic channels that is hemodynamically isolated from the

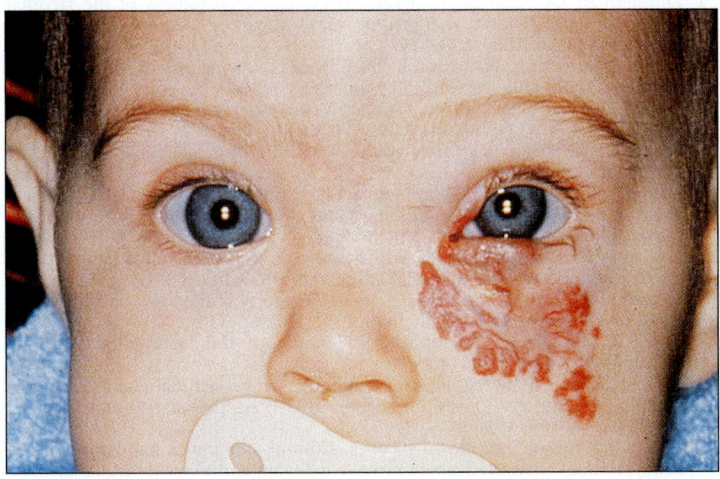

FIG. 95-18 ■ Capillary hemangioma of the lower eyelid in a young child.

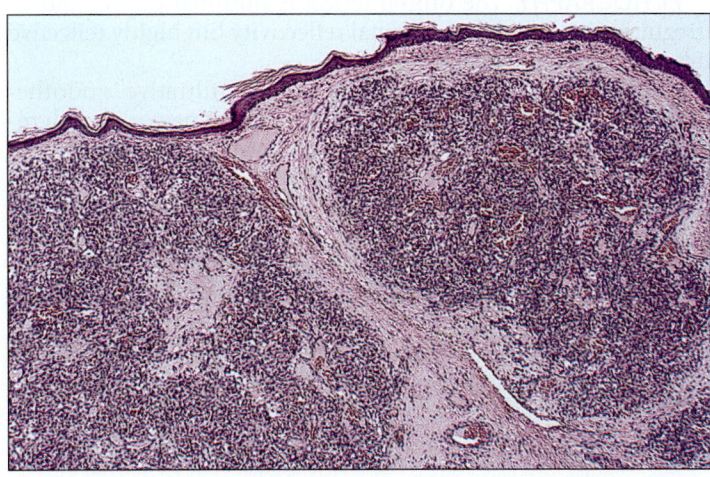

FIG. 95-19 ■ Capillary hemangioma. The tumor is composed of blood vessels of predominantly capillary size. (From Yanoff M, Fine BS. Ocular pathology, ed 5. St. Louis: Mosby, 2002.)

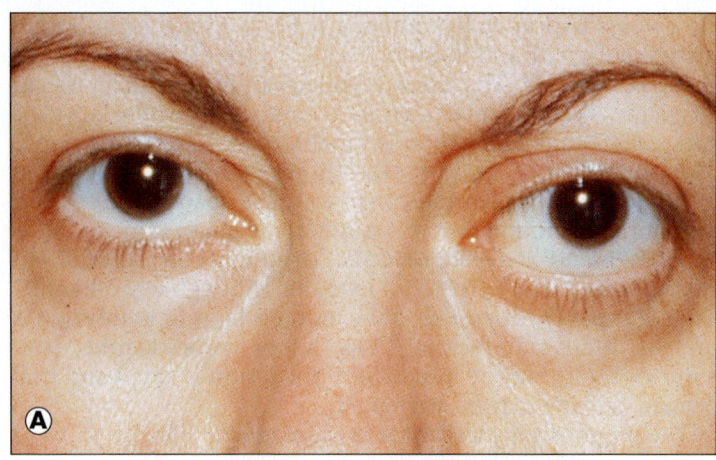

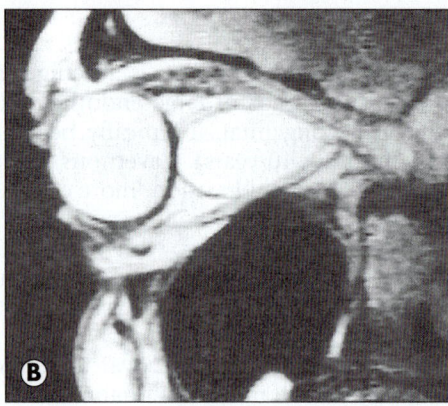

FIG. 95-20 ▌▌ **Cavernous hemangioma. A,** Clinical appearance of left exophthalmos. **B,** MRI shows optic nerve stretched over tumor that "lights up" in the T2-weighted image, characteristic of a hemangioma. (From a presentation by Dr. WC Frayer to the meeting of the Verhoeff Society, 1989.)

vascular system.[65] It occurs in children and teenagers, but most frequently in the first decade of life. The size of the lesion fluctuates with posture and Valsalva's maneuver, and with upper respiratory infections.

SUPERFICIAL LESIONS. Superficial lesions occur in the conjunctiva or lid and are visible as cystic spaces with clear fluid; they may be partially filled with blood.

DEEP LESIONS. Symptoms with deep lesions are proptosis and diplopia. Spontaneous hemorrhage may lead to sudden enlargement and orbital pain and possible visual loss, with the formation of "chocolate cysts."

ORBITAL IMAGING. The orbital lesion is seen as a low-density cystic, intra- and extraconal mass, with variable enhancement. There is no vascular component on angiography. On MRI the lesion is hypointense on T1; on T2 the signal is hyperintense but may be variable, depending on the state of hemoglobin degeneration.

ECHOGRAPHY. The orbital lesion is outlined poorly and of irregular shape, with low internal reflectivity but highly reflective internal septa.

PATHOLOGY. Lymphangiomas show infiltrative endothelium-lined channels, with a sparse cellular framework and lymphocytes. Lymphatic follicles often are seen in the walls of the tumor. Red blood cells are not present.

TREATMENT AND PROGNOSIS. Observation is justified in most cases. Surgery may be hazardous and lead to poor cosmetic results. If acute hemorrhage causes severe symptoms, the lymphangioma may be evacuated and partial resection or ligation attempted. Recurrences are common. The lesion shows limited radiosensitivity. The prognosis is variable. Amblyopia is common from globe compression and recurrent hemorrhage.

Arteriovenous Fistula

KEY POINTS. Arteriovenous fistulas can be traumatic (more common in males than females, age range 15–30 years) or spontaneous (more common in females than males, age range 30–60 years).[1,2] Symptoms depend on blood flow rate—most fistulas are associated with venous dilatation, fluid transudation, sludging, and thrombosis.

LOW-FLOW TYPE. Low-flow fistulas usually result from dural artery–to–cavernous sinus shunts. Symptoms are chemosis, increased episcleral venous pressure, and venous dilatation.

HIGH-FLOW TYPE. High-flow fistulas usually result from carotid artery–to–cavernous sinus shunts. Symptoms are chemosis, orbital edema, proptosis, pulsatile exophthalmos, audible bruit, secondary glaucoma, retinal vascular dilatation, papilledema, afferent pupillary defect, decreased vision, and cranial nerve palsies (third and sixth nerves most common).

PRIMARY SHUNT. Primary shunts (mainly congenital malformations) are rare in the orbit and are usually associated with syndromes (e.g., Wyburn-Mason and Osler-Weber-Rendu).

SECONDARY SHUNTS. Secondary shunts are located outside the orbit, usually in the cavernous sinus. Retrograde blood flow is directed forward into the orbital veins. Secondary shunts may be spontaneous (from venous thrombosis or hypertension) or secondary (from trauma). The latter are usually of the high-flow type, 40–50% causing visual loss.

ORBITAL IMAGING. A dilated superior ophthalmic vein with enlargement of the superior orbital fissure is seen; erosion of the anterior clinoid processes occurs.

ECHOGRAPHY. Echography shows a dilated superior ophthalmic vein and mild thickening of the extraocular muscles, with medium to high internal reflectivity from edema.

TREATMENT AND PROGNOSIS. Resolution of small, spontaneous low-flow shunts frequently occurs from thrombosis and is seen in up to 40% of cases. Embolization is not indicated unless visual loss, glaucoma, or severe pain is present. With traumatic, high-flow shunts, spontaneous resolution is less common. The rate of visual loss is 40–50%, and intervention is therefore required. Balloon or other embolization is the treatment of choice.

With treatment, the prognosis is generally good for vision.

REFERENCES

1. Rootman J. Diseases of the orbit. A multidisciplinary approach. Philadelphia: JB Lippincott; 1988:119–39.
2. Shields JA. Metastatic cancer to the orbit. In: Shields JA, ed. Diagnosis and management of orbital tumors. Philadelphia: WB Saunders; 1989:291–315.
3. Ferry AP, Font RL. Carcinoma metastatic to the eye and orbit. I. A clinicopathologic study of 227 cases. Arch Ophthalmol. 1974;92:276–86.
4. Hart WM. Metastatic carcinoma to the eye and orbit. In: Zimmerman LE, ed. Tumors of the eye and adnexa. Int Ophthalmol Clin. 1962;2:465–82.
5. Shields CL, Shields JA, Peggs M. Metastatic tumors to the orbit. Ophthal Reconstr Plast Surg. 1988;4:73–80.
6. Font RL, Gamel JW. Epithelial tumors of the lacrimal gland: an analysis of 265 cases. In: Jakobiec FA, ed. Ocular and adnexal tumors. Birmingham: Aesculapius; 1978:787.
7. Forrest AW. Lacrimal gland tumors. In: Jones IS, Jakobiec FA, eds. Diseases of the orbit. Hagerstown: Harper & Row; 1979:355.
8. Goder GJ. Tumours of the lacrimal gland. Orbit. 1982;1:91–6.
9. Zimmerman LA, Sanders TE, Ackerman LV. Epithelial tumors of the lacrimal gland: prognostic and therapeutic significance of histologic types. Int Ophthalmol Clin. 1962;2:337–67.
10. Lemke AJ, Hosten N, Neumann K, et al. Space occupying lesions of the lacrimal gland in CT and MRI exemplified by four cases. Aktuelle Radiol. 1995;5:363–6.
11. Forrest AW. Pathologic criteria for effective management of epithelial lacrimal gland tumors. Am J Ophthalmol. 1971;71(Suppl):178–92.
12. Milam DF Jr, Heath P. Primary epithelial tumors of the lacrimal gland. Am J Ophthalmol. 1956;41:996–1006.
13. Sanders TE, Ackerman LV, Zimmerman LE. Epithelial tumors of the lacrimal gland. A comparison of the pathologic and clinical behavior with those of the salivary glands. Am J Surg. 1962;104:657–65.
14. Shields JA, Shields CL, Eagle RC, et al. Pleomorphic adenoma ("benign mixed tumor") of the lacrimal gland. Arch Ophthalmol. 1987;105:560–1.
15. Mercado GJ, Grunduz K, Shields CL, et al. Pleomorphic adenoma of the lacrimal gland in a teenager. Arch Ophthalmol. 1998;116:962–3.
16. Rose GE, Wright JE. Pleomorphic adenoma of the lacrimal gland. Br J Ophthalmol. 1992;76:395–400.
17. Font RL, Gamel JW. Adenoid cystic carcinoma of the lacrimal gland. A clinicopathologic study of 79 cases. In: Nicholson DH, ed. Ocular pathology update. New York: Masson; 1980:277–83.
18. Shields JA, Nelson LB, Brown JF, et al. Clinical, computed tomographic, and histopathologic characteristics of juvenile ossifying fibroma with orbital involvement. Am J Ophthalmol. 1983;96:650–3.
19. Jakobiec FA, Jones IS. Mesenchymal and fibro-osseous tumors. In: Jones IS, Jakobiec FA, eds. Diseases of the orbit. New York: Harper & Row; 1979:461–502.

20. Liakos GM, Walker CB, Carruth JAS. Ocular complications in cranial fibrous dysplasia. Br J Ophthalmol. 1979;63:611–6.
21. Moore RT. Fibrous dysplasia of the orbit. Review. Surv Ophthalmol. 1969;13:321–34.
22. Blodi FC. Pathology of orbital bones. The XXXII Edward Jackson Memorial Lecture. Am J Ophthalmol. 1976;81:1–26.
23. Dhir SP, Munjal VP, Jain IS, et al. Osteosarcoma of the orbit. J Pediatr Ophthalmol Strabismus. 1980;17:312–4.
24. Mortada A. Fibroma of the orbit. Br J Ophthalmol. 1971;55:350–2.
25. Stokes WH, Bowers WF. Pure fibroma of the orbit. Report of a case and review of the literature. Arch Ophthalmol. 1934;11:279–82.
26. Eifrig DE, Foos RY. Fibrosarcoma of the orbit. Am J Ophthalmol. 1969;67:244–8.
27. Weiner JM, Hidayat AA. Juvenile fibrosarcoma of the orbit and eyelid. Arch Ophthalmol. 1983;101:253–9.
28. Yanoff M, Scheie HG. Fibrosarcoma of the orbit. Report of two patients. Cancer. 1966;19:1711–6.
29. Kojima K, Kojima K, Sakai T. Leiomyosarcoma. Acta Soc Ophthalmol Jpn. 1972;76:74–7.
30. Meekins B, Dutton JJ, Proia AD. Primary orbital leiomyosarcoma: a case report and review of the literature. Arch Ophthalmol. 1988;106:82–6.
31. Wojno T, Tenzel RR, Nadji M. Orbital leiomyosarcoma. Arch Ophthalmol. 1983;101:1566–8.
32. Font RL, Hidayat AA. Fibrous histiocytoma of the orbit. A clinicopathologic study of 150 cases. Hum Pathol. 1982;13:199–209.
33. Ros PR, Kursunoglu S, Batle JF, et al. Malignant fibrous histiocytoma of the orbit. J Clin Neuro-Ophthalmol. 1985;5:116–9.
34. Jones IS, Reese AB, Kraut J. Orbital rhabdomyosarcoma: an analysis of sixty-two cases. Trans Am Ophthalmol Soc. 1965;63:223–55.
35. Knowles DM II, Jakobiec FA. Rhabdomyosarcoma of the orbit. Am J Ophthalmol. 1975;80:1011–8.
36. Shields JA. Rhabdomyosarcoma of the orbit. In: Hornblass A, ed. Ophthalmic plastic and reconstructive surgery. Baltimore: Williams & Wilkins; 1987.
37. Abramson DH, Notis CM. Visual acuity after radiation for orbital rhabdomyosarcoma. Am J Ophthalmol. 1994;118:808–9.
38. Gurland JE, Tenner M, Hornblass A, et al. Orbital neurofibromatosis. Arch Ophthalmol. 1976;94:1723–5.
39. Korbin EA, Blodi FC, Weingeist TA. Ocular and orbital manifestations of neurofibromatosis. Surv Ophthalmol. 1984;188:118–27.
40. Della Rocca RC, Roen J, Labay JR, et al. Isolated neurofibroma of the orbit. Ophthalmic Surg. 1985;16:634–8.
41. Farris SR, Grove AS Jr. Orbital and eyelid manifestations of neurofibromatosis: a critical study and literature review. Ophthal Plast Reconstr Surg. 1996;12:245–59.
42. Konrad GB, Thiel HJ. Schwannoma of the orbit. Ophthalmologica. 1984;188:118–27.
43. Rootman J, Goldberg C, Robertson W. Primary orbital schwannomas. Br J Ophthalmol. 1982;66:194–204.
44. Jakobiec FA, Font RL, Zimmerman LE. Malignant peripheral nerve sheath tumors of the orbit. A clinicopathologic study of eight cases. Trans Am Ophthalmol Soc. 1985;83:332–66.
45. Dutton JJ, Tawfik HA, DeBacker CM, et al. Multiple recurrences in malignant peripheral nerve sheath tumor of the orbit: a case report and review of the literature. Ophthal Plast Reconstr Surg. 2001;17:293–9.
46. Traboulsi EI, Shammas IV, Massad M, et al. Ophthalmological aspects of metastatic neuroblastoma. Report of 22 consecutive cases. Orbit. 1984;3:247–54.
47. Alfano J. Ophthalmological aspects of neuroblastoma: a study of 53 verified cases. Trans Am Acad Ophthalmol Otolaryngol. 1968;72:830–48.
48. Dutton JJ. Gliomas of the anterior visual pathways. Surv Ophthalmol. 1993;38:427–52.
49. Listernick R, Louis DN, Packer RJ, Gutman DH. Optic nerve gliomas in children with NF-1: consensus statement for the NF-1 Optic Pathway Glioma Task Force. Ann Neurol. 1997;141:143–9.
50. Dutton JJ. Optic nerve sheath meningiomas. Surv Ophthalmol. 1994;37:167–83.
51. Knowles DM II, Jakobiec FA. Ocular adnexal lymphoid neoplasms: clinical, histopathologic, electron microscopic, and immunologic characteristics. Hum Pathol. 1982;13:148–62.
52. Ellis JH, Banks PM, Campbell RJ, et al. Lymphoid tumors of the ocular adnexa. Clinical correlation with the working formulation, classification and immunoperoxidase staining of paraffin sections. Ophthalmology. 1985;92:1311–24.
53. Shields JA. Lymphoid tumors and leukemias. In: Shields JA, ed. Diagnosis and management of orbital tumors. Philadelphia: WB Saunders; 1989:316–40.
54. Dutton JJ, Byrne SF, Proia A. Diagnostic atlas of orbital diseases. Philadelphia: WB Saunders; 2000.
55. Jakobiec FA, Iwamoto T, Knowles DM II. Ocular adnexal lymphoid tumors. Correlative ultrastructural and immunologic marker studies. Arch Ophthalmol. 1982;100:84–98.
56. Arnow SJ, Notz RG. Eosinophilic granuloma of the orbit. Trans Acad Ophthalmol Otolaryngol. 1983;36:41–8.
57. Kennerdell JS, Dresner SC. The nonspecific orbital inflammatory syndromes. Surv Ophthalmol. 1984;29:93–103.
58. Weinstein GS, Dresner SC, Slamovits TL, et al. Acute and subacute orbital myositis. Am J Ophthalmol. 1983;96:209–17.
59. Sergott RC, Glaser JS. Graves' ophthalmopathy. A clinical and immunological review. Surv Ophthalmol. 1981;26:1–21.
60. Bergin DJ, Wright JE. Orbital cellulitis. Br J Ophthalmol. 1986;70:174–8.
61. Koornneef L, Melief CJM, Peterse HL, et al. Wegener's granulomatosis of the orbit. Orbit. 1983;2:1–10.
62. Sherman RP, Rootman J, LaPointe JS. Orbital dermoids: clinical presentation and management. Br J Ophthalmol. 1986;101:726–9.
63. Avery G, Tang RA, Close LG. Ophthalmic manifestations of mucoceles. Ann Ophthalmol. 1983;15:734–7.
64. Jakobiec FA, Jones IS. Vascular tumors, malformations and degenerations. In: Jones IS, Jakobiec FA, eds. Diseases of the orbit. Hagerstown: Harper & Row; 1979:269–308.
65. Rootman J, Hay E, Graebo D, et al. Orbital-adnexal lymphangiomas: a spectrum of hemodynamically isolated vascular hamartomas. Ophthalmology. 1986;93:1558–70.

96 Orbital Surgery

JONATHAN J. DUTTON

DEFINITION
- Orbital surgery involves tissues bounded by the bony orbital walls posteriorly and by the orbital septum anteriorly.

KEY FEATURES
- Surgical approaches to the orbit may be anterior, lateral, medial, or superior, depending on the location of the lesion and the exposure needed.
- Meticulous attention to anatomical detail, hemostasis, and gentle manipulation of tissues is mandatory to avoid devastating complications.
- The most important complications are loss of vision, injury to extraocular muscles with diplopia, hemorrhage, and cerebrospinal fluid leak and possible meningitis.

INTRODUCTION

Orbital and lacrimal gland surgery is indicated for the evaluation or treatment of orbital disease, restoration of anatomical relationships following trauma, or cosmetic improvement of congenital or acquired deformities. Biopsy of mass lesions is an important technique. Although some authors advocate fine-needle aspiration biopsy of orbital mass lesions under computed tomographic or echographic guidance,[1-3] cytological evaluation on such specimens may be inaccurate.[4] For most orbital lesions, an open biopsy is preferred.

The removal of orbital masses may be indicated when these are well defined and cause either functional compromise or cosmetic deformity. Benign tumors, such as hemangiomas, schwannomas, dermoid cysts, and mixed lacrimal gland tumors, and some malignant lesions usually can be dissected away from adjacent structures. More infiltrative lesions, such as lymphangiomas, usually are impossible to extirpate completely. When not amenable to medical therapy and when it is necessary to restore function, these tumors may be carefully debulked.

Orbital abscesses, either following surgical or nonsurgical trauma or associated with sinusitis, may require direct drainage and antibiotic therapy. When they are loculated within the orbit, drainage to the surface is appropriate.

Nonsurgical traumatic injury to the orbit frequently involves bony fracture or hemorrhage. Orbital rim fractures are easily accessible through anterior approaches; they may be repaired with miniplate fixation of the displaced fragments. Orbital wall fractures, often associated with soft tissue injury or incarceration, must be carefully explored and realigned when it is necessary to restore function or orbital volume. The exact surgical approach depends on the nature and location of the fractures.

Diffuse orbital hemorrhage following trauma may produce massive proptosis and, occasionally, increased intraocular pressure or optic nerve compression. Orbital decompression with a lateral canthotomy is usually sufficient to manage the potential visual loss. If this fails, drainage of loculated pockets or bony decompression may be necessary. Progressive loss of vision associated with proptosis and downward displacement of the globe suggests a subperiosteal hematoma. The diagnosis is confirmed using orbital echography or computed tomography (CT), and immediate drainage via an anteromedial orbitotomy usually reverses the visual loss.

Massive proptosis associated with Graves' orbitopathy may require orbital decompression for the treatment of threatened visual function or cosmetic disfigurement. This is achieved by removal of the inferior or medial orbital walls or, more commonly, both. Decompression also may be indicated for other expanding lesions of the orbit that cannot be surgically extirpated.

Removal of the globe and part or all of the normal orbital contents may be necessary to manage neoplastic processes or to control chronic pain. It is also useful for the cosmetic improvement of congenital or traumatic ocular or orbital deformities. When only the globe is involved, enucleation or evisceration is indicated (see Chapter 97). Cure of neoplasms that extend into the orbit from the globe or eyelids may require more radical exenteration of all the orbital soft tissues.

HISTORICAL REVIEW

The history of orbital and lacrimal gland surgery predates the Christian era—references can be found in writings from antiquity. In 1583, Bartish provided one of the earliest complete descriptions of an orbital procedure (exenteration) for the eradication of orbital disease.[5] The evolution of more modern surgical techniques has paralleled both the accumulation of anatomical knowledge since the middle of the nineteenth century and the development of more sophisticated surgical instruments. Surgical loupes and the operating microscope, fiberoptic illumination, and better methods of hemostatic control have each contributed to safer and more effective procedures. Of particular importance has been the introduction of modern imaging techniques, including CT, magnetic resonance imaging, and orbital echography, which have permitted more precise diagnosis and better surgical planning.

PREOPERATIVE EVALUATION AND DIAGNOSTIC APPROACH

Before a decision is made about the need for orbital or lacrimal gland surgery, a complete evaluation of the patient is mandatory.[6] A careful medical and ophthalmic history uncovers any possible local and systemic diseases that may contribute to the presenting orbital symptoms.

Measurement of visual acuity and current refraction is mandatory. A visual field test is required on all patients who have suspected orbital disease, especially if visual loss occurs.

The presence of periorbital edema or erythema, chemosis, ptosis, and decreased corneal or facial sensation is noted. The degree of proptosis, if any, and the direction of globe displacement are important to help localize orbital pathology. Ocular motility should be carefully measured and, if abnormal, a forced traction test performed to distinguish between paralytic and restrictive causes. The anterior orbit should be palpated for any abnormal masses behind the bony rim.

Modern orbital imaging techniques provide critical information on the specific location of lesions, as well as their relationship to adjacent structures (see Chapter 84). Echography allows the determination not only of topographical contours and surface characteristics but also of the consistency, gross internal structure, and vascularity, which may be difficult to detect with other techniques.[7,8] High-resolution orbital CT with contrast provides superb topographical data and structural details that often can pinpoint the diagnosis without further work-up; it is essential if there is any suggestion of bony involvement.[9] Orbital CT should be obtained in both axial and coronal orientations, with contrast enhancement and bone windows when indicated. Key information, not available with CT alone, may be provided by magnetic resonance imaging, particularly with surface coil technology and fat suppression techniques.

GENERAL TECHNIQUES

General techniques in orbital and lacrimal gland surgery require a thorough understanding of orbital anatomy and the relationships with paraorbital structures. More than for other ophthalmic procedures, orbital and lacrimal gland surgery demands strict respect for fascial planes, adequate exposure and visualization, a planned approach appropriate to the expected pathology, and concern for postoperative cosmesis. The surgeon must be well versed in both gross and microsurgical techniques and must not hesitate to involve other surgical subspecialists when appropriate. Gentle dissection is essential to avoid injury to delicate neurovascular structures; meticulous hemostasis is critical to prevent complications and even potential blindness.

The orbit may be approached through several surgical routes, all generally grouped under the term *orbitotomy*—literally, to cut into the orbit (Box 96-1). Since this term has no particular reference to bone, it may be applied to anterior incisions through the eyelid and lateral or other approaches through the orbital walls. Since the orbital septum represents the anatomically anteriormost layer of the orbital fascial system, any transeyelid surgery that is carried through the septum represents orbital surgery. The major approaches to the orbit are:
- Anterior transcutaneous orbitotomy;
- Lateral orbitotomy; and
- Superior orbitotomy.
The specific approach taken for each orbital procedure is determined primarily by:
- The nature of the pathology;
- The ultimate goals of surgery—whether diagnostic biopsy, palliative debulking, or complete excision;
- The location and size of the lesion; and
- The age or general medical condition of the patient.

For biopsy alone, a palpable anterior lesion usually can be reached through a small transcutaneous or transconjunctival incision. Removal of such a lesion, however, may require a much broader exposure, which may necessitate removal of the lateral orbital wall. Posterior or apical lesions, even when small, usually can be safely reached only via a craniotomy approach. Medial lesions are best approached from the medial side so as not to risk injury to the optic nerve and muscle cone by instruments passed through a lateral orbitotomy incision. The approach to malignant tumors must be carefully planned to avoid contaminating adjacent tissue fields. The biopsy site must be placed so as not to transcend uninvolved closed compartments and must be located within the zone of subsequent excision. When complete exci-

---

BOX 96-1

Orbital Surgery: General Techniques

ANTERIOR ORBIT
Anterior orbitotomy
Inferior orbitotomy

MID-ORBIT
Lateral orbitotomy
Medial orbitotomy

ORBITAL APEX
Superior orbitotomy-craniotomy

---

sion is required, the surgeon must be prepared to remove a wide section of normal tissue, including adjacent bone.

SPECIFIC TECHNIQUES

The orbitotomy procedures include a number of operations for access into the various orbital soft tissue compartments. The specific approach selected depends on the following[10,11]:
- The working diagnosis;
- The location of the pathology;
- Involvement of adjacent bone or paraorbital areas;
- The need for wide surgical margins; and
- The requirements for adequate exposure.

Three surgical spaces are of interest to the orbital surgeon, each of which requires specific consideration for appropriate visualization.[12] The subperiosteal compartment lies between the orbital bony walls and periorbita. Access to this space is necessary to repair orbital wall fractures or to decompress expanding orbital volume, as in Graves' orbitopathy. This is the location where subperiosteal hematomas, expanding mucoceles, and some intracranial lesions, such as sphenoid wing meningiomas, occur. Also, bone lesions, such as aneurysmal bone cysts, cholesteatomas, and eosinophilic granulomas, frequently are confined to the subperiosteal space.

The extraconal or peripheral orbital space lies between the periorbita and the fascial septa that interconnect the extraocular muscles. This septal system is far more complex than once believed[13,14]; it is unusual for lesions to be confined precisely to the extraconal space alone. Access to the peripheral space may be through a transcutaneous trans-septal orbitotomy, if in the anterior orbit, or through a lateral or transconjunctival medial orbitotomy, if deeper.

The intraconal or central orbital space is delimited by the extraocular muscle cone from the annulus of Zinn to the posterior Tenon's capsule. It is not a clearly defined compartment, however, since the intermuscular septum is largely incomplete posteriorly and poorly defined anteriorly. Lesions frequently extend between the extraconal and intraconal compartments without regard to these artificial boundaries.[6] Optic nerve gliomas and sheath meningiomas are located primarily within the muscle cone. The surgical approach is via a lateral orbitotomy for deep lesions and via a transconjunctival medial or lateral orbitotomy for lesions immediately behind the globe. Other types of approaches have been introduced for access to the orbital apex and posterior orbit.[15,16]

The specific surgical procedures described here are designed to give direct access to certain structures and to minimize trauma to adjacent tissues. The anterior orbitotomies are used to reach lesions in the anterior orbit to the level of the posterior globe. The transconjunctival route allows entrance directly into the extraconal space anywhere around the perimeter of the eye. With removal of an extraocular muscle and opening of Tenon's capsule, the intraconal compartment immediately behind the globe also becomes available.

Lateral orbitotomy involves removal of the lateral orbital rim and various amounts of the greater sphenoid wing. It allows

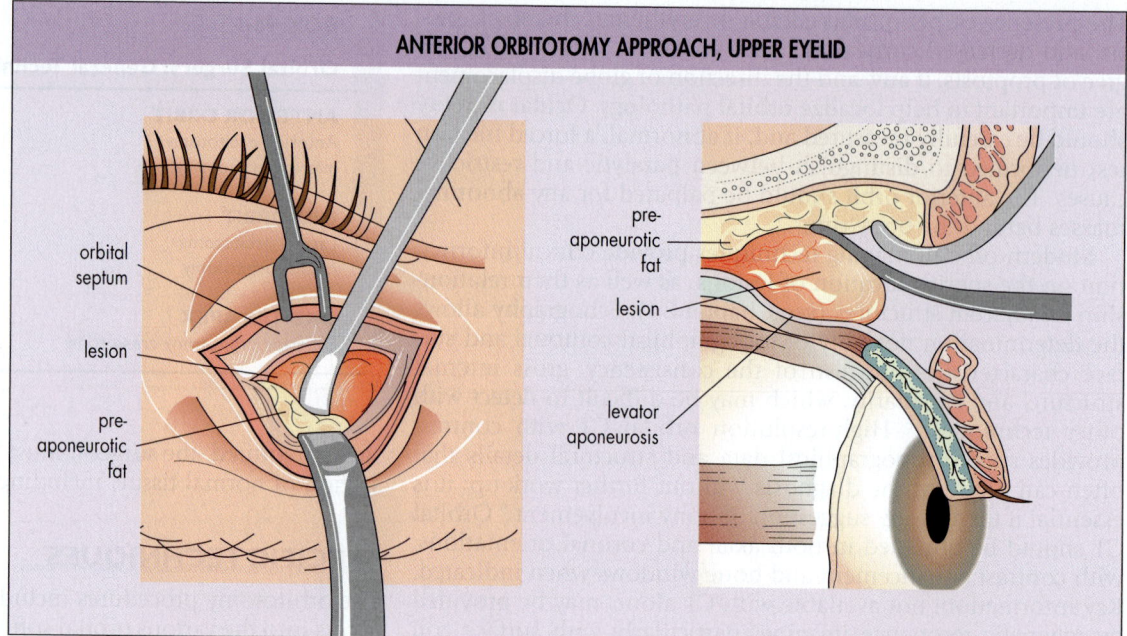

FIG. 96-1 ■ **Anterior orbitotomy approach, upper eyelid.** A lid crease incision is cut, and the orbital septum is opened. Fat is then retracted, and the lesion is identified for biopsy or removal. The anterior view is the inverted image as seen by the surgeon. (Adapted with permission from Dutton JJ. Atlas of ophthalmic surgery, vol II. Oculoplastic, lacrimal, and orbital surgery. St Louis: Mosby–Year Book; 1991.)

wide access to the deep orbital contents and optic nerve; it is preferred for most retrobulbar lesions. Extension of the superior bony cut gives better exposure to the lacrimal gland for *en bloc* excision within its fossa. The lateral orbitotomy may be combined with other approaches, for example, the medial orbitotomy, for better visualization of the deep medial wall.

Meticulous attention to hemostasis must be ensured throughout for visualization. After adequate exposure has been achieved, the dissection must proceed slowly and with great deliberation. Magnification and microdissection instruments are used to gently separate the lesion from adjacent normal structures. Light traction on the lesion usually is necessary to allow posterior dissection. This may be achieved with forceps, but for more vascular lesions, a cryoprobe allows traction without surface bleeding. Dissection around the optic nerve is particularly hazardous because of the delicate pial vessels that penetrate its surface and the close approximation of the posterior ciliary nerves.

Transcutaneous Anterior Orbitotomy

Transcutaneous anterior orbitotomy is used to access the anterior extraconal orbital space (see Chapter 83) to biopsy or excise small lesions located beneath the orbital rims.[17] With care and the use of retractors, deeper lesions to the level of the posterior globe are accessible.

An incision line is marked in the upper eyelid crease to access the superior orbit, or 2mm below the lower eyelid lash line to access the inferior orbit. The skin and orbicularis muscle are opened with scissors to enter the postorbicular fascial plane. A horizontal cut is made with a scalpel or scissors through the orbital septum to enter the extraconal orbital space. If the lesion is not visible immediately, careful palpation through the wound usually locates the structure.

The fat lobules are gently separated with narrow malleable retractors and a Freer periosteal elevator, taking care not to injure vascular structures (Fig. 96-1). In the upper eyelid, the levator muscle lies toward the superior side of the wound. In the lower eyelid, the inferior oblique and rectus muscles lie on the inferior side of the wound.

The lesion then may be biopsied or dissected carefully away from adherent tissues. All bleeding points are cauterized meticulously with bipolar electrode forceps; care is taken to avoid excessive traction on the orbital fat. The cutaneous wound is closed with a running suture of 6–0 nylon or silk or with interrupted stitches of 7–0 Vicryl or chromic gut.

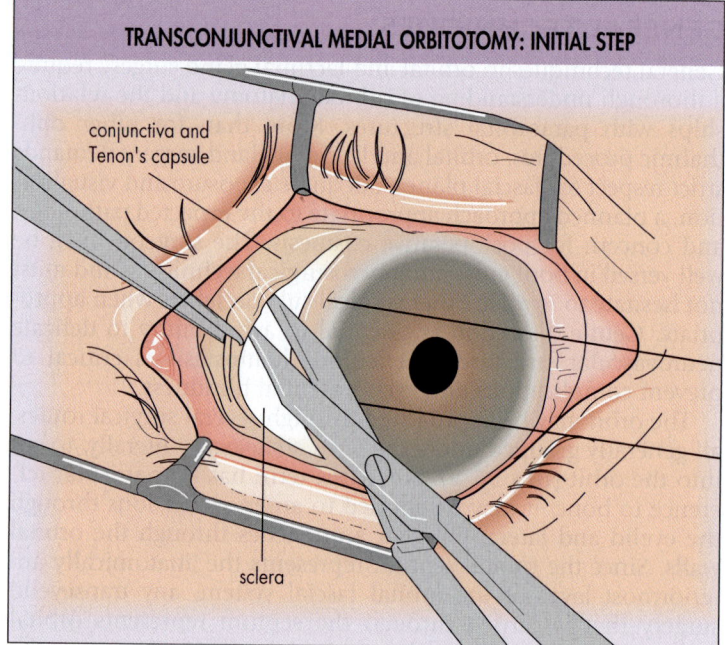

FIG. 96-2 ■ **Transconjunctival medial orbitotomy approach.** The conjunctiva is opened just anterior to the muscle insertion, and Tenon's capsule is separated from the sclera. (Adapted with permission from Dutton JJ. Atlas of ophthalmic surgery, vol II. Oculoplastic, lacrimal, and orbital surgery. St Louis: Mosby–Year Book; 1991.)

Transconjunctival Anterior Orbitotomy

The transconjunctival approach to the anterior orbit is useful for lesions close to the globe, for that portion of the optic nerve immediately posterior to the globe, and for most anteriorly situated intraconal lesions. It also avoids skin incisions that may be cosmetically objectionable in some patients.

An incision is made through conjunctiva and anterior Tenon's capsule, and the dissection is carried in the episcleral space to the posterior globe (Fig. 96-2). Disinsertion of one rectus muscle will facilitate deeper dissection (Fig. 96-3). The location of the incision depends on the location of the orbital lesion. Posterior Tenon's is opened to access the retrobulbar compartment. Malleable retractors and rotation of the globe will provide adequate visualization. In small orbits, however, working room and visualization may be very limited.

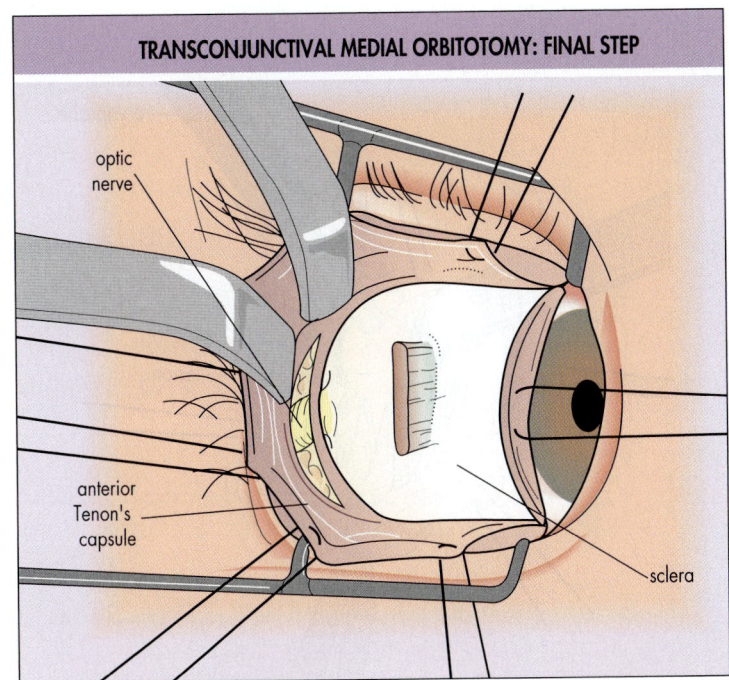

FIG. 96-3 ■ **Transconjunctival medial orbitotomy approach.** The globe is rotated, and malleable retractors are used to visualize the posterior Tenon's capsule. Opening of this layer gives access to the retrobulbar space. (Adapted with permission from Dutton JJ. Atlas of ophthalmic surgery, vol II. Oculoplastic, lacrimal, and orbital surgery. St Louis: Mosby–Year Book; 1991.)

FIG. 96-4 ■ **Lateral orbitotomy approach.** The lateral orbital rim is exposed, and the periorbita is elevated from the lateral orbital wall. (Adapted with permission from Dutton JJ. Atlas of ophthalmic surgery, vol II. Oculoplastic, lacrimal, and orbital surgery. St Louis: Mosby–Year Book; 1991.)

Lateral Orbitotomy

The lateral approach is used for deeper orbital lesions that cannot be reached through an anterior incision or that require wider exposure for excision. This gives excellent access to the midintraconal compartment, except for the extreme medial side.

A variety of skin incisions can be used, including an S-shaped rim incision, a horizontal canthal crease incision, or an eyelid crease incision.[18] The skin is cut with a scalpel blade, and the dissection is extended through orbicularis muscle and deep fascia to the periosteum of the orbital rim. Periosteum along the lateral orbital rim is cut and elevated from the lateral orbital wall for a distance of 3–4cm (Fig. 96-4). Similarly, periosteum is elevated from the temporal fossa to expose the zygomatic bone and greater wing of the sphenoid (see Chapter 83). Wide, malleable retractors are inserted on either side of the bony orbital rim at the level of the frontozygomatic suture line to protect the soft tissues. The bone is cut with an oscillating saw, angling the cut slightly inferiorly and parallel to the orbital roof. The cut is made about 1cm deep, into the thin bone along the sphenozygomatic suture line. A second cut is made through the orbital rim just above the zygomatic arch (Fig. 96-5). Small holes can be drilled on either side of each cut near the rim to facilitate later replacement of the bone. The bony rim is grasped with a sturdy rongeur between the cuts and fractured outward. The thin bone of the greater sphenoid wing is removed with rongeurs to provide adequate retrobulbar exposure (Fig. 96-6). The lateral rectus muscle is identified by grasping its insertion at the globe and rotating the eye medially. The periorbita is then opened with scissors by making a vertical cut just inferior or superior to the muscle.

The orbital fat is dissected gently by blunt separation of the interlobular capsules with a Freer elevator or dissectors. Once the lesion has been identified, it is dissected carefully from adjacent structures, with meticulous hemostasis maintained with gentle cautery or application of neuropathies moistened with epinephrine or thrombin. Traction on the lesion may be achieved with the use of a cryoprobe (Fig. 96-7). After biopsy or removal of the lesion, the periorbita is closed with interrupted sutures of 6–0 Vicryl, with several gaps left in the closure for drainage. The lateral orbital rim is replaced and secured with mi-

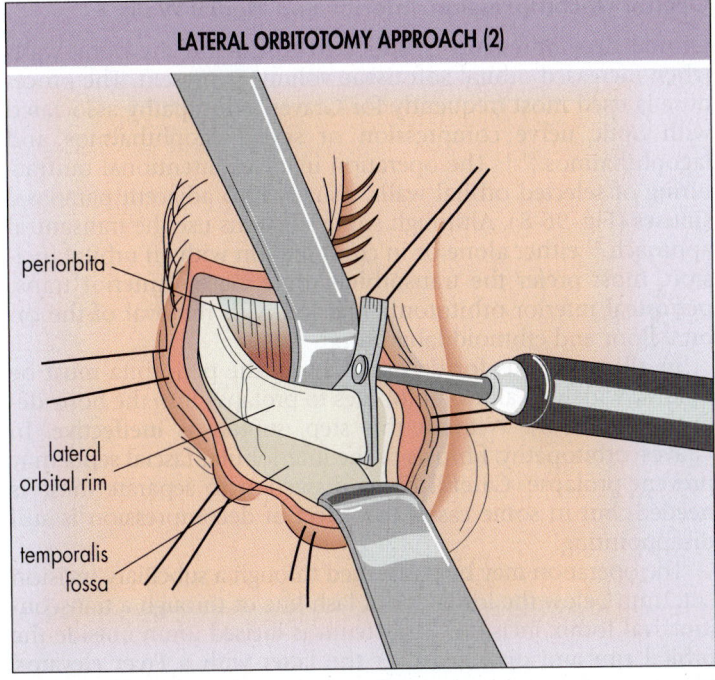

FIG. 96-5 ■ **Lateral orbitotomy approach.** After periosteum has been elevated from the temporal fossa, the lateral rim is cut. (Adapted with permission from Dutton JJ. Atlas of ophthalmic surgery, vol II. Oculoplastic, lacrimal, and orbital surgery. St Louis: Mosby–Year Book; 1991.)

croplate fixation or with 4–0 Prolene or nylon sutures passed through the predrilled holes. Periosteum is closed over the orbital rim with interrupted stitches of 4–0 Vicryl. The orbicularis muscle is approximated with 6–0 chromic gut and the skin with 6–0 nylon or silk vertical mattress sutures.

A firm, but not tight, dressing is placed over the orbit for 24 hours. Systemic corticosteroids may be administered for several days, especially if any manipulation around the optic nerve was carried out. Antibiotic ointment is applied to the suture line four times daily for 1 week. The skin sutures are removed after 5–7 days.

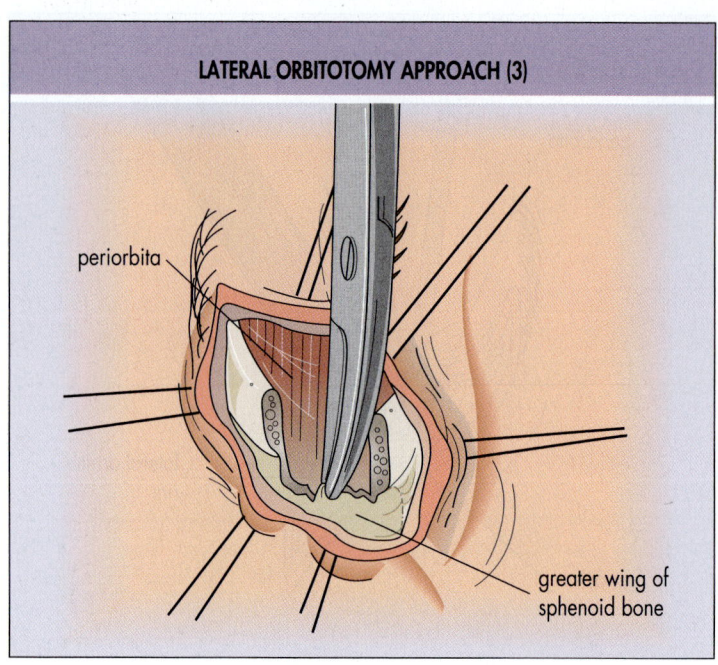

FIG. 96-6 ■ **Lateral orbitotomy approach.** The greater sphenoid wing is removed to provide adequate exposure of the deep orbit. (Adapted with permission from Dutton JJ. Atlas of ophthalmic surgery, vol II. Oculoplastic, lacrimal, and orbital surgery. St Louis: Mosby–Year Book; 1991.)

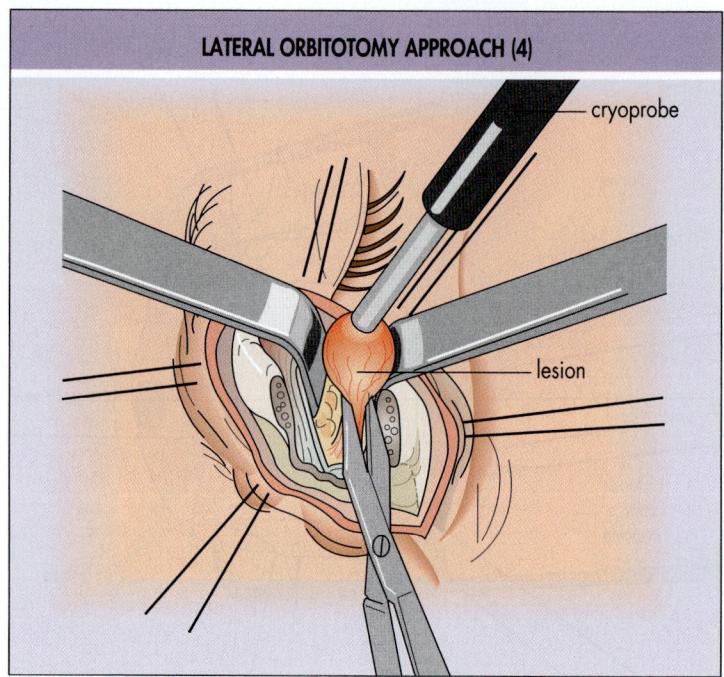

FIG. 96-7 ■ **Lateral orbitotomy approach.** The periorbita is opened, and the lesion is located using gentle dissection. A cryoprobe facilitates removal without surface bleeding. (Adapted with permission from Dutton JJ. Atlas of ophthalmic surgery, vol II. Oculoplastic, lacrimal, and orbital surgery. St Louis: Mosby–Year Book; 1991.)

Orbital Decompression: Inferior and Medial Walls

Orbital decompression is indicated to expand the bony walls when increased orbital soft tissue volume is present. The procedure is used most frequently for Graves' orbitopathy associated with optic nerve compression or severe exophthalmos and lagophthalmos.[19–22] The operation involves intentional outfracturing of selected orbital walls, usually into adjacent paranasal sinuses (Fig. 96-8). Although some surgeons use the transantral approach,[23] either alone or in combination with an orbital incision, most prefer the transorbital route via an anterior transperiosteal inferior orbitotomy incision with removal of the orbital floor and ethmoid labyrinth.[20]

In all operations for decompression, the periorbita must be opened widely to allow fat lobules to prolapse into the bony defects (Fig. 96-8). Without this step, surgery is ineffective. In Graves' orbitopathy, fibrosis of the interlobular fascial septa may prevent prolapse. Careful blunt dissection to separate these is needed, but in some cases, the effect of decompression is still disappointing.

The operation may be performed through a subciliary incision cut 2mm below the lower eyelid lash line or through a transconjunctival fornix incision. Periosteum is incised 2mm outside the orbital rim and dissected over the latter with a Freer elevator. Elevation of periorbita is continued along the orbital floor for a distance of 3.5–4cm posterior to the rim (Fig. 96-9). The thinnest part of the floor is located medial to the infraorbital canal; a small hole is punched through this area with a hemostat. The orbital floor medial to the infraorbital canal is removed with rongeurs (Fig. 96-10). Additional bone is removed back to the posterior wall of the maxillary sinus, medially to the maxillary-ethmoid suture, and laterally to the edge of the infraorbital tissue. The author prefers to leave a narrow bridge of bone over the infraorbital nerve to prevent postoperative injury from displaced orbital contents.

The periorbita is sutured to periosteum over the inferior orbital rim with interrupted sutures of 4–0 Vicryl. Skin and conjunctiva are closed with a running suture.

A firm dressing is applied for 24 hours. Antibiotic ointment is placed on the suture line four times daily for 7 days. Systemic antibiotics and nasal decongestants are prescribed for 1 week. The skin sutures are removed after 5–7 days.

Repair of Orbital Floor Fractures

Blowout fractures of the orbital floor result from hydraulic compression of orbital contents[24] and perhaps from deformation forces transmitted directly from the orbital rims. These occur most frequently just medial to the infraorbital canal, where the bone is thinnest.[25,26] Paresthesias of the cheek and upper gum suggest a more central fracture with injury to the infraorbital nerve. Spontaneous recovery of sensation usually occurs after several months. Vertical diplopia and a positive forced traction test suggest mechanical restriction, with entrapment of the inferior rectus muscle or, more likely, of its fascial attachments in the inferior orbit.[27] However, vertical diplopia and a positive forced traction test also may be seen with contusion injuries to the muscle,[28] in which case motility function typically improves over several weeks as the hematoma resolves.[29,30] Failure to improve over several weeks suggests mechanical restriction that requires surgical exploration.

Early enophthalmos is caused by outward displacement of the orbital contour with an increase in volume of the orbital cavity. It may be associated with downward displacement of the globe when the fracture site involves primarily the orbital floor. Enophthalmos or hypo-ophthalmos alone usually does not cause diplopia, but it may be of cosmetic consequence. When significant, this is an indication for early surgical intervention.[31,32] Associated orbital hemorrhage initially can mask enophthalmos, which may become manifest only after several weeks, when the hematoma resolves. Late enophthalmos, which may occur over several years or even over several decades, results from progressive fat atrophy. This is repaired using volume augmentation of the orbital contents.

Medial wall fractures are often associated with those of the orbital floor and most often result in orbital emphysema. Medial rectus muscle entrapment is uncommon, but it may produce a horizontal diplopia. Enophthalmos may be significant even with pure ethmoid fractures. Injury to the lacrimal drainage system may be seen with more anterior medial rim or nasomaxillary fractures.

Before contemplating any surgical intervention, radiographic imaging is essential. In most cases, CT in both the axial and coronal planes and with bone window settings helps determine which

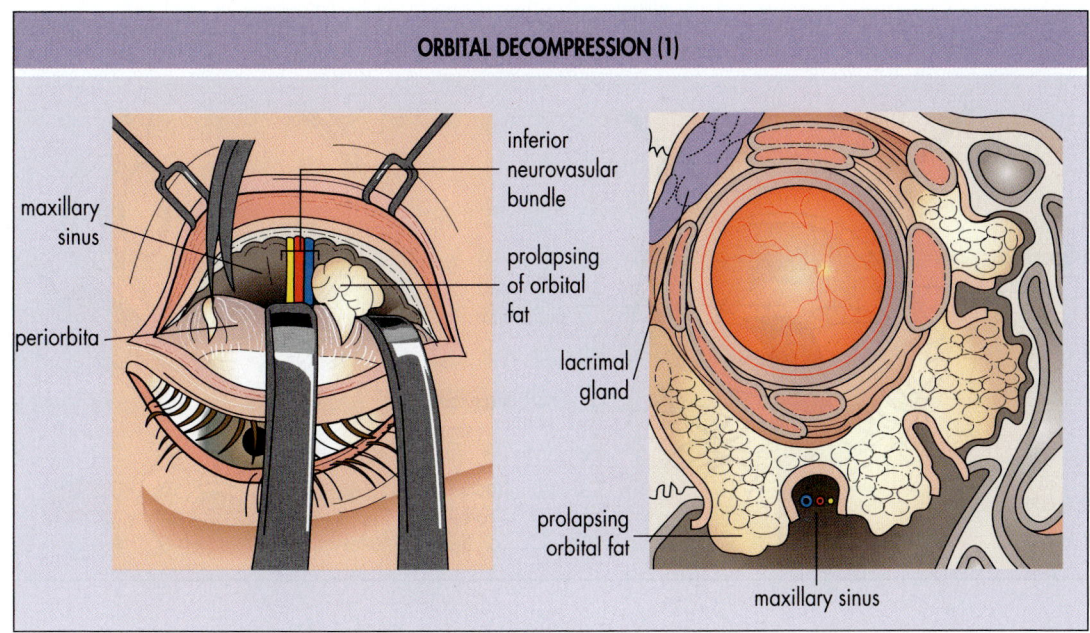

ORBITAL DECOMPRESSION (1)

maxillary sinus

periorbita

inferior neurovasular bundle

prolapsing of orbital fat

lacrimal gland

prolapsing orbital fat

maxillary sinus

FIG. 96-8 ■ Orbital decompression. The orbital floor and medial wall are removed. The periorbita is then opened to allow fat to prolapse into the adjacent sinuses. The anterior view is the inverted image as seen by the surgeon. (Adapted with permission from Dutton JJ. Atlas of ophthalmic surgery, vol II. Oculoplastic, lacrimal, and orbital surgery. St Louis: Mosby–Year Book; 1991.)

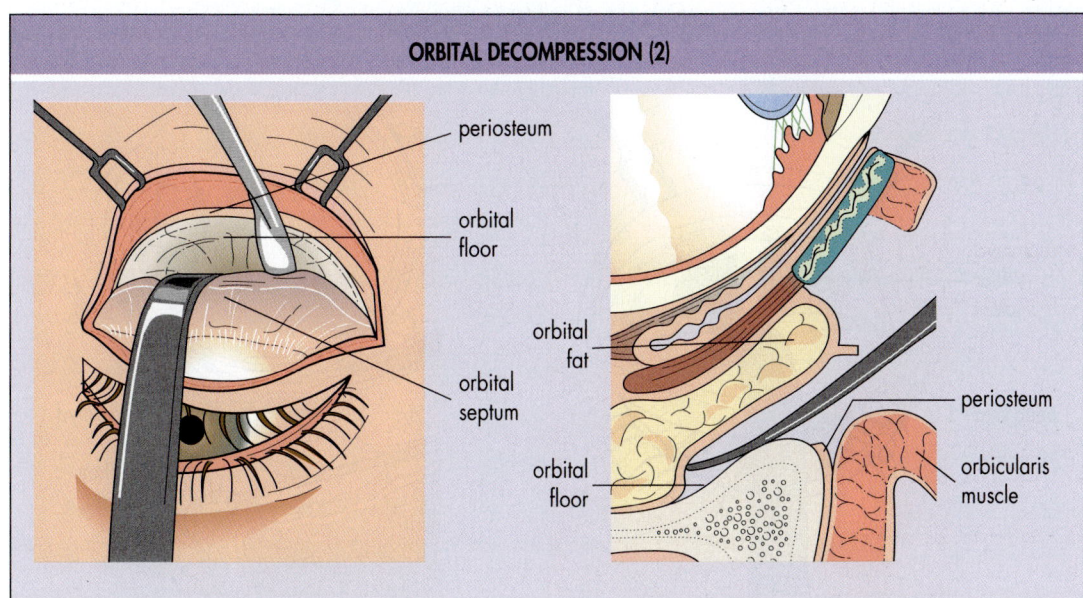

ORBITAL DECOMPRESSION (2)

periosteum

orbital floor

orbital septum

orbital fat

orbital floor

periosteum

orbicularis muscle

FIG. 96-9 ■ Orbital decompression. A skin or conjunctival incision is used to expose the inferior orbital rim. The periorbita is elevated to expose the orbital floor. The anterior view is the inverted image as seen by the surgeon. (Adapted with permission from Dutton JJ. Atlas of ophthalmic surgery, vol II. Oculoplastic, lacrimal, and orbital surgery. St Louis: Mosby–Year Book; 1991.)

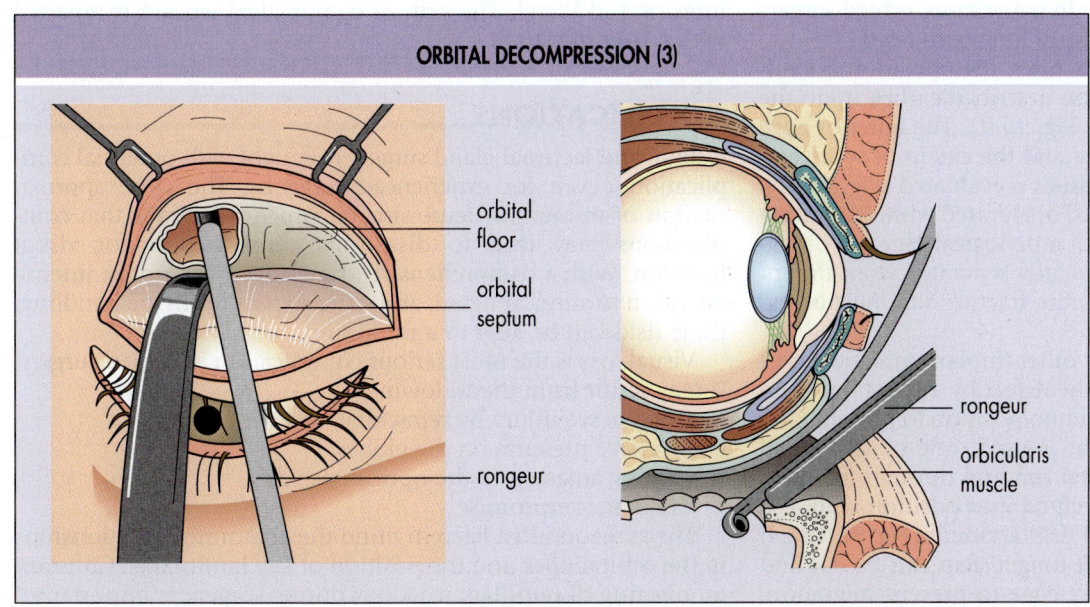

ORBITAL DECOMPRESSION (3)

orbital floor

orbital septum

rongeur

rongeur

orbicularis muscle

FIG. 96-10 ■ Orbital decompression. The floor is removed using rongeurs. The maxillary sinus is then exposed. The anterior view is the inverted image as seen by the surgeon. (Adapted with permission from Dutton JJ. Atlas of ophthalmic surgery, vol II. Oculoplastic, lacrimal, and orbital surgery. St Louis: Mosby–Year Book; 1991.)

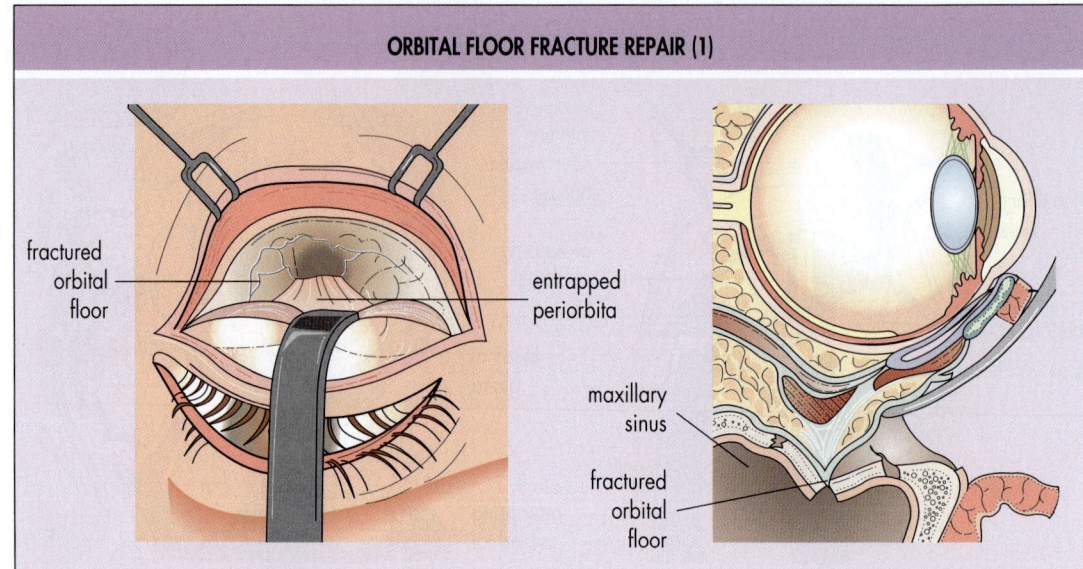

FIG. 96-11 ■ Orbital floor fracture repair. The floor is exposed as for orbital decompression. The fracture site is identified, and any soft tissue incarceration is freed. The anterior view is the inverted image as seen by the surgeon. (Adapted with permission from Dutton JJ. Atlas of ophthalmic surgery, vol II. Oculoplastic, lacrimal, and orbital surgery. St Louis: Mosby–Year Book; 1991.)

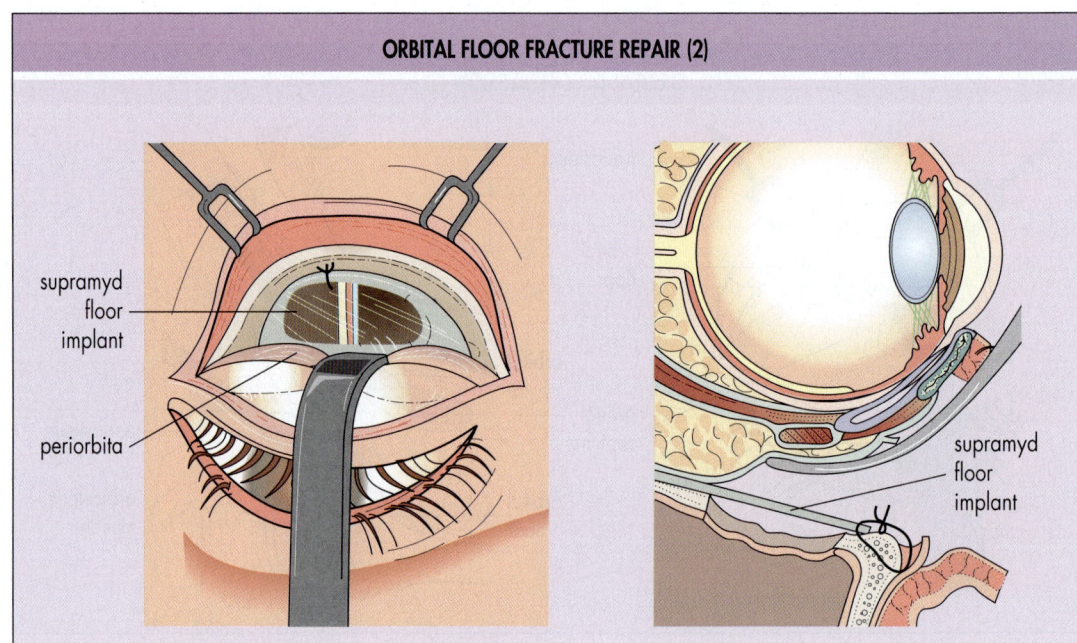

FIG. 96-12 ■ Orbital floor fracture repair. A suitable floor implant is placed over the defect and fixed in position. The anterior view is the inverted image as seen by the surgeon. (Adapted with permission from Dutton JJ. Atlas of ophthalmic surgery, vol II. Oculoplastic, lacrimal, and orbital surgery. St Louis: Mosby–Year Book; 1991.)

cases require immediate repair and which are likely to improve using medical management alone.[33,34] In many cases, orbital surgery can be avoided, with no compromise of long-term results.[35,36]

For the repair of orbital floor fractures, the operation is similar to that for orbital decompression described earlier, up to the stage of exposure of the floor (see Fig. 96-9). The anterior edge of the fracture site is then exposed, and the extent of incarceration of the periorbita and fascial tissues is evaluated (Fig. 96-11). Bony fragments are gently depressed or elevated while periorbita and fat lobules are teased free with a periosteal elevator or microdissector. Orbital tissues are carefully separated from the infraorbital nerve and vessels. The entire fracture site must be exposed to its posterior limit.

A piece of Supramyd, Teflon, or other implant material is cut to a size large enough to overlap the defect by at least 5mm on all sides. It is best to fix the implant into position to prevent later migration.[37] If a full floor implant is used, one or two small holes are drilled through the orbital rim and through the front of the implant, and the latter is secured into position with 4–0 Prolene sutures to prevent forward displacement (Fig. 96-12). If a smaller implant is used, a small tongue flap can be cut and pushed beneath the anterior defect edge to prevent migration.

Periosteum is closed over the orbital rim with interrupted sutures of 4–0 Vicryl. The skin or conjunctival wound is repaired with a running stitch.

COMPLICATIONS

Orbital and lacrimal gland surgery is fraught with potential complications, even for experienced surgeons. The close approximation of numerous neurovascular structures means that complications may lead to disastrous consequences for visual function. With a comprehensive knowledge of anatomy, intense attention to surgical detail, and strict respect for tissue handling, these risks can be kept to a minimum.

Visual loss is the most serious complication of orbital surgery. It may result from the following:
- Optic nerve injury by retractors;
- Excessive pressure on the globe;
- Cautery adjacent to the optic nerve; or
- Vascular compromise.

The surgeon must keep in mind the anatomical relationships in the orbital apex and the position of key landmarks. Constant monitoring of pupillary reactions during surgery is important.

Postoperative orbital hemorrhage is a rare complication that largely can be avoided by meticulous attention to hemostasis during surgery. Excessive traction on orbital fat should be avoided, and bone wax must be applied to any vessels retracted into bony canals. An expanding postoperative hematoma is heralded by progressive proptosis, deep orbital pain, and decreasing vision. The combination of CT and echography helps localize the blood pocket. Treatment may require immediate surgical decompression, either through the original surgical wound or through an alternative, more direct route to the hematoma.

A cerebrospinal fluid (CSF) leak may occur with any surgery on the anterior medial orbital wall carried above the level of the frontoethmoid suture line and causing injury to the cribriform plate. If minimal, it may be treated conservatively, as for CSF rhinorrhea. Alternatively, the leakage site may be packed with fat or sealed with cyanoacrylate glue, and a lumbar drain may be placed. The patient should be provided with appropriate antibiotics.

Diplopia is a constant risk with any surgery adjacent to extraocular muscles or their motor nerves. Muscle sheaths should be left intact whenever possible, and traction sutures across the muscle bellies must be avoided. The inferior oblique muscle is particularly vulnerable where it lies immediately behind the orbital septum, just inside the inferior orbital rim. It may not be recognized by an inattentive orbital surgeon. In the superior medial orbit, the superior oblique trochlea is injured easily by overly aggressive periorbital dissection. When extraocular muscle dysfunction fails to resolve over 3–4 months, strabismus surgery may be required.

Upper eyelid ptosis occurs almost universally following most surgery on the orbit. In most cases, this is transient and usually resolves over days to weeks. Permanent ptosis may result from injury to the aponeurosis, Whitnall's ligament, or the superior division of the oculomotor nerve. If the ptosis does not resolve within 3–4 months, surgical repair may be necessary.

Lower eyelid ectropion, epiblepharon, and other eyelid malpositions may result from injury to the capsulopalpebral fascia or scarring of the orbital septum. These disorders are rarely seen in younger individuals but are more common in older patients who have preexisting eyelid laxity. The appropriate dissection planes should be maintained in all dissections carried through these structures, similar to the techniques applied in eyelid surgery.

OUTCOME

With appropriate planning and surgical technique, orbital surgery yields a high degree of success and few permanent complications. Visual function usually is improved, cosmetic appearance is enhanced, and life-threatening conditions can be eliminated. In some cases, however, vision or cosmesis must be compromised in favor of preservation of life. Such decisions should always be made with the complete understanding and participation of the patient. Occasionally, less radical surgery may be undertaken, even in the face of serious pathology, as dictated by the patient's age, physical condition, and visual status of the contralateral eye.

REFERENCES

1. Kennerdell JS, Slamovitz TL, Dekker A, Johnson DL. Orbital fine needle aspiration biopsy. Am J Ophthalmol. 1985;99:547–51.
2. Dresner SC, Kennerdell JS, Dekker A. Fine needle aspiration biopsy of metastatic tumors. Surv Ophthalmol. 1983;27:397–8.
3. Spoor TC, Kennerdell JS, Dekker A, et al. Orbital fine needle aspiration biopsy with B-scan guidance. Am J Ophthalmol. 1980;89:274–7.
4. Krohel GB, Tobin DR, Chavis RM. Inaccuracy of fine-needle aspiration biopsy (FNAB). Ophthalmology. 1985;92:666–70.
5. Henderson JW. Orbital tumors. Philadelphia: WB Saunders; 1973.
6. Rootman J. Diseases of the orbit. A multidisciplinary approach. Philadelphia: JB Lippincott; 1988.
7. Byrne SF. Standardized echography in the differentiation of orbital lesions. Surv Ophthalmol. 1984;29:226–8.
8. Levine RA. Orbital ultrasonography. Radiol Clin North Am. 1987;25:447–69.
9. Dutton JJ. Radiographic evaluation of the orbit. In: Doxanas MT, Anderson RL, eds. Clinical orbital anatomy. Baltimore: Williams & Wilkins; 1984:8035–56.
10. Leone CR Jr. Surgical approaches to the orbit. Ophthalmology. 1979;86:930–41.
11. Krohel GB. Orbital surgery. In: Smith BC, Della Rocca RC, Nesi FA, Lisman RD, eds. Ophthalmic plastic and reconstructive surgery. St Louis: CV Mosby; 1987.
12. Dutton JJ. Atlas of clinical and surgical anatomy. Philadelphia: WB Saunders; 1994.
13. Koornneef L. Details of the orbital connective tissue system in the adult. Acta Morphol Neerl Scand. 1977;15:1–34.
14. Koornneef L. Orbital septa: anatomy and function. Ophthalmology. 1979;86:876–80.
15. Goldberg RA, Shorr N, Arnold AC, Garcia GH. Deep transorbital approach to the apex and cavernous sinus. Ophthal Plast Reconstr Surg. 1998;14:336–41.
16. Kennerdell JS, Maroon JC, Celin SF. The posterior inferior orbitotomy. Ophthal Plast Reconstr Surg. 1998;14:277–80.
17. Dutton JJ. Atlas of ophthalmic surgery, vol II. Oculoplastic, lacrimal, and orbital surgery. St Louis: Mosby–Year Book; 1991.
18. Harris GJ, Logani SC. Eyelid crease incision for lateral orbitotomy. Ophthal Plast Reconstr Surg. 1999;15:9–16.
19. Linberg JV, Anderson RL. Transorbital decompression: indications and results. Arch Ophthalmol. 1981;99:113–9.
20. Anderson RL, Linberg JV. Transorbital approach to decompression in Graves' disease. Arch Ophthalmol. 1981;99:120–4.
21. Kennerdell JS, Maroon JC. An orbital decompression for severe dysthyroid exophthalmos. Ophthalmology. 1982;89:467–72.
22. McCord CD. Orbital decompression for Graves' disease. Ophthalmology. 1981;88:533–41.
23. Ogura JH, Thawley SC. Orbital decompression for exophthalmos. Otolaryngol Clin North Am. 1980;13:29–38.
24. Smith B, Regan WFJ. Blow-out fracture of the orbit. Mechanism and correction of internal orbital fracture. Am J Ophthalmol. 1957;44:733–8.
25. Gilbard SM, Mafee MF, Lagouros PA, Langer BG. Orbital blowout fractures. The prognostic significance of computed tomography. Ophthalmology. 1985;92:1523–8.
26. Greenwald HS, Keeney AR, Shannon GM. A review of 128 patients with orbital fractures. Am J Ophthalmol. 1974;78:655–64.
27. Koornneef L. Current concepts on the management of orbital blow-out fractures. Ann Plast Surg. 1982;9:185–200.
28. Putterman AM, Stevens T, Urist MJ. Nonsurgical management of blow-out fractures of the orbital floor. Am J Ophthalmol. 1974;77:232–9.
29. Putterman AM. Late management of blow-out fractures of the orbital floor. Trans Am Acad Ophthalmol Otolaryngol. 1977;83:650–9.
30. Putterman AM. Management of blow-out fractures of the orbital floor. III. The conservative approach. Surv Ophthalmol. 1991;35:292–5.
31. Wilkins RB, Havins WE. Current treatment of blow-out fractures. Ophthalmology. 1982;89:464–6.
32. Manson PN, Iliff N. Management of blow-out fractures of the orbital floor. II. Early repair for selected injuries. Surv Ophthalmol. 1991;35:280–92.
33. Grove AS Jr, Tadmore R, New PF, Momose KJ. Orbital fracture evaluation by coronal computed tomography. Am J Ophthalmol. 1978;85:679–85.
34. Dutton JJ. Management of blow-out fractures of the orbital floor. I. Editorial comment. Surv Ophthalmol. 1991;35:279–80.
35. Emery JM, von Noorden GK, Schlernitzauer DA. Orbital floor fractures: long-term follow-up of cases with and without surgical repair. Trans Am Acad Ophthalmol Otolaryngol. 1971;75:802–12.
36. Putterman AM. Dr. Alan M. Putterman on the subject of blow-out fractures of the orbital floor. Ophthal Plast Reconstr Surg. 1985;1:73–74.
37. Smith B, Putterman AM. Fixation of orbital floor implants: description of a simple technique. Arch Ophthalmol. 1970;83:598.

97

Enucleation, Evisceration, and Exenteration

MYRON TANENBAUM

DEFINITIONS
- Enucleation: surgical removal of the entire globe
- Evisceration: surgical removal of the entire contents of the globe leaving a scleral shell
- Exenteration: removal of the entire orbit including the globe, eyelid, and orbital contents—usually performed for malignant tumors

INTRODUCTION

Enucleation, evisceration, and exenteration surgery all involve the permanent removal of the patient's eye. In this chapter the important aspects of each procedure are emphasized, including:
- Indications for surgery
- Preoperative patient counseling
- Surgical techniques
- Postoperative management
- Complications of surgery

PREOPERATIVE EVALUATION AND DIAGNOSTIC APPROACH

Indications for Surgery

Enucleation or evisceration surgery may be indicated for a blind painful eye, endophthalmitis, or cosmetic improvement of a deformed eye. In cases of intraocular neoplasms or the treatment of severe ocular trauma with a ruptured globe, where sympathetic ophthalmia is a concern, enucleation is appropriate and evisceration is contraindicated. Other indications for enucleation may include progressive phthisis bulbi and severe microphthalmia.

In the vast majority of situations, the indication for exenteration surgery is to eradicate life-threatening malignancy or life-threatening orbital infection. The extent of the procedure should be explained to the patient, especially which tissues are to be removed (this includes the eyeball, orbital soft tissues, and part or all of the eyelid structures). The surgeon should avoid lengthy discussions regarding the "mutilating" nature of the procedure but rather should help support the patient to remain focused on the treatment of this potentially life-threatening problem through the life-saving nature of the exenteration surgery.

A summary of the indications for surgery is given in Box 97-1.

Preoperative Counseling

Faced with the permanent loss of an eye, a patient requires the physician's reassurance, caring explanations, and psychological support, both before and after the surgery. The patient (and family) should understand that evisceration and enucleation surgery involve the complete, permanent removal of the diseased or deformed eye. The general nature of the anophthalmic socket should be explained to the patient, who must be informed that an ocular prosthesis will be fitted secondarily approximately 6 weeks following the surgery. The indication for surgery, whether it is pain, poor visual prognosis, the risk of sympathetic ophthalmia, or the presence of an intraocular neoplasm, should be clearly explained. The patient should be informed of the choices between enucleation and evisceration surgery and of the availability of a variety of orbital implants, including common alloplastic implants[1,2] (e.g., polymethyl methacrylate sphere), newer implants designed to maximize ultimate ocular prosthesis motility[3-6] (e.g., hydroxyapatite implants), or autologous tissue orbital implants[7-10] (e.g., dermis-fat grafts).

The patient should understand the risks and benefits of wrapping orbital implants with either autologous tissues or preserved donor tissue and that donor tissues may carry the risks of communicable diseases, such as syphilis, hepatitis, and human immunodeficiency virus. It should be explained to the patient that if a hydroxyapatite implant is used in primary enucleation or evisceration surgery, a delayed second-stage procedure (i.e., second-stage drilling of the hydroxyapatite implant with placement of the motility peg) may be needed in order to maximize the ocular prosthesis motility. A thorough explanation allows the patient and family to make a well-informed decision regarding surgery. Although the specific decision for surgery is to be made by the patient and family, it is reasonable for the surgeon to make a best-judgment recommendation to help with the myriad of choices available (e.g., enucleation versus evisceration and the variety of types of orbital implants).

Following enucleation or evisceration, most patients undergo a grief reaction to varying degrees. The patient, therefore, requires psychological support from the physician. The exenteration candidate must also be informed of the nature of the surgery and the more radical amount of tissue to be resected. Although the patient must be given a full and truthful explanation regarding exenteration surgery, the surgeon should avoid overly gruesome details so as not to deter inadvertently the patient from receiving necessary treatment, such as for a potentially life-threatening neoplasm.

Removal of the Wrong Eye

Removal of the wrong eye presents one of the greatest disasters that can occur to the ophthalmic surgeon and patient. Every ophthalmologist and surgeon must be aware of this possibility, no matter how remote. Preoperatively, the surgeon may mark the forehead or trim the lashes on the appropriate side. These methods, however, are not foolproof. In the operating room, the surgeon should thoroughly review the chart, including the operative permit and the examination notes. It is important, then, that the surgeon him- or herself prepares and drapes the patient. Traquair[11] suggested the use of local anesthesia to prevent removal of the wrong eye, although not even this method is fail-safe. It must never, never happen that a surgeon hurries into the

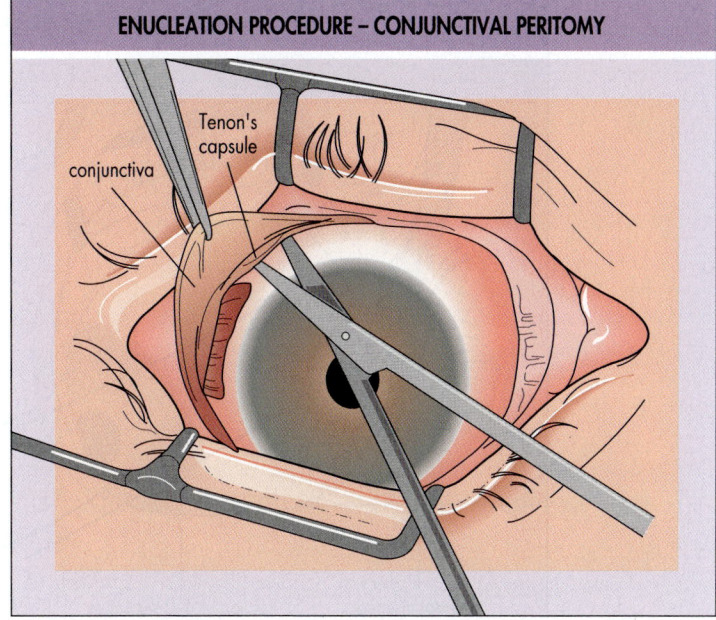

ENUCLEATION PROCEDURE – CONJUNCTIVAL PERITOMY

Tenon's capsule

conjunctiva

FIG. 97-1 ■ **Enucleation procedure.** Following a 360° conjunctival peritomy, a small pair of tenotomy scissors is used to dissect bluntly Tenon's fascia in all four quadrants.

operating room where the patient is already under general anesthesia and begins the operation without an appropriate review of the situation.

Once a sterile operative field is set up, the surgeon must again verify that the correct eye is about to undergo enucleation. Following severe trauma, the correct eye is often externally deformed. In cases where the external appearance of both eyes is normal, the surgeon must compulsively reexamine the fundus to verify the pathology.

The finality of the enucleation procedure cannot be overstressed. No degree of thoroughness is excessive in order to avoid removal of the wrong eye.

ANESTHESIA

Enucleation surgery usually is performed using local anesthesia. For psychological reasons, and occasionally for medical reasons, general anesthesia may be employed. Under any circumstance, agents should be used that maximize intraoperative hemostasis, suppress the oculocardiac reflex,[12] and minimize postoperative pain. The author's choice is to instill 10% phenylephrine eyedrops into the conjunctival cul-de-sac to achieve intense vasoconstriction, and to infiltrate extensive retrobulbar and peribulbar bupivacaine 0.5% with epinephrine (adrenaline) 1:100,000 and hyaluronidase. After adequate time, an excellent anesthetic and vasoconstrictive effect is achieved.

Most evisceration surgeries are also performed under local anesthesia with intravenous sedation. A mixture of lidocaine (lignocaine) 2% with epinephrine 1:100,000, bupivacaine 0.5% with 1:100,000 epinephrine, and hyaluronidase is injected in retrobulbar fashion into the muscle cone. The use of intravenous anesthetic sedatives prevents either the local anesthetic injection or the surgical procedure itself from being unpleasant or producing anxiety. Exenteration surgery is usually performed under general anesthesia, which may be combined with bupivacaine and epinephrine infiltration to aid hemostasis and provide postoperative analgesia.

SPECIFIC TECHNIQUES

Enucleation

The indications for enucleation surgery and important aspects of preoperative counseling have already been discussed. Here two surgical techniques are described:

- Enucleation with placement of a simple sphere implant

- Enucleation with placement of a sclera-wrapped hydroxyapatite implant for improved motility

Before describing the specifics of enucleation surgery, a few aspects in regard to Tenon's fascia must be mentioned. Tenon's capsule is the fibroelastic tissue that surrounds the eye and extraocular muscles in the anterior orbit (see Chapter 83). Anteriorly, Tenon's fascia fuses with the conjunctiva near the corneal limbus. At its posterior extent, Tenon's fascia encircles and fuses with the dura over the optic nerve. The four recti muscles originate from the annulus of Zinn and extend anteriorly to the eyeball. Posterior to the equator of the globe, the rectus muscles penetrate through Tenon's capsule before inserting into the sclera. That part of Tenon's fascia anterior to the rectus muscles is anterior Tenon's, and that part of Tenon's fascia posterior to the site of the rectus muscle penetrations is posterior Tenon's. It is critically important to understand this anatomical concept in order to achieve the proper, desirable orbital implant placement during enucleation surgery.

ENUCLEATION WITH SIMPLE SPHERE IMPLANT. A self-retaining lid speculum is placed to expose the entire epibulbar surface. A 360° conjunctival peritomy is performed (Fig. 97-1). Tenon's fascia is bluntly dissected away from the sclera in all four quadrants. Each of the four rectus muscles is sequentially gathered on a muscle hook, secured with double-armed 6-0 Vicryl suture, and detached from the globe. The superior oblique tendon is severed and detached from the globe. The inferior oblique muscle should be hooked and secured with a 6-0 Vicryl suture, detached, and saved for later attachment to the inferior border of the lateral rectus muscle. This use of the inferior oblique muscle is perhaps more important as an eventual "hammock" for the orbital implant than to enhance meaningfully anophthalmic socket motility.

After the extraocular muscles are detached, the surgeon is ready to sever the optic nerve. Anterior traction on the globe is useful when cutting the optic nerve and can be achieved with a curved hemostat applied to the medial rectus tendon or with a double-armed 4-0 silk suture sewn through the medial and lateral tendon insertions. In most cases it is the author's preference to clamp the optic nerve with a curved hemostat inserted behind the globe in the superonasal direction (Fig. 97-2). With the hemostat in place, a slender curved Metzenbaum scissors is used to

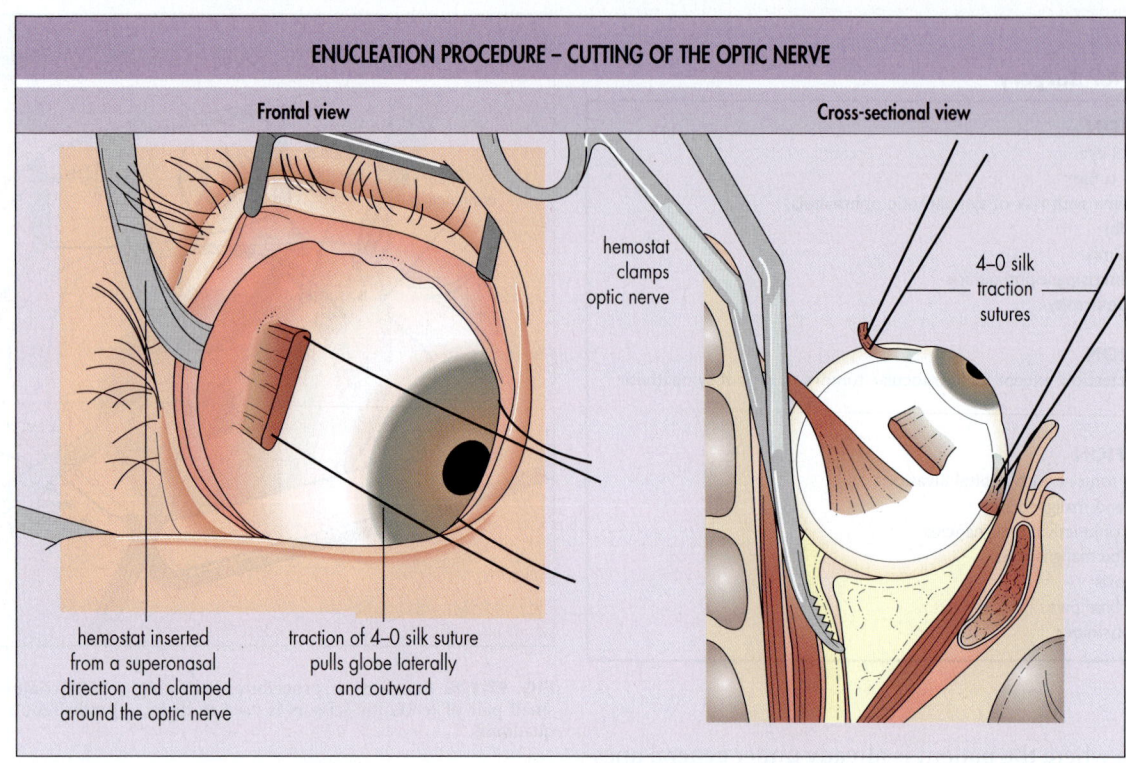

ENUCLEATION PROCEDURE – CUTTING OF THE OPTIC NERVE

Frontal view

Cross-sectional view

hemostat clamps optic nerve

4–0 silk traction sutures

hemostat inserted from a superonasal direction and clamped around the optic nerve

traction of 4–0 silk suture pulls globe laterally and outward

FIG. 97-2 ■ **Each of the four rectus muscles is tagged with a double-armed 6-0 Vicryl suture and detached from the globe.** Some 4-0 silk sutures may be placed through the medial and lateral recti muscle stumps to provide anterior traction on the globe, as a slender curved hemostat is used to clamp the optic nerve.

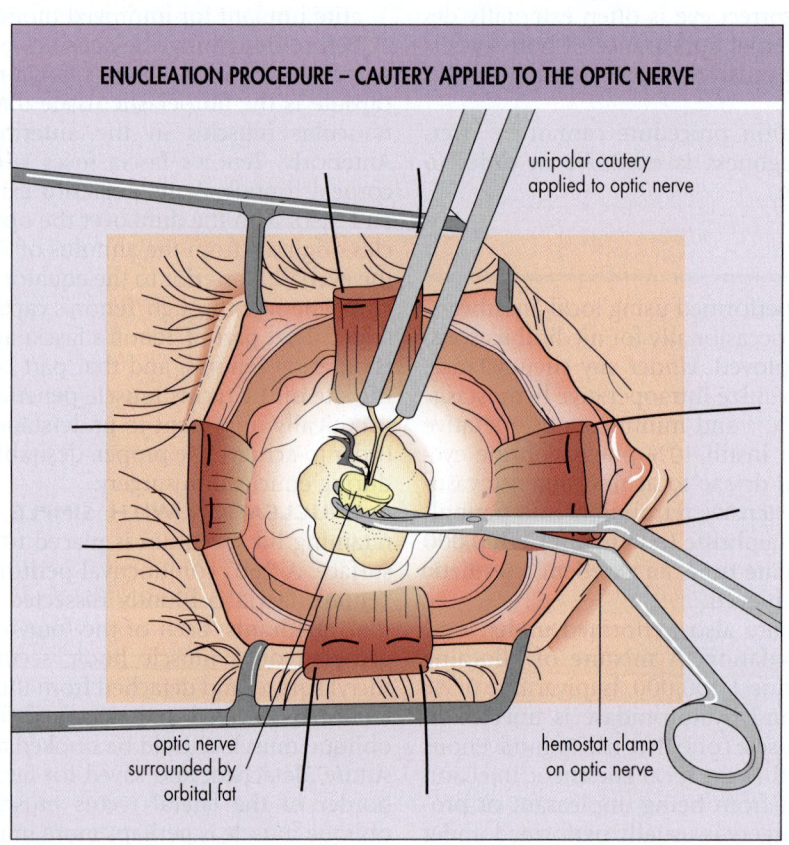

ENUCLEATION PROCEDURE – CAUTERY APPLIED TO THE OPTIC NERVE

unipolar cautery applied to optic nerve

optic nerve surrounded by orbital fat

hemostat clamp on optic nerve

FIG. 97-3 ■ The globe has been removed and cautery is applied to the optic nerve stump to maintain meticulous hemostasis.

transect the optic nerve, and the entire eyeball is removed. The surgeon should inspect the entire globe for intactness and/or unusual findings before submitting the specimen for histopathological examination. Malleable retractors are placed so as to visualize directly the still clamped cut edge of the optic nerve, and the central retinal vessels are cauterized to obtain meticulous hemostasis before removing the clamp (Fig. 97-3). If

the optic nerve is not clamped, such as for intraocular tumors, orbital packing with direct pressure for 5–10 minutes can be applied to achieve adequate hemostasis. In select enucleations, as with tumors in contact with the optic disc, it may be necessary to obtain a long segment of optic nerve.[13,14]

For the average-sized adult orbit a 20mm polymethyl methacrylate orbital implant is usually adequate. The implant

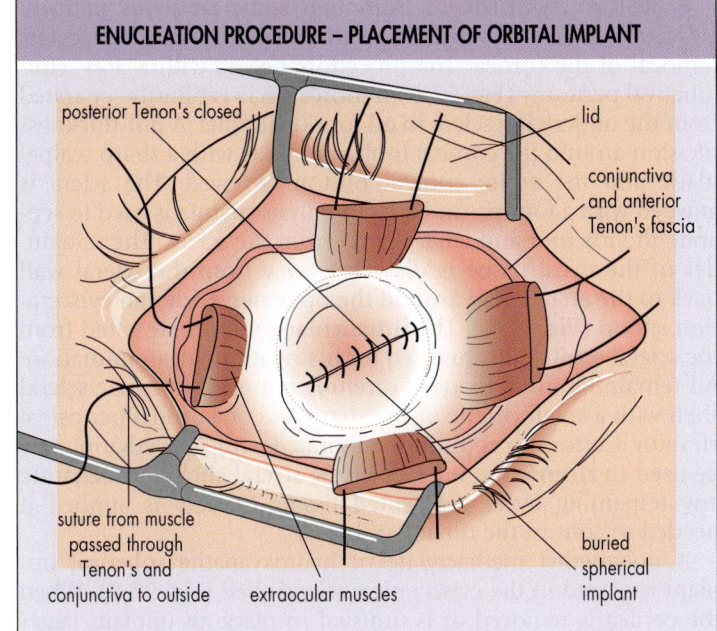

ENUCLEATION PROCEDURE – PLACEMENT OF ORBITAL IMPLANT

posterior Tenon's closed

lid

conjunctiva and anterior Tenon's fascia

suture from muscle passed through Tenon's and conjunctiva to outside

extraocular muscles

buried spherical implant

FIG. 97-4 ■ An orbital implant has been placed behind posterior Tenon's fascia. This layer is then closed with multiple, interrupted 6-0 Vicryl sutures. The four rectus muscle stumps remain free with the 6-0 Vicryl sutures attached.

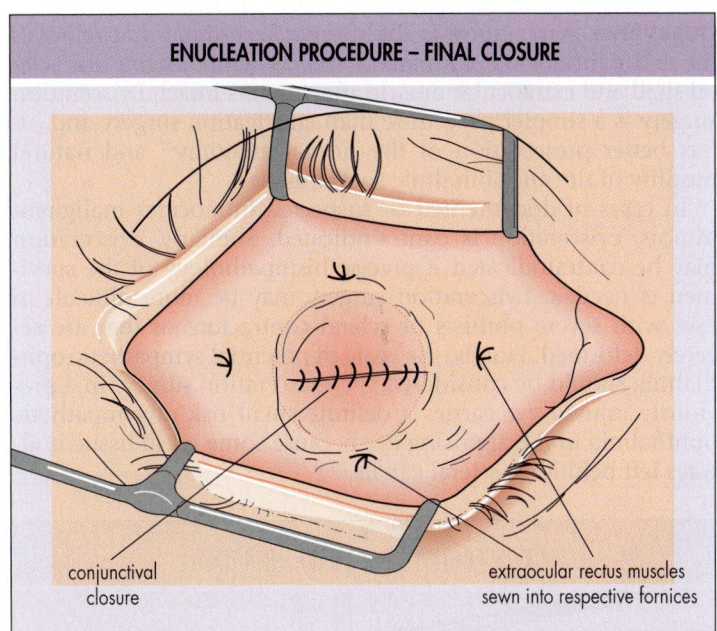

ENUCLEATION PROCEDURE – FINAL CLOSURE

conjunctival closure

extraocular rectus muscles sewn into respective fornices

FIG. 97-5 ■ Enucleation surgery—final closure. The 6-0 Vicryl rectus sutures are sewn onto their respective fornices by passing the sutures through Tenon's fascia and conjunctiva. The anterior Tenon's is closed with 6-0 Vicryl and the conjunctiva with a running 6-0 plain suture.

type and size can, of course, vary, and it may also be wrapped in either autologous fascia or donor sclera. The orbital implant is inserted behind posterior Tenon's fascia, through the central rent left by cutting the optic nerve. Multiple interrupted 6-0 Vicryl sutures securely close posterior Tenon's fascia that overlies the orbital implant.

Each of the four rectus muscles is sutured to the adjacent fornix by passing the previously placed double-armed Vicryl sutures full-thickness through Tenon's fascia and conjunctiva[15] (see Fig. 97-4). This will provide motility to the ocular prosthesis. Care should be taken to avoid advancing the superior rectus suture too close to the midline to avoid inadvertent tension or traction on the superior rectus muscle, which could induce an upper lid ptosis. After anterior Tenon's fascia is closed in the midline with 6-0 Vicryl sutures (Fig. 97-5),[16] the conjunctival edges are loosely reapproximated with a 6-0 plain gut running suture.

At the end of the procedure an additional deep orbital injection with bupivacaine 0.5%, epinephrine, and hyaluronidase is given. A broad-spectrum ophthalmic antibiotic ointment is applied to the conjunctiva. A medium-sized clear acrylic lid conformer is placed and a firm pressure bandage applied over the socket.

The pressure bandage remains intact for 3–4 days postoperatively and, upon removal, the patient uses topical cool compresses with crushed ice. Pain medication is prescribed as appropriate. This perioperative and postoperative management regimen allows the large majority of enucleation procedures to be performed as outpatient procedures, with adequate control of postoperative pain.

ENUCLEATION WITH HYDROXYAPATITE IMPLANT. The purpose of the hydroxyapatite implant is to allow the potential for maximum motility of the ocular prosthesis. Coralline hydroxyapatite contains 500m diameter pores that are similar to the structure of the haversian systems of cancellous bone. The microstructure of this implant allows fibrovascular ingrowth of the host tissues in the anophthalmic socket.[3,4] Once the hydroxyapatite implant is well vascularized, it can be secondarily drilled and fitted with a motility peg implant. This motility peg is then coupled to the ocular prosthesis to enhance maximally prosthesis motility.

A standard enucleation technique is performed, as already described. The socket may be "sized" using sterile trial spheres, but in most cases an 18mm or a 20mm hydroxyapatite implant is appropriate. Keep in mind that wrapping the implant with sclera or fascia adds approximately 1–1.5mm to the overall diameter of the implant.

In most situations, the hydroxyapatite implant is wrapped in donor sclera. The scleral shell should be cut to the appropriate size and shape to enclose the implant securely. Multiple interrupted 6-0 Vicryl sutures are suitable for securely closing the sclera. The hexagonal rosettes of the hydroxyapatite exoskeleton should be aligned in the anterior-posterior direction and an open scleral window should be present at the posterior apex of the hydroxyapatite implant, corresponding to the site of the corneal button removal. Rectangular windows, approximately 2–4mm, are cut through the sclera located within 8–10mm from the anteriormost apex of the implant. To promote further fibrovascular ingrowth into the implant, a handheld 20-gauge needle is used to create drill holes in the hydroxyapatite at the site of each window and at the site of the posterior round corneal window.[17]

The wrapped hydroxyapatite implant is placed into the anophthalmic orbit and the four rectus muscles are secured to the anterior lip of the corresponding rectangular scleral window. Anterior Tenon's fascia is sutured with multiple interrupted 6-0 Vicryl sutures. The conjunctiva can be closed with a loosely running 6-0 plain suture, which is tied and cut on each end. Some authors report a higher exposure rate with hydroxyapatite[18–21] compared with alloplastic sphere implants,[22] thus emphasizing the need for meticulous closure. As is the case with any enucleation procedure, a polymethyl methacrylate lid conformer is placed in the conjunctival cul-de-sac with broad-spectrum antibiotic ointment and a pressure bandage applied.

The unique properties of a hydroxyapatite implant allow fibrovascular ingrowth and integration of the implant with the ocular prosthesis. Without placement of the motility peg, no demonstrable motility difference exists between a sclera-wrapped hydroxyapatite implant and a similarly wrapped polymethyl methacrylate implant.[23] Thus hydroxyapatite implantation is most appropriate for patients who express a strong interest in eventual second-stage drilling of the implant to maximize prosthesis motility. These titanium motility pegs are surgically inserted after adequate fibrovascular ingrowth into the hydroxyapatite implant has occurred.[24–26]

755

Evisceration

OVERVIEW. Evisceration is the surgical technique that removes the entire intraocular contents of the eye while leaving the scleral shell and extraocular muscle attachments intact. Evisceration surgery is a simpler procedure than enucleation surgery and offers better preservation of the orbital anatomy[27] and natural motility of the anophthalmic socket tissues.

In cases of documented or suspected intraocular malignant tumors, evisceration is contraindicated. Similarly, evisceration may be contraindicated if precise histopathology of the specimen is needed. Evisceration surgery may be more difficult in eyes with severe phthisis or scleral contracture or that are severely deformed. Finally, the issue of potential sympathetic ophthalmia should be considered.[28–31] Evisceration surgery in a previously injured eye carries a definite small risk of sympathetic ophthalmia in the apposing eye because some uveal tissue is always left behind in scleral canals.[28]

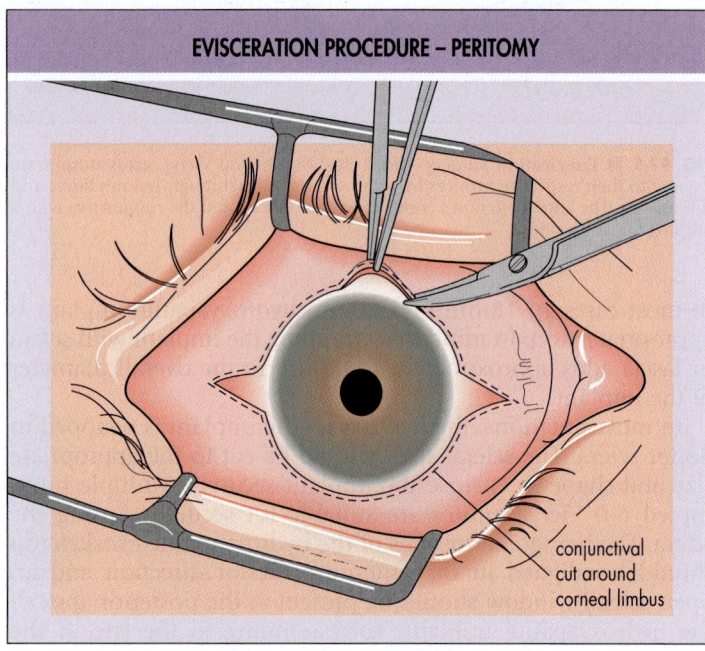

EVISCERATION PROCEDURE – PERITOMY

conjunctival cut around corneal limbus

FIG. 97-6 ▓ Evisceration procedure. A 360° conjunctival peritomy is made, followed by complete excision of the corneal button.

SURGICAL TECHNIQUE. Although some surgeons perform evisceration with preservation of the cornea, this author prefers removal of the cornea. The procedure begins with a 360° conjunctival peritomy (Fig. 97-6). Tenon's fascia is bluntly separated from the underlying sclera in all four quadrants. A full-thickness incision around the corneal limbus is made with a sharp scalpel blade and the entire corneal button removed. The sclera is grasped with a forceps, and a cyclodialysis spatula is used to separate the iris root and ciliary body from the sclera. The remainder of the uveal tissue is dissected away from the scleral wall back to the attachment around the optic nerve with an evisceration spoon (Fig. 97-7). The intraocular contents are lifted from the scleral shell and submitted for histopathologic examination. All remaining uveal tissue is carefully removed from the scleral shell with a small curette or the sharp end of a caudal periosteal elevator. Cotton-tip applicators saturated with 70% ethanol may be used to cleanse the interior of the scleral shell and denature any remaining uveal pigmented tissue. Cautery is applied if needed to control the oozing of blood.

A polymethyl methacrylate or hydroxyapatite spherical implant is placed in the evisceration scleral shell (Fig. 97-8). When the cornea is removed, it is unusual to place an implant larger than 14–16mm. The scleral edges are closed with multiple interrupted 6-0 Vicryl sutures, with the medial and lateral scleral edges cut to reduce any dog ears (Fig. 97-9). The conjunctiva is gently closed with a running 6-0 plain gut suture. If a larger implant is desired, it is necessary to perform radial relaxing sclerotomy incisions posteriorly[32] between the rectus muscles (Fig. 97-10). If a hydroxyapatite implant is used, such sclerotomy openings are necessary to enhance vascular ingrowth.[33]

Dressing and postoperative care are as for enucleation.

Exenteration

OVERVIEW. Exenteration surgery involves complete removal of the eyeball, the retrobulbar orbital soft tissues, and most or all of the eyelids. The most common indication for exenteration surgery is for the treatment of epithelial malignancy with orbital invasion.[34,35]

When exenteration is performed for orbital malignancies, periorbita is usually excised to remove completely all potentially involved tissues. The bare orbital bone can slowly heal by sec-

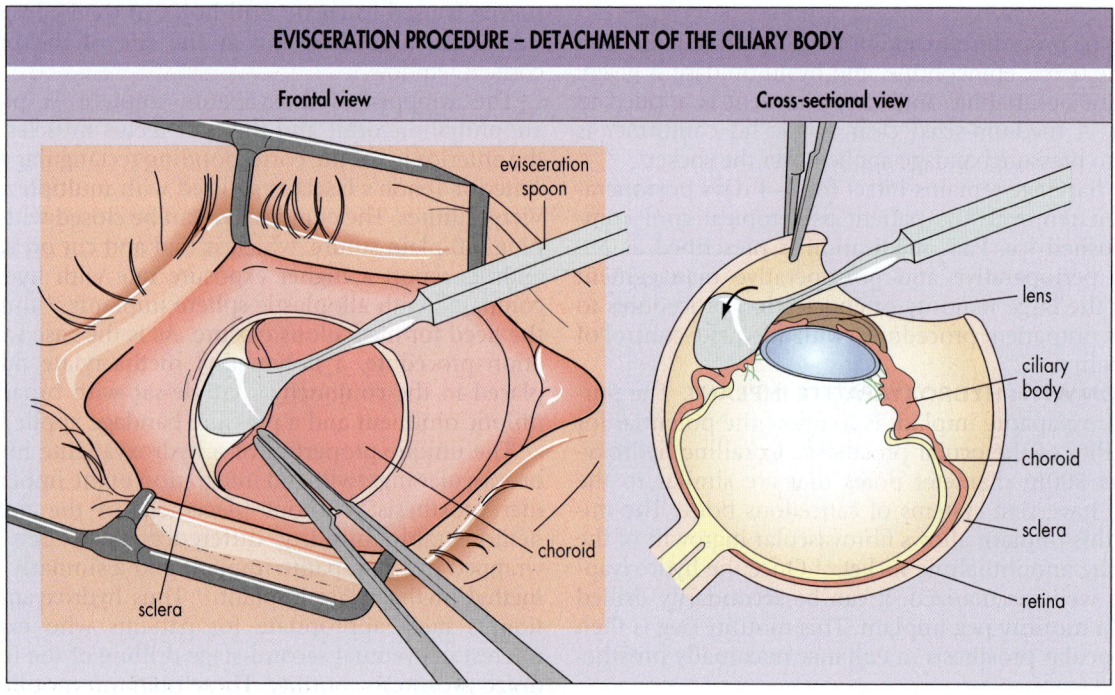

EVISCERATION PROCEDURE – DETACHMENT OF THE CILIARY BODY

Frontal view

Cross-sectional view

evisceration spoon

sclera

choroid

lens

ciliary body

choroid

sclera

retina

FIG. 97-7 ▓ An evisceration spoon is used to detach the ciliary body and bluntly elevate the choroid from the scleral wall.

ondary intent, but in most situations the exenterated orbit is covered with a split-thickness skin graft at the time of the procedure. As there is potential for recurrent tumor, reconstruction with thick, bulky tissue grafts, which could obscure recurrence, is avoided. In very select situations, however, a variety of ancillary reconstructive techniques may be of use, such as those involving ipsilateral temporalis muscle flaps,[36] free dermis-fat grafts,[37] latissimus dorsi myocutaneous free flaps,[38] osseointegrated implant techniques,[39] and other procedures.[40-43]

SURGICAL TECHNIQUE. The area of the proposed exenteration incision is marked with adequate wide margins where necessary for tumors, yet with preservation of as much normal periocular soft tissue as possible (Fig. 97-11). If necessary, adjacent areas of the medial canthus, temple, or forehead are included in the excision site. When surgery is necessary for a conjunctival or deep orbital tumor, a subciliary incision around the eyelid margins and wrapping around the inner canthus preserve the eyelid skin and orbicularis muscle, which can be used for reconstruction.[43]

The skin is incised along the mark and any orbicularis muscle to be spared dissected in a suborbicular plane. The dissection is carried down through periorbita to expose the orbital rim. A periosteal elevator is used to elevate periosteum over the orbital rim and periorbita from the orbital walls (Fig. 97-12). Firm attachments to bone are encountered at the lateral orbital tubercle, the superior oblique trochlea, the medial canthal tendon, the distal lacrimal sac as it enters the bony nasolacrimal canal, the inferior oblique origin near the posterior lacrimal crest, and the superior and inferior orbital fissure attachments (Fig. 97-13; see Chapter 83). Except for these sites of resistance, the periorbita can be elevated quite easily. Medially, the surgeon should use particular care when elevating periorbita so as to avoid inadvertent penetration of the lamina papyracea into the ethmoid sinus air cells, which could result in a chronic sino-orbital fistula.

Superiorly, the superior orbital bone may be quite attenuated in elderly patients and atrophic bony defects may be present. Monopolar cautery to the orbital roof should be avoided, as this may cause inadvertent cerebrospinal fluid leakage.[44] It is generally safe to use bipolar cautery along the orbital roof and deep orbital tissues without the risk of cerebrospinal fluid leakage.

The periorbital lining is mobilized along all orbital walls toward the orbital apex. The dissection and mobilization of soft tissues must extend posteriorly beyond the extent of tumor invasion. A thin curved hemostat can be used to clamp the api-cal tissues while a slender pair of Metzenbaum scissors are used to excise the exenteration specimen anterior to the clamp (Fig. 97-14). An enucleation snare may also be used to incise the apical stump to complete the severing of the exenteration specimen.[45] When necessary, frozen section pathology analysis of the apical stump tissues should be used to verify that the margins of resection are free and clear of neoplasm. The orbital bone should be carefully inspected for subtle bone pitting or other signs of bone erosion or destruction.

In patients who have very bulky or massive orbital neoplasms, exenteration may be difficult, with little space in which to separate periorbita from orbital bone. It may be helpful here first to enucleate the eyeball to make enough room for access to the deeper apical soft tissues under good visualization.

In most patients the orbit will be lined with a split-thickness skin graft harvested from the anterior surface of the thigh. It is

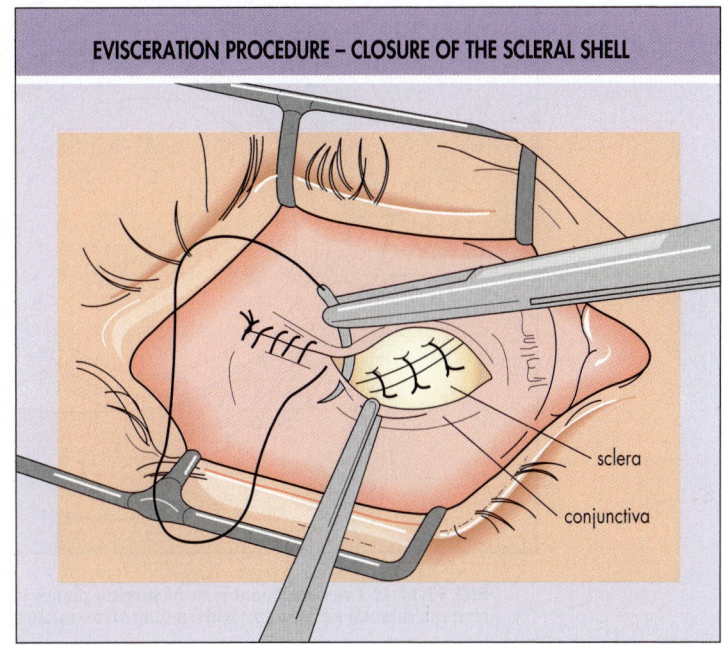

FIG. 97-9 ■ The scleral opening is closed with multiple, interrupted 6-0 Vicryl sutures. Conjunctiva is subsequently closed over the scleral wound using running 6-0 plain gut sutures.

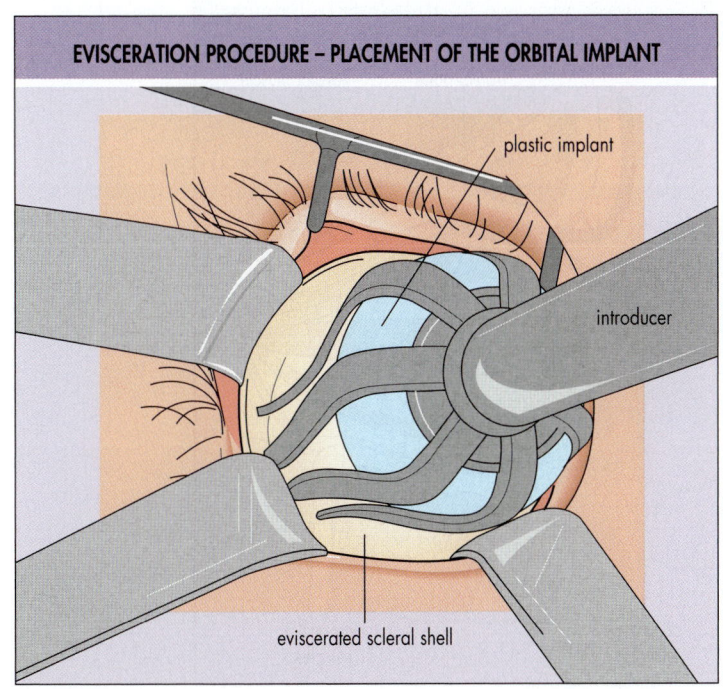

FIG. 97-8 ■ A sphere introducer is used to place the orbital implant into the evisceration scleral shelf.

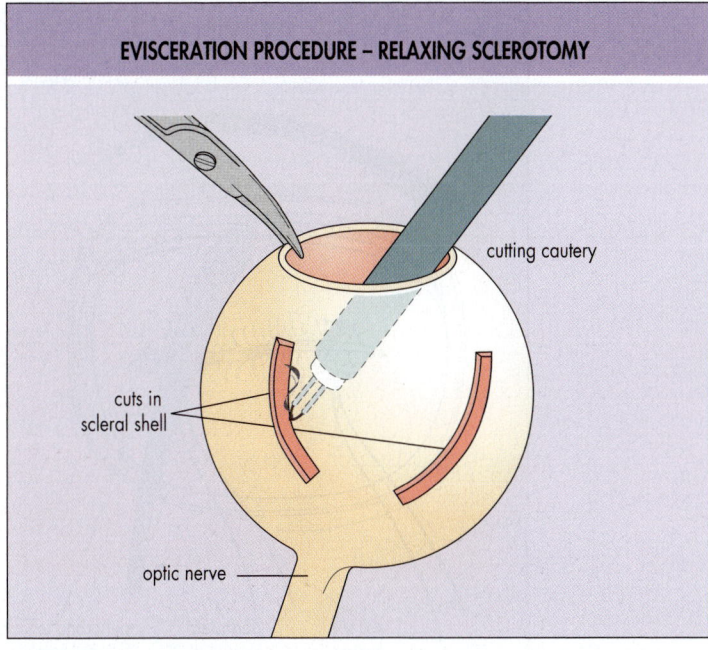

FIG. 97-10 ■ A unipolar cautery is used to incise relaxing sclerotomy slits to expand the scleral shell. This sclerotomy technique to enlarge the scleral shell volume is "optional" with polymethyl methacrylate sphere implants. Sclerotomy slits are "mandatory" when using hydroxyapatite spheres in order to facilitate vascular ingrowth.

usually preferable to expand the skin graft in a mesher. Multiple interrupted 6-0 Vicryl sutures secure all residual host skin edges to the meshed skin graft. The graft is tamponaded within the orbit with a Telfa dressing and Xeroform gauze packing under pressure.

If the upper lid and lower eyelid skin and muscle are preserved, it may be possible in elderly patients with a lot of loose eyelid skin simply to suture the skin edges together and then place a pressure dressing to tamponade the myocutaneous edges against the bare bone.

POSTOPERATIVE MANAGEMENT. The orbital pack and pressure dressing should remain in place for approximately 5–7 days. Following removal of the dressing, the patient can use gen-

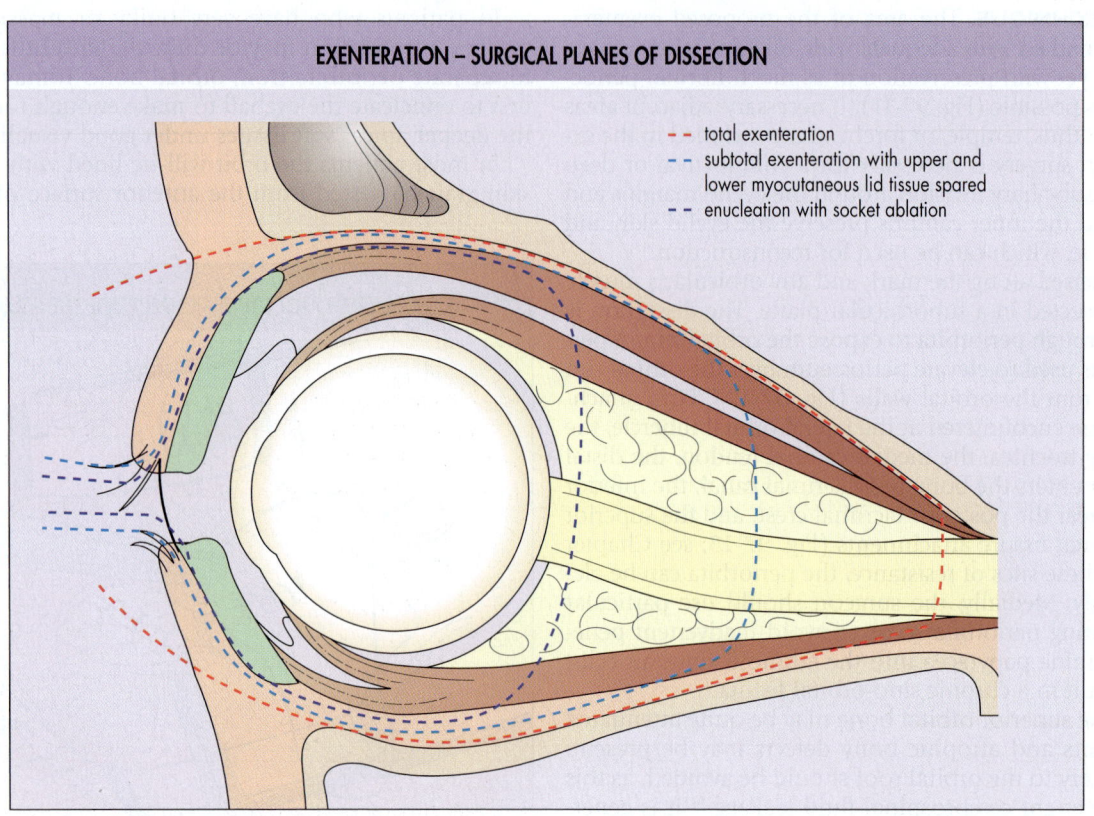

FIG. 97-11 ■ **Cross-sectional view of surgical planes of dissection for exenteration surgical techniques:** total exenteration, subtotal exenteration with sparing of myocutaneous eyelid tissue, and enucleation with partial socket ablation.

EXENTERATION – SURGICAL PLANES OF DISSECTION

- - - total exenteration
- - - subtotal exenteration with upper and lower myocutaneous lid tissue spared
- - - enucleation with socket ablation

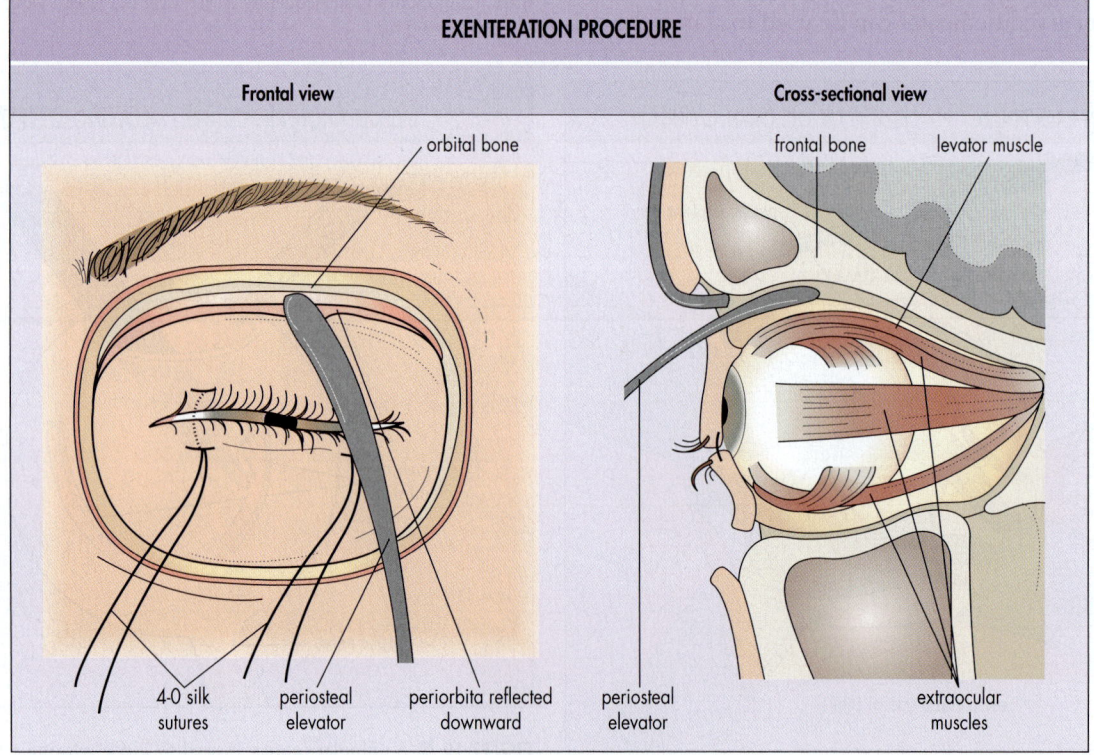

EXENTERATION PROCEDURE

Frontal view

Cross-sectional view

orbital bone

frontal bone   levator muscle

4-0 silk sutures   periosteal elevator   periorbita reflected downward

periosteal elevator   extraocular muscles

FIG. 97-12 ■ **Exenteration procedure.** A 360° skin incision is made down to the periosteum of the orbital rim. A periosteal elevator is used to begin reflecting the superior periorbita downward.

tle hydrogen peroxide rinses to cleanse the socket. Generally, these orbits heal best when left open to the air, so the patients should wear a patch only when going out in public. The surgeon should remain vigilant to the possibility of infection of the skin graft, especially by *Pseudomonas, Staphylococcus,* or *Streptococcus.* Systemic antibiotics may be necessary if these infections arise. In some patients, the exenterated orbit retains chronic, moist, ulcerated areas intermixed with areas of healthy keratinizing epidermis. The use of a gentle handheld hair dryer can help "cure" these slower healing areas.

A combined eyelid-ocular prosthesis can be made by an anaplastologist. Many exenteration patients prefer simply to wear a black patch.

COMPLICATIONS

Evisceration

Postoperative infection is always of concern when evisceration surgery is performed in the setting of endophthalmitis or panophthalmitis. The use of broad-spectrum systemic antibiotics usually minimizes this risk, and the surgeon can generally use a primary orbital implant. Postoperative extrusion of the orbital implant is a complication of evisceration surgery that may be related to postoperative scleral shell shrinkage, to poor wound healing of the scleral edges, or to improper selection of the orbital implant size. Postoperative pain is more common when the cornea is retained.

Enucleation

Orbital implant extrusion is also a complication of enucleation surgery. Meticulous attention to careful Tenon's fascia wound closure and the proper selection of implant size are important principles in avoiding this outcome. Risk of implant extrusion is increased with prior irradiation treatment of the eye and orbit, severe traumatic injuries to the eye and orbit, and severe eye and orbital infections. Long-term complications of the anophthalmic socket are numerous, including generalized volume deficiency of the anophthalmic socket, lower eyelid laxity with poor prosthesis support, orbital implant migration, upper eyelid ptosis, and chronic conjunctivitis and mucoid discharge.

Exenteration

Exenteration surgery carries the risk of severe blood loss. It is important preoperatively to discontinue aspirin and all other medicines that could adversely affect blood clotting. Other complications unique to exenteration surgery include cerebrospinal fluid leakage via orbital roof transgression of the dura and chronic sino-orbital fistulas through the region of the lamina papyracea and ethmoid sinus air cells. During the first few weeks of healing, free skin grafts are susceptible to infection. Patients may require treatment with broad-spectrum systemic antibiotics for coverage of *Staphylococcus, Streptococcus, Pseudomonas,* and

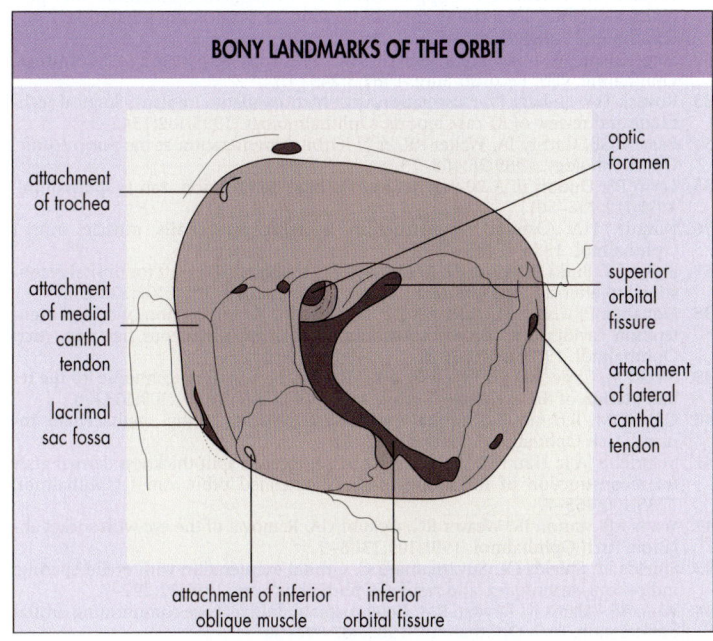

BONY LANDMARKS OF THE ORBIT

attachment of trochea
attachment of medial canthal tendon
lacrimal sac fossa
attachment of inferior oblique muscle
inferior orbital fissure
optic foramen
superior orbital fissure
attachment of lateral canthal tendon

FIG. 97-13 ◼ Bony orbit demonstrating the normal sites of increased resistance to dissection during orbital exenteration.

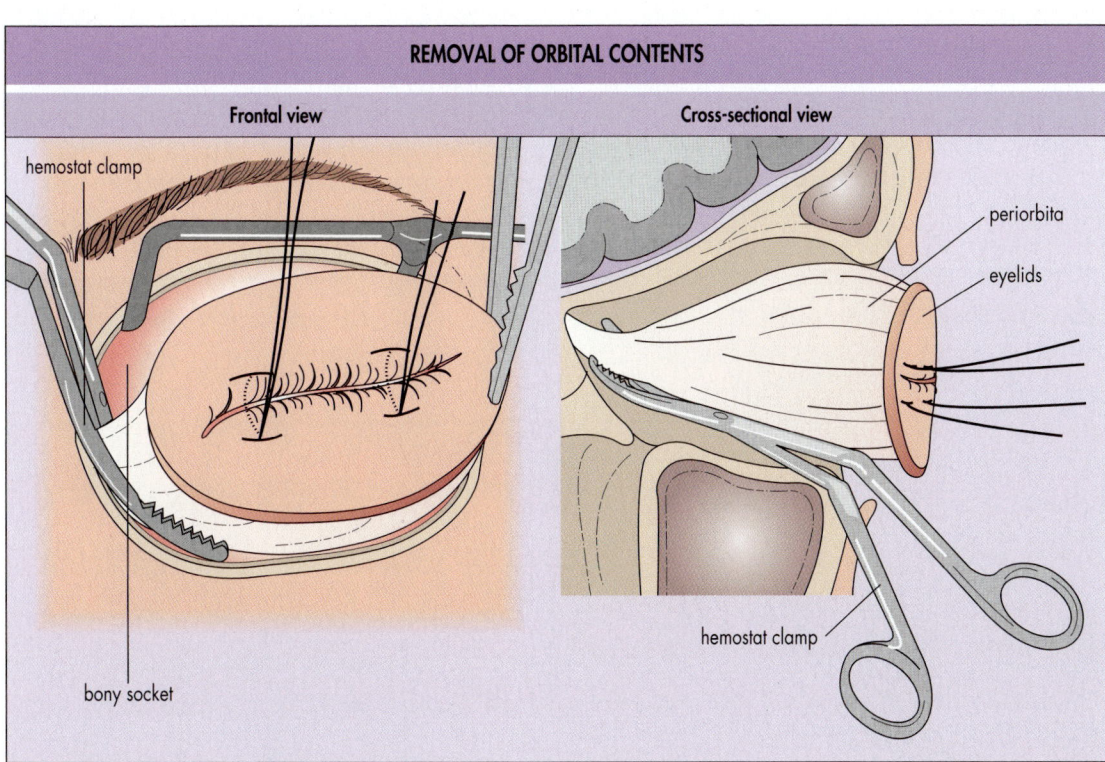

REMOVAL OF ORBITAL CONTENTS

Frontal view | Cross-sectional view

hemostat clamp
bony socket
periorbita
eyelids
hemostat clamp

FIG. 97-14 ◼ Periorbita has been elevated for 360°. Forward traction is applied to the orbital contents as a hemostat is used to clamp the apical orbital tissues.

other bacteria. The administration of systemic antibiotics is combined with maintenance of vigorous topical hygiene of the split-thickness skin graft using hydrogen peroxide rinses. Long term, the surgeon should always remain vigilant for the possible recurrence of tumor.

REFERENCES

1. Mules PH. Evisceration of the globe, with artificial vitreous. Trans Ophthalmol Soc UK. 1885;5:200-6.
2. Coston TO. The spherical implant. Trans Am Acad Ophthalmol Otolaryngol. 1970;74:1284-6.
3. Perry AC. Integrated orbital implants. Adv Ophthalmic Plast Reconstr Surg. 1990;8:75-81.
4. Perry AC. Advances in enucleation. Ophthalmol Clin North Am. 1991;4:173-7.
5. Dutton JJ. Coralline hydroxyapatite as an ocular implant. Ophthalmology. 1991;98:370-7.
6. Shields CL, Shields JA, DePotter P. Hydroxyapatite orbital implant after enucleation. Arch Ophthalmol. 1992;110:333-8.
7. Smith B, Petrelli R. Dermis-fat graft as a movable implant within the muscle cone. Am J Ophthalmol. 1978;85:62-6.
8. Smith B, Bosniak S, Nesi F, Lisman R. Dermis-fat orbital implantation: 118 cases. Ophthalmic Surg. 1983;14:941-3.
9. Nunery WR, Hetzler KJ. Dermal-fat graft as a primary enucleation technique. Ophthalmology. 1985;92:1256-61.
10. Migliori ME, Putterman AM. The doomed dermis-fat graft orbital implant. Ophthalmic Plast Reconstr Surg. 1991;7:23-30.
11. Traquair HM. Local anesthesia in enucleation of the eyeball. Ophthalmic Rev. 1916;35:75-89.
12. Munden PM, Carter KD, Nerad JA. The oculocardiac reflex during enucleation. Am J Ophthalmol. 1991;111:378-9.
13. Havre DC. Obtaining long sections of the optic nerve at enucleation: a new surgical technique based on the anatomy of the posterior fascia bulbi. Am J Ophthalmol. 1965;60:272-7.
14. Karcioglu ZA, Haik BG, Gordon RA. Frozen section of the optic nerve in retinoblastoma surgery. Ophthalmology. 1988;95:674-6.
15. Chen WP. Enucleation with myoconjunctival attachment: biomechanics of socket and prosthetic motility. Atlanta, American Society of Ophthalmic Plastic and Reconstructive Surgery, Thesis for Fellowship Candidacy, 1981.
16. Nunery WR, Hetzler KJ. Improved prosthetic motility following enucleation. Ophthalmology. 1983;90:1110-15.
17. Ferrone PJ, Dutton JJ. Rate of vascularization of coralline hydroxyapatite ocular implants. Ophthalmology. 1992;99:375-9.
18. Buettner H, Bartley GB. Tissue breakdown and exposure associated with orbital hydroxyapatite implants. Am J Ophthalmol. 1992;113:669-73.
19. Goldberg RA, Holds JB, Ebrahimpour J. Exposed hydroxyapatite orbital implants, reports of six cases. Ophthalmology. 1992;99:831-6.
20. Nunery WR, Heinz GW, Bonnin JM, et al. Exposure rate of hydroxyapatite spheres in the anophthalmic socket: histopathologic correlation and comparison with silicone sphere implants. Ophthalmic Plast Reconstr Surg. 1993;9:96-104.
21. Remulla HD, Rubin PA, Shore JW, et al. Complications of porous spherical orbital implants. Ophthalmology. 1995;102:586-93.
22. Nunery WR, Cepela MA, Heinz GW, et al. Extrusion rate of silicone spherical anophthalmic socket implants. Ophthalmic Plast Reconstr Surg. 1993;9:90-5.
23. Frueh BR, Felker GV. Baseball implant: a method of secondary insertion of an intraocular implant. Arch Ophthalmol. 1979;94:429-30.
24. Shields CL, Shields JA, Eagle RC, DePotter P. Histopathologic evidence of fibrovascular ingrowth four weeks after placement of the hydroxyapatite orbital implant. Am J Ophthalmol. 1991;111:363-6.
25. DePotter P, Shields CL, Shields JA, et al. Role of magnetic resonance imaging in the evaluation of the hydroxyapatite orbital implant. Ophthalmology. 1992;99:824-30.
26. Spirnak JP, Nieves N, Hollsten DA, et al. Gadolinium-enhanced magnetic resonance imaging assessment of hydroxyapatite orbital implants. Am J Ophthalmol. 1995;119:431-40.
27. Afran SI, Budenz DL, Albert DM. Does enucleation in the presence of endophthalmitis increase the risk of post-operative meningitis? Ophthalmology. 1987;94:235-7.
28. Green WR, Maumenee AE, Sanders TE, Smith ME. Sympathetic uveitis following evisceration. Trans Am Acad Ophthalmol Otolaryngol. 1972;76:625-44.
29. Marak GE. Recent advances in sympathetic ophthalmia. Surv Ophthalmol. 1979;24:141-6.
30. Rubin JR, Albert DM, Weinstein M. Sixty-five years of sympathetic ophthalmia: a clinicopathologic review of 105 cases (1913-1978). Ophthalmology. 1980;87:109-21.
31. Croxatto JE, Galentine P, Cupples HP, et al. Sympathetic ophthalmia after pars plana vitrectomy-lensectomy for endogenous bacterial endophthalmitis. Am J Ophthalmol. 1984;91:342-6.
32. Stephenson CM. Evisceration of the eye with expansion sclerotomies. Ophthalmic Plast Reconstr Surg. 1987;3:249-51.
33. Kostick DA, Linberg JV. Evisceration with hydroxyapatite implant. Surgical technique and review of 31 case reports. Ophthalmology. 1995;102:1542-9.
34. Bartley GB, Garrity JA, Waller RR, et al. Orbital exenteration at the Mayo Clinic. Ophthalmology. 1989;96:468-73.
35. Levin PS, Dutton JJ. A 20-year series of orbital exenteration. Am J Ophthalmol. 1991;112:496-501.
36. Naquin HA. Orbital reconstruction utilizing temporalis muscle. Am J Ophthalmol. 1956;41:519-21.
37. Shore JW, Burks R, Leone CR Jr, McCord CD Jr. Dermis-fat graft for orbital reconstruction after subtotal exenteration. Am J Ophthalmol. 1986;102:228-36.
38. Donahue PJ, Liston SL, Falconer DP, Manlove JC. Reconstruction of orbital exenteration cavities: the use of the latissimus dorsi myocutaneous free flap. Arch Ophthalmol. 1989;107:1681-6.
39. Nerad JA, Carter KD, La Velle WE, et al. The osseointegration technique for the rehabilitation of the exenterated orbit. Arch Ophthalmol. 1991;109:1032-8.
40. Gass JDM. Technique of orbital exenteration utilizing methyl methacrylate implant. Arch Ophthalmol. 1969;82:789-91.
41. Mauriello JA Jr, Han KH, Wolfe R. Use of autogenous split-thickness dermal graft for reconstruction of the lining of the exenterated orbit. Am J Ophthalmol. 1985;100:465-7.
42. Yeatts RP, Marion JR, Weaver RG, Orkubi GA. Removal of the eye with socket ablation. Arch Ophthalmol. 1991;109:1306-9.
43. Shields JA, Shields CL, Suvarnamani C. Orbital exenteration with eyelid sparing: indications, techniques, and results. Ophthalmic Surg. 1991;22:292-7.
44. Wulc AE, Adams JL, Dryden RM. Cerebrospinal fluid leakage complicating orbital exenteration. Arch Ophthalmol. 1989;107:827-30.
45. Buus DR, Tse DT. The use of the enucleation snare for orbital exenteration. Arch Ophthalmol. 1990;108:636-7.

The Lacrimal Drainage System

JEFFREY J. HURWITZ

DEFINITION
- The tear disposal system of the eye.
- The orbicularis muscle and eyelids provide a lacrimal pump mechanism.

KEY FEATURES
- Punctum.
- Canaliculi.
- Lacrimal sac.
- Nasolacrimal duct.

ASSOCIATED FEATURES
- Congenital obstruction is usually due to an imperforate membrane at the nasal end of the lacrimal duct.
- Acquired obstruction may result from chronic fibrosis of the duct, trauma, or previous nasal or sinus surgery.
- Stenosis or occlusion results in epiphora.
- Testing procedures are designed to localize the site of obstruction.
- Correction of congenital obstruction is typically achieved with a simple probing procedure.
- For acquired obstructions, a dacryocystorhinostomy is usually required for permanent resolution.

INTRODUCTION

Under normal circumstances, the quantity of tears secreted should equal the quantity eliminated. In this way, neither a dry eye nor symptoms of a watery eye occur. Tearing (a watery eye) may be due to hypersecretion of tears or to decreased elimination (Table 98-1). Hypersecretion may result from an increased production of tears from any stimulation of the neurophysiological pathway, either centrally or locally. Decreased elimination is caused by reduced passage of tears into or through the lacrimal drainage system.

ANATOMY AND PHYSIOLOGY

Tears are secreted by the lacrimal gland, with a 24-hour secretory volume of approximately 10ml.[1] With blinking, the palpebral aperture closes from lateral to medial, and tears are pumped along the marginal tear strips of the upper and lower lids toward the lacrimal lake at the inner canthus. In the normal resting state, most of the tears are lost by evaporation, and only a small percentage of the volume passes down through the nasolacrimal passageways.

Tears pass from the lacrimal lake into the canaliculi through the puncta mainly by capillarity. It is important that the puncta of each lid contact the opposite lid on closure and thereby become physiologically occluded. When the lids separate, capillarity draws the tears into the empty canaliculi. Tears then flow to

TABLE 98-1

CAUSES OF TEARING

Lacrimation (hypersecretion)	Epiphora (decreased tear elimination)	
	ANATOMIC FACTORS	**PHYSIOLOGICAL DYSFUNCTION**
Corneal foreign bodies		
Corneal irritation with dry spots	Strictures	Orbicularis muscle weakness
Ocular surface inflammation	Obstructions	Punctal or eyelid malpositions
Refractive errors	Foreign bodies (e.g., stones)	Nasal obstruction with normal lacrimal pathway
Thyroid dysfunction	Tumors	
Nasal irritation and inflammation		

the common canaliculus and lacrimal sac due to a combination of factors[2-5]:
- A change in the caliber of these passages
- A change in pressure within the canalicular passages
- A pumping function (lacrimal pump) of the orbicularis muscle that surrounds these passages

Tears flow into the inferior meatus of the nose through the effect of the lacrimal pump, gravity, and, to a lesser extent, pressure changes within the nose due to respiration. Valves within the drainage system permit only one-way flow of tears.

EVALUATION OF EPIPHORA

Clinical History

The history of symptoms associated with tearing is important. Pain at the side of the nose suggests dacryocystitis, but pain in the eye itself may be due to foreign bodies, keratitis, recurrent corneal erosion, iritis, or glaucoma. Itchiness is suggestive of an allergic problem rather than a lacrimal obstruction. Grittiness and burning of the eyes associated with tearing suggest a tear film problem, such as occurs in keratitis sicca, or dysthyroid eye disease.

A history of medication such as echothiophate iodide (Phospholine Iodide), epinephrine (adrenaline), or pilocarpine is important, since all these drugs may produce lacrimal obstruction. Chemotherapy and radiotherapy also can cause obstruction in the canaliculi.

Physical Examination

EYELIDS. Poor orbicularis muscle tone and lacrimal pump dysfunction may be presumed if the lid can be pulled more than 8mm away from the globe, if there is decreased snap-back, or if there is frank ectropion. The puncta normally should be directed backward into the lacrimal lake. Lesions of the caruncle may interfere with the proper drainage of tears. Blepharitis may cause secondary oversecretion of tears.

LACRIMAL PASSAGES. Facial asymmetry suggests congenital or traumatic anatomical blockage of the nasolacrimal canal. Any mass at the inner canthus should be palpated to determine whether it is soft (indicating mucus) or firm (suggesting a possible tumor) and whether it is compressible or noncompressible. Orbital signs such as proptosis, displacement of the globe, diplopia, and ptosis could indicate that the lacrimal lesion involves the orbit, or vice versa.

NOSE. The nasal examination is an essential part of every lacrimal evaluation. Nasal and sinus conditions, which range from infections and inflammations to tumors, may result in epiphora. Symptoms include anosmia (loss of smell), epistaxis, anesthesia around the roof of the nose, and nasal obstruction.

Clinical Diagnostic Tests

SECRETORY TESTS

Schirmer's Test. The amount of wetting on a strip of filter paper over 5 minutes helps assess tear production. In the normal nonanesthetized eye, 15mm of wetting is expected in a patient younger than 40 years of age, and at least 10mm of wetting is expected in a patient older than 40 years. If anesthetic is placed onto the eye, the basal secretion is expected to be 10mm of wetting in a normal patient younger than 40 years and at least 5mm in a patient older than 40 years.

EXCRETORY TESTS

Lacrimal Syringing. In syringing, a lacrimal irrigation cannula is passed into the punctum and advanced through the canaliculus to the medial wall of the lacrimal sac fossa (see Chapter 83). If the cannula hits bone (hard stop), the canaliculus is open, so the obstruction is probably in the sac or the duct. If it does not hit bone (soft stop), the obstruction is probably in the common canaliculus, especially if the medial angle of the palpebral aperture shifts medially as the cannula is advanced toward lacrimal bone.

Clear water or saline is then gently irrigated through a cannula. If fluid passes into the nose without reflux out of the opposite canaliculus, the system is totally patent. If fluid passes into the nose with resistance and reflux occurs through the opposite canaliculus, the system is anatomically patent but physiologically stenotic (partially occluded). If no fluid passes into the nose but it all comes back through either punctum, complete nasolacrimal duct obstruction is present.

Jones Fluorescein Dye Test. The Jones[6] dye test is used to determine whether the lacrimal drainage system is fully patent or, if partially obstructed, whether the problem is in the upper system (lids, puncta, canaliculi, common canaliculus) or in the lower system (sac, duct, nose).

A drop of fluorescein is placed into the conjunctival cul-de-sac. The nose is examined after 5 minutes to determine whether the dye has passed through the lacrimal system spontaneously, which indicates that it is functionally patent. This test may be facilitated by looking into the nose with a flashlight or an endoscope, or by having the patient blow the nose.

In the second part of the test, the cannula is placed in the sac, and the system is irrigated. Any fluid that passes into the nose during irrigation must be recovered and examined. If no fluorescein is present in the recovered fluid, this suggests that it did not pass into the sac during the initial fluorescein test, so the problem is likely in the upper (canalicular) system. If fluorescein is present in the fluid, this indicates that it reached the sac during the initial test and that the upper system is probably normal, meaning that the problem is in the lower (sac, duct) system. Although many surgeons find these tests useful, other tests and radiological investigation may be necessary for diagnosis or surgical planning.

Diagnostic Imaging

DACRYOCYSTOGRAPHY. Dacryocystography (DCG), an anatomical test, is extremely useful to determine the exact site of ob-

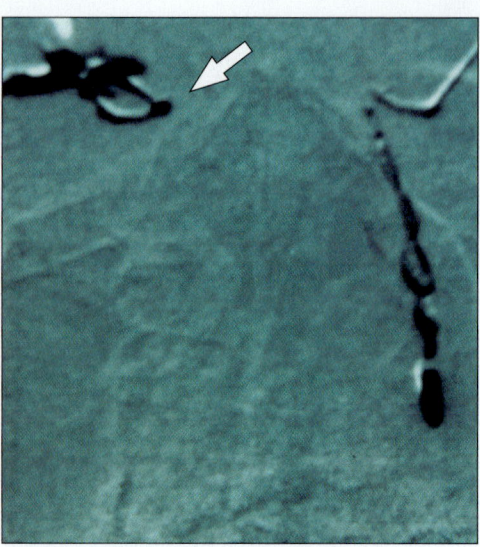

FIG. 98-1 ▪▪
Dacryocystogram. Complete obstruction of the lacrimal drainage pathways at the medial common canalicular level on the right side.

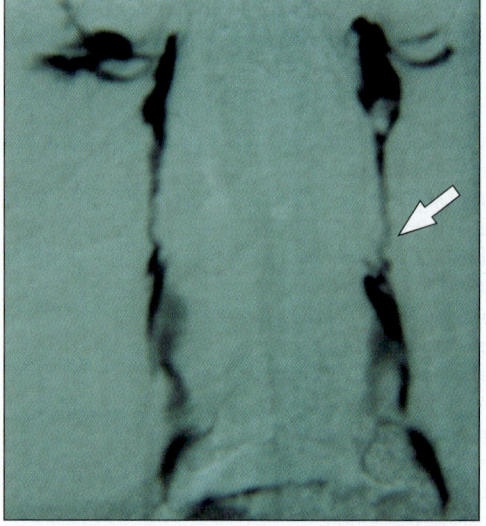

FIG. 98-2 ▪▪
Dacryocystogram. Stenosis at the sac-duct junction is greater on the left side than on the right.

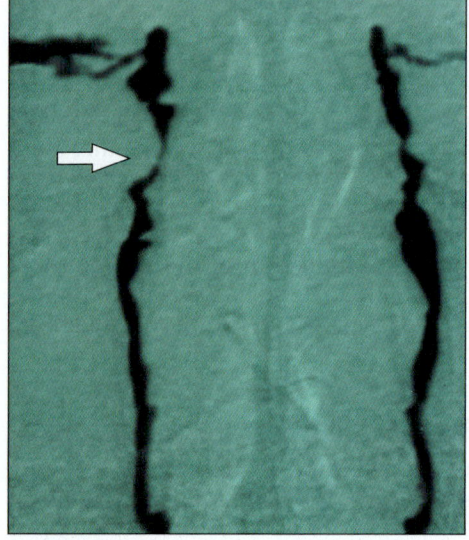

FIG. 98-3 ▪▪
Dacryocystogram. Medial deflection of contrast material within the right sac indicates sac stones.

struction or stenosis within the system (Figs. 98-1 and 98-2) and to visualize any deflection of the passages by diseases of the surrounding structures (Fig. 98-3; Box 98-1). Injection of either a viscous oil (conventional macrodacryocystography)[7] or a water-soluble contrast material (digital subtraction dacryocystography)[8] through a catheter demonstrates the lacrimal drainage pathways and outlines any anatomical abnormalities. This test does not evaluate physiological function.

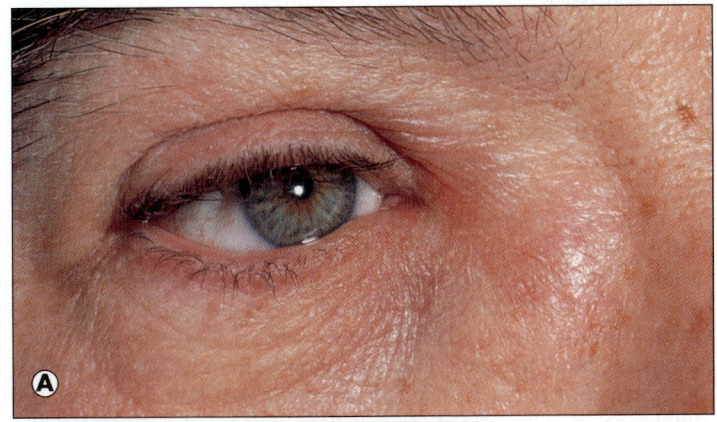

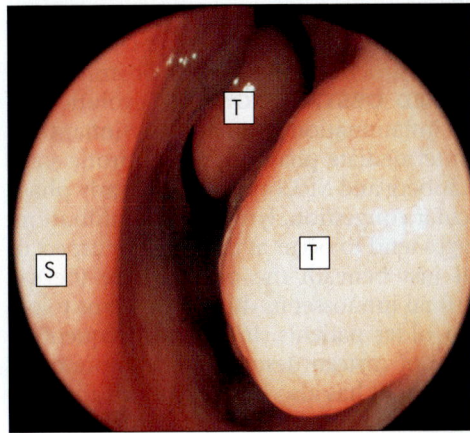

FIG. 98-5 ▮ Endoscopy. Endoscopic view of the nose demonstrates the nasal septum (S), lateral wall, and turbinates (T).

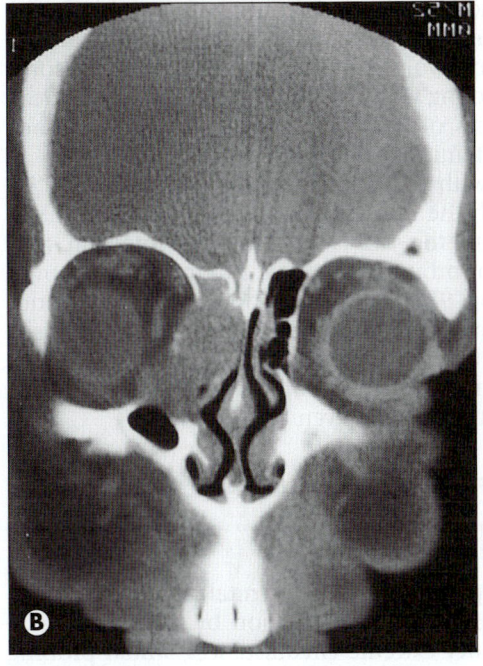

FIG. 98-4 ▮ Tearing secondary to neoplasm. A, Patient with right-sided tearing and a mass at the inner canthus. The system was fully patent to syringing. B, CT scan in this patient demonstrates an ethmoidal orbital plasmocytoma with compression of the lacrimal sac.

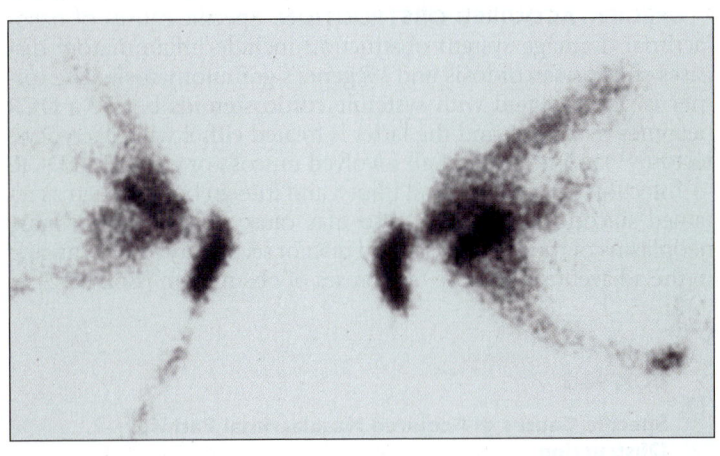

FIG. 98-6 ▮ Lacrimal scan. Complete obstruction on the left side and stenosis on the right side.

BOX 98-1

Uses of Dacryocystography

Complete obstruction where the site of block (canalicular vs sac) cannot be determined clinically

Incomplete obstruction where the area of stenosis cannot be localized on clinical testing

In cases of suspected lacrimal sac tumors to visualize a filling defect

In adnexal disease, to image compression or deflection of the sac or duct

---

COMPUTED TOMOGRAPHY. High-resolution computed tomography (CT) in the axial and coronal planes is a useful anatomical study to assess those patients who have diseases in the structures adjacent to the nasolacrimal drainage pathways (Fig. 98-4). Injection of the canaliculi with contrast provides simultaneous visualization of the lacrimal drainage system (CT–DCG).[9]

ULTRASONOGRAPHY. Conventional ultrasonography of the lacrimal drainage pathways may have a role in demonstrating anatomical abnormalities such as an enlarged lacrimal sac (solid lesion or mucocele).[10] It may also be helpful in patients who have common canalicular obstruction and in whom the sac cannot be demonstrated on DCG. New advances such as ultrasound biomicroscopy, with resolution of the subsurface structures up to 4mm, allow visualization of the canaliculi.[11] This technique may prove to be of value in the assessment of canalicular diseases.

ENDOSCOPY. Nasal endoscopy using a rigid telescope is useful to observe the anatomy of the opening of the nasal lacrimal duct in the inferior meatus and to diagnose any disease within the nose itself (Fig. 98-5). If a lacrimal drainage operation is contemplated, the endoscope is the best method to assess the future surgical site. Should tearing persist following lacrimal surgery, it is useful to view the size and location of the previous dacryocystorhinostomy (DCR) opening using an endoscope to determine whether the opening is obstructed by fibrous tissue, polyps, granuloma, or foreign bodies.

Canalicular endoscopy is in its infancy. In the future, it may play a role in imaging along the canaliculus and into the sac and duct.[12]

NUCLEAR LACRIMAL SCAN. This is an adjunctive physiological test of lacrimal function; it does not demonstrate anatomical structures. A drop of technetium-99m pertechnetate is placed into the palpebral aperture, and a pinhole collimator of a gamma camera is used to record its transit to the nose. The lacrimal scan can help determine the extent of stenosis from a physiological point of view (Fig. 98-6). It also can help evaluate the flow of tears to determine whether lid or punctal malpositions contribute to drainage dysfunction.

OBSTRUCTIONS OF THE LACRIMAL SAC AND DUCT

Congenital Obstruction

Congenital nasolacrimal obstruction is due to an imperforate membrane, which usually opens spontaneously at the time of birth. Sometimes, this may persist into adult life. If spontaneous resolution does not occur by 1 year of age, the patient may be treated by probing through the membrane. If a child has passed the age of 5 or 6 years, the success rate of probing decreases to such an extent that it is preferable to treat the obstruction with a DCR.

Acquired Obstruction

Acquired obstructions of the sac and duct may be classified as nonspecific (idiopathic) obstructions and specific obstructions.

NONSPECIFIC ACQUIRED OBSTRUCTION. The evolution of nonspecific lacrimal sac inflammation from an early inflammatory stage through an intermediate phase to a late fibrotic stage has been proposed by Linberg and McCormick.[13] The early phase is characterized by vascular congestion, lymphocytic infiltration, and edema. These changes tend to occur at the superior aspect of the nasolacrimal canal just beneath the point where the sac passes into the nasolacrimal intraosseous duct. This seems to occur more commonly in older patients. It is more frequent in Caucasians than in those of African descent and is more common in women than in men; it has also been suggested that it is more common in people from lower socioeconomic levels.[14] Inflammatory conditions that affect the inferior meatus of the nose also may involve the respiratory-like mucosa of the inferior aspect of the nasolacrimal canal, thereby leading to obstruction.

SPECIFIC ACQUIRED OBSTRUCTION. Specific causes of nasolacrimal drainage system obstruction include inflammatory diseases such as sarcoidosis and Wegener's granulomatosis. The former is often treated with systemic corticosteroids before a DCR becomes necessary, and the latter is treated either with dacryocystectomy[15] and removal of all involved mucosa or with a full DCR.

Infection, trauma, surgical injury, and foreign bodies, such as retained silicone or eyelashes, also may cause obstruction. Primary neoplasms of the lacrimal sac and duct or secondary tumors arising in the adjacent sinuses are rare causes of obstruction (Box 98-2).

BOX 98-2

Specific Causes of Acquired Nasolacrimal Pathway Obstruction

INFLAMMATORY DISEASES	TRAUMA AND POSTSURGICAL
Sarcoidosis	Nasoethmoid fractures
Wegener's granulomatosis	Nasal and endoscopic sinus surgery
	Rhinoplasty
INFECTIONS	Orbital decompression
Staphylococcus	
Actinomyces	**NEOPLASMS**
Streptococcus	Primary lacrimal sac tumors
Pseudomonas	Benign papillomas
Infectious mononucleosis	Squamous and basal cell carcinoma
Human papillomavirus	Transitional cell carcinoma
Ascaris	Fibrous histiocytoma
Leprosy	Midline granuloma
Tuberculosis	Lymphoma

Dacryocystitis

Dacryocystitis may be classified as acute, subacute, or chronic. It may be localized in the sac, extend to include a pericystitis, or progress to orbital cellulitis. When dacryocystitis is localized to the sac, a palpable painful mass occurs at the inner canthus (Fig. 98-7), and obstruction is present at the junction of the nasolacrimal sac and duct. A preexisting dacryocystocele may or may not be present. When the infection develops, the lateral expansion of the nasolacrimal sac tends to push on the common canaliculus and produce a kink within it, with the result that the sac is no longer reducible. This allows a buildup of material within the sac and a chronic stasis, which leads to an exacerbated infection and more stasis. Approximately 40% of initial attacks do not recur, but in the other 60% of patients, repeated attacks occur. Chronic dacryocystitis may be the end stage of acute or subacute dacryocystitis, but it may present initially as a subclinically infectious cause of nasolacrimal duct obstruction. A common organism involved is *Staphylococcus aureus*. In some cases, especially in young women, stones may develop that lead to intermittent attacks of dacryocystitis; this has been termed acute dacryocystic retention syndrome.

In dacryocystitis with pericystitis, there is percolation of infected debris through the mucosal lining of the wall of the sac, and infection around the sac is present. The infection may spread to the anterior orbit and produce a tremendous amount of eyelid swelling (Fig. 98-8). If the infection proceeds posterior to the orbital septum, as might occur in immunocompromised patients, a true orbital cellulitis may occur, resulting in globe proptosis or displacement, afferent pupillary defect, motility disturbance, optic neuropathy, and even blindness.

TREATMENT OF LACRIMAL SAC AND DUCT OBSTRUCTION

Congenital Nasolacrimal Obstruction

More than 90% of patients with congenital nasolacrimal obstruction undergo spontaneous resolution by 1 year of age.[16] Therefore, except under extreme circumstances, initial probing should be postponed until this age. Congenital amnioceles usually resolve on their own and rarely require probing.

Probings are performed more easily with the patient under general anesthesia. The probe is passed into the lower canaliculus with the lid stretched laterally. The probe is turned past the 90° angulation and advanced inferiorly until it perforates the membrane. Fluorescein-tinted irrigation saline is introduced to see whether it passes into the inferior meatus, and metal-to-metal contact may be obtained by inserting a probe into the nose. The success rate of probing is greater than 90%. If this fails, however, one should wait 3 months before doing another pro-

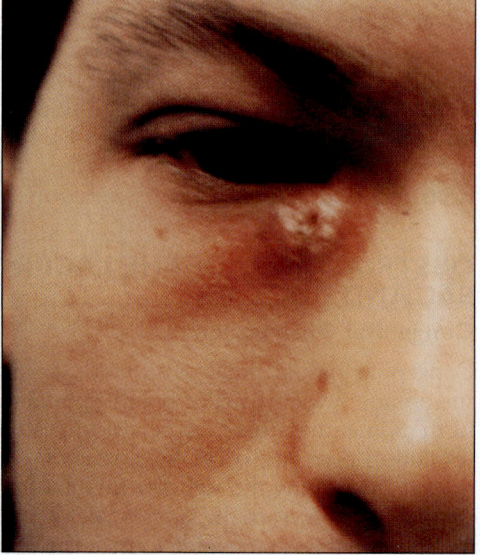

FIG. 98-7 ▮ A patient who has dacryocystitis localized to the lacrimal sac. Mild pericystitis exists.

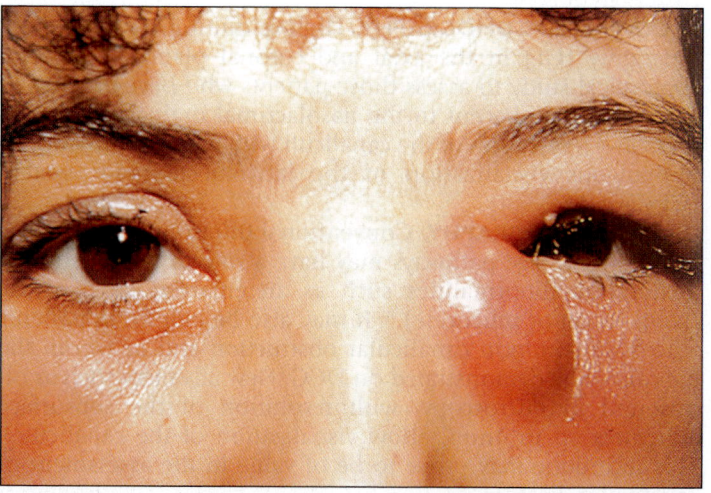

FIG. 98-8 ▮ A patient who has dacryocystitis and orbital cellulitis. Ocular mobility is limited, indicating infection posterior to the orbital septum.

cedure, during which time most cases of seemingly failed probing resolve spontaneously.

If the repeat probing does not proceed easily, Silastic tubes should be placed and left for at least 3 months (preferably 6 months). If these tubes fail and the child is still tearing, a DCR is performed at a later date. However, one may perform a primary DCR on a 1-year-old patient when no nasolacrimal system has developed inferior to the lacrimal sac. Complications of silicone include cheese-wiring into the nose, with destruction of the punctum and proximal canaliculus, and dislocation of the tubes laterally over the cornea. In this latter situation, it is better to reposition the tubes than to remove them.

If the probe cannot be passed through to the nose, a DCR should be performed.

Acquired Nasolacrimal Obstruction

After an attack of dacryocystitis or obstruction, a period of observation is useful. Occasionally, if a mucous plug develops in the system, symptoms may resolve spontaneously. Medication such as naphazoline nasal spray shrink the nasal mucosa and may be used for a short period (no more than 5 days, for fear of atrophic rhinitis developing).

Medications such as antihistamines, either topical or local, and botulinum toxin have been reported to decrease lacrimal secretion. Surgical removal of the palpebral lobe of the lacrimal gland has been attempted, but there is a risk of producing a dry eye.

In the presence of frank dacryocystitis, the cardinal rule is to first treat the infection. The antibiotic of choice is an antistaphylococcal one, such as oral cloxacillin. If postseptal orbital cellulitis is present, a CT scan is obtained to rule out an abscess, and intravenous antibiotics are used. If the infection does not resolve and perforation is impending, a dacryocystotomy should be performed. After injecting lidocaine (lignocaine), an incision is made directly over the lacrimal sac, and the debris within the sac is curetted. Transcutaneous aspiration of sac contents for culture may be done with a No. 22 needle.

If epiphora persists after resolution of the infection, probing and syringing may be attempted before bypass surgery. Also, insertion of silicone tubes to hold the passage open may be attempted, but neither technique is very successful. More recently, attempts to dilate the sac and duct have been undertaken with a balloon catheter passed through the normal system or via an opening made through the lacrimal fossa into the nose.[17] Two successive dilatations using a 5mm-diameter balloon for 60 seconds and then 30 seconds have been reported to permanently dilate the system. Success rates for long-term patency are problematical.

Dacryocystorhinostomy

DCR is an operation whereby the lacrimal sac is drained into the nose. The classic transcutaneous procedure of Toti[18] has undergone many minor modifications, but the basic operation has withstood the test of time and has a high success rate of 93–95%.[19] It may be performed with the patient under general or local anesthesia.[20] In either case, the nose is premedicated with naphazoline nasal spray at 2 hours, 1 hour, and 30 minutes before surgery.

The surgical goal is to make an epithelium-lined tract between the sac and the nasal mucosa. It is important that the epithelium of the sac and the epithelium of the nasal mucosa become continuous, with minimal trauma produced in the epithelium of each structure. It seems logical that this goal is most likely to be achieved by directly suturing both posterior flaps and anterior flaps. A Silastic tube is inserted to hold the passage open if adequate separation of the anterior flaps from the posterior flaps cannot be achieved. Any foreign body or stent within the system can produce complications, so intubation should be avoided if at all possible without compromising the ultimate success of the operation.

The procedure is well described elsewhere.[21] An incision as small as 8mm is made on the side of the nose below the medial canthal tendon, and the dissection is carried down to bone. The periosteum is reflected from the anterior lacrimal crest to reveal the lacrimal sac fossa. The anterior limb of the medial canthal tendon may be cut without compromising the medial canthus because of the tight attachments of the posterior limb of the tendon. The sac is then reflected laterally.

The nose is entered by pushing a blunt instrument through the suture line between the lacrimal bone and the frontal process of the maxilla. Kerrison punches are used to remove bone between the sac fossa and the nose, to create an opening large enough to anastomose the sac and nasal mucosa. Flaps are created in the medial sac wall and in the adjacent nasal mucosa. The posterior flaps and then the anterior flaps of the sac and nasal mucosa are sutured together to form a mucosa-lined tunnel across the ostium (Fig. 98-9). Silicone tubes are usually not necessary, but if desired, they can be placed at this time and left in for 6–12 weeks.[22] Nasal packing is not necessary unless pro-

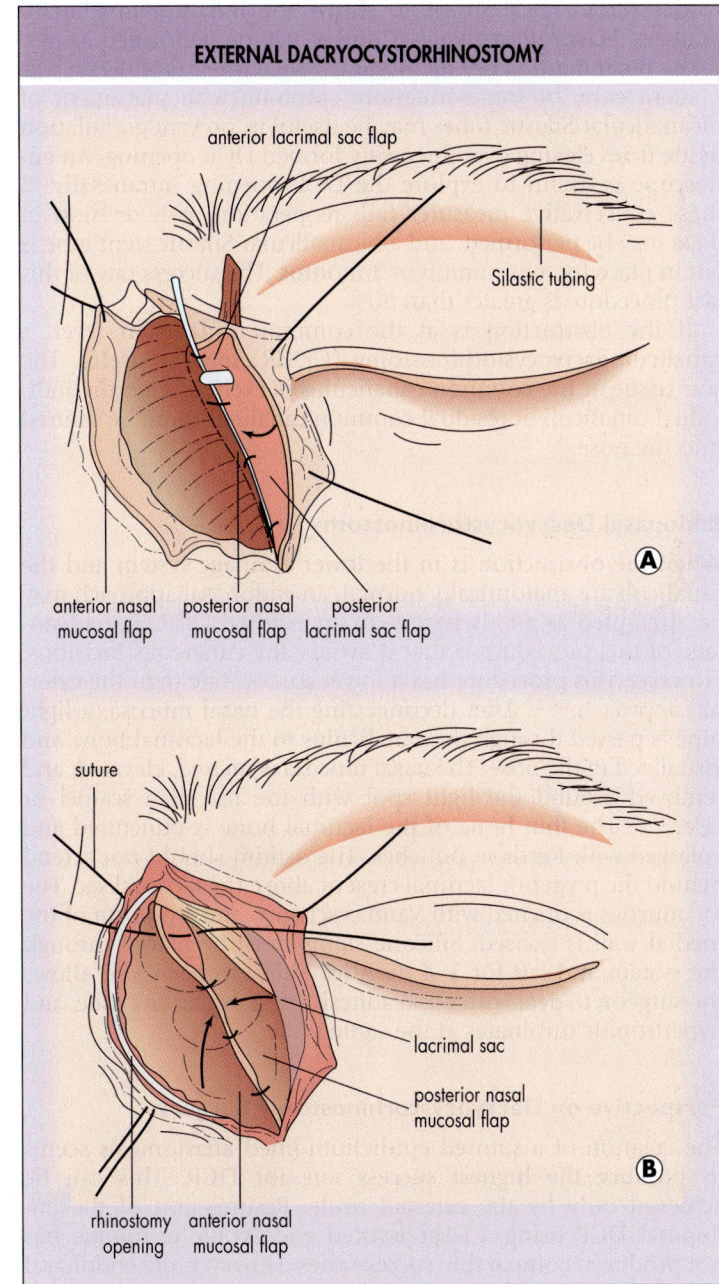

EXTERNAL DACRYOCYSTORHINOSTOMY

anterior lacrimal sac flap

Silastic tubing

anterior nasal mucosal flap   posterior nasal mucosal flap   posterior lacrimal sac flap

Ⓐ

suture

lacrimal sac

posterior nasal mucosal flap

Ⓑ

rhinostomy opening   anterior nasal mucosal flap

FIG. 98-9 ▮ **External dacryocystorhinostomy. A,** Posterior flaps of the sac (*small arrow*) and nasal mucosa (*large arrow*) being sutured. **B,** Anterior flaps of the sac (*small arrow*) and nasal mucosa (*large arrow*) being anastomosed. (Adapted with permission from Hurwitz JJ. Diseases of the sac and duct. In: Hurwitz JJ, ed. The lacrimal system. Philadelphia: Lippincott-Raven; 1996. Artwork courtesy of Terry Tarrant, London.)

fuse bleeding occurs at the end of the operation. Postoperative antibiotics should be considered, even if the patient did not have dacryocystitis preoperatively.

Complications of hemorrhage within the first 24 hours should be controlled by lowering the blood pressure to normal values and by nasal packing. Delayed hemorrhage 4–7 days after surgery is due to clot retraction, comparable to an eight-ball hemorrhage following an initial hyphema. Vaseline gauze packs soaked with thrombin are useful and should be left in place for 48 hours. If all else fails, embolization may be helpful.[23] Orbital hemorrhage may occur, but this is extremely rare.[24]

A hypertrophic cutaneous scar is unusual, but if present, it usually settles quite well with massage. Triamcinolone also may be injected into the scar.

Surgical failure may result from closure of the anastomosis between the sac and the nasal mucosa, or an obstruction may occur at the common canaliculus, either undiagnosed preoperatively or developing postoperatively. Whether the obstruction is within the common canaliculus or at the entrance of the lacrimal sac into the nose can be determined by DCG. Initial treatment is conservative, consisting of decongestants or corticosteroid nasal sprays to shrink the inflammatory membrane or granulation tissue. A probe may be performed to perforate the inflammatory membrane, which often produces a permanent cure. In some situations, probing with placement of bicanalicular Silastic tubes may be useful to prevent granulation tissue from closing over the newly formed DCR opening. An endoscope is useful to explore the DCR opening intranasally. If these conservative measures fail, reoperation with revision of flaps may be performed, and a bicanalicular Silastic stent tube is left in place for a minimum of 3 months. The success rate of this last procedure is greater than 80%.

If the obstruction is at the common canalicular level, a canaliculodacryocystorhinostomy (CDCR) may be useful. The scar tissue at the common canaliculus is excised; then the individual canaliculi or residual common canaliculus can be sutured into the nose.[25]

Endonasal Dacryocystorhinostomy

When the obstruction is in the lower drainage system and the canaliculi are anatomically normal, an endonasal approach may be attempted as an alternative to an external DCR. The advantage of this procedure is that it avoids any cutaneous incisions. However, this procedure has a lower success rate than the external approach.[26, 27] After decongesting the nasal mucosa, a light pipe is passed through the canaliculus to the lacrimal bone and visualized in the nose. The nasal mucosa is incised, elevated, and removed around the light spot with the use of a scalpel or laser.[28-30] The thin bone of the lacrimal bone is punctured and enlarged with Kerrison punches. The ostium should not extend behind the posterior lacrimal crest or above the lacrimal sac. The sac mucosa is opened with Vannas scissors, and a portion of the medial wall is excised. Silicone stents must be placed through the system and left for 3–4 months. This approach also allows the surgeon to deal with nasal adhesions, granulation tissue, and hypertrophic turbinates at the same time.

Perspective on Dacryocystorhinostomy Surgery

The creation of a sutured epithelium-lined anastomosis seems to produce the highest success rate for DCR. This can be achieved only by the external route. Resurrection of the endonasal DCR using a laser-assisted endoscopic technique has not produced comparable success rates. However, the endonasal approach without the laser has better success rates than the endonasal procedure with the laser.

Whatever the surgeon's preference with respect to the indications for surgery in a particular patient, both external and endonasal approaches should be in his or her armamentarium.

TUMORS OF THE LACRIMAL SAC

Primary lacrimal sac tumors present as masses at the medial canthus. Depending on the age of the patient, there may or may not be symptoms of tearing. These patients often exhibit patency to syringing because the tumor usually arises in the epithelium and only later grows toward the lumen. Bloody tears may be present. Lacrimal sac tumors may be benign or malignant, epithelial or nonepithelial.[31] DCG and CT are useful to demonstrate the location of the mass and its extent, as well as associated involvement of the lacrimal drainage pathways. Bony erosion is often present in these cases.

DISEASES OF THE CANALICULI

Canalicular obstruction may have inflammatory, traumatic, idiopathic, or suppurative (canaliculitis—usually actinomycotic) causes. Whereas some diseases certainly involve both the punctum and the canaliculus, many involve either one or the other and so should be considered separately.[32]

PUNCTAL STENOSIS

Punctal stenosis can be congenital or acquired.[33] Congenital obstruction may be caused by a membrane overlying the punctal papilla. In such situations, the rest of the punctum and the canaliculus are patent, so merely perforating the membrane with a 25-gauge needle may be sufficient to achieve permanent patency. If the papilla of the punctum is absent, the distal canaliculus often has not developed either, so affected patients usually require the placement of a Jones tube. Marsupialization of the remaining canaliculus into the lacrimal lake does not offer a good solution.

Acquired obstructions may result from antiviral or antiglaucoma medications, cicatrizing diseases of the conjunctiva, various infections, radiation, and chemotherapeutic agents, which may also obstruct the canaliculi. Intrinsic tumors, such as papillomas and skin malignancies (e.g., basal cell and squamous carcinoma), also may obstruct the puncta. Most acquired punctal obstructions, however, are secondary to punctal eversion, which may be related to eyelid laxity or to cicatrizing diseases of the skin.

REFERENCES

1. Norn MS. Tear secretion in normal eyes. Acta Ophthalmol. 1965;43:567–77.
2. Jones LT. The lacrimal secretory system and its treatment. Am J Ophthalmol. 1966;62:47–64.
3. Jones LT, Wobig JL. Surgery of the eyelids and lacrimal system. Birmingham: Aesculapius; 1976.
4. Ahl NC, Hill JC. Horner's muscle and the lacrimal system. Arch Ophthalmol. 1982;100:488–93.
5. Becker BB. Tricompartment model of the lacrimal pump mechanism. Ophthalmology. 1992;99:1139–45.
6. Jones LT. An anatomical approach to problems of the eyelids and lacrimal apparatus. Arch Ophthalmol. 1961;66:111–20.
7. Lloyd GAS, Welham RAN. Subtraction macrodacryocystography. Br J Radiol. 1974;47:379–91.
8. Galloway JE, Kavic TA, Raflo GT. Digital subtraction macrodacryocystography. Ophthalmology. 1984;91:956–68.
9. Ashenhurst ME, Hurwitz JJ. Combined computed tomography and dacryocystography for complex lacrimal obstruction. Can J Ophthalmol. 1991;26:27–37.
10. Dutton JJ. Standardized echography in the diagnosis of lacrimal drainage dysfunction. Arch Ophthalmol. 1989;107:1010–2.
11. Pavlin CJ, Sherar MD, Foster FS. Subsurface ultrasound biomicroscopic imaging of the intact eye. Ophthalmology. 1990;97:244–50.
12. Ashenhurst ME, Hurwitz JJ. Lacrimal canaliculoscopy: development of the instrument. Can J Ophthalmol. 1991;26:306–9.
13. Linberg JV, McCormick SA. Primary acquired nasolacrimal duct obstruction: a clinical pathological report and biopsy technique. Ophthalmology. 1986;93:1055–62.
14. Hurwitz JJ. Diseases of the sac and duct. In: Hurwitz JJ, ed. The lacrimal system. Philadelphia: Lippincott-Raven; 1996:117–48.
15. Holds JD, Anderson RL, Wolin MJ. Dacryocystectomy for the treatment of dacryocystitis patient with Wegener's granulomatosis. Ophthalmic Surg. 1989;20:443–8.
16. Welham RAN, Bergin DJ. Congenital lacrimal fistulas. Arch Ophthalmol. 1985;103:545–8.
17. Becker BB, Berry FD. Balloon catheter dilatation and lacrimal surgery. Ophthalmic Surg. 1989;20:193–200.
18. Toti A. Dacryocystorhinostomia. Magophthalmology. 1910;23–38.
19. Hurwitz JJ, Rutherford S. Computerized survey of lacrimal surgery patients. Ophthalmology. 1986;93:14–21.

20. Ananthanaryan CR, Hew EM, Hurwitz JJ. Anesthesia for lacrimal surgery. In: Hurwitz JJ, ed. The lacrimal system. Philadelphia: Lippincott-Raven; 1996:247–56.
21. Hurwitz JJ. Dacryocystorhinostomy. In: Hurwitz JJ, ed. The lacrimal system. Philadelphia: Lippincott-Raven; 1996:261–96.
22. Archer K, Hurwitz JJ. An alternative method of canalicular stent tube placement in lacrimal drainage surgery. Ophthalmic Surg. 1988;19:510–20.
23. Elder L, Montanara W, Terbrugge K, *et al.* Angiographic embolisation for the treatment of epistaxis: a review of 108 cases. Otolaryngol Head Neck Surg. 1994; 111:44–54.
24. Hurwitz JJ, Eplett CJ, Fliss D, Freeman JL. Orbital hemorrhage during dacryocystorhinostomy. Can J Ophthalmol. 1992;29:139–44.
25. Doucet TW, Hurwitz JJ. Canaliculodacryocystorhinostomy in the management of unsuccessful lacrimal surgery. Arch Ophthalmol. 1982;100:619–24.
26. Talbet KJ, Custer PL. External dacryocystorhinostomy: surgical success, patient satisfaction and economic costs. Ophthalmology. 1995;102:1065–70.
27. Hartikaine J, Seppa H, Grenman R. External DCR [letter]. Ophthalmology. 1996;103:200.
28. Massaro EM, Gonnering RS, Harris GJ. Endonasal laser dacryocystorhinostomy: new approach to lacrimal duct obstruction. Arch Ophthalmol. 1990;108:1172–8.
29. Silkiss RZ. Nd–YAG nasolacrimal duct recanalization. Ophthalmic Surg. 1993;24:772–6.
30. Bush GA, Lemke BN, Dortzbach RK. Results of endonasal laser assisted dacryocystorhinostomy. Ophthalmology. 1994;101:995–61.
31. Howarth D, Hurwitz JJ. Lacrimal sac tumours. In: Hurwitz JJ, ed. The lacrimal system. Philadelphia: Lippincott-Raven; 1996:187–94.
32. Hurwitz JJ. Canalicular diseases. In: Hurwitz JJ, ed. The lacrimal system. Philadelphia: Lippincott-Raven; 1996:139–47.
33. Hurwitz, JJ. Diseases of the punctum. In: Hurwitz JJ, ed. The lacrimal system. Philadelphia: Lippincott-Raven; 1996:149–53.

RETINA AND VITREOUS

Jay S. Duker

SECTION I BASIC SCIENCE

CHAPTER

99

Structure and Function of the Neural Retina

HERMANN D. SCHUBERT

INTRODUCTION

The primary purpose of the corneoscleral and uveal coats of the eye is to focus light on the retina; they also provide protection and nourishment and enable movement. The retina is derived embryologically from the optic vesicle, an outpouching of the embryonic forebrain.[1] The bilayered neuroepithelial structure of the mature retina reflects the apex-to-apex arrangement of the original optic cup. It also forms the wall of a cavity, the vitreous cavity, which is filled with glycosaminoglycans and collagen. The ocular cavity is homologous to a leptomeningeal cistern,[2] in that both vitreous and choroid are derived from mesenchyme that sandwiches the neuroepithelium on its path away from the brain. The ocular neuroepithelial cyst has two openings. Anteriorly lies the pupil, which is a full-thickness aperture, and posteriorly lies the optic nerve in which, similar to a coloboma, only derivatives of the inner retinal layers are found. Since the cell apices are oriented inwardly, the two layers of the optic cup and their derivatives are enveloped externally by basement membrane (Fig. 99-1).

The relationship of the epithelial layers to each other is modified from anterior to posterior. Anterior to the ora serrata, the pigmented and nonpigmented epithelia of the iris and ciliary body are joined at their apices by a system of intercellular junctions (Fig. 99-2), which is continuous with the external limiting layer of the neural retina and the apical junctional girdles of the retinal pigment epithelium (RPE; Fig. 99-3). At the ora serrata, the pigmented epithelium is continued as RPE; its basement

membrane becomes Bruch's membrane. The nonpigmented epithelium of the ciliary body and pars plana is continued posteriorly as the neural retina; its basement membrane becomes the internal limiting membrane. The union of the epithelial layers delimits the anterior cul-de-sac of the subretinal space.[3]

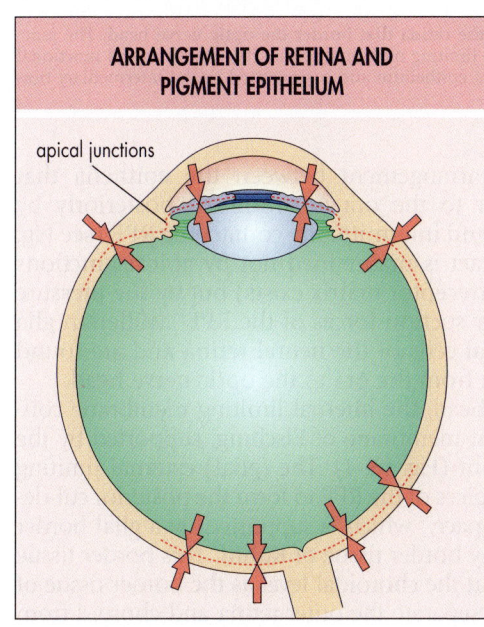

ARRANGEMENT OF RETINA AND PIGMENT EPITHELIUM

apical junctions

FIG. 99-2 ■ Apex-to-apex arrangement of retina and pigment epithelium. Apical attachments connect the iris and ciliary body epithelia (red line).

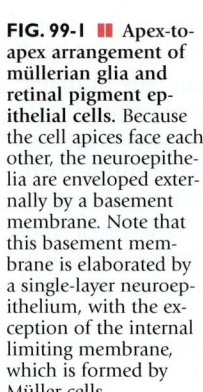

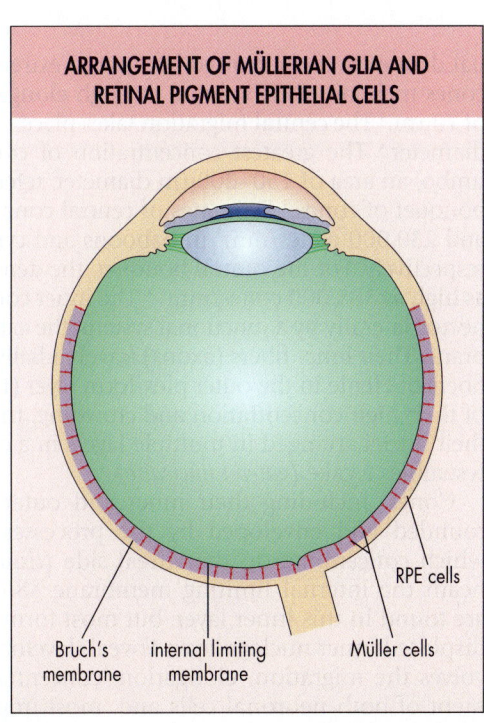

ARRANGEMENT OF MÜLLERIAN GLIA AND RETINAL PIGMENT EPITHELIAL CELLS

Bruch's membrane

internal limiting membrane

Müller cells

RPE cells

FIG. 99-1 ■ Apex-to-apex arrangement of müllerian glia and retinal pigment epithelial cells. Because the cell apices face each other, the neuroepithelia are enveloped externally by a basement membrane. Note that this basement membrane is elaborated by a single-layer neuroepithelium, with the exception of the internal limiting membrane, which is formed by Müller cells.

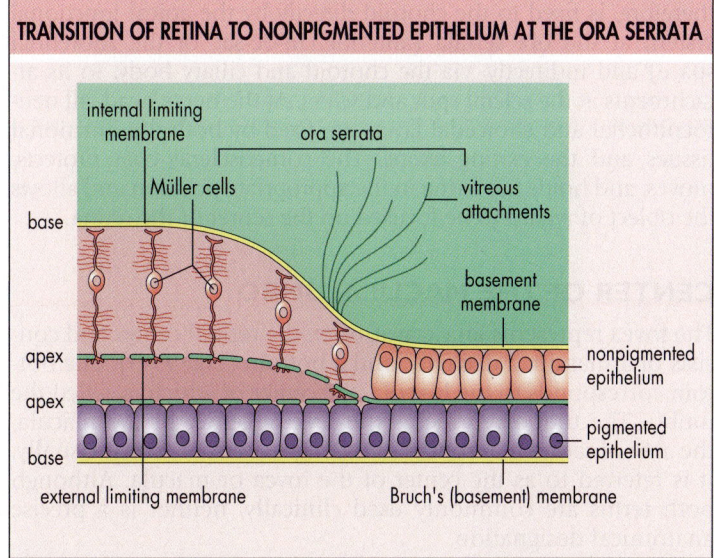

TRANSITION OF RETINA TO NONPIGMENTED EPITHELIUM AT THE ORA SERRATA

internal limiting membrane

ora serrata

Müller cells

vitreous attachments

basement membrane

nonpigmented epithelium

pigmented epithelium

base

apex

apex

base

external limiting membrane

Bruch's (basement) membrane

FIG. 99-3 ■ Transition of neural retina to nonpigmented epithelium at the ora serrata. The external limiting membrane, which consists of the attachment sites of photoreceptors and Müller cells, transforms into the apical junctional system of the pars plana epithelia. The internal limiting membrane becomes the basement membrane of the nonpigmented epithelium.

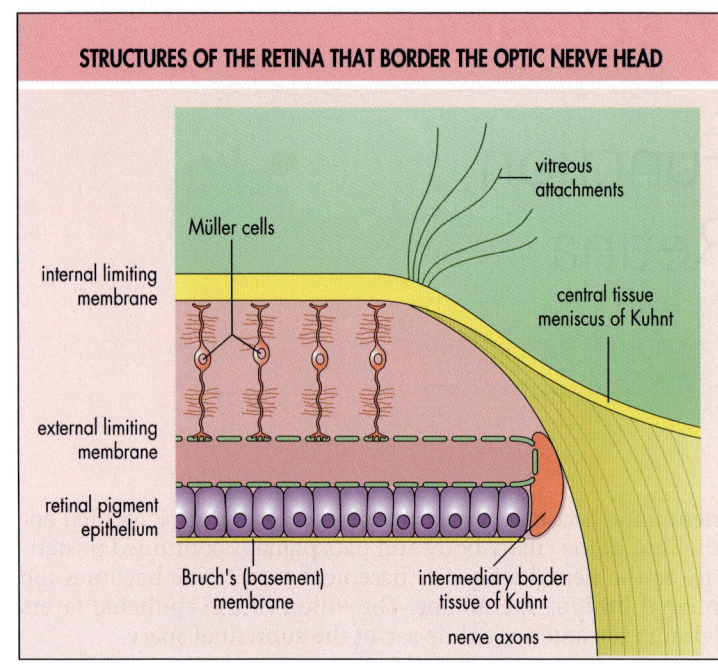

FIG. 99-4 ■ **Structures of the retina that border the optic nerve head.** The junctional system of the external limiting membrane connects with the apical junctional system of the retinal pigment epithelium and is supported by the intermediary border tissue of Kuhnt.

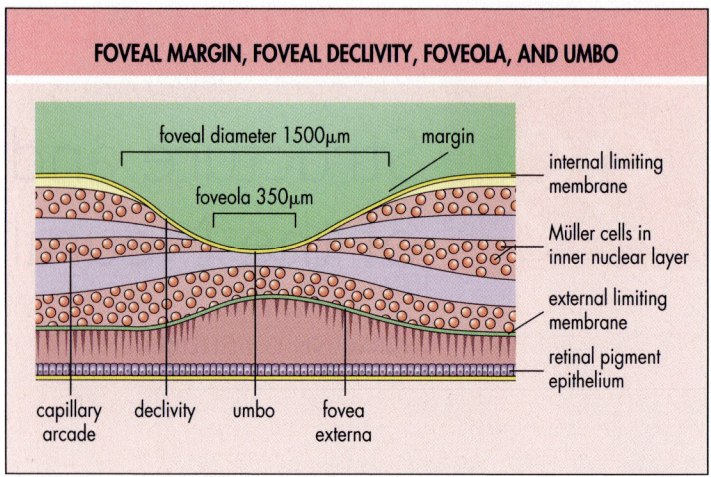

FIG. 99-5 ■ **Foveal margin, foveal declivity, foveola, and umbo.** The foveal diameter (from margin to margin) measures 1500μm, and the foveola is 350μm in diameter. The foveal avascular zone is slightly larger (500μm) and is delimited by the capillary arcades at the level of the inner nuclear layer. The foveal excavation represents the fovea interna, which is lined by the internal limiting membrane. The fovea externa is represented by the junctional system of the external limiting membrane. Both Henle's fibers and the accompanying glia assume a horizontal and radial arrangement in the fovea.

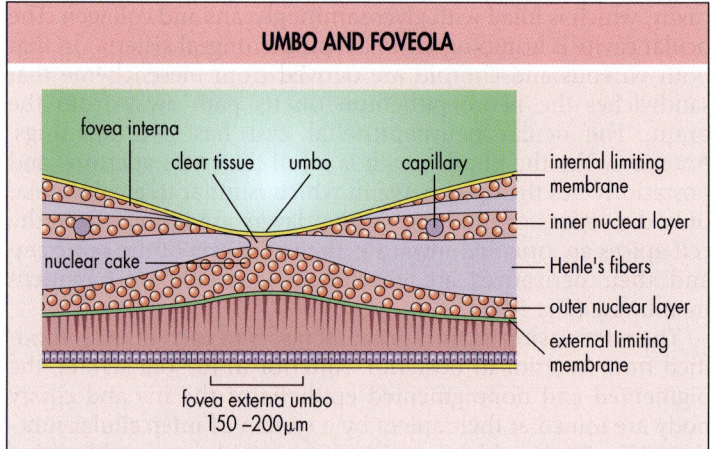

FIG. 99-6 ■ **Umbo (center) and foveola.** The outer nuclear layer is separated from the inner nuclear layer by the horizontal-oblique fibers of Henle. Umbo and foveola between few nuclei feature clear müllerian fibers (clear tissue), delimited by Henle's fibers externally and by the internal limiting membrane internally. The central 150–200μm represents the umbo, where cone concentration is maximal.

The apex-to-apex arrangement between the epithelia that clearly exists anterior to the ora is continued posteriorly by Müller cells that face and intermittently contact the RPE (see Fig. 99-1). Here, the contact is maintained not by apical junctions (even though an interreceptor matrix exists) but by the pressure of the vitreous and by suction forces of the RPE. Müllerian glia are the main structural cells of the neural retina and are found throughout the retina from the ora to the optic nerve head.

At the optic nerve head, the internal limiting membrane continues as the basement membrane of Elschnig, supported by the glial meniscus of Kuhnt (Fig. 99-4). The (glial) external limiting membrane joins the apices of the RPE to form the posterior cul-de-sac of the subretinal space,[3] which is supported by a glial border tissue, the intermediary border tissue of Kuhnt. This border tissue continues posteriorly at the choroidal level as the border tissue of Elschnig; both tissues separate the outer retina and choroid from the axons of the inner retina. The axons in turn fixate the posterior retina to the scleral lamina cribrosa and its glial system. The retina, therefore, is fixed to the choroid directly by the apical junctional system at the ora serrata (anterior cul-de-sac of the subretinal space) and indirectly, via the choroid and ciliary body, to its attachments at the scleral spur and sclera. At the nerve head, all neuroepithelial and choroidal layers are fixed by both the junctional tissues and the exiting axons. The corneoscleral coat protects, moves, and holds the retina in the appropriate position and allows the object of regard to be focused on the center of the retina.

CENTER OF THE MACULA: UMBO

The fovea represents an excavation in the retinal center and consists of a margin, a declivity, and a bottom (Fig. 99-5). The bottom corresponds to the foveola, the center of which is called the umbo. The umbo represents the precise center of the macula, the area of retina that results in the highest visual acuity. Usually, it is referred to as the center of the fovea or macula. Although both terms are commonly used clinically, neither is a precise anatomical designation.

The predominant photoreceptor of the foveola and umbo is the cone. The foveal cones result from the centripetal migration of the first neuron and the centrifugal lateral displacement of the second and third neurons during foveal maturation, which occur 3 months before and 3 months after term.[4] Although their individual diameters are narrowed because of extreme crowding, central cones maintain their volume through elongation, up to a length of 70μm.[5] The central migration takes place in an area of 1500μm diameter.[4] The greatest concentration of cones is found in the umbo, an area of 150–200μm diameter, referred to as the central bouquet of cones.[5] Estimates of central cone density are 113,000 and 230,000 cones/mm² in baboons and cynomolgus monkeys, respectively. For the central bouquet, the density of cones may be as high as 385,000 cones/mm².[6] The inner cone segments are connected laterally by a junctional system, the external limiting membrane. Their inner fibers (axons) travel radially and peripherally as fibers of Henle in the outer plexiform layer (Fig. 99-6). As a result of their high concentration and crowding, the central cones have their nuclei arranged in multiple layers in a circular shape, which resembles a cake (*gateau nucleaire*).[5]

Cones, including their inner and outer segments, are surrounded and enveloped by the processes of müllerian glia, which concentrate on the vitreal side (*tissu clair*),[5] just underneath the internal limiting membrane.[7] Some glial cell nuclei are found in this inner layer, but most form part of the laterally displaced inner nuclear layer. Foveal development, therefore, involves the migration, elongation, concentration, and displacement of both neuronal cells and, most importantly, glial cells, the main structural element of the retina. Radiating striae found in the foveal internal limiting membrane are related to Henle's fibers but are probably mediated by glia that elaborate and are connected to the internal limiting membrane. The density of the foveal glia has been measured as 16,600–20,000 cells/mm[2].[6]

FOVEOLA

The bouquet of central cones is surrounded by the foveal bottom, or foveola, which measures 350μm in diameter and 150μm in thickness (see Fig. 99-5). This avascular area consists of densely packed cones that are elongated and connected by the external limiting membrane. As a result of the elongation of the outer segments, the external limiting membrane is bowed vitreally, a phenomenon that has been termed *fovea externa*. Both umbo and foveola represent the most visible part of the outer retina; however, to the level of the external limiting membrane, all cones and their axons are enveloped by the processes of Müller cells, which form the vitreal inner layer and elaborate and support the internal limiting membrane. Thus, the apex-to-apex arrangement of the optic cup is maintained by the processes of müllerian glia that face the apices of the pigment epithelial cells in the foveola. The high metabolic demands of central cones are met by direct contact with the pigment epithelium, as well as through the processes of glia whose nuclei lie more peripheral in the inner nuclear layer and closer to the perifoveal vascular arcades (see Fig. 99-6).

In pathological conditions, loss of the normal foveolar reflex may indicate a glial disturbance (acute nerve cell damage, cloudy swelling) either primarily or mediated by the vitreous, which is tightly adherent to the thin internal limiting membrane. Loss of the foveal reflex may thus indicate traction or edema of glial cells and, secondarily, of cones. The inner glial layer may separate from the nuclear layer, which results in cystlike schisis.

FOVEA

The fovea consists of the thin bottom, a 22° declivity (the clivus),[3] and a thick margin (see Figs. 99-5 to 99-7). The bottom, or foveola, was described earlier. The declivity of 22° denotes the lateral displacement of the second and third neurons in the inner nuclear layer, which includes most of the nuclei of its müllerian glia. The avascular foveola is surrounded by the vascular arcades, a circular system of capillaries. These vessels are located at the level of the internal nuclear layer and leave an avascular zone of 250–600μm between them. The declivity also is associated with an increase in basement membrane thickness, which reaches a maximum at the foveal margin. Internal limiting membrane thickness and strength of vitreal attachment are inversely proportional; that is, adhesions are strongest in the foveola.[3] Not surprisingly, the foveal center is most affected in traumatic macular holes in which glial opercula suggest anterior-posterior traction as the cause. The margin of the fovea (*margo foveae*) is often seen biomicroscopically as a ring-like reflection of the internal limiting membrane, which measures 1500μm (disc size) in diameter and 0.55mm in thickness (see Fig. 99-7).

PARAFOVEA

The parafovea is a belt that measures 0.5mm in width and surrounds the foveal margin (see Fig. 99-7). At this distance from the center, the retina features a regular architecture of layers, which includes 4–6 layers of ganglion cells and 7–11 layers of bipolar cells.[8]

PERIFOVEA

The perifovea surrounds the parafovea as a belt that measures 1.5mm wide (see Fig. 99-7). The region is characterized by several layers of ganglion cells and six layers of bipolar cells.[8]

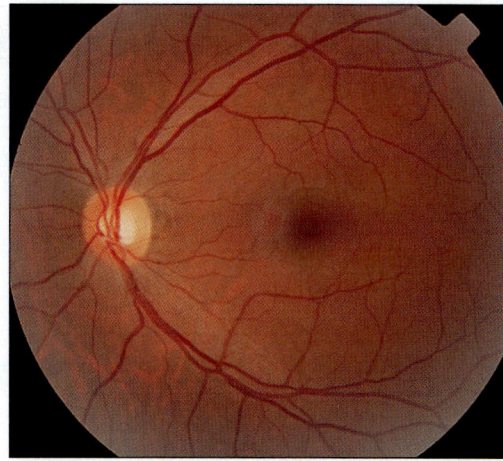

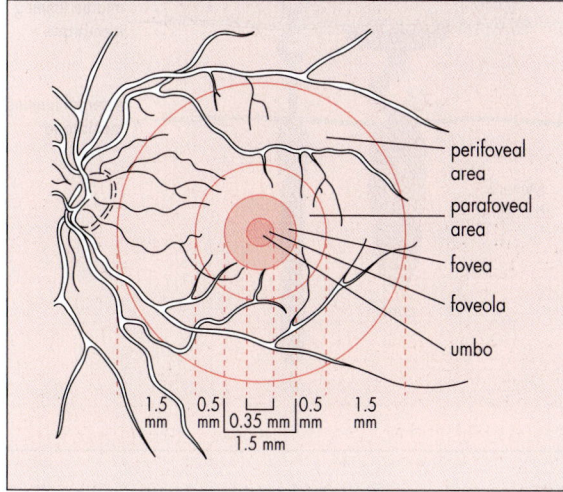

FIG. 99-7 ■ Normal fundus with macula encompassed by major vascular arcades. The macula, or central area, has the following components from center to periphery: umbo, foveola, fovea, parafovea, and perifovea.

MACULA, OR CENTRAL AREA

The umbo, foveola, fovea, parafovea, and perifovea together constitute the macula, or central area.[9] The central area can be differentiated from the extra-areal periphery by the ganglion cell layer. In the macula, the ganglion cell layer is several cells thick; however, in the extra-areal periphery, it is only one cell thick. The macular border coincides with the course of the major temporal arcades and has an approximate diameter of 5.5mm (see Fig. 99-7), which comprises the diameter of the fovea (1.5mm), twice the width of the parafovea (2 × 0.5 = 1mm), and twice the width of the perifovea (2 × 1.5 = 3mm).[10]

EXTRA-AREAL PERIPHERY

The peripheral retina is divided arbitrarily into belts of near, middle, far, and extreme periphery.[9] The belt of the near periphery is 1.5mm wide, and the belt of the middle periphery, or equator, is 3mm wide. The far periphery extends from the equator to the ora serrata. The width of this belt varies, depending on ocular size and refractive error. The average circumference of the eye is 72mm at the equator and 60mm at the ora serrata, and the average width of this belt is 6mm. Since peripheral retinal pathology is usually charted in clock hours, 1 clock hour corresponds to 5–6mm of far peripheral circumference. Therefore, the far periphery of the retina may be divided into 12 segments that measure approximately 6 × 6mm. As a result of the insertion of the posterior vitreous base, most peripheral pathology falls into these segments. The ora serrata and pars plana are referred to as the extreme periphery.[9]

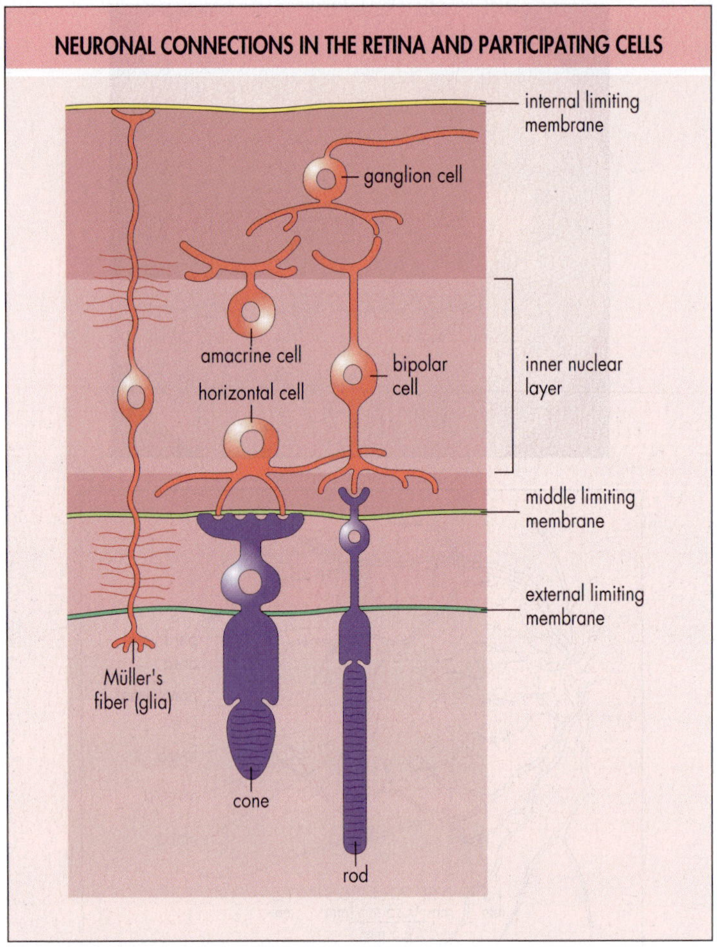

NEURONAL CONNECTIONS IN THE RETINA AND PARTICIPATING CELLS

internal limiting membrane

ganglion cell

amacrine cell

horizontal cell

bipolar cell

inner nuclear layer

middle limiting membrane

external limiting membrane

Müller's fiber (glia)

cone

rod

FIG. 99-8 ■ Neuronal connections in the retina and participating cells. The inner nuclear layer contains the nuclei of the bipolar cells (second neuron) and müllerian glia. The amacrine cells are found on the inside and the horizontal cells on the outside of this layer, next to their respective plexiform connections.

LAYERS OF THE NEURAL RETINA

With the exception of the fovea, ora serrata, and optic disc, the neural retina is organized in layers, dictated by the direction of the müllerian glia, its organizational backbone. Essentially, there is the photoreceptor layer plus the bipolar and ganglion cell layer, which represent the outer first neuron and inner second neuron of the visual pathway. The müllerian glia elaborate the internal limiting membrane as its basement membrane and extend to the external limiting membrane, where it communicates with the apices of the RPE (Fig. 99-8).

The inner nuclear layer is home to the nuclei of the müllerian glia, the bipolar cells, and the horizontal and amacrine cells. The amacrine cells lie on the inside of the inner nuclear layer, and the horizontal cells lie on the outside (see Fig. 99-8). The inner nuclear layer has plexiform layers on either side, which connect it to the outer photoreceptor layer and the (inner) ganglion cell layer. From this simple anatomical consideration, it follows that rods and cones synapse with bipolar and horizontal cells in the outer plexiform layer. As a result of the increased length of Henle's fibers, the junctional system (the middle limiting "membrane") is found in the inner third of the outer plexiform layer, which is the only truly plexiform portion of this layer. The bipolar cells and amacrine cells of the inner nuclear layer synapse

with the dendrites of the ganglion cells in the inner plexiform layer. In embryogenesis, müllerian glia, along with their internal limiting membrane and orientation, antedate photoreceptor differentiation; this is analogous to the rest of the central nervous system, in which structural development precedes individual cell differentiation.

PHOTOTRANSDUCTION AND VISUAL PROCESSING

The retina's function is to both capture external light and process the resultant stimuli. Both these tasks are highly complex and incompletely understood. Despite its relatively small size and compact structure, the morphology of the neural retina is extraordinarily complicated, a reflection of the complexity of its basic tasks.

The capture of a photon of light and its conversion into an electrical signal is called phototransduction, and it is accomplished within the outer segments of the photoreceptors—the rods and cones. The photopigment molecules that are the biochemical basis for phototransduction reside in the membranes of the photoreceptors' outer segment discs. In the rods, rhodopsin is the primary photopigment, and it best absorbs photons with a wavelength of 500nm (blue–green). Cone pigments are referred to collectively as iodopsin; there are three types, with absorption peaks in the blue, green, and yellow parts of the spectrum. Each cone normally contains only one of the three varieties of pigment molecules. Various stimulatory combinations of these three types of pigments are responsible for color vision perception.

All the photoreceptor cells respond to the capture of light energy with a hyperpolarization. The bipolar and horizontal cells represent the site of second-order information processing and communicate with the photoreceptors via the exchange of chemical neurotransmitters. In the dark-adapted state, photoreceptors are depolarized and release neurotransmitters. Hyperpolarization brought on by the capture of light energy results in a reduction in the release of neurotransmitters. As in other parts of the central nervous system, glutamate represents the major excitatory neurotransmitter, but it is likely that many others exist.

Higher-order processing in the neural retina is accomplished via the ganglion cells, the dendrites of which connect to bipolar cells within the inner plexiform layer. Amacrine cells further process the signal. Neuromodulation is probably accomplished via extracellular influences of the Müller cells.

REFERENCES

1. Mann I. The development of the human eye. New York: Grune & Stratton; 1950.
2. Gaertner I. The vitreous, an intraocular compartment of the leptomeninx. Doc Ophthalmol. 1986;62:205–22.
3. Fine BS, Yanoff M. Ocular histology. A text and atlas. New York: Harper & Row; 1979:111–24.
4. Hendrickson AE, Yuodelis C. The morphological development of the human fovea. Arch Ophthalmol. 1969;82:151–9.
5. Rochon-Duvigneaud A. Recherches sur la fovea de la retine humaine et particulierement sur le bouquet des cones centraux. Arch Anat Microsc. 1907;9:315–42.
6. Krebs W, Krebs I. Quantitative morphology of the central fovea in the primate retina. Am J Anat. 1989;184:225–36.
7. Yamada E. Some structural features of the fovea central in the human retina. Arch Ophthalmol. 1969;82:151–9.
8. Spitznas M. Anatomical features of the human macula. In: l'Esperance FA, ed. Current diagnosis and management of retinal disorders. St Louis: CV Mosby; 1977.
9. Polyak SL. The retina. Chicago: University of Chicago Press; 1941.
10. Hogan MJ, Alvarado JA, Wedell JE. Histology of the human eye. Philadelphia: WB Saunders; 1971:491–8.

CHAPTER
100 Retinal Pigment Epithelium

MICHAEL F. MARMOR

DEFINITION

- A melanin-containing epithelial layer that lies between the neural retina and choroid.

KEY FEATURES

- Absorption of scattered light.
- Control of fluid and nutrients in the subretinal space (blood-retinal barrier function).
- Visual pigment regeneration and synthesis.
- Synthesis of growth factors to modulate adjacent structures.
- Maintenance of retinal adhesion.
- Phagocytosis and digestion of photoreceptor wastes.
- Electrical homeostasis.
- Regeneration and repair after injury or surgery.

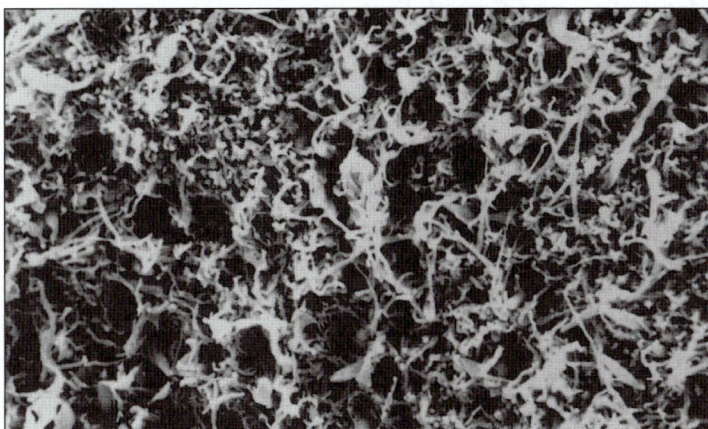

FIG. 100-1 ▌▌ Apical surface of human retinal pigment epithelium as seen through a scanning electron microscope. Fine microvilli cover the surface and reach up between the photoreceptor outer segments (which have been peeled away in this view).

INTRODUCTION

The retinal pigment epithelium (RPE) is a vital tissue for the maintenance of photoreceptor function.[1, 2] It is also affected by many diseases of the retina and choroid. Indeed, much of the pigmentary change that is visible clinically in retinal disorders takes place in the RPE (which is pigmented) rather than in the retina (which is transparent). Embryologically, the RPE is derived from the same neural tube tissue that forms the neural retina, but the cells differentiate into a transporting epithelium, the main functions of which are to metabolically insulate and support the overlying neural retina.

STRUCTURE

Cellular Architecture and Blood-Retinal Barrier

The RPE is a monolayer of cells that are cuboidal in cross section and hexagonal when viewed from above. The interlocking hexagonal cells are joined by tight junctions (zonulae occludens), which block the free passage of water and ions. This junctional barrier is the equivalent of the blood-retinal barrier formed by the capillary endothelium of the intrinsic retinal vasculature.

Cells of the RPE vary in size and shape across the retina. In the macular region, they are small (roughly 10–14μm in diameter), whereas toward the periphery, they become flatter and broader (diameter up to 60μm). The density of photoreceptors also varies across the retina, but the number of photoreceptors that overlie each RPE cell remains roughly constant (about 45 photoreceptors per RPE cell). This constancy has physiological relevance, in that each RPE cell is metabolically responsible for providing support functions to the overlying receptors.

In cross section, the RPE cell is differentiated into apical and basal configurations. On the apical side (facing the photoreceptors), long microvilli reach up between (and envelop) the outer segments of the photoreceptors (Fig. 100-1). Melanin granules are concentrated in the apical end of the cell. The midportion of the cell contains the nucleus and synthetic machinery (e.g., Golgi apparatus, endoplasmic reticulum) and digestive vesicles (lysosomes). The basal membrane lacks microvilli but has numerous convoluted infolds to increase the surface area for the absorption and secretion of material. The two membranes also have different ion channels and pumps.

Pigments

The pigment that gives the RPE its name is melanin, which is present within cytoplasmic granules called melanosomes. Developmentally, the RPE is the first tissue in the body to become pigmented, and melanogenesis continues to some degree throughout life. However, in older age, melanin granules often fuse with lysosomes and break down, so the elderly fundus typically appears less pigmented. The role of melanin in the eye remains somewhat speculative. The pigment serves to absorb stray light and minimize scatter within the eye, which has theoretical optical benefits. However, visual acuity is not degraded in very blond fundi relative to heavily pigmented ones, so the magnitude of this effect is unclear. Further, the appearance of the fundus can be misleading with respect to the RPE, since the greatest racial differences are a result of choroidal pigmentation rather than RPE pigmentation. Melanin also serves as a free radical stabilizer, and it can bind toxins and retinotoxic drugs such as chloroquine and thioridazine, although it is unclear whether this effect is beneficial or harmful. Albino eyes lack melanin, but the poor visual acuity of most albinos is a result of foveal aplasia rather than optical scatter.

The other major RPE pigment is lipofuscin, which accumulates in RPE cells gradually with age. However, lipofuscin is found throughout the nervous system, and its significance within the eye remains to be determined. Some lipofuscin is present in childhood, but by old age, the cells can be severely clogged with the golden, autofluorescent pigment. Lipofuscin is thought to be derived from outer segment lipids that have been ingested and then digested by the RPE; it may represent membrane fragments that have been damaged by light or oxidation. Because the substance accumulates in older eyes and these eyes may show RPE breakdown, as evidenced by drusen formation, RPE atrophy, and choroidal neovascularization, the question has been raised whether excess lipofuscin damages the RPE (or at least is a marker for cellular damage).[3] However, most elderly eyes have a considerable quantity of RPE lipofuscin, whereas only a few have clinically significant macular degeneration. A lipofuscin-like substance also accumulates in the RPE in Stargardt's disease, fundus flavimaculatus, and Best's vitelliform dystrophy, and may play a role in their pathogenesis.

METABOLISM AND MEMBRANE FUNCTION

Metabolism and Growth Factors

RPE cells are packed with mitochondria and engage actively in oxidative metabolism. Enzymes are synthesized for functions such as membrane transport, visual pigment metabolism, and digestion of wastes. The RPE contains the antioxidant enzymes superoxide dismutase and catalase, which minimize the formation of free radicals that can damage lipid membranes. The RPE contributes to the formation and maintenance of the interphotoreceptor matrix, which is critical for retinal adhesion, and to the elaboration of growth factors that modulate nearby tissues.

A number of growth factors are elaborated by RPE cells and serve to modulate not only the behavior of the RPE but also the behavior of surrounding tissues such as the choriocapillaris. Knowledge of these interactions is growing rapidly, and it is now recognized that the RPE is part of a complex system of cellular cross-talk that controls vascular supply, permeability, growth, repair, and other processes vital to retinal function. Factors produced by the RPE (though not necessarily exclusively) include platelet-derived growth factor (PDGF), which modulates cell growth and healing; pigment epithelium–derived factor (PEDF),[4] which acts as a neuroprotectant and vascular inhibitor; vascular endothelial growth factor (VEGF),[5] which can stimulate normal or neovascular growth; fibroblast growth factor (FGF), which can be neurotropic; and transforming growth factor (TGF), which moderates inflammation.

Membrane Properties and Fluid Transport

The RPE membrane contains a number of selective ion channels, as well as a number of active or facilitative transport systems for ions and for metabolites such as glucose and amino acids (e.g., taurine, which is essential to the photoreceptors). Different channels and transporters are present on the apical and basal membranes. For example, an electrogenic sodium-potassium pump occurs only on the apical membrane, whereas a chloride-bicarbonate exchange transporter occurs only on the basal membrane. The net effects of the asymmetrical transport systems are a movement of water across the RPE in the apical-to-basal direction and the generation of voltage across the RPE. It is important to recognize that both the movement of water and the transcellular potential are the sum of several transport systems that are moving ions and water in either direction. Thus, water transport can be diminished either by blocking a transporter that moves ions in the basal direction or by stimulating a transporter that moves ions in the apical direction.

The ability of the RPE to transport water is very powerful, and the RPE can pump fluid against a substantial gradient of hydrostatic or osmotic pressure. However, if the RPE barrier function is broken, fluid will leave the subretinal space more quickly (Fig. 100-2) because of intraocular pressure and osmotic suction from the choroid.[6] In other words, tight junctions are required to protect the neural environment of the retina, and because they are present, active transport by the RPE (and the expenditure of metabolic energy) is needed to keep the subretinal space dry.

These physiological observations have relevance for clinical disorders such as serous detachments. The unusual thing about a serous detachment is not that fluid gets in (given that a break

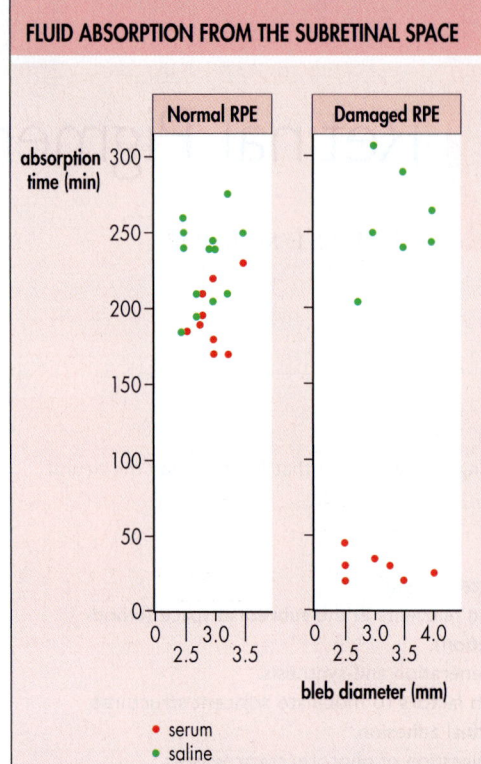

FLUID ABSORPTION FROM THE SUBRETINAL SPACE

Normal RPE | Damaged RPE

absorption time (min)

bleb diameter (mm)

● serum
● saline

FIG. 100-2 ■ Fluid absorption from the subretinal space. These results are from rabbit experiments in which either serum or saline was injected beneath the retina to form fluid blebs. Over normal retinal pigment epithelium (RPE), serum was absorbed nearly as fast as saline, since the water was being absorbed actively. When the RPE barrier was broken (by the toxin sodium iodate), saline fluid was absorbed much more quickly than normal, and the absorption of serum hardly changed, since the absorption now was osmotic. (Adapted from Negi A, Marmor MF. The resorption of subretinal fluid after diffuse damage to the retinal pigment epithelium. Invest Ophthalmol Vis Sci. 1983;24:1475–9.)

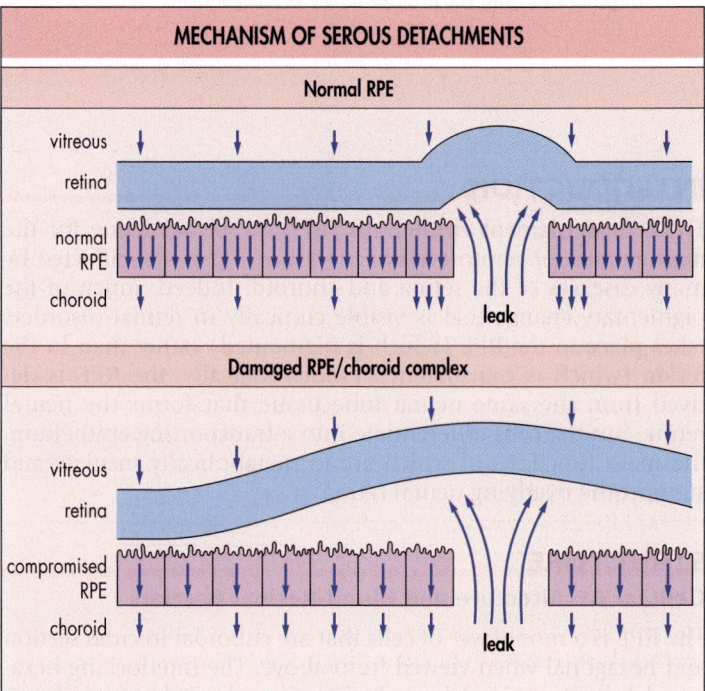

MECHANISM OF SEROUS DETACHMENTS

Normal RPE

vitreous
retina
normal RPE
choroid
leak

Damaged RPE/choroid complex

vitreous
retina
compromised RPE
choroid
leak

FIG. 100-3 ■ Mechanism of serous detachment. When the retinal pigment epithelium (RPE) is normal, no serous detachment occurs beyond a focal site of leakage. When the RPE is compromised by choroidal or RPE disease that impairs outward fluid transport, a serous detachment forms until absorption across the exposed RPE balances the inward leak.

is present in the RPE barrier) but that fluid accumulates and persists (since the powerful RPE would be expected to pump it right back out). Disorders such as central serous chorioretinopathy probably involve diffuse pathological changes of the RPE-choroid complex that impair fluid absorption[7] (Fig. 100-3).

Electrical Activity

The RPE is not a photoreceptive cell, and it generates no direct response to light. However, the asymmetrical transport properties of the apical and basal membranes generate a transepithelial voltage (called the standing potential), which can be modified

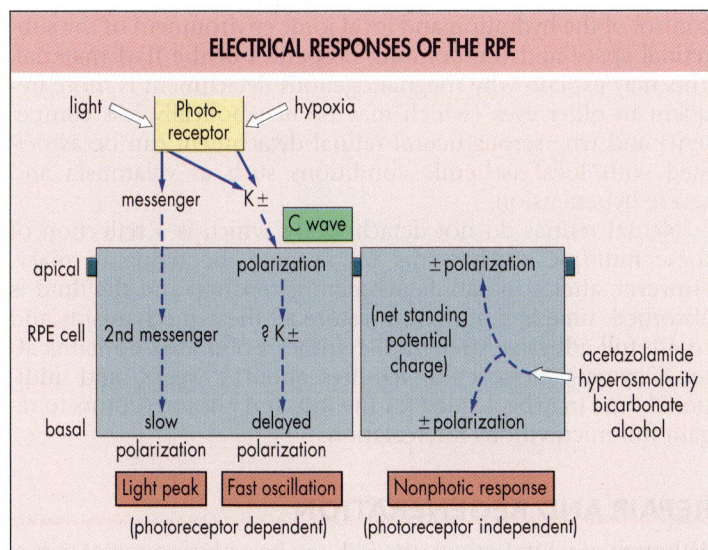

ELECTRICAL RESPONSES OF THE RPE

FIG. 100-4 ■ Electrical responses of the retinal pigment epithelium (RPE). Light induces the c wave, fast oscillation, and light peak (on electro-oculogram). Hypoxia and systemic drugs also modulate the voltage across the RPE. (Adapted from Marmor MF. Clinical electrophysiology of the retinal pigment epithelium. Doc Ophthalmol. 1991;76:301–13.)

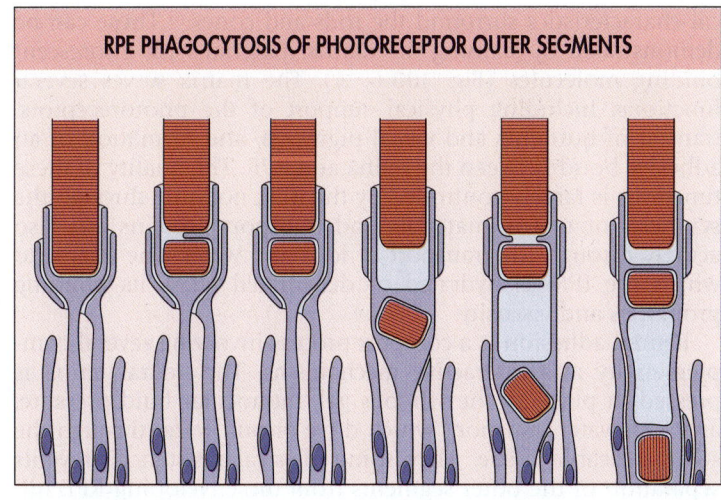

RPE PHAGOCYTOSIS OF PHOTORECEPTOR OUTER SEGMENTS

FIG. 100-5 ■ Retinal pigment epithelium (RPE) phagocytosis of photoreceptor outer segments. The phagosome, containing the ingested material, enters the RPE cytoplasm, where it merges with lysosomes to facilitate digestion of the outdated membranes. (Adapted from Steinberg RH, Wood I, Hogan MJ. Pigment epithelial ensheathment and phagocytosis of extrafoveal cones in human retina. Philos Trans R Soc Lond. 1977;277:459–74.)

secondarily by photoreceptor activity or by endogenously supplied substances[8] (Fig. 100-4).

When the photoreceptors respond to light, the potassium concentration falls for a few seconds in the subneural retinal space. The apical membranes of the RPE and the Müller cells respond by hyperpolarizing, which produces the c wave of the electroretinogram. This potassium change is transmitted slowly through the RPE cell, and roughly 1 minute later, a hyperpolarization appears at the basal membrane, which accounts for the fast oscillation of the electro-oculogram (EOG). This response involves basal chloride channels and is abnormal in some patients who have cystic fibrosis. Light activation of photoreceptors also causes the release of an unknown messenger substance that causes a basal RPE depolarization 5–10 minutes after the onset of light activation. This late basal depolarization is recorded clinically as the light response of the standing potential in the clinical EOG.

The basal membrane of the RPE can be activated independent of light, by chemical agents. For example, it hyperpolarizes several minutes after an intravenous injection of a hyperosmolar agent or acetazolamide, and it depolarizes after an oral dose of alcohol.[9] The clinical significance of these nonphotic responses of the RPE remains to be determined.

PHOTORECEPTOR–RETINAL PIGMENT EPITHELIUM INTERACTIONS
Visual Pigment Regeneration

In 1877, Kuhne demonstrated that visual pigments regenerate to maintain the visual process.[10] The primary rod pigment, rhodopsin, consists of a vitamin A aldehyde molecule bonded to a large protein (opsin); it is sensitive to light only when the vitamin A has the 11-*cis* conformation. Absorption of a photon converts the vitamin A to the all-*trans* form, which initiates the process of transduction and begins a series of regenerative chemical changes that are independent of vision. Vitamin A is split off from the opsin molecule and carried by a transport protein to the RPE. In the RPE, vitamin A may be stored in an ester form, but eventually it is isomerized back to the 11-*cis* form and recombined with opsin. The RPE is vital for this process and for the capture of vitamin A from the bloodstream to maintain its concentration within the eye.

The significance of this regenerative process is apparent in the time it takes to adjust to indoor lighting after a walk on a sunny beach or to the darkness inside a movie theater. In an unusual night-blinding disorder, fundus albipunctatus, this visual pigment regeneration process is severely prolonged,[11] most often as

a result of defects in the retinal dehydrogenase (RDH) gene. Affected individuals may require 3–4 hours, instead of 30 minutes, to fully adapt to the dark. Defects in other regeneration cycle genes can cause retinitis pigmentosa, such as the gene for retinaldehyde binding protein (RLBP) and the RPE65 gene (involved in 11-*cis* retinol metabolism), which is responsible for severe early-onset disease.[12]

Photoreceptor Renewal and Phagocytosis

Photoreceptors, like skin, are continually exposed to radiant energy (light) and oxygen (from the choroid), which facilitates the production of free radicals that can damage membranes over time. Thus, a process of cellular renewal is needed. Every day, upward of 100 discs at the distal end of the photoreceptors are phagocytosed by the RPE (Fig. 100-5), while new discs are synthesized.[13] The cellular renewal process has a circadian rhythm. The rods shed discs most vigorously in the morning at the onset of light, whereas cones shed more vigorously at the onset of darkness. The complete outer segments are renewed roughly every 2 weeks. Within the RPE, the phagocytosed discs become encapsulated in vesicles called phagosomes,[14] which merge with lysosomes so that the material can be digested. Necessary fatty acids are retained for recycling into outer segment synthesis, and waste products or damaged membrane material is digested across the basal RPE membrane. This is an impressive metabolic task for the RPE, since each cell must ingest and digest upward of 4000 discs daily. Some of this membranous material may persist within the RPE cell and contribute to the formation of lipofuscin.

That RPE phagocytosis is important is shown by a peculiar strain of rat (RCS) that lacks the ability to phagocytose outer segments. Within weeks after the birth of these animals, outer segment debris begins to accumulate in the subretinal space, and the photoreceptors degenerate. This is not the problem in most cases of retinitis pigmentosa, however, because eyes examined histologically have had shortened rather than lengthened outer segments. The general process of RPE phagocytosis and its relationship to lipofuscin formation may be more relevant to the process of aging within the RPE cell and the development of age-related macular degeneration.

Interphotoreceptor Matrix and Retinal Adhesion

The interphotoreceptor matrix (IPM) is not simply a sticky glue. It contains complex molecules, such as glycosaminoglycans, and has an elaborate structure in which domains of distinct chemical characteristics surround the rods and cones.[15] These can be demonstrated by staining the matrix material with fluorescent binding molecules (Fig. 100-6, *A*). The matrix serves several functions, including physical support of the photoreceptors, transfer of nutrients and visual pigments, and formation of an adhesive bond between the retina and RPE. The quality of these functions is largely controlled by the RPE, not only through the synthesis of matrix materials and transport proteins but also acutely through the transport of ions and water. The degree to which the IPM is hydrated or dehydrated alters its bonding properties and viscosity.

Retinal adhesion is a complex process involving several complementary and interactive mechanisms. The neural retina is pressed in place by the vitreous gel, intraocular fluid pressure, and RPE water transport, which drive or pull water through the semipermeable tissue. Also, some physical resistance prevents separation of the outer segments from the enveloping RPE microvilli. The strongest mechanism for bonding the retina to the RPE space appears to be the IPM. When neural retina is freshly peeled from the RPE, the IPM material stretches dramatically before it breaks, which shows that it is firmly attached to both neural retinal and RPE surfaces (Fig. 100-6, *B*). It is also important to recognize that, despite these physical forces of adhesion, the strength of neural retinal adhesion is constantly and acutely dependent on metabolism.[16] For example, the retinal adhesive force drops to near zero within minutes after death, and adhesive strength can be reversibly restored or enhanced by tissue oxygenation. The likely basis of these metabolic effects is RPE

control of the hydration and local ionic environment of the subretinal space and the bonding properties of the IPM material. This may explain why rhegmatogenous detachment is more frequent in older eyes (which may be metabolically less competent) and why serous neural retinal detachment can be associated with local ischemic conditions such as eclampsia and severe hypertension.

Neural retinas do not detach easily, which is a reflection of these multiple mechanisms for keeping the retina in place. However, after a retinal detachment is repaired and the fluid is absorbed, time is required to restore all these mechanisms and regain full adhesive strength. Resynthesis of matrix domains after enzymatic destruction requires about 2 weeks, and additional time may be needed for the RPE and photoreceptors to regain full microvillous intercalation.

REPAIR AND REGENERATION

Although of neural origin, the RPE can be a pluripotential tissue. In amphibians, RPE cells can regenerate lens, neural retina, and other components of the eye; mercifully, this does not take place in humans. Nevertheless, the RPE is capable of local repair (unlike the neural retina), and cells may migrate and take on altered characteristics. After a laser burn, for example, the RPE cells that surround the burn begin to divide, and small cells fill the defect to form a new blood-retinal barrier within 1–2 weeks.[17] In degenerative disease, such as retinitis pigmentosa, RPE cells migrate into the injured neural retina and sometimes come to rest around vessels to contribute to the characteristic bone spicule appearance. An overly vigorous RPE response can lead to duplicated layers of RPE cells and RPE scarring, which may be part of a macular degenerative process. In the extreme, RPE cells contribute to proliferative vitreoretinopathy. Growth factors from the RPE may, at times, help contain unwanted proliferation, and at other times they may stimulate vascular or fibrous growth. Functionally, the most useful RPE repair characteristic is the ability to heal defects. The value of photocoagulation for macular edema and proliferative diabetic retinopathy may, in part, depend on the ability of RPE cells to seal laser scars, reestablish a degree of normal transport, and avoid unnecessary leakage of proteins into the subretinal space.

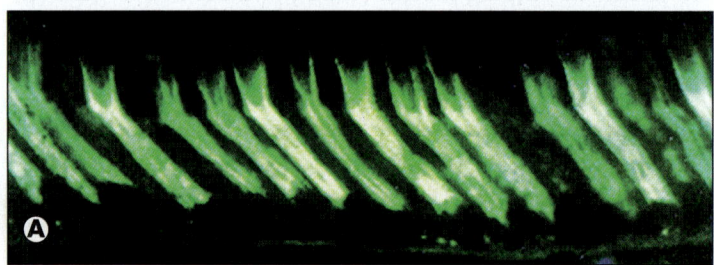

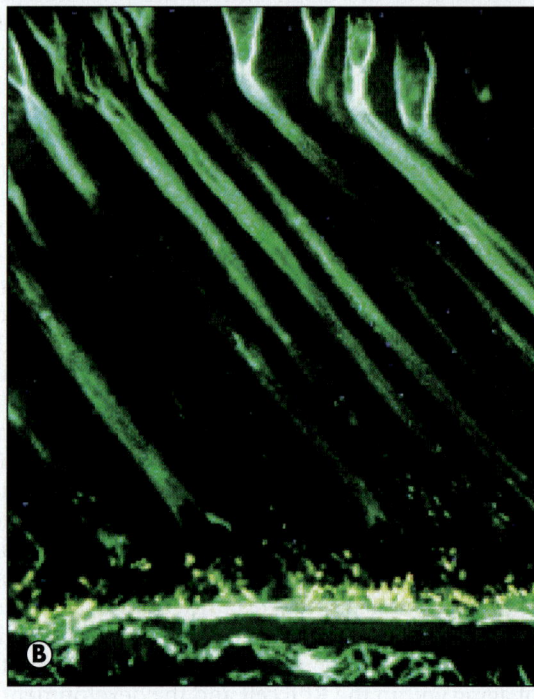

FIG. 100-6 ▓ **Cone sheaths of the interphotoreceptor matrix, shown by fluorescent staining with peanut agglutinin.** Cone tips indent the sheaths from above; the retinal pigment epithelium (RPE) is on the bottom. **A,** The matrix sheaths are short in a normal eye. **B,** They stretch dramatically before breaking as the retina is peeled from the RPE. This shows that matrix material bonds across the subretinal space. (Reproduced with permission from Hageman GS, Marmor MF, Yao X-Y, Johnson LV. The interphotoreceptor matrix mediates primate retinal adhesion. Arch Ophthalmol. 1995;113:655–60.)

REFERENCES

1. Zinn K, Marmor MF, eds. The retinal pigment epithelium. Cambridge: Harvard University Press; 1979.
2. Marmor MF, Wolfensberger TW, eds. The retinal pigment epithelium. Current aspects of function and disease. New York: Oxford University Press; 1998.
3. Boulton M, Dayhaw-Parker P. The role of the retinal pigment epithelium: topographical variation and aging changes. Eye. 2001;15:384–89.
4. Ogata N, Tombran-Tink J, Nishikawa M, et al. Pigment epithelium-derived factor in the vitreous is low in diabetic retinopathy and high in rhegmatogenous retinal detachment. Am J Ophthalmol. 2001;132:378–82.
5. Witmer AN, Vrensen GF, Van Noorden CJ, Schlingemann RO. Vascular endothelial growth factors and angiogenesis in eye disease. Prog Retin Eye Res. 2003;22:1–29.
6. Negi A, Marmor MF. The resorption of subretinal fluid after diffuse damage to the retinal pigment epithelium. Invest Ophthalmol Vis Sci. 1983;24:1475–9.
7. Marmor M, On the cause of serous detachments and acute central serous chorioretinopathy. Br J Ophthalmol. 1997;81:812–3.
8. Marmor MF. Clinical electrophysiology of the retinal pigment epithelium. Doc Ophthalmol. 1991;76:301–13.
9. Arden GB, Wolf JE. The human electro-oculogram: interaction of light and alcohol. Invest Ophthalmol Vis Sci. 2000;41:2722–9.
10. Marmor MF, Martin LJ. 100 Years of the visual cycle. Surv Ophthalmol. 1978;22:279–85.
11. Marmor MF. Long-term follow-up of the physiologic abnormalities and fundus changes in fundus albipunctatus. Ophthalmology. 1990;97:380–4.
12. Sharma RK, Ehinger B. Management of hereditary retinal degenerations: present status and future directions. Surv Ophthalmol. 1999;43:427–44.
13. Young RW. Visual cells and the concept of renewal. Invest Ophthalmol. 1976;15:700–25.
14. Steinberg RH, Wood I, Hogan MJ. Pigment epithelial ensheathment and phagocytosis of extrafoveal cones in human retina. Philos Trans R Soc Lond. 1977;277:459–74.
15. Hageman GS, Marmor MF, Yao X-Y, Johnson LV. The interphotoreceptor matrix mediates primate retinal adhesion. Arch Ophthalmol. 1995;113:655–60.
16. Marmor MF, Yao X-Y. The metabolic dependency of retinal adhesion in rabbit and primate. Arch Ophthalmol. 1995;113:232–8.
17. Negi A, Marmor MF. Healing of photocoagulation lesions affects the rate of subretinal fluid resorption. Ophthalmology. 1984;91:1678–83.

CHAPTER
101

Retinal and Choroidal Circulation

SHIYOUNG ROH • JOHN J. WEITER

INTRODUCTION

The normal clarity of the ocular media allows the retinal circulatory system to be observed *in vivo*. Because many of the important diseases of the retina are related to or associated with changes in the vasculature of the retina and choroid, it is important to understand the circulatory systems involved to better recognize disease states of the posterior segment. In this chapter, the basic anatomy and physiology—gross anatomy, microscopic anatomy, blood flow, regulation of blood flow, and the blood-retinal barrier—of these circulatory systems are outlined.

GROSS ANATOMY

The retina receives its nutrition from two discrete circulatory systems—the retinal blood vessels and the uveal or choroidal blood vessels. Both are derived from the ophthalmic artery, which is the first branch of the internal carotid artery. The major branches of the ophthalmic artery are the central retinal artery, the posterior ciliary arteries, and the muscular branches.[1] Typically two posterior ciliary arteries exist—a medial and a lateral—but occasionally a third superior posterior ciliary artery is seen.[2] The choroidal watershed area, which represents the area between the supply of each posterior ciliary artery, is usually a vertically oriented zone situated between the optic disc and macula (Fig. 101-1). The posterior ciliary arteries further divide into two long posterior ciliary arteries and numerous short posterior ciliary arteries. The posterior choriocapillaris is supplied by these short posterior ciliary arteries, which enter the choroid in the peripapillary and submacular region. The anterior choriocapillaris is supplied by recurrent branches from the long ciliary arteries as well as by recurrent branches from the anterior ciliary arteries. The watershed zone of the anterior and posterior choroidal circulatory systems is at the equator.

The choroid is drained through the vortex venous system, which usually has between four and seven (usually six) major vessels, one or two in each quadrant, located at the equator. In pathological conditions such as high myopia, posterior vortex veins may be observed to drain at the edge of the optic disc. The vortex veins drain into the superior and inferior orbital veins, which drain into the cavernous sinus and pterygoid plexus, respectively. Collateralization between the superior and inferior orbital veins usually exists. The central retinal vein drains the retina and the prelaminar aspect of the optic nerve into the cavernous sinus. Thus, both the retinal and choroidal circulatory systems are in communication with the cavernous sinus.

MICROSCOPIC ANATOMY

The retinal blood vessels provide nourishment for the inner retinal layers and carry off waste products from them. The outer retinal layers are avascular and are supplied by diffusion from the choriocapillaris. Despite this dual circulation to the retina, functionally little overlap occurs, with the watershed zone at the outer plexiform layer. The central retinal artery is an end artery that has no significant anastomoses. In the area of the lamina cribrosa, its lumen measures about 170μm in diameter. Typically, just before

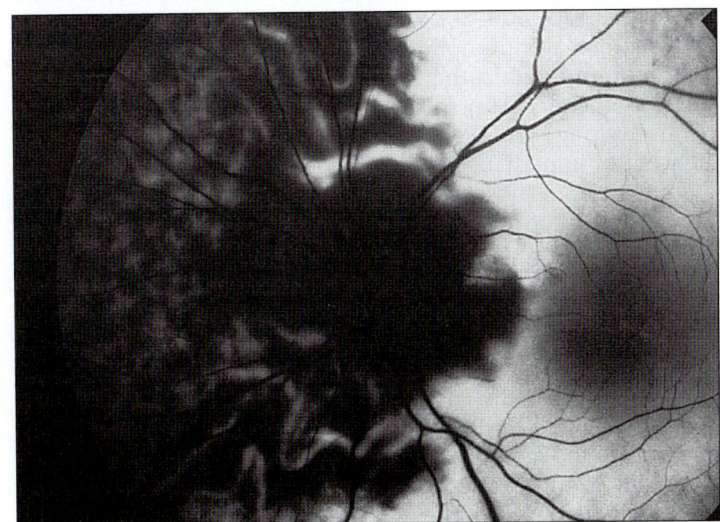

FIG. 101-1 ■ Fluorescein angiogram of a combined medial posterior ciliary artery obstruction and central retinal artery obstruction. The hyperfluorescence results from intact circulation of the lateral posterior ciliary artery. The watershed area between the circulation of the two choroidal vessels is the scalloped vertical line that crosses the temporal peripapillary area.

its exit from the optic nerve the central retinal artery divides into the superior and inferior papillary arteries, which in turn divide into nasal and temporal quadrantic branches. The anatomical division of the retinal arteries into superior and inferior halves is usually maintained throughout the retina because normal retinal vessels rarely cross the horizontal raphe. Collaterals across the midline are a common finding in retinal venous obstructive disease. The major branch arteries are about 110μm in diameter as they cross the disc margin. They course within the nerve fiber layer and ganglion cell layer of the retina.

Usually, after the first branch, the retinal arteries contain no elastic fibers and no internal elastic membrane, criteria for arteries, and thus the term arterioles is more appropriate. No nerve fibers have been found in the media or adventitia of human retinal vessels. Although the ophthalmic artery contains sympathetic nerve fiber endings and therefore is under the control of the autonomic nervous system, apparently no central regulation of the blood flow occurs in the retina itself. The retinal arteries and arterioles remain in the inner retina, and only capillaries are found as deep as the inner nuclear layer. The retinal venous drainage of the retina generally follows the arterial supply. The retinal veins (mainly venules) are present in the inner retina, where they occasionally interdigitate with their associated arteries. When two vessels cross, the artery usually lies anterior (vitriad) to the vein, and the two vessels share a common adventitial coat. Many more arteriovenous crossings occur temporally than nasally because the nasal vessels assume a much straighter course. The crossings are important because they represent the most common site of branch retinal vein obstructions. The retinal veins drain into the central retinal vein, which also acts as the major efferent channel for the vessels of the optic nerve. Near the disc, the retinal veins are approximately 150μm in diameter.[3]

Throughout the retina, the capillaries are arranged in laminar meshworks.[4] Depending on the thickness of the retina, the laminar meshwork can vary from three layers at the posterior pole to one layer in the periphery. Like capillary networks elsewhere in the body, the retinal capillaries assume a meshwork configuration to ensure adequate perfusion to all retinal cells. The deeper layer has a mesh diameter of about 50μm (15–130μm) and the more superficial layer has a slightly larger meshwork of about 65μm (16–150μm) diameter. Besides the laminar characteristic of the retinal capillaries, they also show other variations.

A capillary-free zone is present around each of the larger retinal arteries and veins, but it is more prominent around arteries, where it measures up to 100μm in diameter. In the fovea and the far retinal periphery, retinal capillaries are absent. The foveal avascular area is 400–500μm in diameter.

A distinct layer of capillaries, the radial peripapillary capillaries, are found within the inner aspect of the nerve fiber layer; these are the most superficial of all retinal capillaries. They have relatively long, straight paths and have few anastomoses with adjacent or underlying capillary beds. Their distribution around the optic nerve and superior and inferior temporal arcades reflects the thickest distribution of the nerve fiber layer and suggests some anatomical correlation with various diseases—cotton-wool spots and the arcuate scotoma of glaucoma correspond to this distribution.

Retinal capillaries are 5–6μm in diameter and consist of two layers—endothelial cells and a surrounding layer of pericytes. The pericyte:endothelial ratio is 1:1, which is relatively high compared with elsewhere in the central nervous system or body in general. The capillary basement membrane between the pericytes and endothelial cells is much thinner than the basement membrane that covers the two types of cells, which probably allows increased communications between the cells. The retinal capillary endothelial cells are the major component of the blood-retinal barrier. The retinal pericytes appear to be involved directly in the local control of retinal blood flow and may affect endothelial cell proliferation as well.

The choroid is by far the most vascular portion of the eye and by weight one of the most vascular tissues in the body.[5] The choroidal circulatory system is responsible for the nourishment of the photoreceptor–retinal pigment epithelium (RPE) complex. The choroidal circulatory system's paramount task is to provide nutrition to the retina, but it has other functions as well. As a heat sink, it removes the large amount of heat that develops as a result of the metabolic processes initiated when photons strike the photopigments and the melanin of the RPE and choroid.[6] It probably also serves as a mechanical cushion for the internal structures of the eye.

The blood supply to the choroid is from branches of the anterior and posterior ciliary arteries.[2] The overall structure of the choroid is segmental; this segmental distribution of blood begins at the level of the posterior ciliary branches and is mirrored in the vortex drainage system. As a result of the segmental distribution, the large and medium-sized choroidal arteries act as end arteries. Unlike the situation in the retina, the choroidal arteries and veins do not run parallel to each other. Each terminal choroidal arteriole supplies an independent polygonal segment of the choriocapillaris, referred to as a lobule, which is in turn drained by a venule.[2,7] Thus, although the choriocapillaris is anatomically a single, interconnected layer of capillaries, functionally the lobular anatomy results in a segmental filling pattern (Fig. 101-2). The transition from arteriole to choriocapillaris to venule is abrupt.

The pattern of the choriocapillaris varies from the posterior pole to the ora serrata. At the posterior pole, the lobular pattern is at its most marked, with each unit being approximately 300μm in diameter. In the equator and periphery the pattern changes to less structured and larger units of approximately 1500μm. The choriocapillaris has large diameters of 20–25μm, which allow the passage of multiple red blood cells at any mo-

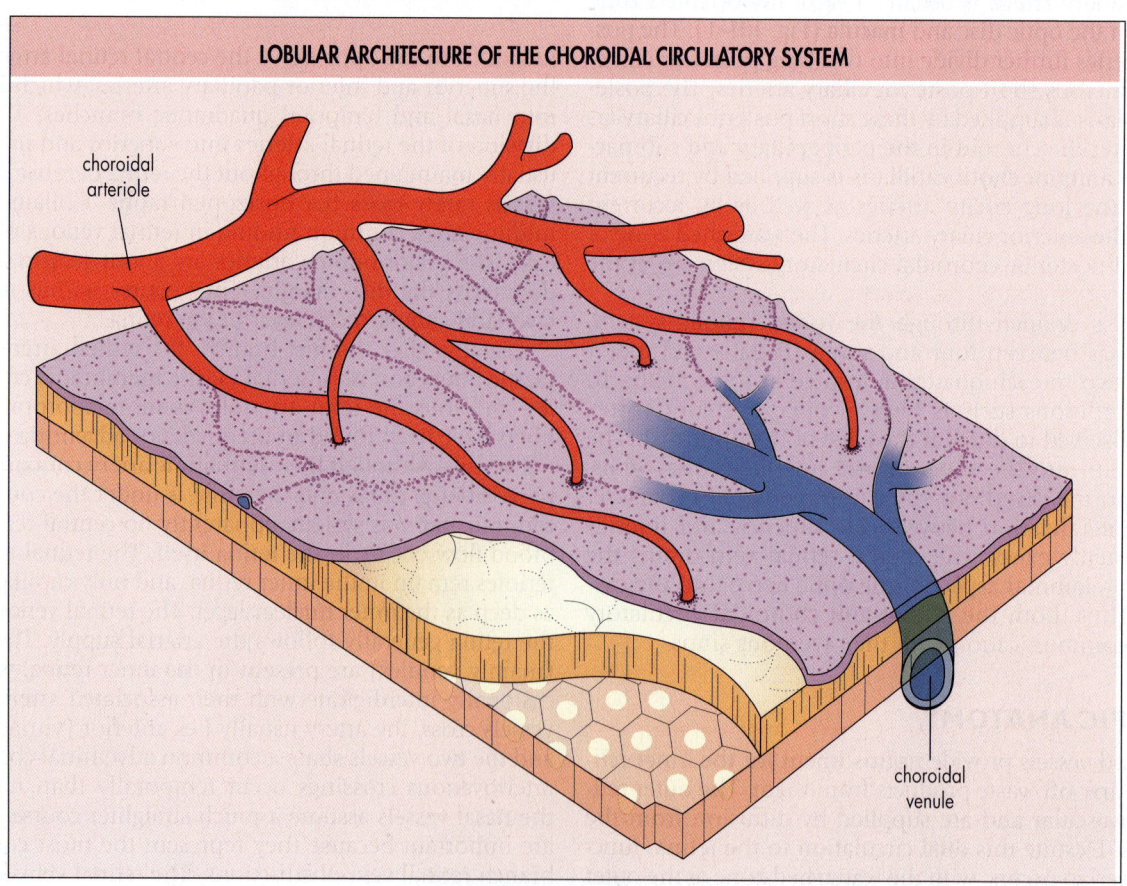

LOBULAR ARCHITECTURE OF THE CHOROIDAL CIRCULATORY SYSTEM

choroidal arteriole

choroidal venule

FIG. 101-2 ■ **The lobular architecture of the choroidal circulatory system.** (Adapted with permission from Duker J, Weiter JJ. Ocular circulation. In: Tasman W, Jaeger EA, eds. Duane's foundations of clinical ophthalmology. New York: JB Lippincott; 1991:1–34.)

ment in time. Larger diameters of up to 50mm are sometimes reported in the literature, but these larger sizes represent venules that lie in the plane of the choriocapillaris.

Unlike the retinal capillaries, the choriocapillaris has fenestrations of 700–800nm diameter, which allows more rapid transport of molecules (leakage). The fenestrations predominantly face the RPE but under pathological conditions may migrate toward the scleral side.

Blood-Retinal Barrier

The blood-retinal barrier is formed by both the retinal vasculature and the RPE.[8] The barrier function depends on tight junctions, which restrict intercellular movement of all water-soluble molecules and thus prevent these molecules from entering the retina. Electron microscopy has shown particularly extensive zonular occludentes surrounding the retinal capillary endothelial cells and the apicolateral aspects of the RPE cells. The glial cells that surround the retinal capillaries, for a time, were thought to have a role in the blood-retinal barrier. Although the endothelium of the retinal capillaries is where the barrier resides, the glial cells may play a role as metabolic intermediaries between the retinal capillaries and retinal neurons. Thus, macromolecules and ions do not passively diffuse into the retina from the circulation but are associated with selective active transport into the retina. The choriocapillaris, with its numerous fenestrations, pinocytic vesicles, and lack of tight junctions, is fairly permeable to macromolecules and does not appear to have much significance in the blood-retinal barrier. Bruch's membrane, located between the choriocapillaris and RPE, acts as a diffusion barrier only to large molecules. The functional significance of having the outer blood-retinal barrier at the level of the RPE, rather than the choriocapillaris, is a subject of unresolved speculation.[9]

The existing pattern allows the RPE, which is a metabolic factory, to have ample access to necessary nutrients such as vitamin A and to be better able to remove waste products. In addition, the high protein permeability of the choriocapillaris results in greater oncotic pressure in the choroid than in the retina. The resultant differences in osmotic pressure facilitate the absorption of fluid from the retinal extracellular spaces into the choroid; this may be a mechanism that helps to keep the retina attached to the RPE. It is interesting to note that no intraocular lymphatic channels exist. Although the retina is protected by blood-retinal barriers, some leakage probably occurs. Most likely this protein leakage is transported across the RPE into the choroid or removed through Schlemm's canal. Choroidal proteins exit the eye through emissary canals (openings in the sclera for vessels and nerves) or through the sclera, probably facilitated by the relatively high tissue pressure of the eye (the intraocular pressure).

RETINAL AND CHOROIDAL BLOOD FLOW

Accurate measurement of retinal blood flow is difficult because of the problems of access to the retinal circulation. Past studies indicate that retinal blood flow represents 5% of total ocular blood flow.[10] Retinal blood flow has been shown, using fluorescein angiography, to be laminar in both the arteries and veins. With laser Doppler velocimetry, the average rate of blood flow for the entire human retina is calculated to be about 80ml/min. Blood flow to the temporal retina is approximately three times larger than that to the nasal retina, with no difference between the superior and inferior retina.[11] The large temporal-nasal difference is a reflection of the large posterior pole (macular) component. In arteries, pulsatile flow is noted. Such measurements also show that the average center blood velocity in the major retinal arteries is 7cm/sec and in the major retinal veins is approximately 3.5cm/sec. Color Doppler imaging suggests that the average blood flow velocity in the central retinal artery is about 10cm/sec.

The mean retinal circulation time in humans has been reported to be 4–5 seconds.[12] The presence of similar, large regional differ-

ences was found in monkeys, where the blood flow to the peripapillary and macular region was approximately four times larger than the flow to the intermediate and peripheral retina.[13]

Unlike the retinal arteries, the retinal veins show no pulsations in blood velocity except at the point of exit from the globe.[14] The venous pressure of the intraocular veins exiting the eye depends upon intraocular pressure (IOP) and coincides with the pulse, which results in a pulsating venous perfusion pressure. The retinal venous outflow resistance is located mainly at the lamina cribrosa. The closed nature of the eye means that the pulsatile choroidal arterial inflow results in a pulse-related change in IOP, which causes a venous pulse. Depending upon the relationship between IOP and venous pressure, this may result in a clinically visible pulse of the veins at their point of exit from the globe.

Widespread discrepancies are found in the values for uveal blood flow, which reflects the complexities inherent in the measurement of flow through relatively inaccessible vessels. In monkeys, uveal blood flow is distributed as follows: 1% iris, 12% ciliary body, 83% choroid.[13] The distribution of blood flow in cats is 5% iris, 28% ciliary body, and 65% choroid.[10] If numerous studies on different species are averaged, it appears that the choroid receives 65–85% and the retina 5% or less of the ocular blood flow.

Using monkey choroidal blood flow values and assuming that the human and monkey eyes are relatively similar, one can derive a retinal blood flow of 80ml/min and a choroidal blood flow of 800ml/min, a 10:1 choroid:retinal blood flow ratio. Indeed, the choroidal blood flow is so high that the arteriovenous oxygen difference for choroidal blood is approximately 3% versus 40% for retinal blood. Despite the low oxygen extraction from choroidal blood, the choroid is of great importance for the supply of nutrients to the retina. Of the oxygen and glucose consumption of the retina, 65–75% is supplied by the choroid.[5] The salient features of the retinal and choroidal circulatory systems are shown in Table 101-1 and the major differences in Table 101-2.

Regulation of Retinal and Choroidal Blood Flows

Regulation of blood flow through the choroid, as in the body in general, is under the control of the autonomic nervous system. Stimulation of the cervical sympathetic chain decreases choroidal flow, and sympathectomy increases it.[5,15] The choroid does not show evidence of autoregulation,[5] the lack of which may have serious consequences. Changes in IOP are not reflected by compensatory changes in the choroidal vascular pressure,[15] and sudden changes in IOP, such as occur in the opening of the eye during surgery, can induce uveal effusion.

Because the autonomic tonus probably protects the eye from transient elevations in the systemic blood pressure under nor-

TABLE 101-1

SALIENT FEATURES OF THE RETINAL AND CHOROIDAL CIRCULATORY SYSTEMS

Choroidal blood flow	Total flow	800–1000 ml/min
Retinal blood flow	Total flow	80ml/min
	Regional flow	
	temporal versus nasal ratio	3:1
	posterior pole and peripapillary versus remainder of retina ratio	4:1
	superior versus inferior ratio	1:1
Retinal blood velocity	Major arteries	7cm/s.
	Major veins	3.5cm/s.
Mean retinal circulation time		4–5sec
Retinal vasculature diameters	Arteries at margin of optic nerve	110μm
	Veins at margin of optic nerve	150μm
	Capillaries	5–6μm
	Choriocapillaris	20–25μm

TABLE 101-2

MAJOR DIFFERENCES BETWEEN THE RETINAL AND CHOROIDAL CIRCULATORY SYSTEMS

Property	Retinal	Choroidal
Blood flow	Normal for tissue	Highest in body
Tissue perfused	Inner two thirds of retina	Photoreceptor–retinal pigment epithelium complex
Cellular junctions	Tight junctions in capillaries	Fenestrations in choriocapillaris
Location of blood–retinal barrier	Tight junctions in capillaries	Tight junctions in the retinal pigment epithelium
Regulation of blood flow	Autoregulation	Controlled by the autonomic nervous system
Nature of vasculature	End artery system	Functionally end artery system in spite of anatomical continuity of the choriocapillaris

mal circumstances,[16] if the nervous regulation breaks down in the presence of systemic hypertension, fluid may be forced through the retinal pigment epithelial barrier into the retina.[17] Such changes hypothetically could contribute to the pathology of central serous chorioretinopathy, cystoid macular edema, and hypotony maculopathy. The ophthalmic artery and its branches are innervated richly with adrenergic fibers until the lamina cribrosa is reached.

From that point on, no nervous system control of the retinal circulation occurs.[18] Thus, the retinal circulation must depend upon local autoregulation to maintain a constant metabolic environment. The process of autoregulation in a vascular bed maintains constant or nearly constant blood flow through a wide range of perfusion pressures. Autoregulation of the retina is commonly used today in a much broader sense, to encompass the local homeostatic blood flow mechanisms that provide a constant metabolic environment in the retina despite various conditions that tend to upset this equilibrium. Blood flow in the retina appears to be primarily controlled by metabolic needs, especially the need for oxygen,[5,19] and the accumulation of metabolic by-products such as carbon dioxide and changes in pH. It is necessary to understand the factors that can influence autoregulation of the retinal circulation as these may have important clinical implications.[20]

External and internal factors that can alter retinal circulation offer exciting new therapeutic possibilities. Studies of cellular biology are uncovering growth factors and an array of cellular receptors that are undoubtedly important in the control of ocular circulation. Furthermore, animal studies show changes in retinal blood flow as a result of various medications, which may have application to the human retinal circulation. These studies are still preliminary and need to be verified by human studies.

REFERENCES

1. Hayreh SS. The ophthalmic artery, Part III. Branches. Br J Ophthalmol. 1962; 46:212–47.
2. Weiter JJ, Ernest JT. Anatomy of the choroidal vasculature. Am J Ophthalmol. 1974;78:583–90.
3. Duker J, Weiter JJ. Ocular circulation. In: Tasman W, Jaeger EA, eds. Duane's foundations of clinical ophthalmology. New York: JB Lippincott; 1991:1–34.
4. Shimizu K, Kazuyoshi U. Structure of ocular vessels. New York: Igaku-Shoin; 1978.
5. Alm A. Ocular circulation. In: Hart WM, ed. Adler's physiology of the eye. St Louis: Mosby–Year Book; 1992:198–227.
6. Parver LM, Auker C, Carpenter DO. Choroidal blood flow as a heat dissipating mechanism in the macula. Am J Ophthalmol. 1980;84:641–6.
7. Torczynski E, Tso MOM. The architecture of the choriocapillaris at the posterior pole. Am J Ophthalmol. 1976;81:428–40.
8. Cunha-Vaz J. The blood-ocular barriers. Surv Ophthalmol. 1979;23:279–96.
9. Bill A. Blood circulation and fluid dynamics in the eye. Physiol Rev. 1975; 55:383–417.
10. Weiter JJ, Schachar RA, Ernest JT. Control of intraocular blood flow, I. Intraocular pressure. Invest Ophthalmol. 1973;12:327–31.
11. Feke GT, Tagawa H, Deupree DM, et al. Blood flow in the normal human retina. Invest Ophthalmol Vis Sci. 1989;30:58–65.
12. Eberli B, Riva CE, Feke GT. Mean circulation time of fluorescein in retinal vascular segments. Arch Ophthalmol. 1979;97:145–8.
13. Alm A, Bill A. Ocular and optic nerve blood flow at normal and increased intraocular pressures in monkeys (Macaca irus): a study with radioactively labelled microspheres including flow determinations in brain and some other tissues. Exp Eye Res. 1973;15:15–29.
14. Michelson G, Jarazny J. Relationship between ocular pulse pressures and retinal vessel velocities. Ophthalmology. 1997;104:664–71.
15. Weiter JJ, Schachar RA, Ernest JT. Control of intraocular blood flow. II Effects of sympathetic tone. Invest Ophthalmol. 1973;12:332–4.
16. Potts AM. An hypothesis on macular disease. Trans Am Acad Ophthalmol Otolaryngol. 1966;70:1058–62.
17. Ernest JT. The effect of systolic hypertension on rhesus monkey eyes after ocular sympathectomy. Am J Ophthalmol. 1977;84:341–4.
18. Laties AM, Jacobwitz D. A comparative study of the autonomic innervation of the eye in monkey, cat and rabbit. Anat Rec. 1966;156:383–96.
19. Feke GT, Zuckerman R, Green GJ, Weiter JJ. Responses of human retinal blood flow to light and dark. Invest Ophthalmol Vis Sci. 1983;24:136–41.
20. Weiter JJ, Zuckerman R. The influence of the photoreceptor-RPE complex on the inner retina: an explanation for the beneficial effects of photocoagulation. Ophthalmology. 1980;87:1133–9.

SECTION 2 BASIC PRINCIPLES OF RETINAL SURGERY

CHAPTER

102

Laser Photocoagulation

MICHAEL S. IP • CARMEN A. PULIAFITO

DEFINITION
- LASER: Light amplification by stimulated emission of radiation.

KEY FEATURES
- Lasers named for their active medium.
- Choice of optimal wavelength depends on absorption spectrum of target tissue.
- Indicated for treatment of retinal and choroidal abnormalities.
- Recent applications exploit the subthreshold effects of laser.

HISTORY

The history of retinal photocoagulation dates to 400 BC, when Plato described the dangers of direct sun gazing during an eclipse. Czerny and Deutschmann, in 1867 and 1882, respectively, focused sunlight through the dilated pupils of rabbits and created thermal burns in the animals' retinas. Meyer-Schwickerath[1] undertook the study of retinal photocoagulation in humans in 1946 using the xenon arc lamp. Xenon arc lamps, commercially available in 1956, rapidly became popular for retinal photocoagulation because of their strong visible and near infrared emission.

The first functioning laser was demonstrated by Maiman[2] in 1960. The active laser material was a ruby—a crystalline sapphire that contained a small percentage of chromium oxide. The chromium ions absorb radiation in the green–blue part of the spectrum and emit radiation of 649nm (red light). The ruby crystal is pulsed with a xenon flash lamp.

The first clinical ophthalmic use of a laser in humans was reported by Campbell et al.[3] in 1963 and Zweng et al.[4] in 1964. They found that laser photocoagulation was efficient and effective and did not require anesthesia or akinesia. The ruby laser they employed operated in a pulsed mode because the thermal characteristics of the ruby crystal prohibited continuous operation at the power levels required for retinal photocoagulation. Use of the pulsed laser often led to the formation of retinal hemorrhages. In addition, the ruby laser was poorly absorbed by hemoglobin.

The argon laser, developed in 1964, provides an emission spectrum that is absorbed well by hemoglobin when the laser is used in a continuous mode. L'Esperance[5] conducted the first human photocoagulation trial for ophthalmic disease using the argon laser in 1968; he also introduced the frequency-doubled neodymium:yttrium-aluminum-garnet (Nd:YAG) and krypton lasers in 1971 and 1972, respectively. The use of the Q-switched and mode-locked Nd:YAG lasers in 1980 and 1981, respectively, allowed transparent membranes (e.g., posterior capsule, vitreous) to be cut using extremely short bursts of laser energy. The tunable dye laser was introduced in 1981 and provided the theoretical advantage of a variable output wavelength to match the absorption spectra of specific ocular tissue.

The semiconductor infrared diode laser was developed in 1962. Since then, the diode laser has been employed in multiple delivery modes—transpupillary slit lamp, transpupillary laser indirect, trans-scleral, and endophotocoagulation. It has been used to treat choroidal neovascularization (CNVM), proliferative retinopathy, retinopathy of prematurity, macular edema, and choroidal melanoma.[6,7]

LASER PRINCIPLES

Laser is an acronym for light amplification by stimulated emission of radiation. The basic laser cavity consists of an active medium in a resonant cavity with two mirrors placed at opposite ends. One of the mirrors allows partial transmission of laser light out of the laser cavity, toward the target tissue. A pump source introduces energy into the active medium and excites a number of atoms. In this manner, amplified, coherent, and collimated light energy is released as laser energy through the mirror that partially transmits. The various lasers differ mainly in the characteristics of the active medium and the way this active medium is pumped.

The properties of laser light that make it useful to ophthalmologists and allow laser energy to be directed at specific target tissue in a controlled manner are monochromaticity, spatial coherence, temporal coherence, collimation, ability to be concentrated in a short time interval, and ability to produce nonlinear tissue effects.

LASER MEDIA

Lasers are named for their active medium. Solid-state lasers include the ruby laser and the Nd:YAG laser. The organic dye laser contains a liquid laser medium that consists of a fluorescent organic compound dissolved in a liquid solvent. As a result, the dye laser can produce multiple wavelengths, because dyes are made up of large molecules that have various structures and complex spectra. Gas lasers include the ion laser and carbon dioxide laser. Ion lasers contain an ionized rare gas, such as argon or krypton, as the active medium. In a carbon dioxide laser, nitrogen and helium are typically present in the gas mixture also. Diode lasers have semiconductor materials as the laser medium. Different semiconductor materials are available that provide a range of wavelengths, such as gallium arsenide (660–900nm) or indium phosphide (1300–1550nm).

In gas or Nd:YAG lasers, only 2% of the energy used to generate the laser emission is converted into laser light. The remaining 98% of energy becomes heat, which is removed by extensive, bulky cooling mechanisms. In contrast, approximately 20% of the input power is converted to laser energy in an infrared diode laser. The infrared wavelength enables increased transmission through lens opacity, hemorrhage, and macular xanthophyll pigment. Additionally, the sclera is transparent to infrared wavelengths, so the diode laser may be used for trans-scleral applications (e.g., cyclodestructive procedures, trans-scleral retinopexy).

DELIVERY SYSTEMS

Clinical laser delivery systems consist of the laser medium, the fiber-optic cable or a mirror arm to take laser light to the delivery system, and the delivery system to direct the treatment beam to the target tissue.

In the slit-lamp biomicroscope, the most common method, the delivery is transcorneal, with or without the aid of contact lenses. The indirect ophthalmoscope with a condensing lens also may be used transcorneally to photocoagulate the posterior segment.[8] Other methods include endolaser and exolaser probes, in which treatment is delivered by fiber-optic probes used within the eye or trans-sclerally, respectively.

PARAMETERS AND TECHNIQUES

Wavelength

The choice of optimal wavelength depends on the absorption spectrum of the target tissue. Blue light is absorbed by macular xanthophyll and is a poor choice for macular photocoagulation. Light scatter also affects wavelength selection. Blue light, with its shorter wavelength, is scattered more than is light of longer wavelengths and thus has a greater potential to produce photochemical retinal damage in nearby untreated retina. Blue light also is scattered by the senescent crystalline lens, requiring more irradiation than longer-wavelength light for the clinical end point of retinal photocoagulation to be achieved.

Green light is absorbed well by melanin and hemoglobin. Red light also is absorbed well by melanin but is absorbed poorly by hemoglobin. Since the radiation of krypton red has a longer wavelength (647nm) than that of argon green, it is absorbed more deeply; therefore, treatment using krypton red may be more uncomfortable. Hemorrhage is difficult to treat using krypton red, because hemoglobin poorly absorbs radiation of this wavelength. However, krypton red radiation penetrates through hazy media better than does radiation of shorter wavelengths. In general, the irradiation required to achieve an ophthalmoscopically visible lesion is most dependent on fundus pigmentation, where the bulk of the absorption occurs. The principal wavelengths of some common photocoagulation lasers are listed in Table 102-1.

Power

Retinal lesion size is strongly dependent on laser power. Most photocoagulation laser systems are controlled by changes in power level, whereas most photodisruptive lasers (Nd:YAG) are controlled by changes in energy level.

Exposure Time

Short exposures may lead to photodisruptive effects, whereas exposures of longer duration lead to photocoagulation or photochemical effects. However, within the realm of photocoagulation, the power used affects lesion size to a greater extent than exposure time does.

Spot Size

Focal laser treatment is optimized by using spots of small size (50–100μm diameter), and panretinal photocoagulation, which requires coverage of large areas of the retina, is facilitated by the use of larger spots (200–500μm diameter). Small spots may result in complications such as choroidal rupture and secondary CNVM when high irradiance levels are used.

Several commercially available contact lens systems may be used to deliver laser energy to the posterior segment. To choose the correct lens and spot size for various clinical problems, it is important to understand the effect of different contact lens systems on spot size. For the Goldmann lens, spot size correlates closely with the actual size of the retinal lesion produced. However, for the Mainster lens, Rodenstock panfundoscope lens, and Krieger lens, the retinal spot size is actually larger than the set spot size by approximately 35–50%. This disparity between set spot size and actual spot size must be kept in mind when using these lenses.

INDICATIONS

The indications for laser photocoagulation in the treatment of ophthalmic disease are myriad and include diabetic retinopathy, branch vein occlusion, and CNVM.[9–11]

Other indications for laser photocoagulation include retinopexy of retinal tears for the prevention of retinal detachment. In most cases, slit-lamp delivery systems provide adequate access to all but the most peripheral retinal tears. Far peripheral tears are treated more effectively using laser indirect ophthalmoscopy, a method likewise preferred for the treatment of peripheral neovascularization. Laser photocoagulation using the indirect ophthalmoscope also is effective for the treatment of certain small ocular tumors. Additionally, argon or diode laser photocoagulation has proved effective in the treatment of threshold retinopathy of prematurity.

COMPLICATIONS

As with all procedures, patients must be given appropriate preoperative education about the potential risks of laser photocoagulation. Inadvertent photocoagulation of the fovea, cornea, iris, or lens can be minimized using careful technique and appropriate spot size. Choroidal effusions are seen most often after extensive panretinal photocoagulation, a complication that may be minimized if the treatments are spread over multiple sessions. Secondary CNVM is thought to result from damage to Bruch's membrane caused by heavy laser treatment. Decreases in intensity and duration, along with the avoidance of smaller spot sizes (50μm), may help minimize this complication.

Retinal pigment epithelium rips have been noted, particularly with the use of the krypton red laser in the treatment of CNVM. Sudden contraction of the neovascular membrane as a result of the thermal effects of the laser may produce a shearing force that causes a rip in the retinal pigment epithelium.

NEW DEVELOPMENTS IN LASER THERAPY

The most recent clinical applications of laser therapy have exploited the nonphotocoagulative and subthreshold effects of

TABLE 102-1

PRINCIPAL WAVELENGTHS OF COMMONLY USED LASERS

Laser	Wavelength (nm)
Argon (blue–green)	488.0
Argon (green)	514.5
Frequency doubled Nd:YAG	532.0
Krypton (yellow)	568.2
Krypton (red)	647.1
Tunable dye	Variable (most 570–630nm), depending on dye
Diode	Variable (most 780–850nm), depending on diode
Nd:YAG	1,064.0

laser. Photodynamic therapy utilizes a low-intensity laser of appropriate wavelength to activate an exogenous photosensitizing agent.[12] The interaction between the laser light and the photosensitizing agent produces a photochemical reaction that results in cellular damage and vascular thrombosis of target tissue such as CNVMs. Thermal damage to adjacent retinal tissue is lessened, because the laser energy used in this technique is insufficient to result in coagulative damage. Subthreshold effects of laser therapy are currently under investigation for the treatment of CNVM (transpupillary thermotherapy) and prophylaxis of CNVM in patients with nonexudative age-related macular degeneration.[13,14]

REFERENCES

1. Meyer-Schwickerath G. Development of photocoagulation. In: March WF, ed. Ophthalmic lasers: a second generation. Thorofare: Slack; 1990:13–19.
2. Maiman TH. Stimulated optical radiation in ruby. Nature. 1960;187:493–7.
3. Campbell CJ, Rittler MC, Koester CJ. The optical maser as a retinal coagulator: an evaluation. Trans Am Acad Ophthalmol Otolaryngol. 1963;67:58–67.
4. Zweng HC, Flocks M, Kapany NS, et al. Experimental laser photocoagulation. Am J Ophthalmol. 1964;58:353–62.
5. L'Esperance FA Jr. An ophthalmic argon laser photocoagulation system: design, construction and laboratory investigations. Trans Am Ophthalmol Soc. 1968;66:827–904.
6. Puliafito CA, Deutsch TF, Boll J, et al. Semiconductor laser endophotocoagulation of the retina. Arch Ophthalmol. 1987;105:424–7.
7. McHugh JDA, Marshall J, Ffytche TJ, et al. Initial clinical experience using a diode laser in the treatment of retinal vascular disease. Eye. 1989;3:516–27.
8. Mizuno K. Binocular indirect argon laser photocoagulation. Br J Ophthalmol. 1981;65:425–8.
9. Early Treatment Diabetic Retinopathy Study Research Group. Photocoagulation for diabetic macular edema. Arch Ophthalmol. 1985;103:1796–806.
10. Branch Vein Occlusion Study Group. Argon laser photocoagulation for macular edema in branch vein occlusion. Am J Ophthalmol. 1984;98:271–82.
11. Macular Photocoagulation Study Group. Argon laser photocoagulation for neovascular maculopathy: five-year results from randomized clinical trials. Arch Ophthalmol. 1991;109:1109–14.
12. Miller JW, Walsh AW, Kramer M, et al. Photodynamic therapy of experimental choroidal neovascularization using lipoprotein-derived benzoporphyrin. Arch Ophthalmol. 1995;113:810–8.
13. Mainster MA, Reichel E. Transpupillary thermotherapy for age-related macular degeneration: long-pulse photocoagulation, apoptosis, and heat shock proteins. Ophthalmic Surg Lasers. 2000;31:359–73.
14. Olk RJ, Friberg TR, Stickney KL, et al. Therapeutic benefits of infrared (810-nm) diode laser macular grid photocoagulation in prophylactic treatment of nonexudative age-related macular degeneration. Ophthalmology. 1999;106:2082–90.

GEORGE A. WILLIAMS

DEFINITION
- Repair of rhegmatogenous retinal detachment via closure of retinal breaks by scleral indentation.

KEY FEATURES
- Identification, localization, and treatment of retinal breaks.
- Scleral imbrication.

INTRODUCTION

The primary surgical procedure for the repair of rhegmatogenous retinal detachment is scleral buckling, which can be accomplished using a variety of techniques and materials. The goal of scleral buckling is to close retinal breaks by indenting the eye wall and thus prevent the passage of liquefied vitreous into the subretinal space. A flexible approach that incorporates the benefits and advantages of different techniques can maximize the rate of anatomical and visual success while minimizing potential complications.

HISTORICAL REVIEW

Recognition of the importance of vitreoretinal traction and retinal breaks in the pathogenesis of retinal detachment by Gonin in 1919 ushered in a new era of repair in which both drainage of subretinal fluid and treatment of retinal breaks were employed. It was not until 1949 that Custodis introduced the concept of scleral buckling—the closure of retinal breaks by scleral indentation. The introduction of the binocular indirect ophthalmoscope by Schepens in 1951, along with the technique of scleral depression, revolutionized the localization of peripheral retinal pathology. Schepens further advanced scleral buckling techniques by combining scleral dissection, diathermy, and intrascleral implantation of silicone buckles. Lincoff and coworkers refined Custodis's procedure by using silicone sponge explants and cryotherapy.[1]

PREOPERATIVE EVALUATION AND DIAGNOSTIC APPROACH

The diagnosis of rhegmatogenous retinal detachment is suggested by complaints of floaters, photopsia, peripheral visual field loss, and decreased visual acuity. In patients who have clear media, the diagnosis is confirmed by indirect ophthalmoscopy with scleral depression. Slit-lamp biomicroscopy with a three-mirror contact lens often is helpful. Identification and precise localization of all retinal pathology are prerequisites of successful scleral buckling surgery. The location and type of retinal breaks, as well as the size and duration of retinal detachment, are factors that help determine the timing and type of scleral buckling to be performed.

In patients who have opaque media, the retinal status may not be determinable with ophthalmoscopy. Diagnostic ultra-sonography is critical in establishing retinal detachment. Bright-flash electroretinography can also be used. An extinguished electroretinogram in conjunction with compatible ultrasonographic findings is strongly indicative of extensive retinal detachment.

DIFFERENTIAL DIAGNOSIS

Not all retinal detachments are rhegmatogenous. Other causes need to be ruled out before retinal detachment repair is performed. Other causes include traction retinal detachments without retinal tears, Harada's disease, eclampsia of pregnancy, tumors (e.g., choroidal hemangiomas and melanomas), and uveal effusion.

ALTERNATIVES TO SCLERAL BUCKLING

Rhegmatogenous retinal detachment can be repaired by surgical techniques other than scleral buckling. Pneumatic retinopexy involves injection of an expansible gas bubble into the vitreous cavity and postoperative positioning so that the gas bubble closes the retinal break.[2] The retinal break is treated with either cryopexy or laser photocoagulation. Usually, pneumatic retinopexy is reserved for mobile retinal detachments in the superior 8 clock hours of the retina that have no retinal break or group of breaks larger than 1 clock hour. The indications for scleral buckling versus pneumatic retinopexy remain controversial among vitreoretinal surgeons.

Vitrectomy techniques also can be used to repair rhegmatogenous retinal detachment. Vitrectomy surgery is described in Chapter 104.

Alternatives to surgery include observation, which is usually reserved for chronic, inferior retinal detachments that are asymptomatic. Acute, symptomatic retinal detachments rarely achieve this status, so unless the patient is severely ill or refuses surgery, observation typically is not recommended in the acute setting.

Barrier laser photocoagulation to surround the detached area of retina can be used in both the acute and chronic settings. Unlike scleral buckling, pneumatic retinopexy, or vitrectomy, it is not curative. The goal is to "wall off" the detachment to preserve macular function. In acute, symptomatic retinal detachment, barrier laser photocoagulation may delay progression but is rarely successful in the long term.

ANESTHESIA

Scleral buckling can be performed with the patient under either local or general anesthesia. The anesthetic technique used is a matter of surgeon preference, but increasingly, local anesthesia is chosen. The advantages of local anesthesia include shorter operating time, quicker postoperative recovery, and possibly decreased morbidity and mortality in select cases. However, retrobulbar placement of local anesthetic is not without risk to the eye or the patient's general health. Perforation of the globe, particularly in myopic patients, and damage to the optic nerve may result in permanent visual loss. Respiratory arrest and grand mal seizures also have been reported. These complications can be minimized by use of either a subconjunctival or a peribulbar technique.[3,4] Subconjunctival or peribulbar infiltration with lidocaine (lignocaine) allows a limbal peritomy and dissection of Tenon's capsule. Additional lidocaine and bupivacaine can then be administered by way of retrobulbar irrigation via a blunt cannula.

GENERAL TECHNIQUES

Conjunctival opening can be performed either at the limbus or several millimeters posterior to it. The conjunctiva is manipulated considerably during scleral buckling, so radial relaxation incisions are suggested to prevent tearing. In patients who have filtering blebs or recent limbal wounds, the peritomy can be extended posteriorly to avoid the area of concern. If only one or two quadrants are to be buckled, a 360° peritomy is not necessary. Conjunctiva and Tenon's capsule can be reflected in the required quadrants only, and the appropriate muscles isolated.

After the peritomy, the space between Tenon's capsule and sclera is entered. The muscle insertion is then engaged with a muscle hook, and the connections to Tenon's capsule are identified and separated from the muscle. A traction suture is placed around the muscle. After all recti have been isolated, the surface of the sclera is inspected for evidence of thinning (most common superotemporally), staphyloma, and anomalous vortex veins. The locations of any abnormalities are noted before scleral depression is started or retinal breaks are marked.

No aspect of scleral buckling is more critical than accurate placement of the buckle on the sclera. This requires precise localization of retinal breaks on the scleral surface. Several instruments with which to localize and mark the sclera are available. For small flap tears or atrophic holes, a single mark on the posterior edge of the break is sufficient. Larger flap tears and nonradial tears require localization of both the anterior and posterior extent of the break (Fig. 103-1).

Treatment of Retinal Breaks

The rationale for the treatment of breaks of the retina is to create an adhesion between the retinal pigment epithelium and the retina, and so prevent liquefied vitreous from entering the subretinal space. This is accomplished by inducing a thermal injury using one of three energy sources: diathermy, cryotherapy, or laser. The morphological and cellular response of the retina and retinal pigment epithelium to each of these energy sources is essentially similar. After 2 weeks, all three modalities show comparable effects on the retinal adhesive force.[5]

SPECIFIC TECHNIQUES

Explant Techniques

Explant techniques allow the surgeon to place scleral buckling material to support retinal pathology.[6] The ability to effectively treat retinal pathology without the need for scleral dissection has resulted in explant surgery becoming the procedure of choice for most retinal surgeons. Explants are made of either solid silicone rubber or silicone sponges and come in a variety of sizes and shapes.

Explants are secured to the sclera with partial-thickness scleral sutures. For most detachments, the actual element selected is not as important as the accurate localization and proper placement of the element with respect to the retinal break(s). Proper placement of the element requires an effective suturing technique that involves the use of a spatula needle with a 5–0 nonabsorbable suture such as polyester, nylon, or polypropylene. Sutures are placed a minimum of 2mm farther apart than the width of scleral contact for a given element (e.g., 9mm apart for a 7mm element). To ensure that the most posterior edge of the retinal break is supported, the posterior suture is placed a minimum of 2–3mm posterior to the scleral localization mark (Figs. 103-2 and 103-3).

The placement of explant material can be either segmental or encircling. Segmental buckles usually are reserved for detachments with single or closely spaced retinal breaks less than 1 clock hour in total extent. Although segmental buckles close isolated tears effectively, they are less useful in preventing new breaks, since they provide little retinal support elsewhere. Encircling procedures are particularly indicated in patients who have the following:
- Multiple breaks in different quadrants,
- Aphakia,

SCLERAL MARKING TECHNIQUE FOR FLAP RETINAL TEARS

retinal tear

localizing marker

FIG. 103-1 ▮ Scleral marking technique for smaller and larger flap retinal tears.

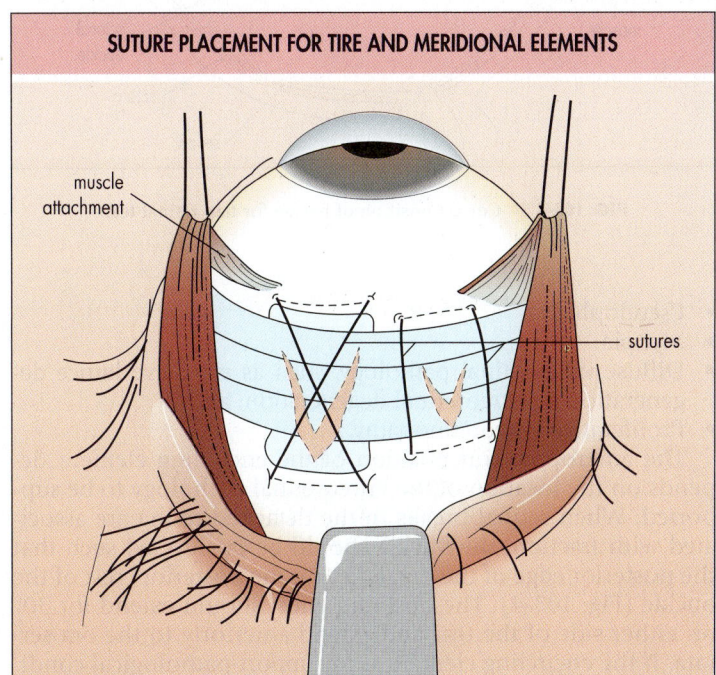

SUTURE PLACEMENT FOR TIRE AND MERIDIONAL ELEMENTS

muscle attachment

sutures

FIG. 103-2 ▮ Suture placement for both tire and meridional elements.

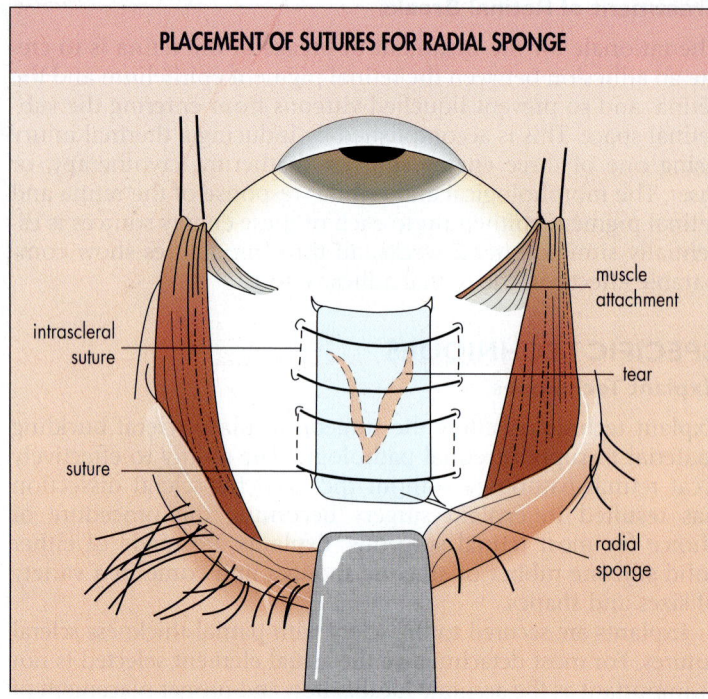

FIG. 103-3 ■ Placement of sutures for radial sponge.

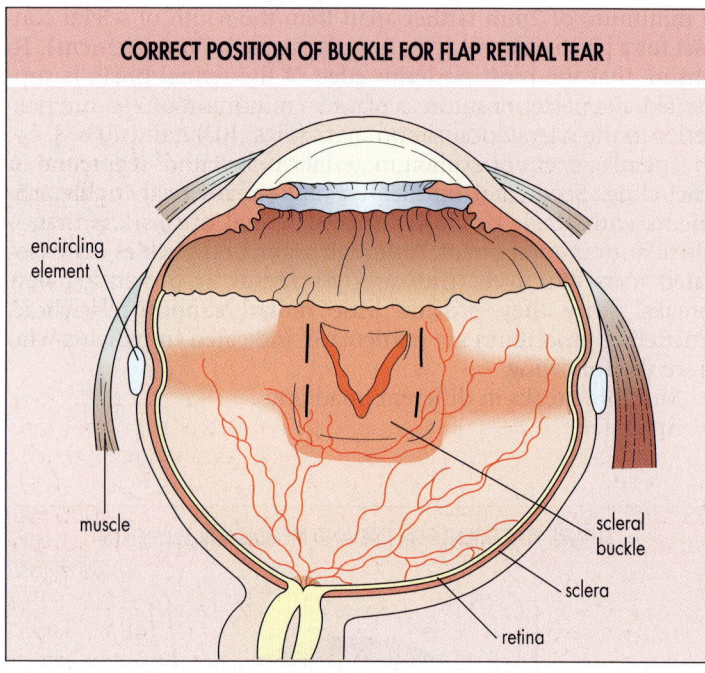

FIG. 103-4 ■ Correct position of buckle for flap retinal tear.

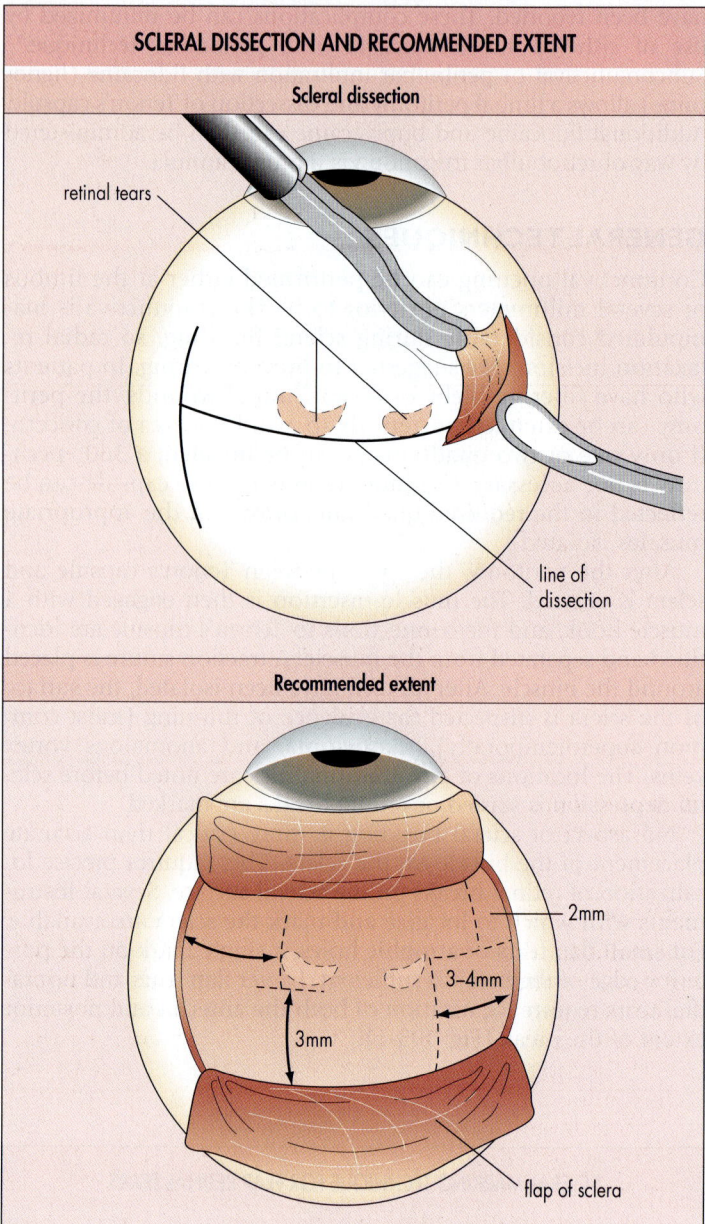

FIG. 103-5 ■ Technique for scleral dissection.

- Pseudophakia,
- Myopia,
- Diffuse vitreoretinal pathology, such as extensive lattice degeneration or vitreoretinal degeneration, and
- Proliferative vitreoretinopathy.

The anteroposterior position of the encircling element depends on the location of the vitreoretinal pathology to be supported. When retinal breaks in the detached retina are associated with traction, the buckle should be positioned such that the posterior edge of the break lies on the posterior crest of the buckle (Fig. 103-4). The buckling effect should extend for 30° on either side of the tear and extend anteriorly to the ora serrata. If the encircling element is to support pathological conditions in an attached retina, such as a retinal break, it should be positioned to reinforce the most posterior aspect of the condition. If no specific pathological factor is to be supported, the encircling element should buttress the posterior margin of the vitreous base.

The buckle height of encircling elements can be obtained in two ways. For thin encircling elements, such as solid silicone bands, the explant can be shortened in relation to the circumference of the globe. The second method to obtain buckle height is via suture placement. This technique is used with wider and thicker explants and does not require the element to be shortened in relation to the ocular circumference. The farther apart the bites of the mattress suture are placed, the greater the height of the buckle when the sutures are tightened.[6]

Implant Techniques

The current system of scleral buckling using implant techniques for rhegmatogenous retinal detachment was begun in 1960 by Schepens and associates with their description of scleral dissection, intrascleral placement of silicone buckles (implants), and diathermy. Subsequently, modifications and refinements of the technique have been described (Figs. 103-5 and 103-6).[1,7]

SCLERAL DISSECTION – PLACEMENT OF IMPLANT AND CLOSURE OF FLAPS

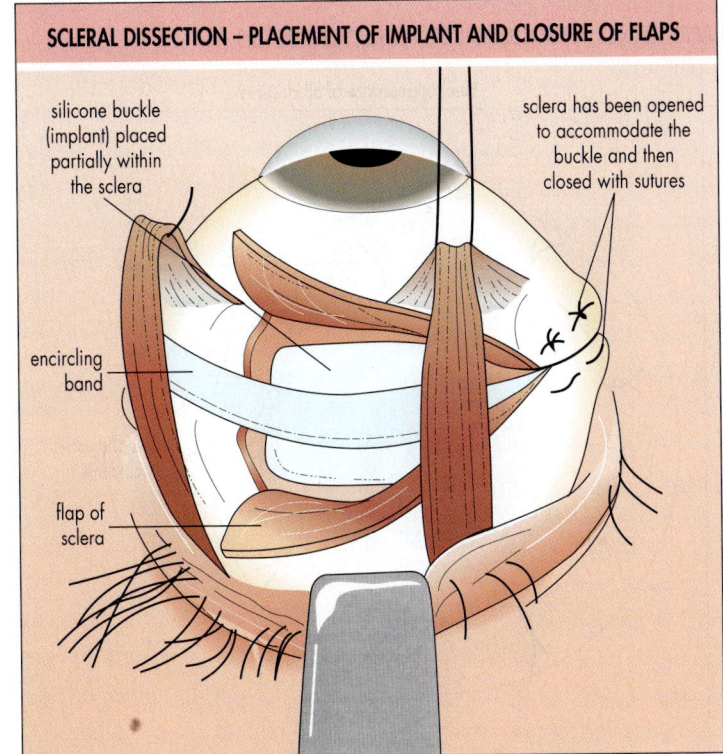

silicone buckle (implant) placed partially within the sclera

sclera has been opened to accommodate the buckle and then closed with sutures

encircling band

flap of sclera

FIG. 103-6 ▮ **Scleral dissection.** Placement of implant in scleral dissection and closure of scleral flaps.

LOCATION OF PREFERRED DRAINAGE SITES

retinal tear

X X X X

X preferred drainage sites

FIG. 103-7 ▮ Location of preferred drainage sites.

Drainage of Subretinal Fluid

Indications for drainage of subretinal fluid during scleral buckling remain controversial. Some authors believe that most cases can be managed without drainage of subretinal fluid, whereas others believe that drainage is a crucial aspect of the procedure.[6,8] The rationale for drainage of subretinal fluid is twofold:
- To diminish intraocular volume so as to allow elevation of the buckle without elevating intraocular pressure (IOP),
- To allow the retina to settle on the elevated buckle by removing fluid from the subretinal space.

Effective drainage of subretinal fluid places the retinal breaks in juxtaposition to the buckle, thereby facilitating closure of the breaks.

The selection of an external drainage site is affected by several factors. Clearly, the location of subretinal fluid is a primary concern. It is not necessary to drain where the amount of fluid is greatest, but rather where there is adequate fluid to safely enter the subretinal space. Whenever possible, it is preferable to drain just above or below the horizontal meridian, either temporally or nasally (Fig. 103-7). This location avoids the major choroidal vessels and vortex veins.

Again, whenever possible, it is preferable to drain in the posterior third of the bed of the buckle. This provides adequate support of the drainage site in the event of a complication such as retinal incarceration or choroidal hemorrhage, and it also provides immediate closure of the drainage site when the buckle is tightened. If, because of the configuration of the detachment or the position of the buckle, it is not possible to drain in the bed of the buckle, closure of the drain site with a mattress suture should be considered. Drainage outside the bed of the buckle allows the buckle to be pulled up as drainage proceeds. Entry through the choroid and into the subretinal space is performed with a needle (27–30 gauge). Usually, the presence of fluid around the needle signifies entry into the subretinal space. As the fluid drains, it is important to maintain a relatively normal and constant IOP to prevent retinal incarceration and choroidal hemorrhage.

After successful subretinal fluid drainage and closure of the drainage site, the buckle is positioned with the appropriate pre-placed scleral sutures to support the retinal pathology. Any suture that overlies a retinal break is tightened first, followed by the remainder of the sutures. The encircling band, if present, is then adjusted with a silicone sleeve. As the sutures are tightened, they are secured with temporary ties, and the optic nerve is inspected to confirm arterial perfusion. Once the buckle is positioned and the band adjusted, the fundus is inspected again to determine the status of the retinal breaks and the perfusion of the optic nerve. The temporary ties allow easy adjustment of the buckle height or position if necessary.

Nondrainage procedures can be used to reattach the retina, with success rates comparable to those of drainage procedures. The primary advantage of a nondrainage procedure is that it avoids the potential complications associated with transchoroidal drainage. In eyes with relatively shallow detachments, the eye may soften enough after scleral depression and cryopexy to allow placement of the buckle without IOP problems. Waiting several minutes between tightening of the scleral sutures also may soften the eye. However, nondrainage techniques often require the IOP to be lowered by additional medical or surgical means.

Closing

After final adjustment of the buckle, the sutures are tied and the knots rotated to the posterior edge of the buckle. Tenon's capsule and the globe can then be irrigated with an antibiotic solution. Retrobulbar irrigation with 0.50% bupivacaine significantly decreases postoperative pain after both general and local anesthesia.

Tenon's capsule is then identified in all quadrants. A layered closure, initially closing Tenon's capsule to the muscle insertions in all quadrants, has advantages (Fig. 103-8). This ensures that the explant and the nonabsorbable sutures are covered by the thick Tenon's capsule and also removes tension on the conjunctival closure, which minimizes the possibility of buckle erosion. During conjunctival closure, the relaxation incisions are closed with a running 6–0 plain gut suture. The conjunctiva is secured at the limbus with one or more sutures.

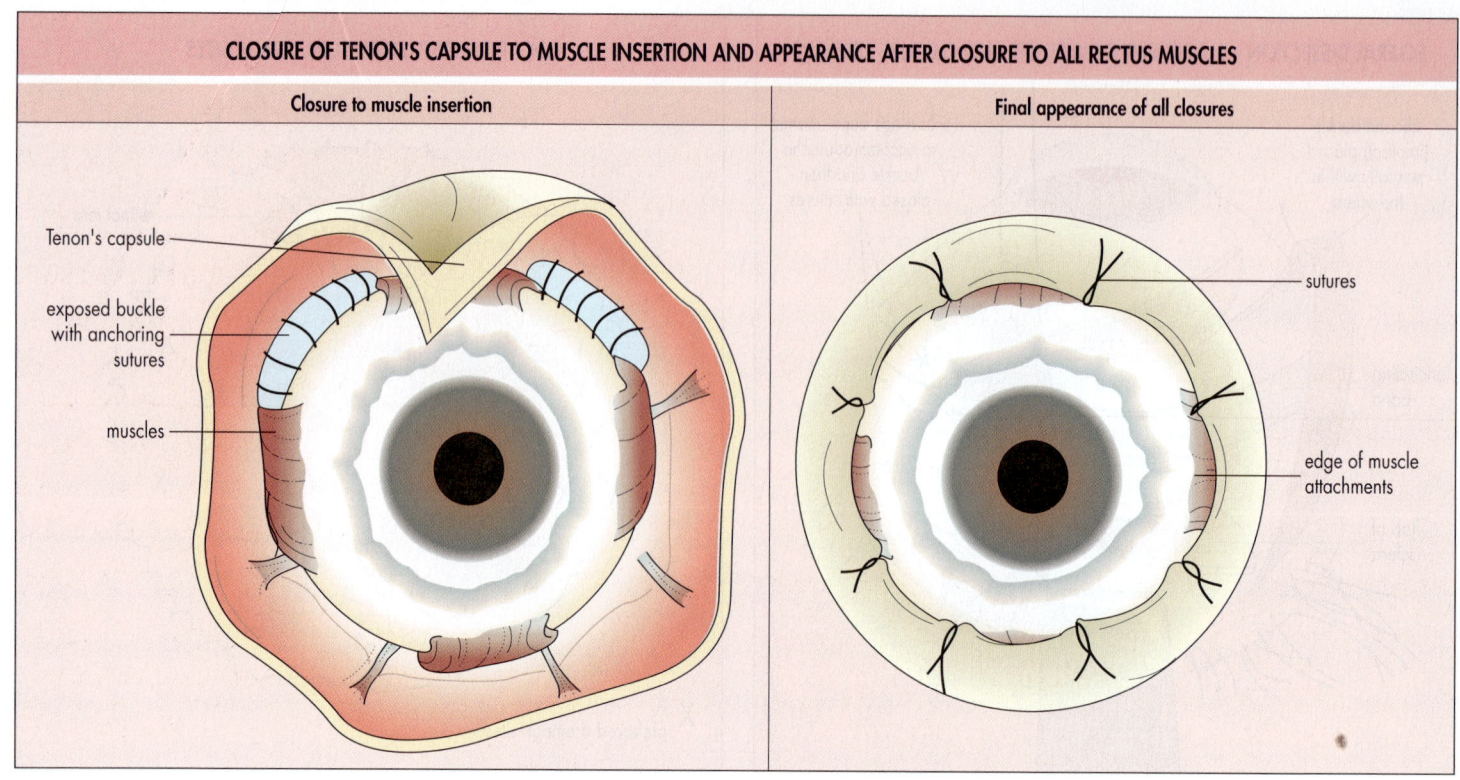

CLOSURE OF TENON'S CAPSULE TO MUSCLE INSERTION AND APPEARANCE AFTER CLOSURE TO ALL RECTUS MUSCLES

Closure to muscle insertion	Final appearance of all closures

Tenon's capsule

exposed buckle with anchoring sutures

muscles

sutures

edge of muscle attachments

FIG. 103-8 ■ Closure of Tenon's capsule to all rectus muscles.

COMPLICATIONS

Intraoperative Complications

SCLERAL PERFORATION. Scleral perforation during placement of scleral sutures is a potentially disastrous complication. Perforation usually is noticed at the time of suture placement and is heralded by the presentation of blood, pigment, or subretinal fluid through the suture tract.

DRAINAGE COMPLICATIONS. The most common drainage complications are retinal incarceration and choroidal or subretinal hemorrhage.[9] Retinal incarceration may occur despite attempts to avoid large fluctuations in IOP during drainage. It is identified by the characteristic dimpled appearance of the retina over the drainage site. Minimal degrees of incarceration rarely result in retinal breaks, but large amounts of incarceration require support with a buckle.

Choroidal (or subretinal) hemorrhage is perhaps the most feared complication of subretinal fluid drainage; it usually occurs at the time of choroidal perforation and is marked by the appearance of blood at the drainage site. If this occurs, the drainage site should be closed as quickly as possible with either the buckle or a sclerotomy suture and the IOP elevated above the systolic perfusion pressure. If the drainage site is temporal, the eye should be positioned to place the located site as inferiorly as possible to prevent gravitation of the subretinal blood to the fovea.

Postoperative Complications

GLAUCOMA. A variety of secondary glaucomas may develop after scleral buckling. Angle closure after scleral buckling may take place with or without pupillary block. When pupillary block is present, accompanying iris bombé occurs; usually, however, pupillary block does not occur. One presumed mechanism of the angle closure in these cases is shallow detachment of the ciliary body, which results in anterior displacement of the ciliary body and occlusion of the angle. Anterior segment ischemia also may cause glaucoma.

INFECTION AND EXTRUSION. Scleral buckling materials constitute foreign bodies and therefore carry the risk of infection and are at risk for extrusion. The incidence of explant infection and extrusion is about 1%. Effective management of infected scleral buckling material usually requires removal of any soft silicone sponge or large solid silicone elements. Topical and systemic antibiotics occasionally result in symptomatic improvement, but they are rarely curative. Removal of the scleral buckling material carries a redetachment risk of 4–33%.[10]

CHOROIDAL DETACHMENT (CHOROIDAL EDEMA). Accumulation of serous or serosanguineous fluid in the suprachoroidal space is relatively common after scleral buckling and is referred to as choroidal detachment or choroidal edema, even though it is truly a choroidal (or ciliary body) effusion. Choroidal detachment occurs after both implant diathermy procedures and explant cryotherapy procedures. The overall incidence of choroidal detachment is about 40%.[11]

CYSTOID MACULAR EDEMA. Using cryotherapy and explant techniques, the incidence of angiographic cystoid macular edema 4–6 weeks after surgery in phakic eyes is 25–28%.[12]

MACULAR PUCKER. Macular pucker is a major cause of decreased vision after scleral buckling. The incidence of macular pucker formation is in the range of 3–17%. Risk factors identified include preoperative proliferative vitreoretinopathy of grade B or greater, age, total retinal detachment, and vitreous loss during drainage.[13]

DIPLOPIA. The incidence of postoperative diplopia is low. In a series of 750 patients whose retinas were reattached with scleral buckling, 3.3% complained of diplopia postoperatively.[14] The incidence of diplopia is greater after reoperations.

CHANGES IN REFRACTIVE ERROR. The extent and direction of change in refractive error after scleral buckling depend on the surgical technique employed. Segmental buckles, whether implants or explants, have little effect on refractive error. However, large radial elements, such as full-thickness sponges that extend anteriorly beyond the ora serrata, may induce an irregular astigmatism. Encircling procedures induce the greatest change in refractive error. This change is greater for phakic than for aphakic eyes because of anterior displacement of the lens, which results in an increased myopic shift.[15]

OUTCOME

The anatomical results following scleral buckling for rhegmatogenous retinal detachments are impressive. An overall reattachment rate of at least 90% is achievable. Unfortunately, the visual results after scleral buckling do not parallel the anatomical results. Multiple factors correlate with visual and anatomical prognosis after scleral buckling. Detachments with the macula attached (macula-on) at the time of surgery have a significantly better anatomical and visual prognosis than do detachments in which the macula has become detached preoperatively. Cumulative data from three series demonstrate successful anatomical reattachment in 99% of cases of macula-on retinal detachment.[16-18] However, despite this high anatomical success rate, decreased visual acuity can occur. Usually this is caused by postoperative macular changes, such as cystoid macular edema or macular pucker. Approximately 10% of patients who have macula-on detachments suffer a visual loss of two Snellen lines or greater with respect to their preoperative vision.

Detachment of the macula results in a variable degree of permanent photoreceptor damage that correlates with the duration of the macular detachment.[6] Macula-off detachments are usually larger and of greater duration than are macula-on detachments. Therefore it is not surprising that retinal detachments that involve the macula have a lower rate of anatomical and visual success than do retinal detachments with macular involvement. The overall anatomical success rate for macula-off detachments is at least 90%, but despite this high rate of reattachment, only 40–60% of patients have a final visual acuity of 20/50 or better.[19-23]

REFERENCES

1. Wilkinson CP, Rice TA, eds. History of retinal detachment surgery. In: Michels RG. Retinal detachment, ed 2. St Louis: Mosby; 1997:251–334.
2. Hilton GF, Grizzard WS. Pneumatic retinopexy. A two-step outpatient operation without conjunctival incision. Ophthalmology. 1986;93:626–41.
3. Mein CE, Woodcock MG. Local anesthesia for vitreoretinal surgery. Retina. 1990;10:47–9.
4. Orgel IK, Williams GA. Peribulbar anesthesia for scleral buckling surgery. Vitreoretinal Surg Technol. 1992;1:4–5.
5. Kita M, Negi A, Kawano S, Honda Y. Photothermal cryogenic and diathermic effects on retinal adhesive force in vivo. Retina. 1991;11:441–4.
6. Williams GA, Aaberg TM Sr. Techniques of scleral buckling. In: Ryan SJ, ed. Retina, vol 3. St Louis: Mosby; 2001:2010–46.
7. Schepens CL. Retinal detachment and allied disease. Philadelphia: WB Saunders; 1983.
8. Sasoh M. The frequency of subretinal fluid drainage and the reattachment rate in retinal detachment surgery. Retina. 1992;12:113–7.
9. Burton RL, Cairns JD, Campbell WG, et al. Needle drainage of subretinal fluid: a randomized clinical trial. Retina. 1993;13:13–6.
10. Wiznia RA. Removal of solid silicone rubber exoplants after retinal detachment surgery. Am J Ophthalmol. 1983;95:495–7.
11. Packer AJ, Maggiano JM, Aaberg TM, et al. Serous choroidal detachment after retinal detachment surgery. Arch Ophthalmol. 1983;101:1221–4.
12. Meredith TA, Reeser FH, Topping TM, Aaberg TM. Cystoid macular edema after retinal detachment surgery. Ophthalmology. 1980;87:1090–5.
13. Lobes LA, Burton TC. The incidence of macular pucker after retinal detachment surgery. Am J Ophthalmol. 1978;85:72–7.
14. Smiddy WE, Loupe DN, Michels RG, et al. Extraocular muscle imbalance after scleral buckling surgery. Ophthalmology. 1989;96:1485–90.
15. Smiddy WE, Loupe DN, Michels RG, et al. Refractive changes after scleral buckling surgery. Arch Ophthalmol. 1989;107:1469–71.
16. Tani P, Robertson DM, Langworthy A. Rhegmatogenous retinal detachment without macular involvement treated with scleral buckling. Am J Ophthalmol. 1980;90:503–8.
17. Wilkinson CP. Visual results following scleral buckling for retinal detachments sparing the macula. Retina. 1981;1:113–6.
18. Girard P, Mimoun G, Karpouzas I, Moutefiove G. Clinical risk factors for proliferative vitreoretinopathy after retinal detachment surgery. Retina. 1994;14:417–24.
19. Tani P, Robertson DM, Langworthy A. Prognosis for central vision and anatomic reattachment in rhegmatogenous retinal detachment with macula detached. Am J Ophthalmol. 1981;92:611–20.
20. Burton TC. Preoperative factors influencing anatomic success rates following retinal detachment surgery. Trans Am Acad Ophthalmol Otolaryngol. 1977;83:499–505.
21. Burton TC, Lambert RW Jr. A predictive model for visual recovery following retinal detachment surgery. Ophthalmology. 1978;85:619–25.
22. Girard P, Karpouzas I. Visual recovery after scleral buckling surgery. Ophthalmologica. 1995;209:323–8.
23. Hussan TS, Sarrafizadeh R, Ruby A, et al. The effect of duration of macular detachment on results after the scleral buckle repair of primary macula-off retinal detachments. Ophthalmology. 2002;109:146–152.

104 Vitrectomy

STANLEY CHANG

INTRODUCTION

In the 30 years since its genesis, remarkable advances in vitreous surgery have established this microsurgical procedure as the most common intraocular operation after cataract extraction. Progress in two major areas fueled the extraordinarily rapid growth in vitreous surgical techniques:

- Understanding of the pathoanatomical changes that affect the retina;
- Introduction of new technology and instrumentation.

In the early years, vitrectomy was used to restore ambulatory vision in eyes that were destined to become blind. Both removal of opacified vitreous and removal of fibrovascular tissue in diabetic retinopathy often resulted in restoration of functional vision. Eyes that had complicated retinal detachments, such as those associated with proliferative vitreoretinopathy or that resulted from severe penetrating injury, were regarded as inoperable previously. As refinements in technique continued and the safety of the procedure was established, the focus shifted to newer applications (e.g., macular surgery). The goals of this surgery are to restore central visual function in such conditions as macular pucker, macular hole, and choroidal neovascularization.

HISTORICAL REVIEW

Until the 1960s, it was believed dogmatically that the vitreous body should not be violated deliberately. In 1970, Machemer and Parel introduced the first instrument to cut and remove vitreous, and the first planned vitrectomy procedure was performed in a diabetic patient who had a long-standing vitreous hemorrhage.

PREOPERATIVE EVALUATION AND DIAGNOSTIC APPROACH

The preoperative evaluation of patients who are to undergo vitrectomy includes a careful examination of the clinical situation as well as assessment of the patient's medical status and anesthetic risk. The surgeon and surgical team review the goals of the planned procedure with the patient and explain the potential benefits and risks.

Slit-lamp examination is carried out to evaluate the anterior segment structures; indirect biomicroscopy is used to determine the vitreoretinal relationships. When a gas bubble tamponade is to be used, the depth of the anterior chamber is examined to assess the possibility of postoperative angle-closure glaucoma. The cornea, size of the dilated pupil, and clarity of the lens are noted to ensure that, intraoperatively, the retina can be visualized adequately. In pseudophakic eyes, the type of intraocular lens (IOL) and its composition are studied. As a consequence of its hydrophobic properties, a silicone IOL may develop condensation on its surface during fluid-air exchange, and the placement of silicone oil intravitreally may result in adhesion of oil droplets to the implant surface, which adversely affects the clarity of the optical zone. Gonioscopic evaluation is carried out in diabetic patients and those who have inflammatory conditions.

The status of the vitreous is best studied using indirect biomicroscopy—a 78D or 90D lens may be used. The absence or presence of separation of the posterior hyaloid surface is determined first, as this finding is critical to the surgical approach in macular conditions. These findings are supplemented by those of careful indirect ophthalmoscopy, which provides information about the severity of epiretinal membrane proliferation, the location of retinal breaks, and anatomical changes in vitreous base and peripheral retinal structures.

In cases of media opacity, ultrasonographic evaluation provides an accurate map of the vitreoretinal relationships. In particular, the mobility of retinal detachment, delineation of tractional regions, and localization of vitreous or subretinal hemorrhage may be depicted. The location and dimensions of prior scleral buckling elements may be determined. In traumatic situations, ancillary tests using computed tomography or orbital radiographic analysis may be necessary to aid in the localization of foreign bodies and damage to periocular structures.

INDICATIONS AND ALTERNATIVES TO SURGERY

The surgical indications for vitrectomy are given in Box 104-1. These include a wide range of conditions, some of which involve the vitreous or retina focally, whereas others represent more diffuse processes. Other chapters in this book describe the alternative medical approaches for many of the listed conditions.

ANESTHESIA

The majority of vitrectomies are carried out under local, infiltrative anesthetic (retrobulbar block, peribulbar block, or subconjunctival irrigation) with monitored anesthetic care. In instances of extreme patient apprehension or an inability to cooperate, general anesthetic is required. When using general anesthetic and intraoperative gas, it is important to discontinue inhalation of nitrous oxide at least 20 minutes prior to the final injection of gas. Otherwise, elevated intraocular pressure or an inadequate gas fill may result.

GENERAL TECHNIQUES

A three-port (sclerotomy) vitrectomy is the routine approach, using separate 20-gauge incisions through the pars plana. The incisions are usually located 3.5–4.0mm posterior to the limbus in phakic eyes and approximately 0.5mm more anteriorly in aphakic or pseudophakic eyes. An infusion cannula is sutured to the sclera, typically inferotemporally, to allow saline to replace the excised tissue and thereby maintain the intraocular pressure. The two additional sclerotomies allow instrumentation to be placed—usually, one of the instruments is connected to a light source for endoillumination. Such an approach allows bimanual control of eye movement and the use of two hands to engage tissue. The surgical incisions may vary depending on the clinical situation.

In general, a surgical microscope is used to view the fundus during surgery. A planoconcave contact lens is used most com-

BOX 104-1

Indications for Vitrectomy

DIABETIC RETINOPATHY
Nonclearing or repeated vitreous hemorrhage
Traction retinal detachment
Combined traction and rhegmatogenous retinal detachment
Progressive fibrovascular proliferation
Macular distortion by fibrovascular proliferation
Macular edema that results from a taut posterior hyaloid

RETINAL DETACHMENT
Retinal detachment with proliferative vitreoretinopathy
Giant retinal tears
Retinal detachment with posterior retinal breaks
Selected primary retinal detachments

COMPLICATIONS OF ANTERIOR SEGMENT SURGERY
Dislocated lens fragments
Dislocated intraocular lens
Aphakic or pseudophakic cystoid macular edema
Endophthalmitis
Choroidal hemorrhage
Epithelial downgrowth
Anesthetic needle perforation

TRAUMA
Hyphema evacuation
Traumatic cataract or dislocated lens
Posterior penetration injuries with vitreous
    hemorrhage and/or retinal detachment
Reactive intraocular foreign body
Subretinal membranes or hemorrhage
Traumatic macular holes

MACULAR SURGERY
Macular pucker
Macular hole
Choroidal neovascularization
Massive subretinal hemorrhage
Vitreomacular traction syndrome
Macular translocation
Serous retinal detachment secondary to optic pit
Transplantation of retinal photoreceptors or retinal pigment epithelium

PEDIATRIC RETINAL DISORDERS
Retinopathy of prematurity
Persistent hyperplastic primary vitreous
Familial exudative vitreoretinopathy
Giant retinal tears/dialysis
Juvenile retinoschisis
Juvenile rheumatoid arthritis
Retinal detachment secondary to choroidal coloboma
Retinal detachment in "morning glory" syndrome or optic nerve colobomas

TUMORS
Choroidal melanoma
Complications of retinal angiomatosis
Combined hamartoma of the retina and retinal pigment epithelium
Intraocular lymphoma
Diagnostic vitrectomy

UVEITIS
Viral retinitis—cytomegalovirus, acute retinal necrosis
Intraocular infections—bacterial, viral, fungal, parasitic
Ophthalmomyiasis
Inflammatory conditions—sarcoidosis, Behçet's syndrome, uveal effusion
Pars planitis
Whipple's disease
Familial amyloidosis
Hypotony

---

monly, but additional surgical viewing lenses (e.g., prism lenses, lenses of higher refractive index) have been developed to improve intraoperative visualization. Of increasing acceptance is the use of wide-field or panoramic viewing systems based on the principles of binocular indirect ophthalmoscopic visualization. Such systems offer an expanded visualization area and increased depth of focus but require that an image inverter be mounted on the microscope. Similarly, it is possible to perform pars plana vitrectomy using the binocular indirect ophthalmoscope rather than an operating microscope for illumination and observation.

SPECIFIC TECHNIQUES

Lensectomy

Lensectomy is indicated when cataract prevents visualization of the fundus or when the lens is subluxated. Also, the lens is removed if vitreoretinal traction located at or anterior to the vitreous base must be dissected, which is most frequently seen in proliferative vitreoretinopathy (PVR) and trauma. Ultrasonic fragmentation of the lens is usually approached from the pars plana with the lens equator entered by the fragmenter probe. If no IOL is to be placed, the capsule is excised completely using the vitreous cutter or removed en bloc with forceps.

In some clinical situations, it has become increasingly common to combine standard phacoemulsification, using an acrylic foldable IOL, with vitrectomy.[1] Such an approach should not be employed when extensive anterior membrane dissection is required.

Vitreous Cutters

The main types of vitreous cutting technology employed are the guillotine and rotary cutters. The guillotine cutter is a 20-gauge blunt instrument with a side port through which tissue is aspirated and cut by an inner sleeve that moves along the long axis of the probe. Currently, cutting speeds of up to 2500 cuts/minute are attainable. Higher cutting speeds result in less traction on the tissue and, theoretically, fewer iatrogenic tears. Rotary cutters have a port closer to the tip of the probe and cut tissue using an inner cutting blade that spins inside the outer needle. Because the port is closer to the tip of the instrument, it is possible to cut closer to the surface of the retina. However, rotary cutters are more costly to produce and are not available as disposable instruments.

Epiretinal Membrane Dissection

Two types of epiretinal proliferation are encountered:
• Fibrovascular proliferation, which contains neovascularization, most commonly seen in proliferative diabetic retinopathy (PDR);
• Nonvascular membranes, found in PVR and macular pucker.
The surgical goals are to separate the posterior hyaloid from the retinal surface peripherally and to remove the epiretinal proliferative tissue or release its tractional effects centrally (Fig. 104-1, A). Surgical techniques employed to remove the proliferative tissue are:
• Segmentation;
• Delamination; and
• En bloc dissection.
The dissections are achieved using microsurgical instruments such as scissors that cut perpendicularly across fibrovascular tissue or scissors that have curved or horizontally oriented blades to cut between the retinal attachments of the proliferative tissue. The use of lit, multifunction instruments allows bimanual delamination of tissue, which can be carried out more safely and

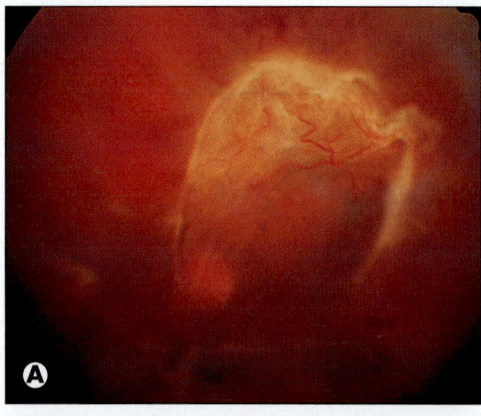

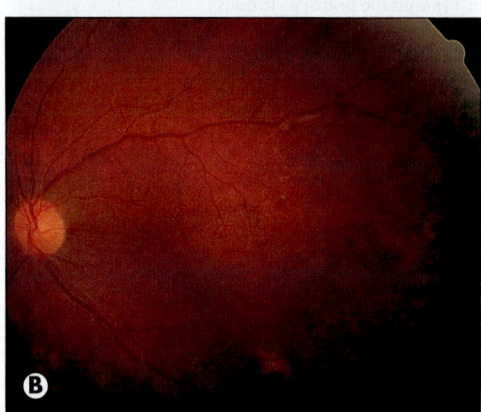

FIG. 104-1 ■ Proliferative diabetic retinopathy. **A,** Severe tractional retinal detachment with vitreous hemorrhage secondary to proliferative diabetic retinopathy. **B,** After vitrectomy and epiretinal membrane removal, the retinal anatomy is restored.

MECHANICAL REATTACHMENT OF POSTERIOR RETINA USING PERFLUOROCARBON LIQUIDS

FIG. 104-2 ■ Ability of perfluorocarbon liquids to reattach mechanically posterior retina in proliferative vitreoretinopathy. Simultaneously, subretinal fluid is displaced anteriorly and out through peripheral retinal breaks.

with less bleeding. Attainment of the surgical objectives results in a stabilization of the retinopathy and vision (Fig. 104-1, *B*).

Nonvascular epiretinal membranes are found in PVR and, in a less severe form, macular pucker. Such membranes may adhere strongly to the surface of the retina and are best removed using end-gripping membrane forceps; a bimanual approach using an illuminated membrane pick and forceps reduces the possibility of the formation of iatrogenic retinal tears.

It is recognized now that mechanical effects of the posterior hyaloid at the vitreoretinal interface may result in macula hole formation and central visual loss. The actual structural changes within this layer of cortical vitreous that cause retinal pathology are unclear. A critical step in the surgical management is separation of the posterior hyaloid from the retina. After a central vitrectomy has been performed, the adherent layer of cortical vitreous at the vitreoretinal interface is engaged and elevated using a silicone tip cannula at high aspiration levels. The posterior hyaloid is most adherent at the optic disc and at the macular region. After separation of the hyaloid, noted by observation of the Weiss ring, the vitreous layer is excised out to the periphery.

Perfluorocarbon Liquids

Perfluorocarbon liquids are useful as an intraoperative mechanical tool. The various perfluorocarbon liquids currently used in vitreous surgery have different physical and optical properties. Perfluoro-*n*-octane, because of the better visibility it allows, low viscosity, and high vapor pressure, is the most commonly used perfluorocarbon liquid. Giant retinal tears with large, inverted posterior flaps can be repositioned easily into their normal anatomical position, which allows the successful management of this condition without the use of special equipment to rotate the patient intraoperatively.[2]

In PVR, as perfluorocarbon liquid flattens the posterior retina, retinal folds are opened and allow traction and visualization of additional membranes (Fig. 104-2). A posterior retinotomy for internal drainage of subretinal fluid is no longer necessary. The retina is stabilized as membrane dissection proceeds, and large retinotomies, when necessary, can be carried out more safely.

Other applications of perfluorocarbon liquids are to float dislocated lens fragments or dislocated IOLs anteriorly, to provide intraocular hemostasis by localization of bleeding, and to express liquefied subretinal blood from under the retina.

Endophotocoagulation

Laser photocoagulation is applied around retinal breaks and circumferential retinotomies; in general, two to three rows of treatment are adequate. In more advanced cases of retinal detachment, such as PVR, laser spots may be placed contiguously in two or three rows on the anterior slope of the scleral buckle. In PDR, scatter photocoagulation is applied peripherally to reduce the risk of neovascular glaucoma. Recent experience with submacular surgery suggests that small, posterior retinotomies do not require laser photocoagulation.

Gas and Silicone Oil Tamponade

The final step in vitreous surgery is to decide whether it is necessary to fill the vitreous space using a tamponade agent. An automated air-infusion pump is used to perform the fluid-air exchange. A flute needle is used actively or passively to aspirate the intraocular fluid as air is infused through the infusion line. The entry of an air bubble into the vitreous results in an altered optical power of the eye and, as a consequence, different contact lenses are required to compensate for these changes.

BOX 104-2

Potential Complications of Vitreous Surgery

INTRAOPERATIVELY
Posterior retinal breaks
Peripheral retinal breaks
Choroidal hemorrhage (rare)

POSTOPERATIVELY
Retinal breaks
Rhegmatogenous retinal detachment
Elevated intraocular pressure (multiple potential causes)
• neovascular glaucoma
• angle-closure glaucoma
• inflammatory debris
• corticosteroid response
• overfill with gas
Anterior hyaloidal fibrovascular proliferation
Fibrin deposition in the anterior chamber (not rare, especially in diabetics)
Progressive nuclear sclerosis (almost universal in phakic eyes)
Corneal decompensation
Hypotony
Endophthalmitis (rare — I in 2000)

TABLE 104-I

SURGICAL OUTCOMES IN VITREOUS SURGERY

Vitreoretinal Disorder	Outcome
Diabetic vitreous hemorrhage	89% improvement with clear vitreous[5]
Diabetic traction retinal detachment	66–95% retinal reattachment rate[6]
Proliferative vitreoretinopathy	94% final retinal reattachment rate[7]
Giant retinal tears	96% final retinal reattachment rate[2]
Macular pucker	78–87% visual improvement by 2 Snellen lines[8]
Idiopathic macular hole	80–94% holes closed[9]
Choroidal neovascularization (idiopathic, presumed histoplasmosis)	58–63% visual improvement if ingrowth site is juxtafoveal or extrafoveal 72% no change in visual acuity if ingrowth site is subfoveal[10]
Dislocated lens fragments	68% final visual acuity 20/40 (6/12) or better[11]

In case no retinal detachment exists, a bubble tamponade may be unnecessary; but in some of these eyes, air is used to smooth out retinal folds or to allow visualization through a hemorrhagic medium postoperatively. In macular hole surgery, a longer lasting gas bubble is useful as its buoyant force may help close the hole. When retinal detachment is present, the subretinal fluid must be evacuated to achieve a complete fill with gas and ensure that the retina flattens without posterior folds. Perfluorocarbon liquid may be injected to flatten the retina up to the level of peripheral retinal breaks—the posterior subretinal fluid is expressed anteriorly. Internal drainage of the remaining subretinal fluid is accomplished by placement of the aspirating needle through the retinal break as air enters the eye. The descending air bubble flattens the anterior retinal detachment and forces the anterior subretinal fluid through the retinal break. When the subretinal fluid has been aspirated completely or nearly completely, the perfluorocarbon liquid may be removed.

The type of gas used is dependent on the individual clinical situation.[3] In eyes that have a simple retinal detachment, the role of the gas bubble is to allow adequate time for the chorioretinal adhesion from laser treatment to form. Usually, air or sulfur hexafluoride, which persists for 10–14 days, may be used. For more complex retinal detachments, such as PVR, trauma, and giant retinal tears, a longer lasting gas bubble is usually required. Perfluorohexane or perfluoropropane gases are chosen frequently for these situations.

Silicone oil tamponade may also be used as a long-term tamponade agent. This clear viscous liquid, which is immiscible with water, replaces the vitreous. Its surface tension and mild buoyant force mechanically hold the retina against the choroid. The advantage of silicone oil is that the patient has vision through the oil bubble and that extensive prone-head positioning (required with gas bubbles) is unnecessary. However, silicone oil may require surgical removal months after the retina has been reattached. The results of a multicenter, randomized clinical trial, in which the use of perfluoropropane gas was compared with the use of silicone oil for the treatment of severe PVR, found no statistically significant difference in the final retinal reattachment rate between the two modalities.[4]

COMPLICATIONS

Many of the potential complications of vitreous surgery may be realized later. The rate of complications has decreased gradually as improvements in technology have been introduced. However, experience, surgical skill, and training are also significant factors that can reduce the rate of complications. The more widely described intraoperative and postoperative complications encountered with vitreous surgery are given in Box 104-2.

OUTCOMES

The introduction of new surgical techniques and instrumentation and improved knowledge of the pathophysiology of abnormal vitreoretinal structural changes have resulted in a steady improvement in the anatomical and visual results of vitreous surgery. Some of the results reported for the most common indications of vitrectomy are given in Table 104-1 and represent significant advances in the surgical treatment of retinal disorders.

REFERENCES

1. Koenig SB, Mieler WF, Han DP, *et al.* Combined phacoemulsification, pars plana vitrectomy, and posterior chamber intraocular lens insertion. Arch Ophthalmol. 1992;110:1101–4.
2. Chang S, Lincoff H, Zimmerman NJ, *et al.* Giant retinal tears: surgical techniques and results using perfluorocarbon liquids. Arch Ophthalmol. 1989;107:761–6.
3. Chang S. Intraocular gases. In: Ryan S, Glaser BM, eds. Retina, ed 2. St Louis: Mosby; 1994.
4. Abrams GW, Azen SP, McCuen BW II, *et al.* Vitrectomy with silicone oil or long-acting gas in eyes with severe proliferative vitreoretinopathy: results of additional and long term follow-up. Silicone Study Report #11. Arch Ophthalmol. 1997;115: 335–44.
5. Thompson JT, de Bustros S, Michels RG, *et al.* Results and prognostic factors in vitrectomy for diabetic vitreous hemorrhage. Arch Ophthalmol. 1987;105:191–5.
6. Gardner T, Blankenship GW. Proliferative diabetic retinopathy: principles and techniques of surgical treatment. In: Ryan S, Glaser BM, eds. Retina, ed 2. St Louis: Mosby; 1994.
7. Coll GE, Chang S, Sun J, *et al.* Perfluorocarbon liquid in the management of retinal detachment with proliferative vitreoretinopathy. Ophthalmology. 1994;102: 630–8.
8. Sjaarda RN, Michels RG. Macular pucker. In: Ryan S, Glaser BM, eds. Retina, ed 2. St Louis: Mosby; 1994.
9. Freeman W, Macular Hole Study Group. Vitrectomy for the treatment of full-thickness stage 3 or stage 4 macular holes: results of a multicentered randomized clinical trial. Arch Ophthalmol. 1997;115:11–21.
10. Melberg NS, Thomas MA, Dickinson JD, *et al.* Surgical removal of subfoveal choroidal neovascularization: ingrowth site as a predictor of visual outcome. Retina. 1996;16:190–5.
11. Borne MJ, Tasman W, Regillo C, *et al.* Outcomes of vitrectomy for retained lens fragments. Ophthalmology. 1996;103:971–6.

CHAPTER

105

SECTION 3 ANCILLARY TESTS

Contact B-Scan Ultrasonography

YALE L. FISHER • HANNA RODRIGUEZ-COLEMAN • ANTONIO P. CIARDELLA • NICOLE E. GROSS

DEFINITION

- Diagnostic technique useful in the evaluation of intraocular and orbital contents.

KEY FEATURES

- It uses high-frequency sound waves emitted and received by a handheld transducer probe.
- Images are processed and displayed on a video monitor.

ASSOCIATED FEATURES

- Adequate interpretation for diagnoses of posterior segment disease depends on three concepts: real time, gray scale, and three-dimensional analysis.

INTRODUCTION

Ophthalmic ultrasonography is one of the most useful diagnostic techniques for intraocular and orbital evaluation, especially in the setting of opaque media. It involves pulse-echo technology in which high-frequency sound waves are emitted from a handheld transducer probe. Returning echoes are processed and displayed on video monitors or oscilloscopes.

In ophthalmology, two modes of display are common:
- A-scan mode (time-amplitude), used predominantly for interpretation of tissue reflectivity—the returning echoes form a graph-like image seen as vertical deflections from a baseline.
- B-scan mode (intensity modulation), used predominantly for anatomical information—it shows cross-sectional images of the globe and orbit.

Both types of sonographic display are complementary. This chapter focuses on B-scan information.

Developed in the mid-1950s with water immersion techniques, B-scan ultrasonography initially required a laboratory setting. In the early 1970s, contact devices were introduced. They utilized methylcellulose, or a similar sound-coupling agent, and rapidly increased B-scan availability and popularity. Subsequent improvements in image quality and scanning rates made interpretation easier for the examiner.[1-7]

DEVICES

Commercially available contact instruments for ocular and orbital B-scan ultrasonography usually employ 10MHz (megacycles/s) transducer probes enclosed in a handheld container. A small motor within the handpiece moves the ultrasonic probe in a rapid sector scan to create cross-sectional B-scan images. In general, these devices have resolution capacities of approximately 0.4mm axially and 1mm laterally. Higher resolution ophthalmic instru-ments are available (20–50 MHz), but limited signal penetration renders them ineffective in the examination of posterior portions of the globe and orbit. Most contact B-scan machines are freestanding and relatively mobile; they consist of a detachable transducer probe, a signal processing box, and a display screen.

TECHNIQUE OF EXAMINATION

The handheld ultrasonic probe is placed gently against the eyelid or sclera using a sound-coupling agent such as methylcellulose. The ultrasonographer can move the probe systematically to scan the globe and orbit. Lateral or medial displacement of the probe can be used to avoid the lens system and thus prevent image artifacts.

CONCEPTS OF B-SCAN INTERPRETATION

Interpretation of a B scan for accurate diagnoses of posterior segment disease depends on three concepts:
- Real time
- Gray scale
- Three-dimensional analysis

Real Time

Ultrasound B-scan images can be visualized at approximately 32 frames/s, allowing motion of the globe and vitreous to be easily detected. Characteristic real-time movements can often identify imaged tissues such as detached retina or mobile vitreous, thus increasing diagnostic capability. Real-time ultrasonic information frequently aids in vitreoretinal surgery.

Gray Scale

A variable gray-scale format is used to display the returning echoes as a two-dimensional image. Strong echoes, such as those seen from sclera or detached retina, are displayed brightly at high instrument gain and remain visible even when the gain is reduced. Weaker echoes, such as those from a vitreous hemorrhage, are seen as a lighter shade of gray that disappears when the gain is reduced. Comparing the echo strengths during ultrasonic examination is the basis for qualitative tissue analysis. This can enhance diagnostic accuracy provided that the strongest possible echoes from each tissue type are being evaluated. Diagnostic accuracy is achieved by ensuring that the probe remains perpendicular to the tissues of interest at all times.

Three-Dimensional Analysis

Developing a mental three-dimensional image or topographic anatomical map from multiple two-dimensional B-scan images is the most difficult concept to master. It is essential because it provides the vital architectural information that is the basis for B-scan diagnosis. Three-dimensional understanding of ultrasound images is especially critical in the preoperative evaluation of complex retinal detachments and also intraocular or orbital tumors.

DISPLAY PRESENTATION AND DOCUMENTATION

B-scan images displayed on a screen are presented horizontally. Areas that are closest to the probe are imaged to the left of the screen and those farthest away are imaged to the right. The top of the screen correlates with a mark located on the examining probe that represents the initial transducer position for each sector scan.

Although contact B-scan ultrasonography is a dynamic examination, documentation and preservation of individual, "frozen" cross-sectional images are possible by photographic techniques. These illustrative images should not be used for interpretation.

Normal Vitreous Cavity

The normal vitreous space is almost clear of echogenic tissue. Occasional small dots or linear echoes can be seen at the highest gain settings (90dB), but they fade rapidly as the gain is reduced. Real-time scanning during voluntary eye movement usually shows some motion of these fine echoes.

Vitreous Hemorrhage

Intravitreal hemorrhage produces easily detectable diffuse dots and blob-like vitreal echoes that correlate with the amount of blood present. Reduction of gain to 70dB results in rapid fading of all but the densest areas of reflectivity. Real-time evaluation usually shows a characteristic rapid, staccato motion with eye movement. This occurs because vitreous hemorrhage induces a general vitreous gel liquefaction and separation from the retina.

Retinal Detachment

Detached retina appears as a highly reflective sheet-like tissue within the vitreous space (Fig. 105-1). Small detachments often appear dome-like on imaging. The appearance of total retinal detachment, which anatomically is cone shaped, varies depending upon the position of the examining probe. Axial images are funnel shaped with attachment to the optic nerve head. Coronal images show a cross section of the cone, that is, a circular image.

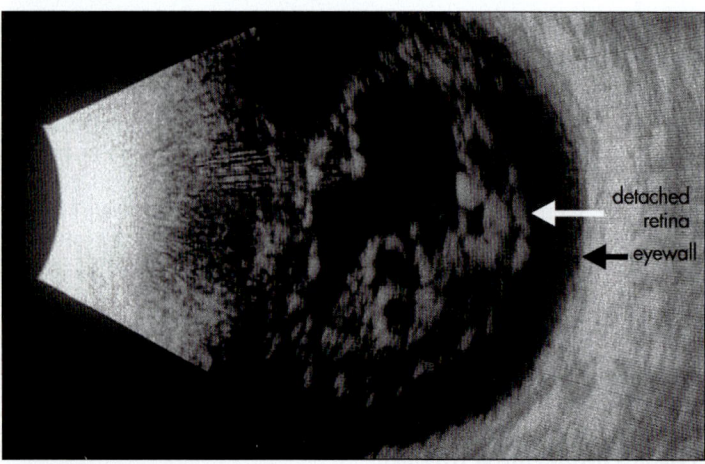

FIG. 105-1 ■ **Contact B-scan image of a retinal detachment.** This axial section of a total retinal detachment reveals a highly reflective sheet-like membrane in the vitreous space, detached from the posterior eye wall *(arrows)* and attached only to the optic nerve head.

Real-time evaluation varies; recent detachments have a characteristic undulating movement, which is slower than that of the vitreous gel. Long-standing detachments appear stiffer with less motion because of proliferation of scar tissue on the retinal surface.

Tumors

Ultrasound evaluation of intraocular tumors requires not only topographic localization but also interpretation of acoustic grayscale characteristics. Malignant choroidal melanomas, for example, have the most characteristic appearance. They are mostly dome or mushroom shaped, and on gray scale their anterior borders are strongly reflective, whereas the progressively deeper portions of the tumor are less reflective. This is due to cellular homogeneity that provides a false hollowing appearance. Tissues, such as orbital fat, localized behind these tumors are often shadowed (they appear less reflective) because of the absorption of sound by the tumor.

DIGITAL AND THREE-DIMENSIONAL CONTACT ULTRASOUND

A series of advances in electronics such as digital techniques and the development of high-capacity storage devices allows documentation of contact ultrasonography to become more than static photographs. Real-time kinetic movie recordings and playback of a B-scan examination with simultaneous amplitude information have made possible the recall of complete examinations. This is invaluable when comparison at a later date is of essence, for example, in tumor evaluation. Also, three-dimensional ultrasound systems allow the examiner to view horizontal, vertical, and diagonal aspects of the pathology at the same time in less than 2 seconds (Fig. 105-2). This is done by collecting a series of two-dimensional scans in a preset fashion and transforming them into a volumetric image that can be processed, using multiplanar reconstruction. This new technique is particularly useful to inexperienced examiners when first learning three-dimensional thinking, and it is also helpful because it provides accurate linear and volume measurements within the context of the contact technique.

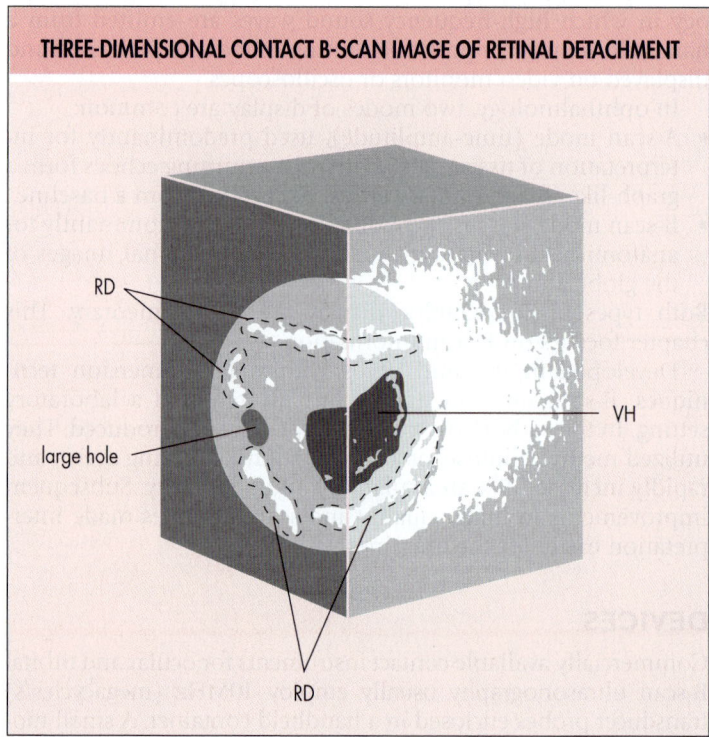

THREE-DIMENSIONAL CONTACT B-SCAN IMAGE OF RETINAL DETACHMENT

FIG. 105-2 ■ **Three-dimensional contact B-scan image of a retinal detachment.** Axial and sagittal views of a total retinal detachment *(RD)* are seen simultaneously. Notice the appreciation of a wide cone-shaped funnel. Also distinguishable are the large hole in the retina and vitreous hemorrhage *(VH)*.

SUMMARY

Contact B-scan ultrasound provides a convenient, noninvasive means for the evaluation of intraocular structures in situations where clinical examination is not possible because of opaque ocular media; it also allows a dynamic examination of the vitreoretinal relationship. Newly developed three-dimensional and digital contact techniques expand teaching capability and clinical availability of contact ultrasonography to a larger audience. Ultrasound studies should be used in conjunction with detailed clinical examination and other investigational modalities.

REFERENCES

1. Purnell EW. Intensity modulated (B-scan) ultrasonography. In: Goldberg RE, Sarin LK, eds. Ultrasonics in ophthalmology: diagnostic and therapeutic applications. Philadelphia: WB Saunders; 1967, 102–123.
2. Coleman DJ. Reliability of ocular and orbital diagnosis with B-scan ultrasound. 1. Ocular diagnosis. Am J Ophthalmol. 1972;73:501–16.
3. Coleman DJ, Koenig WF, Katz L. A hand operated ultrasound scan system for ophthalmic evaluation. Am J Ophthalmol 1969;68:256–63.
4. Coleman DJ, Lizzi FL, Jack RL. Ultrasonography of the eye and orbit. Philadelphia: Lea & Febiger; 1977.
5. Bronson NR. Quantitative ultrasonography. Arch Ophthalmol. 1969;81:400–72.
6. Bronson NR, Fisher YL, Pickering NC, Traynor E. Ophthalmic contact B-scan ultrasonography for the clinician. Baltimore: Williams & Wilkins; 1980.
7. Fisher YL. Contact B-scan ultrasonography: a practical approach. Int Ophthalmol Clin. 1979;19:103–25.

CHAPTER
106 Fluorescein and ICG Angiography

NARESH MANDAVA • ELIAS REICHEL • DAVID R. GUYER • LAWRENCE A. YANNUZZI

DEFINITION

- Fluorescein angiography is an imaging test that highlights the retinal and choroidal circulation and is useful in the diagnosis of retinal, choroidal, and optic nerve disorders. Progression of various disease entities and treatment decisions, as well as guidance during laser treatment, often are based on fluorescein angiography.
- ICG is an infrared-based imaging technique used to detect choroidal abnormalities and is specifically most useful for the detection of occult, poorly defined forms of choroidal neovascularization and can increase the number of patients potentially treatable, using laser photocoagulation.

FLUORESCEIN ANGIOGRAPHY

INTRODUCTION

Fluorescein angiography (FA) has contributed greatly to the diagnosis and treatment of many common chorioretinal diseases. In addition, its use has helped to elucidate previously poorly understood retinal and choroidal diseases and has served as an interesting research modality. Technological advances in digital imaging and computer analysis have further expanded the clinical and research applications of fluorescein angiography.

HISTORICAL REVIEW

Henry Noyes in the late 1800s was the first to attempt fundus photography of rabbits, with limited results. In 1926, Karl Zeiss and Nordensen produced the first reliable commercial fundus camera, and clinical photography of the human ocular fundus became possible. It was not until 1955, when Zeiss introduced the electronic flash, that the modern fundus camera was born.

In 1960, MacLean and Maumenee[1] were the first to perform fluorescein angioscopy in humans to visualize a hemangioma of the choroid, using a slit lamp and cobalt blue filter. Unfortunately, their technique was useful for diagnosis alone, because they were unable to document or to study the fluorescein angioscopy. Flocks, Miller, and Chao[2] attempted to capture angiography on motion picture film but had limited success. Novotny and Alvis[3] were the first to perform successful fluorescein angiography on a human. Using a combination of masked filters, Zeiss optics, electronic flash, and high-speed, high-resolution film, Novotny and Alvis were able to make a careful study of the retinal circulation. These early contributions were crucial to the advancement of fluorescein angiography as an imaging modality in retinal diseases.

Recently, digital imaging has made possible the convenient archiving of images as well as the ability to send images to other locations quickly.

PURPOSE OF THE TEST

Imaging of both the retinal and choroidal circulations is possible with fluorescein angiography; however, the information provided by images of the retinal vasculature is the greatest contribution of fluorescein angiography. Common diseases, such as diabetic retinopathy, cystoid macular edema, central serous chorioretinopathy, and venous occlusive disease, are managed with the assistance of fluorescein imaging. For diagnosis, no substitute exists for a thorough ophthalmologic examination and, in most cases, ophthalmoscopy alone is needed, but fluorescein angiography may be useful to confirm the diagnosis. In addition, fluorescein imaging is used routinely to evaluate the progression of disease and to guide the ophthalmologist in the decision and method of treatment.

PROPERTIES OF SODIUM FLUORESCEIN DYE

Several biochemical characteristics of the sodium fluorescein molecule are fundamental in its use for ophthalmic imaging. The first is fluorescence—the ability to absorb a photon of light of one wavelength and emit a photon of light of a second wavelength. Sodium fluorescein is yellow–red in color, with a molecular weight of 376.67D. Its narrow spectra of absorption (465–490nm [blue]) and excitation (520–530nm [yellow–green wavelength]) makes it ideal for the selective imaging of fluorescein dye. Sodium fluorescein dye usually is available as aliquots of 2–3ml of 25% or 5ml of 10% sodium fluorescein in a sterile aqueous solution. No evidence exists to date of increased side effects with the higher concentration,[4,5] so many practitioners prefer to use the smaller volume of the more concentrated solution. Approximately 80% of fluorescein dye binds to plasma proteins, principally albumin, while the remainder stays in the free state. The dye is metabolized by both the liver and kidneys and is eliminated in the urine within 24–36 hours.

PROCEDURE

Modern fundus cameras are reliable and relatively easy to operate, but the photographer must understand the various camera controls to obtain high-quality photographs. The most common cause of poorly focused fundus photographs is operator error. The fundus camera produces an aerial image, which exists at infinity. Cross hairs in the eyepiece reticle allow the photographer to correct for spheric refractive error. To produce a well-focused fundus photograph, the photographer must see both the cross hairs and the fundus in good focus at the same time. The focusing wheel is used only for fine focus of the retinal pathology.

Unlike with the slit lamp, the joy stick of the fundus camera is used to align critically the camera to the patient's eye only. The photographer looks for even illumination of the image to determine the proper alignment of the camera. Misalignment causes peripheral or central artifacts in the images. Small, careful, lateral movements with the joystick are used to eliminate these before the photographs are taken. Many cameras provide variable magnification options, in the range of 20–60 degrees. It is important to select a magnification that is appropriate to the pathology being photographed.

Communication with the patient is critical to achieve excellent images. The best way to avoid the common errors or pitfalls of fundus photography is to develop and follow a standard photographic protocol, which helps the photographer to avoid mistakes in a busy clinical setting. A sample photographic procedure is given in Box 106-1.

The dye is injected, usually rapidly, into the antecubital vein to maximize the contrast of the early filling phase of the angiography. Precautions should be taken to avoid extravasation of the dye, because infiltration is painful and (rarely) may lead to tissue necrosis. The urine may have an orange hue for a few days. In addition, skin may turn a slight yellow for a few hours, especially in lightly pigmented patients.

COMPLICATIONS

Patients must be cautioned with regard to ultraviolet light exposure, because photosensitivity reactions seem to increase proportionately to the degree of yellowness of skin. Although no adverse reactions or risks to the pregnant woman or fetus have been reported, pregnancy, especially during the first trimester, is a relative contraindication to fluorescein angiography.[6,7]

Adverse reactions to intravenous fluorescein angiography range from mild to severe.[5,8-12] Mild reactions are defined as transient and resolve spontaneously; most commonly these are nausea (approximately 3–15%), vomiting (up to 7%), and pruritus.

TABLE 106-1

INCIDENCE OF ADVERSE REACTIONS TO INTRAVENOUS FLUORESCEIN ANGIOGRAPHY

	Reaction	Incidence
Mild	Incidence of 0–5% (based on 87% of respondents)	
Moderate	Urticaria	1:82
	Syncope	1:337
	Other	1:769
	Overall	1:63
Severe	Respiratory	1:3800
	Cardiac	1:5300
	Seizures	1:13,900
	Death	1:221,781
	Overall	1:1900

Moderate adverse reactions resolve with medical intervention; these include urticaria, syncope, thrombophlebitis, pyrexia, local tissue necrosis, and nerve palsy. Severe reactions are those that require intensive intervention and the patients may have poor recovery; these include laryngeal edema, bronchospasm, anaphylaxis, shock, myocardial infarction, cardiac arrest, tonic-clonic seizures, and death.[5] The incidence of adverse reactions has been reported in a multicenter, collaborative study (Table 106-1).

INTERPRETATION OF RESULTS
Normal Fluorescein Angiogram

Factors that influence the rapidity of onset of fluorescence include the speed of injection, and the age and cardiovascular condition of the patient. Dye first enters the short posterior ciliary arteries and is visualized in the choroid and optic nerve head 10–15 seconds after injection into the antecubital vein. The choroidal flush and patchy filling of the choroid are the hallmarks of the choroidal circulation. Choroidal flush is represented by the mottled fluorescence of the choriocapillaris and is attributed to the variable blockage of the retinal pigment epithelium (RPE). On the other hand, patchy filling of the choroid anatomically represents perfusion of the choriocapillaris lobules sequentially, rather than simultaneously. During the early phases of the angiogram, leakage of dye from the choriocapillaris and staining of Bruch's membrane eclipse the choroidal vascular detail. A cilioretinal artery is continuous with the choroidal circulation in 10–15% of patients and, in such cases, fluoresces simultaneous to the choroid.

The retinal circulation begins to fluoresce at 11–18 seconds, 1–3 seconds after the onset of choroidal filling. The retinal arterial system should fill completely in about 1 second. The early arteriovenous phase is characterized by the passage of fluorescein dye through the central retinal arteries, the precapillary arterioles, and the capillaries, while the late arteriovenous phase is characterized by the passage of dye through the veins in a laminar pattern. During the late arteriovenous phase, maximal fluorescence of the arteries occurs, with early laminar filling of the veins. Laminar filling of veins is caused by the preferential concentration of unbound fluorescein along the vessel walls. Several factors are responsible for the laminar pattern of venous filling; these include the more rapid flow of plasma along the vessel wall, as well as the higher concentration of erythrocytes in the central vascular lumen.

Maximal fluorescence is achieved in the juxtafoveal or perifoveal capillary network after 20–25 seconds (Fig. 106-1). The normal capillary-free zone, or foveal avascular zone, is approxi-

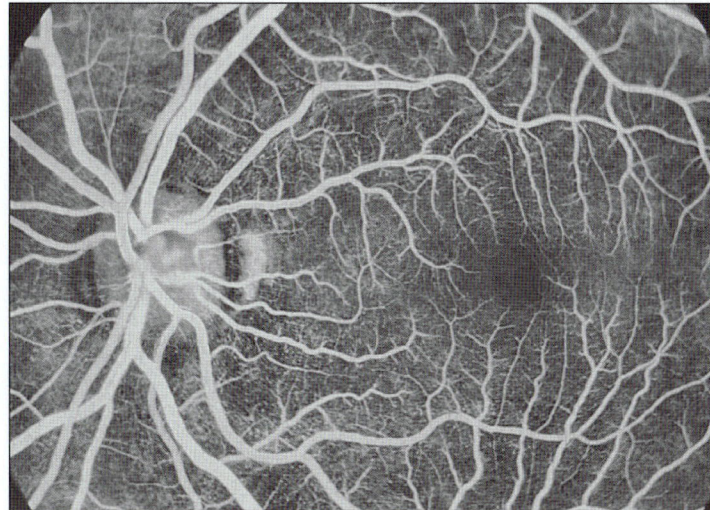

FIG. 106-1 ■ **Peak phase angiogram.** Approximately 25 seconds after injection, the maximal fluorescence of the retinal circulation is evident. Both the arterial and venous circulations fluoresce. In particular, the perifoveal capillary network is shown with intricate detail.

mately 300–500μm in diameter. A dark background to this capillary-free zone in the macula is created through blockage of choroidal fluorescence by both xanthophyll pigment and a high density of RPE cells in the central macula. This phase of the angiogram has been termed the *peak phase* as maximal fluorescence of the capillaries and enhanced resolution of capillary detail occur. The management of microvascular diseases of the retinal capillaries, such as diabetic macular edema, requires excellent peak-phase imaging.

The first pass of fluorescein through the retinal and choroidal vasculature is complete after 30 seconds. The recirculation phases, characterized by intermittent mild fluorescence, follow. After approximately 10 minutes, both the retinal and choroidal circulations generally are devoid of fluorescein. Many normal anatomical structures continue to fluoresce during the late angiogram, such as the disc margin and optic nerve head. The staining of Bruch's membrane, choroid, and sclera is more visible in patients who have lightly pigmented RPE.

Abnormal Fluorescein Angiography

A basic understanding of the anatomy of both the retinal and choroidal circulations and the complex anatomical relationships between the layers of the retina, RPE, and choroid is crucial in the interpretation of fluorescein angiography. The terms *hypofluorescence* and *hyperfluorescence* are used routinely in the interpretation of fluorescein angiograms.[13–19] Hypofluorescence is a reduction or absence of normal fluorescence (Box 106-2), whereas hyperfluorescence is increased or abnormal fluorescence (Box 106-3).

Hypofluorescence

Hypofluorescence can be categorized into blockage (masking of fluorescence) or vascular filling defects. Blocked fluorescence can provide clues as to the level of the blocking material, such as vit-

real, retinal, or subretinal. Only structures or material anterior to the area of fluorescence can block fluorescence.

Blocked retinal fluorescence may be caused by any element that diminishes the visualization of the retina and its circulation. Media opacities secondary to corneal pathology or cataract can block or reduce retinal fluorescence. In addition, hemorrhage on the surface of the retina (preretinal) or debris in the vitreous cavity, such as inflammatory cells or cells from hemorrhage, can mask fluorescence.

Blockage of retinal fluorescence also may localize the pathology to the inner retina. The retinal circulation is unique in that the large retinal vessels and precapillary, first-order arterioles lie in the nerve fiber layer, while the capillaries and postcapillary venules are located in the inner nuclear layer. Flame-shaped hemorrhages are superficial and block all retinal vascular fluorescence, while deeper dot or blot hemorrhages (or intraretinal lipid) block capillary fluorescence but do not block larger superficial vessels.

Blockage of choroidal fluorescence can occur with any of the previously described pathological entities located anterior to the choroid. In addition, subretinal material in pathological states, such as hemorrhage, melanin, lipofuscin, lipid, fibrin, and inflammatory material, can block choroidal fluorescence (Fig. 106-2). As noted previously, the normal fluorescein angiogram displays blockage of choroidal fluorescence as evidenced by early, patchy choroidal filling and a consistently darker macular region. Xanthophyll and a high density of RPE (melanin) are responsible for blockage of fluorescence in the macula. Melanin can accumulate in RPE cells in many disease processes. It is not uncommon for blockage of choroidal fluorescence to surround a scar secondary to accumulation of melanin, as a result of a rim of RPE hypertrophy surrounding the scar. Choroidal nevi and choroidal melanomas represent classic examples of the blockage of choroidal fluorescence. Also, lipofuscin deposits block choroidal fluorescence and are seen in fundus flavimaculatus (Stargardt's disease) and Best's disease. The most common causes of blocked choroidal fluorescence are subretinal hemorrhage and turbid serosanguineous fluid be-

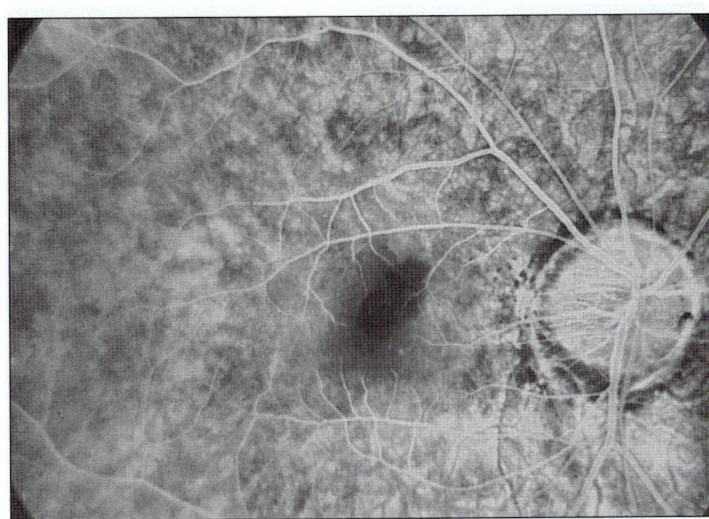

FIG. 106-2 ▪ **Blockage of choroidal fluorescence.** Hypofluorescence is seen in the fovea of this patient who has age-related macular degeneration and a subretinal hemorrhage, which blocks the choroidal circulation. Note that the retinal vessels that overlie the hemorrhage are not blocked, because the pathology is subretinal.

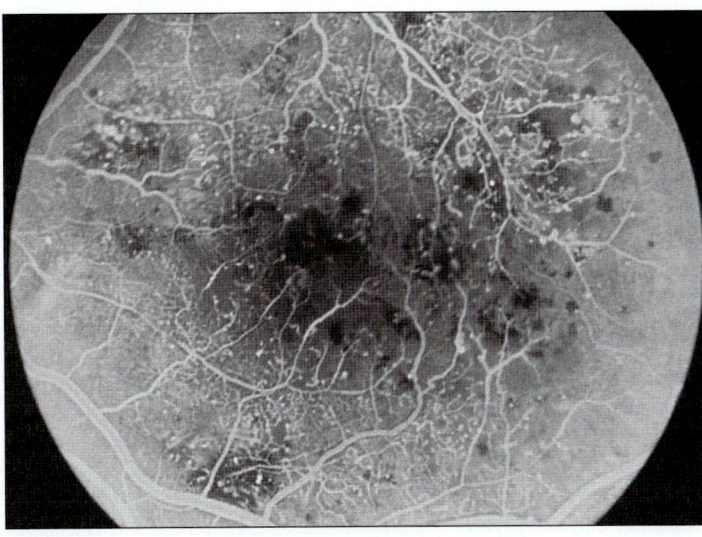

FIG. 106-3 ▪ **Vascular filling defect.** Hypofluorescence in the region of the perifoveal capillary network secondary to nonperfusion of the capillary circulation in diabetic retinopathy. Temporal to the macula, hypofluorescence secondary to blockage by intraretinal hemorrhage also is evident.

neath a RPE detachment, as seen in choroidal neovascularization (CNV) secondary to age-related macular degeneration.

Vascular filling defects produce hypofluorescence because of the reduced or absent perfusion of tissues. Retinal vascular filling defects can involve large-, medium-, or small-caliber vessels. Central or branch retinal artery occlusions show hypofluorescence in the distribution of the arterial tree involved in the occlusion. The zones of capillary nonperfusion manifest as vascular filling defects and appear hypofluorescent on fluorescein angiography. This form of vascular filling defect is seen in common disease processes such as diabetic retinopathy and central retinal vein occlusions (Fig. 106-3).

Choroidal vascular filling defects are more difficult to visualize, because the native RPE prevents adequate visualization of the choroidal circulation. The anatomy of the choroidal vasculature is more complex than that of the retina. Imaging of the choriocapillaris and other structures within the choroid is limited by the difficult visualization of the choroidal circulation as well as by the hyperpermeability of choroidal vessels to fluorescein dye. In general, occlusive diseases that involve isolated, larger choroidal vessels manifest as sectorial, wedge-shaped areas of hypofluorescence. However, it is more common for choroidal hypoperfusion to manifest with diffuse involvement of the choriocapillaris. Systemic diseases, including malignant hypertension, toxemia of pregnancy, and lupus choroidopathy, produce zones of hypofluorescence secondary to focal choroidal nonperfusion. During the late phases of the angiogram, normally perfused choriocapillaris may leak into the area of hypofluorescence. Atrophy or degeneration of the choriocapillaris also is noted in choroideremia.

Also, vascular filling defects of the optic nerve head may be noted by fluorescein angiography. Ischemic optic neuropathy manifests as sectorial or complete optic disc hypofluorescence, while other atrophic or hereditary anomalies of the optic nerve head have diffuse hypofluorescence. Congenital anomalies, including optic nerve head colobomas, optic nerve hypoplasia, and optic pits, also may be associated with hypofluorescence.

Hyperfluorescence

Hyperfluorescence is defined as an abnormal presence of fluorescence or an increase in normal fluorescence in the fluorescein angiogram. Normally, a blue exciter filter allows light of blue wavelength to pass into the eye, while a green barrier filter allows fluorescent yellow–green light to return to the fluorescein camera. Filter mismatch is the inadvertent overlap of the wave-

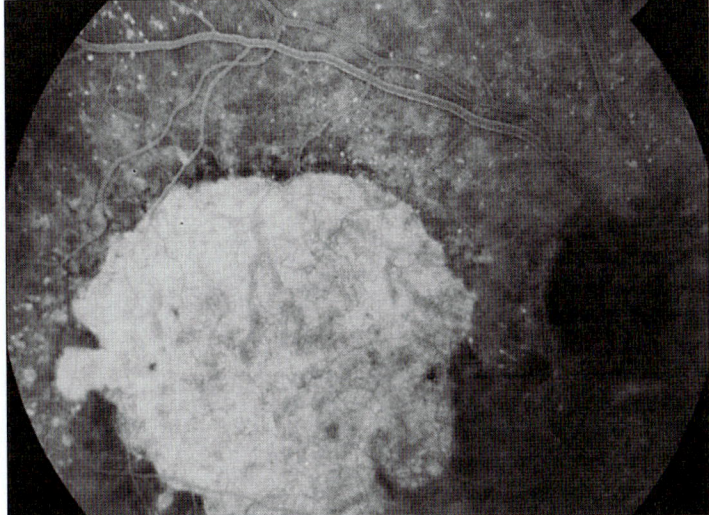

FIG. 106-4 ▪ **Transmitted fluorescence.** Well-demarcated area of retinal pigment epithelium atrophy that produces hyperfluorescence of the choroidal circulation (window defect). The hyperfluorescent spots, mostly outside of the retinal vascular arcades, are drusen.

lengths of light allowed to pass through the camera. It causes white or brighter structures in the fundus to have false fluorescence or pseudofluorescence. The frequent inspection and exchange of barrier and excitation filters avoids the complication of pseudofluorescence.

Autofluorescence is a natural phenomenon seen when lesions physiologically behave like fluorescein dye. By reflecting blue light and emitting yellow–green light, optic nerve head calcified drusen, astrocytic hamartomas, and large deposits of lipofuscin may exhibit autofluorescence.

Frequently hyperfluorescence is seen with transmission window defects and with abnormal blood vessels. A window defect refers to the choroidal fluorescence produced by a relative decrease or absence of pigment in the RPE or an absence of RPE. Transmitted fluorescence is seen with common pathological processes such as chorioretinal atrophic scars, full-thickness macular holes, the atrophic form of macular degeneration, and drusen (Fig. 106-4). Hyperfluorescence attributed to the presence of abnormal blood vessels is seen in the retina, choroid, and optic disc. Retinal vascular anomalies, such as capillary angiomas, arterial venous malformations, and Coats' disease, commonly cause hyperfluorescence in the distribution of the vascu-

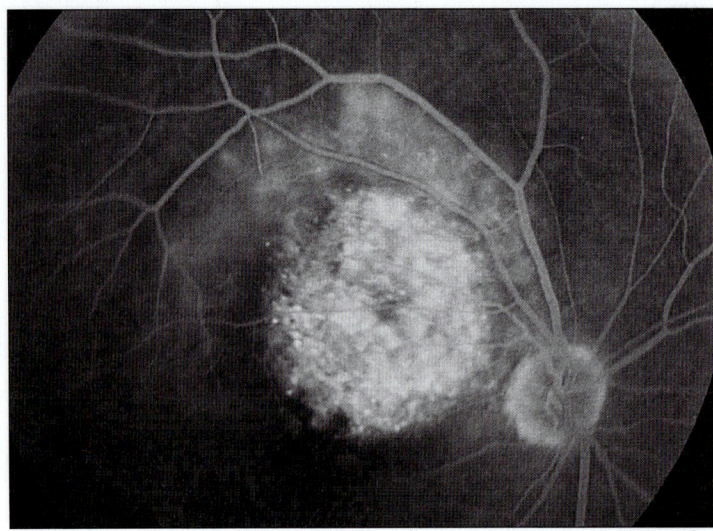

FIG. 106-5 ▌ **Choroidal hemangioma.** Late-phase angiogram that shows the intense hyperfluorescence of the vascular tumor, as well as moderate leakage into the larger neurosensory retinal detachment.

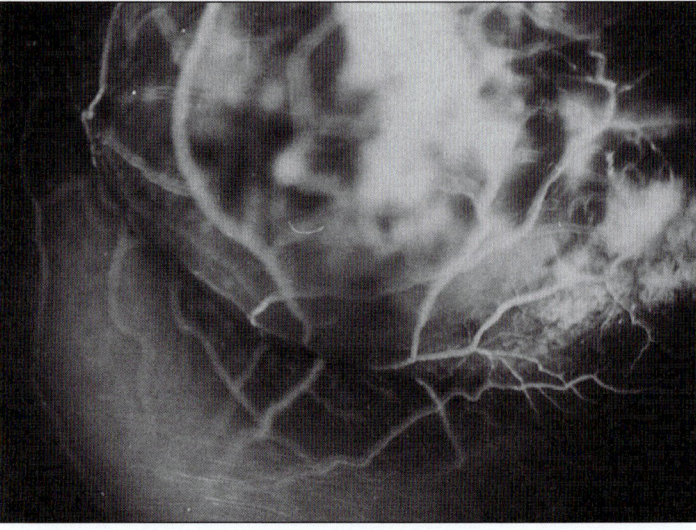

FIG. 106-6 ▌ **Choroidal melanoma.** Late-phase angiogram that illustrates the simultaneous presence of the retinal circulation (overlying the tumor) and the more permeable choroidal vasculature (intrinsic to the tumor). This is referred to as the *double circulation pattern* of choroidal melanoma.

lar pathology. Hyperfluorescence is seen in common abnormalities of native blood vessels; these include telangiectasias, aneurysms, anastomoses, dilation, and tortuosity, which are seen in common retinal vascular diseases such as venous occlusive disease and diabetes. Classically, neovascularization within the retina and choroid manifests with late leakage of fluorescein dye or hyperfluorescence; however, neovascularization also may be associated with early hyperfluorescence in the distribution of new pathological blood vessels. Finally, choroidal tumors, such as melanomas or choroidal hemangiomas, may cause hyperfluorescence on fluorescein angiography (Figs. 106-5 and 106-6). The degree of vascularity and flow through the lesion determine the degree of hyperfluorescence.

Leakage of fluorescein dye is defined as hyperfluorescence of fluorescein in the extravascular space. Typically the area of fluorescence increases in both size and intensity as the study progresses. As discussed earlier, retinal neovascularization manifests with late leakage of fluorescein dye into the vitreous cavity and often is located adjacent to an area of capillary nonperfusion (Fig. 106-7). Often, fluorescein angiography is used to detect neovascularization that is subclinical or cannot be identified by ophthalmoscopy. Other retinal vascular abnormalities, such as vasculitis or inflammatory lesions, can cause leakage of fluorescein into the retina or vitreous because of the increased permeability of blood vessels. The classic appearance of intraretinal leakage is seen with macular edema. The two most common causes of macular edema are diabetes, which is associated with focal parafoveal microaneurysms; and postoperative cystoid macular edema, which is associated with late leakage (in a petaloid pattern) of fluorescein dye into the cystoid spaces of the outer plexiform layer (see Fig. 106-7). Optic nerve pathology, such as seen in papilledema and ischemic optic neuropathy, produces profound leakage of the optic nerve head during the late phase of the angiogram as a result of capillary leakage. Importantly, the normal optic disc also has some minimal leakage along its margins secondary to leakage from adjacent choroidal capillaries. Often, both the distribution of leakage on the optic nerve head and the intensity of hyperfluorescence help in the diagnosis.

Hyperfluorescence secondary to subretinal and choroidal pathology is more difficult to correlate histopathologically; however, the timing, pattern, and location of hyperfluorescence are reproducible in many diseases. Pooling refers to the accumulation of fluorescein dye into an anatomical space, while staining indicates the deposition of fluorescein into tissues. Pooling is seen in both neural retina and RPE detachments. Its

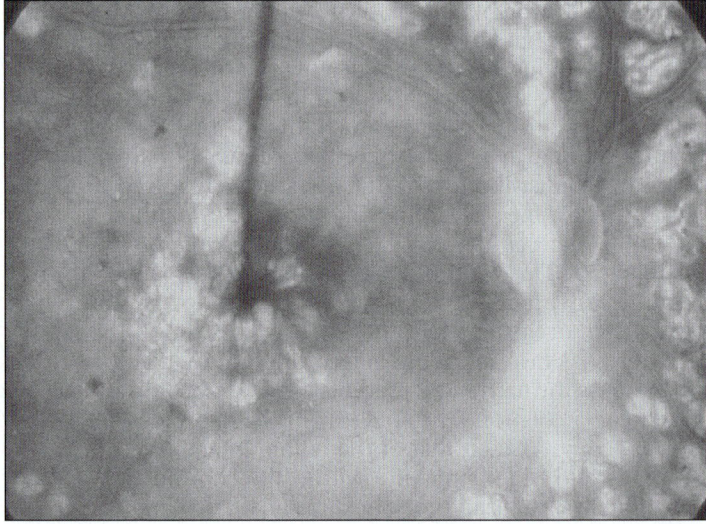

FIG. 106-7 ▌ **Leakage.** Fluorescein dye leaks from an area of neovascularization of the disc along the inferotemporal arcade. Evidence also exists of macular edema secondary to incompetence of the microvascular circulation in this diabetic eye.

rapidity and pattern are important in their differentiation. For example, in central serous chorioretinopathy, neural retinal detachments fluoresce slowly, if at all, because fluorescein must pass through small leaks in the RPE (Fig. 106-8). On the other hand, RPE detachments in macular degeneration are characterized by the rapid pooling of fluorescein under the dome of the detachment, because no barrier exists to the permeability of the choriocapillaris. Note that imaging of the underlying choroid is hampered by this phenomenon.

Staining in fluorescein angiography refers to the deposition of fluorescein dye within the involved tissue and occurs in both normal and pathological states. Normal structures, such as the optic disc and sclera, may stain. Scleral staining is seen more easily in high myopes and patients who have lightly pigmented fundi, because enhancement of transmission occurs through atrophic or absent RPE. Diseases that result in widespread chorioretinal atrophy, such as gyrate atrophy and serpiginous choroidopathy, demonstrate significant scleral staining. The degree of staining is dependent on the competence of the choriocapillaris, because severe atrophy limits the amount of fluorescein that leaks from the choroidal vessels. Finally, staining also is seen in disciform scars and damaged RPE tissue.

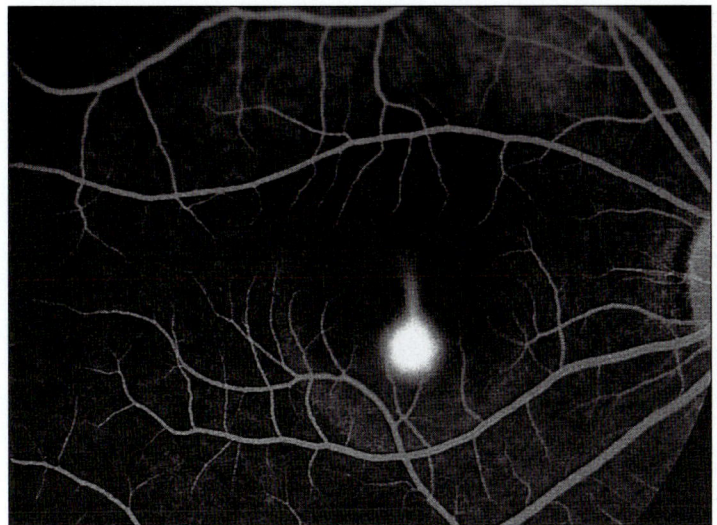

FIG. 106-8 ■ **Central serous chorioretinopathy.** Localized serous detachment of the retinal pigment epithelium with focal leak of fluorescein superiorly into the subretinal space. A later frame of the angiogram would show a classic smokestack pattern.

Fluorescein angiography is indispensable in the management of many retinal and choroidal disorders. The major limitation of fluorescein angiography is the inability to visualize the choroidal circulation accurately. New diagnostic techniques, such as indocyanine green (ICG) angiography, have become complementary to the evaluation of choroidal diseases.

INDOCYANINE GREEN ANGIOGRAPHY

INTRODUCTION

ICG angiography is an infrared-based, dye-imaging technique that is most useful for the evaluation of patients who have exudative changes from CNV. Specifically, patients who have age-related macular degeneration and who are found to have occult (obscured by hemorrhage, exudate, or pigment) or poorly defined CNV via fluorescein angiography may be evaluated using ICG angiography to delineate any CNV that may be treatable with laser photocoagulation. Because 85% of patients who have CNV caused by age-related macular degeneration fall into these categories, ICG angiography enables additional patients to be treated. In addition, ICG angiography is used to detect occult recurrences of CNV following laser photocoagulation.

With respect to other choroidal disorders, which include tumors and inflammatory disorders, ICG angiography is of some diagnostic value. Rarely, ICG is used in individuals who are allergic to fluorescein dye and need imaging because of a retinal vascular disorder.

HISTORICAL REVIEW

Flower and Hochheimer[20] first studied ICG angiography in depth, reported in 1972. The utility of these early experiments was limited by the photographic media used to record the angiographic images. Because ICG has a fluorescent efficiency 25 times less than that of sodium fluorescein, the infrared film used for ICG angiography in these initial studies was insufficient to yield angiograms of acceptable quality. Orth et al.[21] in 1976 used a movie camera to record the angiographic images, but even at speeds of 20 frames per second the filming technique was insufficient to study the choroidal circulation effectively. In addition, the apparatus did not enable the investigators to view the fundus while the angiography was performed.

During the 1980s, major technological advances paved the way for clinically useful ICG angiography. First, the quality of ex-

citatory and emission barriers was improved greatly. These filters, which selectively limit the passage of light to the appropriate infrared wavelengths, decreased the overlap transmission to 0.5%. The second major technological advance was the introduction of videoangiography by Destro and Puliafito.[22] Videoangiography employs an infrared-sensitive videocamera and videocassette recorder to record the fluorescent images obtained during angiographic procedures. The videocamera proved to be much more sensitive than infrared film for the capture of ICG's fluorescence and enabled satisfactory imaging of the choroidal circulation. The quality of angiograms stored on videocassette was limited to 320 lines of resolution. Modern ICG imaging systems use digital videoangiography, in which fluorescent images of ICG dye are recorded from the fundus via an infrared-sensitive analog videocamera attached to a computer, improving image resolution substantially.

PURPOSE OF THE TEST

Abnormalities of the choroidal circulation are detected using ICG angiography, particularly CNV. The early phase of ICG is characterized as the first appearance of ICG dye in the choroidal circulation, which occurs within 1 minute after injection of ICG. Large choroidal arteries and veins are highlighted, as well as the retinal vasculature. Between 5 and 15 minutes after injection the middle phase is entered, during which the choroidal veins become less distinct and a diffuse, homogeneous choroidal fluorescence is observed. The hyperfluorescence of the retinal blood vessels diminishes. During this phase, hyperfluorescent lesions begin to appear in contrast against the fading background fluorescence. During the late phase, which occurs approximately 15 minutes after injection of ICG, no details of the retinal or choroidal vasculature are observable. The optic disc is dark and the large choroidal vessels become hypofluorescent. During this phase, choroidal abnormalities stand out in contrast to the markedly diminished background fluorescence. It is during the late phase that CNV is detected as a hyperfluorescent lesion.

Terms specifically related to ICG imaging of CNV include *focal CNV* (sometimes referred to as a *hot spot*), which often represents an area of occult CNV. Hot spots, by definition, are less than one disc diameter in size and are well delineated (Fig. 106-9). Typically these lesions are not obscured by hemorrhage or exudate. *Placoid hyperfluorescence* is another term that relates to findings on ICG angiography and describes an area of occult CNV that is larger than one disc area in size (Fig. 106-10) that may or may not be well defined during the early phase of the ICG angiogram. During the late phase of the ICG angiogram, the staining of CNV may be well defined and is not obscured by hemorrhage or exudate. If the borders are not distinct because of late leakage of ICG or the borders are obscured by hemorrhage or exudate, the lesion is not considered to be well defined by ICG angiography. For CNV that is well defined or classic in appearance on fluorescein angiography, the appearance on ICG angiography is variable.[23]

UTILITY OF THE TEST

The greatest utility for ICG angiography is in the identification and delineation of poorly defined or occult CNV.[24]

For the imaging of choroidal circulation, ICG angiography has several advantages over fluorescein angiography. After intravenous injection, ICG is bound readily and rapidly to serum proteins. In fact, 98% of ICG is transported in the blood bound to serum proteins, which compares with only 60–80% of fluorescein that is protein bound. The advantage of being more protein bound is that the amount of leakage through the fenestrations of the choriocapillaris is reduced, which results in enhanced definition of larger choroidal vascular channels, the normal choroidal circulation, and CNV. Fluorescein angiography normally does not demonstrate the choroidal circulation

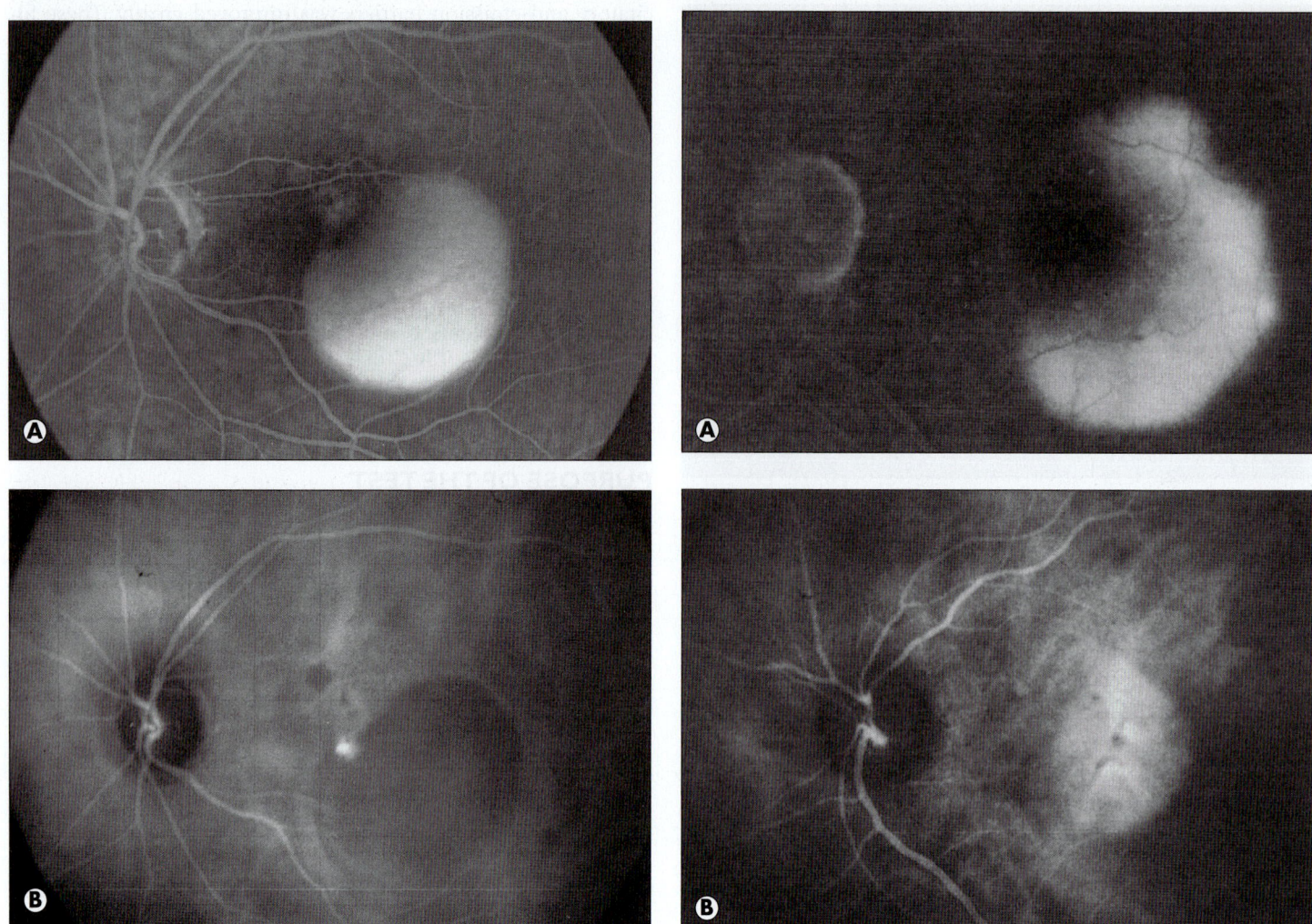

FIG. 106-9 ▌ **Serous retinal pigment epithelial detachment associated with a hot spot. A,** Late-phase fluorescein angiogram illustrates filling of a serous pigment epithelial detachment. No well-defined or classic choroidal neovascularization is observed. **B,** Corresponding midphase ICG angiogram showing a hot spot at the margin of the pigment epithelial detachment.

FIG. 106-10 ▌ **Retinal pigment epithelial detachment and placoid area of hyperfluorescence. A,** Late-phase fluorescein angiogram illustrates a large area of hyperfluorescence consistent with a retinal pigment epithelial detachment. **B,** Corresponding midphase indocyanine green angiogram shows a placoid area of hyperfluorescence.

well, because the unbound fluorescein molecule is very small and rapidly leaks from the choriocapillaris, obscuring the underlying choroidal vessels. Poorly defined or occult CNV appears to be stained by ICG during the late phase of the ICG angiogram. Late leakage from abnormal blood vessels probably causes fibrous tissue to be stained with ICG.

Another advantage of ICG angiography is its fluorescence in the near-infrared spectrum. The RPE and choroid absorbs approximately two thirds of light at 500nm but only one third of light at 800nm. Therefore, light at wavelengths in the near infrared are able to penetrate the pigmented layers of the fundus much better than light in the visible spectrum used by fluorescein angiography. Similarly, near-infrared light is able to penetrate lipid deposits, serous exudate, and hemorrhage better than visible light.[25,26]

Also, ICG angiography is useful for the detection of occult forms of persistent or recurrent CNV.[27,28] Fluorescein angiography is considered the ancillary test of choice for the identification of recurrent CNV. In some cases, however, recurrent CNV may be suspected on clinical examination, yet clear evidence of new vessels may not be ascertained using fluorescein angiography. In such situations, ICG angiography has proved to be a useful adjunct, because it may delineate hot spots consistent with recurrent, poorly defined CNV. When recurrent CNV is suspected but not observed on fluorescein angiography, well-defined (and potentially treatable) recurrent CNV can be detected in an additional 15% of cases using ICG angiography.

Well-defined or classic CNV has a variable appearance on ICG angiography. When the late leakage is associated with a well-defined CNV on fluorescein angiography (type II occult CNV), ICG angiography may delineate more completely the extent of the lesion. Therefore, in eyes suspected to harbor classic and type II occult CNV, ICG angiography may delineate more completely both well-defined and ill-defined lesions and serve as a guide for treatment.[29]

Studies of ICG angiography in patients who are affected acutely with central serous chorioretinopathy reveal diffuse hyperfluorescence during the early stage of the angiogram, presumably caused by hyperpermeability of the choroid (Fig. 106-11). RPE detachments are observed more readily on ICG angiography and are characterized as a ring of hyperfluorescence that surrounds a hypofluorescent spot. Areas of ICG hyperfluorescence can be seen in eyes that have inactive disease or in the inactive or "normal" fellow eye, and they may indicate higher risk of involvement of the fellow eye not seen with fluorescein.[30]

For the assessment of choroidal tumors and inflammatory conditions, ICG angiography appears to be of limited value. Idiopathic polypoidal choroidal vasculopathy has a characteristic appearance on ICG angiography (Fig. 106-12), which is useful for the differentiation of this condition from occult CNV.[31]

PROCEDURE

The technical aspects of the capture of images described herein relate to the use of intravenous doses of 25mg of ICG. Higher dosages typically result in larger degrees of hyperfluorescence and thereby change excitation; gain also may vary. The ICG dye

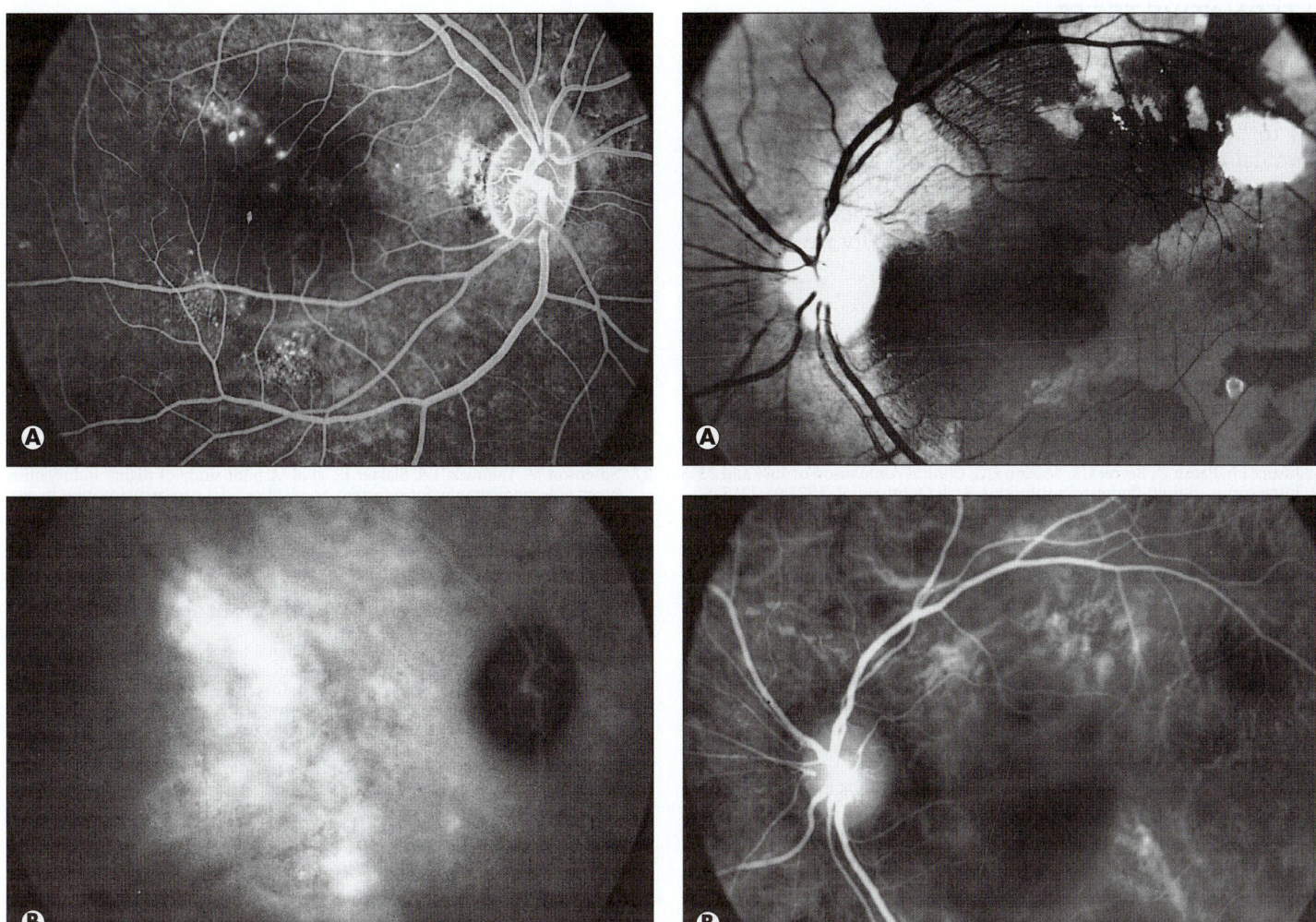

FIG. 106-11 ■ **Idiopathic central serous choroidopathy.** The corresponding late-phase indocyanine green angiogram demonstrates a large area of diffuse hyperfluorescence.

FIG. 106-12 ■ **Idiopathic polypoidal vasculopathy. A,** Red-free image illustrates multiple hemorrhagic pigment epithelial detachments. **B,** Indocyanine green angiography reveals saccular dilations of choroidal vessels consistent with idiopathic polypoidal vasculopathy.

is dissolved in the manufacturer's diluent and administered intravenously as a bolus, after which a normal saline flush is given. If both fluorescein and ICG angiography are performed sequentially, an intravenous catheter may be placed to save the patient from multiple needle sticks.

Excitation illumination should be at a maximum, with a video gain of +6db. Approximately 10 images are acquired over the initial 30 seconds, starting immediately after injection. The video gain and excitation illumination levels should not be changed during the transit phase unless image bloom occurs (an increased fluorescence that obscures images). If this happens, the excitation level is reduced. The best images are retained and, ideally, the transit of ICG through the choroidal vasculature is captured again every 15 seconds. Late images at 5, 10, 15, and 20 minutes after injection also are obtained. Alteration of the excitation level can be increased during the late phase of the ICG angiogram if signal intensity is reduced. During the very late stages, both excitation and video gain can be increased; however, a concomitant reduction in detail results.

COMPLICATIONS

ICG has proved to be a safe and well-tolerated dye for diagnostic imaging. Minor adverse reactions are uncommon following ICG injection but include discomfort, nausea, vomiting, and extravasation of dye. True, life-threatening anaphylactic reactions are very rare but occur in equal incidence following ICG and fluorescein injection (1:1900). Current contraindications to ICG

angiography include prior anaphylactic reaction to ICG dye or contrast agents that contain iodide, liver disease, uremia, and pregnancy. Approximately 5% of current commercial ICG dyes contain iodide and, therefore, ICG is contraindicated in patients who have iodide allergies.

INTERPRETATION OF RESULTS

Software available with the ICG system enables the user to manipulate the angiographic images. For example, the "trace" function allows areas to be copied from the ICG angiogram and placed at the precise location on a red-free photograph. This is helpful when ICG angiography is used as a guide for laser photocoagulation.

For the evaluation of occult or obscured forms of CNV, the images obtained are examined for abnormal areas of hyperfluorescence. Comparison of the ICG angiogram is made against the fluorescein angiogram and slit-lamp biomicroscopy images of the fundus in an attempt to correlate the findings. Although no randomized studies have been carried out to prove the efficacy of ICG-guided laser treatment, practitioners in general treat focal hot spots that are not subfoveal in location. Hot spots that are associated with serous RPE detachments have a less favorable prognosis and may not be treated.[32–35] Therefore, an additional 10–20% of patients who have exudative, age-related macular degeneration may be eligible for laser treatment if ICG angiography is used, compared with those studied with fluorescein angiography alone.

ALTERNATIVE TESTS

ICG angiography also may be performed using the scanning laser ophthalmoscope or by directly obtaining videoangiograms without digitization. These techniques allow for continuous images to be produced that, therefore, allows flow through the choroidal circulation to be imaged. Results similar to those of digital videoangiography can be obtained using these systems. High-speed ICG angiography may be useful in identifying feeder vessels to the choroidal neovascular complex for treatment with conventional laser.

REFERENCES

1. MacLean AL, Maumenee AE. Hemangioma of the choroid. Am J Ophthalmol. 1960;50:3–11.
2. Flocks M, Miller J, Chao P. Retinal circulation time with the aid of fundus cinematography. Am J Ophthalmol. 1959;48:3–6.
3. Novotny HR, Alvis DL. A method of photographing fluorescence in circulating blood in the human retina. Circulation. 1961;24:82–6.
4. Justice J Jr, Paton D, Beyrer CR, Seddon GG. Clinical comparison of 10% and 25% intravenous sodium fluorescein solutions. Arch Ophthalmol. 1977;95:2015–6.
5. Yannuzzi LA, Rohrer MA, Tindel LJ, et al. Fluorescein angiography complication survey. Ophthalmology. 1986;93:611–7.
6. Halperin LS, Olk J, Soubrane G, Coscas G. Safety of fluorescein angiography during pregnancy. Am J Ophthalmol. 1990;109:563–6.
7. Greenberg F, Lewis RA. Safety of fluorescein angiography during pregnancy [Letter]. Am J Ophthalmol. 1990;110:323–5.
8. Amalric P, Biau C, Fenies MT. Incidents et accidents au cours de l'angiographie fluoresceinique. Bull Soc Ophtalmol Fr. 1968;68:968–72.
9. Stein MR, Parker CW. Reactions following intravenous fluorescein. Am J Ophthalmol. 1971;72:861–8.
10. Levacy R, Justice J Jr. Adverse reactions to intravenous fluorescein. Int Ophthalmol Clin. 1976;16:53–61.
11. Butner RW, McPherson AR. Adverse reactions in intravenous fluorescein angiography. Ann Ophthalmol. 1983;15:1084–6.
12. Marcus DF, Bovino JA, Williams D. Adverse reactions during intravenous fluorescein angiography. Arch Ophthalmol. 1984;102:825–33.
13. Delori F, Ben-Sira I, Trempe C. Fluorescein angiography with an optimized filter combination. Am J Ophthalmol. 1976;82:559–66.
14. Gass JDM. Stereoscopic atlas of macular diseases: diagnosis and treatment, ed 4. St Louis: Mosby–Year Book; 1997.
15. Gitter KA, Schatz H, Yannuzzi LA, McDonald HR, eds. Laser photocoagulation of retinal disease. San Francisco: Pacific Medical Press; 1988.
16. Justice J Jr, ed. Ophthalmic photography. Boston: Little, Brown; 1982.
17. Rabb MF, Burton TC, Schatz H, Yannuzzi LA. Fluorescein angiography of the fundus: a schematic approach to interpretation. Surv Ophthalmol. 1978;22:387–403.
18. Schatz H. Flow sheet for the interpretation of the fluorescein angiograms. Arch Ophthalmol. 1976;94:687–94.
19. Schatz H, Burton TC, Yannuzzi LA, Rabb MF. Interpretation of fundus fluorescein angiography. St Louis: Mosby–Year Book; 1978.
20. Flower RW, Hochheimer BF. Clinical infrared absorption angiography of the choroid [Letter]. Am J Ophthalmol. 1972;73:458–9.
21. Orth DH, Patz A, Flower RW. Potential clinical applications of indocyanine green choroidal angiography—preliminary report. Eye Ear Nose Throat Mon. 1976;55:15–28.
22. Destro MC, Puliafito CA. Indocyanine green videoangiography of choroidal neovascularization. Ophthalmology. 1989;96:846–53.
23. Reichel E. Choroidal neovascularization associated with age-related macular degeneration. In: Reichel E, Puliafito CA, eds. Atlas of indocyanine green angiography. New York: Igaku-Shoin; 1996:12–43.
24. Guyer DR, Yannuzzi LA, Slakter JS, et al. Digital indocyanine green videoangiography of occult choroidal neovascularization. Ophthalmology. 1994;101:1727–35.
25. Cohen SM, Shen JH, Smiddy WE. Laser energy and dye fluorescence transmission through blood in vitro. Am J Ophthalmol. 1995;119:452–7.
26. Reichel E, Duker JS, Puliafito CA. Indocyanine green angiography and choroidal neovascularization obscured by hemorrhage. Ophthalmology. 1995;102:1871–6.
27. Sorenson JA, Yannuzzi LA, Slakter JS, et al. A pilot study of digital indocyanine green videoangiography for recurrent occult choroidal neovascularization in age-related macular degeneration. Arch Ophthalmol. 1994;112:473–84.
28. Reichel E, Pollock D, Duker JS, et al. Indocyanine green angiography in the detection of marginal persistence and recurrence of choroidal neovascularization. Ophthalmic Surg. 1995;26:513–8.
29. Avvad FK, Duker JS, Reichel E, et al. The digital indocyanine green videoangiography characteristics of well-defined choroidal neovascularization. Ophthalmology. 1995;102:401–5.
30. Guyer DR, Yannuzzi LA, Slakter JS, et al. Digital indocyanine green videoangiography of central serous chorioretinopathy. Arch Ophthalmol. 1994;112:1057–62.
31. Spaide RF, Yannuzzi LA, Slakter JS, et al. Indocyanine green videoangiography of idiopathic polypoidal choroidal vasculopathy. Retina. 1995;15:100–10.
32. Slakter JS, Yannuzzi LA, Sorenson JA, et al. A pilot study of indocyanine green videoangiography-guided laser photocoagulation of occult choroidal neovascularization in age-related macular degeneration. Arch Ophthalmol. 1994;112:465–72.
33. Regillo CD, Benson WE, Maguire JI, et al. Indocyanine green angiography and occult choroidal neovascularization. Ophthalmology. 1994;101:280–8.
34. Lim JI, Sternberg PS, Capone A Jr, et al. Selective use of indocyanine green angiography for occult choroidal neovascularization. Am J Ophthalmol. 1995;120:75–82.
35. Baumal C, Reichel E, Duker JS, et al. Indocyanine green hyperfluorescence associated with serous retinal pigment epithelial detachment in age-related macular degeneration. Ophthalmology. 1997;104:761–9.

107 Electrophysiology

ELIAS REICHEL

DEFINITIONS

- The electroretinogram records the electrical response evoked from the entire retina by a brief flash of light and consists of an "A" wave, a photoreceptor response, and a "B" wave that emanates from the Müller and bipolar cells.
- The electro-oculogram records the standing electrical potential generated by the retinal pigment epithelium.
- The focal electroretinogram records the central retinal function and represents an isolated foveal cone response.

INTRODUCTION

Electrophysiology encompasses several tests that measure the function of the various components of the retina. In this section, the focus is on full-field electroretinography (ERG), because this is the most useful of these techniques in the assessment of retinal function to help establish retinal diagnoses.[1] Full-field ERG is useful, particularly, in the determination of the abnormal nature of what appears to be a retina of "normal" appearance. It is useful, also, to determine the existence of retinal degeneration that may arise from hereditary, toxic, metabolic, retinal vascular, or inflammatory causes. Only in conjunction with careful history, ophthalmic examination, and laboratory testing can exact diagnoses be made. Therefore, ERG is useful as an adjunct in establishing loss of function; diagnoses should be made only in conjunction with a complete medical and ophthalmic evaluation. Electro-oculography (EOG) and focal ERG are discussed briefly.

HISTORICAL REVIEW

As early as 1865, Holmgren showed that an alteration in electrical potential occurred when light fell on the retina. In 1877, Dewar recorded a light-evoked electrical response, ERG, from humans for the first time. In 1941, Riggs introduced a contact lens electrode for human use. Modern adaptations to ERG testing included Ganzfeld or full-field diffuse illumination to elicit a response from the entire retina. More recently, computer averaging and narrow bandpass filters have enabled the detection of ERG responses below 1mV.

It was Holmgren, again in 1865, who identified a constant standing or resting potential between the cornea and the back of the eye that was altered by changes in retinal illumination. Marg,[2] in 1951, coined the term *electro-oculogram* for the measurement of this potential.

PURPOSE OF THE TEST

Full-field ERG measures a mass response generated by cells from the entire retina. Under dark-adapted conditions, a single flash

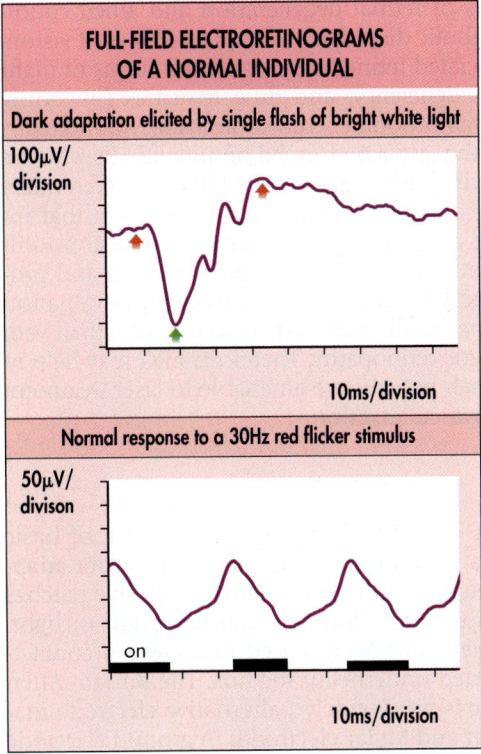

FULL-FIELD ELECTRORETINOGRAMS OF A NORMAL INDIVIDUAL

Dark adaptation elicited by single flash of bright white light

100µV/ division

10ms/division

Normal response to a 30Hz red flicker stimulus

50µV/ divison

on

10ms/division

FIG. 107-1 ■ Full-field electroretinograms, normal individual. Dark adaptation is elicited by a single flash of bright white light after 30 minutes. This stimulus elicits both cone-mediated and rod-mediated responses. The *green arrow* denotes the "A" wave and the *red arrows* the "B" wave. The small wavelets on the ascending limb of the "B" wave are oscillatory potentials. Normal response to a 30Hz red flicker stimulus after testing with the bright white flash. This represents a pure cone response.

of light results in a response that is both rod and cone mediated. Of this response, 80% is attributable to rods and the remainder results from cones. The photoreceptors generate the initial cornea-negative component, or "A" wave, in the ERG, whereas Müller cells and bipolar cells are responsible for the later, cornea-positive, "B" wave (Fig. 107-1). The full-field ERG is useful for establishing generalized loss of rod or cone function, or both. Patients who have focal macular disorders do not have abnormalities of full-field ERG amplitude, nor do patients who have optic nerve or cortical conditions.

Mild reductions in cone amplitudes can be observed when macular scarring covers four or more disc areas. In contrast, individuals who have early retinitis pigmentosa typically display delayed cone "B" wave implicit times; amplitudes are subnormal, although they may not be reduced markedly during the early stages of the disease.

The full-field ERG can be affected by a variety of pathological states unrelated to the function of the retina.[1,3,4] It is important to be aware of these conditions in which the normalcy or abnormalcy of the test is established. Media opacities, which include cataract, vitreous hemorrhage, and vitreous debris, may cause a reduction in ERG amplitude and lengthen the implicit time. Age and myopia also affect the ERG amplitude, but implicit time appears to be unaffected. Pupil size also can affect the amplitude of the ERG, which may account for the decline in ERG amplitude associated with age.

UTILITY OF THE TEST

ERG establishes the loss of retinal function. Specific patient complaints that may warrant the use of ERG include loss of peripheral vision and night blindness. Determination of retinal function when the media is obscured is another important use of full-field ERG. Not only is ERG useful for establishing pathological conditions, it also provides solace to the patient and reassurance to the physician when normalcy of retinal function is established. For situations in which the retina is deemed to be normal, the optic nerve and central nervous system must be evaluated.

Many conditions display loss of retinal function and, therefore, a careful history and ophthalmoscopic examination are necessary to establish a diagnosis. Further, laboratory tests often are necessary to confirm metabolic conditions or rule out the possibility of cancer-associated retinopathy. A test of retinal function is important for the diagnosis of retinal degeneration and allied conditions (including metabolic disorders), unexplained loss of vision, siderosis, cancer-associated retinopathy, stationary forms of night blindness, vitamin A deficiency, and drug toxicities (including chloroquine, hydroxychloroquine, chlorpromazine, thioridazine, and quinine). When the test is performed on individuals who are considered to have retinal degeneration, the ERG can differentiate between an isolated cone abnormality and a condition that involves both the cones and the rods. In addition, the test can differentiate between stationary forms of night blindness and progressive degenerations. Also, ERG can play a role in the evaluation of retinal ischemia, specifically with respect to central retinal vein obstruction and diabetic retinopathy. Therefore, ERG may help in the decision as to which patients are amenable to laser treatment to prevent retinal neovascularization.

PROCEDURE

Standards have been established for the performance of basic clinical ERG. Patients who are to be tested undergo dark adaptation for approximately 30 minutes. Multiple adhesive patches are placed over both eyes to allow for total occlusion of light. After a topical anesthetic has been placed in the eye, a contact-lens electrode is inserted underneath the lids. The Burian–Allen contact lens electrode is used widely[5]; alternative electrode materials include ERG-jet and Mylar electrodes. A ground electrode is placed on the patient's earlobe using electrode paste. A reference, or "inactive," electrode is placed centrally on the patient's forehead. The Grass xenon-arc photostimulator, with flash duration of 10 microseconds, commonly is used to obtain electroretinograms over a range of stimulus intensities. A Ganzfeld stimulus is necessary to standardize the flash stimulus.

The corneal contact lens serves as the active electrode and connects to a junction box along with the ground and reference electrodes. The difference in voltage between the active corneal electrode and the reference electrode is recorded by a differential amplifier.

A series of electroretinograms are obtained using different light intensities. Typically, a white or red 30Hz flicker is obtained to isolate a cone response.

COMPLICATIONS

Difficulty in placement of the contact lens electrode may result in mild corneal abrasions. In individuals who have small palpebral fissures, a pediatric contact lens may be used to avoid this complication.

INTERPRETATION OF RESULTS

When evaluating patients who have retinal degeneration, it is important to quantify the function of both the rod and cone systems. The rod-isolated response is achieved by dark adaptation of the patient's eye and a dim white or blue flash, below cone threshold, is used to stimulate the retina. A waveform results

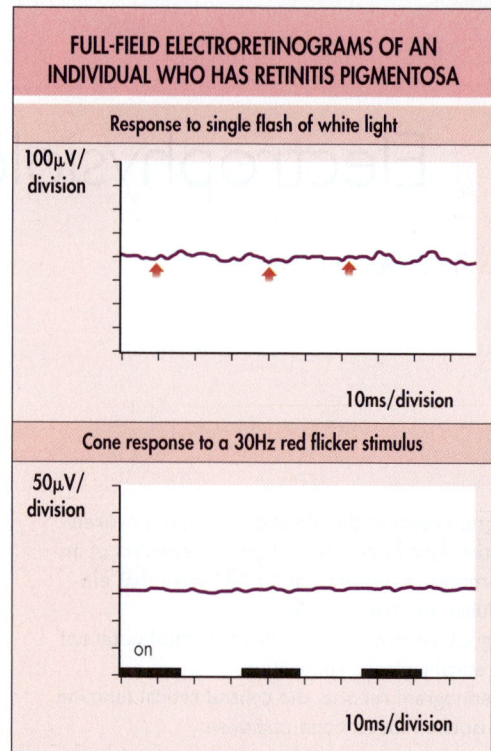

FULL-FIELD ELECTRORETINOGRAMS OF AN INDIVIDUAL WHO HAS RETINITIS PIGMENTOSA

Response to single flash of white light

100μV/division

10ms/division

Cone response to a 30Hz red flicker stimulus

50μV/division

on

10ms/division

FIG. 107-2 ■ Full-field electroretinograms, retinitis pigmentosa. Response to a single flash of bright white light is diminished markedly, consistent with the diagnosis of a retinal degeneration. The cone response to 30Hz red flicker is not recordable.

that has almost no detectable "A" wave but a large "B" wave. A bright, white flash used in the dark-adapted state causes maximal stimulation of both rods and cones and results in large "A" and "B" waves, with oscillatory potentials in the ascending "B" wave (see Fig. 107-1). Oscillatory potentials are believed to be the result of inhibitory influences from amacrine cell input. Oscillatory potentials are diminished when retinal ischemia is present. Cone responses are obtained when the eye is in a light-adapted state (i.e., after a white flash), and the signal is evoked using a red light flash. Cone responses also can be elicited using a flickering stimulus light at 30–40Hz (see Fig. 107-1). Markedly reduced rod and cone responses to a bright flash and markedly reduced cone responses to a 30Hz flicker are typical of a patient who has retinitis pigmentosa (Fig. 107-2).

Normal values for ERG results depend upon stimulus conditions and patient variables and must be considered when normalcy is established. As a rough approximation, a bright, white flash intensity results in a dark-adapted "B" wave amplitude of at least 350mV in individuals less than 50 years of age. The normal value of the 30Hz flicker stimulus is an amplitude of at least 50mV.

ALTERNATIVE TESTS

EOG has been used to evaluate a variety of retinal diseases. It appears to be useful in the evaluation of Best's macular dystrophy and pattern dystrophies. It appears to have little value in the assessment of patients who have retinal photoreceptor degenerations or stationary night blindness.

Focal foveal cone ERG may be used to measure the electrical response of the most central cone photoreceptors.[6] Full-field ERG represents a mass response of the entire retina and, therefore, focal ERG may have practical diagnostic value in the evaluation of patients who have localized macular disease and in patients who have loss of vision and otherwise normal full-field electroretinograms and normal ophthalmic examination findings.

Multifocal ERG (MFERG) is a relatively recent development in recording the ERG and variable evoked potential response and is gaining acceptance as a useful tool for retinal disease evaluation. This technique relies on obtaining multiple samples of ERG responses from different parts of the retina. Fourier transform analysis results in topographical localization of the ERG responses. Therefore, a response can be obtained that encompasses 1 to 5 degrees of the retina, dependent upon photoreceptor density. Localized structural abnormalities can be identified using this functional assessment tool.[7]

REFERENCES

1. Berson EL. Electrical phenomena in the retina. In: Moses RA, Hart WM, eds. Adler's physiology of the eye: clinical application. St Louis: CV Mosby; 1987:506–67.
2. Marg E. Development of electro-oculography. Arch Ophthalmol. 1951;45:169–85.
3. Marmor MF, Arden GB, Nilsson SE, et al. Standard for clinical electroretinography. Arch Ophthalmol. 1989;107:816–9.
4. Carr RE, Siegel IM. Electrodiagnostic testing of the visual system: a clinical guide. Philadelphia: FA Davis; 1990.
5. Burian HM, Allen L. A speculum contact lens electrode for electroretinography. Electroencephalogr Clin Neurophysiol. 1954;6:509–11.
6. Sandberg MA, Ariel M. A hand-held two channel stimulator ophthalmoscope. Arch Ophthalmol. 1977;95:1881–2.
7. OM, Miyake Y, Horiguchi M, et al. Clinical evaluation of the multifocal electroretinogram. Invest Ophthalmol Vis Sci. 1955;36:2146–50.

CHAPTER

108

Retinitis Pigmentosa and Related Disorders

PAUL A. SIEVING

DEFINITION
- Retinitis pigmentosa and the related rod-cone and cone-rod dystrophies constitute a broad set of disorders that generally result in progressive visual dysfunction because of death of the photoreceptors.

KEY FEATURES
- Progressive photoreceptor dysfunction and death.
- Clinical degeneration of the outer retina.
- Intraneural retinal "bone-spicule" pigment.
- Visual field constriction.
- Night blindness.
- Loss of rod and cone electroretinography responses.

ASSOCIATED FEATURES
- Variable degrees of initial visual acuity loss.
- Poor correlation between acuity and extent of "tunnel vision."
- Slowed adaptation to decreased or increased lighting.
- Retinal arteriolar narrowing.
- "Waxy nerve pallor" from reactive gliosis.
- Progressive chorioretinal atrophy.
- Highly variable geographic involvement.
- Posterior subcapsular cataracts in middle age.
- Frequently, but not always, a family history.
- Associated systemic abnormalities uncommon but important.

INTRODUCTION

The term retinitis pigmentosa encompasses a set of diverse hereditary disorders that affect the photoreceptors and retinal pigment epithelium (RPE) diffusely across the entire fundus but begin with initial geographic involvement in either the periphery or the macula. These conditions typically, but not always, progress over many years to an advanced stage and result in global reduction or loss of vision. As a group, the majority of forms of retinitis pigmentosa lead to death of the rod photoreceptors, which impairs vision in dim light and causes loss of peripheral vision, that is, "tunnel vision." However, some of the allied forms primarily cause cone photoreceptor loss and initially manifest with a reduction in central visual acuity.

Such conditions are determined genetically, with rare exception, and are inherited within families. All genetic types are represented. Not infrequently, a patient represents an isolated case in a kindred with no known affected relatives, which makes the condition difficult to differentiate from inflammatory or infectious retinal insults. The possibility of genetic diagnosis is rapidly becoming feasible, with identification of individual genes and the various defects within the genes that result in

these conditions. New treatment options are becoming available and others are anticipated in the years ahead because of a new understanding of the pathophysiology of the disease.

EPIDEMIOLOGY AND PATHOGENESIS

Familial retinal degeneration with intraneural retinal pigmentation was described as early as 1855 by Donders.[1] Although "retinitis" implies an inflammatory or infectious cause, histopathology shows no evidence of macrophage invasion or other inflammatory response in the photoreceptor layer or elsewhere in the retina. Now it is understood that the majority of cases have a genetic basis[2] and involve photoreceptor cell death through apoptosis. No racial or ethnic predisposition exists. Men may be affected slightly more than women because of X-linked conditions.

The term retinitis pigmentosa refers to a broad category of disease that includes many different forms of primary photoreceptor abnormality—some affect rods first and cones later (termed rod-cone dystrophy) or the reverse (cone-rod dystrophy). The key features of the rod-cone type of disease are progressive night blindness and tunnel vision, symptoms that become more severe as more rods die. Because the maximal rod density occurs in the midperiphery, the appearance of midperipheral ring scotomas during progressive stages of visual field loss is not uncommon. Typically, both eyes are affected similarly.

Specific diagnosis of disease subtype results in the best targeted prognoses. In the absence of such diagnosis, however, careful electroretinography (ERG) studies frequently identify cone-rod or rod-cone dystrophy. The cone-rod type of dystrophy causes day-vision problems of reduced acuity, color-vision impairment, and photoaversion. It is more likely that at least some peripheral vision is retained in patients who have cone-rod dystrophy as opposed to those who have rod-cone dystrophy.

The incidence of primary photoreceptor degeneration is in the range 1:3000–1:5000.[3] The carrier state for recessive retinitis pigmentosa is approximately 1:100, based on the incidence of recessive retinitis pigmentosa. These numbers are very approximate and elastic because of the complexity of the many different forms of retinitis pigmentosa now identified by gene cloning. In most cases, these diseases are thought to be simple mendelian traits that result from DNA alteration in single genes.

OCULAR MANIFESTATIONS
Typical Retinitis Pigmentosa

The key features of typical retinitis pigmentosa normally found are:
- "Bone-spicule" intraneural retinal pigment;
- Thinning and atrophy of the RPE in the mid- and far-peripheral retina;
- Relative preservation of the RPE in the macula;
- Gliotic "waxy pallor" of the optic nerve head;
- Attenuation of retinal arterioles.

The extent of bone-spicule pigmentation is highly variable—many involved retinas have some, even if very little, of this pigment. Normally, pigment clumping is not found in typical retinitis pigmentosa. The severity of the features increases with age, such as the amount of pigment, the extent of disc gliosis, and the degree of arteriolar narrowing. Major deviations from this clinical picture suggest atypical retinitis pigmentosa. In particular, several of the X-chromosome retinal dystrophies (described subsequently) deviate widely from this standard picture. The identification of typical retinitis pigmentosa is particularly important for clinical trials because this diagnosis implies the exclusion of other retinitis pigmentosa subtypes that may have unusual rates of progression.

Symptoms of typical retinitis pigmentosa include a prolonged time to adjust to dim lighting. Many retinitis pigmentosa patients are able to drive at night on well-lit streets. The worst problem for driving is at dusk or in rain or fog. Patients complain of problems in dimly lit restaurants and theaters and are symptomatic for slow adaptation when they come indoors from bright sunlight. Dark stairwells cause difficulty. By the midstage of the disease, visual field constriction results, for example, in bruised shins because coffee tables are bumped into at knee height. Patients may appear clumsy because they collide with a door frame or a friend who walks alongside because of unrecognized tunnel vision.

Typically, both eyes are affected to a comparable extent,[4] although some degree of difference between each eye is expected normally. Highly asymmetric differences are described as "unilateral retinitis pigmentosa," in which one eye lags in degeneration by the equivalent of many years, although both eyes invariably show involvement on careful testing.[5] Such apparent unilateral retinitis pigmentosa cases may also result from postinfectious causes or blunt trauma to one eye.[6]

Later manifestations of the disease include cataracts, especially of the posterior subcapsular variety, and cystoid macular edema. Both these complications may reduce the central acuity, even when the underlying disease process affects the peripheral retina only.

Molecular identification of the causative gene is possible for some cases, as for the pro-23-his rhodopsin mutation (Fig. 108-1). A long-sought goal is to correlate a specific gene with a specific phenotype, but this is accomplished rarely because most retinitis pigmentosa mutations result in a similar phenotype. Some unique conditions exist, such as the mutations in the RDS/peripherin gene, which may cause a peculiar maculopathy in addition to peripheral retinal degeneration.[7] In general, however, it is not yet possible to predict the specific causative gene from the clinical presentation.

Further, even within the retinitis pigmentosa cases attributed to a particular gene, such as that which codes for rhodopsin, major variations in the clinical features and disease severity are caused by mutations at different positions within the gene. In rhodopsin retinitis pigmentosa, the pro-23-his mutation causes fairly typical retinitis pigmentosa[8]; the cys-187-tyr mutation follows a rapid course of degeneration[9]; and the thr-58-met mutation results in sectoral involvement and a slow and mild clinical course.[10] The clinical course may vary even within a single family with a single genotype. Consequently, it is impossible to summarize retinitis pigmentosa as a single definition or clinical picture. In general, however, typical retinitis pigmentosa progresses slowly, such that a period of 1–3 years is needed to document changes.[11]

X-Linked Recessive Retinal Dystrophies

X-linked recessive retinal dystrophies warrant separate descriptions because a positive family history directs attention to an X-chromosomal disease. Such patients are identified primarily by pedigree analysis, but, in addition, many of the dystrophies have fairly unique clinical features, which provide the clinical suspicion that results in careful determination of the family history.

X-Linked Retinitis Pigmentosa

X-linked retinitis pigmentosa (XLRP) has features of typical retinitis pigmentosa, although prominent parafoveal atrophy may be present. Affected boys shows subtle or modest RPE granularity, but frank, intraneural retinal bone-spicule pigment typically does not appear until the teenage years. Acuity is good during childhood, but by 20 years of age acuity loss and field constriction rule out the acquisition of a driver's license, and dark-adapted thresholds are elevated by as much as 3 log units (1000-fold sensitivity loss). Night blindness is severe by the midteenage years. Rate of vision decline is rapid, and major functional loss is expected by 30 years of age; blindness by 40 years of age is common.

The clinical features of three different forms of XLRP (RP2, RP3, and RP15) overlap extensively, and all progress to severe vision disability by young adulthood. All those affected show typical characteristics of retinitis pigmentosa, although cone vision is affected to a greater degree than in many autosomal forms of retinitis pigmentosa, particularly in those who have RP15. ERG reveals a major reduction of both the rod and cone responses even in young boys and is essential to stage the disease.

Choroideremia

Choroideremia results in a characteristic choriocapillaris loss with bare sclera and scalloped edges in the peripheral fundus.[12] Wide pigmentary variations occur, but the pigment usually forms in clumps rather than in bone-spicule shapes. Despite only a small central island of vision, a surprising degree of local macular preservation and adequate acuity may occur well into middle age. Choroideremia may be confused with gyrate atrophy, a rare autosomal recessive condition that elevates serum ornithine levels 10- to 20-fold.[13] Diagnosis is by clinical experience and may be confirmed by biochemical assay for Rab escort protein (REP-1) production in a blood sample. Choroideremia carriers show very coarse RPE granularity across major regions of the fundus and clinically are identified readily (see Chapter 110).

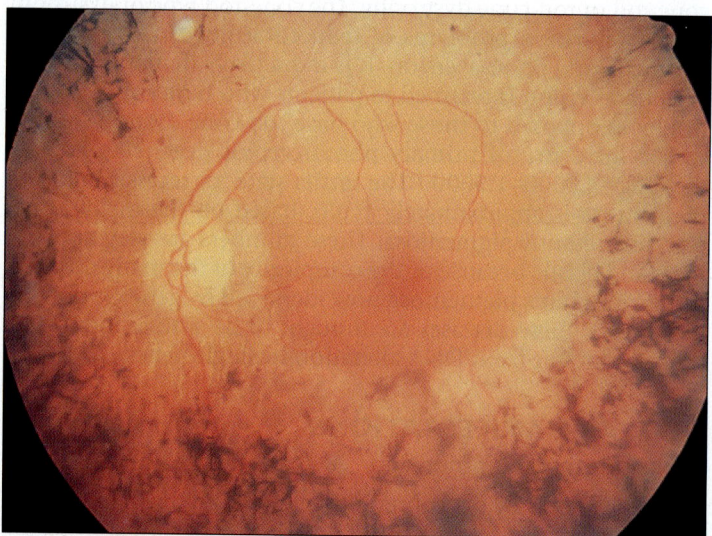

FIG. 108-1 ■ "Typical" retinitis pigmentosa changes in a 73-year-old woman who had a pro-23-his rhodopsin autosomal dominant mutation. Visible are extensive, intraneural, retinal, bone-spicule pigmentation, severely constricted retinal arteries, waxy pallor of the disc, and extensive retinal pigment epithelium atrophy in the macula and midperiphery (which reveals underlying choroidal vessels). Her visual acuity was 20/50 (6/15), but she made no errors on Ishihara color testing; her fields were severely constricted to 17° tunnel vision with the Goldmann V4e target.

Congenital Stationary Night Blindness

X-linked congenital stationary night blindness (CSNB) may be confused with XLRP at first presentation in young boys because both conditions cause complaints of difficult vision at night and show alterations in the fundus pigmentation (see Chapter 111). Differentiation between these two forms is critical because in CSNB vision remains "stationary."[14] In CSNB, night blindness is severe from birth, but visual acuity may be reduced only slightly and color discrimination is unaffected. High myopia is common. The fundus pigmentation is frequently mottled. Both ERG and visual field tests are critical in the diagnosis of CSNB. The photopic ERG provides a diagnostic clue—CSNB shows a characteristically wide cone a-wave trough. Visual fields are full for CSNB, whereas they are constricted to the Goldmann I4e target even in early XLRP and choroideremia.

Juvenile Retinoschisis

Diagnosis is determined by the characteristic spoke wheel pattern of foveal and parafoveal intraretinal cysts and an X-linked family history. The ERG hallmark is a healthy rod a-wave but reduced rod b-wave with bright stimuli.[15] Visual acuity is typically between 20/25 (6/7.5) and 20/80 (6/24) in teenagers but declines further to 20/200 (6/60) during the sixth decade because of secondary atrophy of the RPE in the macula.[16] Despite the reduced rod b-wave, patients rarely complain of night blindness and dark-adapted visual thresholds may be nearly normal (see Chapter 112)

Blue Cone Monochromatism

Boys and men affected by blue cone monochromatism (BCM) have normal nighttime rod vision but poor day vision as a result of the loss of both red and green cone function.[17] Also, BCM causes small-amplitude nystagmus, reduced acuity, and photosensitivity. The acuity is between 20/80 (6/24) and 20/200 (6/60) and this may go unrecognized until school years. The fundus may show minimal RPE pigmentary mottling. Color vision is absent or at least severely limited, but differences in bluish hues are detectable. Some preschoolers affected by BCM correctly identify red-, green-, and blue-colored pencils, whereas achromats (rod monochromats) totally lack color vision. Because rod monochromacy is autosomal recessive, both sexes are affected. Both BCM patients and achromats fail the Ishihara and American Optical color plate tests and the Farnsworth D-15 and 100 Hue tests. Differentiation between achromats and BCM patients is aided by specially designed "blue arrow" color plate tests,[18] which boys and men affected by BCM pass but achromats fail. The dark-adapted ERG b-wave amplitude is normal or slightly subnormal for BCM patients, but rod psychophysical threshold sensitivity remains normal, which differentiates BCM from degenerative rod disease cases. The light-adapted cone ERG single flash and flicker responses are reduced by >80–95%. Only 1% of cones are blue cones, and no blue cones are found within the human fovea, which accounts for the poor acuity in BCM patients. All other aspects of vision remain stable in BCM, and acuity may even improve slightly and reach 20/70 (6/21) by the age of 20 years, by which time the nystagmus is barely detectable. Some older BCM men have progressive macular atrophy. Only boys and men are affected by BCM; female carriers show no changes. Red and green opsins occur on the X chromosome, and BCM is an X-linked recessive trait. An X-linked family history helps differentiate BCM from autosomal recessive, early age, progressive cone dystrophy.

Congenital Red-Green Color Deficiency

Total red (protanopia) or green (deuteranopia) color blindness affects 2–3% of men. Partial forms are termed anomalous color perception (e.g., protanomaly). Tritanopia (total blue blindness) is exceedingly rare. For all forms together, 4–7% of men manifest some type of congenital color deficiency. Given this frequency, some men who are affected by other retinal degenera-

tions are also "color blind," and the congenital condition must be differentiated from the acquired disease. Progressive cone dystrophy also impairs color discrimination but is differentiated by abnormal visual acuity and/or peripheral fields, both of which are usually normal in the congenital color deficiencies. Female carriers manifest no clinical signs.

Ocular Albinism

Ocular albinism occurs in several forms and follows all the inheritance patterns, including an X-linked recessive type. All forms are evident from birth and cause moderate-amplitude nystagmus, which the parents notice quite early. The fundus is hypopigmented and the iris may transilluminate. Acuity is between 20/70 (6/21) and 20/200 (6/60) but is difficult to test precisely during infancy. Color vision remains normal and nyctalopia does not occur. The foveal reflex may be muted or hypoplastic. The electroretinogram is normal or even supranormal because of enhanced intraocular light reflection. Cutaneous involvement accompanies systemic forms. Diagnosis is made by clinical examination. Vision remains stable. Confusion arises in the differentiation of ocular albinism from the "blond fundus" of patients who have pale skin and hair tones but normal acuity.

Female Carriers of X-Chromosomal Retinal Dystrophies

Female carriers of X-chromosomal retinal dystrophies may manifest retinal pigmentary changes and have functional vision impairment that present special difficulty in diagnosis. Recognition of the carrier state is important to establish the correct inheritance pattern for family genetic counseling. Some carriers have a severe vision abnormality, which may lead to a misdiagnosis of autosomal dominant disease. In female carriers, one of the two X chromosomes has a mutant gene. As a result of random X-chromosome inactivation, only one gene is active in each cell (the Lyon hypothesis). Because the mutant gene is retained in some retinal cells during early development, clusters of neighboring cells have the disease, and patches of clinical disease occur that mimic a mild form of the fully expressed male condition in choroideremia, XLRP, and X-linked ocular albinism. Carriers of juvenile retinoschisis, blue cone monochromacy, CSNB, and color-vision dichromacy show no fundus changes and experience no functional vision abnormality. Carriers of autosomal recessive disease rarely show retinal changes or have visual symptoms.

Female carriers of XLRP (Fig. 108-2) show one or more small or large retinal patches of typical, intraneural retinal, bone-

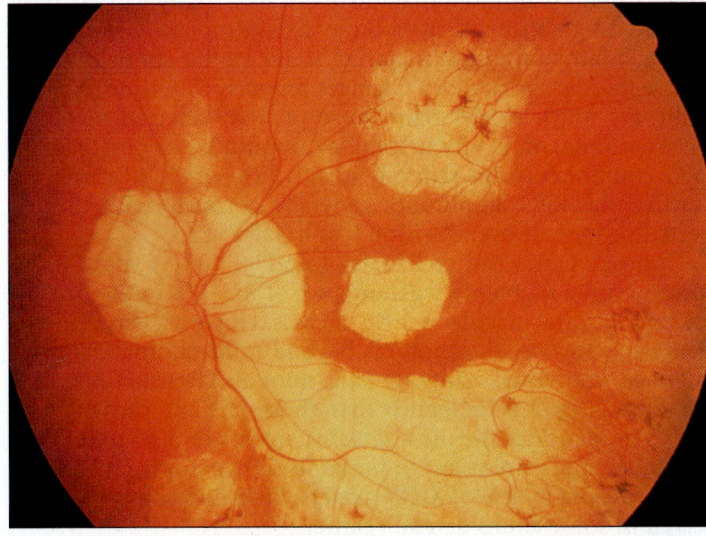

FIG. 108-2 ■ X-linked female retinitis pigmentosa carrier affected by lacunae of disease. Atrophy of retinal pigment epithelium and intraneural retinal bone-spicule pigment result. Acuity is 20/200 (6/60) because of macular atrophy.

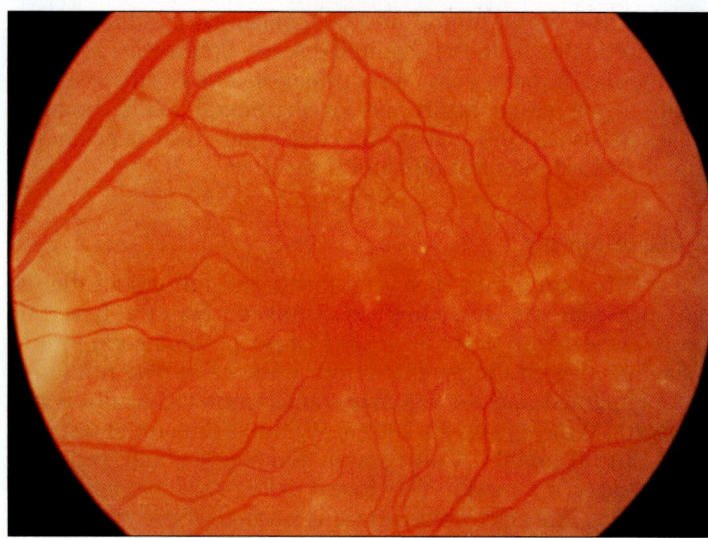

FIG. 108-3 ■ Macular and parafoveal gross pigmentary retinal pigment epithelium mottling in a female choroideremia carrier. Despite such mottling, female choroideremia carriers are asymptomatic.

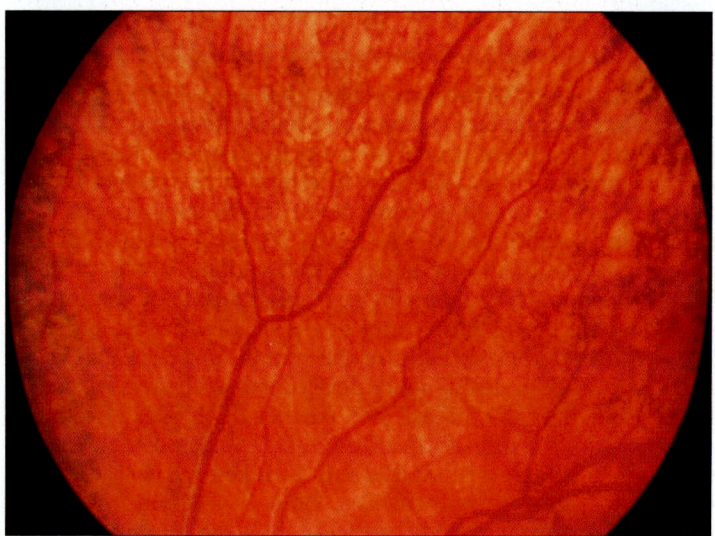

FIG. 108-4 ■ Punctate granularity and attenuation of the normally uniform pigmentation of the retinal pigment epithelium in an X-linked female carrier of ocular albinism.

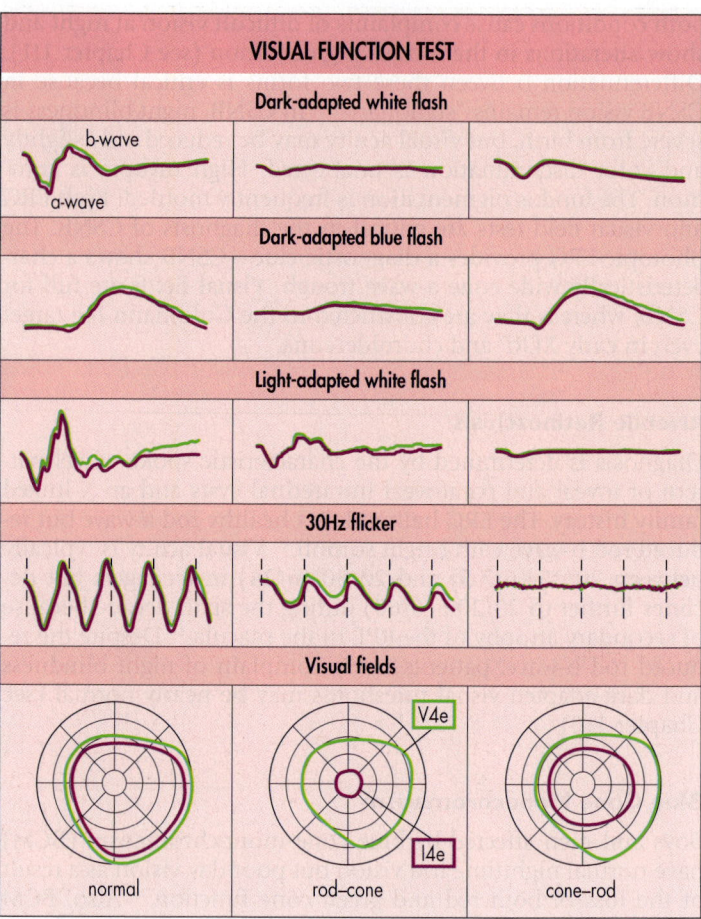

FIG. 108-5 ■ Visual function test. For normal subjects, dark-adapted rod a- and b-waves result from bright, white flashes and, primarily, b-waves from dimmer blue flashes; cone responses are elicited by a single, light-adapted, white flash (a- and b-waves) and by 30Hz flickers. For rod-cone patients, rod responses are reduced proportionally more than cone responses. For cone-rod patients, major losses in light-adapted and 30Hz responses occur, with relative preservation particularly of the rod b-wave, to dim, dark-adapted, blue flash. Goldmann visual field tests using the small I4e target show major tunnel vision in rod-cone patients.

spicule pigmentation and atrophy of the underlying RPE and choriocapillaris in more than 50% of cases. Many carriers have myopic astigmatism at an oblique axis. Although vision is involved minimally in the majority, some are functionally blind by late middle age or older. Changes progress with time but generally are much slower than those in XLRP-affected men. An electroretinogram is very helpful, as amplitudes of one or more ERG components are reduced in 80–95% of XLRP carriers.[19] Further, the ERG amplitudes generally correlate with the expected severity of overall vision loss in later years.

Choroideremia carrier females (see Fig. 108-3) show widespread retinal pigmentary disturbance of the RPE in the periphery and into the macula in 90% of cases. However, very few carriers have any visual symptoms beyond mild photoaversion in later age, and visual acuity remains normal. Electroretinograms are affected far less frequently than those of XLRP carriers; fundus examination is the most sensitive means of detection. Most choroideremia carriers are emmetropic or hyperopic, in contrast to the myopia typical of XLRP carriers. Progression has been observed in some choroideremia carriers.[20]

X-linked ocular albinism female carriers (Fig. 108-4) show punctate RPE pigmentation across the entire fundus and RPE thinning in the periphery (a mild version of changes found in the affected men), which may mimic the "salt-and-pepper" appearance of congenital rubella retinopathy. Visual acuity is not affected, and ERG is normal. Symptoms do not extend beyond mild photoaversion to bright light. Carriers of non–X-linked albinism rarely show fundus changes.

Rod-Cone and Cone-Rod Disease: When Subtyping Fails

Accurate subtyping of the disease provides the best information about prognosis, but if subtyping fails the patient is assessed for rod-cone disease or cone-rod disease, two conditions that carry quite different prognoses. Rod-cone degeneration is the more severe–the long-term prognosis is loss of most or all vision by later years. Cone-rod degeneration affects central vision quite early and peripheral vision only later. Because the human retina has 120 million rods and only 6 million cones, it may survive well without cones, as exemplified by achromatopsia. The prognosis in cone-rod dystrophy is good for at least some future vision, even though central vision is jeopardized. Retinal function studies, particularly ERG, are required to differentiate rod-cone from cone-rod degenerations.

Rod-Cone Dystrophy

Rod-cone dystrophy manifests clinically with typical retinitis pigmentosa and affects the rod photoreceptors earlier and more severely than it does the cones. Severe cone involvement occurs in the end stage of the disease, when total vision loss ensues. End-stage rod-cone disease results in loss of both peripheral and

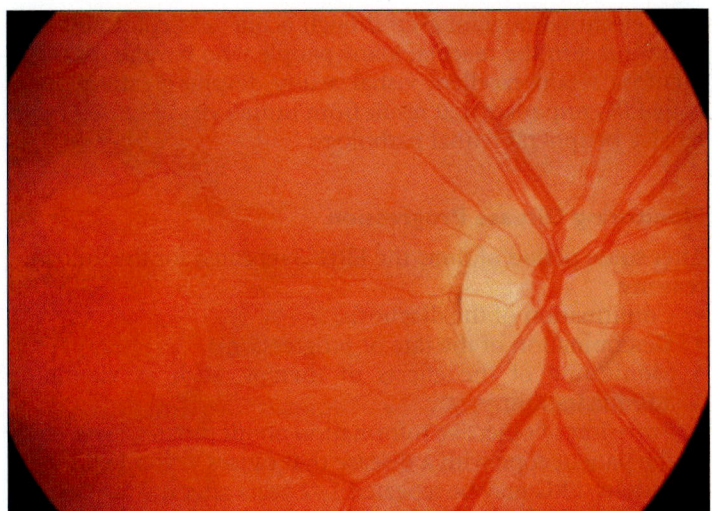

FIG. 108-6 ■ The bull's-eye maculopathy in this 5-year-old male who has a cone-rod dystrophy is not found in all cases of this entity.

central vision. Many patients have only barely functional central vision by late middle age and lose all vision later. However, the changes occur slowly, and the young patient may be reassured that some vision is most likely to persist for many years or decades, even though they must accept that the long-term prognosis is grim. Photoaversion to bright light occurs in end-stage rod-cone dystrophy, when the diseased cones saturate in bright light.

The functional profile of early-stage rod-cone dystrophy is shown in Figure 108-5. The rod ERG amplitude loss is worse than that for cones (light-adapted and 30Hz flicker). Goldmann visual fields are still relatively large with the large V4e target but considerably constricted to the small I4e target—such disparity between the ratio of field to V4e versus I4e is typical for rod-cone dystrophy. Visual acuity is initially affected minimally and typically remains near 20/20 (6/6) for many years despite progressive field loss to severe tunnel vision. Careful history taking reveals some night blindness, even in early-stage rod-cone disease. Tests of dark-adapted thresholds show 1–3 log units of rod sensitivity loss, which equates with 10–1000 times more light to see anything at night. The disease does not act uniformly across the retina, and rod threshold should be tested at multiple points of vision to give a sensitivity profile across the central and peripheral vision.

As visual fields constrict further, even to the large V4e target, dark-adapted thresholds become worse because only cones remain to mediate vision, even in dim light. At this stage the patient suffers from severe night blindness. With time, the cone ERG responses deteriorate further until eventually both the rod and cone responses are reduced profoundly, and all ERG responses are termed "nonrecordable." By this time, visual acuity is typically less than 20/40 (6/12), color discrimination is impaired, and fields are greatly constricted.

Cone-Rod Dystrophy

Cone-rod patients complain of poor acuity, reduced color vision, and photoaversion to bright sunlight. Fundus changes are quite variable, and not all patients show "bull's-eye" maculopathy (Fig. 108-6). Particularly in the early stages, the fundus may appear benign, with minimal diffuse retinopathy and normal vessels and disc. Visual fields initially remain full with the Goldmann V4e target but may be constricted slightly with the I4e target. Electroretinograms show that cone amplitudes (30Hz flicker and photopic single flashes) are reduced proportionally more than the dark-adapted rod b-wave (see Fig. 108-5). Although the rod b-wave amplitudes may be subnormal technically, rod dark-adapted threshold sensitivity remains nearly normal when tested

using a Goldmann-Weekers dark adaptometer after 45 minutes in the dark. Such a combination of ERG and psychophysical rod threshold tests is the best way to diagnose cone-rod dystrophy. Patients who have the least rod involvement carry the best prognosis for intermediate-term vision. Infrequently, a cone-rod patient has an essentially normal rod electroretinogram but a very reduced cone electroretinogram and is considered to have "cone dystrophy." Such patients have a good prognosis for vision into later age. Some cone-rod patients are first symptomatic after the age of 50 years or more and may progress quickly to considerable vision loss.[21] Such patients are a diagnostic challenge because of the later age of presentation; initially, ERG results may be marginally normal, but the results of repeat ERGs after 6–12 months progress to subnormal.

DIAGNOSIS AND ANCILLARY TESTING

The preceding brief descriptions indicate that, for diagnosis, visual function tests are an important adjunct to retinal examination. Tests may also help identify correctly the clinical subtype of the disease. Accurate subtyping provides the basis for counseling about expectations for school and career choices and for the provision of genetic information to the extended family.

Before any tests are carried out, listen carefully to what the patient has to say. Complaints of "night blindness" may indicate a total lack of vision in very dim light or a diminished acuity as ambient light dims. Also, night blindness from rod photoreceptor disease:

- Prolongs the time required to adjust to changes in light, as when dark theaters or dim restaurants are entered or even when moving from sunlight into room light;
- Causes problems at dusk, when the normal switch from daytime to nighttime vision occurs; and
- Results in visual-field constriction in dimmer light.

Tunnel vision may be suggested by recent automobile accidents or clumsiness in the narrow spaces of elevators or doorways. Any family history of slowly progressive unexplained vision loss must be sought. The retina and macula must be examined carefully for RPE granularity that precedes intraneural retinal pigment accumulation or outright atrophy. When the history and clinical features have been assessed together, and if a retinal or macular dystrophy is suspected, formal retinal function tests must be considered, which include ERG, visual field tests, and dark adaptometry.

Retinal function tests have value far beyond simple diagnosis because they give insight into the nature of the disease, inform about the severity or stage, and provide information for genetic counseling. Results of the examination must be communicated to the patient because subtyping and staging the disease provide information about expectations for the course of future vision and the genetic implications for the family.

Results of functional tests must be integrated with knowledge of the clinical state. Although flagrant and advanced retinal degeneration may be diagnosed without extensive tests, tests serve to subtype the disease and establish the severity. Disease progression is monitored by yearly visual field measurements and by repeated ERG every few years. Future clinical trials to treat photoreceptor degenerations are likely, and for this, yearly ERG will be important to establish a baseline rate of progression.

Electroretinography

The electroretinogram is quite sensitive to even mild photoreceptor impairment. Rod b-wave amplitudes are reduced in the earliest stages of disease, when the retina may appear clinically normal and vision complaints are minimal. For the diagnosis of genetically at-risk younger patients who have otherwise minimal retinal pigmentation, ERG is essential. Also, ERG helps in the diagnosis of patients of any age who have unclear visual symptoms. Finally, ERG helps in the diagnosis of the disease in relatives when a retinitis pigmentosa pedigree is established. Good clinical sense and careful ophthalmoscopic examination prevail in most cases, but definitive ERG normal results may allay parents' fears that their child is affected.

Analysis and Interpretation

Initially, ERG is used to test the rod system after 45 or more minutes in the dark (the "scotopic ERG"). The cone system is tested using single, bright flashes superimposed on a bright background that suppresses activity of rods (the "photopic ERG") and also using a 30Hz flicker to which cones respond but rods do not. Many complex and analytic schemes of ERG analysis are employed in special circumstances, but the most useful initial measures of ERG abnormality are[22]:

- Scotopic (dark-adapted condition, rod driven) and photopic (light-adapted, cone driven) b-wave amplitudes—these provide the first index of disease severity and help differentiate rod-cone from cone-rod disease;
- Scotopic b-waves reduced by 50% or more—this indicates progressive disease rather than a variant of "stationary" disease;
- Early cone system disease—this frequently reduces the amplitudes of 30Hz flicker before photopic b-wave responses to single flashes;
- Delayed flicker implicit time (from flash to response peak)—this is a highly sensitive measure of abnormality,[23] and implicit times may be prolonged even with normal flicker amplitude; implicit times are very robust and relatively immune to artifacts caused when the patient squeezes on the ERG contact lens electrode (which reduces flicker amplitude but does not change timing);
- Photopic oscillatory potentials (high-frequency wavelets of small amplitude that originate in the proximal retina)—these are generally reduced earlier or by more than the photopic, single-flash b-wave, and oscillatory potentials may be reduced in retinal vascular diseases;
- Relative preservation of the scotopic a-wave amplitude (from rod photoreceptors) but reduced scotopic b-wave (from signaling by second-order bipolar cells)—this is highly suggestive of CSNB or X-linked juvenile retinoschisis (the ERG change indicates faulty synaptic signaling from rods to bipolar cells, deficient bipolar responsivity, or Müller cell disease);
- Broad and flat bottom trough to the photopic a-wave—this is highly suggestive of CSNB;
- The full-field (termed Ganzfeld) ERG—this reflects global retinal activity and is insensitive to macular scars; thus, it does not correlate with visual acuity determined solely by foveal function.

Disease Staging

Staging of the disease is based on the current visual acuity, dark-adapted rod thresholds, peripheral fields, color discrimination, and rod and cone ERG status. Normally, reduced rod ERG amplitudes correspond to impaired, dark-adapted rod thresholds. If the rod b-wave is reduced greatly but the dark-adapted thresholds are elevated only slightly, it suggests that only a few functioning peripheral rods remain and that vision loss will progress rapidly when these few rods are lost. Rates of visual acuity change are less predictable than changes in peripheral field constriction.

Full-field ERG and visual acuity are quite different measures of vision. Full-field ERG is dominated by a large expanse of the peripheral retina rather than by the macula, whereas visual acuity is determined exclusively by foveal cones, which are only 1% of the total number of cones.

The peripheral retina outside the macular arcade vessels contains 60% of the rods and 60% of the cones. The macula contains about 40% of the total cone population. Loss of peripheral cones as retinitis pigmentosa progresses reduces the full-field

cone electroretinogram even though acuity and color vision remain intact in the macula. Many people who have retinitis pigmentosa retain excellent visual acuity despite greatly reduced cone ERG responses that result from tunnel vision caused by extensive peripheral retinal pathology.

Monitoring Disease Progression

After some period of time, the ERG is repeated for the following reasons:
- Confirmation of the diagnosis;
- Determination of the rate of progression;
- Monitoring of the effects of therapy, such as vitamin A administration;
- Provision of objective information about progression to help the patient cope with a disease that causes vision loss.

For adults, ERG may be repeated 1–2 years after the first test just to confirm the findings, or serial yearly tests may be used to estimate progression. More frequent ERGs are rarely warranted for adults. In younger children, however, retinal dysfunction may progress more rapidly, and yearly repeated ERGs are warranted to guide school decisions and anticipate future vision needs. Exceptionally rapid cone ERG loss in a child may raise suspicion of atypical forms of retinitis pigmentosa, which include neuronal ceroid lipofuscinosis and indicate the need for a neurological evaluation, particularly if seizure activity is reported.

Visual Field Testing

Goldmann perimetry is preferable for retinitis pigmentosa field testing out to 90° in the far temporal periphery, which is involved first in the rod-cone type of disease. Even moderate stages of rod disease typically show extensive peripheral field loss to the small, I4e Goldmann target, whereas cone-rod disease leaves peripheral fields more intact, the I4e target. Retinitis pigmentosa subjects may respond poorly to automated perimeters—careful studies using a Goldmann perimeter are more successful for obtaining reproducible fields. Macular dysfunction may be tracked excellently using the Humphrey Visual Field Analyzer 24-2 or 10-2 programs. Many retinitis pigmentosa patients are unaware of lost peripheral vision or a ring scotoma even after several suggestive events (i.e., recent automobile accidents). The patient will appreciate the physician who simply takes the time to explain visual field test results and may immediately recall instances of previous problems with everyday activities.

Dark-Adaptation Testing

Night-vision symptoms occur early in the course of retinitis pigmentosa disease and must be evaluated using dark-adaptation studies. The most commonly used instrument is the Goldmann-Weekers dark adaptometer. The patient is placed in darkness and asked to detect the dimmest possible light that is made progressively dimmer as time proceeds. Final absolute threshold sensitivity is normally reached after 30–40 minutes in the dark. An alternative test strategy is to determine only the final thresholds after 45–60 minutes in the dark. Thresholds are tested in several different retinal locations to sample the distribution of disease. Some patients who complain of difficulty seeing at night are found to have normal dark-adapted thresholds. Such patients may have undercorrected myopia, and the complaint is really of blurred vision in dimmer light. Other patients may have maculopathy and notice worse acuity in dimmer light, even though normal rod, absolute dark sensitivity is maintained.

Color Vision Tests

In degenerative retinopathy, color testing is a useful adjunct to visual acuity tests because it provides additional information about the condition of the macular cones. Retinitis pigmentosa patients rarely volunteer problems with color vision because nearly all can differentiate readily the major colors of red, green, and blue. However, in rod-cone dystrophies, tritanopic ("blue") color discrimination loss on the Farnsworth D-15 panel is a sensitive index of early foveal cone involvement and may presage acuity loss within the next few years. In cone dystrophies, loss of color discrimination normally parallels visual acuity loss. The D-15 test, which consists of 15 color chips that must be arranged in color sequence, is simple, rapid, does not tire the patient, and is easy to score. More than two minor neighbor errors in the D-15 test indicates pathology. The Farnsworth 100-Hue test is more elaborate but seems to be no more sensitive for detecting maculopathy. The Ishihara and American Optical color plates were designed specifically to detect congenital red-green abnormal individuals and are less useful than the D-15 test for the evaluation of early macular dysfunction that results from a retinal dystrophy.

Fluorescein Angiography

Fluorescein angiography rarely provides novel information in diffuse retinopathy beyond that found by careful retinal examination. It is most useful for hereditary maculopathies, such as Stargardt's disease and Best's disease, or in suspected toxic maculopathy from hydroxychloroquine, chloroquine, or psychotropic agents. A fluorescein angiogram should be obtained for patients who have diminished acuity without any clinically apparent maculopathy or when macular edema is suspected. Cone dystrophies frequently show subtle, foveal RPE window defects early in the course. A fluorescein angiogram provides objective verification of macular pathology in children who might otherwise be considered to suffer from psychogenic vision problems.

Electro-Oculography

Electro-oculography (EOG) is abnormal whenever the ERG is abnormal and thus provides useful information only when the ERG is normal. Therefore, EOG is not performed automatically with every ERG examination. One of the very few current uses for EOG is to track the genetic pattern in Best's vitelliform macular dystrophy, in which the expressivity is highly variable.

Visual-Evoked Cortical Potential

Visual-evoked cortical potential (VECP) monitors visual signals that reach the cortex and is dominated heavily by macular function, with a far smaller contribution from the peripheral retina. Any disturbance of retinal function, altered optic nerve conduction, or visual cortex processing alters the VECP. Retinal, and particularly macular, dystrophies affect the VECP, but these conditions are nearly always identified and followed better by other visual function tests.

DIFFERENTIAL DIAGNOSIS

Toxic Retinopathy

Thioridazine retinal toxicity causes widespread retinal pigmentary degeneration and affects visual acuity; the visual symptoms overlap those of retinitis pigmentosa. Toxicity generally occurs within months of the initiation of thioridazine use, although retinal degeneration is also reported to occur late after use has ceased[24] (see Chapter 143).

Chloroquine causes bull's-eye maculopathy (Fig. 108-7); it binds to melanin in the RPE and causes cytotoxicity, which begins preferentially around the fovea. Visual acuity initially remains excellent, despite parafoveal metamorphopsia and difficulty in reading because of the paracentral scotoma. Because it is far less retinotoxic, hydroxychloroquine has supplanted chloroquine except for those who travel in malarial areas. Only a few cases of hydroxychloroquine toxicity have been reported, but these cause vision pathology similar to that seen in bull's-eye

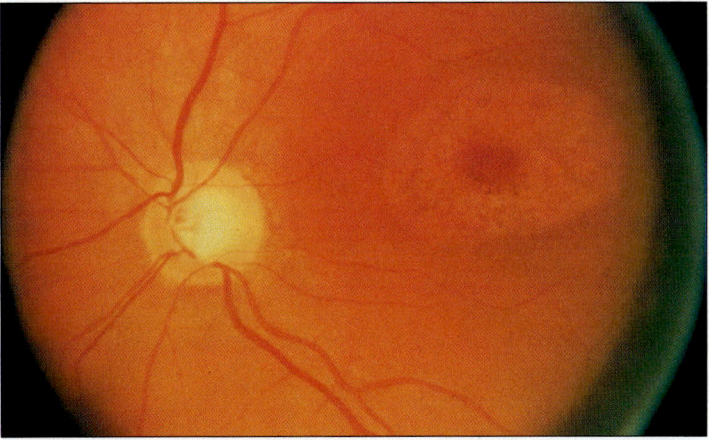

FIG. 108-7 ■ Chloroquine bull's-eye parafoveal atrophy.

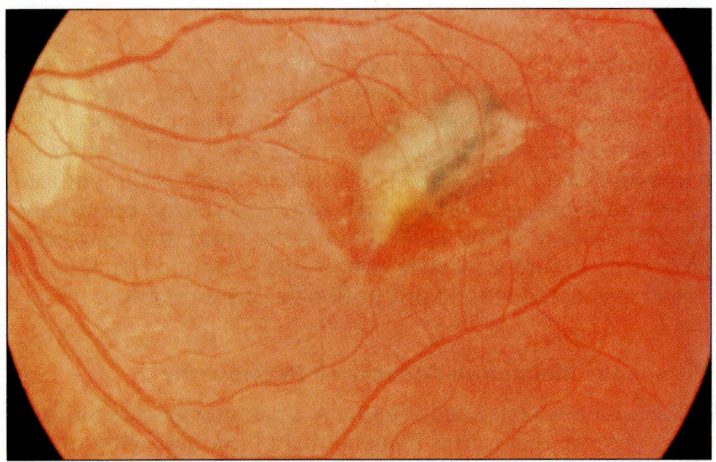

FIG. 108-8 ■ Rubella maculopathy in a young individual who has 20/60 (6/18) visual acuity.

maculopathy. The initial change is parafoveal and is picked up by macular field tests using a Humphrey Visual Field Analyzer Program 10-2, with careful attention paid to sensitivity threshold changes. Field sensitivity changes may even precede changes on fluorescein angiography. Careful examination of the parafoveal RPE using a 90D lens shows RPE disturbance with a sensitivity comparable to that of fluorescein angiography.

Postinfectious Retinopathy

Congenital rubella infection causes coarse pigmentary spots and tiny clumps on the retina, termed salt-and-pepper retinopathy.[25] However, visual fields remain full, and ERG remains essentially normal. The complaint at presentation may involve decreased visual acuity because of maculopathy from a yellowish, fibrotic macular scar (Figs. 108-8 and 108-9). Peripheral vision remains stable, although visual acuity may worsen through young adulthood, and the patient may be predisposed to presenile macular degeneration.

Syphilitic retinitis may result in pigmentary retinopathy and progressive vision impairment that mimics retinitis pigmentosa.[26] It may also cause asymmetric disease that mimics unilateral retinitis pigmentosa.[27] Screening serology tests should be carried out on patients who have retinitis pigmentosa but whose family history is negative.

Cancer-Associated Retinopathy

Cancer-associated retinopathy syndrome results in acute onset of rapid and progressive bilateral vision loss without much ini-

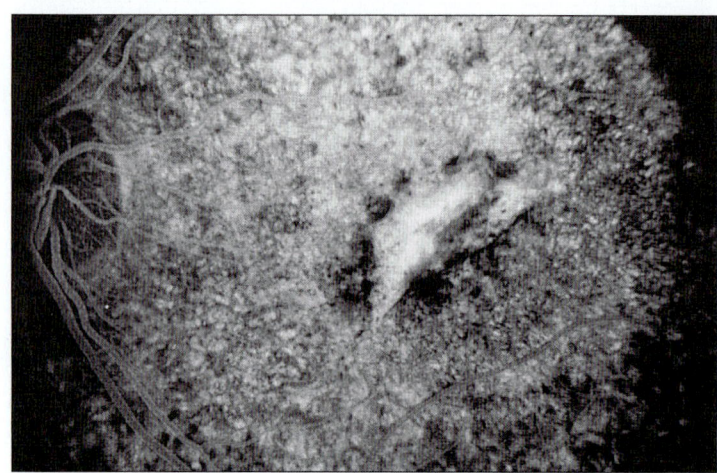

FIG. 108-9 ■ Fluorescein angiogram of patient in Fig. 108-8 who has rubella retinopathy. Marked granularity of the retinal pigment epithelium can be seen.

tial pigmentary retinopathy. Small-cell lung cancer is the most common cause, although many other cancers are also implicated, including endometrial, breast, and prostatic cancer. The mechanism involves production of autoantigens that enter the retina and cause apoptosis. The apparent target is the photoreceptor molecule recoverin, which is integral to the phototransduction cascade.[28] The clinical course is rapid and inexorably progresses toward complete vision loss. Commercial tests for cancer-associated retinopathy antibodies are available.

Cutaneous Melanoma-Associated Retinopathy

Melanoma-associated retinopathy is a paraneoplastic syndrome of acute onset that causes bilateral night blindness without visible retinopathy. Antibodies generated against the cutaneous melanoma cross the blood-retinal barrier and target the retinal bipolar cells, which impairs function but apparently does not cause cell death.[29] Visual symptoms include photopsias and shimmering patches of color.[30] The scotopic ERG is reduced preferentially. Although the retinal course is usually otherwise benign with minimal progression, severe intraocular inflammation has been reported.[31]

SYSTEMIC ASSOCIATIONS

Retinitis pigmentosa is associated with many systemic conditions, of which the following warrant particular attention either because of their incidence (e.g., Usher's syndrome) or because the diagnosis, which may be recognized by the ophthalmologist first, has major medical implications.

Usher's Syndrome

The hearing loss in Usher's syndrome ranges from congenital and total to middle-age onset and partial. Usher's syndrome is nearly always autosomal recessive, and typically no affected relatives are identified in previous generations. If the spouse has normal hearing, the risk of any affected children is small although never absolutely zero. The prevalence of Usher's syndrome within the deaf population is estimated to be as high as 3–6%.[32]

Type I Usher's syndrome results in profound congenital deafness—hearing aids are ineffective. Vestibular dysfunction causes affected infants to walk late, at 18–20 months, because of balance problems; late walking enables the clinical diagnosis of siblings without any need for extensive tests. The vestibular dysfunction again causes problems during the teenage years when visual field loss combines with deafness to make the patient more clumsy at routine school sports that involve running or

jumping. Vision impairment is severe by late teenage years, and functional blindness typically occurs before 40 years of age.

Type II Usher's syndrome results in hearing impairment that may be corrected partially using hearing aids. Vision loss is less rapid than that in the type I disease but at any given age may be more severe than that in most retinitis pigmentosa patients. Vestibular function is normal, and walking begins at a normal age.

Type III Usher's syndrome results in progressive hearing loss that is first apparent in middle age. Progression of retinitis pigmentosa is no faster than that in patients who have retinitis pigmentosa and whose hearing is not impaired.

Not all retinitis pigmentosa patients affected by impaired hearing have Usher's syndrome. Possibly as many as 5–10% of retinitis pigmentosa patients also experience mild, progressive, high-tone hearing loss that begins in middle age, of which only some cases may represent type III Usher's syndrome. Consequently, it cannot be presumed categorically that the inheritance pattern is autosomal recessive when counseling retinitis pigmentosa patients who have hearing loss. Familial hearing loss is not an uncommon genetic trait and may be autosomal recessive or dominant. Occasionally, families have autosomal dominant hearing loss and a sporadic case of retinitis pigmentosa in the same family that is merely coincidental. Any patient with retinal degeneration for whom there is a suspicion of even slight hearing loss must receive audiologic evaluation and treatment to minimize the effect of major sensory problems that arise from combined hearing and vision deficits.

Bardet-Biedl Syndrome

Bardet-Biedl syndrome is an autosomal recessive entity that involves pigmentary retinopathy with polydactyly, renal dysfunction, and short stature in association with truncal obesity. The fingers are thick but taper to fine tips. Because extra digits are often removed surgically during infancy, finger surgery must be asked about specifically. Intelligence is frequently subnormal. Hypogenitalism occurs in more than half of patients. The peripheral fundus pigmentation may appear typical for retinitis pigmentosa or have only very coarse RPE granularity, and progressive parafoveal macular atrophy impairs visual acuity by the teenage years (Fig. 108-10). Both visual acuity loss and field constriction are very severe by middle age. Renal disease frequently causes premature death by middle age, and patients may suffer renal failure that requires transplantation even during the teenage years. A full renal evaluation is suggested when the ophthalmic diagnosis is made. The similar Laurence-Moon syndrome, in addition, features paraplegia.

Kearns-Sayer Syndrome

Kearns-Sayer syndrome is a mitochondrial myopathy that results in external ophthalmoplegia, lid ptosis, cardiac conduction block, and mild retinitis pigmentosa. Such patients present as young adults with modest night blindness and modest peripheral-field constriction. The fundus appearance is atypical for retinitis pigmentosa, as only very coarse RPE granularity is found with little intraneural retinal pigment accumulation. Visual field constriction is modest, but visual acuity may be impaired. The progression of visual symptoms is rather slow. Typically, ERG rod and cone amplitudes are reduced only modestly. Referral for cardiac evaluation is required because the conduction abnormalities may result in life-threatening arrhythmias.

Neuronal Ceroid Lipofuscinosis

Neuronal ceroid lipofuscinosis is a devastating condition that involves progressive neurological failure, mental deterioration, seizures, and visual acuity loss from cone degeneration that causes bull's-eye maculopathy. Several subtypes affect different age groups, from infants to teenagers, and death occurs by the

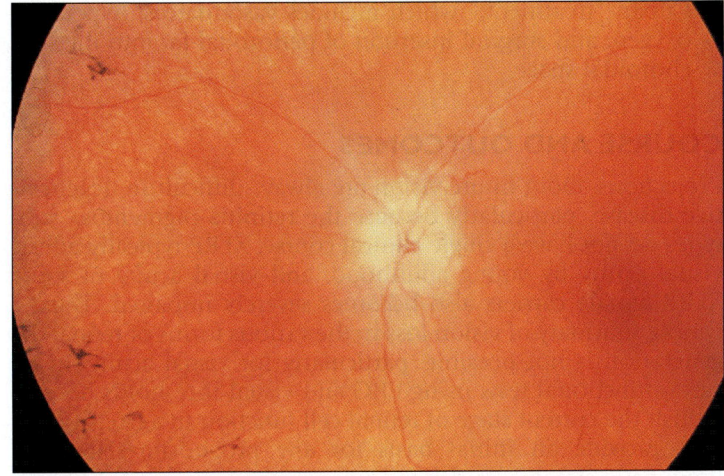

FIG. 108-10 ■ Bardet-Biedl syndrome with extensive peripheral retinal pigment epithelium thinning and parafoveal retinal pigment epithelium atrophy.

Control	pro-23-his RP

FIG. 108-11 ■ Histology of the parafoveal retina of a 73-year-old woman who had a pro-23-his rhodopsin mutation (same patient and eye as in Fig. 108-1). Only the macula retained any photoreceptors. The eyes were fixed about 1 hour postmortem. *INL,* Inner nuclear layer; *ONL,* outer nuclear layer; *IS,* inner segments; *OS,* outer segments; *RPE,* retinal pigment epithelium.)

second decade. The ophthalmologist may be among the first to suspect the diagnosis in the context of maculopathy, recent new seizure activity, and subtle mental deterioration judged by progressive difficulties at school (which initially may be blamed on the subnormal vision). Although the presentation is as a maculopathy, ERG shows widespread cone disease. Skin biopsy shows characteristic "fingerprint inclusions" under electron microscopy. If a neurologist is already involved, the diagnosis of a widespread cone dystrophy must be communicated because this may clarify the differential diagnosis. The vision loss is quite rapid and progresses to blindness within only a few years. Alternative terms include Batten-Mayou and Vogt-Spielmeyer disease.

PATHOLOGY

Gene identification has progressed rapidly since the late 1980s, and currently more than 20 different altered genes have been identified that result in retinitis pigmentosa and allied diseases. Rhodopsin was the first major retinitis pigmentosa gene to be identified.[33] As with rhodopsin, the majority of the retinitis pigmentosa genes identified thus far involve components of the phototransduction cascade within the rod photoreceptor, which include transducin, phosphodiesterase (a- and b-*PDE*), arrestin, recoverin, and the G protein–coupled Na^+/K^+ light-activated channel on the rod membrane. A second set of genes code for structural proteins in rod cells and include *RDS/peripherin*[34] and *ROM1*.[35] Developmental genes are also implicated, such as the homeobox gene *CRX* in the development of a cone-rod degeneration.[36]

The molecular mechanisms by which these genetic mutations eventually cause rod-cell death are unclear, although ample evidence indicates that apoptosis is involved in the final pathway of cell death.[37] Currently, three hypotheses are under investigation:
- Abnormal trafficking because of defective protein folding;
- Cellular metabolic disturbances; and
- "Constitutive activity" of transduction because of rhodopsin mutations.

That the cone photoreceptors ultimately die from a disease that begins with rod-cell disease remains a puzzle. One hypothesis invokes common elements of the RPE that are involved intimately in the diurnal cycle of phagocytosis of the outer-segment discs shed daily by both rods and cones. In the case of rhodopsin-mutation retinitis pigmentosa, rhodopsin is the major protein in the rod outer segments and the diurnal process of phagocytosis of the shed rod-disc membrane by the RPE may eventually result in secondary RPE pathology. With time, the RPE cannot properly service the cone photoreceptors, which subsequently die as "innocent bystanders."

Histological examination of the retina from a 73-year-old woman who had autosomal dominant retinitis pigmentosa from a pro-23-his rhodopsin mutation showed major loss of the photoreceptors (Fig. 108-11). She had 20/50 (6/15) visual acuity several months before death, and her fields were only 17°. Her fundus had typical retinitis pigmentosa changes of heavy bone-spicule pigmentation across the entire 360° periphery, and the underlying RPE was atrophic. Tissue from the parafoveal region of the left eye in the region of relative preserved retina showed:
- Photoreceptor outer segments shortened greatly, such that they are nearly absent, and the inner segments shortened;
- Number of photoreceptor nuclei (outer nuclear layer) decreased greatly, the majority of those left being multinucleated cone nuclei—nearly no rod photoreceptors remain in this end-stage retinitis pigmentosa retina;
- RPE swollen grossly by intraretinal debris, with loss of melanosomes and dispersion of pigment granules.

TREATMENT

Current treatments for retinitis pigmentosa are not highly effective, although new research developments suggest that it may be possible to slow disease progression, possibly to the extent that vision may persist for a lifetime.

Vitamin A

A long-term study of oral vitamin A palmitate supplementation (15,000IU daily) administered to 600 patients who had typical retinitis pigmentosa showed a modest but positive slowing of vision loss.[38] For all cases in aggregate, vision loss slowed to a decline of 8.3% per year compared with 10% per year in controls. Such a slight slowing of degeneration is rarely noticeable to an individual patient over a short period, but it may provide additional years of vision when spread over a lifetime. The rescue mechanism is unknown, but vitamin A is essential for the formation of light-sensitive rhodopsin. Opsin alone, in the absence of vitamin A, may exhibit a small degree of toxicity and possibly cause photoreceptor demise over a lifetime. In the same study,[38] the administration of vitamin E (400IU daily) without vitamin A speeded the degeneration by a small but statistically significant amount. However, when combined with vitamin A, vitamin E did not substantially alter the slowing of progression afforded by vitamin A palmitate alone, and thus the modest amount of vitamin E in multivitamin formulations may not be detrimental when taken along with vitamin A. If this treatment is suggested, the patient is advised to use vitamin A for the long term and to expect no immediate benefit in vision. Yearly checks of serum liver enzymes and/or vitamin A levels are advisable while vitamin A is taken in high dosage, and discontinuation is necessary if pregnancy is expected.

Acetazolamide for Cystoid Macular Edema

In some patients, retinitis pigmentosa results in cystoid macular edema (CME), possibly because the efficiency with which fluid is pumped across the RPE is compromised or because of slow retinal vascular leakage. Some studies show that treatment with acetazolamide may be of benefit,[39] with an initial dose of 250mg daily, increased to 500mg daily if no effect is apparent. A trial of several weeks is warranted, with successful outcome judged by improved visual acuity on careful repeated measurements or by decreased CME on fluorescein angiography. If decreased CME is observed by fluorescein angiography after several weeks of use, the continuation of acetazolamide may be considered even if visual acuity has not improved, provided the patient is able to tolerate the drug.

Docosahexaenoic Acid

Docosahexaenoic acid (DHA), a 22:6 fatty acid, is the major lipid component of rod photoreceptor membranes and is important for the maintenance of membrane fluidity required for rods to function. Abnormal cholesterol and serum lipid levels have been reported in some retinitis pigmentosa patients,[40] and DHA levels are particularly and somewhat consistently low in XLRP patients.[41] On the basis that insufficient DHA may affect photoreceptor survival, trials are under way to determine whether DHA dietary supplementation slows progression in retinal degeneration. Because neither the benefit nor the possible detriment of any substance can be known without formal and rigorous scientific evaluation of efficacy, it is not wise to advise patients to use DHA until the outcome of these ongoing studies is known.

Neurotrophic Factors

A report in 1990 showed that intraocular injection of basic fibroblast growth factor effectively slowed photoreceptor degeneration in the RCS rat model of retinal degeneration.[42] Although no practical current therapy employs growth factors, the results demonstrate that effective therapies may be developed to slow the rate of degeneration radically in these diseases.[43]

Disproved "Treatment" Strategies

Many treatments for retinitis pigmentosa have been tried and discarded now that they have been proved ineffective. Such discredited attempts at therapy are:
- Placental implants along the sclera;
- ENCAD (daily periocular and intramuscular injections of mushroom RNA extract) treatment in Russia;
- Vasodilator drugs; and

- Cuban "treatment," which includes vasodilators, hyperbaric oxygen, and surgical insertion of periorbital fat into the subchoroidal space.

COURSE AND OUTCOMES

Projections about future vision are always difficult in degenerative disease, particularly because the retinitis pigmentosa subtypes do not have a single clinical course. XLRP typically affects visual acuity by young adulthood, and visual acuity of some XLRP female carriers also becomes severely impaired. Thus, a simple summary of vision loss in the various forms of retinal degeneration is not possible, particularly for visual acuity. In all cases, functional tests using ERG and visual thresholds best establish the current stage of retinal cell function in aggregate and thus provide an initial basis for any prognostic statement. Prognostic statements depend upon careful disease subtyping. When subtyping is elusive, analysis of whether the patient has rod-cone disease or cone-rod disease provides vision estimates that may be used for general prognosis.

REFERENCES

1. Donders FC. Beiträge zur pathologischen Anatomie des Auges. Graefes Arch Clin Exp Ophthalmol. 1855;1:106–18.
2. Nettleship E. On retinitis pigmentosa and allied diseases. R Lond Ophthalmol Hosp Rep. 1907;17:1–56.
3. Boughman JA, Conneally PM, Nance WE. Population genetic studies of retinitis pigmentosa. Am J Hum Genet. 1980;32:223–35.
4. Massof RW, Finkelstein D, Starr SJ. Bilateral symmetry of vision disorders in typical retinitis pigmentosa. Br J Ophthalmol. 1979;63:90–6.
5. Henkes HE. Does unilateral retinitis pigmentosa really exist? An ERG and EOG study of the fellow eye. In: Burian HM, Jacobson JH, eds. Clinical electroretinography. Proceedings 3rd ISCERG Symposium. London: Pergamon Press; 1966:327–50.
6. Cogan DG. Pseudoretinitis pigmentosa. Arch Ophthalmol. 1969;81:45–53.
7. Weleber RG, Carr RE, Murphy WH, et al. Phenotypic variation including retinitis pigmentosa, pattern dystrophy, and fundus flavimaculatus in a single family with a deletion of codon 153 or 154 of the peripherin/RDS gene. Arch Ophthalmol. 1993;111:1531–42.
8. Berson EL, Rosner B, Sandberg MA, Dryja TP. Ocular findings in patients with autosomal dominant retinitis pigmentosa and a rhodopsin gene defect (pro-23-his). Arch Ophthalmol. 1991;109:92–101.
9. Richards JE, Scott KM, Sieving PA. Disruption of conserved rhodopsin disulfide bond by Cys187Tyr mutation causes early and severe autosomal dominant retinitis pigmentosa. Ophthalmology. 1995;102:669–77.
10. Richards JE, Kuo C-Y, Boehnke M, Sieving PA. Rhodopsin Thr58Arg mutation in a family with autosomal dominant retinitis pigmentosa. Ophthalmology. 1991;98:1797–805.
11. Berson EL, Sandberg MA, Rosner B, et al. Natural course of retinitis pigmentosa over a three-year interval. Am J Ophthalmol. 1985;99:240–51.
12. McCulloch C, McCulloch RJP. A hereditary and clinical study of choroideremia. Trans Am Acad Ophthalmol Otolaryngol. 1948;542:160–90.
13. Simmel O, Takki K. Raised plasma-ornithine and gyrate atrophy of the choroid and retina. Lancet. 1973;2:1031–3.
14. Carr RE. Congenital stationary night blindness. Trans Am Ophthalmol Soc. 1974;LSXXII:448–85.
15. Murayama K, Sieving PA. Different rates of growth of human and monkey photopic ERG suggests two sites of light adaptation. Clin Vis Sci. 1992;7:385–92.
16. George NDL, Yates JRW, Moore AT. X-linked retinoschisis. Br J Ophthalmol. 1995;79:679–702.
17. Nathans J, Davenport CM, Maumenee IH, et al. Molecular genetics of human blue cone monochromacy. Science. 1989;245:831–4.
18. Berson EL, Sandberg MA, Rosner B, Sullivan PL. Color plates to help identify patients with blue cone monochromatism. Am J Ophthalmol. 1983;95:741–7.
19. Berson EL, Rosen JB, Simonoff EA. Electroretinographic testing as an aid in detection of carriers of X-chromosome–linked retinitis pigmentosa. Am J Ophthalmol. 1979;87:460–8.
20. Sieving PA, Niffennager J, Berson EL. The electroretinogram in selected pedigrees with choroideremia. Am J Ophthalmol. 1986;101:361–7.
21. Rowe SE, Trobe JD, Sieving PA. Idiopathic photoreceptor dysfunction causes unexplained visual acuity loss in later adulthood. Ophthalmology. 1990;97:1632–7.
22. Marmor MF, Arden GB, Nilsson SE, Zrenner E. International Standardization Committee: standards for clinical electroretinography. Arch Ophthalmol. 1989;107:816–19.
23. Berson EL, Guras P, Hoff M. Temporal aspects of the electroretinogram. Arch Ophthalmol. 1969;81:207–14.
24. Meredith TA, Aaberg TM, Willerson D. Progressive chorioretinopathy after receiving thioridazine. Arch Ophthalmol. 1978;96:1172–6.
25. Yanoff M. The retina in rubella. In: Tasman W, ed. Retinal disease in children. New York: Harper & Row; 1971:223–32.
26. Boldi FC, Hervouet F. Syphilitic chorioretinitis. Arch Ophthalmol. 1968;79:294–6.
27. Skalka W. Asymmetric retinitis pigmentosa, luetic retinopathy and the question of unilateral retinitis pigmentosa. Acta Ophthalmol. 1979;57:351–7.
28. Matsubara S, Yamaji Y, Sato M, et al. Expression of a photoreceptor protein, recoverin, as a cancer-associated retinopathy autoantigen in human lung cancer cell lines. Br J Cancer. 1996;74:1419–22.

29. Milam AH, Saari JC, Jacobson SG, et al. Autoantibodies against retinal bipolar cells in cutaneous melanoma-associated retinopathy. Invest Ophthalmol Vis Sci. 1993;34:91–100.

30. Kim RY, Retsas S, Fitzke FW, et al. Cutaneous melanoma-associated retinopathy. Ophthalmology. 1994;101:1837–43.

31. Kellner U, Bornfeld N, Foerster MH. Severe course of cutaneous melanoma associated paraneoplastic retinopathy. Br J Ophthalmol. 1995;79:746–52.

32. Boughman JA, Vernon M, Shaver KA. Usher syndrome: definition and estimate of prevalence from two high-risk populations. J Chronic Dis. 1983;36:595–603.

33. Dryja TP, McGee TL, Reichel E, et al. A point mutation of the rhodopsin gene in one form of retinitis pigmentosa. Nature. 1990;343:364–6.

34. Farrar GJ, Kenna P, Jordan SA, et al. A three-base-pair deletion in the peripherin-RDS gene in one form of retinitis pigmentosa. Nature. 1991;354:478–80.

35. Kajiwara K, Berson EL, Dryja TP. Digenic retinitis pigmentosa due to mutations at the unlinked peripherin/RDS and ROM1 loci. Science. 1994;264:1604–8.

36. Swain PK, Wang Q-L, Chen S, et al. Mutations in the cone-rod homeobox gene are associated with the cone-rod dystrophy photoreceptor degeneration. Neuron. 1997; 19:1329–36.

37. Chang G-Q, Hao Y, Wong F. Apoptosis: final common pathway of photoreceptor death in rd, rds, and rhodopsin mutant mice. Neuron. 1993;11:595–605.

38. Berson EL, Rosner B, Sandberg MA, et al. A randomized trial of vitamin A and vitamin E supplementation for retinitis pigmentosa. Arch Ophthalmol. 1993;111: 761–72.

39. Steinmertz RL, Fitzke FW, Bird ZC. Treatment of cystoid macular edema with acetazolamide in a patient with serpiginous choriodopathy. Retina. 1991;11:412–15.

40. Converse CA, McLachlan T, Hammer HM. Hyperlipidemia in retinitis pigmentosa. In: LaVail MM, Anderson RE, Hollyfield JG, eds. Retinal degenerations. New York: Alan R Liss; 1985:63–74.

41. Hoffman DR, Birch DG. Docosahexaenoic acid in red blood cells of patients with X-linked retinitis pigmentosa. Retina. 1995;36:1009–18.

42. Faktorovich EG, Steinberg RH, Yasumura D, et al. Photoreceptor degeneration in inherited retina dystrophy delayed by basic fibroblast growth factor. Nature. 1990; 347:83–6.

43. Steinberg RH. Survival factors in retinal degenerations. Curr Opin Neurobiol. 1994;4:515–24.

109 Macular Dystrophies

KIMBERLY DRESNER • KENT W. SMALL

DEFINITION

- The process of premature retinal cell aging and cell death, generally confined to the macula, in which no clear demonstrable extrinsic cause is evident, and a heritable genetically determined enzymatic defect is implicated.

KEY FEATURES

- Yellowish material within or beneath the retinal pigment epithelium.
- Loss of macular photoreceptors and retinal pigment epithelial cells.
- Loss of central vision.

ASSOCIATED FEATURES

- Neural retinal, retinal pigment epithelial, and choroidal atrophy commonly limited to the macula.
- Bull's-eye appearance seen rarely.
- Pigment clumps in the posterior pole, midperiphery, or far periphery seen rarely.
- Optic atrophy, retinal vascular attenuation, macular edema, and choroidal neovascularization seen rarely.

INTRODUCTION

The intricate anatomy of the retina is paralleled, perhaps, only by its complex physiology. Certainly, to have such a well-orchestrated, form-following function, many genes must be involved in the development of the macula. Modern genetics has helped to identify a few genetic defects implicated in some of the various macular dystrophies. Unfortunately, until more information is available as to which genetic problem leads to a specific macular dystrophy, classification of the various disorders will not be perfect. The difficulty is that many of the disorders exhibit histological abnormalities in all layers of the neural retina, retinal pigment epithelium (RPE), and choroids. Different genetic disorders may have overlapping phenotypes and, in the end stages, many diseases can appear identical. Conversely, the same genetic abnormality may show different phenotypes, even within the same pedigree. Therefore, to determine a specific macular dystrophy, a constellation of clinical characteristics and ancillary tests must be relied upon.

Most macular dystrophies share the clinical manifestation of accumulated yellowish material within the macular region. The course of each particular disease, however, can be quite different. It, therefore, is important to differentiate clinically among the disorders to be able to give the patient the best genetic counseling and advice on visual prognosis.

No treatment is available for any of the disorders discussed in this chapter. Laser therapy may be used in an attempt to halt the progression of choroidal neovascularization, when present. In this chapter the focus is specifically on macular dystrophies not associated with other systemic abnormalities.

STARGARDT'S DISEASE AND FUNDUS FLAVIMACULATUS

EPIDEMIOLOGY AND PATHOGENESIS

Usually, Stargardt's disease is inherited as an autosomal recessive trait; however, affected families that have autosomal dominance have been described.[1] Stargardt's disease is the most prevalent inherited macular dystrophy and accounts for roughly 7% of all retinal dystrophies.

The autosomal recessive form of the disease was mapped to the short arm of chromosome 1.[1,3] An adenosine triphosphate–binding cassette, the *ABCR* gene (now called *ABCA4*), has been identified as the causative gene. Fundus flavimaculatus and Stargardt's disease are now known to be allelic. However, only about 60% of patients with these diseases have a detected mutation in this gene. This locus has also been implicated in age-related macular degeneration and autosomal recessive retinitis pigmentosa.[2] A knock-out mouse model of Stargardt's disease has been created.[3] The heterozygous mouse also has an accumulation of lipofuscin, supporting the role of *ABCA4's* in age-related macular degeneration.

Autosomal dominant Stargardt's disease originally was mapped to chromosome 13 as *STGD2*. More recently, this has been found to be in error, and dominant Stargardt's disease maps to chromosome 6q16.6 in association with the mutation found on the *ELOVL4* gene.[1] This finding lumps autosomal dominant Stargardt's with several other retinal diseases mapping to chromosome 6.[4]

OCULAR MANIFESTATIONS AND DIAGNOSIS

The term *fundus flavimaculatus* is used when the characteristic flecks that accumulate at the level of the RPE are distributed throughout the fundus and onset is in adulthood. The term *Stargardt's disease* is applied when the flecks are confined mostly to the posterior pole and are present early in life.

An accumulation of discrete "pisciform" flecks at the level of the RPE is a hallmark of the disease (Fig. 109-1).[5,6] The distribu-

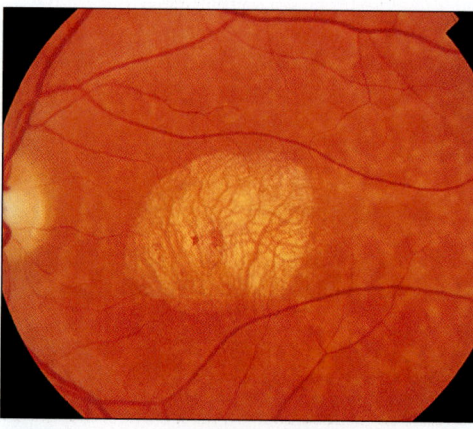

FIG. 109-1
Stargardt's disease

tion of the flecks and the time of their appearance can vary, but the flecks seen in Stargardt's disease are found mostly at the posterior pole and macula. Patients often may have minimal ophthalmoscopic abnormalities early in the disease, but later many flecks, along with patches of central atrophy, can develop. In other patients, particularly those who have fundus flavimaculatus, peripheral flecks only may be seen with a macula of a reasonably normal appearance. Geographical, atrophic RPE patches often coalesce to give the macula a "beaten bronze" appearance.

The most characteristic finding on fluorescein angiography is the phenomenon known as the "dark" or "silent" choroids, which appears as a prominent retinal circulation against hypofluorescent choroids. Although this finding helps to make the diagnosis, it is not seen in up to one fourth of the cases of Stargardt's disease.[7] The flecks, themselves, do not stain with fluorescein.

The electroretinogram findings are normal early but may be reduced moderately in more advanced cases. Also, the electrooculogram (Arden ratio) may be reduced mildly when there are extensive RPE changes. Patients who have Stargardt's disease can exhibit delayed dark adaptation.[8] The differential diagnosis of Stargardt's disease and fundus flavimaculatus is given in Table 109-1.

TABLE 109-1
DIFFERENTIAL DIAGNOSIS OF MACULAR DYSTROPHIES

Disease	Differential Diagnosis
Stargardt's disease and fundus flavimaculatus	Cone dystrophy
	Neuronal ceroid lipofuscinosis
	Pattern dystrophy
Best's disease and vitelliform dystrophy	Age-related macular degeneration
	Pattern dystrophy
Adult vitelliform degeneration	Best's disease
	Pattern dystrophy
	Age-related macular degeneration
Familial (dominant) drusen	Flecked retinal syndromes
	Sorsby's fundus dystrophy
	Age-related macular degeneration
Dominant cystoid macular edema	Dominantly inherited retinitis pigmentosa with cystoid macular edema
	X-linked juvenile retinoschisis
	Goldmann-Favre syndrome
North Carolina macular dystrophy	Toxoplasmosis
	Age-related macular degeneration
Progressive bifocal chorioretinal atrophy	Atrophea areata
	North Carolina macular dystrophy
	Myopic macular degeneration
Atrophea areata	Serpiginous choroiditis
	Peripapillary pigment epithelial dystrophy
	Angioid streaks
	Progressive bifocal chorioretinal atrophy
	Myopic macular degeneration
Cone degeneration (dystrophy)	Stargardt's disease
	Hereditary optic atrophies
	Toxic maculopathy
Central areolar choroidal dystrophy	Sorsby's fundus dystrophy
	North Carolina macular dystrophy
	Angioid streaks
	Stargardt's disease
	Cone dystrophy
	Progressive bifocal chorioretinal atrophy
	Serpiginous choroiditis
	Acute multifocal placoid pigment epitheliopathy

PATHOLOGY

Pathological evaluation shows an accumulation of lipofuscin-like pigment throughout the RPE, although its origin and significance remain unknown[9] (Fig. 109-2). The mouse model (abcr–/–) also has accumulation of a lipofuscin material, the toxic bis-retinoid, N-retinylidene-N retinylethanolamine (A2E) suggesting a significant role in the pathophysiology of the disease.[3]

TREATMENT, COURSE, AND OUTCOME

Tremendous variability occurs in course and outcome among the various pedigrees and even within individual families. Decreased visual acuity is the main symptom and may appear as early as the first decade or much later in middle age.

The visual acuity ranges between 20/50 and 20/200, depending on the degree of macular atrophy. Most patients retain a visual acuity of between 20/70 and 20/100 in at least one eye. The prognosis is worse for patients with fundus flavimaculatus, and the duration predicts the severity more accurately.[6,7] Less commonly, patients who have severe peripheral atrophy manifest visual field loss that may be difficult to differentiate from a rod–cone dystrophy. As with all the retinal dystrophies, no known treatment exists for the disease.

Because ABCA4 is involved in vitamin A processing within the photoreceptors, it is suspected that vitamin A supplements might make the disease worse. Therefore the authors do not recommend vitamins A or B-carotene vitamin supplements.

BEST'S DISEASE AND VITELLIFORM DYSTROPHY

EPIDEMIOLOGY AND PATHOGENESIS

Best's disease is extremely rare—the actual incidence is unknown. The disease is autosomal dominantly inherited and shows highly variable clinical expression. Furthermore, some individuals who carry the defective gene have completely normal vision and fundus examination findings.[10] Such individuals have been referred to as carriers of Best's disease, but this is a misnomer. The gene for Best's disease was mapped to chromosome 11q13 and mutations found in the bestrophin (VMD2) gene. This is a transmembrane protein of undetermined function.[11,12] The protein is expressed in the RPE. Several mutations within the bestrophin gene have been identified and are associated with both Best's and adult vitelliform diseases.[13]

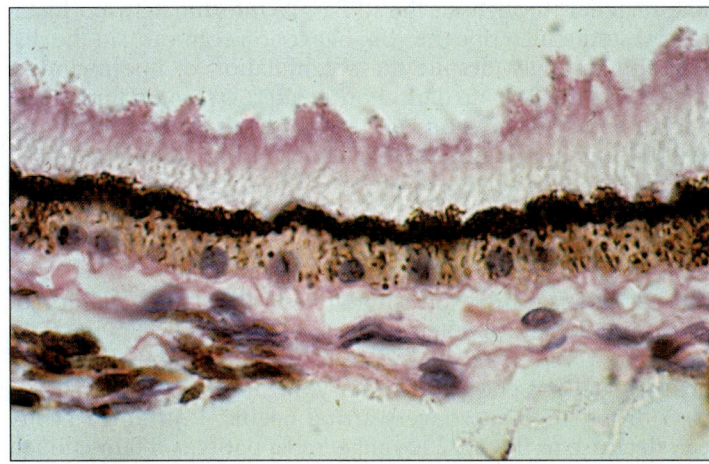

FIG. 109-2 ■ Stargardt's disease (fundus flavimaculatus). Note the fluorescein effect caused by enlarged lipofuscin-containing retinal pigment epithelial cells, which act as a fluorescent filter. (Case reported by Eagle RC Jr, et al. Ophthalmology. 1980;7:1189.)

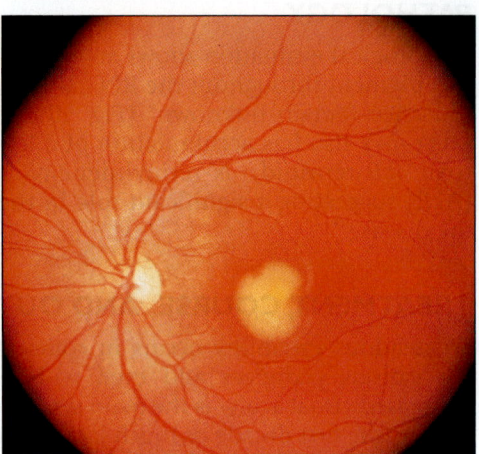

FIG. 109-3 ■ Best's disease. Typical vitelliform lesion from an 11-year-old girl. (Courtesy of Ola Sandgren, University Hospital of Umeå, Sweden.)

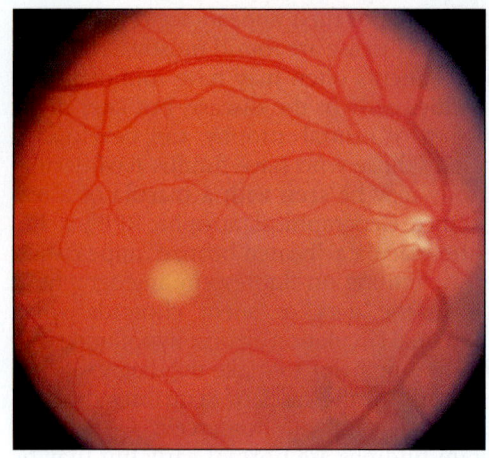

FIG. 109-4 ■ Adult vitelliform degeneration. (Reproduced with permission from Feist RM, White MF Jr, Skalka H, Stone BM. Choroidal neovascularization in a patient with adult foveomacular dystrophy. Am J Ophthalmol. 1994;118:259–60.)

OCULAR MANIFESTATIONS AND DIAGNOSIS

Best's disease is typified by a large, yellow, yolk-like (vitelliform) lesion (Fig. 109-3) that is bilateral and symmetrical in the central macula and appears during childhood. The diameter is in the range 1–5mm. Later in life, the lesion breaks down, with resultant scarring and atrophy. Late lesions often are difficult to diagnose correctly on the basis of their clinical appearance alone. Less commonly, the lesions may be multifocal.[14,15] Choroidal neovascularization can arise adjacent to old vitelliform scars.[15,16]

Early in the disease process, vitelliform dystrophy has such a characteristic "egg yolk" appearance that the diagnosis is not difficult to make. In longstanding cases, or when a fundus of normal appearance is seen, the definitive diagnosis is made on the basis of abnormal electro-oculogram findings. Specifically, a severe loss of the light response of the standing potential occurs. All affected individuals, whether they have funduscopic manifestations or not, have a light-to-dark (or Arden) ratio of less than 1.5 and frequently near 1.1. For this reason, the electro-oculogram is used to evaluate individuals who have a poorly defined macular lesion.

Electroretinographic studies show a reduced "C" wave but are otherwise normal. This is the only disease with relatively normal electroretinographic results associated with abnormal electro-oculographic findings. The differential diagnosis is shown in Table 109-1.

PATHOLOGY

Histopathological studies show an accumulation of lipofuscin-like material throughout the RPE.[17–20] Unfortunately, no histological studies describe the yolk-like lesion seen early in the disease. Interestingly, despite the accumulation of lipofuscin-like material in the RPE, no dark choroid effect is seen on fluorescein angiography. Furthermore, decreased visual acuity results from atrophy and scarring in the macula, not from accumulated material in the RPE.

TREATMENT, COURSE, AND OUTCOME

The age of onset and expression of Best's disease is variable. For most individuals, manifestation of the disease occurs in childhood; however, occasionally onset is in adulthood. The visual acuity usually is good when the "yolk" remains intact. The vision drops, however, once scarring begins.[14] Although acuity can decrease to the 20/200 range, most patients retain enough vision in at least one eye to read and drive. Choroidal neovascular membrane formation is infrequent but may arise from an old scar.[14]

ADULT VITELLIFORM DEGENERATION

EPIDEMIOLOGY AND PATHOGENESIS

This rare dystrophy usually does not have a discernible inheritance pattern. Some patients with adult foveomacular dystrophies, however, have an autosomal dominant trait with mutations in the peripherin/RDS gene.[21] Mutations in the bestrophin gene, VMD2, have also been associated with adult vitelliform degeneration.[11] Some authors consider the foveomacular dystrophy to be a variant of the pattern dystrophies (see later).

OCULAR MANIFESTATIONS AND DIAGNOSIS

Affected individuals show symmetrical, yellowish foveal deposits that resemble the lesions of Best's disease but are smaller (Fig. 109-4). The phenotype can vary from small "yolks" as seen in adults who have widespread, fine, cuticular drusen, to only subtle accumulations of yellowish material in the central fovea.

Examples of the adult vitelliform degenerations include foveomacular dystrophy of Gass, and adults who have coalescent, widespread, cuticular drusen that form vitelliform lesions in the macula.[22]

These disorders usually are distinguished from Best's disease on the basis of a normal or only minimally reduced electro-oculogram. The full-field electroretinogram is normal, but the foveal electroretinogram may be reduced (Arden ratio <1.7). Also, by definition, adult vitelliform macular dystrophies have a presumed adult onset, although this has not been well documented in most reports. The differential diagnosis is given in Table 109-1.

It should be noted that VMD1 (also called *atypical vitelliform macular dystrophy*) no longer exists as a genetic locus and probably as a disease entity. The original mapping of VMD1 to a chromosome 8 locus has recently been shown to be excluded by newer, more informative genetic markers.[23]

PATHOLOGY

Histopathological analyses of these patients' eyes have demonstrated damage at the level of the RPE. Focal loss of the photoreceptors overlie atrophic RPE cells in the fovea. Pigmented material is seen to lie between the retina and Bruch's membrane. Gass[22] found no abnormal accumulation of lipofuscin in RPE cells. Patrinely et al.[17] on the other hand, found high concentrations of lipofuscin in RPE cells and postulated that this accumulation is responsible for the foveal lesion.

TREATMENT, COURSE, AND OUTCOME

The onset of these disorders usually is during the fourth to sixth decade, with visual symptoms generally limited to metamorphopsia or mildly blurred vision. The overall prognosis of adult vitelliform dystrophy is similar to that of Best's disease, in that as the yolk-like accumulations break down, atrophy and gliotic scarring occur, leading to decreased visual acuity. It is important to distinguish adult vitelliform dystrophy from Best's disease because of the potential genetic implications and need for appropriate genetic counseling.

FAMILIAL DRUSEN

EPIDEMIOLOGY AND PATHOGENESIS

Familial (dominant) drusen is a rare autosomal dominant disease with variable expression and age-dependent penetrance.[24] A mutation from an arginine to a tryptophan at amino acid 345 in the *EFEMP1* locus has been associated with both Doyne's and malattia leventinese, which are, therefore, the same disease.[25] Another locus on chromosome 6q14 adjacent to the cone–rod dystrophy gene *(CORD7)* and the North Carolina dystrophy gene *(NCMD)* has also been identified in those with dominant drusen.[26-29] However, these cases are more consistent with North Carolina macular dystrophy with only drusen present and were misdiagnosed as dominant drusen. The various phenotypic patterns have resulted in a number of different names in the older literature, such as Doyne's honeycomb dystrophy, malattia leventinese, and guttate choroiditis.

This disease is thought to arise from an inborn error of metabolism localized to the RPE. One hypothesis is that the defect is in an intercellular matrix protein or a structural protein, which leads to the development of abnormal basement membranes. Although diffuse drusen often are described as being inherited dominantly, to identify a significant family history is difficult because affected individuals usually are not recognized until middle age, when other potentially affected family members are very old or deceased.

OCULAR MANIFESTATIONS AND DIAGNOSIS

Patients exhibit widespread drusen that extend beyond the macula, in a pattern distinct from age-related drusen (Fig. 109-5).[30,31] Typically, diffuse drusen extend peripherally to the macula and involve retina nasal to the optic disc. The drusen, themselves, may be large and sparse or form a constellation of tiny dots, called *cuticular* or *basal laminar drusen*. Sometimes, basal laminar drusen coalesce to form a vitelliform lesion.[32] The drusen usually first appear around the third or fourth decade of life and become quite numerous by middle age. In the late stages, pigmentations occur, along with atrophy of the RPE, choriocapillaris, and large choroidal vessels. Flecks in this disorder are whiter and more sharply delineated than those in fundus flavimaculatus.

Fluorescein angiography often highlights atrophy of the RPE, and the drusen appear more extensive than seen clinically. In advanced cases, a central scotoma is seen on visual field examination. Dark adaptation is usually normal, as are the electroretinographic findings. The electro-oculographic findings are normal in the initial stages, but they become subnormal depending on the degree of macular involvement. The differential diagnosis is shown in Table 109-1.

PATHOLOGY

Histopathological examinations show round accumulations of hyaline in the pigment epithelium that are continuous with the inner layer of Bruch's membrane.[33] The choroids and neural

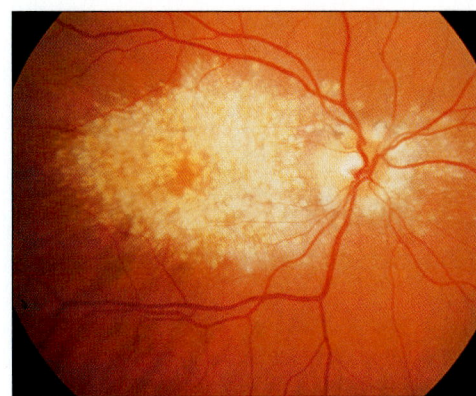

FIG. 109-5 ■ Familial drusen. (Reproduced with permission from Evans K, Gregory CY, Wijesuriya SD, *et al.* Assessment of the phenotypic range seen in Doyne honeycomb retinal dystrophy. Arch Ophthalmol. 1997;115:904–10.)

retina may show atrophy later on, although they appear normal in the earlier stages of the disease.

TREATMENT, COURSE, AND OUTCOME

No known effective treatment exists for diseases in this category. If choroidal neovascularization ensues, laser treatment may stabilize vision, but rarely.

As long as the drusen are relatively discrete and do not affect the fovea markedly, central vision usually is good. Some suggestions exist that affected patients may be at greater risk for degenerative changes in the macula as a result of aging. When basal laminar drusen coalesce to form a vitelliform cyst, a marked degradation in visual acuity can occur if the yolk degenerates into an atrophic scar. Choroidal neovascularization may occur occasionally.

PATTERN DYSTROPHY

EPIDEMIOLOGY AND PATHOGENESIS

The incidence of the pattern dystrophies is unknown; however, they are fairly rare. A number of hereditary patterns are documented. Some autosomal dominant forms of the disease are associated with mutations in peripherin, a retinal protein encoded by a gene located on chromosome 6p.[34] Interestingly, some forms of retinitis pigmentosa, as well as other macular dystrophies (such as the adult foveomacular dystrophy of Gass), are attributed to mutations in this same protein.[35,36] Within a family, some affected patients may manifest retinitis pigmentosa, while others phenotypically appear to have a macular dystrophy. Some patients with butterfly dystrophy have a mutation located at the peripherin/*RDS* gene, although most patients who have pattern dystrophy do not have mutations in the peripherin gene.[37,38]

Current hypotheses as to how mutations in the peripherin protein result in the disease suggest that the abnormal peripherin molecules, which normally are present in photoreceptor outer segments, interfere with RPE metabolism after phagocytosis of the outdated outer-segment material.

OCULAR MANIFESTATIONS AND DIAGNOSIS

This heterogeneous group of disorders is characterized by reticular pigmentation at the level of the RPE.[39,40] Yellow flecks and drusen typically are not found. The clinical phenotypes often take on a characteristic pattern (Fig. 109-6) and, thus, some of these disorders have acquired descriptive names such as *butterfly dystrophy*. Often, no specific pattern exists, and many individuals within affected families have different patterns of pigmentation. Sjögren's reticular dystrophy, an autosomal recessive–pattern dystrophy, is characterized by a network of pigmented lines that surround the macula. Butterfly dystrophy, on the other hand, can

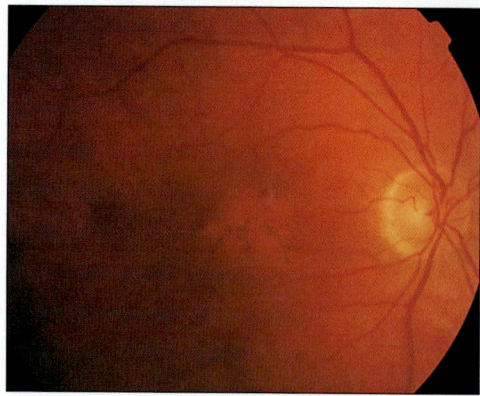

FIG. 109-6 ■ Pattern dystrophy.

be autosomal dominant and demonstrates pigment deposits that radiate from the fovea in the pattern of butterfly wings. However, we now recognize the error of "splitting" these diseases based on such findings as a butterfly shape of pigment in a single individual when findings in other family members have a different appearance. Less commonly, yellowish deposits similar to those found in foveomacular dystrophy or Stargardt's disease are seen.

The diagnosis often is based on the characteristic findings discovered on ophthalmoscopy or angiography, as described above. Electrophysiological testing results usually are normal, but a borderline electro-oculogram result is consistent with a diffuse RPE disorder. Late in the disease, the electroretinogram result may be mildly subnormal as a result of diffuse damage to the photoreceptors.

PATHOLOGY

To the authors' knowledge, a histological study has not been performed for this disease, but it is thought to be a primary abnormality of the RPE in the macula.[40]

TREATMENT, COURSE, AND OUTCOME

The usual initial symptom is slightly diminished visual acuity or mild metamorphopsia. However, many patients who have the disorder are asymptomatic and disease is discovered during routine ophthalmoscopy. Visual acuity usually is good through the first five or six decades of life. The prognosis for maintaining good visual acuity is excellent, except in those patients who develop geographical macular atrophy, which mimics age-related macular degeneration, in old age. A small risk exists of developing choroidal neovascularization later in life.

DOMINANT CYSTOID MACULAR EDEMA

EPIDEMIOLOGY AND PATHOGENESIS

This is an extremely rare autosomal dominant disease that was mapped to chromosome 7q using linkage analysis.[41] Interestingly, autosomal dominant retinitis pigmentosa, known as RP9, also maps to this region.

In contrast to other diseases that affect the macula, this disorder appears to be unique in that the inner nuclear layer of the retina is the site primarily affected. Müller's cells are the specific cellular constituents thought to be involved, based on histopathological evidence.[42]

OCULAR MANIFESTATIONS AND DIAGNOSIS

Ophthalmoscopy reveals multilobulated cysts in the macula. Later in the course of the disease, macular disease of an atrophic appearance develops. Peripheral pigmentary changes may be present.

Ancillary testing with fluorescein angiography shows capillary leakage, with petaloid dye accumulation in the macula. Electrophysiology shows normal electroretinographic findings, but subnormal electro-oculographic light peak–to–dark trough ratios have been found, and abnormal dark-adaptation studies have been documented.[42] The differential diagnosis is given in Table 109-1.

PATHOLOGY

Histopathological studies demonstrate macular cysts, disorganized and gliotic inner nuclear layer, focal Müller's cell necrosis, epiretinal membrane formation, and abnormal deposition of basement membrane in the perivascular space. Degenerative changes also have been seen in the RPE and photoreceptors of the macula.[43] Histopathological features seen in dominantly inherited cystoid macular edema, namely the involvement of Müller's cells, are quite different from those features seen in cystoid macular edema secondary to other causes.

TREATMENT, COURSE, AND OUTCOME

Patients first begin to notice decreasing visual acuity at about 30 years of age, with slowly progressive worsening to a moderate or severe level years later. Advanced cases have maculae of atrophic appearance, with window defects seen on fluorescein angiography. As in all the macular dystrophies, no known effective treatment exists.

SORSBY'S MACULAR DYSTROPHY

EPIDEMIOLOGY AND PATHOGENESIS

This is an extremely rare, dominantly inherited disorder, with many clinical similarities to age-related macular degeneration. A gene for Sorsby's dystrophy that codes for a tissue inhibitor metalloproteinase, TIMP-3, has been identified.[44] TIMP-3 has been cloned and linked to chromosome 22.[45,46] Several mutations of TIMP-3 have been identified in patients with Sorsby's dystrophy. The gene product is an important enzyme in the regulation and composition of the extracellular matrix and is critical for wound healing, bone adaptation, and organ hypertrophy. This enzyme is expressed in the RPE.[47] No association exists between TIMP-3 mutations and age-related macular degeneration.

OCULAR MANIFESTATIONS AND DIAGNOSIS

Early in the disease process, several very fine drusen or a large confluent plaque of yellowish material may be noted beneath the central RPE. Then, typically at around 40 years of age, patients develop bilateral exudative maculopathy, which leaves heavily pigmented macular scars and areas of geographical atrophy.[48]

The electroretinogram and electro-oculogram results usually are normal, but decreased photopic and scotopic electroretinographic amplitudes can be seen late in the disease.

PATHOLOGY

Light and electron microscopic studies show lipid-containing deposits between the basement membrane and the pigment epithelium and the inner collagenous layers of Bruch's membrane.[49]

TREATMENT, COURSE, AND OUTCOME

Patients typically develop bilateral choroidal neovascularization at an early age. Severe loss of central visual acuity results from extensive macular scarring related to the choroidal neovascular membranes. Attempts at laser treatment have had poor results.[50]

Later, vision can decrease to light perception only. Nyctalopia also is a symptom late in the course of disease.[48]

NORTH CAROLINA MACULAR DYSTROPHY

EPIDEMIOLOGY AND PATHOGENESIS

North Carolina macular dystrophy is an autosomal dominant macular degeneration first discovered in a large family in North Carolina, after which the disease was inappropriately named. It has a rare incidence but is found worldwide in over 25 families (Small, personal communication). Several separate affected families have been discovered in the United States, Europe, and Central America. This disorder is now known as MCDR1 (macular dystrophy, retinal subtype, first one mapped). Linkage analysis of the large family from North Carolina mapped the diseased gene to chromosome 6q16.[51,52] Further genetic analysis reveals that families reported to have central areolar pigment epithelial dystrophy and central pigment and choroidal degeneration are branches of the same family from North Carolina.[53] Indeed, reports of various branches of the single family from North Carolina have resulted in this one disease being given 7 different names during the last 25 years. Again, "lumping" diseases has proven to be more accurate than "splitting."

OCULAR MANIFESTATIONS AND DIAGNOSIS

The most striking feature in about one third of affected individuals is a macular coloboma (Fig. 109-7), with well-demarcated atrophy of the RPE and choriocapillaris. A highly variable phenotypic expression occurs from family member to family member. Some individuals express only a few drusen, while others have disciform scars of the central macular area. Choroidal neovascularization can occur. The electroretinogram and electrooculogram results are normal, as is color vision. The differential diagnosis is given in Table 109-1.

PATHOLOGY

Recently Small *et al.*[54] have studied the histopathology of a mildly affected family member who had bilaterally symmetrical confluent drusen in the central macula. Light microscopy demonstrated a discrete macular lesion characterized by focal absence of photoreceptor cells and RPE. Bruch's membrane was attenuated in the center of the lesion and associated with marked atrophy of the choriocapillaris. Adjacent to the central lesion, some lipofuscin was identified in the RPE.

TREATMENT, COURSE, AND OUTCOME

The onset is congenital and nonprogressive. Visual acuity is usually much better than the appearance of the macula suggests. In general, vision is in the 20/20 to 20/200 range, with a median of 20/60. Some individuals may develop progressive worsening of vision secondary to choroidal neovascularization.

PROGRESSIVE BIFOCAL CHORIORETINAL ATROPHY

EPIDEMIOLOGY AND PATHOGENESIS

Progressive bifocal chorioretinal atrophy is a rare (reported only in the United Kingdom) degeneration that is inherited in an autosomal dominant fashion with complete penetrance. The pigment epithelium is thought to be the primary site of involvement. This disease has been mapped to a region overlapping *MCDR1* on chromosome 6.[55,56]

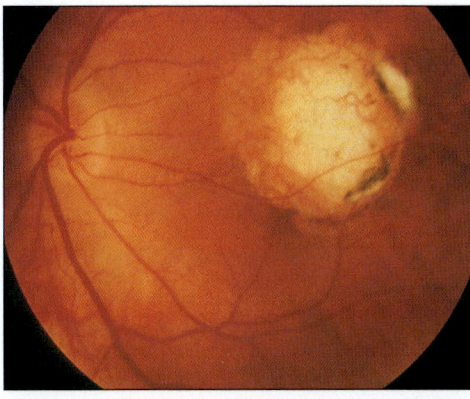

FIG. 109-7 ■ North Carolina macular dystrophy. Macular coloboma in an 18-year-old woman with visual acuity of 20/40 (6/12).

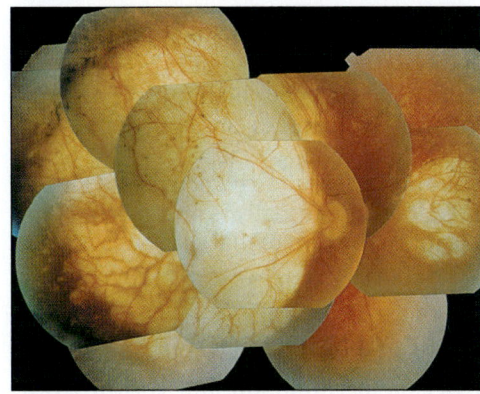

FIG. 109-8 ■ Progressive bifocal chorioretinal atrophy. (Reproduced with permission from Godley BF, Tiffin PA, Evans K, et al. Clinical features of progressive bifocal chorioretinal atrophy: a retinal dystrophy linked to chromosome 6q. Ophthalmology. 1996;103:893–8.)

OCULAR MANIFESTATIONS AND DIAGNOSIS

An initial focus of atrophic retina and choroids is seen temporal to the disc. The focus enlarges in all directions, and the temporal border typically has a serrated edge. Although the atrophy extends to the equator, it does not cross the vertical midline. Later in the disease process, a second nasal atrophic site appears that also slowly and progressively enlarges in all directions, but it also does not cross the vertical midline. The end-stage funduscopic appearance has the unusual image of two separate foci of chorioretinal atrophy, with an intervening segment of normal retina (Fig. 109-8). The diagnosis is made chiefly on the basis of the unusual clinical appearance.[57]

TREATMENT, COURSE, AND OUTCOME

Progressive bifocal chorioretinal atrophy usually is already present at birth and is progressive. Visual acuity loss corresponds to the level and proximity of chorioretinal atrophy of the fovea. Visual loss is usually severe and frequently nystagmus is found. No treatment is effective.

ATROPHIA AREATA

EPIDEMIOLOGY AND PATHOGENESIS

Atrophia areata is a rare autosomal dominant disease reported only in Icelandic families. This disorder, also referred to as helicoid peripapillary chorioretinal degeneration, has been mapped to chromosome 11p15.[58] Although no histological studies exist, it appears that the RPE and choroid are the primary sites affected.

OCULAR MANIFESTATIONS AND DIAGNOSIS

As with most inherited retinal diseases, atrophia areata is a bilateral, symmetrical maculopathy and has an early onset.[58] Marked choroidal atrophy radiates from the optic disc, with two or more

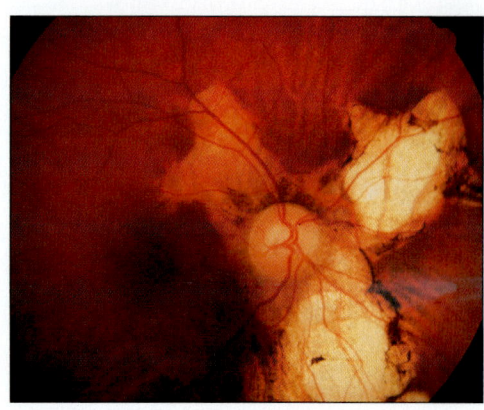

FIG. 109-9 ■ **Atrophia areata in a 37-year-old man.** (Courtesy of Fridbert Jonasson, University Department of Ophthalmology, Landspítalinn, Iceland.)

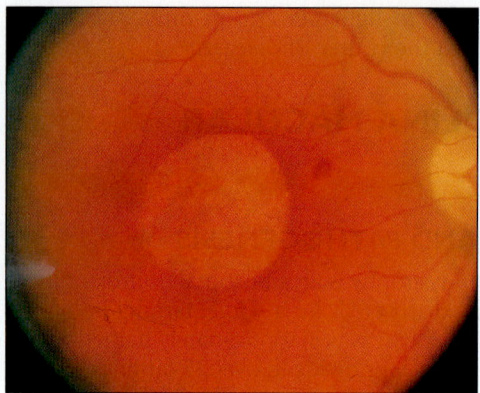

FIG. 109-10 ■ Cone degeneration. (Reproduced with permission from Small KW, Gehrs K. Clinical study of a large family with autosomal dominant progressive cone degeneration. Am J Ophthalmol. 1996;121:1–12.)

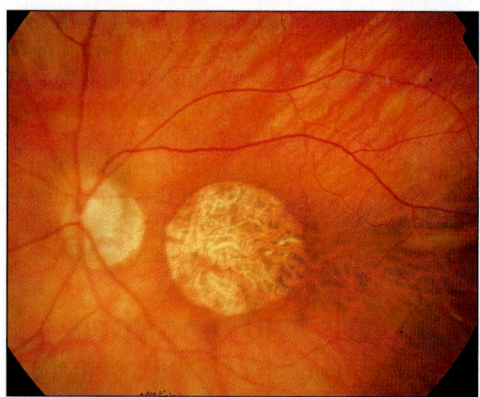

FIG. 109-11 ■ Central areolar choroidal dystrophy. (Courtesy of Giuliani Silvestri.

ring-shaped extensions that do not follow the major retinal vessels (Fig. 109-9). The choroidal vessels drop out in areas of atrophy. This disorder often is associated with high myopic astigmatism. Anterior polar cataracts sometimes are seen in affected persons.

The funduscopic appearance is quite characteristic, particularly in advanced cases. Color vision usually is normal, and high myopia is a consistent feature. The differential diagnosis is given in Table 109-1.

TREATMENT, COURSE, AND OUTCOME

Chorioretinal atrophy begins in childhood and is slowly progressive throughout life. Young patients usually have good visual acuity, but a gradual decline occurs in central vision as macular atrophy ensues.

CONE DEGENERATION

EPIDEMIOLOGY AND PATHOGENESIS

Cone degenerations are a heterogeneous group of disorders characterized by an inherited selective degeneration of cone photoreceptor cells. The mode of inheritance is autosomal dominant in most described cases, but sporadic, sex-linked, and autosomal recessive forms occur as well. Small et al.[59,60] found a single large family from eastern Tennessee with autosomal dominant cone degeneration (designated CORD 5 by Human Genome Organization) and mapped it to chromosome 17p12-13. A similar disease, CORD 6, was subsequently mapped nearby. Eventually, both CORD 5 and CORD 6 were found to be caused by the same mutations in retinal guanylate cyclase 1 (GUCY2D).[61,62] Again, "lumping" is better than "splitting." Mutations in the cone–rod homeobox (CRX) as well as the ABCR gene have also been associated with cone degeneration.[2]

OCULAR MANIFESTATIONS AND DIAGNOSIS

Hallmarks of cone degeneration include the triad of progressive central acuity loss, color vision disturbances, and photophobia.[55,56] Ophthalmoscopic findings can be highly variable. Fundus findings can range from a subtle, diffuse macular granularity only, to a well-demarcated, circular atrophic area in the macular region[55] (Fig. 109-10).

Special color vision testing with the Farnsworth-Munswell 100-Hue test or Hardy–Rand–Rittler plates almost always reveals variable degrees of dyschromatopsia. The electroretinogram is most useful for the definitive diagnosis.[55] Full-field electroretinographic studies show selective diminution of the photopic "B" wave and decreased amplitudes of the 30Hz flicker. The dark-adapted rod responses, on the other hand, are usually normal or mildly attenuated. Focal macular electroretinograms

show abnormally low amplitudes or an abnormal foveal-to-parafoveal ratio, which supports disease involvement of the cone photoreceptors. The electro-oculogram shows abnormalities in severe cases. Perimetry reveals full peripheral fields with bilateral central scotomata. The differential diagnosis is given in Table 109-1.

TREATMENT, COURSE, AND OUTCOME

Typically, cone degenerations begin to manifest symptoms during the first or second decades of life. In contrast to other macular dystrophies, patients with cone degeneration experience color vision problems early in the course of the disease. Individuals with early symptoms tend to have a more severe manifestation of the disease. Visual acuity can range from 20/20 to hand movements. Patients experience progressive worsening of their disease with age.

CENTRAL AREOLAR CHOROIDAL DYSTROPHY

EPIDEMIOLOGY AND PATHOGENESIS

Central areolar choroidal dystrophy is a rare autosomal dominant macular disease that has been mapped to chromosome 17p13.[58,59] Several genes map to this same region and may be potential candidates in the development of the disease; they include phosphatidylinositol transfer protein, retinal guanylate cyclase, β-arrestin 2, pigment epithelium–derived factor, and recoverin. Interestingly, several other inherited retinal diseases have been mapped to chromosome 17p, including autosomal dominant cone dystrophy, Leber's congenital amaurosis, and autosomal dominant retinitis pigmentosa.[63] A mutation in the peripherin gene on chromosome 6 also has been associated with central areolar choroidal dystrophy, linking it with the chromosome 6 retinopathies, as well.[34,64] This disease appears to be a primary dystrophy of either the choroidal vessels or of the pigment epithelium, with secondary involvement of the choroids.

OCULAR MANIFESTATIONS AND DIAGNOSIS

Fundus examination early in the course of the disease reveals nonspecific granular hyperpigmentation of the fovea, which is indicative of pigment epithelial dystrophy. Gradually, a sharply demarcated area of RPE atrophy with underlying loss of choriocapillaris leaves intermediate and large choroidal vessels visible (Fig. 109-11). As the disease progresses, the macular atrophic area expands in a slow, centrifugal manner. This can appear clinically similar to CORD 5 findings.

Fluorescein angiography early in the course of the disease shows background hyperfluorescence from RPE atrophy. When the choriocapillaris becomes lost, this hyperfluorescence disappears, and the intermediate and large choroidal vessels are outlined sharply. The margins of the lesion show hyperfluorescence because of leakage from choriocapillaris at the edges.

The electroretinogram and electro-oculogram findings usually are normal.

PATHOLOGY

Histological analysis of the affected area shows an atrophic, fibrosed area, with loss of RPE as well as photoreceptor cells and the underlying choriocapillaris.[65] The rest of the retina and choroid is normal outside of the atrophic zone. The differential diagnosis is shown in Table 109-1.

TREATMENT, COURSE, AND OUTCOME

Patients begin to complain of symptoms of central vision loss during the third to fourth decades of life. Progressive atrophy leads to severe visual dysfunction and absolute scotoma formation by the seventh decade. Atrophy and fibrosis is noted in the avascular zone, although no arteriosclerosis is present. Some patients, however, may exhibit macular sparing with 20/20 visual acuity.

REFERENCES

1. Donoso LA, Frost AT, Stone EM, et al. Autosomal dominant Stargardt-like macular dystrophy: founder effect and reassessment of genetic heterogeneity. Arch Ophthalmol. 2001;119(4):564–70.
2. Van Driel MA, Maugeri A, Klevering BJ, et al. ABCR unites what ophthalmologists divide(s). Ophthalmic Genet. 1998;19:117–22.
3. Mata NL, Weng J, Travis GH. Biosynthesis of a major lipofuscin fluorophore in mice and humans with ABCR-mediated retinal and macular degeneration. Proc Natl Acad Sci U S A. 2000;97:7154–9.
4. Kaplan J, Gerber S, Larget-Piet D, et al. A gene for Stargardt's disease maps to the short arm of chromosome 1. Nat Genet. 1993;5:308–11.
5. Welber RG. Stargardt's macular dystrophy. Arch Ophthalmol. 1994;112:752–4.
6. Noble KG, Carr RE. Stargardt's disease and fundus flavimaculatus. Arch Ophthalmol. 1979;97:1281–5.
7. Fishman GA, Farber M, Patel S, Derlacki DJ. Visual acuity loss in patients with Stargardt's macular dystrophy. Ophthalmology. 1987;94:809–14.
8. Stavrou P, Good PA, Misson GP, Kritzinger EE. Electrophysiological findings in Stargardt's-fundus flavimaculatus disease. Eye. 1998;12:953–8.
9. Eagle RC Jr, Lucier AC, Bernardino VB Jr, Yanoff M. Retinal pigment abnormalities in fundus flavimaculatus: a light and electron microscope study. Ophthalmology. 1980;87:1189–200.
10. Maloney WF, Robertson DM, Duboff SM. Hereditary vitelliform macular degeneration. Arch Ophthalmol. 1977;95:979–83.
11. Bakall B, Marknell T, Ingvast S, et al. The mutation spectrum of the bestrophin protein—functional implications. Hum Genet. 1999;104:383–9.
12. Stone EM, Nichols BE, Stre LM, et al. Genetic linkage of vitelliform macular degeneration (Best's disease) to chromosome 11q13. Nat Genet. 1992;1:246–50.
13. White K, Marquardt A, Weber BH. VMD2 mutations in vitelliform macular dystrophy (Best disease) and other maculopathies. Hum Mutat. 2000;15:301–8.
14. Mohler CW, Fine SL. Long-term evaluation of patients with Best's vitelliform dystrophy. Ophthalmology. 1981;88:688–92.
15. Noble KG, Scher BM, Carr RE. Polymorphous presentations in vitelliform macular dystrophy: subretinal neovascularization and central choroidal atrophy. Br J Ophthalmol. 1978;62:561–70.
16. Feist RM, White MF Jr, Skalka H, Stone BM. Choroidal neovascularization in a patient with adult foveomacular dystrophy. Am J Ophthalmol. 1994;118:259–60.
17. Patrinely JR, Lewis RA, Foni RL. Foveomacular vitelliform dystrophy, adult type. A clinicopathologic study, including electron microscopic observations. Ophthalmology. 1985;92:1712–8.
18. Weingeist TA, Kobrin JL, Watzke RC. Histopathology of Best's macular dystrophy. Arch Ophthalmol. 1982;100:1108–14.
19. Frangich GT, Green WR, Fine SL. A histopathologic study of Best's macular dystrophy. Arch Ophthalmol. 1982;100:1115–21.
20. O'Gorman S, Flaherty WA, Fishman GA, Benson EL. Histopathologic findings in Best's vitelliform macular dystrophy. Arch Ophthalmol. 1988;106:1261–8.
21. Felbor U, Schilling H, Weber BH. Adult vitelliform macular dystrophy is frequently associated with mutations in the peripherin/RDS gene. Hum Mutat. 1997;10:301–9.
22. Gass JD. A clinicopathologic study of a peculiar foveomacular dystrophy. Trans Am Ophthalmol Soc. 1974;72:139–56.
23. Sohocki M, Sullivan LJ, Mintz-Hittner H, et al. Exclusion of atypical vitelliform macular dystrophy (VMD1) from 8q24.3 and from other known macular degenerative loci. Am J Hum Genet. 1997;61:239–40.
24. Evans K, Gregory CY, Wijesuriya SD, et al. Assessment of the phenotypic range seen in Doyne honeycomb retinal dystrophy. Arch Ophthalmol. 1997;115:904–10.
25. Matsumoto M, Traboulsi EI. Dominant radial drusen and Arg345Trp EFEMP1 mutation. Am J Ophthalmol. 2001;131:810–2.
26. Kniazeva M, Traboulsi EI, Yu Z. A new locus for dominant drusen and macular degeneration maps to chromosome 6q14. Am J Ophthalmol. 2000;130:197–202.
27. Heon E, Piguet B, Munier F. Linkage of autosomal dominant radial drusen (malattia leventinese) to chromosome 2p16-21. Arch Ophthalmol. 1996;114:193–8.
28. Gregory CY, Evans K, Wijesuriya SD, et al. The gene responsible for autosomal dominant Doyne's honeycomb dystrophy (DHRD) maps to chromosome 2p16. Hum Mol Genet. 1996;7:1055–9.
29. Pearce WC. Genetic aspects of Doyne's honeycomb degeneration of the retina. Ann Hum Genet. 1967;31:173–80.
30. Deutman AF, Hansen LMAA. Dominantly inherited drusen of Bruch's membrane. Br J Ophthalmol. 1970;34:373–82.
31. Marmor MF. Dominant drusen. In: Heckenlively JR, Arden GB, eds. Principles and practice of clinical electrophysiology of vision. St. Louis: Mosby–Year Book; 1991:664–8.
32. Gass JD, Jallow S, Davis B. Adult vitelliform macular detachment occurring in patients with basal laminar drusen. Am J Ophthalmol. 1985;99:445–59.
33. Wolter JR. Hyaline bodies of ganglion-cell origin in the human retina. Arch Ophthalmol. 1959;61:127–34.
34. Small KW. High tech meets low tech on chromosome 6. Arch Ophthalmol. 2001;119:573–5.
35. Sohocki MM, Daiger SP, Bowne SJ, et al. Prevalence of mutations causing retinitis pigmentosa and other inherited retinopathies. Hum Mutat. 2001;17:42–51.
36. Wells J, Wroblewski, Keen J, et al. Mutations in the human retinal degenerations slow (RDS) gene can cause either retinitis pigmentosa or macular dystrophy. Nat Genet. 1993;3:213–8.
37. Fossarello M, Bertini C, Galantuomo MS, et al. Deletion in the peripherin/RDS gene in two unrelated Sardinian families with autosomal dominant butterfly-shaped macular dystrophy. Arch Ophthalmol. 1996;114:448–56.
38. Nichols BE, Sheffield VC, Vandenburgh K, et al. Butterfly-shaped pigment dystrophy of the fovea caused by a point mutation in codon 167 of the RDS gene. Nat Genet. 1993;3:202–7.
39. Marmor MF, Byers B. Pattern dystrophy of the pigment epithelium. Am J Ophthalmol. 1977;84:32–44.
40. Hsieh RC, Fine BS, Lyons JS. Pattern dystrophies of the retinal pigment epithelium. Arch Ophthalmol. 1977;95:429–35.
41. Kremer H, Pinkers A, van den Helm B, et al. Localization of the gene for dominant cystoid macular dystrophy on chromosome 7p. Hum Mol Genet. 1994;3:299–302.
42. Pinkers A, Deutman AF, Notting JG. Retinal functions in dominant cystoid macular dystrophy (DCMD). Acta Ophthalmologica. 1976;54:579–90.
43. Loeffler KU, Li ZL, Fishman GA, Tso MO. Dominantly inherited macular edema. A histopathologic study. Ophthalmology. 1992;99:1385–92.
44. Weber BH, Vogt G, Pruett RC, et al. Mutation in the tissue inhibitor of metalloproteinase-3 (TIMP3) in patients with Sorsby's fundus dystrophy. Nat Genet. 1994;8:352–6.
45. Weber BH, Vogt G, Wolz W, et al. Sorsby's fundus dystrophy is genetically linked to chromosome 22q13-d. Nat Genet. 1994;7:158–61.
46. Della NG, Campochiaro PA, Zack DJ. Localization of TIMP-3 mRNA expression to the retinal pigment epithelium. Invest Ophthalmol Vis Sci. 1996;37:1921–4.
47. Felbor U, Doepner D, Schneider U, et al. Evaluation of the gene encoding the tissue inhibitor of metalloproteinases-3 in various maculopathies. Invest Ophthalmol Vis Sci. 1997;38:1054–9.
48. Hamilton WK, Ewing CC, Ives EJ, et al. Sorsby's fundus dystrophy. Ophthalmology. 1989;96:1755–62.
49. Capon MR, Marshall J, Krafft JI, et al. Sorsby's fundus dystrophy. A light and electron microscopic study. Ophthalmology. 1989;96:1769–77.
50. Sieving PA, Boskovich S, Bingham E, et al. Sorsby's fundus dystrophy in a family with a Ser-181-CVS mutation in the TIMP-3 gene: poor outcome after laser photocoagulation. Trans Am Ophthalmol Soc. 1996;94:275–94.
51. Small KW, Weber JL, Roses A, et al. North Carolina macular dystrophy is assigned to chromosome 6. Genomics. 1992;13:681–5.
52. Small KW, Udar N, Yelchits S, et al. North Carolina macular dystrophy (MCDR1) locus: a fine resolution genetic map and haplotype analysis. Mol Vision. 1999;5:38.
53. Small KW, Hermsen V, Gurney N, et al. North Carolina macular dystrophy and central areolar pigment epithelial dystrophy: one family, one disease. Arch Ophthalmol. 1992;110:515–8.
54. Small KW, Voo I, Glasgow B, et al. Clinicopathologic correlation of North Carolina macular dystrophy. Trans Am Ophthalmol Soc. 2001;99:233–8.
55. Kelsell RE, Godley BF, Evans K, et al. Localization of the gene for progressive bifocal chorioretinal atrophy (PBCRA) to chromosome 6q. 1995;4:1653–6.
56. Gehrig A, Felbor U, Kelsell RE, et al. Assessment of the interphotoreceptor matrix proteoglycan-1 (IMPG1) gene localised to 6q13-q15 in autosomal dominant Stargardt-like disease (ADSTGD), progressive bifocal chorioretinal atrophy (PBCRA), and North Carolina macular dystrophy (MCDR1). J Med Genet. 1998;35:641–5.

57. Godley BF, Tiffin PA, Evans K, *et al.* Clinical features of progressive bifocal chorioretinal atrophy: a retinal dystrophy linked to chromosome 6q. Ophthalmology. 1996;103:893–8.

58. Fossdal R, Manusson L, Weber JL, Jensson O. Mapping the locus of atrophia areata, a helicoids peripapillary chorioretinal degeneration with autosomal dominant inheritance, to chromosome 11p15. Hum Mol Genet. 1995;4:479–83.

59. Small KW, Gehrs K. Clinical study of a large family with autosomal dominant progressive cone degeneration. Am J Opthalmol. 1996;121:1–12.

60. Small KW, Syrquin M, Mullen Y, Gehrs K. Mapping of autosomal dominant progressive cone degeneration to chromosome 17p. Am J Ophthalmol. 1996;121:13–8.

61. Wilkie SE, Newbold RJ, Deery E, *et al.* Functional characterization of missense mutations at codon 838 in retinal guanylate cyclase correlates with disease severity in patients with autosomal dominant cone-rod dystrophy. Hum Mol Genet. 2000;9:3065–73.

62. Udar N, Yelchits S, Chalukya M, *et al.* Identification of *GUCY2D* gene mutations in CORD5 families and evidence of incomplete penetrance. Hum Mutat. 2003;21:170–1.

63. Lotery AJ, Ennis KT, Silvestri G, *et al.* Localization of a gene for central areolar choroidal dystrophy to chromosome 17p. Hum Mol Genet. 1996;5:705–8.

64. Hoyng CB, Heutink P, Testers L, *et al.* Autosomal dominant central areolar choroidal dystrophy caused by a mutation in codon 142 in the peripherin/*RDS* gene. Am J Ophthalmol. 1996;121:623–9.

65. Ashton N. Central areolar choroidal sclerosis: a histopathologic study. Br J Ophthalmol. 1953;37:140–7.

CHAPTER 110

Choroidal Dystrophies

SANDEEP GROVER • GERALD A. FISHMAN

DEFINITION
- Choroideremia is a progressive, diffuse, bilateral chorioretinal dystrophy with an X-linked recessive mode of inheritance.
- Gyrate atrophy of the choroid and retina is a progressive, diffuse, bilateral chorioretinal dystrophy with an autosomal recessive mode of inheritance.

KEY FEATURES
- Choroideremia: involvement of the choroid, retinal pigment epithelium, and retinal photoreceptors; nyctalopia; midperipheral and, subsequently, far peripheral visual field loss.
- Gyrate atrophy: chorioretinal lesions of atrophic appearance with scalloped margins; nyctalopia; midperipheral and peripheral visual field loss.

ASSOCIATED FEATURES
- Choroideremia: often initial macular sparing; characteristic findings in female carriers.
- Gyrate atrophy: systemic hyperornithinemia.

INTRODUCTION

Choroidal dystrophies are a group of progressive, hereditary disorders that are characterized by clinically apparent retinal pigment epithelial (RPE) and choroidal atrophy. Krill and Archer[1] classified such dystrophies into two groups, one with a more regional involvement and the other with a diffuse involvement of the fundus. The regional dystrophies are subclassified further on the basis of the initial or predominant site of the degenerative changes (macular, peripapillary, paramacular, or a combination) and the severity of involvement (involving only the choriocapillaris or, in addition, the larger choroidal vessels). Choroideremia and gyrate atrophy of the choroid and retina represent diffuse forms of choroidal dystrophies.

CHOROIDEREMIA

Choroideremia is a progressive, bilateral dystrophy of the retina and choroid. It is an X-linked recessive disease, transmitted on the long arm of the X chromosome, that is characterized by a marked loss of vision at night and progressive loss of peripheral visual fields. Although encountered relatively infrequently, this disease is probably the second most common cause, after retinitis pigmentosa, of progressive, hereditary night blindness.

EPIDEMIOLOGY AND PATHOGENESIS

The exact pathogenesis for the degenerative changes observed in patients with and the cells primarily affected in choroideremia is yet to be defined with certainty. In the past this disease was thought to be caused primarily by degeneration of RPE cells or choroid, or both, with photoreceptors degenerating secondarily. However, recently it has been suggested that the primary defect may be in the rod photoreceptor cells of the retina.[2]

The gene that causes choroideremia was isolated by positional cloning techniques and localized to the long arm of the X chromosome (Xq21).[3,4] The choroideremia gene (CHM) encodes the Rab escort protein-1 (REP-1)[5] of Rab geranylgeranyl transferase, a two-component enzyme (components REP-1 and REP-2) that modifies Rab proteins. Rab proteins are low–molecular-weight guanosine triphosphatases that regulate intracellular vesicular transport. Rab proteins probably exist in two forms: one, the inactive, guanosine diphosphate–bound state, and the other, the active, guanosine triphosphate–bound state. For Rab proteins to bind to membranes, they undergo lipid modification with the addition of 20 carbon units to the carboxy terminal of the protein, a process known as geranylgeranylation. This, then, probably acts as a chaperon to deliver the prenylated Rab protein to the cellular membrane. Of interest, the CHM gene is expressed not only in ocular tissues but also in various cells of nonocular origin. However, CHM gene dysfunction affects only the retina. The proteins REP-1 and REP-2 are 75% identical, and their functions are mutually redundant.[6] The functioning of the majority of the cells in the body, which have a REP-1 deficiency, can be taken over by REP-2 and, hence, can function adequately. However, the retina has a major Rab protein, Rab 27, which is prenylated more efficiently by REP-1 than REP-2.[7] Since all mutations known so far in the CHM gene create stop codons and, hence, an absence of the gene product REP-1, there is a progressive chorioretinal degeneration in patients with CHM.[8]

OCULAR MANIFESTATIONS

Impairment of night vision, which progresses over time, is the initial symptom in most patients who have choroideremia. It usually starts in the first decade of life, although the onset may be delayed. Some patients can, however, have midperipheral visual field loss. The clinical features, including the rate of progression, can show both interfamilial and intrafamilial variability.

The ocular findings in the anterior segment are unremarkable. The crystalline lens remains clear until the later stages of the disease.[9] However, posterior subcapsular changes in the lens develop more frequently than in the general population.[10] The vitreous shows fine, fibrillar degeneration at an early age.

Initial fundus changes most often begin in the midperipheral retina in the form of patches of pigment mottling and hypopigmentation. Nummular areas of patchy RPE and choroidal atrophy can develop subsequently in the midperipheral retina

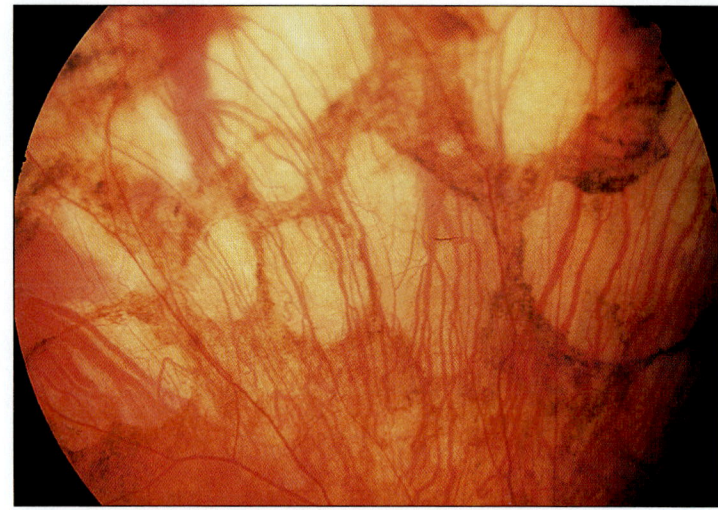

FIG. 110-1 ▐▌ Fundus changes found in choroideremia. Nummular areas of retinal pigment epithelial and choroidal atrophy in the midperipheral retina are shown.

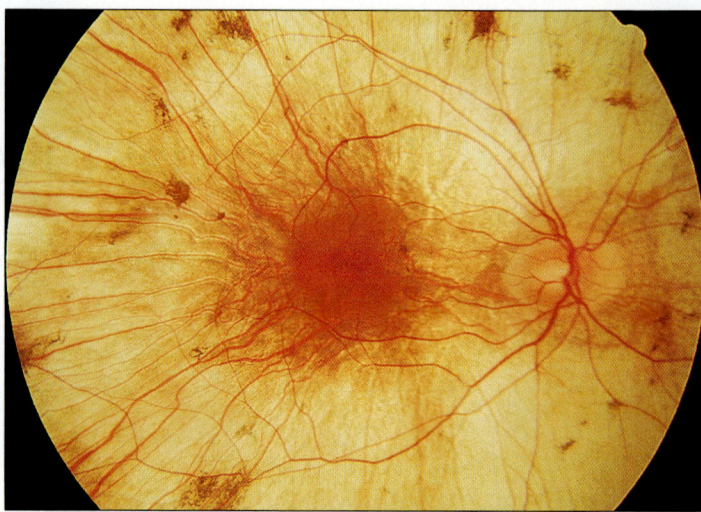

FIG. 110-3 ▐▌ Fundus changes in the right eye in a patient with late-stage choroideremia.

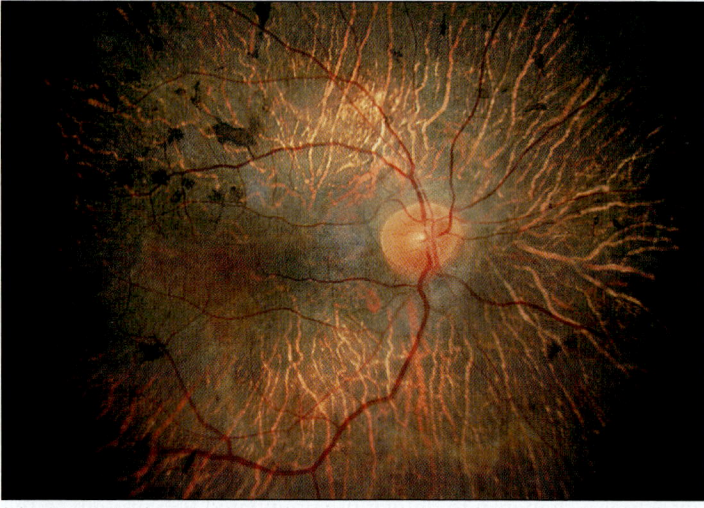

FIG. 110-2 ▐▌ Fundus changes of the right eye in a patient with an intermediate stage of choroideremia. Note the diffuse changes of the retinal pigment epithelium and prominent choroidal vessels.

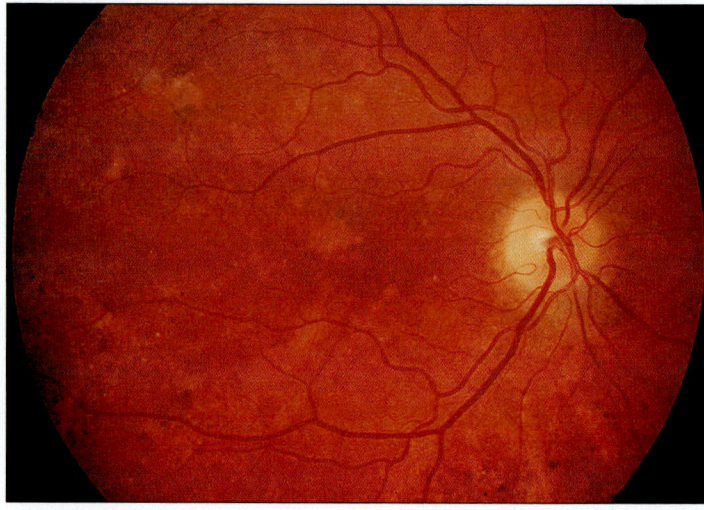

FIG. 110-4 ▐▌ Posterior fundus changes in the right eye in a carrier of choroideremia.

(Fig. 110-1). In the intermediate stages of the disease, the atrophy of the RPE and choriocapillaris become more diffuse, while the intermediate and the larger choroidal vessels remain relatively more preserved (Fig. 110-2). As the disease progresses, both the intermediate-size and large choroidal vessels become more atrophic, which exposes the underlying sclera. The macula initially is spared relatively often and is visible as a remaining island of choriocapillaris in the midst of surrounding white sclera (Fig. 110-3). The macula can be relatively well preserved even in the late stages of the disease. Only in the more advanced stages do the retinal arterioles become attenuated, while the optic disc does not tend to become as pale or waxy pale as occurs in patients with retinitis pigmentosa.[9]

The loss of visual field often corresponds to the clinically discernible areas of chorioretinal atrophy. Visual field examination initially shows a slightly restricted peripheral field or midperipheral scotomas or both. With time, these scotomas coalesce to form a ring scotoma.[11] The fields progressively constrict and finally leave a small central island. The visual acuity often is not notably affected until the fifth decade of life or even later. Visual acuity may be decreased because of degenerative maculopathy or the development of posterior subcapsular cataracts. A careful refraction is prudent, because such patients may have various degrees of myopia.

The female carriers are typically asymptomatic. There is a wide spectrum of clinical fundus appearance, which ranges from a fundus of normal appearance to a full-blown picture of choroideremia, as in an affected male. Characteristically, however, pigmentary changes in the fundus, described as *moth-eaten* in appearance, occur predominantly in the midperipheral retina.[12] Pigmentary atrophy, mottling, and clumping also may be discernible more posteriorly (Fig. 110-4). Areas of hyperpigmentation may be present as radial bands that extend from the midperiphery toward the ora serrata (Fig. 110-5). The visual acuity may be decreased and visual fields reduced, depending on the extent of involvement of the photoreceptors. Usually these defects appear late, if at all, and are often mild. Most carriers do not show any electroretinographic amplitude reductions, although those who have more advanced fundus degenerative changes can show appreciable amplitude reductions.[13] Vitreous fluorophotometry shows a normal blood–retinal barrier in carriers of choroideremia.[14]

DIAGNOSIS AND ANCILLARY TESTING

The clinical fundus features usually are diagnostic in the intermediate and late stages of the disease. Good central visual acuity and slowly progressive visual field changes aid in the diagnosis.

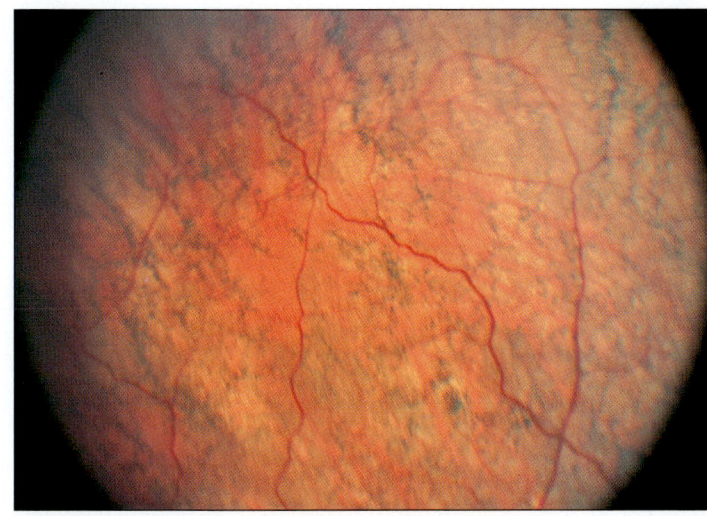

FIG. 110-5 ■ Peripheral fundus changes in a carrier of choroideremia. Note the radial bands of hyperpigmentation and some pigment clumping.

Both the electroretinogram and electro-oculogram can show marked impairment.[12] The electroretinogram may rarely be normal in amplitude initially (Fig. 110-6) or occasionally show only mild impairment in the very early stages. The fundus findings initially may be only normal or minimally abnormal (Fig. 110-7). Once fundus changes become discernible, however, the electroretinogram is affected, usually notably. It often shows markedly reduced isolated rod responses with prolongation of rod b-wave implicit times in affected men. However, the isolated cone responses are initially either normal or moderately reduced in amplitude, with a delayed b-wave implicit time. There is a wide intrafamilial and interfamilial variability in electroretinographic amplitudes with age.[13] The electro-oculogram is markedly abnormal in men with choroideremia[1]; the degree of electro-oculogram abnormality in carriers, although usually normal, varies. In one study the ratio of light–peak to dark–trough was abnormal in about one fourth of carriers; this ratio significantly decreased with increasing age.[15]

Dark-adaptation testing often shows elevated thresholds. In the early stages only the rod portion of the curve is affected, while cone thresholds subsequently also become elevated.

Fluorescein angiography is not useful in the diagnosis of choroideremia. It can, however, define the extent of choriocapillaris atrophy more accurately than ophthalmoscopy. Fluorescein angiography also may be superior to ophthalmoscopy in defining the extent of degenerative changes of the RPE, evident from hyperfluorescence seen on the angiogram.

The clinical diagnosis of CHM in the majority of male patients can be confirmed by an immunoblot analysis with anti–REP-1 antibody.[16] The basis, again, is that all genetic mutations identified so far create stop codons that result in the absence of REP-1. The predictive value of this test, however, has not yet been established.[16] Also, female carriers of CHM cannot be identified with this technique, because their REP-1 expression is not totally absent.

DIFFERENTIAL DIAGNOSIS

The differential diagnosis for choroideremia includes other night-blinding disorders, particularly retinitis pigmentosa. Fundus features of a pale optic disc, attenuated retinal arterioles, typical bone-spicule–like pigmentation, and a higher prevalence of posterior subcapsular cataracts associated with retinitis pigmentosa usually help differentiate the latter disease from choroideremia. Nevertheless, some patients who have the X-linked form of retinitis pigmentosa, who can show higher degrees of myopia and prominent choroidal vessels, may have a

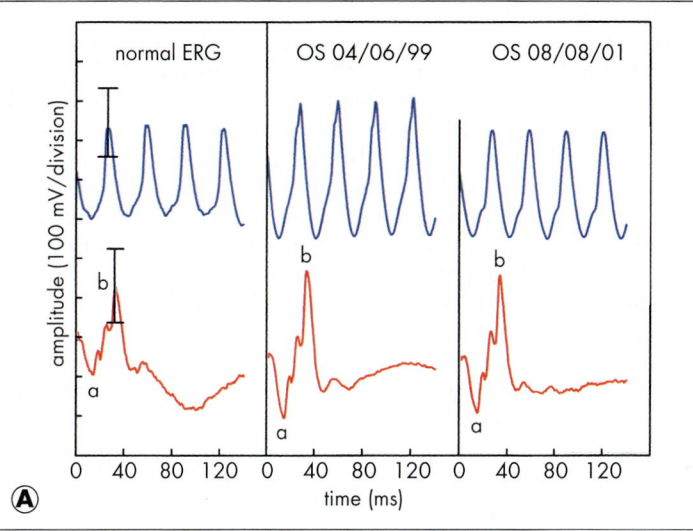

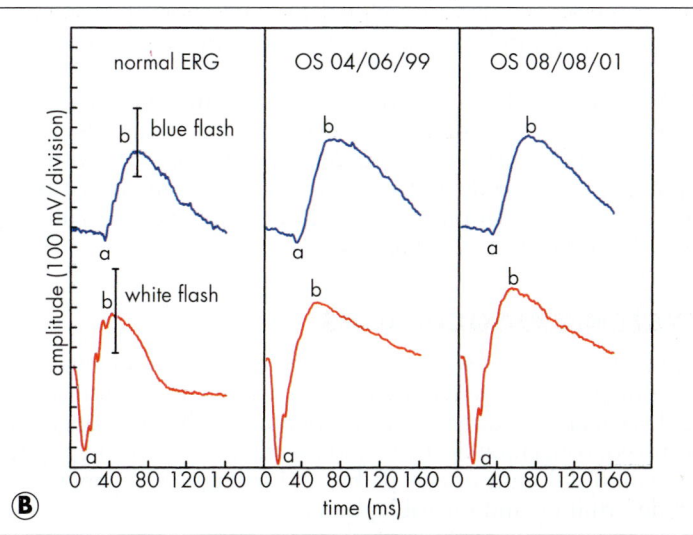

FIG. 110-6 ■ Electroretinographic recordings from a male patient with choroideremia at ages 9 and 11 years showing normal light-adapted flicker and single flash (**A**) and dark-adapted rod-isolated and maximal (**B**) responses.

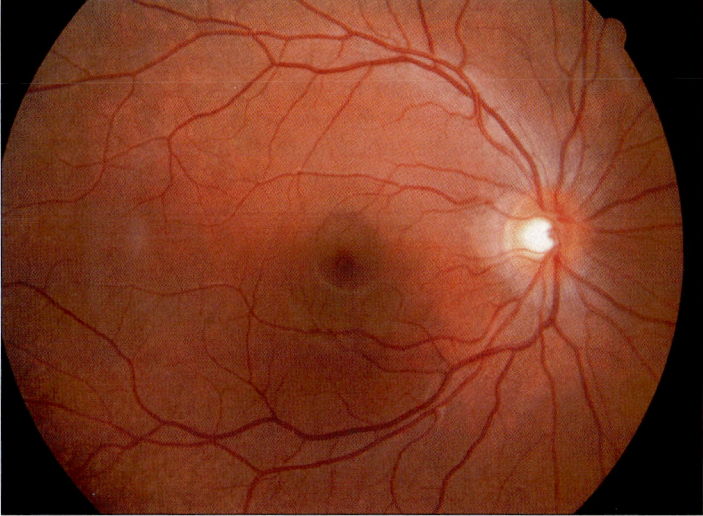

FIG. 110-7 ■ Fundus photograph of the right eye of the same patient as in Figure 110-6 at age 11 years, showing normal optic discs and retinal vessels. Also shown is a mild-to-moderate degree of pigment mottling anterior to the vascular arcades.

phenotypic similarity to patients who have choroideremia. However, patients who have X-linked retinitis pigmentosa have a reduction in central acuity early in the course of their disease, while patients with choroideremia do not characteristically manifest bone-spicule–like pigment clumping.

Patients who have ocular albinism may show some degree of phenotypic similarity to those with choroideremia; however, absence of nyctalopia, decreased vision, nystagmus, iris transillumination defects, and normal electroretinographic amplitudes help to differentiate these two disorders.

Features distinguishing gyrate atrophy of the choroid and retina from choroideremia include autosomal recessive inheritance, well-demarcated, scalloped areas of chorioretinal atrophy, and association of hyperornithinemia with the former. It sometimes may be difficult to differentiate end-stage gyrate atrophy from an advanced case of choroideremia.

Generalized choroidal atrophy, which may show phenotypic similarities to an intermediate stage of choroideremia, is inherited in an autosomal dominant or occasionally autosomal recessive fashion. The various regional types of choroidal atrophies usually cause a milder visual dysfunction and can be differentiated easily.

Myopic retinal degeneration sometimes may mimic choroideremia. However, the myopic degeneration usually is not as diffuse as the lesions of choroideremia, and patients with myopic degeneration do not characteristically complain of night blindness. Examination of other family members, especially carriers, helps facilitate the diagnosis.

SYSTEMIC ASSOCIATIONS

Isolated reports show the association of a choroideremia-like phenotype with mental deficiency, acrokeratosis, anhidrosis, and skeletal deformity; uveal coloboma; obesity and congenital deafness; congenital deafness and mental retardation; hypopituitarism; distal motor neuropathy; and nystagmus, myopia, dental deformities, and microblepharia.

PATHOLOGY

In male patients with choroideremia, light microscopy shows a widespread chorioretinal atrophy, especially the choriocapillaris, along with degenerative changes in the RPE, outer retinal layers (especially the photoreceptors), and larger choroidal vessels (Fig. 110-8). A graded atrophy occurs: The equatorial area is most affected while the macular, peripapillary, and ora serrata areas are relatively spared. In the late stages, the far periphery and the central regions also may be severely involved. Retinal bipolar and ganglion cells appear normal.[9] Electron microscopy shows extensive loss of photoreceptors and RPE, especially away from the macula (Fig. 110-8). End-stage disease can show widespread neural retinal gliosis and atrophy.

A recent histopathological study[2] in an 88-year-old choroideremia carrier showed patchy areas of degeneration of photoreceptors and RPE cells which were not necessarily concordant. The choriocapillaris was normal except corresponding to areas of severe retinal degeneration, as reported previously.[17,18] However, immunofluorescence analysis localized the CHM gene product, REP-1 with a mouse monoclonal antibody, to the rod cytoplasm and amacrine cells but not in the cones.[2] This suggests that the primary site of this disease may be in the rods rather than RPE or choroid. This labeling, which was seen in small vesicles in the rod cytoplasm, is consistent with the association of REP-1 with intracellular vesicular transport.

TREATMENT, COURSE, AND OUTCOME

At present there is no treatment for choroideremia. The disease is invariably progressive, but the rate of progression can be highly variable.

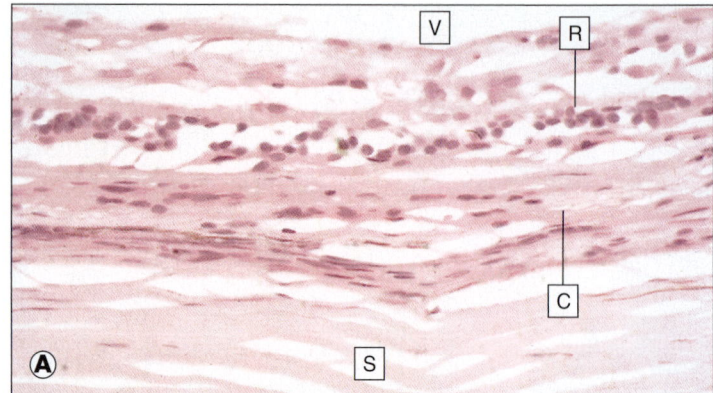

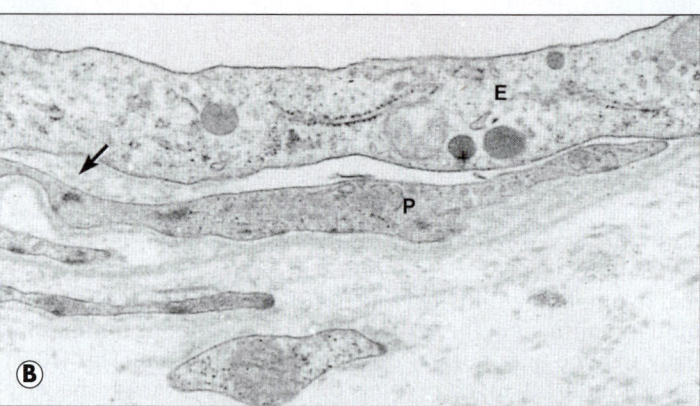

FIG. 110-8 ■ Choroideremia. **A,** Histological section showing absence of retinal pigment epithelium and atrophy of both the overlying neural retina and the underlying choroid (*V,* vitreous; *R,* atrophic retina; *S,* sclera; *C,* atrophic choroid). **B,** Electron micrograph shows choroidal vessel deep to choriocapillaris. Both endothelial (*E*) and pericyte (*P*) basement membranes are absent centrally. A small amount of fragmented basement membrane (*arrow*) persists on the left. (**A,** Presented by Dr. WS Hunter at AOA-AFIP meeting, 1969; **B,** from Cameron JD, et al. Ophthalmology. 1987;94:187.)

GYRATE ATROPHY

INTRODUCTION

Gyrate atrophy of the choroid and retina is a slowly progressive chorioretinal dystrophy. Like many metabolic disorders, it is inherited in an autosomal recessive manner. Gyrate atrophy is characterized by discrete areas of chorioretinal atrophy in the midperipheral retina. These are sharply demarcated from the more posterior retina, which is initially of normal appearance. This dystrophy is associated with hyperornithinemia to levels 10–15-fold above normal, shown to be caused by a deficiency of ornithine ketoacid aminotransferase, also known as ornithine aminotransferase (OAT). This enzyme depends on a cofactor, pyridoxal phosphate (vitamin B$_6$).

EPIDEMIOLOGY AND PATHOGENESIS

Simell and Takki[19] in 1973 were the first to report the finding of hyperornithinemia with gyrate atrophy. Sengers et al.[20] first reported a deficiency of the mitochondrial matrix enzyme OAT in patients who have gyrate atrophy. Ornithine, a nonessential amino acid, is an intermediate compound in the formation of urea (Fig. 110-9). The major pathway for utilization of ornithine is by enzymatic conversion into glutamic-γ-semialdehyde by OAT, a vitamin B$_6$-dependent enzyme, and subsequently to proline. OAT has been found with high activity in the retina, liver, and kidney. An experimental model that resembles gyrate atrophy has been found in animals injected with intravitreous ornithine.[21]

Since OAT is dependent on cofactor B$_6$, treatment with oral vitamin B$_6$ has been tried. Patients who have gyrate atrophy are categorized into two groups, depending on a lowering of plasma ornithine levels in response to vitamin B$_6$. The vitamin

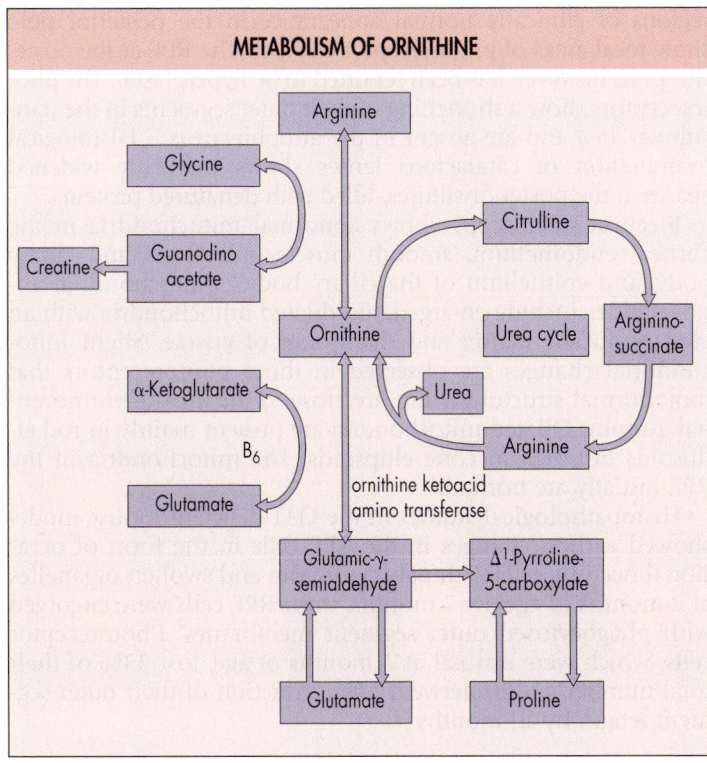

FIG. 110-9 ■ Pathway of ornithine metabolism.

METABOLISM OF ORNITHINE

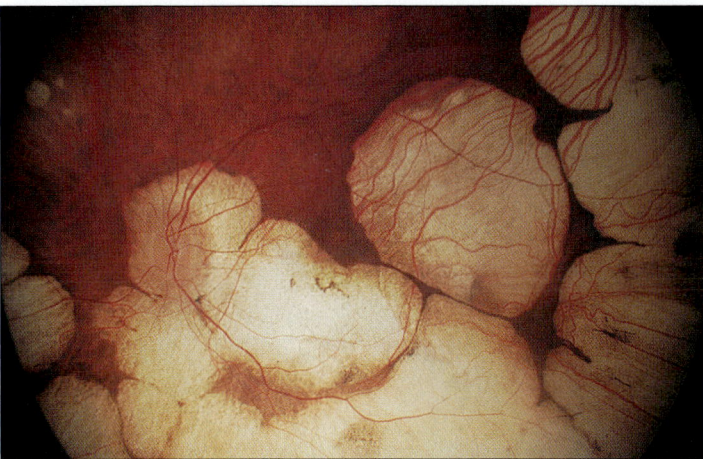

FIG. 110-10 ■ Fundus changes in the left eye of a patient with an intermediate stage of gyrate atrophy of the choroid and retina. Note the well-demarcated, scalloped areas of atrophy.

B_6–responsive patients, although considerably fewer in number than nonresponders, appear to have a milder disease and better visual function than the nonresponsive group.

The human OAT gene has been cloned and mapped to 10q26,[22] and more than 60 mutations have been identified. An OAT-deficient mouse model (Oat–/–) has been developed by gene targeting that has hyperornithinemia levels 10–15 times the normal, as in patients with gyrate atrophy.[23] This has improved the potential for a better understanding of the pathogenesis and possible therapeutic outcome of this disease.

OCULAR MANIFESTATIONS

Patients with gyrate atrophy of the choroid and retina develop nyctalopia during the second to third decade of life. Initially it is mild to moderate in severity and slowly progressive. The earliest appearance may occur in the form of a restriction in peripheral field. Usually visual acuity is preserved until a later stage. Visual acuity may be decreased from involvement of the macula by the disease itself or secondarily from cystoid macular edema or cataracts.

The fundus shows atrophy of the RPE and choriocapillaris during the earlier and intermediate stages, with sharply demarcated scalloped areas of atrophy (Fig. 110-10) and a tendency for pigment clumping to occur at the margins. The atrophy usually starts in the midperipheral and peripheral areas, often referred to as a *garland-shaped* fashion, and then progresses centrally as well as peripherally. Ultimately it involves the entire fundus, including the peripapillary area, with relative sparing of the macula. Fine granular and velvety pigmentation may be observed in the macula area and retinal periphery, respectively, in a number of patients.[24,25] With progressive atrophy, the larger choroidal vessels are also involved. The optic disc and retinal arterioles usually are normal until the later stages.[12] Vitreous changes, such as posterior vitreous detachment, and development of epiretinal membranes with cystoid macular edema, have been observed with gyrate atrophy of the choroid and retina.[26,27]

Visual field defects correspond to the atrophic areas in the choroid. The field loss begins in the midperipheral area as regionally dense scotomas, which eventually coalesce to form a ring scotoma. Progressive field loss ultimately leaves the patient with only small residual central fields. Usually by 40 years of age, the visual fields are substantially restricted.[24]

Moderate-to-marked myopia is found in most patients,[26] and lens changes are seen in almost all patients who have this disease.[28] Posterior sutural and subcapsular cataracts and, in isolated cases, anterior subcapsular plaque-like cataracts have been described.[29]

DIAGNOSIS AND ANCILLARY TESTING

A history of night blindness and the typical fundus feature of scalloped areas of atrophy of the RPE and choroid are suggestive of the diagnosis. The electroretinogram is subnormal in the early stages, with marked reduction or nondetectable a-wave and b-wave responses in the later stages. The rod responses are affected more severely in the early stages, but later both rods and cones become affected.[30] Some patients also have a delayed cone implicit time response when tested using a 30Hz flicker stimulus.[30,31] The electro-oculogram is affected mildly or not at all in very early stages of the disease.[30] However, with progression of the disease, electro-oculogram light-peak to dark-trough ratios become markedly reduced. Overall, the electroretinographic responses, including oscillatory potentials, and electro-oculogram light-peak to dark-trough ratios are better maintained in vitamin B_6–responsive patients.[30] Dark-adaptation curves may show a slightly prolonged cone–rod break time. Again, in a vitamin B_6 responder or in early childhood, when the disease is not as severe, notably less extensive changes occur in dark-adaptation function. However, in later stages of the disease, more marked elevation of cone or rod, or both, thresholds develop.[30]

Fluorescein angiography, not unexpectedly, shows RPE transmission defects in the areas of chorioretinal atrophy. These areas of transmission defects often are larger than the clinically visible atrophic areas.

High ornithine levels are found in the urine, plasma, aqueous humor, and cerebrospinal fluid of these patients, often elevated to 10–20 times the normal levels. No evidence exists of any correlation of age or severity of involvement with the concentration of ornithine in plasma.[32] The 24-hour urine creatine excretion is normal.

DIFFERENTIAL DIAGNOSIS

Gyrate atrophy of the choroid and retina is diagnosed by means of the typical fundus feature of scalloped areas of retinal and choroidal atrophy, an autosomal recessive inheritance, and hyperornithinemia. However, a gyrate atrophy–like fundus phenotype

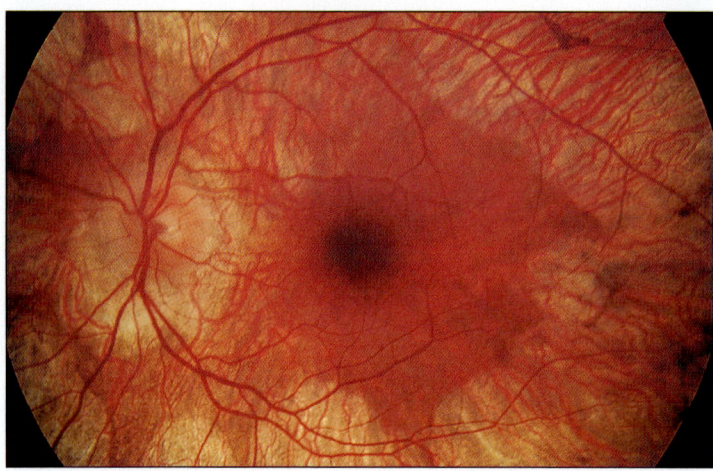

FIG. 110-11 ▮▮ Fundus changes in the left eye of a patient with choroideremia. The scalloped areas of atrophy resemble the lesions found in gyrate atrophy of choroid and retina.

with a possible autosomal dominant inheritance pattern and normal plasma ornithine levels has also been described.[33] Gyrate atrophy also can show certain phenotypic similarities to choroideremia, myopic degeneration, and hereditary choroidal atrophy. It is mainly in its later stages that gyrate atrophy of the choroid and retina clinically may most resemble the retinal findings seen in choroideremia. However, in earlier stages of the disease, patients who have choroideremia may show scalloped or nummular areas of RPE and choroidal atrophy (Fig. 110-11). Typical retinitis pigmentosa usually can be differentiated from gyrate atrophy, but atypical retinitis pigmentosa sometimes may show certain phenotypic similarities. Bone-spicule pigment in the retina and attenuated retinal arterioles at an earlier stage aid in the diagnosis of retinitis pigmentosa. In gyrate atrophy, the pigment clumps usually are more dense and associated with the atrophic lesions.[32]

SYSTEMIC ASSOCIATIONS

Electromyograms are abnormal in most tested patients,[34,35] although only a few complain of slight muscle weakness. Electromyographic observations include a myopathic pattern of short-duration, low-amplitude motor unit action potentials, and increased polyphasic potentials.[34] Muscle biopsy shows atrophic type 2 muscle fibers with tubular aggregates visible on electron microscopy.[34] Abnormal electrocardiographic features may include a broad P-wave, prolonged QT interval, and flattening of the T-wave. Electroencephalograms also may be abnormal in some patients.[25,31,32] The changes include an increase in slow activity, focal slow-wave abnormalities, and focal sharp waves.[32]

Various rare associations of a clinical picture that resembles gyrate atrophy have been seen with microcephaly, spinocerebellar ataxia, subluxation of the lens, pituitary dysfunction, and congenital muscular dystrophy. All of these associations were found with normal levels of plasma ornithine.

Reports exist of fine, sparse hair with patches of alopecia, skeletal muscle abnormalities, hepatic mitochondrial changes, and subnormal intelligence. Massive cystinuria and lysinuria with hypermetropia and diabetes also have been observed with gyrate atrophy. Chorioretinal lesions that resemble gyrate atrophy with vitreochorioretinal degeneration, associated trichomegaly, and normal plasma ornithine levels also have been reported.[36]

PATHOLOGY

Limited information on pathological findings is available on patients with gyrate atrophy.[37] The atrophic areas in the midperipheral retina show a marked atrophy of the choroidal vessels, including the choriocapillaris, RPE, and photoreceptors. The

regions of clinically normal appearance in the posterior pole show focal areas of photoreceptor cell loss. The RPE at the posterior pole, however, has been reported to be hyperplastic. The photoreceptors show a shortening of their outer segments in the transitional area and are absent in the atrophic areas.[37] Histological examination of cataractous lenses shows markedly widened spaces at the posterior sutures, filled with denatured proteins.[28]

Electron microscopy shows abnormal mitochondria in the corneal endothelium, smooth muscle of the iris and ciliary body, and epithelium of the ciliary body.[37] Mitochondrial abnormalities include enlarged and dilated mitochondria with an electron-lucent matrix and disruption of cristae. Slight mitochondrial changes are observed in those photoreceptors that look normal structurally but are close to the area of chorioretinal atrophy. Dilated mitochondria are present mainly in rod ellipsoids but also in cone ellipsoids. The mitochondria in the RPE initially are normal.[37]

Histopathological studies in the OAT-deficient mouse model showed earliest changes in the RPE cells in the form of occasional necrotic cells with pale cytoplasm and swollen organelles at 2 months of age. By 7 months, these RPE cells were engorged with phagocytosed outer segment membranes. Photoreceptor cells, which were normal at 2 months of age, lost 33% of their total number and underwent 60% reduction of their outer segment length by 10 months.[23]

TREATMENT, COURSE, AND OUTCOME

Since ornithine is produced from other amino acids, mainly arginine, some investigators advocate that patients be restricted to a rigid schedule of a low-protein diet, including near-total elimination of arginine, with supplementation of essential amino acids. Administration of high doses of vitamin B$_6$ has reduced the plasma ornithine level in a limited number of such patients. These forms of treatment, although useful to reduce the elevated levels of plasma ornithine, have not convincingly improved or arrested the chorioretinal degeneration.[38,39] A long-term study of an arginine-restricted diet in six pairs of affected siblings was encouraging,[40] because it showed that a substantial reduction of ornithine levels occurred when such patients were fed an arginine-restricted diet over a period of 5–7 years. Also, the younger of the sibling pairs, who were started on this diet at an earlier age, showed markedly fewer signs of the disease compared with the older siblings. The study suggests that an arginine-restricted diet may cause a decrease in the progress of the chorioretinal degeneration. Consistent with this observation, correction of ornithine accumulation by an arginine-restricted diet in the Oat–/– mouse model entirely prevented retinal degeneration.[41] This suggests that it may not be necessary to restore the activity of OAT enzyme to metabolize the accumulating ornithine for treating this condition but, instead, restrict the substrate, arginine, from which ornithine is formed.[41]

As with other inherited retinal degenerative disorders, a better understanding of the pathogenetic mechanisms by which the retinal cells degenerate in patients who have various choroidal dystrophies will ultimately lead to more effective treatment strategies in the future.

REFERENCES

1. Krill AE, Archer D. Classification of the choroidal atrophies. Am J Ophthalmol. 1971;72:562–85.
2. Syed N, Smith JE, John SK, et al. Evaluation of retinal photoreceptors and pigment epithelium in a female carrier of choroideremia. Ophthalmology. 2001;108: 711–20.
3. Cremers FP, van de Pol DJ, van Kerkhoff LP, et al. Cloning of a gene that is rearranged in patients with choroideremia. Nature. 1990;347:674–7.
4. Merry DE, Janne PA, Landers JE, et al. Isolation of a candidate gene for choroideremia. Proc Natl Acad Sci U S A. 1992;89:2135–9.
5. Seabra MC, Brown MS, Goldstein JL. Retinal degeneration in choroideremia: deficiency of Rab geranylgeranyl transferase. Science. 1993;259:377–81.
6. Cremers FPM, Ropers HH. Choroideremia. In: Wright AF, Jay B, eds. Molecular genetics of inherited eye disorders. Chur: Harwood Academic Publishers; 1994:303–19.

7. Seabra MC, Ho YK, Anant JS. Deficient geranylgeranylation of Ram/Rab27 in choroideremia. J Biol Chem. 1995;270:24420–7.

8. Seabra MC. New insights into the pathogenesis of choroideremia: a tale of two REPs. Ophthalmic Genet. 1996;17:43–6.

9. McCulloch C. Choroideremia and other choroidal atrophies. In: Newsome DA, ed. Retinal dystrophies and degenerations. New York: Raven Press; 1988:285–95.

10. Heckenlively J. The frequency of posterior subcapsular cataract in the hereditary retinal degenerations. Am J Ophthalmol. 1982;93:733.

11. Krill AE. Diffuse choroidal atrophies. In: Krill's hereditary retinal and choroidal diseases, vol 2, clinical characteristics. Hagerstown: Harper & Row; 1977:979–1041.

12. Fishman GA. Hereditary retinal and choroidal diseases: electroretinogram and electro-oculogram findings. In: Peyman GA, Sanders DR, Goldberg MF, eds. Principles and practice of ophthalmology, vol 2. Philadelphia: WB Saunders; 1980:857–904.

13. Sieving PA, Niffenegger JH, Berson EL. Electroretinographic findings in selected pedigrees with choroideremia. Am J Ophthalmol. 1986;101:361–7.

14. Rusin MM, Fishman GA, Larson JA, et al. Vitreous fluorophotometry in carriers of choroideremia and X-linked retinitis pigmentosa. Arch Ophthalmol. 1989;107:209–12.

15. Pinckers A, van Aarem A, Brink H. The electrooculogram in heterozygote carriers of Usher syndrome, retinitis pigmentosa, neuronal ceroid lipofuscinosis, Senior syndrome and choroideremia. Ophthalmic Genet. 1994;15:25–30.

16. MacDonald M, Mah DY, Ho YK, et al. A practical diagnostic test for choroideremia. Ophthalmology. 1998;105:1637–40.

17. Ghosh M, McCulloch C, Parker JA. Pathological study in a female carrier of choroideremia. Can J Ophthalmol. 1988;23:181–6.

18. Flannery JG, Bird AC, Farber DB, et al. A histopathologic study of a choroideremia carrier. Invest Ophthalmol Vis Sci. 1990;31:229–36.

19. Simell O, Takki K. Raised plasma-ornithine and gyrate atrophy of the choroid and retina. Lancet. 1973;ii:1031–3.

20. Sengers RCA, Trijbels JMF, Brusaart JH, et al. Gyrate atrophy of the choroid and retina and ornithine ketoacid aminotransferase deficiency. Paediatr Res. 1976;10:894(abst).

21. Kuwabara T, Ishikawa Y, Kaiser-Kupfer MI. Experimental model of gyrate atrophy in animals. Ophthalmology. 1981;88:331–4.

22. O'Donnell J, Cox D, Shows T. The ornithine aminotransferase gene is on human chromosome 10. Invest Ophthalmol Vis Sci. 1985;26:128(abst).

23. Wang T, Milam AH, Steel G, et al. A mouse model of gyrate atrophy of the choroid and retina: early retinal pigment epithelium damage and progressive retinal degeneration. J Clin Invest. 1996;97:2753–62.

24. Takki KK, Milton RC. The natural history of gyrate atrophy of the choroid and retina. Ophthalmology. 1981;88:292–301.

25. McCulloch JC, Arshinoff SA, Marliss EB, et al. Hyperornithinemia and gyrate atrophy of the choroid and retina. Ophthalmology. 1978;85:918–28.

26. Weleber RG, Kennaway NG. Gyrate atrophy of the choroid and retina. In: Heckenlively JR, ed. Retinitis pigmentosa. Philadelphia: JB Lippincott; 1988:198–220.

27. Feldman RB, Mayo SS, Robertson DM, et al. Epiretinal membranes and cystoid macular edema in gyrate atrophy of the choroid and retina. Retina. 1989;9:139–42.

28. Kaiser-Kupfer M, Kuwabara T, Uga S, et al. Cataract in gyrate atrophy: clinical and morphological studies. Invest Ophthalmol Vis Sci. 1983;24:432–6.

29. Steel D, Wood CM, Richardson J, et al. Anterior subcapsular plaque cataract in hyperornithinemia gyrate atrophy: a case report. Br J Ophthalmol. 1992;76:762–3.

30. Weleber RG, Kennaway NG. Clinical trial of vitamin B_6 for gyrate atrophy of the choroid and retina. Ophthalmology. 1981;88:316–24.

31. Raitta C, Carlson S, Vannas-Sulonen K. Gyrate atrophy of the choroid and retina: ERG of the neural retina and the pigment epithelium. Br J Ophthalmol. 1990;74:363–7.

32. Takki K. Gyrate atrophy of the choroid and retina associated with hyperornithinemia. Br J Ophthalmol. 1974;58:3–23.

33. Kellner U, Weleber RG, Kennaway NG, et al. Gyrate atrophy–like phenotype with normal plasma ornithine. Retina 1997;17:403–13.

34. Sipila I, Simell O, Rapola J, et al. Gyrate atrophy of the choroid and retina with hyperornithinemia: tubular aggregates and type 2 fiber atrophy in muscle. Neurology. 1979;29:996–1005.

35. Kaiser-Kupfer MI, Kuwabara T, Askansas V, et al. Systemic manifestations of gyrate atrophy of the choroid and retina. Ophthalmology. 1981;88:302–6.

36. Fishman GA, Fried W, Jednock N. Vitreochorioretinal degeneration associated with trichomegaly. Ann Ophthalmol. 1976;8:811–5.

37. Wilson DJ, Weleber RG, Green WR. Ocular clinicopathologic study of gyrate atrophy. Am J Ophthalmol. 1991;111:24–33.

38. Berson EL, Shih VE, Sullivan PL. Ocular findings in patients with gyrate atrophy on pyridoxine and low-protein, low-arginine diets. Ophthalmology. 1981;88:311–5.

39. Berson EL, Hanson AH, Rosner B, Shih VE. A two year trial of low protein, low arginine diets or vitamin B_6 for patients with gyrate atrophy. Birth Defects Orig Artic Ser. 1982;18:209–18.

40. Kaiser-Kupfer MI, Caruso RC, Valle D. Gyrate atrophy of the choroid and retina— long-term reduction of ornithine slows retinal degeneration. Arch Ophthalmol. 1991;109:1539–48.

41. Wang T, Steel G, Milam AH, et al. Correction of ornithine accumulation prevents retinal degeneration in a mouse model of gyrate atrophy of the choroid and retina. Proc Natl Acad Sci U S A. 2000;97:1224–9.

DEFINITION
• Nonprogressive poor night vision present since birth.

KEY FEATURES
• Normal fundus (inherited as autosomal dominant, autosomal recessive, or X-linked recessive).
• Abnormal fundus (Oguchi's disease, fundus albipunctatus).

ASSOCIATED FEATURES
• The pathology has an anatomical locus, as revealed by visual function tests.
• Molecular genetic studies suggest pathogenetic mechanisms in certain types.

INTRODUCTION

Nowhere in ophthalmology does the name of a disorder so aptly and completely describe all the essentials of the disease as congenital stationary night blindness (CSNB). The early onset of nonprogressive night vision difficulty is the hallmark of CSNB. However, CSNB is not a single disease but rather encompasses diverse disorders that share this common feature. None of the variants is currently treatable. The disorders of CSNB are divided conveniently into two groups: those with a fundus of normal appearance and those with an abnormal fundus.

NORMAL FUNDUS

A fundus of normal appearance with CSNB is inherited as autosomal dominant, autosomal recessive, or X-linked recessive. Because the clinical appearance of these eyes is normal, diagnosis is based on history and ancillary testing.

Diagnosis

The paradigm for autosomal dominant inheritance is exemplified by the complete genealogical records of two large pedigrees with CSNB, which began in the seventeenth century and span 11 generations—the Nougaret family of France[1] and the Danish family studied by Rambusch.[2] Patients who have autosomal dominant CSNB almost invariably have normal vision without a significant refractive error. This is in contradistinction to a significant number of patients in whom CSNB is inherited in the recessive mode (autosomal and X-linked), and who seek treatment for night blindness in association with poor vision, nystagmus, and high-grade myopia. When present, these features can muddle the diagnosis of CSNB.

Specific psychophysical and electrophysiological studies are useful for understanding these diseases and confirming the diagnosis. The initial distinction was based on two different electroretinographic (ERG) findings, named after the investigators who first described them. In 1952, Schubert and Bornschein described a progressive increase in the initial negative response (a wave) during dark adaptation, but without a corresponding increase in the subsequent positive response (b wave).[3] This electronegative ERG finding in CSNB is known as the Schubert–Bornschein response and is seen mostly in autosomal recessive and X-linked recessive CSNB. In 1954, Riggs published the finding of a reduction in amplitude but normal waveform of the photopic response which, under scotopic conditions, manifested only a slight increase in amplitude.[4] The Riggs ERG finding is seen mostly in autosomal dominant CSNB, including members of both the Nougaret and Rambusch families. However, either ERG response may occur in families with the various inheritance patterns.

In the initial studies, rhodopsin pigment concentrations and kinetics measured by fundus reflectometry were found to be normal in patients with CSNB who had a fundus of normal appearance.[5] This finding places the site of pathology proximal to the rod outer segments. In the Schubert–Bornschein response, with a deep a wave of normal appearance, the abnormality is hypothesized to be in the midretinal layer. The abnormal a wave seen in the Riggs response suggests the inner segments of the photoreceptors as the primary site. However, a subsequent study of fundus reflectometry identified a group of patients with CSNB who had abnormal rhodopsin kinetics.[6]

Another classification, complete and incomplete CSNB, is suggested on the basis of visual function studies performed on patients with autosomal recessive and X-linked recessive CSNB who manifested the Schubert–Bornschein electronegative ERG findings.[7] The complete type of CSNB manifests no detectable rod function, with only a slight reduction in cone function in association with diminished vision and myopia. The incomplete type of disease manifests some remaining rod function, more severe cone dysfunction, visual acuity loss, and no specific refractive error. There are now reports confirming a genetic basis for the distinction, because participating family members were found to have either the complete or incomplete type of CSNB.[8]

The incomplete type of X-linked CSNB is associated with a gene that affects the L-type voltage-gated calcium channels.[9] The pathogenetic mechanism is not clear, but it may affect photoreceptor cell neurotransmission or midretinal neural receptors and their responses. The complete type of X-linked CSNB is found at a different locus on the X chromosome.

Studies of molecular genetics have been informative, as well, for dominant CSNB. The possibility that CSNB and retinitis pigmentosa may be allelic suggested candidate genes for study. A heterozygous missense mutation in the rhodopsin gene (Ala292Glu) was confirmed in one patient with CSNB in whom the mode of inheritance could not be determined.[10] Subsequently, studies in families who have dominant inheritance revealed two additional missense mutations in the rhodopsin gene (Gly90Asp) (Thr94Ile).[11,12]

Linkage analysis in a large Danish family (Rambusch pedigree) showing autosomal dominant inheritance of CSNB assigned the locus to the distal chromosome 4p near the gene that encodes the subunit of rod photoreceptor cGMP-phosphodiesterase (βPDE).[13] Because a homozygous nonsense mutation in β-phosphodiesterase had been described recently in autosomal recessive retinitis pigmentosa, this gene was sequenced in the Rambusch pedigree and a heterozygous missense mutation (His258Asp) was identified in affected family members.[14] In the Nougaret family a missense mutation resulting in one amino acid substitution (Gly38Asp) in the α subunit of transducin has been identified.[15] In summary, three different proteins (rhodopsin, the subunit of rod cGMP-phosphodiesterase, and the α subunit of rod transducin), each with one missense mutation and one amino acid substitution, result in autosomal dominant CSNB. Each of these proteins participates in the phototransduction cascade.

A hypothetical pathogenetic model called *constitutive activation* has been proposed to account for the clinical findings. With abnormalities in a protein that participates in phototransduction, there is a continuous ever-present low level of illumination even in the absence of light or the chromophore. This does not allow for full dark adaptation of the rods, which are constantly desensitized, especially in low illumination. This pathophysiological process may be a common final pathway when the phototransduction cascade is affected (see Oguchi's disease).

Pathology

Histopathology studies of these disorders are quite rare. Two well-documented cases, of the Riggs[16] and Schubert–Bornschein[17] types, respectively, agreed that the rod and cone photoreceptors are histopathologically normal. A recent study (Schubert–Bornschein type) remarked on disorganization of the outer plexiform, outer nuclear, and inner nuclear layers.[18]

ABNORMAL FUNDUS

A fundus of abnormal appearance in association with CSNB includes Oguchi's disease and fundus albipunctatus. These two diseases have very little in common, save early-onset nonprogressive night blindness.

Oguchi's Disease

A series of articles in the early twentieth century by the Japanese ophthalmologist C. Oguchi stamped his name on this most unusual disease. The characteristic yellowish metallic sheen of the posterior pole places the retinal vessels in stark relief and serves to establish the diagnosis on a clinical basis (Fig. 111-1, *A*). After prolonged dark adaptation the yellowish fundus appearance reverts to normal, a phenomenon described by and named after Oguchi's countryman, Mizuo (Fig. 111-1, *B*). Reexposure to light results in the return of the metallic sheen.

The abnormal fundus color and the reversion to normal after dark adaptation suggest an abnormality in the rod photopigment, rhodopsin. However, the delay in dark adaptation (normal rod thresholds reached only after several hours) does not correlate with the Mizuo phenomenon.[19] In addition, fundus reflectometry studies document both normal rhodopsin concentrations and normal regeneration kinetics.[20]

Cone function seems normal because cone adaptation, final cone thresholds, and the photopic ERG response are normal. Rod function is abnormal, with normal rod thresholds reached only after 4 hours or longer (normal is 30 minutes) and scotopic ERG showing only a small electronegative response, even when the rod thresholds have reached normal.

Rhodopsin kinase and arrestin are both responsible for terminating the phototransduction cascade. A null allele in the genes for each of these proteins is responsible for Oguchi's disease.[21,22] Therefore, in a similar fashion as discussed with other forms of CSNB, the persistent low level of light may desensitize the rods continually.

Pathology

There are several conflicting histopathological reports, which include the identification of a pigmented cellular layer interposed

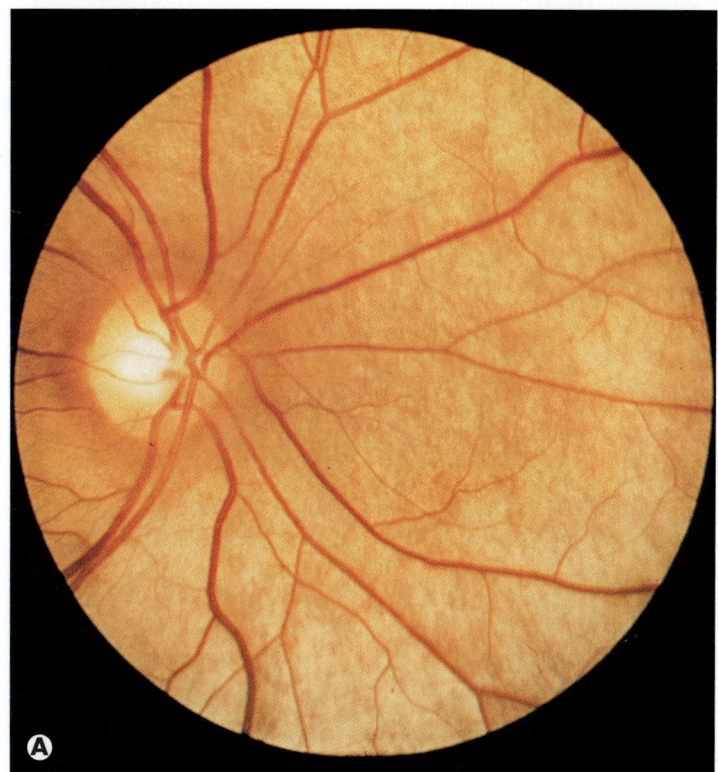

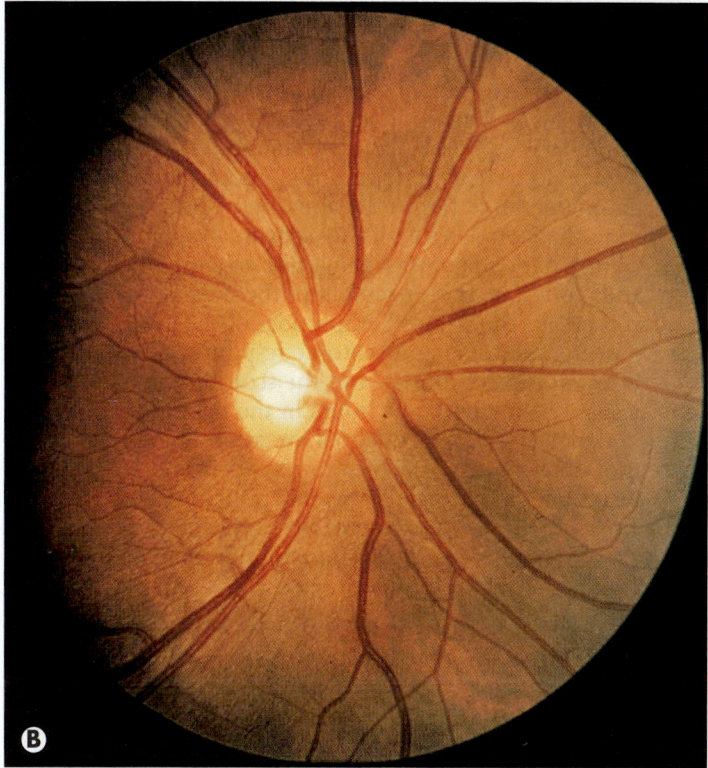

FIG. 111-1 ■ Oguchi's disease. **A,** The yellowish metallic sheen is apparent nasal to the optic disc. **B,** After 3 hours of dark adaptation the fundus reverts to the normal coloration (Mizuo phenomenon).

between the normal retinal pigment epithelium and photoreceptors,[23] an abnormal layering of lipofuscin between the retinal pigment epithelium and photoreceptors,[24] and abnormal numbers, arrangement, and structure of the cones.[25]

Fundus Albipunctatus

Like Oguchi's disease, fundus albipunctatus has a distinctive fundus appearance which should immediately suggest the diagnosis. There are multiple tiny white dots that are monotonous in their

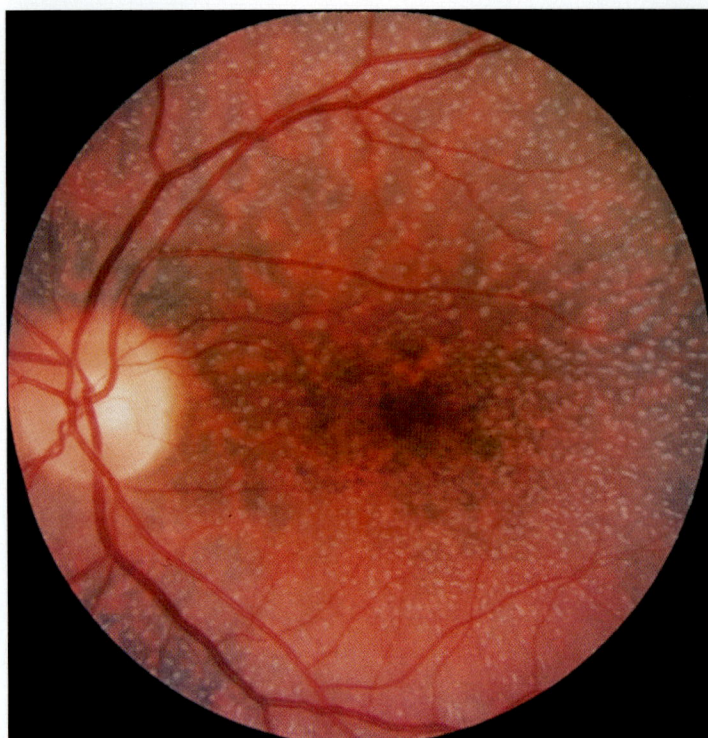

FIG. 111-2 ▉ **Fundus albipunctatus.** The posterior pole and beyond shows multiple small, discrete, round, white dots which spare the fovea.

perfect regularity. They involve the posterior pole, spare the macula, and extend into the midperiphery (Fig. 111-2). Fluorescein angiography shows focal areas of transmission hyperfluorescence, which do not correlate with the fundus pathology.

Visual pigments of both rods and cones show a delay in regeneration that correlates with the delay in visual function studies.[26] During dark adaptation the return to normal of both the rods and cones is prolonged, and there is a delay in the cone–rod break. The reduced amplitudes of the ERG a wave and b wave of the photopic and scotopic responses are diminished under normal test conditions, but the scotopic response slowly returns to normal after a few hours in the dark. The prolonged delay in dark adaptation is due to a mutation in the gene for 11-cis retinol dehydrogenase.[27] This enzyme converts 11-cis retinol to 11-cis retinal in the retinal pigment epithelium, and it then is transported to the photoreceptor to combine with opsin as rhodopsin. The delays in both adaptation and the ERG are consistent with a mutation in this enzyme.

CONCLUSION

The term *congenital stationary night blindness* comprises a heterogeneous group of disorders that have a common history but differ considerably in terms of clinical pictures and visual function studies. An awareness of the distinguishing findings should suggest the correct diagnosis. For a more thorough discussion of this subject the reader is referred to the LVII Edward Jackson Memorial lecture by Thaddeus P. Dryja, MD, entitled *Molecular Genetics of Oguchi Disease, Fundus Albipunctatus, and Other Forms of Stationary Night Blindness.*[28]

REFERENCES

1. Nettleship E. A history of congenital stationary night blindness in nine consecutive generations. Trans Ophthalmol Soc U K. 1907;27:269–93.
2. Rosenberg TR, Haim M, Piczenik Y, et al. Autosomal dominant stationary night-blindness. A large family rediscovered. Acta Ophthalmol. 1991;69:694–702.
3. Schubert G, Bornschein H. Bietrag zur analyse des menschichen elektroretinogramms. Ophthalmol. 1952;123:396–413.
4. Riggs LA. Electroretinography in cases of nightblindness. Am J Ophthalmol. 1954;38:70–8.
5. Carr RE, Ripps H, Siegel IM, et al. Rhodopsin and the electrical activity of the retina in congenital night blindness. Invest Ophthalmol. 1966;5:497–508.
6. Keunen JEE, van Meel GJ, van Norren D. Rod densitometry in congenital stationary night blindness. Appl Optics. 1988;27:1050–6.
7. Miyake Y, Yagasaki K, Horiguchi M, et al. Congenital stationary night blindness with negative electroretinogram. A new classification. Arch Ophthalmol. 1986;104:1013–20.
8. Boycott KM, Pearce WG, Musarella MA, et al. Evidence for genetic heterogeneity in X-linked congenital stationary night blindness. Am J Hum Genet. 1998;62:865–75.
9. Strom TM, Nyakatura G, Apfelstedt-Sylla E, et al. An L-type calcium-channel gene mutated in incomplete X-linked congenital stationary night blindness. Nat Genet. 1998;19:260–3.
10. Dryja TP, Berson EL, Rao VR, et al. Heterozygous missense mutation in the rhodopsin gene as a cause of congenital stationary night blindness. Nat Genet. 1993;4:280–3.
11. Sieving PA, Richards JE, Naarendorp F, et al. Dark-light: model for nightblindness from the human rhodopsin Gly90→Asp mutation. Proc Natl Acad Sci U S A. 1995;92:880–4.
12. Al-Jandal N, Farrar GF, Kiang AS, et al. A novel mutation within the rhodopsin gene (Thr–94–Ile) causing autosomal dominant congenital stationary night blindness. Hum Mutat. 1999;13:75–81.
13. Gal A, Xu S, Pizenik Y, et al. Gene for autosomal dominant congenital stationary night blindness maps to the same region as the gene for the α-subunit of the rod photoreceptor cGMP phosphodiesterase (PDEB) in chromosome 4p16.3. Hum Mol Genet. 1994;3:323–5.
14. Gal A, Orth U, Baehr W, et al. Heterozygous missense mutation in the rod cGMP phosphodiesterase α-subunit gene in autosomal dominant stationary night blindness. Nat Genet. 1994;7:64–7.
15. Dryja TP, Hahn LB, Reboul T, et al. Missense mutation for the gene encoding the α subunit of rod transducin in the Nougaret form of congenital stationary night blindness. Nat Genet. 1996;13:358–60.
16. Vaghefi A, Vaghefi HA, Green WR, et al. Correlation of clinicopathologic findings in a patient. Congenital night blindness, branch retinal vein occlusion, cilioretinal artery, drusen of the optic nerve head, and intraretinal pigmented lesion. Arch Ophthalmol. 1978;96:2097–104.
17. Watanabe I, Taniguchi Y, Morioka K, et al. Congenital stationary night blindness with myopia: a clinicopathologic study. Doc Ophthalmol. 1986;63:55–62.
18. Yamaguchi K, Yamada T, Tamai M. Histological examination of the human retina with congenital stationary night blindness (Japanese). Nippon Ganka Gakkai Zasshi. 1995;99:440–4.
19. Carr RE, Gouras P. Oguchi's disease. Arch Ophthalmol. 1965;73:646–56.
20. Carr RE, Ripps H. Rhodopsin kinetics and rod adaptation in Oguchi's disease. Invest Ophthalmol. 1967;6:426–36.
21. Fuchs S, Nakazawa M, Maw M, et al. A homozygous 1-base pair deletion in the arrestin gene is a frequent cause of Oguchi disease in Japanese. Nat Genet. 1995;10:360–2.
22. Cideciyan AV, Zhao XY, Nielsen L, et al. Null mutation in the rhodopsin kinase gene slows recovery kinetics of rod and cone phototransduction in man. Proc Natl Acad Sci U S A. 1998;95:328–33.
23. Yamanaka T. Existence of pigment displacement in the human eye. The first autopsy of Oguchi's disease. Klin Monatsbl Augenheilkd. 1924;73:742–52.
24. Kuwabara Y, Ishihara K, Akiya S. Histopathological and electron microscopic studies on the retina in Oguchi's disease. Acta Soc Ophthalmol Jpn. 1963;67:1323–51.
25. Oguchi C. Zur anatomie der sogenannten Oguchischen krankheit. Graefes Arch Klin Ophthalmol. 1925;115:234–45.
26. Carr RE, Ripps H, Siegel IM. Visual pigment kinetics and adaptation in fundus albipunctatus. Doc Ophthalmol Proc Ser. 1974;4:193–9.
27. Yamamoto H, Simon A, Eriksson U, et al. Mutations in the gene encoding 11-cis retinol dehydrogenase cause delayed dark adaptation and fundus albipunctatus. Nat Genet. 1999;22:188–91.
28. Dryja TP. Molecular genetics of Oguchi disease, fundus albipunctatus, and other forms of stationary night blindness. Am J Ophthalmol. 2000;130:547–63.

CHAPTER

112 Hereditary Vitreoretinopathies

ALAN E. KIMURA

DEFINITION
- A group of rare, inherited disorders with primary manifestations that include vitreous and retinal degeneration.

KEY FEATURES
- Premature vitreous syneresis.
- Retinal degeneration.
- Abnormal acquired retinal pigmentation.

ASSOCIATED FEATURES
- Autosomal dominant or X-linked recessive inheritance patterns.
- Loss of b wave on electroretinography.
- Retinal pigment epithelial hyperplasia or atrophy.
- Retinal vascular abnormalities.
- Vitreous bands.
- Retinal detachment.

INTRODUCTION

The hereditary vitreoretinopathies are a diverse group of disorders that comprise numerous conditions. Although rare, these diseases are intriguing. Several newly described conditions are included in this chapter, in addition to the diseases classically chosen for discussion. Also, relevant reports concerning molecular diagnostic methods are incorporated.

Patients who are affected by hereditary vitreoretinopathies may have a dramatic clinical picture with characteristic ophthalmoscopic findings, often accompanied by severe visual sequelae that require extensive vitreoretinal surgery. Some diseases feature premature vitreous degeneration with high rates of retinal detachment. Other hereditary vitreoretinopathies manifest secondary vitreous degeneration that arises from primary retinal disease. Some share unusual electroretinographic (ERG) abnormalities, which include an unexplained selective loss of the b wave amplitude. This is not to imply that a single cause exists for selective b wave loss in the hereditary vitreoretinopathies. More likely, multiple links occur in the chain, which, if broken, produce the waveform abnormality of selective b wave loss (Box 112-1). All but two of the diseases in this chapter are inherited in an autosomal dominant fashion, the exceptions being X-linked recessive inheritance in juvenile retinoschisis and X-linked recessive inheritance in some pedigrees of familial exudative vitreoretinopathy (FEVR).

The exact role of the vitreous body in these diseases is unknown and has received little attention. Sebag[1] studied the anatomy of the vitreous body and hypothesized on its role in retinal diseases. Historically, it was felt to play a passive role in the maintenance of the volume of the eye and was inviolate because of poor surgical outcomes. However, therapeutic vitrectomy became safe with refinements in modern guillotine cutters.

As a result of considerable surgical experience, our understanding of the role of vitreoretinal traction in hereditary retinal diseases is now expanding.

For each of the entities discussed below, a McKusick identification number is given. *McKusick's Mendelian Inheritance in Man* is a textbook that is a catalog of genes and genetic disorders in man.[2] Each disease is coded with a number, and the book is updated constantly. The book is a central reference for the discussion of genetic diseases among researchers and clinicians. Recent advances in molecular biology have increased the utility of this work tremendously, and it is now available on the Internet.[2]

STICKLER'S SYNDROME

INTRODUCTION

Stickler's syndrome also is known as hereditary arthro-ophthalmopathy. It is of autosomal dominant inheritance, and the penetrance is complete but the expressivity is widely variable. It is a progressive disorder with a high risk of both ocular problems and systemic morbidity. The clinical spectrum of affected patients who have Stickler's syndrome includes high myopia, retinal detachments, and premature degenerative changes of cartilage.

EPIDEMIOLOGY AND PATHOGENESIS

Stickler's syndrome is the most common autosomal dominantly inherited connective tissue disorder in the American Midwest.[3] The strongest case for the argument that vitreous body abnormalities cause retinal pathology arises primarily in Stickler's syndrome. It is hypothesized that the vitreous degeneration is a direct effect of mutations in a structural protein, procollagen II. A significant advance in our understanding of Stickler's syndrome (McKusick No. 120140) was the discovery of a type II collagen gene (*COL2A1*) mutation on the long arm of chromosome 12 in affected pedigrees. The gene product is a building block in various types of tissue. Structural alterations in the highly ordered

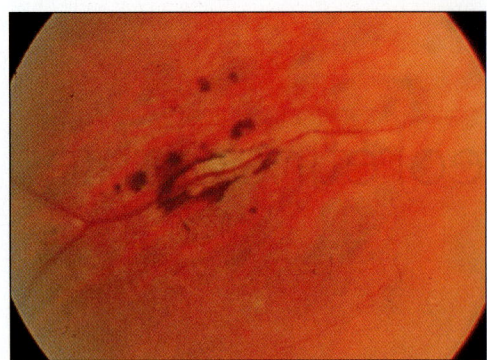

FIG. 112-1 ■ Fundus view of the eye of a patient with Stickler's syndrome. Note the radial perivascular pigmentary changes.

vitreous body that arise from *COL2A1* gene mutations cause vitreous degeneration and a high rate of complex retinal detachments.[4,5] Translational frameshift mutations are a common pathway by which disease is produced in patients with Stickler's syndrome.[6] The original family of the Wagner's syndrome (early-onset cataracts, lattice degeneration of the retina, retinal detachment without involvement of nonocular tissues) is not linked to the *COL2A1* gene and may be called Wagner's syndrome type I.

OCULAR MANIFESTATIONS

High myopia (−8 to −18D) is very common, as is an optically empty vitreous with membranes and strands. The optically empty vitreous refers to the presence of early onset, large lacunae of syneretic gel. It is best seen at the slit lamp through a widely dilated pupil. Dilated fundus examination typically reveals perivascular hyperpigmentary changes (Fig. 112-1). Retinal breaks are common and may lead to complicated retinal detachments (50% of eyes in patients with Stickler's syndrome). Giant retinal tears also may occur. Stickler's syndrome–associated retinal detachments are notoriously difficult to repair, probably because of the underlying abnormal adherence between the vitreous and the retina.

Other ocular manifestations include presenile cataracts (in those patients less than 45 years of age, with peripheral, comma-shaped, cortical opacities). Open-angle glaucoma and ocular hypertension are additional problems found in patients with Stickler's syndrome.

DIAGNOSIS AND ANCILLARY TESTING

Based on the ocular findings alone, the diagnosis can be difficult. When coupled with one or more of the systemic abnormalities, especially with a positive family history, the diagnosis is more assured. Tests for the underlying gene defect are available in some centers and can confirm the diagnosis.

The ERG changes are commensurate with axial myopia reducing b wave amplitudes. No intrinsic abnormality of the generators of the waveforms in the ERG appears to occur. Similarly, the perimetric abnormalities, if any, occur secondary to retinal detachments and do not result from abnormalities in the visual pathway directly. For the differential diagnosis of Stickler's syndrome, see Box 112-2.

SYSTEMIC ASSOCIATIONS

Of all the diseases discussed in this chapter, Stickler's syndrome is unique in its wide-ranging systemic complications. Generalized epiphyseal dysplasia occurs, with premature degenerative changes in weight-bearing joints. Abnormalities of collagen that affect the head include submucous clefting of the palate and bifid uvula (75%; palpation with a gloved finger may be necessary to diagnose a submucous cleft). Midfacial flattening and the Pierre–Robin anomaly often are subtle, and radiographic studies may be required for diagnosis.[7] Sensorineural hearing loss often may be overlooked, as well as mitral valve prolapse (50%),[8] unless sought after in the systemic evaluation. The hearing loss is progressive and affects most individuals by middle age.

TREATMENT, COURSE, AND OUTCOME

Early in life, corrective lenses based on a cycloplegic refraction are prescribed to prevent amblyopia. A multidisciplinary evaluation (otolaryngology, orthopedics) and genetic tests (*COL2A1* gene) with genetic counseling are important components of a global approach to the family with Stickler's disease. A national organization, Stickler Involved People, has branches in England and the Netherlands and plans to expand to Canada and Australia. (The organization can be reached at 316-775-2993 [U.S.].) Annual to semiannual retinal evaluation through dilated pupils with prophylactic treatment of new retinal tears is suggested for longitudinal follow-up. If retinal detachment does not occur, the visual morbidity is minimal. Low-vision evaluation may be beneficial for all patients who develop a serious loss of vision that affects activities of daily living.

EROSIVE VITREORETINOPATHY

INTRODUCTION

Erosive vitreoretinopathy is an autosomal dominantly inherited disease named after its unusual thinning of the retinal pigment epithelium, which produces a characteristically enhanced visualization of the fine choroidal vasculature.[9] In erosive vitreoretinopathy, a striking distortion of the retina occurs, apparently from tangential tractional forces transmitted thorough the vitreous. Pathological vitreoretinal forces are further indicated by the high rate of rhegmatogenous retinal detachments (50%) and severe retinal breaks, such as giant retinal tears. The pathological sequence of events at the molecular level is not yet known.

EPIDEMIOLOGY AND PATHOGENESIS

Erosive vitreoretinopathy is quite rare. The disease (ERVR; McKusick No. 143200) has been mapped to a genetic locus similar to that for Wagner's syndrome on chromosome 5q13–14. These two diseases represent different alleles, however.[10]

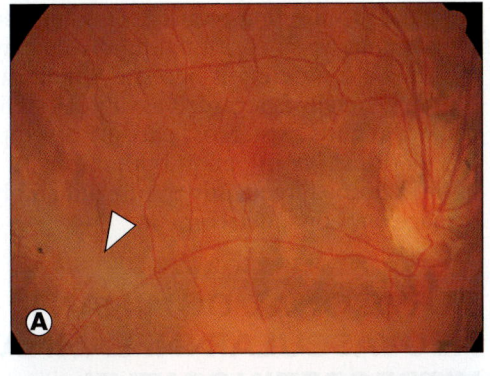

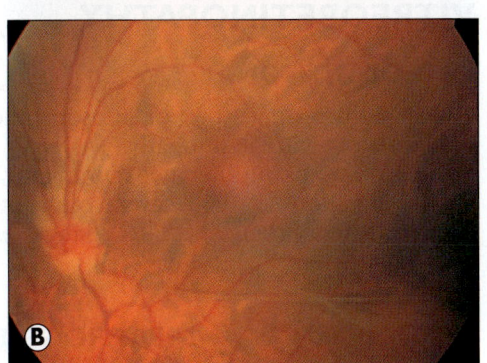

FIG. 112-2 ▮ Fundus view of the eyes of a patient with erosive vitreoretinopathy. Note the vitreous band (*arrow*) and unusual vitreoretinal traction, which has dragged the retinal vasculature superiorly in each eye. **A**, Right eye; **B**, left eye.

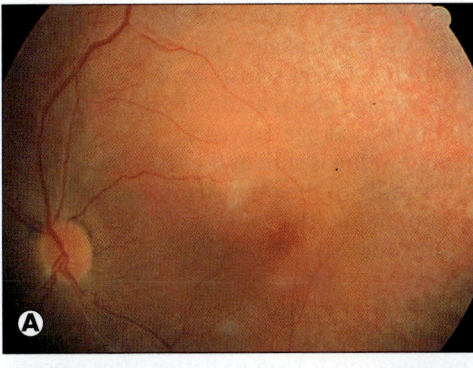

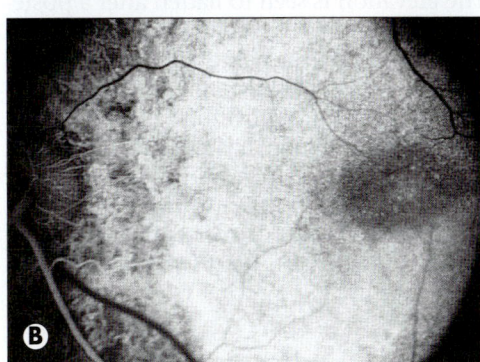

FIG. 112-3 ▮ Eye of a teenage boy with erosive vitreoretinopathy. **A**, Fundus view. **B**, Fluorescein angiogram. Note the unusual thinned retina and retinal pigment epithelium along the superotemporal arcade, which evokes the term *erosive*. Also, note the abnormal hypofluorescence in the macula and thinning of the retinal pigment epithelium adjacent to the optic nerve head.

OCULAR MANIFESTATIONS

Early in the course of the disease premature vitreous syneresis occurs, with traction bands and multiple foci of vitreoretinal traction (Fig. 112-2). Retinal detachments that arise from this atypical vitreous traction are common (50%). Similar to those occurring in patients with Stickler's syndrome, giant tears are difficult problems for the vitreoretinal surgeon to repair. Indeed, 20% of patients are left with no light perception as a result of complex retinal detachments. Even without macular detachment, progressive retinal pigment epithelial thinning may lead to profound choroidal atrophy, or "cratering," in the posterior pole (Figs. 112-3 and 112-4).

DIAGNOSIS AND ANCILLARY TESTING

The diagnosis can be suspected strongly on the basis of the clinical findings of premature vitreous syneresis and choroidal atrophy. Dark adaptometry demonstrates progressive nyctalopia with progressive deterioration of the retina. Ring scotomas develop during the course of the disease, with loss of the central island from central choroidal atrophy later. ERG shows progressive deterioration of both rods and cones, in a similar fashion to that found with the group of diseases called retinitis pigmentosa. Patients with Goldmann–Favre disease typically progress to nonrecordable ERGs much earlier in life than do patients with erosive vitreoretinopathy. There are no known systemic associations (i.e., patients have normal bone survey findings). For the differential diagnosis of erosive vitreoretinopathy, see Box 112-2.

TREATMENT, COURSE, AND OUTCOME

As in other conditions with a high rate of detachments (e.g., Stickler's syndrome), annual to semiannual dilated retinal examination is prudent. Prophylactic treatment of symptomatic retinal breaks is indicated. Given the extremely high incidence of retinal detachment, similar treatment for asymptomatic, traction-related lesions appears prudent, albeit the value is unproved. Family members should be screened for retinal pathology in all diseases of known autosomal dominant inheritance. In the long term, the visual prognosis is poor because of progressive atrophy and retinal detachment.

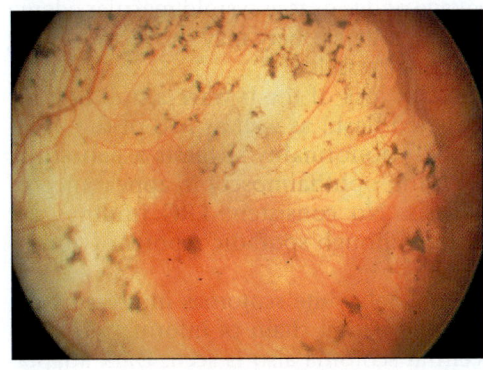

FIG. 112-4 ▮ Fundus view of the eye of the oldest member of a family affected by erosive vitreoretinopathy. Note the extensive full-thickness atrophy in the posterior pole in the form of a "crater."

X-LINKED JUVENILE RETINOSCHISIS

INTRODUCTION

X-linked juvenile retinoschisis is a vitreoretinal degeneration affecting males. The cystic, spoke-like foveal changes, visual acuity deterioration, peripheral retinoschisis, and loss of ERG b wave are bilateral. Despite mutation heterogeneity, there are relatively uniform clinical characteristics, albeit with intrafamilial variation in onset and severity.

EPIDEMIOLOGY AND PATHOGENESIS

The disease is quite rare. X-linked juvenile retinoschisis (XLRS; McKusick No. 312700) has been localized to the short arm of the X chromosome in the region Xp22.1–p22.2. Sauer et al.[11] identified a candidate gene for XLRS comprising six exons encoding a 224–amino acid protein. The predicted protein sequence contains a highly conserved discoid domain, implicated in cell–cell adhesion and phospholipid binding. This may explain the splitting of the retina in XLRS. Because the disease is X-linked, affected patients are almost exclusively men. Loss-of-function mutations may result from mutations involving or creating cysteine residues, which alter tertiary protein folding or protein–protein interactions.

OCULAR MANIFESTATIONS

Cystic-like, stellate maculopathy, or foveal schisis, is present almost universally in XLRS and may be the only abnormality in

845

one half the cases (Fig. 112-5). Similar to the findings in Goldmann–Favre disease, no late leakage occurs on fluorescein angiography. In older patients, foveal schisis evolves into an atrophic maculopathy. The average visual acuity is 20/60 (6/18) at age 20 years and 20/200 (6/60) at age 60 years.[12]

In retinoschisis the inner retina is split at the level of the nerve fiber layer (Fig. 112-6), typically in the inferotemporal quadrant, and bilaterally in 40% of patients. The inner layer balloons into the vitreous cavity, and unsupported retinal vessels may lead to recurrent vitreous hemorrhages from associated vitreous traction. Vitreous veils may overlie the retinoschisis.[13] In XLRS, the vitreous exerts an effect upon the bullous nature of the retinoschisis lesion. The elevation is seen to flatten after a posterior vitreous detachment has produced a separation between the vitreous face and the internal limiting membrane. It is as if the vitreous releases the inner layers of the retina, which allows them to settle back into an anatomical position.

The Mizuo–Nakamura phenomenon has been described in four unrelated men who suffered from X-linked recessive retinoschisis.[14] Originally described in patients who had autosomal recessive Oguchi's disease, a form of congenital stationary night blindness, this phenomenon also occurs in patients who have an X-linked cone dystrophy.[15]

DIAGNOSIS AND ANCILLARY TESTING

The diagnosis is based on clinical examination, because ancillary testing is not particularly helpful. Fluorescein angiography generally shows no leakage of dye or true cystoid macular edema in the posterior pole, while the periphery may show slow filling of opacified, dendritic retinal vessels.[16]

The ERG shows selective loss of the b wave amplitude for the scotopic, nonattenuated flash, as well as loss of the oscillatory potentials. This ERG abnormality suggests a panretinal dysfunction, in spite of the ophthalmoscopic appearance of only foveal retinal schisis. No consistent ERG findings are found in female carriers, although sporadic reports of abnormalities exist.

Visual fields demonstrate absolute scotomas in areas of peripheral schisis, because the neural chain of information is interrupted. A relative central scotoma also is seen. Dark adaptation is normal or only minimally affected in X-linked retinoschisis. There are no known systemic associations. For the differential diagnosis of XLRS, see Box 112-2.

TREATMENT, COURSE, AND OUTCOME

Prophylactic treatment of retinoschisis or holes in schisis is not recommended, whereas secondary retinal detachment necessitates intervention. Combined retinal detachment and retinoschisis requires intervention to close the outer layer holes and full-thickness retinal breaks by vitrectomy, perfluorocarbon reattachment, and panretinal photocoagulation to areas of schisis and detachment, with scleral buckling of the retinal periphery. In young patients who are unable to comply with rigorous post-

operative positioning requirements imposed by instillation of long-acting gas, silicone oil tamponade may be preferable.

Genetic counseling is necessary in all cases. Carrier state detection generally is regarded as difficult in this disease, although isolated reports exist. Most patients develop a significant loss of macular function in one or both eyes with time. Children need to be examined frequently to rule out amblyopia, vitreous hemorrhage, or retinal detachment.

AUTOSOMAL DOMINANT NEOVASCULAR INFLAMMATORY VITREORETINOPATHY

INTRODUCTION

The most interesting aspect of autosomal dominant neovascular inflammatory vitreoretinopathy (ADNIV) is that it combines features of uveitis, proliferative retinopathy, and progressive retinal degeneration.[17] As with several of the other diseases grouped in this chapter, progressive ERG changes begin with selective b wave loss.

EPIDEMIOLOGY AND PATHOGENESIS

All patients who are afflicted with the condition are part of a large, multiple-generation pedigree concentrated in the

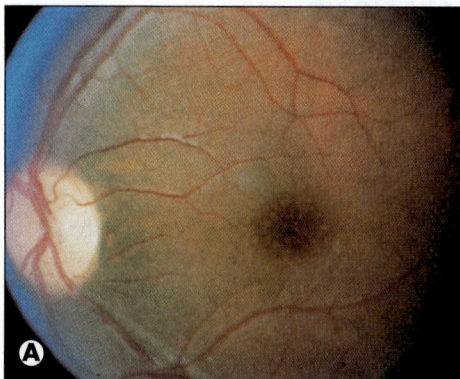
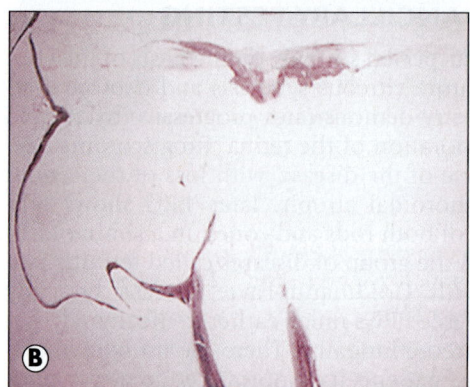
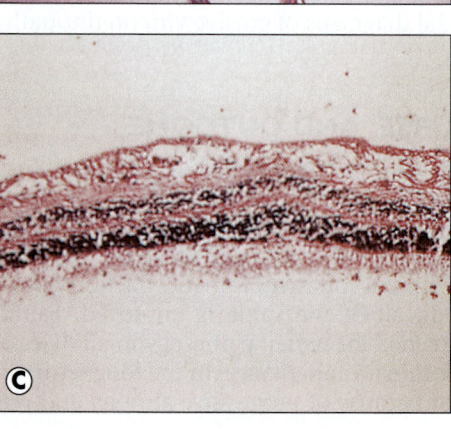

FIG. 112-6 ■ Juvenile retinoschisis. **A,** The characteristic foveal lesion, resembling a polycystic fovea, is shown. Typically, no leakage is present when fluorescein angiography is performed. **B,** A histological section of another eye shows a large temporal peripheral retinoschisis cavity. **C,** A histological section of another area of the same eye shows a splitting in the ganglion and nerve fiber layers of the retina on the earliest finding in juvenile retinoschisis. This pathology of the inner retinal layers is the same as that seen in reticular microcystoid degeneration and retinoschisis. (**A,** Courtesy of Dr. AJ Brucker. In: Yanoff M, Fine BS. Ocular pathology, ed 4. London: Mosby; 1996.)

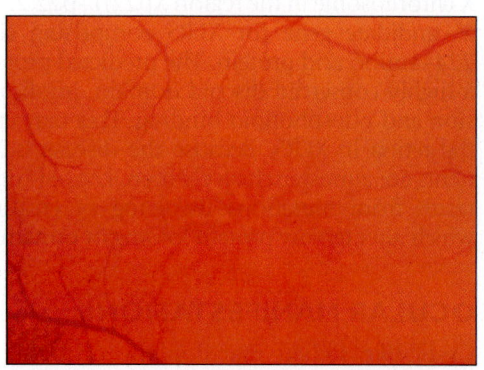

FIG. 112-5 ■ Fundus view of foveal schisis seen in a man who has X-linked juvenile retinoschisis. This lesion should not be confused with cystoid macular edema.

American Midwest. As the name implies, autosomal dominant inheritance is a critical feature of the condition. Genetic linkage for ADNIV (VRNI; McKusick No. 193235) has been established to chromosome 11q13 with a maximal logarithm of the odds (LOD), score of 11.9, centered on marker D11S527.[18]

OCULAR MANIFESTATIONS

Vitreous cells occur alone as the first manifestation of ADNIV, at which stage ERG b wave loss also is noted. These changes occur typically in the teenage years and early twenties. Pigmentary changes appear in the retina, with clumping but not the bone-spicule type of hyperpigmentation seen in retinitis pigmentosa. As the disease progresses, prominent cystoid macular edema with generalized retinal vascular incompetence may be seen. With full-blown disease, a sequence of peripheral retinal vascular closure, peripheral retinal neovascularization, and vitreous hemorrhage occurs (Fig. 112-7). Only minor syneretic vitreous changes, which appear to be secondary to retinal degeneration, occur in ADNIV. As a result, rhegmatogenous retinal detachment is not a common sequela. Traction retinal detachments are the most likely reason for vitreoretinal intervention. Neovascular glaucoma results from tractional changes in the retina or may occur as the end stage of retinal degeneration without detachments.

DIAGNOSIS AND ANCILLARY TESTING

ERG helps to establish the diagnosis of ADNIV. The characteristic selective loss of b wave amplitude (scotopic, 0dB attenuated standard flash) is seen at the earliest stages of disease, when the diagnosis of the condition is most in doubt. An abnormally low b wave–to–a wave ratio of amplitude is another characteristic of the ERG of affected patients. This may help in pedigree analysis to determine which family members are likely to be affected. With advancing age, progressive deterioration of all ERG responses occurs. No known systemic associations exist.

DIFFERENTIAL DIAGNOSIS

Unlike autosomal dominant vitreoretinochoroidopathy (ADVIRC), ADNIV has no distinct border to the peripheral pigmentary changes. Uveitis, proliferative disease, and ERG b wave changes are different from those of ADVIRC. The early ERG b wave loss is unlike that seen in retinitis pigmentosa–type diseases, although end-stage disease leads to progressive deterioration of the ERG a waves and b waves in both diseases.

TREATMENT, COURSE, AND OUTCOME

With advancing pathology, vitrectomy with membranectomy for traction retinal detachments may be necessary. Scatter photocoagulation may influence the course of inflammatory vascular closure and subsequent proliferative disease. It is important to note that, in the past, cataract surgery was often followed by intense postoperative uveitis. It is not known whether more modern techniques of cataract extraction and lens implantation will prove to cause less inflammation.

AUTOSOMAL DOMINANT VITREORETINOCHOROIDOPATHY

OCULAR MANIFESTATIONS

The classic finding of ADVIRC is a sharply defined posterior border to an area of abnormal hypopigmentation or hyperpigmentation for 360 degrees bilaterally between the ora serrata and the equator (Fig. 112-8).[19,20] Within this abnormally pigmented area are narrowed retinal arterioles, vascular incompetence, retinal neovascularization, punctate white retinal opacities, and later retinochoroidal atrophy. Cystoid macular edema, if present, is the most significant morbidity, although vitreous hemorrhage and epiretinal membranes also may affect the visual acuity. Profound alterations in the vitreous body are not described, although small numbers of vitreous cells and early posterior vitreous detachments may occur. The condition is slowly progressive and is not associated with retinal detachments. Histopathology has been described in an 88-year-old patient. Similar features to retinitis pigmentosa were found, along with some differences.[21] No linkage disequilibrium or gene has been identified to date for ADVIRC (VRCP; McKusick No. 193220).

DIAGNOSIS AND ANCILLARY TESTING

Patients who have ADVIRC have no nyctalopia, and ERG findings are normal in younger affected individuals and only moderately depressed in older patients. No known systemic associations exist. For the differential diagnosis of ADVIRC, see Box 112-2.

TREATMENT, COURSE, AND OUTCOME

Annual or biannual dilated fundus examination is suggested unless the disease is symptomatic. The long-term visual prognosis is good.

FAMILIAL EXUDATIVE VITREORETINOPATHY

INTRODUCTION

FEVR, reported initially in 1969 by Criswick and Schepens,[22] has been called dominant exudative vitreoretinopathy, also. Both eyes are affected, but usually asymmetrically.

EPIDEMIOLOGY AND PATHOGENESIS

Linkage of several northern European families with FEVR (EVR; McKusick 133780) has been established on chromosome 11 (11q13), and in a large consanguineous Asian family linkage to

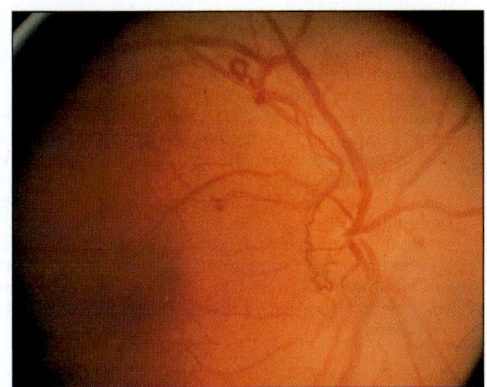

FIG. 112-7 ■ Fundus view of a patient who has autosomal dominant neovascular inflammatory vitreoretinopathy. Note the proliferative retinopathy along the superotemporal arcade.

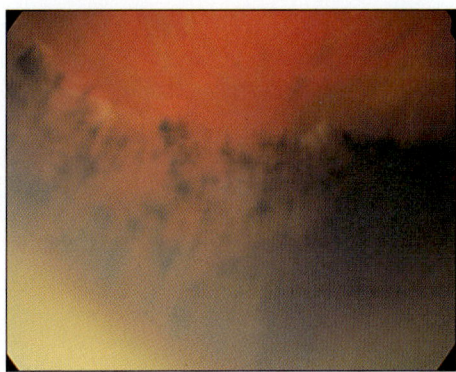

FIG. 112-8 ■ Fundus view of retinal periphery in autosomal dominant vitreoretinochoroidopathy. Note sharply demarcated posterior border to the hyperpigmented peripheral lesion. This border is a useful defining feature of autosomal dominant vitreoretinochoroidopathy.

D11S533 has been shown.[23] The locus of the disease in Schepens'[24,25] original reported family (Criswick–Schepens) also has been mapped to the long arm of chromosome 11. The gene that causes the disease has not been found to date.

Like retinitis pigmentosa, FEVR is genetically heterogeneous. It was believed at one time that FEVR was transmitted only as an autosomal dominant disease; however, independent reports now exist of X-linked recessive inheritance.[26,27] Although rare, FEVR accounts for a significant percentage of all retinal detachments in juvenile and infant patients.

OCULAR MANIFESTATIONS

The prominent feature is the abrupt cessation of peripheral retinal vessels in a scalloped pattern at the temporal equator (Figs. 112-9 and 112-10). Dilated retinal vessels may result in peripheral neovascularization with adjacent preretinal hemorrhage and may later evolve into a fibrovascular scar.[28] Subretinal exudates occur in 10–15% of eyes and can become massive, resembling Coats' disease.

The majority of retinal detachments occur in the first decade of life, with little progression after 10 years of age.[29,30] Vitreous abnormalities include posterior vitreous detachment and vitreous bands or sheets attached to avascular retina, although milder cases may not show any visible vitreous change. An ectopic macula may be found in 50% of patients. A positive-angle kappa or strabismus is common.

DIAGNOSIS AND ANCILLARY TESTING

The diagnosis is based on typical clinical findings, a positive family history, the lack of significant prematurity, and the exclusion of other possible causes of peripheral retinal pathology. Fluorescein angiography can be quite helpful because it highlights peripheral, nonperfused retina and shows the characteristic straightening of peripheral retinal vessels.

No significant ERG findings are noted. Even patients who have enough avascular peripheral retina to produce peripheral retinal neovascularization show only minor reductions in b wave amplitude. No known systemic associations occur. For the differential diagnosis of FEVR, see Box 112-2.

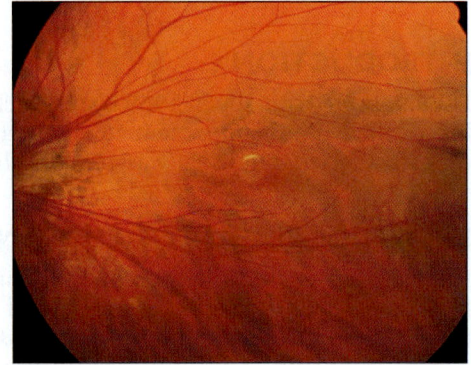

FIG. 112-9 ■ **Fundus view of a patient who has familial exudative vitreoretinopathy.** Note abnormally straightened retinal vasculature.

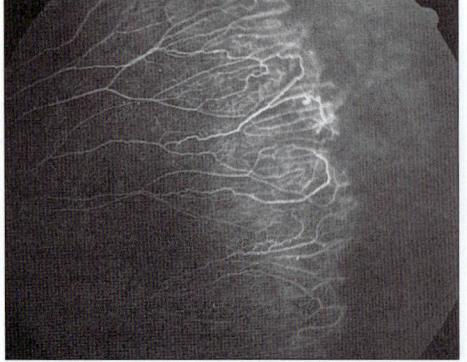

FIG. 112-10 ■ **Fluorescein angiogram of a patient who has familial exudative vitreoretinopathy.** Fluorescein angiography is an excellent tool to define the abnormal retinal vasculature in familial exudative vitreoretinopathy. Fluorescein angioscopy, if available, is particularly useful for peripheral retinal vascular examination.

TREATMENT, COURSE, AND OUTCOME

Early screening of individuals at risk is useful to identify nonperfused peripheral retina. Fluorescein angiography or angioscopy using the indirect ophthalmoscope and appropriate filters may be very useful in the identification of large areas of avascular peripheral retina.

Strabismus from dragged retina must be identified early. Retinal detachments primarily are tractional early in life and combined tractional and rhegmatogenous in the second decade (4–30% incidence).

REFERENCES

1. Sebag J. The vitreous. Structure, function, and pathobiology. New York: Springer-Verlag; 1989.
2. McKusick VA. Mendelian inheritance in man: catalogs of human genes and genetic disorders, ed 11. Baltimore: Johns Hopkins University Press; 1994; (http://www.ncbi.nlm.nih.gov/Omim).
3. Herrmann J, France TD, Spranger JVV, et al. The Stickler syndrome (hereditary arthroophthalmopathy). Birth Defects Orig Artic Ser. 1975;11:76–103.
4. Francomano CA, Liberfarb RM, Hirose T, et al. The Stickler syndrome: evidence for close linkage to the structural gene for type II collagen. Genomics. 1987;1:293–6.
5. Knowlton RG, Weaver EJ, Struyk AF, et al. Genetic linkage analysis of hereditary arthro-ophthalmopathy (Stickler syndrome) and the type II procollagen gene. Am J Hum Genet. 1989;45:681–8.
6. Ahmad NN, Ala KL, Knowlton RG, et al. Stop codon in the procollagen II gene (COL2A1) in a family with the Stickler syndrome (arthro-ophthalmopathy). Proc Natl Acad Sci U S A. 1991;88:6624–7.
7. Weingeist TA, Hermsen V, Hanson JVV, et al. Ocular and systemic manifestations of Stickler's syndrome: a preliminary report. In: Cotlier E, Maumenee IH, Berman ER, eds. Genetic eye diseases: retinitis pigmentosa and other inherited eye disorders; proceedings of the International Symposium on Genetics, September 1981. New York: Alan R Liss; 1982:539–60.
8. Liberfarb R, Goldblatt A. Prevalence of mitral-valve prolapse in the Stickler syndrome. Am J Hum Genet. 1986;24:387–92.
9. Brown DM, Kimura AK, Weingeist TA, Stone EM. Erosive vitreoretinopathy—a new clinical entity. Ophthalmology. 1994;101:694–704.
10. Brown DM, Graemiger RA, Hergersberg M, et al. Genetic linkage of Wagner disease and erosive vitreoretinopathy to chromosome 5q13–14. Arch Ophthalmol. 1995;113:671–5.
11. Sauer CG, Gehring A, Warneke-Wittsock R, et al. Positional cloning of the gene associated with X-linked juvenile retinoschisis. Nat Genet. 1997;17:164–70.
12. Forsius H, Krause U, Helve J, et al. Visual acuity in 183 cases of X-chromosomal retinoschisis. Can J Ophthalmol. 1973;8:385–93.
13. Tolentino FI, Schepens CL, Freeman HM. Vitreoretinal disorders: diagnosis and management. Philadelphia: WB Saunders; 1976:242–68.
14. deJong PT, Zrenner E, van Meel GJ, Keunen JE. Mizuo phenomenon in X-linked retinoschisis: pathogenesis of the Mizuo phenomenon. Arch Ophthalmol. 1991; 109:1104–8.
15. Heckenlively JR, Weleber RG. X-linked recessive cone dystrophy with tapetal-like sheen: a newly recognized entity with Mizuo–Nakamura phenomenon. Arch Ophthalmol. 1986;104:1322–8.
16. Green JL, Jampol LM. Vascular opacification and leakage in X-linked (juvenile) retinoschisis. Br J Ophthalmol. 1979;63:368–73.
17. Bennett SR, Folk JC, Kimura AK, et al. Autosomal dominant neovascular inflammatory vitreoretinopathy. Ophthalmology. 1990;97:1125–36.
18. Stone EM, Kimura AK, Folk JC, et al. Genetic linkage of autosomal dominant neovascular inflammatory vitreoretinopathy to chromosome 11q13. Hum Mol Genet. 1992;1:685–9.
19. Kaufman SJ, Goldberg ME, Orth DH, et al. Autosomal dominant vitreoretinochoroidopathy. Arch Ophthalmol. 1982;100:272–8.
20. Blair NP, Goldberg MF, Fishman GA, Salzano T. Autosomal dominant vitreoretinochoroidopathy (ADVIRC). Br J Ophthalmol. 1984;68:2–9.
21. Goldberg MF, Lee FL, Tso MOM, Fishman GA. Histopathologic study of the autosomal dominant vitreoretinochoroidopathy: peripheral annular pigmentary dystrophy of the retina. Ophthalmology. 1989;96:1736–46.
22. Criswick VG, Schepens CL. Familial exudative vitreoretinopathy. Am J Ophthalmol. 1969;68:578–94.
23. Price SM, Periam N, Humphries A, et al. Familial exudative vitreoretinopathy linked to D11S533 in a large Asian family with consanguinity. Ophthalmic Genet. 1996;17:53–7.
24. Li Y, Muller B, Fuhrmann C, et al. The autosomal dominant familial exudative vitreoretinopathy locus maps on 11q and is closely linked to D11S533. Am J Hum Genet. 1992;51:749–54.
25. Li Y, Fuhrmann C, Schwinger E, et al. The gene for autosomal dominant familial exudative vitreoretinopathy (Criswick–Schepens) on the long arm of chromosome 11. Am J Ophthalmol. 1992;113:712–3.
26. Plager DA, Orgel I, Ellis FD, et al. X-Linked recessive familial exudative vitreoretinopathy. Am J Ophthalmol. 1992;114:145–8.
27. Shastry BS, Hartzer MK, Trese MT. Familial exudative vitreoretinopathy: multiple modes of inheritance [Letter]. Clin Genet. 1993;44:275–6.
28. Gow J, Oliver GL. Familial exudative vitreoretinopathy. An expanded view. Arch Ophthalmol. 1971;86:150–5.
29. Miyakubo H, Inohara N, Hashimoto K. Retinal involvement in familial exudative vitreoretinopathy. Ophthalmologica. 1982;185:125–35.
30. van Nouhuys CE. Dominant exudative vitreoretinopathy and other vascular developmental disorders of the peripheral retina [Thesis]. Doc Ophthalmol. 1982; 54:1–415.

SECTION 5 VASCULAR DISORDERS

CHAPTER
113 Hypertensive Retinopathy

ADAM H. ROGERS

Chronic Hypertensive Retinopathy

DEFINITION
- Retinal vascular changes occurring from chronically elevated systemic arterial hypertension.

KEY FEATURES
- Narrowing and irregularity of retinal arteries.
- Arteriovenous nicking (narrowing of retinal veins at arteriovenous crossing sites).
- Blot retinal hemorrhages.
- Microaneurysms.
- Cotton-wool spots.

ASSOCIATED FEATURES
- Retinal venous obstruction.
- Retinal neovascularization.
- Retinal arterial emboli.

Malignant Acute Hypertensive Retinopathy

DEFINITION
- Retinal, choroidal, and optic nerve changes secondary to acutely elevated systemic arterial blood pressure.

KEY FEATURES
- Retinal arteriolar spasm.
- Superficial retinal hemorrhages.
- Cotton-wool spots.
- Serous retinal detachment.
- Optic disc edema.

ASSOCIATED FEATURES
- Choroidal ischemia.
- Retinal pigment epithelial changes.
- Optic neuropathy.
- Cortical blindness.
- Proteinuria, stroke, kidney failure, encephalopathy.

INTRODUCTION

Hypertensive retinopathy represents the ophthalmic findings of end-organ damage secondary to systemic arterial hypertension. Although its name implies only retinal involvement, changes in both the choroid and the optic nerve are observed, depending on the chronicity and severity of the disease. Ocular changes in malignant hypertension can be striking, with optic neuropathy, choroidopathy, and retinopathy. Changes from essential hypertension are subtler, affecting primarily the retinal vasculature. Because hypertension is so prevalent in industrialized countries, hypertensive retinopathy is a common condition encountered by all ophthalmologists and health care professionals.

EPIDEMIOLOGY AND PATHOGENESIS

Systemic arterial hypertension is one of the most common diseases of adults in industrialized countries. Although the medical literature subdivides hypertension into multiple groups, only essential (primary) and malignant hypertension are relevant to a discussion of hypertensive retinopathy. Essential hypertension is of unknown cause and is diagnosed when the average blood pressure measures greater than 140mmHg systolic or 90mmHg diastolic on at least two subsequent visits. In the United States alone, it is estimated that more than 25% of all adults and 60% of persons older than 60 years are affected. Blacks have a higher prevalence of hypertension than whites, and men are affected more than women.[1] However, over age 50, women have a higher prevalence than men.[2] Elevated blood pressure is rare in agrarian societies and in individuals who are physically active.[1]

Because high blood pressure is an asymptomatic disease, most patients remain undiagnosed or inadequately treated despite the relative ease of detection. In the National Health and Nutrition Study (NHANES III) that evaluated hypertensive adults aged 18 to 74 years, 68.4% were aware of their hypertension, 53.6% were receiving treatment, and only 27.4% had their hypertension under control.[3] Untreated or inadequately treated hypertension carries significant cardiovascular mortality. In patients with borderline hypertension, the relative risk of cardiovascular disease and end-stage renal disease is nearly double compared with patients with "optimal" blood pressure.[4]

The incidence of hypertensive retinal changes is variable and is often confounded by the presence of other retinal vascular disease, such as diabetes. In the Beaver Dam Eye Study,[5] which evaluated hypertensive patients without coexisting, confounding vascular diseases, the overall incidence of hypertensive retinopathy was about 15%; specifically, 8% showed retinopathy, 13% showed arteriolar narrowing, and 2% showed arteriovenous nicking. The predictive value of diagnosing systemic hypertension from ophthalmic findings on examination was only 47–53%, demonstrating that measurement of blood pressure is a more accurate means of diagnosis. The highest frequency of hypertensive retinopathy in the study population was identified in subjects with poor blood pressure control.

Malignant hypertension is a rare syndrome consisting of rapid and severe elevation of blood pressure, with the systolic component above 200mmHg or the diastolic blood pressure greater than 140mmHg. Although the absolute blood pressure measurement is important, the presence of systemic findings defines malignant hypertension. These include ocular, cardiac, renal, and cerebral injury. Persistently elevated malignant hypertension can lead to a rapidly fatal course, with heart failure, myocardial infarction, stroke, or renal failure.[1]

Nearly 1% of hypertensive patients develop malignant hypertension, and it is rare for patients to present initially with this form of elevated blood pressure. Most have a preexisting diagnosis of either primary or secondary hypertension. Malignant hypertension rarely occurs in individuals receiving treatment for hypertension. The average age at diagnosis is 40 years, with men affected more than women. With the advent of effective antihypertensive treatment, nearly 50% of patients survive more than 5 years.[6]

Heredity and environmental factors have been implicated in the pathogenesis of essential hypertension. In the elderly, an increase in basal smooth muscle tone occurs as a result of sympathetic overactivity with increases in the renin-angiotensin system. Other factors include salt sensitivity, low systemic calcium, and insulin resistance with hyperinsulinemia.[7] Secondary hypertension is due to an identifiable cause, usually related to an alteration in hormone secretion or renal function. With correction of the underlying cause, this form of hypertension can be cured.[6] The pathogenesis of malignant hypertension, similar to essential hypertension, is unknown. Research has focused on overactivity of the renin-angiotensin-aldosterone system, with high plasma renin-angiotensin levels as the cause.[7]

OCULAR MANIFESTATIONS

Chronic Hypertensive Retinopathy

Patients with hypertensive retinopathy are usually asymptomatic. Common clinical findings include focal constriction and dilatation of the retinal arterioles, tortuosity of the retinal arterioles, an increase in the arteriolar light reflex, and loss of transparency of the intra-arterial blood column (Fig. 113-1). Arteriovenous nicking is a highly specific finding and the hallmark of chronic hypertensive retinopathy. At the arteriovenous crossings in the retina, the vessels share a common adventitial sheath. Arteriovenous nicking is diagnosed when the crossing retinal vein becomes less apparent or even disappears on either side of the artery (Fig. 113-2). The course of the vein may change to a more perpendicular direction as well. If there is impedance to flow, the segment of the vein distal to the constriction appears larger, darker, and more tortuous. Additional signs of impedance to flow are retinal hemorrhages, macular edema, and cotton-wool spots (Fig. 113-3). In areas of frank obstruction, the presence of venous–venous collaterals may be long-standing. Secondary ocular complications of chronic systemic arterial hypertension include retinal vascular occlusive disease, macroaneurysm formation, and nonarteritic anterior ischemic optic neuropathy.[8] For the differential diagnosis, see Box 113-1.

The appearance of the ocular fundus in hypertension is related directly to the status of the retinal arteries and the rate of rise and degree of systemic blood pressure. The age of the patient may complicate interpretation of the clinical fundus changes. Although arteriolar sclerosis is a finding of long-standing hypertension, these changes, categorized as involutional sclerosis, also occur in the normal aging population.[9] With atherosclerosis alone, mild thickening of the arteriolar wall occurs. Clinically, focal narrowing and straightening of the retinal arterioles are seen in the absence of arteriovenous crossing changes.[10] Because the chronic effects of elevated systemic blood pressure occur along with arteriosclerotic thickening of the blood vessel walls, it can be difficult to categorize fundus changes solely on the basis of elevated blood pressure.

Malignant Hypertensive Retinopathy

Visual disturbances are common in malignant hypertension. Symptoms include headache, scotoma, diplopia, dimness in vision, and photopsia.[11] Ocular findings in malignant arterial hypertension are divided into three distinct categories: hypertensive retinopathy, hypertensive choroidopathy, and hypertensive optic neuropathy. The cause of these clinical findings includes

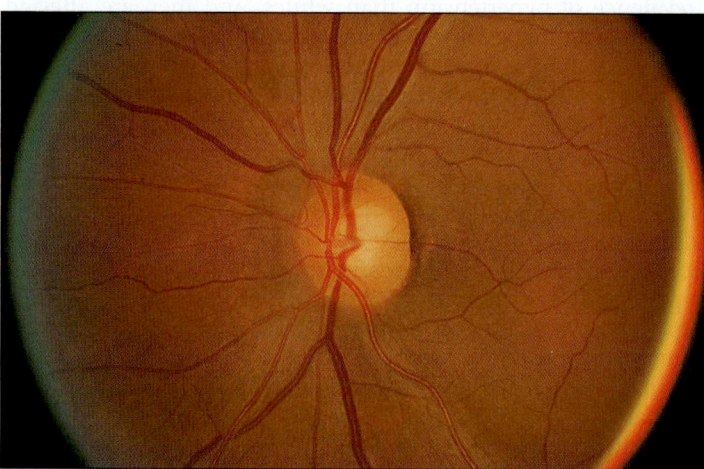

FIG. 113-1 ▌ **Mild to moderate chronic hypertensive retinopathy.** Note the color change in the retinal arterioles and the early arteriovenous crossing changes.

> **BOX 113-1**
>
> **Differential Diagnosis of Chronic Hypertensive Retinopathy**
>
> Diabetic retinopathy
> Retinal venous obstruction
> Hyperviscosity syndromes
> Congenital hereditary retinal arterial tortuosity
> Ocular ischemic syndrome

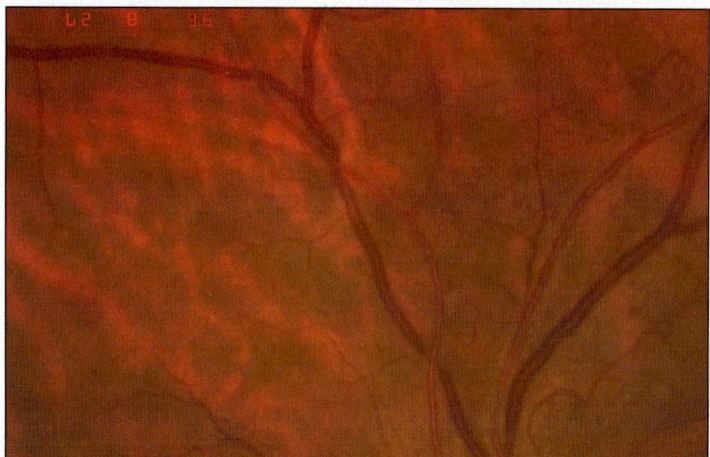

FIG. 113-2 ▌ In this 15° view, note the arteriovenous crossing changes, presence of collateral vessels, and dilated capillary bed.

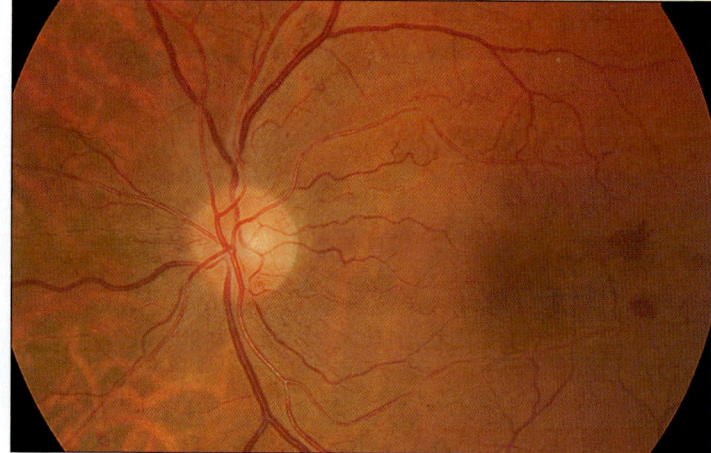

FIG. 113-3 ▌ A 60° view of the same patient as shown in Figure 113-2. Note the telangiectatic vessels on the optic nerve head and intraretinal hemorrhages temporal to the macula.

constriction of vascular beds from circulating catecholamines, obstruction of arterioles, and breakdown in the blood-retina barrier. Ophthalmic findings in acute malignant hypertensive retinopathy include focal arteriolar narrowing, cotton-wool spots, intraretinal transudates, macular edema, and retinal hemorrhages. Retinal hemorrhages are linear, occurring in the nerve fiber layer in the peripapillary region. Cystoid macular edema, lipid deposits, and arteriolar changes are signs of more chronic malignant hypertensive retinopathy.[12]

Arteriolar narrowing observed on ophthalmoscopy has been challenged by Hayreh, who refers to this clinical finding as "pseudonarrowing" secondary to retinal edema creating a visual effect of narrowing of the retinal arteriole. Fluorescein angiography performed in rhesus monkeys with acute malignant hypertension has demonstrated normal retinal arteriolar caliber, casting doubt on the long-standing belief that arteriolar spasm occurs.[13] Cotton-wool spots are fluffy, elevated, tan-white areas of retinal opacity occurring within a few disc diameters of the optic nerve, caused by occlusion of terminal retinal arterioles. Capillary nonperfusion is present on angiography (Fig. 113-4). Cotton-wool spots typically resolve in 3–6 weeks and are associated with permanent nerve fiber layer loss in the vicinity of the lesion.[12] Periarteriolar intraretinal transudates are tan-white retinal lesions occurring in the vicinity of an arteriole. The lesions measure about one quarter of the disc area but are clinically larger, as they coalesce with adjacent lesions. Intraretinal transudates occur secondary to focal areas of arteriolar leakage identified on angiography and resolve without residual retinal damage in 2–3 weeks.[14] Macular edema and subretinal fluid are retinal findings related to hypertensive choroidal changes affecting the retinal pigment epithelium (RPE), with alterations in the blood-retina barrier.

Clinical changes from hypertensive choroidopathy are directly related to the release of endogenous vasoconstrictor agents (e.g., angiotensin II, epinephrine, vasopressin) during systemic hypertension. Angiographically, there is delayed, patchy choroidal filling.[12] Gitter et al.[15] demonstrated through the use of fluorescein angiography that the delay in choroidal filling is followed by late leakage from choroidal vessels into the subretinal space. The leakage is enhanced by infarction and damage to the RPE cells or transudation of fluid into the subretinal space in response to increased pressure in the choroidal vessels.[16,17] Focal occlusion of the choriocapillaris leads to necrosis and atrophy of the RPE, forming Elschnig's spots (Fig. 113-5).[18,19] Acutely, Elschnig's spots are punctate, tan-white lesions that leak on fluorescein and indocyanine green angiography from breakdown in the blood-retina barrier. Subretinal fluid accumulates, with the eventual formation of macular edema, a common finding associated with hypertensive choroidopathy[14] (Fig. 113-6). With time, the focal RPE lesions become confluent and more extensive. Diffuse pigmentary changes with atrophy give a mottled appearance on ophthalmoscopy. Linear configurations of pigmentation along choroidal arteries are known as Siegrist's streaks.[19]

Hypertensive optic neuropathy presents clinically as disc edema (Fig. 113-7). This occurs from vasoconstriction of the posterior ciliary arteries supplying the optic nerve head, resulting from the release of angiotensin II and other vasoconstricting agents. Ischemia occurs in the optic nerve, leading to stasis of axoplasmic flow, which is a form of anterior ischemic optic neuropathy.[20] For the differential diagnosis, see Box 113-2.

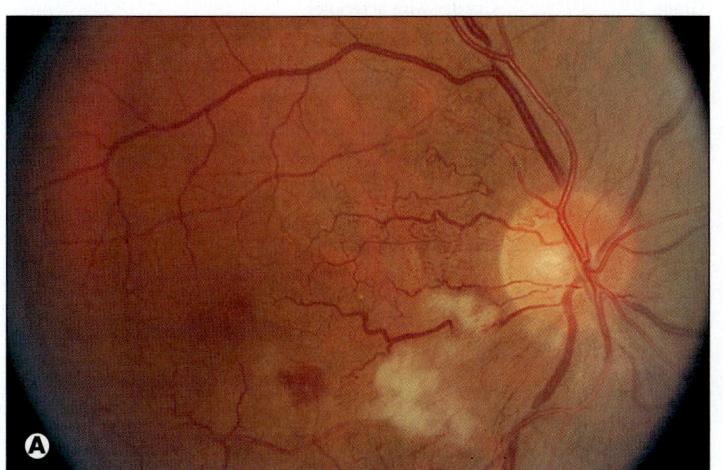

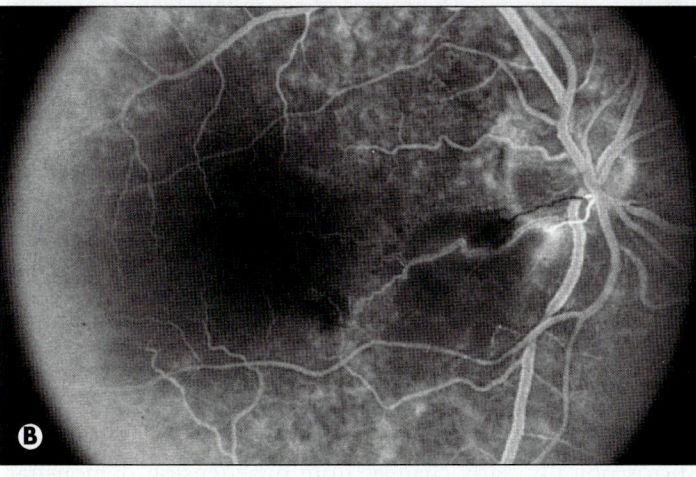

FIG. 113-4 ▮ The right eye of the same patient as shown in Figures 113-2 and 113-3. **A,** A prominent cotton-wool spot in the papillomacular bundle is seen, with an adjacent intraretinal hemorrhage. **B,** Fluorescein angiography shows capillary nonperfusion in the area corresponding to the cotton-wool patch; note the hypofluorescence of the intraretinal hemorrhage, caused by blockage.

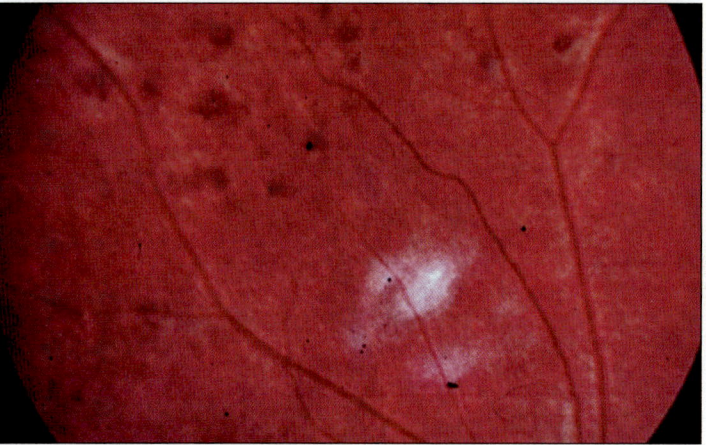

FIG. 113-5 ▮ Elschnig's spots.

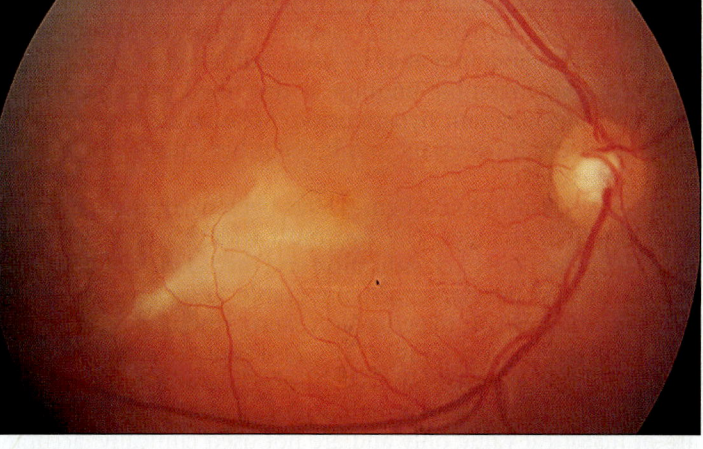

FIG. 113-6 ▮ Serous detachment of the retina in a 27-year-old patient who has pregnancy-induced hypertension, 3 days postpartum. Blood pressure measured 158/100mmHg. Note the subretinal fibrin and folds in the retina. (Courtesy of Franklin L Myers.)

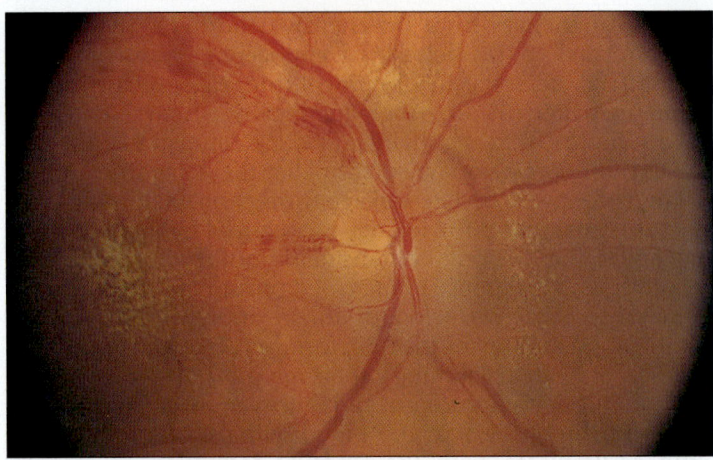

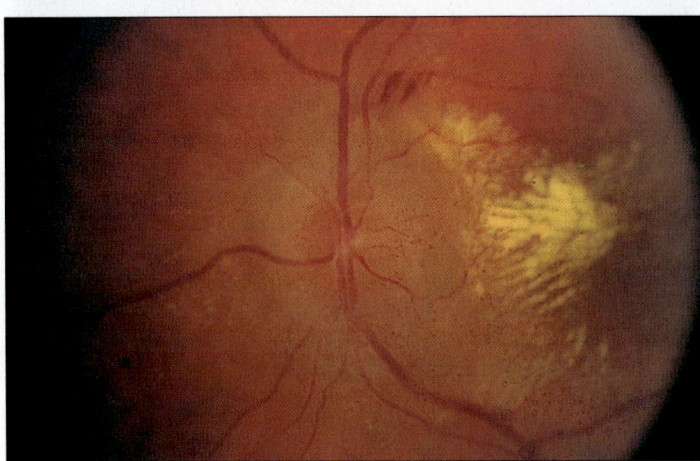

FIG. 113-7 ■ **Bilateral optic nerve edema.** Associated subretinal fluid, flame-shaped hemorrhages, and lipid exudation in a macular star configuration are evident in this patient with malignant hypertensive retinopathy.

TABLE 113-1

KEITH-WAGENER-BARKER CLASSIFICATION

Group 1	Mild-to-moderate narrowing or sclerosis of the arterioles
Group 2	Moderate to marked narrowing of the arterioles Local and/or generalized narrowing of arterioles Exaggeration of the light reflex Arteriovenous crossing changes
Group 3	Retinal arteriolar narrowing and focal constriction Retinal edema Cotton-wool patches Hemorrhage
Group 4	As for Group 3, plus papilledema

(Adapted from Walsh JB. Hypertensive retinopathy. Description, classification and prognosis. Ophthalmology. 1981;89:1127–31.)

TABLE 113-2

SCHEIE CLASSIFICATION

HYPERTENSION

Grade 0	No changes
Grade 1	Barely detectable arteriolar narrowing
Grade 2	Obvious arteriolar narrowing with focal irregularities
Grade 3	Grade 2 plus retinal hemorrhages and/or exudates
Grade 4	Grade 3 plus papilledema

ARTERIOLAR SCLEROSIS

Grade 0	Normal
Grade 1	Barely detectable light reflex changes
Grade 2	Obvious increased light reflex changes
Grade 3	Copper-wire arterioles
Grade 4	Silver-wire arterioles

BOX 113-2

Differential Diagnosis of Acute Hypertensive Retinopathy

Bilateral bullous central serous chorioretinopathy
Bilateral central retinal vein obstruction
Collagen vascular diseases
Diabetic retinopathy (especially in the setting of diabetic papillopathy)

DIAGNOSIS AND ANCILLARY TESTING

Hypertensive retinopathy is a clinical diagnosis made when the characteristic fundus findings are visualized on slit-lamp biomicroscopy in a patient with systemic arterial hypertension. Fluorescein angiography may be used, but it is not crucial in the diagnosis. Angiographic findings as described earlier are more common in malignant hypertension. Measurement of systemic blood pressure is necessary to rule out other causes with similar clinical pictures.

Several classification schemes have been used to stage hypertensive retinal changes. The two most widely accepted are the Keith-Wagener-Barker classification and the Scheie classification. The Keith-Wagener-Barker scheme (Table 113-1) combines the clinical findings of hypertension and atherosclerosis.[21] The Scheie classification (Table 113-2) keeps the two disease processes separate.[22] Unfortunately, no classification is satisfactory because of the high variability of clinical findings.[23] They are of historical value only and are not used clinically; accurate description of the ocular findings is more valuable than any classification system.

Although newer imaging techniques, such as scanning laser ophthalmoscopy, allow quantification of retinal capillary den-sity and flow velocity in patients who have essential hypertension, these results are still preliminary in terms of their application to the long-term prevention of retinal disease.[21] Optical coherence tomography may be used to evaluate cross-sectional images of the retina and subretinal fluid collections.[24]

SYSTEMIC ASSOCIATIONS

Essential hypertension is the most common cause of chronically elevated blood pressure and is typically of unknown cause. Screening for secondary systemic causes is not pursued unless other symptoms are present or the hypertension is resistant to treatment. The causes of secondary hypertension include pheochromocytoma, renovascular stenosis, and primary hyperaldosteronism.[1,7]

In nearly all cases of malignant hypertension, a systemic cause can be elucidated via systemic evaluation. Potential causes include renal disease, such as polycystic kidney or renovascular stenosis; pheochromocytoma; and pregnancy. Rarely, untreated essential hypertension may lead to an acute hypertensive crisis. Systemic abnormalities accompany accelerated hypertension with evidence of end-organ damage, including acute left ventricular heart failure, myocardial infarction, pulmonary edema, dissecting aortic aneurysm, stroke, encephalopathy, and intracranial hemorrhage.[1,7]

PATHOLOGY

Microscopically, early changes from hypertension demonstrate sclerosis and thickening of the arteriolar walls with luminal narrowing. These findings become more prominent with long-standing systemic hypertension. Arteriole thickening in the choroidal vessels is typically more severe than in the retinal arterioles and more closely resembles systemic arterial changes.[19] In malignant hypertension, the arterioles are similarly thickened, but necrosis and fibrinoid deposition in the vessel wall occur. Electron micrographs of retinal arterioles in malignant hypertension eventually demonstrate dilatation of the lumen, with focal breaks in the endothelium surrounded by lipid and fibrin, as the autoregulatory mechanisms of the arterioles are exceeded.[14,19] Other pathological findings include optic nerve edema, cotton-wool spots, microaneurysms, and focal infarcts.[19]

TREATMENT, COURSE, AND OUTCOME

By itself, chronic hypertensive retinopathy rarely, if ever, results in significant loss of vision. Treatment of the underlying systemic condition can halt the progress of the retinal changes, but arteriolar narrowing and arteriovenous nicking usually are permanent.

Treatment of malignant hypertensive retinopathy, choroidopathy, and optic neuropathy consists of lowering blood pressure in a controlled fashion to a level that minimizes end-organ damage. The actual level of blood pressure is less important in gauging the urgency of the situation than is the ongoing end-organ damage. In hypertensive patients, the autoregulatory mechanism that maintains constant blood flow to tissues is elevated to a higher level. This allows for the tolerance of higher blood pressures, and lowering blood pressure below the regulatory range can prevent adequate blood flow from reaching vital organs.[12] Therefore, blood pressure should be lowered in a slow, deliberate, controlled fashion to prevent end-organ damage. Too rapid a decline can lead to ischemia of the optic nerve head, brain, and other vital organs, resulting in permanent damage. Medications used to treat hypertensive emergencies include sodium nitroprusside, nitroglycerin, calcium channel blockers, β-blockers, and angiotensin-converting enzyme inhibitors. Treatment should be initiated in a controlled, monitored setting under the auspices of a physician skilled in the use of antihypertensive medications.

From a systemic viewpoint, the diagnosis of a malignant hypertensive crisis represents a medical emergency. Untreated, the mortality rate is 50% at 2 months and 90% at 1 year.[25,26] Most patients resume normal vision. On the rare occasion when vision loss occurs, this may result from retinal pigment changes secondary to retinal detachment or from optic atrophy due to prolonged papilledema.

REFERENCES

1. Oparil S. Arterial hypertension. In: Goldman L, Bennett JC, eds. Cecil textbook of medicine. Philadelphia: Saunders; 2000:258–73.
2. Joint National Committee on Prevention, Detection, Evaluation, and Treatment of High Blood Pressure. Sixth report of the Joint National Committee on Prevention, Detection, Evaluation, and Treatment of High Blood Pressure (JNC VI). Arch Intern Med. 1997;157:2413.
3. Burt VL, Cutler JA, Higgins M. Trends in the prevalence, awareness, treatment and control of hypertension in the adult US population: data from the Health Examination Surveys, 1960–1991. Hypertension. 1995;26:60.
4. National High Blood Pressure Education Program Working Group report on primary prevention of hypertension. Arch Intern Med. 1993;153:186.
5. Klein R, Klein BE, Moss SE, Wang Q. Hypertension and retinopathy, arteriolar narrowing, and arteriovenous nicking in a population. Arch Ophthalmol. 1994; 112:92–8.
6. Laragh J. Laragh's lessons in pathophysiology and clinical pearls for treating hypertension. Am J Hypertens. 2001;14:186–94.
7. Williams GH. Hypertensive vascular disease. In: Iselbacher KJ, et al, eds. Harrison's textbook of internal medicine. New York: McGraw-Hill;1994:1116–31.
8. Panton RW, Goldberg MF, Farber MD. Retinal arterial macroaneurysm: risk factors and natural history. Br J Ophthalmol. 1990;74:595–660.
9. Leishman R. The eye in general vascular disease: hypertension and arteriosclerosis. Br J Ophthalmol. 1957;41:641–701.
10. Stokoe NL. Fundus changes in hypertension: a long-term clinical study. In: Cant JS, ed. The William Mackenzie centenary symposium on the ocular circulation in health and disease. London: Kimpton; 1969:117–35.
11. Bosco JA. Spontaneous nontraumatic retinal detachment in pregnancy. Am J Obstet Gynecol. 1961;82:208–12.
12. Hayreh SS. Hypertensive fundus changes. In: Guyer DR, ed. Retina-vitreous-macula. Philadelphia: Saunders; 1999:345–71.
13. Hayreh SS, Servais GE, Virdi PS. Retinal arteriolar changes in malignant arterial hypertension. Ophthalmologica. 1989;198:178–96.
14. Hayreh SS, Servais GE, Virdi PS. Fundus lesions in malignant hypertension. IV. Focal intraretinal periarteriolar transudates. Ophthalmology. 1986;93:60–73.
15. Gitter KA, Houser BP, Sarin LK, Justice J. Toxemia of pregnancy. An angiographic interpretation of fundus changes. Arch Ophthalmol. 1968;80:449–54.
16. Fastenberg DM, Fetkenhour CL, Choromolos E, Shoch DE. Choroidal vascular changes in toxemia of pregnancy. Am J Ophthalmol. 1980;89:362–8.
17. Kenny GS, Cerasoli JR. Color fundus angiography in toxemia of pregnancy. Arch Ophthalmol. 1972;87:383–8.
18. Schmidt D, Loffler KU. Elschnig's spots as a sign of severe hypertension. Ophthalmologica. 1993;206:24–8.
19. Green WR. Systemic diseases with retinal involvement. In: Spencer WH, ed. Ophthalmic pathology, an atlas and textbook. Philadelphia: Saunders; 1985: 1034–45.
20. Hayreh SS, Servais GE, Virdi PS. Fundus lesions in malignant hypertension V. Hypertensive optic neuropathy. Ophthalmology. 1986;93:74–87.
21. Wolf S, Arind O, Schulte K, et al. Quantification of retinal capillary density and flow velocity in patients with essential hypertension. Hypertension. 1994;23:464–7.
22. Sheie HG. Evaluation of ophthalmoscopic changes of hypertension and arteriolar sclerosis. Arch Ophthalmol. 1953;49:117–38.
23. Walsh JB. Hypertensive retinopathy. Description, classification and prognosis. Ophthalmology. 1982;89:1127–31.
24. Puliafito CA, Hee MR, Lin CP, et al. Imaging of macular disease with optical coherence tomography. Ophthalmology. 1995;102:217–29.
25. Keith NM, Wagener HP, Barker NW. Some different types of essential hypertension: their course and prognosis. Am J Med Sci. 1939;197:332–43.
26. Kincaid-Smith P, McMichael J, Murphy EA. The clinical course and pathology of hypertension with papilloedema (malignant hypertension). Q J Med. 1958; 27: 117–53.

114 Retinal Arterial Obstruction

JAY S. DUKER

Central Retinal Artery Obstruction

DEFINITION
- An abrupt diminution of blood flow through the central retinal artery severe enough to cause ischemia of the inner retina.

KEY FEATURES
- Abrupt, painless, severe loss of vision.
- Cherry-red spot.
- Box-carring of blood flow in the retinal vessels.
- Ischemic retinal whitening of the posterior pole.

ASSOCIATED FEATURES
- Amaurosis fugax.
- Visible embolus (25%).
- Carotid artery disease (33%).
- Giant cell arteritis (5%).
- Neovascularization of the iris (18%).
- Arterial collaterals on the optic disc.

Branch Retinal Artery Obstruction

DEFINITION
- An abrupt diminution of blood flow through a branch of the central retinal artery severe enough to cause ischemia of the inner retina in the territory of the affected vessel.

KEY FEATURES
- Retinal whitening in the territory of the obstructed vessel.
- Embolus (66%).
- Visual field defect that corresponds to the territory of the obstructed vessels.

ASSOCIATED FEATURES
- Carotid artery disease.
- Cardiac valvular disease.
- Cardiac myxoma, long-bone fracture, endocarditis, depot drug injection (rare).
- Systemic clotting disorder or vasculitis (rare).

CENTRAL RETINAL ARTERY OBSTRUCTION

INTRODUCTION

Retinal arterial obstructions are divided into the categories central and branch, depending on the precise site of obstruction. A central retinal artery obstruction occurs when the blockage is within the optic nerve substance itself and therefore the site of obstruction is generally not visible on ophthalmoscopy. A branch retinal artery obstruction occurs when the site of blockage is distal to the lamina cribrosa of the optic nerve.

Obstructions more proximal to the central retinal artery, in the ophthalmic artery, or even in the internal carotid artery may produce visual loss as well. Ophthalmic artery obstructions may be difficult to differentiate from central retinal artery obstruction. More proximal obstructions usually cause a more chronic form of visual problem—the ocular ischemic syndrome (see Chapter 118).

The majority of retinal arterial obstructions are either thrombotic or embolic in nature. The potential sources and various types of emboli generally do not differ between central retinal artery obstruction and branch retinal artery obstruction; however, a branch retinal artery obstruction is far more likely to be embolic than is a central retinal artery obstruction. It has been determined that over two thirds of branch retinal artery obstructions are caused by emboli, whereas probably less than one third of central retinal artery obstructions result from emboli.

The retina has a dual circulation with little to no anastomoses. The inner retina is supplied by the central retinal artery, which is an end artery. The outer retina receives its nourishment via diffusion from the choroidal circulation (see Chapter 101). Retinal artery obstructions selectively affect the inner retina only.

Because the accompanying visual loss tends to be severe and permanent, it is fortunate that retinal artery obstructions are rare occurrences. As there is a strong association with systemic disease, all patients who suffer retinal artery obstructions should undergo a systemic evaluation.

EPIDEMIOLOGY AND PATHOGENESIS

Central retinal artery obstruction is a rare event—it has been estimated to account for about 1 in 10,000 outpatient visits to the ophthalmologist.[1] Men are affected more commonly than women in the ratio 2:1. The mean age at onset is about 60 years, with a range of reported ages from the first to the ninth decade of life. Right eyes and left eyes appear affected with equal incidence. Bilateral involvement occurs in 1–2% of cases.

In central retinal artery obstruction, the site of obstruction is not usually visible on clinical examination and, in general, the central retinal artery is too small to image with most techniques; therefore, the precise cause is speculative. It is currently believed that the majority of central retinal artery obstructions are caused by thrombus formation at or just proximal to the lamina cribrosa. Atherosclerosis is implicated as the inciting event in most cases, although congenital anomalies of the central retinal artery, systemic coagulopathies, or low-flow states from more proximal arterial disease may also be present and render certain individuals more susceptible.

In only 20–25% of cases are emboli visible in the central retinal artery or one of its branches, suggesting that an embolic cause is not frequent. A more detailed discussion of embolus types is given later in the section on branch retinal artery obstruction. Further indirect evidence against emboli as a frequent cause of central retinal artery obstruction is the 40% or less probability of finding a definitive embolic source on systemic evaluation and the small incidence (approximately 10%) of confirmed associated ipsilateral cerebral emboli in affected patients.[2]

Inflammation in the form of vasculitis (e.g., varicella infection), optic neuritis, or even orbital disease (e.g., mucormycosis) may cause central retinal artery obstruction.[3,4] Local trauma that results in direct damage to the optic nerve or blood vessels may lead to central retinal artery obstruction.[5] Arterial spasm or dissection rarely produces retinal arterial obstruction. In addition, systemic coagulopathies may be associated with both central and branch retinal artery obstructions.[6]

Other rare causes include radiation retinopathy,[7] emboli associated with depot medication injection around the eye,[8] optic disc drusen, and prepapillary arterial loops. Medical examinations and manipulations (e.g., carotid angiography, angioplasty, chiropractic neck manipulation) rarely result in emboli to the central retinal artery.[9,10] Although elevated intraocular pressure has been implicated as a cause of central retinal artery obstruction, unless the underlying perfusion of the eye is impaired markedly or prolonged external pressure is placed on the globe, it is unlikely that intraocular pressure can be raised high enough to block arterial inflow to the eye.

OCULAR MANIFESTATIONS

The hallmark symptom of acute central retinal artery obstruction is abrupt, painless loss of vision.[11] Pain is unusual and suggests associated ocular ischemic syndrome. Amaurosis fugax precedes visual loss in about 10% of patients. Rarely, in cases associated with arterial spasm, a relapsing and remitting course of visual loss precedes central retinal artery obstruction.[12]

Examination typically reveals a visual acuity of 20/800 (6/240) or worse.[13] Hand motion or light perception vision can occur, but no light perception vision is uncommon except in the setting of an ophthalmic artery obstruction or temporal arteritis. If a patent cilioretinal artery is present and perfuses the fovea, normal central acuity may occur. An afferent pupillary defect on the affected side is the rule.

Anterior segment examination is normal except in the setting of concurrent ocular ischemic syndrome with neovascularization of the iris.

Within the first few minutes to hours after the obstruction, the fundus may appear relatively normal (Fig. 114-1, A and B).[1] Eventually, the decreased blood flow results in ischemic whitening of the retina in the territory of the obstructed artery, which is most pronounced in the posterior pole (where the nerve fiber

layer of the retina is thickest). Acutely, the arteries appear thin and attenuated. In severe blockages, both veins and arteries may manifest "box-carring" or segmentation of the blood flow (Fig. 114-2).

A cherry-red spot of the macula is typical and arises in this area because the nerve fiber layer is thin. Transmission of the normal choroidal appearance, therefore, is not diminished, which contrasts distinctly with the surrounding area of intense retinal whitening that blocks transmission of the normal choroidal coloration. Although other conditions may be associated with a macular cherry-red spot (Box 114-1), these are usually differentiated easily from central retinal artery obstruction. Splinter retinal hemorrhages on the disc are common, but more extensive retinal hemorrhaging suggests an alternative diagnosis. If pallid swelling is present, temporal arteritis must be suspected. A patent cilioretinal artery results in a small area of retina that appears normal (Fig. 114-3).

By 4–6 weeks after obstruction, the retinal whitening is usually resolved, the optic disc develops pallor, and arterial collaterals may form on the optic disc. No foveolar light reflex is apparent, and fine changes in the retinal pigment epithelium may be visible.

Secondary ocular neovascularization is not uncommon after central retinal artery obstruction. Iris neovascularization occurs in about 18% of patients,[14,15] with many of these eyes going on to neovascular glaucoma. Panretinal photocoagulation appears to reduce the risk of neovascular glaucoma moderately.[16] Neovascularization of the optic disc occurs after about 2% of

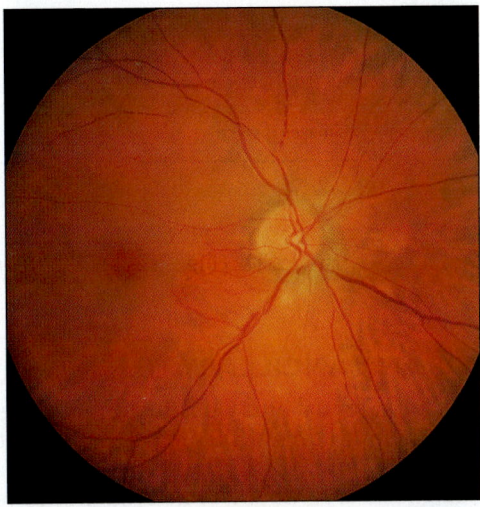

FIG. 114-2 ■ **Central retinal artery obstruction.** The right eye of a 68-year-old woman. Note box-carring of the blood column in the superotemporal arteries and superior veins. Cilioretinal artery sparing is apparent just temporal to the optic disc.

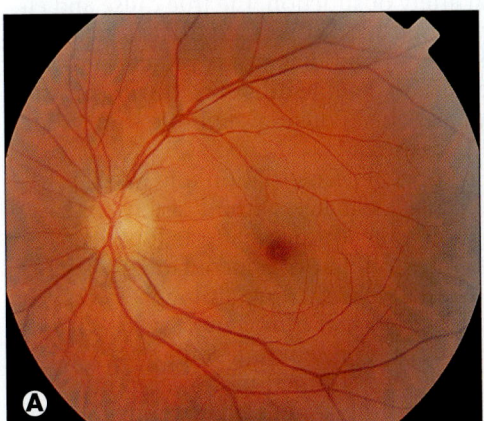
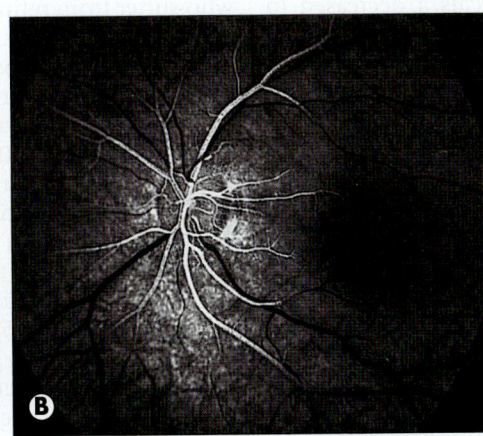
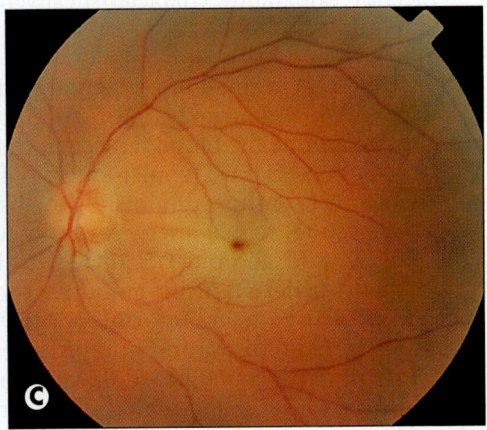

FIG. 114-1 ■ **The left eye of a healthy 37-year-old man.** The patient had a 3-hour history of visual loss and a visual acuity of 20/60 (6/18). **A,** Retinal whitening is very subtle and the retinal vessels appear normal. **B,** Fluorescein angiography reveals abnormal arterial filling with a leading edge of dye that confirms central retinal artery obstruction. **C,** The same eye 24 hours later. Despite intravenous urokinase, visual acuity dropped to hand movements, and intense retinal whitening with a cherry-red spot is present. Note the interruption in the blood column of the retinal arteries.

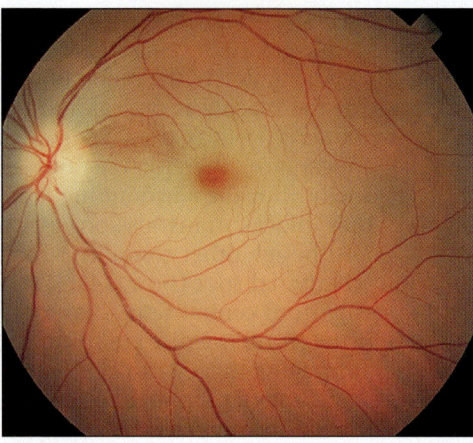

FIG. 114-3 ■ **A central retinal artery obstruction.** A prominent cherry-red spot with cilioretinal artery sparing in the papillomacular bundle.

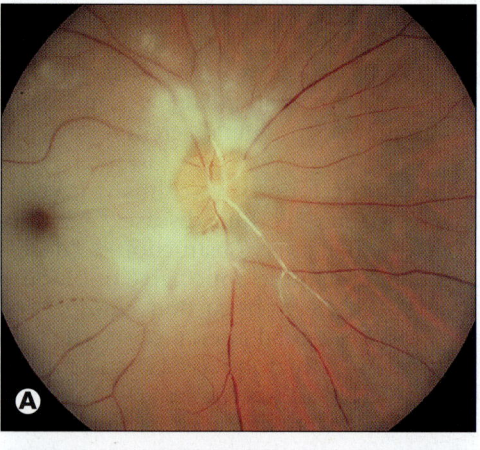

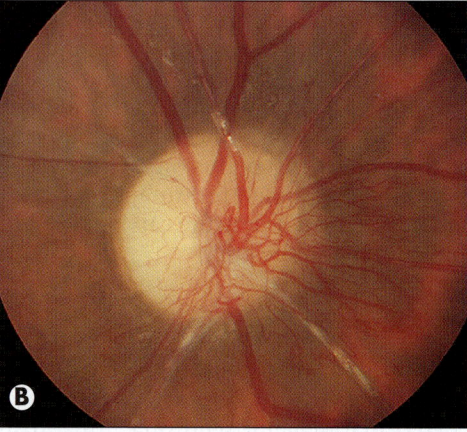

FIG. 114-4 ■ **A 26-year-old diabetic man. A,** Central retinal artery obstruction caused by a platelet-fibrin embolus. **B,** After 3 months, extensive neovascularization of the disc is present. (Courtesy of Larry Magargal, MD.)

BOX 114-1

Other Causes of a Cherry-Red Spot

Tay–Sachs disease
Farber's disease
Sandhoff's disease
Niemann–Pick disease
Goldberg's syndrome
Gaucher's disease
Gangliosidase GM1, type 2
Hurler's syndrome (mucopolysaccharidosis I H)
β-Galactosidase deficiency (mucopolysaccharidosis VII)
Hallevorden-Spatz disease
Batten–Mayou–Vogt–Spielmeyer disease

---

central retinal artery obstruction (Fig. 114-4).[17] Vitreous hemorrhage may ensue.

DIAGNOSIS AND ANCILLARY TESTING

Diagnosis of central retinal artery obstruction is straightforward when diffuse ischemic retinal whitening is present in the setting of abrupt, painless visual loss. Fluorescein angiography may help if the diagnosis is in doubt. A delayed arm-to-retina time with a leading edge of dye visible in the retinal arteries is typical (see Fig. 114-1, *B*). In some cases, it may be minutes before the retinal arterial tree fills with fluorescein. Arteriovenous transit is delayed as well, and late staining of the disc is common.

Electroretinography characteristically reveals a decreased to absent b-wave with intact a-wave. Visual fields show a remaining temporal island of peripheral vision. If a patent cilioretinal artery is present, a small intact central island is found as well.

Color Doppler imaging is a form of ultrasonography that can help to determine the blood flow characteristics of the retrobulbar circulation. Color Doppler studies of acute central retinal artery obstruction show diminished to absent blood flow velocity in the central retinal artery, generally with intact flow in the ophthalmic and choroidal branches. Color Doppler imaging can be used to detect calcific emboli at the lamina cribrosa and also may be used to monitor blood flow changes induced by therapy. In addition, carotid artery studies may be carried out concurrently with ocular blood flow determinations to evaluate the possible causes of the central retinal artery obstruction.

DIFFERENTIAL DIAGNOSIS

The differential diagnosis of central retinal artery obstruction is given in Box 114-2.

BOX 114-2

Differential Diagnosis of Central Retinal Artery Obstruction

Single or multiple branch retinal artery obstruction
Cilioretinal artery obstruction
Severe commotio retinae
Necrotizing herpetic retinitis

SYSTEMIC ASSOCIATIONS

Although systemic diseases are found commonly in patients who suffer from retinal artery obstruction, the true cause and effect may not be clear. About 60% of patients have concurrent systemic arterial hypertension, and diabetes is present in 25%. Systemic evaluation reveals no definite cause for the obstruction in over 50% of affected patients. Potential embolic sources are found in less than 40% of cases.[1,14,18]

The most common pathogenetic association uncovered is hemodynamically significant ipsilateral carotid artery disease, which is present in about one third of affected patients.[1,14] Carotid noninvasive testing should be considered for all patients who have central retinal artery obstruction, although disease in those younger than 50 years of age is quite rare (Fig. 114-5). An embolic source from the heart is present in less than 10% of patients with central retinal artery obstruction; however, echocardiography and Holter monitoring should be performed, especially in younger patients. In some cases, transesophageal echocardiography is necessary to reveal embolic sources.[19]

Even though it is present in less than 5% of cases, it is of paramount importance that temporal arteritis be ruled out in all patients older than 50 years who have a central retinal artery obstruc-

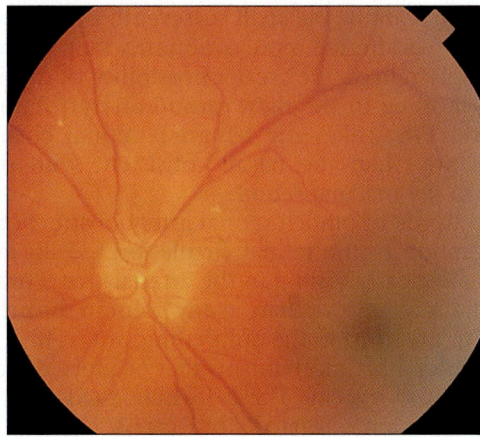

FIG. 114-5 ■ **Acute central retinal artery obstruction.** Secondary to an embolus at the lamina cribrosa. Note two other emboli in the superior retinal vessels. Ipsilateral carotid artery disease was present.

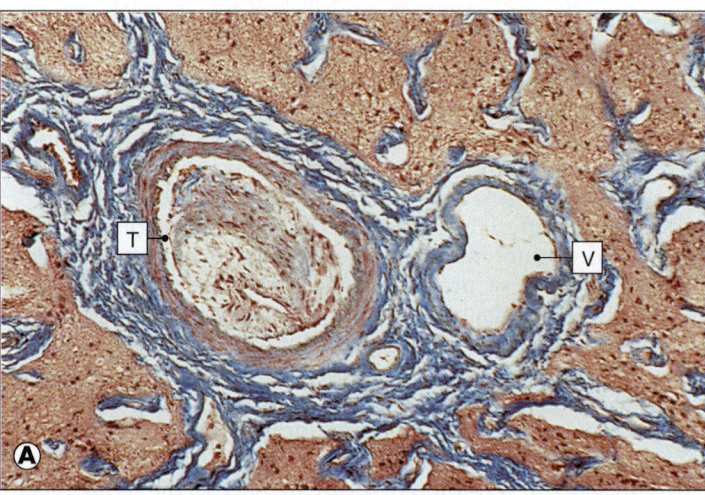

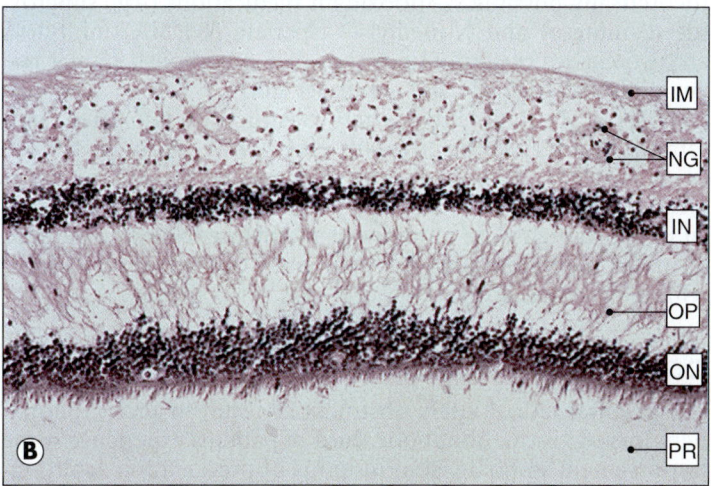

FIG. 114-6 ■ **Central retinal artery occlusion. A,** A trichrome-stained section shows an organized thrombus *(T)* that occludes the central retinal artery within the optic nerve *(V,* vein). **B,** A histological section at the early stage shows edema of the inner neural retinal layers and ganglion cell nuclei pyknosis. Patient had a cherry-red spot in fovea at time of enucleation. *IM,* Internal limiting membrane; *IN,* inner nuclear layer; *NG,* swollen nerve fiber and ganglion layers; *ON,* outer nuclear layer; *OP,* outer plexiform layer; *PR,* photoreceptors. (From Yanoff M, Fine BS. *Ocular pathology,* ed 5. St. Louis: Mosby, 2002.)

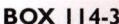
PATHOLOGY

Histopathological examination shows coagulative necrosis of the inner retina. Acute, early, intracellular edema is followed by complete loss of the inner retinal tissue. Chronically, a diffuse acellular zone replaces the nerve fiber layer, ganglion cell layer, and inner plexiform layer. The outer retinal cells remain relatively intact. Sections of the obstructed central retinal artery may reveal a thrombus or embolus that is often recanalized (Fig. 114-6).

TREATMENT

No proved treatment exists for central retinal artery obstruction, but treatment strategies center around the following goals:
- Increase retinal oxygenation
- Increase retinal arterial blood flow
- Reverse arterial obstruction,
- Prevent hypoxic retinal damage

Theoretically, retinal oxygenation can be increased by breathing carbogen (95% oxygen, 5% carbon dioxide). Investigationally, the high concentration of oxygen has been shown to elevate oxygen tension at the inner retina via diffusion through the intact choroidal circulation. The carbon dioxide prevents the normal retinal autoregulatory mechanisms from inducing constriction of the retinal arteries. No clinical study indicates efficacy for carbogen therapy, and one retrospective study suggests that it has no beneficial effect.[22] In most centers, it is no longer used.

tion. An immediate erythrocyte sedimentation rate must be obtained, and if it is elevated or if clinical suspicion exists, corticosteroid therapy and a temporal artery biopsy should be considered.

Other rare associated systemic diseases include blood-clotting abnormalities such as antiphospholipid antibodies, protein S deficiency, protein C deficiency, and antithrombin III deficiency.[20,21] A list of systemic associations for retinal artery obstructions is given in Box 114-3.

An increase in retinal arterial blood flow is attempted by lowering intraocular pressure. This is accomplished by ocular massage, paracentesis, and the administration of ocular antihypertensive medications. Medical attempts to dilate retinal arteries or block vascular spasm have been tried as well. Sublingual nitroglycerin, pentoxifylline (oxpentifylline), calcium channel blockers, and β-blockers have all been used with no proof of efficacy.[11,23]

Reversal of arterial obstruction through the use of anticoagulation and fibrinolytic mediations has been reported. To date, the utility of these mediations has not been proved by controlled clinical trials; however, anecdotal reports of success with intravenous heparin, tissue plasminogen activator, streptokinase, and urokinase exist. In addition, an intra-arterial injection of tissue plasminogen activator, streptokinase, or urokinase during selective catheterization of the ophthalmic artery has been attempted, with reported success in some selected cases.[24,25]

At present, prevention of hypoxic damage to the retina is only theoretically possible.[26] Antioxidant medications (e.g., superoxide dismutase) and N-methyl-D-aspartate (NDMA) inhibitors are two classes of compounds that may accomplish retinal rescue pharmacologically and are under study.

Cases of central retinal artery obstruction associated with temporal arteritis are treated emergently with high-dose corticosteroids. Without therapy, the risk to the second eye is great. Although the first-affected eye rarely recovers, instances exist in which high-dose intravenous methylprednisolone induced visual recovery from central retinal artery obstruction associated with temporal arteritis.[27]

COURSE AND OUTCOME

Most central retinal artery obstructions result in severe, permanent loss of vision. About one third of patients experience some improvement in final vision in terms of presentation acuity, either with or without conventional treatment. Three or more Snellen lines of improved visual acuity occur in only about 10% of patients, whether treated by current methods or untreated. On occasion, some patients experience significant restoration of normal vision.

Experimentally, if an obstruction exists in the primate retina for more than 100 minutes, complete irreversible death of the inner retina occurs.[28] In practice, a rare patient has experienced total spontaneous recovery even after several days of documented visual loss.[29] Spontaneous recovery may be more common in young children.[6,8]

BRANCH RETINAL ARTERY OBSTRUCTION

INTRODUCTION

Branch retinal artery obstruction represents a rarely encountered retinal vascular disorder. Although current treatments are not effective, in the majority of cases the source of the obstruction can be determined. As associated systemic implications occur, diagnosis and systemic evaluation of these patients are critical.

EPIDEMIOLOGY AND PATHOGENESIS

Branch retinal artery obstruction is a rare event, even less common than central retinal artery obstruction overall. The exception to this comparative incidence is with young patients, in whom branch retinal artery obstruction is the more common type of retinal artery obstruction.[30] Overall, men are more affected than women by a 2:1 ratio, which reflects the higher incidence of vasculopathic disease in men. In the subset of young patients (less than 50 years of age), women and men are affected equally. The mean age of affected patients is 60 years, with a range from the second decade of life to the tenth. The great ma-

jority of patients are in the sixth or seventh decade of life. The right eye (60%) is affected more commonly than the left (40%), which probably reflects the greater possibility of cardiac or aortic emboli traveling to the right carotid artery.[11] Branch retinal artery obstruction strikes the temporal retinal circulation far more frequently than the nasal, consistent with the greater blood flow to the macular retina.

Over two thirds of branch retinal artery obstructions are secondary to emboli to the retinal circulation.[1,11,31] In most cases, the emboli are clearly visible in the arterial tree. Emboli to the retinal circulation may originate at any point in the proximal circulation from the heart to the ophthalmic artery. Risk factors reflect the vasculopathic mechanisms that produce disease within the cardiovascular system. These include predisposing family history, hypertension, elevated lipid levels, cigarette smoking, and diabetes mellitus.

Three main types of retinal emboli have been identified:
- Cholesterol (Hollenhorst plaque)
- Platelet-fibrin
- Calcific.

Cholesterol emboli typically emanate from atheromatous plaques of the ipsilateral carotid artery system, although the aorta or heart valves may also be a source. They are yellow-orange in color, refractile, and globular or rectangular in shape. They may be small and do not always result in blockage of blood flow. Platelet-fibrin emboli are long, smooth, white-colored, intra-arterial plugs that may be mobile or break up over time. Usually, they are associated with carotid or cardiac thromboses. Calcific emboli are solid, white, nonrefractile plugs associated with calcification of heart valves or the aorta.

Less commonly seen embolic types include tumor cells from atrial myxoma[32] or a systemic metastasis, septic emboli associated with septicemia or endocarditis, fat emboli associated with large bone fractures, emboli dislodged during angioplasty or angiography, and depot drug preparations from intra-arterial injections around the eye or face.

Rarely, local ocular conditions produce branch retinal artery obstruction. These include inflammatory diseases, such as toxoplasmosis or acute retinal necrosis, or structural problems, such as optic disc drusen or prepapillary arterial loops.[1,11]

Systemic hematological or clotting problems may induce isolated branch retinal artery obstruction or even multiple recurrent branch retinal artery obstruction.[33,34] Systemic vasculitides, such as polyarteritis nodosa or local vasculitis associated with varicella infection, may be associated with branch retinal artery obstruction. Oral contraceptive use and cigarette smoking have been implicated as possible risk factors, especially in young, otherwise healthy women.[18,30]

OCULAR MANIFESTATIONS

Abrupt, painless loss of vision in the visual field corresponding to the territory of the obstructed artery is the typical history of presentation. Unlike the situation in retinal venous obstruction, patients can typically define the time and extent of visual loss precisely. Amaurosis fugax occurs in about one fourth of patients prior to frank obstruction, especially in the setting of carotid disease. Rarely, patients develop bilateral simultaneous branch retinal artery obstruction, which can mimic homonymous field defects.

Acutely, examination reveals intact central acuity in about 50% of patients. A relative afferent pupillary defect is common, the presence of which is determined by the extent of retinal involvement.

Retinal whitening that corresponds to the areas of ischemia is the most notable finding. The whitening stops at adjacent retinal veins, as these vessels mark the extent of the territory of the retinal arteries (Fig. 114-7). Retinal emboli are seen in over two thirds of branch retinal artery obstructions. Flame hemorrhages at the margins of the retinal ischemia are not uncommon, and

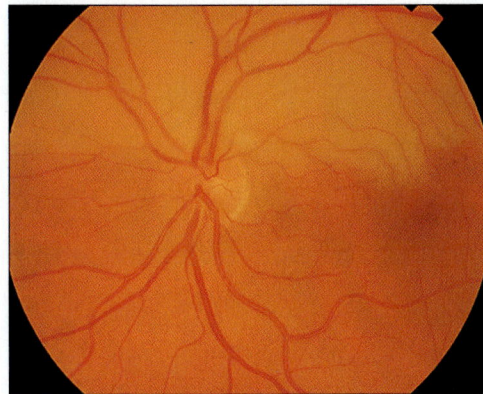

FIG. 114-7 ■ **Superior hemispheric branch retinal artery obstruction.** The site of obstruction is probably within the optic nerve substance itself. Note that the dual trunk of the central retinal artery obstruction has separated proximal to the lamina. Only the superior trunk was affected.

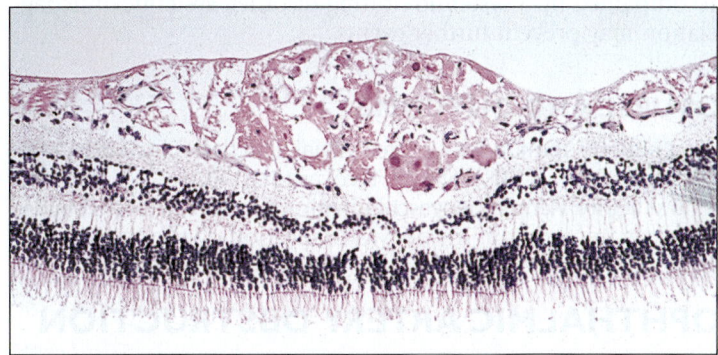

FIG. 114-8 ■ Cytoid body formation in neural retinal nerve fiber layer. Histological counterpart of the clinical cotton-wool spot. (From Yanoff M, Fine BS. Ocular pathology, ed 5. St. Louis: Mosby, 2002.)

BOX 114-4

Differential Diagnosis of Branch Retinal Artery Obstruction

Cotton-wool spot(s)
Central retinal artery obstruction
Cilioretinal artery obstruction
Retinal astrocytoma
Inflammatory or infectious retinitis

---

local areas of more intense inner retinal whitening that resemble scattered cotton-wool spots can develop.

A syndrome of multiple, recurrent, bilateral branch retinal artery obstruction in young, otherwise healthy patients has been reported. A few of the patients also manifest vestibuloauditory symptoms.[35] Although the underlying pathology in this subset of patients is probably heterogeneous, some probably have Susac's syndrome, a rare disorder that manifests as a microangiopathy of the central nervous system. Others probably have various types of systemic clotting abnormalities.[36]

In the chronic phase, when the retinal whitening has diminished, a loss of the nerve fiber layer in the affected area may be apparent. In most instances, the affected retina appears normal. At the site of obstruction, localized sheathing of the arteriole is common. Arteriolar collaterals on the optic disc or at the site of obstruction may develop.

DIAGNOSIS AND ANCILLARY TESTING

Ancillary testing is not usually necessary to make the diagnosis. Fluorescein angiography reveals an abrupt diminution in dye at the site of the obstruction and distally. Filling in the adjacent retinal veins is slow to absent, and late staining or even leakage from the embolus site may occur.

Visual field testing can confirm the extent of visual loss and may pick up contralateral field loss from previous emboli or other associated conditions.

DIFFERENTIAL DIAGNOSIS

The differential diagnosis of branch retinal artery obstruction is given in Box 114-4.

SYSTEMIC ASSOCIATIONS

Systemic evaluation of patients who have branch retinal artery obstruction discloses evidence of an embolic source from the carotid arteries or the heart in many cases. Other rare systemic conditions associated with branch retinal artery obstruction include amniotic fluid embolism, pancreatitis, sickle cell disease, homocystinuria, and Kawasaki disease. Young patients, especially those who have multiple or recurrent branch retinal artery obstruction, should be evaluated for systemic clotting abnormalities such as protein S deficiency, protein C deficiency, antithrombin III deficiency, platelet abnormalities ("sticky platelet syndrome"), and antiphospholipid antibodies.

Branch retinal artery obstruction associated with temporal arteritis is exceedingly uncommon.[37] It is not usually necessary to obtain an erythrocyte sedimentation rate unless other evidence of temporal arteritis exists. Box 114-3 lists the systemic conditions most commonly associated with retinal artery obstructions.

PATHOLOGY

Early, coagulative necrosis of the inner layers of the neural retina, which are supplied by the retinal arterioles, is manifest by edema of the neuronal cells during the first few hours after arterial occlusion and becomes maximal within 24 hours. The intracellular swelling accounts for the gray, retinal opacity seen clinically. If the area of coagulative necrosis is small and localized, it appears as a cotton-wool spot, the clinical manifestation of a microinfarct of the nerve fiber layer of the neural retina. The cytoid body observed microscopically (Fig. 114-8) is a swollen, interrupted axon in the neural retinal nerve fiber layer. Histologically, the swollen end bulb superficially resembles a cell, hence the term cytoid body. A collection of many cytoid bodies, along with localized edema, marks the area of the microinfarct. A cotton-wool spot represents a localized accumulation of axoplasmic debris in the neural retinal nerve fiber layer and results from interruption of the orthograde or retrograde organelle transport in ganglion cell axons, that is, obstruction of axoplasmic flow.

The outer half of the neural retina is well preserved. The inner half of the neural retina, however, becomes "homogenized" into a diffuse, relatively acellular zone, which generally contains thick-walled retinal blood vessels. Because the glial cells die along with the other neural retinal elements, gliosis does not occur.

TREATMENT

No proved treatment exists for branch retinal artery obstruction. Because the visual prognosis is much better for branch retinal artery obstruction than for central retinal artery obstruction, invasive therapeutic maneuvers of dubious utility are not typically performed. On occasion, ocular massage or paracentesis is successful in dislodging an embolus. Laser photocoagulation has been employed to "melt" an embolus, without improvement in the vision.[38]

One report suggests that hyperbaric oxygen therapy may improve the visual loss associated with multiple branch retinal artery obstruction in Susac's syndrome.[39]

In the rare patient who has branch retinal artery obstruction accompanied by a systemic clotting disorder, systemic anticoagulation may prevent further events.

COURSE AND OUTCOME

Most patients remain with a fixed visual field defect but intact central acuity. About 80% of eyes recover to 20/40 (6/12) or better central acuity. Retinal neovascularization has been reported but is distinctly uncommon. Iris neovascularization does not occur.[11]

OPHTHALMIC ARTERY OBSTRUCTION

Acute simultaneous obstruction of both the retinal and choroidal circulations is referred to as an ophthalmic artery obstruction. In some cases a single site of blockage in the ophthalmic artery is present, and in others simultaneous interruption of the retinal and posterior choroidal circulations with multiple blockage sites is found.

Ophthalmic artery obstructions can be differentiated clinically from central retinal artery obstruction by the following features[40]:
- Severe visual loss—bare or no light perception;
- Intense ischemic retinal whitening that extends beyond the macular area;
- Little to no cherry-red spot;
- Marked choroidal perfusion defects on fluorescein angiography;
- Nonrecordable electroretinogram; and
- Late retinal pigment epithelium alterations.

Cases of ophthalmic artery obstruction usually have associated local orbital or systemic diseases, which include orbital mucormycosis, orbital trauma, retrobulbar anesthesia, depot corticosteroid injection, atrial myxoma, or carotid artery disease. Temporal arteritis usually does not produce ophthalmic artery obstruction in the absence of ipsilateral ischemic optic neuropathy.

As with central retinal artery obstruction, no proved therapy exists and significant visual recovery usually does not occur. In the absence of local causes, systemic evaluation must include testing for temporal arteritis, carotid artery disease, and cardiac disease.

CILIORETINAL ARTERY OBSTRUCTION

A cilioretinal artery exists in about 30% of individuals. It is a vessel that perfuses the retina and is derived directly from the posterior ciliary circulation rather than from the central retinal artery. For this reason, it may remain patent in the setting of a central retinal artery obstruction. Such vessels are usually observed to emanate from the temporal disc margin. They may be multiple and can also perfuse the nasal retina. On fluorescein angiography, they fill 1–3 seconds prior to the retinal circulation. Cilioretinal artery obstruction exists in three clinical variations:
- Isolated
- Cilioretinal artery obstruction combined with central retinal vein obstruction
- Cilioretinal artery obstruction combined with ischemic optic neuropathy

Isolated cilioretinal artery obstructions usually occur in young patients in the setting of collagen vascular disorders. They carry a good visual prognosis, with 90% of eyes left with 20/40 (6/12) or better vision.[41]

Cilioretinal artery obstruction combined with central retinal vein obstruction is not an uncommon variant in young patients (Fig. 114-9). It generally behaves as a nonischemic central retinal vein obstruction with a good central visual prognosis. The scotoma from the artery obstruction is usually permanent. Although the mechanism of this association is unclear, it is hypothesized that some eyes harbor a primary optic disc vasculitis (papillophlebitis) that affects both the arterial and venous circulation.[42] It is more common in men than in women and pa-

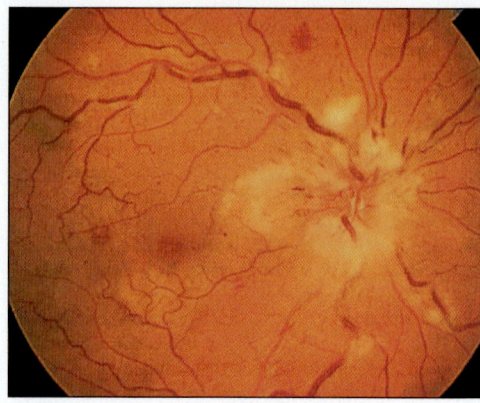

FIG. 114-9 ■ **Cilioretinal artery obstruction.** In conjunction with mild nonischemic central retinal vein obstruction. Note the retinal whitening just inferior to the fovea in the distribution of the cilioretinal artery.

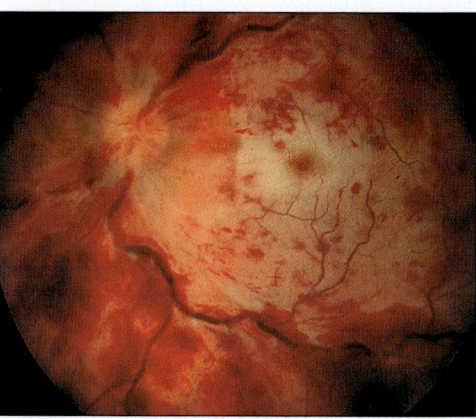

FIG. 114-10 ■ **Combined central retinal artery obstruction and central retinal vein obstruction.** Visual acuity in this 21-year-old woman who had lupus was light perception, and neovascularization of the iris ensued.

tients are generally healthy; however, this entity has been seen in conjunction with inflammatory bowel disease and leukemia.

In contrast to the first two groups discussed before, cilioretinal artery obstruction with ischemic optic neuropathy carries a grim visual prognosis and a strong association with temporal arteritis.

COMBINED ARTERY AND VEIN OBSTRUCTIONS

Central retinal artery obstruction combined with simultaneous central retinal vein obstruction rarely occurs. Such patients present with acute, severe loss of vision, usually to bare or no light perception. Examination shows a cherry-red spot combined with features of a central retinal vein obstruction, which include dilated, tortuous veins that have retinal hemorrhages in all four quadrants (Fig. 114-10).[43] Associated systemic or local disease is the rule—collagen vascular disorders, leukemia, orbital trauma, retrobulbar injections, and mucormycosis have been implicated. The visual prognosis is generally poor and the risk of neovascularization of the iris is about 75%. Exceptionally, a patient may manifest spontaneous improvement.[44]

Branch retinal artery obstruction combined with simultaneous central retinal vein obstruction has also been reported.[45] This rare entity behaves as a central retinal vein obstruction. Neovascularization of the iris is possible, but systemic associations other than hypertension and diabetes have not been confirmed.

REFERENCES

1. Brown GC. Retinal arterial obstructive disease. In: Schachat AP, Murphy RB, Patz A, eds. Medical retina, Vol 2 of Ryan SJ, ed. Retina. St Louis: CV Mosby; 1989:73: 1361–77.

2. Sharma S, Naqvi A, Sharma SM, et al. Transthoracic echocardiographic findings in patients with acute retinal artery obstruction. Arch Ophthalmol. 1996;114:1189–92.

3. Cho NC, Han HJ. Central retinal artery occlusion after varicella. Am J Ophthalmol. 1992;114:235–6.

4. Solomon SM, Solomon JH. Bilateral central retinal artery occlusions in polyarteritis nodosa. Ann Ophthalmol. 1978;10:567–9.

5. Sullivan KL, Brown GC, Forman AR, et al. Retrobulbar anesthesia and retinal vascular obstruction. Ophthalmology. 1983;90:373–7.

6. Cohen RG, Hedges TR, Duker JS. Central retinal artery occlusion in a child with T-cell lymphoma. Am J Ophthalmol. 1995;120:118–20.

7. Noble KG. Central retinal artery occlusion: the presenting sign in radiation retinopathy. Arch Ophthalmol. 1994;112:1409–10.

8. Egbert JE, Schwartz GS, Walsh AW. Diagnosis and treatment of an ophthalmic artery occlusion during an intralesional injection of corticosteroid into an eyelid capillary hemangioma. Am J Ophthalmol. 1996;121:638–42.

9. Jumper JM, Horton JC. Central retinal artery occlusion after manipulation of the neck by a chiropractor. Am J Ophthalmol. 1996;121:321–6.

10. Mames RN, Snady-McCoy L, Guy J. Central retinal and posterior ciliary artery occlusion after particle embolization of the external carotid artery system. Ophthalmology. 1991;98:527–31.

11. Sanborn GE, Magargal LE. Arterial obstructive disease of the eye. In: Tasman WS, Jaegar EA, eds. Clinical ophthalmology, Vol 3. Philadelphia: Lippincott; 1993;14:1–29.

12. Werner MS, Latchaw R, Baker L, Wirtschafter JD. Relapsing and remitting central retinal artery occlusion. Am J Ophthalmol. 1994;118:393–5.

13. Brown GC, Magargal LE. Central retinal artery obstruction and visual acuity. Ophthalmology. 1982;89:14–19.

14. Duker JS, Sivalingam A, Brown GC, Reber R. A prospective study of acute central retinal artery obstruction. Arch Ophthalmol. 1991;109:339–42.

15. Hayreh SS, Podhajsky P. Ocular neovascularization with retinal vascular occlusion. Arch Ophthalmol. 1982;100:1585–96.

16. Duker JS, Brown GC. The efficacy of panretinal photocoagulation for neovascularization of the iris after central retinal artery obstruction. Ophthalmology. 1989;96:92–5.

17. Duker JS, Brown GC. Neovascularization of the optic disc associated with obstruction of the central retinal artery. Ophthalmology. 1989;96:87–91.

18. Brown GC, Magargal LE, Shields JA, et al. Retinal artery obstruction in children and young adults. Ophthalmology. 1981;88:18–25.

19. Greven CM, Weaver RG, Harris WR, et al. Transesophageal echocardiography for detecting mitral valve prolapse with retinal artery occlusions. Am J Ophthalmol. 1991;111:103–4.

20. Glacet-Bernard A, Bayani N, Chretien P, et al. Antiphospholipid antibodies in retinal vascular occlusions. Arch Ophthalmol. 1994;112:790–5.

21. Golub BM, Sibony PA, Coller BS. Protein S deficiency associated with central retinal artery occlusion. Arch Ophthalmol. 1990;108:918–19.

22. Atebara NH, Brown GC, Cater J. Efficacy of anterior chamber paracentesis and carbogen in treating nonarteritic central retinal artery obstruction. Ophthalmology. 1995;102:2029–35.

23. Kuritzky S. Nitroglycerin to treat acute loss of vision. N Engl J Med. 1990;323:1428.

24. Rossman H. Treatment of retinal vascular occlusion by means of fibrinolysis. Postgrad Med J. 1973;Suppl:105–8.

25. Schmidt D, Schumacher M, Wakhloo AK. Microcatheter urokinase infusion in central retinal artery obstruction. Am J Ophthalmol. 1992;113:429–34.

26. Blair NP, Shaw WE, Dunn R, et al. Limitation of retinal injury by vitreoperfusion initiated after onset of ischemia. Arch Ophthalmol. 1991;109:113–18.

27. Matzkin DC, Slamovitz TL, Sachs R, Burde RM. Visual recovery in two patients after intravenous methylprednisolone treatment of central retinal artery occlusion secondary to giant cell arteritis. Ophthalmology. 1992;99:68–71.

28. Hayreh SS, Weingeist TA. Experimental occlusion of the central artery of the retina. Br J Ophthalmol. 1989;64:896–912.

29. Duker JS, Brown, GC. Recovery following acute obstruction of the retinal and choroidal circulations. Ophthalmology. 1988;8:257–60.

30. Greven CM, Slusher MM, Weaver RG. Retinal arterial occlusions in young adults. Am J Ophthalmol. 1995;120:776–83.

31. Arruga J, Sanders MD. Ophthalmologic findings in 70 patients with evidence of retinal embolism. Ophthalmology. 1982;89:1336–47.

32. Lewis JM. Multiple retinal occlusions from a left atrial myxoma. Am J Ophthalmol. 1994;117:674–5.

33. Greven CM, Weaver RG, Owen J, Slusher MM. Protein S deficiency and bilateral branch retinal artery occlusion. Ophthalmology. 1991;98:33–4.

34. Nelson ME, Talbot JF, Preston FE. Recurrent multiple-branch retinal arteriolar occlusions in a patient with protein C deficiency. Graefes Arch Clin Exp Ophthalmol. 1989;227:443–7.

35. Gass JDM, Tiedeman J, Thomas MA. Idiopathic recurrent branch retinal arterial occlusions. Ophthalmology. 1986;93:1148–57.

36. Johnson MW, Thomley ML, Huang SS, Gass JDM. Idiopathic recurrent branch retinal arterial occlusion. Ophthalmology. 1994;101:480–9.

37. Fineman MS, Savino PJ, Federman JL, Eagle RC. Branch retinal artery occlusion as the initial sign of giant cell arteritis. Am J Ophthalmol. 1996;112:428–30.

38. Dutton GN, Craig G. Treatment of a retinal embolus by photocoagulation. Br J Ophthalmol. 1988;72:580–1.

39. Li HK, Dejean BJ, Tand RA. Reversal of visual loss with hyperbaric oxygen treatment in a patient with Susac syndrome. Ophthalmology. 1996;103:2091–8.

40. Brown GC, Magargal LE, Sergott R. Acute obstruction of the retinal and choroidal circulations. Ophthalmology. 1986;93:1373–82.

41. Brown GC, Moffat K, Cruess A, et al. Cilioretinal artery obstruction. Retina. 1983;3:182–7.

42. Keyser BJ, Duker JS, Brown GC, et al. Combined central retinal vein occlusion and cilioretinal artery occlusion associated with prolonged retinal arterial filling. Am J Ophthalmol. 1994;117:308–13.

43. Richards RD. Simultaneous occlusion of the central retinal artery and vein. Trans Am Ophthalmol Soc. 1979;77:191–209.

44. Jorizzo PA, Klein ML, Shults WT, Linn ML. Visual recovery in combined central retinal artery and central retinal vein occlusion. Am J Ophthalmol. 1987;104:358–63.

45. Duker JS, Cohen MS, Brown GC, et al. Combined branch retinal artery and central retinal vein obstruction. Retina. 1990;10:105–12.

CHAPTER

115

Venous Obstructive Disease of the Retina

MICHAEL G. MORLEY • JEFFREY S. HEIER

Central Retinal Vein Obstruction

DEFINITION
- Obstruction of the central retinal vein at the lamina cribrosa.

KEY FEATURES
- Retinal hemorrhages in all four quadrants.
- Dilated, tortuous veins in all four quadrants.

ASSOCIATED FEATURES
- Optic disc edema.
- Macular edema.
- Cotton-wool spots.
- Capillary nonperfusion.
- Neovascularization of the iris, retina, or optic disc.
- Neovascular glaucoma.
- Optic disc venous–venous collateral vessels (opticociliary shunt vessels).
- Exudative retinal detachment in severe cases.

Branch Retinal Vein Obstruction

DEFINITION
- Obstruction of a branch retinal vein.

KEY FEATURE
- Retinal hemorrhages in the distribution of the obstructed branch retinal vein.

ASSOCIATED FEATURES
- Macular edema.
- Retinal neovascularization.
- Vitreous hemorrhage.
- Dilated, tortuous retinal vein.
- Capillary nonperfusion.
- Cotton-wool spots.
- Venous–venous retinal collateral vessels.
- Sheathing of vessel.
- Lipid exudates.
- Microvascular changes including microaneurysms and collateral vessels.
- Pigmentary macular disturbances.
- Subretinal fibrosis.

CENTRAL RETINAL VEIN OBSTRUCTION

INTRODUCTION

Venous obstructive disease of the retina is a relatively common retinal vascular disorder, second only to diabetic retinopathy in incidence. It typically affects patients who are 50 years of age or older. Usually, retinal vein obstructions are recognized easily and treatment options have been investigated thoroughly using large, multicenter, randomized clinical trials.

Retinal vein obstructions are classified according to whether the central retinal vein or one of its branches is obstructed. Central retinal vein obstruction and branch retinal vein obstruction differ with respect to pathophysiology, underlying systemic associations, average age of onset, clinical course, and therapy.

Central retinal vein obstructions can be divided further into ischemic and nonischemic varieties. This distinction among central retinal vein obstructions, although somewhat arbitrary, is important because up to two thirds of patients who have the ischemic variety develop iris neovascularization and neovascular glaucoma.

EPIDEMIOLOGY AND PATHOGENESIS

Central retinal vein obstruction is found most commonly in individuals over 50 years old.[1–2] Diabetes mellitus, systemic arterial hypertension, and atherosclerotic cardiovascular disease are the most frequently associated underlying medical diseases; however, their direct relationship to pathogenesis remains speculative.[2–5] Completely normal medical and laboratory evaluation results are found in about one fourth of patients.[3,6] A significant inverse association with central retinal vein obstruction, which represents decreasing risk, is present with alcohol consumption, education, physical activity and, in women, exogenous estrogen use.[2]

Open-angle glaucoma is a relatively common finding in patients who have central retinal vein obstruction. Patients who have a history of glaucoma are about 5 times more likely to have central retinal vein obstruction than those who do not, presumably because of structural alterations of the *lamina cribrosa* induced by elevated intraocular pressure. Acute angle-closure glaucoma may precipitate central retinal vein obstruction.

The precise pathogenesis of central retinal vein obstruction remains obscure. The obstruction is believed to be the result of a thrombus in the central retinal vein at, or posterior to, the lamina cribrosa. Arteriosclerosis of the neighboring central retinal artery that causes turbulent venous flow and then endothelial damage often is implicated. Also, endothelial cell proliferation has been suggested. An alternative theory is that thrombosis of the central retinal vein is an end-stage phenomenon, induced by a variety of primary lesions. Such lesions could include compressive or inflammatory optic nerve or orbital problems, structural abnormalities in the lamina cribrosa, or hemodynamic changes.

Because the retinal venous circulation represents a relatively high-resistance, low-flow system it is particularly sensitive to hematological factors. Along with an elevated erythrocyte sedimentation rate and antithrombin III levels, other studies indicate that an elevated hematocrit level, elevated homocysteine level, elevated fibrinogen level, increased blood viscosity, the presence of a lupus anticoagulant or another antiphospholipid antibody, and a deficiency in activated protein C may be associated with retinal venous disease.[7-9] Whether these hematological factors alone can initiate a central retinal vein obstruction or whether their role is to function as cofactors remains unknown.

OCULAR MANIFESTATIONS

Both types of central retinal vein obstruction, ischemic and nonischemic, share similar findings—dilated, tortuous retinal veins and retinal hemorrhages in all four quadrants. The distinction between the two varieties is important, because it assists the clinician in the following:

- Prediction of the risk of subsequent ocular neovascularization
- Identification of patients who have poorer visual prognosis
- Determination of the likelihood of spontaneous visual improvement
- Decision as to appropriate follow-up intervals

The distinction between the two types of vein obstructions remains somewhat arbitrary and is based on the total area of nonperfusion on fluorescein angiography. Most investigators accept that nonischemic and ischemic central retinal vein obstructions represent varying severity of the same underlying disease continuum. Other investigators suggest, however, that these are two distinct clinical entities with different pathogenesis. The ischemic variety is associated with concurrent, severe retinal arterial disease, while the milder, nonischemic type results from a thrombosis located more distally, behind the lamina cribrosa.[10]

Nonischemic Central Retinal Vein Obstruction

Alternative names include partial, incomplete, imminent, threatened, incipient, or impending vein obstruction, as well as venous stasis retinopathy.[11] Of the patients who have central retinal vein obstruction, 75–80% can be classified as having this milder form. Patients usually have mild to moderate decreased visual acuity, although this can vary from normal to as poor as difficulty with finger counting. Intermittent blurring or transient visual obscuration also may be a complaint. Pain is rare.

Pupillary testing rarely reveals an afferent defect which, if present, is only slight. Ophthalmoscopy reveals a variable number of dot and flame retinal hemorrhages, present in all four quadrants (Fig. 115-1). Optic nerve head swelling is common, and engorgement and tortuosity of the retinal veins are characteristic. Cotton-wool spots, if present, are few in number and located posteriorly. When vision is decreased, this is usually the result of macular hemorrhage or edema, which may be in the form of cystoid macular edema, diffuse macular thickening, or both.

Neovascularization of either the anterior or posterior segment is rare in a true nonischemic central retinal vein obstruction (less than 2% incidence), although conversion from an initially nonischemic vein obstruction to the ischemic variety is fairly common. The Central Vein Occlusion Study Group noted that 34% of nonischemic central retinal vein occlusions (CRVOs) progressed to become ischemic within 3 years,[12] and 15% of the study group converted within the first 4 months.

Many or all of the pathological retinal findings may resolve over the 6–12 months following diagnosis. Retinal hemorrhages can resolve completely. The optic nerve may appear normal, but opticociliary collateral vessels are common. Macular edema also may resolve, to leave a normal appearance. However, persistent cystoid macular edema can linger and result in permanent visual loss, often leading to pigmentary changes, epiretinal membrane formation, or subretinal fibrosis.

Ischemic Central Retinal Vein Obstruction

Ischemic central retinal vein obstructions are referred to as severe, complete, or total vein obstruction, and hemorrhagic retinopathy[11]; they account for 20–25% of all central retinal vein obstructions. Acute, markedly decreased visual acuity is the usual initial complaint. Vision usually ranges from 20/200 (6/60) to hand-motion acuity. A prominent afferent pupillary defect is typical. Pain at the time of evaluation may occur if neovascular glaucoma has developed.

The ophthalmoscopic picture of an ischemic central retinal vein obstruction may be confused with other entities, but rarely. It is characterized by extensive retinal hemorrhages in all four quadrants, most notably centered in the posterior pole (Fig. 115-2). Hemorrhages can be so extensive that the retinal and choroidal details are obscured. Bleeding may break through the internal limiting membrane, which results in vitreous hemorrhage. The optic disc usually is edematous, and the retinal veins are markedly engorged and tortuous. Cotton-wool spots are usually present and may be numerous. Macular edema is often severe but may be obscured by hemorrhage. Massive lipid exudation in the

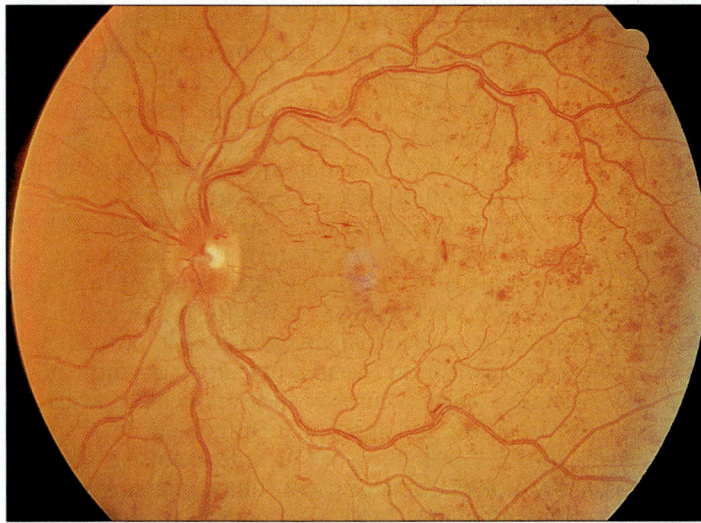

FIG. 115-1 ▌ **Nonischemic central retinal vein obstruction.** Fundus view of diffuse retinal hemorrhages, optic nerve head edema, dilated and tortuous veins, and a cotton-wool spot.

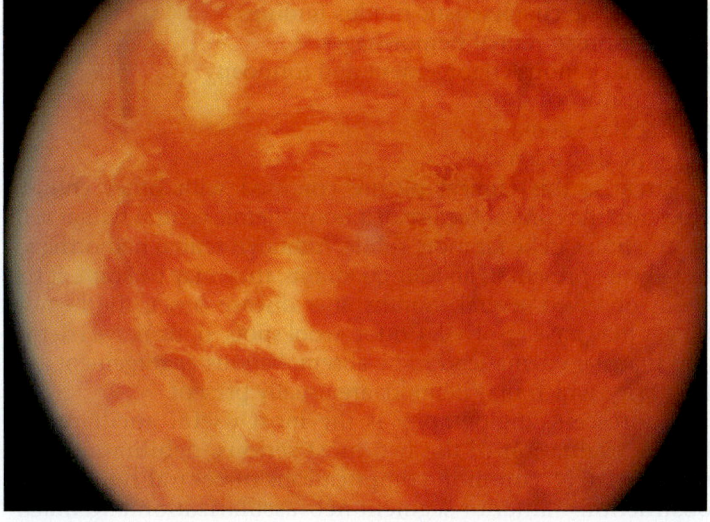

FIG. 115-2 ▌ **Ischemic central retinal vein obstruction.** Fundus view of extensive retinal hemorrhages, venous dilation and tortuosity, and scattered cotton-wool spots.

macular region can occur, especially in patients who have elevated triglyceride levels. Exudative retinal detachment may develop and is associated with a poor visual prognosis. Secondary, non-neovascular angle-closure glaucoma may occur.

The incidence of anterior segment neovascularization in ischemic central retinal vein obstruction is 60% or higher and has been documented as early as 9 weeks after onset.[3,13] Neovascularization of the angle and neovascular glaucoma may occur within 3 months of disease onset (90-day glaucoma), and it can result in intractably elevated pressure. Neovascularization of the optic disc and retinal neovascularization may be seen as well, but they are less common. As with nonischemic central retinal vein obstruction, the findings may decrease or resolve 6–12 months after diagnosis.

During the resolution phase, the optic nerve shows pallor and opticociliary collateral vessels more often than it does in the mild form of central retinal vein obstruction. Permanent macular changes can develop that include pigmentary changes, epiretinal membrane formation, and subretinal fibrosis that resembles disciform scarring. Macular ischemia may be present, as well.

HEMICENTRAL RETINAL VEIN OBSTRUCTION. In about 20% of eyes, the central retinal vein enters the optic nerve as two separate branches, the superior and inferior, prior to merging as a single trunk posterior to the lamina cribrosa. In these eyes, obstruction of one of the dual trunks within the substance of the optic nerve results in a hemicentral retinal vein obstruction. Although only one half of the retina is involved, these obstructions act more like central retinal vein obstructions than a branch retinal vein obstruction in terms of visual outcome, risk of neovascularization, and response to laser treatment.

Papillophlebitis or Optic Disc Vasculitis

Some mild central retinal vein obstructions in patients younger than 50 years have been referred to as papillophlebitis or optic disc vasculitis—terms that suggest a benign course. An inflammatory optic neuritis or vasculitis is hypothesized as the cause. These eyes tend to have optic disc edema out of proportion to the retinal findings, cotton-wool spots that ring the optic disc, and occasionally cilioretinal artery obstructions or even partial central retinal artery obstructions. Although spontaneous improvement is common, the course is not always benign. Up to 30% of these patients may develop the ischemic type of occlusion, a final visual acuity of 20/200 (6/60) or worse occurs in nearly 40%, and neovascular glaucoma has been reported.[14]

DIAGNOSIS AND ANCILLARY TESTING

The diagnosis of an ischemic central retinal vein obstruction is based on the characteristic fundus findings:

- Widespread retinal hemorrhages
- Retinal venous engorgement and tortuosity
- Cotton-wool spots
- Macular edema
- Optic disc edema

Rarely is this clinical picture confused with other entities. However, the clinical picture of a nonischemic central retinal vein obstruction can be far more subtle. Although retinal hemorrhages usually are present in all four quadrants, they may be scant. If the eye is observed several months after disease onset, the hemorrhages may have resolved. Cotton-wool spots, optic nerve edema, and macular edema tend to be absent. Venous engorgement and tortuosity, which may be mild, are usually present.

Fluorescein angiography is the most useful ancillary test for the evaluation of the two most serious, debilitating and, unfortunately, common complications of central retinal vein obstruction—anterior segment neovascularization and macular edema. Studies suggest that eyes with 10 disc areas or greater of nonperfusion noted on fluorescein angiography are at increased risk for the development of anterior segment

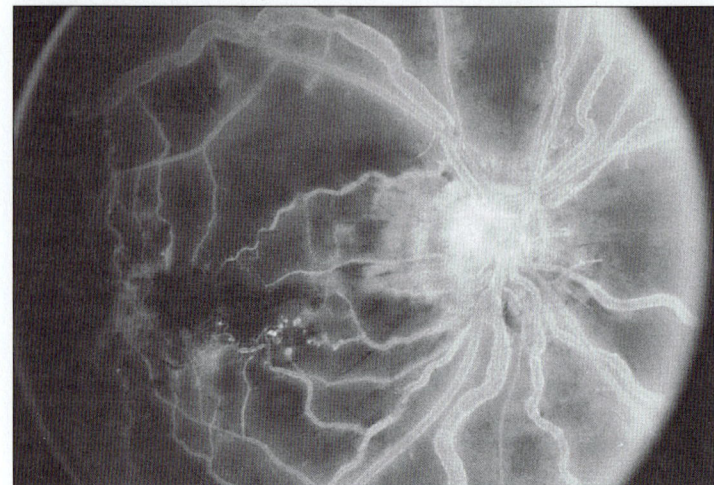

FIG. 115-3 ■ **Ischemic central retinal vein obstruction.** Fluorescein angiography reveals marked hypofluorescence secondary to widespread capillary nonperfusion. The venous system shows marked dilation with focal areas of constriction, and the vessel walls stain in areas of ischemia.

neovascularization and, therefore, should be classified as ischemic.[15,16] The Central Vein Occlusion Study found the greatest risk was in patients with worse than 20/200 (6/60) visual acuity or 30 or more disc areas of nonperfusion.[12] Electroretinography is used occasionally to help determine the prognosis of a CRVO.[17,18]

Fluorescein angiography in ischemic central retinal vein obstruction may show marked hypofluorescence (Fig. 115-3), which may be secondary to blockage from extensive hemorrhages or to retinal capillary nonperfusion. When extensive hemorrhages are present, little information is gained from the angiogram. However, as the hemorrhages clear over several months, the degree of capillary nonperfusion may become apparent. Most eyes (80%) that have this degree of hemorrhage eventually are classified as ischemic.

Macular edema is the most common cause of visual loss in central retinal vein obstruction. It is present almost universally in ischemic cases and frequently is severe. It may manifest as large cystoid spaces or diffuse leakage on fluorescein angiography. Macular edema may be obscured by hemorrhage, but as the hemorrhage and edema resolve, macular ischemia may become apparent. Angiography also reveals optic nerve head leakage and perivenous staining. In the late stages of the disease, generalized extensive retinal capillary nonperfusion, arteriovenous collateral vessels, and microaneurysms are seen. The macular region shows persistent edema or pigmentary degeneration.

With a nonischemic central retinal vein obstruction, fluorescein angiography reveals staining along the retinal veins, microaneurysms, and dilated optic nerve head capillaries. Retinal capillary nonperfusion (Fig. 115-4) is minimal or absent. As the nonischemic central retinal vein obstruction resolves, angiography may become normal. If macular edema persists, or if pigmentary changes occur, these become evident.

The Central Vein Occlusion Study Group reported that 37% of ischemic central retinal vein obstructions demonstrated anterior segment (iris or angle or both) neovascularization at or before the 4-month follow-up.[19] Although the results of fluorescein angiography help to differentiate patients at high risk for the development of neovascularization, visual acuity alone is a more powerful, less expensive, and less invasive measurement by which to determine the prognosis and appropriate follow-up.[12]

A general medical evaluation, to include extensive medical history and physical examination with blood pressure evaluation, is recommended (Box 115-1). Laboratory evaluation may include a complete blood count, glucose tolerance test, lipid profile, serum protein electrophoresis, chemistry profile, and syphilis serology. Additional testing, based upon the above find-

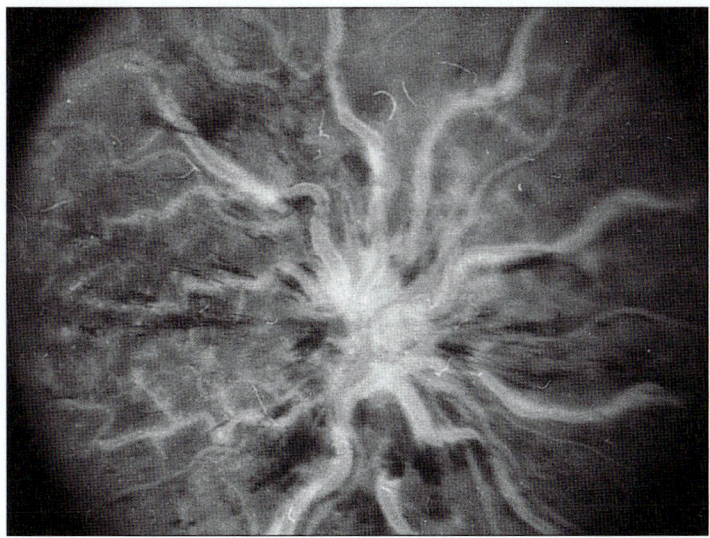

FIG. 115-4 ■ Nonischemic central retinal vein obstruction. Fluorescein angiography shows marked venous dilation and tortuosity, optic nerve head edema, and staining of vessel walls. Capillary nonperfusion is absent.

BOX 115-1

Medical and Ophthalmic Work-Up for Central Retinal Vein Obstruction and Branch Retinal Vein Obstruction

CENTRAL RETINAL VEIN OBSTRUCTION
Complete history and physical examination
Complete ophthalmic examination
Fluorescein angiography
Gonioscopy to look for iris and/or angle neovascularization
Blood pressure
Complete blood count
Prothrombin time
Partial thromboplastin time
Antinuclear antibodies
Serum protein electrophoresis
Erythrocyte sedimentation rate

BRANCH RETINAL VEIN OBSTRUCTION
Complete history and physical examination
Complete ophthalmic examination
Fluorescein angiography
Blood pressure

---

ings, may be necessary. If a history of systemic clotting diathesis exists, further hematological tests such as lupus anticoagulant level, anticardiolipin antibody, and protein S and protein C levels should be considered. Diagnosis and treatment of an associated disease is not expected to improve the visual outcome in the affected eye, but it may help to prevent subsequent obstruction in the fellow eye.

DIFFERENTIAL DIAGNOSIS

As stated above, rarely is the full-blown picture of an ischemic central retinal vein obstruction confused with other disease entities. However, nonischemic or long-standing central retinal vein obstructions can appear similar to the retinopathy of carotid occlusive disease—the ocular ischemic syndrome(s). A great deal of confusion existed in the past over these two entities, not only because of their similar clinical pictures, but also because each has been referred to in the literature as *venous stasis retinopathy*.[11,20] Both conditions are associated with blurred vision, and both may have transient visual loss. Blurring of vision when a darker room is entered after being in a brighter area is suggestive of carotid artery disease.[21] Although disc edema al-

---

ways is present in ischemic central retinal vein obstruction, and may be present in nonischemic central retinal vein obstruction, it is quite rare in carotid occlusive disease. Although the veins are engorged in both diseases, they are generally *not* tortuous in the ocular ischemic syndrome. The retinal hemorrhages seen in carotid disease tend to localize to the midperiphery, instead of the posterior pole as seen in central retinal vein obstruction.

Hyperviscosity syndromes may produce a bilateral retinopathy similar to central retinal vein obstruction and may, in fact, induce a true central retinal vein obstruction with thrombus formation. Simultaneous bilateral disease is an unusual finding in central retinal vein obstructions but occurs more commonly in hypercoagulable and hyperviscous states. Diseases such as sickle cell disease, polycythemia vera, leukemia, and multiple myeloma are but a few of the possibilities. When a patient seeks treatment for bilateral central retinal vein obstructions, especially simultaneous, the medical and laboratory evaluation should include a search for evidence of hyperviscous and hypercoagulable syndromes. Improvement in the affected eye is possible when a hyperviscosity syndrome is responsible and plasmapheresis is performed.[22] Severe anemia with thrombocytopenia can masquerade as a central retinal vein obstruction, and it is differentiated from a central retinal vein obstruction by a complete blood count with platelets. In addition, acute hypertensive retinopathy with disc edema may resemble bilateral central retinal vein obstruction.

SYSTEMIC ASSOCIATIONS

Central retinal vein obstruction has been associated with systemic vascular disease such as hypertension, diabetes mellitus, and cardiovascular disease; blood dyscrasias such as polycythemia vera, lymphoma, and leukemia; paraproteinemias and dysproteinemias including multiple myeloma and cryoglobulinemia; vasculitis of syphilis and sarcoidosis; and autoimmune disease such as systemic lupus erythematosus.[23] Blood dyscrasias and dysproteinemias result in hyperviscosity syndromes, which may appear similar to central retinal vein obstruction but possibly represent curable disease (as discussed under differential diagnosis above). Oral contraceptive use in women may be associated with both thromboembolic disease and central retinal vein obstruction.[24]

PATHOLOGY

Green *et al.*[13] evaluated histological sections of 29 eyes in 28 patients who had central retinal vein obstruction. All 29 eyes had the formation of a fresh or recanalized thrombus at or just posterior to the lamina cribrosa. Within the thrombi, a mild lymphocytic infiltration with prominent endothelial cells was seen. Loss of the inner retinal layers consistent with inner retinal ischemia was a common finding.

Alterations in blood flow, hyperviscosity, and vessel wall abnormalities may produce central retinal vein obstructions by enabling a thrombus of the central retinal vein to form. Local factors can predispose to central retinal vein obstruction. Glaucoma has been associated with central retinal vein obstruction. It has been hypothesized that glaucoma causes stretching and compression of the lamina cribrosa, which results in vessel abnormalities, increased resistance to flow and, ultimately, thrombosis.[13]

TREATMENT

No treatment has been proven to reverse the pathology seen in central retinal vein obstruction. Aspirin; systemic anticoagulation with coumarin, heparin, and alteplase; local anticoagulation with intravitreal alteplase; corticosteroids; anti-inflammatory agents; isovolemic hemodilution; plasmapheresis; and optic nerve sheath decompression all have been advocated but without definitive proof of efficacy. Certain complications of central retinal vein obstruction may be preventable or reversible, however (Box 115-2).

Neovascular Glaucoma

Neovascular glaucoma is a devastating complication of ischemic central retinal vein obstruction. Intractable glaucoma, blindness, and pain that culminates in enucleation can occur. The Central Vein Occlusion Study Group determined whether prophylactic panretinal photocoagulation (PRP) was an effective method with which to prevent the development of iris neovascularization or angle neovascularization in patients who had ischemic central retinal vein obstruction, or whether it was more appropriate to apply PRP after the development of anterior segment neovascularization.[25] The study found that prophylactically treated ischemic eyes developed iris neovascularization less frequently than ischemic eyes that were followed (20% in the early treatment group versus 35% in the no-early-treatment group), although the difference was not statistically significant. However, PRP is more likely to result in prompt regression of neovascularization of the iris in the previously untreated group versus the prophylactically treated group (56% versus 22%, respectively, after 1 month). As a result, for ischemic central retinal vein obstructions, frequent follow-up examinations during the early months and prompt PRP if iris neovascularization develops is the recommended treatment strategy.

Treatment should be applied in all four quadrants to give medium-white burns of diameter 400–500μm (a total of 1000–2000 burns). Identification of early iris neovascularization at the pupillary border is critical—examination of the undilated pupil is recommended. Routine gonioscopy also is suggested, because angle neovascularization can occur without iris neovascularization.

Macular Edema

Macular edema and subsequent permanent macular dysfunction occur in virtually all patients with ischemic central retinal vein obstruction, and in many patients with nonischemic central retinal vein obstruction. The Central Vein Occlusion Study evaluated the efficacy of macular grid photocoagulation in patients with central retinal vein obstruction and macular edema.[26] Patients with both ischemic and nonischemic central retinal vein obstruction were studied. Although macular grid laser treatment conclusively reduced angiographic macular edema, the study did not find a difference in visual acuity between the treated and untreated eyes at any stage of the follow-up period. As a result, currently it is not recommended that macular grid photocoagulation be employed in the setting of central retinal vein obstruction. Intravitreal triamcinolone is being studied as a treatment for cystoid macular edema.

COURSE AND OUTCOME

The prognosis for visual recovery is highly dependent upon the subtype of central retinal vein obstruction. In general, the visual prognosis can be predicted from the visual acuity during evaluation. Patients who have nonischemic central retinal vein ob-

structions may experience a complete recovery of vision, although this occurs in less than 10% of cases.[6] Although patients with nonischemic disease may retain acuity of 20/60 (6/18) or better, as many as 50% deteriorate to levels of 20/200 (6/60) or worse.[3,6] Conversion of nonischemic to ischemic occlusions is seen in about one third of cases and typically occurs during the first 6–12 months after evaluation.[3,6,12,28] Of the patients who have ischemic central retinal vein obstructions, more than 90% have a final visual acuity of 20/200 (6/60) or worse.

As many as 7% of patients with central retinal vein obstruction develop a nonsimultaneous venous occlusion of the fellow eye within 2 years.[29] Contralateral branch retinal vein and retinal arterial obstructions also may be seen. The risk of any vascular occlusion in the fellow eye is estimated to be 0.9% per year.[12]

Based on the Central Vein Occlusion Study, the recommended follow-up examinations in patients who have central retinal vein obstruction are given in Box 115-3.[12,19,25]

If visual acuity deteriorates to less than 20/200 (6/60) at any time during the disease course, the patient should be treated as a patient with a new CRVO who has an acuity of that level and assessed monthly.

BRANCH RETINAL VEIN OBSTRUCTION

INTRODUCTION

Branch retinal vein obstruction is a common retinal vascular disorder of the elderly. Visual loss from a branch retinal vein occlusion usually is caused by macular edema, macular ischemia, or vitreous hemorrhage. In some patients, laser treatment can help stabilize or even improve vision.

EPIDEMIOLOGY AND PATHOGENESIS

Branch retinal vein obstructions occur approximately 3 times more commonly than central retinal vein obstructions. Men and women are affected equally, with the usual age of onset between 60 and 70 years. Most epidemiological and histopathological evidence implicates arteriolar disease as the underlying pathogenesis. Branch retinal vein obstruction almost always occurs at an arteriovenous crossing, where the artery and vein share a common adventitial sheath. The artery nearly always is anterior (innermost) to the vein.[30] It is postulated that a rigid, arteriosclerotic artery compresses the retinal vein, which results in turbulent blood flow and endothelial damage, followed by thrombosis and obstruction of the vein. Most branch retinal vein obstructions occur superotemporally, probably because this is where the highest concentration of arteriovenous crossings lie.

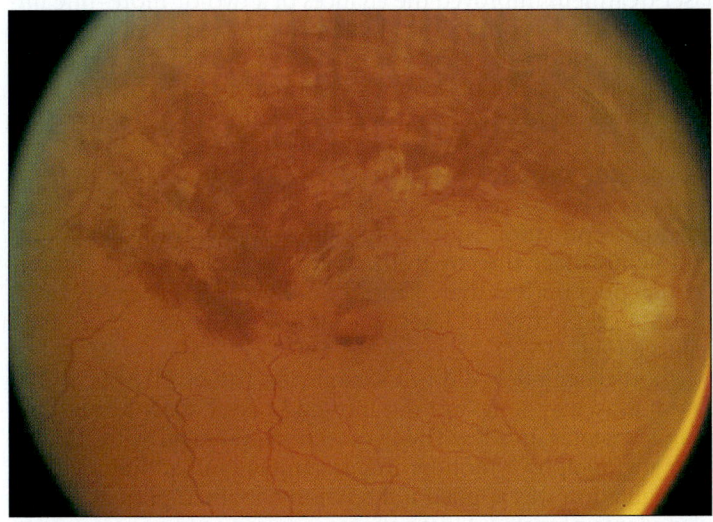

FIG. 115-5 ■ **Branch retinal vein obstruction.** Fundus view of extensive retinal hemorrhages in segmental distribution of a superotemporal retinal vein. Dilated, tortuous veins, cotton-wool spots, and macular edema also can be seen.

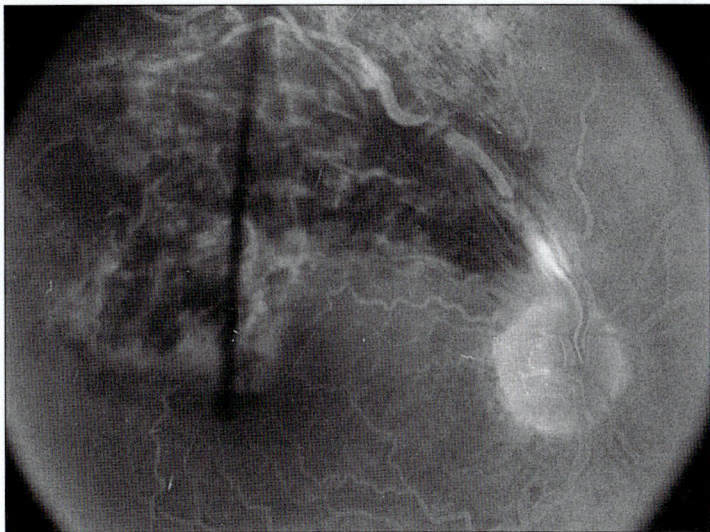

FIG. 115-6 ■ **Branch retinal vein obstruction.** Fluorescein angiography of the patient shown in Figure 115-4. Marked hypofluorescence is present secondary to extensive hemorrhage in the distribution of a superotemporal branch vein. Vessel dilation, tortuosity, and staining is seen in the same distribution.

Rarely, local ocular diseases, especially of an inflammatory nature, can result in a secondary branch retinal vein obstruction. This has been reported in diseases such as toxoplasmosis, Eales' disease, Behçet's syndrome, and ocular sarcoidosis. Also, macroaneurysms, Coats' disease, retinal capillary hemangiomas, and optic disc drusen are linked to branch retinal vein obstruction. Glaucoma is also a risk factor for the development of branch retinal vein occlusion. Branch retinal vein occlusion is usually unilateral, with only 9% of patients having bilateral involvement.

OCULAR MANIFESTATIONS

Patients with branch retinal vein occlusion usually complain of sudden onset of blurred vision or a visual field defect. Retinal hemorrhages confined to the distribution of a retinal vein are characteristic for branch retinal vein obstruction (Fig. 115-5). As a result of the distribution, the hemorrhages usually assume a triangular configuration with the apex at the site of blockage. Flame-shaped hemorrhages predominate. Mild obstructions are associated with a relatively small amount of hemorrhage. Complete obstructions result in extensive intraretinal hemorrhages, cotton-wool spot formation, and widespread capillary nonperfusion. If the macular region is involved, macular edema or hemorrhage occurs, which causes decreased visual acuity. Visual acuity may range from 20/20 (6/6) to counting fingers. If the macula is spared, a branch retinal vein obstruction may be asymptomatic, found only on routine examination of the fundus. Occasionally a partial branch retinal vein occlusion with little hemorrhage and edema may progress to a completely occluded vein, with an increase in hemorrhage and edema and a corresponding decrease in visual acuity. Retinal neovascularization occurs in approximately 20% of cases. The incidence of retinal neovascularization rises with increasing area of retinal nonperfusion. Retinal neovascularization typically develops within the first 6–12 months but may occur years later. Vitreous hemorrhage can ensue and may require vitrectomy. Anterior segment neovascularization rarely is seen in patients with branch retinal vein obstruction, unless other ischemic conditions co-exist (e.g., diabetes). With time, the dramatic picture of an acute branch retinal vein obstruction can become much more subtle. Hemorrhages fade with time so that the fundus can look almost normal. Collateral vessels and microvascular abnormalities develop to help drain the affected area. The collateral vessels often cross the horizontal raphe. Proximal to the site of blockage, the retinal vein may become sclerotic. The reti-

nal artery that feeds the affected zone may become narrowed and sheathed, as well. Microaneurysm formation occurs and lipid exudation may be present. Capillary nonperfusion is seen best in the later stages, after the hemorrhages have cleared. Epiretinal membrane and macular retinal pigment epithelial changes as a result of chronic cystoid macular edema sometimes are seen in the late phase of a branch retinal vein obstruction. Retinal detachment, either rhegmatogenous or tractional, is uncommon but may be seen. Exudative localized retinal detachment in the distribution of the branch retinal vein occlusion also is seen if there is severe ischemia.

DIAGNOSIS AND ANCILLARY TESTING

The diagnosis of an acute branch retinal vein obstruction is made by finding retinal hemorrhages in the distribution of an obstructed retinal vein. Usually the retinal vein is dilated and tortuous (Fig. 115-6). The obstruction almost always occurs at an arteriovenous crossing site, with the artery anterior to the vein.[30]

Fluorescein angiography is a helpful adjunct for both establishment of the diagnosis and guidance for the treatment of branch retinal vein obstruction. Arteriolar filling is usually normal, but venous filling in the affected vessel usually is delayed in the acute phase. Hypofluorescence caused by hemorrhage and capillary nonperfusion are common findings, and dilated, tortuous capillaries are seen. Collateral vessels may cross the horizontal raphe. The retinal vessels, particularly the vein walls, may stain with fluorescein. Neovascular fronds may leak fluorescein profusely. In contrast, collateral vessels do not leak fluorescein. Retinal vessels, particularly the vein walls, may stain with fluorescein, especially at the site of the occlusion. Macular edema, which is noted clinically but not angiographically, may indicate ischemia. Classic petaloid cystoid macular edema may involve the entire fovea or just several clock hours, depending on the distribution of the obstruction.

DIFFERENTIAL DIAGNOSIS

The differential diagnosis of branch retinal vein obstructions is shown in Box 115-4. Hypertensive retinopathy with marked arteriovenous crossing changes and retinal hemorrhages may look like a branch retinal vein occlusion. A chronic branch retinal vein obstruction with telangiectatic capillaries may be confused with juxtafoveal retinal telangiectasia. Asymmetrical diabetic retinopathy can have a picture similar to a branch vein obstruction or, conversely, obscure the diagnosis of a branch vein obstruction.

SYSTEMIC ASSOCIATIONS

Hypertension is the condition most commonly associated with branch retinal vein obstruction. The Eye Disease Case Control Study clearly demonstrated the important association of hypertension with vein obstructions.[2] In that study, more than 50% of branch retinal vein obstructions were associated with hypertension. The study also found an association between vein obstructions and a history of cardiovascular disease, increased body mass index at 20 years of age, glaucoma, and higher serum levels of α_2-globulin. A reduced risk of branch retinal vein obstruction was found with alcohol consumption and increasing levels of high-density lipoprotein cholesterol levels.

PATHOLOGY

A histopathological study of nine branch vein occlusions showed a fresh or recanalized thrombus at the site of the vein occlusion in all eyes.[31] Ischemic atrophy of the retina was found in the distribution of the occlusion in most of the eyes. All eyes showed varied degrees of arteriosclerosis. No thrombus was noted in any of the arteries. Neovascularization of the disc and retina was noted in four eyes and cystoid macular edema was present in five.

TREATMENT

The Branch Vein Occlusion Study represented a major advance in the understanding of the treatments for two of the most significant complications of branch vein occlusions, namely macular edema and neovascularization.[27,32,33] The study found that a grid pattern laser treatment helped to reduce macular edema and improved visual acuity. In patients who have 20/40 (6/12) or worse vision and macular edema on fluorescein angiography,

laser treatment improved the chances of a two-or-more–line improvement in vision on the Snellen chart when compared with untreated controls[32,33] (65% versus 37%). Because visual acuity and macular edema may improve spontaneously, patients were not treated with laser for at least 3 months after the development of the vein obstruction, to allow for spontaneous improvement. Also, treatment was delayed if the intraretinal hemorrhage was too dense to allow either photocoagulation or adequate evaluation with fluorescein angiography. Patients who had hemorrhage directly in the fovea were excluded. A fluorescein angiogram less than 1 month old was used to guide treatment. A grid pattern of laser was applied to the area of capillary leakage (Fig. 115-7).

Photocoagulation did not extend closer than the edge of the foveal avascular zone, nor did it extend peripherally beyond the major vascular arcades. The eyes were reevaluated with fluorescein angiography 4 months after treatment, and additional photocoagulation was applied if the vision remained poor and macular edema persisted. Most patients required only one treatment. Typically, a 100μm spot size is used and medium-white burns, each of 0.1-second duration, are applied to the area of edema. In both treated and controlled groups, patients who had hypertension tended to respond less favorably to laser treatment.

The Branch Vein Occlusion Study Group also evaluated the efficacy and timing of sectorial PRP for retinal neovascularization and vitreous hemorrhage.[32] In patients with neovascularization treated with laser, only 29% developed vitreous hemorrhage, versus 61% of those untreated. The data showed no advantage with treatment before neovascularization occurred, even if extensive capillary nonperfusion existed. If laser is applied to all nonperfused branch retinal vein obstructions, a large percentage of patients will be treated unnecessarily (Boxes 115-5 and 115-6). Fluorescein angiography can be helpful in guiding laser treatment, because it will help define areas of capillary nonperfusion. A scatter pattern of laser is performed in the affected sector. Typically, 500μm–sized medium-white burns are applied, extending from the arcade out to the periphery. Fill-in PRP may be applied if neovascularization progresses or if vitreous hemor-

---

> **BOX 115-4**
>
> **Differential Diagnosis of Branch Retinal Vein Obstruction**
>
> Hypertensive retinopathy
> Diabetic retinopathy
> Ocular ischemic syndrome
> Juxtafoveal retinal telangiectasia
> Combined branch retinal artery and branch retinal vein occlusion
> Radiation retinopathy

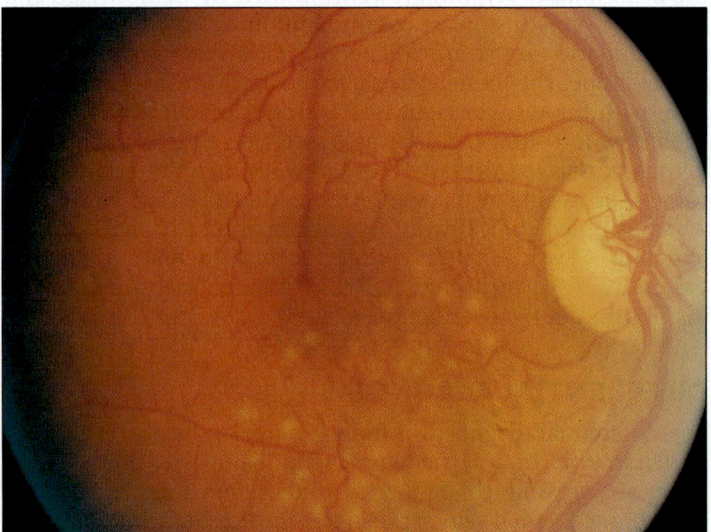

FIG. 115-7 ▪ Branch retinal vein obstruction. Immediate posttreatment view of grid laser treatment for macular edema secondary to a branch retinal vein obstruction.

> **BOX 115-5**
>
> **Treatment Guidelines for Branch Retinal Vein Occlusion and Macular Edema**
>
> **FOR MACULAR EDEMA, VISUAL ACUITY OF 20/40 (6/12) OR WORSE**
> Wait for clearance of retinal hemorrhage to allow adequate fluorescein angiography
> Determine if decreased visual acuity is caused by macular edema (versus macular nonperfusion)
> If macular edema explains visual loss, and no spontaneous improvement has occurred by 3 months, grid macular photocoagulation is recommended
> If capillary nonperfusion explains decreased visual acuity, laser treatment is not advised

> **BOX 115-6**
>
> **Treatment Guidelines for Branch Retinal Vein Occlusion and Neovascularization**
>
> Good quality fluorescein angiography is obtained after retinal hemorrhages have cleared sufficiently.
> If more than five disc diameters of nonperfusion are present, the patient should be followed at 4-month intervals to seek the development of neovascularization.
> If neovascularization develops, panretinal photocoagulation to the involved retinal sector should be applied using argon laser to achieve "medium" white burns, 200–500mm in diameter—one burn width apart to cover the entire involved segment.

rhage occurs. Vitreous surgery is employed occasionally for non-clearing vitreous hemorrhages, epiretinal membrane, or tractional retinal detachment with macular involvement. The outcomes are generally favorable, although preexisting pathology frequently limits recovery of good vision.[34]

COURSE AND OUTCOME

Without treatment, one third of patients who have branch retinal vein occlusion end up with visual acuity better than 20/40 (6/12). However, two thirds have decreased visual acuity secondary to macular edema, macular ischemia, macular hemorrhage, or vitreous hemorrhage. As noted above, laser treatment for macular edema significantly enhances the chance that the patient's baseline visual acuity will improve by two lines (65% versus 37%). The mean number of lines of improvement in visual acuity averages 1.33 in treated patients versus 0.23 in the control group. Poor visual prognostic factors include advancing age, male sex, worse baseline visual acuity, and an increased number of risk factors.[35] Good prognosis is associated with a younger age, female sex, and fewer risk factors. Patients should be followed up every 3–4 months.

Approximately 20% of patients with branch retinal vein occlusion will develop neovascularization. Of these patients, about 60% will have episodic vitreous hemorrhages. Fortunately, laser treatment (sector PRP) can reduce this by one half to 30%.

NEW TREATMENTS FOR BRANCH RETINAL VEIN OCCLUSION

New treatments for branch retinal vein occlusion that are being evaluated include sheathotomy[36–38] and intravitreal steroid injection G triamcinolone for treatment of cystoid macular edema resulting from branch retinal vein occlusion.

REFERENCES

1. Hayreh SS, Zimmerman MB, Podhajsky P. Incidence of various types of retinal vein occlusion and their recurrence and demographic characteristics. Am J Ophthalmol. 1994;117:429–41.
2. The Eye Disease Case-Control Study Group. Risk factors for branch retinal vein occlusion. Am J Ophthalmol. 1993;116:286–96.
3. Zegarra H, Gutman FA, Conforto J. The natural course of central retinal vein occlusion. Ophthalmology. 1979;86:1931–8.
4. Rath EZ, Frank RN, Shin DH, Kim C. Risk factors for retinal vein occlusions. A case-control study. Ophthalmology. 1992;99:509–14.
5. Hayreh SS, Zimmerman B, McCarthy MJ, Podhajsky P. Systemic diseases associated with various types of retinal vein occlusion. Am J Ophthalmol. 2001;131:61–77.
6. Quinlan PM, Elman MJ, Bhatt AK, et al. The natural course of central retinal vein occlusion. Am J Ophthalmol. 1990;110:118–23.
7. Dhote R, Bachmeyer C, Orellou MH, et al. Central retinal vein thrombosis associated with resistance to activated protein C. Am J Ophthalmol. 1995;120:388–9.
8. Glacet-Bernard A, Chabanel A, Lelong F, et al. Elevated erythrocyte aggregation in patients with central retinal vein occlusion and without conventional risk factors. Ophthalmology. 1994;101:1483–7.
9. Vine, AK. Hyperhomocystinemia: a new risk factor for central retinal vein occlusion. Trans Am Ophthalmol Soc. 2000;98:453–503.
10. Hayreh SS. Retinal vein occlusion. Indian J Ophthalmol. 1994;42:109–32.
11. Hayreh SS. Classification of central retinal vein occlusion. Ophthalmology. 1983;90:458–74.
12. The Central Vein Occlusion Study Group. Natural history and clinical management of central retinal vein occlusion. Arch Ophthalmol. 1997;115:486–91.
13. Green WR, Chan CC, Hutchins GM, et al. Central retinal vein occlusion: a prospective histopathologic study of 29 eyes in 28 cases. Retina. 1981;1:27–55.
14. Fong ACO, Schatz H, McDonald HR, et al. Central retinal vein occlusion in young adults (papillophlebitis). Retina. 1991;11:3–11.
15. May DR, Klein ML, Peyman GA, et al. Xenon arc panretinal photocoagulation for central retinal vein occlusion: a randomized prospective study. Br J Ophthalmol. 1979;63:735–43.
16. Magargal LE, Brown GC, Augsburger JJ, et al. Neovascular glaucoma following central retinal vein obstruction. Ophthalmology. 1981;88:1095–101.
17. Sabates R, Hirose T, McMeel JW. Electroretinography in the prognosis and classification of central retinal vein occlusion. Arch Ophthalmol. 1983;101:232–5.
18. Barber C, Galloway NR, Reacher M, et al. The role of the electroretinogram in the management of central retinal vein occlusion. Doc Ophthalmol Proc Ser. 1984;40:149–59.
19. Central Vein Occlusion Study Group. Baseline and early natural history report: the Central Vein Occlusion Study. Arch Ophthalmol. 1993;11:1087–95.
20. Kearns TP. Differential diagnosis of central retinal vein obstruction. Ophthalmology. 1983;90:475–80.
21. Furlan AJ, Whisnant JP, Kearns TP. Unilateral visual loss in bright light; an unusual symptom of carotid artery occlusive disease. Arch Neurol. 1979;36:675–6.
22. Schwab PJ, Okun E, Fahey FL. Reversal of retinopathy in Waldenström's macroglobulinemia by plasmapheresis. Arch Ophthalmol. 1960;64:515–21.
23. Gutman FA. Evaluation of a patient with central retinal vein occlusion. Ophthalmology. 1983;90:481–3.
24. Stowe GC, Zakov ZN, Albert DM. Central retinal vascular occlusion associated with oral contraceptives. Am J Ophthalmol. 1978;86:798–801.
25. The Central Vein Occlusion Study Group. A randomized clinical trial of early panretinal photocoagulation for ischemic central vein occlusion: the Central Vein Occlusion Study Group N Report. Ophthalmology. 1995;102:1434–44.
26. The Central Vein Occlusion Study Group. Evaluation of grid pattern photocoagulation for macular edema in central vein occlusion: the Central Vein Occlusion Study Group M Report. Ophthalmology. 1995;102:1425–33.
27. McAllister IL, Constable IJ. Laser-induced chorioretinal venous anastomosis for treatment of non-ischemic central retinal vein occlusion. Arch Ophthalmol. 1995;113:456–62.
28. Mitchell P, Smith W, Chang A. Prevalence and associations of retinal vein occlusion in Australia. Arch Ophthalmol. 1996;114:1243–7.
29. Hayreh SS, Zimmerman MMB, Podhajsky P. Incidence of various types of retinal vein occlusion and their recurrence in demographic characteristics. Am J Ophthalmol. 1994;117:429–41.
30. Duker JS, Brown GL. Anterior location of the crossing artery in branch retinal vein occlusion. Arch Ophthalmol. 1989;107:998–1000.
31. Frangieh GT, Green WR, Barraquer-Somers E, Finkelstein D. Histopathologic study of nine branch retinal vein occlusions. Arch Ophthalmol. 1982;100:1132–40.
32. Branch Vein Occlusion Study Group. Argon laser scatter photocoagulation for prevention of neovascularization and vitreous hemorrhage in branch vein occlusion. Arch Ophthalmol. 1986;104:34–41.
33. Finkelstein D. Argon laser photocoagulation for macular edema in branch vein occlusion. Ophthalmology. 1986;93:975–7.
34. Amirikia A, Sioh IV, Murray TG, et al. Outcomes of vitreoretinal surgery for complications of branch retinal vein occlusion. Ophthalmology. 2001;108:372–6.
35. Glacet-Bernard A, Coscas G, Chabanel A, et al. Prognostic factors for retinal vein occlusion. A prospective study of 175 cases. Ophthalmology. 1996;103:551–60.
36. Opremcak EM, Bruce RA. Surgical decompression of branch retinal vein occlusions via arteriovenous crossing sheathotomy: a prospective review of 15 cases. Retina. 1999;19:1–5.
37. Ostelah MD, Charles S. Surgical decompression of branch retinal vein occlusions. Arch Ophthalmol. 1998;106:1469–71.
38. Shah GK, Sharma S, Fineman MS, et al. Arteriovenous adventitial sheathotomy for the treatment of macular edema associated with branch retinal vein occlusion. Am J Ophthalmol. 2000;129:104–6.

CHAPTER

116 Retinopathy of Prematurity

FRANCO M. RECCHIA • ANTONIO CAPONE

DEFINITION

- A disorder of premature, low-birth-weight infants featuring abnormal proliferation of developing retinal blood vessels at the junction of vascularized and avascular retina.

KEY FEATURES

- Avascular, peripheral retina.
- A demarcation line lying within the plane of the retina between the vascular and avascular retina.
- Progression of the demarcation line into an elevated ridge or mesenchymal shunt.
- Extraretinal proliferation of blood vessels above the ridge, into the vitreous, with fibrous membrane development.
- Significant shunting of blood through the proliferative ridge (plus disease) with venous dilation adjacent to the optic nerve.

ASSOCIATED FEATURES

- Low birth weight.
- Low gestational age.
- Myopia.
- Macular dragging.
- Traction retinal detachment.
- Retinal fold.
- Retrolental fibroplasia.
- Glaucoma.

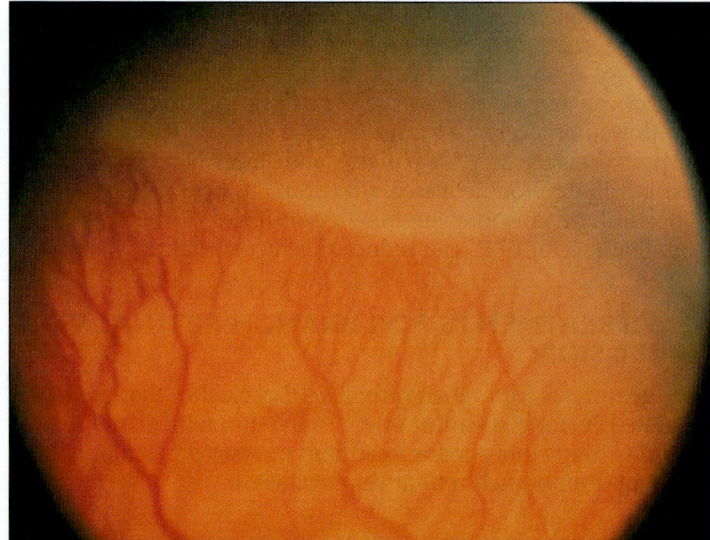

FIG. 116-1 ▍ **Stage I retinopathy of prematurity.** The flat, white border between avascular and vascular retina seen superiorly is called a demarcation line. (Reproduced with permission of Earl A. Palmer, MD and the Multicenter Trial of Cryotherapy for Retinopathy of Prematurity.)

INTRODUCTION

First described in 1942,[1] retinopathy of prematurity (ROP) is a proliferative retinopathy affecting premature infants of low birth weight and young gestational age. Despite improvements in detection and treatment, ROP remains a leading cause of lifelong visual impairment among premature children in developed countries. Basic research into the pathogenesis of ROP continues to provide a greater understanding of retinal development, angiogenesis, and intraocular neovascularization.

CLINCAL FEATURES AND CLASSIFICATION

During normal retinal development, vessels migrate from the optic disc to the ora serrata beginning at about 16 weeks of gestation.[2] Vasculogenesis transforms precursor mesenchymal spindle cells into capillary networks. Mature vessels differentiate from these networks and extend to the nasal ora serrata by 36 weeks of gestation and to the temporal ora serrata by 39–41 weeks. The fundamental process underlying the development of ROP is incomplete vascularization of the retina, and the ophthalmoscopic findings stem from this arrested development. The location of the interruption of normal vasculogenesis is related to the time of premature birth.

The International Classification of Retinopathy of Prematurity (ICROP) was established in 1984, and revised in 1987, to provide standards for the clinical assessment of ROP on the basis of the severity (stage) and anatomical location (zone) of disease.[3,4] According to this classification, the first sign of ROP (stage I) is the appearance of a thin, flat, white structure (termed a demarcation line) at the junction of vascularized retina posteriorly and avascular retina anteriorly (Fig. 116-1). Stage II ROP occurs as the demarcation line develops into a pink or white elevation (ridge) of thickened tissue (Fig. 116-2); small tufts of vessels may be seen posterior to the ridge. Vessel growth into and above the ridge (extraretinal fibrovascular proliferation) characterizes stage III ROP (Figs. 116-3 and 116-4). This fibrovascular proliferation may extend into the overlying vitreous and cause vitreous hemorrhage. With progressive growth into the vitreous, contraction of fibrovascular proliferation exerts traction on the retina, leading to partial retinal detachment (stage IV ROP), either without foveal involvement (stage IVa) or with foveal involvement (stage IVb) (Fig. 116-5). Stage V ROP denotes a total retinal detachment (Fig. 116-6). Because stage V detachments are always funnel shaped, the configuration of such detachments can be further described as open or closed anteriorly and open or closed posteriorly. Leukokoria resulting from fibrovascular proliferation and advanced retinal detachment is termed retrolental fibroplasia.

During the acute phases of ROP, progressive vascular insufficiency at the edge of the abnormally developing vasculature may

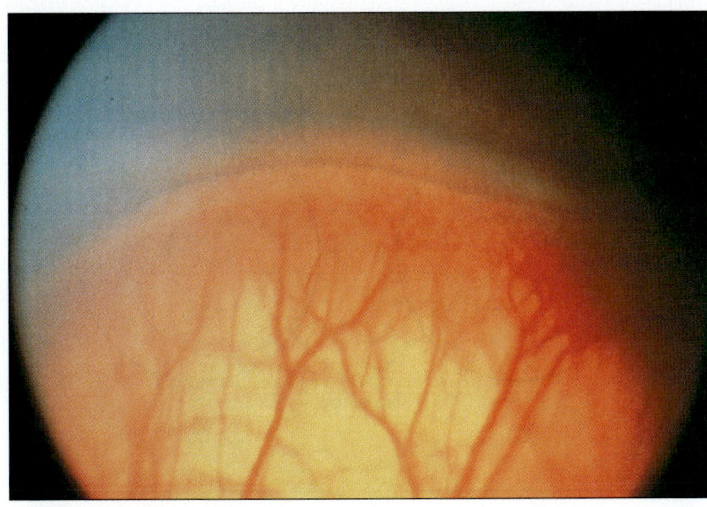

FIG. 116-2 ■ **Stage II retinopathy of prematurity.** The elevated mesenchymal ridge has height. Highly arborized blood vessels from the vascularized retina dive into the ridge. (Reproduced with permission of Earl A. Palmer, MD and the Multicenter Trial of Cryotherapy for Retinopathy of Prematurity.)

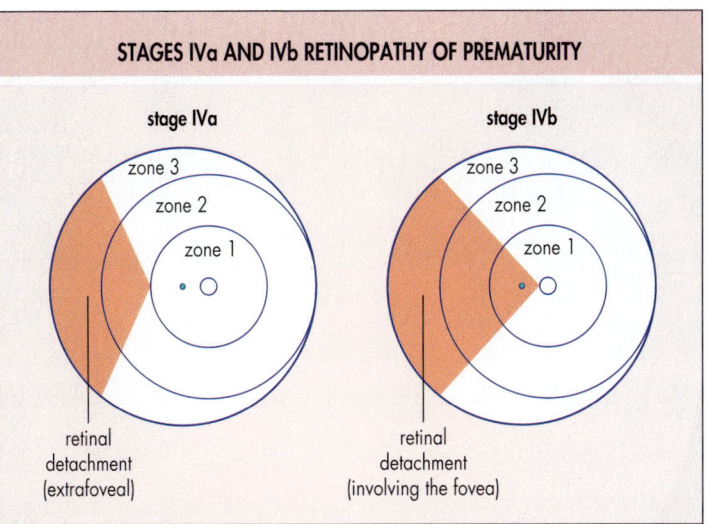

FIG. 116-5 ■ **Stage IV. A,** Stage IVa detachment spares the fovea. **B,** Stage IVb detachment involves the fovea.

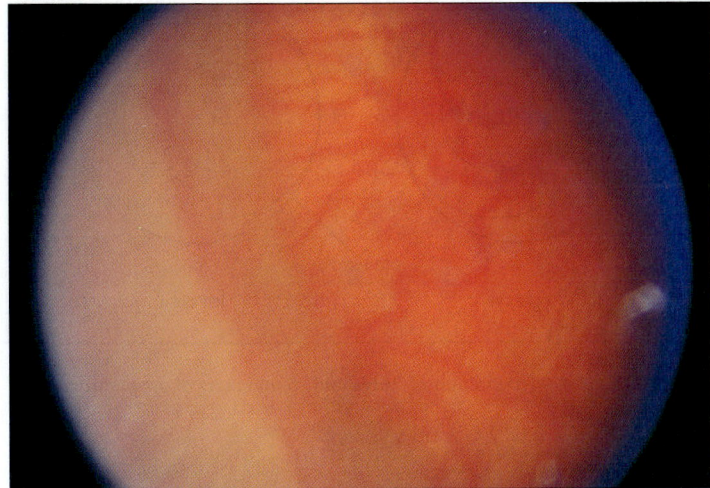

FIG. 116-3 ■ **Stage III retinopathy of prematurity.** Vessels on top of the ridge project into the vitreous cavity. This extraretinal proliferation carries with it a fibrovascular membrane. Note the opalescent avascular retina anterior to the ridge.

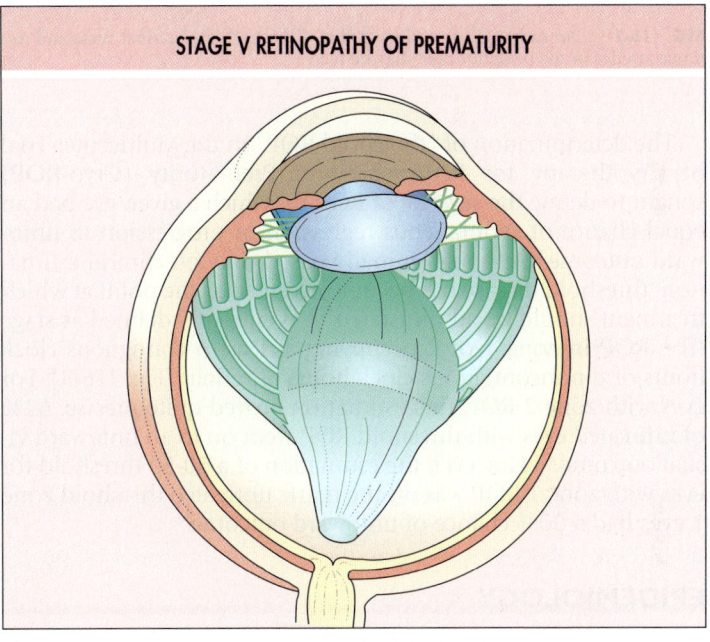

FIG. 116-6 ■ **Stage V retinal detachment.** Depiction of an open anterior configuration secondary to fibrovascular proliferation that pulls the peripheral retina anteriorly.

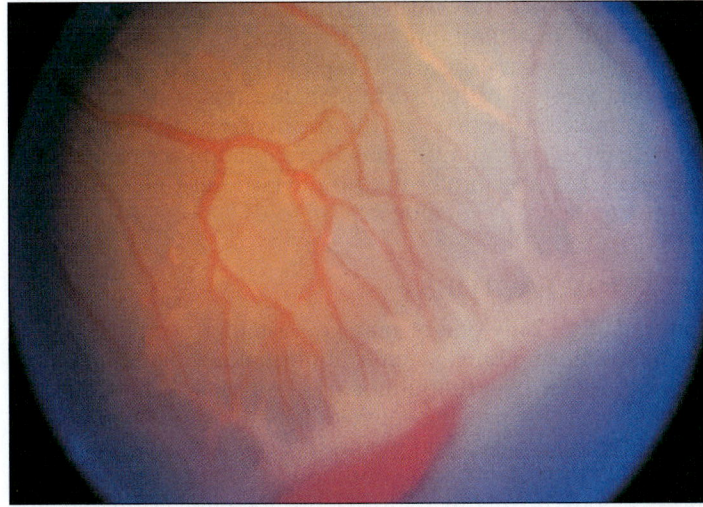

FIG. 116-4 ■ **Stage III retinopathy of prematurity.** Note finger-like projections of extraretinal vessels into the vitreous cavity. Hemorrhage on the ridge is not uncommon.

lead to increasing dilation and tortuosity of peripheral retinal vessels, engorgement of iris vessels, pupillary rigidity, and vitreous haze. These findings were defined by the ICROP as progressive vascular disease.[4] "Plus disease" occurs when the peripheral vascular shunting of blood is so overwhelming that it leads to marked venous dilation and arterial tortuosity in the posterior pole (Fig. 116-7). Plus disease is the hallmark of rapidly progressive ROP and is notated by adding a plus sign after the number of the ROP stage.

ROP is also classified by anatomical location, by identifying the anterior extent of retinal vascularization (Fig. 116-8). Because there is a direct correlation between severity of disease and amount of avascular retina, the location of the border between vascularized and avascular retina is an important prognostic sign. Zone 1 is defined as a circle, the center of which is the disc and the radius of which is twice the distance of the disc to the fovea. Zone 2 is a doughnut-shaped region that extends from the anterior border of zone 1 to within one disc diameter of the ora serrata nasally and to the anatomical equator temporally. Zone 3 encompasses the residual temporal retina. Appropriate description of an eye with ROP includes both a stage and the posteriormost zone containing disease.

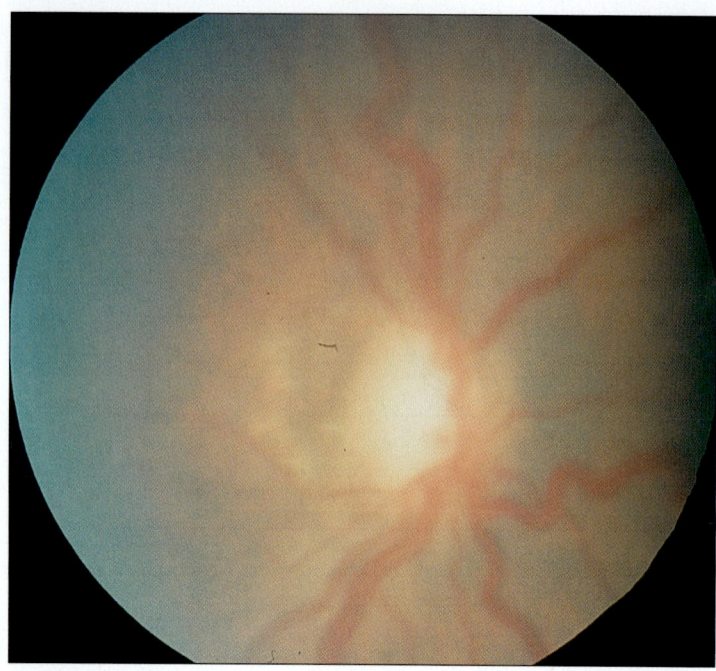

FIG. 116-7 ■ **An example of moderate plus disease.** Dilated retinal veins and tortuous arteries in the posterior pole may be seen.

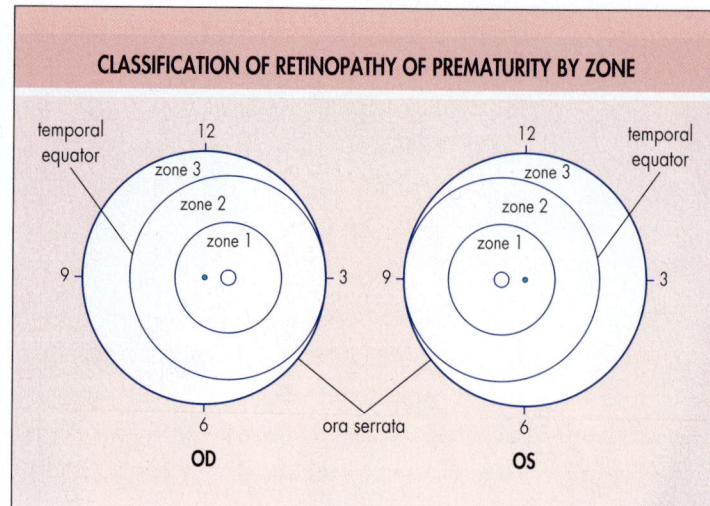

FIG. 116-8 ■ **Classification of retinopathy of prematurity by zone.** The temporal edge of zone 2 coincides with the equator.

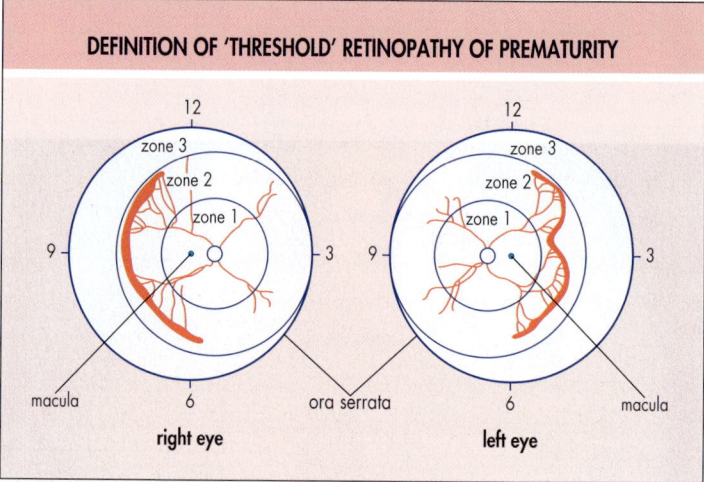

FIG. 116-9 ■ Definition of "threshold" retinopathy of prematurity.

The determination of "threshold ROP" in the Multicenter Trial of Cryotherapy for Retinopathy of Prematurity (Cryo-ROP) sought to define the severity of ROP for which a given eye had an equal chance of spontaneous regression or progression to untoward outcome.[5] Although initially based only on clinical estimation, threshold disease has become accepted as the point at which treatment should be administered. It is currently defined as stage III+ ROP in zone 1 or 2 occupying at least 5 contiguous clock hours or 8 noncontiguous clock hours of retina[5] (Fig. 116-9). For eyes with zone 2 ROP, this estimation proved quite precise: 62% of untreated eyes with threshold ROP went on to an untoward visual outcome.[6,7] However, the estimation of a 50-50 threshold for eyes with zone 1 ROP was off the mark: untreated threshold zone 1 eyes had a 90% chance of untoward outcome.[6]

EPIDEMIOLOGY

Valuable information regarding the incidence, clinical course, and natural history of ROP was gleaned from the CRYO-ROP trial.[8] This prospective trial, initiated in 1986, included 4009 infants weighing less than 1251g (2lb, 13oz). These infants received an initial examination by an experienced examiner at 4 to 7 weeks after birth and at defined intervals thereafter. Overall, 65.8% of infants developed some degree of ROP and 6% reached threshold. Gender was not associated with progression to threshold disease, and African-American infants appeared less susceptible to progression (3.2% versus 7.8%). Multiple births and birth outside a study hospital were associated with an increased risk of severe disease.[8,9]

The incidence and severity of disease were closely correlated with lower birth weights and earlier gestational (postconceptional) age. Whereas the incidence of ROP was 47% in infants with birth weights between 1000 and 1251g (2lb, 3oz to 2lb, 13oz), it rose to 81.6% for infants weighing less than 1000g (2lb, 3oz) at birth. Over 80% of infants born at less than 28 weeks' gestational age developed ROP, but only 60% of infants born at 28–31 weeks developed ROP.[8] Similar findings were reported in a more recent study involving 2528 infants: no infant born after 32 weeks of gestation developed ROP, and stage III disease was not seen in infants with birth weights greater than 1500g (3lb, 5oz).[10] The CRYO-ROP investigators stressed that the timing of pathological vascular events correlated more closely with postconceptional age than chronological age, independent of birth

weight. The median onset of stage I ROP was 34 weeks after conception. The median onset of threshold disease was 37 weeks, with a range of 33.6 to 42 weeks, after conception.[8]

It has been estimated that ROP causes visual loss in 1300 children and severe visual impairment in 500 children born each year in the United States.[11] As technological advances have made possible increased survival for extremely premature infants, it seems likely that the number of infants with ROP will rise.[12] Several studies have suggested, however, that although there is increased survival of high-risk neonates, this is not associated with a universal increase in the incidence of ROP.[10,13–15] This trend may reflect improvements in ventilation techniques and perinatal care, specifically the prophylactic use of surfactant[15] and the maternal use of antenatal steroids.[16]

SYSTEMIC FACTORS

Retinopathy is only one of many devastating complications of premature birth. Other systemic abnormalities that afflict these infants include bronchopulmonary dysplasia, anemia, cardiac defects, sepsis, necrotizing enterocolitis, intraventricular hemorrhage, cerebral palsy, and neurodevelopmental delay.[17–19] As with ROP, these associated conditions are more prevalent and more serious in infants of lower birth weight. Moreover, the severity of neonatal ROP is a marker for functional disability later in life.[19]

A relationship between oxygen levels and ROP has been suspected for half a century.[1] In recent years, results of experiments with animal models and epidemiological studies have brought the complexity and paradox of this relationship to light. In 1948, Michaelson[20] proposed that a progressive oxygen deficit within the retina during normal differentiation can induce angiogenesis in neighboring vessels through secretion of a chemical messenger (so-called factor X). In the 1950s, therapeutic administration of supplemental oxygen to premature infants, in an effort to relieve the putative stimulus for retinal neovascularization, thus seemed rational. This practice was abandoned after the Cooperative Study of Retrolental Fibroplasia disclosed a threefold risk of ROP in neonates without lung disease who had been given prolonged oxygen supplementation.[21] However, the concept of a hypoxic stimulus for neovascularization remained biologically plausible, and the issue of supplementary oxygen regained attention. This renewed interest was based in part on several case-control studies in which infants who developed severe ROP had hospital courses complicated by lower arterial oxygenation and greater fluctuation in blood oxygen levels.[22,23]

The Supplemental Therapeutic Oxygen for Prethreshold ROP (STOP-ROP) was a multicenter clinical trial begun in 1994 to determine the efficacy and safety of supplemental oxygen administered to premature infants to reduce the progression to threshold ROP.[24] Six hundred forty-nine premature infants with prethreshold ROP in at least one eye were randomly assigned to a "conventional" arm (with pulse oximetry targeted at 89–94% oxygen saturation) or to a "supplemental" arm (96–99% oxygen saturation). The progression to threshold ROP was lower in the supplemental arm (41% versus 48%) but not to a statistically significant degree. Subgroup analysis did show, however, that infants without plus disease and without severe lung disease may benefit from supplemental oxygen (32% progression in the supplemental arm versus 46% progression in the conventional arm).[24]

Several authors have suggested that candidemia may be independently associated with severe ROP in babies weighing less than 1000g (2lb, 3oz).[25,26] A large cohort study of 449 infants, however, failed to show a strong correlation and suggested instead that much of the observed association of these two clinical conditions is linked more to young postconceptional age.[27]

Hospital nursery lighting is an additional variable that has been suspected to contribute to ROP. In the Light Reduction in Retinopathy of Prematurity (LIGHT-ROP) study, involving 361 infants weighing less than 1251g, a reduction in exposure to ambient light did not alter the incidence of ROP.[28]

Genetic factors may play a role in the development of severe ROP in a subset of premature infants. Prompted by the observation that some clinical features of ROP noted in near-term and full-term infants may resemble those seen in familial exudative vitreoretinopathy (FEVR), the X-linked form of which is associated with mutations in the Norrie disease (ND) gene,[29] Shastry et al.[30] investigated a cohort of 16 premature infants with ROP for mutations in the ND gene. Missense mutations were found in four, all of whom had advanced disease, and in none of the parents or 50 healthy control subjects.[30] A larger scale study demonstrated the presence of ND mutations in 2% of infants with ROP.[31]

PATHOLOGY AND PATHOPHYSIOLOGY

Histologically, stage I ROP is characterized by hyperplasia of the primitive spindle-shaped cells of the vanguard mesenchymal tissue at the demarcation line.[32] The ridge of stage II consists of further hyperplasia of the spindle cells, along with proliferation of the endothelial cells of the rearguard mesenchymal tissue. In stage III, extraretinal vascular tissue emanates from the ridge. Proliferation of endothelial cells and small, thin-walled vessels occurs. Equally important is the condensation of vitreous into sheets and strands oriented anteriorly toward the equator of the lens. Vitreous tractional forces draw the retina anteriorly and may lead to retinal detachment.

Hypoxia is a common precursor to the abnormal neovascularization seen in many retinal diseases. Michaelson's hypothesis of an angiogenic chemical messenger secreted in response to tissue hypoxia has led to the identification of numerous angiogenic factors, among them basic fibroblast growth factor (bFGF),[33] transforming growth factor–α (TGF-α),[34] and tumor necrosis factor–α (TNF-α).[35] Increasing attention, however, has been focused on vascular endothelial growth factor (VEGF), formerly called vascular permeability factor (VPF).[36] Vitreous levels of VEGF are elevated in patients with a variety of proliferative retinopathies, including ROP, and vitreous fluid from these patients stimulates growth of endothelial cells in vitro.[37]

DIAGNOSIS

Ophthalmoscopic evaluation of the premature infant may be performed in the nursery or in the office. Two drops each of 2.5% phenylephrine and 0.5% tropicamide are applied, and a lid speculum is inserted between the lids. Examination of the anterior segment is performed with a hand light, with specific attention to the iris vessels, lens, and tunica vasculosa lentis. Funduscopy is performed with an indirect ophthalmoscope and a 28D or 30D condensing lens. The posterior pole is examined without depression for the presence of absence of plus disease. Scleral depression is then used to examine the temporal retina, followed by the nasal retina, to establish the proximity of retinal vessels to the ora serrata. Scleral depression is appropriate in all cases.

Given the progressive nature of ROP as well as the proven benefits of early diagnosis and timely intervention to minimize the risk of severe visual loss, a joint statement outlining the principles of a screening program for ROP has been set forth[38]:

1. Screening for ROP should be performed in all infants with a birth weight less than 1500g (3lb, 4oz) or a gestational age of 28 weeks or less, as well as in infants weighing between 1500 and 2000g (4lb, 6 oz) with an unstable clinical course and who are believed to be at high risk.
2. In most cases, at least two examinations should be performed. One examination may suffice if it shows unequivocally that retinal vascularization is complete bilaterally. The first examination should be performed between 4 and 6 weeks of chronological (postnatal) age or between the 31st and 33rd weeks of postconceptional age (calculated as gestational age plus chronological age), whichever is later.
3. Infants at high risk for progression to threshold disease should be examined weekly. Included are infants with any zone 1 disease, stage II+ or stage III disease in zone 2, or stage III+ disease occupying fewer clock hours than defined as threshold.
4. Infants with less severe disease in zone 2 or disease restricted to zone 3 should be examined every 2 weeks until the fundus matures.
5. Infants with threshold ROP should receive peripheral ablative therapy within 72 hours of diagnosis.

DIFFERENTIAL DIAGNOSIS

The differential diagnosis of ROP is given in Box 116-1. In a premature infant of low birth weight with characteristic findings of immature retinal development, the diagnosis is often straightforward. On the other hand, if a premature infant has not been screened or treated appropriately, a white retrolental fibrous mass may develop, and the only presenting sign may be leukokoria. In such cases, the treating ophthalmologist must first suspect and evaluate for retinoblastoma, which often displays calcification on ultrasonography or computed tomography. Other causes of leukokoria in an infant include exudative retinal detachment, most commonly from Coats' disease (usually unilateral and more common in boys) or diffuse choroidal hemangioma; persistent fetal vasculature syndrome, formerly called persistence of primary hyperplastic vitreous[34] (usually uni-

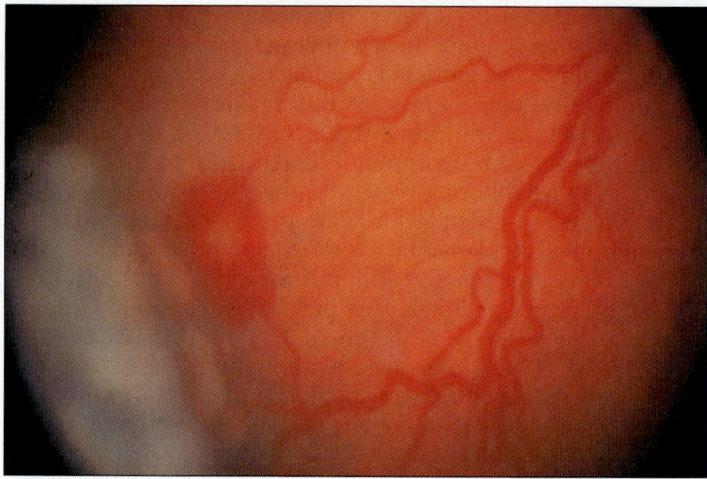

FIG. 116-10 ■ **Threshold retinopathy of prematurity.** Immediate postoperative appearance of indirect laser photocoagulation.

lateral and associated with microphthalmia and prominent ciliary processes); infectious causes such as endogenous endophthalmitis, toxocariasis, or toxoplasmosis (all of which may be diagnosed by appropriate microbiological and immunological testing); coloboma of the optic disc or choroid; cataract; and genetic syndromes, such as trisomy 13, Norrie disease, Warburg syndrome, and incontinentia pigmenti (all of which may be diagnosed by genetic testing and/or characteristic systemic physical findings). Finally, congenital retinoschisis and FEVR may be suggested by family history or examination of relatives.

TREATMENT

The ultimate goals of treatment of threshold ROP are prevention of any retinal detachment or scarring and optimization of visual outcome. Treatment involves ablation of avascular retina by either cryotherapy or laser photocoagulation.

The laser has become the instrument of choice of ophthalmologists throughout the world and has long been the standard of treatment in the management of other vasoproliferative retinopathies associated with diabetes, sickle cell disease, and retinal vascular occlusion. Few indications remain for utilizing cryopexy over the laser in the management of ROP: poor fundus visibility, lack of availability of a laser, and a treating physician's unfamiliarity with indirect laser retinopexy techniques.

Cryotherapy

Cryotherapy has been used to treat ROP since 1972.[39] It may be performed under topical, local, or general anesthesia, either transconjunctivally or transsclerally following a conjunctival peritomy (as is necessary for posterior disease). The probe should be removed periodically for several minutes to avoid prolonged ocular hypertension. A favorable response usually occurs within 1 week.

The Cryo-ROP trial was a multicenter clinical trial in which eyes of premature infants (birth weight less than 1251g) with threshold ROP were randomly assigned to either cryotherapy or observation to establish whether treatment reduced the occurrence of an unfavorable visual outcome (20/200 or worse) or unfavorable structural outcome (retinal fold, retinal detachment, or retrolental fibroplasia).[5,6] At 10-year follow-up, eyes treated with cryotherapy were less likely to be legally blind (44% versus 62%), and were less likely to have an unfavorable structural outcome. Total retinal detachment still occurred in 22% of treated eyes, however.[40] Cryotherapy did not appear to cause a significant detriment to visual field or contrast sensitivity.[41,42]

Laser Photocoagulation

Since the inception of the Cryo-ROP study, argon laser and diode laser indirect ophthalmoscope systems have been developed. Advantages of photocoagulation include ease of treatment, portability, and fewer systemic complications. Photocoagulation is delivered through a dilated pupil with a 20D or 28D condensing lens. The end point is near-confluent ablation, with burns spaced one-half burn width apart, from the ora serrata up to, but not including, the ridge for 360°.[43] The retina should be inspected for skip areas, and the infant should be reexamined within 1 week. Persistent plus disease and fibrovascular prolifer-

ation are indications for additional treatment. Complications of laser treatment include anterior segment ischemia, cataract, and burns of the cornea, iris, or tunica vasculosa lentis.[44,45]

Laser photocoagulation has been shown to be at least as effective as[46-48] if not more effective than[49,50] cryotherapy for threshold disease. In one series of 61 eyes treated exclusively with a diode laser, only 3 eyes (5%) progressed to stage IV disease.[51] In another series of 120 eyes observed for at least 12 months, 91% had favorable structural outcomes (Fig. 116-10).[49] In the largest, prospective, randomized comparison of laser photocoagulation with cryotherapy (25 infants observed for at least 4 years), eyes treated with cryotherapy were significantly more likely to have visual acuity of 20/50 or better and were significantly less myopic.[50] Laser photocoagulation is most effective for posterior (zone 1) disease: favorable anatomical results have been reported in 83–85% of eyes.[52,53] Cryotherapy, by contrast, provided favorable outcomes in only 25% of eyes with zone 1 disease.[54]

Surgery

Although retinal ablation is effective in a majority of cases of threshold ROP, a significant number of these eyes progress to retinal detachment. Detachment is most commonly tractional, originating at the ridge in a circumferential, purse-string pattern that draws the retina anteriorly and centrally (Fig. 116-11).

The advanced stages of ROP (stages IVa, IVb, and V) are poorly understood. Common misconceptions are that macula-sparing (stage IVa) partial retinal detachments are largely benign, that surgery should be deferred until the macula is detached, that scleral buckle is the preferred retinal reattachment procedure, and that useful vision cannot be obtained in eyes with total (stage V) detachments.

ROP-related detachments may appear stable in the first few weeks or months after peripheral retinal ablation. Yet neither the stability of partial detachment[6] nor visual acuity[55] is predictable from the retinal appearance in infants with ROP. This is particularly true for untreated eyes[6] or those with incomplete peripheral retinal ablation. Visual outcome of eyes with even partial ROP-related retinal detachment is generally poor by 4½ years of age: in the cohort of 61 eyes from the Cryo-ROP study with partial retinal detachment 3 months after threshold, only 6 eyes had vision of 20/200 or better at age 4½.[8,56]

The goal of intervention for ROP-related retinal detachments varies with the severity of the detachment. The goal for extramacular retinal detachment (stage IVa ROP) is an undistorted or minimally distorted posterior pole, total retinal reattachment, and preservation of the lens and central fixation vision. Scleral buckling[57,58] and vitrectomy[59] have been used to manage stage IVa ROP. Vitreous surgery can interrupt progression of ROP from

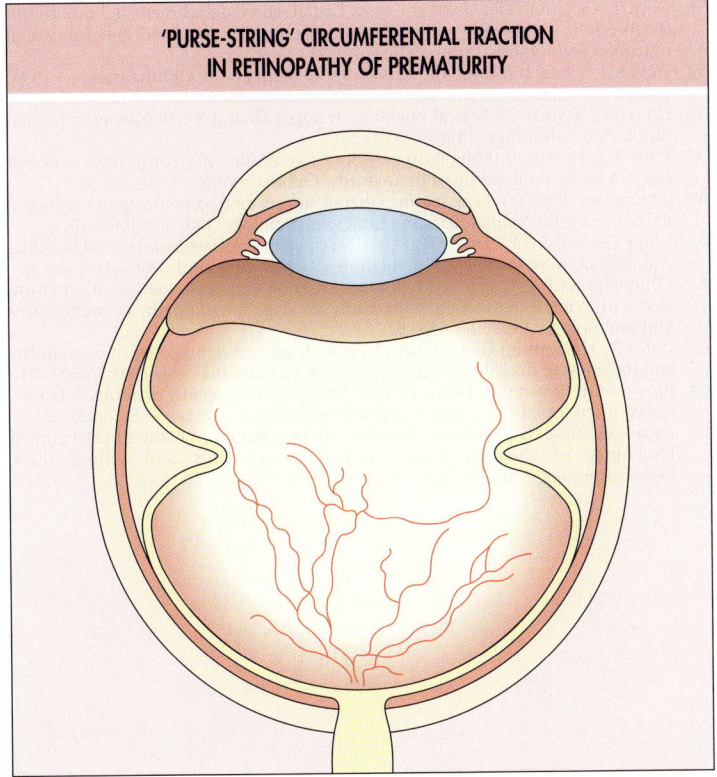

'PURSE-STRING' CIRCUMFERENTIAL TRACTION IN RETINOPATHY OF PREMATURITY

FIG. 116-11 ■ **"Purse-string" circumferential traction.** This causes retinal detachment in retinopathy of prematurity.

stage IVa to stage 4b or 5 by directly addressing transvitreal traction resulting from fibrous proliferation.[60] Disadvantages of scleral buckling for stage IVa ROP are the dramatic anisometropic myopia and the second intervention required for transection or removal so that the eye may continue to grow.[61]

Surgery for tractional retinal detachments involving the macula (stage IVb ROP) is performed to minimize retinal distortion and prevent total detachment (stage V). The functional goal is ambulatory vision. In earlier studies, visual outcome for retinal detachment beyond stage IVa was quite poor. More recent reports demonstrate that form-vision can be obtained by vitrectomy for stage V ROP.[59,62] Maximal recovery of vision following the insult of macula-off retinal detachment and interruption of visual development in infants may take years.

LONG-TERM COURSE

As infants afflicted with ROP have matured, the ophthalmic community has gained experience with "adult ROP." Early nuclear sclerotic cataract, glaucoma,[63] exudative retinopathy,[64] and rhegmatogenous retinal detachment[65] are but a few of the sequelae of ROP prompting the need for lifelong ophthalmic monitoring of formerly premature adults.

REFERENCES

1. Terry TL. Extreme prematurity and fibroblastic overgrowth of persistent vascular sheath behind each crystalline lens. I. Preliminary report. Am J Ophthalmol. 1942;25:203–4.
2. Ashton N. Retinal angiogenesis in the human embryo. Br Med Bull. 1970;26:103–6.
3. Committee for the Classification of Retinopathy of Prematurity. An international classification of retinopathy of prematurity. Arch Ophthalmol. 1984;106:471–9.
4. International Committee for the Classification of the Late Stages of Retinopathy of Prematurity. An international classification of retinopathy of prematurity. II. The classification of retinal detachment. Arch Ophthalmol. 1987;105:906–12.
5. Cryotherapy for Retinopathy of Prematurity Cooperative Group. Multicenter trial of cryotherapy for retinopathy of prematurity. Preliminary results. Arch Ophthalmol. 1988;106:471–9.
6. Cryotherapy for Retinopathy of Prematurity Cooperative Group. Multicenter trial of cryotherapy for retinopathy of prematurity: 3½-year outcome—structure and function. Arch Ophthalmol. 1993;111:339–44.
7. Cryotherapy for Retinopathy of Prematurity Cooperative Group. The natural ocular outcome of premature birth and retinopathy. Status at 1 year. Arch Ophthalmol. 1994;112:903–12.
8. Palmer EA, Flynn JT, Hardy RJ, et al. Incidence and early course of retinopathy of prematurity. Ophthalmology. 1991;98:1628–40.
9. Schaffer DB, Palmer EA, Plotsky DF, et al. Prognostic factors in the natural course of retinopathy of prematurity. Ophthalmology. 1993;100:230–7.
10. Hussain N, Clive J, Bhandari V. Current incidence of retinopathy of prematurity, 1989–97. Pediatrics. 1999;104(3):e26.
11. Phelps DL. Retinopathy of prematurity: an estimate of vision loss in the United States—1979. Pediatrics. 1981;67:924–6.
12. Hack M, Fanaroff AA. Outcomes of extremely-low-birth-weight infants between 1982 and 1988. N Engl J Med. 1989;321:1642–7.
13. Vyas J, Field D, Draper ES, et al. Severe retinopathy of prematurity and its association with different rates of survival in infants less than 1251g birth weight. Arch Dis Child Fetal Neonatal Ed. 2000;82:F145–9.
14. Rowlands E, Ionides ACW, Chinn S, et al. Reduced incidence of retinopathy of prematurity. Br J Ophthalmol. 2001;85:933–5.
15. Pennefather PM, Tin W, Clarke MP, et al. Retinopathy of prematurity in a controlled trial of prophylactic surfactant treatment. Br J Ophthalmol. 1996;80:420–4.
16. Bullard SR, Donahue SP, Feman SS, et al. The decreasing incidence and severity of retinopathy of prematurity. J AAPOS. 1999;3:46–52.
17. Wood NS, Marlow N, Costeloe K, et al. Neurologic and developmental disability after extremely preterm birth. EPICure Study Group. N Engl J Med. 2000;343:378–84.
18. O'Keefe M, Kafil-Hussain N, Flitcroft I, Lanigan B. Ocular significance of intraventricular hemorrhage in premature infants. Br J Ophthalmol. 2001;85:357–9.
19. Msall ME, Phelps DL, DiGaudio KM, et al. Severity of neonatal retinopathy of prematurity is predictive of neurodevelopmental functional outcome at age 5.5 years. Pediatrics. 2000;106:998–1005.
20. Michaelson IC. The mode of development of the vascular system of the retina: with some observations on its significance for certain retinal diseases. Trans Ophthalmol Soc UK. 1948;68:137–80.
21. Kinsey VE, Jacobus JT, Hemphill F. Retrolental fibroplasias: cooperative study of retrolental fibroplasia and the use of oxygen. Arch Ophthalmol. 1956;56:481–547.
22. Kinsey VE, Arnold HJ, Kalina RE, et al. PaO₂ levels and retrolental fibroplasia: a report of the cooperative study. Pediatrics. 1977;60:655–68.
23. Katzman G, Satish M, Krishnan V. Hypoxemia and retinopathy of prematurity. Pediatrics. 1987;80:972.
24. The STOP-ROP Multicenter Study Group. Supplemental therapeutic oxygen for prethreshold retinopathy of prematurity (STOP-ROP), a randomized, controlled trial. I: Primary outcomes. Pediatrics. 2000;105:295–310.
25. Mittal M, Dhanireddy R, Higgins R. Candida sepsis and association with retinopathy of prematurity. Pediatrics. 1998;101:654–7.
26. Noyola DE, Bohra L, Paysse EA, et al. Associations of candidemia and retinopathy of prematurity in very low birthweight infants. Ophthalmology. 2002;109:80–4.
27. Karlowicz MG, Giannone PJ, Pestian J, et al. Does candidemia predict threshold retinopathy of prematurity in extremely low birth weight (1000g) neonates? Pediatrics. 2000;105:1036–40.
28. Reynolds JD, Hardy RJ, Kennedy KA, et al. Lack of efficacy of light reduction in preventing retinopathy of prematurity. Light reduction in retinopathy of prematurity (LIGHT-ROP) study group. N Engl J Med. 1998;338:1572–6.
29. Chen ZY, Battinelli EM, Fielder A, et al. A mutation in the Norrie disease gene (NDP) associated with X-linked familial exudative vitreoretinopathy. Nat Genet. 1993;5:180–3.
30. Shastry BS, Pendergast SD, Hartzer MK, et al. Identification of missense mutations in the Norrie disease gene associated with advanced retinopathy of prematurity. Arch Ophthalmol. 1997;115:651–5.
31. Hiraoka M, Berinstein DM, Trese MT, Shastry BS. Insertion and deletion mutations in the dinucleotide repeat region of the Norrie disease gene in patients with advanced retinopathy of prematurity. J Hum Genet. 2001;46:178–81.
32. Foos RY. Pathologic features of clinical stages of retinopathy of prematurity. In: Flynn JT, Tasman WS, eds. Retinopathy of prematurity. New York: Springer-Verlag; 1992:23–36.
33. Gospodarowicz D. Purification of a basic fibroblast growth factor from bovine pituitary. J Biol Chem. 1975;250:2505–10.
34. Schreiber AB, Winkler ME, Derynk R. Transforming growth factor alpha: a more potent angiogenic mediator than epidermal growth factor. Science. 1986;232:1250–3.
35. Frater-Schroder M, Risau W, Hallman R, et al. Tumor necrosis factor alpha, a potent inhibitor of endothelial cell growth in vitro is angiogenic in vivo. Proc Natl Acad Sci U S A 1987;84:5277–81.
36. Shweki D, Itin A, Soffer D, Keshet E. Vascular endothelial growth factor induced by hypoxia may mediate hypoxia-initiated angiogenesis. Nature. 1992;358:843–5.
37. Aiello LP, Avery RL, Arrigg PG, et al. Vascular endothelial growth factor in ocular fluid of patients with diabetic retinopathy and other retinal disorders. N Engl J Med. 1994;331:1480–7.
38. Screening examination of premature infants for retinopathy of prematurity. Pediatrics. 2001;108:809–11.
39. Yamashita Y. Studies on retinopathy of prematurity: III. Cryocautery for retinopathy of prematurity. Jpn J Ophthalmol. 1972;26:385–93.
40. Cryotherapy for Retinopathy of Prematurity Cooperative Group. Multicenter trial of cryotherapy for retinopathy of prematurity: ophthalmological outcomes at 10 years. Arch Ophthalmol. 2001;119:1110–8.
41. Cryotherapy for Retinopathy of Prematurity Cooperative Group. Effect of retinal ablative therapy for threshold retinopathy of prematurity: results of Goldmann perimetry at the age of 10 years. Arch Ophthalmol. 2001;119:1120–5.
42. Cryotherapy for Retinopathy of Prematurity Cooperative Group. Contrast sensitivity at age 10 years in children who had threshold retinopathy of prematurity. Arch Ophthalmol. 2001;119:1129–33.
43. Banach MJ, Ferrone PJ, Trese MT. A comparison of dense versus less dense diode laser photocoagulation patterns for threshold retinopathy of prematurity. Ophthalmology. 2000;107:324–8.
44. Lambert SR, Capone A Jr, Cingle KA, Drack AV. Cataract and phthisis bulbi after laser photoablation for threshold retinopathy of prematurity. Am J Ophthalmol. 2000;129:585–91.
45. Kaiser RS, Trese MT. Iris atrophy, cataracts, and hypotony following peripheral ablation for threshold retinopathy of prematurity. Arch Ophthalmol. 2001;119:615–7.

46. Shalev B, Farr A, Repka MX. Randomized comparison of diode laser photocoagulation versus cryotherapy for threshold retinopathy of prematurity: seven-year outcome. Am J Ophthalmol. 2001;132:76–80.

47. Pearce IA, Pennie FC, Gannon LM, et al. Three year visual outcome for treated stage 3 retinopathy of prematurity: cryotherapy versus laser. Br J Ophthalmol. 1998;82:1254–9.

48. O'Keefe M, O'Reilly J, Lanigan B. Longer term visual outcome of eyes with retinopathy treated with cryotherapy or diode laser. Br J Ophthalmol. 1998;82:1246–8.

49. Foroozan R, Connolly BP, Tasman WS. Outcomes after laser therapy for threshold retinopathy of prematurity. Ophthalmology. 2001;108:1644–6.

50. Connolly BP, McNamara JA, Sharma S, et al. A comparison of laser photocoagulation with trans-scleral cryotherapy in the treatment of threshold retinopathy of prematurity. Ophthalmology. 1998;105:1628–31.

51. DeJonge MH, Ferrone PJ, Trese MT. Diode laser ablation for threshold retinopathy of prematurity. Short-term structural outcome. Arch Ophthalmol. 2000;118: 365–7.

52. Capone A Jr, Diaz-Rohena R, Sternberg P Jr, et al. Diode-laser photocoagulation for zone 1 threshold retinopathy of prematurity. Am J Ophthalmol. 1993;116:444–50.

53. Axer-Siegel R, Śnir M, Cotlear D, et al. Diode laser treatment of posterior retinopathy of prematurity. Br J Ophthalmol. 2000;84:1383–6.

54. Cryotherapy for Retinopathy of Prematurity Cooperative Group. Multicenter trial of cryotherapy for retinopathy of prematurity. Three-month outcome. Arch Ophthalmol. 1990;108:195–204.

55. Reynolds J, Dobson V, Quinn GE, et al. Prediction of visual function in eyes with mild to moderate posterior pole residua of retinopathy of prematurity. Cryotherapy for Retinopathy of Prematurity Cooperative Group. Arch Ophthalmol. 1993;111:1050–6.

56. Gilbert WS, Quinn GE, Dobson V, et al. Partial retinal detachment at 3 months after threshold retinopathy of prematurity. Long-term structural and functional outcome. Arch Ophthalmol. 1996;114:1085–91.

57. Trese MT. Scleral buckling for retinopathy of prematurity. Ophthalmology. 1994; 101:23–6.

58. Greven C, Tasman W. Scleral buckling in stages 4B and 5 retinopathy of prematurity. Ophthalmology. 1990;97:817–20.

59. Trese MT, Droste PJ. Long-term postoperative results of a consecutive series of stages 4 and 5 retinopathy of prematurity. Ophthalmology. 1998;105:992–7.

60. Capone A Jr, Trese MT. Lens-sparing vitreous surgery for tractional stage 4A retinopathy of prematurity retinal detachments. Ophthalmology. 2001;108:2068–70.

61. Chow DR, Ferrone PJ, Trese MT. Refractive changes associated with scleral buckling and division in retinopathy of prematurity. Arch Ophthalmol. 1998;116:1446–8.

62. Mintz-Hittner HA, O'Malley RE, Kretzer FL. Long-term form identification vision after early, closed, lensectomy-vitrectomy for stage 5 retinopathy of prematurity. Ophthalmology. 1997;104:454–9.

63. Gallo JE, Holmstrom G, Kugelberg U, et al. Regressed retinopathy of prematurity and its sequelae in children aged 5–10 years. Br J Ophthalmol. 1991;75:527–31.

64. Brown MM, Brown GC, Duker JS, et al. Exudative retinopathy of adults: a late sequela of retinopathy of prematurity. Int Ophthalmol. 1994–95;18(5):281–5.

65. Kaiser RS, Trese MT, Williams GA, Cox MS Jr. Adult retinopathy of prematurity. Outcomes of rhegmatogenous retinal detachments and retinal tears. Ophthalmology. 2001;108:1647–53.

117 Diabetic Retinopathy

BRETT J. ROSENBLATT • WILLIAM E. BENSON

DEFINITION
- Progressive dysfunction of the retinal vasculature caused by chronic hyperglycemia.

KEY FEATURES
- Microaneurysms.
- Retinal hemorrhages.
- Retinal lipid exudates.
- Cotton-wool spots.
- Capillary nonperfusion.
- Macular edema.
- Neovascularization.

ASSOCIATED FEATURES
- Vitreous hemorrhage.
- Retinal detachment.
- Neovascular glaucoma.
- Premature cataract.
- Cranial nerve palsies.

INTRODUCTION

Successful management of diabetic retinopathy via a combination of glucose control, laser therapy, and vitrectomy represents one of the most striking achievements of modern ophthalmology. If fundus examinations are initiated prior to the development of significant retinopathy and repeated periodically, and if the recommendations of the Early Treatment Diabetic Retinopathy Study (ETDRS) are followed with respect to the management of subsequent diabetic macular edema or neovascularization, the risk of severe visual loss is less than 5%. Despite this, diabetic retinopathy remains the number one cause of new blindness in most industrialized countries. The vast majority of diabetic individuals who lose vision do so, not because of an inability to treat their disease, but rather due to a delay in seeking medical attention. The key to sight preservation for diabetic patients is routine examinations to detect the earliest signs of retinopathy.

EPIDEMIOLOGY

The best predictor of diabetic retinopathy is the duration of the disease.[1] Patients who have had type 1 for 5 years or less rarely show any evidence of diabetic retinopathy. However, 27% of those who have had diabetes for 5–10 years and 71–90% of those who have had diabetes for longer than 10 years have diabetic retinopathy.[2] After 20–30 years, the incidence rises to 95%, and about 30–50% of these patients have proliferative diabetic retinopathy (PDR).

Yanko et al.[3] described the prevalence of retinopathy in patients with type 2 diabetes. They found that the prevalence of retinopathy 11–13 years after the onset of type 2 diabetes was 23%; after 16 or more years, it was 60%; and 11 or more years after the onset, 3% of the patients had PDR. Klein et al.[2] found that 10 years after the diagnosis of type 2 diabetes, 67% of patients had retinopathy and 10% had PDR.

The most important determinant of retinopathy is the duration of diabetes after the onset of puberty. For example, the risk of retinopathy is roughly the same for two 25-year-old patients, of whom one developed diabetes at the age of 6 and the other at the age of 12 years.[4]

The Diabetes Control and Complications Trial showed emphatically that patients with type 1 diabetes who closely monitored their blood glucose (four measurements per day = tight control) do far better than patients treated with conventional therapy (one measurement per day).[5] The former had a 76% reduction in the rate of development of any retinopathy (primary prevention cohort) and a 54% reduction in progression of established retinopathy (secondary intervention cohort) as compared with the conventional treatment group. For advanced retinopathy, however, even the most rigorous control of blood glucose may not prevent progression. The value of intensive treatment has been demonstrated for type 2 diabetes, as well. The United Kingdom Prospective Diabetes Study (UKPDS) revealed a 21% reduction in the 1-year rate of progression of retinopathy.[6]

Renal disease, as evidenced by proteinuria, elevated blood urea nitrogen levels, and elevated blood creatinine levels, is an excellent predictor of the presence of retinopathy.[1] Even patients with microalbuminuria are at high risk of developing retinopathy.[7] Similarly, 35% of patients with symptomatic retinopathy have proteinuria, elevated blood urea nitrogen values, or elevated creatinine levels. Systemic hypertension appears to be an independent risk factor for diabetic retinopathy.[1]

In women who begin a pregnancy without retinopathy, the risk of developing nonproliferative diabetic retinopathy (NPDR) is about 10%. Those with NPDR at the onset of pregnancy and those who have or who develop systemic hypertension tend to show progression, with increased hemorrhages, cotton-wool spots, and macular edema.[8] Fortunately, there is usually some regression after delivery. About 4% of pregnant women with NPDR progress to PDR. Those with untreated PDR at the onset of pregnancy frequently do poorly unless they are treated with panretinal photocoagulation (PRP). However, previously treated PDR usually does not worsen during pregnancy. There is no doubt that women who maintain good metabolic control during pregnancy have fewer spontaneous abortions and fewer children with birth defects. Therefore, obstetricians strive for strict control. Women who begin pregnancy with poorly controlled diabetes who are suddenly brought under strict control frequently have severe deterioration of their retinopathy and do not always recover after delivery.[8]

PATHOGENESIS

The final metabolic pathway that causes diabetic retinopathy is unknown. There are several theories.

Aldose Reductase

Aldose reductase converts sugars into their alcohols. For example, glucose is converted to sorbitol and galactose is converted to galactitol. Because sorbitol and galactitol cannot easily diffuse out of cells, their intracellular concentration increases. Osmotic forces then cause water to diffuse into the cell, resulting in electrolyte imbalance. The resultant damage to lens epithelial cells, which have a high concentration of aldose reductase, is responsible for the cataract seen in children and in experimental animals with galactosemia and in animals with experimental diabetes mellitus.[9] Because aldose reductase is also found in high concentration in retinal pericytes and Schwann cells, some investigators suggest that diabetic retinopathy and neuropathy may be caused by aldose reductase–mediated damage. Despite all of these theoretical benefits, clinical trials have thus far failed to show a reduction in the incidence of diabetic retinopathy or of neuropathy by aldose reductase inhibitors, possibly because an effective aldose reductase inhibitor with few systemic side effects has yet to be developed.[9]

Vasoproliferative Factors

Currently intense interest exists in vasoproliferative factors released by the retina itself, retinal vessels, and the retinal pigment epithelium, which are felt to induce neovascularization. Vascular endothelial growth factor (VEGF), which inhibits the growth of the retinal endothelial cells *in vitro*, has been implicated in diabetic retinopathy. Considerable evidence suggests that VEGF has a direct role in the retinal vascular abnormalities that are found in diabetes. Animal models demonstrate that VEGF expression correlates with the development and regression of neovascularization.[10] The concentration of VEGF is higher in the vitreous of eyes with PDR as compared with eyes with NPDR.[11] Furthermore, inhibitors of VEGF have been successful in suppressing hypoxia-induced neovascularization in animal models.[12] Although the release of growth factors may explain the neovascular response to ischemia, growth factors themselves may or may not represent a direct link between hyperglycemia and retinal vasculopathy.

Platelets and Blood Viscosity

Diabetes is associated with abnormalities of platelet function. It has been postulated that platelet abnormalities or alterations in blood viscosity in diabetics may contribute to diabetic retinopathy by causing focal capillary occlusion and focal areas of ischemia in the retina which, in turn, contribute to the development of diabetic retinopathy.[13]

OCULAR MANIFESTATIONS

The earliest stage of diabetic retinopathy is nonproliferative (NPDR). In some patients, there is progression to proliferative retinopathy (PDR).

Early Nonproliferative Diabetic Retinopathy

Microaneurysms are the first ophthalmoscopically detectable change in diabetic retinopathy (Fig. 117-1, *A*), seen as small red dots in the middle retinal layers. When the wall of a capillary or microaneurysm is weakened enough, it may rupture, giving rise to an intraretinal hemorrhage. If the hemorrhage is deep (i.e., in the inner nuclear layer or outer plexiform layer), it usually is round or oval ("dot or blot") (see Fig. 117-1, *A*). It is very difficult to distinguish a small dot hemorrhage from a microaneurysm by ophthalmoscopy. Fluorescein angiography helps to distinguish patent microaneurysms because they leak dye (Fig. 117-1, *B*). However, angiography cannot distinguish a hemorrhage from a microaneurysm filled with clotted blood. If the

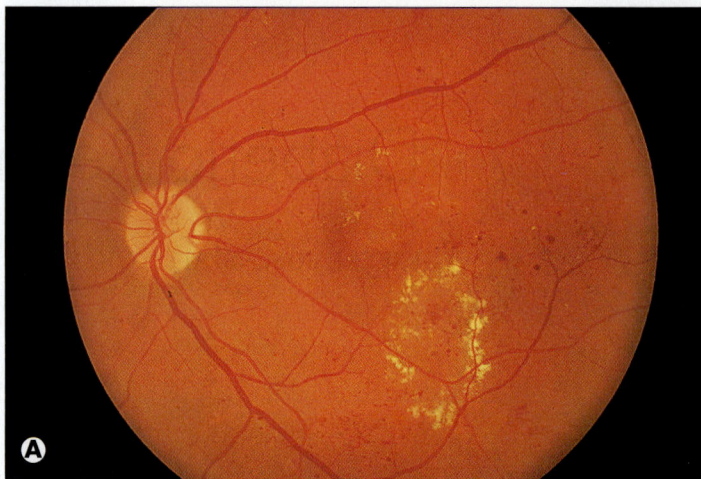

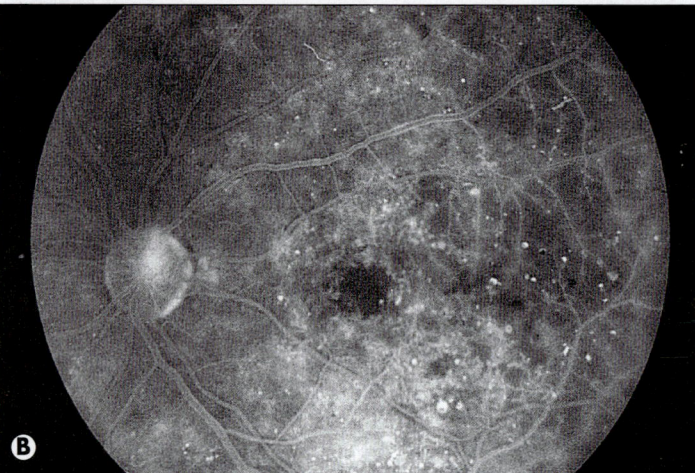

FIG. 117-1 ■ Nonproliferative diabetic retinopathy with microaneurysms. **A,** Small dot hemorrhages, microaneurysms, hard (lipid) exudates, circinate retinopathy, an intraretinal microvascular abnormality, and macular edema. **B,** Fluorescein angiography of the eye shown in **A.** Microaneurysms are seen as multiple dots of hyperfluorescence, but the dot hemorrhages do not fluoresce. The foveal avascular zone is minimally enlarged.

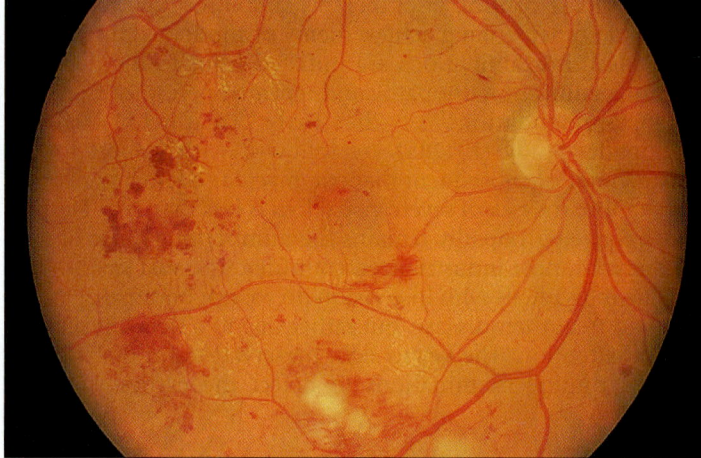

FIG. 117-2 ■ Nonproliferative retinopathy with some blot hemorrhages, splinter hemorrhages, and cotton-wool spots.

hemorrhage is superficial, in the nerve fiber layer, it takes a flame or splinter shape indistinguishable from a hemorrhage seen in hypertensive retinopathy (Figs. 117-2 and 117-3). Diabetics who have normal blood pressure may have multiple splinter hemorrhages. Nevertheless, the presence of numerous splinter hemorrhages in a diabetic patient should prompt a blood pressure

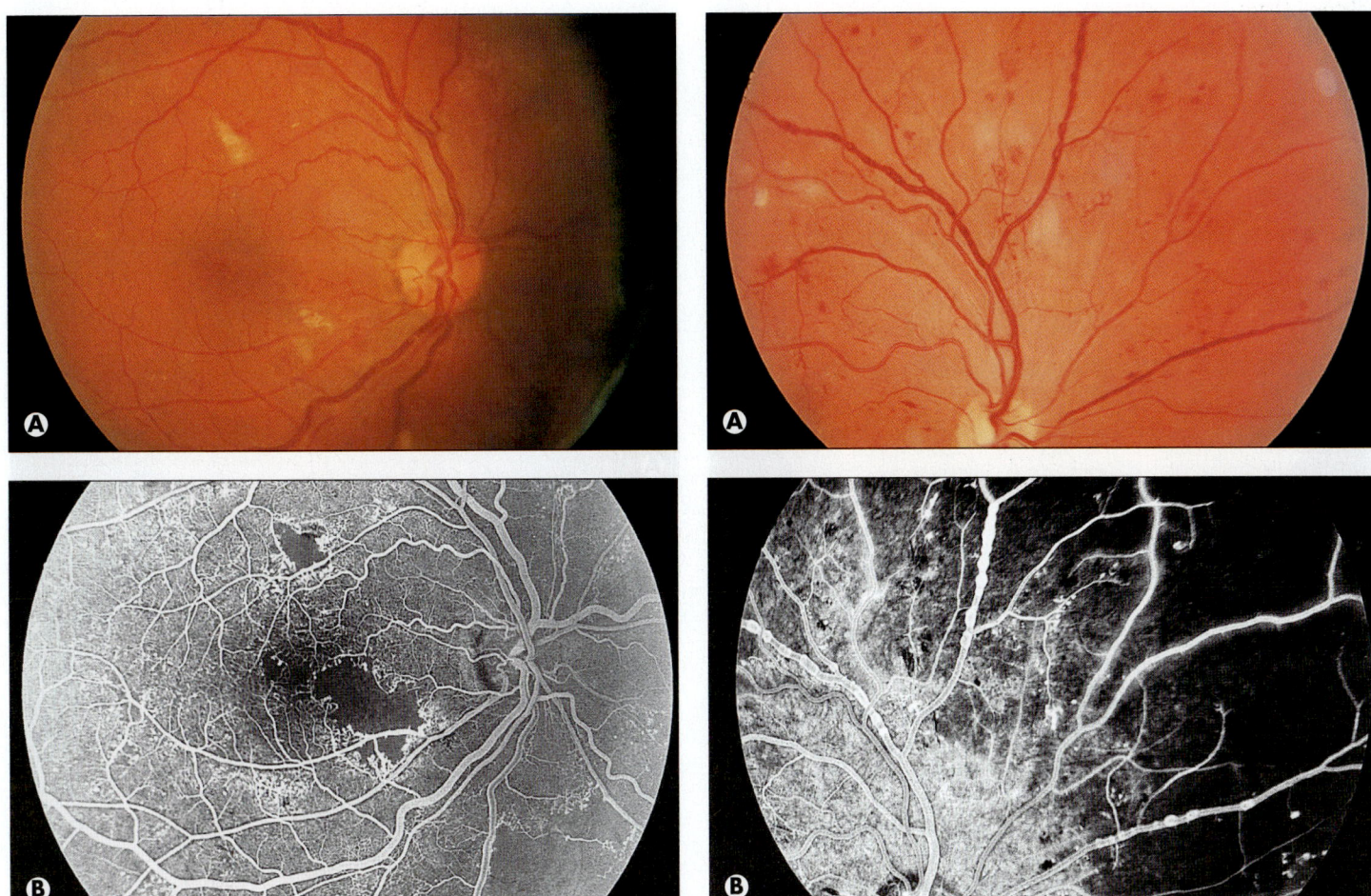

FIG. 117-3 ▌▌ **Nonproliferative retinopathy. A,** With soft exudates. **B,** Fluorescein angiography shows capillary nonperfusion in the area of the superior cotton-wool spot and a larger area just inferonasal to the foveal avascular zone.

FIG. 117-4 ▌▌ **Severe nonproliferative retinopathy. A,** With cotton-wool spots, intraretinal microvascular abnormalities, and venous beading. **B,** Fluorescein angiography shows severe capillary nonperfusion.

check, because a frequent complication of diabetes is systemic hypertension.

Macular edema, or retinal thickening (see Fig. 117-1, *A*), is an important manifestation of NPDR and represents the leading cause of legal blindness in diabetics. The intercellular fluid comes from leaking microaneurysms or from diffuse capillary incompetence. Clinically, macular edema is best detected by biomicroscopy with a 60-diopter or contact macular lens. The edema causes scattering of light by the multiple interfaces it creates in the retina by separated retinal cells. This decreases the retina's translucency such that the normal retinal pigment epithelial and choroidal background pattern is blurred (see Fig. 117-1, *A*). Finally, the pockets of fluid in the outer plexiform layer, if large enough, can be seen as cystoid macular edema. Usually cystoid macular edema is seen in eyes that have other signs of severe NPDR such as numerous hemorrhages or exudates. In rare cases, cystoid macular edema due to generalized diffuse leakage from the entire capillary network can be seen in eyes that have very few other signs of diabetic retinopathy.

If the leakage of fluid is severe enough, lipid may accumulate in the retina (see Fig. 117-1, *A*); again, the outer plexiform layer is first to be affected. In some cases, lipid is scattered through the macula. In others, it accumulates in a ring around a group of leaking microaneurysms, or around microaneurysms surrounding an area of capillary nonperfusion. This pattern is called circinate retinopathy (see Fig. 117-1, *A*).

Advanced Nonproliferative Diabetic Retinopathy

In advanced NPDR, signs of increasing inner retinal hypoxia appear, including multiple retinal hemorrhages, cotton-wool spots (see Fig. 117-3), venous beading and loops (Fig. 117-4), intraretinal microvascular abnormalities (IRMA) (see Figs. 117-1, *A* and 117-4), and large areas of capillary nonperfusion depicted on fluorescein angiography.

Cotton-wool spots, also called soft exudates or nerve fiber infarcts, result from ischemia, not exudation. Local ischemia causes effective obstruction of axoplasmic flow in the normally transparent nerve fiber layer; the subsequent swelling of the nerve fibers gives cotton-wool spots their characteristic white fluffy appearance. Fluorescein angiography shows no capillary perfusion in the area corresponding to a cotton-wool spot. Microaneurysms frequently surround the hypoxic area (see Fig. 117-3).

Venous beading (see Fig. 117-4) is an important sign of sluggish retinal circulation. Venous loops nearly always are adjacent to large areas of capillary nonperfusion. IRMAs are dilated capillaries, which seem to function as collateral channels. They frequently are difficult to differentiate from surface retinal neovascularization. Fluorescein dye, however, does not leak from IRMAs but leaks profusely from neovascularization. Capillary hypoperfusion often surrounds IRMA (see Fig. 117-4).

The ETDRS found that IRMA, multiple retinal hemorrhages, venous beading and loops, widespread capillary nonperfusion, and widespread leakage on fluorescein angiography were all significant risk factors for the development of proliferative retinopathy. Interestingly, cotton-wool spots were not.[14]

Proliferative Diabetic Retinopathy

Although the macular edema, exudates, and capillary occlusions seen in NPDR often cause legal blindness, affected patients usually maintain at least ambulatory vision. PDR, on the other hand,

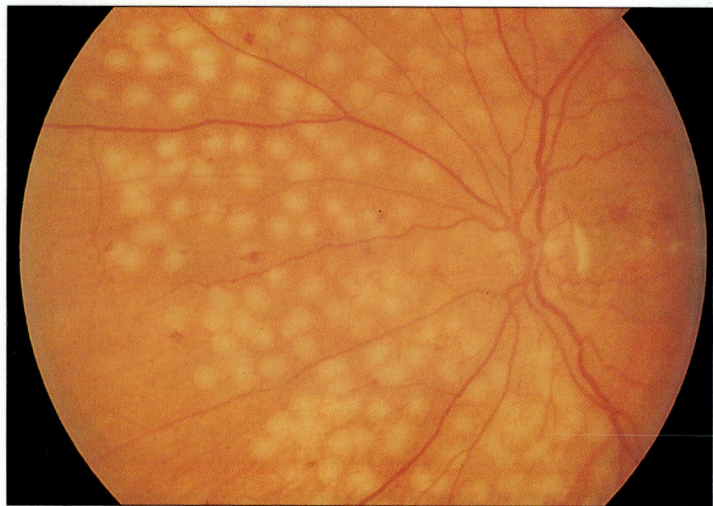

FIG. 117-5 ▌ Approximately one half the disc area shows neovascularization of the disc and initial, incomplete panretinal photocoagulation.

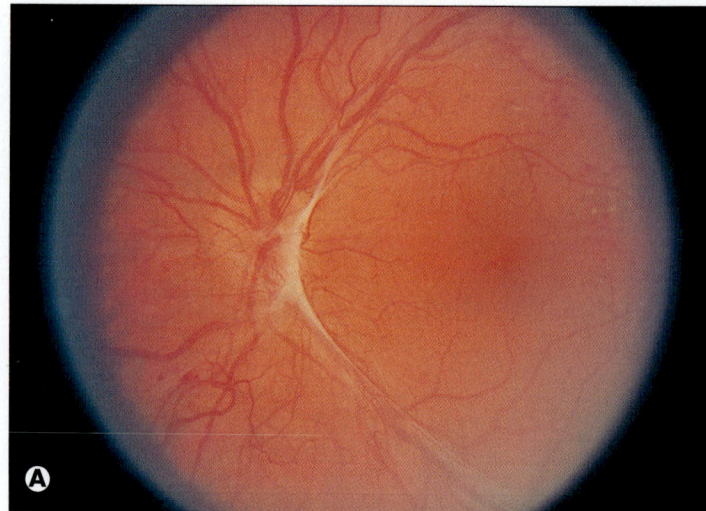

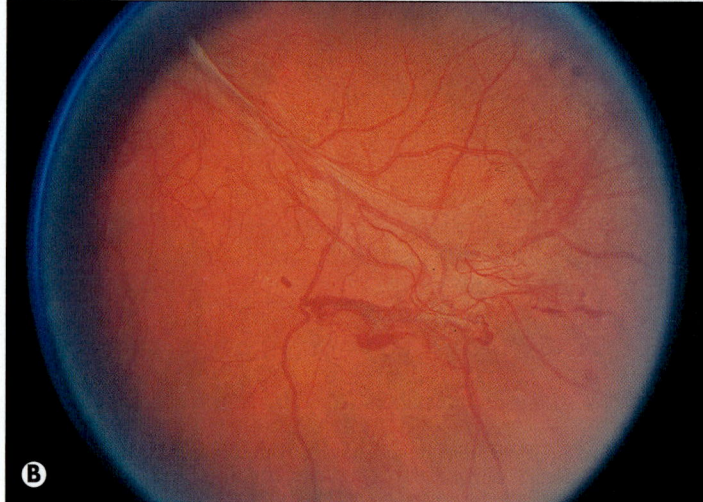

FIG. 117-6 ▌ Neovascularization. **A,** Neovascularization of the disc with some fibrous proliferation. **B,** Neovascularization elsewhere.

may result in severe vitreous hemorrhage or retinal detachment, with hand-movements vision or worse. Approximately 50% of patients with very severe NPDR progress to proliferative retinopathy within 1 year.[15] Proliferative vessels usually arise from retinal veins and often begin as a collection of multiple fine vessels. When they arise on or within one disc diameter of the optic nerve head they are referred to as NVD (neovascularization of the disc) (Figs. 117-5 and 117-6). When they arise further than one disc diameter away, they are called NVE (neovascularization elsewhere) (see Fig. 117-6, *B*). Unlike normal retinal vessels, NVD and NVE both leak fluorescein into the vitreous.

Once the stimulus for growth of new vessels is present, the path of subsequent growth taken by neovascularization is along the route of least resistance. For example, the absence of a true internal limiting membrane on the disc could explain the prevalence of new vessels at that location. Also, neovascularization seems to grow more easily on a preformed connective tissue framework. Thus, a shallowly detached posterior vitreous face is a frequent site of growth of new vessels.

The new vessels usually progress through a stage of further proliferation, with associated connective tissue formation. As PDR progresses, the fibrous component becomes more prominent, with the fibrotic tissue being either vascular or avascular. The fibrovascular variety usually is found in association with vessels that extend into the vitreous cavity or with abnormal new vessels on the surface of the retina or disc. The avascular variety usually results from organization or thickening of the posterior hyaloid face. Vitreous traction is transmitted to the retina along these proliferations and may lead to traction retinal detachment.

NVE nearly always grows toward and into zones of retinal ischemia until posterior vitreous detachment occurs (see Fig. 117-6). Then, the vessels are lifted into the vitreous cavity. The end stage is characterized by regression of the vascular systems. No further damage may take place, but there may be contraction of the connective tissue components, development of subhyaloid bands, thickening of the posterior vitreous face, and the appearance of retinoschisis, retinal detachment, or formation of retinal breaks.

Posterior vitreous detachment in diabetics is characterized by a slow, overall shrinkage of the entire formed vitreous rather than by the formation of cavities caused by vitreous destruction. Davis *et al.*[16] have stressed the role of the contracting vitreous in the production of vitreous hemorrhage, retinal breaks, and retinal detachment. Neovascular vessels do not "grow" forward into the vitreous cavity; they are pulled into it by the contracting vitreous to which they adhere. Confirmation of the importance of the vitreous in the development and progression of proliferative retinopathy comes from the long-term follow-up of eyes that have undergone successful vitrectomy. The existent neovascular-

ization shrinks, leaks less fluorescein, and new areas of neovascularization rarely arise.

It has long been assumed that sudden vitreous contractions tear the fragile new vessels, causing vitreous hemorrhage. However, the majority of diabetic vitreous hemorrhages occur during sleep, possibly because of an increase in blood pressure secondary to early morning hypoglycemia or to rapid eye movement sleep. Because so few hemorrhages occur during exercise, it is not necessary to restrict the activity of patients with proliferative retinopathy. When a hemorrhage occurs, if the erythrocytes are all behind the posterior vitreous face, they usually quickly settle to the bottom of the eye and are absorbed. However, when erythrocytes break into the vitreous body, they adhere to the gel and clearing may take months or years.

A large superficial hemorrhage may separate the internal limiting membrane from the rest of the retina. Such hemorrhages usually are round or oval but also may be boat shaped. The blood may remain confined between the internal limiting membrane and the rest of the retina for weeks or months before breaking into the vitreous. Sub-internal limiting membrane hemorrhages were formerly thought to occur between the internal limiting membrane and the cortical vitreous and were called subhyaloid or preretinal hemorrhages. It is now felt that true subhyaloid hemorrhages probably are quite rare. Tight sub-internal limiting membrane hemorrhages are dangerous, because they may progress rapidly to traction retinal detachment.

As the vitreous contracts, it may pull on the optic disc, causing traction striae involving the macular area, or actually drag the macula itself, both of which contribute to decreased visual acuity.[17]

Two types of diabetic retinal detachments occur, those which are caused by traction alone (nonrhegmatogenous) and those caused by retinal break formation (rhegmatogenous). Characteristics of nonrhegmatogenous (traction) detachment in PDR include the following:

- The detached retina usually is confined to the posterior fundus and infrequently extends more than two thirds of the distance to the equator.
- The detached retina has a taut and shiny surface.
- The detached retina is concave toward the pupil.
- No shifting of subretinal fluid occurs.

Occasionally, a spontaneous decrease in the extent of a traction detachment may occur, but this is the exception rather than the rule. Traction on the retina also may cause focal areas of retinoschisis, which may be difficult to distinguish from full-thickness retinal detachment; in retinoschisis the elevated layer is thinner and more translucent.

When a detachment is rhegmatogenous, the borders of the elevated retina usually extend to the ora serrata. The retinal surface is dull and grayish and undulates because of retinal mobility due to shifting of subretinal fluid. Retinal breaks are usually in the posterior pole near areas of fibrovascular change. The breaks are oval in shape and appear to be partly the result of tangential traction from the proliferative tissue, as well as being due to vitreous traction. Determination of the location of retinal holes may be complicated by many factors, particularly poor dilatation of the pupil, lens opacity, increased vitreous turbidity, vitreous hemorrhage, intraretinal hemorrhage, and obscuration of the breaks by overlying proliferative tissue.

OTHER OCULAR COMPLICATIONS OF DIABETES MELLITUS

Cornea

Corneal sensitivity is decreased in proportion to both the duration of the disease and the severity of the retinopathy.[18] Corneal abrasions are more common in people with diabetes, presumably because adhesion between the basement membrane of the corneal epithelium and the corneal stroma is not as firm as that found in normal corneas. Hyperglycemia and the aldose reductase pathway probably play a major role in epithelial abnormalities, because aldose reductase inhibitors may accelerate healing of corneal abrasions.[19] Following vitrectomy, recurrent corneal erosion, striate keratopathy, and corneal edema are more common in diabetics than in nondiabetics.

Glaucoma

The relationship between diabetes and primary open-angle glaucoma is unclear. Some population-based studies have found an association[20] but others have not.[21]

Neovascularization of the iris (NVI) usually is seen only in diabetics who have PDR. Panretinal photocoagulation not only has protective value against NVI, it also is an effective treatment against established NVI.[22] If the media are clear, PRP should be performed prior to any other treatment for NVI, even in advanced cases, because regression and permanent pressure control in patients who have extensive angle closure and intraocular pressures as high as 60mm Hg have been documented.[22] If the media are too cloudy for PRP, trans-scleral laser or peripheral retinal cryoablation are alternative means of treatment (see below).

Lens

The risk of cataract is 2–4 times greater in diabetics than in nondiabetics and may be 15–25 times greater in diabetics under 40 years old.[23]

Patients with diabetes mellitus who have no retinopathy have excellent results from cataract surgery, with 90–95% having a final visual acuity of 20/40 or better, but chronic cystoid macular edema is about 14 times more common in diabetics than in nondiabetics.[24] The best-known predictor of postoperative success is the preoperative severity of retinopathy.[25] The most dreaded anterior complication is NVI. It was hoped that modern surgery, which leaves an intact posterior capsule, would protect the eye from NVI by reducing the diffusion of vasoproliferative factors into the anterior chamber, but several studies have shown that it does not. Furthermore, an Nd:YAG laser capsulotomy does not increase the risk.[26] Other anterior segment complications which are more common in diabetics than in nondiabetics are pupillary block, posterior synechiae, pigmented precipitates on the implant, and severe iritis.[24]

Posterior complications of cataract surgery include macular edema, proliferative retinopathy,[27] vitreous hemorrhage,[26] and traction retinal detachment. Studies from the early 1990s suggested that patients with NPDR were likely to develop or have worsening of macular edema. Recent reports suggest that modern, uncomplicated cataract surgery may not accelerate progression of diabetic retinopathy in type 2 diabetics with NPDR.[28] Caution should be observed when considering cataract surgery in patients who have diabetic retinopathy; however, up to 70% of these patients can attain a final visual acuity of 20/40 or better.[29]

Cataract surgery in patients with active PDR often results in still poorer postoperative visual outcome because of the high risk of both anterior and posterior segment complications. In one series, no patient with active PDR or preproliferative diabetic retinopathy achieved better than 20/80. Most experts recommend aggressive preoperative PRP.[24,25]

Optic Neuropathy

As demonstrated by increased latency and decreased amplitude of the visual evoked potential, many diabetic patients without retinopathy have subclinical optic neuropathy. They have an increased risk for anterior ischemic optic neuropathy. In addition, diabetics are susceptible to diabetic papillopathy, which is characterized by acute disc edema without the pale swelling of anterior ischemic optic neuropathy. It is bilateral in one half of cases and may not show an afferent pupillary defect.[30] Macular edema is a common concurrent finding and is the most common cause of failure of visual recovery in these patients.[30] Visual fields may be normal or show an enlarged blind spot or other nerve fiber defects. The prognosis is excellent, because most patients recover to 20/50 or better.

Cranial Neuropathy

Extraocular muscle palsies may occur in diabetics secondary to neuropathy involving the third, fourth, or sixth cranial nerves. The mechanism is believed to be a localized demyelinization of the nerve secondary to focal ischemia. Pain may or may not be experienced, and not infrequently extraocular muscle palsy may be the initial clue to a latent diabetic condition. Recovery of extraocular muscle function in diabetic cranial nerve palsies generally takes place within 1–3 months.[31] When the third cranial nerve is involved, pupillary function is usually normal. This pupillary sparing in the diabetic third cranial nerve palsy is an important diagnostic feature, helping to distinguish it from an intracranial tumor or aneurysm.

DIAGNOSIS AND ANCILLARY TESTING

In nearly all instances, diabetic retinopathy is diagnosed easily via ophthalmoscopic examination. The hallmark lesions are microaneurysms, which usually develop in the posterior pole. Without microaneurysms, the diagnosis of diabetic retinopathy is in doubt. Fasting blood sugar testing, a glucose tolerance test, and hemoglobin A_{1c} determinations all can be used to confirm the presence of systemic hyperglycemia.

Although further diagnostic testing rarely is indicated, intravenous fluorescein angiography is a widely administered ancillary test. Fluorescein angiography is most helpful to assess the severity of diabetic retinopathy, to determine sites of leakage in macular edema, to judge the extent of capillary nonperfusion, and to confirm neovascularization. It is a useful preoperative test to evaluate the extent of retinopathy in patients who are to undergo cataract surgery and have media opacity. Optical coherence tomography is a noninvasive imaging technique that accurately measures retinal thickness. Diabetic patients often show psychophysical abnormalities. One of the early symptoms of diabetic retinopathy is poor night vision (dark adaptation) and poor recovery from bright lights (photostress).[32] Diabetics, even those without retinopathy, are more likely to have abnormal color vision than are nondiabetics matched for age.[33] Blue-yellow discrimination is affected earlier and more severely than is red-green discrimination. As retinopathy advances, color vision deteriorates.

One of the earliest electrophysiological abnormalities seen in diabetic patients without ophthalmoscopically visible retinopathy is diminution of the amplitude of the oscillatory potentials of the electroretinogram at a time when both the A and B waves are normal. This abnormality probably reflects ischemia in the inner nuclear layer of the retina. Diminished oscillatory potentials are a good predictor of progression of retinopathy.[34] As the severity of diabetic retinopathy increases, the amplitude of the B wave decreases.

DIFFERENTIAL DIAGNOSIS

The differential diagnosis is listed in Box 117-1.

PATHOLOGY

The earliest histopathological abnormalities in diabetic retinopathy are thickening of the capillary basement membrane and pericyte dropout. Microaneurysms begin as a dilatation in the capillary wall in areas where pericytes are absent; microaneurysms initially are thin walled. Later, endothelial cells proliferate and lay down layers of basement membrane material around themselves. Fibrin may accumulate within the aneurysm, and the lumen of the microaneurysm actually may be occluded (Fig. 117-7). In early cases, microaneurysms are present mostly on the venous side of the capillaries, but later they are seen on the arterial side as well. Despite the multiple layers of basement membrane, they are permeable to water and large molecules, allowing the accumulation of water and lipid in the retina. Because fluorescein passes easily through them, many more microaneurysms are seen on fluorescein angiography than are apparent on ophthalmoscopy (see Figs. 117-1 and 117-3).

TREATMENT

Medical Therapy

ANTIPLATELET THERAPY. The ETDRS reported that aspirin 650 mg daily does not influence the progression of retinopathy, affect visual acuity, or influence the incidence of vitreous hemorrhages. However, there was a significant decrease in cardiovascular morbidity in the aspirin-treated group compared with the placebo cohort.[35] Ticlopidine (Ticlid), like aspirin, inhibits adenosine diphosphate–induced platelet aggregation. It has been shown to decrease the risk of stroke in patients with transient ischemic attacks, but there is no clear evidence showing an impact on diabetic retinopathy.

ANTIHYPERTENSIVE AGENTS. The Hypertension in Diabetes Study, part of the United Kingdom Prospective Diabetes Study, evaluated the effect blood pressure control on the progression of diabetic retinopathy. Patients were treated with angiotensin-converting enzyme inhibitors (ACEIs) or β-blockers to achieve "tight" control of blood pressure (<150/85 mm Hg) or "less tight" control (<180/105 mm Hg). The group with better blood pressure control had a 37% risk reduction in microvascular changes. There was no difference in effect between the two agents used.[36] Lisinopril, an ACEI, has been shown to decrease the progression of NPDR and PDR in normotensive diabetics, as well. The patients in this study with the better glycemic control benefited more from lisinopril.[37]

ANTIANGIOGENESIS AGENTS. Novel approaches to the prevention and treatment of diabetic retinopathy are based on the hypothesis that local growth factors stimulate retinal vascular alterations. Inhibition of protein kinase C, a compound critical in the cascade that activates VEGF expression, is being pursued actively. An oral inhibitor of protein kinase C has been shown to suppress retinal neovascularization in animal models.[38] Currently a multicenter, randomized, placebo-controlled study is under way to evaluate this compound in diabetic patients.

Surgical Therapy

PANRETINAL PHOTOCOAGULATION. The Diabetic Retinopathy Study proved that both xenon arc and argon laser PRP significantly decrease the likelihood that an eye with high-risk characteristics (HRC) will progress to severe visual loss.[39] Eyes with HRC are defined as those with NVD greater than one fourth to one third the disc area, those with any NVD and vitreous hemorrhage, or those with NVE greater than one half the disc area and vitreous or preretinal hemorrhage.

The exact mechanism by which PRP works remains unknown. Some investigators feel that PRP decreases the production of vasoproliferative factors by eliminating some of the hypoxic retina or by stimulating the release of antiangiogenic factors from the retinal pigment epithelium. An alternative hypothesis suggests that by thinning the retina, PRP increases oxygenation of the remaining retina by allowing increased diffusion of oxygen from the choroid. Yet another hypothesis is that PRP leads to an increase in vasoinhibitors by directly stim-

---

BOX 117-1

Differential Diagnosis of Diabetic Retinopathy

Radiation retinopathy
Hypertensive retinopathy
Retinal venous obstruction (central retinal vein occlusion [CRVO], branch retinal vein occlusion [BRVO])
The ocular ischemic syndrome
Anemia
Leukemia
Coats' disease
Idiopathic juxtafoveal retinal telangiectasia
Sickle cell retinopathy

FIG. 117-7 Microaneurysms, pericyte dropout, and acellular capillaries are seen.

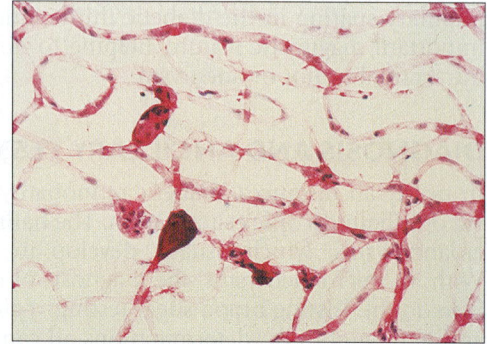

ulating the retinal pigment epithelium to produce inhibitors of vasoproliferation.[40]

The goal of PRP is to arrest or to cause regression of the neovascularization. The recommended therapy is 1200–2000 burns 500μm in diameter delivered through the Goldmann lens, or the same number of 200μm burns delivered through the Rodenstock panfundoscope lens or Volk Superquad lens. The burns should be intense enough to whiten the overlying retina, which usually requires a power of 200–600mW and duration of 0.1 second (see Fig. 117-5). Most ophthalmologists use the argon blue-green or green laser, but a large clinical trial has shown that krypton red is equally effective.[41]

The number of burns necessary to achieve these goals has not been established. Some retinal specialists feel that there is no upper limit to the total number of burns and that treatment should be continued until regression occurs.[42] The only prospective, controlled study found that eyes which received supplementary PRP treatment had no improved outcome over those which received standard PRP only.[43] About two thirds of eyes with HRC that receive PRP have regression of their HRC by 3 months after treatment.

The ETDRS found that PRP significantly retards the development of HRC in eyes with very severe NPDR and macular edema.[15] After 7 years of follow-up, 25% of eyes that received PRP developed HRC as compared with 75% of eyes in which PRP was deferred until HRC developed. Nevertheless, the ETDRS concluded that treatment of severe NPDR and PDR short of HRC was not indicated for three reasons. First, after 7 years of follow-up 25% of eyes assigned to deferral of PRP had not developed HRC. Second, when patients are closely monitored and PRP is given as soon as HRC develops, severe visual loss can be prevented. After 7 years of follow-up, 4.0% of eyes that did not receive PRP until HRC developed had a visual acuity of 5/200 or less, as compared with 2.5% of eyes assigned to immediate PRP. The difference was neither clinically nor statistically significant. Third, PRP has significant complications. It often causes decreased visual acuity by increasing macular edema or by causing macular pucker.[44] Fortunately, the edema frequently regresses spontaneously over 6 months, but the visual field usually is moderately, but permanently, decreased. Color vision and dark adaptation, which often are already impaired, also are worsened by PRP.[32]

PERIPHERAL RETINAL CRYOTHERAPY. Peripheral retinal cryotherapy is used to treat HRC in eyes with media too hazy for PRP. Reported benefits include resorption of vitreous hemorrhages and regression of NVD, NVE, and NVI. The main complication is the development or acceleration of traction retinal detachment in 25–38% of eyes.[44,45] Therefore, this treatment should be avoided in patients with known traction retinal detachment, and all patients must be monitored carefully.

TREATMENT OF MACULAR EDEMA. Patz[46] was the first to show that argon laser photocoagulation decreases or stabilizes macular edema. Later, the ETDRS confirmed his results. The ETDRS defined clinically significant macular edema as:
- Retinal thickening involving the center of the macula
- Hard exudates within 500μm of the center of the macula (if associated with retinal thickening)
- An area of macular edema greater than one disc area but within one disc diameter of the center of the macula

The treatment strategy is to photocoagulate all leaking microaneurysms further than 500μm from the center of the macula (see

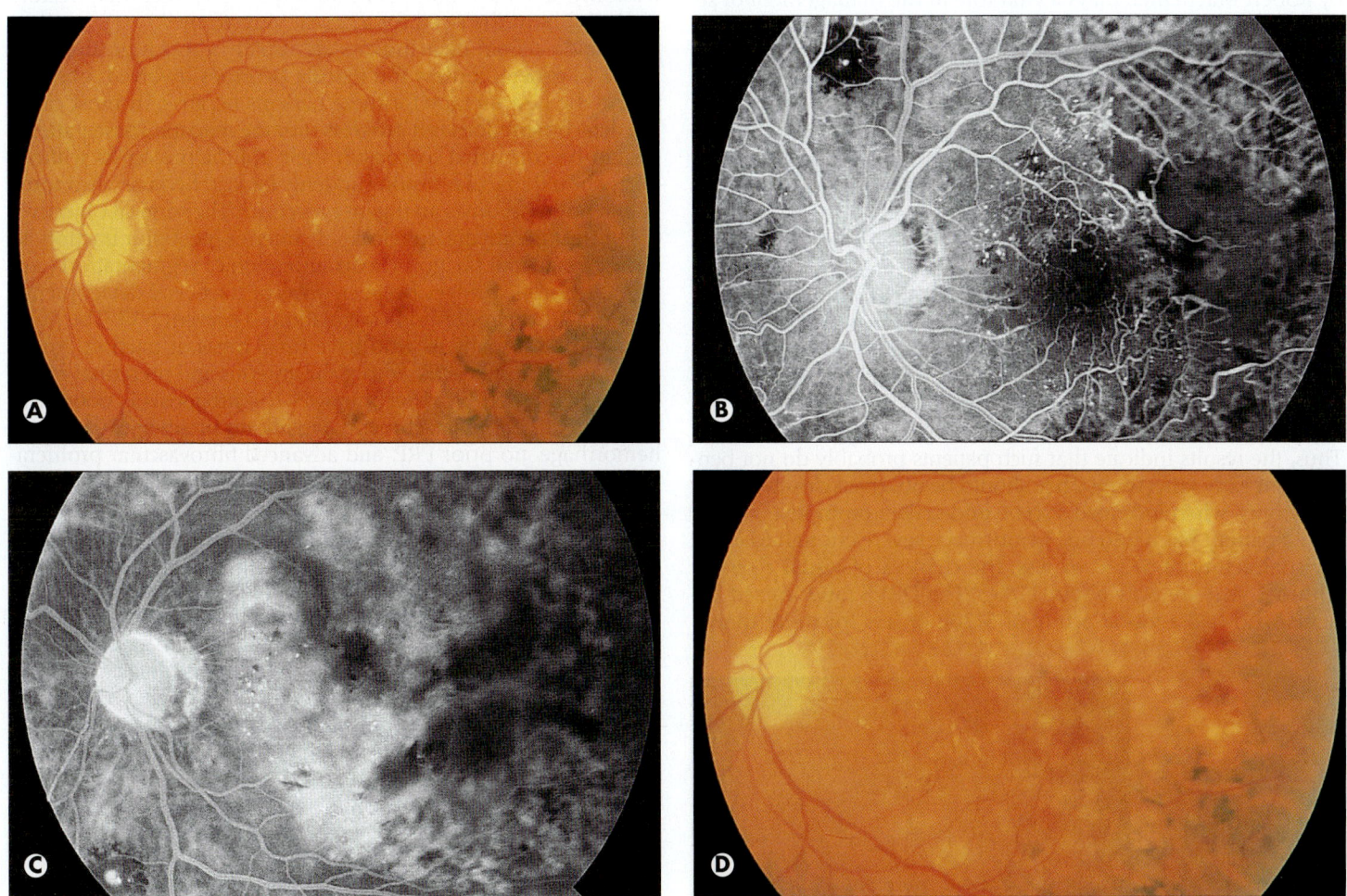

FIG. 117-8 ▮ **Macular edema. A,** In an eye previously treated with panretinal photocoagulation. **B,** Midphase of fluorescein angiography showing microaneurysms, large areas of capillary nonperfusion, and slight enlargement of the foveal avascular zone. **C,** Late phase of fluorescein angiography showing diffuse capillary leakage. **D,** Grid pattern of focal macular photocoagulation in same eye.

Fig. 117-8) and to place a grid of 100–200μm burns in areas of diffuse capillary leakage and in areas of capillary nonperfusion (Fig. 117-8). After 3 years of follow-up, 15% of eyes with clinically significant macular edema had doubling of the visual angle as opposed to 32% of untreated control eyes.[47] The ETDRS also showed that PRP should not be given to eyes with clinically significant macular edema unless HRC are present.[15] Patients with macular edema who have the best prognosis for improved vision have circinate retinopathy of recent duration or focal, well-defined leaking areas and good capillary perfusion surrounding the avascular zone of the retina. Patients with an especially poor prognosis have dense lipid exudate in the center of the foveola (Fig. 117-9). Other poor prognostic signs include diffuse edema with multiple leaking areas, extensive central capillary nonperfusion, increased blood pressure, and cystoid macular edema.[46] Nevertheless, the ETDRS found that even eyes with these adverse findings still benefited from treatment when compared with control eyes.[47] Small, uncontrolled studies have shown encouraging results with intravitreal injection of triamcinolone acetonide, a corticosteroid, in patients who have refractory diabetic edema.[48,49] Long-term efficacy and potential side effects have yet to be clarified.

In summary, the Diabetic Retinopathy Study and the ETDRS conclusively proved that timely laser photocoagulation of diabetic retinopathy can reduce severe visual loss by 95%.[50] Such treatment makes sense, not only from the humanitarian point of view, but also from a cost-effectiveness view. It has been estimated that ETDRS-style therapy saves $250–500 million per year in the United States by enabling patients to avoid disability and welfare.[51] Nevertheless, fully one half of Americans with diabetes do not receive annual eye examinations that include dilatation.

VITRECTOMY IN DIABETIC PATIENTS. Vitrectomy, introduced by Robert Machemer, plays a vital role in the management of severe complications of diabetic retinopathy. The major indications are nonclearing vitreous hemorrhage, macular-involving or macular-threatening traction retinal detachment, and combined traction–rhegmatogenous retinal detachment. Less common indications are macular edema with a thickened and taut posterior hyaloid, macular heterotopia, epiretinal membrane, severe preretinal macular hemorrhage, and neovascular glaucoma with cloudy media.[52]

To evaluate whether early vitrectomy (in the absence of vitreous hemorrhage) might improve the visual prognosis by eliminating the possibility of later traction macular detachment, the Diabetic Retinopathy Vitrectomy Study (DRVS) randomized 370 eyes with florid neovascularization and visual acuity of 20/400 or better to either early vitrectomy or to observation.[53] After 4 years of follow-up, approximately 50% of both groups had 20/60 or better, and approximately 20% of each group had light perception or worse. Thus, the results indicate that such patients probably do not benefit from early vitrectomy. They should be observed closely so that vitrectomy, when indicated, can be undertaken promptly.

If a patient has a vitreous hemorrhage severe enough to cause a visual acuity of 5/200 or less, the chances of visual recovery within 1 year are only about 17%.[54] The DRVS randomized patients who had a visual acuity of 5/200 or less for more than 6

months into two groups, those who received an immediate vitrectomy and those whose vitrectomy was deferred for a further 6 months.[54] The goals of surgery were to release all anterior–posterior vitreous traction and to perform a complete PRP to reduce the incidence of recurrent hemorrhage. Of those who had a deferred vitrectomy, 15% had a final visual acuity of 20/40 or better, as opposed to 25% of those who had an immediate vitrectomy. In patients with type 1 diabetes, 12% of those who had a deferred vitrectomy had a final visual acuity of 20/40 or better, as opposed to 36% of those who had an immediate vitrectomy. The reason for this discrepancy is thought to be excessive growth of fibrovascular proliferation during the waiting period. For this reason, the DRVS concluded that strong consideration should be given to immediate vitrectomy, especially in type 1 diabetics (in type 2 diabetics, the final visual results were similar). Nevertheless, many clinicians feel that in most cases vitrectomy should be deferred for about 6 months or longer if the retina is attached, to give a chance for spontaneous clearing to occur. Some patients will not need the surgery but, more importantly, 25% of the patients in the DRVS who received an immediate vitrectomy had a final visual acuity of no light perception. Exceptions to this general rule are patients who have bilateral visual loss because of vitreous hemorrhage, with chronically recurring hemorrhage, and known traction retinal detachment close to the macula. If surgery is deferred, ultrasonography and electroretinography should be performed at regular intervals to make sure that traction retinal detachment is not developing behind the hemorrhage.

The results of vitrectomy for nonclearing vitreous hemorrhage using this plan are excellent.

In patients who have recurrent vitreous hemorrhage after vitrectomy, a simple outpatient air–liquid exchange may restore vision without the need for a repeat vitrectomy.[55]

Traction retinal detachments are usually a much greater challenge. In general, unless the macula becomes involved, observation is the best therapy for these patients because, in most cases, the detachment does not progress into the macula. These patients should be counseled to consult their ophthalmologists without delay should macular vision suddenly be lost, because vitrectomy at that point becomes an urgent procedure. The surgical objectives are to clear the media, to release all anterior–posterior traction, to release tangential traction via delamination or segmentation (cutting the fibrotic bridges between areas of tractional detachment), and to perform endophotocoagulation to prevent NVI. The prognosis is best in patients who have small areas of traction. An alternative technique is to remove the vitreous and preretinal membranes by the "en bloc" technique.[56] The prognosis is poorest in eyes with table-top detachments, significant preoperative vitreous hemorrhage, no prior PRP, and advanced fibrovascular proliferation. If a lensectomy is required or if iatrogenic breaks are created, the results also are poorer.[57] Approximately 60–70% of patients have improved visual acuity and a final visual acuity of 20/800 or better, but 20–35% have decreased vision after vitrectomy. Cases with severe peripheral fibrovascular proliferation also may require a scleral buckling procedure.[58] Repeated operations are required in about 10% of patients, most commonly for rhegmatogenous retinal detachment and recurrent vitreous hemorrhage.[59]

In traction–rhegmatogenous retinal detachments, the objectives are to find all of the retinal breaks and to release all vitreous traction. After air–fluid exchange to flatten the retina, endolaser photocoagulation is used to treat retinal breaks. Approximately one half of such detachments can be cured. In severe cases, silicone oil is required to maintain reattachment of the retina.

The most common cause of failure following an otherwise successful vitrectomy is NVI resulting in neovascular glaucoma. The risk is higher if there is preoperative NVI (33% versus 17%), if there is persistent retinal detachment after surgery, if the lens is removed during surgery, and if there is florid NVD and retina. In

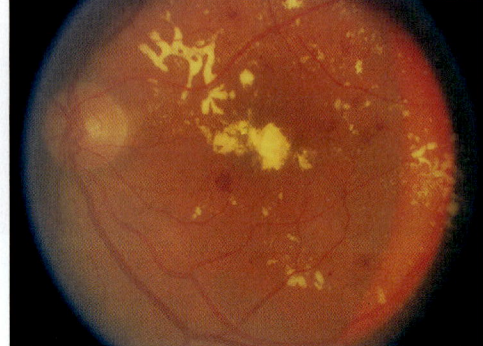

FIG. 117-9 Hard exudate plaque in the center of the macula.

eyes without these factors, the incidence of neovascular glaucoma is only about 2%. The pathogenesis of this complication is unknown. Some investigators feel that removal of the vitreous allows vasoproliferative factors produced in hypoxic retina to diffuse forward to the iris. Others feel that following vitrectomy increased oxygen diffusion occurs posteriorly out of the anterior chamber, thereby lowering its oxygen tension too far. Fortunately, if an eye does not develop iris neovascularization during the first 4–6 months after vitrectomy, it rarely does so later.[60]

Another vision-threatening complication is neovascularization that originates from the anterior retina and extends along the anterior hyaloid to the posterior lens surface (anterior hyaloidal fibrovascular proliferation).[61] This is more common in young, phakic diabetics who have extensive capillary nonperfusion.

CONCLUSIONS

The prognosis for diabetic retinopathy used to be dismal. Today, using timely laser photocoagulation as advocated by the Diabetic Retinopathy Study and the ETDRS, severe visual loss can be reduced by 95%. Nevertheless, many diabetics still become legally blind, because they are not examined regularly by an ophthalmologist. Prevention offers the most hope to diabetics. If blood glucose levels are controlled aggressively, both the onset of retinopathy and the pace of its progression are delayed significantly.

Although all agree that screening of asymptomatic diabetic patients is critical, the most cost-effective timing remains controversial. It generally is agreed that type 2 diabetics should be examined at the onset of their disease, then yearly thereafter. Type 1 diabetics do not have to be examined until 5 years into their disease course, but no sooner than puberty, then yearly thereafter. If retinopathy is detected, the frequency of examinations should be increased appropriately.

REFERENCES

1. Klein R, Klein B. Epidemiology of proliferative diabetic retinopathy. Diabetes Care. 1992;15:1875–91.
2. Klein R, Klein B, Moss S, et al. The Wisconsin epidemiologic study of diabetic retinopathy. XIV. Ten-year incidence and progression of diabetic retinopathy. Arch Ophthalmol. 1994;112:1217–28.
3. Yanko L, Goldbourt U, Michaelson C, et al. Prevalence and 15-year incidence of retinopathy and associated characteristics in middle-aged and elderly diabetic men. Br J Ophthalmol. 1983;67:759–65.
4. Kostraba JN, Dorman JS, Orchard TJ, et al. Contribution of diabetes duration before puberty to the development of microvascular complications in IDDM subjects. Diabetes Care. 1989;12:686–93.
5. Diabetes Control and Complications Trial Research Group. The effect of intensive diabetes treatment on the progression of diabetic retinopathy in insulin-dependent diabetes mellitus. Arch Ophthalmol. 1995;113:36–51.
6. United Kingdom Prospective Diabetes Study Group. Intensive blood-glucose control with sulfonylureas or insulin compared with conventional treatment and risk of complications in patients with type 2 diabetes. UKPDS 33. Lancet. 1998;352:837–53.
7. Klein R, Klein BEK, Moss SE, et al. The Wisconsin epidemiologic study of diabetic retinopathy. II. Prevalence and risk of diabetic retinopathy when age is less than 30 years. Arch Ophthalmol. 1984;102:520–6.
8. Rosenn B, Miodovnik M, Kranias G, et al. Progression of diabetic retinopathy in pregnancy: association with hypertension in pregnancy. Am J Obstet Gynecol. 1992;166:1214–8.
9. Frank RN. The aldose reductase controversy. Diabetes. 1994;43:169–72.
10. Pierce E, Foley E, Smith L. Regulation of vascular endothelial growth factor by oxygen in a model of retinopathy of prematurity. Ophthalmology. 1996;114:1219–28.
11. Aiello L, Avery R, Arrigg P, et al. Vascular endothelial growth factor in ocular fluid of patients with diabetic retinopathy and other retinal disorders. N Engl J Med. 1994;331:1480–7.
12. Adamis A, Shima D, Tolentino M, et al. Inhibition of VEGF prevents retinal ischemia associated iris neovascularization in non-human primate. Arch Ophthalmol. 1996;114:66–71.
13. Colwell J, Winocour P, Halushka P. Do platelets have anything to do with diabetic microvascular disease? Diabetes. 1983;32(suppl):14–9.
14. Early Treatment Diabetic Retinopathy Study Research Group. Fundus photographic risk factors for progression of diabetic retinopathy. ETDRS Report No. 12. Ophthalmology. 1991;98:823–33.
15. Early Treatment Diabetic Retinopathy Study Research Group. Early photocoagulation for diabetic retinopathy. ETDRS Report No. 9. Ophthalmology. 1991;98:766–85.
16. Davis M, Fisher M, Gangnon R. Vitreous contraction in proliferative diabetic retinopathy. Arch Ophthalmol. 1965;74:741–51.
17. Bresnick G, Haight B, deVenecia G. Retinal wrinkling and macular heterotopia in diabetic retinopathy. Arch Ophthalmol. 1979;97:1890–5.
18. Schwartz D. Corneal sensitivity in diabetics. Arch Ophthalmol. 1974;91:174–8.
19. Ohashi Y, Matsuda M, Hosotai H, et al. Aldose reductase inhibitor (CT-112) eye drops for diabetic corneal epitheliopathy. Am J Ophthalmol. 1988;105:223.
20. Klein B, Klein R, Jensen S. Open-angle glaucoma and older-onset diabetes: the Beaver Dam Eye Study. Ophthalmology. 1994;101:1173–7.
21. Tielsch J, Katz J, Quigley H, et al. Diabetes, intraocular pressure, and primary open-angle glaucoma in the Baltimore Eye Survey. Ophthalmology. 1995;102:48–53.
22. Jacobson D, Murphy R, Rosenthal A. The treatment of angle neovascularization with panretinal photocoagulation. Ophthalmology. 1979;86:1270–5.
23. Bernth-Peterson P, Bach E. Epidemiologic aspects of cataract surgery. III: Frequencies of diabetes and glaucoma in a cataract population. Acta Ophthalmol. 1983;61:406–16.
24. Krupsky S, Zalish M, Oliver M, et al. Anterior segment complications in diabetic patients following extracapsular cataract extraction and posterior chamber intraocular lens implantation. Ophthalmic Surg. 1991;22:526–30.
25. Hykin P, Gregson R, Stevens J, et al. Extracapsular cataract extraction in proliferative diabetic retinopathy. Ophthalmology. 1993;100:394–9.
26. Benson W, Brown G, Tasman W, et al. Extracapsular cataract extraction with placement of a posterior chamber lens in patients with diabetic retinopathy. Ophthalmology. 1993;100:730–8.
27. Pollack A, Leiba H, Bukelman A, et al. The course of diabetic retinopathy following cataract surgery in eyes previously treated by laser photocoagulation. Br J Ophthalmol. 1992;76:228–31.
28. Squirrell D, Bhola R, Bush J, et al. A prospective, case controlled study of the natural history of diabetic retinopathy and maculopathy after uncomplicated phacoemulsification cataract surgery in patients with type 2 diabetes. Br J Ophthalmol. 2002;86(5):565–71.
29. Krepler K, Biowski R, Schrey S, et al. Cataract surgery in patients with diabetic retinopathy: visual outcome, progression of diabetic retinopathy, and incidence of diabetic macular oedema. Graefes Arch Clin Exp Ophthalmol. 2002;240(9):735–8.
30. Regillo C, Brown G, Savino P, et al. Diabetic papillopathy: patient characteristics and fundus findings. Arch Ophthalmol. 1995;113:889–95.
31. Burde R. Neuro-ophthalmic associations and complications of diabetes mellitus. Am J Ophthalmol. 1992;114:498–501.
32. Pender P, Benson W, Compton H, et al. The effects of panretinal photocoagulation on dark adaptation in diabetics with proliferative retinopathy. Ophthalmology. 1981;88:635–8.
33. Kinnear P, Aspinall P, Lakowski R. The diabetic eye and colour vision. Trans Ophthalmol Soc U K. 1972;92:69–78.
34. Bresnick G, Palta M. Oscillatory potential amplitudes. Arch Ophthalmol. 1987;105:929–33.
35. Chew E, Klein M, Murphy R, et al. Effects of aspirin on vitreous/preretinal hemorrhage in patients with diabetes mellitus. ETDRS Report No. 20. Arch Ophthalmol. 1995;113:52–5.
36. United Kingdom Prospective Diabetes Study Group. Tight blood pressure control and risk of macrovascular and microvascular complications in type 2 diabetes. UKPDS 38. BMJ. 1998;317:703–13.
37. Chaturvedi N, Sjolie A, Stephenson J, et al. Effect of lisinopril on progression of retinopathy in normotensive people with type 1 diabetes. The EUCLID Study Group. EURODIAB controlled trial of lisinopril in insulin-dependent diabetes mellitus. Lancet. 1998;351:28–31.
38. Danis R, Bingaman D, Jirousak M, et al. Inhibition of intraocular neovascularization caused by retinal ischemia in pigs by PKC with LY333531. Invest Ophthalmol Vis Sci. 1998;39:171–9.
39. Diabetic Retinopathy Study Research Group. Four risk factors for severe visual loss in diabetic retinopathy: the third report from the Diabetic Retinopathy Study. Arch Ophthalmol. 1979;97:654–65.
40. Stefansson E, Machemer R, de Juan E, et al. Retinal oxygenation and laser treatment in patients with diabetic retinopathy. Am J Ophthalmol. 1992;113:36–8.
41. Krypton Argon Regression Neovascularization Study Research Group. Randomized comparison of krypton versus argon scatter photocoagulation for diabetic disc neovascularization. Ophthalmology. 1993;100:1655–64.
42. Reddy V, Zamora R, Olk R. Quantification of retinal ablation in proliferative diabetic retinopathy. Am J Ophthalmol. 1995;119:760–6.
43. Doft B, Metz D, Kelsey S. Augmentation laser for proliferative diabetic retinopathy that fails to respond to initial panretinal photocoagulation. Ophthalmology. 1992;99:1728–35.
44. Ferris F, Podgor M, Davis M, et al. Macular edema in diabetic retinopathy study patients. Diabetic Retinopathy Study Report No. 12. Ophthalmology. 1987;94:754–60.
45. Daily M, Gieser R. Treatment of proliferative diabetic retinopathy with panretinal cryotherapy. Ophthalmic Surg. 1984;15:741–5.
46. Patz A, Schatz H, Berkow J, et al. Macular edema: an overlooked complication of diabetic retinopathy. Trans Am Acad Ophthalmol Otolaryngol. 1973;77:34–42.
47. Early Treatment Diabetic Retinopathy Study Research Group. Focal photocoagulation treatment of diabetic macular edema. Relationship of treatment effect to fluorescein angiographic and other retinal characteristics at baseline: ETDRS Report No. 19. Arch Ophthalmol. 1995;113:1144–55.
48. Martidis A, Duker JS, Greenberg PB, et al. Intravitreal triamcinolone for refractory diabetic macular edema. Ophthalmology. 2002;109(5):920–7.
49. Jonas JB, Kreissig I, Sofker A, Degenring RF. Intravitreal injection of triamcinolone for diffuse diabetic macular edema. Arch Ophthalmol. 2003;121(1):57–61.
50. Ferris F. How effective are treatments for diabetic retinopathy? JAMA. 1993;269:1290–1.
51. Javitt J, Aiello L, Bassi L, et al. Detecting and treating retinopathy in patients with type I diabetes mellitus. Ophthalmology. 1991;98:1565–74.
52. Lewis H, Abrams G, Blumenkranz M, et al. Vitrectomy for diabetic macular traction and edema associated with posterior hyaloidal traction. Ophthalmology. 1992;99:753–9.

53. Diabetic Retinopathy Vitrectomy Study Research Group. Early vitrectomy for severe proliferative diabetic retinopathy in eyes with useful vision. Results of a randomized trial—diabetic retinopathy vitrectomy study report 3. Ophthalmology. 1988;95:1307–20.

54. Diabetic Retinopathy Vitrectomy Study Research Group. Early vitrectomy for severe vitreous hemorrhage in diabetic retinopathy. Two-year results of a randomized trial. Diabetic retinopathy vitrectomy study report 2. Arch Ophthalmol. 1985;103:1644–54.

55. Martin D, McCuen II B. Efficacy of fluid–air exchange for postvitrectomy diabetic vitreous hemorrhage. Am J Ophthalmol. 1992;114:457–63.

56. Williams D, Williams G, Hartz A. Results of vitrectomy for diabetic traction retinal detachments using the en bloc excision technique. Ophthalmology. 1989;96:752–8.

57. Thompson J, deBustros S, Michels R, et al. Results and prognostic factors in vitrectomy for diabetic vitreous hemorrhage. Arch Ophthalmol. 1987;105:191–5.

58. Han D, Pulido J, Mieler W, et al. Vitrectomy for proliferative diabetic retinopathy with severe equatorial fibrovascular proliferation. Am J Ophthalmol. 1995;119:563–70.

59. Brown G, Tasman W, Benson W, et al. Reoperation following diabetic vitrectomy. Arch Ophthalmol. 1992;110:506–10.

60. Schachat A, Oyakawa R, Michels R, et al. Complications of vitreous surgery from diabetic retinopathy. II. Postoperative complications. Ophthalmology. 1983;90:522.

61. Lewis H, Aarberg T, Abrams G. Causes of failures after repeat vitreoretinal surgery for recurrent proliferative vitreoretinopathy. Am J Ophthalmol. 1991;111:15–9.

118 Ocular Ischemic Syndrome

MATTHEW T.S. TENNANT • ARUNAN SIVALINGAM • GREGORY M. FOX • GARY C. BROWN

DEFINITION
- Ocular signs and symptoms secondary to severe, chronic arterial hypoperfusion.

KEY FEATURES
- Visual loss.
- Blot retinal hemorrhages.
- Dilated, beaded retinal veins.
- Decreased ocular perfusion pressure.
- Ocular neovascularization.
- Severe ipsilateral or bilateral carotid artery obstruction.

ASSOCIATED FEATURES
- Pain or ocular angina.
- Neovascular glaucoma.
- Corneal edema and striae.
- Mild anterior uveitis.
- Cherry-red spot in macula.
- Cotton-wool spots.
- Spontaneous pulsations of retinal arteries.
- Ischemic optic neuropathy.

INTRODUCTION

Ocular ischemic syndrome is a condition that has a variable spectrum of signs and symptoms that result from chronic ocular hypoperfusion, usually secondary to severe carotid artery obstruction. Ocular signs and symptoms secondary to severe carotid artery obstruction, described in 1963 by Kearns and Hollenhorst,[1] initially was called *venous stasis retinopathy*. Because other authors employed same the term to describe nonischemic central retinal vein occlusion,[2] an entirely different condition, this nomenclature is best avoided. Additional names given to this condition include hypoperfusion retinopathy, hypotensive retinopathy, ischemic ocular inflammation,[3] and ischemic oculopathy.[4]

EPIDEMIOLOGY AND PATHOGENESIS

The ocular ischemic syndrome occurs at a mean age of 65 years and generally does not develop before 50 years of age. Men who have this condition outnumber affected women by a ratio of 2:1, which reflects the higher incidence of atherosclerotic cardiovascular disease in men. No racial predilection exists. Bilateral involvement occurs in 20% of cases.[5] The incidence of ocular ischemic syndrome is not known precisely but is estimated at 7.5 cases per million population annually based on the work of Sturrock and Mueller.[6] Approximately 5% of patients who have hemodynamically significant carotid artery disease develop ocular ischemic syndrome.

The pathogenesis of the syndrome is decreased arterial inflow on a chronic basis. The period and extent of the impaired blood flow necessary to develop this syndrome still is not clear. Using color Doppler imaging, Ho et al.[7] were able to study blood flow velocity and vascular resistance in the ocular circulation. Reversal of ophthalmic artery flow was demonstrated in 12 of 16 eyes studied, and all the studied eyes that had ocular ischemic syndrome had decreased peak systolic flow velocities of the central retinal artery. Reversal of flow within the ophthalmic artery represents collateralization through the external carotid artery system in response to obstructions in the internal carotid artery system. Moreover, Ho et al.[7] were able to show that eyes that have significant visual loss demonstrate posterior ciliary artery hypoperfusion. Therefore, secondary ischemia of the optic nerve, choroid, retinal pigment epithelium, and outer segments of the photoreceptors is likely to result in the visual loss seen in ocular ischemic syndrome. Experimental blood flow studies of McFadzean et al.[8] corroborate these findings, which suggest that posterior ciliary arterial hypoperfusion results in visual loss in ocular ischemic syndrome. In rare cases, color Doppler imaging detects isolated ophthalmic artery stenosis in patients who have ocular ischemic syndrome but no carotid artery disease.

OCULAR MANIFESTATIONS

Symptoms

Loss of vision is present in over 90% of affected patients at the time of evaluation.[5] The visual loss generally occurs gradually, over a period of weeks to months, but can occur abruptly. Approximately 5% of patients have a previous history of amaurosis fugax.

The severity of the visual loss is variable.[5] About 35% of affected eyes at the time of evaluation have a visual acuity of 20/40 (6/12) or better, while 30% range from 20/50 (6/15) to 20/400 (6/120). In the remaining 35%, acuity is sufficient to count fingers or worse. The absence of light perception is an uncommon finding initially but may develop as a sequela of severe posterior segment ischemia, often in combination with neovascular glaucoma. A prolonged time for recovery of vision after exposure to bright lights may occur in patients who have posterior segment ischemia.

A dull ache over the eye or brow is reported by up to 40% of patients who have ocular ischemic syndrome.[5] The pain results from either ischemia of the globe or elevated intraocular pressure (IOP) caused by neovascular glaucoma. The pain associated with ocular ischemic syndrome, especially when IOP is normal, has been called ocular angina.

Anterior Segment

Anterior segment findings in ocular ischemic syndrome are common. Corneal edema and striae may not be present unless an increased pressure from neovascular glaucoma also is present. Approximately two thirds of eyes that have ocular ischemic syndrome have neovascularization of the iris at the time of initial examination by the ophthalmologist.[5] However, this percentage may be deceptively high, because those who have asymptomatic milder involvement may not visit the ophthalmologist. In severe cases, ectropion uvea may develop. Flare in the anterior chamber commonly accompanies iris neovascularization. Iris neovas-

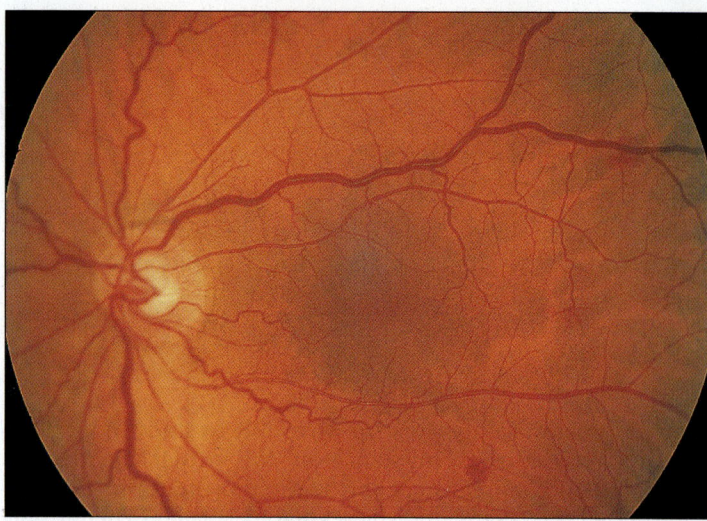

FIG. 118-1 ■ **Retinal vascular changes in ocular ischemic syndrome.** Narrowed retinal arteries; dilated, minimally tortuous retinal veins; and blot retinal hemorrhages are present in an eye that is affected by ocular ischemic syndrome.

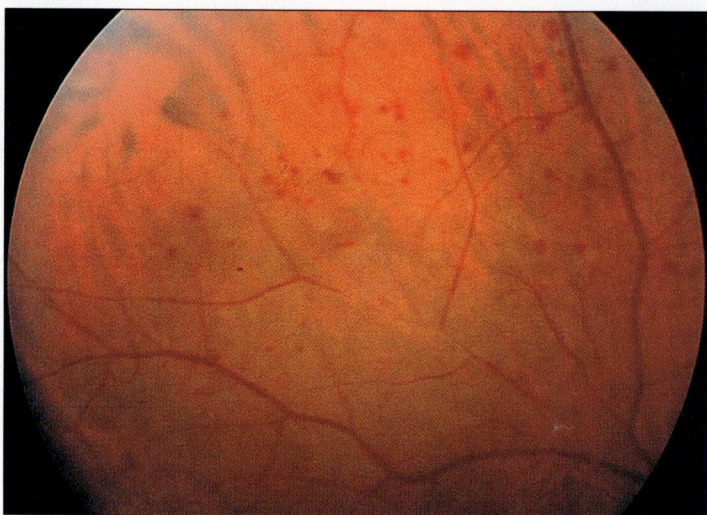

FIG. 118-2 ■ **Retinal hemorrhages in ocular ischemic syndrome.** Dot and blot hemorrhages, as well as microaneurysms, are seen commonly in the midperiphery of eyes that are affected by ocular ischemic syndrome.

cularization in the eye of a nondiabetic, with no evidence of venous occlusive disease or other predisposing cause, is suggestive of ocular ischemic syndrome.

Neovascular glaucoma, defined as neovascularization of the iris and an IOP greater than 22mmHg, is seen in only one half of the patients with ocular ischemia who have neovascularization of the iris.[5] Some patients who have neovascularization of the iris may develop complete closure of the anterior chamber angle with fibrovascular tissue, but the IOP remains normal. This phenomenon probably results from impaired ciliary body perfusion and decreased aqueous humor production as a consequence of carotid stenosis.

Anterior uveitis in eyes that have ocular ischemic syndrome has been described well.[3] Iritis, present in 20% of these eyes, is generally mild. Flare is a more prominent feature than the cellular response, and keratitic precipitates are seen infrequently. In patients over 50 years of age who have new-onset iritis, the possibility of ocular ischemic syndrome must be considered.

Lens opacification, even formation of a mature cataract, may occur in the end stages of ocular ischemic syndrome. However, often at the time of evaluation little difference exists in the incidence of cataract between affected eyes and fellow eyes.[5]

Posterior Segment

Signs in the posterior segment provide important clinical clues that suggest this diagnosis. Numerous signs can be seen in the fundus, which include the following:

• Retinal arterial narrowing
• Retinal venous dilation without tortuosity
• Retinal hemorrhages and microaneurysms
• Neovascularization of the optic disc or retina
• Cherry-red spot
• Cotton-wool spots
• Spontaneous pulsations of the retinal arteries

Retinal arterial narrowing and straightening, commonly associated with areas of focal constriction, are seen in eyes that have ocular ischemic syndrome. These signs can be difficult to differentiate from the narrowed vessels commonly seen in the elderly. Dilated retinal veins are seen frequently in eyes that display ocular ischemic syndrome. In ocular ischemic syndrome retinal veins also may have significant beading, similar to eyes that have preproliferative or proliferative diabetic retinopathy. In contrast to eyes that have central retinal venous occlusion, retinal venous tortuosity is not a prominent feature (Fig. 118-1). Retinal hemorrhages are seen in 80% of eyes, most characteristically of a dot and blot variety located in the midperiphery, but they can extend into the posterior pole (Fig. 118-2). Microaneurysms also

are seen in the same locations. Neovascularization, which ranges from mild to severe, may occur on the optic disc in over one third of patients who have ocular ischemic syndrome.[5] Retinal neovascularization has been described in 8% of eyes.

During examination, a cherry-red spot is seen in 12% of eyes that display ocular ischemic syndrome.[5] This finding most commonly occurs as the IOP from neovascular glaucoma exceeds the central retinal artery's perfusion pressure. Cotton-wool spots and spontaneous pulsations of the retinal arteries are each found in 5% of eyes that have the syndrome.[5] When not present spontaneously, retinal arterial pulsations can be elicited easily by minimal pressure on the globe, because of the severe diminution in ocular perfusion pressure. In contrast, eyes that have nonischemic central retinal venous occlusion require a normal amount of digital pressure to induce retinal arterial pulsations.[9] In the past, ocular plethysmography was performed to assess ocular perfusion pressure quantitatively. It rarely is used now.

Ischemic optic neuropathy, which appears with acute, pale swelling of the disc, has been reported in an eye affected by ocular ischemic syndrome.[10] Otherwise, the optic disc tends to be normal in appearance, unlike the disc edema seen with central retinal vein obstruction.

DIAGNOSIS AND ANCILLARY TESTING

In addition to clinical examination, fluorescein angiography can help to establish the diagnosis of ocular ischemic syndrome. Ideally, a delay in arm-to-choroid and arm-to-retina circulation times is demonstrated by fluorescein angiography, but variation in the location and speed of injection may make these times difficult to assess. However, demonstration of a well-demarcated leading edge of fluorescein dye within a retinal artery is very unusual for a normal eye and suggests ocular hypoperfusion (Fig. 118-3). Patchy filling of the choroid that lasts more than 5 seconds is seen in about 60% of eyes affected by ocular ischemic syndrome (Fig. 118-4).[5]

Other findings on fluorescein angiography include an increased arteriovenous transit time, staining of the retinal vessels, macular edema, retinal capillary nonperfusion, and evidence of microaneurysms (especially in the periphery). The arteriovenous transit time exceeds 11 seconds in approximately 95% of affected eyes.[5] Late staining of retinal vessels, more prominent in arterioles than in venules, is present in about 85% of cases (Fig. 118-5).[5]

Electroretinography demonstrates a decrease in both the a waves and b waves in eyes that are affected by ocular ischemic syndrome, in contrast to the sparing of the a wave found in central retinal artery occlusions.[11] The choroidal and outer retinal ischemia of eyes that have ocular ischemic syndrome accounts for this difference.

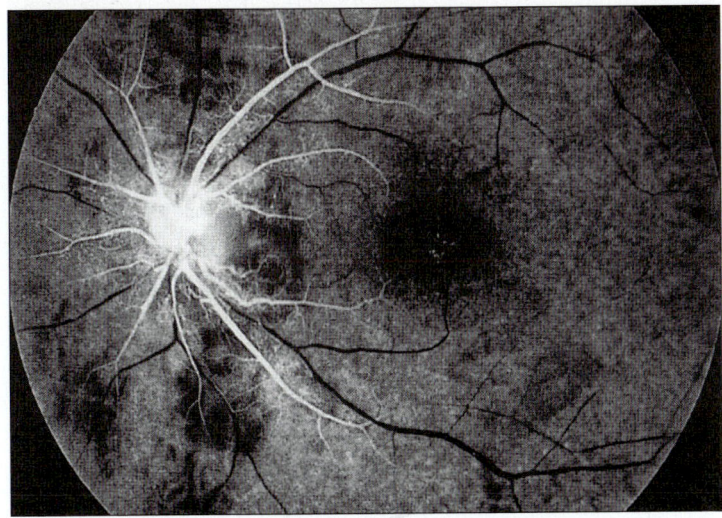

FIG. 118-3 ■ **Fluorescein angiography, ocular ischemic syndrome.** A distinctly abnormal finding in a fluorescein angiogram of eyes that are affected by ocular ischemic syndrome is a well-demarcated leading edge of dye within the retinal arteries.

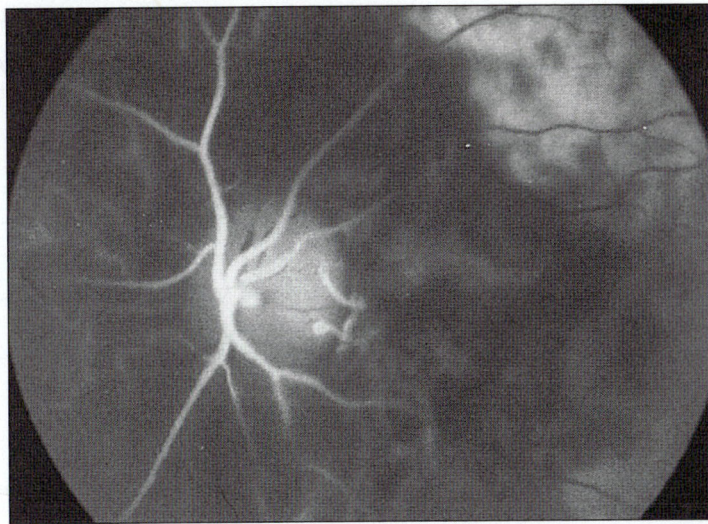

FIG. 118-4 ■ **Patchy choroidal filling, ocular ischemic syndrome.** Patchy choroidal filling that lasts more than 5 seconds occurs in about 60% of eyes affected by ocular ischemic syndrome.

Color Doppler imaging is an excellent noninvasive means by which to assess the velocity of blood flow in the retrobulbar circulation. Diminution of blood flow velocities in the central retinal artery, choroidal vessels, and ophthalmic artery is typical. Reversal of flow in the ophthalmic artery is common, as well. Color Doppler imaging may be used to assess the carotid arteries simultaneously.

Carotid arteriography discloses generally a 90% or greater obstruction of the ipsilateral carotid artery in patients who have ocular ischemic syndrome. If noninvasive carotid artery evaluation is unremarkable in an eye that shows signs suggestive of ocular ischemia, conventional carotid arteriography or digital subtraction angiography may be required to demonstrate possible chronic obstruction of the ophthalmic artery.[11-13] Rarely, cases of ocular ischemia may be induced by a more distal obstruction in the ophthalmic artery itself.

DIFFERENTIAL DIAGNOSIS

Nonischemic central retinal venous occlusions and diabetic retinopathy are conditions most likely to be confused with ocular ischemic syndrome. Various ocular signs help to differentiate these conditions, as given in Table 118-1. One particularly useful differentiating feature is a swollen optic disc, which typically is seen in nonischemic vein occlusions and not in ocular ischemic syndrome. In addition, central retinal vein occlusions typically have dilated and tortuous retinal veins. Although microaneurysms may occur in both diabetes and ocular ischemic syndrome, in diabetes they tend to involve the posterior pole preferentially. On rare occasions, giant cell arteritis may induce findings similar to those of ocular ischemic syndrome. In general, however, giant cell arteritis has a much more dramatic clinical picture, with ischemic optic neuropathy or retinal artery occlusion, or both.

Takayasu's Arteritis

Takayasu's arteritis, also known as aortic arch syndrome or pulseless disease, is an idiopathic inflammation of larger elastic and muscular arteries—the aorta is affected in particular. It is primarily a disease of young adults, especially women, and is most prevalent in the Far East. Constitutional symptoms are common, including fever, fatigue, and weight loss.

The ocular manifestations can mimic those of ocular ischemic syndrome. Retinal arterial narrowing, large arteriovenous anastomoses, and peripheral microaneurysms are common. Retinal neovascularization with vitreous hemorrhage may occur. Systemic corticosteroids are the treatment of choice.

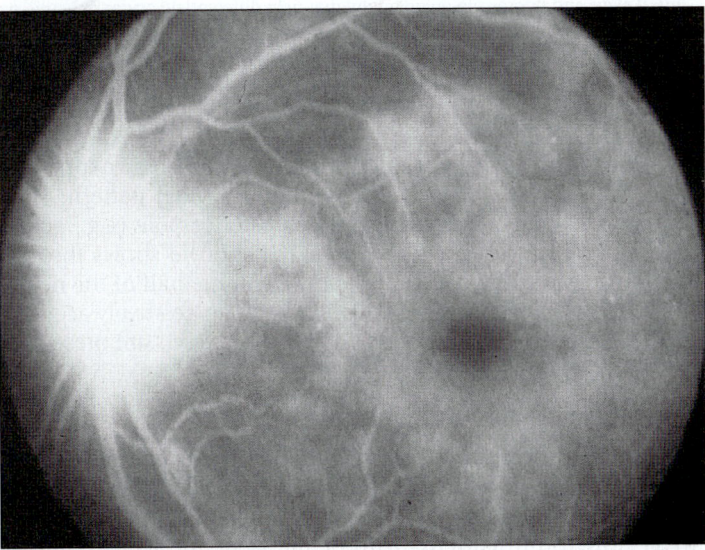

FIG. 118-5 ■ **Staining of retinal arteries, ocular ischemic syndrome.** Prominent staining of retinal arteries, rather than venules, can help to differentiate an eye that has ocular ischemic syndrome from an eye that is affected by a nonischemic central retinal vein occlusion (which shows more prominent staining of the venules).

SYSTEMIC ASSOCIATIONS

The atherosclerosis that affects the carotid artery sufficiently to cause ocular ischemic syndrome generally is widespread. Of patients who have ocular ischemic syndrome, 50% show evidence of ischemic heart disease; and 25% have a history of previous cerebrovascular accidents.[14]

Additional risk factors for both atherosclerosis and arteriosclerosis are found in these patients, such as systemic hypertension, which is found in two thirds of patients who have ocular ischemic syndrome, and diabetes mellitus, which is observed in more than 50% of these patients.[14]

A 5-year mortality of 40% in patients who have ocular ischemic syndrome reflects the severity of their systemic vascular disease. The main cause of death in these patients is ischemic heart disease, with stroke the second most common cause.

PATHOLOGY

In the early stage of the ocular ischemic syndrome, the neural retina shows coagulative necrosis of its inner layers, which are supplied by the retinal arterioles. If the area of coagulative necrosis is small and localized, it appears clinically as a cotton-wool spot, a microinfarct of the nerve fiber layer. Histologically, the

TABLE 118-1

FEATURES THAT DISTINGUISH OCULAR ISCHEMIC SYNDROME

Feature	Ocular Ischemic Syndrome	Nonischemic Central Retinal Vein Occlusion	Diabetic Retinopathy
Laterality	80% unilateral	Unilateral	Bilateral
Age (years)	50–80	50–80	Variable
FUNDUS SIGNS			
Veins	Dilated, nontortuous	Dilated, tortuous	Dilated, beaded
Optic disc	Normal	Swollen	Normal
Retinal artery perfusion pressure	Decreased	Normal	Normal
Retinal hemorrhages	Mild	Mild to severe	Mild to moderate
Microaneurysms	Midperiphery	Variable	Posterior pole
Hard exudates	Absent unless in association with diabetes	Rare	Common
FLUORESCEIN ANGIOGRAPHY			
Choroidal filling	Delayed, patchy	Normal	Normal
Arteriovenous transit time	Prolonged	Prolonged	Normal
Retinal vessel staining	Prominent arterial staining	Prominent venous staining	Absent (usually)

Clinical signs and fluorescein angiography that help differentiate ocular ischemic syndrome from nonischemic central retinal vein occlusions or diabetic retinopathy.

swollen end-bulbs of the infarcted nerve fiber layer superficially resemble cells, hence the term *cytoid body*. If the area of coagulative necrosis is extensive, it appears clinically as a gray neural retinal area, blotting out the background choroidal pattern. With complete coagulative necrosis of the posterior pole (e.g., after a central retinal artery occlusion), the red choroid shows through the central fovea as a cherry-red spot. The inner half of the neural retina becomes "homogenized" into a diffuse, relatively acellular zone. Generally, thick-walled retinal blood vessels are present.

TREATMENT, COURSE, AND OUTCOME

Patients who have mild ocular ischemic syndrome may maintain excellent vision, but the natural course of eyes that have the full-blown syndrome is quite poor.[15] Assessment of carotid artery function in patients with ocular ischemic syndrome is of utmost importance. The North American Symptomatic Carotid Endarterectomy Trial demonstrated that carotid endarterectomy was beneficial for patients with carotid stenosis of 70–99% with a recent history of amaurosis fugax, a hemispheric transient ischemic attack, or a nondisabling stroke. The cumulative risk of ipsilateral stroke was 26% after 2 years for patients receiving antiplatelet treatment, while the cumulative risk of stroke was 9% 2 years after endarterectomy.[16] The benefit of endarterectomy was tempered by a 2.1% risk of severe stroke or death during the immediate postoperative period in the patients who underwent surgery versus 0.9% in the antiplatelet group. In symptomatic patients with carotid artery stenosis of 50–69%, only a moderate reduction in risk of stroke was identified after carotid endarterectomy.[17]

Stabilization or improvement in vision has been reported in about 25% of eyes after endarterectomy.[15] Doppler color imaging has shown postoperative normalization of preoperative retrograde ophthalmic artery flow following endarterectomy.[18] Electroretinogram a waves and b waves have improved with increased amplitude following endarterectomy.[19] Occasionally, in eyes that have ciliary body hypoperfusion, complete angle closure, and normal IOP, carotid endarterectomy has resulted in severe glaucoma immediately after surgery. In cases in which 100% obstruction and distal propagation of a thrombus has occurred, bypass procedures, such as superficial temporal artery to middle cerebral artery, have been attempted. Although the vision improves transiently in 20% of such eyes, it usually deteriorates within 1 year of surgery.[15]

In cases that have iris neovascularization in which the anterior chamber angle is open, panretinal photocoagulation may induce regression of the rubeosis. Unfortunately, the regression is not as prominent as that seen in patients who have iris neovascularization after central retinal vein occlusion.[20] Elevated IOP from neovascular glaucoma may require cyclodestructive therapies or filtering procedures.

REFERENCES

1. Kearns TP, Hollenhorst RW. Venous stasis retinopathy of occlusive disease of the carotid artery. Mayo Clin Proc. 1963;38:304–12.
2. Hayreh SS. So-called "central retinal vein occlusion." Venous stasis retinopathy. Ophthalmologica. 1976;172:14–37.
3. Knox DL. Ischemic ocular inflammation. Am J Ophthalmol. 1965;60:995–1002.
4. Young LHY, Appen RE. Ischemic oculopathy: a manifestation of carotid artery disease. Arch Neurol. 1981;38:358–61.
5. Brown GC, Magargal LE. The ocular ischemic syndrome: clinical, fluorescein angiographic and carotid angiographic features. Int Ophthalmol. 1988;11:239–51.
6. Sturrock GD, Mueller HR. Chronic ocular ischaemia. Br J Ophthalmol. 1984;68:716–23.
7. Ho AC, Lieb WE, Flaharty PM, et al. Color Doppler imaging of the ocular ischemic syndrome. Ophthalmology. 1992;99:1453–62.
8. McFadzean RM, Graham DI, Lee WR, Mendelow AD. Ocular blood flow in unilateral carotid stenosis and hypotension. Invest Ophthalmol Vis Sci. 1989;30:487–90.
9. Kearns TP. Differential diagnosis of central retinal vein obstruction. Ophthalmology. 1983;90:475–80.
10. Brown GC. Anterior ischemic optic neuropathy occurring in association with carotid artery obstruction. J Clin Neurol Ophthalmol. 1986;6:39–42.
11. Brown GC, Magargal LE, Simeone FA, et al. Arterial obstruction and ocular neovascularization. Ophthalmology. 1982;89:139–46.
12. Bullock JD, Falter RT, Downing JE, Snyder HE. Ischemic ophthalmia secondary to ophthalmic artery occlusion. 1972;74:486–93.
13. Madsen PH. Venous-stasis retinopathy insufficiency of the ophthalmic artery. Acta Ophthalmol. 1966;44:940–7.
14. Sivalingham A, Brown GC, Magargal LE, Menduke H. The ocular ischemic syndrome. II. Mortality and systemic morbidity. Int Ophthalmol. 1990;13:187–91.
15. Sivalingham A, Brown GC, Magargal LE. The ocular ischemic syndrome. III. Visual prognosis and the effect of treatment. Int Ophthalmol. 1991;15:15–20.
16. North American Symptomatic Carotid Endarterectomy Trial Collaborators. Beneficial effect of carotid endarterectomy in symptomatic patients with high-grade carotid stenosis. N Engl J Med. 1991;325:445–53.
17. Barnett HJM, Taylor DW, Eliasziw M, et al. Benefit of carotid endarterectomy in patients with symptomatic moderate or severe stenosis. N Engl J Med. 1998;339:1415–25.
18. Kawaguchi S, Okuno S, Sakaki T, Nishikawa N. Effect of carotid endarterectomy on ocular ischemic syndrome due to internal carotid artery stenosis. Neurosurgery. 2001;48:328–33.
19. Story JL, Held KS, Harrison JM, et al. The ocular ischemic syndrome in carotid artery occlusive disease: ophthalmic color Doppler flow velocity and electroretinographic changes following carotid endarterectomy reconstruction. Surg Neurol. 1995;44:534–5.
20. Eggleston TF, Bohling CA, Eggleston HC, Hershey FB. Photocoagulation for ocular ischemia associated with carotid artery occlusion. Ann Ophthalmol. 1980;12:84–7.

CHAPTER 119

Hemoglobinopathies

ALLEN C. HO

DEFINITION
- A spectrum of ocular abnormalities, including peripheral "sea fan" retinal neovascularization, that results from an inherited defect in the synthesis of the hemoglobin molecule.

KEY FEATURES
- Macular ischemia.
- Retinal vascular peripheral nonperfusion.
- Retinal hemorrhages: "salmon patches," "iridescent spots," and "black sunbursts."
- Peripheral retinal neovascularization: "sea fans."

ASSOCIATED FEATURES
- Conjunctival comma-shaped capillaries.
- Iris atrophy and posterior synechiae.
- Sickle disc sign.
- Macular depression sign.
- Arteriovenous anastomoses.
- Vitreous hemorrhage.
- Retinal detachment.

INTRODUCTION

Normal red blood cell hemoglobin comprises four polypeptide globin chains, each associated with a central heme ring (ferroprotoporphyrin).[1] The globin chains consist of an identical pair of β polypeptide chains and an identical pair of β polypeptide chains. The sickle-cell hemoglobinopathies are characterized by a genetic error in β chain synthesis, which results in abnormal function of the hemoglobin molecule. Under certain circumstances, the imperfect globin chains induce pathological alterations in red blood cell morphology. These occur particularly in conditions of ischemia and metabolic stress. Owing to their crescent shape, the altered red blood cells are labeled "sickle cells."

Systemic and ocular sequelae are well described. Interestingly, the severity of systemic symptoms does not typically correlate with the severity of ocular manifestations. The most severe systemic complications are observed in sickle SS disease, while severe ocular features are most commonly noted in patients with sickle SC or sickle thalassemia (S-Thal) disease. In general, vision-threatening sequelae of the sickle hemoglobinopathies are secondary to ischemia or peripheral retinal neovascularization.

EPIDEMIOLOGY AND PATHOGENESIS

Hemoglobinopathies can be characterized electrophoretically as well as by the genetic mutations that lead to abnormal amino acid substitutions in the β globin chain. Normal adult hemoglobin with two normal α and β chains is termed hemoglobin A. Sickle hemoglobin, known as S, was initially described by Pauling and others in 1949 as a single point mutation that results in substitution of the amino acid valine for glutamic acid at the sixth position. The substitution of lysine for glutamic acid at this position results in the manufacture of hemoglobin C. The sickle hemoglobinopathies are caused by qualitative errors in globin chain synthesis. Inadequate production of either normal or abnormal globin chains, a quantitative error in globin synthesis, is referred to as thalassemia (Thal).

Because these mutations are inherited, heterozygous and homozygous conditions exist. For example, normal hemoglobin comprises normal homozygous AA globin chains. Classic sickle cell anemia, or SS disease, usually arises when two parents who have sickle trait (AS) disease each pass on their single abnormal S globin chain mutation. If hemoglobin S is inherited from one parent and hemoglobin C from another, a double heterozygous form of hemoglobin, known as sickle SC disease, is created.

Thalassemia mutations can coexist with normal hemoglobin A or with various abnormal hemoglobin chains to produce double heterozygotes, such as those with S-Thal disease. In the United States, African-Americans account for the majority of patients afflicted by the hemoglobinopathies. In this population, the prevalence of sickle trait disease is estimated to be in the range of 5–10%. Clinical sickle AC disease is believed to afflict up to 5% of this group; double heterozygotes—such as those with SS (afflicting approximately 0.4%), SC (approximately 0.1–0.3%), and S-Thal (approximately 0.5–1.0%)—are all less common than those who have at least one normal globin A chain.[2]

Normal hemoglobin confers pliability to the oval-shaped red blood cells, which allows them to pass easily through the microvasculature, where they deliver oxygen. Sickle hemoglobins, such as hemoglobin SS, result in red blood cells with a crescentic, elongated shape, particularly under conditions of hypoxia or acidosis. This causes the blood cells to stack, which further exacerbates local ischemia. A vicious circle of ischemia, red blood cell sickling, tissue hypoxia, and necrosis is set in motion.

Although sickle SS disease has the most severe systemic manifestations, hemoglobin SC and S-Thal have the most severe ocular manifestations. The reasons for this discrepancy are not clear. The more severe anemia of SS disease is associated with red blood cell counts lower than those in hemoglobin SC and S-Thal disease. Relative anemia may leave the remaining red blood cells less disposed to sludging in the circulation.

Because many of the ocular complications of sickle disease are time dependent, their overall prevalence is unknown. From a cross-sectional study, the incidence of proliferative sickle retinopathy (PSR) has been estimated. Approximately 40% of hemoglobin SC patients and 20% of hemoglobin SS patients can be expected to develop PSR.[3]

The hemoglobinopathies described here constitute only a small sampling of the reported mutants of hemoglobin production. Originally, the abnormal hemoglobin chains were described with letters such as S and C. The subsequent explosion of descriptions of globin chain mutants has led to other names, including some that use the geographical location where the hemoglobin was discovered (e.g., hemoglobin Zurich).[1]

OCULAR MANIFESTATIONS

Nearly all ocular or periocular structures can be affected by the sickle hemoglobinopathies. Classic anterior segment findings include conjunctival comma-shaped capillaries that represent intravascular sludging of sickling red blood cells[4] (Fig. 119-1). Sectorial iris atrophy represents areas of anterior uveal ischemia. Associated anterior or posterior synechiae may occur. A mild anterior chamber cell and flare reaction may be observed secondary to incompetence of the blood-ocular barrier. The anterior segment manifestations generally do not pose significant risks for vision loss.

Posterior segment manifestations of sickle hemoglobinopathies may be observed in the vitreous body, optic disc, retina, and subretinal structures. Vitreous hemorrhage secondary to peripheral retinal neovascularization may develop. The optic disc may demonstrate sludging red blood cells within prepapillary retinal capillaries, which appear as small, dark spots or vascular lines on the surface of the optic disc head.[5] The "macular depression sign" presumably represents atrophy and thinning of the neural macula, which results in an oval depression of the bright central reflex[6] (Fig. 119-2, A). Red-free illumination highlights the macular depression sign; this area of macular ischemia may be associated with a decrease in vision. More debilitating macular ischemia can result in frank macular infarction with an enlarged foveal avascular zone secondary to multiple retinal arteriolar occlusions.[7-9] This type of macular ischemia may have an insidious, progressive course. Fluorescein angiography reveals irregularity in or enlargement of the foveal avascular zone, with adjacent areas of retinal capillary nonperfusion and retinal vascular remodeling (see Fig. 119-2, B). Retinal arterial microaneurysms are less commonly observed, although cotton-wool spots in the posterior segment are not uncommon.

Both nonproliferative and proliferative forms of sickle retinopathy may be observed, including nonspecific, nonproliferative retinal vascular changes, such as retinal arteriolar sclerosis and venous tortuosity. Retinal arteriolar sclerosis may be observed in areas where there is diffuse capillary nonperfusion that reflects prior retinal vascular occlusion. Venous tortuosity is observed in as many as half of all patients who have SS disease and in one third of patients who have SC disease. Neither of these retinal findings is pathognomonic of sickle retinopathy, since they are observed in a variety of other conditions. Angioid streaks are described in association with sickle-cell disease.

Other nonproliferative retinal findings are more characteristic of sickle hemoglobinopathies.[10-12] Salmon-colored retinal hemorrhages are preretinal or superficial intraretinal hemorrhages that occur adjacent to a retinal arteriole and are often found in the equatorial retina (Fig. 119-3). Histopathologically, they dissect into the vitreous cavity or into the subretinal space.[13] The salmon hue is attributed to an evolution of color changes; the initial presentation is bright red. These hemorrhages are believed to result from the rupture of a medium-sized retinal arteriole due to ischemic vasculopathy. They usually resolve with few sequelae, although a retinoschisis cavity lined with iridescent refractile yellow particles may persist. The schisis cavity is created by resorption of the intraretinal hemorrhage, and the iridescent particles represent macrophages that have engulfed hemoglobin and blood breakdown products.[14]

If the intraretinal hemorrhage dissects into the subneural retinal space and disturbs the retinal pigment epithelium, a black sunburst lesion may result (Fig. 119-4). These dark, irregularly shaped, spiculated or stellate lesions are the result of retinal pigment epithelial hyperplasia and intraretinal migration.[13,14] Because they are secondary to equatorial retinal hemorrhages, they are located in the same area and generally do not result in significant visual symptoms.

Because PSR can lead to severe vision loss, it was classified into five stages by Goldberg.[2,12,15] This progression of retinopathy typically occurs in the third or fourth decade of life but has been noted as early as the second decade. The five stages are as follows:
1. Peripheral arteriolar occlusions
2. Arteriolar-venular anastomoses
3. Neovascular proliferation
4. Vitreous hemorrhage
5. Retinal detachment

Peripheral retinal arteriolar occlusion can leave large areas of anterior retinal capillary nonperfusion, which is highlighted well by fluorescein angiography. Curiously, retinal venous occlusion is uncommon in patients who have sickle-cell disease. Occluded arterioles initially appear dark red but subsequently evolve into "silver wire" vessels. Peripheral arteriolar-venular

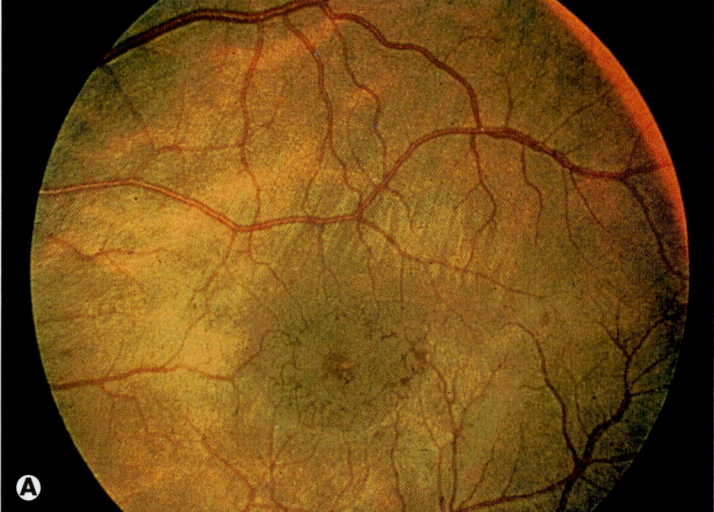

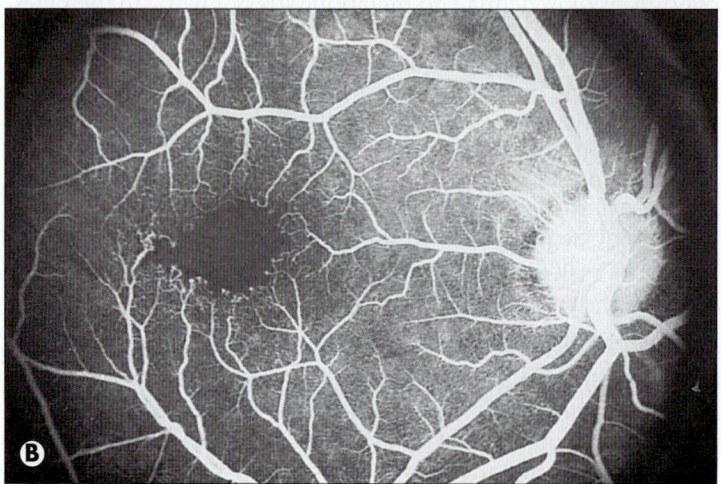

FIG. 119-1 ■ **A classic anterior segment finding in sickle eye disease is comma- or S-shaped conjunctival capillaries.** These vessels represent areas of red blood cell sickling or sludging within the capillary bed. (Courtesy of William Tasman, MD.)

FIG. 119-2 ■ **Sickle SC disease. A,** Macular ischemia with the macular depression sign and perifoveal vascular remodeling. **B,** Fluorescein angiogram of the same patient demonstrating an irregular and moth-eaten perifoveal capillary network and vascular telangiectasia. (Courtesy of William Tasman, MD.)

anastomoses evolve, so retinal arterial blood is shunted into retinal venules. These abnormal arteriolar-venular anastomoses can be seen at the junction of perfused and nonperfused retina, typically just peripheral to the equator. These changes often are difficult to observe ophthalmoscopically but are seen easily with fluorescein angiography.

Retinal neovascularization in a sea-fan configuration is the hallmark of PSR (Fig. 119-5). The neovascularization extends from the border zone of perfused and nonperfused retinae (Fig. 119-6). Initially, a sea fan is supplied by one major feeding retinal arteriole and one major draining retinal venule. Over the course of time, an arborization of the neovascular complex occurs in the peripheral retina. Growth typically is circumferential along the border of perfused and nonperfused retina, rather than radial. Sea fans most commonly are observed in patients who have SC disease or S-Thal disease and are rare in patients who have other hemoglobinopathies.[12,15] Fluorescein angiography demonstrates massive leakage of dye into the vitreous. Generally, the sea fans represent a progressive proliferative retinopathy, which exposes the patient to the risks of vitreous

hemorrhage and retinal detachment. Sea fans may spontaneously involute, resulting in areas of grayish white fibrovascular tissues that often have residual perfused retinal vessels at their base. About 40–50% of sea fans may undergo some degree of autoinfarction during their course.[3]

Vitreous hemorrhage is a common complication of retinal sea-fan formation; it may be spontaneous or induced by minor ocular trauma, and it may be limited or dense. Before this occurs, a patient who has PSR may be entirely visually asymptomatic. Patients who have limited vitreous hemorrhage experience floaters, while those who have dense vitreous hemorrhage have sudden severe vision loss. These hemorrhages may clear spontaneously with time or may persist to give ochre-colored vitreous membranes. It is not uncommon for a patient who has suffered one vitreous hemorrhage to experience recurrent vitreous hemorrhages.

Retinal sea fans may induce fibrovascular tissue on the surface of the retina that causes traction or rhegmatogenous retinal detachments (Fig. 119-7). Circumferential sea-fan involvement can cause peripheral traction retinal detachment through areas of

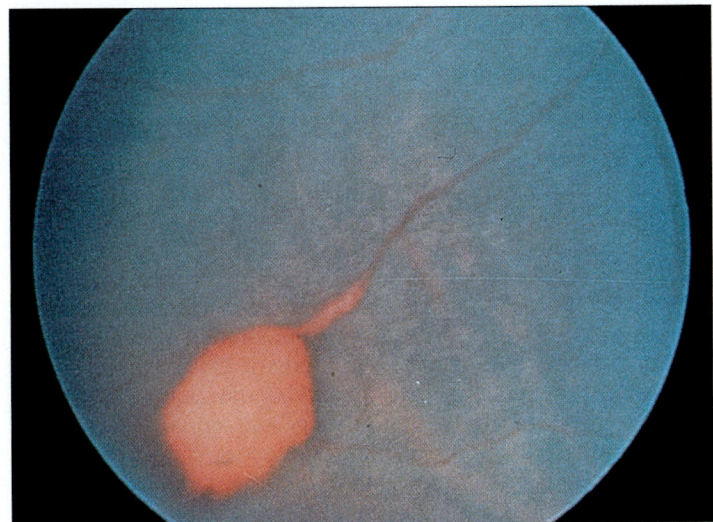

FIG. 119-3 ■ An equatorial "salmon patch" intraretinal hemorrhage with periarteriolar hemorrhage. These peripheral hemorrhages may lead to retinoschisis cavities lined with iridescent particles that comprise hemoglobin degradation products. The vision is 20/20 (6/6). (Courtesy of William Tasman, MD.)

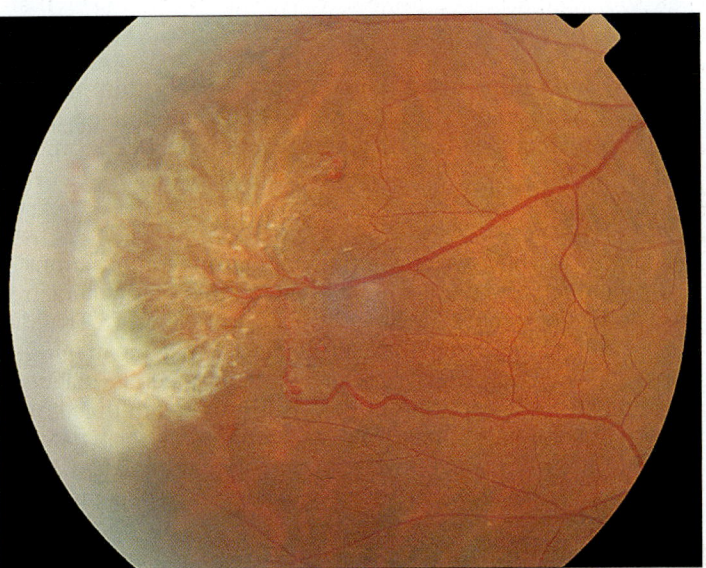

FIG. 119-5 ■ Neural retina in a sickle SC patient. Note the partially regressed peripheral retinal neovascularization at the junction of the perfused retina *(right)* and the nonperfused retina *(far left)*.

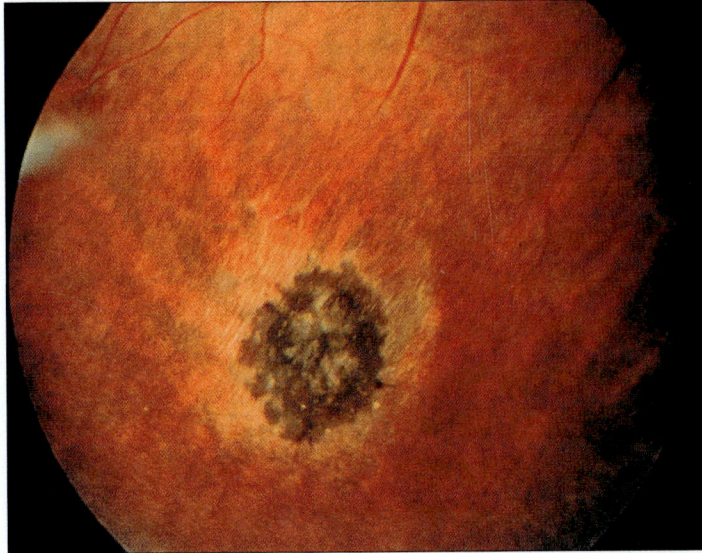

FIG. 119-4 ■ A black "sunburst" retinal lesion. This is caused by a hemorrhage that dissected into the subneural retinal space and disrupted the retinal pigment epithelium, which culminated in pigmentary migration. Note the spiculated borders. (Courtesy of William Tasman, MD.)

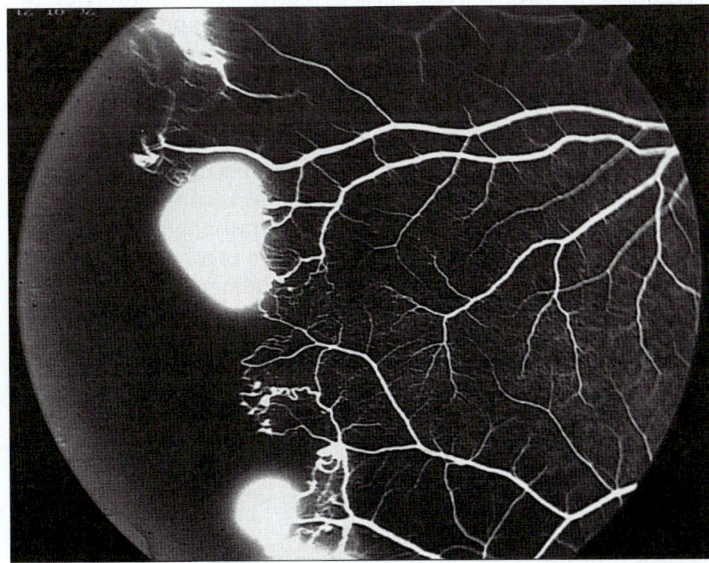

FIG. 119-6 ■ Fluorescein angiography. This demonstrates profound peripheral capillary nonperfusion *(far left)*, retinal vascular remodeling, arteriovenous communications, and extensive leakage of fluorescein dye into the vitreous cavity from the sites of neovascularization.

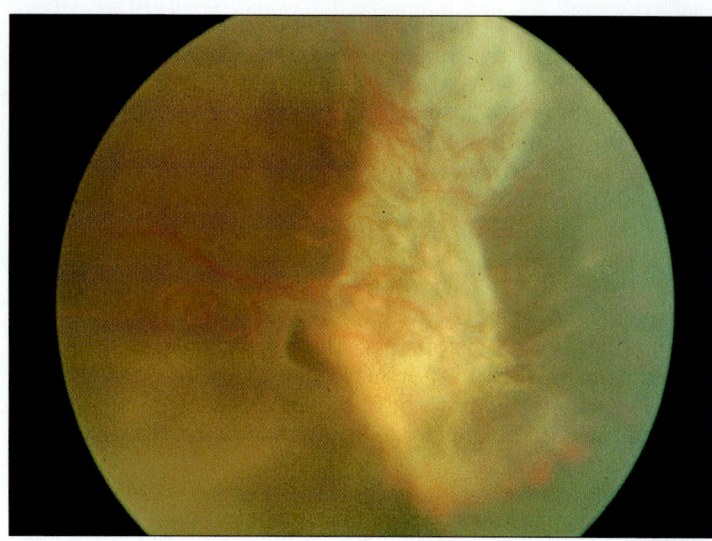

FIG. 119-7 ■ **Traction-rhegmatogenous retinal detachment.** A retinal tear has developed at the site of peripheral neovascularization and fibrosis, leading to a combined traction-rhegmatogenous retinal detachment. (Courtesy of William Tasman, MD.)

perfused and nonperfused retina. In the areas of thin, nonperfused retina, atrophic, stretched retinal holes can develop to create combined traction and rhegmatogenous retinal detachments.

DIAGNOSIS

Most patients who present with the ophthalmic complications of sickle hemoglobinopathies are aware of their underlying red blood cell abnormality. However, patients with SC and S-Thal disease who have milder anemias and minimal systemic manifestations may be completely unaware of their systemic diagnosis when the ocular complications flare. A history of multiple hospitalizations secondary to painful crises, chronic end-organ damage, multiple infections, and bony abnormalities may be absent. These findings are more characteristic of hemoglobin SS patients.

Hemoglobin electrophoresis is necessary to characterize the abnormal globin chain type. A positive test for sickling, such as the metabisulfite preparation (sickle preparation) or the solubility test, indicates the presence of hemoglobin S but does not distinguish among SS, AS, and double heterozygotes such as S-Thal and SC.[1]

Diagnosis of the ophthalmic manifestations of the sickle hemoglobinopathies is enhanced by careful examination of the conjunctiva, iris, anterior chamber, optic disc, and macula, with special attention paid to the subtle ocular manifestations of sickle-cell disease. Indirect ophthalmoscopy and peripheral retinal contact lens biomicroscopy are helpful to delineate retinal hemorrhages and proliferative changes.

Fluorescein angiography characterizes macular perfusion and peripheral retinal perfusion. Early sea-fan formation is highlighted well by fluorescein leakage. Diagnostic ultrasonography can characterize posterior segment anatomy when a media opacity occurs, such as from vitreous hemorrhage or ochre membranes.

DIFFERENTIAL DIAGNOSIS

Other causes of macular ischemia and peripheral retinal neovascularization, vitreous hemorrhage, and neural retinal detachment are given in Box 119-1.

SYSTEMIC ASSOCIATIONS

Patients who have classic sickle SS disease manifest a variety of systemic abnormalities, including anemia, bone marrow infarcts, bony sclerosis (e.g., vertebral "fishmouthing"), aseptic necrosis of the femoral head, ischemia of visceral organs, short-ness of breath caused by pulmonary infarcts, and an increased susceptibility to bacterial infections, particularly salmonellosis caused by reticuloendothelial cell dysfunction.

Other hemoglobinopathies result in less severe systemic disease. In some, a mild anemia may be the only manifestation.

TREATMENT

Despite an understanding of the molecular pathogenesis of sickle hemoglobinopathies, there is currently no effective form of therapy that prevents the sickling of red blood cells or the ensuing ocular complications. For example, no intervention has been shown definitively to halt the progression of macular ischemia, although case reports exist of improvement after exchange transfusion and oxygenation[7,9,13,16] or hyperbaric oxygenation.

Most treatment efforts focus on altering the course of PSR to reduce the chance of vitreous hemorrhage and retinal detachment.[11] Cryotherapy, diathermy, xenon arc photocoagulation, and argon laser photocoagulation have all been employed to treat peripheral retinal neovascularization. Cryotherapy has been used to treat peripheral retinal neovascularization in the presence of vitreous hemorrhage when the neovascular proliferation is visualized only partially and when vitreous hemorrhage precludes treatment with laser photocoagulation. Both single freeze-thaw and triple freeze-thaw techniques have been described. However, cryotherapy has been largely abandoned because of the significant complication rate. Ocular diathermy treatment to obliterate peripheral retinal neovascularization and associated feeder vessels has been reported, but it too is saddled with a high rate of complications.

Various methods of laser photocoagulation effectively induce regression of peripheral neovascularization.[9,17–21] Feeder-vessel laser photocoagulation requires intensive treatment with high energy and is more likely to be complicated by chorioretinal or choriovitreal neovascularization, retinal detachment, and vitreous hemorrhage.[22]

Scatter laser photocoagulation of areas that surround sea-fan proliferation and associated areas of ischemic retina induces regression of these lesions. The rationale is to ablate areas of ischemic retina that are stimulating neovascular proliferation. Two laser techniques have been described, and both can induce successful regression of neovascularization. The first is a localized treatment confined to areas anterior to the patent neovascular fronds.[21] The second uses a 360° peripheral, circumferential retinal scatter technique to the anterior retina.[18,20] The rationale of the 360° scatter treatment is to induce regression of existing peripheral retinal neovascularization and to prevent the formation of any future neovascularization. In general, these techniques can be performed with light- to moderate-intensity burns approximately 500mm in diameter placed approximately one burn width apart. At this time, scatter laser photocoagulation, either localized or circumferential, is the treatment of choice to prevent complications secondary to peripheral sea-fan proliferation.

Vitreous hemorrhage secondary to PSR may be followed for up to 6 months to await spontaneous clearing. If areas of retinal neovascularization can be identified through the vitreous hemorrhage, the associated anterior retina should be treated with scatter laser photocoagulation. Fluorescein angiography or fluorescein angioscopy using an indirect ophthalmoscope and a blue light filter may be used to identify retinal neovascularization in cases of limited vitreous hemorrhage. When the retina is not well visualized, it is important to follow these eyes with ultrasonography to rule out retinal detachment. A minority of patients progress to retinal detachment with or without laser treatment.

Surgery on patients who have sickle hemoglobinopathies is fraught with ocular and systemic pitfalls. A preoperative work-up to assess the severity of anemia, hemoglobin electrophoretic status, and overall systemic condition is critical. Intraoperative and postoperative systemic complications include thromboembolic events such as pulmonary or cerebral embolism. The role of exchange transfusions in reducing the risk of a sickle-cell crisis precipitated by general anesthesia remains unclear. These exchange transfusions are performed to achieve 50–60% hemoglobin A, as indicated by electrophoresis, with a hematocrit of 35–40%. Exchange transfusions may reduce the rate of anterior segment ischemia and optic nerve and macular infarcts, which can occur with intraocular pressures (IOPs) as low as 25mmHg. Currently, however, no compelling reason exists to perform transfusions.[23]

Although the role of exchange transfusions is in question, adequate hydration and supplemental oxygen are often administered during the perioperative and operative periods. If possible, surgery should be performed under monitored local anesthesia; vasoconstrictive agents, such as epinephrine (adrenaline) in the anesthetic block and pupillary dilating agents, should be avoided. Many advocate lowered IOP to both maximize intraocular perfusion and avoid hemoconcentration. Single doses of carbonic anhydrase inhibitors or intravenous mannitol may be administered to lower the IOP, but these agents should not be used repetitively. Even transient elevations in IOP should be avoided, particularly if a scleral buckle is used, to avert vitreous hemorrhage and macular ischemia.

The possibility of anterior segment ischemia is reduced by avoiding treatments in the horizontal meridians, which harbor the long posterior ciliary arteries. For the same reason, manipulation of horizontal and vertical rectus muscles should be performed with care; transection of these muscles should be avoided. Drainage of subretinal fluid is often desirable, since this may minimize the elevation of IOP if a scleral buckle is employed. With current vitrectomy instrumentation, fluctuations in IOP during vitrectomy surgery are less common. A current ultrasonogram to elucidate the intraocular anatomy is important in cases of vitreous hemorrhage. The peripheral vitreous may be firmly attached to shallow areas of traction retinal detachment at the sites of fibrovascular proliferation and may not be well visualized intraoperatively, particularly when ochre-colored membranes are present.

In cases of combined traction-rhegmatogenous retinal detachment, the surgical goals include the release of areas of traction that elevate the retina and the removal of fibrovascular proliferation that may prevent the retinal tear from settling flat. Once this is achieved, scatter endolaser photocoagulation is performed. Postoperatively, the patient's IOP must be monitored closely, particularly if intraocular gas is used.

Anterior segment ischemia does not usually occur if care is taken to avoid elevations of IOP and if the anterior ciliary circulation is not violated.[24] Anterior segment necrosis results in persistent red eye, corneal decompensation, uveitis, and synechiae formation.

Patients who have sickle hemoglobinopathies and who develop postoperative or posttraumatic hyphema are at risk for posterior segment ischemia or infarction, even at mildly elevated IOPs. Low oxygen tension and high ascorbic acid levels in the anterior chamber promote sickling of red blood cells, which can obstruct the trabecular meshwork and lead to a greater elevation of IOP. Macular infarction has been reported with IOPs as low as 25mmHg. Therefore, aggressive lowering of IOP to less than this level is indicated. Some authors recommend early paracentesis to reduce the IOP in acute situations.

COURSE AND OUTCOME

The course for patients who have ocular complications secondary to sickle hemoglobinopathies is variable.[25,26] Untreated, the incidence of blindness from PSR is about 12%.[3] Clearly, with modern laser and vitrectomy techniques, the risk in treated eyes is less. Patients who require intraocular surgery for vitreous hemorrhage or retinal detachment have a higher risk of systemic and postoperative ocular complications, including anterior segment ischemia and optic disc or macular infarction. Patients whose PSR is rendered quiescent with laser photocoagulation may enjoy excellent vision in the long term. In one study of long-term follow-up following laser photocoagulation, only 4% of treated eyes had a repeat vitreous hemorrhage, versus 66% of untreated eyes. Fortunately, severe visual loss was rare in both groups.[26]

REFERENCES

1. Rifkind RA, Bank A, Marks PA, et al. Fundamentals of hematology. Chicago: Year Book Medical Publishers; 1980.
2. Goldberg MF. Sickle cell retinopathy. In: Duane TD, Jaeger EA, Goldberg MF, eds. Clinical ophthalmology. Philadelphia: JB Lippincott; 1989:1–45.
3. Condon PI, Serjeant GR. Behaviour of untreated proliferative sickle retinopathy. Br J Ophthalmol. 1980;64:404–11.
4. Paton D. Conjunctival sign of sickle cell disease. Arch Ophthalmol. 1961;66: 90–4.
5. Goldbaum MH, Jampol LM, Goldberg MF. The disc sign in sickling hemoglobinopathies. Arch Ophthalmol. 1978;96:1597–1600.
6. Goldbaum MH. Retinal depression sign indicating a small retinal infarct. Am J Ophthalmol. 1978;86:45–55.
7. Asdourian GK, Goldberg MF, Rabb MF. Macular infarction in sickle cell B+ thalassemia. Retina. 1982;2:155–8.
8. Merritt JC, Risco JM, Pantell JP. Bilateral macular infarction in SS disease. J Pediatr Ophthalmol Strabismus. 1982;19:275–8.
9. Sanders RJ, Brown GC, Rosenstein RB, Magargal L. Foveal avascular zone diameter and sickle cell disease. Arch Ophthalmol. 1991;109:812–5.
10. Goldberg MF. Retinal vaso-occlusion in sickling hemoglobinopathies [review]. Birth Defects: Original Article Ser. 1976;12:475–515.
11. Cohen SB, Fletcher ME, Goldberg MF, Jednock NJ. Diagnosis and management of ocular complications of sickle hemoglobinopathies: Part V [review]. Ophthalmic Surg. 1986;17:369–74.
12. Goldberg MF. Classification and pathogenesis of proliferative sickle retinopathy. Am J Ophthalmol. 1971;71:649–65.
13. Romayananda N, Goldberg MF, Green WR. Histopathology of sickle cell retinopathy. Trans Am Acad Ophthalmol Otolaryngol. 1973;77:642–76.
14. van Meurs JC. Evolution of a retinal hemorrhage in patient with sickle cell–hemoglobin C disease. Arch Ophthalmol. 1995;113:1074–5.
15. Goldberg MF, Charache S, Acacio I. Ophthalmologic manifestations of sickle cell thalassemia. Arch Intern Med. 1971;128:33–43.
16. Khwarg SG, Feldman S, Ligh J, Straatsma BR. Exchange transfusion in sickling maculopathy. Retina. 1985;5:227–9.
17. Jampol LM, Condon P, Farber M, et al. A randomized clinical trial of feeder vessel photocoagulation of proliferative sickle cell retinopathy. I. Preliminary results. Ophthalmology. 1983;90:540–5.
18. Kimmel AS, Magargal LE, Stephens RF, Cruess AF. Peripheral circumferential retinal scatter photocoagulation for the treatment of proliferative sickle retinopathy. An update. Ophthalmology. 1986;93:1429–34.
19. Fox PD, Minninger K, Forshaw ML, et al. Laser photocoagulation for proliferative retinopathy in sickle haemoglobin C disease. Eye. 1993;7:703–6.
20. Cruess AF, Stephens RF, Magargal LE, Brown GC. Peripheral circumferential retinal scatter photocoagulation for treatment of proliferative sickle retinopathy. Ophthalmology. 1983;90:272–8.
21. Rednam KR, Jampol LM, Goldberg MF. Scatter retinal photocoagulation for proliferative sickle cell retinopathy. A long-term follow-up. Ophthalmology. 1982;98:594–9.
22. Dizon-Moore RV, Jampol LM, Goldberg MF. Chorioretinal and choriovitreal neovascularization: their presence after photocoagulation of proliferative sickle retinopathy. Arch Ophthalmol. 1981;99:842–9.
23. Pulido JS, Flynn HW, Clarkson JG, Blankenship GW. Pars plana vitrectomy in the management of complications of proliferative sickle retinopathy. Arch Ophthalmol. 1988;106:1553–7.
24. Ryan SJ, Goldberg MF. Anterior segment ischemia following scleral buckling in sickle cell hemoglobinopathy. Am J Ophthalmol. 1971;72:35–50.
25. Goldberg MF. Natural history of untreated proliferative sickle retinopathy. Arch Ophthalmol. 1971;85:428–36.
26. Jacobson MS, Gagliano DA, Cohen SB, et al. A randomized clinical trial of feeder vessel photocoagulation of sickle cell retinopathy. Ophthalmology. 1991;98:581–5.

120

Coats' Disease and Retinal Telangiectasia

JULIA A. HALLER

DEFINITION

- A localized, congenital, retinal vascular disorder that consists of abnormal telangiectatic segments of blood vessels that result in leakage.

KEY FEATURES

- Retinal telangiectasia.
- Retinal capillary nonperfusion.
- Dilated intercapillary spaces.
- Lipid exudate.
- Subretinal fluid.

ASSOCIATED FEATURES

- Usually unilateral.
- Male predominance.
- Fibrovascular macular scars.
- Leukokoria.

INTRODUCTION

Retinal telangiectasia is found in a wide range of ocular disease processes. Most retinal telangiectases are acquired secondary to local or systemic conditions, as, for example, in branch retinal vein occlusion and diabetic retinopathy. These disorders should be considered in the differential diagnosis when alterations are seen in the retinal vasculature and should be excluded before primary retinal telangiectasia is diagnosed. Primary retinal telangiectasia is found in Coats' disease, Leber's miliary aneurysms (a localized, less severe form of Coats' disease), idiopathic juxtafoveal telangiectasia, and other angiomatous diseases.

Coats' disease, an idiopathic condition characterized by retinal vascular changes and exudation, was first described by Coats[1] in 1908. In 1912 Leber reported his series of patients who had multiple miliary aneurysms and retinal degeneration. In 1915 Leber wrote two more articles and concluded that the disease he had described in 1912 was a variant of Coats' disease.[2]

EPIDEMIOLOGY

Coats' disease is characterized by discrete zones of alteration in the retinal vascular structure with aneurysmal dilatation, capillary dropout, and leakage. Vision may decrease as a result of leakage from the abnormal vascular channels that are formed, with consequent edema, lipid deposition, and exudative retinal detachment. The disease affects men three times as often as women, has no reported racial or ethnic predilection, and is usually unilateral, although as many as 10–15% of cases may be bilateral. The average age at diagnosis is 8–16 years, although the disease has been described in patients as young as 4 months. About two

thirds of juvenile cases present before age 10 years; approximately one third of patients are 30 years or older before symptoms begin.[3] Coats' disease does not appear to be inherited.

OCULAR MANIFESTATIONS

The typical ophthalmoscopic picture of Coats' disease is one of retinal vascular abnormalities associated with localized lipid deposition and varying degrees of subneural retinal exudate (Fig. 120-1). Vessels may appear sheathed and telangiectatic, and they may have aneurysms that are grape-like, clustered, or lightbulb shaped; often, the vessels are adjacent to areas that lack normal capillaries (Fig. 120-2). The severity of vascular malformation parallels the degree of surrounding neural retinal thickening, exudation, hemorrhage, and destruction of small vessels. Aberrant arteriovenous communicating channels are frequently present, and occasionally true retinal neovascularization occurs. Leakage from the abnormal vascular bed produces a cloudy subretinal exudate, which gravitates toward the posterior pole. As the serous component of the exudate is resorbed by retinal vessels, the lipid-rich yellowish component is left beneath and within the outer neural retinal layers.[4] Over long periods, this yellow exudate may stimulate the ingrowth of blood vessels and fibrous scar tissue (Fig. 120-3). The vascular abnormalities occur more commonly superotemporally; they also are found in the macular and paramacular areas. On average, two quadrants of retina are found to be affected at the initial diagnosis in older patients, but young patients may have more serious disease and more extensive retinal involvement. In more advanced and severe cases

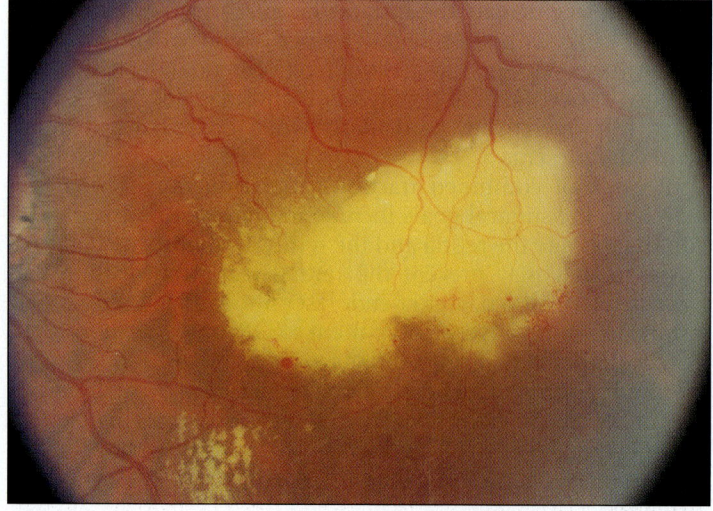

FIG. 120-1 ■ **Coats' disease.** Note the typical vascular abnormalities with aneurysmal dilatation, telangiectasia, exudation, and severe lipid deposition in the macula.

of Coats' disease, exudative retinal detachment develops (Fig. 120-4).[5] Cells in the vitreous are common.

The clinical course is variable but generally progressive. Acute exacerbations of the disease may be interspersed with more quiescent stages. Spontaneous remissions have been reported, with spontaneous occlusion of the vessels and resorption of the exudate, but these are the exception. Choroidal neovascularization may occur in areas of lipid deposition. Secondary complications include neovascularization, vitreous hemorrhage, cataract, rubeosis iridis, and neovascular glaucoma, with phthisis bulbi in severe cases.[3,6,7]

DIAGNOSIS

In children, Coats' disease is typically diagnosed as a result of the recognition of poor vision, strabismus, or leukokoria. In patients with leukokoria, a white pupillary reflex on photographs may be the initially noted abnormality. (The disorder is picked up most frequently by parents or pediatricians or on routine school vision screening.) In these cases, the disease is usually advanced already, with extensive lipid deposition and retinal detachment (see Fig. 120-4). In adults, the most common presenting complaint with Coats' disease is poor vision; in these cases, the disease may be much more limited in extent.

The anterior segment examination findings are normal in all but the most advanced cases of Coats' disease, in which rubeosis iridis, angle-closure glaucoma, and cataract may be present. The diagnosis is confirmed ophthalmoscopically when the typical vascular abnormalities are seen in association with lipid deposition and subretinal exudate. The retinal vascular abnormalities occur in small clusters and include kinked, looped, tortuous, and sheathed vessels of varied and irregular caliber.

Fluorescein angiography is a useful tool for delineating the nature and extent of the vascular abnormalities present in this disease. Most commonly, numerous areas of telangiectasia and micro- and macroaneurysm formation are seen, with beading of blood vessel walls and anomalous vascular communicating channels (Fig. 120-5). Early and persistent dye leakage documents the source of exudation and hemorrhage.[4,8,9] The microvasculature may be diffusely absent, with areas of complete capillary nonperfusion.

DIFFERENTIAL DIAGNOSIS

The severe juvenile form of Coats' disease, which presents with exudative retinal detachment, must be differentiated from other diseases that cause leukokoria in childhood, including retinoblas-

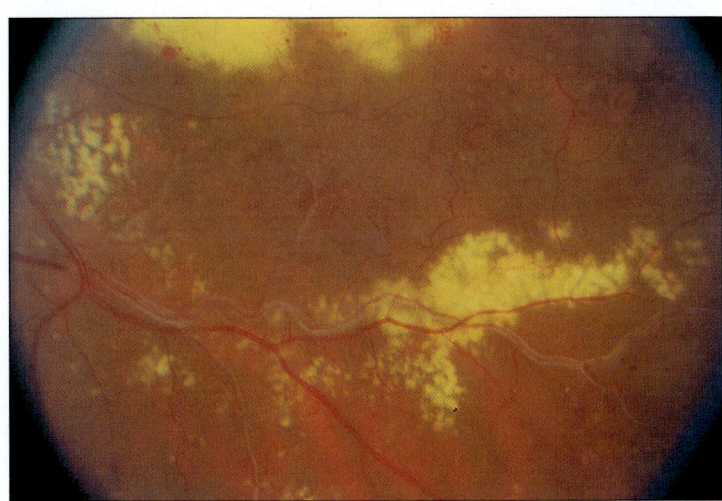

FIG. 120-2 ▮▮ Vessels may appear sheathed, dilated, and telangiectatic or feature grape-like bunches of aneurysms. Vascular changes that are saccular and lightbulb shaped may be seen as well.

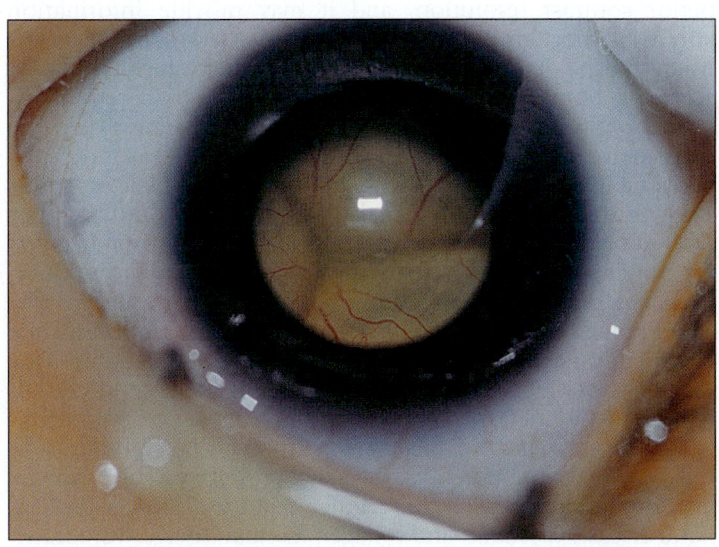

FIG. 120-4 ▮▮ In children, Coats' disease may present as leukokoria, with advanced lipid deposition and exudative retinal detachment. In this eye, the anterior chamber is shallowed slightly, and the retina is immediately behind the lens.

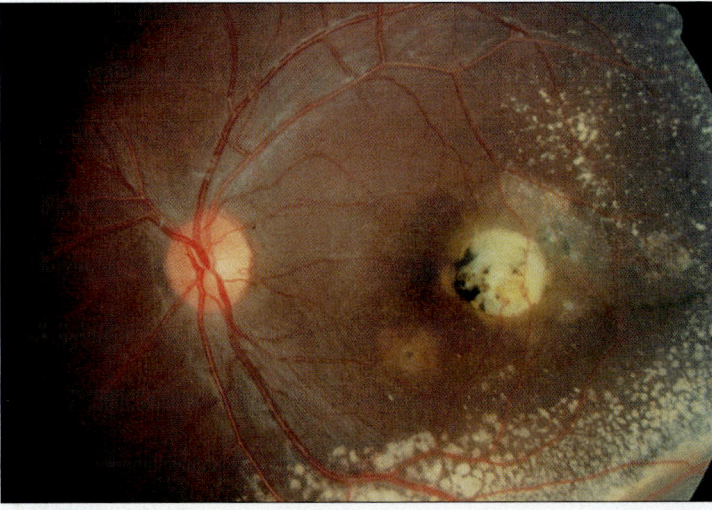

FIG. 120-3 ▮▮ Long-standing submacular exudate. This may stimulate ingrowth of blood vessels or fibrous tissue, with retinal pigment epithelium migration and hyperplasia and the formation of fibrous scars.

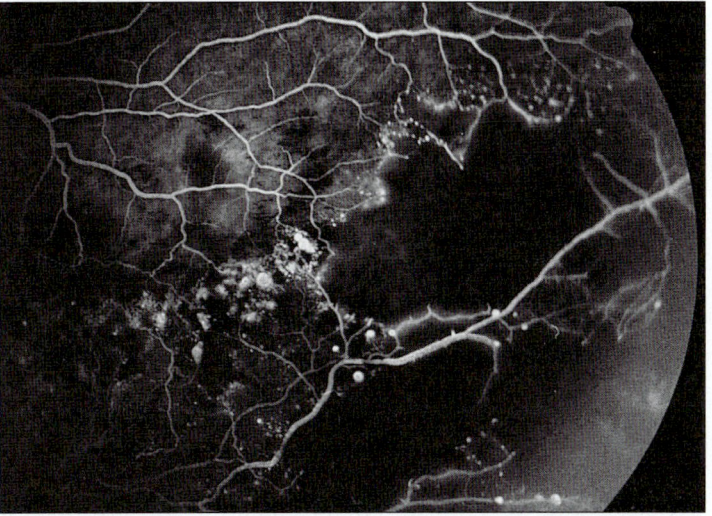

FIG. 120-5 ▮▮ Fluorescein angiography of Coats' disease. In this eye, extensive vascular changes are seen to extend temporally from the macula, with zones of telangiectasia and aneurysm formation adjacent to a large area of capillary nonperfusion. Beading of the blood vessel walls and anomalous vascular communicating channels are present.

toma, retinopathy of prematurity, retinal detachment, persistent hyperplastic primary vitreous, congenital cataract, toxocariasis, incontinentia pigmenti, Norrie's disease, and familial exudative vitreoretinopathy. Gass[4] has pointed out that telangiectatic vessels may appear on the surface of both retinoblastomas and Coats' disease lesions. In retinoblastoma, these dilated vessels are continuous with the large vascular trunks that extend into the tumor; in Coats' disease, the dilated vessels do not extend into the subretinal mass.[4] Fluorescein angiography may help differentiate the two entities. The diagnostic modalities used most commonly are ultrasonography and computed tomography (CT), because of their ability to pick up calcium deposits in retinoblastomas.

Ultrasonography is a convenient, noninvasive test that may distinguish between Coats' disease and retinoblastoma, as well as other entities. The retinal detachment in Coats' disease typically is exudative in appearance, with an absence of the calcifications seen in retinoblastoma. CT may help characterize intraocular morphology, quantify subretinal densities, and identify vascularity within the subretinal space, through the use of contrast enhancement. Also, CT may help detect other abnormalities within the orbit or intracranial space. For optimal resolution, multiple thin slices before and after contrast induction are recommended. Magnetic resonance imaging (MRI) is a useful ancillary test because it permits multiplanar imaging and superior contrast resolution, and it may provide information about the biochemical makeup of tissues. However, MRI is less useful for the detection of calcium than either ultrasound or CT scanning, but it has been shown to help differentiate retinoblastoma from Coats' disease, toxocariasis, and persistent hyperplastic primary vitreous. High-resolution Doppler ultrasonography occasionally may be of use as an adjunctive diagnostic modality. This technique provides real-time imaging; duplex pulse Doppler evaluation may delineate structural abnormalities that are not shown by other testing modalities. Serum lactate dehydrogenase and isoenzyme levels have not proved useful in distinguishing between Coats' disease and retinoblastoma. Examination of subretinal fluid is used rarely, but it confirms the diagnosis of Coats' disease on the basis of cholesterol crystals and pigment-laden macrophages in the absence of tumor cells.[3]

Less severe stages of Coats' disease, especially in adults, must be differentiated from other disorders that produce vascular changes and exudation; these include inflammatory disorders such as Eales disease, vasculitis, and collagen vascular disease. Tumors accompanied by exudation may mimic Coats' disease, as may diabetic vasculopathy with lipid deposition, branch retinal vein occlusion with vascular remodeling and edema, rhegmatogenous retinal detachment, radiation retinopathy, idiopathic juxtafoveal telangiectasia, von Hippel's disease, angiomatosis of retina, exophytic capillary hemangioma, and sickle-cell retinopathy. In these cases, a thorough review of the systems and medical and family histories usually help differentiate primary from secondary disorders. Fluorescein angiography and, occasionally, echography also may be of use.[3,4,10]

Idiopathic Juxtafoveal Retinal Telangiectasia

Idiopathic juxtafoveal retinal telangiectasia is a group of disorders initially described by Gass and Oyakawa[11] in 1982. The disease is characterized by onset in adulthood and presentation with mild blurring of central acuity caused by exudate from ectatic retinal capillaries in the juxtafoveal region of one or both eyes. They divided these patients into four categories: groups 1A, 1B, 2, and 3.[11,12]

GROUP 1A. Group 1A disease consists of unilateral congenital parafoveal telangiectasia, which typically occurs in men and affects only one eye. Retinal vascular abnormalities are present in a small area, one to two disc areas in diameter, in the temporal half of the macula. Onset of symptoms, with visual loss in the 20/40 (6/12) or better range, typically develops at a mean age of 40 years. Photocoagulation of areas of leakage may help restore acuity.

GROUP 1B. Group 1B disease consists of unilateral idiopathic parafoveal telangiectasia, usually found in middle-aged men who have blurring caused by a tiny area of capillary telangiectasia confined to one clock hour at the edge of the foveal avascular zone. Vision is usually 20/25 (6/7) or better. Photocoagulation usually is not considered for these eyes because of the proximity of the leakage to the fovea and the good prognosis without treatment. The lesion may be acquired or may simply be a very small focus of congenital telangiectasia.

GROUP 2. Group 2 disease consists of bilateral, acquired, idiopathic parafoveal telangiectasia. This variant affects patients in the fifth and sixth decades; mild blurring of vision occurs in one or both eyes. The patients typically have small, symmetrical areas of capillary dilatation, usually the size of one disc area or less, in both eyes. The vascular changes may be temporal only or may include all or part of the parafoveolar nasal retina as well. No lipid is deposited, and minimal serous exudation is present. A hallmark is the characteristic gray appearance of the lesions on biomicroscopic examination, with occasional glistening white dots in the superficial retina. Red-free photography often highlights these findings best (Figs. 120-6 and 120-7). These patients also commonly have right-angled retinal venules that drain the capillary abnormalities and are present in the deep or outer retinal layers. Retinal pigment epithelial hyperplasia eventually

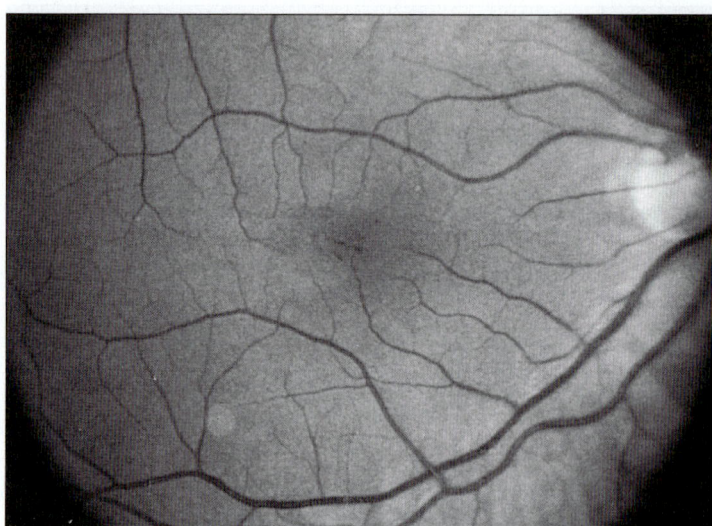

FIG. 120-6 ▮▮ Bilateral idiopathic parafoveal telangiectasia can often best be demonstrated with red-free photography. This eye features capillary abnormalities present for virtually 360° in the parafoveal area.

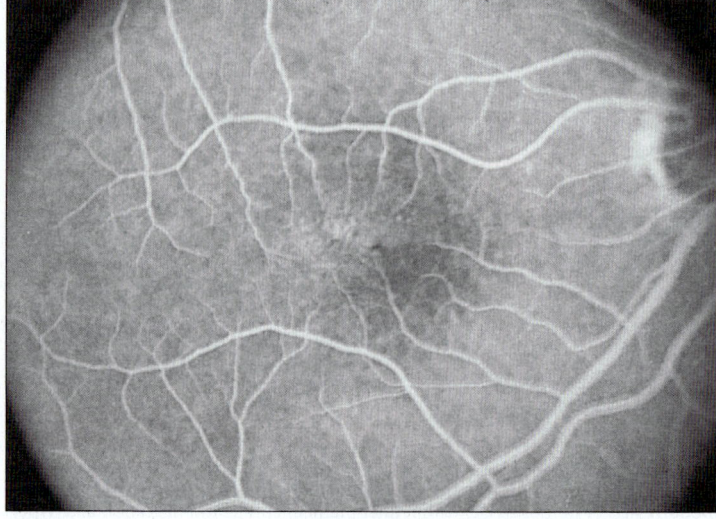

FIG. 120-7 ▮▮ Early transit of the eye shown in Figure 120-6 demonstrates a plexus of capillary abnormalities ringing the fovea.

tends to develop along these venules. In these patients, slow loss of visual acuity over many years is produced by atrophy of the central fovea; patients also may develop choroidal neovascularization, hemorrhagic macular detachment, and retinochoroidal anastomosis. Photocoagulation may be of benefit, but in most cases, the abnormal lesions are so close to the fovea that treatment is problematical, and choroidal neovascularization, if it develops, is often subfoveal.

GROUP 3. Bilateral idiopathic perifoveal telangiectasia with capillary occlusion is a rare variant in which adults experience loss of vision because of progressive obliteration of the capillary network, which begins with telangiectasia. The capillaries' aneurysmal malformations are more marked than in the other, milder forms of the disease; no leakage occurs from the capillary bed.

SYSTEMIC ASSOCIATIONS

Isolated case reports have described a number of other diseases that occurred simultaneously in patients with Coats' disease. In many cases, it is doubtful that an actual causal association exists. These diseases include retinitis pigmentosa, muscular dystrophy, deafness, mental retardation, central nervous system dysfunction, Senior-Loken syndrome, the ichthyosis hystrix variant of epidermal nevus syndrome, and Turner's syndrome. Gass[4] described a patient who had a facial angioma and typical retinal telangiectasia, and another who had bilateral retinal disease and progressive facial hemiatrophy. Bilateral telangiectasia and Coats' syndrome have been reported in multiple family members who have facioscapulohumeral muscular dystrophy and deafness. No definite connection, however, has been made between other systemic or ocular conditions and Coats' disease, and no clear evidence exists of genetic transmission. The adult form of the disease has been described as frequently associated with hypercholesterolemia, although such an association does not occur in the juvenile form.[2,13]

PATHOLOGY

Histopathologically, Coats' disease has been studied intensively because of the number of enucleations formerly performed for suspected intraocular tumors. Eyes with Coats' disease demonstrate marked thickening of the basement membrane of the telangiectatic vessels, as demonstrated by deposition of periodic acid-Schiff (PAS)–positive material. Irregular dilatation of the retinal vessels is seen, often associated with massive exudation of PAS-positive material into the outer neural retinal layers (Fig. 120-8). This exudate produces variable amounts of degeneration and disruption of the neural retinal architecture. Lipid-laden macrophages are present beneath and in the outer layers of the neural retina. Glial cells and retinal pigment epithelium cells may migrate in, surround, and wall off the lipid-laden subretinal exudate, which results in the formation of macular and subretinal nodules. Marked retinal endothelial proliferation and hemorrhagic infarction may occur.[3,7]

TREATMENT

The major goal of treatment in Coats' disease is to preserve or improve visual acuity or, when this is impossible, to preserve the anatomical integrity of the eye. Intervention is contemplated when exudation is extensive and progressive, threatens central acuity, or produces significant peripheral retinal detachment. In severe, untreated cases, total retinal detachment, iris neovascularization with glaucoma, and phthisis bulbi can result. Treatment of Coats' disease is directed toward closure of the abnormal, leaking retinal vessels to allow resorption of exudate. Restoration of vision may be a difficult goal to achieve; in many cases, the visual results are poor even with successful treatment, especially when the macula is involved initially in the exudative process.[2,6,10,14,15]

Laser photocoagulation is the treatment of choice in mild to moderate cases of exudation from Coats' disease. Fluorescein angiographic guidance allows precise, localized treatment of the leaking aneurysms and vessels. Early photocoagulation trials used the xenon arc laser to produce resolution of exudate. The most extensive clinical experience has been with the argon blue-green laser, but more recently, clinicians have employed wavelengths of light better absorbed by hemoglobin, such as the argon green-yellow and the diode green. Lesions that leak are treated directly with relatively large (200–500μm) applications of moderate-intensity light (Fig. 120-9).[3] Scatter photocoagulation to areas of extensive nonperfusion are of unproved value but may lessen the chance of secondary neovascularization. Peripheral lesions may be treated with the indirect laser if they are inaccessible via the contact lens and slit-lamp delivery system. The indirect laser is also a useful modality in children, who frequently need to be treated under general anesthesia.

Cryotherapy and diathermy are of use in the ablation of abnormal retinal vessels in Coats' disease. In cases of exudative detachment, a trans-scleral mode of energy delivery is preferred; cryotherapy is the modality most commonly used. Where subretinal fluid is present, cryotherapy to the anomalous vessels is recommended using a single freeze or freeze-refreeze technique.

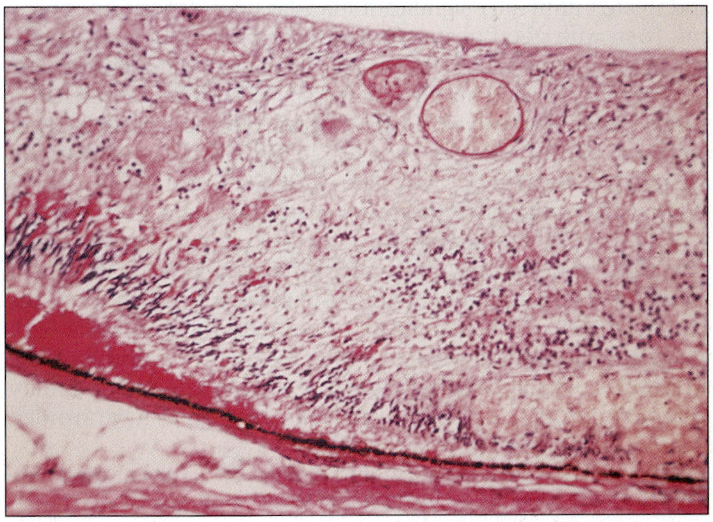

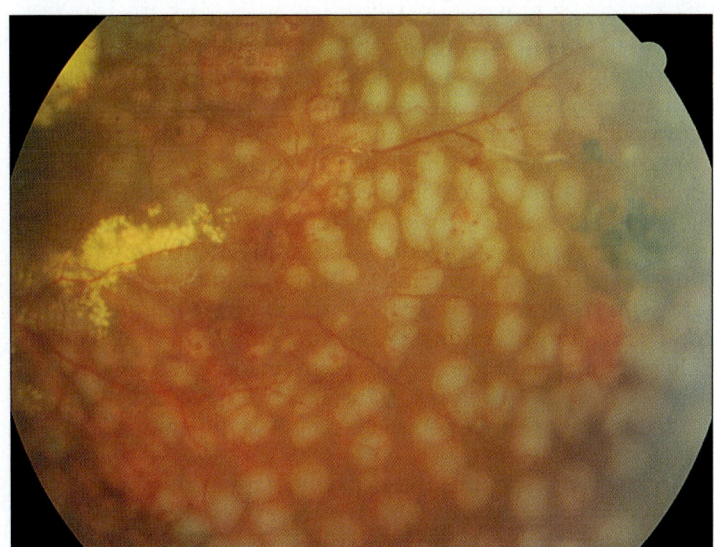

FIG. 120-8 ■ **Histopathological section of an eye with Coats' disease.** Note the marked neural retinal edema, dilated and aneurysmal vascular channels (with PAS-positive material in their walls), and intra- and subneural retinal exudate. (Courtesy of W. R. Green, MD.)

FIG. 120-9 ■ **Initial photocoagulation of the eye shown in Figure 120-5.** Large, medium-intensity spots have been placed on leaking aneurysms, sparing the foveal avascular zone at first. More peripherally, photocoagulation covers temporal aneurysms and is also placed in a scatter pattern in zones of nonperfusion.

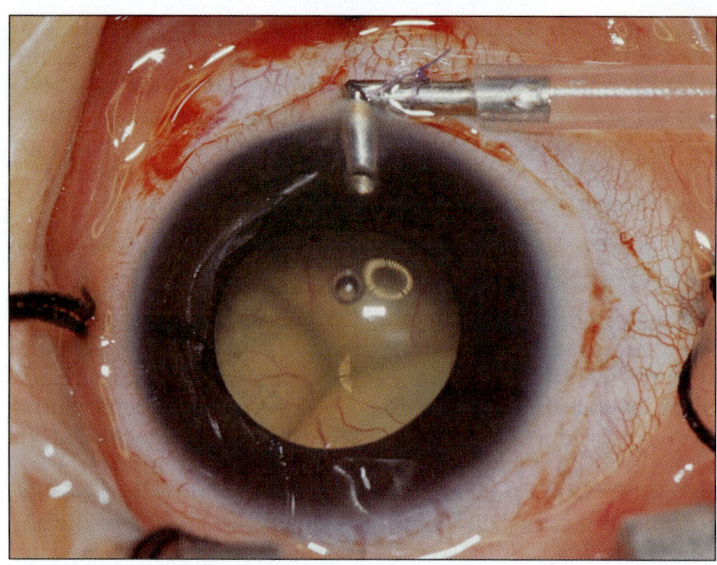

FIG. 120-10 ■ **Technique used for drainage of subretinal fluid in eyes with extensive exudative detachment.** The pediatric infusion cannula is sutured into the anterior chamber through a limbal stab incision with a single Vicryl suture. This is placed in a convenient quadrant so that the eye can be rotated and a posterior draining sclerotomy fashioned. The infusion runs into the anterior chamber and around intact lens zonules, keeping the eye formed as voluminous quantities of thick, yellow subretinal fluid are drained; this subretinal fluid is speckled with cholesterol and lipid deposits.

If the retina is highly elevated, it may be necessary to drain subretinal fluid in order to flatten the retina and allow sufficient freeze to reach the retinal vessels. In these cases, the retina is flattened, the eye reformed, and cryotherapy or laser applied (Fig. 120-10). Subretinal pigmentation and fibrosis usually ensue and follow the lipid resolution. If this involves the macula, visual return is commensurately poor.[3]

Another approach to eyes that have significant retinal detachment is to perform a scleral buckling procedure, which involves dissection of a scleral bed in the area of the abnormal vessels, application of diathermy with drainage of subretinal fluid in the bed, and silicone buckle implantation. In all four of the cases so treated, successful reattachment was achieved, and the exudation gradually resorbed as the abnormal vasculature disappeared, without, however, any return of vision.[2] Harris[14] reported that a scleral buckle sometimes aids the application of postoperative photocoagulation, because it can be oriented beneath the abnormal vessels, and anomalies at the apex of the buckle can be treated effectively, with residual subretinal fluid remaining elsewhere. Siliodor et al.[10] reported a series of 13 children (who had blind eyes and bullous exudative detachments) followed either after no treatment or after surgery that involved intraocular infusion, drainage of subretinal fluid, and cryotherapy on one or more occasions. Of the six untreated eyes, four developed painful neovascular glaucoma and underwent enucleation. The seven treated with surgery all remained cosmetically acceptable and comfortable; none developed neovascular glaucoma.

In selected cases of Coats' disease with intravitreal proliferation and traction detachment, vitreous surgery may improve the clinical course. Machemer and Williams[16] reported successful results with surgical removal of vitreal and preretinal membranes and destruction of leaking vessels in a small series of patients. Other authors have also reported some success, again in end-stage eyes, with vitrectomy, transvitreal drainage of subretinal fluid, and extensive photocoagulation or cryotherapy to prevent neovascular glaucoma.

Repeated therapeutic laser or cryotherapy treatments may be required in eyes that have Coats' disease. Most patients require at least two treatments. Exudate typically begins to resorb within 6 weeks of treatment, if the abnormal vasculature has been eliminated. Depending on the amount of lipid accumulation, in many cases, it takes months to more than a year for complete resolution. Successful treatment is accomplished more easily in eyes that have fewer quadrants with affected vasculature. Recurrence of exudate after initially successful treatment signals the development of new abnormal leaking vessels; these must be searched out meticulously. Contact lens biomicroscopy with a three-mirror lens sometimes is a useful adjunct to indirect ophthalmoscopy in these cases, as is fluorescein angiography with careful sweeps of the retinal periphery. Recurrences may occur years after initially successful treatment, so it is particularly important to follow juvenile patients who may develop significant problems if left unattended. Egerer et al.[2] recommended that all patients who have Coats' disease should be examined at least twice a year to catch any early recurrent problems that may develop in a small percentage of these patients.

COMPLICATIONS OF TREATMENT

Complications of photocoagulation and cryotherapy for Coats' disease include inflammation; hemorrhage; chorioretinal anastomosis formation; and retinal, chorioretinal, and subretinal fibrosis. Macular distortion secondary to epiretinal membrane formation and contraction has been reported following photocoagulation for Coats' disease and may occur even if the disease is untreated. Gass[4] reported one adult patient who developed total retinal detachment and proliferative vitreoretinopathy after cryotherapy for peripheral retinal telangiectasia that was discovered late in life; the eye initially had 20/20 (6/6) acuity.

With intraocular surgical intervention, additional risks include cataract formation, choroidal hemorrhage, retinal detachment, endophthalmitis, glaucoma, and phthisis.

COURSE AND OUTCOME

The clinical course in Coats' disease is variable, but it is usually progressive if left untreated. Continued exudation from abnormal vascular channels produces a gradual accumulation of lipid and serous retinal detachment. The downhill course is more rapid in eyes with more extensive vascular abnormalities. Acute exacerbations of the disease may occur, with intervening periods of relative stability. Occasional remissions, produced by spontaneous occlusion of the vessels, have been reported. The end stage of the exudative process, seen in eyes with severe Coats' disease and particularly in young patients who have an early onset of symptoms, is total retinal detachment, which may be followed by rubeosis iridis, neovascular glaucoma, and eventually phthisis bulbi.

The ultimate prognosis for eyes with Coats' diseases can be measured in terms of two end points: visual acuity and anatomical stability. Unfortunately, central visual acuity is frequently poor in eyes with Coats' disease, because the disease is not diagnosed and treated until after significant macular lipid deposition is present. Even with good treatment and resolution of the macular deposits, significant subretinal fibrosis and macular impairment are present. Despite this, amblyopia therapy should be considered in young patients who have Coats' disease. Optical penalization or occlusion of the better eye can result in significant visual improvement in the diseased eye, with gains in acuity to the 20/60–20/100 (6/18–6/30) range after resorption of macular exudate.

Visual acuity results may be quite good in patients who have very mild vascular anomalies that do not require treatment or are discovered and treated before the macula is involved by the exudative process. It is difficult to estimate the frequency with which this situation develops in the general population, because reported series discuss only more severe cases referred to tertiary treatment centers, and the disease is rare enough to have avoided scrutiny in population-based studies.

Eyes with severe exudation and retinal detachment rarely retain vision better than 20/400 (6/120), and many see much worse than this. Nevertheless, successful treatment of leaking vascular channels may salvage some vision, and this has the advantage of stabilizing the eye anatomically. Occasionally an eye may be saved structurally without light perception.[17]

The prognosis for retaining anatomical integrity of the globe is much better. The worst outcomes are in juvenile cases of total retinal detachment. With modern diagnostic improvements, these eyes are now rarely removed when a tumor is suspected, but some cannot be rehabilitated and go on to phthisis or enucleation. Most eyes with Coats' disease, however, can be saved. Despite chorioretinal scarring, most eyes are cosmetically acceptable, grow and develop otherwise normally, and in many cases have useful vision. Amblyopia therapy, strabismus surgery, and other types of ancillary rehabilitation may be useful and should not be neglected as part of the total treatment of these patients.

REFERENCES

1. Coats G. Forms of retinal dysplasia with massive exudation. Royal London Ophthalmol Hosp Rep. 1908;17:440–525.
2. Egerer I, Tasman W, Tomer TL. Coats' disease. Arch Ophthalmol. 1974;92:109–12.
3. Haller JA. Coats' disease. In: Ryan SJ, ed. Retina. St Louis: CV Mosby; 1989:1453–60.
4. Gass JDM. Stereoscopic atlas of macular diseases. St Louis: CV Mosby; 1987:384–9.
5. Reese AB. Telangiectasis of the retina and Coats' disease. Am J Ophthalmol. 1956;42:1–8.
6. Morales AG. Coats' disease. Natural history and results of treatment. Am J Ophthalmol. 1965;60:855–65.
7. Tarkkanen A, Laatikainen L. Coats' disease: clinical angiographic, histopathological findings and clinical management. Br J Ophthalmol. 1983;67:766–76.
8. Yannuzzi LA, Gitter KA, Schatz H. The macula: a comprehensive text and atlas. Baltimore: Williams & Wilkins; 1979:118–26.
9. Theodossiadis GP. Some clinical, fluorescein-angiographic, and therapeutic aspects of Coats' disease. J Pediatr Ophthalmol Strabismus. 1979;16:257–62.
10. Siliodor SW, Augsburger JJ, Shields JA, Tasman W. Natural history and management of advanced Coats' disease. Ophthalmol Surg. 1988;19:89–93.
11. Gass JDM, Oyakawa RT. Idiopathic juxtafoveal retinal telangiectasis. Arch Ophthalmol. 1982;100:769–80.
12. Gass JDM. Stereoscopic atlas of macular diseases. St Louis: CV Mosby; 1987:390–7.
13. Woods AC, Duke J. Coats' disease. 1. Review of the literature, diagnostic criteria, clinical findings, and plasma lipid studies. Br J Ophthalmol. 1963;47:385–412.
14. Harris GS. Coats's disease, diagnosis and treatment. Can J Ophthalmol. 1970;5:311–20.
15. Ridley ME, Shields JA, Brown GC, Tasman W. Coats' disease. Evaluation of management. Ophthalmology. 1982;89:1381–7.
16. Machemer R, Williams JH Sr. Pathogenesis and therapy of traction detachments in various retinal vascular diseases. Am J Ophthalmol. 1988;105:173–81.
17. Shields JA, Shields CL, Honavar SG, et al. Classification and management of Coats' disease: the 2000 Proctor Lecture. Am J Ophthalmol. 2001;131(5):572–83.

Radiation Retinopathy and Papillopathy

DESMOND B. ARCHER

DEFINITION
- A chronic, progressive retinal and papillary vasculopathy induced by suprathreshold doses of ionizing radiation.

KEY FEATURES
- Retinal microaneurysms.
- Retinal hemorrhages.
- Retinal telangiectatic vessels.
- Retinal hard exudates.
- Macular edema.
- Cotton-wool spots.
- Optic disc swelling.

ASSOCIATED FEATURES
- Intraretinal microvascular abnormalities.
- Retinal neovascularization.
- Vitreous hemorrhage.
- Traction retinal detachment.
- Rubeosis iridis.
- Optic atrophy.
- Occlusive choroidal vasculopathy.

INTRODUCTION

Although Röntgen discovered X-rays more than a century ago, it was not until the mid-1930s that consistent reports of a retinal vasculopathy following radiotherapy began to emerge.[1] It was soon appreciated that the clinical retinopathy and the less frequent papillopathy were dose related and had a characteristic, although variable, latent period.[2]

In more recent years, a better understanding of the biological effects of ionizing radiation and more accurate targeting of radiation energy to the index tissue have reduced the incidence of collateral damage to the retina and optic nerve. Nevertheless, the posterior eye may be unavoidably exposed to excessive radiation in the treatment of cephalic malignancies by external beam irradiation (teletherapy) or in the treatment of retinal and choroidal tumors by teletherapy or plaque therapy (brachytherapy), and a sight-threatening vasculopathy can develop.[3,4] Careful monitoring of the developing vasculopathy and institution of therapy when required often serve to preserve vision in patients who have established and severe retinopathy.

EPIDEMIOLOGY AND PATHOGENESIS
Radiation Dose

The key determinants in the development of radiation retinopathy are the total dose of radiation administered to the retina and the fraction size in the case of teletherapy. In brachytherapy for

choroidal melanoma or retinoblastoma, local retinal and choroidal changes are universal and the severity of retinopathy is directly proportional to the dose of radiation. Brachytherapy for posterior melanomas, especially within 5mm of the macula, carries a significant risk of maculopathy and loss of vision.[5,6] The minimum dose of brachytherapy to induce maculopathy is unknown, although one study of brachytherapy for posteriorly located retinoblastomas recorded maculopathy in 7 of 18 eyes that received an estimated macular dose of 6000rad (60Gy) and in 9 of 10 eyes that received a macular dose of 7500rad (75Gy) or more.[7] The threshold dose of teletherapy for clinical retinopathy is also unknown; estimates fall in the range 1500–6000rad (15–60Gy). The incidence of radiation retinopathy steadily increases with doses greater than 4500rad (45Gy).[8] Dose fractions, the field design, and the type and rate of administration of radiation also have to be taken into account. A general rule is that patients whose eyes receive radiation doses of less than 2500rad (25Gy) in fractions of 200rad (2Gy) or less are unlikely to develop significant retinopathy.

The precise incidence of radiation retinopathy is not known but is probably underestimated because many patients with early or mild retinopathy have few or no symptoms and some patients with established disease are so gravely ill that the ocular pathology goes unreported. One study of patients who received cephalic radiation for orbital, paranasal, and nasopharyngeal malignancies showed that, despite modern radiotherapeutic screening techniques, 55% developed clinical retinopathy and of these almost 50% progressed to sight-threatening vascular complications. Roughly one third of patients who received treatment for midline tumors (e.g., nasopharyngeal carcinomas) developed bilateral retinopathy.[4]

Risk Factors

Several different chemotherapeutic drugs used in tumor therapy may potentiate the injurious effects of ionizing radiation on the retinal and papillary microvasculatures by their effects on DNA synthesis and vascular endothelial cell repair and division.[3,9] Also experimental and clinical evidence suggests that coexisting diabetes mellitus is a risk factor for the development of radiation retinopathy and that patients who have diabetes are more likely to develop extensive retinal ischemia and neovascularization.[10] Patients who have systemic vascular disease (e.g., hypertension, collagen disease, and acute leukemias) also seem more vulnerable to radiation in terms of retinopathy. Concurrent chemotherapy is a risk factor for the development of optic neuropathy.

Latency

The length of time from radiotherapy to development of retinopathy is highly variable and unpredictable. Many patients who receive substantial radiotherapy develop only minor microvascular changes that do not materially affect vision—this probably accounts for the great variation in reported latencies, 1 month to 15 years. The most commonly reported latent intervals are from 6 months to 3 years; the latent period is shorter for eyes with severe ischemia and proliferative retinopathy.[11] The characteristic latent period to retinopathy is probably related to the turnover cycle of retinal vascular endothelial cells, which on average is about once every 2–3 years.[12]

Radiobiology

All retinal cells are relatively radioresistant, and the nonreplicating neural cells are highly radioresistant. The relative radiosensitivity of the retinal vascular cells seems to be related to the conformation of their nuclear chromatin. The heterochromatic nuclear DNA of retinal vascular endothelial cells and pericytes is less accessible to repair enzymes than the loosely arranged euchromatic DNA characteristic of neurons. Hence, the vascular cells are more vulnerable to ionizing radiation "hits," which cause single- or double-stranded DNA breaks. Dividing retinal vascular cells are exquisitely sensitive to radiation as the chromatin of the mitotic cell is in the ultimate state of condensation. The differential sensitivity of retinal vascular endothelial cells with respect to pericyte and smooth muscle cells is probably a function of their particular exposure to high ambient oxygen and blood transition metals, such as iron, which induces free radical formation and cell membrane damage.[12]

Pathogenesis

Good histopathological and ultrastructural evidence indicates that the retinal vascular endothelial cell is the first and prime casualty of retinal irradiation and that its malfunction or demise is the starting point for the development of radiation retinopathy and its complications.[10] With each radiation insult, it is likely that a small and scattered population of vascular endothelial cells that are undergoing mitosis suffer mitotic death. A few cells that absorb sufficient radiation may also suffer immediate interphase death. The first wave of cell death initiates division and migration of adjacent cells to establish endothelial continuity; however, some of these cells will have suffered sufficient radiation damage to cause mitotic death when compelled to replicate. This initiates a further round of division, and so on, until the vascular endothelium is unable to maintain its integrity and the clotting cascade is initiated.

Capillary occlusion leads to the formation of small dilated collateral channels that bypass the area of ischemia and assume a telangiectatic-like form. Microvascular abnormalities, such as microaneurysms, intraretinal microvascular abnormalities, and incompetent capillaries, develop in response to hemodynamic events and alteration in the local metabolism. Where areas of capillary closure are extensive, preretinal and papillary new vessels may form. The events that lead to radiation papillopathy are less certain, although the superficial retinal capillaries probably suffer the same fate as the peripapillary retinal vasculature. High doses of radiation cause an occlusive vasculopathy of the choroidal circulation.[13] It is likely, but unproved, that the posterior ciliary-derived microcirculation of the optic nerve head is similarly compromised. The retinal ganglion cells are highly radioresistant and, although axoplasmic stasis is a feature of acute radiation papillopathy, it is probably secondary to ischemic changes at the optic nerve head.

OCULAR MANIFESTATIONS

The earliest clinical features of radiation retinopathy are discrete foci of occluded capillaries and irregular dilatation of the neighboring microvasculature at the posterior fundus. Fluorescein angiography confirms the extent of capillary dropout and the general capillary competence at this stage.[14] As the retinopathy develops, microaneurysms and telangiectatic channels appear,

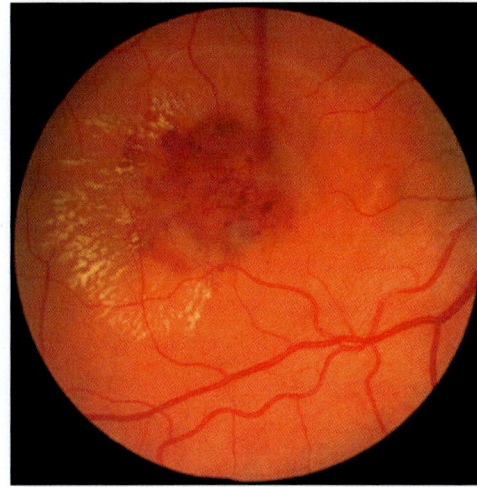

FIG. 121-1 ▮ **Exudative radiation retinopathy of right posterior fundus.** A 45-year-old patient who received 6400rad (64Gy) of radiation and chemotherapy for a nasopharyngeal tumor.

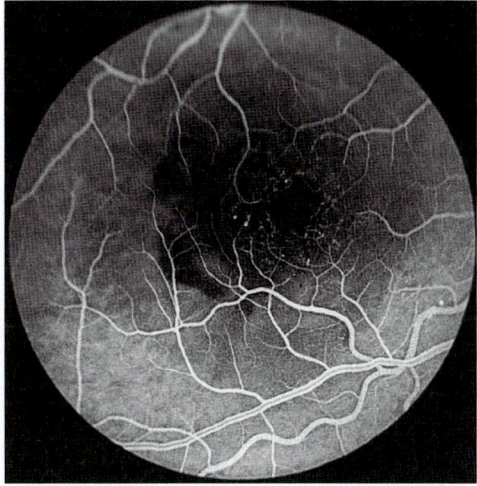

FIG. 121-2 ▮ **Fluorescein angiogram of fundus shown Figure 121-1.** Note the microaneurysms, capillary fallout, and hypofluorescent area of retinal hemorrhage and exudation.

particularly in areas of depleted capillaries, and with time become incompetent. Retinal exudation and small intraretinal or nerve fiber hemorrhages may be superimposed on the gradually evolving ischemic retinopathy; however, with modest radiation damage the retinopathy and vision may change little over a period of years.

More substantial radiation injury is associated with diffuse capillary closure and microvascular incompetence that leads to macular exudation, edema, and decline in vision (Figs. 121-1 and 121-2). An acute form of ischemic retinopathy may follow intense retinal irradiation, as in the course of eradicating a nasopharyngeal or orbital tumor, during which eye protection is limited. The clinical picture is one of ischemic retinal necrosis with widespread arteriolar occlusion, cotton-wool spots, and superficial and deep retinal hemorrhages, which affect both central and peripheral neural retina[3] (Figs. 121-3 and 121-4). Some resolution of hemorrhage and absorption of axoplasmic debris and edema typically occur, and a very limited reperfusion of ischemic areas may be evident. Intraretinal microvascular abnormalities are commonly observed in ischemic retinopathy, and, where vascular occlusion is extensive, preretinal and papillary neovascular membranes form. Most patients who have proliferative retinopathy develop the new vessels within 2 years of diagnosis of retinopathy.[11] Vitreous hemorrhage, traction detachment, rubeosis iridis, and phthisis bulbi are end-stage complications of severe radiation damage to the eye.

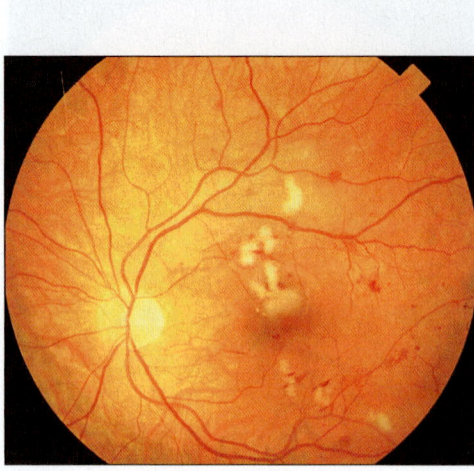

FIG. 121-3 ■ **Ischemic radiation retinopathy of left posterior fundus.** Note the retinal hemorrhages, cotton-wool spots, and optic atrophy, which followed 5500rad (55Gy) of radiation for an anterior meningeal tumor.

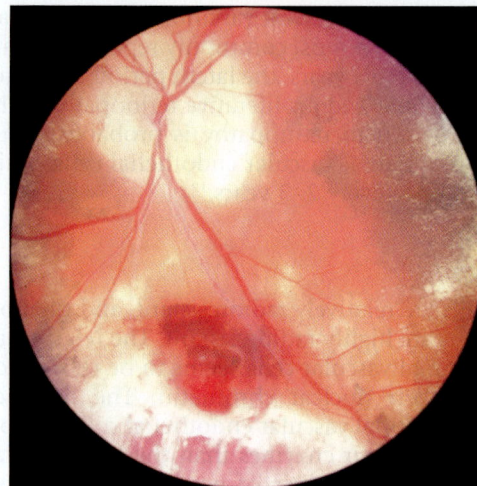

FIG. 121-5 ■ **Proliferative and exudative radiation retinopathy following brachytherapy for retinoblastoma.** Note the chorioretinal atrophy at a prior tumor site inferior to left optic disc. There is hemorrhage and exudation from new and incompetent vessels that border the scar.

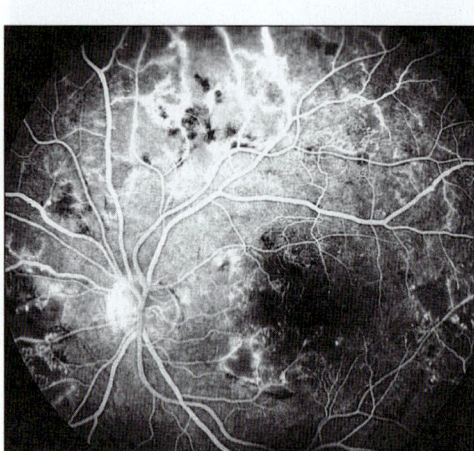

FIG. 121-4 ■ **Fluorescein angiogram of fundus shown in Figure 121-3.** Widespread capillary, arteriolar, and venular occlusion is seen, as well as staining of the vessels and nasal disc with dye.

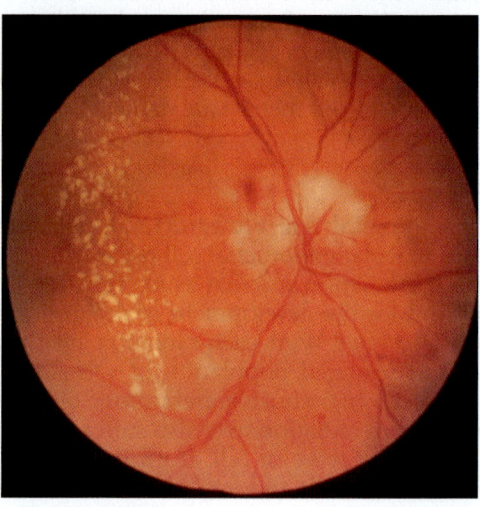

FIG. 121-6 ■ **Radiation papillopathy.** Swollen ischemic right optic nerve head with peripapillary hemorrhage exudation and cotton-wool spots: 27 months following 64Gy for nasopharyngeal tumor.

The retinal pigment epithelium and choroid also display clinical and angiographic signs of radiation damage adjacent to radioactive plaques (Fig. 121-5); this is also seen in patients who receive high-dosage teletherapy. These signs include scattered areas of hypo- and hyperpigmentation, evidence of choroidal vascular stasis and occlusion, serous detachment of the macula, and, very occasionally, choroidal neovascularization.[13]

Radiation optic neuropathy may complicate either brachytherapy or teletherapy—most patients who suffer neuropathy have accompanying retinopathy. In the acute phase disc hyperemia and swelling occur, usually in association with peripapillary edema, hard exudates, hemorrhage, and cotton-wool spots (Fig. 121-6). Fluorescein angiography demonstrates microvascular incompetence, together with areas of capillary nonperfusion of the disc and nearby neural retina. Optic nerve-head swelling may persist for weeks or months but eventually leads to a severe and striking optic atrophy. Vision loss is characteristically severe. The dose of radiation and latent period for clinical optic neuropathy are similar to those for retinopathy; diabetes and concurrent chemotherapy are also risk factors.[15]

DIAGNOSIS

A history of cephalic radiotherapy and the presence of an ischemic retinopathy usually suffice to secure a diagnosis of radiation retinopathy. Macular telangiectatic vessels are a fea-

ture, if not a hallmark, of radiation damage and all the microvascular alterations can be displayed vividly by fluorescein angiography. Indocyanine green angiography may identify areas of choroidal hypoperfusion, precapillary arteriolar occlusion, and abnormal staining of the affected choroid. Electroretinographic (ERG) responses are depressed following acute retinal radiation—pattern ERG and visual evoked response abnormalities confirm inner retinal damage or the presence of a maculopathy. Visual fields show a spectrum of changes, which depend on the extent of ischemic retinopathy and neuropathy and usually correlate with the area of retina exposed to radiotherapy.

DIFFERENTIAL DIAGNOSIS

The differential diagnosis is given in Box 121-1. The diagnosis of radiation retinopathy is usually self-evident, given the history of radiotherapy. However, for diabetic patients who receive radiotherapy for midline cephalic tumors it may be difficult to decide the exact nature of the retinopathy.

The presence of dilated telangiectatic channels at the macula and relative paucity of microaneurysms, venous beading, and vasoproliferative changes (despite sufficient inner neural retinal ischemia) suggest that radiation damage is predominant and may reflect relative sparing of pericytes and smooth muscle cells at the histological level.

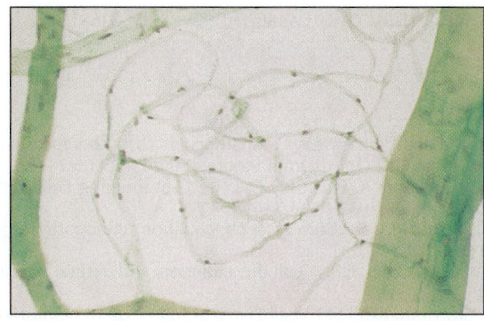

FIG. 121-7 ■ Vascular endothelial cell loss in irradiated retina—5000rad (50Gy). Note the severe depletion of capillary endothelial cells but preservation of pericytes, that is, most of the residual capillary nuclei.

Radiation optic neuropathy in the absence of retinopathy may mimic the clinical picture of anterior ischemic optic neuropathy but tends to occur in younger, normotensive patients and little or no involvement of the short posterior ciliary vessels is seen on angiography. Elderly patients who have ischemic optic neuropathy merit an erythrocyte sedimentation rate or C-reactive protein assessment, despite a history of radiotherapy, to rule out temporal arteritis.

The interpretation of continuing visual loss after neurosurgery and radiotherapy for tumors of the sellar region is often difficult. A diagnosis of radiation-induced optic neuropathy may be facilitated by magnetic resonance imaging with gadolinium–pentetic acid and the presence of altitudinal field defects.[16]

PATHOLOGY

Most histopathological studies show preferential preservation of the outer retina compared with the inner retina and alterations to the nerve fiber layer attributable to inner retinal ischemia. Trypsin digest preparations from irradiated eyes with vasculopathy show an early and unequivocal loss of retinal vascular endothelial cells with relative sparing of the pericyte population (Fig. 121-7). Associated changes include microaneurysms and fusiform dilatation of capillaries, which predominate on the arterial side of the circulation. Acellular, nonperfused, and collapsed capillaries are a feature of ischemic retina and are associated with varying degrees of neuronal degeneration and gliosis. Large thin-walled channels with dense collagenous adventitia are the histopathological correlates of the telangiectatic-like vessels observed clinically.[17] With intense radiation, such as 6000rad (60Gy) for an orbital rhabdomyosarcoma, widespread loss of photoreceptors, retina pigment epithelial cells, and choriocapillaries and atrophy of the associated inner retina and optic nerve may occur.[18]

TREATMENT

Photocoagulation

Only a few patients develop advanced radiation retinopathy, and to date no randomized controlled study exists to assess properly the value of photocoagulation in either limiting macular edema or containing the vasoproliferative response. Anecdotal and small group studies suggest that focal or grid laser photocoagulation, given as for diabetic retinopathy, has a favorable effect on radiation macular edema, particularly in the absence of severe macular ischemia or cystoid degeneration and where vision remains 20/80 (6/24) or better. Cataract, vitreous hemorrhage, prior panretinal photocoagulation or detachment, and optic neuropathy are all factors that may limit visual recovery.[19] Focal photocoagulation may also prove beneficial for retinal and choroidal neovascularization that occurs at tumor sites following either plaque or external beam therapy.[14] Panretinal photocoagulation, given as for proliferative diabetic retinopathy, has been used to contain preretinal and papillary neovascularization and reduce the incidence of vitreous hemorrhage and neural retinal detachment. In general, less intense photocoagulation is required to contain radiation retinopathy compared with that required for diabetic retinopathy. Retinal cryoablation has also been used to contain neovascularization in the presence of dense vitreous hemorrhage.[20]

Vitrectomy—Retinal Detachment Surgery

Persistent vitreous hemorrhage and retinal traction that affect the macula respond to pars plana vitrectomy and rhegmatogenous retinal detachments yield to conventional detachment surgery.

COURSE AND OUTCOME

Clinically significant radiation retinopathy or papillopathy usually follows teletherapy for nasopharyngeal, paranasal sinus, or orbital tumors, during which only limited protection can be afforded during the eradication of the tumor. Plaque therapy for retinal and choroidal neoplasms causes severe damage to the immediate retina and choroid and secondary alterations to the surrounding tissues for a distance of several millimeters. With teletherapy it is often difficult to compute precisely how much radiation the retina and optic disc will receive or the exact dose of radiation that will precipitate clinical retinopathy. Doses in excess of 3400rad (34Gy) are likely to induce retinopathy, especially if fraction doses exceed 200rad (2Gy) and other risk factors are present. Minor degrees of retinopathy, characterized by subtle capillary fallout and occasional dilated channels and microaneurysms, may not affect vision and may remain stable for years. No treatment is required, but such patients merit annual follow-up as the disease is slowly progressive. Macular exudation that causes significant retinal thickening and visual symptoms requires prompt laser photocoagulation. Treatment reduces edema and, in the absence of severe macular ischemia, improves or stabilizes visual acuity. Recurrent treatment may be required if fresh leaking foci develop. Patients who have nonproliferative retinopathy, on average, can expect to retain a visual acuity of 20/50 (6/15) for at least 4 years.[19]

Severe ischemic retinopathy typically follows direct orbital irradiation for lymphoma, rhabdomyosarcoma, or lacrimal gland carcinomas; visual loss is attributable to macular or optic nerve ischemia. New vessels that may bleed profusely develop in some of these patients, who should be observed at regular intervals. Panretinal photocoagulation is effective in the long term in containing the vasoproliferative process. Patients who have proliferative radiation retinopathy have a poor prognosis for retaining good central vision, with a high proportion (86%) achieving only 20/200 (6/60) vision or worse after 6 years.[11]

It is important that the ophthalmologist and radiotherapist liaise closely when patients receive cephalic radiation that involves the eye in the treatment field. Careful monitoring of the patient and judicious photocoagulation can help preserve vision in patients who may otherwise be severely disabled for a variety of reasons.

REFERENCES

1. Stallard HB. Radiant energy as (a) a pathogenic (b) a therapeutic agent in ophthalmic disorders. Br J Ophthalmol Monogr Suppl. 1993;6:1–126.
2. Merriam GR, Szechter A, Focht EF. The effects of ionizing radiations on the eye. Front Radiat Ther Oncol. 1972;6:346–85.
3. Brown GC, Shields JA, Sanborn G, et al. Radiation retinopathy. Ophthalmology. 1982;89:1494–501.
4. Amoaku WMK, Archer DB. Cephalic radiation and retinal vasculopathy. Eye. 1990;4:195–203.
5. Char DH, Castro JR, Kroll SM, et al. Five year follow-up of helium ion therapy for uveal melanoma. Arch Ophthalmol. 1990;108:209–14.
6. Lommatzsch PK. Results after beta-irradiation (106Ru/106Rh) of choroidal melanomas: 20 years' experience. Br J Ophthalmol. 1986;70:844–51.
7. Ehlers N, Kaae S. Effects of ionizing radiation on retinoblastoma and on the normal ocular fundus in infants: a photographic and fluorescein angiographic study. Acta Ophthalmol (Copenh). 1987;65(Suppl 181):1–84.
8. Parsons JT, Bova FJ, Fitzgerald CR, et al. Radiation retinopathy after external-beam irradiation: analysis of time-dose factors. Int J Radiat Oncol Biol Phys. 1994;30:765–73.
9. Griffin JD, Garnick MB. Eye toxicity of cancer chemotherapy: a review of the literature. Cancer. 1981;48:1539–49.
10. Archer DB. Doyne lecture. Responses of retinal and choroidal vessels to ionising radiation. Eye. 1993;7:1–13.
11. Kinyoun JL, Lawrence BS, Barlow WE. Proliferative radiation retinopathy. Arch Ophthalmol. 1996;114:1097–100.
12. Archer DB, Gardiner TA. Ionizing radiation and the retina. Curr Opin Ophthalmol. 1994;5(111):59–65.
13. Midena E, Segato T, Valenti M, et al. The effect of external eye irradiation on choroidal circulation. Ophthalmology. 1996;103:1651–60.
14. Amoaku WMK, Archer DB. Fluorescein angiographic features, natural course and treatment of radiation retinopathy. Eye. 1990;4:657–67.
15. Brown GC, Shields JA, Sanborn G, et al. Radiation optic neuropathy. Ophthalmology. 1982;89:1489–93.
16. Guy J, Mancuso A, Beck R, et al. Radiation-induced optic neuropathy: a magnetic resonance imaging study. J Neurosurg. 1991;74:426–32.
17. Archer DB, Amoaku WMK, Gardiner TA. Radiation retinopathy: clinical, histopathological, ultrastructural and experimental correlations. Eye. 1991;5:239–51.
18. Krebs IP, Krebs W, Merriam JC, et al. Radiation retinopathy: electron microscopy of retina and optic nerve. Histol Histopathol. 1992;7:101–10.
19. Kinyoun JL, Zamber RW, Lawrence BS, et al. Photocoagulation treatment for clinically significant radiation macular oedema. Br J Ophthalmol. 1995;79:144–9.
20. Kinyoun JL, Chittum ME, Wells CG. Photocoagulation treatment of radiation retinopathy. Am J Ophthalmol. 1988;105:470–8.

CHAPTER
122 Proliferative Retinopathies

DANIEL A. EBROON • SRILAXMI BEARELLY • LEE M. JAMPOL

DEFINITION
- A heterogeneous group of disorders that features preretinal and optic disc neovascularization.

KEY FEATURES
- Retinal new blood vessels.
- Optic disc new blood vessels.

ASSOCIATED FEATURES
- Retinal ischemia.
- Retinal capillary nonperfusion.
- Posterior segment inflammation.
- Neoplasia.
- Vitreous hemorrhage and fibrous proliferation.
- Retinal detachment.

INTRODUCTION

The proliferative retinopathies are defined as diseases associated with preretinal or disc neovascularization.[1] These diseases can be divided into two major categories (Box 122-1), each with its own subset of hereditary disorders:

- Systemic diseases
- Retinal vascular and ocular inflammatory diseases

The topic of retinal angiogenesis is first reviewed, after which specific entities with retinal neovascularization are described, along with treatment options. Finally, an approach is suggested for the management of a patient who has neovascularization of unknown cause.

RETINAL ANGIOGENESIS

Current models of neovascularization of the retina are based on the concept of chemoattractants. The initiating event in the retina may be ischemic, inflammatory, or neoplastic.

A critical level of hypoxia or inflammation may stimulate retinal tissue to release potent chemical mediators, which have corresponding receptors in the retinal vasculature that initiate neovascularization. There are numerous chemical mediators, which may be stimulatory or inhibitory. Some stimulatory mediators act directly on endothelial cells to cause migration and proliferation. Other stimulatory mediators act indirectly by the release of sequestered direct-acting factors or by the activation of macrophages.

Factors that act directly on endothelial cells include fibroblast growth factor, transforming growth factor-α, platelet-derived endothelial cell growth factor, angiotropin, angiotensin II, insulin-like growth factor-1, and vascular endothelial growth factor (VEGF). Factors that act indirectly on endothelial cells include transforming growth factor-β, tumor necrosis factor-α, and certain prostaglandins. Numerous animal and laboratory models have demonstrated that VEGF is a significant stimulant of retinal and choroidal neovascularization. In these models, increased expression of VEGF in the retina stimulates neovascularization within the retina, while antagonists of VEGF receptor signaling inhibit retinal and choroidal neovascularization.[7] VEGF has been shown to be upregulated by hypoxia, and its levels are elevated in the retina and vitreous of patients and laboratory animals with ischemic retinopathies.[8] Investigations of antiangiogenic agents such as pigment epithelium–derived factor may prove useful in curtailing aberrant growth of ocular endothelial cells.[9]

Neovascularization has the potential to cause loss of vision because the vessels are fragile and rupture more easily than do normal retinal vessels. Patients may develop vitreous hemorrhage, fibrovascular scarring, epiretinal membranes, retinal traction, and both rhegmatogenous and tractional retinal detachments. Early detection of neovascularization and appropriate treatment may help minimize the risks of such complications.

ENTITIES ASSOCIATED WITH RETINAL NEOVASCULARIZATION

Systemic Diseases

DIABETES MELLITUS. The vast majority of neovascularization in diabetes occurs posterior to the equator (Fig. 122-1), but peripheral neovascularization may occur also. Both panretinal and local scatter photocoagulation are effective in the regression of neovascular tissue. A program of tight blood sugar control helps to prevent the development of neovascular tissue. The extent of hyperglycemia and, therefore, blood sugar control, over both the short and long term, may be ascertained by the measurement of blood glucose levels and the hemoglobin A_{1c} values, respectively. (For a more detailed description of diabetic retinopathy, see Chapter 117.)

HYPERVISCOSITY SYNDROMES. Patients who have disease processes such as chronic myelogenous leukemia, essential thrombocytosis, or polycythemia vera may have dramatic elevations in their leukocyte, platelet, or red blood cell counts, respectively. Elevations may increase blood viscosity, causing a sludging of blood flow in the peripheral retina. The consequences of this abnormal flow include venular dilation, perivenous sheathing, capillary dropout, and microaneurysm formation. Neovascularization develops at the border of perfused and nonperfused retina.[10]

AORTIC ARCH SYNDROMES AND OCULAR ISCHEMIC SYNDROMES. Patients who have atherosclerosis that involves the carotid artery or aortic arch, arteritis (e.g., Takayasu's disease), or syphilitic aortic involvement may develop disc or peripheral retinal neovascularization.[11] Such patients have in common extensive narrowing of the large arteries that supply blood to the eye. The resultant ischemia may cause neovascularization of the disc and iris, in addition to peripheral retinal neovascularization. Although both cryopexy and scatter photocoagulation are helpful, they are less successful in these syndromes than others, perhaps because the vasoproliferative stimulus is so intense and diffuse within the eye (see Chapter 118).

CAROTID–CAVERNOUS FISTULA. In a carotid–cavernous fistula, carotid arterial blood enters the cavernous sinus venous system directly, bypassing the eye, and consequent ischemia may stimulate retinal neovascularization.[12] Panretinal photocoagula-

BOX 122-1

Retinal Neovascularization

SYSTEMIC DISEASE
Diabetes mellitus*
Hyperviscosity syndromes*
Aortic arch syndromes and ocular ischemic syndromes*
Carotid–cavernous fistula*
Multiple sclerosis*
Retinal vasculitis†
- Systemic lupus erythematosus
- Arteriolitis with SS-A autoantibody
- Acute multifocal hemorrhagic vasculitis
- Vasculitis resulting from infection
- Vasculitis resulting from Behçet's disease
Sarcoidosis†
Coagulopathies*

SYSTEMIC DISEASES WITH A STRONG HEREDITARY COMPONENT
Sickling hemoglobinopathies*
- SC, SS, Sβ thalassemia, SO Arab
Other hemoglobinopathies*
- AC and C-β thalassemia
Small vessel hyalinosis*
Incontinentia pigmenti‡
Familial telangiectasia, spondyloepiphyseal dysplasia, hypothyroidism, neovascularization, and tractional retinal detachment‡

RETINAL VASCULAR AND OCULAR INFLAMMATORY DISEASE
Eales' disease*
Branch retinal artery or vein occlusion*
Frosted branch angiitis*,2
Idiopathic retinal vasculitis, aneurysms, and neuroretinitis*,†,3
Retinal embolization* (e.g., talc)
Retinopathy of prematurity*
Encircling buckling operation*
Uveitis including pars planitis†
Acute retinal necrosis†
Birdshot retinochoroidopathy†
Long-standing retinal detachment*
Choroidal melanoma, choroidal hemangioma‡
Cocaine abuse‡
Optic nerve aplasia,*,4 myelinated nerve fiber layer*,5
Radiation retinopathy*,6

RETINAL DISEASES WITH A STRONG HEREDITARY COMPONENT
Familial exudative vitreoretinopathy*
Inherited retinal venous beading*
Retinoschisis†
Retinitis pigmentosa‡
Autosomal dominant vitreoretinochoroidopathy‡

*Vascular disease with ischemia.
†Inflammatory disease with possible ischemia.
‡Stimulus for neovascularization is unclear.

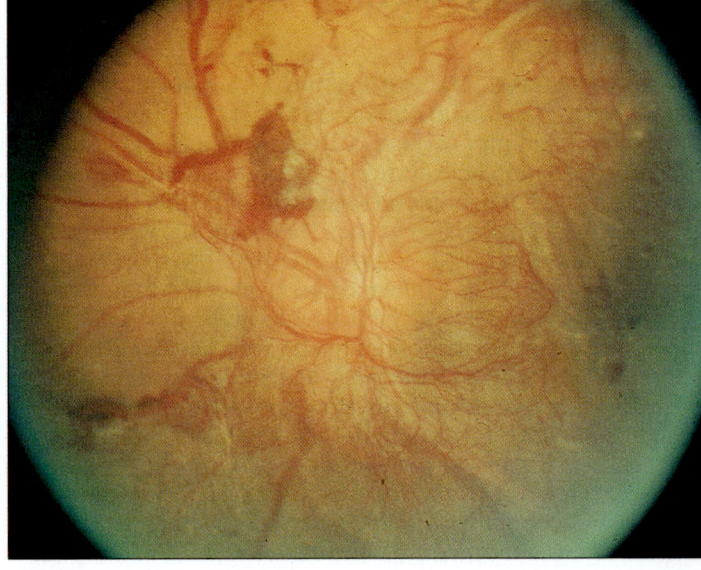

FIG. 122-1 ■ **Diabetes mellitus.** A large area of neovascularization of the disc seen in a patient who has long-standing insulin-dependent diabetes mellitus.

tion has been used effectively to cause regression of neovascular tissue in patients who have carotid–cavernous fistulas.

MULTIPLE SCLEROSIS. Patients who have multiple sclerosis demonstrate focal neurological deficits such as optic neuritis. Neuroimaging reveals characteristic central nervous system plaques. Such patients may develop uveitis, peripheral retinal venous inflammatory sheathing (Rucker's sign), or arteriolar sheathing, which occurs less frequently. If the vasculitis affects blood flow, ischemia and neovascularization may ensue.[13] Local scatter photocoagulation has been shown to halt neovascularization in these patients.

RETINAL VASCULITIS. Neovascularization may result from ocular inflammation. The neovascular signal may be from ischemia, because blood flow is impaired, or may be the result of

vasoproliferative factors induced by the inflammatory response. Specific vasculitic entities that cause retinal neovascularization include systemic lupus erythematosus (SLE),[14] arteriolitis with SS-A autoantibody, acute multifocal hemorrhagic vasculitis, and vasculitis that occurs with infection (e.g., herpes viruses, toxoplasmosis, and cytomegalovirus[15]).

In SLE, vascular proliferation may occur despite normal antinuclear antibody (ANA) or complement levels. Patients who have a constellation of findings that resemble SLE, and whose blood studies are ANA negative and SS-A autoantibody positive, also may develop proliferative changes. Patients affected by acute multifocal hemorrhagic vasculitis have decreased visual acuity, retinal hemorrhages, posterior retinal infiltrates, vitritis, and papillitis, and they also may develop retinal neovascularization.[16] It is recommended that neovascularization in such conditions be treated with panretinal scatter photocoagulation. Treatment of the underlying vasculitis with anti-inflammatory agents or immune suppression also may be beneficial.

SARCOIDOSIS. Sarcoidosis is an idiopathic granulomatous disorder that affects multiple organ systems. The ocular manifestations are disparate and include uveitis with periphlebitis. Inflammation may stimulate neovascularization either by the direct liberation of an angiogenic stimulus or indirectly by blocking blood flow, which results in ischemia.[17] Both anti-inflammatory therapy (e.g., corticosteroids) and scatter laser photocoagulation are recommended for the treatment of retinal neovascularization (see Chapter 175).

Systemic Diseases That Have a Strong Hereditary Component

HEMOGLOBINOPATHIES. Sickle-cell disease has been studied extensively as a cause of retinal neovascularization. As a result of this and its relatively high prevalence, it may serve as a model by which to understand and treat the proliferative retinal vasculopathies (see Chapter 119).

The sickling hemoglobinopathies are blood diseases that share the characteristic of erythrocytes that can assume the shape of an elongated crescent or sickle. Point mutations result in amino acid substitutions within the hemoglobin molecule that change its tertiary structure under conditions of low oxygen tension, acidosis, or hypercapnia. These abnormally shaped erythrocytes become trapped in precapillary arterioles or capillaries and disrupt circulation. Common tissues affected are those of the spleen, bones, lungs, and eyes. African-Americans, as well as people from Mediterranean countries, Africa, India, and Saudi Arabia, have a high prevalence of the sickling hemoglobinopathies.

Proliferative changes in the retinal periphery account for much of the morbidity from sickle-cell disease. Sickling of erythrocytes and changes of the vascular endothelium in the retinal periphery result in capillary nonperfusion. Ischemic signals lead to peripheral neovascularization that takes the shape of a sea fan, a type of coral.[18] Although the term *sea fan* is associated with sickle-cell retinopathy most commonly, almost any type of peripheral retinal neovascularization may assume this configuration. Recent investigations of angiogenic factors in proliferative sickle-cell retinopathy have demonstrated VEGF and basic fibroblast growth factor to be associated with sea fan formations.[19]

The likelihood of neovascularization depends on the type of sickling hemoglobinopathy. For example, patients who have hemoglobin SC disease are 10 times more likely to develop peripheral neovascularization than patients affected by hemoglobin SS disease. This difference may be partly secondary to the higher hematocrit and blood viscosity in hemoglobin SC disease.

Peripheral retinal neovascularization leads to loss of vision if fragile neovascular tissue hemorrhages into the vitreous. With repeated hemorrhages and vitreous degeneration, fibrovascular elements of the vitreous may exert traction on the retina, and tractional or rhegmatogenous retinal detachment may ensue. Fibrovascular proliferation or nonvascular epiretinal membranes that affect the macula can further degrade vision by the formation of macular pucker or macular holes.

The treatment of peripheral ischemic retina with scatter photocoagulation results in the regression of sea fans in the majority of cases.[20] Rarely, vitrectomy may be necessary.

Hemoglobinopathies other than sickle-cell disease may be associated with peripheral retinal neovascularization. For example, patients who have hemoglobin AC and C-β thalassemia have rarely been reported to develop peripheral neovascularization.

INCONTINENTIA PIGMENTI. Incontinentia pigmenti is a rare X-linked dominant disorder that tends to be lethal for male fetuses *in utero*, so nearly all affected patients are female. Patients have dermatological, neurological, dental, and ophthalmologic findings.

One third of patients with incontinentia pigmenti have ophthalmologic findings including cataracts, strabismus, optic atrophy, and foveal hypoplasia. The peripheral retinal vasculature often is poorly developed (Fig. 122-2), and at the junction of normal and abnormal vasculature, arteriovenous anastomoses, microvascular anomalies, and neovascularization may develop.[21] Vitreous hemorrhage, retinal tears, and retinal detachment may ensue. Although a predilection for peripheral involvement of vascular changes is well established, the posterior pole can be affected by similar findings. Neovascularization has been treated effectively in some cases using cryopexy or laser.

Retinal Vascular and Ocular Inflammatory Diseases

EALES' DISEASE. Strictly defined, Eales' disease is a bilateral disorder of young (20–45 years old), otherwise healthy adults in developing countries (especially India). These patients have periphlebitis and develop peripheral retinal capillary nonperfusion, often superotemporally. The etiology remains unknown. The designation of Eales' disease sometimes is used for any patient who has peripheral neovascularization and no clinical or laboratory features that identify another specific entity.

The general principle that neovascularization occurs at the border of perfused and nonperfused retina applies to Eales' disease.[22] Scatter photocoagulation of ischemic retina has been

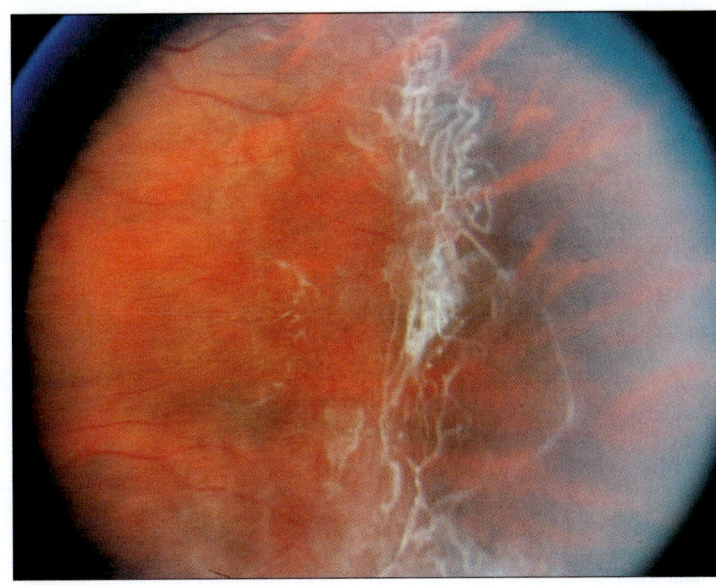

FIG. 122-2 ■ **Incontinentia pigmenti.** The peripheral retina of a patient who has incontinentia pigmenti demonstrates somewhat elevated vessels with white vessel walls. The majority of these vessels show nonperfusion. The more posterior retina was perfused and the anterior retina was ischemic.

shown to cause regression of neovascular tissue, presumably by a modulation of the ischemic signal for neovascularization. Direct feeder-vessel treatment also has been used.

Overall, the visual prognosis in Eales' disease is good, although patients may develop complications such as vitreous hemorrhage, tractional or rhegmatogenous retinal detachment, rubeosis irides, secondary glaucoma, or cataract.

BRANCH RETINAL VEIN OCCLUSION. Retinal neovascularization can occur with branch retinal vein occlusion.[23] Complications include vitreous hemorrhage, epiretinal membranes, and tractional or rhegmatogenous retinal detachments. Local scatter photocoagulation may cause regression of neovascular tissue and prevent vitreous hemorrhage (see Chapter 115).

RETINAL EMBOLIZATION. Intravenous drug abusers who intravenously inject chopped pills that contain talc may develop retinal neovascularization.[24] The talc reaches the ocular arterial system after passage through capillaries or collaterals in the pulmonary vascular system. The talc wedges in smaller caliber arterioles, such as those found in the macula and retinal periphery. Ischemia and neovascularization may ensue (Fig. 122-3). The neovascularization is responsive to either local scatter photocoagulation or cryopexy.

RETINOPATHY OF PREMATURITY. Retinopathy of prematurity (ROP) affects the peripheral vasculature of the retina. Normal vascularization of the retina commences at 4 months of gestation and usually is completed by 9 months. In some instances of low birth weight, prematurity, and supplemental administration of oxygen, the normal process of vascularization is interrupted. How this occurs is understood poorly, but it is thought that hyperoxia from supplemental oxygen may further interrupt normal vascular development, and hypoxia associated with maturing avascular retina may result in liberation of angiogenic stimuli. Some infants progress to neovascularization and its complications, which include tractional, exudative, or rhegmatogenous retinal detachment.[25]

Treatment of ROP hinges on its recognition. Risk factors for ROP must trigger careful examination and follow-up. Treatment involves the use of cryotherapy or scatter laser photocoagulation to the avascular peripheral retina. The object is to arrest actively proliferative lesions by treatment of presumably ischemic avascular retina, which helps to preserve an attached macula (see Chapter 115).

UVEITIS. Some patients who have uveitis, especially intermediate uveitis (pars planitis), may develop neovascularization of the disc or peripheral retina. Uveitic neovascularization appears

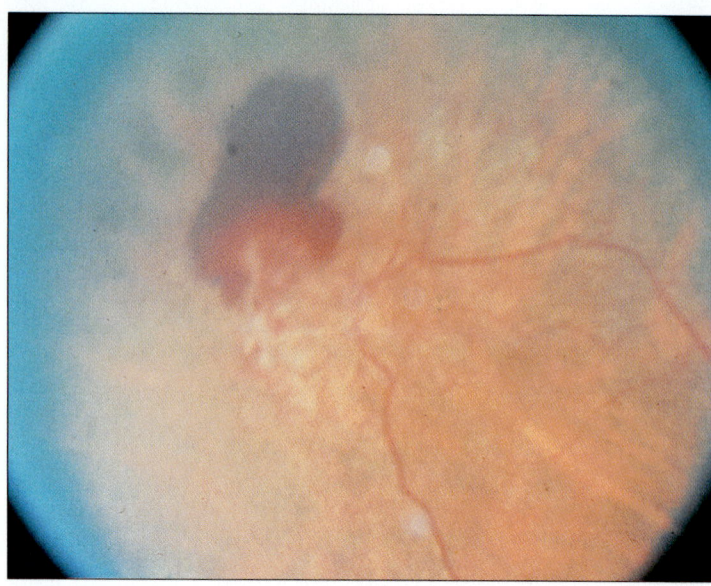

FIG. 122-3 ■ **Talc retinopathy.** An area of sea-fan neovascularization, with a small overlying vitreous hemorrhage is shown, in an intravenous drug abuser. Talc retinopathy is demonstrated elsewhere in the fundus.

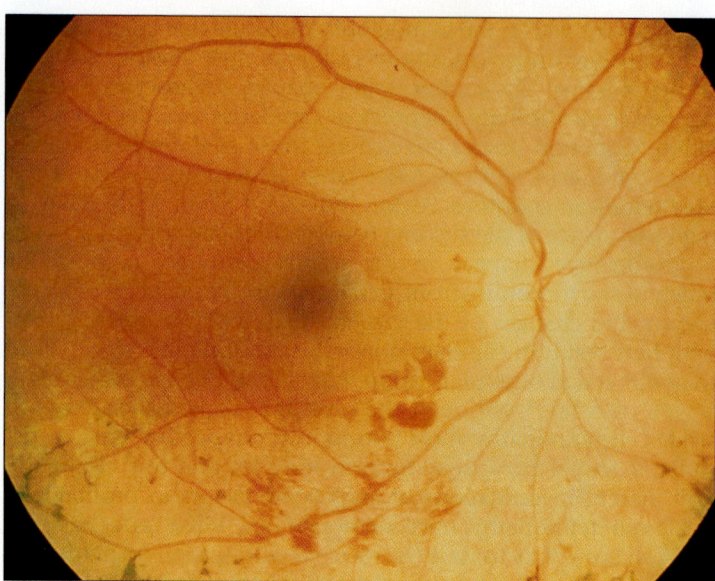

FIG. 122-4 ■ **Retinitis pigmentosa.** This fundus view demonstrates neovascularization of the disc, neovascularization elsewhere, and a small vitreous hemorrhage in a patient who has autosomal dominant retinitis pigmentosa.

to be determined by the severity of inflammation and presence of retinal nonperfusion. A trial of systemic steroids may be attempted and if ineffective, local scatter photocoagulation can be considered[26] (see Chapter 181).

ACUTE RETINAL NECROSIS. Both herpes simplex and herpes zoster cause the acute retinal necrosis syndrome, with findings that include anterior uveitis, vitritis, retinal vasculitis, necrotizing retinitis, and retinal detachment. The inflammation and ischemia may stimulate vascular proliferation[27] (see Chapter 173).

BIRDSHOT CHORIORETINOPATHY. Birdshot chorioretinopathy is characterized by white lesions in the deep retina or retinal pigment epithelium, and by vitritis, papillitis, and macular edema. Closure of peripheral retinal vessels may lead to vasoproliferation.[28] Local scatter photocoagulation has been shown to be beneficial.

LONG-STANDING RETINAL DETACHMENT. Retinal ischemia in a patient who has a prolonged retinal detachment may result from disruption of either the retinal or choroidal supply of oxygen or nutrients to the retina. The neovascularization may appear angiomatous or may take the shape of a sea fan. Surgical repair of a rhegmatogenous detachment can cause regression of the neovascularization.[29]

CHOROIDAL MELANOMA AND HEMANGIOMA. Both choroidal melanoma[30] and hemangioma,[31] perhaps by the release of a tumor angiogenic factor or secondary to retinal detachment over the tumor, can promote neovascularization that overlies the tumor. Treatment of a choroidal melanoma with radiation or scatter photocoagulation can cause regression of the neovascularization. Ocular tumors are covered in Part 9.

Hereditary Retinal Diseases

FAMILIAL EXUDATIVE VITREORETINOPATHY. Familial (dominant or X-linked) exudative vitreoretinopathy (FEVR) is a group of vascular disorders of the peripheral retina with findings on retinal examination that are very similar to those of ROP. However, FEVR differs from ROP in that patients usually are born at full term, have normal birth weight, and have not had supplemental oxygenation. In addition, a positive family history often is found. A demarcation line that separates vascular from avascular retina may occur in the retinal periphery. Peripheral retinal vessels assume a characteristic straightened course.

Presumably, an ischemic signal from the avascular retina stimulates neovascularization. These vessels may leak, form intraretinal or subretinal exudates, and result in exudative retinal

detachment. Some eyes develop cicatricial changes, which include straightened retinal vessels, foveal ectopia, meridional folds, tractional retinal detachment, or rhegmatogenous retinal detachment. Other complications include cataract, band keratopathy, rubeosis iridis, neovascular glaucoma and, in some eyes, phthisis bulbi.[32] Patients with the X-linked variety of FEVR may have abnormalities in the same gene that causes Norrie's disease.

As in ROP, treatment depends on early recognition. Cryotherapy and panperipheral photocoagulation of avascular retina have been shown to halt vasoproliferation in some patients.

INHERITED RETINAL VENOUS BEADING. This rare entity has an autosomal dominant inheritance pattern. Findings on retinal examination include venous beading, microaneurysms, hemorrhages, exudates, neovascularization, and vitreous hemorrhage.[33] Panretinal scatter photocoagulation is advocated as treatment for neovascularization.

RETINOSCHISIS. Patients who have X-linked (juvenile) retinoschisis, degenerative retinoschisis, or acquired retinoschisis with shaken baby syndrome[34] can develop retinal neovascularization. In X-linked retinoschisis, whitish deposits may be seen at the point where peripheral vessels appear to be occluded. Consequent to vascular occlusion, ischemia may promote neovascularization.[35]

RETINITIS PIGMENTOSA. Patients who have retinitis pigmentosa can have neovascularization of the disc and retina (Fig. 122-4).[36] The pathogenesis of the neovascularization is unknown but may be related to the inflammation seen in this disorder. These patients have diffuse loss of retinal pigment epithelial cells, so laser photocoagulation burns are difficult to create. Cryopexy has proved beneficial. Full details are given in Chapter 108.

AUTOSOMAL DOMINANT VITREORETINOCHOROIDOPATHY. Autosomal dominant vitreoretinochoroidopathy is a rare disorder in which the ocular findings include abnormal peripheral chorioretinal pigmentation that has a characteristic sharp demarcation near the equator. Patients also may manifest cataract, macular edema, retinal neovascularization, vitreous hemorrhage, and selective b wave reduction on an electroretinogram.[37]

OVERVIEW ON DIAGNOSING AND TREATING NEOVASCULARIZATION

If retinal neovascularization is identified and the cause is unknown (Fig. 122-5), the physician should obtain a detailed

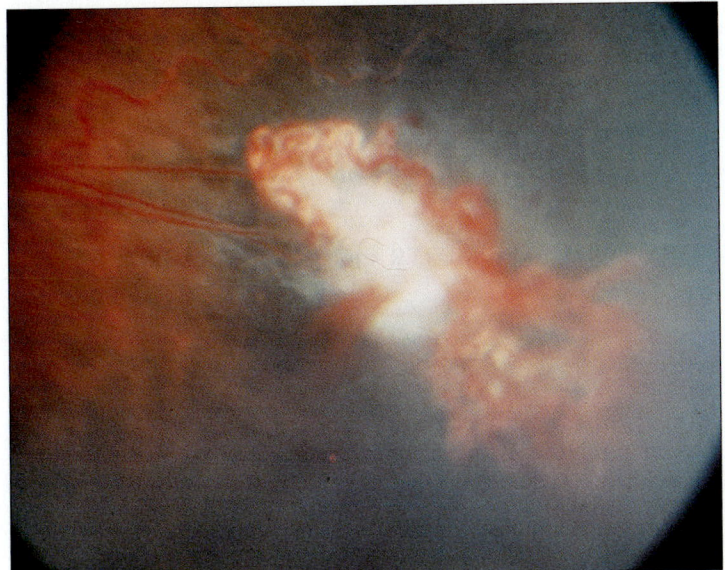

FIG. 122-5 ▪ **Idiopathic proliferative retinopathy.** The temporal periphery of the left retina demonstrates an elevated fibrovascular lesion like a sea fan in an African-American who was otherwise completely healthy. Tests for sickle-cell disease were negative and no causative factor for the neovascularization could be determined. The other eye has no peripheral fundus abnormalities.

medical, family, birth, and social history. ROP, talc retinopathy, diabetes, and familial exudative vitreoretinopathy all are diagnoses that a thorough history will help to uncover. Furthermore, with a detailed review of systems and a family history, disorders can be grouped quickly into one of the categories outlined in Box 122-1. Finally, laboratory tests can be directed toward specific disorders suggested by the history and examination. For example, a suspected diagnosis of a hemoglobinopathy may be confirmed by hemoglobin electrophoresis.

When retinal neovascularization is identified, treatment often is given to prevent complications such as vitreous hemorrhage and rhegmatogenous retinal detachment. In addition to treatment of the underlying systemic condition, the neovascular tissue itself should be treated, if possible, by photocoagulation, cryopexy, or vitreoretinal surgery.

The rationale of treatment is to alter ischemic or inflammatory tissues so that the neovascular stimulus is suppressed. The argon laser may be used to create retinal burns. When hemorrhage or dense nuclear sclerotic cataracts are present, a red or diode laser may be used because these wavelengths penetrate such media better, or the cataract may be removed. In general, laser spots are scattered about one burn-width apart in areas of the retina thought to be ischemic. The power and duration settings on the laser are adjusted so that the laser burn appears as a moderate-intensity gray–white lesion.

If the retinal ischemic process seems to affect the entire retina diffusely, such as in diabetes mellitus, scatter photocoagulation should be placed throughout the peripheral retina (panretinal photocoagulation). Direct treatment of vessels flat on the retina that feed or drain neovascular tissue (feeder-vessel coagulation) is effective. However, such treatment has a greater incidence of complications, which include retinal tears or breaks in Bruch's membrane, than does scatter treatment. Direct treatment of elevated neovascular tissue is not effective.

If neovascular tissue cannot be treated with the laser (e.g., because of a media opacity), then cryopexy may be useful. Similar to the laser, it is applied to peripheral ischemic retina and affects the neovascular tissue indirectly. Alternatively, vitreoretinal surgery is indicated for long-standing vitreous hemorrhage, for repair of rhegmatogenous or tractional retinal detachment, and when epiretinal membrane removal is needed. Removal of the posterior vitreous face also removes the scaffolding for further neovascularization. Furthermore, vitrectomy may remove angiogenic factors affecting the retinal vasculature.

REFERENCES

1. Jampol LM, Ebroon DA, Goldbaum MH. Peripheral proliferative retinopathies: an update on angiogenesis, etiologies, and management. Surv Ophthalmol. 1994;38:519–40.
2. Borkowski LM, Jampol LM. Frosted branch angiitis complicated by retinal neovascularization. Retina. 1999;19:454–5.
3. Chang TS, Aylward GW, Davis JL, et al. Idiopathic retinal vasculitis, aneurysms, and neuro-retinitis. Ophthalmology. 1995;102:1089–97.
4. Lee BL, Bateman JB, Schwartz SD. Posterior segment neovascularization associated with optic nerve aplasia. Am J Ophthalmol. 1996;122:131–3.
5. Leys AM, Leys MJ, Hooymans JM, et al. Myelinated nerve fibers and retinal vascular abnormalities. Retina. 1996;16:89–96.
6. Kinyoun JL, Lawrence BS, Barlow WE. Proliferative radiation retinopathy. Arch Ophthalmol. 1996;114:1097–100.
7. Kwak N, Okamoto N, Wood JM, et al. VEGF is a major stimulator in model of choroidal neovascularization. Invest Ophthalmol Vis Sci. 2000;41:3158–64.
8. Aiello LP, Avery RL, Arrigg PG, et al. Vascular endothelial growth factor in ocular fluid of patients with diabetic retinopathy and other retinal disorders. N Engl J Med. 1994;331:1480–7.
9. Stellmach V, Crawford SE, Zhou W, et al. Prevention of ischemia-induced retinopathy by the natural ocular antiangiogenic agent pigment epithelium-derived factor. Proc Natl Acad Sci U S A. 2001;98:2593–7.
10. Frank RN, Ryan SJ Jr. Peripheral retinal neovascularization with chronic myelogenous leukemia. Arch Ophthalmol. 1972;87:585–9.
11. Brown GC, Magargal LE, Simeone FA, et al. Arterial obstruction and ocular neovascularization. Ophthalmology. 1982;89:139–46.
12. Kalina RE, Kelly WA. Proliferative retinopathy after treatment of carotid–cavernous fistulas. Arch Ophthalmol. 1978;96:2058–60.
13. Vine AK. Severe periphlebitis, peripheral retinal ischemia, and preretinal neovascularization in patients with multiple sclerosis. Am J Ophthalmol. 1992;113:28–32.
14. Kayazawa F, Honda A. Severe retinal vascular lesions in systemic lupus erythematosus. Ann Ophthalmol. 1981;13:1291–4.
15. Bogie GJ, Nanda SK. Neovascularization associated with cytomegalovirus retinitis. Retina. 2001;21:85–7.
16. Blumenkranz MS, Kaplan HJ, Clarkson JG, et al. Acute multifocal hemorrhagic retinal vasculitis. Ophthalmology. 1988;95:1663–72.
17. Asdourian GK, Goldberg MF, Busse BJ. Peripheral retinal neovascularization in sarcoidosis. Arch Ophthalmol. 1975;93:787–91.
18. Goldberg MF. Classification and pathogenesis of proliferative sickle retinopathy. Am J Ophthalmol. 1971;71:649–65.
19. Cao J, Mathews MK, McLeod DS, et al. Angiogenic factors in human proliferative sickle cell retinopathy. Br J Ophthalmol. 1999;83:838–46.
20. Farber MD, Jampol LM, Fox P, et al. A randomized clinical trial of scatter photocoagulation of proliferative sickle cell retinopathy. Arch Ophthalmol. 1991;109:363–7.
21. Goldberg MF, Custis PH. Retinal and other manifestations of incontinentia pigmenti. Ophthalmology. 1993;100:1645–54.
22. Elliot AJ. 30-year observation of patients with Eales' disease. Am J Ophthalmol. 1975;12:404–8.
23. Orth DH, Patz A. Retinal branch vein occlusion. Surv Ophthalmol. 1978;22:357–76.
24. Tse DT, Ober RR. Talc retinopathy. Am J Ophthalmol. 1980;90:624–40.
25. Kingham JD. Acute retrolental fibroplasia. Arch Ophthalmol. 1977;95:39–47.
26. Kuo IC, Cunningham ET Jr. Ocular neovascularization in patients with uveitis. Int Ophthalmol Clin. 2000;40:111–26.
27. Wang CL, Kaplan HJ, Waldrep JC, et al. Retinal neovascularization associated with acute retinal necrosis. Retina. 1983;3:249–52.
28. Barondes MJ, Fastenberg DM, Schwartz PL, et al. Peripheral retinal neovascularization in birdshot retinochoroidopathy. Ann Ophthalmol. 1989;21:306–8.
29. Felder KS, Brockhurst RJ. Retinal neovascularization complicating rhegmatogenous retinal detachment of long duration. Am J Ophthalmol. 1982;93:773–6.
30. Lee J, Logani S, Lakosha H, et al. Preretinal neovascularization associated with choroidal melanoma. Br J Ophthalmol. 2001;85:1309–12.
31. Leys AM, Bonnet S. Case report: associated retinal neovascularization and choroidal hemangioma. Retina. 1993;13:22–5.
32. Ober RR, Bird AC, Hamilton AM, et al. Autosomal dominant exudative vitreoretinopathy. Br J Ophthalmol. 1980;64:112–20.
33. Stewart MW, Gitter KA. Inherited retinal venous beading. Am J Ophthalmol. 1988;106:675–81.
34. Brown SM, Shami M. Optic disc neovascularization following severe retinoschisis due to shaken baby syndrome. Arch Ophthalmol. 1999;117:838–9.
35. Pearson R, Jagger J. Sex linked juvenile retinoschisis with optic disc and peripheral retinal neovascularization. Br J Ophthalmol. 1989;73:311–3.
36. Uliss AE, Gregor ZJ, Bird AC. Retinitis pigmentosa and retinal neovascularization. Ophthalmology. 1986;93:1599–603.
37. Blair NP, Goldberg MF, Fishman GSA, et al. Autosomal dominant vitreoretinochoroidopathy (ADVIRC). Br J Ophthalmol. 1984;68:2–9.

123 Retinal Arterial Macroaneurysms

JANICE E. CONTRERAS • ROBERT A. MITTRA • WILLIAM F. MIELER • JOHN S. POLLACK

DEFINITION
- Localized fusiform or saccular dilation of a retinal arterial vessel within the first three orders of bifurcation.

KEY FEATURES
- Retinal hemorrhage (intraretinal, subretinal, preretinal, and vitreous).
- Protein and lipid exudation.
- Macular edema.

ASSOCIATED FEATURES
- Leaking, telangiectatic vessels in the capillary bed that surrounds the macroaneurysm.
- Retinal artery occlusion.
- Retinal vein occlusion.

INTRODUCTION

Although aneurysms of the retinal arteries have been noted since the early 1900s, Robertson[1] in 1973 was the first to coin the term *macroaneurysm* to describe a distinct clinical entity that consisted of an acquired focal dilation of a retinal artery within the first three orders of bifurcation. Macroaneurysms vary from 100–250μm in diameter, are saccular or fusiform in shape, and are differentiated readily from capillary microaneurysms, which are usually less than 100μm in diameter. Retinal arterial macroaneurysms can be further differentiated from the vessel dilations seen in Coats' disease, which are multiple saccular outpouches of predominantly the venous and capillary system, associated with marked telangiectasia and lipid exudation, primarily found in young males.

Although the clinical course of a retinal arterial macroaneurysm is often benign, in some cases significant visual morbidity results from macular hemorrhage, exudate, or edema, or from the development of a vitreous hemorrhage.

EPIDEMIOLOGY AND PATHOGENESIS

Retinal arterial macroaneurysms tend to occur in older people; most case series include subjects over the age of 60 years.[2–7] Multiple studies conclusively confirm a marked female preponderance, in the range of 60–100%.[2–8] Macroaneurysms typically occur in one eye, with bilaterality in less than 10%.[9] The most consistent systemic association of retinal arterial macroaneurysms is with hypertension—a large controlled study reported it in 79% of patients.[7]

The exact pathogenesis of a macroaneurysm is unknown, but several authors have developed compelling theories. Many have compared retinal arterial aneurysms to cerebral arterial aneurysms, which are generally 100–300μm in diameter, are also more common in women than men, and occur in patients over

50 years of age with a history of hypertension.[1,6,10] Chronic hypertension, along with the replacement of arterial smooth muscle by collagen associated with aging, may effect a focal dilation of the arterial wall in an area of weakness or prior damage. Lavin *et al.*[6] postulated that macroaneurysms are detected more frequently at arteriovenous crossings, because at these locations the arterial and venous walls are in contact without an adventitial layer, which results in an area of limited structural support. Other investigators have noted the development of macroaneurysms at the sites of previously detected emboli.[4,11] They hypothesize that focal arterial damage secondary to embolization can lead to aneurysm formation. Gass now believes that the focal, yellow arterial plaques present are actually atheromas that occur at the site of defects in the arterial wall.[12] He proposes that the previously reported emboli were, in fact, atheromas.

Abdel-Khalek and Richardson[5] detected specific differences between aneurysms that led to hemorrhagic complications and those that resulted in lipid exudation. They found that saccular or "blowout" aneurysms were more prone to bleed, possibly as a result of a thin, stretched aneurysmal sac. This type of lesion develops closer to the optic nerve head, where perfusion pressures are higher.[6] In addition, systolic blood pressures above 200mmHg are more common in patients who have bleeding macroaneurysms. Fusiform dilations, on the other hand, are more prone to result in exudation and to be associated with venous occlusions.[5,6] It is possible that the cause of those aneurysms that eventually lead to hemorrhagic complications is more dependent on hypertension and vessel wall damage, while the cause of those that lead to exudation is more contingent upon local vascular factors.

OCULAR MANIFESTATIONS

The clinical picture of macroaneurysms can be highly variable, dependent on whether the macroaneurysm is hemorrhagic or exudative in nature. Hemorrhagic macroaneurysm can result in acute loss of vision with evidence of subretinal, intraretinal, or preretinal hemorrhage on ocular examination (Fig. 123-1). Often the hemorrhage obscures the site of the aneurysm, but the presence of a localized preretinal and subretinal hemorrhage over a major retinal artery should suggest the possibility of its presence. A nonclearing vitreous hemorrhage without evidence of retinal tear or posterior vitreous detachment may be the result of a macroaneurysm. Because bleeding tends to thrombose the aneurysm, detection once the hemorrhage has cleared may be difficult. The involved artery often retains a focal tortuosity or Z-shaped kink at the location of the involuted aneurysm, which lends indirect evidence in support of the diagnosis.

Patients also can experience a more gradual decline in vision secondary to serous fluid and lipid accumulation in the macula (Fig. 123-2). Exudative macroaneurysms most often are located on the temporal vascular arcades, although rarely macroaneurysms can occur on the optic nerve head, cilioretinal artery, and nasal vessels.[13,14] They frequently demonstrate a circinate lipid pattern (see Fig. 123-2). Finally, asymptomatic macro-

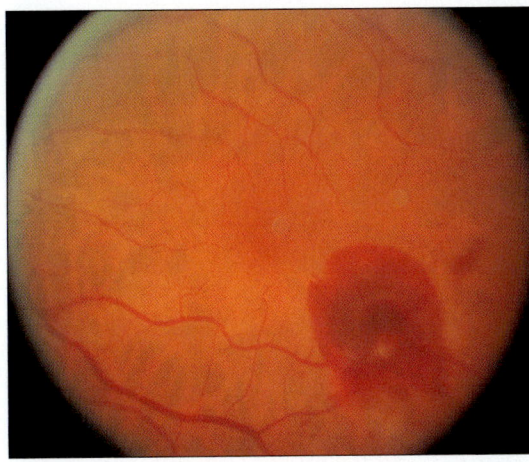

FIG. 123-1 ▮ **Hemorrhagic macroaneurysm.** Note the preretinal and subretinal hemorrhages directly above and below the artery.

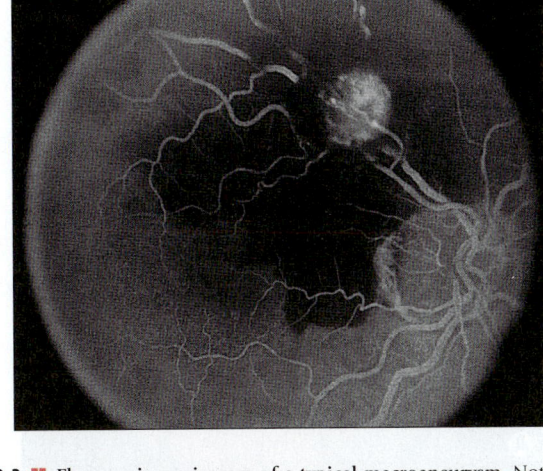

FIG. 123-3 ▮ **Fluorescein angiogram of a typical macroaneurysm.** Note the complete early filling of the macroaneurysm with fluorescein dye.

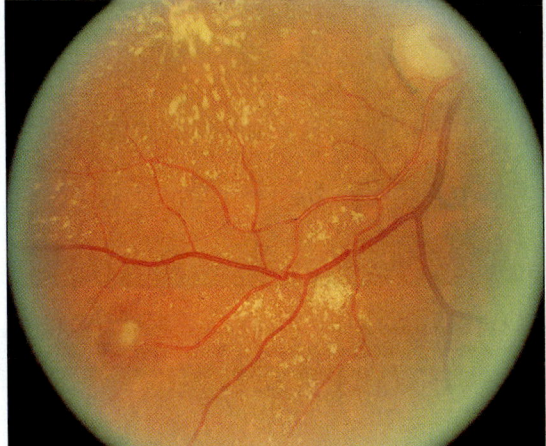

FIG. 123-2 ▮ **Exudative macroaneurysm.** Note the aneurysm along the superotemporal arcade, with marked lipid exudation that extends into the central macula.

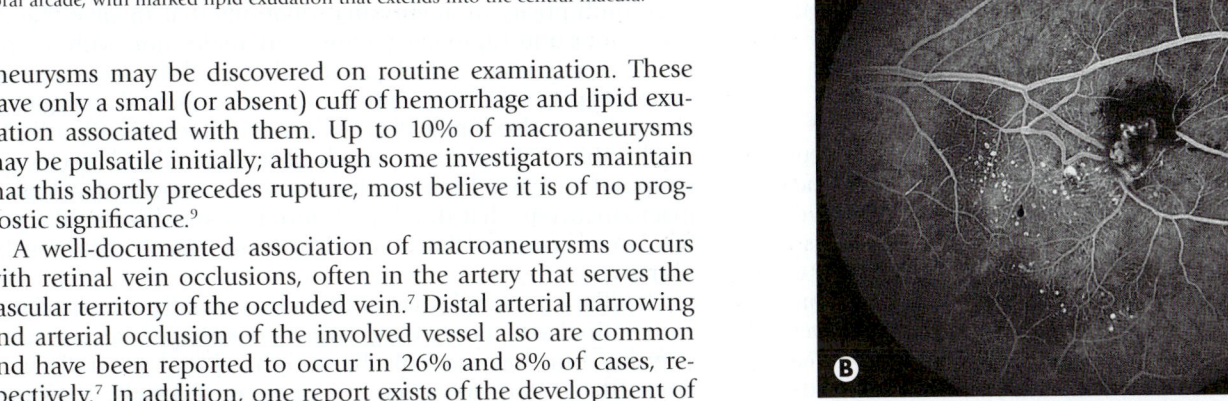

FIG. 123-4 ▮ **Macroaneurysm with surrounding dilated and telangiectatic capillary bed. A,** Note the large bilobed macroaneurysm with surrounding circinate lipid. **B,** The fluorescein angiogram shows dilated, tortuous capillaries and microaneurysms surrounding the macroaneurysm. (Courtesy of Susan Fowell, MD.)

aneurysms may be discovered on routine examination. These have only a small (or absent) cuff of hemorrhage and lipid exudation associated with them. Up to 10% of macroaneurysms may be pulsatile initially; although some investigators maintain that this shortly precedes rupture, most believe it is of no prognostic significance.[9]

A well-documented association of macroaneurysms occurs with retinal vein occlusions, often in the artery that serves the vascular territory of the occluded vein.[7] Distal arterial narrowing and arterial occlusion of the involved vessel also are common and have been reported to occur in 26% and 8% of cases, respectively.[7] In addition, one report exists of the development of retinal macroaneurysms in a 62-year-old patient who has a history of congenital arteriovenous communications.[15]

DIAGNOSIS AND ANCILLARY TESTING

Diagnosis of lesions is based on the characteristic fundus appearance, as described above. Macroaneurysms which have undergone closure may be recognized by Z-shaped deformities in the involved vessel (see above).

Fluorescein angiography may reveal or confirm the presence of a macroaneurysm, usually demonstrating immediate, complete filling of the aneurysm (Fig. 123-3). In some cases, irregular and incomplete filling may be associated with partial thrombosis, and a faint shell (or no) fluorescence may be displayed with a completely involuted macroaneurysm.[9] Leakage from the wall of the aneurysm is common in active lesions. Evidence of arteriolar narrowing usually is present proximal and distal to the macroaneurysm.[12] In many cases, microvascular abnormalities

surround the aneurysm, including a wider capillary-free zone, capillary dilation, capillary nonperfusion, microaneurysms, and intra-arterial collateral vessels[12] (Fig. 123-4).

In cases with dense hemorrhage when fluorescein angiography does not provide definitive evidence of a retinal arterial macroaneurysm, indocyanine green angiography may be a useful adjunct.[16] Because the absorption and emission spectra are in the near-infrared range, the dye can better penetrate through dense hemorrhages, revealing structures that may otherwise be obscured. Additionally, in treatment of a macroaneurysm, indocyanine green dye may leak less than fluorescein, thus providing well-defined images.[16]

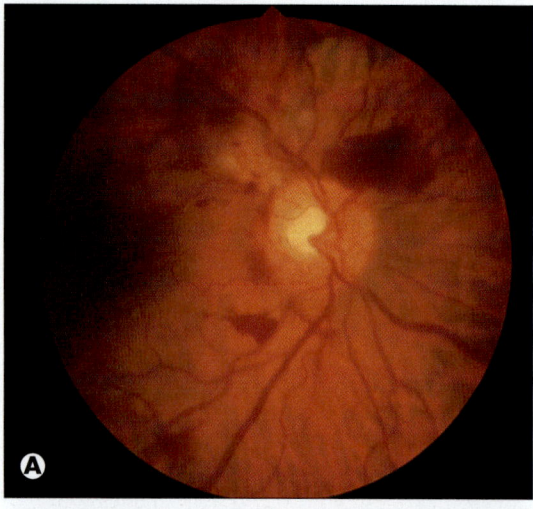

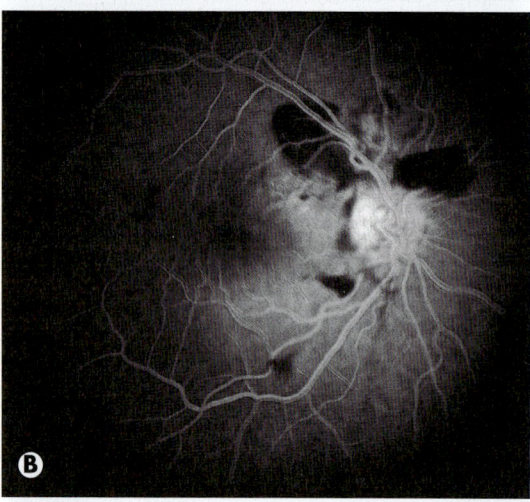

FIG. 123-5 ■ **Venous macroaneurysm secondary to branch retinal vein occlusion.** **A,** Note the venous aneurysm superior to the disc occurring in the setting of a branch retinal vein occlusion. **B,** Fluorescein angiogram showing hyperfluorescence in the venous aneurysm. There was no late leakage from this lesion. (Courtesy of Susan Anderson-Nelson.)

DIFFERENTIAL DIAGNOSIS

Many clinical entities simulate retinal arterial macroaneurysms. Schulman et al.[17] reported large-capillary aneurysms secondary to retinal venous obstruction. These aneurysms are similar in dimension to macroaneurysms, but they originate from the venous side of the capillary bed and may result in visual loss from macular edema, serous elevation of the macula, and circinate lipid exudation.

Venous macroaneurysms also are seen after retinal vein obstruction[18,19] (Fig. 123-5). Cousins et al.[19] recently reviewed their patients involved in the Branch Vein Occlusion Study and noted four types of aneurysms in the area of the vein occlusion:

- Arterial macroaneurysms
- Capillary macroaneurysms (Schulman et al.[17])
- Venous macroaneurysms
- Collateral-associated macroaneurysms

All four types were associated with hemorrhagic and lipid exudation and were found in areas of capillary nonperfusion.

Kimmel et al.[20] reported a case of a temporal branch retinal vein obstruction that masqueraded as a macroaneurysm with the Bonet sign, which consists of hemorrhage at an arteriovenous crossing that indicates an incipient branch vein occlusion. Given the similar patient characteristics and that these two entities are seen together often, differential diagnosis can be difficult. One patient was reported to have had a Valsalva episode that resulted in rupture of a retinal arterial macroaneurysm.[21] In another report, a lesion that simulated an optic nerve head tumor associated with a branch retinal arterial obstruction was eventually diagnosed as a macroaneurysm after 6 months of follow-up.[13]

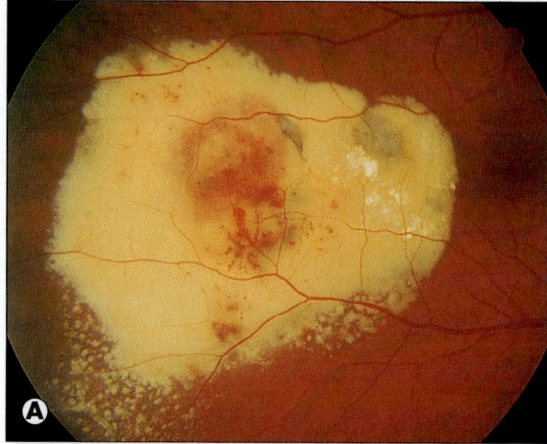

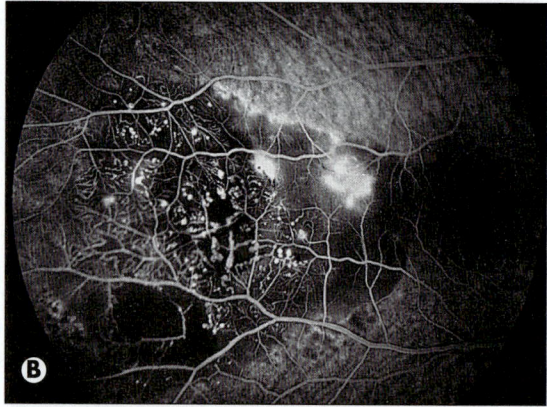

FIG. 123-6 ■ **Coats' disease. A,** The classic fundus picture of Coats' disease with massive lipid exudation causing an exudative retinal detachment. **B,** Fluorescein angiogram from the same patient with large telangiectatic vessels and numerous leaking aneurysms.

Retinal telangiectasia of Coats' disease can be differentiated from a macroaneurysm based on age of onset, gender predilection, multiplicity of aneurysmal dilations that involve mainly the venous and capillary systems, and association with a large net of telangiectatic vessels, as revealed on fluorescein angiography (Fig. 123-6). The adult–Coats' or juxtafoveal telangiectasis syndrome also can be distinguished on the basis of multiple, small-caliber telangiectatic vessels observed in the characteristic temporal macular location; however, one report of a typical macroaneurysm that developed into a Coats' disease–like picture demonstrates that the distinction can sometimes be blurred.[8]

Capillary hemangiomas of the retina usually are associated with retinal edema, exudate, and hemorrhage-like macroaneurysms, but they are typically peripheral and generally have large dilated, tortuous afferent and efferent vessels. Angiomas also can occur on the optic nerve head, where differentiation from macroaneurysms may be particularly difficult. Capillary hemangiomas usually are inherited and often are seen as part of Von Hippel–Lindau disease, which is autosomal dominant with multiple systemic findings that include cerebellar hemangioblastoma, renal cell carcinoma, and pheochromocytoma. A nonfamilial form of acquired angioma, however, which lacks the characteristic large dilated vessels, has been described and more easily can be confused with macroaneurysm[22] (Fig. 123-7). The acquired lesions are either primary, idiopathic, or secondary to a variety of underlying ocular conditions, most commonly retinitis pigmentosa and uveitis.[23] These lesions, or vasoproliferative tumors, can display considerable growth seen on long-term follow-up, which further differentiates them from macroaneurysms.[24]

The accumulation of a subretinal hemorrhage in the macula from a macroaneurysm in an elderly patient with evidence of drusen and pigmentary changes may be confused with a choroidal

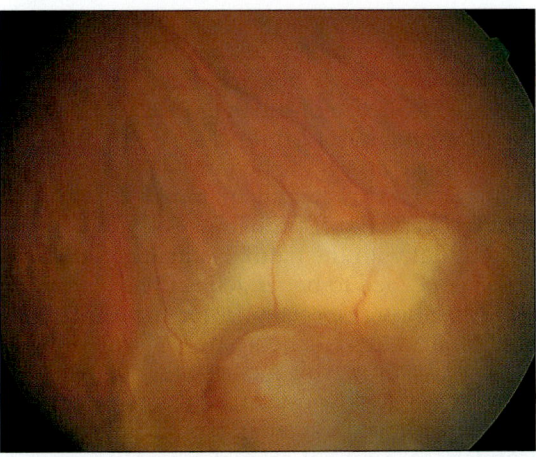

FIG. 123-7 ■ **Idiopathic retinal vasoproliferative tumor.** A typical inferiorly located lesion with conspicuous lack of dilated feeder and drainage vessels. (From McCabe CM, Mieler WF. Arch Ophthalmol. 1996;114[5]:617.)

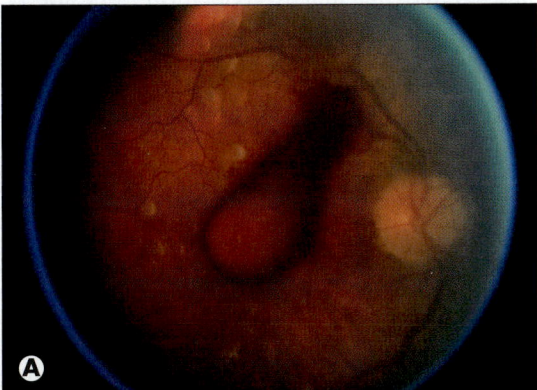

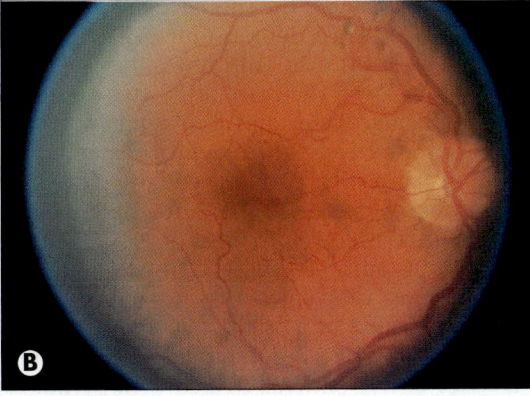

FIG. 123-8 ■ **Submacular hemorrhage simulating choroidal neovascularization.** **A,** Prominent submacular hemorrhage in an elderly patient simulating choroidal neovascular membrane. **B,** Same patient 3 months later following spontaneous resolution of hemorrhage.

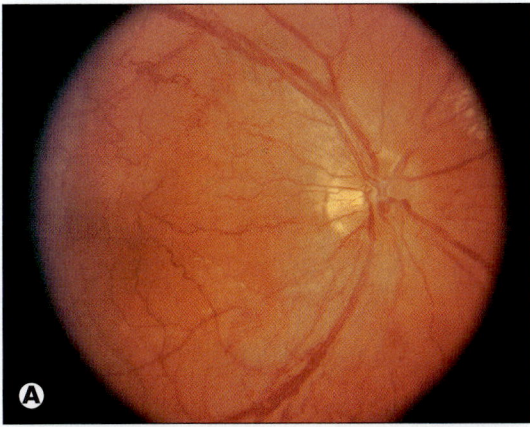

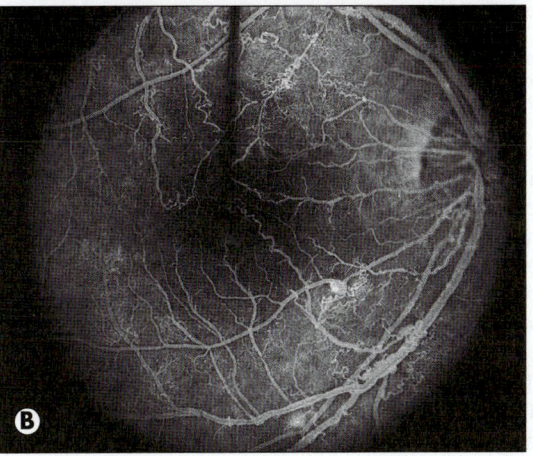

FIG. 123-9 ■ **IRVAN syndrome. A,** Multiple arterial dilations in a patient with IRVAN syndrome. **B,** Fluorescein angiogram readily documents the numerous aneurysms in the juxtapapillary region.

SYSTEMIC ASSOCIATIONS

The only consistent systemic association with retinal arterial aneurysms is systemic arterial hypertension. In a case-control series this was observed in 79% of patients with macroaneurysm and 55% of controls. The difference was found to be statistically significant. The evaluation of a patient who has a macroaneurysm but who has no previous history of hypertension should include the measurement of blood pressure.

PATHOLOGY

Gold *et al.*[28] described a pathology specimen from a patient with a single macroaneurysm and a large ring of circinate lipid in the macula. They found a macroaneurysm located at an arteriovenous crossing, surrounded by dilated capillaries and a heterogeneous accumulation of collagen, hemosiderin, and lipid, with a paramacular deposition of lipid and proteinaceous exudate in the outer plexiform layer. It was proposed that the dilated capillary network that surrounded the macroaneurysm was the source of serous and lipid exudation into the macula. Other reports of ruptured aneurysms have shown evidence of a break in the artery covered by a dense fibrin–platelet clot that contains blood, exudate, lipid-laden macrophages, hemosiderin, and fibroglial reaction products in amounts that vary among patients[29] (Fig. 123-10).

TREATMENT, COURSE, AND OUTCOME

Although treatments using the xenon arc[4,5] and argon[6,10,30] and dye yellow[30–33] lasers, both directly at and around the macroaneurysm, have been described, a laser approach remains controversial. Most authors agree that hemorrhagic macroaneurysms, especially those which cause vitreous or preretinal hemorrhage, tend to thrombose and ultimately result in a better visual outcome than do exudative macroaneurysms, which may

neovascular membrane from age-related macular degeneration (Fig. 123-8). If suspicion of a macroaneurysm exists, then careful examination of the nearby artery and fluorescein angiography are indicated.

There are several reported cases of retinal arterial macroaneurysms with massive subretinal hemorrhage appearing as a dark mass simulating choroidal melanoma.[25] Fluorescein angiography and ultrasonography can aid in the diagnosis.

A distinct entity of multiple aneurysms that involve all the major retinal vessels in both eyes, with neuroretinopathy, vitreous and anterior chamber inflammation, and angiographic evidence of arteritis, has been called the IRVAN (*i*diopathic *r*etinal *v*asculitis, *a*neurysms, and *n*euroretinitis) syndrome[12,26,27] (Fig. 123-9). The cause of this rare disorder is unknown. The disparate clinical findings and the young age range of the patients readily differentiate it from macroaneurysms.

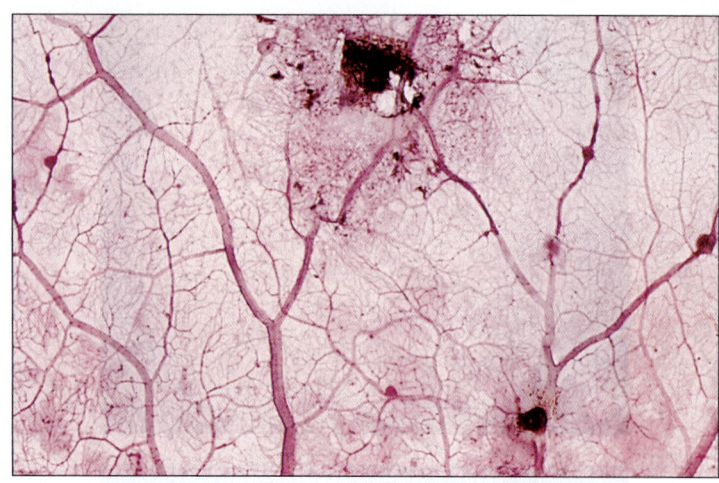

FIG. 123-10 ■ **Retinal arteriolar macroaneurysm.** PAS-stained trypsin-digest preparation. (Courtesy Streeten BW. In: Yanoff M, Fine BS. Ocular pathology, ed 4. London: Mosby; 1995.)

eventually cause macular edema.[2,3,5,10] Therefore, patients who have decreased acuity secondary to retinal or vitreous hemorrhage probably should be followed for several months to enable spontaneous clearance. Many investigators believe that patients who have exudative macroaneurysm and significant macular involvement should undergo photocoagulation treatment, either directly to the lesion[4,5,32,33] or to the surrounding capillary bed,[10] in an effort to close the macroaneurysm and the leaking perianeurysmal vessels. The rationale is that the poorest visual outcomes are observed when macular edema and lipid are allowed to remain for many months.

However, no prospective trial of laser therapy for macroaneurysm has been performed, and the several small uncontrolled clinical series demonstrate mixed results. Abdel-Khalek and Richardson[5] treated 10 eyes and noted visual improvement in two, with no change in seven, and a visual decrease in one. Palestine et al.[10] were unable to show a visual benefit using laser for eyes with macular pathology in six treated eyes versus five controls. Joondeph et al.[33] reported improvement in visual acuity in 8 of 12 cases using the dye yellow laser, while another recent case-control study showed that direct laser treatment resulted in a significantly greater risk for a visual acuity of less than 20/80 when compared with controls.[30] Laser surgery also is associated with an increased threat of arteriolar occlusion, which theoretically may be amplified when using the dye yellow laser.[7,31] Until further definitive studies are performed to elucidate the proper role of and method for using lasers in the treatment of macroaneurysms, laser therapy should be reserved for select exudative macroaneurysms that involve the macula and threaten the fovea with the progressive accumulation of lipid. When employing laser, argon green or dye yellow lasers can be used with long-duration burns (0.2–0.5 seconds) and large spot sizes (500μm in diameter).

Several additional modalities have been advocated for treatment of premacular and submacular hemorrhage associated with retinal arterial macroaneurysms. The neodymium: yttrium–aluminum–garnet laser (Nd:YAG) has been employed in the treatment of dense premacular hemorrhage in order to speed visual recovery and potentially limit tractional macular detachment.[34–36] Nd:YAG photodisruption creates a focal opening in the anterior surface of the preretinal hemorrhage to allow for drainage of entrapped hemorrhage into the vitreous cavity. In a study of six eyes with preretinal hemorrhage secondary to macroaneurysm formation, all eyes showed improvement of vision within 1 week of Nd:YAG photodisruption.[35] In a retrospective review of 21 eyes with premacular hemorrhage secondary to various causes, visual improvement occurred within 1 month in 16 of 21 eyes.[36] However, seven patients required an additional vitrectomy for nonclearing vitreous hemorrhage and

complications including a macular hole and retinal detachment. The macular hole occurred in an eye with a premacular subhyaloid hemorrhage of only one disc diameter. The authors postulated that the small size of the hemorrhage did not provide a sufficient dampening effect for the laser burst, and they recommend laser drainage only if the hemorrhage is beyond three disc diameters in size.[36] This treatment modality can be used for rapid visual recovery, but it probably results in visual outcome no better than that with the natural course of the disease. Long-term studies are needed to better define the risks and benefits of laser photodisruption, especially in for hemorrhage associated with a retinal macroarterial aneurysm.

Pars plana vitrectomy with the use of tissue plasminogen activator (t-PA) has been advocated for the removal of dense, thick subretinal hemorrhage.[37,38] Patients with submacular hemorrhage secondary to a retinal arterial macroaneurysm have had generally favorable visual outcomes with this technique.[3] However, it appears that patients with submacular hemorrhage secondary to retinal arterial macroaneurysms may obtain better visual outcomes than those with hemorrhage from other causes, such as age-related macular degeneration. McCabe et al.[39] recently reviewed the cases of 41 patients with macular hemorrhage secondary to retinal artery macroaneurysms managed with observation alone and found that good visual outcomes often could be achieved with observation alone (see Fig. 123-9). Furthermore, visual outcomes were similar to those of reported cases of patients with submacular hemorrhage secondary to retinal arterial macroaneurysm treated surgically.

Most recently, investigators have treated submacular hemorrhage using pneumatic displacement both with and without the adjunct of intravitreous t-PA.[40–42] Pneumatic displacement is a technique initially suggested by Heriot[40] for subfoveal hemorrhage. It consists of pretreatment with intravitreal t-PA followed by injection of perfluoropropane or sulfur hexafluoride gas, with prone positioning for at least 24 hours in order to compress the macula directly and displace the submacular hemorrhage inferiorly. His initial experience demonstrated displacement of the hemorrhage in 19 of 20 eyes with few complications. Hassan and colleagues[41] reviewed the cases of 15 eyes treated with t-PA and pneumatic displacement and found that subfoveal blood can be displaced effectively, often with substantial initial improvement in visual acuity. Because retinal toxic effects from t-PA have been observed in animal studies, investigators recommend avoiding intravitreous injections of t-PA in concentrations greater than 25μg/0.1ml.[41] Likewise, caution was advised in the use of intravitreous t-PA injection in patients with arterial macroaneurysm because of a possible increased risk of vitreous hemorrhage. Amid concerns of the toxicity of t-PA, Ohji et al.[42] reported a series of five patients treated with perfluoropropane gas followed by prone positioning, without pretreatment with t-PA. Vision improved and blood was displaced from the fovea partially or completely in all five patients. Nevertheless, they speculate that solid blood clots present longer than 1 week may not be displaced with gas compression alone.[42]

In summary, the preferred treatment for patients with macular hemorrhage secondary to retinal arterial macroaneurysm remains controversial. The precise role of these advanced vitreoretinal techniques in the treatment of macroaneurysm will be clarified only with further study.

REFERENCES

1. Robertson DM. Macroaneurysms of the retinal arteries. Trans Am Acad Ophthalmol Otolaryngol. 1973;77:OP55–67.
2. Cleary PE, Kohner EM, Hamilton AM, Bird AC. Retinal macroaneurysms. Br J Ophthalmol. 1975;59:355–61.
3. Nadel AJ, Gupta KK. Macroaneurysms of the retinal arteries. Arch Ophthalmol. 1976;94:1092–6.
4. Lewis RA, Norton EW, Gass JDM. Acquired arterial macroaneurysms of the retina. Br J Ophthalmol. 1976;60:21–30.
5. Abdel-Khalek MN, Richardson J. Retinal macroaneurysm: natural history and guidelines for treatment. Br J Ophthalmol. 1986;70:2–11.
6. Lavin MJ, Marsh RJ, Peart S, Rehman A. Retinal arterial macroaneurysms: a retrospective study of 40 patients. Br J Ophthalmol. 1987;71:817–25.

7. Panton RW, Goldberg MF, Farber MD. Retinal arterial macroaneurysms: risk factors and natural history. Br J Ophthalmol. 1990;74:595–600.
8. Asdourian GK, Goldberg MF, Jampol LM, Rabb M. Retinal macroaneurysms. Arch Ophthalmol. 1977;95:624–8.
9. Rabb MF, Gagliano DA, Teske MP. Retinal arterial macroaneurysms. Surv Ophthalmol. 1988;33:73–96.
10. Palestine AG, Robertson DM, Goldstein BG. Macroaneurysms of the retinal arteries. Am J Ophthalmol. 1982;93:164–71.
11. Wiznia RA. Development of a retinal artery macroaneurysm at the site of a previously detected retinal artery embolus. Am J Ophthalmol. 1992;114:642–3.
12. Gass JDM. Stereoscopic atlas of macular diseases: diagnosis and treatment, vol 1, ed 4. St Louis: Mosby–Year Book; 1997:472–6.
13. Brown GC, Weinstock F. Arterial macroaneurysm on the optic disk presenting as a mass lesion. Ann Ophthalmol. 1985;17:519–20.
14. Giuffre G, Montalto FP, Amodei G. Development of an isolated retinal macroaneurysm of the cilioretinal artery. Br J Ophthalmol. 1987;71:445–8.
15. Tilanus MD, Hoyng C, Deutman AF, et al. Congenital arteriovenous communications and the development of two types of leaking retinal macroaneurysms. Am J Ophthalmol. 1991;112:31–3.
16. Townsend-Pico WA, Meyers SM, Lewis H. Indocyanine green angiography in the diagnosis of retinal arterial macroaneurysms associated with submacular and pre-retinal hemorrhages: a case series. Am J Ophthalmol. 2000;129:33–7.
17. Schulman J, Jampol LM, Goldberg MF. Large capillary aneurysms secondary to retinal venous obstruction. Br J Ophthalmol. 1981;65:36–41.
18. Sanborn GE, Magargal LE. Venous macroaneurysm associated with branch retinal vein obstruction. Ann Ophthalmol. 1984;16:464–8.
19. Cousins SW, Flynn HW, Clarkson JG. Macroaneurysms associated with retinal branch vein occlusion. Am J Ophthalmol. 1990;109:567–74.
20. Kimmel AS, Magargal LE, Morrison DL, Robb-Doyle E. Temporal branch retinal vein obstruction masquerading as a retinal arterial macroaneurysm: the Bonet sign. Ann Ophthalmol. 1989;21:251–2.
21. Avins LR, Krummenacher TK. Valsalva maculopathy due to a retinal arterial macroaneurysm. Ann Ophthalmol. 1983;15:421–3.
22. Shields JA, Decker WL, Sanborn GE, et al. Presumed acquired retinal hemangiomas. Ophthalmology. 1983;90:1292–300.
23. Shields CL, Shields JA, Barrett J, DePotter P. Vasoproliferative tumors of the ocular fundus. Arch Ophthalmol. 1995;113:615–23.
24. McCabe CM, Mieler WF. Six-year follow-up of an idiopathic retinal vasoproliferative tumor. Arch Ophthalmol. 1996;114:617.
25. Fritsche PL, Flipsen E, Polak BCP. Subretinal hemorrhage from retinal arterial macroaneurysm simulating malignancy. Arch Ophthalmol. 2000;118:1704.
26. Kincaid J, Schatz H. Bilateral retinal arteritis with multiple aneurysmal dilations. Retina. 1983;3:171–8.
27. Chang TS, Aylward W, Davis JL, et al. Idiopathic retinal vasculitis, aneurysms, and neuro-retinitis. Ophthalmology. 1995;102:1089–97.
28. Gold DH, La Piana FG, Zimmerman LE. Isolated retinal arterial aneurysms. Am J Ophthalmol. 1976;82:848–57.
29. Fichte C, Steeten BW, Friedman AH. A histopathologic study of retinal arterial aneurysms. Am J Ophthalmol. 1978;85:509–18.
30. Brown DM, Sobol WM, Folk JC, Weingeist TA. Retinal arteriolar macroaneurysms: long term visual outcome. Br J Ophthalmol. 1994;78:534–8.
31. Russel SR, Folk JC. Branch retinal artery occlusion after dye yellow photocoagulation of an arterial macroaneurysm. Am J Ophthalmol. 1987;104:186–7.
32. Mainster MA, Whitacre MM. Dye yellow photocoagulation of retinal arterial macroaneurysms. Am J Ophthalmol. 1988;105:97–8.
33. Joondeph BC, Joondeph HC, Blair NP. Retinal macroaneurysms treated with the dye yellow laser. Retina. 1989;9:187–92.
34. Raymond LA. Neodymium:YAG laser treatment for hemorrhages under the internal limiting membrane and posterior hyaloid face in the macula. Ophthalmol. 1995;102:406–11.
35. Ijima H, Satoh S, Tsukahara S. Nd:YAG laser photodisruption for preretinal hemorrhage due to retinal macroaneurysm. Retina. 1998;18:430–4.
36. Ulbig MW, Mangouritsas G, Rothbacher HH, et al. Long-term results after drainage of premacular subhyaloid hemorrhage into the vitreous with a pulsed ND:YAG laser. Arch Ophthalmol. 1998;116:1465–9.
37. Ibanez HE, Williams DF, Thomas MA, et al. Surgical management of submacular hemorrhage: a series of 47 consecutive cases. Arch Ophthalmol. 1995;113:62–9.
38. Humayun M, Lewis H, Flynn HW, et al. Management of submacular hemorrhage associated with retinal arterial macroaneurysms. Am J Ophthalmol 1998;126:358–61.
39. McCabe CM, Flynn HW, McLean WC, et al. Nonsurgical management of macular hemorrhage secondary to retinal artery macroaneurysms. Arch Ophthalmol. 2000;118:780–5.
40. Heriot WJ. Intravitreal gas and tPA: an outpatient procedure for submacular hemorrhage. Paper presented at: American Academy of Ophthalmology Annual Vitreoretinal Update; Chicago; October 1996.
41. Hassan AS, Johnson MW, Schneiderman TE, et al. Management of submacular hemorrhage with intravitreous tissue plasminogen activator injection and pneumatic displacement. Ophthalmology. 1999;106:1900–7.
42. Ohji M, Saito Y, Hayashi A, et al. Pneumatic displacement of subretinal hemorrhage without tissue plasminogen activator. Arch Ophthalmol. 1998;116:1326–32.

CHAPTER

124

Choroidal Neovascularization

RICHARD F. SPAIDE

DEFINITION

- Choroidal neovascularization is an inappropriate ingrowth of blood vessels and accompanying cellular infiltrate originating in the choroid, which extends through Bruch's membrane to proliferate under the retina, the retinal pigment epithelium, or both. It is a common end-stage process leading to severe visual loss in a number of different diseases.

KEY FEATURES

- Decreased central visual acuity.
- Metamorphopsia.
- Intraretinal, subretinal, subretinal pigment epithelial hemorrhage.
- Macular edema.
- Subretinal fluid.
- Hyperfluorescence and leakage of dye during fluorescein angiography.

ASSOCIATED FEATURES

- Lipid exudation.
- Detachment of the retinal pigment epithelium.
- Retinal pigment epithelial tear.
- Scarring.

INTRODUCTION

Choroidal neovascularization (CNV) is an aberrant growth of blood vessels under the macula associated with numerous disorders (Fig. 124-1). The most significant is age-related macular degeneration (AMD).[1] Several other conditions associated with CNV include intraocular inflammation, angioid streaks, choroidal rupture, pathological myopia, chorioretinal scars, or chorioretinal dystrophy. Despite the disparate causes, the techniques for diagnosis and, in most cases, treatment are common to any form of CNV. Vital in patient management is a thorough understanding of the principles of ocular angiography to establish the diagnosis, categorize the underlying disease process, and plan management strategies. The Macula Photocoagulation Study group (MPS) provided clinicians with valuable information and guidelines in order to make informed and rational decisions about laser photocoagulation by means of randomized clinical trials. More recently, photodynamic therapy (PDT) using verteporfin has been effective for a number of types of CNV in randomized clinical trials. Further investigation of treatment techniques includes pilot studies using laser photocoagulation, PDT, surgery and, more recently, pharmacological therapy. The guidelines provided by these studies are vital to optimal disease management.

EPIDEMIOLOGY AND PATHOGENESIS

CNV may occur in response to virtually any disturbance of the retinal pigment epithelium (RPE) or Bruch's membrane, or by loci of inflammation adjacent to these structures. The incidence of specific etiologies varies with the age of the individual. Traumatic causes may lead to rupture of Bruch's membrane and are seen frequently in younger individuals. Inflammation may lead directly to CNV or may cause scarring and disruption of the normal ocular architecture, which predisposes an individual to later vascular ingrowth. Most, but certainly not all, inflammation-related CNV occurs in young to middle-aged patients. AMD typically is seen in patients over 50 years of age. Pathological myopia is associated with fractures of Bruch's membrane, known as *lacquer cracks*, and also areas of atrophy which may facilitate the growth of CNV, which can occur at any age. By definition, idiopathic CNV is found in individuals less than 50 years of age who do not have evidence of intraocular inflammation, trauma, pathological myopia, chorioretinal scars, or chorioretinal dystrophy.

Theories to explain the growth of CNV include the following pathways:
- Release of cytokines (e.g., vegetative epithelial growth factor [VEGF])
- Rupture of Bruch's membrane
- Inflammation
- Oxidative stress of the RPE
- Abnormal accumulation of lipid by-products
- Vascular insufficiency

OCULAR MANIFESTATIONS

The invading vessels cause visually significant effects through a variety of mechanisms. The physical presence of the vessels causes direct mechanical distortion of the macular tissue. The neovascularization often can be seen as a grayish discoloration under the retina. The vessels are typically incompetent and display varying degrees of leakage. The excessive fluid released manifests as accumulation within tissue or between tissue planes. Detachments of the RPE, macula, and intraretinal edema are the result. Tensile stress from the contracting fibrovascular membrane and excessive hydrostatic pressure may lead to rips of the RPE. Chronic leakage is associated with deposition of lipid and degenerative changes within the detached retina. The newly growing vessels display a peculiar tendency to bleed, which may result in hemorrhages under the RPE or retina or, in extreme cases, may result in breakthrough hemorrhages into the vitreous cavity. Eventually proliferation of RPE, fibroblasts, and glial cells results in the deposition of scar tissue, leading to a whitish accumulation under the macula.

The source for CNV, as implied by the name, is the choroid. The choroid is not the only source of blood flow in some patients, however. Retinal vessels may dive down into the subretinal space and contribute to the neovascular process. The most obvious examples of this tendency are frank chorioretinal anastomosis, which can be seen in inflammatory conditions such as toxoplasmosis and in AMD. Hartnett and coworkers[3] were the first to identify a group of patients with subretinal proliferation of vessels derived solely from the retina; they termed this entity *deep retinal vascular complexes.* Although subsequent investigators have found this entity to be relatively common, the presence of

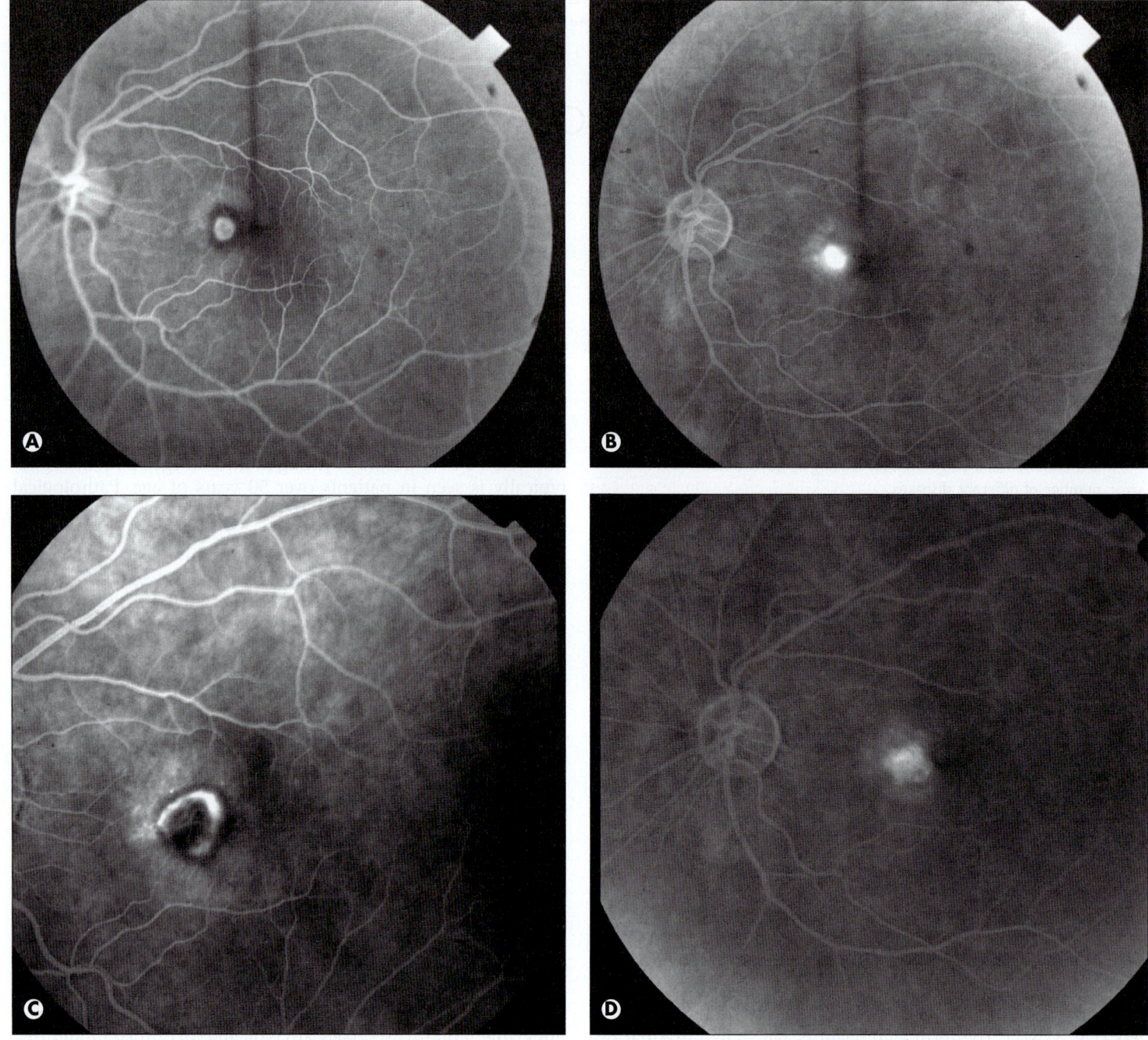

FIG. 124-1 ■ **A 66-year-old patient with metamorphopsia and a visual acuity of 20/40.** She had a small focus of classic choroidal neovascularization that appeared early (**A**) and showed prominent leakage late (**B**) in the fluorescein angiogram. She was treated with laser photocoagulation, but 6 months later she developed recurrent neovascularization (**C**) that extended under the center of the fovea. She was treated with photodynamic therapy and had a resolution of her exudative manifestations. Three months after her only photodynamic therapy session, she showed staining but no leakage from the lesion (**D**). Two years later her acuity was 20/20.

retinal contribution to the exudative process, curiously, has not been mentioned by any large randomized trial of CNV.

DIAGNOSIS AND ANCILLARY TESTING

Patients suspected of having CNV require ancillary testing to establish the diagnosis and to plan and monitor their subsequent treatment. The principal test to diagnose CNV is fluorescein angiography, with indocyanine green (ICG) angiography useful in a limited number of cases.[1]

Angiographic Findings of Choroidal Neovascularization

Vascular ingrowth causes remarkable physiological alteration in the macular region, and this alteration can be detected and evaluated with angiography. The vessels usually grow in the inner portion of Bruch's membrane, although they may penetrate into the subretinal space. The angiographic appearance of CNV is governed by the location, density, and maturity of the new vessels, as well as the amount and character of the intervening tissue. Relatively acute growth of vessels in the inner portion of Bruch's membrane, or even in the subretinal space, with minimal accompanying tissue results in a vascular network that shows hyperfluorescence soon after the appearance of the dye. In this pattern of vascular ingrowth, the vessels themselves often are easily visualized during the early phases of the angiogram. These vessels show prominent leakage during the course of the angiogram, and the vessels often are obscured by the overlying fluorescein which has leaked from the vessels. This topographical and temporal pattern defines *classic CNV*. In classic CNV there is early hyperfluorescence with late leakage. Vessels in classic CNV can appear as a "brush" or "cartwheel" early in the angiogram. This pattern as a pure component is seen in only about 10% of patients with AMD but in a much higher proportion of patients with other causes of CNV.

Obscuration of the fibrovascular ingrowth by intervening tissue alters the fluorescein appearance of the lesion. In such lesions we can observe the fluorescein characteristics of the vessels indirectly. Because we don't see the vessels directly but, instead, infer their presence through more indirect effects, this type of CNV is called *occult CNV*. There are two fluorescein angiographic types of occult CNV,[2] and the differentiation depends on the relative elevation of the leaking lesion. Fibrovascular ingrowth leads to elevation of the RPE, producing a fibrovascular PED. After injection of fluorescein, the fluorescence within the fibrovascular PED slowly increases, often in a heterogeneous manner. Retention of dye within the fibrovascular PED late in the angiogram leads to the appearance of staining. Leakage from the fibrovascular PED can result in the appearance of hypofluorescence internal to the fibrovascular elevation, into the subretinal space, or even into the retina. This leakage can blur the outer margins of the fibrovascular PED. A second form of occult CNV is called *late leakage of undetermined source*. In this form of occult CNV, there is little or no early hyperfluorescence and leakage emanating from poorly defined areas later in the angiogram. Late leakage of undetermined source is not elevated, as is a fibrovascular PED. On occasion the term *poorly defined CNV* is used synonymously for occult CNV, but this is not correct terminology. Some forms of occult CNV, particularly fibrovascular PEDs, can be well defined even though they show occult characteristics.

ICG offers additional insights into characterizing CNV. Generally, CNV seen as classic during fluorescein angiography is not imaged as dramatically by ICG angiography. Classic CNV does not show prominent leakage during ICG angiography, probably because of the higher protein binding of ICG. Occult CNV, either fibrovascular PEDs or late leakage of undetermined source, shows a variety of patterns during ICG angiography. Curiously, areas of CNV which appear very poorly defined during fluorescein angiography can be well defined during ICG angiography. Most regions of occult CNV appear as relatively large plaques during ICG angiography. On occasion, there may be focal areas of intense hyperfluorescence. These may be due to a limited number of conditions, in particular polypoidal choroidal vasculopathy[22] and deep retinal vascular anomalous complexes.[3] Polypoidal choroidal vasculopathy was first described in black women but subsequently has been found in all races. Patients with polypoidal choroidal vasculopathy have a slowly progressive vascular proliferation, which has characteristic findings during ICG angiography. The lesion is composed of nodular, aneurysmal dilatations at the outer border of the lesion, with intervening vascular channels. It is not uncommon to see plaque-like changes typically seen in occult CNV in older patients with polypoidal choroidal vasculopathy.

Disciform Scar

With time, continued exudation, bleeding, proliferation of vessels, hyperplasia of REP cells, and invasion of fibroblasts and inflammatory cells, a sizable scar may form in the macular region. On occasion the scar becomes white and fibrous in appearance, being almost completely devoid of visible vessels. This typical end-stage manifestation is called a *disciform scar*, although certain studies have used slightly differing definitions based on fluorescein angiography. Disciform scars are a common end-stage development in AMD but may be seen in a number of different diseases causing CNV.

DIFFERENTIAL DIAGNOSIS

Only a limited number of diseases may be mistaken for typical CNV:
- Acute posterior multifocal placoid pigment epitheliopathy
- Serpiginous choroidopathy
- Unilateral acute idiopathic maculopathy
- Central serous chorioretinopathy
- Cystoid macular edema
- Epiretinal membrane

SYSTEMIC RISK FACTORS

Systemic risk factors vary with the cause of the CNV. Patients with angioid streaks usually have a predisposing cause, the most common being pseudoxanthoma elasticum. Those with inflammatory lesions in the eye may have generalized systemic conditions. The interaction among systemic risk factors and CNV has been studied most in patients with AMD. Interestingly, many of the AMD studies identified differing risk factors depending on the populations studied. One risk factor common to most studies for the development of CNV in AMD was cigarette smoking. Other risk factors identified in some studies include hypertension and hypercholesterolemia. The Eye Disease Case-Control study had only a handful of women using estrogen replacement, but these patients seemed to have had a lower risk for neovascularization than women not using estrogen.[4] Hypertension appears to be a risk factor for poor response to thermal laser among patients with juxtafoveal CNV.

PATHOLOGY

The fundamental pathological change in CNV is the invasion of blood vessels through the outer portion of Bruch's membrane.[5] Along with the invasion of blood vessels, there are usually a varying proportion of inflammatory cells including lymphocytes and macrophages. Once Bruch's membrane is breached, the vessels may proliferate in the inner portion of Bruch's membrane, may proliferate in the subretinal space, or may do both. There is an unusual tendency for the proliferating fibrovascular tissue to hemorrhage. The free blood may accumulate under the RPE, in the subretinal space, or may even break through into the vitreous cavity. Organization of the blood can lead to scarring. The RPE cells in the regions surrounding the CNV may show hyperplasia and fibrous metaplasia, also. Admixture of these tissue elements produces a fibrocellular scar known as a *disciform scar*. The inner portion of the scar is characteristically less vascular than the outer portion. Serous, serosanguineous, or frankly hemorrhagic detachment of the retina may occur. Chronic exudation of fluid commonly is accompanied by the deposition of yellowish subretinal material referred to as *lipid*. This material probably is composed of lipid and lipoprotein and appears to accumulate, because the aqueous phase of the exudation is resorbed faster than lipid and lipoproteins, which are removed from the subretinal space through differing transport mechanisms.

TREATMENT

The strategies for treating CNV are constrained by the location of the proliferating tissue, the close proximity of this proliferating tissue to delicate, easily damaged structures critical for detailed vision and, chiefly, by the lack of understanding of why and how the body makes these vessels grow. Much of our conceptualization of the condition, which leads directly to terminology and ultimately to management approaches, was derived from angiography, principally fluorescein angiography. The vascular ingrowth appears to be the hallmark of the disease (and its name). It is logical that management approaches attacked the vessels with heat, light, ionizing radiation and, more recently, photodynamic effects. Newer pharmacological approaches have attempted to block cytokines or the induced effects of cytokines.

Laser Photocoagulation

The investigation of the effect of laser photocoagulation on CNV was one of the first multicenter randomized trials organized in ophthalmology. The extrafoveal study investigators examined patients aged 50 years or older, who had CNV located

200–2500μm from the center of the foveal avascular zone, with a best-corrected acuity of 20/100 or better and drusen in the study or fellow eye. The juxtafoveal study enrolled patients aged 50 years or greater with (1) CNV located 1–199μm from the center of the foveal avascular zone or (2) more than 200μm if there was blood or pigment extending to within 200μm of the center of the foveal avascular zone with a best-corrected acuity of 20/400 or better and drusen in the study or fellow eye. The Subfoveal New CNV study enrolled patients with recent CNV less than 3.5 MPS standard disc areas located under the geometrical center of the fovea who had a visual acuity from 20/40 to 20/320. (An MPS standard disc area is an arcane measurement bearing only an approximate correlation with the typical size of the optic nerve head. One MPS standard disc area = 1.77mm².) The Recurrent Subfoveal CNV study enrolled patients with recurrent CNV located under or within 150μm of the geometrical center of the fovea who had an acuity of 20/40 to 20/320. For both subfoveal studies, most of the lesion had to be composed of CNV.

For extrafoveal CNV, the lesion was treated using green or blue-green argon laser, with the goal of uniform whitening of the lesion extending 100–125μm around the lesion.[6] The enrollment for the extrafoveal study was stopped after 18 months because of a large difference between the treatment and control groups. After 18 months, 60% of untreated patients sustained a severe visual loss, which was defined as a 6-line visual acuity loss, while only 25% of treated patients did. At the end of the follow-up period of 5 years, 64% of untreated patients and 46% of treated patients had severe visual loss.[6] The main cause of decreased visual acuity was recurrent CNV, which occurred in 54% of treated patients and usually was seen on the foveal side of the treated lesion. Patients who smoked cigarettes were more likely to have recurrent neovascularization. The mean acuity of patients with recurrent neovascularization was 20/250, while patients without recurrence had a mean acuity of 20/50. In the juxtafoveal study, patients were treated with krypton red laser, which has the theoretical advantage of less damage to the overlying retina.[7,8] After 3 years of follow-up, 58% of untreated eyes versus 49% of treated eyes had severe visual loss, which was defined as 6 lines or more of visual acuity loss. After 5 years, 65% of untreated and 55% of treated eyes sustained severe visual loss.[8] Persistent neovascularization was defined as *neovascularization seen within the first 6 weeks after photocoagulation* and was seen in 32% of patients. Recurrent neovascularization was seen in 47% of patients by the 5-year follow-up point. Patients with hypertension did not seem to show a treatment benefit in the juxtafoveal study. Thermal laser treatment of new and recurrent subfoveal CNV demonstrated immediate loss of visual acuity in the treatment groups, with moderate treatment benefit demonstrated with extended follow-up.

Photodynamic Therapy

RANDOMIZED STUDIES. Large randomized trials were performed to evaluate the efficacy of PDT with verteporfin for CNV secondary to AMD. Each patient in the study received 6mg of verteporfin per square meter of body surface area intravenously over 10 minutes.[9,10] Fifteen minutes after the start of the infusion, a diode laser at 689nm delivered 50J/cm² at an intensity of 600mW/cm² over 83 seconds using a spot size diameter of 1000μm larger than the greatest linear dimension of the neovascular lesion. Patients were re-evaluated at 3-month intervals. Patients showing leakage during fluorescein angiography at the 3-month return visit were retreated. Patients in the Treatment of Age-related Macular Degeneration with Photodynamic Therapy (TAP) Study Group showed 1- and 2-year treatment benefit results for patients with predominantly classic CNV.[9,10]

Patients with occult CNV who had less than 50% classic findings did not show a treatment benefit. Patients were retreated a mean of 3.3 times during the first year and 2.2 times during the second year. At the end of the first year of follow-up, the patients treated with verteporfin showed a pronounced treatment effect

when their neovascular lesions comprised 50% or more of classic CNV, with 67% versus 39% ($P < .001$) showing fewer than 15 letters of visual acuity lost. This trend continued at the second year follow-up, when 59% of those treated and 31% of control patients lost fewer than 3 lines of acuity. Verteporfin therapy of occult subfoveal CNV in AMD was studied in the Verteporfin In Photodynamic Therapy (VIP) study.[11] The entry criteria for this study were somewhat elaborate, in that patients had to have either occult with no classic CNV and a history of recent visual acuity loss, or they had to have classic CNV with a visual acuity of 20/40 or better. Clearly, evaluation of the results of the study required extensive subgroup analysis. After 1 year of follow-up, treated patients did not fare better than untreated controls. After 2 years of follow-up, there was a statistically significant treatment benefit, with 55% of treated patients versus 68% of control patients experiencing at least 15 letters of acuity decline. Further subgroup analysis (which was already of a subgroup of the recruited patients) showed that eyes with smaller lesions (4 disc areas or less) or lower levels of visual acuity (approximately Snellen equivalent of 20/50 or worse) at baseline did better than did eyes not having these characteristics. Patients who had occult with no classic CNV required a mean of 3.1 treatments during the first year and 1.8 during the second.

PDT for pathological myopia was studied in a multicenter randomized trial.[12] After 1 year of follow-up, 72% of the verteporfin-treated patients compared with 44% of the placebo-treated patients lost fewer than 8 letters of visual acuity (which corresponds to approximately 11/2 lines). A lower threshold was chosen, because pathological myopia frequently doesn't cause as profound a visual loss as does AMD. Among treated patients, 32% improved by 5 letters, yet a different threshold, as compared with 15% of control patients. Two-year follow-up data had a less impressive difference with a loss of statistical significance.

NON-COMPARATIVE STUDIES. Patients with CNV 5400m or smaller secondary to ocular histoplasmosis syndrome were treated with PDT using verteporfin.[13] Analysis of data from 25 patients followed for 1 year showed a median improvement of 7 letters, and 56% of patients gained 7 or more letters, while 16% lost 8 or more letters. No ocular or systemic side effects were noted. Additional non-comparative studies have been performed independently of pharmaceutical company support and have examined idiopathic CNV, polypoidal choroidal vasculopathy, and CNV associated with multifocal choroiditis and panuveitis. A study of PDT using verteporfin for idiopathic subfoveal CNV in eight eyes of eight patients with a mean age of 34.6 years found that the mean improvement was of 3.6 lines of Snellen acuity after a mean of 13.5 months of follow-up.[14] The difference in visual acuity at the end of the follow-up period was significantly different than the baseline acuity ($P = .027$). Visual acuity improvement, defined as a halving of the visual angle, was seen in five of the eight patients. Some patients had a remarkable improvement of visual acuity. The mean number of treatments was 2.9. No patient had any treatment-related side effects. The incidence of side effects in alternative methods of treatment, such as vitrectomy, would be expected to be much higher.

Patients with polypoidal choroidal vasculopathy have a slowly progressive vascular growth associated with exudative manifestations typically seen in CNV, such as leakage and hemorrhage. However, the disease process seems to progress over a period of what may be many years. Sixteen patients with subfoveal involvement were treated with PDT, and they were followed for a mean of 12 months.[15] The mean age of the patients involved was 70.5 years. The visual acuity improved (defined as a halving of the visual angle) in nine (56.3%), remained the same in five (31.3%), and decreased (defined as doubling of the visual angle) in two (12.5 %). The mean change in visual acuity was an improvement of 2.38 lines, a difference that was highly significant. The mean number of treatments given was 2.3. One patient had an exudative detachment that resolved after 5 days. No patient had any permanent ocular or systemic side effects. Although the short-term results for treatment of polypoidal choroidal vasculopathy appear to be favorable, the long-term outcome is unknown. CNV secondary to AMD often will "burn out" and leave a fibrotic scar that sometimes appears to be devoid of vessels. Polypoidal choroidal vasculopathy almost never burns out. The vessels continue to expand, albeit slowly, with the threat of exudation and hemorrhage looming larger in lockstep. Although patients with polypoidal choroidal vasculopathy have a lessening of the exudation after PDT, the vessels, particularly the larger vascular channels, persist.

Multifocal choroiditis and panuveitis causes recurrent inflammation associated with punched-out chorioretinal atrophic spots and usually occurs in myopic young to middle-aged women. Subfoveal neovascularization sometimes may respond to corticosteroids but often will not. In a study of seven patients with subfoveal CNV, the mean change in acuity after a follow-up period of 10 months was an improvement of 0.86 lines, a change that was not statistically significant from the baseline acuity.[16] However, three patients (42.8%) had an improvement in visual acuity representing at least a halving of their visual angle, while the other four patients remained stable. The patients required a mean of 1.9 treatments. Four of the seven were being treated with corticosteroids at baseline, and by the end of the follow-up period none of the patients was using corticosteroids. No patient had any ocular or systemic side effects. Although the neovascularization showed good anatomical response, many patients with MCP have underlying abnormalities of the RPE and choroid that may limit visual recovery.

A curious complication of verteporfin infusion is the incidence of pain associated with the infusion. This pain usually starts a few minutes after the infusion is begun and stops a few minutes after the infusion is stopped. The pain usually occurs in the back, chest, or groin. Its incidence has been estimated from a little more than 2% to up to 9.6% of patients receiving an infusion.[17] The pain during infusion has been linked to transient neutropenia, most likely representing massive neutrophil margination, induced by infusion of the verteporfin.[17]

Additional Treatment Modalities

RADIATION. CNV has been treated with a variety of dosages and types of ionizing radiation. Initial reports suggested that external beam radiotherapy was a beneficial treatment for CNV secondary to AMD.[18] Subsequent case series also reported what the authors believed was a favorable treatment effect from radiation. A larger series which compared 91 patients treated with 10Gy (2Gy in 5 fractions) of external beam photons and an historical control group recruited with similar entry criteria found no treatment benefit.[19] A multicenter parallel, randomized, double-masked clinical trial with sham controls administered 16Gy (2Gy in 8 fractions) of external beam photons to treated patients.[20] After 1 year, 51.1% of treated patients and 52.6% of control subjects lost 3 or more lines ($P = .88$). Analysis of classic versus occult disease showed no apparent treatment benefit in either subgroup. A prospective randomized trial using 14Gy (2Gy × 7) found no statistically significant differences in changes in visual acuity, contrast sensitivity, or fluorescein angiographic progression from baseline between groups after any follow-up period.[21] A randomized trial using a higher dosage of radiation, 24Gy (6Gy in 4 fractions), found a treatment benefit.[22] At follow-up after 12 months, 52.2% of the observation group versus 32.0% of the irradiation group had lost 3 or more lines of visual acuity (Snellen acuity was used), a significant result ($P = .03$). No complication, particularly radiation retinopathy, was seen in the short term of the follow-up. The number of patients lost to follow-up was significant.

SURGERY. Submacular surgery has been used as an approach for a number of types of CNV. Surgical removal did not appear to have any benefit for most cases of CNV secondary to AMD, and most researchers have focused on other forms of CNV. Surgical technique has been refined over time, with a reduction in the number of complications. Unavoidable complications are expected with any vitrectomy surgery, such as the progression of nuclear sclerosis. A particularly difficult problem with surgical excision of CNV is the high rate of recurrence, which in large series has been reported as 57% in those with pathological myopia[23] and 52% of patients with ocular histoplasmosis[24] after 24 months. The Submacular Surgery Trials have been initiated to study the efficacy of sumacular surgery. The trials have recruited patients fully, but the Data and Safety Monitoring Committee has not come out with any recommendations yet.

Macular translocation involves moving the macula and varying amounts of adjacent retina to a new location, away from the ingrowth of the new vessels. This may be accomplished by limited translocation, in which a limited retinal detachment is made and the scleral wall is shortened by imbrication or outpouching, or there may be a 360-degree retinotomy, with a rotation of the entire retina. Some patients having translocation have had large amounts of acuity improvement. The complication rate is very high. In a series of 100 eyes with AMD undergoing limited inferior translocation follow-up, information was available for 86 eyes that were followed for 1 year.[25] The mean visual acuity at baseline was 20/160 and at the end of the follow-up period was 20/150. Of these, 52 (60.4%) achieved what the authors considered effective translocation and laser photocoagulation. Of those 52, an estimated 34.6% had recurrence of their neovascularization by the 12-month follow-up visit. The main complications included retinal detachment in 11.6%, retinal breaks in 4.7%, and macular fold in 3.5%. The incidence of cataract was not listed. The results of translocation surgery will probably improve with refinement in technique, but the complication rate is very high given the modest acuity results.

Pharmacological Therapy

Intravitreal triamcinolone has been studied in case series reports and in a randomized trial involving 27 patients. In the randomized trial, patients treated with intravitreal triamcinolone had better acuity after 3 and 6 months than did untreated controls, but they still suffered an acuity loss. Increased intraocular pressure was seen in 25% of treated patients.[26] In a recent study of combination intravitreal triamcinolone with PDT using verteporfin, the mean change in acuity for newly treated patients with any type of CNV secondary to AMD was an improvement of 1.9 lines after 3 months and an improvement of 2.4 lines after 6 months.[27] The need for retreatment because of recurrent leakage was much less than would be expected from PDT alone. Patients treated with the combination therapy had a statistically significant improvement in visual acuity, as compared with the expected decline in acuity for those treated with PDT alone. Anecortave acetate is an angiostatic steroid with no corticosteroid effects, which is being investigated using a posterior sub-Tenon injection every 6 months. The results of a phase II study are awaiting publication. An aptamer directed against $VEGF_{165}$ has been investigated in a phase IA trial.[28] Of 15 patients treated with intravitreal injections, four improved by 3 or more lines with no apparent complications. A phase III trial is under way. An antibody fragment that binds to all isoforms of VEGF has undergone phase I study and is expected to undergo phase III study shortly.

REFERENCES

1. Spaide RF. Fluorescein angiography. In: Spaide RF. Diseases of the retina and vitreous. Philadelphia, WB Saunders; 1999:29–38.
2. Macular Photocoagulation Study Group. Subfoveal neovascular lesions in age-related macular degeneration. Guidelines for evaluation and treatment in the macular photocoagulation study. Arch Ophthalmol. 1991;109:1217–8.
3. Hartnett ME, Weiter JJ, Staurenghi G, Elsner AE. Deep retinal vascular anomalous complexes in advanced age-related macular degeneration. Ophthalmology. 1996; 103:2042–53.
4. Risk factors for neovascular age-related macular degeneration. The Eye Disease Case-Control Study Group. Arch Ophthalmol. 1992;110:1701–8.
5. Green WR, Enger C. Age-related macular degeneration histopathologic studies. The 1992 Lorenz E. Zimmerman Lecture. Ophthalmology. 1993;100:1519–35.
6. Argon laser photocoagulation for neovascular maculopathy. Five-year results from randomized clinical trials. Macular Photocoagulation Study Group. Arch Ophthalmol. 1991;109:1109–14.

7. Macular Photocoagulation Study Group. Krypton laser photocoagulation for neovascular lesions of age-related macular degeneration. Results of a randomized clinical trial. Arch Ophthalmol. 1990;108:816–24.

8. Macular Photocoagulation Study Group. Laser photocoagulation for juxtafoveal choroidal neovascularization. Five-year results from randomized clinical trials. Arch Ophthalmol. 1994;112(4):500–9.

9. Photodynamic therapy of subfoveal choroidal neovascularization in age-related macular degeneration with verteporfin: one-year results of 2 randomized clinical trial—TAP report 1. Treatment of age-related macular degeneration with photodynamic therapy (TAP) study group. Arch Ophthalmol. 1999;117:1329–45.

10. Bressler NM. Photodynamic therapy of subfoveal choroidal neovascularization in age-related macular degeneration with verteporfin: two-year results of 2 randomized clinical trials—TAP report 2. Arch Ophthalmol. 2001;119:198–207.

11. Verteporfin In Photodynamic Therapy Study Group. Verteporfin therapy of subfoveal choroidal neovascularization in age-related macular degeneration: two-year results of a randomized clinical trial including lesions with occult with no classic choroidal neovascularization—verteporfin in photodynamic therapy report 2. Am J Ophthalmol. 2001;131:541–60.

12. Verteporfin In Photodynamic Therapy Study Group. Photodynamic therapy of subfoveal choroidal neovascularization in pathologic myopia with verteporfin. 1-year results of a randomized clinical trial—VIP report no. 1. Ophthalmology. 2001;108:841–52.

13. Saperstein DA, Rosenfeld PJ, Bressler NM, et al. Photodynamic therapy of subfoveal choroidal neovascularization with verteporfin in the ocular histoplasmosis syndrome: one-year results of an uncontrolled, prospective case series. Ophthalmology. 2002;109:1499–50.

14. Spaide RF, Martin ML, Slakter J, et al. Treatment of idiopathic subfoveal choroidal neovascular lesions using photodynamic therapy with verteporfin. Am J Ophthalmol. 2002;134:62–8.

15. Spaide RF, Donsoff I, Lam DL, et al. Treatment of polypoidal choroidal vasculopathy with photodynamic therapy. Retina. 2002;22:529–35.

16. Spaide RF, Freund KB, Slakter J, et al. Treatment of subfoveal choroidal neovascularization associated with multifocal choroiditis and panuveitis with photodynamic therapy. Retina. 2002;22:545–9.

17. Spaide RF, Maranan L. Neutrophil margination as a possible mechanism for verteporfin infusion-associated pain. Am J Ophthalmol. 2003. In press.

18. Chakravarthy U, Houston RF, Archer DB. Treatment of age-related subfoveal neovascular membranes by teletherapy: a pilot study. Br J Ophthalmol. 1993;77:265–73.

19. Spaide RF, Guyer DR, McCormick B, et al. External beam radiation therapy for choroidal neovascularization. Ophthalmology. 1998;105:24–30.

20. A prospective, randomized, double-masked trial on radiation therapy for neovascular age-related macular degeneration (RAD Study). Radiation therapy for age-related macular degeneration. Ophthalmology. 1999;106:2239–47.

21. Marcus DM, Sheils W, Johnson MH, et al. External beam irradiation of subfoveal choroidal neovascularization complicating age-related macular degeneration: one-year results of a prospective, double-masked, randomized clinical trial. Arch Ophthalmol. 2001;119:275–6.

22. Bergink GJ, Hoyng CB, van der Maazen RW, et al. A randomized controlled clinical trial on the efficacy of radiation therapy in the control of subfoveal choroidal neovascularization in age-related macular degeneration: radiation versus observation. Graefes Arch Klin Exp Ophthalmol. 1998;236:321–5.

23. Uemura A, Thomas MA. Subretinal surgery for choroidal neovascularization in patients with high myopia. Arch Ophthalmol. 2000;118:344–50.

24. Holekamp NM, Thomas MA, Dickinson JD, Valluri S. Surgical removal of subfoveal choroidal neovascularization in presumed ocular histoplasmosis: stability of early visual results. Ophthalmology. 1997;104:22–6.

25. Fujii GY, de Juan E Jr, Pieramici DJ, et al. Inferior limited macular translocation for subfoveal choroidal neovascularization secondary to age-related macular degeneration: 1-year visual outcome and recurrence report. Am J Ophthalmol. 2002;134:69–74.

26. Danis RP, Ciulla TA, Pratt LM, Anliker W. Intravitreal triamcinolone in exudative age-related macular degeneration. Retina. 2000;20:244–50.

27. Spaide RF, Sorenson J, Maranan L. Combined photodynamic therapy with verteporfin and intravitreal triamcinolone acetonide for choroidal neovascularization. Ophthalmology. In press.

28. The Eyetech Study Group. Preclinical and phase 1A clinical evaluation of an anti-VEGF pegylated aptamer (EYE001) for the treatment of exudative age-related macular degeneration. Retina. 2002;22:143–52.

CHAPTER

125 Age-Related Macular Degeneration

ADAM MARTIDIS • MATTHEW T. S. TENNANT

DEFINITION

- A common, chronic degenerative disorder of unknown pathogenesis that affects older individuals and features central visual loss as a result of geographical atrophy, serous detachment of the retinal pigment epithelium, and choroidal neovascularization.

KEY FEATURES

- Age older than 50 years.
- Bilateral.
- Drusen.
- Geographical atrophy.
- Serous retinal pigment epithelial detachment.
- Choroidal neovascularization.

ASSOCIATED FEATURES

- Retinal pigment epithelial clumping or loss.
- Subretinal fluid.
- Subretinal hemorrhage.
- Lipid exudation.
- Subretinal fibrosis (disciform scarring).
- Generally progressive.

INTRODUCTION

Age-related macular degeneration (AMD) is the leading cause of central visual loss among individuals 65 years of age and older in developed countries.[1-4] The disease primarily affects the choriocapillaris, Bruch's membrane, and retinal pigment epithelium (RPE). However, visual loss typically results from photoreceptor dysfunction due to underlying atrophy or choroidal neovascularization (CNV), with its corresponding fluid accumulation, hemorrhage, lipid exudation, and fibrosis.[5] Despite the profound clinical impact of this disorder and the extensive research regarding its prevention and treatment, the cause remains unclear, treatment is largely unsatisfactory, and prevention is usually not possible.

EPIDEMIOLOGY

AMD can be classified broadly into two categories: non-neovascular (dry) and neovascular (wet). Although non-neovascular AMD accounts for approximately 80% of all diagnosed cases, neovascular AMD is responsible for nearly 80% of significant visual disability associated with this disease. Geographical atrophy, the most severe non-neovascular manifestation of AMD, causes approximately 21% of the cases of legal blindness in North America.[3]

The average age at onset of visual loss is about 75 years. After the age of 50, the incidence steadily increases, with more than one third of people in the ninth decade of life affected. Estimates show that approximately 315,000 Americans aged 75 and older will develop AMD over a 5-year period.[2] The visual impact is significant; the Salisbury Eye Evaluation Study reported the prevalence of blindness (visual acuity 20/200 or worse) associated with AMD as 0.38% in individuals aged 70–79 years and 1.15% in individuals aged 80–84 years.[6]

Many studies have reported the prevalence of AMD in various populations using multiple definitions. The Framingham Eye Study cited a prevalence of approximately 2% in Americans aged 52–64 years, 11% in those 65–74 years, and 28% in those 75 years and older.[3] In the Netherlands, severe atrophic or neovascular AMD was identified in 1.7% of the population.[7] In a U.S. study of Chesapeake Bay watermen, 3% of the subjects older than 70 years had geographical atrophy, and 2% had neovascular AMD.[8] The Baltimore Eye Survey reported the overall prevalence of AMD as 0.32% in individuals aged 70–79 and 2.9% in individuals aged 80 and older.[4]

No significant gender predilection has been identified for AMD. The Framingham Eye Study showed a slightly higher incidence of moderate to severe AMD in Caucasian women compared with men.[3] The Health and Nutrition Examination Survey (HANES), which included milder cases, found no difference.[9]

Historically, it was believed that increased skin pigmentation decreased the risk of neovascular AMD, but recent studies are inconsistent. A study of elderly British individuals found that 3.5% had choroidal neovascularization, while a comparative, age-matched group of black African patients manifested only a 0.1% incidence. A study of an African-Caribbean population from Barbados found neovascular AMD in 0.5% of the population, a percentage possibly lower than that found in Caucasian Americans.[10] The HANES study noted a comparable prevalence of AMD consisting primarily of cases of non-neovascular AMD in Caucasian and African-American participants.[9]

PATHOGENESIS

The causes of AMD and choroidal neovascularization are currently unknown. One theory postulates that abnormalities in the enzymatic activity of aged RPE cells lead to accumulation of metabolic by-products. Engorgement of RPE cells interferes with their normal cellular metabolism, leading to extracellular excretions.[1, 5] In addition, lipids are deposited in Bruch's membrane, possibly from failure of the RPE to process cellular debris associated with outer segment turnover. The resulting hydrophobic barrier may impede the passage of fluid from the retina to the choroid, causing detachment of the RPE. Breaks in Bruch's membrane are thought to be responsible for neovascular ingrowth from the choriocapillaris.[11]

A more recent theory suggests that hemodynamic alteration in the choroidal circulation is an important pathophysiological mechanism.[12] Atherosclerotic changes in the ocular vasculature lead to increased ocular rigidity and decreased vascular compliance. The resulting increased postcapillary resistance causes elevated hydrostatic pressure, with exudation of extracellular proteins and lipids; these manifest as basal deposits and drusen. Corresponding degeneration of elastin and collagen causes calcification and fragmentation of Bruch's membrane. An angiogenic stimulus induced by relative choroidal ischemia results in increased levels of vascular endothelial growth factor (VEGF).

This, in turn, incites neovascular ingrowth from the choriocapillaris through a calcified, fractured Bruch's membrane. In support of this theory, Doppler imaging has confirmed choroidal vascular compromise in AMD patients relative to age-matched controls in several studies.[13-15]

Regardless of the mechanism of deposition, drusen are generally accepted to be precursor lesions for AMD when they are "soft" or "indistinct" ($\geq 63\mu m$). Small drusen ($< 63\mu m$) are extremely common, with approximately 80% of the general population older than 30 years manifesting at least one. The number and confluence of drusen increase with age. After the age of 70 years, 26% of individuals have large or soft drusen, and 17% have confluent drusen.[8]

Risk factors for the development of AMD have been identified despite a limited understanding of the exact pathophysiology. Various researchers have implicated atherosclerosis, oxidative damage, photic toxicity, inflammation, diet, and genetics. Systemic arterial hypertension and cigarette smoking are associated with an increased risk of neovascular AMD.[16,17] Although early studies suggested a relationship between light and AMD, more recent publications suggest that exposure to visible light is not a risk factor for AMD.[16,18]

The extent to which heredity can be implicated in the pathogenesis of AMD is not clear, but it may be substantial[10,19]; autosomal dominant inheritance with variable penetrance has been suggested.[1] Nearly one fourth of parents, siblings, and offspring of patients who have AMD manifest the disease concurrently.[20] The relative roles of genetic and environmental influences need to be delineated further.[21-23] In studies of monozygotic twins with AMD and common environmental and dietary influences, the fundus appearance and degree of visual loss were strikingly similar (89–100%). Clinical concordance in dizygotic twins reared in a shared environment was markedly less but still substantial (46%).[22,23] The search for one or more AMD genes continues; AMD may ultimately prove to be a group of distinct diseases that manifest a similar clinical appearance.

OCULAR MANIFESTATIONS

Individuals affected with AMD typically report blurred vision or metamorphopsia in one or both eyes, but they may be asymptomatic. Decreased reading ability, especially in dim light, and difficulty with dark adaptation are other common complaints. The onset is subacute, except in some cases of neovascular AMD in which abrupt visual loss is noted. Neovascular AMD typically shows a more rapid progression of visual loss relative to its nonneovascular counterpart.

Non-Neovascular Age-Related Macular Degeneration

GEOGRAPHICAL ATROPHY. Visual loss from non-neovascular AMD is generally due to geographical atrophy involving the foveal region. This is seen clinically as one or more well-delineated areas of hypopigmentation or depigmentation due to absence or severe attenuation of the underlying RPE (Fig. 125-1). The larger, deep choroidal vessels are more readily visualized through the atrophic patches. These areas are usually small (less than a disc area) and may surround the fovea in a petalloid pattern; they typically coalesce over time or manifest as one large central lesion up to 7mm in diameter. If the foveal center is spared, good visual acuity may be preserved, although reading vision may remain poor. At times, even in the presence of severe atrophy, visual acuity is only mildly affected. Most, but not all, eyes that have geographical atrophy also exhibit drusen. In fact, most cases of geographical atrophy occur in a pattern corresponding to the regression of prior, significant drusen. Alterations in the RPE consisting of focal hyper- or hypopigmentation are also associated with AMD, distinct from geographical atrophy.

DRUSEN AND FOCAL HYPERPIGMENTATION. Clinically, drusen appear as focal, whitish yellow excrescences deep to the

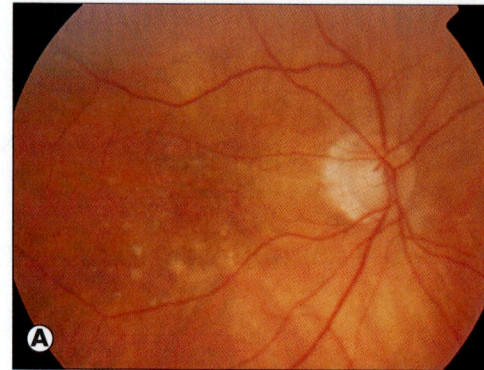
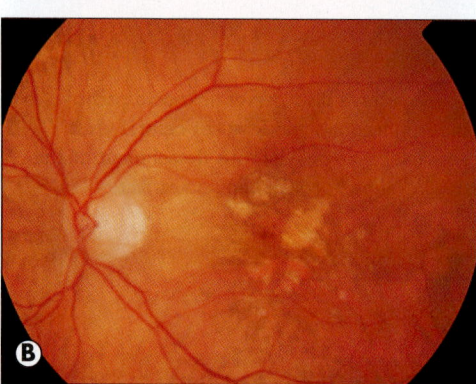

FIG. 125-1 ■ Non-neovascular age-related macular degeneration with drusen and geographical atrophy. A, Right eye. B, Left eye. Visual acuity measures 20/30 (6/9) in both eyes, with corresponding metamorphopsia

retina. Generally, they cluster in the posterior pole but can occur anywhere in the fundus. Drusen in an extramacular location are of no visual consequence. They vary widely in number, size, shape, and distribution. Most drusen are 20–100μm in diameter. They may disappear with time, while new ones develop elsewhere in the macula. For the most part, drusen alone do not cause visual loss; mild metamorphopsia, loss of reading speed, and impaired contrast sensitivity may occur. They do represent a significant risk factor for subsequent geographical atrophy and CNV.

Drusen may be categorized into hard and soft varieties. Hard drusen are round, discrete, yellow-white deposits measuring less than 63m. These drusen are commonly identified in many populations; they are not age related and do not carry an increased risk for the development of CNV. In contrast, soft drusen are ill defined, with nondiscrete borders, measuring 63μm or greater. They are age related and have been associated with the development of CNV. The Macular Photocoagulation Study (MPS) reported that the 5-year risk of CNV in fellow eyes of individuals with unilateral neovascular AMD was 10% in those without large drusen and 30–46% in those with large drusen.[24]

Focal hyperpigmentation of the RPE is another important clinical feature of non-neovascular AMD. The risk of developing soft drusen and geographical atrophy increases in its presence. The MPS showed that in patients with unilateral neovascular AMD, the 5-year risk of developing CNV in fellow eyes that manifest both soft drusen and focal hyperpigmentary changes was 58–73%.[24]

Neovascular Age-Related Macular Degeneration

The hallmark of neovascular AMD is the ingrowth of CNV from the choriocapillaris under the macular region (Fig. 125-2). The potential clinical manifestations include the following:
- Subretinal fluid.
- Macular edema.
- Retinal, subretinal, or sub-RPE hemorrhage.
- Retinal or subretinal lipid exudate.
- Plaque-like membrane or gray or yellow-green discrete discoloration.
- Retinal pigment epithelial detachment.
- RPE tear.
- Subretinal fibrosis or disciform scar.

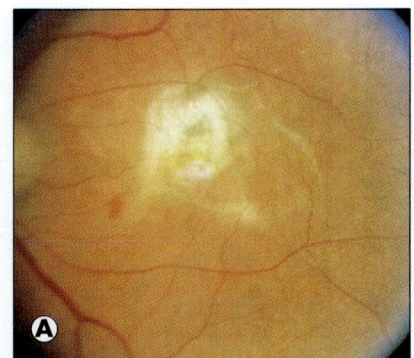

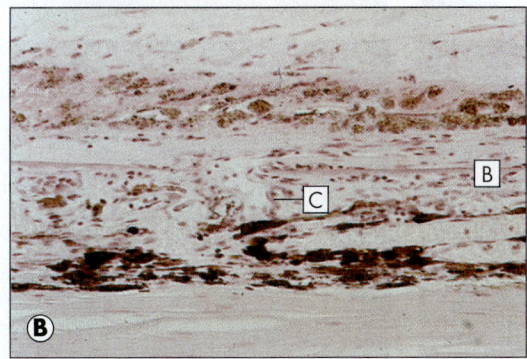

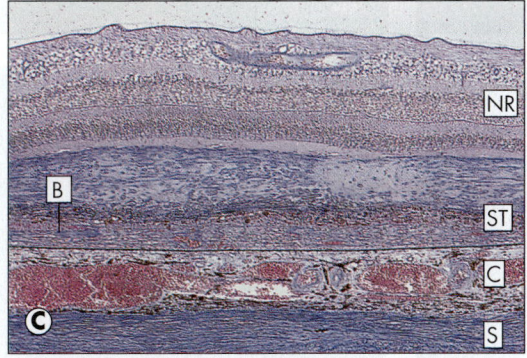

FIG. 125-2 ■ **Neovascular age-related macular degeneration. A,** The patient had choroidal neovascularization followed by numerous episodes of hemorrhage, resulting in an organized scar. **B,** A small vessel (*C,* capillary) has grown through Bruch's membrane *(B)* into the sub–retinal pigment epithelial space, resulting in hemorrhage and fibroplasia. **C,** The end stage shows a thick, fibrous scar between the choroid and the outer retinal layers (trichrome stain). Note the preservation of the retina, except for complete degeneration of the photoreceptors (*B,* Bruch's membrane; *C,* choroid; *NR,* neural retina; *S,* sclera; *ST,* scar tissue). (**B,** Courtesy of WC Frayer. **C,** From Yanoff M, Fine BS. Ocular pathology, ed 5. St. Louis: Mosby, 2002.)

Associated features of non-neovascular AMD, including drusen, RPE atrophy, and focal pigmentary changes, are typically present in eyes manifesting CNV, as well as fellow eyes. However, CNV secondary to AMD may occur without any of these precursor lesions; if they are not present, other possible causes of CNV must be evaluated.

Histopathologically, patients affected by AMD may develop nonmacular peripheral CNV, especially in the temporal retina. Occasionally, such lesions result in clinically evident postequatorial subretinal hemorrhage and fluid accumulation. These peripheral disciform detachments rarely require therapy but may lead to breakthrough vitreous hemorrhage.

RETINAL PIGMENT EPITHELIAL DETACHMENT. A retinal pigment epithelial detachment (PED) may be caused by fibrovascular tissue, hemorrhage, serous fluid, or coalescence of drusen beneath the RPE. Each has a unique clinical appearance and exhibits specific patterns of fluorescence on angiography. Fibrovascular PED represents a type of occult CNV described later. Hemorrhagic PED manifests as a dark elevation of the RPE due to underlying blood, showing blocked fluorescence throughout all phases of angiography. Serous PED appears as a dome-shaped detachment of the RPE, exhibiting bright diffuse hyperfluorescence with progressive pooling in a fixed space.

Drusenoid PED, caused by coalescence of drusen, shows staining, often with fading fluorescence in the late phase and an absence of leakage.

DIAGNOSIS AND ANCILLARY TESTING

Visual loss from AMD may be diagnosed when an individual older than 50 years has geographical atrophy in the macula, a PED, or CNV. Other clinical findings, such as drusen, RPE hyperpigmentation, and RPE depigmentation help confirm the diagnosis, but their presence alone may not be associated with visual loss. Clinical examination is usually sufficient to establish a diagnosis of AMD. Subtle macular abnormalities, especially subretinal fluid, are best detected by stereoscopic slit-lamp biomicroscopic examination using a contact lens.

Fluorescein angiography is useful in any patient in whom CNV is suspected to determine the characteristics of the lesion and the patient's potential qualification for available therapeutic modalities. It is not a useful screening test for eyes that have drusen or geographical atrophy alone, in which no new symptoms or no clinical evidence of neovascularization is present. Determination of the presence of CNV and evaluation of the extent, location, and composition of its components are critical in deciding whether treatment is indicated and, if so, which therapeutic modality is appropriate.[25,26] This is becoming increasingly important as new treatments are developed, each with its own specific criteria for effective utilization.

If a lesion is well demarcated, its location may be determined by the closest point to the center of the foveal avascular zone (FAZ). Lesion location is classified angiographically as follows:

- Extrafoveal (≥200μm and <2500μm from the center of the FAZ).
- Juxtafoveal (1–199μm from the center of the FAZ).
- Subfoveal (under the center of the FAZ).

Based on angiographic patterns of fluorescence, components of CNV lesions may be categorized as either classic or occult (Fig. 125-3). Classic CNV is characterized by bright, uniform, early hyperfluorescence exhibiting leakage in the late phase and obscuring the boundaries. Occult CNV is recognized angiographically by one of two patterns: fibrovascular PED, or late leakage from an undetermined source.

Fibrovascular PED is characterized by an area of irregular elevation of the RPE (which is neither as bright nor as discrete as in classic CNV), often with stippled hyperfluorescence present in the midphase of the angiogram and leakage or staining by the late phase. Late leakage from an undetermined source usually appears as speckled hyperfluorescence with dye pooled in the subretinal space in the late phase; the source of leakage does not correspond to classic CNV or fibrovascular PED in the early or midphase of the angiogram. Identification of occult CNV is facilitated by late-phase images (up to 10 minutes after dye injection) and stereoscopic images, which may display the irregular elevation of the RPE. Angiograms are also evaluated for the presence of hemorrhage, blocked fluorescence that does not correspond to hemorrhage, or serous detachment of the RPE. Serous PED exhibits bright hyperfluorescence with progressive pooling of fluorescence within a fixed sub-RPE cavity (see Fig. 125-3). Classic or occult CNV within the area of the serous detachment may not be identifiable due to intense hyperfluorescence.

With the introduction of digital imaging systems, the use of indocyanine green (ICG) angiography in AMD has been evaluated. The dye's characteristics enable this mode of angiography to delineate the choroidal circulation better than fluorescein angiography does.[25] Hence, ICG angiography may be useful for the detection of areas of occult CNV. The appearance of CNV based on ICG angiography may be categorized into three types[27,28]: focal spots, plaques, and a combination of the two. Laser treatment based on ICG angiography findings has been advocated but remains unproved in a controlled, prospective study.[29]

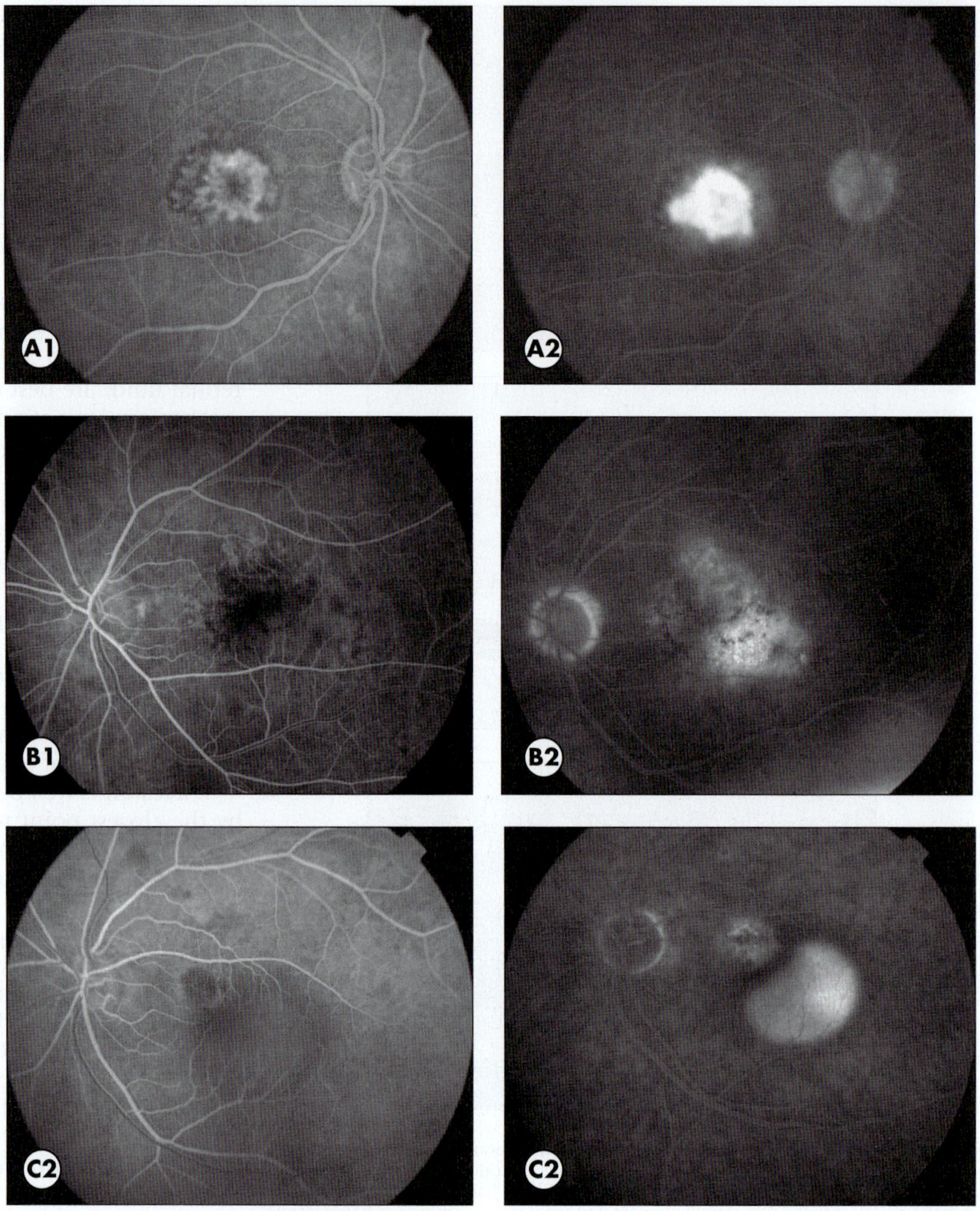

FIG. 125-3 ■ Neovascular age-related macular degeneration. *A1–A2,* Fluorescein angiography of classic choroidal neovascularization showing early, bright, uniform hyperfluorescence with leakage in the late frame. *B1–B2,* Fluorescein angiography of occult choroidal neovascularization (fibrovascular pigment epithelial detachment) showing stippled hyperfluorescence in the earlier frame and late leakage. *C1,* Fluorescein angiography of a serous pigment epithelial detachment showing pooling within a fixed sub–retinal pigment epithelial cavity. *C2,* Optical coherence tomography cross-section demonstrates a dome-shaped elevation of the retinal pigment epithelium by a hyporeflective (serous) fluid collection.

Rarely, ultrasonography is necessary in the diagnosis of neovascular AMD. B-scan ultrasonography may be necessary when the media is obscured by breakthrough vitreous hemorrhage from CNV, precluding a clear ophthalmoscopic view of the fundus. When a hemorrhagic macular lesion simulates a tumor, acoustic properties may assist in the diagnosis.[30]

DIFFERENTIAL DIAGNOSIS

The differential diagnosis of non-neovascular AMD includes other conditions that affect the RPE and choriocapillaris (Box 125-1). CNV has been described in a variety of different ophthalmic conditions (Box 125-2), including pathological myopia, ocular histoplasmosis syndrome, and angioid streaks.[31] Individuals affected by AMD are typically elderly and have drusen present in the involved or fellow eye. When CNV is detected, it is important to determine whether AMD is the cause, since other causes of CNV may carry different prognoses, affecting counseling and treatment decisions.

Other causes of subretinal hemorrhage must be ruled out, including retinal arterial macroaneurysm (which usually shows fluorescein or ICG dye leakage from the aneurysm centered along a retinal arteriole) or choroidal rupture (which usually shows irregular staining of the rupture site). Other causes of subretinal fluid also need to be considered, most commonly central serous chorioretinopathy.

BOX 125-1

Differential Diagnosis for Dry Age-Related Macular Degeneration

Hereditary diseases
*   pattern dystrophy
*   Stargardt's disease
*   Best's disease
*   angioid streaks

Central serous chorioretinopathy

Bilateral idiopathic juxtafoveal telangiectasis

Multifocal choroiditis

Acute posterior multifocal placoid pigment epitheliopathy

Toxic lesions
*   chloroquine
*   phenothiazines
*   canthaxanthin

PATHOLOGY

Histopathologically, drusen appear as focal areas of eosinophilic material between the basement membrane of the RPE and Bruch's membrane (Fig. 125-4).[32] They stain positively with periodic acid-Schiff. Soft drusen are larger and represent detachment of the thickened inner aspect of Bruch's membrane along with the RPE (Fig. 125-5).[32] Generally, little or no photoreceptor degeneration overlies drusen.

Bruch's membrane is a five-layered structure in which the basement membrane of the RPE represents the innermost layer.[33] The outermost layer is a second basement membrane associated with the endothelium of the choriocapillaris. In between is a zone of elastin sandwiched on both sides by an inner and outer collagenous layer. An age-related change is the appearance of basal laminar deposits, which represent type IV collagen, between the RPE plasma and the basement membrane (see Fig. 125-5). Progressive thickening of this inner part of Bruch's membrane is associated with RPE degeneration. Eosinophilic deposits that coalesce between the RPE basement membrane and the inner collagenous zone of Bruch's membrane are called basal linear deposits. By light microscopy, it is difficult to differentiate these two types of deposits.[33] One hypothesis suggests that the material accumulates from damaged RPE cells. Basal linear deposits are most prominent in eyes that have soft drusen and are more common in eyes affected by neovascular AMD.[33,34] Aging also results in increased lipid deposition in Bruch's membrane.[11] Bruch's membrane often shows areas of calcification and fragmentation, changes found more commonly in eyes that harbor CNV due to AMD.[33] The choriocapillaris shows thickened and hyalinized vascular walls, while larger choroidal vessels appear normal. Loss of the RPE in geographical atrophy is accompanied by attenuation of the overlying photoreceptors (see Fig. 125-5). In areas of geographical atrophy, the underlying choriocapillaris is also generally hyalinized.

CNV represents new blood vessel growth from the choriocapillaris through a degenerated Bruch's membrane (see Fig. 125-2). The earliest form of histopathologically evident CNV consists of fine vessels within Bruch's membrane.[33] Occasionally, a low-grade granulomatous inflammation accompanies CNV. Even when CNV is first noted clinically, the histopathology shows a prominent fibrotic component.[35] The fibrotic component may be associated with hyperplasia or metaplasia of the RPE, overlying retinal atrophy, and cystoid macular edema. Hemosiderin from previous hemorrhage may be seen.

NATURAL HISTORY AND PROGNOSIS

The risk of visual loss in eyes that initially manifest drusen or RPE abnormalities varies, depending on the characteristics of the macula and the status of the fellow eye. In eyes of patients older than 65 years that have bilateral drusen but no significant visual loss initially, the risk of a new atrophic lesion or neovascular lesion that results in visual loss has been reported as 9% at 1 year, 16% at 2 years, and 24% at 3 years.[36] Confluent drusen, focal hyperpigmentation of the RPE, and extrafoveal areas of chorioretinal atrophy are three clinical findings that increase the risk for the subsequent development of visual loss.

In individuals who already have neovascular AMD in one eye, the risk of developing CNV in the fellow eye is estimated at about 7–10% per year. If the fellow eye has no large drusen or focal RPE hyperpigmentation, the 5-year risk of developing CNV is only 10%. When both large drusen and RPE hyperpigmentation are present, however, the 5-year risk increases to approxi-

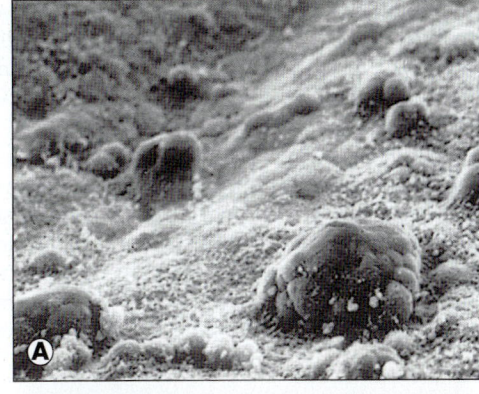
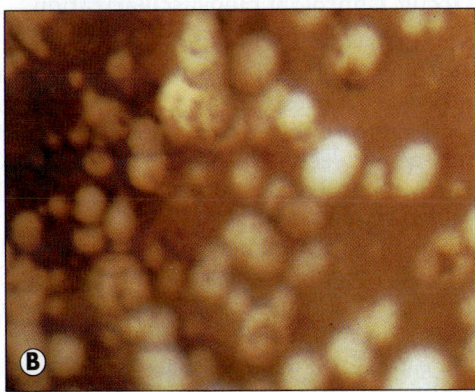
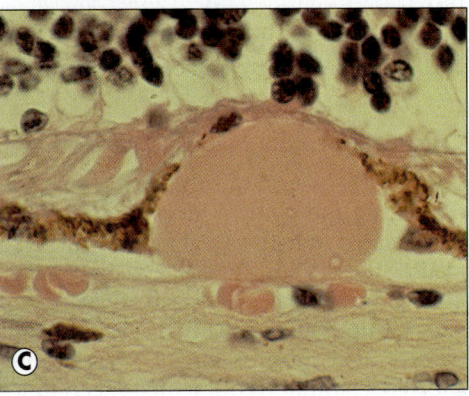

FIG. 125-4 ■ Nodular (hard) drusen. Scanning (A) and gross (B) appearance of nodular drusen. Histological section (C) shows an eosinophilic nodular druse external and contiguous to the original thin basement membrane of the retinal pigment epithelium (RPE), that is, between RPE basement membrane and Bruch's membrane. (A and B, Courtesy of Dr. R. C. Eagle Jr. C, Courtesy of Dr. M. Yanoff.)

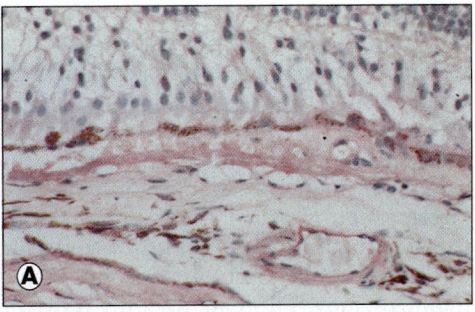
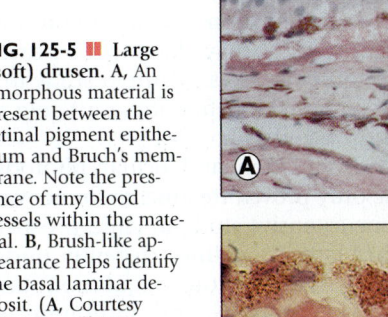
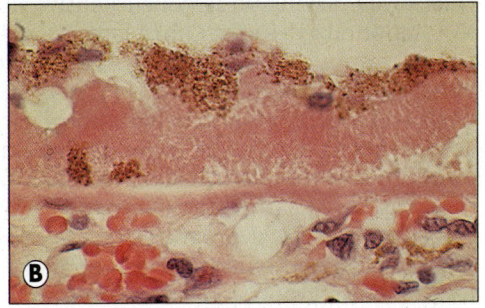

FIG. 125-5 ■ Large (soft) drusen. A, An amorphous material is present between the retinal pigment epithelium and Bruch's membrane. Note the presence of tiny blood vessels within the material. B, Brush-like appearance helps identify the basal laminar deposit. (A, Courtesy of M. Yanoff, MD. B, Courtesy of R.C. Eagle Jr, MD.)

mately 60%.[24] In one study, an individual who has subfoveal or juxtafoveal CNV in one eye, systemic arterial hypertension, and a fellow eye with large, multiple drusen with focal RPE hyperpigmentation was shown to have an 87% risk of developing CNV in the fellow eye over 5 years.[37]

The degree of visual loss associated with CNV can be directly correlated to the most posterior extent of the neovascular complex with respect to the center of the FAZ. The vast majority of CNV lesions associated with AMD are subfoveal in location,[38,39] and most cases of untreated CNV that begin outside the fovea extend under the center of the FAZ with time.[40] The natural history of CNV associated with AMD generally carries a poor visual prognosis.[40,41]

Occult Choroidal Neovascularization

Natural history studies of occult CNV demonstrate a poor visual outcome associated with these lesions. One retrospective study reviewed 84 eyes with occult CNV and showed a 63% rate of moderate visual loss over an average of 28 months; average visual acuity declined from 20/80 to 20/250 over this interval.[42] The MPS observed 26 eyes with occult subfoveal CNV and reported severe visual loss in 41% of eyes at 12 months and 64% at 36 months; median visual acuity declined from 20/50 to 20/200 over 36 months.[43] The Verteporfin in Photodynamic Therapy (VIP) Study followed 93 eyes with purely occult subfoveal CNV in a placebo control arm. At 12 months, 73% of these eyes experienced visual loss from baseline, with 32% manifesting severe visual loss. At 24 months, 79% experienced visual loss from baseline, with a 43% rate of severe visual loss. Mean loss of visual acuity from baseline was four and five lines at 12 and 24 months, respectively.[44,45]

Classic Choroidal Neovascularization

The natural history of subfoveal classic CNV can be discerned by evaluating the control arms of the MPS and the Treatment of Age-Related Macular Degeneration with Photodynamic Therapy (TAP) Study.[46,47] In the MPS, visual acuity in untreated eyes harboring classic CNV decreased an average of 1.9 lines at 3 months and 4.4 lines at 24 months. Severe visual loss was noted in 11% of eyes at 3 months and 37% at 24 months. The TAP Study showed a similar trend, with a mean loss of 2 lines at 3 months, 3.5 lines at 12 months, and 3.9 lines at 24 months. Severe visual loss was identified in 36% of control eyes at 24 months.

TREATMENT AND PREVENTION

No proven treatment exists for the visual loss associated with non-neovascular AMD. Laser therapy to drusen to prevent visual loss from the development of CNV is currently under study.[48–52] Initial trials evaluated fovea-sparing laser treatment for soft drusen using low-intensity burns in a grid fashion. Results indicate that this method can speed resorption of drusen and may improve visual acuity. However, CNV may develop in treated eyes more frequently than in untreated eyes.[48] Further study in a larger, randomized trial will attempt to define the exact role of this treatment modality in non-neovascular AMD.

Conventional laser photocoagulation and ocular photodynamic therapy (OPT) are the only proven treatments for neovascular AMD, having undergone extensive study in large, prospective, randomized trials. Other laser modalities currently under consideration include feeder vessel photocoagulation and transpupillary thermotherapy. Pharmacological inhibition of neovascularization is also being studied, targeting VEGF. Surgical approaches to the disease include submacular excision, macular translocation, macular rotation, and RPE transplantation.

As discussed earlier, the natural history of neovascular AMD carries a poor visual prognosis. Traditionally, the goal of treatment has been to reduce the risk of additional visual loss, with restoration of vision expected in only a minority of treated eyes.

Conventional Laser Photocoagulation

For many years, laser photocoagulation was the only proven treatment for CNV associated with AMD. Every controlled study that showed a benefit from laser photocoagulation in this condition included only CNV lesions with well-demarcated boundaries. Unfortunately, no more than 15–20% of neovascular AMD cases present with well-defined CNV, limiting the utility of this treatment modality.

Lesions considered eligible for photocoagulation by MPS criteria should contain some classic CNV but may manifest occult CNV. There may be associated blood, blocked fluorescence not corresponding to visible blood, or serous PED, provided the total area of these components is less than the area of any classic and occult CNV. Laser photocoagulation is performed using initial treatment settings of 200μm spot size, 0.2–0.5 second duration, and 100–200mW power. The lesion is treated so that the end result is a uniform, confluent, yellow-white laser burn. Photocoagulation should cover the entire lesion and extend 100μm beyond the peripheral boundaries of all lesion components except blood.[25] For recurrent lesions, treatment should extend 100μm beyond the perimeter of the lesion, except at the interface of the recurrence and the previous area of photocoagulation, where the laser treatment should extend 300μm into the area of previous laser treatment.[25] Feeder vessels, when identified, should be treated for at least 100μm on both sides, and 300μm radially at the origin of the feeder vessel. Complications associated with laser photocoagulation include hemorrhage, perforation of Bruch's membrane, RPE tear, and arteriolar narrowing.[53–55] Persistent or recurrent CNV after photocoagulation is common.

MACULAR PHOTOCOAGULATION STUDY. The MPS consisted of eight multicenter, randomized clinical trials designed to determine whether laser photocoagulation reduces the risk of severe vision loss associated with CNV from AMD, ocular histoplasmosis syndrome, and idiopathic causes. Eligible patients were randomized to laser treatment or observation. Two randomized clinical trials studied subfoveal CNV due to AMD; one evaluated new lesions with no prior laser treatment, and the other evaluated recurrent lesions with prior laser treatment that did not involve the fovea.

Overall, for patients who had new, small (3.5 MPS disc areas), well-demarcated subfoveal lesions containing classic CNV, laser-treated eyes retained better levels of visual acuity, reading speed, and contrast sensitivity when compared with untreated eyes.[54] These benefits were sustained for at least 4 years.[56] However, an immediate and substantial decrease in visual acuity averaging three lines occurred after treatment. Eyes treated with photocoagulation had worse visual acuity, on average, than did untreated eyes at 3 and 6 months after enrollment. Even though both groups lost visual acuity at 4 years, the majority of treated eyes maintained visual acuity better than 20/400, whereas the majority of untreated eyes had a final visual acuity of 20/400 or worse. The treatment benefit is affected by the size of the CNV complex and by the initial visual acuity.[57] Eyes that harbor smaller lesions typically obtain a greater treatment benefit. In contrast, a better initial visual acuity is associated with greater immediate visual loss from treatment.

After initial treatment of new subfoveal CNV, 13% of treated eyes demonstrated persistent neovascularization, and an additional 31% developed recurrent CNV within 2 years. In addition, a new, distinct area of CNV developed in 3% of treated eyes over 3 years. Mean visual acuity at 3 years after treatment was 20/400 for treated eyes that had persistent CNV, 20/250 for treated eyes that had recurrent CNV, and 20/320 (6/100) for treated eyes that had no peripheral leakage.[58] Approximately half of all treated eyes were retreated in the study. The MPS recommended that retreatment be considered when the lesion is relatively small with well-demarcated boundaries; the size of the persistent or recurrent CNV and the previous laser-treated area was required to be equivalent to six or fewer MPS disc areas.

The MPS also demonstrated a long-term benefit of laser photocoagulation in reducing visual loss associated with extrafoveal

Ocular Photodynamic Therapy

OPT is a more recent technology that uses low-energy light to activate an intravenously injected photosensitizing agent and induce closure of a choroidal neovascular complex. The goal of OPT is to specifically target neovascular tissue while sparing surrounding and overlying retinal structures. No immediate, permanent laser-induced scotoma is produced, and there is no corresponding RPE defect.[39] It was hoped that the narrow eligibility requirements and high recurrence rates of conventional photocoagulation would be improved with OPT (Fig. 125-6).

The mechanism of action of OPT involves delivery of a photosensitizing agent to its site of action, followed by activation with wavelength-specific light. Theoretically, current photosensitizers have an affinity for proliferating neovascular tissue due to the increased expression of low-density lipoprotein (LDL) receptors on neovascular endothelium. The LDL-bound photosensitizer complex is preferentially transported across the vascular endothelium and localized within the CNV. Activation of the photosensitizer with specific nonthermal light produces a triplet state; this reacts with oxygen, ultimately producing singlet oxygen. The resulting local cytotoxicity causes an acute inflammatory response with production of cytokines. Occlusion of the vascular bed occurs from endothelial damage, platelet adhesion and aggregation, and subsequent thrombus formation.[61–64]

Benzoporphyrin derivative monoacid (Verteporfin) is the only approved photosensitizer for OPT at the time of this publication. Dosage is determined by body surface area ($6mg/m^2$). The drug is infused intravenously over 10 minutes, followed by a 5-minute accumulation phase. It is then activated with low-energy laser light for 83 seconds using a wavelength corresponding to its peak absorption at 689nm and a fluence of $600mW/cm^2$. A treatment spot size is chosen 1000m larger than the greatest linear dimension of the lesion to ensure complete coverage of the neovascular complex.

After treatment, individuals are advised to avoid direct sunlight or bright illumination for 5 days to prevent phototoxicity to exposed body surfaces. The treatment is generally safe, but serious adverse events have been reported, including severe vision loss and extravasation of the photosensitizer. The most common side effects include visual disturbances (blurred vision, decreased vision, visual field defect) and injection site events (extravasation, rash). Allergic reaction and back pain have also been reported. Overdosage of the drug or light may result in nonperfusion of the retinal vasculature, with subsequent severe visual loss from macular infarction.

Two large, prospective trials have evaluated Verteporfin for the treatment of subfoveal CNV due to AMD: the TAP Study and the VIP Study.

TAP STUDY. The TAP Study[46,47] enrolled 609 eyes with subfoveal CNV secondary to AMD and randomized them in a double-blind fashion to treatment with Verteporfin or a placebo control. Best-corrected visual acuity at study entry was 20/40 to 20/200 equivalent, measured on an early treatment diabetic retinopathy study (ETDRS) chart. The lesion was required to be subfoveal in location, be less than or equal to 5400m in greatest linear dimension (nine MPS disc areas), and contain a classic component. The main outcome measure was moderate visual loss, defined as a loss of 15 letters or doubling of the visual angle (e.g., from 20/80 to 20/160).

At 24 months, outcomes were reported for 351 (87%) in the Verteporfin group and 178 (86%) in the placebo group. A statistically significant treatment benefit was identified for a specific subgroup of individuals with predominantly classic CNV. A predominantly classic lesion is defined as one that contains a classic component occupying 50% or more of the entire neovascular complex; the remainder of the lesion may consist of PED, occult CNV, or blocked fluorescence from hemorrhage or other cause. For this subgroup of patients, moderate visual loss occurred in 41% of eyes treated with Verteporfin, compared with 69% treated with placebo, at 24 months. Severe visual loss (loss

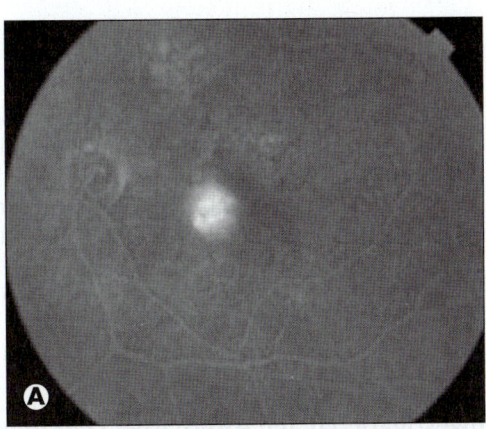
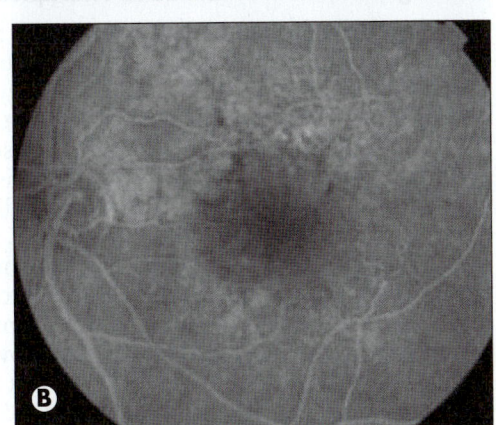

FIG. 125-6 ▪ **A,** Classic choroidal neovascularization prior to ocular photodynamic therapy (OPT). **B,** Same lesion 2 weeks following OPT, demonstrating hypofluorescence in the area of the treatment spot and corresponding hypoperfusion of the neovascular complex; no laser scotoma is induced. Reperfusion of the choroidal circulation after several weeks will determine whether retreatment is required or the lesion has regressed to an inactive, fibrotic scar.

CNV.[59] Approximately 46% of treated eyes, compared with 64% of untreated eyes, had severe visual loss by 5 years after study entry. Recurrence after laser treatment of extrafoveal CNV developed in 54% of eyes during the 5-year follow-up period. Most of these recurrences occurred in the first 2 years after treatment. They tended to occur on the foveal side of the original neovascular lesion, resulting in significant loss of visual acuity.

The MPS demonstrated the efficacy of laser photocoagulation for juxtafoveal CNV associated with AMD as well.[53, 60] At 5 years, almost no eyes with juxtafoveal CNV showed improvement in vision over baseline levels. However, 25% of treated eyes, compared with 15% of untreated eyes, maintained their baseline visual acuity. The mean visual acuity of laser-treated eyes was 20/200, compared with 20/250 for untreated eyes. Despite this small difference in final visual acuity, more than twice as many treated eyes retained visual acuity of 20/40 or better. Similarly, 25% of treated eyes had visual acuity of 20/400 or worse, compared with 40% of untreated eyes.[60] Rates of severe vision loss were 52% among treated eyes and 61% among untreated eyes. Treated eyes lost 1.2 fewer lines of visual acuity on average than did untreated eyes. Disappointing long-term visual results for treated juxtafoveal lesions can be explained by the high frequency of persistent or recurrent CNV. Persistent CNV was identified in 32% of treated eyes, and recurrent CNV occurred in an additional 42% within the follow-up period.

The MPS also showed a treatment benefit for subfoveal recurrences that received prior laser photocoagulation for juxtafoveal or extrafoveal CNV.[55,56] At 3 years after randomization, laser-treated eyes had better visual acuity than did untreated eyes, although both groups had limited distance visual acuity. Twice as many treated eyes as untreated eyes had visual acuity better than 20/200 at the 3-year examination, and fewer than half as many treated eyes as untreated eyes had visual acuity of 20/400 or worse.

Laser photocoagulation is limited by restrictive eligibility criteria, immediate visual loss due to laser-induced scotoma, and high recurrence rates. These shortcomings have prompted research into alternative therapies with broader applicability and higher success in preserving or improving vision and maintaining closure of CNV.

of 30 letters or quadrupling of the visual angle) occurred in 15% of treated eyes versus 36% of controls. Legal blindness resulted in 44% and 68%, respectively; mean final visual acuities were 20/160 and 20/200 in the two groups. Statistically significant benefits of Verteporfin were also demonstrated for preservation of contrast sensitivity and limitation of final lesion size, progression, and leakage.

Retreatment rates were documented for the Verteporfin and placebo groups. Lesions were eligible for retreatment at 3-month intervals if they showed any evidence of leakage on fluorescein angiography. In the first year, retreatment was performed an average of 3.4 times in the Verteporfin group, compared with 3.7 times in the placebo group. The Verteporfin group required an average of 2.1 retreatments in the second year, for a mean total of 5.5 treatments over 2 years.

VIP STUDY. The second VIP report[44,45] focused primarily on AMD patients with occult subfoveal CNV and no classic component. The study enrolled 225 eyes in the Verteporfin treatment group and 114 in the placebo control group. Eligibility required a visual acuity of at least 20/100 and a lesion size of 5400m or less. Occult lesions were required to have associated hemorrhage or show deterioration within 3 months of enrollment. Deterioration was defined as a loss of 1 ETDRS line or a 10% increase in the greatest linear dimension of the lesion.

At 12 months, no statistically significant difference was detected between the Verteporfin and placebo groups with respect to the primary outcome measure, moderate visual loss. At 24 months, however, a statistically significant benefit was identified, with 54% in the Verteporfin group experiencing moderate visual loss, compared with 67% in the placebo group. Severe visual loss occurred in 30% of treated cases versus 46% of controls. Legal blindness resulted in 28% and 45%, respectively; mean final visual acuities were 20/126 and 20/160 in the two groups.

Four percent of Verteporfin-treated eyes experienced acute visual loss, defined as loss of 20 or more letters within 7 days of treatment. Causes included hemorrhagic PED, neurosensory detachment, and idiopathic visual loss.

ONGOING RESEARCH. OPT has generally replaced conventional laser photocoagulation for the treatment of predominantly classic subfoveal CNV due to AMD. The treatment of occult CNV is currently not universally agreed on, and results of other ongoing studies may definitively determine the treatment of choice. OPT technology in its current form is still limited by restrictive eligibility criteria and the need for multiple retreatments. Research is ongoing to evaluate newer photosensitizers in an attempt to address these issues. Other studies are combining OPT with different therapeutic modalities, such as pharmacological inhibition of VEGF, to enhance the effect. The timing of retreatment is also being altered to determine the most appropriate interval. Regardless, OPT represents a major advance in the treatment of CNV resulting from AMD.

Nutritional Supplementation

The Age-Related Eye Disease Study[65] is the first large, prospective trial to show a benefit of antioxidant and zinc supplementation on the progression of AMD and associated visual loss. The study enrolled 3640 participants followed for an average of 6.3 years. Individuals were randomized to receive daily oral nutritional supplementation in the following subgroups:

1. Antioxidants (500mg vitamin C, 400IU vitamin E, 15mg beta-carotene)
2. Zinc (80mg zinc oxide, 2mg cupric oxide)
3. Antioxidants plus zinc
4. Placebo

The study recommended antioxidants plus zinc for the subset of AMD patients with extensive intermediate-size drusen ($\geq$63μm but <125μm), at least one large druse ($\geq$125μm), noncentral geographical atrophy in one or both eyes, or advanced AMD in one eye. Advanced AMD was defined as photocoagula-

tion or other treatment for CNV, central geographical atrophy, nondrusenoid PED, serous or hemorrhagic retinal detachment, hemorrhage under the retina or RPE, or subretinal fibrosis.

Primary outcome measures included progression to advanced AMD and moderate visual acuity loss from baseline (loss of $\geq$15 letters or doubling of the visual angle). For the subset defined above, 28% assigned to the placebo arm progressed to advanced AMD, compared with 23% assigned to antioxidants, 22% assigned to zinc, and 20% assigned to antioxidants plus zinc. In this same subset, 29% assigned to placebo experienced moderate visual loss, compared with 26%, 25%, and 23% in the respective arms. These results were statistically significant.

Investigational and Alternative Therapies

Transpupillary thermotherapy is currently the focus of a large, randomized, prospective trial for the treatment of occult subfoveal CNV due to AMD. This technology uses subthreshold laser irradiation with a long exposure duration and a large spot size to thermally treat CNV. The induced tissue temperature rise is estimated at 10° C, well below the 42° rise encountered with laser photocoagulation. Using an 810nm-diode laser, transmitted energy penetrates the RPE and choroid, minimizing absorption by the neurosensory retina. Proposed mechanisms of CNV closure include vascular thrombosis, apoptosis, and thermal inhibition of angiogenesis. A pilot study enrolling 16 eyes followed for 1 year showed that 16% improved by two or more Snellen lines, 56% stabilized, and 25% lost two or more lines.[66]

Pharmacological inhibition of angiogenesis is currently being studied using anecortave acetate and other specific agents that target VEGF, a known promoter of CNV. Feeder vessel photocoagulation guided by high-speed ICG angiography has been advocated but has yet to be studied in a large, controlled trial. Radiation therapy has also been suggested, but it failed to show a benefit relative to sham treatment in the prospective, randomized Radiation Therapy for Age-Related Macular Degeneration Study; the authors suggested that an alternative radiation dosage might have yielded a significantly different outcome.[67] Surgical approaches to subfoveal CNV have been attempted using subfoveal excision and macular translocation. The Submacular Surgery Trial compared surgical excision of recurrent subfoveal CNV to laser photocoagulation and found no benefit after 2 years of follow-up.[68] Macular translocation involves surgical displacement of the fovea overlying subfoveal CNV to a healthier area of RPE and choroid. Results have been reported in small series, but a larger, controlled trial has yet to be organized.

Low-Vision Aids

Low-vision aids should be considered in any individual who experiences untreatable visual loss that affects his or her ability to perform activities of daily living. Various devices exist for different tasks, such as reading, writing, computer work, driving, and distance vision. Reading lamps and simple magnifiers may be of significant benefit. Closed-circuit television and scanning devices are available to provide electronic magnification and contrast enhancement.

CONCLUSION

Age-related macular degeneration continues to be the leading cause of visual loss in developed countries, despite extensive resources dedicated to research involving its prevention and treatment. New therapeutic strategies continue to be developed and tested. Laser-based technologies remain the mainstay of current treatment. Pharmacological approaches appear promising in thwarting angiogenesis, and refinements in advanced surgical techniques may offer better outcomes in the future. Treatment of AMD in the next decade will likely be very different from its treatment a decade ago.

REFERENCES

1. Gass JD. Stereoscopic atlas of macular disease: diagnosis and treatment, ed 4. St Louis: CV Mosby; 1997:70–2.

2. Klein R, Klein BE, Jensen SC, Meuer SM. The five-year incidence and progression of age-related maculopathy: the Beaver Dam Eye Study. Ophthalmology. 1997;104:7–21.

3. Leibowitz HM, Krueger DE, Maunder LR, et al. The Framingham Eye Study monograph: an ophthalmological and epidemiological study of cataract, glaucoma, diabetic retinopathy, macular degeneration, and visual acuity in a general population of 2631 adults, 1973–1975. Surv Ophthalmol. 1980;24:335–610.

4. Rahmani B, Tielsch JM, Katz J, et al. The cause-specific prevalence of visual impairment in an urban population. The Baltimore Eye Survey. Ophthalmology. 1996;103:1721–6.

5. Young RW. Pathophysiology of age-related macular degeneration. Surv Ophthalmol. 1987;31:291–306.

6. Munoz B, West SK, Rubin GS, et al. Causes of blindness and visual impairment in a population of older Americans: The Salisbury Eye Evaluation Study. Arch Ophthalmol. 2000;118:819–25.

7. Vingerling JR, Dielemans I, Hofman A, et al. The prevalence of age-related maculopathy in the Rotterdam Study. Ophthalmology. 1995;102:205–10.

8. Bressler NM, Bressler SB, West SK, et al. The grading and prevalence of macular degeneration in Chesapeake Bay watermen. Arch Ophthalmol. 1989;107:847–52.

9. Klein BE, Klein R. Cataracts and macular degeneration in older Americans. Arch Ophthalmol. 1982;100:571–3.

10. Schachat AP, Hyman L, Leske MC, et al.. Features of age-related macular degeneration in a black population. The Barbados Eye Study Group. Arch Ophthalmol. 1995;113:728–35.

11. Pauleikhoff D, Harper CA, Marshall J, Bird AC. Aging changes in Bruch's membrane. A histochemical and morphologic study. Ophthalmology. 1990;97:171–8.

12. Friedman E. The role of the atherosclerotic process in the pathogenesis of age-related macular degeneration. Am J Ophthalmol. 2000;130:658–63.

13. Ciulla TA, Harris A, Kagemann L, et al. Choroidal perfusion perturbations in non-neovascular age related macular degeneration. Br J Ophthalmol. 2002;86:209–13.

14. Friedman E, Krupsky S, Lane AM, et al. Ocular blood flow velocity in age-related macular degeneration. Ophthalmology. 1995;102:640–6.

15. Grunwald JE, Hariprasad SM, DuPont J, et al. Foveolar choroidal blood flow in age-related macular degeneration. Invest Ophthalmol Vis Sci. 1998;39:385–90.

16. Risk factors for neovascular age-related macular degeneration. The Eye Disease Case-Control Study Group. Arch Ophthalmol. 1992;110:1701–8.

17. Seddon JM, Willett WC, Speizer FE, Hankinson SE. A prospective study of cigarette smoking and age-related macular degeneration in women. JAMA. 1996;276: 1141–6.

18. West SK, Rosenthal FS, Bressler NM, et al. Exposure to sunlight and other risk factors for age-related macular degeneration. Arch Ophthalmol. 1989;107:875–9.

19. Hyman LG, Lilienfeld AM, Ferris FL 3rd, Fine SL. Senile macular degeneration: a case-control study. Am J Epidemiol. 1983;118:213–27.

20. Francois J. L'heredite des degenerescences maculaires seniles. Ophthalmologica. 1977;175:67–72.

21. Klein ML, Mauldin WM, Stoumbos VD. Heredity and age-related macular degeneration. Observations in monozygotic twins. Arch Ophthalmol. 1994;112:932–7.

22. Meyers SM, Greene T, Gutman FA. A twin study of age-related macular degeneration. Am J Ophthalmol. 1995;120:757–66.

23. Seddon JM, Ajani UA, Mitchell BD. Familial aggregation of age-related maculopathy. Am J Ophthalmol. 1997;123:199–206.

24. Bressler SB, Maguire MG, Bressler NM, Fine SL. Relationship of drusen and abnormalities of the retinal pigment epithelium to the prognosis of neovascular macular degeneration. The Macular Photocoagulation Study Group. Arch Ophthalmol. 1990;108:1442–7.

25. Subfoveal neovascular lesions in age-related macular degeneration. Guidelines for evaluation and treatment in the Macular Photocoagulation Study. Macular Photocoagulation Study Group. Arch Ophthalmol. 1991;109:1242–57.

26. Chamberlin JA, Bressler NM, Bressler SB, et al. The use of fundus photographs and fluorescein angiograms in the identification and treatment of choroidal neovascularization in the Macular Photocoagulation Study. The Macular Photocoagulation Study Group. Ophthalmology. 1989;96:1526–34.

27. Guyer DR, Yanuzzi LA, Slakter J, et al. Classification of choroidal neovascularization by digital indocyanine green videoangiography. Ophthalmology. 1996;103: 2054–60.

28. Regillo CD, Benson WE, Maguire JI, Annesley WH Jr. Indocyanine green angiography and occult choroidal neovascularization. Ophthalmology. 1994;101:280–8.

29. Bressler NM, Bressler SB. Indocyanine green angiography. Can it help preserve the vision of our patients? Arch Ophthalmol. 1996;114:747–9.

30. Valencia M, Green RL, Lopez PF. Echographic findings in hemorrhagic disciform lesions. Ophthalmology. 1994;101:1379–83.

31. Green WR, Wilson DJ. Choroidal neovascularization. Ophthalmology. 1986;93: 1169–76.

32. Green WR, McDonnell PJ, Yeo JH. Pathologic features of senile macular degeneration. Ophthalmology. 1985;92:615–27.

33. Spraul CW, Grossniklaus HE. Characteristics of drusen and Bruch's membrane in postmortem eyes with age-related macular degeneration. Arch Ophthalmol. 1997;115:267–73.

34. Bressler NM, Silva JC, Bressler SB, et al. Clinicopathologic correlation of drusen and retinal pigment epithelial abnormalities in age-related macular degeneration. Retina. 1994;14:130–42.

35. Bressler SB, Silva JC, Bressler NM, et al. Clinicopathologic correlation of occult choroidal neovascularization in age-related macular degeneration. Arch Ophthalmol. 1992;110:827–32.

36. Holz FG, Wolfensberger TJ, Piguet B,et al. Bilateral macular drusen in age-related macular degeneration. Prognosis and risk factors. Ophthalmology. 1994;101:1522–8.

37. Risk factors for choroidal neovascularization in the second eye of patients with juxtafoveal or subfoveal choroidal neovascularization secondary to age-related macular degeneration. Macular Photocoagulation Study Group. Arch Ophthalmol. 1997;115:741–7.

38. Bressler NM, Bressler SB, Gragoudas ES. Clinical characteristics of choroidal neovascular membranes. Arch Ophthalmol. 1987;105:209–13.

39. Freund KB, Yannuzzi LA, Sorenson JA. Age-related macular degeneration and choroidal neovascularization. Am J Ophthalmol. 1993;115:786–91.

40. Bressler SB, Bressler NM, Fine SL, et al. Natural course of choroidal neovascular membranes within the foveal avascular zone in senile macular degeneration. Am J Ophthalmol. 1982;93:157–63.

41. Guyer DR, Fine SL, Maguire MG, et al. Subfoveal choroidal neovascular membranes in age-related macular degeneration. Visual prognosis in eyes with relatively good initial visual acuity. Arch Ophthalmol. 1986;104:702–5.

42. Bressler NM, Frost LA, Bressler SB, et al. Natural course of poorly defined choroidal neovascularization associated with macular degeneration. Arch Ophthalmol. 1988;106:1537–42.

43. Occult choroidal neovascularization. Influence on visual outcome in patients with age-related macular degeneration. Macular Photocoagulation Study Group. Arch Ophthalmol. 1996;114:400–12.

44. Verteporfin therapy of subfoveal choroidal neovascularization in age-related macular degeneration: two-year results of a randomized clinical trial including lesions with occult with no classic choroidal neovascularization. Verteporfin in Photodynamic Therapy report 2. Am J Ophthalmol. 2001;131:541–60.

45. Bressler NM. Verteporfin therapy of subfoveal choroidal neovascularization in age-related macular degeneration: two-year results of a randomized clinical trial including lesions with occult with no classic choroidal neovascularization. Verteporfin in Photodynamic Therapy report 2. Am J Ophthalmol. 2002;133:168–9.

46. Photodynamic therapy of subfoveal choroidal neovascularization in age-related macular degeneration with Verteporfin: one-year results of 2 randomized clinical trials—TAP report. Treatment of Age-Related Macular Degeneration with Photodynamic Therapy (TAP) Study Group. Arch Ophthalmol. 1999;117:1329–45.

47. Bressler NM. Photodynamic therapy of subfoveal choroidal neovascularization in age-related macular degeneration with Verteporfin: two-year results of 2 randomized clinical trials—TAP report 2. Arch Ophthalmol. 2001;119:198–207.

48. Laser treatment in eyes with large drusen. Short-term effects seen in a pilot randomized clinical trial. Choroidal Neovascularization Prevention Trial Research Group. Ophthalmology. 1998;105:11–23.

49. Figueroa MS, Regueras A, Bertrand J. Laser photocoagulation to treat macular soft drusen in age-related macular degeneration. Retina. 1994;14:391–6.

50. Guymer RH, Gross-Jendroska M, Owens SL, et al. Laser treatment in subjects with high-risk clinical features of age-related macular degeneration. Posterior pole appearance and retinal function. Arch Ophthalmol. 1997;115:595–603.

51. Little HL, Showman JM, Brown BW. A pilot randomized controlled study on the effect of laser photocoagulation of confluent soft macular drusen. Ophthalmology. 1997;104:623–31.

52. Sigelman J. Foveal drusen resorption one year after perifoveal laser photocoagulation. Ophthalmology. 1991;98:1379–83.

53. Krypton laser photocoagulation for neovascular lesions of age-related macular degeneration. Results of a randomized clinical trial. Macular Photocoagulation Study Group. Arch Ophthalmol. 1990;108:816–24.

54. Laser photocoagulation of subfoveal neovascular lesions in age-related macular degeneration. Results of a randomized clinical trial. Macular Photocoagulation Study Group. Arch Ophthalmol. 1991;109:1220–31.

55. Laser photocoagulation of subfoveal recurrent neovascular lesions in age-related macular degeneration. Results of a randomized clinical trial. Macular Photocoagulation Study Group. Arch Ophthalmol. 1991;109:1232–41.

56. Laser photocoagulation of subfoveal neovascular lesions of age-related macular degeneration. Updated findings from two clinical trials. Macular Photocoagulation Study Group. Arch Ophthalmol. 1993;111:1200–9.

57. Visual outcome after laser photocoagulation for subfoveal choroidal neovascularization secondary to age-related macular degeneration. The influence of initial lesion size and initial visual acuity. Macular Photocoagulation Study Group. Arch Ophthalmol. 1994;112:480–8.

58. Persistent and recurrent neovascularization after laser photocoagulation for subfoveal choroidal neovascularization of age-related macular degeneration. Macular Photocoagulation Study Group. Arch Ophthalmol. 1994;112:489–99.

59. Argon laser photocoagulation for neovascular maculopathy. Five-year results from randomized clinical trials. Macular Photocoagulation Study Group. Arch Ophthalmol. 1991;109:1109–14.

60. Laser photocoagulation for juxtafoveal choroidal neovascularization. Five-year results from randomized clinical trials. Macular Photocoagulation Study Group. Arch Ophthalmol. 1994;112:500–9.

61. Henderson BW, Donovan JM. Release of prostaglandin E2 from cells by photodynamic treatment in vitro. Cancer Res. 1989;49:6896–900.

62. Rutledge JC, Curry FE, Blanche P, Krauss RM. Solvent drag of LDL across mammalian endothelial barriers with increased permeability. Am J Physiol. 1995;268: 1982–91.

63. Bown SG, Tralau CJ, Smith PD. Photodynamic therapy with porphyrin and phthalocyanine sensitization: quantitative studies in normal rat liver. Br J Cancer. 1986;54:43–52.

64. Henderson BW, Dougherty TJ. How does photodynamic therapy work? Photochem Photobiol. 1992;55:145–57.

65. A randomized, placebo-controlled, clinical trial of high-dose supplementation with vitamins C and E, beta carotene, and zinc for age-related macular degeneration and vision loss: AREDS report no. 8. Arch Ophthalmol. 2001;119:1417–36.

66. Reichel E, Berrocal AM, Ip M, et al. Transpupillary thermotherapy of occult subfoveal choroidal neovascularization in patients with age-related macular degeneration. Ophthalmology. 1999;106:1908–14.

67. Marcus DM, Sheils W, Johnson MH, et al. External beam irradiation of subfoveal choroidal neovascularization complicating age-related macular degeneration: one-year results of a prospective, double-masked, randomized clinical trial. Arch Ophthalmol. 2001;119:171–80.

68. Submacular surgery trials randomized pilot trial of laser photocoagulation versus surgery for recurrent choroidal neovascularization secondary to age-related macular degeneration. I. Ophthalmic outcomes. Submacular Surgery Trials pilot study report number 1. Am J Ophthalmol. 2000;130:387–407.

126 Degenerative Myopia

BRAD J. BAKER • RONALD PRUETT

DEFINITION
- A poorly understood form of excessive axial myopia that can be associated with potentially blinding complications.

KEY FEATURES
- Progressive global expansion with posterior staphyloma formation and secondary macular degeneration.

ASSOCIATED FEATURES
- Premature cataract formation.
- Vitreous syneresis, rhegmatogenous retinal detachment, and glaucoma.

BOX 126-1

Ocular Manifestations of Degenerative Myopia

ANATOMICAL MANIFESTATIONS	FUNCTIONAL MANIFESTATIONS
Corneal astigmatism	Image minification
Deep anterior chamber	Anisometropic amblyopia
Angle iris processes	Subnormal visual acuity
Zonular dehiscences	Visual field defects
Vitreous syneresis	Impaired dark adaptation
Lattice retinal degeneration	Abnormal color discrimination
Scleral expansion and thinning	Suboptimal binocularity
Decreased ocular rigidity	
Increased axial length	
Posterior staphyloma	
Tilted disc	
Temporal crescent or halo atrophy	
Macular lacquer cracks	
Pigment epithelial thinning	
Choroidal attenuation	

INTRODUCTION

Myopia is a common optical aberration. Physiological myopia, by far the most prevalent, is less than $-6D$ in magnitude and is considered a normal biological variation. Eyes that have errors greater than $-6D$ are said to have high myopia. The greater the myopia, the more likely are complications that can threaten vision. A subgroup of high myopes have axial lengths that fail to stabilize during young adulthood. The pathophysiology of this progressive, degenerative form of myopia is unknown.

EPIDEMIOLOGY AND PATHOGENESIS

Not all eyes that have myopia greater than $-6D$ progress; nor does every eye that has progressive myopia develop degenerative complications. The worldwide distribution of those who have truly degenerative myopia is unknown, but the prevalence of progressive "pathological" myopia was surveyed by Fuchs[1] more than 40 years ago. Among 15 countries in the study, progressive myopia was found in 0.3% (Egypt) to 9.6% (Spain) of their populations. Asians are known to have a high prevalence of myopia. That of progressive myopia in Japan was 8.4%. This wide variation implies that there is a genetic influence.

In the multiethnic United States, the prevalence was estimated at 2.1% in a U.S. Public Health Service study.[2] Women are affected twice as commonly as men, and black Africans infrequently have progressive myopia. It is the seventh leading cause of blindness in the United States, and its effects generally occur at an earlier average age than those of diabetic retinopathy and age-related macular degeneration.

The pathogenesis of myopia in general, and progressive myopia in particular, is unclear, but both heredity and environment play a role.[3] The mode of inheritance may be autosomal recessive or dominant, but it also can appear sporadically. Progressive myopia occurs commonly in association with

Marfan's, Ehlers–Danlos, and Stickler's syndromes, and twin studies confirm its genetic basis.

The most widely accepted environmental influences are excessive near work and increasing formal education. Sustained accommodation and intraocular pressure (IOP), both basal and phasic, are suspected to influence axial elongation in eyes that have decreased scleral resistance,[4,5] but recent evidence questions both of these hypotheses. Topical atropine slows the progression of myopia in children,[6] but this may be via a mechanism independent of accommodation. Further, it appears that at least some degree of active scleral growth and remodeling appears to be involved in pathological myopia. This may be regulated by various local growth factors, independent of central nervous system control. Experimentally, ocular growth can be governed by the application of plus or minus spectacles,[7] and children who have threshold retinopathy of prematurity develop less myopia following peripheral retinal ablation.[8] Understanding of these and other influences upon development of myopia is still too fragmentary to permit therapeutic application.

OCULAR MANIFESTATIONS

The more important anatomical and functional abnormalities found in extremely myopic individuals are listed in Box 126-1.[9]

Patients who have excessive myopia often have strabismus, especially exophoria and exotropia, and are more likely to develop premature nuclear sclerosis or, in some cases, posterior subcapsular lens opacities. Glaucoma is more common among highly myopic eyes and is particularly insidious. Its prevalence is related to the degree of myopia. Curtin[10] found glaucoma in 3% of eyes that had axial lengths less than 26.5mm, in 11% that had

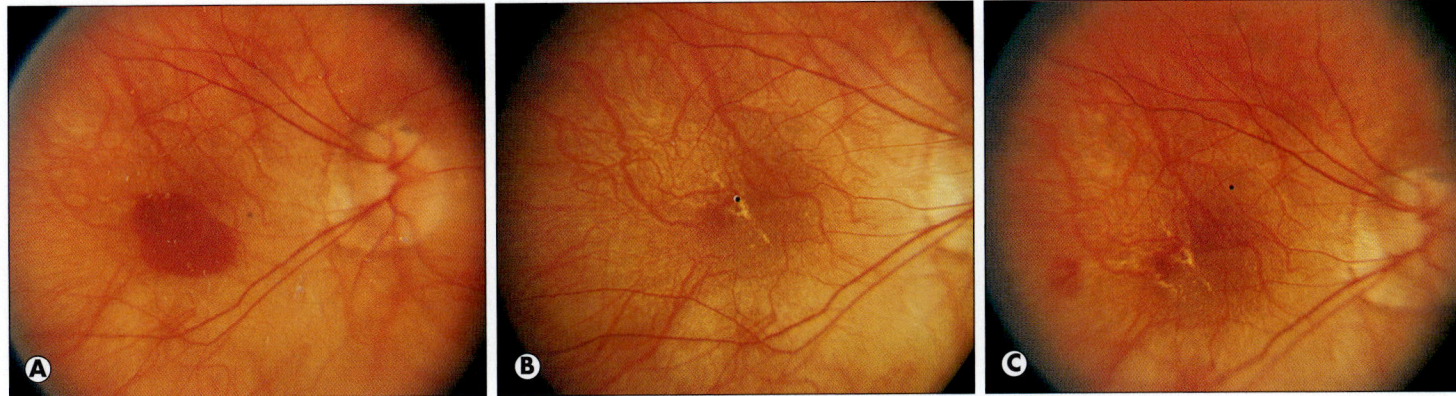

FIG. 126-1 ■ A 28-year-old Caucasian woman experienced a central light flash followed by blurred vision in her −23.50D right eye. **A,** A subretinal hemorrhage is present in the fovea. **B,** A small wishbone-shaped lacquer crack was observed 13 months later. **C,** At 27 months from the original bleed, another such crack was noted along a temporal extension of the growing lacquer crack pattern. This was asymptomatic and the corrected acuity was 20/60 (6/18).

axial lengths in the range 26.5–33.5mm, and in 28% of eyes that had axial lengths over 33.5mm. Determination of glaucomatous changes are especially difficult in highly tilted optic discs, with posterior staphyloma adjacent to the myopic disc complicating the evaluation of visual field defects. Also, pigmentary and normal-tension glaucoma occurs more frequently in myopes.

Among the other serious complications of progressive myopia are vitreous syneresis and rhegmatogenous retinal detachment that results from peripheral tears. Such detachments usually are spontaneous, but they may occur after blunt ocular trauma or subsequent to cataract surgery, especially when complicated by capsular rupture and vitreous loss.

The abnormality seen in the myope that justifies use of the term *degenerative* is posterior staphyloma (ectasia), with its devastating secondary effects in the posterior pole. The progressively myopic eye expands in all its posterior dimensions, and the formation of an equatorial staphyloma with scleral dehiscence is not uncommon, especially in the superotemporal quadrant. Visual loss is most often due to macular involvement of a posterior pole staphyloma.[11] The deformity occurs in various locations, described by Curtin[12] as posterior polar (disc and macula central), macula centered with the disc at the margin, peripapillary, inverse (in which the depression extends nasally from the optic nerve head), and an inferior type that involves the lower portion of the disc and the fundus below it. Complex patterns are termed *compound staphylomata*. Usually, the edge of the defect is sharper closer to the disc and more blended away from it. Staphylomata that are clear edged and deep in a young person may occasionally lose some definition as the scleral envelope enlarges with age.[11]

As the scleral shell expands, the neural retina, pigment epithelium, and choroid stretch and thin to accommodate the area they cover. Tissue attenuation causes the fundus to have a pale, tessellated appearance. The pigment epithelial cells are flattened, and a reduction occurs in the thickness of the choriocapillaris and in the larger vessel layers and pigment of the choroid. This is evident especially within the staphyloma itself, where the fundus pallor is exaggerated by the increased visibility of the underlying sclera.

With time and progression, traction and tension phenomena are observed. The first is a pale, temporal crescent at the disc as the pigment epithelium and choriocapillaris are retracted from the disc's margin toward the deepest area of the staphyloma. Bruch's membrane is noncellular and elastic but has a limited capacity to stretch. If its elastic limit is exceeded, the internal tension is relieved by formation of microdehiscences called lacquer cracks. Acute lacquer crack formation near the fovea occasionally is signaled by photopsias and metamorphopsia (Fig. 126-1). Defects in the overlying pigment epithelium may appear punc-

tate, but eventually a linear pattern develops that coincides with the breaks in Bruch's membrane. Continued break formation results in a reticular pattern that usually is most obvious in the deepest recess of the staphyloma and portends a guarded prognosis for central vision.

The lacquer crack defects usually slowly increase in width and grow in number. Other isolated, round, or irregular pigment epithelial and choriocapillaris defects may develop along the margin or within the staphyloma. If a choroidal neovascular membrane invades a crack, an abrupt macular hemorrhage may be produced. Although usually self-limited, the hyperpigmented fibrovascular scar that evolves (Förster–Fuchs' spot) causes a central or paracentral scotoma. An area of choroidal and pigment epithelial atrophy develops and surrounds the scar (Fig. 126-2). This extends and coalesces with areas of atrophy that advance from other lacquer cracks, eventually to produce large geographical areas of destruction in which sclera can be seen through the transparent neural retina. The process is usually bilateral and insidious. As paracentral fixation areas diminish, even low-vision aids become useless and ambulatory sight is all that remains.

Macular hole formation in extreme myopes may occur, but the exact mechanism is unknown. Whether attenuation of the neural retina and its supportive pigment epithelium and choroid are responsible is speculative. Vitreous syneresis and posterior vitreous detachment are more common and occur at an earlier age among high myopes than among others[13]; usually they are not accompanied by vitreomacular traction or an epiretinal membrane and only rarely produce a posterior rhegmatogenous retinal detachment.

DIAGNOSIS AND ANCILLARY TESTING

Myopes are recognized easily by their poor distance visual acuity that is improved by negative-power lenses. Degenerative myopia is a diagnosis made when clinical findings and extreme axial length occur together, as cause and effect.

The need for ancillary diagnostic testing is dictated by the preliminary findings. If a posterior staphyloma is detected or questioned, A and B scan ultrasonography can confirm its presence. Fluorescein angiography and, in some cases, indocyanine green angiography may demonstrate more extensive lacquer crack formation than is detected by ophthalmoscopy and can be used to rule out choroidal neovascularization.

DIFFERENTIAL DIAGNOSIS

The clinician who has taken a careful history and performed a meticulous examination will have no difficulty in diagnosing

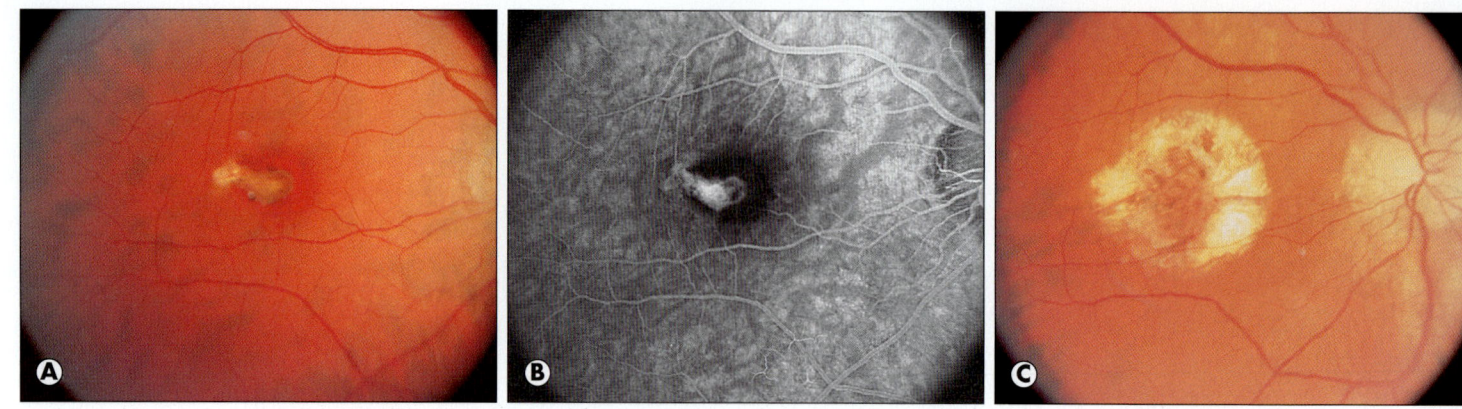

FIG. 126-2 ■ **Sudden loss of vision.** This male Caucasian myope (right eye, −8.00D; left eye, −9.00D) suddenly lost vision to 20/400 (6/120) in the right eye at 35 years of age. **A,** A choroidal neovascular membrane invades the fovea. **B,** Fluorescein angiography demonstrates the central membrane that had not been treated. **C,** The patient underwent a scleral reinforcement procedure on both eyes. Fifteen years later the area of central choriocapillary atrophy has enlarged, but corrected visual acuity is a surprising 20/80 (6/24).

progressive myopia. Its signature deformity is posterior staphyloma. Although patients who have retinitis pigmentosa are frequently myopic, show secondary cataract and vitreous liquefaction, can develop macular degeneration, and have peripheral visual field defects, these are easily distinguished by other findings in most cases. Peripapillary atrophic changes, punched-out defects in the pigment epithelium, and macular neovascular lesions are seen in ocular histoplasmosis syndrome. Myopes are unprotected from acquiring this infection, but its characteristics are not easily confused with those of degenerative myopia.

SYSTEMIC ASSOCIATIONS

Myopia of different degrees and incidence may be associated with a wide variety of disorders. Many of these are hereditary and all forms of inheritance are represented.[14,15] A selected listing is presented in Box 126-2. Environmental factors also determine expression, but because the complex development of the eye can be misdirected by a number of code sequence errors leads to an unavoidable conclusion—no single "myopia gene" exists.

Some systemic disorders are diagnosed easily, conditions such as albinism and trisomy 21; others are more subtle. Because the cardiovascular complications of Marfan's syndrome and congenital rubella and the orthopedic disabilities associated with Ehlers–Danlos and Stickler's syndromes may produce morbidity and even mortality, prompt referral to medical and surgical colleagues is indicated if the patient has not been referred already.

PATHOLOGY

Typically, the extremely myopic eye is enlarged in all its posterior dimensions, but particularly in its axial length. Anteriorly, the cornea may be slightly thinner and flatter than normal, with a deeper anterior chamber, and the angle recess shows iris processes attached to the trabeculum. The lens has a tendency to show early nuclear sclerosis. Defects in the zonular membrane are common and may present a challenge during cataract surgery. The ciliary body may be smaller than normal, although considerable variability exists.

Generalized scleral thinning is associated with increased scleral elasticity, or decreased ocular rigidity. Especially when combined with zonular dehiscence, this results in rapid vitreous fluid egress and global collapse when the eye is opened to atmospheric pressure. Sudden hypotony can result in a serous or hemorrhagic choroidal detachment during intraocular surgery. Anatomically, the sclera is not only thin but also has an abnormal constitution. The classic electron microscopic findings of Garzino[16] have been corroborated by others. The collagen fibers are of much smaller average diameter than in a normal eye.

BOX 126-2

Systemic Associations of Degenerative Myopia

Albinism
Congenital rubella
de Lange's syndrome
Down's syndrome
Ehlers–Danlos syndrome
Fetal alcohol syndrome
Gyrate atrophy—hyperornithinemia
Laurence–Moon–Bardet–Biedl syndrome
Marfan's syndrome
Pierre Robin's syndrome
Stickler's syndrome

Further, the fibrils show greater interfibrillar separation and the normally tightly opposed and interwoven architecture of the collagen bundles[17] gives way to a more uniformly lamellar and eventually amorphous appearance.[18] Choroidal neovascularization may be evident through Bruch's membrane dehiscences.[19]

TREATMENT

The ultimate goal is to prevent myopia progression and posterior staphyloma with its associated visual loss, but currently no proven method exists by which to accomplish this.

In children, topical atropine can effectively slow enlargement of the myopic eye and the effect is sustained even after the drug has been withdrawn.[6] However, the possibility of long-term light damage to eyes that have dilated pupils has been investigated insufficiently. If this method is chosen, a thorough informed consent is required, and sun shielding and filters are advised. The effectiveness of atropine in eyes genomically destined to become pathologically myopic is unknown. Other approaches presumed to act via modification of accommodation include the use of bifocals, undercorrection of myopia, and part-time spectacle wear. Clinical trials report contradictory results,[20] but the regulation of young primate eye growth has proved possible by using plus and minus lenses to blur the retinal image.[7]

Because highly myopic eyes have reduced scleral resistance plus a tendency to develop glaucoma, many investigators have postulated that scleral expansion is caused by raised IOP.[4] Pärssinen[21] found a significant correlation between raised IOP and myopic progression among boys, but not among girls, while Quinn et al.[5] noted that ocular tension is higher in children who have myopia than in nonmyopes. Controlled trials of IOP reduction have been reported.[22-24] Timolol maleate was employed, all the subjects were children, and the focus was not on progressive degenerative myopia. Goldschmidt's pilot study of 10 children showed a tendency for the children who had a reduction in IOP to slow in their progression of myopia,[23] but Jensen's 2-year study of 94 children did not prove timolol to be effective.[24] The possibility remains that optical and pharmacological methods, alone or in concert, may be devised to retard axial elongation.

If advancing myopia in children continues beyond pubertal years, follow-up at least yearly is indicated. A stereoscopic, indirect ophthalmoscopic, and biomicroscopic search for staphyloma formation is important and, if suspected, staphyloma formation is investigated further using A and B scan ultrasonography. Some of these eyes eventually stabilize as highly myopic but with no posterior complications. The ongoing evaluation of any peripheral lattice degeneration lesions that may be evident, especially in the event of blunt trauma or an acute posterior vitreous separation, is critical.

If staphyloma formation is detected, further caution is warranted. Biannual examinations may reveal lacquer crack development that is not heralded by a photopsia or blurred central vision. Once lacquer crack formation or areas of choriocapillary and pigment epithelial atrophy are present in a young adult, it becomes likely that the central vision will be threatened in time by advancing atrophy, choroidal neovascularization, or both. The traditional option in the United States at this stage has been to continue observation, while ophthalmologists in some eastern European countries advocate the use of various tissue extract injections, vasodilators, and scleral reinforcement. Although the value of reinforcement surgery is unproved,[25,26] it may have application in selected and obviously endangered eyes in which the disease continues to advance.[27]

One step short of surgery, or in addition to it, is to lower IOP. No controlled trial has been used to confirm efficacy or assured safety. Until such information is available, and in the absence of other contraindications, the use of a tension-reducing agent in "normal" eyes seems not unreasonable and has been recommended.[27] Relative ocular hypotension in eyes prone to develop tears in Bruch's membrane may help to prolong central vision.

Other conservative measures include avoidance of eye rubbing, trauma, Valsalva exertion, and regular use of anticoagulants such as aspirin (unless required for systemic disease). Because topical corticosteroids frequently provoke a rise in IOP in the highly myopic eye, these also should be used with caution and with frequent tension checks.

Myopia-related choroidal neovascularization is a major cause of visual loss, especially when located in a subfoveal location. Photodynamic therapy has shown a statistically significant reduction in visual loss when compared with a placebo group after 1 year for subfoveal choroidal neovascularization associated with pathological myopia.[28] The lesion could be classic or occult on fluorescein angiography if either was at least 50% of the total area. The median visual acuity following treatment was 20/64+2 in the treatment group and 20/80−2 in the control group, with 77% of treated patients losing fewer than 8 letters compared with 44% of the placebo group at 12 months. The average patient received 3.4 treatments during the study. Extrafoveal choroidal neovascularization may also be treated with argon laser photocoagulation. Confluent argon laser burns of diameter 100–200μm delivered over 0.2–0.4 seconds are most effective. Whether laser treated or allowed to involute spontaneously, the cicatricial lesion eventually becomes surrounded by a zone of atrophy that slowly enlarges with time. This atrophy typically is relentless and may progress to compromise the central vision.

Macular hole formation and the less frequently encountered detachment of the posterior retina are problems that confront those who care for patients who have degenerative myopia. Even for those patients who are attended by surgeons trained and practiced in modern vitreoretinal surgical skills, these complications result in a poorer prognosis and increased risk. Modern vitreoretinal surgical techniques can restore vision in select cases.

COURSE AND OUTCOME

Because the degenerative form of progressive myopia is among the leading causes of legal blindness is testimony that today's treatment methods do not offer a cure. Affected individuals cannot share in the optimism of the more numerous patients with low myopia that the development of keratorefractive techniques will help them, because the fundamental nature of their disease, axial elongation and posterior staphyloma, is not altered by such techniques. Hopefully, laboratory and clinical evidence will provide practical methods by which to reduce the risk of progressive myopia. Meanwhile, the management of degenerative myopia is that of its complications and the prognosis for patients is guarded.

REFERENCES

1. Fuchs A. Frequency of myopia gravis. Am J Ophthalmol. 1960;49:1418–9.
2. Roberts J, Slaby D. Refraction status of youths 12–17 years. Pub No (HRA) 75–1630. Washington, DC: US Dept Health, Education and Welfare; 1974.
3. Mutti DO, Zadnik K, Adams AJ. Myopia, the nature versus nurture debate goes on. Invest Ophthalmol Vis Sci. 1996;37:952–7.
4. Pruett RC. Progressive myopia and intraocular pressure: what is the linkage? Acta Ophthalmol. 1988;185:117–27.
5. Quinn GE, Berlin JA, Young TL, et al. Association of intraocular pressure and myopia in children. Ophthalmology. 1995;102:180–5.
6. Kennedy RH. Progression of myopia. Trans Am Ophthalmol Soc. 1995;93:755–800.
7. Hung LF, Crawford MLJ, Smith EL. Spectacle lenses alter eye growth and the refractive status of young monkeys. Nat Med. 1995;1:761–5.
8. Algawi K, Goggin M, O'Keefe M. Refractive outcome following diode laser versus cryotherapy for eyes with retinopathy of prematurity. Br J Ophthalmol. 1994;78:612–4.
9. Curtin BJ. The myopias, basic science and clinical management. Philadelphia: Harper & Row; 1985:277–385.
10. Curtin BJ. Myopia: a review of its etiology, pathogenesis and treatment. Surv Ophthalmol. 1970;15:1–17.
11. Steidl SM, Pruett RC. Macular complications associated with posterior staphyloma. Am J Ophthalmol. 1997;123:181–7.
12. Curtin BJ. The posterior staphyloma of pathologic myopia. Trans Am Ophthalmol Soc. 1977;75:67–86.
13. Morita H, Funata M, Tokoro T. A clinical study of the development of posterior vitreous detachment in high myopia. Retina. 1995;15:117–24.
14. Curtin BJ. The myopias, basic science and clinical management. Philadelphia: Harper & Row; 1985:72–97.
15. Fong DS, Pruett RC. Systemic associations with myopia. In: Albert DM, Jakobiec FA, eds. Principles and practices of ophthalmology. Philadelphia: WB Saunders; 1994:3142–51.
16. Garzino A. Modificazione del collagene scleralae nella miopia maligna. Ross Ital Ottal. 1956;25:241–74.
17. Komai Y, Ushiki T. The three-dimensional organization of collagen fibrils in the human cornea and sclera. Invest Ophthalmol Vis Sci. 1991;32:2244–58.
18. Curtin BJ, Teng CC. Scleral changes in pathological myopia. Trans Am Acad Ophthalmol Otolaryngol. 1957;62:777–90.
19. Pruett RC, Weiter JJ, Goldstein RB. Myopic cracks, angioid streaks, and traumatic tears in Bruch's membrane. Am J Ophthalmol. 1987;103:537–43.
20. Goss DA. Effect of spectacle correction on the progression of myopia in children, a literature review. J Am Optom Assoc. 1994;65:117–28.
21. Pärssinen O. Intraocular pressure in school myopia. Acta Ophthalmol. 1990;68:559–63.
22. Goldschmidt E, Jensen H, Marushak D, et al. Can timolol maleate reduce the progression of myopia? Acta Ophthalmol. 1985;63(Suppl):90.
23. Jensen H. Timolol maleate in the control of myopia. Acta Ophthalmol. 1988;185:128–9.
24. Jensen H. Myopia progression in young school children. A prospective study of myopia progression and the effect of a trial with bifocal lenses and β blocker eye drops. Acta Ophthalmol. 1991;69:1–79.
25. Curtin BJ. The myopias, basic science and clinical management. Philadelphia: Harper & Row; 1985:415–21.
26. Thompson FB. Scleral reinforcement. In: Thompson FB, ed. Myopia surgery: anterior and posterior segments. New York: MacMillan; 1990:267–97.
27. Pruett RC. Posterior segment. In: Roy FH, ed. Master techniques in ophthalmic surgery. Philadelphia: Williams & Wilkins; 1995:994–1006.
28. Photodynamic therapy of subfoveal choroidal neovascularization in pathologic myopia with verteporfin. 1-year results of a randomized clinical trial—VIP report No 1. Verteporfin in Photodynamic Therapy Study Group. Ophthalmology. 2001;108:841–52.

CHAPTER 127

Central Serous Chorioretinopathy

WILLIAM J. WIROSTKO • JOSE S. PULIDO

DEFINITION
- An idiopathic chorioretinal disorder characterized by serous detachment of the neural retina in the macular region.

KEY FEATURES
- One or more focal areas of subretinal fluid in the macula.
- One or more focal leaks at the level of the retinal pigment epithelium.

ASSOCIATED FEATURES
- Retinal pigment epithelial detachment.
- Mottling of the retinal pigment epithelium.
- Yellowish white subretinal deposits.
- Unilateral or bilateral involvement.
- Recurrences.
- Dependent, bullous retinal detachment.

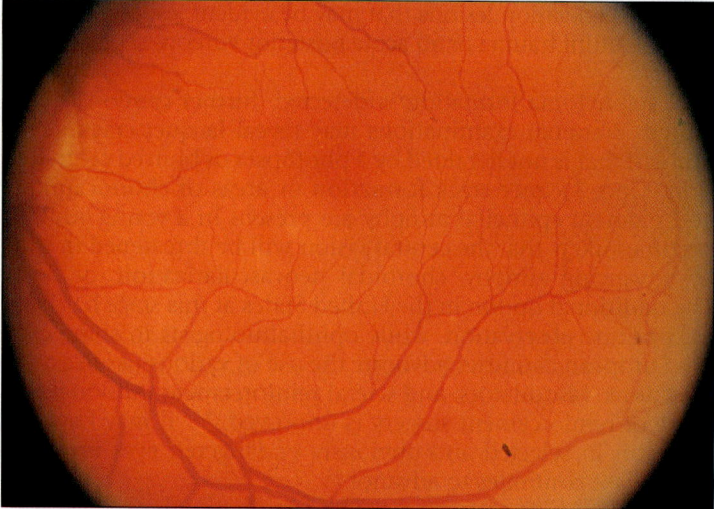

FIG. 127-1 ▮▮ Fundus photograph of central serous chorioretinopathy. Note the neural retinal detachment the size of two disc diameters in the macular region, the pigment epithelial abnormalities inferonasal to the fovea, and the numerous tiny yellow dots on the undersurface of the retina. (Courtesy of T.C. Burton, MD.)

INTRODUCTION

Central serous chorioretinopathy (CSC) is a common retinal disorder characterized by an idiopathic serous neural retinal detachment in the macular region (Fig. 127-1). Since its initial description as relapsing central syphilitic retinitis by von Graefe in 1866, it has been referred to by many names, including central serous retinopathy, central serous pigment epitheliopathy, and central serous retinitis. The most common symptoms of CSC include metamorphopsia, blurred vision, and micropsia. Visual disturbances typically take several months to resolve. The most surprising aspect of the disease is the relative preservation of retinal function despite prolonged separation from the retinal pigment epithelium (RPE). Occasionally, the macular detachment may fail to resolve spontaneously; for these eyes, laser photocoagulation appears to be beneficial, as it accelerates the resorption of subretinal fluid and improves vision.[1-3]

EPIDEMIOLOGY AND PATHOGENESIS-11

Typically, CSC affects men aged 20 to 50 years. No case has been reported in a person younger than 20 years. In patients older than 50 years, CSC does occur, but it can be difficult to distinguish from age-related macular degeneration. An increased frequency may exist in intelligent individuals engaged in visually demanding work who display type A personality traits or who are experiencing physical strain or emotional stress.[4] A history of migraine-type headaches may be elicited.[1] Also, CSC has been associated with vasoconstrictive agents,[4] endogenous hypercortisolism,[5] smoking,[6] and the systemic use of corticosteroids (oral, intranasal, and inhaled),[7,8] psychopharmacological agents,[8] alcohol,[6] antibiotics (oral),[6] and antihistamines (oral).[6] It can be produced in animals by repeated intravenous epinephrine (adrenaline) injections.[4]

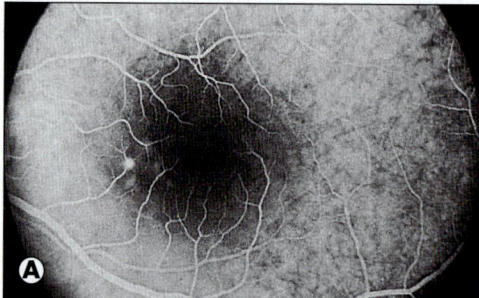

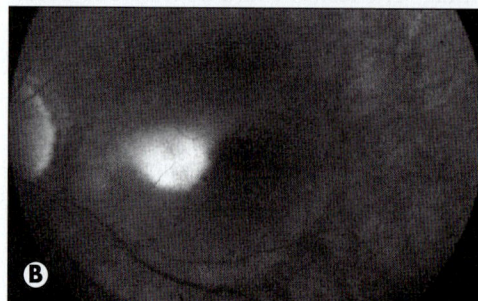

FIG. 127-2 ▮▮ Fluorescein angiogram of central serous chorioretinopathy. A, Early phase reveals focal leakage nasal to the macula. B, Late phase demonstrates pooling of the dye within the subneural retinal space.

The understanding of the pathogenic accumulation of subneural retinal fluid in the macular region is limited. Few pathological studies have been performed, and the observations from angiographic, clinical, and experimental models are subject to interpretation. It is well known, however, that the subneural retinal fluid originates from the choroid. The leakage of dye through an abnormal focal defect at the level of the RPE and its

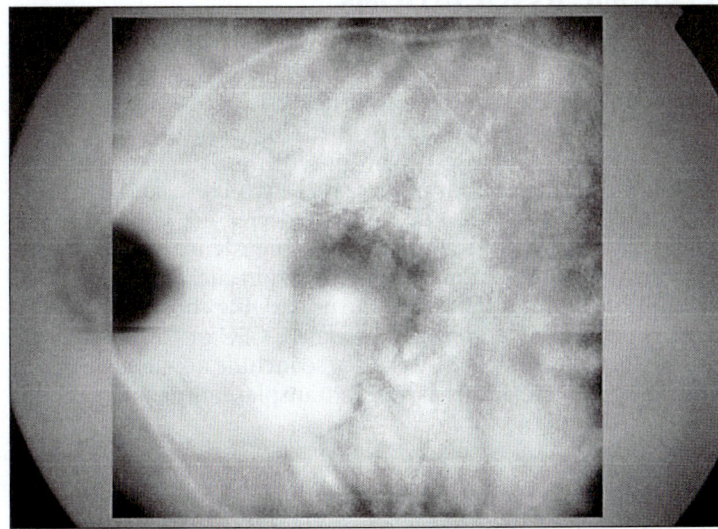

FIG. 127-3 ▮ Indocyanine green angiogram of central serous chorioretinopathy. Contrast enhancement reveals a focal area of hyperfluorescence during the midphase of the study. Fluorescein angiography demonstrated no leakage in the corresponding area.

accumulation in the subneural retinal space are seen clearly on fluorescein angiography[1] (Fig. 127-2).

The cause of the focal RPE leak is unclear. At first it was believed that a simple breakdown of the blood-retinal barrier at the RPE level was responsible for the leak. However, this theory does not explain the beneficial effect of the permanent RPE barrier breakdown produced during laser photocoagulation. Later, it was suggested that the subneural retinal fluid pooled secondary to a collection of pathologically hypersecreting RPE cells, but this theory fails to explain the widespread choroidal hyperpermeability seen with indocyanine green angiography[4] (Fig. 127-3).

Increasing evidence implicates an abnormal choroidal circulation as the cause of CSC. Using indocyanine green angiography, Prunte and Flammer[4] showed delayed choroidal capillary lobular filling in areas of hyperpermeability. They proposed that localized capillary and venous congestion in the affected lobules impaired the circulation, produced ischemia, and allowed increased choroidal exudation and a focally hyperpermeable choroid. This allows excess choroidal fluid to accumulate and produces a retinal pigment epithelial detachment (RPED). As the detachment grows, the target junctions between RPE cells are broken, and a focal defect of the blood-retinal barrier develops. Choroidal fluid passes through this opening and produces a neural retinal detachment.[9] Interestingly, recent studies reveal that corticosteroids can influence the production of nitric oxide, prostaglandins, and free radicals within the choroidal circulation. All three participate in the autoregulation of blood flow within the choroid.[8]

OCULAR MANIFESTATIONS

Although unilateral metamorphopsia is the classic symptom of CSC, patients also may present with unilateral blurred vision, micropsia, impaired dark adaptation, color desaturation, delayed retinal recovery time to bright light, and relative scotoma. Visual acuity ranges from 20/15 (6/5) to 20/200 (6/60) but averages 20/30 (6/9). The visual acuity may improve with hyperopic correction. Symptoms typically resolve after several months but may linger even after the fluid resolves; only rarely do they persist indefinitely. Permanent sequelae include metamorphopsia, decreased brightness perception, and altered color vision.[1]

Also, CSC can present as a bullous, inferior nonrhegmatogenous peripheral retinal detachment. The presence of RPE atrophic tracts from the macular region to the peripheral detachment, seen best with fluorescein angiography, reveals the true diagnosis and source of the subretinal fluid.[10]

A chronic form of CSC exists as well. It occurs in about 5% of cases, most commonly in older individuals and in patients receiving corticosteroids.[8,11] The use of psychopharmacological agents may also predict its development.[8] Chronic CSC is characterized by a diffuse retinal pigment epitheliopathy that progresses in conjunction with persistent or intermittent subretinal fluid. The retinal detachments tend to be shallow and more diffuse than in the classic form. The visual prognosis is more guarded.

DIAGNOSIS

The diagnosis of CSC is clinical, with confirmation by fluorescein angiography. Although in most cases the diagnosis can be made confidently without ancillary testing, the information derived from angiography is critical to detect the extent of the retinal abnormalities and to exclude the presence of other pathology.

Biomicroscopically, a transparent blister in the posterior pole between the neural retina and the RPE is observed. This is best seen through a fundus contact lens with a wide light beam, set slightly off axis. Signs that suggest the presence of a retina-RPE separation include beam splitting as the light traverses the serous space, an increased distance between the retinal vessels and their shadows, and an absent foveal reflex. Shallow detachments may be difficult to demonstrate clinically.[1]

The subretinal serous fluid within the blister often is transparent. This fluid may have protein and fibrin and be turbid or yellowish, especially in patients who are pregnant or have increased pigmentation, concurrent diabetes, or RPED.[1,11] It is believed that the small dotlike deposits that form on the posterior surface of the retina or on the anterior surface of the RPE cells under the area of the detachment represent precipitates of this protein. This is noted best when the fluid component is resolving. Diffuse deposits of serous proteins can produce a whitish retinal appearance that mimics intraretinal edema. A normal retinal thickness and transparency help distinguish this from true retinal edema.[1]

Oval yellow-gray elevations beneath the detachment also may be seen. These are generally less than one fourth of a disc diameter in size and are surrounded by a faint grayish halo. Fluorescein angiography identifies them as RPEDs and frequently demonstrates the focal RPE leaks responsible for the neural retinal detachment within their borders. Because subretinal exudative fluid may track inferiorly in response to gravity, a leaking RPED may lie beyond the superior margin of its retinal detachment. Numerous factors can help differentiate an elevated RPED from a shallow focal retinal detachment:

- An RPED obscures the choroidal pattern (this characteristic may abate as the RPE cells in the RPED atrophy).
- The boundary of the RPED typically is better defined than the edge of the retinal detachment.
- The light beam reflex is bowed forward toward the observer, preventing visualization of the sub-RPE space.

A large RPED must also be differentiated from an amelanotic melanoma or metastatic lesion to the choroid. Both can appear dome-shaped, solid, and nontranslucent and produce an overlying neurosensory detachment.[1]

The presence of cystic retinal degeneration, fine RPE mottling, or RPE clumping suggests chronicity of the present episode or a history of a previous CSC episode (Fig. 127-4). Additional ophthalmoscopic findings, such as lipid or hemorrhage, are rare and should call into question the diagnosis of idiopathic CSC.[1] The fellow eye may show evidence of either concurrent or previously resolved CSC, manifested as focal areas of RPE rarefaction or small asymptomatic RPEDs.

Fluorescein angiography plays an important role in the evaluation of CSC. It is used to exclude the presence of other pathologies that produce neural retinal detachments and to confirm the diagnosis. Classically, dye from the choroid leaks through a focal RPE defect and pools in the subretinal space. In

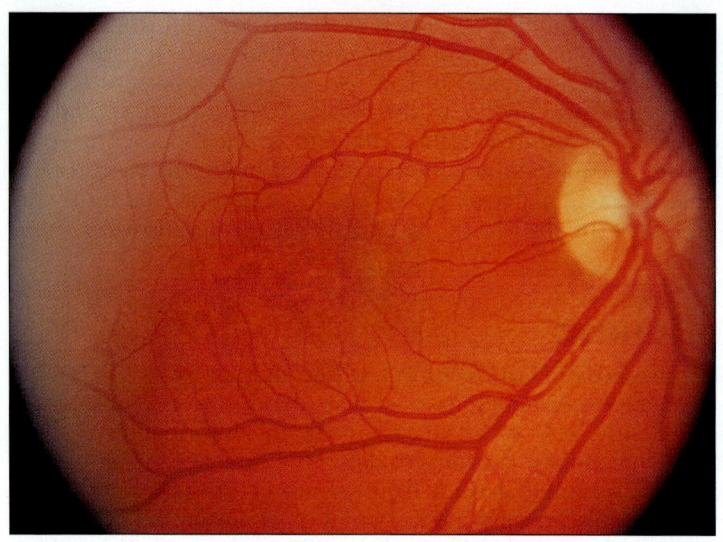

FIG. 127-4 ▮▮ Fundus photograph of an eye with resolved central serous chorioretinopathy showing chronic pigmentary changes. (Courtesy of W.F. Mieler, MD.)

more than 75% of patients, this pooling occurs within 1 disc diameter of the fovea.[12] Less pooling may be observed in older lesions in which the RPE exudate has become inspissated.[1] When fluorescein angiography is atypical, indocyanine green angiography can help exclude the presence of other pathology. Indocyanine green angiography of CSC classically reveals bilateral multifocal hyperfluorescence in affected and unaffected areas of the choroid. These appear during the midphase of the angiogram and are later silhouetted against larger choroidal vessels as the dye diffuses through the choroid.[13]

Optical coherence tomography is a new, noninvasive technique that can demonstrate the presence of subretinal fluid. In cases of CSC, optical coherence tomography has been used successfully to quantify the amount and extent of subretinal fluid and to demonstrate thickening of the neurosensory retina.[14]

DIFFERENTIAL DIAGNOSIS

Serous elevations of the neurosensory retina in the macular region can be produced by numerous diseases of the choroid, RPE, and retina. These include choroidal neovascularization, optic disc pits, polypoidal choroidal vasculopathy, choroidal melanoma, choroidal metastasis, and peripheral retinal breaks. Choroidal hemangioma, uveitis, Harada's disease, optic neuritis, papilledema, vitreous traction, macular holes, and systemic hypertension can produce neural retinal detachments as well.[1]

In particular, CSC must be differentiated from a neural retinal detachment secondary to subretinal choroidal neovascularization, polypoidal choroidal vasculopathy, or an optic disc pit. These three diseases mimic CSC by producing similar clinical findings, including neural retinal detachment, RPE changes, RPED, and subretinal exudate, but they have a significantly different pathophysiology, prognosis, and treatment. Consequently, their presence should be excluded with fluorescein angiography in all cases of presumed CSC. If fluorescein angiography is inconclusive, one can perform indocyanine green angiography. Indocyanine green angiography of subretinal choroidal neovascularization usually reveals only one area of hyperfluorescence that progressively enlarges during the later frames of the study. Indocyanine green angiography of polypoidal choroidal vasculopathy demonstrates small-caliber, polypoidal choroidal vascular lesions and no areas of choroidal hyperpermeability.[15] If the possibility of a choroidal neovascular membrane remains despite angiography, it may be prudent to observe the patient and repeat angiography 2 weeks later. An area of CSC leakage should remain constant or regress with time, whereas a choroidal neovascular membrane will likely grow.

SYSTEMIC ASSOCIATIONS

Usually, CSC is an isolated idiopathic ocular disorder. Patients may, however, exhibit various CSC risk factors, including type A personality traits or a recent episode of stress.[1]

Also, CSC has been associated with hypercortisolism and systemic corticosteroid use.[5,7] The observation of increased CSC symptoms during periods of increased steroid use, and their subsequent resolution when dosages are decreased, led to this discovery. Bouzas et al.[5] reported a CSC prevalence of 5% among patients with endogenous Cushing's syndrome.

Multiple diseases that share the underlying choroidal vascular dysfunction have been linked to classic CSC or to a visual syndrome that mirrors the disease. These include accelerated hypertension, pregnancy, dialysis, organ transplantation, and systemic lupus erythematosus.[16-20]

PATHOLOGY

The benign course of CSC and the low incidence among the elderly have limited the number of pathological studies. In those few performed, the RPE, choroid, and retinal vessels appear normal. The only histopathological changes observed include serous RPEDs, serous detachments of the cuticular portion of Bruch's membrane, and cystic degeneration in the outer layers of the detached neural retina.[1]

TREATMENT

The treatment of CSC is laser photocoagulation to the site of fluorescein leakage. Although this has been proved to reduce the duration of the serous detachment, it has no effect on the final visual prognosis and consequently is reserved for select patients.[2,3] It is the only therapy proved beneficial by large clinical trials.

The technique of laser photocoagulation involves using a green-wavelength laser to produce a light scar over the focal RPE leak. Typically, 6–12 laser burns of 50–200μm spot size at 0.1-second duration and 75–200mW are used. Permanent RPE change is induced at the site of the laser scar. It has been suggested that while the scar facilitates the absorption of subretinal fluid via the choroid, it also destroys an area of abnormally hypersecreting RPE cells. The absence of any beneficial effect when the laser scar does not overlie the focal choroidal leak suggests the presence of a focal RPE abnormality.[3]

The only definite benefit from laser therapy is its ability to decrease the duration of the neurosensory detachment. This has been documented in numerous studies.[2,3] In 1974, Watzke et al.[2] demonstrated that the median duration of disease decreased from 23 weeks in untreated eyes to 5 weeks in treated eyes. Whether laser therapy is of benefit in decreasing the risk of recurrence remains an unresolved question. The 0% rate of recurrence obtained by Yap and Robertson[21] disagrees with the 34% recurrence rate obtained by Watzke et al.[2] Both figures compare favorably with the 45% recurrence rate found by Klein et al.[12] for untreated eyes.

Complications from laser photocoagulation include choroidal neovascularization and central scotoma. Although rare, they can be visually devastating (Fig. 127-5). Complications may be reduced by using larger spots sizes, employing lower intensities, and avoiding the capillary-free zone.[3] The rapid development of a choroidal neovascular membrane following laser photocoagulation suggests the possibility of an initial misdiagnosis.[22] Subfoveal choroidal neovascularization associated with CSC may be treated with submacular surgery.[23]

Because most CSC episodes resolve spontaneously, laser treatment is reserved for patients who fail to improve after 4–6 months, demonstrate permanent changes from CSC in the other eye, demonstrate multiple recurrences, or require improved vision for work. Treatment should be avoided if the leak occurs within 200μm of the center of the foveal avascular zone.[3] Eyes with chronic CSC unresponsive to laser treatment may benefit from photodynamic therapy.[24]

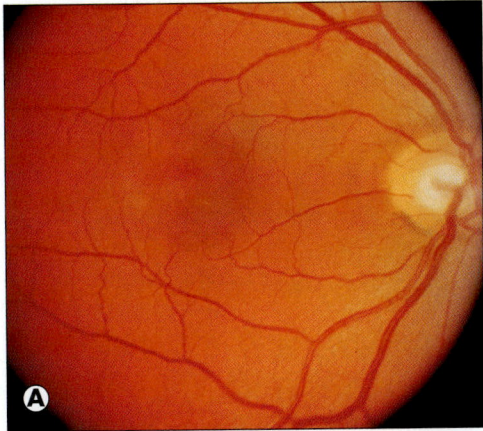

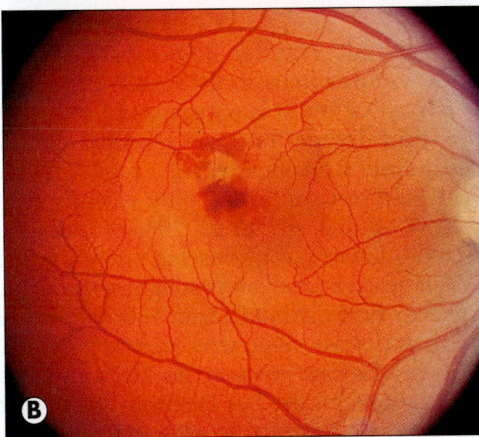

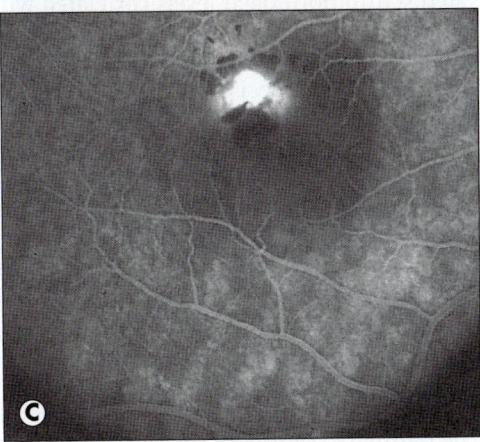

FIG. 127-5 ■
Choroidal neovascular
membrane after laser
photocoagulation for
central serous chori-
oretinopathy. **A,** Fundus
of an eye with a 2-year
history of recurrent CSC.
Note the neurosensory
detachment and the nu-
merous fine yellow de-
posits under the retina.
B, Fundus showing
subretinal blood at the
treatment site. **C,** Late-
frame fluorescein an-
giogram demonstrating
dye leakage from a
choroidal neovascular
membrane. (Courtesy
of W.F. Mieler, MD.)

Despite isolated reports, no medical therapy is of proven value. Ongoing studies are still investigating the beneficial role of systemic β-blockers.[25] The association of corticosteroids with CSC suggests that dosages should be reduced if a patient is receiving exogenous supplementation.[8]

COURSE AND OUTCOME

Generally, the visual prognosis is good. The majority of patients suffer no significant permanent visual loss. In a series of 34 eyes with CSC followed for an average of 23 months without treatment,[12] visual acuity was no worse than 20/40 in any eye. This was despite large neural retinal detachments, multiple RPE leaks, cystoid macular changes, persistent RPEDs, and marked visual loss during acute episodes. The persistent Amsler's chart changes present in 24 of 27 eyes were described as visually insignificant and causing no difficulty. Although visual acuity usually improves, patients may continue to have persistent meta-

morphopsia. After resolution of an episode of CSC, multifocal electroretinogram may be helpful for suggesting the risk of recurrence.[26]

Rarely, CSC can produce significant visual damage, usually caused by the chronic form of the disease. RPE atrophy, a metallic sheen at the level of the RPE, drusen, and choroidal neovascularization have also been described in eyes with untreated CSC.[14] Cases called "CSC" exist in which bullous neurosensory detachments extend from the posterior pole to the most dependent part of the retina.

Follow-up fluorescein angiography of eyes with CSC suggests that, in certain patients, CSC may herald a bilateral progressive RPE disturbance known as chronic CSC.[27] It remains unresolved whether a history of CSC exacerbates the natural course of age-related macular degeneration. However, recent studies suggest that CSC in older individuals is more frequently associated with the formation of choroidal neovascularization than in younger patients.[11]

REFERENCES

1. Gass JDM. Pathogenesis of disciform detachment of the neuroepithelium. II. Idiopathic central serous choroidopathy. Am J Ophthalmol. 1967;63:587–615.
2. Watzke RC, Burton TC, Leaverton PE. Hruby laser photocoagulation therapy of central serous retinopathy. Trans Am Acad Ophthalmol Otolaryngol. 1974;78:205–11.
3. Robertson DM, Illstrup D. Direct, indirect, and sham laser treatment in the management of central serous choroidopathy. Am J Ophthalmol. 1983;95:457–66.
4. Prunte C, Flammer J. Choroidal capillary and venous congestion in central serous choroidopathy. Am J Ophthalmol. 1996;121:26–34.
5. Bouzas EA, Scott MH, Mastorakos G, et al. Central serous chorioretinopathy in endogenous hypercortisolism. Arch Ophthalmol. 1993;111:1229–33.
6. Haimovici R, Koh SS, Lehrfeld T, et al. Systemic factors associated with central serous chorioretinopathy: a case-control study. Paper presented at the annual meeting of the American Academy of Ophthalmology, New Orleans, 2001.
7. Polak BCP, Baarsma GS, Snyers B. Diffuse retinal pigment epitheliopathy complicating systemic corticosteroid treatment. Br J Ophthalmol. 1995;79:922–5.
8. Tittl MK, Spaide RF, Wong D, et al. Systemic findings associated with central serous chorioretinopathy. Am J Ophthalmol. 1999;128:63–8.
9. Marmor MF. New hypothesis on the pathogenesis and treatment of serous retinal detachment. Graefes Arch Clin Exp Ophthalmol. 1988;226:548–52.
10. Sahu DK, Namperumalsamy P, Hilton GF, et al. Bullous variant of idiopathic central serous chorioretinopathy. Br J Ophthalmol. 2000;84:485–92.
11. Spaide RF, Campeas L, Haas A, et al. Central serous chorioretinopathy in younger and older adults. Ophthalmology. 1996;103:2070–80.
12. Klein ML, Van Buskirk EM, Freidman E, et al. Experience with non-treatment of central serous choroidopathy. Arch Ophthalmol. 1974;91:247–50.
13. Guyer DR, Yannuzzi LA, Slakter JS, et al. Digital indocyanine-green videoangiography of central serous chorioretinopathy. Arch Ophthalmol. 1994;112:1057–62.
14. Iida T, Hagimura N, Sato T, et al. Evaluation of central serous chorioretinopathy with optical coherence tomography. Am J Ophthalmol. 2000;129:16–20.
15. Yannuzzi LA, Freund KB, Goldbaum M, et al. Polypoidal choroidal vasculopathy masquerading as central serous chorioretinopathy. Ophthalmology. 2000; 107:767–77.
16. Venecia G, Jampol LM. The eye in accelerated hypertension. II. Localized serous detachments of the retina in patients. Arch Ophthalmol. 1984;102:68–73.
17. Sunness JS, Baller JA, Fine SL. Central serous chorioretinopathy and pregnancy. Arch Ophthalmol. 1993;111:360–4.
18. Gass JDM. Bullous retinal detachment and multiple retinal pigment epithelial detachments in patients receiving hemodialysis. Graefes Arch Clin Exp Ophthalmol. 1992;230:454–8.
19. Gass JDM, Slamovits TL, Fuller DG, et al. Posterior chorioretinopathy and retinal detachment after organ transplantation. Arch Ophthalmol. 1992;110:1717–22.
20. Cunningham ET, Alfred PR, Irvine AR. Central serous retinopathy in patients with systemic lupus erythematosus. Ophthalmology. 1996;103:2081–90.
21. Yap EY, Robertson DM. The long term outcome of central serous chorioretinopathy. Arch Ophthalmol. 1996;114:689–92.
22. Schatz H, Yannuzzi LA, Gitter KA. Subretinal neovascularization following argon laser photocoagulation treatment for central serous chorioretinopathy. Complications or misdiagnosis? Trans Am Acad Ophthalmol Otolaryngol. 1977;83:893.
23. Cooper BA, Thomas MA. Submacular surgery to remove choroidal neovascularization associated with central serous chorioretinopathy. Am J Ophthalmol. 2000;130:187–91.
24. Chen JC. Photodynamic therapy in the treatment of chronic central serous chorioretinopathy. Paper presented at the annual meeting of the American Academy of Ophthalmology, New Orleans, 2001.
25. Avci R, Deutmann AF. Die Behandlung der zentralen serosen choroidopathie mit dem betarezeptorenblocker Metoprolol (Vorlaufige Ergebnisse). Klin Monatsbl Augenheilkd. 1993;202:199–205.
26. Chappelow AV, Marmor MF. Multifocal electroretinogram abnormalities persist following resolution of central serous chorioretinopathy. Arch Ophthalmol. 2000;118:1211–5.
27. Levine R, Brucker AJ, Robinson F. Long-term follow-up of idiopathic central serous chorioretinopathy by fluorescein angiography. Ophthalmology. 1989;96:854–9.

128 Macular Hole

JAY S. DUKER

DEFINITION
- A full-thickness depletion of the neural retinal tissue in the center of the macula.

KEY FEATURES
- Central scotoma.
- Round, central neural retinal tissue defect.
- Cystic retinal changes in the perifoveolar area that surrounds the macular hole.
- Yellow spots in the base of the macular hole.
- Small surrounding cuff of subretinal fluid.

ASSOCIATED FEATURES
- Attached posterior hyaloid initially.
- Epiretinal membrane.
- Occasionally bilateral (10–20%).
- Retinal detachment (rare), previous trauma (rare), previous macular edema (rare).

INTRODUCTION

Idiopathic macular holes were identified as a unique clinical entity more than 100 years ago,[1,2] and Ogilvie[3] is credited with introducing the term *macular hole*. Until recently, ophthalmologists paid little attention to macular holes, because the pathogenesis was obscure and cure impossible. Recently, interest in this entity has increased dramatically. Although the pathogenesis remains incompletely understood, a new classification has emerged that accounts for premacular hole clinical appearances and gives insight into the intraocular processes that lead to macular hole formation.[4–6] In addition, some new ancillary tests are now available to assist in the diagnosis.[7–9] Most importantly, there is now surgical therapy to reverse the visual loss in most cases.[10,11]

EPIDEMIOLOGY AND PATHOGENESIS

The majority of macular holes are idiopathic, occurring in eyes that have no previous ocular pathology. Exceptionally, a pathological process can induce secondarily the formation of a macular hole. A macular hole can form immediately after blunt trauma—the initial published description of a macular hole by Herman Knapp[2] in 1869 was of one in a previously traumatized eye. Besides trauma, other ocular problems have been associated with macular hole formation including cystoid macular edema, epiretinal membrane, vitreomacular traction syndrome, rhegmatogenous retinal detachment, inadvertent exposure to laser energy, Best's disease, high myopia with posterior staphyloma, lightning strike injury, hypertensive retinopathy, and proliferative diabetic retinopathy.[1,12–14]

Idiopathic macular hole most commonly affects otherwise healthy individuals in their sixth or seventh decade of life. The mean age of onset is 65 years, but onset in patients as young as the third decade has been reported. Women are affected more commonly than men by a 2:1 ratio, an observation made many years ago but confirmed only recently by a well-designed case-control study.[15] About 10–20% of individuals eventually are affected bilaterally, but onset is rarely simultaneous.[1,16,17]

For years, investigators sought systemic reasons why idiopathic macular holes should form. Previous studies implicated cardiovascular disease, hypertension, and previous hysterectomy as possible risk factors; however, no confirming evidence supports these associations. In the Eye Disease Case-Control study, many possible systemic risk factors were examined prospectively. Only elevated serum fibrinogen levels correlated with an increased risk of idiopathic macular hole.[15] Macular holes are rare conditions, estimated to occur in the vicinity of 1 in 5000 patients.

Although the precise pathogenesis of idiopathic macular hole remains speculative, evidence suggests that abnormal tractional forces of the vitreous on the macula are directly responsible. Such tractional forces can be observed clinically with contact lens examination, with ultrasonography, and with newer imaging techniques like optical coherence tomography and laser biomicroscopy.[6–9] The success of vitreous surgery for macular holes provides strong evidence for a direct role of the vitreous in pathogenesis.[10]

OCULAR MANIFESTATIONS

The hallmark complaint of idiopathic macular hole formation is painless central visual distortion or blur of an acute or subacute nature. Quite typically, when only one eye is involved, the visual loss goes undetected unless cross-covering is performed. Central visual acuity initially may be diminished only mildly; however, as the hole progresses over weeks to months, the acuity usually deteriorates, then stabilizes around the 20/200–20/800 (6/60–6/240) level.

A currently accepted system of stages based on biomicroscopic observations was reported initially by Gass in 1988 and then revised in 1995; it explains the clinically observed appearances of macular holes and their precursor lesions. The hallmark inciting event of idiopathic macular hole formation is hypothesized to be focal shrinkage of the vitreous cortex in the foveal area.[4–6] Clinically, four stages occur in idiopathic macular hole development. Although Gass' biomicroscopic interpretations of the various stages are accepted widely, newer imaging techniques imply that the pathological processes that occur in stage 1 holes may differ slightly from the accepted classification.[8–10]

In idiopathic macular hole, impaired visual function is probably multifactorial. Photoreceptor loss from the central foveal area may occur in some cases, although a true retinal operculum rarely is evident. The central scotoma that results from foveal dehiscence is made significantly larger by the surrounding localized retinal detachment. Cystic changes develop in the intact perifoveal retina, as well, and some eyes develop epiretinal membranes. All the factors combine to decrease the central vision. Rhegmatogenous retinal detachment beyond the macula occurs secondary to a macular hole only if abnormal vitreous traction or extreme myopia with staphyloma is present concurrently.

Stage 1 Macular Hole

With a unilateral stage 1 macular hole, the patient typically is asymptomatic with both eyes open. For this reason and because they are evanescent lesions, stage 1 macular holes are not observed commonly and their diagnosis can be difficult. When symptoms are present, they consist of painless metamorphopsia or decreased vision or both. Stage 1 macular holes also have been referred to as *premacular holes, macular cysts,* or *involutional macular thinning.*

In a stage 1 macular hole, no true neural retinal defect is present, the photoreceptor layer is believed to be intact, and no vitreofoveal separation has occurred. Tangential or oblique vitreous traction on the fovea is hypothesized to be the inciting event. Stage 1 holes are further divided into stage 1a and stage 1b, based on clinical appearance. In a stage 1a macular hole, a small central yellow spot is seen on ophthalmoscopy. The fovea may be thickened along with a loss of the normal foveal contour. In a stage 1b macular hole, a yellow ring is visible in the foveal area.[4-6]

Gass suggests that the yellow spot of a stage 1a macular hole results from a small foveal detachment. Other observers, bolstered by ancillary testing, conclude that a stage 1a macular hole actually represents a cystic change in the fovea, rather than a true photoreceptor detachment from the retinal pigment epithelium.[8-10] In a stage 1b macular hole, the cyst-like space or foveal detachment enlarges to a point just short of actual dehiscence.

Stage 1 holes spontaneously resolve in about 50% of eyes with no visual sequelae (Fig. 128-1). The worse the initial visual acuity, the less likely is spontaneous resolution.

Stage 2 Macular Hole

When continued shrinkage of the perifoveal vitreous cortex occurs, a stage 1 hole advances to a stage 2 hole. Stage 2 holes have a small (100–200μm), full-thickness neural retinal defect, either centrally or eccentrically. The defect can be round, oval, crescentic, or horseshoe shaped (Fig. 128-2). The visual acuity typically is diminished and a pseudo-operculum, which represents condensed vitreous, may overlie the hole. It is believed that once a stage 2 hole occurs, it nearly always progresses to stage 3, with little hope for spontaneous visual improvement. The visual acuity with a stage 2 hole varies between 20/50 (6/15) and 20/400 (6/120).

Stage 3 Macular Hole

Stage 3 macular hole is the end result of continued vitreofoveal traction on a stage 2 hole. At stage 3, the hole is developed fully and has the classic appearance of an idiopathic macular hole. This consists of a round, 350–600μm full-thickness neural retinal defect with smooth edges, and a small, surrounding, doughnut-shaped rim of subretinal fluid (see Fig. 128-1, A). This fluid rarely progresses to cause a widespread retinal detachment. Yellow deposits can be seen in the base of the defect, and perifoveal cystic retinal changes are present. With time, retinal pigment epithelial alterations (pigmented demarcation line) may develop at the leading edge of the subretinal fluid cuff. The visual acuity typically is 20/200–20/800 (6/60–6/240); however, visual acuity as good as 20/40 (6/12) may be seen with a stage 3 hole, but rarely. Vitreofoveal separation still has not occurred.

Stage 4 Macular Hole

A stage 4 macular hole has all the features of a stage 3 hole, but with complete posterior separation of the vitreous from the fovea.

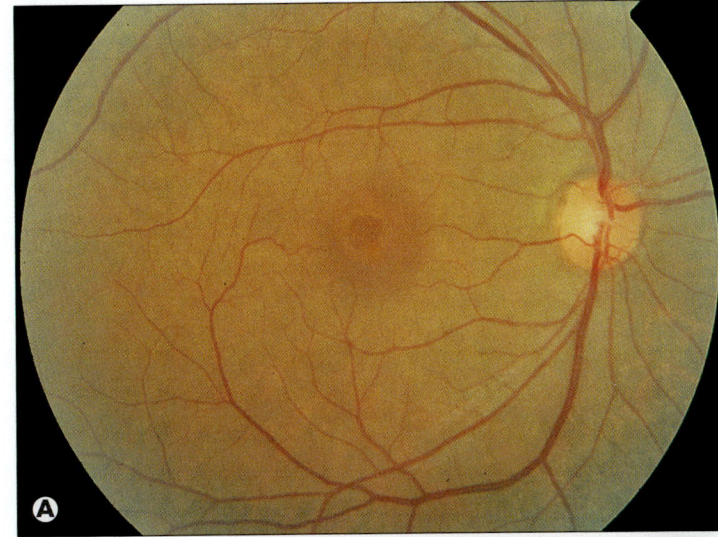

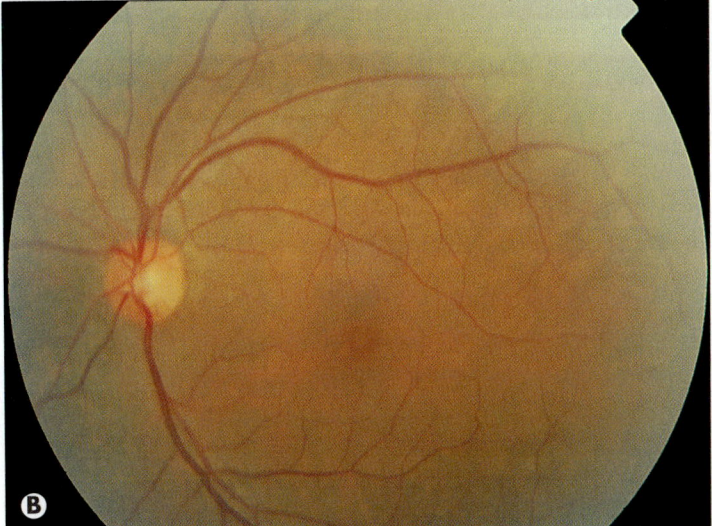

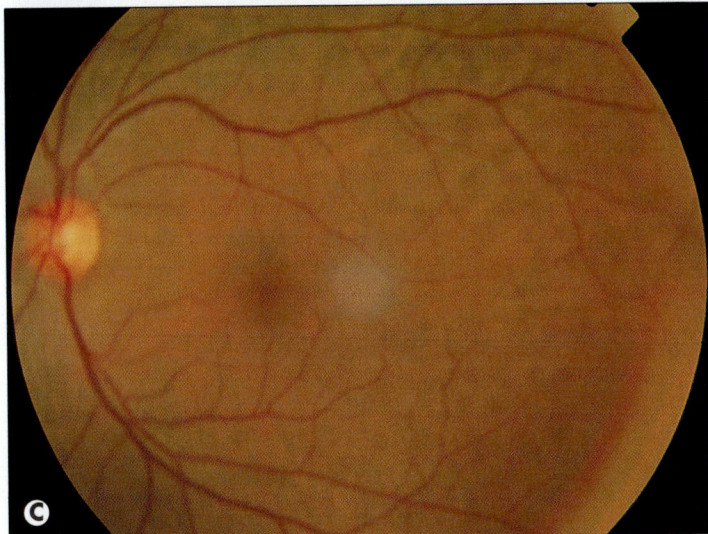

FIG. 128-1 ▪ **Spontaneous resolution of a macular hole. A,** Full-thickness stage 3 macular hole in the right eye of a 62-year-old woman who has a visual acuity of 20/200 (6/60). **B,** Stage 1a macular hole of several weeks' duration in the left eye of the same patient as shown in A. Visual acuity was 20/70 (6/21). Note central yellow spot. **C,** Several weeks later, spontaneous vitreofoveal separation has occurred in the eye shown in B, the stage 1a hole has resolved, and visual acuity is 20/30 (6/9).

Lamellar Macular Hole

A lamellar macular hole represents an aborted macular hole. Clinically, a round central inner retinal defect is found, with no thickening, cystic change, or subretinal fluid. An overlying operculum is common. Vitreofoveal separation occurs with loss of

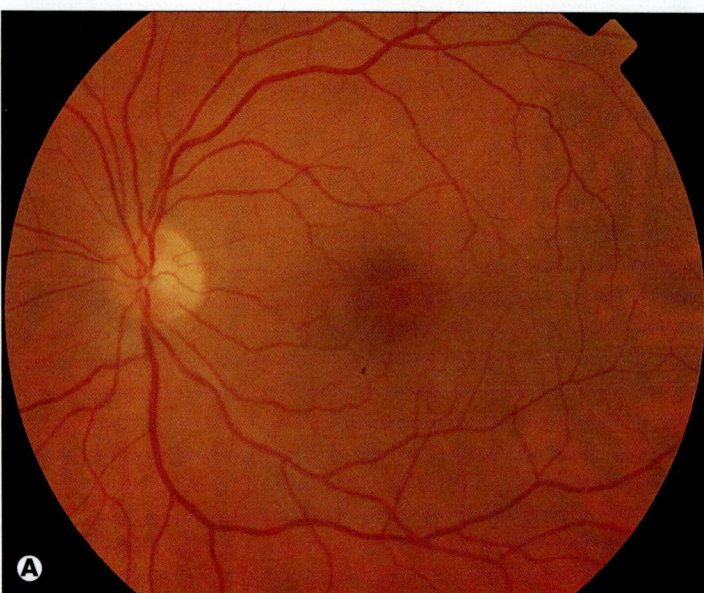

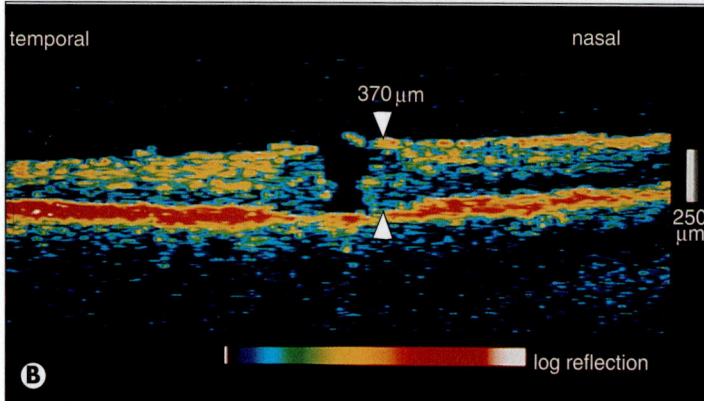

FIG. 128-2 ■ **Stage 2 macular hole. A,** Eccentric stage 2 macular hole with a vision of 20/80 (6/24). **B,** Optical coherence tomography of same eye as in **A,** showing full-thickness defect with eccentric opening of inner retina, consistent with a stage 2 macular hole.

the inner retinal layers; however, the outer, photoreceptor layer is intact. The vision usually is good (20/20–20/30 [6/6–6/9]) and many patients are asymptomatic. Fluorescein angiography typically shows no abnormal fluorescence. It is believed that, because vitreofoveal separation has occurred, the risk of continued progression to a macular hole is insubstantial.

DIAGNOSIS AND ANCILLARY TESTING

The diagnosis of idiopathic macular hole is a clinical one, made at the slit lamp with a handheld or fixed lens, used in either a contact or noncontact fashion. At times, the diagnosis can be difficult, especially when a unilateral stage 1 or stage 2 hole is present.[18,19]

Ancillary testing can be helpful in certain cases. Fluorescein angiography is not diagnostic, although it can help to rule out other entities that mimic macular hole. In stage 1 macular holes, fluorescein angiography commonly is normal or reveals only a small window defect. Some stage 2 macular holes show an intense, small, central window defect, while others manifest normal angiography or a mild window defect. In a stage 3 or 4 macular hole, the window defect tends to be mild and corresponds in size and location to the retinal defect.

The slit-beam test (Watzke–Allen sign) usually is reliable to test subjectively for a full-thickness retinal defect. In this test, a thin, vertically oriented slit beam is focused on the macula and the patient is asked to describe the line of light. In a full-thickness defect, a break or thinning of the beam is seen centrally.[18] The

scotoma associated with a macular hole can be mapped using the scanning laser ophthalmoscope or with the aiming beam of a laser.

Imaging tests of the retina and vitreous, such as ultrasonography, optical coherence tomography, and scanning laser biomicroscopy, are used to confirm the diagnosis and to assess the attachment of the vitreous to the fovea.[7–9,20] Optical coherence tomography appears to be the most clinically useful ancillary test.

DIFFERENTIAL DIAGNOSIS

Macular holes are most apt to be confused with epiretinal membranes, cystoid macular edema, or the vitreomacular traction syndrome. For the differential diagnosis of macular hole, an isolated ocular condition, see Box 128-1.

PATHOLOGY

Histopathological examination shows a round, full-thickness defect through all neural retinal layers. The underlying retinal pigment epithelium is intact. Associated intraretinal edema and perifoveal photoreceptor atrophy are common. Epiretinal membrane formation is also common.

In the few reported eyes that have undergone histopathological evaluation after successful vitreous surgery to close macular holes, fibroglial proliferation across the retinal defect has been observed.[21]

TREATMENT

Prior to 1989, idiopathic macular holes were considered untreatable. Kelly and Wendel[10] were the first to report that vitreous surgery can improve the visual acuity in some eyes with acute, idiopathic macular holes. Since then, vitrectomy for idiopathic macular holes rapidly has become a widely performed procedure throughout the world.

Most surgeons do not advocate operating on stage 1 holes for three reasons:

- Stage 1 macular holes have a 50% rate of spontaneous improvement.
- Surgical intervention does not prevent macular hole formation universally, and intraoperative macular hole can occur.
- Vitrectomy for a stage 2 hole of recent onset has a very high (>90%) success rate.

Macular hole surgery typically is performed under local anesthesia, unless general anesthesia is requested by the patient. A standard three-port core vitrectomy is completed. Following this, the intact posterior cortical vitreous is engaged gently, using a silicone-tipped extrusion needle attached to the suction line of the vitrectomy instrument. Alternatively, the vitreous cutting instrument, a bent needle, or a pick can be used to engage the cortical vitreous. The posterior cortical vitreous is usually invisible until it is elevated off the retina. At that point, it appears as a diaphanous membrane that may insert on the edges of the macu-

lar hole, the optic disc, or the midperipheral retina. Gentle elevation of the cortical vitreous and posterior hyaloid is carried out until complete separation of the vitreous is achieved. The remainder of the posterior vitreous is removed with the vitrectomy cutting instrument. At this juncture, epiretinal membrane, if present, is peeled using a bent, sharp needle or fine (ILM) forceps. If internal limiting membrane peeling is felt to be beneficial, it is performed at this stage. The internal limiting membrane can be stained with indocyanine green dye to make its surgical removal technically simpler. An air–fluid exchange follows, and if an adjunctive agent (e.g., transforming growth factor β or autologous serum) is to be used, it is applied at this point. Air, dilute sulfur hexafluoride (SF_6) gas, or dilute perfluoropropane (C_3F_8) gas is placed in the vitreous cavity, and the sclerostomy sites are closed. The surgery can be performed safely in an outpatient setting. Patients usually are instructed to maintain strict face-down positioning for at least 7 days postoperatively.

As in any invasive surgical procedure, intraoperative and postoperative complications can occur[22]; some are unique to macular hole surgery, while others may develop during any vitreoretinal procedure. The most common complication after the surgery is cataract formation. It has long been known that vitrectomy in a phakic eye leads to accelerated nuclear sclerosis; the addition of intravitreal gas probably speeds the process. Over 50% of phakic eyes that undergo vitrectomy for a macular hole suffer significant nuclear sclerosis during the subsequent 2-year follow-up. In successful cases, eventual removal of the cataract by standard techniques can be performed without undue risk. Some surgeons advocate removal of clear lenses or minimal cataracts at the time of macular hole surgery to eliminate the need for a second procedure.

Retinal tears or retinal detachment or both may be seen in up to 10% of eyes that undergo vitreous surgery for an idiopathic macular hole. This incidence is relatively high, because an intraoperative and, therefore, traumatic creation of a posterior vitreous detachment is a critical step in the procedure. Intraoperative recognition of retinal tears with prompt treatment using either laser or cryotherapy can keep the occurrence of retinal detachment low. Some retinal tears develop during the immediate postoperative period, so vigilant postoperative fundus observation is necessary. Most retinal detachments can be repaired with standard scleral buckling, vitrectomy, or pneumatic retinopexy techniques.

Other, less common complications include intraoperative light or mechanical toxicity to the macular retinal pigment epithelium, intraoperative enlargement of the macular hole, and late reopening of successfully closed holes.[22-24] Late reopening occurs in 5% of once-successfully treated holes and can occur years after the initial surgery. Second operations to close the reopened holes may be successful in some cases. Some investigators have observed dense, temporal visual field defects in eyes that have undergone vitrectomy for macular holes. The cause and incidence is still unclear.[25]

COURSE AND OUTCOME

Premacular holes (stage 1 holes) have a spontaneous rate of improvement of about 50%. A lamellar macular hole represents an abortive macular hole and is stable with good vision. Once a stage 2 hole occurs, without surgery visual loss is nearly always permanent. Spontaneous closure of full-thickness macular holes occurs in 2–4% of eyes, probably secondary to epiretinal membrane formation.[26,27] Visual improvement does not always occur concurrently.

Without surgery, macular holes tend to stabilize with a visual acuity of 20/200–20/800 (6/60–6/240) and a diameter of about 500μm. With surgery, visual improvement is possible. Anatomical success can be determined 2–4 weeks after surgery, when the gas bubble has resorbed enough to be no longer in contact with the macular hole in the upright position.

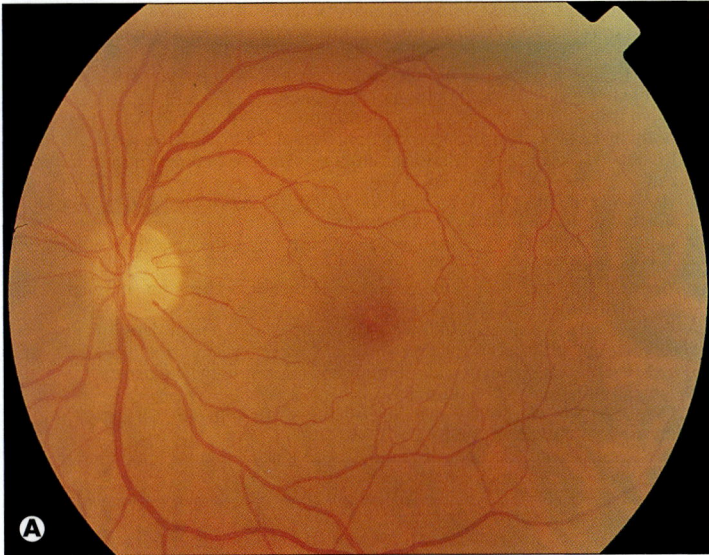

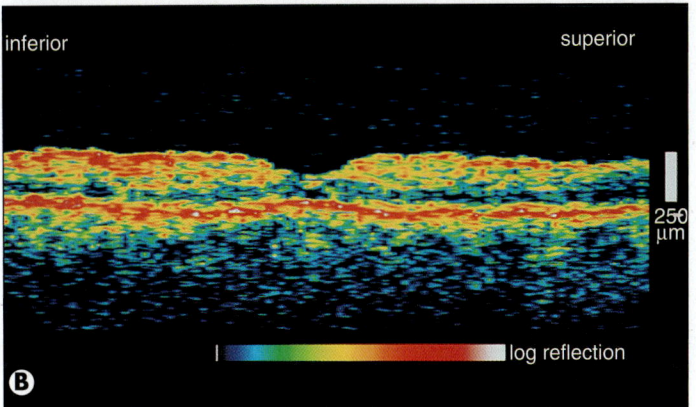

FIG. 128-3 ▮▮ Stage 2 macular hole. A, The same eye as in Figure 128-2, 2 weeks after surgery. The hole is closed and the vision is 20/20 (6/6). The gas bubble is still visible superiorly. B, Optical coherence tomography postoperatively of same eye as in Figures 128-2 and A showing normal foveal architecture after surgery.

Anatomical success usually is defined as complete disappearance of the cuff of subretinal fluid that surrounds the macular hole. In most instances, when this occurs the edges of the macular hole are opposed firmly to the retinal pigment epithelium, which renders identification of the macular hole difficult (Fig. 128-3). Visual success is defined as an improvement in postoperative visual acuity of at least two or more Snellen lines over preoperative acuity.

In their initial series of 52 treated eyes, Kelly and Wendel[10] found that 42% showed a visual acuity improvement of two or more Snellen lines following surgery. A higher percentage, 58% of eyes, were considered anatomical successes. Their subsequent series showed that anatomical success could be achieved in 73% of eyes, with an improvement of two or more Snellen lines in 55%.[11] Best results were obtained when surgery was performed within 6 months of visual loss. A randomized, multicenter trial achieved a closure rate of 69%.[26]

The results of two recent series of vitrectomy on early, small, stage 2 macular holes suggest a success rate of 90% or greater for anatomical closure, with visual improvement in 80% (see Fig. 128-3).[28,29]

REFERENCES

1. Aaberg TM. Macular holes: a review. Surv Ophthalmol. 1970;15:139–62.
2. Knapp H. Ueber isolirte zerreissungen der aderhaut in folge von traumen auf dem augapfel. Arch Augenheilkd. 1869;1:6–29.
3. Ogilvie FM. On one of the results of concussive injuries of the eye ("holes" at the macula). Trans Ophthalmol Soc U K. 1900;20:202–29.
4. Gass JDM. Idiopathic senile macular hole: its early stages and pathogenesis. Arch Ophthalmol. 1988;106:629–39.

5. Johnson RN, Gass JDM. Idiopathic macular holes: observations, stages of formation, and implications for surgical intervention. Ophthalmology. 1988;95: 917–24.
6. Gass JDM. Reappraisal of biomicroscopic classification of stage of development of a macular hole. Arch Ophthalmol. 1995;119:752–9.
7. Kiryu J, Shahidi M, Ogura Y, et al. Illustration of the stages of idiopathic macular holes by laser biomicroscopy. Arch Ophthalmol. 1995;113:1156–60.
8. Kokame GT. Clinical correlation of ultrasonographic findings in macular holes. Am J Ophthalmol. 1995;119:441–51.
9. Hee MR, Puliafito CA, Wong C, et al. Optical coherence tomography of macular holes. Ophthalmology. 1995;102:748–56.
10. Kelly NE, Wendel RT. Vitreous surgery for idiopathic macular holes. Arch Ophthalmol. 1991;109:654–9.
11. Wendel RT, Patel AC, Kelly NE, et al. Vitreous surgery for macular holes. Ophthalmology. 1993;100:1671–6.
12. Brown GC. Macular hole following rhegmatogenous retinal detachment repair. Arch Ophthalmol. 1988;106:765–6.
13. Cohen SM, Gass JDM. Macular hole following severe hypertensive retinopathy. Arch Ophthalmol. 1994;112:878–9.
14. Flynn HW. Macular hole surgery in patients with proliferative diabetic retinopathy. Arch Ophthalmol. 1994;112:877–8.
15. The Eye Disease Case-Control Study Group. Risk factors for idiopathic macular hole. Am J Ophthalmol. 1994;118:754–61.
16. Bronstein MA, Trempe CL, Freeman HM. Fellow eyes of eyes with macular holes. Am J Ophthalmol. 1981;92:757–61.
17. Lewis ML, Cohen SM, Smiddy WE, Gass JDM. Bilaterality of idiopathic macular holes. Graefes Arch Klin Exp Ophthalmol. 1996;234:241–5.
18. Fisher YL, Slakter JS, Yannuzzi LA, Guyer DR. A prospective natural history study and kinetic ultrasound evaluation of idiopathic macular holes. Ophthalmology. 1994;101:5–11.
19. Martinez J, Smiddy WE, Kim J, Gass JDM. Differentiating macular holes from macular pseudoholes. Am J Ophthalmol. 1994;117:762–7.
20. Gass JDM, Joondeph BC. Observations concerning patients with suspected impending macular holes. Am J Ophthalmol. 1990;109:638–46.
21. Rosa RH, Glaser BM, de la Cruz Z, Green WR. Clinicopathologic correlation of an untreated macular hole and a macular hole treated by vitrectomy, transforming growth factor-2 and gas tamponade. Am J Ophthalmol. 1996;122:853–63.
22. Park S, Marcus DM, Duker JS, et al. Posterior segment complications after vitrectomy for macular hole. Ophthalmology. 1995;102:775–81.
23. Poliner LS, Tornambe PE. Retinal pigment epitheliopathy after macular hole surgery. Ophthalmology. 1992;99:1671–7.
24. Duker JS, Wendel R, Patel A, Puliafito CA. Late reopening of macular holes following initially successful vitreous surgery. Ophthalmology. 1994;101:1373–8.
25. Boldt HC, Munden PM, Folk JC, Mehaffey MG. Visual field defects after macular hole surgery. Am J Ophthalmol. 1996;122:371–81.
26. Freeman WR, Azen AP, Kim JW, et al. Vitrectomy for the treatment of full-thickness stage 3 or 4 macular holes. Arch Ophthalmol. 1997;115:11–21.
27. Lewis H, Cowan GM, Straatsma BR. Apparent disappearance of a macular hole associated with development of an epiretinal membrane. Am J Ophthalmol. 1986;102:172–5.
28. Ryan EH, Gilbert HD. Results of surgical treatment of recent-onset full-thickness idiopathic macular holes. Arch Ophthalmol. 1994;112:1545–53.
29. Ip MS, Baker BJ, Duker JS, et al. Anatomical outcomes of surgery for idiopathic macular hole as determined by optical coherence tomography. Arch Ophthalmol. 2002;120:29–35.

CHAPTER

129

Epiretinal Membrane

MARK W. JOHNSON

DEFINITION
- An avascular, fibrocellular membrane that proliferates on the inner surface of the retina to produce various degrees of macular dysfunction

KEY FEATURES
- Transparent, translucent, opaque, or pigmented membrane on the inner retinal surface
- Tangential traction on the macula
- Partial or complete posterior vitreous separation

ASSOCIATED FEATURES
- Central vision loss with or without metamorphopsia
- Glistening light reflex
- Retinal distortion
- Macular edema
- Retinal whitening (axoplasmic stasis)
- Intraretinal or preretinal hemorrhage
- Macular hole or pseudohole

INTRODUCTION

The proliferation of fibrocellular membranes on the inner retinal surface in the macular area may occur in otherwise healthy eyes or secondary to retinal breaks and rhegmatogenous retinal detachment, retinal vascular diseases, intraocular inflammation, blunt or penetrating trauma, and other ocular disorders. Common synonyms applied to epiretinal membranes include macular pucker, premacular fibrosis or gliosis, cellophane maculopathy, surface wrinkling retinopathy, and epimacular membrane. Visual symptoms associated with epiretinal membranes range in severity, depending on the opacity of the membrane and the amount of macular distortion induced by the contracting fibrocellular tissue. Surgical peeling of epiretinal membranes in patients who have significant visual symptoms typically results in improved visual acuity and reduced metamorphopsia.

EPIDEMIOLOGY AND PATHOGENESIS

The majority of patients who have idiopathic epiretinal membranes are over 50 years old; however, children and young adults occasionally are affected.[1,2] The prevalence of idiopathic epiretinal membrane in consecutive patients seen for eye examination and aged 50 years or older is approximately 6%.[3] Similarly, epiretinal membranes are found in approximately 6% of eyes examined at autopsy, with increasing prevalence in advancing age groups.[4,5] Many large series suggest a higher incidence of epiretinal formation in women than in men.[1,6–8] Although idiopathic epiretinal membranes are bilateral in 20–30% of cases,[1,3,4] significant bilateral loss of central vision is uncommon.

The incidence of symptomatic epimacular membrane formation is 4–8% after repair of rhegmatogenous retinal detachment[9–11] and 1–2% after prophylactic treatment of peripheral retinal breaks.[12] Risk factors for the development of macular epiretinal membranes after conventional retinal detachment surgery include older age, preoperative vitreous hemorrhage, macular detachment, preoperative signs of proliferative vitreoretinopathy, large retinal breaks, intraoperative use of cryotherapy, and multiple operations.[9–11,13]

Mild epiretinal membrane formation occurs commonly in association with blunt or penetrating ocular trauma, vitreous inflammatory conditions, retinal vascular diseases that cause chronic intraretinal edema, and long-standing vitreous hemorrhage.[13,14] Apart from penetrating trauma, these are uncommon clinical contexts in which to find significant macular dysfunction as a result of epiretinal membrane contracture.

A clue to the pathogenesis of epiretinal membrane formation is the observation that posterior vitreous detachment is present in approximately 90% of eyes that have idiopathic membranes,[1,7,15–17] and in virtually all eyes that have epiretinal membranes that develop after retinal breaks or rhegmatogenous retinal detachment. It is believed widely that idiopathic epiretinal membranes are produced by retinal glial cells that migrate through defects in the internal limiting membrane to proliferate and contract on the inner retinal surface.[4,18,19] In most patients, such dehiscences in the internal limiting membrane probably are created at the time of vitreous separation.[19] However, idiopathic epiretinal membrane formation is well documented in eyes that have no evidence of posterior vitreous detachment, suggesting that cellular migration may sometimes occur through preexisting defects or thinning in the internal limiting membrane.[20] An alternative proposed mechanism for idiopathic epiretinal membrane formation involves proliferation, fibrous metaplasia, and contraction of hyalocytes left behind on the inner retinal surface after posterior vitreous detachment.[13]

Epiretinal membranes that develop in eyes that have retinal breaks most likely represent a mild form of proliferative vitreoretinopathy caused by retinal pigment epithelial cells that are liberated into the vitreous cavity and proliferate, along with other cellular constituents, to form contractile membranes on the retinal surface.[21] Cellular proliferation stimulated by vitreous inflammation or breakdown of the blood–retinal barrier is a plausible pathogenic mechanism for the remaining types of secondary epiretinal membranes.

OCULAR MANIFESTATIONS

The clinical appearance of an epiretinal membrane depends on its thickness and the extent to which it has undergone shrinkage or contraction. In its mildest form, sometimes called *cellophane maculopathy*, the membrane is thin and transparent, produces no distortion of the inner retinal surface, and leaves the patient asymptomatic. It is detectable on biomicroscopic examination only by an abnormal glistening light reflex from the inner retinal surface (Fig. 129-1).

Thin membranes that have undergone limited contraction or shrinkage produce a series of fine, irregular striations or wrinkles that are confined to the internal limiting membrane and

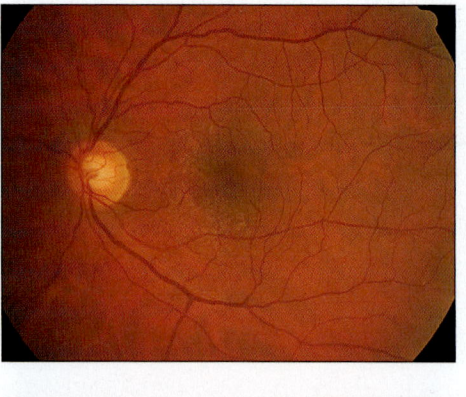

FIG. 129-1 ■ Mild asymptomatic epiretinal membrane. This thin, transparent membrane is detectable only from an irregular, glistening (cellophane) light reflex from the inner retinal surface.

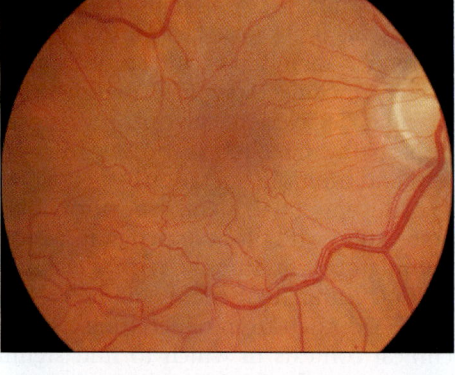

FIG. 129-2 ■ Transparent epiretinal membrane here seen to produce significant retinal vascular distortion.

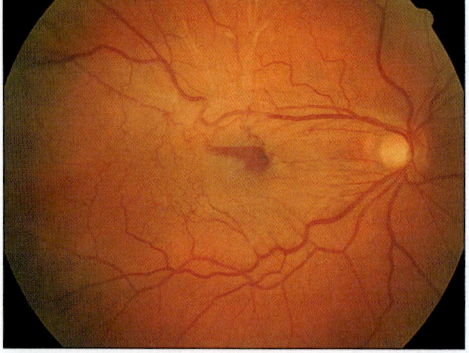

FIG. 129-4 ■ Severe macular puckering by an opaque epiretinal membrane after retinal detachment surgery. Much of the apparent opacity is due to inner retinal whitening from axoplasmic stasis.

FIG. 129-5 ■ Preretinal hemorrhage induced by traction from an epiretinal membrane.

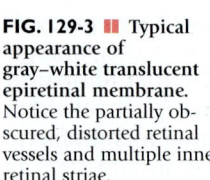
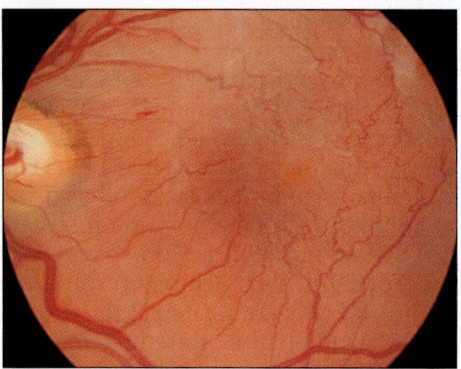
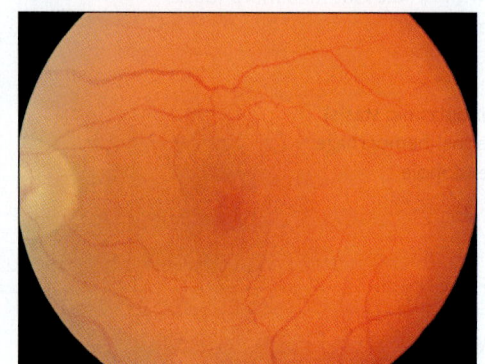

FIG. 129-3 ■ Typical appearance of gray–white translucent epiretinal membrane. Notice the partially obscured, distorted retinal vessels and multiple inner retinal striae.

FIG. 129-6 ■ Epiretinal membrane with macular pseudohole. The visual acuity is 20/25 (6/8) and slit-lamp biomicroscopy shows retinal tissue in the base of the apparent macular hole.

inner retinal tissue. The inner retinal striae typically are most apparent where they radiate out from the margins of the membrane, but they also may develop in a radiating pattern around one or more epicenters of membrane contraction. The fine macular capillaries may be tortuous, even in the absence of large-vessel displacement. Patients who have such membranes may be asymptomatic and have normal visual acuity. Others may complain of vague visual disturbance or mild metamorphopsia, or both. Thicker, more contracted epiretinal membranes produce tangential traction on the full-thickness neural retina, which results in more severe degrees of macular dysfunction. The membrane itself may remain largely invisible, despite significant underlying retinal vascular tortuosity or straightening (Fig. 129-2). In other cases, the membrane is visible as a gray–white translucent membrane that partially obscures visualization of retinal vessels (Fig. 129-3). Some membranes, particularly those that develop subsequent to retinal breaks or rhegmatogenous retinal detachment, are thick and opaque, usually white in color, but occasionally darkly pigmented. Often, a significant component of the membrane's apparent opacity is whitening of the inner retina that underlies the membrane; presumably this results from traction-induced axoplasmic stasis in the nerve fiber layer (Fig. 129-4).

Patients who have epiretinal membranes that produce full-thickness macular distortion, folding, or puckering typically complain of marked metamorphopsia, loss of visual acuity, and occasionally central photopsia. The tractional effects of the membrane on the retina may cause macular edema, preretinal

or intraretinal hemorrhage (Fig. 129-5), or traction macular detachment. Traction-induced detachments of the macula may be subtle, shallow, "tabletop" elevations visible only by contact lens biomicroscopy, or obvious ridges of detachment that pass through the macula. In some patients, an eccentrically located epiretinal membrane may cause lateral displacement of the fovea without detachment from the pigment epithelium (foveal ectopia); this results in relative preservation of visual acuity and symptoms of central binocular diplopia. Other patients who have epiretinal membranes that do not result in severe acuity loss complain of macropsia, presumably because of the crowding of photoreceptors caused by tangential retinal traction.

A defect in the prefoveolar portion of an epiretinal membrane may simulate the appearance of a full-thickness macular hole (Fig. 129-6). A macular pseudohole is a result of the defect in the epiretinal tissue itself, as well as of the anterior and central displacement of the perifoveolar retina (clivus) during contraction of the epiretinal membrane.[13] In some cases, a pseudohole also involves an inner lamellar macular defect that developed at the time of vitreofoveolar separation. Unlike eyes that have true macular holes, those with pseudoholes usually are minimally symptomatic and have normal or near-normal visual acuities. Biomicroscopic clues that help differentiate a macular pseudohole from a true macular hole include the following:

- Wrinkling of the inner retinal surface that surrounds the hole
- Retinal tissue in the base of the pseudohole
- Absence of characteristic features of full-thickness macular holes, such as yellow retinal pigment epithelium (RPE) de-

posits in the base of the hole, a halo of neural detachment, and an overlying operculum or pseudo-operculum.

In equivocal cases, optical coherence tomography usually can distinguish between a full-thickness macular hole and a macular pseudohole. Additionally, fluorescein angiography of pseudoholes typically shows either no or only mild hyperfluorescence, in contrast to the prominent transmission defect seen in full-thickness macular holes. Although it is an uncommon mechanism, tangential foveal traction from contraction of an eccentric epiretinal membrane occasionally causes full-thickness macular hole formation. On the other hand, mild degrees of cellophane epiretinal membrane commonly form around idiopathic macular holes, presumably as a wound-healing response.

Rarely, contracture of an epiretinal membrane with a central dehiscence causes anterior prolapse of foveal tissue through the hole in the membrane.[22] Long-standing macular traction or retinal vascular leakage induced by epiretinal membranes may cause atrophic or hypertrophic RPE alterations. Such changes generally are considered poor prognostic signs for visual recovery after surgical removal of the epiretinal membrane. Occasionally, intraretinal lipid (hard) exudates and microvascular changes, such as microaneurysms, are produced by the retinal vascular traction and leakage caused by idiopathic epiretinal membranes. Such findings, however, also may signal the presence of associated pathology, such as a choroidal neovascular membrane or long-standing branch retinal vein occlusion, which may require different management approaches and alter the visual prognosis.

DIAGNOSIS AND ANCILLARY TESTING

The diagnosis of epiretinal membranes is clinical, based on biomicroscopic observation of the physical features detailed in the previous section. In patients who have obvious membranes and clear media, ancillary testing generally is unnecessary. Contact lens biomicroscopy frequently is helpful in the detection of subtle transparent or translucent epiretinal membranes, particularly in eyes that have corneal surface irregularities or media opacities. Furthermore, the excellent resolution and stereopsis afforded by the fundus contact lens permit detailed assessment of the extent to which the macula is distorted, thickened, displaced, or detached by the membrane. Detection of subtle membrane edges by contact lens examination may help to plan the surgical approach. Examination or photography, or both, of the macula with red-free light may highlight glistening reflexes and thereby assist in assessment of the extent of the membrane. The Watzke–Allen (slit-beam) test or aiming beam laser perimetry occasionally may help to differentiate a macular pseudohole from a full-thickness macular hole that complicates an epiretinal membrane. Optical coherence tomography is probably the most reliable ancillary test for distinguishing between full-thickness macular holes and pseudoholes, and for confirming a component of vitreomacular traction.

In eyes that have media opacities that preclude adequate macular examination, fluorescein angiography often is helpful diagnostically, because it demonstrates the retinal vascular distortion that underlies an epiretinal membrane. Although not necessary in every case, angiography also may be valuable to assess the degree of retinal vascular distortion, confirm the presence of foveal ectopia, detect associated macular edema, differentiate pseudoholes from full-thickness macular holes, and highlight underlying RPE changes. Macular edema caused by an epiretinal membrane often can be differentiated angiographically from pseudophakic cystoid macular edema by the irregular and asymmetrical pattern of leakage typically induced by epiretinal membranes. Finally, fluorescein angiography may be critical in the exclusion of associated macular pathology, such as choroidal neovascularization or venous obstructive disease (Fig. 129-7).

DIFFERENTIAL DIAGNOSIS

The differential diagnosis of epiretinal membranes is given in Box 129-1. The most common diagnoses that must be differenti-

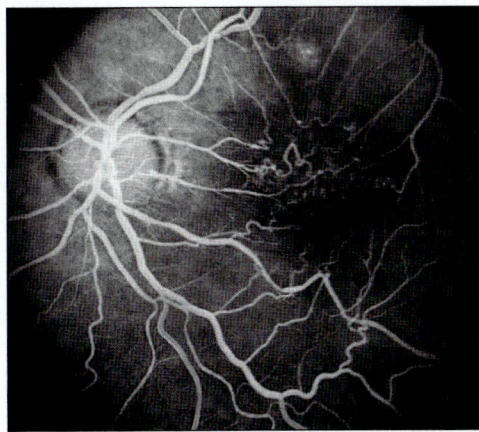

FIG. 129-7 ▉ Fluorescein angiography of an epiretinal membrane that complicates an old branch retinal vein occlusion. Notice the collateral vessel formation, in addition to the marked vascular distortion.

ated from epiretinal membrane and its associated features include the vitreomacular traction syndrome, postoperative cystoid macular edema, and full-thickness macular hole (as opposed to epiretinal membrane with macular pseudohole). Such differentiations are important to make because each of these clinical entities (discussed in detail in the chapters listed) differs from epiretinal membrane in its management and prognosis.

PATHOLOGY

Histopathological and ultrastructural studies have shown that epiretinal membranes consist of a fibrocellular sheet of varying thickness, in which both native vitreous and newly synthesized collagen have been found.[4,5,13,18–21,23,24] Fragments of internal limiting membrane are seen commonly in surgical specimens,[24] which suggests that the inadvertent or intentional removal of this membrane does not preclude good visual outcomes.

The cellular elements of most epiretinal membranes include one or more of the following: RPE cells, fibrous astrocytes, fibrocytes, and macrophages. The cell types found in a particular membrane may depend in part on the associated ocular disorders.[4,21,23,24] Furthermore, the precise identification of the cells of origin within epiretinal membranes is hampered by the ability of each of the common constituent cells to transform into cells with similar morphology and function.[13] The observation that RPE cells are the main cell type in many cases of idiopathic epiretinal membrane is poorly understood[24] but possibly may involve transretinal migration of RPE cells in response to biochemical stimuli.[25] Most of the cell types found in epiretinal membranes have the capacity to assume myofibroblastic properties, which allows them to change shape and cause the membrane to contract.[13]

TREATMENT

No treatment is indicated for mild epiretinal membranes that produce minimal symptoms. Patients whose membranes have more severe characteristics and produce significant visual loss and metamorphopsia usually benefit from vitreous surgery, with peeling of the epiretinal membrane from the surface of the macula. The goal of membrane peeling is to reduce or eliminate the most common mechanisms of visual loss, including macular distortion, traction macular detachment, foveal ectopia, tissue that covers the fovea, retinal vascular leakage with macular edema, and traction-induced obstruction of axoplasmic flow.

Surgical membrane peeling generally is recommended for patients who have substantial visual acuity loss, marked metamorphopsia, or disabling central binocular diplopia. Because epiretinal membranes often show little or no progression after the initial diagnosis, surgery is not performed prophylactically on membranes that cause only mild symptoms. The best candidates for surgery are those who have had membranes for a relatively short time, because the potential for visual recovery decreases with increasing duration of preoperative symptoms.[8] However, excellent visual recovery is not necessarily precluded

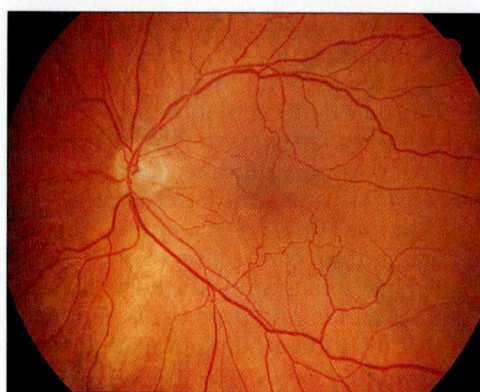

FIG. 129-8 Postoperative appearance of the eye shown in Figure 129-4. After membrane peeling, the retinal whitening and most of the macular distortion has resolved. The visual acuity improved from 20/100 (6/30) to 20/30 (6/9).

in patients who have symptoms that have lasted longer than 1 year. Careful preoperative evaluation of all eyes should exclude additional causes of vision loss, such as choroidal neovascularization, macular ischemia from previous retinal vascular occlusion, or other preexisting macular disease.

Conventional pars plana vitreous surgical techniques are used to remove the vitreous gel, which in most cases has separated previously from the posterior retina. An edge of the epiretinal membrane is engaged with a vitreoretinal pick or forceps, or created with a sharp bent-tip needle. After the edge has been developed, the membrane typically is peeled from the retina with forceps, usually as a single piece. Rarely, sites of firm adhesion to the retina are encountered; at these the membrane may be amputated in preference to the creation of retinal breaks in the macular area. Some vitreoretinal surgeons use indocyanine green dye intraoperatively to stain the internal limiting membrane, thereby clarifying the extent of the epiretinal membrane or facilitating the intentional removal of the internal limiting membrane.

The most common surgical complication is progressive nuclear sclerotic cataract, which occurs in 60–70% of eyes within 2 years of surgery, with a much lower incidence in patients under 50 years of age.[8,26] Other less common complications include peripheral retinal breaks, rhegmatogenous retinal detachment, posterior retinal breaks, photic maculopathy, and endophthalmitis. Late postoperative recurrence of symptomatic epiretinal tissue occurs in approximately 5% of patients.[6,8]

COURSE AND OUTCOMES

Most patients who have epiretinal membranes experience little or no symptom progression after the initial diagnosis, which implies that membrane contraction usually occurs soon after its formation and then stabilizes. Only 10–25% of eyes show a decline in visual acuity over time—rates of progression vary from over several months to many years.[6,13,15] Rarely, epiretinal membranes separate spontaneously from the retina, which results in visual improvement.[13] Approximately 20% of patients who develop macular pucker after scleral buckling experience spontaneous improvement in visual acuity as a result of resolution of the macular edema and relaxation or partial peeling of the epiretinal membrane.[9]

Following surgical removal of epiretinal membranes, most of the macular distortion and all of the retinal whitening resolves, typically within days or weeks of the operation (Fig. 129-8). Associated cystoid macular edema may resolve or persist chronically. Visual improvement of two or more Snellen lines occurs in 60–85% of eyes and may continue for 6–12 months after surgery.[6,8,17] A small number of eyes (2–15%) have worse visual acuity postoperatively.[6,8,17]

Although visual acuity improves and metamorphopsia is reduced significantly in most eyes after epiretinal membrane peeling, the visual function rarely returns to normal. Patients commonly are advised to expect improvement in visual acuity that is approximately halfway between the preoperative acuity and that before the membrane developed. Preoperative factors prognostic of the final visual acuity include the level of preoperative visual acuity, duration of symptoms before surgery, and nature of previous macular damage (such as by retinal detachment involving the macula).[8,27] Eyes that have lower levels of preoperative visual acuity typically improve by the greatest number of lines but tend

to have lower final acuities than eyes that had better preoperative vision.[27] Although the prognostic value of preoperative macular edema is controversial, fluorescein angiography probably does not help to predict the visual outcome in patients who undergo surgery for idiopathic epiretinal membrane.[8,28]

REFERENCES

1. Wise GN. Clinical features of idiopathic preretinal macular fibrosis. Am J Ophthalmol. 1975;79:349–57.
2. Barr CC, Michels RG. Idiopathic nonvascularized epiretinal membranes in young patients: report of six cases. Ann Ophthalmol. 1982;14:335–41.
3. Pearlstone AD. The incidence of idiopathic preretinal macular gliosis. Ann Ophthalmol. 1985;17:378–80.
4. Roth AM, Foos RY. Surface wrinkling retinopathy in eyes enucleated at autopsy. Trans Am Acad Ophthalmol Otolaryngol. 1971;75:1047–58.
5. Foos RY. Surface wrinkling retinopathy. In: Freeman HM, Hirose T, Schepens CL, eds. Vitreous surgery and advances in fundus diagnosis and treatment. New York: Appleton-Century-Crofts; 1977:23–38.
6. Margherio RR, Cox MS Jr, Trese MT, et al. Removal of epimacular membranes. Ophthalmology. 1985;92:1075–83.
7. Appiah AP, Hirose T, Kado M. A review of 324 cases of idiopathic premacular gliosis. Am J Ophthalmol. 1988;106:533–5.
8. Pesin SR, Olk RJ, Grand MG, et al. Vitrectomy for premacular fibroplasia: prognostic factors, long-term follow-up, and time course of visual improvement. Ophthalmology. 1991;98:1109–14.
9. Hagler WS, Aturaliya U. Macular puckers after retinal detachment surgery. Br J Ophthalmol. 1971;55:451–7.
10. Lobes LA Jr, Burton TC. The incidence of macular pucker after retinal detachment surgery. Am J Ophthalmol. 1978;85:72–7.
11. Uemura A, Ideta H, Nagasaki H, et al. Macular pucker after retinal detachment surgery. Ophthalmic Surg. 1992;23:116–9.
12. Michels RG, Wilkinson CP, Rice TA. Retinal detachment. St Louis: CV Mosby; 1990:1096–8.
13. Gass JDM. Stereoscopic atlas of macular diseases; diagnosis and treatment, ed 4. St Louis: CV Mosby; 1997:938–51.
14. Appiah AP, Hirose T. Secondary causes of premacular fibrosis. Ophthalmology. 1989;96:389–92.
15. Sidd RJ, Fine SL, Owens SL, Patz A. Idiopathic preretinal gliosis. Am J Ophthalmol. 1982;94:44–8.
16. Hirokawa H, Jalkh AE, Takahashi M, et al. Role of the vitreous in idiopathic preretinal macular fibrosis. Am J Ophthalmol. 1986;101:166–9.
17. de Bustros S, Thompson JT, Michels RG, et al. Vitrectomy for idiopathic epiretinal membranes causing macular pucker. Br J Ophthalmol. 1988;72:692–5.
18. Bellhorn MB, Friedman AH, Wise GN, Henkind P. Ultrastructure and clinicopathologic correlation of idiopathic preretinal macular fibrosis. Am J Ophthalmol. 1975;79:366–73.
19. Foos RY. Vitreoretinal juncture; epiretinal membranes and vitreous. Invest Ophthalmol Vis Sci. 1977;16:416–22.
20. Heilskov TW, Massicotte SJ, Folk JC. Epiretinal macular membranes in eyes with attached posterior cortical vitreous. Retina. 1996;16:279–84.
21. Cherfan GM, Smiddy WE, Michels RG, et al. Clinicopathologic correlation of pigmented epiretinal membranes. Am J Ophthalmol. 1988;106:536–45.
22. Zarbin MA, Michels RG, Green WR. Epiretinal membrane contracture associated with macular prolapse. Am J Ophthalmol. 1990;110:610–8.
23. Clarkson JG, Green WR, Massof D. A histopathologic review of 168 cases of preretinal membrane. Am J Ophthalmol. 1977;84:1–17.
24. Smiddy WE, Maguire AM, Green WR, et al. Idiopathic epiretinal membranes; ultrastructural characteristics and clinicopathologic correlation. Ophthalmology. 1989;96:811–21.
25. Smiddy WE, Michels RG, Green WR. Morphology, pathology, and surgery of idiopathic vitreoretinal macular disorders: a review. Retina. 1990;10:288–96.
26. Cherfan GM, Michels RG, de Bustros S, et al. Nuclear sclerotic cataract after vitrectomy for idiopathic epiretinal membranes causing macular pucker. Am J Ophthalmol. 1991;111:434–8.
27. Rice TA, deBustros S, Michels RG, et al. Prognostic factors in vitrectomy for epiretinal membranes of the macula. Ophthalmology. 1986;93:602–10.
28. Maguire AM, Margherio RR, Dmuchowski C. Preoperative fluorescein angiographic features of surgically removed idiopathic epiretinal membranes. Retina. 1994;14:411–6.

CHAPTER
130 Vitreomacular Traction Syndrome

WILLIAM E. SMIDDY

DEFINITION
- Incomplete posterior vitreous separation with preretinal tissue proliferation and associated macular traction distributed in the zone of persistent vitreous attachment.

KEY FEATURES
- Prominent vitreoretinal attachment at the posterior pole.
- Peripheral vitreous detachment.
- Epiretinal membrane proliferation.

ASSOCIATED FEATURES
- Distortion of the internal limiting membrane with retinal striae and vascular tortuosity.
- Macular edema.
- Localized traction-related macular retinal detachment.
- Retinal vascular and optic disc staining on fluorescein angiography.

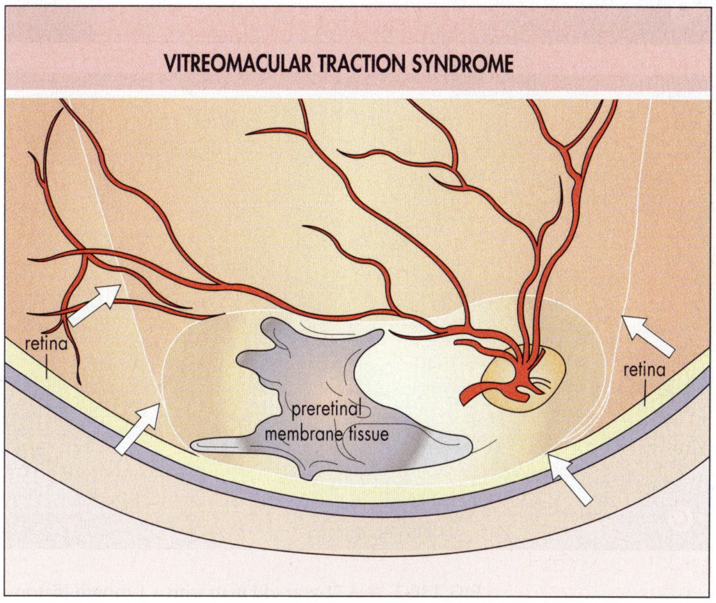

FIG. 130-1 ∎∎ Schematic representation of vitreomacular traction syndrome which depicts the peripheral posterior vitreous separation *(arrows)* and vitreomacular attachment in the zone that involves the macula. It is uncertain whether the macular traction impedes completion of the posterior vitreous separation or whether the aborted posterior vitreous separation stimulates preretinal tissue proliferation.

INTRODUCTION

The effects of vitreous-induced traction on the neural retina are dependent upon the site, extent, and cause of the traction. Anterior vitreoretinal traction may induce peripheral retinal breaks and lead to retinal detachment.[1] Vitreoretinal traction at the macula may induce a broad range of effects, including retinoschisis, cystoid macular edema, and preretinal traction effects.[2–8] Although debated, vitreomacular traction may be the initiating cause of macular hole formation.[7,9,10]

Macular traction induced by preretinal tissue of a typical macular pucker most commonly is associated with complete posterior vitreous detachment. Vitreomacular traction syndrome has been differentiated from idiopathic macular pucker by virtue of the association of the preretinal tissue with persistent vitreomacular attachment.[1] Persistent vitreomacular attachment may assume a multiplicity of configurations. Ophthalmoscopically, the condition commonly mimics idiopathic macular pucker or macular hole syndromes, but specific clinical, angiographic, ultrasonographic, prognostic, and intraoperative features distinguish it. These factors should be recognized by the physician to deliver optimal management.

EPIDEMIOLOGY AND PATHOGENESIS

Vitreomacular traction syndrome was described first by Reese *et al.*, both clinically[11] and histopathologically,[12] as a condition characterized by persistent vitreous attachment in the center of the macula, causing a cystoid configuration and decreased vision. More commonly described is broad-based vitreoretinal attachments.[13–18] Jaffe[13,14] described several cases; most resolved spontaneously as completion of a posterior vitreous detachment was observed. These probably represent mild cases in a clinical

spectrum, with delayed posterior separation of an unusually prominent posterior vitreous surface. Others have described cases with vitreomacular traction features in the class of macular hole precursors,[7] while still others include this entity in idiopathic macular pucker cases.[19] Rarely, preretinal membranes may peel spontaneously,[20–23] a sequence that may be mimicked by or possibly represented by vitreomacular traction syndrome if the persistent posterior vitreous attachment releases, as apparently occurred in many of Jaffe's cases.

No known racial predilection exists for vitreomacular traction syndrome. Most reported studies include about 65% women.[12–18] The reported age range is 26–85 years, but most patients are in their sixth or seventh decade.

The pathogenesis of vitreomacular traction syndrome is unknown. Possibly, the unusually firm posterior hyaloid attachment stimulates cell proliferation. Alternatively, primary preretinal tissue proliferation may limit the normal process of posterior vitreous separation (Fig. 130-1).

OCULAR MANIFESTATIONS

The typical clinical picture of a patient who has vitreomacular traction syndrome involves decreased central vision with some degree of metamorphopsia (Fig. 130-2). Even patients who have 20/20 (6/6) vision may manifest fairly extensive preretinal tissue and moderate symptoms. Symptoms usually develop over several weeks and patients seek sreatment after persistence of such

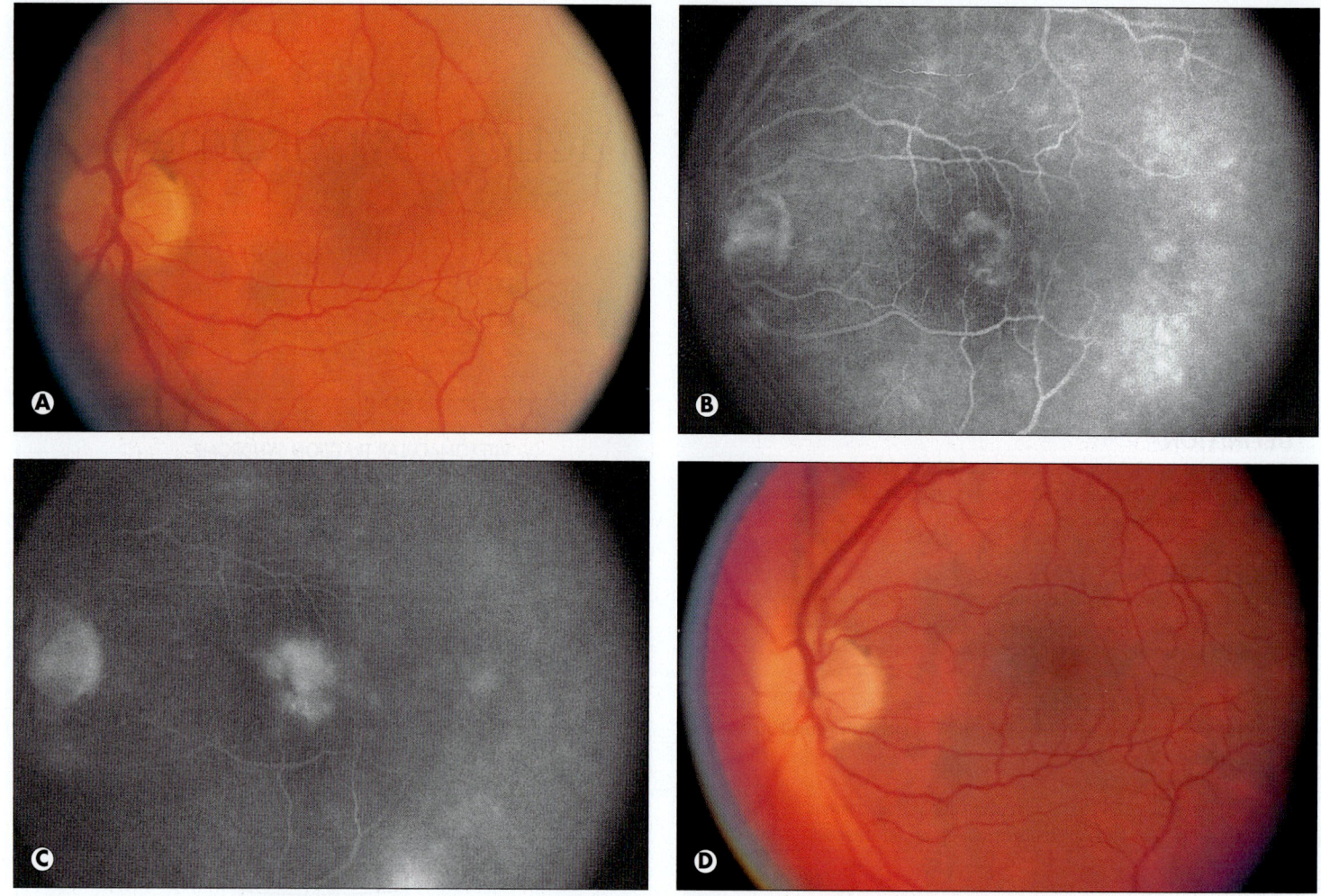

FIG. 130-2 ■ **A 71-year-old man with a 1-month history of decreased vision in the left eye to 20/80 (6/26).** The vision in the right eye was 20/40 (6/13) with an preretinal membrane and pseudohole configuration. **A,** Clinical appearance of the patient's eye, with features of bilateral vitreomacular traction syndrome, left eye. Fluorescein angiogram preoperatively shows (**B**) early and (**C**) late cystoid pattern of leakage. **D,** The macular appearance is improved markedly 3 months following surgery for vitreomacular traction syndrome. After 2.5 years postoperatively (and after cataract extraction), vision was 20/25 (6/8) in the left eye. Typical features of fibrous astrocytes include a multilayered growth pattern with a base of membrane *(arrowheads)* and characteristic 10mm diameter intracytoplasmic filaments. (From Greven GM, Slusher MM, Weaver RG. Epiretinal membrane release and posterior vitreous detachment. Ophthalmology. 1988;95:902–5.)

symptoms. On Watzke-Allen testing, patients may report "thinning" of the beam, without total central disappearance.[16]

In many patients, the disease will not progress and symptoms may remain fairly mild. A subset of patients progress from minimal to severe symptoms and disproportionately visit a retina specialist, usually with visual acuity of 20/50 (6/16) or worse. The natural history of such patients is usually continued slow progression of traction, with moderate cystoid macular edema changes, and visual loss stabilizing around the level of 20/200 (6/60). The hallmark of vitreomacular traction syndrome is persistent anterior-to-posterior traction on the macula, which usually is directly observable[24] (see Fig. 130-2, *A*). Often, a segment of the attachment is visible as a curvilinear attachment site, but the entire perimeter of the attachment may not be visible. Indeed, entire peripheral quadrants of persistent vitreous attachment may be demonstrable intraoperatively but may be difficult to observe preoperatively by clinical examination.[17] The profile of the vitreous against the optically clear retrohyaloid space usually is most prominent immediately anterior to its attachment site. The zone of vitreoretinal attachment typically involves a region of several disc areas centered on the fovea and frequently extends nasally to encompass the optic nerve head.

Associated cystoid macular changes are present in up to 95% of cases.[17] In many cases, the cystoid spaces accumulate fluorescein dye on angiography (see Fig. 130-2, *B* and *C*); this may mimic postoperative cystoid macular edema in pseudophakic eyes. The extent of premacular fibrous proliferation usually corresponds to the zone of macular vitreous attachment. Rarely, the traction is extreme enough to induce focal tractional retinal detachment and has been distinguished as a separate diagnostic entity.[25,26]

DIAGNOSIS AND ANCILLARY TESTING

The diagnosis of the condition rests primarily on the observation of the preretinal tissue in association with the vitreomacular traction attachment, as described above. Fluorescein angiography may help to confirm the diagnosis by revealing dye leakage from the affected posterior pole vessels and, on occasion, from the optic disc. A "B" scan ultrasonic examination may demonstrate the peripheral detached posterior hyaloid with the attached hyaloid over the posterior pole, differentiating the vitreomacular traction syndrome from idiopathic macular pucker, in which a completely separated, mobile posterior vitreous surface is present (Fig. 130-3, *A*). Ocular coherence tomography (OCT) also demonstrates the pathognomonic vitreoretinal attachment (Fig. 130-3, *B*).[31]

DIFFERENTIAL DIAGNOSIS

Idiopathic macular pucker is the most commonly encountered condition that may mimic vitreomacular traction syndrome. With macular pucker, however, Weiss' ring usually is present, which indicates complete posterior vitreous detachment. Stage 1 macular hole and lamellar macular holes also may mimic vitreomacular traction syndrome (see Fig. 130-2, *B*) but, in these, neither the vitreomacular attachment nor the preretinal tissue is

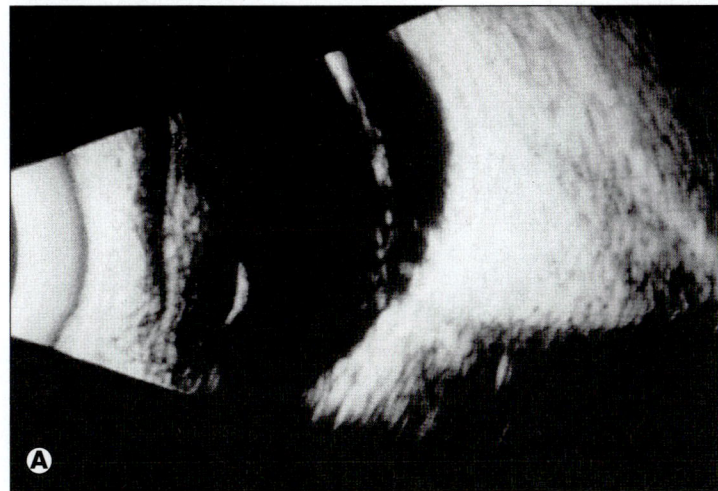

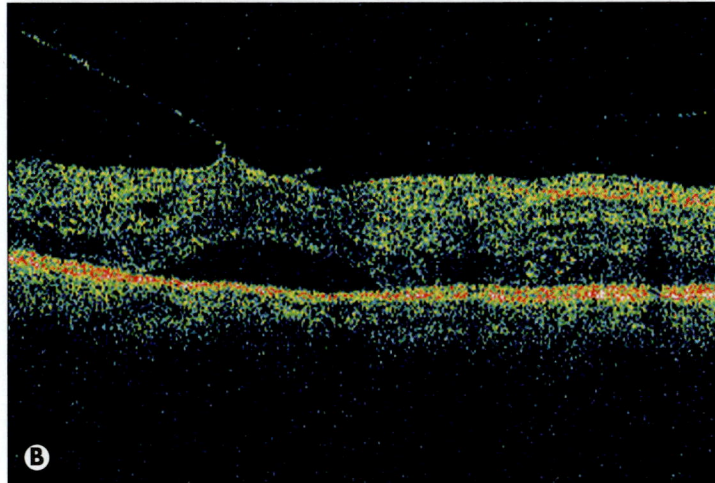

FIG. 130-3 ▮▮ A, Ultrasonographic feature of patient who has vitreomacular traction syndrome. The insertion of vitreous into the posterior pole is demonstrated. **B,** A 67-year-old female with central metamorphopsia and visual loss to 20/200 has visible vitromacular insertion, causing macular distortion.

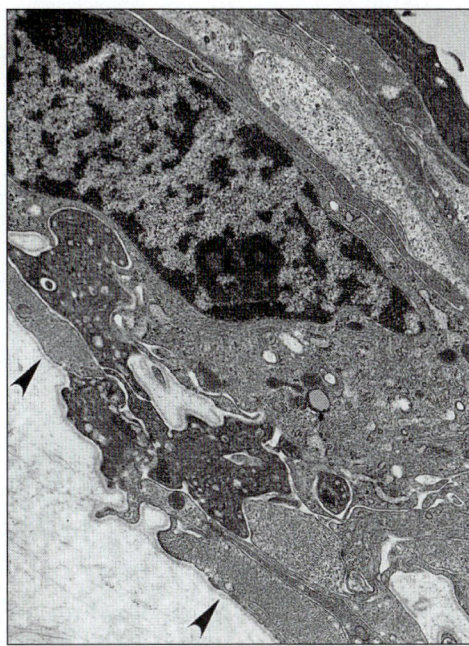

FIG. 130-4 ▮▮ Histopathology of membrane specimen removed from a patient who has vitreomacular traction syndrome. Typical features of fibrous astrocytes include a multilayered growth pattern with a base of membrane *(arrowheads)* and characteristic 10nm diameter intracytoplasmic filaments. (From Greven GM, Slusher MM, Weaver RG. Epiretinal membrane release and posterior vitreous detachment. Ophthalmology. 1988;95:902–5.)

as prominent. Prominent internal limiting membrane stippling due to pseudophakic cystoid macular edema also may mimic the surface wrinkling appearance and, especially in the absence of posterior vitreous detachment, may resemble vitreomacular traction syndrome. Also, early stages of macular hole may mimic vitreomacular traction syndrome, but the risk of developing a full-thickness macular hole is extremely low in these patients (although it has been observed).

PATHOLOGY

The original case described by Reese *et al.*[12] was studied postmortem; vitreous attachment at the fovea and cystoid macular changes were found. A review of the electron microscopic features of the preretinal membrane tissue removed from eyes with vitreomacular traction syndrome showed a high prevalence of fibroglial tissue[27] (Fig. 130-4). Retinal pigment epithelial cells were notably absent. This contrasts sharply to the retinal pigment epithelial cells that dominate idiopathic macular pucker specimens[28] and suggests a separate pathogenic mechanism. Also, thickened internal limiting lamina, astrocyte elements, and myofibrocytes have been identified in an electron microscopy and immunohistochemical study.[29] These findings bespeak a tighter vitreoretinal adhesion and may explain the clinical finding of petechial hemorrhages seen intraoperatively after removing the preretinal tissue component.

TREATMENT

Most cases do not require treatment. Patients often have relatively good visual acuity and only mild metamorphopsia, which

usually remains stable. Some cases may resolve spontaneously, with completion of the posterior vitreous separation,[13,14,30] which has been demonstrated by OCT,[31] but this sequence is observed infrequently and a substantial proportion have progressive traction and visual loss.[32] Once the visual acuity drops to 20/60 (6/20) or worse, surgical treatment should be considered.

The surgical treatment involves three-port pars plana vitrectomy and utilizes standard vitreous surgical techniques[15–18,33] (Fig. 130-5). Removal of anterior-to-posterior traction has been advocated with secondary removal of preretinal tissue. An edge is identified with a sharp needle or pick; a more generalized dissection is then made with a pick to elevate the preretinal tissue from the retinal surface, and ultimately removal is by intraocular forceps as for cases of macular pucker. An alternative strategy uses an *en bloc* approach, with initial release of the posterior vitreous attachment so as to utilize the support and stability that anterior-to-posterior vitreous orientation offers.[17]

A unique finding in the surgical anatomy is a "double layer" of preretinal proliferation in about 15% of cases. The anterior layer may represent simply a thickened posterior hyaloid. Deep to that on the internal surface of the neural retina, a second, preretinal layer may be found in up to 15% of cases.[17] In cases of macular pucker there is not a second layer, but opacities of the nerve fiber layer due to traction-induced axoplasmic stasis may mimic a second layer and should not be dissected.

COURSE AND OUTCOME

The results in the three reported series that involved surgical intervention are summarized in Table 130-1.[15,17,18,33] An additional reported series includes similar cases, but the data were not presented separately from other cases.[16] The preoperative visual acuity was <20/100 (6/33) in 60–78%, improved by at least two lines in 44–70%, and had a final visual acuity of >20/100 (6/30) in 44–80% of cases. The visual results are better with earlier surgical intervention.[33] Scanning laser ophthalmoscopic microperimetry studies have demonstrated a small central scotoma that resolves postoperatively.[34] The characteristic cystoid macular edema[26] has been demonstrated to resolve using ocular coherence tomography[35,36] and fluorescein angiography,[37] as has the vitreomacular traction.

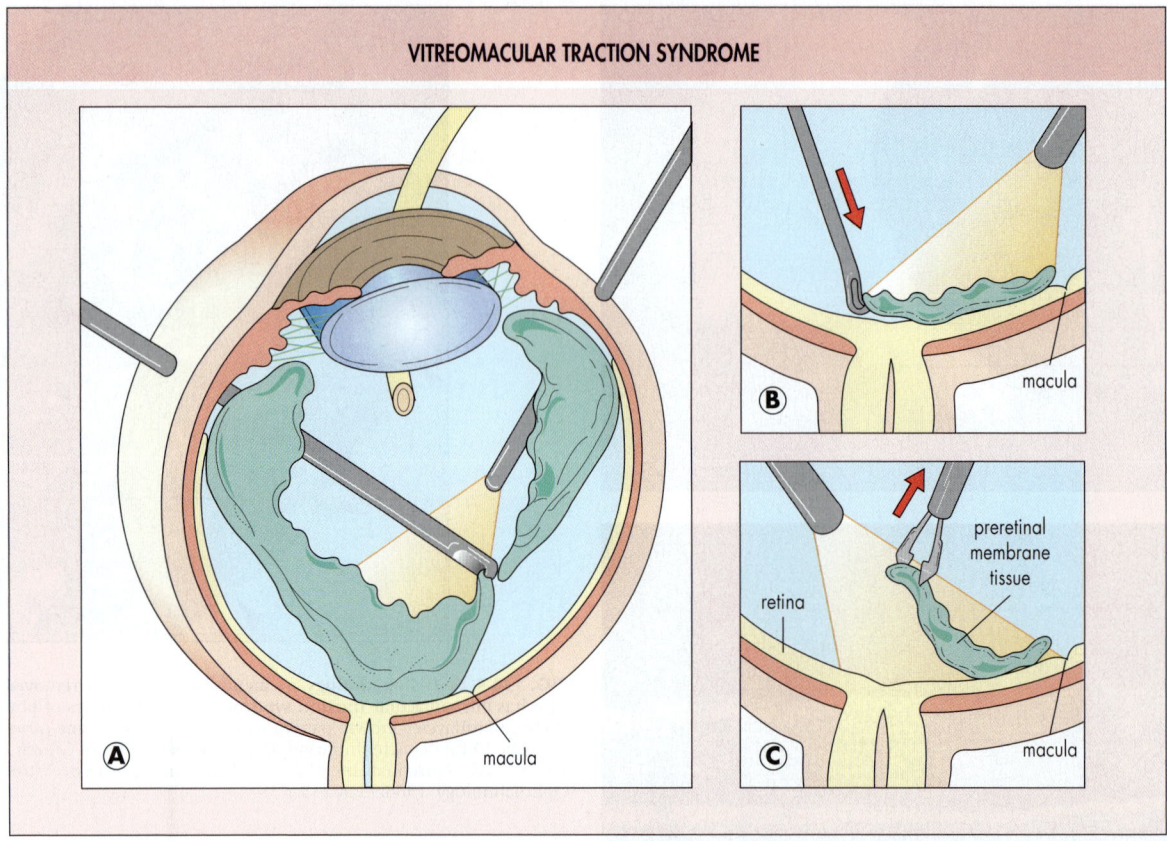

VITREOMACULAR TRACTION SYNDROME

FIG. 130-5 ■ Surgical features of vitreomacular traction syndrome. **A,** Removal of anterior-to-posterior traction by incision of the posterior hyaloid. **B,** Development of surgical plane for removal of preretinal membrane. **C,** Removal of preretinal tissue with forceps. (From Jaffe NS, ed. Atlas of ophthalmic surgery. St Louis: Mosby; 1996:209.)

TABLE 130-1

SUMMARY OF SERIES OF VITREOMACULAR TRACTION SYNDROME

Series	Number of Eyes	Percentage Width Visual Activity >20/100 (6/33)		% >2 Lines	Complications
		Preoperatively	Postoperatively		
Smiddy *et al.*	16	63	69	63	—
MacDonald *et al.*	20	60	80	70	4 with breaks
Melberg *et al.*	9	78	44	44	1 with break; 1 postoperative retinal detachment

Data from Smiddy WE, Michels RG, Glaser BM, deBustros S. Vitrectomy for macular traction caused by incomplete vitreous separation. Arch Ophthalmol. 1988;106:624–8. *RD,* Retinal detachment.

Surgical complication rates are expected to be similar to rates generally extrapolated from those for macular pucker, which include a postoperative retinal detachment rate of 5% or less and a high frequency of induced accelerated nuclear sclerosis. Only about 90 cases have been reported, so accurate data are not available, but acceptably low complication rates have been found.[15–18,33] Of note, however, is that the series with the *en bloc* technique had a slightly higher rate of intraoperative peripheral breaks, but all were successfully controlled with retinal cryopexy and fluid–gas exchange.[17]

REFERENCES

1. Green WR. Vitreoretinal juncture. In: Ryan SJ, ed. Retina. St Louis: Mosby; 1989:13–69.
2. Sebag J, Balazs EAC. Pathogenesis of cystoid macular edema: an anatomic consideration of vitreoretinal adhesions. Surv Ophthalmol. 1984;28:495–8.
3. Boniuk M. Cystoid macular edema secondary to vitreoretinal traction. Surv Ophthalmol. 1968;13:118–21.
4. Nasrallah FP, Jalkh AE, van Coppenolle F, et al. The role of the vitreous in diabetic macular edema. Ophthalmology. 1988;95:1335–9.
5. Lewis HL, Abrams GW, Blumenkranz MS, Campo RV. Vitrectomy for diabetic macular traction and edema associated with posterior hyaloid traction. Ophthalmology. 1992;99:753–9.
6. Michels RG. Macular pucker. In: Ryan SJ, ed. Retina. St Louis: Mosby; 1989:419–30.
7. Gass JDM. Vitreous traction maculopathy in stereoscopic atlas of macular diseases. St Louis: Mosby; 1987:678–83.
8. Falcone PM. Vitreomacular traction syndrome confused with pseudophakic cystoid macular edema. Ophthalmic Surg Lasers. 1996;27:392–4.
9. Gaudric A, Haouchine B, Massin P, et al. Macular hole formation. Arch Ophthalmol. 1999;117:744–51.
10. Kakehashi A, Schepens CL, Trempe CL. Vitreomacular observations. II. Data on the pathogenesis of idiopathic macular breaks. Graefes Arch Klin Exp Ophthalmol. 1996;234:425–33.
11. Reese AB, Jones IR, Cooper WC. Macular changes secondary to vitreous traction. Am J Ophthalmol. 1967;51:544–9.
12. Reese AB, Jones IR, Cooper WC. Vitreomacular traction syndrome confirmed histologically. Am J Ophthalmol. 1970;69:975–7.
13. Jaffe NS. Vitreous traction at the posterior pole of the fundus due to alterations in the vitreous posterior. Trans Am Acad Ophthalmol Otolaryngol. 1967;71:642–52.
14. Jaffe NS. Macular retinopathy after separation of vitreoretinal adherence. Arch Ophthalmol. 1967;78:585–91.
15. Smiddy WE, Michels RG, Glaser BM, deBustros S. Vitrectomy for macular traction caused by incomplete vitreous separation. Arch Ophthalmol. 1988;106:624–8.
16. Margherio RR, Trese MT, Margherio AR, Cartright K. Surgical management of vitreomacular traction syndromes. Ophthalmology. 1989;96:1437–45.
17. MacDonald HR, Johnson RN, Schatz H. Surgical results in the vitreomacular traction syndrome. Ophthalmology. 1994;101:1397–403.
18. Melberg N, Williams DF, Balles MW, et al. Vitrectomy for vitreomacular traction syndrome with macular detachment. Retina. 1995;15:192–7.
19. Hirokawa H, Jalk AE, Takahashi M, et al. Role of vitreous in independent preretinal macular fibrosis. Am J Ophthalmol. 1989;101:166–9.
20. Byer NE. Spontaneous disappearance of early postoperative preretinal traction. Arch Ophthalmol. 1973;90:133–5.
21. Messner KH. Spontaneous separation of preretinal macular fibrosis. Am J Ophthalmol. 1977;83:9–11.

22. Sumers KD, Jampol LM, Goldberg MS, Huamonte FU. Spontaneous separation of epiretinal membranes. Arch Ophthalmol. 1980;98:318–20.
23. Greven GM, Slusher MM, Weaver RG. Epiretinal membrane release and posterior vitreous detachment. Ophthalmology. 1988;95:902–5.
24. Smiddy WE, Michels RG, Greene WR. Morphology, pathology, and surgery for idiopathic macular disorders. Retina. 1990;10:288–96.
25. Thomas EL, Michels RG, Rice TA, et al. Idiopathic progressive unilateral vitreous fibrosis and secondary traction retinal detachment. Retina. 1982;2:134–44.
26. Hashimoto E, Hirakata A, Hotta K, et al. Unusual macular retinal detachment associated with vitreomacular traction syndrome. Br J Ophthalmol. 1998;82:326–7.
27. Smiddy WE, Green WR, Michels RG, de la Cruz Z. Ultrastructural studies of vitreomacular traction syndrome. Am J Ophthalmol. 1989;107:177–85.
28. Smiddy WE, Maguire AM, Green WR, et al. Idiopathic epiretinal membranes. Ultrastructural characteristics in clinical pathologic correlation. Ophthalmology. 1989;96:811–21.
29. Shinoda K, Hirakata A, Hida T, et al. Ultrastructural and immunohistochemical findings in five patients with vitreomacular traction syndrome. Retina. 2000;20:289–93.
30. Kakehashi A, Schepens C, Akiba J, et al. Spontaneous resolution of foveal detachments and macular breaks. Am J Ophthalmol 1995;120:767–75.
31. Sulkes D, Ip M, Baumal C, et al. Spontaneous resolution of vitreomacular traction documented by optical coherence tomography. Arch Ophthalmol. 2000;118:286–7.
32. Hikichi T, Yoshida A, Trempe C. Course of vitreomacular traction syndrome. Am J Ophthalmol. 1995;119:55–61.
33. Koerner F, Garweg J. Vitrectomy for macular pucker and vitreomacular traction syndrome. Doc Ophthalmol. 1999;97:449–58.
34. Goto M, Nishimura A, Shirao Y. Scanning laser ophthalmoscopic microperimetry on idiopathic epiretinal membrane and vitreomacular traction syndrome. Jpn J Ophthalmol. 2001;45:115.
35. Kusaka S, Saito Y, Okada A, et al. Optical coherence tomography in spontaneously resolving vitreomacular traction syndrome. Ophthalmologica. 2001;215:139–41.
36. Ito Y, Terasaki H, Mori M, et al. Three-dimensional optical coherence tomography of vitreomacular traction syndrome before and after vitrectomy. Retina. 2000;20:403–5.
37. Pournaras CJ, Kapetanios AD, Donati G. Vitrectomy for traction macular edema. Doc Ophthalmol. 1999;97:439–47.

CHAPTER

131 Cystoid Macular Edema

ARTHUR FU • IRMA AHMED • EVERETT AI

DEFINITION

- A pathological response consisting of fluid accumulation in the outer plexiform layer of the central macula that results in the formation of visible cystic spaces.

KEY FEATURES

- Serous fluid accumulation in multiple cystoid spaces.
- Thickening of the central macula.
- Loss of the normal foveal depression.
- Best detected by slit-lamp biomicroscopy with a contact or handheld lens.
- A petalloid pattern of dye leakage from the perifoveal capillaries on fluorescein angiography.

ASSOCIATED FEATURES

- Conjunctival injection.
- Aqueous and/or vitreous cell and flare.
- Optic disc edema.
- A variety of ocular conditions, including aphakia, pseudophakia, inflammation, tumors, vascular abnormalities, dystrophies, medication usage, and foveal traction.

BOX 131-1

Ocular Conditions Associated with Cystoid Macular Edema

POSTOPERATIVE
- Cataract surgery
- Penetrating keratoplasty
- Astigmatic corneal incisions
- Scleral buckling
- Laser iridotomy
- Cryotherapy for retinal break
- Panretinal photocoagulation

INHERITED/DYSTROPHIES
- Retinitis pigmentosa
- Autosomal dominant cystoid macular edema

MEDICATIONS
- Topical epinephrine
- Nicotinic acid

TUMORS
- Choroidal melanoma
- Choroidal hemangioma
- Retinal capillary hemangioma

TRACTIONAL
- Idiopathic epiretinal membrane
- Vitreomacular traction syndrome

INFLAMMATORY CONDITIONS
- Eales' disease
- Cytomegalovirus retinitis
- Pars planitis
- Behçet's syndrome
- Birdshot choroidopathy
- Sarcoidosis
- Idiopathic vitritis
- Scleritis
- Toxoplasmosis

VASCULAR
- Diabetic retinopathy
- Retinal vein obstruction
- Ocular ischemic syndrome
- Idiopathic juxtafoveal telangiectasias
- Choroidal neovascularization
- Coats' disease
- Acute hypertensive retinopathy
- Radiation retinopathy
- Retinal arterial macroaneurysm

INTRODUCTION

Cystoid macular edema (CME) represents a "final common pathway" response of the retina to a variety of possible insults. It has been reported in association with vascular problems (such as diabetes and retinal vein obstruction), inflammatory conditions (such as pars planitis), inherited diseases (such as retinitis pigmentosa or dominant CME), tractional problems (such as vitreomacular traction syndrome), and use of medication such as epinephrine (adrenaline) or latanoprost, but its most common setting is following cataract surgery (Box 131-1).

Postcataract CME was initially reported in 1953 by Irvine.[1] It represents a common clinical problem that, for the most part, is self-limited. The management challenge arises in the chronic and persistent case, for which a stepwise therapeutic approach is optimal. The clinician must always be alert to the possible side effects of the many effective, but potentially toxic, pharmaceutical agents used to treat this entity. In addition, surgical management should be considered for unremitting cases of CME.

EPIDEMIOLOGY AND PATHOGENESIS

CME is a common condition associated with intraocular inflammation, vitreoretinal traction, and vascular incompetence; CME following cataract surgery is known as the Irvine-Gass syndrome.[1,2] Intracapsular cataract extraction is associated with angiographically evident CME in 60% of uncomplicated cases. Extracapsular cataract extraction is associated with angiographically evident CME in 20% of uncomplicated cases.[2] In the ma-jority of these eyes, no retinal thickening is apparent and no decrease in the visual acuity occurs. Clinically significant CME with decreased visual acuity following modern cataract surgery is seen in only 0.2 to 1.4% of eyes.[3,4] Although planned posterior capsulorrhexis at the time of phacoemulsification does not lead to an increased prevalence of CME,[5] those with inadvertent rupture of the posterior capsule and/or persistent vitreous traction to anterior segment structures are at highest risk. Neodymium:yttrium-aluminum-garnet (Nd:YAG) capsulectomy, when performed at least 3 months after cataract surgery, does not appear to increase the incidence of CME. Diabetics who have any degree of retinopathy have an increased incidence of postcataract CME.

Also, CME can occur after other types of intraocular surgery. It is especially common after penetrating keratoplasty in eyes that require concurrent vitrectomy.[2,6] In a retrospective study, 6 of 14 eyes (43%) receiving a posterior chamber intraocular lens (PCIOL) implantation with scleral fixation had angiographic macular edema that was a cause of low final visual acuity.[7] It has been reported following retinal detachment repair and glaucoma filtering procedures as well.[8] In phakic eyes it nearly always resolves spontaneously.

The mechanisms by which postoperative CME has been postulated to occur include vitreomacular traction, vascular compromise, and prostaglandin (PG) secretion and inflammation, although the exact cause remains unknown. Regardless of the initial insult(s), the fluid accumulation in CME is the direct con-

PROSTAGLANDIN SYNTHESIS PATHWAY AND INHIBITORY AGENTS

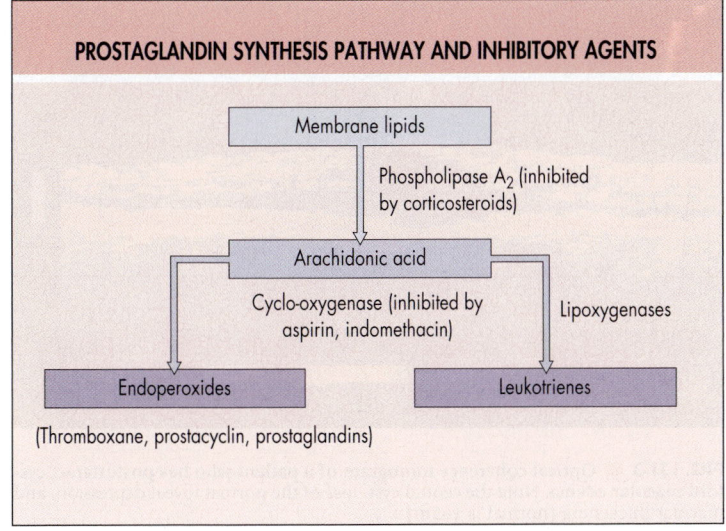

FIG. 131-1 ■ Prostaglandin synthesis pathway and inhibitory agents.

sequence of damage to the retinal vascular endothelium. When extracellular fluid in the central macula accumulates in the outer plexiform layer, cystoid spaces can develop due to the horizontally loose intracellular adhesions.

Although many mechanisms may be active in the genesis of CME, the most important is intraocular inflammation. It is clear that many affected patients exhibit signs and symptoms of intraocular inflammation that may respond to anti-inflammatory agents. Figure 131-1 illustrates the synthesis of PGs and the sites of action of corticosteroids and cyclo-oxygenase inhibitors (COIs). The formation of the end product in this pathway, PGs, can be blocked at the outset by corticosteroids. Step two in this pathway, which leads to the formation of endoperoxidases, can be blocked by COIs.

Aside from the postcataract patient, CME occurs most commonly in the setting of diabetic retinopathy, in which case associated microaneurysms and hard exudates are often evident. In most diabetics, CME occurs along with diffuse macular edema; however, rarely it is an isolated problem. While the Early Treatment Diabetic Retinopathy Study[9] demonstrated the visual benefit of focal photocoagulation for clinically significant macular edema, the CME component does not respond as well to laser photocoagulation. Panretinal photocoagulation for high-risk characteristics in diabetics can result in CME, which is usually self-limited.[10]

Retinal vein obstructions represent another common retinal vascular cause of CME. Both branch and central vein occlusions can result in severe macular edema. In these conditions it is due to hypoxic capillary endothelial damage secondary to increased intravascular hydrostatic pressure.[11] Branch vein occlusions are associated acutely with a sectoral pattern of dilated and tortuous blood vessels, flame and dot-and-blot hemorrhages, and cotton-wool spots. In the chronic phase, persistent CME, venous sheathing, microaneurysms, collateral vessels, shunts, and hard exudates are seen. The Branch Vein Occlusion Study[12] demonstrated a visual benefit following the application of a grid pattern of photocoagulation to the area of chronic macular edema. Acutely in central retinal vein obstruction, retinal hemorrhages and dilated retinal veins are prominent. In the chronic phase, vascular sheathing, absorption of retinal hemorrhages, and optociliary collateral vessels may develop. The macula may demonstrate CME, epiretinal membrane, and lamellar hole formation. The Central Retinal Vein Occlusion Study[13] showed no visual benefit in the use of grid macular photocoagulation for the treatment of associated macular edema. However, a possible benefit may be seen in younger patients who undergo treatment.

It is not unusual for CME to overlie a choroidal neovascular membrane or a serous retinal detachment. Often it goes unnoticed in light of the accompanying severe subretinal and/or intraretinal abnormalities.

Other, more unusual retinal vascular conditions produce CME. Retinal telangiectasis (also known as Leber's miliary aneurysms or Coats' disease) is a unilateral condition that occurs more commonly in males. The retinal vasculature is anomalous and produces leakage with resultant cystoid and diffuse macular edema. The vascular anomalies may be local or widespread. Cryotherapy or laser treatment is applied if these lesions threaten macular function. Idiopathic juxtafoveal telangiectasis can occur in either a unilateral or bilateral pattern. Exudation and CME result in visual loss. Photocoagulation may help to improve vision if there is no spontaneous improvement.

Patients who receive radiation treatment involving the head and neck may develop signs of radiation retinopathy 6 months to 3 years following this treatment. The incidence depends on total dose and the daily fraction, with changes developing most commonly after doses of 3000–3500 rads (30–35 Gy). A bilateral retinopathy occurs in almost one third of patients treated with external beam irradiation. Local plaque therapy requires higher doses than external beam therapy to produce damage. The clinical features of radiation retinopathy mirror those of diabetic retinopathy and include CME. Although no therapy is proved, grid laser photocoagulation is believed to lessen the macular edema.

Acquired retinal arterial macroaneurysms are often multiple and may thrombose and close spontaneously. This entity is treated if lipid exudate threatens the macula or if CME develops. Two modalities of laser treatment to be considered are direct laser treatment to close off the lesions and indirect laser treatment in a tight grid pattern around the macroaneurysm.

Also, CME with choroidal tumors, such as nevi, malignant melanomas, and cavernous hemangiomas, can occur. Intraretinal cystoid changes occur over the tumor and at sites distant from the tumor as a result of lack of oxygenation of retinal tissue.[6]

A multitude of ocular inflammations and infections can result in CME. These include idiopathic uveitis, intermediate uveitis, birdshot retinochoroidopathy, sarcoidosis, toxoplasmosis, posterior scleritis, Harada's syndrome, and Behçet's syndrome. The common underlying cause is an inflammatory-mediated breakdown in the blood-retina barrier.

Medications such as epinephrine, nicotinic acid, and latanoprost cause CME rarely. In one study, angiographically visible macular edema occurred in 28% of aphakic eyes under treatment with epinephrine drops for glaucoma versus a 13% incidence in aphakic eyes that did not receive epinephrine. These findings were reversed with cessation of the medication.[14] The mechanism of epinephrine maculopathy may be reduced blood flow in the retina and choroids.[15] Nicotinic acid, a treatment for hypercholesterolemia, is a rarer cause of CME. Tiny cysts are seen in a regular pattern in the foveal region, sparing the anatomical fovea, with no leakage from retinal vessels on fluorescein angiography and a small scotoma near the point of fixation.[15] The fundus findings resolve upon discontinuation of nicotinic acid. Latanoprost in various studies has been associated with CME. As a PG analog, latanoprost is thought to contribute to the disruption of the blood-aqueous barrier and angiographic CME formation in early postoperative pseudophakes.[16–20]

Patients who have retinitis pigmentosa can also have CME. Although the precise pathophysiology is not clearly defined, it is felt that the perifoveal capillaries demonstrate increased permeability in such cases. An inherited form of CME exists as well.

The presence of epiretinal membranes and the vitreomacular traction syndrome are associated with CME, particularly in areas of greatest traction and distortion of retinal blood vessels. Management of this condition is to remove the membrane surgically.

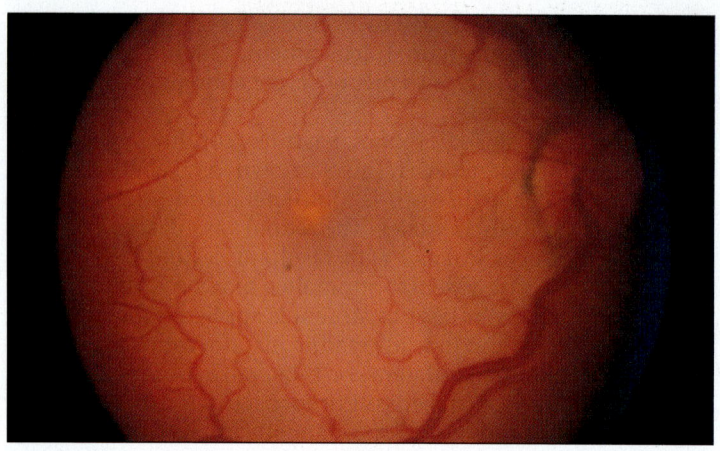

FIG. 131-2 ■ Cystoid macular edema in the Irvine-Gass syndrome. Note the radial cystoid changes centered in the fovea causing a "yellow spot."

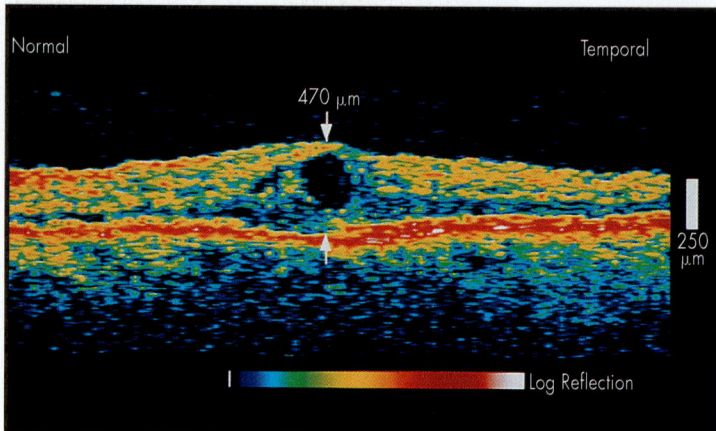

FIG. 131-3 ■ Optical coherence tomogram of a patient who has postcataract cystoid macular edema. Note the central cyst, loss of the normal foveal depression, and macular thickening (normal is 165m).

OCULAR MANIFESTATIONS

The major symptom of CME is decreased central visual acuity. Accompanying symptoms may include metamorphopsia, micropsia, scotomata, ocular irritation, photophobia, and conjunctival injection. Presenting visual acuities usually range from 20/25 (6/8) to 20/80 (6/26) but may be as poor as 20/400 (6/133).

Clinically, CME is seen best using the slit lamp and either a contact lens (e.g., Goldmann lens) or a handheld, noncontact lens (e.g., 78D, 60D). The edema results in light scattering due to the multiple interfaces created by the separated retinal cells. This light scattering decreases the neural retina's translucency so that the normal retinal pigment epithelial and choroidal background patterns are blurred. Individual pockets of fluid in the outer plexiform layer are seen, with the largest pockets centrally and progressively smaller cysts peripherally. Retroillumination can help to delineate the polycystic spaces. As these changes can be subtle and media opacity can affect the view, clinical confirmation of CME may be difficult in certain eyes. A yellow spot, believed to be due to diffusion of the luteal pigment, may be evident in the central macula (Fig. 131-2). Small intraretinal and intracystic hemorrhages, microaneurysms, and telangiectasias may be seen as well.

The underlying cause of CME does not alter its appearance, but the associated ocular findings vary widely depending on etiology.

After cataract surgery, aqueous and/or vitreous cell and flare, optic nerve head swelling, and a ruptured anterior hyaloid face may be evident. Other patients show vitreous traction to anterior chamber structures. Epiretinal membranes are concurrently present in about 10% of eyes. Inflammatory, vascular, tractional, inherited, and tumor-related causes result in the corresponding associated ocular findings.

As a result of CME, a rupture of the inner retinal cyst can occur to give a lamellar macular hole. Prolonged CME may induce atrophy of the macular photoreceptors—visual acuity is poor, but clinical examination and fluorescein angiography may be grossly normal with the exception of a blunting of the foveal reflex.

Fluorescein angiography is much better than clinical examination to show CME. It has been demonstrated that a close relationship exists between mean macular thickening and visual acuity.[21] However, fluorescein angiography yields only qualitative information. Quantitative data on retinal thickness can be derived only with newer techniques such as optical coherence tomography (Fig. 131-3).[22]

The majority of cases occur between 4 weeks and 12 weeks after cataract surgery.[23,24] Rarely, cases can occur years after surgery. Most instances of CME (approximately 75%) resolve spontaneously within 6 months. Two thirds of patients who have intracapsular cataract extraction with CME regain 20/30 (6/10) or better vision 3–12 months after surgery.[24] If, however, the surgery is complicated by vitreous loss or incarceration, resolution may be hindered.

DIAGNOSIS AND ANCILLARY TESTING

In eyes with clear media, clinical examination usually yields the diagnosis. Fluorescein angiography is the best ancillary test to assist in the diagnosis—in eyes with hazy media it is especially useful. It reveals a typical petalloid pattern in the central macula secondary to dye leakage from the perifoveal capillaries (Fig. 131-4). The dye accumulates in cyst-like spaces within the outer plexiform layer (Henle's layer).[23] Late fluorescein angiographic pictures should be taken (up to 30 minutes following injection) to allow time for the dye to accumulate within the anatomical fovea. Also seen on fluorescein angiography is leakage from the disc and retinal vessels.

In cases of aphakic and pseudophakic CME it is critical to perform gonioscopy, which is helpful in diagnosing structural problems of the wound, such as in the iris, capsule, or vitreous, that may be playing a role.

Other methods proposed to quantify macular edema include confocal scanning laser ophthalmoscopy (SLO), retinal thickness analyzers, and optical coherence tomography (OCT). The axial resolution of SLOs has been estimated at 300μm versus 50μm for retinal thickness analyzers. OCT provides high-resolution cross-sectional imaging of the retina analogous to B-scan ultrasonography using optical rather than acoustic reflection. Its theoretical axial resolution is 10–14μm and has been shown to be as effective at detecting CME as fluorescein angiography.[22,25–27]

DIFFERENTIAL DIAGNOSIS

The differential diagnosis is summarized in Box 131-2.

PATHOLOGY

Electron microscopy shows that an intracellular accumulation of fluid produces cystoid areas and swelling of Müller's cells, a condition that is reversible. If excess fluid is present, it may break through cell membranes and accumulate extracellularly, at which stage the condition becomes irreversible.[23] Histologically, large cystic spaces are seen in the outer plexiform layer (Fig. 131-5).

TREATMENT

Medical Treatment (Box 131-3)

CORTICOSTEROIDS. Corticosteroids act by inhibiting phospholipase A_2, preventing the conversion of membrane lipids into arachidonic acid. Locally, they decrease intracellular and inter-

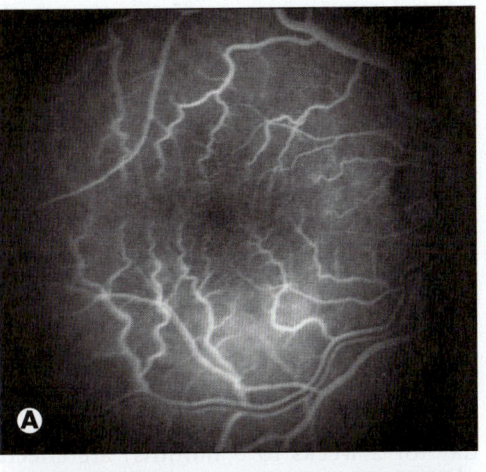
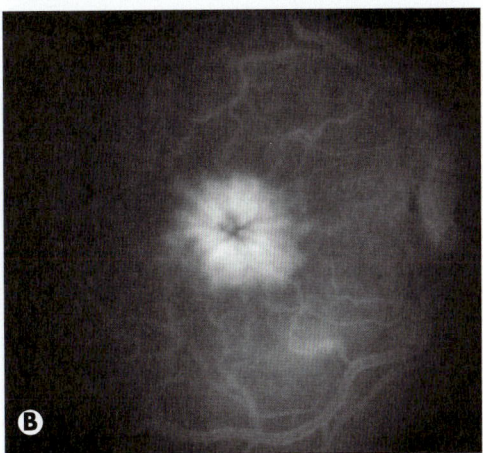
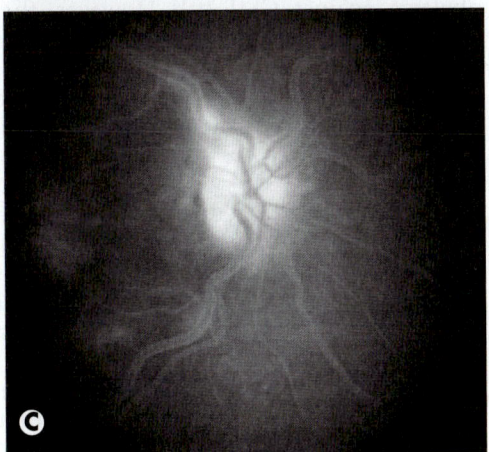

FIG. 131-4 ■ Fluorescein angiography demonstrates cystoid macular edema very well. **A,** In the early stage of the angiography, minimal leakage is seen. **B,** The petalloid leakage pattern, present in the late stages of the angiography, is diagnostic of CME. **C,** Note the profuse leakage from the optic nerve head in the late stages.

BOX 131-2

Differential Diagnosis of Cystoid Macular Edema

Stage I macular hole	Solar retinopathy
Lamellar macular hole	Rhegmatogenous retinal detachment
Idiopathic epiretinal membrane	X-linked juvenile retinoschisis
Vitreomacular traction syndrome	Diffuse macular edema
Pattern dystrophy	

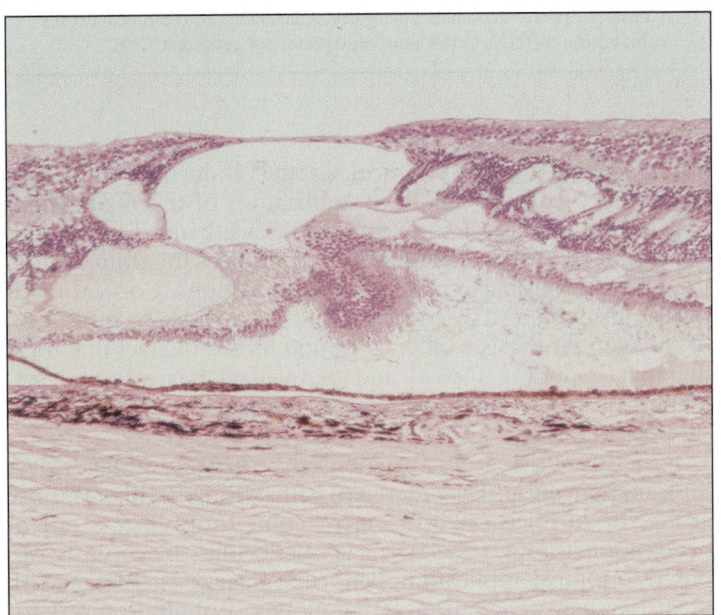

FIG. 131-5 ■ Typical pathological appearance of cystoid macular edema. Large cystoid spaces in the outer plexiform layer of the retina are demonstrated. (Courtesy of Dr W. Spencer.)

---

cellular edema, suppress macrophage activity, and decrease lymphokine production. Systemically, they sequester T cells out of circulation (inhibiting cytotoxic and recruitment functions) and decrease the enzymatic and phagocytic activity of polymorphonuclear leukocytes.[28] No well-controlled trial has been undertaken to evaluate corticosteroids in the treatment of chronic aphakic or pseudophakic macular edema.

Topical corticosteroids composed of lipophilic acetate suspensions of prednisolone penetrate the intact corneal epithelium and reach the anterior chamber in higher concentration than water-soluble forms, such as dexamethasone.[28] The relative potency of steroids tested in decreasing order is as follows: dexamethasone 0.1%, prednisolone 1%, fluorometholone 0.1%, rimexolone 1%, loteprednol 0.5%, and medrysone 1%. Phosphate preparations are water soluble and available as solutions—acetate and alcohol preparations are marketed as suspensions.[29]

Significant potential complications of topical corticosteroid therapy include glaucoma, posterior subcapsular cataracts, exacerbations of infections, and corneal problems.

Potent topical corticosteroids such as prednisolone, dexamethasone, and betamethasone, applied four times a day for 6 weeks, cause an elevation of intraocular pressure (IOP) to over 31 mmHg (4.13 kPa) in 5% of the general population (steroid responders). A rise in the range 22–30 mmHg (29.3–3.9 kPa) is ex-

hibited by 35% and the remaining population show no pressure response. Less potent steroids, such as fluorometholone, have a lower likelihood of elevating IOP. Of note, anecdotal evidence indicates that the visual acuity of "corticosteroid responders" with postcataract CME improves more than that of patients whose IOP remains normal. This may be explained by a hydrostatic effect.

Posterior subcapsular cataracts can be induced by local (topical and periocular) and systemic corticosteroid administration, with systemic medication being associated with a greater propensity for this complication. Cataract induction varies with the potency and the length of application of the medication. Application of topical corticosteroids exacerbates external herpes simplex virus infections and compromises the immunological resistance to bacterial and fungal infections. Corneal melting can be enhanced by corticosteroid therapy due to inhibition of collagen synthesis.[11] Of great importance is the fact that local therapy (including topical and periocular) has minimal systemic side effects but can perpetuate already existing adrenal suppression.[29]

Posterior sub-Tenon's injections may have advantages over topical application. They exert a maximal, long-lasting response at the site of injection, and water-soluble drugs have excellent penetration through the sclera via periocular injection as opposed to topical application. Periocular injections carry the risk of inadvertent penetration of the globe. Contraindications for patients receiving posterior sub-Tenon's injections include steroid-induced glaucoma, hypersensitivity to components of the injected steroid preparation, active necrotizing scleritis, and active ocular toxoplasmosis.[30]

Intravitreal triamcinolone for the treatment of CME secondary to uveitis has been described. A single intravitreal injection of triamcinolone induced clinical and angiographic resolution of CME. The side effects of treatment were similar to those of periocular injection including IOP rise and increased rate of cataract formation.[31]

Systemic corticosteroids used for CME are administered orally or intravenously.[32,33] Numerous potential side effects occur. Ocular complications include elevated IOP, posterior subcapsular cataract, increased incidence of viral ocular infections, ptosis, mydriasis, scleral melt, and lid skin atrophy.

Potential short-term systemic effects include peptic ulcer disease, aseptic necrosis of the femoral head, and mental changes consisting of euphoria, insomnia, and psychosis. Long-term systemic side effects include osteoporosis, a cushingoid state, electrolyte imbalance, reactivation of latent infections such as tuberculosis, myopathy, suppression of the pituitary-adrenal axis, and increased severity of preexisting diabetes and hypertension. Patients should be observed by an internist and informed of all risks and complications associated with systemic corticosteroid use.

CYCLO-OXYGENASE INHIBITORS. Cyclo-oxygenase is inhibited by COI drugs, which prevents the conversion of arachidonic acid into endoperoxides and, hence, inhibits PG synthesis. Clinically, COIs decrease capillary leakage.

Topical COIs (e.g., topical indomethacin 1% three times per day for 2 weeks to 9 months) are effective in achieving prophylaxis against CME.[34-36] However, these studies included concurrent corticosteroid treatment and no significant long-term benefit in vision was documented. A synergistic effect with corticosteroids may play a role in the improvement, particularly as corticosteroids inhibit the generation of PGs. It was shown by Flach et al.[37] that treatment with topical ketorolac tromethamine (0.5%) with no concurrent corticosteroid treatment resulted in a reduction in postoperative angiographic CME but no significant difference in visual acuity. A later study using topical ketorolac tromethamine (0.5%) versus prednisolone versus combination therapy indicated improvement in vision with the use of combination therapy over monotherapy with either agent alone.[38]

Complications associated with the use of topical anti-inflammatory agents include ocular irritation and discomfort following application, conjunctival injection, mild punctate keratopathy, and mydriasis. In addition, allergic and hypersensitivity reactions have been reported.

Topical COIs are used to treat symptomatic CME. Two studies indicate their efficacy in this situation. In a study in which 1% topical fenoprofen was used three times a day for 8 weeks, only two patients showed an improvement in vision and this improvement ceased with discontinuation of treatment but returned when treatment was reinstituted.[39] A multicenter study conducted by Flach et al.[40] demonstrated a statistically significant improvement in visual acuity of two Snellen lines in a group treated with a topical ketorolac 0.5% compared with a placebo-treated group. This improvement remained statistically significant 1 month following cessation of treatment.

Systemic absorption of COIs can occur following topical application. Whether this is clinically important is unknown. No study has shown that the use of these drugs topically before or after ocular surgery increases bleeding tendencies in ocular tissues. It is prudent to keep in mind the possibility of increased bleeding time.[41]

Yannuzzi et al.[42] studied a systemic COI (oral indomethacin 25mg three times a day) for its effect on postoperative CME. No significant effect was noted on visual acuity or the presence of chronic CME.

Systemic COIs are associated with multiple side effects. Gastrointestinal side effects include nausea, vomiting, diarrhea, anorexia, abdominal discomfort, ulceration, and gastrointestinal bleeding. These agents can interfere with platelet function and clotting. Bone marrow suppression, hepatotoxicity, impaired renal function, and central nervous system symptomatology, including headache, dizziness, somnolence, depression, fatigue, insomnia, and confusion, have been reported. Hypersensitivity and induction of asthmatic attacks can occur. Indomethacin can be deposited in the cornea in a whorl-like pattern. Association with optic nerve dysfunction has been reported. Finally, dermatologic reactions include rash, dermatitis, and Stevens-Johnson syndrome can occur.

The availability of topical formulations that provide good ocular penetration of the drug make it unnecessary to recommend

TABLE 131-1

SURGICAL TREATMENT OF CHRONIC APHAKIC AND PSEUDOPHAKIC CYSTOID MACULAR EDEMA

Situation	Recommendations/Options
Intracameral lens (within the pupil; iris suspended).	Remove, consider exchange for flexible AC IOL, or suture-fixated PC IOL.
Anterior chamber IOL with distorted pupil and vitreous strands in AC.	Vitrectomy to restore normal pupil. Leave IOL if flexible, remove if not. Would a sulcus-fixated PC IOL be safe? Omitting IOL is another option, as is a suture-fixated PC IOL.
AC IOL without distorted pupil or vitreous in AC.	Remove, especially if rigid IOL; replace with flexible IOL or would sulcus-fixated PC IOL be safe? Omit IOL; use contact lens or place a suture-fixated PC IOL.
Elevated, isolated vitreous strand distorting pupil with AC or PC IOL.	Consider YAG vitreolysis.
PC IOL with pupillary capture.	Free capture.
PC IOL with moderate pupillary distortion from vitreous strands.	Anterior vitrectomy for restoring pupil to normal and consider leaving lens.
PC IOL, sulcus fixation, normal pupil.	Consider removing IOL; possibly exchange for flexible AC IOL, or leave IOLs out, or use a suture-fixated PC IOL.
PC IOL; "in-the-bag," normal pupil.	Pars plana vitrectomy if evidence of traction on macula (rare). Rule out other causes of CME.

AC, Anterior chamber; PC, posterior chamber.

systemic therapy for ophthalmic indications, particularly in view of the many serious side effects of systemic administration.[41]

ACETAZOLAMIDE. Acetazolamide is a carbonic anhydrase inhibitor. It has been shown to facilitate the transport of water across the retinal pigment epithelium from the subretinal space to the choroids.[43] A case report suggests a direct correlation of resolution of pseudophakic CME with acetazolamide therapy.[44]

A study conducted by Cox et al.[45] demonstrated that 16 of 41 patients responded to acetazolamide treatment with partial or complete resolution of edema and improved vision. These patients had macular edema secondary to a host of other conditions, including the Irvine-Gass syndrome.

The complications and side effects of acetazolamide[11] include paresthesias, which occur almost universally. Fatigue, depression, anorexia, weight loss, and loss of libido, as well as nausea, diarrhea, cramps, and gastric irritation, may occur. Hematologic complications consist of Stevens-Johnson syndrome and blood dyscrasias. Finally, renal stone formation is a well-known and potentially serious complication.

HYPERBARIC OXYGEN. Improvement in aphakic CME with hyperbaric oxygen therapy was reported by Ploff and Thom.[46] The dosage given was 2.2atm (222.92kPa) oxygen for 1.5h twice a day for 7 days, followed by 2h daily for 14 days. The mechanism was hypothesized to be macular capillary contraction.

Surgical Treatment

Surgical management is directed toward reducing vitreomacular traction, which may play a role in the development of CME. However, it is not as important in the pathogenesis of this condition as is inflammation. Eyes that continue to have depressed central vision, photophobia, conjunctival injection, and discomfort almost always have vitreous strands adherent to the undersurface of the cataract wound, the iris, or the intraocular lens (IOL) implant. This may be accompanied by a peaked pupillary margin, which results from vitreous emerging from the posterior chamber to the cataract wound or from formed vitreous that has condensed on the anterior surface of the iris.[47]

If medical management fails and evidence exists of vitreous adhesions to the cataract wound, consideration should be given to the application of the YAG laser to sever these connections. In cases of persistent and unremitting CME, consideration can also be given to performing a vitrectomy or removing the IOL. The vitrectomy should eliminate any vitreous in the anterior chamber. Anterior chamber lenses, in particular, may require removal if they appear to be associated with chronic uveitis. Table 131-1 summarizes the surgical treatment of chronic aphakic and pseudophakic CME present in a variety of situations.

COURSE AND OUTCOME

The majority of patients who have aphakic or pseudophakic CME attain vision of 20/30 (6/9) or better 3–12 months following surgery. In unrelenting cases, medical or surgical management may be indicated.

REFERENCES

1. Irvine SR. A newly defined syndrome following cataract surgery, interpreted according to recent concepts of the structure of the vitreous. Am J Ophthalmol. 1953;36:599–619.
2. Gass JDM. Stereoscopic atlas of macular diseases: diagnosis and treatment, 3rd ed. St Louis: CV Mosby; 1987:333–453.
3. Norregaard JC, Bernth-Petersen P, Bellen L, et al. Intraoperative clinical practice and risk of early complications after cataract extraction in the United States, Canada, Denmark, and Spain. Ophthalmology. 1999;106:42–8.
4. Wegener M, Alsbirk PH, Hojgaard-Olsen K. Outcome of 1000 consecutive clinic- and hospital-based cataract surgeries in a Danish county. J Cataract Refractive Surg. 1998;24:1152–60.
5. Zaczek A, Petrelius A, Zetterstrom C. Posterior continuous curvilinear capsulorhexis and postoperative inflammation. J Cataract Refract Surg. 1998;24:1339–42.
6. Fung WE. Other causes of cystoid macular edema and retinal trauma after surgery. In: Ryan SJ, ed. The retina, 2nd ed. St Louis: Mosby; 1994:1811–25.
7. Lanzetta P, Menchini U, Virgili G, et al. Scleral fixated intraocular lenses. An angiographic study. Retina. 1998;18:515–20.
8. Carter J, Barron BA, McDonald MB. Cystoid macular edema following cornea-relaxing incision. Arch Ophthalmol. 1987;105:70–2.
9. Early Treatment Diabetic Retinopathy Study Group. Photocoagulation for diabetic macular edema. Arch Ophthalmol. 1985;103:1796–806.
10. McDonald HR, Schatz H. Macular edema following panretinal photocoagulation. Retina. 1985;5:5–10.
11. Kanski JJ. Clinical ophthalmology, 2nd ed. London: Butterworths; 1989:300–37.
12. Branch Vein Occlusion Study Group. Argon laser photocoagulation for macular edema in branch vein occlusion. Am J Ophthalmol. 1984;98:271–82.
13. Central Vein Occlusion Study Group. Evaluation of grid pattern photocoagulation for macular edema in central vein occlusion. Ophthalmology. 1994;102:1425–33.
14. Thomas JV, Gragoudas ES, Blair NP, et al. Correlation of epinephrine use and macular edema in aphakic glaucomatous eyes. Arch Ophthalmol. 1978;96:625–8.
15. Grant WM, Schuman JS. Toxicology of the eye: effects on the eyes and visual system from chemicals, drugs metals and minerals, plants, toxins and venoms; also, systemic side effects from eye medications, 4th ed. Springfield, IL: Charles C Thomas; 1993:629–40, 1040–1.
16. Warwar RE, Bullock JD, Ballal D. Cystoid macular edema and anterior uveitis associated with latanoprost use. Ophthalmology. 1998;105:263–8.
17. Callanan D, Fellman RL, Savage JA. Latanoprost-associated cystoid macular edema. Am J Ophthalmol. 1998;126:134–5.
18. Miyake K, Ota I, Maekubo K, et al. Latanoprost accelerates disruption of the blood aqueous barrier and the incidence of angiographic cystoid edema in early postoperative pseudophakias. Arch Ophthalmol. 1999;117:34–40.
19. Moroi SE, Gottfredsdottir MS, Schteingart MT, et al. Cystoid macular edema associated with latanoprost therapy in a case series of patients with glaucoma and ocular hypertension. Ophthalmology. 1999;106:1024–9.
20. Ayyala RS, Cruz DA, Margo CE, et al. Cystoid macular edema associated with latanoprost in aphakic and pseudophakic eyes. Am J Ophthalmol. 1998;126;602–4.
21. Nussenblatt RB, Kaufman SC, Palestine AG, et al. Macular thickening and visual acuity: measurement in patients with cystoid macular edema. Ophthalmology. 1987;94:1134–9.
22. Hee MR, Puliafito CA, Wong C, et al. Quantitative assessment of macular edema with optical coherence tomography. Arch Ophthalmol. 1995;113:1019–29.
23. Yanoff M, Fine BS. Ocular pathology: a text and atlas, 3rd ed. Philadelphia: JB Lippincott; 1989:102–63.

24. Gass JDM, Norton EWD. Cystoid macular edema and papilledema following cataract extraction: a fluorescein funduscopic and angiographic study. Arch Ophthalmol. 1966;76:646–62.

25. Zeimer R, Shahidi M, Mori M, et al. A new method for mapping of the retinal thickness at the posterior pole. Ophthalmol Vis Sci. 1996;37:1994–2001.

26. Woon WH, Fitzke FW, Bird AC, Marshall J. Confocal viewing of the fundus using a scanning laser ophthalmoscope. Ophthalmology. 1992;76:470–4.

27. Puliafito CA, Hee MR, Lin CP, et al. Imaging of macular diseases with optical coherence tomography. Ophthalmology. 1995;102:217–29.

28. Wilson FM. Intraocular inflammation and uveitis, Section 9: basic and clinical sciences course. San Francisco: American Academy of Ophthalmology; 1991.

29. McGee CNJ. Pharmacokinetics of ophthalmic corticosteroids. Br J Ophthalmol. 1992;76:681–4.

30. Min DI, Monaco AP. Complications associated with immunosuppressive therapy and their management. Pharmacotherapy. 1991;5:119–25.

31. Young S, Larkin G, Branley M, Lightman S. Safety and efficacy of intravitreal triamcinolone for cystoid macular edema in uveitis. Clin Exp Ophthalmol. 2001; 29:2–6.

32. Wakefield D, McCluskey P, Penny R. Intravenous pulse methylprednisolone therapy in severe inflammatory eye disease. Arch Ophthalmol. 1986;104:847–51.

33. Abe T, Hayasaka S, Nagaki Y, et al. Pseudophakic cystoid macular edema treated with high-dose intravenous methylprednisolone. J Cataract Refract Surg. 1999;25:1286–8.

34. Kraff MC, Sanders DR, Jampol LM, et al. Prophylaxis of pseudophakic cystoid macular edema with topical indomethacin. Ophthalmology. 1982;89:885–90.

35. Miyake K, Sakamura S, Miura H. Long-term follow-up study on the prevention of aphakic cystoid macular edema by topical indomethacin. Br J Ophthalmol. 1980;64:324–8.

36. Yannuzzi A, Landau AN, Turta AL. Incidence of aphakic cystoid macular edema with the use of topical indomethacin. Ophthalmology. 1981;88:947–54.

37. Flach AJ, Stegman RC, Graham J. Prophylaxis of aphakic cystoid macular edema without corticosteroids. Ophthalmology. 1990;97:1253–8.

38. Heier JS, Topping TM, Baumann W, et al. Ketorolac versus prednisolone versus combination therapy in the treatment of acute pseudophakic cystoid macular edema. Ophthalmology. 2000;107:2034–9.

39. Burnett J, Tessler H, Isenberg S, et al. Double-masked trial of fenoprofen sodium: treatment of chronic aphakic cystoid macular edema. Ophthalmic Surg. 1983;14:150–2.

40. Flach AJ, Jampol LM, Weinberg D, et al. Improvement in visual acuity in chronic aphakic and pseudophakic cystoid macular edema after treatment with topical 0.5% ketorolac tromethamine. Am J Ophthalmol. 1991;112:514–19.

41. Flach AJ. Cyclo-oxygenase inhibitors in ophthalmology. Surv Ophthalmol. 1992;36:259–84.

42. Yannuzzi LA, Klein RM, Wallyn RH. Ineffectiveness of indomethacin in the treatment of chronic cystoid macular edema. Am J Ophthalmol. 1977;84:517–19.

43. Fung WE. Cystoid macular edema. In: Fraunfelder FT, Roy FH, eds. Current ocular therapy 4. Philadelphia: WB Saunders; 1995:714–18.

44. Tripathi RC, Fekrat S, Tripathy BJ, Ernest JT. A direct correlation of the resolution of pseudophakic cystoid macular edema with acetazolamide therapy. Ann Ophthalmol. 1991;23:127–9.

45. Cox SN, Hay E, Bird AC. Treatment of chronic macular edema with acetazolamide. Arch Ophthalmol. 1988;106:1190–5.

46. Ploff DS, Thom SR. Preliminary report on the effect of hyperbaric oxygen on cystoid macular edema. J Cataract Refract Surg. 1987;13:136–40.

47. Fung WE, Custis PH. Aphakic and pseudophakic cystoid macular edema. In: Ryan SJ, ed. The retina, 2nd ed. St Louis: Mosby; 1994:1797–810.

132 Coexistent Optic Nerve and Macular Abnormalities

GARY C. BROWN • MELISSA M. BROWN

DEFINITION
- A heterogeneous group of optic nerve disorders that have secondary pathological effects on the macular retina.

KEY FEATURES
- Structural changes of the optic nerve.
- Secondary retinal detachment, retinoschisis, or macular edema.

ASSOCIATED FEATURES
- Optic nerve pit.
- Morning glory optic disc anomaly.
- Optic nerve coloboma.
- Optic nerve edema.
- Choroidal neovascularization.
- Optic nerve abnormalities may be associated with macular abnormalities, the most common being detachment of the macular retina. Choroidal neovascularization, macular edema, retinoschisis, and lipid exudation also may be found.

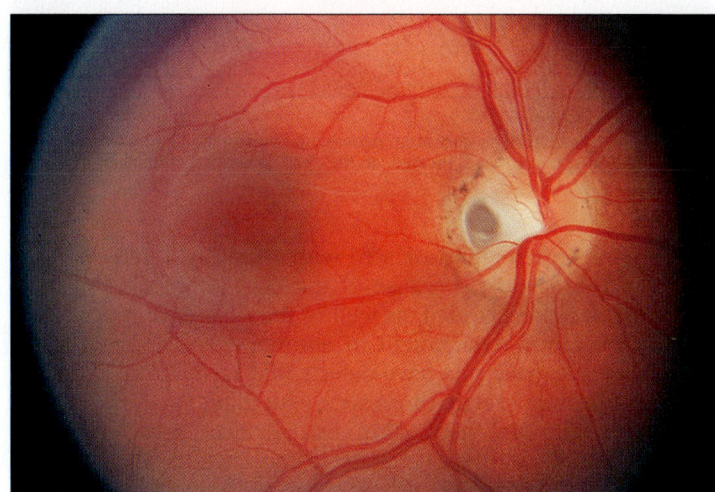

FIG. 132-1 ■ Temporally located congenital optic pit associated with a localized retinal detachment in the macula in the eye of a 15-year-old girl. Peripapillary retinal pigment epithelial changes are seen adjacent to the pit. The visual acuity was 20/60 (6/18).

CONGENITAL PIT OF THE OPTIC DISC

INTRODUCTION

Congenital pits of the optic disc are localized excavations that typically measure less than one half a disc diameter in width.[1] Although over 50% are located on the temporal aspect of the optic disc (Fig. 132-1), they can be located anywhere on the nerve head. Approximately one third are located centrally (Fig. 132-2). Those located centrally on the optic disc are not associated with retinal detachment.

EPIDEMIOLOGY AND PATHOGENESIS

Optic pits are believed to be secondary to a disturbance in the development of the primitive epithelial papilla, but the exact cause is uncertain. In some instances they can be associated with classic retinochoroidal colobomas, as well. In these instances it is possible that they are secondary to a defect in closure of the embryonic fissure.

Kranenburg[2] found pits in approximately 1 per 11,000 patients. Because approximately 40% of pits are or have been associated with retinal detachment (see Fig. 132-1),[3] about 1 per 25,000 examined patients demonstrate an optic pit with evidence of a previous or present serous detachment of the neural retina. Pits are unilateral in 95% of cases, and in 85% of unilateral instances the optic disc on the side of the pit is larger than the contralateral optic disc.[1] Occasionally, more than one pit can be seen on a single optic disc.

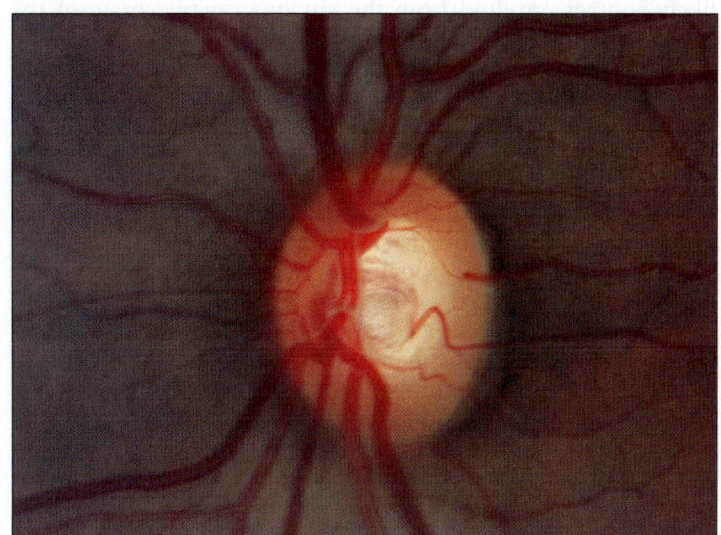

FIG. 132-2 ■ Centrally located congenital pit of the optic disc.

OCULAR MANIFESTATIONS

The pits vary in color. Approximately 60% are gray, 30% are yellow, and 10% are black.[2] The depth is variable and usually ranges from less than a diopter to several diopters. Peripapillary retinal pigment epithelial changes or choroidal atrophy or both are seen in 95% of eccentrically located pits (see Fig. 132-1). It is believed that this peripapillary disturbance may predispose to peripapillary choroidal neovascularization in rare instances (Fig. 132-3).

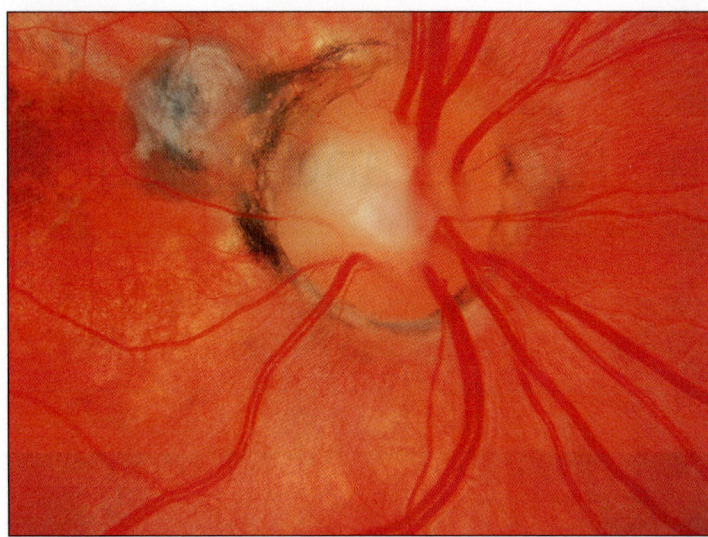

FIG. 132-3 ■ Peripapillary choroidal neovascularization adjacent to a congenital pit of the optic nerve head located at the 9:30 position. (Courtesy of Dr. W. Jackson.)

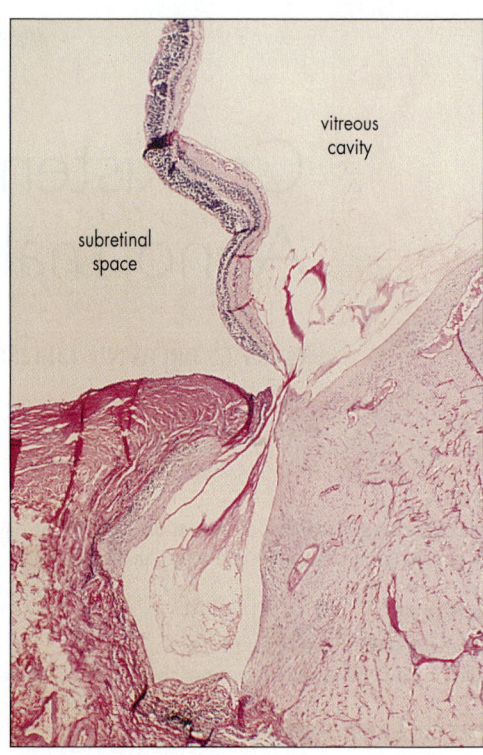

FIG. 132-4 ■ Histopathology of a collie dog eye with a congenital optic pit and associated serous retinal detachment. Vitreous gel has entered the pit from the vitreous cavity, and a connection exists between the pit and the subretinal space (periodic acid–Schiff).

Optic pits often are associated with visual field defects. If the enlarged blind spots (because of the large optic disc) seen in 85% of cases are excluded, as well as the defects that occur secondary to retinal detachment in another 40%, about 60% of eyes that have optic pits have defects that result from the pits.[3] These can mimic exactly those seen with glaucoma and include nasal and temporal steps, altitudinal defects, paracentral scotomas, arcuate scotomas, generalized constriction, and localized constriction. Centrally located pits, as well as eccentrically located pits, may be associated with field defects.

Although an associated maculopathy was noted first by Reis[4] in 1908, it was not until 1958 that Petersen[5] emphasized the relationship between congenital optic pits and a central serous chorioretinopathy–like picture.

The cause of the subretinal fluid remains debatable. The most likely sources are fluid from the vitreous cavity[1,6] or from the subarachnoid space.[7,8] Leakage from the choroid, from vessels at the base of the optic pit, and through macular holes also have been suggested, although these probably are less likely sources of the subretinal fluid. Experimental evidence from collie dogs shows a connection among the vitreous cavity, the pit, and the subretinal space in eyes that have congenital nerve head pits and retinal detachment (Fig. 132-4). In addition, active transport of India ink from the vitreous cavity into the pit and subretinal space has been shown. Convincing similar histopathology has not been demonstrated in humans. Nevertheless, in most human eyes that have associated retinal detachment, a small fenestration can be seen in the membrane that often overlies congenital optic pits. It is thought that intravitreal traction on the optic pit by an anomalous Cloquet's canal may play a role in the development of macular detachment.[9]

The retinal detachments usually extend into the macular region or slightly beyond. They typically are shallow, only rarely are bullous, and may be associated with subretinic precipitates that occur secondary to macrophages that have imbibed retinal pigment epithelial cells and deposited on the undersurface of the retina. Cystic changes are seen frequently in the foveal region of the detached retina, and apparent macular holes develop in about 25% of eyes that have macular retinal detachment. The macular holes seen with optic pits differ from idiopathic macular holes in that the former often appear to have an intact, overlying internal limiting membrane. If a macular hole develops, the prognosis for visual return to better than 20/200 with treatment is poor. Macular holes can develop within 2 weeks of the onset of retinal detachment.[3]

A splitting of the retinal layers occurs in many eyes that have optic pit and macular retinal detachment. This was noted first by Lincoff et al.[10] and has been referred to as a *retinoschisis*, although it is unrelated to either the typical juvenile or senile retinoschisis. The area of schisis tends to be larger than the area of subretinal fluid.

The mean age at the time of onset of retinal detachment is about 30 years, although it can occur as early as the first decade of life or as late as the ninth decade. Larger pits and temporal location appear to be predisposing factors to the development of retinal detachment.

SYSTEMIC ASSOCIATIONS

Systemic associations typically are not seen in conjunction with congenital optic pits. Nevertheless, an association with basal encephalocele has been described.[11]

TREATMENT, COURSE, AND OUTCOME

Retinal detachments associated with optic pits may fluctuate and occasionally resolve without therapy. The natural course of untreated macular retinal detachment, however, is poor. The Wills eye series showed that among untreated eyes that had an optic pit and macular retinal detachment, 55% had a visual acuity of 20/100 (6/30) or less after at least 1 year of follow-up.[1] Data from a more recent series from Iowa showed that 80% of such affected eyes eventually dropped to a visual acuity of 20/200 (6/60) or worse.[12] Although there have been no clinical trials to study the effect of treatment, a somewhat comparable 44% of laser-treated eyes have vision less than 20/100 (6/30) after 1 year.[3] Furthermore, among laser-treated eyes, only 16% have subretinal fluid at the end of 1 year, versus 75% of those that have not undergone photocoagulation.[3]

It is agreed generally that peripapillary laser therapy should be considered for cases of congenital optic pit associated with macular retinal detachment. The most widely used technique is to place two to three rows of 200μm spot-size burns in a peripapillary distribution temporally (Fig. 132-5).[13] The treatment is extended into flat retina, both superiorly and inferiorly to the subretinal fluid, to allow the retina to adhere to the retinal pig-

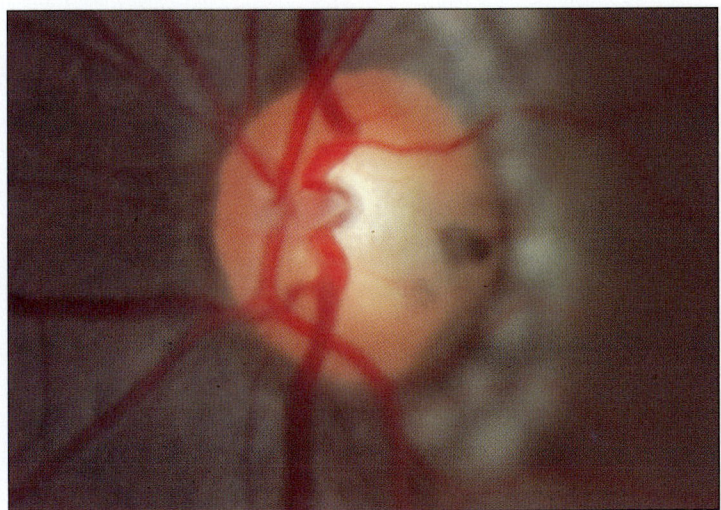

FIG. 132-5 ▌▌ Two rows of 200μm spot-size laser burns applied to the peripapillary fundus in an eye with a congenital optic pit and macular retinal detachment. The treatment is carried into flat retina superiorly and inferiorly to the area of detachment, so the retinal pigment epithelium can adhere to the retina and, hopefully, to continue that adherence centrally.

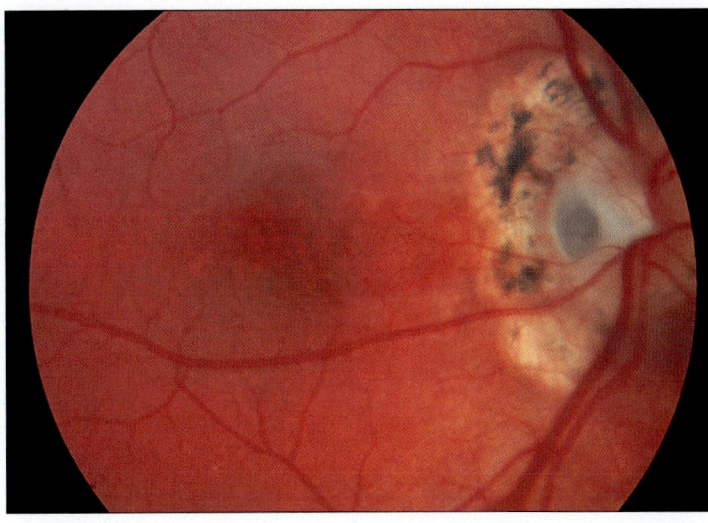

FIG. 132-6 ▌▌ The same eye as shown in Figure 132-1 almost 3 years after laser therapy. The subretinal fluid is gone and the visual acuity is 20/25 (6/8).

ment epithelium (RPE), starting at the edges of the area of detachment. It is undesirable to produce burns that traverse the full thickness of the retina, especially in areas of flat retina, because these may create arcuate scotomas because of the close proximity to the optic disc.

The subretinal fluid resolves in 50% of cases after laser therapy, typically within several weeks (Fig. 132-6).[3,14] If the treatment is ineffective, it can be repeated several months later. The greater the separation of the peripapillary retina from the underlying RPE, the less the chance of the treatment being successful.

If laser therapy does not flatten the retina after a second application, the possibility of additional laser treatment in combination with a pars plana vitrectomy and air–gas fluid exchange can be considered.[15,16] Because the retinal detachment generally is shallow, internal drainage of subretinal fluid usually is not necessary. It may actually be undesirable, because the vitreous gel can be very difficult to separate from the retina in young people. An inability to separate the gel may result in later retinal detachment as the remaining vitreous contracts.

Vitrectomy flattens the retina in an additional 80% of eyes that do not respond to laser therapy. Thus, the subretinal fluid can be eradicated with some form of treatment in at least 90% of eyes that have a macular retinal detachment (50% initially with laser, and 80% of the remaining 50% of recalcitrant cases with subsequent vitrectomy). The subretinal fluid initially may be displaced peripherally to the macular region with vitrectomy and require several weeks or longer to resolve after the intravitreal gas has dissipated. Laser therapy in combination with a perfluoropropane (C_3F_8) gas injection into the vitreous cavity without concurrent vitrectomy (pneumatic retinopexy) also has been successful in ultimately flattening the retina in approximately 90% of eyes that have a macular detachment.[17]

Subretinal fluid present in the macula for several months does not preclude good visual return if the retina is flattened and a macular hole has not developed. Subretinic precipitates typically resolve once the detached macular retina is flattened.

OPTIC NERVE COLOBOMA

Colobomas of the eye can arise anywhere along the line of fusion of the embryonic fissure, which extends from the optic disc posteriorly to the inferior pupillary frill of the iris anteriorly. The fissure begins to close centrally at 5–6 weeks of gestation. Failure of closure of the superior end produces an optic nerve

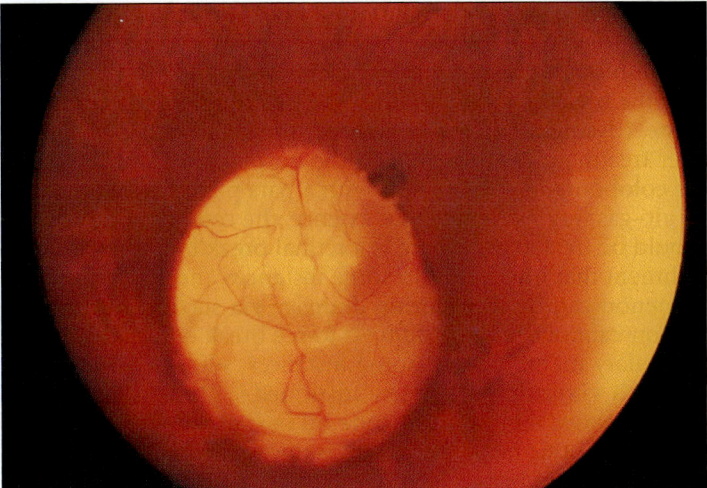

FIG. 132-7 ▌▌ Equator-plus photograph of a retinochoroidal coloboma. The embryonic fissure has closed partially, as shown by the normal rim of peripheral fundus inferiorly.

coloboma, whereas more widespread failure to close causes a retinochoroidal coloboma (Fig. 132-7), sometimes in combination with an iris coloboma. In eyes with iris and retinochoroidal colobomas, it is not uncommon to see a normal fundus appearance anteriorly where the embryonic fissure started to close.

Both retinochoroidal and optic nerve colobomas may be associated with systemic abnormalities. Included among these are abnormalities of the central nervous, cardiovascular, genitourinary, musculoskeletal, gastrointestinal, and nasopharyngeal systems. One syndrome found in conjunction with retinochoroidal colobomas that has received particular attention is the CHARGE syndrome (coloboma, heart disease, atresia choanae, retarded growth, genital hypoplasia, ear anomalies, with or without deafness).[18] Renal hypoplasia also has been associated with optic nerve coloboma, retinochoroidal coloboma, congenital optic pit, and the morning glory optic disc anomaly. This has been referred to as the *renal coloboma syndrome*.[19] A mutation of the *PAX2* gene has been noted in 50% of such cases.

Among the ocular abnormalities associated with both optic nerve and retinochoroidal coloboma is retinal detachment. Retinochoroidal colobomas also have been associated with choroidal neovascularization of the macula that originates at the edge of the colobomatous defect.[20]

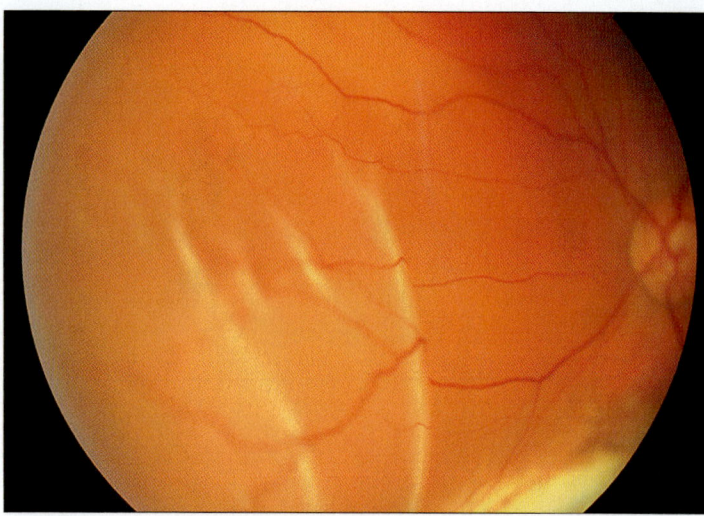

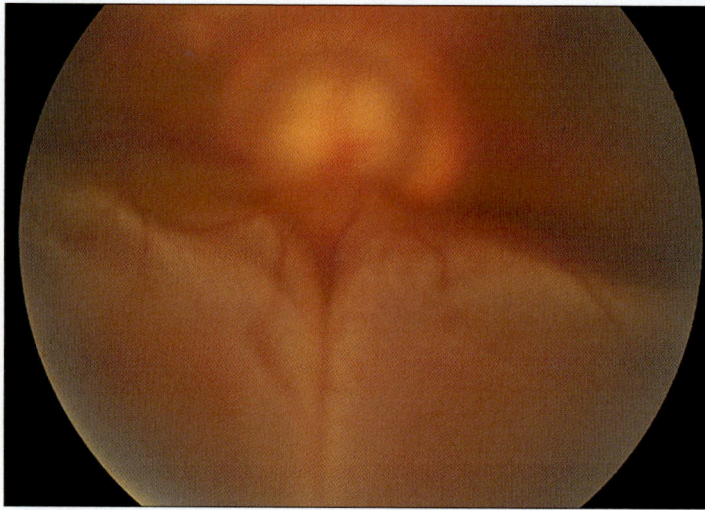

FIG. 132-8 ■ **Rhegmatogenous detachment in an eye with a retinochoroidal coloboma.** A peripheral retinal break was noted and the detachment was repaired successfully using a scleral buckling procedure.

FIG. 132-9 ■ **Optic nerve coloboma associated with a bullous retinal detachment.** After multiple vitrectomies, including one that employed the injection of intravitreal silicone oil, the retina eventually was flattened with an air–gas fluid exchange.

The retinal detachments associated with retinochoroidal colobomas can be rhegmatogenous (Fig. 132-8) or non-rhegmatogenous. If the retinal break is located peripherally, scleral buckling surgery may be effective.

If the break is located within the detached intercalary membrane (dysplastic retina) overlying the colobomatous defect, laser treatment can be given to the normal retina surrounding the coloboma in conjunction with a pars plana vitrectomy and an air–gas fluid exchange.[21] In essence, the colobomatous defect should be treated as if there is a retinal break in any area of detachment that involves it. In some instances, the Schliering phenomenon can be seen during drainage via suction with an extrusion cannula, when a difficult-to-see break occurs within the intercalary membrane. In some instances, silicone oil tamponade with vitrectomy has been advocated.[22] There is some controversy about the use of silicone oil in eyes with excavated defects of the optic nerve, because it is uncertain whether there is a communication between colobomatous optic nerve defects and cerebrospinal fluid in some eyes. Little is known about possible adverse effects of silicone oil if it gains access to the subarachnoid space.

The success rate for repair of retinal detachment associated with retinochoroidal colobomas was poor prior to the advent of vitrectomy.[23] Using buckling and vitrectomy techniques, the retina remains flattened after 1 year in about 81% of cases, with approximately 70% of all eyes recovering vision to 20/400 or better.[22] It should be noted, however, that the vision in eyes with optic nerve or retinochoroidal colobomas may be poor even without retinal detachment.

Retinal detachments associated with solely optic nerve colobomas typically are nonrhegmatogenous (Fig. 132-9). Overall, the entity is less well described in the literature than detachment associated with optic pits.[3,24] The origin of the subretinal fluid in this colobomatous variant is unclear. These detachments are treated in a manner similar to retinal detachments associated with congenital optic pits. If the subretinal fluid seen in conjunction with an optic nerve coloboma is minimal and borders only a portion of the optic disc, laser therapy alone to the peripapillary area of retinal elevation and adjacent flat retina can be considered. Unfortunately, these detachments often are more pronounced than those associated with optic pits and, therefore, cause more severe visual loss. If the detachment is bullous, it is usually necessary to perform a pars plana vitrectomy, with internal drainage of subretinal fluid and laser therapy to the peripapillary region of the detached retina. If the subretinal fluid completely surrounds the optic disc, 360-degree laser ther-

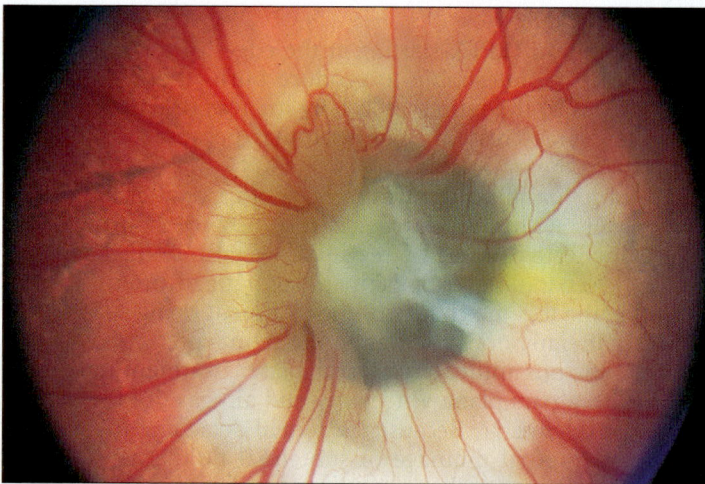

FIG. 132-10 ■ **Morning glory optic disc in this left eye is associated with a shallow retinal detachment.** The yellow pigment that overlies the area of subretinal fibrosis at the 3 o'clock position is due to the xanthophyll pigment in the fovea, which is abnormally close to the disc.

apy should be given lightly to minimize the chance of damaging the short posterior arteries that supply the prelaminar portion of the optic nerve head.

MORNING GLORY OPTIC DISC ANOMALY

The morning glory optic disc[3,25–27] is characterized ophthalmoscopically by:

- An enlarged disc with central excavation
- A central tuft of dysplastic white retina
- Peripapillary subretinal fibrosis
- Straightened retinal vessels that often are sheathed and emanate from the edge of the disc (Fig. 132-10)

The entity is most commonly unilateral but also can be bilateral. As is the case with both congenital pit of the optic disc and optic nerve coloboma, basal encephalocele has been described in association with the morning glory disc anomaly.[28]

Approximately one third of reported cases of the morning glory disc anomaly have been associated with nonrhegmatogenous retinal detachment that is connected to the optic disc.[24] Retinal detachment can occur later but most typically occurs during the first and second decades of life. The origin of the subretinal fluid is unclear.[8]

The detachments can be shallow (see Fig. 132-10) or bullous. Peripapillary laser therapy alone can be considered for shallow, localized retinal detachment, but with bullous retinal detachment, pars plana vitrectomy in combination with peripapillary laser therapy and internal drainage of subretinal fluid may be necessary to flatten the retina.[15] Therapy for bullous detachments, especially in children, may not be successful. Optic nerve sheath decompression also has been reported to treat this form of retinal detachment, but its exact role is uncertain.[29]

OTHER OPTIC NERVE ABNORMALITIES ASSOCIATED WITH MACULAR PATHOLOGY

ABNORMALITIES ASSOCIATED WITH CHOROIDAL NEOVASCULARIZATION

A number of optic nerve abnormalities have been associated with peripapillary choroidal neovascularization. Among these are drusen of the optic disc (Fig. 132-11), papilledema, papillitis associated with multifocal choroiditis, and congenital pits of the optic nerve head. It is believed that these abnormalities, in some way, disrupt the peripapillary Bruch's membrane, which predisposes to the development of new vessel growth.

Laser therapy is often of benefit in the eradication of peripapillary choroidal neovascularization. When the membrane extends to within 2500 μm from the center of the foveola, it often falls into the extrafoveal group studied in the Macular Photocoagulation Study.[30] In this instance, laser photocoagulation has been shown statistically to be of benefit. If the membrane has not grown into the subfoveal region, the visual prognosis with laser therapy is reasonable. The authors usually treat temporally located, peripapillary choroidal neovascularization even if it has not extended to within 2500 μm from the center of the foveola. The morbidity associated with such treatment is low, although the morbidity associated with choroidal neovascular membranes that eventually reach the central macula is high.

ABNORMALITIES ASSOCIATED WITH EXUDATION

Abnormalities that cause papillitis can lead to severe chronic leakage of plasma and lipid products that extends into the central macula.[31] The lipid is located within the outer plexiform layer (Henle's fiber layer) and often has the configuration of a hemi-macular star or a full macular star. When this hard exudate is present, retinal thickening (macular edema) often is seen concomitantly.

Among the specific entities that can cause papillitis and subsequent hard exudation into the macula are idiopathic optic neuritis, radiation optic neuropathy (Fig. 132-12), malignant hypertension, and anterior ischemic optic neuropathy. An idiopathic form of anterior optic neuropathy with stellate exudate is referred to as *Leber's stellate optic neuropathy*. It is likely that almost any cause of acute optic neuropathy can produce the clinical picture of optic disc edema and hard exudation into the macular retina.

No specific treatment is indicated for these exudative maculopathies other than amelioration of the underlying problem when possible. When the underlying cause is systemic arterial hypertension, resolution of the hard exudate usually occurs within weeks to months after the blood pressure returns to normal.

Recently, systemic infection with *Bartonella henselae* has been associated with unilateral or bilateral optic disc edema and secondary serous macular detachment.[32,33] *B. henselae* is the causative organism of cat-scratch disease and a history of close

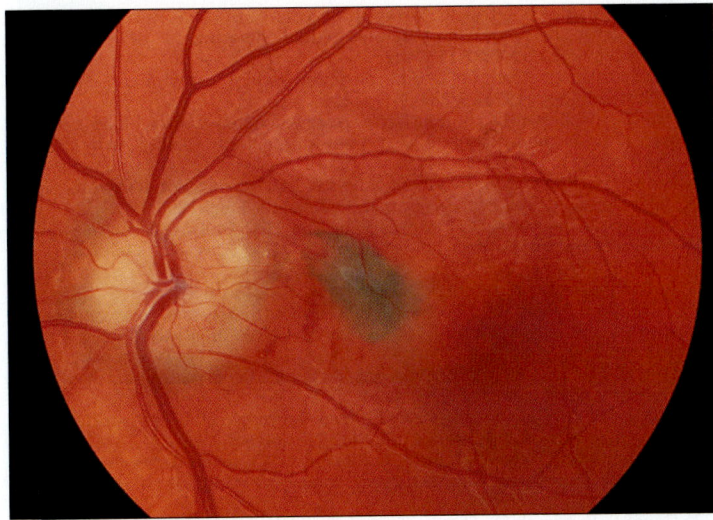

FIG. 132-11 ■ Pigmented peripapillary choroidal neovascular membrane developing in an eye with optic nerve head drusen.

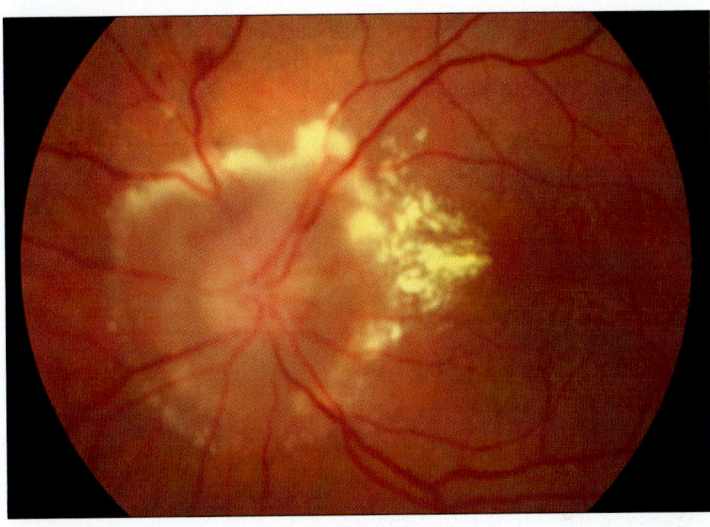

FIG. 132-12 ■ Macular hard exudate secondary to marked chronic leakage of plasma from the optic nerve head in an eye with radiation-induced optic neuropathy.

contact with cats, especially kittens, may be elicited. Diagnosis is made by measuring serum antibody titers for *B. henselae*. Treatment with systemic tetracycline or ciprofloxacin may be successful.

REFERENCES

1. Brown GC, Shields JA, Goldberg RE. Congenital pits of the optic nerve head. II. Clinical studies in humans. Ophthalmology. 1980;87:51–65.
2. Kranenburg EW. Crater-like holes in the optic disc and central serous retinopathy. Arch Ophthalmol. 1960;64:912–28.
3. Brown GC, Tasman WS. Congenital anomalies of the optic disc. New York: Grune & Stratton; 1983:95–191.
4. Reis W. Eine wenig bekannte typische missbildung an Sehnerveneintritt. Unschreibene Grubenbildung aufder Papilla n. optici. Augenheilkd. 1908;19: 505–28.
5. Petersen HP. Pits or crater-like holes in the optic disc. Arch Ophthalmol. 1958;36:435–43.
6. Brown GC, Shields JA, Patty B, Goldberg RE. Congenital pit of the optic nerve head. I. Experimental studies in collie dogs. Arch Ophthalmol. 1979;97:1341–4.
7. Regenbogen L, Stein R, Lazar M. Macular and juxtapapillary serous retinal detachment associated with pit of the optic disc. Ophthalmologica. 1964;148: 247–51.
8. Irvine AR, Crawford JB, Sullivan JH. The pathogenesis of retinal detachment with morning glory disc and optic pit. Retina. 1986;6:146.
9. Akiba J, Kakehashi A, Hikichi T, Trempe CL. Vitreous findings in cases of optic nerve pits and serous macular detachment. Am J Ophthalmol. 1993;116:38–41.
10. Lincoff H, Lopez R, Kreissig I, *et al.* Retinoschisis associated with optic pits. Arch Ophthalmol. 1988;106:61–7.
11. Van Nouhuys JM, Bruyn G. Nasopharyngeal transsphenoidal encephalocele, crater-like hole in the optic disc and agenesis of the corpus callosum, pneumoencephalographic visualisation in a case. Psychiatr Neurol Neurochir. 1964;67:243–58.

12. Sobol WM, Blodi CF, Folk JC, Weingeist TA. Long-term visual outcome in patients with optic nerve pit and serous retinal detachment of the macula. Ophthalmology. 1990;97:1539–42.
13. Brockhurst RJ. Optic pits and posterior retinal detachment. Trans Am Ophthalmol Soc. 1975;73:264–91.
14. Annesley W, Brown GC, Bolling J, et al. Treatment of retinal detachment with congenital optic pit by krypton laser photocoagulation. Graefes Arch Klin Exp Ophthalmol. 1987;225:311–4.
15. Brown GC, Brown MM. Treatment of retinal detachment associated with congenital excavated defects of the optic disc. Ophthalmic Surg. 1995;26:11–5.
16. Cox MS, Witherspoon CD, Morris RE, Flynn HW. Evolving techniques in the treatment of macular detachment caused by optic nerve pits. Ophthalmology. 1988;95:889–96.
17. Bonnet M. Personal communication. Ahmedabad, India, 1994.
18. Pagon RA, Graham JM, Zonana J, et al. Coloboma congenital heart disease, and choanal atresia with multiple anomalies. CHARGE association. J Pediatr. 1981;99:223–7.
19. Dureau P, Attie-Bitach T, Salomon R, et al. Renal coloboma syndrome. Ophthalmology. 2001;108:1912–6.
20. Leff S, Britton WA, Brown GC, et al. Retinochoroidal coloboma associated with subretinal neovascularization. Retina. 1985;3:154–6.
21. MacDonald HR, Lewis H, Brown GC, Sipperly GO. Vitreous surgery for retinal detachment associated with choroidal coloboma. Ophthalmology. 1991;109:1399–402.
22. Gopal L, Badrinath SS, Sharma T, et al. Surgical management of retinal detachments related to coloboma of the choroids. Ophthalmology. 1998;105:804–9.
23. Jesburg DO, Schepens CL. Retinal detachment associated with coloboma of the choroid. Arch Ophthalmol. 1961;65:163–73.
24. Savell J, Cook JR. Optic nerve colobomas of autosomal-dominant heredity. Arch Ophthalmol. 1976;94:395–400.
25. Kindler P. Morning glory syndrome. Unusual congenital optic disc anomaly. Am J Ophthalmol. 1970;69:376–84.
26. Beyer WB, Quencer RM, Osher RH. Morning glory syndrome. A functional analysis including fluorescein angiography, ultrasonography, and computerized tomography. Ophthalmology. 1982;100:1361–7.
27. Steinkuller PG. The morning glory disc anomaly. Case report and literature review. J Pediatr Ophthalmol. 1980;17:81–7.
28. Pollock JA, Newton TH, Hoyt WF. Transsphenoidal and transethmoidal encephaloceles. Radiology. 1968;90:442–53.
29. Irvine AR, Crawford JB, Sullivan JH. The pathogenesis of retinal detachment with morning glory disc and optic pit. Retina. 1986;6:146–50.
30. Macular Photocoagulation Study Group. Argon laser photocoagulation for neovascular maculopathy. Five year results from randomized clinical trials. Arch Ophthalmol. 1991;109:1109–14.
31. Grand G, Bressler NM, Brown GC, et al. Retina and vitreous, basic and clinical course, section 12. San Francisco: American Academy of Ophthalmology. 1996–1997:68–127.
32. Golnik KC, Marotto ME, Fanous MM, et al. Ophthalmic manifestations of Rochalimaea species. Am J Ophthalmol. 1994;118:145–51.
33. Zacchei AC, Newman N, Sternberg P. Serous retinal detachment of the macula with cat scratch disease. Am J Ophthalmol. 1995;120:796–7.

CHAPTER
133 Angioid Streaks

JAMES F. VANDER

DEFINITION
- Irregular, jagged breaks in an abnormal, calcified Bruch's membrane.

KEY FEATURES
- Narrow, jagged lines deep to the retina.
- Radiating out from the optic disc in a fashion similar to the retinal vessels.

ASSOCIATED FEATURES
- Choroidal neovascularization.
- Optic disc drusen.
- "Peau d'orange."
- Retinal hemorrhages.
- Systemic diseases: pseudoxanthoma elasticum, Paget's disease, sickle hemoglobinopathies.

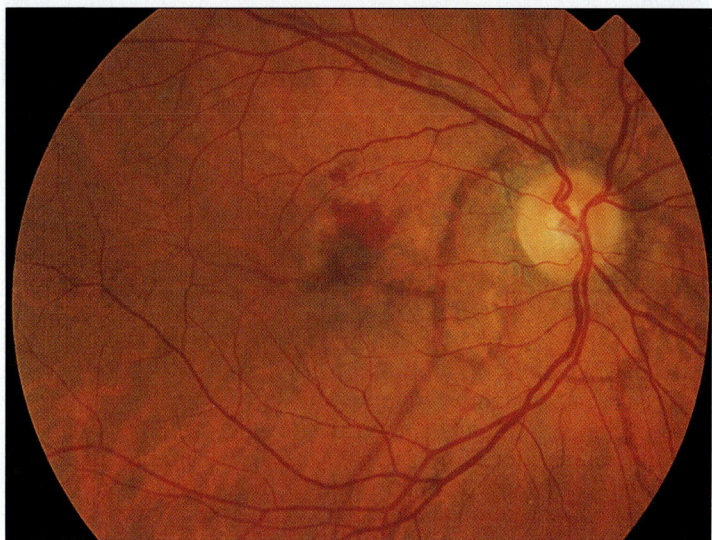

FIG. 133-1 ■ **Peripapillary angioid streaks.** Classical ophthalmoscopic appearance associated with a choroidal neovascular membrane.

INTRODUCTION

Angioid streaks were initially reported in 1889 by Doyne,[1] who described angioid streaks in a patient who had retinal hemorrhages secondary to trauma. Knapp[2] first coined the term "angioid" streaks because their appearance suggested a vascular origin. Not until 1917 did Kofler[3] correctly determine that angioid streaks represented changes at the level of Bruch's membrane. Clinical examination with subsequent histopathological correlation later confirmed that the underlying abnormality was not vascular in nature but rather a structural alteration in Bruch's membrane.[4,5]

EPIDEMIOLOGY AND PATHOGENESIS

Angioid streaks have been documented in early childhood but are not thought to be present at birth. Angioid streaks represent breaks or dehiscences in a thickened, calcified, and abnormally brittle Bruch's membrane.[6] Whether the breaks occur spontaneously or are caused only by trauma, even if minor, is not known. The initiating stimulation for the calcification and degeneration of Bruch's membrane in patients who have angioid streaks is not yet known. No known sex or race predilection exists.

OCULAR MANIFESTATIONS

Angioid streaks appear as narrow, jagged lines deep to the retina, almost always bilaterally. They can closely resemble blood vessels because of their size, shape, color, and course (Fig. 133-1). Angioid streaks typically radiate out in a cruciate pattern from an area of peripapillary pigment alterations, although they may circumferentially ring the peripapillary area as well. Generally, they taper and fade a few millimeters away from the optic disc; however, they have been reported to extend farther anteriorly.[7] Very rarely they occur in a random distribution throughout the posterior pole.[8] The number of streaks can be variable. Progression of the streaks with time has been observed.

The color of angioid streaks depends on the background coloration of the fundus and the degree of atrophy of the overlying retinal pigment epithelium (RPE). In lightly colored fundi, angioid streaks are red, reflecting the pigmentation of the underlying choroid. In patients who have darker background pigmentation, angioid streaks are usually a medium to dark brown.[7–9] A gray color also occurs. The RPE on either side of an angioid streak often manifests pigment alterations as well. Some patients have mottled RPE, either locally or diffusely throughout the macular area; this is referred to as peau d'orange ("skin of an orange"; Fig. 133-2). Although most commonly seen with angioid streaks related to pseudoxanthoma elasticum, the peau d'orange fundus is also seen in patients who have other underlying systemic diseases.[7]

The factors responsible for the characteristic radiating configuration of angioid streaks are not clear. It has been suggested that the pull of the extraocular muscles creates stress forces against the fixed point of the optic nerve, which results in the characteristic pattern.

Optic disc drusen have been associated with angioid streaks. As many as 25% of patients who have angioid streaks have clinical or echographic evidence of disc drusen.[10]

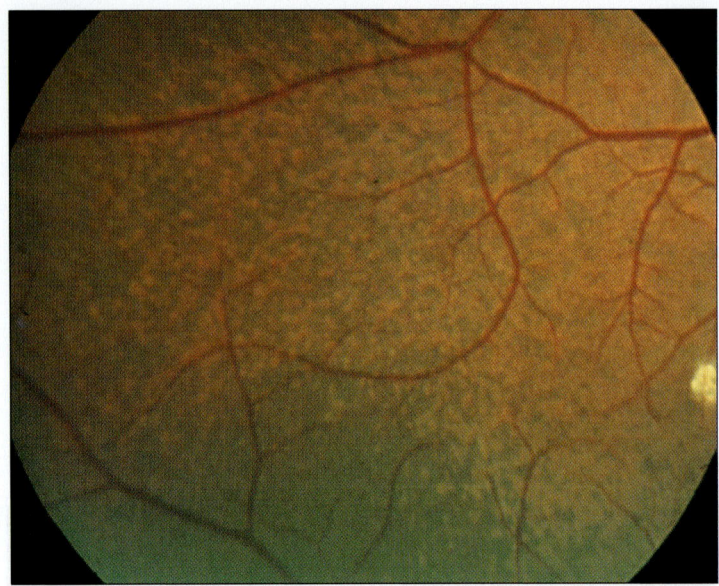

FIG. 133-2 ■ Mottled pigmentation of the fundus, known as "peau d'orange."

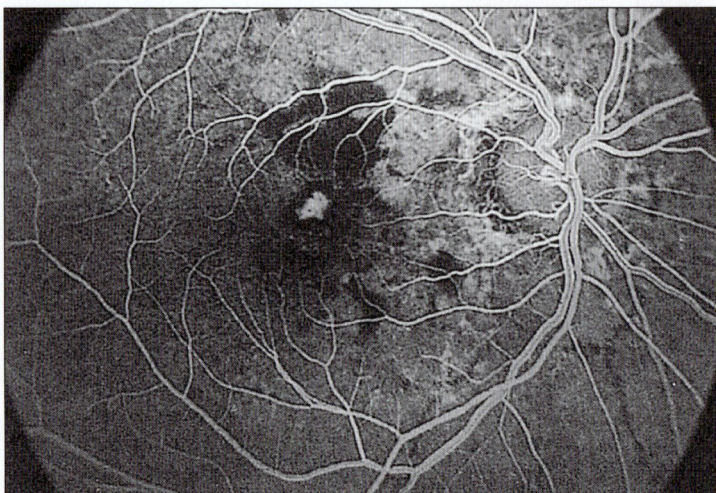

FIG. 133-3 ■ Fluorescein angiogram of the same patient as in Figure 133-1. Hyperfluorescence of radiating angioid streaks, along with a well-defined choroidal neovascular membrane.

DIAGNOSIS

Although the diagnosis of angioid streaks is usually made on the basis of ophthalmoscopic observations, intravenous fluorescein angiography can help to delineate the presence of angioid streaks when the ophthalmoscopic appearance is subtle. With fluorescein angiography, angioid streaks are variably hyperfluorescent depending on the condition of the overlying RPE (Fig. 133-3). Adjacent to the streaks, the RPE can be irregularly clumped, which results in a mottled appearance. When present, a choroidal neovascular membrane shows the classical increase in both size and intensity of the fluorescence as the angiogram progresses (Figs. 133-4 and 133-5).

Indocyanine green (ICG) angiography shows hyperfluorescent lines that are larger and more numerous than those see on fluorescein angiography or red-free photography (Fig. 133-6).[11] In some eyes with suspected choroidal neovascularization, ICG angiography demonstrates the membrane more clearly than fluorescein angiography.

DIFFERENTIAL DIAGNOSIS

The differential diagnosis consists of:
- Choroidal rupture
- Lacquer cracks
- Myopic degeneration
- Age-related macular degeneration

SYSTEMIC ASSOCIATIONS

The most common systemic disease associated with angioid streaks is pseudoxanthoma elasticum. In one large series, approximately 50% of the patients who had angioid streaks also had pseudoxanthoma elasticum.[12] Pseudoxanthoma elasticum is a systemic disease whose hallmark feature is abnormal skin and subcutaneous tissue, but the clinical spectrum may include arterial insufficiency secondary to calcification of blood vessels as well as gastrointestinal bleeding. The skin findings are classical and most commonly seen in the neck, axillary, inguinal, and periumbilical areas. They are said to resemble the skin of a plucked chicken (Fig. 133-7). No sex or race predilection exists, and both autosomal dominant and recessive inheritance modes have been described. A primary disorder of elastic tissue is the underlying pathophysiology.

Angioid streaks are seen in 80–87% of all patients who have pseudoxanthoma elasticum.[7] Aside from angioid streaks, other

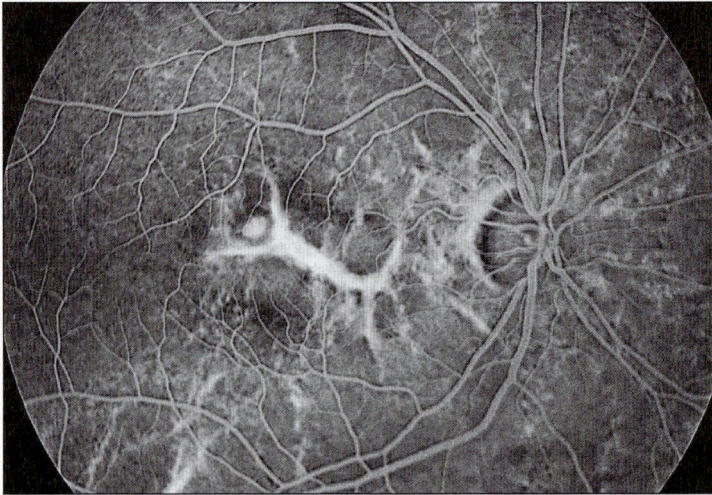

FIG. 133-4 ■ Fluorescein angiogram. Choroidal neovascularization is secondary to angioid streaks. The early transit phase demonstrates hyperfluorescence at the level of pigment epithelium.

associated ocular findings with pseudoxanthoma elasticum include peau d'orange, as described earlier, and "punched out" peripheral chorioretinal lesions, similar to those seen with presumed ocular histoplasmosis.

Of patients who have Paget's disease of bone (osteitis deformans), 2–15% have angioid streaks as well.[7,13] Paget's disease is characterized by heavy calcification of bones. The pelvis, skull, femur, and humerus are most commonly affected. The underlying pathogenesis is an exuberant osteoclastic reaction with a secondary osteoblastic response. Some evidence exists that a slow virus is responsible.[7] Diagnosis is made most readily on the basis of an elevated serum alkaline phosphatase level, with confirmation using radiography or a bone scan.

Patients who have sickle cell disease and other hemoglobinopathies can develop angioid streaks. Various studies have found the incidence to be in the range 0–6%. A strong correlation exists between age and the development of angioid streaks, which explains why studies that have looked at patients who have sickle disease, most of whom are younger than 40 years, show a low incidence of angioid streaks. Angioid streaks are rarely seen in patients younger than 25 years.

Many other systemic diseases have been linked to the presence of angioid streaks (Box 133-1); some of these associations

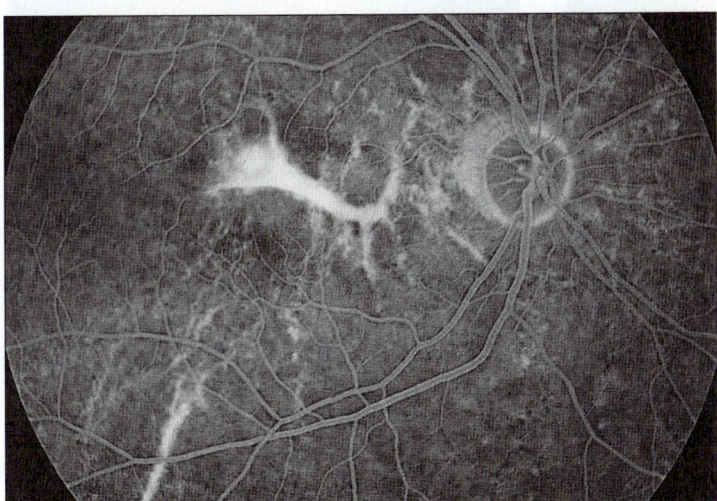

FIG. 133-5 ▌ Late phase angiogram of the same patient as in Figure 133-4. Leaking hyperfluorescence typical of choroidal neovascularization is seen.

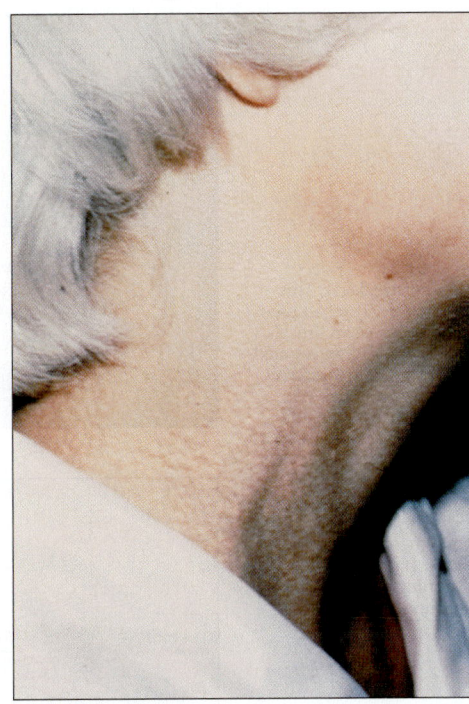

FIG. 133-7 ▌ Plucked chicken skin appearance on neck is characteristic of pseudoxanthoma elasticum.

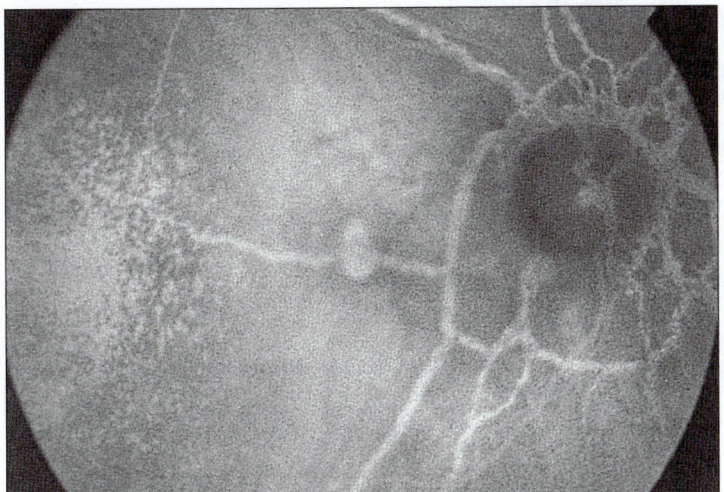

FIG. 133-6 ▌ An indocyanine green angiogram of choroidal neovascularization secondary to angioid streaks. The streaks are starkly hyperfluorescent.

BOX 133-1

Systemic Conditions Associated with Angioid Streaks

Abetalipoproteinemia
Acromegaly
Ehlers–Danlos syndrome
Diabetes
Facial angiomatosis
Hemochromatosis
Hemolytic anemia (acquired)
Hereditary spherocytosis
Hypercalcinosis
Hyperphosphatemia
Lead poisoning
Myopia
Neurofibromatosis
Paget's disease of bone
Pseudoxanthoma elasticum
Senile elastosis
Sickle cell disease/hemoglobinopathies
Sturge–Weber syndrome
Tuberous sclerosis

---

may represent coincidental occurrences. Because angioid streaks are often an acquired manifestation of systemic disease, studies that attempt to document population prevalences are strongly age dependent. Work-up for systemic disease in patients with angioid streaks should include skin biopsy, serum alkaline phosphatase, serum calcium and phosphate, and hemoglobin electrophoresis. About 40% of all patients who have angioid streaks do not have an underlying, causative systemic problem.

PATHOLOGY

The elastic lamina that occupies the midsegment of Bruch's membrane is primarily affected, which results in disintegration and fraying of the elastic fibers (Fig. 133-8). Diffuse and extensive basophilic stains caused by the deposition of calcium are commonly seen with routine hematoxylin and eosin. The choriocapillaris and RPE are minimally affected initially; however, with progression these structures become secondarily degenerated. Eventually, neovascular vessels from the choroid may penetrate through the breaks in Bruch's membrane, which results in subretinal hemorrhage, exudation, and edema followed by the fibrovascular deposition that is typical of a disciform scar. All cases of angioid streaks studied histopathologically have shown identical changes despite different underlying systemic diseases.[7]

TREATMENT, COURSE, AND OUTCOME

Because angioid streaks are generally asymptomatic and not visually significant, no treatment is warranted. Patients who have angioid streaks should be advised to avoid activities that increase the likelihood of a blow to the eye because of the increased risk of subretinal hemorrhage from relatively minor trauma.

If a choroidal neovascular membrane develops with secondary serous or hemorrhagic detachment of the retina, laser photocoagulation should be considered. The efficacy of photocoagulation for choroidal neovascularization has not been the subject of controlled, clinical trials. Some evidence exists that laser photocoagulation for well-defined extrafoveal or juxtafoveal membranes is beneficial. Singerman and Hatem[14] reported long-term successful

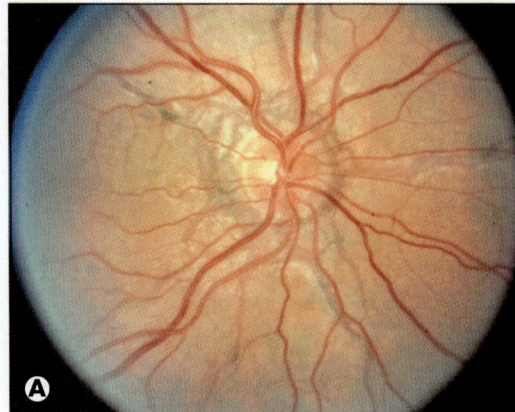
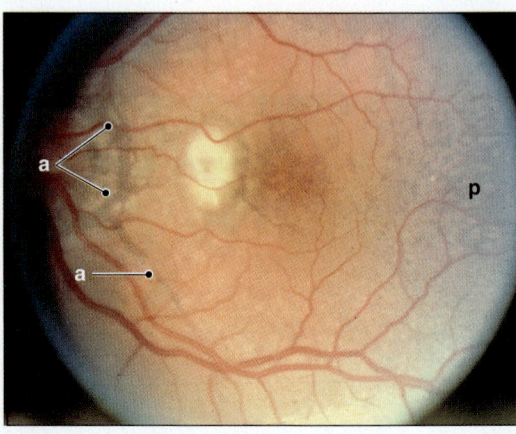

FIG. 133-8 ■ Angioid streaks. A, This patient with angioid streaks also had pseudoxanthoma elasticum. Breaks in Bruch's membrane around the optic nerve resulted in angioid streaks. B, Similar breaks away from the optic nerve have resulted in "peau d'orange" appearance (a, angioid streaks; p, peau d'orange). The yellow area just temporal to the optic nerve represents subretinal neovascularization. C, A histologic section of another case, from a patient with Paget's disease, also shows streaks caused by an interruption (break) in Bruch's membrane. (From Yanoff M, Fine BS. Ocular pathology, ed 5. Philadelphia: WB Saunders; 2002.)

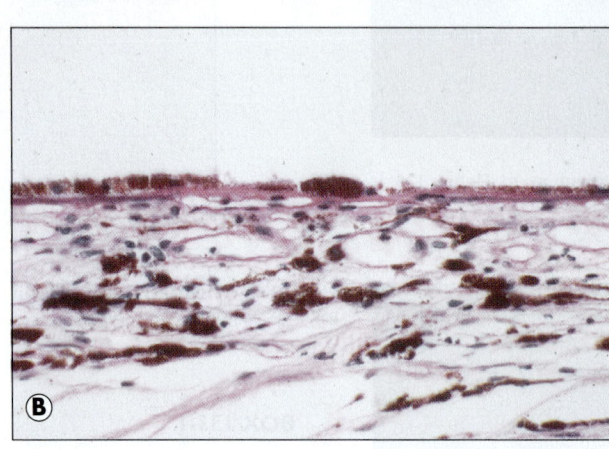

treatment with seven out of eight membranes. A subsequent study of 30 eyes treated using light photocoagulation showed that the vision remained stable or was improved in 16 eyes and that vision in 14 eyes worsened, although 12 of the patients concerned retained 20/200 visual acuity or better. In a group of patients with 11 untreated eyes showing subretinal neovascularization, all had the visual acuity of counting fingers.[15] Lim et al.[16] found either recurrence or persistence of 14 out of 24 well-defined choroidal neovascular membranes. The presence of a disciform scar or choroidal neovascularization in the fellow eye is a poor prognostic factor for successful laser treatment. Repeated treatment may be necessary, as the recurrence rate appears to be high. No role exists for prophylactic photocoagulation of angioid streaks.

Photodynamic therapy is a technique for treatment of subfoveal choroidal neovascularization using a photosensitizing intravenous dye followed by low-energy infrared laser. Initially approved for use in age-related macular degeneration, photodynamic therapy has been shown to have some promise in treatment of subfoveal neovascularization in angioid streaks.[17]

REFERENCES

1. Doyne RW. Choroidal and retinal changes that result from blows on the eye. Trans Ophthalmol Soc UK. 1889;9:128.
2. Knapp H. On the formation of angioid streaks as an unusual metamorphosis of retinal hemorrhages. Arch Ophthalmol. 1892;21:289–92.
3. Kofler A. Beitraege zur Kenntnis der angioid Streaks (Knapp). Arch Augenheilkd. 1917;82:134–49.
4. Bock J. Zur Klinik und Anatomic der gefaessehnlichen Streifen im Augenhintergrund. Z Augenheilkd. 1938;95:1–50.
5. Hagedoorn A. Angioid streaks. Arch Ophthalmol. 1939;21:746–74.
6. Smith JJ, Gass JDM, Justice J. Fluorescein fundus photography of angioid streaks. Br J Ophthalmol. 1964;48:517–21.
7. Clarkson JG, Altman RD. Angioid streaks. Surv Ophthalmol. 1982;26:235–46.
8. Terry TL. Angioid streaks and osteitis deformans. Trans Am Ophthalmol Soc. 1934;32:555–73.
9. Schatz H. Other retinal pigment epithelial diseases. Int Ophthalmol Clin. 1975; 15:181–97.
10. Pierro L, Brancato R, Minicucci M, et al. Echographic diagnosis of drusen of the optic nerve head in patients with angioid streaks. Ophthalmologica. 1994;208:239–42.
11. Quaranta M, Cohen SY, Krott R, et al. Indocyanine green videoangiography of angioid streaks. Am J Ophthalmol. 1995;119:136–42.
12. Shields JA, Federman JL, Tomer TL, Annesley WH. Angioid streaks. I. Ophthalmoscopic variations and diagnostic problems. Br J Ophthalmol. 1975;59:257–66.
13. Dabbs TR, Skjodt K. Prevalence of angioid streaks and other ocular complications of Paget's disease of bone. Br J Ophthalmol. 1990;74:579–82.
14. Singerman LJ, Hatem G. Laser treatment of choroidal neovascular membranes in angioid streaks. Retina. 1981;1:75–83.
15. Geliske O, Hendrikse F, Deutman AF. A long-term follow-up study of laser coagulation of neovascular membranes in angioid streaks. Am J Ophthalmol. 1988;105:299–303.
16. Lim JI, Bressler NM, Marsh MJ, et al. Laser treatment of choroidal neovascularization in patients with angioid streaks. Am J Ophthalmol. 1993;116:414–23.
17. Sickenberg M, Schmidt-Erfurth U, Miller JW, et al. A preliminary study of photodynamic therapy using verteporfin for choroidal neovascularization in pathologic myopia, ocular histoplasmosis syndrome, angioid streaks, and idiopathic causes. Arch Ophthalmol. 2000;118:327–36.

SECTION 7 RETINAL DETACHMENT

CHAPTER

134

Peripheral Retinal Lesions

WILLIAM S. TASMAN

DEFINITION AND KEY FEATURES

- A heterogeneous group of anatomical variations, degenerative changes, and pathological processes that can be observed ophthalmoscopically in the anterior neural retina and ora serrata region.

ASSOCIATED FEATURES

- Best observed with indirect ophthalmoscopy and scleral depression.
- Contact lens examination may assist.
- Possible association with premature vitreous collapse and retinal detachment.
- Usually stable over time.

INTRODUCTION AND ANATOMY

Many variations occur in the ophthalmoscopic appearance of the peripheral neural retina. In most cases, these variations are not of clinical significance; however, certain anatomical changes can render eyes at higher risk for retinal breaks and rhegmatogenous retinal detachment. In order to detect and diagnose pathology versus normal variation in the anterior retina accurately, it is of critical importance to be aware of the normal anatomical appearance of this area.

The fundus may be roughly separated into central (posterior) and peripheral (anterior) portions by a circle that passes through the posterior edge of the scleral entrance of each vortex vein ampulla. The anatomical equator is located approximately two disc diameters (3mm) anterior to the entrance of the scleral canals. Thus, the vortex veins become important landmarks when separating the peripheral fundus from the posterior pole.

The fundus also may be divided by natural features into superior and inferior halves by the long ciliary nerves and arteries that form a horizontal boundary nasally and temporally.[1]

In the peripheral fundus it often is difficult or impossible to distinguish between arterioles and venules on the basis of size, color, or pattern.[2] The most practical method of identification is to trace the vessels back to the posterior fundus. The retinal arterioles and venules generally do not course together but are evenly distributed throughout the periphery. The majority become very small and disappear before reaching a distance of 0.5 disc diameter from the ora serrata. The arteries disappear first, whereas the venules tend to extend closer toward the ora serrata.

Ora Serrata

In the ora serrata region, the retina becomes opalescent and often is marked by small rows of cystoid cavities.[3] This is normal—extensive cystoid changes do not represent pathology. The un-

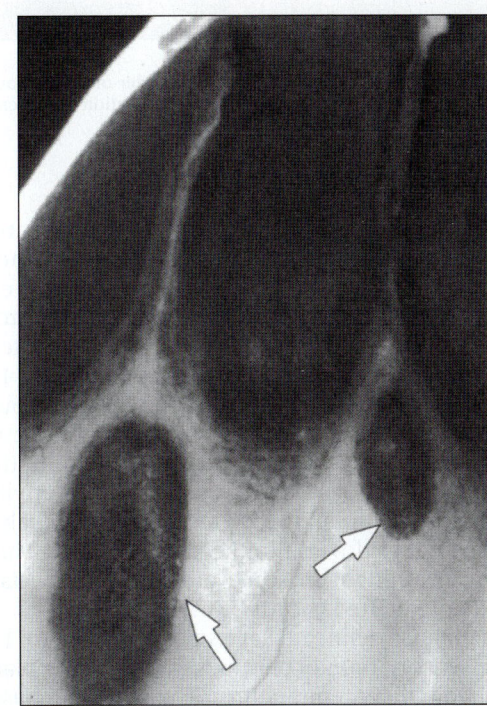

FIG. 134-1 ■ Enclosed oral bays. The dentate processes connect with ciliary processes to form a meridional complex.

derlying pigment epithelium appears darker and more granular than that seen posteriorly. The neural retina stops abruptly at the ora serrata and is continued by the nonpigmented ciliary epithelium, which appears considerably thinner than the retina. The pars plana corporis ciliaris is more deeply pigmented than the peripheral retina and, thus, the choroidal pattern is obscured by that of the pigment epithelium. The development of the ora serrata is incomplete at birth and continues during early life.[4,5]

Because ora bays and teeth (or dentate processes) frequently are difficult to identify temporally, the exact number of ora teeth is not easy to calculate. Salzmann[5] in 1912 identified 48, whereas Straatsma et al.[6] noted 16 dentate processes along the average ora serrata. In the author's experience the number varies, but usually between 20 and 30 dentate processes can be counted reliably, corresponding in position to the intervals between the ciliary processes. Occasionally, two oral teeth join to form an enclosed oral bay, which may be confused with a retinal hole (Fig. 134-1). Oral bays do not carry an increased risk for rhegmatogenous retinal detachment.

Vitreous Base

One of the most significant structures in the peripheral fundus is the vitreous base. It is of clinical importance because retinal

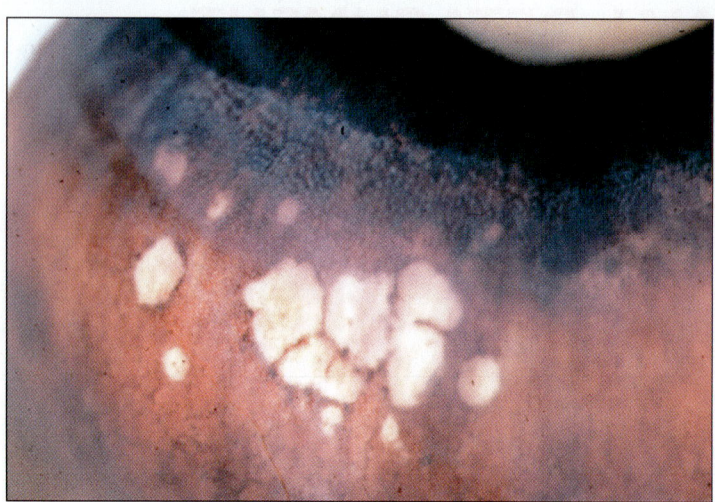

FIG. 134-2 ■ The anterior border and posterior border of the vitreous base. The posterior border is irregular. Areas of paving stone degeneration that extend across the ora serrata into the pars plana can also be seen.

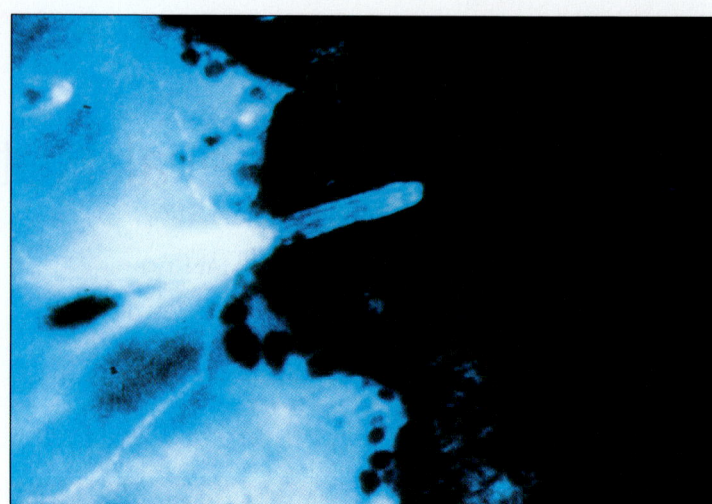

FIG. 134-3 ■ Meridional fold with a small break at the base of the fold.

breaks frequently occur along its posterior border and, in the case of traumatic detachment, occasionally along the anterior border, as well.[7] The vitreous base involves the full circumference of the peripheral fundus and measures approximately 3.2mm in width. Generally, it is wider nasally than temporally and may have an irregular posterior border (Fig. 134-2). It represents an area in the fundus in which the vitreous, neural retina, and pigment epithelium all are firmly adherent, one to the other. It is for this reason that in some cases of traumatic detachment the vitreous base is avulsed with its underlying neural retina and pigment epithelium, to create a retinal dialysis and a "garland" that hangs down into the vitreous cavity. The vitreous base may be prominent in some individuals, especially those with a darkly pigmented choroid.

The pars plana is delineated at its posterior margin by the ora serrata. The sensory retina continues into the pars plana as the nonpigmented ciliary epithelium. The vitreous base, which straddles the ora serrata, has its anterior border in the pars plana, where it parallels the configuration of the ora serrata.

OCULAR MANIFESTATIONS AND DIAGNOSIS OF PERIPHERAL RETINAL LESIONS

Meridional Folds or Radial Folds

Meridional folds, or radial folds, which usually involve all neural retinal layers, are a common, normal variant seen in the peripheral fundus. As a rule, a meridional fold begins in the ora serrata and runs posteriorly and perpendicularly to it in a meridional fashion. It is a radially aligned elevation of the peripheral retina and may be associated with retinal breaks (Fig. 134-3). Meridional folds are found significantly more often nasally than temporally and especially in the upper nasal quadrant.[3,8] They occur in 20% of eyes examined during autopsy.[9] In cases of rhegmatogenous retinal detachment, the posterior edges of meridional folds must be examined carefully for retinal breaks.

Meridional Complex

Occasionally, meridional folds extend to the posterior aspect of a ciliary process. The configuration is called a meridional complex (see Fig. 134-1). The fundamental and consistent feature of a meridional complex is an atypical dentate process that aligns with a ciliary process. Both meridional folds and meridionally aligned complexes can be the sites of small retinal breaks and require careful examination in patients who have retinal detachment (see Fig. 134-3).

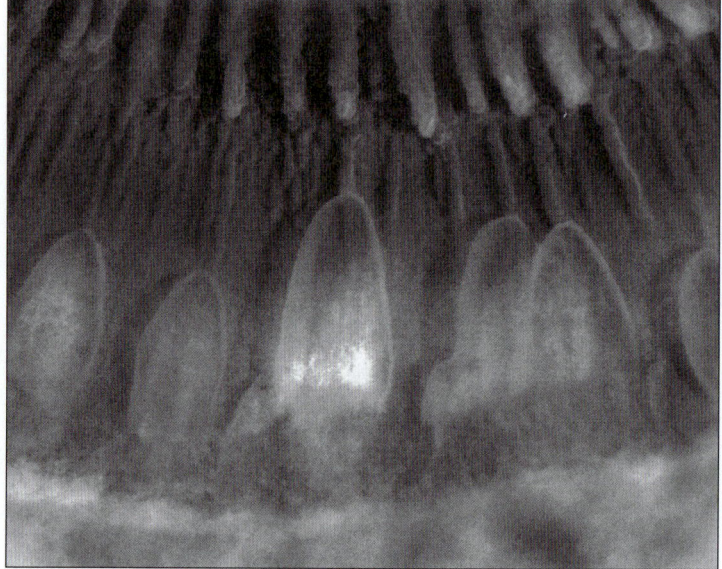

FIG. 134-4 ■ Pars plana cysts. The radial striations can also be seen directed between the ciliary processes. (Courtesy of Dr. Ralph Eagle, Jr.)

Pars Plana Cysts

Cysts of the pars plana corporis ciliaris are another variant seen in the fundus periphery.[10] These consist of a clear cystoid space between the pigmented and nonpigmented epithelium located anterior to the ora serrata (Fig. 134-4). The cysts, which have the appearance of half-inflated balloons, lie between the pars plana radiations. Generally, the overlying vitreous and its surrounding ciliary pigment epithelium remain unchanged. Occasionally, highly myopic patients demonstrate a marked degree of cyst formation along the entire pars plana.

Ora Serrata Pearls

Still another change that may be noted in the fundus periphery is the ora serrata pearl. This glistening opacity (Fig. 134-5), which usually forms over an oral tooth, varies from pinpoint to pinhead in size.[11] It appears in all age groups but increases significantly in incidence with advancing age.[12] Pearls are not related to other fundus pathology and are probably of developmental origin. They occur throughout the ora serrata region and

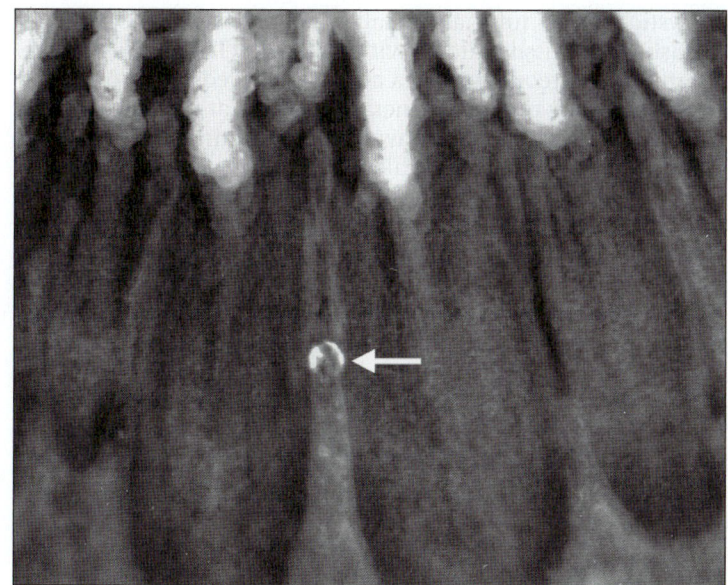

FIG. 134-5 ■ Ora serrata pearl *(arrow)*. The pearl lies on an oral tooth. Again, radial striations are directed between the ciliary processes.

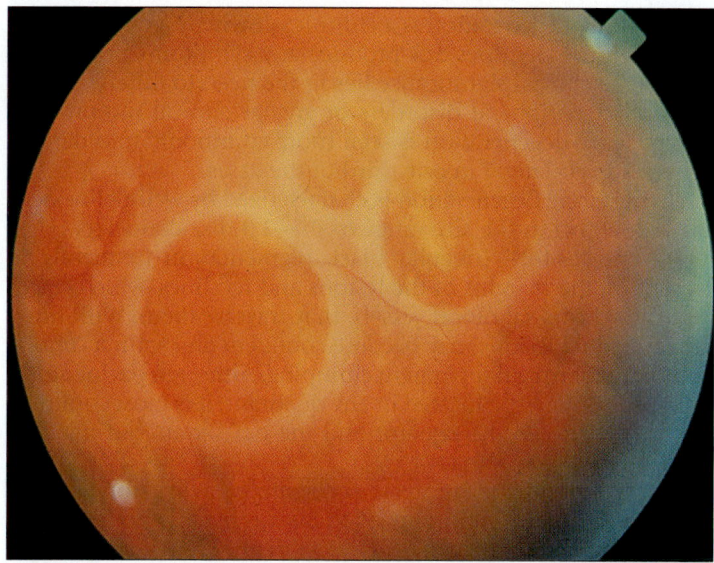

FIG. 134-6 ■ Multiple outer layer breaks. Over a 3-year period, this eye developed multiple outer layer breaks.

are drusen-like structures that, on pathological examination, show the staining qualities of an acid carbohydrate.

Degenerative Adult Retinoschisis

Degenerative retinoschisis, in most cases, is asymptomatic and has little clinical significance. However, in rare instances it can progress to retinal detachment. Types of retinoschisis that occur include:

- Degenerative (or adult acquired)
- X-linked
- Reticular
- Secondary

Several ocular diseases may show degrees of secondary retinoschisis; of these, diabetes, retinopathy of prematurity, and familial exudative vitreoretinopathy are three of the most important.[13]

Degenerative retinoschisis usually is bilateral, often symmetrical, and commonly bullous. It frequently first appears in the inferotemporal quadrant and may be slowly progressive.

Bullous types of retinoschisis appear clinically as thin, elevated layers of tissue, best observed in the inferotemporal periphery. The retinal vessels often are sheathed terminally, and fine white spots may occur on the inner surface. These represent the Müller fibers that traverse the schisis cavity.

Larger outer layer holes may develop over time, often with a rolled edge (Fig. 134-6). A small rim of fluid, located between the outer layer and the retinal pigment epithelium, occasionally may be present. Pigmented demarcation lines are not a clinical feature of bullous retinoschisis—if present, they usually indicate longstanding nonprogressive retinal detachment.

The major complication of retinoschisis is retinal detachment. In 987 patients with retinal detachment followed up by Pecold *et al.*,[14] retinoschisis was present in 25, an incidence of about 2.5%.

Retinal detachment occasionally may occur when holes exist in the outer layer of the schisis. In many cases inner layer holes also occur, but these need not be present for retinal detachment to develop. The detachment begins around the outer layer holes and may progress gradually to extend beyond the area of the retinoschisis, itself. In an advanced stage it may closely resemble a typical rhegmatogenous detachment secondary to vitreous traction.[15] When progression of the schisis toward the posterior pole extends posterior to the equator, perimetry reveals an ab-

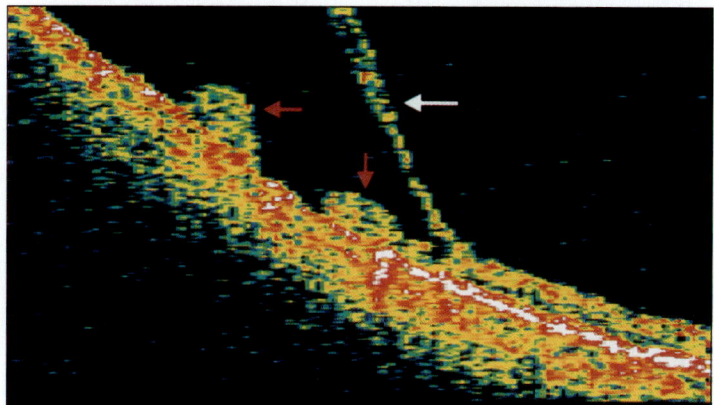

FIG. 134-7 ■ Optical coherence tomography picture showing elevated inner retinal layers *(white arrow)* and edges of outer retinal breaks *(red arrow)*.

solute field defect, whereas the defect associated with retinal detachment is relative.

Optical coherence tomography can be helpful, as well, in differentiating retinoschisis from retinal detachment.[16] Optical coherence tomography images of retinal detachment show separation of full-thickness neurosensory retina from the retinal pigment epithelium, while retinoschisis shows the splitting within the neurosensory retina (Fig. 134-7).

Byer[17] conducted a long-term natural history study of 123 consecutive, unselected patients (218 eyes) who had suffered acquired retinoschisis for from 1 to 21 years (average, 9.1 years), to ascertain the natural behavior and prognosis of this disease and formulate reasonable recommendations for its management. The quadrant of maximal involvement was the inferior temporal, and 74% of the lesions had postequatorial posterior borders. Most importantly, degenerative retinoschisis was found to be primarily asymptomatic and nonprogressive. No case of symptomatic progressive retinal detachment occurred, but 14 cases of localized, nonprogressive, and asymptomatic schisis–detachment were noted.

Byer[17] concludes that the only indication for treatment of a schisis is the symptomatic or progressive schisis–retinal detachment which threatens the macula. Laser demarcation of a schisis or treatment of the borders of outer layer retinal breaks should be avoided.[17,18]

Paving Stone Degeneration

Paving stone degeneration is a chronic, slowly progressive disorder which usually does not produce any symptoms or complications. Its clinical significance lies in the need to differentiate it from other peripheral disorders of greater clinical importance. Paving stone degeneration is seen more commonly in older patients and is bilateral in one third of the cases.[19]

Paving stone degeneration is characterized by well-delineated, flat yellow foci in the size range of 0.5–2.0 disc diameters (Figs. 134-2 and 134-8). Irregular black pigmentation frequently is present on the margins of the lesions and red lines, which correspond to choroidal blood vessels, may traverse them. With time, the individual lesions may become confluent and form a continuous band of irregular pigment clumping. Although paving stone degeneration may be located in any quadrant, it is most common inferiorly between the equator and the ora serrata but may extend into the pars plana.

Several fundus conditions may resemble paving stone degeneration. The most important of these are inactive toxoplasmic retinochoroiditis, lattice degeneration, retinal holes, and benign hypertrophy of the retinal pigment epithelium. Toxoplasmosis is more likely to show lesions of variable size and shape, with posterior pole involvement and overlying vitreous changes.

Lattice degeneration (see below) also occurs in the peripheral retina. In contrast to paving stone degeneration, it is more common superiorly and is more likely to be equatorial, rather than adjacent to the ora serrata.

Round retinal holes may resemble focal areas of paving stone degeneration. The yellow appearance of the latter condition, with its traversing blood vessels and absence of subretinal fluid, differentiate it from a retinal hole.

Benign hypertrophy of the retinal pigment epithelium usually is located more posteriorly in the fundus and typically is pigmented more diffusely and darkly. Lacunae may be present, but only in longstanding cases in which the pigment has disappeared would it resemble paving stone degeneration.

Paving stone degeneration does not increase the risk of retinal detachment and does not require prophylactic therapy.

Retinal Tufts

Retinal tufts can be classified into three types:
- Cystic retinal tuft
- Noncystic retinal tuft
- Traction tuft

Cystic retinal tufts are small, pyramid-like projections of whitish retinal tissue into the vitreous cavity. They almost always occur in the vitreous base area and are believed to be congenital in origin. Cystic retinal degeneration occurs at the base of tufts. Severe vitreous traction may avulse a cystic retinal tuft; this leads to a full-thickness retinal break.

Noncystic retinal tufts are smaller, acquired, and much more common. Up to three fourths of adults manifest one or more. These tufts look like small, pointed retinal bumps within the vitreous base, most commonly in the nasal quadrants. They do not increase the risk of retinal detachment.

Traction retinal tufts project more anteriorly into the vitreous cavity because of their creation by zonular traction. These also are believed to be congenital and occur more commonly nasally, but usually develop close to the ora serrata. Small retinal breaks can occur at their base, even in the absence of a posterior vitreous separation.

Lattice Degeneration

In contrast to the degenerations previously described, lattice degeneration has greater clinical significance.[20] It is especially important because of its relationship to rhegmatogenous retinal detachment.

Ophthalmoscopically, lattice degeneration appears as one or more linear bands of retinal thinning located in the equatorial region (Fig. 134-9). Fine white lines, which account for the term *lattice degeneration*, are present in only about 9% of lesions.[21] Pigmentary disturbances within the band of retinal thinning, however, are present in most cases. Lattice degeneration is more common superiorly and occurs less frequently near the inferior equator. It is considerably less common in the horizontal meridians. In most cases, the lesions of lattice degeneration are arranged parallel to the ora serrata.

More rarely, the lesions are orientated obliquely or even radially along retinal vessels, as in Stickler's syndrome (Fig. 134-10).

Lattice in myopic eyes may be influenced by axial elongation. Using "A" scan axial length measurement, the prevalence of lattice was greater in eyes without staphyloma in which the whole eye was elongated, versus eyes with staphyloma in which only the posterior pole was elongated.[21]

Biomicroscopy of the vitreous adjacent to lattice degeneration may reveal rather typical changes. The vitreous gel is attached

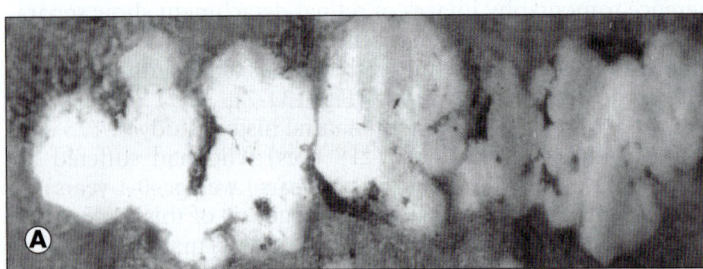
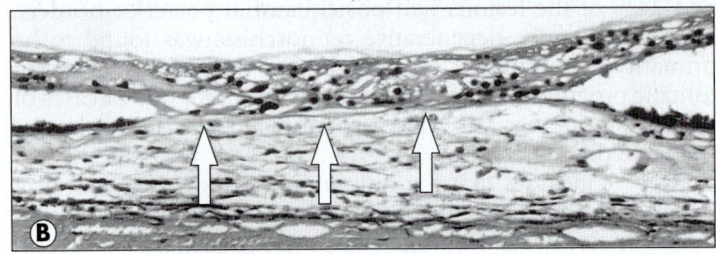

FIG. 134-8 ■ **Paving stone degeneration. A,** Clinical appearance. **B,** Light microscopy showing a chorioretinal adhesion to Bruch's membrane with no retinal pigment epithelium or choriocapillaris present. (Courtesy of Dr. Ralph Eagle, Jr.)

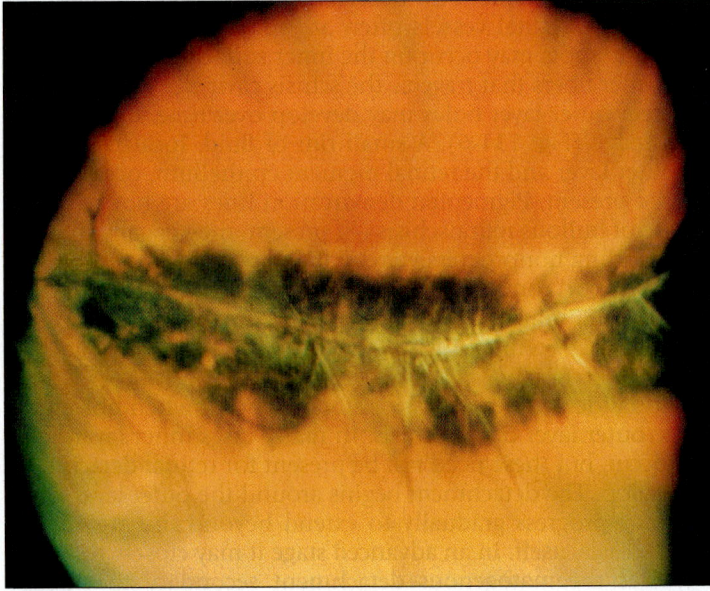

FIG. 134-9 ■ **Clinical picture of lattice degeneration showing the typical white lines.** These lines represent hyalinized vessels.

firmly to the margin of the lesion. Usually a clear pocket of liquid vitreous exists over the central thin portion of each lesion.

Retinal holes often can be observed in lattice degeneration. Two types of breaks have been recognized. Round or atrophic holes usually are found centrally within the thin portion of the lesion and usually are not associated with vitreous traction. These may lead to retinal detachment in young myopes. Horseshoe-shaped breaks occur most commonly on the posterior edge of the lesion and are associated with severe vitreous traction (Fig. 134-11). In many cases, multiple breaks of both types are present. Horseshoe breaks often lead to retinal detachment.[22]

Lattice degeneration of the retina is present in about 7–8% of adult eyes.[23–25] Burton[22] has shown that patients with lattice degeneration, between 40 and 60 years of age, and with low to moderate degrees of myopia tend to develop detachments caused by premature posterior vitreous separation and traction tears. However, he points out that prophylaxis for this group is not warranted, because only 5–10% will experience detachments during their lives. On the other hand, this study verified the previous suspicions that those with myopia exceeding −5.0D and lattice degeneration have an increased risk of detachment during their lives. Detachments in this group tend to cluster in the second, third, and fourth decades, typically are caused by atrophic holes, are slowly progressive, and often are simultaneously bilateral. Enhanced vigilance is certainly appropriate during this time, but prophylactic treatment would be no small task because, as Burton points out, within a population of 1 million persons there are about 1150 aged 10–39 years with myopia exceeding −5.0D and lattice degeneration. Only 4 detachments annually and 40 detachments in 10 years would be expected in this highest risk group.

In an evidence-based analysis of prophylactic treatment of asymptomatic retinal breaks and lattice degeneration, a panel of vitreoretinal experts reviewed the literature published in English.[26] They concluded that there was insufficient information to strongly support prophylactic treatment of lesions other than symptomatic flap tears.

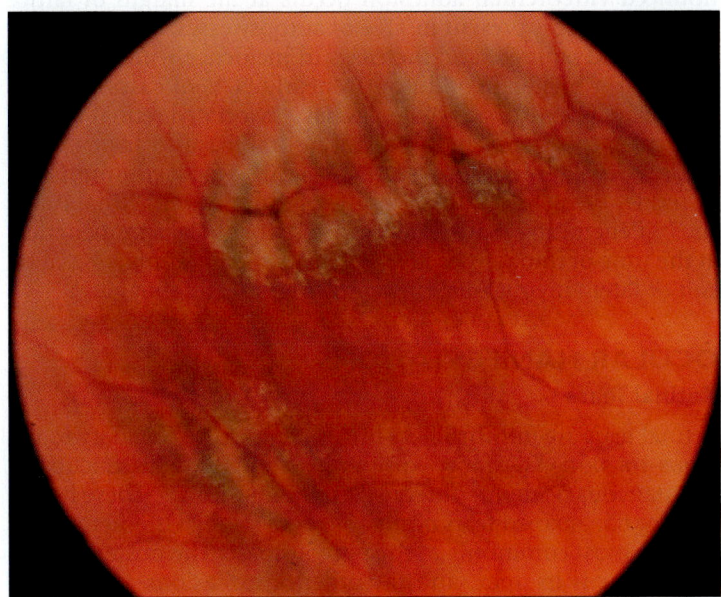

FIG. 134-10 ■ **Perivascular lattice in a patient with Stickler's syndrome.** Affected patients also have optically empty vitreous cavities, cataracts, glaucoma, loss of hearing, flattened facies, cleft palates, and arthritis.

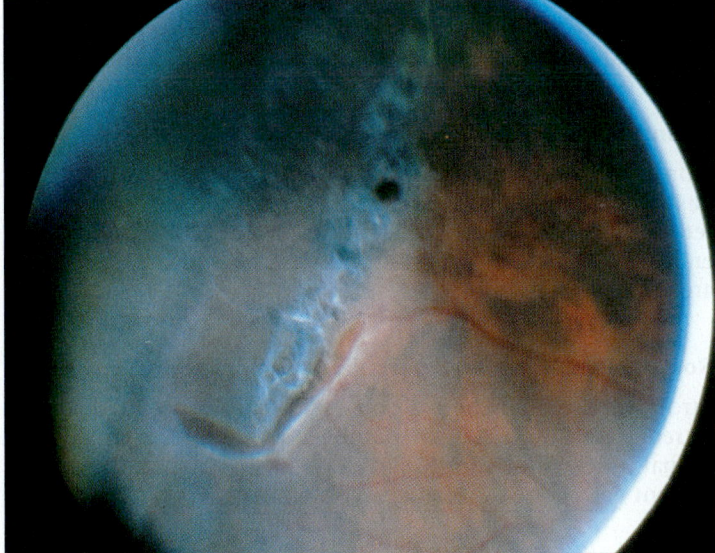

FIG. 134-11 ■ **Horseshoe tear on the posterior and inferior edge of lattice degeneration.**

REFERENCES

1. Rutnin U. Fundus appearance in normal eyes. I. The choroid. Am J Ophthalmol. 1967;64:821–39.
2. Foos RY. Vitreoretinal juncture: topographical variations. Invest Ophthalmol II. 1972;11:801–8.
3. Rutnin U, Schepens CL. Fundus appearance in normal eyes. II. The standard peripheral fundus and development variations. Am J Ophthalmol. 1967;64:840–52.
4. Maggiore L. L'ora serrata nell'occhilio uman. Ann Otol Rhinol Laryngol. 1924;53:625–723.
5. Salzmann M. The anatomy and history of the human eyeball in the normal state: its development and senescence. Chicago:1912.
6. Straatsma BR, Landers MB, Kreiger AE. The ora serrata in the adult human eye. Arch Ophthalmol. 1968;80:3–20.
7. Foos R. Vitreous base, retinal tufts, and retinal tears: pathogenic relationships. In: Pruett RC, Regan CDJ, eds. Retina Congress. New York: Appleton–Century–Crofts; 1974:259–80.
8. Spencer LM, Foos RY, Straatsma BM. Meridional folds, meridional complexes, and associated abnormalities of the peripheral retina. Am J Ophthalmol. 1970; 70:697–714.
9. Spencer LM, Foos RY, Straatsma BR. Enclosed bays of the ora serrata. Arch Ophthalmol. 1970;83:421–5.
10. Teng CC, Katzin HM. An anatomic study of the retina, part I. Nonpigmented epithelial cell proliferation and hole formation. Am J Ophthalmol. 1951;34:1237–40.
11. Rutnin U, Schepens CL. Fundus appearance in normal eyes, IV. Retinal breaks and other findings. Am J Ophthalmol. 1967;64:1063–78.
12. Lonn LI, Smith TR. Ora serrata pearls. Arch Ophthalmol. 1967;77:809–13.
13. Madjarov B, Hilton GF, Brinton DA, Lee SS. A new classification of the retinoschises. Retina. 1995;15(4):282–5.
14. Pecold K, Czaplicka E, Bernardczyk J. Retinoschisis vs. retinal detachment—diagnosis and treatment. Klin Oczna. 1993;95(1):32–4.
15. Hagler WS, Woldoff HS. Retinal detachment in relation to senile retinoschisis. Trans Am Acad Ophthalmol Otolaryngol. 1973;77:99–113.
16. Ip M, Garaza-Karren C, Duker JS, et al. Differentiation of degenerative retinoschisis from retinal detachment using optical coherence tomography. Ophthalmology. 1999;106(3):600–5.
17. Byer NE. Long-term natural history study of senile retinoschisis with implications for management. Ophthalmology. 1986;93(9):1127–37.
18. Clemens S, Busse H, Gerding H, Hoffmann P. Treatment guidelines in various stages of senile retinoschisis. Klin Monatsbl Augenheilkd. 1995;206(2):83–91.
19. O'Malley P, Allen RA, Straatsma BR, O'Malley CC. Paving stone degeneration of the retina. Arch Ophthalmol. 1965;73:169–82.
20. Straatsma BR, Zeegen PD, Foos RY, et al. Lattice degeneration of the retina. XXX Edward Jackson Memorial Lecture. Am J Ophthalmol. 1974;77:619–49.
21. Byer NE. Clinical study of lattice degeneration of the retina. Trans Am Acad Ophthalmol Otolaryngol. 1965;69:1064–77.
22. Burton TC. The influence of refractive error and lattice degeneration on the incidence of retinal detachment. Trans Am Ophthalmol Soc. 1989;87:143–55,155–7.
23. Yura T. The relationship between the types of axial elongation and the prevalence of lattice degeneration of the retina. Acta Ophthalmol Scand. 1998;76(1):90–5.
24. Tillery WV, Lucier AC. Round atrophic holes in lattice degeneration—an important cause of phakic retinal detachment. Trans Am Acad Ophthalmol Otolaryngol. 1976;81:509–18.
25. Byer NE. Lattice degeneration of the retina. Surv Ophthalmol. 1979;23:213–47.
26. Wilkinson CP. Evidence-based analysis of prophylactic treatment of asymptomatic retinal breaks and lattice degeneration. Ophthalmology. 2000;107(1):12–5.

135 Retinal Breaks

CRAIG M. GREVEN

DEFINITION
- A full-thickness defect in the neural retina.

KEY FEATURES
- A round, oval, or horseshoe-shaped defect.
- Typical location near the vitreous base, but can occur anywhere.
- Subcategories are holes, tears, or dialyses.

ASSOCIATED FEATURES
- Pigmented cells in the vitreous (tobacco dust).
- Vitreous traction.
- Vitreous hemorrhage.
- Pigmentary changes in the adjacent retina.
- Localized abnormal vitreoretinal interface (lattice degeneration).

INTRODUCTION

Retinal breaks are full-thickness defects in the neurosensory retina. Although they typically occur in the equatorial and ora serrata regions of the retina, such defects can develop more posteriorly. Peripheral retinal breaks alone do not cause loss of vision, but the associated conditions of vitreous hemorrhage and rhegmatogenous retinal detachment can culminate in severe visual loss. The first goal in the management of retinal breaks is to differentiate those that are not likely to cause severe visual sequelae from those that are more likely to lead to visual loss and retinal detachment. In this chapter the identification of "high-risk" retinal breaks is discussed and appropriate management strategies are suggested.

EPIDEMIOLOGY AND PATHOGENESIS

The pioneering works of ophthalmic giants such as deWecker, Leber, and Gonin pointed out the significance of retinal breaks in the pathophysiology of rhegmatogenous retinal detachment. The importance of prophylaxis of retinal breaks to help prevent detachments became popular after the introduction of the binocular indirect ophthalmoscope.

The incidence of retinal breaks at autopsy in individuals over 20 years of age is in the range 6–11%.[1,2] The prevalence of retinal breaks in clinical series of routine patients aged 10 years or more with no known antecedent ocular disease is in the range 6–14%.[3,4] The annual incidence of retinal detachment is approximately 12 per 100,000 population per year.[5,6] From these data, it is intuitive that the majority of retinal breaks do not lead to retinal detachment. Therefore, it has been the goal of clinicians to determine which breaks may benefit from prophylaxis.

The occurrence of retinal breaks is age dependent, with increasing incidence accompanying increasing age. However, no statistical difference exists between men and women in the incidence of retinal breaks.[1,3] The prevalence of retinal breaks in myopic eyes is similar to that in eyes of the general population, about 11%.[7] However, myopes account for 42% of all phakic retinal detachments, and, therefore, myopia is considered a risk factor for retinal breaks that lead to retinal detachment.[8]

Lattice degeneration of the retina is another risk factor for the development of a retinal break. Lattice degeneration is a condition in which peripheral retinal thinning is associated with liquefaction and separation of the overlying vitreous. A pronounced vitreoretinal adhesion occurs at the margin of lattice lesions. Lattice is present in 11% of autopsy cases, occurs equally in men and women, and increases in incidence with increasing age.[9] It is a bilateral condition in nearly 50% of cases, and approximately 25% of affected eyes have associated retinal breaks.

Ocular contusion and penetrating trauma also increase the risk for development of a retinal break. The most common type of retinal break after ocular contusion injuries is a retinal dialysis.[10,11] Penetrating trauma may cause retinal breaks immediately at the time of impact, because of direct retinal trauma, or as a result of later vitreous traction on the peripheral retina.

OCULAR MANIFESTATIONS

Retinal Tears

Retinal tears are full-thickness breaks that occur secondary to vitreous traction. The most common inciting vitreous traction is spontaneous posterior vitreous detachment (PVD). These horseshoe or flap-shaped tears occur at sites of strong vitreoretinal adhesion, most commonly at the vitreous base. The posterior edge of the tear is its apex, and the anterior extensions are its base (Figs. 135-1 and 135-2). Symptoms associated with acute retinal horseshoe tears include floaters secondary to vitreous debris (hemorrhage, retinal pigment epithelium cells) and flashes that result from persistent vitreous traction.

Firm vitreoretinal adhesions are present at the margins of lattice degeneration. When a PVD occurs, traction at the margin of the lattice degeneration can lead to retinal tears. These tears typically occur at the posterior margin or posterior lateral margin of a patch of lattice.

Round Holes with Opercula

Horseshoe or flap tears with persistent traction often avulse the base of the tear to leave a small, round defect in the neural retina with an overlying operculum of retinal tissue. This generally indicates complete relief of vitreoretinal traction in this area (Fig. 135-3).

Round Holes without Opercula (Atrophic Holes)

Atrophic holes in the retina occur secondary to retinal thinning. Vitreous traction is not the pathogenic mechanism of atrophic retinal holes. Although these can occur in isolation, they often present within areas of lattice degeneration.

Traumatic Retinal Breaks

Blunt trauma to the globe can induce many varieties of retinal breaks, which include horseshoe tears, retinal dialysis, and macu-

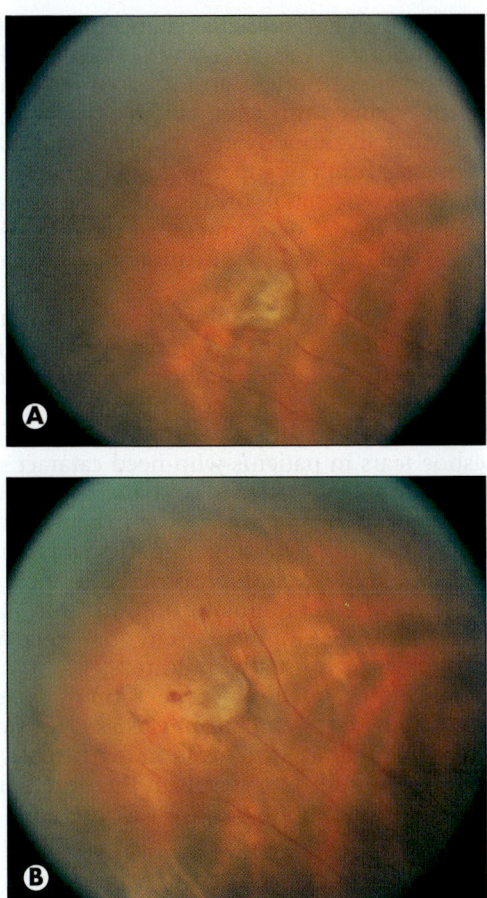

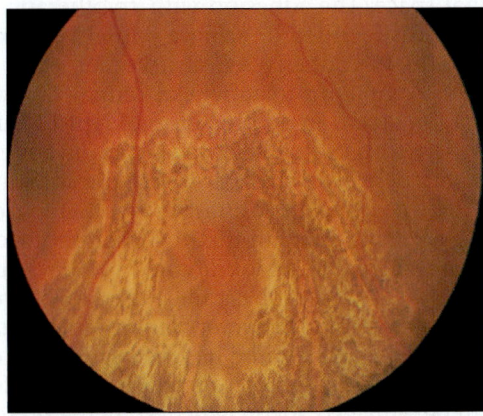

FIG. 135-1 ▮▮ Symptomatic acute, superotemporal horseshoe tear anterior to the equator in the right eye. **A,** At presentation. Note the hemorrhage at its margins. **B,** The same eye 1 week after cryopexy. Note the affectation of retinal pigment epithelium adjacent to the tear.

FIG. 135-2 ▮▮ Symptomatic inferior horseshoe tear 6 weeks after cryopexy.

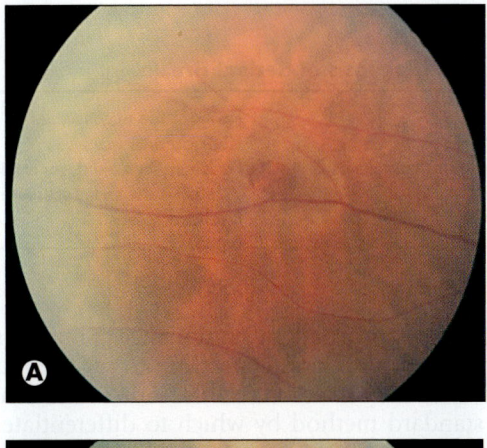

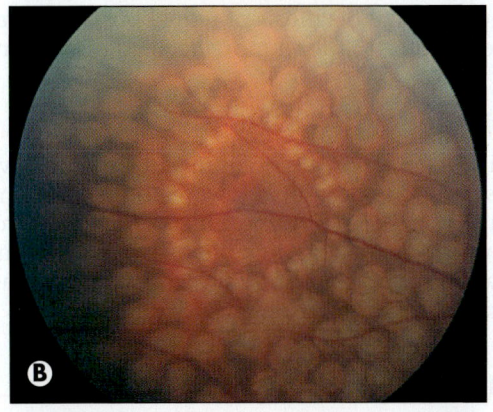

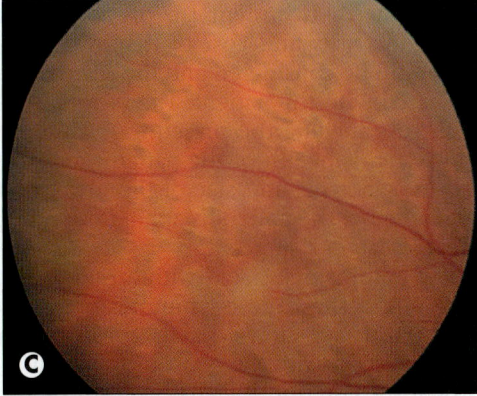

FIG. 135-3 ▮▮ Symptomatic operculated hole. **A,** At presentation. **B,** Immediately after laser treatment. **C,** 1 month postoperatively. Operculum is best seen in **C.**

Macular Breaks

Macular holes occur secondary to tangential traction on the retina from the precortical vitreous. They also are well-recognized sequelae of blunt trauma. A more complete discussion of macular holes is presented in Chapter 128.

DIAGNOSIS AND ANCILLARY TESTING

With clear media, the diagnosis of retinal break is straightforward. In the setting of cloudy media, ultrasonography helps to rule out associated retinal detachment. In some cases, experienced ultrasonographers are able to detect the presence of larger retinal breaks in attached retina when cloudy media prevents direct observation.

DIFFERENTIAL DIAGNOSIS

Many conditions exist in the peripheral fundus that can mimic full-thickness retinal breaks. Obstacles to an accurate diagnosis being made include inadequate pupillary dilatation, cataract, anterior and posterior capsular opacities in pseudophakic eyes,

lar holes. The major mechanism of peripheral break formation is hypothesized to be compression of the globe with subsequent distortion and expansion at the area of the ora serrata and equator. This expansion produces an acute increase in vitreoretinal traction, which often results in a retinal dialysis.[11] Traumatic retinal dialyses most commonly occur inferotemporally and superonasally.[12] They can occur at the anterior margin of the vitreous base in the pars plana, at the junction of the ciliary epithelium and neural retina, or in the retina at the posterior margin of the vitreous base. Occasionally, a "ribbon" of avulsed vitreous base is seen adjacent to a dialysis. This finding is considered diagnostic of previous trauma. Direct contusion injury to the globe can lead to disruption of the retina and necrotic breaks. The retinal defects are typically irregular and located in the region of the vitreous base.

vitreous opacities, and patient compliance. Binocular indirect ophthalmoscopy with scleral depression to see the retina in relief, supplemented by Goldmann three-mirror examination, remains the standard method by which to differentiate these lesions. The differential diagnosis of retinal breaks is given in Box 135-1. (See Chapter 134 for a more detailed discussion.)

SYSTEMIC ASSOCIATIONS

The majority of retinal breaks occur in patients who have no predisposing systemic association. However, certain systemic conditions, such as Marfan's syndrome, Ehlers-Danlos syndrome, and homocystinuria, as well as hereditary hyaloideoretinopathies such as Wagner's syndrome and Stickler's syndrome can predispose to retinal break formation (see Chapter 112).

TREATMENT

Upon the discovery of a retinal break, the initial decision is whether the benefits of treatment (to prevent retinal detachment) outweigh the risks and cost of treatment. In each case many factors should be considered and the risks and benefits of treatment discussed with the patient. The factors under consideration in each case include the presence or absence of symptoms; age and systemic health of the patient; refractive error of the eye; location, age, type, and size of the break; status of the fellow eye; and whether the patient is aphakic, pseudophakic, or will soon undergo cataract surgery.

The typical symptoms associated with an acute retinal break are new floaters and flashes. These symptoms occur secondary to an acute PVD. Studies have shown that the presence or absence of symptoms in association with the onset of the break is the most important prognostic criterion for progression to retinal detachment.[13,14] In a prospective follow-up study of 359 asymptomatic retinal breaks in 231 phakic eyes of 196 patients, no clinical retinal detachment had occurred after a minimum of 1 year follow-up.[13] Included in this study were 276 round atrophic holes, 50 tears with attached flaps, and 33 tears with free opercula. In phakic patients who have no previous history of retinal disease or of high myopia and who develop asymptomatic horseshoe tears, atrophic holes, or holes with opercula, prophylactic treatment is rarely indicated. In each case, the patient should be made aware of the symptoms of vitreous traction and retinal detachment and should be instructed on how to assess the peripheral visual field.

In contrast, the rate of retinal detachment in phakic patients who have symptomatic breaks is 35%.[14] Therefore, it is recommended that nearly all acute, symptomatic retinal breaks be treated prophylactically to prevent retinal detachment.

Age and systemic health status of the patient are other variables to be considered in the management of a retinal break. As an example, a superotemporal horseshoe tear in a 27-year-old patient is more likely to cause a subsequent retinal detachment than is one in an 80-year-old patient who has metastatic lung cancer.

Refractive error is another variable to consider in the management of retinal breaks. The increased incidence of retinal detachment in patients who have greater than 6D of myopia may increase the likelihood for treatment of an asymptomatic retinal tear.

The age, location, and size of a retinal break are also considered when its management is determined. Long-standing tears

often have retinal pigment epithelial changes adjacent to them. These changes indicate to the clinician the decreased likelihood of retinal detachment. Although no increased incidence of retinal detachment occurs with a retinal break in any particular quadrant, a greater likelihood of a macula-off retinal detachment is present as a result of superotemporal breaks than of either inferior breaks or nasal breaks. Although small retinal breaks can lead to retinal detachment, most ophthalmologists agree that in general larger breaks are more likely to cause a retinal detachment.

The type of break should also be a consideration in whether prophylactic treatment is offered. A horseshoe tear with persistent traction or a retinal dialysis is much more likely to result in a detachment than is an atrophic hole.

Some controversy exists about the management of asymptomatic horseshoe tears in patients who need cataract surgery, in aphakic or pseudophakic patients, and in patients who have retinal detachments in their fellow eye.[15,16] In general, because of the increased incidence of detachment in these scenarios, strong consideration should be given to prophylaxis in these cases.

Retinal dialyses, whether traumatic or idiopathic, have a high association with the development of retinal detachment. In these cases, prophylaxis is usually indicated.

Asymptomatic holes in lattice degeneration rarely lead to detachment and usually receive no prophylaxis.[17] However, retinal tears at the margin of lattice degeneration, particularly in symptomatic eyes, are more likely to result in the development of a retinal detachment and require prophylactic therapy.

Retinopexy

Two main modalities are utilized in the treatment of retinal breaks—cryopexy and laser photocoagulation. Cryotherapy is delivered transconjunctivally. It destroys the choriocapillaris, retinal pigment epithelium (RPE), and outer retina to provide a chorioretinal adhesion between the tear and the adjacent retina, which prevents liquid vitreous access through the hole and into the subretinal space. The adhesion with cryotherapy is not immediate; 1 week is required to achieve partial adhesion and up to 3 weeks for the full adhesive effects to occur.

Laser photocoagulation treatment of retinal breaks typically utilizes the argon green, argon blue-green, krypton red, or diode laser. No evidence exists that one wavelength is better than another. Two main delivery systems are used, the slit lamp and the indirect ophthalmoscope. In contrast to cryotherapy, chorioretinal adhesion occurs the instant that the laser photocoagulation is applied, but maximal adhesion occurs 7–10 days later.

Often, either of the techniques can be used for successful prophylaxis of retinal breaks. However, certain circumstances dictate which modality is easiest and has the best chance of success. Cryopexy has the advantage of not requiring a perfectly clear media; it can be delivered adequately despite the presence of extensive cataract, anterior or posterior capsular opacity, or relatively dense vitreous hemorrhage. Media opacity can make adequate treatment of retinal breaks by laser nearly impossible.

In general, retinal cryopexy and indirect ophthalmoscopic laser photocoagulation are preferred for anterior retinal breaks because of difficulty in treatment of the anterior margin at the slit lamp. Similarly, posterior breaks are difficult to reach with the cryoprobe unless a conjunctival incision is made. These breaks can be managed more easily with the slit lamp or an indirect laser delivery system. Occasionally, breaks with a large anteroposterior extent require both cryopexy to the anterior and photocoagulation to the posterior margins of the break.

Patients who have a retinal tear and no detachment may have an avulsed retinal vessel with persistent traction and recurrent vitreous hemorrhage. In these cases, scleral buckling or vitrectomy may be necessary to relieve traction and prevent further hemorrhage.[18]

Anesthesia

Eyes that undergo laser photocoagulation with the slit-lamp delivery system can often be treated with topical anesthesia alone. If multiple large breaks are present and the patient is unable to tolerate the treatment, retrobulbar anesthesia may facilitate completion of the procedure.

In patients treated with transconjunctival cryotherapy or indirect laser photocoagulation with scleral depression, topical anesthesia supplemented with cotton-tipped applicators soaked in 4% lidocaine (lignocaine) or 10% cocaine placed on the conjunctiva that overlies the retinal breaks is usually adequate. In some cases, 2% lidocaine injection subconjunctivally via a 30 gauge needle may be necessary. Approximately 0.2cm³ of anesthetic is necessary per quadrant.

Cryopexy

Under indirect ophthalmoscopic visualization, the cryoprobe is placed on the conjunctiva that overlies the break and cryotherapy is delivered until the retina adjacent to the tear becomes gray-white. Approximately 2mm of retinal whitening should be obtained around the entire break. Multiple applications are placed until the break is surrounded completely with confluent treatment (see Figs. 135-1 and 135-2). An attempt should be made not to treat the choroid and RPE directly beneath the break, especially in large tears, because of disruption and displacement of RPE cells into the vitreous cavity and concerns of macular pucker and proliferative vitreoretinopathy. In horseshoe tears, the anterior retina between the tear and the ora serrata should be treated, as anterior extension of the tear secondary to continuous vitreous traction can lead to retinal detachment.

Photocoagulation

The Goldmann three-mirror lens or panfundoscope lens is used when treatment is with the slit-lamp delivery system. The tear should be surrounded completely by three to four rows of laser burns. Although the spots need not be confluent, there should be no more than half a spot size of untreated retina between burns. Typically, the settings are 200–500μm spot size and 0.1–0.2 seconds application at the power necessary to generate a gray-white burn.

The indirect laser delivery system can also be used to treat retinal breaks. An advantage of this technique is that simultaneous scleral depression allows treatment of anterior tears and even dialysis.

As with cryopexy, care should be taken to treat thoroughly the anterior margin of horseshoe tears to prevent anterior traction that reopens the break.

COURSE AND OUTCOMES

The eye may be patched for a few hours after treatment. If a subconjunctival injection has been utilized, a topical antibiotic corticosteroid preparation may be used for the first 2–3 days. Subsequently, the eye is reexamined after approximately 7 days. Although vigorous patient activity is often discouraged initially, no clinical study has suggested that diminished activity improves treatment results. A firm chorioretinal adhesion is present by 3 weeks after either technique.

Failure rates for prophylactically treated retinal breaks depend on many factors, which include the type of retinal break, indications for treatment, length of follow-up, and definition of failure. Reported failure rates are in the range 0–22%.[19,20] In one large series of prophylactically treated retinal breaks, 22% of eyes required an additional procedure to prevent or repair a retinal detachment.[20] Retinal detachment occurred in 9% of treated eyes, 4% from the original break and 5% from a new retinal break. A new break without detachment or an inadequate chorioretinal adhesion around the original break that required additional treatment occurred in 14% of eyes. Risk factors for failure in this series included aphakic or pseudophakic status, acute symptoms, retinal detachment in the fellow eye, and male gender. Nearly 90% of eyes treated in this series had a final visual acuity of 20/50 (6/17) or better.

Epiretinal membrane and macular pucker are the most frequent visually significant complications associated with prophylactic treatment of a retinal break; they occur in 1–5% of treated eyes.[20,21] As epiretinal membranes occur in eyes that have retinal breaks and receive no treatment, it is not entirely clear whether the macular pucker is exacerbated by the treatment modality or is solely a result of the disease process itself.

Additional, more rare, complications that can occur include Adie's pupil, subretinal and vitreous hemorrhage, and breaks in Bruch's membrane. An exceedingly rare, but potentially devastating, complication in patients who have staphylomatous sclera and eyes treated with cryotherapy is scleral rupture.

In eyes that fail prophylactic therapy, retinal detachment repair by pneumatic retinopexy, scleral buckling, or vitrectomy is usually successful in the anatomical reattachment of the retina.

REFERENCES

1. Okun E. Gross and microscopic pathology in autopsy eyes. Part III. Retinal breaks without detachment. Am J Ophthalmol. 1961;51:369–91.
2. Foos RY, Allen RA. Retinal tears and lesser lesions of the peripheral retina in autopsy eyes. Am J Ophthalmol. 1967;64:643–55.
3. Byer NE. Clinical study of retinal breaks. Trans Am Acad Ophthalmol Otolaryngol. 1967;71:461–73.
4. Rutnin U, Schepens CL. Fundus appearance in normal eyes. IV. Retinal breaks and other findings. Am J Ophthalmol. 1967;64:1063–78.
5. Haiman MH, Burton TC, Brown CK. Epidemiology of retinal detachment. Arch Ophthalmol. 1982;100:289–92.
6. Wilkes SR, Beard CM, Kurland LT, et al. The incidence of retinal detachment in Rochester Minnesota, 1970–1978. Am J Ophthalmol. 1982;94:670–3.
7. Hyams SW, Neumann E. Peripheral retina in myopia with particular reference to retinal breaks. Br J Ophthalmol. 1969;53:300–6.
8. Ashrafadeh MT, Schepens CL, Elzeneiny II, et al. Aphakic and phakic retinal detachment. I. Preoperative findings. Arch Ophthalmol. 1973;89:476–83.
9. Straatsma BR, Zeegan PD, Foos RY, et al. Lattice degeneration of the retina. XXX Edward Jackson Memorial Lecture. Am J Ophthalmol. 1974;77:619–49.
10. Cox MS, Schepens CL, Freeman HM. Retinal detachment due to ocular contusion. Arch Ophthalmol. 1966;76:678–85.
11. Cox MS. Retinal breaks caused by blunt nonperforating trauma at the point of impact. Trans Am Ophthalmol. Soc. 1980;78:414–66.
12. Hagler WS, North AW. Retinal dialyses and retinal detachment. Arch Ophthalmol. 1968;79:376–88.
13. Byer NE. The natural history of asymptomatic retinal breaks. Ophthalmology. 1982;89:1033–9.
14. Davis MD. Natural history of retinal breaks without detachment. Arch Ophthalmol. 1974;92:183–94.
15. Benson WE, Grand MG, Okun E. Aphakic retinal detachments. Management of the fellow eye. Arch Ophthalmol. 1975;93:245–9.
16. McPherson A, O'Malley R, Beltangady SS. Management of the fellow eyes of patients with rhegmatogenous retinal detachment. Ophthalmology. 1981;88:922–34.
17. Byer NE. Long-term natural history of lattice degeneration of the retina. Ophthalmology. 1989;96:1396–402.
18. Robertson DM, Curtin VT, Norton EWD. Avulsed retinal vessels with retinal breaks. Arch Ophthalmol. 1971;85:669–72.
19. Morse PH, Scheie HG. Prophylactic cryoretinopexy of retinal breaks. Arch Ophthalmol. 1974;92:204–7.
20. Smiddy WE, Flynn HW, Nicholson DH, et al. Results and complications in treated retinal breaks. Am J Ophthalmol. 1991;112:623–31.
21. Robertson DM, Norton EWD. Long-term follow-up of treated retinal breaks. Am J Ophthalmol. 1973;75:395–404.

CHAPTER

136 Rhegmatogenous Retinal Detachment

CHARLES P. WILKINSON

DEFINITION
- A condition in which fluid from the vitreous cavity passes through a full-thickness retinal defect into the subretinal space to cause separation of the neural retina from the underlying retinal pigment epithelium (RPE).

KEY FEATURES
- Seen clinically as an elevation and separation of the neural retina from the underlying RPE.
- One or more retinal breaks (holes, tears, or dialyses).

ASSOCIATED FEATURES
- Vitreous liquefaction.
- Posterior vitreous detachment.
- Vitreoretinal traction.
- Vitreous cells (pigment and/or hemorrhage).
- Flashes (photopsia) and floaters.
- Scotoma corresponds to the area of retinal elevation.

FIG. 136-1 ■ **Classical pathogenesis of rhegmatogenous retinal detachment.** The detached vitreous gel has caused a retinal tear by exerting traction upon the retina at the site of a vitreoretinal adhesion. Liquid in the vitreous cavity passes through the break into the subretinal space.

INTRODUCTION

Rhegmatogenous retinal detachments are an important potential cause of reduced visual acuity, particularly in the subgroup of individuals who are predisposed to the development of retinal tears. Nearly all symptomatic rhegmatogenous retinal detachments progress to total blindness unless they are repaired successfully. Timely recognition of the symptoms and signs of retinal detachment is important to maximize the chances of a favorable surgical outcome and preserve visual acuity.

EPIDEMIOLOGY AND PATHOGENESIS

The essential requirements for a rhegmatogenous retinal detachment include a neural retinal break (rhegma = rent or rupture) and vitreous liquefaction sufficient to allow vitreous fluid to pass through the break into the subretinal space. The usual pathological sequence that results in retinal detachment is vitreous liquefaction followed by a posterior vitreous detachment (PVD), which in turn causes a retinal tear at the site of a significant vitreoretinal adhesion (Fig. 136-1). All ocular conditions that are associated with an increased prevalence of vitreous liquefaction and PVD or with an increased number or extent of vitreoretinal adhesions are associated with a higher incidence of retinal detachment.

Factors That Cause Retinal Detachment

The major factors associated with the development of retinal detachment include retinal breaks, vitreous liquefaction and de-

tachment, traction on the retina (vitreoretinal traction), and intraocular fluid currents associated with movement of liquid vitreous and subretinal fluid. The majority of eyes with retinal breaks do not develop retinal detachment because the physiological forces present are sufficient to hold the retina in place. Retinal attachment is usually maintained by[1]:
- An adhesive-like mucopolysaccharide in the subretinal space
- Oncotic pressure differences between the choroid and subretinal space
- Hydrostatic or hydraulic forces related to intraocular pressure
- Metabolic transfer of ions and fluid by the retinal pigment epithelium (RPE)

Retinal detachment occurs when the combination of factors that promote retinal detachment overwhelms the normal attachment forces.

RETINAL BREAKS. Retinal breaks are traditionally classified as holes, tears, or dialyses. Retinal holes are full-thickness retinal defects that are not associated with persistent vitreoretinal traction in their vicinity. They usually occur as a result of localized atrophic intraretinal abnormalities.

Retinal tears are usually produced by PVD and subsequent vitreoretinal traction at the site of a significant vitreoretinal ad-

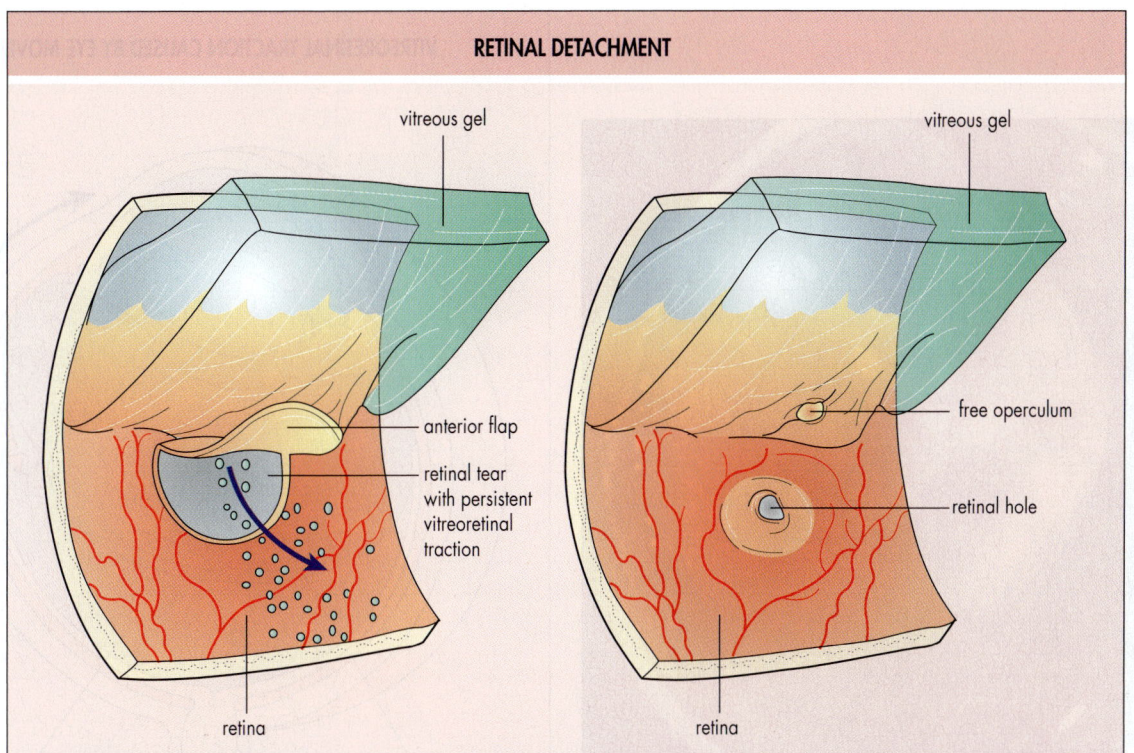

RETINAL DETACHMENT

vitreous gel

vitreous gel

anterior flap

free operculum

retinal tear with persistent vitreoretinal traction

retinal hole

retina

retina

FIG. 136-2 ▌▌ **Retinal detachment.** Retinal tears are due to vitreoretinal traction. Persistent traction frequently causes extensive retinal detachment (on left). If the traction results in a break that is not associated with persistent vitreoretinal traction (on right), the tear acts as a retinal hole and detachment is quite unlikely.

hesion (Figs. 136-1 and 136-2). Vitreous traction usually persists at the edge of a tear, which promotes progression of the retinal detachment.

Dialyses are linear retinal breaks that occur along the ora serrata. Although most are strongly associated with blunt ocular trauma, dialyses can occur spontaneously in certain individuals.

VITREOUS LIQUEFACTION AND DETACHMENT. Aging of the human vitreous (synchysis senilis) is characterized by liquefaction of the vitreous gel and the occurrence of progressively enlarging pools of fluid (lacunae) within the gel. These optically empty liquid spaces continue to coalesce as age advances; extensive liquefaction within the vitreous cavity leads to a reduction in both the shock-absorbing capabilities and the stability of the gel. Accelerated vitreous liquefaction is associated with significant myopia, surgical and nonsurgical trauma, intraocular inflammation, and a variety of other congenital, inherited, or acquired ocular disorders.

Posterior vitreous detachment, routinely termed PVD, usually occurs as an acute event after significant liquefaction of the vitreous gel. The precipitating event is probably a break in the posterior cortical vitreous in the region of the macula.[2] This is followed by the immediate passage of intravitreal fluid into the space between the cortical vitreous and retina (Fig. 136-3). Characteristically, this rapid movement of fluid and the associated collapse of the remaining structure of the gel result in extensive separation of the vitreous gel and retina posterior to the vitreous base, especially in the superior quadrants. Partial PVDs usually progress rapidly (within days) to become complete (Fig. 136-4).

TRACTION ON THE RETINA. Vitreoretinal traction has a number of causes, which range from simple action of gravitational force on the vitreous gel to prominent transvitreal fibrocellular membranes. Gravitational force is important and probably accounts for the high percentage of superior retinal tears (80%). However, rotational eye movements, which exert strong forces on all vitreoretinal adhesions, are probably more important causes of ongoing vitreoretinal traction.[3] When the eye rotates, the inertia of the detached vitreous gel causes it to lag behind the rota-

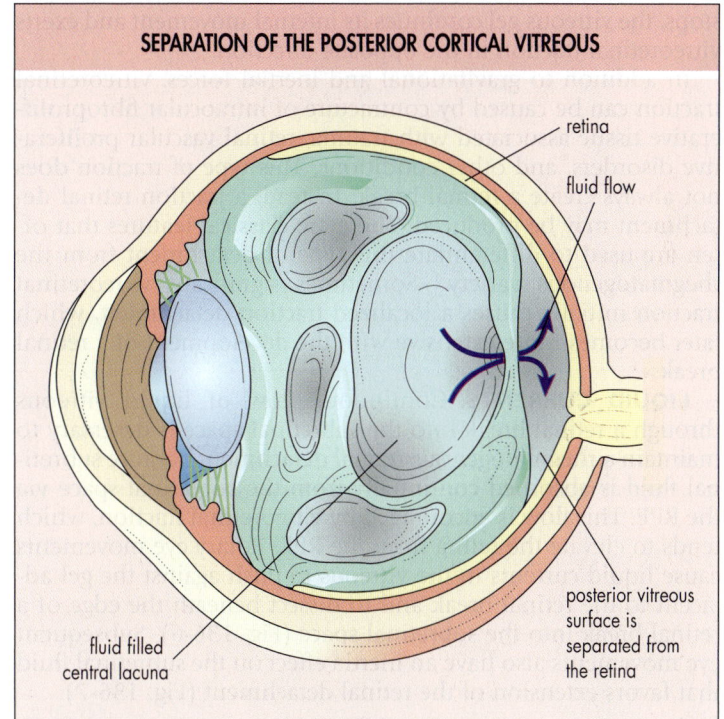

SEPARATION OF THE POSTERIOR CORTICAL VITREOUS

retina

fluid flow

posterior vitreous surface is separated from the retina

fluid filled central lacuna

FIG. 136-3 ▌▌ **Separation of the posterior cortical vitreous.** An acute event, posterior vitreous detachment usually begins with an apparent break in the cortical vitreous that overlies the macula. Fluid from a central lacuna flows through this hole and separates the cortical vitreous from the retina.

tion of the eye wall and, therefore, the attached retina. The retina at the site of a vitreoretinal adhesion exerts force on the vitreous gel, which causes the adjacent vitreous to rotate. The vitreous gel, because of its inertia, exerts an equal and opposite force on the retina, which can cause a retinal break or separate the neural retina farther from the pigment epithelium if subretinal fluid is already present (Fig. 136-5). When the rotational eye movement

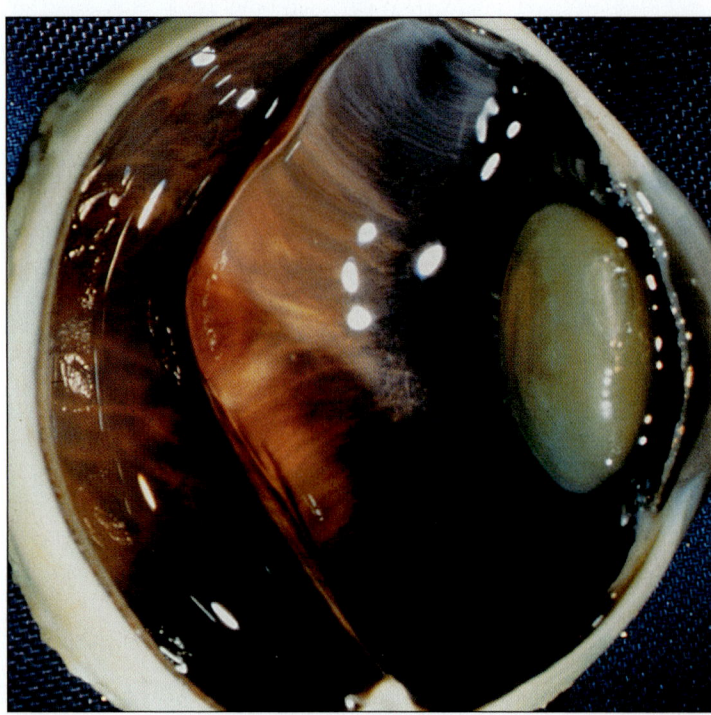

FIG. 136-4 ■ **Gross pathological appearance of a total posterior vitreous detachment.** The cortical vitreous has separated from the retina except at the vitreous base. (Courtesy of W. Richard Green, MD.)

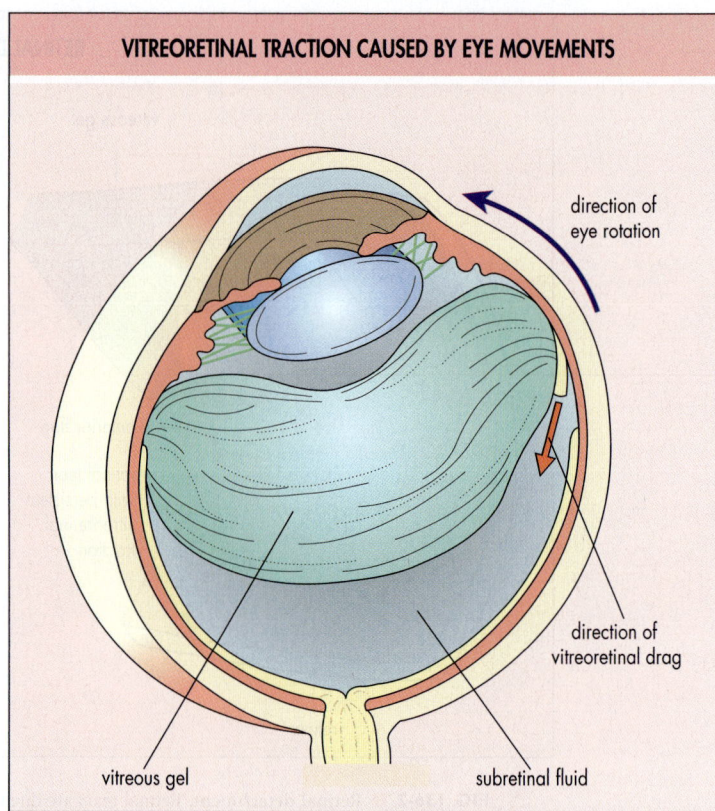

VITREORETINAL TRACTION CAUSED BY EYE MOVEMENTS

direction of eye rotation

direction of vitreoretinal drag

vitreous gel

subretinal fluid

FIG. 136-5 ■ **Vitreoretinal traction caused by eye movements.** When the eye rotates, the inertia of the vitreous gel causes it to lag behind the eye movement, which effectively causes vitreoretinal traction ("drag") in the opposite direction and the production of a retinal tear.

stops, the vitreous gel continues its internal movement and exerts vitreoretinal traction in the opposite direction.

In addition to gravitational and inertial forces, vitreoretinal traction can be caused by contracture of intraocular fibroproliferative tissue associated with trauma, retinal vascular proliferative disorders, and other conditions. This type of traction does not always create a retinal break. Instead, a traction retinal detachment may be produced. There are classical features that often are used to differentiate this type of detachment from the rhegmatogenous variety.[4] Sometimes significant vitreoretinal traction initially causes a localized traction detachment, which later becomes more extensive with the development of a retinal break.

LIQUID CURRENTS. Continuous flow of liquid vitreous through a retinal break into the subretinal space is necessary to maintain a rhegmatogenous retinal detachment because subretinal fluid is absorbed continually from the subretinal space via the RPE. This flow is encouraged by vitreoretinal traction, which tends to elevate the retina from the RPE. Rotary eye movements cause liquid currents in the vitreous to push against the gel adjacent to the retinal break and to dissect beneath the edge of a retinal break into the subretinal space (Fig. 136-6). Subsequent eye movements also have an inertia effect on the subretinal fluid that favors extension of the retinal detachment (Fig. 136-7).

Conditions That Predispose an Eye to Retinal Detachment

Retinal detachments are relatively unusual in the general population—the accepted annual incidence figure is approximately 1:10,000.[5] However, a variety of ocular and systemic disorders are associated with pathological vitreous liquefaction, premature vitreous detachment, and extensive sites of vitreoretinal adhesion. These conditions, therefore, are also associated with increased chances of retinal detachment. Particularly important predisposing entities include high myopia, pseudophakia and aphakia, blunt and penetrating ocular trauma, and cytomegalovirus retinitis associated with acquired immunodeficiency syndrome.

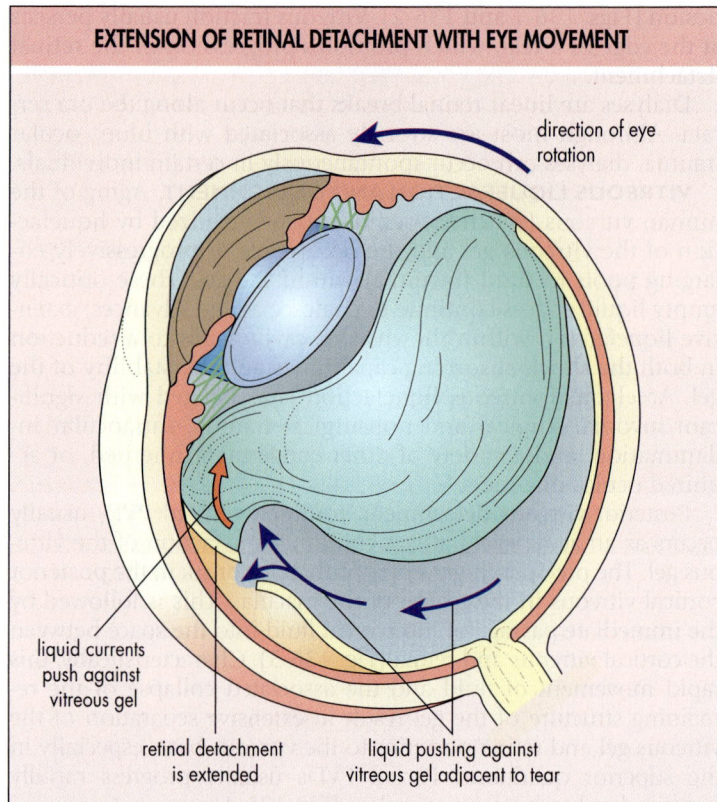

EXTENSION OF RETINAL DETACHMENT WITH EYE MOVEMENT

direction of eye rotation

liquid currents push against vitreous gel

retinal detachment is extended

liquid pushing against vitreous gel adjacent to tear

FIG. 136-6 ■ **Extension of retinal detachment associated with eye movements.** Rotary eye movement causes movement of the vitreous gel, which increases traction upon the retinal break. In addition, liquid currents dissect beneath the edge of the retinal tear and push against the vitreous gel adjacent to the tear. All three factors promote extension of the retinal detachment.

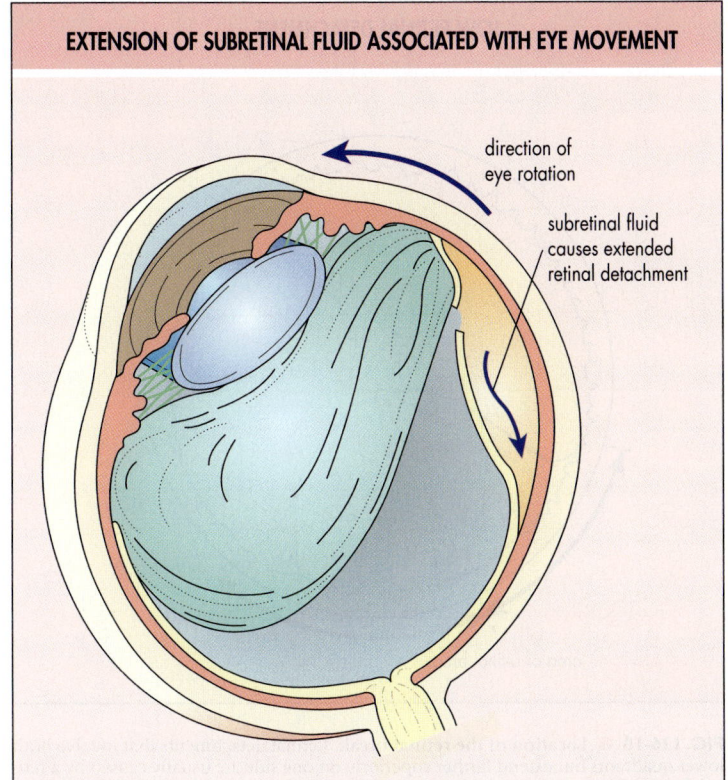

EXTENSION OF SUBRETINAL FLUID ASSOCIATED WITH EYE MOVEMENT

direction of eye rotation

subretinal fluid causes extended retinal detachment

FIG. 136-7 ■ **Extension of subretinal fluid associated with eye movements.** In addition to exacerbating vitreoretinal traction, rotary eye movement has an inertia effect upon subretinal fluid that causes it to dissect further between the retina and pigment epithelium.

Although cataract surgery has been performed on only approximately 3% of the general population, up to 40% of eyes with retinal detachment have had prior cataract surgery.[6] Retinal detachment represents the most significant potential postsurgical complication of cataract surgery, as it occurs in nearly 1% of pseudophakic eyes.[7] Removal of the natural lens is believed to increase the risk of retinal detachment because of its effect on vitreous liquefaction and subsequent premature PVD.[8] The status of the posterior capsule determines the rapidity of vitreous liquefaction. It is clear that opening the posterior capsule, either surgically or with a neodymium:yttrium-aluminum-garnet laser, significantly increases the incidence of retinal detachment.[9]

High myopia (>6.0D myopia) is associated with at least a threefold increased incidence of retinal detachment.[10] Severe ocular trauma is believed to be responsible for 10–15% of retinal detachments, and up to 50% of patients who have a diagnosis of cytomegalovirus retinitis develop a rhegmatogenous retinal detachment within 1 year.[11]

Risk factors for retinal detachment are not mutually exclusive and may be additive. For example, prior cataract extraction and nonsurgical trauma are more likely to be complicated by retinal detachment in myopic eyes. Pathological vitreoretinal changes often occur bilaterally—patients who have a retinal detachment in one eye usually have a substantially increased risk of retinal detachment in the fellow eye, provided that additional acquired risk factors are comparable.

OCULAR MANIFESTATIONS

The early symptoms of acute retinal detachment are the same as those of acute PVD—the sudden onset of tiny dark floating objects, frequently associated with photopsia (flashes). Photopsia flashes are usually brief, in the temporal visual field, and are best seen in the dark immediately following eye movement. Loss of visual field does not occur until sufficient fluid has passed through the retinal break(s) to cause a retinal detachment pos-

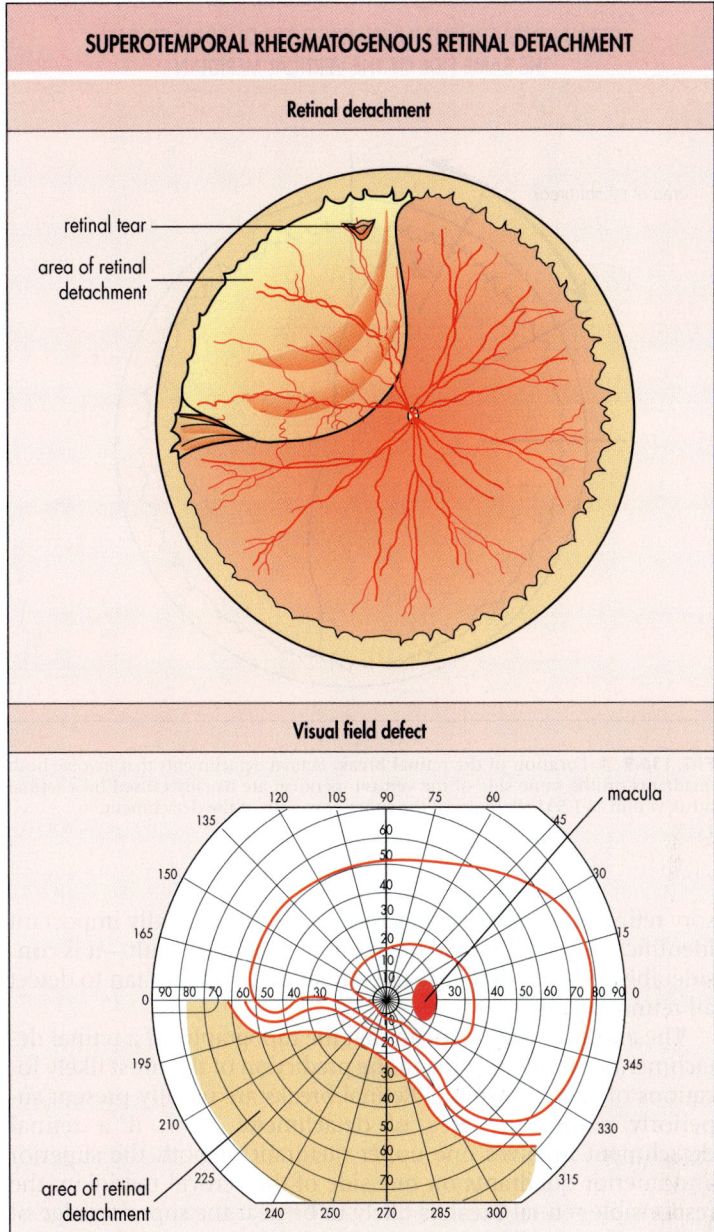

SUPEROTEMPORAL RHEGMATOGENOUS RETINAL DETACHMENT

Retinal detachment

retinal tear

area of retinal detachment

Visual field defect

macula

area of retinal detachment

FIG. 136-8 ■ **Superotemporal rhegmatogenous retinal detachment.** The neural retina is elevated in the area of detachment and the macula remains uninvolved. Visual field defect associated with retinal detachment shows that peripheral vision is lost inferonasally, corresponding to the area of detachment. The visual defect is an inverted image of the retinal detachment.

terior to the equator. Retinal detachments with a relatively small amount of subretinal fluid (less than two disc diameters from the break) are often not accompanied by visual field loss; these are termed subclinical detachments. Rarely, but especially in young female myopes, asymptomatic retinal detachment can occur. This is most common inferiorly and usually occurs as a result of atrophic holes in lattice degeneration.[12]

The vast majority of retinal breaks are located at the equator or more anteriorly; subretinal fluid initially accumulates in the retinal periphery, where it causes a corresponding loss of peripheral vision in the area that is related inversely to the location of the retinal detachment (Fig. 136-8). The loss of peripheral vision (a "curtain effect") increases as the detachment enlarges; central visual acuity is lost when subretinal fluid passes beneath the macula. Frequently, patients do not notice any symptoms until the macula becomes involved.

Retinal breaks associated with small amounts of subretinal fluid are difficult to detect; however, the diagnosis becomes more obvious as the retinal detachment increases in size. A stereoscopic vitreoretinal examination typically reveals an elevated sen-

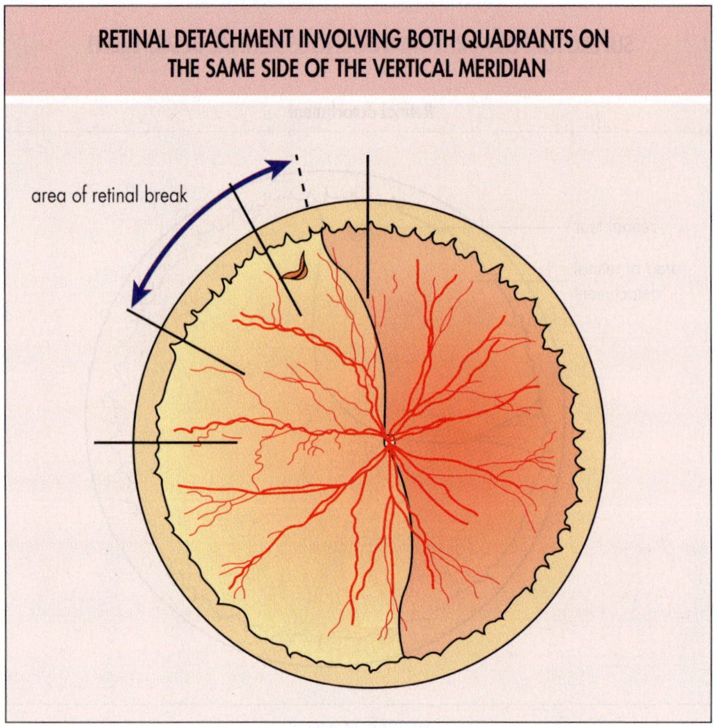

RETINAL DETACHMENT INVOLVING BOTH QUADRANTS ON THE SAME SIDE OF THE VERTICAL MERIDIAN

area of retinal break

FIG. 136-9 ■ **Location of the retinal break.** Retinal detachments that involve both quadrants on the same side of the vertical meridian are usually caused by a retinal break within 1–1.5 clock hours of the superior margin of the detachment.

LOW RETINAL DETACHMENT

area of retinal break

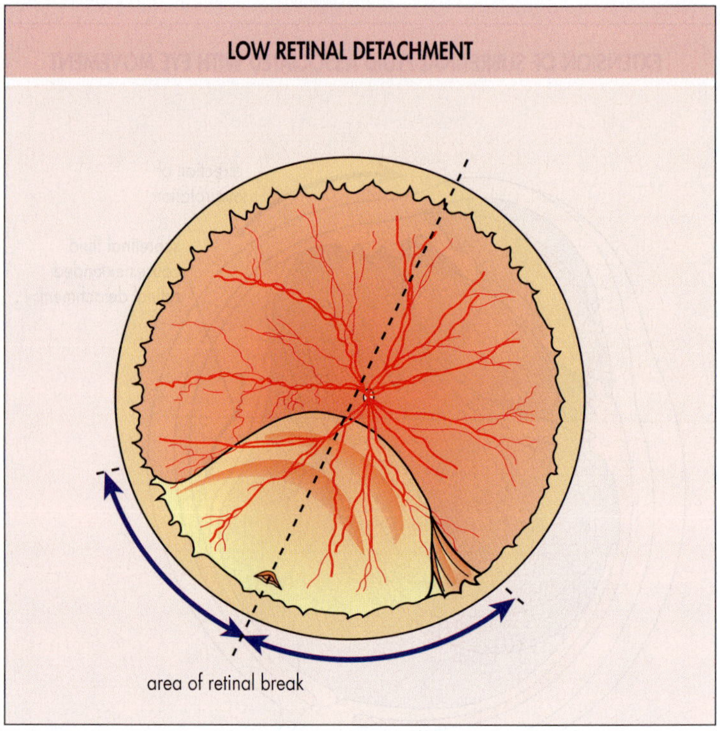

FIG. 136-10 ■ **Location of the retinal break.** Retinal detachments that involve both lower quadrants but extend farther superiorly on one side are usually caused by a retinal break within 1–1.5 clock hours of the superior margin of the retinal detachment or by a break in a meridian that bisects the margins of the retinal detachment.

sory retina in the area of detachment, but the critically important identification of all retinal breaks may remain difficult—it is considerably easier to diagnose the retinal detachment than to detect all retinal breaks.

The effects of gravity mean that the topography of a retinal detachment is of major value in the prediction of the most likely locations of retinal breaks.[13] Retinal breaks are usually present superiorly within the area of detachment. Thus, if a retinal detachment involves one upper quadrant or both the superior and inferior quadrants on one side of the vertical meridian, the responsible retinal break is likely to be near the superior edge of the detachment (Fig. 136-9). Retinal detachments that involve the inferior quadrants tend to follow the same rules, but the progression of the detachment is often much slower, and symmetrical spread of subretinal fluid may occur on both sides of the break. Therefore, detachments that involve one or both inferior quadrants may have a break near the superior margin of the detachment or in the meridian that bisects the area of detachment (Fig. 136-10). Nevertheless, because multiple retinal breaks are common, the entire periphery of the detached retina must be meticulously examined.

DIAGNOSIS

If the retina can be visualized well, the diagnosis of rhegmatogenous retinal detachment is made on the basis of clinical examination. In eyes with opaque media, the presence of a retinal detachment is usually determined ultrasonographically; the location and identification of the causative retinal breaks are based upon the configuration of the detachment as well as on the patient's history and associated findings.

The vast majority of retinal detachments are diagnosed easily with a binocular stereoscopic evaluation of the entire retina. Areas of retinal detachment are recognized by elevation of the neural retina from the RPE and loss of pigment epithelial and choroidal detail beneath the elevated retina (Fig. 136-11). Retinal breaks are also discovered by direct visualization. Indentation of the peripheral retina (scleral depression) is employed to visualize the entire anterior retina and to view the

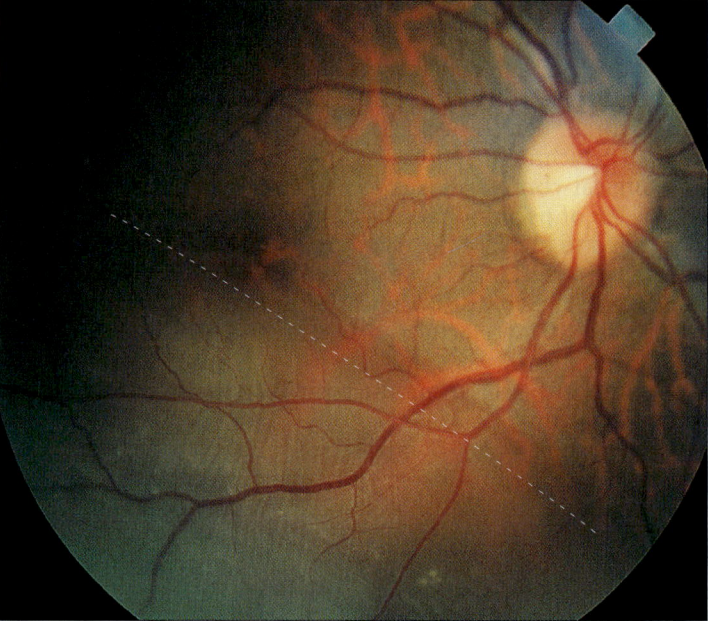

FIG. 136-11 ■ **Rhegmatogenous retinal detachment.** The inferior temporal portion of the retina is detached and the subretinal fluid makes visualization of the pigment epithelium and choroid relatively difficult.

retinal surface at different angles, which facilitates the identification of full-thickness retinal defects.

DIFFERENTIAL DIAGNOSIS

Retinal detachments that occur as a result of retinal breaks must be distinguished from several conditions in which retinal blood vessels are clearly separated from the pigment epithelium. These include retinal detachments from other causes and retinoschisis (see Box 136-1). Choroidal lesions that elevate the overlying retina and intravitreal pathology that simulates an elevated retina may also be confused with retinal detachment.

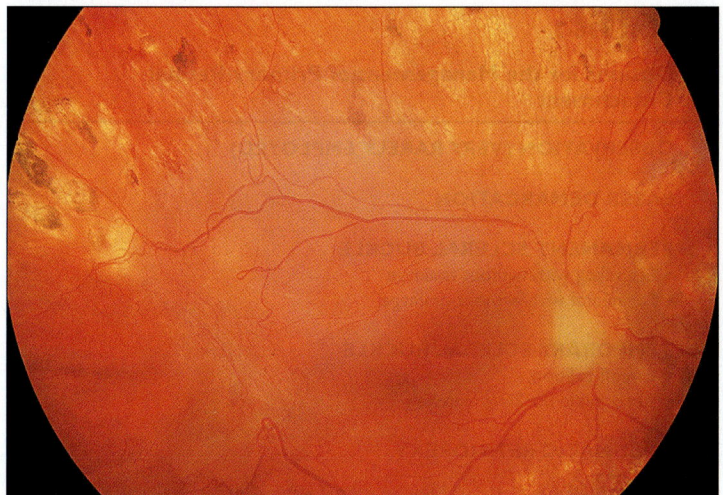

FIG. 136-12 ▪▪ **Traction retinal detachment.** The central area of retinal elevation is localized and due to areas of visible vitreoretinal traction associated with proliferative diabetic retinopathy.

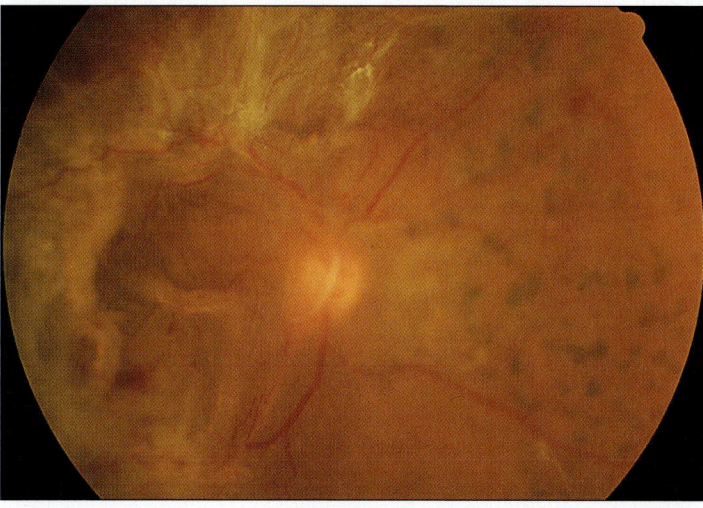

FIG. 136-13 ▪▪ **Combined retinal detachment.** Vitreoretinal traction associated with proliferative diabetic retinopathy has caused a tiny retinal break; the area of retinal elevation is more extensive and more convex than usually found in a pure traction detachment.

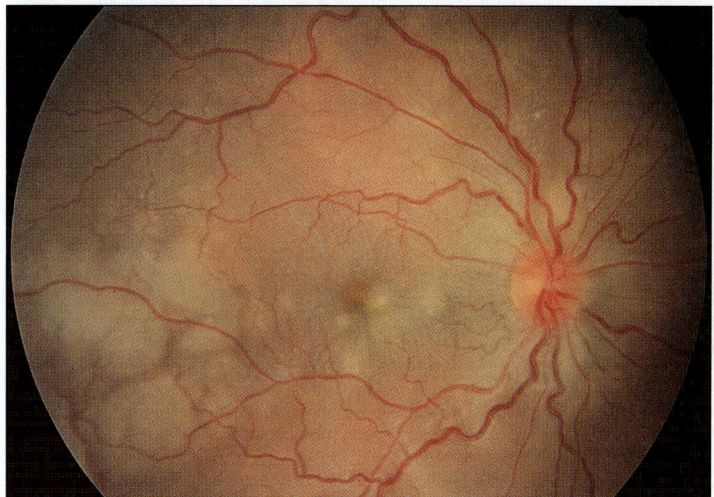

FIG. 136-14 ▪▪ **Exudative retinal detachment.** The small amounts of subretinal fluid (note the retinal striae) are due to leakage from an inflammatory process that involves the choroid and retinal pigment epithelium.

BOX 136-1

Differential Diagnosis of Rhegmatogenous Retinal Detachment

TRACTION RETINAL DETACHMENT
• Proliferative diabetic and other retinopathies
• Following penetrating trauma

EXUDATIVE RETINAL DETACHMENT
• Inflammatory disorders
• Choroidal neoplasms
• Retinal vascular tumors and other disorders

RETINOSCHISIS
• Age-related
• Congenital sex-linked

ELEVATED CHOROIDAL LESIONS
• Choroidal detachments
• Choroidal tumors

INTRAVITREAL OPTICAL ILLUSIONS
• Vitreous hemorrhage

The distinction between different types of retinal detachment can be difficult to make in eyes with small or undetectable retinal breaks and features associated with intraocular proliferation or exudation. In some cases, both a rhegmatogenous and a traction or exudative component may be important in the pathogenesis of the detachment. This is particularly common in eyes with proliferative diabetic retinopathy and retinal detachment. Pure traction detachments usually have a concave surface, and the shape, location, and extent of the detachment can be accounted for by the evident vitreous traction (see Fig. 136-12). Diabetic retinal detachments with a rhegmatogenous component are usually more extensive and often have a convex contour (see Fig. 136-13). Exudative detachments from a variety of causes are characterized by shifting subretinal fluid, which assumes a dependent position beneath the retina. In most cases, the fluid is located inferiorly and its source within or beneath the retina is apparent (see Fig. 136-14).

SYSTEMIC ASSOCIATIONS

A variety of systemic disorders are associated with rhegmatogenous retinal detachment. In the most important situations, the ocular disorder is either an additional manifestation of a hereditary systemic abnormality (usually an inherited disorder of collagen) or the result of complications of a systemic disease. The most important entity in the former group is Stickler's syndrome, in which a predisposition to retinal detachment is associated with a variety of facial and skeletal abnormalities. The most important systemic diseases associated with the complication of retinal detachment are diabetes mellitus and acquired immunodeficiency syndrome.

PATHOLOGY

The initial research of Jules Gonin,[14] which culminated in a proven pathogenesis and therapy of retinal detachment, was devoted to the pathological examination of eyes with this disorder. Retinal breaks, liquefaction and collapse of the vitreous gel, and visible vitreoretinal adhesions were all well documented prior to the first surgical cure. Nutrition of the outer retina is lost during retinal detachment, so the first visible pathological retinal changes occur in the outer segments of the photoreceptors.[15] Long-standing retinal detachments are associated with further atrophy of the photoreceptor layer and cystic degeneration within the retina (Fig. 136-15).[16] The vitreous macromolecular changes that result in liquefaction of the gel have not been identified.

Successfully repaired retinal detachments show a variety of histopathological abnormalities. There is a high incidence of epiretinal membrane formation (76%).[17] Cystoid macular

987

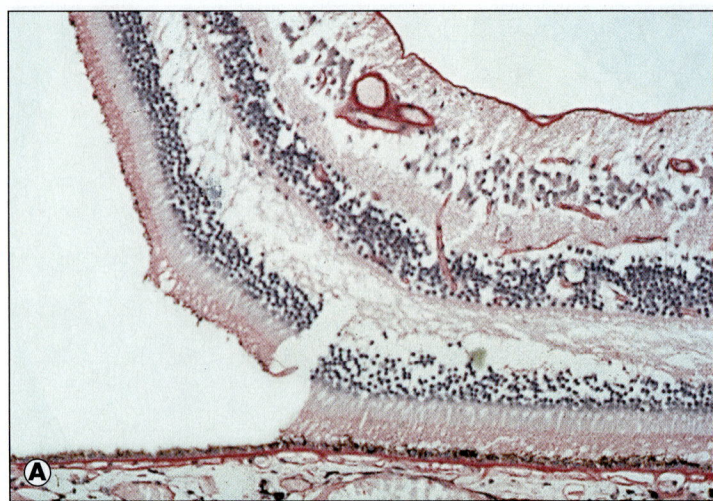

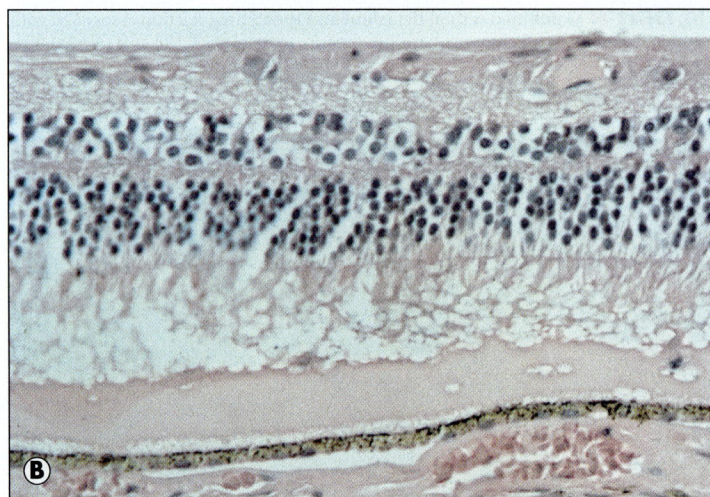

FIG. 136-15 ■ **Retinal detachment. A,** An artifactitious neural retinal detachment shows no fluid in the subneural retinal space, pigment adherent to the tips of the photoreceptors, and good preservation of the normal retinal architecture in all layers. **B,** A true retinal detachment shows material in the subneural retinal spaces and degeneration of the outer retinal layers. (From Yanoff MS, Fine S, eds: Ocular pathology, ed 5. Philadelphia: 2002; WB Saunders.)

edema (10%) is common as well, along with significant photoreceptor atrophy in about 27% of eyes.

TREATMENT

The aim of retinal detachment therapy is to counter the factors and forces that cause retinal detachment and to reestablish the physiological conditions that normally maintain contact between the neural retina and pigment epithelium. The main goal of surgery (i.e., to close each retinal break) usually is sufficient to reattach the retina. Long-term closure of retinal breaks also may require permanent reduction or elimination of vitreoretinal traction, accompanied by maneuvers designed to offset the harmful effects of fluid currents in the vitreous cavity.

At present, most retinal surgeons use scleral buckling techniques and the creation of a chorioretinal adhesion around each break to eliminate and counteract vitreoretinal traction.[18] These procedures are discussed in Chapter 103. Vitrectomy techniques are performed in selected cases; these are discussed in Chapter 104. Contemporary options in the management of primary rhegmatogenous retinal detachment are given in Box 136-2, and one of these (pneumatic retinopexy) has become more popular in the past few years.[19]

COURSE AND OUTCOME

Rhegmatogenous retinal detachment was an essentially incurable disorder until approximately 80 years ago. Surgical success

rates have now improved to such a degree that, with one or more surgical procedures, approximately 95% of all retinal detachments can be successfully repaired (i.e., the retina is returned to its normal anatomical position with no residual subretinal fluid). The two most common reasons for failure of retinal detachment surgery are:
- Failure to identify and/or close all retinal breaks
- Proliferative vitreoretinopathy

Unfortunately, visual results after anatomically successful surgery do not necessarily reflect this high rate of success.

Postoperative visual acuity is most dependent upon the extent of damage to the macula caused by the retinal detachment. If the macula becomes detached by subretinal fluid, some degree of permanent damage to vision usually occurs in spite of surgical reattachment. In eyes with no macular detachment present, 85% can be expected to have 20/40 vision or better. Conversely, about 10% of eyes with normal or near-normal vision undergo visual loss after successful repair of a macula-sparing detachment.[20] Of eyes with macular detachment, only 50% have 20/40 vision or better. Of those with preoperative visual acuity worse than 20/200, fewer than 15% achieve 20/50 or better vision.[21] Some investigators believe that eyes treated with pneumatic retinopexy finally gain better vision than comparable eyes treated with scleral buckling, but this point remains highly controversial.

In addition, sometimes responsible for disappointing postoperative vision are complications caused by:
- The pathophysiology of retinal detachment,
- The subsequent reattachment surgery, or
- Progressive ischemic or infectious retinal damage.

The most common of such entities, other than macular damage from the detachment, are cystoid macular edema (5–10%) and epiretinal membrane formation (5%).[22]

REFERENCES

1. Wilkinson CP, Rice TA. Michels retinal detachment, Ch 8. Philadelphia: Mosby–Year Book; 1997:471–516.
2. Eisner G. Biomicroscopy of the peripheral fundus: an atlas and textbook. New York: Springer-Verlag; 1993:45.
3. Rosengren B, Osterlin S. Hydrodynamic effects in the vitreous space accompanying eye movements: significance for the pathogenesis of retinal detachment. Ophthalmologica. 1976;173:513–24.
4. Wilkinson CP, Rice TA. Michels retinal detachment, Ch 6. Philadelphia: Mosby–Year Book; 1997:335–90.
5. Haimann NH, Burton TC, Brown CK. Epidemiology of retinal detachment. Arch Ophthalmol. 1982;100:289–92.
6. Goldberg MF. Clear lens extraction for axial myopia. An appraisal. Ophthalmology. 1987;94:571–82.
7. Javitt JC, Street DA, Tielsch JM, et al. Retinal detachment and endophthalmitis after outpatient cataract surgery. Ophthalmology. 1994;101:100–6.

8. Duker JS. In: Steinert RF, ed. Cataract surgery: technique, complications, and management. Philadelphia: WB Saunders; 1995:434–8.

9. Tielsch JM, Legro MW, Cassard SD, *et al.* Risk factors for retinal detachment after cataract surgery. A population-based case control study. Ophthalmology. 1996;103:1537–45.

10. Austin KL, Palmer JR, Seddon JM, *et al.* Case-control study of idiopathic retinal detachment. Int J Epidemiol. 1990;19:1045–50.

11. Wilkinson CP, Rice TA. Michels retinal detachment, Ch 4. Philadelphia: Mosby–Year Book; 1997:175–250.

12. Brod RD, Flynn HW, Lightman DA. Asymptomatic rhegmatogenous retinal detachments. Arch Ophthalmol. 1995;113:1030–32.

13. Lincoff H, Geiser R. Finding the retinal hole. Arch Ophthalmol. 1971;85:565–9.

14. Gonin J. Le décollement de la rétine. Lausanne: Librairie Payot and Co; 1934:13–52.

15. Kroll AJ, Machemer R. Experimental retinal detachment in the owl monkey. III. Electron microscopy of the retina and pigment epithelium. Am J Ophthalmol. 1968;66:410–27.

16. Green WR. Retina. In: Spencer WH, ed. Ophthalmic pathology. An atlas and textbook, Vol 2. Philadelphia: WB Saunders; 1985:905–13.

17. Wilson DJ, Green WR. Histopathologic study of the effect of retinal detachment on 49 eyes obtained post mortem. Am J Ophthalmol. 1987;103:167–79.

18. American Academy of Ophthalmology. The repair of rhegmatogenous retinal detachment. Ophthalmology. 1996;103:1313–24.

19. Wilkinson CP. What is the 'best' way to fix a routine retinal detachment? In: Lewis H, Ryan SJ, eds. Medical and surgical retina. St Louis: Mosby; 1994:85–102.

20. Wilkinson CP. Visual results following scleral buckling for retinal detachments sparing the macula. Retina. 1981;1:113–16.

21. Burton TC. Recovery of visual acuity after retinal detachment involving the macula. Trans Am Ophthalmol Soc. 1982;80:475–82.

22. Greven CM, Sanders RJ, Brown GC, *et al.* Pseudophakic retinal detachments. Anatomic and visual results. Ophthalmology. 1992;99:257–62.

137 Serous Detachment of the Neural Retina

RAJIV ANAND

DEFINITION
- An elevation of the neural retina due to the accumulation of subretinal fluid in the absence of a retinal break or significant preretinal traction.

KEY FEATURES
- Dependent subretinal fluid that shifts with change in head position.
- Lack of a rhegmatogenous or tractional component.
- Secondary to local ocular or systemic etiology.

ASSOCIATED FEATURES
- A breakdown in the blood–retina barrier.
- Absence of corrugated or fixed retinal folds.
- Clear or lipid-rich exudative subretinal fluid.
- Local ocular-associated disease, such as tumor, inflammation, vasculopathy.
- Systemic associated disease, such as hypertension, acute fluid retention.

INTRODUCTION

Serous detachment of the neural retina (serous retinal detachment) has been the subject of intense experimental scrutiny as the mechanisms that keep the neural retina attached to the underlying retinal pigment epithelium have become better understood. Normal retina is kept dehydrated and in apposition to the choroid by the blood–retina barrier and active cellular transport. Serous or exudative retinal detachment develops secondarily when the blood–retina barrier is damaged. In the absence of a retinal break, the diagnosis of serous, non-rhegmatogenous retinal detachment may be fairly straightforward; however, management often is fraught with difficulty. A wide variety of local and systemic pathology can cause secondary subretinal fluid accumulation. In this chapter the important clinical entities are discussed briefly and an attempt is made to summarize the pathogenic mechanisms in a logical fashion.

EPIDEMIOLOGY AND PATHOGENESIS

The cellular and fluid flow mechanisms that keep the neural retina attached to the retinal pigment epithelium (RPE) have been investigated fairly thoroughly. It is accepted that the vitreous gel and interdigitations between the photoreceptor outer segments and the RPE provide very little mechanical support for the retina. On the other hand, fluid flow dynamics play a major part in providing a suction force that keeps the retina attached to the RPE.[1] A significant suction force is generated by ionic flow from the RPE to the choriocapillaris. This is demonstrated in freshly enucleated animal eyes and also in human eyes, in which detaching healthy retina is difficult. The colloidal osmotic forces in the choriocapillaris provide an additional unidirectional flow of fluid from the posterior segment of the eye toward the vortex veins and then to the orbital venous system. The retina is kept dehydrated by tight junctions between the capillary endothelial cells. In addition, tight junctions also exist between the adjacent RPE cells, which provide a barrier between the sensory retina and the highly vascularized choroid.

The pump and metabolic functions of the RPE cells play the predominant role in keeping the neural retina attached as well as dehydrated. Experimental studies by Marmor and colleagues[2,3] show that damage to the RPE barrier is necessary before large molecules such as albumin can diffuse into the subretinal space from both the vitreous and the bloodstream. Even when a breakdown in the blood–retina barrier occurs, as long as the RPE cells are capable of pumping out the extra fluid, subretinal fluid does not accumulate. If the function of the RPE is impaired and a breach in Bruch's membrane occurs, such as in choroidal tumors or choroiditis, fluid accumulates in the subretinal space. At this stage, destructive procedures (e.g., radiotherapy, cryotherapy, or laser) work by obliterating the primary site of blood–retinal barrier breakdown and provide adhesion to the underlying choroid. Also, the surrounding healthy RPE cells resume their active outward transport and thereby reattach the retina. Figure 137-1 illustrates the major forces involved in keeping normal retina attached.

Three major pathological mechanisms are implicated in the accumulation of subretinal fluid:
- A net increase in fluid flow into the subretinal space (e.g., a vascularized tumor with incompetent vasculature)
- An impaired outflow that disrupts the normal anterior-to-posterior egress of fluid (e.g., choroidal inflammation or orbital infiltration)
- A breakdown of the blood–retina barrier with impairment of the RPE fluid pump (e.g., central serous chorioretinopathy, inflammation)

Only one mechanism need be present for serous detachment of the neural retina to occur, but all three mechanisms may coexist simultaneously in various disease entities. Figure 137-2 shows the pathological mechanisms of serous subretinal fluid accumulation.

The common and rare conditions that can cause serous detachment of the neural retina are summarized in Box 137-1.

OCULAR MANIFESTATIONS

Serous, or exudative, retinal detachment typically causes decreased visual function that corresponds to the area of involved retina. Central visual acuity may be intact or may be diminished markedly, and the visual complaints may wax and wane. Patients may complain of metamorphopsia or scotomas accompanied by other complaints such as pain, photophobia, and redness. Photopsias are common and do not necessarily indicate a

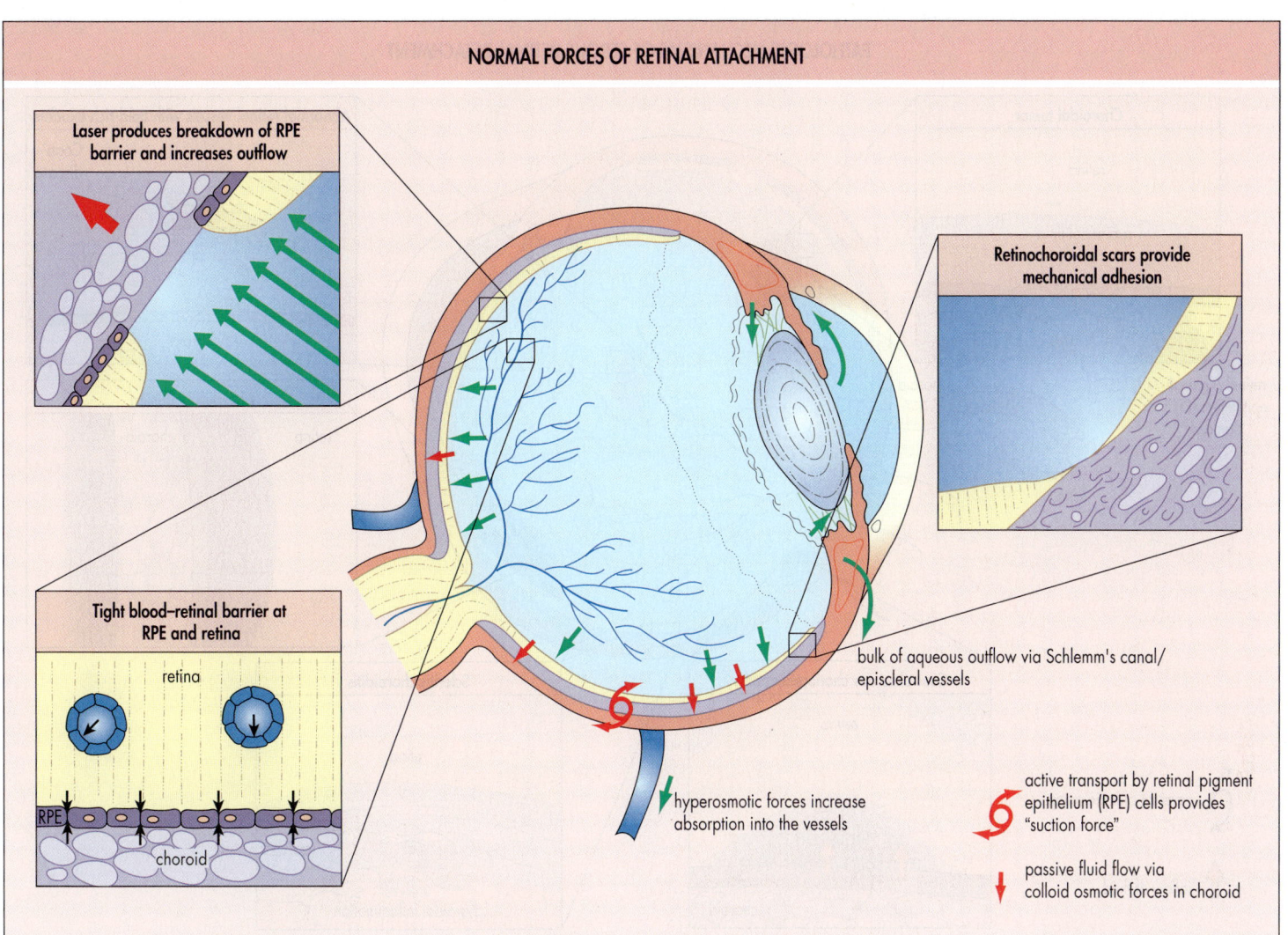

NORMAL FORCES OF RETINAL ATTACHMENT

Laser produces breakdown of RPE barrier and increases outflow

Retinochoroidal scars provide mechanical adhesion

Tight blood–retinal barrier at RPE and retina

retina

RPE

choroid

bulk of aqueous outflow via Schlemm's canal/episcleral vessels

hyperosmotic forces increase absorption into the vessels

active transport by retinal pigment epithelium (RPE) cells provides "suction force"

passive fluid flow via colloid osmotic forces in choroid

FIG. 137-1 ■ The normal forces of neural retinal attachment.

retinal break; however, a rhegmatogenous break always must be excluded by careful ophthalmoscopy.

Clinically, serous detachment results in a smooth elevation of the neural retina above the retinal pigment epithelium (RPE). The exudative fluid may be clear or cloudy, shallow or bullous. When bullous, shifting subretinal fluid may occur as the patient's head position changes, whereas rhegmatogenous retinal detachment does not shift its pattern that readily. This is visualized best with the help of the indirect ophthalmoscope, allowing patients to lie in a dependent position for a few minutes. Sometimes shallow retinal detachments can be observed more easily when a green filter is used on the examining light (Fig. 137-3). In shallow detachments, the fluid may not extend all the way to the ora serrata, although in severe cases, the retina may be so bullous as to contact the posterior lens surface (Fig. 137-4).

Serous detachment of the neural retina caused by local ocular pathology is accompanied by signs of the underlying disease. Vitreous or anterior segment inflammatory cells, external signs of scleritis, exophthalmos, retinal or choroidal vascular abnormalities, congenital disc or retinal abnormalities, choroidal detachments, or intraocular masses may be found along with the exudative fluid.

Below, various disease entities that result in exudative retinal detachment are described. For an in-depth discussion, the reader is referred to the appropriate sections within this book.

Coats' Disease

Coats' disease is an idiopathic, presumed congenital disorder of pathological retinal vessel formation that affects predominantly

boys during the first two decades of life. Abnormal retinal vessels can occur either in the periphery or the central retina and produce extravasation of lipid-rich serum into the surrounding tissues. As increasing leakage occurs, intraretinal and subretinal fluid accumulates. The retina may become bullously detached or, in milder cases, hard exudates accumulate in the macular area. If the retina is detached only shallowly, the characteristic dilated telangiectatic vessels can be confirmed easily with indirect ophthalmoscopy. Fluorescein angiography may be helpful in identifying the "light bulb" appearance of the abnormal vessels and in directing treatment.[4] However, if the retina has elevated bullously with lipid-rich accumulation of subretinal fluid, the diagnosis may be difficult and a differential diagnosis of retinoblastoma should be considered, sometimes necessitating a computed tomography scan if the media are opaque. The features that differentiate Coats' disease from retinoblastoma are that, in the former disease, the patients are somewhat older, calcium deposition is not seen within the eye, and characteristic retinal vascular abnormalities are present.

In Coats' disease, destructive therapy directed to the abnormal vessels via trans-scleral cryotherapy or transpupillary laser is effective in inducing gradual resolution of the subretinal fluid.[4] Surgical drainage of the subretinal fluid may be needed simultaneously if the retina is detached bullously. Newer methods of treatment such as radiation therapy, intraocular steroids, and photodynamic therapy are being considered, also, for this disease, although experience is anecdotal. Although the retinal exudates are absorbed completely with time in treated cases, the accompanying amblyopia may limit visual recovery, especially if the condition remains undetected until the child is in school.

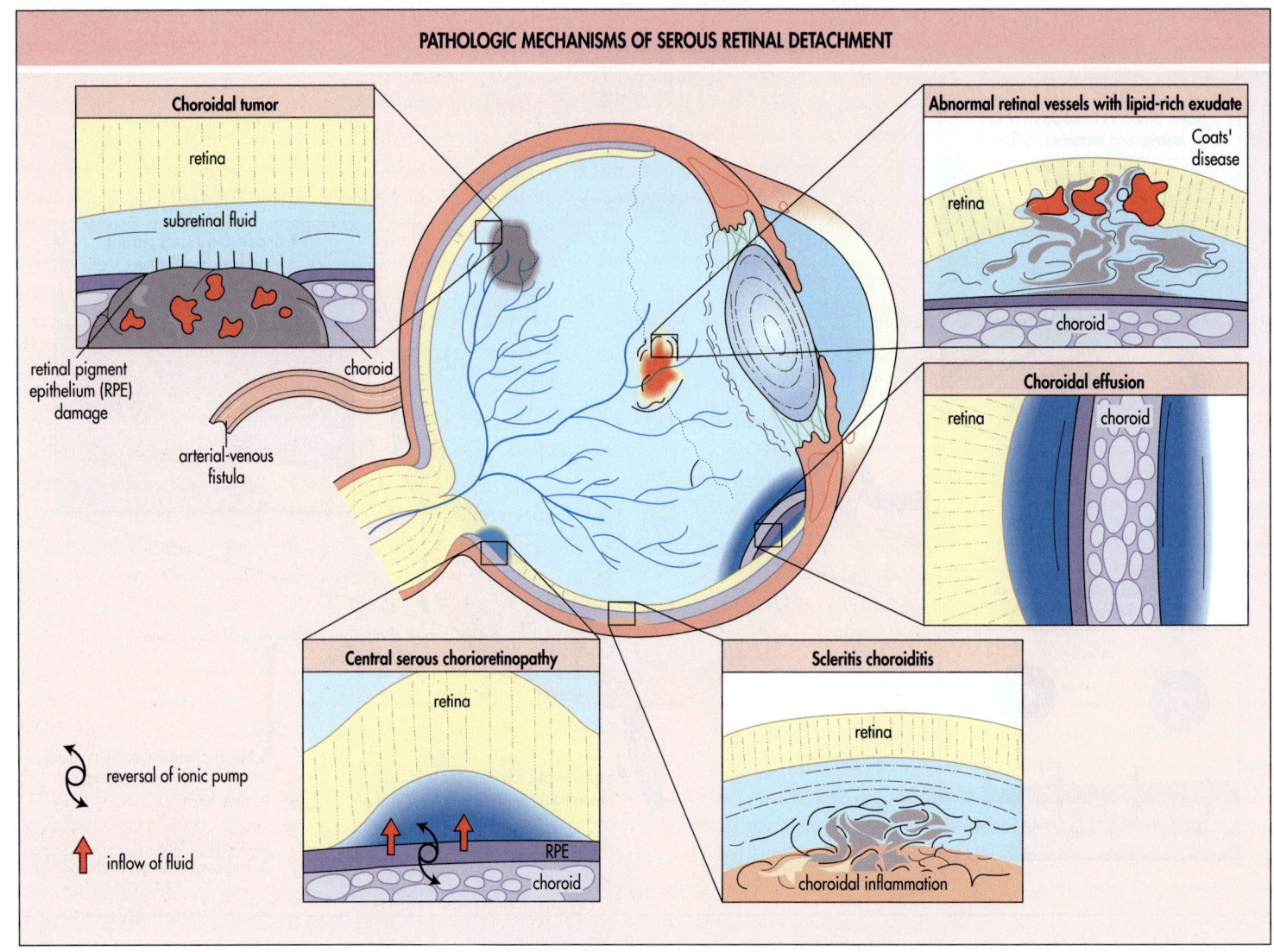

PATHOLOGIC MECHANISMS OF SEROUS RETINAL DETACHMENT

FIG. 137-2 ■ Pathological processes that result in serous detachment of the neural retina. *RPE,* Retinal pigment epithelium.

BOX 137-1

Common and Uncommon Causes of Serous Detachment of the Neural Retina

COMMON CONDITIONS
Coats' disease
Central serous chorioretinopathy
Choroidal tumors
Postsurgical (associated with choroidal detachments)
Vogt–Koyanagi–Harada syndrome
Posterior scleritis
Exudative age-related macular degeneration

UNCOMMON CONDITIONS
Nanophthalmos
Uveal effusion syndrome
Familial exudative vitreoretinopathy
Orbital inflammation (pseudotumor, cellulitis)
Infectious retinochoroiditis ((toxoplasmosis, syphilis, cytomegalovirus)
Sympathetic ophthalmia
Vasculitis (polyarteritis nodosa, Goodpasture's syndrome, systemic lupus erythematosus)
Acute vascular/hemodynamic (hypertensive crisis, toxemia of pregnancy, renal failure)
Optic nerve pits and colobomas (including morning glory syndrome)

Central Serous Chorioretinopathy (see Chapter 127)

Central serous chorioretinopathy (CSR) generally affects patients from the third to fourth decades of life. An association has been found with periods of high stress in people with type A, highly anxious personalities. The patients complain of distortion, decreased color sensation, and loss of central vision. The accumulation of subretinal fluid takes place in the macula with secondary pigmentary and RPE changes. Fluorescein angiography often reveals a classic focal point of hyperfluorescence, which may appear like an inverted smoke stack or ink blot. Variations of this classic clinical picture include bullous elevation of the retina with extra macular subretinal fluid and the "hanging teardrop" appearance, in which fluid tracks to the inferior periphery of the eye.

The pathogenesis of CSR has been the subject of debate and conjecture. Fluorescein angiography clearly reveals a focal spot of leakage that originates at the level of the RPE, and fluorescein dye leaks into the subretinal space. However, some reabsorption of fluid must take place from the subretinal space, because the detachment does not enlarge progressively. One theory suggests that the ionic flow is reversed in certain RPE cells and that passive movement of water molecules follows the ions from the choriocapillaris to the subretinal space.[5] Additionally, surrounding RPE cells are not able to absorb all the fluid as rapidly. Focal laser treatment certainly is effective in resolving the detachment associated with CSR, with destruc-

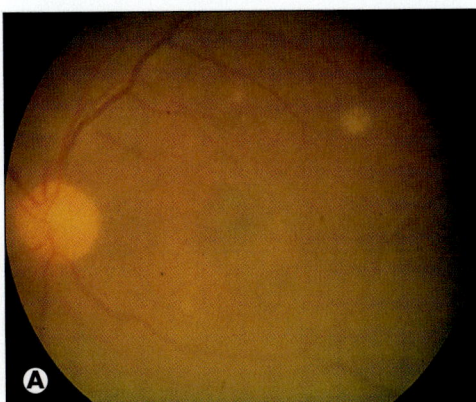
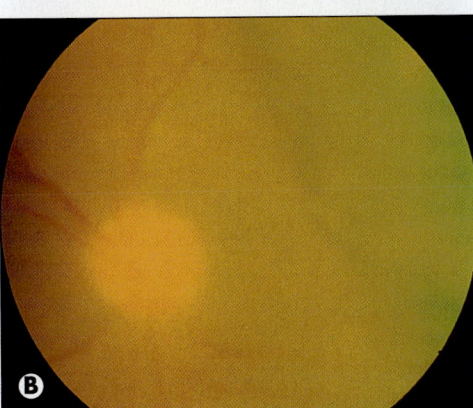

FIG. 137-3 ▮▮ Serous detachment of the neural retina photographed with green filtered light. A, With the patient in the upright position, fluid is seen along the inferior retinal periphery. B, With the patient in the reclining position, the fluid shifts posteriorly to detach the macula.

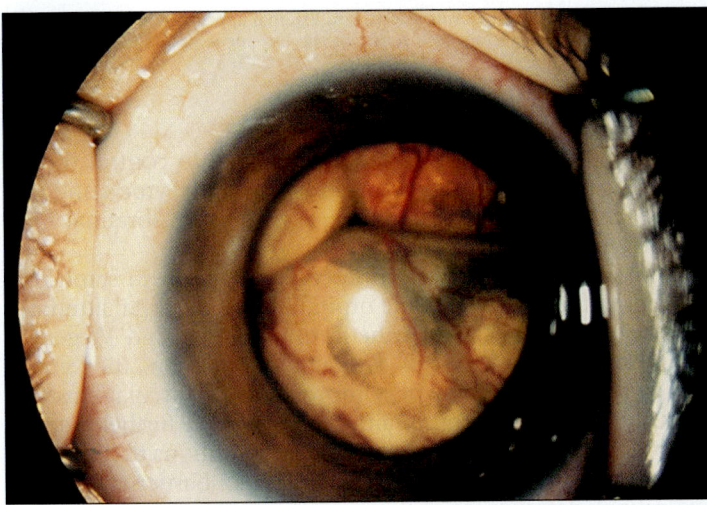

FIG. 137-4 ▮▮ Serous detachment of the neural retina secondary to retinoblastoma. A totally detached retina is visible behind the crystalline lens in an eye with an exophytic retinoblastoma. Subretinal tumor foci can be distinguished under the detached retina.

Postsurgical Serous Detachment

Fortunately, the incidence of postsurgical serous detachment of the neural retina has decreased substantially due to modern meticulous wound closure. Exudative retinal detachment with associated choroidal detachment currently is seen most frequently in glaucoma procedures that employ a secondary drainage implant, or injection of an antimetabolite, such as mitomycin C, during trabeculectomy.[6] Generally, the retinal detachment subsides with reabsorption of the suprachoroidal fluid; however, detachments associated with a suprachoroidal hemorrhage may take much longer to settle. The pathogenesis of subretinal fluid accumulation is decreased transport of fluid out of the suprachoroidal space. In mild cases, management consists of observation alone, although leaking surgical wounds need to be repaired immediately with drainage of suprachoroidal fluid and restoration of the ocular integrity. Secondary complications, such as corneal endothelial touch, iris prolapse, or choroidal hemorrhage, may have to be corrected with subsequent staged surgery.

Vogt–Koyanagi–Harada Syndrome

The Vogt–Koyanagi–Harada syndrome of ocular inflammation can vary from bilateral iridocyclitis to the full-blown syndrome of choroidal effusion, accumulation of subretinal fluid, optic neuropathy, and meningeal irritation. This entity is seen more commonly in Asians and can prove to be a management dilemma. In one large series, posterior uveitis was present in 75–80% of the eyes that showed evidence of retinal detachment.[7] Systemic corticosteroids are the mainstay of treatment, and early initiation can help to abort the attack. The pathogenesis in this entity, as well as in other types of posterior segment inflammation, is choroidal infiltration with inflammatory cells, destruction of the blood–retina barrier, and vascular leakage into the subretinal space. Immune suppressive agents such as cyclosporin A and methotrexate have been employed successfully in this chronic disease of remissions and flare-ups.

Choroidal Tumors

Solid tumors of the choroid commonly are associated with accumulation of subretinal fluid that produces localized exudative or bullous detachment of the retina. In choroidal melanoma, fluorescein angiography reveals a significant lack of capillary blood supply to the overlying retina along with damage to the RPE cells. Some authors suggest that the metabolic needs of a rapidly growing choroidal tumor outstrip its blood supply, which results in localized ischemia and induced damage in adjacent structures.[8] This explains why subretinal fluid can be associated with a growing choroidal mass and is considered by some to represent a sign of a malignancy in a nevus.

A circumscribed hemangioma of the choroid is a highly vascularized, congenital tumor located close to the disc and macula in most eyes. It manifests during the third to fourth decades of life, with significant leakage associated with its rich vascular supply. Destruction of the overlying RPE impairs the blood–retina barrier, which then allows the large, incompetent choroidal vessels from within the substance of the tumor to leak into the surrounding tissues. Focal grid laser treatment to the surface of a choroidal hemangioma can dry out the associated subretinal fluid by allowing the choriocapillaris to absorb the fluid and by providing a barrier around the margins of the lesion.[9] The benefit of laser therapy is temporary, because the leakage recurs and vision is affected by chronic detachment of the macula. Current means of therapy include low-dose radiation and photodynamic therapy.[9,10] The diffuse choroidal hemangioma associated with Sturge–Weber's disease can be extremely difficult to treat, because there is a total exudative detachment of the retina in these eyes and secondary glaucoma is a common complication.

Surface laser treatment of a small choroidal melanoma or nevus to dry out the serous fluid should be contemplated with

tion of the source of leakage allowing rapid absorption of the accumulated fluid.

The role of laser in this entity has been debated. Generally, it is accepted that treatment of classic CSR be delayed for a period of 3–4 months to allow for spontaneous resolution, because laser treatment does produce a paracentral scotoma. Additionally, laser treatment does not prevent a recurrence from an adjacent source of leakage. In atypical cases or in recurrences, vision may be impaired markedly, with loss of contrast sensitivity and color discrimination. Earlier focal laser treatment can be contemplated in patients who require rapid rehabilitation, or where the focal area of leakage is located outside the central macula.

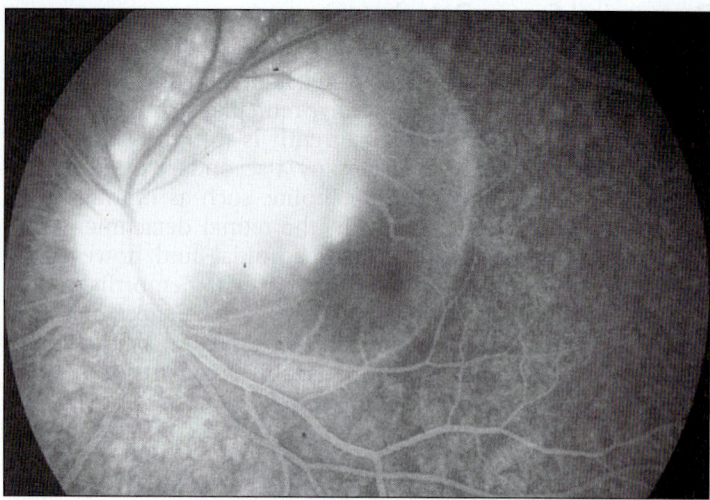

FIG. 137-5 ▓ An intravenous fluorescein angiogram highlights a serous detachment of the neural retina associated with choroidal metastasis. The metastatic tumor to the choroid is visualized along the superotemporal vessels; the fluid extends into the fovea. Note the extensive hyperfluorescence from the surface of the choroidal tumor.

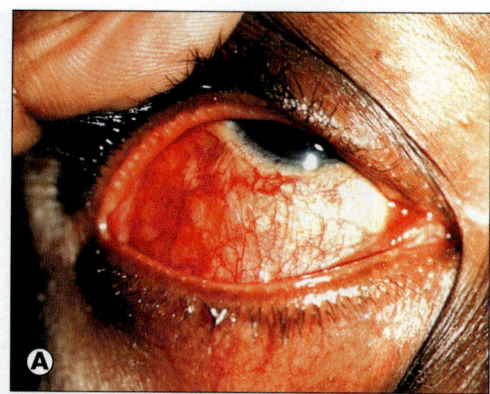

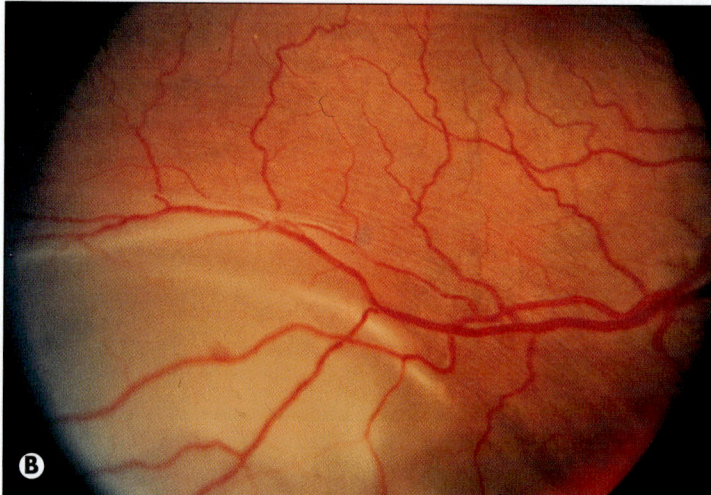

FIG. 137-6 ▓ Nodular posterior scleritis. A, External appearance. B, The accompanying serous retinal detachment is noted in the inferior retina. (Courtesy of Rand Spencer, MD.)

great caution, because rupture of the Bruch's membrane can lead to a rapid mushroom-shaped growth of the tumor.

Retinoblastomas, especially of the exophytic growth pattern, can produce early, highly bullous detachments of the retina due to the rich vascular supply and rapid increase in size (see Fig. 137-4). Systemic chemotherapy with adjuvant local tumor destruction is the treatment of choice and has salvaged many eyes and preserved ambulatory vision.[11,12] However, if there is vitreous seeding and total retinal detachment, some of these eyes may still need to be enucleated.

The most common primary sites of metastatic carcinoma to the choroid are the breast in female patients and the lung in male patients.[8] Choroidal metastases appear as creamy yellow multi-lobulated lesions and are almost invariably associated with accumulation of subretinal fluid (Fig. 137-5). Physical examination with appropriate ancillary testing spearheaded by an internist is indicated to identify the primary malignancy. If non-invasive testing proves unrewarding in the identification of a primary lesion, then a local choroidal biopsy using a fine-needle aspiration may be employed to determine the cells of origin. Treatment is directed toward the primary tumor with chemotherapy with additional local ocular irradiation. Although radiotherapy may be effective in resolving the subretinal fluid and limiting the growth of the choroidal tumors, the visual prognosis may be limited by the scarring or pigmentary changes in the macula.

Macular Degeneration and Diabetic Retinopathy

Both of these conditions may lead, rarely, to massive exudation from multiple leaking vessels into the subretinal space. The additional presence of elevated serum lipid levels results in a chronic accumulation of fluid with the formation of a macular serous detachment of the neural retina. Treatment is directed toward the choroidal neovascular membrane with thermotherapy or photodynamic laser therapy. In diabetic macular edema, focal laser photocoagulation accompanied by aggressive glycemic and lipid control may help in re-absorption of the exudative fluid.

Rare Conditions That Produce Serous Detachment of the Neural Retina

Nodular or diffuse posterior scleritis consists of painful inflammation of the sclera and associated serous detachment of the choroid and neural retina (Fig. 137-6). This condition can be extremely difficult to treat; fortunately, it is rare. Oral corticoste-

roids and anti-metabolites may be indicated to control the inflammation. Other posterior uveitides such as Lyme's and cat-scratch disease can also produce peri-papillary subretinal fluid accumulation.[13,14]

Other less common conditions that can result in serous detachment of the retina include orbital cellulitis, orbital arteriovenous malformations, sympathetic ophthalmia, and Wegener's granulomatosis. In cases of orbital inflammation, the venous outflow from the eye may be compromised by vascular engorgement. This results in exophthalmus, and thereby further vascular compromise. Other systemic circulatory conditions that can produce a rapid breakdown of the blood–retina barrier and exudative retinal detachment include accelerated hypertension, toxemia of pregnancy, and renal failure with acute fluid retention.[15]

Nanophthalmos and idiopathic uveal effusion are rare entities associated with impaired posterior fluid outflow. As a result of thickening of the sclera, the scleral outflow channels become impaired significantly, with a marked decrease in transmission of fluid through the posterior segment. The management of both of these conditions is surgical and consists of making scleral windows to decompress the vortex veins.

Other developmental disorders, such as optic nerve colobomas, morning glory disc, and optic nerve pits, are associated with a combination of retinoschisis and serous detachment of the neural retina.[16,17] For shallow detachments, demarcating laser treatment can be effective, whereas for larger detachments vitrectomy and gas tamponade may be necessary.

DIAGNOSIS AND ANCILLARY TESTING

Serous separation of the retina can be diagnosed fairly easily with indirect ophthalmoscopy, provided the ocular media is clear. When the media is hazy due to hemorrhage or inflammation, ancillary testing using ophthalmic ultrasonography or computed tomography scans may provide additional information. Blood tests for a uveitis workup to rule out an infectious cause such as Lyme's borreliosis, *Bartonella* infection, and syphilis testing should be considered.

Clinically, the examiner must look carefully for a retinal break to rule out a rhegmatogenous detachment. The vitreous cavity and preretinal surface should be studied for associated traction. A detachment with a rhegmatogenous component has corrugated folds and an opaque appearance of the retina, whereas a serous detachment is smooth and convex in nature. The color of the non-rhegmatogenous detached retina may appear more pink and healthy; however, this feature is difficult to distinguish in long-standing cases. Ocular inflammation, external signs of scleritis, local vascular changes, and lipid-rich subretinal fluid are also helpful in differentiating serous detachment of the neural retina. In longstanding serous detachment of the neural retina, especially when the fluid has waxed and waned, underlying RPE changes—"leopard skin"—are common. Patients who have systemic diseases, such as toxemia of pregnancy and acute renal failure, have the systemic signs associated with these conditions.

Diagnostic Ultrasonography

A diagnostic ultrasonographic evaluation using the "B" scan mode may be extremely helpful for opaque media. Improved tissue resolution with newer ultrasound machines and the ability to image retrobulbar tissues have enhanced diagnostic capabilities. Ultrasonography reveals a convex, dome-shaped collection of subretinal fluid, as well as subretinal fluid that shifts with changes in head position. Local pathology, such as choroidal tumors and scleral inflammation, can be defined fairly easily, and subretinal hemorrhage or other opacities may be better defined, as well.

Computed Tomography and Magnetic Resonance Imaging

These methods of radiological examination of the head and orbits become necessary if retrobulbar orbital pathology is suspected. Radiological investigations may be ordered for an orbital tumor, arteriovenous anastomosis, or exophthalmos. Gadolinium-enhanced magnetic resonance images offer a significant improvement in resolution of the tissue characteristics and may be beneficial in differentiating vascular from infiltrative orbital lesions.

Fluorescein Angiography

Retinal photography and fluorescein angiography can be extremely helpful to establish a source of the subretinal fluid and are necessary if focal laser treatment is contemplated. However, hazy media, vitreous hemorrhage, and bullous retinal detachment may limit the ability of fundus photography to distinguish the cause.

Indocyanine Green Angiography

Digital angiography using indocyanine green dye is a relatively recent innovation. It can be especially helpful to delineate the choroidal vasculature and to detect choroidal pathology in posterior uveitis and central serous chorioretinopathy.[18] In addition, it is possible that the combination of indocyanine green angiography with high-speed video digital imaging may identify abnormal choroidal feeder vessels in vascularized lesions.

Optical Coherence Tomography

Optical coherence tomography (OCT) is an exciting new, noninvasive technique that allows tissue resolution at a cellular level and, thereby, a cell layer–by–cell layer analysis of the ocular tis-

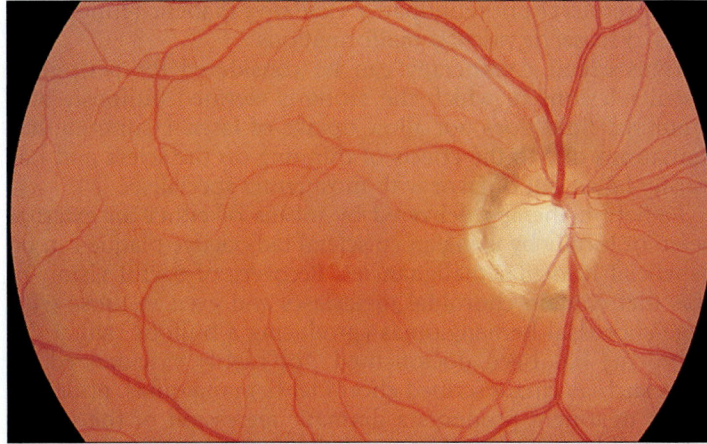
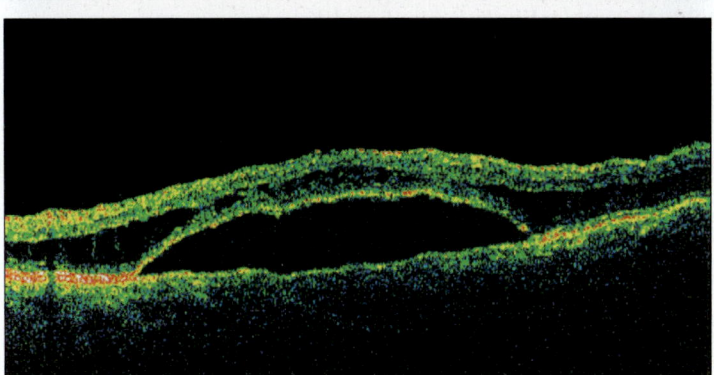

FIG. 137-7 ■ An optic nerve pit with serous detachment of the neural retina involving the central macula. **A,** A larger area of retinoschisis is present between the arcade vessels. **B,** Optical coherence tomography of the same eye shows the subretinal fluid under the macula with the larger area of inner retinoschisis.

> **BOX 137-2**
>
> **Differential Diagnosis of Serous Detachment of the Neural Retina**
>
> Retinoschisis
> Traction retinal detachment
> Rhegmatogenous retinal detachment
> Choroidal detachment
> Retinal or subretinal cyst
> Choroidal or retinal tumor

sues. The ability to resolve the tissue characteristics is helpful in differentiating the hemorrhagic from serous component of age-related macular degeneration. In serous detachment of the neural retina associated with optic nerve pits and colobomas, OCT has shown that no communication exists between the vitreous and the subretinal space.[17] Although the origin of the fluid is yet to be elucidated clearly, tomography findings (Fig. 137-7) do support the hypothesis that the initial elevation of the retina is a schisis-like cavity, followed by a later communication with the subarachnoid fluid. OCT also is helpful in sequential examination of subretinal fluid and to measure the extent of retinal edema.

DIFFERENTIAL DIAGNOSIS

The differential diagnosis is given in Box 137-2.

TREATMENT

The choice of treatment to resolve the secondary subretinal accumulation of fluid should be directed toward the primary pathology. As discussed above, laser treatment may be effective to treat focal breakdown of the blood–retina barrier, as seen in central serous chorioretinopathy, exudative diabetic retinopathy, Coats' disease, or vascular malformations.

Trans-scleral cryotherapy can be considered for peripheral vascular lesions in which the retina is elevated bullously and subretinal fluid does not allow uptake of laser. Diathermy has limitations due to the effects of thinning on the sclera and has mostly fallen out of favor with most retina specialists.

Radiation therapy delivered by means of either an external beam or locally by using an episcleral radioactive plaque can be beneficial in ocular malignancies. Recovery of useful vision in eyes that contain choroidal metastases and even in those with large choroidal hemangiomas (producing a bullous retinal detachment) has been documented. For highly vascularized lesions such as circumscribed choroidal hemangiomas, photodynamic treatment produces a dramatic regression of the tumor and would seem to be the logical choice.[10] However, experience with this modality is limited and long-term outcomes are unknown. Photodynamic therapy is also effective in reducing leakage from occult choroidal neovascularization and capillary hemangiomas, although its visual benefits remain controversial.[19] Trans-pupillary thermotherapy (TTT) is a useful adjunctive therapy for choroidal melanomas after radioactive plaque therapy, as well as for capillary and choroidal hemangiomas, and produces a rapid resolution of accumulated subretinal fluid associated with these tumors. TTT also is being investigated for the treatment of age-related macular degeneration and related occult neovascularization and RPE detachments.

Intra-vitreal steroids delivered by intraocular injection are effective in stabilizing the blood–retina barrier, and various trials have shown their efficacy in macular edema and chronic retinal edema. Similarly, sustained release steroid devices may prove beneficial for chronic conditions such as posterior uveitis and pars planitis.

Systemic treatment with oral or intravenous steroids may be required in cases with bilateral involvement or severe inflammation. Occasionally, systemic anti-metabolite agents may be necessary. Glucocorticoids, anti-inflammatory agents, cyclosporin A, and FK506 (tacrolimus) are powerful drugs with significant systemic toxic effects and, thus, should be used cautiously.

Medical management of a local ocular condition must be carefully coordinated—a physician experienced in the use of oral anti-metabolites and anti-inflammatory agents should be involved in the continued care of the patient.

COURSE AND OUTCOME

The visual outcome and success of therapy for serous detachment of the neural retina is highly dependent on the primary cause. Age of the patient and underlying systemic disease are other important factors. Persistent subretinal fluid does not bode well for long-term visual function. In general, however, the retina seems to tolerate exudative subretinal fluid better than fluid from rhegmatogenous retinal detachment. Therefore, provided the mechanism of fluid accumulation can be altered, good visual outcome can result, even for relatively longstanding macular detachments.

REFERENCES

1. Anand R, Tasman WS. Non-rhegmatogenous retinal detachment. In: Ryan SJ, ed. Retina, vol 3. Surgical retina, ed 3. St Louis: Mosby; 2001.
2. Marmor MF, Yao XY. Conditions necessary for the formation of serous detachment. Experimental evidence from the cat. Arch Ophthalmol. 1994;112:830–8.
3. Takeuchi A, Kricorian G, Yao XY, et al. The rate and source of albumin entry into saline filled experimental retinal detachments. Invest Ophthalmol Vis Sci. 1994; 35:3792–8.
4. Silidor SW, Augsburger JJ, Shields JA, Tasman WS. Natural history and management of advanced Coats' disease. Ophthalmic Surg. 1988;19:89–93.
5. Spitznas M. Pathogenesis of central serous retinopathy: a new working hypothesis. Graefe Arch Klin Exp Ophthalmol. 1986;224:321–4.
6. Kokame GT, de Leon MD, Tanji T. Serous retinal detachment and cystoid macular edema in hypotony maculopathy. Am J Ophthalmol. 2001;131:384–6.
7. Ohno S, Char DH, Kimura SJ, O'Connor GR. Vogt–Koyanagi–Harada syndrome. Am J Ophthalmol. 1977;83:735–40.
8. Shields JA, Shields CL. Intraocular tumors. A text and atlas. Philadelphia: WB Saunders; 1992.
9. Shields CL, Honavar SG, Shields JA, et al. Circumscribed choroidal hemangioma: clinical manifestations and factors predictive of visual outcome in 200 consecutive cases. Ophthalmology. 2001;108:2237–48.
10. Robertson DM. Photodynamic therapy for choroidal hemangioma associated with serous retinal detachment. Arch Ophthalmol. 2002;120:1155–61.
11. Shields CL, Shields JA. Editorial: chemotherapy for retinoblastoma. Med Pediatr Oncol. 2002;38:377–8.
12. Shields CL, Shields JA. Recent developments in the management of retinoblastoma. J Pediatr Ophthalmol Strabismus. 1999;36:8–18.
13. Krist D, Wenkel H. Posterior scleritis associated with Borrelia burgdorferi (Lyme disease) infection. Ophthalmology. 2002;109:143–5.
14. Wade NK, Levi L, Jones MR, et al. Optic disk edema associated with peripapillary serous retinal detachment: an early sign of systemic Bartonella henselae infection. Am J Ophthalmol. 2000;130:327–34.
15. Hayreh SS. Systemic arterial blood pressure and the eye. Eye. 1996;10:5–28.
16. Lincoff H, Lopez R, Kreissig I. Retinoschisis associated with optic nerve pits. Arch Ophthalmol. 1988;106:61–7.
17. Krivoy D, Gentile R, Leibmann JM, et al. Imaging congenital optic disc pits and associated maculopathy using optical coherence tomography. Arch Ophthalmol. 1996;114:165–70.
18. Oshima Y, Harino S, Hara Y, Tano Y. Indocyanine green angiographic findings in Vogt–Koyanagi–Harada disease. Am J Ophthalmol. 1996;122:58–66.
19. Schmidt-Erfurth UM, Kusserow C, Barbazetto IA, Laqua H. Benefits and complications of photodynamic therapy of papillary capillary hemangiomas. Ophthalmology. 2002;109:1256–66.

138 Choroidal Hemorrhage

MICHAEL A. KAPUSTA • PEDRO F. LOPEZ

DEFINITION
- A hemorrhage in the suprachoroidal space that occurs spontaneously, intraoperatively, or traumatically, or is associated with intraocular vascular anomalies.

KEY FEATURES
- One or more dome-shaped choroidal protrusions.
- Forward movement of the iris, lens, and vitreous body.
- Elevated intraocular pressure.

ASSOCIATED FEATURES
- Darkening of the red reflex.
- Excessive bleeding of conjunctiva and episcleral tissues.
- Severe pain, even under local anesthetic.
- Breakthrough vitreous hemorrhage.
- Rhegmatogenous, exudative, or tractional retinal detachment.

INTRODUCTION

Choroidal hemorrhage is a serious ocular condition, which may be associated with permanent loss of visual function. Both limited and massive choroidal hemorrhages may occur as complications of most forms of ocular surgery, as well as from trauma. Intraoperative choroidal hemorrhage may progress to expulsion of intraocular tissues through the surgical wound. In some cases, expedient wound closure and appropriate application of pressure can prevent total loss of the globe. Despite modern vitreoretinal techniques, choroidal hemorrhage is associated with visual loss in most cases.

EPIDEMIOLOGY AND PATHOGENESIS

Choroidal hemorrhage may occur in a limited form or as a massive event. Massive choroidal hemorrhage is of sufficient volume to cause extrusion of intraocular contents outside the eye or to move retinal surfaces into or near apposition ("kissing"). Massive choroidal hemorrhage may be expulsive or nonexpulsive, immediate (intraoperative), or delayed hours to weeks postoperatively; it may occur spontaneously, with choroidal mass lesions (e.g., choroidal hemangioma), or with surgical or noniatrogenic trauma.[1-3]

Limited choroidal hemorrhage occurs in over 3% of intracapsular cataract extractions and in 2.2% of nucleus-expression extracapsular cases.[1] Massive choroidal hemorrhage has complicated 0.2% of cataract extractions and 0.73% of glaucoma filtering procedures[2]; it may occur even more frequently with keratoplasty.[3] Scleral buckling procedures, as well as pars plana vitrectomy, may be complicated by either limited or massive choroidal hemorrhage.

Choroidal hemorrhage may occur when a fragile vessel is exposed to sudden compression and decompression events. An intact posterior lens capsule may serve as a tamponade against such intense intraocular decompression during surgery.[3] Retrobulbar anesthetic injection, retrobulbar hemorrhage, or excessive pressure on the globe during surgery may impede vortex venous outflow and lead to choroidal effusion and hemorrhage.[4] Decompression hypotony, created when the eye is entered, and repeated fluctuations in intraocular fluid dynamics may add further insult to these fragile vessels. The resultant suprachoroidal effusion progresses to stretch the suprachoroidal space and cause further tension on the ciliary vessels. Alternatively, chronic hypotony may facilitate the extension of a pre-existing suprachoroidal effusion toward the anterior ciliary arteries. Either pathway may result in vessel wall rupture and suprachoroidal hemorrhage.

Systemic conditions which may serve as risk factors for expulsive choroidal hemorrhage include advanced age, arteriosclerosis, hypertension, diabetes mellitus, blood dyscrasias, and obesity. Ocular risk factors include previous surgery, aphakia, glaucoma, uveitis, high myopia, trauma, vitreous removal, laser photocoagulation, and choroidal sclerosis. A scleral buckle placed during vitrectomy is a risk factor for postoperative choroidal hemorrhage. A history of choroidal hemorrhage serves as a risk factor for surgery on either eye. Intraoperative risk factors include increased intraocular pressure, increased axial length, open-sky procedures, and Valsalva maneuvers. Intraoperative tachycardia has been identified as a significant risk factor or an early symptom of expulsive hemorrhage.[5] It is unclear whether local anesthetic agents pose more risk than general anesthesia.

The risks of choroidal hemorrhage may be minimized by control of known risk factors. Preoperative massage and a Honan balloon may be used to control intraocular pressure. Intraoperative temporary security sutures may be placed before expression delivery of the lens. The water-tight wound created for phacoemulsification helps to maintain intraocular turgor; it may reduce the incidence and limit the severity of suprachoroidal hemorrhage. Blood pressure and heart rate should be monitored carefully.

OCULAR MANIFESTATIONS

Both serous and hemorrhagic choroidal detachments usually cause decreased vision. Serous choroidal detachment may be asymptomatic; however, hemorrhagic choroidal detachment often is extremely painful. Slit-lamp examination reveals a shallow anterior chamber with mild cells and flare. Ophthalmoscopy demonstrates a smooth, bullous, orange-brown elevation of the retina and choroid. Choroidal detachment that occurs anterior to the equator often extends in an annular fashion around the globe; whereas postequatorial choroidal detachment often is unilobulated or multilobulated, secondary to the periequatorial attachment of the choroid at the vortex vein ampullae. Visualization of the ora serrata without scleral depression may be a sign of pre-equatorial choroidal detachment (Fig. 138-1).

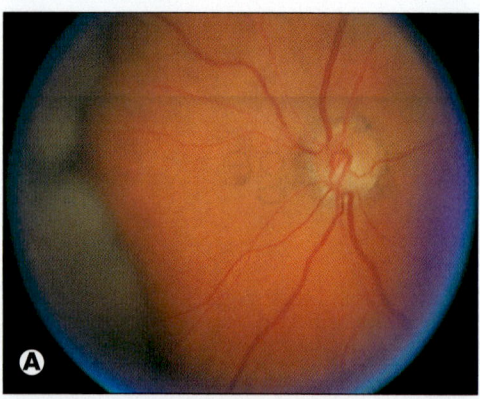

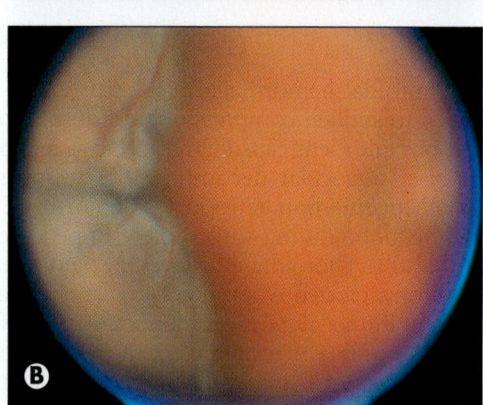

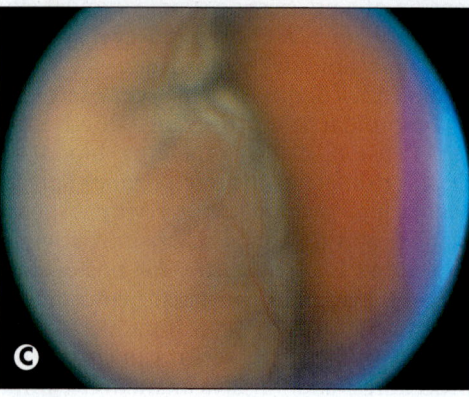

FIG. 138-1 ▥ Hemorrhagic choroidal detachment viewed ophthalmoscopically. **A,** The extent of choroidal protrusion, as evidenced by a fundus photograph focused on the optic nerve. **B,** The dome-shaped lobules and orange-brown color of a choroidal detachment. **C,** A closer view demonstrates no subretinal fluid, helping to establish that this is a choroidal detachment, not a retinal detachment.

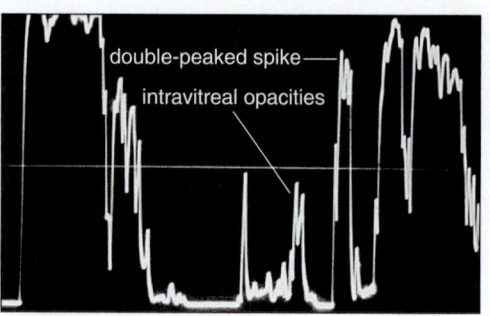

FIG. 138-2 ▥ A-scan echogram. This demonstrates intravitreal opacities and the highly reflective, double-peaked, wide spike characteristic of choroidal detachment.

Serous choroidal detachment, or effusion, occurs most frequently after recent glaucoma surgery. It also may develop, however, under the same conditions that lead to hemorrhagic choroidal detachment. Serous choroidal detachments are more frequent and generally subside within 3 weeks without alteration in vision. Serous choroidal detachment may be differentiated from rhegmatogenous retinal detachment by the absence of retinal breaks or outer retinal hydration lines and usually can be differentiated from hemorrhagic choroidal detachment by the low intraocular pressure and ready transillumination of serous choroidal detachment. Eyes with limited and massive (delayed) hemorrhagic choroidal detachments generally have elevated intraocular pressure and the detachments do not transilluminate. Serous choroidal detachments often are confined to the pre-equatorial suprachoroidal space, with limited postequatorial extension. Hemorrhagic choroidal detachments may extend to the posterior pole and are more voluminous posterior to the equator.

The initial intraoperative symptoms of massive choroidal hemorrhage may be paroxysmal onset of severe intraoperative pain despite akinesia and previously adequate analgesia. Classically, the pain radiates from the brow to the vertex of the head along the V1 dermatome and is often refractory to further retrobulbar analgesia. The intraoperative signs of massive choroidal hemorrhage may include tachycardia and excessive iris movement or prolapse. This usually is accompanied by forward movement of the lens and vitreous body, as the globe tenses. Darkening of the red reflex may precede or accompany a choroidal elevation that protrudes into the operative field. Expulsion of intraocular contents may ensue.

DIAGNOSIS AND ANCILLARY TESTING

The intraoperative diagnosis of massive choroidal hemorrhage is based on recognition of early signs and changing ocular dynamics. Such recognition requires a high index of suspicion. Similarly, the diagnoses of delayed massive choroidal hemorrhage and limited choroidal hemorrhage are made after recent ocular surgery by consideration of the risk factors, symptoms, and signs. Measurement of intraocular pressure, gonioscopy, slit-lamp biomicroscopy, and dilated fundus examination, comparing both eyes, lead the examiner toward the diagnosis. Transillumination may be employed to differentiate serous from hemorrhagic choroidal detachment.

When the media is opaque or clear, echography may help to establish an accurate diagnosis.[6] An A-scan echogram demonstrates a lesion with medium–high internal reflectivity and a steeply rising, 100% high spike. At low gain, this is observed to be a double-peaked wide spike characteristic of choroidal detachment (Fig. 138-2). The first peak may represent the surface of the overlying detached retina or the anterior surface of the choroid. Alternatively, the double peak may represent both the anterior and posterior surfaces of the choroid. On B-scan echograms, a choroidal detachment typically appears as a smooth, thick, dome-shaped membrane in the periphery that exhibits little, if any, aftermovement on kinetic evaluation. Fresh blood clots are seen echographically as a high-reflective, solid-appearing mass, with irregular internal structure and irregular shape.[7] Serial ultrasonography may demonstrate liquefaction of hemorrhage; the suprachoroidal space is filled with low-reflective mobile opacities, which have replaced the hemorrhagic clot.[6] Serous elevation of the retina may accompany choroidal detachment and often resolves spontaneously. Choroidal melanoma may be distinguished from choroidal hemorrhage by its low–medium reflectivity on A-scan echography and its typical collarbutton configuration and decreased reflectivity at the tumor base on B-scan echography.

DIFFERENTIAL DIAGNOSIS

Differential diagnosis consists of choroidal effusion, rhegmatogenous retinal detachment, and melanoma or metastatic tumor of choroid or ciliary body.

TREATMENT

Primary Management

The management of serous choroidal detachment usually is conservative. Postoperative serous choroidal detachments often resolve on their own within days. Cycloplegia and topical corticosteroids are general management measures. Most commonly, serous choroidal detachments occur after excessive leakage from a wound or after glaucoma filtering surgery. These cases usually respond to measures that reduce over-filtration and consequent hypotony, such as pressure patching and glue or bandage contact lens use. Surgical management of serous choroidal detachment may be indicated for refractory progressive shallowing or flattening of the anterior chamber—particularly in association with marked inflammation, which may promote the formation of peripheral anterior synechiae. The threat of corneal decompensation after lens–cornea touch or the apposition of retinal surfaces in kissing choroidal detachment are other potential indications for surgical intervention.

Delayed nonexpulsive limited choroidal hemorrhage generally carries a good prognosis. Limited choroidal hemorrhage usually resolves spontaneously within 1–2 months without ophthalmoscopic evidence of damage.[8] Management remains conservative in this situation and includes the use of cycloplegics and topical corticosteroids. The management of delayed, nonexpulsive, massive choroidal hemorrhage, by contrast, remains controversial. Systemic corticosteroids are employed by some investigators.[9] Some reports suggest that massive choroidal hemorrhage that follows glaucoma surgery can be observed, with spontaneous resolution to preoperative vision levels.[10] Others suggest that delayed massive choroidal hemorrhage after filtering or seton surgery may result in irreversible loss of vision when intervention does not take place within 1 week.[11] Surgical drainage should be considered in the following circumstances:

- Massive choroidal hemorrhage associated with severe pain
- Elevated intraocular pressure
- Persistently flat anterior chamber
- Suprachoroidal hemorrhage under the macula
- Extension of hemorrhage into the subretinal space or vitreous cavity

Significant vitreous incarceration in the surgical wound and kissing choroidal detachments, which may lead to secondary subacute traction or rhegmatogenous detachment after resolution of the suprachoroidal hemorrhage and its classic "buckle-like" effect, also are potential indications for surgical drainage.[12]

In 1915, Voerhoeff introduced posterior sclerotomy to release suprachoroidal blood for the management of massive choroidal hemorrhage. Intraoperative massive choroidal hemorrhage is managed by tamponade of the eye with direct digital pressure and rapid wound closure. After penetrating keratoplasty, a Cobo temporary keratoprosthesis may be useful to prevent expulsion of intraocular contents. Posterior sclerotomy may be necessary, at the time of surgery, to permit adequate wound closure. Sclerotomies should be performed by careful cut-down incisions to the suprachoroidal space, beginning posterior to the muscle insertions. The vortex veins and long posterior ciliary vessels should be avoided, to minimize the risks of recurrent choroidal hemorrhage postoperatively.[6,9] The goal of rapid wound closure is to prevent expulsion or loss of the intraocular contents and incarceration of vitreous or retina in the surgical wound.

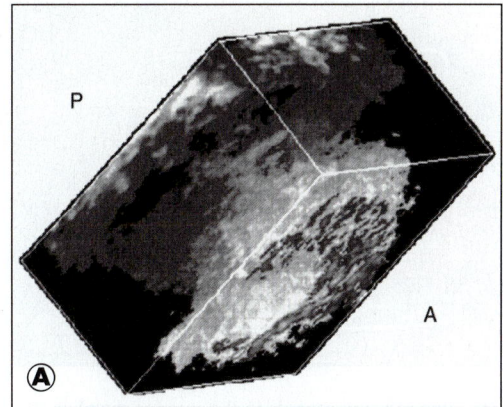

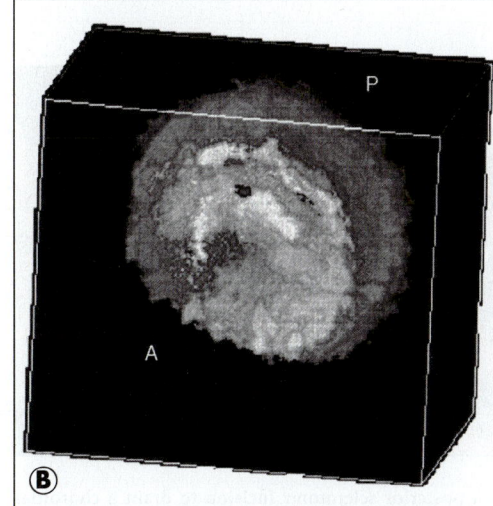

FIG. 138-3 ■ A 3D ultrasonogram of choroidal hemorrhage.

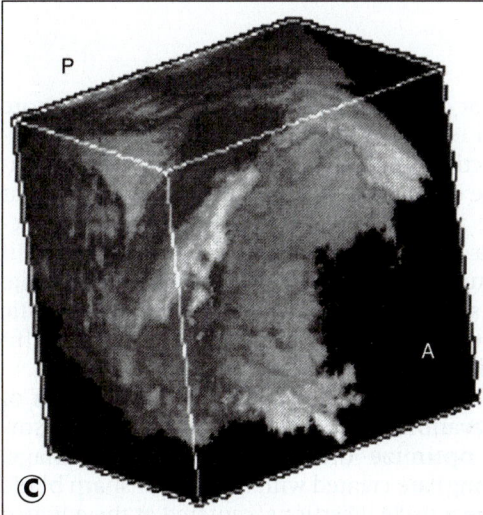

Secondary Management

Choroidal hemorrhage that occurs postoperatively, recurs, or meets indications for further surgical intervention should be managed by a vitreoretinal surgeon. The successful management of affected eyes requires that vitreous or retinal incarceration be relieved completely. Patients who have vitreous incarceration are at high risk of developing retinal detachment. Eyes with concurrent vitreous and retinal detachment, at the time of diagnosis, may not be amenable to surgical repair or may be at high risk for proliferative vitreoretinopathy. Surgical intervention to drain choroidal hemorrhage ideally is conducted after liquefaction of the suprachoroidal hemorrhage, which may be assessed by serial echography.[6,7] Three-dimensional reconstruction of the B scan is possible with modern ultrasonography. This may assist in localization of the best sites for surgical drainage (Fig. 138-3).

The timing of such intervention may be altered by the presence of rhegmatogenous retinal detachment.

The primary surgical goal is to separate any kissing choroidal detachments to prevent secondary traction or rhegmatogenous retinal detachment. Additional surgical goals include posterior rotation of the lens–iris diaphragm, which results in a deepened anterior chamber and, thus, prevents peripheral anterior synechiae and secondary angle-closure glaucoma, as well as corneal endothelial damage from lens–cornea contact. Surgical goals should also include the separation of kissing choroidal detachments by one half of their original height.

The initial stages of surgical drainage of massive choroidal hemorrhage include conjunctival peritomy and isolation of the relevant rectus muscles with bridle sutures. Often, all four rectus muscles are isolated to enable exposure if posterior drainage sclerotomies are needed in multiple quadrants to evacuate adequately the suprachoroidal hemorrhage.

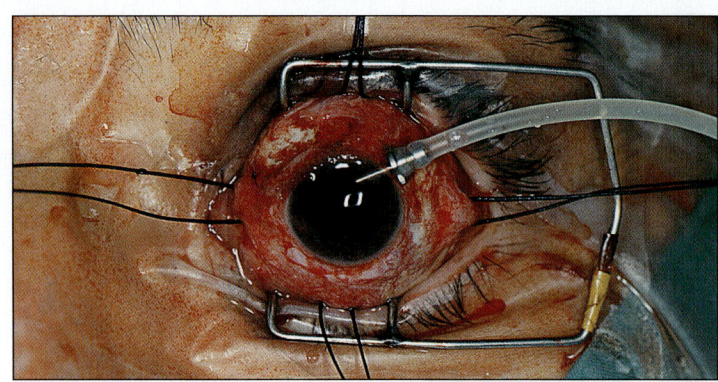

FIG. 138-4 ■ A self-retaining infusion cannula in the anterior chamber.

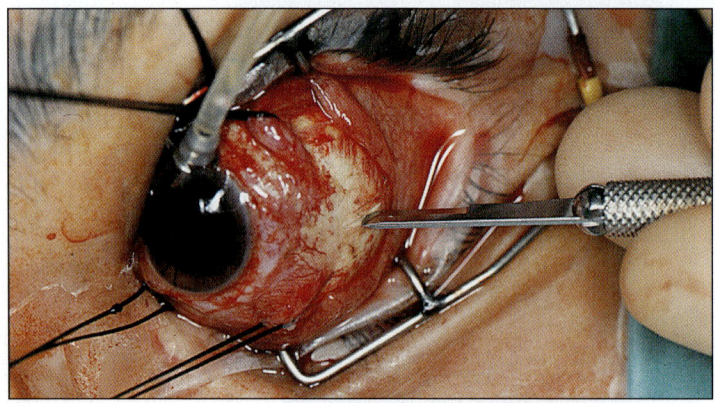

FIG. 138-5 ■ Creation of a posterior sclerotomy incision to drain a choroidal hemorrhage.

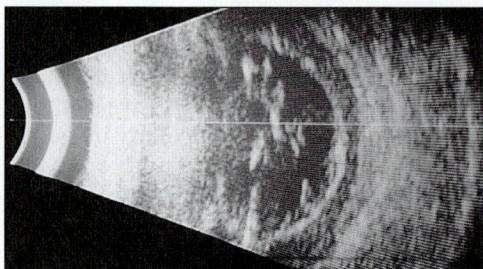

FIG. 138-6 ■ Transverse B-scan of an eye after repair of a ruptured globe. The annular, flat, and diffuse hemorrhagic choroidal detachment is typical of trauma.

Infusion of fluid or air to pressurize the eye and allow more complete evacuation of the suprachoroidal hemorrhage generally is a useful adjunctive procedure. The anterior chamber is entered with a 25-guage or smaller needle, bent posteriorly, so that the bevel directs the infusion away from the corneal endothelium. Alternatively, a micro–vitreo-retinal blade may be used if a self-retaining or sutured infusion cannula is to be inserted (Fig. 138-4). Again, flow should be directed posteriorly. Viscoelastic agents may be employed to deepen the anterior chamber sufficiently to insert the infusion cannula.

Posterior sclerotomy sites generally are created in the area of greatest choroidal elevation, with the patient in the supine (surgical) position to optimize drainage of the hemorrhage. Incisions (4–6mm long) are created with a round or sharp blade posterior to the rectus muscle insertions, centered at the equator of the globe. Exposure is best in the inferotemporal quadrant, but other quadrants may be incised to achieve optimal drainage, as judged by inspection and ophthalmoscopy (Fig. 138-5). The sclerotomy sites may be sutured closed to restore anatomical integrity and stability, or left open if further spontaneous drainage is felt likely or necessary.

If vitreous is incarcerated in the original surgical wound, a vitrectomy probe may be introduced through a second limbal incision and an anterior vitrectomy performed to minimize vitreoretinal traction during the choroidal drainage procedure. Anterior chamber lens remnants similarly may be removed. Once adequate initial drainage has been achieved, a posterior vitrectomy with scleral depression may be performed to remove residual lens fragments, cortex, and vitreous adhesion to the iris.[13] In the absence of retinal detachment, this may be deferred to later surgical intervention. For rhegmatogenous retinal detachment, a more extensive posterior vitrectomy in conjunction with drainage of the choroidal hemorrhage usually is necessary.

In these cases, the insertion of a 6mm infusion cannula through the anterior pars plana may be necessary to prevent suprachoroidal infusion. Relaxing peripheral retinotomy or retinectomy may be necessary to relieve incarceration of the retina or severe anterior vitreous traction.[14] The use of perfluorocarbon liquids may facilitate the drainage of suprachoroidal hemorrhage and facilitate reattachment of the retina.[15] Scleral buckling or long-term intraocular tamponade with silicone oil may minimize the chances of recurrent retinal detachment in these eyes.

Central retinal apposition in retinal detachment that follows drainage of choroidal fluid poses a unique surgical challenge. Perfluorocarbon liquids may be used to stabilize the posterior retina. A taper-tip endocautery can preserve hemostasis as the retinal surfaces are teased or cut apart to separate them. The perfluorocarbon level can be raised further to flatten the now-separated surfaces. Endolaser treatment and gas or oil tamponade may then be used.

Eyes for which the outcomes are successful through observation, conservative measures, or surgical intervention may be considered for intraocular lens implantation for visual rehabilitation.[16] The reduction of risk factors for choroidal hemorrhage should achieve foremost attention at the time of secondary lens implant.

Choroidal Hemorrhage in Trauma

Choroidal hemorrhage that occurs with noniatrogenic trauma or rupture of the globe may be associated with intraocular structural damage. In addition to contusive injury, fibrocellular proliferation with membrane formation may limit the visual rehabilitation of the eye.[17] The management of these cases must take into consideration the high likelihood of retinal detachment and associated proliferative vitreoretinopathy. Surgery may require evacuation of hyphema. Corneal blood staining may necessitate the use of a temporary keratoprosthesis. The choroidal hemorrhage is drained as described above. Scleral buckling and long-term tamponade with silicone oil may be required to effect repair of an associated rhegmatogenous retinal detachment. The echographic characteristics of choroidal hemorrhages that result from trauma differ from those that arise from other causes. In general, traumatic choroidal hemorrhages tend to be more diffuse and less elevated (Fig. 138-6).[6]

Choroidal Hemorrhage in Other Conditions

Choroidal hemorrhage may occur in association with hemoglobinopathies, with anticoagulants, or spontaneously (Fig. 138-7). In one series, patients developed acute angle-closure glaucoma from forward displacement of the lens–iris diaphragm, which resulted from massive hemorrhagic detachment of the choroid and retina. Affected patients often have associated systemic hypertension or a primary or anticoagulant-induced clotting disorder.[18] The source of "spontaneous" hemorrhage in these patients is choroidal neovascularization in a disciform lesion.

Sturge–Weber syndrome is characterized by a flat, facial hemangioma that follows the distribution of the fifth cranial nerve. Occasionally, meningeal hemangiomas may be present and can produce seizures. Choroidal and episcleral hemangiomas are

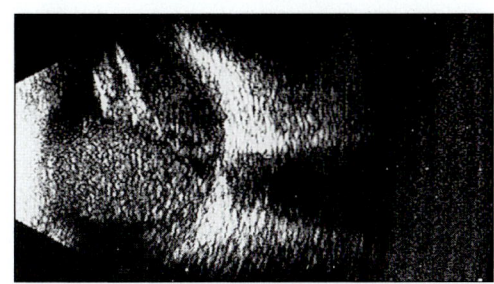

FIG. 138-7 ■ A hemorrhagic choroidal detachment seen in a patient using warfarin. (Courtesy of Jeffrey L. Marx, MD.)

seen commonly—leakage from the choroidal hemangioma can cause retinal edema. Glaucoma may be present when the facial hemangioma involves the lid or conjunctiva. Trabeculectomy in these cases is complicated by rapid expansion of the hemangioma, with effusion of fluid into the suprachoroidal and subretinal space in 17% of cases. Some surgeons recommend placement of two or three posterior sclerotomies to prevent such expansion. Definitive management includes posterior drainage sclerotomy followed by reformation of the anterior chamber.[19]

Limited choroidal hemorrhage can be mistaken for a choroidal melanoma, particularly when it appears as a discrete, dark, posterior mass. Failure to differentiate these lesions can lead to unnecessary treatment or enucleation. Recent ocular surgery, trauma, or use of anticoagulants should alert the clinician to consider choroidal hemorrhage when malignant melanoma is suspected. Fluorescein angiography and ultrasonography may help to differentiate these entities. Serial examination by ophthalmoscopy or ultrasonography reveals diminishing size of choroidal hemorrhage, over a period of several weeks, and little or no growth of malignant melanoma.[20] Suprachoroidal hemorrhage has been reported to occur with systemic tissue plasminogen activator. In one case, this complication occurred days after administration of the agent to a patient with acute myocardial infarction.[21]

COURSE AND OUTCOME

Delayed, nonexpulsive, limited choroidal hemorrhage generally carries a good prognosis. Choroidal hemorrhages in cataract surgery tend to fare better than those in other forms of ocular surgery or in trauma. Retinal detachment in an eye with choroidal detachment or with choroidal hemorrhage in all four quadrants correlates with a poor visual outcome.[2,22] The extension of suprachoroidal hemorrhage into the posterior pole has been associated with worse visual and anatomical outcomes.[23] Vitreous and, especially, retinal incarceration is associated with

a poorer prognosis.[24] In the absence of retinal adherence, however, kissing choroidal detachments may not portend a worse outcome—the natural history of this condition has not been delineated precisely.

REFERENCES

1. Bukelman A, Hoffman P, Oliver M. Limited choroidal hemorrhage associated with extracapsular cataract extraction. Arch Ophthalmol. 1987;105(3):338–41.
2. Welch JC, Spaeth GL, Benson WE. Massive suprachoroidal hemorrhage. Ophthalmology. 1988;95(9):1202–6.
3. Ingraham HJ, Donnenfeld ED, Perry HD. Massive suprachoroidal hemorrhage in penetrating keratoplasty. Am J Ophthalmol. 1989;108(6):670–5.
4. Beyer CF, Peyman GA, Hill JM. Expulsive choroidal hemorrhage in rabbits. Arch Ophthalmol. 1989;107(11):1648–53.
5. Speaker MG, Guerriero PN, Met JA, et al. A case-control study of risk factors for intraoperative suprachoroidal expulsive hemorrhage. Ophthalmology. 1991;98(2):202–10.
6. Chu TG, Cano MR, Green RL, et al. Massive suprachoroidal hemorrhage with central retinal apposition. Arch Ophthalmol. 1991;109(11):1575–81.
7. Chu TG, Green RL. Suprachoroidal hemorrhage. Surv Ophthalmol. 1999;43:471–86.
8. Wheeler TM, Zimmerman TJ. Expulsive choroidal hemorrhage in the glaucoma patient. Ann Ophthalmol. 1987;19(5):165–6.
9. Lambrou FH, Meredith TA, Kaplan HJ. Secondary surgical management of expulsive choroidal hemorrhage. Arch Ophthalmol. 1987;105(9):1195–8.
10. Ariano ML, Ball SF. Delayed nonexpulsive suprachoroidal hemorrhage after trabeculectomy. Ophthalmic Surg. 1987;18(9):661–6.
11. Canning CR, Lavin M, McCartney ACE, et al. Delayed suprachoroidal hemorrhage after glaucoma operations. Eye. 1989;3(3):327–31.
12. Davidson JA. Vitrectomy and fluid infusion in the treatment of delayed suprachoroidal hemorrhage after combined cataract and glaucoma filtering surgery. Ophthalmic Surg. 1987;18(5):334–6.
13. Lakhanpal V, Schocket SS, Elman MJ, et al. A new modified vitreoretinal surgical approach in the management of massive suprachoroidal hemorrhage. Ophthalmology. 1989;96(6):793–800.
14. Iverson DA, Ward TG, Blumenkranz MS. Indications and results of relaxing retinotomy. Ophthalmology. 1990;97(10);1298–304.
15. Desai UR, Peyman GA, Chen CJ, et al. Use of perfluoroperhydrophenanthrene in the management of suprachoroidal hemorrhages. Ophthalmology. 1992;99(10):1542–7.
16. Awan KJ. Intraocular lens implantation following expulsive choroidal hemorrhage. Am J Ophthalmol. 1988;106(3):261–3.
17. Liggett PE, Mani N, Green RL, et al. Management of traumatic rupture of the globe in aphakic patients. Retina. 1990;10:S59–S64.
18. Pepsin SR, Katz J, Augsburger JJ, et al. Acute angle-closure glaucoma from spontaneous massive hemorrhagic retinal or choroidal detachment. Ophthalmology. 1990;97(1):76–84.
19. Hoskins HD Jr, Kass MA. Developmental and childhood glaucoma. In: Becker–Shaffer's diagnosis and therapy of the glaucomas, ed 6. St Louis: Mosby; 1989:355–403.
20. Morgan CM, Gragoudas ES. Limited choroidal hemorrhage mistaken for a choroidal melanoma. Ophthalmology. 1987;94(1):41–6.
21. Khawly JA, Ferrone PJ, Holck DEE. Choroidal hemorrhage associated with systemic tissue plasminogen activator. Am J Ophthalmol. 1996;121(5):577–8.
22. Reynolds MG, Haimovici R, Flynn HW, et al. Suprachoroidal hemorrhage. Clinical features and results of secondary surgical management. Ophthalmology. 1993;100(4):460–5.
23. Tabandeh H, Sullivan PM, Smahliuk P. Suprachoroidal hemorrhage during pars plana vitrectomy. Ophthalmology. 1999;106:236–42.
24. Wirostko WJ, Han DP, Mieler WF, et al. Suprachoroidal hemorrhage: outcome of surgical management according to hemorrhage severity. Ophthalmology. 1998;105:2271–5.

CHAPTER
139 Proliferative Vitreoretinopathy

G. WILLIAM AYLWARD

DEFINITION
- The proliferation of avascular fibrocellular retinal membranes associated with rhegmatogenous retinal detachment.

KEY FEATURES
- Epiretinal and subretinal fibrous proliferation.
- Contraction of membranes.
- Recurrent or persistent retinal detachment.
- Retinal shortening.
- Reopening of preexisting retinal breaks.
- Formation of new retinal breaks.

ASSOCIATED FEATURES
- Hypotony.
- Vitreous opacity.
- Aqueous flare.
- Iris neovascularization.
- Macular pucker.

INTRODUCTION

Proliferative vitreoretinopathy (PVR) is the most common cause of ultimate failure after surgical treatment for rhegmatogenous retinal detachment.[1,2] A wound-healing response, PVR is characterized by the formation of surface membranes in the posterior segment. Membranes most commonly form on the inner surface of the neural retina but can also be found in the subretinal space and on the ciliary body. Contraction of these membranes may cause macular pucker, new retinal breaks, recurrent retinal detachment, and ocular hypotony.

EPIDEMIOLOGY AND PATHOGENESIS

PVR occurs following surgical repair of retinal detachment but can develop in untreated cases, particularly those that are long-standing or with large breaks. It may also occur following large choroidal detachments or in eyes with large, treated retinal tears but no previous retinal detachment. It occurs in 5–10% of treated rhegmatogenous retinal detachment cases and represents the major cause of ultimate surgical failure.[1]

Certain types of retinal detachments are more likely to develop PVR than others. For example, those associated with giant retinal tears (greater than 3 clock hours) have a high incidence of postoperative PVR, probably because of the large area of bare retinal pigment epithelium (RPE) that is exposed. Other risk factors have been identified in several studies that used multivariate regression analysis. These include the number and size of retinal breaks, the number of previous operations,

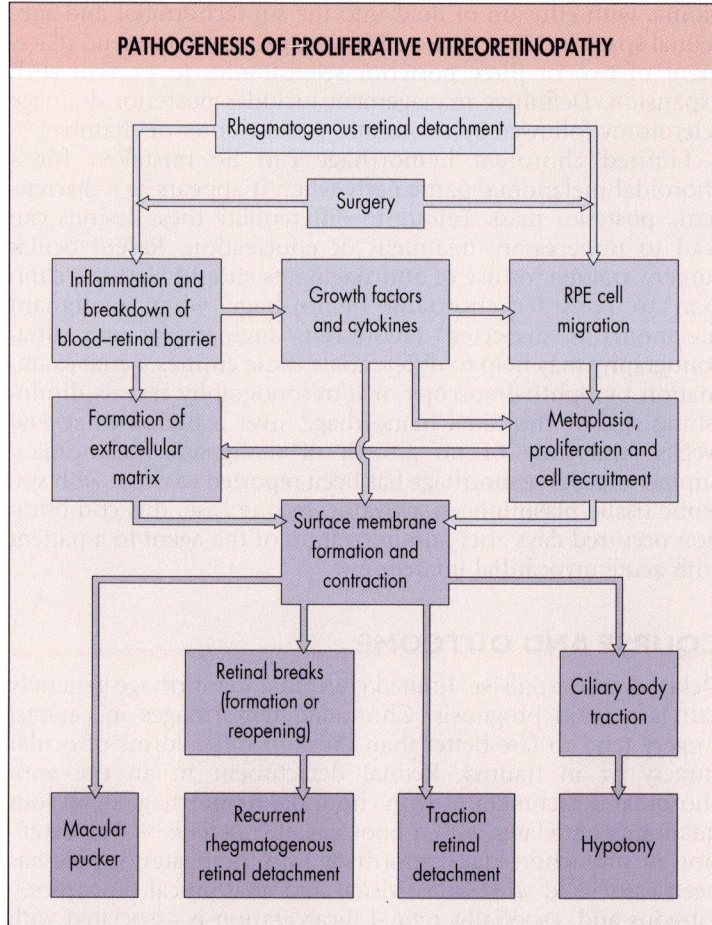

PATHOGENESIS OF PROLIFERATIVE VITREORETINOPATHY

FIG. 139-1 ■ Pathogenesis of proliferative vitreoretinopathy. The flow chart illustrates the interaction of various factors in the pathogenesis of proliferative vitreoretinopathy, from the initial retinal detachment to the serious complications of recurrent detachment and hypotony.

the presence of choroidal effusions, the use of cryotherapy, intraocular hemorrhage, aphakia, high vitreous protein levels, and the severity of preoperative PVR.[2–4] Young patients who have penetrating trauma, especially double perforating injuries, also have a very high risk of PVR.

The pathogenesis of PVR is multifactorial and is summarized in Figure 139-1. The primary event is the formation of a retinal break. It is thought that RPE cells then migrate through the break into the preretinal space, where they settle on the retinal surface. Most of the fibrocellular tissue develops inferiorly, which suggests that gravity influences the distribution of the RPE cells. Glial cell proliferation follows, and an extracellular matrix is laid down. These cells take on the characteristics of myofibroblasts in that they have contractile elements and deposit collagen.[2] While the cellular origins of PVR are critical, the extracellular environment plays a decisive role as well. Inflammation

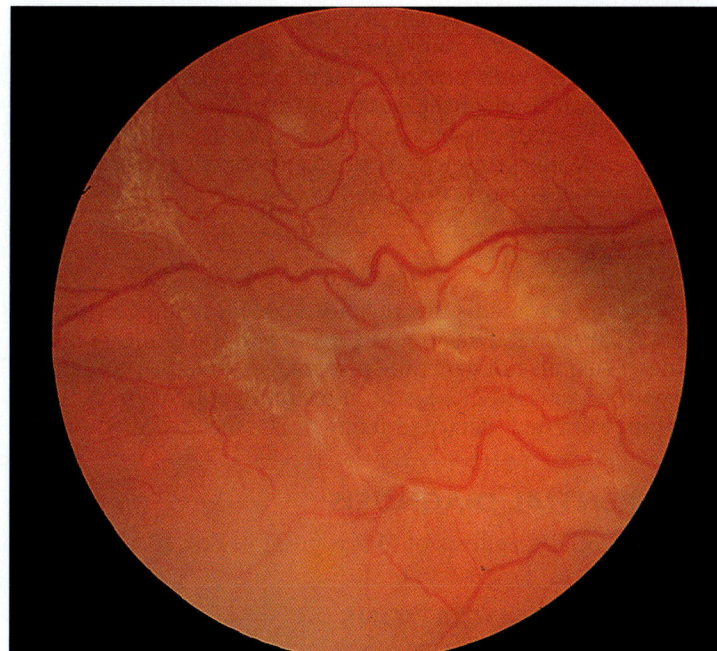

FIG. 139-2 ▌ **Macular pucker following retinal detachment surgery.** Contraction of a surface membrane at the macula produces symptoms of distortion and reduced visual acuity. Such epiretinal membranes are identical histologically to those removed from elsewhere on the retina in proliferative vitreoretinopathy.

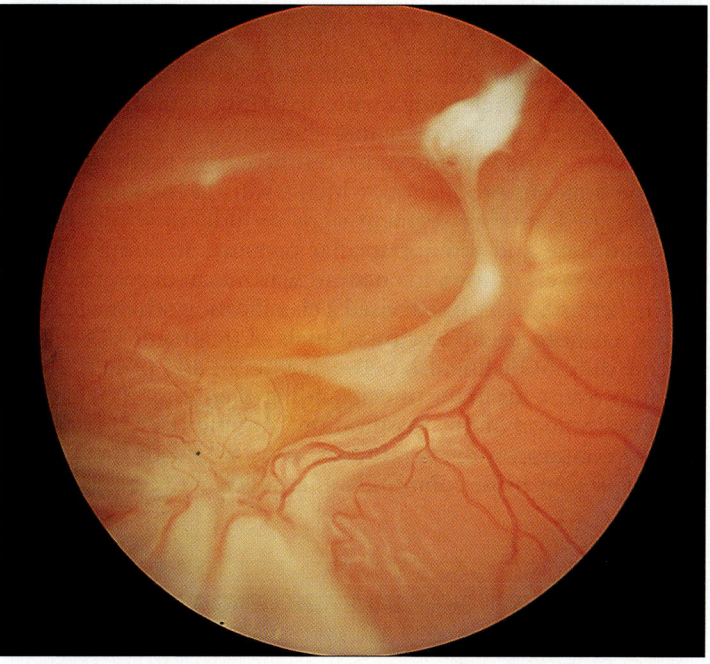

FIG. 139-3 ▌ **Star fold from proliferative vitreoretinopathy.** Contraction of a focal retinal surface membrane has resulted in the formation of a star fold. In this case, membranes can also be seen on the posterior surface of the partially detached hyaloid face.

and breakdown of the blood-retina barrier are associated with further cellular recruitment, modulated by inflammatory mediators and the formation of extensive fibrous membranes.[5] Collagen is produced and the membranes then contract. It is the contraction of surface membranes that produces the clinical features described below. The cycle of cell dispersion, inflammation, membrane formation, and contraction with eventual redetachment of the retina has a typical time scale of 4–6 weeks after the initial repair.

OCULAR MANIFESTATIONS

The clinical spectrum of PVR varies according to the extent and location of membranes and the presence and position of retinal breaks. Macular pucker after successful retinal detachment surgery can be considered a mild form of PVR (Fig. 139-2). In its most severe form, membrane contraction produces a total, funnel-shaped detachment with retina adherent anteriorly to the ciliary body and even to the iris, which results in hypotony and phthisis bulbi.

Surface membranes can be difficult to diagnose when the retina is attached. Many successfully repaired retinal detachments show surface membrane formation if examined histopathologically. Occasionally, surface membranes can result in localized traction retinal detachments, often seen just posterior to a scleral buckle. These localized traction detachments tend to be stable and should be differentiated from recurrent rhegmatogenous detachments associated with open retinal breaks. Traction retinal detachments have a concave surface generated by the RPE pump pulling against traction, in contradistinction to the convex profile of rhegmatogenous detachments. Should a new retinal break develop acutely or a preexisting break reopen, already present but unsuspected membranes may result in dramatic contraction of the newly redetached retina to give the clinical impression of sudden development of severe PVR.

The earliest signs of PVR include marked vitreous flare and clumps of pigment in the vitreous. Increased stiffness of the detached retina often occurs, which can be detected with indirect ophthalmoscopy while the patient's eye is making saccades. A fresh retinal detachment without PVR appears to undulate under these conditions, an undulation that is reduced if significant sur-

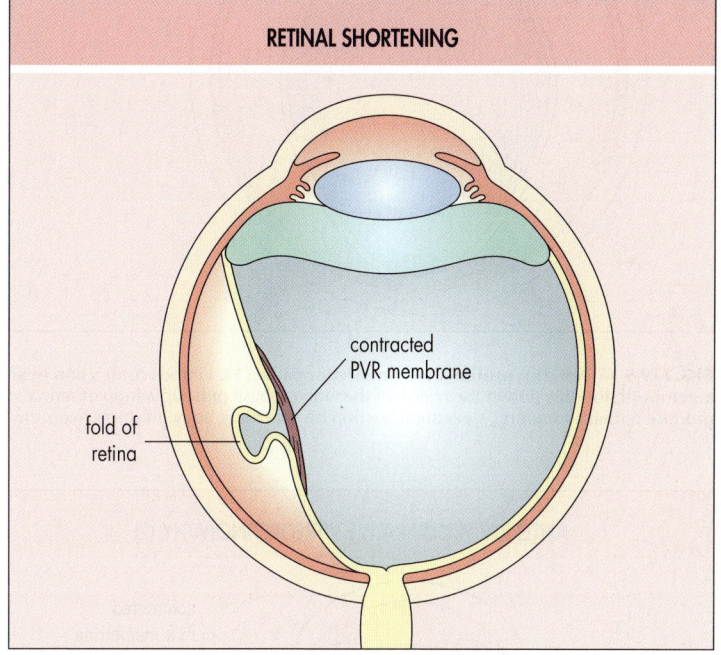

FIG. 139-4 ▌ **Retinal shortening.** Surface membrane contraction can result in retinal shortening, which prevents break closure and retinal reattachment.

face membranes are present. The edges of retinal breaks may be rolled over, as a result of contraction on one surface only, and retinal breaks may appear stretched open. Star folds represent localized areas of puckering in detached retina after focal, localized contraction (Fig. 139-3).

Subretinal fibrosis may accompany surface membranes to give a "Swiss cheese" appearance to the subretinal space. Some of the subretinal sheets of membrane coil together, which results in broad, subretinal strands. A subretinal "napkin ring" of membrane can surround the peripapillary retina to produce a tight posterior funnel configuration and obscure the optic nerve. Significant amounts of surface traction produce retinal shortening, which makes break closure and retinal reattachment impossible (Fig. 139-4). More severe contraction may pull the anterior retina inward, which leads to an anterior funnel appearance. In severe cases, closure of the anterior end of the funnel may make it impossible to visualize the optic disc even if the posterior retina is relatively unaffected. Contraction of the vitreous base leads to circumferential shortening and anterior loop contraction. Surface membranes on the ciliary body may compromise aqueous production, which results in hypotony.

Associated anterior segment signs include anterior chamber cells and flare and low intraocular pressure. In some eyes, dilated iris vessels or even iris neovascularization develops.

The Retina Society has devised a classification scheme for PVR, which has been useful in clinical trials of treatment.[6] The initial scheme did not distinguish between anterior and posterior PVR, and improvements in the understanding of anterior PVR have led to a modification of the classification.[7] Anterior PVR is characterized by contraction of membranes associated with the vitreous base; it is seen most commonly after failed vitrectomy and gas

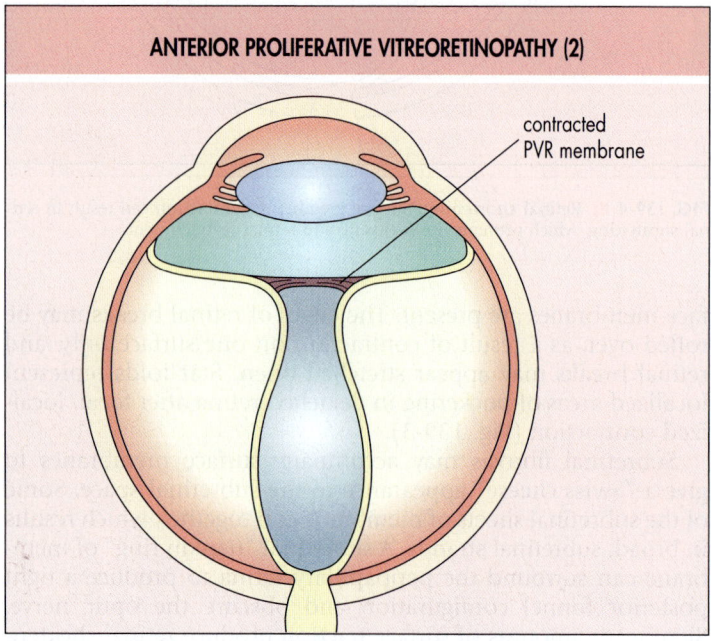

FIG. 139-5 ■ Anterior proliferative vitreoretinopathy (1). Fibrous contraction in an anteroposterior direction in the region of the vitreous base pulls up a loop of retina to produce retinal shortening. Coexistent traction on the ciliary body produces hypotony.

FIG. 139-6 ■ Anterior proliferative vitreoretinopathy (2). Contraction of the anterior vitreous produces a funnel configuration.

tamponade for retinal detachment or after penetrating trauma.[8] Anteroposterior traction can pull a fold of retina forward to produce a "trough" with posterior shortening (Fig. 139-5), which can be difficult to diagnose preoperatively. Circumferential contraction of the vitreous base produces radial folds in the retina, and perpendicular contraction of the anterior vitreous leads to an anterior funnel-shaped configuration (Fig. 139-6).

DIAGNOSIS

In eyes with clear media, the diagnosis of PVR is straightforward. A history of retinal detachment surgery and the clinical features just described do not generally present a diagnostic problem. In eyes with opaque media, B-scan ultrasonography is necessary to reveal the stiffened, detached retina and associated membranes.

DIFFERENTIAL DIAGNOSIS

The differential diagnosis of PVR is given in Box 139-1.

SYSTEMIC ASSOCIATIONS

Although no direct, significant systemic associations exist, patients who have Stickler's syndrome have an increased risk of retinal detachment because of large and/or multiple retinal breaks that make subsequent PVR likely.

PATHOLOGY

A large body of pathologic information exists that confirms the role of RPE cells, inflammation, breakdown of the blood-ocular barrier, macrophages, growth factors, cytokines, clotting cascade proteins, adhesion molecules, and extracellular matrices in the development of PVR. In histological specimens, RPE cells are uniformly present, and evidence shows that they can undergo metaplastic change to macrophages or fibroblasts.[9] Glial cells are a major component of PVR membranes and may arise from retinal astrocytes.[10] Lymphocytes have been identified in excised PVR membranes,[11] although the role of humoral immunity in PVR remains unclear.

The behavior of the RPE cell may be stimulated by several different growth factors. For example, platelet-derived growth factor stimulates chemotaxis,[12] and fibroblast growth factor and insulin-like growth factor-1 stimulate RPE cell proliferation.[13] In contrast, transforming growth factor-β has an inhibitory effect on cell proliferation in tissue culture.[14] Interleukins (ILs) also play a role. Elevated levels of IL-1 and IL-6 have been detected in the vitreous of patients with PVR.[15] Many of these growth factors and cytokines are also known to play a significant part in the wound-healing process in general.

The extracellular matrix associated with PVR consists of various types of collagen, particularly types I and III. Other components include fibronectin and the basal lamina proteins, heparan sulfate, laminin, and collagen type IV.[16] Recent work suggests that the matrix metalloproteinases may play a role in the pathogenesis of PVR.[17]

The mechanism of membrane contraction remains poorly understood. Some of the cell types found in membranes are capable of contraction, including fibroblasts and RPE cells.[18] Cytoplasmic

---

BOX 139-1

Differential Diagnosis of Proliferative Vitreoretinopathy

Proliferative diabetic retinopathy with traction retinal detachment
Chronic retinal detachment with retinal edema and/or cyst formation
Severe choroidal detachments
Severe vitreomacular traction syndrome with traction retinal detachment
Severe ocular hypotony

myofilaments have been seen in some fibroblastic cells, but simple motility of cells through a collagen matrix may be sufficient to produce shortening.

TREATMENT

In the absence of open retinal breaks, PVR does not require treatment unless the macula is involved. Localized traction detachments posterior to a scleral buckle are stable and asymptomatic. Macular pucker after otherwise successful retinal detachment surgery may be responsible for reduced visual acuity and distortion. Such cases often benefit from membrane peeling.

In rhegmatogenous retinal detachment, the choice of treatment is based on the severity and location of the PVR and the location of the retinal break or breaks. Scleral buckling alone may be successful if the surface membranes do not prevent break closure. For example, the presence of inferior star folds does not prevent successful closure of a single superior retinal break by means of a scleral buckle. However, it can be difficult to judge the extent of retinal shortening and, therefore, the influence of a star fold on a remote break. If surface membranes occur in close association with retinal breaks, closed intraocular microsurgery with membrane peeling is required to enable break closure, although occasionally a substantial inferior buckle can be used successfully to close breaks associated with a moderate degree of surface contraction (Fig. 139-7).

With an internal approach, a complete pars plana vitrectomy is followed by peeling of surface membranes, using a combination of a retinal pick and microforceps (Fig. 139-8).[19] The ease with which membranes can be removed varies, but it is important to relieve traction associated with breaks if surgery is to succeed. Perfluorocarbon liquids may assist the process as they highlight the membranes and act as a "third hand" to assist in membrane removal.[20] If long-term intravitreal tamponade with silicone oil is to be used, the membranes may be more visible after oil injection and so are peeled at that stage. If not already present, a circumferential scleral buckle is usually applied to support the vitreous base, which typically is shortened circumferentially. Occasionally, peeling of posterior membranes is insufficient to relieve retinal shortening. In such cases, further dissection of the vitreous base may be successful. Alternatively, a relaxing retinectomy can be performed (Fig. 139-9).[21]

Rarely, subretinal membranes may be present, usually in a band-like configuration. These can tent up the retina, although in most cases simple closure of the break results in complete reattachment. If necessary, the bands can be divided through a small retinotomy or pulled out hand over hand, as they tend to be only loosely adherent to the overlying retina.

After membrane removal, the retina is reattached by means of internal drainage of subretinal fluid, usually accompanied by a fluid-air exchange. Retinopexy with cryotherapy or laser photocoagulation is applied to all breaks. Laser retinopexy is often preferred because of the theoretically increased risk of further PVR associated with the use of cryotherapy.

A long-acting gas or silicone oil is injected for tamponade; the choice of agent depends on a number of factors. In the Silicone

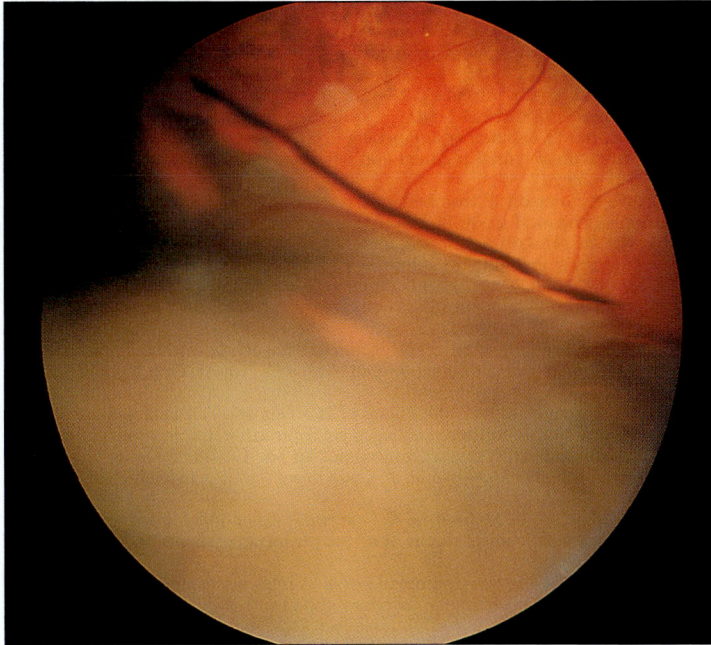

FIG. 139-7 ▮▮ **Scleral buckling in proliferative vitreoretinopathy.** The large inferior buckle seen here was used to support inferior breaks associated with proliferative vitreoretinopathy. Recurrent gray proliferative vitreoretinopathy membranes can be seen on the surface of the buckle, but the retina remains attached posteriorly. Note the dark line on the edge of the buckle, which is an optical effect of the silicone oil fill.

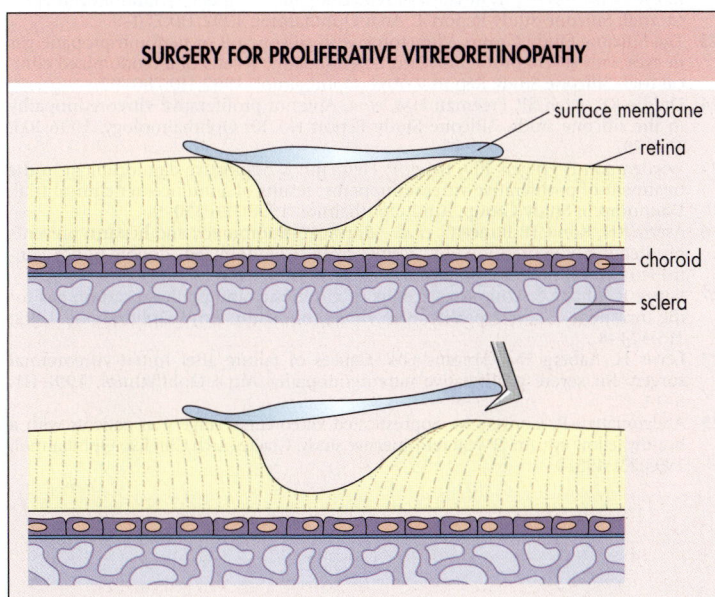

FIG. 139-8 ▮▮ **Surgery for proliferative vitreoretinopathy.** A pick is used to elevate surface membranes prior to removal with forceps.

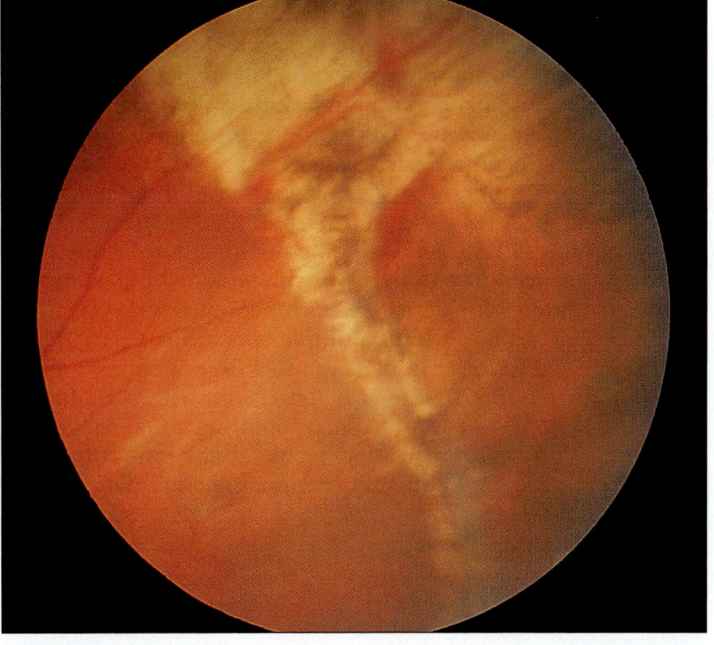

FIG. 139-9 ▮▮ **A severe case of anterior proliferative vitreoretinopathy treated with a 270° relaxing retinectomy.** The line of laser retinopexy at the edge of the retinectomy can be seen to join with an area of chorioretinal adhesion from cryotherapy.

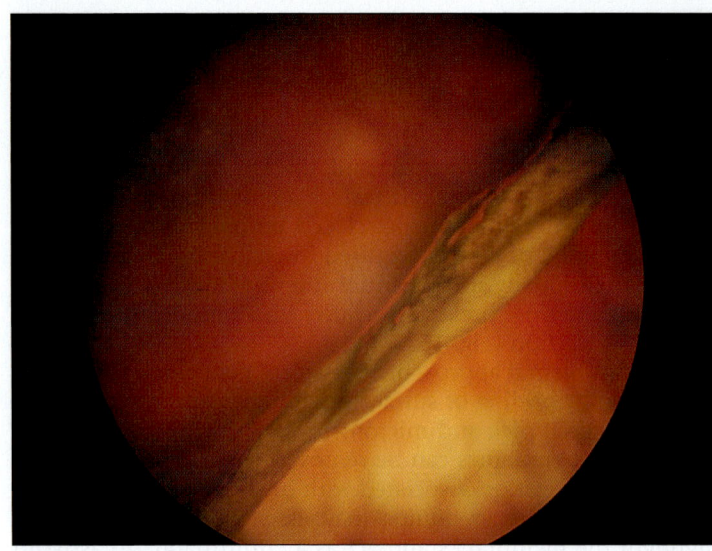

FIG. 139-10 ■ **Reproliferation and failed retinectomy for proliferative vitreo-retinopathy.** Reproliferation of membranes along the edge of a relaxing retinectomy has resulted in elevation of the posterior edge.

Study, the effect of the choice of long-term retinal tamponade on final surgical outcome in PVR cases was examined. The study indicated that both C_3F_8 gas and silicone oil were of similar benefit in PVR, and both are superior to SF_6.[22,23] In anterior PVR, silicone oil has been shown to yield a better visual outcome than C_3F_8.[24] Silicone oil has certain intraoperative and postoperative advantages over gas, which include improved visualization for retinopexy, less need for positioning, and better vision in the immediate postoperative period.

Despite successful treatment, PVR can recur, which results in the formation of new breaks or the reopening of treated breaks (Fig. 139-10). The tendency of PVR to recur has generated much interest in the use of pharmacological agents for adjuvant therapy to surgery. Figure 139-1 shows that many potential pharmacological targets exist for such therapy. A large-scale randomized controlled trial has shown a weak beneficial effect for perioperative daunomycin.[25] A combination of adjuvant 5-hydroxyuracil and low-molecular-weight heparin has been shown to reduce the incidence of PVR in high-risk cases undergoing vitrectomy.[26]

COURSE AND OUTCOME

Untreated, PVR inevitably leads to severe loss of vision, hypotony, and sometimes phthisis bulbi. Success rates for surgical treatment vary and depend on the severity of PVR and the surgical techniques employed.[27,28] Prior to the introduction of closed intraocular microsurgery, success rates were poor. With modern techniques, anatomic success is being achieved in an increasing number of cases. Most recent series report final anatomic success rates of around 70%.[23,27,28] Using perfluorocarbon liquid as an intraoperative tool in conjunction with wide-field viewing systems, success rates for retinal reattachment after one operation can be as high as 78%.[20] With multiple operations, up to 91% of all PVR-affected retinas can be reattached. In one series, 74% of eyes ended up with 20/400 or better vision, with 30% having 20/80 or better.[20] The continued disappointing visual results, despite quite high anatomic reattachment, are the result of a combination of macular dysfunction from previous detachment,

macular pucker, and hypotony. The majority of patients who have PVR have a normal fellow eye. Functional vision in these cases may not be useful to the patient; often the operated eye is considered a "spare."[29]

REFERENCES

1. Rachal WF, Burton TC. Changing concepts of failure after retinal detachment surgery. Arch Ophthalmol. 1979;97:480–3.
2. Ryan SJ. The pathophysiology of proliferative vitreoretinopathy in its management. Am J Ophthalmol. 1985;100:188–93.
3. Cowley M, Conway BP, Campochiro PA, et al. Clinical risk factors for proliferative vitreoretinopathy. Arch Ophthalmol. 1989;107:1147–51.
4. Kon CH, Asaria RH, Occleston NL, et al. Risk factors for proliferative vitreoretinopathy after primary vitrectomy: a prospective study Br J Ophthalmol 2000;84:506–11.
5. Campochiaro PA, Bryan JA, Conway BP, Jaccoma EH. Intravitreal chemotactic and mitogenic activity. Implication of blood-retinal barrier breakdown. Arch Ophthalmol. 1986;104:1685–7.
6. Retina Society Terminology Committee. The classification of retinal detachment with proliferative vitreoretinopathy. Ophthalmology. 1983;90:121–5.
7. Machemer R, Aaberg TM, MacKenzie Freeman H, et al. An updated classification of retinal detachment with proliferative vitreoretinopathy. Am J Ophthalmol. 1991;112:159–65.
8. Lewis H, Aaberg TM, Abrams GW. Anterior proliferative vitreoretinopathy. Am J Ophthalmol. 1988;105:277–84.
9. Mandelcorn MS, Machemer R, Fineberg E, Hersch SB. Proliferation and metaplasia of intravitreal retinal pigment epithelial cell autotransplants. Am J Ophthalmol. 1975;80:227–37.
10. Hiscott PS, Grierson I, Trombetta CJ, et al. Retinal and epiretinal glia—an immunohistochemical study. Br J Ophthalmol. 1984;68:698–707.
11. Charteris DG, Hiscott P, Grierson I, Lightman SL. Proliferative vitreoretinopathy: lymphocytes in epiretinal membranes. Ophthalmology. 1992;99:1364–7.
12. Baudouin C, Fredj Reygrobellet D, Brignole F, et al. Growth factors in vitreous and subretinal fluid cells from patients with proliferative vitreoretinopathy. Ophthalmic Res. 1993;25:52–9.
13. Leschey KH, Hackett SF, Singer JH, Campochiaro PA. Growth factor responsiveness of human retinal pigment epithelial cells. Invest Ophthalmol Vis Sci. 1990;31:839–46.
14. Pena RA, Jerdan JA, Glaser BM. Effects of TGF beta and TGF beta neutralizing antibodies on fibroblast induced collagen gel contraction; implications for proliferative vitreoretinopathy. Invest Ophthalmol Vis Sci. 1994;35:2804–8.
15. Limb GA, Little BC, Meager A, et al. Cytokines in proliferative vitreoretinopathy. Eye. 1991;5:686–93.
16. Morino I, Hiscott PS, McKechnie N, Grierson I. Variation in epiretinal membrane components with clinical duration of the proliferative tissue. Br J Ophthalmol. 1990;74:393–9.
17. Kon CH, Occlestone NL, Charteris D, et al. A prospective study of matrix metalloproteinases in proliferative vitreoretinopathy. Invest Ophthalmol Vis Sci. 1998;39:1524–9.
18. Hiscott PS, Grierson I, McLeod D. Retinal pigment epithelial cells in epiretinal membranes; an immunohistochemical study. Br J Ophthalmol. 1984;68:708–15.
19. Aaberg TM. Management of anterior and posterior proliferative vitreoretinopathy. Am J Ophthalmol. 1988;5:519–32.
20. Coll GE, Chang S, Sun J, et al. Perfluorocarbon liquid in the management of retinal detachment with proliferative vitreoretinopathy. Ophthalmology. 1995;102:630–8.
21. Bovey EH, De Ancos E, Gonvers M. Retinotomies of 180 degrees or more. Retina. 1995;15:394–8.
22. The Silicone Study Group. Vitrectomy with silicone oil or sulfur hexafluoride gas in eyes with severe proliferative vitreoretinopathy; results of a randomized clinical trial. Silicone Study Report 1. Arch Ophthalmol. 1992;110:770–9.
23. The Silicone Study Group. Vitrectomy with silicone oil or perfluoropropane gas in eyes with severe proliferative vitreoretinopathy; results of a randomized clinical trial. Silicone Study Report 2. Arch Ophthalmol. 1992;110:780–92.
24. Diddie KR, Azen SP, Freeman HM, et al. Anterior proliferative vitreoretinopathy in the silicone study. Silicone Study Report No 10. Ophthalmology. 1996;103:1092–9.
25. Wiedemann P, Hilgers RD, Bauer P, Heimann K Adjunctive daunorubicin in the treatment of proliferative vitreoretinopathy: results of a multicenter clinical trial. Daunomycin Study Group. Am J Ophthalmol. 1998;126:550–9.
26. Asaria RH, Kon CH, Bunce C, et al. Adjuvant 5-fluorouracil and heparin prevents proliferative vitreoretinopathy: results from a randomized, double-blind, controlled clinical trial Ophthalmology. 2001;108:1179–83.
27. Lopez R, Chang S. Long term results of vitrectomy and perfluorocarbon gas for the treatment of severe proliferative vitreoretinopathy. Am J Ophthalmol. 1992;113:424–8.
28. Lewis H, Aaberg TM, Abrams GW. Causes of failure after initial vitreoretinal surgery for severe proliferative vitreoretinopathy. Am J Ophthalmol. 1991;111:8–14.
29. Andenmatten R, Gonvers M. Sophisticated vitreoretinal surgery in patients with a healthy fellow eye. An 11-year retrospective study. Graefes Arch Clin Exp Ophthalmol. 1993;231:495–9.

SECTION 8 TRAUMA

CHAPTER

140

Posterior Segment Ocular Trauma

PATRICK E. RUBSAMEN

DEFINITION
- Damage to the posterior intraocular structures secondary to unplanned external physical contact.

KEY FEATURES
- Blunt, contusive injury, with or without globe rupture.
- Sharp, penetrating injury.
- High-velocity foreign body injury.

ASSOCIATED FEATURES
- Hemorrhage.
- Retinal detachment.
- Proliferative vitreoretinopathy.
- Choroidal rupture.
- Endophthalmitis.
- Cataract.

INTRODUCTION

Ocular trauma is an important cause of visual loss and disability. With modern diagnostic techniques, surgical approaches, and rehabilitation, many eyes can be salvaged with retention of vision.[1-4] Despite advances in medical and surgical management, penetrating trauma continues to be a complicated and challenging condition.

Posterior segment trauma is divided, to aid evaluation and management, into the categories nonpenetrating and penetrating injuries. Nonpenetrating injuries that involve the posterior segment are often the result of severe, blunt, concussive blows to the globe and result in special types of ocular damage.

Penetrating injuries are further divided into subcategories based upon the type and extent of damage. Penetrating wounds may be classified into rupture secondary to blunt injury (such as being struck by a rock or associated with a fall), lacerating injuries (involved in, for instance, a knife stab wound or a glass cut), and injuries related to intraocular foreign bodies. A clarification of the definitions related to penetrating injuries has been proposed by Kuhn *et al.*[5]

OCULAR MANIFESTATIONS

Penetrating ocular injuries may result in ocular damage of various degrees and may present with a wide array of clinical findings. It is important to perform an initial ophthalmic evaluation of the patient who has ocular trauma as thoroughly as possible. One needs to determine whether a penetrating or nonpenetrating injury is present, the extent of the clinical injury, and whether any associated extraocular injuries exist. The general status of the patient who has what appears to be an isolated ocular trauma should not be overlooked by the ophthalmologist, as this initial evaluation may be the first encounter for the patient with the medical system.

Clinical history is important, and as much information about the details of the injury should be obtained as possible. The history related to the injury may provide clues to the nature of the ocular injury (e.g., hammering metal on metal or struck in the eye with a wire). The history can also provide clues to the likelihood of other associated extraocular injuries (e.g., fall in an elderly patient that resulted in head trauma and subdural hemorrhage or orthopedic injury) that need to be evaluated concurrently. Prior history of ocular surgery, such as prior cataract extraction, should prompt a search for an occult cataract wound rupture. It is important to document the setting of the injury as well, as this may have long-term implications. Was the patient assaulted, did the injury occur during work, was the patient wearing protective eyewear, what were the circumstances of the injury? Documentation of prior visual function and the degree of visual loss is important and can play a role in management decisions.

The initial clinical examination should be as complete as possible, but any further injury to the globe should be avoided. In some settings after penetrating trauma, it may be difficult to assess precisely the patient's visual acuity; however, assessment of visual acuity is important. The level of vision at presentation is an accurate predictor of the long-term visual prognosis.[6,7] The pupils should be examined carefully for the presence of an afferent pupillary defect. The presence or absence of an afferent pupillary defect provides important information about the extent of intraocular injury and may provide information as to the visual prognosis of the patient.

A careful slit-lamp and external examination should be performed to ensure that any open lacerations to the cornea or sclera are found. A search for periocular lacerations that involve the lids or for any evidence of orbital fracture is important. Occult rupture of the sclera should be considered, especially if extensive hemorrhagic chemosis of the conjunctiva is present. Occult rupture often originates under one of the rectus muscle insertions and may extend posteriorly along the globe without evidence of external prolapse of any intraocular tissue. A low intraocular pressure may be an indication of an occult rupture; however, the intraocular pressure can be normal or elevated in this setting.

The presence or absence of anterior chamber hemorrhage, cataract, or irregularity of the pupil should be noted. Patients who have undergone previous cataract extraction are predisposed to rupture of their prior cataract wound, and this area should be examined carefully. Ruptured cataract incisions may be overlooked as they may "self-seal," even if extrusion of the intraocular lens has occurred (Fig. 140-1). Laceration, puncture, or dislocation of the crystalline lens should be noted. Signs of early or established infection, such as undue inflammation or hypopyon, retinal vasculitis, or purulent discharge, should be assessed. Early intervention in this setting may enable the salvage of some eyes that have traumatic endophthalmitis.[8,9]

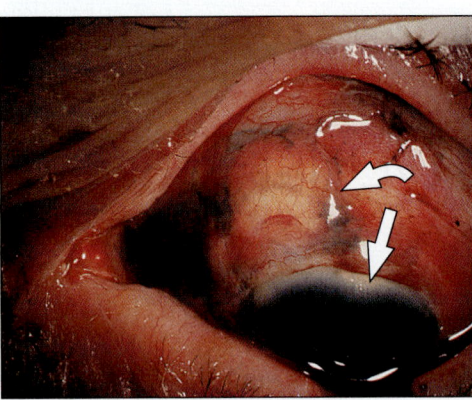

FIG. 140-1 ■ **The patient underwent cataract surgery 2 years before suffering a blunt injury to the eye.** Note the self-sealing wound in the area of the prior cataract surgery incision *(arrow)* and the extruded intraocular lens underneath the conjunctiva *(curved arrow).*

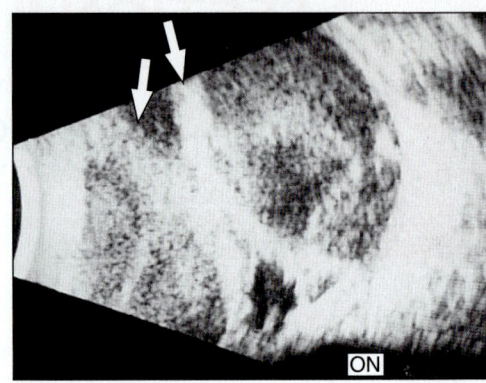

FIG. 140-3 ■ **Massive "kissing" hemorrhagic choroidal detachments** *(arrows).* Note the classical dome shape seen with choroidal detachment and internal echoes consistent with blood. *(ON,* Optic nerve.)

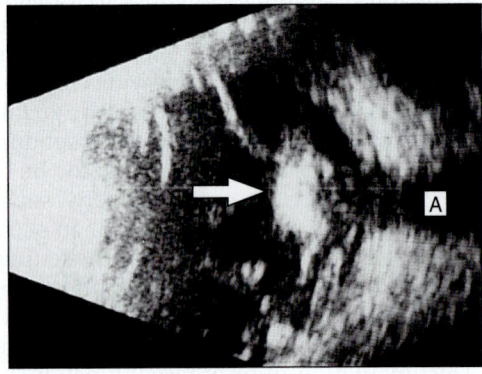

FIG. 140-2 ■ **Radiopaque intraocular foreign body** *(arrow).* Note the characteristic acoustic shadowing *(A)* behind it.

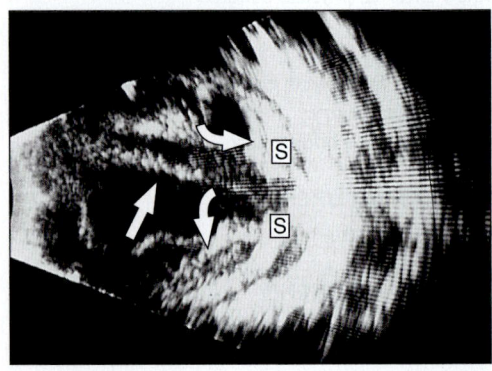

FIG. 140-4 ■ **Perforating ocular injury from a nail.** Note the discontinuity of the sclera *(S).* A retinal detachment with subretinal blood is present *(curved arrows),* as well as a hemorrhagic vitreous track *(arrow).*

If the fundus can be visualized, the presence of retinal detachment, retina tears, choroidal hemorrhage, or intraocular foreign body should be sought. Early in the course following injury it is, at times, possible to obtain a view of the fundus using indirect ophthalmoscopy; this information may prove useful in subsequent management decisions.

DIAGNOSIS AND ANCILLARY TESTING

Ancillary testing is sometimes used to assist the evaluation of patients who have penetrating injuries. Radiopaque foreign bodies are usually evident on standard, orbital, plain film radiographs. Computed tomography is helpful in the evaluation of both intraocular and periocular structures.[10] Also, computed tomography may help to determine the presence of a metallic intraocular foreign body or to ascertain the presence or degree of periocular damage. Furthermore, it may show whether a patient has sustained an intracranial injury, such as subdural hemorrhage. Although computed tomography provides a helpful diagnostic adjunct in penetrating ocular trauma, it may not be sensitive enough to be relied upon as the sole means of evaluating an open globe injury.[11]

Diagnostic ultrasound can also provide useful information about the status of intraocular structures.[12,13] Ultrasound can localize intraocular foreign bodies (Fig. 140-2) and may provide some advantage over other imaging techniques when the presence or location of a nonmetallic intraocular foreign body needs to established. After the initial primary closure, ultrasound may be used to evaluate the extent of intraocular injury and to plan secondary surgical intervention.[12,13] Ultrasound accurately detects choroidal hemorrhage, posterior scleral rupture, retinal detachment, and subretinal hemorrhage.

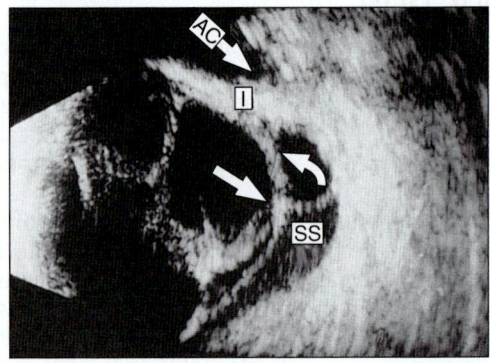

FIG. 140-5 ■ **Anterior proliferative vitreoretinopathy following trauma.** A cross section of the iris *(I),* ciliary body, and anterior chamber *(AC)* is seen. Note the traction detachment of the anterior retina *(arrow)* caused by the fibrous membrane *(curved arrow).* *(SS,* Subretinal space.)

On echography, choroidal hemorrhage appears as a dome-shaped elevation with echodense fluid in the suprachoroidal space (Fig. 140-3). In the early period after trauma the hemorrhage in the suprachoroidal space appears relatively homogeneous; however, later (7–14 days) liquefaction occurs, as indicated by the appearance of a fluid level in the suprachoroidal space. Retinal detachment is seen as a highly reflective, mobile membrane that inserts into the optic nerve. With the onset of proliferative vitreoretinopathy, the retina may become less mobile or assume a funnel-shaped configuration. A posterior scleral defect with vitreous that streams to the exit wound may be seen when a posterior exit site is present (Fig. 140-4).

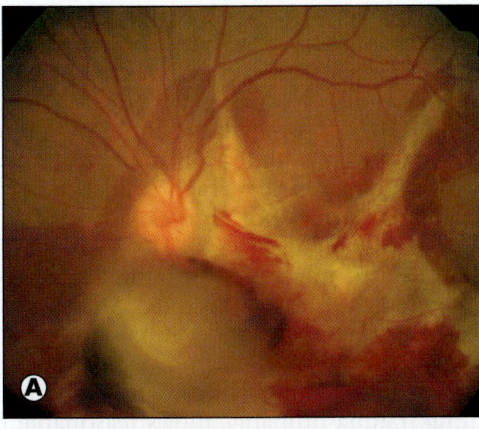

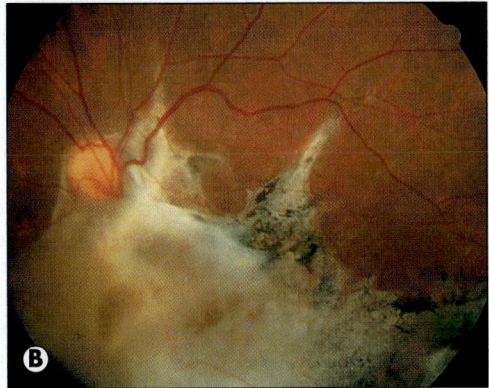

FIG. 140-6 ▮▮ **Gunshot wound to the periocular region. A,** Sclopetaria manifests as subretinal and choroidal hemorrhage; also note marked disruption and necrosis of the choroid and retina. **B,** After 6 months and no surgical intervention, the retina remains attached and marked chorioretinal scarring is present.

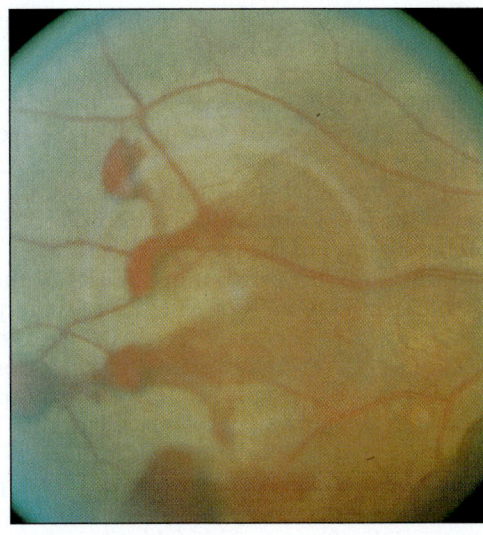

FIG. 140-7 ▮▮ **Berlin's edema (commotio retinae) in a patient after blunt ocular trauma.** Note the gray opacification of the retina; vitreous hemorrhage is also present.

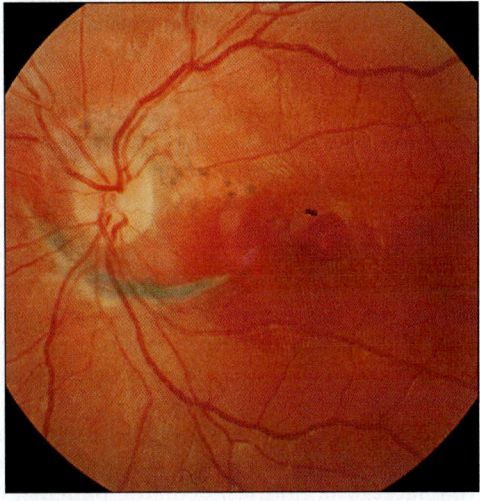

FIG. 140-8 ▮▮ **Choroidal rupture after blunt trauma with a tennis ball.** Note the concentric area of choroidal injury; also visible is a full-thickness, post-traumatic macular hole.

Ultrasound may also be used to evaluate more anterior regions of the globe, such as occult ruptures of the sclera that underlie the rectus muscle insertions or the anterior epiretinal membrane formation seen with anterior proliferative vitreoretinopathy (Fig. 140-5). A water-immersion technique can be used to detect posterior lens rupture, especially when anterior chamber blood precludes visualization of the crystalline lens.

TREATMENT

Nonpenetrating Injury

Blunt injury to the globe can result in subluxation or dislocation of the crystalline lens. A subluxated lens that becomes cataractous or interferes with the patient's vision (because of malposition) can be removed either using an anterior limbal approach, with careful attention to the anterior vitreous, or via the pars plana. Completely dislocated, nonruptured lenses may be observed in some cases. If removal is necessary, pars plana lensectomy is preferable. Concurrent vitreous hemorrhage can also be removed via the pars plana.

A variety of retinal injuries may occur with blunt injury to the globe; these include macular hole, peripheral retinal tear, giant retinal tear, retinal dialysis, and avulsion of the vitreous base.[14] Management of these injuries depends on the nature of the retinal injury and on the presence of retinal detachment and/or vitreous hemorrhage; it may include prophylactic laser photocoagulation or cryopexy, scleral buckling, and pars plana vitrectomy. Improved surgical techniques have increased the success rate for repair of retinal detachment after both penetrating and nonpenetrating trauma.[1-4,13] The use of perfluorocarbon liquids during surgical repair has also improved the prognosis for eyes that have a giant retinal tear or retinal detachment.[15]

Hemorrhagic necrosis of the retina (chorioretinitis sclopetaria) is a special circumstance that results from severe contusion injury of the globe (e.g., missile injury). Despite widespread injury to the retina, retinal pigment epithelium, and choroid, the retina often remains attached, even with no treatment, as a result of chorioretinal scarring and the subsequent adhesion between the retina and underlying tissues (Fig. 140-6).

A common finding with blunt injuries, which may lead to acute visual loss, is Berlin's edema (commotio retinae; Fig. 140-7); this manifests as a widespread or localized whitening of the retina. Recovery of vision is common; however, some patients may sustain some degree of permanent visual loss often accompanied by subretinal pigmentary changes in the macula.

Chorioretinal rupture may occur as a result of the compressive forces generated by a blunt injury. These ruptures tend to occur in a concentric fashion relative to the optic nerve and may result in severe visual loss if the central macula is involved (Fig. 140-8). Delayed visual loss may also occur as a result of the development of choroidal neovascularization. Laser photocoagulation or subretinal surgical extraction of the neovascular membrane may be indicated in some cases.[16] Direct or indirect trauma to the optic nerve or avulsion of the nerve itself may result in profound loss of vision.

Penetrating Trauma

Management of penetrating injuries varies widely according to the severity, extent, and location of the injury. Several general principles of management apply to all penetrating ocular injuries; these include the following:

- Primary closure of the penetrating wound
- Removal of any foreign body material
- Prevention of further or secondary injury to the eye (infection)
- Anatomical and visual rehabilitation of the eye
- Protection of the fellow uninvolved eye (protective eyewear)
- General rehabilitation of the patient.

INITIAL CLOSURE. With penetrating injuries of the eye, primary closure of the laceration is the first goal of surgery. Wounds isolated to the cornea can generally be closed with interrupted 10-0 nylon sutures. Occasionally, with irregular wounds that cannot be closed in a watertight fashion with sutures, closure may be obtained by application of cyanoacrylate glue. Prolapsed intraocular tissue may be reposited into the globe if the tissue appears viable. Iris that has been externalized for a protracted period, appears necrotic, or is epithelialized should be excised. Viscoelastic materials often prove useful in the reformation and maintenance of the anterior chamber and to separate adhesions between tissues in the anterior chamber. In general, repair of a scleral laceration is accomplished most easily by an initial closure at the limbus and then progressive closure posteriorly. Closure should be performed as meticulously as possible to prevent extrusion of intraocular contents. Knots from sutures in the cornea should be buried if possible.

For posterior penetrating injuries that violate the vitreous base, an encircling scleral buckle may be considered. Previous investigators found that prophylactic placement of an encircling scleral buckle at the time of repair of a penetrating injury may reduce the risk of subsequent retinal detachment.[2,3] Placing the scleral buckle at the time of the initial repair also eliminates the need to reopen the tissues in the area of the prior laceration at a subsequent operation. Furthermore, in eyes with posterior scleral injuries, many eyes that do not have a scleral buckle placed at the time of the initial surgical closure ultimately require scleral buckle surgery.[17]

ANESTHESIA. General anesthesia is used most commonly in the repair of penetrating ocular wounds. This is particularly the case for severe lacerating injuries, pediatric patients, or patients who are uncooperative because of alcohol or drug intoxication. Succinylcholine, which can cause contraction of the rectus muscles, should not be used as a paralyzing agent as this can result in extrusion of intraocular contents. In some cases, local anesthesia can be used safely, especially in the setting of limited corneal lacerations where the risk of prolapse of intraocular tissue is minimal. As an alternative, local irrigation of anesthetic may be performed via a blunt cannula through an incision of the conjunctiva and Tenon's capsule in order to decrease the risk of retrobulbar hemorrhage. Use of local anesthesia may be particularly helpful in elderly or debilitated patients in whom a significant risk may occur with general anesthesia.

INTRAOCULAR FOREIGN BODIES. Intraocular foreign bodies should be removed if at all possible at the time of initial closure. The presence of an intraocular foreign body increases the risk of endophthalmitis in the acute setting, and surgical extraction may be associated with a decreased risk of clinical infection.[8,18,19] Metallic foreign bodies that contain iron and are left within the eye may result in chronic visual loss (siderosis). Posterior segment foreign bodies may be removed internally via a pars plana approach. If lens damage with cataract formation is present, lensectomy followed by pars plana vitrectomy may be necessary. The foreign body may be grasped using intraocular forceps and delivered through the pars plana or, if large, may be delivered through a limbal incision. Some metallic intraocular foreign bodies can be removed externally by use of an external electromagnet. This may be a particularly useful technique with foreign bodies located in the anterior vitreous cavity or in the region of the pars plana.

PROPHYLAXIS AGAINST INFECTION AND SECONDARY OCULAR INJURY. Prior to primary closure, care must be taken to ensure that no subsequent injury to the already traumatized eye occurs. It is important to limit the transfer of the patient as much as possible and to place a protective eye shield when the eye is not under examination.

The role and utility of prophylactic antibiotics in penetrating trauma without confirmed infection are still to be evaluated completely. Although a relatively high incidence of inoculation with organisms may occur, not all eyes that have positive cultures go on to develop infection.[8,20] However, the devastating impact of infection in the setting of trauma suggests that prophylactic systemic treatment is warranted. Studies that involved management of postoperative endophthalmitis raise questions about the need for intravenous antibiotics in some types of endophthalmitis.[21] However, the damage sustained by the eye that has penetrating trauma probably allows reasonable intraocular penetration in this setting, and continued use of systemic antibiotics, both prophylactic and in the treatment of documented infection, appears to be justified. The potential toxicity and the problem of where to inject in some severely traumatized eyes indicate that the use of intraocular antibiotics probably should be reserved for patients who have a clinical diagnosis of endophthalmitis or a high risk of infection.

SECONDARY REHABILITATION—SURGICAL TIMING. Timing and approach to surgical repair of disrupted intraocular structures after penetrating injury are somewhat dependent upon the nature and severity of the initial trauma. Two general approaches toward timing of surgery have been suggested. One is to complete the initial closure of the cornea and/or scleral injury with a secondary repair of intraocular structures at a later date. Some authors suggest a period of 4–10 days between the initial repair and the vitrectomy,[1] which may provide the benefit of easier visualization through the cornea and less chance of further intraocular bleeding. A second approach is to close the initial injury and repair intraocular damage either at the time of the initial repair or shortly after the initial closure (24–72 hours). Removal of lens remnants, vitreous, and intraocular blood early may lessen the risk of complicated retinal detachment as a result of intraocular scarring with proliferative vitreoretinopathy.[22]

The timing of subsequent intervention, however, may be dictated by associated findings, such as endophthalmitis, retinal detachment, or the presence of an intraocular foreign body. Early removal of subretinal blood theoretically may decrease the severity of photoreceptor damage and provide the potential for better visual recovery (Fig. 140-9). Successful results following removal of subretinal hemorrhage after penetrating trauma have been documented, but a guarded visual prognosis is the case for most of these patients.[23] Which of the approaches to use depends upon the surgeon's preference and the nature of the injury, as each approach may provide certain advantages depending on the clinical setting.

Two settings in which deferral of secondary repair may be the preferred management are posterior exit wounds and massive hemorrhagic choroidal detachments. Large, posterior penetrating wounds are often best managed with primary closure of the anterior wound and no closure of the exit site. The exit sites are usually sealed enough to allow vitrectomy within 1 week of the initial injury.[24] Often, it is useful to delay surgery in patients who have massive choroidal hemorrhage as well because adequate drainage of blood may be difficult in the first few days following the injury.

SECONDARY REHABILITATION—TECHNIQUE. Pars plana vitrectomy now permits the rehabilitation of many eyes that previously would have been lost after penetrating injuries.[1–4] A three-port approach is used most commonly in this setting. An infusion cannula is placed through the pars plana and then additional sclerotomies are placed, usually near the 2 and 10 o'clock positions to accommodate the vitrectomy cutter and fiberoptic light pipe or other intraocular instruments. Areas of scleral laceration must be avoided when sclerotomy sites are chosen. In addition, confirmation that the infusion port is not trapped under an area of

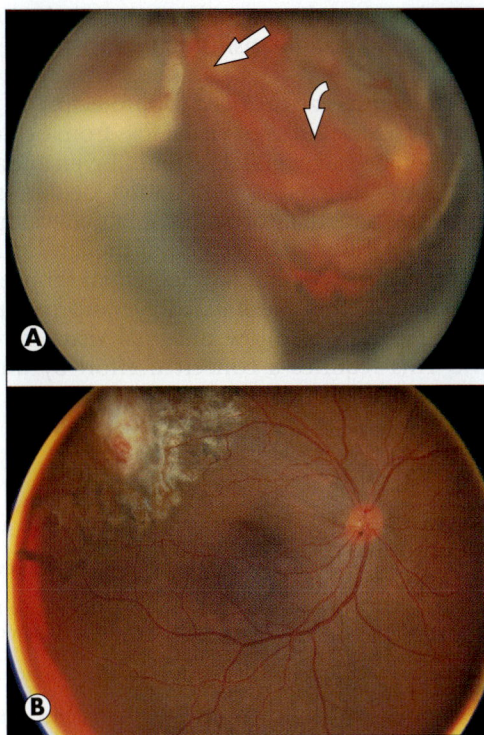

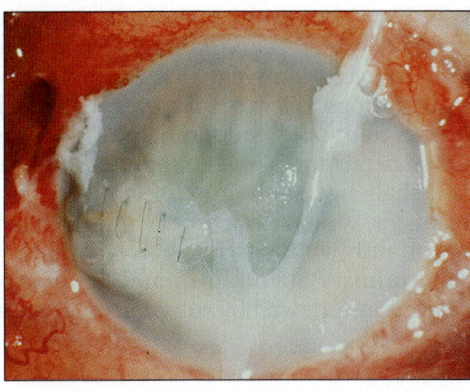

FIG. 140-9 ▮ Hemorrhagic retinal detachment in a patient after an ice-pick stab wound. **A,** Note the incarceration of the retina in the posterior impact site *(arrow)* and the subretinal blood *(curved arrow)*. A localized choroidal hemorrhage is seen in the foreground on the left. **B,** Postoperative appearance after vitrectomy, removal of subretinal blood, and extraction of retina from the area of incarceration (scar).

FIG. 140-10 ▮ Traumatic endophthalmitis (*Streptococcus faecalis*) at presentation after penetrating trauma. Note the marked anterior chamber fibrin, early ring infiltrate of the cornea, peripheral hypopyon, and purulent material in the area of corneal laceration.

choroidal elevation or retinal detachment is critical to prevent infusion of irrigation fluid into the suprachoroidal or subretinal space.

As much vitreous as possible should be removed, but also iatrogenic damage to crucial intraocular structures, such as the retina, must be avoided. If a posterior vitreous detachment is not present at the time of surgery, it is preferable to create one. This may be performed using suction on the posterior cortical vitreous with a vitreous cutter or an extrusion needle or by incision of the posterior hyaloid with a microvitreoretinal blade. When peripheral retinal tears, peripheral scleral laceration, or retinal detachment is present, it is usually advisable to place an encircling scleral buckle.

Cataract

When there has been injury to the lens that involves cataract formation or laceration to the lens capsule, lensectomy is often necessary and can be performed via the pars plana or through an anterior approach. In selected patients who have limited corneal injuries and cataract formation, lensectomy can be performed along with primary intraocular lens implantation. This is not advisable if there is significant posterior segment trauma, scleral laceration, or undue intraocular inflammation.[25]

Complicated Retinal Detachment and Proliferative Vitreoretinopathy

Complicated retinal detachment with proliferative vitreoretinopathy may occur in some eyes after penetrating ocular injury. Proliferative vitreoretinopathy may manifest as severe, widespread membrane contraction with retinal detachment or as localized macular pucker. In the setting of complicated retinal detachment, general principles for the repair of retinal detachment with proliferative vitreoretinopathy should be used; these include the following:

- Release of all traction by meticulous membrane dissection;
- Placement of an encircling scleral buckle to support the vitreous base and peripheral retinal breaks;

- Reapplication of the retina under gas or silicone oil; and
- Production of chorioretinal adhesion with endolaser photocoagulation.

Special circumstances unique to penetrating injury include retinal incarceration through posterior extension of scleral lacerations or posterior exit sites and large retinal tears with possible loss of retinal tissue. It is occasionally necessary to perform a relaxing retinotomy to allow reattachment of the retina, especially if the retina is incarcerated or if extensive areas of retinal atrophy or necrosis are present. Intraocular tamponade is obtained with long-acting gas or silicone oil.

Traumatic Endophthalmitis

Endophthalmitis in the setting of penetrating trauma is usually associated with a poor outcome.[26,27] This results from both the associated tissue injury of the trauma and the damage caused by infection. Contributory factors may be delay in treatment because an early diagnosis is difficult to make and the frequency of infection by virulent organisms (e.g., *Bacillus cereus*) that are associated with penetrating trauma. Traumatic endophthalmitis occurs in approximately 7% of cases of penetrating trauma. An increased risk of infection has been found with retained intraocular foreign bodies,[8,18,19] rural injury,[28] and injury to the crystalline lens.[19] Eyes with severe injuries that result from blunt ocular trauma may have a lower risk of infection than those with lacerating injuries or injuries related to foreign bodies. Endophthalmitis may be difficult to diagnose but should be suspected when unusual inflammation is present—this includes hypopyon, retinal vasculitis, and vitritis (Fig. 140-10). Pain out of proportion to the injury can be a useful indicative symptom.

Cultures may be obtained from the anterior chamber and vitreous cavity. Cultures obtained in the setting of a clinical diagnosis of infection are useful to direct subsequent management. Screening cultures obtained without a concurrent high index of suspicion of infection do not usually alter management decisions.[20] Treatment should not be delayed if endophthalmitis is suspected. Generally, intraocular antibiotics are used together with systemic and topical treatment. Broad-spectrum coverage, such as vancomycin plus ceftazidime or an aminoglycoside antibiotic, is suggested and treatment should cover *Bacillus* species (vancomycin and/or clindamycin), which are found in association with penetrating trauma with relatively high frequency.[26,27] Ceftazidime provides an alternative to gentamicin injection, which can be associated with toxicity because of macular infarction. The use of intraocular corticosteroid injection is controversial. Intraocular corticosteroids probably should not be used if fungal infection is suspected.

The utility of vitrectomy in the setting of traumatic endophthalmitis is uncertain. Mieler *et al.*[8] found that eyes that have positive cultures that undergo vitrectomy have a low incidence of clinical infection. Vitrectomy may play a therapeutic role in this setting as it débrides the vitreous abscess. Care must be taken, however, to avoid iatrogenic tears or retinal detachment as a very guarded prognosis exists for eyes that develop retinal detachment after traumatic endophthalmitis. Management of coexistent retinal detachment and endophthalmitis can prove to be a significant challenge. With mild infection as a result of low-virulence organisms, retinal detachment and infection might be managed concurrently with success; however, in the setting of severe infection primary attention should be directed to treatment of the infection followed by subsequent attempts at repair of retinal detachment.

COURSE AND OUTCOMES

Prognosis is related to the severity of the initial penetrating injury. Several variables are associated with long-term visual prognosis, which include the following[6,7]:

- Initial visual acuity;
- Presence of an afferent pupillary defect;
- Injuries associated with blunt trauma;
- Large corneoscleral laceration; and
- Presence of infection.

The presence of massive hemorrhagic choroidal detachment and posterior exit wounds, retinal detachment, or subretinal hemorrhage is associated with a worse visual outcome.[13,24] Exit wounds that involve the macula or optic nerve usually give rise to poor vision. Intraocular BB injuries are often associated with a poor outcome because of the extent of injury to intraocular tissues. Diagnostic ultrasound may provide useful information for both management and prognosis determination. In an attempt to correlate injury characteristics and visual outcome, a system by which to grade the extent of intraocular injury has been proposed.[29] This scoring system may provide an improved means by which to determine prognosis in eyes that have penetrating ocular injuries and thus to optimize management decisions.

Sympathetic Uveitis and Enucleation

Sympathetic uveitis (sympathetic ophthalmia) is a rare, but potentially severe, complication after penetrating injury.[30] It manifests as a bilateral granulomatous inflammatory condition, presumed to be caused by sensitization of the immune system to uveal antigens. Although 80% occur between 3 weeks and 3 months of initial injury, patients may present even years after the initial traumatic insult with symptoms of pain, photophobia, loss of vision, or difficulty with accommodation. Bilateral inflammation with keratic precipitates, vitreous cells, choroidal infiltration, and occasional exudative retinal detachment may be seen. Treatment is directed at immune suppression using systemic corticosteroids and/or cytotoxic agents and may be prolonged (e.g., months).[30] Early enucleation (prior to 2 weeks) after trauma is thought to prevent the development of sympathetic uveitis and should be considered for severely traumatized eyes that have no visual potential and in which cosmetic ocular deformity is present. Once sympathetic uveitis develops, however, removal of the inciting traumatized eye in an attempt to decrease the inflammatory reaction in the fellow eye is controversial, especially if useful vision is present in the inciting eye.[30] Despite the relative rarity of the condition, the patient should be advised of it in the early period after penetrating trauma.

Visual Rehabilitation

In patients who have lost the crystalline lens or in whom an intraocular lens has been lost, rehabilitation with secondary intraocular lens implantation or contact lens correction is possible occasionally. The use of an anterior chamber intraocular lens should be reserved only for eyes that do not have significant damage to the angle structures after the initial injury. Contact lens correction has the advantage that it may help compensate for irregular corneal astigmatism that may result following corneal laceration.

It is critical to emphasize the need for protection of the fellow eye in patients who have suffered visual loss from ocular trauma. Use of polycarbonate safety glasses should be encouraged in all patients who have suffered a penetrating ocular injury.[31] In young children the potential for amblyopia to develop exists after a period of visual loss or after loss of the lens as a result of penetrating trauma. In eyes that have potential for useful vision, aphakic correction of the traumatized eye and patches for the fellow eye are necessary to allow maximal visual recovery and development. This requires a concerted effort by the surgeon, the family, and a pediatric ophthalmologist.

REFERENCES

1. Ryan SL, Allen AW. Pars plana vitrectomy in ocular trauma. Am J Ophthalmol. 1979;88:483–91.
2. Brinton GS, Aaberg TA, Reeser FH, et al. Surgical results in ocular trauma involving the posterior segment. Am J Ophthalmol. 1982;93:271–8.
3. Hutton WI, Fuller DG. Factors influencing final visual results in severely injured eyes. Am J Ophthalmol. 1984;97:715–22.
4. Liggett PE, Gauderman J, Moreira CM, et al. Pars plana vitrectomy for acute retinal detachment in penetrating ocular injuries. Arch Ophthalmol. 1990;108:1724–8.
5. Kuhn F, Morris R, Witherspoon D, et al. A standardized classification of ocular trauma. Ophthalmology. 1996;103:240–3.
6. de Juan E, Sternberg P, Michels RG. Penetrating ocular injuries: types of injuries and visual results. Ophthalmology. 1983;90:1318–22.
7. Sternberg P, de Juan E, Michels RG. Multivariate analysis of prognostic factors in penetrating ocular injuries. Am J Ophthalmol. 1984;98:467–72.
8. Mieler WF, Ellis MK, Williams DF, Han DP. Retained intraocular foreign bodies and endophthalmitis. Ophthalmology. 1990;97:1532–8.
9. Foster RE, Martinez JA, Murray TG, et al. Useful visual outcomes after treatment of Bacillus cereus endophthalmitis. Ophthalmology. 1996;103:390–7.
10. Maguire AM, Enger C, Eliott D, Zinreich SJ. Computerized tomography in the evaluation of penetrating ocular injuries. Retina. 1991;1:405–11.
11. Joseph DP, Pieramici DJ, Beauchamp NJ Jr. Computed tomography in the diagnosis and prognosis of open-globe injuries. Ophthalmology 2000;107:1899–906.
12. Coleman DJ, Jack RL, Franzen LA. Ultrasonography in ocular trauma. Am J Ophthalmol. 1973;75:279–88.
13. Rubsamen PE, Cousins SW, Winward KE, Byrne SF. Diagnostic ultrasound and pars plana vitrectomy in penetrating ocular trauma. Ophthalmology. 1994;101:809–14.
14. Cox MS, Schepens CL, Freeman HM. Retinal detachment due to ocular contusion. Arch Ophthalmol. 1966;76:678–85.
15. Chang S, Lincoff H, Zimmerman NJ, Fuchs W. Giant retinal tears. Surgical techniques and results using perfluorocarbon liquids. Arch Ophthalmol. 1989;107:761–6.
16. Gross JG, King LP, de Juan E Jr, Powers T. Subfoveal neovascular membrane removal in patients with traumatic choroidal rupture. Ophthalmology. 1996;103:579–85.
17. Stone TW, Siddiqui N, Arroyo JG, et al. Primary scleral buckling in open-globe injury involving the posterior segment. Ophthalmology. 2000;107:1923–6.
18. Thompson JT, Parver LM, Enger CL, et al, for the National Eye Trauma System. Infectious endophthalmitis after penetrating injuries with retained intraocular foreign bodies. Ophthalmology. 1993;100:1468–74.
19. Thompson WS, Rubsamen PE, Flynn HW Jr, et al. Endophthalmitis following penetrating ocular trauma: risk factors and visual acuity outcomes. Ophthalmology. 1995;102:1696–701.
20. Rubsamen PE, Cousins SW, Martinez J. Impact of cultures on management decisions following surgical repair of penetrating ocular trauma. Ophthalmic Surg Lasers. 1997;28:43–9.
21. Endophthalmitis Vitrectomy Study Group. Results of the Endophthalmitis Vitrectomy Study: a randomized trial of immediate vitrectomy and of intravenous antibiotics for the treatment of postoperative bacterial endophthalmitis. Arch Ophthalmol. 1995;113:1479–96.
22. Coleman DJ. Early vitrectomy in the management of the severely traumatized eye. Am J Ophthalmol. 1982;93:543–51.
23. Han DP, Mieler WF, Schwartz DM, Abrams GW. Management of traumatic hemorrhagic retinal detachment with pars plana vitrectomy. Arch Ophthalmol. 1990;108:1281–6.
24. Martin DF, Meredith TA, Topping TM, et al. Perforating (through-and-through) injuries of the globe: surgical results with vitrectomy. Arch Ophthalmol. 1991;109:951–6.
25. Rubsamen PE, Irvine WD, McCuen BW II, et al. Primary intraocular lens implantation in the setting of penetrating ocular trauma. Ophthalmology. 1995;102:101–7.
26. Affeldt JC, Flynn HW Jr, Foster RK, et al. Microbial endophthalmitis resulting from ocular trauma. Ophthalmology. 1987;94:407–13.
27. Brinton GS, Topping TM, Hyndiuk RA, et al. Posttraumatic endophthalmitis. Arch Ophthalmol. 1984;102:547–50.
28. Boldt HC, Pulido JS, Blodi CF, et al. Rural endophthalmitis. Ophthalmology. 1989;96:1722–6.
29. Aaberg TM, Capone A Jr, de Juan E Jr, et al. A system for classifying mechanical injuries of the eye. Am J Ophthalmol. 1997;123:820–31.
30. Nussenblatt RB, Whitcup SM, Palestine AG. Sympathetic ophthalmia. In: Nussenblatt RB, Whitcup SM, Palestine AG, eds. Uveitis. Fundamentals and clinical practice. St Louis: Mosby; 1996:299–311.
31. Simmons ST, Krohel GB, Hay PB. Prevention of ocular gunshot injuries using polycarbonate lenses. Ophthalmology. 1984;91:977–83.

CHAPTER 141

Distant Trauma with Posterior Segment Effects

CARL D. REGILLO

Terson's Syndrome

DEFINITION
- Intraocular hemorrhage associated with acute intracranial hemorrhage.

KEY FEATURES
- Bilateral, multiple posterior segment hemorrhages.
- Intraretinal, preretinal, or intravitreal location.

ASSOCIATED FEATURES
- Spontaneous or trauma-induced intracranial blood (usually subarachnoid).
- Decreased vision with good spontaneous recovery.

Purtscher's Retinopathy

DEFINITION
- Peripapillary retinal infarctions associated with severe trauma or various systemic conditions (e.g., acute pancreatitis).

KEY FEATURES
- Bilaterally symmetrical peripapillary cotton-wool spots.
- Bilateral retinal hemorrhages.

ASSOCIATED FEATURES
- Severe head, chest, or long bone injury.
- Amniotic fluid embolism.
- Pancreatitis.
- Other rare systemic conditions.
- Decreased vision with variable or limited recovery.

Shaken Baby Syndrome

DEFINITION
- Intraocular hemorrhage that results from whiplash-like child abuse.

KEY FEATURES
- Bilateral retinal or vitreous hemorrhage.
- No evidence for direct eye trauma.

ASSOCIATED FEATURES
- Intracranial hemorrhage (usually subdural).
- Cerebral edema or atrophy.
- Decreased vision.
- Variable recovery as a result of ocular or central nervous system damage.

TERSON'S SYNDROME

INTRODUCTION

In 1900, Terson reported the association of vitreous hemorrhage with an acute subarachnoid hemorrhage. The syndrome that now bears his name, however, has evolved to include cases with any type of intraocular hemorrhage present after spontaneous or trauma-induced intracranial bleeding.[1]

EPIDEMIOLOGY AND PATHOGENESIS

Intraocular hemorrhage is seen in approximately 20% of patients with acute intracranial bleeding.[1,2] Significant vitreous hemorrhage occurs in a smaller percentage of these patients, being observed with an incidence of 3–5% of all patients who have intracranial bleeding. The intracranial hemorrhage can be subdural, subarachnoid, or intracerebral in location. Subarachnoid bleeding from a cerebral aneurysm, in particular an aneurysm of the anterior communicating artery, is the most common underlying cause.[2]

The pathogenesis of Terson's syndrome has been a controversial subject for many years. Some investigators, early on, assumed that the intraocular hemorrhage resulted from direct dissection of the subarachnoid hemorrhage down the optic nerve sheath and into the eye.[1] The lack of communication between the subarachnoid space of the optic nerve and the vitreous renders this mechanism unlikely. Furthermore, the retinal hemorrhages are often not contiguous with the optic nerve and autopsy studies have not shown that the optic nerve sheath hemorrhage extends to the globe.

It is believed now that the sudden rise in intracranial pressure that occurs at the time of the intracranial bleed is the primary event that leads to intraocular bleeding.[2] In support of this theory is the observation that the amount of ocular hemorrhage correlates directly with the rapidity and magnitude of intracranial pressure elevation. How increased intracranial pressure translates into intraocular bleeding remains unclear. Increased orbital venous pressure translated directly through the cavernous sinus or compression of both the ophthalmic vein and adjacent retinochoroidal anastomoses—because of a rapid effusion of cerebrospinal fluid or of blood into the optic nerve sheath—could explain the phenomenon.[1–3] In either scenario, an acute obstruction to the retinal venous circulation results and leads to the rupture of superficial retinal vessels.

OCULAR MANIFESTATIONS

Terson's syndrome consists of multiple, usually bilateral, retinal hemorrhages in the posterior pole (see Fig. 141-1). Visual acuity is often diminished, but this may not be easily quantified when the neurological manifestations predominate. The amount of acute vision loss is typically related to the extent of ocular hem-

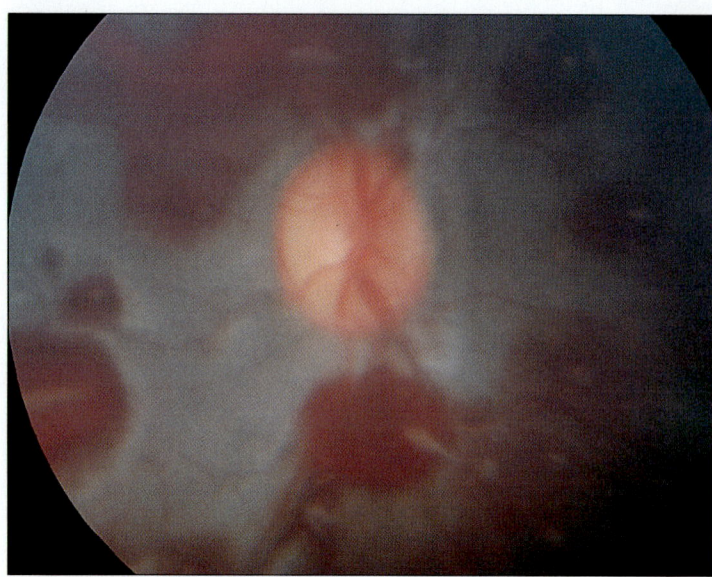

FIG. 141-1 ■ **Terson's syndrome.** Multiple superficial intraretinal hemorrhages and preretinal hemorrhage in an eye of a patient who had suffered intracranial bleeding from head trauma. (Courtesy of Lon S. Poliner, MD.)

BOX 141-1

Differential Diagnosis of Terson's Syndrome

Purtscher's retinopathy
Shaken baby syndrome
Valsalva retinopathy
Blood dyscrasia

---

orrhage. Although hemorrhages can be subretinal and deep intraretinal in location, they are usually more superficial, being just under the internal limiting membrane or preretinal (subhyaloid). Significant vitreous hemorrhage is possible, probably from intraretinal blood that breaks through the internal limiting membrane or posterior hyaloid face into the vitreous gel. Late complications include epiretinal membrane formation, perimacular retinal folds, and, rarely, traction or rhegmatogenous retinal detachments.[4]

DIAGNOSIS AND ANCILLARY TESTING

The typically devastating consequences of acute intracranial hemorrhage, rather than the intraocular consequences, bring the patient to seek medical attention. In such patients, the diagnosis of Terson's syndrome is generally obvious on initial ophthalmic evaluation. It may be an important diagnosis to establish as some series suggest that the presence of intraocular hemorrhage in this setting may be associated with a higher mortality than when no ocular involvement occurs.[5] In suspected cases without established intracranial hemorrhage, emergency neuroimaging with either tomography or magnetic resonance imaging is indicated.

DIFFERENTIAL DIAGNOSIS

The differential diagnosis for Terson's syndrome is given in Box 141-1.

TREATMENT AND OUTCOME

In Terson's syndrome, the blood typically clears completely and the visual acuity returns to normal.[1,2] However, in some cases the vision remains decreased from persistent vitreous hemorrhage or epiretinal membrane formation. In such situations, vitrectomy to clear the hemorrhage or remove mem-

branes can improve the visual outcome.[5,6] The rare, associated retinal detachment requires surgical intervention. Even in cases without these significant complications, occasionally some degree of visual acuity loss may persist indefinitely because subretinal hemorrhage has resulted in disruption of the retinal pigment epithelium or direct damage to the outer retina in the foveal area.

PURTSCHER'S RETINOPATHY

INTRODUCTION

In 1910, Purtscher described the occurrence of bilateral patches of retinal whitening and hemorrhage around the optic disc in patients who suffered massive head trauma.[7] Subsequently, this fundus appearance was observed to be associated with other types of trauma, along with a variety of nontraumatic systemic diseases such as acute pancreatitis, systemic lupus erythematosus, thrombotic thrombocytopenic purpura, and chronic renal failure.[8–10]

EPIDEMIOLOGY AND PATHOGENESIS

There are both clinical and experimental data to suggest that Purtscher's retinopathy results from the occlusion of small arterioles by intravascular microparticles generated by the underlying systemic condition.[1,8,9,11] These microparticles may consist of fibrin clots, platelet-leukocyte aggregates, fat emboli, air emboli, or other particles of similar size that block the arterioles in the peripapillary retina. It has been shown experimentally that fibrin clots 0.15–1.0 mm in size injected into the ophthalmic artery of pigs can produce a fundus appearance that mirrors Purtscher's retinopathy.[11]

OCULAR MANIFESTATIONS

Subjectively, patients experience acute, painless, loss of central vision in one or both eyes. The visual acuity loss is often marked. Ophthalmoscopy reveals multiple, variably sized cotton-wool spots and intraretinal hemorrhages around the optic nerve head (Figs. 141-2 and 141-3). Some degree of asymmetry is often seen, but a unilateral picture is rare. Acutely, the optic nerve head and peripheral retina are usually of normal appearance, although commonly the disc exhibits pallor over time (Fig. 141-3, *B*).

DIAGNOSIS AND ANCILLARY TESTING

Classically, Purtscher's retinopathy occurs in conjunction with severe head or chest trauma. It can also be seen after extensive fracture injury of long bone.[10] For trauma-related cases, the diagnosis is apparent after fundus examination and no further evaluation is needed. However, for cases associated with a systemic medical condition, the underlying cause may not be readily recognizable by either patient or physician. Such patients may present to the ophthalmologist first if the ocular symptoms predominate.[9] Therefore, the fundus appearance of Purtscher's retinopathy without a history of recent trauma or an already known causative medical condition requires a comprehensive medical evaluation performed in conjunction with an internist. Fluorescein angiography shows areas of capillary dropout corresponding to the patches of retinal whitening and blocked fluorescence from intraretinal blood.[9] Angiographic evidence for a lack of retinal capillary around the fovea may be present in cases with decreased visual acuity.

SYSTEMIC ASSOCIATIONS

Systemic conditions associated with Purtscher's retinopathy are listed in Box 141-2.

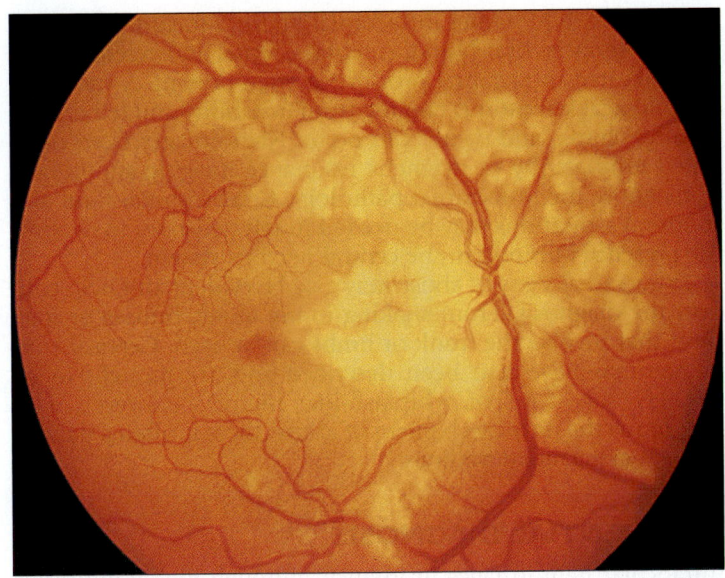

FIG. 141-2 ■ Purtscher's retinopathy. Near-confluent cotton-wool spots clustered around an otherwise normal optic nerve head in an eye of a patient who had sustained a severe blunt injury to the head and chest. (Courtesy of Jeffrey G. Gross, MD.)

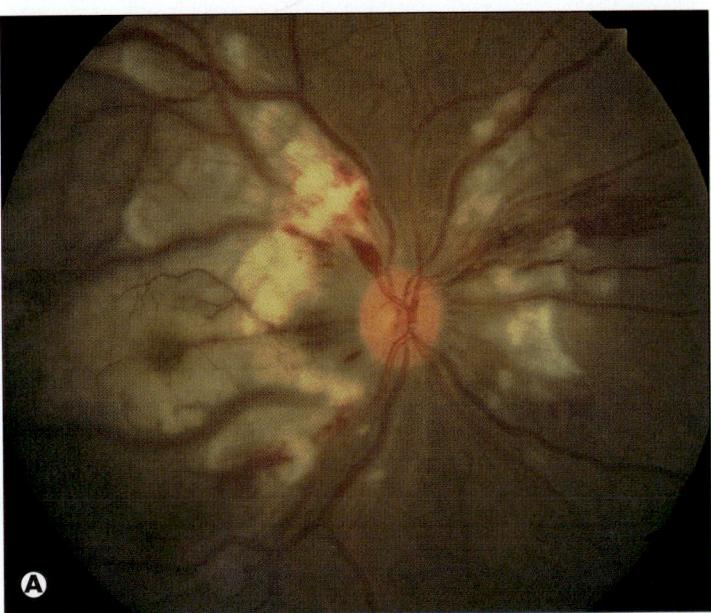

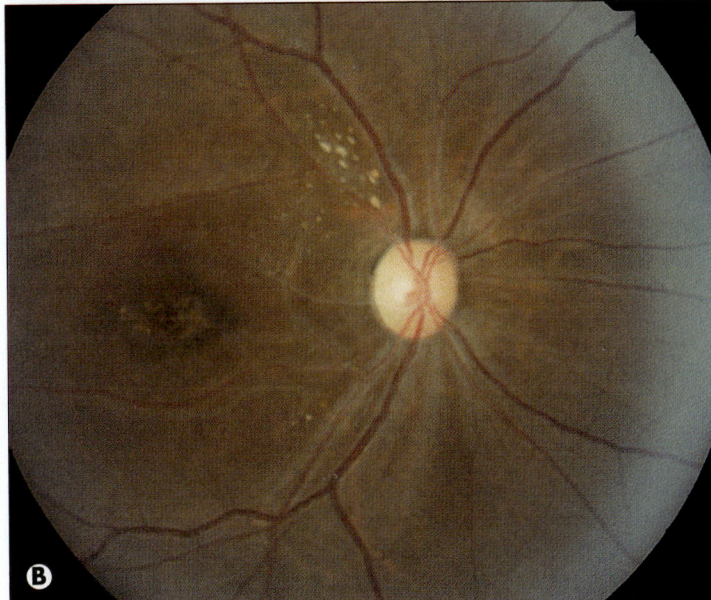

FIG. 141-3 ■ Purtscher's retinopathy associated with thrombotic thrombocytopenic purpura. (A, At presentation. B, After 4 months of follow-up. Peripapillary retinal whitening and hemorrhage slowly resolved to leave macular pigment mottling and optic disc pallor. Visual acuity remained unchanged in the counting fingers range. (Copyright 1997, American Medical Association. With permission from Power MH, Regillo CD, Custis PH. Thrombotic thrombocytopenic purpura associated with Purtscher retinopathy. Arch Ophthalmol. 1997;115:128–9.)

PATHOLOGY

Histopathologically, evidence exists for retinal capillary obliteration and inner retinal atrophy in areas of clinically observed retinal whitening. These findings are relatively nonspecific, being consistent with cotton-wool spots of a variety of causes.[8] As noted clinically, the pathology is confined mainly to the retina posterior to the equator. Optic atrophy is typically present to various degrees.

TREATMENT AND COURSE

No known treatment exists for Purtscher's retinopathy. Although retinal whitening and retinal hemorrhages slowly disappear over weeks or months, usually no significant recovery of vision occurs. The visual acuity remains decreased on the basis of infarction of either the foveal retina or optic nerve. Macular pigmentary alterations and optic atrophy are typical late findings. Medical or surgical therapy directed at the underlying condition, however, should help to prevent additional retinal or optic nerve damage by eliminating or reducing the potential for new emboli to form.

SHAKEN BABY SYNDROME

INTRODUCTION

In the 1970s, the radiologist John Caffey proposed a whiplash-like mechanism of child abuse to explain the association of ocular and intracranial bleeding in infants who lacked external signs of direct head trauma.[12] These are now recognized as hallmark findings of the shaken baby syndrome. Unfortunately, this syndrome represents a common form of child abuse that often results in significant morbidity and mortality. As the name implies, it is encountered almost exclusively in children younger than 2 years of age, most of whom are younger than 12 months.[13]

EPIDEMIOLOGY AND PATHOGENESIS

The age predilection is thought to be due to certain anatomical features that make the infant more likely to suffer from intracranial and intraocular bleeding as a result of shaking.[12] The head of an infant is proportionately larger and heavier relative to the body than that of an older child or adult and is not as well sta-

---

BOX 141-2

Systemic Conditions Associated with Purtscher's Retinopathy

Severe head, chest, or long bone trauma
Acute pancreatitis
Systemic lupus erythematosus (SLE)
Fat embolism syndrome
Thrombotic thrombocytopenic purpura (TTP)
Chronic renal failure
Amniotic fluid embolism
Scleroderma
Dermatomyositis

bilized by neck muscles. The average adult is also able to generate relatively larger acceleration-deceleration forces when shaking an infant than when shaking a larger person.

Intracranial bleeding in this setting is believed to result primarily from the delicate vessels that bridge the cerebral cortices and venous sinuses being torn when the brain quickly shifts within the cranium during the forceful shaking. Direct contusion effects probably also occur. Blood, edema, and intracranial pressure elevation all play a role in the often permanent neurological damage.

The pathogenesis of the ocular hemorrhage is not as well understood. Although a mechanism akin to that of Terson's syndrome may be a possible explanation, it is likely that the movement of the vitreous gel within the globe contributes to secondary traction on the internal limiting membrane and superficial retinal vessels. Increased venous pressure transmitted to the retina, such as in Valsalva retinopathy, may also occur, especially with a firm grip on the chest with shaking or even from direct choking of the victim.

OCULAR MANIFESTATIONS

The most common ocular finding in shaken baby syndrome is intraocular hemorrhage in various locations—subretinal, intraretinal, preretinal (subhyaloid), and intravitreal.[13-16] Intraretinal and preretinal hemorrhages predominate (Fig. 141-4). As in Terson's syndrome, the hemorrhages are concentrated in the posterior pole region and are usually bilateral. In many cases, the amount of intraocular blood correlates with the degree of acute neurological damage. Cotton-wool spots, white-centered hemorrhages, macular edema, papilledema, and retinoschisis are less common findings at presentation.[1,12] After the abuse has stopped, hemorrhages and other acute changes resolve within several months. Late manifestations include perimacular retinal folds, chorioretinal atrophy or scarring, optic atrophy, and retinal detachment.[13,17,18]

DIAGNOSIS AND ANCILLARY TESTING

The diagnosis of shaken baby syndrome is made when the ocular findings just discussed are present in conjunction with certain systemic features and a history of shaking abuse. As a history of physical abuse may be difficult or impossible to elicit with certainty, especially at first, the clinician must maintain a high index of suspicion based on the constellation of clinical findings. The hallmark nonocular sign in shaken baby syndrome is intracranial hemorrhage. Unlike that in Terson's syndrome, this is usually subdural in location and often involves both sides

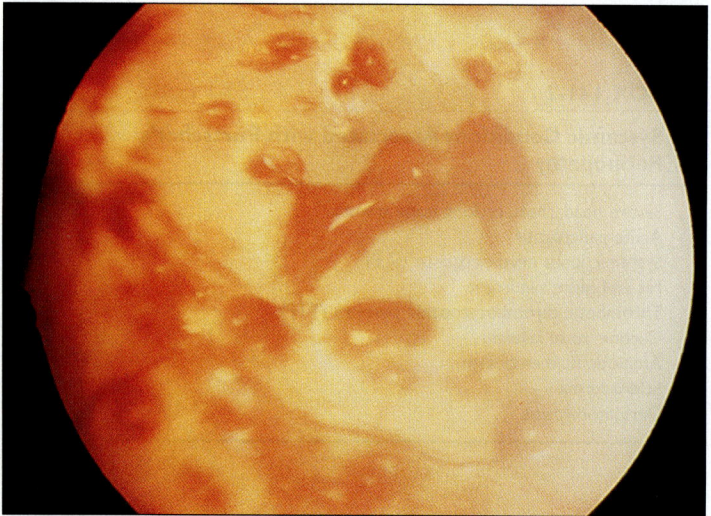

FIG. 141-4 ■ Shaken baby syndrome. Numerous superficial retinal hemorrhages (many with white centers) in the posterior pole of an infant who had been the subject of shaking abuse. (Courtesy of Dennis P. Han, MD.)

of the brain.[12,14,19] Other intracranial findings include subarachnoid or intracerebral blood, cerebral edema, and cerebral atrophy. Elevated intracranial pressure is often present. A variety of neurological symptoms, ranging from irritability and lethargy to seizures, coma, and death, can occur. Neuroimages from computed tomography or magnetic resonance imaging are utilized to diagnose the intracranial pathology. Cerebrospinal fluid and subdural aspirations may be needed in selected cases to confirm the presence of blood in the central nervous system.

Extracranial signs of abuse may also be evident and help confirm the diagnosis. From shaking injury alone, bruises or fractures that involve the trunk or limbs can be seen. Cervical cord hematomas have also been described and are thought to be strongly suggestive of whiplash-like injury.[19] However, with shaking as the only mechanism of abuse, there is often a paucity of overt extracranial findings.

DIFFERENTIAL DIAGNOSIS

Intraocular hemorrhages in infancy, although highly indicative of shaken baby syndrome, are not specific for child abuse as they can be seen in a variety of other conditions during infancy (Box 141-3).[13] Direct trauma to the head or a spontaneous subarachnoid hemorrhage can result in intraocular bleeding, as described in the section on Terson's syndrome. Retinal hemorrhages can also be seen after vaginal delivery and cardiopulmonary resuscitation. Finally, a number of systemic conditions, such as arterial hypertension, hematological disorders (e.g., leukemia), sepsis, meningitis, and vasculitis, can cause various degrees of intraretinal hemorrhage.

PATHOLOGY

As observed clinically, the most common histopathological finding is intraocular hemorrhage with the blood observed in all layers of the retina, between the retina and the retinal pigment epithelium (RPE), and in the vitreous.[15,16] Intraorbital optic nerve sheath hemorrhage with blood is observed frequently and may cause or contribute to optic disc edema or optic atrophy.[13,15,16] Intraretinal edema, retinal folding, and RPE alterations are other, not uncommon, ocular findings. Other pathological changes of the globe are unusual in a case of shaken baby syndrome alone.

TREATMENT, COURSE, AND OUTCOME

Some degree of permanent visual loss is common in shaken baby syndrome, and, therapeutically, little can be done to alter the visual outcome. Irreversible damage to the macula, optic nerve, occipital cortex, or some combination of these is responsible for the decreased vision.[12,13,17,18] Signs indicative of at least a fair potential for visual function are good pupillary reflexes, clear ocular media, retinal findings that are limited to intraretinal hemorrhages, and a normal optic nerve head.[12] In patients who have vitreous hemorrhage dense enough to obscure the

---

BOX 141-3

Causes of Retinal Hemorrhages in Infancy

Birth trauma (neonates only)
Shaken baby syndrome
Spontaneous intracranial hemorrhage (Terson's syndrome)
Acute hypertension
Direct eye, head, or chest trauma (accidental or nonaccidental)
Cardiopulmonary resuscitation
Systemic infections and meningitis
Viral retinitis
Hematologic disorders (e.g., malignancies, coagulopathies)
Systemic (or retinal) vasculitis

macula, vitrectomy surgery to clear the blood can be performed. In this setting, electroretinography should be utilized preoperatively as surgery is not likely to be of benefit if there is no significant bright flash response.[12] Unfortunately, although the visual pathway may be relatively well preserved, the patient's overall function may still be very limited as a result of severe neurological damage.

MISCELLANEOUS CONDITIONS

WHIPLASH INJURY

A whiplash injury to the head in adults produces a unique ocular problem referred to as whiplash maculopathy.[20] In this disorder, the patient usually reports bilateral, mild blurring of vision that begins immediately after a significant head and neck flexion-extension injury. Automobile accidents with rapid deceleration are the most common cause. Visual acuity is found to be slightly decreased, rarely worse than 20/30, and ocular examination is notable only for a faint gray haze to the foveal retina accompanied by a small depression. A shallow posterior vitreous separation may also be seen. Fluorescein angiography is usually normal. Within days, the vision returns to normal and the gray retinal discoloration fades, but the small, foveal depression appears to persist indefinitely. Similar foveal changes can be seen after direct eye trauma with mild commotio retinae of the central macula and after sun gazing (solar retinopathy).

FAT EMBOLISM SYNDROME

Distinct posterior segment changes are also seen in the fat embolism syndrome. Within a few days of sustaining significant fractures of medullated bones, a variety of systemic and ocular signs can be manifest. Retinal changes are observed in as many as 60% of patients who meet the diagnostic criteria of fat embolism syndrome but in only about 5% of the patients who present with long bone fractures, with or without other systemic signs.[10]

The classical eye findings are bilateral cotton-wool spots and intraretinal hemorrhages.[1,10] Although the syndrome may resemble Purtscher's retinopathy, the white retinal infarcts and hemorrhages are usually smaller, less numerous, and more peripheral.[8] Moreover, it differs from Purtscher's retinopathy in that most patients are either asymptomatic or have only minor visual complaints.

The associated systemic manifestations of fat embolism syndrome include petechial rash, central nervous system alterations, respiratory compromise, fever, tachycardia, anemia, and elevated erythrocyte sedimentation rate. The condition is fatal in 20% of cases.[1] The ophthalmologist is rarely involved during the acute phase of fat embolism syndrome as ocular symptoms are usually minimal. However, some patients notice persistent paracentral scotomata and the ophthalmologist may be in a position to evaluate these and other ocular symptoms at some point during or after the acute phase of the syndrome.[10]

No treatment is currently available for ocular manifestations associated with fat embolism syndrome.

VALSALVA RETINOPATHY

Valsalva retinopathy occurs when increased intrathoracic or intra-abdominal pressure is transmitted to the eye, which results in intraocular bleeding. The hemorrhage is usually unilateral or bilaterally asymmetrical and located in the macula. Subinternal limiting membrane hemorrhage is most common, but subretinal, retinal, and/or intravitreal bleeding can occur as well. Coughing, vomiting, sneezing, straining at stool, lifting, and sexual intercourse are all possible causes. Valsalva retinopathy typically clears without sequelae. The neodymium: yttrium-aluminum-garnet laser has been used to disrupt preretinal hemorrhage in selected cases to speed the clearance. In most cases, however, laser or surgical intervention is rarely ever needed.

REFERENCES

1. Williams DF, Mieler WF, Williams GA. Posterior segment manifestations of ocular trauma. Retina. 1990;10:S35–S44.
2. Garfinkle AM, Danys IR, Nicolle DA, et al. Terson's syndrome: a reversible cause of blindness following subarachnoid hemorrhage. J Neurosurg. 1992;76:766–71.
3. Ogawa T, Kitaoka T, Dake Y, Amemiya T. Terson syndrome. A case report suggesting the mechanism of vitreous hemorrhage. Ophthalmology. 2001;108:1654–6.
4. Schultz PN, Sobol WM, Weingiest TA. Long-term visual outcome in Terson syndrome. Ophthalmology. 1991;98:1814–19.
5. Kuhn F, Morris R, Witherspoon CD, Mester V. Terson syndrome. Results of vitrectomy and the significance of vitreous hemorrhage in patients with subarachnoid hemorrhage. Ophthalmology. 1998;105:472–7.
6. Gnanaraj L, Tyagi AK, Cottrell DG, et al. Referral delay and ocular surgical outcome in Terson syndrome. Retina. 2000;20:374–7.
7. Purtscher O. Angiopathia retinae traumatica. Lymphorrhagien des Augengrundes. Arch Ophthalmol. 1912;56:244–7.
8. Gass JDM. Stereoscopic atlas of macular disease: diagnosis and treatment, 3rd ed. St Louis: Mosby–Year Book; 1997:452–5, 746–7.
9. Power MH, Regillo CD, Custis PH. Thrombotic thrombocytopenic purpura associated with Purtscher retinopathy. Arch Ophthalmol. 1997;115:128–9.
10. Chuang EL, Miller FS, Kalina RE. Retinal lesions following long bone fractures. Ophthalmology. 1985;92:370–4.
11. Behrens-Baumann W, Scheurer G, Schroer H. Pathogenesis of Purtscher's retinopathy: an experimental study. Graefes Arch Clin Exp Ophthalmol. 1992; 230:286–91.
12. Greenwald MJ. The shaken baby syndrome. Semin Ophthalmol. 1990;5:202–14.
13. Levin AV. Ocular manifestations of child abuse. Ophthalmol Clin North Am. 1990;3:249–64.
14. Kivlin JD. Manifestations of the shaken baby syndrome. Curr Opin Ophthalmol. 2001;12:158–63.
15. Munger CE, Peiffer RL, Bouldin TW, et al. Ocular and associated neuropathologic observations in suspected whiplash shaken infant syndrome: a retrospective study of 12 cases. Am J Forensic Med Pathol. 1993;14:193–200.
16. Riffenburgh RS, Sathyavagiswaran L. Ocular findings at autopsy of child abuse victims. Ophthalmology. 1991;98:1519–24.
17. McCabe CF, Donahue SP. Prognostic indicators for vision and mortality in shaken baby syndrome. Arch Ophthalmol. 2000;118:373–7.
18. Han DP, Wilkinson WS. Late ophthalmic manifestations of the shaken baby syndrome. J Pediatr Ophthalmol Strabismus. 1990;27:299–303.
19. Hadley MN, Sonntag VKH, Rekate HL, Murphy A. The infant whiplash-shake injury syndrome: a clinical and pathologic study. Neurosurgery. 1989;24:536–40.
20. Kelley JS, Hoover RE, George T. Whiplash maculopathy. Arch Ophthalmol. 1978; 96:834–5.

142 Light Toxicity and Laser Burns

CAROLINE R. BAUMAL

DEFINITION
- Damage to the retina produced by any type of light source.

KEY FEATURES
- Mechanism of damage is usually photochemical.
- Thermal enhancement of retinal damage is possible.
- Potential causes of photic retinopathy include solar eclipse, welding arc, lightning, ophthalmic instruments, laser.

ASSOCIATED FEATURES
- Delayed appearance of the lesion after the injury by hours to days.
- Variable recovery of vision.
- Severity of damage proportional to increased duration and intensity of exposure.

INTRODUCTION

There are a variety of methods to prevent damage to structures of the eye, which may be induced by light sources. Breakdown of the intrinsic ocular protective mechanisms or exposure to external high-risk conditions can produce light or photic damage to the retina. The development and degree of photic damage to the retina depends on numerous factors including the preexisting ocular anatomy and the parameters of the light source (including wavelength, duration, and power).

LIGHT INTERACTION WITH THE RETINA

The electromagnetic spectrum encompasses a broad range of radiation (Fig. 142-1). The eye primarily perceives radiation in the optical spectrum, which is comprised of visible (400–760nm), ultraviolet (UV, 200–400nm), and infrared (IR, >760nm) wavelengths. Radiation in this region can be produced by many sources such as the sun, artificial lighting, ophthalmic instruments, and lasers.

The tissue effects of light may be classified as mechanical, thermal, or photochemical. These effects are determined by the irradiance (W/cm^2) from the light source, the wavelength of incident light, the duration of exposure, and the absorption of target tissue.[1] Mechanical injury results from high irradiance, short-duration exposures in the nanosecond (10^{-9}sec) to picosecond (10^{-12}sec) range. The energy produced strips electrons from molecules and disintegrates the target tissue into a collection of ions and electrons, known as *plasma*. This is the mechanism of photodisruption produced by the neodymium: yttrium–aluminum–garnet (Nd:YAG) laser. At a moderate irradiance and exposure duration greater than 1µsec, thermal effects result from a critical temperature rise in the target tissue. An elevation of retinal temperature by 10–20°C produces protein denaturation and enzyme inactivation, which results in coagulation, cellular necrosis, and hemostasis.[2,3] Long visible wavelengths and IR radiation produce

thermal injury to the retina and choroid during retina laser photocoagulation. Photochemical or phototoxic effects occur with low-to-moderate irradiances below coagulation thresholds and with short wavelengths, in particular UV and visible blue wavelengths. Damage to cellular components occurs at temperatures too low to cause thermal destruction, which may account for a delay of 24–48 hours before the appearance of a lesion. Absorption of a photon by the outer electrons produces an excited molecular state, which can drive a chemical reaction. Because the energy per photon is inversely proportional to its wavelength, short-wavelength photons have more energy to induce a photochemical reaction. Long-wavelength visible light also can induce photochemical changes when tissues are sensitized by an exogenous photosensitizer. At intermediate values of irradiance and exposure, more than one of the above mechanisms may be in effect to produce tissue damage.

Light must penetrate the ocular media in order to interact with the retina. The ocular media transmit 75–90% of electromagnetic radiation in the range of 400–1064nm.[4] Several mechanisms exist to reduce retinal light exposure. The cornea absorbs most UV-B (280–315nm) and UV-C (<280nm), as well as some IR radiation, and reflects up to 60% of incident light that is not perpendicular to its surface.[4] The lens absorbs most UV-A (315–400nm) and visible blue wavelengths. Intrinsic ocular defenses against retinal light damage include xanthophyll absorption of near-UV and blue light to protect the photoreceptors, temperature control by the choroidal circulation, intracellular molecular detoxification of free radicals and toxic molecules, and retinal pigment epithelium (RPE)-mediated photoreceptor renewal.[5] Physiological protective mechanisms include the eyebrow ridge, squint and blink reflexes, the aversion response, and pupillary miosis. Light damage to the retina may occur when protective mechanisms are impaired, such as with surgical alterations to the eye or with deliberate gazing at a light source. Young patients may be at increased risk due to more efficient transmission of light through the ocular media.

PHOTIC RETINOPATHY

Photic retinopathy is a nonspecific term that refers to light-induced retinal damage. It is most often due to inadvertent exposure. Retinal damage induced by solar viewing and the operating microscope is typically photochemical and may be enhanced by elevated tissue temperature and increased blood oxygen tension.[6] Increased chorioretinal pigmentation facilitates light absorption in the RPE and choroid, which may elevate the background retinal temperature and thermally enhance photochemical damage. It has been hypothesized that retinal defenses against toxic free radicals from light and oxygen are overwhelmed by supranormal light exposure. Damage manifests as a disorder of RPE and photoreceptor outer segments.[7] Retinal phototoxic injury originally was believed to be permanent; however, visual recovery has been noted in cases of solar retinopathy, welding arc maculopathy, and operating microscope phototoxicity. Mild photochemical damage may not be symptomatic or visible ophthalmoscopically, so clinical reports appear to represent the more severe

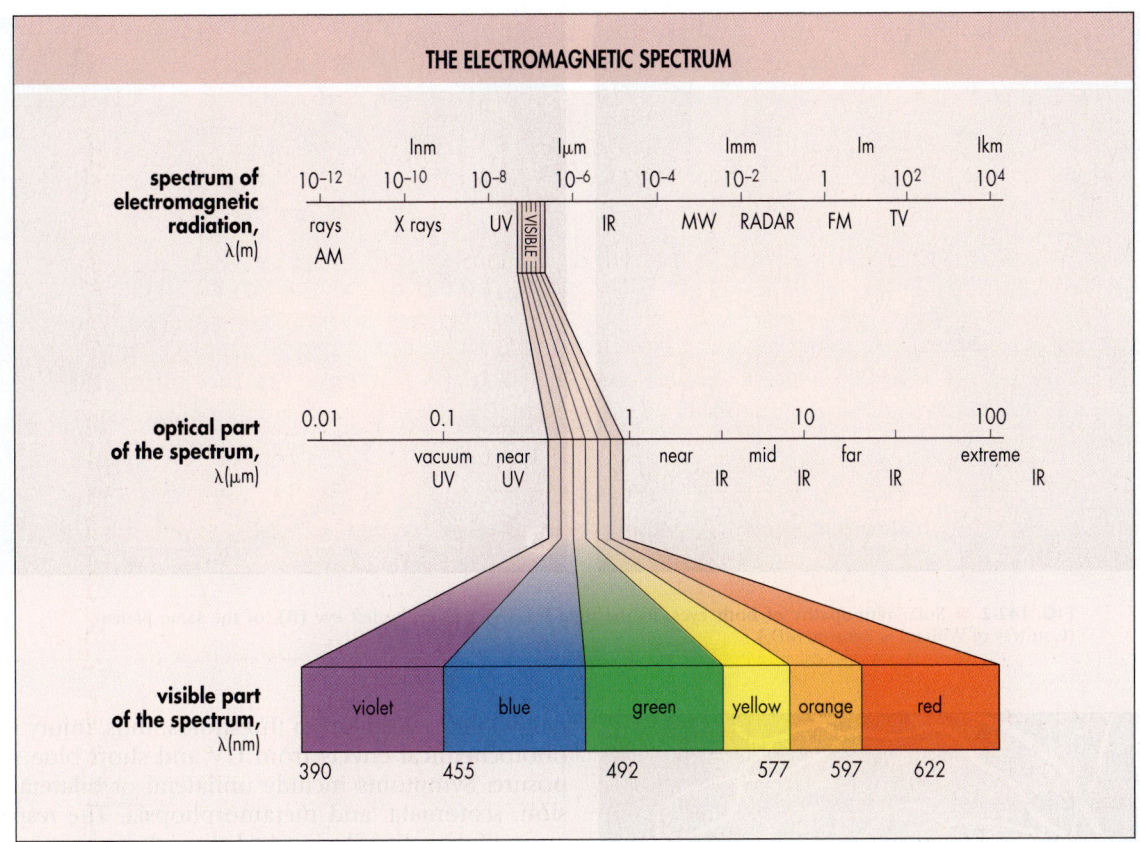

FIG. 142-1 ■ **The electromagnetic spectrum.** This includes the spectrum of electromagnetic radiation, the optical part of the spectrum and the visible part of the spectrum.

injuries. The extent of retinal injury and the likelihood of visual recovery depend on multiple factors, including the location and area of exposed retina, the duration, intensity, and spectrum of the light source, and host susceptibility factors, such as age, nutritional status, ocular pigmentation, and core temperature.

Solar Retinopathy

Solar retinopathy refers to retinal injury induced by direct or indirect solar viewing. Other names for this entity include foveomacular retinitis, photoretinitis, photomaculopathy, and eclipse retinopathy. The harmful effects of solar viewing have been recognized for centuries. Foveomacular retinitis was characterized initially as a syndrome of bilateral decreased vision and foveal lesions in military persons. A history of solar viewing was elicited subsequently from most of these patients.[8] Solar retinopathy also has been associated with religious sun gazing, solar eclipse observing, telescopic solar viewing, sunbathing, psychiatric disorders, and the use of psychotropic drugs.[9] Solar radiation damages the retina through photochemical effects, which may be enhanced by elevated tissue temperature. Direct solar observation through a 3mm pupil produces a 4°C temperature rise, which is below thermal damage thresholds.[3] Sustained solar viewing for more than 90 seconds through a constricted pupil exceeds the threshold for photochemical retinal damage.[10] Solar observation through a dilated 7mm pupil produces a 22°C increase in retinal temperature, which is above photocoagulation thresholds.[3]

Symptoms usually develop 1–4 hours after solar exposure and include unilateral or bilateral decreased vision, metamorphopsia, central or paracentral scotomata, chromatopsia, photophobia, afterimage, and periorbital ache. Visual acuity ranges from 20/40 to 20/200 acutely. A small yellow spot with a gray margin may be noted in the foveolar or parafoveolar area shortly after exposure (Fig. 142-2). This discoid lesion measures up to

200μm in diameter and corresponds to the retinal image of the sun.[3,9] In mild cases, a lesion may not be visible ophthalmoscopically. Histopathology of the acute solar lesion demonstrates injury to the RPE with necrosis, detachment, irregular pigmentation, and minimal change to the photoreceptors.[11] Fluorescein angiography may be normal or reveal transmission defects due to RPE irregularities (Fig. 142-3). Leakage of fluorescein rarely is noted during the acute stage.

The yellow lesion is replaced by a permanent focal depression, with RPE mottling or a lamellar hole during the weeks following injury. Vision usually improves to 20/20–20/40 within 6 months, although scotomata and metamorphopsia can persist. Multiple areas of RPE mottling may represent previous episodes of sun gazing.

Numerous factors may affect and increase the susceptibility of the retina to photic damage. These include the interval and spectrum of solar exposure, a reduction in the ozone layer, atmospheric conditions, the distance from the sun, telescopic viewing, pupil dilatation, elevated body temperature, increased chorioretinal pigmentation, clarity of the ocular media, and preexisting retinal disease. Emmetropes and hyperopes may be at increased risk caused by effective focusing of light on the retina.[5] Systemic photosensitizing agents, such as tetracycline, hematoporphyrins, and psoralen, may predispose to photochemical damage.

The term *eclipse retinopathy* specifically describes macular damage that occurs as a result of viewing a solar eclipse. The visual morbidity associated with the full solar eclipse on August 11, 1999, was evaluated. The majority of patients sought treatment within 2 days of viewing the eclipse. An abnormal macular appearance was reported in 84% of those evaluated. The visual morbidity is usually, but not always, temporary. There were no cases of continued visual loss or symptoms after 6 months in a series of 70 cases.[12] In another report, four patients had persistent symptoms 7 months after eclipse viewing.[13] Evaluation of the mechanism of retinal damage following eclipse and excessive light exposure in albino rats demonstrated irreversible neu-

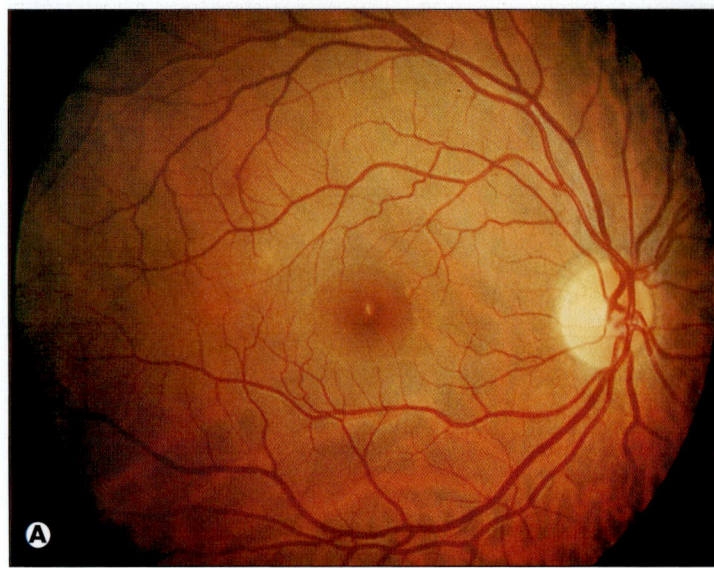
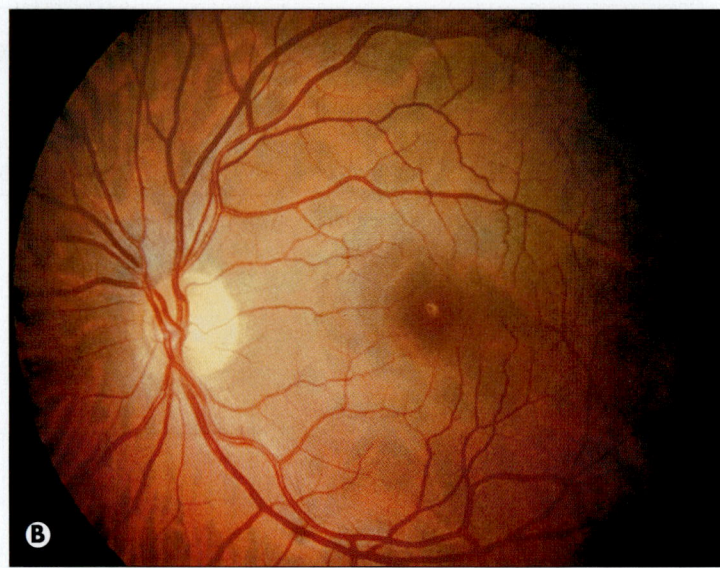

FIG. 142-2 ■ **Solar retinopathy of both eyes.** In the right eye **(A)** and in the left eye **(B)**, of the same patient. (Courtesy of William E. Benson, MD.)

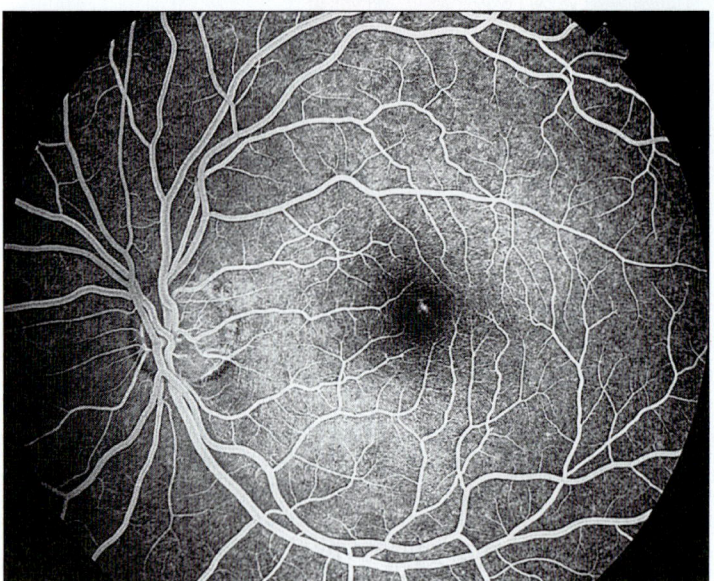

FIG. 142-3 ■ Fluorescein angiography of solar retinopathy in the left eye. Transmission hyperfluorescence corresponds to the retinal pigment epithelium defect. (Courtesy of William E. Benson, MD.)

ronal apoptosis of retinal cells and gliovascular responses.[14] Cellular apoptosis is an irreversible process, which could account for permanent visual impairment, while the activation of the non-neuronal glial and endothelial cells may be responsible for the more transient clinical symptoms.

No specific therapy exists for solar retinopathy. Further episodes of solar viewing should be discouraged. Eclipse viewing should be discouraged unless there is adequate use of the proper protective eyewear. Commercially available tested solar filters with high-quality absolute visible, UV, and IR light are recommended for eclipse observation. Public health education may reduce visual morbidity. Oral corticosteroids have been used to treat acute lesions, but a beneficial effect has not been demonstrated conclusively because vision often improves spontaneously.

Welding Arc Exposure

Welding arcs emit radiation, and the most common injury produced is keratitis due to UV absorption by the cornea. Retinal injury is rare but can occur after a welding arc is viewed without proper ocular protection.[15] The retinal temperature increase is below photocoagulation thresholds; thus, injury is produced by photochemical effects from UV and short blue wavelength exposure. Symptoms include unilateral or bilateral decreased vision, scotomata, and metamorphopsia. The respective appearances of the retinal lesion and clinical course are similar to those of solar retinopathy. A yellow edematous lesion occurs acutely in the fovea, which is replaced over time by an RPE irregularity or a pseudomacular hole. No effective therapy exists. Vision usually improves with time, although some patients experience a permanent loss of vision.

Lightning Retinopathy

Lightning maculopathy describes acute visual loss and macular changes that occur after one is injured by lightning. The visual loss to light perception may be severe. Lesions described include macular edema, macular hole, cyst, or a solar retinopathy-like picture, cataract, retinal detachment, retinal artery occlusions, and relative afferent pupillary defect.[16] Visual recovery often occurs over time, even with severe maculopathy. High-dose intravenous methylprednisolone treatment may play a role in recovery of vision, because its use has been associated with reversal of lightning-induced blindness in two cases.[17]

Retinal Phototoxicity From Ophthalmic Instruments

Ophthalmologists use a variety of powerful light sources for diagnostic and therapeutic purposes. Retinal injury in humans has been described following exposure to light produced by the operating microscope and fiberoptic endoillumination. Iatrogenic phototoxicity has been reported after cataract extraction, epikeratophakia, combined anterior segment procedures, and vitreous surgery.[7] The most frequently cited cause of ophthalmic instrument phototoxicity is the operating microscope. The associated injury was described initially after uncomplicated extracapsular cataract extraction.[18] A wide range in the incidence of operating microscope phototoxicity has been reported, up to 28% in a prior study. In one series, 7% of 135 patients having cataract operations demonstrated operating microscope phototoxicity, while there were no cases in a prospective study of 37 cataract surgeries.[19,20] This range is likely due to variations in the intensity of microscope illumination, surgical technique, cataract density, and duration of surgery. The mechanism of intraoperative phototoxicity is photochemical but may be thermally enhanced. Because operating microscopes generate little UV radiation, photochemical damage probably is caused by short-wavelength visi-

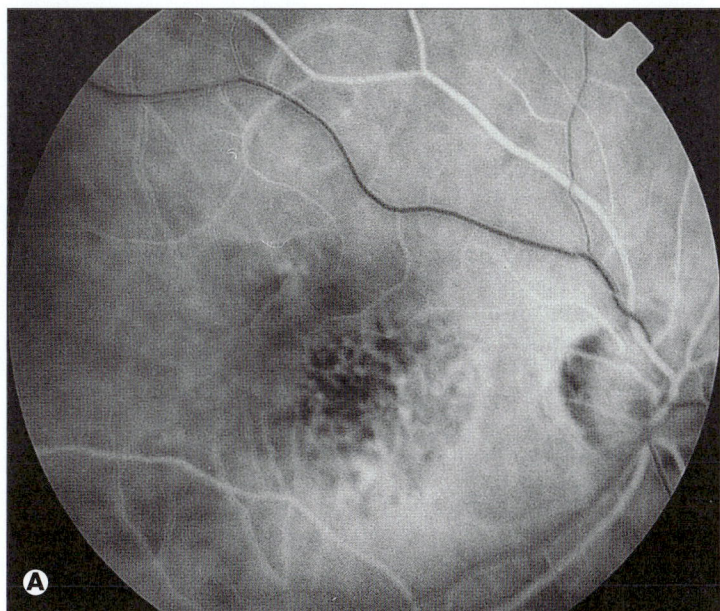

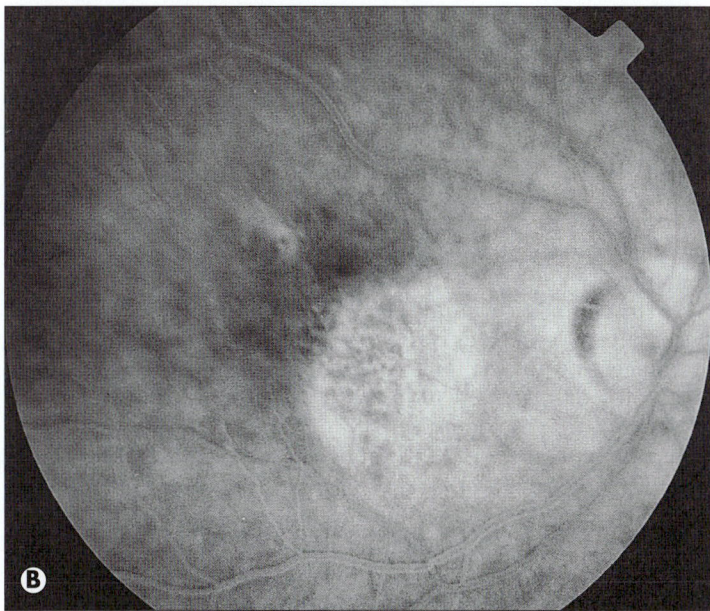

FIG. 142-4 ■ **Acute retinal phototoxicity 2 weeks after cataract surgery. A,** Perifoveal fluorescein mottling in the early stage angiogram. **B,** Modest fluorescein leakage and retinal pigment mottling in the late phase. Visual acuity is 20/60. (Courtesy of Gordon A. Byrnes, MD.)

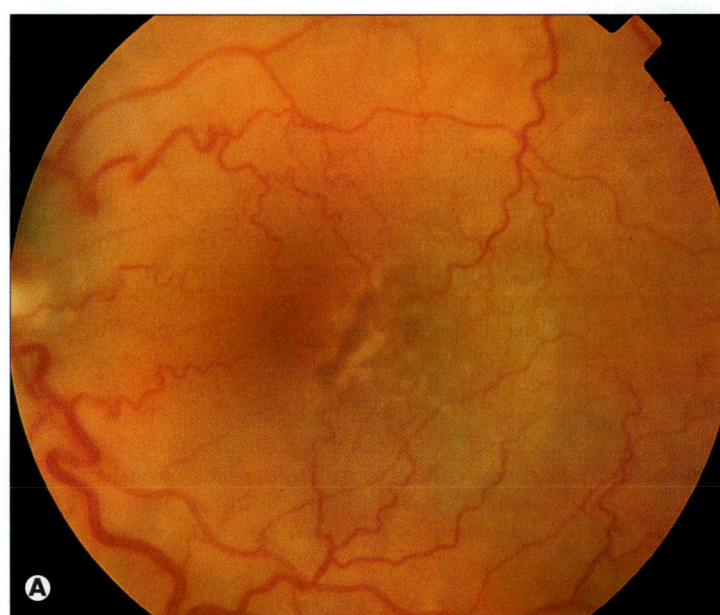

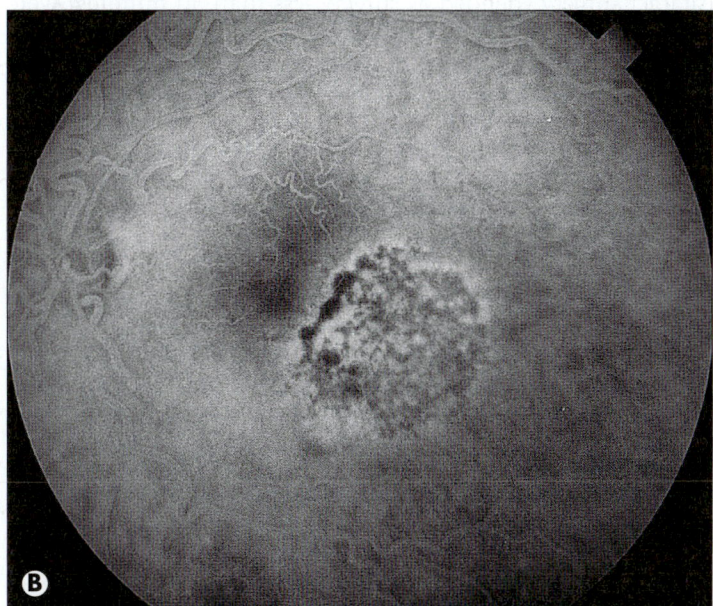

FIG. 142-5 ■ **Chronic retinal phototoxicity in the left eye. A,** Visual acuity is 20/50 (6/15). A well-defined area of retinal pigment epithelium mottling is present. The patient also has congenital retinal venous tortuosity. **B,** Fluorescein angiogram reveals blocking and transmission defects without late fluorescein leakage. (Both courtesy of Gordon A. Byrnes, MD.)

ble blue and green light. The incorporation of UV and IR filters in the intraocular lens (IOL) and microscope may reduce the risk of photic and thermal effects, respectively. Human photic retinal injury has been produced in a blind phakic eye after 60 minutes of operating microscope light exposure, despite the presence of UV and IR filters, which demonstrates that filters do not prevent damage completely.[21]

Few patients manifest symptoms after operating microscope damage, and the level of vision depends on the size and location of the lesion. A foveal lesion can produce severe permanent vision loss, while an eccentric lesion is compatible with good vision and a pericentral scotoma that corresponds to the lesion's location. Immediately after exposure, there is little to no clinical evidence of macular pathology. Within 24–48 hours, a yellow lesion measuring 0.5–2.0 disc diameters at the level of the RPE is found and retinal edema may be present. Retinal damage often

is inferior to the fovea due to rotation of the globe by a superior rectus bridle suture, microscope tilt, and displacement of the microscope field over the superior limbus. Injury may occur at or superior to the fovea during vitreous surgery or when a superior rectus bridle suture is not used. The shape of the lesion matches that of the surgical illuminating source. A tungsten filament in the operating microscope produces a horizontal, oval lesion, while the fiberoptic illuminator produces a round lesion. Fluorescein angiography of the acute lesion reveals fluorescein leakage at the level of the RPE (Fig. 142-4), which may simulate the appearance of choroidal neovascularization. Over subsequent weeks, the yellow lesion fades and is replaced by permanent areas of RPE clumping and atrophy (Fig. 142-5, *A*), which correspond angiographically to blocking and transmission defects, respectively (Fig. 142-5, *B*). Other long-term sequelae include postoperative erythropsia and retinal surface wrinkling.

Choroidal neovascularization has been reported adjacent to an area of operating microscope photic damage at 18 months after cataract surgery.[22] In primates, sub-RPE neovascularization in areas of photic damage has been reported after 2–5 years.[23] Mild light-induced retinal injuries may be overlooked, because subtle postoperative pigmentary changes may be attributable to other causes. Operating microscope light exposure has been implicated in the development of post–cataract extraction cystoid macular edema, but this association has not been demonstrated conclusively.[7]

Histopathological studies of acute human photic lesions produced after 60 minutes of operating microscope exposure prior to enucleation for malignant melanoma revealed RPE and photoreceptor damage.[24] In primates, early photic lesions demonstrate photoreceptor damage and disruption of RPE tight junctions; the latter is noted clinically by fluorescein leakage through the RPE.[23] Regeneration of photoreceptor outer segments was noted in primates 3–5 months after injury. This may account for the recovery of vision after phototoxic injury noted in some human eyes.

Operating microscope phototoxicity has been associated with multiple surgical factors, including increased microscope brightness, wavelength of light exposure, prolonged surgical duration, and surgical technique. Although the duration of surgery has decreased with phacoemulsification, phototoxic retinal lesions still may occur. Retinal phototoxic lesions after short-duration cataract surgery (defined as surgery less than 30 minutes) were associated with a final refraction within 1.0D of emmetropia and with diabetic retinopathy.[25] The risk of photic damage may increase after IOL insertion, which can focus the incoming light on the retina; however, photic injury has been described without IOL insertion. Patient susceptibility factors include increased body temperature and blood oxygenation, chorioretinal pigmentation, preexisting maculopathy, pupillary dilatation, diabetes mellitus, retinal vascular disease, deficiencies of either ascorbic acid or vitamin A, and hydrochlorothiazide use.

No specific treatment is available for acute lesions, but spontaneous visual improvement usually occurs within a few months. The prognosis for visual recovery appears to be good, even when phototoxic lesions involve the macula. Various methods recommended to decrease the risk of phototoxicity include reduction of microscope coaxial illumination and operative time, use of IR and UV filters in the microscope and IOL, placement of an air bubble in the anterior chamber to defocus the light, and use of an eclipse filter or corneal cover to block light from entering the pupil when the incision is sutured.

The irradiance produced by the indirect ophthalmoscope and fundus camera are lower than experimentally determined retinal injury thresholds.[26] The total energy delivered to the eye is less under nonoperative than operative conditions. These instruments have not been shown to produce acute retinal injury in humans; however, prolonged exposure to the indirect ophthalmoscope has produced lesions in primates. The cumulative effect of repeated examination is unknown, and it is recommended that retinal examinations be performed with the minimal illumination required.

LIGHT EXPOSURE AND AGE-RELATED MACULAR DEGENERATION

The relationship between environmental light exposure and age-related macular degeneration (AMD) remains speculative. It has been suggested that the cumulative effect of repeated mild photic injury during life may contribute to retinal and RPE degeneration in AMD. An association between long-term solar exposure and AMD was suggested when AMD was found to be less common in patients who have nuclear cataract formation.[27] Histopathological studies of acute photic injury in animals reveal damage to the RPE and photoreceptors in the macular region, which is at the same tissue depth and geographical loca-

tion as changes observed in AMD.[23] Solar observation in humans acutely damages the RPE and produces RPE pigmentary irregularities, which are similar in appearance to those in AMD, although the diffuse thickening of Bruch's membrane noted in AMD does not occur with solar damage.[11] The relationship between light and AMD has been evaluated using epidemiological studies. In a population-based study of Chesapeake Bay watermen, no association was found between cumulative UV-A or UV-B exposure and mild or advanced AMD.[28] An association was noted between blue or visible light exposure over the preceding 20 years and the risk of developing advanced AMD (defined as exudative neovascular disease or geographical atrophy).[29] In the Beaver Dam Eye Study, no association was found between the estimated ambient UV-B exposure and AMD.[30] The amount of outdoor leisure time in summer was associated with increased retinal pigmentation in men and late AMD in both men and women. The use of hats and sunglasses was inversely associated with the prevalence of soft, indistinct drusen.

Although some association may exist between visible light exposure and AMD, no study has yet demonstrated conclusively a relationship between long-term UV light exposure and AMD. Until the relationship between light and AMD is more clearly defined, sunglasses to filter UV and blue light may be considered for individuals, especially those at risk, such as pseudophakes and aphakes without UV-protective intraocular lenses and individuals with decreased ocular pigmentation or at risk of developing AMD.[5]

LASER BURNS

Laser applications in industrial, military, and laboratory situations account for a number of cases of accidental retinal injury. Retinal damage results from either direct exposure to the laser or its reflections. It usually occurs when the laser is fired inadvertently and an individual without ocular protection is in the vicinity of the laser. Although this type of injury often can be avoided by wearing proper eye protection, goggles may impair vision and the ability to perform fine tasks, such as alignment of the laser. The type of retinal damage depends on the laser parameters; the mechanism may be thermal, mechanical, or photochemical. Damage ranges from a small, subtle lesion to extensive hemorrhage and disruption of the retina and choroid. Accidental foveal photocoagulation can produce immediate loss of vision up to 20/200, with a foveal cyst or yellow discoloration of the RPE (Fig. 142-6). Long-term evaluation may reveal RPE irregularities,

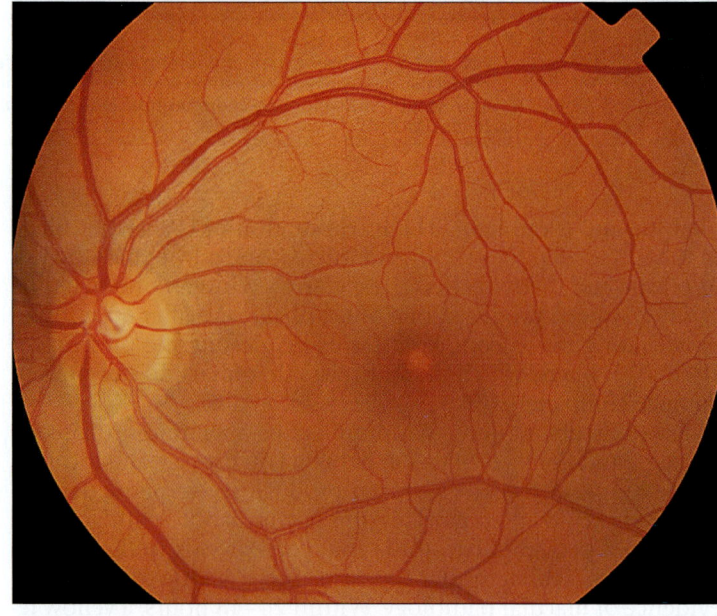

FIG. 142-6 ■ Inadvertent foveal laser burn from an Nd:YAG laser. Snellen visual acuity is 20/200. (Courtesy of Carmen A. Puliafito, MD.)

epiretinal membrane, macular hole, and gliosis. Recovery of vision is variable and is related to the extent and location of the initial injury.[31] Corticosteroids have been used to treat laser-induced retinal injuries, although their benefit is unproved.

In the ophthalmology setting, laser operators and persons in the laser area are at risk from laser light scattered from optical interfaces, such as contact lenses and mirrors. Lasers for photocoagulation contain filters to protect the operator and are positioned in the slit lamp or operating microscope before laser energy is produced. The risk to others in the vicinity of the laser is related to the distance from the laser—protective goggles should be worn by all. Decreased color discrimination in a tritan color-confusion axis has been noted in ophthalmologists who use the argon blue–green laser.[32] This may be due to long-term exposure to reflections from the argon blue aiming beam. Many photocoagulators now employ either a red or green aiming beam to minimize operator risk.

LASER POINTERS

Laser pointers are low-energy lasers with output powers either less than 1 milliwatt (mW) (class 2 devices) or between 1 and 5 mW (class 3A devices). Most of the common class 3A laser pointers have power outputs that are 2mW or less. In contrast, class 3B lasers used by ophthalmologists for retinal therapy have output powers up to or greater than 100mW. The use and availability of laser pointers to the general public has become quite common. There is a potential for misuse of and inadvertent ocular exposure to these handheld lasers. As well, the emitted red beam may produce visual distraction or simulate a weapon-aiming beam. There are very few reports of presumed retinal damage caused by laser pointers.[33-36] The mechanism of injury is not clear, but it appears due to thermal chorioretinal damage, because the longer red 650nm- or 635nm-wavelength light emitted from a laser pointer should not produce significant retinal phototoxicity.[37] Damage manifests as transient visual abnormalities and macular RPE disturbances that correspond to window defect hyperfluorescence on fluorescein angiography.[33] Acute uniocular reduction in vision to 20/40 with two small pericentral scotomata and a hypopigmented ring-shaped foveal lesion was described in a 19-year-old woman after deliberate staring into a commercial class 2 laser pointer for 10 seconds.[33] Visual acuity improved to 20/20 and visual field returned to normal within 8 weeks, but a subjective decrease in brightness and foveal RPE disturbances persisted. Retinal injury was not demonstrated in three patients after class 3A laser pointer retinal exposure (parameters 1mW, 2mW, or 5mW for up to 15 minutes' duration to foveal and juxtafoveal locations) prior to enucleation for uveal melanoma. Other than transient afterimages for minutes, there was no specific laser-induced ocular damage noted with ophthalmoscopy, angiography, or histology.[38] Thus, it appears to be difficult to produce ocular injury with a laser pointer without deliberate inappropriate, prolonged, foveal exposure. Factors such as patient age, preexisting maculopathy, and clarity of the ocular media likely play a role in determining retinal susceptibility to damage.

REFERENCES

1. Mainster MA, Ham WT, DeLori FC. Potential retinal hazards. Instrument and environmental light sources. Ophthalmology. 1983;90:927–32.
2. Priebe LA, Cain CP, Welch AJ. Temperature rise required for the production of minimal lesions in the *Macaca mulatta* retina. Am J Ophthalmol. 1975;79:405–43.
3. White TJ, Mainster MA, Wilson PW, Tips JH. Chorioretinal temperature increases from solar observation. Bull Math Biophys. 1971;33:1–17.
4. Boettner EA, Wolter JR. Transmission of the ocular media. Invest Ophthalmol. 1962;1:776–83.
5. Mainster M. Light and macular degeneration: a biophysical and clinical perspective. Eye. 1987;1:304–10.
6. Lanum J. The damaging effects of light on the retina. Empirical findings. Theoretical and practical implications. Surv Ophthalmol. 1978;22:221–49.
7. Michels M, Sternberg P Jr. Operating microscope-induced retinal phototoxicity: pathophysiology, clinical manifestations and prevention. Surv Ophthalmol. 1990;34:237–52.
8. Cordes FC. A type of foveo-macular retinitis observed in the U.S. Navy. Am J Ophthalmol. 1944;27:803–16.
9. Yannuzzi LA, Fisher YL, Krueger A, Slatker J. Solar retinopathy; a photobiological and geophysical analysis. Trans Am Ophthalmol Soc. 1987;85:120–58.
10. Sliney DH, Wolbarsht ML. Safety with lasers and other optical sources. A comprehensive handbook. New York: Plenum; 1980.
11. Tso MOM, LaPiana FG. The human fovea after sungazing. Trans Am Acad Ophthalmol Otolaryngol. 1975;79:788–95.
12. Michaelides M, Rajendram R, Marshall J, Keightley S. Eclipse retinopathy. Eye. 2001;15:148–151.
13. Wong SC, Eke T, Ziakas NG. Eclipse burns: a prospective study of solar retinopathy following the 1999 solar eclipse. Lancet. 2001;357:199–200.
14. Thanos S, Heiduschka P, Romann I. Exposure to a solar eclipse causes neuronal death in the retina. Graefes Arch Klin Exp Ophthalmol. 2001;239(10):794–800.
15. Naidoff MA, Sliney DH. Retinal injury from a welding arc. Am J Ophthalmol. 1974;77:663–8.
16. Lee MS, Gunton KB, Fischer DH, Brucker AJ. Ocular manifestations of a remote lightning strike. Retina. Am J Ophthalmol. 2002;22:808–10.
17. Norman ME, Younge BR. Association of high-dose intravenous methylprednisolone with reversal of blindness from lightning in two patients. Ophthalmology. 1999;106:743–5.
18. McDonnell HR, Irvine AR. Light-induced maculopathy from the operating microscope in extracapsular cataract extraction and intraocular lens implantation. Ophthalmology. 1983;90:945–51.
19. Khwarg SG, Linstone FA, Daniels SA, et al. Incidence, risk factors, and morphology in operating microscope light retinopathy. Am J Ophthalmol. 1987;103:255–63.
20. Byrnes GA, Chang B, Loose I, et al. Prospective incidence of photic maculopathy after cataract surgery. Am J Ophthalmol. 1995;119:231–2.
21. Robertson DM, McLaren JW. Photic retinopathy from the operating microscope. Arch Ophthalmol. 1989;107:373–5.
22. Leonardy NJ, Dabbs CK, Sternberg P Jr. Subretinal neovascularization after operating microscope burn. Am J Ophthalmol. 1990;109:224–5.
23. Tso MOM, Woodford BJ. Effect of photic injury on the retinal tissues. Ophthalmology. 1983;90:952–63.
24. Green WR, Robertson DM. Pathologic findings of photic retinopathy in the human eye. Am J Ophthalmol. 1991;112:520–7.
25. Kleinmann G, Hoffman P, Schechtman E, Pollack A. Microscope-induced retinal phototoxicity in cataract surgery of short duration. Ophthalmology. 2002;109:334–8.
26. Robertson DM, Erikson GJ. The effect of prolonged indirect ophthalmoscopy on the human eye. Am J Ophthalmol. 1979;87:652–60.
27. Sperduto RD, Hiller R, Seigel D. Lens opacities and senile maculopathy. Arch Ophthalmol. 1981;99:1004–8.
28. West SK, Rosenthal FS, Bressler NM, et al. Exposure to sunlight and other risk factors for age-related macular degeneration. Arch Ophthalmol. 1989;107:875–9.
29. Taylor HR, West S, Munoz B, et al. The long-term effects of visible light on the eye. Arch Ophthalmol. 1992;110:99–104.
30. Cruickshanks KJ, Klein R, Klein BEK. Sunlight and age-related macular degeneration. The Beaver Dam Eye study. Arch Ophthalmol. 1993;111:514–8.
31. Thach AB, Lopez PF, Snady-McCoy LC, et al. Accidental Nd:YAG laser injuries to the macula. Am J Ophthalmol. 1995;119:767–73.
32. Berninger TA, Canning CR, Gunduz K, et al. Using argon laser blue light reduces ophthalmologists color contrast sensitivity. Arch Ophthalmol. 1989;107:1453–8.
33. Sell CH, Bryan JS. Maculopathy from handheld diode laser pointer. Arch Ophthalmol. 1999;117:1557–8.
34. Zamir E, Kaiserman I, Chowers I. Laser pointer maculopathy. Am J Ophthalmol. 1999;127:728–9.
35. McGhee CNJ, Crain JP, Moseley H. Laser pointers can cause permanent retinal injury if used inappropriately. Br J Ophthalmol. 2000;84:229–230.
36. Mainster MA, Timberlake GT, Warren KA, Sliney DH. Pointers on laser pointers. Ophthalmology. 1997;104:1213–4.
37. Mainster MA, Reichel E. Transpupillary thermotherapy for age-related macular degeneration: long-pulse photocoagulation, apoptosis and heat shock proteins. Ophthalmic Surg Lasers. 2000;31:359–73.
38. Robertson DM, Lim TH, Salomao DR, et al. Laser pointers and the human eye: a clinicopathologic study. Arch Ophthalmol. 2000;118:1686–91.

143 Toxic Retinopathies

DAVID V. WEINBERG

DEFINITION
- Retinal injury resulting from systemically administered drugs.

KEY FEATURES
- Retinal pigmentary epithelial irregularities.
- Atrophy of the retina, retinal pigment epithelium, and/or choroid.
- Bull's-eye maculopathy.
- Crystalline deposition.

ASSOCIATED FEATURES
- Rheumatoid arthritis.
- Collagen vascular diseases.
- Psychiatric illness.
- Acquired immunodeficiency syndrome.
- Breast cancer.

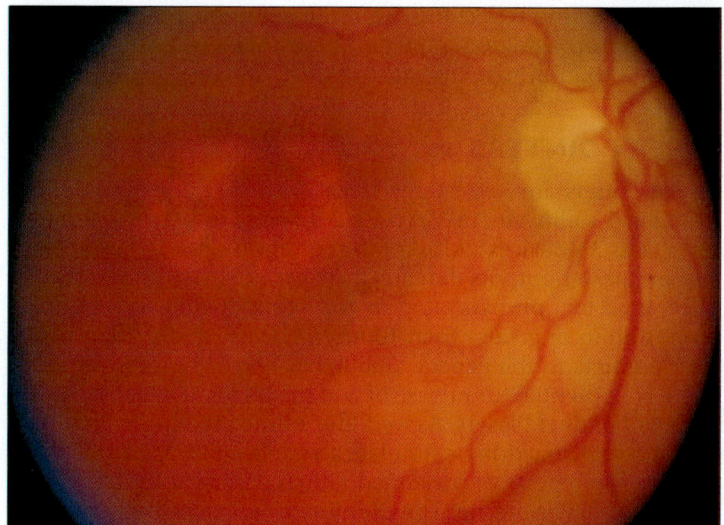

FIG. 143-1 ■ Chloroquine and hydroxychloroquine maculopathy. Note the concentric zone of depigmentation, more prominent inferiorly. (From Weinberg DV, D'Amico DJ. Retinal toxicity of systemic drugs. In: Albert DM, Jakobiec FA, eds. Principles and practice of ophthalmology. Philadelphia: WB Saunders; 1994:1042–50.)

INTRODUCTION

The toxic retinopathies form a diverse group of conditions that result from retinal damage caused by a systemically administered drug. Although they are relatively rare, these conditions should be considered whenever an "unknown" retinopathy is evaluated, particularly when features of macular pigmentary disturbance or retinal crystal deposition are present. Recognition of a toxic retinopathy may spare the patient from future exposure to the noxious agent.

CHLOROQUINE AND HYDROXYCHLOROQUINE

Chloroquine was popularized first for the prophylaxis and treatment of malaria. Later, chloroquine was recognized as an effective treatment for various connective tissue diseases, especially rheumatoid arthritis and systemic lupus erythematosus. Treatment of these diseases required higher doses and longer duration of therapy than employed for malaria. In the late 1950s and early 1960s, descriptions of a toxic retinopathy that resulted from chloroquine use began to appear.[1-3] Currently, hydroxychloroquine, a closely related drug, has largely replaced chloroquine for the treatment of connective tissue diseases. Chloroquine and hydroxychloroquine differ in their therapeutic and toxic dose ranges but can produce identical retinopathy.

Patients who have retinopathy may be asymptomatic. When symptoms do occur, the earliest complaints are usually difficulty with reading or with other fine visual tasks because of central or paracentral scotomas.

The earliest scotomas are subtle, usually within 10° of fixation, and are more common superiorly than inferiorly to fixation.[4] With time, the scotomas enlarge, multiply, and may involve fixation, which reduces visual acuity.

The fundus appearance may remain entirely normal even after scotomas have developed. The earliest fundus findings are irregularity in the macular pigmentation and blunting of the foveal re-

flex. With time, the central irregular pigmentation may become surrounded by a concentric zone of hypopigmentation, usually horizontally oval and more prominent inferiorly to the fovea (Fig. 143-1).[5] This paracentral depigmentation results in the classical bull's-eye maculopathy. With continued exposure to the drug, there may be more generalized pigmentary changes. The end-stage appearance may be indistinguishable from that of retinitis pigmentosa, with peripheral pigment irregularity and bone spicule formation, vascular attenuation, and optic disc pallor.

Fluorescein angiography highlights the macular pigmentary changes seen in established chloroquine and hydroxychloroquine maculopathy but rarely enhances the accuracy of the diagnosis.[6] Occasionally, it may be used to help differentiate toxic maculopathy from other macular abnormalities.

The reported incidences of retinopathy with these two drugs vary widely in the literature because of variations in the definition of retinopathy and changes in the dosages used in clinical practices. The incidence of retinopathy has consistently been reported to increase with both the dose and duration of treatment. For chloroquine, daily doses of ≤250mg, cumulative doses of <100g, and duration of treatment of less than a year are associated with a very low incidence of retinopathy. For hydroxychloroquine, a dose of 400mg/day or less has been associated with low risk of retinopathy.[7]

To avoid toxicity with long-term therapy, the most important factor appears to be the daily dose. If the daily dose is kept below a safe threshold, no limit seems to exist to the duration of dosage or cumulative dose that can be given safely.[8] This threshold dose has been reported as 3.5mg/kg/day for chloroquine and 6.5mg/kg/day for hydroxychloroquine. These dosages are based upon lean body weight. Using these criteria, the com-

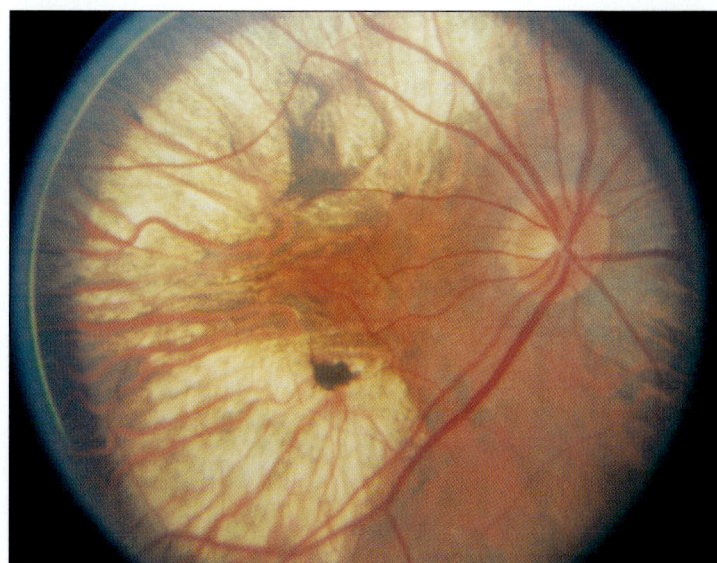

FIG. 143-2 ■ **Thioridazine retinopathy.** Large areas of atrophy are seen in advanced retinopathy. (From Weinberg DV, D'Amico DJ. Retinal toxicity of systemic drugs. In: Albert DM, Jakobiec FA, eds. Principles and practice of ophthalmology. Philadelphia: WB Saunders; 1994:1042–50.)

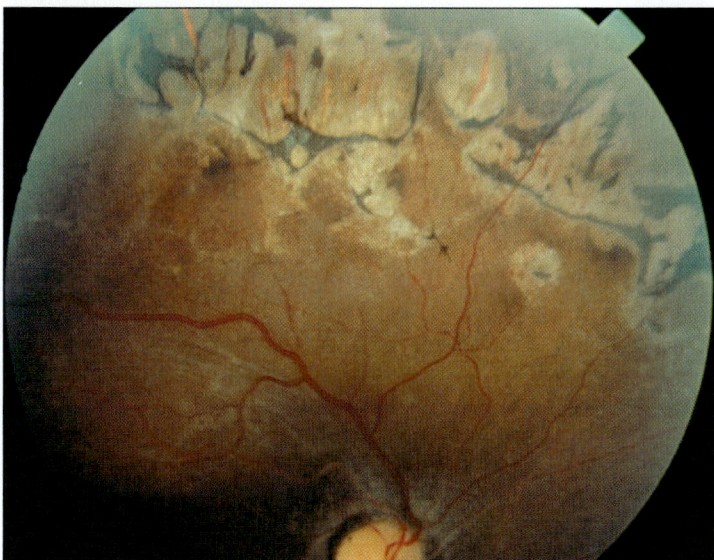

FIG. 143-3 ■ **Thioridazine retinopathy associated with chronic use (nummular retinopathy).** (From Weinberg DV, D'Amico DJ. Retinal toxicity of systemic drugs. In: Albert DM, Jakobiec FA, eds. Principles and practice of ophthalmology. Philadelphia: WB Saunders; 1994:1042–50.)

monly administered dose of 400mg/day of hydroxychloroquine is excessive for patients who have a lean body weight <62kg (<136 pounds). Dose adjustment is also necessary for patients with impaired renal function. It has been demonstrated that well-documented cases of maculopathy are virtually nonexistent for patients who have normal renal function and take <6.5 mg/kg/day of hydroxychloroquine for less than 10 years.[9–11]

Because the earliest macular changes are nonspecific and may be indistinguishable from age-related changes, a baseline examination that includes measurement of the central visual field and the use of color photographs is valuable. For asymptomatic patients who take <6.5mg/kg/day of hydroxychloroquine, annual or semiannual examinations that include detailed questions about visual symptoms, dilated fundus examination, and central visual field testing should reveal rare cases of maculopathy at a very early stage. Amsler grid testing may be useful for home monitoring between visits.

The toxicity of these drugs may be related to their affinity for pigmented structures, especially in the eye. In animal models, the ganglion cells show the earliest histological evidence of toxicity, followed by other neural elements of the retina and the retinal pigment epithelium.

THIORIDAZINE

Thioridazine is a phenothioridazine antipsychotic drug that became popular in the late 1950s because of a favorable side-effect profile. It was used in doses of up to several grams per day. At these doses, a subacute, dramatic form of retinopathy could appear.[12–14] After 2 weeks or more of therapy, patients complained of the development of visual symptoms, which included blurring, nyctalopia, and a brownish visual discoloration; vision was normal to profoundly reduced. At the onset of symptoms, the fundus could appear normal, but within a couple of weeks characteristic changes evolved. Pigment granularity developed posterior to the equator and became more coarse over time. Eventually, geographic areas of depigmentation and loss of choriocapillaris developed (Fig. 143-2). If the drug was withdrawn early after the onset of symptoms, the patients usually reported improvement in vision; however, the pigmentary changes in the fundus often progressed.

At the lower doses used today, this dramatic type of retinopathy rarely, if ever, occurs. A variant referred to as nummular retinopathy has been described in patients taking chronic doses of thioridazine. These patients are much less likely to have symptoms. Multiple, large, round areas of depigmentation and atrophy develop posterior to the equator, with relative sparing of the macula (Fig. 143-3). Over time, the areas of atrophy may enlarge and become confluent. Fluorescein angiography demonstrates loss of pigment epithelium and choriocapillaris within the areas of depigmentation.[15,16] Visual field changes are nonspecific, but most characteristically show paracentral scotomas or ring scotomas.

The manufacturers' current recommendation is that the dose be titrated to a minimal effective dose of 300mg/day or less, with an absolute maximum of 800mg/day for limited periods of time. Cases of retinopathy among patients treated according to these guidelines are rare.

NIACIN

Niacin (nicotinic acid, vitamin B_6) is used at pharmacological doses to lower serum cholesterol. Rarely, patients who take 1.5g or more daily develop maculopathy.

The patients develop central visual changes weeks or months after the initial administration of the drug. Visual acuity is usually reduced mildly to moderately.[17,18] The patients develop a bilateral maculopathy that has the clinical appearance of cystoid macular edema, but there is no dye accumulation with fluorescein angiography. The subjective and objective findings are partially or wholly reversible after the drug is withdrawn.

CANTHAXANTHINE

Canthaxanthine is a carotenoid drug that, when taken orally, causes bronzing of the skin. Although it has been used for treatment of certain dermatologic disorders, its main use has been as an artificial tanning agent. The risk of retinopathy is dose related. At cumulative doses of greater than 60g, the majority of patients are found to have retinopathy. Patients who have canthaxanthine retinopathy are usually asymptomatic. The fundus appearance is bilateral, dramatic, and distinctive. A wreath formation of highly refractile yellow crystals is found in the inner retinal layers that surround the fovea (Fig. 143-4).[19,20]

Although the patients are usually asymptomatic, central perimetry demonstrates reduced sensitivity in patients who have retinopathy. After administration of the drug has been stopped, the number of visible crystals decreases slowly over many years.[21]

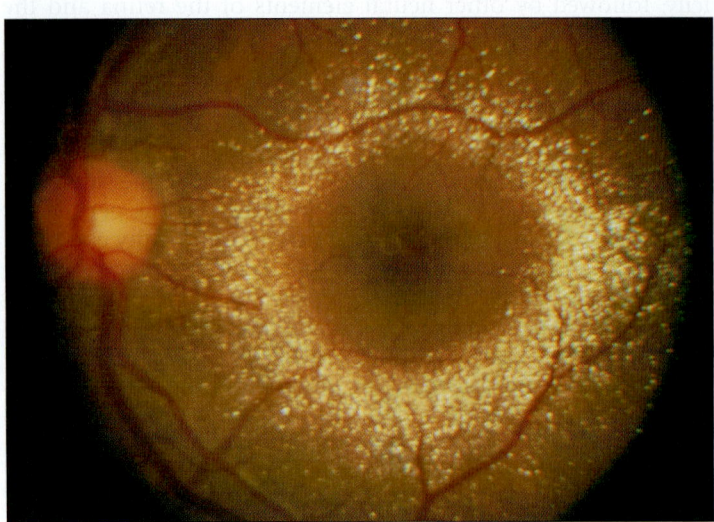

FIG. 143-4 ■ Canthaxanthine retinopathy. Large yellow crystals are distributed in a prominent macular ring. (From Weinberg DV, D'Amico DJ. Retinal toxicity of systemic drugs. In: Albert DM, Jakobiec FA, eds. Principles and practice of ophthalmology. Philadelphia: WB Saunders; 1994:1042–50.)

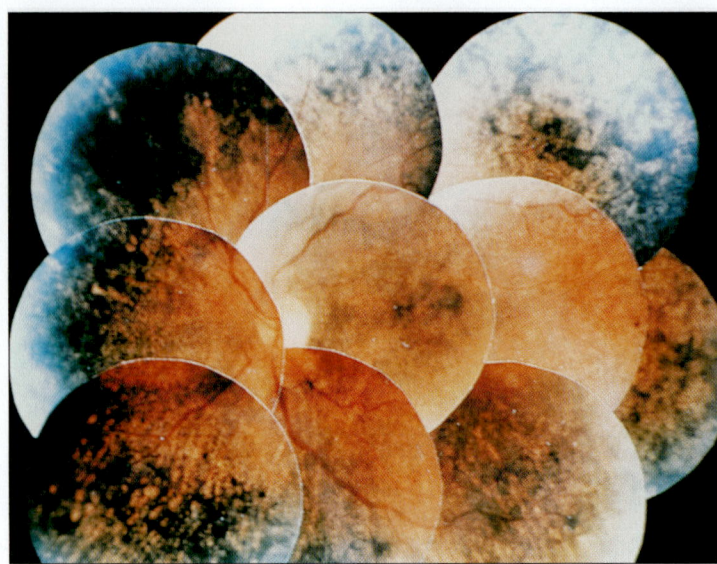

FIG. 143-6 ■ Deferoxamine retinopathy. (From Lakhanpal V, Schocket SS, Jiji R. Deferoxamine (Desferal)-induced toxic retinal pigmentary degeneration and presumed optic neuropathy. Ophthalmology. 1984;91:443–51.)

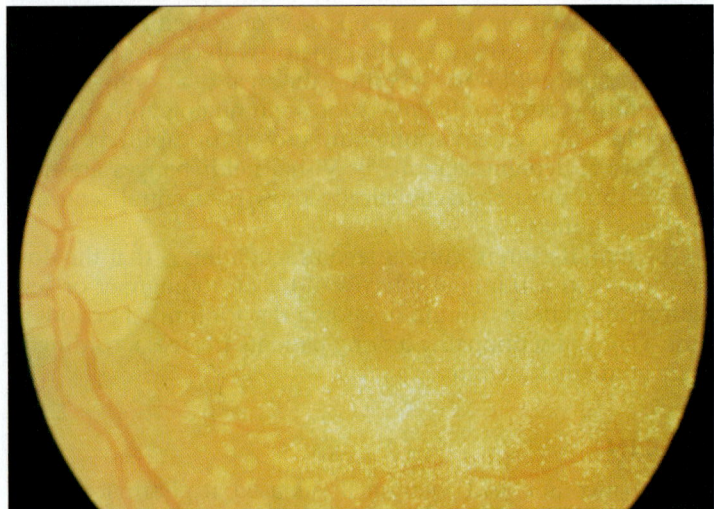

FIG. 143-5 ■ Severe tamoxifen retinopathy. (From McKeown CA, Swartz M, Blom J, Maggiano JM. Tamoxifen retinopathy. Br J Ophthalmol. 1981;65:177–9 and the BMJ Publishing Group.)

TAMOXIFEN

Tamoxifen is a nonsteroidal estrogen antagonist that is used in treatment of breast cancer. Retinopathy was first described among women treated with more than 180mg/day for longer than a year.[22] These patients usually had a symptomatic decrease in vision. The characteristic fundus findings were small white refractile deposits in the inner retina, particularly in the perimacular area. Associated pigmentary irregularity occurred (Fig. 143-5).[23] Fluorescein angiography demonstrated macular edema in most cases.

Currently, the drug is used at much lower doses. Conflicting data exist in the literature as to the incidence and significance of retinopathy at these lower doses.[24–26] Although mild crystal deposition with or without macular edema may be possible with low doses, it is probably quite rare. This is supported by the large number of patients treated with this drug and the relative paucity of well-documented cases in the literature. The most recent study of 135 patients who took 20mg/day found two patients with questionable, but visually insignificant, maculopathy.[26] The authors concluded that it was not necessary to screen patients who take low doses of tamoxifen.

METHOXYFLURANE

Methoxyflurane is an inhalation anesthesia agent. Rare reports exist of crystalline retinopathy as a result of calcium oxalate deposition following methoxyflurane inhalation after prolonged surgical procedures with methoxyflurane anesthesia or after illicit methoxyflurane abuse.[27,28]

DEFEROXAMINE

Deferoxamine mesylate is a chelating agent used to remove toxic levels of heavy metals from the body. Its primary use is to reduce iron levels in patients who have transfusion-dependent anemias. Also, it has been used to treat aluminum toxicity in patients receiving chronic renal dialysis. The drug is given as a slow intravenous or subcutaneous infusion or by intramuscular injection. The onset of visual symptoms from deferoxamine toxicity may be relatively acute. Patients usually complain of blurred vision, nyctalopia, color vision abnormalities, or visual field restriction. At the time of onset, the fundus may appear normal or subtle pigment mottling may be found. Color vision is frequently abnormal, typically with a tritan dyschromatopsia. Visual field testing usually shows central or centrocecal scotomas and, less commonly, peripheral restriction. Electroretinography may show decreased amplitude and prolonged implicit times. Visually evoked potentials may also show low voltage and delayed conduction times. If deferoxamine is withdrawn promptly, partial or complete functional recovery is usually seen. The maculopathy may progress, however, and develop into coarse macular pigmentary changes (Fig. 143-6) and, occasionally, peripheral pigmentary clumping as well.[29–31]

Whether this represents a purely retinal toxicity or has a component of optic neuropathy is somewhat unclear from the literature.

DIDANOSINE

Didanosine (2',3'-dideoxyinosine) is an antiretroviral drug used for the treatment of patients who have human immunodeficiency virus infection. A peripheral retinal degeneration has been observed in a subset of children who were treated with this drug. Of 43 children receiving didanosine followed prospectively, 3 (7%) developed an asymptomatic peripheral retinal degeneration first noted after 9–19 months of therapy. The findings consisted of small, sharply demarcated areas of retinal and

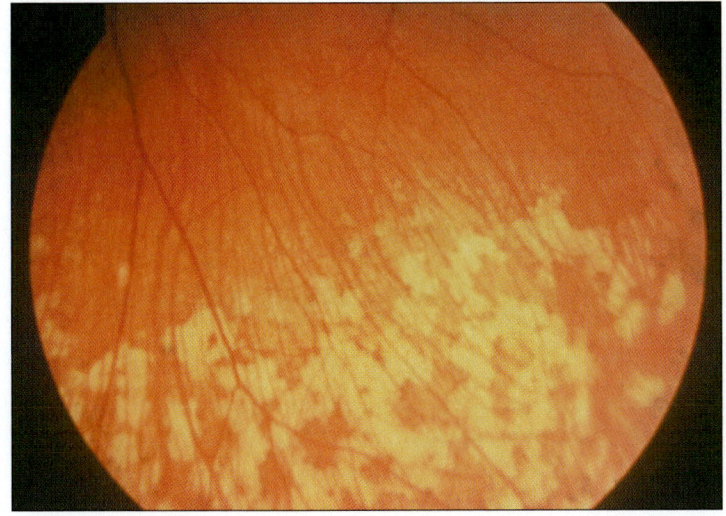

FIG. 143-7 ■ Didanosine retinopathy in a child. (Courtesy of Scott M. Whitcup.)

retinal pigment epithelial atrophy around the midperiphery (Fig. 143-7). The degeneration appeared to progress with continued exposure to the drug. Visual acuity remained normal in all patients. One patient who was able to undergo reliable testing demonstrated mild restriction of the peripheral visual field.[32]

CLOFAZIMINE

Clofazimine is an iminophenazine dye with antimycobacterial and anti-inflammatory activity. Retinal toxicity in the form of a bull's-eye maculopathy has been reported in patients who were given clofazimine for *Mycobacterium avium* complex infections associated with acquired immunodeficiency syndrome. The patients developed a bilateral pattern of parafoveal pigmentary irregularity and atrophy. This was visible clinically and appeared as an irregular parafoveal transmission defect on fluorescein angiography. In contrast to other bull's-eye maculopathies, the pigment changes in these patients were more extensive and extended outside the major vascular arcades.[33,34]

REFERENCES

1. Hobbs HE, Sorsby A, Freedman A. Retinopathy following chloroquine therapy. Lancet. 1959;2:478–80.
2. Hobbs HE, Eadie SP, Somerville F. Ocular lesions after treatment with chloroquine. Br J Ophthalmol. 1961;45:284–97.
3. Henkind P, Rothfield NF. Ocular abnormalities in patients treated with synthetic antimalarial drugs. N Engl J Med. 1963;269:433–9.
4. Hart WM, Burde RM, Johnston GP, Drews RC. Static perimetry in chloroquine retinopathy. Perifoveal patterns of visual field depression. Arch Ophthalmol. 1984;102:377–80.
5. Weinberg DV, D'Amico DJ. Retinal toxicity of systemic drugs. In: Albert DM, Jakobiec FA, eds. Principles and practice of ophthalmology. Philadelphia: WB Saunders; 1994:1042–50.
6. Cruess AF, Schachat AP, Nicholl J, Augsburger JJ. Chloroquine retinopathy. Is fluorescein angiography necessary? Ophthalmology. 1985;92:1127–9.
7. Scherbel AL, Mackenzie AH, Nousek JE, Atdjian M. Ocular lesions in rheumatoid arthritis and related disorders with particular reference to retinopathy. A study of 741 patients treated with and without chloroquine drugs. N Engl J Med. 1965; 273:360–6.
8. Johnson MW, Vine AK. Hydroxychloroquine therapy in massive total doses without retinal toxicity. Am J Ophthalmol. 1987;104:139–44.
9. Bernstein HN. Ocular safety of hydroxychloroquine sulfate (Plaquenil). South Med J. 1992;85:274–9.
10. Easterbrook M. The ocular safety of hydroxychloroquine. Semin Arthritis Rheum. 1993;23(Suppl):62–7.
11. Rynes RI, Bernstein HN. Ophthalmologic safety profile of antimalarial drugs. Lupus. 1993;2(Suppl):S17–S19.
12. May RH, Selymes P, Weekley RD, Potts AM. Thioridazine therapy: results and complications. J Nerv Ment Dis. 1960;130:230–4.
13. Weekley RD, Potts AM, Reboton J, May RH. Pigmentary retinopathy in patients receiving high doses of a new phenothiazine. Arch Ophthalmol. 1960;64:65–76.
14. Hagopian V, Stratton DB, Busiek RD. Five cases of pigmentary retinopathy associated with thioridazine administration. Am J Psychiatry. 1966;123:97–100.
15. Meredith TA, Aaberg TM, Willerson WD. Progressive chorioretinopathy after receiving thioridazine. Arch Ophthalmol. 1978;96:1172–6.
16. Kozy D, Doft BH, Lipkowitz J. Nummular thioridazine retinopathy. Retina. 1984; 4:253–6.
17. Gass JDM. Nicotinic acid maculopathy. Am J Ophthalmol. 1973;76:500–10.
18. Millay RH, Klein ML, Illingworth DR. Niacin maculopathy. Ophthalmology. 1988;95:930–6.
19. Ros AM, Leyon H, Wennersten G. Crystalline retinopathy in patients taking an oral drug containing canthaxanthine. Photodermatology. 1985;2:183–5.
20. Boudreault G, Cortin P, Corriveau LA, et al. La rétinopathie á la canthaxanthine. I. Etude clinique de 51 consommateurs. Can J Ophthalmol. 1983;18:325–8.
21. Harnois C, Samson J, Malenfant M, Rousseau A. Canthaxanthin retinopathy. Anatomic and functional reversibility. Arch Ophthalmol. 1989;107:538–40.
22. Kaiser-Kupfer MI, Lippman ME. Tamoxifen retinopathy. Cancer Treat Rep. 1978;62:315–20.
23. McKeown CA, Swartz M, Blom J, Maggiano JM. Tamoxifen retinopathy. Br J Ophthalmol. 1981;65:177–9.
24. Pavlidis NA, Petris C, Briassoulis E, et al. Clear evidence that long-term low-dose tamoxifen treatment can induce ocular toxicity. Cancer. 1992;69:2961–4.
25. Longstaff S, Sigurdsson H, O'Keefe M, et al. A controlled study of the ocular effects of tamoxifen in conventional dosage in the treatment of breast carcinoma. Eur J Cancer Clin Oncol. 1989;25:1805–8.
26. Heier JS, Dragoo RA, Enzenauer RW, Waterhouse WJ. Screening for ocular toxicity in asymptomatic patients treated with tamoxifen. Am J Ophthalmol. 1994;117:772–5.
27. Bullock JD, Albert DM. Flecked retina. Appearance secondary to oxalate crystals from methoxyflurane anesthesia. Arch Ophthalmol. 1975;93:26–31.
28. Novak MA, Roth AS, Levine MR. Calcium oxalate retinopathy associated with methoxyflurane abuse. Retina. 1988;8:230–6.
29. Lakhanpal V, Schocket SS, Jiji R. Deferoxamine (Desferal)-induced toxic retinal pigmentary degeneration and presumed optic neuropathy. Ophthalmology. 1984;91:443–51.
30. Olivieri NF, Buncic JR, Chew E, et al. Visual and auditory neurotoxicity in patients receiving subcutaneous deferoxamine infusions. N Engl J Med. 1986;314:869–73.
31. Cases A, Kelly J, Sabater F, et al. Ocular and auditory toxicity in hemodialyzed patients receiving desferrioxamine. Nephron. 1990;56:19–23.
32. Whitcup SM, Butler KM, Caruso R, et al. Retinal toxicity in human immunodeficiency virus–infected children treated with 2',3'-didoxyinosine. Am J Ophthalmol. 1992;113:1–7.
33. Craythorn JM, Swartz M, Creel DJ. Clofazimine-induced bull's-eye retinopathy. Retina. 1986;6:50–2.
34. Cunningham CA, Friedberg DN, Carr RE. Clofazimine-induced generalized retinal degeneration. Retina. 1990;10:131–4.

FIG. 147-2 Bull's-eye retinopathy in a child. (Courtesy of Scott Newman.)

References listing (mirror-reversed, largely illegible)

Final pigment deposition around the midperiphery (Fig. 147-2). The deterioration appeared to progress with continued exposure to the drug. Visual acuity remained normal in all patients. One patient who was able to undergo reliable testing demonstrated mild narrowing of the peripheral visual field.

CLOFAZIMINE

Clofazimine is an iminophenazine dye with antimycobacterial and anti-inflammatory activity. Retinal toxicity in the form of a bull's-eye maculopathy has been reported in patients who were given clofazimine for *Mycobacterium avium* complex infections associated with acquired immunodeficiency syndrome. The patients developed a typical pattern of perifoveal pigmentation in regularity and atrophy. There was visible, clinically and appreciated as irregular or numerous or transmission defect on fluorescein angiography. In contrast to other bull's-eye maculopathies, the pigment changes in these patients were more extensive and extended outside the major vascular arcades.[1,2]

REFERENCES

1. (illegible)
2. (illegible)

CHAPTER

144

Vitreous Anatomy and Pathology

JERRY SEBAG

DEFINITIONS

- Vitreous is an extended extracellular matrix of approximately 4.0 ml in volume and 16.5 mm in axial length (emmetropia) that is situated between the lens and retina.

KEY FEATURES

- The clear vitreous gel fills the center of the eye, modulates growth of the eye, maintains media transparency, and during aging detaches away from the retina, in most cases innocuously.

ASSOCIATED FEATURES

- Anomalous posterior vitreous detachment is the fundamental cause of rhegmatogenous retinal detachment and vitreo-maculopathies, and plays an important role in proliferative diabetic vitreo-retinopathy.

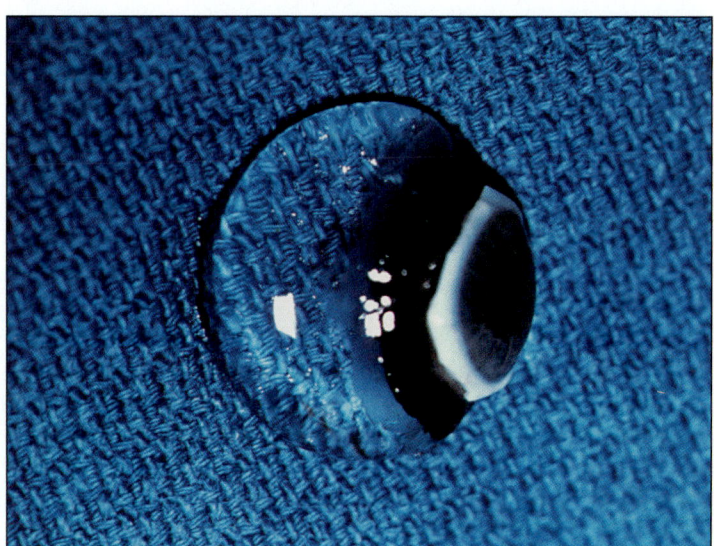

FIG. 144-1 ■■ **Vitreous obtained at autopsy from a 9-month-old child.** The sclera, choroid, and retina were dissected off the transparent vitreous, which remains attached to the anterior segment. A band of gray tissue can be seen posterior to the ora serrata. This is neural retina that was firmly adherent to the vitreous base and could not be dissected. The vitreous is almost entirely gel (because of the young age of the donor) and thus is solid and maintains its shape, although situated on a surgical towel exposed to room air. (Courtesy of the New England Eye Bank, Boston, MA.)

INTRODUCTION

Although vitreous is the largest structure within the eye, constituting 80% of the ocular volume, investigators of vitreous anatomy are hampered by two fundamental difficulties:

- Any attempts to define vitreous morphology are efforts to "visualize" a tissue that is invisible by design (Fig. 144-1).
- The various techniques that were employed previously to define vitreous structure were flawed by artifacts induced by tissue fixatives, which caused precipitation of hyaluronan (formerly called hyaluronic acid), a glycosaminoglycan.

The development of slit-lamp biomicroscopy by Gullstrand in 1912 was expected to enable clinical investigation of vitreous structure without the introduction of the aforementioned artifacts. Yet, a widely disparate set of descriptions resulted because of the first of the inherent difficulties just described; that is, the vitreous body, by design, is largely invisible. This problem even persists in so-called modern investigations. Consider, for example, that in the 1970s Eisner[1] described "membranelles" and Worst[2] "cisterns," in the 1980s Sebag and Balazs[3,4] identified "fibers," and in the 1990s Kishi and Shimizu[5] found "pockets" in the vitreous body. The discrepant observations of the last-mentioned group have now been explained largely as an age-related phenomenon with no relevance to the inherent macromolecular structure or anatomy.[6,7]

In the following, vitreous anatomy is characterized in terms of its molecular constituents and their macromolecular organization, the resultant macroscopic morphology, and the effects of major disease processes on vitreoretinal pathology.

MOLECULAR CONSTITUENTS

Collagens

As shown in Fig. 144-2, individual vitreous collagen fibrils are organized as a triple helix of three alpha chains. The major collagen fibrils of the vitreous body are heterotypic, consisting of more than one collagen type. Studies of pepsinized forms of collagen confirm that the vitreous body contains collagen type II, a hybrid of types V and XI, and type IX.[8] Considerable similarities exist between vitreous collagen, the major collagen fibrils of articular cartilage, and the nucleus pulposus of the spine. This may explain why some clinical phenomena occur simultaneously in these different tissues.

TYPE II COLLAGEN. Total vitreous collagen is 75% type II collagen.[9] It is a homotrimer, composed of three identical alpha chains designated as $[1(II)]_3$. When first synthesized as a procollagen and secreted into the extracellular space, type II collagen is highly soluble. The activity of *N*-proteinase and *C*-proteinase enzymes reduces the solubility and enables type II collagen molecules to cross-link covalently in a quarter-staggered array. Within this array are likely to be *N*-propeptides, which probably extend outward from the surface of the forming fibril.[10] This may influence the interaction of the collagen fibril with other components of the extracellular matrix. That type IIA procollagen propeptides[11] specifically bind transforming growth factor-β1 and BMP-2[12] supports the concept that in certain circumstances such growth factors and cytokines interact with vitreous fibrils to promote the cell migration and proliferation that result in proliferative diabetic retinopathy and proliferative vitreoretinopathy.

TYPE IX COLLAGEN. Type IX collagen is a heterotrimer that is disulfide bonded with an $[\alpha1(IX)\alpha2(IX)\alpha3(IX)]$ configuration. This heterotrimer is oriented regularly along the surfaces of the major collagen fibrils in a "D periodic" distribution, where it is cross-linked onto the fibril surface. Type IX is not a typical

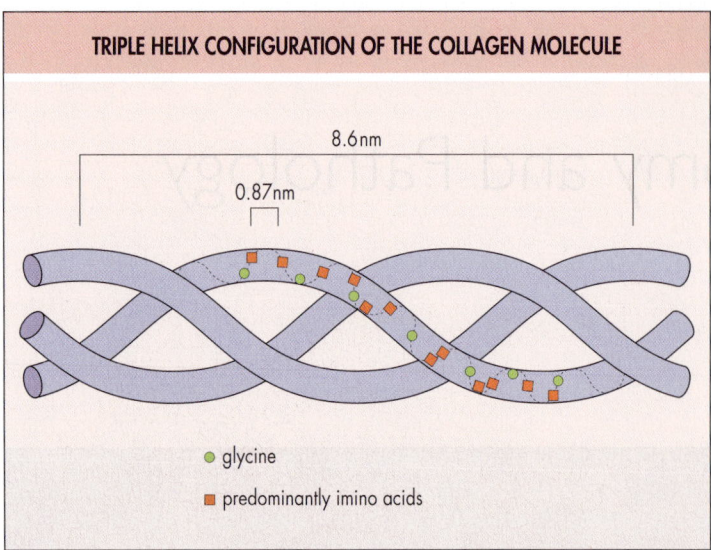

TRIPLE HELIX CONFIGURATION OF THE COLLAGEN MOLECULE

8.6nm

0.87nm

● glycine
■ predominantly imino acids

FIG. 144-2 ■ The triple helix configuration of the collagen molecule. Individual alpha chains are left-handed helices with approximately three residues per turn. The chains themselves, however, are coiled around each other in a right-handed twist. The triple helix configuration is stabilized by hydrogen bonds, which form between opposing residues in different chains (interpeptide hydrogen bonding). (Reprinted with permission from Nimni ME, Harkness RD. Molecular structure and functions of collagen. In: Nimni ME, ed. Collagen, Vol 1. Boca Raton, FL: CRC Press; 1988.)

collagen but is a member of the FACIT (fibrillar-associated collagens with interrupted triple helixes) group of collagens. It contains collagenous regions described as COL1, COL2, and COL3 interspersed between noncollagenous regions called NC1, NC2, NC3, and NC4.[9,10] In vitreous (as opposed to cartilage) the NC4 domain is small and, therefore, not highly charged and not likely to exhibit extensive interaction with other extracellular matrix components.[13] In vitreous, type IX collagen always contains a chondroitin sulfate glycosaminoglycan chain,[9,10] which is linked covalently to the $\alpha2(IX)$ chain at the NC3 domain; this enables the molecule to assume a proteoglycan form. Duplexing of glycosaminoglycan chains from adjacent collagen fibrils may result in a "ladder-like" configuration.[14]

TYPE V/XI COLLAGEN. Ten percent of vitreous collagen is a hybrid V/XI collagen that is believed to constitute the central core of the major collagen fibrils of vitreous.[15] Type V/XI is a heterotrimer that contains 1(XI) and 2(V) in two chains; the nature of the third chain is not yet known.[15] Along with type II collagen, type V/XI is a fibril-forming collagen. Although, in cartilage, the interaction of the fibril with other extracellular matrix components is probably influenced by a retained *N*-propeptide[15] that protrudes from the surface of the fibril, it is not known whether this is the case in vitreous.

TYPE VI COLLAGEN. Although there are only small amounts of type VI collagen in vitreous, the ability of this molecule to bind both type II collagen and hyaluronan suggests that it could be important in organizing and maintaining the supramolecular structure of vitreous gel.[16]

Glycosaminoglycans

HYALURONAN. Hyaluronan is found throughout the body, but it was first isolated from bovine vitreous. In human vitreous, hyaluronan first appears after birth and is believed to be synthesized primarily by hyalocytes,[4] although other plausible candidates exist, such as the ciliary body and retinal Müller cells. Whereas the synthesis of hyaluronan seems to stabilize at a constant level in the adult, no extracellular degradation occurs. Levels of hyaluronan remain constant because it escapes from vitreous via the anterior segment of the eye[17] and because of reuptake by hyalocytes.

Hyaluronan is a long, unbranched polymer of repeating disaccharide (glucuronic acid-1,3-*N*,*N*-acetylglucosamine) linked by 1–4 bonds.[18] It is a linear, left-handed, three-fold helix with a rise per disaccharide on the helix axis of 0.98nm.[19] Rotary shadowing electron microscopy of human and bovine vitreous demonstrates lateral aggregates of hyaluronan that form an anastomosing three-dimensional network. This periodicity varies depending on whether the helix is in a "compressed" or "extended" configuration.[20]

The sodium salt of hyaluronan has a molecular weight of $3-4.5 \times 10^6$ in normal human vitreous. Recent studies used dynamic light scattering in bovine vitreous and found a weight-averaged molecular weight of 170,000. Although there is no evidence that adjacent hyaluronan chains bind to one another, rotary shadowing electron microscopy of bovine and human vitreous found lateral aggregates of hyaluronan that formed three-dimensional lattice-like networks.[20]

The volume of the unhydrated hyaluronan molecule is about $0.66cm^3/g$, whereas the hydrated specific volume is 2000–3000cm^3/g.[17] Thus, the degree of hydration has a significant influence on the size and configuration of the molecular network.[21] Furthermore, as a result of its entanglement and immobilization in tissue, hyaluronan interacts with the surrounding mobile ions and thus undergoes changes in its conformation.[22] A decrease in surrounding ionic strength can cause the anionic charges on the polysaccharide backbone to repel one another, which results in an extended configuration of the macromolecule. In this way, changes in the ionic milieu of vitreous may be converted into mechanical energy through extension or contraction of the hyaluronan macromolecule and, in turn, swelling or shrinkage of the vitreous body. This can be important in certain pathological conditions, such as diabetes.[23]

Another important property of hyaluronan is that of steric exclusion.[24] Hyaluronan, with its flexible linear chains and random coil conformation, occupies a large volume and resists the penetration of this volume by other molecules to a degree dependent upon their size and shape.[20] This "excluded volume" effect can influence equilibria between different conformational states of macromolecules and alter the compactness or extension of these molecules.[22] Steric exclusion also causes an excess of osmotic pressure when such compounds as albumin and hyaluronan are mixed because the resultant osmotic pressure is greater than the sum of the two components. This could be important in diabetes, in which vascular incompetence can increase vitreous concentrations of serum proteins such as albumin. Thus, osmotic effects can induce contraction and expansion of the vitreous body, which can in turn play an important role in neovascularization and vitreous hemorrhage.[23] An increase in the chemical activity of a compound because of steric exclusion can cause its precipitation if the solubility limit is reached. This could be important in the formation of pathological vitreous opacities, such as asteroid hyalosis and amyloidosis.[4]

CHONDROITIN SULFATE. Vitreous contains two chondroitin sulfate proteoglycans. The minor type is actually type IX collagen, which has already been described. The majority of vitreous chondroitin sulfate is in the form of versican.[25] This large proteoglycan has a globular N-terminal that binds hyaluronan via a 45kDa link protein. In human vitreous, versican is believed to form complexes with hyaluronan as well as microfibrillar proteins such as fibulin-1 and fibulin-2.

Noncollagenous Structural Proteins

FIBRILLINS. Fibrillin-containing microfibrils are more abundant than the type VI collagen microfibrils described earlier. They are found in vitreous gel as well as the zonules of the lens. This fact explains why in Marfan's syndrome the defects in the gene encoding fibrillin-1 (*FBN1* on chromosome 15q21) result in both ectopia lentis and vitreous liquefaction. The latter probably plays a role in the frequent occurrence of rhegmatogenous retinal detachment in these patients, through anomalous posterior vitreous detachment.

OPTICIN. The major noncollagenous protein of vitreous is a leucine-rich repeat (LRR) protein that is bound to the surface of the heterotypic collagen fibrils, known as opticin.[26] Formerly called vitrican, opticin is believed to be important in collagen fibril assembly and in preventing the aggregation of adjacent collagen fibrils into bundles. Thus, a breakdown in this property or activity may play a role in the age-related changes described later in this chapter.

VIT1. Another novel vitreous protein is VIT1, a collagen-binding macromolecule. Because of its propensity to bind collagen, this highly basic protein may play an important role in maintaining vitreous gel structure.[27]

Miscellaneous Molecular Components

Amino acids are present in vitreous, perhaps to serve as a metabolic repository for lens and/or retinal protein metabolism. Albumin, transferrin,[28] and metalloproteinases[29] are also present. Glycoproteins, which are heteropolysaccharides as opposed to the homogeneous, repeating disaccharide units of glycosaminoglycans, are found in relatively large quantities.[17] Cartilage oligomeric protein (COMP), an acidic glycoprotein with a characteristic five-armed structure, is present in vitreous, although its function is unknown.

Vitreous ascorbic acid may serve as a free radical scavenger to protect the retina and lens from the untoward effects of metabolic and light-induced singlet oxygen generation and oxidative damage as a result of inflammation.[30] Lipids, phospholipids, and many different low-molecular-weight components, as well as several ions, are present in vitreous.[4,31]

MOLECULAR ANATOMY

Supramolecular Organization

Vitreous is composed of a dilute meshwork of collagen fibrils with interspersed extensive arrays of long hyaluronan molecules. The collagen fibrils provide a solid structure that is "inflated" by the hydrophilic hyaluronan. If collagen is removed, the remaining hyaluronan forms a viscous solution; if hyaluronan is removed, the gel shrinks[22] but is not destroyed. Physiological observations also suggest the existence of an important interaction between hyaluronan and collagen.[32] It has been hypothesized that the hydroxylysine amino acids of collagen mediate polysaccharide binding to the collagen chain through O-glycosidic linkages.[17] These polar amino acids are present in clusters along the collagen molecule, which perhaps explains why proteoglycans attach to collagen in a periodic pattern.[33]

Hyaluronan-collagen interaction in the vitreous body may be mediated by a third molecule. In cartilage, "link glycoproteins" have been identified that interact with proteoglycans and hyaluronan.[34] Supramolecular complexes of these glycoproteins are believed to occupy the interfibrillar spaces. Bishop[16] has elegantly described the potential roles of type IX collagen chondroitin sulfate chains, hyaluronan, and opticin in the short-range spacing of collagen fibrils and how these mechanisms might break down in aging and disease.

Many investigators believe that hyaluronan-collagen interaction occurs on a "physicochemical" rather than a "chemical" level.[22] Reversible formation of complexes of an electrostatic nature between solubilized collagen and various glycosaminoglycans occurs. Electrostatic binding in vitreous could occur between negatively charged hyaluronan and positively charged collagen.[22]

VITREOUS ANATOMY

Macroscopic Morphology

In an emmetropic adult human eye the vitreous body is approximately 16.5mm in axial length with a depression anteriorly just behind the lens (patellar fossa). The hyaloideocapsular ligament of Weiger is the annular region (1–2mm in width and 8–9mm

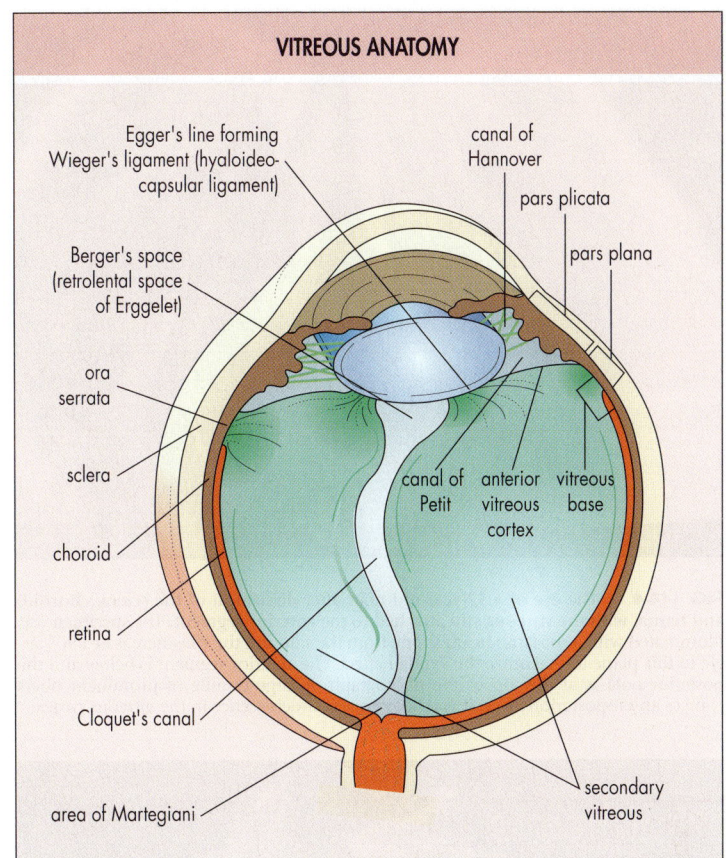

FIG. 144-3 ■ Vitreous anatomy according to classical anatomical and histological studies. (Reprinted with permission from Schepens CL, Neetens A, eds. The vitreous and vitreoretinal interface. New York: Springer-Verlag; 1987:20.)

in diameter) where the vitreous body is attached to the posterior aspect of the lens. Erggelet's or Berger's space is at the center of the hyaloideocapsular ligament. The canal of Cloquet arises from this space and courses posteriorly through the central vitreous (Fig. 144-3), which is the former site of the hyaloid artery in the embryonic vitreous.[35] The former lumen of the artery is an area devoid of collagen fibrils and surrounded by multifenestrated sheaths that were previously the basal laminae of the hyaloid artery wall.[4] Posteriorly, Cloquet's canal opens into a funnel-shaped region anterior to the optic disc, known as the area of Martegiani.

Within the adult human vitreous fine, parallel fibers course in an anteroposterior direction, are continuous, and do not branch (Fig. 144-4). The fibers arise from the vitreous base, where they insert anterior and posterior to the ora serrata. Various concepts are used to explain the connection between the peripheral anterior vitreous fibers and the retina and pars plana,[4] but all agree that the pathophysiology of retinal tears is vitreous traction upon foci of strong adhesion at the vitreoretinal interface in these locations.

As the central fibers near the vitreous cortex course posteriorly, they are circumferential with the vitreous cortex, while central fibers "undulate" in a configuration parallel to Cloquet's canal. Ultrastructural studies demonstrate that collagen, organized in bundles of packed, parallel fibrils, is the only microscopic structure that corresponds to these fibers.[3] It is hypothesized that visible vitreous fibers form when hyaluronan molecules no longer separate the microscopic collagen fibrils, which results in the aggregation of collagen fibrils into bundles from which hyaluronan molecules are excluded.[3,4,36] The areas adjacent to these large fibers have a low density of collagen fibrils and a relatively high concentration of hyaluronan molecules. Composed primarily of "liquid vitreous," these areas scatter very little incident light and, when prominent, constitute "lacunae" seen in aging (see Fig. 144-5).

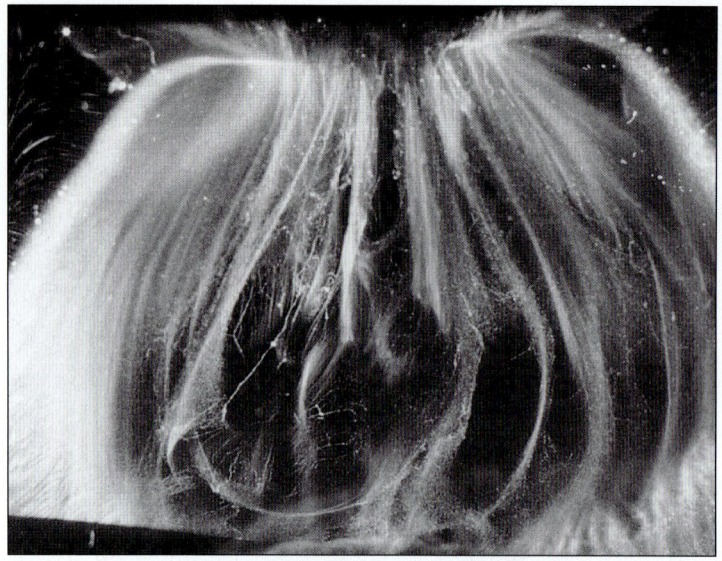

FIG. 144-4 ■ **The eye of a 57-year-old man after dissection of the sclera, choroid, and retina, with the vitreous still attached to the anterior segment.** The specimen was illuminated with a slit-lamp beam shone from the side and the view here is at a 90° angle to this plane to maximize the Tyndall effect. The anterior segment is below and the posterior pole is at the top of the photograph. A large bundle of prominent fibers courses anteroposteriorly to exit via the premacular dehiscence in the vitreous cortex.

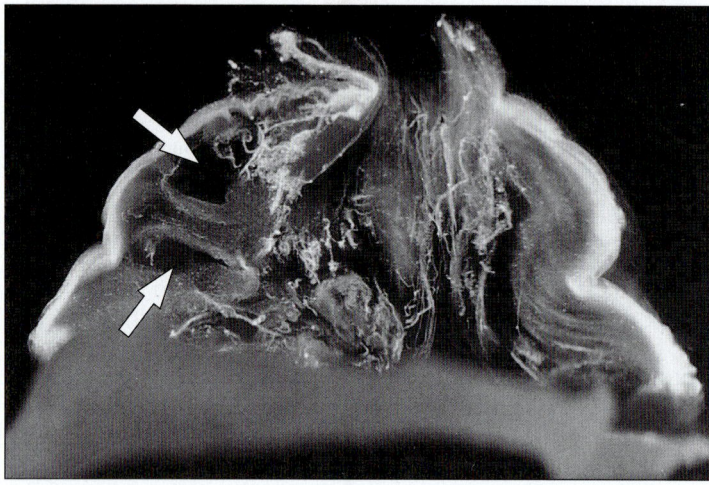

FIG. 144-5 ■ **Human vitreous in old age.** The central vitreous has thickened, tortuous fibers. The peripheral vitreous has regions devoid of any structure, which contain liquid vitreous. These regions correspond to "lacunae," as seen clinically using biomicroscopy *(arrows)*.

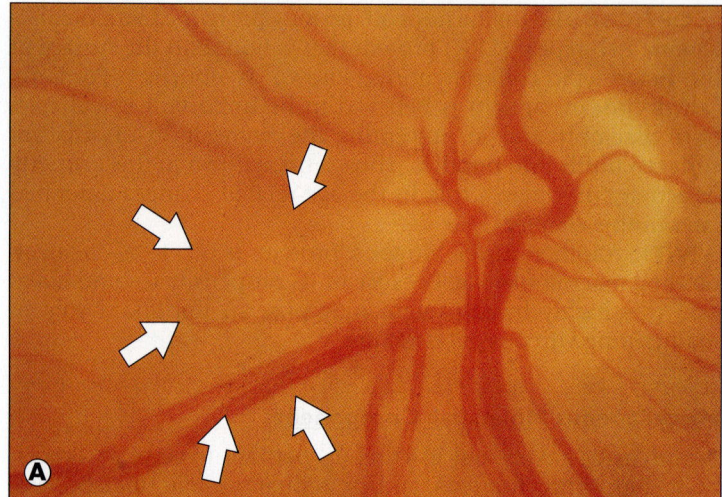

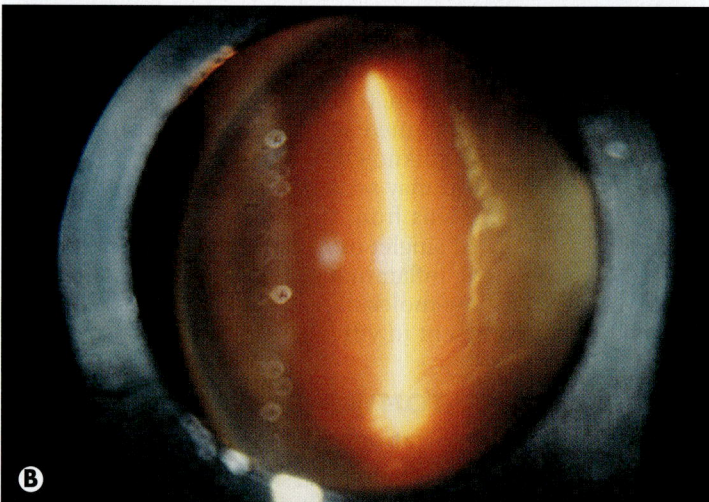

FIG. 144-6 ■ **Fundus view of posterior vitreous detachment. A,** The posterior vitreous in the left eye of this patient is detached and the prepapillary hole in the posterior vitreous cortex is anterior to the optic disc *(arrows, slightly below and to the left of the optic disc here)*. **B,** A slit beam illuminates the retina and optical disc *(at bottom)* in the center. To the right is the detached vitreous. The posterior vitreous cortex is the dense, whitish gray, vertically oriented linear structure to the right of the slit beam. *(Courtesy of CL Trempe, MD.)*

Microscopic Morphology

The vitreous cortex is defined as the peripheral "shell" of the vitreous body that courses forward and inward from the anterior vitreous base, the "anterior vitreous cortex," and posteriorly from the posterior border of the vitreous base, the "posterior vitreous cortex." The posterior vitreous cortex is 100–110μm thick and consists of densely packed collagen fibrils.[4,37] Although no direct connections exist between the posterior vitreous and the retina, the posterior vitreous cortex is adherent to the internal limiting lamina of the retina, which is actually the basal lamina of retinal Müller cells. The exact nature of the adhesion between the posterior vitreous cortex and the internal limiting lamina is not known, but it most probably results from the action of various extracellular matrix molecules.[38]

A hole in the prepapillary vitreous cortex can sometimes be visualized clinically when the posterior vitreous is detached from the retina (Fig. 144-6). If peripapillary glial tissue is torn away during posterior vitreous detachment and remains attached to the vitreous cortex about the prepapillary hole, it is referred to as Vogt's or Weiss' ring. Vitreous can extrude through the prepapillary hole in the vitreous cortex but does so to a lesser

extent than through the premacular vitreous cortex. Various vitreomaculopathies can result.[39] Other mechanisms, particularly tangential vitreo-macular traction,[40] are implicated in the pathogenesis of macular holes.

Embedded within the posterior vitreous cortex are hyalocytes. These mononuclear cells are spread widely apart in a single layer situated 20–50μm from the internal limiting membrane of the retina. The highest density of hyalocytes is in the vitreous base, followed next by the posterior pole, with the lowest density at the equator. Hyalocytes are oval or spindle shaped, 10–15μm in diameter, and contain a lobulated nucleus, a well-developed Golgi complex, smooth and rough endoplasmic reticula, many large lysosomal granules (periodic acid–Schiff positive), and phagosomes (Fig. 144-7). Balazs[17] pointed out that hyalocytes are located in the region of highest hyaluronan concentration and suggested that these cells are responsible for hyaluronan synthesis. Hyalocyte capacity to synthesize collagen was first demonstrated by Newsome *et al.*[41] Thus, in a similar fashion to the chondrocyte metabolism in the joint, hyalocytes may be responsible for vitreous collagen synthesis at some point(s) during life. The phagocytic capacity of hyalocytes is consistent with the presence of pinocytic vesicles and phagosomes and the presence of surface receptors that bind immunoglobulin G and complement.[37] It is intriguing to consider that hyalocytes are among the first cells to be exposed to any migratory or mitogenic stimuli during various disease states, particularly proliferative vitreo-

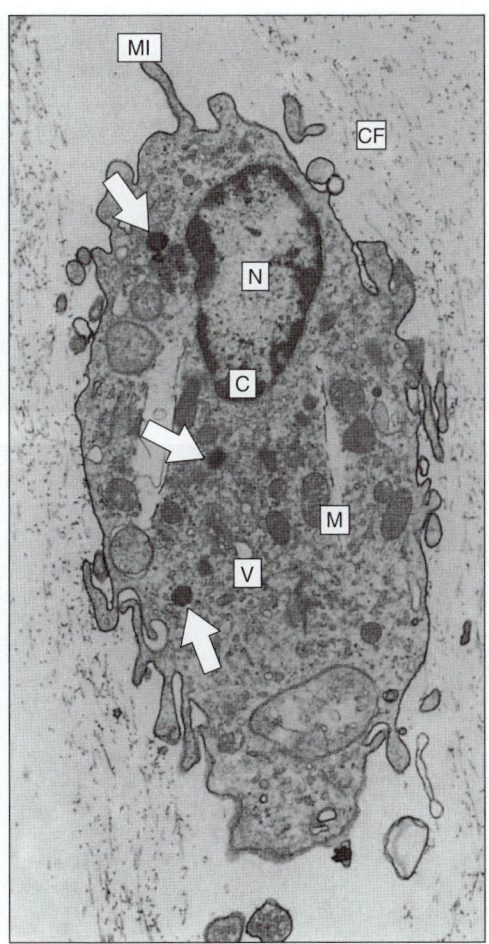

FIG. 144-7 ▪ Ultrastructure of human hyalocyte. A mononuclear cell is embedded within the dense collagen fibril *(CF)* network of the vitreous cortex. There is a lobulated nucleus *(N)* with a dense marginal chromatin *(C)*. In the cytoplasm there are mitochondria *(M)*, dense granules *(arrows)*, vacuoles *(V)*, and microvilli *(MI)*. (Courtesy of Joe Craft and DM Albert, MD.)

near the optic disc in proliferative diabetic retinopathy and premacular membranes with macular pucker.

The vitreous is known to be most firmly attached at the vitreous base, disc, and macula and over retinal blood vessels. The posterior aspect (retinal side) of the internal limiting lamina demonstrates irregular thickening the farther posteriorly from the ora serrata.[4,37] So-called attachment plaques between the Müller cells and the internal limiting lamina have been described in the basal and equatorial regions of the fundus but not in the posterior pole, except for the fovea.[4,37] It has been hypothesized that these develop in response to vitreous traction upon the retina. The thick internal limiting lamina in the posterior pole dampens the effects of this traction, except at the fovea, where the internal limiting lamina is thin. The thinness of the internal limiting lamina and the purported presence of attachment plaques at the central macula could explain the predisposition of this region to changes induced by traction. An unusual vitreoretinal interface overlies retinal blood vessels. Physiologically, this may provide a shock-absorbing function to dampen arterial pulsations. However, pathologically, this structural arrangement could also account for the proliferative and hemorrhagic events upon retinal blood vessels that are associated with vitreous traction.

AGE-RELATED CHANGES

Embryology and Postnatal Development

Early in embryogenesis, the vitreous body is filled with blood vessels, the vasa hyaloidea propria. It is not known what stimulates regression of this hyaloid vascular system, but studies have identified a protein native to vitreous that inhibits angiogenesis in experimental models.[43] Teleologically, this seems necessary not only to induce regression of the vascular primary vitreous but also to inhibit subsequent cell migration and proliferation and thereby minimize light scatter and achieve transparency. Identifying the phenomena inherent in this transformation may reveal how to control pathological angiogenesis.

Developmental Anomalies

Proper vitreous biosynthesis during embryogenesis depends upon normal retinal development because at least some of the vitreous structural components are synthesized by retinal Müller cells.[41] A clear gel, typical of normal "secondary vitreous," appears only over normally developed retina. Thus, in various developmental anomalies, such as retinopathy of prematurity (ROP), familial exudative vitreoretinopathy, and related entities, vitreous that overlies undeveloped retina in the peripheral fundus is a viscous liquid and not a gel. The extent of this finding depends, at least in ROP, upon the gestational age at birth, because the younger the individual the less developed retina is present in the periphery, especially temporally. In other, truly congenital conditions, there are inborn errors of collagen metabolism that have now been elucidated. In Stickler syndrome, defects in specific genes have been associated with particular phenotypes,[44] thus enabling the classification of patients with Stickler syndrome into four subgroups. Patients in the subgroups with vitreous abnormalities are found to have defects in the genes coding for type II procollagen and type V/XI procollagen.

Ongoing synthesis of both collagen and hyaluronan occurs during development to the adult. Because the synthesis of collagen keeps pace with increasing vitreous volume, the overall concentration of collagen within the vitreous body is unchanged during this period of life. Total collagen content in the gel vitreous decreases during the first few years of life and then remains at about 0.05mg until the third decade.[45] Because collagen concentration does not increase appreciably as the size of the vitreous increases, the network density of collagen fibrils effectively decreases. This potentially could weaken the collagen network and destabilize the gel. However, as net synthesis of hyaluronan

retinopathy. Therefore, the role of these cells must be considered when the pathophysiology of all proliferative disorders at the vitreoretinal interface is considered, including premacular membrane formation.

The basal laminae about the vitreous body are composed of type IV collagen closely associated with glycoproteins.[37] At the pars plana, the basal lamina has a true lamina densa. The basal lamina posterior to the ora serrata is the internal limiting lamina of the retina. The layer immediately adjacent to the Müller cell is a lamina rara, which is 0.03–0.06μm thick. The lamina densa is thinnest at the fovea (0.01–0.02μm) and disc (0.07–0.1μm). It is thicker elsewhere in the posterior pole (0.5–3.2μm) than at the equator or vitreous base.[4,37] The anterior surface of the internal limiting lamina (vitreous side) is normally smooth, whereas the posterior aspect is irregular, as it fills the spaces created by the irregular surface of the subjacent retinal glial cells. This feature is most marked at the posterior pole, whereas in the periphery both the anterior and posterior aspects of the internal limiting lamina are smooth. The significance, if any, of this topographic variation is not known. At the rim of the optic disc the retinal internal limiting lamina ceases, although the basal lamina continues as the "inner limiting membrane of Elschnig."[42] This membrane is 50μm thick and is believed to be the basal lamina of the astroglia in the papilla. At the central-most portion of the optic disc the membrane thins to 20μm, follows the irregularities of the underlying cells of the optic nerve head, and is composed only of glycosaminoglycans with no collagen.[42] This structure is known as the "central meniscus of Kuhnt." The thinness and chemical composition of these structures may account for, among other phenomena, the frequency with which abnormal cell proliferation arises from or

occurs during this time, the dramatic increase in hyaluronan concentration "stabilizes" the thinning collagen network.[17]

Aging of the Vitreous Body

Substantial rheological, biochemical, and structural alterations occur in the vitreous body during aging.[46] After 45–50 years of age a significant decrease occurs in the gel volume and an increase in the liquid volume of human vitreous. These findings were confirmed qualitatively in postmortem studies of dissected human vitreous, and liquefaction was observed to begin in the central vitreous.[1,4–6] Vitreous liquefaction actually begins much earlier than the ages at which clinical examination or ultrasonography detects changes. Postmortem studies found evidence of liquid vitreous in eyes at 4 years of age and observed that by the time the human eye reaches its adult size (age 14–18 years) approximately 20% of the total vitreous volume consists of liquid vitreous.[45] In these postmortem studies of fresh, unfixed human eyes it was observed that after the age of 40 years a steady increase occurs in liquid vitreous simultaneously with a decrease in gel volume. By 80–90 years of age more than half the vitreous body is liquid. The finding that the central vitreous is where fibers are first observed is consistent with the concept that breakdown of the normal hyaluronan-collagen association results in the simultaneous formation of liquid vitreous and aggregation of collagen fibrils into bundles of parallel fibrils, seen as large fibers (see Fig. 144-4).[1,4–6] In the posterior vitreous such age-related changes often form large pockets of liquid vitreous, recognized clinically as lacunae,[4–6] and mistakenly described as anatomic structures.[5–7]

The mechanism of vitreous liquefaction is not understood. Gel vitreous can be liquefied *in vivo* through the removal of collagen by enzymatic destruction of the collagen network.[47] Endogenous liquefaction may be the result of changes in the minor glycosaminoglycans and chondroitin sulfate profile of vitreous. It has been shown that the injection of chondroitinase ABC can induce liquefaction and "disinsertion" of the vitreous body.[48] Plasmin is another agent being developed as an adjunct to vitreoretinal surgery[49] because of its purported ability to induce liquefaction of the central vitreous and dehiscence at the vitreoretinal interface. Another possible mechanism of vitreous liquefaction is a change in the conformation of hyaluronan molecules with aggregation or cross-linking of collagen molecules. Singlet oxygen can induce conformational changes in the tertiary structure of hyaluronan molecules. Free radicals generated by metabolic and photosensitized reactions could alter hyaluronan and/or collagen structure and trigger a dissociation of collagen and hyaluronan molecules, which ultimately results in liquefaction.[30] This is plausible because the cumulative effects of a lifetime of daily exposure to light may influence the structure and interaction of collagen and hyaluronan molecules by the proposed free radical mechanism(s).

Biochemical studies support the rheologic observations. Total vitreous collagen content does not change after 20–30 years of age. However, in studies of a large series of normal human eyes obtained at autopsy, the collagen concentration in the gel vitreous at 70–90 years of age (approximately 0.1mg/ml) was greater than at 15–20 years of age (approximately 0.05mg/ml).[45] Because the total collagen content does not change, this finding most likely reflects the decrease in the volume of gel vitreous that occurs with aging and consequent increase in the concentration of the collagen that remains in the gel. The collagen fibrils in this gel become packed into bundles of parallel fibrils,[3,4,36,46] perhaps with cross-links between them. Abnormal collagen cross-links have been identified in the vitreous body of humans who have diabetes,[41] and the findings are consistent with "precocious senescence" of vitreous collagen, a phenomenon that has been described for other organs and tissue in diabetes.[19]

The structural changes that derive from the aforementioned biochemical and rheologic changes consist of a transition from

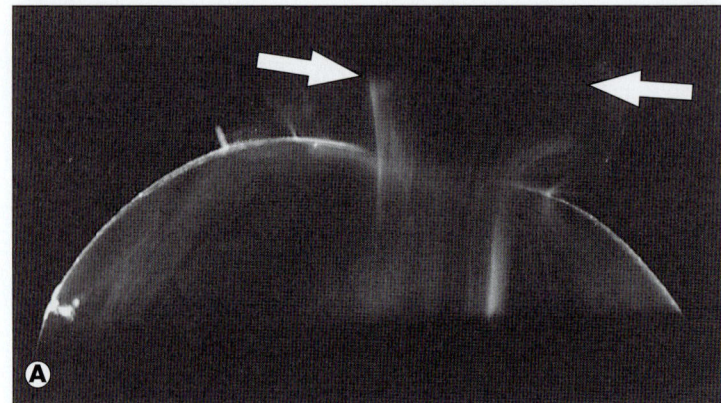

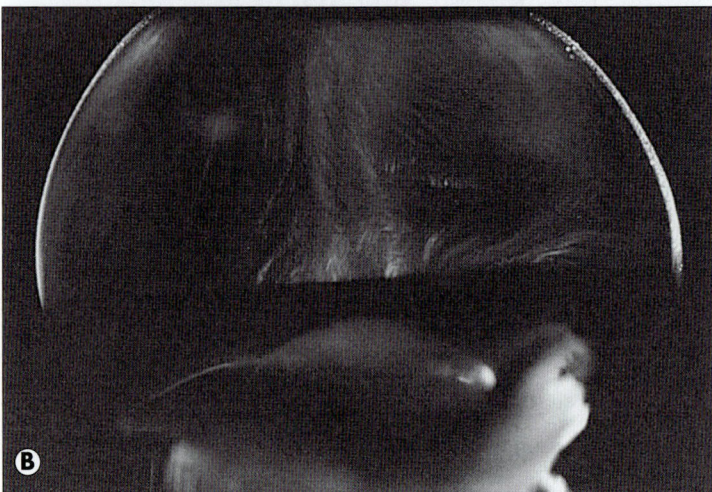

FIG. 144-8 ▌▌ **Vitreous structure in childhood. A,** The posterior and central vitreous in a 4-year-old child has a dense vitreous cortex with hyalocytes. A substantial amount of vitreous extrudes into the retrocortical (preretinal) space through the premacular vitreous cortex. However, no fibers are present in the vitreous. **B,** Central vitreous structure in an 11-year-old child has hyalocytes in a dense vitreous cortex *(arrows)*. No fibers are seen within the vitreous.

a clear vitreous in youth (Fig. 144-8), the consequence of a homogeneous distribution of collagen and hyaluronan, to a fibrous structure in the adult (see Fig. 144-4), which results from aggregation of collagen fibrils. In old age advanced liquefaction (see Fig. 144-5) occurs with ultimate collapse of the vitreous body and posterior vitreous detachment (PVD).

The vitreous base posterior to the ora increases in size with increasing age to nearly 3.0mm, to bring the posterior border of the vitreous base closer to the equator.[50] This widening of the vitreous base was found to be most prominent in the temporal portion of the globe. The posterior migration of the vitreous base probably plays an important role in the pathogenesis of peripheral retinal breaks and rhegmatogenous retinal detachment. Within the vitreous base, a "lateral aggregation" of the collagen fibrils is present in older individuals,[51] similar to aging changes within the central vitreous.[36] Recent studies[52] have confirmed posterior migration of the posterior border of the vitreous base during aging. There is also intraretinal synthesis of collagen fibrils that penetrate the internal limiting of the retina and "splice" with vitreous collagen fibrils. These aging changes at the vitreous base could contribute to increased traction on the peripheral retina and to the development of retinal tears and detachment.

Posterior Vitreous Detachment (PVD)

The most common age-related event in the vitreous is PVD.[53] True PVD can be defined as a separation between the posterior vitreous cortex and the internal limiting lamina of the retina; PVD can be localized, partial, or total (up to the posterior border of the vitreous base). Autopsy studies reveal that the incidence of PVD is 63% by the eighth decade,[54] and it is more common in myopic eyes, in which it occurs on average 10 years earlier than in emmetropic and hyperopic eyes. Cataract extraction in myopic patients introduces additional effects, which caused PVD to develop in all but 1 of 103 myopic (greater than −6D) eyes.[4]

Rheologic changes within the vitreous produce liquefaction, which, in conjunction with weakening of the vitreous cortex–internal limiting laminar adhesion, results in PVD. It is likely that dissolution of the posterior vitreous cortex–internal limiting laminar adhesion at the posterior pole allows liquid vitreous to enter the retrocortical space via the prepapillary hole and perhaps also the premacular vitreous cortex. With rotational eye movements, liquid vitreous can dissect a plane between the vitreous cortex and the internal limiting lamina, which results in true PVD. This volume displacement from the central vitreous to the preretinal space causes the observed collapse of the vitreous body (syneresis). Glare may be induced by PVD because of light scattering by the dense collagen fibril network in the posterior vitreous cortex.

"Floaters" are the most common complaint of patients who have PVD. These usually result from entoptic phenomena caused by condensed vitreous fibers, glial tissue of epipapillary origin (which adheres to the posterior vitreous cortex), and/or intravitreal blood. Floaters move with vitreous displacement during eye movement and scatter incident light, which casts a shadow on the retina that is perceived as a gray, "hair-like" or "fly-like" structure. In 1935, Moore[55] described "light flashes" as a common complaint that results from PVD. Wise[56] noted that light flashes occurred in 50% of cases at the time of PVD; they were usually vertical and temporally located. Voerhoeff[57] suggested that the light flashes result from the impact of the detached vitreous cortex upon the retina during eye movement.

Anomalous Posterior Vitreous Detachment

In addition to the symptoms already described, various untoward effects of PVD can develop if the aforementioned sequence of events occur in an anomalous manner. These anomalies can be grouped into two categories: disruption of retinal tissue and disruption of vitreous.

RETINAL DISRUPTION. Vitreous traction upon retinal structures can induce damage to various tissues; the resultant pathology depends upon the type of tissue involved. Lindner[58] found that minimal vitreous hemorrhage occurred in 13–19% of cases with PVD. This finding is generally considered to be an important risk factor for the presence of a retinal tear. Retinal tears result from lesions with firm vitreoretinal adhesion, such as lattice degeneration and rosettes, as well as in areas of the peripheral fundus with no obvious lesions.

VITREOUS DISRUPTION. A relatively unrecognized form of vitreoretinal separation that can mimic true PVD is called vitreoschisis. It features forward displacement of the anterior portion of the posterior vitreous cortex to leave part or all of the posterior layer of the vitreous cortex still attached to the retina. Vitreoschisis occurs in proliferative diabetic retinopathy[59] and may play an important role in its pathophysiology.[23] Cases of macular pucker and macular holes may also result from persistent attachment of part or all of the posterior vitreous cortex to the macula while the more anterior and central vitreous detaches forward.

METABOLIC DISORDERS OF VITREOUS

Diabetic Vitreopathy

In humans who have diabetes, there is an increase in vitreous glucose levels.[60] These elevated levels of glucose are associated with increased nonenzymatic glycation products in human vitreous collagen and elevated levels of the enzyme-mediated cross-link dihydroxylysinonorleucine.[23] Also, considerable diabetic effects may involve hyaluronan. In the daily management

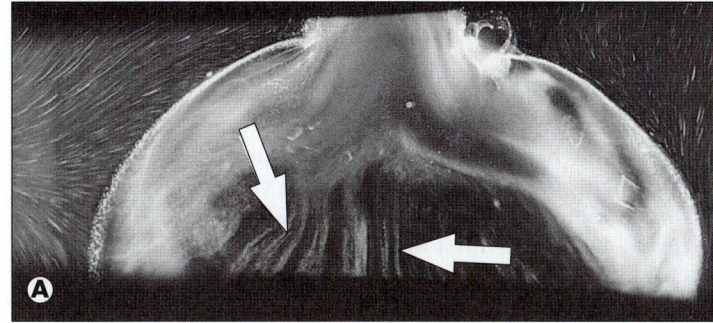
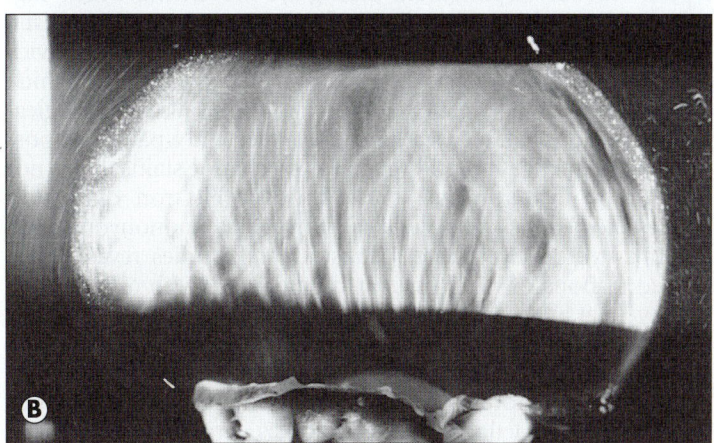

FIG. 144-9 ■ Diabetic vitreopathy. A, Right eye of a 9-year-old girl who has a 5-year history of type I diabetes shows extrusion of central vitreous through the posterior vitreous cortex into the retrocortical (preretinal) space. The subcortical vitreous appears very dense and scatters light intensely. Centrally, there are vitreous fibers *(arrows)* with an anteroposterior orientation and adjacent areas of liquefaction. B, Central vitreous in the left eye of the same patient shows prominent fibers that resemble those seen in nondiabetic adults (see Fig. 144-5). (Reprinted with permission from Sebag J. Abnormalities of human vitreous structure in diabetes. Graefes Arch Clin Exp Ophthalmol. 1993;231:257–60.)

of diabetes, significant fluctuations in the systemic concentrations of a variety of molecules may occur, which can alter the ionic milieu of the vitreous body. Shifts in systemic metabolism, and in turn osmolarity and hydration of the vitreous body, could result in periodic swelling and contraction of the entire vitreous body, with consequent traction upon structures attached to the posterior vitreous cortex, such as new blood vessels that have grown out of the optic disc and/or retina.[61] These events could influence the course of diabetic retinopathy as they may contribute to the proliferation of neovascular frond and perhaps even induce rupture of the new vessels and cause vitreous hemorrhage.

Such molecular effects of diabetes result in morphological changes within the vitreous body,[62] which represent precocious senescence in the vitreous structure (Fig. 144-9). The roles of these and other pathological changes, such as posterior vitreoschisis,[23] are being investigated at present. It is hoped that the future will see therapy designed to inhibit diabetic vitreopathy. Alternatively, the induction of innocuous PVD early in the course of diabetic retinopathy may have long-term salubrious effects in patients at great risk.

Synchysis Scintillans

This condition features vitreous opacification as a consequence of chronic vitreous hemorrhage. These vitreous opacities are noted when frank hemorrhage is no longer present. They appear as flat, refractile bodies, golden brown in color, and are freely mobile. Associated with liquid vitreous, they settle to the most dependent portion of the vitreous body when eye movement stops. The vitreous about these opacities is degenerated so that collagen is displaced peripherally. Chemical studies demonstrate the presence of cholesterol crystals in these opacities, and the condition is sometimes referred to as "cholesterolosis bulbi."[63] Free hemoglobin spherules can occur within the vitreous body.[64]

Asteroid Hyalosis

This generally benign condition is characterized by small yellow-white spherical opacities throughout the vitreous. The prevalence of this condition in the general population is 0.042–0.5%, and it affects all races but with a male-to-female ratio of 2:1. Curiously, asteroid hyalosis is unilateral in over 75% of cases. Asteroid bodies are associated intimately with the vitreous gel and move with typical vitreous displacement during eye movement, which suggests a relationship with collagen fibril degeneration.[65] However, PVD, either complete or partial, occurs less frequently in individuals with asteroid hyalosis than in age-matched controls,[66] which does not support age-related degeneration as a cause. Histological studies demonstrate a crystalline appearance and a pattern of positive staining to fat and acid mucopolysaccharide stains that is not affected by hyaluronidase pretreatment.[57] Electron diffraction studies showed the presence of calcium oxalate monohydrate and calcium hydroxyphosphate. Ultrastructural studies reveal intertwined ribbons of multilaminar membranes (with a 6nm periodicity) that are characteristic of complex lipids, especially phospholipids, that lie in a homogeneous background matrix.[67] In these investigations, energy-dispersive X-ray analysis showed calcium and phosphorus to be the main elements in asteroid bodies. Electron diffraction structural analysis demonstrated calcium hydroxyapatite and possibly other forms of calcium phosphate crystals.

Reports exist that suggest an association between asteroid hyalosis and diabetes mellitus.[68,69] Other investigators dispute such an association.[70] Asteroid hyalosis appears to be associated with certain pigmentary retinal degenerations,[71] although it is not known whether this is related to the presence of diabetes in these patients. Yu and Blumenthal[72] proposed that asteroid hyalosis results from aging collagen, whereas other studies[73] suggested that asteroid formation is preceded by depolymerization of hyaluronan.

Amyloidosis

Amyloidosis can result in the deposition of opacities in the vitreous of one or both eyes. Bilateral involvement can be an early manifestation of the dominant form of familial amyloidosis, although rare cases of vitreous involvement in nonfamilial forms have been reported. The opacities first appear in the vitreous adjacent to retinal blood vessels and later appear in the anterior vitreous. Initially, the opacities are granular with wispy fringes and later take on a "glass wool" appearance. When the opacities form strands, they appear to attach to the retina and the posterior aspect of the lens by thick footplates.[66] Following PVD, the posterior vitreous cortex is observed to have thick, linear opacities that follow the course of the retinal vessels. The opacities seem to aggregate by "seeding" on vitreous fibrils and along the posterior vitreous cortex.[66]

Histopathological specimens contain star-like structures with dense, fibrillar centers. The amyloid fibrils are 5–10nm in diameter and are differentiated from the 10–15nm vitreous fibrils by stains for amyloid and by the fact that the vitreous fibrils are very straight and long.[66] Electron microscopy can confirm the presence of amyloid, and immunocytochemical studies identified the major amyloid constituent as a protein that resembles prealbumin.[74] Streeten[67] proposed that hyalocytes could perform the role of macrophage processing of the amyloid protein before its polymerization. This may further explain why the opacities initially appear at the posterior vitreous cortex where hyalocytes reside.

REFERENCES

1. Eisner G. Biomicroscopy of the peripheral fundus. New York: Springer-Verlag; 1973.
2. Worst JGF. Cisternal systems of the fully developed vitreous body in the young adult. Trans Ophthalmol Soc UK. 1977;97:550–4.
3. Sebag J, Balazs EA. Morphology and ultrastructure of human vitreous fibers. Invest Ophthalmol Vis Sci. 1989;30:187–91.
4. Sebag J. The vitreous—structure, function, and pathobiology. New York: Springer-Verlag; 1989.
5. Kishi S, Shimizu K. Posterior precortical vitreous pocket. Arch Ophthalmol. 1990;108:979–82.
6. Sebag J. Letter to the editor. Arch Ophthalmol. 1991;109:1059–60.
7. Kakehashi A. Age-related changes in the premacular vitreous cortex. Invest Ophthalmol Vis Sci. 1996;37:2253.
8. Seery CM, Davison PF. Collagens of the bovine vitreous. Invest Ophthalmol Vis Sci. 1990;32:1540–50.
9. Bishop PN, Crossman MV, McLeod D. Extraction and characterization of the tissue forms of collagens type II and IX from bovine vitreous. Biochem J. 1994;299:497–505.
10. Bishop PN, Reardon AJ, McLeod D, Ayad S. Identification of alternatively spliced variants of type II procollagen in vitreous. Biochem Biophys Res Commun. 1994;203:289–95.
11. Reardon A, Sandell L, Jones CJP, et al. Localization of pN-type IIA procollagen on adult bovine vitreous collagen fibrils. Matrix Biol. 2000;19:169–73.
12. Zhu Y, Oganesian A, Keene DR, Sandell LJ. Type IIA procollagen containing the cysteine-rich amino propeptide is deposited in the extracellular matrix of prechondrogenic tissue and binds to TGFbeta-1 and BMP-2. J Cell Biol. 1999;144:1069–80.
13. Brewton RG, Ouspenskaia MV, Van der Rest M, Mayne R. Cloning of the chicken alpha 3 (IX) collagen chain completes the primary structure of type IX collagen. Eur J Biochem. 1992;205:443–9.
14. Scott JE. The chemical morphology of the vitreous. Eye. 1992;6:553–5.
15. Zhidkova NI, Justice S, Mayne R. Alternative in RNA processing occurs in the variable region of the pro-peptide. J Biol Chem. 1995;270:9485–93.
16. Bishop PN. Structural macromolecules and supramolecular organization of the vitreous gel. Prog Retinal Eye Res. 2000;19:323–44.
17. Balazs EA. The vitreous. In: Davson H, ed. The eye, Vol la. London: Academic Press; 1984:533–89.
18. Swann DA. Chemistry and biology of the vitreous. Int Rev Exp Pathol. 1980;22:1–63.
19. Sheehan JK, Atkins EDT, Nieduszynski IA. X-ray diffraction studies on the connective tissue polysaccharides. Two dimensional packing scheme for threefold hyaluronic chains. J Mol Biol. 1975;91:153–63.
20. Chakrabarti B, Park JW. Glycosaminoglycans. Structure and interaction. CRC Crit Rev Biochem. 1980;8:225–313.
21. Brewton RG, Mayne R. Mammalian vitreous humor contains networks of hyaluronan molecules. Exp Eye Res. 1992;198:237–49.
22. Comper WD, Laurent TC. Physiological function of connective tissue polysaccharides. Physiol Rev. 1978;58:255–315.
23. Sebag J. Diabetic vitreopathy. Ophthalmology. 1996;103:205–6.
24. Ogston AG, Phelps CF. The partition of solutes between buffer solutions and solutions containing hyaluronic acid. Biochem J. 1961;78:827–33.
25. Reardon A, Heinegard D, McLeod D, et al. The large chondroitin sulphate proteoglycans versican in mammalian vitreous. Matrix Biol. 1998;17:325–33.
26. Reardon AJ, LeGoff M, Briggs MD, et al. Identification in vitreous and molecular cloning of opticin, a novel member of the family of leucine-rich repeat proteins of the extracellular matrix. J Biol Chem. 2000;275:2123–9.
27. Mayne R, Ren Z-X, Liu J, et al. VIT1—the second member of a new branch of the von Willebrand A domain superfamily. Biochem Soc Trans. 1999;27:832–5.
28. Laicine EM, Haddad A. Transferrin, one of the major vitreous proteins, is produced within the eye. Exp Eye Res. 1994;59:441–5.
29. Brown D, Hamdi H, Bahri S, Kenney MC. Characterization of an endogenous metalloproteinase in human vitreous. Curr Eye Res. 1994;13:639–47.
30. Ueno N, Sebag J, Hirokawa H, Chakrabarti B. Effects of visible light irradiation on vitreous structure in the presence of a photosensitizer. Exp Eye Res. 1987;44:863–70.
31. Mayne R. The eye. In: Connective tissue and its heritable disorders. New York: Wiley-Liss; 2001:131–41.
32. Tokita M, Fujiya Y, Hikichi K. Dynamic viscoelasticity of bovine vitreous body. Biorheology. 1984;21:751–65.
33. Asakura A. Histochemistry of hyaluronic acid of the bovine vitreous body as studied by electron microscopy. Acta Soc Ophthalmol Jpn. 1985;89:179–91.
34. Hardingham TE. The role of link-protein in the structure of cartilage-proteoglycan aggregates. Biochem J. 1979;177:237–47.
35. Schepens CL, Neetens A, eds. The vitreous and vitreoretinal interface. New York: Springer-Verlag; 1987:20.
36. Sebag J. Age-related changes in human vitreous structure. Graefes Arch Clin Exp Ophthalmol. 1987;225:89–93.
37. Sebag J. Surgical anatomy of vitreous and the vitreo-retinal interface. In: Tasman W, Jaeger E, eds. Clinical ophthalmology, Vol 6. Philadelphia: JB Lippincott; 1994:Ch 51;1–36.
38. Sebag J. Age-related differences in the human vitreo-retinal interface. Arch Ophthalmol. 1991;109:966–71.
39. Sebag J. Anatomy and pathology of the vitreo-retinal interface. Eye. 1992;6:541–52.
40. Gass JDM. Reappraisal of biomicroscopic classification of stages of development of a macular hole. Am J Ophthalmol. 1995;119:752–9.
41. Newsome DA, Linsemayer TF, Trelstad RJ. Vitreous body collagen. Evidence for a dual origin from the neural retina and hyalocytes. J Cell Biol. 1976;71:59–67.
42. Heergaard S, Jensen OA, Prause JU. Structure of the vitreal face of the monkey optic disc. Graefes Arch Clin Exp Ophthalmol. 1988;226:377–83.
43. Lutty GA, Mello RF, Chandler C, et al. Regulation of cell growth by vitreous humor. J Cell Sci. 1985;76:53–65.
44. Snead MP, Yates JRW. Clinical and molecular genetics of Stickler syndrome. J Med Genet. 1999;36:353–9.
45. Balazs EA, Denlinger JL. Aging changes in the vitreous. In: Aging and human visual function. New York: Alan R Liss; 1982:45–57.
46. Sebag J. Ageing of the vitreous. Eye. 1987;1:254–62.
47. Aguayo J, Glaser BM, Mildvan A, et al. Study of vitreous liquefaction by NMR spectroscopy and imaging. Invest Ophthalmol Vis Sci. 1985;26:692–7.

48. Hageman G, Russel S. Chondroitinase-mediated disinsertion of the primate vitreous body. Invest Ophthalmol Vis Sci. 1994;35:1260.

49. Verstraeten TC, Chapman C, Hartzer M, et al. Pharmacologic induction of posterior vitreous detachment in the rabbit. Arch Ophthalmol. 1993;111:849–54.

50. Teng CC, Chi HH. Vitreous changes and the mechanism of retinal detachment. Am J Ophthalmol. 1957;44:335.

51. Gartner J. Electron microscopic study on the fibrillar network and fibrocyte-collagen interactions in the vitreous cortex at the ora serrata of human eyes with special regard to the role of disintegrating cells. Exp Eye Res. 1986;42:21–33.

52. Wang J, McLeod D, Henson DB, Bishop PN. Age-dependent changes in the basal retinovitreous adhesion. Invest Ophthalmol Vis Sci. 2003;44(5):1793–800.

53. Sebag J. Classifying posterior vitreous detachment—a new way to look at the invisible. Br J Ophthalmol. 1997;81:521.

54. Foos RY. Posterior vitreous detachment. Trans Am Acad Ophthalmol Otolaryngol. 1974;76:480–96.

55. Moore RF. Subjective 'lightening streak.' Br J Ophthalmol. 1935:545–50.

56. Wise GN. Relationship of idiopathic preretinal macular fibrosis to posterior vitreous detachment. Am J Ophthalmol. 1975;79:358–61.

57. Voerhoeff FH. Are Moore's lightening streaks of serious portent? Am J Ophthalmol. 1956;41:837–41.

58. Lindner B. Acute posterior vitreous detachment and its retinal complications. Acta Ophthalmol. 1966;87(Suppl):1–108.

59. Chu T, Lopez PF, Cano MR, et al. Posterior vitreoschisis. An echographic finding in proliferative diabetic retinopathy. Ophthalmology. 1996;103:315–22.

60. Lundquist O, Osterlin S. Glucose concentration in the vitreous of nondiabetic and diabetic human eyes. Graefes Arch Clin Exp Ophthalmol. 1995;232:71–4.

61. Faulborn J, Bowald S. Microproliferations in proliferative diabetic retinopathy and their relation to the vitreous. Graefes Arch Clin Exp Ophthalmol. 1985;223:130–8.

62. Sebag J. Abnormalities of human vitreous structure in diabetes. Graefes Arch Clin Exp Ophthalmol. 1993;231:257–60.

63. Andrews JS, Lynn C, Scobey JW, Elliot JH. Cholesterolosis bulbi—case report with modern chemical identification of the ubiquitous crystals. Br J Ophthalmol. 1973;57:838–44.

64. Grossniklaus HE, Frank KE, Farbi DC, et al. Hemoglobin spherulosis in the vitreous cavity. Arch Ophthalmol. 1988;106:961–2.

65. Rodman HI, Johnson FB, Zimmerman LE. New histopathological and histochemical observations concerning asteroid hyalitis. Arch Ophthalmol. 1961;66:552–63.

66. Wasano T, Hirokuwa H, Tagawa H, et al. Asteroid hyalosis—posterior vitreous detachment and diabetic retinopathy. Am J Ophthalmol. 1987;19:255–8.

67. Streeten BA. Disorders of the vitreous. In: Garner A, Klintworth GK, eds. Pathobiology of ocular disease—a dynamic approach, Part B. New York: Marcel Dekker; 1982:1381–419.

68. Smith JL. Asteroid hyalitis—incidence of diabetes mellitus and hypercholesterolemia. JAMA. 1958;168:891–3.

69. Bergren RC, Brown GC, Duker JS. Prevalence and association of asteroid hyalosis with systemic disease. Am J Ophthalmol. 1991;111:289–93.

70. Hatfield RE, Gastineau CF, Rucke CW. Asteroid bodies in the vitreous—relationship to diabetes and hypercholesterolemia. Mayo Clin Proc. 1962;37:513–14.

71. Sebag J, Albert DM, Craft JL. The Alström syndrome—ocular histopathology and retinal ultrastructure. Br J Ophthalmol. 1984;68:494–501.

72. Yu SY, Blumenthal HT. The calcification of elastic tissue. In: Wagner BM, Smith DE, eds. The connective tissue. Baltimore: Williams & Wilkins; 1967:17–49.

73. Lamba PA, Shukla KM. Experimental asteroid hyalopathy. Br J Ophthalmol. 1971;55:279–83.

74. Doft BH, Rubinow A, Cohen AS. Immunocytochemical demonstration of prealbumin in the vitreous in heredofamilial amyloidosis. Am J Ophthalmol. 1984;97:296–300.

145 Persistent Fetal Vasculature Syndrome

A. BAWA DASS • MICHAEL T. TRESE

DEFINITION
- A developmental ocular anomaly in which the primary vitreous and hyaloid vasculature fail to involute completely.

KEY FEATURES
- Leukokoria.
- Cataract.
- Microphthalmia.
- Retrolenticular fibrovascular tissue.
- Elongated ciliary processes.
- Usually unilateral.

ASSOCIATED FEATURES
- Late-onset angle-closure glaucoma.
- Intraocular hemorrhage.
- Optic nerve hypoplasia.
- Retinal detachment.
- Amblyopia.

INTRODUCTION

Persistent fetal vascular syndrome (PFV) is an uncommon congenital ocular anomaly in which the hyaloid vasculature system and primary vitreous fail to involute. This was initially described in detail by Reese[1] in his 1955 Jackson Memorial Lecture, at which time it was described as persistent hyperplastic primary vitreous (PHPV). Although the visual outcomes historically have been poor, advances in clinical evaluation and surgical technique have resulted in more frequent preservation of the affected eyes and vision.

EPIDEMIOLOGY AND PATHOGENESIS

PFV appears sporadically in the vast majority of cases. One report exists of possible vertical transmission with both a mother and son affected, which suggests autosomal dominant inheritance.[2] In two other reports, autosomal recessive inheritance was suggested; these included one case of fraternal twins, both of whom had PFV.[3,4]

Although no definite risk factors or confirmed systemic associations occur, maternal cocaine use during pregnancy of affected newborns has been reported.[5,6] Rarely, PFV occurs in conjunction with other ocular or systemic abnormalities, for example, microcephaly, mental retardation, spasticity, cleft palate, and short stature in the oculopalatocerebral dwarfism syndrome.[7] One case of PFV associated with bilateral megalocornea[8] and another with optic nerve coloboma[9] have been noted. No sex predilection occurs.

The cause of PFV remains obscure. During ocular development, the primary vitreous fills the vitreous cavity as a fibrillar meshwork of mesenchymal tissue and serves as structural support for the hyaloid vasculature. The hyaloid vessels emerge

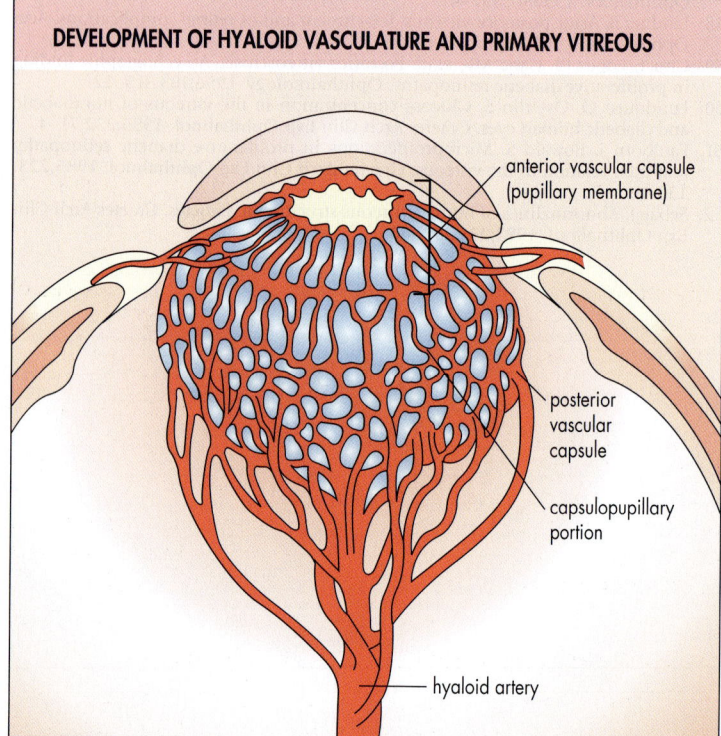

DEVELOPMENT OF HYALOID VASCULATURE AND PRIMARY VITREOUS

anterior vascular capsule (pupillary membrane)

posterior vascular capsule

capsulopupillary portion

hyaloid artery

FIG. 145-1 ▮▮ Hyaloid vasculature and primary vitreous during embryologic ocular development.

from the optic nerve and course anteriorly to nourish the developing lens and anterior segment structures (Fig. 145-1). The hyaloid vessels and primary vitreous normally begin to involute in the second month of gestation, giving way to the secondary vitreous. If this regression does not occur completely, subsequent contraction and opacification of the primary vitreous along the hyaloid vascular system lead to the clinical presentation of PFV. This mechanism of maldevelopment has led to the term to describe this disease coined by Goldberg,[10] persistent fetal vasculature syndrome. The specific insults that prevent regression of the primary vitreous remain unknown.

OCULAR MANIFESTATIONS

Failure of regression of the primary vitreous and hyaloid vasculature can result in a broad spectrum of findings.[11] Pupillary strands and a Mittendorf's dot represent the mildest manifestations and leukokoria with a dense retrolenticular membrane and/or retinal detachment the most severe. Depending on which intraocular structures are involved, the designation of anterior PFV, posterior PFV, or both can be assigned.

Anterior PFV consists of retrolenticular fibrovascular tissue that attaches to the ciliary processes and draws them centrally (Fig. 145-2). Often, the elongated ciliary processes are visible readily through the dilated pupil. As the fibrous tissue contracts and remodels, cataract formation, shallowing of the anterior

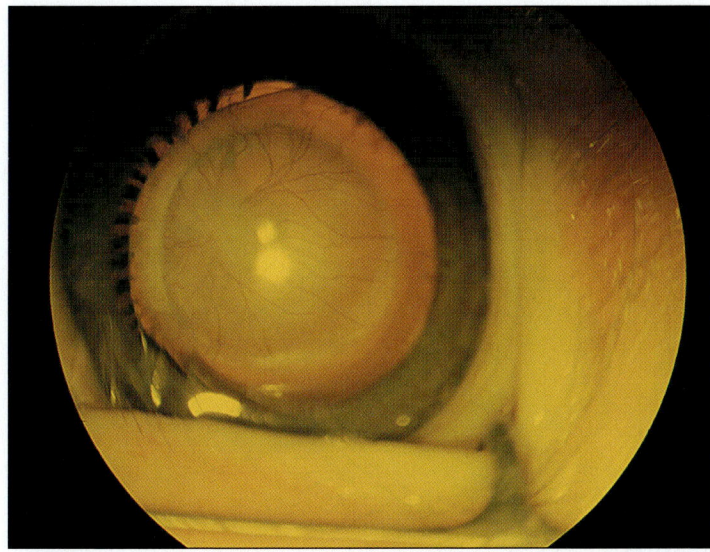

FIG. 145-2 ■ **Typical appearance of persistent fetal vasculature syndrome.** An opacified retrolenticular fibrovascular membrane is attached to drawn-in ciliary processes.

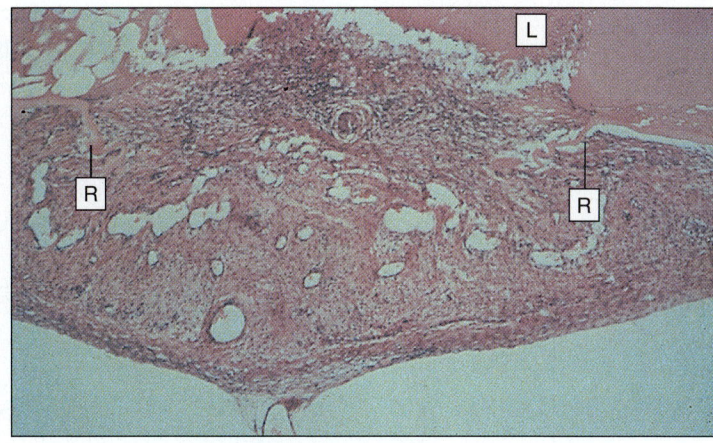

FIG. 145-3 ■ **Persistent fetal vasculature.** Abundant mesenchymal fibrovascular tissue can be seen just behind and within the posterior lens *(L)*. Note the ends of the ruptured lens capsule *(R)*. A persistent hyaloid vessel. (From Caudill JW, Streeten BW, Tso MO: Ophthalmology. 1985;92:1153.)

chamber, and angle-closure glaucoma may develop. Iris vessel engorgement and recurrent intraocular hemorrhage can occur, which result in pain and possibly eventual phthisis bulbi. Microphthalmia is a prominent finding.

Posterior PFV consists of a prominent vitreous fibrovascular stalk that emanates from the optic nerve and courses anteriorly. Preretinal membranes at the base of the stalk are common. Tractional retinal folds and traction retinal detachment may be present. Retinal dysplasia and optic nerve hypoplasia have also been described. Various degrees of microphthalmia and leukokoria may occur in both anterior and posterior PFV.[12]

DIAGNOSIS AND ANCILLARY TESTING

The diagnosis of PFV is frequently a clinical one. The young age at which affected patients are usually diagnosed means that an examination under anesthesia to confirm the diagnosis and to examine the fellow eye is often indicated. When the full constellation of clinical findings is present unilaterally, the diagnosis is usually straightforward. True cases of bilaterality have rarely arisen. It is in these cases of bilaterality, as well as in those that have atypical clinical presentations, that further history and ancillary testing may be beneficial. Positive family history, complicated birth history, and bilaterality, as seen in retinoblastoma, Norrie's disease, and retinopathy of prematurity, are usually absent in PFV. Computed tomographic scanning can be used to evaluate the presence of intraocular calcification, which is seen frequently in retinoblastoma but not in PFV. Conversely, microphthalmia is a consistent feature of PFV but not most other causes of leukokoria. Bilateral axial length measurements with ultrasonography, therefore, are helpful. In addition, B-scan ultrasonography and computed tomographic scanning can be used to determine the extent of posterior segment involvement, namely retinal detachment, when not visible on examination.

DIFFERENTIAL DIAGNOSIS

The differential diagnosis of PFV is shown in Box 145-1. The differential diagnosis of PFV includes the differential diagnosis of leukokoria. It is most important to exclude the diagnosis of retinoblastoma. Although retinoblastoma is usually seen in an average-size eye and PFV in a smaller eye, the diagnosis of retinoblastoma must be carefully ruled out. Bilaterality of leukokoria is also a possible point of confusion for retinoblastoma, Norrie's disease, retinopathy of prematurity, and other

---

BOX 145-1

Differential Diagnosis of Persistent Fetal Vasculature Syndrome

Retinoblastoma
Retinopathy of prematurity
Coats' disease
Toxocariasis
Norrie's disease
Familial exudative vitreoretinopathy
Congenital cataract
Uveitis
Incontinentia pigmenti

---

causes of leukokoria. Coats' disease and PFV tend to be unilateral, but bilateral PFV certainly does occur. Once the diagnosis of PFV has been established, therapeutic considerations can proceed.

PATHOLOGY

The histopathology of PFV illustrates the preceding clinical findings (Fig. 145-3). The primary vitreous is a plaque of numerous spindle cells in a collagen matrix. Fragile blood vessels are supplied by a patent hyaloid artery. The plaque is attached to drawn-in ciliary processes. Cataract formation may occur should a defect be present in the adjacent posterior capsule.

TREATMENT

Controversy exists as to which patients should undergo surgery, especially because visual results are often poor and the fellow eye is usually normal. However, the natural course of severe anterior PFV typically culminates in angle-closure glaucoma and intraocular hemorrhage, seen most frequently in the first 3 years of life, often occurring suddenly. Consequently, many have advocated early surgical intervention to preserve the globe.[1,13,14]

When treatment for anterior PFV is considered, surgical intervention should be performed as soon as possible to shorten the duration of deprivational amblyopia. Reese[1] originally described a two-stage procedure, which consisted of needling the lens and a later dissection of the retrolental membrane. With the advent of vitreous cutting instruments and fine intraocular forceps, a closed system, single-stage procedure has become the standard of care (Fig. 145-4).[13-16] Posterior segment abnormalities can also be addressed with this instrumentation. The cataract and

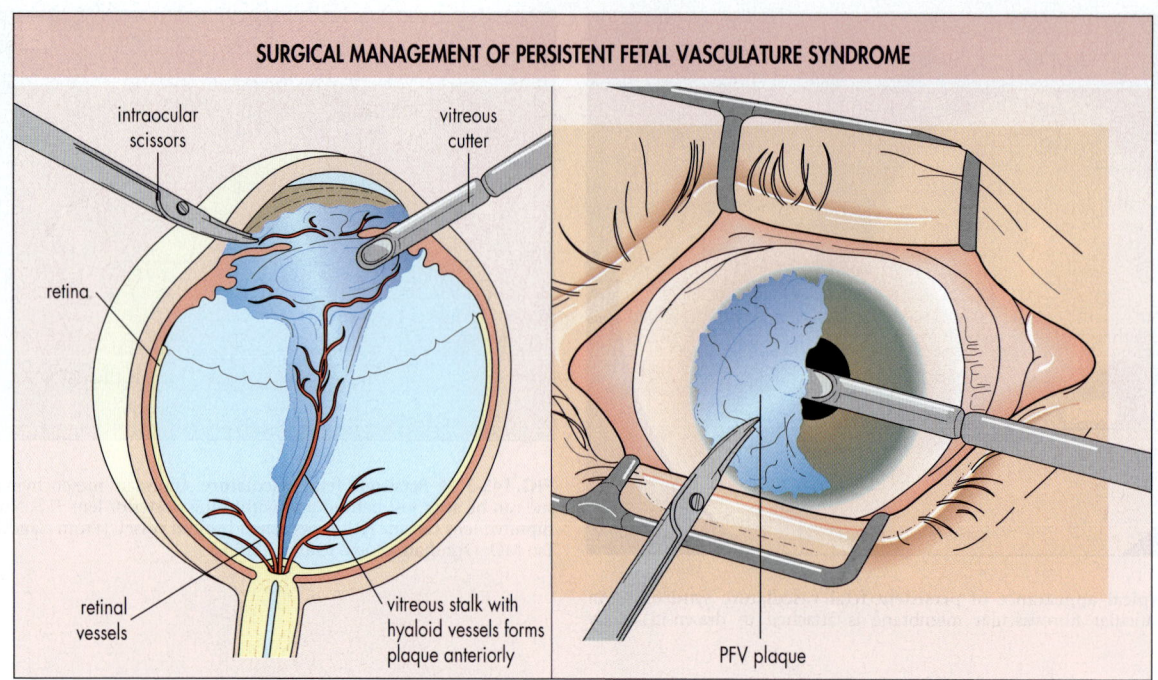

SURGICAL MANAGEMENT OF PERSISTENT FETAL VASCULATURE SYNDROME

intraocular scissors

vitreous cutter

retina

retinal vessels

vitreous stalk with hyaloid vessels forms plaque anteriorly

PFV plaque

FIG. 145-4 ■ **Surgical management of persistent fetal vasculature syndrome (PFV).** Vitreous cutting instruments are used to remove carefully lens and retrolenticular material. Anterior incisions at the limbus or pars plicata are often used to avoid the vitreous base and peripheral retina, which may be present anteriorly in PFV.

retrolental tissue can be reached by either a limbal or a pars plicata approach. The posterior approach is potentially hazardous if the peripheral retina is pulled up into the ciliary processes. Aggressive postoperative amblyopia therapy is critical.[14]

Surgery for severe isolated posterior PFV is rarely undertaken. Although the fibrovascular tissue can be dissected and the accompanying retinal detachment may reapproximate to the retinal pigment epithelium, visual outcomes are quite poor. This is a result of the associated retinal detachment, retinal dysplasia, and, most critically, the normal fellow eye causing dense amblyopia.

COURSE AND OUTCOME

Visual results after treatment for PFV are generally poor, with affected eyes frequently manifesting hand motion or light perception vision only. The early two-stage approaches rarely achieved vision of 20/400 (6/121) or better.[1] With modern surgical techniques, outcomes of 20/40 (6/12) to 20/200 (6/60), although uncommon, are possible. Posterior segment involvement is a poor prognostic sign for ambulatory vision.[1,13,14,16] However, visual acuities of 20/60 (3/18) to 20/800 (6/266) in some eyes that have posterior PFV have been reported.[6] This review again supported aggressive amblyopia therapy as being critical to successful visual outcomes but noted that final vision is limited eventually by the degree of maldevelopment.

REFERENCES

1. Reese AB. Persistent hyperplastic primary vitreous. Am J Ophthalmol. 1955; 30:317–31.
2. Lin AE, Biglan AW, Garver KL. Persistent hyperplastic primary vitreous with vertical transmission. Ophthalmic Paediatr Genet. 1990;11:121–2.
3. Wang MK, Phillips CI. Persistent hyperplastic primary vitreous in non-identical twins. Acta Ophthalmol (Copenh). 1973;51:434–7.
4. Menchini U, Pece A, Alberti P, et al. Vitre primitif hypérplastique avec persistence de l'artère hyaloide, chez deux frères non jumeaux. J Fr Ophthalmol. 1987; 3:241–5.
5. Teske M, Trese MT. Retinopathy of prematurity-like fundus and persistent hyperplastic primary vitreous associated with maternal cocaine use. Am J Ophthalmol. 1987;103:719–20.
6. Dass AB, Trese MT. Surgical results of persistent hyperplastic primary vitreous. Presented at the 1995 annual meeting of the American Academy of Ophthalmology.
7. Frydman M, Kauschansky A, Leshem I, Savir H. Oculo-palato-cerebral dwarfism: a new syndrome. Clin Genet. 1985;27:414–19.
8. Burke JP, O'Keefe M. Megalocornea and persistent hyperplastic primary vitreous masquerading as congenital glaucoma. Acta Ophthalmol (Copenh). 1988;66:731–3.
9. Shami M, McCartney D, Benedict W, Barnes C. Spontaneous retinal reattachment in a patient with persistent hyperplastic primary vitreous and an optic nerve coloboma. Am J Ophthalmol. 1992;114:769–71.
10. Goldberg M. Persistent fetal vasculature syndrome (PFV): an integrated interpretation of signs and symptoms associated with persistent hyperplastic primary vitreous (PHPV). LIV Edward Jackson Memorial Lecture. Am J Ophthalmol. 1997;124:587–626.
11. Haddad R, Font RL, Reeser F. Persistent hyperplastic primary vitreous. A clinicopathologic study of 62 cases and review of the literature. Surv Ophthalmol. 1978;23:123–40.
12. Rubinstein K. Posterior hyperplastic primary vitreous. Br J Ophthalmol. 1980; 64:105–11.
13. Federman JL, Shields JA, Altman B, Koller H. The surgical and non-surgical management of persistent hyperplastic primary vitreous. Ophthalmology. 1982;89:20–4.
14. Karr DJ, Scott WE. Visual acuity results following treatment of persistent hyperplastic primary vitreous. Arch Ophthalmol. 1986;104:662–7.
15. Stark W, Lindsey P, Fagadau W, Michels R. Persistent hyperplastic primary vitreous, surgical treatment. Ophthalmology. 1983;90:452–7.
16. Pollard Z. Results of treatment of persistent hyperplastic primary vitreous. Ophthalmic Surg. 1991;22:48–52.

PART

9

INTRAOCULAR TUMORS

James J. Augsburger

SECTION 1 MALIGNANT INTRAOCULAR TUMORS

CHAPTER

146 Retinoblastoma

JAMES J. AUGSBURGER • NORBERT BORNFELD • MICHAEL E. GIBLIN

DEFINITION
- Primary malignant neoplasm of the retina that arises from immature retinal cells.

KEY FEATURES
- Affects infants and children.
- Leukokoria in one or both eyes.
- White retinal tumor fed and drained by dilated, tortuous retinal blood vessels.
- Well-established tendency to invade optic nerve and choroid, extend extrasclerally, invade the brain, and metastasize.
- Unilateral (60–70%) or bilateral (30–40%) ocular involvement; most unilateral cases are unifocal, and most bilateral cases are multifocal in both eyes.
- Germinal (heritable, 40%) and somatic (nonheritable, 60%) forms.
- Autosomal dominant inheritance pattern in germinal cases.
- Attributable to loss or inactivation of both alleles of retinoblastoma gene, a tumor suppressor gene on the long arm of chromosome 13.

ASSOCIATED FEATURES
- Seeding of viable tumor cells into vitreous or subretinal space.
- Neovascular glaucoma in infancy or childhood.
- Nonrhegmatogenous retinal detachment.
- Intralesional calcification detectable by ultrasonography and computed tomography in most cases.
- Second (nonretinoblastoma) malignancy in substantial proportion of survivors of germinal disease.

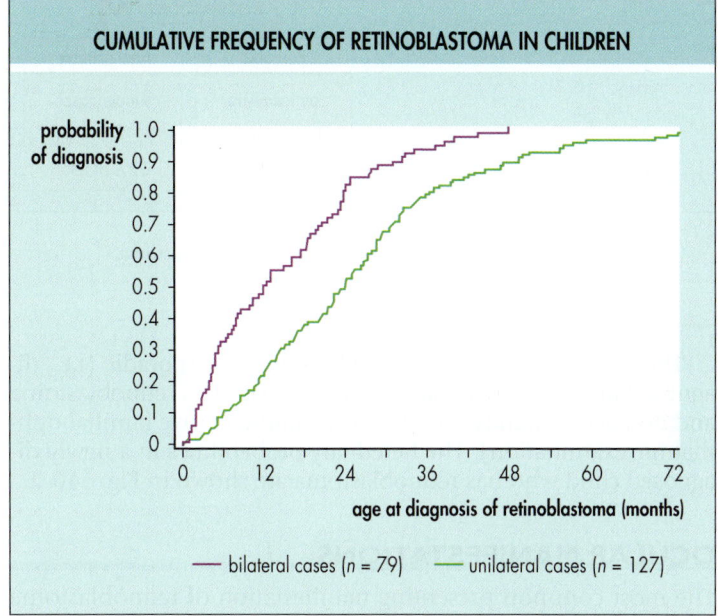

FIG. 146-1 ■ **Cumulative frequency of retinoblastoma diagnosis.** Frequency is shown as a function of age at diagnosis in subgroups of unilateral versus bilateral disease. The data from which these curves are derived come from the private practice of James J. Augsburger, M.D.

INTRODUCTION

Retinoblastoma is a primary malignant intraocular neoplasm that arises from immature retinoblasts within the developing retina. It is the most common primary intraocular malignancy of childhood in all racial groups. The neoplasm has strong tendencies to invade the brain via the optic nerve and to metastasize widely. Untreated children typically die of their disease within 2–4 years of the onset of symptoms.

EPIDEMIOLOGY AND PATHOGENESIS

Retinoblastoma has a cumulative lifetime incidence of approximately 1 in 15,000 individuals.[1] Its annual incidence is highest in the first few months of life; thereafter, the yearly incidence decreases steadily and is extremely low by 6 years of age. In spite of its early onset in most children, retinoblastoma is rarely diagnosed congenitally or even within the first 3 months of life, except in familial cases. The median age at the time of diagnosis is approximately 12 months in children who have bilateral retinoblastoma and 24 months in those who suffer unilateral disease (Fig. 146-1).[1] Retinoblastoma affects boys and girls with equal frequency and has no known racial predilection.

Approximately 60–70% of retinoblastoma cases are unilateral, and the remaining 30–40% are bilateral.[1] In unilateral cases, only a single tumor is usually present in the affected eye. In bilateral cases, multifocal tumors in both eyes are the rule. Retinoblastoma is generally a sporadic condition (i.e., no previously affected family members exist). Most children who have the sporadic form of retinoblastoma are affected unilaterally. A small number of patients have a prior family history of retinoblastoma, in which case one of the parents is probably a survivor of the disease. In hereditary cases, the affected child usually, but not always, has multiple tumors in both eyes. Transmission of the disease in such families follows genetic rules of autosomal dominant inheritance.[2]

Retinoblastoma appears to result from loss or inactivation of both normal alleles of the retinoblastoma gene,[2] a DNA sequence localized to a small segment of the long arm (the q14 region) of chromosome 13 (see Chapter 1). The timing of the loss or inactivation of the two normal alleles determines whether the disease is germinal (i.e., can be inherited by the offspring of an affected person) or somatic (i.e., cannot be inherited by the offspring of an affected person). In germinal retinoblastoma, at least one normal allele must be lost or inactivated prior to the first mitotic division of embryogenesis. This circumstance arises if the sperm or the egg contains defective DNA from an affected or carrier parent or develops that defect by means of spontaneous mutation prior to fertilization. In somatic retinoblastoma, both alleles are present and active beyond the stage of the fertilized egg, but one or more subsequent mutations occur to delete or inactivate both alleles in at least one immature retinal cell (retinoblast).

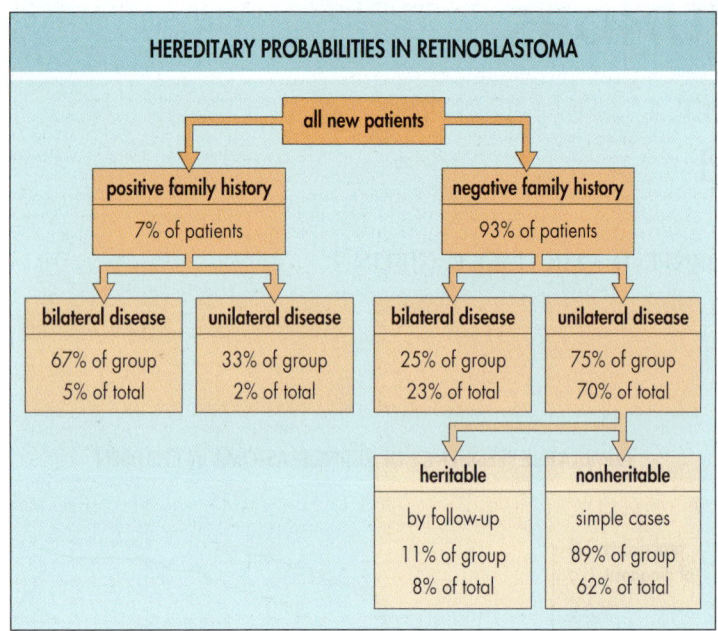

FIG. 146-2 ■ Hereditary probabilities in retinoblastoma.

HEREDITARY PROBABILITIES IN RETINOBLASTOMA

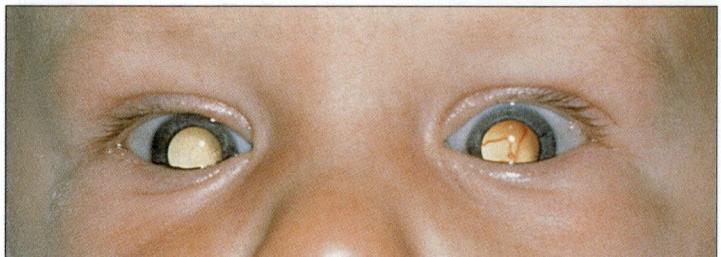

FIG. 146-3 ■ Bilateral leukokoria as a result of retinoblastoma. Note the white pupillary reflection in each eye.

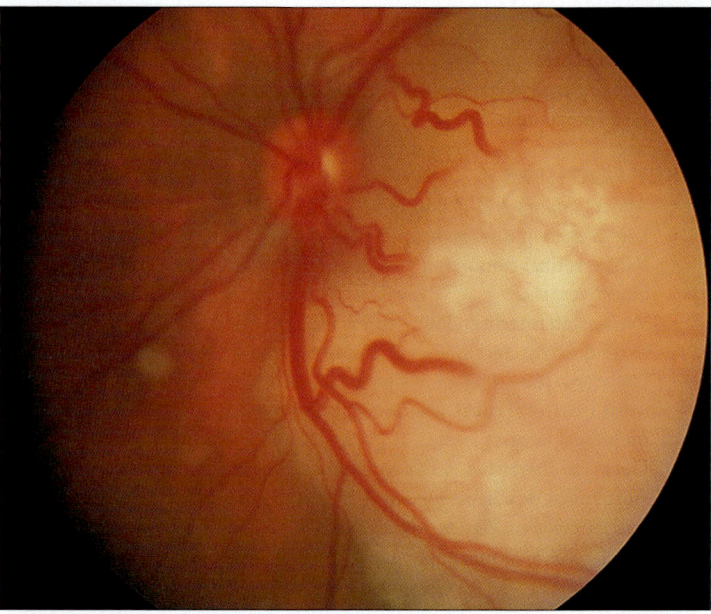

FIG. 146-4 ■ Typical appearance of intraretinal retinoblastoma. Opaque, yellow-white macular tumor fed and drained by dilated, tortuous retinal blood vessels.

The majority of cases of retinoblastoma are sporadic (i.e., diagnosed in patients who have no family history of retinoblastoma and no affected family members on comprehensive familial ophthalmic examination). The hereditary probabilities in a newly diagnosed child who has retinoblastoma are shown in Fig. 146-2.

OCULAR MANIFESTATIONS

The most common presenting manifestation of retinoblastoma is a white glow in the pupil (leukokoria) (Fig. 146-3). This appearance is caused by reflection of light from the white intraocular tumor. Depending on the intraocular extent of the tumor and its laterality, one or both eyes may exhibit this appearance. The second most common presenting manifestation is strabismus, which may be either esotropia or exotropia. Because of the association between retinoblastoma and strabismus, every child who has strabismus must undergo a complete ophthalmic examination to rule out retinoblastoma (as well as other potentially treatable ocular diseases). Presenting manifestations of retinoblastoma encountered less frequently include a red eye, excessive tearing, globe expansion (buphthalmos) and corneal clouding that result from elevated intraocular pressure, discoloration of the iris in the involved eye (usually caused by neovascularization of the iris), loss of the fundus reflection in the affected eye due to intraocular bleeding from the tumor, clumping or layering of white tumor cells on the iris or in the aqueous humor, spontaneous hyphema, and orbital cellulitis.

Although slit-lamp biomicroscopy of young children is frequently quite difficult, every effort should be made to perform this examination in the office at the time of initial patient assessment. This examination allows one to assess the anterior chamber and iris for evidence of tumor cells and iris neovascularization and to evaluate the clarity of the lens and retrolental vitreous. In almost all children with retinoblastoma, even those who have advanced intraocular tumor that fills most of the globe, the lens is completely clear. Slit-lamp biomicroscopy may also disclose finely dispersed cells or tumor cell clumps (seeds) in the vitreous.

Using indirect ophthalmoscopy, the extent of the intraocular tumor, the presence and extent of retinal detachment, and the presence and extent of intravitreal or subretinal tumor seeds can be determined. In eyes that have less advanced disease, well-defined individual tumors may be identified, often in association with dilated, tortuous retinal blood vessels (Fig. 146-4).

Small tumors along the ora serrata and finely dispersed vitreous cells may also be detected during such an examination. In infants and cooperative older children, indirect ophthalmoscopy with scleral depression can be performed in the office; however, in toddlers and uncooperative older children, this examination almost always requires anesthesia.

Discrete intraretinal tumors appear as white, round to oval, dome-shaped retinal masses (see Fig. 146-4). Even relatively small tumors tend to attract retinal blood vessels, which ramify prominently on the surface of the lesion. Very small tumors sometimes appear as translucent, insubstantial thickenings of the retina. Examination of the fundus using a green filter (red-free light) often accentuates such subtle lesions. Larger tumors are frequently associated with a nonrhegmatogenous retinal detachment, which may become bullous and involve the entire retina. This tends to occur with tumors that grow from the retina toward the retinal pigment epithelium and choroid (exophytic growth pattern). In other cases, finely dispersed tumor cells or cell clumps accumulate in the gelatinous vitreous that overlies tumors growing from the retina toward the vitreous (endophytic growth pattern). Many tumors exhibit elements of both endophytic and exophytic growth. A small proportion of eyes with retinoblastoma exhibit generalized thickening of the retina by the tumor, a growth pattern referred to as diffuse infiltrating retinoblastoma.[3] This form of retinoblastoma is commonly associated with diffuse vitreous seeding and is sometimes associated with extension of tumor cells into the anterior chamber aqueous.

Occasionally, a retinoblastoma stops growing spontaneously and loses its malignant character. Such a tumor is called a retinoma.[4] Tumors of this type tend to appear virtually identical to regressed retinoblastoma lesions following successful radia-

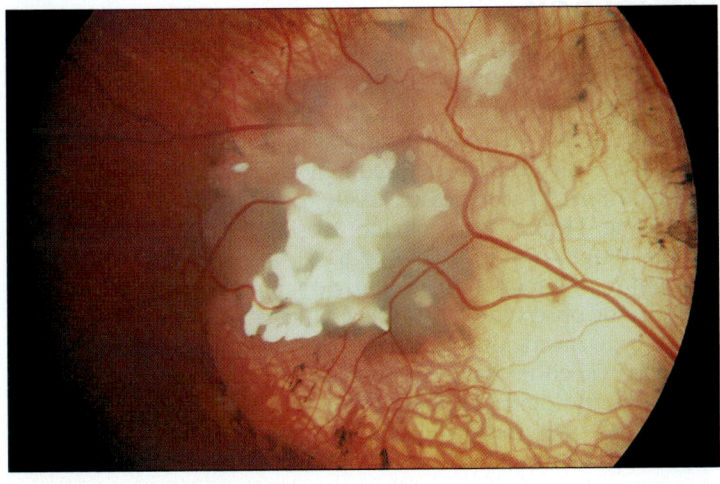

FIG. 146-5 ■ Retinoma (spontaneously arrested retinoblastoma).

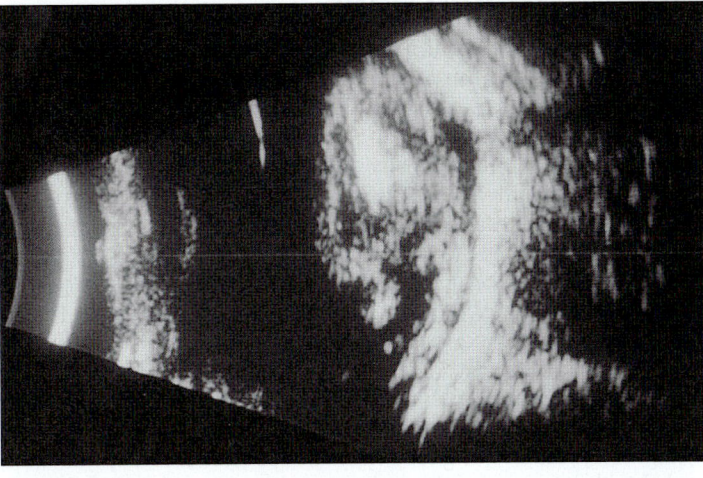

FIG. 146-6 ■ B-scan ultrasonography of retinoblastoma. Solid, posterior intraocular mass contains strong particulate reflections attributable to intralesional calcification.

tion therapy (Fig. 146-5). In other cases, massive intraocular retinoblastomas occasionally undergo spontaneous necrosis, which results in phthisis bulbi.[4]

DIAGNOSIS AND ANCILLARY TESTING

Ultrasonography frequently provides helpful differential diagnostic information in cases of suspected retinoblastoma. Most relatively large tumors (>10–15mm in diameter) contain multiple foci of intralesional calcification. B-scan ultrasonography of such a tumor shows the lesion to be strongly sonoreflective because of the intralesional calcification (Fig. 146-6). In addition, the calcific mass shadows the sclera and orbital soft tissues posteriorly. When the examiner reduces the gain of the instrument, the reflections from the calcific particles within the tumor persist. Standardized A-scan ultrasonography typically shows multiple highly reflective intralesional foci.

Computed tomography (CT) helps confirm the diagnosis, especially in cases of tumor-filled eyes in which there is uncertainty whether the leukokoria results from retinoblastoma or a simulating disorder such as Coats' disease.[5] Because retinoblastoma tumors are characteristically calcified, they usually show up brightly on CT images (Fig. 146-7). However, intralesional calcification is not always present in retinoblastoma. Particularly important in this category are children who suffer diffuse infiltrating retinoblastoma.[3] Children with this clinical form of retinoblastoma characteristically develop tumors multicentrically within the retina and exhibit extensive seeding into the vitreous but no associated intratumoral calcification.

Magnetic resonance imaging (MRI) is the most useful and informative tool for evaluating the sellar and parasellar regions of the brain (to rule out ectopic intracranial retinoblastoma)[5] and for studying the orbital optic nerve. At the same time, however, MRI appears to be less valuable than CT in assessing the intraocular tumor because it does not show the intralesional calcification characteristic of this malignancy.

Fluorescein angiography is usually not performed as a diagnostic aid in suspected retinoblastoma. If this technique is performed on a discrete intraretinal retinoblastoma, the angiogram shows rapid filling of the feeder artery, prompt filling of the intralesional vasculature, and rapid draining via the efferent vein. The intralesional capillaries tend to leak fluorescein, so the tumor characteristically stains brightly in the late frames.

DIFFERENTIAL DIAGNOSIS

The differential diagnosis of retinoblastoma is given in Box 146-1. Coats' disease is the disorder most frequently mistaken for retinoblastoma.

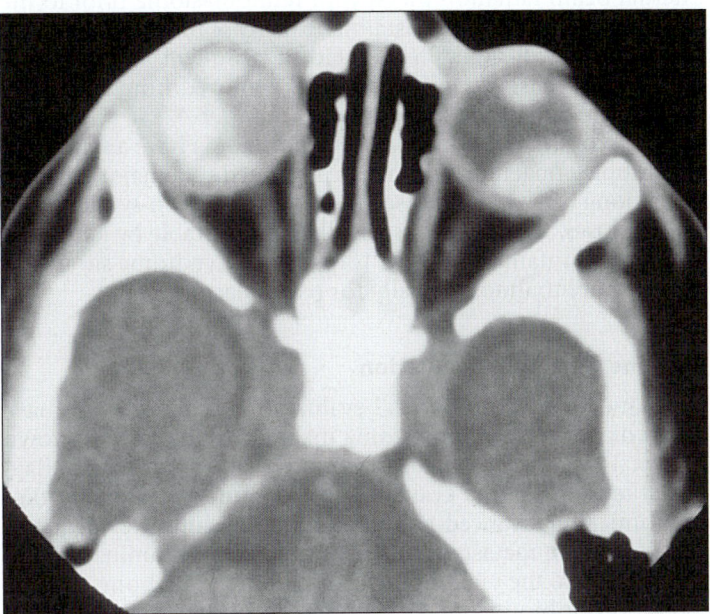

FIG. 146-7 ■ Computed tomography of bilateral intraocular retinoblastoma. Intraocular masses appear bright because of intralesional calcification.

BOX 146-1

Differential Diagnosis of Retinoblastoma

DIFFERENTIAL DIAGNOSIS OF LEUKOKORIA
Coats' disease
Persistent hyperplastic primary vitreous
Ocular toxocariasis
Cicatricial retinopathy of prematurity
Familial exudative vitreoretinopathy
Incontinentia pigmenti retinopathy
Norrie's disease

DIFFERENTIAL DIAGNOSIS OF VITREOUS SEEDS
Pars planitis (intermediate uveitis)
Microbial endophthalmitis or retinitis
Leukemic infiltration

DIFFERENTIAL DIAGNOSIS OF DISCRETE RETINAL TUMORS
Astrocytoma of retina
Medulloepithelioma
Retinal capillary hemangioma
Focal patches of myelinated retinal nerve fibers

SYSTEMIC ASSOCIATIONS

Children who have germinal retinoblastoma have a strong tendency to develop nonretinoblastoma malignancies.[6–9] Around the time of diagnosis of the intraocular disease, a primary nonretinoblastoma intracranial malignancy (which is usually categorized histopathologically as either a pineoblastoma or an ectopic intracranial retinoblastoma) is the most common neoplasm encountered.[6] Presenting features of such a tumor include somnolence, headache, and other neurological symptoms. Central nervous system imaging studies show a solid tumor that involves the suprasellar or parasellar regions of the brain. Ophthalmoscopy frequently reveals papilledema. Because this type of tumor usually occurs in children who have germinal retinoblastoma and bilateral disease, this association is commonly referred to as trilateral retinoblastoma.[10] The intracranial malignancy has a strong tendency to seed the cerebrospinal fluid and thereby spawn implantation tumors along the spinal cord. This malignancy is usually fatal.[6,9] Later in life, various sarcomas of bone and soft tissues represent the most frequent nonretinoblastoma malignancies in these patients.[6,9] Oculo-orbital external beam radiation therapy for retinoblastoma prior to the age of 1 year appears to substantially increase the likelihood that such tumors will occur in the field of treatment later in life,[7,8] but they may also occur in tissues far removed from and unrelated to the radiation.

Some children who develop retinoblastoma have a syndrome of multiple congenital anomalies attributed to a major deletion in the long arm of chromosome 13 (13q deletion syndrome).[11] In such cases, the deletion is usually demonstrable by karyotype analysis. All infants who have 13q deletion syndrome should be screened ophthalmoscopically for retinoblastoma.

Baseline Systemic Evaluation

The standard baseline clinical evaluation of children who have newly diagnosed retinoblastoma includes all the studies shown in Box 146-2. However, most children who have newly diagnosed retinoblastoma evaluated in the United States and other economically advanced countries have no clinical evidence of extraocular or metastatic disease at baseline examination. In such children, the yield of positive findings from bone marrow aspiration or biopsy, lumbar puncture, and bone scan is low.[12] Consequently, these ancillary studies are generally not recommended, except for children who have advanced intraocular disease or clinical evidence of extraocular tumor extension at baseline.

Genetic testing should be considered for all children who have bilateral or familial retinoblastoma.[2] Modern molecular biology techniques enable investigators to determine the precise genetic defect in a given individual or family and to assess the risk that a particular individual may transmit the disease to offspring. Children with germinal retinoblastoma and unaffected carriers of the disease must be advised of their potential to transmit the disease when they reach reproductive age.

BOX 146-2

Baseline Systemic Evaluation in Retinoblastoma

Complete pediatric history and physical examination
Blood for complete blood count (CBC)
MRI or CT of brain, especially in bilateral or familial cases to look for ectopic intracranial retinoblastoma
Lumbar puncture for cerebrospinal fluid analysis*
Bone marrow aspiration or biopsy*
Bone scan*

*Currently advocated only for children with advanced intraocular disease or clinically extraocular disease at baseline.

PATHOLOGY

Retinoblastoma is characterized histopathologically by malignant neuroepithelial cells (retinoblasts) that arise within the immature retina.[13] The retinoblasts typically appear to have a large basophilic nucleus and scanty cytoplasm. Cellular necrosis and intralesional calcification are frequent associations, especially in larger tumors. In some cases, tissue differentiation occurs, often producing Flexner-Wintersteiner rosettes (Fig. 146-8, A) or Homer Wright rosettes (Fig. 146-8, B). In occasional cases, photoreceptor differentiation of individual retinoblasts (fleurettes) may also be observed (Fig. 146-8, C). Retinoblastoma has a strong tendency to invade the optic nerve and choroid and extend out of the globe via either the optic nerve or the scleral emissary canals.

Histopathological studies of eyes that contain clinical retinomas show such tumors to be composed entirely of benign-appearing neuronal cells with photoreceptor differentiation, most notably in the form of fleurettes.[14] Necrosis and mitotic ac-

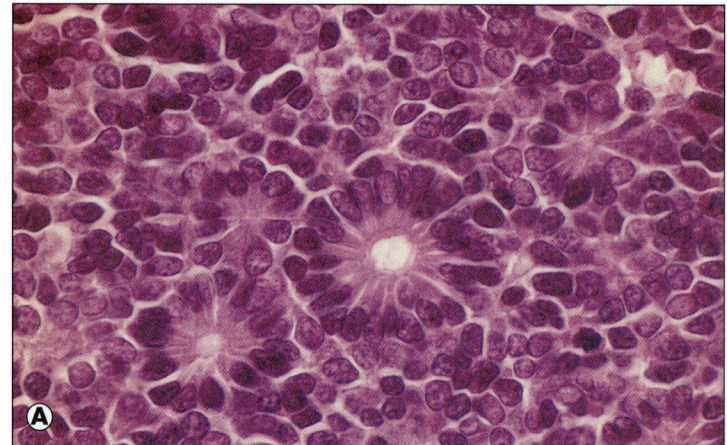

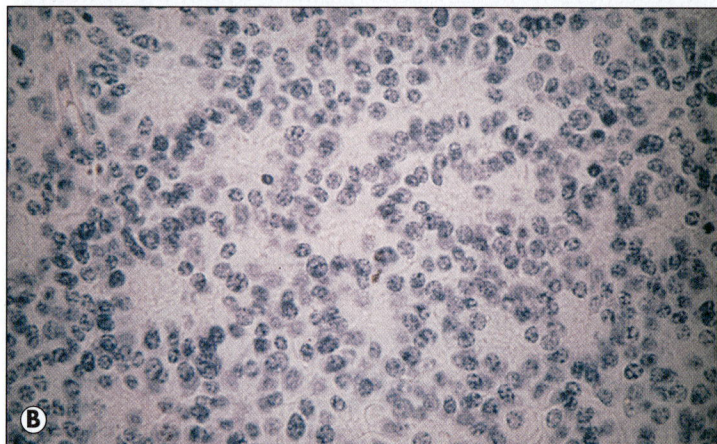

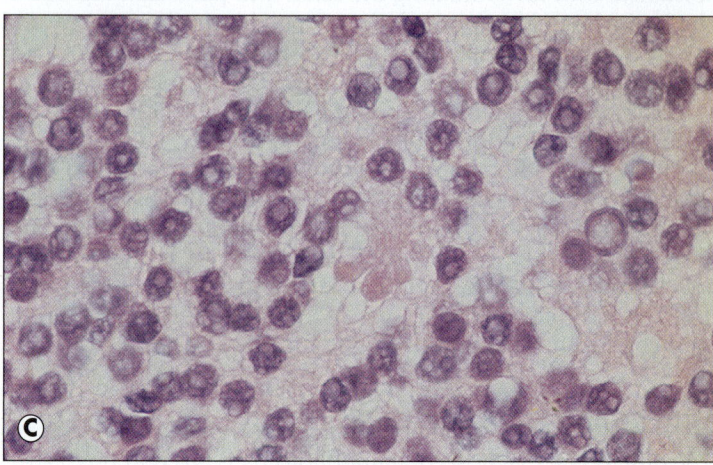

FIG. 146-8 ■ **Histopathology of retinoblastoma. A,** Flexner-Wintersteiner rosettes. **B,** Homer Wright rosettes. **C,** Fleurettes.

tivity are absent, but limited amounts of calcification are present in some of these lesions. The histopathological term applied to such tumors is retinocytoma.

TREATMENT

Currently employed treatment options for retinoblastoma are listed in Box 146-3. Factors that influence the management recommendations for children who have retinoblastoma include the size of the tumor or tumors, the location of the tumors, the laterality of the disease, the vision or visual potential in the affected eye, and the vision or visual potential in the unaffected eye (assuming the disease is unilateral). Any associated ocular problems such as retinal detachment, vitreous hemorrhage, neovascularization of the iris, and secondary glaucoma are also taken into account. Finally, the age and general health of the child must be considered, as well as personal preferences of the child's parents or legal guardians.

Chemotherapy

Chemotherapy is currently the primary therapeutic option in children with bilateral retinoblastoma.[15] It is also employed as initial treatment in some children with unilateral disease when the affected eye is believed to be salvageable. The most common chemotherapeutic regimen in use around the world today consists of a combination of carboplatin, etoposide or a related drug, and vincristine. In some centers, cyclosporine is added to this regimen to reduce the multidrug resistance that occurs in many retinoblastomas.[16] Chemotherapy must be supervised by a pediatric oncologist who is familiar with the side effects and complications of the drugs and can monitor the child closely during treatment. If chemotherapy is employed, it is given as a cyclic treatment every 3 to 4 weeks for six or more cycles. Most intraocular retinoblastoma lesions (including vitreous seeds) regress substantially within the first two cycles (Fig. 146-9). Partially regressed tumors that are still viable following the second cycle of chemotherapy and any new tumors that develop during the course of chemotherapy must be treated by local therapies such as cryotherapy, laser therapy, and episcleral plaque radiation therapy[17-19] (see later for details). Residual or recurrent vitreous seeds following chemotherapy usually require external beam radiation therapy[18,19] if the eye is to be salvaged.

Chemotherapy is also used to treat children with extraocular tumor extension at presentation[20] or detected on histopathological study of an enucleated eye,[21] orbital tumor recurrence after enucleation,[22] intracranial invasion by tumor,[23] and metastatic disease.[24] Unfortunately, most children who develop metastatic or intracranial retinoblastoma ultimately die of this disease.[23,24]

Enucleation

In spite of the current popularity of chemotherapy as the primary treatment for retinoblastoma, enucleation remains an important therapeutic option for this disease. This treatment is par-

ticularly applicable to children who have unilateral advanced intraocular disease. Enucleation is sometimes recommended for both eyes in children who have bilateral far-advanced disease not amenable to any eye-preserving therapy and for the more severely affected eye in markedly asymmetrical bilateral cases. If enucleation is performed, the ophthalmic surgeon must attempt to obtain a long section of optic nerve during surgery. The principal route of exit of tumor cells from the eye is along the optic nerve. Prior pathological studies have shown that enucleation is usually curative in retinoblastoma if an optic nerve section longer than 5mm is obtained with the globe.[13] If possible, the ophthalmic surgeon should attempt to obtain an optic nerve section 10–15mm long in every case.

Contrary to some popular recommendations, insertion of an orbital implant at the time of enucleation appears to be appropriate except when there is a strong likelihood of residual tumor in the orbit. The cosmetic results of enucleation are generally quite satisfactory as long as the child does not also undergo orbital radiation therapy.

External Beam Radiation Therapy

Prior to the development of effective chemotherapy for retinoblastoma, the most commonly employed regional eye-preserving therapy for this disease was external beam radiation therapy.[25] This treatment is usually performed using a linear accelerator in

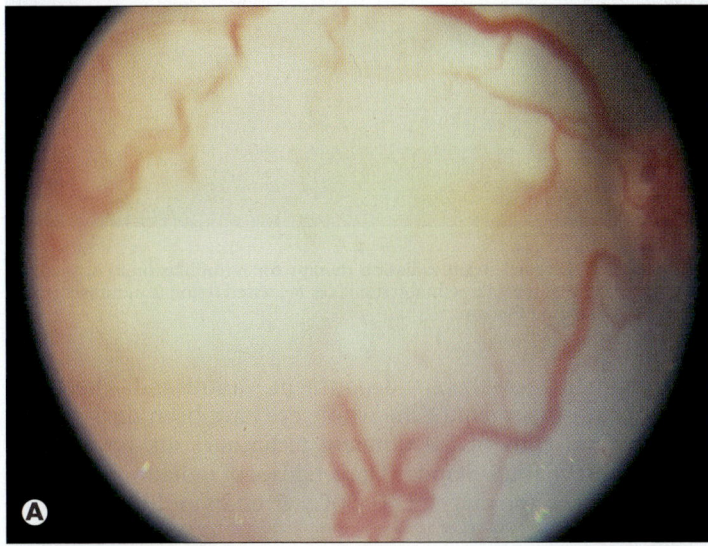

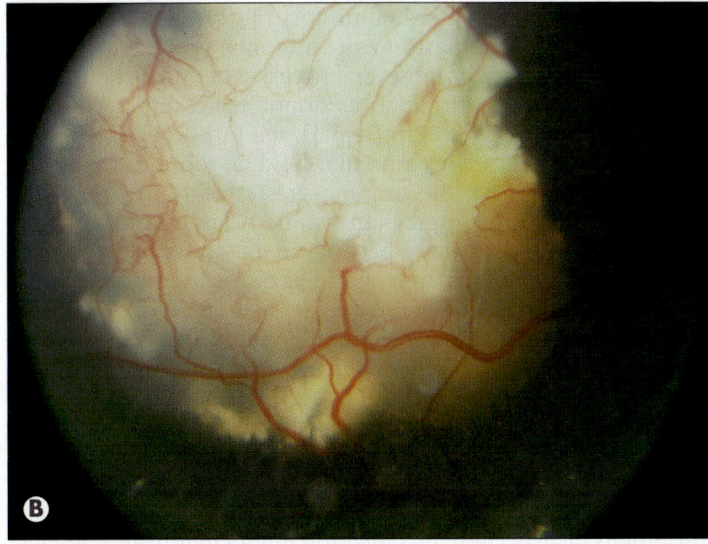

FIG. 146-9 ■ Chemotherapy for retinoblastoma. **A,** Pretreatment appearance of macular retinoblastoma. **B,** Same lesion after two cycles of chemotherapy using vincristine, etoposide, and carboplatin.

BOX 146-3

Treatment Options for Intraocular Retinoblastoma

Intravenous chemotherapy
Enucleation
Radiation therapy
• External beam radiation therapy
• Plaque radiotherapy
Photocoagulation and laser therapy
Cryotherapy
Observation (for spontaneously arrested retinoblastoma, retinoma)

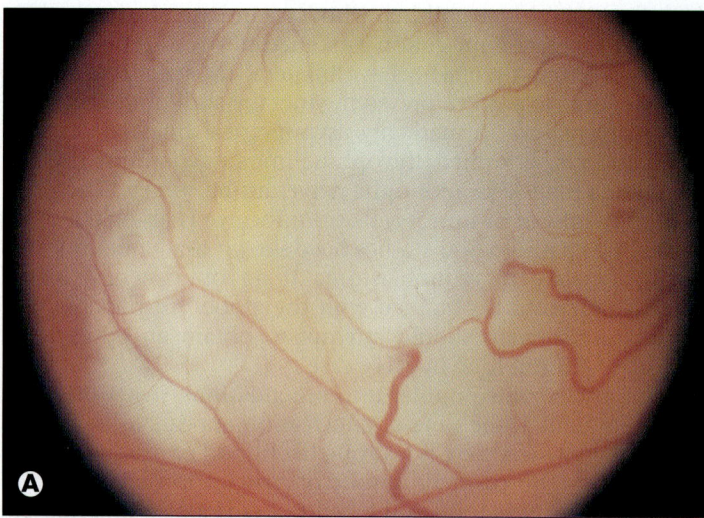

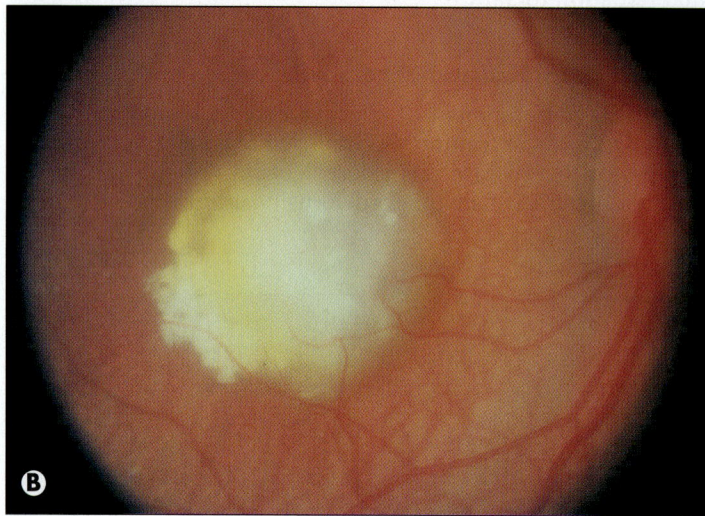

FIG. 146-10 ■ External beam radiation therapy for retinoblastoma. A, Pretreatment appearance of macular retinoblastoma. B, Regressed lesion 2 months after external beam radiation therapy.

a hospital radiation therapy department. Various radiotherapeutic setups for treatment of the whole eye have been devised, but the pros and cons of the different techniques are beyond the scope of this chapter. Standard target doses of radiation to the eye and orbit are in the range of 40–50Gy given in multiple fractions of 150–200cGy over 4–5 weeks.

External beam radiation therapy results in highly effective regression of vascularized retinal tumors (Fig. 146-10). Even very large, cohesive retinoblastomas commonly show pronounced clinical regression within several weeks after treatment. Two main patterns of postirradiation tumor regression have been identified. In the first pattern (type I), the tumor regresses to an almost exclusively calcific, avascular residual mound. In the second pattern (type II), the tumor regresses without prominent calcification but with a gray-tan fish-flesh appearance. The dilated retinal vessels usually become markedly attenuated with both regression patterns. In type III regression, a combination of both regression patterns occurs (Fig. 146-10, B).

External beam radiation therapy is applicable to eyes containing one or more tumors that involve the optic disc, eyes that show diffuse vitreous seeding, and eyes for which prior chemotherapy or local treatments, such as photocoagulation, laser therapy, cryotherapy, or plaque radiotherapy, failed. Vitreous seeds generally do not respond well to radiation therapy, presumably because of their relatively hypoxic status. As also might be expected, the larger the intraocular tumor, the less predictable the successful local response to treatment.

If the whole eye is treated by external beam radiation therapy, a radiation-related cataract is likely to result.[25] Such a cataract

typically begins as posterior subcapsular clouding. In some children, the cataract remains limited and stable in extent after development. In other children, it becomes progressively more pronounced and gradually obscures details of the fundus and worsens vision. In such situations, cataract extraction is usually required.[26] Fortunately, the cataract usually does not form for at least 6 months after radiation therapy and is often delayed for as much as 1–1.5 years after treatment. At the radiation levels mentioned earlier, other significant intraocular complications such as radiation retinopathy and neovascular glaucoma are extremely uncommon. External beam radiation therapy also causes orbital bone growth arrest, which results in a cosmetic facial deformity in many children who have retinoblastoma.[27] This complication is most pronounced in children who undergo treatment prior to the age of 1 year. Fortunately, the resultant deformities associated with current radiation doses and instrumentation are generally not as severe as those associated with higher doses of radiation therapy and electron beam therapy used in the past. External beam radiation therapy also increases the risk of nonretinoblastoma malignancies in the field of treatment in survivors of germinal retinoblastoma[7,8] (see Course and Outcome section later). This effect also appears most pronounced in children irradiated before the age of 1 year. Because of this, most ocular oncologists currently recommend delaying external beam radiation therapy until the child is 1 year old if possible.

Plaque Radiation Therapy

In some children who have relatively large but localized retinoblastomas, even in the presence of limited localized vitreous seeding, plaque radiation therapy may be employed successfully.[28] The principal isotopes used in radioactive eye plaques at present are iodine-125 and ruthenium-106. When such plaques are used to treat retinoblastoma, a target dose of 40–45Gy to the tumor apex is generally employed. As a result of the physical dose-distribution considerations of the plaques, the base of the tumor always receives a substantially higher dose than the apex. In contrast, the orbital tissues receive only a small fraction of the radiation dose because a metallic layer on the outer surface of the plaque effectively shields the emissions in that direction. Plaque radiation therapy typically produces prompt regression of treated tumors (Fig. 146-11). This form of therapy seems particularly applicable to eyes that contain a solitary medium to large tumor that does not involve the optic disc or macula and is associated with no more than a limited amount of adjacent vitreous seeding. It may also be used in eyes for which prior local therapy, such as photocoagulation, laser therapy, or cryotherapy, failed, as well as in some eyes that failed prior external beam radiation therapy locally.

Photocoagulation

Photocoagulation has been used for a number of years to treat eyes that contain one or a few small tumors, clear optical media, and no vitreous seeds.[29] Such treatments are generally not advocated for tumors that involve the optic disc or macula. Tumors most amenable to this form of therapy are quite small, usually less than 7mm in basal diameter and 2–3mm thick, and posterior to the ocular equator. Until recently, xenon arc photocoagulation was the modality employed in almost all retinoblastoma management. The technique consisted of the creation of intense burns that overlapped in a complete circle around the base of the tumor. These burns were intended to block the tumor's retinal vascular supply. The treatment had to be repeated every 3–4 weeks until all that remained was an atrophic chorioretinal lesion. Unless the entire tumor was so small that it could be totally encompassed in a single photocoagulation burn, treatment was usually not directed at the tumor itself, in case the internal limiting membrane ruptured and released viable tumor cells

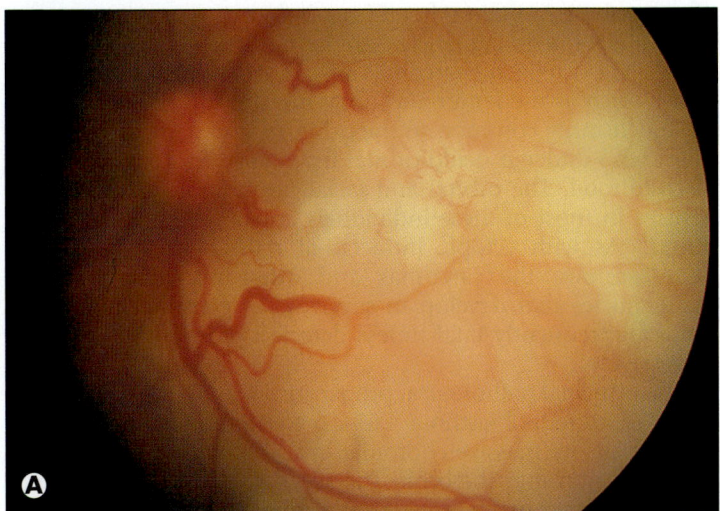

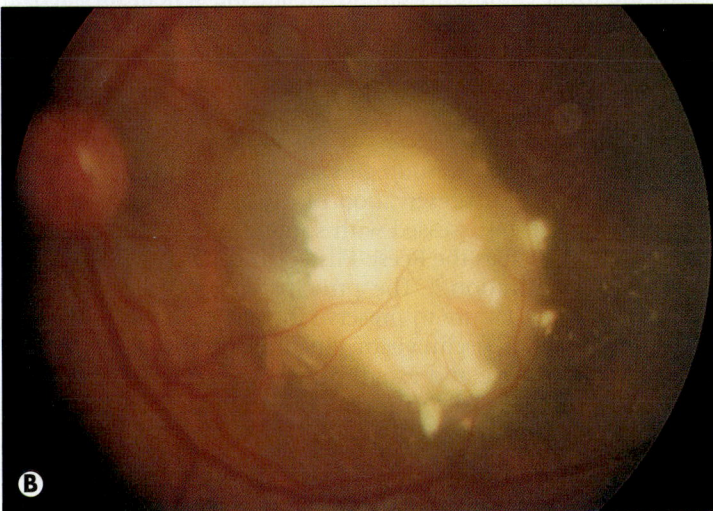

FIG. 146-11 ▪▪ **Plaque radiation therapy for retinoblastoma. A,** Pretreatment appearance of macular retinoblastoma. **B,** Regressed lesion 6 weeks following iodine-125 notched plaque radiotherapy.

into the overlying vitreous. Photocoagulation can also be performed using various lasers (see the next section).

Laser Therapy

Since the advent of laser systems that can deliver the treatment beam via an indirect ophthalmoscope or operating microscope, many small to medium retinoblastoma tumors that would have been difficult or impossible to treat effectively using xenon arc photocoagulator can now be treated using laser therapy. Initially, laser therapy was performed using a technique similar to that described for the xenon arc photocoagulator. Later, some clinicians found that they could create an effective, intense confluent burn (as opposed to the overlapping burns of xenon arc photocoagulation) two to three spot diameters wide around the tumor base by using continuous or long-duration exposures.[30] More recently, low-power, long-duration, long-wavelength laser therapy (commonly referred to as transpupillary thermotherapy) has gained popularity as a treatment for selected retinoblastomas.[31] In this therapy, a diode laser (wavelength in the infrared range) is focused on the tumor using a slit lamp, operating microscope, or indirect ophthalmoscope. Large spot sizes (generally 2–3 mm in diameter) are used if the pupil can be dilated widely. Individual exposures of at least 60 seconds are employed at sufficiently low power settings to produce a dull white discoloration of the tumor during treatment. The entire lesion is treated with a series of overlapping spots. The effectiveness of laser therapy is usually checked within 2–4 weeks, and treatment is repeated if necessary until the entire tumor is gone.

Cryotherapy

Trans-scleral cryotherapy under indirect ophthalmoscopic visualization may be used to treat one to a few equatorial or preequatorial retinoblastoma tumors of small to medium size,[32] but it should not be used to treat eyes that have vitreous seeding. A double or triple freeze-thaw technique is usually employed, and the ice ball is allowed to encompass the entire tumor and overlying vitreous during each freezing cycle. As with photocoagulation and laser therapy, this form of treatment is generally repeated every 2–4 weeks until the entire tumor is gone.

Multimodality Therapy

Most children with bilateral retinoblastoma, multifocal retinoblastoma, or both, and occasional children with unilateral retinoblastoma, are currently managed by multimodality therapy. If a child has small intraretinal tumors without vitreous seeding and the macula and optic disc are not involved by tumor, he or she is typically treated by a combination of laser therapy and cryotherapy (laser for the more posterior tumors, and cryotherapy for the more peripheral tumors). If the child has larger tumors or ones that involve the central macula or optic disc, he or she is frequently treated initially by chemotherapy in an effort to shrink the tumors. Once partial regression of the tumors has been achieved, sequential locally destructive therapies (laser therapy, cryotherapy, plaque radiotherapy) are used to destroy the residual lesions. In some instances, laser therapy or cryotherapy is performed shortly after intravenous administration of chemotherapy. Such treatments are frequently referred to as photochemotherapy, chemothermotherapy, and chemocryotherapy. Accumulated laboratory and clinical experience indicates that these combination therapies produce greater local destructive effects than the same therapies applied sequentially on separate dates.

Observation

In view of the recognized natural history of retinoblastoma, observation with no therapeutic intervention is usually not advocated. However, a number of circumstances exist in which such an approach is almost certainly warranted. The most important circumstance is that of a spontaneously arrested retinoblastoma. As mentioned earlier (see Ocular Manifestations), a spontaneously arrested retinoblastoma (retinoma) appears similar to a regressed retinoblastoma after irradiation (see Fig. 146-5); however, such tumors are detected in eyes that have received no prior radiation therapy or other treatment. Although retinomas have the same implications for inheritance of retinoblastoma as do viable lesions,[4] such tumors usually remain dormant clinically and appear to have limited malignant potential.[33] Consequently, they should simply be monitored on a regular basis, with no intervention unless they show evidence of renewed clinical activity. A second circumstance in which continued observation may be appropriate is that of true spontaneous regression of retinoblastoma.[4] Spontaneous regression is characterized by phthisis bulbi of the involved eye.

COURSE AND OUTCOME

As many as 45% of eyes treated initially by some form of eye-preserving therapy eventually require subsequent therapy by the same or another modality because of the development of new or recurrent intraocular tumors.[34] In spite of the need for secondary sequential treatments, the great majority of eyes that have small to medium-sized tumors and no vitreous seeding are salvaged with useful vision.

Following local obliterative treatment of retinoblastoma, children must be re-examined within 2–4 weeks to assess treatment efficacy. Supplemental local treatment is performed at those evaluations if the prior therapy appears inadequate. Once treatment appears to have totally eradicated all intraocular tumors, children are monitored every 3 months for at least 2 years. Thereafter, children should be followed at 6-month intervals until they are at least 6 years old, after which they should be followed at yearly intervals.

Some children have substantial orbital extension of tumor at the time of their initial diagnosis and treatment,[20] and others develop orbital recurrence after enucleation.[22] Although such cases were almost invariably fatal in the past, current evidence suggests that at least some of these children can now be saved by an aggressive regimen of tumor debulking, supplemental orbital irradiation, and systemic multidrug chemotherapy.[20,22] Unfortunately, the prognosis for children who have intracranial extension or widespread metastasis remains dismal.

Untreated, children who have retinoblastoma almost always die of intracranial extension or widely disseminated disease within approximately 2 years of tumor detection. Recognized adverse clinical prognostic factors for retinoblastoma-related death include larger size of the intraocular tumor, older age of the child at detection and diagnosis, and, most important, evidence of retrobulbar optic nerve expansion by tumor or trans-scleral extraocular tumor extension on CT or other imaging studies. The survival rate for both unilaterally and bilaterally affected children who have retinoblastoma in developed countries is currently about 90–95% (Fig. 146-12).[1] Most retinoblastoma-related deaths occur within 2–3 years of the initiation of treatment; few deaths attributable directly to retinoblastoma occur thereafter.

As mentioned previously, children with germinal retinoblastoma who survive their intraocular retinoblastoma have a substantially increased risk of death from one or more nonretinoblastoma malignancies over the course of their lifetimes.[9] The exact probability of such an event is somewhat controversial, but the best available evidence suggests that at least 20% of survivors of germinal retinoblastoma develop such malignancies within 25 years of their retinoblastoma treatment.[8,9] During the period from just before diagnosis of the intraocular cancer to about 2 years after, the most common nonretinoblastoma malignancies that arise are pineoblastoma and ectopic intracranial retinoblastoma involving the suprasellar or parasellar tissues (trilateral retinoblastoma).[10] Such lesions can cause obstructive hydrocephalus as well as seeding into the cerebrospinal fluid and implantation metastasis along the spinal cord. Unfortunately, most cases of ectopic intracranial retinoblastoma are fatal in spite

of aggressive treatment. After this period, the most common non-retinoblastoma malignancies are bony and soft tissue sarcomas.[7–9] The osteogenic sarcomas arise most frequently in the long bones, such as the femur and tibia, but the soft tissue sarcomas are much more common in the orbit or face, particularly in patients who undergo oculo-orbital irradiation for retinoblastoma in childhood. The orbital and facial nonretinoblastoma malignancies in most of these individuals appear to be radiation induced.[7] As with ectopic intracranial retinoblastomas and pineoblastomas, the sarcomas and other nonretinoblastoma malignancies that develop in survivors of germinal retinoblastoma are frequently fatal unless detected promptly and treated aggressively.

The principal pathological prognostic factors for tumor-related mortality in retinoblastoma[13] appear to be the presence of optic nerve invasion, massive choroidal invasion, and trans-scleral tumor extension into the orbit. The severity of anaplasia does not appear to have much impact on survival prognosis. In recent years, the most commonly employed staging system for survival in retinoblastoma is one that categorizes affected children as those who have tumor confined to the eyes (stage 1), those who have local extraocular extension into the optic nerve or orbit (stage 2), and those who have metastatic disease (stage 3). The tumor-node-metastasis (TNM) system is also used in some centers to group children according to survival prognosis.

The prognosis for preservation of the eye with at least some useful vision can be assessed with some degree of success using classifications such as the Reese-Ellsworth system[35] and the Essen prognosis classification.[36] The principal prognostic factors for ocular mortality (failure to preserve the eye) and visual mortality (failure to retain useful vision) include the size of intraocular tumors, the presence and extent of vitreous seeds, the presence and extent of retinal detachment, and the locations of the tumors within the eye.

REFERENCES

1. Sanders BM, Draper GJ, Kingston JE. Retinoblastoma in Great Britain 1969–80: incidence, treatment and survival. Br J Ophthalmol. 1988;72:576–83.
2. Smith BJ, O'Brien JM. The genetics of retinoblastoma and current diagnostic testing. J Pediatr Ophthalmol Strabismus. 1996;33:120–3.
3. Bhatnagar R, Vine AK. Diffuse infiltrating retinoblastoma. Ophthalmology. 1991;98:1657–61.
4. Gallie BL, Phillips RA, Ellsworth RM, et al. Significance of retinoma and phthisis bulbi for retinoblastoma. Ophthalmology. 1982;89:1393–9.
5. Mafee MF, Goldberg MF, Cohen SB, et al. Magnetic resonance imaging versus computed tomography of leukocoric eyes and use of in vitro proton magnetic resonance spectroscopy of retinoblastoma. Ophthalmology. 1989;96:965–76.
6. Draper GJ, Sanders BM, Kingston JE. Second primary neoplasms in patients with retinoblastoma. Br J Cancer. 1986;53:661–71.
7. Roarty JD, McLean IW, Zimmerman LE. Incidence of second neoplasms in patients with bilateral retinoblastoma. Ophthalmology. 1988;95:1583–7.
8. Mohney BG, Robertson DM, Schomberg PJ, Hodge DO. Second nonocular tumors in survivors of heritable retinoblastoma and prior radiation therapy. Am J Ophthalmol. 1998;126:269–77.
9. Eng G, Li FP, Abramson DH, et al. Mortality from second tumors among long-term survivors of retinoblastoma. J Natl Cancer Inst. 1993;85:1121–8.
10. Amoaku WMK, Willshaw HE, Parkes SE, et al. Trilateral retinoblastoma. A report of five patients. Cancer. 1996;78:858–63.
11. Seidman DJ, Shields JA, Augsburger JJ, et al. Early diagnosis of retinoblastoma based on dysmorphic features and karyotype analysis. Ophthalmology. 1987;94:663–6.
12. Karcioglu ZA, Al-Mesfer SA, Abboud E, et al. Workup for metastatic retinoblastoma. A review of 261 patients. Ophthalmology. 1997;104:307–12.
13. Khelfaoui F, Validire P, Auperin A, et al. Histopathologic risk factors in retinoblastoma. A retrospective study of 172 patients treated in a single institution. Cancer. 1996;77:1206–13.
14. Margo C, Hidayat A, Kopelman J, Zimmerman LE. Retinocytoma. A benign variant of retinoblastoma. Arch Ophthalmol. 1983;101:1519–31.
15. Gombos DS, Kelly A, Coen PG, et al. Retinoblastoma treated with primary chemotherapy alone: the significance of tumor size, location, and age. Br J Ophthalmol. 2002;86:80–3.
16. Chan HS, DeBoer G, Thiessen JJ, et al. Combining cyclosporin with chemotherapy controls intraocular retinoblastoma without requiring radiation. Clin Cancer Res. 1996;2:1499–508.
17. Murphree AL, Villablanca JG, Deegan WF, et al. Chemotherapy plus local treatment in the management of intraocular retinoblastoma. Arch Ophthalmol. 1996;114:1348–56.
18. Wilson MW, Rodriguez-Galindo C, Haik BG, et al. Multiagent chemotherapy as neoadjuvant treatment for multifocal intraocular retinoblastoma. Ophthalmology. 2001;108:2106–14.
19. Shields CL, Honavar SG, Shields JA, et al. Factors predictive of recurrence of retinal tumors, vitreous seeds, and subretinal seeds following chemoreduction for retinoblastoma. Arch Ophthalmol. 2002;120:460–4.

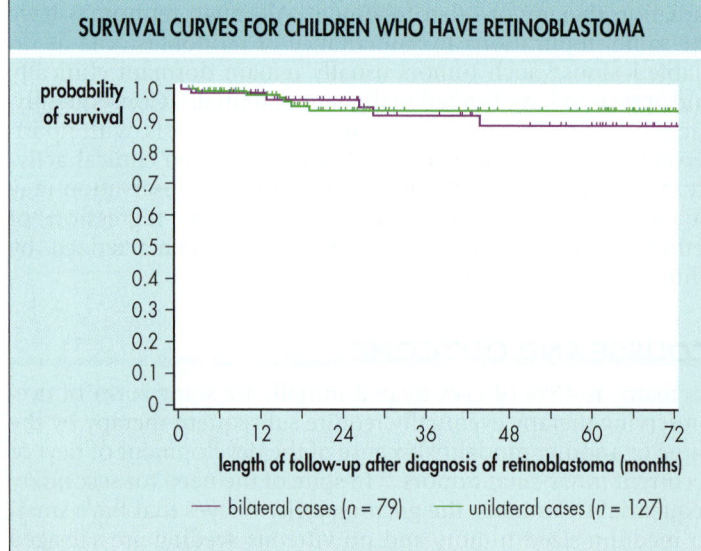

SURVIVAL CURVES FOR CHILDREN WHO HAVE RETINOBLASTOMA

probability of survival (y-axis: 0 to 1.0)
length of follow-up after diagnosis of retinoblastoma (months) (x-axis: 0, 12, 24, 36, 48, 60, 72)

— bilateral cases (n = 79)　　— unilateral cases (n = 127)

FIG. 146-12 ■ **Survival of children with retinoblastoma.** Separate curves are plotted for children with unilateral and bilateral disease. These curves are based on deaths from retinoblastoma only. Other causes of death, including deaths due to second malignancies, are not considered in the computation of these curves. The data from which these curves are derived come from the private practice of James J. Augsburger, M.D.

20. Kiratli H, Bilgic S, Ozerdem U. Management of massive orbital involvement of intraocular retinoblastoma. Ophthalmology. 1998;105:322–6.
21. Mustafa MM, Jamshed A, Khafaga Y, et al. Adjuvant chemotherapy with vincristine, doxorubicin, and cyclophosphamide in the treatment of postenucleation high risk retinoblastoma. J Pediatr Hematol Oncol. 1999;21:364–9.
22. Goble RR, McKenzie JE, Kingston JE, et al. Orbital recurrence of retinoblastoma successfully treated by combined therapy. Br J Ophthalmol. l990;74:97–8.
23. Namouni F, Doz F, Tanguy ML, et al. High-dose chemotherapy with carboplatin, etoposide and cyclophosphamide followed by hematopoietic stem cell rescue in patients with high-risk retinoblastoma: a SFOP and SFGM study. Eur J Cancer. 1997;33:2368–75.
24. Saleh RA, Gross S, Cassano W, Gee A. Metastatic retinoblastoma successfully treated with immunomagnetic purged autologous bone marrow transplantation. Cancer. 1988;62:2301–2.
25. Hungerford JL, Toma NMG, Plowman PN, Kingston JE. External beam radiotherapy for retinoblastoma: I. Whole eye technique. Br J Ophthalmol. 1995;79:109–11.
26. Brooks HL, Meyer D, Shields JA, et al. Removal of radiation-induced cataracts in patients treated for retinoblastoma. Arch Ophthalmol. 1990;108:1701–8.
27. Egbert PR, Donaldson SS, Moazed K, et al. Visual results and ocular complications following radiotherapy for retinoblastoma. Arch Ophthalmol. 1978;96:1826–30.
28. Shields CL, Shields JA, De Potter P, et al. Plaque radiotherapy in the management of retinoblastoma. Use as a primary and secondary treatment. Ophthalmology. 1993;100:216–24.
29. Shields JA, Shields CL, Parsons H, et al. The role of photocoagulation in the management of retinoblastoma. Arch Ophthalmol. 1990;108:205–8.
30. Augsburger JJ, Faulkner CB. Indirect ophthalmoscope argon laser treatment of retinoblastoma. Ophthalmic Surg. 1992;23:591–3.
31. Shields CL, Santos MCM, Diniz W, et al. Thermotherapy for retinoblastoma. Arch Ophthalmol. 1999;117:885–93.
32. Shields JA, Parsons H, Shields CL, et al. The role of cryotherapy in the management of retinoblastoma. Am J Ophthalmol. 1989;108:260–4.
33. Eagle RC, Shields JA, Donoso L, et al. Malignant transformation of spontaneously regressed retinoblastoma, retinoma/retinocytoma variant. Ophthalmology. 1989;96:1389–95.
34. Messmer EP, Sauerwein W, Heinrich T, et al. New and recurrent tumor foci following local treatment as well as external beam radiation in eyes of patients with hereditary retinoblastoma. Graefes Arch Clin Exp Ophthalmol. 1990;228:426–31.
35. Reese AB, Ellsworth RM. The evaluation and current concept of retinoblastoma therapy. Trans Am Acad Ophthalmol Otolaryngol. 1963;67:164–72.
36. Höpping W. The new Essen prognosis classification for conservative sight saving treatment of retinoblastoma. In: Lommatzsch PK, Blodi FC, eds. Intraocular tumors. Berlin: Akademie-Verlag; 1983:497–505.

147 Uveal Melanoma

JAMES J. AUGSBURGER • BERTIL E. DAMATO • NORBERT BORNFELD

DEFINITION
- Primary acquired malignant neoplasm of uveal melanocytes.

KEY FEATURES
- Dark brown to golden tumor of choroid, ciliary body, or iris.
- Choroidal and ciliary body tumors are usually more than 7mm in basal diameter and more than 2mm thick at the time of diagnosis; iris tumors are much smaller at diagnosis.
- Unilateral, unifocal in almost all affected patients.
- Well-established tendency to metastasize, especially to liver.
- Much more common in lighter-skinned races.

ASSOCIATED FEATURES
- Nonrhegmatogenous retinal detachment with shifting subretinal fluid, frequently associated with choroidal and ciliary body melanomas.
- Prominent clumps of orange pigment lipofuscin commonly present on surface of choroidal tumors.
- Eruption of some choroidal tumors through Bruch's membrane to achieve a mushroom-like shape.
- Extrascleral extension.

INTRODUCTION

Uveal melanoma is a malignant neoplasm that arises from neuroectodermal melanocytes within the choroid, ciliary body, or iris. It is the most common primary malignant intraocular neoplasm of Caucasian adults. This neoplasm has a well-documented capacity to metastasize hematogenously and kill the patient. Its favored metastatic site is the liver. It can arise from any portion of the uveal tract, but choroidal involvement is by far the most common. Uveal melanomas confined to the iris appear to be substantially less malignant in terms of their potential to kill the host than are melanomas confined to the choroid and ciliary body. Furthermore, the extent of the tumor at the time of detection and the methods of management employed are substantially different for iris melanoma than for choroidal and ciliary body melanomas. For this reason, these two general forms of uveal melanoma are discussed separately in this chapter.

EPIDEMIOLOGY AND PATHOGENESIS

Uveal melanoma has a cumulative lifetime incidence of approximately 1 in 2000–2500 Caucasian individuals.[1,2] It is between 15 and 50 times less common in African blacks and intermediate in frequency in other racial groups. The average annual incidence in Caucasians older than 30 years has been estimated to be approximately seven to eight new cases per million persons. The annual incidence increases with advancing age. Before age 30 years, the annual incidence is less than one new case per million. In contrast, by age 70 years, the annual incidence is approximately 50 new cases per million.

The average age at detection of melanomas of the choroid or ciliary body is about 55–60 years in most large series.[1] The average age at detection of melanomas of the iris is 10–20 years younger. As indicated earlier, uveal malignant melanoma is rare in persons younger than 30 years and increases in frequency with each decade of life. The cumulative lifetime incidence of primary uveal melanoma is slightly higher in men than in women.[2]

Patients who have a history of intense, sustained, recurrent sunlight exposure sometime during life appear to be more likely to develop a uveal melanoma than those without such exposure.[1] A generalized congenital ocular hyperpigmentation known as ocular melanocytosis appears to predispose patients to the development of uveal melanoma. The dermatological condition dysplastic nevus syndrome is also associated with an increased risk of uveal melanoma. However, reproductive factors, estrogen therapy, and cigarette smoking do not appear to increase the risk of uveal melanomas appreciably.

Although uveal malignant melanoma occurs in more than one member of a family more frequently than one would expect by chance alone, no strong familial inheritance pattern exists for this neoplasm. Several somatic cytogenetic abnormalities have been encountered rather frequently in uveal melanoma cells,[3] and these chromosomal abnormalities may be responsible in some way for the development of the malignancy. The most commonly encountered chromosomal abnormalities to date include monosomy of chromosome 3, a duplication of a portion of the long (q) arm of chromosome 8, partial deletion of the short (p) arm of chromosome 9, and complementary gains of material on chromosome 6p and loss of material from chromosome 6q.

IRIS MELANOMAS

OCULAR MANIFESTATIONS

The usual symptom of an iris melanoma is a visible spot on the iris or a discoloration of the iris in one eye. Many patients with an iris melanoma have no symptoms, and the lesion in these patients usually is detected on routine eye examination.

The typical iris melanoma is a localized, dark brown to tan iris tumor (Fig. 147-1). Features of a tumor that help the ophthalmologist assess its malignant potential include size of the lesion, its apparent cohesiveness, its intrinsic vascularity, and its effects on the adjacent ocular tissues.[4,5] As one would expect, the larger the lesion, the greater the concern about its potential malignancy. Thickness of the lesion greater than 0.5–1mm is of particular concern in such cases. Prominent intralesional blood vessels frequently develop within iris melanomas (Fig. 147-2). Such blood vessels are occasionally the source of spontaneous hyphema. Most iris melanomas appear well circumscribed and relatively cohesive, but others appear shaggy with dispersion of tumor cells, free pigment, or both onto the adjacent iris and trabecular meshwork. If tumor cells, liberated pigment, or macrophages clog the trabecular meshwork in such a case, a substantial rise in intraocular pressure can occur. Other features

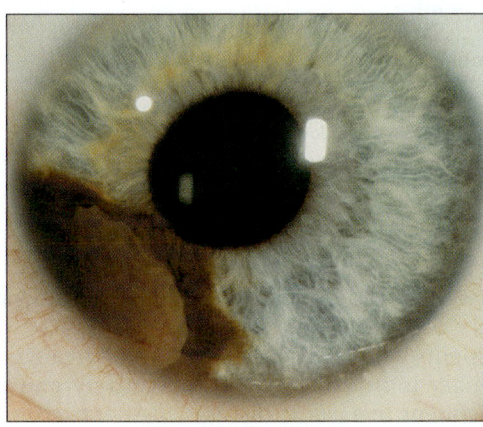

FIG. 147-1 ▪ Iris melanoma. Darkly melanotic iris tumor has a thick central nodule.

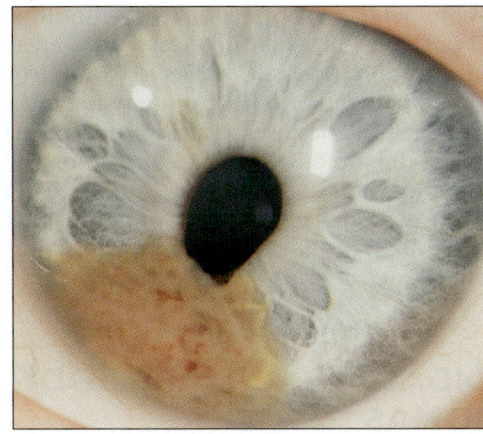

FIG. 147-2 ▪ Iris melanoma. A melanotic iris tumor contains prominent intrinsic blood vessels. Note peaking of the pupil toward the tumor and focal ectropion iridis.

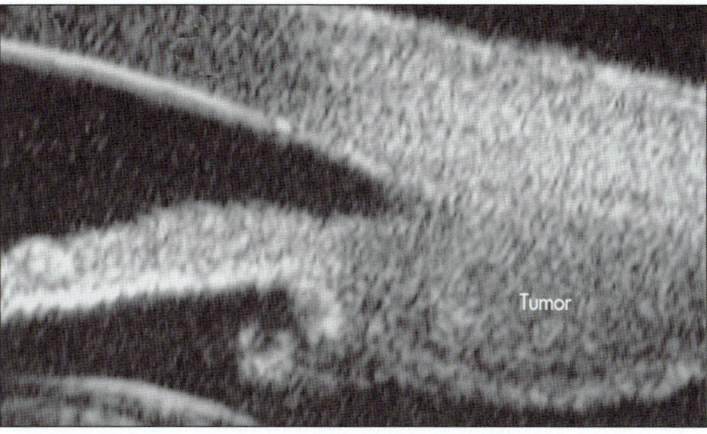

FIG. 147-3 ▪ Ultrasound biomicroscopy of iridociliary melanoma. Image shows the solid nature of the lesion and involvement of the ciliary body.

frequently associated with a melanocytic iris tumor include pupillary peaking (see Fig. 147-2), ectropion iridis, and iris splinting (failure to dilate fully in the zone of involvement); however, because all these features can also occur with benign nevi,[5] none of them should be regarded as a reliable indicator of malignancy.

DIAGNOSIS AND ANCILLARY TESTING

Transpupillary or transconjunctival trans-scleral transillumination of the eye is a relatively simple method that can be used to assess the posterior extent of melanocytic iris tumors. If the tumor is confined to the iris, transillumination will project no shadow in the pars plicata region. In contrast, if the tumor involves both the iris and the ciliary body, transillumination will reveal a shadow that extends into the pars plicata or even pars plana region. Because darkly melanotic uveal tissue blocks light transmission, this technique is usually unsuccessful in darkly pigmented eyes, including those affected by ocular melanocytosis.

Anterior segment photography, including goniophotography, is frequently used to document the size, extent, color, surface texture, vascularity, and location of melanocytic iris lesions. Such photographs are most useful in patients who are followed for documentation of lesion enlargement or other signs of possible malignant behavior in lieu of biopsy or treatment. Fluorescein angiography is used occasionally to assess the intralesional vascularity and filling pattern of presumed melanocytic iris tumors. Although some authors suggest that the angiographic findings help distinguish between benign nevi and malignant melanomas, most experienced ocular tumor experts believe that angiograms provide little if any useful diagnostic or prognostic information in

such cases. In some centers, indocyanine green angiography is now used as a diagnostic tool for iris tumors. There is no convincing evidence that this test provides any better diagnostic or prognostic information than does fluorescein angiography.

Ultrasound biomicroscopy enables clinicians to assess the size, cross-sectional shape, and internal characteristics of suspected iris melanomas (Fig. 147-3).[6] It allows reliable differentiation between solid and cystic lesions of the iris and also provides a baseline for future assessment of lesion enlargement in the case of tumors that are observed rather than treated. In most cases, it shows clearly whether the tumor is confined to the iris or involves the ciliary body as well.

Biopsy can be performed on melanocytic iris lesions that are larger or more worrisome than typical benign nevi but are not convincingly malignant melanomas in terms of their clinical features. For such tumors, either incisional biopsy or fine-needle aspiration biopsy can be performed.[7] Advantages of incisional biopsy include the relatively large tumor specimen that can be obtained and the ability to process the obtained tissue by standard histopathological methods. Disadvantages of incisional biopsy include the need for a corneal or limbal incision that must be closed surgically and the possibility of hyphema, postoperative glare, and other less common problems. Advantages of fine-needle aspiration biopsy include the relative simplicity of the technique and the possibility that several portions of the tumor may be sampled. Disadvantages of fine-needle aspiration biopsy include the limited number of cells obtained and the inability to evaluate tissue architecture on fine-needle aspirates of the tumor. If biopsy is performed and malignant melanoma is confirmed pathologically, one can justifiably advise the patient to undergo excision of the lesion or other intervention and risk the visual consequences of that treatment.

Baseline Systemic Evaluation

Unless the tumor is relatively large, has a substantial ciliary body component, causes pronounced elevation of intraocular pressure, or shows clinical evidence of extrascleral tumor extension, an extremely limited likelihood exists of detection of any clinical metastatic disease at the time of ocular tumor diagnosis. Consequently, a systemic metastatic search before treatment is probably unwarranted in most patients who have an iris melanoma. In patients who have any or all of the higher-risk characteristics mentioned earlier, however, a baseline metastatic search similar to the type suggested for patients with a choroidal or ciliary body melanoma (see later) is probably appropriate.

DIFFERENTIAL DIAGNOSIS

A list of the pertinent lesions in the differential diagnosis of iris melanomas is presented in Box 147-1.

PATHOLOGY

Iris melanoma is composed of atypical melanocytic cells that occupy and replace normal iris stroma. These cells tend to have a larger nuclear-to-cytoplasmic ratio, more prominent nucleoli, a higher likelihood of multiple nucleoli, and more frequent mitotic figures than do nevus cells. Tumor cells that have a fusiform shape and relatively mild atypia are termed spindle melanoma cells, and those that have a more spherical shape and more pronounced anaplasia are called epithelioid melanoma cells. The majority of iris melanomas are composed either exclusively of spindle melanoma cells or of an admixture of spindle melanoma cells and benign nevus cells.[8] Most of the remaining iris melanomas consist of an admixture of spindle and epithelioid melanoma cells. Relatively few iris melanomas are composed exclusively of epithelioid melanoma cells. In comparison with choroidal and ciliary body melanomas, iris melanomas are more likely to be composed exclusively of spindle melanoma cells and to be smaller at the time of detection and treatment. Consequently, the survival prognosis of patients who have iris melanomas is generally substantially better than that of patients who have choroidal or ciliary body melanomas.[9]

TREATMENT

Many suspected iris melanomas, especially those that are small, should be observed without intervention unless unequivocal enlargement occurs within a short time. Currently, no compelling evidence exists that prompt excision of small suspected iris melanomas improves the survival prognosis over that expected with observation alone.[5] Treatment of iris melanomas, when warranted, usually consists of excision of the tumor (iridectomy or iridocyclectomy; Box 147-2). Surgical techniques for such procedures have been described in detail by other authors.[10] Plaque radiotherapy and proton beam irradiation have been performed in a small number of cases and appear to be effective in short-term follow-up.[11] Enucleation is occasionally required for large iris melanomas that cannot be resected, diffuse iris melanomas associated with extensive seeding into the aqueous, iris melanomas extending transsclerally, and eyes rendered blind and painful by complications related to the tumor.[12]

COURSE AND OUTCOME

The typical iris melanoma grows relatively slowly but eventually replaces a substantial proportion of the iris and ciliary body. It can cause secondary glaucoma by invading the peripheral iris and trabecular meshwork in a ring growth pattern or by clogging the trabecular meshwork with macrophages that contain phagocytosed cellular debris. Tumor cells can extend extrasclerally along the scleral vascular and neural foramina in the anterior cil-

iary body region. The eye can become blind and painful as a consequence of tumor progression.

Most patients who have an iris melanoma treated by excision of the primary tumor do well postoperatively and do not develop subsequent metastatic disease.[9,13] After excision of an iris melanoma, the patient must be monitored on a regular basis for tumor recurrence in the adjacent iris or ciliary body and for development of satellite lesions caused by tumor cell dispersion before or during surgery. Ophthalmic follow-up evaluations are generally recommended at approximately 6-month intervals for the first 3–5 postexcision years and every year thereafter for life.

Important clinical prognostic factors for death from metastatic melanoma in patients who have primary iris melanoma and no evidence of metastatic disease at the time of diagnosis include the size of the tumor (the bigger the tumor, the worse the prognosis), the location of the tumor (tumors that involve the ciliary body are associated with a worse prognosis than are those confined to the iris), a diffuse or ring growth pattern, and extrascleral tumor extension.[5,13]

CHOROIDAL AND CILIARY BODY MELANOMAS

OCULAR MANIFESTATIONS

Although some choroidal and ciliary body melanomas are detected on ophthalmic evaluations prompted by the development of visual symptoms (e.g., blurred vision, visual field defect, flashes, floaters), many patients who have such a tumor are asymptomatic at the time of detection of the lesion on routine ophthalmic examination. Pain is unusual, although some advanced cases are associated with severe ocular and periocular pain (usually due to secondary glaucoma or spontaneous tumor necrosis). Virtually all ciliary body melanomas stimulate the development of dilated episcleral sentinel blood vessels (Fig. 147-4, A), extend through the sclera to form a melanotic epibulbar nodule (Fig. 147-4, B), or both.

The typical choroidal melanoma appears as a dark brown to golden solid tumor and has a biconvex, lenticular cross-sectional shape (Fig. 147-5, A). About 20% of choroidal malignant melanomas eventually break through the overlying Bruch's membrane and retinal pigment epithelium to form a nodular eruption beneath the retina. As this nodular eruption enlarges, the tumor commonly takes on a mushroom-like configuration (Fig. 147-5, B). This particular configuration is highly characteristic of choroidal melanoma.

Darkly melanotic choroidal melanomas commonly exhibit prominent clumps of orange lipofuscin pigment on their surface. These pigment clumps are not specific for choroidal melanomas and can be observed over some choroidal nevi and other benign choroidal tumors.[12] However, choroidal melanomas are much more likely to have prominent clumps of orange pigment on their surface than are benign simulating lesions.

Choroidal melanomas are commonly associated with secondary nonrhegmatogenous retinal detachment characterized by clear, serous, shifting subretinal fluid. In some cases, the fluid extends over and a short distance around the base of the lesion. In others, it accumulates to the extent that the retina is exten-

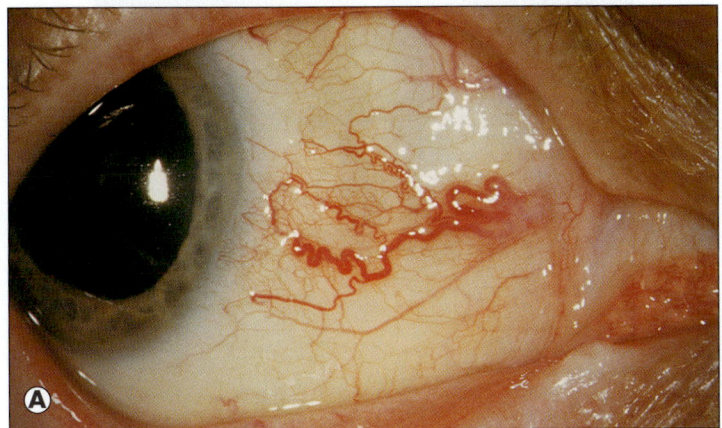

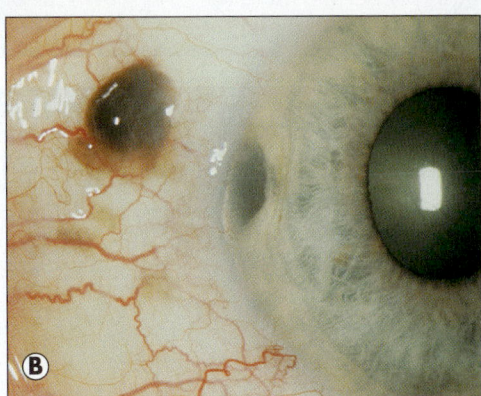

FIG. 147-4 ■ External indicators of underlying ciliary body melanoma. **A,** Sentinel blood vessels on the sclera overlying a ciliary body melanoma. **B,** Transscleral extension of an iridociliary melanoma. Note that the anterior margin of the intraocular tumor is in the peripheral iris.

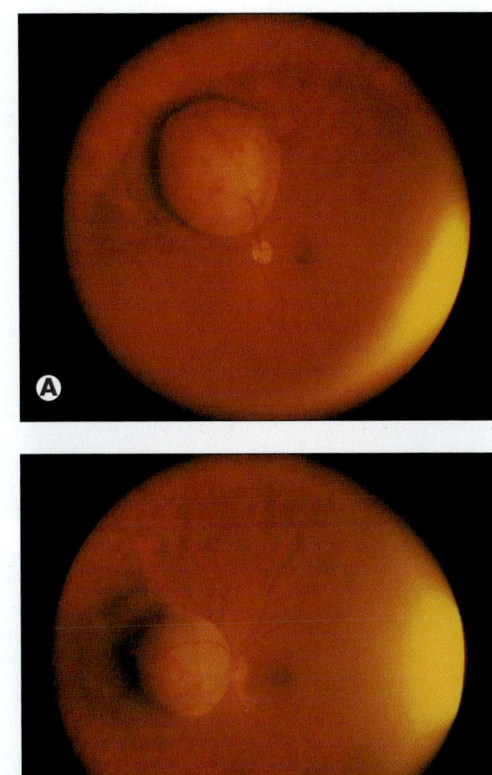

FIG. 147-5 ■ Typical shapes of choroidal melanomas. **A,** Dome-shaped choroidal melanoma. **B,** Mushroom-shaped choroidal melanoma.

sively or even totally detached. In some cases, the subretinal fluid is bloody, almost exclusively in eyes that have tumor eruption through Bruch's membrane. In still other cases, vitreous hemorrhage is a presenting manifestation, sometimes precluding a clear view of the intraocular tumor. In most if not all such cases, the choroidal or ciliary body melanoma has not only erupted through Bruch's membrane but also invaded the retina.

The typical ciliary body melanoma appears as a highly elevated, nodular, dark brown lesion in the peripheral fundus. Some of these tumors are thick enough to indent the lens in its equatorial region.

DIAGNOSIS AND ANCILLARY TESTING

B-scan ultrasonography of a choroidal or ciliary body malignant melanoma usually reveals a solid, acoustically dark (relatively sonolucent) mass that has a biconvex cross-sectional shape (Fig. 147-6, *A*). Choroidal melanomas that have erupted through Bruch's membrane show the more characteristic mushroom-like cross-sectional shape (Fig. 147-6, *B*). These tumors often have relative acoustic brightness in their caps but almost always show the characteristic relative internal sonolucency in their basal aspects.

Standardized A-scan ultrasonography of choroidal and ciliary body melanomas typically reveals low-amplitude internal reflectivity with a characteristic stepwise decremental reduction in echo spike amplitude from the front to the back of the lesion. Choroidal melanomas that have erupted through Bruch's membrane typically show high-amplitude internal reflectivity corresponding to the apical cap but low-amplitude internal reflectivity corresponding to the basal region. In many tumors, A-scan also reveals fluctuations in the height of some of the intralesional echoes coincident with the pulse. These fluctuations are indicative of the presence of prominent intralesional blood vessels fed from choroidal or posterior ciliary arteries.

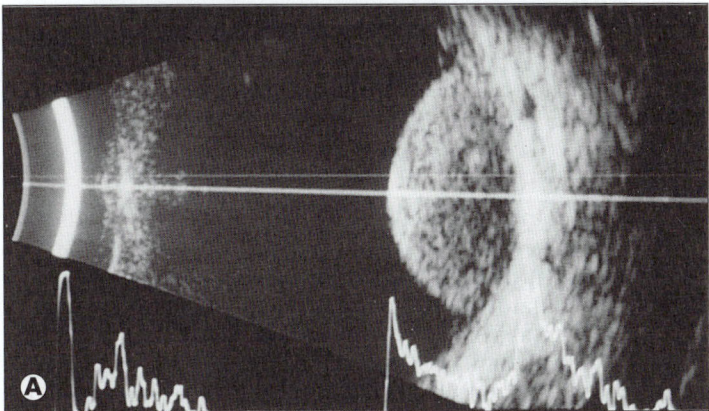

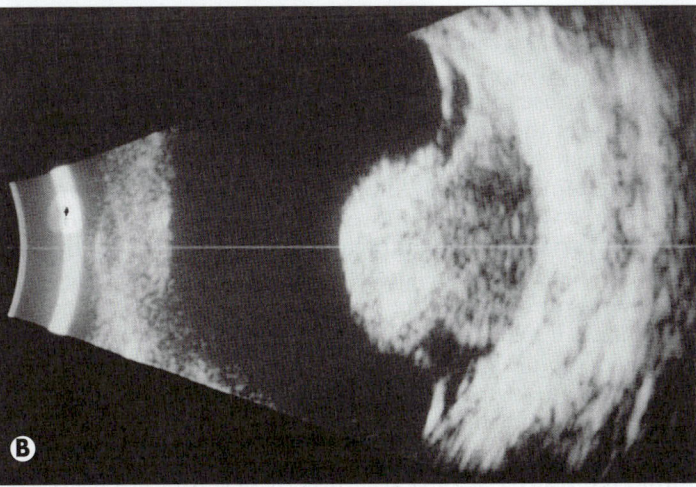

FIG. 147-6 ■ Ultrasonography of choroidal melanoma. **A,** B-scan of dome-shaped choroidal melanoma. **B,** B-scan of mushroom-shaped choroidal melanoma.

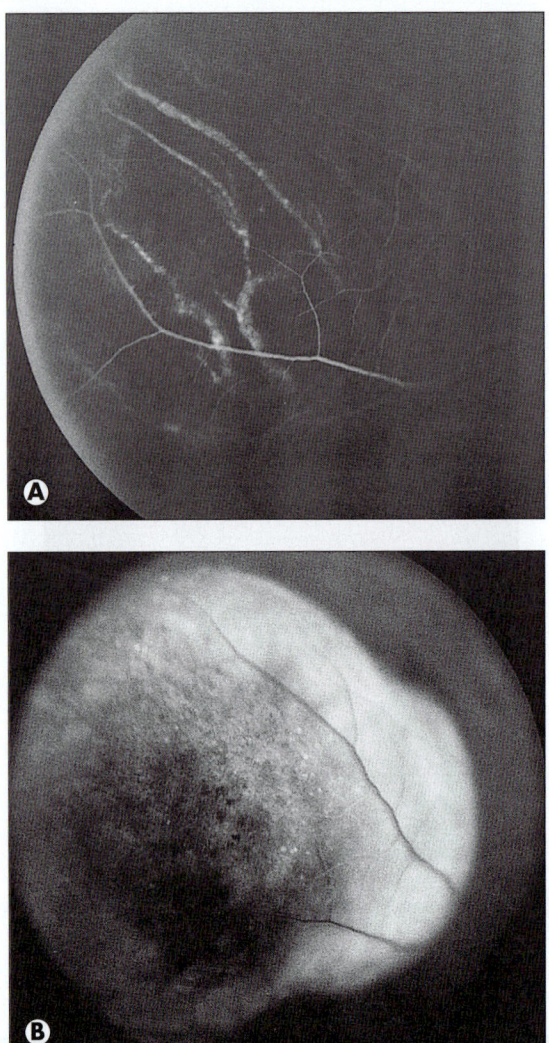

FIG. 147-7 ■ Fluorescein angiography of dome-shaped choroidal melanoma. **A,** Early phase frame shows filling of both retinal and intratumoral arteries. **B,** Late phase frame shows nonuniform hyperfluorescent staining of tumor.

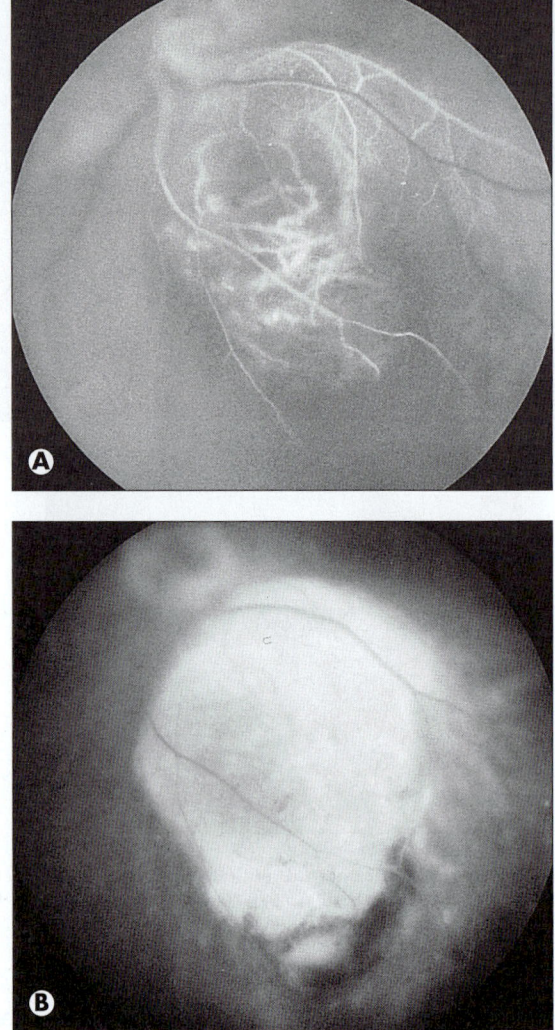

FIG. 147-8 ■ Fluorescein angiography of mushroom-shaped choroidal melanoma. **A,** Early laminar venous phase frame shows filling of intratumoral blood vessels. **B,** Late phase frame shows intense generalized staining of apical nodule and associated subretinal fluid.

Fluorescein angiography of choroidal melanomas yields several distinct patterns that depend on the cross-sectional shape of the tumor, its intrinsic and overlying pigmentation, the presence or absence of healthy overlying retinal pigment epithelium, and the presence or absence of retinal invasion and retinal detachment. The typical dark brown choroidal melanoma that has not broken through Bruch's membrane characteristically appears hypofluorescent throughout the early phases of the study (Fig. 147-7, *A*). A few large-caliber intralesional blood vessels can be detected in many cases in the early phase frames. Blood vessels of this type usually become ill defined and smudgy within a few seconds because of profuse fluorescein leakage into the extracellular space of the tumor. By the late frames of the study, the fluorescein that has leaked from the intralesional blood vessels stains the tumor intensely, along with any associated subretinal fluid (Fig. 147-7, *B*). Fluorescein also tends to accumulate in pinpoint foci at the retinal pigment epithelial level by the late phase of the study. Amelanotic melanomas show less lesional hypofluorescence and more prominent intralesional blood vessels than their melanotic counterparts but otherwise appear similar angiographically.

Fluorescein angiography of choroidal melanomas that have erupted through Bruch's membrane typically reveals prominent apical intralesional blood vessels that fill slowly but intensely during the study (Fig. 147-8). These vessels leak profusely and result in intense late staining of the tumor and any associated subretinal fluid. If a melanoma has invaded the overlying retina, the retinal blood vessels at the area of invasion can be masked by an overlying plaque of pigmented tumor cells. In such cases, the area of retinal invasion may appear completely nonfluorescent throughout the entire study. The small retinal blood vessels at the margins of an area of retinal invasion commonly leak fluorescein by the late phase of the study.

Indocyanine green angiography of choroidal melanomas shows most tumors to be quite hypofluorescent throughout the study.[14] However, large-caliber intralesional blood vessels usually are better defined on indocyanine green angiography than on fluorescein angiography, particularly if the study is performed using a scanning laser ophthalmoscope.

Computed tomography (CT) is capable of imaging most choroidal and ciliary body melanomas. Virtually all melanomas of the choroid and ciliary body (except for those that are totally necrotic) exhibit pronounced contrast enhancement. However, because almost all other viable intraocular tumors also show contrast enhancement, this feature is not usually of any differential diagnostic importance. Subretinal fluid associated with a choroidal or ciliary body melanoma appears almost isodense with the tumor on both nonenhanced and contrast-enhanced images.

Magnetic resonance imaging (MRI) is also used occasionally to image choroidal and ciliary body melanomas.[15] It appears to have greater differential diagnostic value than CT for differentiating melanomas from simulating lesions. The great majority of malignant melanomas of the choroid and ciliary body appear bright (hyperintense) relative to the dark vitreous on T1-weighted images and dark (hypointense) relative to the bright vitreous on T2-

Differential Diagnosis of Choroidal and Ciliary Body Melanomas

Choroidal nevus (including melanocytoma of optic disc)
Metastatic carcinoma to choroid or ciliary body
Disciform lesion (central or peripheral)
Subretinal or subpigment epithelial hematoma
Localized suprachoroidal hematoma
Circumscribed choroidal hemangioma
Nodular posterior scleritis
Choroidal osteoma
Congenital hypertrophy of retinal pigment epithelium
Reactive hyperplasia of retinal pigment epithelium
Syndrome of bilateral diffuse uveal melanocytic proliferation associated with systemic carcinoma
Massive gliosis of retina
Ocular melanocytosis

weighted images. Few intraocular tumors of other types have consistently shown this particular pattern. Unfortunately, some atypical choroidal and ciliary body melanomas, most notably ones that are almost completely amelanotic, do not yield this characteristic MRI pattern. Another important use of MRI is the detection of posterior extrascleral tumor extension.

Open surgical biopsy is not generally advised for suspected malignant melanomas of the choroid and ciliary body (unless the biopsy is intended to achieve complete tumor resection). Previous experience with incisional biopsy techniques for suspected choroidal and ciliary body melanomas showed unacceptably high rates of local tumor recurrence and death from metastatic disease after the biopsy.[16] In recent years, however, fine-needle aspiration biopsy methods have been used before treatment in selected choroidal and ciliary body melanomas.[17] Although implantation of a few melanoma cells along the scleral needle tract has been documented pathologically after fine-needle aspiration biopsy,[18] this type of biopsy has not been associated with any clinical tumor recurrence along the needle tract to date in eyes preserved by some modality after biopsy.

Baseline Systemic Evaluation

A standard baseline systemic assessment of the extent of disease generally consists of a complete physical examination; selected blood tests, which usually include at least a complete blood count and a serum liver enzyme panel; chest radiograph; and CT scan (with contrast), MRI, or ultrasound evaluation of the abdominal organs (especially the liver).[19] The great majority of patients (approximately 98%) who have a choroidal or ciliary body malignant melanoma have no detectable extraocular or metastatic disease at the time of detection and diagnosis of the ocular tumor.[20] Those who have concurrent clinically detectable metastatic uveal melanoma at baseline evaluation usually have a very large intraocular tumor and frequently have nodular extrascleral tumor extension.

DIFFERENTIAL DIAGNOSIS

The most important lesions in the differential diagnosis of choroidal and ciliary body melanomas are listed in Box 147-3.

PATHOLOGY

As mentioned earlier in the section on iris melanomas, all uveal melanomas are composed of anaplastic melanocytic cells that have a relatively large nuclear-to-cytoplasmic ratio and one or more prominent nucleoli.[21] Most tumors of this type also have relatively frequent mitotic figures. Tumor cells that have less pronounced anaplasia are termed spindle melanoma

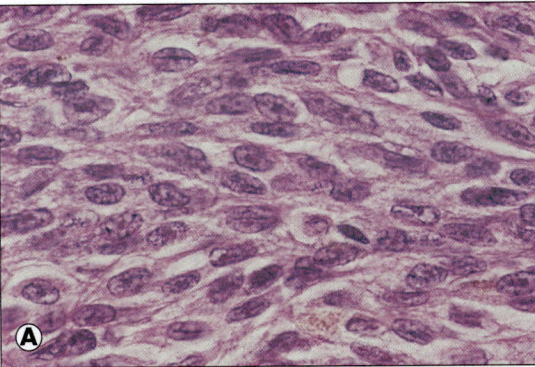

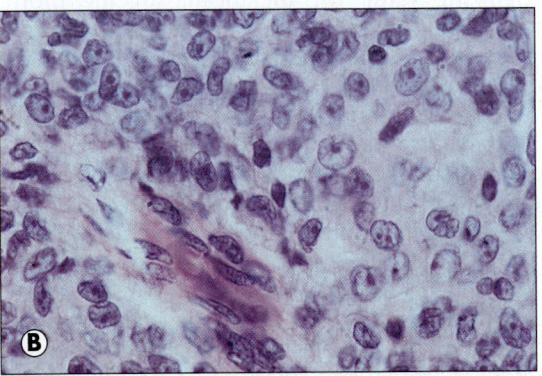

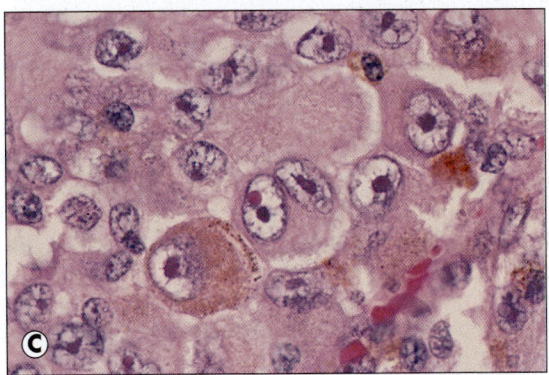

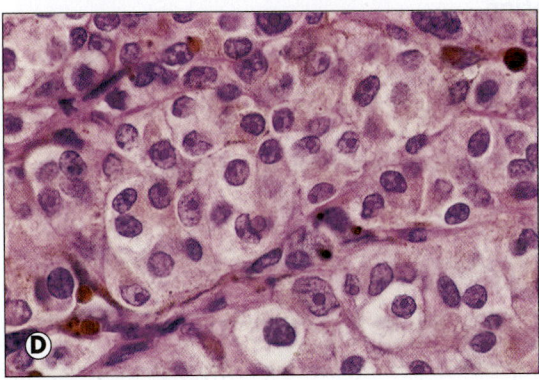

FIG. 147-9 ■ Histopathology of posterior uveal melanoma. **A,** Spindle cell melanoma. **B,** Mixed-cell melanoma. **C,** Epithelioid cell melanoma. **D,** Vascular loops and networks that separate lobules of choroidal melanoma.

cells (Fig. 147-9, A), and those that exhibit more pronounced anaplasia are called epithelioid melanoma cells (Fig. 147-9, C). Precise morphological criteria for the two cell types have not been established. Uveal melanomas are generally classified as spindle cell melanomas if they contain only spindle cells (see Fig. 147-9, A), mixed-cell melanomas if they are composed of an admixture of spindle cells and epithelioid cells without a preponderance of epithelioid cells (see Fig. 147-9, B), and epithelioid cell melanomas if they are composed entirely or predominantly of epithelioid cells (see Fig. 147-9, C). In many independent studies, spindle cell melanomas have been shown to be associated with the most favorable survival prognosis, epithelioid cell melanomas with the least favorable survival prognosis, and mixed-cell melanomas with an intermediate survival prognosis.[21] Some choroidal and ciliary body melanomas contain only necrotic cells on histopathological study, and a cell type cannot be determined for such tumors.

In comparison with iris melanomas, choroidal and ciliary body melanomas are more likely to be composed of epithelioid melanoma cells and to be substantially larger at the time of detection and treatment. Consequently, the survival prognosis for patients who have choroidal or ciliary body melanomas is much worse than that for patients who have iris melanomas.[22]

Many pathological features other than melanoma cell type have prognostic value for melanoma-specific mortality.[21-23] Unfavorable pathological prognostic factors include larger tumor size, presence of fibrovascular loops and networks within the tumor (see Fig. 147-9, D), larger calculated values of various cytomorphometric parameters of the tumor (mean nuclear diameter and area, standard deviation of nuclear area, mean nucleolar diameter and area, standard deviation of nucleolar area), presence of scleral invasion, presence of trans-scleral tumor extension, involvement of the ciliary body, higher mitotic index of the tumor, and greater level of pigmentation of tumor cells. Specific cytogenetic abnormalities (monosomy 3, partial duplication of chromosome 8, and others) have also been associated with increased risk of metastasis and metastatic death in patients with primary choroidal and ciliary body melanomas.[24,25]

TREATMENT

Many therapeutic options are available for choroidal and ciliary body melanomas (Box 147-4). Factors that influence the therapeutic decision include the size and extent of the intraocular tumor, location of the tumor within the eye, presence or absence of extrascleral tumor extension, presence or absence of clinically detectable metastasis to other organs, visual status of the affected eye, visual status of the unaffected eye, age and general health of the patient, availability of the various treatments, and personal preferences and biases of the patient and physician.

Enucleation

At present, enucleation of the eye containing the tumor is still one of the more commonly employed therapeutic methods for patients who have choroidal or ciliary body melanomas. Enucleation is an aggressive local treatment designed to rid the body of the cancer. It has been in use longer than any of the al-

---

BOX 147-4

Treatment Options for Choroidal and Ciliary Body Melanomas

Enucleation
Radiation therapy
• Plaque radiotherapy (iodine-125, ruthenium-106, palladium-103)
• Proton beam irradiation
• Gamma knife and stereotactic radiosurgery
Microsurgical resection
• External trans-scleral resection
• Transvitreal endoresection
Photocoagulation and laser therapy
Photodynamic therapy
Hyperthermia
Cryotherapy
Observation (appropriate only for patients with small or dormant-appearing tumors or poor general health)
Exenteration
Chemotherapy (currently employed only as palliative therapy for metastatic disease)

---

ternative treatments, and it is certainly the simplest of the available treatments. Surprisingly, there are no reliable natural history data on the outcomes of untreated patients with choroidal and ciliary body melanomas. Because of this, there is no convincing evidence that enucleation improves the survival prognosis of affected patients compared with no treatment at all. More disturbingly, a substantial body of evidence obtained from the analysis of survival distributions of patients undergoing enucleation suggests that enucleation may actually worsen rather than improve a patient's survival prognosis.[26] The hypothesis that enucleation worsens the survival prognosis of patients who have choroidal or ciliary body melanomas (Zimmerman-McLean hypothesis) has been neither proved nor disproved.

Although all patients who have choroidal or ciliary body melanomas can be managed by enucleation, this method of treatment is most strongly indicated for those with tumors that cause the eye to be blind and painful, extremely large intraocular tumors, or tumors that surround or invade the optic disc. For such patients, especially those whose tumor has extended transsclerally into the orbit, pre-enucleation radiation therapy (20Gy dose in five fractions of 4Gy each over 5–7 days immediately before enucleation) is employed occasionally as adjuvant therapy.[27] Results from the Collaborative Ocular Melanoma Study and several nonrandomized comparative survival studies indicate that pre-enucleation radiation therapy does not improve survival appreciably compared with enucleation alone.[28] However, pre-enucleation radiation therapy may lessen the recurrence rate of melanoma in the anophthalmic orbit in such patients.[29]

As long as uveal melanoma cells have not metastasized via the bloodstream to distant organs before or at the time of removal of the eye, enucleation is curative; however, microscopic metastasis cannot be detected reliably by currently available methods. Consequently, failure of baseline medical tests to show metastatic disease before enucleation does not guarantee that metastasis will not develop in the future. Unfortunately, approximately half of all patients who have a choroidal or ciliary body melanoma treated by enucleation eventually die of metastatic melanoma.[22] Cosmetic results with an ocular prosthesis are quite satisfactory. Most patients adapt well to their monocular status within a few months.

Radiation Therapy

Radiation therapy is probably the most commonly employed method of management for choroidal and ciliary body melanomas today. Two principal methods of irradiation are currently in use for such tumors. In plaque radiotherapy, a radioactive device (plaque) is sutured to the episcleral surface of the eye directly exterior to the tumor. The radioisotopes used most commonly in episcleral plaques are ruthenium-l06 (mostly in Europe) and iodine-125 (in the United States). A plaque that is generally at least 3mm larger in diameter than the measured maximal basal diameter of the tumor is selected for the treatment. Plaques are constructed in such a way that they typically deliver a radiation dose of 80–100Gy to the apex of the tumor during a treatment interval of about 3–5 days. Implantation and removal of the radioactive plaque are generally performed under local anesthesia. Depending on national, regional, and local radiation safety guidelines, patients may have to remain in the hospital during the period of plaque treatment, but they can usually be discharged on the day the plaque is removed.

The second method of local tumor irradiation currently in use is proton beam irradiation. This treatment modality is much less widely available than plaque radiotherapy. Charged particle beam radiotherapy consists of surgical localization of the tumor base, suturing of radiopaque markers (tantalum rings) to the sclera around the tumor base, computer-assisted treatment simulation, and, finally, tumor treatment with the charged particle beam while the eye is maintained in a stable direction of gaze.

The treatment is generally given in four or five equivalent fractions over 4–7 days starting several days after the placement of the tantalum rings. The standard target dose is in the range of 50–70Gy.

Plaque and charged particle beam radiation therapy appear to be most appropriate for patients who have relatively small tumors (preferably <15mm at greatest diameter and <8mm thick) located 3mm or more from the optic disc and fovea. Older patients are more likely to be advised to undergo treatment by plaque or charged particle bea radiotherapy than are younger patients.

Plaque radiotherapy has been used extensively in Europe and the United States during the past 25 years. Charged particle beam radiotherapy has been used in a small number of centers since the mid-1970s. Both methods of local tumor radiotherapy cause substantial clinical regression of most treated tumors (Fig. 147-10). Several nonrandomized comparative survival studies that included statistical adjustment for recognized differences in baseline prognostic clinical variables have shown that plaque and charged particle beam radiotherapy are essentially equivalent to enucleation in terms of their success in preventing death from metastatic disease.[30-34] The recently published results of the randomized Collaborative Ocular Melanoma Study of enucleation versus iodine-125 plaque radiotherapy confirmed the equivalency of these two treatments.[35]

Vision in the treated eye usually remains the same as before treatment or even improves for several months to several years after uveal melanoma radiation therapy; however, many treated eyes eventually lose a substantial amount of vision as a consequence of radiation retinopathy, optic papillopathy, cataract, or neovascular glaucoma (Fig. 147-11).[36,37] Factors that influence how much vision will be lost and how soon the vision will de-

teriorate include the location of the posterior edge of the tumor relative to the optic disc and fovea, the visual acuity before treatment, the presence or absence of macular retinal detachment, and the thickness of the tumor. Some systemic factors, such as diabetes mellitus, may also worsen a patient's prognosis for retention of useful vision in the treated eye. Some eyes treated by plaque or proton beam radiotherapy eventually become severely painful as a complication of the treatment, usually because of neovascular glaucoma. Furthermore, 10–15% of patients treated initially by plaque radiotherapy and 3–5% of those treated by charged particle irradiation experience local tumor relapse.[38-40] Patients who develop a blind, painful eye or local tumor relapse must undergo supplemental treatment, which usually consists of enucleation.[41,42]

Gamma knife radiotherapy[43] and stereotactic radiosurgery[44] are alternative radiation therapies being used in several centers to treat selected patients with choroidal and ciliary body melanomas. No long-term results of these treatments are yet available.

Observation

At the other extreme of treatment from enucleation is observation (i.e., periodic re-evaluation of the tumor with appropriate documentation of its size and appearance to permit the detection of abrupt enlargement or other signs of malignant potential).[45,46] Observation without intervention is probably an appropriate option for patients in whom the differentiation between nevus and melanoma cannot be made with reasonable certainty, and it is almost certainly advisable for those who have coexistent life-threatening medical conditions that preclude surgical intervention. However, observation is not deemed advis-

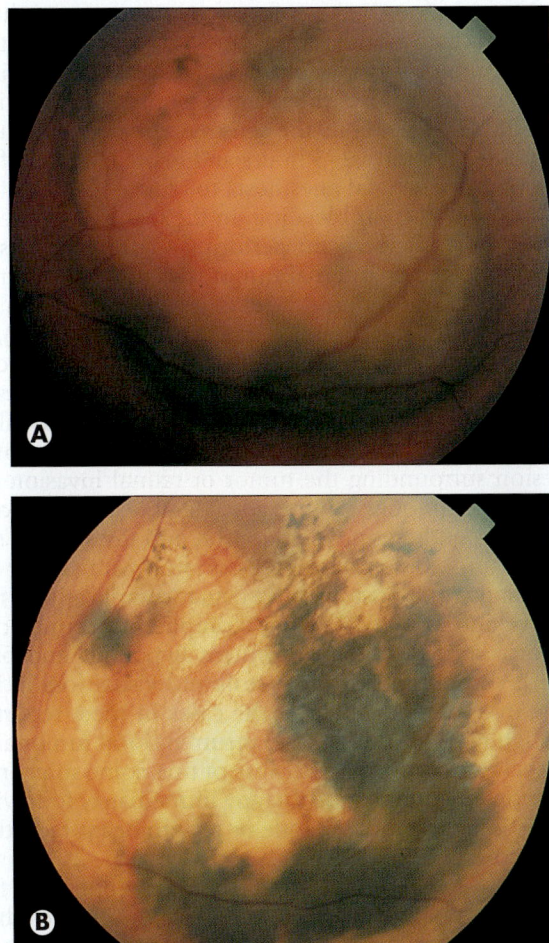

FIG. 147-10 ■ **Plaque radiotherapy of choroidal melanoma. A,** Choroidal melanoma before treatment. **B,** Partially regressed lesion 24 months after iodine-125 plaque radiotherapy.

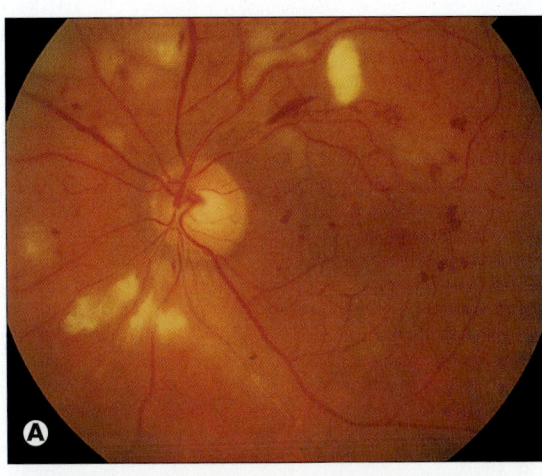

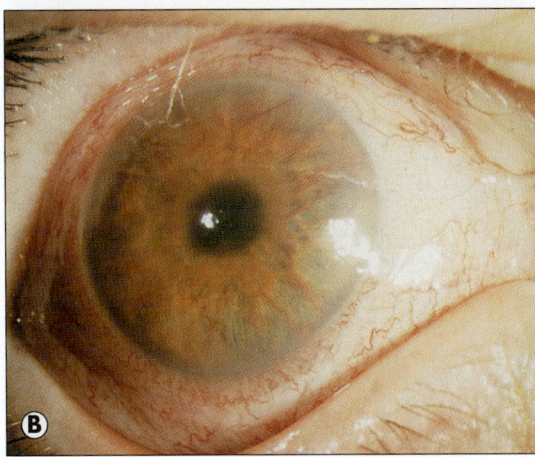

FIG. 147-11 ■ **Ocular complications of plaque radiotherapy for uveal melanoma. A,** Radiation retinopathy. **B,** Radiation-induced neovascular glaucoma with prominent rubeosis iridis.

able by most ocular tumor experts for most patients who have an unequivocal malignant melanoma. The obvious concern about observation is that a patient whose tumor enlarges substantially during observation may have an increased risk of death from metastatic melanoma.[47]

Photocoagulation

Photocoagulation is a treatment that attempts to destroy a choroidal tumor with high-intensity light energy (Fig. 147-12). It is applicable only to relatively small tumors (<3mm thick and <7mm in basal diameter). In this treatment, the clinician uses either a xenon arc photocoagulator or a laser to burn the tumor.[48] Treatment is usually provided first around the margin of the tumor to cause a strong chorioretinal adhesion. At subsequent sessions, the tumor itself is treated, usually in a concentric fashion from the periphery toward the center. Multiple photocoagulation sessions are required, typically at 2–4-week intervals, until the tumor is totally eradicated. Because relatively high power settings are required for such treatments, retrobulbar or periocular anesthesia is required before each treatment session. Sometimes an audible pop and the appearance of a small gas bubble accompany an intense burn, especially one created with a laser using a very short exposure time. If successful, photocoagulation causes total destruction not only of the tumor and its blood supply but also of the retina overlying the tumor. Consequently, this treatment produces a permanent scotoma or sectorial defect in the field of vision. If the tumor is located a substantial distance away from the macular region and optic disc, reasonably good visual acuity can be retained after successful photocoagulation. Conversely, if the tumor is located next to the optic disc or in the central macular region, vision in the affected eye is likely to be poor immediately after treatment.

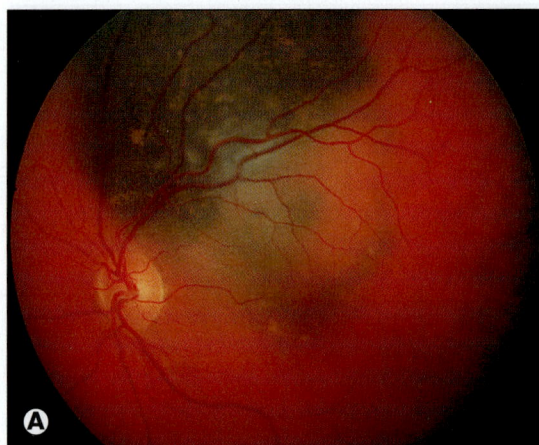

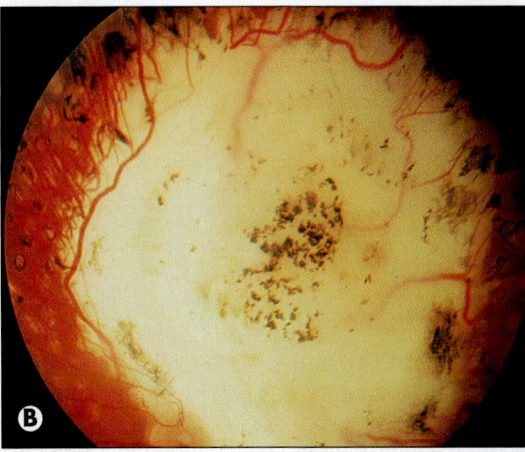

FIG. 147-12 ■ **Photocoagulation of choroidal melanoma. A,** Pretreatment appearance of a small but growing choroidal melanoma. **B,** Regressed lesion 34 months after initial treatment.

Unfortunately, follow-up studies have shown relatively high rates of local treatment failure and delayed local tumor relapse following photocoagulation alone.[48]

Noncoagulative Laser Therapy

Laser therapy can be performed using various low-power, long-duration methods that are quite different from photocoagulation. In low-power, long-duration laser therapy, the tumor is heated to subcoagulative levels with transpupillary laser light.[49,50] Because of this, some clinicians refer to this treatment as laser hyperthermia or transpupillary thermotherapy (TTT). A diode infrared laser (810nm) is employed for deep penetration of the laser energy. The laser treatment is delivered using a slit lamp, operating microscope, or indirect ophthalmoscope delivery system. Relatively large spot sizes of 2–3mm are commonly employed for this treatment. The duration of each exposure is generally at least 60 seconds. The appropriate endpoint of each spot is a dull white discoloration of the tumor without visible effects on the large, overlying retinal blood vessels. Overlapping spots are applied until the entire tumor has been treated. Although the temperature is not monitored during treatment, animal experiments have shown that low-power, long-duration laser therapy can produce sustained intralesional temperatures in the range of 45–60°C (113–140°F). Unfortunately, follow-up studies after TTT alone have shown relatively high rates of local tumor failure and late tumor relapse,[49,50] including some instances of extrascleral tumor extension into the orbit.[51]

Microsurgical Resection

Microsurgical resection (surgical excision of the tumor) has been used for many years to treat selected patients who have choroidal or ciliary body melanomas. In the commonly employed trans-scleral resection technique,[52] the surgeon creates a partial-thickness scleral flap directly over the tumor; cuts the tumor out of the eye, along with some of the adjacent normal uveal tissue, using microscissors; and then closes the scleral opening with multiple interrupted sutures. If possible, the sensory retina is left intact. The surgery routinely requires 2–3 hours and is preferably performed under hypotensive general anesthesia to reduce the risk of major intraoperative intraocular bleeding. In the less common endoresection method,[53] the surgeon performs a complete pars plana vitrectomy, followed by internal tumor resection using vitreoretinal instruments. The retina that overlies the tumor can be resected along with the tumor (transretinal technique), or a retinotomy can be created some distance from the tumor, and the retina reflected away from the lesion before tumor resection (subretinal technique). The transretinal technique is usually employed in eyes that already have a firm, laser-induced chorioretinal adhesion surrounding the tumor or retinal invasion by the tumor. These techniques require considerable surgical skill and experience. Depending on case selection and the surgeon's experience, these procedures may be associated with highly varied rates of operative and postoperative ocular complications, including massive intraocular bleeding, complicated retinal detachment, choroidal detachment, persistent hypotony, and phthisis bulbi. Such complications cause profound visual loss in the affected eye in approximately half the cases in most reported series.[52,53] High rates of residual and recurrent local tumor also occur after such procedures.[54,55] Because of this, some surgeons now perform supplemental plaque therapy immediately following external resection and advise plaque or proton beam radiotherapy prior to endoresection.[55,56]

Trans-scleral resection appears to be most applicable for patients who are relatively young and systemically healthy and who have rather thick malignant melanomas of the ciliary body or peripheral choroid that are no more than 12–13mm in basal dimension. Endoresection appears to be most applicable for patients who have relatively small choroidal melanomas adjacent to or partly overlying the optic disc. In these patients, the best alternative would probably be enucleation of the eye rather than radiation therapy. For patients whose eyes tolerate the surgery well, there is an excellent chance for long-term stability of the postoperative visual acuity and field. The survival prognosis of patients who have similar tumors treated by primary enucleation versus local resection appears to be nearly equal.[57]

Exenteration

Exenteration of the orbit is occasionally performed for patients who have choroidal or ciliary body melanomas associated with massive extrascleral tumor extension or orbital recurrence after enucleation. However, survival data on such patients suggest that this radical surgery does not improve their survival chances compared with more conservative management approaches.[58,59] In view of this, clinicians generally are advised not to perform a mutilating exenteration for limited extraocular melanoma extension or localized orbital recurrence. Many patients who have such limited orbital disease can be managed at least as effectively in terms of survival prognosis by enucleation of the eye or debulking of the orbital tumor, coupled with preoperative or postoperative orbital external beam radiation therapy (usually about 50Gy in multiple fractions over 4–5 weeks).

Hyperthermia Therapy

Hyperthermia therapy entails treatment of a lesion by the application of local heat. When the temperature of a tumor is raised by several degrees Centigrade for even a few minutes, marked cellular damage and subsequent tumor regression usually result. The local heating is provided with a focused external ultrasonic beam[60] or a plaque that generates microwaves.[61] Very few patients with malignant melanoma of the choroid or ciliary body have been treated using hyperthermia, and most of those who have undergone hyperthermia treatment have done so in conjunction with plaque radiation therapy. True hyperthermia therapy employs a temperature-measuring instrument (thermocouple) to determine the temperature in (or at least on the surface of) a tumor during therapy. Some clinicians have suggested that tumor laser therapy using a relatively low power setting, long-duration exposures, and a laser of long-wavelength (infrared) light (i.e., TTT) is a form of hyperthermia treatment. Although some of the effect of this therapy is likely to be attributable to tumor heating, temperature is not monitored during this treatment. Consequently, it is inappropriate to regard TTT as true hyperthermia treatment.

Photodynamic Therapy

Photodynamic therapy employs a sensitizing drug and a subsequent low-power laser treatment to cause tumor destruction by means of a photochemical reaction.[62] Few patients worldwide have undergone this treatment for choroidal melanoma, and most ophthalmologists currently consider photodynamic therapy an unproven treatment for such tumors.

Cryotherapy

Cryotherapy has been used extensively to treat retinoblastomas but has not gained wide acceptance for the treatment of choroidal and ciliary body melanomas. However, several case reports have indicated that this treatment is effective against selected tumors of this type.[63]

Chemotherapy

Chemotherapy is not currently advocated as treatment for patients who have choroidal or ciliary body melanomas confined to the eye. This is because no currently available chemotherapy regimen has produced clinical regression of the intraocular tumor on a consistent basis. Patients who develop clinical metastatic disease are likely to be advised about various chemotherapy regimens and approaches that might be used in an attempt to control the disease.[64] Unfortunately, no chemotherapy regimen has been able to eradicate malignant melanoma once it has metastasized.

Multimodal Therapy

Several of the previously mentioned treatment methods are used in combination for choroidal and ciliary body melanomas. The most common multimodal therapies are combined plaque radiotherapy and laser treatment,[65,66] combined plaque radiotherapy and hyperthermia treatment,[61] and combined microsurgical resection and plaque radiotherapy.[55] These combined treatments appear to increase the rate and extent of local tumor regression and decrease the rate of local tumor relapse compared with single-modality therapy. However, they also cause more early post-treatment visual impairment than do single-method treatments. At present, there is no evidence that such combined modalities significantly improve a patient's survival prognosis compared with single-method treatment.

Randomized Clinical Trials

The Collaborative Ocular Melanoma Study was a multicenter study of uveal melanoma management sponsored by the National Eye Institute of the United States.[67] It recruited patients from 1986 through 1999. This study evaluated pre-enucleation radiation therapy versus enucleation alone for large choroidal melanomas and iodine-125 plaque radiotherapy versus enucleation for medium-sized choroidal melanomas. Neither trial showed any clinically important difference in survival.[2,35,48] Both clinical trials confirmed the results of previously published, nonrandomized clinical trials that included statistical adjustment for recognized intergroup differences in baseline clinical prognostic factors.[30,33,34,68]

COURSE AND OUTCOME

As surprising as it may seem, the natural history of untreated choroidal and ciliary body melanomas is not well documented. Relatively few patients with presumed choroidal or ciliary body melanomas have been followed for long periods without intervention when progressive tumor enlargement has occurred. Furthermore, relatively few untreated patients with choroidal or ciliary body melanomas have ever been documented to develop metastatic disease and die of metastatic melanoma.[20] Most of the patients with presumed choroidal or ciliary body melanomas who have been followed without treatment have had either small tumors (i.e., a large nevus versus a small melanoma) or clinically dormant tumors. These highly selected patients are not representative of the total spectrum of patients with choroidal and ciliary body melanomas, and their clinical course under observation without intervention cannot be extrapolated to the larger group of more typical patients who have larger and actively growing tumors.

Important clinical prognostic factors for death from metastatic melanoma in patients who have primary choroidal or ciliary body melanomas but no clinical evidence of metastatic disease at the time of diagnosis include the size of the tumor (the bigger the tumor, the worse the prognosis), the location of the tumor (tumors within the ciliary body are associated with a worse prognosis than are those confined to the choroid), the age of the patient at the time of diagnosis (the older the patient, the worse the short-term survival prognosis), and extrascleral tumor extension.[69] Choroidal and ciliary body melanomas are generally categorized on the basis of largest linear tumor dimension into small (10mm in maximal linear dimension), medium (10–15mm in maximal linear dimension), and large (>15mm in maximal linear dimension) groups.

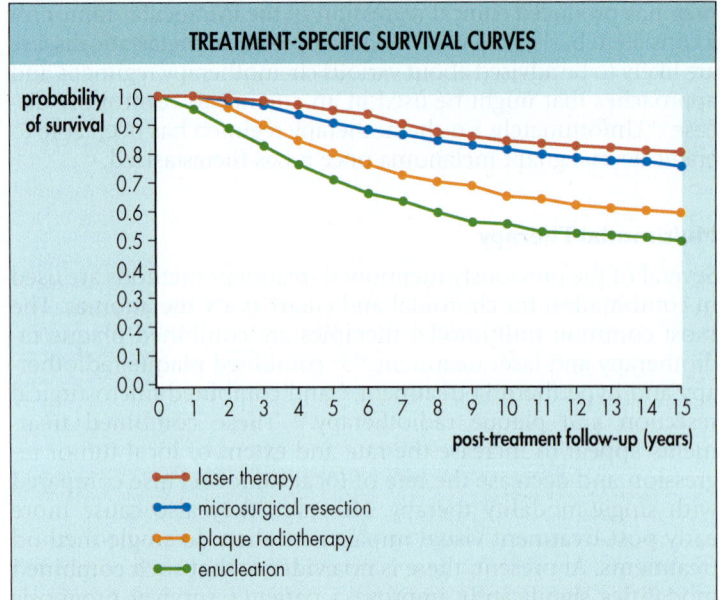

FIG. 147-13 ■ **Survival curves of patients with primary choroidal or ciliary body melanoma as a function of initial treatment method.** These curves are based on deaths from metastatic uveal melanoma only. The differences among the curves reflect baseline differences in susceptibility to uveal melanoma metastasis related to criteria used to select patients for each treatment; they are not intended to imply the relative effectiveness of the treatments for equivalent tumors. (Data from private practice of James J. Augsburger, M.D.)

Patients who have choroidal or ciliary body melanomas are routinely advised to undergo periodic physical examinations, blood tests for liver enzyme levels, and imaging studies such as chest radiographs and ultrasonography or MRI of the liver. The cost-benefit ratio of such testing for metastatic uveal melanoma, a condition for which there is currently no effective therapy, is high; consequently, the appropriateness of such testing is controversial.[19]

A patient's prognosis for survival after detection and treatment of a primary choroidal or ciliary body melanoma is a function of many factors, including absence versus presence and extent of metastatic disease at the time of intraocular tumor detection, age at the time of treatment, size of the intraocular tumor, absence versus presence and extent of extrascleral tumor extension, absence versus presence of ciliary body involvement, and many histopathological and cytogenetic features of the tumor (which are not determinable unless the tumor is biopsied prior to treatment or treated by enucleation of the eye or en bloc tumor resection). At present, no compelling scientific evidence exists that one form of locally effective treatment is substantially better than any other in terms of preventing metastatic disease or prolonging survival. In spite of this, comparison of survival curves in patient subgroups treated by different methods reveals substantial differences (Fig. 147-13); however, these differences are caused mainly by inequalities in baseline prognostic factors (such as tumor size and patient age) among the subgroups and not by differential effectiveness of the various forms of treatment. Fortunately, the vast majority of patients who have choroidal or ciliary body melanomas retain good vision in at least one eye for the remainder of their lives. Furthermore, most patients who undergo one of the conservative treatments mentioned earlier retain the affected eye, and at least some of these patients also retain good vision in the treated eye.

REFERENCES

1. Egan KM, Seddon JM, Glynn RJ, et al. Epidemiologic aspects of uveal melanoma. Surv Ophthalmol. 1988;32:239–51.
2. Iskovich J, Ackerman C, Andrew H, et al. An epidemiological study of posterior uveal melanoma in Israel, 1961–1989. Int J Cancer. 1995;61:291–5.
3. Singh AD, Boghosian-Sell L, Wary KK, et al. Cytogenetic findings in primary uveal melanoma. Cancer Genet Cytogenet. 1994;72:109–15.
4. Shields JA, Sanborn GE, Augsburger JJ. The differential diagnosis of malignant melanoma of the iris. A clinical study of 200 patients. Ophthalmology. 1983; 90:716–20.
5. Harbour JW, Augsburger JJ, Eagle RC. Initial management and follow-up of melanocytic iris tumors. Ophthalmology. 1995;102:1987–93.
6. Pavlin CJ, McWhae JA, McGowan HD, Foster FS. Ultrasound biomicroscopy of anterior segment tumors. Ophthalmology. 1992;99:1220–8.
7. Midena E, Segato T, Piermarocchi S, Boccato P. Fine needle aspiration biopsy in ophthalmology. Surv Ophthalmol. 1985;29:410–22.
8. Jakobiec FA, Silbert G. Are most iris "melanomas" really nevi? A clinicopathologic study of 189 lesions. Arch Ophthalmol. 1981;99:2117–32.
9. Geisse LJ, Robertson DM. Iris melanomas. Am J Ophthalmol. 1985;99:638–48.
10. Naumann GO, Rummelt V. Block excision of tumors of the anterior uvea. Report on 68 consecutive patients. Ophthalmology. 1996;103:2017–27.
11. Finger PT. Plaque radiation therapy for malignant melanoma of the iris and ciliary body. Am J Ophthalmol. 2001;132:328–35.
12. Shields JA, Rodrigues MM, Sarin LK, et al. Lipofuscin pigment over benign and malignant choroidal tumors. Trans Am Acad Ophthalmol Otolaryngol. 1976; 81:OP-871–81.
13. Shields CL, Shields JA, Materin M, et al. Iris melanoma: risk factors for metastasis in 169 consecutive patients. Ophthalmology. 2001;108:172–8.
14. Sallet G, Amoaku WMK, Lafaut BA, et al. Indocyanine green angiography of choroidal tumors. Graefes Arch Clin Exp Ophthalmol. 1995;233:677–89.
15. Bond JB, Haik BG, Mihara F, Gupta KL. Magnetic resonance imaging of choroidal melanoma with and without gadolinium contrast enhancement. Ophthalmology. 1991;98:459–66.
16. Sanders TE, Smith ME. Biopsy of intraocular tumors: a reevaluation. Int Ophthalmol Clin. 1972;12:163–76.
17. Augsburger JJ, Shields JA, Folberg R, et al. Fine needle aspiration biopsy in the diagnosis of intraocular cancer. Cytologic-histologic correlations. Ophthalmology. 1985;92:39–49.
18. Karcioglu ZA, Gordon RA, Karcioglu GL. Tumor seeding in ocular fine needle aspiration biopsy. Ophthalmology. 1985;92:1763–7.
19. Albert DM, Wagoner MD, Smith ME. Are metastatic evaluations indicated before enucleation of ocular melanoma? Am J Ophthalmol. 1980;90:429–31.
20. Rankin SJA, Johnston PB. Metastatic disease from untreated choroidal and ciliary body melanomas. Int Ophthalmol. 1991;15:75–8.
21. McLean IW, Foster WD, Zimmerman LE, Gamel JW. Modifications of Callender's classification of uveal melanoma at the Armed Forces Institute of Pathology. Am J Ophthalmol. 1983;96:502–9.
22. Gamel JW, McCurdy JB, McLean IW. A comparison of prognostic covariates for uveal melanoma. Invest Ophthalmol Vis Sci. 1992;33:1919–22.
23. Folberg R, Rummelt V, Parys-Van Ginderdeuren R, et al. The prognostic value of tumor blood vessel morphology in primary uveal melanoma. Ophthalmology. 1993;100:1389–98.
24. Sisley K, Rennie IG, Parsons MA, et al. Abnormalities of chromosomes 3 and 8 in posterior uveal melanoma correlate with prognosis. Genes Chromosomes Cancer. 1997;19:22–8.
25. Patel KA, Edmondson ND, Talbot F, et al. Prediction of prognosis in patients with uveal melanoma using fluorescence in situ hybridization. Br J Ophthalmol. 2001;85:1440–4.
26. Zimmerman LE, McLean IW, Foster WD. Does enucleation of the eye containing a malignant melanoma prevent or accelerate the dissemination of tumour cells? Br J Ophthalmol. 1978;62:420–5.
27. Char DH, Phillips TL. The potential for adjuvant radiotherapy in choroidal melanoma. Arch Ophthalmol. 1982;100:247–8.
28. Collaborative Ocular Melanoma Study Group. The Collaborative Ocular Melanoma Study (COMS) randomized trial of pre-enucleation radiation of large choroidal melanoma II: initial mortality findings. COMS Report No. 10. Am J Ophthalmol. 1998;125:779–96.
29. Collaborative Ocular Melanoma Study Group. The Collaborative Ocular Melanoma Study (COMS) randomized trial of pre-enucleation radiation of large choroidal melanoma III: local complications and observations following enucleation. COMS Report No. 11. Am J Ophthalmol. 1998;126:362–72.
30. Augsburger JJ, Gamel JW, Lauritzen K, Brady LW. Cobalt-60 plaque radiotherapy vs enucleation for posterior uveal melanoma. Am J Ophthalmol. 1990;109: 585–92.
31. Guthoff R, Frischmuth J, Jensen OA, et al. Das Aderhautmelanoma. Eine retrospektive randomisierte Vergleichsstudie Ruthenium-Bestrahlung vs Enukleation. Klin Monatsbl Augenheilkd. 1992;200:257–67.
32. Seddon JM, Gragoudas ES, Egan KM, et al. Relative survival rates after alternative therapies for uveal melanoma. Ophthalmology. 1990;97:769–77.
33. Augsburger JJ, Corrêa ZM, Freire J, Brady LW. Long-term survival in choroidal and ciliary body melanoma after enucleation versus plaque radiation therapy. Ophthalmology. 1998;105:1670–8.
34. Augsburger JJ, Schneider S, Freire J, Brady LW. Survival following enucleation versus plaque radiotherapy in statistically matched subgroups of patients with choroidal melanomas: results in patients treated between 1980 and 1987. Graefes Arch Clin Exp Ophthalmol. 1999;237:558–67.
35. Diener-West M, Earle JD, Fine SL, et al. The COMS randomized trial of iodine 125 brachytherapy for choroidal melanoma III: initial mortality findings. COMS Report No. 18. Arch Ophthalmol. 2001;119:969–82.
36. Markoe AM, Brady LW, Kalsson UL, et al. Eye. In: Perez CA, Brady LW, eds. Principles and practice of radiation oncology, 2nd ed. Philadelphia: Lippincott; 1992:595–609.
37. Seddon JM, Gragoudas ES, Polivogianis L, et al. Visual outcome after proton beam irradiation of uveal melanoma. Ophthalmology. 1986;93:666–74.
38. Karlsson UL, Augsburger JJ, Shields JA, et al. Recurrence of posterior uveal melanoma after 60Co episcleral plaque therapy. Ophthalmology. 1989;96: 382–8.
39. Gragoudas ES, Egan KM, Seddon JM, et al. Intraocular recurrence of uveal melanoma after proton beam irradiation. Ophthalmology. 1992;99:760–6.
40. Char DH, Quivey JM, Castro JR, et al. Helium ions versus iodine 125 brachytherapy in the management of uveal melanoma. A prospective, randomized, dynamically balanced trial. Ophthalmology. 1993;100:1547–54.
41. Shields CL, Shields JA, Karlsson UL, et al. Reasons for enucleation after plaque radiotherapy for posterior uveal melanoma. Ophthalmology. 1989;96:919–24.
42. Egan KM, Gragoudas ES, Seddon JM, et al. The risk of enucleation after proton beam irradiation of uveal melanoma. Ophthalmology. 1989;96:1377–83.

43. Mueller AJ, Talies S, Schaller UC, *et al.* Stereotactic radiosurgery of large uveal melanomas with the gamma-knife. Ophthalmology. 2000;107:1381–8.
44. Bellmann C, Fuss M, Holz FG, *et al.* Stereotactic radiation therapy for malignant choroidal tumors. Preliminary, short-term results. Ophthalmology. 2000; 107:358–65.
45. Gass JDM. Observation of suspected choroidal and ciliary body melanomas for evidence of growth prior to enucleation. Ophthalmology. 1980;87:523–8.
46. Augsburger JJ. Is observation really appropriate for small choroidal melanomas? Trans Am Ophthalmol Soc. 1994;91:147–68.
47. Augsburger JJ, Vrabec TR. Impact of delayed treatment in growing posterior uveal melanomas. Arch Ophthalmol. 1993;111:1382–6.
48. Shields JA, Glazer LC, Mieler WF, *et al.* Comparison of xenon arc and argon laser photocoagulation in the treatment of choroidal melanomas. Am J Ophthalmol. 1990;109:647–55.
49. Oosterhuis JA, Journée-de Korver HG, Keunen JE. Transpupillary thermotherapy: results in 50 patients with choroidal melanoma. Arch Ophthalmol. 1998;116:157–62.
50. Shields CL, Shields JA, Perez N, *et al.* Primary transpupillary thermotherapy for small choroidal melanoma in 256 consecutive cases: outcomes and limitations. Ophthalmology. 2002;109:225–34.
51. Finger PT, Lipka AC, Lipkowitz JL, *et al.* Failure of transpupillary thermotherapy (TTT) for choroidal melanoma: two cases with histopathological correlation. Br J Ophthalmol. 2000;84:1075–6.
52. Damato BE, Paul J, Foulds WS. Predictive factors of visual outcome after local resection of choroidal melanoma. Br J Ophthalmol. 1993;77:616–25.
53. Peyman GA, Charles H. Internal eye wall resection in the management of uveal melanoma. Can J Ophthalmol. 1988;23:219–23.
54. Robertson DM, Campbell RJ, Weaver DT. Residual intrascleral and intraretinal melanoma: a concern with lamellar sclerouvectomy for uveal melanoma. Am J Ophthalmol. 1991;112:590–3.
55. Damato BE, Paul J, Foulds WS. Risk factors for residual and recurrent uveal melanoma after trans-scleral local resection. Br J Ophthalmol. 1996;80:102–8.
56. Bornfeld N, Talies S, Anastassiou G, *et al.* Proton beam irradiation of large posterior uveal melanomas prior to endoresection. Ophthalmologe. 2002;99:338–44.
57. Foulds WS, Damato BE, Burton RL. Local resection versus enucleation in the management of choroidal melanoma. Eye. 1987;1:676–9.
58. Kersten RC, Tse T, Anderson RL, *et al.* The role of orbital exenteration in choroidal melanoma with extrascleral extension. Ophthalmology. 1985;92:436–43.
59. Pach JM, Robertson DM, Taney BS, *et al.* Prognostic factors in choroidal and ciliary body melanomas with extrascleral extension. Am J Ophthalmol. 1986;101:325–31.
60. Coleman DJ, Lizzi FL, Eng SD, *et al.* Ultrasonic hyperthermia and radiation in the management of intraocular malignant melanoma. Am J Ophthalmol. 1986;101:635–42.
61. Finger PT. Microwave thermoradiotherapy for intraocular melanoma. Am J Clin Oncol. 1996;19:281–9.
62. Favilla I, Barry WR, Gosbell A, *et al.* Phototherapy of posterior uveal melanomas. Br J Ophthalmol. 1991;75:718–21.
63. Klein ML, Wilson DJ. Cryotherapy for the treatment of small growing choroidal melanomas (abstract). Invest Ophthalmol Vis Sci. 1996;37:S242.
64. Albert DM, Niffenegger AS, Willson JKV. Treatment of metastatic uveal melanoma: review and recommendations. Surv Ophthalmol. 1992;36:429–38.
65. Augsburger JJ, Kleineidam M, Mullen D. Combined iodine-125 plaque irradiation and indirect ophthalmoscope laser therapy of choroidal malignant melanomas: comparison with iodine-125 and cobalt-60 plaque radiotherapy alone. Graefes Arch Clin Exp Ophthalmol. 1993;231:500–7.
66. Seregard S, Landau I. Transpupillary thermotherapy as an adjunct to ruthenium plaque radiotherapy for choroidal melanoma. Acta Ophthalmol Scand. 2001; 79:19–22.
67. Straatsma BR, Fine SL, Earle JD, *et al.* Enucleation versus plaque irradiation for choroidal melanoma. Ophthalmology. 1988;95:1000–4.
68. Augsburger JJ, Lauritzen K, Gamel JW, *et al.* Matched group study of preenucleation radiotherapy versus enucleation alone for primary malignant melanoma of the choroid and ciliary body. Am J Clin Oncol. 1990;13:382–7.
69. Augsburger JJ, Gamel JW. Clinical prognostic factors in patients with posterior uveal malignant melanoma. Cancer. 1990;66:1596–600.

148 Metastatic Cancer to the Eye

JAMES J. AUGSBURGER • RUDOLF GUTHOFF

DEFINITION
- Primary extraophthalmic neoplasm that spreads hematogenously to the eye.

KEY FEATURES
- Choroidal masses are most common; individual choroidal lesions typically appear as relatively thin, amelanotic, round to oval choroidal masses.
- Infiltrative amelanotic masses of iris or optic disc are less common.
- Unifocal and unilateral in 80% of cases; multifocal, bilateral, or both in 20% of cases.

ASSOCIATED FEATURES
- Clinically evident primary extraophthalmic neoplasm.
- Other clinically detectable metastatic foci.
- Nonrhegmatogenous retinal detachment that surrounds and overlies choroidal tumor.

INTRODUCTION

Patients who have a cancer (usually a carcinoma) that arises in some bodily organ or tissue other than the eye occasionally develop implantation tumors (metastases) within the eye. Most intraocular metastatic tumors involve the choroid, but similar lesions also affect the iris, ciliary body, optic nerve, neural retina, and vitreous in some patients. About 80% of affected persons present with a single tumor in only one eye. The other 20% have multiple tumors, bilateral tumors, or both. The presence of metastatic cancer in the eye poses a substantial risk to the patient for visual deterioration and possibly total blindness in the affected eye. Fortunately, treatment of such tumors is usually highly effective in terms of both local tumor control and preservation of sight. Unfortunately, metastatic cancer to the eye is a poor prognostic sign for long-term survival.

EPIDEMIOLOGY AND PATHOGENESIS

Metastatic carcinoma to the eye is generally regarded as the most common intraocular malignant neoplasm. Recent tables of vital statistics for the United States indicate that 20–25% of all deaths are attributable to cancer.[1] Microscopic metastatic intraocular lesions are demonstrable in at least one eye in 5–10% of these individuals.[2] This means that 1–2.5% of all people have metastatic carcinoma in at least one eye at the time of death. About 10% of these persons have one or more metastatic intraocular lesions detected clinically before death. Thus, the cumulative lifetime incidence of clinically detected metastatic intraocular tumors is approximately 0.1% (1 in 1000) to 0.25% (1 in 400). Of course, some of these tumors are not detected until shortly before death, when the patient is already in a terminal stage of cancer. Annual age-adjusted incidence rates of ocular metastatic lesions for various types of primary cancer have not been reported.

The obvious principal risk factor for the occurrence of metastatic carcinoma to the eye is a prior history of cancer.[3] In women, the most common malignancy that gives rise to metastatic carcinoma to the eye is breast cancer. In men, the most common primary cancer type appears to be lung cancer. Most patients who develop metastatic carcinoma to the eye have a known prior cancer and frequently other known sites of metastasis as well. However, approximately 25% of individuals who are found to have metastatic carcinoma in the eye develop that condition as the initial manifestation of their cancer.

OCULAR MANIFESTATIONS

The principal symptom caused by metastatic carcinoma to the eye is blurred or distorted vision. Such visual impairment may be present in one or both eyes, depending on the laterality and extent of involvement. Pain is usually not a sign of metastatic cancer to the eye, except in patients who have extensive intraocular tumor and marked visual impairment, frequently in association with bullous retinal detachment and secondary glaucoma. Metastatic carcinoma to the intraocular tissues is often detected by an ophthalmologist who is consulted because of the visual symptoms. Occasionally, if a tumor develops in the iris, it may actually become apparent to the patient, spouse, relative, or friend as a visible discoloration or spot.

The typical metastatic carcinoma to the choroid from breast, lung, or gastrointestinal tract appears as a golden yellow to yellowish white round to oval lesion (Figs. 148-1 and 148-2). It is often associated with a nonrhegmatogenous retinal detachment that is out of proportion to the size of the tumor. In contrast to the typical amelanotic metastatic carcinoma, cutaneous malignant melanoma that metastasizes to the eye commonly appears intensely melanotic.[4] Other neoplasms that tend to have a characteristic color include renal cell carcinoma (typically reddish orange), follicular carcinoma of the thyroid (also reddish orange to pink), and carcinoid from the gastrointestinal tract or lung (usually pink or golden orange).[3]

Metastatic carcinoma to the optic disc can appear either as a swollen disc without a distinct mass or as a discohesive cellular infiltration of the superficial aspects of the optic disc (Fig. 148-3).[5] A metastatic carcinoma to the optic disc is often associated with profound visual loss, which may or may not be reversible.

Metastatic carcinoma to the iris typically appears as a solid, amelanotic iris mass (Fig. 148-4).[6] Some metastases to the iris are quite discohesive and shed cells that form a pseudohypopyon in the anterior chamber. The shed tumor cells can clog the trabecular meshwork and cause a secondary open-angle glaucoma. Metastatic iris tumors can also cause spontaneous hyphema.

Ciliary body metastatic carcinoma occasionally presents as diffuse and sometimes multinodular masses, often associated with extensive retinal detachment and occasionally severe ocular pain. The precise mechanism for the pain in this sort of ocular metastatic carcinoma is not clear.

Exceptional presentations of metastatic carcinoma to the eye include infiltrative lesions of the neural retina (Fig. 148-5)[7] and dispersed cells in the vitreous.[8]

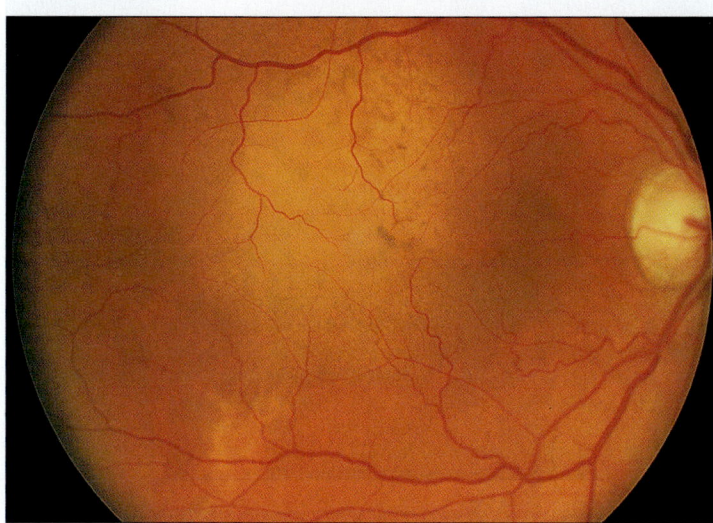

FIG. 148-1 ■ Unifocal metastatic carcinoma to choroid. The patient was a 58-year-old woman who had primary breast carcinoma.

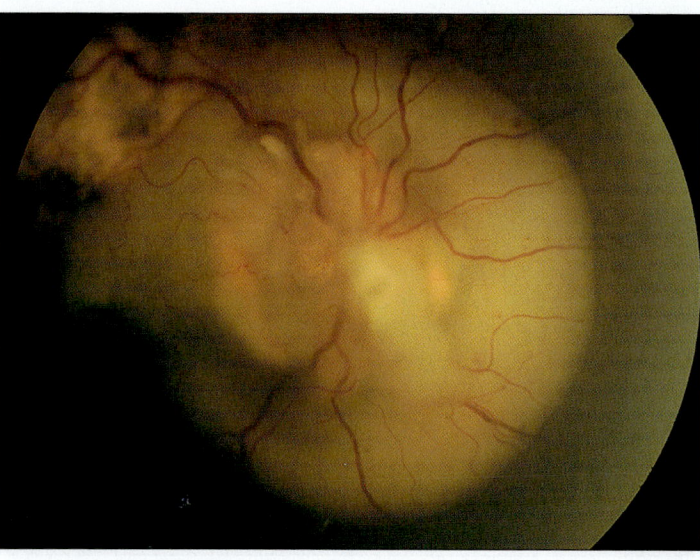

FIG. 148-3 ■ Metastatic carcinoma to optic disc. The patient was a 67-year-old woman who had breast carcinoma.

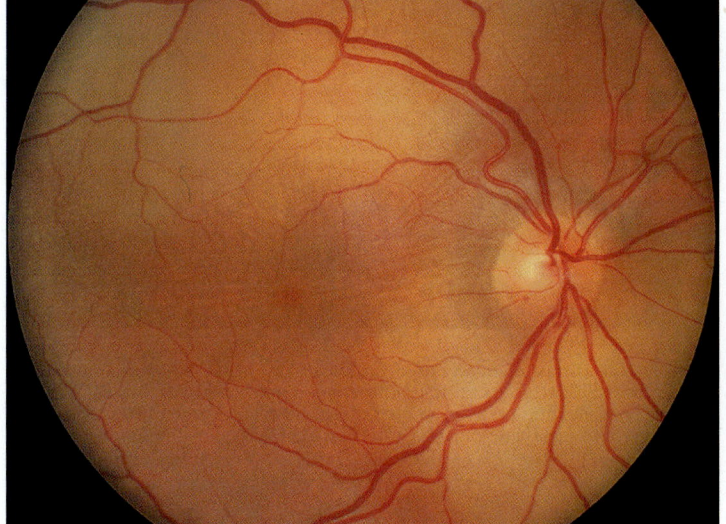

FIG. 148-2 ■ Multifocal metastatic tumors to choroid. The patient was a 43-year-old woman who had primary breast carcinoma.

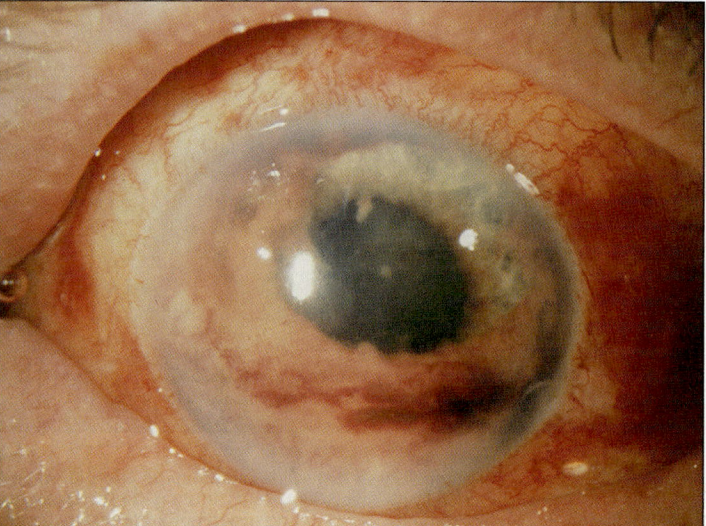

FIG. 148-4 ■ Metastatic carcinoma to iris. The patient was a 56-year-old man who had a primary cancer of unknown type and site.

DIAGNOSIS AND ANCILLARY TESTING

Fluorescein angiography of metastatic carcinoma to the choroid typically shows few or no large-caliber intralesional vessels, relative hypofluorescence of the lesion in the early frames, and diffuse hyperfluorescence of the lesion in the late frames (Fig. 148-6). In some cases, multiple hyperfluorescent dots are evident on the surface of the lesion in the venous phase and late phase frames (see Fig. 148-6). The dots appear to be foci of microcystic alteration in the overlying retinal pigment epithelium. Fluorescein angiography of metastatic carcinoma to the optic disc, retina, or iris also shows the lesion to be hypofluorescent early but hyperfluorescent late.

Indocyanine green angiography of metastatic carcinoma to the choroid[9] frequently reveals subtle metastatic lesions that are not evident on fluorescein angiography. Most metastatic tumors appear hypofluorescent throughout the study.

B-scan ultrasonography of metastatic carcinoma to the choroid shows the typical tumor to have a relatively flat cross-sectional shape compared with its basal diameters (Fig. 148-7). In contrast to choroidal melanomas, metastatic choroidal tumors usually appear relatively sonoreflective (bright) rather than sonolucent internally. However, certain metastatic tumors, in-

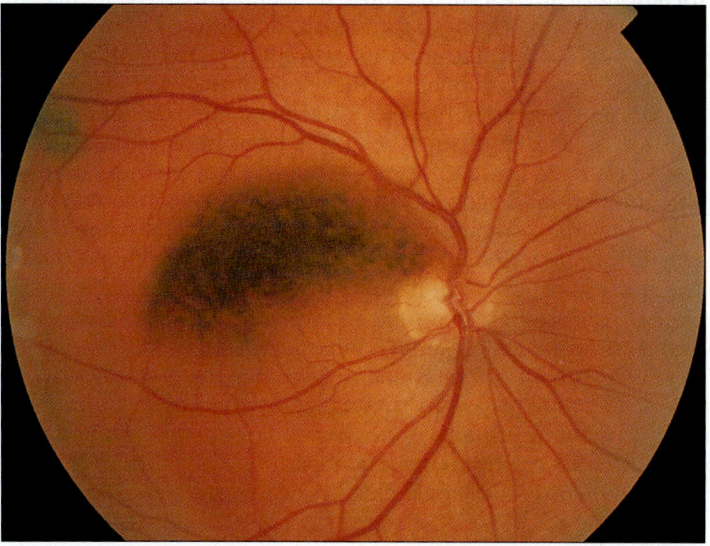

FIG. 148-5 ■ Metastatic cutaneous melanoma to retina and choroid. The patient was a 33-year-old man. Note the small choroidal metastasis temporal to the fan-shaped retinal lesion.

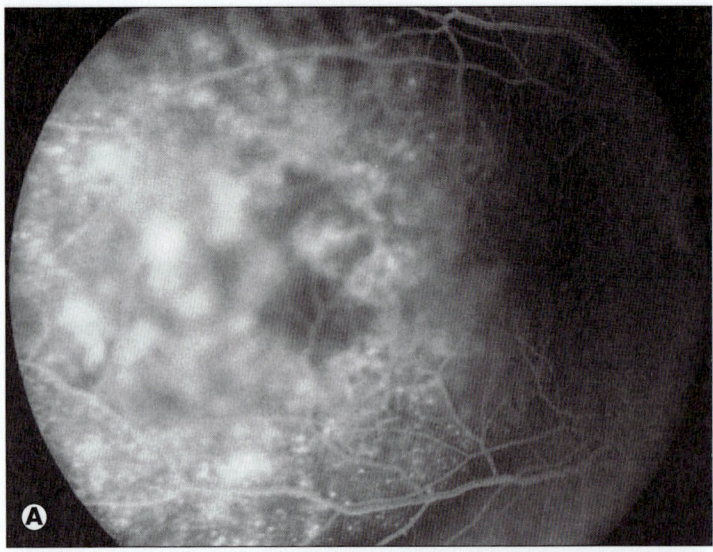

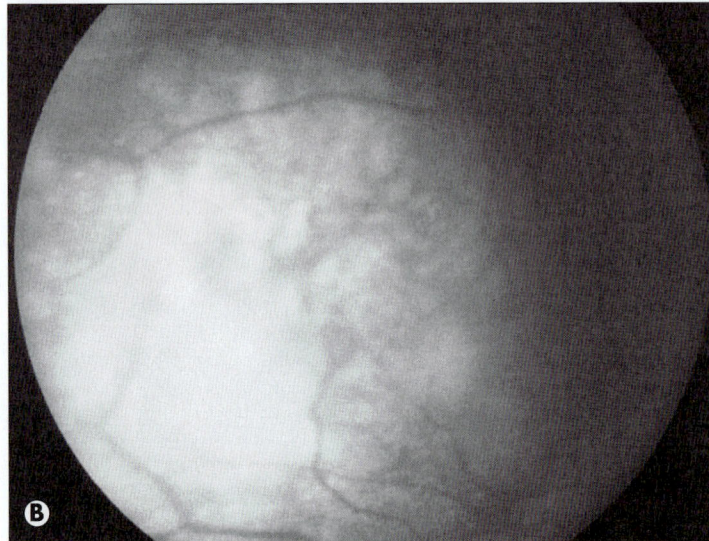

FIG. 148-6 ▌▌ Fluorescein angiogram of metastatic carcinoma to choroid. A, Full venous phase frame shows multiple hyperfluorescent dots on the surface of a choroidal lesion. B, Late phase frame shows diffuse hyperfluorescence of the entire choroidal tumor.

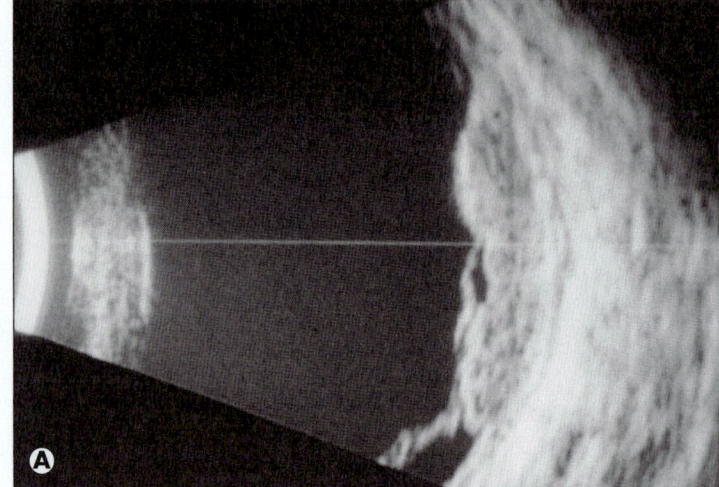

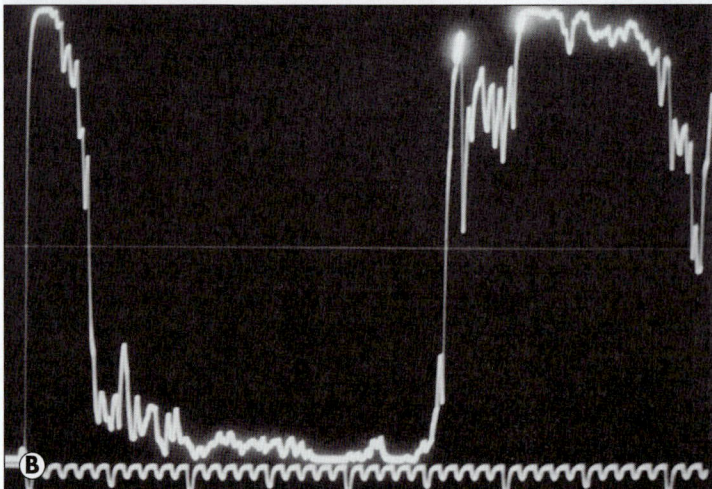

FIG. 148-7 ▌▌ Ultrasonography of metastatic carcinoma to choroid. A, B-scan image of metastatic carcinoma to choroid from lung. Note the brightness of the intralesional echoes and the presence of secondary retinal detachment. B, Standardized A-scan image of metastatic carcinoma to choroid shows high-amplitude internal reflectivity of the mass.

cluding metastatic cutaneous melanomas and some oat cell carcinomas, appear virtually identical to primary choroidal melanomas on B-scan. In most patients who have metastatic carcinoma to the choroid, standardized A-scan ultrasonography reveals high-amplitude internal reflectivity and no prominent, spontaneous intralesional vascular pulsations.

Computed tomography (CT) and magnetic resonance imaging (MRI) can demonstrate relatively large intraocular metastatic carcinomas; however, these studies do not provide any reliable differential diagnostic information about such lesions.

Fine-needle aspiration biopsy appears to be a reliable and safe technique for establishing the diagnosis in selected cases.[10,11] The most appropriate indication for such a procedure is suspicion of metastatic carcinoma in a patient with no history of prior nonocular cancer or no concurrent extraophthalmic foci of possible primary or metastatic malignancy that would be more amenable to biopsy than the ocular lesion. For iris tumors, a limbal puncture usually is employed. For choroidal metastatic tumors, either a direct trans-scleral puncture or an indirect transvitreal puncture in the pars plana region is employed.

DIFFERENTIAL DIAGNOSIS

The principal lesions and disorders in the differential diagnosis of intraocular metastatic carcinoma are listed in Box 148-1. The

most important of these is amelanotic choroidal melanoma, which can closely resemble unilateral, unifocal metastatic carcinoma to the choroid. Ultrasonography is usually helpful in making this distinction. A metastatic carcinoma typically appears relatively bright (sonoreflective) internally, but an amelanotic choroidal melanoma usually appears relatively dark (sonolucent). The lesions that most closely resemble multifocal, bilateral metastatic carcinoma to the choroid are multifocal vitelliform fundus lesions and the multifocal lesions of idiopathic sclerochoroidal calcification. Fortunately, the former can usually be distinguished by fluorescein angiography (individual vitelliform lesions usually block fluorescence) and the latter by ultrasonography (calcific sclerochoroidal lesions are extremely bright and shadow the orbital soft tissues).

SYSTEMIC ASSOCIATIONS

The principal systemic associations in patients who have metastatic carcinoma to the eye are primary extraocular cancers and metastatic tumors in other organs. In recognition of these systemic associations, every patient who has presumed metastatic carcinoma to the eye must be evaluated thoroughly for clinical evidence of extraocular cancer before biopsy of the ocular tumor or any ocular treatment (assuming that there is no indication for urgent intervention).

BOX 148-1

Differential Diagnosis of Intraocular Metastatic Carcinoma

METASTATIC TUMORS TO CHOROID
Amelanotic nevus
Amelanotic malignant melanoma
Circumscribed choroidal hemangioma
Choroidal osteoma
Primary intraocular lymphoma
Astrocytoma of retina
Idiopathic sclerochoroidal calcification
Bullous central serous choroidopathy
Uveal effusion syndrome
Vitelliform dystrophy (especially if multifocal)
Posterior scleritis
Harada's disease
Tuberculoma

METASTATIC TUMORS TO IRIS
Nonmicrobial inflammatory granuloma (sarcoidosis, juvenile xanthogranuloma)
Microbial abscess
Iris cyst
Amelanotic nevus
Amelanotic malignant melanoma
Leiomyoma of iris
Focally nodular peripheral anterior synechia
Lisch nodules
Intraocular foreign body

METASTATIC TUMORS TO OPTIC DISC
Leukemic infiltration
Lymphomatous infiltration
Microbial infiltrate (toxocariasis, toxoplasmosis, viral)
Nonmicrobial inflammatory granuloma (sarcoid)

METASTATIC TUMORS TO RETINA
Leukemic or lymphomatous lesion
Microbial retinitis, choroiditis, vitritis

BOX 148-2

Baseline Systemic Evaluation of Patients Who Have Presumed Intraocular Metastatic Carcinoma

PATIENTS PREVIOUSLY AFFECTED BY KNOWN EXTRAOPHTHALMIC MALIGNANCY:
Staging examination pertinent to presumed underlying malignancy

PATIENTS WHO HAVE NO KNOWN PRIOR EXTRAOPHTHALMIC MALIGNANCY:
Complete physical examination
  • Breast examination (women)
  • Prostate examination (men)
  • Regional lymph node palpation
  • Dermatologic survey (especially if metastatic melanoma is suspected)
Laboratory studies
  • Mammography
  • Chest radiograph
  • Computed tomography or magnetic resonance imaging of chest and abdomen
  • Bone survey or scan

BOX 148-3

Treatment Options for Metastatic Carcinoma to the Eye

Chemotherapy
Hormonal therapy
Radiation therapy
  • External beam radiation therapy
  • Plaque radiotherapy (iodine-125, ruthenium-106, palladium-103)
Enucleation

Baseline Systemic Evaluation

The systemic testing appropriate for a patient with suspected metastatic intraocular carcinoma is summarized in Box 148-2. In women with no prior history of cancer, breast examination and mammography should be undertaken first. In men with no prior history of cancer and in women with no evidence of breast carcinoma, a chest radiograph and abdominal and thoracic CT or MRI are most likely to lead to a diagnosis.

PATHOLOGY

The pathology of intraocular metastatic carcinoma depends largely on the type of metastasizing cancer, the intraocular tissues involved, and the size and extent of the intraocular tumor. Involved tissues are replaced by malignant cells that have cytological features consistent with the primary neoplasm. Unfortunately, the degree of cellular dedifferentiation frequently makes identification of the source of neoplasm difficult or impossible. Immunohistochemical stains are frequently helpful for identifying the type of cancer and its probable source.

TREATMENT

The principal management options for patients who have metastatic carcinoma to the eye include radiotherapy, chemotherapy, and hormonal therapy (Box 148-3).[3] Radiotherapy for intraocular metastatic carcinoma is generally given as an outpatient course of linear accelerator beam treatment.[12] This form of treatment can be used to deliver a relatively uniform dose of radiation (usually in the range of 35–50Gy) to all affected portions of the eye while giving a limited radiation dose to other tissues. To max-

imize treatment effectiveness and minimize complications, such treatment is usually given in multiple fractions over 3–5 weeks. External beam radiation therapy is particularly applicable to patients who have large tumors that involve the optic nerve or macula and cause substantial visual disturbance or affect multiple areas in both eyes.

In contrast, individuals who have single small to medium-sized tumors can occasionally be treated effectively by radioactive plaque therapy.[13] This treatment consists of suturing a radioactive device (plaque) to the sclera directly overlying the intraocular tumor. The plaque is left in place for several days, generally until a radiation dose of 40–50Gy has been delivered to the apex of the tumor, and then removed.

Most metastatic carcinomas are responsive to the doses of radiation given by external beam and plaque methods. Metastatic intraocular tumors generally show rapid regression (shrinkage) after radiation therapy (Fig. 148-8), and vision in the eye is frequently stabilized if not improved (especially if the cause of visual disturbance was subretinal fluid that involved the macula).

If vision is not severely affected, and particularly if other sites are found to have concurrent metastatic tumors, chemotherapy or hormonal therapy may be recommended as a first-line treatment.[3] In patients already on chemotherapy or hormonal therapy at the time of detection of metastatic carcinoma to the eye, a change in that regimen may be recommended. In any event, an appropriate drug regimen often produces satisfactory regression of all tumors and preservation or recovery of useful vision in the affected eye or eyes (Fig. 148-9).

Many patients who develop metastatic carcinoma to the eye are managed by both radiation therapy and chemotherapy.[3] The

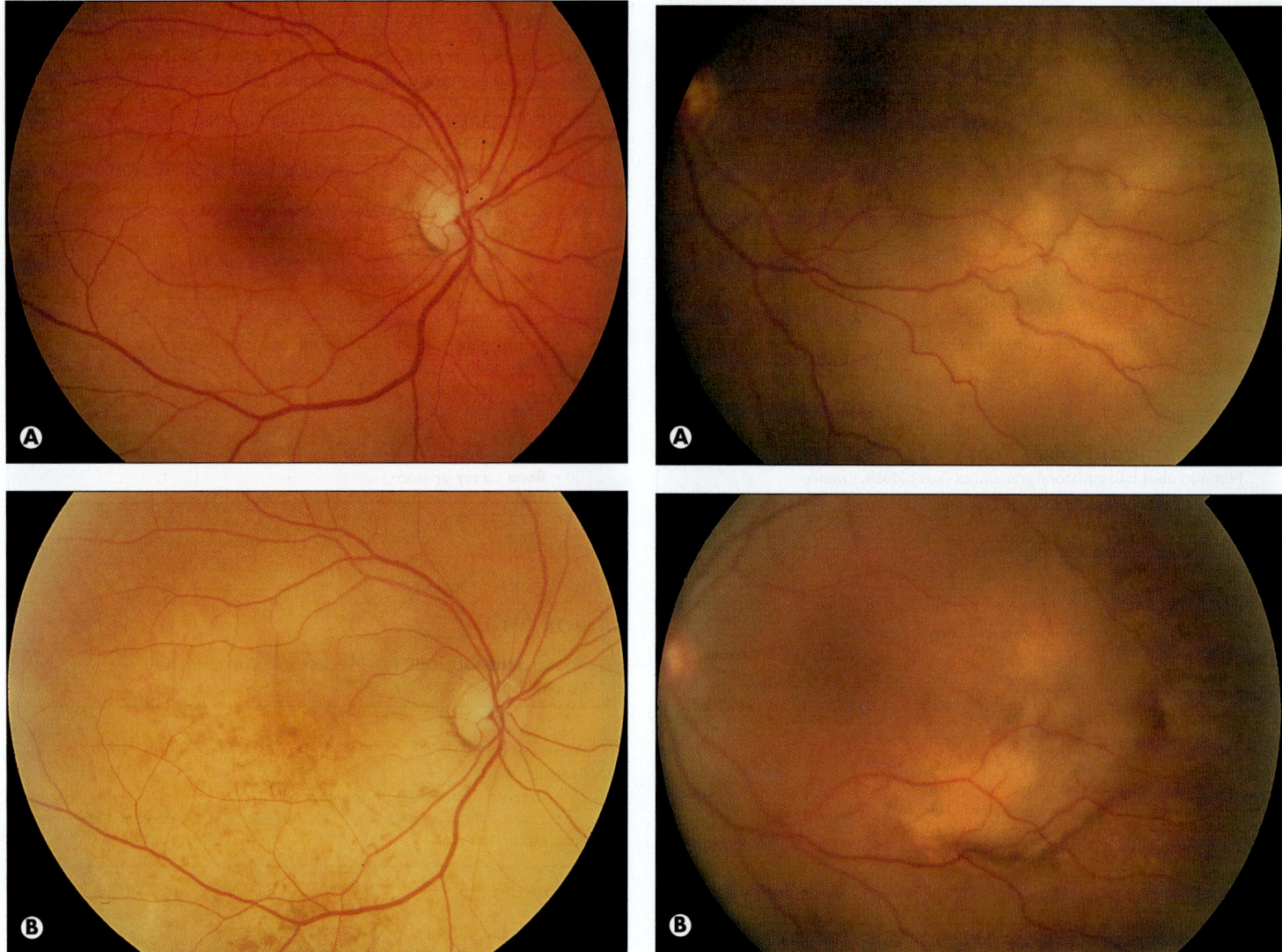

FIG. 148-8 ■ External beam radiation therapy for choroidal metastasis. A, Pretreatment appearance of macular choroidal tumor. B, Fully regressed lesion 8 months after external beam radiation therapy. Note that a larger area of the fundus appears depigmented than would have been predicted from the pretreatment size of the tumor. Also note clumps of pigment on the surface of the regressed tumor.

FIG. 148-9 ■ Chemotherapy for choroidal metastasis. A, Ill-defined amelanotic choroidal metastatic tumor with overlying retinal detachment prior to treatment in a 66-year-old woman with breast carcinoma. B, Partially regressed lesion 1 month after the start of chemotherapy.

particular treatment regimen advocated for an individual depends on the type of tumor; the size, extent, and location of the intraocular tumor; the number of tumors; the laterality of involvement; the effects on associated intraocular tissues; the visual status of the affected eye or eyes; the visual status of the fellow eye in unilateral cases; the extent of extraocular disease; and the age and general health of the patient.

COURSE AND OUTCOME

Most metastatic carcinomas to the eye are relentlessly progressive if untreated. Such tumors tend to grow faster on average than do primary malignant intraocular neoplasms. Choroidal tumors give rise to bullous retinal detachment, which can cause forward displacement of the lens and iris and lead to secondary angle-closure glaucoma. Optic disc metastases often produce rapid, profound visual loss. Iris metastases frequently cause secondary open-angle glaucoma when the trabecular meshwork becomes clogged with tumor cells. Provided that the patient survives long enough, many if not most eyes that have untreated metastatic carcinoma ultimately progress to a blind, painful condition.

Factors used to predict the potential for preservation or recovery of vision in the affected eye or eyes include the number and size of tumors, their locations relative to the optic disc and fovea, the severity of their effects on the retina and other ocular tissues, and their responsiveness to the selected therapy. The responsiveness of a tumor is dependent on the site of origin of the original tumor and its pathological nature.

Metastatic carcinoma to the interior of the eye is not a threat to survival, because the eye is not a vital structure. The prognosis for a patient's survival is dependent on the pathological nature, anatomical site, and size of the source tumor; the presence and extent of metastatic tumors in vital organs; and the responsiveness of the carcinoma to radiotherapy and chemotherapy. The impact of tumor type on survival is shown in Figure 148-10. As revealed by this figure, the median survival time for patients with metastatic breast carcinoma is substantially longer than that for patients with the other specified metastatic neoplasms.

The ophthalmologist's role in treating patients who have metastatic carcinoma to the eye is to establish the intraocular diagnosis, work out treatment modalities to preserve or restore vision in the affected eye or eyes, and help monitor treatment by evaluating the status of the intraocular tumor after treatment. Ophthalmologists must work as part of a team with internists, medical oncologists, and radiation therapists to ensure optimal care of patients who have metastatic carcinoma to the eye.

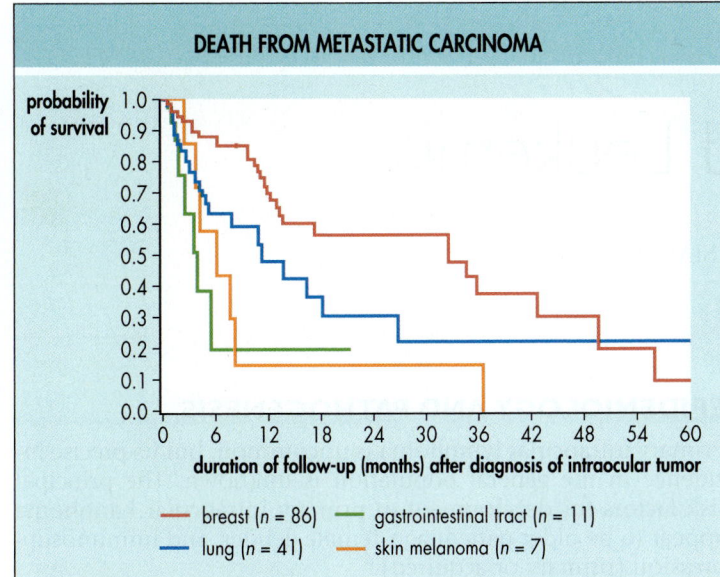

DEATH FROM METASTATIC CARCINOMA

duration of follow-up (months) after diagnosis of intraocular tumor

— breast (*n* = 86)   — gastrointestinal tract (*n* = 11)
— lung (*n* = 41)   — skin melanoma (*n* = 7)

FIG. 148-10 ▉ **Actuarial survival curves of patients with specified types of primary cancer metastatic to the eye.** These curves are based on deaths from metastatic carcinoma only.

REFERENCES

1. Parker SL, Tong T, Bolden S, Wingo PA. Cancer statistics, 1997. CA Cancer J Clin. 1997;47:5–27.
2. Nelson CG, Hertzberg BS, Klintworth GK. A histopathologic study of 716 unselected eyes in patients with cancer at the time of death. Am J Ophthalmol. 1983;95:788–93.
3. Shakin EP, Shields JA, Augsburger JJ. Metastatic cancer to the uvea and optic disk: analysis of 200 patients. In: Bornfeld N, Gragoudas ES, Höpping W, *et al.*, eds. Tumors of the eye. Amsterdam: Kugler; 1991:623–31.
4. deBustros S, Augsburger JJ, Shields JA, *et al.* Intraocular metastases from cutaneous malignant melanoma. Arch Ophthalmol. 1985;103:937–40.
5. Allaire GS, Corriveau C, Arbour JD. Metastasis to the optic nerve: clinicopathological correlation. Can J Ophthalmol. 1995;30:306–11.
6. Shields JA, Shields CL, Kiratli H, de Potter P. Metastatic tumors to the iris in 40 patients. Am J Ophthalmol. 1995;119:422–30.
7. Leys AM, VanEyck LM, Nuttin BJ, *et al.* Metastatic carcinoma to the retina. Clinicopathologic findings in two cases. Arch Ophthalmol. 1990;108:1448–52.
8. Spraul CW, Martin DF, Hagler WS, Grossniklaus HE. Cytology of metastatic cutaneous melanoma to the vitreous and retina. Retina. 1996;16:328–32.
9. Harino S, Miyamoto K, Okada M, *et al.* Indocyanine green videoangiographic findings in choroidal metastatic tumor. Graefes Arch Clin Exp Ophthalmol. 1995;233:339–46.
10. Scholz R, Green WR, Baranano EC, *et al.* Metastatic carcinoma to the iris. Diagnosis by aqueous paracentesis and response to irradiation and chemotherapy. Ophthalmology. 1983;90:1524–7.
11. Augsburger JJ. Fine needle aspiration biopsy of suspected metastatic cancers to the posterior uvea. Trans Am Ophthalmol Soc. 1988;86:499–560.
12. McCormick B, Harrison LB. Radiation therapy or choroidal metastases. In: Alberti WE, Sagerman RH, eds. Radiotherapy of intraocular and orbital tumors. Berlin: Springer-Verlag; 1993:93–7.
13. Shields CL, Shields JA, De Potter P, *et al.* Plaque radiotherapy for the management of uveal metastasis. Arch Ophthalmol. 1997;115:203–9.

Lymphoma and Leukemia

JAMES J. AUGSBURGER • WILLIAM G. TSIARAS

DEFINITION
• Leukocytic malignancies that infiltrate ocular tissues in some affected patients.

KEY FEATURES
• Diffuse, whitish cellular infiltrates that involve retina, vitreous, or optic disc.
• Geographical amelanotic subpigment epithelial infiltrates characteristic of primary intraocular lymphoma.

ASSOCIATED FEATURES
• Central nervous system involvement.
• Hemorrhagic retinopathy.
• Propensity to develop opportunistic retinitis.

INTRODUCTION

Lymphoma and leukemia are distinct neoplastic disorders that are linked by their common leukocytic basis. Both entities may be associated with various intraocular lesions. Of the two, lymphoma produces intraocular tumors much more commonly. One particularly important subtype of lymphoma that has a strong propensity to produce intraocular tumors is known as primary intraocular lymphoma. Some intraocular lymphomas are metastatic tumors from a solid visceral lymphoma. Tumors of this type exhibit the same general features described in Chapter 148 and are not discussed in this chapter.

PRIMARY INTRAOCULAR LYMPHOMA

INTRODUCTION

Primary intraocular lymphoma is an uncommon but important lymphocytic neoplasia that arises diffusely or multicentrically within the retina or uvea of one or both eyes. Two principal subtypes of primary intraocular lymphoma are currently recognized.[1] Primary vitreoretinal lymphoma is characterized by vitreous cells and geographical subretinal pigment epithelial infiltrative masses. This subtype is regularly associated with independent nonmetastatic foci of primary central nervous system (CNS) lymphoma. Primary uveal lymphoma is characterized by diffuse or multifocal creamy yellow choroidal infiltrates in one or both eyes. This subtype is usually associated with independent foci of visceral non-Hodgkin's lymphoma. Correct clinical diagnosis of the intraocular disease and awareness of the links with CNS and visceral lymphoma may lead to earlier detection and more effective treatment of this malignancy.

EPIDEMIOLOGY AND PATHOGENESIS

Primary intraocular lymphoma is uncommon, but its precise incidence in the general population is unknown. The principal risk factors for development of primary intraocular lymphoma appear to be older patient age, female gender, and immunosuppression (primary or acquired).[2]

OCULAR MANIFESTATIONS

Characteristic clinical manifestations of primary vitreoretinal lymphoma include diffuse cellular infiltration of the vitreous and accumulations of lymphomatous cells in the subpigment epithelial space of the retina (Fig. 149-1).[3-5] The subretinal pigment epithelial lesions are yellowish white, geographical infiltrates with clumping of the overlying retinal pigment epithelium. Smaller satellite-type lesions of a similar color and texture often are present adjacent to the principal lesion. Bilateral involvement is present in 80–90% of affected patients. Other less common presenting features of primary vitreoretinal lymphoma include a pattern of chorioretinal spots simulating the multiple evanescent white dot syndrome,[6] retinal infiltrates with associated intraretinal hemorrhage that resemble cytomegalovirus retinitis,[2,7] and retinal artery obstruction.[2,7]

The characteristic clinical manifestation of primary uveal lymphoma is a creamy yellow thickening of the choroid diffusely or multifocally (Fig. 149-2).[8,9] Few if any vitreous cells are present in this form of primary intraocular lymphoma. Less common features of primary uveal lymphoma include a fundus pattern of orange spots resembling fundus flavimaculatus[10] and disruption and clumping of the retinal pigment epithelium overlying an ill-defined area of uveal thickening.[10]

DIAGNOSIS AND ANCILLARY TESTING

Fluorescein angiography of a typical subretinal pigment epithelial lesion in primary vitreoretinal lymphoma characteristically shows the mass to be hypofluorescent early in the study and hyperfluorescent late. Indocyanine green angiography of such lesions has not yet been reported. Fluorescein angiography of primary uveal lymphoma typically shows an irregular pattern of fluorescence blockage by the orange pigment clumps or disrupted retinal pigment epithelium. Ultrasonography can show diffuse uveal thickening, prominent infiltrative subretinal retinal masses, and intravitreal cells in primary intraocular lymphoma, but these findings are not diagnostic.

Because several non-neoplastic conditions can simulate primary intraocular lymphoma quite closely, biopsy of an appropriate tissue is usually performed to confirm the diagnosis before treatment. If a cellular infiltrate in the vitreous is a prominent aspect of the disorder, the diagnosis can be confirmed by cytological examination of vitreous fluid removed by pars plana vitrectomy.[11-13] Occasionally, the vitreous specimen from the initial vitrectomy contains only activated lymphocytes.[11,12] If primary intraocular lymphoma is still strongly suspected, a second vitrectomy should be considered. The second vitrectomy specimen may contain lymphoma cells even when none were present in the orig-

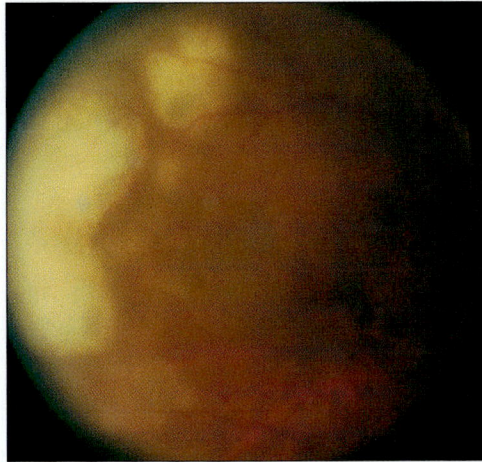

FIG. 149-1 ■ **Primary vitreoretinal lymphoma.** Typical geographical subretinal pigment epithelial lesion. This eye had relatively few vitreous cells.

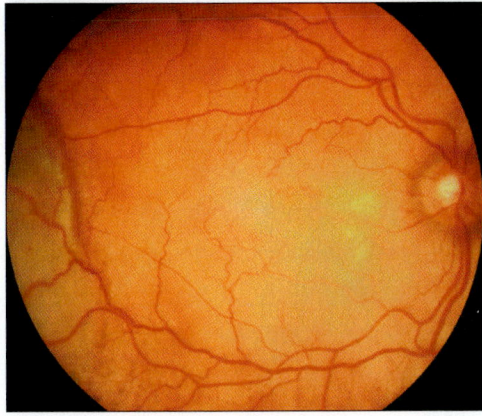

FIG. 149-2 ■ **Primary uveal lymphoma.** Diffuse, creamy uveal infiltration with focal nodular accentuation inferotemporal to macula.

inal one. In patients with a subretinal pigment epithelial lesion or infiltrative choroidal or retinal lesion, the diagnosis of lymphoma can be confirmed pathologically by examination of a fine-needle aspirate or incisional chorioretinal biopsy specimen.[13] An alternative method that may be useful for confirming primary intraocular lymphoma in uncertain cases is determination of the relative concentrations of interleukin-10 and interleukin-6 in the fluid specimen.[14] An interleukin-10–to–interleukin-6 ratio substantially greater than 1.0 is strongly suggestive of lymphoma, while a ratio substantially less than 1.0 is more suggestive of intraocular inflammation.

DIFFERENTIAL DIAGNOSIS

Several of the more important lesions and disorders in the differential diagnosis of primary intraocular lymphoma are listed in Box 149-1.

SYSTEMIC ASSOCIATIONS

As noted earlier, patients with primary vitreoretinal lymphoma frequently develop independent primary foci of lymphoma within the CNS.[3,4,11,12] The lymphomatous brain tumors can appear before, concurrent with, or after the development of primary intraocular lymphoma. Unfortunately, these brain lesions frequently prove fatal. In contrast, patients with primary uveal lymphoma are unlikely to have associated primary CNS lymphoma but are highly likely to have or develop visceral non-Hodgkin's lymphoma in the abdomen or pelvis.[8,9] Not surprisingly, some overlap of these subtypes has been reported.[15,16]

PATHOLOGY

The infiltrative subretinal pigment epithelial and retinal lesions of primary vitreoretinal lymphoma are usually composed of malignant lymphoid cells that have the cytological features of diffuse large cell lymphoma.[17,18] The cells that infiltrate the vitreous appear in cytological preparations as lymphoid cells that have pleomorphic nuclei and scanty cytoplasm.[13,17] These cells occur singly or in small clusters and are frequently associated with many necrotic lymphocytes. Immunocytochemical stains and flow cytometry can be used to identify the cell of origin in most cases. Most of the abnormal lymphoid cells in such cases appear to be B-cell derived.

The tumor cells that infiltrate the uvea in primary uveal lymphoma are more likely to be well-differentiated small lymphoma cells than cells of diffuse large cell lymphoma.[19,20] The lymphoid cells in such cases may be either B-cell or T-cell derived.

TREATMENT

Treatment of the intraocular lesions of primary intraocular lymphoma generally consists of whole eye irradiation by fractionated external beam radiation therapy (Box 149-2).[12,21,22] The typical target dose of radiation is 30–45Gy. The fundus lesions usually respond promptly to radiotherapy (Fig. 149-3). If concurrent CNS lymphoma exists, aggressive intravenous and intrathecal chemotherapy[12,21,22] and occasionally whole brain irradiation are usually recommended.[21] Bone marrow transplantation has been used with some success in selected patients.[22] The role of chemotherapy in primary intraocular lymphoma without evidence of CNS lymphoma or visceral lymphoma is controversial. Intravitreal chemotherapy has been given to a few patients with residual or recurrent vitreoretinal lymphoma after conventional therapy[23] and has reportedly been effective, at least through short-term follow-up.

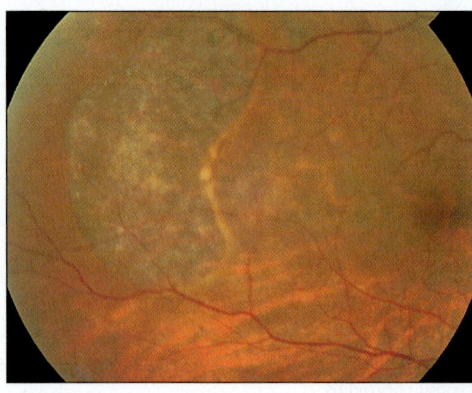

FIG. 149-3 ▉ **External beam radiation therapy for primary vitreoretinal lymphoma.** The same lesion shown in Figure 149-1 underwent complete regression 2 months after radiation therapy.

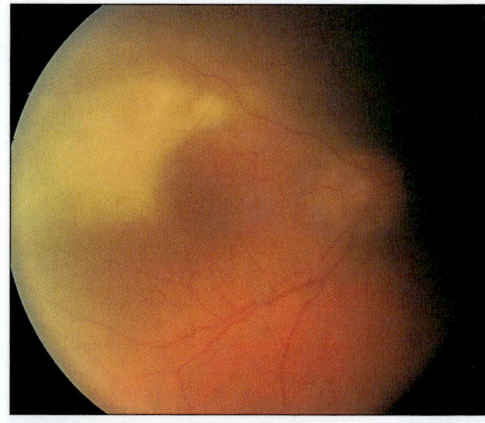

FIG. 149-4 ▉ **Leukemic retinal infiltrate.** The patient was a 76-year-old woman who had chronic myelogenous leukemia.

COURSE AND OUTCOME

Primary intraocular lymphoma has a highly variable clinical course that ranges from an indolent waxing and waning to an aggressive progression that results in a completely blind eye. Patients who develop primary intraocular lymphoma in the context of the acquired immunodeficiency syndrome (AIDS) tend to have an extremely virulent and rapidly progressive form of the disease.[24]

Following chemotherapy or ocular irradiation, subretinal pigment epithelial lesions of primary vitreoretinal lymphoma typically become totally atrophic (see Fig. 149-3), and the vitreous infiltration usually clears. Unfortunately, the vitreous cellular infiltration sometimes relapses within a few months after initially effective therapy. Diffuse uveal infiltrates also typically regress completely following chemotherapy, radiation therapy, or a combination of these therapies. Extensive retinal pigment epithelial degeneration and pigment clumping are usually evident at sites of prior uveal infiltration.

Patients with primary intraocular lymphoma must be followed on a regular basis after their treatment to monitor for local ocular relapse or the development of extraophthalmic disease in the CNS or elsewhere. If primary CNS lymphoma develops, the patient's prognosis for long-term survival is poor.[10,25] The survival prognosis of patients with visceral non-Hodgkin's lymphoma is generally substantially better than that of patients with primary CNS lymphoma[20]; however, patients with aggressive forms of non-Hodgkin's lymphoma also have substantially shortened survival.

INTRAOCULAR LEUKEMIA

INTRODUCTION

Intraocular leukemia is an uncommon ophthalmic disorder due to accumulation of circulating leukemic cells in the uvea, neural retina, optic disc, vitreous, or other intraocular tissues and fluids. Although leukemic patients frequently develop hemorrhagic retinopathy and occasionally develop microbial intraocular lesions, true leukemic intraocular lesions occur in only a small proportion of patients who have leukemia. Unfortunately, leukemic intraocular infiltrates are a poor prognostic sign for survival.

EPIDEMIOLOGY AND PATHOGENESIS

The cumulative lifetime incidence of intraocular leukemic infiltration in the general population of the United States, based on published data on the annual incidence of new cases of leukemia

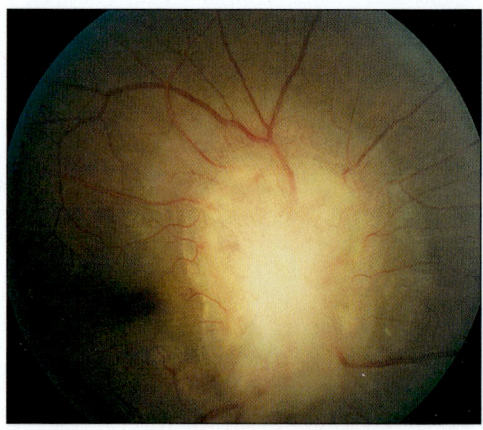

FIG. 149-5 ▉ **Leukemic optic disc infiltration.** The patient was a 37-year-old man who had chronic myelogenous leukemia.

and death from leukemia[26] and the percentage of leukemic patients dying of the disease who have intraocular lesions (infiltrative or other) at the time of death,[27] is approximately 1 case per 2000–2500 persons. Because only about one out of every six patients dying of leukemia develops ophthalmic symptoms that necessitate referral to an ophthalmologist,[27] and because only about 10% of all clinically detected intraocular lesions in leukemic patients are infiltrative in nature,[28] one can further estimate that the incidence of clinically important intraocular infiltrative leukemic lesions is 1 per 12,000–13,000 persons.

Infiltrative intraocular lesions can occur in individuals of any age, but peaks of incidence mirror those of leukemia in general. Intraocular leukemic lesions are usually not a presenting feature of the disease but are more likely to occur during leukemic relapse.

OCULAR MANIFESTATIONS

The most characteristic clinical intraocular lesion of leukemia is the leukemic retinal infiltrate. The typical lesion of this type is a fuzzy, flat, white retinal patch (Fig. 149-4) that is frequently associated with retinal hemorrhages and overlying intravitreal cells. Leukemic retinal infiltrates can be unifocal or multifocal and can present in one eye or both eyes. Other recognizable intraocular infiltrative lesions of leukemia include cells in the vitreous, sheathing of retinal blood vessels, optic disc infiltration (Fig. 149-5), retinal pigment epithelial detachment, nonrhegmatogenous retinal detachment, localized or diffuse choroidal infiltration, neoplastic pseudohypopyon, and iris infiltration.[28,29]

Hemorrhagic retinal lesions are much more common in leukemic patients than are true malignant infiltrates.[28] These lesions are frequently multifocal and bilateral. They are usually attributable to associated anemia and thrombocytopenia rather than to the leukemia per se. Larger intraretinal hemorrhages sometimes have prominent white centers (Roth's spots). If the anemia and thrombocytopenia are addressed, the extravasated blood gradually resolves in most patients.

Because patients who have leukemia are commonly immunosuppressed (either because of their malignancy or, more often, because of the effects of chemotherapy), it is sometimes difficult, if not impossible, to tell clinically whether a fundus lesion is truly a leukemic infiltration or a microbial focus caused by an opportunistic organism. In such cases, fine-needle aspiration biopsy or another specimen-generating technique may be of great value in establishing the correct diagnosis.

In patients who have chronic myelogenous leukemia, peripheral retinal capillary obstruction and microaneurysm formation have been observed.[30] In a few patients who have leukemia, neovascularization of the optic disc and retina has been reported.

DIAGNOSIS AND ANCILLARY TESTING

All patients who have suspected leukemic intraocular infiltration should be evaluated thoroughly from a hematological perspective. This evaluation should include a complete blood count with differential, bone marrow aspiration or biopsy, complete systemic staging evaluation, and probably lumbar puncture for cerebrospinal fluid cytology. If monocular or binocular optic disc edema or infiltration is present, computed tomography or magnetic resonance imaging of the orbits and brain is indicated (see Systemic Associations below). If uncertainty still exists about the ocular diagnosis, and if vitreous cells and retinal infiltrates are prominent features of the clinical presentation, one should consider pars plana vitrectomy or fine-needle aspiration biopsy to confirm the diagnosis. Biopsy is most appropriate if the patient has no clinical evidence of leukemic relapse elsewhere and is believed to be in clinical remission.

DIFFERENTIAL DIAGNOSIS

The principal lesions in the differential diagnosis of intraocular leukemia are listed in Box 149-3.

SYSTEMIC ASSOCIATIONS

Concurrent CNS leukemia is common in patients who develop an intraocular leukemic infiltrate. This relationship is particularly strong in patients who have infiltrative lesions of the optic disc.[29] Consequently, CNS imaging and lumbar puncture are especially indicated in any patient suspected of having leukemic relapse in the eye.

BOX 149-3

DIFFERENTIAL DIAGNOSIS OF INTRAOCULAR LEUKEMIA

Microbial infiltrate (e.g., *Candida, Nocardia, Cryptococcus*)
Nonmicrobial intraocular inflammation (e.g., sarcoid granuloma, pars planitis)
Primary vitreoretinal lymphoma

BOX 149-4

TREATMENT OPTIONS FOR INTRAOCULAR LEUKEMIA

Chemotherapy (regimen appropriate to specific type of leukemia)
Radiotherapy (fractionated low-dose external beam radiation therapy)

PATHOLOGY

Pathologically, the infiltrated uvea, optic disc, retina, and overlying vitreous contain leukemic cells in various quantities. In reported autopsy series, choroidal infiltration is much more frequent than infiltration of any other intraocular tissue. Leukemic cells are also commonly observed in the lumina of choroidal and retinal blood vessels.

TREATMENT

Infiltrative intraocular leukemia is generally treated by a combination of systemic chemotherapy appropriate to the particular type of leukemia and external beam radiation therapy to the involved eye or eyes (Box 149-4).[29,31] The dose of radiation required is usually much less than that recommended for intraocular lymphoma and may be as low as 12–20Gy.

COURSE AND OUTCOME

Untreated leukemic infiltrates usually progress relentlessly and ultimately cause profound visual loss in the affected eye or eyes. Fortunately, most retinal lesions respond promptly and completely to low-dose external beam radiation therapy, appropriate chemotherapy, or both. Massive optic disc infiltration that causes visual loss also commonly responds to this treatment, but the vision in such eyes often does not improve. Unfortunately, the survival prognosis of leukemic patients who develop intraocular infiltrative tumors is extremely poor.[32] The median survival time after detection of infiltrative intraocular lesions in most series is 3–5 months.

REFERENCES

1. Augsburger JJ, Greatrex KV. Intraocular lymphoma: clinical presentations, differential diagnosis and treatment. Trans Pa Acad Ophthalmol Otolaryngol. 1989;40:797–808.
2. Gill MK, Jampol LM. Variations in the presentation of primary intraocular lymphoma: case reports and a review. Surv Ophthalmol. 2001;45:463–71.
3. Peterson K, Gordon KB, Heinemann MH, DeAngelis LM. The clinical spectrum of ocular lymphoma. Cancer. 1993;72:843–9.
4. Whitcup SM, de Smet MD, Rubin BI, et al. Intraocular lymphoma. Clinical and histopathologic diagnosis. Ophthalmology. 1993;100:1399–406.
5. Gass JDM, Sever RJ, Grizzard WS, et al. Multifocal pigment epithelial detachments by reticulum cell sarcoma: a characteristic funduscopic picture. Retina. 1984;4:135–43.
6. Shah GK, Kleiner RC, Augsburger JJ, et al. Primary intraocular lymphoma seen with transient white fundus lesions simulating the multiple evanescent white dot syndrome. Arch Ophthalmol. 2001;119:617–20.
7. Ridley ME, McDonald R, Sternberg P, et al. Retinal manifestations of ocular lymphoma (reticulum cell sarcoma). Ophthalmology. 1992;99:1153–61.
8. Jakobiec FA, Sacks E, Kronish JW, et al. Multifocal static creamy choroidal infiltrates. An early sign of lymphoid neoplasia. Ophthalmology. 1987;94:397–406.
9. Ciulla TA, Bains RA, Jakobiec FA, et al. Uveal lymphoid neoplasia: a clinical-pathologic correlation and review of the early form. Surv Ophthalmol. 1997;41:467–76.
10. Gass JDM, Weleber RG, Johnson DR. Non-Hodgkin's lymphoma causing fundus picture simulating fundus flavimaculatus. Retina. 1987;7:209–14.
11. Char DH, Ljung BM, Deschênes J, Miller TR. Intraocular lymphoma: immunological and cytological analysis. Br J Ophthalmol. 1988;72:905–11.
12. Akpek EK, Ahmed I, Hochberg FH, et al. Intraocular–central nervous system lymphoma: clinical features, diagnosis, and outcomes. Ophthalmology. 1999;106:1805–10.
13. Blumenkranz M, Ward T, Murphy S, et al. Applications and limitations of vitreoretinal biopsy techniques in intraocular large cell lymphoma. Retina. 1992;12(Suppl 3):S64–70.
14. Whitcup SM, Stark-Vancs V, Wittes RE, et al. Association of interleukin 10 in vitreous and cerebrospinal fluid and primary central nervous system lymphoma. Arch Ophthalmol. 1997;115:1157–60.
15. Cursiefen C, Holbach LM, Lafaut B, et al. Oculocerebral non-Hodgkin's lymphoma with uveal involvement. Development of an epibulbar tumor after vitrectomy. Arch Ophthalmol. 2000;118:1437–40.
16. Hunyor AP, Harper CA, O'Day J, McKelvic PA. Ocular–central nervous system lymphoma mimicking posterior scleritis with exudative retinal detachment. Ophthalmology. 2000;107:1955–9.
17. Green WR. Diagnostic cytopathology of ocular fluid specimens. Ophthalmology. 1984;91:726–49.
18. Dean JM, Novak MA, Chan CC, Green WR. Tumor detachments of the retinal pigment epithelium in ocular/central nervous system lymphoma. Retina. 1996;16: 47–56.
19. Grossniklaus HE, Martin DF, Avery R, et al. Uveal lymphoid infiltration. Report of four cases and clinicopathologic review. Ophthalmology. 1998;105:1265–73.
20. Cockerham GC, Hidayat AA, Bijwaard KE, Sheng ZM. Re-evaluation of "reactive lymphoid hyperplasia of the uvea." An immunohistochemical and molecular analysis of 10 cases. Ophthalmology. 2000;107:151–8.

21. Valluri S, Moorthy RS, Khan A, Rao NA. Combination treatment of intraocular lymphoma. Retina. 1995;15:125–9.

22. Soussain C, Suzan F, Hoang-Xuan K, et al. Results of intensive chemotherapy followed by hematopoietic stem-cell rescue in patients with refractory or recurrent primary CNS lymphoma or intraocular lymphoma. J Clin Oncol. 2001;19:742–9.

23. Fishburne BC, Wilson DJ, Rosenbaum JT, Neuwelt EA. Intravitreal methotrexate as an adjunctive treatment of intraocular lymphoma. Arch Ophthalmol. 1997;115:1152–6.

24. Rivero ME, Kuppermann BD, Wiley CA, et al. Acquired immunodeficiency syndrome–related intraocular B-cell lymphoma. Arch Ophthalmol. 1999;117:616–22.

25. Freeman LN, Schachat AP, Knox DL, et al. Clinical features, laboratory investigations, and survival in ocular reticulum cell sarcoma. Ophthalmology. 1987;94:1631–9.

26. Parker SL, Tong T, Bolden S, Wingo PA. Cancer statistics, 1997. CA Cancer J Clin. 1997;47:5–27.

27. Leonardy NJ, Rupani M, Dent G, Klintworth GK. Analysis of 135 autopsy eyes for ocular involvement in leukemia. Am J Ophthalmol. 1990;109:436–44.

28. Schachat AP, Markowitz JA, Guyer DR, et al. Ophthalmic manifestations of leukemia. Arch Ophthalmol. 1989;107:697–700.

29. Kaikov Y. Optic nerve head infiltration in acute leukemia in children: an indication for emergency optic nerve radiation therapy. Med Pediatr Oncol. 1996;26:101–4.

30. Wiznia RA, Rose A, Levy A. Occlusive microvascular retinopathy with optic disc and retinal neovascularization in acute lymphocytic leukemia. Retina. 1994;14:253–5.

31. Brady LW, Shields JA, Augsburger JJ, et al. Malignant intraocular tumors. In: Mansfield CM, ed. Therapeutic radiology, 2nd ed. New York: Elsevier; 1989:181–97.

32. Ohkoshi K, Tsiaras WG. Prognostic importance of ophthalmic manifestations in childhood leukemia. Br J Ophthalmol. 1992;76:651–5.

CHAPTER 150

Medulloepithelioma

JAMES J. AUGSBURGER • SUSAN SCHNEIDER

DEFINITION
- Primary intraocular neoplasm derived from immature medullary epithelial cells of embryonic optic cup.

KEY FEATURES
- Amelanotic tumor that arises mainly in the ciliary body.
- Affects infants and young children preferentially.
- Occurs in both benign and malignant forms.

ASSOCIATED FEATURES
- Neuroepithelial cysts on surface of tumor.
- Coloboma or notch of lens in some eyes.
- Neovascular glaucoma in childhood.

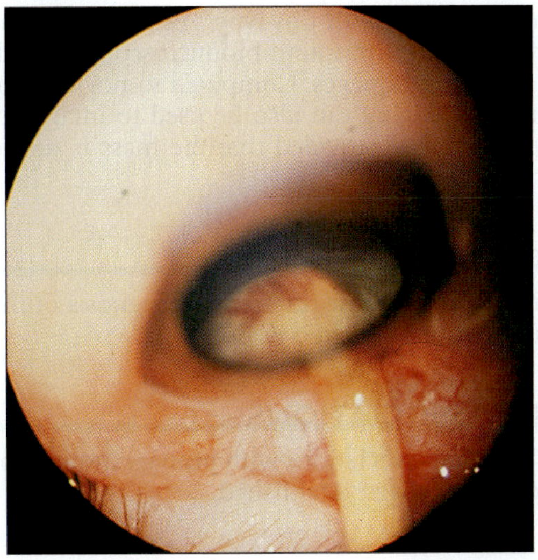

FIG. 150-1 ■ **Medulloepithelioma of ciliary body.** White ciliary body tumor is revealed by scleral depression.

INTRODUCTION

Intraocular medulloepithelioma is a rare primary intraocular neoplasm derived from neuroectoderm. This type of tumor characteristically arises from the nonpigmented epithelium of the ciliary body. On rare occasions, medulloepithelioma also arises from the iris, retina, or optic disc. The tumors range from benign proliferations to malignant neoplasms with unequivocal invasive capacity but limited metastatic potential.

EPIDEMIOLOGY AND PATHOGENESIS

Medulloepithelioma is uncommon, but its precise incidence is unknown. Based on relative prevalence data from multiple clinical and pathological case series, however, its incidence can be estimated at approximately one thirtieth to one fiftieth that of retinoblastoma. This would correspond to a cumulative lifetime incidence of approximately 1 case per 450,000–1,000,000 persons. Intraocular medulloepithelioma is usually a congenital or infantile tumor,[1] but juvenile- and even adult-onset cases have been reported. The average age of the affected individual at diagnosis is about 5 years in most series. Medulloepithelioma affects all ethnic groups and both sexes equally. It does not appear to be transmitted genetically. No known risk factors exist for this tumor.

OCULAR MANIFESTATIONS

The usual presenting symptoms of medulloepithelioma are a red eye, change in color of the iris, visible mass in the iris, and (in adults and some older children) visual impairment.[1] Medulloepithelioma of the ciliary body typically appears as a tan to white lesion of the extreme peripheral fundus. Because of its peripheral location, the tumor may be detectable only by binocular indirect ophthalmoscopy with scleral depression during ophthalmic examination under anesthesia (Fig. 150-1). A tumor of this type frequently appears intrinsically cystic or has prominent neuroepithelial cysts on its surface.[1,2] In occasional patients, localized absence of the zonule and resultant abnor-

malities of lens curvature (lens coloboma), lens subluxation, and cataract have been observed.[1–3]

An intraocular medulloepithelioma that involves the iris usually appears as a tan to pink mass that replaces the peripheral iris and fills the angle.[1,2] Such tumors often have prominent intrinsic blood vessels.

A common complication of medulloepitheliomas of the ciliary body is development of neovascular glaucoma.[1,4] In some cases, glaucoma of this type develops even when the tumor is limited in extent. In other cases, non-neovascular angle closure develops in response to the ciliary body tumor.[5] Because the eye in such cases is extremely firm, it may not be possible to depress the sclera sufficiently during indirect ophthalmoscopy at examination under anesthesia to visualize the tumor. Also, the far peripheral location of the lesion may preclude the use of conventional contact B-scan to detect the tumor. In the face of unexplained neovascular glaucoma or angle closure and a posterior fundus of essentially normal appearance, the ophthalmologist should strongly consider the possibility of medulloepithelioma and evaluate the eye further by alternative methods of ocular imaging (computed tomography, magnetic resonance imaging, or ultrasound biomicroscopy) or perform a paracentesis followed by re-examination of the peripheral fundus with scleral depression.

In exceptional cases, intraocular medulloepithelioma arises from the retina or optic disc. All reported cases of this type have occurred in children younger than 7 years. Because of this, such tumors have uniformly been misdiagnosed clinically as retinoblastoma.

DIAGNOSIS AND ANCILLARY TESTING

B-scan ultrasonography is frequently able to image a relatively large ciliary body medulloepithelioma.[6] However, conventional contact B-scan ultrasonography is often unable to demonstrate a small ciliary body tumor of this type. For such a lesion, either a water bath B-scan or ultrasound biomicroscopy should be used to obtain satisfactory images. Computed tomography and magnetic resonance imaging can also be used to image intraocular medulloepitheliomas, provided that the mass is not too small and the scan slices are thin.

DIFFERENTIAL DIAGNOSIS

The principal lesions in the differential diagnosis of intraocular medulloepithelioma are listed in Box 150-1.

SYSTEMIC ASSOCIATIONS

As yet, no systemic associations with primary intraocular medulloepithelioma have been established.

Baseline Systemic Evaluation

Because medulloepithelioma tends to be locally invasive but not metastatic in most patients, no systemic evaluation is generally indicated at baseline before initial ocular treatment.

PATHOLOGY

The characteristic histopathological feature of intraocular medulloepithelioma is a structural arrangement of cells that closely resembles that of neural medullary epithelium (Fig. 150-2). The degree of cellular differentiation differs widely from case to case. Many well-differentiated medulloepitheliomas contain prominent rosettes and cystic spaces filled with hyaluronic acid. Medulloepitheliomas that contain heterotopic elements such as hyaline cartilage, striated muscle, or brain are referred to as teratoid medulloepitheliomas. Those that do not contain such elements are termed nonteratoid medulloepitheliomas. About two thirds of intraocular medulloepitheliomas are categorized as malignant pathologically,[1,2] largely on the basis of invasiveness and extraocular extension of the tumor, especially if associated with numerous mitotic figures and undifferentiated cells.

TREATMENT

Although iridocyclectomy and episcleral plaque radiotherapy have both been employed in some cases of iridociliary or ciliary body medulloepithelioma (Box 150-2), such treatments have frequently failed to eradicate the tumor. In fact, local failure of such treatments appears to be almost the rule in medulloepitheliomas judged to be malignant by histopathological criteria. Eyes that have an extremely large intraocular tumor at presentation, those

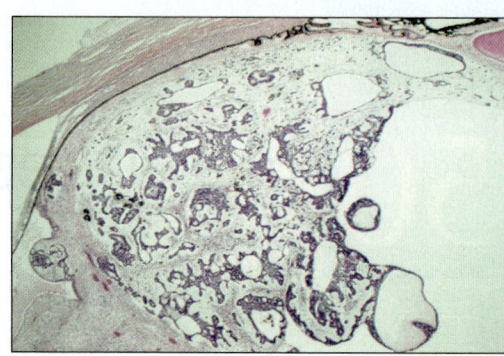

FIG. 150-2 ■ **Pathology of medulloepithelioma.** Photomicrograph of nonteratoid medulloepithelioma (hematoxylin-eosin stain, original magnification 100×) showing cords and tubules of tumor cells and prominent associated cysts.

that are blind and painful as a result of tumor-related complications, and most eyes that develop local recurrence of medulloepithelioma after primary attempted resection or plaque radiotherapy eventually require enucleation. Patients who have massive orbital extension may even require exenteration.

COURSE AND OUTCOME

Medulloepithelioma, even in its benign varieties, tends to be a relentlessly progressive tumor. This can lead ultimately to destruction of the eye, profound visual loss, and even trans-scleral tumor extension. As long as the tumor is still contained within the eye at the time of enucleation, survival generally is assured.

In eyes that have a well-defined, histologically benign medulloepithelioma, surgical resection of the lesion by iridocyclectomy is frequently curative.[2] If local recurrence develops after such surgery, it usually becomes evident within about 6 months. As long as a medulloepithelioma is completely contained within the eye, it is unlikely to produce metastatic disease. However, if a malignant medulloepithelioma extends through the sclera and invades the orbit, it occasionally proves fatal due to invasive intracranial extension, widespread metastasis, or both.

REFERENCES

1. Canning CR, McCartney CE, Hungerford J. Medulloepithelioma (diktyoma). Br J Ophthalmol. 1988;72:764–7.
2. Shields JA, Eagle EC, Shields CL, De Potter P. Congenital neoplasms of the nonpigmented ciliary epithelium (medulloepithelioma). Ophthalmology. 1996;103:1997–2006.
3. Gupta NK, Simon JW, Walton DS, Augsburger JJ. Bilateral ectopia lentis as a presenting feature of medulloepithelioma. J AAPOS. 2001;5:255–7.
4. Singh A, Singh AD, Shields CL, Shields JA. Iris neovascularization in children as a manifestation of underlying medulloepithelioma. J Pediatr Ophthalmol Strabismus. 2001;38:224–8.
5. Katsushima H, Suzuki J, Adachi J, et al. Non-rubeotic angle-closure glaucoma associated with ciliary medulloepithelioma. Jpn J Ophthalmol. 1996;40:244–50.
6. Orellana J, Moura RA, Font RL, et al. Medulloepithelioma diagnosed by ultrasound and vitreous aspirate. Ophthalmology. 1983;90:1531–9.

SECTION 2 BENIGN INTRAOCULAR TUMORS

CHAPTER 151

Uveal Nevus

JAMES J. AUGSBURGER • J. WILLIAM HARBOUR • JOHN R. GONDER

DEFINITION
- Primary benign acquired melanocytic tumor of uvea.

KEY FEATURES
- Brown or fleshy iris mass usually 3mm or less in diameter and 0.5mm or less in thickness.
- Gray to brown (melanotic) or tan (amelanotic) choroidal mass usually 5mm or less in diameter and 1mm or less in thickness.

ASSOCIATED FEATURES
- Anterior uveal nevi: ectropion iridis and pupillary peaking.
- Posterior uveal nevi: drusen and retinal pigment epithelial alterations on surface of choroidal tumor; occasional shallow non-rhegmatogenous retinal detachment that overlies and surrounds choroidal tumor.

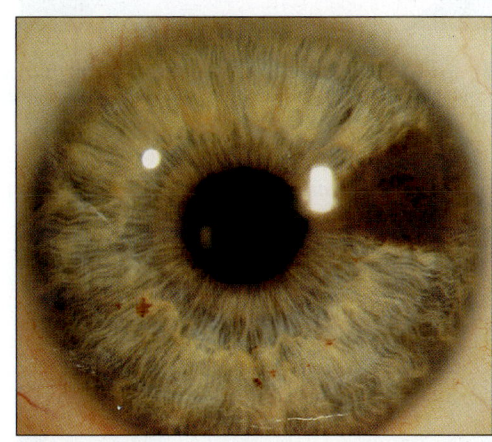

FIG. 151-1 ▥ **Typical iris nevus.** Thin, dark brown iris lesion does not cause pupillary irregularity.

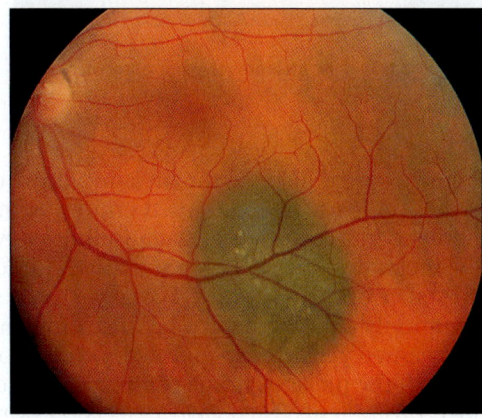

FIG. 151-2 ▥ **Typical choroidal nevus.** Thin gray-brown choroidal lesion has a few small drusen on its surface.

INTRODUCTION

The uveal nevus is a benign tumor that arises from melanocytic cells derived from the neural crest. Uveal nevi occur most commonly in the choroid, but similar lesions also occur in the iris, ciliary body, and optic disc.

EPIDEMIOLOGY AND PATHOGENESIS

The uveal nevus is unquestionably the most common primary intraocular tumor. In Caucasians, it has been estimated that approximately 20% of persons older than 50 years have at least one choroidal nevus.[1] If small melanocytic iris lesions are counted as nevi, 30–50% of eyes have at least one uveal nevus. Most uveal nevi are likely to be congenital in nature, but they usually do not become pigmented and detectable clinically until after childhood. The frequency of clinically evident uveal nevi increases with advancing age.[2] Uveal nevi are much more common in persons of lightly pigmented races. They appear to be equally common in men and women.

Uveal nevi are commonly regarded as precursor lesions to uveal malignant melanoma.[3] Although some uveal nevi unquestionably undergo malignant change, comparative age-specific prevalence estimates for uveal nevi and uveal melanomas suggest that only about 1 in 4000–5000 uveal nevi actually does so.[2]

OCULAR MANIFESTATIONS

Most uveal nevi are asymptomatic. Macular choroidal nevi, however, can cause visual loss in the affected eye.[4]

The typical iris nevus appears as a localized melanotic stromal lesion of the iris (Fig. 151-1). It can involve any portion of the iris from the pupillary margin to the iris root. The typical iris nevus is 3mm or less in diameter and 0.5mm or less in thickness; how-ever, larger iris nevi are documented from time to time. Iris nevi can cause pupillary peaking, focal ectropion iridis, or both, but they are rarely associated with abnormal iris vasculature.

The typical choroidal nevus appears as a small gray to brown choroidal tumor with a bland surface appearance (Fig. 151-2). Many choroidal nevi exhibit characteristic surface alterations such as drusen and retinal pigment epithelial pigment clumping (Fig. 151-3). Most choroidal nevi are 5mm or less in basal diameter and 1mm or less in thickness, but occasional lesions of this type attain a basal diameter of 10mm or more, a thickness of 3mm or more, or both. Blurred or distorted vision attributable to a choroidal nevus may be the result of an accumulation of serous subretinal fluid,[5] cystic degeneration of the retina overlying a macular choroidal nevus,[4] or choroidal neovascularization.[6] Occasional choroidal nevi have a halo appearance characterized by a golden orange marginal zone that surrounds the typically gray to brown central zone.

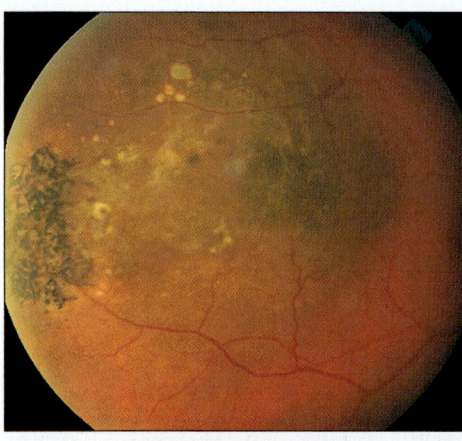

FIG. 151-3 ▮▮ **Large choroidal nevus.** This mildly elevated (thickness 1.5mm) melanotic choroidal tumor has prominent drusen and retinal pigment epithelial pigment clumps on its surface.

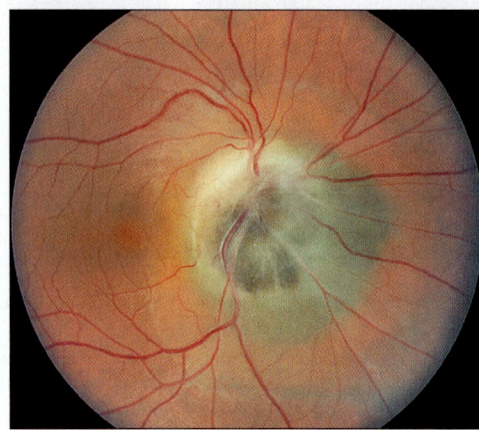

FIG. 151-4 ▮▮ Melanocytoma of optic disc.

A special type of uveal nevus is the melanocytoma of the optic disc.[7] This lesion is usually composed entirely of maximally pigmented, polyhedral nevus cells (magnocellular nevus cells). Clinically, the melanocytoma is a brown to black tumor that involves the substance of the optic disc (Fig. 151-4). The surface of the lesion commonly appears striated because of insinuation of the darkly pigmented cells of the tumor between axons in the nerve fiber layer. If the melanocytoma compresses the optic disc, it can produce prominent visual field defects. Lesion enlargement can occur but is usually slow.[8] Magnocellular nevi also occur in the choroid, ciliary body, and iris, but such nevi cannot be differentiated clinically from nevi of other histopathological types.

DIAGNOSIS AND ANCILLARY TESTING

Suspected melanocytic lesions of the iris are usually documented photographically shortly after detection and then monitored for subsequent enlargement or other worrisome changes that might signal malignant behavior. Fluorescein angiography and indocyanine green angiography have little differential diagnostic or prognostic value. Ultrasound biomicroscopy is used to measure the size and extent of an iris tumor.

Suspected melanocytic tumors of the choroid (i.e., nevi versus melanomas) are generally evaluated by ultrasonography and fluorescein angiography. Ultrasonography allows the ophthalmologist to assess the precise thickness of the lesion, identify its reflectivity pattern, and rule out scleral invasion and trans-scleral tumor extension. Fluorescein angiography and indocyanine green angiography assess the presence or absence of prominent blood vessels within the tumor. Most benign choroidal nevi do

not have prominent intralesional blood vessels, but most choroidal melanomas do. Consequently, most choroidal nevi appear totally hypofluorescent throughout the angiogram except at sites of drusen and retinal pigment epithelial depigmentation. With indocyanine green angiography, most choroidal nevi appear totally nonfluorescent throughout the study. The full basal extent of a choroidal nevus is defined better by indocyanine green angiography than by fluorescein angiography. For worrisome lesions, fine-needle aspiration biopsy can be used to determine the pathological nature of the tumor before therapeutic intervention.[9] Melanotic choroidal lesions more than 1.5mm thick can usually be biopsied successfully using a transvitreal, bent-needle technique.

DIFFERENTIAL DIAGNOSIS

Most of the important lesions in the differential diagnosis of uveal nevi are listed in Box 151-1. Uveal melanoma is unquestionably the most important lesion in the differential diagnosis.

SYSTEMIC ASSOCIATIONS

Two important systemic disorders are associated with melanocytic choroidal nevi. In some patients who have neurofibromatosis type 1, multiple uveal nevi develop in both eyes. These lesions must be differentiated from the small, tan, melanocytic iris lesions (Lisch nodules) that arise multifocally from the anterior surface of the iris. Lisch nodules appear to be nodular aggregates of dendritic melanocytes and not true nevi. They usually become evident by the age of 10–15 years and are highly characteristic of neurofibromatosis type 1.

In patients who have the syndrome of bilateral diffuse melanocytic proliferation associated with systemic carcinoma,[10] multiple acquired melanocytic uveal nevi frequently arise in both eyes in response to some as yet undetermined substance elaborated by an underlying but often occult systemic cancer.

Baseline Systemic Evaluation

Because uveal nevi are benign lesions, baseline systemic evaluation is generally not recommended in patients who have such lesions. If changes in a presumed uveal nevus prompt its reclassification as a probable malignant melanoma, a baseline systemic evaluation appropriate to a uveal melanoma (see Chapter 147) becomes warranted.

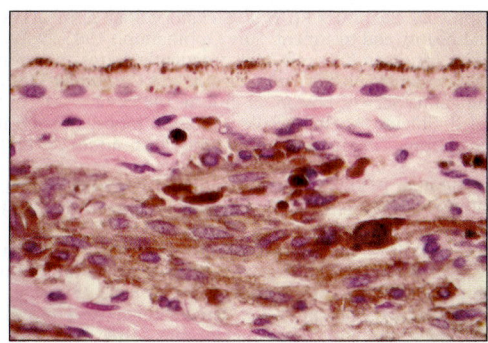

FIG. 151-5 ■ **Histopathology of choroidal nevus.** Note the spindle-shaped nuclei, absent and prominent nucleoli, uniformity of tumor cells, and prominent intracytoplasmic melanin that characterize spindle cell choroidal nevus.

BOX 151-2

Treatment Options for Uveal Nevi

Observation (unless lesion enlarges abruptly or substantially or otherwise changes and is reclassified as uveal melanoma)
Treatment of subretinal fluid involving macula
• Focal laser therapy to angiographically localized leak sites
• Barrier laser around nevus to wall off subretinal fluid
Biopsy or excision of worrisome lesions
• Fine-needle aspiration biopsy
• Incisional biopsy or excision (iridectomy for iris lesions)

PATHOLOGY

The uveal nevus is composed of atypical melanocytic cells that are benign by histopathological criteria (Fig. 151-5). Several different types of uveal nevus cells are known.[11] Spindle nevus cells are fusiform melanocytes that typically have a relatively small nucleus and either no nucleolus or a small nucleolus. Spindle nevus cells usually contain relatively few small, intracytoplasmic melanin granules. Magnocellular nevus cells are plump polyhedral melanocytes that typically contain numerous large, intracytoplasmic melanin granules but have completely benign-appearing nuclei. Epithelioid nevus cells are relatively large, spherical melanocytes that contain a variable amount of intracytoplasmic melanin but do not have the nuclear and nucleolar pleomorphism that characterizes epithelioid melanoma cells. Balloon nevus cells are relatively large, spherical melanocytes characterized by a substantial amount of foamy, vacuolated cytoplasm.

The predominant cell type in most iris nevi is the spindle nevus cell. In contrast, the predominant cell type in most choroidal and ciliary body nevi is the magnocellular nevus cell.[11] Many uveal nevi consist of an admixture of more than one cell type. Balloon nevus cells typically occur in the yellow-orange halo that surrounds some choroidal nevi.

Dendritic melanocytes, which occur in some uveal nevi, in Lisch nodules of neurofibromatosis type 1, and in the iris nodules of the Cogan-Reese syndrome and iridocorneal endothelial syndrome, appear to be normal uveal melanocytes and not nevus cells.

TREATMENT

The standard management of patients who have choroidal nevi is photographic documentation of the tumor's appearance, ultrasonographic documentation of its thickness, and periodic re-evaluation to make sure that it remains dormant (Box 151-2). The recommended frequency of follow-up is largely a function of the level of diagnostic certainty and concern about potential malignancy. For very small nevi that appear nonsuspicious, the ophthalmologist may simply recommend re-evaluation within 1–2 years. For slightly larger nevi, the ophthalmologist may recommend re-evaluation within 6–12 months. If concern exists that the lesion may actually be a small malignant melanoma, the patient may be re-examined within 1–3 months. If re-evaluation over that short interval shows no appreciable change in the lesion, subsequent re-evaluations are usually scheduled at increasingly longer intervals. In general, nevi that are suspicious must be followed relatively closely for at least 3–5 years. If no substantial change occurs in the nevus over that interval, most ophthalmologists recommend future follow-up evaluations at approximately yearly intervals. If the nevus remains stable, periodic follow-up examinations will reassure both the patient and the ophthalmologist about the continued dormancy and benign status of the tumor.

Focal laser therapy can be considered for presumed choroidal nevi that are associated with serous macular retinal detachment and distorted or blurred vision.[5] If the fluid fails to disappear or increases, or the visual acuity in the affected eye deteriorates substantially, focal laser treatment to the angiographic leak sites can be used to stimulate fluid reabsorption.[12] If no focal angiographic leak sites are evident and the lesion does not extend beneath the fovea, laser treatment in the form of a barrier of overlapping or confluent laser burns between the nevus and the fovea sometimes walls off the subretinal fluid from the central macula. Alternatively, if the angiogram reveals a choroidal neovascular membrane that overlies the nevus, focal obliterative laser therapy can be employed to eradicate the vascular network.[6] Although some small choroidal melanomas with associated serous subretinal fluid develop nodular eruption through Bruch's membrane after focal laser treatment to the retinal pigment epithelial leak sites or to a suspected choroidal neovascular membrane that overlies the lesion,[12] no compelling evidence exists that such laser treatment ever induces malignant change in a benign choroidal nevus.

COURSE AND OUTCOME

Most uveal nevi change very little over the course of several years.[13] At the same time, however, many nevi exhibit slight changes in color and surface features or enlarge slightly over long periods of follow-up. Such minor changes should not be considered indicative of malignancy but rather should be considered manifestations of normal growth and aging. Conversely, some benign-appearing melanocytic uveal tumors that are initially diagnosed as nevi eventually exhibit clinical features suggesting that they are in fact malignant melanomas. In such cases, one can never be certain whether the change in the lesion represents more pronounced enlargement of a benign nevus than usually occurs,[14] malignant transformation of a benign nevus to a malignant melanoma, or activation of a malignant melanoma that had been dormant. Substantial tumor enlargement, especially if it occurs over a relatively short time (e.g., 6 months or less), must be regarded as strong circumstantial evidence of the malignancy of the lesion.[13] Such a change usually prompts the ophthalmologist to reclassify the tumor as a malignant melanoma and recommend intervention accordingly.

Features of a melanocytic choroidal lesion that help assure the ophthalmologist of its benign nature[15] include small size (basal diameter <5mm, thickness <1mm), homogeneous gray-brown surface coloration, feathered margins that blend almost imperceptibly into the surrounding normal choroid, drusen and retinal pigment epithelial pigment clumping and migration on the surface of the lesion, absence of prominent clumps of orange lipofuscin pigment on the surface of the lesion, absence of overlying serous subretinal fluid, and clinical dormancy of the lesion over long-term follow-up. As with presumed iris nevi, the greater the number of unfavorable features, the greater the concern that the lesion is in fact a melanoma rather than a benign uveal nevus.

By definition, uveal nevi are benign lesions. Therefore, unless malignant change occurs within such a lesion, the affected patient's risk of metastasis and tumor-related death is effectively zero. Because the likelihood of malignant transformation by classic uveal nevi appears to be exceptionally low, obliterative treatment of such lesions to prevent possible future malignant transformation is inappropriate.

REFERENCES

1. Gass JDM. Choroidal nevi or benign melanomas. In: Gass JDM, ed. Differential diagnosis of intraocular tumors. A stereoscopic presentation. St. Louis: Mosby; 1974:14.
2. Ganley JP, Comstock GW. Benign nevi and malignant melanomas of the choroid. Am J Ophthalmol. 1973;76:19–23.
3. Yanoff M, Zimmerman LE. Histogenesis of malignant melanomas of the uvea. II. Relationship of uveal nevi to malignant melanomas. Cancer. 1967;20:493–507.
4. Gonder JR, Augsburger JJ, McCarthy EF, et al. Visual loss associated with choroidal nevi. Ophthalmology. 1982;89:961–5.
5. Pro M, Shields JA, Tomer TL. Serous detachment of the macula associated with presumed choroidal nevi. Arch Ophthalmol. 1978;96:1374–7.
6. Callanan DG, Lewis ML, Byrne SF, Gass JD. Choroidal neovascularization associated with choroidal nevi. Arch Ophthalmol. 1993;111:789–94.
7. Reidy JJ, Apple DJ, Steinmetz RL, et al. Melanocytoma: nomenclature, pathogenesis, natural history and treatment. Surv Ophthalmol. 1985;29:319–27.
8. Augsburger JJ, Lauritzen K, Pon D. How frequently do melanocytomas of the optic disc really enlarge? Abstract presented at the Combined Meeting of Macula Society and Retina Society, Boston, 21–5 June 1989:172.
9. Augsburger JJ, Shields JA. Fine needle aspiration biopsy of solid intraocular tumors: indications, instrumentations and techniques. Ophthalmic Surg. 1984;15:34–40.
10. Mooy CM, de Jong PTVM, Strous C. Proliferative activity in bilateral paraneoplastic melanocytic proliferation and bilateral uveal melanoma. Br J Ophthalmol. 1994;78:483–4.
11. Naumann G, Yanoff M, Zimmerman LE. Histogenesis of malignant melanomas of the uvea: I. Histopathologic characteristics of nevi of the choroid and ciliary body. Arch Ophthalmol. 1966;76:784–96.
12. Folk JC, Weingeist TA, Coonan P, et al. The treatment of serous macular detachment secondary to choroidal melanomas and nevi. Ophthalmology. 1989;96:547–51.
13. Harbour JW, Augsburger JJ, Eagle RC. Initial management and follow-up of melanocytic iris tumors. Ophthalmology. 1995;102:1987–93.
14. MacIlwaine WA, Anderson B, Klintworth GK. Enlargement of histologically documented choroidal nevus. Am J Ophthalmol. 1979;87:480–6.
15. Augsburger JJ, Schroeder RP, Territo C, et al. Clinical parameters predictive of enlargement of melanocytic choroidal lesions. Br J Ophthalmol. 1989;73:911–7.

152 Choroidal Hemangiomas

JAMES J. AUGSBURGER • RAJIV ANAND • GEORGE E. SANBORN

DEFINITION
- Benign congenital vascular hamartoma of choroid.

KEY FEATURES
- Red-orange, ill-defined, disc-shaped choroidal tumor located 3mm or less from optic disc, foveola, or both.
- Diffuse or circumscribed growth patterns.

ASSOCIATED FEATURES
- Congenital, infantile, or juvenile glaucoma.
- Serous nonrhegmatogenous retinal detachment.
- Metaplasia of retinal pigment epithelium overlying tumor.
- Cystic degeneration of sensory retina overlying tumor.
- Other features of Sturge-Weber syndrome in patients who have diffuse choroidal hemangioma.

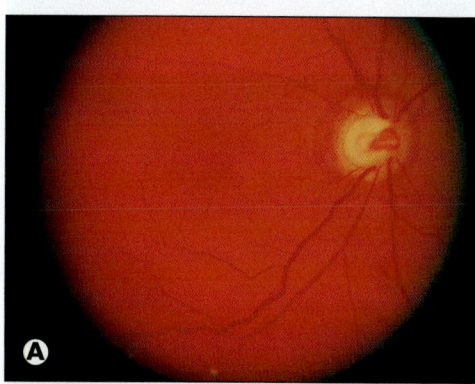

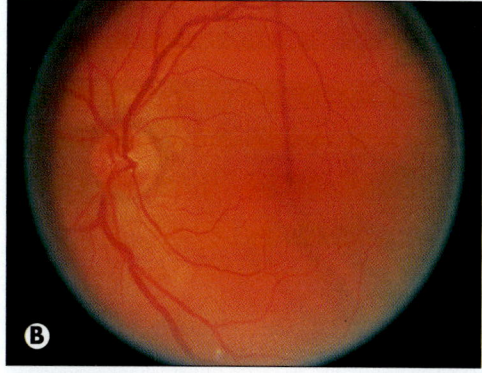

FIG. 152-1 ■ Asymmetric fundus appearance in patient with diffuse choroidal hemangioma. A, Right fundus has saturated red color caused by diffuse choroidal hemangioma. Note large deep cup of optic disc. B, Uninvolved left fundus has more orange choroid than right. Note normal appearance of optic disc.

INTRODUCTION

The choroidal hemangioma is a benign vascular tumor of the choroid. It occurs in two distinct clinical forms: a circumscribed form that is almost always isolated and nonsyndromic and a diffuse form that is usually part of the Sturge-Weber syndrome of encephalofacial hemangiomatosis.

EPIDEMIOLOGY AND PATHOGENESIS

Choroidal hemangiomas appear to be vascular birthmarks. They are relatively uncommon, but their precise incidence in the general population is unknown. They affect both sexes and all ethnic groups. Although probably congenital in most if not all patients, they are frequently not detected until the second through fourth decades of life.[1] No cause has ever been identified. Neither form of the disease appears to be hereditary.

OCULAR MANIFESTATIONS

Most circumscribed choroidal hemangiomas are noted first when they produce visual symptoms caused by accumulation of serous subretinal fluid, degenerative changes in the macular retina, or both. Diffuse choroidal hemangiomas are usually detected at baseline ophthalmic evaluation of patients who have a facial nevus flammeus before the onset of symptoms. Visual impairment in eyes that have either diffuse or circumscribed choroidal hemangioma ranges from none to total blindness.

The *diffuse choroidal hemangioma*, usually part of the Sturge-Weber syndrome, is generally identified ipsilaterally to a facial nevus flammeus. The fundus on the affected side typically has a much more saturated red appearance than does the fundus on the uninvolved side (Fig. 152-1). The choroid tends to be thickened diffusely by the hemangiomatous vascular lesion, but accentuated and sometimes nodular thickening occurs frequently in the macular and circumpapillary regions. The choroidal hemangioma becomes progressively thinner peripherally and gradually blends into the normal peripheral choroid. The choroidal thickening around the optic disc commonly results in prominent disc cupping that resembles glaucomatous optic neuropathy. Because elevated intraocular pressure, which is usually caused by elevated episcleral and orbital venous pressure, angle malformation, or both, is a feature of many eyes that have diffuse choroidal hemangioma, the optic disc can also exhibit true glaucomatous cupping. Although the retinal vasculature is sometimes normal in eyes that have a diffuse choroidal hemangioma, marked retinal vascular tortuosity is observed frequently in such eyes. The retinal pigment epithelium that overlies thicker portions of a diffuse choroidal hemangioma often undergoes fibrous metaplasia. The fibrous tissue on the surface of the hemangioma gives a whitish appearance to that part of the lesion. The neurosensory retina that overlies thicker portions of a diffuse choroidal hemangioma typically becomes thickened and cystic. Serous nonrhegmatogenous retinal detachment, either partial or total, is an eventual complication in many eyes that have diffuse choroidal hemangioma.

The *circumscribed choroidal hemangioma* is a reddish-orange, round to oval choroidal tumor located largely if not completely in the posterior half of the fundus (Fig. 152-2). The typical lesion ranges from approximately 3–7mm in diameter and 1–3mm in thickness at the time of detection and diagnosis, but larger lesions

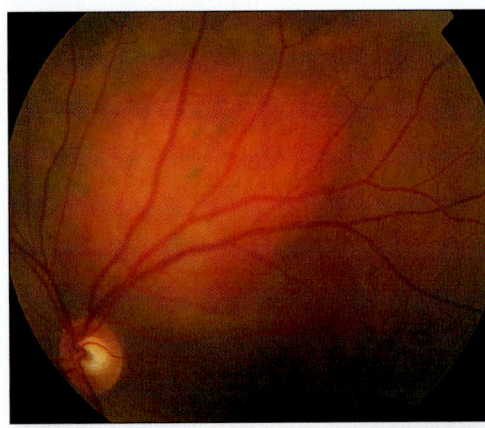

FIG. 152-2 ∎ Clinical appearance of circumscribed choroidal hemangioma. Juxtapapillary reddish choroidal tumor is associated with shallow serous subretinal fluid that involves the central macula.

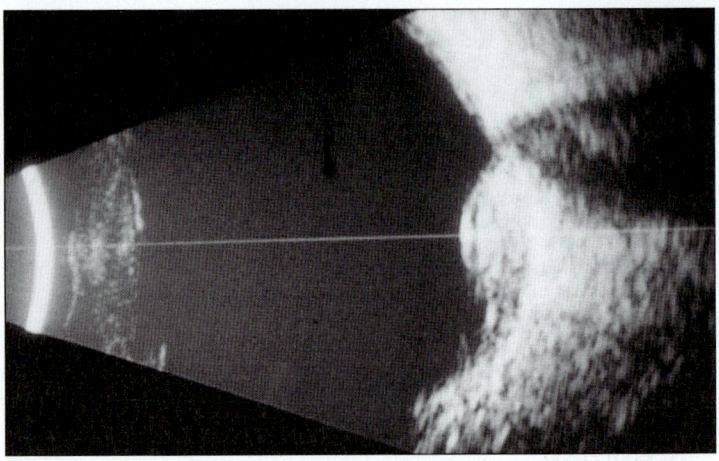

FIG. 152-4 ∎ B-scan ultrasonography of circumscribed choroidal hemangioma. Lesion appears fusiform in cross-sectional shape and is almost as sonoreflective as orbital fat. Note localized retinal detachment overlying tumor.

FIG. 152-3 ∎ Indocyanine green angiography of circumscribed choroidal hemangioma (same lesion shown in Fig. 152-2). A, Early phase frame shows filling of prominent large-caliber intralesional blood vessels. B, Intermediate phase frame shows intense diffuse hyperfluorescence of hemangioma. C, Late phase frame shows central washout of fluorescence from tumor but persistent hyperfluorescence at margins of tumor.

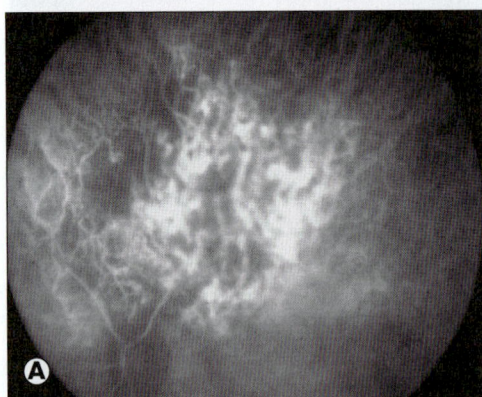

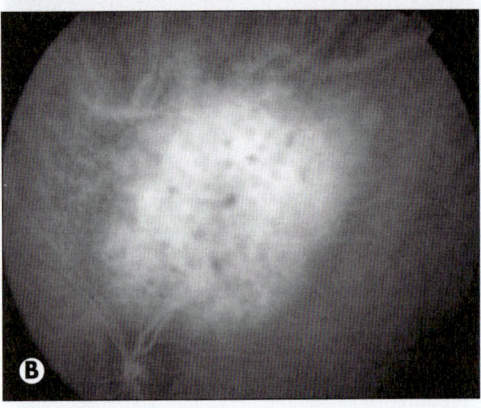

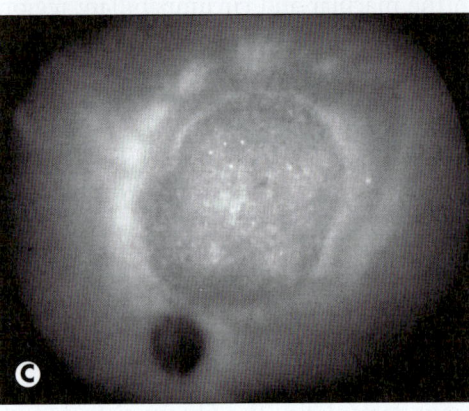

tion of circumscribed choroidal hemangiomas, but massive accumulation of subretinal or intraretinal exudates, as occurs with retinal capillary hemangiomas and Coats' disease, is rare.

DIAGNOSIS AND ANCILLARY TESTING

Fluorescein angiography of circumscribed choroidal hemangiomas typically reveals very early fluorescence of large-caliber choroidal blood vessels either before or simultaneously with the initial filling of the retinal arterioles. The entire lesion usually becomes diffusely fluorescent within several seconds after initial vascular filling. By the late frames, fluorescein commonly stains the entire lesion and any associated subretinal fluid.

Indocyanine green angiography of a circumscribed choroidal hemangioma[2] typically shows early filling of the intralesional vascular channels, intense hyperfluorescence of the lesion by the intermediate frames, and late washout of the central portion of the lesion (Fig. 152-3). The full extent of a circumscribed choroidal hemangioma is usually revealed much more clearly by indocyanine green angiography than by fluorescein angiography.

B-scan ultrasonography of a circumscribed choroidal hemangioma typically shows a fusiform, biconvex cross-sectional shape of the lesion and internal brightness similar to that of orbital fat (Fig. 152-4). B-scan ultrasonography of a diffuse choroidal hemangioma characteristically reveals generalized choroidal thickening by sonoreflective soft tissue and prominent optic disc cupping. On standardized A scan, both types of choroidal hemangioma tend to exhibit high-amplitude, broad-based echo spikes.

DIFFERENTIAL DIAGNOSIS

The principal lesions and disorders in the differential diagnoses of circumscribed and diffuse choroidal hemangiomas are listed in Box 152-1.

SYSTEMIC ASSOCIATIONS

For patients who have a diffuse choroidal hemangioma and ipsilateral facial nevus flammeus, the Sturge-Weber syndrome or a related multisystem syndrome must be suspected. Circumscribed choroidal hemangiomas are rarely associated with other features of the Sturge-Weber syndrome.

Baseline Systemic Evaluation

Because of the benign nature of choroidal hemangiomas, baseline systemic evaluation to look for evidence of metastatic disease is not appropriate.

occur occasionally. Almost all circumscribed choroidal hemangiomas are located within two disc diameters from the optic disc, foveola, or both at their posterior margins.[1] Such tumors almost never extend anterior to the equator unless they are extremely large. The retinal pigment epithelium that overlies a circumscribed choroidal hemangioma commonly undergoes degenerative changes, including fibrous metaplasia and occasionally bone formation, and the neurosensory retina overlying such lesions frequently becomes thickened and cystic. Partial or total nonrhegmatogenous retinal detachment occurs frequently as a complica-

TREATMENT

The currently employed treatment options for circumscribed choroidal hemangiomas are listed in Box 152-2. Because choroidal hemangiomas are benign tumors without malignant potential, treatment is directed toward limitation or reversal of visual loss related to secondary retinal detachment, glaucoma, or other complications. Until recently, photocoagulation by means of a xenon arc photocoagulator or argon, krypton, or dye laser was the mainstay of treatment for most circumscribed choroidal hemangiomas and occasional diffuse choroidal hemangiomas associated with nonrhegmatogenous retinal detachment.[4,5] An intense, confluent photocoagulation of the entire lesion in an attempt to obliterate it was used for some tumors of this type, but a less intense treatment with spaced burns to the surface of the lesion in an attempt to reduce or block accumulation of subretinal fluid and promote its reabsorption was employed more extensively.[4] Both methods led to partial or complete reabsorption of the subretinal fluid, but the former technique usually caused profound visual loss and the latter was frequently associated with subsequent fluid reaccumulation and progressive visual impairment. As an alternative to photocoagulation, a noncoagulative infrared laser therapy employing relatively large spot sizes and long-duration exposures (transpupillary thermotherapy) has been used to treat such tumors in several centers.[6,7] The long-term effectiveness of this therapy is unknown. Photodynamic therapy using verteporfin has been used with considerable success as treatment of small to medium-size circumscribed choroidal hemangiomas in recent years[8,9] and is currently regarded as the treatment of choice for such lesions.

In patients who have an extremely thick choroidal hemangioma, extensive nonrhegmatogenous retinal detachment, or a diffuse or circumscribed choroidal hemangioma that failed to respond to photocoagulation, noncoagulative laser therapy, or photodynamic therapy, low-dose ocular irradiation appears to be an effective therapeutic option (Fig. 152-6). Several different radiation therapy methods (external beam photon radiotherapy,[5,10] plaque radiotherapy,[11] and proton beam irradiation[12]) have been employed with good success in selected patients. When external beam radiotherapy or proton beam irradiation is used, the eye is usually treated to a target dose of approximately 12–20Gy.[5,10,12] When plaque radiotherapy is employed, the tumor is usually treated to an apex dose of approximately 20–30Gy.[11] These forms of radiation therapy induce partial or total tumor regression, stimulate gradual reabsorption of subretinal fluid that is usually sustained for many months to years, and provide better visual results than obliterative or repeated scatter photocoagulation.[5]

COURSE AND OUTCOMES

If a circumscribed choroidal hemangioma involves the central macula or if a diffuse hemangioma is particularly thick in the macula, progressive degeneration of the overlying retinal pigment epithelium and sensory retina often occurs. These degenerative

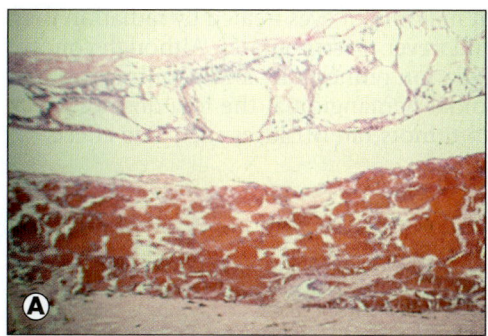

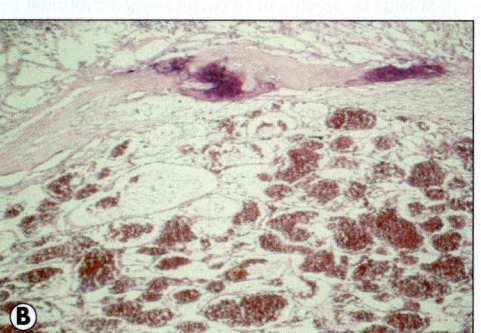

FIG 152-5 ■
Histopathology of circumscribed choroidal hemangioma. A, Low-power photomicrograph (H&E, original magnification 100×) shows large choroidal vascular channels constituting choroidal hemangioma, overlying serous retinal detachment, and partially degenerated cystic overlying retina.
B, Higher power photomicrograph (H&E, original magnification 200×) shows metaplastic thickening with partial calcification of retinal pigment epithelium overlying circumscribed choroidal hemangioma.

PATHOLOGY

Choroidal hemangiomas usually consist in large part of cavernous vascular channels lined by mature endothelial cells and supported by thin intervascular fibrous septa (Fig. 152-5, A–B).[3] Some choroidal hemangiomas, especially those of the diffuse type, also contain a prominent component of small, capillary-type vessels. Circumscribed choroidal hemangiomas appear to end rather abruptly at their margins and to cause some compression of the adjacent normal choroid. In contrast, diffuse choroidal hemangiomas terminate indistinctly in the periphery and do not have abrupt margins. Fibrous transformation of the retinal pigment epithelium occurs frequently over circumscribed choroidal hemangiomas (Fig. 152-5, B) and thick posterior regions of diffuse choroidal hemangiomas, and ossification of the transformed pigment epithelium develops in some eyes. The sensory retina that overlies a choroidal hemangioma frequently appears thickened and cystic. Eyes that have a diffuse choroidal hemangioma often have numerous other abnormalities, including dilated episcleral and intrascleral blood vessels, malformation or synechial closure of the anterior chamber angle, and massive cupping of the optic disc.

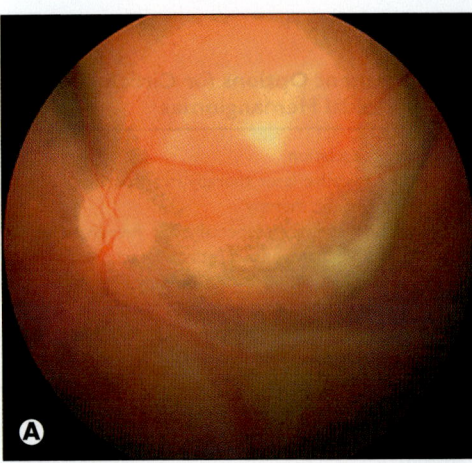

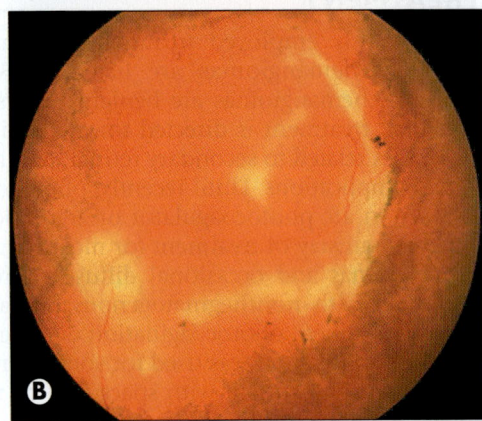

FIG 152-6 ■
Radiation therapy of larger circumscribed choroidal hemangioma. A, Pretreatment appearance of choroidal hemangioma. Note secondary serous retinal detachment involving macula and fibrous metaplasia of overlying retinal pigment epithelium. B, Post-treatment appearance of same eye 1 year following I-125 plaque radiotherapy. Note pronounced tumor regression and retinal reattachment. Unfortunately, vision in the eye was only hand motion perception because of extensive retinal degeneration and optic atrophy.

usually resolves within a few weeks.[4] The lesion proper typically shows minimal if any change in size. Unfortunately, the subretinal fluid frequently reaccumulates after a few months to a few years. Additional scatter laser therapy can be provided, but each supplemental laser treatment of this type appears less likely to produce a favorable effect on the fluid.[13] The long-term course after laser thermotherapy is currently unknown.

Following photodynamic therapy, prompt clinical regression of the tumor generally occurs.[8,9] Associated subretinal fluid usually disappears promptly. Sustained local tumor regression and lack of reaccumulation of subretinal fluid have been reported.

Following external beam radiation therapy or proton beam irradiation, the hemangioma undergoes partial regression and the subretinal fluid slowly goes away.[5,10,12] Even a total bullous retinal detachment usually resolves, but it may take up to 6 months or more for this to happen. The greater the amount of subretinal fluid and the longer it has been present at the time of irradiation, the longer it usually takes for it to go away after that treatment. After plaque radiotherapy, the hemangioma usually undergoes more rapid and more extensive clinical regression than after external beam radiation therapy.[11] Any associated subretinal fluid is reabsorbed slowly, just as occurs after external beam treatment. In the great majority of eyes treated by radiation therapy, the subretinal fluid never reaccumulates. Although concern always exists about radiation retinopathy and papillopathy after irradiation of a choroidal hemangioma, the low dose of radiation used to treat such tumors rarely causes such side effects.

REFERENCES

1. Anand R, Augsburger JJ, Shields JA. Circumscribed choroidal hemangiomas. Arch Ophthalmol. 1989;107:1338–42.
2. Schalenbourg A, Piguet B, Zografos L. Indocyanine green angiographic findings in choroidal hemangiomas: a study of 75 cases. Ophthalmologica. 2001;214:246–52.
3. Witschel H, Font RL. Hemangioma of the choroid. A clinicopathologic study of 71 cases and a review of the literature. Surv Ophthalmol. 1976;20:415–31.
4. Sanborn GE, Augsburger JJ, Shields JA. Treatment of circumscribed choroidal hemangiomas. Ophthalmology. 1982;89:1374–80.
5. Madreperla SA, Hungerford JL, Plowman PN, et al. Choroidal hemangiomas: visual and anatomic results of treatment by photocoagulation or radiation therapy. Ophthalmology. 1997;104:1773–8.
6. Garcia-Aruni J, Ramsay LS, Guraya BC. Transpupillary thermotherapy for circumscribed choroidal hemangiomas. Ophthalmology. 2000;107:351–6.
7. Kamal A, Watts AR, Rennie IG. Indocyanine green enhanced transpupillary thermotherapy of circumscribed choroidal hemangioma. Eye. 2000;14:701–5.
8. Barbazetto I, Schmidt-Erfurth U. Photodynamic therapy of choroidal hemangioma: two case reports. Graefes Arch Clin Exp Ophthalmol. 2000;238:214–21.
9. Madreperla SA. Choroidal hemangioma treated with photodynamic therapy using verteporfin. Arch Ophthalmol. 2001;119:1606–10.
10. Schilling H, Sauerwein W, Lommatzsch A, et al. Long-term results after low dose ocular irradiation for choroidal haemangiomas. Br J Ophthalmol. 1997;81:267–73.
11. Zografos L, Bercher L, Chamot L, et al. Cobalt-60 treatment of choroidal hemangiomas. Am J Ophthalmol. 1996;121:190–9.
12. Zografos L, Egger E, Bercher L, et al. Proton beam irradiation of choroidal hemangiomas. Am J Ophthalmol. 1998;126:261–8.
13. Augsburger JJ, Shields JA, Moffat KP. Circumscribed choroidal hemangiomas: long term visual prognosis. Retina. 1981;1:56–61.

changes can, and commonly do, result in progressive visual loss.[13] In addition, secondary serous retinal detachment can cause profound visual impairment, especially if the subretinal fluid becomes bullous and persists chronically. Chronic, bullous retinal detachment is frequently followed by neovascularization of the iris and neovascular glaucoma. Many patients who have diffuse choroidal hemangioma and facial nevus flammeus also develop primary congenital, infantile, or juvenile glaucoma in the affected eye, and this condition can also impair vision in the eye.

Following obliterative laser therapy, most circumscribed choroidal hemangiomas shrink considerably and develop fibrous scarring on their surface. The associated retinal detachment is usually reabsorbed within a few weeks. Unfortunately, such treatment is often associated with persistent macular retinal traction, chronic cystoid macular edema, or both. After scatter laser therapy to the surface of the tumor, the subretinal fluid

CHAPTER
153 Choroidal Osteoma

JAMES J. AUGSBURGER • RUDOLF GUTHOFF

DEFINITION
• Acquired benign bony tumor of choroid.

KEY FEATURES
• Orange to pale yellow, geographic, plate-like juxtapapillary or circumpapillary choroidal lesion.
• Bone density of tumor detectable by ultrasonography or computed tomography.
• Bilateral in at least 20% of affected patients but unifocal in each affected eye.

ASSOCIATED FEATURES
• Progressive retinal degeneration that overlies the lesion.
• Secondary macular choroidal neovascularization.

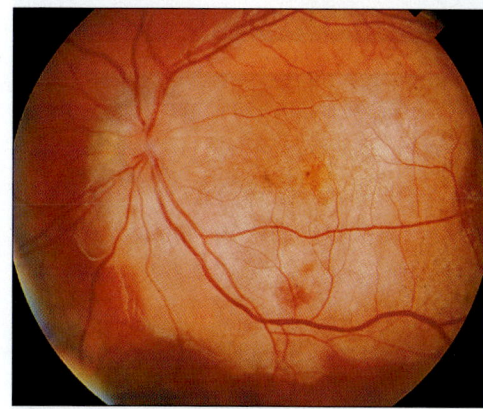

FIG. 153-1 ■ Clinical appearance of choroidal osteoma. Note juxtapapillary location of tumor, its yellow-orange color, and prominent ramifying blood vessels on surface of lesion. The patient was a 12-year-old girl.

INTRODUCTION

The choroidal osteoma is an uncommon benign acquired bony tumor of the choroid. It was classified originally as a choristoma (a benign congenital tumor composed of normal tissue elements that do not normally occur at that site), but it is currently regarded as an acquired benign choroidal neoplasm. Its cause is unknown.

EPIDEMIOLOGY AND PATHOGENESIS

Choroidal osteoma appears to be extremely rare, but its precise frequency is unknown. It usually makes its appearance between the middle of the second decade and the end of the third decade of life.[1] Lesions of this type occur in all ethnic groups, but over 90% of them occur in women. The stimulus for development of choroidal osteomas is not known. Affected patients do not appear to have abnormalities of calcium and phosphorus metabolism more frequently than would be expected in an unselected population of similar age and sex distribution.[1] The fact that the vast majority of affected individuals are women suggests, however, that endocrine or hormonal factors may have a role in the development of these lesions. Occasionally, familial cases have been reported.[2] In affected families, an autosomal dominant inheritance pattern has been observed.

OCULAR MANIFESTATIONS

Patients who have a choroidal osteoma usually present to the eye care professional with either painless progressive loss of vision over several months or years or abrupt recent blurring of central vision with micropsia and distortion. Some lesions of this type are detected initially on routine eye examination.

The typical choroidal osteoma appears as a yellowish to orange, well-defined, juxtapapillary or circumpapillary choroidal tumor (Fig. 153-1). It involves one eye only in 70–80% of cases

and both eyes in 20–30%. The surface of the tumor may be relatively flat or visibly uneven with depressions and elevations. The margins of the lesion are typically somewhat irregular in contour and sometimes have localized extensions that resemble pseudopods. Prominent inner choroidal blood vessels frequently ramify on the surface of the lesion.

If the lesion involves the macula, the visual acuity can be impaired on the basis of degeneration of the overlying retinal pigment epithelium and sensory retina. In other cases, a choroidal neovascular membrane arises from the inner surface of the lesion and produces a serous or serosanguineous macular retinal detachment that results in loss of vision.[3]

DIAGNOSIS AND ANCILLARY TESTING

Ultrasonography and computed tomography are of particular value for confirming a presumptive diagnosis of choroidal osteoma.[3] Because choroidal osteomas are composed of dense bone, they appear as highly reflective plate-like lesions that shadow the orbit on B-scan ultrasonography (Fig. 153-2). Computed tomography accentuates the plate-like thickening of the posterior ocular wall, which is isodense with normal skeletal bone (Fig. 153-3).[3] Fluorescein angiography typically shows patchy early hyperfluorescence and late diffuse hyperfluorescence of choroidal osteomas.[1] Indocyanine green angiography reveals generalized hypofluorescence of the mass with superimposed hyperfluorescent intralesional blood vessels in the early phase frames and diffuse hyperfluorescence of the mass in the late phase frames.[4]

DIFFERENTIAL DIAGNOSIS

The most important lesions in the differential diagnosis of choroidal osteoma are listed in Box 153-1.

SYSTEMIC ASSOCIATIONS

Occasional patients with choroidal osteoma have been found to have hyperparathyroidism with secondary alterations of serum calcium and phosphorus levels. However, most individuals who

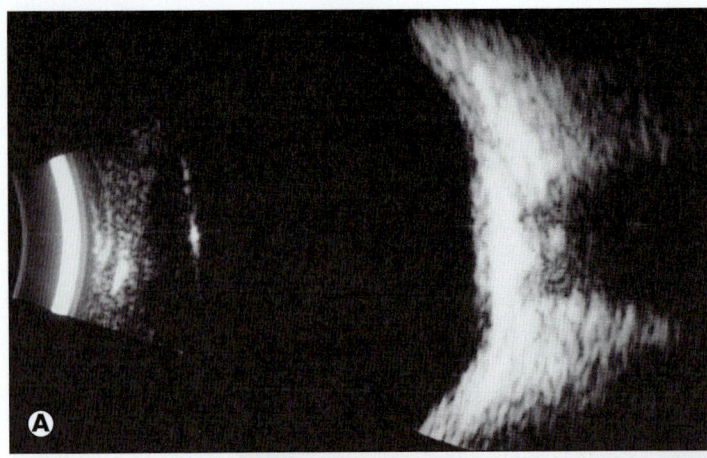

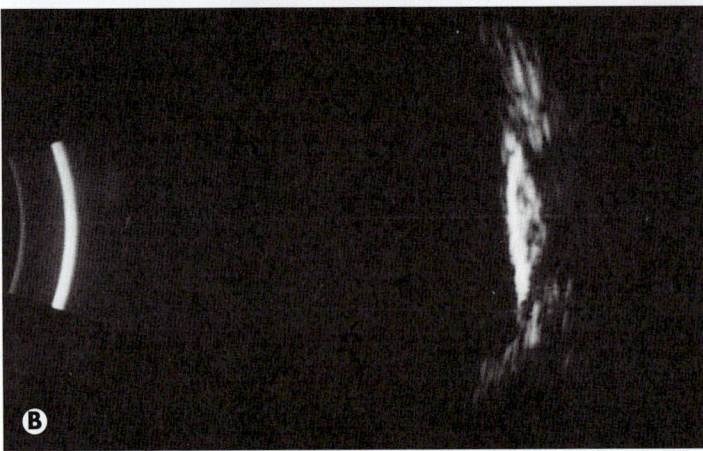

FIG. 153-2 ■ B-scan ultrasonography of choroidal osteoma. **A,** At 77dB the osteoma appears as an intensely bright plate in the posterior eye wall. Note orbital shadowing behind mass. **B,** At 55dB the lesion persists while most of the normal tissues are no longer evident.

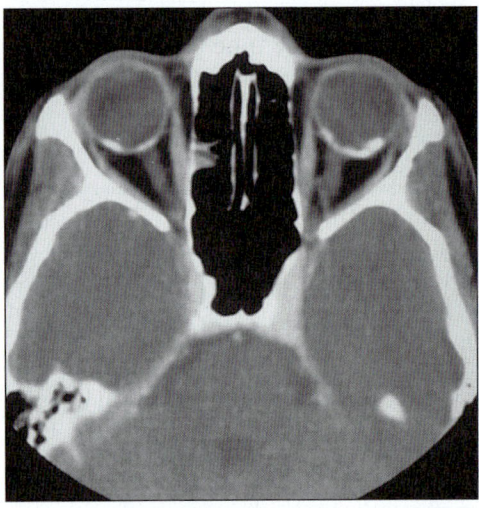

FIG. 153-3 ■ Computed tomography of bilateral choroidal osteoma. Note bilateral bone-dense plate involving posterior pole of each eye. The patient was a 39-year-old woman.

BOX 153-1

Differential Diagnosis of Choroidal Osteoma

Circumscribed choroidal hemangioma
Metastatic carcinoma to choroid
Amelanotic choroidal nevus or melanoma
Neurilemoma (schwannoma) of choroid
Idiopathic or dystrophic sclerochoroidal calcification
Vitelliform macular dystrophy
Bone formation in phthisical eyes
Intrascleral cartilage in linear sebaceous nevus syndrome
Fundus lesions of Aicardi's syndrome

BOX 153-2

Treatment Options for Choroidal Osteoma

No treatment available for tumor per se
Photocoagulation or photodynamic therapy for choroidal neovascularization associated with choroidal tumor

have a choroidal osteoma have no abnormalities of calcium and phosphorus metabolism.

Baseline Systemic Evaluation

Because of the occasional association with hyperparathyroidism, patients with choroidal osteoma should probably undergo blood testing for serum calcium and phosphorus levels.

PATHOLOGY

The choroidal osteoma is composed of mature bone that replaces full-thickness choroid in a plate adjacent to or around the optic disc. The overlying choriocapillaris is sometimes preserved, but the retinal pigment epithelium and sensory retina overlying the lesion are typically disrupted. When choroidal neovascularization is present, ingrowth of a neovascular complex derived from the choroid is sometimes identified.

TREATMENT

Lesions of this type appear to have no malignant potential. Consequently, patient management is directed at preservation of vision and, if possible, restoration of vision impaired by reversible mechanisms (Box 153-2). If the mechanism of visual loss is a choroidal neovascular membrane causing an exudative macular retinal detachment, the vascular lesion may be treatable by focal retinal laser photocoagulation[5] or photodynamic therapy.[6] No known effective management exists for the retinal pigment epithelial and sensory retinal degeneration that occurs over macular lesions.

COURSE AND OUTCOMES

Choroidal osteomas have been recognized to enlarge slightly during several years of observation.[7,8] However, malignant transformation has not been reported.

REFERENCES

1. Shields CL, Shields JA, Augsburger JJ. Choroidal osteoma. Surv Ophthalmol. 1988;33:17–27.
2. Cunha SL. Osseous choristoma of the choroid. A familial disease. Arch Ophthalmol. 1984;102:1052–4.
3. Guthoff R, Abramo F. Osteome der bulbuswand. Erscheinungsformen in abhängigkeit von Lage und Ausdehnung. Klin Monatsbl Augenheilkd. 1991;198:124–8.
4. Lafaut BA, Mestdagh C, Kohno T, et al. Indocyanine green angiography in choroidal osteoma. Graefes Arch Clin Exp Ophthalmol. 1997;235:330–7.
5. Grand MG, Burgess DB, Singerman LJ, et al. Choroidal osteoma. Treatment of associated subretinal neovascular membranes. Retina. 1984;4:84–9.
6. Battaglia Parodi M, Da Pozzo S, Toto L, et al. Photodynamic therapy for choroidal neovascularization associated with choroidal osteoma. Retina. 2001;21:660–1.
7. Augsburger JJ, Shields JA, Rife CJ. Bilateral choroidal osteoma after nine years. Can J Ophthalmol. 1979;14:281–4.
8. Aylward GW, Chang TS, Pautler SE, Gass JD. A long-term follow-up of choroidal osteoma. Arch Ophthalmol. 1998;116:1337–41.

CHAPTER 154
Astrocytoma of Retina

JAMES J. AUGSBURGER • ALAN F. CRUESS

DEFINITION
- Benign neuroglial tumor that arises from retinal astrocytes.

KEY FEATURE
- Translucent to opaque white inner retinal tumor.

ASSOCIATED FEATURE
- Tuberous sclerosis in many affected individuals, especially those who have bilateral, multifocal retinal lesions.

INTRODUCTION

The retinal astrocytoma is a benign acquired neoplasm that arises from astrocytes of the sensory retina. Lesions of this type occur in a multifocal bilateral pattern that is frequently associated with tuberous sclerosis and in a unilateral, unifocal pattern that usually represents a sporadic nonsyndromic disorder.

EPIDEMIOLOGY AND PATHOGENESIS

Astrocytoma of the retina appears to be rare, but its precise frequency in the general population has not been determined. The tumor tends to arise early in life and is frequently detected during childhood or adolescence. However, some lesions are not noted until adulthood. Astrocytoma of the retina affects all ethnic groups and both sexes equally. Recognized risk factors for development of an astrocytoma of the retina include tuberous sclerosis and possibly neurofibromatosis (see Systemic Associations).

OCULAR MANIFESTATIONS

Patients who have one or more retinal astrocytomas usually have no visual symptoms unless the tumor involves the macula. Occasionally, a retinal astrocytoma remote from the fovea causes a nonrhegmatogenous retinal detachment that involves the macular retina and abruptly blurs the vision in that eye.

The retinal astrocytoma usually appears as a white, superficial retinal mass.[1,2] The clinical spectrum of retinal astrocytomas characteristically ranges from faint translucent intraretinal patches (Fig. 154-1) through more distinctly nodular, opaque white, inner-retinal lesions to dense partially calcified mulberry-like tumors (Fig. 154-2). Lesions of these three types may be present simultaneously in the same eye. The lesion is vascularized from the retina, but its afferent and efferent blood vessels are usually not particularly dilated or tortuous. Retinal astrocytomas can arise from any location in the retina, from the optic disc and macula to the oral zone. Patients who have tuberous sclerosis or neurofibromatosis and develop retinal astrocytomas are more likely to have multiple and more peripheral lesions than patients with the nonsyndromic disease.

An atypical type of retinal astrocytoma is the isolated nonsyndromic lesion that occurs unilaterally in otherwise unaffected individuals (Fig. 154-3).[3] Lesions of this type can attain a relatively large size and cause profound visual loss, usually on the basis of their macular location or accumulation of exudative subretinal fluid. Unless the possibility of an astrocytoma is considered clinically, eyes that have this sort of tumor usually come to enucleation because amelanotic choroidal melanoma or another malignant neoplasm is suspected.

DIAGNOSIS AND ANCILLARY TESTING

In most cases, conventional diagnostic testing does not help in diagnosis or treatment planning. Fluorescein angiography of a classical retinal astrocytoma typically shows relatively slow filling of the intralesional vasculature, absence of dilated afferent

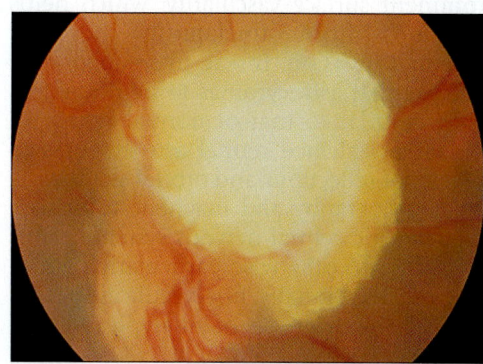

FIG. 154-2 ∎∎ Calcified mulberry-like retinal astrocytoma partially overlying optic disc. The patient had tuberous sclerosis.

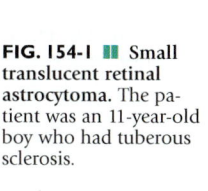
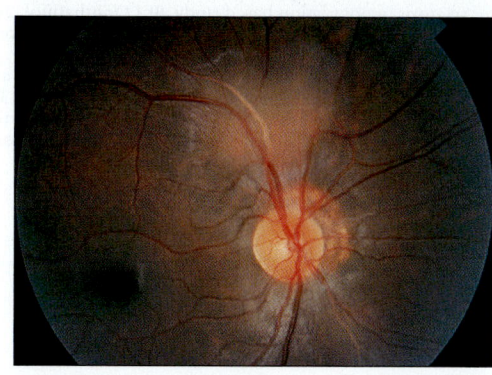

FIG. 154-1 ∎∎ Small translucent retinal astrocytoma. The patient was an 11-year-old boy who had tuberous sclerosis.

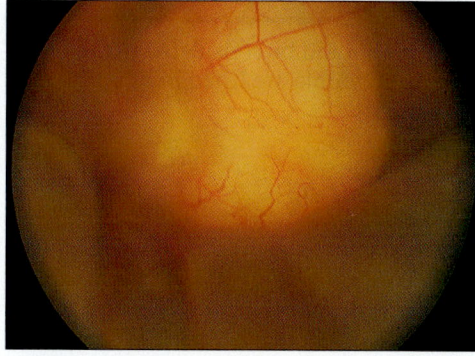

FIG. 154-3 ∎∎ Isolated nonsyndromic retinal astrocytoma with secondary retinal detachment. The patient was a 35-year-old woman.

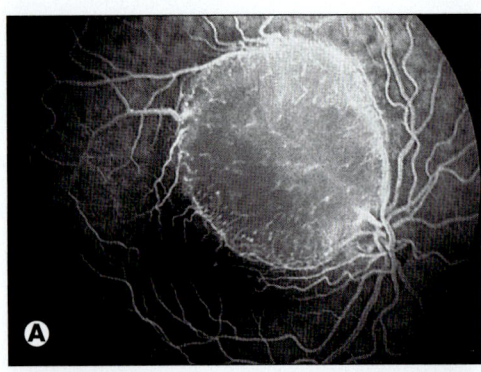

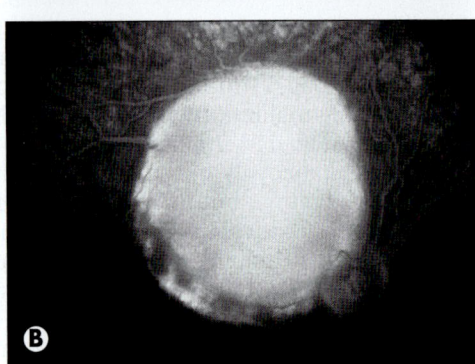

FIG. 154-4 ▌▌
Fluorescein angiography of retinal astrocytoma. A, Retinal venous phase frame showing multitude of fluorescent small blood vessels within generally hypofluorescent mass. B, Late phase frame showing diffuse staining of astrocytoma and associated serous subretinal fluid.

SYSTEMIC ASSOCIATIONS

As indicated previously, multifocal bilateral retinal astrocytomas usually occur in the context of tuberous sclerosis.[1,2] In contrast, most unilateral unifocal retinal astrocytomas occur as isolated lesions in patients who have no underlying systemic disorder.

Baseline Systemic Evaluation

Because of the benign nature of the retinal astrocytoma, a baseline systemic evaluation for malignancy is not warranted. However, an assessment aimed at the detection of other features of tuberous sclerosis or neurofibromatosis is appropriate.

PATHOLOGY

The typical retinal astrocytoma consists of a mass of interlacing spindle-shaped fibrous astrocytes that contain small bland elongated oval nuclei and have indistinct wavy cytoplasmic borders. Larger lesions frequently contain foci of calcification. Many retinal astrocytomas, especially those that occur in tuberous sclerosis or neurofibromatosis, also contain plump, polygonal cells having eosinophilic cytoplasm that have been termed giant astrocytes.[5] The retinal astrocytoma is regarded by many ophthalmic pathologists as a hamartoma (a benign congenital tumor composed of tissue elements that are normal for the location in which they occur) rather than as an acquired neoplasm.

TREATMENT

For most retinal astrocytomas, no treatment is required (Box 154-2). For patients whose intraocular tumor enlarges progressively and eventuates in a blind, painful eye, enucleation seems to be the only effective treatment. Radiotherapy by plaque or charged particle beam has not been shown to be effective.

COURSE AND OUTCOMES

Astrocytomas of the retina tend to develop early in childhood and show some tendency for limited progression during the childhood years. However, these tumors have extremely limited malignant potential and do not metastasize. If they occur in or adjacent to the foveola, they can cause visual loss on the basis of progressive retinal degeneration. In most cases, however, they are associated with normal visual acuity.

REFERENCES

1. Nyboer JH, Robertson DM, Gomez MR. Retinal lesions in tuberous sclerosis. Arch Ophthalmol. 1976;94:1277–80.
2. Rowley SA, O'Callaghan FJ, Osborne JP. Ophthalmic manifestations of tuberous sclerosis: a population based study. Br J Ophthalmol. 2001;85:420–3.
3. Lee JA, Harvey P, Finlay RD, Berry PJ. Solitary astrocytoma of the retina in a child. Br J Ophthalmol. 1996;80:673–4.
4. Shields JA, Shields CL, Ehya H, et al. Atypical retinal astrocytic hamartoma diagnosed by fine-needle biopsy. Ophthalmology. 1996;103:949–52.
5. Ulbright TM, Fulling KH, Helveston EM. Astrocytic tumors of the retina. Differentiation of sporadic tumors from phakomatosis-associated tumors. Arch Pathol Lab Med. 1984;108:160–3.

and efferent retinal vascular channels, and limited late staining of the tumor (Fig. 154-4). Isolated retinal astrocytomas characteristically exhibit prominent surface vascularity, which helps differentiate these lesions from amelanotic choroidal melanomas that have retinal invasion. B-scan ultrasonography shows small noncalcified retinal astrocytomas to be ill-defined lesions having reflectivity similar to that of normal retina. In contrast, B scan shows larger calcified retinal astrocytomas to have focal strong intralesional reflections and orbital shadowing by the mass. Computed tomography and magnetic resonance imaging can reveal characteristic central nervous system lesions of tuberous sclerosis but are not otherwise particularly helpful in the differential diagnosis. Occasionally, fine-needle aspiration biopsy can help to establish the diagnosis of an atypical retinal astrocytoma.[4]

DIFFERENTIAL DIAGNOSIS

The lesions and disorders that should be considered in the differential diagnosis of retinal astrocytoma are listed in Box 154-1.

CHAPTER
155 Hemangiomas of Retina

JAMES J. AUGSBURGER • NORBERT BORNFELD • ZÉLIA MARIA S. CORRÊA

DEFINITION
- Benign primary blood vessel tumors of retina in two distinct types: retinal capillary hemangiomas (von Hippel tumors) and retinal cavernous hemangiomas.

KEY FEATURES
- Capillary hemangioma of retina: spherical bright red intraretinal tumor associated with dilated afferent artery and efferent vein.
- Cavernous hemangioma of retina: sessile intraretinal lesion composed of cluster of dark red vascular saccules.

ASSOCIATED FEATURE
- Distinct ophthalmic and systemic features that correspond to specific type of retinal hemangioma.

CAPILLARY HEMANGIOMA OF RETINA

INTRODUCTION

The retinal capillary hemangioma (von Hippel tumor) is a benign vascular tumor that arises from the blood vessels of the retina or optic disc. It develops unifocally or multifocally and unilaterally or bilaterally, tends to enlarge progressively, and frequently leads to exudative or tractional retinal complications that impair vision in the affected eye or eyes. This lesion occurs in both syndromic and isolated clinical settings. In the syndromic form, retinal capillary hemangiomas occur as manifestations of the von Hippel–Lindau syndrome (VHLS). In the isolated nonsyndromic form of the disease, a single retinal capillary hemangioma is usually detected in only one eye of an otherwise healthy individual. If a patient has only the characteristic retinal lesion and its associated ocular complications, that patient is said to have von Hippel's disease (angiomatosis retinae) and not VHLS.

EPIDEMIOLOGY AND PATHOGENESIS

The retinal capillary hemangioma is uncommon, but its precise frequency in the general population is unknown. Men and women are affected equally, without any racial predilection. The age at the time of initial detection of the retinal lesion can range from younger than 10 years to older than 80 years; however, the average age at initial detection is usually between 15 and 35 years.[1] The lesions can occur unilaterally or bilaterally and unifocally or multifocally in affected persons. The precise relative incidences of unilateral, unifocal lesions versus bilateral, multifocal retinal capillary hemangiomas are unknown.

The principal recognized risk factor for development of one or more retinal capillary hemangiomas is presence of the gene for VHLS. Most individuals who have multifocal bilateral retinal capillary hemangiomas have this syndrome, whereas most persons who have a single tumor in one eye do not.

OCULAR MANIFESTATIONS

Blurred vision in the affected eye or loss of visual field is the usual presenting symptom. In families known to contain members who have VHLS, ophthalmic screening examinations frequently identify asymptomatic small tumors in one or both eyes.

The typical retinal capillary hemangioma appears as a reddish spherical lesion fed and drained by dilated tortuous retinal blood vessels (Fig. 155-1). Prominent afferent and efferent vessels of this type are commonly associated with tumors as small as 1mm in diameter.[2] In many cases, the feeding arteries and draining veins also become irregularly segmented with fusiform dilations along their course. Intraretinal and subretinal exudation overlying and surrounding a retinal capillary hemangioma is common, particularly when the tumor is more than 2–3mm in diameter. In many eyes, the accumulation of intraretinal and subretinal exudates is accentuated in the macular region even if the hemangioma is remote from the macula. An exudative retinal detachment may occur and become chronic, frequently leading to iris neovascularization and neovascular glaucoma. Some eyes that have one or more retinal capillary hemangiomas develop proliferative vitreoretinopathy as a prominent feature. The vitreous membranes are strongly adherent to the hemangioma; consequently, contraction of the membranes often leads to a tractional retinal detachment.

Capillary hemangiomas can also arise from the optic disc. Lesions of this type usually retain the reddish color of extrapapillary retinal capillary hemangiomas but frequently appear less well defined than their extrapapillary counterparts.[3] The development of exudative intraretinal and subretinal fluid around the lesion and disc can obscure the margins of the lesion.

DIAGNOSIS AND ANCILLARY TESTING

Fluorescein angiography of a typical retinal capillary hemangioma shows rapid filling of the afferent artery, brisk filling of the retinal vascular tumor, intense hyperfluorescence of the entire vascular lesion shortly thereafter, and subsequent rapid fill-

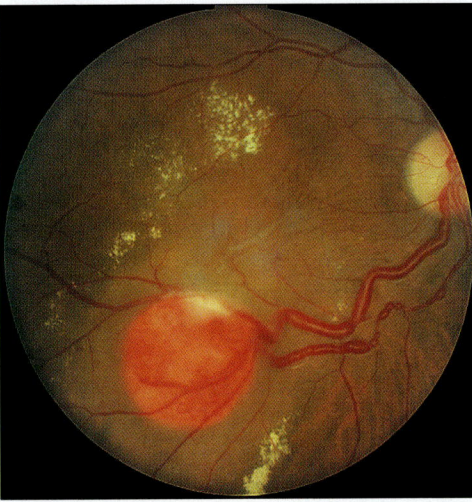

FIG. 155-1 ■ Typical retinal capillary hemangioma. Note associated intraretinal exudates and shallow exudative retinal detachment. The patient was a 62-year-old man who did not have the von Hippel–Lindau syndrome.

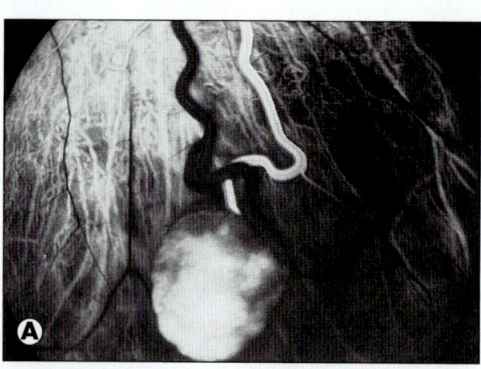

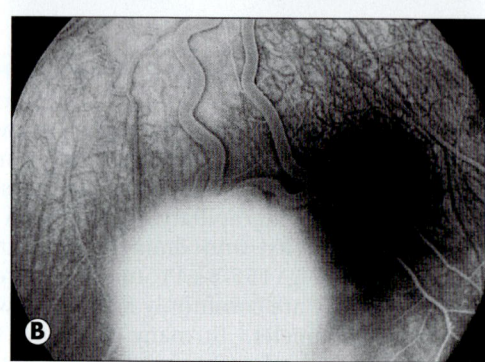

FIG. 155-2 ■
Fluorescein angiography of retinal capillary hemangioma.
A, Retinal arterial phase frame shows early hyperfluorescence of entire mass. **B,** Late phase frame that shows intense generalized hyperfluorescence of hemangioma plus leakage of fluorescein into adjacent vitreous.

BOX 155-2

Treatment Options for Retinal Capillary Hemangiomas

Photocoagulation
Cryotherapy
Diathermy
Radiation therapy
   • Plaque radiotherapy
   • Proton beam irradiation
Microsurgical resection
Enucleation (blind painful eyes due to tumor-related complications)

---

retina, vascular CNS tumors, or renal cell carcinoma should be considered to have VHLS until proved otherwise.[1,2] These individuals should undergo comprehensive evaluation for features of VHLS.[1] If possible, family members should also be examined ophthalmoscopically to see if any other affected individuals can be identified.

PATHOLOGY

The von Hippel tumor consists of small capillary-like blood vessels lined by endothelial cells and a delicate stroma of vacuolated fibrous astrocytes. Although vascular components of von Hippel tumors are much more prominent clinically than the stromal elements, cytogenetic studies have shown the stromal cells to be the ones with chromosome 3p25-26 abnormalities.

TREATMENT

Management decisions for capillary hemangiomas of the retina should be based on the desire to preserve or restore vision in affected eyes (Box 155-2). The most commonly employed method of management is photocoagulation of the vascular tumor.[4] This treatment is particularly effective against tumors that are up to about 3mm in diameter. Treatment usually entails creation of a confluent white burn that encompasses the entire hemangioma. Large spot sizes and relatively long-duration exposures are generally recommended. Multiple treatment sessions are usually required to eradicate the hemangioma. Laser treatment of the retinal arteriole that supplies the hemangioma is sometimes performed in an attempt to occlude that vessel and thereby enhance the direct treatment effect.[5] Also, scatter laser treatment is frequently given to the retina surrounding the capillary hemangioma in an effort to prevent post-treatment extension of any exudative retinal detachment. In successfully treated patients, the hemangioma becomes atrophic and involuted, the feeding and draining retinal vessels lose their dilation and tortuosity, and associated exudates disappear gradually. Depending on the extent of macular retinal degeneration and scarring, the vision may or may not recover.

For peripheral retinal capillary hemangiomas and some larger postequatorial lesions of this type, transconjunctival or transscleral cryotherapy can be employed as an alternative to photocoagulation.[6] Double or even triple freeze-thaw therapy is applied to the tumor; during treatment, the ice ball is allowed to come completely through the lesion into the overlying vitreous. This form of treatment must be repeated at intervals of about 4–6 weeks until the lesion is totally obliterated and the retinal feeder and drainer vessels are back to normal caliber.

In some eyes that contain an extremely large retinal capillary hemangioma, a few experienced ophthalmic surgeons have employed aggressive surgical techniques such as penetrating diathermy[7] and microsurgical tumor resection[8] in an attempt to salvage the eye. A relatively new method for the treatment of selected retinal capillary hemangiomas associated with massive exudative retinal detachment is focal tumor irradiation using either a radioactive plaque or charged particle beam.[9] Plaque ra-

---

BOX 155-1

Differential Diagnosis of Retinal Capillary Hemangioma

Retinoblastoma
Astrocytoma of retina
Idiopathic retinal telangiectasis (Coats' disease and Leber's retinal aneurysms)
Acquired fibrovascular retinal hemangiomatous lesion

---

ing of the efferent vein (Fig. 155-2). An active retinal capillary hemangioma characteristically leaks fluorescein exuberantly into the overlying vitreous, often causing the late phase frames to be extremely hazy because of diffuse vitreous fluorescence. Fluorescein also leaks into the subretinal fluid of an associated exudative retinal detachment.

Ultrasonography is not particularly helpful for the identification and delineation of the extent of individual retinal capillary hemangiomas. Computed tomography and magnetic resonance imaging are effective for the detection of concurrent central nervous system (CNS) vascular lesions of VHLS.

DIFFERENTIAL DIAGNOSIS

The important lesions in the differential diagnosis of retinal capillary hemangioma are listed in Box 155-1.

SYSTEMIC ASSOCIATIONS

As already indicated, there is a strong association between retinal capillary hemangiomas and VHLS. However, the precise proportions of isolated and syndromic cases are unknown. In general, patients who have VHLS are likely to develop retinal capillary hemangioma at an earlier age and are more likely to have multiple, bilateral retinal tumors than patients who have sporadic retinal capillary hemangioma.[1,2]

Baseline Systemic Evaluation

Individuals who have multifocal or bilateral retinal capillary hemangiomas, a family history of capillary hemangiomas of the

diotherapy appears to work well for medium-sized to large retinal capillary hemangiomas located 3mm or more from the optic disc, and charged particle beam irradiation is particularly appropriate for juxtapapillary and epipapillary tumors. Some eyes that contain a large retinal capillary hemangioma or multiple capillary hemangiomas of the retina can also be managed by pars plana vitrectomy coupled with endophotocoagulation or endodiathermy of the tumors.[10] Finally, some eyes that become blind and painful or phthisical eventually come to enucleation.

Patients who have a small retinal capillary hemangioma that causes no exudative phenomena and those who have one or more previously treated regressed retinal capillary hemangiomas must continue to be monitored periodically for local tumor reactivation or new tumor formation.

COURSE AND OUTCOMES

The natural history of retinal capillary hemangiomas is highly varied. Although some retinal capillary hemangiomas have been observed to remain stable for months to even years and others to regress spontaneously without resultant exudative phenomena,[11] many if not most capillary hemangiomas of the retina enlarge to at least a limited degree during follow-up. Some cases progress to a blind painful eye. Visual prognosis in eyes that have retinal capillary hemangioma depends on the size, location, and number of lesions, the extent of intraretinal and subretinal exudation that occurs, and the amount of vitreoretinal fibroplasia that develops in response to the lesion. Fortunately, most retinal capillary hemangiomas can now be controlled, if not eradicated, by local obliterative therapy. Unfortunately, many affected eyes still suffer mild to profound uncorrectable visual impairment.

CAVERNOUS HEMANGIOMA OF RETINA

INTRODUCTION

Cavernous hemangioma of the retina is a benign retinal vascular hamartoma. It is generally asymptomatic and visually insignificant unless it involves the macula or causes intravitreal bleeding. Although occasionally associated with cutaneous vascular lesions and minimal nonprogressive intracranial vascular lesions, the retinal cavernous hemangioma usually appears to be nonsyndromic in nature. It is most frequently identified in a unifocal nonfamilial situation, but occasional bilateral familial cases have been reported. The lesion has no recognized malignant potential.

EPIDEMIOLOGY AND PATHOGENESIS

Cavernous hemangioma of the retina is uncommon, but its precise frequency in the general population is unknown. It affects both sexes and occurs in all ethnic groups. The lesion is congenital but may not be detected until relatively late in life. Most affected patients have a single lesion in one eye and no evidence of a multisystem syndrome; however, occasional patients have multiple retinal lesions and some have a familial disorder characterized by benign cavernous hemangiomas or telangiectatic vascular lesions of the skin and CNS.

OCULAR MANIFESTATIONS

Most patients are asymptomatic, and their tumor is detected on routine ophthalmic examination. In some cases, vision is blurred because of the macular location of the lesion. In other cases, the patient reports floaters attributable to intravitreal bleeding from the hemangioma.

The typical retinal cavernous hemangioma appears as a cluster of vascular saccules within the sensory retina in association

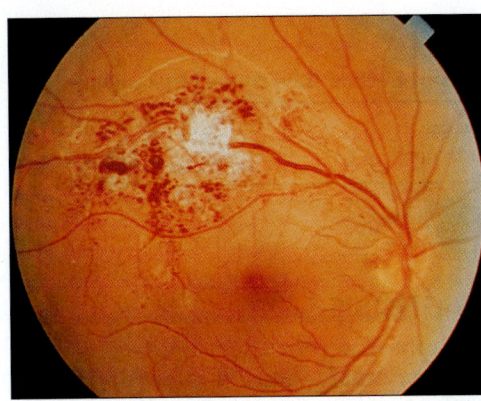

FIG. 155-3 ■ Typical cavernous hemangioma of the retina.

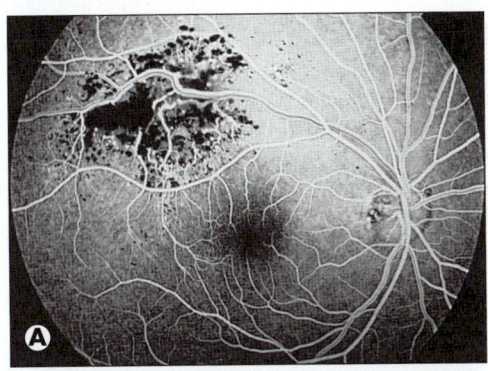

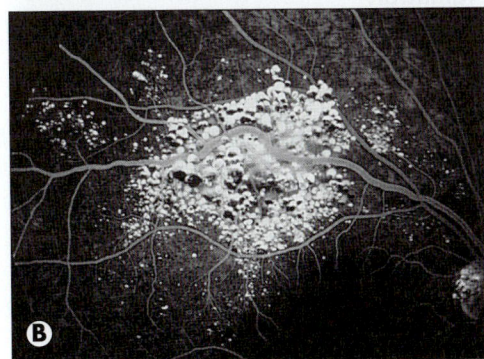

FIG. 155-4 ■ Fluorescein angiography of cavernous hemangioma of retina. A, Laminar venous phase frame shows most vascular saccules that comprise the lesion to be nonfluorescent. B, Late phase frame shows hyperfluorescence of most vascular saccules. Note the plasma-erythrocyte separation in some larger vascular saccules.

with a retinal vein of anomalous appearance that is neither dilated nor tortuous (Fig. 155-3).[12,13] The individual intraretinal lesion typically measures approximately 1–4 disc areas in size, and the component vascular saccules generally range from microaneurysmal size to about 0.1mm in diameter. In some of the larger vascular saccules, gravitational plasma-erythrocyte separation can sometimes be observed. Larger lesions commonly have associated whitish glial proliferation on their surface, which can be mistaken for intraretinal exudates. True subretinal and intraretinal exudates are extremely uncommon in association with such lesions. Occasional cavernous hemangiomas of the retina give rise to spontaneous vitreous hemorrhage, which may be recurrent and massive.

Cavernous hemangiomas of the retina can arise from all regions of the retina and also from the optic disc.[14]

DIAGNOSIS AND ANCILLARY TESTING

Fluorescein angiography (Fig. 155-4) typically shows hypofluorescence of the entire lesion in the early phase frames and slow filling of the lesion as the study progresses. The component vascular saccules accumulate fluorescein gradually and then remain brightly fluorescent long after normal intravascular fluorescence has faded. Fluorescein leakage into the retina or vitreous is usually not evident, even in late phase frames.

Ultrasonography is generally not helpful in the diagnostic assessment of retinal cavernous hemangiomas.[14]

DIFFERENTIAL DIAGNOSIS

The only lesions that resemble cavernous hemangioma of retina clinically are the microaneurysmal lesions of idiopathic retinal telangiectasia and retinal arterial macroaneurysms (Box 155-3).

SYSTEMIC ASSOCIATIONS

Most patients who have a cavernous hemangioma of the retina have no associated systemic disorder. However, occasional patients have small hemangiomas and telangiectases of the skin and similar lesions in the CNS.[15–17] In some families, this multisystem disorder appears to be inherited as an autosomal dominant syndrome.[15] Individuals who have this syndrome are more likely to have multifocal retinal cavernous hemangiomas, bilateral retinal cavernous hemangiomas, or both than persons who have sporadic nonfamilial disease.

Baseline Systemic Evaluation

If the family history or examination of family members suggests an autosomal dominant inheritance pattern and examination of affected individuals reveals multifocal or bilateral retinal cavernous hemangiomas or cutaneous hemangiomas and telangiectases, baseline CNS imaging and even periodic follow-up imaging are probably advisable.[17]

PATHOLOGY

The cavernous hemangioma of the retina consists of a cluster of large-caliber thin-walled intraretinal vascular saccules lined by normal vascular endothelial cells.[18] The tumor thickens and replaces the sensory retina at the affected site. Because it is a congenital tumor composed of benign tissue elements that occur normally in the retina, the retinal cavernous hemangioma is generally considered to be a hamartoma.

TREATMENT

Most eyes that contain a cavernous hemangioma of the retina or optic disc have no visual problems and require no treatment (Box 155-4). If recurrent massive vitreous hemorrhage from a cavernous hemangioma of the retina occurs, transscleral cryotherapy or pars plana vitrectomy with endophotocoagulation may be required.[19]

COURSE AND OUTCOMES

Most retinal cavernous hemangiomas that have been observed for prolonged periods of time remain stable in size and clinical appearance. Occasional hemangiomas of this type bleed repeatedly into the vitreous over the course of many years. The visual prognosis of the affected eyes is good unless the hemangioma involves the macular retina.

REFERENCES

1. Hardwig P, Robertson DM. von Hippel–Lindau disease: a familial, often lethal, multi-system phakomatosis. Ophthalmology. 1984;91:263–70.
2. Schmidt D, Neumann HPH. Retinal vascular hamartoma in von Hippel–Lindau disease. Arch Ophthalmol. 1995;113:1163–7.
3. Gass JD, Braunstein R. Sessile and exophytic capillary angiomas of the juxtapapillary retina and optic nerve head. Arch Ophthalmol. 1980;98:1790–7.
4. Lane CM, Turner G, Gregor ZJ, et al. Laser treatment of retinal angiomatosis. Eye. 1989;3:33–8.
5. Blodi CF, Russell SR, Pulido JS, et al. Direct and feeder vessel photocoagulation of retinal angiomas with dye yellow laser. Ophthalmology. 1990;97:791–7.
6. Watzke RC. Cryotherapy for retinal angiomatosis. Arch Ophthalmol. 1974;92:399–401.
7. Cardoso RD, Brockhurst RJ. Perforating diathermy coagulation for retinal angiomas. Arch Ophthalmol. 1976;94:1702–15.
8. Peyman GA, Rednam KRV, Mottow-Lippa L, Flood T. Treatment of large von Hippel tumors by eye wall resection. Ophthalmology. 1983; 90:840–7.
9. Augsburger JJ, Freire J, Brady LW. Radiation therapy for choroidal and retinal hemangiomas. In: Wiegel T, Bornfeld N, Foerster MH, Hinkelbein W, eds. Radiotherapy of ocular disease. In the series: Frontiers of Radiation Therapy and Oncology. Basel: Karger; 1997;30:265–80.
10. Schwartz PL, Fastenberg DM, Shakin JL. Management of macular puckers associated with retinal angiomas. Ophthalmic Surg. 1990;21:550–6.
11. Whitson JT, Welch RB, Green WR. von Hippel–Lindau disease: case report of a patient with spontaneous regression of a retinal angioma. Retina. 1986;6:253–9.
12. Colvard DM, Robertson DM, Trautmann JC. Cavernous hemangioma of the retina. Arch Ophthalmol. 1978;96:2042–4.
13. Messmer E, Laqua H, Wessing A, et al. Nine cases of cavernous hemangioma of the retina. Am J Ophthalmol. 1983;95:383–90.
14. Ruhswurm I, Zehetmayer M, Till P, et al. Kavernöses Hämangiom der Papille: klinische und echographische Befunde. Klin Monatsbl Augenheilkd. 1996;209:380–2.
15. Goldberg RE, Pheasant TR, Shields JA. Cavernous hemangioma of the retina. A four-generation pedigree with neurocutaneous manifestations and an example of bilateral retinal involvement. Arch Ophthalmol. 1979;97:2321–4.
16. Schwartz AC, Weaver RG, Bloomfield R, Tyler ME. Cavernous hemangioma of the retina, cutaneous angiomas, and intracranial vascular lesion by computed tomography and nuclear magnetic resonance imaging. Am J Ophthalmol. 1984;98:483–7.
17. Pancurak J, Goldberg MF, Frenkel M, Crowell RM. Cavernous hemangioma of the retina. Genetic and central nervous system involvement. Retina. 1985;5:215–20.
18. Messmer E, Font RL, Laqua H, et al. Cavernous hemangioma of the retina. Immunohistochemical and ultrastructural observations. Arch Ophthalmol. 1984; 102:413–18.
19. Haller JA, Knox DL. Vitrectomy for persistent vitreous hemorrhage from a cavernous hemangioma of the optic disk. Am J Ophthalmol. 1993;116:106–7.

CHAPTER 156

Combined Hamartoma of Retina

JAMES J. AUGSBURGER • SANFORD M. MEYERS

DEFINITION
- Benign congenital tumor composed of retinal pigment epithelium, retinal astrocytes, and retinal blood vessels.

KEY FEATURES
- Gray, deep retinal mass that has superficial gliotic component and tortuous intralesional blood vessels.
- Juxtapapillary tumor location.

ASSOCIATED FEATURE
- Other features of neurofibromatosis type 2 in substantial proportion of cases.

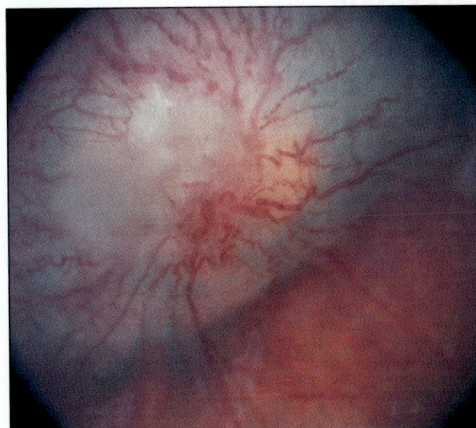

FIG. 156-1 ■ Typical combined hamartoma of retina. Note typical juxtapapillary and epipapillary location of lesion. The patient was a child who was subsequently found to have bilateral acoustic neuromas and other features of neurofibromatosis type 2.

INTRODUCTION

The combined hamartoma of the retina is an unusual benign congenital retinal tumor composed of sensory retina, retinal pigment epithelium, retinal blood vessels, and vitreoretinal membranes. It tends to be unilateral and unifocal in most cases. It characteristically involves the juxtapapillary retina, macula, or both and frequently causes moderate to profound visual impairment in the affected eye. Fortunately, the combined hamartoma of the retina has no recognized malignant potential.

EPIDEMIOLOGY AND PATHOGENESIS

The combined hamartoma is an uncommon lesion, but its precise frequency in the general population is unknown. It is presumably congenital, but most cases have not been detected before the age of 6 years.[1] It appears to affect men and women equally, and it has been reported to occur in various racial groups. The only currently recognized risk factor for development of combined hamartoma of the retina appears to be the presence of neurofibromatosis (usually type 2; see Systemic Associations).

OCULAR MANIFESTATIONS

The most common presenting feature is painless loss of vision or amblyopia in the involved eye caused by macular involvement.[1] Other presenting symptoms include strabismus, floaters, and leukokoria. Patients who have an extramacular lesion of this type generally have no symptoms related to the mass.

The typical combined hamartoma of the retina is characterized by a whitish superficial appearance caused by epiretinal and intraretinal gliosis, marked tortuosity of the involved retinal arterioles and venules, and deep grayish-black pigmentation (Fig. 156-1). The lesion is usually located in a juxtapapillary or circumpapillary position.[1] It frequently achieves a size of 4–6mm in diameter, but smaller and larger lesions have been encountered. Combined hamartomas of the retina occur occasionally in extrapapillary and peripheral fundus locations (Fig. 156-2).[1]

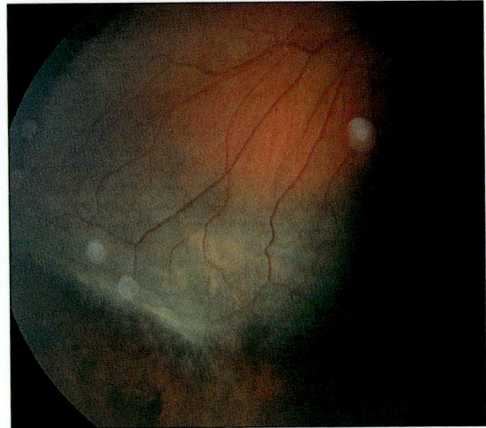

FIG. 156-2 ■ Atypical combined hamartoma of retina. Lesion is located in inferotemporal periphery of right eye.

DIAGNOSIS AND ANCILLARY TESTING

Fluorescein angiography in the typical case reveals relative hypofluorescence of the lesion caused by the intrinsic retinal pigment epithelial pigmentation in the early phase frames. The prominent intralesional blood vessels fluoresce brightly in the arterial and venous phase frames and accentuate the ophthalmoscopically evident intralesional vascular tortuosity. By the late phase of the study, the lesion often appears diffusely hyperfluorescent because of fluorescein leakage from the abnormal intralesional blood vessels.

B-scan ultrasonography can image thicker lesions but is not particularly helpful in differential diagnosis. Computed tomography and magnetic resonance imaging can reveal bilateral acoustic neuromas (the characteristic feature of neurofibromatosis type 2) in patients who have that syndromic association (see Systemic Associations).

DIFFERENTIAL DIAGNOSIS

The several lesions that should be considered in the differential diagnosis of combined hamartoma of the retina are listed in Box 156-1.

SYSTEMIC ASSOCIATIONS

Although most cases of combined hamartoma of the retina appear to be sporadic and nonsyndromic, a considerable number of individuals with such a lesion have been found to have neurofibromatosis type 2 (central neurofibromatosis).[2–4] A weaker but still noteworthy association with neurofibromatosis type 1 has also been reported by some authors.[5] Because of these associations, all patients who have a combined hamartoma of the retina should be evaluated for the presence of other clinical manifestations of neurofibromatosis types 1 and 2.

Baseline Systemic Evaluation

Because this lesion has no recognized malignant potential, baseline systemic evaluation to look for extraophthalmic malignancies is not warranted. However, newly diagnosed children should be evaluated for neurofibromatosis, especially neurofibromatosis type 2.

PATHOLOGY

The few pathological specimens that have been reviewed and reported have been composed of interlacing cords of hyperplastic retinal pigment epithelial cells, blood vessels within disorganized and thickened sensory retina, and a proliferation of benign glial cells on the vitreal surface of the lesion.[6]

TREATMENT

No treatment is generally indicated. Pars plana vitrectomy has been employed in a few cases to remove the epiretinal membrane, but such procedures have generally not resulted in improved vision.[7]

COURSE AND OUTCOMES

Most such lesions are minimally progressive after detection. In the cases that appear to change during follow-up, the progression is frequently caused by contraction of the vitreoretinal surface of the lesion and not by cellular proliferation of the lesion per se. Malignant transformation of a combined hamartoma of the retina has never been documented.

REFERENCES

1. Schachat AP, Shields JA, Fine SL, et al. Combined hamartomas of the retina and retinal pigment epithelium. Ophthalmology. 1984;91:1609–15.
2. Sivalingam A, Augsburger J, Perilongo G, et al. Combined hamartoma of the retina and retinal pigment epithelium in a patient with neurofibromatosis type 2. J Pediatr Ophthalmol Strabismus. 1991;28:320–2.
3. Good WV, Brodsky MC, Edwards MS, Hoyt WF. Bilateral retinal hamartomas in neurofibromatosis type 2. Br J Ophthalmol. 1991;75:190.
4. Meyers SM, Gutman FA, Kaye LD, Rothner AD. Retinal changes associated with neurofibromatosis 2. Trans Am Ophthalmol Soc. 1995;93:245–52.
5. Tsai P, O'Brien JM. Combined hamartoma of the retina and retinal pigment epithelium as the presenting sign of neurofibromatosis-1. Ophthalmic Surg Lasers. 2000;31:145–7.
6. Font RL, Moura RA, Shetlar DJ, et al. Combined hamartoma of sensory retina and retinal pigment epithelium. Retina. 1989;9:302–11.
7. McDonald HR, Abrams GW, Burke JM, et al. Clinicopathologic results of vitreous surgery for epiretinal membranes in patients with combined retinal and retinal pigment epithelial hamartomas. Am J Ophthalmol. 1985;100:800–13.

CHAPTER 157

Hypertrophy of Retinal Pigment Epithelium

JAMES J. AUGSBURGER • JAMES P. BOLLING

DEFINITION
- Benign congenital lesion of retinal pigment epithelium.

KEY FEATURES
- Gray to black, well-defined, thin, circular, oval or geographic lesion deep to sensory retina.
- Unifocal or multifocal, typical and atypical forms.

ASSOCIATED FEATURES
- Loss of retinal pigment epithelial cells with formation of depigmented lacunae within central regions of larger lesions.
- Marginal pseudoshadowing of many larger lesions.
- Atypical, multifocal, bilateral lesions occur as markers of familial adenomatous polyposis–carcinoma syndrome.

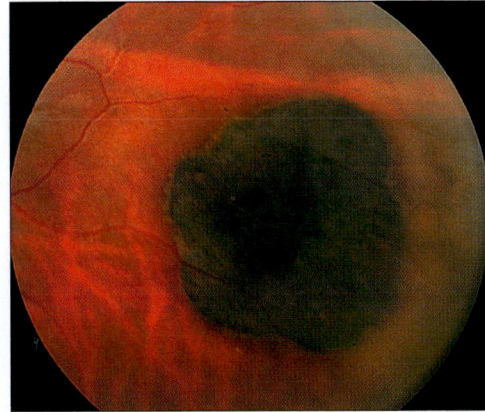

FIG. 157-1 ■ Typical unifocal, unilateral hypertrophy of retinal pigment epithelium.

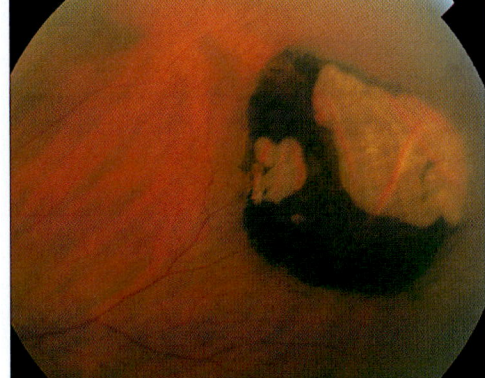

FIG. 157-2 ■ Unifocal unilateral hypertrophy of retinal pigment epithelium with prominent depigmented lacunae.

INTRODUCTION

Hypertrophy of the retinal pigment epithelium (RPE) is an uncommon benign fundus lesion that is probably always congenital in nature. Three varieties occur: the typical unifocal unilateral lesion, the typical multifocal unilateral lesion (grouped pigmentation of the retina), and the atypical multifocal bilateral lesion, the last of which is an indicator of familial colonic adenomatous polyposis–carcinoma syndrome.

EPIDEMIOLOGY AND PATHOGENESIS

Unilateral, multifocal clustered lesions of congenital hypertrophy of the RPE (CHRPE) are the most common type, occurring in about 1% of individuals. Unilateral, unifocal CHRPE lesions are slightly less common, occurring in about 0.5% of individuals. The atypical, bilateral, multifocal CHRPE lesions associated with familial adenomatous polyposis (FAP) of the colon are relatively uncommon, occurring in only about 1 in 100,000 persons.[1] Men and women are affected equally. All racial groups appear susceptible to these lesions. No recognized risk factors exist for typical unilateral unifocal and multifocal grouped CHRPE, but autosomal dominant colonic adenomatous polyposis–carcinoma syndrome predisposes individuals to develop multifocal atypical and bilateral lesions (see Systemic Associations).

OCULAR MANIFESTATIONS

CHRPE lesions are usually asymptomatic and detected on routine ophthalmic examination. The typical unifocal CHRPE is a gray to black, well-defined, minimally elevated fundus lesion having a diameter in the range of 2–5mm (Fig. 157-1). A narrow zone of granular gray pigmentation or depigmentation is frequently evident around the margins of the lesion. The lesion frequently undergoes at least partial depigmentation with aging, developing discrete intralesional atrophic foci (lacunae, Fig. 157-2) that tend to enlarge and coalesce over the years. Slight lesion enlargement has been documented in some patients.[1]

The typical multifocal congenital hypertrophy of the RPE is characterized by multiple flat gray to black retinal pigment epithelial lesions clustered in one region of the fundus (Fig. 157-3). The individual foci within the lesion cluster are usually round to oval and range in size from approximately 0.1–2.0mm in diameter; however, some larger and smaller lesions and occasional foci that have curvilinear or irregular shapes are frequently present in the clusters. This form of CHRPE is often referred to as congenital grouped pigmentation of the retina or bear tracks of the ocular fundus.

The CHRPE lesions in patients who have familial colonic adenomatous polyposis syndrome (see Systemic Associations) tend to be oval or irregularly shaped, variable in size (usually between 0.1 and 2.0mm in maximal diameter), multifocal, widely separated rather than clustered, and usually present in both eyes.[2]

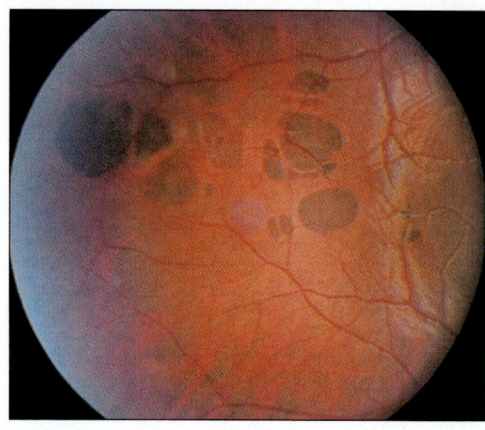

FIG. 157-3 ■ Typical multifocal clustered hypertrophy of retinal pigment epithelium (grouped pigmentation of retina).

Larger lesions frequently exhibit irregular retinal pigment epithelial disruption adjacent to one or more of the margins and well-defined areas of partial depigmentation of the lesion proper.

DIAGNOSIS AND ANCILLARY TESTING

No diagnostic studies are generally indicated for characterization of these retinal lesions. Fluorescein angiography and indocyanine green angiography show a well-defined blocking defect at the retinal pigment epithelial level.[3] Transmission of choroidal fluorescence takes place through lacunae in the lesion.

DIFFERENTIAL DIAGNOSIS

The important lesions and disorders in the differential diagnosis of congenital hypertrophy of the RPE are listed in Box 157-1.

SYSTEMIC ASSOCIATIONS

Atypical, multifocal, bilateral CHRPE lesions are strongly associated with several familial colonic adenomatous polyposis–carcinoma syndromes. The most frequently associated disorder, Gardner's syndrome, is an autosomal dominant cancer syndrome characterized by colonic adenomatous polyposis, bone cysts, hamartomas, and soft tissue tumors (desmoid tumors).[4–6] The risk of developing colon cancer during adult life in affected individuals is virtually 100%. When associated with neuroepithelial tumors of the central nervous system, familial colonic adenomatous polyposis–carcinoma syndrome is called Turcot's syndrome.[7] Autosomal dominant colonic adenomatous polyposis that occurs in the absence of extracolonic features is simply termed familial adenomatous polyposis (FAP). Gardner's syndrome, Turcot's syndrome, and FAP are believed to be variable phenotypic expressions of the same genotypic disorder.[5] The gene for familial colonic adenomatous polyposis in these disorders has been localized to chromosome 5q21-q22. The precise site of the mutation in the gene seems to correlate with the presence or absence

of CHRPE lesions.[8] In kindreds who have linkage between FAP and atypical CHRPE lesions, almost all at-risk individuals in the family have at least one characteristic fundus lesion as a marker of the disease. Most of the affected individuals have multiple lesions in both eyes, and the total number of such lesions in those patients is frequently as high as 20–30. In contrast, approximately one third of families who have FAP do not have CHRPE lesions as markers of the disease.

Typical unifocal unilateral CHRPE lesions and the lesions of grouped pigmentation are not linked to any of the FAP syndromes.[9]

Baseline Systemic Evaluation

In any individual who has multifocal, bilateral, atypical hypertrophy of the RPE, the ophthalmologist should review the family history for information about colon polyps, colon carcinoma, and colectomy and arrange for comprehensive colonic evaluation.

PATHOLOGY

The lesions of hypertrophy of the RPE consist of well-defined foci of taller than normal retinal pigment epithelial cells that contain an increased number of melanin granules.[10] In classic unifocal unilateral CHRPE, the intracytoplasmic melanin granules tend to be large and oval in shape. In areas of lacunar depigmentation, the hypertrophic retinal pigment epithelial cells are absent. The retinal photoreceptors overlying such lesions typically appear degenerated, at least in adult eyes. Grouped pigmentation of the retina has similar pathology.

TREATMENT

No treatment is warranted for these retinal lesions. They are typically photographed and then monitored periodically for enlargement or other changes.

COURSE AND OUTCOMES

Most retinal lesions of this type change minimally if at all over extended periods of follow-up.[1] Malignant change of a classical unifocal hypertrophy of the RPE has been reported[11] but appears to be rare.

REFERENCES

1. Boldrey EE, Schwartz A. Enlargement of congenital hypertrophy of the retinal pigment epithelium. Am J Ophthalmol. 1982;94:64–6.
2. Romania A, Zakov ZN, McGannon E, et al. Congenital hypertrophy of the retinal pigment epithelium in familial adenomatous polyposis. Ophthalmology. 1989;96:879–84.
3. Cohen SY, Quentel G, Guiberteau B, Coscas GJ. Retinal vascular changes in congenital hypertrophy of the retinal pigment epithelium. Ophthalmology. 1993;100: 471–4.
4. Traboulsi EI, Maumenee IH, Krush AJ, et al. Congenital hypertrophy of the retinal pigment epithelium predicts colorectal polyposis in Gardner's syndrome. Arch Ophthalmol. 1990;108:525–6.
5. Rossato M, Rigotti M, Grazia M, et al. Congenital hypertrophy of the retinal pigment epithelium (CHRPE) and familial adenomatous polyposis (FAP). Acta Ophthalmol Scand. 1996;74:338–42.
6. Valanzano R, Cama A, Volpe R, et al. Congenital hypertrophy of the retinal pigment epithelium in familial adenomatous polyposis. Novel criteria of assessment and correlations with constitutional adenomatous polyposis coli gene mutations. Cancer. 1996;78:2400–10.
7. Munden PPM, Sobol WM, Weingeist TA. Ocular findings in Turcot syndrome (glioma-polyposis). Ophthalmology. 1991;98:111–14.
8. Bunyan DJ, Shea-Simonds J, Reck AC, et al. Genotype-phenotype correlations of new causative APC gene mutations in patients with familial adenomatous polyposis. J Med Genet. 1995;32:728–31.
9. Shields JA, Shields CL, Shah PG, et al. Lack of association among typical congenital hypertrophy of the retinal pigment epithelium, adenomatous polyposis, and Gardner's syndrome. Ophthalmology. 1992;99:1709–13.
10. Regillo CD, Eagle RC, Shields JA, et al. Histopathologic findings in congenital grouped pigmentation of the retina. Ophthalmology. 1993;100:400–5.
11. Shields JA, Shields CL, Eagle RC, Singh AD. Adenocarcinoma arising from congenital hypertrophy of retinal pigment epithelium. Arch Ophthalmol. 2001;119: 597–602.

Phakomatoses

JAMES J. AUGSBURGER • JAMES P. BOLLING

DEFINITION
- Group of multisystem syndromes that have characteristic ophthalmic manifestations:
  - neurofibromatosis type 1 (von Recklinghausen's disease) and type 2 (central neurofibromatosis).
  - tuberous sclerosis.
  - von Hippel–Lindau syndrome.
  - Sturge-Weber syndrome.
  - Wyburn-Mason syndrome.

KEY FEATURES
- Characteristic retinal or uveal lesions.

ASSOCIATED FEATURES
- Characteristic cutaneous lesions in several of the syndromes.
- Characteristic central nervous system lesions in all of the syndromes.
- Miscellaneous other systemic features specific to syndrome.

INTRODUCTION

The phakomatoses are a group of complex multisystem disorders linked, at least in a historical sense, by various attributes of the component lesions, the organs involved, and the pattern of clinical inheritance observed in some cases. Although the term phakomatoses was coined by van der Hoeve in 1923 in a paper concerned with the similarities between von Recklinghausen's neurofibromatosis (NF) and Bourneville's tuberous sclerosis (TS), this term has never been defined satisfactorily. Absolute inclusion criteria were not presented by van der Hoeve, and a consensus about such criteria has not been reached in the years since. Some authors define the phakomatoses as neuro-oculo-cutaneous syndromes with autosomal dominant inheritance. Others believe that one or more characteristic skin lesions must be present in a substantial number of patients who have a neuro-ocular syndrome to warrant its classification as a phakomatosis. Still others believe that the essential element of a phakomatosis is the presence or development of multiorgan hamartomas.

For the purposes of this chapter, the authors define the phakomatoses as a group of independent clinical syndromes characterized by multiple tumors or tumor-like lesions, some of which are or can become malignant and arise in disparate organs of the body, including the eye in a substantial proportion of patients. Three syndromes are consistently classified as phakomatoses by most authors and also meet our definitional criteria: NF, TS, and von Hippel–Lindau syndrome (VHLS). Two other syndromes are classified as phakomatoses by many authors, but these do not conform precisely to our definition: Sturge-Weber syndrome (SWS) and Wyburn-Mason syndrome (WMS). These five syndromes are reviewed briefly in this chapter. Other syndromes that are occasionally grouped with the

phakomatoses by some authors [e.g., Louis-Bar syndrome (ataxia telangiectasia) and Weskamp-Cotlier syndrome (retinal-neuro-cutaneous cavernous hemangioma syndrome)] are not reviewed in this chapter.

NEUROFIBROMATOSIS

The syndrome of NF consists of two distinct genetic diseases with considerable phenotypic overlap. Both are characterized by neuroectodermal tumors that arise within multiple organs and autosomal dominant inheritance. These two forms of NF are termed NF-1 and NF-2.

EPIDEMIOLOGY AND PATHOGENESIS

Neurofibromatosis is the most common phakomatosis, having a frequency of approximately 1 case per 3500 persons in the general population.[1] NF-1 is by far the more common of the two types, affecting approximately 1 person per 3500–4000 persons in the general population. In contrast, NF-2 affects no more than 1 person per 40,000–50,000 persons. Men and women appear to be affected with equal frequency, and there is no racial predilection for either type of the disease.

Many features of these syndromes do not appear until late childhood or early adulthood.[2] The severity of the syndrome varies markedly from patient to patient. Many patients who have limited forms of NF are probably not identified.

The gene for NF-1 has been localized to chromosome 17q11,[3] and that for NF-2 has been localized to chromosome 22q12.[4]

EXTRAOPHTHALMIC MANIFESTATIONS

Neurofibromatosis type 1 (peripheral NF, von Recklinghausen's disease) is characterized by cutaneous café-au-lait spots, axillary and inguinal freckling, Lisch nodules of the iris, several types of cutaneous neurofibromas, optic nerve gliomas, and neurofibromas or other solid neoplasms of the central nervous system (CNS).[1] Currently accepted diagnostic criteria for NF-1 are listed in Box 158-1. The café-au-lait spots in this syndrome tend to be multiple. Many are larger than 0.5cm in diameter in childhood and enlarge to 1.5cm in diameter by the postpubertal years. Six or more café-au-lait spots larger than 1.5cm in diameter in postpubertal individuals are generally considered diagnostic of NF-1.[5] Axillary freckling and inguinal freckling are present in 90–95% of affected individuals.[6] Subcutaneous neurofibromas in NF-1 tend to arise multifocally and can be either pedunculated nodules or diffuse plexiform lesions. CNS neurofibromas can cause hemiparesis, hemiatrophy, and seizures in some affected individuals. Because of bone abnormalities related to the syndrome, some individuals develop severe scoliosis. About one half of the patients affected by NF-1 have some sort of learning disability, but most are of normal intelligence. In older patients, systemic hypertension appears to be more frequent than it is in the general population.

Neurofibromatosis type 2 (central NF) is typified by bilateral vestibular schwannomas (acoustic neuromas) and widely scat-

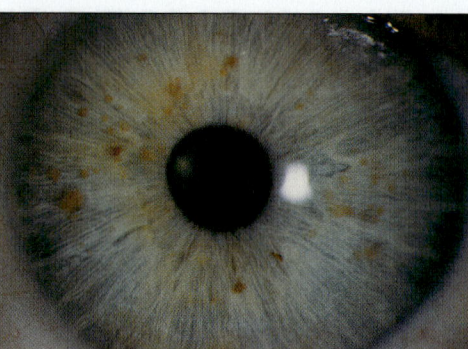

FIG. 158-1 ■ Lisch nodules in neurofibromatosis type 1.

10–15% of affected patients.[10] They can occur unilaterally or bilaterally and frequently involve the optic chiasm. Optic nerve gliomas in the orbit cause progressive proptosis and optic atrophy and frequently result in unilateral or bilateral blindness. Those that arise within the brain and involve the chiasm can cause bilateral visual loss as well as intracranial mass effects. Some patients affected by NF-1 have pulsating exophthalmos caused by anomalous development of the sphenoid bone.[7] Congenital and infantile glaucomas appear to be common in patients who have this syndrome.[7] Some affected patients develop multifocal choroidal nevi bilaterally,[8] and these patients appear to have an increased cumulative lifetime risk for the development of an uveal melanoma.[11]

Ophthalmologic findings in NF-2 are relatively uncommon.[12] Lisch nodules of the iris, eyelid neurofibromas, and optic nerve gliomas occur occasionally but are not generally present. The most consistent ocular findings in patients who have NF-2 are combined hamartomas of the retina[13] and juvenile posterior subcapsular or cortical lens opacities.[5]

SYSTEMIC EVALUATION

Detailed recommendations for systemic evaluation of patients who have suspected NF-1 or NF-2 have been published.[5] For patients who have suspected NF-1, the basic diagnostic evaluation should consist of a complete history and comprehensive physical examination, including an ophthalmic examination. The history and physical examination should attempt to identify the diagnostic criteria listed in Box 158-1. Ancillary studies such as computed tomography (CT) and magnetic resonance imaging (MRI) should be performed in NF-1 if the history or findings revealed by physical examination suggest that they might be helpful. For patients who have suspected NF-2, the basic diagnostic evaluation should consist of a complete history and physical examination, including an ophthalmic examination, and high-resolution MRI or CT imaging of the brain and spinal cord. The history and physical examination should attempt to identify the diagnostic criteria listed in Box 158-2, and the imaging studies should address the presence or absence of vestibular schwannomas. Other studies in suspected NF-2 are obtained as indicated by the findings detected during the basic evaluation.

TREATMENT

Treatment of optic nerve gliomas in NF is covered in Chapter 96. Treatment of neurofibromas of the eyelids and conjunctiva is covered in Chapter 92. Treatment of the intracranial lesions of NF-1 and NF-2 is beyond the scope of this book.

COURSE AND OUTCOMES

Life expectancy is reduced substantially in patients who have NF-1 or NF-2.[14,15] The principal causes of early death in persons who have NF-1 are complications of systemic hypertension, cancer, and expansive growth of benign intracranial neoplasms. Several types of cancer, including neurofibrosarcoma, other sar-

tered neurofibromas, meningiomas, gliomas, and schwannomas. Currently accepted diagnostic criteria for NF-2 are listed in Box 158-2. The most consistent extraophthalmic problem suffered by patients affected by NF-2 is sensorineural deafness caused by the vestibular schwannomas.

OCULAR MANIFESTATIONS

Ophthalmologic findings in NF-1 include Lisch nodules of the iris, subcutaneous pedunculated and plexiform neurofibromas of the eyelids, optic nerve gliomas, multifocal choroidal nevi, and occasionally retinal tumors indistinguishable from the retinal astrocytic hamartomas found in TS.[7,8] Lisch nodules have been described as melanocytic hamartomas of the iris stroma. These lesions appear as tan to light brown nodules that stud the iris surface (Fig. 158-1). They are rarely present at birth but tend to develop by the second to third decade of life in over 95% of persons who have NF-1.[9] Histopathologically, Lisch nodules consist of closely packed dendritic or spindle-shaped melanocytes within the anterior layers of iris stroma. Because these cells are normal uveal melanocytes and not nevus cells, these lesions are not true nevi. Neurofibromas of the eyelids can be either nodular or plexiform in nature. They tend to develop early in life and can enlarge progressively. Gliomas of the optic nerve develop in

comas, leukemias, and lymphomas, occur with increased frequency in patients who have NF-1. In patients with NF-2, the main cause of early death is expansion of a CNS neoplasm. Unilateral or bilateral blindness occurs in some individuals affected by NF-1 or NF-2, usually because of glioma of the optic nerves or chiasm (especially in NF-1) but occasionally because of expansile intracranial growth of a vestibular schwannoma or an apoplectic episode (NF-2).

TUBEROUS SCLEROSIS

TS is a multiorgan tumor syndrome that is characterized by multifocal, bilateral retinal astrocytic hamartomas, astrocytic tumors of the CNS, several unusual cutaneous lesions, mental retardation, seizures, and a variety of cysts and tumors of other organs. The clinical spectrum is extremely broad and ranges from minimal to marked in affected individuals. Many persons who have limited forms of the disease are probably not recognized as TS sufferers.

EPIDEMIOLOGY AND PATHOGENESIS

The prevalence of TS in the general population has been estimated to be approximately 1 case per 10,000 persons.[16] About one third of cases are familial and two thirds are sporadic. No recognized racial predilection exists, and the sexes are affected equally. Signs and symptoms of TS usually begin by the time the patient is 6 years of age.

TS genes have been identified on loci on the long arm of chromosome 9 (9q32-34), on the long arm of chromosome 11, on the short arm of chromosome 16 (16p13), and on the long arm of chromosome 12 (12q22-24).[16] Of these loci, the 9q32-34 locus has been the most consistent, being associated with between one third and one half of all familial cases.

EXTRAOPHTHALMIC MANIFESTATIONS

Central nervous system tumors that occur in TS are generally low-grade astrocytomas. These CNS lesions can become calcified and detectable on skull radiographs; however, they are revealed much more effectively by CT (Fig. 158-2) or MRI.[17] Complications associated with such lesions include mental deficiency and seizures, both of which can range from mild to severe. Many individuals who have TS have normal intellectual abilities.

The cutaneous lesions characteristically associated with TS include adenoma sebaceum, ash leaf spots, shagreen patches, and subungual fibromas.[18] Adenoma sebaceum is an unusual facial dermatological eruption characterized by pinhead to pea-sized yellowish to reddish-brown papules distributed in a butterfly fashion over the nose, cheeks, and nasolabial folds (Fig. 158-3). Histopathologically, the individual skin lesions are angiofibromas. Ash leaf spots are congenital white or hypomelanotic skin macules ranging in size from about 1mm to several centimeters in diameter and having a configuration that resembles an ash leaf. These lesions usually show up prominently when the skin is viewed under ultraviolet light. The shagreen patch is a thickened patch of skin with the texture of pigskin or sharkskin and usually occurs over the lower back. Subungual fibromas are benign fibrous tumors that develop at the sides of the nail beds in some patients.

A variety of unusual tumors develop in the heart, kidney, lungs, thyroid, and other visceral organs in some patients who have TS. The most common visceral tumor in TS appears to be the angiomyolipoma of the kidney.[19] Probably the most distinctive visceral tumor in TS is the benign cardiac rhabdomyoma. In some patients who have TS, an unusual lung disease (pulmonary lymphangioleiomyomatosis) develops.[19] In addition, benign cysts develop multifocally in various visceral organs, including the kidneys, liver, and lungs, in many patients who have TS.

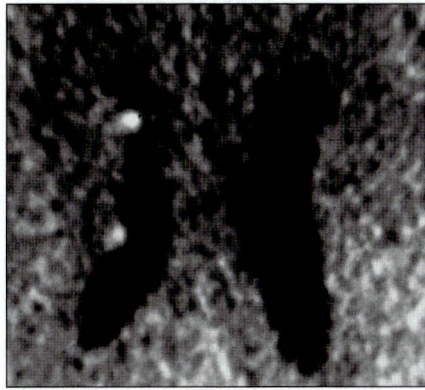

FIG. 158-2 ■ Computed tomography of paraventricular astrocytomas in a patient who has tuberous sclerosis.

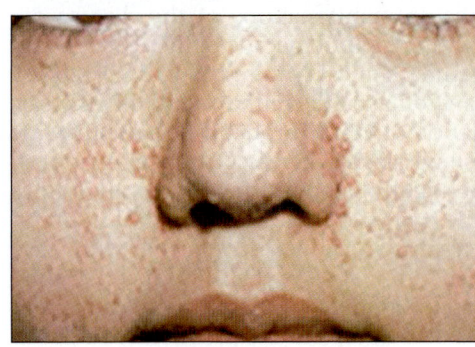

FIG. 158-3 ■ Adenoma sebaceum of face in a patient who has tuberous sclerosis.

OCULAR MANIFESTATIONS

The classical ophthalmoscopic feature of TS is the retinal astrocytoma (astrocytic hamartoma).[20] Lesions of this type are described in detail and illustrated in Chapter 154. Approximately one half of all patients affected by TS develop at least one retinal astrocytoma in one eye.[20] In the individuals who have TS and develop retinal astrocytomas, multiple lesions in both eyes occur in 40–50% of cases.[21] Malignant transformation of retinal astrocytomas occurs in TS but is rare.

SYSTEMIC EVALUATION

Systemic evaluation of individuals for whom TS is suspected should include fundus examination, dermatological evaluation to identify characteristic skin lesions, CT or MRI of the CNS, and CT or MRI of the abdominal viscera.[21] Examination of family members to look for a familial pattern is also appropriate.

TREATMENT

Treatment of affected individuals is purely symptomatic at present. Periodic physical examination and imaging of the CNS and abdominal-thoracic viscera by CT or MRI are appropriate to identify potentially treatable problems such as cardiac rhabdomyomas, cysts and tumors of the kidney, and enlarging CNS astrocytomas.

COURSE AND OUTCOMES

The life expectancy of individuals who have TS is reduced substantially compared with that expected in the normal population.[22] The most common cause of early death in this syndrome is renal failure secondary to angiomyolipomas, cysts, or both. The second most common cause of death is obstructive hydrocephalus or other CNS problems caused by enlargement of one or more of the CNS astrocytomas. Other important but less frequent causes of death are cardiac conduction defects and heart failure from cardiac rhabdomyoma and chronic pulmonary insufficiency associated with lymphangioleiomyomatosis of the lung. In patients who have profound mental retardation and severe seizures, death occurs frequently as a result of status epilepticus or pneumonia.

VON HIPPEL–LINDAU SYNDROME

VHLS is a multiorgan disorder characterized by retinal capillary hemangiomas, CNS hemangioblastomas, various solid and cystic visceral hamartomas and hamartias, and malignant neoplasms, including renal cell carcinomas and pheochromocytomas. The full-fledged syndrome commonly runs in families that have a clear autosomal dominant inheritance pattern. Affected individuals are at substantial risk of early death, usually on the basis of their intracranial hemangiomatous lesion or renal cell carcinoma.

EPIDEMIOLOGY AND PATHOGENESIS

VHLS appears to be rare, but its precise incidence has not been determined.[23] In patients who have full-fledged VHLS, one or more clinically identifiable manifestations of the disease are usually present by or before the third decade of life. The median age at detection of the first clinical features of VHLS is 20–25 years.[23] Capillary hemangiomas of the retina are usually the earliest detected manifestation of VHLS (probably because they are easiest to detect at a small size), whereas CNS hemangioblastomas typically appear slightly later and renal cell carcinomas substantially later in life. However, the timing of clinical emergence of the various lesions in individual patients who have VHLS varies greatly. The cumulative probability of developing retinal capillary hemangiomas and CNS hemangioblastomas in a patient who has VHLS is >80%, and the probability of developing renal cell carcinoma is >60%.

VHLS affects both sexes equally and occurs in all racial groups. Molecular biological studies have localized the VHLS gene to chromosome 3p25-26.[24]

EXTRAOPHTHALMIC MANIFESTATIONS

Important extraocular features of VHLS include hemangioblastomas (capillary hemangiomas) of the brain and spinal cord, renal cell carcinoma, pheochromocytoma, several other less common solid neoplasms and related lesions, and cystic lesions of various visceral organs. The classical CNS lesions of VHLS are solid and cystic cerebellar hemangioblastomas (Fig. 158-4),[25] which occur in about 40% of affected individuals by the age of 30 years and in about 70% of them by the age of 60 years.[23] The component cells in these tumors appear benign by histopathological criteria. Similar vascular lesions also occur in the medulla and spinal cord in 10–15% of patients who have VHLS.

Renal cell carcinoma is an acquired malignant neoplasm of the kidney that occurs in about 5% of VHLS patients by the age of 30 years but in >40% by the age of 60 years.[23] The renal cell carcinomas that occur in VHLS are bilateral in approximately 75% of cases.[23] This tumor can metastasize, so it must be recognized early and treated aggressively if a fatal outcome is to be avoided. Other visceral neoplasms that develop in some patients who have VHLS include pheochromocytoma, islet cell carcinoma of the pancreas, and cyst-adenomas of the pancreas and epididymis.[23] Also, those affected by VHLS have a strong tendency to develop multifocal cysts in the kidneys, pancreas, and ovaries.[23] Unlike NF and TS, VHLS does not have dermatological lesions as part of the syndrome.

OCULAR MANIFESTATIONS

The classic ocular lesion of VHLS is the retinal capillary hemangioma, which is described in detail in Chapter 155. Approximately 50–60% of patients who have VHLS develop retinal capillary hemangiomatosis during their lifetimes, and about one half of these individuals have multiple retinal capillary hemangiomas in both eyes.[26]

SYSTEMIC EVALUATION

As a result of the frequency and severity of the various multiorgan lesions in VHLS, a comprehensive protocol of periodic reexamination and ancillary testing of affected patients and at-risk relatives in identified VHLS families has been developed (Box 158-3).

A challenging clinical situation occurs in patients who have a single retinal capillary hemangioma, a single CNS hemangioblastoma, or renal cell carcinoma and no family history of VHLS at the time of initial diagnosis. More aggressive baseline evaluation and follow-up are probably appropriate for such patients who present with CNS or retinal vascular lesion or kidney tumor early in life than for those who have a lesion first detected at age 40 years or older.

First- and second-degree relatives of patients with VHLS are at risk for VHLS. The only way to determine with certainty whether someone has VHLS is though DNA testing. This testing is performed on blood, which must be processed at a clinical testing laboratory that has the necessary equipment and appropriate DNA probes. A list of clinical laboratories that offer genetic testing for VHLS is currently available on the Internet at http://www.vhl.org/healthcare/dna-src.htm.

TREATMENT

Signs and symptoms of VHLS and the necessity for treatment depend on the nature of the lesion, the location and size of the lesions, and the symptoms that result. Treatment of retinal capillary hemangiomas is covered in Chapter 155. Treatment of the CNS and visceral lesions of this disease is generally surgical and is beyond the scope of this book.

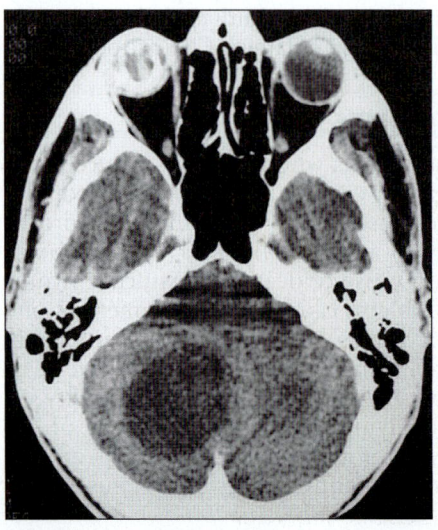

FIG. 158-4 ■ Computed tomography of cerebellar hemangioblastoma in von Hippel–Lindau syndrome. Note cystic lesion in cerebellum and increased intraocular density ipsilaterally (related to advanced retinal capillary hemangiomatosis causing phthisis bulbi).

BOX 158-3

Screening Protocol for von Hippel–Lindau Syndrome

AFFECTED PATIENTS
Annual physical examination
Annual comprehensive fundus examination
Magnetic resonance imaging or computed tomography of brain every 3 years to age 50 years and every 5 years thereafter
Annual renal ultrasound scan, with computed tomography scan every 3 years (more frequently if multiple renal cysts are present)
Annual 24-hour urine collection for vanillylmandelic acid

AT-RISK RELATIVES
Annual physical examination
Annual comprehensive fundus examination from age 5 years
Magnetic resonance imaging or computed tomography of brain every 3 years from age 15 to 50 years and then every 5 years until age 60 years
Annual renal ultrasound scan, with computed tomography scan every 3 years from age 20 to 65 years
Annual 24-hour urine collection for vanillylmandelic acid

COURSE AND OUTCOMES

Progression of retinal capillary hemangiomas in VHLS is highly variable, but tumor enlargement, intraretinal and intravitreal bleeding, exudation, gliosis, and retinal detachment may develop. These complications can result in profound visual loss or even phthisis bulbi of one or both eyes. Fortunately, ophthalmic treatment is usually able to preserve good vision in at least one eye. If the associated renal tumors and intracranial vascular tumors are not detected at an early stage or are not controlled by aggressive intervention, they commonly prove fatal to the affected individuals.[23,25] Consequently, the life expectancy of patients who have VHLS is reduced considerably compared with that of unaffected persons in the general population. The median age at death in patients who have VHLS is 45–50 years in most series.[23]

STURGE-WEBER SYNDROME

SWS is a dermato-oculo-neural syndrome characterized by cutaneous facial nevus flammeus in the distribution of the branches of the trigeminal nerve, ipsilateral diffuse cavernous hemangioma of the choroid, and ipsilateral meningeal hemangiomatosis. The lesions in the eye, skin, and brain are always present at birth (i.e., they are birthmarks or congenital anomalies rather than acquired neoplasms such as those that occur in the three syndromes already covered in this chapter).

EPIDEMIOLOGY AND PATHOGENESIS

The frequency of the complete SWS and its formes fruste is unknown. Men and women appear to be affected equally. No recognized racial predilection occurs. The vast majority of patients affected by SWS have sporadic nonfamilial disease. Only a few familial clusters of the syndrome have been reported, and most of these have not exhibited the clear-cut autosomal dominant inheritance pattern that typifies NF, TS, and VHLS.

EXTRAOPHTHALMIC MANIFESTATIONS

The classical cutaneous feature of SWS is the facial nevus flammeus (Fig. 158-5), a flat to moderately thick zone of dilated telangiectatic cutaneous capillaries lined by a single layer of endothelial cells in the dermis.[27] The lesion is usually unilateral and most frequently involves the regions of the face innervated by the first, occasionally the first and second, and rarely all three branches of the trigeminal nerve. The ipsilateral nasal and buccal mucosa is involved in some patients, and localized hypertrophy of the involved tissues may be present. The characteristic CNS manifestation of SWS is ipsilateral leptomeningeal hemangiomatosis, which causes atrophy of the cortical parenchyma of the brain, seizures, and frequently mental retardation.[28] The CNS lesions are present at birth and are detectable by MRI or CT.[29] They tend to be progressive throughout life. In many patients, the affected meninges become irregularly calcified during life, in which case the CNS vascular lesion can be detected on routine skull radiographs.

OCULAR MANIFESTATIONS

The classical ocular manifestation of SWS is the diffuse choroidal hemangioma, which is described in detail in Chapter 152. Other ocular abnormalities that have been described in patients who have SWS include telangiectasia of the conjunctiva and episclera (Fig. 158-6) and ipsilateral congenital, infantile, or juvenile glaucoma.[27] These features and their potential sequelae are also discussed in Chapter 152.

SYSTEMIC EVALUATION

Because patients affected by SWS do not have any recognized propensity to develop benign or malignant neoplasms, they do not require periodic systemic or CNS screening tests for such lesions. However, patients who have SWS and develop seizures or progressive mental deterioration probably need periodic neurological evaluation and intermittent evaluation by CT or MRI of the brain to rule out treatable lesions or disorders. Regular ophthalmological evaluations are appropriate in all patients who have suspected or confirmed SWS to screen for treatable ocular complications such as glaucoma and exudative retinal detachment.

TREATMENT

Treatment of patients who have SWS is generally symptomatic and directed toward complications caused by the vascular lesions of the brain and eyes. Seizures are treated medically unless that therapy proves unsuccessful. Intractable seizures and progressive mental deterioration are sometimes treated surgically by techniques such as subtotal hemispherectomy.[30] The facial nevus flammeus can be treated by dermatological laser therapy. This treatment frequently results in marked regression of the vascular birthmark and substantial cosmetic improvement. Treatment of the ophthalmic lesions and complications of SWS are discussed in Chapter 152.

COURSE AND OUTCOMES

The life expectancy of patients who have SWS appears to be reduced substantially compared with that of persons in the general population.[31] However, most early deaths occur in individuals who have profound mental retardation and intractable seizures and not in those who have a limited form of the disease, normal intellectual ability, and no seizures.

WYBURN-MASON SYNDROME

WMS is characterized by arteriovenous malformations (AVMs) of the retina and ipsilateral CNS. Because the abnormal lesions are not distinct tumors but rather anomalous arteriovenous communications, this syndrome is not a true phakomatosis by the definition used herein. Furthermore, most patients who have

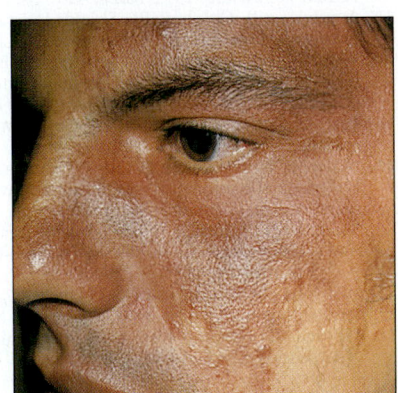

FIG. 158-5 ◼◼ Facial nevus flammeus in a patient with Sturge-Weber syndrome.

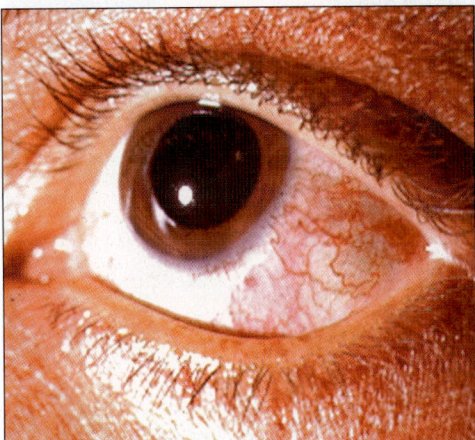

FIG. 158-6 ◼◼ Episcleral telangiectasis ipsilateral to facial nevus flammeus and diffuse choroidal hemangioma in a patient with Sturge-Weber syndrome.

WMS have unilateral nonfamilial disease. A hereditary pattern has not been identified.

EPIDEMIOLOGY AND PATHOGENESIS

This syndrome is very uncommon. The retinal and intracranial AVMs of WMS are congenital. However, they are usually incompletely developed at birth but progress during growth and aging.[32,33] Consequently, the vascular malformations in the retina and CNS are often undetected until the second through fourth decades of life. The more extensive the congenital vascular lesions, the earlier the presentation in most patients. Men and women appear to be affected equally. No racial predilection occurs. No hereditary pattern has been identified.[34]

EXTRAOPHTHALMIC MANIFESTATIONS

Complex AVMs occur in the orbit, in the periorbital soft tissues and bones, and in the midbrain ipsilateral to the retinal AVM.[33,34] Not all patients who have a retinal AVM have or develop extraretinal AVMs, and only the patients who have both retinal and CNS AVMs should be considered to have WMS. In general, the more complex the retinal vascular anomalies, the higher the likelihood of associated CNS AVMs.[34]

OCULAR MANIFESTATIONS

The classic ophthalmic abnormality of WMS is the AVM of the retina (Fig. 158-7).

SYSTEMIC EVALUATION

Baseline assessment of patients who have a complex retinal AVM should probably include MRI and possibly magnetic resonance angiography of the ipsilateral orbit and brain.[35] Such investigation is probably not indicated in patients who have small, limited retinal AVMs unless they have neurological symptoms. Currently, no consensus exists about what constitutes appropriate follow-up of affected patients.

TREATMENT

No effective treatment is currently available for retinal AVM. Complex, symptomatic intracranial AVMs can sometimes be managed effectively by intracranial resection, arterial ligation, arterial embolization,[36] stereotactic radiosurgery,[37] or charged particle beam irradiation.

COURSE AND OUTCOMES

Life expectancy is reduced in patients who have WMS because of early deaths attributable to spontaneous bleeding from the intracranial AVMs[38] and strokes related to their treatment. In addition, the affected eye is sometimes blinded as a result of spontaneous or post-therapeutic occlusion of the retinal AVM.

REFERENCES

1. Riccardi VM. Neurofibromatosis: past, present, and future. N Engl J Med. 1991; 324:283–5.
2. North K. Neurofibromatosis type 1: review of the first 200 patients in an Australian clinic. J Child Neurol. 1993;8:395–402.
3. O'Connell P, Cawthon R, Xu GF, et al. The neurofibromatosis type 1 (NF1) gene: identification and partial characterization of a putative tumor suppressor gene. J Dermatol. 1992;19:881–4.
4. MacCollin M, Mohney T, Trofatter J, et al. DNA diagnosis of neurofibromatosis 2. Altered coding sequence of the merlin tumor suppressor in an extended pedigree. JAMA. 1993;170:2316–20.
5. Guttmann DH, Aylsworth A, Carey JC, et al. The diagnostic evaluation and multidisciplinary management of neurofibromatosis 1 and neurofibromatosis 2. JAMA. 1997;278:51–7.
6. Crowe FW. Axillary freckling as a diagnostic aid in neurofibromatosis. Ann Intern Med. 1964;61:1142–3.
7. Huson S, Jones D, Beck L. Ophthalmic manifestations of neurofibromatosis. Br J Ophthalmol. 1987;71:235–8.
8. Destro M, D'Amico DJ, Gragoudas ES, et al. Retinal manifestations of neurofibromatosis. Arch Ophthalmol. 1991;109:662–6.
9. Lewis RL, Riccardi VM. von Recklinghausen neurofibromatosis. Incidence of iris hamartomata. Ophthalmology. 1981;88:348–54.
10. Lewis RL, Gerson LP, Axelson KA, et al. von Recklinghausen neurofibromatosis. II. Incidence of optic gliomata. Ophthalmology. 1984;91:929–35.
11. Wiznia RA, Freedman JK, Mancini AD, et al. Malignant melanoma of choroid in neurofibromatosis. Am J Ophthalmol. 1978;86:684–7.
12. Kaye LD, Rothner AD, Beauchamp GR, et al. Ocular findings associated with neurofibromatosis type II. Ophthalmology. 1992;99:1424–9.
13. Sivalingam A, Augsburger JJ, Perilongo G, et al. Combined hamartoma of the retina and retinal pigment epithelium in a patient with neurofibromatosis type 2. J Pediatr Ophthalmol Strabismus. 1991;28:320–2.
14. Zoller M, Rembeck B, Akesson HO, Angervall L. Life expectancy, mortality and prognostic factors in neurofibromatosis type 1. A twelve-year follow-up of an epidemiological study in Goteborg, Sweden. Acta Derm Venereol. 1995;75:136–40.
15. Evans DG, Huson SM, Donnai D, et al. A clinical study of type 2 neurofibromatosis. Q J Med. 1992;84:603–18.
16. Northrup H. Tuberous sclerosis complex: genetic aspects. J Dermatol. 1992; 19:914–19.
17. Truhan AP, Filipek PA. Magnetic resonance imaging. Its role in the neuroradiologic evaluation of neurofibromatosis, tuberous sclerosis, and Sturge-Weber syndrome. Arch Dermatol. 1993;129:219–26.
18. Webb DW, Clarke A, Fryer A, Osborne JP. The cutaneous features of tuberous sclerosis: a population study. Br J Ophthalmol. 1996;135:1–5.
19. Maziak DE, Kesten S, Rappaport DC, Mauer J. Extrathoracic angiomyolipomas in lymphangioleiomyomatosis. Eur Res J. 1996;9:402–5.
20. Nyboer JH, Robertson DM, Gomez MR. Retinal lesions in tuberous sclerosis. Arch Ophthalmol. 1976;94:1277–80.
21. Roach ES, Smith M, Huttenlocher P, et al. Diagnostic criteria: tuberous sclerosis complex. Report of the Diagnostic Criteria Committee of the National Tuberous Sclerosis Association. J Child Neurol. 1992;7:221–34.
22. Shepherd CW, Gomez MR, Lie JT, Crowson CS. Causes of death in patients with tuberous sclerosis. Mayo Clin Proc. 1991;66:792–6.
23. Maher ER, Yates JR, Harries R, et al. Clinical features and natural history of von Hippel–Lindau disease. Q J Med. 1990;77:1151–63.
24. Glenn GM, Linehan WM, Hosoe S, et al. Screening for von Hippel–Lindau disease by DNA polymorphism analysis. JAMA. 1992;267:1226–36.
25. Neumann HP, Eggert HR, Scheremet R, et al. Central nervous system lesions in von Hippel–Lindau syndrome. J Neurol Neurosurg Psychiatry. 1992;55:898–901.
26. Hardwig P, Robertson DM. von Hippel–Lindau disease. A familial, often lethal, multi-system phakomatosis. Ophthalmology. 1984;91:263–70.
27. Sullivan TJ, Clarke MP, Morin JD. The ocular manifestations of the Sturge-Weber syndrome. J Pediatr Ophthalmol Strabismus. 1992;29:349–56.
28. Pascual-Castroviejo I, Diaz-Gonzalez C, Garcia-Melian RM, et al. Sturge-Weber syndrome: study of 40 patients. Pediatr Neurol. 1993;9:283–8.
29. Marti-Bonmati L, Menor F, Poyatos C, Cortina H. Diagnosis of Sturge-Weber syndrome: comparison of the efficacy of CT and MR imaging in 14 cases. AJR Am J Roentgenol. 1992;158:867–71.
30. Ito M, Sato K, Ohnuki A, Uto A. Sturge-Weber disease: operative indications and surgical results. Brain Dev. 1990;12:473–7.
31. Oakes WJ. The natural history of patients with the Sturge-Weber syndrome. Pediatr Neurosurg. 1992;18:287–90.
32. Augsburger JJ, Goldberg RE, Shields JA, et al. Changing appearance of retinal arteriovenous malformation. Graefes Arch Clin Exp Ophthalmol. 1980;215:65–70.
33. Willinsky RA, Lasjaunias P, Terbrugge K, Burrows P. Multiple cerebral arteriovenous malformations (AVMs). Review of our experience from 203 patients with cerebral vascular lesions. Neuroradiology. 1990;32:207–10.
34. Patel U, Gupta SC. Wyburn-Mason syndrome. A case report and review of the literature. Neuroradiology. 1990;31:544–6.
35. Nussel F, Wegmuller H, Huber P. Comparison of magnetic resonance angiography, magnetic resonance imaging and conventional angiography in cerebral arteriovenous malformation. Neuroradiology. 1991;33:56–61.
36. Morgan MK, Johnston IH, de Silva M. Treatment of ophthalmofacial-hypothalamic arteriovenous malformation (Bonnet-Dechaume-Blanc syndrome). Case report. J Neurosurg. 1985;63:794–6.
37. Lunsford LD, Kondziolka D, Flickinger JC, et al. Stereotactic radiosurgery for arteriovenous malformations of the brain. J Neurosurg. 1991;75:512–24.
38. Wilkins RH. Natural history of intracranial vascular malformations: a review. Neurosurgery. 1985;16:421–30.

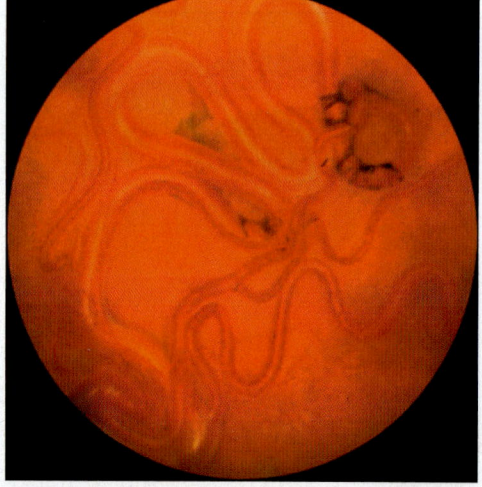

FIG. 158-7 ▮
Complex arteriovenous malformation of retina in a young woman with Wyburn-Mason syndrome.

UVEITIS AND OTHER INTRAOCULAR INFLAMMATIONS

Narsing A. Rao

CHAPTER
159

SECTION I BASIC PRINCIPLES

Mechanisms of Uveitis

GEETA PARARAJASEGARAM

DEFINITION
- Uveitis is a complex intraocular inflammatory process that primarily involves the uveal tract.

KEY FEATURES
- The disease is characterized by the classical signs of inflammation, including inflammatory exudates and cells in the anterior chamber and/or vitreous.

ASSOCIATED FEATURES
- In most instances the cause is unknown.
- When identified, the causative agents and/or mechanisms include infectious agents, trauma, and autoimmunity.

INTRODUCTION

Uveitis is an inflammatory condition of the uvea and adjacent structures that affects mainly children and young adults. In the majority of patients, the cause of uveitis remains obscure even after extensive investigation. The inflammation might be induced by infectious agents or trauma, but in most cases the underlying mechanisms appear to be autoimmune in nature. Many excellent publications address the basic elements involved in the circuitry of the immune system and the induction of autoimmunity.[1,2] The following includes an overview only of the main elements involved in immunity-autoimmunity and emphasizes the factors that have been shown to be involved in uveitis.

The immune response is an intricate event that is regulated by a number of different types of cells and the soluble factors secreted by some of these cells. The cells fall into two main categories, leukocytes and tissue cells. The former subclass comprises lymphocytes (T and B), phagocytes, and auxiliary cells (basophils, mast cells, and platelets). Tissue cells include in situ antigen-presenting cells (APCs), some of the functions of which have been elucidated in vivo; others are putative APCs, based on in vitro studies.

CELLS OF THE IMMUNE SYSTEM

B and T Lymphocytes

Both B and T lymphocytes are capable of participating in specific responses to a particular antigen and are derived from stem cells in the bone marrow. In mammals, B cells mature in the bone marrow, whereas T cells are "educated" through a sojourn in the thymus. B cells play a role in the immune system by producing specific antibodies to an antigen that is encountered. The antibodies belong to a group of extensively studied proteins called immunoglobulins (Igs), of which five different types occur— IgD, IgM, IgG, IgA, and IgE. When the antibody response requires the aid of T cells, the antigen against which this type of antibody is formed is termed a T cell–dependent antigen. The antibody produced by the differentiated B cell or plasma cell is

inserted into the surface of the same cell, where it acts as a specific antigen receptor. Whereas B cells have the ability to recognize native antigen that is not processed or presented by other cells, T cells require the presence of a compatible APC for this recognition phase.

T cells express various surface molecules, which play a significant role in antigen recognition. These include the T-cell antigen receptor (TCR), surface molecules (CD4 and CD8), and others. The TCR is a disulfide-linked glycoprotein that allows T cells to recognize a wide range of antigens.[3] Two forms of TCRs ($\alpha\beta$ TCR and $\gamma\delta$ TCR) exist, based on the structure of the heterodimeric glycoproteins, and the two types have distinct anatomical locations. The $\alpha\beta$ TCR is present on more than 90% of peripheral T cells and on the majority of thymocytes that express TCRs. The preponderance of T cells present in the epithelium and substantia propria of the normal conjunctiva express the $\alpha\beta$ TCR.[4] The T cells that express the $\gamma\delta$ receptor occur in abundance in the epithelia of the intestine, uterus, and tongue. TCR $\gamma\delta$ T cells have also been detected in inflamed conjunctiva and isolated and cultured from inflamed vitreous.[4,5]

Role of T Cells

Different groups of T cells occur, determined by the role played by each type. These functions are determined by surface receptors on the various subsets. Helper T cells (TH cells), of which further subsets exist, act in conjunction with other immune cells to produce a response. The TH cells in one subset activate B cells to produce antibodies, and those in another subset interact with phagocytes in the destruction of pathogens. Cytotoxic T cells (TC cells) attack foreign cells and host cells infected with viruses. TH cells are identified most commonly by their surface receptor CD4, and the CD8 marker distinguishes TC cells. TH cells can be divided into two subsets, TH1 and TH2, on the basis of the pattern of production of various soluble mediators called cytokines.[6] TH1 cells produce cytokines such as interleukin-2 (IL-2), interferon (IFN)-γ and tumor necrosis factor (TNF)-α and TNF-β. They are the major effectors in delayed-type hypersensitivity, cytotoxicity, and macrophage activation and are also implicated in autoimmune diseases. TH2 cells preferentially produce IL-4, IL-5, IL-6, IL-10, and IL-13 and are responsible for the immune response against extracellular pathogens, allergens, and parasites.

Other Cells

Although the role of T and B lymphocytes in immune responses has been discussed, it must be stressed that these cells alone are not capable of achieving the wide range of responses involved in the initiation, perpetuation, and termination of an inflammatory reaction. In addition to B and T cells, a third population of lymphocytes exists, referred to as natural killer (NK) cells. These cells lack both immunoglobulins, which are characteristic of B cells, and TCRs, which are the hallmark of T cells, and constitute about 15% of blood lymphocytes. The role of these cells, although not fully understood, appears to lie in their ability to recognize and kill certain tumor cells and virus-infected cells.

Mononuclear phagocytes, to which group belong the APCs, are derived from the bone marrow. Macrophages (mononuclear phagocytes in tissues) are found in many organs and participate predominantly in the removal of particulate antigens. These cells bind microorganisms through specialized receptors on their surface and ingest the invading organism. Neutrophils, also termed polymorphonuclear neutrophils (PMNs), are a hallmark of an acute inflammatory response. Their ability to ingest and kill invading organisms is based largely on the presence of two types of granules within the cell, the primary or azurophilic granules and the secondary or specific granules. Eosinophils also appear to be capable of phagocytosing and killing ingested microbes, although they play a more specialized role in the immunity to parasitic worms through the extracellular release of a toxin referred to as major basic protein. Eosinophils are also important participants in the termination or damping of an immune response. This is effected through the secretion of molecules such as histaminase and aryl sulfatase, which inactivate soluble products of mast cells.

Mast cells, functionally similar to basophils, play a role in the body's response to an allergen by the release of mediators such as histamine. This reaction occurs through an interaction of the allergen with IgE molecules present on the surface of the mast cells and basophils. Mast cells, which have been demonstrated in the conjunctiva, play a pivotal role in allergic conjunctivitis.[7]

Processing of Antigens

As stated before, T cells require processing and presentation of antigen by APCs prior to being activated. Antigen recognition by T cells is dependent on two steps. One occurs through a TCR,[3] and the second involves binding of accessory molecules present on the APC to appropriate receptors on the T cell (Fig. 159-1). In the absence of antigen, a T cell is not reactive. However, antigen alone cannot stimulate the cell. In fact, this first signal received alone will "turn off" the T cell, resulting in one mechanism in which a response to autoantigens is prevented. T-cell proliferation or stimulation requires signaling between costimulatory molecules on the APC and cell surface molecules on the T cell. The best studied costimulatory molecules for T-cell activation are B7-1 (CD80), B7-2 (CD86), and CD40 and their respective receptors on the T cell, namely CD28, CTLA4, and CD40L (CD40 ligand).[8] Compatibility of the APC and T cell is a pivotal step in antigen presentation. This recognition, also termed "restriction," is determined by the proteins of the major histocompatibility complex (MHC).

The human MHC system, known as the human leukocyte antigen (HLA) system, consists of three classes of molecules, class I, class II, and class III. Class I molecules in the human system are further subdivided into A, B, C, E, F, and G. These molecules, which are present on the surface of almost all nucleated cells in the body, are required for activation of CD8+ cells. Class II molecules, which are derived from the genes located in the D region of the human HLA complex, are also referred to as the HLA-DP, DQ, and DR molecules. CD4+ T cells respond to peptides (antigens) when presented with MHC class II or HLA-D region molecules. The latter are constitutively present only on cells involved in immune responses, such as APCs, which include dendritic cells, macrophages, and B cells. Their expression can, however, be induced in a variety of cell types following stimulation by cytokines. Studies have demonstrated MHC class II molecule expression on activated CD4+ and CD8+ cells, which allows them to act as APCs to themselves or to other autologous T cells.[9] Class III molecules are encoded by over 20 genes, some of which encode complement system products whereas others are responsible for the production of molecules involved in antigen processing.

Antigen is processed by APCs via a complex intracellular system, which includes proteolytic enzymes, peptide transporters, and molecular chaperones.[2] The processed antigen is then bound to MHC molecules on the surface of the APC. For antigen recognition by T lymphocytes, the MHC molecule must present the antigenic peptide to the TCR, which is associated with a molecule termed CD3 on the T cell. Various types of T cells require different MHC molecules for antigen presentation. Once the initial antigen presentation has occurred, the T cells respond by either acting directly with other cells or generating soluble factors that act on other cells. As more information becomes available, it appears that these soluble factors or cytokines are pivotal in the maintenance of balance of the immune system.

Importance of Antigen Presentation

The importance of antigen presentation in immunity cannot be overstated. This presumed first step in the induction of an im-

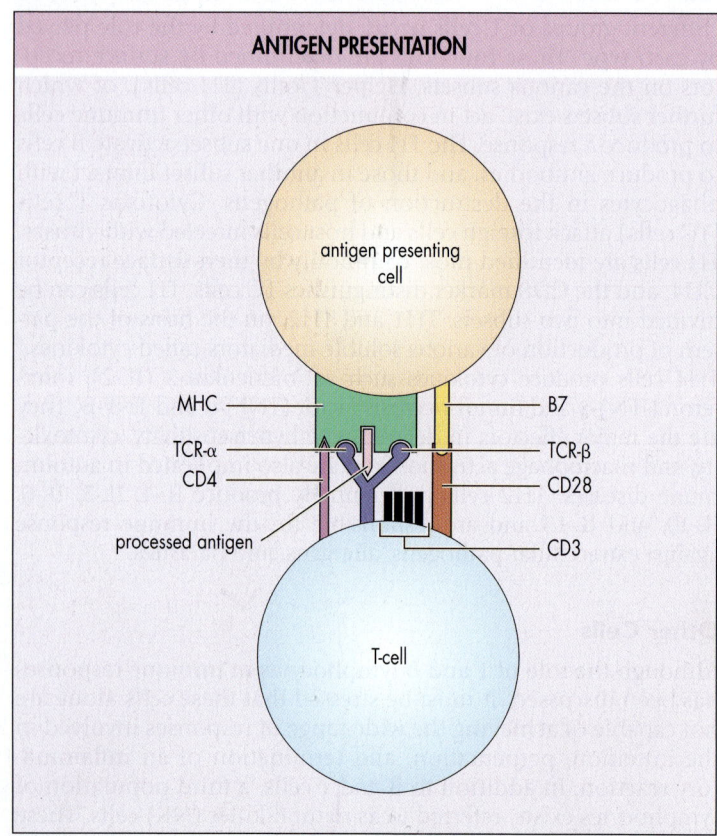

ANTIGEN PRESENTATION

antigen presenting cell

MHC
TCR-α
CD4
processed antigen

B7
TCR-β
CD28
CD3

T-cell

FIG. 159-1 ■ Diagrammatic representation of antigen presentation to CD4 marker positive T cells. *MHC,* Major histocompatibility complex; *TCR,* T-cell antigen receptor.

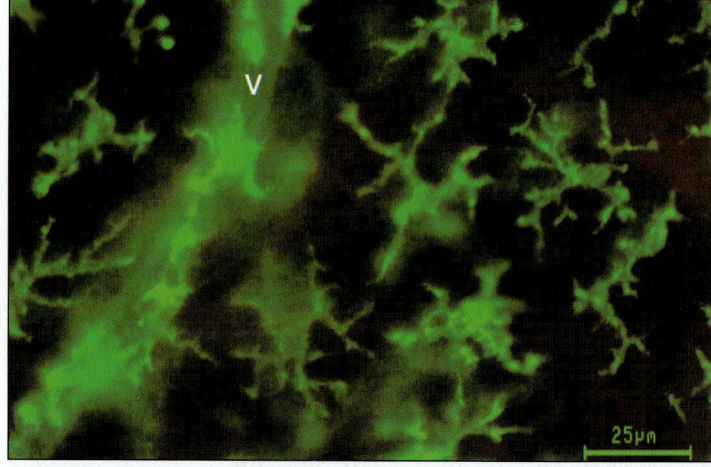

FIG. 159-2 ■ Fluorescent antibody–labeled microglial cells in a rat retina. A whole mount of rat retina was stained with antibody to Ox42, a marker for microglia and/or monocytes. The microglial cells are observed both perivascularly and in locations distant from the vessel. Microglial cells are thought to be the local antigen-presenting cells (APCs) in the retina. *V,* Vessel.

mune reaction is responsible for the protection afforded against microbes, parasites, and other infectious agents. The established APCs in the eye include Langerhans' cells (which are dendritic cells) and macrophages in the peripheral cornea and bone marrow–derived cells in the uvea[10] and retina (Fig. 159-2).[11]

TOLERANCE AND AUTOIMMUNITY

The delicate balance afforded by the interaction of the various types of cells and their soluble products results in an almost perfect immune system. However, even slight aberrations of this self-regulating balance can lead to disastrous consequences. A reaction that could certainly lead to deleterious effects for the host concerned is the mounting of an immune response to autoantigens. This phenomenon is referred to as autoimmunity. However, nature, to a large extent, has prevented this from occurring through a mechanism referred to as tolerance. Immunological tolerance to autoantigens is a basic property of the immune system and is a feature by which the immune system can differentiate between self and nonself. Antigens that induce tolerance are termed tolerogens; they are distinct from immunogens, which are antigens that produce an immune response. Under normal conditions, all autoantigens act as tolerogens.

TOLERANCE

Tolerance to self is an active process, and there are two well-established mechanisms by which it is achieved (Box 159-1). These are termed central and peripheral tolerance.[12] Central tolerance occurs during T-cell development, when immature T cells migrate from the bone marrow to the thymus. In the thymus, these T cells encounter autoantigens presented by APCs in conjunction with the MHC. The T cells with high affinity for au-

---

BOX 159-1

Mechanisms of Tolerance Induction

CENTRAL TOLERANCE
- Usually occurs in the thymus during T-cell development
- Death of immature T cells that express a TCR that recognizes autoantigens
- Process referred to as negative selection
- Autoreactive T cells undergo clonal deletion by apoptosis

PERIPHERAL TOLERANCE
Mechanisms by which mature autoreactive T cells are kept in check include anergy, deletion, suppression, and ignorance

Anergy
- Occurs when antigen presentation to T cell occurs in absence of co-stimulatory molecules
- Mediated by block in IL-2 transcription

Deletion
- Autoreactive cells may be deleted by apoptosis
- Also referred to as *programmed cell death*
- Mediated via Fas and FasL

Suppression
- Mediated by antigen-specific T cells, natural suppressor (NS) cells, and veto cells
- Antigen-specific T cells suppress the response of autoreactive T cells
- NS cell–mediated suppression is antigen nonspecific
- Veto cells present negative signals to CD4+ cells, causing inactivation of effector T cells
- May be due to TH subset that produces transforming growth factor-β

Ignorance
- Nonrecognition of antigen by autoreactive T cells
- May be due to presentation of autoantigen by cells that do not possess co-stimulatory molecules or autoantigens that are anatomically sequestered
- Autoreactive cells recognize only "cryptic" determinants on the autoantigen

---

toantigens are programmed to die through a process termed apoptosis. This mechanism of clonal deletion occurs through a process referred to as negative selection and ensures that a large number of autoreactive T cells are deleted. Elimination of autoreactive B-cell clones also occurs through clonal deletion of immature B cells and takes place in the bone marrow. Not all the self-peptides that T and B cells might encounter during their lifetime are present in the thymus and bone marrow; hence, it is possible that occasional autoreactive cells may escape the process of negative selection. Peripheral tolerance comes into play, to ensure that regulatory mechanisms exist to curb the activity of these cells that have the potential to cause autoimmune disease. Mechanisms that prevent mature autoreactive cells in the periphery from causing autoimmune disease include anergy, deletion, suppression, and ignorance.

ANERGY. Anergy, which is defined as the functional inactivation of lymphocytes without their elimination, is induced when an autoreactive T cell is presented antigen in the absence of a costimulatory molecule or "second" signal, thus preventing further activation of the T cell. Thus, although autoreactive cells are present, they are incapable of responding to antigen. The process is thought eventually to be due to a block in the transcription of the gene for IL-2.[13]

DELETION. Peripheral autoreactive T cells may also be deleted through apoptosis. It is mediated by a cell surface protein termed Fas (CD95), which is expressed on many cell types, including hemopoietic and epithelial cells.[14] Following antigen receptor-mediated activation, the expression of Fas on T and B cells has been shown to increase. The distribution of the Fas ligand FasL is much more restricted; it is induced on CD4+ and CD8+ lymphocytes following activation but not expressed on any other hemopoietic cells. Interactions between FasL and Fas play an obligatory role in apoptosis of T cells. Studies that demonstrate the constitutive expression of FasL in the eye have led to the theory that the interaction of Fas and FasL could be significant in the immune privilege of the eye.[15] In other studies, it has been shown that memory T cells in the aqueous humor of patients with uveitis preferentially express Fas antigen, which suggests that this increase in the number of Fas+ T cells may be involved in the pathogenesis of uveitis.[16]

SUPPRESSION. Another potential mechanism of peripheral tolerance is suppression, in which a reactive T cell is actively kept from carrying out its function by another cell. T cells that belong to the TH2 subgroup appear to be one of the principal regulatory cell types in this mechanism, based on their ability to produce cytokines that suppress immune responses associated with autoimmune diseases. Whereas antigen-specific T suppressor cells inhibit the responsiveness of autoreactive effector T cells, another population of suppressor cells termed natural suppressor cells mediate suppression in a manner that is not antigen specific and does not require MHC restriction. Yet another subset of T cells, termed veto cells, has also been identified. Veto cells are T cells that have an APC function, present antigen to CD4+ T cells, and deliver negative signals to produce inactivation of the effector T cell. This form of anergy seems to be unrelated to the absence of costimulatory molecules. Studies have implicated a separate population of TH cells, which elaborate large amounts of the cytokine transforming growth factor-β, an effective inhibitor of lymphocyte proliferation. As a result of the difficulty encountered in cloning suppressor cells and the lack of a suppressor-specific surface marker, the role of suppressor cells in tolerance is still largely unknown.

IGNORANCE. Autoreactive T cells do not initiate disease if they ignore or are protected from autoantigens. In this form of peripheral tolerance, autoreactive cells may ignore autoantigens either because the antigen is present on cells that do not possess costimulatory molecules or because the antigen is anatomically sequestered. In addition, the amount of antigen available may be below the threshold necessary for activation of the T cell. Only a small portion of any antigen, known as the dominant determinant, is usually presented to T cells. If an autoreactive T cell recognizes only a region of an autoantigen that is not normally accessible during presentation (a cryptic determinant), the antigen may be ignored by peripheral autoreactive cells. The mechanism of tolerance by ignorance is considered a passive one because it leads to neither deletion nor anergy of autoreactive cells.

Breakdown of Tolerance and Autoimmunity

Even as there are several ways in which tolerance to autoantigens is established and maintained, there are also multiple mechanisms through which this tolerance can break down (Box 159-2). The selection of nonautoreactive clones in the thymus could be flawed in individuals who have certain MHC genotypes, which leads to either the presence of autoreactive T cells or the absence of immunoregulatory T cells that are necessary to inhibit the former. Any factor that causes the release of previously sequestered autoantigens could potentially lead to a breakdown of tolerance to those antigens. Mechanisms that overcome the maintenance of peripheral tolerance could also lead to autoimmunity. For example, the absence of costimulatory molecules on APCs in antigen recognition by T cells leads to tolerance. However, if conditions exist that lead to the expression of these molecules by APCs, loss of T-cell tolerance results. Clonal anergy is ultimately thought to be due to a block in transcription of IL-2. Certain studies indicate that the responsiveness of these anergic T cells can be restored by culture with IL-2; this leads to the suggestion that local production of IL-2 during T-cell responses to nonautoantigens may overcome the peripheral tolerance of autoreactive T cells present at the site and so lead to autoimmunity.[13]

Autoimmunity may also result from a stimulation of autoreactive lymphocytes not deleted during development. This stimulation by polyclonal activators, which stimulate many T- and B-cell clones, occurs irrespective of their antigenic specificity. Bacterial lipopolysaccharide is a well-known polyclonal B-cell activator, and polyclonal T-cell stimulation by bacterial "superantigens" has been proposed as another mechanism of autoimmunity. T cells that express the $\gamma\delta$ TCR are thought to be involved in this response to superantigens. The polyclonal activation of B cells may be induced by bacterial products that act like lipopolysaccharide and may give some insight into the possible link between infection and autoimmunity. In some cases, a response to a foreign antigen that has determinants in common with autoantigens could potentially lead to an autoimmune reaction.

CAUSES OF UVEITIS

In the various types of uveitis encountered in humans in which the mechanism is known, three main underlying causes occur:
- Reaction to trauma
- Autoimmune reaction
- Response to an infectious agent

Uveitis related to trauma could follow a penetrating injury (see Chapter 179). In the case of the autoimmune component, this could be either a direct response to autoantigens as a consequence of tolerance breakdown, as discussed earlier, or a secondary reaction to autoantigens that results from damage to ocular structures from other causes. In the matter of infectious uveitis, *Toxoplasma* and other infectious agents have been implicated in many cases. The inflammatory response observed in infectious uveitis could result from two scenarios—first, a reaction to noxious agents such as toxins produced by pathogens, and second, an immune response to the pathogen itself. In some cases, a response to a particular pathogen could lead to a reaction against autoantigens because of similarity or cross-reaction in antigenic structure between the two. This cross-reaction or homology is termed molecular mimicry and is postulated to be one mechanism by which an autoimmune response could be initiated. Although many examples of molecular mimicry are found in viruses, bacteria, protozoa, and helminths, its biological relevance to human disease is yet to be confirmed. In experimental studies, microbial (nonself) proteins that have sequence homology to certain uveitogenic self-peptides have been shown to induce autoimmune uveitis in rats and subhuman primates. These nonself proteins include sequences from hepatitis B virus, Moloney murine leukemia virus, baker's yeast, and *Escherichia coli*, among others.[17–19]

There has been some speculation about molecular mimicry playing a role in certain diseases with a genetic predisposition. Correlations between the expression of various HLAs and certain autoimmune diseases have been noted for antigens of HLA class I and II (Table 159-1). For example, anterior uveitis is strongly associated with the presence of HLA-B27. Uveitis in Behçet's disease has an association with HLA-B51 and birdshot choroidopathy with HLA-A29.[20] Because MHC class II molecules are involved in the selection and activation of CD4+ T cells and these T cells play an integral part in the regulation of the immune response, much work has been done on the association of MHC class II antigens and disease prevalence. This is demonstrated in studies of sympathetic ophthalmia, Vogt-Koyanagi-Harada syndrome, rheumatoid arthritis, insulin-dependent diabetes mellitus, and Sjögren's disease, to name a few.[21,22] Although it is apparent that the presence of certain haplotypes predisposes an individual to some diseases, it is still unclear how the disease process in these instances is initiated. Cross-reactivity between microbial proteins and certain HLA antigens might result in an autoimmune response. Although examples of such molecular mimicry have been noted, their significance in pathogenesis is unclear. Studies have analyzed disease induction by HLA peptides that have a homology in their sequence to certain retinal antigens.[23] Although the expression of a particular HLA gene product may not by itself be the cause

---

BOX 159-2

Possible Mechanisms of Tolerance Breakdown and Autoimmunity

Presence of certain MHC genotypes that could lead to:
- Presence of autoreactive T cells
- Absence of immunoregulatory T cells

Release of normally sequestered autoantigens due to:
- Trauma
- Infection

Alteration of autoantigen structure resulting from:
- Tissue injury
- Inflammation

Expression of costimulators on APCs can overcome peripheral tolerance

Polyclonal stimulation of self-reactive lymphocytes by:
- LPS (for B cells)
- Bacterial 'superantigens' (for T cells)

Both are characterized by antigen-independent stimulation

Molecular mimicry due to homology between:
- Pathogens and host tissue antigens
- Microbial proteins and certain HLA antigens

TABLE 159-1

ASSOCIATION OF HUMAN LEUKOCYTE ANTIGEN (HLA) AND OCULAR INFLAMMATORY DISEASE

Disease	Associated HLA
Anterior uveitis	HLA-B27
Behçet's syndrome	HLA-51
Birdshot retinopathy	HLA-A29
Intermediate uveitis	HLA-A28[22]
Vogt–Koyanagi–Harada syndrome	HLA-Dw53, HLA-DR4

of any autoimmune disease, it may be one of several factors that contribute to the breakdown of tolerance.

INFLAMMATION AND HYPERSENSITIVITY REACTIONS

Inflammation is a response that causes the influx of leukocytes and plasma molecules to the site of an infection, antigenic challenge, or tissue damage. This process, which involves chemotactic factors and cell migration, adhesion molecules and vascular permeability, and the release of various inflammatory mediators both locally at the site of inflammation and at distant locations, is an exquisitely orchestrated sequence of events (Fig. 159-3). The sequence at an inflammatory site is dependent on the cause of the inciting event. In the case of an infection, leukocytes arrive at the site and produce soluble mediators that regulate subsequent events such as cell accumulation and activation. The inflammation ideally resolves when the causative agent is removed. When the inflammation is elicited by the immune system itself, ensuing events are controlled by the antigen that initiated the original response. This situation usually results in a chronic inflammatory state, either in an infection or in an autoimmune response because the inciting antigen cannot be completely removed.

Chemokines

Cells migrate to sites of subsequent inflammation through the action of mediators known as chemokines released at these locations. Chemokines are chemotactic cytokines and belong to a family of small proteins.[24,25] They can be divided into subgroups, named CC, CXC, C-x3-C, and C chemokines, on the basis of the location of the first two cysteines compared with other amino acids (X) in the structure of the protein. The CXC subgroup is also referred to as α-chemokines and the CC subgroup as β-

chemokines. T lymphocytes produce the chemokine macrophage inflammatory protein 1α (MIP-1α), which causes chemotaxis of naive T cells, B cells, and NK cells.[24] The chemokine RANTES (regulated upon activation normal T cell expressed presumed secreted), which is produced by many cell types in response to specific stimuli, is preferentially chemotactic for memory T cells but also acts on NK cells and so causes activation of both these cell types. RANTES is a chemoattractant for eosinophils and macrophages and causes histamine release from basophils. It is found in very low amounts in normal adult human tissue, but its expression increases dramatically at inflammatory sites.[25]

MIP-1α, RANTES, and monocyte chemoattractant protein 1 (MCP-1) are examples of CC chemokines. IL-8, which is derived from monocytes, lymphocytes, fibroblasts, epithelial cells, and vascular endothelial cells, localizes PMNs and belongs to the CXC subgroup. Fractalkine or neurotactin is a chemokine belonging to the C-x3-C subgroup, and lymphotactin, which is chemotactic for T cells and NK cells, is a member of the C chemokine subgroup. Molecules that are chemotactic for PMNs and macrophages include the complement system–derived factor C5a and leukotriene B4. In addition, studies have indicated that oxidized lipids derived from retinal membranes are chemotactic for PMNs.[26]

Extravasation of Cells

A circulating inflammatory cell must leave the blood in order to reach a tissue site. This transendothelial migration through the vessel wall includes tethering, triggering, and latching of leukocytes to the vascular endothelial cells. These events are mediated by adhesion molecules expressed on vascular endothelial cells, which bind to corresponding molecules on leukocytes (Fig. 159-4). The major endothelial cell adhesion molecules include intercellular adhesion molecule-1 (ICAM-1), ICAM-2, and vascular cell adhesion molecule-1 (VCAM-1). The adhesion molecules present on leukocytes belong to a family of proteins referred to as integrins. Different types of integrins exist, broadly differentiated by their structure. The leukocyte func-

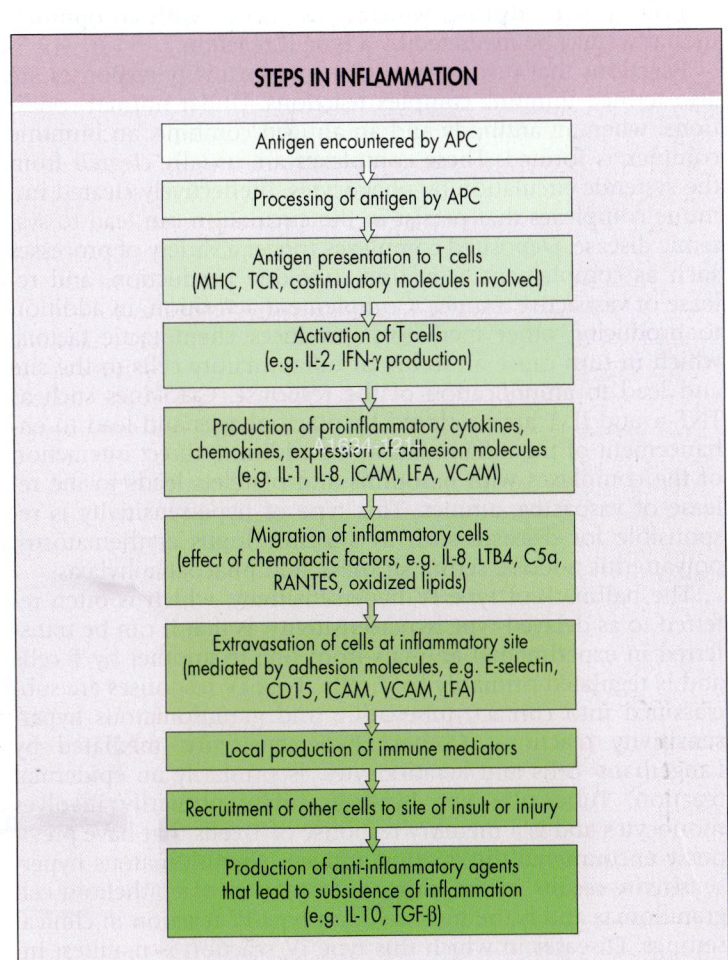

STEPS IN INFLAMMATION

- Antigen encountered by APC
- Processing of antigen by APC
- Antigen presentation to T cells (MHC, TCR, costimulatory molecules involved)
- Activation of T cells (e.g. IL-2, IFN-γ production)
- Production of proinflammatory cytokines, chemokines, expression of adhesion molecules (e.g. IL-1, IL-8, ICAM, LFA, VCAM)
- Migration of inflammatory cells (effect of chemotactic factors, e.g. IL-8, LTB4, C5a, RANTES, oxidized lipids)
- Extravasation of cells at inflammatory site (mediated by adhesion molecules, e.g. E-selectin, CD15, ICAM, VCAM, LFA)
- Local production of immune mediators
- Recruitment of other cells to site of insult or injury
- Production of anti-inflammatory agents that lead to subsidence of inflammation (e.g. IL-10, TGF-β)

FIG. 159-3 ▪ Steps in inflammation.

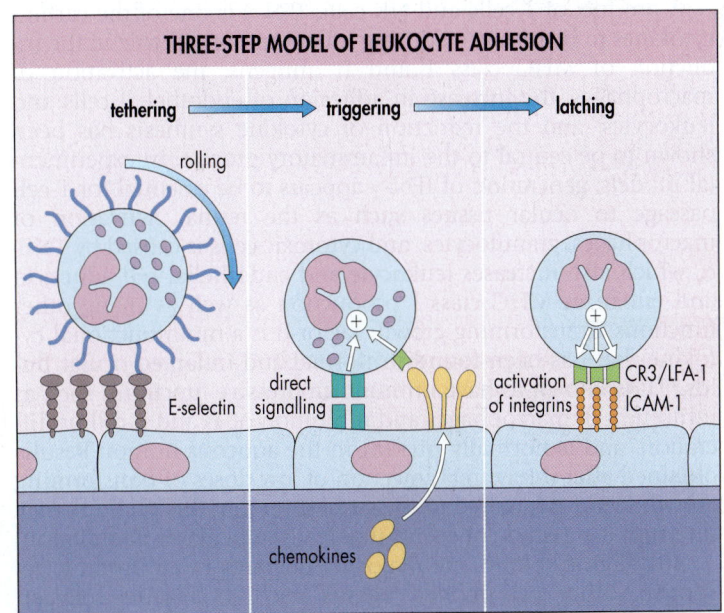

THREE-STEP MODEL OF LEUKOCYTE ADHESION

tethering → triggering → latching

rolling

E-selectin — direct signalling — activation of integrins — CR3/LFA-1 ICAM-1

chemokines

FIG. 159-4 ▪ Steps in leukocyte adhesion. The initial step in adhesion involves the interaction of adhesion molecules (CD15) on leukocytes with molecules present on endothelium. The latter belong to a group of molecules termed selectins, E-selectin being one such transmembrane member, expressed on endothelium. This first stage of attachment is referred to as tethering. In the next phase, the tethered cell is activated or triggered by either direct or indirect signals from molecules on the epithelium or by the action of chemokines. This step is termed triggering. In the final phase, termed latching, there is up-regulation of various molecules, such as integrins, on the leukocytes, which then attach to adhesion molecules such as intercellular adhesion molecules (ICAM)-1 that are generated on the endothelium. The latching stage is induced by triggering. (Adapted from Figure 14.10 of Roitt I, Brostoff J, Male D. Immunology, 4th ed. London: Mosby; 1996.)

tional antigens (LFAS) bind to ICAM-1 and ICAM-2 and are present on most leukocytes. The VLAs (very late antigen), which include the integrin VLA-4, are primarily involved in binding cells to extracellular matrix. In addition, VLA-4 binds to VCAM-1 on the vascular endothelium.

When inflammatory cells reach the tissue to which they are directed, a phenomenon referred to as homing, they participate in the local immune response. This process is controlled by the production of various soluble mediators, termed cytokines, which are proteins involved in the communication between cells. Cytokines have been shown to have autocrine, paracrine, and endocrine functions. Some of these cytokines induce perpetuation of the inflammation through the recruitment of other effector cells to the site, whereas others modulate the process by shutting down the operation of effector cells so that host tissue damage is minimized. A balance between these different cytokines is crucial to the outcome of the response. Ample evidence is available to support the fact that cytokines play a pivotal role in the pathogenesis of uveitis.[25]

Cytokines

Cytokines generated in uveitis include some of the IL family of proteins (IL-1, IL-2, IL-4, IL-6, IL-8, IL-10, and IL-12), IFN-γ and TNF-α.[24] The ILs (IL-1 through IL-18 at the present time) are a major group of cytokines that have been found to have diverse functions in immune responses. Macrophages and B cells produce IL-1, which is important in the stimulation of macrophages, the activation of lymphocytes, and the adhesion of leukocytes to endothelial cells. IL-2 is a potent cytokine produced by T cells, and its primary known physiological effect is its action as a T-lymphocyte growth factor. T cells also produce IL-4, the principal targets of which are B cells and T cells. IL-4 also functions in B-cell growth. T and B cells and macrophages secrete IL-6, which is known to act on B cells during their differentiation. Finally, IL-10 is one of the T cell–derived mediators known to down-regulate an immune response by the inhibition of cytokine synthesis by TH1 cells, and IL-12, a monocyte product, is responsible for the induction of TH1 cells.

A product of T cells and NK cells, IFN-γ is one of the earliest cytokines to be produced during inflammation. Its role in the induction of MHC class I and II antigens, the activation of macrophages, the increase in adhesion of endothelial cells and leukocytes, and the reduction of cytokine synthesis has been shown to be central to the inflammatory process. In experimental models, generation of IFN-γ appears to be essential for T-cell passage to ocular tissues such as the retina. Activation of macrophages, granulocytes, and cytotoxic cells is caused by TNF-α, which also increases leukocyte and endothelial cell adhesion and enhances MHC class I production as well as many other functions. Transforming growth factor-β is a multifunctional cytokine that has been found in normal and inflamed ocular fluids.[27] It is known to have immunosuppressive functions, such as inhibition of macrophages and inhibition of T- and B-cell proliferation, and is normally present in the aqueous humor. Results obtained after intravitreal injection of low doses of transforming growth factor-β have led to the suggestion that this cytokine may interrupt the cascade of events that leads to ocular inflammation.

Although cytokines are major participants in an immune response, other cell-derived agents such as reactive oxygen metabolites and hydrolytic enzymes or proteases are equally important in determining the consequence of an inflammatory reaction. These oxygen free radicals and proteases are produced by phagocytic cells and are a normal part of the armament of these cells in their role against microbes. However, free radicals have also been implicated in uveitis.[28] A reactive radical given prominence in the pathogenesis of several inflammatory diseases is nitric oxide, which is produced endogenously in small amounts. However, certain cytokines can induce the production of large amounts of nitric oxide. Studies in an acute model of uveitis have indicated that nitric oxide may be a key mediator, playing a complex role in ocular inflammation.[29]

Immune Response and Hypersensitivity

A specific immune response involves the interaction of effector mechanisms such as complement, phagocytes, inflammatory cells, and cytokines. However, because these responses are not directed against the inciting agent only, injury to the surrounding host tissue usually occurs as well. Under normal conditions, because of the self-limiting nature of immune responses, these injurious reactions are minimal and dampened when the foreign antigen is eliminated. In addition, because of tolerance to autoantigens, immune responses to autologous tissues do not usually occur. In some cases, however, when a specific immune response is not appropriately controlled, a phenomenon termed hypersensitivity ensues. Hypersensitivity is the result of a beneficial immune response that has gone awry. Four main types of hypersensitivity reactions occur, classified as types I, II, III, and IV.

Type I reactions are the result of an IgE response to a particular antigen termed an allergen, which is the underlying mechanism in allergic reactions. They are mediated by mast cells and their mediators, in particular histamine. A type I reaction is the underlying mechanism for the development of conditions such as allergic conjunctivitis.

Type II hypersensitivity responses are observed in transfusion reactions, hemolytic anemia, Goodpasture's syndrome, pemphigus, and myasthenia gravis. In this category of hypersensitivity, the reaction is a result of antibody binding to cell surface antigens on cells or tissues. As a result, damage is restricted to the cells or tissues that express those antigens. The initial antibody binding, which could be of the IgM or IgG type, leads to activation of the complement system and effector cells and results in ultimate damage to cells and tissues by cytotoxic effects or lysis, or both. Graves' disease, which is associated with an ophthalmopathy, may be mediated by a type II reaction.

Reactions that involve type III hypersensitivity responses are also termed immune complex reactions. Under normal conditions, when an antibody and an antigen combine, an immune complex is formed. These complexes are usually cleared from the systemic circulation by phagocytes. Ineffectively cleared immune complexes that persist in the circulation can lead to systemic disease. Deposited complexes trigger a variety of processes such as complement activation, cytokine production, and release of vasoactive amines. Complement activation, in addition to producing other mediators, produces chemotactic factors, which in turn cause an influx of inflammatory cells to the site and lead to amplification of the response. Cytokines such as TNF-α and IL-1 are produced by macrophages and lead to enhancement of the inflammation. In addition, direct interaction of the complexes with basophils and platelets leads to the release of vasoactive amines. This type of hypersensitivity is responsible for diseases such as systemic lupus erythematosus, polyarteritis nodosa, serum sickness, and phacoanaphylaxis.

The hallmark of type IV hypersensitivity, which is often referred to as delayed-type hypersensitivity, is that it can be transferred in experimental animals from one to another by T cells and is regulated primarily by T cells. Type IV responses are subclassified into contact, tuberculin, and granulomatous hypersensitivity reactions. Contact hypersensitivity, mediated by Langerhans' cells and keratinocytes, is primarily an epidermal reaction. Tuberculin-type hypersensitivity primarily involves monocytes and is a memory response of T cells that have previously encountered the inciting antigen. Granulomatous hypersensitivity results in the ultimate formation of epithelioid cell granulomas and is the most relevant type IV reaction in clinical settings. Diseases in which this type IV reaction is manifest include leprosy, tuberculosis, and sarcoidosis. A common trend in these diseases is that the causative agent persists, generating a chronic antigenic stimulus. The pathogenesis of sympathetic ophthalmia is mediated by a type IV reaction.

ANIMAL MODELS OF UVEITIS

Uveitis in humans is a complex intraocular condition. Notwithstanding the fact that much effort has been spent to elucidate the mechanism of pathogenesis in human cases of uveitis, to date most of the data regarding the possible pathways of disease induction and progression have been obtained from well-established animal models. These models not only allow study of the pathogenesis of uveitis but also in some cases are aimed at modulating the disease process. Investigators have striven to use various inducing agents in developing animal models of uveitis in an effort to mimic the inflammation observed in humans.

Experimental Autoimmune Uveitis

Experimental autoimmune uveitis has been induced in subhuman primates, rats, mice, and guinea pigs using a variety of intraocular antigens. Animals that under normal conditions do not spontaneously develop inflammation do so following immunization with a range of ocular autoantigens. These models provide an understanding of the prevailing mechanisms in the types of human uveitis that may have an autoimmune component. Among these is Vogt-Koyanagi-Harada disease.[30]

Although many ocular antigens have been used to induce uveitis in animal models, the best studied condition is that induced in rats and subhuman primates with the retinal soluble protein S-antigen (Fig. 159-5). Most animal models of uveitis have been shown to be mediated by CD4[+] cells. Some of the antigens that have been utilized are interphotoreceptor retinoid binding protein, melanin protein, rhodopsin, PEP-65 (a protein purified from retinal pigment epithelial cells), phosducin, recoverin (a calcium-binding protein identified in cancer-associated retinopathy), and those belonging to the tyrosinase family of proteins.[30] Whereas most of the antigens used produce a disease that mainly involves the posterior region of the eye, the disease produced with melanin protein is characterized by an inflammation that is predominantly anterior in nature, with essentially no retinal involvement (Fig. 159-6). It is termed experimental autoimmune anterior uveitis and resembles the noninfectious iridocyclitis observed in humans.

S-Antigen Uveitis

The model of S-antigen uveitis is used here to discuss the disease process that occurs in experimental autoimmune uveitis, which develops when S-antigen–reactive lymphocytes are activated. The activation is initiated when TCRs recognize the peptide presented to them by the MHC class II molecule on APCs. It has been postulated that these APCs are present in the eye.[11] The uveoretinitis that ensues as a final consequence of this initial reaction is the result of an immune reaction that occurs when these activated lymphocytes reach the eye and further activate the immunological process. The sensitized lymphocytes trigger this cascade of events, which include the production of cytokines, expression of adhesion molecules, and the recruitment of inflammatory cells to ocular tissue. Studies have demonstrated an increase in the expression of cytokines IL-2, IL-4, lymphotoxin, and IFN-γ.[25] Enhanced expression of adhesion molecules has also been noted in experimental autoimmune uveitis.[31] The expression of the adhesion molecule ICAM-1 occurred prior to the earliest detection of inflammatory cells, indicating a definite pattern in the sequence of events.

Arthus-Type Reaction

An animal model using lens antigen has been extensively analyzed to study the pathogenesis of phacoanaphylactic endophthalmitis in humans, and it has been reported that the inflammation observed in experimental lens-induced uveitis is due to an altered tolerance to lens proteins (Fig. 159-7). Studies by Marak[32] and others have proved that the inflammation in lens-induced uveitis is a result of a type III hypersensitivity reaction. This indicates that the response is an Arthus-type reaction involving antigen-antibody complexes and the subsequent activation of the complement cascade.

IMMUNE PRIVILEGE OF THE EYE

An anatomical site in which immunogenic tissue survives for extended periods of time in an immunocompetent host is referred to as an immune-privileged site.[33] This privilege is thought to have evolved as a protective mechanism in highly specialized organs whose normal function would be disrupted as a consequence of a local immune response; this phenomenon is believed to occur only in organs whose maintenance of normal function is vital to host survival. It has long been known that the eye is such a site of immune privilege, which is evident in the anterior chamber (AC), vitreous cavity, and subretinal space. Some of the features that appear to play a role in this privilege include the presence of a tight blood-ocular barrier, the complete lack of an intraocular lymphatic system, and an intraocular microenvi-

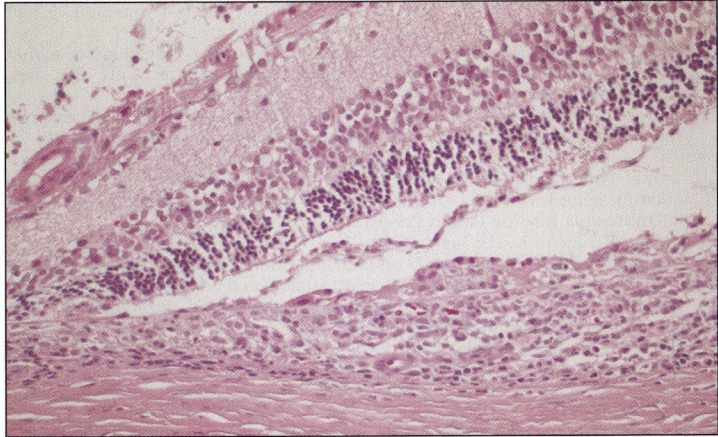

FIG. 159-5 ▪ Histopathology of a rat eye with retinal S-antigen–induced experimental autoimmune uveitis (the prototype animal model for many human cases of uveitis). The intraocular inflammation consists of mononuclear cells and polymorphonuclear leukocytes present at the site of retinal damage, in the outer segment and in the choroid (hematoxylin & eosin).

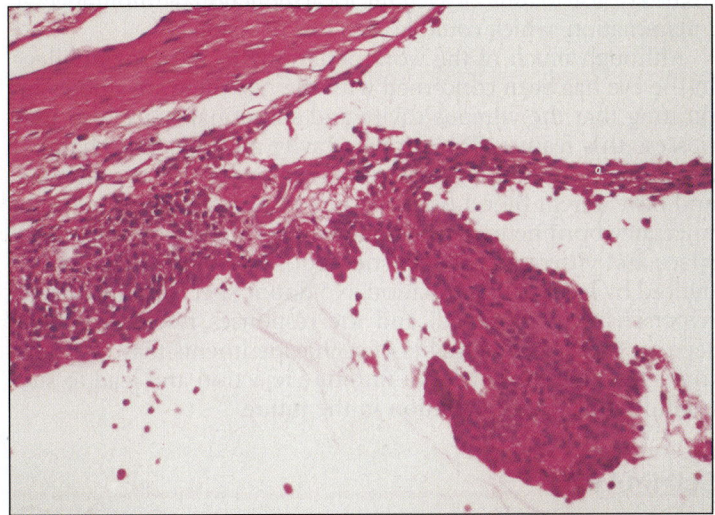

FIG. 159-6 ▪ Histopathology of a rat eye following induction of uveitis with melanin. The disease is characterized by an anterior uveitis with inflammatory cells predominantly infiltrating the iris and ciliary body (hematoxylin & eosin).

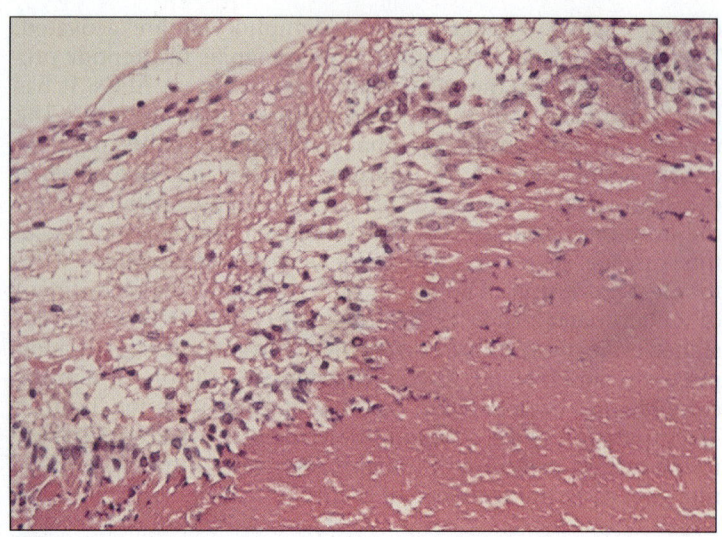

FIG. 159-7 ■ **Histopathology of a rat eye with lens-induced granulomatous uveitis.** The inflammation is distinguished by the presence of multinucleated giant cells and epithelioid cells present around the extruded lens cortex material (hematoxylin & eosin).

ronment that is immunosuppressive. The presence of an intraocular immunosuppressive microenvironment is most apparent in the AC. As a result of this feature, antigens experimentally placed in the eye elicit a stereotypic deviant form of systemic immunity termed AC-associated immune deviation (ACAID). It was originally believed that this phenomenon arose because antigens within the AC failed to escape and therefore could not induce an immune response in the host; the lack of direct access to the lymphatic system supported this belief. Although the human AC has no direct lymphatic drainage, a pathway has been demonstrated in monkeys.

Many studies have demonstrated that various cytokines, neuropeptides, and other factors appear to contribute to intraocular immunosuppression. Some of the better studied of these are transforming growth factor-β1 and 2, α-melanocyte–stimulating hormone, calcitonin gene–related peptide, and cortisol. ACAID may develop through a mechanism in which parenchymal cells within the iris–ciliary body secrete immunosuppressive factors into the aqueous humor. This deviant systemic immunity is selectively deficient in T cells that mediate delayed hypersensitivity reactions as well as in complement-fixing antibodies. The phenomenon has been confirmed by the adoptive transfer of lymphoid cells. It is thought that the immunosuppressive microenvironment observed in the eye acts to limit or avert the local induction of immunogenic inflammation, which could lead to loss of vision.[33]

Although much of the work pertaining to immune privilege in the eye has been concerned with the AC, there are studies indicating that the vitreous cavity and subretinal space also may possess this feature. The vitreous cavity and aqueous chamber are similar in that both sites lack significant lymphatic drainage and have a tight blood-tissue barrier. In experimental studies in mice, newborn neural retinal grafts implanted in the subretinal space and vitreous cavity experienced immune privilege, as evidenced by lack of inflammation. No donor-specific delayed-type hypersensitivity occurred, and the responses resembled those seen in ACAID.[34] The results of such experiments may be useful in overcoming the barrier of immune rejection and lead to successful retinal transplantation in the future.

SUMMARY

Uveitis is a complex intraocular inflammatory process characterized by the classical features of inflammation. Clinically, the disease includes altered vascular permeability, cellular infiltration of the uveal tract and intraocular cavities, and, in severe cases, loss of vision. In the majority of cases the cause of the disease remains elusive. However, in instances in which the cause is known, infection, trauma, and autoimmunity appear to play a role.

In this chapter, the basic immune mechanisms of inflammation and their participation in uveitis, where relevant, are discussed. A better understanding of ocular immune responses would lead to elucidation of the cause and pathophysiology of many uveitides and result in more effective therapy for these potentially blinding diseases.

REFERENCES

1. Roitt I, Brostoff J, Male D. Immunology, 4th ed. London: Mosby; 1996.
2. Parkin J, Cohen B. An overview of the immune system. Lancet 2001;357:1777–89.
3. Klein J, Sato A. The HLA system. First of two parts. N Engl J Med. 2000;343:702–9.
4. Soukiasian SH, Rice B, Foster CS, et al. The T-cell receptor in normal and inflamed human conjunctiva. Invest Ophthalmol Vis Sci. 1992;33:453–9.
5. Liversidge J, Dick A, Cheng YF, et al. Retinal antigen specific lymphocytes, TCR-gamma delta T cells and CD5+ B cells cultured from the vitreous in acute sympathetic ophthalmitis. Autoimmunity. 1993;15:257–66.
6. Del Prete G, Maggi E, Romagnani S. Human Th1 and Th2 cells: functional properties, mechanisms of regulation, and role in disease. Lab Invest. 1994;70:299–306.
7. Foster CS. The pathophysiology of ocular allergy: current thinking. Allergy. 1995;50(Suppl 21):6–9.
8. Greenfield EA, Nguyen KA, Kuchroo VK. CD28/B7 costimulation: a review. Crit Rev Immunol. 1998;18:389–418.
9. Pichler WJ, Wyss-Coray T. T cells as antigen presenting cells. Immunol Today. 1994;15:312–15.
10. Choudhury A, Pakalnis VA, Bowers WE. Characterization and functional activity of dendritic cells from rat choroids. Exp Eye Res. 1994;59:297–304.
11. Ishimoto S-I, Zhang J, Gullapalli V, et al. Antigen-presenting cells in experimental autoimmune uveitis. Exp Eye Res. 1998;67:539–48.
12. Kamradt T, Mitchison NA. Tolerance and autoimmunity. N Engl J Med. 2001;344:655–64.
13. Ring GH, Lakkis FG. Breakdown of self-tolerance and the pathogenesis of autoimmunity. Semin Nephrol. 1999;19:25–33.
14. Nishimura Y, Ishui A, Kobayashi Y, et al. Expression and function of mouse Fas antigen on immature and mature T cells. J Immunol. 1995;154:4395–4403.
15. Griffith TS, Brunner T, Fletcher SM, et al. Fas ligand-induced apoptosis is a mechanism of immune privilege. Science. 1995;270:1189–92.
16. Ohta K, Norose K, Wang XC, et al. Apoptosis-related fas antigen on memory T cells in aqueous humor of uveitis patients. Curr Eye Res. 1996;15:299–306.
17. Eto K, Suzuki S, Singh V-K. Immunization with recombinant Escherichia coli expressing retinal S-antigen induced experimental autoimmune uveitis (EAU) in Lewis rats. Cell Immunol. 1993;147:203–14.
18. Singh V-K, Kalra HK, Yamaki K, et al. Molecular mimicry between a uveitopathogenic site of S-antigen and viral peptides. Induction of experimental autoimmune uveitis in Lewis rats. J Immunol. 1990;144:1282–7.
19. Bora NS, Bora PS, Tandhasetti MT, et al. Molecular cloning, sequencing and expression of the 36kDa protein present in pars planitis. Invest Ophthalmol Vis Sci. 1996;37:1877–83.
20. Davey MP, Rosenbaum JT. The human leukocyte antigen complex and chronic ocular inflammatory disorders. Am J Ophthalmol. 2000;129:235–43.
21. Moorthy RS, Inomata H, Rao NA. Vogt-Koyanagi-Harada syndrome. Surv Ophthalmol. 1995;39:265–92.
22. Nepom GT, Erlich H. MHC class II molecules and autoimmunity. Annu Rev Immunol. 1991;9:493–525.
23. Wildner G, Thurau SR. Cross-reactivity between an HLA-B27–derived peptide and a retinal autoantigen peptide: a clue to major histocompatibility complex association autoimmune disease. Eur J Immunol. 1994;24:2579–85.
24. Wakefield D, Cuello C, Di Girolamo N, et al. The role of cytokines and chemokines in uveitis. Dev Ophthalmol. 1999;31:53–66.
25. Magone MT, Whitcup SM. Mechanisms of intraocular inflammation. Chem Immunol. 1999;73:90–119.
26. Goto H, Wu G-S, Gritz DC, et al. Chemotactic activity of the peroxidized retinal membrane lipids in experimental autoimmune uveitis. Curr Eye Res. 1991;10:1009–14.
27. de Boer JH, Limpens J, Orengo-Nania S, et al. Low mature TGF-beta 2 levels in aqueous humor during uveitis. Invest Ophthalmol Vis Sci. 1994;35:3702–10.
28. Rao NA. Role of oxygen free radicals in retinal damage associated with experimental uveitis. Trans Am Ophthalmol Soc. 1990;738:797–850.
29. Allen JB, Keng T, Privalle C. Nitric oxide and peroxynitrite production in ocular inflammation. Environ Health Perspect. 1998;106(Suppl 5):1145–9.
30. Yamaki K, Gocho K, Hayakawa K, et al. Tyrosinase family proteins are antigens specific to Vogt-Koyanagi-Harada disease. J Immunol. 2000;165:7323–9.
31. Whitcup SM, DeBarge LR, Caspi RR, et al. Monoclonal antibodies against ICAM-1 (CD54) and LFA-1 (CD11a/CD18a) inhibit experimental autoimmune uveitis. Clin Immunol Immunopathol. 1993;67:143–50.
32. Marak GE Jr. Phacoanaphylactic endophthalmitis. Surv Ophthalmol. 1992;36:325–39.
33. Streilein JW. Regional immunity and ocular immune privilege. Chem Immunol. 1999;73:11–38.
34. Jiang LQ, Jorquera M, Streilein JW. Subretinal space and vitreous cavity as immunologically privileged sites for retinal allografts. Invest Ophthalmol Vis Sci. 1993;34:3347–54.

CHAPTER
160

Anatomy of the Uvea

KAY L. PARK

DEFINITION
- The uvea is a pigmented, vascular structure consisting of the iris, ciliary body, and choroid.

KEY FEATURES
- Supplies blood to most of the eye from anterior and posterior ciliary branches of the ophthalmic artery.

ASSOCIATED FEATURES
- Produces aqueous humor in the ciliary processes.
- Controls near accommodation by contraction of ciliary muscles, which relax the zonular fibers to the lens.
- Increases aqueous outflow by contraction of ciliary muscles, which open the trabecular meshwork.

INTRODUCTION

The uvea (from the Latin *uva*, meaning grape) is a pigmented structure that primarily lies between the retina and the sclera and constitutes the vascular portion of the eye. Its blood supply comes from the ophthalmic artery, which nourishes most of the eye through branches of the anterior and posterior ciliary arteries. A separate branch of the ophthalmic artery, the central retinal artery, supplies the inner retinal layers and part of the optic nerve. The uvea also has secretory and mechanical functions including production of aqueous humor, improvement of aqueous outflow, and control of near accommodation. The uvea may become involved in disease processes through inflammation, known as uveitis, neoplasia (e.g., melanoma), and growth of abnormal vessels, known as choroidal neovascularization.

IRIS

The anterior portion of the uvea is called the iris (Fig. 160-1). It is composed primarily of vascular stroma as well as melanocytes, nerves, clump cells, collagen, and hyaluronidase-sensitive acid mucopolysaccharides.[1] The vascular supply to the iris originates in the anterior and long posterior ciliary branches of the ophthalmic artery. These branches join in the ciliary body to form the major arterial circle before entering radially into the iris. The vessels lack an internal elastic lamina and are lined by nonfenestrated endothelial cells.

The anterior surface of the iris is composed of a fibroblast cell layer folded into many ridges and crypts, with a pupillary aperture located slightly inferonasal to the center.[2] Eye color is determined by the number and degree of melanin granules in the stromal melanocytes.[3]

Muscular and pigment epithelial structures are located in the posterior portion of the iris. Smooth muscle is tightly arranged in a circle to form the pupillary sphincter and is primarily innervated by parasympathetic nerves coming from the third cranial nerve nucleus. The radially oriented dilator muscles extend from their cell bodies in the anterior pigment epithelial layer and are innervated by the sympathetic nervous system.

In contrast to the irregular surface of the anterior iris, the posterior iris epithelium is velvety smooth. Here, heavily pigmented columnar cells are arranged apex to apex in two layers, absorbing incident light that does not enter through the pupil.[4] These two layers are continuous with the pigmented and nonpigmented layers of the ciliary body.

CILIARY BODY

The anterior portion of the ciliary body, the pars plicata, is composed of approximately 70 ciliary processes (Fig. 160-1). The ciliary processes are arranged in a radial fashion and consist of vascularized stromal cores surrounded by two layers of epithelium—the inner pigmented layer and the outer nonpigmented layer. The cells of these two layers are arranged apex to apex with tight junctions between them.[5] The zonula occludens near the apices of the nonpigmented epithelial cells form the blood-aqueous barrier. The nonpigmented epithelium is also the site of aqueous secretion. Arterioles regulating blood flow through the ciliary body influence the rate of aqueous formation.

The middle portion of the ciliary body, the pars plana, is a flat structure, 4mm in length, located between the pars plicata and the ora serrata.[6] Surgical access through the pars plana requires entry approximately 3–4mm behind the limbus to avoid trauma to the lens or to the retina. The inner layer of the pars plana is composed of pigmented epithelial cells that are uniformly cuboidal in shape and continuous with the retinal pigment epithelium; the outer layer is made up of nonpigmented epithelial cells that are columnar in shape near the pars plicata and more cuboidal as they near the ora serrata. The nonpigmented epithelium secretes acid mucopolysaccharide, one of the main components of the vitreous.

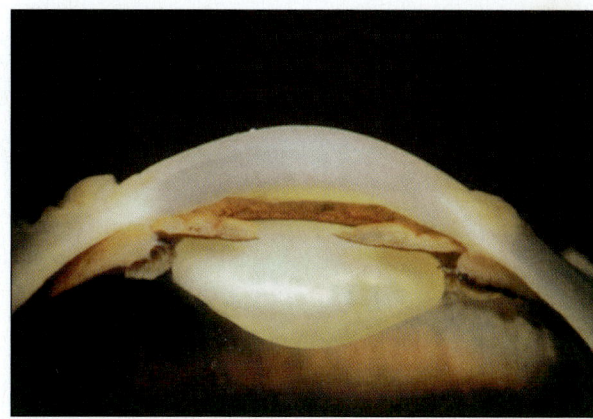

FIG. 160-1 ■ **Iris and ciliary body.** The iris is lined posteriorly by its pigment epithelium, and anteriorly by the avascular anterior border layer. The bulk of the iris is made up of vascular stroma. Considerable pigment is present in the anterior border layer and stroma in this brown iris. (Courtesy of Dr. RC Eagle, Jr.)

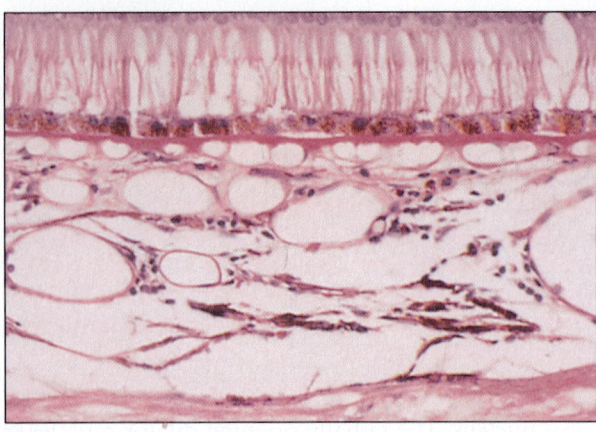

FIG. 160-2 ■ **Choroid.** The choroid is composed, from outside to inside, of the suprachoroidal (potential) space and lamina fusca, the choroidal stroma (which contains uveal melanocytes, fibrocytes, collagen, blood vessels, and nerves), the fenestrated choriocapillaris (the largest capillaries in the body), and the outer aspect of Bruch's membrane. (From Yanoff M, Fine BS. Ocular pathology, ed 5. St. Louis: Mosby; 2002.)

Adjacent to the pars plicata, the ciliary body is composed of three layers of smooth, nonstriated, muscular tissue. The outer longitudinal layer, which makes up the bulk of the tissue, attaches to the scleral spur; the radial and circular muscles originate from the middle and inner ciliary body, respectively. The three layers act as a unit and are innervated primarily by the parasympathetic nervous system with synapses in the ciliary ganglion. Contraction of these muscles relaxes the zonular fibers to the lens, allowing the lens to move forward and assume a more spherical shape for accommodation at near. Miotics also contract the ciliary muscles, opening the trabecular meshwork to increase aqueous outflow.

CHOROID

The choroid, located between the retina and the sclera, extends from the scleral spur anteriorly to the optic nerve posteriorly (Fig. 160-2). Scleral attachments at vortex veins located near the equator account for the characteristic shape of choroidal detachments.[7] The choroid is composed of vessels, melanocytes, and fine connective tissue. The number of pigmented melanocytes in the outermost layer determines the degree of pigmentation in the choroid. Lighter-skinned individuals have less pigmentation in their choroid than those who have darker skin.

The choroid nourishes the outer retina and a portion of the optic nerve. It is the sole vascular supply to the foveal area, manifesting as a cherry-red spot in a central retinal artery occlusion. A cilioretinal branch from the choroid may also supply the fovea in about 10–15% of the population. Blood flow in the choroid is very high, with an oxygen concentration in the venous compartment that is only a few percent less than in the arterial. Drainage of the choroid occurs through four to seven vortex veins.

The choriocapillaris is a continuous vascular sheet of capillaries that lies beneath Bruch's membrane and the retinal pigment epithelium. The architecture of the choriocapillaris differs from one area to the next. In the peripapillary and submacular regions, a dense honeycomb arrangement of capillaries is seen. In the remainder of the posterior pole and near the equator, lobular structures with central postcapillary venules and peripheral precapillary arterioles are found. Finally, peripheral to the choriocapillaris, the pattern of vascular networks is more elongated. Throughout this heterogeneous structure making up the choriocapillaris, angiographic dye has been shown to distribute homogeneously within lobular networks. Differential pressure gradients within the choroidal blood flow may explain these two patterns of lobuli in the choriocapillaris, anatomic versus functional.[8,9]

The choriocapillaris, the largest capillaries in the body, is composed of vessels that are 40–60mm in diameter and contain multiple fenestrations. Small molecules, such as fluorescein, readily pass through these fenestrations and are seen as the choroidal blush on fluorescein angiography. The middle and large choroidal vessels are not fenestrated. Indocyanine green dye has been used more recently to visualize the choroidal circulation because, unlike fluorescein, it is mostly bound to protein and does not leak from the choriocapillaris. Moreover, the longer wavelengths used by indocyanine green (with light absorption and emission at 766nm and 826nm, respectively, versus 485nm and 520nm for fluorescein) allow superior penetration of hazy media, blood, and retinal pigment epithelium. This makes indocyanine green particularly useful for identifying occult choroidal neovascularization, such as in patients with age-related macular degeneration.

REFERENCES

1. Fine BS, Yanoff M, eds. Ocular histology: a text and atlas, 2nd ed. New York: Harper & Row; 1972:168–212.
2. Hogan MJ, Alvarado JA, Weddell JE, eds. Histology of the human eye. Philadelphia: WB Saunders; 1971:202–59.
3. Apple DJ, Rabb MF, eds. Ocular pathology: clinical applications and self-assessment, ed 4. St. Louis: Mosby–Year Book; 1991:201–6.
4. Kardon RH. Anatomy. In: Tripathi RC, ed. Fundamentals and principles of ophthalmology, Section 2. San Francisco: American Academy of Ophthalmology; 1995–1996:49–54.
5. Green WR. The uveal tract. In: Spencer WH. Ophthalmic pathology: an atlas and textbook, 4th ed, Vol 3. Philadelphia: WB Saunders; 1996:1439–60.
6. Aiello AL, Tran VT, Rao NA. Postnatal development of the ciliary body and pars plana. A morphometric study in childhood. Arch Ophthalmol. 1992;110:802–5.
7. Guyer DR, Schachat AP, Green WR. The choroid: structural considerations. In: Ryan SJ, ed. Retina, ed 2. St. Louis: CV Mosby; 1994:18–31.
8. Fryczkowski AW, Sherman MD, Walker J. Observations on the lobular organization of the human choriocapillaris. Int Ophthalmol. 1991;15:109–20.
9. Fryczkowski AW. Anatomical and functional choroidal lobuli. Int Ophthalmol. 1994;18:131–41.

161 General Approach to the Uveitis Patient and Treatment Strategies

DAVID J. FORSTER

DEFINITION
- Uveitis is any condition that involves inflammation of the uveal tract (iris, ciliary body, choroid) or adjacent structures.

KEY FEATURES
- Inflammatory cells in the anterior chamber and/or vitreous cavity.

ASSOCIATED FEATURES
- Pain, redness, photophobia, blurred vision, floaters.
- Localized infiltration of inflammatory cells (e.g., keratic precipitates, iris nodules, retinochoroidal infiltrates).
- Anterior or posterior synechiae.
- Disc or macular edema, sheathing of retinal vessels.
- Secondary cataract or glaucoma.

BOX 161-1

The Classification of Uveitis

ANTERIOR UVEITIS
Iritis, anterior cyclitis, iridocyclitis

INTERMEDIATE UVEITIS (FORMERLY KNOWN AS PARS PLANITIS)
Posterior cyclitis, hyalitis, basal retinochoroiditis

POSTERIOR UVEITIS
Focal, multifocal, or diffuse choroiditis, chorioretinitis, retinochoroiditis, or neurouveitis

PANUVEITIS

INTRODUCTION

Uveitis encompasses a myriad of conditions, all of which are characterized by inflammation of the uveal tract (iris, ciliary body, choroid), either directly or indirectly. The ophthalmologist's goal in treating these potentially blinding conditions is to eliminate the inflammatory reaction within the eye while minimizing the potential risks of therapy to the patient. This is best achieved once an accurate diagnosis has been obtained. To do this most efficiently, an extensive history and ophthalmologic examination are required.

EPIDEMIOLOGY AND PATHOGENESIS

Numerous classification schemes have been used to categorize the various types of uveitis. These are based on such factors as follows:
- Location (e.g., anterior, posterior),
- Course (acute, chronic, recurrent),
- Pathology (granulomatous, nongranulomatous), and
- Causative factors (e.g., infectious, autoimmune, systemic, neoplastic diseases).

The classification scheme recommended by the International Uveitis Study Group is based on anatomical location (Box 161-1).[1]

Large series of uveitis patients show variation in terms of the relative prevalence of different forms of uveitis. In surveys of patients referred to tertiary centers, anterior uveitis has been shown to account for 28–66% of cases, intermediate uveitis for 5–15%, posterior uveitis for 19–51%, and panuveitis for 7–18%.[2,3] However, in a large community-based study, the vast majority of uveitis cases were anterior (71%), followed by posterior uveitis (5%) and intermediate and panuveitis (1% each).[4] As regards specific entities associated with various types of uveitis, the numbers again vary from survey to survey. The most common causes of anterior uveitis are idiopathic (38–56%), the seronegative spondyloarthropathies (21–23%), juvenile rheumatoid arthritis (JRA; 9–11%), and herpetic keratouveitis (6–10%). The vast majority of cases of intermediate uveitis are idiopathic.

Toxoplasmosis is the most common cause of posterior uveitis, and the most common causes of panuveitis are idiopathic (22–45%) and sarcoidosis (14–28%).[2-4]

Because uveitis is frequently associated with other systemic conditions, it is critical that a comprehensive history and review of systems be obtained for every patient who presents with intraocular inflammation (see Box 161-2). This is the first step in the process of appropriately classifying the type of uveitis present and is indispensable in helping to arrive at the correct diagnosis.

OCULAR MANIFESTATIONS

The clinical manifestations of uveitis vary depending on several factors—the primary site of involvement in the eye, the course of the inflammatory process (e.g., acute or chronic), and the presence of secondary complications arising from the uveitis itself.

The symptoms of acute anterior uveitis (e.g., human leukocyte antigen HLA-B27–related entities, such as ankylosing spondylitis) generally include pain, redness, photophobia, and blurred vision, which typically develop over a period of hours or days. On the other hand, patients who have chronic anterior uveitis, such as that seen with JRA or Fuchs' heterochromic iridocyclitis, may present merely with blurring of vision or mild redness, with little pain or photophobia. Patients who have intermediate or posterior uveitis typically present with floaters or impaired vision secondary to cystoid macular edema or chorioretinal involvement. Patients who have panuveitis may present with any or all of these symptoms.

On clinical examination, findings likewise vary depending on the location, course, and pathogenesis of the inflammation. Virtually any ocular tissue may yield findings that may be helpful in the diagnosis. The conjunctiva may show ciliary flush (perilimbal injection characteristic of anterior uveitis) or nodules (e.g., in sarcoidosis). The cornea should be examined for keratic precipitates, which are collections of inflammatory cells on the endothelial surface (Fig. 161-1). Small keratic precipitates are usually seen in nongranulomatous types of uveitis, whereas larger ("mutton fat") keratic precipitates are characteristic of granulomatous uveitis. The normal convection currents of the

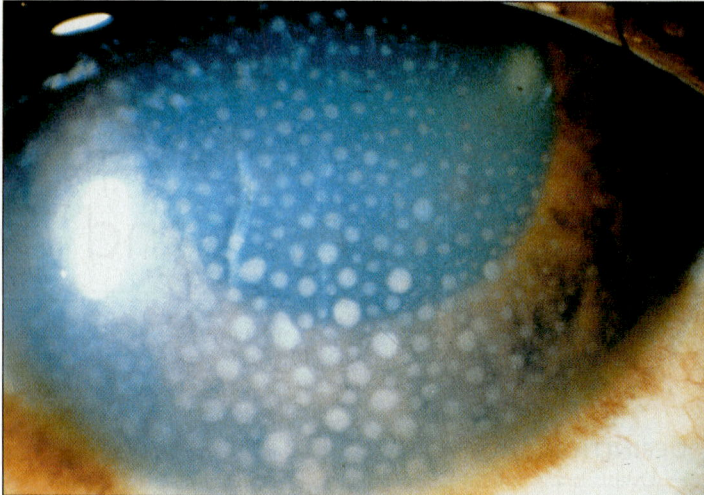

FIG. 161-1 ▌▌ Keratic precipitates in anterior uveitis. These keratic precipitates are granulomatous in appearance, as would be expected with entities such as sarcoidosis, Vogt–Koyanagi–Harada syndrome, and sympathetic ophthalmia.

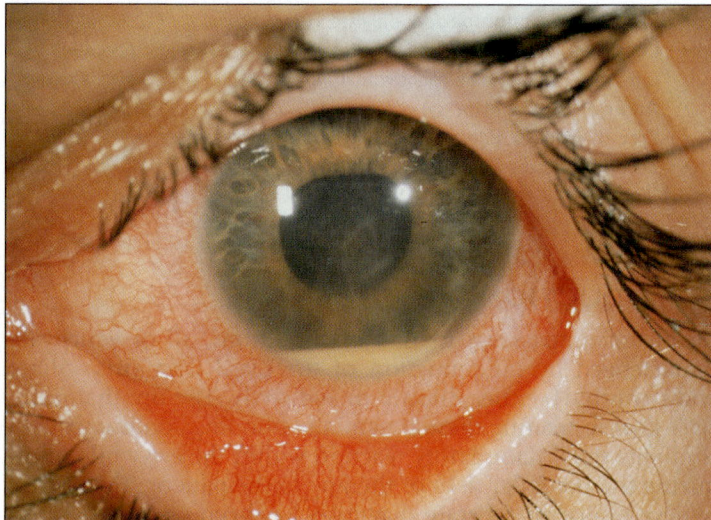

FIG. 161-2 ▌▌ HLA B27–related acute anterior uveitis. This severe case of anterior uveitis demonstrates fibrin clot formation and hypopyon in the anterior chamber.

aqueous humor result in keratic precipitates being typically concentrated on the inferior half of the cornea; a more diffuse pattern of keratic precipitates is frequently seen with Fuchs' heterochromic iridocyclitis or herpetic keratouveitis. If they are new, keratic precipitates are usually white and become more pigmented or shrunken ("crenated") as they age. The cornea may demonstrate epithelial dendrites, geographic ulcers, or stromal scarring in cases of herpetic keratouveitis. Chronic uveitis may result in the formation of band keratopathy, which is a deposition of calcium at the level of Bowman's membrane.

Mechanisms of inflammation that occur at the cellular level (e.g., release of chemotactic factors and mediators that increase vascular permeability) result in the presence of cells and flare (protein) in the aqueous humor. Both of these are graded on a scale of zero to 4+. In severe cases of anterior uveitis, fibrin clot and/or hypopyon formation may be seen (Fig. 161-2). With long-standing uveitis (e.g., that seen with JRA), eyes may have persistent flare from damage to the vasculature of the iris and ciliary body. This does not necessarily represent an active inflammatory process; the presence of cells in the anterior chamber is a more accurate marker of active inflammation.

The iris may show either anterior or posterior synechiae. If advanced, pupillary block, iris bombé, and/or angle-closure glaucoma may result. Iris nodules (Koeppe's nodules at the pupillary border; Busacca's nodules within the iris stroma) or actual granulomas may be seen in cases of granulomatous uveitis (Fig. 161-3). Sectoral iris atrophy is characteristic of herpetic disease.

Cataract is a common complication of long-standing uveitis as well as chronic corticosteroid therapy. Most such cataracts are posterior subcapsular in location, but cortical opacities may also be seen (see Fig. 161-3). Patients who present with post-traumatic or postsurgical inflammation need to be checked carefully for capsular rupture, retained lens material, or intraocular lens (IOL) malposition.

The vitreous may show cellular infiltration, "snowball opacities" (commonly seen in intermediate uveitis and sarcoidosis), fibrosis with resultant traction on the retina, or cyclitic membrane formation behind the lens. It is important to determine where cells are present in the vitreous cavity. In cases of iridocyclitis, cells in the vitreous cavity are found anteriorly, whereas with intermediate or posterior uveitis cells are distributed either throughout the vitreous or more posteriorly.

Posterior segment manifestations of uveitis may include the following:

- Disc eccema
- Macular edema
- Retinal vasculitis
- Perivascular exudates
- Focal or diffuse retinitis or choroiditis
- Pars plana exudates ("snowbanking")
- Serous, tractional, or rhegmatogenous retinal detachment
- Retinochoroidal atrophy
- Choroidal and retinal neovascularization

Intraocular pressure (IOP) can be affected by uveitis in a number of ways. Frequently, patients have low IOP with acute iridocyclitis due to the inflammation-induced decrease in aqueous production. Long-standing uveitis or cyclitic membrane–induced ciliary body detachment may result in hypotony and eventual phthisis bulbi. Conversely, IOP may be elevated by several mechanisms:

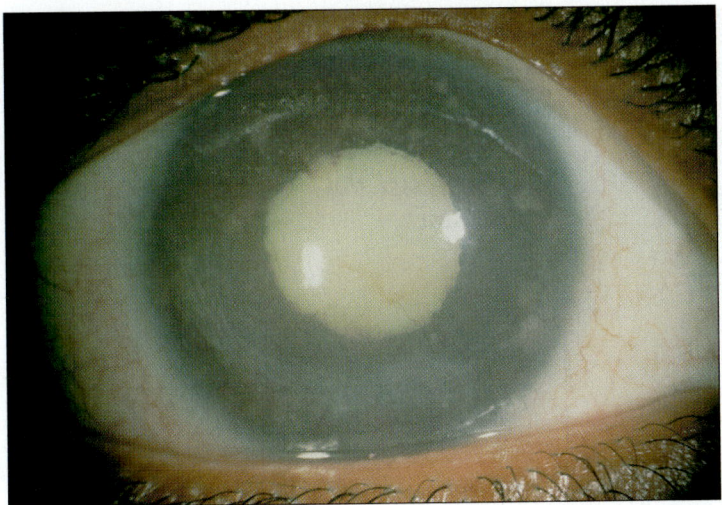

FIG. 161-3 ■ **Chronic granulomatous uveitis.** This patient demonstrates several features of chronic granulomatous uveitis, as may be seen with sarcoidosis, including iris nodules, posterior synechiae, and cataract formation.

- Plugging of trabecular meshwork with inflammatory cells,
- Swelling of meshwork fibers ("trabeculitis"),
- Peripheral anterior synechiae formation,
- Pupillary block from extensive posterior synechiae, and
- Corticosteroid-induced IOP elevation.

Gonioscopy should be performed regularly in patients who have chronic uveitis to check for peripheral anterior synechiae formation and angle closure.

DIAGNOSIS AND ANCILLARY TESTING

Once a list of potential uveitic entities has been developed, ranked from most likely to least likely, a list of laboratory investigations can be formulated that will yield the most useful information with respect to arriving at the final diagnosis. Here, most authorities advocate a "tailored" approach, whereby tests are carried out only for the most likely entities.[5]

Table 161-1 lists the most commonly used laboratory investigations in the work-up of uveitis patients as well as the diseases for which they are useful. These tests are discussed further in the respective chapters for individual uveitic entities.

Most of these uveitis tests are specialized laboratory investigations that should be ordered only when a reasonable chance exists that they will provide useful diagnostic information for a particular patient. No hard-and-fast rules govern when a laboratory work-up should be pursued in patients who have uveitis. Work-up may not be indicated in initial episodes of isolated anterior uveitis. On the other hand, patients who have granulomatous inflammation or posterior uveitis of unclear cause probably merit a work-up because there is more likelihood of finding an underlying disease. The key is to make maximal use of the history, review of systems, and physical examination to tailor the work-up for each patient.

Fluorescein angiography (to assess cystoid macular edema, serous retinal detachments, infiltration of the choroid, and vascular abnormalities) and ultrasonography (to rule out posterior segment pathology in eyes with media opacities) are useful ancillary tests in patients who have uveitis. Diagnostic vitrectomy and/or retinochoroidal biopsy can be of help in suspected cases of infectious uveitis and intraocular neoplasms. Specimens can be sent for culture, antibody testing, electron microscopy, or polymerase chain reaction (PCR) testing.

DIFFERENTIAL DIAGNOSIS

Once a complete history and physical examination have been performed, the next step in the evaluation of the uveitis patient is to develop a detailed list of differential diagnoses. This process be-

gins by first giving the particular type of inflammation present as specific a descriptor as possible, using the previously mentioned classification schemes. For instance, instead of merely naming the entity "anterior uveitis," a much more helpful and descriptive term is one such as "acute nongranulomatous anterior uveitis." The "naming-meshing" system described by Smith and Nozik[5] utilizes this approach to help formulate a list of differential diagnoses. Once the entity is appropriately named, the pattern of uveitis exhibited is matched or meshed with a list of potential types of uveitis that have similar clinical characteristics (see Table 161-1). In the preceding example, the most likely diagnoses would be an HLA-B27–related iridocyclitis, Behçet's syndrome, and herpetic uveitis, whereas diagnoses such as sarcoidosis, JRA, and Fuchs' heterochromic iridocyclitis fall much lower on the list.

TREATMENT

The ultimate goal of the practitioner with respect to the management of the patient with uveitis is to treat effectively the inflammatory process within the eyes while minimizing the complications of both the disease process and the therapeutic regimen selected. To achieve this, the natural history of the particular uveitic entity and its expected impact on visual function need to be fully understood. Certain conditions require the prompt institution of specific therapy (e.g., intravenous acyclovir for the acute retinal necrosis syndrome) or the early institution of immunosuppressive agents (e.g., for Behçet's syndrome) for optimal control of the inflammatory process. On the other hand, instances appear in which the treatment risks may outweigh the benefits (e.g., a patient who has a small peripheral focus of toxoplasmic retinochoroiditis, or patients with Fuchs' heterochromic iridocyclitis, in which chronic corticosteroid therapy may have little impact on the degree of intraocular inflammation but may hasten the formation of cataract or further elevate IOP).

The most common anti-inflammatory medications used in the treatment of uveitis are outlined in Table 161-2. Subsequent chapters detail agents used for specific types of uveitis (e.g., antimicrobial therapy for toxoplasmosis, intravenous acyclovir for acute retinal necrosis syndrome) (see Chapters 169 and 172).

Mydriatic and Cycloplegic Agents

These topical medications are used to treat the ciliary spasm that frequently occurs with acute anterior uveitis and to break recently formed posterior synechiae and/or prevent the development of new synechiae. Longer acting agents, such as homatropine, scopolamine (hyoscine), or atropine, are utilized to relieve ciliary spasm, whereas the shorter acting agents (tropicamide or cyclopentolate) may play a role in preventing new posterior synechiae formation in patients who have chronic iridocyclitis (e.g., secondary to JRA) and minimal photophobia in whom the pupil should be kept relatively mobile.

Corticosteroids

Corticosteroids represent the primary therapeutic modality in patients who have uveitis. These medications produce a broad suppression of the immune system and achieve their anti-inflammatory effect by a number of mechanisms (Table 161-2). Corticosteroids are given topically, by periocular injection, by intravitreal injection, or systemically.

Topical Route

The topical route is useful primarily in patients who have anterior uveitis, as topically applied medications penetrate the posterior segment poorly (unless the patient is pseudophakic or aphakic, in which case topical corticosteroids may have somewhat more effect posteriorly). Prednisolone acetate is generally regarded as the most effective topical corticosteroid for treating anterior uveitis; generic versions may have significantly less anti-

TABLE 161-1

DIFFERENTIAL DIAGNOSIS AND LABORATORY INVESTIGATIONS FOR UVEITIS

Type of Uveitis	Most Common Etiologies	Laboratory Tests
Anterior		
Acute	Seronegative spondyloarthropathies	HLA-B27, sacroiliac films
	Behçet's syndrome	HLA-B5, -B51
	Herpetic (HSV, VZV)	
	Glaucomatocyclitic crisis	
	Idiopathic	
Chronic	Juvenile rheumatoid arthritis	Antinuclear antibodies (ANAs)
	Sarcoidosis	Angiotensin-converting enzyme (ACE), chest x-ray/CT, gallium scan, biopsy
	Fuchs' heterochromic iridocyclitis	
	Syphilis	Rapid plasma reagin (RPR), FTA-ABS (if RPR positive)
	Tuberculosis	PPD, chest x-ray
	Herpetic	
	Idiopathic	
Intermediate	Pars planitis	
	Sarcoidosis	See above
	Lyme disease	ELISA
	Multiple sclerosis	MRI of brain
Posterior	Toxoplasmosis	ELISA
	Toxocariasis	ELISA
	Sarcoidosis	See above
	Syphilis	See above
	Tuberculosis	See above
	Viral (HSV, VZV, CMV, acute retinal necrosis [ARN])	ELISA, vitrectomy/biopsy for PCR
	Birdshot choroidopathy	HLA-A29
	Serpiginous choroidopathy	
	Ocular histoplasmosis	
	Multifocal choroiditis/panuveitis	
Panuveitis	VKH syndrome	Fluorescein angiography (FA), lumbar puncture
	Sympathetic ophthalmia	FA
	Sarcoidosis	See above
	Toxoplasmosis	See above
	Toxocariasis	See above
	Syphilis	See above
	Tuberculosis	See above
	Endophthalmitis	Vitreous culture

See subsequent chapters for detailed description of each entity.
CMV, Cytomegalovirus; *ELISA,* enzyme-linked immunosorbent assay; *FTA-ABS,* fluorescent treponemal antibody absorption; *HLA,* human leukocyte antigen; *HSV,* herpes simplex virus; *MRI,* magnetic resonance imaging; *PPD,* purified protein derivative; *VKH,* Vogt-Koyanagi-Harada; *VZV,* varicella-zoster virus.

inflammatory effect. Rimexolone and loteprednol etabonate, while probably not as potent in terms of anti-inflammatory effect, tend to elevate IOP less than prednisolone.[6]

Periocular Route

The periocular route is effective for administering corticosteroids to patients who have intermediate uveitis, posterior uveitis, or cystoid macular edema, particularly if unilateral. It may also be beneficial in patients who have severe anterior uveitis unresponsive to topical therapy. Injection is usually performed by a sub–Tenon's capsule or trans-septal approach, using only topical anesthesia. The longer acting agents (e.g., triamcinolone acetonide or methylprednisolone acetate) are preferred and are usually given every 3–4 weeks until the desired effect is achieved. Periocular injections of corticosteroids should not be used in cases of infectious uveitis (e.g., acute retinal necrosis syndrome, toxoplasmosis) and should be used with caution in patients who have a history of corticosteroid-induced IOP elevation.

Systemic Route

The systemic route is used in cases of severe posterior uveitis or panuveitis, especially if bilateral, or in cases of severe anterior uveitis poorly responsive to topical and/or periocular corticosteroids. It is better to start at a higher dose (e.g., 1–2mg/kg/day or 60–120mg/day) and taper it as quickly as possible than to start at a low dose and have to increase it repeatedly because of poor response. These agents should be tapered gradually if the patient has been taking them for longer than 2–3 weeks.

Nonsteroidal Anti-Inflammatory Drugs

Nonsteroidal anti-inflammatory drugs (NSAIDs) do not play a primary role in the treatment of most types of uveitis. However, at times the adjunctive use of oral NSAIDs may allow maintenance of the patient on a lower dose of corticosteroids than would be the case otherwise (e.g., in chronic iridocyclitis secondary to JRA). Oral NSAIDs do have a role, however, in the treatment of certain types of scleritis.

TABLE 161-2

ANTI-INFLAMMATORY THERAPY IN THE TREATMENT OF UVEITIS

Medication	Mechanism of Action	Complications
Corticosteroids	Inhibition of cyclo-oxygenase and lipoxygenase pathways	Topical—elevated IOP, cataract exacerbation of infection, corneal or scleral thinning/perforation
	Decreases complement levels	Periocular—same as topical, as well as ptosis, scarring of Tenon's capsule, scleral perforation, hemorrhage, abscess
	Decreased migration of lymphocytes	Systemic—same as topical, as well as weight gain, fluid retention, electrolyte disturbances, peptic ulcer disease, osteoporosis, aseptic necrosis of hip, hypertension, impaired glucose tolerance, mental status changes, impaired wound healing, menstrual irregularities, others
	Decreased production of vasoactive amines and interleukins	
	Decreased circulating monocytes	
	Decreased macrophage activity	
Immunosuppressive medications	Interfere with DNA synthesis and cellular replication	All: bone marrow suppression, teratogenicity, increased risk of infection
Antimetabolites		
Methotrexate	Folate analog; inhibits dihydrofolate reductase	Hepatotoxicity, GI upset, pneumonitis, stomatitis
Azathioprine	Alters purine metabolism	GI upset, hepatitis
Mycophenolate mofetil	Inhibits purine synthesis	Diarrhea, nausea
Alkylating agents		
Cyclophosphamide	Lymphotoxicity, cross-links DNA	Hemorrhagic cystitis, sterility, increased risk of malignancy
Chlorambucil	Lymphotoxicity, cross-links DNA	Sterility, increased risk of malignancy
T-cell inhibitors		
Cyclosporine	Inhibits T cells	Renal toxicity, hypertension, hirsutism, tremor
Tacrolimus	Inhibits T cells	Renal toxicity, hypertension, neurotoxicity, hepatitis, diabetes

As can be seen, the potential complications of such therapy are numerous and must be discussed fully with the patient prior to instituting therapy with these agents.
GI, Gastrointestinal; IOP, intraocular pressure.

Immunosuppressive Therapy

Immunosuppressive medications have generally been reserved for severe, sight-threatening uveitis that has not responded adequately to corticosteroids or for patients who experience severe side effects from corticosteroid therapy.[7] However, evidence suggests that these agents can play an important part in the treatment regimen for uveitis, with potentially less morbidity than long-term corticosteroid use. Although several entities exist for which the early use of immunosuppressive agents is indicated (Behçet's syndrome, Vogt-Koyanagi-Harada (VKH) syndrome, sympathetic ophthalmia, and necrotizing sclerouveitis), they should also be considered in patients who require chronic (e.g., longer than 6 months) corticosteroid therapy at doses greater than 10mg/day.[7]

Several classes of immunosuppressive medications exist. The commonly used agents, their mode of action, and their potential side effects are summarized in Table 161-2. Antimetabolites include methotrexate, azathioprine, and mycophenolate. Methotrexate in particular has been used to treat many types of chronic noninfectious uveitis, including JRA-associated iridocyclitis, sarcoidosis, panuveitis, and scleritis.[7–11] It is given as a weekly dose of 7.5–25mg, either orally, subcutaneously, or intramuscularly, and is generally well tolerated. Azathioprine, which is usually given at a dose of 1–3mg/kg/day, has been shown to be beneficial in patients who have sympathetic ophthalmia, VKH syndrome, intermediate uveitis, and Behçet's syndrome.[7,12] Mycophenolate is usually used at a dose of 1g twice daily and may be an alternative for patients who are intolerant of methotrexate or azathioprine.[7]

Alkylating agents include cyclophosphamide and chlorambucil and have been used in the treatment of Behçet's syndrome, sympathetic ophthalmia, and intermediate uveitis.[13,14] Cyclophosphamide is usually given at a dose of 1–3mg/kg/day and chlorambucil at 0.1–0.2mg/kg/day.

Cyclosporine and tacrolimus are examples of T-cell inhibitors. The primary effect of these medications is inhibition of T-cell activation and recruitment, although the exact mechanism by which this occurs is debated.[15] Cyclosporine has been shown to be effective in various types of posterior uveitis as well as intermediate uveitis.[7,16] It is usually begun at a dose of 2–5mg/kg/day, usually in combination with corticosteroids. The primary side effects are renal toxicity and hypertension, which occur in up to 75% and 25% of patients, respectively.[14] Unlike cytotoxic agents, which can actually kill the cells responsible for inflammatory disease, cyclosporine is cytostatic and merely suppresses the inflammatory cells. Thus, inflammation may recur when the medication is tapered. However, the treatment may be effective long enough to allow the inflammatory activity to subside by the time the medication is withdrawn.

Immunosuppressive medications may have serious and potentially life-threatening side effects (see Table 161-2). Most worrisome are renal or hepatic toxicity, bone marrow suppression, and, particularly with the alkylating agents, the potential for future malignancies (e.g., leukemia or lymphoma).[7] These agents are teratogenic, and therefore patients should take precautions against becoming pregnant while taking them. Patients must be informed of such risks. Regular blood monitoring (complete blood count, hepatic function tests) needs to be performed, and most such patients should be observed closely by an internist or other physician familiar with the potential side effects of these medications.

Newer Therapies

Cytokine inhibitors such as etanercept and infliximab are being studied for treatment of various types of uveitis. In one study, a single intravenous infusion of infliximab resulted in a rapid decrease in intraocular inflammation in patients who have Behçet's syndrome.[17] Intravenous immune globulin and interferon alfa-2b were shown in small studies to have beneficial effects in some patients with uveitis.[18,19] Also, a multicenter trial is ongoing using a sustained-release intravitreal implant that delivers the corticosteroid fluocinolone acetonide directly into the eye. This therapy has the potential advantage of sustained, consistent intraocular therapy without systemic side effects.

COURSE AND OUTCOME

Uveitis is a potentially blinding condition that can result in serious complications in the eyes. Cataracts are one of the most common causes of visual loss in patients who have uveitis.[20] Cataract extraction should ideally be performed only after uveitis has been quiescent for 3–4 months. Phacoemulsification or nuclear expression (NE) extracapsular cataract extraction (ECCE) may be performed, although phacoemulsification is probably associated with fewer complications than NE.[21] Cases associated with vitritis (e.g., intermediate uveitis) often benefit from combined cataract extraction and pars plana vitrectomy.[22,23] With the exception of patients who have JRA-associated uveitis, most patients tolerate a posterior chamber IOL well, provided their inflammation is aggressively treated during the perioperative period.[21,24] However, patients who have inflammation centered around the pars plana region tend to have a higher complication rate than those with other types of uveitis.[25] Acrylic or all-polymethylmethacrylate lenses seem to incite less inflammatory response than lenses containing silicone or polypropylene.[26]

Glaucoma is also a common complication of chronic uveitis. The various mechanisms for the development of glaucoma in uveitic eyes were discussed earlier. Medical therapy is used initially, although miotics should be avoided as they may exacerbate ciliary spasm and predispose to posterior synechiae formation. Also, prostaglandin analogs have been associated with anterior uveitis and cystoid macular edema.[27] In cases of pupillary block, iridectomy should be performed. Laser iridectomies frequently close off with continued inflammation; in such cases surgical iridectomy should be performed. If filtering surgery is necessary, the use of antimetabolites (e.g., mitomycin) or aqueous drainage devices greatly increases the success rate in these patients.[28]

Patients who have uveitis may also have cystoid macular edema, which, if long-standing, can result in irreversible visual loss. Periocular or systemic corticosteroids are usually successful, but, if not, immunosuppressive agents may be helpful. Therapeutic vitrectomy may also be beneficial in some cases as it debulks the vitreous cavity of inflammatory cells and mediators, which may be responsible for chronic vascular leakage.[29]

Retinal detachment can be either serous (e.g., with VKH syndrome), rhegmatogenous (e.g., acute retinal necrosis syndrome), or tractional. Serous detachments usually respond to corticosteroids (either periocular or systemic); rhegmatogenous or tractional detachments may require the use of silicone oil tamponade (especially in cases such as acute retinal necrosis syndrome).

Chronic uveitis may lead to aqueous hyposecretion with decreased nutrient supply to anterior segment structures or cyclitic membrane formation with ciliary body detachment and subsequent hypotony. Cyclitic membranes may be removed through a pars plana approach; such surgery may allow reattachment of the ciliary body and return of normal aqueous production. Chronic hypotony may result in phthisis bulbi.

REFERENCES

1. Bloch-Michel E, Nussenblatt RB. International uveitis study group recommendations for the evaluation of intraocular inflammatory disease. Am J Ophthalmol. 1987;103:234–5.
2. Henderly DE, Genstler AJ, Smith RE, Rao NA. Changing patterns of uveitis. Am J Ophthalmol. 1987;103:131–6.
3. Rodriguez A, Calonge M, Pedroza-Seres M, et al. Referral patterns of uveitis in a tertiary eye care center. Arch Ophthalmol. 1996;114:593–9.
4. McCannel CA, Holland GN, Helm CJ, et al. Causes of uveitis in the general practice of ophthalmology. UCLA Community-Based Uveitis Study Group. Am J Ophthalmol. 1996;121:35–46.
5. Smith RE, Nozik RA. Uveitis: a clinical approach to diagnosis and management, 2nd ed. Baltimore: Williams & Wilkins; 1989:23–6.
6. The Loteprednol Etabonate US Uveitis Study Group. Controlled evaluation of loteprednol etabonate and prednisolone acetate in the treatment of acute anterior uveitis. Am J Ophthalmol. 1999;127:537–44.
7. Jabs DA, Rosenbaum JT, Foster CS, et al. Guidelines for the use of immunosuppressive drugs in patients with ocular inflammatory disorders: recommendations of an expert panel. Am J Ophthalmol. 2000;130:492–513.
8. Holz FG, Krastel H, Breitbart A, et al. Low-dose methotrexate treatment in noninfectious uveitis resistant to corticosteroids. Geriatr J Ophthalmol. 1992;1:142–4.
9. Shah SS, Lowder CY, Schmitt MA, et al. Low-dose methotrexate therapy for ocular inflammatory disease. Ophthalmology. 1992;99:1419–23.
10. Samson CM, Waheed N, Baltatzis S, Foster CS. Methotrexate therapy for chronic noninfectious uveitis. Ophthalmology. 2001;108:1134–9.
11. Dev S, McCallum RM, Jaffe GJ. Methotrexate treatment for sarcoid-associated panuveitis. Ophthalmology. 1999;106:111–8.
12. Yazici H, Pazarli H, Barnes CG, et al. A controlled trial of azathioprine in Behçet's syndrome. N Engl J Med. 1990;322:281–5.
13. Tessler HH, Jennings T. High-dose short-term chlorambucil for intractable sympathetic ophthalmia and Behçet's disease. Br J Ophthalmol. 1990;74:353–7.
14. Nussenblatt RB, Whitcup SM, Palestine AG. Uveitis, fundamentals and clinical practice, 2nd ed. St Louis: Mosby–Year Book; 1996:97–134.
15. Schreiber SL, Crabtree GR. The mechanism of action of cyclosporin A and FK506. Immunol Today. 1992;13:136–42.
16. Whitcup SM, Salvo EC Jr, Nussenblatt RB, et al. Combined cyclosporine and corticosteroid therapy for sight-threatening uveitis in Behçet's disease. Am J Ophthalmol. 1994;118:39–45.
17. Sfikakis PP, Theodossiadis PG, Katsiari CG, et al. Effect of infliximab on sight-threatening panuveitis in Behçet's disease. Lancet. 2001;358:295–6.
18. Rosenbaum JT, George R, Gordon C. The treatment of refractory uveitis with intravenous immunoglobulin. Am J Ophthalmol. 1999;127:545–9.
19. Demiroglu H, Ozcebe OI, Barista I, et al. Interferon alfa-2b, colchicines, and benzathine penicillin versus colchicines and benzathine penicillin in Behçet's disease: a randomized trial. Lancet. 2000;355:605–9.
20. Smith RE. Pars planitis. In: Ryan SJ, ed. Retina, 2nd ed, Vol 2. St Louis: CV Mosby; 1994:1621–31.
21. Estafanous MFG, Lowder CY, Meisler DM, Chauhan R. Phacoemulsification cataract extraction and posterior chamber lens implantation in patients with uveitis. Am J Ophthalmol. 2001;131:620–5.
22. Walker J, Rao NA, Ober RR, et al. A combined anterior and posterior approach to cataract surgery in patients with chronic uveitis. Int Ophthalmol. 1993;17:63–9.
23. Foster RE, Lowder CY, Meisler DM, et al. Combined extracapsular cataract extraction, posterior chamber intraocular lens implantation, and pars plana vitrectomy. Ophthalmic Surg. 1993;24:446–52.
24. Krishna R, Meisler DM, Lowder CY, et al. Long-term follow-up of extracapsular cataract extraction and posterior chamber lens implantation in patients with uveitis. Ophthalmology. 1998;105:1765–9.
25. Foster CS, Stavrou P, Zafirakis P, et al. Intraocular lens removal from patients with uveitis. Am J Ophthalmol. 1999;128:31–7.
26. Hooper PL, Rao NA, Smith RE. Cataract extraction in uveitis patients. Surv Ophthalmol. 1990;35:120–44.
27. Warwar RE, Bullock JD, Ballal D. Cystoid macular edema and anterior uveitis associated with latanoprost use. Ophthalmology. 1998;105:263–8.
28. Forster DJ, Rao NA, Hill RA, et al. Incidence and management of glaucoma in Vogt-Koyanagi-Harada syndrome. Ophthalmology. 1993;100:613–18.
29. Heiligenhaus A, Bornfeld N, Foerster MH, Wessing A. Long-term results of pars plana vitrectomy in the management of complicated uveitis. Br J Ophthalmol. 1994;78:549–54.

CHAPTER 162

Herpes and Other Viral Infections

P. KUMAR RAO

Varicella-Zoster and Herpes Simplex Virus–Induced Acute Retinal Necrosis

DEFINITION
- A necrotizing retinitis caused by infection with VZV or HSV in an immunocompetent host.

KEY FEATURES
- Severe uveitis or vitritis.
- Retinal vasculitis.
- Retinal necrosis.

ASSOCIATED FEATURES
- Keratic precipitates.
- Papillitis.
- Retinal detachment.

Progressive Outer Retinal Necrosis

DEFINITION
- A necrotizing retinitis caused by infection with VZV of HSV in an immunocompromised host.

KEY FEATURES
- Multifocal lesions.
- Outer retinal involvement.
- Minimal or no vasculitis and vitritis.

ASSOCIATED FEATURES
- Rapid progression.
- Poor prognosis.
- Other viruses
  - Epstein-Barr virus
  - Human T-cell lymphotropic virus type I
  - Influenza A virus
  - Measles virus
  - Rubella virus

VARICELLA-ZOSTER AND HERPES SIMPLEX VIRUS

INTRODUCTION

Both varicella-zoster (VZV) and herpes simplex viruses (HSV) can cause devastating intraocular inflammation.

EPIDEMIOLOGY/PATHOGENESIS

In general, transmission is thought to occur through exposure to a person with an actively shedding viral lesion. Most cases of retinal disease are believed to be reactions of previously acquired infection. Along with VZV, two types of HSV (HSV1 and HSV2) can

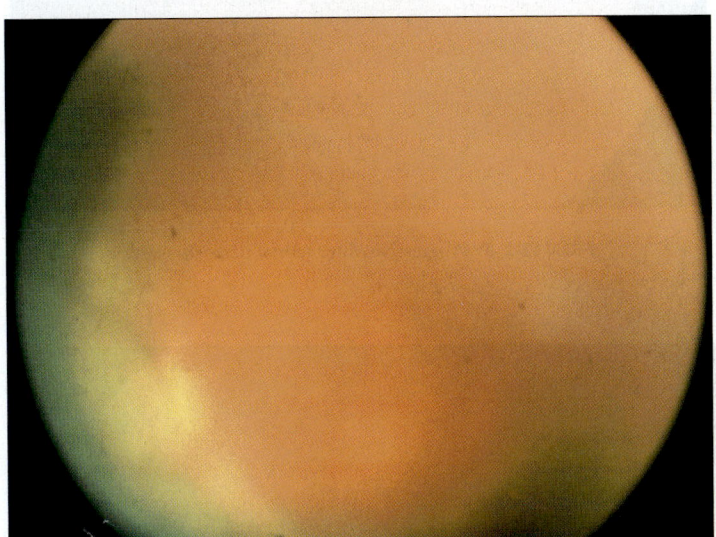

FIG. 162-1 ■ Progressive outer retinal necrosis—early.

cause acute retinal necrosis (ARN).[1] This retinal necrosis is seen in otherwise healthy individuals of both sexes and any age but may occur in immunocompromised persons. Necrotizing herpetic retinopathies represent a spectrum of disease, which may range from ARN to progressive outer retinal necrosis (PORN).

OCULAR MANIFESTATIONS

Both VZV and HSV can affect a variety of ocular tissues and result in manifestations such as blepharitis, conjunctivitis, scleritis, keratitis, anterior uveitis, glaucoma, vitritis, and retinitis. Maternal transmission to a developing fetus can cause serious systemic and ocular disease. Congenital VZV or HSV retinitis may appear as a pigmentary retinopathy in babies born to mothers known to have varicella-zoster or congenital herpes simplex infection during pregnancy.

The most common clinical manifestation of VZV or HSV retinitis has been called the acute retinal necrosis syndrome. Typically, it presents with a severe uveitis, retinal vasculitis, and retinal necrosis in presumably immunocompetent patients. In the early phase, there may be keratic precipitates and vitritis (Fig. 162-1). The retinitis typically begins in the periphery and results in rapid confluence over a week to 10 days and can be associated with an occlusive vasculitis and papillitis. Retinal detachment typically occurs several weeks later. The retinitis may develop in the contralateral eye in over one third of patients. Usually VZV or HSV1 causes ARN in patients older than 25 years, whereas HSV2 causes ARN in younger patients. This viral infection can also present as a variant of retinal vasculitis with a frosted branch angiitis-like picture.[2]

In the immunocompromised patient, the clinical appearance of zoster or simplex retinitis may be similar to that of ARN or may follow a pattern called progressive outer retinal necrosis. PORN differs from ARN in that it may begin in the posterior pole or the periphery and is commonly multifocal (Fig. 162-2). It may not be associated with vasculitis, and vitritis may be min-

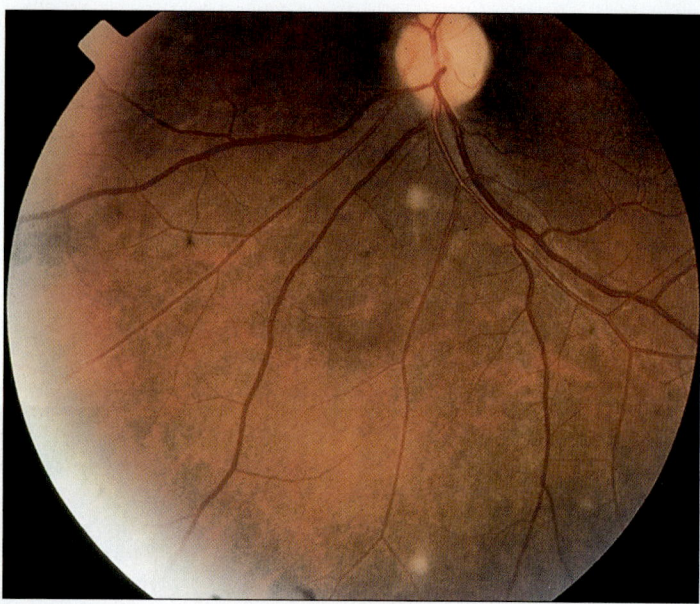

FIG. 162-2 ▌ Progressive outer retinal necrosis—late.

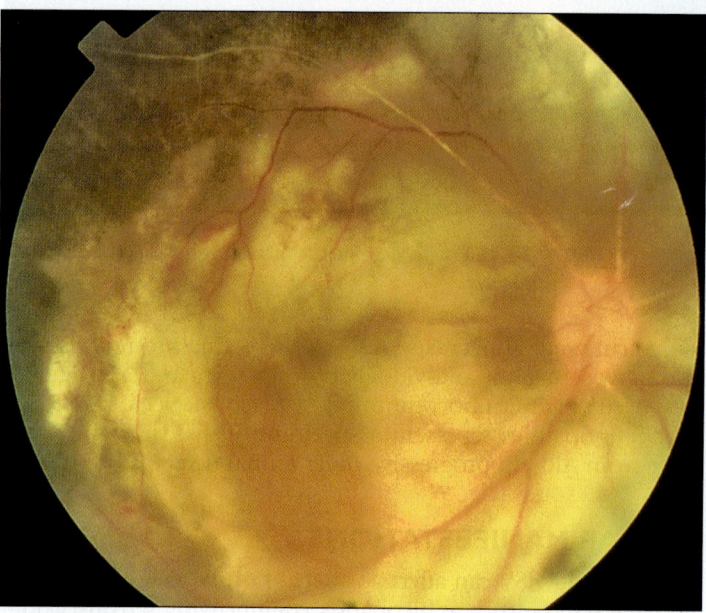

FIG. 162-3 ▌ Acute retinal necrosis.

imal (Fig. 162-3). In general, the rate of progression is rapid. Treatment of PORN is difficult and visual prognosis is poor.

DIAGNOSIS

The diagnosis of ARN is based mainly on its clinical features. Diagnostic dilemmas occur in unusual cases. In these cases, confirmation of the diagnosis is possible through viral culture, detection of antiviral antibodies, and, more recently, polymerase chain reaction (PCR) analysis for viral DNA from ocular samples.[3]

DIFFERENTIAL DIAGNOSIS

The differential diagnosis of ARN includes cytomegalovirus (CMV) retinitis, aspergillosis of the eye, and lymphoma. However, patients with ARN tend to demonstrate more vitritis than those with CMV infection, and the eye tends to be more red or painful than in patients with lymphoma. Aspergillosis is mainly seen in patients with granulocytopenia.

PATHOLOGY

Histopathologically, ARN demonstrates full-thickness retinal necrosis with arteritis. The areas of necrotic retina are demarcated sharply from areas of normal retina. The necrotic retina may contain intranuclear inclusions. Electron microscopic studies may demonstrate viral particles.

TREATMENT

Intravenous acyclovir is given at 1500mg/m² every 8 hours for about 7 days. Because fellow eye involvement may occur within the following few weeks, intravenous acyclovir is usually followed by 4 to 6 weeks of oral acyclovir at 2–4g/day. Occlusive vasculopathy and optic neuropathy have been treated with aspirin and corticosteroids. As retinal detachment may be the most devastating cause of vision loss in these patients, prophylactic laser demarcation has been administered posterior to the advancing border of retinitis. Repair of ARN-associated retinal detachments may be achieved by using vitrectomy, endolaser, and silicone oil techniques. Treatments for PORN include the use of intravenous Acyclovir, and some patients have been treated with intravenous and intravitreal administration of foscarnet and ganciclovir.

COURSE AND OUTCOME

Visual recovery depends upon the extent of retinal involvement. In addition, the presence of vascular occlusion and optic neuropathy may limit the overall visual outcome. Immunosuppressed patients have the worst visual outcomes.

EPSTEIN-BARR VIRUS

INTRODUCTION

The Epstein-Barr virus (EBV) is double-stranded DNA virus. It is transmitted through exchange of saliva or blood transfusions. By adulthood, most people have acquired an infection with the virus. EBV is the causative agent of infectious mononucleosis, and it is also associated with Burkitt's lymphoma and other B-cell malignancies seen in immunosuppressed patients. Various ocular manifestations related to EBV occur primarily in association with infectious mononucleosis.

OCULAR MANIFESTATIONS

The ocular manifestations of EBV infection are varied. Ocular motor nerve palsy, abducens nerve palsy, and optic neuritis have been attributed to EBV infections. Anterior segment manifestations have included conjunctivitis, iritis, mucosa-associated lymphoid tissue (MALT)–related lymphomas, conjunctival Burkitt's lymphoma, iritis, and Parinaud's oculoglandular syndrome. Posterior segment involvement may include multifocal choroiditis characterized by punched-out areas of pigment epithelial changes and vitritis (Table 162-1).[4]

DIFFERENTIAL DIAGNOSIS

The diagnostic entities that may mimic EBV chorioretinitis include presumed ocular histoplasmosis syndrome (POHS), recurrent multifocal choroiditis, multiple evanescent white dot syndrome (MEWDS), acute retinal pigment epitheliitis, and birdshot choroidopathy.

DIAGNOSIS AND ANCILLARY TESTING

Immunoglobulin M (IgM) and IgG antibodies in the serum can be detected and followed. In addition, EBV-related antigen can be quantified in the serum. PCR techniques to detect viral DNA

TABLE 162-1

POSTERIOR SEGMENT FINDINGS IN EBV, HTLV-1, INFLUENZA A, MEASLES, AND RUBELLA VIRAL INFECTIONS

	Vascular Changes	Retinal Changes	Retinal Pigment Epithelium Changes	Optic Nerve Changes
EBV			Punched-out areas	
HTLV-1	Gray-white granular deposits		Retinitis pigmentosa–like	Optic neuritis
Influenza A	Shiny dots at termination of capillaries Sclerotic vasculature	Macular edema Darkened macular area Small retinal hemorrhages		Optic neuritis
Measles	Attenuated vessels	Retinal edema Stellate macular lesions	Depigmented areas Salt-and-pepper changes	Optic neuritis
SSPE		Macular edema White retinal infiltrates Serous detachments	Depigmented areas	Optic neuritis
Rubella		Serous detachments	Salt-and-pepper changes	

in ocular fluids have been successful. In situ hybridization techniques applied to biopsy specimens from the eye have also demonstrated the presence of EBV.

TREATMENT

In general, EBV-related chorioretinitis appears to be fairly self-limiting, but for severe cases acyclovir therapy may be of some value. In general, because the EBV-related disease appears to be fairly self-limited, little documentation exists regarding its most effective therapy.

HUMAN T-CELL LYMPHOTROPIC VIRUS TYPE I

INTRODUCTION

Perinatal infection with human T-cell lymphotropic virus type 1 (HTLV-1) is considered a risk factor for adult T-cell leukemia and of a degenerative neurological disorder known as tropical spastic paraparesis. This viral infection can cause intermediate uveitis.

EPIDEMIOLOGY/PATHOGENESIS

In certain populations, infection with HTLV-1 is considered endemic, such as in areas of southwest Japan. In one study, 0.79% of people tested were seropositive for the HTLV antigens.[5] The Tax protein of HTLV-1 is oncogenic and binds to transcription factors. The interaction of HTLV-1–disregulated cells with various kinds of normal lymphocytes and vascular endothelial cells may determine the type of HTLV-1–associated disease manifestation.[6]

OCULAR MANIFESTATIONS

Ocular manifestations include vitritis and uveitis/vasculitis.[7] A vasculitis composed of gray-white granular deposits scattered on the retinal veins and arteries may be characteristic of HTLV-1–associated retinal disease. Other manifestations include T-cell conjunctival and intraocular lymphomas, interstitial keratitis, Sjögren's syndrome, optic neuritis, and retinal choroidal degeneration similar to retinitis pigmentosa.

DIAGNOSIS AND ANCILLARY TESTING

Tests for viral DNA, including PCR techniques, have proved the presence of the HTLV-1 virus. Serum antibodies against the HTLV-1 proteins have also been used to make the diagnosis of systemic HTLV-1 infection.

DIFFERENTIAL DIAGNOSIS

The differential diagnosis of HTLV-1–associated uveitis includes those uveitic conditions caused by multiple sclerosis, syphilis, sarcoidosis, and Behçet's disease.

TREATMENT

The intraocular inflammation may respond to corticosteroid therapy.[8]

COURSE AND OUTCOME

A single episode of uveitis with resolution over a few weeks occurs in the majority of patients. Only a few patients suffer poor visual outcomes from either steroid-induced cataracts or a retinal choroidal degeneration.

INFLUENZA A VIRUS

INTRODUCTION

The influenza A virus is a single-stranded RNA virus that commonly causes acute respiratory illnesses. The ability of the virus to undergo reassortment of genomic segments between virus strains allows antigenic shifts in the lipid envelope of the virus. This allows new outbreaks every year.

EPIDEMIOLOGY/PATHOGENESIS

The infection is acquired from secretions of the respiratory tract from acutely infected individuals. The virus first infects the respiratory epithelium and respiratory illness ensues, accompanied by headache, fever, chills, malaise, myalgia, cough, and sore throat. The acute illness usually resolves over the following 2 to 3 days, and most patients largely recover in 1 week's time.

OCULAR MANIFESTATIONS

Ocular complications of influenza infection include iridocyclitis, interstitial keratitis, and dacryoadenitis. Posterior segment manifestations include macular edema, macular lesions consisting of shiny dots at the termination of a capillary, absent foveal reflexes, darkening of the macular area, optic neuritis, and small retinal hemorrhages[9] (see Table 162-1). These changes appear reversible.

DIAGNOSIS AND ANCILLARY TESTING

Serological methods to confirm the diagnosis exist but require comparison of antibody titers obtained during the acute illness with those obtained several weeks after the onset of the illness. Virus can be isolated from throat swabs or nasopharyngeal washes and grown in tissue culture. Viral antigens may be detected by the use of indirect immunofluorescent techniques on exfoliated nasopharyngeal cells.

DIFFERENTIAL DIAGNOSIS

Influenza A retinopathy may appear similar to Vogt-Koyanagi-Harada (VKH) syndrome or other viral infections.

TREATMENT

Inactivated influenza vaccination is recommended for patients with chronic cardiovascular or pulmonary disorders, nursing home patients, medical personnel in contact with high-risk patients, or people with chronic metabolic disease as well as immunocompromised individuals. There have been case reports of optic neuropathy and corneal graft rejection after influenza vaccination.[10,11] These complications were treated successfully with steroids.

COURSE AND OUTCOME

Fortunately, influenza viral infection usually resolves without any sequelae. The posterior segment manifestations of influenza A infection appear to be reversible and leave minimal visual effects.

MEASLES VIRUS

INTRODUCTION

The measles virus is another RNA virus classified as a paramyxovirus. Infection with the virus is usually self-limited but can be associated with subacute sclerosing panencephalitis (SSPE).

EPIDEMIOLOGY/PATHOGENESIS

The virus is transferred by nasopharyngeal secretions to the respiratory tract or conjunctiva of susceptible patients. The virus is highly contagious and is typically contracted in childhood. Congenital infections can occur. Prenatal transmission in the first trimester may cause abortion; infection later may result in premature birth or malformations such as cardiomyopathy, cataract, deafness, and pigmentary retinopathy.

OCULAR MANIFESTATIONS

The ocular manifestations of congenital infection include cataract and pigmentary retinopathy.[12] The most common ocular manifestations of acquired infection are a self-limited keratitis or conjunctivitis. Retinopathy can occur with acquired measles infections. During the acute stages of retinal involvement, the fundus vessels may appear attenuated. There may be diffuse retinal edema associated with optic disc swelling, small hemorrhages, and stellate macular lesions. Irregular, flat, depigmented areas may also appear with some decline in vision. As the retinopathy resolves, a secondary pigment retinopathy with a salt-and-pepper appearance may occur (see Table 162-1). Retinal findings associated with SSPE include macular edema, pigment epithelial abnormalities, choroiditis, whitish retinal infiltrates, serous macular detachments, areas of retinal depigmentation, and optic neuritis.[13–15]

DIAGNOSIS AND ANCILLARY TESTING

Fluorescein angiography may demonstrate a diffuse leakage associated with retinal edema or increased transmission of choroidal fluorescence related to the pigment epithelial disease. There may be vascular occlusions, retinal pigment epithelial disturbances,

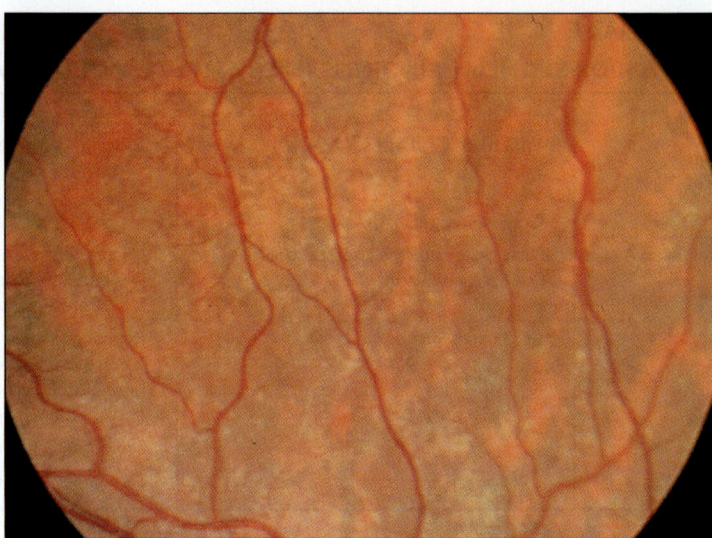

FIG. 162-4 ■ **Rubella retinopathy.** Classic salt-and-pepper appearance of the fundus is seen in this case of congenital rubella retinopathy. (Courtesy of George S. Novalis, MD.)

and cystic areas of hyperfluorescence. Serological tests for measles virus include compliment fixation, enzyme immunoassay, immunofluorescence, and the hemagglutination inhibition test.[15] In addition, PCR techniques may be used for detecting viral RNA.[16]

DIFFERENTIAL DIAGNOSIS

The differential diagnosis of measles retinopathy includes central serous chorioretinopathy, VKH disease, influenza A retinitis, toxoplasmic retinal choroiditis, and retinitis pigmentosa.

PATHOLOGY

Histological specimens from uncomplicated measles cases are rare, but specimens have been documented in patients who have suffered from SSPE. Histologically, there may be areas of focal retinal necrosis with invasion of pigment-laden macrophages. The retinal pigment epithelium may show patchy areas of loss, but the choroid may appear normal. Intranuclear inclusions can be seen in the nuclear layers of the retina.[15]

TREATMENT

No treatment is necessary for uncomplicated measles infections. Measles retinopathy may result in the onset of acute blindness a few weeks following the measles rash and in general resolving over the following months. No therapy for measles-related retinopathy exists.

RUBELLA VIRUS

The ophthalmic manifestations of rubella virus are similar to those of measles virus infections, and both can be seen in congenital and acquired forms. The congenital rubella retinitis may present as a salt-and-pepper fundus appearance (Fig. 162-4). Acquired rubella begins with a classical rash and malaise. Ophthalmic manifestations include conjunctivitis, keratitis, and iritis. A retinitis may appear and can be associated with exudative detachments of the retina and retinal pigment epithelium.[17,18]

SUMMARY

Multiple viruses can cause intraocular inflammation. Many of them can cause decreased vision and can have devastating long-term effects. Ocular manifestations of other viral infections are being discovered. New diagnostic techniques such as PCR may allow testing for the presence of a viral cause for some of the idiopathic intraocular inflammations.

REFERENCES

1. Ganatra JB, Chandler D, Santos C, et al. Viral causes of acute retinal necrosis syndrome. Am J Ophthalmol. 2000;129:166–72.
2. Markomichelakis NN, Barampouti F, Zafirakis P, et al. Retinal vasculitis with frosted branch angiitis-like response due to herpes simplex virus type 2. Retina. 1999;19:455–7.
3. Madhavan HN, Priya K, Anand AR, Therese KL. Detection of herpes simplex virus (HSV) genome using polymerase chain reaction (PCR) in clinical samples comparison of PCR with standard laboratory methods for the detection of HSV. J Clin Virol. 1999;14:145–51.
4. Demols PF, Cochaux PM, Velu T, Caspers-Velu L. Chorioretinal post-transplant lymphoproliferative disorder induced by the Epstein-Barr virus. Br J Ophthalmol. 2001;85:93–5.
5. Goto K, Sato K, Kurita M, et al. The seroprevalence of HTLV-1 in patients with ocular diseases, pregnant woman and healthy volunteers in the Kanto district, central Japan. Scand J Infect Dis. 1997;29:219–21.
6. Uchiyama T. Human T cell leukemia virus type I (HTLV-I) and human diseases. Annu Rev Immunol. 1997;15:15–37.
7. Mochizuki M, Ono A, Ikeda E, et al. HTLV-I uveitis. J Acquir Immune Defic Syndr. 1996;13(Suppl):s50–6.
8. Ishioka M, Goto K, Nakamuara S, et al. Prevalence of HTLV-1-associated uveitis in the Kanto Plain, Japan. Graefes Arch Clin Exp Ophthalmol. 1995;233:476–8.
9. Mathur SP. Macular lesion after influenza. Br J Ophthalmol. 1958;40:702.
10. Ray CL, Dreizin IJ. Bilateral optic neuropathy associated with influenza vaccination. J Neuroophthalmol. 1996;16:182–4.
11. Solomon A, Frucht-Pery J. Bilateral simultaneous corneal graft rejection after influenza vaccination. Am J Ophthalmol. 1996;121:708–9.
12. Foxman SG, Heckenlively JR, Sinclair SH. Rubeola retinopathy and pigmented paravenous retinochoroidal atrophy. Am J Ophthalmol. 1985;99:605–6.
13. De Laey JJ, Hanssens M, Colette P. Subacute sclerosing panencephalitis: fundus changes and histopathologic correlations. Doc Ophthalmol. 1983;56:11–21.
14. Totan Y, Cekic O. Bilateral retrobulbar neuritis following measles in an adult. Eye. 1999;13:383–4.
15. Park DW, Boldt HC, Massicotte SJ, et al. Subacute sclerosing panencephalitis manifesting as a viral retinitis: clinical and histopathologic findings. Am J Ophthalmol. 1997;123:533–42.
16. Tomoda A, Miike T, Miyagawa S, et al. Subacute sclerosing panencephalitis and chorioretinitis. Brain Dev. 1997;19:55–7.
17. Gerstle C, Zinn KM. Rubella-associated retinitis in an adult: report of a case. Mt Sinai J Med. 1976;43:303–8.
18. Hayashi M, Yoshimura N, Kondo T. Acute rubella retinal pigment epitheliitis in an adult. Am J Ophthalmol. 1982;93:285–8.

163 Cytomegalovirus Retinitis (CMVR) in AIDS

EHUD ZAMIR

DEFINITION
- Full-thickness, necrotizing retinitis caused by cytomegalovirus (CMV) in acquired immunodeficiency syndrome (AIDS).

KEY FEATURES
- Slowly progressive, perivascular retinal whitening, hemorrhages, and necrosis.
- "Brushfire" pattern of advancing edge.
- Mild vitreous inflammatory response.
- Profound immune suppression.

ASSOCIATED FEATURES
- Secondary rhegmatogenous retinal detachment.
- Immune recovery uveitis after treatment with highly active antiretroviral therapy (HAART).

INTRODUCTION

Cytomegalovirus retinitis (CMVR) has been the most common opportunistic ocular infection and the leading cause of visual loss in AIDS patients. Despite its well-characterized clinical course and the multitude of high-quality studies on the treatment of this common disease, new forms of CMV infection are being described as immune recovery secondary to combination drug therapy becomes more common. CMVR is still a diagnostic and therapeutic challenge in many patients.

EPIDEMIOLOGY, PATHOGENESIS, AND HISTOPATHOLOGY

CMV is a double-stranded DNA herpesvirus. Serological evidence of past infection can be found in the sera of 60–90% of normal adults. Transmission occurs via infected body fluids, blood, or transplanted organs. Transplacental infection is possible, but most cases are acquired. Seropositivity increases with age and is higher among patients of low socioeconomic status. Typically, acquired CMV infection in immune competent individuals causes a self-limiting, mononucleosis-like febrile illness. Many cases are asymptomatic. However, the virus remains latent and is capable of reactivation if and when the cellular immune status is compromised, as in transplant recipients or in those with AIDS. Extraocular CMV disease in immune compromised patients may include pneumonitis, hepatitis, colitis, and encephalitis.

CMVR is a clinical marker of profound immune deficiency and is therefore one of the disease-defining infections of AIDS. Typically, the disease occurs in AIDS patients with CD4 counts <50 cells/mm3.[1] However, selective loss of anti-CMV CD4 clones may occur, leading to clinical disease despite significantly higher total CD4 counts. This may occur with[2] or without prior use of highly active antiretroviral therapy (HAART).

Histopathological examination of retinas with CMVR shows a full-thickness retinal necrosis. Enlarged cells with two types of CMV inclusions may be seen: basophilic cytoplasmic inclusions and eosinophilic intranuclear inclusions.[3]

CLINICAL PRESENTATION

Depending on its anatomical location and complicating factors, CMVR can be asymptomatic or give rise to a wide range of visual symptoms. Thus, small, asymptomatic peripheral lesions without significant vitreous inflammation can be detected incidentally in routine examination. More posterior lesions, involving the macula or optic nerve, or those associated with significant vitritis can gradually reduce visual acuity and cause floaters, photophobia, or visual field defects. Secondary rhegmatogenous retinal detachment may present with abrupt visual acuity or field loss.

The diagnosis of CMVR can be made clinically in the vast majority of patients and is supported by a favorable response to anti-CMV therapy. However, the differential diagnosis is broad and atypical lesions, or lesions that do not respond to standard therapy, may require tissue diagnosis.

Clinical examination typically reveals necrotizing retinitis, which at its early stages may be as small as a cotton-wool spot. It can occur in any retinal area and may have more than one active focus at a time. Anterior chamber and vitreous reaction is typically minimal, but significant vitritis can occur if CMVR develops in a patient with relatively high CD4 counts or if the area of retinitis is large. The disease progresses along the retinal blood vessels, causing confluent areas of retinal whitening, often associated with intraretinal hemorrhages and hard exudates (Fig. 163-1). The lesions progress in a "brushfire" manner, led by an active border. The rate of progression is typically slow, as opposed to that in other infectious retinitides, such as progressive outer retinal necrosis, acute retinal necrosis, or toxoplasmic retinochoroiditis. The border of the lesion typically advances by 250–350μm per week.[4] The optic nerve head may be directly involved, presenting with hemorrhagic papillitis and adjacent retinitis (Fig. 163-2).[5] Determination of progression may be difficult and should be based on systematic comparison of old and current photographs. In this manner, subtle changes in the area of retinitis can be detected in the most sensitive manner. CMVR in profoundly immunosuppressed patients does not heal spontaneously. It progresses unless treated successfully or unless the immune system recovers. When retinal inflammation subsides, it leaves an atrophic-appearing retina, sometimes with associated pigmentation (Fig. 163-3).

A variant of CMVR may present without much retinal whitening or hemorrhage, having the so-called granular morphology. This type may pose a diagnostic challenge. Another morpholog-

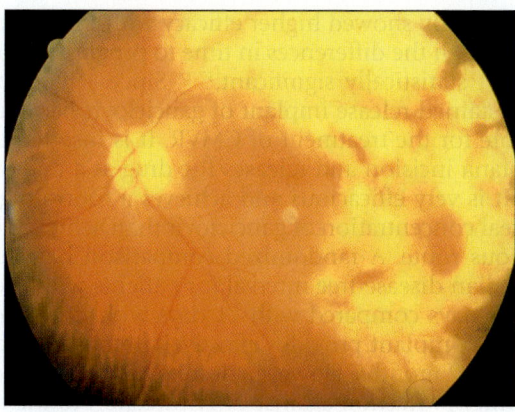

FIG. 163-1 ■ CMV retinitis involving the posterior pole, threatening the fovea. Note confluent areas of necrotizing retinitis. The necrotic retina is yellow-white and few hemorrhages may be seen.

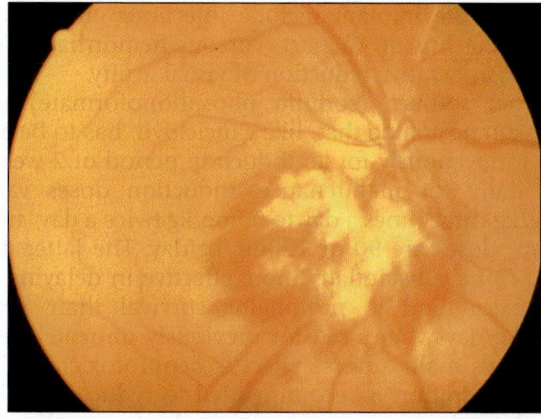

FIG. 163-2 ■ CMV affecting the optic nerve head and the peripapillary retina. The same eye later developed diffuse CMV retinitis leading to retinal detachment.

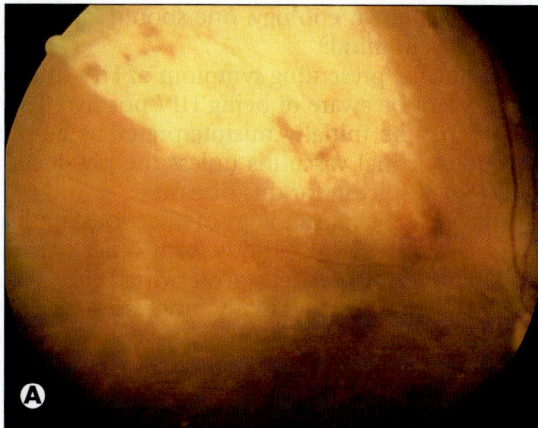

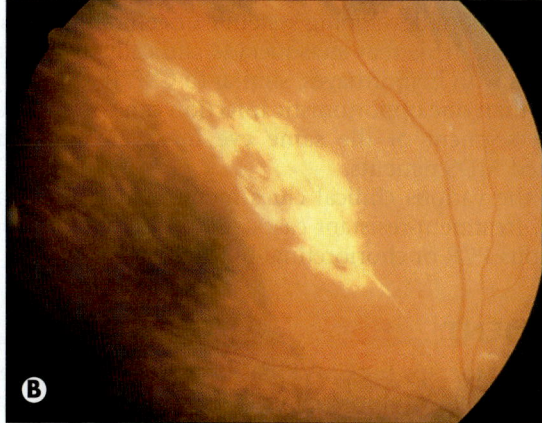

FIG. 163-3 ■ Effect of anti-CMV induction treatment on lesion morphology. **A,** A confluent, triangular area of necrotizing retinitis. **B,** After 4 weeks of intravenous induction therapy with ganciclovir, the same area shows resolving retinitis.

ical variant is "frosted branch" angiitis, in which there is diffuse vascular sheathing.[6] This is not a specific morphology, and it can also be found in toxoplasmosis and other retinal infections.

The area of retinal involvement has been divided into three concentric zones[7]: zone 1 is the posterior pole, defined as the area within 3000μm of the foveal center or 1500μm around the optic nerve head. Zone 2 extends from the borders of zone 1 to the ampullae of the vortex veins, and zone 3 is the retina peripheral to zone 2.

Zone 1 disease threatens the macula, papillomacular bundle, or optic nerve and is therefore immediately vision threatening. The proximity to the posterior pole is a major determinant of the type and urgency of required intervention. Peripheral lesions and high myopia carry an increased risk of rhegmatogenous retinal detachment, which, according to one study,[8] may occur in 38% of patients over the course of 1 year.

CMVR IN THE HAART ERA

Following the introduction of HAART into AIDS management, immune recovery has become an increasingly common phenomenon. HAART is a combination of two drug categories: two or more reverse transcriptase inhibitors, such as zidovudine (a nucleoside analog) or nevirapine (a nonnucleoside reverse transcriptase inhibitor) together with one or more viral protease inhibitors, such as indinavir or ritonavir. HAART often leads to recovery of CD4 counts and a decline in the serum human immunodeficiency virus (HIV) viral RNA load. This is associated with functional immune recovery. The incidence of new CMVR has declined by more than 50% since the introduction of HAART.[9,10] CMVR has become a potentially self-limiting disease, sometimes spontaneously healing after successful HAART. Although the recovering immune system

regains its ability to control CMVR and various other opportunistic infections, clinically significant inflammation may become a new challenge. Eyes with quiet retinal lesions that have previously healed under anti-CMV treatment may now develop uveitis. This syndrome, immune recovery uveitis (IRU), includes vitritis, cystoid macular edema, epiretinal membranes, and variable anterior uveitis. It is presumed to represent a late immune response to the viral antigens in the retina and vitreous rather than active infection. This may become a major source of visual morbidity in AIDS patients with past CMVR.

DIAGNOSIS

The diagnosis of CMVR is usually made clinically. However, in a minority of cases the diagnosis has to be confirmed by laboratory tests. Serological evidence of past infection with CMV (immunoglobulin G) is common in AIDS patients and thus has limited diagnostic value. Blood or urine viral cultures may support the diagnosis and have been shown to be positive in 45% and 71% of new CMVR cases for blood and urine, respectively.[11] However, the predictive value of this indirect test is too low for it to be used for therapeutic decisions. In difficult, atypical cases in which there is an urgent need for correct microbial diagnosis, a polymerase chain reaction (PCR) test from a vitreous or aqueous tap may be highly helpful. Vitreous PCR has been shown to be 95% sensitive and highly specific in untreated cases of CMVR.[12] Similarly, a chorioretinal biopsy can be obtained and examined histopathologically in difficult cases.[13]

DIFFERENTIAL DIAGNOSIS

The differential diagnosis of necrotizing retinitis in AIDS patients includes other infectious, neoplastic, and autoimmune retinal vasculitides. When approaching a patient with necrotizing retinitis of unknown etiology, one should keep several important principles in mind:

1. CMVR may be the presenting symptom of HIV infection. The patient may not be aware of being HIV positive. Thus, atypical lesions may be initially misinterpreted as autoimmune, noninfectious retinal vasculitis unless the physician keeps a high index of suspicion for this disease.
2. In AIDS patients, the morphology of infectious fundus lesions may be misleading. Viral retinitis from other herpes viruses (herpes simplex virus, varicella-zoster virus) may appear similar to CMVR, although it usually progresses faster. Bacterial retinitis/choroiditis can be seen with syphilis or with mycobacterial infections. Toxoplasmic retinitis/retinochoroiditis is usually associated with more vitritis and more anterior segment inflammation. Infections with fungi such as *Aspergillus* should also be kept in mind. Finally, AIDS patients have increased risk of developing systemic or central nervous system lymphoma. This may masquerade clinically as a necrotizing retinitis with hemorrhages, similar to CMVR.
3. More than one opportunistic infection can coexist in the posterior segment of the same eye in severely immunosuppressed AIDS patients.

Despite the various clinical clues mentioned, the diagnosis in atypical, treatment-resistant cases should be based, if possible, on vitreous PCR or chorioretinal biopsy.

TREATMENT

The optimal therapy for CMVR has been the subject of extensive clinical research. Multiple clinical trials have led to evidence-based treatment recommendations. These relate to drugs, drug combinations, treatment regimens, administration routes, and delivery systems. However, because of the introduction of HAART into routine management of AIDS patients in the late 1990s, some of these treatment recommendations are currently being modified. In the pre-HAART era, AIDS patients were profoundly immune suppressed at the time of diagnosis of CMVR. This illness was preterminal, with death occurring in a matter of months. Therefore, lifelong parenteral anti-CMV therapy through a permanent intravenous catheter was recommended. Even then, relapse of the disease occurred in as many as 85% of patients treated by systemic ganciclovir or foscarnet 120 days after initiation of therapy.[14] The remarkable immune recovery that followed HAART in many AIDS patients has changed this approach.

Anti-CMV Drugs and Delivery Routes

The principal antiviral drugs used in the treatment of CMVR are ganciclovir, foscarnet, and cidofovir. All three are virostatic DNA polymerase inhibitors.

1. Ganciclovir (DHPG) is a nucleoside analog available for intravenous infusion, oral therapy, and as an intravitreal, sustained-release implant. It is virostatic against CMV. Resistance to ganciclovir is rare in isolates of CMV obtained from blood or urine of newly diagnosed patients.[15] Therefore, the vast majority of patients with CMVR respond favorably to an induction course of this drug. The drug is infused intravenously twice daily for an induction period of 2–3 weeks (5mg/kg twice a day), then once daily at a maintenance dose of 5mg/kg/day. The main adverse effect is bone marrow toxicity, mainly neutropenia. Alternatively, it may be injected intravitreally, using doses of 200–2000µg in a volume of 0.05–0.1ml once to twice weekly. Oral ganciclovir is available but because of its low bioavailability has to be taken in high doses (3000–4500mg daily). Its prophylactic value against CMV disease is controversial.[16] The Oral Ganciclovir European and Australian Cooperative Study Group and the Syntex Cooperative Oral Ganciclovir Study Group have compared the efficacy of maintenance oral GCV, 500mg six times daily, with that of standard intravenous GCV maintenance. Their re-

sults generally showed higher efficacy with intravenous delivery, although the differences in time to progression of retinitis were not statistically significant.[17,18] Since 1996, an intravitreal, sustained-release implant of ganciclovir has been widely available for the treatment of CMVR. It is inserted through a pars plana incision and releases the drug at a rate of 1µg per hour. It is very efficacious and achieves a fourfold greater intravitreal concentration of ganciclovir than achieved by the intravenous route. A randomized comparison has shown that the median disease-free interval for patients with the implant was 221 days compared with 71 days with intravenous therapy.[19] The implant provides effective vitreous ganciclovir levels for 6–12 months. However, despite its local efficacy, it does not confer protection against CMV infection to the fellow eye or to other organs. This drawback may be overcome by the concomitant use of oral ganciclovir, 3–4.5g daily. In patients who are not receiving HAART, this combination is effective in reducing the incidence of new CMV disease as well as reducing the risk of Kaposi's sarcoma.[20] The complications associated with the implant include infectious endophthalmitis, retinal detachment, cataract, vitreous hemorrhage, and transient, postoperative reduction of visual acuity.

2. Foscarnet sodium (sodium phosphonoformate) is a pyrophosphate analog that, like ganciclovir, has to be administered intravenously for an induction period of 2 weeks, then once daily for maintenance. Induction doses vary from 60mg/kg three times a day to 90mg/kg twice a day, and maintenance doses are 90 or 120mg/kg/day. The latter dose was found to be substantially more effective in delaying retinitis progression and in prolonging survival than a dose of 90mg/kg/day when used for previously untreated retinitis.[21] Foscarnet's main adverse effect is nephrotoxicity, and intravenous hydration is recommended to reduce this risk. Like ganciclovir, foscarnet may be injected intravitreally, at a dose of 1.2–2.4mg in 0.05–0.1ml, once or twice a week.

   Ganciclovir and foscarnet therapies were compared in untreated CMVR with regard to their effect on visual outcomes and survival of patients. Combination therapy with these two agents was assessed in cases of relapse or persistent disease. Although mortality in the foscarnet group was lower than that in the ganciclovir group,[22] a fact that was attributed to foscarnet's antiretroviral properties,[23,24] foscarnet was associated with more adverse effects and was less well tolerated than ganciclovir.[25] Both drugs had equivalent efficacy.[14] Combination therapy was the most effective regimen for controlling persistent or recurrent retinitis under treatment. However, the dosing schedule of such combination therapy is extremely inconvenient.[26]

3. Cidofovir (HPMPC) is a nucleoside analog. It is administered intravenously at a dose of 5mg/kg once weekly and once every 2 weeks for induction and maintenance, respectively. Therefore it does not require a permanent intravenous catheter. Its use is limited by the high risk of nephrotoxicity as well as its tendency to cause potentially severe uveitis and hypotony in 40% of patients.[27] The risk of severe uveitis and chronic hypotony is 3% with local intravitreal injection of cidofovir.[28] To minimize the risk of nephrotoxicity, oral probenecid and adequate intravenous hydration are given with the drug. Also, renal function has to be monitored carefully during therapy. Cidofovir's efficacy is equivalent to that of intravitreal ganciclovir implant plus oral ganciclovir, as shown by the Ganciclovir Cidofovir Cytomegalovirus Retinitis Trial.[29] This study compared the efficacy of these two therapies, neither of which requires a central venous line.

4. Valganciclovir is a valine ester prodrug of ganciclovir. It is rapidly absorbed and hydrolyzed into ganciclovir. Its bioavailability is approximately 10 times higher than that of oral ganciclovir. A once-daily dose of 900mg creates serum concentrations equivalent to those of 5mg/kg intravenous ganciclovir. The drug has been approved by the Food and Drug Administration for this indication.[30] Its main adverse ef-

fects are similar to those of the intravenous form, most commonly neutropenia.

5. Fomivirsen (Vitravene) is an antisense inhibitor of CMV, administered by monthly intravitreal injections. Although it is approved for use in CMVR, currently there is limited information regarding its relative efficacy in the ophthalmologic literature.

Recommended Treatment Strategies in the HAART Era

The therapeutic choices for AIDS patients with CMVR depend on whether or not immune recovery is expected.[31] In HAART-naive patients there is a high probability of a favorable response to HAART. In such cases, systemic therapy is usually appropriate because the immune system may recover in a matter of months, saving the need for intraocular surgery. If severe zone 1 disease is present, a ganciclovir implant is the treatment of choice because of its superior efficacy. Similarly, intravitreal injections of ganciclovir or foscarnet may be used together with systemic therapy. The implant should also be used in patients with contraindications to systemic therapy or in whom a central line is a problem. Either the implant, supplemented by oral ganciclovir, or parenteral systemic therapy is a reasonable choice for patients in whom immune recovery is not expected.

In case of relapse under treatment with ganciclovir or foscarnet, therapy may be switched to or combined with the other drug. Although extremely inconvenient, the combination of ganciclovir and foscarnet has been shown to be more effective than each drug given separately.

Maintenance Therapy after Immune Recovery

The changing patterns of disease associated with immune recovery have raised new therapeutic questions. Patients who were previously expected to need lifelong treatment are now showing resistance to CMVR. Therefore, the need for lifelong treatment is being questioned. Reactivation of treated CMVR is rare in patients responding to HAART while receiving maintenance anti-CMV therapy and tends to occur mostly in the first 100 days after starting HAART.[32] Several studies have shown that chronic anti-CMV therapy can be stopped after immune recovery is sustained for a few months.[33-35] The current recommendations for maintenance therapy for quiescent CMVR in patients receiving HAART are to discontinue such therapy after two conditions are met: (1) the patient has to respond to HAART by increasing the CD4 count by more than 50 cells/mm^3 and to higher than 100–150 cells/mm^3 and (2) this response should be sustained for at least 3–6 months, therefore avoiding the small risk of early reactivation.[35,36] The question of whether or not continued anti-CMV therapy has a role in modifying the incidence and course of IRU is still unanswered. IRU is managed by topical and/or sub-Tenon corticosteroid injections.

REFERENCES

1. Pertel P, Hirschtick R, Phair J, et al. Risk of developing cytomegalovirus retinitis in persons infected with the human immunodeficiency virus. J Acquir Immune Defic Syndr. 1992;5:1069–74.
2. Jacobson MA, Zegans M, Pavan PR, et al. Cytomegalovirus retinitis after initiation of highly active antiretroviral therapy. Lancet. 1997;349:1443–5.
3. Yoser SL, Forster DJ, Rao NA. Systemic viral infections and their retinal and choroidal manifestations. Surv Ophthalmol. 1993;37:313–52.
4. Holland GN, Shuler JD. Progression rates of cytomegalovirus retinopathy in ganciclovir-treated and untreated patients. Arch Ophthalmol. 1992;110:1435–42.
5. Gross JG, Sadun AA, Wiley CA, Freeman WR. Severe visual loss related to isolated peripapillary retinal and optic nerve head cytomegalovirus infection. Am J Ophthalmol. 1989;108:691–8.
6. Spaide RF, Vitale AT, Toth IR, Oliver JM. Frosted branch angiitis associated with cytomegalovirus retinitis. Am J Ophthalmol. 1992;113:522–8.
7. Holland GN, Buhles WC Jr, Mastre B, Kaplan HJ. A controlled retrospective study of ganciclovir treatment for cytomegalovirus retinopathy. Use of a standardized system for the assessment of disease outcome. UCLA CMV Retinopathy Study Group. Arch Ophthalmol. 1989;107:1759–66.
8. Rhegmatogenous retinal detachment in patients with cytomegalovirus retinitis: the Foscarnet-Ganciclovir Cytomegalovirus Retinitis Trial. The Studies of Ocular Complications of AIDS (SOCA) Research Group in Collaboration with the AIDS Clinical Trials Group (ACTG). Am J Ophthalmol. 1997;124:61–70.
9. Jacobson MA, Zegans M, Pavan PR, et al. Cytomegalovirus retinitis after initiation of highly active antiretroviral therapy. Lancet. 1997;349:1443–5.
10. Macdonald JC, Torriani FJ, Morse LS, et al. Lack of reactivation of cytomegalovirus (CMV) retinitis after stopping cytomegalovirus maintenance therapy in AIDS patients with sustained elevations in CD4 T cells in response to highly active antiretroviral therapy. J Infect Dis. 1998;177:1182–7.
11. Cytomegalovirus (CMV) culture results, drug resistance, and clinical outcome in patients with AIDS and CMV retinitis treated with foscarnet or ganciclovir. Studies of Ocular Complications of AIDS (SOCA) in collaboration with the AIDS Clinical Trial Group. J Infect Dis. 1997;176:50–8.
12. McCann JD, Margolis TP, Wong MG, et al. A sensitive and specific polymerase chain reaction–based assay for the diagnosis of cytomegalovirus retinitis. Am J Ophthalmol. 1995;120:219–26.
13. Rutzen AR, Ortega-Larrocea G, Dugel PU, et al. Clinicopathologic study of retinal and choroidal biopsies in intraocular inflammation. Am J Ophthalmol. 1995;119:597–611.
14. Foscarnet-Ganciclovir Cytomegalovirus Retinitis Trial. 4. Visual outcomes. Studies of Ocular Complications of AIDS Research Group in collaboration with the AIDS Clinical Trials Group. Ophthalmology. 1994;101:1250–61.
15. Jabs DA, Dunn JP, Enger C, et al. Cytomegalovirus retinitis and viral resistance. Prevalence of resistance at diagnosis, 1994. Cytomegalovirus Retinitis and Viral Resistance Study Group. Arch Ophthalmol. 1996;114:809–14.
16. Brosgart CL, Louis TA, Hillman DW, et al. A randomized, placebo-controlled trial of the safety and efficacy of oral ganciclovir for prophylaxis of cytomegalovirus disease in HIV-infected individuals. Terry Beirn Community Programs for Clinical Research on AIDS. AIDS. 1998;12:269–77.
17. Drew WL, Ives D, Lalezari JP, et al. Oral ganciclovir as maintenance treatment for cytomegalovirus retinitis in patients with AIDS. Syntex Cooperative Oral Ganciclovir Study Group. N Engl J Med. 1995;333:615–20.
18. Intravenous versus oral ganciclovir: European/Australian comparative study of efficacy and safety in the prevention of cytomegalovirus retinitis recurrence in patients with AIDS. The Oral Ganciclovir European and Australian Cooperative Study Group. AIDS. 1995;9:471–7.
19. Musch DC, Martin DF, Gordon JF, et al. Treatment of cytomegalovirus retinitis with a sustained-release ganciclovir implant. The Ganciclovir Implant Study Group. N Engl J Med. 1997;337:83–90.
20. Martin DF, Kuppermann BD, Wolitz RA, et al. Oral ganciclovir for patients with cytomegalovirus retinitis treated with a ganciclovir implant. Roche Ganciclovir Study Group. N Engl J Med. 1999;340:1063–70.
21. Jacobson MA, Causey D, Polsky B, et al. A dose-ranging study of daily maintenance intravenous foscarnet therapy for cytomegalovirus retinitis in AIDS. J Infect Dis. 1993;168:444–8.
22. Mortality in patients with the acquired immunodeficiency syndrome treated with either foscarnet or ganciclovir for cytomegalovirus retinitis. Studies of Ocular Complications of AIDS Research Group, in collaboration with the AIDS Clinical Trials Group. N Engl J Med. 1992;326:213–20.
23. Reddy MM, Grieco MH, McKinley GF, et al. Effect of foscarnet therapy on human immunodeficiency virus p24 antigen levels in AIDS patients with cytomegalovirus retinitis. J Infect Dis. 1992;166:607–10.
24. Antiviral effects of foscarnet and ganciclovir therapy on human immunodeficiency virus p24 antigen in patients with AIDS and cytomegalovirus retinitis. Studies of Ocular Complications of AIDS Research Group in collaboration with AIDS Clinical Trials Group. J Infect Dis. 1995;172:613–21.
25. Morbidity and toxic effects associated with ganciclovir or foscarnet therapy in a randomized cytomegalovirus retinitis trial. Studies of ocular complications of AIDS Research Group, in collaboration with the AIDS Clinical Trials Group. Arch Intern Med. 1995;155:65–74.
26. Combination foscarnet and ganciclovir therapy vs monotherapy for the treatment of relapsed cytomegalovirus retinitis in patients with AIDS. The Cytomegalovirus Retreatment Trial. The Studies of Ocular Complications of AIDS Research Group in Collaboration with the AIDS Clinical Trials Group. Arch Ophthalmol. 1996;114:23–33.
27. Davis JL, Taskintuna I, Freeman WR, et al. Iritis and hypotony after treatment with intravenous cidofovir for cytomegalovirus retinitis. Arch Ophthalmol. 1997;115:733–7.
28. Taskintuna I, Rahhal FM, Rao NA, et al. Adverse events and autopsy findings after intravitreous cidofovir (HPMPC) therapy in patients with acquired immune deficiency syndrome (AIDS). Ophthalmology. 1997;104:1827–36; discussion 1836–7.
29. The ganciclovir implant plus oral ganciclovir versus parenteral cidofovir for the treatment of cytomegalovirus retinitis in patients with acquired immunodeficiency syndrome: The Ganciclovir Cidofovir Cytomegalovirus Retinitis Trial. Am J Ophthalmol. 2001;131:457–67.
30. Schwetz BA. From the Food and Drug Administration. JAMA. 2001;285:2705.
31. Martin DF, Dunn JP, Davis JL, et al. Use of the ganciclovir implant for the treatment of cytomegalovirus retinitis in the era of potent antiretroviral therapy: recommendations of the International AIDS Society–USA panel. Am J Ophthalmol. 1999;127:329–39.
32. Mitchell SM, Membrey WL, Youle MS, et al. Cytomegalovirus retinitis after the initiation of highly active antiretroviral therapy: a 2 year prospective study. Br J Ophthalmol. 1999;83:652–5.
33. Macdonald JC, Torriani FJ, Morse LS, et al. Lack of reactivation of cytomegalovirus (CMV) retinitis after stopping CMV maintenance therapy in AIDS patients with sustained elevations in CD4 T cells in response to highly active antiretroviral therapy. J Infect Dis. 1998;177:1182–7.
34. Komanduri KV, Viswanathan MN, Wieder ED, et al. Restoration of cytomegalovirus-specific CD4+ T-lymphocyte responses after ganciclovir and highly active antiretroviral therapy in individuals infected with HIV-1. Nat Med. 1998;4:953–6.
35. Whitcup SM. Cytomegalovirus retinitis in the era of highly active antiretroviral therapy. JAMA. 2000;283:653–7.
36. 1999 USPHS/IDSA guidelines for the prevention of opportunistic infections in persons infected with human immunodeficiency virus. MMWR Morb Mortal Wkly Rep. 1999;48:1–66.

CHAPTER

164 HIV-Related Uveitis

PRAVIN U. DUGEL • ALLEN B. THACH

DEFINITION

- In individuals infected by human immunodeficiency virus, most of the ocular infections are caused by opportunistic organisms. The opportunistic infections include cytomegalovirus retinitis, progressive outer retinal necrosis, toxoplasmic retinochoroiditis, fungal chorioretinitis, infectious multifocal choroiditis, molluscum contagiosum, and microsporidia keratopathy.

KEY FEATURES

- The features of the infection depend on the infectious agent and the site of infection.
- Retinal necrosis.
- Chorioretinal lesions.
- Multifocal choroidal lesions.
- Eyelid lesions.
- Epithelial keratopathy.

ASSOCIATED FEATURE

- Retinal microvasculopathy.

INTRODUCTION

The ocular manifestations of acquired immunodeficiency syndrome (AIDS) are protean. They include various opportunistic infections of the retina, choroid, and ocular adnexa and neoplasms that involve the eyelids, conjunctiva, and other ocular and orbital structures. A number of anterior segment diseases, such as herpes simplex, herpes zoster, and ulcerative keratitis, are described in more detail in Chapter 162. A separate class of anterior and posterior segment manifestations that concern ocular neoplasms and AIDS is described in Chapter 183. In AIDS, even though anterior and posterior segments, including orbital tissue, are involved through various infections or neoplastic disorders, the most common visually disabling complications occur primarily in the posterior segment. Cytomegalovirus (CMV) retinitis is the most common intraocular infection in patients with AIDS. This entry is described in detail in Chapter 163. The introduction of highly active antiretroviral therapy (HAART) resulted in a dramatic decline in incidence of CMV retinitis and other opportunistic ocular infections.

PROGRESSIVE OUTER RETINAL NECROSIS

EPIDEMIOLOGY AND PATHOGENESIS

Even though progressive outer retinal necrosis (PORN) is less common than CMV retinitis, the former causes a more rapid destruction of the retina and carries a poor prognosis. Electron microscopy of a retinal biopsy specimen and polymerase chain re-

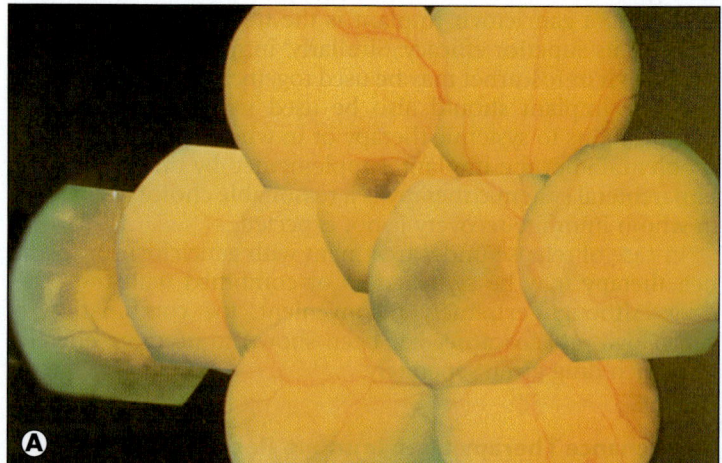

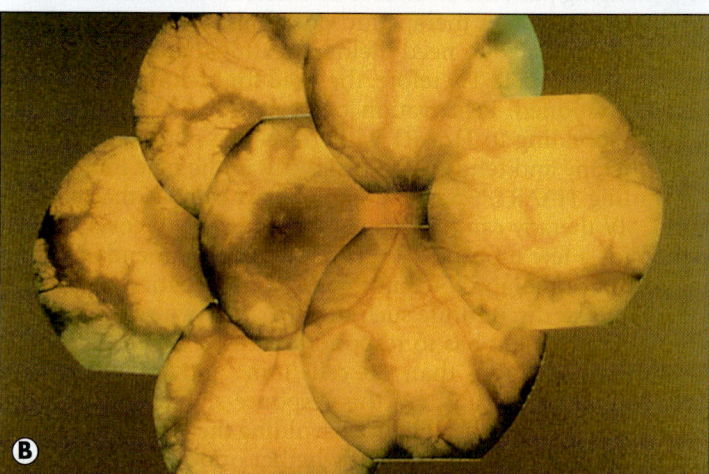

FIG. 164-1 ■ **Progressive outer retinal necrosis. A,** Day 2. **B,** Day 6. Notice the deep, white outer retinal lesions that coalesce and progressively expand in a circumferential manner, with sparing of the perivascular retina and minimal overlying inflammation. (With permission from the American Journal of Ophthalmology.)

action studies show herpes zoster as the causative agent of retinal necrosis.

OCULAR MANIFESTATIONS

In a patient with AIDS, PORN consists of deep outer retinal lesions in a circumferential pattern in the peripheral retina. These lesions tend to coalesce rapidly and progress to full-thickness retinal necrosis in a matter of days, and they continue to progress more posteriorly with a minimal amount of overlying inflammation (Fig. 164-1). A unique feature that characterizes this condition is apparent sparing of the paravascular retina.[1] Within a matter of weeks, vision may deteriorate from 20/20 (6/6) to no light perception. Often the disease starts in one eye and the fellow eye becomes involved within weeks to months. In a variant of PORN the retinitis begins in the posterior pole with little or no clinical evidence of vasculitis.[2,3]

DIAGNOSIS

The diagnosis of PORN is a clinical one in a patient who has human immunodeficiency virus (HIV) infection. A history of recent or concurrent herpes zoster infection in the skin or elsewhere is helpful in the diagnosis. Rapid progression and sparing of retinal vessels and adjacent retina are characteristic. Histopathological and immunohistochemical studies, *in situ* hybridization, and polymerase chain reaction that utilizes varicella-zoster virus primers may reveal a herpes zoster viral process.

DIFFERENTIAL DIAGNOSIS

Progressive outer retinal necrosis must be differentiated from peripheral CMV retinitis and ocular toxoplasmosis. The characteristic and differentiating features of PORN include rapid and relentless progression, circumferential involvement of the outer retina followed by full-thickness retinal necrosis, and initial sparing of the paravascular retina. In CMV retinitis all layers of the retina tend to be affected in a granular fashion in the periphery. The retinal vessels are not spared and, in fact, often have segmented vasculitis. Progression is usually toward the posterior pole in a radial fashion as opposed to a circumferential fashion. Toxoplasmosis tends to cause a vitritis and a significant necrotizing reaction in the retina. The vasculature is not spared and progression does not take place in a circumferential manner.

SYSTEMIC ASSOCIATION

Several HIV-infected individuals who have PORN usually develop cutaneous zoster infection prior to its development. Occasionally, simultaneous development of cutaneous zoster and PORN occurs. Usually, the CD4+ lymphocyte count is low (peripheral CD4+ lymphocyte counts less than 50 cells/mm³).[4] Patients may also develop other manifestations of advanced HIV infection.

PATHOLOGY

Histopathologically, advanced cases of PORN reveal total necrosis of the retina, with both inner and outer retina necrosis. However, sparing of the retinal venules also occurs in such cases. Retinal pigment epithelium may be involved.[4] Viral inclusions could be observed in the retinal cells. Immunohistochemical or *in situ* hybridization that utilizes varicella-zoster virus probes may show positive immunostaining or hybridization in the infected cells. Electron microscopic studies may disclose typical herpes viral particles in the infected cells.

TREATMENT

No treatment has been found to be universally successful. Treatment with more than one antiviral agent (i.e., ganciclovir and foscarnet, ganciclovir and acyclovir, foscarnet and acyclovir, or all three together) may improve the response and final visual outcome.[3,5] Sorivudine, an oral antiviral agent, may be effective.[6] Intravitreal injection of ganciclovir and foscarnet has also been attempted with limited success.[6,7]

COURSE AND OUTCOME

The disease tends to progress rapidly and often results in a retinal detachment within days or weeks. The progression is usually toward the posterior pole in cases that present with peripheral retinitis. The retinal detachment appears to proceed via a rhegmatogenous process.

TOXOPLASMIC RETINOCHOROIDITIS

The incidence of ocular toxoplasmosis in HIV-infected certain individuals varies; it appears to be relatively more common in countries such as Brazil. Ocular toxoplasmosis in many patients who have AIDS is thought to result from an acquired infection by the parasite *Toxoplasma gondii*, which may be surmised from multifocality, bilaterality, and the lack of preexisting scars.[8-10]

Ocular toxoplasmosis associated with AIDS is often seen with no preexisting chorioretinal scar and is frequently bilateral and multifocal. Vitreous inflammation is a common clinical finding. In some patients the clinical picture is quite similar to that of ocular toxoplasmosis observed in immunocompetent individuals. However, some of the HIV patients present with diffuse retinitis that simulates CMV infection, but retinal hemorrhages are not observed in toxoplasmosis. The typical "headlight in a fog" funduscopic picture is also found. Surprisingly, a significant inflammatory reaction is normally present despite the immunosuppression. Almost 25% of patients who have ocular toxoplasmosis have intracranial involvement. In fact, toxoplasmosis is the most common cause of AIDS-associated, nonviral intracranial infection. Therefore, all AIDS patients who have ocular toxoplasmosis should undergo an intracranial imaging study (computed tomography or magnetic resonance imaging with contrast).

Usually, ocular toxoplasmosis is diagnosed on the basis of clinical findings. Serological tests and polymerase chain reaction performed with the intraocular fluids may be helpful, and occasionally a retinal or choroidal biopsy may be required to establish the tissue diagnosis.[10,11] Ocular toxoplasmosis must be distinguished from CMV retinitis and PORN. Characteristic features of the ocular toxoplasmosis in AIDS include significant inflammation despite immunocompromise, multifocal and sometimes bilateral lesions, and lack of preexisting chorioretinal scars. Unlike the finding in PORN, there is no circumferential pattern of progression with sparing of the paravascular retina. Unlike the finding in CMV retinitis, there is a significant amount of overlying inflammation with no significant retinal hemorrhage.

Histopathologically, several cysts of *Toxoplasma* are present at the site of retinitis. In addition, free forms of the organism may be found. The retina is almost always necrotic, and adjacent choroid often contains chronic inflammatory cell infiltration.

Antitoxoplasma therapy similar to that given to patients who are immunocompetent is effective in patients who have AIDS. This consists of a combination of pyrimethamine, sulfadiazine, and folinic acid. However, clindamycin, tetracycline, atovaquone, and spiramycin are also effective. Patients who have AIDS are not given high doses of systemic corticosteroids. Additional immunosuppression in an already immunocompromised patient may bring about severe opportunistic infections, which may be life threatening as well as sight threatening.

FUNGAL CHORIORETINITIS

In individuals infected by HIV, various fungi may cause chorioretinitis and orbital cellulitis. These include *Candida albicans*, *Aspergillus*, *Histoplasma capsulatum*, and others. *Candida* (Chapter 171) and *Aspergillus* result in similar intraocular infection.

Ocular histoplasmosis is an uncommon opportunistic infection in patients who have AIDS. It presents clinically as a creamy white, choroidal lesion with subretinal infiltrates that are approximately one fourth of a disc diameter; the lesions may be bilateral. Scattered intraretinal hemorrhages have been reported. All retinal infiltrates have distinct borders.

The diagnosis of ocular histoplasmosis is often made in the setting of a disseminated infection. The clinical picture is entirely nonspecific, but it does serve to initiate a full evaluation for a systemic infection. As a result of this systemic evaluation, other likely candidates, such as ocular toxoplasmosis, fungal endophthalmitis, and other opportunistic infections that cause a

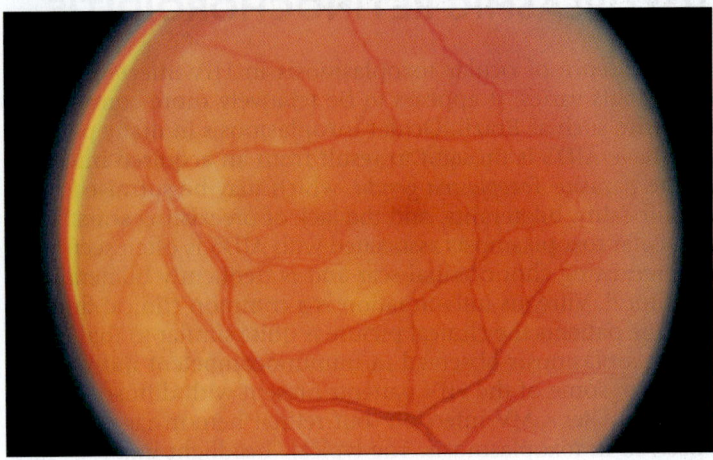

FIG. 164-2 ■ **Pneumocystic choroiditis.** Multiple lesions occur in the choroid.

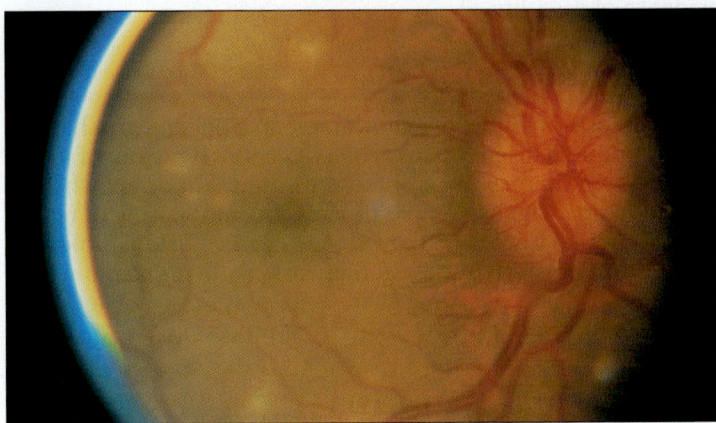

FIG. 164-3 ■ **Infectious multifocal choroiditis.** This is secondary to infection with *Cryptococcus neoformans*.

retinochoroiditis, can be ruled out. In the differential diagnosis of ocular histoplasmosis the following entities are considered: candidal retinitis, toxoplasmic retinochoroiditis, and mycobacterial and pneumocystic choroiditis.

Most patients who have ocular histoplasmosis present with sepsis, and, therefore, the ocular findings occur relatively late in the course of this life-threatening disease. However, if the ocular findings occur earlier, the ophthalmologist must obtain a full systemic evaluation for an opportunistic infection to make this diagnosis.

On pathological evaluation, the retina contains multiple, white-tan lesions that may measure up to 1mm in diameter—many are surrounded by a light tan halo. These lesions are located superficially and deep in the retina, are often perivascular, and contain histoplasmic organisms in all layers. The organisms are free or phagocytosed within histiocytic cells that occur with or without surrounding lymphocytes.

The ocular histoplasmosis is usually treated sufficiently by the intravenous antifungal medications required to treat the systemic infection. However, if necessary, supplemental intravitreal injections may be given concurrently.

INFECTIOUS MULTIFOCAL CHOROIDITIS

About 8–10% of terminally ill patients who have acquired immunodeficiency syndrome develop multifocal choroidal lesions that result from various infectious agents, which include *Pneumocystis carinii* (Fig. 164-2), *Cryptococcus* (Fig. 164-3), mycobacteria, and others.[12–14]

Infectious multifocal choroiditis presents as deep, creamy white to gray lesions below the retinal pigment epithelial layer. These are in a multifocal pattern in the posterior pole and mid-periphery and tend to be more elongated in the far periphery, with very little, if any, overlying inflammation, and the retina may not be involved. These lesions may be caused by *Cryptococcus neoformans*, atypical mycobacteria, *Pneumocystis carinii*, or other infectious agents.

Diagnosis is a clinical one, but the specific diagnosis requires systemic evaluation, which includes imaging studies, blood cultures, biopsy, and histological examination of the affected visceral organs (such as lungs). The differential diagnosis of infectious multifocal choroiditis includes ocular toxoplasmosis and ocular histoplasmosis. These two disorders present with significant intraocular inflammation and lesions that tend to involve the outer retinal layers. Although these lesions may be multifocal, they are usually not arranged in a reg-

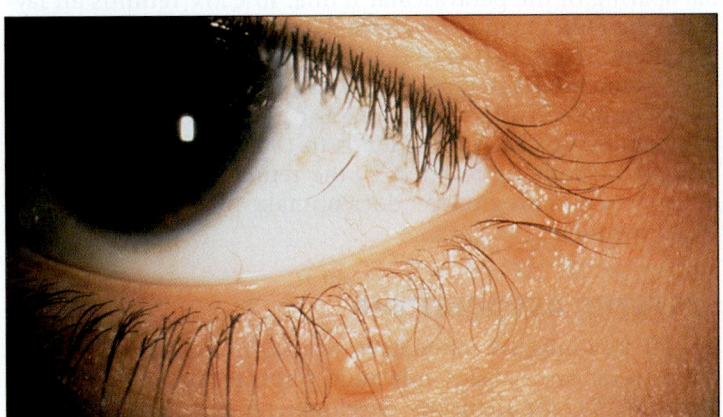

FIG. 164-4 ■ **Molluscum contagiosum.** Typically has raised, 2–3mm diameter eyelid lesions with umbiculated centers.

ular multifocal pattern that reflects the choroidal angioarchitecture. Rarely, deep outer retinal lesions of early PORN may be confused with infectious multifocal choroiditis. However, no progression toward coalescence of these lesions occurs in infectious multifocal choroiditis.[11]

The clinical picture of infectious multifocal choroiditis is entirely nonspecific for a causative organism. Unlike patients who have ocular histoplasmosis, patients who have infectious multifocal choroiditis may be completely asymptomatic, other than the occasional patient who presents with symptoms of blurred vision. Indeed, this may be the first clinical sign of a systemic infection. Therefore, a full systemic evaluation is imperative and must be carried out immediately.

Histopathologically, the causative organisms can be seen vividly using special stains. Usually, the inflammatory cell infiltration is minimal or absent in the choroid. However, individuals receiving HAART may show morbid inflammatory reaction.[13] Treatment of infectious multifocal choroiditis depends on the causative agent. As systemic involvement is the rule, intravenous therapy is required. Over a period of 1–3 months, the multifocal lesions may fade gradually, with minimal overlying retinal pigment epithelial changes.

MOLLUSCUM CONTAGIOSUM

Molluscum contagiosum (Fig. 164-4) consists of raised lesions in the ocular adnexa that are 2–3mm in diameter and typically have an umbiculated center. These lesions often shed viral parti-

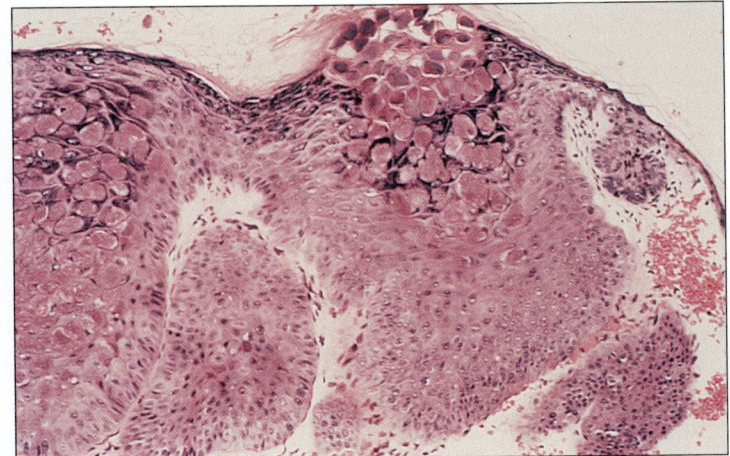

FIG. 164-5 ▪ **Molluscum contagiosum.** Intracytoplasmic, small eosinophilic molluscum bodies occur in the deep layers of epidermis. The bodies become enormous and basophilic near the surface. The bodies may be shed into the tear film, where they cause a secondary, irritative, follicular conjunctivitis. (From Yanoff M, Fine BS. Ocular pathology, ed 5. St. Louis: Mosby; 2002.)

cles in the conjunctival cul-de-sac, which results in a follicular conjunctivitis. In patients who have AIDS these lesions tend to be multiple and bilateral.[15] In immunocompromised patients, the molluscum virus, a DNA virus that belongs to the poxvirus family, tends to spread aggressively to the head and neck areas. Therefore, these lesions can be progressive as well as persistent.

The differential diagnosis of molluscum contagiosum includes ocular neoplasms typically associated with AIDS patients (Chapter 183). Molluscum contagiosum is characterized by an umbiculated center, a lack of vasculature, and a lack of necrosis that differentiates it from a more aggressive neoplastic lesion, such as squamous cell carcinoma, Kaposi's sarcoma, and lymphoma.

Histopathologically, the lesions show multiple, round or oval, eosinophilic and basophilic bodies in the cytoplasmic inclusions. These inclusions are present in the epithelium, and larger basophilic inclusions usually displace the nucleus toward the periphery of the cell (Fig. 164-5). Electron microscopy of these inclusions reveals viral particles that are somewhat rectangular and contain electron-dense nucleoid.

If patients have significant functional difficulties, such as persistent conjunctivitis, that cause irritation or visual symptoms, surgical excision, cautery, or cryotherapy is often effective.

MICROSPORIDIA

Microsporidia are intracellular obligate parasitic protozoa that can cause punctate epithelial keratopathy in individuals infected by HIV. The patient may develop mild conjunctivitis. CD4+ lymphocyte counts in such patients are usually below 50 cells/ml³. Gram staining of the conjunctival and corneal epithelial cells reveals organisms. Some patients respond well to topical fumagillin.

HUMAN IMMUNODEFICIENCY VIRUS MICROVASCULOPATHY

Approximately 75% of individuals infected by HIV develop microvascular abnormalities that involve the conjunctiva and retina. Hematological abnormalities, such as increased red blood cell aggregation, high fibrinogen levels, and above normal levels of plasma viscosity and quantitative immunoglobulin G, have been noted in most HIV-positive patients. Such hematological abnormalities may contribute to vascular damage and ocular ischemic lesions in the conjunctiva and retina. However, the possibility exists that this is a manifestation of an infectious microvasculopathy, perhaps as a result of HIV itself. An increased prevalence of retinopathy was observed in patients coinfected with HIV and hepatitis C compared with patients infected with HIV alone, which may indicate that immune complex deposition may cause vascular occlusion. Hepatitis C infection has a known association with hypergammaglobulinemia and cryoglobulinemia.[15]

Clinically, HIV microvasculopathy may be seen in the anterior segment or the posterior segment of the eye. The conjunctiva may show dilated, short segments of vessels, often in a corkscrew-like, tortuous pattern. In the posterior segment, intraretinal hemorrhage, retinal telangiectasia, cotton-wool spots, retinal vascular tortuosity, and vein or artery occlusions have been described. No known treatment exists for HIV microvasculopathy.

REFERENCES

1. Foster DJ, Dugel PU, Frangieh GT, et al. Rapidly progressive outer retinal necrosis in the acquired immunodeficiency syndrome. Am J Ophthalmol. 1990;110:341–8.
2. Margolis TP, Lowder CY, Holland GN, et al. Varicella zoster retinitis in patients with the acquired immune deficiency syndrome. Am J Ophthalmol. 1991;112:119–31.
3. Engstrom RE Jr, Holland GN, Margolis TP, et al. The progressive outer retinal necrosis syndrome. A variant of necrotizing herpetic retinopathy in patients with AIDS. Ophthalmology. 1994;101:1488–502.
4. Kuppermann BD, Quiceno JI, Wiley C, et al. Clinical and histopathologic study of varicella zoster virus retinitis in patients with the acquired immunodeficiency syndrome. Am J Ophthalmol. 1994;118:589–600.
5. Chulla TA, Rutledge BK, Morley MG, Duker JS. The progressive outer retinal necrosis syndrome: successful treatment with combination antiviral therapy. Ophthalmic Surg Lasers. 1998;29:198–206.
6. Pinnolis MK, Foxworthy D, Kemp B. Treatment and progressive outer retinal necrosis with sorivudine. Am J Ophthalmol. 1995;119:516–17.
7. Morley MG, Duker JS, Zacks C. Successful treatment of rapidly progressive outer retinal necrosis in the acquired immunodeficiency syndrome. Am J Ophthalmol. 1994;117:264–5.
8. Holland GN, Engstrom RE Jr, Glasgow B, et al. Ocular toxoplasmosis in patients with the acquired immunodeficiency syndrome. Am J Ophthalmol. 1988;106:653–67.
9. Cochereau-Massin I, LeHoang P, Lautier-Frau M, et al. Ocular toxoplasmosis in human immunodeficiency virus–infected patients. Am J Ophthalmol. 1992;114:130–5.
10. Moorthy RS, Smith RE, Rao NA. Progressive ocular toxoplasmosis in patients with acquired immunodeficiency syndrome. Am J Ophthalmol. 1993;115:742–7.
11. Fardeau C, Romand S, Rao NA, et al. Diagnosis of toxoplasmic retinochoroiditis with atypical clinical features. Am J Ophthalmol. 2002;134:196–203.
12. Morinelli EN, Dugel PU, Riffenburgh R, Rao NA. Infectious multifocal choroiditis in patients with acquired immune deficiency syndrome. Ophthalmology. 1993;100:1014–21.
13. Zamir E, Hudson H, Ober R, et al. Massive mycobacterial choroiditis during highly active antiretroviral therapy: another immune-recovery uveitis? Ophthalmology. 2002;109:2144–8.
14. Dugel PU, Rao NA, Forster DT, et al. Pneumocystis carinii choroiditis after long-term aerosolized pentamidine therapy. Am J Ophthalmol. 1990;110:113–17.
15. Dugel PU, Rao NA. Ocular infections in the acquired immunodeficiency syndrome. Int Ophthalmol Clin. 1993;33:103–27.

SECTION 3 INFECTIOUS CAUSES OF UVEITIS—BACTERIAL

CHAPTER

165

Syphilitic Uveitis

PRAVIN U. DUGEL • ALLEN B. THACH

DEFINITION

- A complex series of infectious and immunologically mediated intraocular inflammation initiated by *Treponema pallidum*.

KEY FEATURES

- Intraocular inflammation.
- Systemic manifestations.
- Latent intraocular and/or systemic manifestations.

ASSOCIATED FEATURES

- Chancres and gummatous involvement of the conjunctiva.
- Secondary episcleritis or scleritis.
- Interstitial keratitis.
- Congenital and acquired cataracts.
- Secondary glaucoma.
- Argyll Robertson pupil.

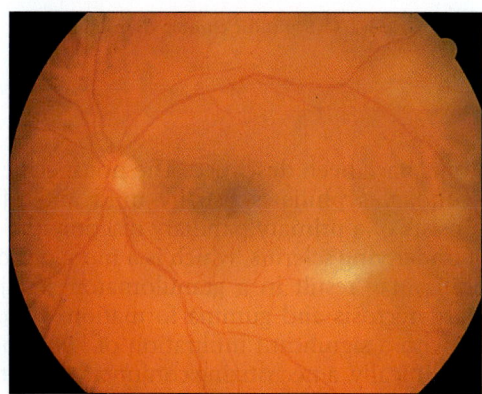

FIG. 165-1 ■ **Ocular retinitis.** This developed in a 38-year-old man who had a positive serology for syphilis.

INTRODUCTION

The ophthalmic manifestations of syphilis are protean and consist of inflammation and its sequelae. New clinical signs have been recognized in patients who also are infected with human immunodeficiency virus (HIV).

EPIDEMIOLOGY AND PATHOGENESIS

Syphilis is caused by the bacterium *Treponema pallidum* (*Tr. pallidum*). It is primarily a sexually transmitted disease but can be spread by transfusion of fresh blood or by accidental contact with an infected lesion. This disease has been a source of social stigma, morbidity, and mortality for centuries. Not until the widespread availability of penicillin after World War II was an appreciable decline in its incidence seen. However, penicillin alone is not the cure. Increasing bacterial resistance, socioeconomic factors, increased high-risk sexual activity, and devastating diseases that result in permanent immunodepression have contributed to a resurgence of syphilis.[1,2]

Perhaps syphilis is one of the difficult infectious diseases to understand and treat because it modulates the host immune system. Once infection takes place, immunity does occur, but it does not confer absolute protection. Humoral antibodies are protective only partially. Cell-mediated immunity, on the other hand, confers some resistance but, more important, may be a key factor in the development of late complications in humans.

Socioeconomic factors along with high-risk sexual behaviors and the HIV infection have resulted in an increased incidence of syphilis. It is therefore recommended that tests for both syphilis and HIV be carried out in patients who test positive for either disease. Because immunomodulation has a significant role in the development of clinical manifestations of syphilis, patients who have the acquired immunodeficiency syndrome (AIDS)

present a new and formidable challenge in the diagnosis and management of syphilis.

OCULAR MANIFESTATIONS

Nonspecific iritis and iridocyclitis are the most commonly associated forms of uveitis and may be the predominant finding in secondary syphilis. The anterior uveitis, however, is nonspecific and may be granulomatous or nongranulomatous. Dilated iris capillaries (roseola) during the second stage of syphilis have been described as a distinctive feature. Some authorities speculated that treponemal emboli may cause secondary vascular tortuosity and dilatation.[3]

The clinical manifestations of syphilis chorioretinitis are diverse. All forms of posterior uveitis have been described—vitritis, vasculitis with or without vascular occlusion, macular edema, stellate maculopathy, disciform macular detachment, pseudoretinitis pigmentosa, retinal detachment, uveal effusion, central retinal vein occlusion, subretinal neovascular membrane formation, retinal necrosis, big blind spot syndrome, and neuroretinitis (Figs. 165-1 to 165-3).[4–8] In HIV-positive individuals, the posterior intraocular inflammation includes large macular or juxtapapillary placoid lesions at the level of the retinal pigment epithelium. These lesions are yellowish or gray with atrophic centers and are flat with no fluid or hemorrhage. The fluorescein angiogram shows early hypofluorescence and late staining in a pattern described as a "leopard spot" hypofluorescence, which is thought to be a distinguishing finding; the condition is named acute syphilitic posterior placoid chorioretinitis.[9] HIV-positive patients may also present with a dense vitritis and no other signs of posterior uveitis (Fig. 165-4).[7]

Other ocular manifestations arise from involvement of the conjunctiva, cornea, sclera, optic nerve, and central nervous system.

Involvement of the conjunctiva may occur in all three stages of syphilis. The chancre of primary syphilis is very similar to that seen systemically. It consists of an ulcerative conjunctival lesion with a rounded edge and surrounding conjunctival injection; no discharge occurs. This chancre is usually asymptomatic, but irri-

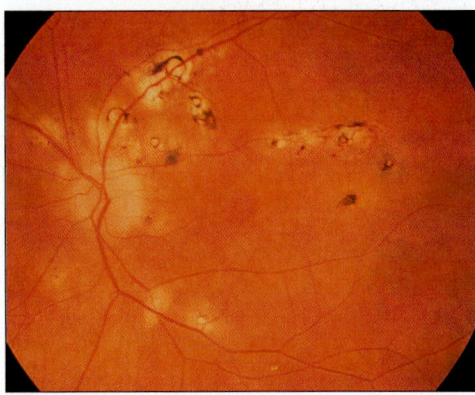

FIG. 165-2 ■ Syphilitic chronic choroiditis.

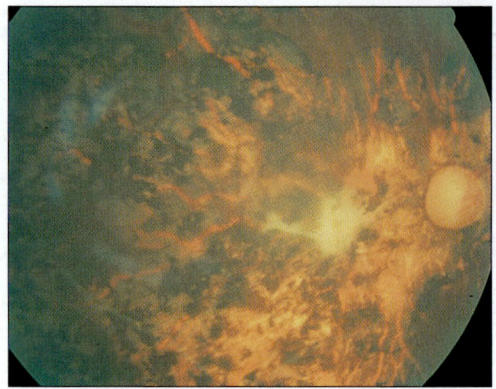

FIG. 165-3 ■ **Extensive chorioretinal damage with hyperplasia of retinal pigment epithelium.** The patient has syphilis.

tative symptoms have been described. The nonspecific conjunctivitis of secondary syphilis is usually mild and often overlooked. It consists of a primary papillary reaction and may be a harbinger of underlying scleritis, which is a more ominous sign. Tertiary syphilis may result in a granulomatous conjunctivitis with secondary necrosis and gumma formation, which can be quite painful with a significant infiltration of lymphocytes and plasma cells. Clinically, a necrotizing conjunctivitis with intense inflammation and pain is found.

Scleritis or episcleritis as part of conjunctivitis is a relatively common finding in secondary syphilis, but isolated episcleritis or scleritis is uncommon at any stage of the disease. When scleritis or episcleritis does occur, it is entirely nonspecific and usually does not progress to necrosis. The involvement of the sclera or episclera may be secondary to an immune complex reaction.

Corneal manifestations of congenital and acquired syphilis are probably the best known of all ocular manifestations. Syphilitic interstitial keratitis usually results from congenital infection but occasionally may be acquired. As there is a delay in the clinical manifestation of congenital infection, the cause of interstitial keratitis is often presumed and not apparent. It is also not clear whether inflammation arises from direct infection or from an immune complex reaction.

Clinically, acquired active interstitial keratitis consists of stromal inflammation, particularly in the peripheral cornea. Marginal infiltrates of the anterior stroma may be seen, which usually occur in association with a secondary anterior uveitis. As the uveal inflammation subsides, corneal scarring develops. Stromal neovascularization, just anterior to Descemet's membrane, is a distinctive feature of interstitial keratitis. However, in inactive interstitial keratitis, ghost vessels may lie within areas of stromal scarring and are difficult to visualize. Inactive interstitial keratitis is usually the clinical presentation of presumed congenital syphilis. Another clinical feature that has been described as being characteristic of interstitial keratitis is alteration in Descemet's membrane with the development of ridges, webs, or thick scrolls.

Cataracts have been described in association with congenital as well as acquired syphilis but are not distinctive. It is not known whether cataract is a direct manifestation of syphilis or a secondary result of intraocular inflammation.

Although numerous types of glaucoma have been described in association with syphilis, the type most often seen is secondary to uveitis and can occur in either congenital or acquired syphilitic iridocyclitis. It is thought that patients who develop interstitial keratitis early in infancy, be it congenital or acquired, may not develop a mature anterior segment and angle. This maldevelopment may cause narrow-angle glaucoma in later life.

The classical pupillary finding in syphilis is the Argyll Robertson pupil, which is most commonly seen in late syphilis

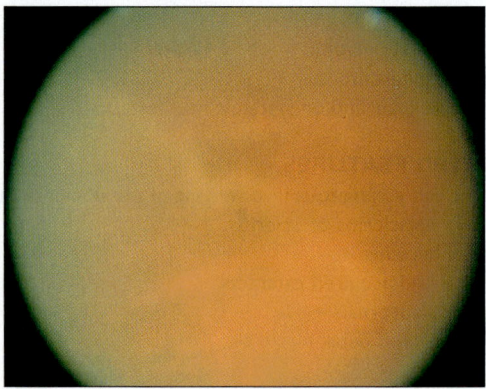

FIG. 165-4 ■ **Acute syphilitic retinitis.** This individual is infected by the human immunodeficiency virus. Note that the media is hazy from collections of inflammatory cells in the vitreous.

but may be seen in early neurosyphilis as well. The pupils are unequal in size, irregular, and miotic, with light-near dissociation (the last may also occur with a normal pupillary size). Interruption of fibers from the Edinger-Westphal nuclei that connect to the pretectal nuclei is thought to result in the light-near dissociation.

The neuro-ophthalmic manifestations of early neurosyphilis are diverse. Early neurosyphilis results in vasculitis and vascular compromise, which often presents as a stroke-like clinical finding. Therefore, any of the cranial nuclei and their pathways may be affected, which results in isolated as well as complicated palsies of the third, fourth, and sixth cranial nerves. Abnormalities of the saccadic systems and smooth pursuit systems may also occur. Other neuro-ophthalmologic manifestations that have been described include the superior orbital fissure syndrome that arises from focal gummas, brainstem infarction, basilar meningitis, homonymous hemianopia, chiasmal syndrome with bitemporal hemianopia, cortical blindness, lateral medullary plate syndrome, Horner's syndrome, and internuclear ophthalmoplegia. Late neurosyphilis may cause a general paresis and tabes dorsalis.[10–12]

DIAGNOSIS

Syphilis is the great masquerader. Therefore, diagnosis requires a high level of clinical suspicion combined with the appropriate laboratory tests. The demonstration of live organisms using dark-field microscopy or an immunofluorescent technique may confirm the diagnosis of syphilis before seroconversion occurs 10–20 days after contact. Although these tests are highly specific, they may not be very sensitive. However, serological tests are the mainstay of diagnosis. Serological tests can be divided into two groups—those that detect antibody to cardiolipin (lecithin) cholesterol antigen (nontreponemal tests) and those that detect antibodies against treponemal antigens (treponemal tests). Venereal Disease Research Laboratory (VDRL) and rapid plasma reagin (RPR) tests are the nontreponemal tests used most commonly. Of the treponemal tests, fluorescent treponemal antibody absorption tests (FTA-ABS), hemagglutination treponemal test for syphilis, hemagglutination assay for *Tr. pallidum*, and microhemagglutination tests are used most commonly. The selection and interpretation of a specific test must take into account its diagnostic sensitivity and specificity at each stage of syphilis as well as the population in which it is being used. For instance, a nontreponemal test may be suited best for general screening (in a population that shows a low prevalence of disease), and any positive results are confirmed using a treponemal test. However, when the likelihood of syphilis is high (such as in patients who have one or more of the systemic and/or ocular manifestations discussed herein), an initial treponemal test is best. Treponemal tests are at least as sensitive as and more specific than nontreponemal tests. Nontreponemal tests may be used to monitor treatment effectiveness, as the titers decrease with appropriate treatment.

In a clinically suspected case of syphilitic uveitis, a screening test such as VDRL or RPR is performed to obtain a quantitative measure of antibody production. An FTA-ABS or hemagglutination assay for *Tr. pallidum* is also obtained, either to confirm a positive screening test or to document a case of tertiary or latent syphilis, in which VDRL or RPR is often negative.

In individuals infected by HIV, both treponemal and nontreponemal tests may be unreliable, and in some patients a normal serological response to syphilis infection may be found. However, a false-negative test may occur because of insufficient antibody production or decreased immunoreactivity. False-positive tests may be encountered, particularly with nontreponemal tests, most likely because of the polyclonal B-cell activation that occurs with HIV infection. In addition, nontreponemal test titers may fail to decline after adequate therapy because of the polyclonal B-cell stimulation.[13]

The Centers for Disease Control and Prevention recommends the use of the cerebrospinal fluid (CSF)–VDRL test to establish the diagnosis of neurosyphilis when serological tests are positive. The role of CSF–FTA-ABS in the diagnosis of neurosyphilis is controversial, as it may be too sensitive. However, no absolute test exists for the diagnosis of neurosyphilis. A CSF leukocytosis and elevated CSF protein concentration present for more than 1 year in a patient at any stage of syphilis who has neurological symptoms are consistent with a diagnosis of neurosyphilis. Such patients are treated accordingly even if the CSF-VDRL test is negative. The advantage of CSF-VDRL is seen in the evaluation of patients who have suspected neurosyphilis when the possibility of previously treated disease cannot be excluded. In this situation, CSF-VDRL is superior to CSF–FTA-ABS in the differentiation of currently active neurosyphilis from past syphilis.

DIFFERENTIAL DIAGNOSIS

The ocular manifestations of syphilis in general are nonspecific. Therefore, the diagnosis always requires serological confirmation when a high index of clinical suspicion exists. The differential diagnosis of uveitis includes sarcoidosis, tuberculosis, and autoimmune uveitis. The most important conditions to rule out in the diagnosis of acute syphilitic posterior chorioretinitis are acute posterior multifocal placoid pigment epitheliopathy and atypical serpiginous choroidopathy.

It must be emphasized, however, that eventual diagnosis always requires serological confirmation. The great masquerader, however, can be uncovered only if a high degree of clinical suspicion exists.

SYSTEMIC ASSOCIATIONS

The systemic manifestations of syphilis have been divided arbitrarily into three clinical stages, which overlap. The primary stage is characterized by an ulcerative lesion called a chancre, which occurs in the site where *Tr. pallidum* penetrates the skin or mucous membrane. The organism enters the lymphatics and blood stream and disseminates shortly after contact. Only rarely is primary dissemination associated with flu-like systemic symptoms. The mean incubation period is approximately 3 weeks, within a range of 3 days to 3 months. The primary lesions heal spontaneously within 2–8 weeks.

The systemic treponemal load is largest in the secondary stage, which usually occurs 2–12 weeks after contact. This stage is characterized by fever, malaise, lymphadenopathy, and mucocutaneous lesions. Clinically apparent secondary syphilis occurs in 60–90% of patients, and one third of patients who have secondary syphilis may have the primary chancre as well. Central nervous system infection may be demonstrated in nearly one fourth of patients who have early syphilis (early syphilis includes primary, secondary, and early latent stages and is usually of less than 1 year's duration). The secondary stage of syphilis resolves in weeks to months but can recur, usually within 1 year and rarely as long as 4 years later.

The tertiary stage of syphilis refers to its late sequelae. Complications include vaso vasorum of the aorta or the central nervous system. Focal inflammatory lesions, known as gummas, may affect any organ. Approximately one third of untreated patients develop tertiary syphilis, and less than 1% develop clinical neurosyphilis. A quaternary stage of syphilis was described occasionally in the older literature, and the term has been revived for a necrotizing encephalitis that occurs in patients who have AIDS. It is useful to differentiate this aggressive form of neurosyphilis (quaternary syphilis) from the tabes dorsalis and general paresis of tertiary syphilis.

The clinical manifestations of congenital syphilis may occur at any time throughout life. An arbitrary division between early and late onset of congenital syphilis has been selected as 2 years of age. The incidence of congenital syphilis may increase as HIV infection permeates into the heterosexual population.

PATHOLOGY

Diffuse or focal lymphocytic infiltration, particularly around the blood vessels, is seen in the iris, ciliary body, or choroid. A chronic granulomatous inflammation contains epithelioid histiocytes and multinucleated giant cells. In selected cases, conjunctival biopsy obtained from patients who have granulomatous anterior uveitis may reveal a granulomatous conjunctival inflammation. In such cases, special stains for spirochetes may reveal organisms consistent with *Tr. pallidum* (Fig. 165-5).

TREATMENT[14]

Penicillin G (benzylpenicillin) is the drug of choice for the treatment of all stages of syphilis.[16] However, the duration of treatment required for various stages of syphilis remains a topic of much debate. It is accepted that early syphilis (primary, secondary, or latent of less than 1 year's duration) in immunocompetent patients may be treated effectively with one intramuscular injection of 2.4 million units of benzathine penicillin G. For patients with a penicillin allergy other antibiotics can be used; however, no other antibiotic is as effective as penicillin, and penicillin skin testing and desensitization are recommended over the use of other antibiotics. Doxycycline (100mg twice a day for 14–28 days) and tetracycline (500mg four times a day for 14–28 days) have been used.

For patients who have failed primary treatment and for patients who have syphilis of more than 1 year's duration and no evidence of central nervous system involvement, three doses of

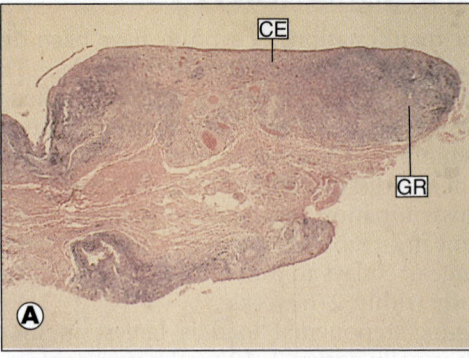

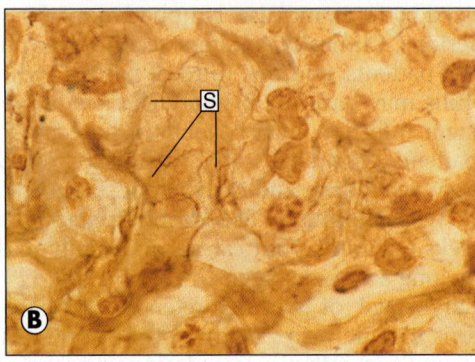

FIG. 165-5 ■ Syphilis. A, The biopsied nodules show numerous granulomas under the conjunctival epithelium (*CE*, surface conjunctival epithelium; *GR*, granulomatous reaction in substantia propria). **B,** A special stain, Dieteria, demonstrates spirochetes (*S*) within the inflammatory infiltrate. (Case reported in Spektor FE *et al.* Ophthalmology. 1981;88:863.)

2.4 million units of benzathine penicillin G intramuscularly at weekly intervals are recommended. Whether such patients need a routine lumbar puncture with examination of the CSF in the presence of a normal neurological examination is not known—asymptomatic neurosyphilis has been described in such a setting. However, the number of patients who fall into this category is not known. Risk factors for asymptomatic neurosyphilis that may justify examination of the CSF include evidence of aortitis, visceral gummas, ocular inflammation, and serum nontreponemal titers greater than 1:32.

The recommended treatment for neurosyphilis consists of intravenous aqueous penicillin G 2–4 million units every 4 hours for 10–14 days. An alternative regimen consists of daily intramuscular procaine penicillin G 2.4 million units plus oral probenecid (500mg four times a day) for 10–14 days. No alternative to penicillin has proved scientifically effective in the treatment of neurosyphilis.

Congenital syphilis has been treated with a 10- to 14-day regimen of either intravenous aqueous penicillin G or procaine penicillin G. Ceftriaxone and ampicillin have also been used as alternative antibiotics. No known optimal treatment exists for congenital syphilis.

Although no specific treatment is known for ocular syphilis, any patient who presents with ocular findings must be evaluated for neurosyphilis. Thereafter, the treatment is as described previously. However, benzathine penicillin G fails to cross the blood-brain barrier, and presumably the blood-ocular barrier, and does not consistently provide measurable levels in the CSF. Patients may need higher doses and longer duration of therapy if the eye is involved.

Treponema pallidum is thought to take a particularly aggressive course in patients who are immunocompromised by HIV. Abnormalities of CSF are known to be present in 40–60% of HIV-infected patients who do not have syphilis. Therefore, the diagnostic evaluation of the CSF in HIV-infected patients is a challenge. In this setting, HIV-infected patients who have syphilis are treated aggressively with a course sufficient to cure neurosyphilis, irrespective of the CSF examination. Certainly, overtreatment of some patients is justified by the prevention of the morbidity and mortality that often occur in immunocompromised patients.[15]

In immunocompetent patients, treatment effectiveness may be evaluated clinically and serologically. Clinical manifestations often improve after effective treatment. Seroconversion or stable low titers of nontreponemal tests also indicate effective treatment. The well-published criteria of fourfold and eightfold decreases in nontreponemal titer that should occur by 3 and 6 months, respectively, in early syphilis may be too stringent. However, evaluation of treatment effectiveness in patients who are affected simultaneously with HIV is difficult if not impossible. Given the inaccuracy of serological tests, resolution of clinical findings is most important. The inability to monitor treatment effectiveness is another reason for aggressive treatment in such patients.

Adjunctive corticosteroid therapy may be useful for some forms of ocular inflammation related to syphilis. Topical steroids are useful in patients with stromal keratitis and anterior uveitis. Prolonged treatment may be necessary to prevent a recurrence. Oral corticosteroids may be useful for scleritis, posterior uveitis, and optic neuritis. Corticosteroids should not be used without concomitant antibiotics.

COURSE AND OUTCOME

Prompt diagnosis and treatment with antimicrobial agents usually result in full visual recovery. Syphilitic intraocular inflammation untreated with penicillin or other appropriate antibiotics may lead to chronic progressive intraocular inflammation. Such an inflammatory process may lead to secondary glaucoma, chronic vitritis, retinal necrosis, and optic atrophy.

REFERENCES

1. Margo CE, Hamed LM. Ocular syphilis. Surv Ophthalmol. 1992;37:203–20.
2. Tamesis RR, Foster CS. Ocular syphilis. Ophthalmology. 1990;97:1281–7.
3. Shalaby IA, Dunn JP, Semba RD, Jabs DA. Syphilitic uveitis in human immunodeficiency virus–infected patients. Arch Ophthalmol. 1997;115:469–73.
4. Pillai S, Dipaolo F. Bilateral panuveitis, sebopsoriasis, and secondary syphilis in a patient with acquired immunodeficiency syndrome. Am J Ophthalmol. 1992;114:773–5.
5. Levy JH, Liss RA, Maquirz AM. Neurosyphilis and ocular syphilis in patients with concurrent human immunodeficiency virus infection. Retina. 1989;9:175–80.
6. Pasco MS, Rosenbaum JT. Ocular syphilis in patients with human immunodeficiency virus infection. Am J Ophthalmol. 1988;106:1–6.
7. Kuo IC, Kapusta MA, Rao NA. Vitritis as the primary manifestation of ocular syphilis in patients with HIV infection. Am J Ophthalmol. 1998;125:306–11.
8. Browning DJ. Posterior segment manifestations of active ocular syphilis, their response to a neurosyphilis regimen of penicillin therapy, and the influence of human immunodeficiency virus status on response. Ophthalmology. 2000;107:2015–23.
9. Gass JDM, Braunstein RA, Chenowith RG. Acute syphilitic posterior placoid chorioretinitis. Ophthalmology. 1990;97:1288–97.
10. Zaidman GW. Neurosyphilis and retrobulbar neuritis in a patient with AIDS. Ann Ophthalmol. 1986;18:260–1.
11. Winward KE, Hamed LM, Glaser JS. The spectrum of optic nerve disease in human immunodeficiency virus infection. Am J Ophthalmol. 1989;107:373–80.
12. Smith JL, Byene SF, Cambson CR. Syphiloma/gumma of the optic nerve and human immunodeficiency virus seropositivity. J Clin Neuroophthalmol. 1990;10:175–84.
13. Johnson PDR, Graves SR, Stewart L, et al. Specific syphilis serological tests may become negative in HIV infection. AIDS. 1991;5:419–23.
14. Centers for Disease Control and Prevention. 1998 sexually transmitted diseases treatment guidelines. MMWR Recomm Rep. 1998;47 (RR1):1–118.
15. Gordon SM, Eaton ME, George R, et al. The response of symptomatic neurosyphilis to high-dose intravenous penicillin G in patients with human immunodeficiency virus infection. N Engl J Med. 1994;331:1469–73.
16. Aldave AJ, King JA, Cunningham ET Jr. Ocular syphilis. Curr Opin Ophthalmol. 2001;12:433–41.

CHAPTER 166

Tuberculosis, Leprosy, and Brucellosis

RAJEEV BUDDI

DEFINITIONS

- Tuberculous uveitis is a granulomatous infection caused by *Mycobacterium tuberculosis* that can involve any part of the uveal tract.
- Leprosy (Hansen's disease) is a chronic granulomatous disease caused by the intracellular acid-fast bacillus *Mycobacterium leprae*.
- Brucellosis is a zoonotic disease caused by members of the genus *Brucella*.

KEY FEATURES

- Tuberculosis
  —Chronic, smoldering granulomatous lesions in the choroid or iris.
- Leprosy
  —Granulomatous infection of the facial and trigeminal nerves, eyelids, and ocular tissue.
  —Lagophthalmos.
  —Exposure keratitis.
  —Chronic anterior uveitis.
- Brucellosis
  —Granulomatous or nongranulomatous uveitis.
  —Optic nerve inflammation.
  —Hypopyon.
  —Rising titers of *Brucella* antibodies.

ASSOCIATED FEATURES

- Tuberculosis—exudative retinal detachment, hyalitis, retinal vasculitis, retinal hemorrhages, scleritis, subretinal abscess, panophthalmitis, chorioretinal atrophy.
- Leprosy—prominent or beaded corneal nerves, corneal hypoesthesia, conjunctivitis, iris pearls, iris atrophy, pinpoint pupils, ptosis, entropion.
- Brucellosis—multifocal choroiditis, chronic anterior uveitis, keratitis, conjunctivitis, posterior uveitis, cranial nerve palsies, endophthalmitis, retinal detachment.

TUBERCULOSIS

INTRODUCTION

In the past decade, tuberculosis (TB) has shown a steady decline in the United States, but the potential for debilitating ocular involvement persists. Also of concern is the emergence of drug resistance and the need for an accurate and early specific diagnosis. Newer molecular diagnostic techniques are available but are not yet standardized or universally available.

EPIDEMIOLOGY AND PATHOGENESIS

The number of tuberculosis cases has decreased during the past decade, with only 18,361 cases (6.8 cases per 100,000 population) being reported to the Centers for Disease Control and Prevention in 1998, a 34% decrease from 1990.[1] Most of these cases occur in human immunodeficiency virus (HIV)–positive individuals or those who have immigrated from countries where TB is endemic. Resistance to the development of TB may be lowered by chronic diseases, such as diabetes mellitus or malignancy, or altered immune status, as found in malnutrition, old age, or with immunosuppressive therapy.

Unlike that of systemic TB, the diagnosis of intraocular TB in most cases is based on clinical features and investigations alone and uncommonly on histological and microbiological evaluation. This, in part, accounts for the variation in the reported incidence of ocular TB in surveys of patients who have intraocular inflammation (0–0.16%) or in those who have systemic TB (0.27–1.4%).[2,3] Some reports include assumed or proven tuberculoprotein hypersensitivity–related ocular lesions, such as phlyctenulosis and retinal vasculitis. Reports of microbiologically or histopathologically proven cases of intraocular TB are relatively rare.[4–6]

Infection with *Mycobacterium* (*M.*) *tuberculosis* occurs primarily by inhalation of aerosolized droplets that contain the organisms. Usually this develops into an asymptomatic, self-limited pulmonary granuloma that resolves and remains dormant but can be reactivated later. With reactivation, the bacilli may disseminate, involve any part of the body, and cause clinically active disease (TB). Sensitization to tuberculoprotein (purified protein derivative [PPD]) develops 2–10 weeks after the initial infection, and a positive skin test may persist in the absence of clinically active disease. Ocular involvement is secondary to a primary focus in the lung or alimentary tract and uncommonly a contiguous spread from adjacent structures (secondary TB). Rarely, the eye may be the portal of entry for the organisms (primary TB).

OCULAR MANIFESTATIONS

Ocular TB may have protean manifestations, as do syphilis and sarcoidosis, and may involve any part of the eye, ocular adnexae, or orbit. Also, ocular TB may present without demonstrable active TB elsewhere in the body. The most common ocular manifestations are anterior uveitis and choroiditis or chorioretinitis.

The anterior uveitis may be granulomatous or uncommonly nongranulomatous. Rarely, tubercles or an exudative mass may occur in the anterior chamber.[4] The intensity of inflammation may vary from a mild acute iritis to a severe granulomatous reaction with granulomatous keratic precipitates and posterior synechiae.

Choroidal TB may present as tubercles or tuberculomas (large solitary masses). Choroidal tubercles occur predominantly in the posterior pole as solitary or multiple lesions (multifocal choroiditis) of various sizes, in the range 0.3–3.0mm in diameter; appear yellowish, grayish, or whitish in color; and may have overlying serous retinal detachment. The anterior segment may be normal with minimal or no hyalitis, particularly in HIV-positive individuals.[7] On fluorescein angiography (FA), these lesions are hypofluorescent initially with progressive hyperfluorescence in the late phases. Indocyanine green angiography may sometimes detect

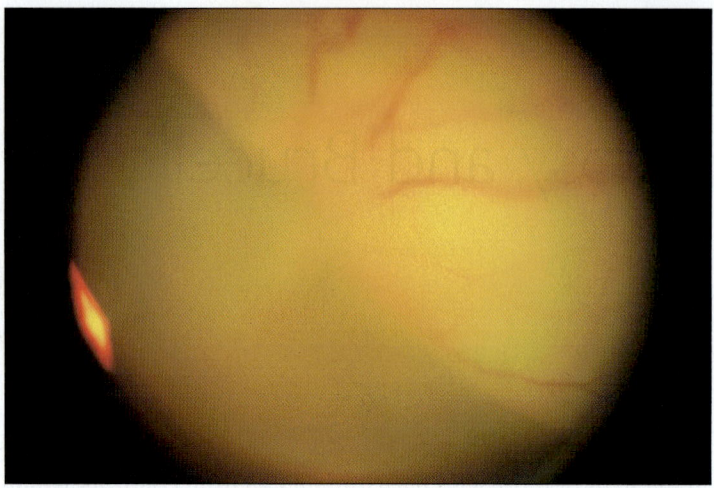

FIG. 166-1 ■ **Choroidal tuberculoma.** A large, yellow-white, subretinal mass occupies almost one quadrant of the retina in this 13-year-old child. A differential diagnosis of subretinal cysticercosis was entertained because of the presence of a coin-shaped lesion in the brain (Fig. 166-2). Chorioretinal biopsy confirmed tuberculosis (Fig. 166-3).

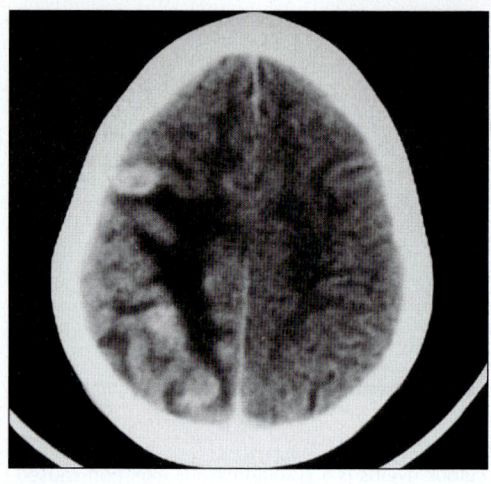

FIG. 166-2 ■ **Tuberculoma of the left temporal lobe.** Coin-shaped hyperdense lesion seen on computed tomographic scan in the same patient as shown in Figure 166-1.

BOX 166-1

Differential Diagnosis of Tuberculosis

Sarcoidosis	Behçet's syndrome
Syphilitic gummas	Cat-scratch disease
Toxoplasmosis	Leprosy
Toxocariasis	Lyme disease
Candidiasis	Leptospirosis
Coccidiomycosis	Chronic granulomatous disease
Nocardiasis	Tumor metastasis
Brucellosis	Subretinal cysticercosis

subclinical lesions or those missed by FA.[8] Choroidal tuberculomas (Fig. 166-1) present as solitary grayish white, raised lesions of area 2–3 disc diameters or larger, with indistinct margins, an overlying exudative retinal detachment, and sometimes intraretinal exudation. FA in choroidal tuberculomas may show early hyperfluorescence, with leakage around the margins in the later phases. Ultrasonography shows an acoustically dense lesion with no choroidal excavation. Low internal reflectivity and high vascularity may simulate a melanoma.[3] Isolated retinal TB is very rare. Retinal involvement is secondary to adjacent choroidal lesions, and subretinal abscess associated with TB has also been reported.[4]

Other intraocular manifestations attributed to TB include retinal vasculitis and Eales' disease. These are not the result of direct invasion by tubercle bacilli but instead are presumed to be an immunological response to the mycobacteria. This association is based on increased prevalence of tuberculoprotein hypersensitivity or concurrent active pulmonary TB in such patients. Reports of retinal vasculitis from direct infection are rare and are based on a positive response to antituberculous therapy or detection of *M. tuberculosis* DNA by polymerase chain reaction (PCR).[9]

DIAGNOSIS

Laboratory evidence of *M. tuberculosis*, using smears, cultures, and histopathology on chorioretinal, iris, or vitreous tissue, is diagnostic. Newer techniques for diagnosis such as PCR[9,10] and serological assays (to detect anticord factor antibodies)[11] are yet to be standardized and not universally available. Other ancillary tests, such as tuberculin skin testing, chest radiography, and therapeutic trials, provide only presumptive evidence for a clinical diagnosis of intraocular TB, particularly in areas endemic for TB. In immunosuppressed individuals, other species of *Mycobacterium* (e.g., *M. avium-intracellulare*) may cause opportunistic infection.

Interpretation of the diagnostic value of the Mantoux test using PPD is difficult,[2,3] but a negative reaction is more important than a positive one. Induration >5mm indicates prior exposure rather than an active infection, and indurations >10mm in a high-risk population and >15mm in a low-risk population are significant. The specificity of the PPD skin test is interpreted from the size of the reaction, contact history, regional prevalence of TB, and age and immune status of the patient. Because TB is a rare cause of uveitis, a positive PPD in a patient who has uveitis but no other signs of TB is more misleading than helpful.

DIFFERENTIAL DIAGNOSIS

Various entities that may mimic tuberculous uveitis are given in Box 166-1.

SYSTEMIC ASSOCIATIONS

In addition to the eye, TB can involve any part of the body. Choroidal tubercles indicate hematogenous spread of bacilli and may be associated with miliary TB.[2,3] Uncommonly, ocular involvement may occur with concurrent extraocular TB, such as pulmonary TB, tuberculous lymphadenitis, TB of the alimentary tract, and tuberculoma of the brain (Fig. 166-2).

PATHOLOGY

A characteristic caseating, granulomatous inflammation results from infection by *M. tuberculosis* (Fig. 166-3), which consists of a central caseation surrounded by epithelioid cells, multinucleated giant cells of the Langerhans type, and lymphocytes. Absence of giant cells and caseation, however, does not exclude the diagnosis of TB. In immunocompromised individuals, histopathology may reveal mononuclear cells only, with no epithelioid cells and giant cells, but with abundant acid-fast bacilli (nonreactive TB).[12]

TREATMENT

Treatment of intraocular TB is often problematic because it is difficult to establish the cause conclusively, particularly for the patient who has uveitis compatible with TB, a positive PPD, and no other systemic evidence of TB. In such cases the use of a 2- to 3-week therapeutic trial with single or multiple drugs is recommended, with ocular evaluation each week. If ocular inflammation improves, the patient is considered to have a positive test response and a full course of anti-TB therapy is advised. However,

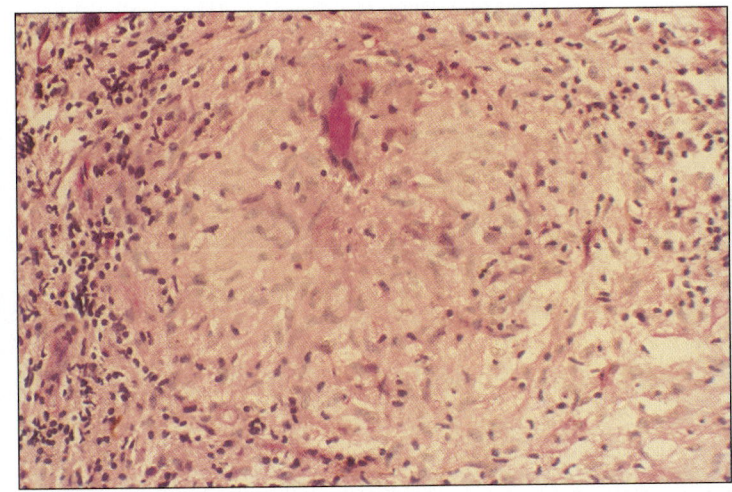

FIG. 166-3 ■ **Tuberculous granuloma with central caseation.** Chorioretinal biopsy from the choroidal lesion shown in Figure 166-1. Hematoxylin-eosin–stained sections show multiple granulomas with caseation and multinucleated giant cells. Acid-fast stains did not reveal any organisms.

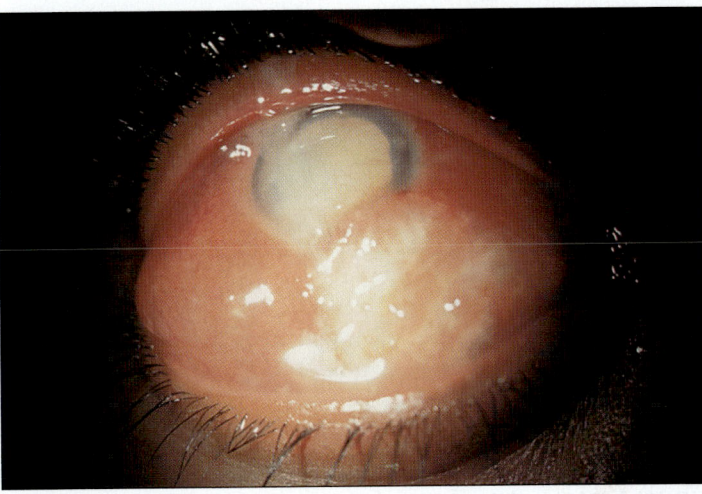

FIG. 166-4 ■ **Tuberculous panophthalmitis.** Conjunctival granuloma with chemosis and yellow-white pupillary reflex in an 11-year-old girl, initially treated as infective endophthalmitis. Conjunctival biopsy showed multiple caseating granulomas and giant cells. The inflammation responded positively to a three-drug antituberculosis regimen.

concurrent use of anti-inflammatory agents or a natural temporary regression of inflammation may reduce the value of this test. Alternatively, if anti-inflammatory therapy alone fails to control the inflammation, an anterior chamber tap, vitreous aspirate, or chorioretinal biopsy may be carried out to obtain a definitive laboratory diagnosis.

Multidrug anti-TB therapy is preferably administered by an internist well versed in current treatment recommendations and drug resistance. The duration of therapy and drug combination depend on the type of extraocular TB, immune status of the individual, and drug resistance. The concomitant use of corticosteroids is still controversial because of fear of exacerbation of the infection, but in vision-threatening cases corticosteroid may be used in low doses with a careful follow-up.

COURSE AND OUTCOME

Early diagnosis and treatment appears to be associated with a good prognosis. One series reported a good response to anti-TB treatment in only 3 of 12 patients who had suspected intraocular TB,[13] whereas others noted improvement in only 2 of 5[4] and 2 of 4[6] histologically or microbiologically proved cases. Spread of TB choroiditis to involve the retina may occur, and iridocyclitis (if untreated) may involve the sclera with a resultant uveal tissue prolapse and glaucoma. Extraocular spread may result in panophthalmitis (Fig. 166-4).

LEPROSY

EPIDEMIOLOGY AND PATHOGENESIS

Leprosy affects 10 million to 12 million people worldwide, 3–7% of whom are blind.[14] A total of 108 cases of Hansen's disease were reported in the United States in 1998.[1] The highest prevalence of leprosy occurs in the Indian subcontinent, sub-Saharan Africa, and Southeast Asia.

Mycobacterium (M.) leprae has a tropism for body areas that have low temperatures, particularly the skin, peripheral nerves, nasal mucosa, and the eye. The mode of transmission is probably through the mucous membrane of the upper respiratory tract or the skin. Leprosy is divided into two major subtypes on the basis of the host immune response.[15] In the tuberculoid type, an active, cell-mediated immune response is seen, whereas in the lepromatous type patients have a poor cellular immune response. In addition to this, acute reactional states (type I and type II) that arise from acute changes in the immune status are

described. Intraocular inflammatory disease occurs more commonly in the lepromatous type. Ocular manifestations depend on the duration of infection, the immune response, and the time of initiation and type of treatment. Paralysis of the trigeminal and facial nerve results in lid abnormalities and corneal hypoesthesia, which results in corneal damage. Direct bacterial invasion of the external eye results in keratitis, scleritis, and iritis, which may also occur during the reactional stages of the disease. Destruction of the autonomic nerve fibers that supply the eye results in pinpoint pupil and a low-grade iridocyclitis.

OCULAR MANIFESTATIONS

Comprehensive ocular evaluations of leprosy patients show that uveitis occurs in about 7%,[14,16] whereas other reports indicate an incidence of 5.3–63%.[17] Iritis or iridocyclitis is the main complication. Acute anterior iridocyclitis is uncommon, occurs bilaterally, and develops during the reactional state (type II), especially with therapy or sometimes after cessation of therapy. This granulomatous anterior uveitis may be associated with a hyphema or hypopyon. A chronic, low-grade bilateral uveitis with minimal or no symptoms until late in the disease process is more common. It is associated with few, scattered, fine, white keratic precipitates, few anterior chamber cells, mild to moderate flare, and minimal ciliary or conjunctival congestion. Posterior synechiae are uncommon. If not aggressively treated, pinpoint pupils, glaucoma or hypotony, iris atrophy, ciliary body damage, and cataract occur insidiously and result in loss of vision. Iris pearls are characteristic of leprosy (Fig. 166-5) and are seen on the anterior surface of the iris or at the pupillary border as creamy white particles. After several years, they may coalesce and drop into the inferior angle, where they may be observed by gonioscopy.[15] Rarely, choroiditis, pars planitis, and uveal effusion associated with overlying scleral inflammation have been reported.[15]

DIAGNOSIS

Diagnosis is usually made easily on the basis of a thorough clinical evaluation but must be confirmed by histology of the skin lesions or skin biopsy. Iris pearls are characteristic. Skin tests with lepromin may be highly positive (Mitsuda reaction) in the tuberculoid type.

DIFFERENTIAL DIAGNOSIS

The differential diagnosis of leprosy-associated uveitis is given in Box 166-2.

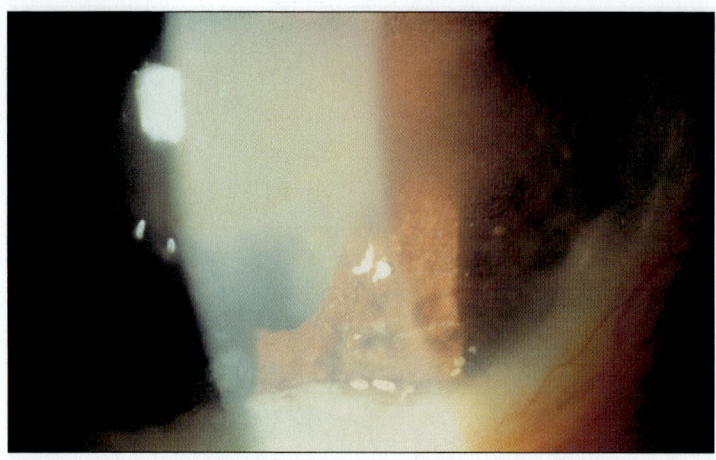

FIG. 166-5 ■ Iris pearls in a patient who has leprosy. (Courtesy of Dr. G.C. Sekhar.)

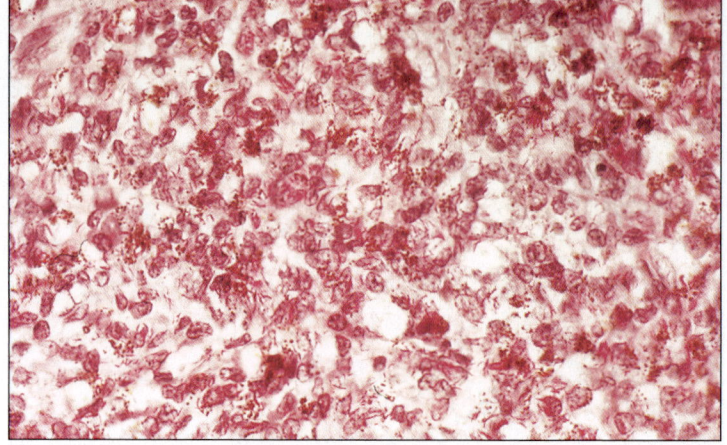

FIG. 166-6 ■ Cells teem with acid-fast leprous organisms (red color), seen with the Ziehl-Neelsen method. The patient had lepromatous leprosy. (Courtesy of Dr. P. Henkind. In Yanoff M, Fine BS. Ocular pathology, ed 4. London, Mosby, 1996.)

BOX 166-2

Differential Diagnosis of Leprosy-Associated Uveitis

Tuberculosis	Idiopathic anterior uveitis
Sarcoidosis	Syphilis

SYSTEMIC ASSOCIATIONS

The common systemic manifestations of leprosy consist of hypopigmented skin lesions, skin anesthesia, thickened peripheral nerves, deformed hands and feet, and leonine facies.

PATHOLOGY

The tuberculoid form of disease is characterized by granuloma formation and the lack of a large number of bacilli because of an active cell-mediated immune response. In contrast to this, lesions in the lepromatous form are composed predominantly of macrophages with numerous acid-fast bacilli (Fig. 166-6). Iris pearls consist of macrophages filled with bacilli.

TREATMENT

Because of the chronicity and insidious nature of this anterior uveitis, early screening for ocular complications, to detect asymptomatic disease, is advisable. Once detected, regular (every 1–6 months) eye examinations are advisable, depending on the severity of the uveitis and its response to therapy. Supervision of continuous corticosteroid and mydriatic therapy at home is necessary,[17] along with appropriate antimicrobial therapy. Multidrug treatment (MDT) instituted in 1982 by the World Health Organization has resulted in sustained high microbiological cure rates. However, leprosy-related ocular pathology such as lagophthalmos, posterior synechiae, and keratitis continues to develop after a microbiological cure and therefore regular monitoring is required.[18]

BRUCELLOSIS

EPIDEMIOLOGY AND PATHOGENESIS

The disease has a very low incidence in the United States (total of 79 cases reported in 1998),[1] with higher rates in the less developed countries. *Brucella* (*Bru.*) is a bacterium that infects the genitourinary tract of domestic animals such as sheep (*Bru. melitensis*), cattle (*Bru. abortus*), swine (*Bru. suis*), and dogs (*Bru.*

canis). Human beings become infected by direct contact or by airborne spread after exposure to infected animals, contaminated meat, or dairy products. Infection occurs mostly among farmers and abattoir workers.

OCULAR MANIFESTATIONS

Brucellosis may affect all the ocular structures, but uveitis with or without optic nerve involvement appears to be the most common result.[19,20] The uveitis may be granulomatous or nongranulomatous and unilateral or bilateral. Anterior, intermediate, and posterior uveitis may occur in patients who have brucellosis. Anterior uveitis may result in hypopyon, which responds well to topical corticosteroids. Rarely, acute brucellosis may manifest as endophthalmitis with sudden loss of vision.[21] Choroiditis that results from brucellosis is usually multifocal and either nodular or geographic.[19] Optic nerve involvement appears as hyperemia, retrobulbar neuritis, papilledema, or arachnoiditis of the chiasm.[19] Vitreous exudates, cystoid macular edema, and retinal detachment have also been reported.

DIAGNOSIS

For a definitive etiological diagnosis, laboratory investigations are necessary in addition to the ocular and systemic clinical manifestations. Blood, vitreous, or aqueous cultures may give positive results in the acute stages. In chronic stages, it is more difficult to isolate the organisms. To be cultured, *Brucella* species require careful laboratory processing.[19] Serological investigations for the detection of brucella antibodies vary in sensitivity and specificity.[19] Serum antibody titers are high in chronic stages, whereas recent infections are associated with low titers. The standard agglutination test can also be carried out using vitreous and aqueous samples.[19,22]

DIFFERENTIAL DIAGNOSIS

The entities listed in Box 166-3 are considered in the differential diagnosis of brucellosis.

SYSTEMIC ASSOCIATIONS

In the acute stage, systemic infection is characterized by fever, headache, arthralgia, generalized aches, chills, sweating, malaise, anorexia, and weight loss. More than 90% of patients have intermittent fever with a characteristic diurnal variation as the fever tends to peak daily in the afternoon.[19,21] Splenomegaly and diffuse lymphadenopathy occur in as many as 30% of patients.[19] Pneumonia, hepatitis, splenic abscess, epididymo-orchitis, prostatitis, endocarditis, arthritis, osteomyelitis, and meningoencephalitis have been reported.

TREATMENT

It is not clear whether antibiotic therapy is helpful for uveitis associated with brucellosis. The treatment of brucellosis requires more than one agent to decrease the incidence of relapses. Therapy with combinations of tetracyclines, cephalosporins, rifampin, trimethoprim-sulfamethoxazole, and aminoglycosides has been employed.[19] Effective treatment often requires prolonged therapy (4–8 weeks).

COURSE AND PROGNOSIS

The severity and chronicity of disease in humans vary with the species and strain. Most of the infections with *Bru. abortus* involve a self-limited disease, whereas *Bru. melitensis* or *Bru. suis* may cause more severe or chronic disease. As with tuberculosis, the disease may become chronic and the organism may persist in tissue for years.[19]

REFERENCES

1. Summary of notifiable diseases, United States, 1998. MMWR Morb Mortal Wkly Rep. 1999;53:1–93.
2. Copeland RA Jr. The classics: tuberculosis, syphilis, and sarcoidosis. Ophthalmol Clin North Am. 1993;6:69–80.
3. Helm CJ, Holland GN. Ocular tuberculosis. Surv Ophthalmol. 1993;38:229–56.
4. Biswas JB, Madhavan HN, Gopal L, Badrinath SS. Intraocular tuberculosis. Clinicopathologic study of five cases. Retina. 1995;15:461–8.
5. Morinelli EN, Dugel RU, Riffenburgh R, Rao NA. Infectious multifocal choroiditis in patients with acquired immune deficiency syndrome. Ophthalmology. 1993;100:1014–21.
6. Sheu SJ, Shyu SJ, Chen LM, et al. Ocular manifestations of tuberculosis. Ophthalmology. 2001;108:1580–5.
7. DiLoreto DA Jr, Rao NA. Solitary nonreactive choroidal tuberculoma in a patient with acquired immune deficiency syndrome. Am J Ophthalmol. 2001;131:138–40.
8. Wolfensberger TJ, Piguet B, Herbort CP. Indocyanine green angiographic features in tuberculous chorioretinitis. Am J Ophthalmol. 1999;127:350–3.
9. Madhavan HN, Therese KL, Gunisha P, et al. Polymerase chain reaction for detection of *Mycobacterium tuberculosis* in epiretinal membrane in Eales' disease. Invest Ophthalmol Vis Sci. 2000;41:822–5.
10. Kotake S, Kimura K, Yoshikawa K, et al. Polymerase chain reaction for the detection of *Mycobacterium tuberculosis* in ocular tuberculosis. Am J Ophthalmol. 1994;117:805–6.
11. Sakai J, Matsuzawa S, Usui M, et al. New diagnostic approach for ocular tuberculosis by ELISA using the cord factor as antigen. Br J Ophthalmol. 2001;85:130–3.
12. Croxatto JO, Mestre C, Puente S, Gonzalez G. Nonreactive tuberculosis in a patient with acquired immune deficiency syndrome. Am J Ophthalmol. 1986;102:659–60.
13. Rosen PH, Spalton DJ, Graham EM. Intraocular tuberculosis. Eye. 1990;4:486–92.
14. Dana MR, Hochman MA, Viana MAG, et al. Ocular manifestations of leprosy in a noninstitutionalized community in the United States. Arch Ophthalmol. 1994;112:626–9.
15. Schwab IR, Ostler HB, Dawson CR. Hansen's disease of the eye (ocular leprosy). In: Tasman W, Jaeger EA, eds. Duane's clinical ophthalmology, Vol 5. Philadelphia: JB Lippincott; 2000.
16. Sekhar GC, Vance G, Otton S, et al. Ocular manifestations of Hansen's disease. Doc Ophthalmol. 1994;87:211–21.
17. Espiritu CG, Gelber R, Ostler HB. Chronic anterior uveitis in leprosy: an insidious cause of blindness. Br J Ophthalmol. 1991;75:273–5.
18. Lewallen S, Tungpakorn NC, Kim SH, et al. Progression of eye disease in "cured" leprosy patients: implications for understanding the pathophysiology of ocular disease and for addressing eyecare needs. Br J Ophthalmol. 2000;84:817–21.
19. Al-Kaff AS. Ocular brucellosis. In: Tabbara KF, ed. Posterior uveitis—Part II. Int Ophthalmol Clin. 1995;35:139–45.
20. Puig-Solanes M, Heatley J, Arenas F, et al. Ocular complications in brucellosis. Am J Ophthalmol. 1953;36:675–89.
21. Al-Faran MF. *Brucella melitensis* endogenous endophthalmitis. Ophthalmologica. 1990;201:19–22.
22. Akduman L, Or M, Hasenreisoglu B, Kurtark K. A case of ocular brucellosis: importance of ocular specimen. Acta Ophthalmol. 1993;71:130–2.

Spirochete Infections: Lyme Disease and Leptospirosis

SOMASHEILA I. MURTHY • NARSING A. RAO

Lyme Disease

DEFINITION
• Lyme disease is characterized by dermatological, neurological, cardiac, rheumatic, and ophthalmic manifestations that result from tick-borne transmission of the spirochete *Borrelia burgdorferi*.

KEY FEATURES
• Three chronological stages:
  1. Primary or initial phase—rash at the site of tick bite (erythema chronicum migrans) and flu-like symptoms.
  2. Secondary or dissemination stage—further dermatological, cardiac, and neurological manifestations.
  3. Tertiary or late stage—arthritis, meningoencephalitis, cranial neuropathy, peripheral neuropathy, carditis.

ASSOCIATED FEATURES
• Conjunctivitis, most common manifestation in stage 1.
• Cranial nerve palsies, optic nerve inflammation can occur in stage 2.
• Corneal, uveal, and retinal inflammation can occur in stage 3.

Leptospirosis

DEFINITION
• Leptospirosis is a zoonotic infection of worldwide distribution caused by pathogenic *Leptospira* species.

KEY FEATURES
• Biphasic disease.
• Leptospiremic phase—severe headache, fever, myalgia.
• Immune phase—high fever, meningismus, central and peripheral nervous system manifestations.
• Ocular manifestations occur in the majority of patients.
• Conjunctivitis, uveitis, subconjunctival hemorrhages.

ASSOCIATED FEATURE
• Weil's disease—severe disease with hemorrhages, renal failure, and jaundice.

LYME DISEASE

INTRODUCTION

Lyme disease has a worldwide distribution with a growing incidence. It is the most common arthropod-borne disease in the United States and Europe,[1] and endemic areas are distributed throughout North America, Europe, and northern Asia. The endemic areas support a reservoir for the spirochete in a host (such

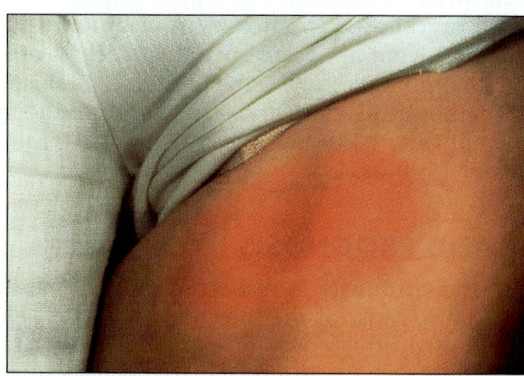

FIG. 167-1 ■ Note a single large erythematous lesion involving the skin known as erythema chronicum migrans. (Adapted with permission of the American Academy of Ophthalmology from Basic and clinical science course. San Francisco: American Academy of Ophthalmology; 1998–1999.)

as deer) and the critical arthropod vector, an *Ixodes* tick. The disease takes its name from the town of Lyme, Connecticut, where an outbreak of chronic arthritis in children occurred in 1975.[1] The infectious agent was identified in 1982 as a spirochete and named *Borrelia burgdorferi*.[2,3]

EPIDEMIOLOGY AND PATHOGENESIS

In the United States, it is endemic in the northeast in Connecticut, Westchester, and Long Island; in the midwest in Minnesota and Wisconsin; and in the northwest in Washington, Oregon, and northern California. It has also been reported as the most frequent vector-borne disease in Germany, Austria, Sweden, France, and Switzerland as well as in Asia and Australia.[4]

As with syphilis, the disease usually progresses in three phases. Stage 1 disease is thought to be due to spirochetemia, whereas stages 2 and 3 may be due to the immunological response of the host to parasitic invasion or due to a vasculitis.[5] The initial or early phase usually includes the pathognomonic rash, called erythema migrans, at the site of the tick bite. It is characterized by an annular, expanding erythematous margin, often with a central area of clearing. The size of the skin lesion is at least 5cm (Fig. 167-1). This stage begins days to weeks after the bite and may also include fever, flu-like symptoms, and arthralgias. However, the history of tick bite or rash may be absent in over 50% of individuals.[6]

The second phase is the phase of dissemination of the spirochete. It occurs within days, weeks, or even months after infection and reflects the spread of the organism to multiple organ systems, especially the skin, heart, joints, and the nervous system.[7,8] Neurological manifestations are typical of this stage and consist of meningoencephalitis, cranial neuropathy (especially Bell's palsy), and peripheral neuropathy.[8] Carditis (especially conduction defects) and chronic arthritis may also develop.[9] The initial skin lesion fades and then reappears. Another skin lesion, the lymphocytoma, may develop as a purplish nodule, especially on the earlobe or breast.[8]

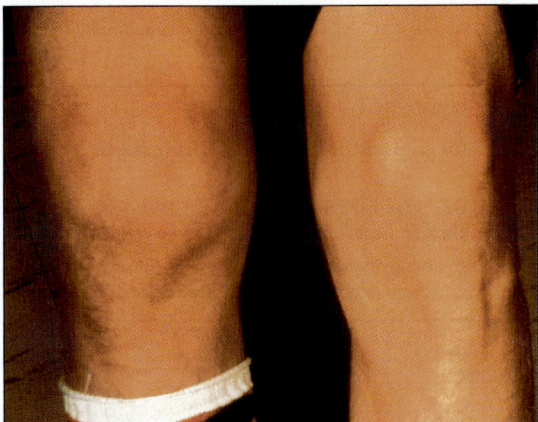

FIG. 167-2 ■ Inflammation involving knee joint in Lyme disease. (Adapted with permission of the American Academy of Ophthalmology from Basic and clinical science course. San Francisco: American Academy of Ophthalmology; 1998–1999.)

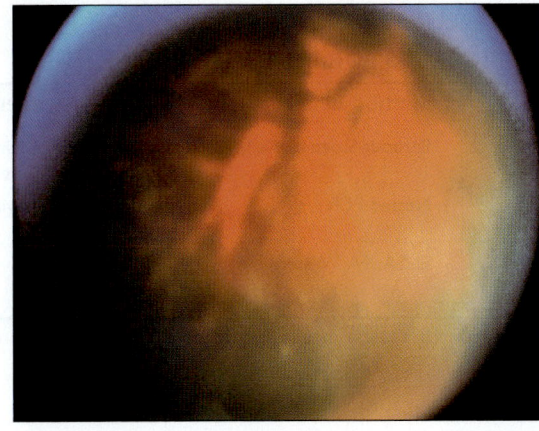

FIG. 167-3 ■ Moderate degree of vitritis is noted in Lyme disease. The vitritis can simulate pars planitis. (Adapted with permission of the American Academy of Ophthalmology from Basic and clinical science course. San Francisco: American Academy of Ophthalmology; 1998–1999.)

TABLE 167-1

OCULAR MANIFESTATIONS IN LYME DISEASE

Stage 1	Stage 2	Stage 3
Conjunctivitis, photophobia, periorbital edema	Iridocyclitis, vitritis, choroiditis, panophthalmitis, exudative retinal detachment, retinal vasculitis, macular edema, papilledema Optic neuritis and motility abnormalities	Stromal keratitis, episcleritis, symblepharon, orbital myositis

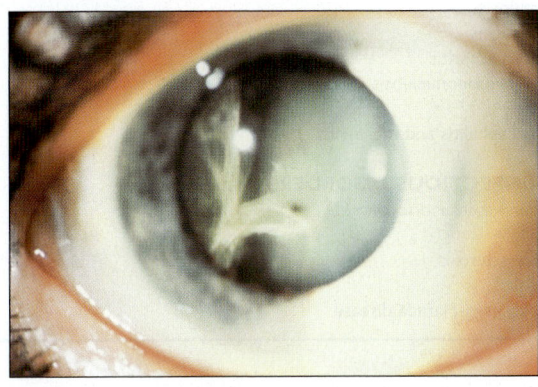

FIG. 167-4 ■ Ocular Lyme disease showing dense vitreous debris. (Adapted with permission of the American Academy of Ophthalmology from Basic and clinical science course. San Francisco: American Academy of Ophthalmology; 1998–1999.)

The third or late stage of disease can occur after a long disease-free period, which can be months to years, and may involve recurrent manifestations. Late stage can occur in spite of early antibiotic treatment. The hallmark manifestation of this stage is chronic, relapsing arthritis.[1,7–10] The knee is the joint most commonly affected (Fig. 167-2). Skin changes include a rash known as acrodermatitis chronica atrophicans, which eventually resolves, leaving atrophy of the skin and underlying structures. Late neurological manifestations in this stage include encephalopathy, demyelination, and dementia. The ocular manifestations occur in all three stages, and they are summarized in Table 167-1.

OCULAR MANIFESTATIONS

Unlike the significant cutaneous, neurological, and rheumatologic manifestations in Lyme disease, ocular findings are generally not prominent.[7] Conjunctivitis is the most common ocular manifestation of Lyme disease; it is present in approximately 11% of patients who have early Lyme disease.[1,10] The conjunctivitis is a nonspecific conjunctival inflammation and resolves on its own. Photophobia and periorbital edema are also mild and self-limiting.[1] Neuro-ophthalmic complications can be commonly seen in stage 2, as part of the neurological involvement. These include ocular motility problems and diplopia due to cranial nerve palsies; optic nerve inflammation, papilledema, and pseudotumor cerebri occur in association with meningoencephalitis.[7,10–13]

Intraocular inflammations in the form of chorioretinitis and other forms of uveitis, especially vitreous inflammation (Figs. 167-3 and 167-4), have been described in Lyme disease.[14–16] Vitreous organization that results in the appearance of a "spiderweb" vitritis has been described.[17] Patchy, stromal keratitis, episcleritis, and symblepharon have also been reported in stage 3 disease.[18–20]

DIAGNOSIS AND ANCILLARY TESTING

Clinical diagnosis of Lyme disease is based on the appearance of the pathognomonic skin rash—erythema chronicum migrans (EM)—in a patient either with a history of tick bite or in an area endemic for Lyme disease (or both). In patients unaware of the tick bite or in a nonendemic area, appearance of EM as well as involvement of two organ systems is adequate for diagnosis. The diagnostic criteria for Lyme disease recommended by the Centers for Disease Control and Prevention[21,22] are listed in Box 167-1.

Definitive diagnosis of Lyme disease is made with a culture of *B. burgdorferi* in Barbour-Stoenner-Kelly medium.[21] Spirochetes can be isolated from peripheral blood,[23] areas of skin rash,[24] and

TABLE 167-2

DIAGNOSTIC TESTS FOR LYME DISEASE

Test type	Method details	Specimens	Diagnostic value
Culture	Barbour-Stoenner-Kelly medium	Plasma, skin lesion, synovial fluid, and cerebrospinal fluid (CSF)	100% diagnostic, high yield only in early stages
PCR	Nested PCR	CSF, synovial fluid, vitreous	Highly diagnostic, technically difficult, low yield, useful for chronic stage
Serology	ELISA, IFA, Western blot	Serum	High sensitivity, low specificity, negative in stage 1, 90% positive in stages 2 and 3 (Western blot 100% in stages 2 and 3)[4]

ELISA, Enzyme-linked immunosorbent assay; *IFA,* immunofluorescent antibody assay.

BOX 167-2

Differential Diagnosis of Lyme Disease

INFECTIOUS DISORDERS
Syphilis
Tuberculosis
Viral keratitis
Infectious arthritis
Infectious mononucleosis
Mumps
Viral encephalitis and meningitis

NONINFECTIOUS DISORDERS
Collagen vascular disorders
Sarcoid
Multiple sclerosis
Vasculitis
Vogt-Koyanagi-Harada disease

BOX 167-3

Treatment for Lyme Disease

EARLY INFECTION—LOCAL OR DISSEMINATED
Adults   Doxycycline 100mg orally twice daily for 14 to 21 days
          Amoxicillin 500mg orally three times a day for 14 to 21 days
In case of doxycycline/amoxicillin allergy:
          Cefuroxime 500mg orally twice daily for 14 to 21 days
          Erythromycin 250mg orally four times daily for 14–21 days
Children   Amoxicillin 50mg per kilogram of body weight per day in three divided doses for 14 to 21 days
In case of penicillin allergy:
          Cefuroxime 30mg per kg per day in two divided doses for 14 to 21 days

NEUROLOGICAL AND/OR OCULAR ABNORMALITIES (EARLY OR LATE)
Adults   Ceftriaxone 2g IV once a day for 14 to 28 days
          Cefotaxime 2g IV every 8 hours for 14 to 28 days
In case of ceftriaxone or penicillin allergy:
          Doxycycline 100mg orally 3 times a day for 30 days
Children   Ceftriaxone 75 to 100mg per kg per day (maximum 2g) IV once a day for 14 to 28 days
          Cefotaxime 150mg per kg per day in 3 to 4 divided doses (maximum 6g) for 14 to 28 days

Adapted from Steere AC. Lyme disease. N Engl J Med. 2001;345:115–25.
Avoid doxycycline in pregnant women.

---

cerebrospinal fluid samples.[25] However, these positive cultures have been obtained only in the early stages of the disease. In the chronic stages, polymerase chain reaction (PCR)[26] testing has been used in detection of the spirochete.

The ocular manifestations of Lyme disease are protean and can occur several years after the initial tick bite; therefore, serological tests are often the only aids for diagnosis. The enzyme-linked immunosorbent assay (ELISA) and indirect immunofluorescent antibody (IFA) assay are the most commonly employed tests. These tests detect the presence of antibodies (both immunoglobulin G [IgG] and IgM) specific for *B. burgdorferi.* However, serodiagnostic tests are insensitive during the first few weeks of infection. After 1 month, the majority of patients have IgG antibody responses, even after treatment with antibiotics.[25]

Although these tests are highly sensitive for *B. burgdorferi,* the specificity is low and cross-reactivity with other spirochetes is often seen.[27,28] Approximately 10% of the population has a falsely positive serological test for Lyme disease. Screening all patients with uveitis for possible Lyme disease would result in many more false-positive results relative to true positive results.[29] Occasionally, patients who have well-documented Lyme disease also have a negative serological study for Lyme disease. It is recommended that serological testing for Lyme disease be reserved for patients who have uveitis of unknown cause and at least one other manifestation of the disease, such as a knee arthritis or an encephalitis within the spectrum of Lyme disease. Other diagnostic tests include Western blot analysis, lymphocyte antigen stimulation, antibody capture enzyme immunoassay, and detection of antibodies in urine.

The various diagnostic tests are summarized in Table 167-2.

DIFFERENTIAL DIAGNOSIS

The differential diagnosis is summarized in Box 167-2.

PATHOLOGY

The mechanisms[8,9,30,31] underlying the multisystem presentations are thought to be due to direct invasion of tissues by the *Borrelia* spirochete in stage 1. In the later stages, perivascular infiltration of plasma cells leading to small-vessel obliteration and vasculitis has been observed.

TREATMENT AND PREVENTION

Medical treatment for Lyme disease is summarized in Box 167-3. Although there is some consensus on the systemic treatment for Lyme disease, because of the less frequent occurrence of ocular manifestations, the most effective treatment strategy for ocular disease is unclear.[4] Generally, patients benefit from systemic treatment as outlined in Box 167-3. The use of corticosteroids is controversial, with reports of a higher incidence of relapses.[7] Topical corticosteroids have been used beneficially in keratitis and episcleritis.[18–20] However, treatment failures have been reported with all regimens[32] and clinical response can take as long as 1 year. Inadequate early treatment can lead to relapses and facilitate late manifestations.[7]

Preventive measures in endemic areas include use of protective clothing, repellents, and acaricides; tick checks; and landscape modifications.[33] Vaccination is considered for those between the ages of 15 to 70 who live in or are likely to visit endemic areas.[33,34] Three injections of the vaccine are recommended at intervals of 0, 1, and 12 months, with booster injections given every 1 to 3 years.[35] In case of tick bite, a single dose

TABLE 167-3

SYSTEMIC MANIFESTATIONS IN LEPTOSPIROSIS

Stage	Leptospiremic	Immune
Onset	First week of disease, abrupt onset	Second week
Duration	4 to 9 days	Undetermined
Manifestations—common	Severe headaches, fever with spikes, chills, myalgia, abdominal pain, skin rash, arthralgia	High fever, meningismus, encephalitis, cranial nerve palsies of 6th, 7th, and 8th cranial nerves, peripheral neuropathy
Manifestations—rare	Jaundice, altered consciousness, cardiac	Spontaneous abortion during pregnancy

TABLE 167-4

OCULAR MANIFESTATIONS OF LEPTOSPIROSIS

Anterior	Posterior	Miscellaneous
Conjunctivitis	Pars planitis	Periorbital pain
Subconjunctival hemorrhage	Vitritis	Facial palsy
	Periphlebitis	Palpebral herpes
Scleral icterus	Retinal exudates	
Keratitis	Choroiditis	
Iridocyclitis	Papillitis	
	Optic neuritis	
	Macular edema	
	Retinal hemorrhages	
	Retinal arteritis	

BOX 167-4

Differential Diagnosis of Leptospirosis

HLA-B27–related uveitis	Syphilis
Behçet's disease	Leprosy
Eales' disease	Sarcoidosis
Endophthalmitis	Toxoplasmosis
Tuberculosis	

of 200mg of doxycycline can prevent Lyme disease when given within 72 hours of the tick bite.[36]

COURSE AND OUTCOME

Untreated disease can have a chronic relapsing course for several years, with late neurological sequelae similar to those seen in syphilis. The majority of patients respond well to systemic antibiotic therapy. However, posterior segment manifestations (vitritis), late occurring stromal keratitis, and neurotrophic keratitis are slow to respond to treatment.

LEPTOSPIROSIS

INTRODUCTION

Leptospirosis is a zoonotic infection of worldwide distribution caused by spirochetes of the genus *Leptospira*.[37] It manifests as an acute febrile illness or a flu-like syndrome, with ocular involvement, commonly in the form of uveitis. Adolf Weil[38] first reported a severe form of leptospirosis in 1886, which was subsequently called Weil's disease. The etiological agent of Weil's disease was discovered in 1915.[39]

EPIDEMIOLOGY AND PATHOGENESIS

Leptospirosis is a worldwide disease with higher incidence and prevalence in the tropical and subtropical regions, where exposures to infected animals and contaminated water are common.[40] The natural reservoir for pathogenic leptospira is wild animals, especially rodents, as well as domestic animals including livestock and dogs.[41] Humans are accidental hosts, and infection is due to contact with infected urine, tissues, or water.[41] People at high risk for the disease include farmers, veterinarians, abattoir workers, miners, and sewer workers.[42] Pathological leptospira belong to the species *Leptospira interrogans*.[43]

CLINICAL MANIFESTATIONS

The disease is often biphasic, with varying severity. The two phases are summarized in Table 167-3. Weil's disease is a severe form of leptospirosis, with jaundice and hepatomegaly, azotemia, hemorrhages, anemia, persistent fever, and altered mental status. Hepatic and renal dysfunction occurs early, with high mortality in untreated cases.[41]

OCULAR MANIFESTATIONS

Ocular complications can occur from 2 weeks to 6 months after the febrile stage and can lead to decreased vision and blindness.[37,39,44] The ocular manifestations are summarized in Table 167-4.

DIAGNOSIS AND ANCILLARY TESTING

Culture of the organism from body fluids (blood or cerebrospinal fluid) is the "gold standard" for diagnosis. Serological testing includes the microscopic slide agglutination test. This is considered to be the reference test for the serological diagnosis of leptospirosis[45]; however, this test may not be practical in establishing the diagnosis in a timely manner.[44–46]

Specific combined PCR hybridization assay of the *Leptospira* 16S ribosomal ribonucleic acid (rRNA) gene, as well as conventional PCR, is now widely used for detection of *Leptospira* DNA in various samples (blood, urine, aqueous humor, cerebrospinal fluid).[47] PCR assay is highly sensitive and specific and allows early diagnosis.[44]

DIFFERENTIAL DIAGNOSIS

Systemic leptospirosis has protean manifestations and may not be easily diagnosed (except for Weil's disease). Ophthalmic manifestations are variable (Table 167-4). The systemic disease mimics influenza and other acute febrile illnesses. The differential diagnosis for ocular disease is summarized in Box 167-4.

TREATMENT AND PREVENTION

The penicillin group of drugs (penicillin 1.5 million units intravenously or ampicillin 500 to 1000mg 6 hourly for 10 days) is the mainstay in treatment for systemic disease. For ocular disease, combination therapy with quinolones and cyclins has been recommended[44] in the doses of amoxicillin plus clavulanic acid (1.5g/day) and pefloxacin (800mg/day) for 3 weeks. Corticosteroids, both systemic and topical, have also been recommended for the control of intraocular inflammation.

Preventive measures include elimination of cattle-associated leptospirosis and protection for workers at risk. Doxycycline 200mg orally once a week has been used as prophylaxis for high-risk individuals.[41]

COURSE AND OUTCOME

Anicteric leptospirosis is associated with a better outcome; Weil's disease is associated with a fatal outcome in 5 to 30% of untreated patients.[41] The prognosis for patients with ocular disease is generally good, with one large series reporting that more than 50% of patients regained 20/20 vision.[46]

REFERENCES

1. Steere AC, Bartenhagen NH, Craft JE, et al. The early clinical manifestations of Lyme disease. Ann Intern Med. 1983;99:76–82.
2. Burgdorfer W, Barbour AG, Hayes SF, et al. Lyme disease—a tick borne spirochetosis? Science. 1982;216:1317–19.
3. Lebech AM, Hansen K, Wilske B, Theisen M. Taxonomic classification of 29 Borrelia burgdorferi strains isolated from patients with Lyme borreliosis: a comparison of five different phenotypic and genotypic typing schemes. Med Microbiol Immunol. 1994;183:325–41.
4. Zaidman GW. The ocular manifestations of Lyme disease. Int Ophthalmol Clin. 1997;37(2):13–28.
5. Lesser RL, Kornmehl EW, Pachner AR, et al. Neuro-ophthalmologic manifestations of Lyme disease. Ophthalmology. 1990;97:699–706.
6. Reik L Jr, Burgdorfer W, Donaldson JO. Neurologic abnormalities in Lyme disease without erythema chronicum migrans. Am J Med. 1986;81:73–8.
7. Winterkorn JM. Lyme disease: neurologic and ophthalmic manifestations. Surv Ophthalmol. 1990;35:191–204.
8. Duray PH, Steere AC. Clinical pathologic correlations of Lyme disease by stage. Ann N Y Acad Sci. 1988;539:65–79.
9. Steere AC. Lyme disease. N Engl J Med. 1989;321:586–98.
10. Rahn DW. Lyme disease: clinical manifestations, diagnosis, and treatment. Arthritis Rheum. 1991;20:201–18.
11. Aaberg TM. The expanding ophthalmologic spectrum of Lyme disease. Am J Ophthalmol. 1989;107:77–80.
12. Jacobson DM, Frens DB. Pseudotumor cerebri syndrome associated with Lyme disease. Am J Ophthalmol. 1989;107:81–2.
13. Karma A, Seppala I, Mikkila H, et al. Diagnosis and clinical characteristics of ocular Lyme borreliosis. Am J Ophthalmol. 1995;119:127–35.
14. Bialasiewicz AA, Ruprecht KW, Naumann GOH, Blenk H. Bilateral diffuse choroiditis and exudative retinal detachment with evidence of Lyme disease. Am J Ophthalmol. 1988;105:419–20.
15. Breeveld J, Kuiper H, Spanjaard L, et al. Uveitis and Lyme borreliosis. Br J Ophthalmol. 1993;77:480–1.
16. Kuiper H, Koelman JH, Jager MJ. Vitreous clouding associated with Lyme borreliosis. Am J Ophthalmol. 1989;108:453–4.
17. Rothova A, Kuiper H, Spanjaard L, et al. Spiderweb vitritis in Lyme borreliosis. Lancet. 1991;337:490–1.
18. Flach AJ, Lavoie PE. Episcleritis, conjunctivitis, and keratitis as ocular manifestations of Lyme disease. Ophthalmology. 1990;97:973–5.
19. Orlin SE, Lauffer JL. Lyme disease keratitis. Am J Ophthalmol. 1989;107:678–9.
20. Zaidman GW. Episcleritis and symblepharon associated with Lyme keratitis. Am J Ophthalmol. 1990;109:487–8.
21. Case definitions for public health surveillance. MMWR Morb Mortal Wkly Rep. 1990;39(RR-13):1–43.
22. Recommendations for test performance and interpretations from the Second National Conference on Serological Diagnosis of Lyme Disease. MMWR Morb Mortal Wkly Rep. 1995;44:590–1.
23. Wormser GP, Bittker S, Cooper D, et al. Comparison of the yields of blood cultures using serum or plasma from patients with early Lyme disease. J Clin Microbiol. 2000;38:1648–50.
24. Berger BW, Johnson RC, Kodner C, et al. Cultivation of Borrelia burgdorferi from erythema migrans lesions and perilesional skin. J Clin Microbiol. 1992;30:359–61.
25. Steere AC. Lyme disease. N Engl J Med. 2001;345:115–25.
26. Molloy PJ, Persing DH, Berardi VP. False-positive results of PCR testing for Lyme disease. Clin Infect Dis. 2001;33:412–13.
27. Isogai E, Isogai H, Kotake S, et al. Detection of antibodies against Borrelia burgdorferi in patients with uveitis. Am J Ophthalmol. 1991;112:23–30.
28. Corpuz M, Hilton E, Lardis P, et al. Problems in the use of serologic tests for the diagnosis of Lyme disease. Arch Intern Med. 1991;151:1837–40.
29. Rosenbaum JT, Rahn DW. Prevalence of Lyme disease among patients with uveitis. Am J Ophthalmol. 1991;112:462–3.
30. Steere AC. Pathogenesis of Lyme arthritis: implications for rheumatic disease. Ann N Y Acad Sci. 1988;539:87–92.
31. Habicht GS, Beck G, Benach JL. The role of interleukin-1 in the pathogenesis of Lyme disease. Ann N Y Acad Sci. 1988;539:80–6.
32. Berger BW. Treatment of erythema chronicum migrans of Lyme disease. Ann N Y Acad Sci. 1988;539:346–51.
33. Recommendations for the use of Lyme disease vaccination: recommendations of the Advisory Committee on Immunization Practices (ACIP). MMWR Morb Mortal Wkly Rep. 1999;48(RR-7):1–17, 21-5. [Erratum Morb Mortal Wkly Rep. 1999;48:883.]
34. Steere AC, Sikand VK, Meurice F, et al. Vaccination against Lyme disease with recombinant Borrelia burgdorferi outer surface lipoprotein A with adjuvant. N Engl J Med. 1998;339:209–15.
35. Schoen RT, Sikand VK, Caldwell MC, et al. Safety and immunogenicity profile of a recombinant outer-surface protein A Lyme disease vaccine: clinical trial of a 3-dose schedule at 0, 1, and 2 months. Clin Ther. 2000;22:315–25.
36. Nadelman RB, Nowakowski J, Fish D, et al. Prophylaxis with single dose doxycycline for the prevention of Lyme disease after an Ixodes scapularis tick bite. N Engl J Med. 2001;345:79–84.
37. Faine S. Leptospira and leptospirosis. Boca Raton, FL: CRC Press; 1994.
38. Weil A. Uber eine eigentumliche, mit milztumor, Ikterus and nephritis einhergehende, acute infektionskrankheit. Dtsch Arch Klin Med. 1886;39:209–32.
39. Barkay S, Garzozi H. Leptospirosis and uveitis. Ann Ophthalmol. 1984;16:164–8.
40. Rathinam SR, Namperumalswamy P, Cunningham ET Jr. Spontaneous cataract absorption in patients with leptospiral uveitis. Br J Ophthalmol. 2000;84:1135–41.
41. Nussenblat RB, Whitcup SM, Palestine AG. Uveitis fundamentals and clinical practice, 2nd ed. Chicago: Mosby–Year Book; 1996:175–81.
42. Watkins SA. Update on leptospirosis. BMJ. 1985;290:1502–3.
43. Palmer MF. Laboratory diagnosis of leptospirosis. Med Lab Sci. 1988;45:174–5.
44. Mancel E, Merien F, Pesenti L, et al. Clinical aspects of ocular leptospirosis in New Caledonia (South Pacific). Aust N Z J Ophthalmol. 1999;27:380–6.
45. Sulzer CR, Jones WL. Leptospirosis: methods in laboratory diagnosis, rev ed. Atlanta: Centers for Disease Control; 1978. Washington, DC: US Department of Health, Education, Welfare, Public Health Service. Publication CDC 79-8275.
46. Rathinam SR, Rathnam S, Selvaraj S, et al. Uveitis associated with an epidemic outbreak of leptospirosis. Am J Ophthalmol. 1997;124:71–9.
47. Merien F, Perolat P, Baranton G. Comparison of polymerase chain reaction with microagglutination test and culture for the diagnosis of leptospirosis. J Infect Dis. 1995;172:281–5.

CHAPTER
168 Cat-Scratch and Whipple's Diseases

ROBERT C. WANG

DEFINITION
- Cat-scratch and Whipple's diseases are caused by *Bartonella henselae* and *Tropheryma whippelii*, respectively, and the ocular inflammation induced by these agents may be associated with systemic signs and symptoms.

KEY FEATURES
Cat-scratch disease
- Cat-scratch disease most commonly manifests as a unilateral granulomatous conjunctivitis with regional lymphadenopathy.
- The more sight-threatening malady includes neuroretinitis with macular star formation. Retinitis may also occur.
- It is typically a self-limited disease, rarely requiring treatment.

Whipple's disease
- Gastrointestinal symptoms include diarrhea and weight loss.
- Panuveitis may occur, with or without systemic symptoms.
- Multifocal choroiditis, retinitis, and retinal vascular occlusions are observed.

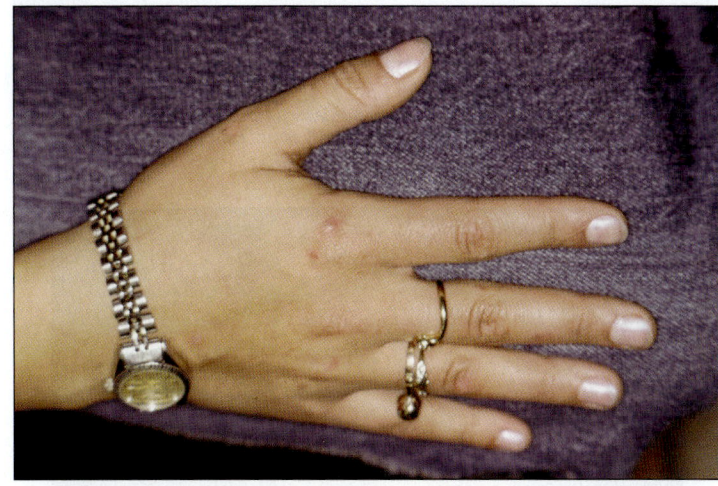

FIG. 168-1 ■ **Erythematous papule at site of cat scratch.** Appearance of erythematous papule at the base of the right index finger after multiple scratches from 1-month-old kitten. (Courtesy of Ehud Zamir, Hadassah University Hospital, Jerusalem, Israel.)

INTRODUCTION

Of the many infectious conditions that cause uveitis, cat-scratch, and Whipple's disease are less-frequent causes of intraocular inflammation. However, they remain important entities in the diagnostic acumen of the ophthalmologist. Cat-scratch disease has been associated with Parinaud's oculoglandular syndrome. Only recently has it been linked to neuroretinitis and macular star formation. Whipple's disease is a less-frequent cause of ocular inflammation that is mainly associated with gastrointestinal symptoms including diarrhea.

CAT-SCRATCH DISEASE: *BARTONELLA HENSELAE*–ASSOCIATED UVEITIS

EPIDEMIOLOGY AND PATHOGENESIS

Bartonella spp. are gram-negative bacilli which have been associated with a clinical manifestation of self-limited lymphadenopathy associated with a cat scratch or bite. The disease has been reported to affect 22,000 patients in the United States but has a worldwide distribution, commonly affecting children and young adults.[1] There is a higher prevalence in the autumn and winter during the seasonal breeding of the domestic cat. In 1992 the organism previously classified as *Rochalimaea henselae*, currently classified as *B. henselae*, was identified as the causative agent of cat-scratch disease (CSD).[2]

In humans, a small erythematous papule occurs in 25–60% at the site of inoculation, followed by systemic symptoms during the following days to weeks (Fig. 168-1). Fever, malaise, fatigue, and lymphadenopathy are seen. Typically symptoms are self-limited.

However, more serious complications can occur, such as splenomegaly, splenic abscess, encephalopathy, granulomatous hepatitis, pneumonia, bacillary angiomatosis, and osteomyelitis.[3]

Ocular manifestations typically occur following systemic symptoms. Conjunctival reactions such as Parinaud's oculoglandular syndrome and follicular conjunctivitis have been seen. More vision-threatening disorders include neuroretinitis, optic neuritis, focal chorioretinitis, exudative maculopathy, serous retinal detachment, and vitritis.[4–6]

Fleas have been implicated as a vector for CSD. Higher incidence of cat infestation by *B. henselae* is seen in areas with more fleas. However, the direct role of the fleas is still unknown.[1] Human infection has been speculated to occur from direct inoculation of open wounds or mucous membranes, possibly from contact with flea feces, which remain infectious for prolonged periods.[7,8]

OCULAR MANIFESTATIONS

The eye is the most commonly infected nonlymphatic organ in patients with CSD.[9] However, not all patients demonstrate prodromal symptoms or a history of cat or flea exposure. This can make diagnosis difficult and requires a high clinical suspicion, when there are clinical signs, and careful history taking.

Parinaud's oculoglandular syndrome is the most common manifestation of *Bartonella* infection.[10] Patients have a unilateral granulomatous conjunctivitis and regional lymphadenopathy (Fig. 168-2). They demonstrate symptoms of unilateral conjunctiva injection, foreign body sensation, and epiphora. Preauricular, submandibular, and cervical lymph nodes typically are enlarged.[10] Conjunctival epithelium ulcerations and necrosis commonly are seen and produce a purulent discharge.[11]

More sight-threatening effects of CSD include optic nerve swelling with a complete or partial macular star formation (Fig. 168-3). In 1984 Gass termed this appearance as neuroretinitis to

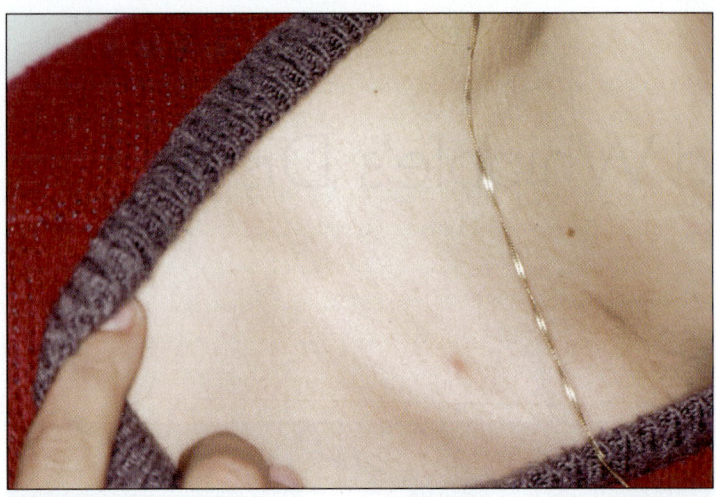

FIG. 168-2 ■ **Supraclavicular lymphadenopathy.** Onset of tender supraclavicular lymphadenopathy in same patient. (Courtesy of Ehud Zamir, Hadassah University Hospital, Jerusalem, Israel.)

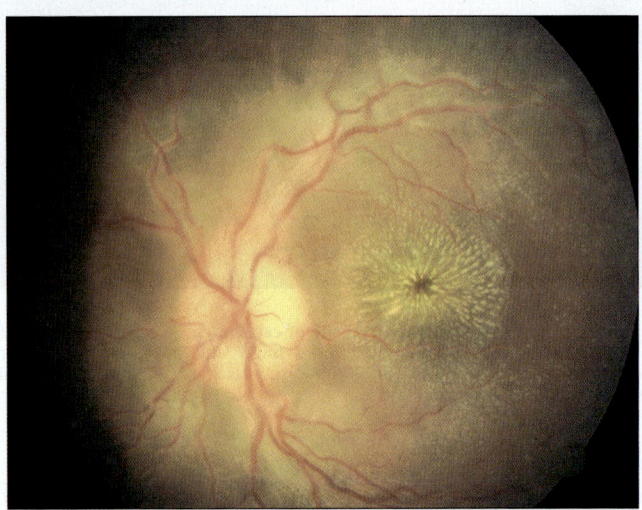

FIG. 168-3 ■ **Neuroretinitis with complete macular star formation.** (Courtesy of Ehud Zamir, Hadassah University Hospital, Jerusalem, Israel.)

distinguish this entity from primary inflammation of the optic nerve head.[12] In addition, macular star formation is not a primary maculopathy. Instead it results from vascular leakage from the optic nerve head. Despite resolution of neuroretinitis, the macular star may persist for months. An afferent pupillary defect typically is present in unilateral cases and a cecocentral scotoma is present on visual field testing.

Similar to Parinaud's oculoglandular syndrome, prodromal symptoms may or may not be present. Patients typically experience a unilateral decline in vision (mean 20/80) with systemic symptoms in 67% of patients.[6] Ocular examination typically demonstrates a mild vitritis and mild blurring of the disc margins. Macular star formation is seen in approximately 43% of cases.[6]

Multifocal retinitis and choroiditis typically is seen in conjunction with disc swelling. Foci of retinochoroiditis also can be observed in the absence of disc edema and macular star formation.[9] Accompanying multifocal retinitis or choroiditis, branch retinal artery and vein occlusion, and local serous retinal detachments have been observed.[11] Focal retinal lesions have a predilection for retinal vessels, particularly arteries, causing secondary occlusions.[13] In addition these lesions occasionally are associated with angiomatous-like proliferation of capillaries.[13,14]

DIAGNOSIS

Diagnosis of CSD is straightforward when there is typical neuroretinitis and macular star formation. Typical history of pro-

dromal symptoms, lymphadenopathy, and cat exposure helps strengthen the diagnosis, especially in young adults or children. In addition, the presence of chorioretinitis supports the clinical suspicion.[9] However, isolated neuroretinitis can make the diagnosis challenging. Serological evaluation for anti–B. henselae antibodies can aid in the diagnosis with a sensitivity and specificity of 62% and 100%, respectively.[15,16] Occasionally, Bartonella bacilli can be isolated from the affected.[17]

DIFFERENTIAL DIAGNOSIS

The differential diagnosis includes inflammatory and infiltrative processes such as optic neuritis and sarcoid papillitis. Infectious etiologies such as syphilitic perineuritis and, rarely, toxoplasmosis can also produce a similar clinical appearance. Pseudotumor cerebri can mimic bilateral CSD.[18] Finally, diabetic papillopathy with macular star formation can appear similar to the neuroretinitis.[19]

PATHOLOGY

Bartonella organisms typically invade and colonize erythrocytes, although endothelial cells are also a target for the organisms. Endothelial invasion leads to a proinflammatory response and formation of vasoproliferative tumors.[20] It is unclear if this is the same mechanism that takes place in the ocular lesions. In animal models, γ-interferon–activated macrophages have been documented to aid in clearing of B. henselae and may explain the self-limited nature of the infection.[21]

TREATMENT

CSD tends to be a self-limited disease. Usually no treatment is recommended. However, in immunocompromised patients antibiotic treatment has led to dramatic clinical responses.[9] Currently, no controlled trial has demonstrated efficacy in immunocompetent patients. However, in patients with severe ocular or systemic complications a course of antibiotics can be attempted. Doxycycline (100mg twice daily) has good intraocular and central nervous penetration. However, in patients 8–12 years of age, erythromycin is recommend due to the risk of tooth discoloration. Gentamicin and azithromycin also have been used for systemic CSD.[1] Azithromycin administration has been shown to result in rapid resolution of lymphadenopathy.[22] However, the distribution of azithromycin appears to be higher in conjunctival tissue and lower in intraocular fluids.[23,24]

WHIPPLE'S DISEASE: *TROPHERYMA WHIPPELII*–ASSOCIATED UVEITIS

EPIDEMIOLOGY AND PATHOGENESIS

Whipple's disease is a rare, multisystemic disease caused by the bacillus *T. whippelii*. It was first described in 1907 as an intestinal lipodystrophy.[25] It has been associated with a clinical syndrome of migratory arthritis, diarrhea, and weight loss. The disease most commonly affects white males in the fourth to sixth decades, although it has been reported to occur at any age.[26]

Arthritis is typically the first symptom experienced. The arthritis is migratory, occurring in 80% of patients. Gastrointestinal symptoms occur in approximately 75% of cases, producing abdominal pain with diarrhea, steatorrhea, and intestinal malabsorption.[26] Weight loss with pitting edema is also common due to protein-losing enteropathy. However, when gastrointestinal symptoms are not present, diagnosis can be difficult and often can be delayed for several years. Cardiac involvement can occur, with myocardial or valvular involvement with secondary heart failure or valvular regurgitation. Low-grade fever is present in 50%. Central nervous system involvement occurs in 10% of cases. Clinical symptoms include dementia, coma, and seizures.[26]

Cranial nerves can be involved also, producing ophthalmoplegia and nystagmus.[27]

Ocular manifestations typically occur following systemic symptoms. These include vitritis, keratitis, retinitis, and retinal hemorrhages.[27,28] The source of infection in humans is unknown. Additional, no human-to-human spread has been documented.

OCULAR MANIFESTATIONS

Ocular involvement is estimated to occur in less than 5% of patients with Whipple's disease.[29] In most reported cases of Whipple's disease, ocular involvement typically is secondary to central nervous system involvement. Symptoms include nystagmus, oculomasticatory myorhythmia, and a progressive supranuclear-like palsy.[27]

Inflammation can be bilateral, with panuveitis and retinal vasculitis. Both anterior uveitis and moderate vitritis are present. In a reported case, unique white granular crystalline deposits were seen at the pupillary margin.[30] Diffuse chorioretinal inflammation has been observed also. Diffuse vasculitis, typically in the perifoveal and midperipheral areas, are accompanied by hemorrhages and retinal vascular occlusions.[27–29] Optic nerve involvement can occur, with prolonged involvement leading to optic atrophy.

DIAGNOSIS

Diagnosis of Whipple's disease can be difficult in the absence of systemic signs. Duodenal biopsy remains the gold standard for diagnosis of Whipple's disease. The presence of strongly positive periodic acid-Schiff bacillus within macrophages is virtually pathognomonic for the disease.[26] Occasionally, biopsy results have been reported to be negative despite multiple attempts. Diagnosis was confirmed after polymerase chain reaction (PCR) analysis of peripheral blood DNA.[31,32] In addition, PCR analysis has been demonstrated to identify *T. whippelii* DNA in vitreous samples.[33,34]

DIFFERENTIAL DIAGNOSIS

Differential diagnosis includes entities that have multisystemic involvement and retinal vasculitis. These include systemic lupus erythematosus (SLE), polyarteritis nodosa (PAN), and Behçet's disease. Unlike Whipple's disease, SLE rarely produces intestinal malabsorption. Similarly SLE and PAN tend to cause more vasculitic manifestations, with gastrointestinal hemorrhage or ischemia. Oral and genital ulcers seen in patients with Behçet's disease differentiates patients with Whipple's disease. Sarcoidosis can cause retinal vasculitis and ocular inflammation, however severe gastrointestinal findings are seen less frequently. In immunocompromised patients, *Mycobacterium avium intracellulare* (MAI) can produce similar systemic symptoms and histological picture (PAS-positive histiocytes). However, MAI tends to produce a multifocal choroiditis rather than a primary vasculitis.[35]

PATHOLOGY

Currently *T. whippelii* has been difficult to culture and no animal models of the infection currently exist. However, periodic acid-Schiff–positive rod-shaped bacilli have been identified within macrophages, which has been considered pathognomonic for the disease. However, laboratory techniques have identified metabolically active *T. whippelii* outside of cells in intestinal villi specimens, suggesting that *T. whippelii* is not an obligate intracellular pathogen.[36] Recently culture for these bacteria has been possible, hopefully leading to further understanding of infection and the host immune response of this disease.[37]

TREATMENT

Whipple's disease is a chronic, recudescent disease that can be fatal. Intestinal symptoms typically resolve within 1–3 months with treatment. However, relapses can occur in up to one third of patients, requiring prolonged treatment for up to 1 year.[26] With ocular involvement, drugs that cross the blood–brain barrier are preferred. Double-strength oral trimethoprim-sulfamethoxazole is the preferred first-line therapy. In sulfonamide-allergic patients, ceftriaxone or chloramphenicol can be tried. Retinal vasculitis typically responds to antibiotic treatment.[27] However, antibiotic treatment seldom resolves neurological signs and they frequently become permanent.

REFERENCES

1. Windsor JJ. Cat-scratch disease: epidemiology, aetiology and treatment. Br J Biomed Sci. 2001;58:101–10.
2. Karem KL, Paddock CD, Regnery RL. *Bartonella henselae, B. quintana,* and *B. bacilliformis:* historical pathogens of emerging significance. Microbes Infect. 2000;2:1193–205.
3. Massei F, Messina F, Talini I, et al. Widening of the clinical spectrum of *Bartonella henselae* infection as recognized through serodiagnostics. Eur J Pediatr. 2000;159:416–9.
4. Ormerod LD, Skolnick KA, Menosky MM, et al. Retinal and choroidal manifestations of cat-scratch disease. Ophthalmology. 1998;105:1024–31.
5. Zacchei AC, Newman NJ, Sternberg P. Serous retinal detachment of the macula associated with cat scratch disease. Am J Ophthalmol. 1995;120:796–7.
6. Solley WA, Martin DF, Newman NJ, et al. Cat scratch disease: posterior segment manifestations. Ophthalmology. 1999;106:1546–53.
7. Chomel BB, Kasten RW, Floyd-Hawkins K, et al. Experimental transmission of *Bartonella henselae* by the cat flea. J Clin Microbiol. 1996;34:1952–6.
8. Foil L, Andress E, Freeland RL, et al. Experimental infection of domestic cats with *Bartonella henselae* by inoculation of *Ctenocephalides felis* (Siphonaptera: Pulicidae) feces. J Med Entomol. 1998;35:625–8.
9. Cunningham ET, Koehler JE. Ocular bartonellosis. Am J Ophthalmol. 2000;130:340–9.
10. Huang MC, Dreyer E. Parinaud's oculoglandular conjunctivitis and cat-scratch disease. Int Ophthalmol Clin. 1996;36:29–36.
11. Ormerod LD, Dailey JP. Ocular manifestations of cat-scratch disease. Curr Opin Ophthalmol. 1999;10:209–16.
12. Dreyer RF, Hopen G, Gass JD, Smith JL. Leber's idiopathic stellate neuroretinitis. Arch Ophthalmol. 1984;102:1140–5.
13. Gray AV, Reed JB, Wendel RT, Morse LS. *Bartonella henselae* infection associated with peripapillary angioma, branch retinal artery occlusion, and severe vision loss. Am J Ophthalmol. 1999;127:223–4.
14. Fish RH, Hogan RN, Nightingale SD, Anand R. Peripapillary angiomatosis associated with cat-scratch neuroretinitis. Arch Ophthalmol. 1992;110:870.
15. Tsuneoka H, Fujii R, Fujisawa K, et al. Clinical evaluation of commercial serological test for *Bartonella* infection. Kansenshogaku Zasshi. 2000;74:387–91.
16. Suhler EB, Lauer AK, Rosenbaum JT. Prevalence of serologic evidence of cat scratch disease in patients with neuroretinitis. Ophthalmology. 2000;107:871–6.
17. Del Prete R, Fumarola D, Fumarola L, Miragliotta G. Detection of *Bartonella henselae* and *Afipia felis* DNA by polymerase chain reaction in specimens from patients with cat scratch disease. Eur J Clin Microbiol Infect Dis. 2000;19:964–7.
18. Friedman DI. Papilledema and pseudotumor cerebri. Ophthalmol Clin North Am. 2001;14:129–47, ix.
19. Regillo CD, Brown GC, Savino PJ, et al. Diabetic papillopathy. Patient characteristics and fundus findings. Arch Ophthalmol. 1995;113:889–95.
20. Dehio C. *Bartonella* interactions with endothelial cells and erythrocytes. Trends Microbiol. 2001;9:279–85.
21. Musso T, Badolato R, Ravarino D, et al. Interaction of *Bartonella henselae* with the murine macrophage cell line J774: infection and proinflammatory response. Infect Immun. 2001;69:5974–80.
22. Conrad DA. Treatment of cat-scratch disease. Curr Opin Pediatr. 2001;13:56–9.
23. O'Day DM, Head WS, Foulds G, et al. Ocular pharmacokinetics of orally administered azithromycin in rabbits. J Ocul Pharmacol. 1994;10:633–41.
24. Tabbara KF, al-Kharashi SA, al-Mansouri SM, et al. Ocular levels of azithromycin. Arch Ophthalmol. 1998;116:1625–8.
25. Maiwald M, Relman D. Whipple's disease and *Tropheryma whippelii:* secrets slowly revealed. Clin Infect Dis. 2001;32:457–63.
26. Puechal X. Whipple disease and arthritis. Curr Opin Rheumatol. 2001;13:74–9.
27. Avila MP, Jalkh AE, Feldman E, et al. Manifestations of Whipple's disease in the posterior segment of the eye. Arch Ophthalmol. 1984;102:384–90.
28. Leland TM, Chambers JK. Ocular findings in Whipple's disease. South Med J. 1978;71:335–8.
29. Nishimura JK, Cook BE Jr, Pach JM. Whipple disease presenting as posterior uveitis without prominent gastrointestinal symptoms. Am J Ophthalmol. 1998;126:130–2.
30. Williams JG, Edward DP, Tessler HH, et al. Ocular manifestations of Whipple disease: an atypical presentation. Arch Ophthalmol. 1998;116:1232–4.
31. Kelly P. PCR for *Tropheryma whippelii*. Lancet. 1999;354:1476–7.
32. Coria F, Cuadrado N, Velasco C, et al. Whipple's disease with isolated central nervous system symptomatology diagnosed by molecular identification of *Tropheryma whippelii* in peripheral blood. Neurologia. 2000;15:173–6.
33. Sommer S, Rozot P, Wagner M, et al. Uveitis in Whipple disease: identification of *Tropheryma whippelii* by PCR. J Fr Ophthalmol. 1998;21:588–90.
34. Durant WJ, Flood T, Goldberg MF, et al. Vitrectomy and Whipple's disease. Arch Ophthalmol. 1984;102:848–51.
35. Rao NA. Acquired immunodeficiency syndrome and its ocular complications. Indian J Ophthalmol. 1994;42:51–63.
36. Fredricks DN, Relman DA. Localization of *Tropheryma whippelii* rRNA in tissues from patients with Whipple's disease. J Infect Dis. 2001;183:1229–37.
37. Raoult D, La Scola B, Lecocq P, et al. Culture and immunological detection of *Tropheryma whippelii* from the duodenum of a patient with Whipple disease. JAMA. 2001;285:1039–4.

DEFINITION
- Inflammation within the anterior or posterior segment, or both, traditionally occurs with concurrent partial-thickness involvement of an adjacent ocular wall. Endophthalmitis may be either infectious or noninfectious.

KEY FEATURES
- Decreased vision.
- Anterior chamber or vitreous cellular reaction.
- Hypopyon.
- Pain.

ASSOCIATED FEATURES
- Conjunctival hyperemia.
- Lid edema.

INTRODUCTION

Endophthalmitis is a potentially severe intraocular inflammation which may occur as a complication of intraocular surgery or as a result of nonsurgical trauma or systemic infection. Endophthalmitis is not necessarily an infectious process, therefore lens-induced inflammation and severe noninfectious postoperative inflammations may be termed *sterile endophthalmitis*. In common usage, however, the term *endophthalmitis* indicates an infectious cause.

EPIDEMIOLOGY AND PATHOGENESIS

Endophthalmitis can be classified as in Box 169-1. Organisms causing infectious endophthalmitis usually originate from an exogenous source, entering the eye following intraocular surgery including cataract extraction, secondary lens implantation, *pars plana* vitrectomy, glaucoma filter, penetrating keratoplasty, and others. Infection may also follow a penetrating ocular injury or occur as a result of hematogenous spread from a systemic infection.

Acute Infectious Postoperative Endophthalmitis

Acute endophthalmitis typically is defined as occurring within 6 weeks of surgery. The incidence of endophthalmitis following intraocular surgery has decreased steadily during the twentieth century. Studies published within the last 10 years have reported an incidence of acute endophthalmitis following cataract extraction of between 0.072% and 0.13%.[1–4]

The most common infecting organisms following cataract extraction are the coagulase-negative *Staphylococcus* spp., especially *S. epidermidis*.[5,6] Gram-negative bacteria and anaerobes are much less frequent causative agents. The most likely source of infectious agents is the patient's own lid and conjunctival flora, with entry at the time of surgery. One study showed a 29% incidence of positive aqueous culture results taken at the time of cataract extraction.[7] Because the incidence of endophthalmitis is much lower than 29%, factors other than the presence of bacteria in the eye must be at play. Infection may occur due to an overwhelming of intrinsic ocular defense mechanisms such as clearance of organisms by aqueous outflow, complement activation, and phagocytosis.[8] Preoperative risk factors include active ocular surface infections or colonization, such as blepharitis, conjunctivitis, lacrimal drainage system infection or obstruction, and contaminated eyedrops. Operative risks include wound abnormalities, vitreous loss,[9] prolonged surgery, and contaminated irrigation solutions. Thus careful preoperative evaluation and correction of preexisting risk factors, application of topical povidone-iodine (5%) solution prior to surgery,[10] careful draping to isolate the lid margin and lashes from the surgical wound, and careful surgical technique should reduce the risk of endophthalmitis. The issue of perioperative antibiotic use is one of great controversy and is yet to be resolved.

Delayed-Onset Infectious Endophthalmitis

Delayed-onset endophthalmitis is defined as that occurring more than 6 weeks following surgery. Persistent or recurrent uveitis following cataract extraction is difficult to differentiate from a smoldering or delayed-onset postoperative infection. Thus the clinician must have a high index of suspicion. Typically organisms of lower virulence, such as *Propionibacterium acnes, S. epidermidis,* and fungi are involved.

Bleb-Associated Infectious Endophthalmitis

Bleb-associated endophthalmitis following a glaucoma filtering procedure may range from blebitis to frank purulent endophthalmitis and may occur during the early or late postoperative periods. The incidence of acute infectious endophthalmitis following glaucoma filtering surgery has been reported to be 0.061–0.3%.[4] The most common causative organisms are *Streptococcus* spp.[11] The reported incidence of delayed bleb-related endophthalmitis is in the range of 0.2–18%.[12] The most common causative organisms may differ from those found in acute-onset disease and include *Streptococcus* spp. and *Haemophilus influenzae.*[13,14] Local antimetabolite adjunctive therapy further increases the risk of bleb-related endophthalmitis.[15]

Other Intraocular Surgery

Endophthalmitis also can occur, but rarely, following pars plana vitrectomy, penetrating keratoplasty,[1] and pneumatic retinopexy.[16] Corneal transplantation presents a unique opportunity for inoculation of microorganisms via the donor graft tissue.[17] Thus most surgeons submit the donor rim for culture at the time of surgery.

Posttraumatic Infectious Endophthalmitis

The incidence of endophthalmitis following penetrating ocular trauma is approximately 7%,[18] but it may be as high as 30% in

Classification of Endophthalmitis

I. Infectious
   A. Exogenous
      1. Surgical
         a. Acute onset
         b. Delayed onset
         c. Bleb associated
      2. Nonsurgical
         a. Posttraumatic
   B. Endogenous
      1. Hematogenous spread
II. Noninfectious
   A. Lens induced
   B. Sterile

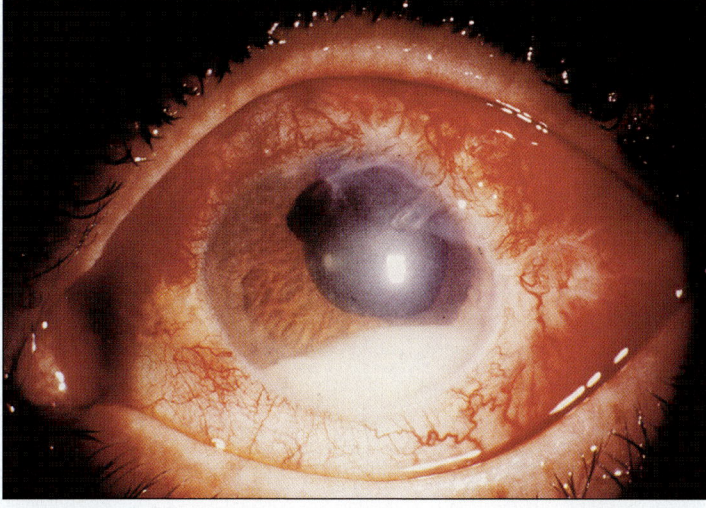

FIG. 169-1 ▌▌ **Hypopyon following cataract extraction.** Note the presence of neovascularization of the iris.

rural locales.[19] Presence of an intraocular foreign body increases the risk.[19] Although gram-positive cocci are still the most common isolates,[20,21] *Bacillus* spp.[22] and other virulent organisms, sometimes polymicrobial, are potential causes.

Endogenous Endophthalmitis

Endogenous endophthalmitis occurs as a result of the hematogenous or direct spread of microorganisms from a site external to the eye and mandates a thorough systemic search for the site of origin. One series reported that organisms causing endocarditis and those in the gastrointestinal tract were the most common primary sources.[23] Organisms may be those common to other types of endophthalmitis, such as streptococcal and staphylococcal spp.,[23] or unusual organisms, including fungi.[24]

OCULAR MANIFESTATIONS

Acute postoperative endophthalmitis by definition occurs within 6 weeks after surgery. Severity may range from mild to severe. Milder forms—usually due to less virulent organisms—tend to become apparent later than the more severe form, which usually occurs within the first 6 postoperative days. The most common symptoms reported in the Endophthalmitis Vitrectomy Study (EVS) were blurred vision, occurring in 94% of patients; a red eye, occurring in 82% of patients; and pain, reported by 74% of patients.[25]

Critical findings on examination include decreased visual acuity, eyelid edema and erythema, conjunctival hyperemia and chemosis, corneal edema and opacification, anterior chamber cell and flare (more than expected for a typical postoperative course) frequently with a hypopyon (found in 86% of patients in the EVS[25]) (Fig. 169-1), vitritis, and scattered retinal hemorrhages and periphlebitis if the retina is visible. In 79% of EVS patients, no view of the retinal vessels was possible with indirect ophthalmoscopy, and a red reflex was present in only 32% of patients.[25]

In delayed-onset endophthalmitis, the clinical picture is frequently indistinguishable from that of anterior uveitis. Patients may complain of photophobia, blurred vision, and mild pain. Keratic precipitates with anterior chamber and vitreous cells and flare can be seen. A capsular plaque is very typical in cases of P. *acnes* endophthalmitis (Fig. 169-2). Endophthalmitis may develop following Nd:YAG laser capsulotomy, presumably due to release of previously sequestered low-virulence organisms into the vitreous.[26]

Endophthalmitis associated with filtering blebs can occur anytime after surgery. Symptoms and signs are similar to those seen with post-cataract extraction endophthalmitis, with the addition of a hypopyon or cellular debris within the bleb. Patients may exhibit the latter signs without vitreous involvement, termed *blebitis*.

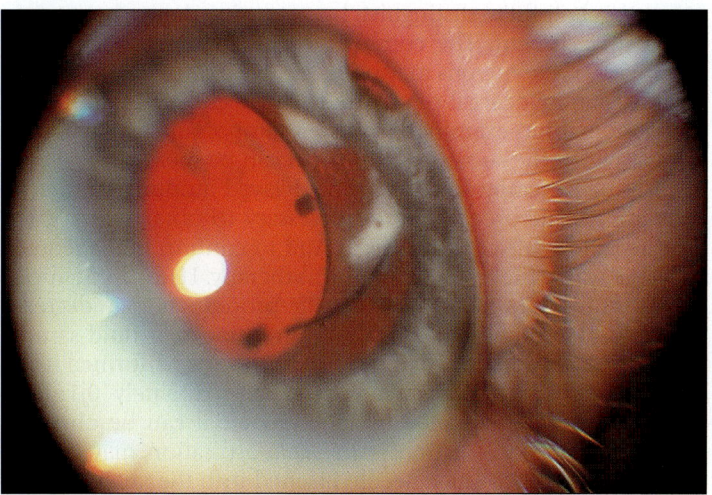

FIG. 169-2 ▌▌ *Propionibacterium acnes* plaque on the posterior capsule following cataract extraction and posterior chamber lens insertion. (Courtesy of Howard H. Tessler.)

In posttraumatic endophthalmitis, the onset may occur anytime from days to weeks following injury. Diagnosis is not uncommonly delayed due to the difficulty inherent in differentiating expected posttraumatic inflammation from infection. As mentioned previously, an intraocular foreign body increases the risk of infection.

Patients who have endogenous endophthalmitis most frequently experience decreased vision and floaters in one or both eyes. They typically experience less inflammation and pain than those with other forms of endophthalmitis. Retinal, subretinal, and choroidal infiltrates are seen (Fig. 169-3). Depending on the timing of diagnosis after onset and degree of immunosuppression present, the vitreous may contain cells and debris overlying these infiltrates. Involvement of both eyes occurs in one fourth of cases, but involvement of the fellow eye may be delayed several days to weeks.

DIAGNOSIS AND ANCILLARY TESTING

Early recognition is critical; therefore a high index of suspicion must be maintained. A complete ocular and medical history is taken and a thorough ophthalmic examination performed. Ultrasonography is helpful, especially in cases with significant anterior-segment media opacity, to confirm the presence of vitreous cells, detect a retinal or choroidal detachment or both, and to search for retained lens remnants in the posterior segment. An

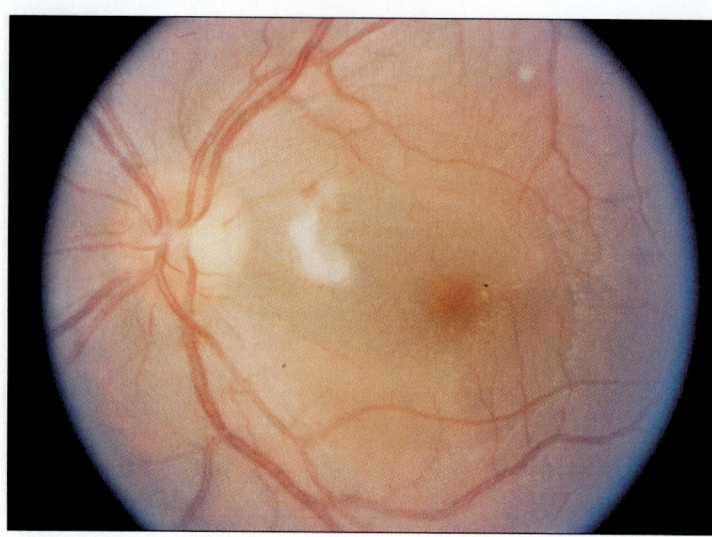

FIG. 169-3 ▮▮ **Candidal retinal infiltrate in an intravenous drug abuser.** Note the small exudative detachment adjacent to the infiltrate.

"A" scan is helpful to distinguish between vitreal membranes and retinal detachment. The combination of hypopyon and echographically clear vitreous may be suggestive of an early coagulase-negative staphylococcal or culture-negative endophthalmitis. An ultrasonographic examination also is important as a baseline against which the success of treatment can be measured.[27]

Although therapy should not be delayed awaiting culture results, diagnostic procedures are necessary to obtain intraocular fluid to guide subsequent therapy and to confirm that adequate coverage was achieved with empirical therapy. Use of systemic or topical antibiotics prior to diagnostic procedures may decrease the yield of culturable organisms from intraocular fluid sample collections. An anterior chamber paracentesis is performed using either a 25- or 27-gauge needle and approximately 0.1ml of aqueous material aspirated. Vitreous material can be obtained via several methods. A trans–*pars plana* aspiration may be performed, using a 23-gauge needle inserted into the anterior vitreous cavity, entering 3mm posterior to the limbus in pseudophakic or aphakic eyes and 4mm posterior to the limbus in phakic eyes. If possible, the needle should be visualized in the vitreous cavity. Approximately 0.2ml of liquid vitreous is aspirated. Small and careful movements of the needle in the vitreous cavity may be necessary to obtain an adequate sample. Small-gauge battery-powered vitreous cutting instruments are available for office use and may decrease the risk of an iatrogenic retinal tear by cutting, rather than pulling, on the vitreous body. Finally, a traditional three-port vitrectomy can be performed. The latter has the advantages of production of a larger sample volume, debulking the vitreous of toxic products, decreasing the infecting agent load, and releasing possible sources of vitreous traction. Comparison between immediate vitrectomy and vitreous sampling, as regards visual acuity and media clarity, was a major goal of the Endophthalmitis Vitreous Study (EVS). This study found that immediate vitrectomy produced a better outcome only in eyes with light perception vision at the time of evaluation.[25]

Aqueous and vitreous samples should be plated on blood agar, chocolate agar, Sabouraud dextrose agar, thioglycollate broth, and anaerobic medium. Gram and Giemsa stains should be performed also. The remainder of the specimen should be mixed with an equal volume of 95% alcohol and submitted for pathological evaluation. The polymerase chain reaction may provide a more rapid method of specific diagnosis by allowing detection of DNA from infecting organisms. Issues with contamination and ability to provide rapid speciation of the amplified DNA products need to be resolved before this methodology can totally supplant culture. Traditional culture results are generally positive within 48 hours, with sensitivities usually available 24 hours later. The EVS yielded a 68.2% incidence of confirmed positive culture results,[25] similar to those found in other series. Reasons for negative culture results include fastidious organisms, insufficient sampling, and "sterile" endophthalmitis.

DIFFERENTIAL DIAGNOSIS

The differential diagnosis of endophthalmitis is detailed in Box 169-2.

SYSTEMIC ASSOCIATIONS

Endogenous endophthalmitis typically occurs with sepsis, an immunocompromised state (such as by the acquired immunodeficiency syndrome; immunosuppressive therapy, including corticosteroid use; long-term antibiotic use; or disseminated cancer), presence of an indwelling catheter (urethral or intravenous), or intravenous drug abuse. Patients with these conditions usually do not have a history of recent intraocular surgery.

PATHOLOGY

Acute endophthalmitis is characterized by the influx of neutrophils. The inflammatory process may be suppurative, as determined by the production of pus, or nonsuppurative. Certain bacteria, such as the *Staphylococci*, have a propensity to produce purulent inflammation and are termed *pyogenic*. Necrosis of the involved ocular structures is common. Neutrophils actively produce reactive oxygen species as one mechanism of host defense, and these toxic substances cause much of the damage and subsequent visual loss that occurs in infectious endophthalmitis. Repair of damaged tissues results in scar formation via the mechanisms of fibrosis and gliosis.

Chronic inflammation is characterized by the presence of lymphocytes and is divided further into granulomatous and nongranulomatous forms. Granulomatous inflammation is characterized by the presence of epithelioid cells and giant cells and may occur with fungal infection.

TREATMENT

Acute infectious endophthalmitis is a true ophthalmic emergency and mandates prompt therapy if visual acuity is to be preserved.

Medical Treatment

Because rapid administration of antibiotics is necessary, waiting for culture results or even a Gram stain is not feasible. Although most studies, including the EVS,[25] have shown a majority of iso-

BOX 169-3

Empirical Medical Therapy of Endophthalmitis

ACUTE ONSET POST–CATARACT EXTRACTION[25]

Intravitreal
Vancomycin hydrochloride 1.0mg in 0.1ml (normal saline) and
Ceftazidime 2.25mg in 0.1ml (normal saline) or Amikacin 200–400μg in 0.1ml (normal saline)
Dexamethasone 400μg in 0.1ml (optional)

Subconjunctival
Vancomycin hydrochloride 25mg in 0.5ml (normal saline) and
Ceftazidime 100mg in 0.5ml (normal saline) or Amikacin 25mg in 0.5ml (normal saline) if β-lactam allergy exists and
Dexamethasone 6mg in 0.25ml (normal saline)

Topical
Vancomycin hydrochloride 50mg/ml and
Amikacin 20mg/ml and
Atropine sulfate 1% or scopolamine hydrobromide 0.25% and
Prednisolone acetate 1%

Oral
Prednisone 30mg twice daily for 5–10 days (optional)

POSTTRAUMATIC[33]
Parallel to those listed for post–cataract extraction, and in addition:
May also consider use of intravitreal clindamycin phosphate (450μg)
Systemic antibiotics still considered standard of care, options include selections from the following:
Clindamycin 600–900mg intravenously every 8 hours
Ceftazidime 2g intravenously every 8 hours
Amikacin 7.5mg/kg intravenously once, then 6mg/kg every 12 hours
Ciprofloxacin 750mg po twice daily
May respond to above topical regimen alone

BLEB-ASSOCIATED ENDOPHTHALMITIS
Parallel to post–cataract extraction, but consider addition of systemic antibiotics as well

---

lates from postsurgical and posttraumatic infections are gram positive, empirical broad spectrum coverage for both gram-positive and gram-negative organisms is necessary. Box 169-3 lists antibiotics and dosages. Vancomycin is widely accepted as the intravitreous agent of choice for gram-positive coverage. Studies have shown that a dose of 1.0mg is well tolerated and nontoxic in a rabbit model. In several series of endophthalmitis, 100% of gram-positive organisms cultured were found to be sensitive to vancomycin. Concerns over resistance developing are probably not realistic when used intravitreally, in sharp contrast to the legitimate concern when a valuable agent such as vancomycin is used indiscriminately as a prophylactic agent.

Gram-negative intravitreous coverage may be provided with a variety of agents, including aminoglycosides and β-lactams. Each has advantages and disadvantages. Aminoglycosides have a synergistic effect with vancomycin for the treatment of enterococci. Aminoglycosides, however, may produce macular infarction. Amikacin appears to present less risk than other aminoglycosides, especially gentamicin. Third-generation cephalosporins, such as ceftazidime 2.25mg, may be used instead, and they provide good coverage for gram-negative organisms without the risk of retinal damage. If aminoglycosides are used, their repeated intravitreal injection over a several-day period should be avoided.

Although gram-positive cocci are the most common cause of posttraumatic endophthalmitis,[20] the risk of infection with organisms such as *Bacillus* must be considered. One study from India showed an 84% sensitivity rate of *Bacillus* to vancomycin, 43% sensitivity rate to ceftazidime, and a 100% sensitivity rate to amikacin, gentamicin, and ciprofloxacin.[20] Another study, also from India, showed an 87% sensitivity to amikacin, 94% sensitivity to gentamicin, and 68% sensitivity to vancomycin. Ciprofloxacin appears to have reasonably good activity against

Bacillus, and studies have shown adequate penetration into the vitreous after a single 750mg oral dose.[28] Other options include clindamycin (see Box 169-3).

Fungal endophthalmitis is treated with intravitreal amphotericin B (5mg in 0.1ml) after a positive culture result is obtained or if there is reason for strong suspicion of fungal infection. Systemic therapy also should be given, but renal toxicity must be monitored closely. Adjunctive corticosteroid therapy should not be given for eyes in which fungal endophthalmitis is suspected.

Clinical studies in bacterial endophthalmitis have reported varied results as regards the use of concurrent intravitreal corticosteroids. In a retrospective review, visual acuity and inflammation were improved in eyes injected with intravitreous dexamethasone.[29] However, in a prospective, randomized trial evaluating vitrectomy with coadministration of intravitreal dexamethasone and antibiotics in exogenous bacterial endophthalmitis (including both postoperative and posttraumatic causes), Das *et al.*[30] found that intravitreal dexamethasone reduced early inflammatory scores but had no influence on the visual outcome as measured at 12 weeks. Because the EVS did not randomize patients to receive glucocorticoids or not, it does not address this issue.

Subconjunctival injection of dexamethasone (12mg) is used commonly, as are topical glucocorticoids. Systemic glucocorticoids can be administered orally (30mg twice a day for 5–10 days[25]) if there are no contraindications.

The role of systemic antibiotic therapy had been controversial in postoperative endophthalmitis, but the EVS[25] reported no difference in final visual acuity and media clarity with or without the use of systemic antibiotics for acute post–cataract extraction endophthalmitis. The role of systemic antibiotics in other forms of endophthalmitis has not been addressed, and many clinicians still consider their use the standard of care in these situations.[31] Systemic antimicrobial usage is mandatory in endogenous endophthalmitis and is tailored to the offending organism. Infectious disease consultation is recommended both for the systemic work-up and systemic treatment of endogenous endophthalmitis. Intravitreal antibiotics are required if the infecting agent has gained access to the vitreous cavity or empirically if any question exists.

Surgical Treatment

In one sense, surgical management of endophthalmitis begins before the infection occurs. Careful operative technique to minimize wound abnormalities, avoidance of vitreous loss during cataract surgery, and careful microsurgical wound management and closure in open globe injuries decrease the risk. Once endophthalmitis has begun, early options primarily center around the method of intraocular fluid sampling and response to therapy (Fig. 169-4).

Later surgery to deal with complications may also be required. The advantages of early therapeutic vitrectomy are clearing of the ocular media, removal of potentially harmful bacterial products, reduction of bacterial load, and removal of the vitreous scaffolding by which traction retinal detachments may occur. Disadvantages include delay in treatment until operating room time is available, iatrogenic retinal holes or detachments, choroidal hemorrhage, and the problem of visualizing the posterior segment in an eye that has had recent surgery. Retinal detachment is difficult to treat in eyes that undergo vitrectomy for endophthalmitis due to the need for air-fluid exchange and injection of aqueous antibiotic. Concentration of antibiotic in the aqueous layer may lead to an increased risk of toxicity. In acute-onset post–cataract extraction endophthalmitis, the EVS[25] showed that no difference exists in visual outcome for eyes with visual acuity of hand motions or better with or without vitrectomy. In the subgroup of patients who have initial light perception, vitrectomy produced a threefold increase in the frequency

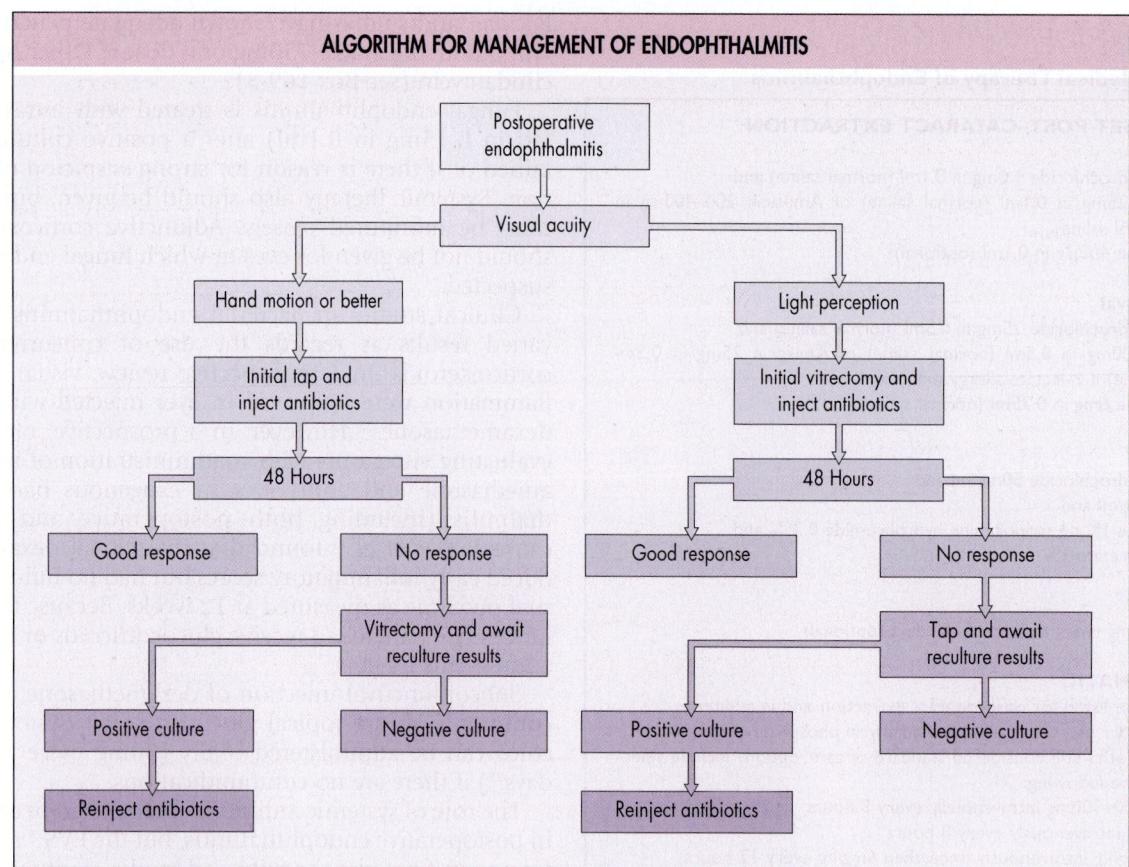

ALGORITHM FOR MANAGEMENT OF ENDOPHTHALMITIS

FIG. 169-4 ■ Algorithm for management of acute endophthalmitis after cataract extraction.

of achieving 20/40 (6/12) vision or better, a twofold increased chance of achieving 20/100 (6/30) vision or better, and a 50% decrease in the frequency of severe visual loss. In addition, no difference was found in the confirmed culture results between the group of patients who had undergone tap versus those with a therapeutic vitrectomy.

Chronic endophthalmitis caused by *P. acnes* frequently requires surgery, not only to confirm the diagnosis but also to remove any sequestered infectious material from the posterior capsule, along with injection of intravitreous antibiotics, usually vancomycin. If this is not successful, removal of the intraocular lens with complete *en bloc* removal of the anterior and posterior capsules may be necessary.

Endogenous endophthalmitis may require surgical intervention in the form of vitreal, retinal, and choroidal biopsies, and culture if there is no obvious primary source and blood cultures and other studies are negative.

COURSE AND OUTCOME

The findings from the EVS[25] that patients with post–cataract surgery endophthalmitis with hand-motion or better acuity had no benefit from either systemic antibiotic therapy or immediate vitrectomy have moved management of this specific category of patients primarily to the outpatient office setting. Regardless, the patient should be monitored on a daily basis. Admission should be considered if a patient cannot return on a frequent basis, has a history of trauma, or is believed to have endogenous endophthalmitis. Cultures usually require 24–48 hours for initial results and need to be checked daily.

The axiom "if it isn't worse, it's better," may apply, because media clarity and visual acuity may not improve initially. Level of pain and lid injection may be helpful in determining an early response. Repeat intravitreous injection of antibiotics may be required if the condition worsens and infection persists as confirmed by repeat culture. Serial ultrasonography may be used to monitor clinical response and detect retinal detachment.

BOX 169-4

Baseline Risk Factors for Decreased Visual Acuity Outcome[34]

Older age
Diabetes
Corneal infiltrate or ring ulcer
Posterior capsule not intact
Intraocular pressure less than 5mm Hg or greater than 25mm Hg
Afferent pupillary defect
Rubeosis irides
Absent red reflex
Visual acuity of light perception, the most important risk factor, with a twofold greater risk of poor visual outcome compared with those with hand-motion or better acuity during initial evaluation

Risk factors for decreased visual acuity outcome found at baseline examination, as determined by the EVS, are detailed in Box 169-4. EVS data showed that 53.1% of patients had a final visual acuity of >20/40 (6/12), 74.4% of >20/100 (6/30), and 88.6% of >5/200 (6/240).[25]

REFERENCES

1. Aaberg TM Jr, Flynn HW Jr, Schiffman J, Newton J. Nosocomial acute-onset postoperative endophthalmitis survey. A 10-yr review of incidence and outcomes. Ophthalmology. 1998;105:1004–10.
2. Powe NR, Schein OD, Gieser SC, et al. Synthesis of the literature on visual acuity and complications after cataract extraction with intraocular lens implantation. Arch Ophthalmol. 1994;112:239–52.
3. Javitt JC, Vitale S, Canner JK, et al. National outcomes of cataract extraction: endophthalmitis after inpatient surgery. Arch Ophthalmol. 1991;109:1085–9.
4. Kattan HM, Flynn HW Jr, Pflugfelder SC, et al. Nosocomial endophthalmitis survey. Current incidence of infection after intraocular surgery. Ophthalmology. 1991;98:227–38.
5. Han DP, Wisniewski SR, Wilson LA, et al. Spectrum and susceptibilities of microbiologic isolates in the Endophthalmitis Vitrectomy Study. Am J Ophthalmol. 1996;122:1–17 [erratum in Am J Ophthalmol. 1996;122:920].
6. Kunimoto DY, Das T, Sharma S, et al. Microbiologic spectrum and susceptibility of isolates: part I. Postoperative endophthalmitis. Endophthalmitis Research Group. Am J Ophthalmol. 1999;128:240–2.

7. Beigi B, Westlake W, Mangelschots E, *et al.* Perioperative microbial contamination of anterior chamber aspirates during extracapsular cataract extraction and phacoemulsification. Br J Ophthalmol. 1997;81:953–5.

8. Maxwell DP, Brent BD, Orillac R, *et al.* A natural history study of experimental *Staphylococcus epidermidis* endophthalmitis. Curr Eye Res. 1993;12:907–12.

9. Driebe WT Jr, Mandelbaum S, Forster RK, *et al.* Pseudophakic endophthalmitis. Diagnosis and management. Ophthalmology. 1986;93:442–8.

10. Bohigian GM. A study of the incidence of culture-positive endophthalmitis after cataract surgery in an ambulatory care center. Ophthalmic Surg Lasers. 1999;30:295–8.

11. Ciulla TA, Beck AD, Topping TM, Baker AS. Blebitis, early endophthalmitis, and late endophthalmitis after glaucoma-filtering surgery. Ophthalmology. 1997;104: 986–95.

12. Mandelbaum S, Forster RK, Gelender H, Culbertson W. Late onset endophthalmitis associated with filtering blebs. Ophthalmology. 1985;92:964–72.

13. Waheed S, Ritterband DC, Greenfield DS, *et al.* New patterns of infecting organisms in late bleb-related endophthalmitis: a ten year review. Eye. 1998;12:910–5.

14. Kangas TA, Greenfield DS, Flynn HW Jr, *et al.* Delayed-onset endophthalmitis associated with conjunctival filtering blebs. Ophthalmology. 1997;104:746–52.

15. Greenfield DS, Suner IJ, Miller MP *et al.* Endophthalmitis after filtering surgery with mitomycin. Arch Ophthalmol. 1996;114:943–9.

16. Hilton GF, Tornambe PE. Pneumatic retinopexy. An analysis of intraoperative and postoperative complications. The Retinal Detachment Study Group. Retina. 1991;11:285–94.

17. Merchant A, Zacks CM, Wilhelmus K, *et al.* Candidal endophthalmitis after keratoplasty. Cornea. 2001;20:226–9.

18. Kresloff MS, Castellarin AA, Zarbin MA. Endophthalmitis. Surv Ophthalmol. 1998;43:193–224.

19. Boldt HC, Pulido JS, Blodi CF, *et al.* Rural endophthalmitis. Ophthalmology. 1989;96:1722–6.

20. Kunimoto DY, Das T, Sharma S, *et al.* Microbiologic spectrum and susceptibility of isolates: part II. Posttraumatic endophthalmitis. Endophthalmitis Research Group. Am J Ophthalmol. 1999;128:242–4.

21. Abu el-Asrar AM, al-Amro SA, al-Mosallam AA, al-Obeidan S. Post-traumatic endophthalmitis: causative organisms and visual outcome. Eur J Ophthalmol. 1999;9:21–31.

22. Duch-Samper AM, Chaques-Alepuz V, Menezo JL, Hurtado-Sarrio M. Endophthalmitis following open-globe injuries. Curr Opin Ophthalmol. 1998; 9:59–65.

23. Okada AA, Johnson RP, Liles WC, *et al.* Endogenous bacterial endophthalmitis. Report of a ten-year retrospective study. Ophthalmology. 1994;101:832–8.

24. Essman TF, Flynn HW Jr, Smiddy WE, *et al.* Treatment outcomes in a 10-year study of endogenous fungal endophthalmitis. Ophthalmic Surg Lasers. 1997;28: 185–94.

25. Endophthalmitis Vitrectomy Study Group. Results of the endophthalmitis vitrectomy study: a randomized trial of immediate vitrectomy and of intravenous antibiotics for the treatment of postoperative bacterial endophthalmitis. Arch Ophthalmol. 1995;113:1479–96.

26. Carlson AN, Koch DD. Endophthalmitis following Nd:YAG laser posterior capsulotomy. Ophthalmic Surg. 1988;19:168–70.

27. Dacey MP, Valencia M, Lee MB, *et al.* Echographic findings in infectious endophthalmitis. Arch Ophthalmol. 1994;112:1325–33.

28. Keren G, Alhalel A, Bartov E, *et al.* The intravitreal penetration of orally administered ciprofloxacin in humans. Invest Ophthalmol Vis Sci. 1991;32:2388–92.

29. Mao LK, Flynn HW Jr, Miller D, Pflugfelder SC. Endophthalmitis caused by *Staphylococcus aureus*. Am J Ophthalmol. 1993;116:584–9.

30. Das T, Jalali S, Gothwal VK, *et al.* Intravitreal dexamethasone in exogenous bacterial endophthalmitis: results of a prospective randomised study. Br J Ophthalmol. 1999;83:1050–5.

31. Sternberg P Jr, Martin DF. Management of endophthalmitis in the post-endophthalmitis vitrectomy study era. Arch Ophthalmol. 2001;119:754–5.

32. Bhagat N, Read RW, Rao NA, *et al.* Rifabutin-associated hypopyon uveitis in human immunodeficiency virus–negative immunocompetent individuals. Ophthalmology. 2001;108:750–2.

33. Aaberg TM Jr, Sternberg P. Trauma: principles and techniques of treatment. In: Ryan SJ, ed. Retina, vol 3, ed 3. St. Louis: Mosby; 2001:2400–26.

34. Doft BH. The endophthalmitis vitrectomy study. In: Kertes PJ, Conway MD, eds. Clinical trials in ophthalmology: a summary and practice guide. Philadelphia: Lippincott, Williams & Wilkins; 1998:97–111.

SECTION 4 INFECTIOUS CAUSES OF UVEITIS—FUNGAL

CHAPTER 170

Histoplasmosis

RAMANA S. MOORTHY • JAMES A. FOUNTAIN

DEFINITION

- Histoplasmosis is a chronic intraocular inflammation induced by *Histoplasma capsulatum*, a diphasic fungus.

KEY FEATURES

- Ocular histoplasmosis can appear as an endophthalmitis or solitary granuloma or, more commonly, as a syndrome characterized by peripheral "punched-out" chorioretinal scars, absence of inflammatory cells in the anterior chamber or vitreous, and positive histoplasmin skin test results.

ASSOCIATED FEATURES

- Peripapillary chorioretinal atrophy, choroidal neovascularization, and hemorrhagic macular lesions occur.
- The disease is endemic in the Ohio and Mississippi river valleys.

INTRODUCTION

Histoplasma capsulatum is a diphasic, soil-borne fungus. Humans and other mammals inhale wind-blown soils and aerosolized bird droppings that contain these organisms and so become infected. These organisms infect the lungs and can be disseminated through the systemic circulation to other organs such as the liver, kidney, spleen, and the eye. *H. capsulatum* is responsible for three different forms of ocular involvement in humans[1]:

- Endophthalmitis with diffuse uveal and retinal involvement from disseminated histoplasmosis
- Solitary chorioretinal granuloma
- Ocular histoplasmosis syndrome (OHS)

The *Histoplasma* organisms have been identified in ocular tissues in all three of these forms.[1]

Histoplasmin endophthalmitis occurs mainly in immunocompromised patients, particularly those who have acquired immunodeficiency syndrome (AIDS). Symptoms can include floaters, decreased vision, and pain in the affected eye. Ophthalmic examination reveals conjunctival injection, anterior chamber flare and cells, yellow iris infiltrates, posterior synechiae, vitreous cells, and multiple, white, creamy foci of retinochoroiditis.[1,2] Diagnosis is based on the presence of active pulmonary or disseminated histoplasmosis and positive cultures from sputum, bronchial washings, and biopsy specimens from the anterior chamber or vitreous cavity. Complement fixation titers are elevated (>1:32) in disseminated disease. Histopathological evaluation of eyes with histoplasmic endophthalmitis demonstrates diffuse granulomatous inflammation that involves the entire uveal tract, focal retinal inflammation, and intracellular and extracellular *H. capsulatum* that are detected with periodic acid-Schiff and Gomori methenamine-silver (GMS) stains.[1,2] Prompt treatment with systemic amphotericin B or itraconazole is recommended in affected patients.

Solitary histoplasmic granuloma is an extremely rare condition found in immunocompromised patients.[1] An identifiable primary source of histoplasmic infection may not be found in these patients who have a white, ill-defined choroidal lesion of variable size in one eye.[1] Inflammation of the vitreous cavity is variable. Histopathological evaluation shows a dense, granulomatous mass that contains lymphocytes and epithelioid and giant cells. Few histoplasma organisms are noted within the granuloma.[1] Treatment with systemic amphotericin B should be considered if a granuloma appears to be growing or is associated with severe vitritis.

OHS is by far the most common form of ocular disease caused by *H. capsulatum*. It continues to be an important cause of central visual loss during the productive years of human life. The syndrome consists of peripapillary chorioretinal atrophy and scarring, peripheral "punched-out" chorioretinal scars, hemorrhagic macular lesions secondary to choroidal neovascularization, absence of anterior segment and vitreous inflammation, and yields a positive histoplasmin skin test result.[3]

EPIDEMIOLOGY AND PATHOGENESIS

OHS is endemic in the Ohio and Mississippi river valleys of the eastern half of the United States. Up to 80 million people are at risk for the development of OHS in this part of the country.[4] In endemic areas, 60% or more of the population may have positive histoplasmin skin tests. Approximately 5% of these patients who have positive skin tests have peripheral atrophic scars and peripapillary atrophy. Additionally, 95% or more of patients who have typical signs of OHS have positive histoplasmin skin test results.[5] Although *H. capsulatum* has not been cultured from peripheral, atrophic chorioretinal scars or disciform macular scars, organisms have been demonstrated histopathologically in both.[6,7] These observations suggest that *H. capsulatum* causes OHS.

Genetic factors may be important in the pathogenesis of OHS, because patients with macular or peripapillary hemorrhagic lesions have a significantly higher prevalence of human lymphocyte antigen B-7 (HLA-B7) than the population at large. No significant increase in HLA-B7 occurs in patients who have only peripheral atrophic spots associated with OHS.[8]

H. capsulatum may cause a subclinical systemic infection in patients in the endemic areas prior to the development of the typical ocular manifestations of OHS. This may be a self-limited upper respiratory tract illness. Subsequent routine radiological studies of patients in endemic areas may disclose asymptomatic pulmonary, hepatic, splenic, and renal granulomas.

OCULAR MANIFESTATIONS

Anterior segment and vitreous inflammation are notably absent. The characteristic fundus findings of OHS include:

- Small, oval to round, "punched-out" chorioretinal scars in the midperiphery or posterior pole (Fig. 170-1)
- A macular lesion that varies from atrophic scar to active choroidal neovascularization (Fig. 170-2) to disciform scar
- Peripapillary atrophy or scarring (Fig. 170-2)

The peripheral chorioretinal lesions are discrete, "punched-out," atrophic scars that are 0.2–0.6 disc diameters in size. They

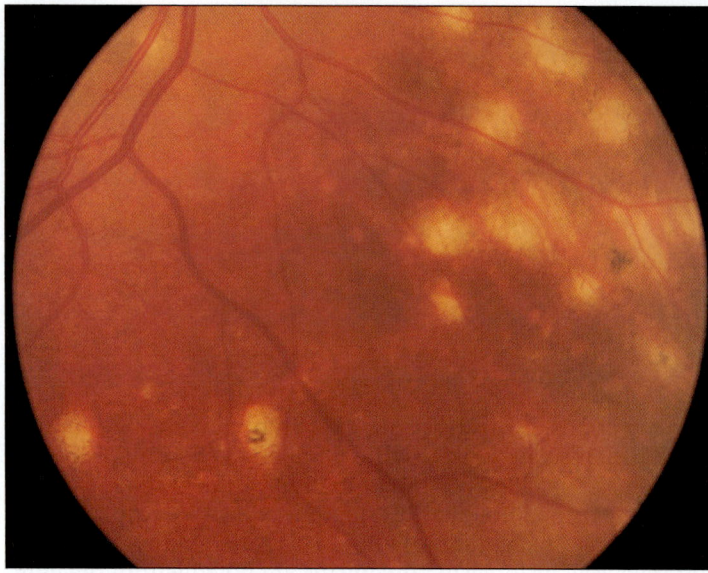

FIG. 170-1 ■ Atrophic "punched-out" chorioretinal scars in the midperiphery in a patient who has ocular histoplasmosis syndrome.

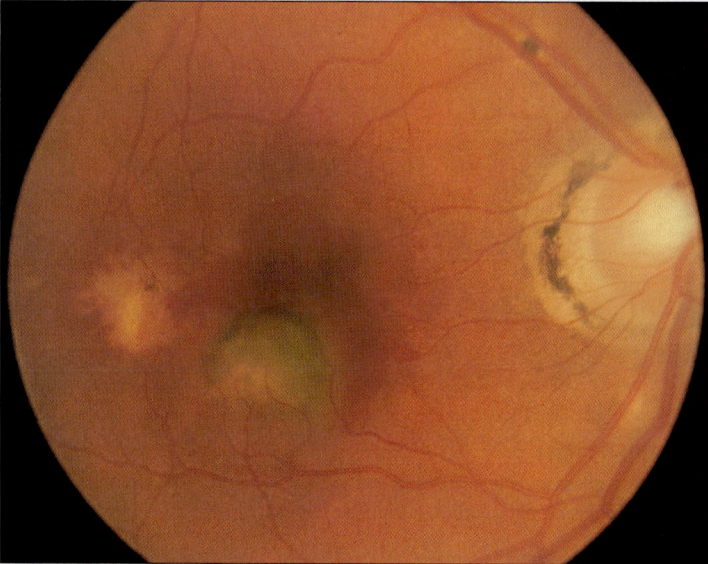

FIG. 170-2 ■ Peripapillary scarring and macular, juxtafoveal choroidal neovascular membrane with surrounding subretinal hemorrhage in the eye of a patient who has ocular histoplasmosis syndrome.

often have pigmented borders and may be located in the midperiphery or in the posterior pole. The macular lesions may be hemorrhagic initially and associated with a pigment ring. An overlying serous retinal detachment or retinal pigment epithelial (RPE) detachment may occur. Subretinal hemorrhaging and fluid accumulation are due to the growth of a choroidal neovascular membrane (CNVM) into the sub-RPE or subretinal space. If untreated these lesions may evolve into disciform scars. The disciform lesion may appear yellowish to whitish, fibrotic, and associated with variable amounts of pigmentation. The size of the disciform macular scar can vary, depending upon the amount of serum and blood in the subretinal space prior to its development.[7] Peripapillary scarring is associated with a thin area of chorioretinal atrophy adjacent to the optic nerve and a peripheral zone of hyperpigmentation at the edge farthest from the optic nerve (see Fig. 170-2). Choroidal neovascularization also may develop in the peripapillary area and result in peripapillary subretinal hemorrhage and serous retinal detachment, which may occasionally involve the macula. In addition to these three characteristic lesions, linear streak lesions at the equator have been found in up to 5% of patients with OHS (Fig. 170-3). Equatorial linear streak lesions, however, also may be seen in idiopathic multifocal choroiditis.[9]

Patients who have OHS generally are asymptomatic unless macular or peripapillary choroidal neovascularization causes metamorphopsia.[10] This usually is followed by visual loss and the development of a small scotoma in the central or paracentral visual field. Patients who have OHS usually seek treatment for these symptoms between their third and sixth decades.[10]

DIAGNOSIS

The diagnosis of OHS may be made by funduscopic examination alone. Skin testing with *H. capsulatum* antigen is not recommended because of the high prevalence of positive results in endemic areas and controversy as to whether the skin test may actually cause activation of otherwise quiet, atrophic chorioretinal scars.[11]

Patients with known, asymptomatic OHS should be instructed to perform frequent Amsler's chart self-monitoring for early detection of choroidal neovascularization.[10] Patients who have OHS who have symptoms of metamorphopsia or scotoma should have fluorescein angiography performed. In asymptomatic patients fluorescein angiographic findings consist of late

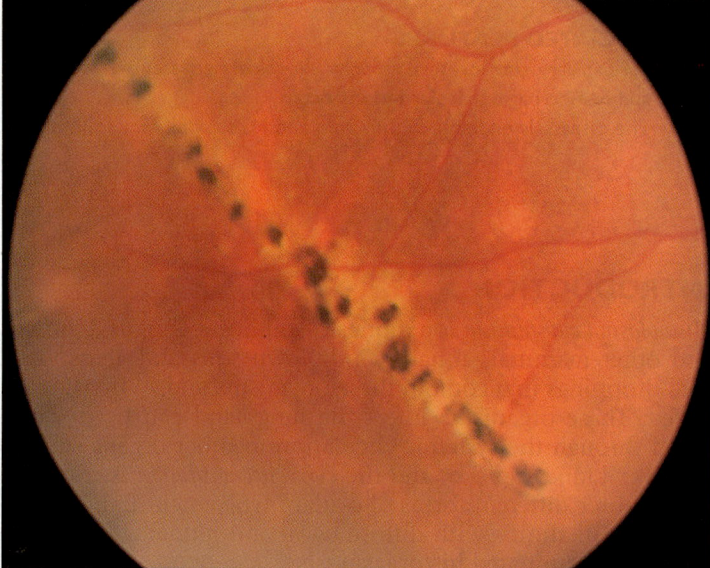

FIG. 170-3 ■ Nasal equatorial linear streak lesion in the eye of a patient who has ocular histoplasmosis syndrome.

staining of the peripapillary scar, midperipheral atrophic spots, and atrophic macular scars. If clinical examination suggests the presence of subretinal fluid or a subretinal hemorrhage (see Fig. 170-2), fluorescein angiography demonstrates early hyperfluorescence and late leakage from a complex of lacy, small blood vessels in the subretinal space or subretinal pigment epithelial space (Fig. 170-4). This is consistent with the diagnosis of choroidal neovascularization. Similar findings are seen on indocyanine green angiography, which may be helpful in delineating the CNVM when it is obscured by subretinal hemorrhage.

DIFFERENTIAL DIAGNOSIS

All of the syndromes listed in Box 170-1, except myopic degeneration, have anterior segment and vitreous inflammation in association with the chorioretinal findings. Peripheral, "punched-out," atrophic scars may be present in all of these syndromes. In sarcoidosis, the atrophic scars may be present throughout the fundus. In Vogt-Koyanagi-Harada syndrome and sympathetic

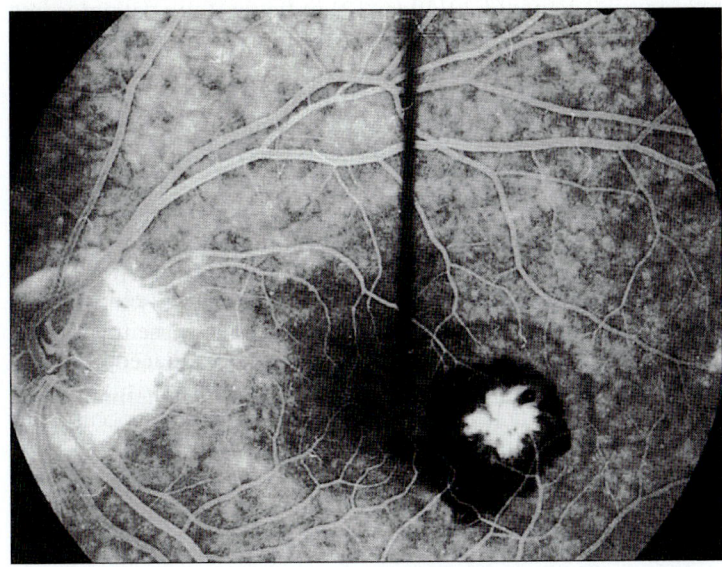

FIG. 170-4 ■ **Arteriovenous phase fluorescein angiogram of extrafoveal choroidal neovascular membrane of the left eye.** Note the leakage of fluorescein from the macular lesion, hypofluorescence due to blockage of choroidal fluorescence by surrounding subretinal hemorrhage, faint ring of subretinal fluid, and peripapillary staining.

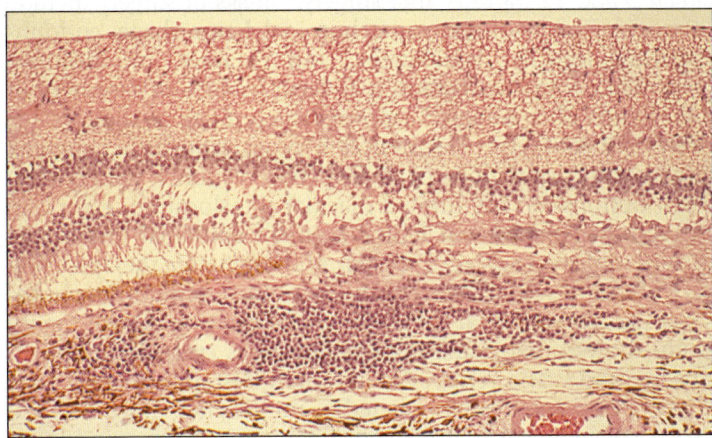

FIG. 170-5 ■ **Histopathology of an "active" atrophic chorioretinal scar in ocular histoplasmosis syndrome.** Note the lymphocytic infiltrate of the choroid, disruption of Bruch's membrane and retinal pigment epithelium, and extension of inflammation from choriocapillaris into the subretinal space. Typical histoplasmin organisms are not demonstrated here but have been isolated from other lesions. (Courtesy of Yanoff M, Fine BS. Ocular pathology: a text and atlas, ed 5. St. Louis: Mosby; 2002:412.)

BOX 170-1

Differential Diagnosis of Ocular Histoplasmosis Syndrome

Sarcoid panuveitis
Vogt-Koyanagi-Harada syndrome
Sympathetic ophthalmia
Idiopathic multifocal choroiditis
Myopic degeneration

---

ophthalmia, these lesions typically are located in the inferior mid- to far-peripheral retina. Atrophic and disciform macular scarring and peripapillary atrophy, scarring, and choroidal neovascularization also may occur in all of these syndromes.

PATHOLOGY

Histopathology of peripheral lesions demonstrates the infiltration of lymphocytes.[12] Caseating granulomatous foci with fibrohyaline scarring may be present.[12] The granulomas may contain structures suggesting *H. capsulatum*.[6,7]

The macular lesions of OHS show disruption of Bruch's membrane with ingrowth of a neovascular complex into the subretinal space (Fig. 170-5).[13] There may be an overlying serous retinal detachment and subretinal hemorrhage. A variable amount of lymphocytic infiltration may be present. The CNVM may appear only loosely adherent to the overlying photoreceptors and underlying native RPE.[13] If left untreated, the subretinal hemorrhage and serum in the subretinal space may lead to proliferation and metaplasia of RPE into fibrovascular tissue that organizes into an inactive disciform plaque.[12] Lymphocytes can sometimes become a prominent feature of the choroid adjacent to the subretinal scar.[12] The peripapillary scar also demonstrates RPE proliferation and replacement of much of the choroid by fibrovascular tissue.[12] Disruption of Bruch's membrane and extensive destruction of the overlying photoreceptors also may occur in this area.[14]

Surgically excised CNVMs demonstrate the expression of various growth factors—basic fibroblast growth factor, transforming growth factor β-1, and procollagen.[15] These growth factors may play a role in the development of choroidal neovascularization.

TREATMENT

Most patients who have OHS are asymptomatic unless they develop choroidal neovascularization in the peripapillary or macular regions. Macular choroidal neovascularization may be subdivided into the following[16]:

- Extrafoveal lesions, when the foveal edge is more than 200mm from the center of the fovea
- Juxtafoveal lesions, when the foveal edge is 1–199mm from the center of the fovea
- Subfoveal lesions, when any part of the membrane has clearly grown underneath the center of the fovea

Argon green or krypton red laser photocoagulation of extrafoveal and juxtafoveal lesions in ocular histoplasmosis is recommended. Untreated eyes with CNVM and ocular histoplasmosis have a 3–6 times greater risk of losing six or more lines of visual acuity than do treated eyes.[16] Recurrent neovascularization has been observed in 26% of treated eyes within 5 years of the initial laser photocoagulation.[16] Treatment using argon green or krypton red laser is equally efficacious with similar visual outcomes.[17] Laser treatment is accomplished by using a 100–200mm spot size of 0.2–0.5sec duration, and enough power to attain a uniform whitening of the entire CNVM defined anatomically by fluorescein angiography. Treatment using laser photocoagulation is reassessed 2–4 weeks after the treatment; and fluorescein angiography is used to look for persistence or recurrence of choroidal neovascularization. Continued Amsler's chart monitoring for the development of new metamorphopsia is important. Follow-up visits should be performed at 2, 3, and 6 months posttreatment.

Treatment of subfoveal CNVMs in OHS is less clear cut.[18] Patients who have good visual acuity with subfoveal choroidal neovascularization should not be treated with laser photocoagulation because an immediate drop in visual acuity occurs, particularly if visual acuity is better than 20/200 (6/60). Up to 14% of eyes with subfoveal CNVMs retain visual acuity of 20/40 (6/12) or better without any treatment.[18] Periocular depot injections of triamcinolone or dexamethasone or a course of oral corticosteroids for 3–4 weeks may be useful to limit the progression of subfoveal choroidal neovascularization in some patients. Subfoveal surgery to remove CNVMs in ocular histoplasmosis appears to be promising. However, surgery requires pars plana vitrectomy, disinsertion and removal of the posterior hyaloid, a small retinotomy, and careful delamination, dissection, and removal of the CNVM from the subretinal space.[19] With successful surgery, 85% of patients have stable vision between 3 and 12 months after surgery.[20] Risks of surgery include intraocular hemorrhage, suprachoroidal hemorrhage, endophthalmitis, retinal detachment, and cataract. In addition, choroidal neovascularization may recur in 44% of cases within 13 months after surgery.[21] Approximately 66% of these recurrences are subfoveal. Recurrences may warrant further surgery, laser photocoagulation, or merely observation.[21] Other treatment options include limited macular translocation, especially in cases when subfoveal retinal pigment epithelial loss occurs during subfoveal surgery.[22] Ocular photodynamic therapy using verteporfin, a second-generation lipophilic-amphiphilic photosensitizer, for subfoveal CNVMs is also promising. A preliminary study showed that visual improvement was even possible with this method.[23] The Verteporfin in Ocular Histoplasmosis (VOH) study group recently completed a multicenter, uncontrolled, prospective clinical trial for choroidal neovascular membranes less than 5400 μm in greatest lesional dimension that extended under the geometric center of the foveal avascular zone.[24] At the end of 1 year of follow-up, 25 patients had received an average of 2.9 treatments and 56% (14) has improved 7 or more ETDRS letters of visual acuity from baseline and 16% (4) had lost 8 or more letters. There are no systemic or ocular adverse events reported.[24] The 2-year results are still pending.

COURSE AND OUTCOME

Patients who have OHS who do not develop macular complications of the disease enjoy excellent visual acuity and visual prognosis. Treatment of extrafoveal and juxtafoveal choroidal neovascularization with argon or krypton laser photocoagulation reduces the risk of serious visual loss by at least 50%.[16] Extrafoveal choroidal neovascularization has an excellent visual prognosis after treatment.[16] However, the visual prognosis for subfoveal choroidal neovascularization is guarded.[18]

Patients who have a disciform scar or choroidal neovascularization in one eye and evidence of macular atrophic scars in the high-risk region (defined vertically between the temporal arcades, nasally by the temporal disc margin, and temporally by disc to fovea distance from the foveal center) in the fellow eye have approximately a 20% risk over a 2–3-year period of developing choroidal neovascularization in the macula of the fellow eye.[18] Patients who do not have macular lesions are at significantly lower risk of developing choroidal neovascularization. However, de novo choroidal neovascularization has been reported in patients with OHS who did not appear to have macular scars.

Reactivation of inflammatory lesions may occur also in patients with OHS.[25] This phenomenon dispels the notion of OHS being a static disease and may explain the development of new lesions and enlargement of old chorioretinal scars in patients with OHS. Patients with reactivation may complain of decreased vision and metamorphopsia. Reactivation usually is not accompanied by vitritis. Clinical examination may demonstrate mild graying of the choroid and/or RPE and thickening of the retina. Fluorescein angiography of reactivated lesions demonstrates progressive leakage with irregular borders without evidence of underlying CNVM.[25] Patients may be treated with systemic itraconazole combined with oral corticosteroids, which also may be used alone.[25] Most lesions improve within 4 to 12 weeks. Choroidal neovascularization only rarely occurs after several months at the site of these reactivated lesions.[25]

Subfoveal choroidal neovascularization generally is associated with a poorer visual prognosis.[18] More than 75% of patients who have subfoveal choroidal neovascularization have visual acuity of 20/100 (6/30) or worse after 3 years.[18] However, up to 14% of eyes with subfoveal choroidal neovascularization may retain visual acuity of 20/40 (6/12) or better if the patient is less than 30 years of age, has small CNVMs, and has no visual loss secondary to OHS in the fellow eye.[18] Patients who are older and who have more than 50% involvement of the foveal avascular zone at the time of diagnosis have a significantly greater likelihood of poorer visual outcomes with subfoveal choroidal neovascularization in OHS.[18]

Spontaneous visual acuity recovery in patients who have central disciform scarring in OHS has been reported only when visual acuity drops to 20/80 (6/24) or worse in the fellow eye.[26] Spontaneous visual recovery occurs more commonly in younger patients and patients who have smaller diameter disciform scars, shorter distances from the foveal center to adjacent normal retina, and shorter intervals of visual loss prior to visual loss in the fellow eye.[26] Such visual acuity recovery also may occur from spontaneous involution of subfoveal choroidal neovascularization in some rare instances.

REFERENCES

1. Weingeist TA, Watzke RC. Ocular involvement by *Histoplasma capsulatum*. Int Ophthalmol Clin. 1983;23:33–47.
2. Specht CS, Mitchell KT, Bauman AE, Gupta M. Ocular histoplasmosis with retinitis in a patient with acquired immune deficiency syndrome. Ophthalmology. 1991;98:1356–9.
3. Schlaegel TF Jr. Ocular histoplasmosis. Proceedings of the ocular histoplasmosis symposium. Int Ophthalmol Clin. 1975;15:285–6.
4. Burgess DB. Ocular histoplasmosis syndrome. Ophthalmology. 1986;93:967–8.
5. Smith RE, Ganley JP. Presumed ocular histoplasmosis. I. Histoplasmin skin test sensitivity in cases identified during a community survey. Arch Ophthalmol. 1972;87:245–50.
6. Khalil MK. Histopathology of presumed ocular histoplasmosis. Am J Ophthalmol. 1982;94:369–76.
7. Roth AM. *Histoplasma capsulatum* in the presumed ocular histoplasmosis syndrome. Am J Ophthalmol. 1977;84:293–8.
8. Meredith TA, Smith RE, Braley RE, et al. The prevalence of HLA-B7 in presumed ocular histoplasmosis in patients with peripheral atrophic scars. Am J Ophthalmol. 1978;86:325–8.
9. Spaide RF, Yannuzzi LA, Freund KB. Linear streaks in multifocal choroiditis and panuveitis. Retina. 1991;11:229–31.
10. Fine SL. Early detection of extrafoveal neovascular membranes by daily central field evaluation. Ophthalmology. 1985;92:603–9.
11. Ganley JP. Epidemiology of presumed ocular histoplasmosis [editorial]. Arch Ophthalmol. 1984;102:1754–6.
12. Makley TA, Craig EL, Werling K. Histopathology of ocular histoplasmosis. Int Ophthalmol Clin. 1983;23:1–18.
13. Gass JD. Biomicroscopic and histopathologic considerations regarding the feasibility of surgical excision of subfoveal neovascular membranes. Am J Ophthalmol. 1994;118:285–98.
14. Yanoff M, Fine BS. Ocular pathology: a text and atlas, ed 4. St. Louis: CV Mosby; 1994:395.
15. Reddy VM, Zamora RL, Kaplan HJ. Distribution of growth factors in subfoveal neovascular membranes in age-related macular degeneration and presumed ocular histoplasmosis syndrome. Am J Ophthalmol. 1995;120:291–301.
16. Anonymous. Argon laser photocoagulation for neovascular maculopathy. Five-year results from randomized clinical trials. Macular Photocoagulation Study Group. Arch Ophthalmol. 1991;109:1109–14 [erratum in Arch Ophthalmol. 1992;110:761].
17. Anonymous. Argon green vs krypton red laser photocoagulation for extrafoveal choroidal neovascularization. One-year results in ocular histoplasmosis. The Canadian Ophthalmology Study Group. Arch Ophthalmol. 1994;112:1166–73 [erratum in Arch Ophthalmol. 1995;113:184].
18. Olk RJ, Burgess DB, McCormick PA. Subfoveal and juxtafoveal subretinal neovascularization in the presumed ocular histoplasmosis syndrome. Visual prognosis. Ophthalmology. 1984;91:1592–602.
19. Thomas MA, Kaplan HJ. Surgical removal of subfoveal neovascularization in the presumed ocular histoplasmosis syndrome. Am J Ophthalmol. 1991;111:1–7.
20. Holekamp NM, Thomas MA, Dickinson JD, Valluri S. Surgical removal of subfoveal choroidal neovascularization in presumed ocular histoplasmosis: stability of early visual results. Ophthalmology. 1997;104:22–6.
21. Melberg NS, Thomas MA, Dickinson JD, Valluri S. Managing recurrent neovascularization after subfoveal surgery in presumed ocular histoplasmosis syndrome. Ophthalmology. 1996;103:1064–7.
22. Fujii GY, de Juan E, Thomas MA, et al. Limited macular translocation for the management of subfoveal retinal pigment epithelial loss after submacular surgery. Am J Ophthalmol. 2001;131:272–5.
23. Sickenberg M, Schmidt-Erfurth U, Miller JW, et al. A preliminary study of photodynamic therapy using verteporfin for choroidal neovascularization in pathologic myopia, ocular histoplasmosis syndrome, angioid streaks, and idiopathic causes. Arch Ophthalmol. 2000;118:327–36.
24. Saperstein DA, Rosenfeld PJ. Bressler NM. Verteporfin in Ocular Histoplasmosis (VOH) study group. Photodynamic therapy of subfoveal choroidal neovascularization with verteporfin in the ocular histoplasmosis syndrome: one-year results of an uncontrolled, prospective case series. Ophthalmology. 2002;109:1499–505.
25. Callanan D, Fish GE, Anand R. Reactivation of inflammatory lesions in ocular histoplasmosis. Arch Ophthalmol. 1998;116:470–4.
26. Jost BF, Olk RJ, Burgess DB. Factors related to spontaneous visual recovery in the ocular histoplasmosis syndrome. Retina. 1987;7:1–8.

CHAPTER

171 Candidiasis, Aspergillosis, and Coccidioidomycosis

SHAILAJA VALLURI • RAMANA S. MOORTHY

DEFINITION
- A chronic intraocular inflammation induced by fungi such as *Candida albicans, Coccidioides immitis,* and *Aspergillus* spp.

KEY FEATURES
- Candidal intraocular infection usually manifests as a fluffy white choroidal or retinal lesion with white snowball-like vitreous opacities.
- *Aspergillus* causes endophthalmitis via hematogenous spread, usually from the lung.
- Coccidioidal intraocular inflammation may appear as chronic iridocyclitis, iris granuloma, choroiditis, or chorioretinitis.

ASSOCIATED FEATURES
Candidal Intraocular Infection
- Usually seen in immunocompromised individuals, presence of candidemia.

Aspergillus Endogenous Endophthalmitis
- Usually seen in immunocompromised individuals but rarely in healthy patients.

Coccidioidal Intraocular Inflammation
- Systemic coccidioidal infection, endemic in American Southwest, including the San Joaquin Valley in California, northern Mexico, and Argentina.

INTRODUCTION

Various fungi can cause chronic granulomatous or nongranulomatous uveitis or other intraocular inflammations. The infectious agent can gain access into the ocular cavity either by traumatic introduction (exogenous) or through hematogenous spread (endogenous). In this chapter clinically significant and varied endogenous fungal intraocular inflammation caused by *Candida albicans, Coccidioides immitis, Aspergillus flavus,* and *Aspergillus fumigatus* are discussed. The exogenous infections are discussed in Chapter 169.

CANDIDA ALBICANS—ENDOGENOUS ENDOPHTHALMITIS

INTRODUCTION

Candida albicans is an important nosocomial, diphasic fungal pathogen. The yeast form is responsible for human disease. The incidence of hospital-acquired candidemia appears to be increasing as the number of immunocompromised patients rises.[1]

EPIDEMIOLOGY AND PATHOGENESIS

Patients who develop endogenous candida endophthalmitis are usually immunocompromised. Most patients either have a chronic underlying systemic illness, an associated septicemia for which broad spectrum systemic antibiotic therapy is being administered, intravenous hyperalimentation with chronic indwelling catheters, or an organ transplantation that requires immunosuppression.[1,2] In addition, intravenous drug abusers and those with acquired immunodeficiency syndrome are also at high risk for candida endophthalmitis.[1]

OCULAR MANIFESTATIONS

Patients who have endogenous candida endophthalmitis seek treatment for ocular pain, decreased vision, and floaters.[1] The typical lesion of candida endophthalmitis is that of a white, fluffy, chorioretinal lesion that has overlying vitreous inflammation and haze (Fig. 171-1). The infection can extend into the vitreous and produce white snowball-like opacities. The retinochoroiditis may progress and satellite lesions may develop adjacent to the primary lesion. Occasionally anterior uveitis, scleritis, or panophthalmitis also may occur.

DIAGNOSIS

Diagnosis usually is based on the typical clinical appearance. Cultures of blood, catheter tips, surgical wounds, and body fluids are often positive for *Candida*. Diagnostic vitreous biopsy and cultures may be required to confirm the diagnosis. Polymerase chain reaction (PCR)–mediated detection of *C. albicans* in vitreous has been performed successfully and may be used to aid in the diagnosis.[3]

DIFFERENTIAL DIAGNOSIS

The differential diagnosis of candida endophthalmitis is given in Box 171-1.

PATHOLOGY

Candidal fungemia can lead to the development of random lesions in the eye, particularly in the vitreous, retina, and choroid.

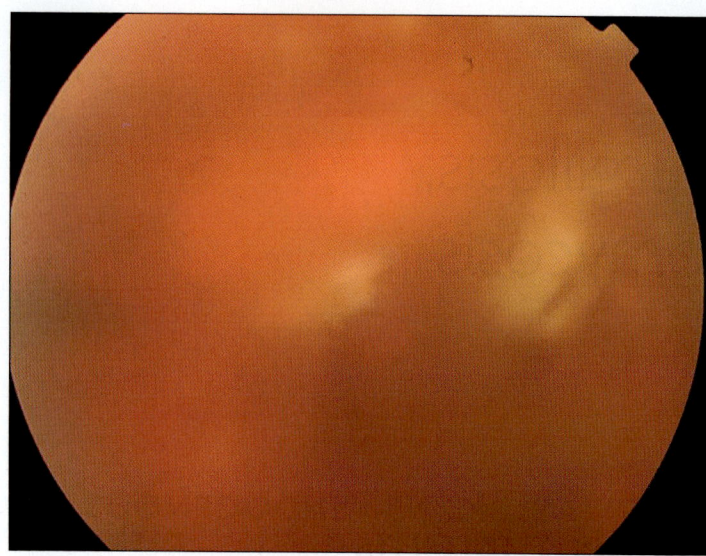

FIG. 171-1 ■ Fifty-year-old patient with endogenous candida endophthalmitis with a history of pancreaticoduodenectomy requiring intravenous hyperalimentation. Note vitreous haze from vitreitis, white chorioretinitis over the optic disc, and a separate focus in macula of the right eye.

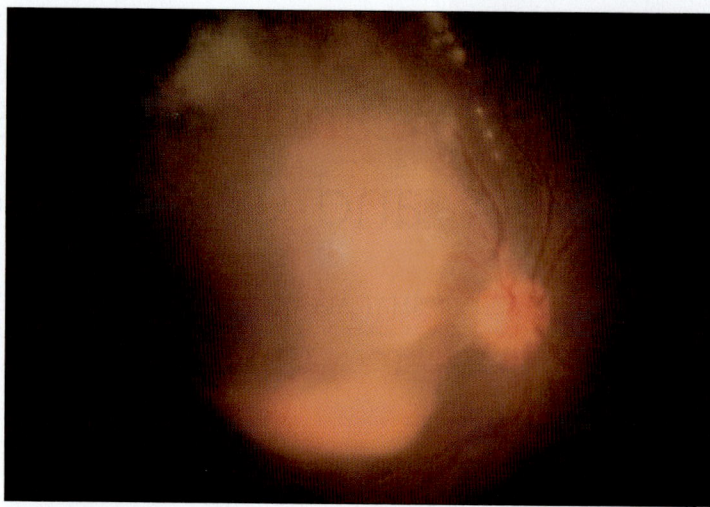

FIG. 171-2 ■ Twenty-seven-year-old patient with endogenous aspergillus endophthalmitis. Fundus photograph demonstrates a posterior hyaloidal hypopyon and a chorioretinitis affecting the macular region.

BOX 171-1

Differential Diagnosis of Candida Endophthalmitis

Endogenous bacterial endophthalmitis
Toxoplasmin retinochoroiditis
Primary intraocular lymphoma
Cytomegalovirus retinitis
Syphilitic chorioretinitis
Aspergillus endophthalmitis

The lesions demonstrate polymorphonuclear leukocytes, lymphocytes, budding yeast, and pseudohyphae. Choroidal and retinal vessel wall invasion is not seen in candida endophthalmitis.[4] The vitreous is the primary focus of infection in candida endophthalmitis.[4] The vitreous inflammatory masses also may contain the organism.

TREATMENT

Because most patients with candida endophthalmitis have concurrent candida septicemia, intravenous amphotericin B therapy is recommended.[1] A total intravenous dose of 1g usually is sufficient to eradicate endogenous candida endophthalmitis when given over a 4–6 week period. 5-Fluorocytosine may be substituted for or given concurrently with amphotericin B in particularly resistant cases.

Persistent candida endophthalmitis that does not respond to systemic intravenous amphotericin B should be treated with pars plana vitrectomy (PPV) and an intravitreal injection of 5μg of amphotericin B. PPV has now become an essential part of the management of most cases of candida endophthalmitis,[5] especially those with marked vitreous infiltration.

Nephrotoxicity is the most serious complication of systemic amphotericin B therapy. Consultation with an infectious disease specialist and careful monitoring of serum creatinine levels are recommended for patients who receive intravenous amphotericin B.

COURSE AND OUTCOME

Rapid diagnosis and induction of systemic amphotericin B therapy are essential for both reduction of mortality and ocular mor-

bidity associated with endogenous candida endophthalmitis.[1] Efficacy of treatment is determined by close ophthalmic follow-up. The patient may need to be examined twice weekly for the first 2 weeks, followed by weekly bilateral dilated fundus examinations. Often, significant visual improvements occur within 1 week of initiating systemic amphotericin B therapy. The visual prognosis for candida endophthalmitis is better than for that caused by *Aspergillus* if properly managed. Approximately 76% of eyes in one series achieved a final visual acuity of 20/400 or better.[5]

ASPERGILLUS FLAVUS AND FUMIGATUS—ENDOGENOUS ENDOPHTHALMITIS

EPIDEMIOLOGY AND PATHOGENESIS

Aspergillus fumigatus is the most common pathogen in human aspergillosis, followed by *A. flavus*, *A. niger*, *A. nidulans*, and *A. terreus*. Endogenous aspergillus endophthalmitis is a rare disorder associated with disseminated aspergillosis and intravenous drug abuse.[6,7] Disseminated aspergillosis appears to be most common among patients with severe chronic pulmonary diseases or those who are severely immunocompromised.[6] It has been reported in particular among patients following orthotopic liver transplantation.[7] The eyes are a common site of infection, in some series second only to the lung. Rarely aspergillus endophthalmitis may occur in immunocompetent patients with no apparent predisposing factors.[8]

Aspergillus spp. commonly grow in soils and decaying vegetation. They are ubiquitous saprophytic spore-forming molds. The spores or conidia become airborne and seed the lungs and paranasal sinuses of humans. Although exposure is very common, human infection is rare. Predisposing conditions of the host combined with virulence of *Aspergillus* spp. affect development of human disease. Hematogenous dissemination of organisms from the lung to the choroid results in ocular disease.[6,7]

OCULAR MANIFESTATIONS

Endogenous aspergillus endophthalmitis has characteristic ocular features. Patients develop rapid onset of pain and visual loss. A confluent yellowish infiltrate is seen in the macula beginning

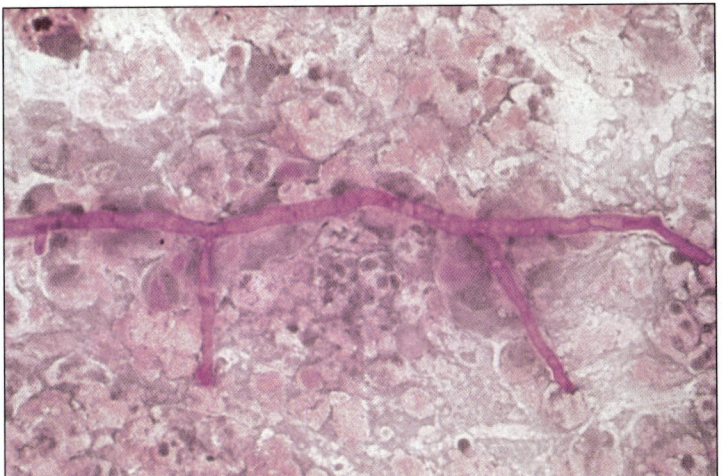

FIG. 171-3 ■ Light micrograph of vitreous aspirate demonstrating large branching septate hyphae of *Aspergillus fumigatus.* Periodic acid-Schiff, ×520.

BOX 171-2

Differential Diagnosis of Endogenous Aspergillus Endophthalmitis

Candida endophthalmitis
Cytomegalovirus retinitis
Toxoplasma retinochoroiditis
Coccidioidomycotic choroiditis/endophthalmitis
Bacterial endophthalmitis

in the choroid and subretinal space. A hypopyon develops in the subretinal or subhyaloidal space (Fig. 171-2). This can progress to retinal vascular occlusion and full-thickness retinal necrosis. Intraretinal hemorrhages usually occur. Eventually the infection spreads into the vitreous, producing dense vitritis and into the anterior segment, producing varying degrees of cell, flare, and hypopyon in the anterior chamber. The macular lesions heal to form a central atrophic scar.[6]

DIAGNOSIS

The diagnosis of endogenous aspergillus endophthalmitis is based on pars plana vitreous biopsy and cultures aided by Gram and Giemsa stains (Fig. 171-3).[6,7] Anterior chamber and vitreous aspirates alone are unreliable. Coexisting systemic aspergillosis may provide obvious clues to the clinical diagnosis, especially among high-risk patients.

DIFFERENTIAL DIAGNOSIS

The differential diagnosis of endogenous aspergillus endophthalmitis is given in Box 171-2.

HISTOPATHOLOGY

Aspergillus endophthalmitis lesions have a predilection for the postequatorial fundus.[6,7] Histologically, these retinal and choroidal lesions are angiocentric.[7] Extensive areas of deep choroiditis and retinitis may be present.[4] Mixed acute (polymorphonuclear leukocytes) and chronic (lymphocytes and plasma cells) inflammatory cells infiltrate the infected areas of the choroid and retina. Hemorrhage is present in all retinal lay-

ers and occasional choroidal hemorrhage occurs.[7] Granulomata contain rare giant cells. Contiguous inflammation of the choroid and retina is present as a rule. Fungal hyphae may be seen spreading on the surface of Bruch's membrane without penetrating it.[7] Vitreous inflammatory cells are composed mainly of polymorphonuclear leukocytes. Fungal hyphae often are surrounded by macrophages and lymphocytes, which form small vitreous abcesses.[7] Unlike candida endophthalmitis, in which the vitreous is the primary focus of infection, aspergillus endophthalmitis is marked by retinal and choroidal vessel invasion and subretinal pigment epithelial and subretinal infection.[4]

TREATMENT

Endogenous aspergillus endophthalmitis must be treated aggressively with diagnostic and therapeutic PPV combined with intravitreal injection of 5–10μg of amphotericin B.[6] The amphotericin B may be reinjected weekly, but the cumulative intravitreal dose should be kept below 25μg. Intravitreal corticosteroids may be used in conjunction with amphotericin B to reduce severe postoperative inflammatory response.[6] Because most patients with endogenous aspergillus endophthalmitis have disseminated aspergillosis, systemic treatment with intravenous amphotericin B is usually required. Other systemic antifungal agents such as itraconazole, miconazole, fluconazole, and ketoconazole may be used also. Systemic aspergillosis is best managed by an infectious disease specialist. The value of systemic antifungal agents in isolated ocular disease is unknown and controversial.

COURSE AND OUTCOME

Despite aggressive treatment, the visual prognosis is dismal. The final visual outcome is poor because of macular involvement. Most eyes have final visual acuity of less than 20/200.[6] Repeated operations to remove cataract, epiretinal membranes, or to control recalcitrant infection are not uncommon.[4,6,7] Close follow-up during the first 3 months after surgery is required.

COCCIDIOIDES IMMITIS—OCULAR COCCIDIOIDOMYCOSIS

INTRODUCTION

Coccidioidal uveitis should be considered for anyone with an apparent idiopathic iritis who has lived or traveled through endemic areas of the American Southwest, specifically southern California and the San Joaquin Valley, northern Mexico, or Argentina.[9]

OCULAR MANIFESTATIONS

Intraocular manifestations of coccidioidomycosis consist of iridocyclitis, iris granuloma (Fig. 171-4, *A*), choroiditis, or chorioretinitis.[9,10]

DIAGNOSIS

Systemic coccidioidal infection usually is present and complement fixation titers are elevated (>1:32). Rarely, the eye may be the only organ involved.[9,10] With isolated anterior segment involvement, an anterior chamber sample may be useful. Culturing for the organism may result in delayed diagnosis. The material from the anterior chamber sample may be examined directly for coccidioidal organisms using the Papanicolaou stain.[10]

DIFFERENTIAL DIAGNOSIS

The differential diagnosis of coccidioidal uveitis is given in Box 171-3.

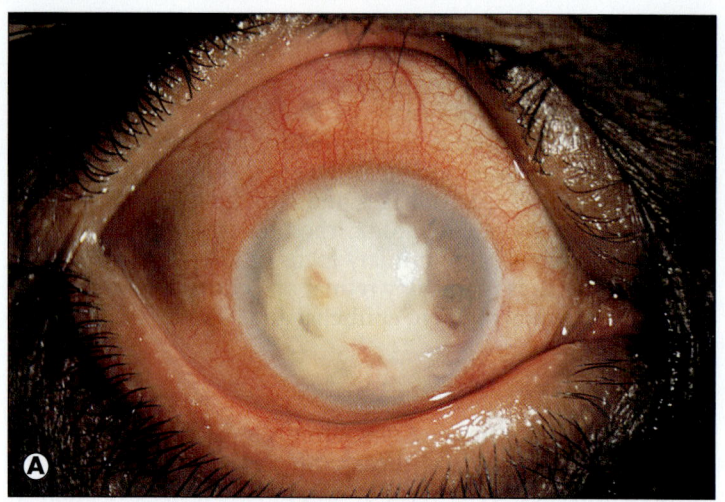

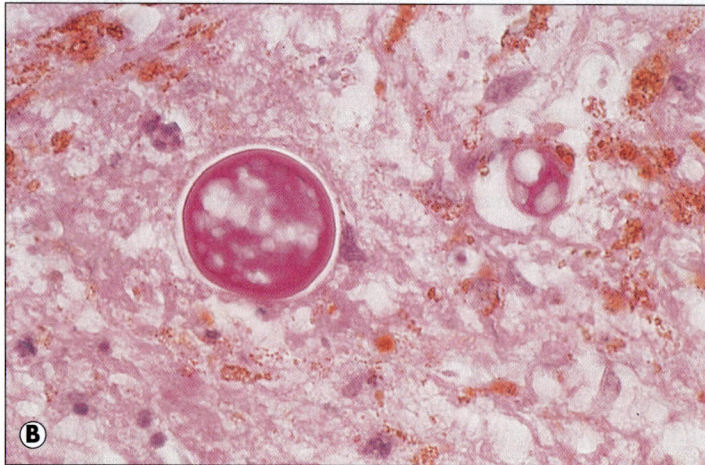

FIG. 171-4 ■ Anterior chamber coccidioidal granuloma causing pupillary block. **A,** Note the fungating nature of the lesion. **B,** Biopsy of the lesion revealed coccidioidal spherules.

BOX 171-3

Differential Diagnosis of Coccidioidal Uveitis

Candida endophthalmitis
Tuberculous uveitis
Aspergillus endophthalmitis
Histoplasma endophthalmitis

PATHOLOGY

Histopathologically, *C. immitis* evokes pyogenic, granulomatous, and mixed reactions. Intraocular lesions from the anterior segment usually demonstrate zonal granulomatous inflammation that involves the uvea and angle structure,[10] and coccidioides organisms usually are seen (Fig. 171-4, *B*).

TREATMENT

The treatment of intraocular coccidioidomycosis consists of administration of intravenous amphotericin B. The role of intraocular injections of this agent remains unclear. With systemic disease, much higher doses of intravenous amphotericin B may be needed. The role of systemic itraconazole in the treatment of intraocular coccidioidomycosis is unclear. Involvement of the infectious disease specialist is essential in these cases, because it is often difficult to determine when systemic therapy may be discontinued.[9,10]

COURSE AND OUTCOME

Prognosis for patients who have ocular coccidioidomycosis is poor. Most eyes require enucleation due to pain and blindness, despite aggressive treatment.[9,10]

OTHER FUNGAL UVEITIS

Endogenous fungal endophthalmitis due to *Cryptococcus neoformans*, *Sporothrix schenckii*, and *Blastomyces dermatitidis* are less common than those due to *Candida* and *Aspergillus*. Cryptococcal retinochoroiditis occurs in immunosuppressed patients, particularly those with acquired immunodeficiency syndrome and lymphoma. It often is associated with meningitis.[11] Both *S. schenckii* and *B. dermatitidis* tend to cause panuveitis, endophthalmitis and, in the case of *Blastomyces*, multifocal chorioretinitis.[12,13] Sporotrichosis often is found in horticulturists.[12] North American systemic blastomycosis usually is concurrently present in cases of blastomycotic panuveitis.[13] These infections often require intraocular as well as systemic therapy with amphotericin B, itraconazole, or ketoconazole.

REFERENCES

1. Menezes AV, Sigesmund DA, Demajo WA, Devenyi RG. Mortality of hospitalized patients with *Candida* endophthalmitis. Arch Intern Med. 1994;154:2093–7.
2. Brooks RG. Prospective study of *Candida* endophthalmitis in hospitalized patients with candidemia. Arch Intern Med. 1989;149:2226–8.
3. Hidalgo JA, Alangaden GJ, Eliot D, *et al.* Fungal endophthalmitis diagnosis by detection of *Candida albicans* DNA in intraocular fluid by use of species-specific polymerase chain reaction assay. J Infect Dis. 2000;181:1198–1201.
4. Rao NA, Hidayat AA. Endogenous mycotic endophthalmitis: variations in clinical and histopathologic changes in candidiasis compared with aspergillosis. Am J Ophthalmol. 2001;132:244–51.
5. Essman TF, Flynn HW, Smiddy WE, *et al.* Treatment outcomes in a 10-year study of endogenous fungal endophthalmitis. Ophthalmic Surg Lasers. 1997;28:185–94.
6. Weishaar PD, Flynn HW Jr, Murray TG, *et al.* Endogenous *Aspergillus* endophthalmitis: clinical features and treatment outcomes. Ophthalmology. 1998;105:57–65.
7. Hunt KE, Glasgow BJ. *Aspergillus* endophthalmitis: an unrecognized endemic disease in orthotopic liver transplantation. Ophthalmology. 1996;103:757–67.
8. Valluri S, Moorthy RS, Rao NA. Endogenous *Aspergillus* endophthalmitis in an immunocompetent individual. Int Ophthalmol. 1993;17:131–5.
9. Rodenbiker HT, Ganley JP. Ocular coccidioidomycosis. Surv Ophthalmol. 1980;24:263–90.
10. Moorthy RS, Sidikaro Y, Foos RY, Rao NA. *Coccidioidomycosis* iridocyclitis. Ophthalmology. 1994;101:1923–8.
11. Crump JR, Elner SG, Elner VM, Kauffman CA. Cryptococcal endophthalmitis: case report and review. Clin Infect Dis. 1992;14:1069–73.
12. Witherspoon CD, Kuhn F, Owens SD, *et al.* Endophthalmitis due to *Sporothrix schenckii* after penetrating ocular injury. Ann Ophthalmol. 1990;22:385–8.
13. Safneck JR, Hogg GR, Napier LB. Endophthalmitis due to *Blastomyces dermatitidis*. Case report and review of the literature. Ophthalmology. 1990;97:212–6.

SECTION 5 INFECTIOUS CAUSES OF UVEITIS: PROTOZOAL AND PARASITIC

CHAPTER 172

Ocular Toxoplasmosis

RALPH D. LEVINSON • SARAH M. RIKKERS

DEFINITION
- Intraocular inflammation due to infection with the parasite *Toxoplasma gondii*.

KEY FEATURE
- Focal retinochoroiditis.

ASSOCIATED FEATURES
- Decreased vision.
- Floaters.
- Anterior uveitis.
- Vitritis.
- Retinal vasculitis and vascular occlusions.
- Retinochoroidal scars.
- Papillitis.

INTRODUCTION

Ocular inflammation caused by infection with the obligate intracellular parasite *Toxoplasma gondii* (ocular toxoplasmosis) is the most common posterior uveitis in immunocompetent individuals.[1,2] Although ocular toxoplasmosis usually consists of a self-limited retinochoroiditis, sight-threatening complications do occur, and in one study it was the foremost cause of unilateral vision loss in patients who have uveitis.[3] In infants and immunosuppressed individuals, ocular toxoplasmosis may be more severe and can also be associated with potentially fatal systemic toxoplasmosis.

Our understanding of ocular toxoplasmosis is changing.[4,5] Traditionally, it was thought that toxoplasmic retinochoroiditis was almost always a reactivation of infection acquired in utero. New evidence has shown that newly acquired infection is more common than previously appreciated. The importance of the pathogenicity of specific strains of *T. gondii*, the role of host factors (including age and immune status), and new techniques for diagnosis and therapy of ocular toxoplasmosis are actively being researched.

ORGANISM AND LIFE CYCLE

T. gondii is an obligate intracellular protozoan parasite that is found worldwide and can infect most mammals and some birds. The life cycle of the organism is complex but helps explain many of the epidemiological and clinical features of the disease.[6] The sexual reproductive cycle of the parasite occurs within the small intestines of felines, the definitive hosts. The major morphological forms of *T. gondii* are the oocyst, tachyzoite, and tissue cyst. The oocyst is the product of sexual reproduction and is shed in the feces of cats. Oocysts can persist in soil for more than a year. Sporulation creates the infectious oocyst (containing sporozoites), which is ingested by cats and

other animals, including humans, with invasion of intestinal epithelial cells and asexual proliferation of the organism as tachyzoites. Tachyzoites can disseminate throughout the host's body in the lymph and hematological systems, carried by macrophages. Tachyzoites can penetrate virtually any nucleated cell. In the cell cytoplasm the organism is found in a parasitophorous vacuole, which protects the organism. In certain tissue types such as brain, heart, skeletal muscle, and retina, slowly metabolizing organisms (bradyzoites) form an argyrophilic, periodic acid-Schiff–positive tissue cyst in which the organism is safely isolated from the host's immune system. When the cyst wall breaks down, bradyzoites develop into tachyzoites and can invade neighboring cells.

EPIDEMIOLOGY

Human infection with *T. gondii* is most often acquired by eating the meat of infected animals, particularly undercooked pork and, less frequently, lamb, chicken, and beef. Exposure can also occur from contact with contaminated cat feces while cleaning a litter box or by playing in public sandboxes or dirt. Other sources of infection include eggs,[7] unpasteurized goat milk,[8] unwashed fruits and vegetables, municipal drinking water,[9] and inhalation of sporulated oocysts.[10] There is increasing evidence that acquired disease is more important as a source of ocular infection than previously recognized.[9–14]

Most individuals who have ocular manifestations of toxoplasmosis are thought to have acquired the disease in utero. Transplacental transmission of *T. gondii* to the fetus occurs only with new-onset maternal infection; chronic maternal infection or recurrent disease is not thought to result in transplacental transmission and congenital infection. Primary maternal infection has been estimated to occur in 0.2–1% of pregnancies.[11] Subsequent congenital infection also depends on the stage of pregnancy in which maternal infection develops. The rate of congenital toxoplasmosis increases from 10–15% following exposure in the first trimester to 60% following third-trimester exposure.[11] Congenital disease is much more severe when acquired early in pregnancy; the low rate of congenital disease with infection in the first trimester may be due to the risk of spontaneous abortion with early infection.

The rate of ocular disease appears to vary widely in different populations. The rate of seropositivity for toxoplasmosis is estimated to be from 3% to as high as 70% of adults in the United States; this varies for different locales and age groups,[6] whereas the prevalence of ocular toxoplasmosis is less than 1%. In areas such as Micronesia, there is a high degree of seropositivity, but ocular disease is very uncommon. This suggests that either host or parasite factors, or both, are important in the development of ocular disease. In evaluating 28 strains from around the world, Sibley and Boothroyd[15] found that virulent strains had the same genotype, whereas nonvirulent strains were polymorphic, implying that specific strains are more likely to cause disease. Host factors that are important in disease pathogenesis include the individual's immune status, which is discussed in the next section.

PATHOLOGY AND PATHOGENESIS

The primary pathological finding in active ocular toxoplasmosis is a well-demarcated coagulative retinal necrosis.[16] Viable tachyzoites and tissue cysts may be found in the infected retina.[17] An intense mononuclear inflammatory cell reaction is seen in the involved retina and vitreous, whereas a granulomatous reaction usually occurs in the contiguous choroid.

It is not known what factors are critical for the establishment of ocular disease or the triggering of recurrences. Tissue cysts may persist for years without causing an inflammatory reaction. The immune status of the host is clearly important, as demonstrated by the severe and prolonged disease course in patients who have acquired immunodeficiency syndrome (AIDS)[18] and in other immunosuppressed individuals, including those receiving corticosteroid therapy.[19,20] Host factors that determine the outcome of infection include multiple components of the immune response to the parasites.[6,21-25] Humoral immunity can play a role in lysis of the parasite when the parasites are extracellular, and antibody-coated parasites may not form a protective membrane, which is important for parasite survival in the host macrophage. However, the cellular immune response appears to be of primary importance for host defense, and both CD4 and CD8 T cells are involved in the immune defenses against *T. gondii*.[6]

There may be a role for autoimmunity in the pathogenesis of the ocular inflammation seen in ocular toxoplasmosis. The inflammatory response in the vitreous and anterior chamber is not associated with viable parasites in these fluids, at least in immunocompetent individuals. Further, the retinitis itself may in part be an autoimmune response and not just a response to the organism.[26,27] Meenken *et al.*[28] found that the HLA-Bw62 antigen correlated with severe ocular involvement in congenital toxoplasmosis. However, despite the frequently reported association of HLA subtypes with specific autoimmune diseases, HLA genes are important in host responses to infectious agents, so an HLA association may not imply an autoimmune pathogenesis.

OCULAR MANIFESTATIONS

Active ocular infection with toxoplasmosis typically manifests as a localized necrotizing retinitis. The classic lesion is a gray-white focus of retinal necrosis at the edge of a pigmented chorioretinal scar (Fig. 172-1). An adjacent choroiditis, retinal vasculitis, vitritis, iritis, and papillitis may also be seen. There is an overlying vitritis that can be so dense as to prohibit an adequate view of the posterior segment. When the white retinal lesion can just be seen through a dense vitritis, it has been described as a "headlight in the fog." The associated iritis can be quite severe, with granulomatous features, and may be associated with increased intraocular pressure.

The patient may present with floaters (vitritis), decreased vision (vitritis, papillitis, retinal necrosis, macular edema, choroidal neovascular membranes, vascular occlusions, retinal detachment), pain, redness, and photophobia (iritis). Complications that can result in permanent loss of vision include macular inflammation resulting in a scar, choroidal neovascular membranes, vascular occlusions, optic nerve involvement, and retinal detachment.

A chorioretinal scar may not be present, particularly with recently acquired disease[14,29] (Fig. 172-2). Holland *et al.*[29] reported 10 patients who presented with vitritis, iritis, and retinal vasculitis without clinically apparent retinal lesions. Four of nine of these patients later developed retinochoroidal scars. The authors thought that this presentation probably represented acquired disease. Conversely, extensive retinal necrosis can be seen in elderly patients with what may also be recently acquired disease.[30]

Other forms of toxoplasmosis have been described in immunocompetent patients. Freidmann and Knox[31] classified 56% of their patients as having "large destructive lesions," 27% as having "punctate inner lesions," and 17% as having "punctate deep lesions." The punctate inner lesions had less vitritis than did the large destructive lesions. The punctate deep lesions were located in the macula and had no significant vitritis. Punctate outer retinal toxoplasmosis[32] was described by Doft and Gass[33] and consists of multiple gray-white lesions less than 1000 μm in diameter at the level of the deep retina or retinal pigment epithelium. Their patients also had little vitritis. Punctate outer toxoplasmosis can be bilateral and may resolve without treatment, leaving fine white dots or small chorioretinal scars.[33] Neuroretinitis has also been attributed to infection with *T. gondii*. Most patients with toxoplasmic neuroretinitis have a good visual outcome with antiparasitic therapy.[34]

The most common manifestation of congenital toxoplasmosis is retinochoroiditis. Chorioretinal scars, often bilateral, are seen in about 80% of patients with congenital toxoplasmosis.[35] There is a moderate predilection for macular involvement, which may relate to fetal vascular patterns. The retinal inflammation in congenital toxoplasmosis tends to be self-limited, and the lesions may already be healed at birth or may develop months or years after birth. Other ocular manifestations include microcornea, microphthalmos, nystagmus, and strabismus.

Presumably, most individuals who are infected in utero and subsequently develop ocular toxoplasmosis do not develop clinical systemic congenital toxoplasmosis. However, acute congenital toxoplasmosis is a systemic disease and may be associated with low birth weight, fever, jaundice, maculopapular rash,

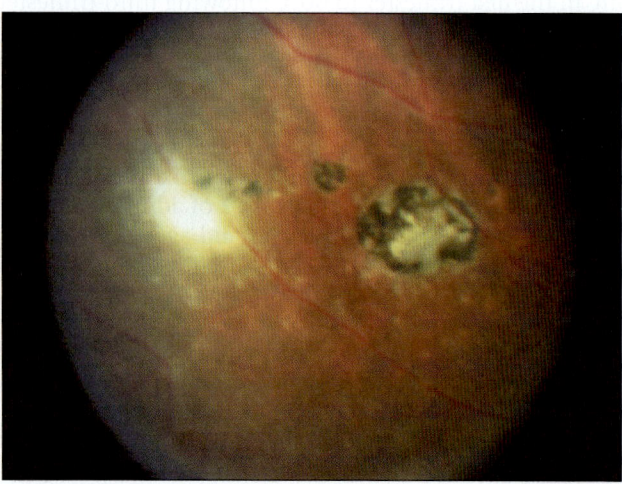

FIG. 172-1 ▮▮ Active ocular toxoplasmosis with an adjacent chorioretinal scar. From Holland GN, O'Connor GR, Belfort R, Remington JS. Toxoplasmosis. In Pepose JS, Holland GN, Wilhelmis KW, eds. Ocular infection and immunity. St. Louis: Mosby; 1996.

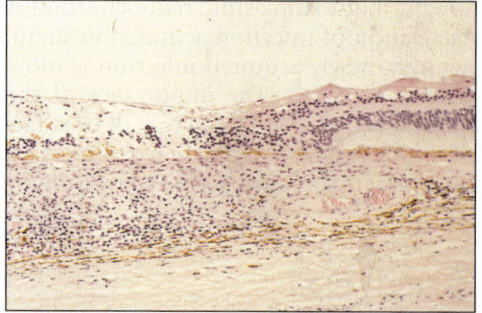

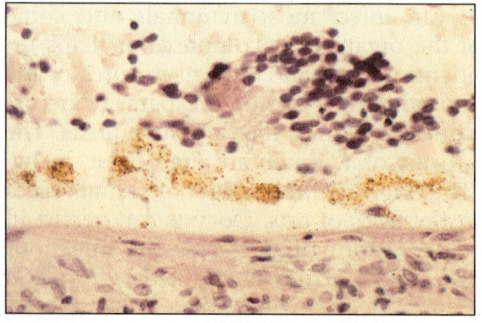

FIG. 172-2 ▮▮
Toxoplasmosis.
A, Histologic section showing an acute coagulative retinal necrosis, whereas the choroid shows a secondary diffuse granulomatous inflammation. **B,** A toxoplasmic cyst is present in the neural retina; note the tiny nuclei in the cyst. (From Yanoff M, Fine BS. Ocular pathology, ed 5. St. Louis: Mosby; 2002.)

pneumonia, and hepatosplenomegaly. Central nervous system involvement portends a poor outcome and may result in microcephaly, hydrocephaly, seizures, disseminated intracranial calcification, and psychomotor retardation. Severely infected infants may die within the first month of life, although infants with less severe forms of the disease may not show any signs of infection for months after birth.

In immunosuppressed and elderly patients, ocular infection can be quite severe, but perhaps more importantly, it can be associated with fatal systemic toxoplasmosis. Toxoplasmosis infection may involve the central nervous system, heart, and lungs in patients after organ transplants and in patients who have lymphomas.[19] In patients with AIDS, ocular toxoplasmosis is less common than toxoplasmic infection of other organs, in particular the central nervous system. Fifteen to 40% of individuals who have AIDS have antitoxoplasmosis antibodies in the United States,[36] and toxoplasmic encephalitis was seen in 25–50% of individuals who have AIDS and positive serologies before the era of immune reconstitution with multidrug regimens.[37] Toxoplasmic encephalitis in AIDS patients is usually a focal disease, but some patients may develop a diffuse encephalitis, which may be rapidly fatal.[38]

Ocular toxoplasmosis in individuals who have AIDS may be unilateral or bilateral, with single or multiple lesions, and it is often chronic or recurrent, requiring prolonged therapy.[18] The retinitis may be slowly progressive or very aggressive, with large areas of full-thickness retinal necrosis and severe vitritis. Patients who have AIDS have been reported to have unusual forms of ocular toxoplasmosis. Ocular toxoplasmosis presenting as an iridocyclitis without retinal involvement was confirmed by polymerase chain reaction techniques in an AIDS patient who had retinitis in the fellow eye.[39] Panophthalmitis with a presumed secondary orbititis has also been reported.[40]

DIAGNOSIS

The diagnosis of ocular toxoplasmosis is often made by the clinical features alone. Serological studies may be helpful in selected cases, but a positive serology does not in itself confirm the diagnosis, given the high rate of seropositive individuals found in many populations. A negative serology can, however, assist in eliminating the disease from the differential diagnosis, although false negatives do occur.

Serial tests for immunoglobulin G (IgG) and immunoglobulin M (IgM) antibodies, spaced at 3-week intervals, can identify a rise in titer levels and help point toward a recently acquired infection. Typically, IgG antibodies are produced within 2 weeks of infection, peak at 2 months, and are present for life. Detection of IgM antibody titers is usually possible within 2 weeks of infection and suggests a recently acquired infection. However, the IgM titer may be only transiently elevated; therefore, a negative titer does not rule out recent infection. Immunoglobulin A (IgA) antibodies are usually detectable for only 7 months and may be helpful in evaluating a patient for a recently acquired infection.[41,42] Because IgM antibodies do not cross the maternal-placental blood barrier, they are especially useful in diagnosing congenital toxoplasmosis. IgA antibodies may also be useful for evaluating infants for congenital toxoplasmosis.

The standard reference study for toxoplasmosis serologies is the Sabin-Feldman dye test. This test requires live *T. gondii* organisms and is not readily available. Most laboratories use enzyme-linked immunosorbent assay (ELISA), immunofluorescent antibody (IFA) test, or related techniques to measure serum anti-*Toxoplasma* antibodies. Serologies performed using Food and Drug Administration–approved ELISA kits for the detection of IgM may vary somewhat in their sensitivity and specificity.[43] False positives in patients with rheumatoid factor or antinuclear antibodies have been reported, but this appears to be less problematic with the newer available techniques.

Diagnosis in difficult cases could require invasive techniques. Ocular tissue sections and intraocular fluids have been examined for toxoplasmic DNA by polymerase chain reaction technology. Polymerase chain reaction has proved useful in the evaluation of some difficult cases.[44,45] Intraocular antibody production can be examined. Calculation of the Witmer Goldman coefficient is a technique used to evaluate intraocular antibody production by comparing the levels of antibody titers found in aqueous humor to those found in serum. In addition, detection of local IgA production increases the diagnostic sensitivity of aqueous humor analysis in early disease.[46]

DIFFERENTIAL DIAGNOSIS

Other diseases that must be considered in the differential diagnosis include acute retinal necrosis, sarcoidosis, pars planitis, endogenous bacterial or fungal infection, syphilis, tubercular chorioretinitis, and intraocular lymphoma. The differential diagnosis in newborn patients should include other congenital infections in the TORCH complex (*t*oxoplasmosis, *o*ther agents, *r*ubella, *c*ytomegalovirus, *h*erpes simplex), toxocariasis, macular coloboma, and retinoblastoma. Lymphocytic choriomeningitis has been described as resulting in macular scars that mimicked ocular toxoplasmosis in two otherwise normal children.[47] In AIDS patients, ocular toxoplasmosis can mimic cytomegalovirus retinopathy[48] (Fig. 172-3). In toxoplasmic retinochoroiditis, the retinitis is often more sharply demarcated, without associated hemorrhage, and there is usually more vitritis than in cytomegalovirus retinitis. Syphilitic uveitis, as well as other infections and lymphoma, must also be considered in AIDS patients.

TREATMENT

Toxoplasmic retinochoroiditis in immunocompetent individuals is often a self-limited process; therefore, not every episode requires therapeutic intervention. The potential benefits of treatment need to be balanced against the risks associated with antimicrobial therapy.[49,50]

Criteria that have been used for the initiation of treatment of immunocompetent patients include a two-line decrease in visual acuity, lesions located within the temporal arcade or affecting the optic nerve, moderate to severe vitreous inflammation. Relative indications for treatment include lesions with active inflammation for greater than 1 month, multiple active lesions, and newly acquired infections. The size of the lesion is thought by some to be a less important criterion for treatment. It is not clear whether punctate outer retinal toxoplasmosis requires therapy.[33,49,50]

Many agents have been used to treat ocular toxoplasmosis (Table 172-1). A triple-therapy regimen of pyrimethamine in conjunction with sulfadiazine and oral corticosteroids, or

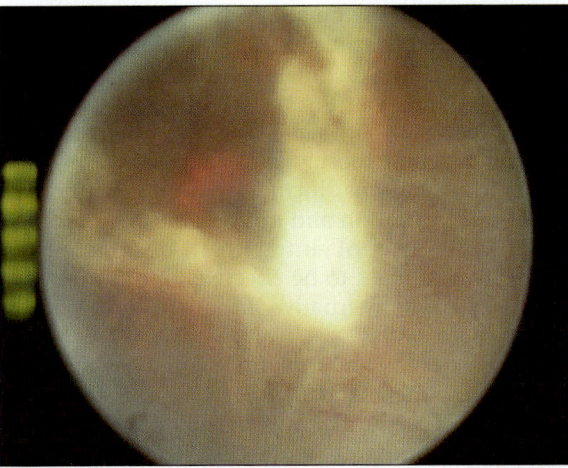

FIG. 172-3 ■ **Progressive toxoplasmic retinal necrosis in an AIDS patient.** From Holland GN, O'Connor GR, Belfort R, Remington JS. Toxoplasmosis. In Pepose JS, Holland GN, Wilhelmis KW, eds. Ocular infection and immunity. St. Louis: Mosby; 1996.

TABLE 172-1

DRUG THERAPY FOR OCULAR TOXOPLASMOSIS

	Triple/Quadruple Therapy*		
	Drug	Loading Dose	Treatment Dose
1	Pyrimethamine	50–100mg	25–50mg qd
2	Sulfadiazine	2–4g	1.0g qid
3	Clindamycin	None	300mg qid
4	Prednisone†	None	20–80mg qd (0.5–1.0mg/kg qd)
	+		
	Folinic acid	None	5mg/3× per week
	Other Agents		
	Atovaquone	None	750mg tid or qid
	Spiramycin	None	400mg tid
	Azithromycin	None	250mg qd
	Minocycline	None	100mg bid

*Numbers 1+2+4 = triple therapy; numbers 1+2+3+4 = quadruple therapy.
†Prednisone is started 24 hours after initiating antimicrobial therapy and is tapered before discontinuing antimicrobial therapy.

quadruple therapy with the addition of clindamycin, has traditionally been used to treat ocular toxoplasmosis. In a treatment survey, triple therapy was the most common single regimen selected; quadruple therapy was a close second.[49,50] A prospective study comparing triple therapy to sulfadiazine, clindamycin and prednisone, trimethoprim-sulfamethoxazole and prednisone, or no treatment found that the duration of ocular inflammation and mean recurrence rate were the same for all groups.[51] Although the first two regimens resulted in smaller lesion size compared with no treatment, the difference was statistically significant only for the triple therapy group.

Sulfonamides and pyrimethamine work by inhibiting folic acid metabolism. Folinic acid is administered concurrently with pyrimethamine to prevent bone marrow suppression. A baseline complete blood count needs to be obtained before initiating treatment, followed by weekly measurements during the duration of treatment to monitor for drug toxicity. Therapy should be discontinued if the white cell count falls below 4000 cells/μl or the platelet count is less than 100,000 cells/μl, or if either decreases 25–50% below baseline.[49]

Other agents that have been used to treat infections with *T. gondii* are included in Table 172-1. Atovaquone, a newer antiparasitic agent recently evaluated in a phase I trial, appears to be a well-tolerated therapeutic option.[52] Azithromycin may also be an effective agent for the treatment of acute disease, but it does not provide preventive benefits. A prospective, randomized trial comparing pyramethamine and sulfadiazine with pyramethamine and azithromycin found similar treatment efficacy but significantly less adverse drug effects with azithromycin.[53] Tetracycline, clarithromycin, and spiramycin also appear to be active against *T. gondii*. Combinations of medications that work by different mechanisms may have a synergistic effect. Such combinations include pyrimethamine and atovaquone or clarithromycin and minocycline.[5] According to a recent report, the use of intravitreal dexamethasone and clindamycin was thought to be effective in four eyes of four patients and may be an alternative in patients who cannot tolerate systemic therapy.[54]

Oral corticosteroids are sometimes used to control the inflammatory component of ocular toxoplasmosis, including any associated vitritis, vasculitis, and macular edema. Because increased ocular inflammation and retinal necrosis may be seen in patients receiving steroids without antimicrobial therapy, it is generally recommended that patients be treated for at least 24 hours with antiparasitic agents before beginning oral steroids.

Topical steroids may be used for the anterior uveitis but have no effect on vitritis or retinochoroiditis.

In immunocompetent individuals, treatment is continued until a significant decrease in inflammation is detected and the retinochoroiditis is no longer active. This is typically in the range of 4–6 weeks, but may be longer. Steroids should be tapered before discontinuing the antimicrobial agents. A recent randomized prospective study demonstrated that in healthy individuals the rate of recurrent toxoplasmic retinochoroiditis may be reduced by the use of long-term, intermittent trimethoprim/sulfamethoxazole therapy.[55]

Treatment of pregnant women is indicated in newly acquired disease and must take into consideration the teratogenicity of standard therapeutic agents. Spiramycin is thought to be the safest agent for use in pregnancy and may reduce the rate of *T. gondii* transmission to the fetus.[11] As noted earlier, recurrent maternal toxoplasmic retinochoroiditis is probably not associated with transmission of the parasite to the fetus and does not require treatment unless the mother's vision is threatened. Consideration could be given to intravitreal therapy, but the safety and effectiveness of this approach, particularly in pregnant women, have not been established. Because of the progressive nature of the ocular disease in immunosuppressed individuals with active ocular toxoplasmosis, treatment is recommended when there is any active disease in this patient population. Assessment for systemic toxoplasmosis, especially central nervous system disease, should also be pursued. The possibility of bone marrow suppression from pyrimethamine and the risk of further immunosuppression with corticosteroids are additional concerns. Long-term maintenance therapy, often with a single agent such as clindamycin, is needed to prevent recurrent disease. The role of immune reconstitution with the new antiretroviral therapies in preventing recurrences and controlling progression of toxoplasmosis in AIDS patients is not well established. It may be that with immune reconstitution it will be possible to forgo long-term therapy.

Surgical treatment with laser photocoagulation, cryotherapy, and vitrectomy has been tried, but efficacy has not been clearly demonstrated. The potential for retinal or vitreous hemorrhage and even retinal detachment when treating the acutely inflamed retina makes surgical intervention less desirable for active disease. In addition, laser or cryotherapy cannot predictably prevent disease recurrence, given that normal-appearing retina can harbor *Toxoplasma* tissue cysts. In cases in which vitrectomy is required to remove dense vitreous opacities, treatment with antimicrobial agents is recommended before and after surgery.

COURSE AND OUTCOME

Ocular toxoplasmosis is a self-limited process in immunocompetent patients, and most episodes resolve over a period of 1–2 months. The course can be prolonged in immunosuppressed patients, and in these individuals, as well as in infants, central nervous system and other systemic involvement may result in significant morbidity and mortality. Vision loss can be permanent from macular infection with a resultant scar or, less commonly, from optic nerve involvement, choroidal neovascular membranes, vascular occlusion, or rhegmatogenous retinal detachment.

REFERENCES

1. Henderly DE, Genstler AJ, Smith RE, Rao NA. Changing patterns of uveitis. Am J Ophthalmol. 1987;103:131–6.
2. McCannel CA, Holland GN, Helm CJ, et al. Causes of uveitis in the general practice of ophthalmology. UCLA Community-Based Uveitis Study Group. Am J Ophthalmol. 1996;121:35–46.
3. Rothova A, Suttorp-van Schulten MS, Frits Treffers W, Kijlstra A. Causes and frequency of blindness in patients with intraocular inflammatory disease. Br J Ophthalmol. 1996;80:332–6.
4. Holland GN. Reconsidering the pathogenesis of ocular toxoplasmosis. Am J Ophthalmol. 1999;128:502–5.
5. Holland GN. Ocular toxoplasmosis: new directions for clinical investigation. Ocul Immunol Inflamm 2000;8:1–7.
6. Holland GN, O'Connor GR, Belfort R Jr, Remington JS. Toxoplasmosis. In: Pepose JS, Holland GN, Wilhelmus KR, eds. Ocular infection and immunity, 1st ed. St. Louis: Mosby-Year Book; 1995:1183–223.
7. Swartzberg JE, Remington JS. Transmission of Toxoplasma. Am J Dis Child. 1975;129:777–9.
8. Sacks JJ, Roberto RR, Brooks NF. Toxoplasmosis infection associated with raw goat's milk. JAMA. 1982;248:1728–32.
9. Bowie WR, King AS, Werker DH, et al. Outbreak of toxoplasmosis associated with municipal drinking water. The BC Toxoplasma Investigation Team. Lancet. 1997;350:173–7.
10. Teutsch SM, Juranek DD, Sulzer A, et al. Epidemic toxoplasmosis associated with infected cats. N Engl J Med. 1979;300:695–9.
11. Wong SY, Remington JS. Toxoplasmosis in pregnancy. Clin Infect Dis. 1994;18:853–61.
12. Burnett AJ, Shortt SG, Isaac-Rentom J, et al. Multiple cases of acquired toxoplasmosis retinitis presenting in an outbreak. Ophthalmology. 1998;105:1032–7.
13. Nussenblatt RB, Belfort RJ. Ocular toxoplasmosis. An old disease revisited [clinical conference]. JAMA. 1994;271:304–7; erratum in JAMA. 1994;272(5):356.
14. Silveira C, Belfort RJ, Muccioli C, et al. A follow-up study of Toxoplasma gondii infection in southern Brazil. Am J Ophthalmol. 2001;131:351–4.
15. Sibley LD, Boothroyd JC. Virulent strains of Toxoplasma gondii comprise a single clonal lineage. Nature. 1992;359:82–5.
16. Zimmerman LE. Ocular pathology of toxoplasmosis. Surv Ophthalmol. 1961;6:832–8.
17. Rao NA, Font RL. Toxoplasmic retinochoroiditis: electron-microscopic and immunofluorescence studies of formalin-fixed tissue. Arch Ophthalmol. 1977;95:273–7.
18. Holland GN, Engstrom REJ, Glasgow BJ, et al. Ocular toxoplasmosis in patients with the acquired immunodeficiency syndrome. Am J Ophthalmol. 1988;106:653–67.
19. Israelski DM, Remington JS. Toxoplasmosis in the non-AIDS immunocompromised host. Curr Clin Top Infect Dis. 1993;13:322–56.
20. Morhun PJ, Weisz JM, Elias SJ, Holland GN. Recurrent ocular toxoplasmosis in patients treated with systemic corticosteroids. Retina. 1996;16:383–7.
21. Sharma SD, Hofflin JM, Remington JS. In vivo recombinant interleukin 2 administration enhances survival against a lethal challenge with Toxoplasma gondii. J Immunol. 1985;135:4160–3.
22. Lyons RE, Anthony JP, Ferguson DJ, et al. Immunological studies of chronic ocular toxoplasmosis: up-regulation of major histocompatibility complex class I and transforming growth factor beta and a protective role for interleukin-6. Infect Immun. 2001;69:2589–95.
23. Nagineni CN, Detrick B, Hooks JJ. Toxoplasma gondii infection induces gene expression and secretion of interleukin 1 (IL-1), IL-6, granulocyte-macrophage colony-stimulating factor, and intercellular adhesion molecule 1 by human retinal pigment epithelial cells. Infect Immun. 2000;68:407–10.
24. Shen DF, Matteson DM, Tuaillon N, et al. Involvement of apoptosis and interferon-gamma in murine toxoplasmosis. Invest Ophthalmol Vis Sci. 2001;42:2031–6.
25. Yap G, Pesin M, Sher A. Cutting edge: IL-12 is required for the maintenance of IFN-gamma production in T cells mediating chronic resistance to the intracellular pathogen, Toxoplasma gondii. J Immunol. 2000;165:628–31.
26. Muino JC, Juarez CP, Luna JD, et al. The importance of specific IgG and IgE autoantibodies to retinal S antigen, total serum IgE, and sCD23 levels in autoimmune and infectious uveitis. J Clin Immunol. 1999;19:215–22.
27. Nussenblatt RB, Mittal KK, Fuhrman S, et al. Lymphocyte proliferative responses of patients with ocular toxoplasmosis to parasite and retinal antigens. Am J Ophthalmol. 1989;107:632–41.
28. Meenken C, Rothova A, de Waal LP, et al. HLA typing in congenital toxoplasmosis 2720. Br J Ophthalmol. 1995;79:494–7.
29. Holland GN, Muccioli C, Silveira C, et al. Intraocular inflammatory reactions without focal necrotizing retinochoroiditis in patients with acquired systemic toxoplasmosis. Am J Ophthalmol. 1999;128:413–20.
30. Johnson MW, Greven GM, Jaffe GJ, et al. Atypical, severe toxoplasmic retinochoroiditis in elderly patients. Ophthalmology. 1997;104:48–57.
31. Friedmann CT, Knox DL. Variations in recurrent active toxoplasmic retinochoroiditis. Arch Ophthalmol. 1969;81:481–93.
32. Matthews JD, Weiter JJ. Outer retinal toxoplasmosis. Ophthalmology. 1988;95:941–6.
33. Doft BH, Gass DM. Punctate outer retinal toxoplasmosis. Arch Ophthalmol. 1985;103:1332–6.
34. Fish RH, Hoskins JC, Kline LB. Toxoplasmosis neuroretinitis. Ophthalmology. 1993;100:1177–82.
35. Mets MB, Holfels E, Boyer KM, et al. Eye manifestations of congenital toxoplasmosis. Am J Ophthalmol. 1996;122:309–24.
36. Luft BJ, Remington JS. Toxoplasmic encephalitis in AIDS. Clin Infect Dis. 1992;15:211–22.
37. Wong SY, Remington JS. Toxoplasmosis in the setting of AIDS. In: Broder S, Merigan TC, Bolognesi D, eds. Textbook of AIDS medicine, 1st ed. Baltimore: Williams & Wilkins; 1994:223–57.
38. Gray F, Gherardi R, Wingate E, et al. Diffuse "encephalitic" cerebral toxoplasmosis in AIDS. Report of four cases. J Neurol. 1989;236:273–7.
39. Cano-Parra JL, Diaz-Lopis ML, Cordoba JL, et al. Acute iridocyclitis in a patient with AIDS diagnosed as toxoplasmosis by PCR. Ocul Immunol Inflamm. 2000;8:127–30.
40. Moorthy RS, Smith RE, Rao NA. Progressive ocular toxoplasmosis in patients with acquired immunodeficiency syndrome. Am J Ophthalmol. 1993;115:742–7.
41. Ongkosuwito JV, Bosch-Driessen EH, Kijlstra A, Rothova A. Serologic evaluation of patients with primary and recurrent ocular toxoplasmosis for evidence of recent infection. Am J Ophthalmol. 1999;128:407–12.
42. Ronday MJ, Ongkosuwito JV, Rothova A, Kijlstra A. Intraocular anti-Toxoplasma gondii IgA antibody production in patients with ocular toxoplasmosis. Am J Ophthalmol. 1999;127:294–300.
43. Wilson M, Remington JS, Clavet C, et al. Evaluation of six commercial kits for detection of human immunoglobulin M antibodies to Toxoplasma gondii. The FDA Toxoplasmosis Ad Hoc Working Group. J Clin Microbiol. 1997;35:3112–5.
44. Figueroa MS, Bou G, Marti-Belda P, et al. Diagnostic value of polymerase chain reaction in blood and aqueous humor in immunocompetent patients with ocular toxoplasmosis. Retina. 2000;20:614–9.
45. Montoya JG, Parmley S, Liesenfeld O, et al. Use of the polymerase chain reaction for diagnosis of ocular toxoplasmosis. Ophthalmology. 1999;106:1554–63.
46. Garweg JG, Jacquier P, Boehnke M. Early aqueous humor analysis in patients with human ocular toxoplasmosis. J Clin Microbiol. 2000;38:996–1001.
47. Brezin AP, Thulliez P, Cisneros B, et al. Lymphocytic choriomeningitis virus chorioretinitis mimicking ocular toxoplasmosis in two otherwise normal children. Am J Ophthalmol. 2000;130:245–7.
48. Elkins BS, Holland GN, Opremcak EM, et al. Ocular toxoplasmosis misdiagnosed as cytomegalovirus retinopathy in immunocompromised patients. Ophthalmology. 1994;101:499–507.
49. Engstrom RE, Holland GN, Nussenblatt RB, Jabs DA. Current practices in the management of ocular toxoplasmosis. Am J Ophthalmol. 1991;111:601–10.
50. Holland GN, Lewis KG. An update on current practices in the management of ocular toxoplasmosis. Am J Ophthalmol. 2002;134:102–14.
51. Rothova A, Meenken C, Buitenhuis HJ, et al. Therapy for ocular toxoplasmosis. Am J Ophthalmol. 1993;115:517–23.
52. Pearson PA, Piracha AR, Sen HA, Jaffe GJ. Atovaquone for the treatment of Toxoplasma retinochoroiditis in immunocompetent patients. Ophthalmology. 1999;106:148–53.
53. Bosch-Driessen LH, Verbaak FD, Suttorp-Schulten MS, et al. A prospective, randomized trial of pyrimethamine and azithromycin vs pyrimethamine and sulfadiazine for the treatment of ocular toxoplasmosis. Am J Ophthalmol. 2002;134:34–40.
54. Kishore K, Conway MD, Peyman GA. Intravitreal clindamycin and dexamethasone for toxoplasmic retinochoroiditis. Ophthalmic Surg Lasers. 2001;32:183–92.
55. Silveira C, Belfort R Jr, Muccioli C, et al. The effect of long-term intermittent trimethoprim/sulfamethoxazole treatment on recurrences of toxoplasmic retinochoroiditis. Am J Ophthalmol. 2002;134:41–6.

JONATHAN D. WALKER

DEFINITION
- Ocular inflammation as a result of infection with a helminthic parasite. The three most common are *Toxocara canis*, *Cysticercus cellulosae*, and microfilariae of *Onchocerca volvulus*.

KEY FEATURES
Toxocariasis
- A result of ingesting eggs of *Toxocara*.
- Intraocular granuloma formation in the posterior pole or periphery.
- Endophthalmitis.

Cysticercosis
- A result of ingestion of tapeworm eggs.
- Ocular cysticercosis may occur anywhere in and around the eye.
- The appearance of cysticercosis is characteristic. It has a spherical, translucent cyst cavity associated with a protoscolex that may evaginate or invaginate in response to examination lights.

Onchocerciasis
- The presence of the microfilaria, alive or dead, in the ocular structures.
- Manifestations include sclerosing keratitis, iridocyclitis, glaucoma, and chorioretinitis.

ASSOCIATED FEATURES
Toxocariasis
- Ocular manifestations occur in systemically asymptomatic older children.
- Traction develops on the macula or optic disk or both.

Cysticercosis
- Death of the organism causes marked intraocular inflammation.
- Central nervous system cysticercosis may occur.

Onchocerciasis
- Onchocerciasis causes punctate keratitis.
- Secondary glaucoma.
- Optic atrophy occurs.

TOXOCARIASIS

EPIDEMIOLOGY AND PATHOGENESIS

The adult dog usually acquires *Toxocara canis* infection by eating eggs or second-stage larvae found in contaminated soil or infected meat or feces. The larvae encyst, and if the animal be-

comes pregnant some of the larvae may reactivate, at which time they can infect the fetal puppies in the uterus. Following birth the larvae then migrate to the puppy's lungs, are coughed up and swallowed, and finally grow to become egg-producing adult worms in the gastrointestinal tract. The eggs begin to be excreted about 4 weeks after birth.[1] Puppies are extremely important in the development and spread of this organism; ascertaining exposure to puppies may be a key part of the clinical history. However, *T. canis* is ubiquitous and soil samples show a rate of contamination in the range 10–92%.[2,3] As a result, human infection can occur fairly easily, especially in people who are exposed to puppies or who have a history of ingesting contaminated soil. Studies on populations demonstrate serological evidence of *T. canis* infection in the range 2–10%, but this may be as high as 80% in endemic areas.[4,5]

Following ingestion of the eggs a systemic *Toxocara* infection, known as *visceral larva migrans*, develops. This generally occurs in patients who are around 2 years old, which is younger than the average age of patients who have ocular disease.[6] The actual clinical picture of patients who have visceral larva migrans may vary, depending on the number of eggs ingested, distribution, and host immune factors. The eggs hatch in the intestines, and the larvae enter the bloodstream and migrate until the narrowing of the vascular lumen blocks progress. At this point the larvae enter the tissue and encyst; they often are found in the brain, liver, and lungs. Patients may have irritability, fever, and pulmonary and dermatological findings. Most cases probably go unrecognized because of few or no symptoms. Typical laboratory findings include a very elevated white blood cell count with a very high percentage of eosinophils.[4] Because the larva is incapable of completing its life cycle in humans, there is no point in checking stool for ova and parasites. It is uncommon for patients who have ocular toxocariasis to report a history suggestive of visceral larva migrans.[6]

OCULAR MANIFESTATIONS

The ocular disease may appear in a number of ways, the most common being in the form of a dense white granuloma in the posterior pole or retinal periphery where the larva has encysted. The inflammatory mass then contracts and draws the retina and vitreous toward the lesion (Fig. 173-1). A common finding with peripheral granulomas is a radial fold in the retina that extends from the optic nerve to the mass (Fig. 173-2). Vision may decrease markedly if the granuloma affects the optic nerve or posterior pole, or if significant dragging of the posterior pole occurs toward a more peripheral lesion. Late development of a rhegmatogenous retinal detachment may develop if holes occur in the atrophic retina that is being elevated by the traction. The granuloma itself often is white and globular, with a size of about one disc diameter. The eye usually is quiet, but low-to-moderate levels of smoldering inflammation may occur, even with what appears to be an old quiescent granuloma.

Patients may have a more marked inflammation that may simulate endophthalmitis, probably due to massive antigen release by dying organisms. Usually a significant vitreous reaction

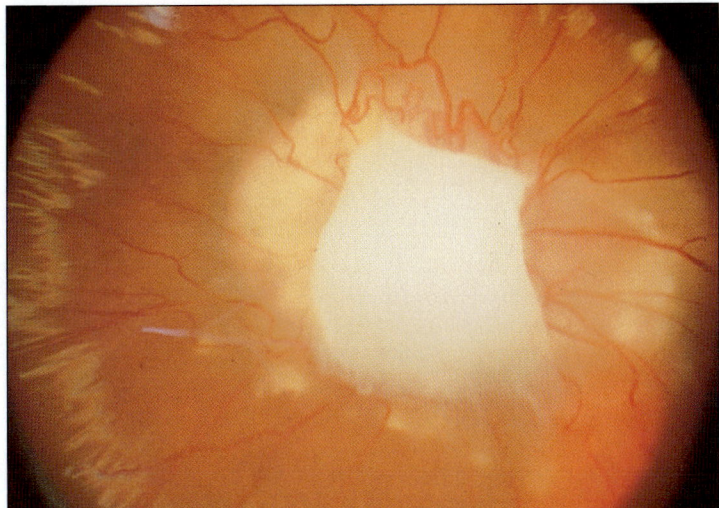

FIG. 173-1 ■ Typical toxocara granuloma located over the optic nerve. Note how the surrounding retina is drawn toward the lesion.

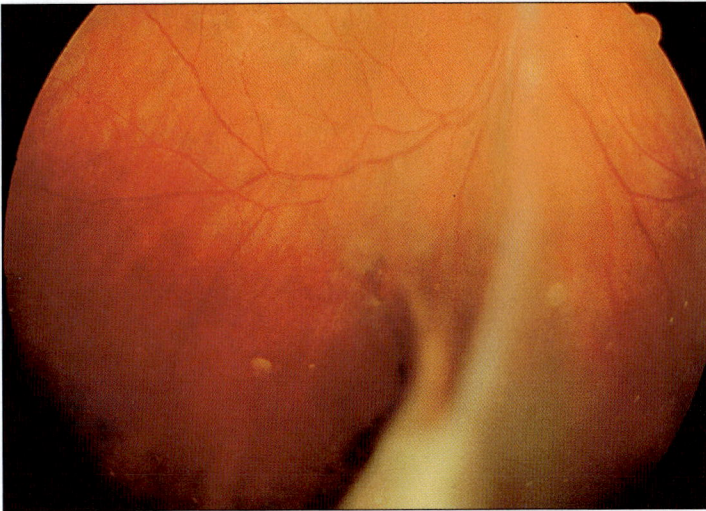

FIG. 173-2 ■ Falciform fold. It extends from the optic nerve *(top)* to a peripheral toxocara granuloma *(bottom)*.

occurs with a variable anterior chamber response. The eye may have surprisingly little injection or discomfort. As the inflammation subsides, it may be possible to identify a typical granuloma. Some eyes, however, may develop severe complications that can lead to phthisis. Another clinical picture consists of living, mobile larvae identified within the eye,[7–9] although this simply may be other nematodes in a patient who also happens to have identifiable *Toxocara* titers. Other more unusual manifestations include optic neuritis, neuroretinitis, and late choroidal neovascularization.[10–13] Also, this disease entity can be acquired in later ages and should be considered in older patients who have new onset of a localized inflammatory granuloma.[14,15]

DIAGNOSIS

The diagnosis usually is straightforward, with the classic features of a whitish granuloma and surrounding vitreoretinal traction. Confirmation usually is by enzyme-linked immunosorbent assay (ELISA) titers. In general, a titer of 1:8 or greater supports a diagnosis of ocular toxocariasis. In the appropriate clinical situation even lower titers may be useful, and there is at least one case of histologically confirmed infection with negative ELISA testing results.[16] The possible seropositivity of a given population to this test must be considered, and any positive results should be viewed only in terms of the overall clinical picture. Other diagnostic approaches include ELISA titers on aqueous or vitreous specimens, or the demonstration of a preponderance of eosinophils on cytological examination of the aspirate.[10,17] Ultrasonography may show characteristic findings, which include a highly reflective peripheral mass, and vitreous bands or retinal folds that extend from the mass.[18] Ultrasonographic biomicroscopy may demonstrate a very unusual pseudocystic appearance in the vitreous base.[19]

DIFFERENTIAL DIAGNOSIS

The differential diagnosis of ocular toxocariasis varies depending on the clinical picture. In the past, perhaps the most common difficult diagnosis was between toxocariasis and retinoblastoma. Retinoblastoma usually is diagnosed earlier in life, and a positive family history often is present. Exophytic retinoblastoma usually has an overlying retinal detachment with clear vitreous, whereas endophytic retinoblastoma may have a hazy vitreous but no evidence of the vitreoretinal traction that occurs around *Toxocara* lesions. Patients who have retinoblastoma also are less likely to develop a cataract. Computed tomography may be useful, especially in demonstrating areas of calcification in retinoblastoma. Although small amounts of calcium have been

described echographically in *Toxocara* lesions, this is more likely to be seen in older patients who have quiet eyes in whom the differentiation of a *Toxocara* granuloma from retinoblastoma is much less problematic.[18]

Other conditions may be confused with toxocariasis. Coats' disease can be differentiated by the lack of discrete granuloma formation, the presence of an exudative detachment, and the abnormal retinal vasculature associated with prominent subretinal fluid. Persistent hyperplastic primary vitreous generally is recognized earlier in life; the characteristic findings include a smaller eye and a retrolental fibrovascular membrane. More posterior persistent hyperplastic primary vitreous usually has an obvious hyaloid artery that extends from the nerve, with no peripheral granuloma. Retinopathy of prematurity, familial exudative vitreoretinopathy, and peripheral trauma may be seen with peripheral traction that superficially may resemble a *Toxocara* lesion. These entities usually are differentiated on the basis of history and clinical appearance. Toxocariasis should also be considered in the differential diagnosis of patients who appear to have a purely unilateral *pars planitis*.[20]

It may be difficult to distinguish between the endophthalmitic manifestation of toxocariasis and other causes of acute endophthalmitis. *Toxocara* endophthalmitis has a tendency to be gradual and indolent; however, it may be fulminant and if the diagnosis is not clear, a vitrectomy with culture and injection of intraocular antibiotics may be necessary.

PATHOLOGY

The pathology of toxocariasis consists of granuloma formation with a predominance of eosinophils (Fig. 173-3). The eosinophilic infiltrate may be so severe as to create an abscess, which is surrounded by a more typical granulomatous response of epithelioid cells, lymphocytes, and plasma cells. The actual identification of a larva may require multiple sections of the tissue; the simple presence of a marked eosinophilic response is essentially diagnostic for toxocariasis.

TREATMENT

Eyes that have active inflammation generally require treatment with systemic or periocular corticosteroids. Patients who have a mild inflammatory component to their toxocariasis may have disease that smolders for some time; therapy should be designed to both control inflammation and minimize systemic side effects. No clear guidelines exist about the use of antihelminthic therapy. If the eye disease is not responsive to corticosteroids, or if it is associated with systemic symptoms or a very high anti-

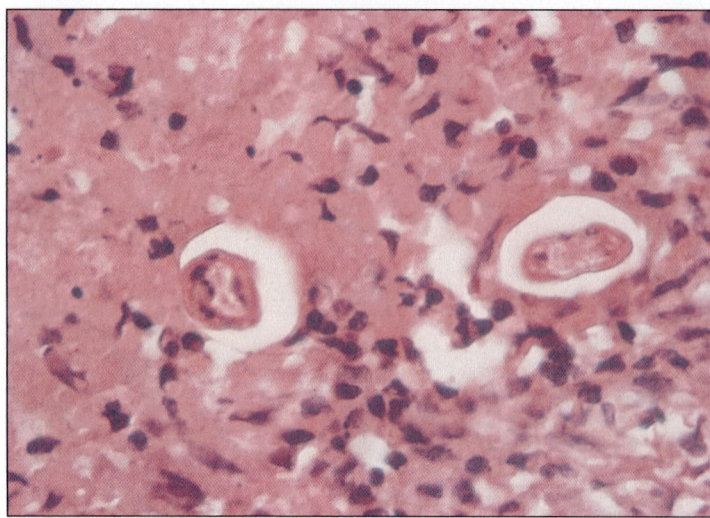

FIG. 173-3 ■ **Histopathology of a toxocara lesion.** Inflammatory infiltrate surrounds the organism.

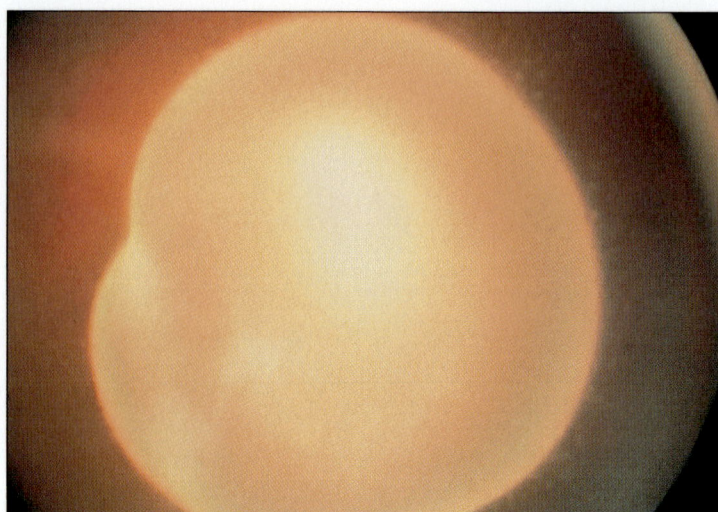

FIG. 173-4 ■ **Cysticercus in the eye.** The large cavity of the cysticercus is visible, as well as the denser white area of the protoscolex.

body titer, it may be more reasonable to treat with an anhelmintic agent such as thiabendazole[21] or albendazole.[21a] Vitrectomy may be required for anatomical abnormalities such as retinal detachment, epiretinal membranes, or macular distortion. The granuloma itself usually is invested in retinal tissue and not removed easily without a retinectomy. Small *et al.*[22] reported a series in which it was shown that improvement in visual function generally occurred only with reasonably good preoperative levels of vision. A poor outcome is associated with a large fold in the macular region, and there is a fairly high risk of late redetachments.[2,22] For cases in which a mobile larva can be identified, photocoagulation has been recommended.[9,10] It is important to destroy the larva completely to avoid a significant inflammatory response; a marked increase in inflammation should be anticipated and the patient treated as needed with corticosteroids.

CYSTICERCOSIS

EPIDEMIOLOGY AND PATHOGENESIS

Cysticercosis is caused by the *Cysticercus cellulosa* larvae of the adult tapeworms *Taenia solium* and *T. saginata*. Although the larvae may be present in many tissues, clinical disease usually is identified only in patients who have cerebral or ocular problems. The term *cysticercosis* implies infestation with the larval stage of the organism and should not be confused with taeniasis, which describes the presence of the adult tapeworm in the intestines.

Humans are the definitive host of *T. solium*. The adult worm lives in the small intestine, where it releases proglottids, which ultimately disintegrate to release eggs. Pigs are the intermediate hosts. They become infected by ingestion of soil contaminated with eggs. The eggs hatch and the organisms spread through the animal and encyst. Human beings are then infected by eating incompletely cooked pork that contains the cysts. The cysts then go on to develop into adult tapeworms in the intestines to complete the cycle. Cysticercosis occurs when human beings ingest the actual eggs; this may occur through fecal-oral contamination or autoinfection from reverse peristalsis. These eggs then hatch and penetrate the gut wall to disseminate throughout the body forming cysts, as normally occurs in the intermediate host.[23,24]

OCULAR MANIFESTATIONS

Any part of the visual system can be affected, from the visual cortex to subconjunctival involvement. Posterior segment involve-

ment appears to be most common.[25,26] Ocular symptoms may vary depending on the location of the infection. They include loss of vision and orbital or even neuro-ophthalmic symptoms. The appearance of the organism is very characteristic; it has a spherical, translucent cyst cavity associated with a protoscolex that may evaginate or invaginate in response to examination lights (Fig. 173-4).

DIAGNOSIS

The diagnosis usually is made by identification of the organism in the eye. Extraocular involvement may require radiological imaging of the orbit and central nervous system. In patients who have opaque media, the ultrasonographic appearance is very characteristic. It shows the spherical area of the cyst associated with the localized solid region of the protoscolex.

SYSTEMATIC ASSOCIATIONS

The clinical manifestations of cysticercosis depend on the location, size, and number of organisms present in the body. Central nervous system symptoms occur in a high percentage of cases, including seizures, focal neurological deficits, hydrocephalus, and mental status changes, and also symptoms of meningitis.[23,24]

PATHOLOGY

A living cysticercus usually induces no significant immune response. There is only mild fibrosis around the cyst. When the cysticercus dies, however, the inflammation becomes much more marked, with an acute granulomatous inflammatory infiltration. Secondary pathological findings then are related to the amount of inflammatory damage, which may include disruption or scarring in the retina, retinal pigment epithelium, or choroid. Glaucoma or cataract also may occur if anterior segment structures are involved.

TREATMENT

Localized ocular or adnexal cysticercosis generally is treated by surgical removal, because death of the organism results in marked inflammation and severe damage to the eye.[25-27] Vitrectomy usually is required for posterior segment involvement. The organism itself can be removed either by aspiration through the vitrectomy handpiece or by extraction through a *pars plana* sclerotomy. If the cyst is ruptured, care should be taken to remove all of the residual debris to prevent severe postoperative inflammation. Orbital involvement may respond to medical therapy alone, but patients may need to be treated with steroids to avoid inflammatory damage around dying cysts.[28] The treatment of neurocysticercosis generally involves observation or use of oral albendazole or praziquantel and supportive measures for neurological problems.[24]

COURSE AND OUTCOME

Reviews of treated cases suggest that early removal of the organism is associated with preservation of visual function.[25–27] If possible, ocular cysts should be removed before systemic treatment is undertaken to prevent damage from death of the intraocular organisms.

ONCHOCERCIASIS

EPIDEMIOLOGY AND PATHOGENESIS

The parasite *Onchocerca volvulus* is transmitted by the blackfly. The geographical distribution of the disease is characterized by local areas where the blackfly breeds most effectively.[29] Onchocerciasis is endemic across equatorial Africa, Yemen, Mexico, and areas of Central America and northern South America.

An infected blackfly deposits several larvae with each bite. Over a year the larvae develop into mature adult worms. The worms remain encapsulated in characteristic nodules from which they release large numbers of microfilariae. These microfilariae then migrate throughout the body and may be taken up by another blackfly when the host is bitten. The result is that people who live in endemic areas are reinfected continually. As long as adult worms are present in the nodules, a constant stream of microfilariae is produced and all susceptible tissues are invaded. The microfilariae themselves may live up to 2 years. Upon their deaths they may stimulate a localized immune reaction in the involved tissues.

OCULAR MANIFESTATIONS

The most significant morbidity associated with onchocerciasis occurs as a result of ocular involvement. The microfilariae can invade all the ocular structures, but the earliest sign of involvement is the presence of microfilariae in the anterior chamber, best demonstrated after the patient has been in a face-down position for several minutes before the examination. Live microfilariae are difficult to identify in the cornea, but a characteristic inflammatory infiltrate and punctate keratitis can surround dead microfilariae. The chronic inflammation brought on by the presence of large numbers of microfilariae in the cornea results in the development of sclerosing keratitis (Fig. 173-5). This initially begins in the peripheral cornea in the intrapalpebral areas and gradually spreads across the entire cornea. A variable amount of anterior uveitis also may occur and patients may develop granulomatous changes, synechiae (leading to angle-closure glaucoma), and irregular iris depigmentation. Chronic, blinding chorioretinitis is another feature of this entity. Patients develop areas of depigmentation that proceed to coalesce and become large areas of geographical atrophy (Fig. 173-6). Patients may develop optic atrophy in excess of the chorioretinal damage either as a function of a microfilaria in the optic nerve or as an inflammatory response caused by death of microfilaria.[29] Occasional patients may have evidence of intraretinal inflammation, such as cotton-wool spots, hemorrhages, or vasculitis. Intraretinal microfilariae also may be identified with careful contact lens examination.[30]

DIAGNOSIS

The diagnosis usually can be made by identification of the microfilariae in tissues. Skin snips can be used to look for the emer-

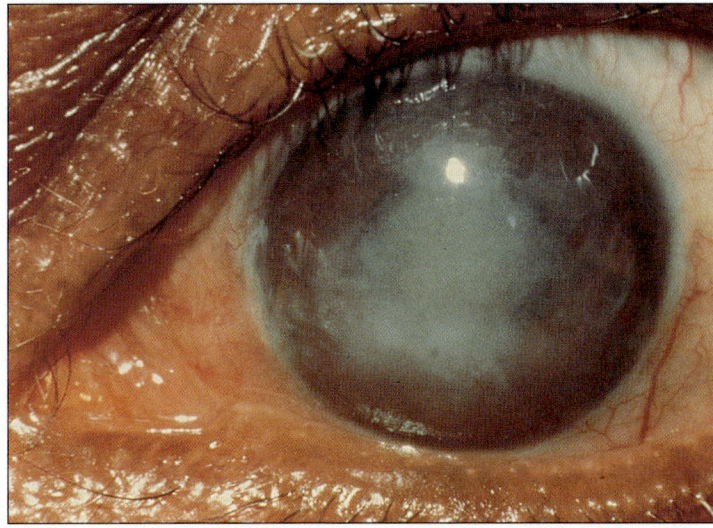

FIG. 173-5 ■ Sclerosing keratitis as a result of onchocerciasis. (Courtesy of Professor HR Taylor.)

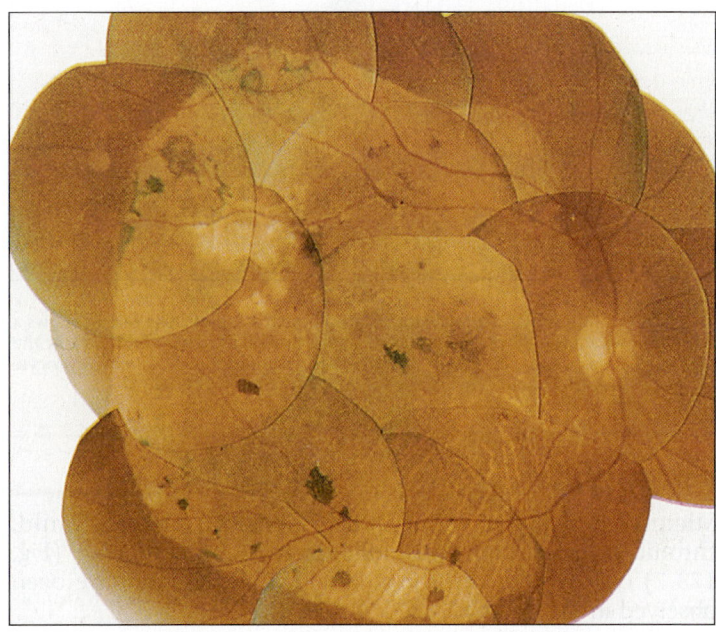

FIG. 173-6 ■ Extensive chorioretinitis as a result of onchocerciasis.

gence of microfilariae from the sample. Skin nodules may be sampled for biopsy to determine the presence of adult worms as well. In endemic areas, a tentative diagnosis can be made based simply on the presence of typical skin nodules and ocular features.[29] Present research is directed at using polymerase chain reaction probes to identify small numbers of organisms to determine whether patients are truly free of disease or simply have a very low organism load.

SYSTEMATIC ASSOCIATIONS

Clinical features are a function of both degree of infection and of immune response. The bite of the blackfly usually resolves in a few days, followed by a latent interval of 6–24 months during which the larvae develop into mature worms, which release microfilariae that migrate and begin to die in tissues. The most common early manifestation is pruritus caused by inflammation around dead microfilariae in the skin. With time, the constant irritation in the skin results in pigment changes, lichenification, and loss of dermal collagen (the last results in the skin hanging loosely, especially around the groin and face). Nodules that contain adult worms (onchocercomas) usually are found around the pelvis or in the head and shoulder region.

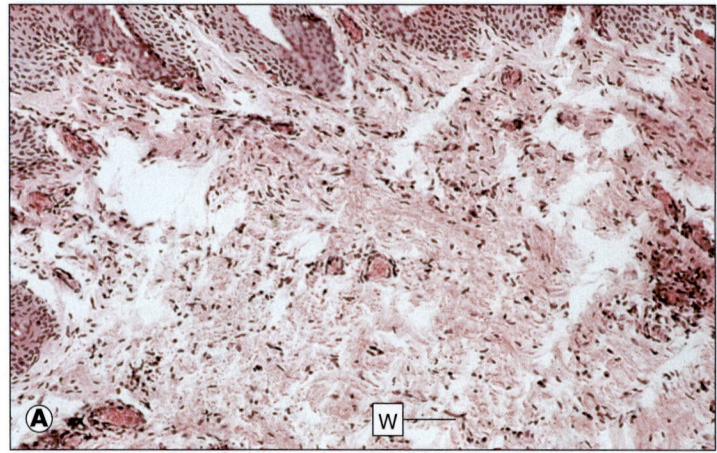

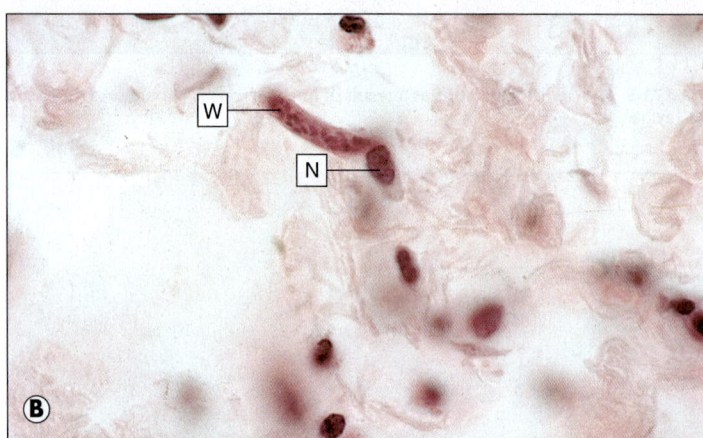

FIG. 173-7 ∎ **Microfilariae. A,** Histological section of a conjunctival biopsy shows a chronic nongranulomatous inflammation and a tiny segment of worm *(W)* in the deep substantia propria. **B,** Shown under higher magnification. *N,* Human fibrocyte nucleus. (Case reported in Scheie HG *et al. Ann Opthalmol.* 1971;3:697.)

PATHOLOGY

Microscopically the iridocyclitis is characterized by mild, chronic nongranulomatous inflammation. Microfilariae (Fig. 173-7) can be found in the stroma; similar lesions have been observed in the choroid.

TREATMENT

The treatment of onchocerciasis has been revolutionized by the development of ivermectin, and tremendous strides have been made because the company that makes the drug has offered it free of charge as long as necessary.[31]

The drug is given at a dosage of 150µg/kg PO and is repeated every 3 months.[32] It is very effective at killing microfilariae, although it is ineffective against the adult worm. As a result, continuous treatment is required to decrease the load of microfilariae in infected individuals. Perhaps the most important treatment approach is to prevent infection. This involves vector control through treatment of areas infested with blackflies, as well as measures against fly bites, such as avoidance of areas known to be infected and the use of protective clothing and insect repellents. However, socioeconomic constraints in infested areas make preventive measures very difficult to implement.

COURSE AND OUTCOME

Blindness is the major disability caused by onchocerciasis and has profound effects on villages in endemic areas.[33] This disease carries a significant toll, because it affects otherwise healthy adults who have the greatest responsibility for supporting families. If individuals are affected to the point of blindness, they have a high risk of death within 10 years.[34] Treatment with iver-

mectin can markedly reverse the anterior segment manifestations of onchocerciasis. Chorioretinitis responds less predictably and may be the result of a combination of infectious damage and possibly autoimmune mechanisms.[35] The overall effect of treatment programs, however, has been a significant decrease in morbidity from the disease and prevention of the devastating socioeconomic consequences of this infection.

REFERENCES

1. Nash T. Visceral larva migrans and other unusual helminth infections. In: Mandell G, Bennett J, Dolin R, eds. Principles and practice of infectious diseases. New York: Churchill Livingstone; 2000;2965–70.
2. Parke DW, Shaver RP. Toxocariasis. In: Pepose JS, Holland GN, Wilhelmus KR, eds. Ocular infection and immunity. St Louis: Mosby; 1996:1225–35.
3. Uga S. Prevalence of *Toxocara* eggs and number of faecal deposits from dogs and cats in sandpits of public parks in Japan. J Helminthol. 1993;67:78–82.
4. Glickman L, Francois-Magnaval J. Zoonotic roundworm infections. Infect Dis Clin North Am. 1993;7:717–32.
5. Thompson DE, Bundy DAP, Cooper ES, et al. Epidemiological characteristics of *Toxocara canis* zoonotic infections of children in a Caribbean community. Bull WHO. 1986;64:283–90.
6. Brown DH. Ocular *Toxocara canis.* II. Clinical review. J Pediatr Ophthalmol. 1970; 7:182–91.
7. Rubin ML, Kaufman HE, Tiemey JP, et al. An intraretinal nematode. Trans Am Acad Ophthalmol Otolaryngol. 1968;72:855–66.
8. Karel I, Peleska M, Uhlikova M, et al. *Larval migrans lentis.* Ophthalmologica. 1977;174:14–19.
9. Sorr EM. Meandering ocular toxocariasis. Retina. 1984;4:90–6.
10. Shields JA. Ocular toxocariasis: a review. Surv Ophthalmol. 1984;28:361–81.
11. Cox TA, Haskins GE, Gangitano JL, et al. Bilateral *Toxocara* optic neuropathy. J Clin Neuro Ophthalmol. 1983;3:267–74.
12. Brown GC, Tasman WS. Retinal arterial obstruction in association with presumed *Toxocara canis* neuroretinitis. Ann Ophthalmol. 1981;13:1385–7.
13. Monshizadeh R, Ashrafzadeh MT, Rumelt S. Choroidal neovascular membrane: a late complication of inactive *Toxocara* chorioretinitis. Retina 2000;20:219–20.
14. Steahly LP, Mader T. Acute ocular toxocariasis in adults. J Ocul Ther Surg. 1985;4:93–9.
15. Yoshida M, Shirao Y, Asai H, et al. A retrospective study of ocular toxocariasis in Japan: correlation with antibody prevalence and ophthalmological findings of patients with uveitis. J Helminthol 1999;73:357–61.
16. Sharkey JA, McKay PS. Ocular toxocariasis in a patient with repeatedly negative ELISA titre to *Toxocara canis.* Br J Ophthalmol. 1993;77:253–4.
17. Felberg NT, Shields JA, Federman JL. Antibody to *Toxocara canis* in the aqueous humor. Arch Ophthalmol. 1981;99:1563–4.
18. Wan WL, Cano MR, Pince KJ, Green RL. Echographic characteristics of ocular toxocariasis. Ophthalmology. 1991;98:28–32.
19. Tran VT, Lumbroso L, LeHoang P, Herbort CP. Ultrasound biomicroscopy in peripheral retinovitreal toxocariasis. Am J Ophthalmol.1999;127:607–9.
20. Gillespie SH, Dinning WJ, Voller A, Crowcroft NS. The spectrum of ocular toxocariasis. Eye. 1993;7:415–8.
21. Dinning W, Gillespie SH, Cooling RJ, et al. Toxocariasis: a practical approach to management of ocular disease. Eye. 1988;2:580–2.
21a. Barisani-Asenbauer T, Maca SM, Hauff W, et al. Treatment of ocular toxocariasis with albendazole. J Ocul Pharmacol Ther. 2001;17:287–94.
22. Small KW, McCuen BW, deJuan E, et al. Surgical management of retinal traction caused by toxocariasis. Am J Ophthalmol. 1989;108:10–14.
23. Kean BH, Sun T, Ellsworth RM. Color atlas/text of ophthalmic parasitology. New York: Igaku-Shoin; 1989:115–22, 173–81.
24. King CH. *Cestodes* (tapeworms). In: Mandell G, Bennett J, Dolin R, eds. Principles and practice of infectious diseases. New York: Churchill Livingstone; 2000: 2960–2.
25. Topilow HW, Yimoyines DI, Freeman HM, et al. Bilateral multifocal intraocular cysticercosis. Ophthalmology. 1981;88;1166–72.
26. Kruger-Leite E, Jalkh AE, Quiroz H, et al. Intraocular cysticercosis. Am J Ophthalmol. 1985;99:252–7.
27. Steinmetz R, Masket S, Sidikaro Y. The successful removal of a subretinal cysticercus by pars plana vitrectomy. Retina. 1989;9:276–80.
28. Tandon R, Sihota R, Dada T, Verma L. Optic neuritis following albendazole therapy for orbital cysticercosis. Aust N Z J Ophthalmol. 1998;26:339–41.
29. Taylor HR, Nutman TB. Onchocerciasis. In: Pepose JS, Holland GN, Wilhelmus KR, eds. Ocular infection and immunity. St Louis: Mosby; 1996:1481–504.
30. Murphy RP, Taylor HR, Greene BM. Chorioretinal damage in onchocerciasis. Am J Ophthalmol. 1984;98:519–21.
31. Abiose A. Onchocercal eye disease and the impact of Mectizan treatment. Ann Trop Med Parasitol. 1998;92(Suppl 1):S11–22.
32. Grove DI. Onchocerciasis. In: Mandell G, Bennett J, Dolin R, eds. Principles and practice of infectious diseases. New York: Churchill Livingstone; 2000:2947–8.
33. Nwoke BEB. The socioeconomic aspects of human onchocerciasis in Africa: present appraisal. J Hyg Epidemiol Microbiol Immunol. 1990;1:37–44.
34. Prost A. The burden of blindness in adult males in the savanna villages of West Africa exposed to onchocerciasis. Trans R Soc Trop Med Hyg. 1986;80:525–7.
35. Mabey D, Whitworth JA, Eckstein M, et al. The effects of multiple doses of ivermectin on ocular onchocerciasis. Ophthalmology. 1996;103:1001–8.

SECTION 6 UVEITIS ASSOCIATED WITH SYSTEMIC DISEASE

CHAPTER 174

Uveitis Related to HLA-B27 and Juvenile Arthritis

JUSTINE R. SMITH • JAMES T. ROSENBAUM

Uveitis Related to HLA-B27

DEFINITION
- Ocular inflammation associated with HLA-B27.

KEY FEATURES
- Recurrent unilateral acute (sudden onset) anterior uveitis.
- Photophobia and ocular redness.
- Ciliary injection.
- Often florid anterior chamber reaction that may include formation of hypopyon and/or anterior chamber fibrin clot.
- Posterior synechiae.

ASSOCIATED FEATURES
- Spondyloarthropathy.
- HLA-B27.

Uveitis Related to Juvenile Arthritis

DEFINITION
- Ocular inflammation associated with juvenile idiopathic arthritis.

KEY FEATURES
- Bilateral chronic (insidious onset) anterior uveitis.
- Usually asymptomatic unless complications have occurred.
- Complications may include band keratopathy, cataract, inflammatory glaucoma.

ASSOCIATED FEATURES
- Oligoarthritis.
- Antinuclear antibodies.

INTRODUCTION

Uveitis may occur in association with a variety of systemic inflammatory diseases. However, by far the most common association is between inflammation of the uvea and inflammation of the joints. In adults, the so-called seronegative spondyloarthropathies, which occur in the context of HLA-B27 and include ankylosing spondylitis and reactive arthritis, may be associated with an acute (sudden onset) anterior uveitis. Patients with psoriatic arthritis and inflammatory bowel disease, some of whom may be HLA-B27 positive, may also develop uveitis. In children, each of these types of arthritis occurs and may be associated with uveitis. However, it is more typical for a child to develop a chronic anterior uveitis in association with juvenile idiopathic arthritis (JIA). The patterns of the different uveitis diagnoses that coexist with these rheumatologic diseases are often typical and, in some cases, may be the key to a previously unsuspected systemic diagnosis.

UVEITIS RELATED TO HLA-B27

In humans, the molecules encoded by the major histocompatibility complex (MHC) are generally referred to as human leukocyte antigens (HLAs). Three classes of HLA are inherited separately and perform different functions that are critical for a normal immune response. HLA-B27 belongs to the group known as the class I molecules. Located on the surface of most nucleated cells, the class I molecules present antigens such as viral peptide fragments to T cells. In this capacity, this molecule facilitates the destruction of cells that are infected with virus. The presence of HLA-B27 predisposes to several diseases, including a specific form of anterior uveitis, often termed acute anterior uveitis, which is of sudden onset and short duration but recurrent.[1] Other HLA-B27–associated diseases include the seronegative spondyloarthropathies, ankylosing spondylitis and reactive arthritis.

HLA-B27 is present in 6 to 8% of the Caucasian population in the United States.[2] It is much more common in certain ethnic groups, such as Finns and specific native North American tribes. Conversely, it is relatively uncommon in some populations, such as Japanese, and is virtually absent among others, including the indigenous Australians. There are at least 20 subtypes of HLA-B27, differing from one another by one or multiple amino acid substitutions and named HLA-B*2701, HLA-B*2702, and so on.[3] HLA-B*2705 has been further subdivided on the basis of a silent nucleotide substitution. It has been proposed that different subtypes of HLA-B27 may imply different disease susceptibility and that this may vary with the ethnic population.[3] HLA-B*27052 is the most common subtype and is definitely associated with disease.

Acute (sudden onset) anterior uveitis is the most common form of uveitis, with a lifetime cumulative incidence estimated at 4 per 1000 in the general population.[4] Approximately 50% of all individuals who have acute anterior uveitis are HLA-B27 positive.[1] In most instances, the uveitis occurs sporadically. However, familial cases of acute anterior uveitis have been described and, in general, affect patients who are HLA-B27 positive.[5] Some patients with HLA-B27–associated uveitis may suffer from a spondyloarthropathy in addition. Psoriasis and inflammatory bowel disease may also be associated with HLA-B27–associated uveitis, although other patterns of uveitis often occur in these groups of patients.

PATHOGENIC MECHANISMS

The pathogenesis of the HLA-B27–associated diseases, including uveitis, remains incompletely understood. A history of infection with gram-negative bacteria, including *Salmonella*, *Shigella*, *Campylobacter*, and *Yersinia* microorganisms, or *Chlamydia trachomatis*, is recorded significantly frequently in patients who suffer from these diseases.[6] This is readily apparent in a case of reactive arthritis that follows an acute intestinal or genitourinary infection or in a patient with inflammatory bowel disease. However, ileocolonoscopy has also demonstrated subclinical bowel inflammation in patients with acute anterior uveitis as well as spondyloarthropathy.[7,8] Some studies suggest that antibiotics that alter gut flora may favorably affect the course of both the joint inflammation and the ocular disease.[9-13]

Work conducted in animal models supports the concept that HLA-B27 and gram-negative bacteria interact to cause these diseases. The expression of HLA-B27 in transgenic rats is associated with a diarrheal illness and joint and skin involvement that mimic spondyloarthritis.[14] Gram-negative flora appear to be a critical part of this disease because it is ameliorated markedly when the rats are reared in a germ-free environment.[15] An anterior uveitis of sudden onset and short duration can be induced in rats by a systemic injection of endotoxin, also known as lipopolysaccharide, which is the major component of the gram-negative bacterial cell wall.[16]

The exact mechanism of the interaction between HLA-B27 and the bacteria is unclear. It is possible that HLA-B27 presents bacterial peptides that first have been processed within the cell.[17] The molecule might also present endogenous peptides that are produced as a consequence of infection. Presentation to a cytotoxic T cell would allow an immune response to proceed. The molecular mimicry theory explains disease occurrence on the basis that there is structural homology between the amino acid structures of HLA-B27 and the implicated microorganisms.[17] Structural homology does exist between amino acid sequences of HLA-B27 and *Klebsiella pneumoniae*, for example. According to this theory, an immune response initially directed against an invading pathogen might subsequently be directed against HLA-B27. It has been suggested that misfolding of the HLA-B27 molecule during assembly may be the key to disease pathogenesis,

possibly by stimulating intracellular signaling pathways that influence cellular immune functioning.[18] Aqueous fluid obtained at the time of anterior chamber paracentesis demonstrates the presence of a heterogeneous cell infiltrate in patients with acute anterior uveitis, including substantial numbers of T cells, granulocytes, and macrophages.[19]

CLINICAL FEATURES AND LABORATORY INVESTIGATIONS

The uveitis that typifies HLA-B27 disease is a unilateral, recurrent, acute, anterior uveitis involving the iris and/or the pars plicata (Fig. 174-1).[20] The inflammation is of sudden onset and usually resolves completely within 2 to 3 months after the onset, but has a strong tendency to recur. Although an attack is almost always unilateral, both eyes may be involved on separate occasions. Other forms of uveitis, such as Behçet's syndrome or Vogt-Koyanagi-Harada syndrome, also tend to be recurrent, but episodes usually subside incompletely such that residual inflammation persists. The complete resolution between attacks is especially suggestive of the HLA-B27 spectrum of disease. In general, the visual prognosis for HLA-B27–associated disease is excellent. So, although the inflammation associated with this illness is often intense, the resolution is usually complete, often with little or no impairment between attacks. Cataract formation has been reported to affect up to 30% of patients.[21] Glaucoma occurs less commonly. In the event that complications do occur, it is not uncommon for these to be multiple in the affected individual.[21]

Typically, the onset of the uveitis is heralded by a short prodrome of vague discomfort followed, within 24 to 48 hours, by intense ocular redness with photophobia and lacrimation, pain, and reduced vision. Visual acuity is variably reduced. There is an intense injection of the limbal vasculature. The anterior chamber may contain 3 to 4 plus aqueous cell and a heavy flare. In severe cases a hypopyon may be present or a fibrin clot may form. Hypopyon is rare, but in North America, HLA-B27–associated disease is easily the most common cause of hypopyon in the setting of a noninfectious cause of uveitis.[22] Posterior synechiae are common. Fine, nongranulomatous keratic precipitates collect on the inferior corneal endothelium. Cells in the anterior vitreous are common in cases that involve the ciliary body, but a marked vitritis is not the rule. According to the largest series, cystoid macular edema occurs in approximately 10% of patients.[21] Optic nerve head hyperemia is another possible manifestation. Intraocular pressure tends to fall in the affected eye. Atypical forms of uveitis have been reported in association with HLA-B27, with prominent involvement of the posterior segment of the eye, including vitritis, retinal vasculitis, and pars plana exudates.[23] Given the common occurrence of HLA-B27 in the general population, this observation may sometimes represent coincidence.

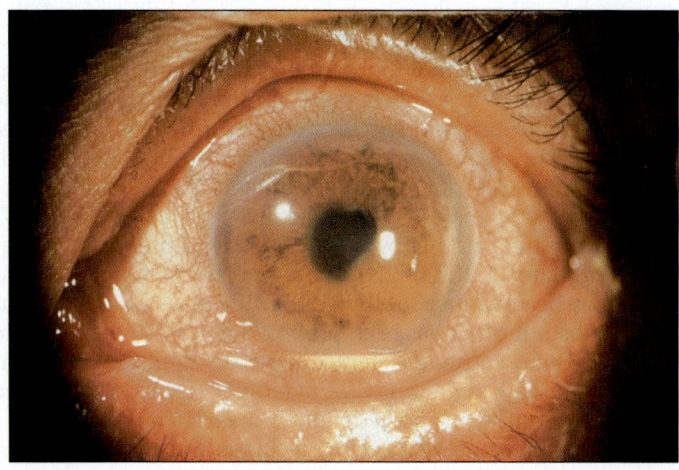

FIG. 174-1 ■ Slit-lamp photograph of left eye of a patient with acute anterior uveitis related to HLA-B27. Limbal injection, a hypopyon, fibrin at the pupil, and posterior synechiae are present. (Photograph provided by NA Rao, MD, Doheny Eye Institute, Los Angeles.)

TABLE 174-1

SUMMARY OF THE CLINICAL FEATURES OF ANKYLOSING SPONDYLITIS, REACTIVE ARTHRITIS, INFLAMMATORY BOWEL DISEASE, AND PSORIATIC ARTHRITIS

Clinical Feature	Disease			
	Ankylosing Spondylitis	Reactive Arthritis (Reiter's Syndrome)	Inflammatory Bowel Disease	Psoriatic Arthritis
Sacroiliitis	Always	Common	Occasional	Occasional
Peripheral arthritis	Common	Common	Occasional	Common
Iritis	Common	Common	Occasional	Occasional
Urethritis	Not associated	Common	Not associated	Not associated
Conjunctivitis	Not associated	Occasional	Occasional	Occasional
Stomatitis	Not associated	Occasional	Occasional	Not associated
Diarrhea	Occasional	Occasional	Almost always	Not associated
Rash/nail changes	Not associated	Occasional	Occasional	Always

In some studies, 80–90% of individuals who have HLA-B27–associated iritis also have systemic disease, either ankylosing spondylitis or reactive arthritis.[20] Conversely, between 20 and 40% of patients who have reactive arthritis or ankylosing spondylitis develop an anterior uveitis during the course of the joint disease.[24] Although not routinely determined in diagnosing these diseases, rheumatoid factor is negative in these patients, hence the descriptive term *seronegative spondyloarthropathy*. The spondyloarthropathies, ankylosing spondylitis, and reactive arthritis (previously termed *Reiter's syndrome*), are similar diseases with many overlapping clinical features, as listed in Table 174-1. In general, reactive arthritis is distinguished from ankylosing spondylitis by the involvement of mucosal surfaces, such as conjunctiva, urethra, mouth, or skin.

The most common form of joint involvement associated with HLA-B27–associated iritis is mild, chronic low back pain. Unlike mechanical low back pain, as associated with intervertebral disc disease, inflammatory low back pain tends to start insidiously, to be associated with morning stiffness, and to respond very well to nonsteroidal anti-inflammatory medications, such as ibuprofen or indomethacin. About two thirds of patients who have HLA-B27–associated iritis present to the ophthalmologist without a diagnosis of inflammatory joint disease.[20] Many, of course, are cognizant of chronic low back pain, but the diagnosis of spondyloarthritis has been overlooked.

Ankylosing spondylitis is more common in men. Symptoms typically begin during the teenage years or twenties. Sacroiliitis is the rule, although other sites, particularly other axial joints, may also be involved in the inflammatory process (Fig. 174-2). Reactive arthritis refers to a peripheral arthritis that may follow infection of the genitourinary or genital tract. The disease is most common in young adult males. In the classical presentation, which is rare, a patient suffers from a bilateral conjunctivitis that occurs after or at the time of the infection, but prior to the onset of the arthritis. The arthritis has an acute onset and is typically asymmetrical and oligoarticular. Lower limb joints are most commonly involved. Enthesitis or inflammation at bone attachments of tendons and ligaments is common, especially involving the calcaneus and causing heel pain. Lower back pain also occurs. Characteristic skin lesions include keratoderma blennorrhagicum, a variant of psoriasis that occurs on the palms and soles, circinate balanitis, and mouth ulceration. Aortitis is an uncommon, but serious, association.

Testing for HLA-B27 is useful in patients with acute anterior uveitis. Not only does it help in suggesting the diagnosis of systemic disease, but it also provides prognostic information. One review of eight studies compared HLA-B27–associated anterior uveitis with HLA-B27–negative anterior uveitis.[25] This study showed that when occurring in the context of HLA-B27, anterior uveitis was relatively more severe, more likely to resolve within 3 months, but also more likely to recur. It was more likely to be unilateral and more likely to be associated with spondyloarthropathy. However, the final visual prognosis was no different between HLA-B27–positive uveitis and HLA-B27–negative disease. A large study from a single group has suggested otherwise, reporting a greater number of complications and a higher incidence of legally blind eyes among patients with HLA-B27–associated anterior uveitis versus HLA-B27–negative patients with anterior uveitis.[26]

In patients with inflammatory lower back pain, a radiograph of the sacroiliac joints may be considered (Fig. 174-3). In the early stages of spondyloarthropathy, the lumbosacral x-ray film demonstrates bilateral sacroiliac juxta-articular bony sclerosis, blurring of the joint margins, and/or erosive changes that may give the margins an irregular, serrated appearance. Erosions may also give the impression of widening of the sacroiliac joint. Later, inflammation leads to ossification. There is loss of joint space and finally ankylosis.

TREATMENT

The uveitis associated with HLA-B27 generally responds to treatment with topical corticosteroids, instilled frequently. The most useful preparation is prednisolone acetate 1%, which penetrates the cornea to achieve high levels within the anterior chamber.[27] Other topical corticosteroids have less tendency to raise the intraocular pressure but are also less potent anti-inflammatory treatments.[28] One randomized controlled clinical trial comparing topical indomethacin with topical dexamethasone indicated that both treatments were effective but that the nonsteroidal anti-inflammatory preparation took significantly longer to work.[29] Generally, eyedrops are instilled as frequently as every hour initially and then tapered as the inflammation begins to decrease in intensity. Most patients require about 6 weeks of treatment. Patients who have recurrent episodes may be instructed to begin treatment at the onset of the prodrome, to abort the attack early and reduce the duration of treatment. Mydriatic-cycloplegic preparations such as topical homatropine or cyclopentolate are useful during an acute attack to prevent formation of posterior synechiae. If posterior synechiae are present, it may be necessary

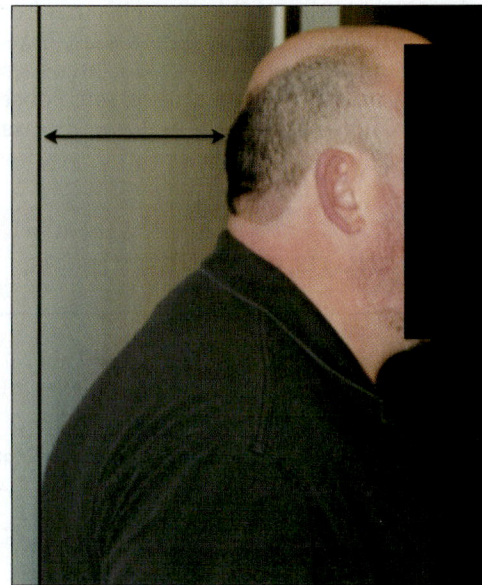

FIG. 174-2 ❚ Patient with advanced ankylosing spondylitis involving the axial skeleton, demonstrating a characteristic posture with forward stoop of the neck. The black lines illustrate the occiput-to-wall measurement, obtained when a patient with back to the wall attempts to touch the wall with his occiput. An unaffected individual performing this test is able to touch the occiput to the wall.

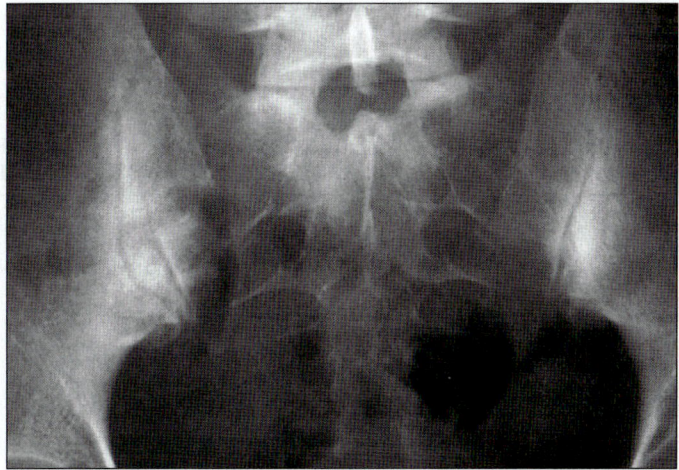

FIG. 174-3 ❚ Radiograph of the sacroiliac joints from a patient with ankylosing spondylitis showing bilateral juxta-articular sclerosis with irregularity of the joint margins.

to use more aggressive treatments, such as a mydriatic cocktail that might include atropine or a subconjunctival injection of Mydricaine (epinephrine, atropine, and procaine). In the early stages, frequent follow-up visits are suggested. For exceptional cases that fail to respond to topical therapy, treatment with a periocular injection of corticosteroid, such as triamcinolone acetonide, or a short (1- to 2-week) course of oral corticosteroid, such as prednisone, may be required to abort the attack. Cataract in a patient with HLA-B27–associated uveitis can be successfully managed with surgical extraction and intraocular lens implantation.[30]

PREVENTION

Prevention of recurrent episodes is a frequent dilemma for the clinician. Although long-term topical corticosteroid use would probably be effective in this regard, the benefit is far outweighed by the risks of corticosteroid-induced cataract and glaucoma as well as susceptibility to infections. The evidence supporting the role of gut infection in the HLA-B27 diseases has led some groups to consider the possibility of using antibiotic prophylaxis to prevent attacks. A 12-month double-blind randomized, placebo-controlled trial conducted in Australia, including patients with reactive arthritis and/or recurrent acute anterior uveitis, failed to demonstrate any difference in outcome between ciprofloxacin-treated and control-treated groups.[31] On the other hand, a number of European studies have suggested a useful role for sulfasalazine as prophylaxis for recurrent anterior uveitis.[10–13]

INFLAMMATORY BOWEL DISEASE AND PSORIATIC ARTHRITIS

Inflammatory bowel disease and psoriatic arthritis are diseases that may also occur in association with HLA-B27, although the association is less strong than for ankylosing spondylitis or reactive arthritis. Of patients who have either ulcerative colitis or Crohn's disease, approximately 5% develop uveitis at some point during their lifetime.[32] Crohn's disease is far more likely than ulcerative colitis to be associated with uveitis, at least in a referral setting.[32] These patients are also at risk for other inflammatory eye diseases, in particular episcleritis and scleritis. Psoriatic arthritis is a condition that affects approximately 5% of persons with psoriasis.[33] It may take various forms, including asymmetric oligoarthritis or monoarthritis, symmetric polyarthritis, and axial arthritis. Ankylosing spondylitis, reactive arthritis, inflammatory bowel disease, and psoriatic arthritis share many features, which include diarrhea, joint involvement and sacroiliitis, skin lesions, and, of course, uveitis. Despite this clinical overlap, which is presented in Table 174-1, the eye manifestations of the latter two conditions are frequently distinct from the ocular presentation of the former two conditions.

Some of the differences between uveitis in association with inflammatory bowel disease and psoriatic arthropathy, and uveitis in association with spondyloarthropathy are highlighted in Table 174-2. Uveitis in association with inflammatory bowel disease or psoriasis is frequently bilateral, often involves prolonged or continuous inflammation, may start insidiously, and commonly has a posterior component.[32,34] However, in some patients with psoriatic arthritis or inflammatory bowel disease, uveitis is identical to that typically observed in patients with ankylosing spondylitis. It is hypothesized that male sex, axial arthritis, and the presence of HLA-B27 are factors that predispose to an acute (sudden onset) anterior uveitis.[34] Interestingly, the rate of complications does not appear to differ substantially between these two forms of uveitis.[34] Uveitis does tend to coexist with other extracolonic manifestations of inflammatory bowel disease, such as joint and skin disease, but the correlation with bowel activity is not particularly strong. In more than half of cases, a diagnosis of uveitis precedes the diagnosis of inflammatory bowel disease.[32] As is true for spondyloarthritis, the uveitis may be a clue to the diagnosis of inflammatory bowel disease. Patients who have iritis of unknown cause should be questioned carefully about bowel habits. In psoriatic arthritis, the diagnosis typically follows the joint diagnosis.[34]

One other form of HLA-B27–associated spondyloarthropathy is known as undifferentiated spondyloarthropathy, implying that the patient does not fit a specific disease category but has one or more features consistent with the diagnosis. Although uveitis may occur in association with undifferentiated spondyloarthropathy, this group of patients has not been systematically studied to define the uveitis phenotype.

UVEITIS RELATED TO JUVENILE ARTHRITIS

Various forms of childhood arthritis may occur in association with uveitis. The group of inflammatory joint diseases implied by the umbrella term juvenile idiopathic arthritis are by far the most common arthritides encountered in pediatric patients with uveitis. Further, these diseases are the most common of all the systemic conditions associated with childhood uveitis, affecting up to approximately 40% of children who present with uveitis and up to approximately 80% of children who present with anterior uveitis.[35] In one large study from a tertiary eye care center, JIA-associated uveitis accounted for almost 6% of the total uveitis population.[36] In other children, uveitis may be associated with various forms of inflammatory joint disease that also occur in adults, including the HLA-B27–associated seronegative arthropathies, inflammatory bowel disease, sarcoidosis, Behçet's disease, and infectious entities such as Lyme disease. In addi-

---

TABLE 174-2

SUMMARY OF UVEITIS OCCURRING IN ASSOCIATION WITH ANKYLOSING SPONDYLITIS, REACTIVE ARTHRITIS, INFLAMMATORY BOWEL DISEASE, AND PSORIATIC ARTHRITIS

Systemic Disease	Average Age at Onset of Uveitis (years)	Gender Ratio (male:female)	HLA-B27 Positivity (%)	Lifetime Incidence of Uveitis (%)	Clinical Pattern of Uveitis
Ankylosing spondylitis and reactive arthritis	33	2:1	89	20–40	Unilateral, anterior, sudden onset, episodic
Inflammatory bowel disease	37	1:4.5	46	3–11	Frequently bilateral, posterior, insidious onset, continuous*
Psoriatic arthritis	39	2.2:1	67	7	Frequently bilateral, posterior, insidious onset, continuous*

Adapted from Paiva ES, Macaluso DC, Edwards A, Rosenbaum JT. Characterisation of uveitis in patients with psoriatic arthritis. Ann Rheum Dis. 2000;59:67–70.
*Some patients with psoriatic arthritis or inflammatory bowel disease have uveitis that follows the pattern seen with ankylosing spondylitis and reactive arthritis. Axial arthritis, male sex, and the presence of HLA-B27 might be factors that predispose to the unilateral, anterior, sudden onset, episodic pattern.

tion, a rare inherited syndrome known as familial juvenile systemic granulomatosis, which includes uveal and joint inflammation, typically presents in childhood.

JUVENILE IDIOPATHIC ARTHRITIS

The term juvenile idiopathic arthritis refers to a collection of different diseases that share three common features—the presence of arthritis, an onset prior to the 16th birthday, and no identifiable cause for the joint inflammation. By definition, the arthritis must have been present for a minimum of 6 weeks. At different times in the past, this group of diseases has been described as Still's disease, juvenile chronic arthritis, and juvenile rheumatoid arthritis. The current nomenclature was suggested by the Task Force for Classification Criteria of the Pediatric Standing Committee of the International League of Associations for Rheumatology, which defined seven subsets of JIA.[37] This classification is presented in Box 174-1. Interestingly, psoriatic arthritis is included within this classification, whereas other HLA-B27–associated arthropathies, ankylosing spondylitis and reactive arthritis, are excluded. As

---

BOX 174-1

Classification Criteria for Juvenile Idiopathic Arthritis

CATEGORIES OF JUVENILE IDIOPATHIC ARTHRITIS
1. Systemic
2. Oligoarthritis
3. Polyarthritis (rheumatoid factor negative)
4. Polyarthritis (rheumatoid factor positive)
5. Psoriatic arthritis
6. Enthesitis-related arthritis
7. Other arthritis
   A. Fits no other category
   B. Fits more than one category

Adapted from Petty RE and the Task Force for Classification Criteria. Revision for the proposed classification criteria for juvenile idiopathic arthritis: Durban, 1997. J Rheumatol. 1998;25:1991–4.

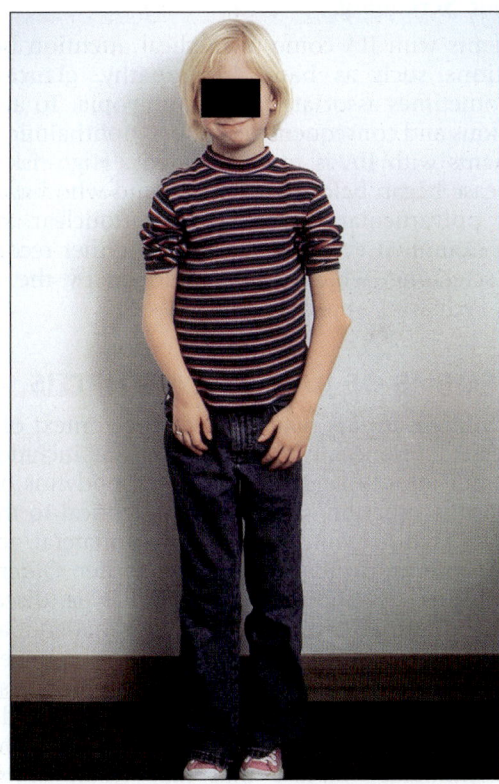

FIG. 174-4 ▊ Patient with juvenile idiopathic arthritis who has bilateral elbow flexion contractures that prevent straightening of the arms.

many as 20% of patients with JIA develop uveitis, usually after, but within 7 years of, the onset of the arthritis.[38]

Clinical Features and Laboratory Findings

Although ocular inflammation may occur in association with any form of JIA, it is most commonly associated with oligoarthritis.[38] This arthritis involves no more than four joints, frequently the large joints such as the knee, and often resolves completely (Fig. 174-4). It may even be absent clinically. Of the patients who present with oligoarthritis, approximately 25% are affected by uveitis.[39] Female gender is a well-documented risk factor for the development of ocular inflammation.[38] Most patients who have JIA and uveitis test positively for circulating antinuclear antibodies and negatively for rheumatoid factor. The presence of the antinuclear antibody in a patient with JIA is considered another risk factor for the development of uveitis.[38]

The uveitis associated with JIA is usually bilateral, anterior, and chronic with an insidious onset (Fig. 174-5).[38] The eye disease behaves independently of the joint disease. Whereas joint inflammation often resolves in childhood, ocular inflammation may persist into adulthood. Characteristically, there is no pain or redness. In most cases, this asymptomatic ocular involvement is detected during a routine screening examination. Visual acuity may be variably affected. Slit-lamp examination reveals an absence of limbal injection. There are often inferiorly located small to medium-sized keratic precipitates. Aqueous cell counts are generally low, in the order of trace to 2 plus cell, and generally associated with a chronic flare. Exacerbations with 4 plus aqueous cell may be observed, but hypopyon formation is rare. Posterior synechiae are frequently present, and, in some cases, a pupillary fibrin membrane may occur. Posterior eye inflammation is unusual.

Band keratopathy, cataract, and glaucoma are frequent complications of JIA, one large series reporting the incidences as 41%, 42%, and 19% of patients, respectively.[40] These complications are the usual cause of reduced visual acuity. The rate of blindness in patients with JIA would appear to be decreasing, from about one third of patients in the 1950s and 1960s to 6% in a survey in 2001, the largest undertaken to date.[41] This recent study indicates that the single most significant risk factor associated with the development of complications is the severity of the uveitis at onset of the disease.[41]

Management of Uveitis

The uveitis associated with JIA is often a considerable therapeutic challenge because of its chronic nature and the unique prob-

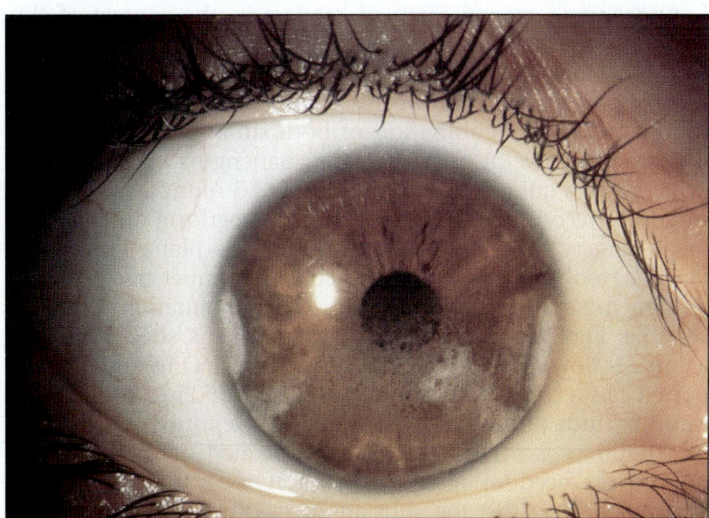

FIG. 174-5 ▊ Slit-lamp photograph of the right eye of a patient with chronic anterior uveitis related to juvenile idiopathic arthritis. As is typical of this condition, the eye appears uninflamed. Band keratopathy is present.

lems presented in the treatment of uveitis in childhood. The aim is to eradicate intraocular inflammation, although some practitioners are stricter with this goal than others. Topical corticosteroid, in the form of prednisolone acetate 1%, is generally effective in controlling the disease. Given the risks of cataract and glaucoma associated with both the therapy and the disease, frequent review is necessary to tailor the frequency of instillation of the eyedrops to the degree of inflammation. A mydriatic is frequently prescribed to avoid the formation of posterior synechiae. For the relatively small number of patients who fail to respond to topical therapy, options include periocular corticosteroid injections, orally administered corticosteroid, and/or systemic immunosuppressive agents. The frequent requirement for general anesthesia to administer a periocular injection to a child makes this form of treatment less appealing than it is for adult patients.

Oral corticosteroid therapy is associated with a multitude of side effects in a patient of any age. However, in children, retardation of growth is an additional concern. For this reason, oral corticosteroid is not favored except in the short term to control a severe exacerbation. Instead, one or a combination of other systemic immunosuppressive therapies is generally used, including the antimetabolites, methotrexate and azathioprine, and the T-cell inhibitor, cyclosporine. Risk of secondary malignancy and variable therapeutic success explain why alkylating agents, such as cyclophosphamide and chlorambucil, are rarely employed in children. The most frequently used drug is methotrexate, which is also effective for the joint disease. Advantages include once-a-week administration, low expense, and high tolerability. Some clinicians advocate the use of nonsteroidal anti-inflammatory agents if local corticosteroid therapy is unsuccessful before opting for a systemic immunosuppressive agent.[42] One small prospective study has reported success in treating 10 patients with JIA-associated uveitis using the new inhibitor of tumor necrosis factor, etanercept.[43] However, a second, retrospective study has been less optimistic,[44] and the results of ongoing larger prospective studies are awaited.

Course and Outcome

Band keratopathy may require treatment when it involves the visual axis and reduces visual acuity. Chelation therapy using ethylenediaminetetraacetic acid is the simplest option. More recently, the excimer laser has been used successfully to remove the calcium by phototherapeutic keratectomy. One large series included a small number of patients with band keratopathy related to JIA-associated uveitis.[45] However, no information about the age at the time of treatment or about the specific outcome for the patients with JIA was included in the report.

Appropriate management of cataract in the context of JIA-associated uveitis is highly controversial. Amblyopia in a patient who is younger than 10 years must be considered. Yet, cataract surgery in a patient with uveitis or a pediatric patient is never routine, and the combination of both situations, a child with JIA-associated uveitis, is particularly challenging. Observing the principle of a quiet eye for a minimum of 3 months prior to the surgery is recommended. Some surgeons perform anterior segment surgery, whereas others include pars plana vitrectomy. Positive results have been published by a number of centers, although the success of intraocular lens implantation has been variable, and it remains unclear whether this should be performed following the extraction of the lens.[46] One study has reported a best corrected vision of 20/20 to 20/50 in 8 of 10 eyes.[47] Another study published in the same year reported visual acuity of 20/200 or worse in 4 of 5 eyes operated on during childhood.[48] The need for aphakic correction needs to be considered and weighed against the substantial risk of membrane formation and posterior capsule opacification. Age of the patient and the presence or absence of amblyopia appear to be important factors in predicting the success of the procedure.

TABLE 174-3

FREQUENCY OF OPHTHALMOLOGIC VISITS FOR CHILDREN WITH JUVENILE IDIOPATHIC ARTHRITIS AND WITHOUT KNOWN IRIDOCYCLITIS*

Juvenile Idiopathic Arthritis Subtype at Onset	Age at Onset of Arthritis	
	7 years†	7 years‡
Pauciarticular (ANA positive)	H§	M
Pauciarticular (ANA negative)	M	M
Polyarticular (ANA positive)	H§	M
Polyarticular (ANA negative)	M	M
Systemic	L	L

Adapted from American Academy of Pediatrics Section on Rheumatology and Section on Ophthalmology. Guidelines for ophthalmologic examinations in children with juvenile rheumatoid arthritis. Pediatrics. 1993;92:295–6.
*High risk (H) patients should have ophthalmologic examinations every 3 to 4 months. Medium-risk (M) patients should have ophthalmologic examinations every 6 months. Low-risk (L) patients should have ophthalmologic examinations every 12 months. ANA indicates the antinuclear antibody test.
†All patients are considered at low risk 7 years after the onset of their arthritis and should have yearly ophthalmologic examinations indefinitely.
‡All patients are considered at low risk 4 years after the onset of their arthritis and should have yearly ophthalmologic examinations indefinitely.
§All high-risk patients are considered at medium risk between 4 and 7 years after the onset of their arthritis.

Although medical therapy, including topical antiglaucoma medications and oral carbonic anhydrase inhibitors, may control intraocular pressure, the largest series of patients with JIA-associated uveitis and glaucoma, which included 41 eyes, demonstrated that surgery was required in approximately two thirds of patients.[49] The increase in availability of different types of antiglaucoma medications may allow control to be achieved medically in a larger number of affected individuals. Although earlier studies gave pessimistic results for glaucoma surgery, one more recent report described a success rate (normalized intraocular pressure with the same or less antiglaucoma medications as preoperatively) by life-table analysis of 90% at 52 months of follow-up after implantation of a valve device.[50]

Ophthalmic Screening

Some patients with JIA come to medical attention because of complications such as band keratopathy, glaucoma, and cataract, sometimes associated with amblyopia. To avoid these complications and consequent visual loss, ophthalmic screening of all patients with JIA is recommended. "High-risk" patients whose disease began before age 7 years and who have pauciarticular or polyarticular disease with antinuclear antibodies should be examined every 3–4 months.[51] Other recommendations for screening, which were developed by the American College of Pediatrics, appear in Table 174-3.

OTHER FORMS OF JUVENILE ARTHRITIS

In some children, uveitis may occur in the context of an HLA-B27–associated seronegative arthropathy not included within the JIA classification, that is, ankylosing spondylitis or reactive arthritis. In this situation, the uveitis is identical to that occurring in adults, in other words, a recurrent, unilateral, acute (sudden onset), anterior uveitis as described earlier. Older children with sarcoidosis develop a typical adult-type disease, with prominent pulmonary involvement, lymphadenopathy, and constitutional symptoms. However, children younger than 4 years have a characteristic presentation including a skin rash, uveitis, and arthritis. A complete description of sarcoid uveitis is presented in Chapter 175. Behçet's disease is one other multisystem inflammatory disease that may result in childhood uveitis and arthritis. Although uveitis appears to occur more commonly in children with Behçet's disease, the disease appears to run a more benign course in this age group.[52] Further infor-

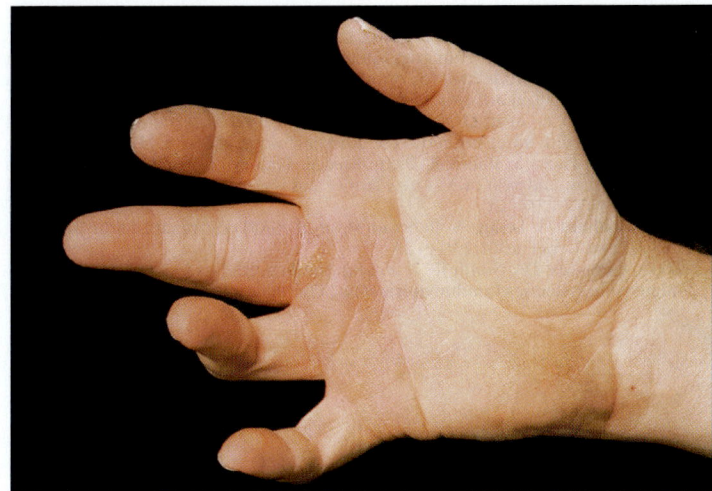

FIG. 174-6 ■ Outstretched hand of a patient with familial juvenile systemic granulomatosis demonstrating the typical finding of camptodactyly or fixed flexion deformity of the fingers.

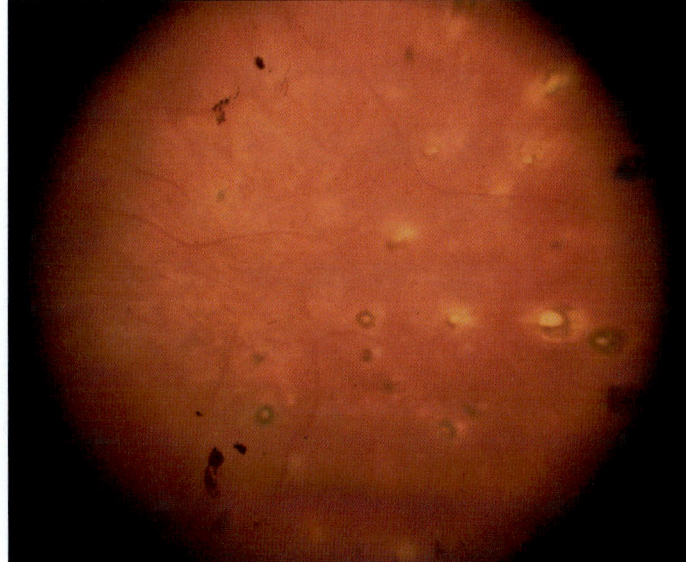

FIG. 174-7 ■ Peripheral fundus photograph from a patient with familial juvenile systemic granulomatosis showing multiple, small, rounded chorioretinal lesions, many of which are pigmented.

mation about the uveitis associated with Behçet's disease may be found in Chapter 176.

Familial juvenile systemic granulomatosis, also referred to as Blau syndrome or Jabs syndrome, is a rare granulomatous inflammatory syndrome that is inherited in an autosomal dominant fashion.[53] The responsible allele was identified as a mutation of a gene known as *CARD15* or *NOD2* that is located on chromosome 16.[54] The protein product of the gene is expressed in monocytes, cells having the capacity to differentiate into the phagocytic cells that are found in granulomas. Interestingly, other mutations of the same gene have been shown to predispose to Crohn's disease. Familial juvenile systemic granulomatosis is characterized by granulomatous uveitis, dermatitis, and an arthritis that most commonly affects the hands and feet (Fig. 174-6). Although initial descriptions indicated that uveitis affected the anterior eye, posterior eye involvement, including vitritis and chorioretinal lesions, has been described more recently (Fig. 174-7).[55]

REFERENCES

1. Brewerton DA, Caffrey M, Nicholls A, *et al.* Acute anterior uveitis and HLA-B27. Lancet. 1973;2:994–6.
2. Khan MA. HLA-B27 and its subtypes in world populations. Curr Opin Rheumatol. 1995;7:263–9.
3. Khan MA. HLA-B27 polymorphism and association with disease. J Rheumatol. 2000;27:1110–13.
4. Linssen A, Rothova A, Valkenburg HA, *et al.* The lifetime cumulative incidence of acute anterior uveitis in a normal population and its relation to ankylosing spondylitis and histocompatibility antigen HLA-B27. Invest Ophthalmol Vis Sci. 1991;32:2568–78.
5. Martin TM, Doyle TM, Smith JR, *et al.* Acute anterior uveitis in families. Invest Ophthalmol Vis Sci. 2001;42:S708.
6. Wakefield D, Montanaro A, McCluskey P. Acute anterior uveitis and HLA-B27. Surv Ophthalmol. 1991;36:223–32.
7. Banares AA, Jover JA, Fernandez-Gutierrez B, *et al.* Bowel inflammation in anterior uveitis and spondyloarthropathy. J Rheumatol. 1995;22:1112–17.
8. Mielants H, Veys EM, Goemaere S, *et al.* A prospective study of patients with spondyloarthropathy with special reference to HLA-B27 and to gut histology. J Rheumatol. 1993;20:1353–8.
9. Dougados M, vam der Linden S, Leirisalo-Repo M, *et al.* Sulfasalazine in the treatment of spondylarthropathy. A randomized, multicenter, double-blind, placebo-controlled study. Arthritis Rheum. 1995;38:618–27.
10. Dougados M, Berenbaum F, Maetzel A, Amor B. Prevention of acute anterior uveitis associated with spondyloarthropathy induced by salazosulfapyridine. Rev Rhum Ed Fr. 1993;60:81–3.
11. Breitbat A, Bauer H, Krastel H, *et al.* Sulfasalazine in recurrent anterior uveitis: a new therapeutical survey. Arthritis Rheum. 1993;36:S225.
12. Benitez-Del-Castillo JM, Garcia-Sanchez J, Iradier T, Banares A. Sulfasalazine in the prevention of anterior uveitis associated with ankylosing spondylitis. Eye. 2000;14:340–3.
13. Munoz-Fernandez S, Hidalgo V, Bonilla G, *et al.* Sulfasalazine improves the number of flares of acute anterior uveitis over a one year period. Arthritis Rheum. 2001;44:S123.
14. Hammer RE, Maika SD, Richardson JA, *et al.* Spontaneous inflammatory disease in transgenic rats expressing HLA-B27 and human beta-2 microglobulin: an animal model of HLA-B27–associated human disorders. Cell. 1990;63:1099–1112.
15. Taurog JD, Richardson JA, Croft JT, *et al.* The germfree state prevents development of gut and joint inflammatory disease in HLA-B27 transgenic rats. J Exp Med. 1994;180:2359–64.
16. Rosenbaum JT, McDevitt HO, Guss RB, Egbert PR. Endotoxin-induced uveitis in rats as a model for human disease. Nature. 1980;286:611–13.
17. Feltkamp TEW, Khan MA, Lopez de Castro JA. The pathogenic role of HLA-B27. Immunol Today. 1996;17:5–8.
18. Colbert RA. HLA-B27 misfolding and spondyloarthropathies: not so groovy after all? J Rheumatol. 2000;27:1107–9.
19. Dick AD, Siepmann K, Dees C, *et al.* Fas-Fas ligand-mediated apoptosis within aqueous during idiopathic acute anterior uveitis. Invest Ophthalmol Vis Sci. 1999;40:2258–67.
20. Rosenbaum JT. Characterization of uveitis associated with spondyloarthritis. J Rheumatol. 1989;16:792–6.
21. Tay-Kearney ML, Schwam BL, Lowder C, *et al.* Clinical features and associated systemic diseases of HLA-B27 uveitis. Am J Ophthalmol. 1996;121:47–56.
22. D'Alessandro LP, Forster DJ, Rao NA. Anterior uveitis and hypopyon. Am J Ophthalmol. 1991;112:317–21.
23. Rodriguez A, Akova YA, Pedroza-Seres M, Foster CS. Posterior segment ocular manifestations in patients with HLA-B27–associated uveitis. Ophthalmology. 1994;101:1267–74.
24. Rosenbaum JT. Acute anterior uveitis and spondyloarthropathies. Rheum Dis Clin North Am. 1992;18:143–51.
25. Linssen A. B27+ disease versus B27– disease. Scand J Rheumatol. 1990;Suppl 87:111–19.
26. Power WJ, Rodriguez A, Pedroza-Seres M, Foster CS. Outcomes in anterior uveitis associated with the HLA-B27 haplotype. Ophthalmology. 1998;105:1646–51.
27. Leibowitz HM, Kupferman A. Bioavailability and therapeutic effectiveness of topically administered corticosteroids. Trans Am Acad Ophthalmol Otolaryngol. 1975;79:OP-78–88.
28. Loteprednol Etabonate US Uveitis Study Group. Controlled evaluation of loteprednol etabonate and prednisolone acetate in the treatment of acute anterior uveitis. Am J Ophthalmol. 1999;127:537–44.
29. Sand BB, Krogh E. Topical indomethacin, a prostaglandin inhibitor, in acute anterior uveitis. A controlled clinical trial of non-steroid versus steroid anti-inflammatory treatment. Acta Ophthalmol (Copenh). 1991;69:145–8.
30. Okhravi N, Lightman SL, Towler HM. Assessment of visual outcome after cataract surgery in patients with uveitis. Ophthalmology. 1999;106:710–22.
31. Wakefield D, McCluskey P, Verma M, *et al.* Ciprofloxacin treatment does not influence course or relapse rate of reactive arthritis and anterior uveitis. Arthritis Rheum. 1999;42:1894–7.
32. Lyons JL, Rosenbaum JT. Uveitis associated with inflammatory bowel disease compared with uveitis associated with spondyloarthropathy. Arch Ophthalmol. 1997;115:61–4.
33. Ruzicka T. Psoriatic arthritis. Arch Dermatol. 1996;132:215–19.
34. Paiva ES, Macaluso DC, Edwards A, Rosenbaum JT. Characterisation of uveitis in patients with psoriatic arthritis. Ann Rheum Dis. 2000;59:67–70.
35. Cunningham ET. Uveitis in children. Ocul Immunol Inflamm. 2000;8:251–61.
36. Rodriguez A, Calonge M, Pedroza-Seres M. Referral patterns of uveitis in a tertiary eye care center. Arch Ophthalmol. 1996;114:593–9.
37. Petty RE and the Task Force for Classification Criteria. Revision for the proposed classification criteria for juvenile idiopathic arthritis: Durban, 1997. J Rheumatol. 1998;25:1991–4.
38. Kanski JJ. Juvenile arthritis and uveitis. Surv Ophthalmol. 1990;34:253–67.
39. Rosenberg AM. Uveitis associated with juvenile rheumatoid arthritis. Semin Arthritis Rheum. 1987;16:158–73.
40. Kanski JJ. Anterior uveitis in juvenile rheumatoid arthritis. Arch Ophthalmol. 1977;95:1794–7.
41. Edelsten C, Lee V, Bentley CR, *et al.* An evaluation of baseline risk factors predicting severity in juvenile idiopathic arthritis associated uveitis and other chronic anterior uveitis in early childhood. Br J Ophthalmol. 2002;86:51–6.
42. Nguyen QD, Foster CS. Saving the vision of children with juvenile rheumatoid arthritis–associated uveitis. JAMA. 1998;280:1133–4.
43. Reiff A, Takei S, Sadeghi S, *et al.* Etanercept therapy in children with treatment-resistant uveitis. Arthritis Rheum. 2001;44:1411–15.

44. Smith JR, Levinson RD, Holland GN, et al. Differential efficacy of tumor necrosis factor inhibition in the management of inflammatory eye disease and associated rheumatic disease. Arthritis Rheum. 2001;45:252–7.

45. O'Brart DPS, Gartry DS, Lohmann CP, et al. Treatment of band keratopathy by excimer laser phototherapeutic keratectomy: surgical techniques and long term follow up. Br J Ophthalmol. 1993;77:702–8.

46. Holland G. Intraocular lens implantation in patients with juvenile rheumatoid arthritis–associated uveitis: an unresolved management issue. Am J Ophthalmol. 1966;122:255–7.

47. Lundvall A, Zetterstrom C. Cataract extraction and intraocular lens implantation in children with uveitis. Br J Ophthalmol. 2000;84:791–3.

48. BenErza D, Cohen E. Cataract surgery in children with chronic uveitis. Ophthalmology. 2000;107:1255–60.

49. Foster CS, Havrlikova K, Baltatzis S, et al. Secondary glaucoma in patients with juvenile rheumatoid arthritis–associated iridocyclitis. Acta Ophthalmol Scand. 2000;78:576–9.

50. Valimaki J, Airaksinen PJ, Tuulonen A. Molteno implantation for secondary glaucoma in juvenile rheumatoid arthritis. Arch Ophthalmol. 1997;115:1253–6.

51. American Academy of Pediatrics Section on Rheumatology and Section on Ophthalmology. Guidelines for ophthalmologic examinations in children with juvenile rheumatoid arthritis. Pediatrics. 1993;92:295–6.

52. Krause I, Uziel Y, Guedj D, et al. Childhood Behçet's disease: clinical features and comparison with adult-onset disease. Rheumatology. 1999;38:457–62.

53. Manouvrier-Hanu S, Puech B, Piette F, et al. Blau syndrome of granulomatous arthritis, iritis, and skin rash: a new family and review of the literature. Am J Med Genet. 1998;76:217–21.

54. Miceli-Richard C, Lesage S, Rybojad M, et al. CARD15 mutations in Blau syndrome. Nat Genet. 2001;29:19–20.

55. Latkany PA, Jabs DA, Smith JR, et al. Multifocal choroiditis in patients with familial juvenile systemic granulomatosis. Am J Ophthalmol. 2002;134(6):897–904.

CLAUDE L. COWAN JR.

DEFINITION
- A multisystem inflammatory disorder characterized histologically by the presence of noncaseating granulomas.

KEY FEATURES
- Anterior and posterior uveitis.
- Bilateral hilar lymphadenopathy and/or pulmonary parenchymal disease.

ASSOCIATED FEATURES
- Cutaneous lesions.
- Neurological abnormalities, including optic neuropathy.
- Cardiomyopathy.
- Orbital and conjunctival infiltration.
- Arthropathy.

INTRODUCTION

Sarcoidosis is a systemic disorder characterized histologically by localized granuloma formation with a concomitant T-cell lymphopenia involving the peripheral blood. Its clinical features can be highly variable and may show considerable differences among individuals, geographical regions, and ethnic groups. The course of the disease demonstrates a similar variability—some patients have an acute, self-limited process, whereas others experience a progressive downhill course that results in severe disability or death. Ocular involvement is common and may precede clinical manifestations of systemic disease. Corticosteroids are the mainstay of treatment for both ocular and systemic disease and can be effective in the prevention of severe functional impairment.

EPIDEMIOLOGY AND PATHOGENESIS

The etiology of sarcoidosis remains unclear, but evidence suggests that it is an immunological response to some exogenous agent. The widespread distribution and diverse clinical presentations of sarcoidosis suggest that many causal agents exist.[1] Bacteria and bacterial DNA fragments have been reported in sarcoid granulomas, but attempts to transmit sarcoid have not been successful.[2-4] Localized and regional granulomatous responses have been produced following inoculation of sarcoid material into experimental animals, but this has not been followed by the development of a systemic disorder compatible with the disease seen in humans.[5] Nevertheless, reports of "transmission" of sarcoidosis through organ transplantation suggest that a transmissible agent may be a factor in some patients.[6] Sarcoidosis incidence has shown an inverse secular trend with tuberculosis, but this finding remains unexplained. If sarcoid is triggered by an infectious agent, it is presumably widely distributed but of low virulence, such that clear time-space relationships have not been established in spite of scattered reports of local clustering.

Noninfectious agents, most notably pine products, have been linked to the development of sarcoidosis, but the geographical diversity that characterizes the distribution of sarcoid argues against a single or predominant causative agent. Familial clustering is well described, and although this is consistent with an infectious or environmental process, the greater prevalence among certain parent-offspring and sibling pairs suggests that genetically determined factors are at least as important as environmental ones.[1,7] The association of several human leukocyte antigen haplotypes with specific clinical courses and racial differences in susceptibility offer further evidence for the role of genetic factors in the development of sarcoidosis.[8] Genetically programmed T-cell antigenic responsiveness may determine which environmental factors will precipitate a sarcoid reaction, with some threshold level of exposure being required to initiate the inflammatory response. More than one candidate gene has been found with increased frequency in individuals with sarcoidosis, raising the possibility that a synergistic response among two or more genes is required to confer disease risk.

Sarcoid is worldwide in distribution, and its prevalence varies widely from one region to another. The prevalence and incidence are probably underestimated, since the disease is often asymptomatic and may be suspected only on the basis of an abnormal chest x-ray. In addition, seasonal variations may affect the calculation of incidence rates. In Europe, there appears to be a north-south gradient, with the highest rates noted in Sweden, Norway, and Ireland. The incidence in the United States is highly associated with race, and the age-adjusted annual incidence is more than three times higher in blacks compared with whites.[9] When stratified by age and race, the highest rate, 107/100,100, is found in African-American women aged 30–39. This is among the highest in the world. A similar predilection for blacks has not been confirmed throughout Africa but has been described in South Africa. The incidence of sarcoid peaks in the 20s and 30s, but presentations in early childhood and later in life are well described. The disease is reported to be more common in women, but some variability may occur based on age at presentation.

OCULAR MANIFESTATIONS

Ocular involvement by sarcoid is common and has been reported in up to 78% of patients.[10] The wide range of reported prevalence reflects differences in study methodology, the demographics of the study population, and the length of follow-up, as well as the transient and asymptomatic nature of many findings.

Anterior uveitis is the foremost cause of ocular morbidity and often presents early in the course of the disease or before the diagnosis is suspected. Although frequently unilateral at the onset, second eye involvement is common at some point during the course of the disease. The uveitis is characteristically granulomatous in nature and accompanied by medium to large "mutton fat" keratic precipitates. Multiple Busacca or Koeppe nodules are not uncommon, and they may achieve considerable size (Fig. 175-1). Nodular deposits may occasionally be seen in the angle and, when extensive, can lead to increased intraocular pressure.

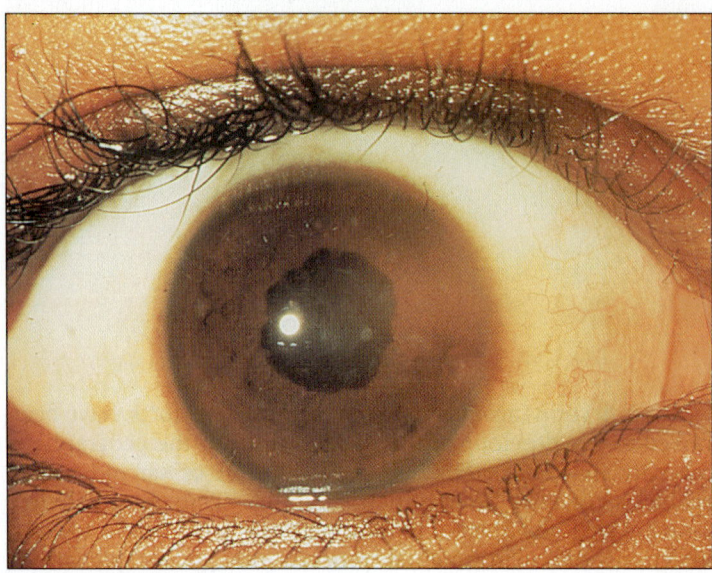

FIG. 175-1 ▌ **Typical appearance of chronic sarcoid uveitis.** Note the multiple Busacca iris nodules and posterior synechiae.

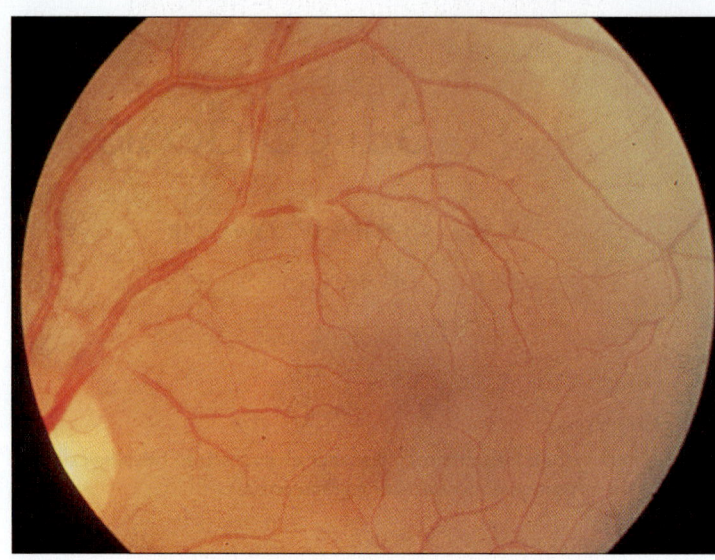

FIG. 175-2 ▌ **Retinal periphlebitis involving the superior temporal arcade.** Note the appearance of focal vascular narrowing associated with the phlebitic foci.

A subacute presentation occurs most frequently, and patients may be relatively asymptomatic until the inflammation is well established. This can lead to the insidious development of anterior and posterior synechiae. Patients who experience a chronic course with multiple exacerbations are at high risk for secondary glaucoma or cataract. Cystoid macular edema may accompany anterior segment inflammation and can serve as a barometer of disease activity, since it often resolves when the inflammation subsides. However, protracted periods of inflammation may lead to chronic macular edema and loss of visual acuity. Acute anterior uveitis occurs relatively infrequently and is less often associated with severe sequelae because its symptomatic nature leads the patient to seek treatment.

Other manifestations of anterior segment sarcoid include conjunctival granulomas, scleritis and episcleritis, a nonspecific conjunctivitis, and interstitial keratitis. These infrequently cause significant ocular morbidity, but conjunctival inflammation occasionally resolves with symblepharon formation. Band keratopathy, though associated with sarcoidosis, is rarely a primary event and is more likely to be a complication of chronic uveitis.

Posterior segment involvement is reported to occur in nearly 30% of patients with ocular disease. This may be an underestimation due to the small size and peripheral location of many lesions and the generally asymptomatic nature of localized disease. Periphlebitis and vitritis are the most common manifestations of posterior uveitis in sarcoidosis. The involved venules are often mid-peripheral or peripheral in location and demonstrate short segments of perivascular cuffing with or without focal vascular narrowing (Fig. 175-2). A cellular reaction in the anterior vitreous may accompany the periphlebitis, and when this is seen on anterior segment examination, it should prompt a careful examination of the peripheral retina. Severe vasculitis may be associated with extensive perivascular exudation, resulting in an appearance that has been likened to candlewax drippings. Periphlebitis is occasionally complicated by retinal neovascularization, and these lesions can simulate the peripheral "sea fans" associated with sickle retinopathy. The report of multifocal arterial ectasias associated with sarcoidosis suggests that a clinically significant arteritis may occasionally accompany posterior segment inflammation.[11]

The vitritis of sarcoidosis may be generalized and nonspecific or characterized by gray-white round opacities in the inferior vitreous. These "snowball" opacities can occur singly, in clusters, or in a linear array or strand, like a "string of pearls." Veil-like vitreous condensations are not uncommon, and although they

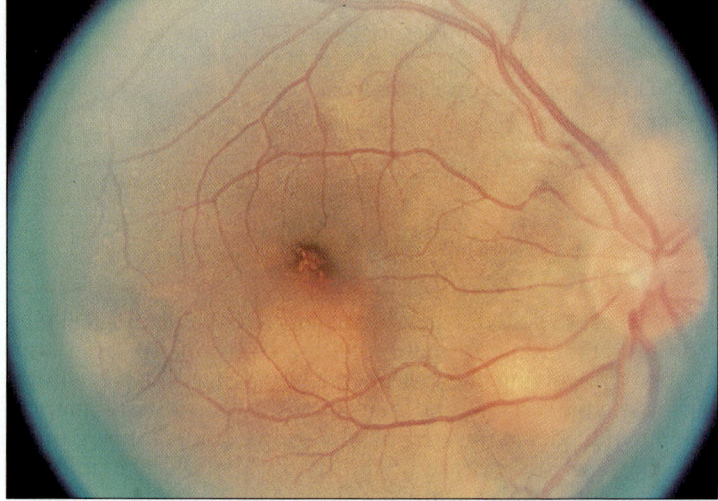

FIG. 175-3 ▌ **Multiple choroidal lesions simulating pneumocystis choroiditis.** These lesions remained unchanged in spite of several courses of systemic corticosteroids.

may cause bothersome symptoms, vision remains good in the absence of severe clouding or macular edema. Retinitis associated with sarcoid may be difficult to distinguish from other causes of retinal inflammation. It can extend into the preretinal vitreous, leading to the appearance of vitreous snowballs.

Choroidal lesions vary considerably in their appearance and often mimic nonsarcoid choroidal disorders (Fig. 175-3). Isolated tumefactions with or without subretinal fluid, clusters of yellow subretinal lesions, and scattered discrete peripheral white lesions occur in one or both eyes. The latter may increase in number over time and evolve into focal atrophic spots. Histologically, choroidal granulomas are seen less frequently than clinical descriptions suggest, since many of these lesions are actually located in the subpigment epithelial space. Fluorescein angiography may demonstrate nonfluorescence, hypofluorescence, early blocking with late staining, or hyperfluorescence throughout. If the eye is otherwise uninvolved, it is usually remarkably quiet. Vision loss may be associated with serous detachment of the macula, pigment epithelial dropout, or subretinal neovascularization.

Sarcoid involves the optic nerve infrequently. Clinically, the nerve may show edema, infiltration, swelling associated with adjacent retinitis, or progressive atrophy. Retrobulbar or chiasmatic involvement can present with progressive vision loss in the face

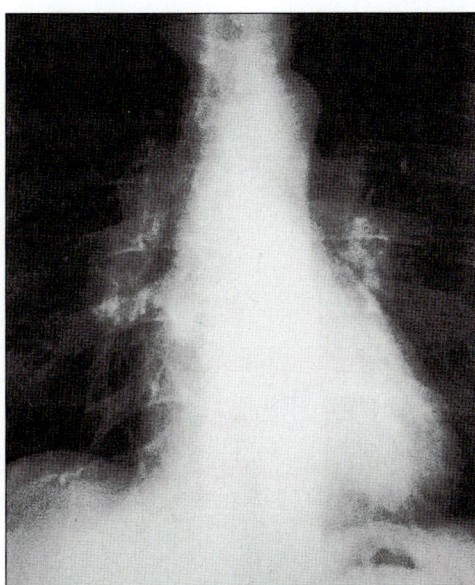

FIG. 175-4 ■ Bilateral hilar adenopathy in a patient without pulmonary symptoms. Note the symmetry of the hilar node enlargement.

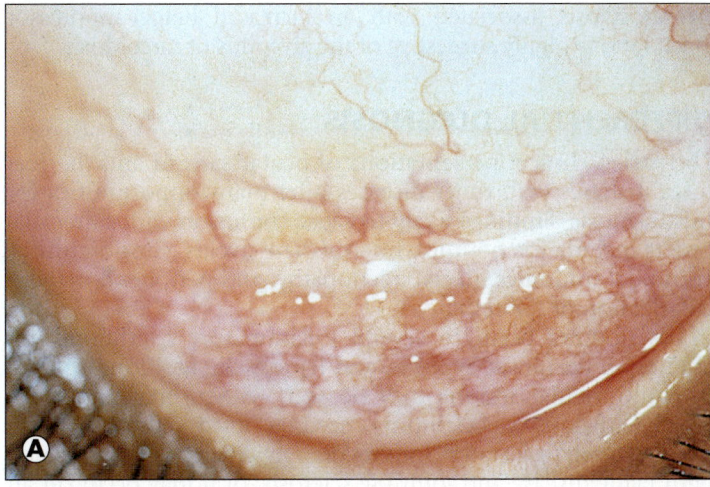

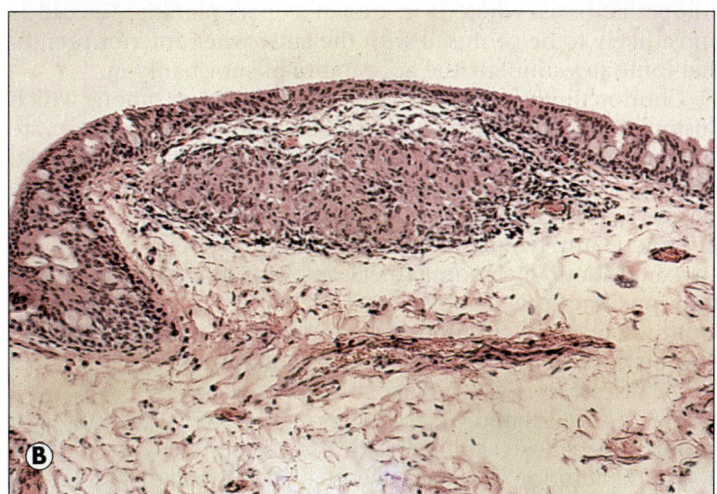

FIG. 175-5 ■ Conjunctival sarcoidosis. **A,** The patient shows numerous small, round nodular lesions and translucent cysts in the conjunctival fornix. **B,** A conjunctival biopsy reveals a discrete granuloma composed of epithelioid cells and surrounded by a rim of lymphocytes and plasms cells. Such granulomas may be found histologically even if no conjunctival nodules are seen clinically. (**A-B,** From Yanoff M, Fine BS. Ocular pathology. St Louis: Mosby; 2002.)

of a normal-appearing nerve. Visual field defects often accompany lesions of the visual pathways and may be indistinguishable from those caused by cerebrovascular accidents or mass lesions.

Dacryoadenitis is often initially suspected on the basis of swelling of the lateral aspect of the upper lids. Though frequently asymptomatic, it can cause pain, proptosis, and exposure keratopathy when severe. Infiltration of the lacrimal gland may also occasionally cause symptoms of keratoconjunctivitis sicca, even in the absence of overt dacryoadenopathy. Rarely, isolated orbital or extraocular muscle granulomas occur. They often lead to misdiagnosis, and the correct diagnosis typically is made only after orbital exploration and biopsy.

DIAGNOSIS

The diagnosis of sarcoidosis is based on the presence of a compatible clinical picture, supportive laboratory findings, and, in most cases, a confirmatory biopsy. Pulmonary involvement occurs at some point in the disease in nearly all cases. Bilateral hilar adenopathy, with or without parenchymal infiltrates, is the radiographical hallmark of the disease (Fig. 175-4). One or more skin lesions occur in approximately 25% of patients, but they can be nonspecific and mimic other dermatological lesions. However, lupus pernio and erythema nodosum, when associated with hilar adenopathy, are sufficiently characteristic of this disorder to be considered supporting diagnostic criteria. Other nonocular extrapulmonary manifestations, although compatible with sarcoidosis, are less reliable as diagnostic criteria. Nevertheless, in the appropriate clinical setting, plaque-like skin lesions, peripheral lymphadenopathy, Bell's palsy, cardiac conduction abnormalities, and childhood arthritis should raise the index of suspicion for sarcoid. Symptoms associated with sarcoidosis are generally nonspecific. Although cough, dyspnea, or chest pain may suggest the presence of pulmonary disease, other symptoms such as weight loss, malaise, fever, night sweats, or fatigue are nonlocalizing.

Laboratory tests, although not specific for sarcoidosis, may provide a high degree of correlation with disease activity. Serum angiotensin-converting enzyme (ACE) is elevated in approximately 60% of patients and correlates well with the degree of pulmonary involvement.[12] Other tests, such as serum and urine calcium, erythrocyte sedimentation rate, immunoglobulin electrophoresis, liver function studies, and serum lysozyme, are less useful as predictors of sarcoid activity because of their lack of sensitivity or specificity. However, when used selectively, they can aid in making the diagnosis.

Gallium scanning is based on the tendency for ^{67}Ga to accumulate at sites of inflammation. It is especially useful in patients who have normal or equivocal chest radiographs but clinical or laboratory findings consistent with sarcoidosis. Bilateral hilar uptake combined with increased uptake in the parotids and orbits is highly characteristic of sarcoid.[13] The greater sensitivity of chest computerized tomography in detecting intrathoracic adenopathy compared with standard radiographs makes it another useful adjunct in the evaluation of suspected pulmonary sarcoidoses. Gallium scanning combined with serum ACE provides increased sensitivity and specificity but should be considered as providing supportive rather than confirmatory evidence. Relative anergy to recall antigens occurs in sarcoidosis because of impaired recruitment of helper cells in the skin. Although testing for tuberculosis is commonly recommended, tests with other antigens, such as *Trichophyton, Candida,* and mumps, may be more useful in patients without known exposure to tuberculosis.

A confirmatory biopsy is usually sought, since some patients require chronic or high-dose corticosteroid therapy. Transbronchial biopsy provides ready access to pulmonary tissue, but conjunctiva, lacrimal glands, peripheral lymph nodes, skin, nasal mucosa, and minor salivary glands can also provide suitable biopsy sites. The lacrimal gland should not be considered a primary biopsy site if it is not easily accessible or appears entirely normal. Conjunctival biopsies, especially when granulomas are present (Fig. 175-5), yield a high percentage of positive biopsies and are relatively easy to do. Analysis of bronchoalveolar lavage fluid is useful for establishing the diagnosis and staging disease activity. The presence of a lymphocytosis associated with an increased helper-suppressor T-cell ratio is highly suggestive of the alveolitis of sarcoidosis.[14]

DIFFERENTIAL DIAGNOSIS

The varied clinical presentations of ocular sarcoid and the features it shares with other diseases offer many opportunities for misdiagnosis. Findings likely to cause confusion with other disorders include iris nodules, intermediate uveitis, chorioretinitis, choroidal infiltrates, dacryoadenopathy, and peripheral neovascularization of the retina.

Iris nodules occur in several inflammatory conditions, including tuberculosis, syphilis, and leprosy. In addition, isolated or multinodular lesions may be seen with primary iris neoplasms, metastatic carcinoma, seeding from retinoblastoma, and leukemic infiltrates. Intermediate uveitis can be associated with Lyme disease and multiple sclerosis, or it may occur on an idiopathic basis, where it is known as pars planitis. Sarcoid is most likely to be confused with the latter when inferior preretinal infiltrates simulate the appearance of snowbanking.

Chorioretinitis is a feature of multiple disorders, among which histoplasmosis, tuberculosis, syphilis, and toxoplasmosis are most likely to be confused with sarcoid. Subretinal or choroidal infiltration occurs in a variety of conditions, including acute posterior multifocal placoid pigment epitheliopathy, birdshot choroidopathy, lymphoid hyperplasia, central serous choroidopathy, amelanotic melanoma, metastatic lesions, Harada's disease, and pneumocystis choroiditis. Differentiating these disorders from sarcoid is often impossible on the basis of the fundus picture alone, and it often requires demonstration of other features of the disease in order to make the correct diagnosis.

Sarcoid-associated dacryoadenopathy and parotitis can mimic tuberculosis, Hodgkin's disease, lymphoma, and brucellosis. In addition, isolated lacrimal gland enlargement may cause confusion with orbital pseudotumor or primary lacrimal gland tumors. Peripheral retinal neovascularization occurs relatively infrequently, but other causes of sea fan–like proliferations, such as sickle retinopathy, venous occlusive disease, and diabetic retinopathy, occur with sufficient frequency that sarcoid may be overlooked as a cause.

Infiltrative disease of the optic nerve, other inflammatory optic neuropathies, ischemic optic neuropathy, optic gliomas, optic disc edema, and optic nerve sheath meningiomas all have features that can be mimicked clinically or radiographically by sarcoidosis. Avoidance of misdiagnosis can be difficult when other signs of sarcoid are absent, but an appropriate index of suspicion may save patients from unnecessary investigations.

SYSTEMIC ASSOCIATIONS

Sarcoidosis is a multisystem disorder that can involve virtually any organ. It is accompanied by abnormalities in cell-mediated and humoral immunity that lead to impaired responsiveness to recall antigens, depressed circulating T-cell levels, elevated globulin levels, and nonspecific elevation of antibody titers.

It involves the lungs and/or thoracic nodes in 90% of patients and is staged according to the severity of radiographical findings:
- Stage I consists of bilateral hilar adenopathy alone.
- Stage II adds parenchymal involvement.
- In stage III, parenchymal disease predominates without prominent hilar involvement.
- Stage IV is a late stage characterized by pulmonary fibrosis.

Upper respiratory tract involvement can be overlooked, as its symptoms may suggest a nonspecific rhinitis. Complaints of nasal stuffiness or congestion warrant examination of the nasal mucosa in any patient who is suspected of having sarcoidosis. Cutaneous manifestations are common and include nodules, plaques, psoriasiform lesions, papules, ulcerations, and erythema nodosum (Fig. 175-6).[15] Lupus pernio, a plaque-like

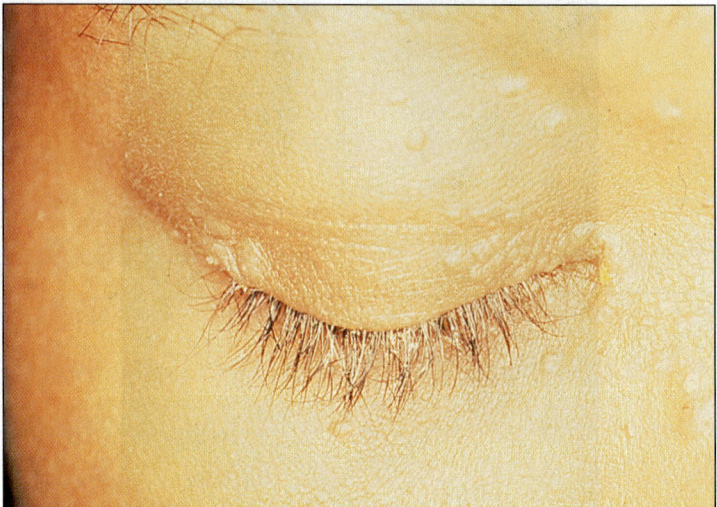

FIG. 175-6 ■ **Multiple cutaneous lesions involving the lid.** Papules, umbilicated lesions, and plaques are evident in this patient.

lesion that involves the face, can be disfiguring and may be of prognostic value because of its association with chronic disease. Eyelid lesions mirror those seen elsewhere and should be considered part of the cutaneous disease.

Peripheral lymphadenopathy is common, but its nonspecificity makes it a poor stand-alone predictor of sarcoidosis. Occasionally, a sarcoid reaction is seen in regional lymph nodes that drain a carcinoma or lymphoma.[16] This can lead to diagnostic confusion and a delay in reaching the correct diagnosis.

Cardiac involvement is apparent clinically in approximately 5% of patients, but its prevalence is reported to be as high as 27% in autopsy series. It is associated with conduction defects and ventricular arrhythmias and can cause sudden death from complete heart block or ventricular tachyarrhythmias. The association with heart block requires that caution be exercised when beta blockers are prescribed for patients who have glaucoma and sarcoidosis.

Neurosarcoidosis occurs in 5–10% of patients and may precede other manifestations of the disease by a year or more.[17,18] It has a predilection for the basal leptomeninges, and cranial nerve involvement is common (Fig. 175-7). Hypothalamic and pituitary involvement can cause significant morbidity, and diffuse hemispheric disease may lead to seizures. Large lesions can mimic intracranial tumors and cause hemianopic or quadrantanopic field defects. Spinal tract lesions are unusual but may result in paralysis. Sarcoid retinitis is often seen with neurosarcoidosis.

Hepatic, splenic, and bone involvement causes symptomatic clinical disease in a minority of patients; however, subclinical liver disease is not uncommon, and liver biopsy for other indications may reveal a diagnosis of sarcoidosis. Hypercalcemia and/or hypercalciuria occur in up to 17% of individuals, and sarcoid is associated with an increased risk for nephrocalcinosis and nephrolithiasis compared with the general population.[19]

Early-onset sarcoid that occurs in children younger than 4 years has a distinct clinical picture—the triad of rash, polyarthritis, and uveitis occurs commonly.[20] The arthritis may initially be mono- or pauciarticular and may lead to a diagnosis of juvenile rheumatoid arthritis. These patients often have multisystem disease, and hepatosplenomegaly, parotid swelling, and cardiac abnormalities are not uncommon.

PATHOLOGY

Sarcoidosis is defined by its histopathology. Characteristically, sarcoid tissue demonstrates granulomas with central nodules of

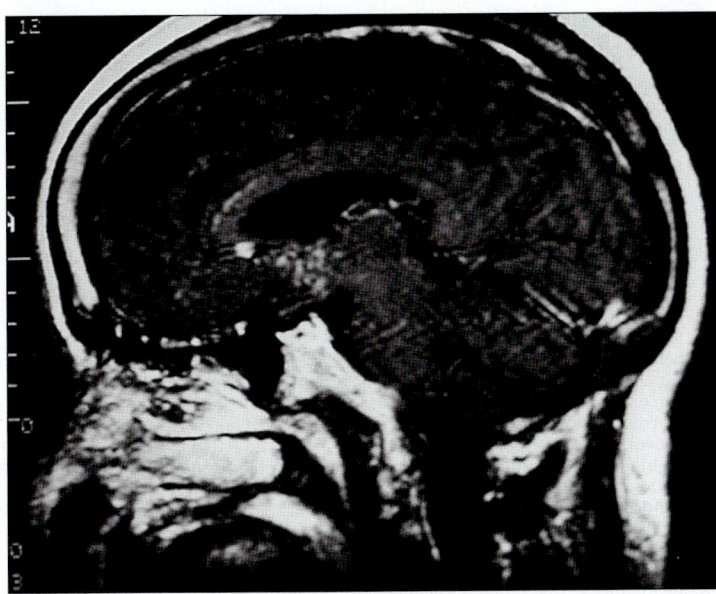

FIG. 175-7 ▪ **Enhancing lesions in a patient with progressive vision loss and seizures.** Involvement of the frontal basal meninges and thalamus can be seen.

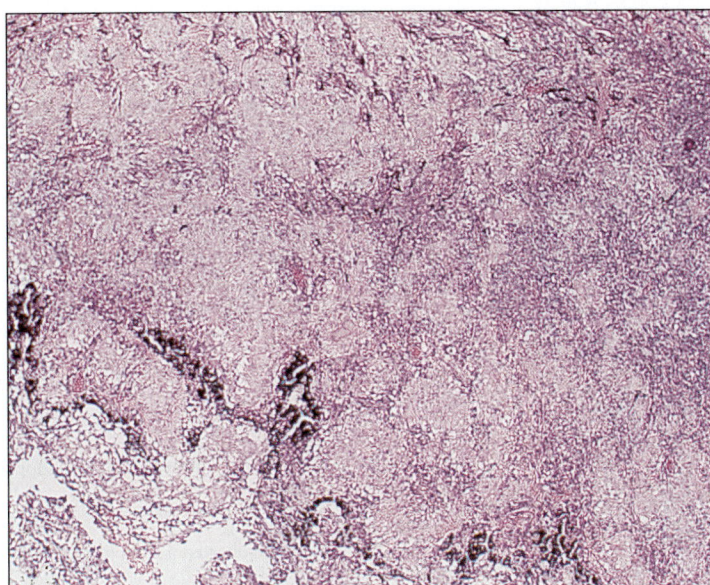

FIG. 175-8 ▪ **Sarcoid granulomas replacing much of the ciliary body.** Lighter-staining epithelioid granulomas are surrounded by darker-staining lymphocytes.

epithelioid cells surrounded by a mantle of lymphocytes and other mononuclear cells (Figs. 175-5, *B* and 175-8). Although mild central necrosis may be seen, caseation is not a feature of sarcoidosis. Fibrosis can be associated with maturation of sarcoid granulomas and may lead to severe pulmonary dysfunction.

TREATMENT

No known cure exists for sarcoidosis. Treatment is intended primarily to reduce the symptoms, lessen disability during periods of activity, and minimize the sequelae of inflammation. Corticosteroids remain the mainstay of treatment for ocular sarcoid, regardless of the site of involvement. Topical administration, when done with sufficient frequency, is effective for most patients who have anterior segment inflammation, but supplementation with periocular steroids may be required for patients who have severe or well-established disease. Occasionally, adequate control can be achieved only with systemic administration.

Chronic or recurrent anterior uveitis may require more aggressive therapy than would be suggested by the level of clinical inflammation. Progressive anterior and posterior synechiae can occur in patients who have frequent episodes of "silent" reactivation. The latter group of patients may be best served by long-term maintenance therapy, even in the absence of clinically active disease.

Posterior uveitis is managed primarily with periocular and/or systemic corticosteroids. Small segments of peripheral periphlebitis or mild vitritis may not require treatment, as the disease can wax and wane without progression. Choroidal infiltrates can be associated with serous elevation of the overlying retina and, rarely, subretinal neovascularization. Systemic steroids can clear choroidal lesions and any accompanying serous retinal detachment, but their effect is variable, and recurrences are not unusual. No clear evidence exists that steroid use prevents subretinal new vessel formation, but the association of prior inflammation with neovascularization in diseases such as presumed ocular histoplasmosis argues strongly for treating choroidal lesions when they involve the macula. Optic nerve involvement can be resistant to even high doses of oral steroids, and "pulsed" intravenous methylprednisolone may be required to achieve a response. Systemic cytotoxic agents are used to supplement steroid therapy for refractory disease or to allow a reduction in steroid dose. Regardless of the site of involvement, treatment should not be considered curative, and relapses should be anticipated.

Indications for the treatment of systemic sarcoidosis include bothersome symptoms, organ dysfunction, and biochemical or radiographical deterioration. Oral corticosteroids remain the primary first-line therapy.[21–23] Inhaled steroids appear to be less effective for pulmonary disease, but they have been shown to be useful as maintenance therapy following an initial course of oral prednisone.[24] High-dose intravenous methylprednisolone, when used in short 2- to 3-day pulses, can be a useful supplement to oral steroids. Steroid therapy has not been proved to provide long-term disease effect modification, but early treatment has been shown to improve 5-year pulmonary function in some patients with newly diagnosed stage II disease.[25,26] Cytotoxic drugs, and less frequently cyclosporin, can be useful for refractive disease or can be used as part of a steroid-sparing strategy.[27] Methotrexate and azathioprine are the preferred cytotoxic agents due to their effectiveness and relative safety. However, like all such agents, they have the potential for hematological and gastrointestinal toxicity, as well as teratogenicity. These drugs may also be carcinogenic, although methotrexate appears to be less problematic in this regard.

Chloroquine and hydroxychloroquine can be very effective for pulmonary and cutaneous disease, but hydroxychloroquine is preferred due to its significantly lower risk for ocular toxicity. Thalidomide is reported to provide another alternative to systemic steroids for cutaneous sarcoid, but caution should be exercised when recommending this drug to women of child-bearing age.[28] Ketoconazole has been useful in the management of hypercalcemia, and radiation therapy may be effective for some patients with refractory neurosarcoid. The successful use of tumor necrosis factor-α in one patient with advanced sarcoidosis suggests that selective manipulation of inflammation may have a future role in sarcoid management.[29]

COURSE AND OUTCOME

The overall prognosis for systemic and ocular sarcoid is good. Most patients recover without significant functional impairment.[30–32] Chronicity increases the risk for complications, as does delay in receiving appropriate therapy,[33] but early recognition and treatment of patients who are prone to recurrences can improve their outlook. Systemic features associated with chronicity or poorer outcomes include central nervous system involvement, lupus pernio, nephrocalcinosis, stage III pulmonary disease, hepatosplenomegaly, and cardiac involvement. Clinical depression may occur in more than 50% of patients and, as with other chronic conditions, can adversely affect adherence to therapy. Multisystem disease and pulmonary symptoms increase the risk for this complication. Black patients may be more likely to have symptomatic disease and ocular involvement, and they have higher rates of severe complications. However, a recent metaanalysis concluded that sarcoid mortality is largely independent of ethnicity.[34] Most patients with sarcoidosis retain normal vision; bilateral vision loss to less than 20/200 is unusual. Chronic uveitis, cystoid macular edema, secondary glaucoma, and retina and optic nerve involvement are associated with poorer visual outcomes and represent difficult therapeutic challenges.

REFERENCES

1. Sharma O. Sarcoidosis. Dis Mon. 1990;9:471–535.
2. Kon OM, du Bois RM. Mycobacteria and sarcoidosis. Thorax. 1997;52(suppl 3):547–51.
3. Popper HH, Klemen H, Hoefler G, et al. Presence of mycobacterial DNA in sarcoidosis. Hum Pathol. 1997;28:796–800.
4. Li N, Bajoghi A, Kubbu A, et al. Identification of mycobacterial DNA in cutaneous lesions of sarcoidosis. J Cutan Pathol. 1999;26:271–8.
5. Ikonomopoulos JA, Gargoulis VG, Kastrinakis NE, et al. Experimental inoculation of laboratory animals with samples collected from sarcoid patients and molecular diagnostic evaluation of the results. In Vivo. 2000;14:761–5.
6. Heyll A, Mechkenstock G, Aul C, et al. Possible transmission of sarcoidosis via allogenic bone marrow transplantation. Bone Marrow Transplant. 1994;14:161–4.
7. Rybicki BA, Maliarik MJ, Major M, et al. Epidemiology, demographics, and genetics of sarcoidosis. Semin Respir Infect. 1998;13:166–73.
8. Martinetti M, Tinelli C, Kolek V, et al. The sarcoidosis map: a joint survey of clinical and immunogenetic findings in two European countries. Am J Respir Crit Care Med. 1995;152:557–64.
9. Rybicki BA, Major M, Popovich J, et al. Racial differences in sarcoidosis incidence: a 5-year study in a health maintenance organization. Am J Epidemiol. 1997;145:234–41.
10. Iwata K, Nanka K, Sobu K, et al. Ocular sarcoidosis: evaluation of intraocular findings. N Y Acad Sci. 1976;278:445–54.
11. Verougstraete C, Snyers B, Leys A, et al. Multiple arterial ectasias in patients with sarcoidosis and uveitis. Am J Ophthalmol. 2001;131:223–31.
12. Poe RH, Utell MJ. Diagnosis and management of pulmonary sarcoidosis. Compr Ther 1989;15:35–42.
13. Israel HL, Albertine KH, Park CH, et al. Whole-body gallium-67 scans: role in diagnosis of sarcoidosis. Am Rev Respir Dis. 1991;144:1182–6.
14. Bienfait MF, Hoogstenders HC, Baarasma GS, et al. Diagnostic value of bronchoalveolar lavage in ocular sarcoidosis. Acta Ophthalmol. 1987;65:745–8.
15. Zax RH. Sarcoidosis. Dermatol Clin. 1989;7:505–15.
16. Brincker H. Interpretation of granulomatous lesions in malignancy. Acta Oncol. 1992;31:85–9.
17. Chapelon C, Ziza JM, Piette JC, et al. Neurosarcoidosis: signs, course, and treatment in 35 confirmed cases. Medicine. 1990;69:261–76.
18. Lower EE, Broderick JP, Brott TE, et al. Diagnosis and management of neurological sarcoidosis. Arch Intern Med. 1997;157:1864–8.
19. Sharma OP. Vitamin D, calcium, and sarcoidosis. Chest. 1996;109:535–9.
20. Hafner R, Voge P. Sarcoidosis of early onset. A challenge for the pediatric rheumatologist. Clin Exp Rheumatol. 1993;11:685–91.
21. Selroos O. Treatment of sarcoidosis. Sarcoidosis. 1994;11:80–3.
22. American Thoracic Society/European Respiratory Society/World Association of Sarcoidosis and Other Granulomatous Disorders. Statement on sarcoidosis. Sarcoidosis Vasc Diffuse Lung Dis. 1999;16:149–73.
23. Newman LS, Rose CS, Maier LA. Sarcoidosis. N Engl J Med. 1997;336:1224–34.
24. Pietnalho A, Tukiainen P, Haahtela T, et al. Oral prednisone followed by inhaled budesonide in newly diagnosed pulmonary sarcoidosis: a double blind, placebo-controlled multicenter study. Finnish Pulmonary Sarcoidosis Study Group. Chest. 1999;116:424–31.
25. Paramothayan S, Jones PW. Corticosteroid therapy in pulmonary sarcoidosis: a systematic review. JAMA. 2002;287:1301–7.
26. Pietinalho A, Tukiaimen P, Haahtela T, et al. Early treatment of stage II sarcoidosis improves 5-year pulmonary function. Chest. 2002;121:24–31.
27. Baughman RP, Lower EE. Steroid-sparing alternative treatments for sarcoidosis. Clin Chest Med. 1997;18:853–64.
28. Baughman RP, Judson MA, Teirstein AS, et al. Thalidomide for chronic sarcoidosis. Chest. 2002;122:227–32.
29. Baughman RP, Lower EE. Infliximab for refractory sarcoidosis. Sarcoidosis Vasc Diffuse Lung Dis. 2001;18:70–4.
30. Yamamoto M, Kosada T, Yanagawa H, et al. Long-term follow-up in sarcoidosis in Japan. ZE Krank Atm-Org. 1977;149:191–6.
31. Peckham DG, Spiteri MA. Sarcoidosis. Postgrad Med J. 1996;72:196–200.
32. Karma A, Hukti E, Poukkula A. Course and outcome of ocular sarcoidosis. Am J Ophthalmol. 1988;106:467–72.
33. Dana MR, Merayo-lloves J, Schaumberg DA, et al. Prognosticators for visual outcome in sarcoid uveitis. Ophthalmology. 1996;103:1846–53.
34. Reich JM. Mortality of intrathoracic sarcoidosis in referral vs population-based settings: influence of stage, ethnicity, and corticosteroid therapy. Chest. 2002;121:32–9.

CHAPTER
176 Behçet's Disease

ANNABELLE A. OKADA • NARSING A. RAO • MASAHIKO USUI

DEFINITION
- A multisystem vasculitis of unknown cause primarily involving the eyes, the mucosal surfaces, and the skin.

KEY FEATURES
- Recurrent anterior and posterior uveitis.
- Recurrent oral ulcers (aphthae).
- Genital ulcers.
- Skin lesions such as erythema nodosum.

ASSOCIATED FEATURES
- Arthritis of large joints.
- Epididymitis.
- Intestinal ulcers.
- Vascular lesions such as thrombophlebitis, arterial occlusions, and aneurysms.
- Central nervous system or cranial nerve involvement.

INTRODUCTION

Behçet's disease is named after Turkish dermatologist Hulusi Behçet, who in 1937 described recurrent oral ulcers, genital ulcers, and uveitis in three patients.[1] Similar cases had been reported earlier by Shigeta in 1924, Adamantiadis in 1931, and Whitwell in 1934.[2] Inflammatory manifestations may also occur in other organ systems including the skin, the joints, the gastrointestinal tract, and the central nervous system.

EPIDEMIOLOGY AND PATHOGENESIS

Although Behçet's disease occurs worldwide, it is a particularly common cause of uveitis in countries that line the ancient Silk Road, including Italy, Turkey, Greece, Israel, Saudi Arabia, Iran, China, Korea, and Japan. Prevalence varies from a high of 80–370/100,000 in Turkey to lower rates of 2–30/100,000 in East Asia.[3] For comparison, the prevalence of Behçet's disease is estimated to be only 0.12–0.33/100,000 in the United States and 0.64/100,000 in the United Kingdom.[3] Isolated pockets of higher prevalence in countries of otherwise low prevalence also exist. For example, while the prevalence among German natives is reported to be 0.42–0.55/100,000, the Turkish community in Berlin is estimated to have a prevalence of 21/100,000.[3] Behçet's disease appears to be rare among Japanese immigrants in Hawaii and California.[4] Furthermore, recent figures indicate that the incidence and severity of Behçet's disease are decreasing in Japan.[5,6] Taken together, these observations suggest that both genetic and environmental factors play a role in the pathogenesis of Behçet's disease. The age of onset of uveitis is usually in the third to fourth decades of life, with men being more commonly affected than women.[7] The uveitis of Behçet's disease is believed to be most severe in young men between 15 and 25 years of age.[7]

The pathogenesis of Behçet's disease remains obscure. The disease has long been associated with the HLA-B51 allele; in Japan, 55% of patients with Behçet's disease are positive for HLA-B51, as opposed to 10–15% of the general population.[3] However, this HLA association appears to be true only in countries of high prevalence. For example, the relative risk of disease among HLA-B51–positive individuals is 6.7 in Japan but only 1.3 in the United States.[3] A recent study analyzing polymorphic microsatellite markers near the HLA-B gene in Japanese, Greek, and Italian patients with Behçet's disease strongly suggests that it is the HLA-B51 gene itself that is related to disease pathogenesis and not other genes located in the vicinity of HLA-B.[8] The manner in which HLA-B51 relates to disease susceptibility is unknown.

It has been suggested that microbial infections may serve as a trigger in the onset of Behçet's disease. For example, a higher proportion of patients who have Behçet's disease have herpes simplex virus DNA and serum antibodies against the virus when compared with controls.[9] *Streptococcus sanguis* and antibodies against the bacteria are also found more commonly in Behçet's patients.[9] Observations such as these have led to the hypothesis that exposure to various microbial antigens may trigger cross-reactive autoimmune responses in genetically susceptible individuals and lead to the onset of Behçet's disease.

OCULAR MANIFESTATIONS

Ocular involvement is seen in about 70% of patients who have Behçet's disease.[10] In most cases, the onset of uveitis follows the onset of recurrent oral ulcers by 3–4 years, although ocular disease is the initial manifestation in about 20% of cases. Initial ocular involvement may be unilateral but progresses to bilateral disease in at least two thirds of cases.

Patients with Behçet's disease often present to the ophthalmologist with decreased vision due to anterior chamber inflammation with or without hypopyon (Fig. 176-1). Pain, redness, and photophobia may be present. The hypopyon typically shifts with changes in head position. A very small hypopyon may be discovered only upon gonioscopic examination. Usually little iris synechia formation occurs initially, although this can subsequently develop after repeated bouts of anterior segment inflammation. The intraocular pressure is often normal or low. Mild vitreous cells or mild to moderate vitreous opacification occurs commonly. Fundus examination may reveal scattered yellow-white retinal exudates, retinal hemorrhages, vascular engorgement, or disc hyperemia. However, the fundus may also appear entirely normal during an episode of anterior segment inflammation. Bouts of posterior segment inflammation can also occur in the absence of any anterior chamber cells.

Typically, the clinical course is one of chronic or recurrent inflammation. Long-term complications in the anterior segment include iris neovascularization, glaucoma, and cataract. In the posterior segment, retinal vascular sheathing or occlusion, retinal or disc neovascularization (Fig. 176-2), vitreous hemorrhage or progressive vitreous opacification, optic atrophy (Fig. 176-3), and phthisis bulbi may ensue.

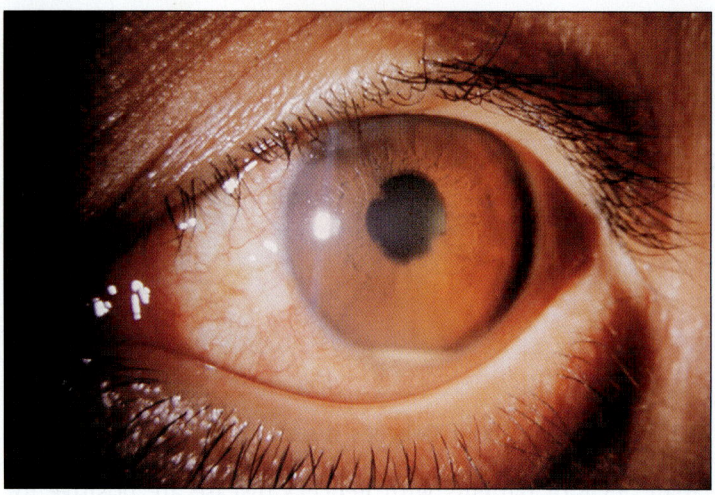

FIG. 176-1 ■ Conjunctival injection, hypopyon, and posterior synechia. The patient, who has Behçet's syndrome, is having an acute inflammatory attack.

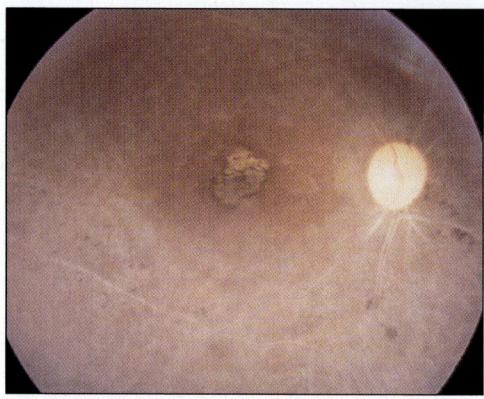

FIG. 176-3 ■ The fundus of a patient who has end-stage ocular Behçet's syndrome. Note the severe retinal atrophy, vascular attenuation with sheathing, and optic atrophy.

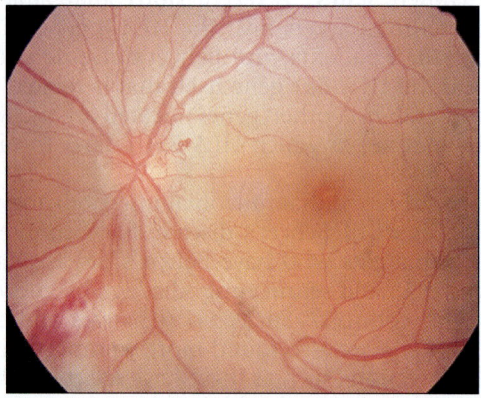

FIG. 176-2 ■ Acute retinal vasculitis with retinal hemorrhages and cotton-wool spots. Neovascularization at the optic disc is also present.

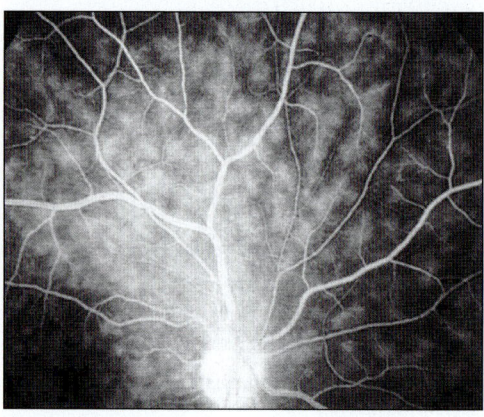

FIG. 176-4 ■ Fluorescein angiogram of a patient who has Behçet's syndrome. Typical findings include widespread ("fern-like") leakage from the capillary tree and secondary vessels.

DIAGNOSIS

The diagnosis of Behçet's disease is based on the constellation of systemic and ocular clinical findings rather than on specific laboratory test results. However, some tests are useful adjuncts in the evaluation of patients. Fundus fluorescein angiography shows marked dilatation or occlusion of retinal vessels. Affected retinal and optic nerve vessels leak fluorescein profusely during early transit, and their walls stain in late transit. Fluorescein leakage from the retinal vasculature may also be seen before any ophthalmoscopic signs of vasculitis. Even during presumably quiescent periods, in the absence of obvious inflammation in the fundus, dilatation of retinal capillaries with dye leakage is commonly observed (Fig. 176-4). Fluorescein angiography may confirm cystoid macular edema or macular ischemia.

During episodes of acute inflammation, patients may have a high erythrocyte sedimentation rate, elevated C-reactive protein, or increased peripheral leukocytes. HLA typing may be helpful, depending on the patient population. In Japan, where Behçet's disease is prevalent, a positive HLA-B51 result supports the diagnosis. However, an association with HLA-B51 has not been shown for some countries of low prevalence, such as the United States.[11]

Infrequently used today, the pathergy test (also referred to as the "skin prick" test or "Behçetine" test) looks for a nonspecific inflammatory reaction to a needle prick or an intradermal injection of saline. This test is positive in 23.8–78.9% of patients, depending on the country,[10,12] and is an indication of cutaneous hypersensitivity, which is characteristic of Behçet's disease. However, a history of cutaneous hypersensitivity may be elicited by careful

questioning, since patients may recall pustular inflammation after accidental skin injury such as that incurred while shaving.

There are two widely used diagnostic criteria for Behçet's disease. The first was initially proposed in 1972 by the Behçet's Disease Research Committee of the Japanese Ministry of Health and Welfare[13] and relies on four major and five minor findings (updated version shown in Box 176-1). Behçet's disease of the "complete type" is diagnosed when all four major findings (with or without minor findings) occur during the course of the disease. Behçet's disease of the "incomplete type" is diagnosed when only three major findings (with or without minor findings) occur, when two major and at least two minor findings occur, or when there is characteristic uveitis with either one other major finding or at least two minor findings. The second diagnostic criterion was proposed in 1990 by the International Study Group for Behçet's Disease (Table 176-1).[14] Using this, the diagnosis of Behçet's disease requires the presence of recurrent oral ulceration plus at least two other findings among recurrent genital ulceration, uveitis, skin lesions, and positive pathergy test result. The major difference between the two criteria is that the Behçet's Disease Research Committee gives more significance to uveitis, while the International Study Group for Behçet's Disease places greater weight on oral ulcers.

DIFFERENTIAL DIAGNOSIS

Because Behçet's disease can present as anterior uveitis, posterior uveitis, or panuveitis, the differential diagnosis must include a variety of diseases. The most common diseases mistaken for Behçet's

BOX 176-1

Behçet's Disease Research Committee Diagnostic Criteria

I. Major findings
  1. Recurrent ulcers of the oral mucosa
  2. Skin lesions
    a. Erythema nodosum
    b. Subcutaneous thrombophlebitis
    c. Follicular rash, acneiform rash (cutaneous hypersensitivity)
  3. Ocular findings
    a. Iridocyclitis
    b. Chorioretinitis
    c. Presence of posterior iris synechia, pigment clumps on the anterior surface of the lens, chorioretinal atrophy, optic atrophy, secondary cataract, secondary glaucoma, or phthisis bulbi
  4. Genital ulcers
II. Minor findings
  1. Arthritis not associated with deformation or rigidity
  2. Epididymitis
  3. Intestinal lesions such as ileocecal ulcer
  4. Vascular lesions
  5. Central nervous system findings
III. Diagnostic criteria
  1. Complete type: all 4 major findings occur
  2. Incomplete type:
    a. 3 major findings, or 2 major and 2 minor findings
    b. Characteristic ocular disease, plus 1 other major finding or 2 minor findings
  3. Diagnosis suspected: some major findings occur, but the criteria for incomplete-type disease are not met, and characteristic minor findings recur or are progressive
  4. Special disease types based on predominance of findings
    a. Intestinal Behçet's
    b. Vascular Behçet's
    c. Neuro-Behçet's
IV. Supportive findings
  1. Skin-prick test positive
  2. Evidence of inflammatory reaction present: elevated erythrocyte sedimentation rate, elevated serum C-reactive protein, increased peripheral white blood cells
  3. HLA-B51 positive

TABLE 176-1

INTERNATIONAL STUDY GROUP CRITERIA FOR THE DIAGNOSIS OF BEHÇET'S DISEASE*

Finding	Definition
Recurrent oral ulceration	Minor aphthous, major aphthous, or herpetiform ulcers observed by physician or patient, which have recurred at least 3 times over a 12-mo period
Plus at least 2 of the following criteria:	
Recurrent genital ulceration	Aphthous ulceration or scarring observed by physician or patient
Eye lesions	Anterior uveitis, posterior uveitis, or cells in vitreous on slit-lamp examination; or retinal vasculitis detected by an ophthalmologist
Skin lesions	Erythema nodosum observed by physician or patient, pseudofolliculitis, or papulopustular lesions; or acneiform nodules observed by physician in postadolescent patients not on corticosteroid treatment
Positive pathergy test	Interpreted by physician at 24–48 hr

*Findings applicable only in absence of other clinical explanations.

disease with hypopyon formation are HLA-B27–associated acute anterior uveitis and infectious endophthalmitis. Diseases often mistaken for Behçet's disease with posterior segment inflammation include sarcoidosis, tuberculosis, and syphilis. Behçet's disease with panuveitis may look like acute retinal necrosis in the early stages. Numerous other noninfectious and infectious disorders can mimic the ocular findings of Behçet's disease. Therefore, careful questioning of the patient for systemic signs or symptoms is crucial to making a diagnosis.

SYSTEMIC ASSOCIATIONS

Oral Ulcers

Recurrent ulcers of the oral mucosa are the most common finding and usually the initial symptom in Behçet's disease, although one must be careful because they also occur commonly in the general population. A 1991 study of 3316 Japanese patients with Behçet's disease found the frequency of recurrent oral ulcers to be 98%.[10] These lesions may appear anywhere in the mouth, including the lips, buccal mucosa, gingiva, tongue, hard palate, uvula, and oral pharynx. They tend to be painful but heal within 10 days, usually without scarring unless the lesion is particularly large. A typical lesion is round, with surrounding erythema and a pseudomembranous covering.

Skin Involvement

Skin lesions are the second most common systemic manifestation of Behçet's disease, occurring in 87% of patients in the 1991 Japanese study.[10] Together with uveitis and genital ulcers, skin lesions tend to occur after the onset of recurrent oral ulcers during the middle course of the disease.[2] Skin manifestations include erythema nodosum, subcutaneous thrombophlebitis, acneiform lesions, and follicular rash. Of these, erythema nodosum appears to occur most frequently and is characterized by a slightly raised red nodule with subcutaneous induration and tenderness. These lesions are usually found on the anterior surfaces of the legs, but they may also occur on the face, arms, and buttocks. They tend to involute in 10–14 days without scarring, although some hyperpigmentation may remain.[2] A history of pustular inflammation after accidental skin injury is usually included as skin involvement in Behçet's disease.

Genital Ulcers

The 1991 Japanese study found genital ulcers in 73% of Behçet's patients,[10] which is similar to the frequency of ocular involvement. As mentioned earlier, genital lesions tend to occur during the middle course of disease, at about the same time as the ocular and skin manifestations. The genital ulcers may have deeper tissue involvement in comparison to oral ulcers, are generally painful, and often leave scars after healing. The lesions usually occur on the scrotum or vulva but may also be found on the penis and the perianal and vaginal mucosa.

Other Manifestations

Other manifestations are myriad. The most common are arthritis, intestinal ulcers, central nervous system disease, and epididymitis, in descending order of frequency. Although rare, myocarditis, various cardiac vascular lesions, pulmonary hypertension, and renal involvement have also been reported in association with Behçet's disease. In general, all these manifestations tend to occur late in the course of the disease.[2] The most debilitating manifestation by far is central nervous system involvement, which can affect both motor and sensory systems and may occur in up to 10% of patients.[2] Signs and symptoms include headache, meningismus, nystagmus, tremor, ataxia, speech disturbances, memory impairment, behavioral changes, and dementia.

PATHOLOGY

Only a few eyes with Behçet's disease have been examined histologically. A characteristic feature is a necrotizing, leukocytoclastic, obliterative vasculitis affecting arteries and veins of all sizes. The vasculitic changes seen in the eyes are similar to those observed in other organs.

During acute inflammation, the iris, ciliary body, and choroid show diffuse infiltration with neutrophils. In the retina, severe vasculitis occurs with marked infiltration of leukocytes in and around blood vessels (Fig. 176-5). During the chronic phase, a lymphocytic and plasma cell infiltration occurs. Retinal vessels develop thickened basement membranes with swollen endothelial cells, which can lead to thrombus formation and vascular obliteration. In late stages, there is neovascularization of the iris and retina, formation of cyclitic membranes, and sometimes hypotony and phthisis bulbi. The phthisical globe may reveal a disrupted lens capsule with histological features of phacoanaphylaxis and intralenticular or vitreous hemorrhage.

TREATMENT

The short-term goal of therapy for ocular involvement in Behçet's disease is to suppress active inflammation. The long-term goals are to reduce the frequency and severity of recurrences, minimize involvement of the retina and the optic nerve, and avoid complications such as cataract, synechia formation, and glaucoma. Treatment must be started early to be effective. Drug selection should be determined based on the clinical history, location of intraocular inflammation, and severity of inflammation. As this disease often involves other organ systems, a multidisciplinary approach is necessary. The drug armamentarium for ocular disease includes colchicine, corticosteroids, immunophylin ligands, and cytotoxic agents.[15]

Colchicine

Colchicine is a plant alkaloid that acts by binding tubulin and inhibiting cell division. It is widely used in Japan as the systemic drug of first choice, based on the results of a retrospective study showing that patients treated with colchicine fared better than historical controls. However, the drug is viewed by many outside of Japan as being ineffective, and a double-blind study from Turkey showed no benefit. Commonly used doses range between 0.5 and 1.5mg/day orally. The major side effects are decreased fertility and azoospermia.

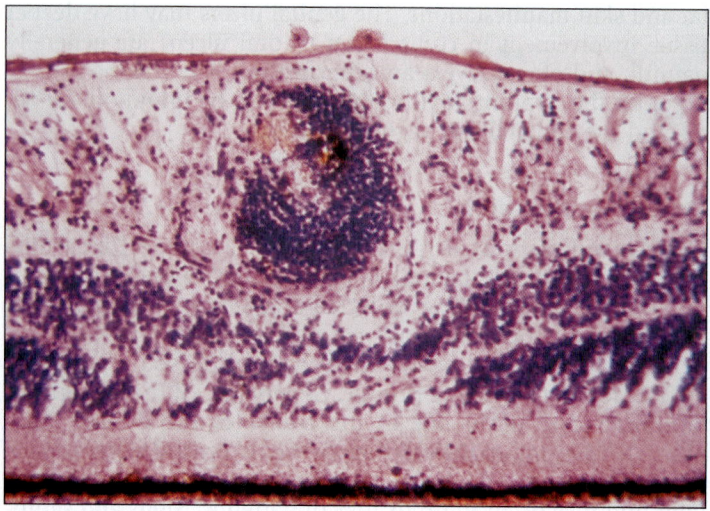

FIG. 176-5 ▪ Behçet's syndrome. Heavy inflammatory cell infiltration around a retinal vessel. (Hematoxylin and eosin.)

Corticosteroids

Corticosteroids are effective in the treatment of acute inflammation in Behçet's disease by means of their potent suppressive effects on the immune system, including neutrophil and macrophage migration and lymphocyte activity. However, they may have limited efficacy in decreasing the frequency of recurrences and preserving visual function.[15] Topical corticosteroids are used for anterior segment inflammation, while periocular injections (e.g., 20–40mg triamcinolone) or systemic corticosteroids (e.g., starting dose of 30–80mg/day prednisolone) are used for posterior segment inflammation. With systemic administration, the corticosteroid dose needs to be tapered slowly, often over years and in combination with a second "steroid-sparing" agent such as cyclosporine, to avoid a rebound effect. The major side effects of local corticosteroid therapy include elevated intraocular pressure, cataract progression, infection, and globe perforation in the case of injections. The major side effects of systemic corticosteroid administration are hypertension, diabetes mellitus, gastrointestinal ulceration, electrolyte abnormalities, osteoporosis, and reduced resistance to infections. Due to the frequency and severity of side effects of systemic corticosteroid treatment, it is unlikely that patients can remain on this therapy for prolonged periods. Other immunosuppressive agents, whether or not given in combination with low-dose corticosteroids, should be considered for long-term treatment in severe cases of uveitis.

Immunophilin Ligands

Cyclosporine and tacrolimus (FK506) are immunophilin ligands that bind to cytoplasmic receptors termed *immunophilins* in T cells, thereby selectively inhibiting T-cell activity. A Japanese study showed that cyclosporine at a dose of 5mg/kg/day was effective in decreasing the frequency of ocular inflammatory attacks in 70% of Behçet's patients who had previously refractory disease.[16] Starting doses of 3–5mg/kg/day for cyclosporine and 0.05–0.2mg/kg/day for tacrolimus are commonly used, depending on the severity of disease and whether other agents are being used in combination.[15] Major side effects of the immunophilin ligands are renal dysfunction, neurological abnormalities, and gastrointestinal upset, and hirsutism for cyclosporine. Because of variable absorption from the gut, periodic measurement of serum drug trough levels should be performed to determine the appropriate dose and help avoid side effects.

Cytotoxic Agents

Both antimetabolites (e.g., azathioprine, methotrexate) and alkylating agents (e.g., cyclophosphamide, chlorambucil) have been used in refractory cases of ocular Behçet's disease, particularly before the widespread use of cyclosporine. One masked trial showed that azathioprine, with or without concomitant corticosteroids, was better than placebo in controlling disease.[17] Triple-drug therapy using corticosteroids, cyclosporine, and azathioprine has also been reported to successfully induce remission in some patients.[18] The side effects of cytotoxic drugs may be serious and include bone marrow suppression, hepatotoxicity, secondary malignancies, and decreased fertility.

Laser and Surgical Treatment

Historically, laser surgery for an eye with Behçet's disease was considered extremely risky, due to the recurrence of uncontrollable inflammation postoperatively. However, with advances in both medical therapies and surgical techniques, recent reports appear to be encouraging. Scatter laser photocoagulation has been used successfully to treat areas of retinal nonperfusion after the development of retinal or optic nerve neovascularization. Furthermore, cataract and even vitreous surgery has been performed safely in selected patients with good control of inflammation, although postoperative inflammatory attacks need to be aggressively treated.

COURSE AND OUTCOME

The natural history of uveitis in Behçet's disease is one of attacks and remissions. A poor visual outcome can be avoided if the frequency of attacks is limited and irreversible complications are prevented. Decades ago, the visual outcome of Behçet's disease was uniformly dismal, with more than half of patients having visual acuity deterioration to worse than 20/200 in 5 years.[19] However, advances in therapeutics since then have improved the prospects for maintaining useful vision.

REFERENCES

1. Behçet H. Über rezidiverende aphthöse, durch ein virus verursachte geschwüre am mund, am auge und an den genitalien. Dermatol Wochenschr. 1937;105:1152–7.
2. Shimizu T, Ehrlich GE, Inaba G, et al. Behçet disease (Behçet syndrome). Semin Arthritis Rheum. 1979;8:223–60.
3. Sakane T, Takeno M, Suzuki N, et al. Behçet's disease. N Engl J Med. 1999;341:1284–91.
4. Hirohata T, Kuratsume M, Nomura A, et al. Prevalence of Behçet's syndrome in Hawaii, with particular reference to the comparison of the Japanese in Hawaii and Japan. Hawaii Med J. 1975;34:244–6.
5. Yokoi H, Goto H, Sakai J, et al. Incidence of uveitis at Tokyo Medical College Hospital. Nippon Ganka Gakkai Zasshi. 1995;99:710–4.
6. Kotake S, Furudate N, Sasamoto Y, et al. Characteristics of endogenous uveitis in Hokkaido, Japan. Graefes Arch Clin Exp Ophthalmol. 1997;235:5–9.
7. Yazici H, Tüzün Y, Pazarli H, et al. Influence of age of onset and patient's sex on the prevalence and severity of Behçet's syndrome. Ann Rheum Dis. 1984;43:783–9.
8. Mizuki N, Ota M, Yabuki K, et al. Localization of the pathogenic gene of Behçet's disease by microsatellite analysis of three different populations. Invest Ophthalmol Vis Sci. 2000;41:3702–8.
9. Lehner T. The role of heat shock protein, microbial and autoimmune agents in the aetiology of Behçet's disease. Int Rev Immunol. 1997;14:21–32.
10. Nakae K, Masaki F, Hashimoto T, et al. A nation-wide epidemiological survey on Behçet's disease, report 2: association of HLA-B51 with clinico-epidemiological features. Report of Behçet's Disease Research Committee. Japan: Ministry of Health and Welfare; 1992:70–82.
11. O'Duffy JD, Taswell HF, Elveback LR. HL-A antigens in Behçet's disease. J Rheumatol. 1976;3:1–3.
12. Koc Y, Gullu I, Akpek G, et al. Vascular involvement in Behçet disease. J Rheumatol. 1992;19:402–10.
13. Shimizu T. Behçet's disease. Jpn J Ophthalmol. 1974;18:291–4.
14. International Study Group for Behçet's Disease. Criteria for diagnosis of Behçet's disease. Lancet. 1990;335:1078–80.
15. Okada AA. Drug therapy in Behçet's disease. Ocul Immunol Inflamm. 2000;8:85–91.
16. Kotake S, Ichiishi A, Kosaka S, et al. Low dose cyclosporin treatment for ocular lesions of Behçet's disease. Nippon Ganka Gakkai Zasshi. 1992;96:1290–4.
17. Yazici H, Pazarli H, Barnes CG, et al. A controlled trial of azathioprine in Behçet's syndrome. N Engl J Med. 1990;322:821–5.
18. Kotter I, Durk H, Saal J, et al. Therapy of Behçet's disease. Ger J Ophthalmol. 1996;5:92–7.
19. Mishima S, Masuda K, Izawa Y, Mochizuki M. Behçet's disease in Japan: ophthalmological aspects. Trans Am Ophthalmol Soc. 1979;57:225–79.

177 Vogt-Koyanagi-Harada Disease

HAJIME INOMATA

DEFINITION

- An idiopathic bilateral uveitis featuring exudative retinal detachment associated with extraocular involvement, including neurological symptoms.

KEY FEATURES

- Bilateral granulomatous panuveitis.
- Exudative retinal detachment.
- Pigmentary changes in the eye in the chronic and recurrent phases (sunset glow fundus).
- Iris atrophy.
- Retinochoroidal atrophy.

ASSOCIATED FEATURES

- Meningitic manifestations: fever, headache, nausea, vomiting, and pleocytosis in cerebrospinal fluid.
- Auditory signs: tinnitus, vertigo, and neurosensory hearing loss.
- Dermal signs: vitiligo, alopecia, and poliosis.

INTRODUCTION

Vogt-Koyanagi-Harada (VKH) disease is a bilateral uveitis of unknown cause. The disease is often associated with extraocular involvement, including pleocytosis in cerebrospinal fluid, dysacousia, alopecia, poliosis, and vitiligo. Histopathology of eyes with VKH disease shows bilateral granulomatous inflammation throughout the uveal tissues. Originally, VKH disease was classified as two separate entities:

1. Vogt-Koyanagi syndrome, characterized by chronic anterior uveitis associated with alopecia, vitiligo, and dysacousia.[1,2]
2. Harada's disease, characterized by bilateral exudative uveitis, primarily in the posterior segment of the eye, accompanied by pleocytosis of cerebrospinal fluid.[3]

These two entities are known to overlap in many aspects, clinically and histopathologically, so are now combined as Vogt-Koyanagi-Harada disease.[4-6]

EPIDEMIOLOGY AND PATHOGENESIS

The occurrence of VKH disease is more frequent in the pigmented races: Asians, Hispanics, Native Americans, and Asian Indians. It is rare in Caucasians. Women seem to be affected more frequently than men. In the author's Eye Clinic at Kyushu University, Japan, 148 new patients (all Japanese) with VKH disease were registered in the 22 years from 1974 to 1995, an incidence of 7 cases per year. Of the 148 patients, 81 (55%) were women and 67 (45%) men. Ages ranged from 15 to 85 years, but the disease occurs mainly in the fourth and fifth decades of life (80 of the 148 cases [54%] were in this age group). In a study from Southern California, of the 65 patients with VKH disease, 78% were Hispanic, 10% were Asian, 6% were African-American, and 3% were white; one patient was an Asian Indian,

and one was a Native American.[5] In this study, 74% of the patients were women, and most patients were in the second to fifth decades of life at the onset of the illness. The age range was 7–71 years, with a mean of 32 years.

There is a genetic link in the development of VKH disease.[7] Evidence of increased risk among those with certain HLA genotypes indicates a genetically determined susceptibility for VKH disease.[8,9]

The cause of the disease remains unknown. Viral infection has been suggested, but no direct evidence exists to support this. From histopathological and immunological studies, an autoimmune reaction to melanocytes has been suggested to play an important role in the pathogenesis. It was recently reported that tyrosinase-related proteins experimentally induced inflammatory changes similar to those seen in patients with VKH disease.[10] However, the trigger that initiates the immune reaction to the melanocytes is yet to be discovered.

OCULAR MANIFESTATIONS

The diagnostic criteria for VKH disease were suggested by the International Committee on Nomenclature of the disease.[11] Clinically, the disease is categorized into prodromal, uveitic, chronic, and recurrent phases.[4]

Prodromal Phase

Patients who have VKH disease may visit internists first because of influenza-like symptoms with fever, headache, and sometimes nausea. Within 1–2 days of the prodromal phase, the patient complains of blurring of vision, photophobia, injection of bulbar conjunctiva, ocular pain, and metamorphopsia. Sensitivity of the hair and skin to touch is another sign during the prodromal phase.

Uveitic Phase

In the early stage of the uveitic phase, cells are present in both anterior chambers, and in typical cases, bilateral exudative retinal detachments are present. Cells in the anterior chamber become more prominent in the later stage. The anterior chamber often is slightly shallow. The blurring of vision is caused mainly by exudative retinal detachment due to inflammation in the choroid (Fig. 177-1). The pattern of the retinal detachment in VKH disease is characteristic. It shows discrete and shallow elevation of the neural retina, with small folds that radiate from the macula. A cloverleaf pattern of detachment often is seen in the posterior fundus. In severe cases, the detachment becomes bullous. The optic disc becomes hyperemic and edematous.

Chronic Phase

After treatment with systemic corticosteroids, elevation of the neural retina gradually disappears with absorption of the subretinal fluid. Cells in the anterior chamber decrease or disappear and the depth of the anterior chamber becomes normal. As in-

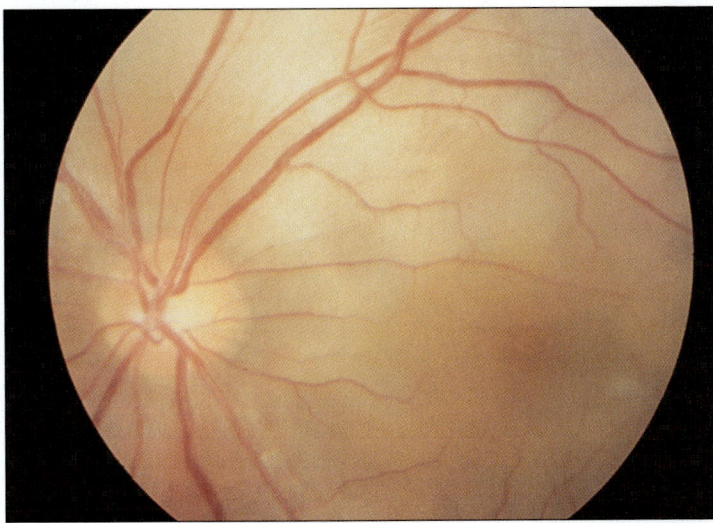

FIG. 177-1 ▓ **Fundus in the uveitic phase of Vogt-Koyanagi-Harada disease.** Note the exudative detachment of the neural retina due to inflammation in the choroid. The retinal detachment appears to be discrete; it can be of various sizes, depending on the amount of accumulated subretinal fluid.

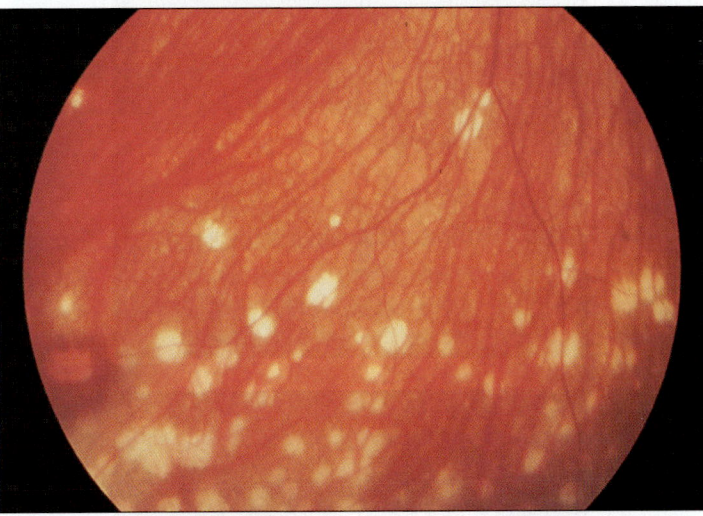

FIG. 177-2 ▓ **Sunset-glow fundus in the chronic phase of Vogt-Koyanagi-Harada disease.** The fundus has a slightly reddish appearance, mainly due to the disappearance of melanocytes in the choroid. Note the numerous small, depigmented dots, most of which are lesions of degenerated or disappeared retinal pigment epithelium (RPE). Only a few of them may represent resolved Dalen-Fuchs nodules.

flammation in the uveal tissue subsides, depigmentation occurs in the fundus to give it the appearance of a sunset glow. Small, discrete, and scattered depigmented lesions are seen within the sunset-glow fundus (Fig. 177-2). Most of these lesions represent degenerated or disappeared retinal pigment epithelium (RPE).[12] Only a few of them may represent resolved Dalen-Fuchs nodules. Depigmentation in the corneal limbus sometimes is noticed about 1 month after the onset and is known as Sugiura's sign.[4]

Recurrent Phase

The uveitis in VKH disease often recurs or becomes chronic. In recurrent cases, anterior uveitis is more predominant than posterior uveitis. Though the neural retina is free from the primary inflammation, retinal vasculitis and arteriovenous anastomosis occur as secondary reactions to the severe or long-standing inflammation in the choroid. Subretinal neovascularization is seen in the peripapillary region and in the macula; it often causes retinal hemorrhage.

The eyes show signs of chronic iridocyclitis. Mutton-fat keratic precipitates, Koeppe iris nodules, and posterior synechiae are signs of the chronic and recurrent phase. The iris becomes atrophic, with less pigmentation. Gonioscopy reveals depigmentation of the ciliary body band. Neovascularization in the chamber angle may occur in recurrent and long-standing cases.

DIAGNOSIS AND ANCILLARY TESTING

Fluorescein Fundus Angiography

In the early, active stage of the disease, subretinal exudation from the choroid can be demonstrated by fluorescein fundus angiography, which shows numerous hyperfluorescent dots located at the level of the RPE that have a tendency to gradually enlarge. The dye leaks through the pigment epithelial layer and accumulates in the subretinal space (Fig. 177-3). When the exudative retinal detachment disappears after treatment, the hyperfluorescent dots and diffuse dye accumulation in the subretinal space no longer can be observed. In the chronic phase, fundus angiography shows diffusely scattered dots of hyperfluorescence due to window defects at the level of the RPE.

Indocyanine Green Fundus Angiography

Indocyanine green fundus angiography is a useful technique to evaluate the choroidal circulation in VKH disease.[13] Circulatory

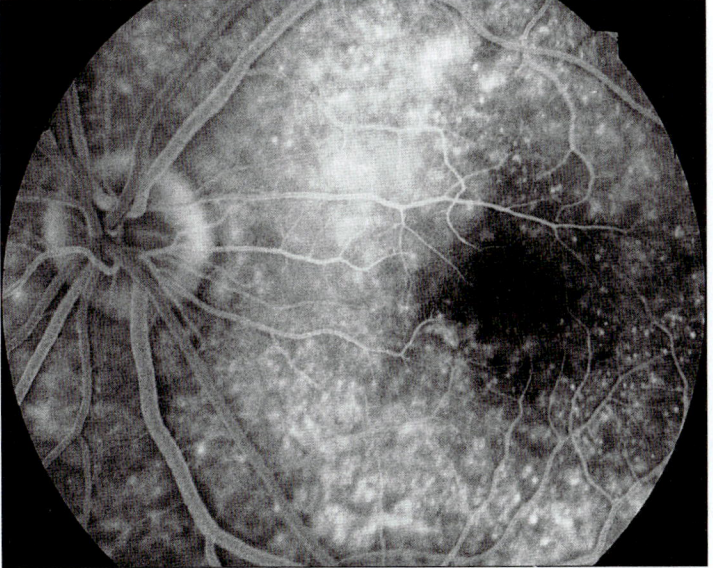

FIG. 177-3 ▓ **Fluorescein fundus angiography in the uveitic phase of Vogt-Koyanagi-Harada disease.** Note the dot-like lesions with dye leakage from the damaged retinal pigment epithelium and fluid accumulation in the subretinal space.

disturbance occurs in the choroid in the early, active stage, with the choroid showing a decrease in the number of large choroidal vessels filled with fluorescein dye. The number of large fluorescent choroidal vessels increases after the exudative retinal detachment subsides. Indocyanine green fundus angiography also may reveal choroidal neovascularization, if present.

Ultrasound Examination

Ultrasound biomicroscopy of the anterior segment of the eye reveals a narrow anterior chamber angle due to accumulation of exudate between the ciliary body and sclera (Fig. 177-4).[14] After treatment with systemic corticosteroids, the supraciliary exudate disappears. Standardized echography is another helpful technique with which to diagnose VKH disease, particularly in patients who have opaque media. The echographic manifestations include diffuse thickening of the posterior choroid, serous detachment of the retina, vitreous opacities, and posterior thickening of the sclera or episclera.[15] Resolution of these findings occurs with systemic corticosteroid therapy.

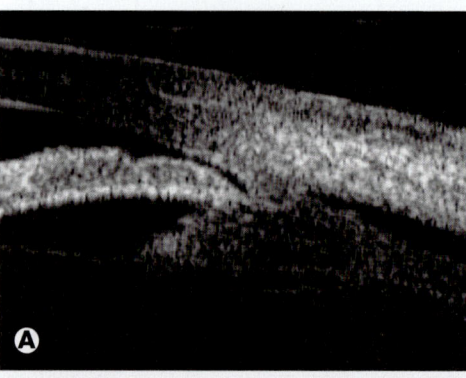

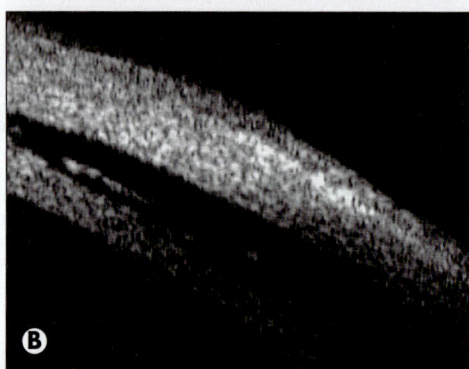

FIG. 177-4 ■ Ultrasound biomicroscopy of the uveitic phase in a patient with Vogt-Koyanagi-Harada disease. **A,** Cross section of the anterior angle. **B,** Posterior section of the anterior segment. The anterior chamber is narrow, and a layer of fluid has accumulated external to the ciliary body and choroid.

Cerebrospinal Fluid Analysis

Pleocytosis is seen in the cerebrospinal fluid in approximately 80% of patients within 1 week and in 97% of patients within 3 weeks of the onset of the disease.[4] Most of the cells in cerebrospinal fluid are small lymphocytes. Protein levels in the cerebrospinal fluid are elevated in about half the patients.

DIFFERENTIAL DIAGNOSIS

Sympathetic uveitis should be differentiated from VKH disease. Clinical manifestations and histopathology of eyes with sympathetic uveitis include bilateral granulomatous uveitis, which resembles that seen in VKH disease. In both diseases, uveal melanocytes are the target of the ocular inflammation. The sunset-glow appearance of the fundus due to depigmentation throughout the choroid is one of the most characteristic features of the chronic phases of both diseases. The only difference between sympathetic uveitis and VKH disease is a history of penetrating ocular injury or intraocular surgery in sympathetic uveitis and the absence of such a history in patients who have VKH disease.

Central serous chorioretinopathy must be differentiated from the uveitic phase of VKH disease. Shallow retinal detachment occurs in the macular area in central serous chorioretinopathy. The retinal detachment in VKH disease, however, is very specific in ophthalmological appearance, with a discrete and sometimes cloverleaf pattern. No inflammatory signs occur in central serous chorioretinopathy.

Posterior scleritis often shows exudative retinal detachment. Computed tomography scans and ultrasonography help make the correct diagnosis, as they reveal thickening of the posterior sclera.

Acute posterior multifocal placoid pigment epitheliopathy may be confused with VKH disease because multiple white-yellow flat to placoid lesions at the level of the RPE are seen. However, acute posterior multifocal placoid pigment epitheliopathy usually shows no cells in the anterior chamber or in the vitreous.

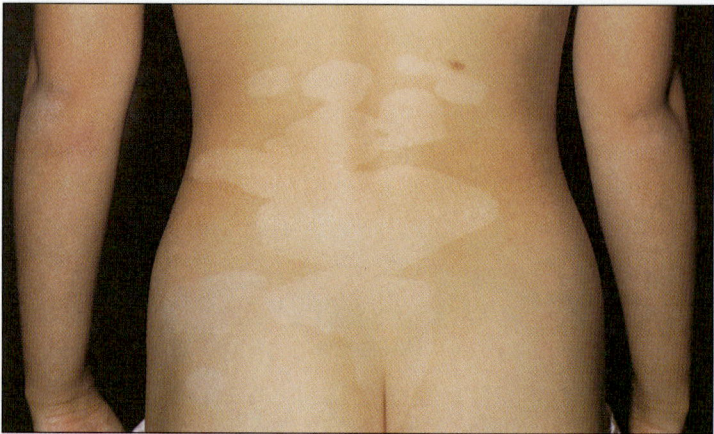

FIG. 177-5 ■ Vitiligo seen during the chronic phase in a patient with Vogt-Koyanagi-Harada disease. The skin on the lower back is one of the preferred sites for vitiligo in this disease.

Bilateral chronic uveitis, as occurs in Behçet's syndrome, needs to be differentiated from VKH disease in the chronic and recurrent phases, but the characteristic sunset-glow fundus does not occur in Behçet's syndrome. Extraocular manifestations of these diseases are the key to differentiating them.

SYSTEMIC ASSOCIATIONS

Auditory Signs

Auditory disturbance in VKH disease consists of a sensory neural hearing loss due to inner ear dysfunction. Some patients complain of tinnitus and vertigo at the onset. An audiogram demonstrates hearing loss in the high-frequency ranges; hearing usually returns to normal within several weeks.

Neurological Signs

Meningitic manifestations at the onset of the disease may include fever, headache, nausea, and vomiting, but in many cases, none of these signs occurs. Examination of the cerebrospinal fluid demonstrates pleocytosis and an increase in protein content. The cells in the cerebrospinal fluid are lymphocytes[16] and disappear after the systemic administration of corticosteroids. However, many cases of VKH disease occur without pleocytosis. Central nervous system involvement in VKH disease has been emphasized, but encephalitic signs occur rarely, if at all.

Dermal Signs

About 2–3 months after onset, vitiligo occurs on the face (around the eyelashes), hands, shoulders, breasts, and back. One site of predilection for vitiligo is the lower back region (Fig. 177-5), where mongolian spots are seen in Asian children. Erythema of the skin sometimes precedes the vitiligo.

Other Signs

Poliosis (whitened hair or canities) and alopecia (loss of hair) often occur.

PATHOLOGY

Uveitic Phase

The pathology of VKH disease is basically the same as that for sympathetic uveitis, with granulomatous inflammation throughout the uveal tissues. The uveal tissues are thickened by diffuse infiltration of lymphocytes, macrophages, and epithelioid cells, and the neural retina is detached from the RPE due to fluid accumulation in the subretinal space (Fig. 177-6). The infiltrating lymphocytes and macrophages are related closely to uveal

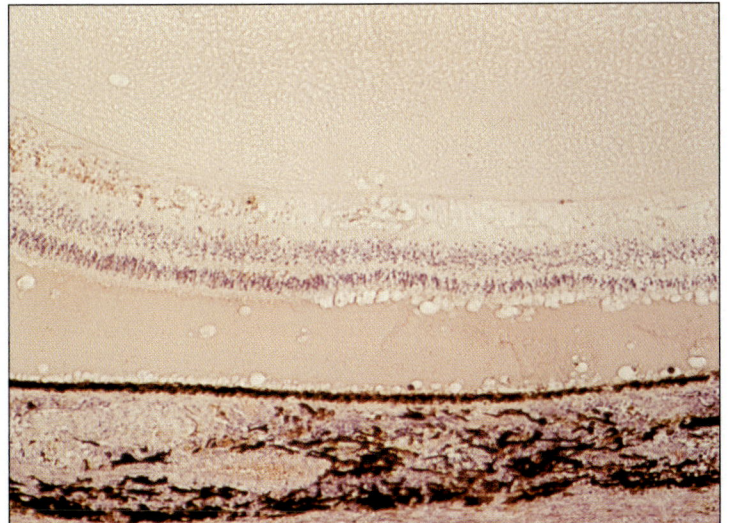

FIG. 177-6 ■ The uveitic phase of Vogt-Koyanagi-Harada disease. The choroid is thickened with inflammatory cell infiltration. Note fluid accumulation in the subneural retinal space secondary to choroidal inflammation.

melanocytes.[17] The peripapillary choroid is the predominant area of lymphocytic infiltration. Inflammation of the ciliary body and iris is essentially the same as that in the choroid.

Granulomatous inflammation also is seen in the perivascular and perineural loose connective tissues in the sclera, because melanocytes are present in these areas. The epithelioid and giant cells contain pigment granules. It appears that the pigment granules of damaged melanocytes are engulfed by activated macrophages, and these histiocytes subsequently transform into epithelioid cells and multinucleated giant cells.

Immunohistochemical techniques reveal that the choroidal infiltrate in VKH disease is composed predominantly of T lymphocytes of the suppressor-cytotoxic subset.[17] Class II major histocompatibility complex antigens are expressed on choroidal melanocytes and on the endothelium of the choriocapillaris.[18] In severe cases, lymphocytic infiltration extends into the choriocapillaris and Bruch's membrane, and even underneath the RPE. Exudative fluid from the choroid accumulates in the subretinal space, which results in exudative retinal detachment. Dalen-Fuchs nodules represent granulomas between the RPE and Bruch's membrane.

Chronic and Recurrent Phases

The melanocytes decrease in number and disappear from the choroid, which results in the sunset-glow appearance of the fundus. The inflammation in the choroid tends to subside with the disappearance of the choroidal melanocytes, but lymphocytic infiltration remains in the ciliary body and iris. In long-standing cases, however, degenerative changes occur in the RPE and neural retina, in association with subretinal neovascularization.[19] Small, depigmented atrophic lesions, which are seen predominantly in the peripheral fundi of the chronic phase, show degeneration or disappearance of the RPE cells.

TREATMENT

Uveitis due to VKH disease is treated effectively by the systemic administration of corticosteroids, and in most cases, a favorable prognosis exists for visual recovery. Inadequate treatment, however, results in recurrent long-standing uveitis, which finally becomes intractable.

In the early, active stage, high doses of corticosteroids should be given intravenously (100–200mg/day prednisolone) for a week. Thereafter, corticosteroids are given orally for 2–3 months, with a gradual tapering dose once an angiogram reveals the disappearance of dye leakage through the RPE. Topical corticosteroids in the form of 0.1% dexamethasone and cycloplegics are administered, the former 2–6 times/day and the latter 2–4 times/day. The eyedrops should be continued for about 3 months, unless the cells in the anterior chamber disappear.

When the intraocular inflammation cannot be controlled with systemic corticosteroids, or when a patient cannot tolerate the side effects of corticosteroids, cytotoxic and/or immunosuppressive agents may be utilized; the latter includes azathioprine, cyclophosphamide, and cyclosporine.[5,20]

COURSE AND OUTCOME

Uveitis due to VKH disease is treated effectively with the systemic administration of corticosteroids. However, as a complication of prolonged uveitis and a side effect of corticosteroids, posterior subcapsular cataract may develop. Other complications include secondary angle-closure glaucoma and subretinal neovascularization in the area of the optic papilla or at the macula and ora serrata.

REFERENCES

1. Vogt A. Frühzeitiges Ergrauen der Zilien und Bemerkungen uber den sogenannten plötzlichen Eintritt dieser Veranderung. Klin Monatsbl Augenheilk. 1906;44:228–42.
2. Koyanagi Y. Dysakusis, Alopecia und Poliosis bei schwerer Uveitis nicht traumatischen Ursprungs. Klin Monatsbl Augenheilk. 1929;82:194–211.
3. Harada E. On the acute diffuse choroiditis. Acta Soc Ophthalmol Jpn. 1926;30:356–78.
4. Sugiura S. Vogt-Koyanagi-Harada disease. Jpn J Ophthalmol. 1978;22:9–35.
5. Moorthy RS, Inomata H, Rao NA. Vogt-Koyanagi-Harada syndrome. Surv Ophthalmol. 1995;39:265–92.
6. Rao NA, Inomata H, Moorthy RS. Vogt-Koyanagi-Harada syndrome. In: Pepose JS, Holland GN, Wilhelmus KR, eds. Ocular infection and immunity. St Louis: Mosby; 1996:734–53.
7. Ohno S. Immunological aspects of Behçet's and Vogt-Koyanagi-Harada's diseases. Trans Ophthalmol Soc UK. 1981;101:335–41.
8. Shindo Y, Inoko H, Tuji K, et al. HLA-DRB1 typing of Vogt-Koyanagi-Harada's disease by PCR-RFLP and the strong association with DRB1*0405 and DRB1*0410. Br J Ophthalmol. 1994;78:223–6.
9. Shindo Y, Ohno S, Nakamura S, et al. A significant association of HLA-DRB1*0501 with Vogt-Koyanagi-Harada's disease results from a linkage disequilibrium with the primarily associated allele, DRB1*0405. Tissue Antigens. 1996;47:344–5.
10. Yamaki K, Kondo I, Nakamura H, et al. Ocular and extraocular inflammation induced by immunization of tyrosinase related protein 1 and 2 in Lewis rats. Exp Eye Res. 2000;71:361–9.
11. Reed RW, Holland GN, Rao NA, et al. Revised diagnostic criteria for Vogt-Koyanagi-Harada disease: report of an International Committee on Nomenclature. Am J Ophthalmol. 2001;131:647–52.
12. Inomata H, Rao NA. Depigmented atrophic lesions in sunset glow fundi of Vogt-Koyanagi-Harada disease. Am J Ophthalmol. 2001;131:607–14.
13. Yuzawa M, Kawamura A, Matsui M. Indocyanine green video-angiographic findings in Harada's disease. Jpn J Ophthalmol. 1993;37:456–66.
14. Kawano Y-I, Tawara A, Nishioka Y, et al. Ultrasound biomicroscopic analysis of transient shallow anterior chamber in Vogt-Koyanagi-Harada syndrome. Am J Ophthalmol. 1996;121:720–3.
15. Foster DJ, Cano MR, Green RL, Rao NA. Echographic features of the Vogt-Koyanagi-Harada syndrome. Arch Ophthalmol. 1996;108:1421–6.
16. Norose K, Yano A, Aosai F, Segawa K. Immunologic analysis of cerebrospinal fluid lymphocytes in Vogt-Koyanagi-Harada disease. Invest Ophthalmol Vis Sci. 1990;31:1210–6.
17. Inomata H, Sakamoto T. Immunohistochemical studies of Vogt-Koyanagi-Harada disease with sunset sky fundus. Curr Eye Res. 1990;9(suppl):35–40.
18. Sakamoto T, Murata T, Inomata H. Class II major histocompatibility complex on melanocytes of Vogt-Koyanagi-Harada disease. Arch Ophthalmol. 1991;109:1270–4.
19. Inomata H, Minei M, Taniguchi Y, Nishimura F. Choroidal neovascularization in a long-standing case of Vogt-Koyanagi-Harada disease. Jpn J Ophthalmol. 1983;27:9–26.
20. Rubsamen PE, Gass JDM. Vogt-Koyanagi-Harada syndrome. Clinical course, therapy, and long-term visual outcome. Arch Ophthalmol. 1991;109:682–7.

CHAPTER
178

Phacoantigenic Uveitis

DAVID J. FORSTER

DEFINITION
- Intraocular inflammation induced by lens protein, usually after surgical or traumatic rupture of the lens capsule.

KEY FEATURE
- Anterior uveitis that occurs days to weeks after capsular disruption.

ASSOCIATED FEATURES
- Acute, more severe cases are associated with redness, pain, photophobia, and possibly hypopyon formation.
- Chronic low-grade inflammation may be seen with milder cases or may be related to intraocular lens, anaerobic infection, or fungal endophthalmitis.

INTRODUCTION

Phacoantigenic, or lens-induced, *uveitis* is a term used to describe several entities that may have overlapping clinical features. All are believed to be caused by immune reaction to lens protein. *Phacoanaphylactic endophthalmitis* is an acute granulomatous anterior uveitis that occurs after surgical or traumatic rupture of the lens capsule. *Phacogenic nongranulomatous uveitis* (previously called "phacotoxic" uveitis) is a more chronic form of uveitis that can be seen after cataract surgery and is the result of immunological reaction to retained lens material. The third entity, *phacolytic glaucoma,* is not a true uveitis but may present clinically as a lens-induced uveitis. It is the result of leakage of lens protein through the intact capsule of a hypermature cataract. Recognition of these entities is important, since prompt removal of lens material is usually curative. In addition, they must be differentiated from postoperative endophthalmitis, which requires prompt intervention and antibiotic treatment to minimize visual loss.

EPIDEMIOLOGY AND PATHOGENESIS

The incidence of phacoantigenic uveitis is low. Most series report that phacoanaphylactic endophthalmitis and phacogenic nongranulomatous uveitis account for less than 1% of all cases of uveitis. Likewise, intraocular lens (IOL)–related uveitis accounts for only about 1% of uveitis cases.[1–3] Postsurgical infectious endophthalmitis, which may mimic phacoanaphylactic endophthalmitis, is rare as well, occurring in 0.10–0.35% of surgical cases.

The pathogenesis of lens-induced uveitis is hypothesized to be an immunological response to lens proteins that occurs after surgical or nonsurgical traumatic rupture of the lens capsule. In the past, it was thought that lens protein was organ specific and that it was sequestered from the immune system in normal individuals by an intact lens capsule.[4,5] However, studies have since shown that the majority of healthy persons have measurable anti-lens antibodies in the circulation, even in the absence

of eye disease.[6] Development of phacoanaphylactic endophthalmitis may depend more on altered tolerance to lens protein than on an immune reaction to "sequestered" lens antigens.[7] Most likely, phacoanaphylactic endophthalmitis represents an immune complex–mediated phenomenon related to traumatically released lens protein, facilitated by B cells that have been stimulated by bacterial lipopolysaccharides.[7,8]

Phacogenic nongranulomatous uveitis was once referred to as phacotoxic uveitis because it was believed that the inflammation was caused by the release of toxic substances into the anterior chamber after disruption of the lens capsule.[4,9] However, there is no evidence to support the hypothesis that lens proteins are directly toxic to ocular tissues.[10,11] Most likely, this type of uveitis, if it exists at all, represents a variant of phacoanaphylactic endophthalmitis, or it may represent undiagnosed cases of IOL-related uveitis or low-grade bacterial endophthalmitis.

Phacolytic glaucoma results from leakage of protein through an intact lens capsule and is generally seen in the setting of a hypermature lens. Protein that leaks into the anterior chamber is engulfed by macrophages, which in turn cause blockage of the trabecular meshwork, resulting in the elevation of intraocular pressure, which is characteristic of this entity (see Chapter 230).[12]

IOL-associated uveitis, though not strictly a subset of phacoantigenic uveitis, is mentioned here because it may be the cause of chronic postoperative inflammation in patients who have undergone cataract extraction. A number of factors can result in IOL-related uveitis, including lens–iris or lens–ciliary body contact, or complement activation in the aqueous by certain types of lens materials (e.g., polypropylene haptics).[13,14] Likewise, chronic uveitis may be seen in patients who have low-grade endophthalmitis postoperatively. Agents responsible for these cases include *Propionibacterium acnes,* *Staphylococcus epidermidis,* *Candida parapsilosis,* and *Torulopsis candida.*[15–17]

OCULAR MANIFESTATIONS

Phacoanaphylactic endophthalmitis usually develops days to weeks (or sometimes months) after surgical or nonsurgical trauma or surgical disruption of the lens capsule. It may occur within 24 hours of cataract surgery in a patient who has been previously sensitized to lens protein (i.e., if the fellow eye has undergone cataract extraction). It typically has an abrupt onset, with a granulomatous type of inflammatory response. Mutton-fat keratic precipitates and posterior synechiae are common. Anterior chamber reaction is moderate to severe, and hypopyon formation may be seen. Lens debris may be seen floating in the anterior chamber, and intraocular pressure may be elevated from blockage of the trabecular meshwork. There may be an associated vitritis, but typically there is no involvement of the retina, choroid, or optic nerve. Some cases, however, have been seen in association with sympathetic uveitis.[18] Visual acuity is usually diminished, but generally less pain occurs than with acute infectious endophthalmitis.

Phacogenic nongranulomatous uveitis may share features of phacoanaphylactic endophthalmitis, but the inflammation is usually less severe or acute than with the latter. It typically develops within 2–3 weeks of lens capsule disruption (either surgical or traumatic). Retained lens material may elicit an ongoing inflammatory response, with cells and flare in the anterior chamber and posterior synechiae formation. Unlike with phacoanaphylactic endophthalmitis, however, the inflammation is nongranulomatous; the mutton-fat keratic precipitates seen with phacoanaphylactic endophthalmitis are absent in this condition. Intraocular pressure may be elevated from plugging of the trabecular meshwork by inflammatory cells or lens material.

Phacolytic glaucoma is seen in patients who have a hypermature lens and an intact lens capsule. Large cells and protein (flare) are seen in the anterior chamber, but keratic precipitates and posterior synechiae are usually absent. Intraocular pressure is elevated, sometimes markedly, and may result in corneal edema.

A chronic form of uveitis may be elicited by IOLs themselves. Patients may have persistent anterior chamber reaction, keratic precipitates, or inflammatory precipitates on the IOL surface. Most types of posterior chamber lenses in use today rarely cause such problems, but the presence of iris chafing by either the optic or haptic portion of the IOL may result in chronic inflammation. This is more common with anterior chamber lenses. As mentioned earlier, certain materials in the prosthesis (e.g., polypropylene) may activate complement, which leads to recruitment of inflammatory cells into the anterior chamber.

In acute cases of postoperative inflammation, the possibility of infectious endophthalmitis must be considered. Generally, these patients present within a week after surgery with pain and visual loss; usually moderate to severe inflammation is seen in the anterior chamber and vitreous cavity, with possible hypopyon formation. Lid edema, chemosis, and corneal clouding also may be present. However, certain types of infectious endophthalmitis may have a much more insidious onset, not manifesting until weeks or months after surgery. Frequently, this is the case with infections caused by *S. epidermidis* or anaerobic bacteria and fungi. This type of infectious endophthalmitis is commonly referred to as delayed or localized endophthalmitis.

One causative organism that has become important in such delayed types of infections is *P. acnes*, an anaerobic bacterium.[15] Infection with *P. acnes* usually manifests as chronic low-grade inflammation postoperatively. Often the inflammation is responsive transiently to topical corticosteroids, but typically it flares up as the corticosteroids are tapered. Findings may include granulomatous keratic precipitates or hypopyon. Frequently, a white fibrous plaque is evident on the posterior capsule or between the capsule and the IOL (Fig. 178-1). It is possible that *P. acnes* organisms become sequestered within this fibrous pocket, which results in the chronic low-grade inflammatory reaction. Cases of exacerbation of intraocular inflammation following neodymium:yttrium-aluminum-garnet capsulotomy have been associated with *P. acnes* infection.[19,20] Presumably, the laser-induced capsular disruption liberates the previously sequestered organisms, which results in an acute increase in inflammation. Other organisms that may produce a picture similar to that seen with *P. acnes* include *S. epidermidis*, *C. parapsilosis*, and *T. candida*.[17]

DIAGNOSIS

Diagnosis of phacoantigenic uveitis is usually made on a clinical basis. However, in cases of acute inflammation after a penetrating injury or surgery, differentiation of an immune-mediated process (e.g., phacoanaphylactic endophthalmitis) from an infectious process (e.g., acute bacterial endophthalmitis) may be difficult or impossible based on clinical findings alone. Characteristically, the inflammation associated with phacoanaphylactic endophthalmitis is granulomatous in nature, with mutton-fat keratic precipitates; these are much less common in bacterial endophthalmitis. Also, the severe pain caused by infec-

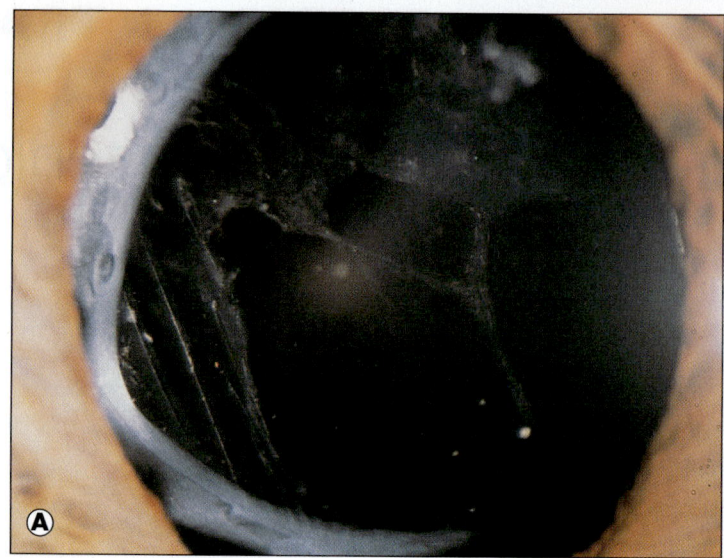

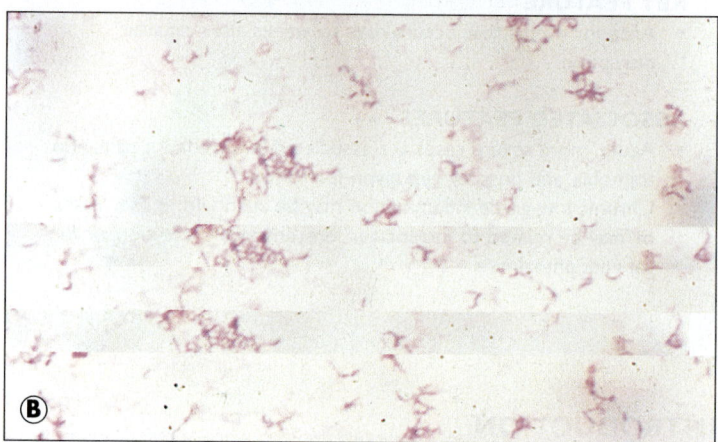

FIG. 178-1 ■ *Propionibacterium acnes* endophthalmitis. **A,** Note the typical fibrous white plaque between the intraocular lens and the posterior capsule. **B,** Examination of a surgically removed plaque shows a mass of *P. acnes*. (Courtesy of Dr. A. H. Friedman.)

tious endophthalmitis is not characteristic of phacoanaphylactic endophthalmitis. Nonetheless, when the diagnosis is unclear, diagnostic vitrectomy should be performed as soon as possible because of the rapidity with which bacterial endophthalmitis can destroy ocular tissues. Culture of vitrectomy specimens is preferred to that of anterior chamber fluid because of the higher yield of positive results with the former.

Cases of delayed bacterial (e.g., *P. acnes*) or chronic fungal endophthalmitis often do not become apparent until months after surgery. In any patient who has ongoing inflammation postoperatively and is only partially responsive to topical corticosteroids, *P. acnes* should be suspected, particularly if hypopyon develops after corticosteroid withdrawal or in the presence of plaque-like material on the posterior capsule. It also should be strongly suspected when the uveitis is exacerbated by laser capsulectomy.[19,20] Diagnosis of *P. acnes* endophthalmitis usually requires vitrectomy; posterior capsulectomy, particularly if any plaques are present, may be necessary to demonstrate the organisms (Fig. 178-2). Since *P. acnes* is very slow growing, the laboratory should be instructed to hold the plates for at least 2 weeks before reading the culture as negative. Fungal endophthalmitis may present with a similar picture of chronic low-grade inflammation and may progress to the point of forming vitreous "fluff balls" or foci of retinochoroiditis. In particular, this entity should be considered in patients who are immunocompromised or iatrogenically immunosuppressed. Diagnosis also is made by culture of vitrectomy specimens; the yield can be increased by first passing the fluid through a Millipore filter and sending the filter for culture as well.

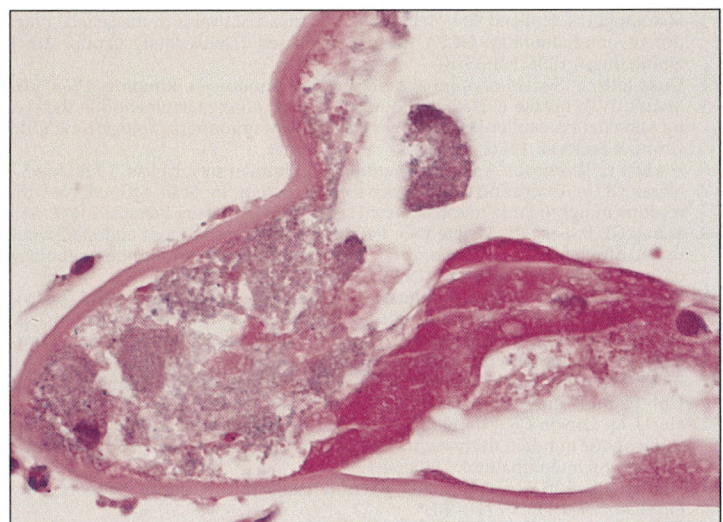

FIG. 178-2 ■ Reaction to *Propionibacterium acnes*. Capsulectomy specimen reveals the presence of bacteria and remnants of lens fibers in the lens capsule.

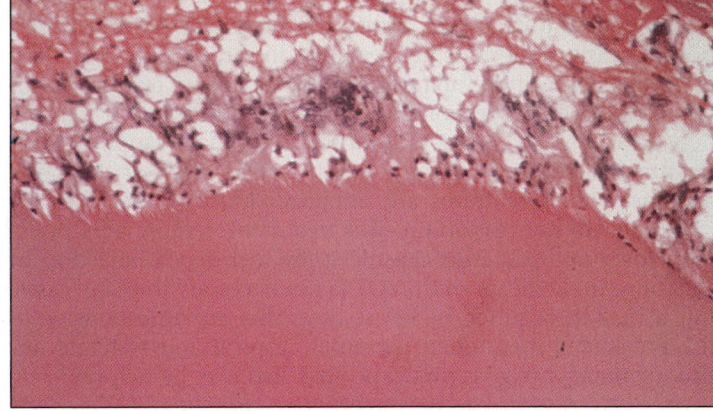

FIG. 178-3 ■ Phacoanaphylactic endophthalmitis. The zonal type of granulomatous inflammation seen in phacoanaphylactic endophthalmitis is evident here. A lens remnant is surrounded by a zone of neutrophils, which in turn is surrounded by a zone of macrophages, epithelioid cells, and giant cells; the outermost layer is composed of lymphocytes and plasma cells.

DIFFERENTIAL DIAGNOSIS

The differential diagnosis of phacoantigenic uveitis is outlined in Box 178-1. The distinguishing features of these entities were discussed earlier. One entity that is not discussed here, although it is covered in detail in Chapter 179, is sympathetic uveitis. This is a rare bilateral granulomatous type of panuveitis that occurs after injury to one eye (the "exciting eye"). After weeks or years, the patient develops inflammation in the fellow ("sympathizing") eye as well. Ninety percent of cases occur between 2 weeks and 1 year after injury. The inflammation is characterized by mutton-fat keratic precipitates, anterior chamber and vitreous cellular infiltration, choroidal thickening, disc edema, serous retinal detachments, and characteristic yellow-white infiltrates at the level of the retinal pigment epithelium (Dalen-Fuchs nodules). Histopathologically, eyes with sympathetic uveitis may show signs of phacoanaphylactic endophthalmitis as well.[18] The key distinguishing features between sympathetic uveitis and the other types of post-traumatic uveitis discussed earlier are that sympathetic uveitis causes a panuveitis as opposed to merely an anterior uveitis, and it is always bilateral, whereas the others usually affect only the traumatized eye. Fluorescein angiography and ultrasonography can be useful in demonstrating the posterior uveal involvement of sympathetic uveitis.

Patients who present with chronic inflammation after penetrating injury also need to be examined carefully for a retained intraocular foreign body. Ultrasonography and computed tomography scanning are helpful in ruling this out as a cause of prolonged post-traumatic uveitis.

SYSTEMIC ASSOCIATIONS

No identified associations exist between post-traumatic uveitis and systemic disease. As mentioned earlier, however, immunocompromised patients who present with persistent inflammation postoperatively should cause an increased level of suspicion of fungal endophthalmitis.

PATHOLOGY

Phacoanaphylactic endophthalmitis is characterized histopathologically by a *zonal* type of granulomatous inflammation centered around lens remnants (Fig. 178-3). Polymorphonuclear leukocytes immediately surround the lens material. These in turn are surrounded by a zone of granulomatous reaction, which consists of macrophages, epithelioid cells, and giant cells. Lymphocytes and plasma cells make up the outermost area of inflammation.

Phacoantigenic nongranulomatous uveitis, as its name implies, typically exhibits a nongranulomatous inflammatory reaction around the lens material.[10] The cellular infiltrate consists of lymphocytes, histiocytes, and polymorphonuclear leukocytes, but epithelioid and giant cells are absent.

Histopathology of specimens taken from eyes infected with *P. acnes* usually shows the presence of neutrophils, admixed with macrophages. However, the inflammatory reaction around pockets of *P. acnes* organisms is often surprisingly minimal (see Fig. 178-2). This may be because of the organism's low virulence.

TREATMENT

Mild postsurgical inflammation is normal in the first few weeks and usually responds well to topical corticosteroids or topical nonsteroidal anti-inflammatory medications. Retained lens material, however, is frequently associated with more severe or prolonged postoperative inflammation. Most of these cases eventually resolve with prolonged corticosteroid therapy. Topical therapy is often sufficient, but in more severe cases, systemic or periocular corticosteroids may be necessary. Cases that persist in spite of such therapy usually require surgical removal of the remaining lens material. Phacoanaphylactic endophthalmitis, in contrast, should be treated as soon as possible with removal of all lens material. Intensive corticosteroid therapy should also be employed, but it is usually insufficient to control the inflammation if the inciting lens material is not removed.

Prolonged topical corticosteroid therapy also may be required for IOL-related uveitis. If the uveitis is persistent, repositioning of the IOL (particularly if there is iris touch or pupillary capture) or complete removal of the IOL may be necessary. Other potential causes of prolonged postoperative inflammation (e.g., iris or vitreous incarceration in the wound) should be corrected surgically if inflammation or secondary cystoid macular edema does not respond to corticosteroid therapy.

Mild cases of *P. acnes* endophthalmitis may respond to intravitreal vancomycin (1mg), which can be given at the same time as vitreous cultures are obtained. More severe cases, or cases that do not respond to this treatment, require pars plana vitrectomy and posterior capsulectomy with repeat injection of vancomycin. Removal of the IOL is not necessary in many cases, but it may be required in severe cases that are unresponsive to the previously mentioned measures. Topical and systemic antibiotic therapy (e.g., cephalosporins) also may be helpful.[21]

COURSE AND OUTCOME

Mild cases of lens-induced uveitis usually do well with corticosteroid therapy. In more severe cases or in cases of phacoanaphylactic endophthalmitis, prompt removal of all lens material is usually curative. The same is true with phacolytic glaucoma. Low-grade endophthalmitis from organisms such as *S. epidermidis* or *P. acnes* often has a favorable outcome if appropriate therapy is instituted in a timely manner. In one series of 16 patients with *P. acnes* endophthalmitis, 11 had final visual acuity of 20/40 (6/13) or better.[6]

REFERENCES

1. Henderly DE, Genstler AJ, Smith RE, Rao NA. Changing patterns of uveitis. Am J Ophthalmol. 1987;103:131–6.
2. Rodriguez A, Calonge M, Pedroza-Seres M, *et al*. Referral patterns of uveitis in a tertiary eye care center. Arch Ophthalmol. 1996;114:593–9.
3. McCannel CA, Holland GN, Helm CJ, *et al*. Causes of uveitis in the general practice of ophthalmology. UCLA Community-Based Uveitis Study Group. Am J Ophthalmol. 1996;121:35–46.
4. Duke-Elder S. System of ophthalmology, vol. 9. London: H. Kimpton; 1966:501.
5. Manski W, Wirostko E, Halbert SSP, *et al*. Autoimmune phenomenon in the eye. In: Miescher PA, Muller-Eberhard, eds. Textbook of immunopathology. New York: Grune & Stratton; 1976.
6. Hackett E, Thompson A. Anti-lens antibody in human sera. Lancet. 1964;2:663.
7. Marak GE Jr. Abrogation of tolerance to lens protein. In: Sears MG, ed. New directions in ophthalmic research. New Haven: Yale University Press; 1981:47–58.
8. Marak GE Jr, Font RL, Weigle WO. Pathogenesis of lens-induced endophthalmitis. In: Silverstein AM, O'Connor GR, eds. Immunology and immunopathology of the eye. New York: Masson; 1978:135–7.
9. Irvine SR, Irvine AR Jr. Lens-induced uveitis and glaucoma. Part II. The "phacotoxic" reaction. Am J Ophthalmol. 1952;35:370.
10. Spencer WH. Lens. In: Spencer WH, ed: Ophthalmic pathology: an atlas and textbook. Philadelphia: WB Saunders; 1985:473–5.
11. Blodi FC. Sympathetic uveitis as an allergic phenomena. Trans Am Acad Ophthalmol Otolaryngol. 1959;63:642–56.
12. Flocks M, Littwin CS, Zimmerman LE. Phacolytic glaucoma: a clinicopathologic study of one hundred thirty-eight cases of glaucoma associated with hypermature cataract. Arch Ophthalmol. 1955;54:37.
13. Hooper PL, Rao NA, Smith RE. Cataract extraction in uveitis patients. Surv Ophthalmol. 1990;35:120–44.
14. Tuberville AW, Galin MA, Perez HD, *et al*. Complement activation by nylon- and polypropylene-looped prosthetic intraocular lenses. Invest Ophthalmol Vis Sci. 1982;22:727–33.
15. Meisler DM, Mandelbaum S. *Propionibacterium*-associated endophthalmitis after extracapsular cataract extraction. Review of reported cases. Ophthalmology. 1989;96:54–61.
16. Piest KL, Apple DJ, Kincaid MC, *et al*. Localized endophthalmitis: a newly described cause of the so-called toxic lens syndrome. J Cataract Refract Surg. 1987;13:498–510.
17. Rao NA, Nerenberg AV, Forster DJ. *Torulopsis candida* (*Candida famata*) endophthalmitis simulating *Propionibacterium acnes* syndrome. Arch Ophthalmol. 1991;109:1718–21.
18. Chan CC. Relationship between sympathetic ophthalmia, phacoanaphylactic endophthalmitis, and Vogt-Koyanagi-Harada disease. Ophthalmology. 1988;95:619–24.
19. Tetz MR, Apple DJ, Price FW Jr, *et al*. Bath phacoanaphylactic endophthalmitis. A newly described complication of neodymium–YAG laser capsulotomy: exacerbation of an intraocular infection. Case report. Arch Ophthalmol. 1987;105:1324–5.
20. Carlson AN, Koch DD. Endophthalmitis following Nd:YAG laser posterior capsulotomy. Ophthalmol Surg. 1988;19:168–70.
21. Zambrano W, Flynn HW, Pflugfelder SC, *et al*. Management options for *Propionibacterium acnes* endophthalmitis. Ophthalmology. 1989;96:1100–5.

CHAPTER
179

Sympathetic Uveitis

GEORGE E. MARAK, JR.

DEFINITION
- A bilateral uveitis that develops after penetrating injury to one eye; believed to be an autoimmune disease.

KEY FEATURES
- Bilateral anterior or posterior uveitis of variable severity with a uniform choroiditis.
- Histopathologically, predominantly consists of mononuclear and epithelioid cells.

ASSOCIATED FEATURES
- Dalen–Fuchs spots.
- Papillitis.
- Dysacousis and tinnitus.
- Alopecia, poliosis, vitiligo.
- Headache.

INTRODUCTION

Sympathetic uveitis (sympathetic ophthalmia) was a fairly common and dreaded disease during the nineteenth century. Many cases of bilateral blindness associated with injury and inflammation were diagnosed as sympathetic uveitis. However, during the 20th century, with the development of accurate clinical and pathological definitions, it became evident that this is a relatively rare disease. MacKenzie gave a detailed clinical description of sympathetic uveitis in 1865. Fuchs established the pathological definition in 1905.[1]

EPIDEMIOLOGY AND PATHOGENESIS

No reliable figures exist for the incidence of sympathetic uveitis because of the unreliability of diagnosis, inherent sampling errors, and medicolegal concerns. Sympathetic uveitis occurs in fewer than 1 in 100 nonsurgical penetrating wounds and in fewer than 1 in 10,000 surgical penetrating wounds. The incidence is higher in men than women, but the difference results from the higher incidence of accidental penetrating wounds in men. The frequency of occurrence is higher in children under 10 years of age because of the higher frequency of injuries; it also increases in those over the age of 60 years because of the increase in eye surgery. There may be a genetic propensity to develop sympathetic uveitis after a penetrating wound, because there is an increased incidence of the same human lymphocyte antigen types in both oriental and occidental populations.[2] No other reliable demographic data exist.

Sympathetic uveitis is believed to represent an autoimmune response to a component or components of the retina, retinal pigment epithelium, or choroid (e.g., retinal "S" antigen tyrosinase-related protein).[1,3]

Experimental models similar to those for sympathetic uveitis have been described but, like experimental models of multiple sclerosis, these do not reproduce exactly the clinical disease.[4] Lymphocytes with both helper (CD4+ and CD4−) and suppressor (CD8+ and CD8−) cell surface markers have been found in sympathetic uveitis.[5] Cell-mediated immune responses to retinal antigens also have been found in patients who have sympathetic uveitis.[6] The specific antigen or antigens involved in sympathetic uveitis have not been identified. A penetrating wound appears to be essential for the development of sympathetic uveitis. Additional insults, such as vitrectomy, and laser or radiation therapy, may increase the incidence.[7] Several studies show a disproportionate incidence of sympathetic ophthalmia after primary or secondary vitrectomy.[3] Although there are periodic reports of sympathetic uveitis developing in the absence of a penetrating histopathological wound, all affected eyes that have been subjected to a careful and complete serial sectioning demonstrate scleral penetrations.[8]

Presumably, a penetrating wound with uveal prolapse permits tolerated ocular antigens to reach dendritic cells, or the so-called *professional antigen-presenting cell*, outside of the eye when there is an inflammatory stimulus. Because the antigen-presenting cells of the eye appear to be functionally suppressed *in situ*, these antigens normally would produce an inactivation signal.[9]

The anterior chamber–associated immune deviation (ACAID) phenomenon has been offered as an explanation for the role of the penetrating wound in sympathetic uveitis. This is a curious laboratory phenomenon, wherein systemic tolerance to an antigen can be produced by injecting large amounts of the antigen into the anterior chamber of the eye. A large antigenic load in the absence of antigen-presenting cells is well known to be tolerogenic. When dendritic cells are added to the anterior chamber inoculum, this becomes an immunogenic stimulus. Because the large antigenic loads required to induce the ACAID phenomenon cannot occur under any conceivable clinical conditions, this curious laboratory phenomenon has limited value in explaining the role of the penetrating wound in the development of sympathetic uveitis.[10] Recent transgenic studies indicate that endogenous ocular immunoregulation differs considerably from this artificial laboratory phenomenon.[11]

Sympathetic uveitis and phacoanaphylactic endophthalmitis frequently were observed to occur together. It was suggested that common pathogenic features may exist. More recent studies, however, show that the concurrent development of these two inflammations is now relatively infrequent. This change is presumably because of improvements in the management of penetrating wounds. Sympathetic uveitis is believed to be an autoimmune response to a retinal, retinal pigment epithelial, or choroidal antigen that involves a cell-mediated immune response.[1] Phacoanaphylactic endophthalmitis is clearly an immune complex reaction to a lens protein. The basis for the association of these two diseases is akin to the correlation between the price of rum and preachers' salaries—it is a fortuitous consequence that the development of both diseases is related to the penetrating wound.

OCULAR MANIFESTATIONS

Sympathetic uveitis may appear with varying degrees of severity, from an anterior uveitis or peripapillary choroiditis to a severe

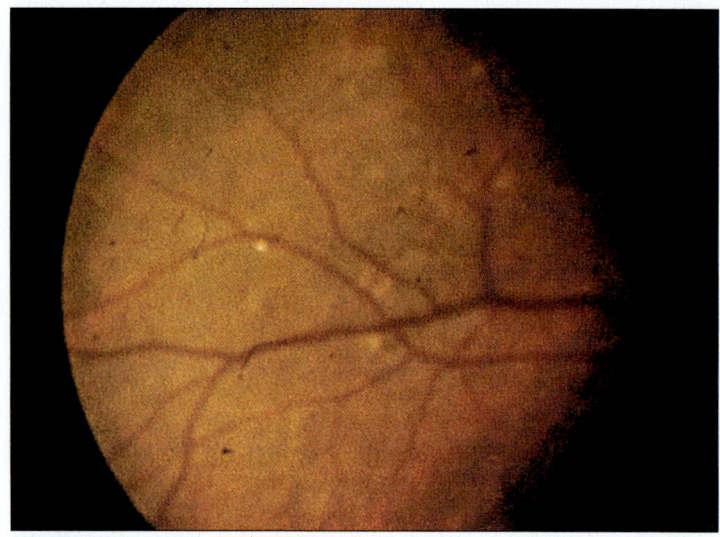

FIG. 179-1 ▌▌ Dalen–Fuchs spot in a patient who has sympathetic ophthalmia.

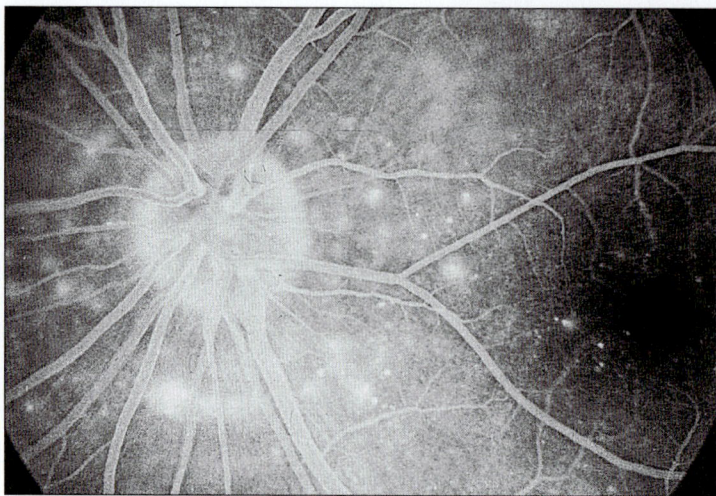

FIG. 179-3 ▌▌ Fluorescein angiography in sympathetic ophthalmia. Note the multiple hyperfluorescent dots.

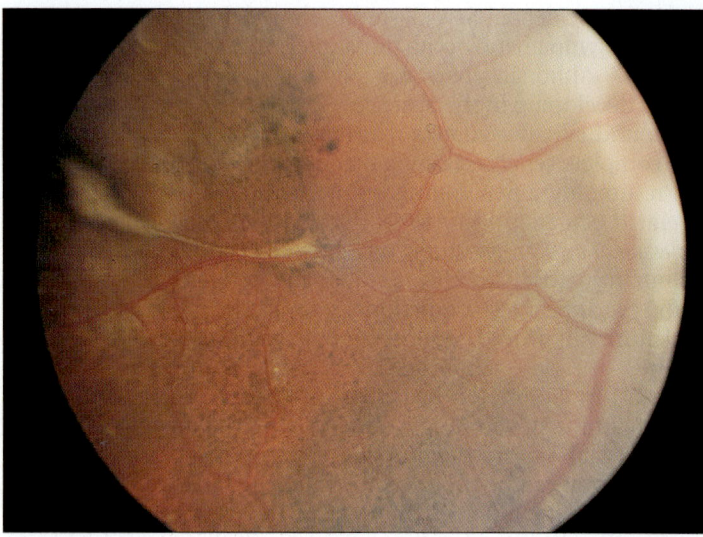

FIG. 179-2 ▌▌ Retinal and macular scarring in sympathetic ophthalmia.

panuveitis with mutton-fat keratic precipitates. Focal, elevated choroid infiltrates are common in the midperiphery. These Dalen–Fuchs spots (Fig. 179-1) represent the Dalen–Fuchs nodules seen on histopathological analysis. Inflammation of the optic nerve, or papillitis, is a common feature of sympathetic uveitis and provides a useful means by which to follow the progress of the disease. Exudative retinal detachment may occur in the more severe cases. Chorioretinal scarring frequently is observed clinically when the inflammation abates (Fig. 179-2). Severe scarring throughout the retina and in the posterior pole and macula may be observed in 25–30% of the cases. The peripheral retina may take on a moth-eaten appearance. The macular scars may be responsible for considerable visual loss. A "sunset glow" fundus appearance, similar to that seen in Harada's syndrome, may be observed.

DIAGNOSIS

Sympathetic uveitis is not easily diagnosed. Only 20% of clinically suspected cases are confirmed histopathologically.[1] In one series, one third of the cases were not diagnosed within 1 year of the time of onset of the symptoms.[12] The time of onset is not reliably known, but clinical diagnosis is made within 3 months of the injury to the exciting eye in most cases. The earliest cases occur within 9–10 days of injury. Some cases are diagnosed many years after injury. Unilateral sympathetic uveitis, based on histopathology of the enucleated eye and absence of clinical inflammation in the sympathizing eye, has been reported.[13] A likely explanation for late-onset or unilateral sympathetic uveitis is that of a mild, overlooked, prior inflammatory episode. One patient followed by the author had a single, brief episode of anterior uveitis in the sympathizing eye. This lasted a few days and cleared spontaneously.[1] The injured eye was enucleated, 1 month after injury, for severe pain and loss of vision. The unexpected histopathological diagnosis was typical sympathetic uveitis. On rare occasions, spontaneous clearance of inflammation in the sympathizing eye may occur.

The history of a penetrating wound and bilateral anterior and posterior uveitis serves as the basis for diagnosis. Along with typical ocular and associated features, fluorescein angiography and ultrasonography may assist in diagnosis. Serological tests and HLA typing are not helpful. The characteristic fluorescein findings consist of multiple, persistent foci of leakage from which the dye may spread (Fig. 179-3). Coalescent pools of dye are seen in areas of exudative retinal detachment. Occasionally, hypofluorescent foci (which stain later) are seen early in the angiogram.[7] Ultrasonography may demonstrate choroidal thickening when the fundus is obscured by severe inflammation, which may be particularly helpful in the differentiation of bilateral phacoanaphylactic endophthalmitis and sympathetic uveitis.

DIFFERENTIAL DIAGNOSIS

Differential diagnosis includes Harada's syndrome, bilateral phacoanaphylactic endophthalmitis, multifocal choroiditis, and other forms of panuveitis or posterior uveitis. A history of penetrating injury helps to differentiate sympathetic uveitis from Harada's syndrome. Bilateral phacoanaphylaxis manifests primarily as severe anterior uveitis. Ultrasonography can differentiate this entity from sympathetic uveitis, because the latter shows marked thickening of the choroid in the posterior segment.

SYSTEMIC ASSOCIATIONS

Sympathetic uveitis may be accompanied by headache, pleocytosis of the spinal fluid, dysacousis, tinnitus, alopecia, poliosis, and vitiligo. The systemic associations are similar to those seen in Harada's syndrome. The principal differentiating feature is the history of a penetrating wound.

Some controversy exists concerning the incidence of systemic associative features and histopathological differences between sympathetic uveitis and Harada's disease. No evidence is known

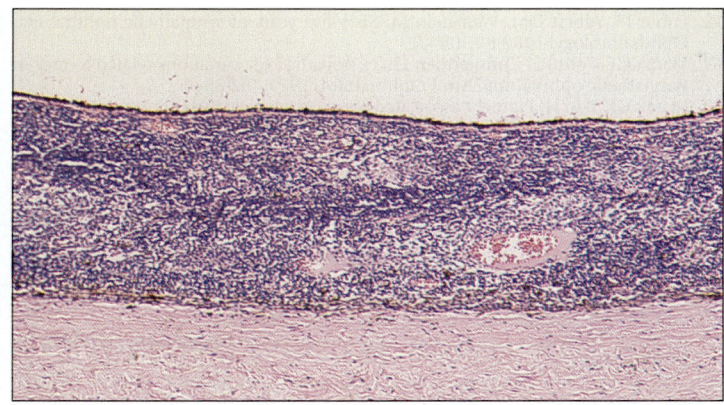

FIG. 179-4 ■ **Diffuse choroidal inflammation in sympathetic ophthalmia.** In this case the retina is detached and is not shown in the illustration.

for a difference in the ocular manifestations, systemic signs, or histopathological characteristics between sympathetic uveitis and Harada's syndrome.[14,15]

PATHOLOGY

The typical histological picture of sympathetic uveitis is a uniform infiltration of the choroid with mononuclear and epithelioid cells (Fig. 179-4). The inflammation has been characterized as non-necrotizing, sparing the choriocapillaris, and not extending into the retina. Cellular collections termed *Dalen–Fuchs nodules* project from the retinal pigment epithelium and are the pathological features that correspond to the spots observed with the ophthalmoscope. The collections of cells contain modified retinal pigment epithelial cells, histiocytes, and lymphocytes.[3] Epithelioid and giant cells that contain pigment are seen in the choroid. Some evidence exists that necrosis of melanocytes occurs and that phagocytic cells are present, but the latter appear very different to other melanophages.[16] Considerable variations from the typical picture are seen,[17,18] such as frequent retinal detachments (50%) and retinal perivasculitis (55%). Obliteration of the choriocapillaris (40%), retinal extension of the inflammation (18%), plasma cell infiltration (60%), eosinophilia (34%), and optic nerve involvement (25%) also are significant variations from the classic histopathology of sympathetic uveitis. With increasing severity of inflammation, there are increased numbers of inflammatory cells in the normal drainage channels, such as the scleral canals and meningeal sheaths of the optic nerves. Uveal pigmentation is related to the severity of the choroidal inflammation.[19,20] Because the pathologist studies only a few sections of the eye, the incidence of chorioretinal scarring probably is underestimated, because this is seen clinically in 25% of the cases.

TREATMENT

Sympathetic uveitis may be prevented by enucleating the injured eye within 2 weeks of injury. Enucleation after that time is not preventive. However, sympathetic uveitis may develop after the injured eye has been removed, so every attempt should be made to save an injured eye if a reasonable expectation exists for useful vision. Careful clinical and ultrasonographic monitoring and possibly an exploratory vitrectomy may save some potentially useful eyes. Those eyes that, in the surgeon's opinion, have little hope of useful vision should be enucleated with the patient's consent. Because evisceration does not protect against sympathetic uveitis, it should not be the procedure of choice. Prophylactic corticosteroids do not prevent the development of sympathetic uveitis. Large, immunosuppressive doses of corticosteroids introduce an unacceptable risk of infection in a recently traumatized eye.

It is not justifiable to remove a potentially functional injured eye in established cases of sympathetic uveitis, for the injured eye may ultimately have the better vision.[21]

Two reports suggest that early enucleation of the exciting eye improves the vision in the sympathizing eye. Both of these reports have statistical problems which vitiate their conclusions. In one report, the patients who had early enucleation also had better vision in the sympathizing eye prior to enucleation. They were compared with patients who had worse vision in the sympathizing eye prior to later enucleation. It, therefore, is not surprising that those who began with better vision before enucleation had better vision after enucleation.[22] The second report is more difficult to evaluate, because the number of cases changes from table to table, new supporting data were found after publication, and regressions were calculated from nonparametric enumeration data. Also, the authors of this report added 9 to 62 and gave a total of 73, so it is difficult to justify sacrifice of a patient's eye on the basis of their statistics.[18,23] If sympathetic uveitis is an autoimmune disease, it is as reasonable to remove an eye as it is to remove half of the brain in a patient with multiple sclerosis to improve the outcome.[24]

The objective of anti-inflammatory treatment is to suppress completely the inflammation as soon as possible and to continue treatment for an extended period. Topical corticosteroids may control very mild cases, but generally large doses (1.0–1.5mg/kg) of prednisone may be required to suppress the inflammation initially. After control has been achieved, the corticosteroid dosage may be tapered and alternate-day therapy started. Treatment should be continued for several months. Treatment for 3–6 months after the inflammation has cleared on alternate-day therapy of 10–20mg of prednisone is desirable.

For those cases in which corticosteroids either do not control the inflammation or produce unacceptable side effects, reduced dosages may be administered with other immunosuppressive agents, such as methotrexate, chlorambucil, azathioprine, or cyclosporine.[25]

COURSE AND OUTCOME

Early, aggressive treatment improves the visual outcome, but one third of the patients in a recent series had visual acuity of worse than 20/200 (6/60).[12] Relapses occur in more than one half the patients and may be delayed for several years. Long-term follow-up is necessary for all patients, including those who have been free of inflammation for several years.[26]

Common complications include band keratopathy, cataract, glaucoma, macular edema, and scarring, retinal detachments (both exudative and rhegmatogenous), hypotony, and phthisis bulbi.

Cataract surgery involves no unusual risks when performed during remission. No reliable data exist for the complications of glaucoma and retinal surgery in patients with sympathetic uveitis.

Although rare, sympathetic uveitis is a serious disease that results in blindness in a significant number of patients. The importance of early, aggressive treatment and regular follow-up cannot be overemphasized.

REFERENCES

1. Marak GE. Recent advances in sympathetic ophthalmia. Surv Ophthalmol. 1979; 24:141–56.
2. Yamaki K, Gocho K, Hayakawa K, *et al.* Tyrosine family proteins are antigens specific to Vogt–Koyanagi–Harada disease. J Immunol. 2000;165:7323–9.
3. Kilmartin DJ, Dick D, Forrester JV. Br J Ophthalmol. 2000;84:259–63.
4. Wacker WB, Rao NA, Marak GE. Experimental sympathetic ophthalmia. In: Silverstein A, O'Connor G, eds. Immunology and immunopathology of the eye. New York: Masson & Cie; 1979;135–7.
5. Chan CC, Benezra D, Rodrigues MM, *et al.* Immunochemistry and electron microscopy of choroidal infiltrates and Dalen–Fuchs nodules in sympathetic ophthalmia. Ophthalmology. 1985;92:580–90.
6. Marak GE, Aye MS, Alepa EP. Cellular hypersensitivity in penetrating eye injuries. Invest Ophthalmol. 1973;12:380–2.
7. Lewis ML, Gass JDM, Spencer WH. Sympathetic uveitis after trauma and vitrectomy. Arch Ophthalmol. 1978;96:263–7.

8. Stafford WR. Sympathetic ophthalmia, report of a case with onset 18 years after contusion with unsuspected scleral rupture. Surv Ophthalmol. 1965;10:232–7.

9. Matzinger P. Tolerance, danger and the extended family. Ann Rev Immunol. 1994; 12:991–1045.

10. Marak GE. Phacoanaphylactic endophthalmitis. Surv Ophthalmol. 1992;4:129–35.

11. Greyerson DC, Dorr C. Spontaneous induction of immunoregulation by an endogenous retinal antigen. Invest Ophthalmol Vision Sci. 2002;43:2984–91.

12. Chan CC, Roberge EG, Whitcop SM, Nussenblatt RB. 32 cases of sympathetic ophthalmia. Arch Ophthalmol. 1995;113:597–600.

13. Kayazama F. A case of sympathetic uveitis. Ann Ophthalmol. 1980;12:1106–8.

14. Kumagi N, Shinda Y, Yamamoto T, et al. Clinical studies on sympathetic ophthalmia. In: Dernouchamps JP, Verougstraetec C, Caspers-Velu C, Tassignon MJ, eds. Recent advances in uveitis. New York: Kugler; 1992:199–200.

15. Rao NA, Marak GE. Sympathetic ophthalmia simulating Vogt–Koyanagi–Harada's disease: clinicopathologic study of four cases. Jpn J Ophthalmol. 1983;27:506–11.

16. Inomata H. Necrotic changes of choroidal melanocytes in sympathetic ophthalmia. Arch Ophthalmol. 1988;106:239–42.

17. Croxato JO, Rao NA, McLean IW, Marak GE. Atypical histopathologic features in sympathetic ophthalmia. Int Ophthalmol. 1981;4:129–35.

18. Lubin JR, Albert DM, Weinstein M. Sixty-five years of sympathetic ophthalmia. Ophthalmology. 1980;87:109–21.

19. Marak GE, Font RL, Zimmerman LE. Histopathologic variations related to race in sympathetic ophthalmia. Am J Ophthalmol. 1974;78:935–8.

20. Marak GE, Ikui H. Pigment associated histopathological variations in sympathetic ophthalmia. Br J Ophthalmol. 1980;64:220–2.

21. Winter EC. Sympathetic ophthalmia: a clinical and pathological study of the visual result. Am J Ophthalmol. 1955;39:340–7.

22. Reynard M, Riffenburg RS, Maes EF. Effect of corticosteroid treatment and enucleation on the visual prognosis of sympathetic ophthalmia. Am J Ophthalmol. 1983;96:290–4.

23. Lubin JR, Albert DM, Weinstein M. Letter to the editor. Ophthalmology. 1982;89: 1291–2.

24. Marak GE. Sympathetic ophthalmia. In: Fraunfelder FT, Roy FH, eds. Current ocular therapy. Philadelphia: WB Saunders; 1995:454–5.

25. Jennings T, Tessler H. Twenty cases of sympathetic ophthalmia. Br J Ophthalmol. 1989;73:140–3.

26. Makey TA, Azar A. Sympathetic ophthalmia. Arch Ophthalmol. 1978;96:257–62.

CHAPTER

180

Idiopathic and Other Anterior Uveitis Syndromes

ROBERT C. WANG • NARSING A. RAO

DEFINITION
- Inflammation in the anterior uvea not associated with defined clinical syndromes.

KEY FEATURES
- Typically a nongranulomatous inflammation associated with cells and flare in the anterior chamber.
- Small-to-medium–size keratic precipitates.

ASSOCIATED FEATURES
- Pain.
- Photophobia.
- Ciliary "flush."
- Posterior synechiae.

INTRODUCTION

Idiopathic anterior uveitis is a frequent cause of acute anterior uveitis encountered in clinical practice. Clinical signs and symptoms such as photophobia and anterior segment cell and flare make the diagnosis straightforward. Treatment with topical corticosteroids and cycloplegics are generally rapid and effective, with few bouts of recurrence. However, frequent recurrences or signs of systemic disease warrant further evaluation. Recognition of the lack of these signs and symptoms and elimination of other disease entities strengthen the accurate assessment of idiopathic disease. However, other distinct syndromes can be mistaken for idiopathic anterior uveitis. These include glaucomatocyclitic crisis (Posner–Schlossman syndrome), Fuchs' heterochromic iridocyclitis (FHI), Schwartz syndrome, and drug-induced anterior uveitis.

IDIOPATHIC ANTERIOR UVEITIS

EPIDEMIOLOGY AND PATHOGENESIS

Idiopathic acute anterior uveitis is the most common cause of uveitis. The prevalence is near 50% (i.e., 50% of uveitis patients have idiopathic uveitis)[1,2] with an annual incidence of 8–15 cases per 100,000 population.[3] Men and women are affected equally.

Although clinical features of acute or chronic anterior uveitis are well described, including associations of the acute process with the HLA-B27 haplotype, there is a lack of clear understanding about the pathogenesis and etiology of iridocyclitis in the vast majority of cases. Such cases are thought to be mediated by an autoimmune process. The latter could be a response to abnormal immune response consisting of recognition of self-protein, possibly induced by an infectious agent.

Recognition of self-protein involves a breakdown in tolerance and recognition of previously sequestered ocular antigens. In animal models sensitization with the ocular antigen, melanin-associated protein, produced an acute recurrent anterior uveitis with a delayed onset but an extended nature.[4] This model mimics human disease closely, with the underlying mechanism primarily from T cell–mediated delayed hypersensitivity. Recently, herpes simplex virus (HSV) antigens and DNA have been found in the aqueous humor of patients with recurrent anterior uveitis and iris atrophy without keratopathy.[5] These lesions have been attributed previously to varicella zoster virus. However in the younger age group, HSV was recovered in the anterior chamber sample. It is interesting to note that the study was performed on patients who have recurrent disease and that HSV was detected after an average of a 14-year follow-up in some cases.

OCULAR MANIFESTATIONS

Idiopathic anterior uveitis appears with an acute onset of pain, photophobia, and decreased vision. Ocular examination typically exhibits limbal vascular injection (ciliary flush) with occasional chemosis. Intraocular pressure is typically normal. However, severe chronic inflammation can lead to elevated intraocular pressure. Slit-lamp evaluation of the anterior chamber demonstrates variable amounts of cell and flare depending on the severity. Severe inflammation can result in fibrin or hypopyon formation (Fig. 180-1). However, the presence of these two signs is atypical for idiopathic disease and more characteristic of the HLA-B27–associated spondyloarthropathy.[6] Precipitates of inflammatory cells can be seen on the inferior endothelial surface of the cornea (Arlt's triangle). Small collections of white-appearing keratic precipitates usually represent a nongranulomatous anterior uveitis. Large, greasy, keratic precipitates are not typical of idiopathic anterior uveitis, and their presence should lead to the consideration of other granulomatous processes such as sarcoidosis, lens-induced uveitis, and others.

Chronic or severe inflammation can lead to secondary complications, including cataract formation and glaucoma. In addition, cystoid macular edema can develop decreasing vision out of proportion to the amount of inflammation.

DIAGNOSIS

Diagnosis of idiopathic disease is generally straightforward. Clinical history is typical, with an acute onset of pain and photophobia in a healthy individual without systemic disease. Examination demonstrates small keratic precipitates, anterior chamber cells, and flare. Usually the inflammation responds rapidly to therapy. However, frequent recurrences, slowly resolving inflammation, systemic symptoms, or granulomatous keratic precipitates should indicate the possibility of an alternative diagnosis.

DIFFERENTIAL DIAGNOSIS

Critical to the diagnosis of idiopathic disease is a thorough and complete history and review of systems. Importantly, review of systems can differentiate HLA-B27–associated disease, which is among the common causes of anterior uveitis. These diseases include Reiter's syndrome, ankylosing spondylitis, psoriatic arthritis, ulcerative colitis, and Crohn's disease. Other possibilities include

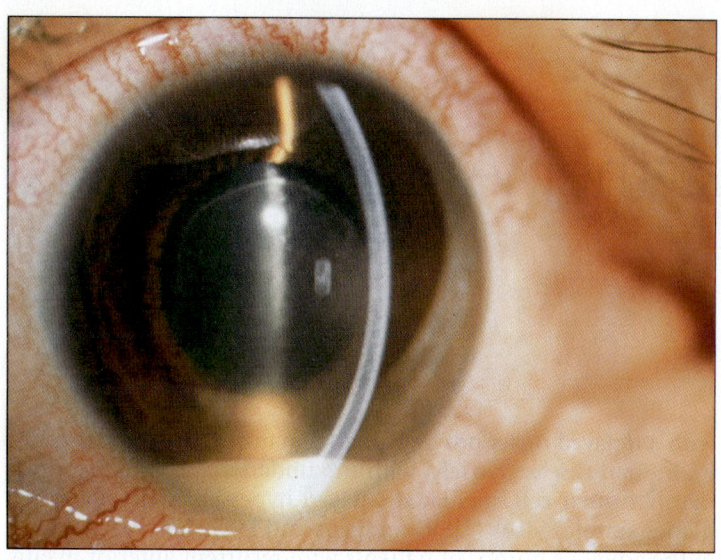

FIG. 180-1 ▮▮ Severe idiopathic anterior uveitis with fibrinoid reaction in a patient with HLA-B27. Extensive anterior segment reaction with posterior synechiae is present. Note large amount of fibrin in the anterior chamber. Typical limbal injection is seen.

TABLE 180-1

DIFFERENTIAL DIAGNOSIS OF ENTITIES WITH ANTERIOR UVEITIS

ANTERIOR SEGMENT SIGNS	
Granulomatous keratic precipitates	Sarcoid, sympathetic ophthalmia, VKH, tuberculosis, toxoplasmosis, infectious etiologies
Hypopyon	HLA-B27, Behçet's, intraocular lymphoma, endophthalmitis
Diffuse keratic precipitates	Fuchs' heterochromic iridocyclitis, herpes simplex virus, cytomegalovirus retinitis
SYSTEMIC DISEASE	
Autoimmune	HLA-B27 (ankylosing spondylitis, Reiter's, psoriasis, ulcerative colitis, Crohn's disease), sarcoid, Behçet's disease, VKH, TINU
Infectious	Syphilis, tuberculosis, herpes simplex virus, Whipple's, fungal, *Propionibacterium acnes*, and others

*HLA-B27, Human lymphocyte antigen B27; TINU, tubulointerstitial nephritis and uveitis; VKH, Vogt-Koyanagi-Harada syndrome.

infectious and noninfectious causes. In addition, diagnosis can be refined in the presence of a granulomatous keratic precipitates. Dilated fundal examination should be performed to eliminate other pathology with secondary anterior uveitis (Table 180-1).

PATHOLOGY

Histologically the inflammatory infiltrate consists of lymphocytes admixed with monocytes.[4] They are seen primarily in the anterior uvea, with spillover of cells into the anterior chamber and vitreous cavity. Monocytes are seen as the earliest cellular infiltrate marginating in the iris vasculature. Chemotactic factors are found in the aqueous humor and contribute to migration of leukocytes. Accumulating evidence suggests that cytokines produced by the uveal macrophages initiate the uveitis.[7]

TREATMENT

Topical corticosteroids remain the mainstay of therapy for idiopathic anterior uveitis. Frequent administration of topical corticosteroids rapidly resolves the inflammation. Although

studies noted differences in efficacy between phosphate and acetate formulations, most have not noticed a difference in treatment outcomes.[8] Addition of a mydriatic agent reduces pain associated with the uveitis, prevents the likelihood of posterior synechiae formation, and attempts to break those that have formed already. Rarely, idiopathic inflammation fails to respond to topical therapy. In these recalcitrant cases, sub-Tenon's injection of corticosteroids delivers a relatively high concentration in a sustained release fashion, resulting in rapid resolution. Additionally, sub-Tenon's injection of corticosteroids is effective in the treatment of cystoid macular edema.[9] Different formulations of injectable corticosteroids are available. In particular, triamcinolone appears to have a better safety profile causing less local fibrosis than other injectable corticosteroid formulations.

Occasionally, topical treatment with corticosteroids produces a rise in intraocular pressure not associated with anterior segment inflammation. Newer formulations of corticosteroids, such as loteprednol, have reduced the steroid-response effect.[10,11] Though both standard topical corticosteroid therapy and corticosteroid-sparing therapy reduced intraocular inflammation, the latter appears less efficacious in reducing inflammation.[12,13]

FUCHS' HETEROCHROMIC IRIDOCYCLITIS

FHI is a rare form of anterior uveitis that accounts for approximately 1.5% of all anterior uveitis.[14,15] Most patients are diagnosed between 35–40 years of age with equal male-to-female predominance. The intraocular inflammation is typically unilateral. However, bilateral involvement is seen in 15% of cases.[16] Ocular toxoplasmosis and herpes simplex virus (HSV) infection have been implicated.[17–19] However, the underlying etiology remains unknown.

Unlike idiopathic anterior uveitis, patients with FHI have minimal symptoms. Typically patients have a noninjected, "quiet-appearing" eye, with decreased vision due to the development of cataract. Slit-lamp evaluation typically demonstrates fine, "stellate" keratic precipitates (KP). Unlike idiopathic uveitis, these KP generally cover the entire corneal endothelium. There is usually a mild anterior chamber cellular reaction with minimal flare, without iris synechiae.[16]

Gonioscopy demonstrates fine vessels crossing the trabecular meshwork in 20–30% of patients. These vessels do not tend to cause neovascular glaucoma. However, they are friable and may cause minute hemorrhages into the anterior chamber. Historically, surgical intervention into the anterior chamber produces hemorrhages from these vessels, termed Amsler's sign.[20]

The classic description of FHI includes diffuse, stellate keratic precipitates with iris heterochromia. Unilateral inflammation causes the involved iris to appear lighter compared with the fellow eye. In lighter color eyes, extensive iris atrophy may produce a paradoxical heterochromia. Bilateral disease is subtle and can be discerned by signs of blurring of the iris stroma and loss of detail of the iris surface. Bilateral, diffuse stellate keratic precipitates are a more specific sign.[16]

Complications of FHI include elevated intraocular pressure, which is seen in 25–60% of the patients.[16] Additionally, cataract formation, most commonly posterior subcapsular cataracts, develops in over 80% of patients.[21] Patients tend to tolerate cataract extraction well. However, glaucoma develops in 6.3–59% of eyes, and 25–60% of these eyes require filtering surgery.[22]

Despite these complications there is currently no indication that treatment with anti-inflammatory agents alters the course or the outcome of the disease. Up to 50% of eyes retain 20/40 or better vision.[16,23] Occasional use of glucocorticoids may be indicated if an exacerbation of inflammation is symptomatic. Periocular glucocorticoids may help to decrease symptomatic vitreous inflammation.

GLAUCOMATOCYCLITIC CRISIS

Glaucomatocyclitic crisis, also known as Posner–Schlossman syndrome, is an entity associated with an acute uniocular elevation of intraocular pressure. Glaucomatocyclitic crisis is rare and reported in 0.5% of cases of uveitis.[1] Studies demonstrate a stronger male predilection, with onset from the third through sixth decade of life.[24] Although recurrent, it rarely occurs later in life. However, in recurrent cases in patients who have the disease for longer than a 10-year period, there is an increased risk of developing glaucoma.[25] The pathogenesis has been suggested to be both immunological and infectious in nature. Association with both HLA-Bw54 and *Borrelia burgdorferi* have been shown.[26,27] Recently DNA fragments of HSV have been recovered in the aqueous humor of patients with acute episodes.[28] However, it is still unclear whether these observations are related directly to the underlying pathogenesis.

Patients typically seek treatment for a blurring of vision and periorbital discomfort. Examination reveals a noninjected eye with a slightly mydriatic pupil. Slit-lamp examination reveals a paucity of anterior chamber cells with occasional, small, nonpigmented keratic precipitates on the corneal endothelium. The intraocular pressure is elevated to 40–60mm Hg, usually despite an open angle.[24]

Diagnosis generally is based on clinical findings. However, herpetic uveitis can mimic this disease. Unlike glaucomatocyclitic crisis, herpetic anterior uveitis typically reveals a heavier anterior chamber reaction with signs of posterior synechiae and iris atrophy.

Therapy of glaucomatocyclitic crises is directed primarily at control of the elevated intraocular pressure. Apraclonidine appears to be especially effective in the reduction of intraocular pressure in glaucomatocyclitic crises; it has been shown in one study to reduce intraocular pressure by 50% over a 4-hour period.[29] However, use of other pressure-lowering agents such as β-blockers and topical carbonic anhydrase inhibitors also may be used. The prostaglandin analog, latanoprost, was associated with an increase in intraocular pressure and worsening of uveitis in a small case series.[30–32] Due to the inflammatory component, anecdotal evidence suggests that therapy with topical glucocorticoids may shorten the duration of the intraocular pressure rise.

DRUG-INDUCED ANTERIOR UVEITIS: RIFABUTIN AND CIDOFOVIR

Rifabutin is used in the treatment or prophylaxis of *Mycobacterium avium* complex (MAC) infections in acquired immunodeficiency syndrome.[33,34] Patients who have human immunodeficiency virus (HIV) at risk of MAC infection tend to have a low CD4 cell count and high viral load. With the advent of highly active antiretroviral therapy (HAART), the incidence of MAC infection has decreased.[35] However, use of rifabutin in doses of 300–1800mg has been associated with the development of a severe hypopyon anterior uveitis in 16% of patients receiving therapy. Rifabutin levels have been demonstrated to increase with the addition of clarithromycin, a macrolide, which inhibits the cytochrome P450 enzymatic pathway, increasing the concentration of rifabutin.[36] The concomitant use of clarithromycin and ethambutol was not associated with increased risk of uveitis.[37] Recently rifabutin-associated anterior uveitis has been observed in immunocompetent individuals, thus making the association between the anterior uveitis and immune status less likely.[38] The exact pathogenesis of the rifabutin-associated uveitis is still unknown.

Patients typically experience an acute onset of uniocular blurring of vision and ocular injection. Examination demonstrates a marked fibrinoid anterior chamber reaction and hypopyon that mimic infectious endophthalmitis (Fig. 180-2). Anterior vitreous

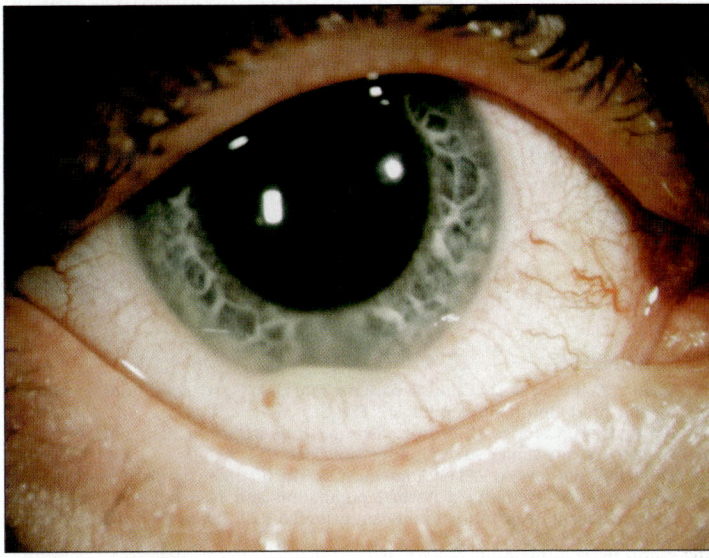

FIG. 180-2 ■ **Rifabutin-associated anterior uveitis.** Severe inflammation with evidence of hypopyon and fibrin formation.

cells are typically present, rarely with diffuse vitreitis. Occasionally, bilateral involvement can occur.[39,40]

Diagnosis is based on clinical findings, history of recent rifabutin treatment, and clinical suspicion. Differential diagnosis includes infectious causes causing endophthalmitis. Differentiation can be especially challenging in an immunocompromised HIV-infected individual, occasionally requiring diagnostic vitrectomy to eliminate an infectious etiology.

Patients typically respond to withdrawal of the rifabutin.[39] Clinical improvement has been seen after reduction of the dosage. In addition, adjunctive use of frequently applied topical steroids and mydriatic agents resolve most of the anterior segment inflammation. Occasionally regional or oral administration of steroids is required for recalcitrant inflammation or vitreitis.

Cidofovir is a nucleotide analog used primarily for the treatment of cytomegalovirus (CMV) retinitis in patients who have HIV.[41,42] Use of cidofovir has been associated with the development of anterior uveitis and hypotony.[43] Cidofovir seems to contribute directly to the development of anterior uveitis.[44]

Cidofovir-associated anterior uveitis typically occurs unilaterally. Patients exhibit signs of anterior uveitis with decreased vision, photophobia, and limbal injection. Anterior segment examination reveals a mild cellular reaction with fibrinous response. Posterior synechiae is occasionally present. Mild amounts of anterior vitreous humor reaction can be seen in 50% of cases.[45]

Diagnosis requires a high clinical suspicion and a recent history of cidofovir treatment. The differential diagnosis includes the entity of immune recovery uveitis (IRU). IRU occurs following immune reconstitution with HAART therapy with CD4 counts of 100 cells/μl or more. In contrast to cidofovir uveitis, IRU typically is associated with a prominent vitreitis.[46] In addition, IRU typically occurs following immune reconstitution with quiescence of the CMV lesion, whereas cidofovir uveitis can occur during an early phase of the infection.

Treatment consists of removal of the drug, if possible, with substitution of ganciclovir or other anti-CMV agents. Ocular hypotony tends to return to normal after cessation of the drug. However, prolonged use can result in ciliary body atrophy and permanent hypotony.[47] The intraocular inflammation tends to clear rapidly and seems to be sensitive to topical glucocorticoid therapy.

SCHWARTZ SYNDROME

Schwartz syndrome was initially described as increased intraocular pressure with an open chamber angle, anterior uveitis, and rhegmatogenous retinal detachment.[48] However, unlike with idiopathic uveitis, patients have a quiet eye and fine anterior chamber reaction. Additionally, retinal examination reveals peripheral retinal detachment.

Predisposition to Schwartz syndrome was found in patients with small oral dialysis with detachments that were flat in height, involved a large area including the macula, and were of long duration.[49–51]

Management is best accomplished by surgical repair of retinal detachment. Topical pressure-lowering agents can control acute IOP rises prior to the surgery.

REFERENCES

1. Weiner A, BenEzra D. Clinical patterns and associated conditions in chronic uveitis. Am J Ophthalmol. 1991;112:151–8.
2. Rodriguez A, Calonge M, Pedroza-Seres M, et al. Referral patterns of uveitis in a tertiary eye care center. Arch Ophthalmol. 1996;114:593–9.
3. Linssen A, Rothova A, Valkenburg HA, et al. The lifetime cumulative incidence of acute anterior uveitis in a normal population and its relation to ankylosing spondylitis and histocompatibility antigen HLA-B27. Invest Ophthalmol Vis Sci. 1991;32:2568–78.
4. Smith JR, Hart PH, Williams KA. Basic pathogenic mechanisms operating in experimental models of acute anterior uveitis. Immunol Cell Biol. 1998;76:497–512.
5. Van der Lelij A, Ooijman FM, Kijlstra A, et al. Anterior uveitis with sectoral iris atrophy in the absence of keratitis: a distinct clinical entity among herpetic eye diseases. Ophthalmology. 2000;107:1164–70.
6. D'Alessandro LP, Forster DJ, Rao NA. Anterior uveitis and hypopyon. Am J Ophthalmol. 1991;112:317–21.
7. Rosenbaum JT, Seymour BW, Raymond W, et al. Similar chemotactic factor for monocytes predominates in different animal models of uveitis. Inflammation. 1988;12:191–201.
8. Musson DG, Bidgood AM, Olejnik O. An in vitro comparison of the permeability of prednisolone, prednisolone sodium phosphate, and prednisolone acetate across the NZW rabbit cornea. J Ocul Pharmacol. 1992;8:139–50.
9. Thach AB, Dugel PU, Flindall RJ, et al. A comparison of retrobulbar versus sub-Tenon's corticosteroid therapy for cystoid macular edema refractory to topical medications. Ophthalmology. 1997;104:2003–8.
10. Whitcup SM, Ferris FL III. New corticosteroids for the treatment of ocular inflammation. Am J Ophthalmol. 1999;127:597–9.
11. Bartlett JD, Horwitz B, Laibovitz R, et al. Intraocular pressure response to loteprednol etabonate in known steroid responders. J Ocul Pharmacol. 1993;9:157–65.
12. Howes JF. Loteprednol etabonate: a review of ophthalmic clinical studies. Pharmazie. 2000;55:178–83.
13. Controlled evaluation of loteprednol etabonate and prednisolone acetate in the treatment of acute anterior uveitis. Loteprednol Etabonate US Uveitis Study Group. Am J Ophthalmol. 1999;127:537–44.
14. La Hey E, de Jong PT, Kijlstra A. Fuchs' heterochromic cyclitis: review of the literature on the pathogenetic mechanisms. Br J Ophthalmol. 1994;78:307–12.
15. Paivonsalo-Hietanen T, Tuominen J, Vaahtoranta-Lehtonen H, et al. Incidence and prevalence of different uveitis entities in Finland. Acta Ophthalmol Scand. 1997;75:76–81.
16. Fearnley IR, Rosenthal AR. Fuchs' heterochromic iridocyclitis revisited. Acta Ophthalmol Scand. 1995;73:166–70.
17. Schwab IR. The epidemiologic association of Fuchs' heterochromic iridocyclitis and ocular toxoplasmosis. Am J Ophthalmol. 1991;111:356–62.
18. La Hey E, Rothova A, Baarsma GS, et al. Fuchs' heterochromic iridocyclitis is not associated with ocular toxoplasmosis. Arch Ophthalmol. 1992;110:806–11.
19. Barequet IS, Li Q, Wang Y, et al. Herpes simplex virus DNA identification from aqueous fluid in Fuchs' heterochromic iridocyclitis. Am J Ophthalmol. 2000;129:672–3.
20. Bloch-Michel E, Frau E, Chhor S, Tounsi Y. Amsler's sign associated significantly with Fuch's heterochromic cyclitis (FHC). Int Ophthalmol. 1995;19:169–71.
21. Jones NP. Cataract surgery in Fuchs' heterochromic uveitis: past, present, and future. J Cataract Refract Surg. 1996;22:261–8.
22. La Hey E, de Vries J, Langerhorst CT, et al. Treatment and prognosis of secondary glaucoma in Fuchs' heterochromic iridocyclitis. Am J Ophthalmol. 1993;116:327–40.
23. Liesegang TJ. Clinical features and prognosis in Fuchs' uveitis syndrome. Arch Ophthalmol. 1982;100:1622–6.
24. Camras CD, Schlossman A, Posner A. Posner–Schlossman syndrome. Ocular infection and immunity. St Louis: Mosby; 1996:529–36.
25. Jap A, Sivakumar M, Chee SP. Is Posner–Schlossman syndrome benign? Ophthalmology. 2001;108:913–8.
26. Isogai E, Isogai H, Kotake S, et al. Detection of antibodies against Borrelia burgdorferi in patients with uveitis. Am J Ophthalmol. 1991;112:23–30.
27. Hirose S, Ohno S, Matsuda H. HLA-Bw54 and glaucomatocyclitic crisis. Arch Ophthalmol. 1985;103:1837–9.
28. Yamamoto S, Pavan-Langston D, Tada R, et al. Possible role of herpes simplex virus in the origin of Posner–Schlossman syndrome. Am J Ophthalmol. 1995;119:796–8.
29. Hong C, Song KY. Effect of apraclonidine hydrochloride on the attack of Posner–Schlossman syndrome. Korean J Ophthalmol. 1993;7:28–33.
30. Warwar RE, Bullock JD. Latanoprost-induced uveitis. Surv Ophthalmol. 1999;43:466–8.
31. Smith SL, Pruitt CA, Sine CS, et al. Latanoprost 0.005% and anterior segment uveitis. Acta Ophthalmol Scand. 1999;77:668–72.
32. Sacca S, Pascotto A, Siniscalchi C, et al. Ocular complications of latanoprost in uveitic glaucoma: three case reports. J Ocul Pharmacol Ther. 2001;17:107–13.
33. Schouten JT, Whittemore S. Recent development in the treatment and prevention of disseminated Mycobacterium avium complex (MAC). STEP Perspect. 1996;8:5–6.
34. MAC management. PI Perspect. 1996:16–7.
35. Tumbarello M, Tacconelli E, de Donati KG, et al. Changes in incidence and risk factors of Mycobacterium avium complex infections in patients with AIDS in the era of new antiretroviral therapies. Eur J Clin Microbiol Infect Dis. 2001; 20:498–501.
36. Kuper JI, D'Aprile M. Drug–drug interactions of clinical significance in the treatment of patients with Mycobacterium avium complex disease. Clin Pharmacokinet. 2000;39:203–14.
37. Shafran SD, Singer J, Zarowny DP, et al. Determinants of rifabutin-associated uveitis in patients treated with rifabutin, clarithromycin, and ethambutol for Mycobacterium avium complex bacteremia: a multivariate analysis. Canadian HIV Trials Network Protocol 010 Study Group. J Infect Dis. 1998;177:252–5.
38. Bhagat N, Read RW, Rao NA, et al. Rifabutin-associated hypopyon uveitis in human immunodeficiency virus–negative immunocompetent individuals. Ophthalmology. 2001;108:750–2.
39. Tseng AL, Walmsley SL. Rifabutin-associated uveitis. Ann Pharmacother. 1995;29:1149–55.
40. Cunningham ET Jr. Uveitis in HIV positive patients. Br J Ophthalmol. 2000;84:233–5.
41. Rougier MB, Neau D, Viallard JF, et al. Anterior uveitis and cidofovir. J Fr Ophthalmol. 2001;24:491–5.
42. The ganciclovir implant plus oral ganciclovir versus parenteral cidofovir for the treatment of cytomegalovirus retinitis in patients with acquired immunodeficiency syndrome: the Ganciclovir Cidofovir Cytomegalovirus Retinitis Trial. Am J Ophthalmol. 2001;131:457–67.
43. Long-term follow-up of patients with AIDS treated with parenteral cidofovir for cytomegalovirus retinitis: the HPMPC Peripheral Cytomegalovirus Retinitis Trial. The Studies of Ocular Complications of AIDS Research Group in collaboration with the AIDS Clinical Trials Group. AIDS. 2000;14:1571–81.
44. Scott RA, Pavesio C. Ocular side-effects from systemic HPMPC (cidofovir) for a non-ocular cytomegalovirus infection. Am J Ophthalmol. 2000;130:126–7.
45. Cochereau I, Doan S, Diraison MC, et al. Uveitis in patients treated with intravenous cidofovir. Ocul Immunol Inflamm. 1999;7:223–9.
46. Karavellas MP, Azen SP, MacDonald JC, et al. Immune recovery vitritis and uveitis in AIDS: clinical predictors, sequelae, and treatment outcomes. Retina. 2001;21:1–9.
47. Taskintuna I, Rahhal FM, Rao NA, et al. Adverse events and autopsy findings after intravitreous cidofovir (HPMPC) therapy in patients with acquired immune deficiency syndrome (AIDS). Ophthalmology. 1997;104:1827–36; discussion 1836–7.
48. Netland PA, Mukai S, Covington HI. Elevated intraocular pressure secondary to rhegmatogenous retinal detachment. Surv Ophthalmol. 1994;39:234–40.
49. Matsuo N, Takabatake M, Ueno H, et al. Photoreceptor outer segments in the aqueous humor in rhegmatogenous retinal detachment. Am J Ophthalmol. 1986;101:673–9.
50. Lambrou FH, Vela MA, Woods W. Obstruction of the trabecular meshwork by retinal rod outer segments. Arch Ophthalmol. 1989;107:742–5.
51. Matsushita M, Matsuo T, Matsuo N. Retinal detachment with oral dialysis: differences in clinical features between cases with and without photoreceptor outer segments in aqueous humor. Jpn J Ophthalmol. 1990;34:338–4.

CHAPTER
181

Pars Planitis and Other Intermediate Uveitis

PAUL L. ZIMMERMAN • THOMAS M. BOYLE

DEFINITION
- Intraocular inflammation centered primarily in the anterior vitreous, peripheral retina, and pars plana ciliaris.

KEY FEATURES
- Inflammatory cells in the anterior vitreous.
- Mild or absent anterior chamber cell and flare.
- Vitreous clumps of inflammatory cells (snowballs).
- An inferior pars plana white exudate (a "snowbank").
- Vascular sheathing (frequently adjacent to the snowbank).
- Cystoid macular edema.
- Vitreous opacity.
- Typically bilateral.

ASSOCIATED FEATURES
- Young age (range 5–40 years). The subclass of intermediate uveitis associated with HTLV-1 may occur in patients up to the seventh and eighth decades.
- No sex predilection exists.
- Floaters or blurry vision and, less frequently, mild pain, photophobia, and redness.
- Less common clinical findings include vitreous detachment, traction or rhegmatogenous retinal detachment, vitreous hemorrhage, posterior subcapsular cataract, glaucoma, inferior endotheliitis, posterior synechiae, peripheral or posterior retinal vasculitis, and retinal or anterior segment neovascularization.

INTRODUCTION

The International Uveitis Study Group has recommended the anatomical designation intermediate uveitis (IU) for the entities that have been called cyclitis, peripheral uveitis, chronic cyclitis, vitritis, and pars planitis.[1–4] Its cause is unknown, but it is likely to be an autoimmune response to vitreous, ciliary body, or peripheral retinal tissue. Herein, the authors refer to idiopathic IU, without systemic disease association and with a pars plana "snowbank," as pars planitis. Pars planitis accounts for the large majority of patients with IU. A significant portion of patients who attend uveitis referral practices have IU; it probably accounts for approximately one fifth of all uveitis in children. In addition to the idiopathic disease, pars planitis, IU occurs in association with multiple sclerosis and with human T-cell lymphoma virus-1 infections. Lyme disease, sarcoidosis, and syphilis can also cause anatomical IU (see Chapters 168 and 175).

EPIDEMIOLOGY AND PATHOGENESIS

In several large series from uveitis referral practices, IU represented 11–15% of patients.[5–9] In exclusively pediatric series the number tends to be slightly higher, typically 17.5–20%.[10] Pars planitis occurs in patients between the ages of 5 and 40 years. It has a bimodal distribution, with a young group in the age range 5–15 years and an older group in the age range 20–40 years; each group constitutes about half the patients. There has been no striking sex predilection, although there seems to be a slight male preponderance in the younger age group and a slight female preponderance in the older age group.

Pars planitis does not have a striking familial tendency. As there are large numbers of pars planitis patients and relatively few familial cases reported, it is unlikely that the disease is inherited. However, there have been numerous reports of families with multiple affected members, suggesting that some heritable or environmental cause may play a role in the disease.

The pathogenesis of IU is largely unknown. In IU associated with multiple sclerosis (MS), an autoimmune cause is suspected. In IU associated with Lyme disease, a combination of infectious and immunologic causes is probable.

The association of IU with human T-cell lymphoma virus type 1 (HTLV-1) is also probably the result of immune disregulation. Vitreous samples from patients who have HTLV-1–associated uveitis contain HTLV-1–infected CD4 lymphocytes.[11] Elevated CD4 lymphocyte levels and lowered CD8 lymphocyte levels, with resultant increased CD4/CD8 ratios, occur.[12] In addition, levels of serum CD25-positive T lymphocytes with interleukin-2 (IL-2) receptors are elevated, as are soluble IL-2 receptors in patients with HTLV-1–associated IU. Other studies show increased levels of IL-6 and tumor necrosis factor-α production from T-cell clones taken from HTLV-1–associated uveitis aqueous samples.[13] The exact nature of the immune dysfunction in this disease is the subject of ongoing investigation.

The pathogenesis of the inflammation in pars planitis has been much debated. Autoimmune reactions against vitreous, peripheral retina, and ciliary body have been proposed. Numerous studies have looked at and reported human leukocyte antigen (HLA) associations in IU.[14–18] Several HLA types have been reported to be present at higher frequencies in IU patients than controls. These include HLA-B8, HLA-B51, HLA-DR17, HLA-DR51, and HLA-DR2. However, HLA-DR15, a suballele of HLA-DR2, has been shown in every study that has included it to have the highest association with IU, present in 64.3–72% of IU patients versus 20–28% of controls. This is the same HLA class II allele that has been associated with MS and may explain the association between IU and MS.

OCULAR MANIFESTATIONS

The clinical findings and complications of IU are listed in Table 181-1.[18–22] The onset of IU is insidious and gradual. Most patients have some bilateral findings, although asymmetry may be marked. Patients complain most commonly of floaters and, in many, blurred vision. Rarely, the initial complaint is of mild pain, photophobia, red eye, or severe visual loss due to vitreous hemorrhage.

The sine qua non of IU is vitritis, which may be mild or very severe (Fig. 181-1). Vitreous snowballs are quite common (Fig. 181-2); they are usually located in the inferior vitreous peripher-

TABLE 181-1

INTERMEDIATE UVEITIS; FINDINGS AND COMPLICATIONS

Finding/Complication	58 eyes[19] (%)	108 eyes[20] (%)	182 eyes[21] (%)	100 patients[22] (%)	53 patients[18] (%)
Cystoid macular edema	52	51	28	21	68
Cataract	40	41	42	36	57
Retinal tear/detachment	13	8	5	22	—
Neovascularization	9	6.5	—	—	8
Vitreous hemorrhage	9	—	3	3	—
Glaucoma	7	—	8	16	—
Band keratopathy	5	—	9	3	2
Retinoschisis	2	—	4	—	—
Dragged disk vessels	2	—	1	—	—

ally but may be found throughout the vitreous cavity. Occasionally, they may be located on the posterior aspect of a detached posterior vitreous face (posterior keratic precipitates). Vitreous strands, sheets, and membranes are common and sometimes have attached snowballs. Posterior vitreous detachment is common when inflammation has been present for some time.

Pars planitis patients frequently have a snowbank along the inferior pars plana, ora serrata, and peripheral retina (Fig. 181-3). In quiescent or "burned-out" pars planitis, the snowbank may be smooth and shiny, whereas in active disease, especially in young patients, it is fluffy, giving a cumulus cloud appearance with attached snowballs.

The snowbank is invariably found to be vascularized on close examination. Where it is markedly vascularized, an increased risk of vitreous hemorrhage is present. Felder and Brockhurst[23] have described "angiomas," tumor-like vascular changes, on the snowbanks of pars planitis patients. Vitreous hemorrhage, although not common in adults, was reported in a retrospective study of 118 consecutive patients to have a prevalence of 28% in children.[24]

Peripheral retinal perivasculitis (especially periphlebitis) and perivascular sheathing are common in pars planitis. These occur most frequently in the inferior retina beneath the vitreous base and adjacent to the snowbank. More posterior perivasculitis and sheathing occur occasionally, more commonly with HTLV-1–associated IU.[16] Obliteration of peripheral venules can also occur. Cotton-wool spots and hemorrhages occur rarely in pars planitis but more commonly in HTLV-1–associated IU.[25]

Cataract is common in protracted pars planitis; it may be caused either by the inflammation or by corticosteroid treatment employed in the management of the disorder.[18–22]

Cystoid macular edema (CME) is common in pars planitis, being the most common cause of decreased visual acuity.[18–22] Inflammation and/or vitreous traction may play a role in CME development. It does not seem to be as common in HTLV-1–associated IU, possibly because the disease is more acute in onset and is treated before becoming chronic.[26] If allowed to remain for months to years, CME can lead to macular degeneration and permanent visual loss.

Neovascularization of the disc (NVD), of the retinal periphery (NVE), or of the iris (NVI) can occur in more severe disease; NVD (or rarely NVE) can lead to vitreous hemorrhage and NVI to neovascular glaucoma.

Papillitis and optic nerve edema are not common but can be striking and thus can prompt investigations for other causes of optic nerve edema and inflammation.

Anterior segment findings are not typical and are usually mild. Anterior chamber cell and flare are absent to mild, rarely as much as 2+. Small to moderate-sized keratic precipitates occur but tend to be scattered and, again, are somewhat unusual. Autoimmune endotheliopathy consisting of clumped keratic precipitates posterior to a discrete endothelial line, with accom-

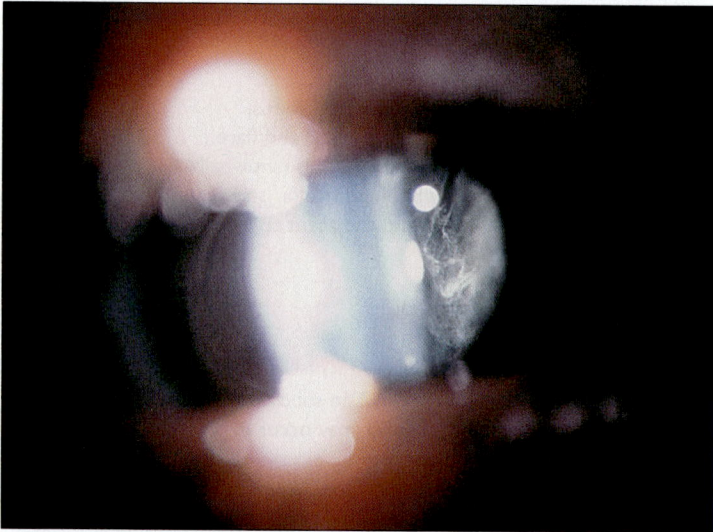

FIG. 181-1 ▌▌ Typical anterior vitreous cells and debris.

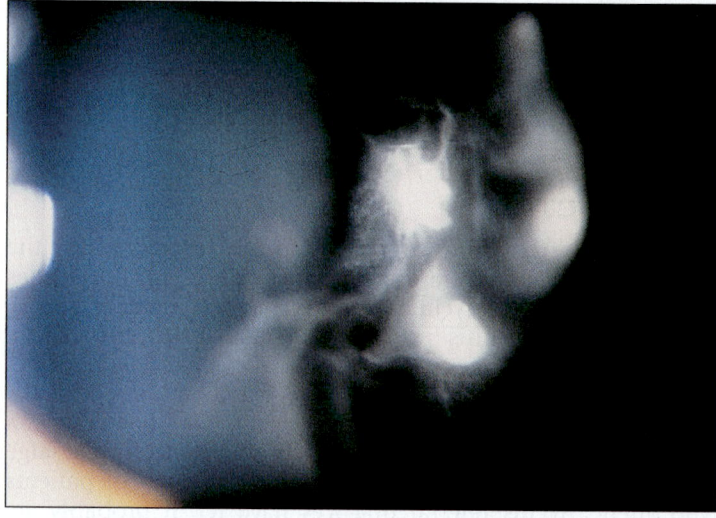

FIG. 181-2 ▌▌ Retrolental snowballs.

panying corneal edema, has been associated with pars planitis[27] (Fig. 181-4) and frequently causes more pain, photophobia, and redness than occur in its absence. Trabecular precipitates are sometimes seen. Endotheliopathy is most common at disease onset but can occur in chronic pars planitis.

Posterior synechiae are relatively uncommon. When they occur they are usually broad based and difficult to break with di-

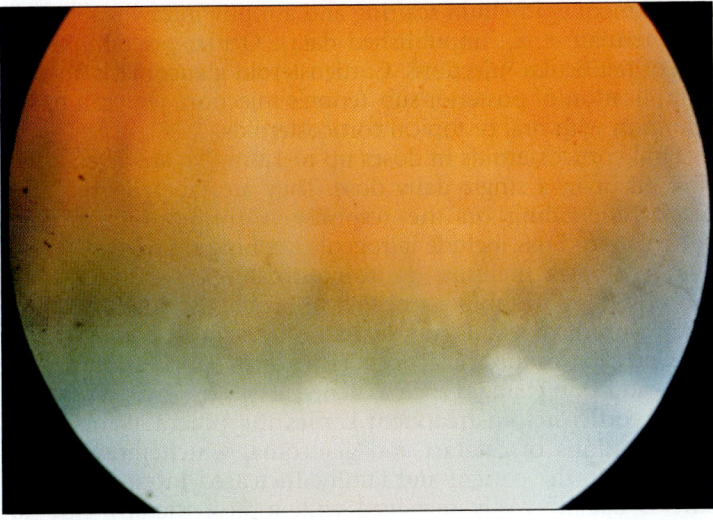

FIG. 181-3 ■ Inferior pars plana snowbank with attached snowballs.

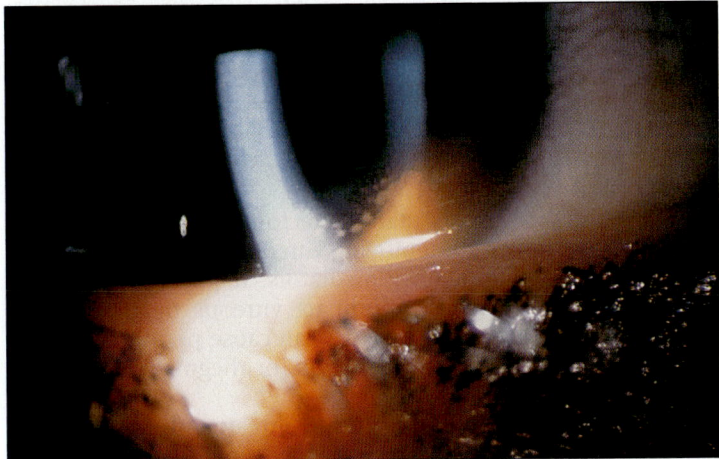

FIG. 181-4 ■ Corneal endotheliopathy in intermediate uveitis. Note the discrete superior border of keratic precipitates and the mild stromal edema that overlies the endotheliopathy.

BOX 181-1

Differential Diagnosis of Intermediate Uveitis

UNILATERAL CONDITIONS

Coats' disease: This is unilateral and a focus or foci of intraretinal angiomatosis are present. Vitreous flare is striking.

Intraocular tumors: Tumors such as a retinoblastoma, malignant melanoma, or medulloepithelioma can disseminate into the vitreous and simulate IU. Atypical-appearing vitreous cells and a mass, detectable by funduscopy or ultrasonography, constitute these diagnoses.

Fuchs' heterochromic iridocyclitis (FHI): Patients can have quite significant vitritis and even CME. There is no snowbank. Stellate or comma-shaped keratic precipitates outside Arlt's triangle and the heterochromia iridis constitute this diagnosis. Usually FHI is unilateral, but it is bilateral in up to 10% of patients. (Posterior synechiae preclude this diagnosis.)

Infection: *Propionibacterium acnes* and other indolent infections can mimic IU, but these are always postoperative.

Intraocular foreign body or chronic retinal detachment: Can cause vitritis, but careful history and examination should make possible these diagnoses.

UNILATERAL OR BILATERAL CONDITIONS

Sarcoidosis should be suspected in all patients with IU. Chest radiograph, angiotensin-converting enzyme, serum lysozyme, and gallium scans support the diagnosis, but only tissue biopsy confirms it. Conjunctival nodules should be biopsied.

Lyme disease can cause IU. Serology should be performed if suspicion is high on the basis of exposure or review of systems, which include erythema migrans–like rash, cardiac conduction defects, and facial or other neuropathy or radiculopathy.

Cat-scratch disease: Infection with *Bartonella henselae* usually causes less vitritis and more retinal vasculitis than IU.

The retinal vasculitis of Wegener's granulomatosis, Behçet's syndrome, or inflammatory bowel disease can involve significant vitritis but no snowbank or snowballs.

Large-cell lymphoma occurs in older patients and must be ruled out by imaging and/or lumbar puncture or by vitreous biopsy in patients who are over 40 years old. Vitreous membranes that stimulate snowbanks occur.

BILATERAL CONDITIONS

Senile vitritis is idiopathic vitritis of older patients. Affected eyes have no retinal vasculitis, no snowbank, and few snowballs but may have CME. This is a diagnosis of exclusion.

Amyloidosis can cause vitropathy/vitritis but not the associated snowbank, vasculitis, or CME.

Whipple's disease can present as IU, but no snowballs are observed.

---

latation. More than three to four total clock hours of posterior synechiae challenges the diagnosis of IU.

Snowbank formation and its accompanying neovascularization can cause peripheral retinal perturbation. Subretinal exudation with serous retinal detachment adjacent to the snowbank is relatively uncommon. Retinal traction can lead to retinal tears and rhegmatogenous retinal detachment or to peripheral retinoschisis. Rarely, retinal traction can be severe and result in proliferative vitreoretinopathy or cyclitic membrane formation. Also, rarely, vitreous hemorrhage can cause massive proliferative vitreoretinopathy that results in retinal detachment.

DIAGNOSIS

The diagnosis of IU is clinical. Tests should include a complete blood count to look for significant white blood cell abnormalities (as in a malignant masquerade syndrome), syphilis serology, and a chest radiograph to screen for sarcoidosis. Review of systems may point to further tests, such as magnetic resonance imaging (MRI) to look for MS-related changes, Lyme disease serology, and angiotensin-converting enzyme, serum lysozyme, or gallium scan if sarcoidosis is strongly suspected. A routine MRI has been suggested by some authors for patients older than 25 because of the higher association between IU and MS in this group. Serum HTLV-1 testing should be performed in patients from endemic areas (southern Japan, Central Africa, and the

Caribbean region). In older patients who have vitritis, cranial imaging with or without lumbar puncture may help to rule out large-cell lymphoma.

Fluorescein angiography can demonstrate staining of or dye leakage from inflamed retinal vessels and often shows some late optic nerve staining if disease is active. Fluorescein angiography is helpful to uncover subtle CME; it shows a classical petaloid leakage with significant CME.

High-frequency ultrasound biomicroscopy may be of value in diagnosis and management, particularly in cases of hypotony or opaque media.

Both unilateral and bilateral conditions that mimic IU are listed in Box 181-1.

SYSTEMIC ASSOCIATIONS

Especially in the younger age group of patients who have pars planitis, asthma and possibly atopy are found in higher incidence than in the general population. In most cases, the associated conditions have been previously diagnosed and so lend circumstantial evidence for pars planitis.

A number of studies strengthen the association between IU and MS.[14,18] Wegemens and Breehaart[28] summarized the association between MS and both retinal vasculitis and IU. Both an increased incidence of MS in IU patients and an increased incidence of IU in MS patients have been shown. In patients who have both diseases, either one can present first. Zierhut and Foster[29] report MS diagnosis as long as 17 years before IU diagnosis in some patients but up to 7 years after in others.

Ohba et al.[26] first described IU associated with HTLV-1 infection. Nakao et al.[30] demonstrated the association of HTLV-1 and ocular disorders serologically. Mochizuki et al.[31] described the characteristic ocular findings of uveitis in patients seropositive for HTLV-1, thus strengthening the association between the diseases. The retrovirus HTLV-1 is implicated in acute T-cell leukemia and lymphoma; chronic myelopathy; tropical spastic paraparesis; lymphadenitis; opportunistic skin, lung, and gastrointestinal infection; monoclonal gammopathy; and chronic lung disease. It is transmitted by breast feeding, blood transfusion, and sexual contact and is endemic in southern Japan and among blacks in central Africa and the Caribbean region.

Patients in the age range 19–75 years have been diagnosed with HTLV-1–associated IU. This group overlaps with the second age peak of incidence of pars planitis but extends to older patients. Other ocular associations with HTLV-1 include Graves' disease, Sjögren's syndrome, anterior uveitis, and retinal pigment epithelial degeneration.

PATHOLOGY

Histopathologic findings in IU included fibrovascular proliferation and lymphocytic infiltration of the vitreous base, perivasculitis of peripheral retinal vessels, and peripheral choroidal lymphocytic infiltration.[32] Vitrectomy specimens showed B lymphocytes and a smaller number of T lymphocytes along with phagocytic cells (some multinucleated) and calcified debris. Electron microscopic ultrastructural evaluation of the snowbank in an evisceration specimen showed collapsed and condensed vitreous, fibrous astrocytes, fibroglial membranes with collagen production, and nonpigmented epithelial cell inclusions. Immunopathology performed on an eye from a family with two affected members further defined these pathological changes.[33] It showed the snowbank to consist mainly of glial elements, with Muller cells being the predominant cell type. The inflammatory cell infiltrate was mostly T lymphocytes with a CD-4$^+$/CD-8$^+$ ratio of 10:1.

TREATMENT

The treatment goal in IU is to eliminate or diminish long-term visual loss. As IU is a chronic inflammatory disease, treatment is not aimed at elimination of all inflammation but at the amelioration of vision-threatening complications. As CME is the major sight-threatening complication of pars planitis, most treatment focuses on the elimination of CME.

Topical corticosteroids should be used for significant anterior chamber reaction, with posterior synechia or endotheliopathy, and for patients who have symptoms of anterior uveitis.

Kaplan[34] outlined a four-step approach to treatment of vision loss secondary to pars planitis. Originally, Kaplan recommended that treatment be instituted when vision drops to 20/40 (6/12). Although most clinicians generally follow the four-step approach, many do not wait to treat CME until visual acuity drops to 20/40 (6/12) but institute treatment for CME with any decreased vision that lasts 1–2 months. Step 1 entails the use of oral corticosteroids or periocular corticosteroid injections. Patient, family, and treating physician must determine the optimal route of corticosteroid administration for each patient. Periocular corticosteroid injections have the advantage of causing minimal systemic corticosteroid complications.[35] Posterior sub-Tenon's corticosteroid injections are given usually every 6–8 weeks until resolution of CME or return of 20/20 (6/6) visual acuity. The author prefers triamcinolone because of its small particle size and the lack of a carrier vehicle (which can cause orbital inflammation). Another benefit of triamcinolone is that it is well tolerated in the vitreous cavity, whereas the vehicle of the methylprednisolone acetate depot preparation causes severe retinal and reti-

nal pigment epithelium scarring and atrophy intravitreally (P. L. Zimmerman et al., unpublished data). Ocular perforation is a risk of periocular injections. Corticosteroid glaucoma is another complication of posterior sub-Tenon's injection, which it has in common with oral or topical corticosteroids.

Oral corticosteroids in doses up to 1.0mg/kg are given either divided or in a single daily dose. They are tapered over 6–12 weeks depending on the response. Complications of oral corticosteroid use include iatrogenic Cushing's syndrome; iatrogenic diabetes mellitus; gastrointestinal upset or ulceration; mood swings, irritability, or other reversible psychiatric difficulties; insomnia; weight gain; hypertension; congestive heart failure; muscle weakness; osteoporosis; growth suppression in children; and skin changes such as acne.

All corticosteroid treatment carries the potential for ocular complications of cataract and glaucoma, which must be discussed with the patient and family. Increased intraocular pressure is usually easily managed with topical therapy, but trabeculectomy with an antimetabolite may be necessary if a long-term or difficult-to-control pressure increase is present.

When corticosteroids fail to eliminate inflammation and CME, most clinicians apply cryotherapy, laser treatment, or both to the snowbank, step 2 in Kaplan's scheme. Aaberg et al.[36] showed decreased CME and increased visual acuity with cryotherapy for patients who have IU in whom corticosteroid treatment had failed. Peripheral laser photocoagulation has also been shown to be effective, causing a significant decrease in the use of corticosteroids and the regression of vitreous base neovascularization.[37]

Step 3 consists of pars plana vitrectomy[38] (PPV), which has the theoretical benefit of removing vitreous antigens, inflammatory cells, and inflammatory mediators. It physically removes vitreous opacities and can eliminate vitreous traction, which may play a role in CME and which can cause peripheral retinal abnormalities such as serous, traction, or rhegmatogenous retinal detachment.

Step 4 involves immunosuppressive treatment. Such therapy has been shown to be effective in patients who have severe uncontrolled disease or who are corticosteroid intolerant and do not respond to other treatment modalities. Methotrexate, azathioprine, chlorambucil, cyclophosphamide, and cyclosporin A have all shown good results in small case reports. Newer agents such as tacrolimus, etanercept, infliximab, and mycophenolate mofetil have been used successfully and may prove useful in selected cases. Combination therapy (prednisone plus immunosuppressives, or two or three different immunosuppressives) can be used for severe cases. All immunosuppressive medications have significant systemic side effects, and their use should be monitored by a physician experienced in evaluating and dealing with these complications.

Although the four-step approach is still the accepted approach to treatment, other approaches are also being used. Often, with cases of mild CME and mild to moderate vision loss, oral nonsteroidal anti-inflammatory drugs have been used successfully. With severe inflammation and CME, intravitreal triamcinolone (0.1ml, 4mg) has been shown to be effective, and its use is becoming more common. Another potentially beneficial therapy is the use of the phenomenon of oral tolerance, which appeared effective in animal studies and is currently undergoing human trial.[39]

Treatment of inflammatory and/or corticosteroid cataract in IU has progressed impressively over the past 15 years. Most surgeons follow the guidelines outlined by Foster et al.[40] for cataract extraction in uveitis patients, namely that eyes are free of active inflammation for 3 months or more preoperatively. Systemic or injected corticosteroid as well as topical corticosteroids are used preoperatively, and both are tapered slowly postoperatively as clinically indicated.

In the past, recommendations have been for extracapsular surgery without intraocular lens (IOL) implantation. Reports of

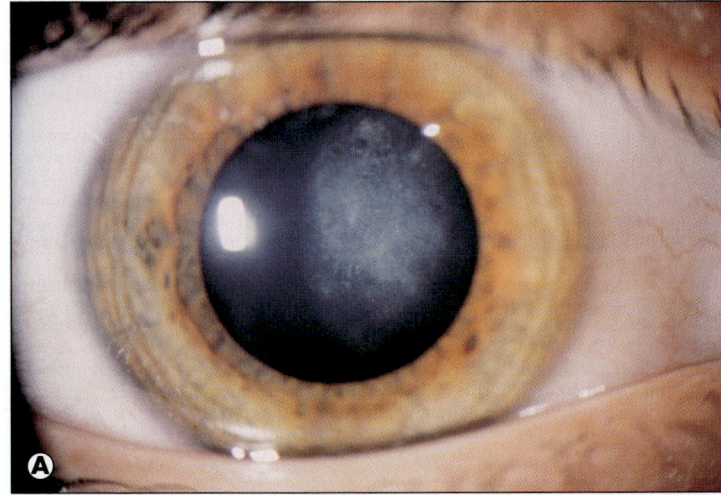

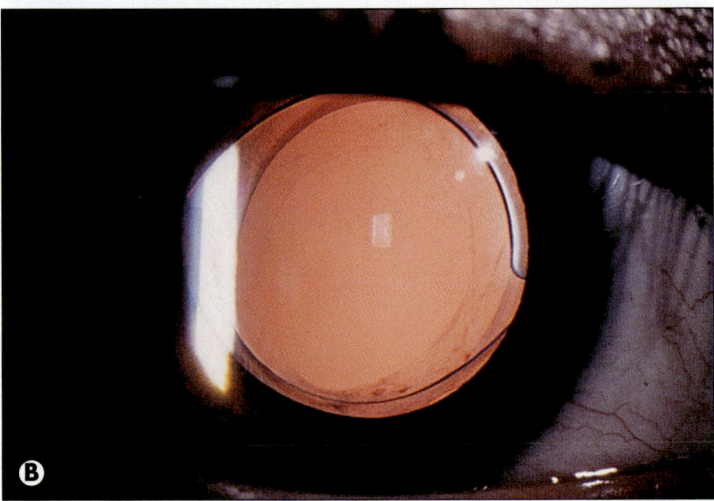

FIG. 181-5 ▌ **Posterior subcapsular cataract secondary to intermediate uveitis.** **A,** Preoperative view. **B,** Postoperative view following phacoemulsification of cataract, IOL implantation, pars plana vitrectomy, and posterior capsulectomy.

combined vitrectomy-lensectomy surgery have been generally favorable. Michelson et al.[41] reported extracapsular cataract extraction (ECCE) and IOL implantation with pars planitis vitrectomy in 15 eyes, 60% of which had 20/40 (6/12) postoperative vision. Kauffman and Foster[42] reported 14 eyes with ECCE or phacoemulsification and IOL, 13 of which improved postoperatively and 11 of which had postoperative vision of 20/40 (6/12) or better. Six of these cases had concomitant PPV. The author's (Zimmerman) personal approach is to use phacoemulsification with an all-polymethyl methacrylate (PMMA) IOL, close the wound, and then perform a PPV and a posterior capsulectomy (PC). We have performed phacoemulsification (Fig. 181-5), IOL, and PPV-PC in 12 eyes with IU. With follow-up of 6 to 58 months (average 38 months), 10 of the 12 eyes have vision of at least 20/40 (6/12) and 7 of the 12 at least 20/25 (6/7.5). One complicated retinal detachment required silicone oil with a best-corrected visual acuity of 20/60 (6/18). This procedure has been successful—all the patients show improved vision and most show significant long-term diminution of inflammation.

Regardless of therapy, the vision of IU patients usually improves slowly. Treatment failure should not be assumed at any step without at least 3–6 months of a given treatment. Beware of treatment complications, which may necessitate treatment change even if a good therapeutic response has been achieved.

COURSE AND OUTCOME

Several studies have attempted to assess the course and outcome of patients who have IU. Henderley et al.[19] stress the relationship

between presence of snowbanks and development of CME in pars planitis.

Brockhurst et al.[22] divided patients into three major categories: 46% of patients had a chronic smoldering course, 28% a benign subsiding course, and 26% complications such as cyclitic membrane formation, vascular occlusion, and retinal detachment. Smith et al.,[21] in their large series, reported 59% of patients with a prolonged disease course, 31% showing a smoldering course with exacerbations and remissions, and 10% having a self-limited course.

In the authors' experience, pars planitis tends to follow a prolonged exacerbating-remitting course. Most patients have inflammation for at least 3 years. The disease tends to "burn out" after 5–15 years and, if the macula can be kept healthy, most eyes ultimately achieve good vision. Of the 173 patients of Smith et al. with at least 4 years' follow-up, 73% had vision of at least 20/50 (6/21)[21]; 67% of the 42 patients of Hirokawa et al., again with at least 4 years' follow-up, had vision of at least 20/50 (6/21)[43]; and 74% of the 43 patients of Chester et al. had vision of at least 20/30 (6/9) after at least 3 years' follow-up.[44] Although most patients do achieve good vision, it is worth noting that children, when considered as a separate group, have worse visual acuity both at initial diagnosis and at follow-up than adults.[45]

Most reports of the new disease entity HTLV-1–associated IU detail good treatment response to oral and topical corticosteroids. Long-term disease course and visual results have not been reported.

REFERENCES

1. Fuchs E. Textbook of ophthalmology. Duane A, trans. Philadelphia: JB Lippincott; 1903.
2. Schepens CL. Examination of the ora serrata region: its clinical significance. International Congress of Ophthalmology, XVI Concilium Ophthalmologicum 1950, Britannica Acta. London: British Medical Association; 1951:1384–93.
3. Kimura SJ, Hogan MJ. Chronic cyclitis. Arch Ophthalmol. 1964;71:193–201.
4. Welch RB, Maumenee AE, Whalen HE. Peripheral posterior segment inflammation, vitreous opacities, and edema of the posterior pole. Arch Ophthalmol. 1960;64:540–9.
5. Henderley DE, Genstler AJ, Smith RE, Rao NA. Changing patterns of uveitis. Am J Ophthalmol. 1987;103:131–6.
6. Wakefield D, Dunlop I, McCluskey PJ, Penny R. Uveitis: aetiology and disease associations in an Australian population. Aust N Z J Ophthalmol. 1986;14:181–7.
7. Tran VT, Auer C, Guex-Crosier V, et al. Epidemiology of uveitis in Switzerland. Ocul Immunol Inflamm. 1994;2:169–76.
8. Pivetti-Pezzi P, Accoriniti M, La Cava M, et al. Endogenous uveitis: an analysis of 1,417 cases. Ophthalmologica. 1996;210:234–8.
9. Merrill PT, Kim J, Cox TA, et al. Uveitis in the southeastern United States. Curr Eye Res. 1997;16:865–74.
10. Cunningham ET. Uveitis in children. Ocul Immunol Inflamm. 2000;8:251–61.
11. Mochizuki M, Watanabe T, Yamaguchi K, et al. Uveitis associated with human T-cell lymphotropic virus type I. Am J Ophthalmol. 1992;114:123–9.
12. Yoshimura K, Mochizuki M, Araki S, et al. Clinical and immunological features of human T-cell lymphotropic virus type I uveitis. Am J Ophthalmol. 1993;116:156–63.
13. Sagawa K, Mochizuki M, Masuoka K, et al. Immunopathogenical mechanisms of human T-cell lymphotropic virus type I (HTLV-I) uveitis. Detection of HTLV-I-infected T-cells in the eye and their constitutive cytokine production. J Clin Invest. 1995;95:852–74.
14. Davis JL, Mittal KK, Nussenblatt RB. HLA in intermediate uveitis. Dev Ophthalmol. 1992;23:35–7.
15. Malinowski SM, Pulido JS, Goeken NE, et al. The association of HLA-B8, B51, DR2, and multiple sclerosis in pars planitis. Ophthalmology. 1993;100:1199–205.
16. Tang WM, Pulido JS, Eckels DD, et al. The association of HLA-DR15 and intermediate uveitis. Am J Ophthalmol. 1997;123:70–5.
17. Oruc S, Duffy BF, Mohanakumar T, Kaplan HJ. The association of HLA class II with pars planitis. Am J Ophthalmol. 2001;131:657–9.
18. Raja SC, Jabs DA, Dunn JP, et al. Pars planitis: clinical features and class II HLA associations. Ophthalmology. 1999;106:594–9.
19. Henderley DE, Genstler AJ, Rao NA, Smith RE. Pars planitis. Trans Ophthalmol Soc UK. 1986;105:227–32.
20. Malinowski SM, Pulido JS, Folk JC. Long-term visual outcome and complications associated with pars planitis. Ophthalmology. 1993;100:818–25.
21. Smith RE, Godfrey WA, Kimura ST. Chronic cyclitis I course and visual prognosis. Trans Am Acad Ophthalmol Otolaryngol. 1973;77:760–8.
22. Brockhurst RJ, Schepens CL, Okamura ID. Uveitis II: peripheral uveitis: clinical description, complications and differential diagnosis. Am J Ophthalmol. 1960;49:1257–66.
23. Felder KS, Brockhurst PJ. Neovascular fundus abnormalities in peripheral uveitis. Arch Ophthalmol. 1982;100:750–4.
24. Lauer AK, Smith JR, Robertson JE, Rosenbaum JT. Vitreous hemorrhage is a common complication of pediatric pars planitis. Ophthalmology. 2002;109:95–8.
25. Nakao K, Ohba N. Clinical features of HTLV-1 associated uveitis. Br J Ophthalmol. 1993;77:274–9.

26. Ohba N, Matsumoto M, Sameshima M, *et al.* Ocular manifestations in patients infected with human T-lymphotropic virus type I. Jpn J Ophthalmol. 1989;33:1–12.
27. Khodadoust AA, Karnama V, Stoessel KM, Puklin JE. Pars planitis and autoimmune endotheliopathy. Am J Ophthalmol. 1986;102:633–9.
28. Wegemens MAJ, Breehaart AC. Association between intermediate uveitis and multiple sclerosis. Dev Ophthalmol. 1992;23:99–105.
29. Zierhut M, Foster CS. Multiple sclerosis, sarcoidosis and other diseases in patients with pars planitis. Dev Ophthalmol. 1992;23:41–7.
30. Nakao K, Matsumoto M, Ohba N. Seroprevalence of antibodies to HTLV-1 in patients with ocular disorders. Br J Ophthalmol. 1993;77:274–9.
31. Mochizuki M, Tajima K, Watanabe T, Yamaguchi K. Human T-lymphotropic virus type I uveitis. Br J Ophthalmol. 1994;78:149–54.
32. Yoser SL, Forster DJ, Rao NA. Pathology of intermediate uveitis. Dev Ophthalmol. 1992;23:67–70.
33. Wetzilg RP, Chan CC, Nussenblatt RB, *et al.* Clinical and immunopathological studies of pars planitis in a family. Br J Ophthalmol. 1988;72:5–10.
34. Kaplan HJ. Intermediate uveitis (pars planitis, chronic cyclitis): a four-step approach to treatment. In: Saari KM, ed. Uveitis update. Amsterdam: Excerpta Medica; 1984:169–72.
35. Smith RE, Nozik RA. Uveitis: a clinical approach to diagnosis and management, 2nd ed. Baltimore: Williams & Wilkins; 1989:63–6.
36. Aaberg TM, Cesarz TJ, Flochenger RR. Treatment of peripheral uveoretinitis by cryotherapy. Am J Ophthalmol. 1973;75:685–9.
37. Pulido JS, Mieler WF, Walton D, *et al.* Results of peripheral laser photocoagulation in pars planitis. Trans Am Ophthalmol Soc. 1998;96:127–37.
38. Meiler WF, Aaberg TM. Vitreous surgery in the management of peripheral uveitis. Dev Ophthalmol. 1992;23:239–50.
39. Nussenblatt RB, Whitcup SM, de Smet MD, *et al.* Intraocular inflammatory disease (uveitis) and the use of oral tolerance: a status report. Ann N Y Acad Sci. 1996;13:325–37.
40. Foster CS, Fong LP, Singh G. Cataract surgery and intraocular lens implantation in patients with uveitis. Ophthalmology. 1989;96:281–8.
41. Michelson B, Friedlander MH, Nozik RA. Lens implant surgery in pars planitis. Ophthalmology. 1990;97:1023–6.
42. Kauffman AH, Foster CS. Cataract extraction in patients with pars planitis. Ophthalmology. 1993;100:1210–17.
43. Hirokawa H, Takahashi M, Tremmpe CL. Vitreous changes in peripheral uveitis. Arch Ophthalmol. 1985;103:1704–7.
44. Chester GH, Black RK, Cleary PE. Inflammation in the region of the vitreous base. Trans Ophthalmol Soc UK. 1976;96:151–7.
45. Guest S, Funkhouser E, Lightman S. Pars planitis: a comparison of childhood onset and adult onset disease. Clin Exp Ophthalmol. 2001;29:81–4.

182 Posterior Uveitis of Unknown Cause

RAMANA S. MOORTHY • LEE M. JAMPOL

DEFINITION
- Inflammatory disorders of unknown cause that involve the outer retina, retinal pigment epithelium, or choroid, or a combination, in one or both eyes of patients in their second to sixth decades of life.

KEY FEATURES
- Unknown cause with negative serological evaluation.
- White or yellow spots in the posterior segment.

ASSOCIATED FEATURES
- Unilateral or bilateral, depending on the disease.
- Second to sixth decades of life.
- Variable inflammatory cells in the anterior chamber and vitreous humor, depending on the disease.
- Usually self-limited course but variable prognosis, depending on the disease.

FIG. 182-1 ▮▮ **Fundus view of the right eye of a 17-year-old man who has acute posterior multifocal placoid pigment epitheliopathy.** Numerous creamy, white-yellow, placoid lesions are seen in the posterior pole. Note the pigmenting lesion in the inferior macula that has started to heal.

INTRODUCTION

Several disorders occur that affect the retina and choroid. They are multifocal in nature, are associated with whitening in the retina, typically affect patients between the second and sixth decades of life, and despite exhaustive evaluation, have no known cause. These entities carry the label *white spot syndromes* or *inflammatory multifocal chorioretinopathies*. The *latter*, more descriptive, term is preferred. These entities include acute posterior multifocal placoid pigment epitheliopathy (APMPPE), multiple evanescent white dot syndrome (MEWDS), birdshot chorioretinopathy, serpiginous choroiditis, multifocal choroiditis and panuveitis, subretinal fibrosis and uveitis, punctate inner choroidopathy, acute macular neuroretinopathy, acute retinal pigment epitheliitis, unilateral acute idiopathic maculopathy, acute zonal occult outer retinopathy (AZOOR) and, more recently, relentless placoid chorioretinitis and unifocal helioid choroiditis. All affect the retina, retinal pigment epithelium (RPE), or choroid. They rarely have signs of anterior uveitis, yet these entities are important causes of decreased vision in young patients. Although some of these disorders are self-limited and have good visual outcomes, others are associated with serious retinal and choroidal sequelae and can result in visual loss. In the future, these entities may be proven to be autoimmune or infectious or both.

ACUTE POSTERIOR MULTIFOCAL PLACOID PIGMENT EPITHELIOPATHY

EPIDEMIOLOGY AND PATHOGENESIS

APMPPE is an inflammatory disease, usually bilateral, that affects the choriocapillaris, RPE, and outer retina of otherwise healthy young adults in the second and third decades of life.

Men and women are affected equally. The disease may be preceded by a viral prodrome.[1]

OCULAR MANIFESTATIONS

After a short viral prodrome, symptoms of mild myelomeningeal encephalitis, namely meningismus, headaches, and transient hearing loss, may develop.[2–4] Patients subsequently develop a sudden, painless loss of vision in one or, more typically, both eyes.[1]

Ocular examination usually shows no evidence of anterior uveitis. Minimal to no vitreous cells occur.[1,5] Yellow, creamy colored, flat-to-placoid lesions of variable size are seen and involve mostly the posterior pole (Fig. 182-1).[1,5] Episcleritis, disc hyperemia and, rarely, exudative neurosensory retinal detachment have been reported.[6,7]

DIAGNOSIS

The characteristic choroidal lesions and fluorescein angiographic pattern are usually sufficient to make the diagnosis of APMPPE. The absence of substantial anterior chamber or vitreous inflammation in a young, healthy patient who has a viral prodrome with typical fundus lesions is highly suggestive of APMPPE. Fluorescein angiography shows early hypofluorescence of these white placoid lesions with late staining of these same lesions (Figs. 182-2 and 182-3).[1] Indocyanine green angiography also shows hypofluorescent lesions. Laboratory evaluation of these patients is usually unrewarding (except for the findings of protein and cells in the spinal fluid, and rare hematuria) and usually not necessary.

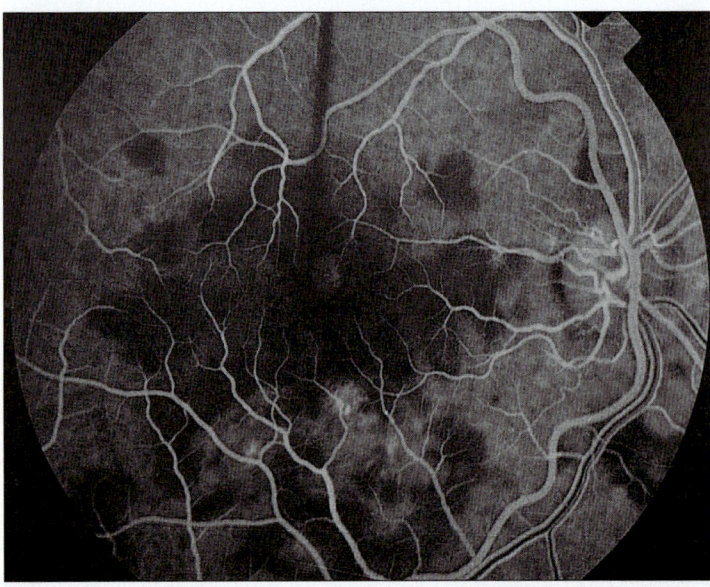

FIG. 182-2 ■ **Hypofluorescence of acute lesions and early hyperfluorescence of healing lesions.** Laminar, venous phase fluorescein angiogram of the right eye of the patient shown in Figure 182-1.

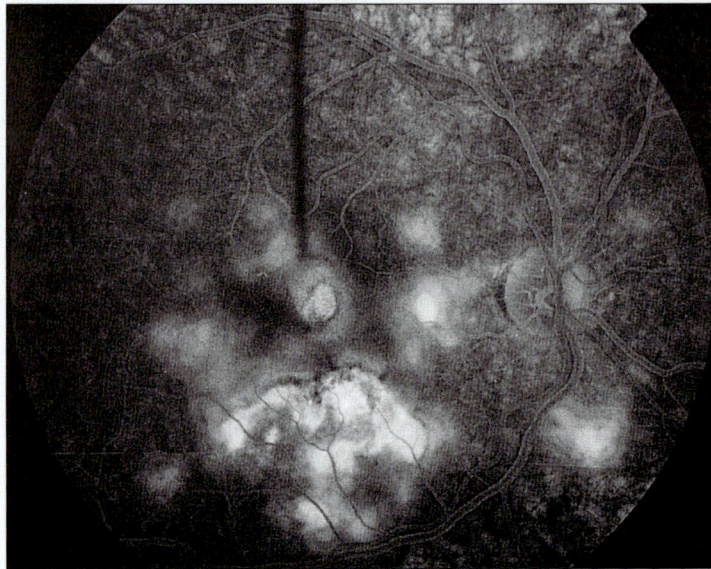

FIG. 182-3 ■ **Late hyperfluorescence of both acute and healing lesions.** Late arteriovenous phase fluorescein angiogram of the same eye as shown in Figures 182-1 and 182-2.

DIFFERENTIAL DIAGNOSIS

The differential diagnosis of APMPPE is given in Box 182-1. The creamy lesions of APMPPE are unique but occasionally may be confused with metastatic tumors, viral retinitis, and toxoplasma retinochoroiditis. In APMPPE, however, the creamy lesions are flat and are not associated with significant vitreitis. Healed APMPPE may leave behind variable amounts of pigmentary changes in the posterior pole, which can be difficult to differentiate from other inflammatory conditions.

SYSTEMIC ASSOCIATIONS

Cerebral vasculitis and cerebrospinal fluid pleocytosis have been reported in patients who have APMPPE.[2-5] Rarely this may be fatal. Acute nephritis occurred concurrently with APMPPE in one patient.[8] It is thought that one or more viruses may be the causative agents of APMPPE.[1] Serological evidence of adenovirus type 5 infection has been documented with APMPPE.[9]

PATHOLOGY

The histopathology of eyes that have APMPPE has not been studied. However, because the placoid lesions result in variable retinal pigment epithelial alterations with usually good visual acuity, it is thought that lesions occur either at the level of the RPE or perhaps the choriocapillaris.

TREATMENT

Usually no treatment is necessary; the disease tends to be self-limited. Some ophthalmologists use systemic corticosteroids, although no convincing evidence exists that corticosteroids speed visual recovery or improve visual outcome.

COURSE AND OUTCOMES

Most patients who have APMPPE have a self-limited course of 2–6 weeks. Visual acuity is usually diminished during the early part of the disease and may vary from 20/20 (6/6) to 20/400 (6/120), depending on the location of the placoid lesions. In most patients vision improves to near-normal levels during the first 2–3 weeks after the onset of symptoms. Patients, however, may continue to complain of difficulty with reading or of sco-

tomas in the central visual field. The placoid lesions resolve over a period of 2–6 weeks. Significant macular retinal pigment epithelial mottling and alterations remain after the resolution of these placoid lesions.[1] Rare cases of persistent, chronic, or recurrent APMPPE have been reported in which severe retinal pigment epithelial alterations may occur.[10] This can result in severe visual loss. Choroidal neovascularization is an uncommon complication of APMPPE but has been reported.[11] Disruption of Bruch's membrane and the choriocapillaris probably occurs less frequently in APMPPE than with serpiginous choroidopathy.

MULTIPLE, EVANESCENT, WHITE DOT SYNDROME

EPIDEMIOLOGY AND PATHOGENESIS

MEWDS is an inflammatory chorioretinopathy that affects mainly young, healthy women in the second to fifth decades of life. A flu-like illness is present in about one half of the patients.[12]

OCULAR MANIFESTATIONS

Patients who have MEWDS have acute, unilateral, painless visual loss.[12] Bilateral cases have been reported, but they tend to be asymmetrical.[13] Patients often complain of a scotoma and associated shimmering photopsias, often in the temporal visual field. Ocular findings include a variable amount of vitreitis, op-

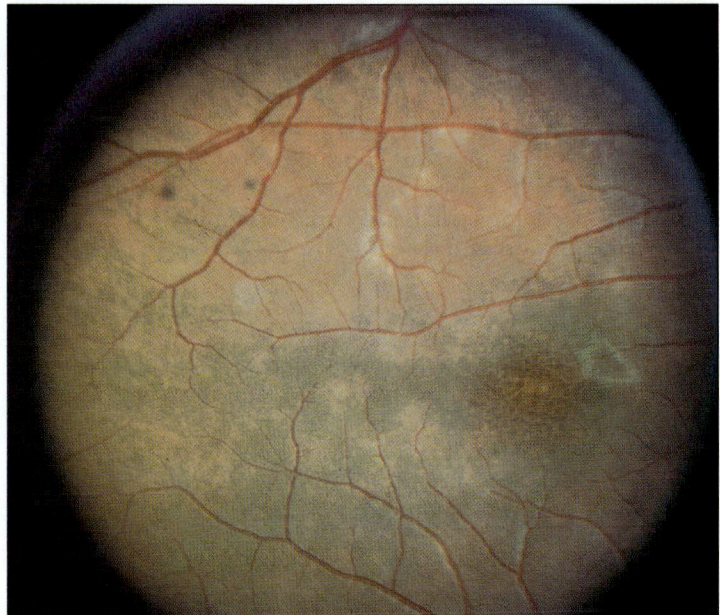

FIG. 182-4 ▪ Right eye of a woman who has multiple, evanescent, white dot syndrome. Note multiple white spots throughout posterior pole and granular appearance to fovea.

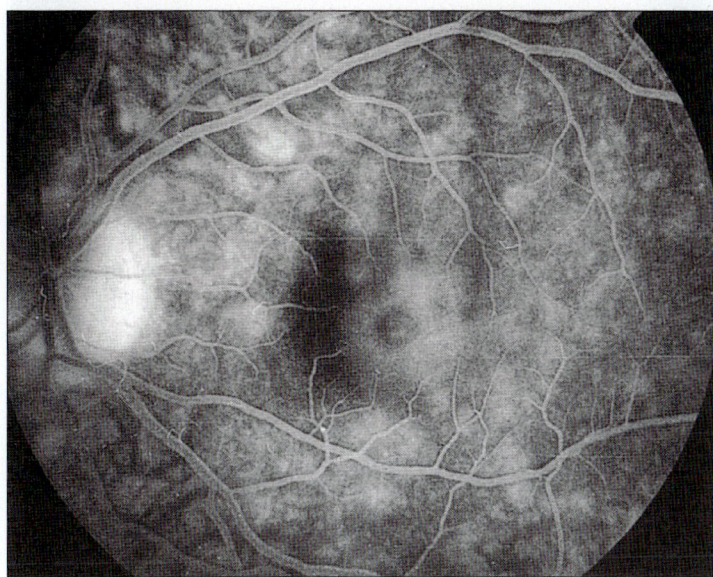

FIG. 182-5 ▪ Disc hyperfluorescence and hyperfluorescence of the corresponding white spots in the posterior pole in multiple, evanescent, white dot syndrome.

tic disc edema and, characteristically, multiple white spots at the level of the RPE or deep retina in the posterior pole (Fig. 182-4). Retinal vascular sheathing may be present also. A characteristic granular appearance to the fovea is present acutely, and the fovea usually does not return to a normal appearance (see Fig. 182-4).[12]

DIAGNOSIS

Diagnosis is made by the typical ocular manifestations of the disease. Visual field testing may reveal enlargement of the blind spot.[12,14] Fluorescein angiography may reveal leakage from disc capillaries and late punctate staining of the RPE, sometimes in the shape of a wreath (Fig. 182-5).[12,14] Indocyanine green angiography demonstrates multiple hypofluorescent areas in the posterior pole. These hypofluorescent areas suggest that MEWDS affects the outer retina or RPE (blockage), or the underlying choroid (nonperfusion).[15] Electrophysiological studies may reveal a profoundly decreased a-wave amplitude on the electroretinogram and early receptor potential amplitudes in the acute phase of the disease, which suggests widespread photoreceptor dysfunction.[16] During the recovery phases, these amplitudes return to normal. In addition, prolonged regeneration kinetics of the RPE also are present in the acute phases of the disorder.[16] The exact mechanisms of visual loss in MEWDS are not understood well but may represent photoreceptor, RPE, and optic nerve dysfunction.

DIFFERENTIAL DIAGNOSIS

Acute idiopathic blind spot enlargement may occur alone or with MEWDS, multifocal choroiditis, or acute macular neuroretinopathy. It is thought that acute idiopathic blind spot enlargement may be either a common factor that links all of these disorders or part of the spectrum of diseases that include all of these inflammatory chorioretinopathies (Box 182-2).[17-19] Systemically, viral prodrome may occur in up to 50% of patients.[12]

COURSE AND OUTCOMES

Because MEWDS has a self-limited course, no specific treatment is necessary.[12] The white dots fade and disc edema gradually resolves, usually within 2–6 weeks of the onset of symptoms and

BOX 182-2

Differential Diagnosis of Multiple, Evanescent, White Dot Syndrome

Acute posterior multifocal placoid pigment epitheliopathy
Acute macular neuroretinopathy
Multifocal choroiditis
Birdshot retinochoroidopathy
Diffuse unilateral subacute neuroretinitis
Lymphoma
Sarcoidosis

ocular findings. Visual acuity gradually returns to baseline levels. The temporal scotoma and photopsias may take considerably longer to resolve (several months).[12] Recurrences are uncommon but have been reported.[13] Visual prognosis is good even among patients who have recurrences. An uncommon association of MEWDS with acute macular neuroretinopathy has been described.[20] Rare instances of choroidal neovascularization following MEWDS have been reported,[21] which may be confused with idiopathic choroidal neovascularization, because the white dots are no longer present.[20]

SERPIGINOUS CHOROIDITIS

EPIDEMIOLOGY

Serpiginous choroiditis has been described under many different names, including helicoid and geographical choroidopathy; current understanding of this disease is limited. The condition affects healthy patients from the second to seventh decades of life. Men and women are affected equally.[22-24]

OCULAR MANIFESTATIONS

Patients who have serpiginous choroiditis typically experience paracentral or central scotomata with vision loss. Some lesions may be asymptomatic. Ocular examination may reveal some inflammatory response in the anterior chamber or vitreous humor.[22-25] The typical lesions begin either in the peripapillary region or macula and eventually affect both eyes.

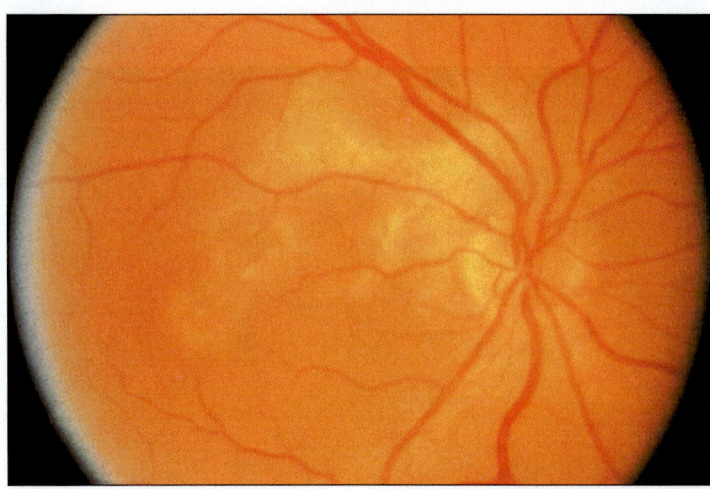

FIG. 182-6 ■ **Fundus view of the right eye of a 57-year-old woman who has early serpiginous choroiditis.** A peripapillary serpentine lesion extends into the fovea. Visual acuity is 20/60 (6/18).

BOX 182-3

Differential Diagnosis of Serpiginous Choroiditis

Acute posterior multifocal placoid pigment epitheliopathy
Relentless placoid chorioretinitis
Multifocal choroiditis and uveitis
Birdshot retinochoroidopathy
Ocular histoplasmosis syndrome

New lesions usually appear at the edges of older ones. The disease has a progressive, step-wise course. New lesions appear slightly yellow to gray in color, and the overlying retina may be thickened. Often these lesions progress in a centripetal, helicoid, or serpentine-like fashion from the peripapillary area or macula into the remainder of the posterior pole (Fig. 182-6).[23,24] With time these lesions become atrophic, with disappearance of the RPE, choriocapillaris, and choroid.[26] In patients who have macular serpiginous choroiditis, the initial lesions are seen in the macula with no initial peripapillary activity.[27] Subretinal hemorrhage and serous retinal detachment as a result of choroidal neovascularization can occur in eyes with serpiginous choroiditis.[22,28]

DIAGNOSIS

Diagnosis is established by the typical clinical appearance of the lesions. Fluorescein angiography demonstrates early hypofluorescence and late hyperfluorescence of active lesions. Indocyanine green angiography also shows hypofluorescent active lesions. Atrophic lesions show diffuse loss of pigment, choroidal vessels, and late staining on fluorescein angiography. Retinal vascular staining also may occur adjacent to active lesions. Associated choroidal neovascularization shows late leakage and often arises from the borders of old scars.[28]

Laboratory evaluation of these patients is invariably unrewarding. An association of serpiginous choroiditis and tuberculosis has been suggested. However, treatment with antimicrobial agents has made no difference to the course of the disease in these patients.[26]

DIFFERENTIAL DIAGNOSIS

The differential diagnosis of serpiginous choroiditis is given in Box 182-3. The peripapillary scarring seen in serpiginous choroiditis may be difficult to differentiate from inactive multifocal choroiditis and uveitis syndrome and ocular histoplasmo-

sis syndrome. However, serpentine centripetal progression is quite characteristic of serpiginous choroiditis.

PATHOLOGY

The few eyes with serpiginous choroiditis that have been studied histopathologically showed extensive loss of RPE, with destruction of the overlying retina and lymphocytic infiltration of the choriocapillaris and other areas of the choroid.[29]

TREATMENT

The inflammatory nature of this disorder means that systemic and periocular glucocorticoids may be of benefit. However, treatment with these medications acutely does not prevent recurrences. Recurrences may result in progressive macular involvement. Cyclosporin, azathioprine, and other cytotoxic agents also have been used to treat serpiginous choroiditis.[22,30,31] Because these medications have associated potential systemic side effects, they should be used with the assistance of a rheumatologist, internist, or oncologist. Choroidal neovascularization has been treated successfully with laser photocoagulation.[28]

COURSE AND OUTCOMES

Many cases of serpiginous choroiditis are relentlessly progressive, and foveal destruction eventually occurs. Central visual acuity is lost in 20% or more of eyes with serpiginous choroiditis.[22,24] Central visual loss also can occur from choroidal neovascularization, which carries a poor visual prognosis. Long-term immunosuppressive therapy with glucocorticoids, azathioprine, cyclophosphamide, and cyclosporin alone or in combination remains unproved as a way to prevent visual loss.[22,30]

BIRDSHOT RETINOCHOROIDOPATHY

EPIDEMIOLOGY AND PATHOGENESIS

Birdshot retinochoroidopathy also has been called vitiliginous chorioretinitis. This syndrome affects healthy patients, usually women, between the third and sixth decades of life.[32] Nearly 90% of patients who have birdshot retinochoroidopathy have positive human lymphocyte antigen A29 (HLA-A29) levels. This is the highest association of any HLA antigen with a human disease. Lymphocyte reactivity to retinal S-antigen is also present in these patients, which suggests an autoimmune pathogenesis.[33]

OCULAR MANIFESTATIONS

Patients complain of blurred vision, floaters, central and peripheral photopsias and, later, nyctalopia and color blindness.[32,34] Vitreous inflammation is present. Multifocal depigmented patches are seen throughout the posterior pole. Disc edema, narrowed retinal vessels, and cystoid macular edema (CME) are present. The creamy lesions typically are small and less than one disc diameter in size; they are scattered throughout the entire fundus, which gives the disease its characteristic name of birdshot retinochoroidopathy (Fig. 182-7). These lesions may be depigmented spots at the level of the pigment epithelium or may represent changes at the level of the photoreceptors or choroid.[32,34]

DIAGNOSIS

The diagnosis of birdshot retinochoroidopathy is based on age of onset combined with the characteristic ocular findings.[32,34] Fluorescein angiography reveals disc staining, vascular leakage, and late CME.[32,34] The hypopigmented patches usually do not

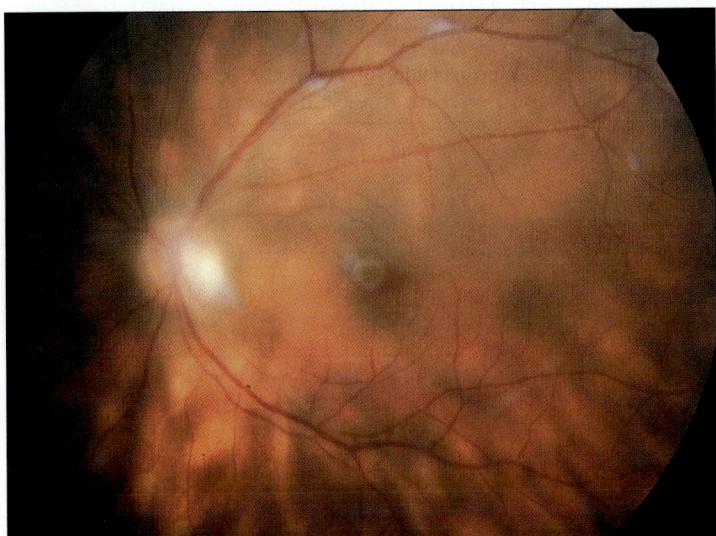

FIG. 182-7 ▮▮ Birdshot retinochoroidopathy. Note optic disc edema, vitritis, and multiple, creamy, yellow choroidal lesions in the midperiphery of the left eye.

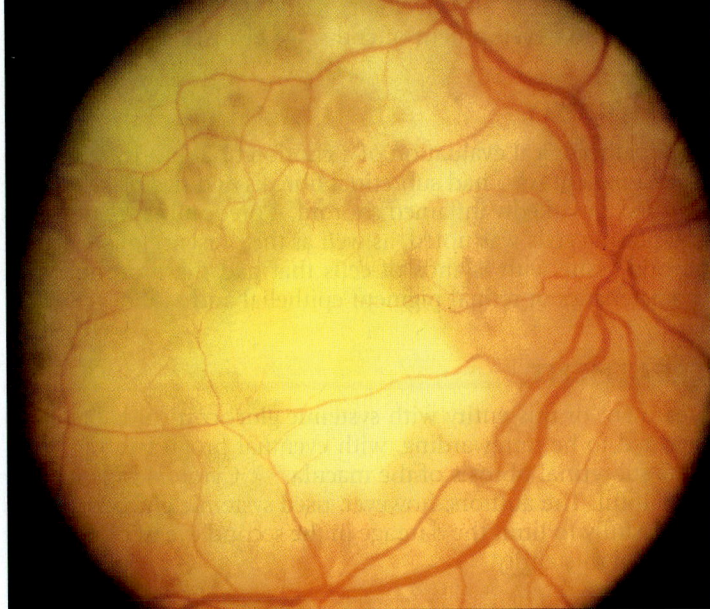

FIG. 182-8 ▮▮ Fundus view of the right eye of a patient who has progressive subretinal fibrosis and uveitis syndrome. Note the extensive submacular fibrosis.

BOX 182-4

Differential Diagnosis of Birdshot Retinochoroidopathy

Pars planitis
Chronic iridocyclitis, idiopathic
Papilledema
Intraocular lymphoma
Vogt–Koyanagi–Harada syndrome
Multiple, evanescent white dot syndrome
Ocular histoplasmosis syndrome
Sympathetic uveitis
Sarcoidosis

BOX 182-5

Differential Diagnosis of Subretinal Fibrosis

Sarcoid panuveitis
Ocular histoplasmosis syndrome
Multifocal choroiditis
Birdshot retinochoroidopathy
Toxoplasmosis

---

show any significant change in normal background choroidal fluorescence. In the late phases of the angiogram, these hypopigmented lesions do appear mildly hyperfluorescent. These patches are more prominent ophthalmoscopically than angiographically.[32,34]

Electroretinography reveals bilateral, moderately to severely depressed rod and cone function. Severe cases often demonstrate a totally extinguished electroretinogram. Electro-oculography usually is normal but can be variably subnormal in some patients.[34]

DIFFERENTIAL DIAGNOSIS

The differential diagnosis of birdshot retinochoroidopathy is given in Box 182-4. Several disorders produce multiple, creamy choroidal lesions. Few are so commonly associated with CME as birdshot retinochoroidopathy. *Pars planitis* and chronic iridocyclitis can produce CME but are not associated with choroidal lesions. Onset of vitreitis and CME in the fifth and sixth decades is quite characteristic of birdshot retinochoroidopathy.

TREATMENT

Periocular and systemic glucocorticoids have been the mainstay of therapy for patients who have birdshot retinochoroidopathy. Treatment should be considered when visual acuity drops below 20/40 (6/12) as a result of CME. However, glucocorticoids are of limited value in many patients. Vision may continue to deteriorate because of chronic CME. As a result systemic cyclosporin, azathioprine, or low-dose methotrexate may be administered judiciously, with the help of an oncologist, rheumatologist, or an internist for patients who have birdshot retinochoroidopathy and are unresponsive to glucocorticoids.

COURSE AND OUTCOME

The long-term visual prognosis for patients who have birdshot retinochoroidopathy is guarded. Retinal vascular attenuation and chorioretinal atrophy eventually occur. Chronic CME may cause permanent visual loss.[32,34]

PROGRESSIVE SUBRETINAL FIBROSIS AND UVEITIS SYNDROME

EPIDEMIOLOGY AND PATHOGENESIS

Progressive subretinal fibrosis and uveitis syndrome is an extremely rare entity that occurs primarily in young women who are in the second and third decades of life and otherwise healthy. The subretinal fibrosis and uveitis syndrome is associated with chronic vitreous inflammation and white, fibrotic subretinal lesions, which enlarge and coalesce in a progressive manner to involve most of the retina and choroid (Fig. 182-8). Diagnosis is based mainly on the characteristic ophthalmoscopic appearance.[35,36]

Ancillary testing reveals markedly decreased electroretinographic amplitudes, which confirms the diffuse retinal involvement. Laboratory evaluation is typically unrewarding.[35]

DIFFERENTIAL DIAGNOSIS

The differential diagnosis of subretinal fibrosis and uveitis is shown in Box 182-5. Sarcoidosis, ocular histoplasmosis syndrome, and toxoplasma retinochoroiditis can be differentiated by appearance, clinical course, and laboratory evaluation from subretinal fibrosis and uveitis syndrome. Often the diagnosis of subretinal fibrosis and uveitis is made only with disease progression and development of end-stage fibrosis.

PATHOLOGY

Histopathological evaluation of a chorioretinal biopsy specimen from a patient who had subretinal fibrosis and uveitis syndrome revealed a markedly inflamed choroid. A predominance of B cells and plasma cells was noted, as well as the presence of subretinal fibrotic tissue with islands of cells that had the morphological characteristics of retinal pigment epithelial and Müller cells.[37]

TREATMENT

Treatment of this entity with systemic glucocorticoids has been reported to be unrewarding, with eventual progression to complete subretinal fibrosis of the macula.[35,36] Cytotoxic agents may be helpful. The authors, however, used systemic glucocorticoids successfully to limit the damage in the second eye of one patient who had this entity.

MULTIFOCAL CHOROIDITIS AND PANUVEITIS

EPIDEMIOLOGY

Multifocal choroiditis with panuveitis is a common inflammatory disease that occurs predominantly in women between the second and sixth decades of life. Most cases are bilateral when diagnosed or become bilateral.[38,39]

OCULAR MANIFESTATIONS

Patients have decreased visual acuity in one or both eyes. Photopsias may be present, and an enlarged blind spot may be symptomatic. Most patients have a variable amount of anterior segment inflammation and vitreitis. The optic discs generally are normal, but the peripapillary RPE usually is disrupted. An area of fibrosis in the shape of a napkin holder may surround the disc. Peripapillary and macular choroidal neovascular membranes can occur.[39] Acute choroidal lesions vary in size in the range of 50–350m. They may vary in number from several to several hundred, and they can occur in linear clusters or as streak lesions.[40] Acute lesions are yellowish to gray in color and located at the level of the RPE. Older lesions appear atrophic and "punched-out," with variable amounts of pigment. Retinal pigment epithelial metaplasia with associated fibrosis may be seen.[38,39]

DIAGNOSIS

Diagnosis is made by clinical examination. The fundus examination findings are reminiscent of ocular histoplasmosis syndrome but with the presence of cells in the vitreous humor. Extensive subretinal proliferation of RPE with fibrosis or clumping is more common with multifocal choroiditis than with ocular histoplasmosis syndrome. Fluorescein angiography reveals early blockage by acute, active, yellow lesions in the choroid, with late staining of these lesions.[39] With progression and atrophy, these lesions show early hyperfluorescence which fades in the late phases of the angiogram. Peripapillary or subfoveal choroidal neovascularization may be seen. CME may be seen in the late phases of the angiogram in some patients.[38] Indocyanine green angiography shows hypofluorescent lesions that may cluster around the optic disc.

The electroretinogram is usually normal or borderline, however in severe cases it may be extinguished. The electro-oculogram is normal.[38]

Visual field testing may reveal an enlarged blind spot and, rarely, other abnormalities.

BOX 182-6

Differential Diagnosis of Multifocal Choroiditis with Panuveitis and Punctate Inner Choroidopathy

Ocular histoplasmosis syndrome
Sarcoidosis
Vogt–Koyanagi–Harada syndrome
Sympathetic uveitis
Subretinal fibrosis and uveitis syndrome
Serpiginous choroiditis
Birdshot retinochoroidopathy
Myopic degeneration maculopathy

DIFFERENTIAL DIAGNOSIS

The differential diagnosis of multifocal choroiditis with panuveitis is shown in Box 182-6. Ocular histoplasmosis and myopic degeneration are not associated with any vitreitis, unlike multifocal choroiditis.[40a] Other disorders may be much more difficult to differentiate from multifocal choroiditis, often a diagnosis of exclusion.[40a]

SYSTEMIC ASSOCIATIONS

An association between multifocal choroiditis and Epstein–Barr virus systemic infection has been suggested.[41] Immunoglobulin M antibodies directed against the viral capsid antigen or the Epstein–Barr early antigen were present in ten patients in one series—similar antibodies were not present in controls. A second investigation could not confirm this.[42] It has been suggested that Epstein–Barr virus triggers an immune response that results in persistent intraocular inflammation. However, the antibodies to viral capsid antigen and Epstein–Barr early antigen may be present in normal individuals who do not have multifocal choroiditis.[41] Some patients who have multifocal choroiditis also have known sarcoidosis or later are diagnosed with sarcoidosis. These cases may be indistinguishable from the group with idiopathic etiology.

TREATMENT

Treatment of multifocal choroiditis with panuveitis is with topical, periocular, or systemic glucocorticoids, which may be used to reduce anterior segment and vitreous inflammatory activity, macular detachment, or edema. Choroidal neovascularization may be treated with laser photocoagulation, photodynamic therapy, or glucocorticoid therapy (which appears to be of some value), although spontaneous involution of choroidal neovascularization is not uncommon. Laser photocoagulation may be associated with an increase in inflammatory response, which in itself may be the underlying initiator of choroidal neovascularization.[38,39] Subfoveal choroidal neovascular membranes may be removed surgically. The value of this intervention for ocular histoplasmosis and idiopathic choroidal neovascularization is being investigated in a randomized trial.

COURSE AND OUTCOMES

Multifocal choroiditis and panuveitis waxes and wanes, but progressive loss of vision may take place. Glucocorticoids alone may become insufficient to control intraocular inflammation. Macular disciform scarring may occur. Severe cases of subretinal fibrosis may develop and resemble subretinal fibrosis uveitis syndrome.[38,39] Thus it is felt by some investigators that multifocal choroiditis with panuveitis and subretinal fibrosis with uveitis represent the same disease but a different intensity of subretinal fibrotic reaction.[38,39]

PUNCTATE INNER CHOROIDOPATHY

EPIDEMIOLOGY AND PATHOGENESIS

Punctate inner choroidopathy is a bilateral, ocular inflammatory disease that affects young, otherwise healthy, myopic women. Initially patients complain of blurred vision, photopsias, or paracentral scotomas.[20,43]

OCULAR MANIFESTATIONS

Usually, little anterior segment or vitreous inflammation occurs. On ophthalmoscopic examination, small, yellow-white lesions at the level of the choroid or pigment epithelium are present in the posterior pole. Often a serous detachment of the retina overlies active lesions (Fig. 182-9). The lesions "heal" to form atrophic scars of variable pigmentation. Choroidal neovascular membranes may develop from these healed, atrophic, or pigmented scars. If choroidal neovascularization occurs in the macula or near the fovea, serious vision loss may result.[43] Vision also may be affected if the acute phase lesions develop underneath the fovea.[43]

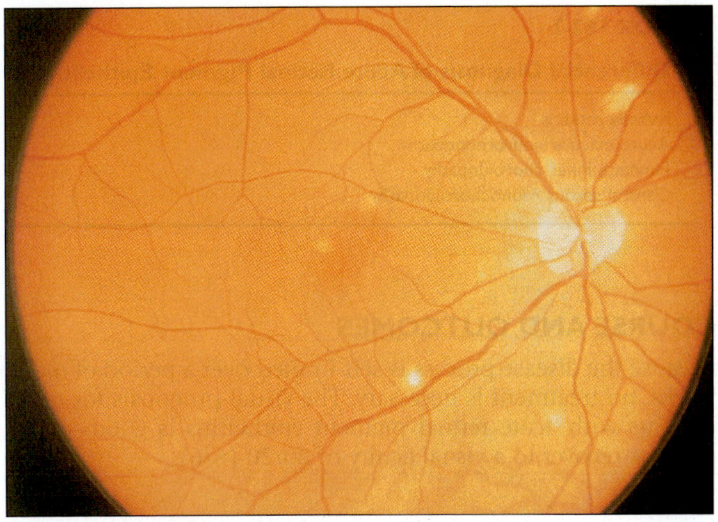

DIAGNOSIS

Diagnosis is based on typical ocular findings; laboratory evaluation is not helpful. Fluorescein angiography of acute lesions reveals early hyperfluorescence and staining, and leakage into the subretinal space if an overlying serous detachment is present. Choroidal neovascularization also shows late leakage.[43]

DIFFERENTIAL DIAGNOSIS

The differential diagnosis is the same as that for multifocal choroiditis and panuveitis (see Box 182-6). The lesions also may resemble myopic macular changes and myopic choroidal neovascularization. Many people believe choroiditis and panuveitis and punctate inner choroidopathy represent the same entity.

TREATMENT

When vision is decreased because of serous retinal detachment, systemic or periocular glucocorticoids may be given. Usually, however, the acute phase of the disease is self-limited and treatment is unnecessary. Treatment of extrafoveal macular choroidal neovascularization using focal laser photocoagulation is often warranted to prevent visual loss.[43] Surgical removal of subfoveal membranes may be helpful in selected cases. Photodynamic therapy may be helpful.

COURSE AND OUTCOMES

The visual prognosis of patients who have punctate inner choroidopathy is guarded. If subfoveal lesions and choroidal neovascularization do not occur, visual acuity is usually better than 20/40 (6/12). Recurrences are common. Because there are similarities between punctate inner choroidopathy, multifocal choroiditis and panuveitis, and subretinal fibrosis and uveitis, all three are believed by some investigators to be part of a spectrum of one or more related diseases.[43]

ACUTE RETINAL PIGMENT EPITHELIITIS

EPIDEMIOLOGY AND PATHOGENESIS

Acute retinal pigment epitheliitis is a rare condition that affects young adults in the second to fourth decades of life.[44] Patients usually report minimal to severe visual loss in one eye. Bilateral involvement can occur.

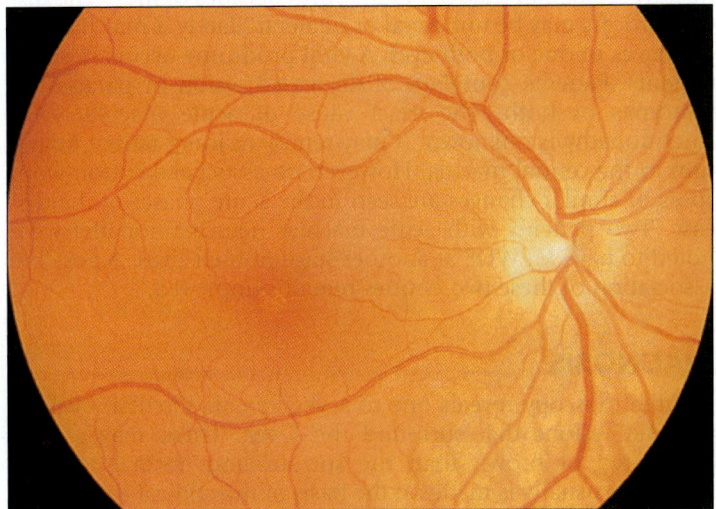

FIG. 182-9 ■ **Punctate inner choroidopathy.** White, punctate chorioretinal lesions in the macula with overlying serous retinal detachment of the fovea in the right eye of a 20-year-old myopic woman. (Courtesy of Richard R. Ober.)

FIG. 182-10 ■ **Retinal pigment epitheliitis.** A discrete cluster of gray-to-yellow, outer retinal lesions in the central macula of the right eye of a 27-year-old woman.

OCULAR MANIFESTATIONS

Anterior segment examination is normal; no vitreous cells are seen. Ophthalmoscopy reveals discrete clusters of small, brown or gray spots in the involved macula (Fig. 182-10). Usually, from two to four spots occur; occasionally, a yellow or white halo may surround some of the spots. Resolution is gradual but usually complete within 6–12 weeks, and visual acuity often returns to normal levels. The acute lesions become blacker. However, some pigmented spots may actually appear faint and be more difficult to see as they resolve.

DIAGNOSIS

A ring of hyperfluorescence is seen on fluorescein angiography to surround the hypofluorescent acute lesions. With resolution, the hyperfluorescence persists and represents window defects from retinal pigment epithelial derangement. Electrophysiological testing results are normal.

DIFFERENTIAL DIAGNOSIS

The differential diagnosis of acute retinal pigment epitheliitis is given in Box 182-7.

COURSE AND OUTCOMES

Because the disease process is self-limited over a period of 6–12 weeks, no treatment is necessary. The visual prognosis for most patients with acute retinal pigment epitheliitis is good—most patients recover to a visual acuity of 20/20 (6/6).

ACUTE MACULAR NEURORETINOPATHY

EPIDEMIOLOGY AND PATHOGENESIS

Acute macular neuroretinopathy occurs mainly in young, healthy women in the second to fourth decades of life.[45] The disease process may be unilateral or bilateral. Rarely it may have recurrences in one or both eyes. A viral prodrome occurs in some patients. Patients complain of decreased vision or paracentral scotomas or both. The exact cause of acute macular neuroretinopathy is unknown. It may represent inner retinal infarction in the central macula. However, no associated cotton-wool spots or similar changes are seen in the acute phases of the disease. Two patients with acute macular neuroretinopathy were noted to have MEWDS at another stage of their lives. A possible association of these two entities remains unproved.

DIAGNOSIS

Ophthalmoscopy reveals one to several small, circular, oval, or petaloid lesions that surround the fovea. These may appear darker red or brown than the surrounding normal macula. Diagnosis usually is made on the basis of the clinical course and appearance of the lesion. Fluorescein angiography is normal. Visual field testing often reveals paracentral scotomas that correspond very accurately to the shape and location of the macular lesions. Electrophysiological testing is normal.

DIFFERENTIAL DIAGNOSIS

The differential diagnosis of acute macular neuroretinopathy is given in Box 182-8.

COURSE AND OUTCOMES

No treatment is effective, but the disease is usually self-limited. Visual acuity improves and the paracentral scotomas decrease in size, however resolution of symptoms may take months. The acute retinal lesions fade but do not resolve completely. The authors have seen one patient who had multiple recurrences in both eyes.

UNILATERAL ACUTE IDIOPATHIC MACULOPATHY

EPIDEMIOLOGY AND PATHOGENESIS

Unilateral acute idiopathic maculopathy is a rare disorder that usually appears in the second to fourth decades of life and affects men and women equally.[46] Most patients have a history of a flu-like prodrome that precedes the onset of visual symptoms.

Patients often complain of sudden, severe, unilateral central visual loss. A central scotoma is often present on visual field testing. Bilateral cases and eccentric (nonfoveal) cases have been described recently. There may be an association of the disease with hand, foot, and mouth disease and coxsackievirus infection (Jampol, work in progress).

DIAGNOSIS

Ophthalmoscopic examination discloses an exudative detachment of the macula with irregular borders. There is typically a wedge configuration to the serous retinal elevation. In addition, white, gray, or yellow subretinal thickening at the level of the pigment epithelium, beneath the neurosensory retinal detachment, is often present. Careful evaluation of the posterior vitreous may detect cells that overlie the serous retinal detachment.

Fluorescein angiography shows alternating areas of hyperfluorescence and hypofluorescence beneath the neurosensory retinal detachment. In the late phases of the angiogram, hyperfluorescence occurs from both staining at the level of the RPE and pooling of fluorescein in the subretinal space.

DIFFERENTIAL DIAGNOSIS

The differential diagnosis of unilateral acute idiopathic maculopathy is given in Box 182-9.

TREATMENT

Treatment of this condition is not necessary. The natural course is a rapid and spontaneous improvement in vision with resolution of the neural retinal detachment. However, retinal pigment epithelial atrophy and hypopigmentation do develop in the area of the neurosensory retinal detachment. Visual acuity usually improves to 20/25 (6/7.5) or better in the affected eye. As a result of the surrounding areas of hypopigmentation, the macula takes on a bull's eye appearance after resolution of the disease.

ACUTE ZONAL OCCULT OUTER RETINOPATHY

EPIDEMIOLOGY

AZOOR is a disorder that predominantly affects young women in the second to fourth decades of life.[47,48] It is characterized by acute loss of zones of outer retinal function. Photopsias are usually present, and the condition may be unilateral or bilateral. Autoimmune disorders such as Hashimoto's thyroiditis are not uncommon among women with AZOOR.[48]

OCULAR MANIFESTATIONS AND DIAGNOSIS

On initial examination minimal to no fundal changes are seen. Narrow retinal vessels and depigmentation of the RPE are found within months of onset of symptoms, in zones that correspond to the visual field loss. Varying vitreitis also has been described in patients with AZOOR.

BOX 182-9

Differential Diagnosis of Unilateral Acute Idiopathic Maculopathy

Idiopathic choroidal neovascularization
Central serous chorioretinopathy
Vogt–Koyanagi–Harada syndrome
Serpiginous choroidopathy
Posterior scleritis
Acute posterior multifocal placoid pigment epitheliopathy
Placoid syphilitic retinitis
Retinal pigment epithelial detachment

BOX 182-10

Differential Diagnosis of Acute Zonal Occult Outer Retinopathy

Cancer-associated retinopathy
Retinal vasculitis
Syphilitic chorioretinitis
Diffuse unilateral subacute neuroretinitis
Retinitis pigmentosa

Visual field testing shows large, superior, temporal and, occasionally, central zones of visual field loss. The scotomas often increase in size within a few days to weeks and then stabilize. Visual field loss often occurs in both eyes, but can be very asymmetrical. Some improvement may occur.

Fluorescein angiographic findings typically are normal during the early phases of the disorder. Once the retinal pigment epithelial changes occur, pigment mottling and window defects develop in the periphery. The outer retinal dysfunction can be documented by visual field testing and electroretinography, which reveals moderate to severe reduction in a-wave amplitude. Laboratory evaluation is noncontributory.

DIFFERENTIAL DIAGNOSIS

The differential diagnosis of AZOOR is given in Box 182-10.

COURSE AND OUTCOME

No specific treatment exists for AZOOR. Glucocorticoids and antiviral agents have been tried but have not reduced the amount of visual field loss.

Although most patients retain visual acuity of better than 20/40 (6/12), permanent and occasionally severe visual field loss can occur.

RELENTLESS PLACOID CHORIORETINITIS

EPIDEMIOLOGY

RPC is a rare, often bilateral ocular inflammatory disease of unknown etiology affecting patients between the second and sixth decades of life.[49] Men and women are equally affected. When seeking treatment, patients complain of decreased vision, pericentral scotomas, photopsias, floaters and, rarely, pain.

OCULAR MANIFESTATIONS

Varying degrees of anterior chamber and vitreous cells may be seen. Active retinal lesions appear placoid, white to yellow, and similar in appearance to those of APMPPE or serpiginous choroiditis. These lesions tend to occur characteristically in multi-

---

BOX 182-11

Differential Diagnosis of Relentless Placoid Chorioretinitis

Acute posterior multifocal placoid pigment epitheliopathy
Serpiginous choroiditis
Multifocal choroiditis
Birdshot retinochoroidopathy
Vogt–Koyanagi–Harada syndrome
Neoplastic infiltration of the choroids
Syphilitic chorioretinitis
Sarcoid panuveitis
Tuberculous choroiditis

---

ples, are one disc diameter or less in size, and may affect the mid- and far periphery prior to involvement of the posterior pole, unlike APMPPE or serpiginous choroiditis.[49] Many of these lesions heal over weeks, resulting in superficial chorioretinal atrophy. However, progressive increase in size of subacute lesions and development of new lesions occurs in all patients. Fifty or more lesions can occur throughout the fundus. These lesions eventually can involve the macular region and acutely result in visual loss, metamorphopsia, or scotoma. Subretinal fluid may be seen in association with the acute lesions. When these lesions heal, visual acuity is often preserved even with macular involvement.[49]

Fluorescein angiography shows early hypofluorescence and late hyperfluorescence of acute lesions.

DIAGNOSIS

Diagnosis is based on clinical appearance of retinal lesions and prolonged clinical course. Laboratory evaluation is not helpful. No consistent systemic association has been found.

DIFFERENTIAL DIAGNOSIS

See Box 182-11.

TREATMENT

In the original report on RPC, glucocorticoids, antiviral agents, and cyclosporine all were used to treat patients. Immune suppression did appear to halt disease activity.[49] With glucocorticoid treatment, healing and improvement in visual acuity are observed, however the disease can recur despite use of glucocorticoids. The best treatment for this condition is unknown.

COURSE AND PROGNOSIS

Growth of subacute lesions and appearance of new lesions occurs from 5 to 24 months after initial diagnosis. Relapses are common. Eventually, most patients develop 50 or more (sometimes hundreds) healed lesions in the periphery and posterior pole. The long-term visual prognosis appears good.[49] Central vision is preserved as a rule.

UNIFOCAL HELIOID CHOROIDITIS

EPIDEMIOLOGY AND PATHOGENESIS

UHC (also called solitary idiopathic choroiditis) is an inflammatory disorder affecting young, healthy, white patients in the first to third decades of life.[50,51] Males and females are affected equally. The disease appears to be common in the midwestern United States where histoplasmosis is endemic. There has been no clear-cut relationship between this disease and systemic histoplasmosis. It is not clear whether these lesions represent a microbial infection or immunological reaction of the choroid.

OCULAR MANIFESTATIONS

All patients acutely developed a one–disc diameter, yellow-white choroidal lesion with overlying subretinal fluid and occasional subretinal hemorrhages. Patients may have decreased vision or metamorphopsia or both, depending upon the location of the lesion and the presence of subretinal fluid. Anterior chamber and vitreous inflammation is usually absent but occasionally can be marked. The acute choroidal lesion may be 1–2mm thick. The lesion may grow slightly in size. The lesions thin slightly and become pigmented as they heal. Overlying subretinal fluid resolves. During the chronic phase the lesions become whiter due to subretinal fibrosis. Fluorescein angiography demonstrated leakage and late staining of the acute inflammatory lesions.[50] Choroidal neovascularization may develop.

DIAGNOSIS

Diagnosis is based on age of the patient, symptoms, and clinical appearance. A uveitis work-up is warranted but may not be helpful.

DIFFERENTIAL DIAGNOSIS

See Box 182-12.

TREATMENT

No treatment for UHC has been proven to be of value.

COURSE AND OUTCOME

Relapses in the disease marked by slight increase in the size of the lesion or increase in subretinal fluid are common and may last from 1 to 18 months. Choroidal neovascularization occasionally may develop. The visual prognosis is variable and guarded, based on the location of the lesion with regard to the macula.[49] Permanent visual loss may occur.

REFERENCES

1. Gass JDM. Acute posterior multifocal placoid pigment epitheliopathy. Arch Ophthalmol. 1968;80:177–85.
2. Clearkin LG, Hung SO. Acute posterior multifocal placoid pigment epitheliopathy associated with transient hearing loss. Trans Ophthalmol Soc U K. 1983;103:562–4.
3. Holt WS, Regan ADJ, Trempe C. Acute posterior multifocal placoid pigment epitheliopathy. Am J Ophthalmol. 1976;81:403–12.
4. Kersten DH, Lessell S, Carlow TJ. Acute posterior multifocal placoid pigment epitheliopathy and late-onset meningo-encephalitis. Ophthalmology. 1987;94:393–6.
5. Ryan SJ, Maumenee AE. Acute posterior multifocal placoid pigment epitheliopathy. Am J Ophthalmol. 1972;81:1066–74.
6. Wright BE, Bird AC, Hamilton AM. Placoid pigment epitheliopathy and Harada's disease. Br J Ophthalmol. 1978;62:609–21.
7. Savino PJ, Weinberg RJ, Yassin JC, Pilkerton AR. Diverse manifestations of acute posterior multifocal placoid pigment epitheliopathy. Am J Ophthalmol. 1974;77:659–62.
8. Laatikainen LT, Immonen IJR. Acute posterior multifocal placoid pigment epitheliopathy in connection with acute nephritis. Retina. 1988;8:122–4.
9. Azar PJ, Gohd RS, Waltman D, Gitter KA. Acute posterior multifocal placoid pigment epitheliopathy associated with an adenovirus type 5 infection. Am J Ophthalmol. 1975;80:1003–5.
10. Damato BE, Nanjiani M, Foulds WS. Acute posterior multifocal placoid pigment epitheliopathy. A follow-up study. Trans Ophthalmol Soc U K. 1983;103:517–22.
11. Isashiki M, Koide H, Yamashita T, Ohba N. Acute posterior multifocal placoid pigment epitheliopathy associated with diffuse retinal vasculitis and late haemorrhagic macular detachment. Br J Ophthalmol. 1986;70:255–9.
12. Jampol LM, Sieving PA, Pugh D, et al. Multiple evanescent white dot syndrome. I. Clinical findings. Arch Ophthalmol. 1984;102:671–4.
13. Aaberg TM, Campo RV, Joffe L. Recurrences and bilaterality in the multiple evanescent white-dot syndrome. Am J Ophthalmol. 1985;100:29–37.
14. Mamalis N, Daily MJ. Multiple evanescent white dot syndrome. A report of eight cases. Ophthalmology. 1987;94:1209–12.
15. Ie D, Glaser BM, Murphy RP, et al. Indocyanine green angiography in multiple evanescent white-dot syndrome. Am J Ophthalmol. 1994;117:7–12.
16. Sieving PA, Fishman GA, Jampol LM, Pugh D. Multiple evanescent white dot syndrome. II. Electrophysiology of the photoreceptors during retinal pigment epithelial disease. Arch Ophthalmol. 1984;102:675–9.
17. Callanan D, Gass JD. Multifocal choroiditis and choroidal neovascularization associated with the multiple evanescent white dot and acute idiopathic blind spot enlargement syndrome. Ophthalmology. 1992;99:1678–85.
18. Khorram KD, Jampol LM, Rosenberg MA. Blind spot enlargement as a manifestation of multifocal choroiditis. Arch Ophthalmol. 1991;109:1403–7.
19. Singh K, de Frank MP, Shults WT, Watzke RC. Acute idiopathic blind spot enlargement. A spectrum of disease. Ophthalmology. 1991;98:497–502.
20. Jampol LM. Inflammatory multifocal chorioretinopathies. In: Freeman WR, ed. Practical atlas of retinal disease and therapy. New York: Raven Press; 1993:71–83.
21. Wyhinny GJ, Jackson JL, Jampol LM, Caro NC. Subretinal neovascularization following multiple evanescent white-dot syndrome [letter]. Arch Ophthalmol. 1990;108:1384–5.
22. Bock CJ, Jampol LM. Serpiginous choroiditis. In: Albert DM, Jakobiec FA, eds. Principles and practice of ophthalmology. Philadelphia: WB Saunders; 1994:517–23.
23. Hamilton AM, Bird AC. Geographical choroidopathy. Br J Ophthalmol. 1974;58:784–97.
24. Laatikainen L, Erkkila H. A follow-up study on serpiginous choroiditis. Acta Ophthalmol. 1981;59:707–18.
25. Masi RJ, O'Connor GR, Kimura SJ. Anterior uveitis in geographic or serpiginous choroiditis. Am J Ophthalmol. 1978;86:228–32.
26. Nussenblatt RB, Palestine AG. Serpiginous choroidopathy (choroiditis). In: Nussenblatt RB, Palestine AG, eds. Uveitis. Fundamentals and clinical practice. Chicago: Year-Book Medical Publishers; 1989:309–14.
27. Mansour AM, Jampol LM, Packo KH, Hrisomalos NF. Macular serpiginous choroiditis. Retina. 1988;8:125–31.
28. Jampol LM, Orth D, Daily MJ, Rabb MF. Subretinal neovascularization with geographic (serpiginous) choroiditis. Am J Ophthalmol. 1979;88:683–9.
29. Gass JDM. Serpiginous choroidopathy. In: Gass JDM, ed. Stereoscopic atlas of macular diseases: diagnosis and treatment. St Louis: CV Mosby; 1987:136–44.
30. Hooper PL, Kaplan HJ. Triple agent immunosuppression in serpiginous choroiditis. Ophthalmology. 1991;98:944–51.
31. Nussenblatt RB, Palestine AG, Chan CC. Cyclosporine A therapy in the treatment of intraocular inflammatory disease resistant to systemic corticosteroids and cytotoxic agents. Am J Ophthalmol. 1983;96:275–82.
32. Ryan SJ, Maumenee AE. Birdshot retinochoroidopathy. Am J Ophthalmol. 1980;89:31–45.
33. Nussenblatt RB, Mittal KK, Ryan SJ, et al. Birdshot retinochoroidopathy associated with HLA-A29 antigen and immune responsiveness to retinal S-antigen. Am J Ophthalmol. 1982;94:147–58.
34. Gass JDM. Vitiliginous chorioretinitis. Arch Ophthalmol. 1981;99:1778–87.
35. Palestine AG, Nussenblatt RB, Parver LM, Knox DL. Progressive subretinal fibrosis and uveitis. Br J Ophthalmol. 1984;68:667–73.
36. Cantrill HL, Folk JC. Multifocal choroiditis associated with progressive subretinal fibrosis. Am J Ophthalmol. 1986;101:170–80.
37. Palestine AG, Nussenblatt RB, Chan CC, et al. Histopathology of the subretinal fibrosis and uveitis syndrome. Ophthalmology. 1985;92:838–44.
38. Dreyer RF, Gass DJ. Multifocal choroiditis and panuveitis. A syndrome that mimics ocular histoplasmosis. Arch Ophthalmol. 1984;102:1776–84.
39. Morgan CM, Schatz H. Recurrent multifocal choroiditis. Ophthalmology. 1986;93:1138–47.
40. Spaide RF, Yannuzzi LA, Freund KB. Linear streaks in multifocal choroiditis and panuveitis. Retina. 1991;11:229–31.
40a. Parnell JR, Jampol LM, Yannuzzi LA, et al. Differentiation between presumed ocular histoplasmosis syndrome and multifocal choroiditis with panuveitis based on morphology of photographed fundus lesions and fluorescein angiography. Arch Ophthalmol. 2001;119:208–12.
41. Tiedeman JS. Epstein–Barr viral antibodies in multifocal choroiditis and panuveitis. Am J Ophthalmol. 1987;103:659–63.
42. Spaide RF, Sugin S, Yannuzzi LA, De Rosa JT. Epstein–Barr virus antibodies in multifocal choroiditis and panuveitis. Am J Ophthalmol. 1991;112:410–13.
43. Watzke RC, Packer AJ, Folk JC, et al. Punctate inner choroidopathy. Am J Ophthalmol. 1984;98:572–84.
44. Krill AE, Deutman AF. Acute retinal pigment epitheliitis. Am J Ophthalmol. 1972;74:193–205.
45. Bos PJM, Deutman AF. Acute macular neuroretinopathy. Am J Ophthalmol. 1975;80:573–84.
46. Yannuzzi LA, Jampol LM, Rabb MF, et al. Unilateral acute idiopathic maculopathy. Arch Ophthalmol. 1991;109:1411–16.
47. Gass JDM. Acute zonal occult outer retinopathy. J Clin Neuro Ophthalmol. 1993;13:79–97.
48. Gass JD, Agarwal A, Scott IU. Acute zonal occult outer retinopathy: a long-term follow-up study. Am J Ophthalmol. 2002;134:329–39.
49. Jones BE, Jampol LM, Yannuzzi LA, et al. Relentless placoid chorioretinitis: a new entity or an unusual variant of serpiginous chorioretinitis? Arch Ophthalmol. 2000;118:931–8.
50. Hong PH, Jampol LM, Dodwel DG, et al. Unifocal helioid choroiditis. Arch Ophthalmol. 1997;115:1007–13.
51. Shields JA, Shields CL, Demirci H, Hanovar S. Solitary idiopathic choroiditis. Arch Ophthalmol. 2002;120:311–19.

SECTION 9 MASQUERADE SYNDROMES

CHAPTER

183 Ocular Neoplasms Related to Human Immunodeficiency Virus

PRAVIN U. DUGEL • ALLEN B. THACH

DEFINITION
- A number of neoplastic disorders that take on an aggressive course in the setting of immunosuppression induced by the human immunodeficiency virus.

KEY FEATURE
- A well-localized or diffuse mass that involves ocular adnexa, orbit, or intraocular structures.

ASSOCIATED FEATURE
- A constellation of ocular, adnexal, intraocular, intraorbital, and intracranial signs and symptoms dependent on the site and nature of the neoplasm.

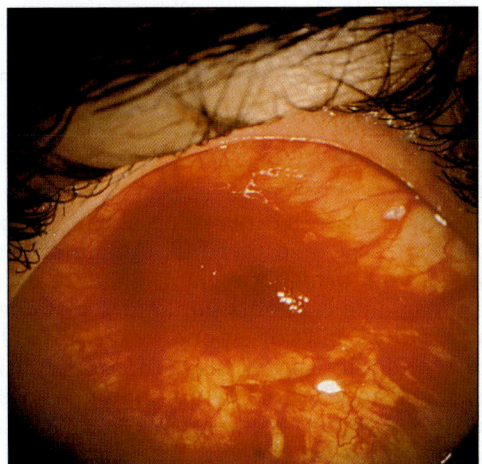

FIG. 183-1 ▌ **Kaposi's sarcoma, stage III lesions.** These are nodular, raised (>3mm) lesions of more than 4 months' duration.

INTRODUCTION

The most common ocular neoplasm in individuals infected by the human immunodeficiency virus (HIV) is Kaposi's sarcoma. Other tumors in such patients include lymphoma and squamous cell carcinomas. Ocular manifestation of Kaposi's sarcoma and lymphoma may be the first sign of systemic dissemination of the neoplasm. Therefore, a thorough systemic evaluation is essential. Kaposi's sarcoma and squamous cell carcinoma develop in the conjunctiva and ocular adnexa. Lymphomas develop at these sites, in the orbit, and intraocularly.

OCULAR ADNEXAL KAPOSI'S SARCOMA

EPIDEMIOLOGY AND PATHOGENESIS

Since the original description of Kaposi's sarcoma in 1872, two aggressive variants of this tumor have been described. The first is an endemic variety found in Africa, especially Kenya and Nigeria, where it accounts for nearly 20% of all malignancies.[1] The second variant, epidemic Kaposi's sarcoma, occurs in about 30% of all patients who have AIDS.[2] Kaposi's sarcoma associated with AIDS is particularly aggressive and disseminates to visceral organs (gastrointestinal tract, lung, and liver) in 20–50% of patients.[2]

The pathogenesis of AIDS-related Kaposi's sarcoma is not known. Recent developments suggest that this tumor may be caused by human herpes virus 8 (HHV-8).[3,4] Transgenic mice that bear the HIV-1 transactivator (*tat*) gene under control of the virus regulatory region (HIV-LTR) produce a protein that has been shown to be a potent mitogen for human Kaposi's sarcoma–derived cell lines.[5] Interestingly, in mice as in humans, Kaposi's

sarcoma occurs predominantly in males, which suggests that the development may be hormonally controlled.

OCULAR MANIFESTATIONS

Typically, AIDS-associated adnexal Kaposi's sarcoma occurs in the eyelids or conjunctiva late in the course of disease.[6–9] However, rarely ocular adnexal Kaposi's sarcoma may be the initial manifestation of AIDS. The clinical features include a vascular lesion that may be flat or raised. In the conjunctiva it is bright red in color and is surrounded by tortuous and dilated vessels. No evidence of necrosis or discharge is seen. Three clinical stages have been described. Clinically, stage I and stage II tumors (clinically indistinguishable, differentiated only by their pathologic features) are patchy and flat (<3mm in vertical height) and of less than 4 months' duration. Stage III tumors are nodular and elevated (>3mm in height; Fig. 183-1) and of more than 4 months' duration.[8]

DIAGNOSIS

The diagnosis of Kaposi's sarcoma may be based on the clinical findings in a patient who has a history of HIV infection. Tortuous and dilated vessels around the mass and the presence of subconjunctival hemorrhages help to make the correct diagnosis. The hemorrhages may be recent or old, and the blood pigment is usually present. Tissue diagnosis may be obtained by local excision of the tumor.

DIFFERENTIAL DIAGNOSIS

The differential diagnosis of ocular adnexal Kaposi's sarcoma includes subconjunctival hemorrhage, hemangioma, foreign body, allergic reaction, infection, and orbital cellulites. Slit-lamp evaluation, with lid eversion and a thorough examination of the entire conjunctival surface, discloses the typical, densely vascular nature of the tumor. Therefore, such an evaluation is undertaken in all patients, especially those known to have AIDS.

SYSTEMIC ASSOCIATIONS

The recognition of ocular adnexal Kaposi's sarcoma by the ophthalmologist is important. Once this tumor has been recognized, a thorough evaluation must be undertaken to rule out systemic Kaposi's sarcoma. Therefore, an immediate referral to a qualified internist or oncologist is necessary. Systemic lesions often precede ocular manifestation, but it is thought that approximately 20% of patients who have systemic Kaposi's sarcoma have an ocular manifestation. Occasionally, patients present to the ophthalmologist with recurrent epithelial defects, irritation, red eyes, or entropion that result from ocular adnexal Kaposi's sarcoma, which may be the first manifestation of a more widespread disease.

PATHOLOGY

The pathological features of ocular adnexal Kaposi's sarcoma are dependent on the size, and therefore duration, of the lesion. They can range from benign vascular changes to the malignant appearance of spindle cell formation. Three histological stages have been described and correspond to the clinical stages already discussed.[8] Histologically, stage I tumors consist of thin, dilated vascular channels lined by flat endothelial cells that are often filled with erythrocytes. Abnormal mitotic figures are usually not seen. A moderate amount of mononuclear cells infiltrate the abnormal vessels, but no spindle cells or slit spaces are seen. Stage II lesions feature plump, fusiform cells that line thin, dilated, empty vascular channels. Many of these cells have hyperchromatic nuclei. Usually, no mitotic cells are noted. A sparse, inflammatory infiltrate, which consists mostly of macrophages, plasma cells, and lymphocytes, is seen. Foci of immature spindle cells and early slit vessels occur. Stage III lesions are characterized by large aggregates of densely packed spindle cells that have hyperchromatic nuclei and occasional mitotic figures. Between these spindle cells are slit spaces, many of which contain erythrocytes (Fig. 183-2). Inflammatory cells are scant. On the basis that recurrences are of an earlier stage than the primary tumor and that all three stages can be present within the same lesion, it is believed that these three stages are part of a continuum.

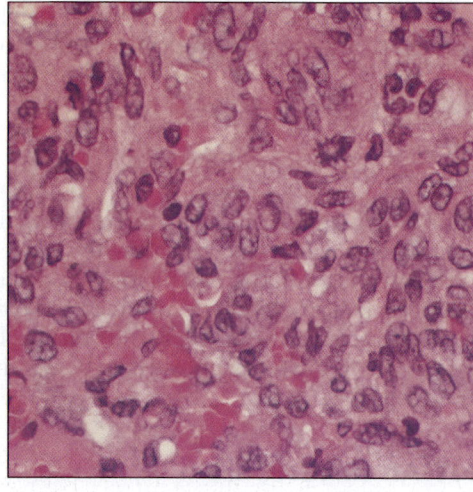

FIG. 183-2 ■ **Kaposi's sarcoma, histopathology.** Stage III lesions show densely packed spindle cells with hyperchromatic nucleus.

TREATMENT

The treatment of ocular adnexal Kaposi's sarcoma depends on the ocular complaints of the patient as well as on the possible systemic manifestations of the tumor. If the patient has no ocular symptoms, no local treatment is required. After systemic evaluation, if the patient is found to have systemic Kaposi's sarcoma that requires chemotherapy, the ocular lesions often regress significantly after systemic chemotherapy. Only if ocular symptoms continue after a full course of systemic chemotherapy or only if significant ocular symptoms occur in a patient who does not have systemic Kaposi's sarcoma should local treatment be considered. Radiotherapy is an effective local treatment,[7] but the expense and complications are significant. Complications specifically reported after irradiation of ocular adnexal Kaposi's sarcoma include skin erythema, hair loss, and possible radiation-induced optic neuropathy. A safer and more effective treatment regimen, based on the clinical and histopathological stage of the tumor and its location, involves surgical excision and cryotherapy.[8] If the tumor is confined to the bulbar conjunctiva and is clinical stage I or stage II, excisional biopsy with 1–2mm of tumor-free margins is considered. Clinical stage III Kaposi's sarcoma of the bulbar conjunctiva is excised surgically, preferably after delineation by fluorescein angiography, which may allow better visualization of tumor-associated vessels. Stage I and stage II Kaposi's sarcoma that involve the eyelid may be treated with cryotherapy. However, stage III Kaposi's sarcoma of the eyelid may require radiotherapy. Injection of intralesional interferon may be effective in some cases.[10]

COURSE AND OUTCOME

Untreated Kaposi's sarcoma may grow and damage the ocular adnexa and ocular surface. Frequent subconjunctival hemorrhage may occur. With surgical intervention, most tumors are excised totally. Ocular morbidity may be prevented by early diagnosis and treatment with either surgical excision, cryotherapy, or intralesional interferon injection. Radiation treatment may result in ocular sicca.

CONJUNCTIVAL INTRAEPITHELIAL NEOPLASIA

In immunocompetent individuals, conjunctival intraepithelial neoplasia (CIN) is the most common neoplasm of the ocular surface. It is a known precursor of squamous cell carcinoma, the most common conjunctival malignant neoplasm. Traditional risk factors for this disease include ultraviolet light exposure, petroleum products, heavy cigarette smoking, light hair and ocular pigmentation, and family history.[11] The most significant risk factor, however, is human papillomavirus infection. Although CIN typically affects men in the sixth and seventh decades of life, this ocular tumor has been observed in young AIDS patients. Cervical intraepithelial neoplasia, increasingly common in women who have AIDS, shares some characteristics with CIN—both involve nonkeratinized epithelium, occur at transitional zones of surface epithelium, and have been associated with human papillomavirus infection.[11]

SQUAMOUS CELL CARCINOMA

EPIDEMIOLOGY AND PATHOGENESIS

In patients who have AIDS, several studies describe an aggressive form of squamous cell carcinoma in the conjunctiva and/or eyelids.[12-16] The pathogenesis of CIN and squamous cell carcinoma in AIDS patients is not clear. Two hypotheses exist. First, a generalized depression of immune surveillance may be present with severe immunosuppression. Second, immunosuppression by

HIV may enable coinfection with the human papillomavirus, which is a known causative agent for CIN as well as squamous cell carcinoma.

OCULAR MANIFESTATIONS

The clinical features include a hyperemic nodular mass with well-defined borders in the conjunctiva or eyelid (Fig. 183-3, *A*). This mass is often more than 2mm in vertical height and may contain areas of necrosis. The overlying epithelium is of a grayish color, which distinguishes it from the surrounding normal epithelium.

DIAGNOSIS

Several epithelial as well as stromal neoplasms may mimic squamous cell carcinomas of the ocular adnexa and conjunctiva. Excisional biopsy in small tumors or incisional biopsy of the larger tumors establishes the tissue diagnosis.

DIFFERENTIAL DIAGNOSIS

The differential diagnosis of squamous cell carcinoma includes basal cell carcinoma, Kaposi's sarcoma, lymphoma, sebaceous carcinoma, and amelanotic melanoma. Squamous cell carcinoma may be differentiated by a lack of the vascularity that occurs with Kaposi's sarcoma, the lack of significant overlying necrosis that occurs with basal cell carcinoma, and the lack of a salmon or a pink color that occurs with lymphoma. A rough, grayish, amorphous, raised epithelial lesion characterizes squamous cell carcinoma. Histological examination of the tumor is essential to rule out other neoplasms.

PATHOLOGY

Extensive squamous cell proliferation is the most prominent histological manifestation. The epithelium shows acanthosis and dyskeratosis (Fig. 183-3, *B*). Stromal invasion is present, with a concentric collection of epithelial and spindle cells that have prominent nuclei and nucleoli. Abnormal mitotic figures are abundant within neoplastic cells. Immunohistologic staining of the spindle cells and other infiltrating carcinoma cells shows positive staining with antibodies to cytokeratin. Polymerase chain reaction studies are often positive for the human papillomavirus.

TREATMENT, COURSE, AND OUTCOME

The only known systemic association of CIN is cervical intraepithelial neoplasia. Both are thought to be caused by the human papillomavirus. Ophthalmologists must be aware of suspicious lesions in the ocular adnexa in AIDS patients. Treatment consists of total excision of the tumor with clear surgical margins documented histologically. The patient is checked frequently thereafter for early detection of any recurrence or invasion into adjacent tissue, or both. One patient who had CIN was treated effectively with topical interferon. Early diagnosis and total excision of the tumor carry a good prognosis against recurrence.

INTRAOCULAR, INTRAORBITAL, AND CENTRAL NERVOUS SYSTEM LYMPHOMA

EPIDEMIOLOGY AND PATHOGENESIS

Non-Hodgkin's lymphoma associated with HIV infection is now recognized more frequently as survival increases in patients who have AIDS. Approximately 20% of patients who are affected with both AIDS and non-Hodgkin's lymphoma have extranodular in-

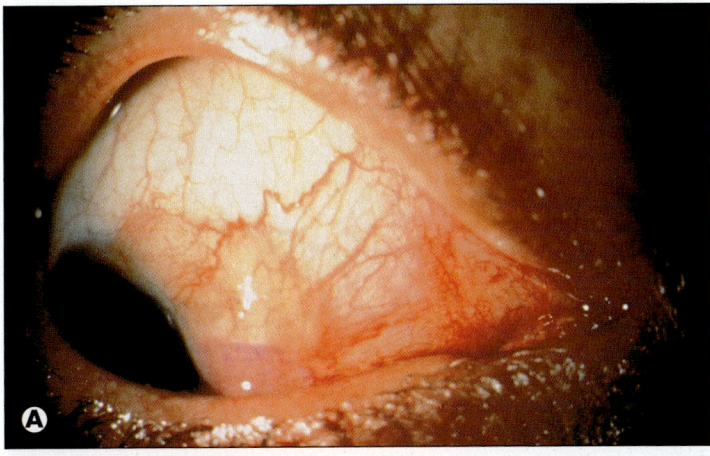

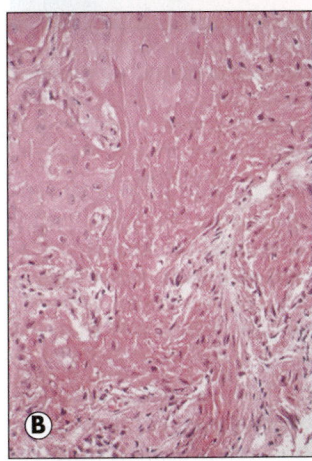

FIG. 183-3 ▮ **Squamous cell carcinoma.** **A,** Raised nodular, hyperemic mass with grayish overlying epithelium. **B,** Extensive squamous cell proliferation with acanthosis, dyskeratosis, and infiltration into the stroma (hematoxylin and eosin). (With permission from Muccioli C, Belfort R, Burnier M, Rao N. Squamous cell carcinoma of the conjunctiva in a patient with the acquired immune deficiency syndrome. Am J Ophthalmol. 1996;121:94–6.)

volvement, especially of the central nervous system (CNS), compared with less than 1% of patients who do not have AIDS but who have non-Hodgkin's lymphoma.[17] The risk for the development of ocular and CNS non-Hodgkin's lymphoma in patients who have AIDS has been estimated to be approximately 100 times that of immunocompetent patients.[17] In AIDS-affected patients, the disease is more likely to be a high-grade B-cell malignancy that can develop in the ocular adnexa or orbit. Nevertheless, intraocular lymphoma in AIDS patients is quite rare.

The pathogenic mechanism of AIDS-associated B-cell lymphoma is not known. Possible hypotheses include the synergistic association between the Epstein-Barr virus and HIV.[18] Immunosuppression induced by HIV may enable the clonal expansion of B cells immortalized by Epstein-Barr virus. With clonal expansion, a small population of B cells may undergo genetic alteration (*c-myc* rearrangement), which transforms these cells into truly monoclonal malignant lymphoma. Interleukins, which are involved in differentiation and maturation of white blood cells, may modulate this process. Another hypothesis proposes the proliferation of B cells because of chronic antigenic stimulation, which may occur by stimulation via retroviral products and which results in a lymphomatous transformation.[19]

OCULAR MANIFESTATIONS

Intraocular involvement of non-Hodgkin's lymphoma in patients who have AIDS is similar to that in patients who do not have AIDS. Patients often present with poor vision, which may be unilateral or bilateral. Minimal to moderate anterior segment inflammation may occur. The primary site of inflammation, however, is the posterior segment. A significant vitritis may be seen with peripapillary infiltrates and often with a marked swelling of the optic disc. Yellow-white, subretinal pigment epithelium lesions (Fig. 183-4) are most characteristic. Most of the lesions represent localized and multiple areas of retinal pigment epithelial detachment that results from tumor infiltration.[20] The

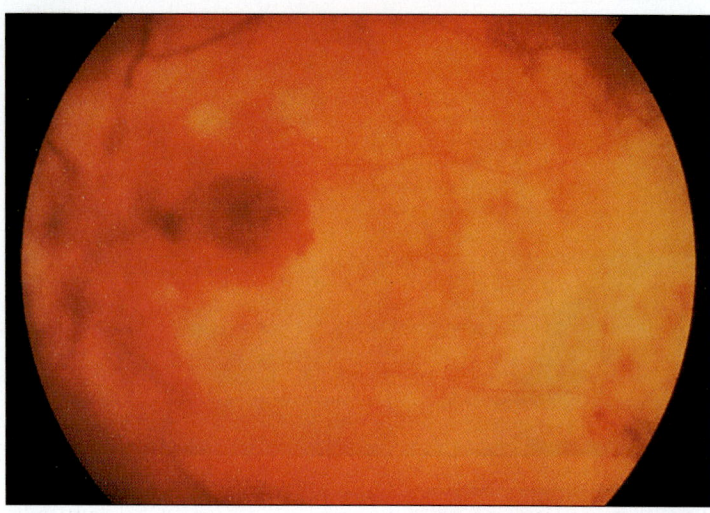

FIG. 183-4 ■ **Intraocular lymphoma.** Peripapillary hemorrhage and subretinal infiltrates.

aggressive nature of this tumor may cause infiltration into retinal vessels, which produces vascular sheathing, vein occlusion, and artery occlusion. Patients who have orbital or sinus involvement may present with facial numbness, proptosis, poor vision, diplopia, and ptosis.[19]

Patients with primary CNS involvement may present with a history of diplopia, ocular motor paresis, and signs and symptoms of increased intracranial pressure.[21] Neuroimaging studies show a typical periventricular, aqueductal position of these lymphomas. However, the diagnosis requires cerebrospinal fluid cytology. Ocular manifestations may be the first and only sign of primary CNS lymphoma. Alternatively, ocular manifestations may occur as a result of metastasis late in the course of systemic lymphoma. However, a full systemic evaluation with particular attention to the CNS must be carried out in patients who have ocular lymphoma.

DIAGNOSIS

The clinical features of lymphoma depend on the location. The diagnosis is best made by a vitrectomy followed by cytologic examination of the specimen.[21] The diagnosis of adnexal or intraorbital lymphoma is made on the basis of fine-needle aspiration or an incisional biopsy. Intracranial lymphoma is diagnosed by neuroimaging studies followed by lumbar puncture and/or craniotomy with a biopsy of the brain.

DIFFERENTIAL DIAGNOSIS

The differential diagnosis of intraocular lymphoma includes infectious multifocal choroiditis, retinal necrosis induced by varicella-zoster virus, ocular toxoplasmosis, ocular histoplasmosis, and cytomegalovirus (CMV) retinitis. The differential diagnosis of orbital lymphoma includes all forms of bacterial and fungal infections. Intraorbital lymphoma tends to be more indolent and slowly progressive than an intraorbital infection. The differential diagnosis of intracranial lymphoma includes toxoplasmosis, AIDS-associated infectious or noninfectious dementia, cryptococcosis, and CMV.

PATHOLOGY

Histopathological studies reveal that the tumor cells are usually large B cells that exhibit prominent nucleoli or multiple nucleoli in a large nucleus. The neoplastic cells may show an eosinophilic cytoplasm and altered nuclear/cytoplasmic ratio. Necrotic foci may be observed. Abnormal mitotic figures are found frequently.[21]

TREATMENT, COURSE, AND OUTCOME

Treatment involves radiation and chemotherapy (see Chapter 184). Despite treatment, patients usually die within 12–18 months.

REFERENCES

1. Templeton AC, Hutt MS. Distribution of tumours in Uganda. Recent Results Cancer Res. 1973;41:1–22.
2. Dugel PU, Rao NA. Ocular infections in acquired immune deficiency syndrome. Int Ophthalmol Clin. 1993;33:103–27.
3. Ablashi DV, Chatlynne LG, Whitman JE Jr, Cesarman E. Spectrum of Kaposi's sarcoma–associated herpesvirus, or human herpesvirus 8, diseases. Clin Microbiol Rev. 2002;15:439–64.
4. Gnann JW Jr, Pellett PE, Jaffe HW. Human herpesvirus 8 and Kaposi's sarcoma in persons infected with human immunodeficiency virus. Clin Infect Dis. 2000;Suppl 2:S72–6.
5. Vogel J, Hinrichs SH, Reynolds PA, et al. The HIV (tat) gene induces dermal lesions resembling Kaposi's sarcoma in transgenic mice. Nature. 1988;335:606–11.
6. Dugel PU, Gill PS, Frengieh GT, Rao NA. Ocular adnexal Kaposi's sarcoma in acquired immune deficiency syndrome. Am J Ophthalmol. 1990;110:500–3.
7. Shuler JD, Holland GN, Miles SA, et al. Kaposi's sarcoma in the conjunctiva and eyelids associated with the acquired immune deficiency syndrome. Arch Ophthalmol. 1989;107:858–62.
8. Dugel PU, Gill PS, Frengieh GT, Rao NA. Treatment of ocular adnexal Kaposi's sarcoma in acquired immune deficiency syndrome. Ophthalmology. 1992;99:1127–32.
9. Brun SC, Jakobiec FA. Kaposi's sarcoma of the ocular adnexa. Int Ophthalmol Clin. 1997;37:25–38.
10. Hummer J, Gass, JD, Huanga JW. Conjunctival Kaposi's sarcoma treated with interferon alpha-2a. Am J Ophthalmol. 1993;116:502–3.
11. Karp CL, Scott IU, Chang TS, Pflugfelder SC. Conjunctival intraepithelial neoplasia. A possible marker for human immunodeficiency virus? Arch Ophthalmol. 1996;114:257–61.
12. Muccioli C, Belfort R, Burnier M, Rao N. Squamous cell carcinoma of the conjunctiva in a patient with the acquired immune deficiency syndrome. Am J Ophthalmol. 1996;121:94–6.
13. Maclean H, Dhillon B, Ironside J. Squamous cell carcinoma of the eyelid and the acquired immune deficiency syndrome. Am J Ophthalmol. 1996;121:219–21.
14. Lewalen S, Shroyer KR, Keyser RB, Liomba G. Aggressive conjunctival squamous cell carcinoma in three young Africans. Arch Ophthalmol. 1996;114:215–18.
15. Margo CE, Mack W, Guffey JM. Squamous cell carcinoma of the conjunctiva and human immune deficiency virus infection. Arch Ophthalmol. 1996;114:349.
16. Kaimbo WA, Kaimbo D, Parys-Van Ginderdeuren R, Missotten L. Conjunctival squamous cell carcinoma and intraepithelial neoplasia in AIDS patients in Congo Kinshasa. Bull Soc Belge Ophtalmol. 1998;268:135–41.
17. Matzkin DC, Slamovits TL, Rosenbaum PS. Simultaneous intraocular and orbital non-Hodgkin lymphoma in acquired immune deficiency syndrome. Ophthalmology. 1994;101:850–5.
18. Mittra RA, Pulido JS, Hanson GA, et al. Primary ocular Epstein-Barr virus–associated non-Hodgkin's lymphoma in a patient with AIDS: a clinicopathologic report. Retina. 1999;19:45–50.
19. Font RL, Laucirica R, Patrinely JR. Immunoblastic B-cell malignant lymphoma involving the orbit and maxillary sinus in a patient with acquired immune deficiency syndrome. Ophthalmology. 1993;100:966–70.
20. Schanzer CM, Font RL, O'Malley RE. Primary ocular malignant lymphoma associated with the acquired immune deficiency syndrome. Ophthalmology. 1991;98:88–91.
21. Read RW, Zamir E, Rao NA. Neoplastic masquerade syndromes. Surv Ophthalmol. 2002;47:81–124.

CHAPTER 184

Masquerade Syndromes: Neoplasms

RUSSELL W. READ

DEFINITION
- Simulation of an inflammatory condition by a neoplastic process

KEY FEATURES
- Usually bilateral, may have asymmetrical involvement
- Cells in aqueous or vitreous humor or both
- Older age or known history of malignancy elsewhere

ASSOCIATED FEATURES
- May respond initially to corticosteroids, but eventually becomes "corticosteroid resistant"
- Usually a lack of inflammatory features such as pain, keratic precipitates and synechiae, but this is not a universal feature
- With primary central nervous system lymphoma: neural retinal infiltration, subretinal pigment epithelial lesions, central nervous system involvement, typically over 50 years of age

INTRODUCTION

A wide variety of entities can produce cells in the intraocular compartments, resulting in what appears to be uveitis. In a review of 828 consecutive patients from a uveitis clinic, Rothova *et al.*[1] diagnosed a neoplastic masquerade syndrome in 19 patients (2.3%), 13 of whom (68%) had intraocular lymphoma, making it the most common neoplastic masquerader. This text will therefore concentrate on this entity, with other neoplasms that could be considered masquerade syndromes detailed in Table 184-1.

PRIMARY CENTRAL NERVOUS SYSTEM LYMPHOMA

INTRODUCTION

Primary central nervous system lymphoma (PCNSL) is usually extranodal, non-Hodgkin's B cell lymphoma involving the central nervous system (CNS) or eye or both. T cell varieties have been reported, but only account for approximately 2% of intraocular lymphomas. Ocular involvement by PCNSL may affect the vitreous humor, retina, subretinal, or subretinal pigment epithelial spaces. Because the ocular and the CNS components show identical cytologic features and phenotypic expression, these two entities are combined under the heading PCNSL. Some clinicians still refer to this entity as reticulum cell sarcoma, an old term used when understanding of this condition was incomplete.

EPIDEMIOLOGY PATHOGENESIS

PCNSL most commonly affects individuals in the sixth to seventh decades of life, although rarely it may affect children and adolescents. PCNSL is a rare condition, but its incidence is increasing, and the increase does not appear to be solely secondary

to the acquired immunodeficiency syndrome (AIDS). It was estimated that PCNSL would occur in 51 of 10 million immunocompetent individuals in 2000.[2]

The site of origin of PCNSL is unknown. Neither the CNS nor intraocular space is known to contain lymphatic tissue. Lymphoma cells might arise in a site external to the CNS or eye, yet they are able to grow only in these two immunologically sequestered locations.[3] Another theory supposes the development of a polyclonal inflammation in which a monoclonal proliferation subsequently develops.[4]

OCULAR MANIFESTATIONS

Patients may seek treatment for either CNS or ocular complaints, or both. Ocular disease has been reported in up to 25% of PCNSL cases affecting the brain or spinal cord.[5] When ocular findings occur first, decreased acuity and floaters are typically present, and the finding of a vitreous cellular infiltration may be the only evidence of disease. In this situation the diagnosis may be missed and an autoimmune or infectious cause presumed. Therapy with corticosteroids or other immunosuppressive agents may result in a decrease in the number of cells, but this response typically does not last, and the "uveitis" becomes resistant to therapy. When the retina is involved, the diagnosis may be more apparent, but it still may be difficult to establish definitively in the absence of CNS findings. The lesions typically are elevated creamy yellow subretinal infiltrates, with overlying retinal pigment epithelial detachments (Fig. 184-1, *A*) and vitreous cells. Keratic precipitates and synechiae may be absent. Findings are usually bilateral but may be asymmetrical.

DIAGNOSIS AND ANCILLARY TESTING

Diagnosis in immunocompetent patients is established by fluid or tissue specimens from the eye (vitreous humor and, rarely, chorioretinal biopsy) or CNS (lumbar puncture or brain biopsy), but ancillary testing can be helpful in supporting the clinical diagnosis.

Ultrasonography may reveal vitreous debris, choroidal-scleral thickening, widening of the optic nerve, elevated chorioretinal lesions, and retinal detachment.[6] Fluorescein angiography may reveal punctate hyperfluorescent window defects, round hypofluorescent lesions, "vasculitis," papilledema, and cystoid macular edema, indicating a disturbance of the retinal pigment epithelium[7] (Figs. 184-1, *B, C*). Computed axial tomography (CAT) scans typically show multiple, diffuse, periventricular lesions with high-density tumor before contrast injection. After contrast injection, dense periventricular enhancement appears and may involve the corpus callosum. Magnetic resonance imaging (MRI) shows isointense lesions on T1, and isointense to hyperintense lesions on T2. Periventricular contrast enhancement is strong. Positron emission tomography and single-photon emission computed tomography (SPECT) may show alterations in brain metabolism, perfusion, and blood–brain barrier permeability. Cerebrospinal fluid (CSF) analysis may allow the diagnosis of

TABLE 184-1

MALIGNANT CONDITIONS THAT MAY PRODUCE MASQUERADE SYNDROMES

Condition	Epidemiology	Ocular Manifestations	Systemic Associations	Comments
PCNSL in IC	98% B cell, 6th–7th decades of life	Vitreitis, creamy yellow retinal, subretinal, sub-RPE infiltrates, cranial nerve palsies	Behavioral changes, hemiparesis, ataxia	Methotrexate-containing regimens have most success to date
PCNSL in AIDS	12% risk	Similar to IC patients	Diffuse cerebral disease, CD4 typically <100	Positive SPECT and EBV PCR of CSF is diagnostic
SYSTEMIC LYMPHOMA/LEUKEMIA				
B cell lymphoma	Rare intraocular involvement, older adults	Vitreitis, retinal vasculitis, necrotizing retinitis, diffuse choroiditis, focal uveal masses, AU, hypopyon	Lymphadenopathy, involvement of retroperitoneum, paranasal sinuses, orbits, meninges, bone marrow	Usually have a known history of systemic lymphoma, but ocular involvement may be initial sign, average longevity of 31 months following ocular diagnosis
T cell lymphoma	2% of intraocular lymphomas	AU, iris thickening, hypopyon, vitreitis, chorioretinitis	May have widespread systemic disease by time of ocular involvement	Ocular involvement usually anterior
Mycosis fungoides	Rare intraocular involvement	AU, vitreitis, KP, papilledema	Typical cutaneous lesions of MF	Reported cases typically had a known history of MF
HTLV-1 lymphoma	Retrovirus endemic in southwest Japan, Caribbean islands, parts of central Africa	Retinal vasculitis, CWS, AU, vitreitis, subretinal infiltrates, retinal hemorrhages, iris nodules, CME	Adult T cell leukemia or lymphoma	
Ki-1 lymphoma	Single case report, 22-month-old male	Hyphema, fibrin in AC	Fever, adenopathy, hepatosplenomegaly	
Hodgkin's disease	Rare intraocular involvement	AU, PU, retinal lesions, CR scarring, optic disc swelling, periphlebitis, chorioretinitis, vitreitis	Lymphadenopathy, fever, nausea, abdominal pain	
Richter's syndrome	Rare intraocular involvement	AU, KP, vitreitis, yellow submacular lesion	Diffuse large cell lymphoma in patients with preexisting chronic lymphocytic leukemia	
Leukemia	Ocular findings in 28–75% with acute leukemia, less with chronic	Intraretinal hemorrhages, CWS, Roth spots, MA, peripheral NV, vitreitis, exudative RD, AU, hypopyon	Markedly high white blood cell count and other features of leukemia	Reed-Sternberg cells found in AC in one reported case

Primary intravascular lymphoma	Older adults	Vitreitis, iridocyclitis, KP, retinal artery occlusion	Tender erythematous nodules on trunk and extremities, CNS disturbances	Commonly fatal within 1 year of diagnosis
Uveal lymphoid proliferations	30-81 years	Multifocal creamy choroidal lesions, AU, KP, hypopyon, serous RD, diffuse choroidal thickening, ocular HTN, epibulbar mass	May be associated with systemic lymphoma	Range from benign to malignant, episcleral biopsy may not be representative[24]
Posttransplantation lymphoproliferative disorder	3% of patients on immunosuppressive agents for liver tx, four cases reported with intraocular involvement	Iris nodules (¾ patients), chorioretinitis (¼)	Most common in GI and CNS	Ranges from benign to aggressive multi-system malignancy; presumed EBV-stimulated B cell proliferation
Uveal melanoma	4.9% of 450 enucleation specimens had ocular inflammation initially[25]	Episcleritis, AU, PU, endophthalmitis, panophthalmitis	May have features of metastatic melanoma	Usually necrotic, diffuse, or plaque-like melanomas
Retinoblastoma	Inflammatory appearance in 1–3%, around 6 years old	Lack of calcification, unilateral, nonfamilial, AU, vitreitis, shifting white hypopyon, diffuse involvement	Typically none	
Juvenile xanthogranuloma	85% of skin lesions present before 1 year of age	Yellowish iris nodule or diffuse thickening, heterochromia, spontaneous hyphema	Raised, reddish-yellowish skin lesions	If eyelid involved, globe usually spared
Metastatic tumors	Most common intraocular malignancy in adults	Usually bilateral, multifocal, plateau-shaped, yellow posterior segment lesions with SRF; anterior segment: AU, iris nodules, NVI	Lung and breast carcinoma most common primary sites	Cutaneous melanoma most common metastasis to retina
PARANEOPLASTIC SYNDROMES				
Carcinoma-associated retinopathy/melanoma-associated retinopathy		Rapid vision loss, nyctalopia, color vision loss, vitreitis, abnormal ERG, attenuated retinal arterioles	Serum antiretinal antibodies, primary malignancy	
Bilateral diffuse uveal melanocytic proliferation		Rapid vision loss, cataract, multiple pigmented and nonpigmented placoid iris and choroidal nodules, serous RD	Primary nonocular malignancy	

AC, Anterior chamber; *AIDS,* acquired immunodeficiency syndrome; *AU,* anterior uveitis; *CME,* cystoid macular edema; *CNS,* central nervous system; *CR,* chorioretinal; *CSF,* cerebrospinal fluid; *CWS,* cotton-wool spots; *EBV,* Epstein–Barr virus; *ERG,* electroretinogram; *GI,* gastrointestinal; *HTLV,* human T cell lymphoma virus; *HTN,* hypertension; *IC,* immunocompetent; *KP,* keratic precipitates; *MA,* microaneurysm; *MF,* mycosis fungoides; *NV,* neovascularization; *NVI,* neovascularization of the iris; *PCNSL,* primary central nervous system lymphoma; *PCR,* polymerase chain reaction; *PU,* posterior uveitis; *RD,* retinal detachment; *RPE,* retinal pigment epithelium; *SPECT,* single-photon emission computed tomography; *SRF,* subretinal fluid; *tx,* transplant.

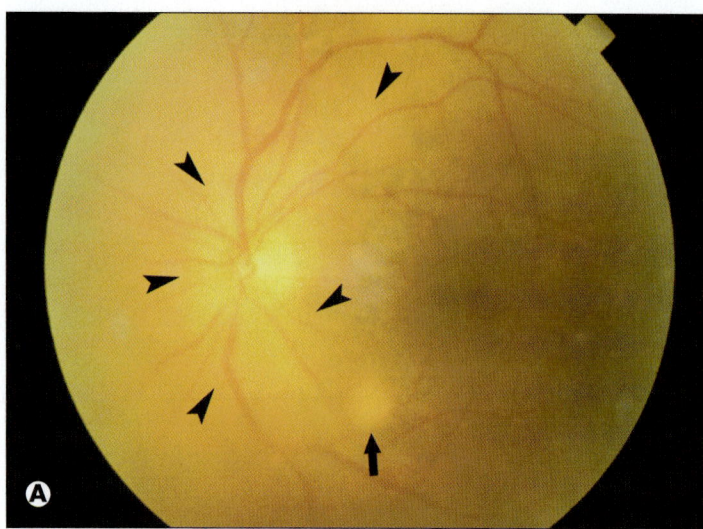

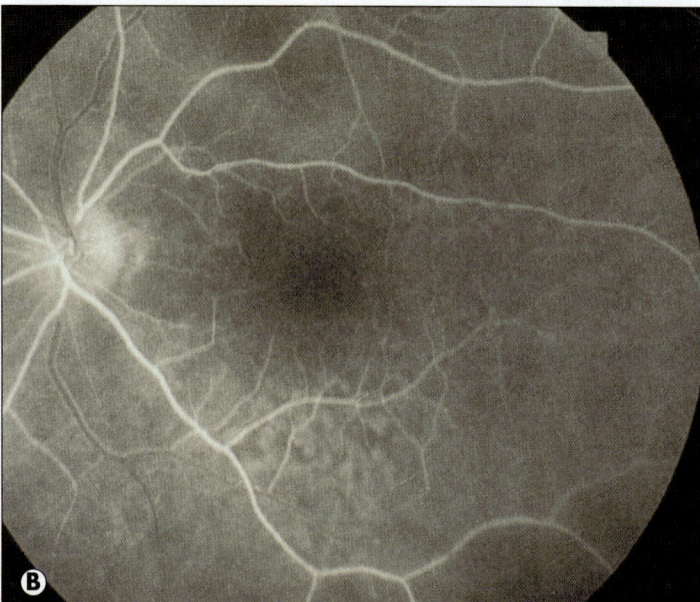

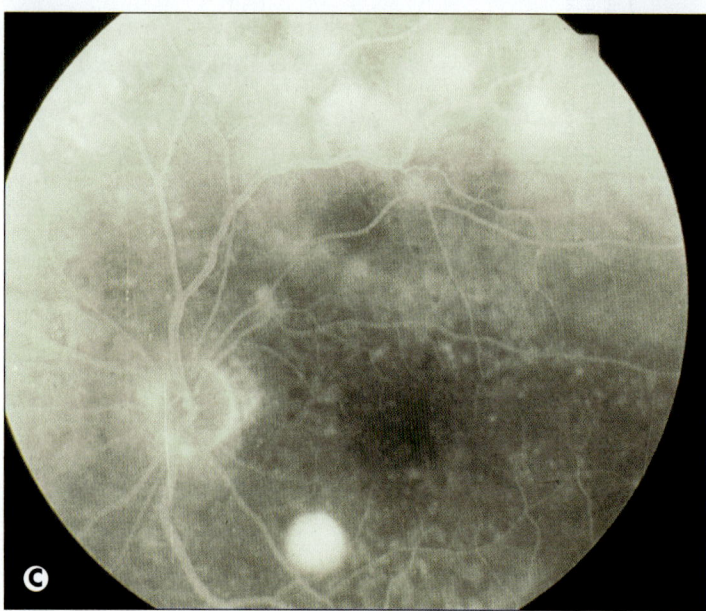

FIG. 184-1 ■ A, Left fundus of patient with primary central nervous system lymphoma involving vitreous and subretinal space. Note cloudiness of view due to vitreous cell, peripapillary involvement *(arrowheads)*, and separate lesion inferotemporal to optic nerve *(arrow)*. *B*, Fluorescein angiogram of left eye during laminar flow phase, revealing early hypofluorescence of lesions noted in A. *C*, Fluorescein angiogram of same eye after 6 minutes, revealing intense staining of infiltrates.

> **BOX 184-1**
>
> **Vitreous Humor Sample Processing Options**
>
> - Filtration through membrane (Millipore) filters, using negative pressure followed by fixation in 95% alcohol and staining of the filter
> - Initial fixation in an equal volume of 95% alcohol followed by
>   - Centrifugation
>   - Concentration of cells onto glass slides, air drying, followed by staining
>   - Paraffin embedding of resultant cellular pellet
>   - Celloidin bag technique: centrifugation of specimen in a celloidin-coated tube, followed by processing of the celloidin "bag," paraffin embedding, and sectioning

PCNSL to be made without the need for vitreous humor biopsy, but multiple samples may be needed.

The diagnosis of intraocular PCNSL may be made by cytological examination of a vitreous specimen. Vitrectomy itself does not result in cellular degradation.[8] To ensure that appropriate special staining and studies are performed, the specimen should be examined by an experienced ophthalmic pathologist and the surgeon must communicate directly with the pathologist before surgery to plan such studies. At the beginning of surgery, a 1ml undiluted vitreous humor sample should be manually aspirated into a syringe before the infusion is started. This sample should be processed rapidly to preserve cellular morphology. Retinal, subretinal, or sub-retinal pigment epithelium (RPE) material biopsy may be required if there is high clinical suspicion but repeatedly negative vitreous biopsy results. Processing options for the vitreous humor sample are detailed in Box 184-1.

One diagnostic algorithm for the evaluation of suspected PCNSL begins with cerebral MRI and lumbar puncture. If a definitive diagnosis is not made by the demonstration of malignant cells in the CSF, then a vitreous humor biopsy is performed. If these techniques fail to yield the diagnosis, repeat vitrectomy, with or without chorioretinal biopsy, is considered. If MRI revealed the presence of brain lesions and the vitreous humor biopsy result is unrevealing yet suspicion remains high, then stereotactic brain biopsy is considered.

DIFFERENTIAL DIAGNOSIS

The differential diagnosis of PCNSL includes all forms of ocular inflammatory disease that produce cells within the eye, including true uveitis and scleritis. Especially difficult to differentiate are those with concurrent retinal lesions, such as toxoplasmosis and acute retinal necrosis, although these two entities tend to have characteristic features described elsewhere in this text. Other neoplastic conditions which may masquerade as uveitis are covered in Table 184-1.

SYSTEMIC ASSOCIATIONS

The finding of intraocular PCNSL mandates a systemic evaluation, because it is the CNS involvement which results in the high mortality rate produced by this condition. When CNS involvement is present, patients may exhibit both general and focal signs and symptoms. The most frequent symptom reported at time of admission is behavioral changes. Focal neurological signs include hemiparesis, cerebellar signs (including ataxia), and cranial nerve palsies.[9] The mnemonic "GUN" syndrome has been proposed to emphasize the frequent occurrence of *glau*coma, *u*veitis, and *n*eurological symptoms in PCNSL.[10]

PATHOLOGY

With increased awareness and better diagnosis based on vitrectomy specimens, enucleation for PCNSL is not common. When enucleation is performed, gross examination reveals vitreous hu-

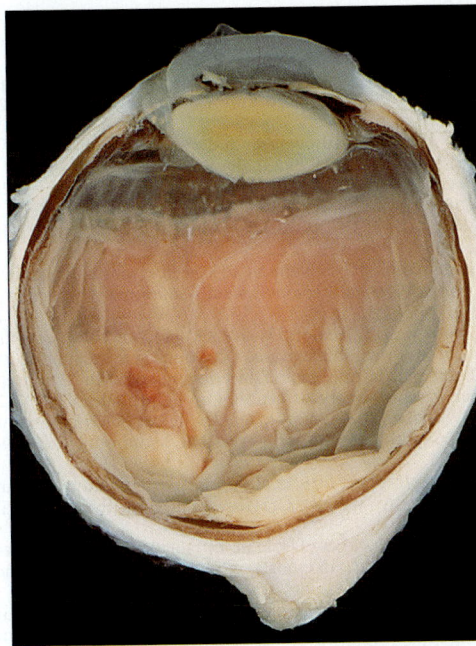

FIG. 184-2 ■ Gross photograph of enucleated globe with primary central nervous system lymphoma, revealing retinal thickening, hemorrhage, and subretinal pigment epithelial involvement.

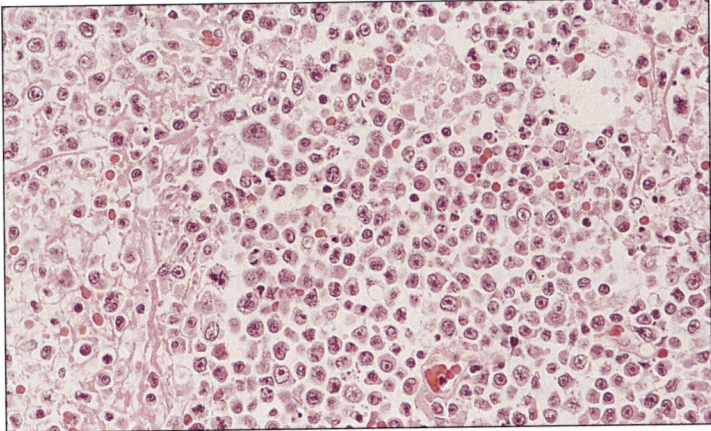

FIG. 184-3 ■ Photomicrograph of primary central nervous system lymphoma, revealing large neoplastic cells with necrosis.

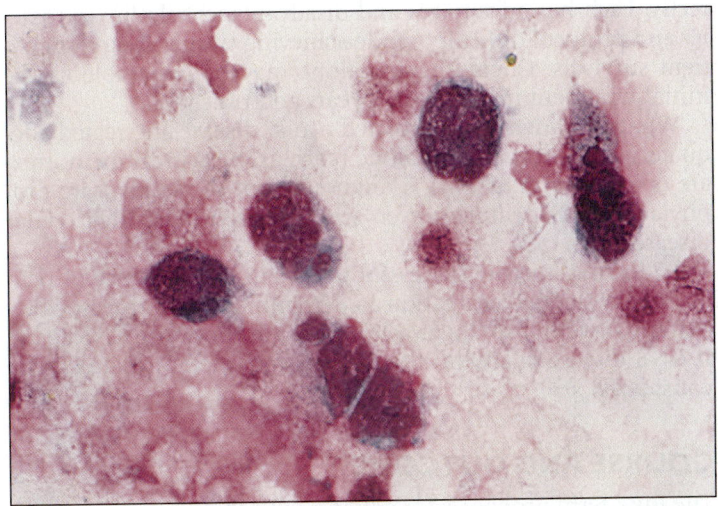

FIG. 184-4 ■ Vitreous cytology in primary central nervous system lymphoma, showing large neoplastic cells.

mor opacification, retinal thickening, and subretinal elevations (Fig. 184-2). Microscopic examination may reveal compartmentalization of malignant B cells from reactive T cells, with the former found in the retina, the latter in the choroid. This is in contrast to pathological findings in ocular involvement in systemic lymphoma, when the malignant infiltrate is within the uvea. Vitreous humor specimens typically produce much less cellular material, with an admixture of neoplastic and reactive lymphocytes. The neoplastic B lymphocytes are pleomorphic cells with hyperchromatic nuclei and an elevated nuclear-to-cytoplasm ratio. Nuclear membranes may show finger-like projections or folds and an irregular contour. Multiple nucleoli may be seen, and nuclear chromatin is coarse (Figs. 184-3 and 184-4). Also typical is the presence of necrotic cellular debris in the background (see Fig. 184-3).

False-negative reports may occur from improper or delayed fixation of the sample, which either damages or alters the staining properties of the neoplastic cells. Other factors that may lead to diagnostic pitfalls include the distribution of variable proportions of neoplastic and inflammatory cells in the vitreous humor. This variable distribution may mask the true pathology. Neoplastic cells may be concentrated in the subretinal and sub-RPE spaces, with the vitreous containing only inflammatory cells. In several reported cases, repeated vitrectomies showed negative cytology findings, and only a later vitrectomy or chorioretinal biopsy of subretinal lesions provided the diagnosis.[11] Prior use of systemic corticosteroids may produce false-negative results due to corticosteroid-induced cell loss.

Molecular pathology with immunophenotypic and genetic tests may be helpful in determining clonality. Although clonal expansion is part of a normal immune response, benign lymphoid lesions generally should not contain one dominant clone. Demonstration of an abnormal κ or λ light chain predominance helps to establish B lymphocyte clonality. Some B cell lymphomas may not express detectable surface immunoglobulins, a finding which itself is correlated with malignancy. Immunophenotyping can be carried out by immunohistochemistry or flow cytometry. Both use antibodies directed against specific cellular markers. Immunohistochemistry uses tissue sections on a microscope slide, while flow cytometry uses fresh cells labeled with fluorescent antibodies which are passed through a computerized cell counter. Gene rearrangement studies may enable determination of the clonality and lineage of lymphoid lesions as well.

An increased ratio of vitreous interleukin-10 to interleukin-6 has been proposed as suggestive of lymphoma,[12] but the diagnostic usefulness of this ratio remains to be verified.[13]

TREATMENT

The evaluation and treatment of PCNSL is best accomplished by practitioners at large centers with extensive experience, because of the condition's relative rarity and the need for coordination with a neuro-oncologist familiar with its treatment. Median survival with supportive care alone is 1.9–3.3 months.[14]

Surgery

PCNSL involvement in the CNS is multifocal, diffuse, and infiltrative in nature, therefore neurosurgical extirpation is not feasible and is indicated only to establish the diagnosis. Median survival following surgery alone ranges from 1–4.6 months.[14] Likewise vitrectomy surgery is indicated only to establish the diagnosis.

Medical Treatment

Isolated radiotherapy for PCNSL achieves a high rate of successful initial control of disease. However, in contrast to the long-term good results in non-Hodgkins lymphomas outside the CNS, radiotherapy produces short survival times when used in PCNSL[15] and is no longer standard as an isolated treatment in immunocompetent patients. For patients with CNS lymphoma who have advanced AIDS, radiotherapy remains a central therapeutic modality.

Multiple chemotherapeutic agents and regimens have been used in PCNSL, including chemotherapy alone and in combination with radiotherapy. Those chemotherapy protocols effective in systemic lymphoma have been found ineffective in PCNSL. Corticosteroids typically provide a dramatic clinical improvement, in part due to their lympholytic action. Regardless of their benefits, corticosteroids should be withheld until the diagnosis is established, due to the adverse impact they have on the establishment of the diagnosis through biopsy. Regimens containing methotrexate have been found to be the most effective. Two routes of methotrexate administration have shown the most promise, one using combination high-dose intravenous plus intrathecal methotrexate with subsequent cytarabine and radiotherapy,[16] and another using mannitol-induced blood–brain barrier disruption followed by intraarterial methotrexate and intravenous cyclophosphamide, with radiotherapy variably used.[17] No studies have been published comparing these regimens directly. Each has advantages and disadvantages relating to toxicity and protocol difficulty, while achieving similar long-term patient survivals. Chemotherapy alone may be preferable as the initial treatment in patients 60 years and older.[18]

Whether patients with isolated ocular disease are treated adequately with local therapy alone (such as intravitreal methotrexate or ocular irradiation) is unknown, but some advocate prophylactic CNS treatment even with apparently isolated ocular disease.[19]

Following initially successful treatment, a recurrence of ocular cells requires reevaluation to determine if CNS disease is recurrent as well. If so, therapy is directed at the entire CNS again. If CNS disease is absent, then intravitreal methotrexate can be considered.[20,21]

COURSE AND OUTCOME

The long-term prognosis for patients with PCNSL remains poor, with the longest median disease-free survivals reported to date of approximately 40 months.[22,23] Multiple factors have been found to be of significance in predicting outcomes and survival in patients with PCNSL, including age, performance status, neurological function, single versus multiple lesions, and superficial cerebral and cerebellar hemisphere lesions versus deep nuclei and periventricular region lesions.

OTHER SYSTEMIC CONDITIONS PRODUCING MASQUERADE SYNDROMES

Multiple other neoplastic conditions may result in confusion with an ocular inflammatory disease. These are detailed in Table 184-1.

REFERENCES

1. Rothova A, Ooijman F, Kerkhoff F, et al. Uveitis masquerade syndromes. Ophthalmology. 2001;108:386–99.
2. Corn BW, Marcus SM, Topham A, et al. Will primary central nervous system lymphoma be the most frequent brain tumor diagnosed in the year 2000? Cancer. 1997;79:2409–13.
3. Paulus W. Classification, pathogenesis and molecular pathology of primary CNS lymphomas. J Neurooncol. 1999;43:203–8.
4. Alderson L, Fetell MR, Sisti M, et al. Sentinel lesions of primary CNS lymphoma. J Neurol Neurosurg Psychiatry. 1996;60:102–5.
5. Hochberg FH, Miller DC. Primary central nervous system lymphoma. J Neurosurg. 1988;68:835–53.
6. Ursea R, Heinemann MH, Silverman RH, et al. Ophthalmic, ultrasonographic findings in primary central nervous system lymphoma with ocular involvement. Retina. 1997;17:118–23.
7. Cassoux N, Merle-Beral H, Leblond V, et al. Ocular and central nervous system lymphoma: clinical features and diagnosis. Ocul Immunol Inflamm. 2000;8:243–50.
8. Conlon MR, Craig I, Harris JF, et al. Effect of vitrectomy and cytopreparatory techniques on cell survival and preservation. Can J Ophthalmol. 1992;27:168–71.
9. Herrlinger U, Schabet M, Clemens M, et al. Clinical presentation and therapeutic outcome in 26 patients with primary CNS lymphoma. Acta Neurol Scand. 1998;97:257–64.
10. Kim EW, Zakov ZN, Albert DM, et al. Intraocular reticulum cell sarcoma: a case report and literature review. Graefes Arch Klin Exp Ophthalmol. 1979; 209:167–78.
11. Akpek EK, Ahmed I, Hochberg FH, et al. Intraocular-central nervous system lymphoma: clinical features, diagnosis, and outcomes. Ophthalmology. 1999; 106:1805–10.
12. Whitcup SM, Stark-Vancs V, Wittes RE, et al. Association of interleukin 10 in the vitreous and cerebrospinal fluid and primary central nervous system lymphoma. Arch Ophthalmol. 1997;115:1157–60.
13. Akpek EK, Maca SM, Christen WG, Foster CS. Elevated vitreous interleukin-10 level is not diagnostic of intraocular-central nervous system lymphoma. Ophthalmology. 1999;106:2291–5.
14. Jellinger K, Radaskiewicz TH, Slowik F. Primary malignant lymphomas of the central nervous system in man. Acta Neuropathol Suppl (Berl). 1975;(Suppl):95–102.
15. Nelson DF. Radiotherapy in the treatment of primary central nervous system lymphoma (PCNSL). J Neurooncol. 1999;43:241–7.
16. Nasir S, DeAngelis LM. Update on the management of primary CNS lymphoma. Oncology (Huntingt). 2000;14:228-34; 237–42; 244.
17. Neuwelt EA, Goldman DL, Dahlborg SA, et al. Primary CNS lymphoma treated with osmotic blood-brain barrier disruption: prolonged survival and preservation of cognitive function. J Clin Oncol. 1991;9:1580–90.
18. Freilich RJ, Delattre JY, Monjour A, DeAngelis LM. Chemotherapy without radiation therapy as initial treatment for primary CNS lymphoma in older patients. Neurology. 1996;46:435–9.
19. Read RW, Zamir E, Rao NA. Neoplastic masquerade syndromes. Surv Ophthalmol. 2002;2:81–124.
20. de Smet MD, Vancs VS, Kohler D, et al. Intravitreal chemotherapy for the treatment of recurrent intraocular lymphoma. Br J Ophthalmol. 1999;83:448–51.
21. Fishburne BC, Wilson DJ, Rosenbaum JT, Neuwelt EA. Intravitreal methotrexate as an adjunctive treatment of intraocular lymphoma. Arch Ophthalmol. 1997;115:1152–6.
22. Abrey LE, DeAngelis LM, Yahalom J. Long-term survival in primary CNS lymphoma. J Clin Oncol. 1998;16:859–63.
23. McAllister LD, Doolittle ND, Guastadisegni PE, et al. Cognitive outcomes and long-term follow-up results after enhanced chemotherapy delivery for primary central nervous system lymphoma. Neurosurgery. 2000;46:51–61.
24. Cockerham GC, Hidayat AA, Bijwaard KE, Sheng ZM. Re-evaluation of "reactive lymphoid hyperplasia of the uvea": an immunohistochemical and molecular analysis of 10 cases. Ophthalmology. 2000;107:151–8.
25. Fraser DJ Jr, Font RL. Ocular inflammation and hemorrhage as initial manifestations of uveal malignant melanoma. Incidence and prognosis. Arch Ophthalmol. 1979;97:1311–4.

NEURO-OPHTHALMOLOGY

Alfredo A. Sadun

CHAPTER

185

Principles of Imaging in Neuro-Ophthalmology

SWARAJ BOSE

DEFINITION

- Computed tomography, magnetic resonance imaging, angiography, and ultrasonography are used in the neuro-ophthalmic evaluation of the anatomical, pathological, vascular, and functional status of the eye, orbit, visual pathways, brain, and ocular motor system.
- Computed tomography
- Magnetic resonance imaging
- Angiography
  Magnetic resonance and computed tomographic angiography
  Conventional catheter angiography and angio-embolization
- Ultrasonography
- Functional imaging
  Positron emission tomography
  Single photon emission computed tomography
  Magnetic resonance spectroscopy
  Functional magnetic resonance imaging

INTRODUCTION

Neuroradiological evaluation of visual disorders using computed tomography and magnetic resonance imaging has advanced dramatically during the past two decades. Plain radiographs, arteriograms, and pneumoencephalograms have been replaced by modern computed imaging using better signal characteristics, resulting in sound clinicopathological and biochemical correlations. Even more exciting is the advent of functional imaging techniques such as positron emission tomography (PET), single photon emission computed tomography (SPECT), and functional magnetic resonance imaging (fMRI) that reveal both pathophysiology and pathology of the visual apparatus. Other techniques such as computed tomographic and magnetic resonance angiography (CTA and MRA), super-selective catheter angiography, use of newer embolization materials, magnetic resonance spectroscopy, carotid and transcranial Doppler, and color-flow imaging provide valuable information to the modern neuro-ophthalmologist and neuro-diagnostician. A word of caution: although modern neuroimaging techniques have improved considerably our diagnostic speed and accuracy, they should not be used as a substitute for an excellent and thorough clinical evaluation.

COMPUTED TOMOGRAPHY

Computed tomography (CT) was developed by Sir Godfrey Hounsfield at Electrical and Musical Industries in England, and he was awarded the Nobel Prize for medicine in 1979.[1] His innovation was to use a computer to improve on the technique of tomography. Tomography is used to concentrate on the object of interest, where the x-ray source and the film move relative to the patient during exposure. The scanning assembly consists of an x-ray detector on one side of the patient, rigidly connected to a collimated source of x-rays on the other side. Thus, the x-ray tube and the detector move around the patient as a single unit and images can be acquired at different levels. The computer then reconstructs the image from data points. These data points are represented as pixels of a numerical value resulting from the attenuation of the x-ray beams. This attenuation coefficient (Hounsfield unit [H]; ranges from −1000H for air, to 0H for water, and to +1000H for dense bone) provides a numerical matrix that helps the computer to reconstruct an image.[2,3]

To display the values of each data point in a meaningful way on photographic film, gray scales are chosen in which each contrast change represents a range of attenuation coefficients. The extent of the gray scale, referred to as the *window width,* and its central value, the *window level,* may be adjusted to emphasize certain aspects of the scanned tissues. Thus, soft tissue windows and bone windows have different central window levels and widths.

The clinical indications for CT scanning are as follows: (1) orbital disorders—thyroid, trauma, drusen, infection and tumor, (2) sinus and lacrimal disorders, (3) calcification, (4) brain imaging—acute bleeds and contraindications of magnetic resonance imaging (MRI), (5) bony abnormalities, and (6) acute hemorrhage. Disadvantages of CT include exposure to radiation, no direct sagittal imaging, possibility of contrast reactions, and dental or bony artifacts. The x-ray dose for a standard scan is 3–5 rads and 10 rads for a high-resolution scan. This is a very small dose as compared with 750–2000 rads needed to induce changes in the crystalline lens. The adjunctive intravenous injection of iodinated contrast provides enhancement in cranial CT to areas of increased vascularity and to areas of blood–brain barrier breakdown, through which seepage of iodinated contrast occurs. Contrast enhancement is used to detect intracranial extension of orbital tumors and evaluation of chiasmal and parachiasmal lesions. The use of intravenous iodinated contrast must be weighed against its risks, which include allergic reactions, nephrotoxicity, and anaphylactic shock that can be life-threatening. CT has the advantage over MRI of being a procedure that takes shorter time, is less expensive, and is useful in patients with contraindications or inability to perform MRI (Box 185-1).

Newer generation scanners employ thinner sections (which may be as small as 1mm thick) with less volume averaging, faster scan times, decreased motion artifact, reduced radiation exposure, more choices of position, and new reconstruction algorithms that enable sagittal and multiplanar reformations. Helical or spiral scanning has reduced imaging time further, because it enables continuous data acquisition as the patient table is moved.

MAGNETIC RESONANCE IMAGING

MRI is based on the concept of nuclear magnetic resonance, in which the nuclei of certain atoms become aligned or polarized when placed in a strong magnetic field.[2,3] Hesselink and Karampekios[4] in 1973 suggested that information from magnetic field gradients could be translated into position-dependent image maps.

By the early 1980s, it became apparent that MRI could identify lesions missed by CT scans, particularly demyelinating

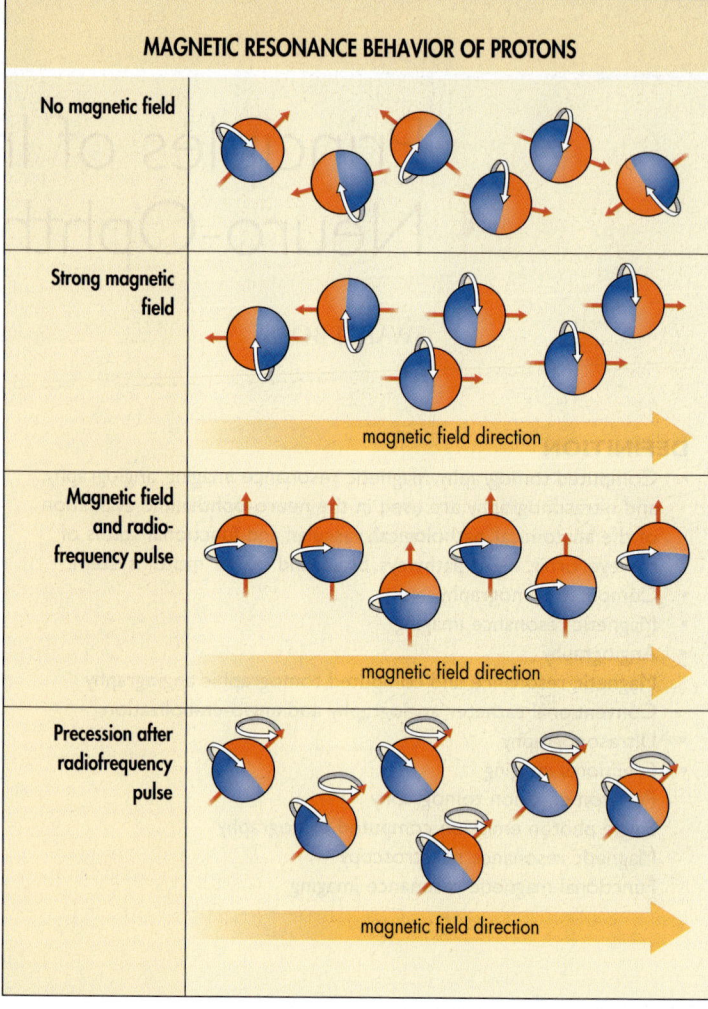

FIG. 185-1 ■ **Magnetic resonance behavior of protons.** In the absence of an external magnetic field, the spin orientation of free protons is random. In a strong magnetic field, the free protons become aligned with their magnetic axis parallel (or, less often, antiparallel) to the magnetic field. Exposure to a brief radiofrequency pulse at the Larmor frequency changes the alignment of the free protons' spin axes. After the radiofrequency pulse, the free protons twirl like tops around the lines of force of the magnetic field with a motion called *precession.*

plaques and posterior fossa pathology. The advantages of MRI and CT are outlined in Box 185-2.

Principles

When body tissue is placed in a strong magnetic field, the magnetic axes of a small percentage of randomly oriented, mobile hydrogen protons (distributed in body water) align parallel (and some antiparallel) to the magnetic field (Fig. 185-1). The lower energy state (parallel) is preferred, so a few more protons align this way. The protons perform a motion that resembles the wobbling of a spinning top that was hit. This motion is called precession. The precession frequency is dependent upon the strength of the external magnetic field. This relationship is described by the Larmor equation, $\omega_0 = \gamma B_0$, where ω_0 is the precession frequency (Hz or MHz), B_0 is the strength of the magnet (Tesla [T]), and γ is the gyro-magnetic ratio (a constant). Thus, the stronger the magnetic field (higher Tesla), the higher is the precession frequency. During this state, there are more protons aligned parallel to the external field, resulting in a net magnetic moment aligned with or longitudinal to the external magnetic field (see Fig. 185-1, second picture from top). An exposure to a brief radiofrequency (RF) pulse at the same frequency as the precessing protons (Larmor frequency) causes resonance or transfer of energy to the protons. This results in more protons being antiparallel and, thus, neutralizing more protons in the opposite direction. The consequence is a decrease in the longitudinal magnetization. The RF pulse can also cause the protons to precess in phase or be synchronous, resulting in a new magnetic vector called the *transversal magnetization.*

Three distinct procedures are used to encode 3-dimensional spatial localization—slice selection, frequency encoding, and phase encoding. Computer analysis of the frequency-encoded and phase-encoded information from each slice can be converted into spatial localization and signal intensity. An image is created using algorithms similar to those used to create CT images.

Imaging Parameters

T1 AND T2. When the RF pulse is switched off, the longitudinal magnetization increases and the transversal magnetization decreases or disappears. The longitudinal relaxation is described by the time constant T1, the longitudinal or spin–lattice relaxation time; the transversal relaxation is described by the time constant T2, the transversal or spin–spin relaxation time. Longitudinal and transversal relaxation times are different, independent processes. These time constants are intrinsic tissue parameters that describe the rate of relaxation of the perturbed nuclei. T1 depends on tissue composition, structure, and surroundings and is an expression of the time it takes for the energy imparted by the RF pulse to be transferred to the lattice of atoms that surround the nuclei. T2 comes about when protons go out of phase due to inhomogeneities of the external and internal magnetic field and is an expression of the time it takes for the loss of coherent precession of the nuclei after the RF pulse.

In T1-weighted images, fluid is dark ("black" vitreous, looks like high-definition CT scan) and fat is bright; this is good for

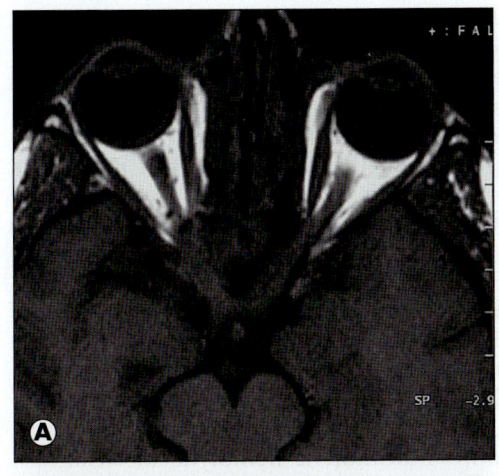
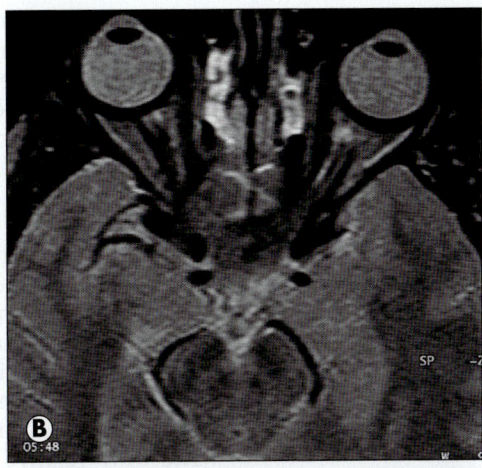
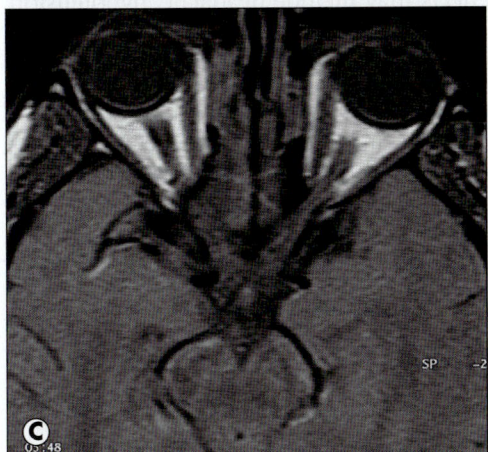
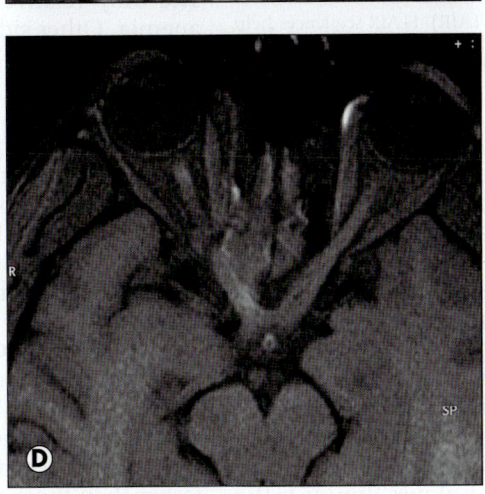

FIG. 185-2 ■ **Comparison of image contrast.** **A,** T1-Weighted image. **B,** T2-Weighted image. **C,** Proton-density image. **D,** Fat suppression reducing the normal bright signal of orbital fat in T1-weighted images and improving contrast between fat, optic nerve, and extraocular muscles. (Courtesy of Dr. Ramon Figueroa.)

TABLE 185-1

IMAGE CONTRAST AS A FUNCTION OF THE REPETITION AND ECHO TIMES

	Short Repetition Time, 300–800ms	Long Repetition Time, 2000–3000ms
Short echo time, 10–40ms	T1-weighted scan	Intermediate scan (proton-density scan)
Long echo time, 60–120ms	Poor signal-to-noise ratio	T2-weighted scan

TABLE 185-2

T1 AND T2 SIGNAL CHARACTERISTICS OF COMMON TISSUES AND MATERIALS

	T1 Signal	T2 Signal
Air Bone Dense calcification	Dark	Dark
High protein Paramagnetic substances (e.g., gadolinium, melanin)	Bright	Dark
Fat	Bright	Dark (bright on fast spin echo)
Water Edema Vitreous Cerebrospinal fluid	Dark	Bright
Very viscous protein Fibrosis Dura mater Ligaments	Dark	Dark
Muscle Nerve	Light gray	Dark gray
Gray matter	Dark gray	Light gray
White matter	Light gray	Gray

delineating anatomy. Contrast-enhanced images are done with T1 weighting. In T2-weighted images, fluid is bright ("white" vitreous) and is good for seeing pathology. As a rule, processes that are dark on CT are bright on T2. In proton-density image, fluid is darker than solid structures, but gray matter is brighter than on T2.

TR AND TE. Extrinsic parameters may be altered to capitalize on various intrinsic tissue parameters and, thereby, highlight or contrast certain tissue characteristics, while other tissue differences may be mitigated. Extrinsic parameters include time between RF pulses or repetition time (TR) and the time between the RF pulse and the signal measurement or echo time (TE). Alteration of TR and TE creates images that depend more on either the T1 or the T2 characteristics of the tissues (Table 185-1). T1-weighted images are created by using relatively short TE and TR, whereas T2-weighted images require a relatively long TE and TR. Images that have a mixture of the T1 and T2 tissue characteristics also may be created by using a long TR and short TE. These balanced or intermediate images sometimes are referred to as *proton-density images* (Fig. 185-2). The T1 and T2 signal characteristics of common tissues and materials are summarized in Table 185-2.

Special Sequences and Techniques

SPIN ECHO, GRADIENT ECHO, FLUID-ATTENUATED INVERSION RECOVERY, FAT SUPPRESSION. Various pulse sequences are used in the production of images. The three most common are the spin echo pulse sequence (SE), gradient echo pulse sequence (GRE), and inversion recovery pulse sequence. The SE technique has the advantage that T2 signal caused by inhomogeneity in the

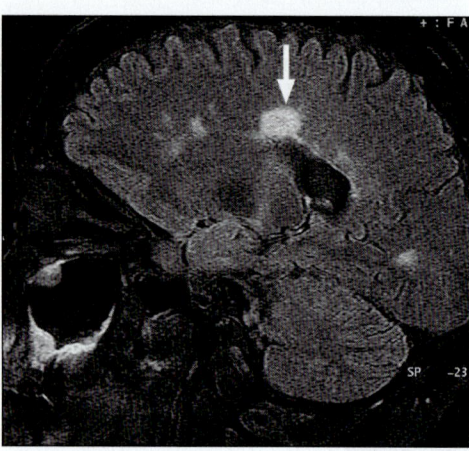

FIG. 185-3 ▌ **Fluid-attenuated inversion recovery (FLAIR).** FLAIR sequences help reveal demyelination in the central nervous system that often is not visible on routine magnetic resonance imaging (*arrow*). (Courtesy of Dr. Ramon Figueroa.)

main magnetic field or by paramagnetic substances is diminished. Fast SE techniques reduce motion artifact but are inferior to SE in the detection of hemorrhage or small lesions that have weak signal strength.[5-7]

Because GRE sequences exaggerate magnetic field inhomogeneities, they enhance the signal from paramagnetic substances, such as iron in an old hemorrhage, and may be used to supplement SE sequences for the detection of hemorrhage. Also, GRE protocols have a shorter TR (which allows faster imaging), a high signal-to-noise ratio (which allows thinner slices), and provide flow-related enhancement (which can be used to form images for MRA).[8,9] Inversion recovery techniques diminish the signal from protons of particular substances that are relaxed only partially to a perpendicular orientation to the main magnetic field, such as fat in short time interval inversion recovery and in spectral presaturation inversion recovery sequences, or cerebrospinal fluid (CSF) in fluid-attenuated inversion recovery (FLAIR). FLAIR sequences help reveal demyelination or multiple sclerosis plaques in the central nervous system, which often is not visible on routine MRI (see Fig. 185-3).[10] In this sequence, the CSF signal is strongly attenuated, accentuating periventricular and extra-axial pathology near the brain surface.

Fat suppression is a technique that deletes the fat in the orbit, allowing visibility of small lesions in the orbit. Two main techniques follow: (1) STIR—short time inversion recovery and (2) CHESS—chemical-shift-based fat suppression, also called *fat-sat*, which is very useful when combined with intravenous contrast. Fat-suppression techniques particularly improve the detection of pathology in the orbit, the pituitary, and around the skull base (which has fat in the bone marrow), but also may introduce artifacts, particularly in the lower aspects of the orbit (Fig. 185-3).[11-14]

DIFFUSION-WEIGHTED IMAGING. To measure the phenomenon of slow water diffusion in tissues (which generally increases in pathological states), diffusion-weighted images help in the evaluation of cytotoxic edema, demyelinating plaques, inflammation, tumors, and early brain infarction, and to define internal tissue architecture.[15-17]

CONTRAST ENHANCEMENT. Paramagnetic substances have large magnetic moments that may be over 1000 times that of a proton because of the presence of at least one unpaired electron. The large magnetic moment allows rapid fluctuations of the local magnetic field, which facilitates energy transfer from nearby protons to their lattice and results in a shortened T1 relaxation time. The T2 relaxation time is shortened, also, but to a much lesser extent. Gadolinium, a toxic metal ion, is chelated with diethylenetriamine pentaacetic acid (DTPA), which reduces its toxicity but retains its paramagnetic properties and gives biodistribution characteristics similar to those of iodinated contrast media used in CT scans.[18] The chelate remains extracellular, does

not cross the intact blood–brain barrier, and is excreted renally. In pathological states, the chelate tends to move from the intravascular to the extracellular space and, thereby, highlights pathological processes.

Because it shortens the T1 relaxation time, gadolinium typically is used for T1-weighted imaging, in which it provides a bright signal. For orbital studies, T1-weighting techniques are combined with a fat-suppression technique to enhance lesions so that they may be differentiated from the otherwise bright orbital fat signal (see Fig. 185-3).[19] Gadolinium–DTPA is administered in current applications as its dimeglumine salt at a dose of 0.1 mmol/kg. Double-dose or triple-dose contrast studies may help in the detection of subtle lesions such as cerebral metastasis.[20,21] Gadolinium has an excellent safety record, with rare serious reactions such as hives, bronchospasm, or asthmatic attack. The only relative contraindication is hemolytic or sickle cell anemia. Other side effects may include headache, hypotension, or a transient rise in serum iron or bilirubin levels.

SURFACE AND HEAD COILS. The placement of receiver coil antennae close to the tissues to be scanned may provide much stronger signal acquisition and, thus, allow thinner sections, better resolution, and shorter scan times. Surface coils for the eyes provide high-resolution visualization of the globe and optic nerve[22,23] but are limited by signal drop-off in and behind the posterior orbit. Suspected disease involvement of the orbital apex, chiasm, or more posterior structures indicates the need for a head coil.

MAGNETIZATION TRANSFER IMAGING. Magnetic transfer imaging capitalizes on the effect large proteins have on the transfer of energy between bound and unbound water protons. The benefits of magnetization transfer are greatest in tissues that have high macromolecular concentrations (e.g., brain, muscle) rather than those that have low macromolecular concentrations (e.g., fat).[24] Magnetic transfer contrast sequences improve the detection of brain lesions such as cerebral metastases, and the best differentiation of demyelinating plaques from edematous lesions is effected with magnetization transfer techniques combined with gadolinium enhancement.[25] Small-vessel visualization may be improved by background suppression in MRA that uses magnetization transfer.

Contraindications and Risks

Long-lasting biohazards from exposure to the large magnetic fields and RF pulses of MRI alone have not been demonstrated yet. However, physical injury may occur in the presence of ferromagnetic foreign bodies because of movement within these strong magnetic fields.[26] Ferromagnetic, metallic, intraocular, intraorbital or intracranial foreign bodies, cochlear implants, intracranial aneurysm clips, cardiac pacemakers, and defibrillators are contraindications to MRI.[27] Most neurosurgical clips are not ferromagnetic, and those placed in other locations (e.g., dura, meninges) are not a contraindication. When the operator is not sure, CT scans may be carried out to screen for such objects. Although unusual, burns have been reported during MRI with the concurrent use of an electrocardiogram lead and a pulse oximeter.[28] Medical personnel must be careful not to bring ferromagnetic objects into the vicinity of the MRI, because these could be transformed into dangerous projectiles that may result in serious injury.

ANGIOGRAPHY

Magnetic Resonance Angiography

The technique MRA, developed over a decade ago, consists of an entire family of new pulse sequences.[1] In MRA, three basic approaches are utilized: time-of-flight (TOF) MRA, phase-contrast angiography (PCA), and gadolinium-enhanced MRA (GDx-MRA). These techniques share two basic steps as follows: (1) acquisition of flow-sensitive image of vessels, with suppression of

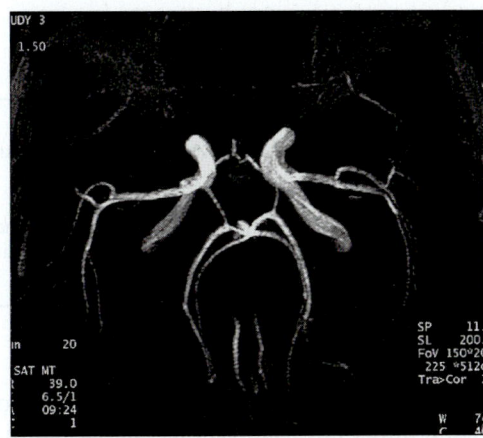

FIG. 185-4 ▌▌ Magnetic resonance angiography of the circle of Willis. (Courtesy of Dr. Ramon Figueroa.)

stationary background to enhance vascular anatomy and (2) production of 2-dimensional images from 3-dimensional volume image data. TOF utilizes a gradient-echo technique that relies on inflow-related signal enhancement of vessels, while PCA utilizes a similar technique to detect velocity-induced phase shifts that distinguish flowing blood from stationary tissues.[29-31] TOF methods capitalize on the fully relaxed protons in flowing blood that move into the imaging slice when stationary protons have been excited to a saturation level (low signal) by very frequent RF pulses. TOF methods have the advantages of less signal loss because of complex flow and better accuracy with high-velocity flow. Disadvantages include insensitivity to slow flow in smaller vessels and limited imaging of a long length of vessel as a result of signal loss from eventual saturation of the protons in the flowing blood. Phase-contrast methods have the advantages of excellent background suppression and sensitivity to slow flow, and the ability to encode direction and velocity information. A newer hybrid technique, multiple overlapping thin slab acquisitions, combines the advantages of 2-dimensional and 3-dimensional modes for TOF acquisitions, because it limits signal drop-off yet retains high resolution.[32]

MRA is not a simple display of vascular anatomy, as in contrast angiography. Instead, MRA extrapolates physiological data obtained from flow characteristics of protons to demonstrate anatomy. Thus, the diameter of the blood vessels sometimes may appear smaller with MRA than with contrast angiography. Clinical applications of MRA in neuro-ophthalmology include the evaluation of the extracranial (carotid stenosis, plaques, and dissections in the evaluation of transient visual loss) and the intracranial circulations (aneurysms, arteriovenous malformations, occlusive disease, and carotid fistulas). The limitations of MRA are as follows: (1) detecting aneurysms less than 5mm in diameter, (2) false-positive results in tightly wound vessel loops, and (3) a tendency to overinterpret vessel stenosis. Conversely, MRA is an excellent noninvasive technique for detecting asymptomatic aneurysms measuring greater than 5mm (Fig. 185-4).

Computed Tomographic Angiography

This is a minimally invasive, relatively new technology that uses an intravenous bolus injection of iodinated contrast, followed by high-speed spiral CT scan with computer-generated 3-dimensional images of medium-sized and large-sized arteries. The advantages of CTA over standard MRA are the rapidity of examination and images of the true lumen (rather than flow within a vessel), and can be performed in patients with claustrophobia, pacemakers, and older aneurysm clips.[33] The advantages of CTA include detection of aneurysms as small as 1.7mm, superior imaging of the neck of the aneurysm, better delineation of surgical anatomy, characterization of mural thrombi, detection of vasospasm, arte-

rial stenosis, and carotid–cavernous fistulas, and provision of rotating 3-dimensional images.[34,35] CTA drawbacks include difficult detection and delineation of cavernous sinus and posterior inferior cerebellar artery aneurysms, feeding vessels for dural carotid–cavernous fistulas, and risks involving radiation exposure and contrast agents. CTA offers distinct advantages over MRA but has not yet replaced conventional angiography.

Conventional Angiography

Conventional percutaneous cerebral angiography (usually via the femoral artery) remains the gold standard for accurate detection and localization of small intracranial aneurysms, with or without subarachnoid hemorrhage.[36] Interventional neuroimaging (synonyms are interventional neuroradiology, endovascular neurosurgery, neuroendovascular therapy) involves the introduction of coaxial systems of extremely flexible microcatheters, balloons, coils, and other devices in the cerebral vascular system for therapeutic purposes. Currently, endovascular treatment is applied commonly for arteriovenous malformations and carotid–cavernous and dural fistulas using GDC coils (Guglielmi detachable coils, Target Therapeutics, Fremont, Calif.).[37-39] The field of endovascular therapy is fascinating and is rapidly growing, making it safe, reliable, and a real alternative to neurosurgical intervention. Some risks and complications include local hematomas (15% of cases), vessel wall dissection (<1% of cases), emboli, and transient ischemic attacks or cerebral infarction (reported to occur in 1.6% of cases).[40]

ULTRASONOGRAPHY

Ultrasonographic technology is based on the reflection of ultrasound waves (5–20MHz) at acoustic interfaces and has the advantages that it does not require ionizing radiation or injection of contrast agents and often is available in an office setting. It also gives a real-time display of moving tissues. It is used in neuro-ophthalmology for the evaluation of orbital pathology such as mass lesions, inflammatory–congestive processes (Chapter 201), and foreign bodies. Dilatation of the optic nerve sheath in papilledema also may be detected, and papilledema may be differentiated from some causes of pseudopapilledema (e.g., disc drusen), which give their own strong acoustic interface.[41] Some disadvantages of orbital ultrasonography are generally poor visualization of the orbital apex (especially at 20MHz) and that expertise and experience are necessary to perform and interpret the study adequately.

Doppler ultrasonographic techniques provide an inexpensive, rapid, and easily tolerated method for the noninvasive investigation of cerebral and orbital vasculature, and they may help to elucidate the cause and guide the treatment of many ocular vascular syndromes. Carotid, vertebral, transcranial, and orbital and color Doppler imaging have been utilized to investigate directly vessel patency, blood flow, and pulsation.[42] The Doppler principle is based on the shift in frequency that occurs when ultrasound waves are reflected off flowing blood cells. The frequency change can be translated into a flow velocity. Doppler flow information may be overlaid onto conventional "B"-mode ultrasonographic images to help localize the vessel and properly assign flow information.

FUNCTIONAL IMAGING

Recent advances in neuroimaging technology have permitted new understandings of the neuroanatomical basis of psychophysical and pathophysiological phenomena of vision. An emergent area is the use of functional imaging techniques that include PET, SPECT, magnetic source imaging, magnetic resonance spectroscopy (MRS), or neurospectroscopy, and fMRI. Current applications of functional imaging include detection of hypermetabolic states associated with tumor, differentiation of tumor from areas of radiation necrosis, localization of seizure foci, detection of ischemic regions, evaluation of biochemical changes associated with cognitive and psychiatric abnormalities and their response to pharmaceutical intervention, and drug localization in the brain.

PET and SPECT

PET and SPECT are performed with systemically administered isotopes (such as 18F-fluoro-2-deoxyglucose [FDG], 13-N ammonia [$^{13}NH_3$], fluoride-18 [^{18}F]) that emit protons to image biological processes that measure regional cerebral blood flow and glucose consumption and thus, indirectly, tissue metabolism.[43,44] In PET, the isotope FDG is injected intravenously. It traces the transport and phosphorylation of glucose, and the glucose-linked positron emits two photons, which strike detectors placed around the head. The greater the glucose metabolism of the tissue, the more photons are emitted, and the blacker is the representation on the PET image. Glucose metabolism provides about 95% of the adenosine triphosphate required for brain function. FDG is taken rapidly into the intracellular compartment but, because its metabolism stops following its phosphorylation to deoxyglucose-6-phosphate, FDG cannot diffuse from the brain. It, therefore, remains trapped intracellularly and, thus, is an excellent agent to use for cerebral metabolism imaging.[45] The PET scanner assays either the changing tissue concentration of the labeled molecule or product over time or the accumulated concentration of the molecule at any given time. Tomographic images are obtained in a manner similar to those for MRI or CT scanning. Cerebral blood flow, oxygen utilization, and glucose utilization may be measured. PET scanning is used mainly for evaluation of stroke, tumors, migraine, blepharospasm, cortical visual loss, and mapping of the visual cortex, among others.[46–48] The shortcoming of PET is its relatively poor resolution of 5–7mm, exorbitant cost, and limited availability because of the requirement for close proximity to a cyclotron to produce the radioisotopes.

In SPECT, isotopes such as iodine-123 iodoamphetamine or technetium-99 are incorporated into biologically active compounds, and CT plots their distribution. The information provided by SPECT is similar to that of PET, but SPECT does not require the use of isotopes produced in a cyclotron. However, resolution is even poorer with SPECT. The future of these technologies is very bright and with the new advent of micro-PET, higher resolution receptor and genetic imaging will provide greater understanding about the workings and abnormalities of the human brain.

Magnetic Resonance Spectroscopy

MRS is used for diagnostic biochemistry *in vivo* and is based on the same principle previously used in analytical chemistry to obtain MR spectra. MRS studies of cerebral ischemia are confined solely to proton (^1H) and phosphorus-31 (^{31}P) because of their intrinsically higher sensitivity compared with other nuclear species. Neurospectroscopy is synonymous with proton MRS (higher sensitivity than ^{31}P MRS), which provides results that are easy to interpret, uses small voxel size ($1cm^3$), and enables the detection of compounds such as *N*-acetylaspartate, creatine, choline, lactate, and inositols.[49] Each metabolite has a "signature" that, when added to the other major metabolites, results in a complex spectrum of overlapping peaks.[50] Acquiring and interpreting spectra form the basis of a clinical report. Pathologies documented by MRS include brain tumor, stroke, focal cerebral lesions, multiple sclerosis, and intracranial hemorrhage.[51] An acutely ischemic brain produces lactate, by anaerobic metabolism during the first 2–3 days after injury, which can be detected by MRS. With the advent of MRS and using multi-MR modalities (MRI, MRA, perfu-

sion MR), it is now possible to evaluate extensively not only regions of cerebral injury but regions at risk of infarction.

The magnetic source imaging technique is an approach to functional imaging that correlates magnetic resonance anatomy with magnetoencephalography, which is a mapping of the magnetic flux, induced by the background or evoked electrical activity of the brain.[52]

Functional Magnetic Resonance Imaging

Compared with PET and SPECT, fMRI is a more recent, less invasive technology for mapping cerebral cortical activation in response to performing specific cognitive, sensory, or motor tasks. The basis for most fMRI done today is pixel-by-pixel measurement of increases in blood oxygenation level during the performance of specific tasks (BOLD imaging: blood oxygen level dependent).[53] This method utilizes the change in magnetic susceptibility of hemoglobin as it changes from oxyhemoglobin (diamagnetic, reduces magnetic field into which it is placed) to deoxyhemoglobin (paramagnetic, increases magnetic field), which results in T2 shortening. Although a weak effect is produced, repeated measurements, data subtraction techniques between resting and activated oxygen content, and sophisticated statistical methods may result in sufficient information to give a topographical representation of perfusion. The advantage of this technique is that no injection is required. fMRI is evolving rapidly as a useful experimental and clinical tool for functional cortical mapping, psychophysical tests, brain tumor mapping, and understanding the basis of higher visual functioning.[54,55]

IMAGING STRATEGIES IN NEURO-OPHTHALMOLOGY

General guidelines for the choice of imaging technique are given in Table 185-3. To improve the diagnostic yield, it is important to order the appropriate neuroimaging technique and communicate clearly with the neuroradiologist (Box 185-3). In brief, CT scan, a relatively less-expensive, easier for patient, and faster imaging technique, is still very useful for the evaluation of orbital pathology (tumor, trauma, thyroid) and in patients with acute intracranial bleeding. It is important to remember that head CT scans should not be used to interpret orbital pathology, and separate orbital scans should be ordered. Orbital scans require negative angulation, parallel to the orbital floor, while head scans require positive angulation.

Gadolinium-enhanced, fat-suppression magnetic resonance techniques generally best demonstrate pathology of the optic nerve, which includes tumors (such as glioma, meningioma, and hemangioma), radiation damage, demyelinating disease, and inflammatory damage (such as sarcoidosis). Papilledema can be evaluated using "B" scan ultrasonography to look for a dilated optic nerve sheath and confirmed by a decrease in the diameter of the sheath with abduction (or adduction) of the eye by 30°.[56] MRI of the brain in papilledema will show slit ventricles, and a different sequence for the veins may reveal a venous thrombosis (MR venogram). Optic nerve drusen, often calcified, may be seen

---

TABLE 185-3

GENERAL GUIDELINES FOR THE CHOICE OF NEUROIMAGING TECHNIQUES IN NEURO-OPHTHALMOLOGY

Anatomical Location	Clinical Condition	Neuroimaging Technique(s)		
Orbit	Tumors	USG (solid vs. cystic), CT (non-contrast) MRI (soft tissue, fat suppression)		
	Thyroid ophthalmopathy, trauma, hemorrhage, foreign body	Non-contrast CT (preferred imaging)		
	Optic nerve tumor, orbital apex tumor	Gd-enhanced, fat-suppressed MRI		
Cavernous sinus, chiasm, parasellar region	Tumor	High-resolution contrast CT (fine cuts), MRI		
	Aneurysm (e.g., CN III palsy)	Gd-enhanced MRI, MRA, catheter angiography		
	Aneurysm with bleeding	Non-contrast CT scan		
Retrochiasmal area and posterior fossa	Aneurysm or AV malformation with bleed	Non-contrast CT scan		
Brain	Intracerebral hemorrhage	CT density	MRI-T1	MRI-T2
	1. Acute (intracellular Fe^{++}/metHb)	Bright	Isodense	Hypodense
	2. Subacute (extracellular Fe^{+++}/metHb)	Isodense	Hyperdense	Hyperdense
	3. Chronic (metHb/hemosiderin)	Dark	Hyperdense	Hyperdense
	Papilledema	"B" scan USG (optic sheath dilatation) Gd-enhanced MRI, MR venogram		
	Multiple sclerosis	Gd-enhanced MRI, T2, FLAIR sequence		
Carotids and vertebrals	Stenosis, dissection, plaques, evaluation of amaurosis	Carotid Doppler (USG), MRA, CT angiography, catheter angiography		
Globe	Optic disc drusen	"B" scan USG, non-contrast CT		
	Tumor, trauma, calcification	Non-contrast CT		

AV, Arteriovenous; *CN*, cranial nerve; *CT*, computed tomography; *Fe⁺⁺*, ferrous iron; *Fe⁺⁺/metHb*, iron-methemoglobin; *Fe⁺⁺⁺*, ferric iron; *FLAIR*, fluid-attenuated inversion recovery; *Gd*, gadolinium; *MR*, magnetic resonance; *MRA*, magnetic resonance angiography; *MRI*, magnetic resonance imaging; *USG*, ultrasonography.

with "B" scan, CT, MRI, or intravenous fluorescein angiography. For most sellar and parasellar lesions, MRI usually is the study of choice. The Optic Neuritis Treatment Trial (ONTT) and the Controlled High-risk Avonex Multiple Sclerosis (CHAMPS) study have found MRI changes to be of diagnostic and predictive value.[57,58] Also, the extent of MRI lesions in the optic nerve in patients with optic neuritis using short-time inversion recovery (STIR) imaging correlated with visual recovery.[59]

REFERENCES

1. Hounsfield G. Computerized transverse axial scanning (tomography): I. Description of the system. Br J Radiol. 1973;46:1016–22.
2. Berman EL, Wirtschafter JD, eds. Imaging: ophthalmology clinics of North America. Philadelphia: Saunders; 1994.
3. Wirtschafter JD, Berman EL, McDonald CS. Magnetic resonance imaging and computed tomography. Ophthalmology Monograph 6. San Francisco: American Academy of Ophthalmology; 1992.
4. Hesselink JR, Karampekios S. Normal computed tomography and magnetic resonance imaging of the globe, orbit, and visual pathways. Neuroimaging Clin North Am. 1996;6:15–27.
5. Ahn SS, Mantello MR, Jones KM, et al. Rapid magnetic resonance imaging of the pediatric brain using the fast spin-echo technique. AJNR Am J Neuroradiol. 1992;13:1169–77.
6. Jolesz FA, Jones KM. Fast spin echo imaging of the brain. Magn Reson Imaging. 1993;5:1–13.
7. Norbash AM, Glover GH, Enzman DR. Intracerebral lesion contrast with spin-echo and fast spin-echo pulse sequences. Radiology. 1992;185:661–5.
8. Taveras JM. Technical considerations. In: JM Taveras. Neuroradiology, ed 3. Baltimore: Williams & Wilkins; 1996:3–30.
9. Elster AD. Gradient-echo magnetic resonance imaging: techniques and acronyms. Radiology. 1993;186:1–8.
10. Takanashi J, Sugita K, Fujii K, et al. Optic neuritis with silent cerebral lesions: availability of FLAIR sequences. Pediatr Neurol. 1995;12:152–4.
11. Tien RD, Hesselink JR, Chu PK, et al. Improved detection and delineation of head and neck lesions with fat suppression spin-echo magnetic resonance imaging. AJNR Am J Neuroradiol. 1991;12:19–24.
12. Tien RD. Fat-suppression magnetic resonance imaging in neuroradiology: techniques and clinical application. AJR Am J Roentgenol. 1992;158:369–79.
13. Anzai Y, Lufkin RB, Jabour BA, Hanafee WN. Fat-suppression failure artifacts simulating pathology on frequency-selective fat-suppression magnetic resonance images of the head and neck. AJNR Am J Neuroradiol. 1992;13:879–84.
14. Takehara S, Tanaka T, Uemura K, et al. Optic nerve injury demonstrated by magnetic resonance imaging with STIR sequences. Neuroradiology. 1994;36:512–4.
15. Mosely ME, Kucharczyk J, Mintoravitch J, et al. Diffusion-weighted magnetic resonance imaging of acute stroke: correlation with T2-weighted and magnetic susceptibility-enhanced magnetic resonance imaging in cats. AJNR Am J Neuroradiol. 1990;11:423–9.
16. Sevick RJ, Kanda F, Mintorovitch J, et al. Cytotoxic brain edema: assessment with diffusion-weighted magnetic resonance imaging. Radiology. 1992;185:687–90.
17. Doran M, Hajnal JV, von Bruggen N, et al. Normal and abnormal white matter tracts shown by magnetic resonance imaging using directional diffusion weighted sequences. J Comput Assist Tomogr. 1990;14:865–73.
18. Carr JJ. Magnetic resonance contrast agents for neuroimaging. Safety issues. Neuroimaging Clin North Am. 1994;4:43–54.
19. Tien RD, Chu PK, Hesselink JR, et al. Intra- and paraorbital lesions: value of fat-suppression magnetic resonance imaging with paramagnetic contrast enhancement. AJNR Am J Neuroradiol. 1991;12:245–53.
20. Yuh WTC, Engelken JD, Muhonen MG, et al. Experience with high-dose gadolinium magnetic resonance imaging in the evaluation of brain metastases. AJNR Am J Neuroradiol. 1992;13:335–45.
21. Haustein J, Laniado M, Niendorf HP, et al. Triple-dose versus standard-dose gadopentetate dimeglumine: a randomized study in 199 patients. Radiology. 1993;186:855–60.
22. Gass A, Barker GJ, MacManus D, et al. High resolution magnetic resonance imaging of the anterior visual pathway in patients with optic neuropathies using fast spin echo and phased array local coils. J Neurol Neurosurg Psychiatry. 1995;58:562–9.
23. Breslau J, Dalley RW, Tsuruda JS, et al. Phased-array surface coil magnetic resonance of the orbits and optic nerves. AJNR Am J Neuroradiol. 1995;16:1247–51.
24. Gillams AR, Fuleihan N, Grillone G, Carter AP. Magnetization transfer contrast magnetic resonance in lesions of the head and neck. AJNR Am J Neuroradiol. 1996;17:355–60.
25. Elster AD, King JC, Matthews VP, et al. Cranial tissues: appearance at gadolinium-enhanced and non-enhanced magnetic resonance imaging with magnetization transfer contrast. Radiology. 1994;190:541–6.
26. Klucznik RP, Carrier DA, Pyka R, Haid RW. Placement of a ferromagnetic intracranial aneurysm clip in a magnetic field with a fatal outcome. Radiology. 1993;187:855–6.
27. Shellock FG, Kanal E. Policies, guidelines, and recommendations for magnetic resonance imaging safety and patient management. J Magn Reson Imaging. 1991;1:97–101.
28. Shellock FG, Slimp G. Severe burn of the finger caused by using a pulse oximeter during magnetic resonance imaging. AJR Am J Roentgenol. 1989;153:1105.
29. Turski PA, Korosec FR. Technical features and emerging clinical applications of phase contrast MRA. Neuroimaging Clin North Am. 1992;2:785–800.
30. Parker DL, Yuan C, Blatter DD. Magnetic resonance angiography by multiple thin slab 3D acquisition. Magn Reson Med. 1991;17:434–51.
31. Kaufman DI, Siebert JE, Pernicone JR, Eggenberger E. The use of magnetic resonance angiography in neuro-ophthalmology. Ophthalmol Clin North Am. 1994; 7:487–508.
32. Polachini I Jr. Magnetic resonance angiography. In: Greenberg JO, ed. Neuroimaging: a companion to Adams and Victor's principles of neurology. New York: McGraw-Hill; 1999:667–725.
33. Katz DA, Marks MP, Napel SA, et al. Circle of Willis: evaluation with spiral computed tomography angiography, magnetic resonance angiography, and conventional angiography. Radiology. 1995;195:445–9.
34. Villablanca JP, Martin N, Jahan R, et al. Volume rendered helical computerized tomography angiography in the detection and characterization of intracranial aneurysms. J Neurosurg. 2000;93:254–64.
35. Coskum O, Hamon M, Catroux G, et al. Carotid cavernous fistulas: diagnosis with spiral CT angiography. AJNR Am J Neuroradiol. 2000;21:712–6.
36. Gomez CR, Zenteno MA. Interventional neuroimaging. In: Greenberg JO, ed. Neuroimaging: a companion to Adams and Victor's principles of neurology. New York: McGraw-Hill; 1999:775–96.
37. Guglielmi G, Vinuela F, Dion J, et al. Electrothrombosis of saccular aneurysms via endovascular approach. J Neurosurg. 1991;75:8–14.
38. Roy D, Raymond J, Bouthillier A, et al. Endovascular treatment of ophthalmic segment aneurysms with Guglielmi detachable coils. AJNR Am J Neuroradiol. 1997;18:1207–15.

39. Nelson PK, Levy D, Masters LT, *et al*. Neuroendovascular management of intracranial aneurysms (review). Neuroimaging Clin North Am. 1997;18:1207–15.

40. Grossman RI, Yousem DM. Techniques in neuroimaging. In: Thrall JH, ed. Neuroradiology: the requisites. St Louis: Mosby–Year Book; 1994:1–23.

41. Jamieson DG, Bosley TM, Sergott RC. Non-invasive vascular imaging in ophthalmology. Ophthalmol Clin North Am. 1994;7:437–48.

42. Williamson TH, Harris A. Color Doppler ultrasound of the eye and orbit. Surv Ophthalmol. 1996;40:225–67.

43. Phelps ME. PET: the merging of biology and imaging into molecular imaging. J Nucl Med. 2000;41:661–81.

44. Thrall JH, Ziessman HA. SPECT and PET. In: Nuclear medicine: the requisites, ed 2. Chicago: Mosby; 2001.

45. Coleman RE. Clinical PET: role in diagnosis and management. J Nucl Med. 2000;41:36–41.

46. Moster ML, Galetta SL, Schatz NJ. Physiologic imaging in 'functional' visual loss. Surv Ophthalmol. 1996;40:395–9.

47. Bernarczyk EM, Remler W, Weikart C. Global cerebral blood flow, blood volume, and oxygen metabolism in patients with migraine headache. Neurology. 1998;50:1736–40.

48. Esmaeli-Gutstein B, Nahmias C, Thompson M, *et al*. PET in patients with benign essential blepharospasm. Ophthal Plast Reconstr Surg. 1999;15:23–7.

49. Ettl A, Fischer-Klein C, Chemelli A, *et al*. Nuclear magnetic resonance spectroscopy: principles and applications in neuroophthalmology. Int Ophthalmol. 1994;18:171–81.

50. Michaelis T, Merboldt KD, Bruhn H, *et al*. Absolute concentrations of metabolites in the adult human brain in vivo: quantification of localized proton MR spectra. Radiology. 1993;187:210–27.

51. Koopmans RA, Li DKB, Zhu G, *et al*. MRS in multiple sclerosis: in vivo detection of myelin breakdown products. Lancet. 1993;341:631–2.

52. George JS, Aine CJ, Mosher JC, *et al*. Mapping function in the human brain with magnetoencephalography, anatomical magnetic resonance imaging, and functional magnetic resonance imaging. J Clin Neurophysiol. 1995;12:406–31.

53. Thulborn KR. A BOLD move for fMRI. Nat Med. 1998;4:155–6.

54. Beauchamp MS. A functional MRI case study of acquired cerebral dyschromatopsia. Neuropsychologia. 2000;38:1170–9.

55. Chen W, Zhu XH, Thulborn KR, Ugurbil K. Retinotopic mapping of lateral geniculate nucleus in humans using functional magnetic resonance imaging. Proc Natl Acad Sci U S A. 1999;96:2430–4.

56. Gans MS, Byrne SF, Glaser JS. Standardized A-scan echography in optic nerve disease. Arch Ophthalmol. 1987;105:1232–6.

57. Beck RW, Arrington J, Murtagh R, *et al*. Brain magnetic resonance imaging in acute optic neuritis. Experience of the optic neuritis study group. Arch Neurol. 1993;50:841–6.

58. Jacobs LD, Beck RW, Simon JH, *et al*. Intramuscular interferon β-1a therapy initiated during a first demyelinating event in multiple sclerosis. N Engl J Med. 2000;343:898–904.

59. Dunker S, Weigand W. Prognostic value of magnetic resonance imaging in monosymptomatic optic neuritis. Ophthalmology. 1996;1013:1768–73.

SECTION 2 THE AFFERENT VISUAL SYSTEM

CHAPTER

186

Anatomy and Physiology

ALFREDO A. SADUN

DEFINITION

- The optic nerve, being a portion of the central nervous system, is really a tract and not a (peripheral) nerve. However, as a convention, the 1.2 million axons that derive from the retinal ganglion cells carry the name the optic nerve until they partially decussate at the optic chiasm.

HISTORICAL REVIEW

Until recently, anatomical tracing techniques, quite useful in animals, could not be applied to delineate the fiber projections in humans. Hence, much of what is taught concerning the visual projections in humans derives from experimental animal studies. Because a great deal of interspecies variation exists in anatomy, some scholars rely largely on the original dissection studies performed on humans.

The optic nerves are obvious—Aristotle described them as joining at the optic chiasm, now so called because it resembles the Greek letter χ (chi). Galen of Pergamon, in about AD 150, gave a more detailed description of the optic nerves as sensory in nature but incorrectly as hollow and continuous with the ventricular system. Little progress in the understanding of the visual pathways occurred between Galen and Gratiolet, 1700 years later.

Using orangewood sticks (soft) for blunt dissection, Gratiolet was able to tease, as much as trace, the retinofugal projection to the pretectum via the brachium of the superior colliculus and to confirm the main pathway from the optic chiasm to the lateral geniculate nucleus and hence to the cerebral cortex.[1]

GENERAL ANATOMY

The optic nerve carries about 1.2 million axons that derive from the retinal ganglion cells and project to the eight primary visual nuclei (Fig. 186-1).[2-5] However, only the anterior part of this heavily myelinated tract is termed the optic nerve. The optic chiasm consists of the partial decussation; the optic tract is the posterior continuation of the same fiber tract to its termination.

Hence, the optic nerve is about 50mm long and extends from the eye to the optic chiasm. It is often described as consisting of four portions (see Fig. 186-2):

- Intraocular portion (the optic disc, 1mm in anterior-posterior length)
- Intraorbital portion (about 25mm long)
- Intracanalicular portion within the optic canal (about 9mm long)
- Intracranial portion (about 16mm long)

Three anatomical zones occur within the 1mm long intraocular optic nerve (optic disc):

- Anteriorly, the retinal or prelaminar zone

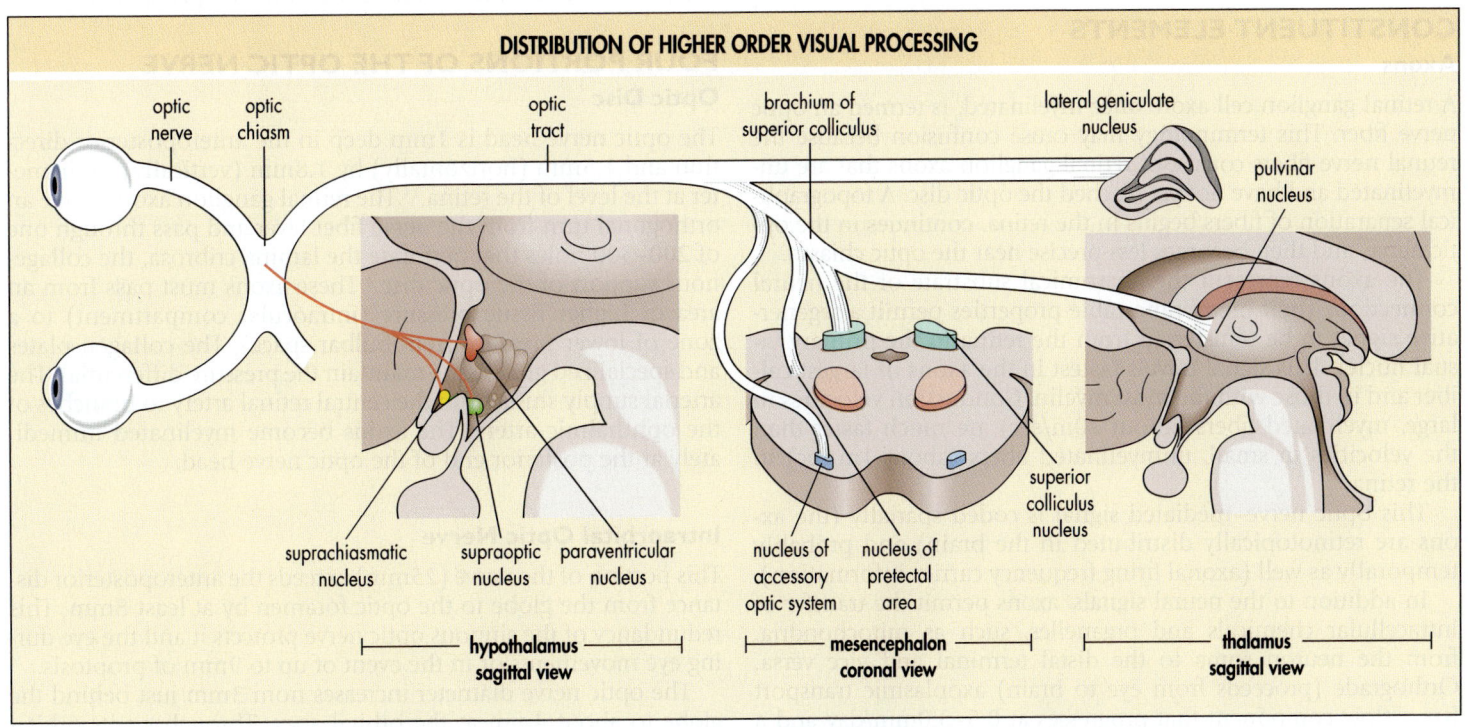

DISTRIBUTION OF HIGHER ORDER VISUAL PROCESSING

optic nerve · optic chiasm · optic tract · brachium of superior colliculus · lateral geniculate nucleus · pulvinar nucleus

suprachiasmatic nucleus · supraoptic nucleus · paraventricular nucleus · nucleus of accessory optic system · nucleus of pretectal area · superior colliculus nucleus

hypothalamus sagittal view · **mesencephalon** coronal view · **thalamus** sagittal view

FIG. 186-1 ■ Retinal projections to the eight primary nuclei, showing distribution of higher order visual processing.

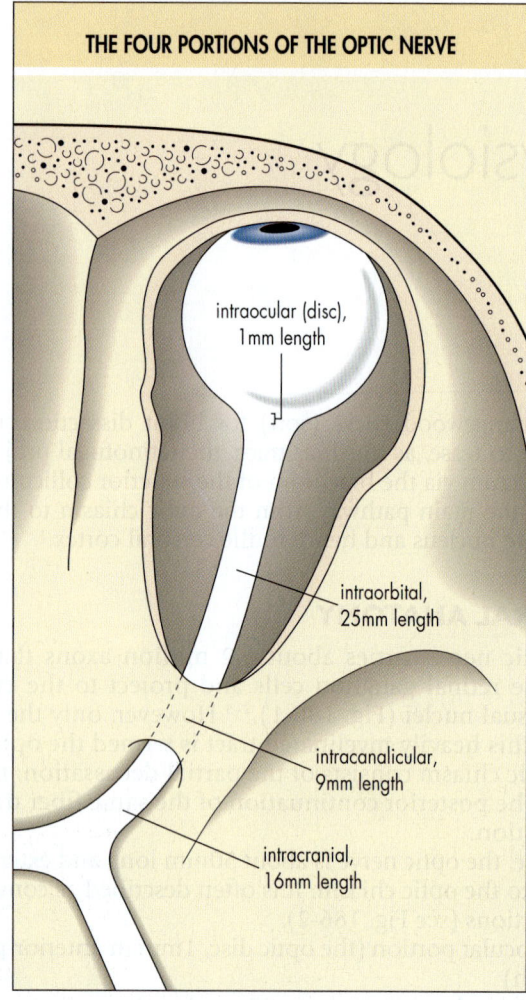

THE FOUR PORTIONS OF THE OPTIC NERVE

intraocular (disc),
1mm length

intraorbital,
25mm length

intracanalicular,
9mm length

intracranial,
16mm length

FIG. 186-2 ■ **The four portions of the optic nerve.** The lengths are given.

- Centrally, the choroidal or laminar zone
- Posteriorly, the scleral or retrolaminar zone

Each zone contains different structures and elements of neuroectoderm and mesoderm.[6,7]

CONSTITUENT ELEMENTS

Axons

A retinal ganglion cell axon, once myelinated, is termed an optic nerve fiber. This terminology may cause confusion because the retinal nerve fibers consist of retinal ganglion axons that are unmyelinated and have not yet reached the optic disc. A topographical separation of fibers begins in the retina, continues in the optic nerve, and then becomes less precise near the optic chiasm.

The axons represent the anatomical substrate of the neural connection. Their membrane cable properties permit a regenerative signal to be transferred from the retina to the primary visual nuclei. This signal travels fastest in the axons of largest caliber and in those with the most myelin. Conduction velocities in large, myelinated fibers (about 20m/sec) are much faster than the velocities in small, unmyelinated fibers (about 1m/sec) in the retina.[8]

This optic nerve–mediated signal is coded spatially (the axons are retinotopically distributed in the brain) and probably temporally as well (axonal firing frequency carries information).

In addition to the neural signals, axons permit the transfer of intracellular chemicals and organelles, such as mitochondria, from the neuron soma to the distal terminal and vice versa. Orthograde (proceeds from eye to brain) axoplasmic transport has a slow component that progresses at 0.5–3.0mm/day and a rapid component that moves at 200–1000mm/day.[9,10] Retrograde (brain to eye) axonal transport also occurs at an intermediate rate.

It has been suggested that, in humans, at least two classes of retinal ganglion cells exist. About 90% of the retinal ganglion cells are relatively small, concentrated in the macula, and contribute axons of small caliber that project to the parvocellular layers of the dorsal lateral geniculate nucleus (the so-called P-cell system). P cells have color-opponent physiology and are thought to subserve high-contrast, high-spatial-frequency resolution. In contradistinction, M cells are larger cells that contain large, fast-conducting axons and make up about 5–10% of the retinal ganglion cells. The M cells may be involved primarily with noncolor information of high temporal and low spatial frequency.[11,12]

Oligodendrocytes

Oligodendrocytes are specialized glia that provide membranes for axonal myelination. Such myelination begins centrally during development and stops at the lamina cribrosa of the optic disc at birth. However, oligodendrocytes may extend anomalously anterior to the lamina to myelinate the peripapillary retinal nerve fiber layer (optic disc medullation) in about 1% of the general population.

Microglia

Microglia and macrophages are cells that derive from the immune system and can move readily into the central nervous system from the vascular beds. These immunocompetent cells probably play a far greater role than simple protection of the optic nerve from infection. For example, the apoptosis (programmed death) of retinal ganglion cells, which occurs during development and in various diseases, is probably modulated by these glial cells.

Astrocytes

Astrocytes have extensive neurofibrillary processes that spread among the nerve fibers. These specialized glial cells line the borders between axons and other tissues, such as capillaries. They form part of the blood-brain barrier and play a role in the nutritional and structural support of axons. Intercellular junctions between cells couple chains of astrocytes electrically and biochemically.[13] When axons are lost because of optic atrophy, astrocytes move and proliferate to fill all the empty spaces.[13]

FOUR PORTIONS OF THE OPTIC NERVE

Optic Disc

The optic nerve head is 1mm deep in the anteroposterior direction and 1.5mm (horizontally) by 1.8mm (vertically) in diameter at the level of the retina.[14] The retinal ganglion axons make an orthogonal turn from the nerve fiber layer and pass through one of 200–300 holes that perforate the lamina cribrosa, the collagenous support of the optic disc.[7] These axons must pass from an area of higher tissue pressure (intraocular compartment) to a zone of lower pressure (retrobulbar space). The collagen plates and specialized glial tissue maintain the pressure differential. The arterial supply shifts from the central retinal artery to branches of the ophthalmic artery. The axons become myelinated immediately at the posterior end of the optic nerve head.

Intraorbital Optic Nerve

This portion of the nerve (25mm) exceeds the anteroposterior distance from the globe to the optic foramen by at least 8mm. This redundancy of the sinuous optic nerve protects it and the eye during eye movements or in the event of up to 9mm of proptosis.

The optic nerve diameter increases from 3mm just behind the globe to about 4mm at the orbital apex. Throughout its orbital course, the nerve is surrounded by dura, arachnoid, and pia mater (Fig. 186-3). The outermost sheath is the dura and is composed of

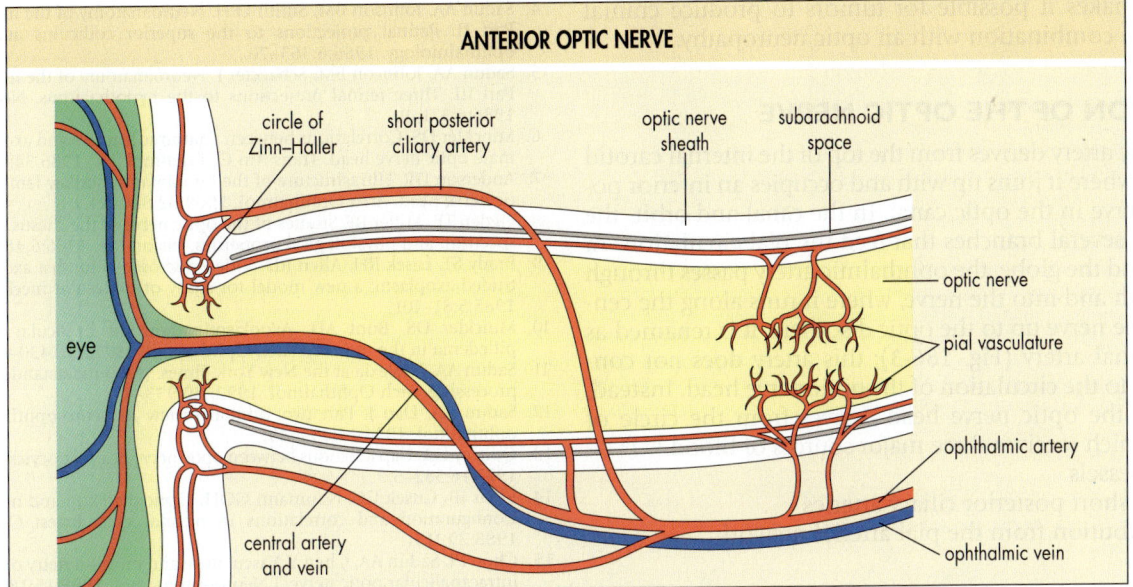

FIG. 186-3 ■ **Anterior optic nerve.** The sheath and the vascular supply to the intraocular and intraorbital portions are shown.

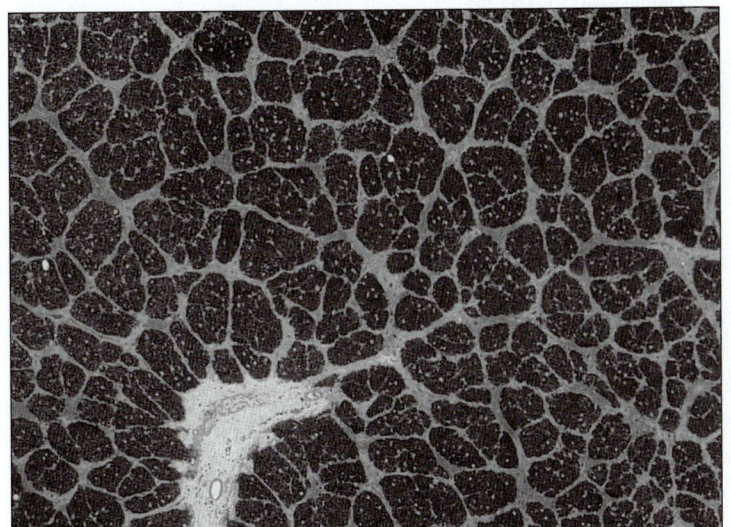

FIG. 186-4 ■ **Retrobulbar optic nerve.** This cross section is approximately 5mm behind the globe and is a 1μm Epon-embedded section stained with *para*-phenylenediamine. The axon fascicles (about 400–600 per nerve) each carry approximately 2000 axons. The fascicles are separated by connective tissue septa. In the lower left, the central artery and vein can be seen. On the right, the pial surface is visible.

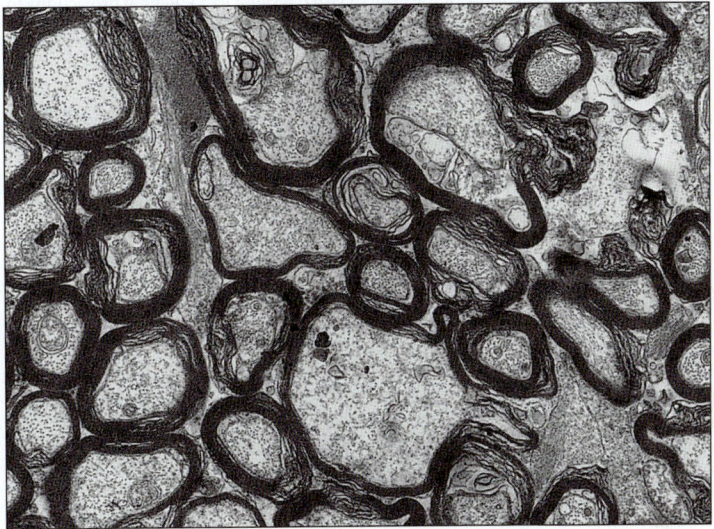

FIG. 186-5 ■ **Axon in the retrobulbar optic nerve.** This is an ultrastructural high-magnification view approximately 5mm behind the globe and is 400× the magnification of Figure 186-4. Note the heavily myelinated axons of various sizes. The smaller axons are 0.6–0.9μm in diameter and are probably of retinal ganglion cells of the P-cell system. The larger axons are 1–2μm in diameter and may be part of the M-cell system. Mitochondria and cellular debris can be seen intra-axonally.

dense collagen. The arachnoid, which lies under the dura, is more cellular and less collagenous. Delicate arachnoidal trabeculae connect this membrane with the dura and underlying pia. The pia is the most delicate and the most vascular of the sheaths that cover the optic nerve. The subarachnoid space is continuous with the intracranial subarachnoid space and carries cerebrospinal fluid.

The optic nerve substance consists of 400–600 fascicles, each of which contain about 2000 fibers (Fig. 186-4). The fascicles are separated by connective tissue septa through which run the smaller blood vessels. The axons are myelinated heavily (Fig. 186-5) by oligodendrocytes.

Intracanalicular Optic Nerve

The optic nerve's intracanalicular portion begins as it enters the optic canal through an opening in the lesser wing of the sphenoid bone at the apex of the orbit known as the optic foramen (Fig. 186-2). The orbital canal opening is elliptic, with its widest diameter oriented vertically. The intracranial opening of the optic canal is also elliptic but with the horizontal width greater than the height.[15] The medial canal wall is the thinnest and most likely to fracture.

Unlike the intraorbital optic nerve, the intracanalicular optic nerve does not move freely and is fixed tightly within the optic canal. Thus, small lesions that arise within the optic canal may compress and significantly damage the optic nerve while still relatively small and not radiologically visible.

Intracranial Optic Nerve

Once past the hard fold of dura above the intracranial opening of the canal, the intracranial optic nerve runs for 12–16mm to reach the optic chiasm. The intracranial optic nerve is now about 4.5mm in average diameter.

Above each nerve lie the gyri recti of the frontal lobes of the brain. On the lateral side of the optic nerve may lie the internal carotid artery, or alternatively the anterior cerebral and middle cerebral arteries may lie immediately adjacent. The ophthalmic artery arises from the carotid and lies to the lateral side and below the nerve within its dural sheath. The proximity of the cav-

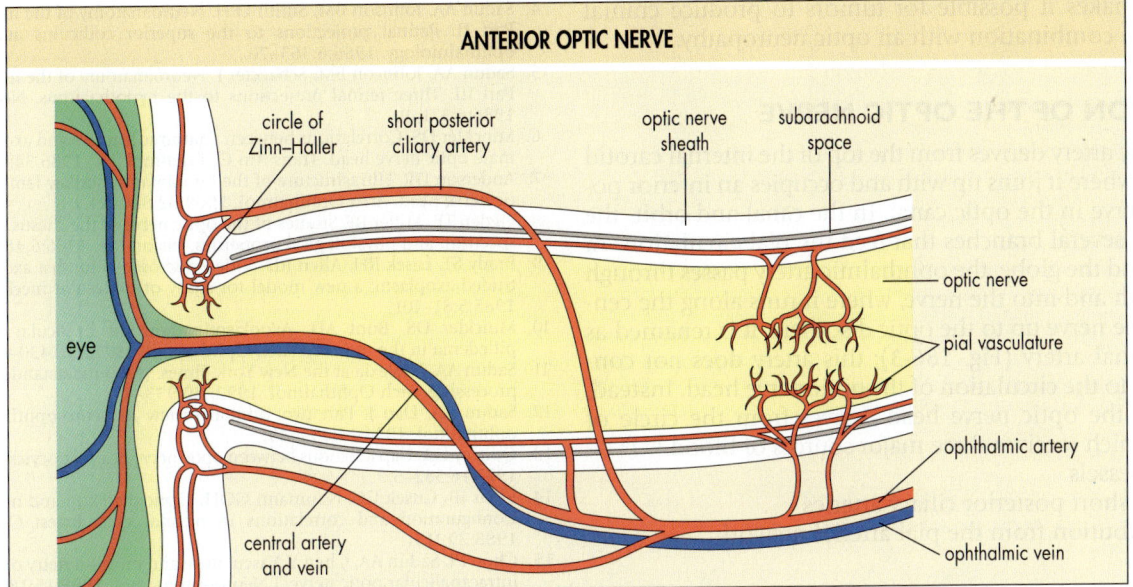
(labels: circle of Zinn–Haller; short posterior ciliary artery; optic nerve sheath; subarachnoid space; optic nerve; pial vasculature; ophthalmic artery; ophthalmic vein; central artery and vein; eye)

ernous sinus makes it possible for tumors to produce cranial nerve palsies in combination with an optic neuropathy.

CIRCULATION OF THE OPTIC NERVE

The ophthalmic artery derives from the top of the internal carotid artery siphon, where it joins up with and occupies an inferior position to the nerve in the optic canal. In the canal and orbit, the artery gives off several branches that feed the pial circulation. At 8–12mm behind the globe, the ophthalmic artery passes through the nerve sheath and into the nerve, where it runs along the central aspect of the nerve up to the optic disc; here, it is renamed as the central retinal artery (Fig. 186-3); this artery does not contribute directly to the circulation of the optic nerve head. Instead, blood flow to the optic nerve head derives from the circle of Zinn-Haller, which receives three major sources of blood.[16-18]

- Choroidal vessels
- Four or five short posterior ciliary arteries
- Small contribution from the pial arterial network

REFERENCES

1. Polyak S. The vertebrate visual system. Chicago: University of Chicago Press; 1957:132–41.
2. Fredericks CA, Giolli RA, Blanks RH, Sadun AA. The human accessory optic system. Brain Res. 1988;454:116–22.
3. Sadun AA. Neuroanatomy of the human visual system: Part I. Retinal projections to the LGN and pretectum as demonstrated with a new stain. Neuroophthalmology. 1986;6:353–61.
4. Sadun AA, Johnson BM, Smith LEH. Neuroanatomy of the human visual system: Part II. Retinal projections to the superior colliculus and pulvinar. Neuro ophthalmology. 1986;6:363–70.
5. Sadun AA, Johnson BM, Schaecter J. Neuroanatomy of the human visual system: Part III. Three retinal projections to the hypothalamus. Neuroophthalmology. 1986;6:371–9.
6. Minckler DS. Correlations between anatomic features and axonal transport in primate optic nerve head. Trans Am Ophthalmol Soc. 1986;34:429–52.
7. Anderson DR. Ultrastructure of the human and monkey lamina cribrosa and optic nerve head. Arch Ophthalmol. 1969;82:800–14.
8. Ogden TE, Miller RF. Studies of the optic nerve of the rhesus monkey: nerve fiber spectrum and physiological properties. Vision Res. 1966;6:485–506.
9. Brady ST, Lasek RH, Allen RD. Video microscopy for fast axonal transport of extruded axoplasm: a new model for study of molecular mechanisms. Cell Motil. 1985:5:81–101.
10. Minckler DS, Bunt AH. Axoplasmic transport in ocular hypotony and papilledema in the monkey. Arch Ophthalmol. 1977;95:1430–6.
11. Sadun AA. Dyslexia at the New York Times. (Mis)understanding of parallel visual processing. Arch Ophthalmol. 1992;110:933–4.
12. Sadun AA, Dao J. Part two: annual review in neuro-ophthalmology. J Neuroophthalmol. 1994;14:234–49.
13. Quigley HA. Gap junctions between optic nerve head astrocytes. Invest Ophthalmol. 1977;16:582–5.
14. Jonas JB, Gusek GC, Naumann GOH. Optic disc, cup and neuroretinal rim size. Configuration and correlations in normal eyes. Invest Ophthalmol Vis Sci. 1988;29:1151.
15. Chou PI, Sadun AA, Chen Y. Vasculature and morphometry of the optic canal and intracanalicular optic nerve. J Neuroophthalmol. 1995;15:186–90.
16. Hayreh SS. Anatomy and physiology of the optic nerve head. Trans Am Acad Ophthalmol Otolaryngol. 1974;78:240–54.
17. Onda E, Cioffi GA, Bacon DR, van Burskirk EM. Microvasculature of the human optic nerve. Am J Ophthalmol. 1995;120:92–102.
18. Cioffi GA, van Burskirk EM. Microvasculature of the anterior optic nerve. Surv Ophthalmol. 1994;38:107–17.

187 Differentiation of Optic Nerve from Retinal Macular Disease

ALFREDO A. SADUN

DEFINITION
- Optic nerve disease involves injury of the retinal ganglion cells and hence the axons that constitute the optic nerve, whereas macular disease involves injury to the retina in the fovea and parafoveal areas.

KEY FEATURES
- Optic nerve lesions generally produce an afferent pupillary defect and a severe dyschromatopsia.
- Macular lesions usually cause severe loss of central acuity and metamorphopsia.

ASSOCIATED FEATURES
- Photostress and electroretinography testing may reveal retinal disease.
- Contrast sensitivity and visually evoked response testing may disclose optic nerve disease.

INTRODUCTION

Optic nerve disease may be severe with profound losses of visual acuity, color vision, and visual field such that the diagnosis is obvious. However, mild optic neuropathies that cause only minimal visual loss may be difficult to diagnose. Optic neuropathies and maculopathies often have overlapping presentations, for example, optic neuritis and central serous retinopathy, both of which can present in a young adult with acute, painless, monocular visual loss. At times the relative absence of fundus findings in patients who have acute visual loss may further frustrate the clinician's ability to make the correct diagnosis.[1,2] Because impairments of vision that result from optic nerve dysfunction may be harbingers of intracranial pathology, which might require neurosurgical intervention, and maculopathies often respond to local treatment,[3] such as laser photocoagulation, the clinician needs to make an early and accurate distinction between an optic neuropathy and a maculopathy.

EPIDEMIOLOGY AND PATHOGENESIS

The most common optic neuropathies in young and older adults are optic neuritis and nonarteritic anterior ischemic optic neuropathy, respectively. Regardless of the nature of the optic neuropathy, the cell that is injured or impaired is the retinal ganglion cell. Once this cell is dead, its axon undergoes anterograde degeneration, resulting in optic atrophy.

Retinal maculopathies may arise from a variety of lesions of the outer or inner retina or choroid and often present somewhat like optic neuropathies.

TABLE 187-1

DIFFERENTIATION OF OPTIC NERVE FROM MACULAR DISEASE BY HISTORY

Feature	Optic Nerve	Macula
Onset	Variable	Variable
Course	Stable, progressive, or transient	Slow changes
Pain	Sometimes with eye movements	Rarely
Description of deficit	Dark or gray cloud	Metamorphopsia
Refractive error	Unchanged	Sometimes toward hyperopia

OCULAR MANIFESTATIONS

Loss of visual acuity from optic nerve disease is usually perceived as a sense of generalized dimness, patchy dark spots, or black curtains across the visual field.[4] Optic neuropathies also cause a darkening or desaturation of colors and objects, which may appear to have less contrast to the point of becoming indistinguishable. Patients with optic neuritis may also describe phosphenes with eye movements. Pain is associated with certain optic neuropathies (Table 187-1).

In contradistinction, patients who have maculopathies complain of metamorphopsia in the central visual field.[5] Micropsia is more common than macropsia. Patients who have maculopathies may experience slight photophobia or complain of glare or even dazzle. Instead of objects that appear dim (as in optic neuropathies), patients may complain that objects appear too bright.

DIAGNOSIS AND ANCILLARY TESTING

History

It is important to elicit from the patient the tempo of the onset and course of symptoms. Optic neuritis usually develops over hours to days, stabilizes, and then shows improvement in the ensuing weeks. Anterior ischemic optic neuropathy causes a sudden loss of vision with very little progression or resolution thereafter.[4] Maculopathies may be acute or insidious in onset.

Physical Examination

Visual acuity is more likely to be affected by macular disease than by diseases of the optic nerve (Table 187-2). Three tests—the measurement of the pupillary response,[6] color vision,[7] and sense of brightness testing[8]—are particularly sensitive to impairments of the optic nerve. A consensual pupillary response that is greater than the direct pupillary response is indicative of an afferent pupillary defect. This is usually judged qualitatively, although Fineberg and Thompson[6] quantitate it using neutral density filters.

TABLE 187-2

DIFFERENTIATION OF OPTIC NERVE FROM MACULAR DISEASE BY CLINICAL EXAMINATION

Visual Function	Optic Nerve	Macula
Visual acuity	Variably reduced	Markedly reduced
Afferent pupillary defect	Present	Absent
Brightness sense	Very reduced	Slightly reduced
Color vision	Very reduced	Slightly reduced
Visual field	Variable	Normal or central scotoma

TABLE 187-3

DIFFERENTIATION OF OPTIC NERVE FROM MACULAR DISEASE BY SPECIAL TESTS AND LABORATORY STUDIES

Test	Optic Nerve	Macular
Amsler chart	Central scotoma	Metamorphopsia
Visual evoked response	Large latency delay	Small latency delay
Contrast sensitivity functions	Greatest losses between 6–12 cycles/degree	Greatest losses around 18 cycles/degree
Photostress	Normal	Abnormal

Although color vision is best assessed using a Farnsworth-Munsell 100-hue test,[7] a more convenient option is the shorter, desaturated form of the Farnsworth-Munsell test, the D-15, which requires the alignment of only 15 color caps. An even easier in-office test of color vision involves the use of pseudoisochromatic plates of the A-O or Ishihara type. Disease of the optic nerve invariably produces dyschromatopsia and a subjective loss of color vividness, which may be compared between eyes.

The third sensitive measure of optic neuropathy is a change in brightness sense, which may be estimated subjectively when the patient is asked which eye sees a light as brighter, or quantitated using neutral density filters or brightness-sense spectacles, consisting of two pairs of cross-polarizing filters.[8]

Extensive retinal disease may produce mild abnormalities in color vision, brightness sense, and pupillary response, but this is usually accompanied by marked visual loss.[8]

Fundus examination may disclose optic disc swelling; however, optic disc elevation itself does not produce significant impairment of visual function.[9] Optic atrophy is generally visualized first about 1 month after acute injury to the nerve. Optic neuropathies may produce diffuse dropout or segmental losses in the nerve fiber layer, and certain lesions can produce slits or rake defects[10] in the nerve fiber layer, which may be seen as early as 1 week after injury to the optic nerve. Sectoral disc edema with flame-shaped hemorrhages (anterior ischemic optic neuropathy), lumps and bumps (optic disc drusen), pathologic cupping (glaucoma), sectoral optic atrophy, secondary optic atrophy, and butterfly optic atrophy are patterns of optic disc change that indicate nerve damage of specific types.

Serous neural retinal or retinal pigment epithelial detachments, retinal edema, vascular abnormalities, and exudates may all be seen by direct or indirect ophthalmoscopy or by stereomicroscopy.

Ancillary Testing

Optic neuropathies may cause a large variety of visual field defects, some of which are specific. For example, toxic or nutritional deficiency optic neuropathies usually cause centrocecal field defects. Diseases of the optic nerve head often produce arcuate or altitudinal field defects.

The visual field defect of a maculopathy is almost invariably a central scotoma with a zone of metamorphopsia that surrounds it.

Tangent visual field testing remains a very effective way to assess the central 20° of visual field and when performed at 6.5ft (2m) may make the identification of a small central scotoma much easier. Amsler chart testing provides a very sensitive assessment of the central 10° of visual field[11] and documents the presence or absence of metamorphopsia, a strong indicator of macular disease.

Several specialized tests are very simple, inexpensive, and easy to perform in the office (Table 187-3). Threshold Amsler chart testing is a method in which the Amsler grid is made far more sensitive.[12] In this approach, the patient wears specialized glasses with cross-polarizers in front of both oculars, which are turned to reduce the patient's perception so that the Amsler chart is barely discerned.

In macular disease a delay usually occurs in the recovery of visual pigments that are bleached by a bright light, but bright light has no effect on optic nerve conduction. Hence, photostress testing may be very helpful in the differentiation between maculopathies and optic nerve disorders.[13] A penlight is used to stress each eye and the recovery time, when compared, is much greater with a maculopathy. Patients who have optic neuropathies show little or no prolongation of this recovery time. Fundus fluorescein angiography may be particularly useful for the characterization of retinal diseases.

The visual evoked response may be used to document optic nerve dysfunction. However, increased latency in the visual evoked response may arise from a variety of other diseases, which include refractive error, a maculopathy, or even feigned visual loss.[14] Nevertheless, the test can be very useful when bilateral disease of the optic nerves makes the diagnosis more difficult or when documentation is desired for medicolegal purposes.

The Pulfrich phenomenon is often elicited in a patient who has unilateral optic nerve conduction block and in whom a latency delay may be noted with visual evoked response. In this test, the patient is asked to observe, with both eyes open, a pendulum that swings in one plane. In the presence of a unilateral conduction delay caused by an optic neuropathy, the patient may have the impression that the pendulum swings through an elliptic arc.

In contrast sensitivity testing, patients are asked to view a series of sinusoidal gratings of different spatial frequencies.[15] Vistech plates may be used. Patients who have optic neuropathies may have deficiencies in the middle to high spatial frequencies; patients who have maculopathies usually have deficiencies only in the highest spatial frequencies.

REFERENCES

1. Nikoskelainen E. Symptoms, signs and early course of optic neuritis. Acta Ophthalmol. 1975;53:254–72.
2. Gass JDM. Stereoscopic atlas of macular diseases: diagnosis and treatment. St. Louis: CV Mosby; 1987:46–59.
3. Early Treatment Diabetic Retinopathy Study Research Group. Photocoagulation for diabetic macular edema: Early Treatment Diabetic Retinopathy Study report number 1. Arch Ophthalmol. 1985;103:1796–806.
4. Glaser JS. Neuro ophthalmology, 2nd ed. Philadelphia: JB Lippincott; 1990:115–17.
5. Fine AM, Elman MJ, Ebert JE, et al. Earliest symptoms caused by neovascular membranes in the macula. Arch Ophthalmol. 1986;104:513–14.
6. Fineberg E, Thompson HS. Quantitation of the afferent pupillary defect. In: Smith JL, ed. Neuro-ophthalmology focus. New York: Masson; 1979:25–9.
7. Hart WM Jr. Acquired dyschromatopsias. Surv Ophthalmol. 1987;32:10–31.
8. Sadun AA, Lessell S. Brightness-sense and optic nerve disease. Arch Ophthalmol. 1985;103:39–43.
9. Hayreh SS. Optic disc edema in raised intracranial pressure. VI. Associated visual disturbances and their pathogenesis. Arch Ophthalmol. 1977;95:1566–79.
10. Stevens RA, Newman NM. Abnormal visual-evoked potentials from eyes with optic nerve head drusen. Am J Ophthalmol. 1981;92:857–62.
11. Amsler M. Earliest symptoms of diseases of the macula. Br J Ophthalmol. 1953;37:521–37.
12. Wall M, Sadun AA. Threshold Amsler grid testing: cross-polarizing lenses enhance yield. Arch Ophthalmol. 1986;104:520–3.
13. Glaser JS, Savino PJ, Sumers KD, et al. The photostress recovery test: in the clinical assessment of visual function. Am J Ophthalmol. 1977;83:255–60.
14. Towle VL, Sutcliffe E, Sokol S. Diagnosing functional visual deficits with the P300 component of the visual evoked potential. Arch Ophthalmol. 1985;103:47–50.
15. Arden GB, Jacobson JJ. A simple grating test for contrast sensitivity: preliminary results indicate value in screening for glaucoma. Invest Ophthalmol Vis Sci. 1978;17:23–32.

CHAPTER 188

Congenital Optic Disc Anomalies

MICHAEL C. BRODSKY

DEFINITION
- Unusual configurations of the optic disc(s) typically present since birth.

KEY FEATURE
- Small, pale, or unusually shaped optic discs may reflect mere curiosities or significant anomalies associated with visual defects.

ASSOCIATED FEATURE
- Abnormalities of the surrounding retina (e.g., in morning glory syndrome), anterior segment (e.g., iris coloboma), face, or brain may occasionally be seen.

INTRODUCTION

The principles outlined here apply to the evaluation and management of children who have congenital optic disc anomalies.[1]

Age Association

Children who have bilateral optic disc anomalies generally present in infancy with poor vision and nystagmus; those who have unilateral optic disc anomalies generally present during the preschool years with sensory esotropia.

Central Nervous System Malformations

Central nervous system malformations are common in patients who have malformed optic discs. Small discs are associated with a variety of malformations that involve the cerebral hemispheres, pituitary infundibulum, and midline intracranial structures (e.g., septum pellucidum, corpus callosum).

Optic discs of the morning glory configuration are associated with the transsphenoidal form of basal encephalocele, whereas optic discs with a colobomatous configuration are associated with systemic anomalies in a variety of coloboma syndromes. Investigation using magnetic resonance imaging (MRI) is advisable for infants who have small optic discs and for infants who have large optic discs who have either neurodevelopmental deficits or midfacial anomalies that are suggestive of basal encephalocele. This generalization applies to patients with unilateral as well as bilateral optic disc anomalies.

Functional Amblyopia

Any structural ocular abnormality that reduces visual acuity in infancy may lead to a superimposed amblyopia. A trial of occlusion therapy is warranted in most young patients who have unilateral optic disc anomalies and decreased vision in the affected eye.

OPTIC NERVE HYPOPLASIA

Optic nerve hypoplasia is a congenital anomaly that has become recognized as a major cause of blindness in children.[1] Histologically, it is characterized by a subnormal number of optic nerve axons with normal mesodermal elements and glial supporting tissue.[2] The ophthalmoscopic appearance is that of a small, gray, or pale optic nerve head, which is often surrounded by a yellowish mottled peripapillary halo, flanked on either side by a ring of pigment (double-ring sign)[2] (Fig. 188-1). Visual acuity may range from 20/20 to no light perception.[2] Because visual acuity depends only on the degree of papillomacular nerve fiber bundle hypoplasia, it does not necessarily correlate with the overall size of the disc.[1]

The term *septo-optic dysplasia* (de Morsier syndrome) describes the constellation of optic nerve hypoplasia, absence of the septum pellucidum, and partial or complete agenesis of the corpus callosum.[2] MRI of the brain in optic nerve hypoplasia frequently shows coexistent cerebral hemispheric abnormalities (most often schizencephaly) and absence of the pituitary infundibulum with or without posterior pituitary ectopia.[3] The presence of an ectopic posterior pituitary gland, which appears as a hyperintense nodule at the median eminence on T1-weighted images, indicates that posterior pituitary function is intact.[3] Cerebral hemispheric abnormalities indicate that neurodevelopmental deficits are likely, and absence of the pituitary infundibulum with an ectopic posterior pituitary gland indicates congenital hypopituitarism. Absence of the septum pellucidum does not place the child at higher risk for neurodevelopmental or en-

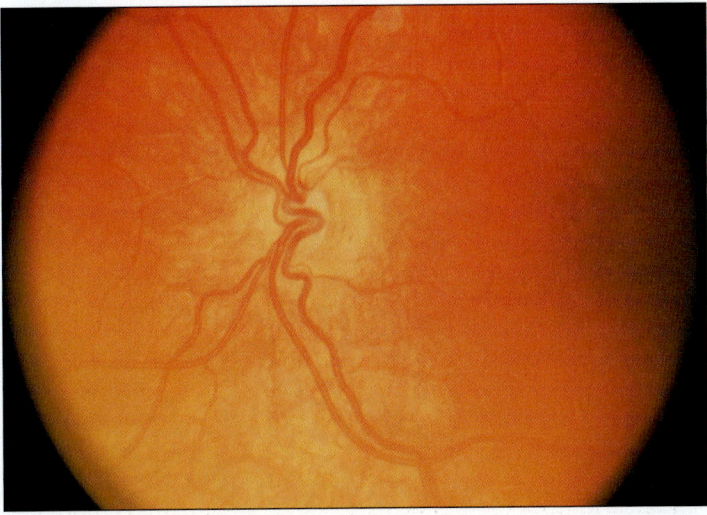

FIG. 188-1 ■ Optic nerve hypoplasia (note double-ring sign).

docrinologic problems unless the cerebral hemispheres or pituitary infundibulum are also abnormal.[3]

A reduction in the diameter of the hypoplastic optic nerve and chiasm is demonstrated reliably by MRI, which establishes the presumptive diagnosis of optic nerve hypoplasia.[1]

The association of septo-optic dysplasia with pituitary hormone deficiencies warrants endocrinologic evaluation in children who have both optic nerve hypoplasia and absence of the pituitary infundibulum on MRI. Growth hormone deficiency is most common, followed by deficiency of thyroid-stimulating hormone, corticotropic hormone, and vasopressin. In infants who have septo-optic dysplasia, a history of neonatal jaundice suggests hypothyroidism and neonatal hypoglycemia indicates corticotropin deficiency. Children who have corticotropin deficiency are at risk for sudden death from hypoglycemia and shock during intercurrent illness; parents should be instructed to administer injectable parenteral corticosteroids at the onset of febrile illness.[4]

MORNING GLORY DISC ANOMALY

The morning glory disc anomaly is a congenital excavation of the posterior globe that involves the optic disc.[5] Embryologically, the morning glory disc anomaly may result from an anomalous, funnel-shaped expansion of the distal portion of the optic stalk, which causes the opening of its lumen into the cavity of the optic vesicle to be abnormally large. Closure of the embryonic fissure occurs normally; however, progression of the closure into the distal portion of the stalk does not obliterate the space within the fissure because of the increased dimensions of this space.[5]

The optic disc is enlarged, orange or pink in color, and either excavated or situated within a funnel-shaped area of excavation (Fig. 188-2).[5] A variably elevated annular zone surrounds the disc with irregular areas of pigmentation and depigmentation. A white tuft of glial tissue overlies the center of the disc. The retinal blood vessels appear increased in number, arise from the periphery of the disc, run an abnormally straight course over the peripapillary retina, and tend to branch at acute angles. It is often difficult to distinguish arteries from veins. The macula may be incorporated into the excavated defect (macular capture).[5] Although mistakenly referred to as a variant of optic disc coloboma, the morning glory disc anomaly is truly a distinct anomaly, as evidenced by its sporadic occurrence, its lack of association with iris or retinal colobomas, and its systemic associations.[5]

The morning glory disc anomaly is associated with transsphenoidal encephalocele,[1] and with hypoplasia of the ipsilateral intracranial vasculature (which can be visualized by magnetic resonance angiography).[5,6] Children who have this occult basal encephalocele have characteristic facies, which consist of mild

hypertelorism with a depressed nasal bridge, a midline notch in the upper lip, and sometimes a midline cleft in the soft palate. Respiratory symptoms of transsphenoidal encephalocele in infancy may include rhinorrhea, nasal obstruction, mouth breathing, or snoring. Most affected children have no overt intellectual or neurologic deficits, but panhypopituitarism is common. Patients who have morning glory discs are also at risk for acquired visual loss. Nonrhegmatogenous retinal detachments develop in approximately one third of eyes with morning glory discs and usually involve the peripapillary retina.[5] Controversy exists about the source of subretinal fluid; however, intraoperative findings in one case showed that the vitreous cavity, subarachnoid space, and subretinal space were all interconnected. (See Chapter 187.)

OPTIC DISC COLOBOMA

In optic disc coloboma, the disc appears enlarged and a sharply demarcated, glistening white, bowl-shaped excavation occurs (Fig. 188-3).[7] The inferior rim of the disc is thinner than the superior rim, which reflects the position of the embryonic fissure relative to the primitive epithelial papilla. The excavation may extend inferiorly to involve the adjacent choroid and retina, in which case microphthalmia is frequently present. In some instances, the entire disc is excavated, but the colobomatous nature of the defect can still be appreciated ophthalmoscopically because the excavation is deeper inferiorly. The excavation is contained within the colobomatous optic disc, as opposed to the morning glory disc anomaly, in which the disc falls within the excavation.[7] Visual acuity may be minimally or severely affected, depending upon the extent of the lesion. Although the optic disc area appears enlarged, optic disc coloboma is actually an inferior segmental form of optic nerve hypoplasia. The only remaining neural tissue lies superiorly in a C-shaped or moon-shaped crescent (Fig. 188-3).

Optic disc coloboma may arise sporadically or be inherited in an autosomal dominant fashion and may be accompanied by iris or retinochoroidal colobomas in the same or fellow eye. Often it is associated with systemic anomalies in a number of genetic syndromes (CHARGE [coloboma of the eye, heart anomaly, choanal atresia, retardation, and genital and ear anomalies] association, Walker-Warburg syndrome, Goltz focal dermal hypoplasia, Goldenhar's syndrome, linear nevus sebaceus syndrome), but rarely is it associated with transsphenoidal encephalocele.[1]

OPTIC PIT

An optic pit appears as a round or oval, gray, white, or yellowish crater-like depression in the optic disc (Fig. 188-4).[7] Optic pits

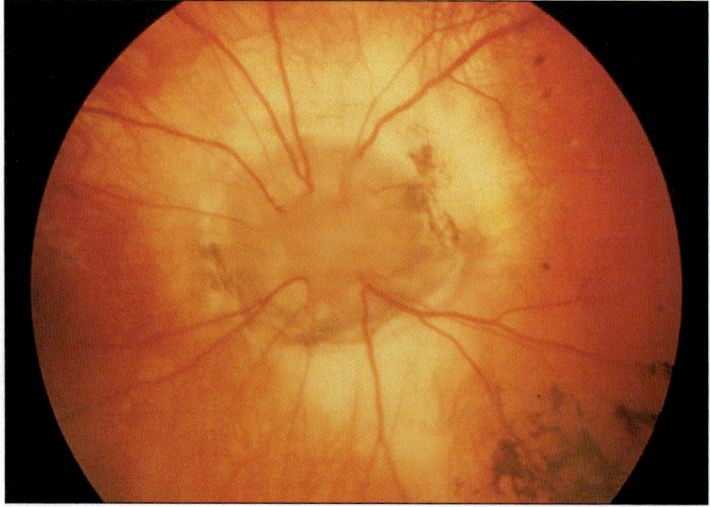

FIG. 188-2 ▌ Morning glory disc anomaly.

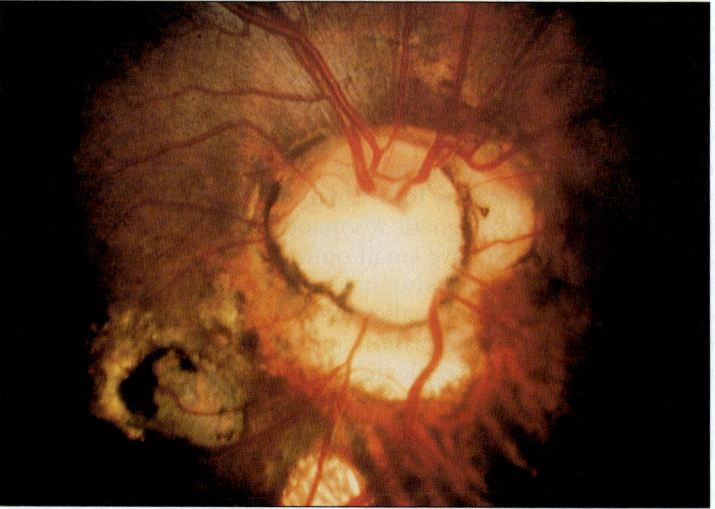

FIG. 188-3 ▌ Optic disc coloboma.

commonly involve the temporal optic disc but may be situated in any sector.[8] Temporal optic pits are often associated with adjacent peripapillary retinal pigment epithelium changes.[8] In unilateral cases, the involved disc is slightly larger than the normal disc.[8]

Visual field defects are variable and often correlate poorly with the location of the pit; the most common defect appears to be a paracentral arcuate scotoma connected to an enlarged blind spot. Acquired depressions in the optic disc that are indistinguishable from optic pits have been documented in eyes with normal-tension glaucoma.[1] Histologically, an optic pit is a herniation of rudimentary neuroectodermal tissue into a pocket-like depression within the nerve substance[8] (Fig. 188-5). Its pathogenesis is unknown.

Optic pits are not associated with brain malformations, and their discovery does not warrant neuroimaging. Approximately 45% of eyes with optic pits develop serous retinal detachments.[6] Some serous retinal detachments associated with optic pits resolve spontaneously, but the visual prognosis remains poor.[8] The subretinal fluid most likely originates from the vitreous cavity or the subarachnoid space that surrounds the optic nerve. Lincoff et al.[9] demonstrated that fluid from the optic pit initially produces an inner layer retinal separation (retinoschisis) that overlies the posterior pole. An outer layer macular hole subsequently develops through which this intraretinal fluid communicates with the subretinal space to form a sensory macular detachment that gradually enlarges.[9] This key observation has changed the preferred surgical therapy of serous macular detachments from photocoag-

ulation at the disc margin (which was performed to block the flow of subretinal fluid from the disc to the macula) to internal gas tamponade (which is used to displace mechanically subretinal fluid from beneath the macula).[1] (See Chapter 187.)

MEGALOPAPILLA

Megalopapilla is a generic term that connotes an abnormally large optic disc that lacks the inferior excavation of optic disc coloboma or the numerous anomalous features of the morning glory disc anomaly.[1] This condition is usually bilateral and often associated with a large cup-to-disc ratio. Patients who have megalopapilla are often suspected to have glaucoma. Unlike the situation in glaucoma, however, the optic cup is usually round or horizontally oval with no vertical notch or encroachment (Fig. 188-6). Visual acuity is generally normal in megalopapilla but may be mildly decreased in some cases. Visual fields are usually normal except for an enlarged blind spot, which enables the examiner to rule out low-tension glaucoma or a compressive lesion. Megalopapilla is only rarely associated with brain anomalies, and neuroimaging is not warranted unless midline facial anomalies are present.

CONGENITAL TILTED DISC SYNDROME

The tilted disc syndrome is a nonhereditary bilateral condition in which the superotemporal optic disc is elevated and the inferonasal disc is displaced posteriorly, which results in an optic disc of oval appearance with its long axis obliquely orientated (Fig. 188-7).[10] This configuration is accompanied by situs inver-

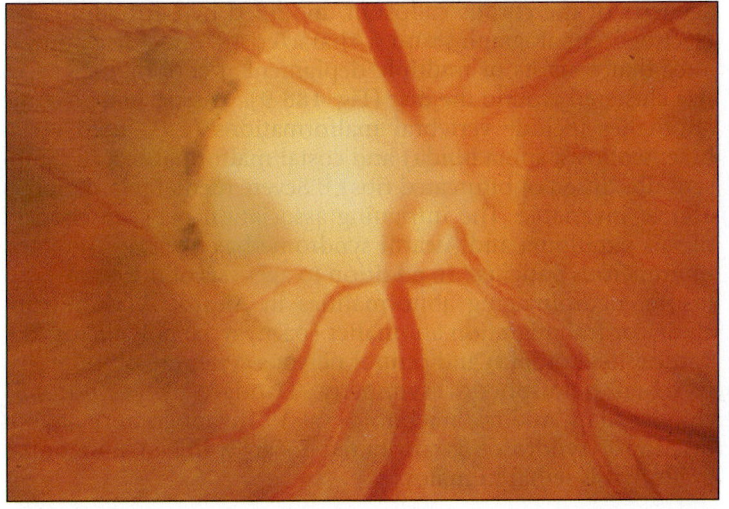

FIG. 188-4 ▐▐ Optic pit.

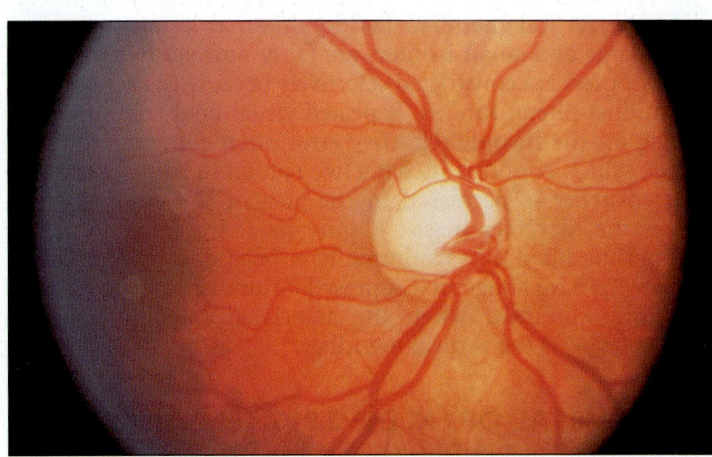

FIG. 188-6 ▐▐ Megalopapilla.

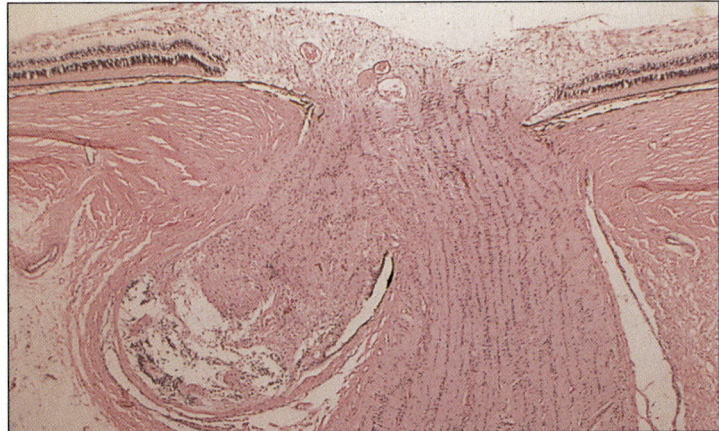

FIG. 188-5 ▐▐ **Optic pit.** Herniation of retinal tissue through an enlarged scleral opening along one side of the optic nerve. (Courtesy of Dr JB Crawford, from Irvine AR, Crawford JB, Sullivan JH. The pathogenesis of retinal detachment with morning glory disc and optic pit. Retina. 1986;6:146–50.)

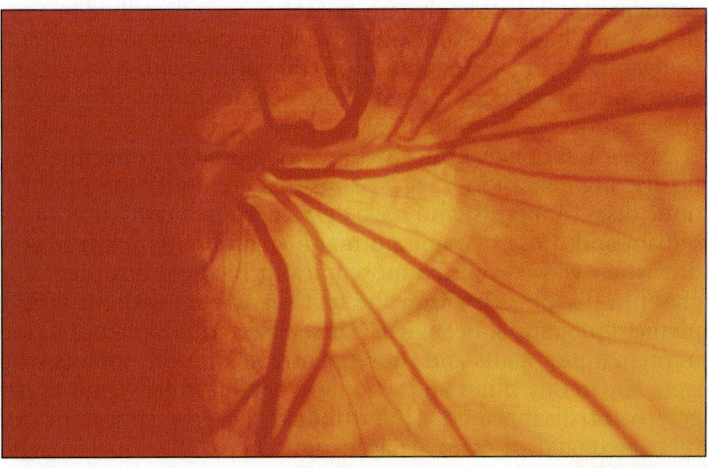

FIG. 188-7 ▐▐ **Congenital tilted right optic disc.** Note the inferonasal retinochoroidal depigmentation. (Left optic disc is the mirror image.)

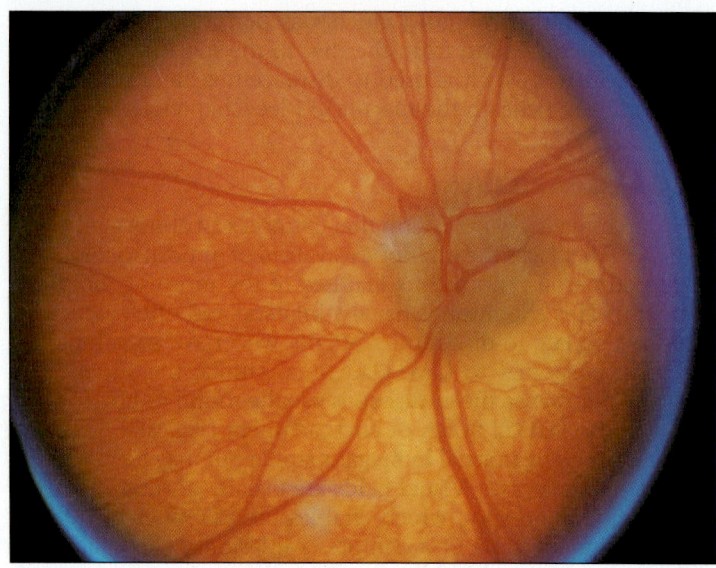

FIG. 188-8 ■ Congenital optic disc pigmentation.

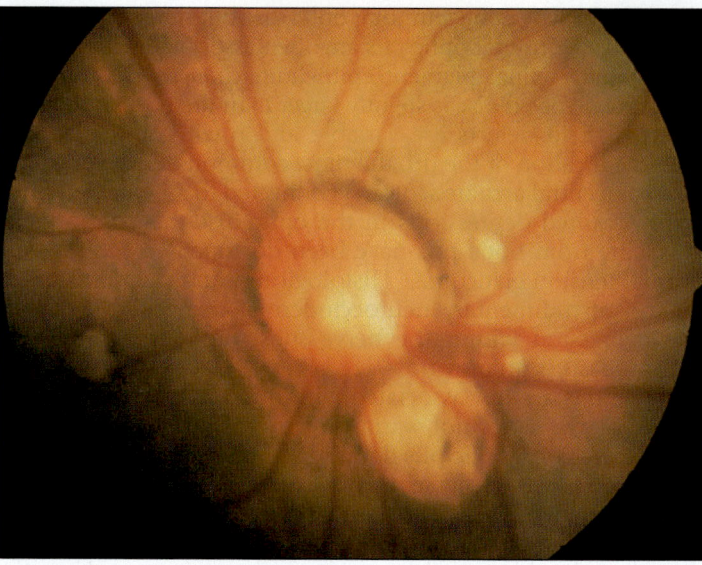

FIG. 188-9 ■ Aicardi syndrome.

sus of the retinal vessels, congenital inferonasal conus, thinning of the inferonasal retinal pigment epithelium and choroid, and myopic astigmatism. These features presumably result from a generalized ectasia of the inferonasal fundus that involves the corresponding sector of the optic disc.

Familiarity with this condition is important because affected patients may present with the suggestion of bitemporal hemianopias, which involve primarily the superotemporal quadrants. However, these field defects, when observed carefully, do not respect the vertical meridian (as do chiasmal lesions). Furthermore, large and small isopters are fairly normal, but medium-sized isopters are constricted selectively because of the ectasia of the midperipheral fundus. Repeated visual field tests after correcting for the myopic refractive error often eliminate the field defect, which confirms its refractive nature. In some cases, retinal sensitivity is decreased in the area of the ectasia, which causes the defect to persist despite refractive correction. Rare cases of the tilted disc syndrome have been documented in patients who have congenital suprasellar tumors; neuroimaging is therefore warranted when the associated bitemporal hemianopia respects the vertical meridian.[10]

CONGENITAL OPTIC DISC PIGMENTATION

Congenital optic disc pigmentation is a condition in which melanin anterior to or within the lamina cribrosa imparts a gray appearance to the disc (Fig. 188-8). True congenital optic disc pigmentation is extremely rare, but it has been described in a patient who had an interstitial deletion of chromosome 17. Congenital optic pigmentation is compatible with good visual acuity but may be associated with coexistent optic disc anomalies that decrease vision.[11]

Most cases of gray optic discs are not caused by congenital optic disc pigmentation.[11] For reasons that are understood poorly, optic discs of infants who have delayed visual maturation or albinism and those of some normal neonates have a diffuse gray tint when viewed ophthalmoscopically. In these disorders, the gray tint disappears within the first year of life without visible pigment migration. Beauvieux[12] first observed this phenomenon in premature infants and subsequently in albinotic infants who were apparently blind and who developed normal vision as the gray color disappeared. He attributed the gray appearance of these neonatal discs to delayed optic nerve myelination with preservation of the "embryonic tint."

Patients who have "optically gray optic discs" have unfortunately been lumped together with those who have congenital

optic disc pigmentation. These two conditions can usually be distinguished ophthalmoscopically because the melanin deposition is often irregular and displays some degree of granularity.[11]

AICARDI SYNDROME

The major features of Aicardi syndrome are infantile spasms, agenesis of the corpus callosum, modified hypsarrhythmia on electroencephalography, and a characteristic optic disc appearance that consists of multiple depigmented chorioretinal lacunae clustered around the disc (Fig. 188-9).[13] Associated systemic anomalies include vertebral malformations (e.g., fused vertebrae, scoliosis, spina bifida) and costal malformations (e.g., absent ribs, fused or bifurcated ribs).[13] Severe mental retardation is almost invariable. The intriguing association between choroid plexus papilloma and Aicardi syndrome has been documented in numerous patients.[1] In addition to agenesis of the corpus callosum, neuroimaging abnormalities in Aicardi syndrome include cortical migration anomalies (pachygyria, polymicrogyria, cortical heterotopia) and central nervous system malformations (cerebral hemispheric asymmetry, Dandy-Walker syndrome, colpocephaly, midline arachnoid cysts).[1] The inheritance pattern of Aicardi syndrome is attributed to an X-linked mutational event that is lethal in males.[1]

REFERENCES

1. Brodsky MC. Congenital optic disc anomalies. Surv Ophthalmol. 1994;39:89–112.
2. Lambert SR, Hoyt CS, Narahara MH. Optic nerve hypoplasia. Surv Ophthalmol. 1987;32:1–9.
3. Brodsky MC, Glasier CM. Optic nerve hypoplasia: clinical significance of associated central nervous system abnormalities on magnetic resonance imaging. Arch Ophthalmol. 1993;111:66–74.
4. Brodsky MC, Conte FA, Hoyt CS, et al. Sudden death in septo-optic dysplasia: report of five cases. Arch Ophthalmol. 1997;115(1):66–70.
5. Pollock S. The morning glory disc anomaly: contractile movement, classification, and embryogenesis. Doc Ophthalmol. 1987;65:442–53.
6. Massaro M, Thorarensen O, Liu GT, et al. Morning glory disc anomaly and moyamoya vessels. Arch Ophthalmol. 1998;116(2):253–4.
7. Brown G, Tasman W. Congenital anomalies of the optic disc. New York: Grune & Stratton; 1983:91–126.
8. Brodsky MC. Magnetic resonance imaging of colobomatous optic hypoplasia. Br J Ophthalmol. 1999;83(6):755–6.
9. Lincoff H, Lopez R, Kreissig I, et al. Retinoschisis associated with optic nerve pits. Arch Ophthalmol. 1988;106:61–7.
10. Young SE, Walsh FB, Knox DL. The tilted disc syndrome. Am J Ophthalmol. 1976;82:16–23.
11. Brodsky MC, Buckley EG, McConkie-Rosell A. The case of the gray optic disc. Surv Ophthalmol. 1989;33:367–72.
12. Beauvieux J. La pseudo-atrophie optique des nouveau-nes (dysénésie myélinque des voies optiques). Ann Ocul (Paris). 1926;163:881–921.
13. Carney SH, Brodsky MC, Good WV, et al. Aicardi syndrome: more than meets the eye. Surv Ophthalmol. 1993;37:419–24.

189 Papilledema and Raised Intracranial Pressure

ALFREDO A. SADUN

DEFINITION
- Optic disc edema, usually bilateral, that results from increased intracranial pressure.

KEY FEATURES
- Blurring of the optic disc margins.
- Anterior extension of the nerve head.
- Venous congestion of arcuate and peripapillary vessels.
- Hyperemia of the optic nerve head.

ASSOCIATED FEATURES
- Gross elevation of the optic nerve head.
- Engorged and dusky veins.
- Peripapillary splinter hemorrhages.
- Choroidal folds.
- Retina striae.

INTRODUCTION

About 1.2 million axons converge at the optic disc to form the optic nerve. The optic nerve follows a 50mm course as it extends from the back of the eye, travels through the orbit, passes through the optic canal, runs intracranially, and partially decussates along with the contralateral optic nerve to form the optic chiasm. Each axon must maintain active axonal transport in both the orthograde (eye to brain) and retrograde directions. The subarachnoid space of the brain is continuous with the optic nerve sheath. An extensive litany of insults may lead to dysfunction or compression of the optic nerve, which may cause a partial arrest of axoplasmic transport and result in optic disc edema. If the compression is caused by raised intracranial pressure, the condition is termed *papilledema*. The term, papilledema, carries neurological and neurosurgical connotations. If the cause of the disc edema is not increased intracranial pressure, the term *optic disc edema* should be used instead of papilledema. Long-standing or severe papilledema, in addition to reflecting intracranial pathology, also may result in bilateral optic nerve dysfunction because of compromise of axonal integrity at the lamina cribrosa.

EPIDEMIOLOGY AND PATHOGENESIS

Tumors of the brain may be benign or malignant, and primary or metastatic. All may cause a rise in intracranial pressure. About 100,000 patients a year in the United States die with intracranial masses (most with metastatic disease). Although tumors of the posterior fossa are very likely to cause obstruction of cerebral spinal fluid flow between the ventricles, most cases of increased intracranial pressure in adults arise from large hemispheric masses.

Patients may suffer from many of the features of intracranial tumors in the absence of any mass lesion. Pseudotumor cerebri (PTC), also termed *idiopathic intracranial hypertension*, requires that neuroimaging prove negative for mass lesions and obstruction of the ventricular system, and that a lumbar puncture prove positive for high pressure although the fluid is normal in composition.

PTC is a syndrome that is much more likely to be a cause of increased intracranial pressure and hence papilledema among young adults than real tumor. This syndrome has several features that characterize it. The only initial symptom may be a headache, which tends to be worst when recumbent. There is usually an absence of any neurological signs other than visual loss, although a sixth cranial nerve palsy is not rare. Irreversible visual loss from chronic papilledema is the all-too-common sequela (about 50% of cases) that must be avoided. PTC is usually idiopathic, but it may be seen in association with certain drugs and agents and in particular types of patients. One well understood cause of PTC is from intracranial venous thrombosis which may be subsequent to head trauma. Historically, a common cause of intracranial venous thrombosis was otitis media with mastoiditis.

Drugs such as tetracycline, nalidixic acid, corticosteroids (or more commonly steroid withdrawal), or vitamin A may produce PTC. Patients with hypoparathyroidism and adrenal adenomas are more likely to develop PTC. Chronic respiratory insufficiency, renal syndrome, and iron deficiency anemia also have been associated with PTC.

In the majority of cases, however, no etiological factor can be found for PTC. Most patients are obese young women, and there is a suggestion that there is an endocrine abnormality at the basis of the disorder.

Like glaucoma, increased intracranial pressure can be consequent to an increased production of fluid or to a decrease in outflow facility. Many investigators feel that most causes of PTC involve increased resistance to cerebrospinal fluid drainage.

Most patients (80–90%) with PTC seek treatment for a headache. Less often, visual disturbances bring the patient to medical attention. The patient may complain of decreased visual acuity, transient obscuration of visions, an enlarged blind spot, or diplopia (due to sixth cranial nerve palsy).

The sixth cranial nerve palsy is a nonspecific sign of increased intracranial pressure and resolves following a decrease in the intracranial pressure. Permanent impairments produced by PTC are those resulting from chronic papilledema.

Obstruction of the ventricular system, or shunt failure in an individual in whom a ventricular or lumbar peritoneal shunt has been placed previously, may lead to a very rapid rise in intracranial pressure and fulminant papilledema.

The principal pathophysiology of optic disc swelling is blockage of axoplasmic transport. Axoplasmic transport is the movement of materials responsible for maintaining the axon, primarily proteins and organelles formed in the neuronal soma and transported along the axon. Axonal transport may depend on the microtubules that act as "railroad tracks." Orthograde axoplasmic transport can be slow or rapid. The former occurs at 0.5–3.0mm per day, and rapid flow at 200–1000mm per day. In addition, retrograde axoplasmic transport also occurs.[1] Mechanical and vascular causes can combine to produce a blockage of optic nerve axoplasmic flow. Such blockage at the level of the lamina choroidalis and lamina scleralis occurs when optic disc edema is produced experimentally through increased intracranial pressure, ocular hypotony, or increased intraocular pressure. It is felt that local factors produce a stasis of axoplasmic flow. Optic disc edema also may be produced by an event that increases venous pressure at or near the lamina cribrosa,[2-5] such as occurs secondary to intrinsic tumors or extrinsic orbital masses, or by abnormalities in blood flow such as central retinal vein occlusion (CRVO).

OCULAR MANIFESTATIONS

Papilledema is observed on fundus examination, usually by direct ophthalmoscopy performed both with the standard (white) and red-free light (to better visualize the nerve fiber layer). Indirect ophthalmoscopy with a 20D lens provides a better stereoscopic view, but it is even better with the higher magnification of the 14D. A 90D lens used in conjunction with biomicroscopy is excellent. It is useful to characterize the changes in the optic nerve head that occur in papilledema as being mechanical or vascular in nature. The five mechanical clinical signs of optic disc edema are:

- Blurring of the optic disc margins
- Filling in of the optic disc cup
- Anterior extension of the nerve head (3D = 1mm of elevation)
- Edema of the nerve fiber layer
- Retinal or choroidal folds (or both)

The five vascular clinical signs of optic disc edema are venous congestion of arcuate and peripapillary vessels, papillary and retinal peripapillary hemorrhages, nerve fiber layer infarcts (cotton-wool spots), hyperemia of the optic nerve head, and hard exudates of the optic disc.

In addition, elements of optic disc swelling can be used to help characterize the papilledema as early, fully developed, chronic, or late. In early papilledema disc hyperemia, disc swelling, blurring of the disc margins, and blurring of the nerve fiber layer are found (Fig. 189-1). In fully developed papilledema gross elevation of the optic nerve head and engorged and dusky

veins appear, peripapillary splinter hemorrhages and sometimes choroidal folds arise, and retina striae are seen (Fig. 189-2). In chronic papilledema fewer hemorrhages occur, the optic disc cup is obliterated completely, less disc hyperemia is seen, and hard exudates occur within the nerve head (Fig. 189-3). In late disc edema secondary optic atrophy occurs, disc swelling subsides, retinal arterioles are narrowed or sheathed, and the optic disc appears dirty gray and blurred, secondary to gliosis (Fig. 189-4).

Symptoms of increased intracranial pressure include headache and brief transient obscurations of vision. Less commonly, the patient may describe blurred vision, constriction of visual fields, dyschromatopsia, and diplopia.

The headache of increased intracranial pressure usually is quite distinctive (see Chapter 204). Cause for concern exists if the headache is particularly severe or associated with nausea and vomiting or a sense of pressure around the ears. This concern is heightened if the headache becomes worse in a recumbent position or is worst in the early morning, when the patient wakes up, but improves during the day. Even more specific are the transient obscurations of vision, usually described as monocular or binocular blackouts, that last 3–4 seconds and most often occur as the patient arises from the recumbent position to sitting or standing.[6] Papilledema may produce visual blurring because of enlargement of the blind spot and adjacent retinal folds or edema; this blurring usually is reversible. However, further injury to the optic nerve may be associated with secondary optic atrophy and be permanent, which results in symptoms such as constricted visual fields and poor color vision. Diplopia usually arises from nonlocalizing sixth cranial nerve palsies, and it often resolves after the increased intracranial pressure has been controlled.

DIAGNOSIS AND TESTING

An index of suspicion for papilledema is provided by the history. A careful fundus examination is mandatory. The optic nerve

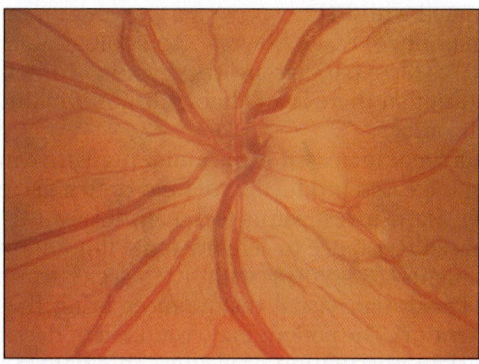

FIG. 189-1 ▮ **Early papilledema.** The optic disc of an 18-year-old man 2 weeks after he had complained of diplopia arising from sixth cranial nerve palsies caused by increased intracranial pressure. Note the minimal evidence of edema.

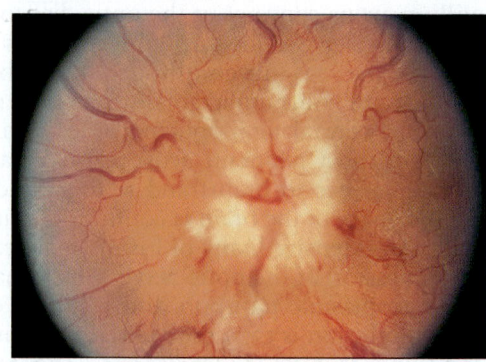

FIG. 189-3 ▮ **Chronic papilledema.** Severe and chronic disc edema in a 27-year-old, very obese woman who has pseudotumor cerebri. Note that the disc cusp is obliterated and hard exudates are present.

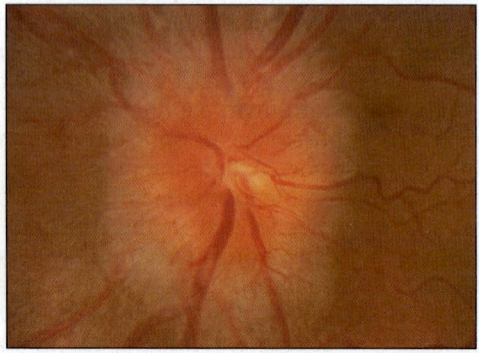

FIG. 189-2 ▮ **Developed papilledema.** The optic disc of a 36-year-old woman who suffered headache and blurred vision for 2 months. Fully developed disc edema present—note the engorged veins and peripapillary hemorrhages.

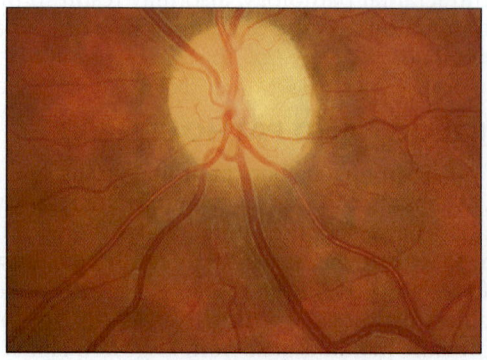

FIG. 189-4 ▮ **Secondary optic atrophy from chronic papilledema.** The same 27-year-old obese female patient 5 months later. Note the secondary optic atrophy has developed fully. The disc margins appear hazy or "dirty."

head is assessed for each of the ten signs of disc edema described above and the papilledema characterized not only as mild, moderate, or severe, but also as early, developed, late, or chronic. A careful procedure is instituted to determine whether the disc edema is, in fact, papilledema; this usually begins with neuroimaging followed by, in most cases, a lumbar puncture with manometry.

DIFFERENTIAL DIAGNOSIS

The differential diagnosis of papilledema is disc edema without increased intracranial pressure and pseudopapilledema. The latter rubric includes all abnormalities of the optic disc that can mimic optic disc edema. The most common of such disc anomalies are optic disc drusen which, especially when deeply buried, may give the disc a lumpy, elevated appearance. However, very few, if any, of the other nine signs of disc edema mentioned above apply. Other causes of optic disc edema without increased intracranial pressure need to be considered—compressive optic neuropathies, papillitis, anterior ischemic optic neuropathy, CRVO, juvenile diabetic papillopathy, and optic disc vasculitis.[7]

Compressive Optic Neuropathies

Compressive optic neuropathies that may produce disc edema often are located in the anterior orbit. Neoplasms of the optic nerve itself (gliomas) or of its sheaths (meningiomas), or masses from the orbital tissues or paranasal sinuses, may impinge on the anterior optic nerve and result in disc edema. Inflammatory and infiltrative lesions also may manifest as masses. Distal malignancies also may involve the optic nerve and its sheaths by metastasis.

Papillitis

Papillitis often has a component of disc edema and frequently follows a prodromal viral illness. The inflammation may extend beyond the confines of the optic disc and may develop into a neuroretinitis. Cells are found frequently in the vitreous humor; retinal exudates may form a star or a half-star figure between the disc and the macula. Both papillitis and neuroretinitis are seen often in young, healthy adults.

Anterior Ischemic Optic Neuropathy

Anterior ischemic optic neuropathy usually demonstrates sectorial disc edema and peripapillary hemorrhages. An acute loss of vision occurs and the visual field deficit may take on an altitudinal shape. Anterior ischemic optic neuropathy is found most often in patients of age 50–75 years and who have hypertension or diabetes.[8]

Central Retinal Vein Occlusion

CRVO or impending CRVO also may result in congestion in the optic nerve heads. However, the extensive hemorrhages found in CRVO usually make the differentiation easy. Generally, CRVOs occur in middle-aged or older individuals who have hypertension or, less often, hyperviscosity syndrome.

Juvenile Diabetic Papillopathy

Juvenile diabetic papillopathy includes unilateral or bilateral disc edema in its manifestations. The loss of vision usually is minimal, and the visual fields may show peripheral constriction or central scotomas. The fundus examination often reveals dilated telangiectatic vessels over the discs, which appears very much like optic disc neovascularization, but these disappear when the disc edema resolves spontaneously 4–8 weeks later.[8]

Optic Disc Vasculitis

Optic disc vasculitis, or (more globally) uveitis, also may result in optic disc edema. Papillophlebitis, optic disc vasculitis, benign retinal vasculitis, and "the big blind-spot syndrome" may be considered variations on this theme. These conditions often develop in young, healthy adults who have only minimal visual impairment. The optic disc edema usually occurs in association with engorged retinal veins and occasionally with retinal hemorrhages.

Other Causes

Other causes of disc edema include advanced Graves' disease, malignant hypertension, and hypotony. Malignant processes, such as carcinoma, lymphoma, or leukemia,[9] as well as uremia[10] and sarcoid granuloma, also may cause swelling of the optic disc. Nutritional optic neuropathies, such as in tropical epidemics, and toxic optic neuropathies often caused by drugs, such as ethambutol, may result in mild disc edema.[11] Orbital or cranial trauma, radiation, and burns also may cause swelling of the optic discs.

SYSTEMIC ASSOCIATIONS

In addition to papilledema and the potential for visual loss, increased intracranial pressure can cause other signs and symptoms. However, the most serious and irreversible problems associated with increased intracranial pressure, *per se*, are visual; hence, the ophthalmologist is a critical member of the clinical team for such patients. Palsies of the sixth cranial nerve, hearing loss, and facial nerve palsies also are found, in decreasing order of frequency, in patients who have increased intracranial pressure. However, the cranial nerve palsies are likely to be self-limiting after reduction of the pressure. More often, patients who have increased intracranial pressure complain of headache, pressure in the ears, tinnitus, and fatigue, and sometimes, if severe, nausea and vomiting.

PATHOLOGY

The histopathology of acute optic disc edema reveals axoplasmic stasis, edema, and vascular congestion (Fig. 189-5). Peripapillary hemorrhages are seen primarily in the retinal nerve fiber layer, but they may overlie the optic disc.[12] The increase in tissue mass fills the physiological cup and causes the optic nerve head to protrude anteriorly. The small blood vessels are engorged and tortuous. Vacuoles of extracellular fluid accumulate in and anterior to the retinal lamina cribrosa, and the subarachnoid space is enlarged with stretching of the subarachnoid strands.[12]

The neural retina is displaced away from the optic disc and the outer layer of the retina may be buckled (retinal folds). The rods and cones are displaced away obliquely from their anchor near Bruch's membrane. A shallow retinal detachment may occur in the peripapillary area.

Engorgement of axons in the laminar portion of the optic nerve is best demonstrated by electron microscopy. The swollen axons are filled with mitochondria primarily anterior to the choroidal lamina cribrosa. The mitochondria themselves appear swollen and disrupted, and the fascicles of microtubules also are in disarray. Importantly, the extracellular accumulation is minimal compared with the intracellular and intraaxonal accumulation.[13]

TREATMENT

The treatment of papilledema associated with visual loss depends in large part on the cause, symptoms, signs, and progression of the problem. Attempts must be made to redress the pathophysiology. However, a few comments on the general concepts are given here.

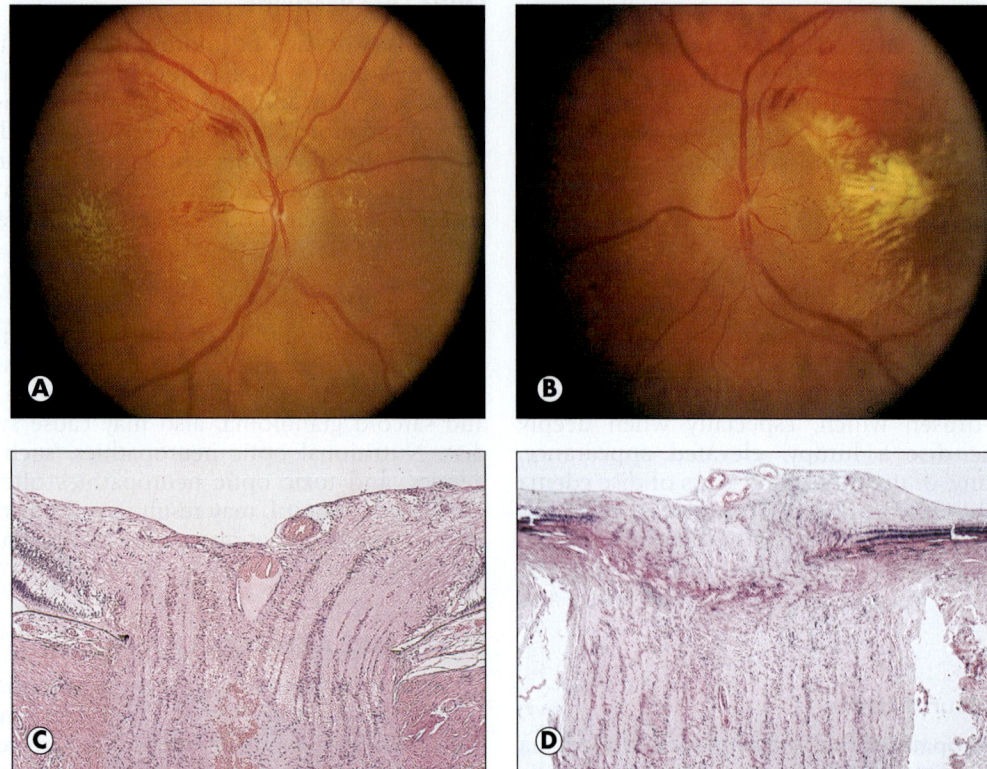

FIG. 189-5 ▪ **Optic disc edema. A** and **B,** Patient has bilateral optic disc edema secondary to grade IV malignant hypertension. **B,** Note exudates in nasal macula. **C,** Histological section shows optic disc edema secondary to ocular hypertension caused by phacolytic glaucoma. **D,** Optic disc edema secondary to ocular hypotony caused by a ruptured globe. Optic disc edema can be caused by increased intracranial pressure or increased or decreased intraocular pressure. The main findings in C and D consist of increased mass of anterior optic nerve caused by axonal swelling, optic nerve head tissue edema and vascular congestion, and lateral displacement of photoreceptors from the end of Bruch's membrane, which terminates in a ring at the optic nerve.

Medical treatment usually consists of repeated lumbar punctures and diuretics, especially carbonic anhydrase inhibitors and, in cases of pseudotumor, weight reduction.[14]

If medical treatment is not sufficient, optic nerve sheath decompression[15,16] or a lumboperitoneal shunt[17] may need to be carried out. It is very important to understand that the decision to treat, or to alter treatment modality, usually is based on the ophthalmologist's descriptions of the extent of both optic disc edema and visual loss, as measured by such parameters as color vision or visual fields. Hence, the ophthalmologist is a crucial member of the clinical team that makes management decisions.

COURSE AND OUTCOMES

The prognosis for papilledema is largely dependent on the cause. Most patients who have metastatic brain tumors do very badly; those who have ventricular obstructive disease may be shunted successfully; patients who have pseudotumor usually can be managed quite well. Two general points warrant emphasis. The diagnosis of papilledema requires a prompt work-up until the most serious pathologies are ruled out. Here, neurological, neurosurgical, or neuroradiological consultation is required usually. However, once the problem has been reduced to that of papilledema only, the ophthalmologist can best determine how aggressive the course of management needs to be. All too often, permanent visual loss occurs in relatively benign diseases such as PTC for lack of appropriate ophthalmologic involvement.[14]

REFERENCES

1. Brady ST, Lasek RJ, Allen RD. Video microscopy for fast axonal transport of extruded axoplasm: a new model for study of molecular mechanisms. Cell Motil. 1985;5:81–101.
2. Minckler DS, Bunt AH. Axoplasmic transport in ocular hypotony and papilledema in the monkey. Arch Ophthalmol. 1977;95:1430–6.
3. Hayreh MS, Hayreh SS. Optic disc edema in raised intracranial pressure. I. Evolution and resolution. Arch Ophthalmol. 1977;95:1237–44.
4. Tso MOM, Hayreh SS. Optic disc edema in raised intracranial pressure. III. A pathologic study of experimental papilledema. Arch Ophthalmol. 1977;95:1448–57.
5. Hayreh SS. Optic disc edema in raised intracranial pressure. V. Pathogenesis. Arch Ophthalmol. 1977;95:1553–65.
6. Sadun AA, Currie JN, Lessell S. Transient visual obscurations with elevated optic discs. Ann Neurol. 1984;16:489–94.
7. Sanders MD, Sennhenn RH. Differential diagnosis of unilateral optic disc edema. Trans Ophthalmol Soc U K. 1980;100:123–31.
8. Glaser J. Neuro-ophthalmology, ed 2. Philadelphia: JB Lippincott; 1990:64–8, 95–7, 107–8, 135–40.
9. Currie JN, Lessell S, Lessell IM, et al. Optic neuropathy in chronic lymphocytic leukemia. Arch Ophthalmol. 1988;106:654–60.
10. Knox DL, Hanneken AM, Hollows FC, et al. Uremic optic neuropathy. Arch Ophthalmol. 1988;106:50–4.
11. Sadun AA, Martone JF, Muci-Mendoza R, et al. Epidemic optic neuropathy in Cuba: eye findings. Arch Ophthalmol. 1994;112:691–9.
12. Sadun AA. Optic atrophy and papilledema. Jakobiec F, Albert D, eds. In: Principles of ophthalmology. Philadelphia: WB Saunders; 1993:2529–38.
13. Minckler DS, Tso MOM. A light microscopic autoradiographic study of axoplasmic transport in the normal rhesus optic nerve head. Am J Ophthalmol. 1976;82:1–15.
14. Corbett JJ, Thompson HS. The rational management of idiopathic intracranial hypertension. Arch Neurol. 1989;46:1049–51.
15. Brourman ND, Spoor TC, Ramocki JM. Optic nerve decompression for pseudotumor cerebri. Arch Ophthalmol. 1988;106:1378–83.
16. Corbett JJ, Nerad JA, Tse DT, et al. Results of optic nerve sheath fenestration for pseudotumor cerebri: the lateral orbitotomy approach. Arch Ophthalmol. 1988;106:1391–7.
17. Tytla ME, Buncic JR. Recovery of spatial vision following shunting for hydrocephalus. Arch Ophthalmol. 1990;108:701–4.

CHAPTER 190

Inflammatory Optic Neuropathies and Neuroretinitis

LAURA J. BALCER • ROY W. BECK

DEFINITION
- Optic neuritis refers to inflammation of the optic nerve. Such inflammation may spare the optic disc (retrobulbar optic neuritis) or may cause optic disc swelling (papillitis).

KEY FEATURES
- Abrupt vision loss.
- Dyschromatopsia.
- Afferent pupillary defect.

ASSOCIATED FEATURES
- Pain, particularly on eye movement.
- Inflammation of the optic disc with adjacent retinal inflammation (referred to as *neuroretinitis*).

INTRODUCTION

Optic neuritis, or primary inflammation of the optic nerve, is referred to as *papillitis* when the optic disc is swollen and *retrobulbar neuritis* when the disc appears normal. The most common form of optic neuritis is acute demyelinating optic neuritis. Much of our current knowledge about acute demyelinating optic neuritis has been derived from the Optic Neuritis Treatment Trial (ONTT). This was a multicenter trial supported by the National Eye Institute that assessed the benefit of corticosteroid treatment of optic neuritis, and investigated the relation between optic neuritis and multiple sclerosis (MS).[1-14] Although numerous autoimmune conditions, such as sarcoidosis, may be associated with acute or chronic optic nerve inflammation, this chapter will focus on acute demyelinating optic neuritis.

EPIDEMIOLOGY AND PATHOGENESIS

The annual incidence of optic neuritis, as estimated in population-based studies, is approximately 5 per 100,000 per year, while the prevalence is 115 per 100,000.[15] The majority of patients who develop optic neuritis are between the ages of 20 and 50 years. Women are affected more commonly than men. In the ONTT, 77% of the patients were women, 85% were white, and the mean age was 32 ± 7 years. In most cases, the pathogenesis of optic neuritis is inflammatory demyelination, whether or not MS is diagnosed clinically.[16,17] It is likely that many cases of monosymptomatic optic neuritis occur as the initial manifestation of MS.[18]

OCULAR MANIFESTATIONS

Loss of vision in patients who have acute demyelinating optic neuritis is usually abrupt and occurs over several hours to days. Progression for a longer period is possible but suggests an alternative underlying cause. Visual loss is usually monocular, although occasionally both eyes are affected, particularly in children.

Mild pain in or around the eye is present in more than 90% of patients. Such pain may precede or occur concomitantly with visual loss, is usually exacerbated by eye movement, and generally lasts no more than a few days. The presence of pain, particularly on eye movement, is a helpful (although not definitive) clinical feature that differentiates acute demyelinating optic neuritis from nonarteritic anterior ischemic optic neuropathy (AION).[19]

On examination of the patient, optic nerve dysfunction is evident. The severity of visual loss varies from a mild visual field defect to severe loss of central acuity (3% of ONTT participants had no light perception).[3] Color vision and contrast sensitivity are impaired in almost all cases, often out of proportion to visual acuity. Among primary visual outcome measures in the ONTT, contrast sensitivity demonstrated the highest percentage of eyes with abnormalities (even after 5 years of follow-up).[8] Visual field loss, which may be diffuse (48% of 415 ONTT patients tested) or focal (52% are nerve fiber bundle defects, central or cecocentral scotomas, hemianopic defects), is also common in acute optic neuritis.[4]

An afferent pupillary defect (APD) is detected in almost all unilateral cases of optic neuritis. If an APD is not present, a preexisting optic neuropathy in the fellow eye must be suspected. In fact, asymptomatic visual dysfunction is fairly common among fellow eyes of patients who have apparent unilateral optic neuritis.[7]

The optic disc appears normal in approximately two thirds of patients who have acute demyelinating optic neuritis (retrobulbar optic neuritis), while disc swelling is present in about one third of cases (papillitis) (Fig. 190-1). Although the clinical features are similar in both forms, optic disc hemorrhages were uncommon in the ONTT (6%), and their presence should suggest an alternative diagnosis.

DIAGNOSIS AND ANCILLARY TESTING

The diagnosis of acute demyelinating optic neuritis is based on an appropriate history (typical versus atypical course) and clinical signs and symptoms as described above. Diagnostic tests, including magnetic resonance imaging (MRI), cerebrospinal fluid (CSF) analysis, and serological studies, usually are performed for the following reasons[10,11]: (1) to determine if the cause of the acute optic neuropathy is noninflammatory (such as a compressive lesion), or a nonidiopathic inflammatory or infectious process in cases that are not typical for acute demyelinating optic neuritis, and (2) to determine the prognosis or risk for subsequent development of clinically definite MS (CDMS) in monosymptomatic cases for which the history and clinical signs are typical.

In patients who have suspected optic neuritis, MRI of the brain and orbits with fat suppression and gadolinium should be performed, even in typical cases, to confirm the diagnosis and to assess for the presence of other white matter lesions.[10,11] Follow-up of the ONTT cohort to 5 years and beyond has confirmed that the number of white matter lesions, specifically two or more, is highly predictive of the development of CDMS in monosympto-

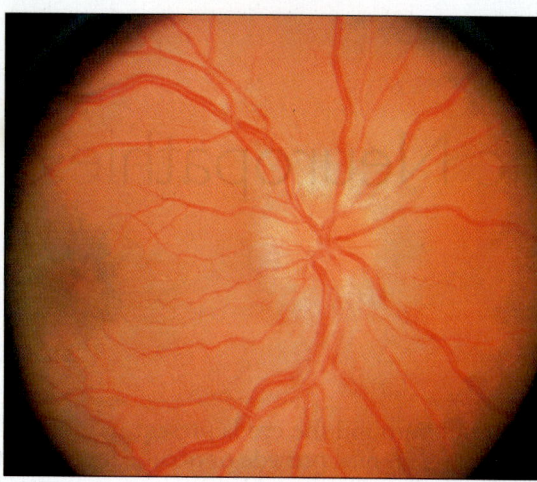

FIG. 190-1 ▪ Optic disc swelling (papillitis) associated with acute optic neuritis.

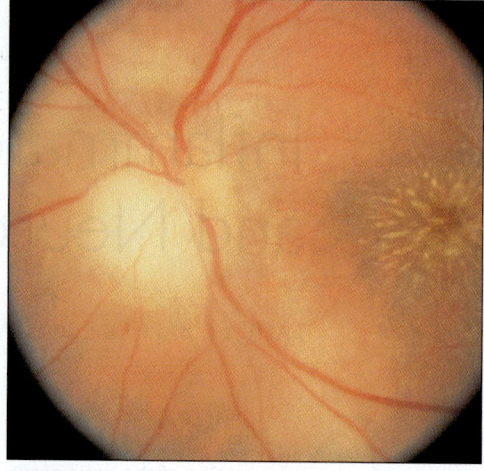

FIG. 190-2 ▪ Optic disc edema and macular star formation. Color fundus photograph from a 13-year-old girl who came to medical attention with counting fingers acuity secondary to cat-scratch (Bartonella) neuroretinitis.

BOX 190-1

Differential Diagnosis of Acute Unilateral Optic Neuropathy

Anterior ischemic optic neuropathy
Tumor
Aneurysm
Vasculitis
Neuroretinitis
Metastatic carcinoma
Lymphoreticular disorder
Sinusitis
Granulomatous inflammation
Leber's hereditary optic neuropathy (although always bilateral, this frequently presents initially with visual loss in only one eye)

---

matic patients (51% for two or more lesions versus 16% for normal MRI findings).[10]

DIFFERENTIAL DIAGNOSIS

The diagnosis of acute visual loss begins with the localization of the involved portion of the visual system. An optic neuropathy is presumed when no ocular cause for visual loss is apparent and an APD is present. The differential diagnosis for acute optic neuropathy is outlined in Box 190-1. Because most cases of optic neuritis produce unilateral visual loss, discussion here is limited to unilateral optic neuropathies. When there is acute visual loss and unilateral optic disc swelling, both optic neuritis and AION must be considered. Although the clinical profiles of these disorders overlap, AION is typically painless, occurs in patients over 50 years of age, and may be associated with optic disc hemorrhages. When the optic disc is normal in patients who have unilateral optic neuropathy, a compressive lesion must be excluded; this usually is differentiated from acute optic neuritis by a history of progressive visual loss beyond the typical period of 1–2 weeks.

Other inflammatory, infectious, and neoplastic disorders may produce infiltration or demyelination, or both, of the optic nerve. These conditions may appear as either acute or progressive visual loss, and include sarcoidosis, systemic lupus erythematosus, syphilis, postviral syndromes, lymphoma, and leukemia.

Neuroretinitis, characterized by optic disc edema and macular exudates, must be differentiated from acute demyelinating optic neuritis (Fig. 190-2). Macular edema is initially diffuse; hard exudates form within days, frequently in a star-shaped pattern. Deep, whitish lesions are noted at the level of the retinal pigment epithelium, scattered throughout the fundus. Both types of retinal findings are important to recognize, because their presence virtually excludes idiopathic demyelination or MS as the cause. Most cases of neuroretinitis are caused by viral syndromes, although cat-scratch disease and toxoplasmosis also must be considered.

Viral and Postviral Syndromes

Parainfectious optic neuritis typically follows the onset of a viral infection by 1–3 weeks, but it also can occur as a postvaccination phenomenon. It is more common in children than adults and likely occurs by an immunological process that produces optic nerve demyelination. Postviral (or parainfectious) optic neuritis may be unilateral but is frequently bilateral. The optic discs may appear normal or swollen; retinal involvement (neuroretinitis) is common when there is optic disc swelling. Associated meningoencephalitis, with MRI changes and CSF pleocytosis, is not unusual. Visual recovery after parainfectious optic neuritis usually is excellent, even with no treatment. Corticosteroids may or may not hasten recovery, but this treatment is reasonable to consider, particularly in cases of bilateral, severe visual loss.

Sarcoidosis

Granulomatous inflammation of the optic nerve is a frequent ocular manifestation of sarcoidosis and may be an initial sign of this disorder. Clinical findings may be similar to those of acute demyelinating optic neuritis. However, the optic disc may have a characteristic lumpy, white appearance, suggestive of granulomatous infiltration. Recovery of vision is rapid in most cases following corticosteroid treatment. In fact, rapid recovery of vision with corticosteroid treatment and subsequent deterioration following taper is atypical for acute demyelinating optic neuritis and should suggest an infiltrative process such as sarcoidosis.

Syphilis

Syphilitic optic neuritis has become more common since the increase in prevalence of human immunodeficiency virus (HIV) infection (see below). Optic nerve involvement may be unilateral or bilateral. Vitreous cellular reaction is a typical feature that differentiates syphilis infection from acute demyelinating optic neuritis, in which the vitreous humor usually is clear. The diagnosis is established with identification of positive syphilis serological and CSF VDRL (Venereal Disease Research Laboratories) test results. Treatment with penicillin produces visual recovery in most cases; however, recurrences are possible.

Lyme Disease

Although optic neuritis has been reported in patients with positive Lyme serological test results or other neurological findings suggestive of Lyme disease, definitive evidence of a causal relationship with *Borrelia burgdorferi* infection or rapid improvement of optic neuropathy following antibiotic treatment has not been established in most cases.[20] Acute demyelinating optic neuritis, particularly in patients with a history of or MRI findings consistent with MS (or two or more white matter lesions suggesting high MS risk in monosymptomatic patients), must be strongly considered in such patients, given the recent recommendations for early interferon treatment (see Treatment). Syphilis infection may produce false-positive Lyme disease serological examination results and, therefore, must also be considered in patients with optic neuropathy or other neurological manifestations.

Optic Neuritis in Human Immunodeficiency Virus Disease

In immunocompromised patients, particularly those with HIV infection, many other infectious diseases may cause optic neuropathy, including tuberculosis, toxoplasmosis, toxocariasis, cytomegalovirus, herpes zoster, *Cryptococcus*, and other fungi. Primary central nervous system lymphoma infiltrating the optic nerves and chiasm has been reported recently in patients who have HIV.[21]

Systemic Lupus Erythematosus and Other Vasculitides

Optic neuritis may occur in patients who have systemic lupus erythematosus (SLE), polyarteritis nodosa, and other vasculitides. Involvement of the optic nerve occurs in about 1% of patients who have SLE. Rarely, the disease manifests with optic neuropathy. The pathogenesis is related to ischemia, which may produce demyelination alone or in combination with axonal necrosis. Clinical manifestations may include those of acute optic neuritis (both papillitis and retrobulbar neuritis), acute ischemic optic neuropathy, or chronic progressive visual loss. The diagnosis of SLE as a cause of optic neuropathy is established by identification of systemic symptoms and signs of the disease, and by serological testing. Treatment with high-dose corticosteroids is indicated and has been demonstrated to reverse severe visual loss.[22]

The term autoimmune optic neuritis has been suggested for cases of steroid-responsive optic neuritis with serological evidence of vasculitis (such as antinuclear antibodies [ANA]) but no signs of systemic involvement.[23] However, the existence of "autoimmune optic neuritis," distinct from either SLE or MS, is unproved. Patients with acute demyelinating optic neuritis or MS also may have positive ANA serological test results. Among ONTT participants, the ANA finding was positive at a titer <1:320 in 13% and >1:320 in 3%; only one patient developed a diagnosable connective tissue disease during the first 2 years of follow-up. Visual outcomes for these patients were similar between the placebo and intravenous methylprednisolone groups.

SYSTEMIC ASSOCIATIONS

Although inflammation of the optic nerve occurs in numerous systemic disorders as outlined above, acute demyelinating optic neuritis occurs most often in MS (among 50% of patients with MS) and frequently represents the first well-documented manifestation of MS (in 20% of patients with MS).[9,10,18,24] The most comprehensive information to date regarding the relation of acute demyelinating optic neuritis to MS has been provided by the ONTT. Follow-up of the ONTT cohort to 5 years and beyond has continued to demonstrate that brain MRI is the most powerful predictor of subsequent CDMS risk in monosymptomatic patients.[9,10] The presence of two or more white matter lesions was associated with a 51% risk of CDMS after 5 years, while the risk was 37% for those with 1 or 2 lesions, and only 16% if the MRI results were normal (excluding optic nerve enhancement).[9,10]

Monosymptomatic patients who have two or more brain white matter lesions seen with MRI therefore, are, considered to be at high risk for the development of CDMS following acute demyelinating optic neuritis. Among patients who have normal brain MRI findings (no white matter lesions) in the ONTT, lack of pain, presence of optic disc swelling, and mild visual acuity loss were features associated with a reduced risk of CDMS.

PATHOLOGY

Although the exact underlying cause is unknown, the pathophysiology of acute optic neuritis and MS is that of primary inflammatory demyelination.[16,17] Very little is written about the pathology of "isolated" optic neuritis, and no autopsy data has been reported. The inflammatory response in MS plaques is marked by perivascular cuffing, T cells, and plasma cells. Although MS, itself, previously was thought to be exclusively a disease of myelin with sparing of nerve axons, neuronal and axonal loss have been demonstrated to occur pathologically.[16]

TREATMENT

The ONTT has been the most comprehensive investigation to date regarding the treatment of acute demyelinating optic neuritis with corticosteroids, and it has had a significant impact on the practice patterns of both ophthalmologists and neurologists.[1-14] The ONTT enrolled 457 patients, aged 18 to 46 years, with acute unilateral optic neuritis. Follow-up data from the ONTT cohort (Longitudinal Optic Neuritis Study [LONS]) has been extensive and has provided important information regarding clinical features, long-term visual outcome, vision-specific health-related quality of life, and the role of brain MRI in determining risk for development of CDMS.

Patients in the ONTT were randomized to one of three treatment groups as follows:

* Oral prednisone (1mg/kg per day) for 14 days with 4-day taper (20mg on day 1, 10mg on days 2 and 4)
* Intravenous methylprednisolone (250mg every 6 hours for 3 days) followed by oral prednisone (1mg/kg per day) for 11 days with 4-day taper
* Oral placebo for 14 days[1]

Visual acuity and contrast sensitivity were primary visual outcome measures in the ONTT, while development of CDMS was a secondary end point. MRI scanning of the brain and orbits with gadolinium was performed for all patients.

Major findings of the ONTT may be summarized as follows: (1) intravenous methylprednisolone treatment hastened recovery of visual function but did not affect long-term visual outcome after 6 months to 5+ years compared with placebo or oral prednisone—this benefit for intravenous methylprednisolone was greatest within the first 15 days, (2) patients treated with oral prednisone alone (without intravenous methylprednisolone) unexpectedly demonstrated an increased risk of recurrent optic neuritis (30% after 2 years versus 16% for the placebo group and 13% for those receiving intravenous steroids) that has persisted throughout the 5+ year follow-up period,[8,10] and (3) monosymptomatic patients in the intravenous methylprednisolone group had a reduced rate of development of CDMS during the first 2 years of follow-up, but this benefit did not persist beyond 2 years and was seen only in patients with brain MRI scans that indicated a high risk for subsequent CDMS (MRI scans with two or more white matter lesions).[9,10]

Among patients at high risk for the development of CDMS as established by MRI criteria from the ONTT (two or more white matter lesions), a recent randomized trial of 383 patients (the Controlled High-Risk Avonex MS Prevention Study [CHAMPS]) demonstrated that treatment with interferon β-1a (Avonex) following acute monosymptomatic demyelinating optic neuritis or other first demyelinating event (including brainstem syndrome or incomplete transverse myelopathy) significantly reduced the

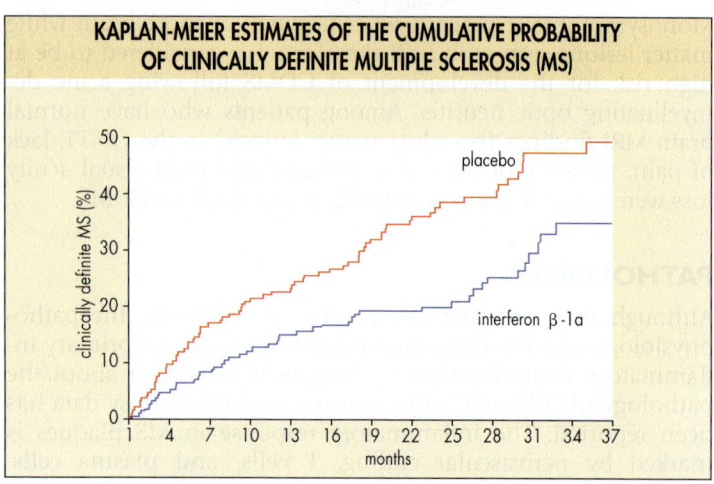

KAPLAN-MEIER ESTIMATES OF THE CUMULATIVE PROBABILITY OF CLINICALLY DEFINITE MULTIPLE SCLEROSIS (MS)

FIG. 190-3 ■ Kaplan-Meier estimates of the cumulative probability of clinically definite multiple sclerosis (MS) according to treatment group in the Controlled High-Risk Avonex MS Prevention Study (CHAMPS).[24] The cumulative probability of the development of clinically definite MS during the 3-year follow-up period was significantly lower in the interferon β-1a group than in the placebo group (P = 0.002 by the Mantel log-rank test). (From Jacobs LD, Beck RW, Simon JH, *et al.* Intramuscular interferon β-1a therapy initiated during a first demyelinating event in multiple sclerosis. N Engl J Med. 2000;343:898–904.)

3-year cumulative probability or CDMS versus placebo (rate ratio 0.56, P = 0.002, Kaplan-Meier analysis/Mantel log-rank test) (Fig. 190-3).[24] CHAMPS participants in the interferon β-1a group also had significantly reduced rates of accumulation of new but clinically silent lesions on brain MRI (P < 0.001 for both T2-enhancing and gadolinium-enhancing lesions after 18 months of follow-up). Results were similar in the subgroup of patients in CHAMPS who experienced optic neuritis as their first demyelinating event (192 patients), supporting the initiation of interferon β-1a in patients at high risk for CDMS by MRI criteria.[25] All patients in CHAMPS (interferon β-1a and placebo groups) also received a 3-day course of intravenous methylprednisolone followed by oral prednisone, as per the ONTT protocol (see above). Although the potential for long-term benefit of interferon β-1a in patients with acute monosymptomatic demyelinating optic neuritis (or other first demyelinating event) and high-risk brain MRI findings is not known, results from CHAMPS provide rationale for early therapy.

Early interferon therapy following a first demyelinating event is likewise supported by results of a randomized trial of interferon β-1a (Rebif) performed in Europe (Early Treatment of Multiple Sclerosis Study [ETOMS]).[26] Patients in ETOMS (n = 308) were randomized to receive interferon β-1a (Rebif) 22µg subcutaneously weekly or placebo; treatments were begun within 3 months following a first demyelinating event. During the 2-year follow-up period, a significantly lower proportion of patients developed CDMS in the interferon β-1a than in the placebo groups (52/154 [34%] versus 69/154 [45%], P = 0.047, chi-square test). Time to occurrence of a second demyelinating event (CDMS) in 30% of patients was also significantly shorter for the treatment group than the placebo group (569 days versus 252 days, hazard ratio 0.65, P = 0.023, Cox proportional hazards model). With respect to MRI parameters, patients in the interferon β-1a group had significantly fewer lesions on T2-weighted images (P <0.001, analysis of covariance).

Other Treatments

In experimental models of MS, intravenous immunoglobulin G (IVIG) has been shown to promote remyelination of the central nervous system.[27] A small pilot study in 1992 suggested that IVIG treatment may have some benefit in patients with resolved optic neuritis who have significant visual deficits.[28] However, a recent randomized trial of IVIG versus placebo in 55 patients with MS and persistent visual acuity loss (20/40 or worse) fol-

lowing optic neuritis did not demonstrate a significant benefit for recovery using visual acuity (logMAR units) as the primary outcome measure.[29]

Management Recommendations

In patients with a typical clinical course and examination findings for acute monosymptomatic demyelinating optic neuritis (first demyelinating event), MRI of the brain (T2-enhanced and gadolinium-enhanced images) should be performed to determine whether they are at high risk for the development of CDMS. Patients whose clinical course is atypical for acute demyelinating optic neuritis should also receive MRI of the orbits with gadolinium and fat saturation. The presence of two or more white matter lesions on MRI (3mm diameter or larger, at least one lesion periventricular or ovoid) should prompt consideration of one of the following treatments based on data from the ONTT, CHAMPS, and ETOMS[1–14,24–26]:

- Intravenous methylprednisolone (1g per day, single or divided doses, for 3 days) followed by oral prednisone (1mg/kg per day for 11 days, then 4-day taper)
- Interferon β-1a (Avonex 30µg intramuscularly once weekly) Rebif (22µg subcutaneously weekly)

In monosymptomatic patients who have fewer than two MRI white matter lesions, and in those for whom a diagnosis of CDMS has been established, intravenous methylprednisolone treatment (followed by oral prednisone as outlined) may be considered on an individual basis to hasten visual recovery, but this has not been demonstrated to improve long-term visual outcome. Based on findings from the ONTT, oral prednisone alone (without prior treatment with intravenous methylprednisolone) may increase the risk of recurrent optic neuritis and should be avoided.

COURSE AND OUTCOMES

At least some visual improvement is expected in all patients who have acute demyelinating optic neuritis. Visual improvement usually begins rapidly in patients treated with intravenous methylprednisolone. Even with no treatment, however, most patients start to recover vision within 2–3 weeks of symptom onset. Once recovery begins, most patients achieve near maximal improvement within 1–2 months, although recovery up to 1 year is possible. Severity of the initial visual loss appears to be the only predictor of visual outcome.[2]

Despite favorable recovery of vision, frequently to 20/20 or better, many patients with acute demyelinating optic neuritis continue to experience subtle visual abnormalities that affect their daily function and quality of life.[12–13] Persistent abnormalities of visual acuity (15–30%), contrast sensitivity (63–100%), color vision (33–100%), the visual field (62–100%), stereopsis (89%), light brightness sense (89–100%), afferent pupillary reaction (55–92%), optic disc appearance (60–80%), and the visual-evoked potential (63–100%) have been demonstrated in such patients. Recurrent episodes of optic neuritis in the initially affected or fellow eye may occur also; approximately 30% of ONTT participants had a second episode in either eye within the 5-year follow-up period.[8,9]

During and even beyond the recovery of vision following acute demyelinating optic neuritis, patients frequently experience transient worsening of symptoms with exposure to heat (Uhthoff's symptom).[30] Positive visual phenomena and photopsias are also common and were reported by 30% of ONTT participants.[1,3]

REFERENCES

1. Beck RW, Cleary PA, Anderson MA, *et al.* A randomized, controlled trial of corticosteroids in the treatment of acute optic neuritis. N Engl J Med. 1992; 326:581–8.
2. Beck RW, Cleary PA, Backlund JC, *et al.* The course of visual recovery after optic neuritis: experience of the Optic Neuritis Treatment Trial. Ophthalmology. 1994; 101:1771–8.

3. Optic Neuritis Study Group. The clinical profile of acute optic neuritis: experience of the Optic Neuritis Treatment Trial. Arch Ophthalmol. 1991;109:1673–8.
4. Arnold AC. Visual field defects in the Optic Neuritis Treatment Trial: central vs. peripheral, focal vs. global. Am J Ophthalmol. 1999;128:632–4.
5. Beck RW, Kupersmith MJ, Cleary PA, et al. Fellow eye abnormalities in acute unilateral optic neuritis: experience of the Optic Neuritis Treatment Trial. Ophthalmology. 1993;100:691–8.
6. Beck RW, Cleary PA. The Optic Neuritis Study Group: Optic Neuritis Treatment Trial: one-year follow-up results. Arch Ophthalmol. 1993;111:773–5.
7. Beck RW. The Optic Neuritis Treatment Trial: three-year follow-up results. Arch Ophthalmol. 1995;113:136–7.
8. Optic Neuritis Study Group. Visual function five years after optic neuritis: experience of the Optic Neuritis Treatment Trial. Arch Ophthalmol. 1997;115:1545–52.
9. Beck RW, Cleary PA, Trobe JD, et al. The effect of corticosteroids for acute optic neuritis on the subsequent development of multiple sclerosis. N Engl J Med. 1993;329:1764–9.
10. Optic Neuritis Study Group. The 5-year risk of multiple sclerosis after optic neuritis: experience of the Optic Neuritis Treatment Trial. Neurology. 1997;49:1404–13.
11. Beck RW, Arrington J, Murtagh FR, et al. Brain MRI in acute optic neuritis: experience of the Optic Neuritis Study Group. Arch Neurol. 1993;8:841–6.
12. Cleary PA, Beck RW, Bourque LB, et al. Visual symptoms after optic neuritis: results from the Optic Neuritis Treatment Trial. J Neuroophthalmol. 1997;17:18–28.
13. Cole SR, Beck RW, Moke PS, et al. The National Eye Institute Visual Function Questionnaire: experience of the ONTT. Invest Ophthalmol Vis Sci. 2000;41:1017–21.
14. Trobe JD, Sieving PC, Guire KE, et al. The impact of the Optic Neuritis Treatment Trial on the practices of ophthalmologists and neurologists. Ophthalmology. 1999;106:2047–53.
15. Rodriguez M, Siva A, Cross SA, et al. Optic neuritis: a population-based study in Olmsted County, Minnesota. Neurology. 1995;45:244–50.
16. Trapp BD, Peterson J, Ransohoff RM, et al. Axonal transection in the lesions of multiple sclerosis. N Engl J Med. 1998;338:278–85.
17. Ulrich J, Groebke-Lorenz W. The optic nerve in multiple sclerosis: a morphological study with retrospective clinico-pathological correlations. Neuro-ophthalmol. 1983;3:149–59.
18. Kurtzke JF. Optic neuritis or multiple sclerosis. Arch Neurol. 1985;42:704–10.
19. Swartz NG, Beck RW, Savino PJ, et al. Pain in anterior ischemic optic neuropathy. J Neuroophthalmol. 1995;15:9–10.
20. Balcer LJ, Winterkorn JMS, Galetta SL. Neuro-ophthalmic manifestations of Lyme disease. J Neuroophthalmol. 1997;17:108–21.
21. Lee AG, Tang RA, Roberts D, et al. Primary central nervous system lymphoma involving the optic chiasm in AIDS. J Neuroophthalmol. 2001;21:95–8.
22. Frohman LP, Frieman BJ, Wolansky L. Reversible blindness resulting from optic chiasmatis secondary to systemic lupus erythematosus. J Neuroophthalmol. 2001;21:18–21.
23. Kupersmith MJ, Burde RM, Warren FA, et al. Autoimmune optic neuropathy: evaluation and treatment. J Neurol Neurosurg Psychiatry. 1988;51:1381–6.
24. Jacobs LD, Beck RW, Simon JH, et al. Intramuscular interferon β-1a therapy initiated during a first demyelinating event in multiple sclerosis. N Engl J Med. 2000;343:898–904.
25. CHAMPS Study Group. Interferon β-1a for optic neuritis patients at high risk for multiple sclerosis. Am J Ophthalmol. 2001;132:463–71.
26. Rodriguez M, Lennon VA. Immunoglobulins promote remyelination in the central nervous system. Ann Neurol. 1990;27:12–7.
27. Comi G, Filippi M, Barkhof F, et al. Effect of early interferon treatment on conversion to definite multiple sclerosis: a randomized study. Lancet. 2001;357:1576–82.
28. van Engelen BG, Mommes OR, Pinckers A, et al. Improved vision after intravenous immunoglobulin in stable demyelinating optic neuritis [Letter]. Ann Neurol. 1992;32:834–5.
29. Noseworthy JH, O'Brien PC, Petterson TM, et al. A randomized trial of intravenous immunoglobulin in inflammatory demyelinating optic neuritis. Neurology. 2001;56:1514–22.
30. Scholl GB, Song HS, Wray SH. Uhthoff's symptom in optic neuritis: relationship to magnetic resonance imaging and development of multiple sclerosis. Ann Neurol. 1991;30:180–4.

191 Ischemic Optic Neuropathy, Diabetic Papillopathy, and Papillophlebitis

ANTHONY C. ARNOLD

DEFINITION
- Acute, painless optic neuropathy occurring predominantly in patients over 50 years of age.
- Additional acute pathologies of the optic disc may be associated with diabetes and venous congestion.

KEY FEATURES
- Optic disc edema, often pale or segmental (in anterior ischemic optic neuropathy).
- Dimming of vision, dyschromatopsia, afferent pupillary defect, and altitudinal or other optic disc–related visual field loss (in anterior ischemic optic neuropathy).
- Minimal optic nerve dysfunction (in diabetic papillopathy).
- Big blind spot with relatively normal optic nerve function (in papillophlebitis).

ASSOCIATED FEATURES
- Peripapillary flame hemorrhages.
- Peripapillary arteriolar narrowing.

ISCHEMIC OPTIC NEUROPATHIES

INTRODUCTION

Optic nerve ischemia most frequently occurs at the optic nerve head, where structural crowding of nerve fibers and reduction of the vascular supply may combine to impair perfusion to a critical degree. Such acute anterior ischemia produces optic disc edema. The most common such syndrome is termed *anterior ischemic optic neuropathy* (AION).[1] Generally, AION is categorized as either arteritic (associated with temporal arteritis) or nonarteritic (Table 191-1). A number of syndromes that share similar characteristics also may be ischemic in origin—diabetic papillopathy, hypertensive papillopathy, "AION of the young," preinfarct disc edema in nonarteritic AION, and migrainous optic neuropathy. Optic nerve ischemia affects the intraorbital portion of the nerve less frequently, with no visible disc edema, and has been termed posterior ischemic optic neuropathy. This rare syndrome has been reported most often in cases of vasculitis, including systemic lupus erythematosus and temporal arteritis, or anemia with hypotension, and is rare.

EPIDEMIOLOGY AND PATHOGENESIS

Nonarteritic anterior ischemic optic neuropathy (NAION) is the most common acute optic neuropathy in patients over 50 years of age, with an estimated annual incidence in the United States of 2.3–10.2 per 100,000 population,[2,3] some 6000–8000 new cases each year. No gender predisposition exists, but the disease occurs with significantly higher frequency in the white than in African-American or Hispanic populations.[2,4] The incidence of arteritic anterior ischemic optic neuropathy (AAION) is significantly lower (0.36 per 100,000 population annually in patients over 50 years of age[2]).

Arteritic Anterior Ischemic Optic Neuropathy

Ample evidence exists that AAION results from short posterior ciliary artery (SPCA) vasculitis and the resultant optic nerve head infarction. Human autopsy studies of acute AAION demonstrate optic disc edema with ischemic necrosis of the prelaminar, laminar, and retrolaminar portions of the nerve and infiltration of the SPCAs by chronic inflammatory cells. Segments of these vessels in some cases have been occluded by inflammatory thickening and thrombus.[5]

Fluorescein angiographic data support the histopathological evidence of involvement of the SPCAs in AAION. Delayed filling of the optic disc and choroid is a consistent feature. Hayreh[6] emphasized a correlation between the delay in filling of an affected segment of disc and the adjacent choroid and related it to a specific branch of the SPCA system. In addition, extremely poor or absent filling of the choroid has been depicted as a characteristic of AAION and has been suggested as one useful factor by which to differentiate AAION from NAION. Delayed completion of choroidal fluorescein filling that averages 30–69 seconds has been reported in AAION, compared with a mean of 5–13 seconds in NAION.[7,8]

Nonarteritic Anterior Ischemic Optic Neuropathy

The rapid onset, stable course with generally poor recovery, association with vasculopathic risk factors, and similarity to AAION have implied a vascular cause for NAION as well, but the direct evidence remains limited. Several histopathological reports document laminar and retrolaminar infarction, but cases of uncomplicated NAION are rare, and none has confirmed vasculopathy within the SPCAs or their distal branches. The most commonly proposed pathogenic theory states that insufficiency of the optic disc circulation, exacerbated by structural crowding of nerve fibers and supporting structures at the nerve head, eventually reaches a point at which inadequate oxygenation produces ischemia and swelling of the disc. These features may be mild and subclinical (no visual loss), reversible to some degree, or irreversible (infarction). In some cases, a cycle of ischemia, axonal swelling, microvascular compression, and further ischemia may lead to progressive nerve damage. Knox *et al.*[9] have recently documented cavernous degeneration within ischemic regions of the optic nerve head, with distortion of adjacent axons, theorizing that this process may be responsible for the progressive course in some cases. Periodic nocturnal systemic hypotension and the location of the optic disc in a watershed zone between distributions of lateral and medial SPCAs may be contributing factors.[10]

Fluorescein angiographic studies in NAION also suggest impaired optic disc perfusion. Detailed quantitative analysis of

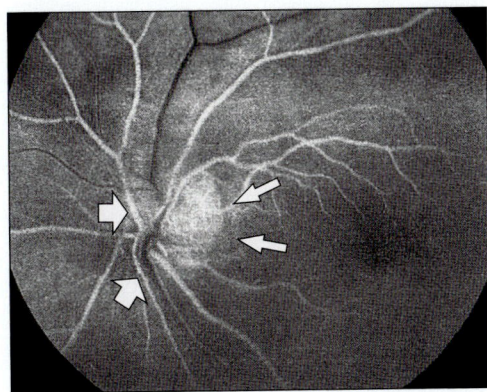

FIG. 191-1 ■ Fluorescein angiogram, early arteriovenous phase, in nonarteritic anterior ischemic optic neuropathy. The temporal portion of the optic disc fills normally (small arrows), but the remaining sectors demonstrate markedly delayed filling (large arrows) approximately 10 seconds later.

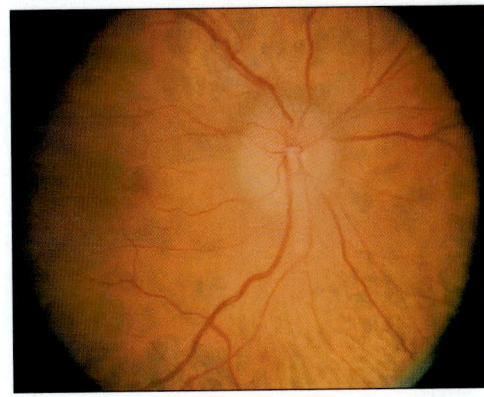

FIG. 191-2 ■ Fundus view, anterior ischemic optic neuropathy. The optic disc demonstrates pale, diffuse edema.

TABLE 191-1

COMPARISON OF MAJOR FEATURES OF ARTERITIC AND NONARTERITIC ANTERIOR ISCHEMIC OPTIC NEUROPATHY (AION)

Feature	Arteritic AION	Nonarteritic AION
Age (mean years)	70	60
Sex ratio	Female > male	Male = female
Associated symptoms	Headache, scalp tenderness, jaw claudication	Pain occasionally noted
Visual acuity	Up to 76% <20/200 (6/60)	Up to 61% >20/200 (6/60)
Disc	Pale > hyperemic edema	Hyperemic > pale edema
	Cup normal	Cup small
Mean erythrocyte sedimentation rate (mm/h)	70	20–40
Fluorescein angiogram	Disc and choroid filling delay	Disc filling delay
Natural history	Improvement rare	Improvement in up to 43%
	Fellow eye in up to 95%	Fellow eye in <30%
Treatment	Corticosteroids	None proved

prelaminar optic disc and peripapillary choroidal filling in NAION confirms significantly delayed disc filling when compared with age-matched controls.[11] Delay in a segment of disc (Fig. 191-1), by at least 5 seconds, was present in 75.6% of such cases.[11] In contrast, peripapillary choroidal filling was not delayed consistently and not significantly more than the degree of segmental delay often found in normal subjects. These findings suggest that the impaired flow to the optic nerve head in NAION is distal to the SPCAs themselves, possibly at the level of the paraoptic branches that supply the optic nerve head directly.

OCULAR MANIFESTATIONS

AION typically becomes apparent with the rapid onset of painless, unilateral visual loss manifested by decreased visual acuity, visual field, or both. The level of visual acuity impairment varies widely, from minimal loss to no light perception, and the visual field loss may conform to any pattern of deficit related to the optic disc. An altitudinal field defect is most common, but generalized depression, broad arcuate scotomas, and cecocentral defects also are seen. A relative afferent pupillary defect invariably is present with monocular optic neuropathy. The optic disc is edematous at onset, and edema occasionally precedes visual loss by weeks to months.[12] Although pallid edema has been described as the hallmark of AION (Fig. 191-2), it is common to see hyperemic swelling (Fig. 191-3), particularly in the nonarteritic form. The disc most often is swollen diffusely, but a segment of more prominent involvement frequently is present (see Fig. 191-3), and

either focal or diffuse surface telangiectasia is not unusual and may be quite pronounced. Commonly, flame hemorrhages are located adjacent to the disc, and the peripapillary retinal arterioles frequently are narrowed.

Arteritic Anterior Ischemic Optic Neuropathy

In 5–10% of cases, AION may occur as a manifestation of the vasculitis associated with temporal arteritis. Patients who have the arteritic form usually note other symptoms of the disease— headache (most common), jaw claudication, and temporal artery or scalp tenderness are those aligned most frequently with a final diagnosis of temporal arteritis. Malaise, anorexia, weight loss, fever, proximal joint arthralgia, and myalgia also are noted commonly; however, the disease occasionally manifests with visual loss in the absence of overt systemic symptoms, so-called *occult temporal arteritis.*

Typically, AAION is exhibited in elderly patients, with a mean age of 70 years, as severe visual loss (visual acuity <20/200 [6/60] in the majority). It may be preceded by transient visual loss similar to that of carotid artery disease; this finding is extremely unusual in the nonarteritic form and, when present, is highly suggestive of arteritis.[13,14] Pallor is associated with the edema of the optic disc more frequently in AAION than in the nonarteritic form. Choroidal ischemia may be associated with the optic neuropathy and produces peripapillary pallor and edema deep to the retina, or it may occur with no optic disc involvement. The disc of the fellow eye is of normal diameter most frequently, with a normal physiological cup (see NAION below).[15]

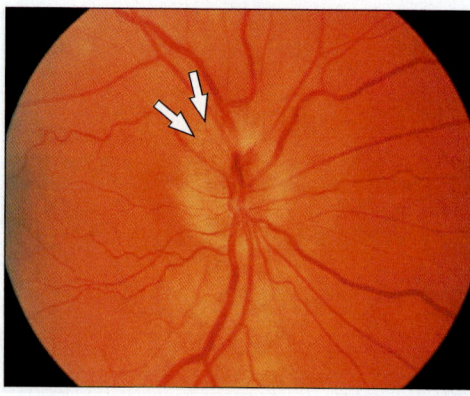

FIG. 191-3 ■ Fundus view, nonarteritic anterior ischemic optic neuropathy. The hyperemic disc edema is more prominent superiorly. Focal surface telangiectasia of disc vessels is seen superotemporally (arrows).

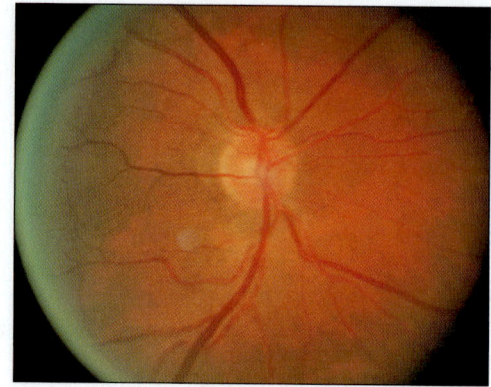

FIG. 191-4 ■ Fellow eye in nonarteritic anterior ischemic optic neuropathy. The optic disc is small in diameter, with absent physiological cup and slight blurring of the nasal margin.

Nonarteritic Anterior Ischemic Optic Neuropathy

In 90–95% of cases, AION is unrelated to temporal arteritis. The nonarteritic form of the disease occurs in a relatively younger age group (mean age of 60 years) and usually is associated with less severe visual loss. Frequently, visual impairment is reported upon awakening, possibly related to nocturnal systemic hypotension.[10] The initial course of visual loss may be static (with little or no fluctuation of visual level after the initial loss) or progressive (with either episodic or visual loss that declines steadily over weeks to months prior to eventual stabilization). The progressive form has been reported in 22%[16] to 37%[17] of NAION cases. Usually no associated systemic symptoms occur, although periorbital pain is described occasionally. Fellow eye involvement is estimated to occur in 12–19% by 5 years after onset.[18] Recurrent episodes of visual loss that result from NAION in the same eye are extremely rare and occur most often in young patients.

The optic disc edema in NAION may be diffuse or segmental, hyperemic or pale, but pallor occurs less frequently than it does in AAION. A focal region of more severe swelling often is seen and typically displays an altitudinal distribution, but it does not correlate consistently with the sector of visual field loss.[11] Diffuse or focal telangiectasia (see Fig. 191-3) of the edematous disc may be present, occasionally prominent enough to resemble a vascular mass or neovascularization. This finding may represent microvascular shunting from ischemic to nonischemic regions of the optic nerve head, so-called *luxury perfusion*. The optic disc in the contralateral eye typically is small in diameter and demonstrates a small or absent physiological cup.[15] The disc appearance in such fellow eyes (Fig. 191-4) has been described as the *disc at risk*, with postulated structural crowding of the axons at the level of the cribriform plate, associated mild disc elevation, and disc margin blurring without overt edema.

DIAGNOSIS AND ANCILLARY TESTING

The most important early step in the management of AION is the differentiation of the arteritic from the nonarteritic form of the disease. Measurement of the erythrocyte sedimentation rate (ESR) is standard. Active temporal arteritis usually is associated with an elevation of ESR to 70–120mm/h, and in acute AION that is associated with other typical features, this finding suggests the arteritic form; in most cases it should prompt immediate corticosteroid therapy and confirmatory temporal artery biopsy (see below). The test has significant limitations, however, with normal measurements found in an estimated 16% of biopsy-proved cases.[19] Conversely, abnormally high readings occur normally with increasing age and with other diseases, most commonly occult malignancy, other inflammatory disease, and diabetes. Measurement of serum C-reactive protein (CRP), another acute-phase plasma protein, may aid in diagnosis. Hayreh

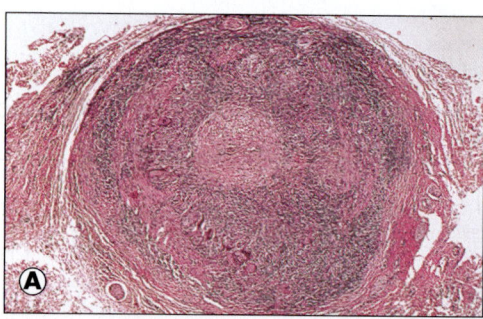

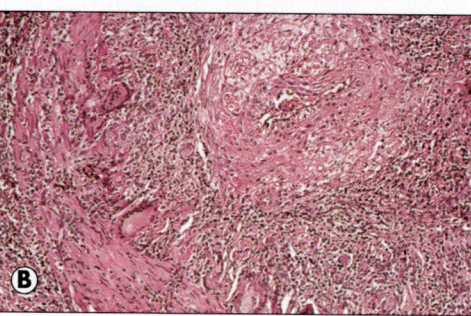

FIG. 191-5 ■ Typical temporal arteritis. A, Histological section shows a vasculitis involving all coats of the temporal artery. B, Increased magnification shows the typical giant cell–granulomatous inflammation. (A-B, courtesy of Dr. MM Rodrigues.)

et al.[20] reported 97% specificity for temporal arteritis in cases of AION in which both ESR >47mm/hr and CRP >2.45mg/dl were found.

Confirmation of the diagnosis of temporal arteritis by superficial temporal artery biopsy is recommended in any case of AION in which a clinical suspicion of arteritis exists based on age, associated systemic symptoms, severity of visual loss, and elevated ESR and CRP levels. Positive biopsy findings, such as intimal thickening, internal limiting lamina fragmentation, and chronic inflammatory infiltrate with giant cells, provides support for long-term systemic corticosteroid therapy (Fig. 191-5). A negative biopsy result, however, does not rule out arteritis; both discontinuous arterial involvement ("skip lesions") and solely contralateral temporal artery inflammation may result in false-negative results. In the face of negative initial biopsy, consideration is given to contralateral biopsy in cases with high clinical suspicion of temporal arteritis. Recent reports indicate a 3–5% false-negative error rate.[21]

DIFFERENTIAL DIAGNOSIS

The differential diagnosis of AION includes idiopathic optic neuritis, particularly in patients under 50 years of age; other forms of optic nerve inflammation, such as those related to syphilis or sarcoidosis; infiltrative optic neuropathies; anterior orbital lesions that produce optic nerve compression; and idiopathic forms of optic disc edema, which include diabetic papillopathy and papillophlebitis. Optic neuritis may resemble AION with regard to rate of onset, pattern of visual field loss, and optic disc appearance. In most cases, however, the patient's age, lack of pain with eye movement, and pallor or segmental configuration of the disc edema enable differentiation. Early disc filling delay on fluorescein angiography may confirm ischemia. Syphilitic or sarcoid-associated optic neuritis often is associated with other intraocular inflammatory signs, which should prompt further testing. Orbital lesions typically produce gradually progressive visual loss. Associated signs of orbital disease, such as mild exophthalmos, lid abnormalities, or eye movement limitation, may suggest the use of neuroimaging to detect anterior orbital inflammation or tumor. Diabetic papillopathy and papillophlebitis are discussed below.

SYSTEMIC ASSOCIATIONS

AAION is known to be a manifestation of temporal arteritis. NAION has been reported in association with a number of diseases that could predispose to reduced perfusion pressure or increased resistance to flow within the optic nerve head. Systemic hypertension has been documented in up to 47% of patients who have NAION[22] and diabetes in up to 24%.[22] Repka et al.[23] indicated that the prevalences of both hypertension and diabetes are increased over those of the control population in NAION patients in the age range 45–64 years, but that in patients over 64 years of age, no significant difference exists from those of the general population. Diabetics in particular show a predisposition to NAION at a young age.

Carotid occlusive disease, itself, does not appear to be associated directly with NAION in most cases. However, indirect evidence shows increased central nervous system, small vessel, ischemic disease in patients who have NAION, based on magnetic resonance imaging (MRI) data.[24] Early reports did not indicate that the incidence of prior or subsequent cerebrovascular or cardiovascular events is increased, but more recent studies indicate that they are both more common than in the normal population, particularly in patients who have hypertension or diabetes.[25] Subsequent mortality, however, is not affected.[25]

Also, NAION has been reported in association with multiple forms of vasculitis, acute systemic hypotension, migraine, optic disc drusen, and idiopathic vaso-occlusive diseases. Other risk factors, such as hyperopia, smoking, the presence of human lymphocyte antigen A29, and hyperlipidemia have been proposed. Recent reports of the association of hyperhomocystinemia with AION, particularly in patients under 50, are inconclusive.[26] Prothrombotic risk factors, such as protein C and S and antithrombin III deficiencies, factor V Leiden mutation, and cardiolipin antibodies, do not seem to be associated with AION.[27]

TREATMENT
Arteritic Anterior Ischemic Optic Neuropathy

Early treatment of AAION is essential and must be instituted immediately in any suspected case of temporal arteritis. High-dose systemic corticosteroids are standard; the use of intravenous methylprednisolone at 1g/day for the first 3 days has been recommended for AAION when the patient is in the acute phase of severe involvement, because this mode of therapy produces higher blood levels of medication more rapidly. Oral prednisone in the range of 60–100mg/day may be used initially and for follow-up to intravenous pulse therapy; alternate day regimens do not suppress the disease effectively. Treatment usually reduces systemic symptoms within several days. A positive response is so typical that if it does not occur, an alternate disease process should be considered.

Nonarteritic Anterior Ischemic Optic Neuropathy

There is no proven effective therapy for NAION. Oral corticosteroids at standard dosage (1mg/kg per day) are not beneficial, and megadose intravenous therapy has not been evaluated systematically. Optic nerve sheath decompression (ONSD) surgery has been attempted, based on the theory that reduction of perineural subarachnoid cerebrospinal fluid pressure might improve local vascular flow or axoplasmic transport in the optic nerve head, and thus reduce tissue injury in reversibly damaged axons. The Ischemic Optic Neuropathy Decompression Trial[4] compared ONSD surgery in 119 patients with no treatment in 125 controls. The study revealed no significant benefit for treatment and a possible, although not proven, harmful effect; it was recommended that ONSD not be performed for NAION. The 2-year follow-up study confirmed the lack of beneficial effect.[28] Hyperbaric oxygen, by marked elevation of the dissolved oxygen content in the blood, provides increased tissue oxygenation that might reduce damage in reversibly injured axons. A controlled clinical pilot study of hyperbaric oxygen in 22 patients who had acute NAION, however, has shown no beneficial effect.[29] Johnson et al.[30] reported a beneficial effect for oral levodopa on the visual outcome for NAION, but the study was controversial,[31] and the effect is considered unproved. Neuroprotective agents have shown a beneficial effect in animal models of optic nerve damage and are currently being studied in NAION. The effect of aspirin in reducing risk of fellow eye involvement is unclear.[32,33] Studies are emerging to test whether pentoxifylline may ameliorate the visual loss following NAION. There is a theoretical basis for assuming that it may increase blood flow in the region by rheological alterations.[34]

COURSE AND OUTCOME
Arteritic Anterior Ischemic Optic Neuropathy

The major goal of therapy in AAION is to prevent visual loss in the fellow eye. Untreated, such involvement occurs in 54–95% of cases,[35,36] typically within 4 months. With corticosteroid therapy, the rate of such breakthrough is reduced to an estimated 13%. Prognosis for visual recovery in the affected eye that has treatment generally is poor, but recent reports suggest a 15–34% improvement rate,[35,37] which is higher with intravenous than with oral therapy. Worsening of vision in spite of therapy has been reported in 9–17% of cases.[35,37]

Nonarteritic Anterior Ischemic Optic Neuropathy

The course of untreated NAION varies considerably. Reports indicate that 24–43% of cases demonstrate spontaneous improvement of visual acuity by three Snellen lines or more.[4,16] Improvement has been reported to occur in roughly 30% of this subgroup, as well. Whether NAION is static or progressive, visual acuity and field stabilize after several months. Within 6 weeks, occasionally sooner, the optic disc becomes visibly atrophic, either in a sectorial (Fig. 191-6) or diffuse pattern. Further progression or recurrent episodes are extremely rare after 2 months and, if present, should prompt evaluation for another cause of optic neuropathy.

LASIK

There are several reports suggesting an association between optic neuropathy and LASIK (laser in situ keratomileusis). The patients in these reports developed acute visual loss following LASIK and all had clinical evidence of optic neuropathy. Unfortunately, none of these patients could experience significant recovery and eventually all developed optic atrophy in the affected eye.

The reason for this association is unknown but may be related to the marked increase in intraocular pressure that occurs during a portion of the procedure.[38,39]

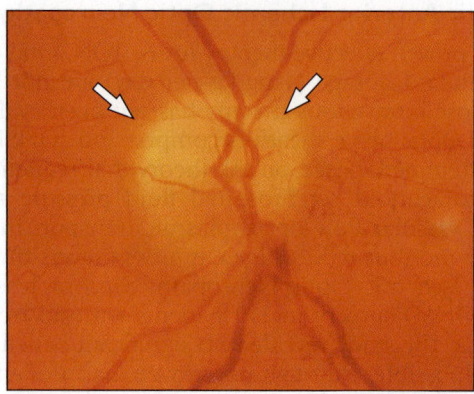

FIG. 191-6 ■ Optic disc, nonarteritic anterior ischemic optic neuropathy. The disc, 2 months after onset of inferior visual field loss, is segmentally atrophic superiorly (arrows), with sparing and resolving edema inferiorly.

POSTERIOR ISCHEMIC OPTIC NEUROPATHY

Posterior ischemic optic neuropathy is caused by infarction of the optic nerve posterior to the lamina cribrosa. This probably reflects a watershed-type infarct, because most patients have low hematocrit levels and hypotension.

The condition is usually of sudden onset with bilateral involvement, following massive bleeding with or without surgery.[40]

Several studies have investigated the risk factors that may predispose to this condition. Prolonged intraoperative hypotension, postoperative anemia, and facial swelling commonly were found.[40]

The incidence of posterior ischemic optic neuropathy might be reduced significantly by compensating for the contributory factors.

DIABETIC PAPILLOPATHY

PATHOGENESIS

The pathogenesis of diabetic papillopathy is unclear. Early investigators postulated either a toxic effect on the optic nerve secondary to abnormal glucose metabolism or a vascular disturbance of the inner disc surface, similar to that which produces retinal edema, with the resultant microvascular leakage into the disc. The most commonly proposed theory suggests diabetic papillopathy to be a mild form of NAION, with reversible ischemia of both the prelaminar and inner surface layers of the optic nerve head.[41] Edema of the optic nerve head in the absence of significant visual dysfunction and not secondary to elevated intracranial pressure occurs in several disorders as follows:

- Asymptomatic optic disc edema, which evolves to typical NAION weeks to months after initial symptoms[13]
- Asymptomatic disc edema of the fellow eye in patients who have NAION, which may either progress to NAION or resolve spontaneously
- Disc edema in association with systemic hypertension, which resolves without sequelae as blood pressure is normalized

Diabetic papillopathy fits this category, as well. The prominent surface telangiectasias may represent vascular shunting from prelaminar to ischemic vascular beds. The frequent occurrence of a crowded optic disc in the fellow eye (see below),[42] as in NAION, also supports an ischemic mechanism.

OCULAR MANIFESTATIONS

Early reports of diabetic papillopathy depicted the acute onset of unilateral or bilateral disc edema in young, type 1 diabetics, without the usual defects in visual field and pupillary function associated with NAION or optic neuritis[41,42]; a recent report included a substantial number of older patients with type 2 diabetes.[43]

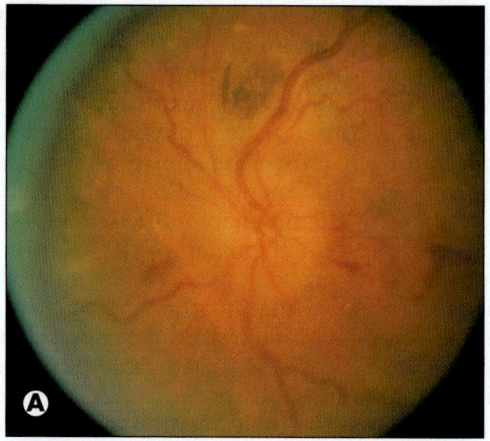

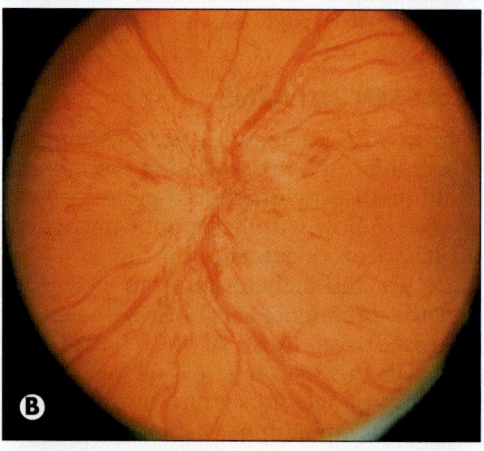

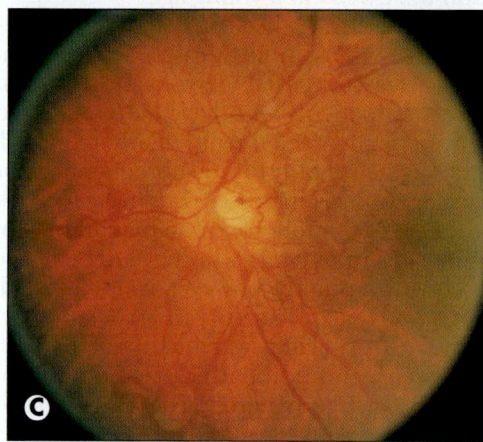

FIG. 191-7 ■ Optic disc in diabetic papillopathy. **A,** Nonspecific hyperemic disc edema. **B,** Surface vessels show marked telangiectasia, in which dilated vessels generally follow a radial distribution. **C,** Contrast with diabetic optic disc neovascularization; note the irregular, random branching pattern of surface vessels.

The currently accepted criteria for the diagnosis of diabetic papillopathy include:

- Presence of diabetes (approximately 70% type 1, 30% type 2)
- Optic disc edema (unilateral in roughly 60%)
- Only mild optic nerve dysfunction

To use visual acuity levels as criteria is difficult, because coexisting maculopathy is a common confounding feature, but over 75% of reported cases measured 20/40 (6/12) or better. The absence of ocular inflammation or elevated intracranial pressure also is essential to the diagnosis.

Although younger patients predominate (approximately 75% of those reported are under the age of 50 years), those affected may be of any age and typically experience either no visual complaints or vague, nonspecific visual disturbance, such as mild blurring or distortion; transient visual obscuration has been reported rarely. Pain is absent, as are other ocular or neurological symptoms.

The involved optic discs may demonstrate either nonspecific hyperemic edema or, in approximately 55% of cases, marked telangiectasia of the inner surface microvasculature (Figs. 191-7, A and B); pale swelling typically has been a criterion for exclusion and suggests AION. The surface telangiectasia is so prominent in many cases that it may be mistaken for neovascularization (Fig. 191-7, C).

True disc neovascularization occasionally is superimposed on the edema of diabetic papillopathy. The fellow eye frequently demonstrates crowding, with a small cup-to-disc ratio similar to the configuration seen in patients who have NAION.[43]

Diabetic retinopathy usually is present (in more than 80% of reported cases) at the time of onset of papillopathy, but it varies in severity. It is associated with cystoid macular edema in about 25% of cases and neovascularization in approximately 9%.

DIFFERENTIAL DIAGNOSIS

Conditions that may simulate diabetic papillopathy include papilledema (elevated intracranial pressure), hypertensive papillopathy, optic disc neovascularization, papillitis, NAION, and papillophlebitis. Symptoms of elevated intracranial pressure usually differentiate papilledema, and in bilateral cases with such symptoms, neuroimaging and lumbar puncture must be considered. Disc edema related to systemic hypertension typically does not demonstrate prominent telangiectasia and usually is associated with hypertensive retinopathy; blood pressure measurement is important in suspected cases. Papillitis and NAION both demonstrate significant optic nerve dysfunction, as evidenced by afferent pupillary defect and visual field loss. Papillophlebitis typically shows more prominent retinal venous congestion, peripheral retinal hemorrhages and, possibly, retinal vascular sheathing (see below).

COURSE AND OUTCOME

Although systemic corticosteroids have been used in isolated cases, no proven therapy exists for this disorder. Untreated, the optic disc edema gradually resolves over a period of 2–10 months, to leave minimal optic atrophy in about 20% of cases and subtle, if any, visual field loss. Visual acuity at the time of resolution of edema is 20/40 (6/12) or better in about 80% of cases; the remainder of patients suffer visual impairment because of maculopathy. The long-term visual prognosis for patients who have diabetic papillopathy, however, is limited by the associated diabetic retinopathy. Proliferative changes, with attendant complications, develop in approximately 25% of cases.

PAPILLOPHLEBITIS

A syndrome of unilateral retinal venous congestion and optic disc edema in healthy young patients was originally termed *papillophlebitis* by Lonn and Hoyt in 1966.[44] Similar clinical entities have been described as *optic disc vasculitis*,[45] *benign retinal vasculitis, mild retinal and papillary vasculitis,* and *big blind-spot syndrome.* The syndrome is a subset of central retinal vein occlusion in the young,[46] in which the disc edema and the retinal venous distention are unusually prominent. Investigators have suggested that it results from central retinal vein inflammation at the disc, with secondary venous occlusion and disc edema. To date, however, histopathological studies have been limited to severe, atypical cases of retinal vasculitis, and proof of phlebitis in this syndrome is not available.

The disorder typically manifests with mild symptoms of unilateral visual blurring, photopsia, or transient visual obscuration, without headache, ocular pain, or other complaints. Visual acuity typically is normal or is diminished mildly on the basis of macular hemorrhage or edema. An afferent pupillary defect is absent, color vision is normal, and visual field testing

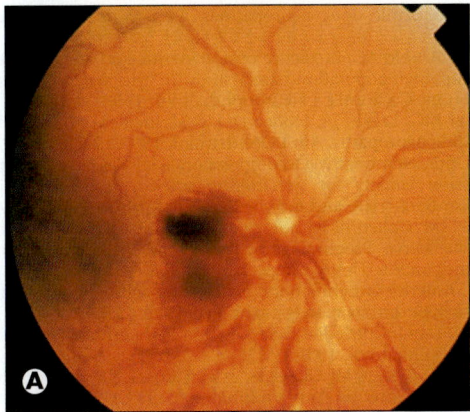

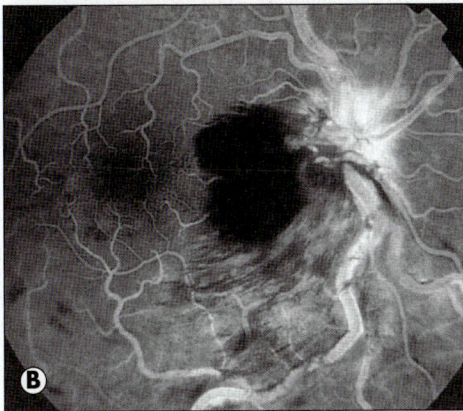

FIG. 191-8 ■ Papillophlebitis. A, Fundus view, which shows marked venous congestion, moderate optic disc edema, and retinal hemorrhages. B, Fluorescein angiography, which illustrates disc leakage associated with retinal venous dilation, filling delay, and staining.

shows enlargement of the physiological blind spot. Minimal additional field abnormality may be present because of retinal involvement. Fundus examination demonstrates marked retinal venous engorgement in association with hyperemic optic disc edema (Fig. 191-8, A). Retinal hemorrhages that extend to the equatorial region are present in many cases, but additional signs of inflammation or ischemia, such as retinal periphlebitis or capillary nonperfusion, are noted only infrequently. Occasionally, a cilioretinal artery obstruction will be present concurrently.

The differential diagnosis of papillophlebitis includes unilateral papilledema, papillitis and optic perineuritis, orbital compressive lesions, diabetic papillopathy, and arteriosclerotic central retinal vein occlusion. The prominent retinal venous distention, involvement of the peripheral retina with hemorrhages, and the lack of symptoms of elevated intracranial pressure, evidence of optic neuropathy or orbitopathy, and the presence of systemic diseases such as diabetes and hypertension all aid in differentiation.

Fluorescein angiography typically demonstrates marked retinal venous dilation,[45] staining, and leakage, in association with circulatory slowing (Fig. 191-8, B); the regions of capillary occlusion seen with diabetic retinopathy and ischemic central retinal vein occlusion are demonstrated only rarely. Late staining and leakage from the disc is common but nonspecific.

On the basis of the presumed inflammatory process, glucocorticoids, both systemic and injected locally, have been used in many of the reported cases. Their value is unproved, however, because the disease tends to follow a benign course if untreated. Retinal and optic disc changes resolve after 6–18 months, usually with no significant sequelae; persistent visual loss is unusual. Retinal venous sheathing and opticociliary collateral vessels are not uncommon on late follow-up examinations, but neovascularization rarely occurs.

REFERENCES

1. Arnold AC. Ischemic optic neuropathies. Ophthalmol Clin North Am. 2001; 14:83–98.

2. Johnson LN, Arnold AC. Incidence of nonarteritic and arteritic anterior ischemic optic neuropathy: population-based study in the state of Missouri and Los Angeles County, California. J Neuroophthalmol. 1994;14:38–44.

3. Hattenhauer MG, Leavitt JA, Hodge DO, et al. Incidence of nonarteritic anterior ischemic optic neuropathy. Am J Ophthalmol. 1997;123:103–7.

4. Ischemic Optic Neuropathy Decompression Trial Research Group. Optic nerve decompression surgery for nonarteritic anterior ischemic optic neuropathy (NAION) is not effective and may be harmful. JAMA. 1995;273:625–32.

5. MacMichael IM, Cullen JF. Pathology of ischaemic optic neuropathy. In: Cant JS, ed. The optic nerve. Proceedings of the Second William MacKenzie Memorial Symposium. London: Henry Kimpton; 1972:108–16.

6. Hayreh SS. Anterior ischemic optic neuropathy. Differentiation of arteritic from non-arteritic type and its management. Eye. 1990;4:25–41.

7. Mack HG, O'Day J, Currie JN. Delayed choroidal perfusion in giant cell arteritis. J Clin Neuroophthalmol. 1991;11:221–7.

8. Siatkowski RM, Gass JDM, Glaser JS, et al. Fluorescein angiography in the diagnosis of giant cell arteritis. Am J Ophthalmol. 1993;115:57–63.

9. Knox DL, Kerrison JB, Green WR. Histopathologic studies of ischemic optic neuropathy. Trans Am Ophthalmol Soc. 2000;98:203–22.

10. Hayreh SS, Zimmerman BM, Podhajsky PA, Alward WLM. Nocturnal arterial hypotension and its role in optic nerve head and ocular ischemic disorders. Am J Ophthalmol. 1994;117:603–24.

11. Arnold AC, Hepler RS. Fluorescein angiography in acute anterior ischemic optic neuropathy. Am J Ophthalmol. 1994;117:222–30.

12. Arnold AC, Badr M, Hepler RS. Fluorescein angiography in nonischemic optic disk edema. Arch Ophthalmol. 1996;114:293–8.

13. Hayreh SS. Anterior ischemic optic neuropathy. V. Optic disk edema an early sign. Arch Ophthalmol. 1981;99:1030–40.

14. Hayreh SS, Podhajsky PA, Zimmerman P. Ocular manifestations of giant cell arteritis. Am J Ophthalmol. 1998;125:509–20.

15. Beck RW, Servais GE, Hayreh SS. Anterior ischemic optic neuropathy. IX. Cup-to-disc ratio and its role in pathogenesis. Ophthalmology. 1987;94:1503–8.

16. Arnold AC, Hepler RS. Natural history of nonarteritic anterior ischemic optic neuropathy. J Neuroophthalmol. 1994;14:66–9.

17. Yee RD, Selky AK, Purvin VA. Outcomes of optic nerve sheath decompression for nonarteritic ischemic optic neuropathy. J Neuroophthalmol. 1994;14:70–6.

18. Beck RW, Hayreh SS, Podhajsky PA, et al. Aspirin therapy in nonarteritic anterior ischemic optic neuropathy. Am J Ophthalmol. 1997;123:212–7.

19. Keltner JL. Giant cell arteritis. Signs and symptoms. Ophthalmology. 1982; 89:1101–10.

20. Hayreh SS, Podhajsky PA, Raman R, et al. Giant cell arteritis: validity and reliability of various diagnostic criteria. Am J Ophthalmol. 1997;123:285–96.

21. Boyev LR, Miller NR, Gree WR. Efficacy of unilateral versus bilateral temporal artery biopsies for the diagnosis of giant cell arteritis. Am J Ophthalmol. 1999;128:211–5.

22. Ischemic Optic Neuropathy Decompression Trial Research Group. Characteristics of patients with nonarteritic anterior ischemic optic neuropathy eligible for the Ischemic Optic Neuropathy Decompression Trial. Arch Ophthalmol. 1996; 114:1366–74.

23. Repka MX, Savino PJ, Schatz NJ, Sergott RC. Clinical profile and long-term implications of anterior ischemic optic neuropathy. Am J Ophthalmol. 1983;96:478–83.

24. Arnold AC, Hepler RS, Hamilton DR, Lufkin RB. Magnetic resonance imaging of the brain in nonarteritic anterior ischemic optic neuropathy. J Neuroophthalmol. 1995;15:158–60.

25. Hayreh SS, Joos KM, Podhajsky PA, Long CR. Systemic diseases associated with nonarteritic anterior ischemic optic neuropathy. Am J Ophthalmol. 1994; 118:766–80.

26. Pianka P, Almog Y, Man O, et al. Hyperhomocystinemia in patients with nonarteritic anterior ischemic optic neuropathy, central retinal artery occlusion, and central retinal vein occlusion. Ophthalmology. 2000;107:1588–92.

27. Salomon O, Huna-Baron R, Kurtz S, et al. Analysis of prothrombotic and vascular risk factors in patients with nonarteritic anterior ischemic optic neuropathy. Ophthalmology 1999;106:739–42.

28. Ischemic Optic Neuropathy Decompression Trial Research Group. Ischemic Optic Neuropathy Decompression Trial. Twenty-four month update. Arch Ophthalmol. 2000;118:793–8.

29. Arnold AC, Hepler RS, Lieber M, Alexander JM. Hyperbaric oxygen therapy for nonarteritic anterior ischemic optic neuropathy. Am J Ophthalmol. 1996;122: 535–41.

30. Johnson LN, Guy ME, Krohel GB, et al. Levodopa may improve visual loss in recent-onset nonarteritic anterior ischemic optic neuropathy. Ophthalmology. 2000;107:521–6.

31. Beck RW, Ferris FL. Does levodopa improve visual function in NAION? Ophthalmology. 2000;107:1431–4.

32. Salomon O, Huna-Baron R, Steinberg DM, et al. Role of aspirin in reducing the frequency of second eye involvement in patients with nonarteritic anterior ischemic optic neuropathy. Eye. 1999;13:357–9.

33. Beck RW, Hayreh SS. Role of aspirin in reducing the frequency of second eye involvement in patients with nonarteritic anterior ischemic optic neuropathy [Letter]. Eye. 2000;14:118.

34. Sebag J, Tang M, Brown S, et al. Effects of pentoxifylline on choroidal blood flow in nonproliferative diabetic retinopathy. Angiology. 1994;45:429–33.

35. Liu GT, Glaser JS, Schatz NJ, Smith JL. Visual morbidity in giant cell arteritis. Ophthalmology. 1994;101:1779–85.

36. Beri M, Klugman MR, Kohler JA, Hayreh SS. Anterior ischemic optic neuropathy. VII. Incidence of bilaterality and various influencing factors. Ophthalmology. 1987;94:1020–8.

37. Aiello PD, Trautmann JC, McPhee TJ, et al. Visual prognosis in giant cell arteritis. Ophthalmology. 1993;100:550–5.

38. Lee AG, Kohnen T, Ebner R, et al. Optic neuropathy associated with laser in situ keratomileusis. J Cataract Refract Surg. 2000;26(11):1581–4.

39. Luna JD, Artal N, Reviglio VE, Juarez CP. LASIK-induced optic neuropathy. Ophthalmology. 2002;109(5):817–8.

40. Dunker S, Hsu HY, Sebag J, Sadun AA. Perioperative risk factors for posterior ischemic optic neuropathy. J Am Coll Surg. 2002;194:705–10.

41. Hayreh SS, Zahoruk RM. Anterior ischemic optic neuropathy. VI. In juvenile diabetics. Ophthalmologica. 1981;182:13–28.

42. Barr CC, Glaser JS, Blankenship G. Acute disc swelling in juvenile diabetes. Clinical profile and natural history of 12 cases. Arch Ophthalmol. 1980; 98:2185–92.

43. Regillo CD, Brown GC, Savino PJ, et al. Diabetic papillopathy. Patient characteristics and fundus findings. Arch Ophthalmol. 1995;113:889–95.

44. Lonn LI, Hoyt WF. Papillophlebitis: a cause of protracted yet benign optic disc edema. Eye Ear Nose Throat Mon. 1966;45:62–8.

45. Hayreh SS. Optic disc vasculitis. Br J Ophthalmol. 1972;56:652–70.

46. Fong ACO, Schatz H. Central retinal vein occlusion in young adults. Surv Ophthalmol. 1993;37:393–417.

Hereditary, Nutritional, and Toxic Optic Atrophies

ALFREDO A. SADUN • SEVGI GURKAN

DEFINITION

- Leber's hereditary optic neuropathy, which arises from an inherited point mutation in mitochondrial DNA, manifests in young adulthood as a distinctive heredodegenerative optic neuropathy.
- Nutritional deficiency states, particularly those that involve the vitamins (e.g., B_{12} or folic acid) and amino acids used in mitochondrial metabolism (e.g., homocysteine or methionine), can result in a stereotypical optic neuropathy, probably by affecting mitochondria on an acquired basis.
- Certain toxins, possibly through interference with mitochondrial metabolism on an acquired basis (e.g., cyanide), may cause a very similar optic neuropathy.

KEY FEATURES

- Fairly symmetrical visual impairments.
- Loss of central visual acuity.
- Dyschromatopsia.
- Centrocecal visual field defects.
- Temporal optic disc pallor.
- Nerve fiber layer loss in the papillomacular bundle.

ASSOCIATED FEATURES

- Loss of hearing.
- Peripheral neuropathy.

INTRODUCTION

Leber's hereditary optic neuropathy (LHON) first was described in 1871 as a disease that produced a subacute onset of dyschromatopsia and bilateral loss of visual acuity, primarily in young men. It was thought originally to be inherited as X-linked with partial penetrance.[1] However, in 1988 Wallace and co-workers[2] described the genetics as a point mutation in the mitochondrial DNA (and hence involves maternal inheritance). Three commonly reported point mutations are involved in the pathogenesis of LHON, all three of which affect complex I of the respiratory chain, and the biochemical defect they induce is still under investigation. Both an impairment of energy production and a chronic increase of reactive oxygen species are the potential consequences of the underlying pathogenic mutations leading to optic nerve degeneration.[3,4] The fundus examination is unusual, because there are characteristic changes in the optic disc and loss of the papillomacular nerve fiber layer.

The peculiar term *tobacco–alcohol amblyopia* refers to one of the most frequently considered toxic or nutritional deficiencies. Traquair[5] emphasized that heavy drinking and smoking could lead to a slow, progressive, bilateral visual field loss. Tobacco–alcohol amblyopia is now thought to result from the relative roles of cyanide from tobacco and low levels of B_{12}, brought about by poor nutrition and poor absorption associated with al-cohol consumption.[6] Deficiencies of B_{12}, other B vitamins and, in particular, folic acid are known to result in a similar clinical picture.[7] Furthermore, a number of toxins, such as ethambutol or methanol, injure the optic nerve and produce a clinical picture that is difficult or impossible to differentiate. Indeed, it is one of the fundamental curiosities of these disorders that they, along with LHON, all have such similar and characteristic clinical manifestations.[8] In considering toxic agents that are best known to cause optic neuropathy, it is remarkable that most are known to interfere with oxidative phosphorylation.[9]

EPIDEMIOLOGY AND PATHOGENESIS

It is said that LHON has a prevalence rate as high as 2% of legally blind individuals in Australia and New Zealand.[10] The age of onset is typically in the late twenties, often at a critical stage in the patient's domestic and professional life. For almost all pedigrees, men are more likely to demonstrate clinical symptoms than women; however, this ratio varies considerably from country to country.[11,11a]

It cannot be overemphasized that the papillomacular bundle is the main site of the problem, and it eventually becomes atrophic. The pathophysiology of this injury to the papillomacular bundle probably begins with impairments in mitochondria that involve oxidative phosphorylation. The resultant decrease in adenosine 5′-triphosphate (ATP) may compromise axonal transport which, paradoxically, is highly energy dependent.[12,13] Hence mitochondria, which arise solely in the soma and have a lifespan of only 7–14 days, may not make it to the distal terminals if the efficiency of transport is compromised due to energy depletion. This situation would be particularly problematic in long fibers, such as those of the peripheral nervous system, or in axons of very narrow caliber, those with minimal or no myelin, and those with a rapid rate of firing. These three latter features are all found in retinal ganglion cells of the papillomacular bundle.[9]

Toxic and nutritional deficiency optic neuropathies are fairly uncommon causes of optic neuropathy in the United States and Western Europe. However, a recent epidemic of optic and peripheral neuropathy in Cuba serves to remind that these types of optic neuropathies may be far more common in the third world than is supposed generally.[14] This family of diseases may be relegated to the background until such times as famine, new application of pharmaceuticals, or changes in the workplace lead to nutritional deficiencies or toxic exposures, which in turn lead to the re-emergence of these diseases.

In terms of deficiencies that result in toxic optic neuropathies, probably the most crucial nutrients are vitamins, particularly vitamin B_{12} (cobalamin), vitamin B_1 (thiamin), vitamin B_2 (riboflavin), and folic acid. Proteins, in particular those that contain the sulfur amino acids, are probably also crucial for efficient mitochondrial oxidative phosphorylation. Toxins established most clearly as producers of an optic neuropathy include ar-sacetin, carbon monoxide, clioquinol, cyanide, ethambutol, hexachlorophene, isoniazid, lead, methanol, plasmocid, and tri-ethyl tin.[15] These agents interfere with mitochondrial oxidative phosphorylation.[16–19] Certain factors, such as impaired renal function in patients on ethambutol, may increase the risk and severity of the toxic optic neuropathy.

A number of important agents also exist that are less clearly toxic to the optic nerve, such as carbon disulfide, chloramphenicol, pheniprazine, quinine, and thallium. A large number of other toxins, such as carbon tetrachloride, cassava, dapsone, and suramin, are suspected, but not proven, as causes of optic neuropathy.[15]

The clinical picture found in a large number of different toxic optic neuropathies is essentially the same. Furthermore, the central visual loss associated with dyschromatopsia, the centrocecal scotomas, and the selective loss of the papillomacular bundle that characterize most toxic optic neuropathies are also common to nutritional deficiencies such as single or mixed vitamin deficiencies of B_{12}, B_2, or folic acid. These findings also have been found in malnourished prisoners of war, frequently with an associated peripheral neuropathy.[20]

It may seem peculiar that so many nutritional deficiency and toxic optic neuropathies produce very similar clinical pictures, yet there are common pathways by which these vitamins work and by which many of these toxins interact. Oxidative phosphorylation within the mitochondria involves the process of electron transfer to oxygen at one end and the production of ATP at the other end. Vitamins such as B_{12} and folic acid are crucial to this process and deficiency therein results in decreased ATP. Similarly, agents such as cyanide or formate (a metabolic product of methanol) block this electron transport. The final common product of these deficiencies and toxins is decreased ATP production by mitochondria within all of the cells of the body and likely the accumulation of reactive oxygen species (ROS).[20a] Compensatory mechanisms may permit most cells in the body, such as muscle cells, to deal with decreased mitochondrial deficiency perhaps via the production of more mitochondria.[21] However, neurons with axons that are very long, very thin, or unmyelinated (such as the papillomacular nerve fiber bundle) are at a great disadvantage.

OCULAR MANIFESTATIONS

LHON typically begins with the sudden onset of painless monocular visual loss, which the patient may describe as a blurring of vision but more often as a central dark or gray cloud. This develops first in one eye and then, soon after (days to several weeks), it occurs in similar fashion in the fellow eye. In contradistinction, most patients who have either toxic or nutritional optic neuropathy experience slowly progressive bilateral loss of central vision. Described below are the ocular manifestations that, on the whole, are quite similar for all three syndromes (LHON, nutritional, and toxic optic neuropathies).

The patient initially may describe an inability to read, see traffic signs, or details in the faces of acquaintances. Patients do not complain of pain or positive visual phenomena, such as photopsias.

On examination, patients generally have bilateral impairments of visual acuity that vary from minimal losses (20/25 [6/7.5]) to hand motion vision (for LHON the usual range is 20/100 [6/30]) to finger counting. The visual acuity loss in the two eyes is usually quite symmetrical. Loss of vision to the light perception or no light perception levels is extremely rare. Loss of color vision is usually more profound than the loss of visual acuity. Very early cases may exhibit isolated dyschromatopsia. The hallmark of this disorder is the visual field defect that consists of a centrocecal scotoma that begins nasal to the blind spot and extends to involve fixation on both sides of the vertical meridian (Fig. 192-1). There is usually an area of relative scotoma that forms a bridge between the two islands of absolute scotoma at fixation and at the blind spot. Often a complete loss of the perception of red occurs, and color perimetry demonstrates a much larger elliptical centrocecal scotoma than found with white light. Pupillary reactions are usually normal, even in the early monocular stages of LHON. There are histopathological findings of a relative preservation of the retinotectal pathway in LHON.[22]

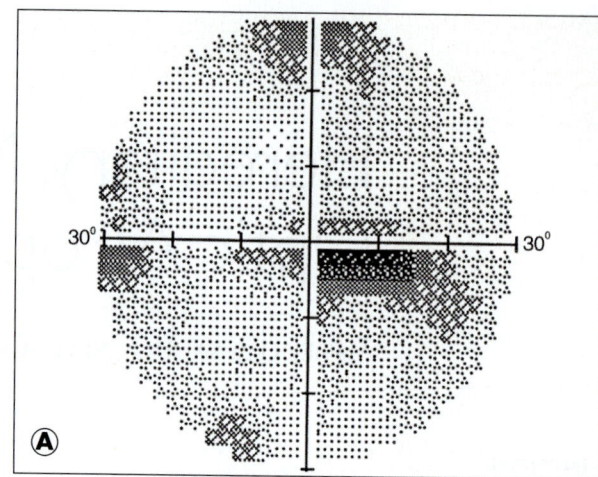

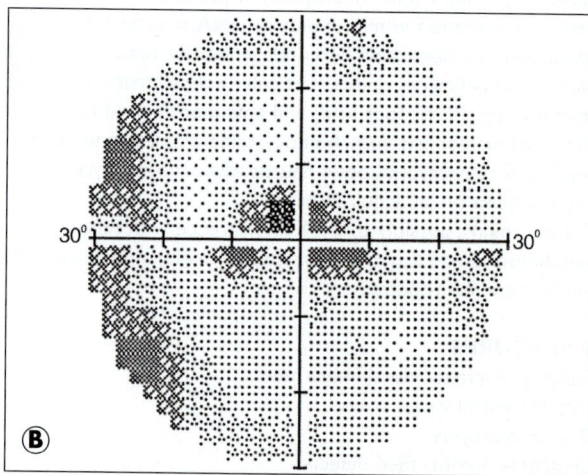

FIG. 192-1 ■ Humphrey visual field strategies 30–2. A large stimulus V was used. A, Note the centrocecal scotoma that bridges fixation to the blind spot of the right eye. B, In the left eye, the scotoma seems a little more centralized around fixation. It is notable that this patient, who had tobacco–alcohol amblyopia (mixed toxic and nutritional deficiency optic neuropathy), also had relatively small central scotomas but visual acuities of 20/400 (6/120) in each eye.

In early LHON, a peripapillary microangiopathy may occur.[11] Telangiectatic or tortuous blood vessels may be seen around the optic disc, but this occurs transiently and often is missed until involvement of the second eye becomes apparent. In nutritional deficiencies and toxic optic neuropathies, the fundus may appear normal initially. However, a careful examination may reveal nerve fiber layer losses in the papillomacular bundle, sometimes associated with swelling of the nerve fiber layer in the arcuate bundles above and below the denuded area.[23] Later in the course of the disease, the temporal optic disc often appears mildly pale (Fig. 192-2). The mismatch between relatively mild temporal disc pallor and severe depression of visual acuity, visual field, and color vision may lead to the misconception that the patient is malingering.

DIAGNOSIS AND ANCILLARY TESTING

A carefully history usually provides enough information to make a presumptive diagnosis of LHON. The patient describes the subacute, painless loss of vision monocularly, possibly followed soon after by involvement of the fellow eye. This slight temporal asymmetry and the family history help to differentiate LHON from nutritional deficiencies and toxic optic neuropathies. Most often, LHON manifests in men in their late teens or early twenties. It can be differentiated from toxic and nutritional optic neuropathies by:

- Family history
- Presence of telangiectatic vessels around the optic nerve head during the acute phase

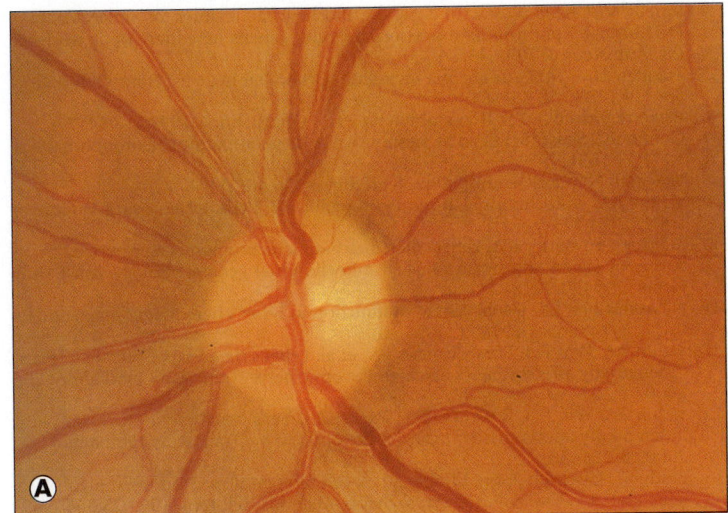

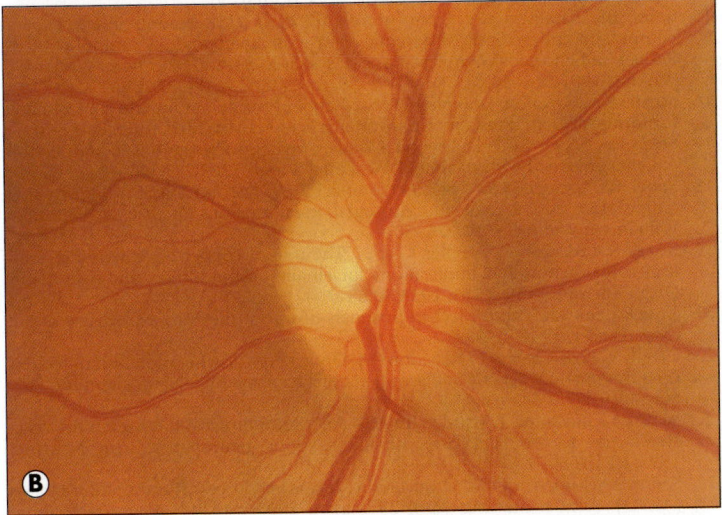

FIG. 192-2 ■ **Fundus views reveal mild temporal optic disc pallor. A,** Right optic disc. **B,** Left optic disc. More interesting, however, is the loss of the nerve fiber layer in the papillomacular bundle. This patient, who had tobacco–alcohol amblyopia (mixed toxic and nutritional deficiency optic neuropathy), also had visual acuities of 20/400 (6/120) in each eye, which recovered to only 20/100 (6/30) after changes in habit and diet, and vitamin therapy. In this class of optic neuropathies, relatively severely compromised visual acuities and dyschromatopsia often are found with minimal optic disc atrophy.

- Likelihood that one eye is affected before the other (not simultaneous occurrence)
- Confirmation by laboratory study of the point mitochondrial DNA mutation

The history is particularly helpful to differentiate LHON from toxic and nutritional optic neuropathies. Care must be taken to explore all possible oddities in terms of diet and exposures, with an emphasis on particulars that have changed recently. Suspected toxicities can be confirmed through serum and urine analysis. In particular, 24-hour urine collection for heavy metal screening may yield unexpected results. In addition to serum vitamin levels for B_1, B_2, B_{12}, and folic acid, it is often useful to obtain serum pyruvate levels as well.

DIFFERENTIAL DIAGNOSIS

The differential diagnosis for toxic and nutritional optic neuropathies includes disorders that cause acute and subacute symmetrical losses in visual acuity and color vision. The similarity between LHON and nutritional deficiency and toxic optic neuropathies has been addressed.

Kjer's autosomal dominant optic atrophy is confused less often with toxic and nutritional optic neuropathies. An autosomal dominant family history often occurs, and the optic neuropathy occurs much more slowly and progressively in late childhood.

Although less commonly confused with toxic and nutritional optic neuropathies, chiasmal syndromes sometimes need to be ruled out. Pituitary adenomas or other lesions that impact on the optic chiasm generally present with bitemporal visual field loss, but without any significant loss of central acuity or color vision. However, in the early stages, bitemporal field losses may appear similar to centrocecal scotomas. It sometimes may be confusing as to whether the visual field defect crosses the vertical meridian. Fortunately, chiasmal syndromes nearly always result from mass lesions that are visualized easily on standard imaging studies.

Occasionally, optic neuritis may occur bilaterally. Because there can be almost any type of visual field defect in optic neuritis, the clinical picture of bilateral optic neuritis may appear like that of toxic and nutritional optic neuropathies. If the patient has multiple sclerosis, a number of plaques may be picked up on magnetic resonance imaging; furthermore, most patients who have optic neuritis show dramatic recovery of visual acuity.

A recent area of controversy pertains to the possibility that amiodarone may cause an optic neuropathy. Amiodarone, a benzofuran derivative with vasodilatory and antiarrhythmic properties, is used for treating supraventricular and ventricular cardiac arrhythmias.[24] Although it is a potent antiarrhythmic, numerous side effects, ranging from mild to life threatening, have been described.[25] Among the mild side effects, corneal microdeposits are very common. This can even be used to ascertain the therapeutic dosage of the therapy. The keratopathy usually does not cause any serious visual disturbance, but occasionally the patients may complain about flares, halos, and mild photosensitivity[26] (Chapter 36). Dermatitis and gastrointestinal disturbances are among the other few mild side effects, whereas hypothyroidism and hyperthyroidism, peripheral neuropathy, ataxia, bone marrow depression, and pulmonary toxicity are several of the more severe side effects that are attributed to use of amiodarone.[24,25,27,28]

Some reports suggest that patients on amiodarone therapy may also be at risk for developing an amiodarone-induced optic neuropathy which is hard to distinguish from nonarteritic anterior ischemic optic neuropathy (AION). The most compelling evidence for the existence of amiodarone-induced AION is the increased incidence of AION among patients receiving amiodarone therapy (1.79%[29]). This is much higher than the incidence of AION in the general population aged 50 or older (which is approximately 0.3%[29]). However, such a comparison fails to consider that patients on amiodarone therapy have cardiac arrhythmias, hypertension, and other potential risk factors for AION.

Others have suggested that amiodarone produces an optic neuropathy that can be distinguished from AION.[30] Purported amiodarone-induced optic neuropathy may be characterized by the insidious onset of bilateral and symmetrical visual loss with slow progression, whereas AION is characterized by an acute, unilateral visual loss that is rarely progressive. Purported amiodarone-induced optic neuropathy causes a protracted disc swelling that tends to stabilize within several months of discontinuation of medication, but AION is characterized by resolution of disc edema over several weeks.[30]

In purported amiodarone-induced optic neuropathy the cup-to-disc ratio is larger than that seen in AION,[29] and these should be bilateral disc edema.

One theoretical mechanism of amiodarone-induced optic neuropathy has been suggested by a primary lipidosis seen ultrastructurally in one human optic nerve.[31] However, the patient in this case had no associated visual loss, and membranous lipid accumulation is nonspecific in the optic nerve.[31,32] Most case reports suggesting amiodarone as inducing a type of AION failed to establish causality.[33,34]

Nonetheless, it may be prudent to perform ophthalmological examinations on patients taking amiodarone. If an amiodarone-induced optic neuropathy is entertained seriously, alternative antiarrhythmic therapy may be considered.[30]

Finally, because the nerve and nerve fiber layer changes in LHON and nutritional and toxic optic neuropathies can sometimes be very subtle, psychogenic visual loss often is considered in the differential diagnosis. Visual evoked potentials may be useful to document the increased latencies seen in organic disease.

SYSTEMIC ASSOCIATIONS

Especially in mixed nutritional optic neuropathies, there may be other associated neurological symptoms, such as paresthesias, ataxia, or hearing impairment. However, these are more characteristic of general nutritional deficiencies sometimes found in clusters in equatorial countries and termed tropical amblyopias, and they usually are not described in cases of toxic exposure or single vitamin deficiency.[35] Visual symptoms may be seen in association with paresthesias and dysesthesias, particularly in the legs, in association with ataxia and hearing loss.[36] This has been described in vitamin deficiencies associated with poor diet, compounded by the ingestion of cassava and by elevated levels of cyanide.[37]

PATHOLOGY

Very little is currently published on the histopathology of these optic neuropathies. However, Sadun et al.,[21,38,39] as well as Kerrison et al.,[40] provided ultrastructural characterizations of the three mutations in LHON from genetically characterized pedigrees. In addition to severe losses of retinal ganglion cells in the macular area and depletion of the nerve fiber layer, these authors described accumulations of mitochondria in other orbital tissues and electron-dense, membrane-bound calcium inclusions in the remaining retinal ganglion cells.

TREATMENT

If the cause of the toxic or deficiency optic neuropathy can be found and treated early (for example, by cessation of smoking and the administration of vitamins in tobacco–alcohol amblyopia), vision generally returns to near normal over several months. However, there often is permanent visual loss in cases of long-standing toxic or nutritional optic neuropathy. Some investigators advocate general nutritional supplementation for any of these optic neuropathies. However, in the absence of a demonstrable deficiency, no good evidence exists that giving B vitamins or folic acid is of any benefit. Nonetheless, it is not uncommon to see cyanocobalamin (vitamin B_{12}) given, not only in suspected cases of tobacco–alcohol amblyopia, but for LHON as well. Idebenone, a quinol analog, has been used recently in a few cases of LHON to ameliorate the net ATP synthesis by providing an alternate pathway, as well as scavenging free radicals with the advantage of concentrating readily in the mitochondria. The results were modest.[41] Patients who have already lost vision in one eye from LHON might be candidates for pharmacological manipulation of mitochondrial metabolism to protect the second eye.[9]

COURSE AND OUTCOMES

In many cases, prompt administration of the deficient nutrient (such as a vitamin) or removal of the toxin (such as ethambutol) results in significant recovery over a period of several weeks, and sometimes months. However, in cases in which the injury is long standing there may be little or no recovery. In LHON, most patients show minimal recovery, although there have been reports of dramatic and late improvements.[42] The worst visual prognosis is for LHON cases that have the 11778 mutation; over 75% become legally blind in both eyes.[11]

REFERENCES

1. Bodis-Wollner I. Leber's hereditary optic neuropathy: a model disease of the decade of the brain. Clin Neurosci. 1994;2:112–4.
2. Wallace DC, Singh G, Lott MT, et al. Mitochondrial DNA mutations associated with Leber's hereditary optic neuropathy. Science. 1988;242:1427.
3. Carelli V, Ghelli A, Ratta M, et al. Leber's hereditary optic neuropathy: biochemical effect of 11778/ND4 and 3460/ND1 mutations and correlation with the mitochondrial genotype. Neurology. 1997;48:1623–32.
4. Carelli V, Ghelli A, Bucchi L, et al. Biochemical features of mtDNA 14484 (ND6/M64V) point mutation associated with Leber's hereditary optic neuropathy. Ann Neurol. 1999;45:320–8.
5. Traquair HM. Toxic amblyopia including retrobulbar neuritis. Trans Ophthalmol Soc U K. 1930;50:351–84.
6. Rizzo JF, Lessell S. Tobacco amblyopia. Am J Ophthalmol. 1993;116:84–7.
7. Golnik KC, Schaible ER. Folate-responsive optic neuropathy. J Neuroophthalmol. 1994;14:163–9.
8. Newman NJ. Optic neuropathy. Neurology. 1996;46(2):315–22.
9. Sadun AA. Mitochondrial optic neuropathies. J Neurol Neurosurg Psychiatry. 2002;72(4):423-5.
10. Mackey DA, Butter RD. Leber's hereditary optic neuropathy characterized by recovery of vision and by an unusual mitochondrial genetic etiology. Am J Hum Genet. 1994;51:1218–28.
11. Nicoskelainen EK. Visual system dysfunction in Leber's hereditary optic neuropathy. Clin Neurosci. 1994;2(2):115–20.
11a. Sadun AA, Win PH, Ross-Cisneros FN, et al. Leber's hereditary optic neuropathy differentially affects smaller axons in the optic nerve. Trans Am Ophthalmol Soc. 2000;98:223–32.
12. Sadun AA, Win PH, Ross-Cisneros FN, et al. Leber's hereditary optic neuropathy differentially affects smaller axons in the optic nerve. Trans Am Ophthalmol Soc. 2000;98:223–35.
13. Brady ST, Lasek RJ. Axonal transport. A cell biological method for studying proteins that associate with the cytoskeleton. Methods Cell Biol. 1982;25:365–98.
14. Sadun AA, Martone JF, Muci-Mendoza R, et al. Epidemic optic neuropathy in Cuba: eye findings. Arch Ophthalmol. 1994;112:691–9.
15. Sobel RS, Yannuzzi RA. Optic nerve toxicity: a classification in retinal and choroidal manifestations of systemic disease. In: Singerman LJ, Jampol LM, eds. Retinal and choroidal manifestations of systemic disease. Baltimore: Williams & Wilkins; 1991:226–50.
16. McMartin KE, Ambre JJ, Tephly TR. Methanol poisoning in human subjects. Role for formic acid accumulation in metabolic acidosis. Am Med. 1980;8:414–8.
17. Sejerstes OM, Jacobsen D, Ovrebo S, et al. Formate concentrations in plasma from patients poisoned with methanol. Acta Med Scand. 1983;213:105–10.
18. Sobel RS, Yanuzzi LA. Optic nerve toxicity. A classification. In: Singerman I, Jampol LM, eds. Retinal and choroidal manifestations of disease. Baltimore: Williams & Wilkins; 1991:226–50.
19. Kozak S, Inderlieb CB, Heller K, et al. The role of copper on ethambutol's antimicrobial action and implications for ethambutol-induced optic neuropathy. Diagn Microbiol Infect Dis. 1998;30:83–7.
20. Cruickshank EK. Painful feet in prisoners-of-war in the Far East. Review of 500 cases. Lancet. 1946;ii:369–72.
20a. Carelli V, Ross-Cisneros FN, Sadun AA. Optic nerve degeneration and mitochondrial dysfunction: genetic and acquired optic neuropathies. Neurochem Int. 2002 May;40(6):573–84.
21. Sadun AA, Kashima Y, Wurdeman AE, et al. Morphological findings in the visual system in a case of Leber's hereditary optic neuropathy. Clin Neurosci. 1994;2(2):165–72.
22. Sadun AA, Kupersmith MJ. Association for research in vision and ophthalmology (ARVO). Annual meeting, April 29–May 4, 2001. #5020. J Neuroophthalmol. 2001;21(3):227–30.
23. Sadun AA, Martone JF, Reyes L, et al. Epidemic of optic neuropathy in Cuba. JAMA. 1994;271(9):663–4.
24. Raeder EA, Podrid PJ, Lown B. Side effects and complications of amiodarone therapy. Am Heart J. 1985;109:975–83.
25. Kudenchuk PJ, Pierson DJ, Greene HL, et al. Prospective evaluation of amiodarone pulmonary toxicity. Chest. 1984;86:541–8.
26. Orlando RG, Dangel ME, Schaal SF. Clinical experience and grading of amiodarone keratopathy. Ophthalmology. 1984;91:1184–7.
27. Hawthorne GC, Campbell NPS, Geddes JS, et al. Amiodarone-induced hypothyroidism: a common complication of prolonged therapy; a report of 8 cases. Arch Intern Med. 1985;145:1016–9.
28. Charness ME, Morady F, Scheinman MM. Frequent neurologic toxicity associated with amiodarone therapy. Neurology. 1984;34:669–71.
29. Feiner LA, Younge BR, Kazmier FJ, et al. Optic neuropathy and amiodarone therapy. Mayo Clin Proc. 1987;62:702–17.
30. Macaluso DC, Shults WT, Fraunfelder FT. Features of amiodarone-induced optic neuropathy. Am J Ophthalmol. 1999;127:610–2.
31. Mansour AM, Puklin JE, O'Grady R. Optic nerve ultrastructure following amiodarone therapy. J Clin Neuroophthalmol. 1988;8:231–7.
32. Sadun AA, Bassi C. Optic nerve damage in Alzheimer's disease. Ophthalmology. 1990;97:1, 9–17.
33. Sadun AA, Dao J. Part two: annual review in neuro-ophthalmology. J Neuroophthalmol. 1994;14(4):234–49.
34. Sedwick LA. Getting to the heart of visual loss: when cardiac medication may be dangerous to the optic nerves. Comments by Hedges TR III, Newman NJ. Surv Ophthalmol. 1992;36:366–72.
35. Miller NR. Retrobulbar toxic and deficiency optic neuropathies. In: Miller NR, ed. Walsh and Hoyt's clinical neuro-ophthalmology, vol 1, ed 4. Baltimore: Williams & Wilkins; 1982:289–307.
36. Osuntokun BO. Ataxic neuropathy in Nigeria. A clinical, biochemical and electrophysiological study. Brain. 1968;91:215–48.
37. Osuntokun BO, Osuntokun O. Tropical amblyopia in Nigerians. Am J Ophthalmol. 1971;72:708–16.
38. Sadun AA. Acquired mitochondrial impairment as a cause of optic nerve disease. Trans Am Ophthalmol Soc. 1998;96:881–923.
39. Saadati HG, Hsu HY, Heller KB, Sadun AA. A histopathological and morphometric differentiation of nerves in optic nerve hypoplasia and Leber hereditary optic neuropathy. Arch Ophthalmol. 1998;116:911–6.
40. Kerrison JB, Howell N, Miller NR, et al. Leber's hereditary optic neuropathy: electron microscopy and molecular genetic analysis of a case. Ophthalmology. 1995;102:1509–16.
41. Carelli V, Ghelli A, Cevoli S, et al. Idebenone therapy in Leber's hereditary optic neuropathy: report of six cases. Neurology. 1998;50:A4.
42. Newman NJ. Leber's hereditary optic neuropathy. New genetic considerations. Arch Neurol. 1993;50:540–8.

193

Prechiasmal Pathways—Compression by Optic Nerve and Sheath Tumors

THOMAS C. SPOOR

DEFINITION

- Optic nerve dysfunction as a result of compression by tumor or aneurysm anywhere along the nerve's course from globe to chiasm.

KEY FEATURES

- Progressive visual field loss.
- Relative afferent pupillary defect.
- Dyschromatopsia.

ASSOCIATED FEATURES

- Proptosis.
- Swollen or atrophic optic disc.
- Retinal and choroidal striae.
- Opticociliary collateral vessels.
- Venous stasis retinopathy or central retinal vein occlusion.

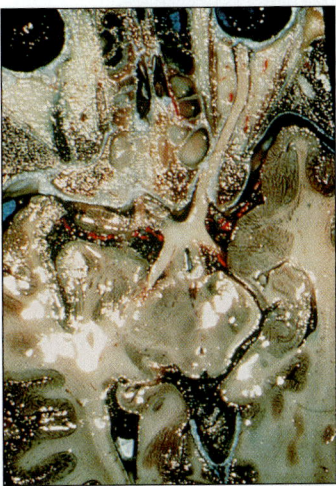

FIG. 193-1 ■ Axial cadaver section that demonstrates the course of the optic nerve from the globe to the optic chiasm. Note the intraorbital, intracanalicular, and intracranial segments of the optic nerve.

The optic nerve extends from the back of the eye, traverses the orbit, passes through the optic canal, and has a variable intracranial course before it joins with the contralateral optic nerve to form the chiasm (Fig. 193-1). Compression by a tumor or an aneurysm may cause optic nerve dysfunction anywhere along its course, from globe to chiasm.

EXTRINSIC ORBITAL OPTIC NERVE COMPRESSION

INTRODUCTION

Extrinsic optic nerve compression by orbital tumors or apical orbital compression by enlarged dysthyroid extraocular muscles represents an uncommon but potentially treatable cause of optic neuropathy. These tumors may compress the optic nerve at the orbital apex (Fig. 193-2).

EPIDEMIOLOGY AND PATHOGENESIS

Compression of the apical orbital optic nerve by enlarged extraocular muscles is an uncommon manifestation of dysthyroid orbitopathy (Fig. 193-3). The vast majority of patients who have hyperthyroidism have mild, noninfiltrative orbitopathy. Clinically, significant infiltrative orbitopathy occurs in only 3–5% of the hyperthyroid population. The most severe infiltrative orbitopathy, dysthyroid optic neuropathy, occurred in 8.6% of 675 patients with dysthyroid orbitopathy in one large series.[1]

Encapsulated orbital tumors are quite uncommon. Of these, cavernous hemangiomas are the most common, neurilemomas are less common, and hemangiopericytomas are rarer still.

OCULAR MANIFESTATIONS

Initially, extrinsic optic nerve compression within the orbit manifests with slowly progressive loss of visual acuity and brightness sensation, and dyschromatopsia. Visual field deterioration and relative afferent pupillary defect are seen with progression. Examination may be entirely normal, and patients who have large tumors with more anterior optic nerve compression also may have a swollen optic disc and choroidal striae. However, anterior orbital tumors more commonly occur with proptosis but without compressive optic neuropathy.

In patients with thyroid eye disease, other manifestations such as eyelid retraction and extraocular motility restriction may be seen. It may be more difficult to diagnose disease in patients who do not have other signs of thyroid eye disease, and they may be followed for months to years with progressive visual field loss and negative neuroimaging study results.

DIAGNOSIS AND ANCILLARY TESTING

The key to the diagnosis is first to consider it and then to obtain appropriate imaging studies to visualize the orbital apex. Computed tomography (CT) scanning differentiates optic nerve compression by orbital tumors from apical orbital optic nerve compression by enlarged, dysthyroid extraocular muscles (see Fig. 193-2). Magnetic resonance imaging (MRI) scans can help differentiate orbital tumor from the compressed optic nerve and facilitate surgical decision making.

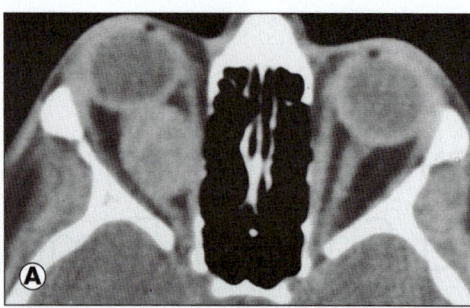

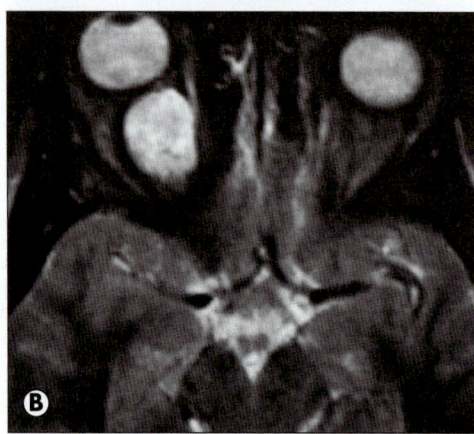

FIG. 193-2 ■ Images of a large orbit mass adjacent or contiguous with the optic nerve. **A,** Computed tomography scan (axial). **B,** Magnetic resonance imaging shows obvious demarcation between the tumor and the adjacent optic nerve.

FIG. 193-3 ■ Computed tomography scans (axial and coronal). The optic nerves are compressed at the orbital apex by enlarged extraocular muscles.

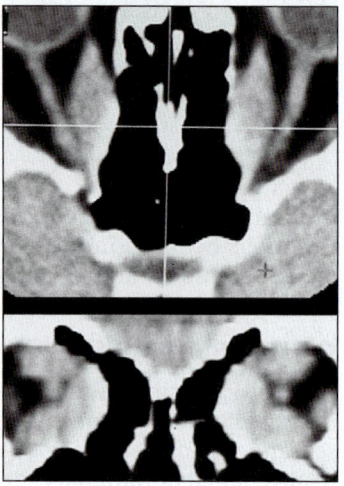

TREATMENT

Treatment of dysthyroid optic neuropathy is to decompress the orbital apex. Extraocular muscles may be shrunk with systemic corticosteroids or low-dose irradiation, and the orbital apex may be expanded by surgical removal of the medial orbital wall—advocates exist for each technique.[2,3] The author favors the initial use of systemic corticosteroids (prednisone 80mg daily), followed by decompression of the medial orbital wall and orbital apex via an external ethmoidectomy. Orbital irradiation is reserved for cases refractory to corticosteroids and surgical decompression or for patients who are unwilling or unable to undergo general anesthesia and surgery. However, contrary to clinical experience, a recent study has found that external beam irradiation is not an effective treatment for Grave's ophthalmopathy.[4]

Treatment of optic nerve compression by an encapsulated orbital tumor entails surgical removal of the tumor. MRI may help to differentiate the tumor from the optic nerve and ascertain the tumor's position in reference to the optic nerve. The latter is important in planning an appropriate surgical approach for tumor excision.

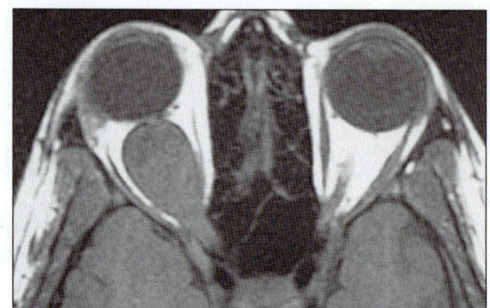

FIG. 193-4 ■ Magnetic resonance imaging of a large optic nerve glioma and optic canal confined to the orbit.

OPTIC NERVE COMPRESSION BY OPTIC NERVE AND SHEATH TUMORS

The optic nerve may be invaded by intrinsic tumors (such as gliomas) arising from the neuroglia or neurons, or compressed by extrinsic tumors arising from the meninges (such as meningiomas). Optic nerve gliomas and optic nerve sheath meningiomas are the most common tumors to involve the optic nerve. Less commonly, the optic nerve also may be involved by lymphomas, leukemias, malignant gliomas, and metastatic cancers.

GLIOMAS AND MALIGNANT GLIOMAS
Epidemiology and Pathogenesis

Gliomas of the anterior visual pathways are the most common tumors of the central nervous system. They account for 2% of all gliomas and 5% of childhood gliomas and occur most commonly during the first two decades of life—65% occur within the first decade, and 90% occur before 20 years of age. Rarely, a glioma may occur in a previously asymptomatic adult as an expanding orbital mass. Gliomas of the anterior visual pathways account for 65% of all intrinsic optic nerve tumors.[5] Malignant gliomas of the optic nerve are rare.[6] Gliomas that involve the intraorbital optic nerve are most common (47%), those that involve the orbital and intracranial optic nerve are second most common (26%), followed by intracranial and chiasmal involvement (12%) and gliomas confined to the optic chiasm (5%).[7]

Ocular Manifestations

Patients who have optic nerve gliomas usually experience exophthalmos, decreased visual function, and dyschromatopsia accompanied by a relative afferent pupillary defect. The optic disc may be normal, swollen, or atrophic. Central retinal vein occlusion may occur.

Patients who have malignant gliomas of the optic nerve have rapidly progressive, painful visual loss accompanied by signs of an optic neuropathy.[6,7] Initial visual loss may be unilateral or bilateral (chiasmal involvement), but rapid progression to bilateral blindness and death are constant features.[5] Depending on the initial location of the tumor, visual loss may be accompanied by exophthalmos, extraocular motility dysfunction, venous stasis retinopathy, and an optic disc that is swollen, atrophic, or of normal appearance.

Diagnosis

Intrinsic enlargement of the optic nerve on MRI is evident in patients who have optic nerve gliomas. The presence and extent of optic nerve gliomas is best demonstrated by MRI (Fig. 193-4).[5] Although rarely missed with high-resolution CT scans, optic nerve enlargement by an intrinsic glioma may be confused with compression by a resectable orbital tumor; MRI may help to differentiate these (see Fig. 193-3).

For patients who have orbital nerve gliomas and neurofibromatosis type 1, MRI demonstrates a typical double-intensity tubular thickening caused by perineural arachnoid gliomatosis, and elongation and downward kinking of the midorbital optic nerves.[8]

Imaging studies of an optic nerve glioma may show enlargement of the optic forearm that arises from secondary meningeal hyperplasia. Consequently, enlargement of the optic forearm is not firm evidence of intracranial extension of an optic nerve glioma.

Imaging studies of malignant gliomas of the optic nerve demonstrate enlargement of the involved regions of the optic nerve and chiasm, although initially normal imaging study results have been reported.[6] The diagnosis of this devastating disease should be confirmed by biopsy of the involved portion of the optic nerve.

Differential Diagnosis

The differential diagnosis of visual loss from optic nerve glioma is the differential diagnosis of any slowly progressive optic neuropathy. Differentiation between gliomas and other causes of optic nerve compression in a child is best accomplished using appropriate imaging studies (see above).

Systemic Associations

Frequently, optic nerve gliomas are found in association with neurofibromatosis type 1 (only rarely with neurofibromatosis type 2), which is present in 25% of patients who have optic nerve gliomas, while 15% of patients with neurofibromatosis have optic nerve gliomas. Increased intracranial pressure and chiasmal and optic tract involvement are more common in patients who do not have neurofibromatosis. Precocious puberty is more common in children who have gliomas and neurofibromatosis.[9,10]

Pathology

Optic nerve gliomas are intrinsic tumors that arise from the neuroglia—usually astrocytes, but occasionally oligodendrocytes (see Fig. 193-3). Three histopathological patterns exist:
- Transitional areas in which the tumor merges with normal optic nerve and which may be difficult to differentiate from reactive gliosis
- Areas of tumor necrosis, which may appear as cystic spaces that contain reticulated, myxomatous material
- Areas where astrocytes may show spindle cell formation and contain cytoplasmic, eosinophilic structures called *Rosenthal fibers* (Fig. 193-5)

These patterns are characteristic but not diagnostic of optic nerve gliomas.[9] Arachnoid hyperplasia, secondary to infiltration by the glioma through the pia, may mimic an optic nerve sheath meningioma.

Biopsy specimens of malignant gliomas of the optic nerve demonstrate bizarre, atypical malignant astrocytes that separate disrupted myelin sheaths.

Treatment

If visual function is good, isolated intraorbital optic nerve gliomas may be observed. Visual function may be followed with serial visual field testing, and MRI should be done every 6–12 months to detect any intracranial extension. If vision is poor, or exophthalmos is excessive and unsightly, the lesion may be removed via a craniotomy and superior orbitotomy. If intracranial extension by a glioma initially confined to the orbit is documented, the tumor should be removed completely via craniotomy in an effort to avoid chiasmal, hypothalamic, or third ventricle involvement.[5]

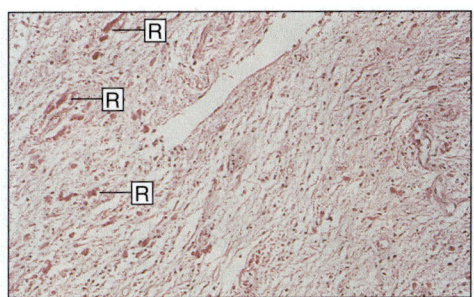

FIG. 193-5 ■ **Optic nerve glioma.** Many astrocytes contain intracytoplasmic eosinophilic structures, called Rosenthal fibers *(R)*.

Unfortunately, no successful treatment exists for malignant gliomas of the optic nerve.

Course and Outcome

Optic nerve gliomas are true neoplasms that characteristically demonstrate early growth followed by long periods of stability in many cases. They have a poor prognosis for vision, but if confined to the optic nerve, long-term survival is excellent. If the chiasm, hypothalamus, or third ventricle are involved, the prognosis for life diminishes. Once the hypothalamus is involved, mortality rises to over 50%. No therapy exists of proven benefit.[5] Spontaneous regression may occur.[11] There is a tendency for vision in the worse eye to deteriorate and vision in the better eye to remain stable regardless of treatment or neurofibromatosis status.[12]

Patients who have malignant gliomas of the optic nerve experience painful visual loss and rapidly progress to bilateral blindness within 6–8 weeks. Death invariably follows within 6–9 months after the initial symptoms.[6]

OPTIC NERVE SHEATH MENINGIOMAS

INTRODUCTION

Meningiomas are benign neoplasms that arise from the meningothelial cells of the meninges. The optic nerve may be compressed by meningiomas confined to the optic nerve or by orbital extension of intracranial tumors. Slowly progressive, relentless visual loss may be accompanied by proptosis and extraocular motility dysfunction.

EPIDEMIOLOGY AND PATHOGENESIS

Optic nerve sheath meningiomas represent 1–2% of all meningiomas. After gliomas, these are the second most common type of optic nerve tumor[13] and primarily affect middle-aged adults, usually women.

OCULAR MANIFESTATIONS

Slowly progressive visual loss is the hallmark of an optic nerve sheath meningioma. A relative afferent pupillary defect and dyschromatopsia invariably are present. The optic disc may be swollen or atrophic. Opticociliary collateral vessels and retinal and choroidal folds may be evident on fundus examination. Extraocular motility dysfunction is present in some cases.

DIAGNOSIS

Neuroimaging confirms the diagnosis of optic nerve sheath meningioma. CT scans demonstrate fusiform, tubular, or irregular enlargement of the optic nerve. The borders of the enlarged optic nerve may enhance after administration of intravenous

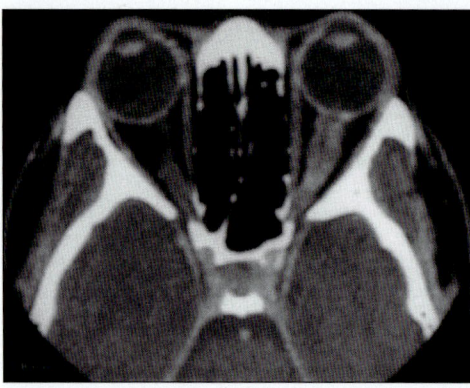

FIG. 193-6 ▌▌ Computed tomography scan of optic nerve sheath meningioma.

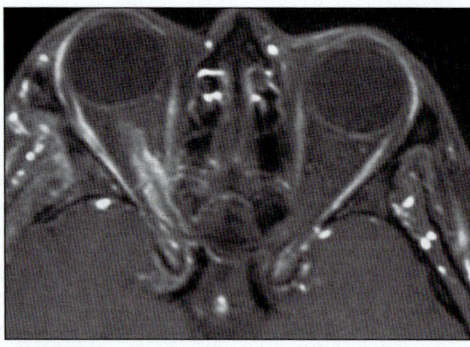

FIG. 193-7 ▌▌ Gadolinium-enhanced magnetic resonance imaging demonstrates the intracranial extension of an optic nerve sheath meningioma.

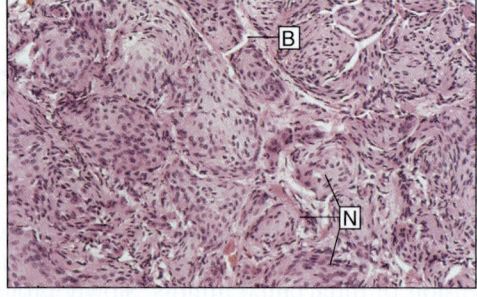

FIG. 193-8 ▌▌ **Meningioma of optic nerve.** This biopsy shows a proliferation of meningothelial cells. As is often the case, no psammoma bodies are present. *B,* blood vessels; *N,* nests of meningothelial cells.

contrast, to leave a central, linear lucency within the optic nerve sheath (tram-track sign; Fig. 193-6). Extensive or segmental calcifications also may be present.

MRI fat suppression and gadolinium–diethylenetriamine-pentaacetic-acid (Gd-DTPA) enhancement can detect and demarcate precisely the degree of intracanalicular and intracranial extension of optic nerve sheath meningiomas (Fig. 193-7). The majority of intraorbital and intracranial meningiomas are detected by CT scans, but only gadolinium-enhanced MRI reliably demonstrates a meningioma that involves the intracanalicular optic nerve (see Fig. 193-7). Studies with high-quality MRI demonstrate that, even with small tumors, intracranial extension is the rule rather than the exception.[14]

PATHOLOGY

Meningiomas arise from the meningothelial cells of the arachnoid villi. Histopathology demonstrates patterns of whorls and sheets of meningothelial cells (Fig. 193-8). A variable amount of fibrous and vascular tissue occurs in fibroblastic pattern menin-

---

BOX 193-1

Intracranial Causes of Compressive Optic Neuropathies

INFLAMMATION
Neurosarcoidosis

INFECTIOUS
Tuberculous meningitis
Syphilis-meningitis or gumma

ANEURYSMS
Supraclinoidal
Ophthalmic

TUMORS
Gliomas
Pituitary adenomas
Meningiomas
• sphenoid ridge
• planum sphenoidale, suprasellar, intrasellar
Craniopharyngiomas
Paranasal sinus tumors
Mucoceles
Fibrous dysplasia

---

giomas, with psammoma bodies present in psammomatous and mixed meningiomas.

TREATMENT

Treatment of optic nerve sheath meningiomas is conservative, because these tumors usually grow very slowly. Observation, serial automated visual fields, and regular MRI scans with gadolinium enhancement are appropriate for patients who have good vision and no evidence of intracranial or intracanalicular extension of tumor. Patients for whom MRI evidence exists of such extension should be offered a neurosurgical opinion, but they should be informed that these tumors may grow very slowly. It may be appropriate to follow a small amount of intracranial extension with serial MRI, with craniotomy reserved for those patients who have documented progressive intracranial extension of tumor.

Intraorbital or intracranial surgical removal of selected tumors or intracranial optic canal decompression may improve vision in some patients, but the improvement rarely lasts. Patients who have blind eyes and severe exophthalmos may benefit from extirpation of intraorbital and intracranial tumor. Documented intracanalicular or intracranial progression of tumor growth warrants neurosurgical removal of the tumor.

A large, recent series in which visual outcome was reviewed in a group of patients who underwent radical tumor resection of cranio-orbital meningiomas reported improved visual function in 27%, stable visual function in 62%, and worsening vision in 11%. The postoperative visual outcome is related to the degree of preoperative visual impairment.[14] These results seem better than those previously described.[15]

Recurrent tumor and progressive visual loss may be treated with radiation. Treatment is controversial. Radiation therapy has been used in patients who have progressive visual loss and good visual function, and in patients who have recurrent tumor. Preliminary results are encouraging, but too few patients have been treated with this modality and its long-term advantage for vision remains unknown and unproved.[12] More recently, excellent results actually reversing visual loss utilizing 3-dimensional conformal radiation have been reported.[16]

COURSE AND OUTCOME

The clinical course of optic nerve sheath meningiomas is slowly progressive, relentless visual loss in the affected eye. The prognosis for life is excellent, with an overall tumor-related mortality of near zero.[12]

INTRACANALICULAR AND INTRACRANIAL COMPRESSIVE LESIONS

The optic nerves may be compressed within the optic canal or intracranially by any entity that can compress the optic chiasm, depending upon the length of the intracranial optic nerves and their position relative to intracranial structures (e.g., pre- or postfixed optic chiasm; see Chapter 195). Aneurysms, tumors, infection, inflammation, mucoceles, and processes that involve the sphenoid bone, such as fibrous dysplasia, may cause a compressive optic neuropathy (Box 193-1). The involved optic nerves may appear normal, atrophic, swollen, or excavated. Optic disc excavation in the absence of elevated intraocular pressure may indicate a compressive optic neuropathy, especially if accompanied by pallor of the neuroretinal rim.[16]

REFERENCES

1. Rootman J. Diseases of the orbit. Philadelphia: JP Lippincott; 1988:243–4.
2. Garrity JA, Fatourechi V, Bergstralh EJ, et al. Results of transantral decompression in 428 patients with severe Grave's ophthalmology. Am J Ophthalmol. 1993;116:533–47.
3. Lloyd WC, Leone CR Jr. Supervoltage orbital radiotherapy in 36 cases of Grave's disease. Am J Ophthalmol. 1992;113:374–80.
4. Gorum CA, Garrity JA, Fatourechi V, et al. A prospective randomized double-blind placebo-controlled study of orbital radiotherapy for Grave's ophthalmology. Ophthalmology. 2001;108:1525–34.
5. Dutton JJ. Gliomas of the anterior visual pathways. Surv Ophthalmol. 1994;38:427–52.
6. Spoor TC, Kennerdell JS, Martinez J, et al. Malignant gliomas of the optic pathways. Am J Ophthalmol. 1980;89:284–90.
7. Yanoff M, Fine B. Ocular pathology. Philadelphia: Mosby; 1996.
8. Imes RK, Hoyt WF. Magnetic resonance imaging signs of optic nerve gliomas in neurofibromatosis 1. Am J Ophthalmol. 1991;111:729–34.
9. Sadun AA, Rubin RM. The anterior visual pathways—part II. J Neuroophthalmol. 1996;16:212–22.
10. Listernick R, Darling C, Greenwald M, et al. Optic pathway tumors in children: the effect of neurofibromatosis type 1 on the clinical manifestations and natural history. J Pediatr. 1995;127:718–22.
11. Passo CF, Hoyt CS, Lesser RL, et al. Spontaneous regression of optic gliomas: 13 cases documented by serial neuroimaging. Arch Ophthalmol. 2001;119:516–29.
12. Gayre GS, Scott IU, Feuer W, et al. Long-term visual outcome in patients with anterior visual pathway gliomas. J Neuroophthalmol. 2001;21:1–7.
13. Dutton JJ. Optic nerve sheath meningiomas. Surv Ophthalmol. 1992;37:167–83.
14. Lindblom B, Truwit CL, Hoyt WF. Optic nerve sheath meningioma definition of intraorbital, intracanalicular, and intracranial components with magnetic resonance imaging. Ophthalmology. 1992;99:560–6.
15. Kennerdell JS, Maroon JC, Malton M, et al. The management of optic nerve sheath meningiomas. Am J Ophthalmol. 1998;106:450–7.
16. Moyer PD, Golnik KC, Breneman J. Treatment of optic nerve sheath meningiomas with 3-dimensional conformal radiation. Am J Ophthalmol. 2000;129:694–6.

CHAPTER
194 Traumatic Optic Neuropathies

THOMAS C. SPOOR

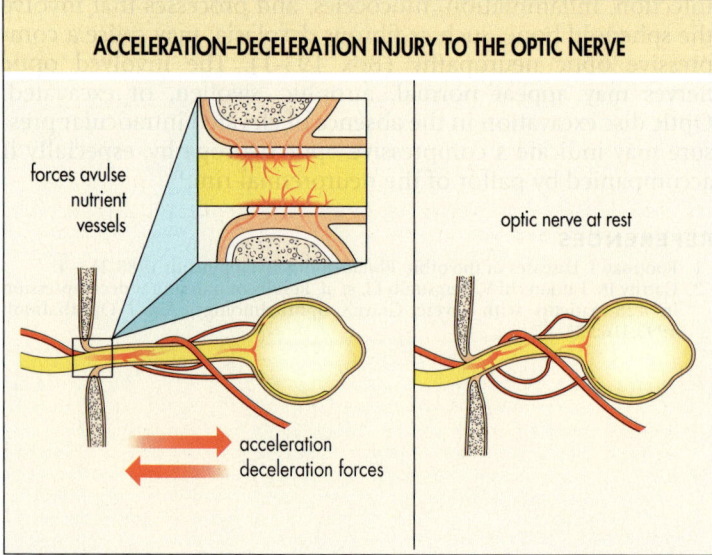

ACCELERATION–DECELERATION INJURY TO THE OPTIC NERVE

forces avulse nutrient vessels

optic nerve at rest

acceleration deceleration forces

FIG. 194-1 ▮ Acceleration–deceleration injury to the optic nerve results in avulsion of its nutrient vessels.

INTRODUCTION

The optic nerve may be damaged directly or indirectly after cranio-orbital trauma. Normal visual acuity and normal visual field and pupillary function are not compatible with the diagnosis of optic nerve injury. Both direct and indirect injury may damage the optic nerve as a result of transection of nerve fibers, interruption of blood supply, or secondary hemorrhage and edema. Primary injury to the optic nerve fibers by transection or infarction at the time of injury results in permanent damage. Neural dysfunction secondary to compression within the optic canal, as a result of edema and hemorrhage, may respond to medical or surgical intervention.

EPIDEMIOLOGY AND PATHOGENESIS

Indirect injury to the optic nerve occurs in 0.5–5% of patients who suffer closed head trauma.[1] The optic nerve is enclosed tightly within the bony optic canal; it may be damaged by shearing and avulsion of its nutrient vessels (Fig. 194-1) or by pressure transmitted along the bone to the optic canal (Fig. 194-2).[2]

OCULAR MANIFESTATIONS

Patients who have optic neuropathy have decreased visual acuity or visual field defects. A relative afferent pupillary defect—the *sine qua non*—of an optic neuropathy often is the ocular abnormality evident. If a relative afferent pupillary defect is not evident, the patient does not have a traumatic optic neuropathy, unless it is bilateral. Patients who have bilateral optic nerve dysfunction demonstrate light–near dissociation of their pupillary reactions. The near response is brisker than the pupillary response to light.

If the anterior optic nerve is injured, infarction, hemorrhage, or a central retinal artery occlusion are evident on ophthalmoscopy. Patients who have a more posterior injury to the nerve may be found to have a normal fundus on examination but have an afferent pupillary defect and visual loss.

Associated ocular injuries should be documented and treated, if possible. If the ocular injuries do not account for the degree of visual loss, a traumatic optic neuropathy should be suspected.

DIAGNOSIS AND ANCILLARY TESTING

High-resolution computed tomography (CT) is the diagnostic procedure of choice for patients who have suspected traumatic optic neuropathy. Treatable causes of optic nerve compression, such as orbital and optic nerve sheath hemorrhages, are detected using CT scans[3]; also, orbital and optic canal fractures may be detected using these scans. The presence of an optic canal fracture is not necessary for the diagnosis of traumatic optic neuropathy. Prior to transethmoidal optic canal decompression, CT scans show the information necessary to plan surgery.[3]

DIFFERENTIAL DIAGNOSIS

Visual loss and an afferent pupillary defect result from optic nerve dysfunction. Traumatic optic nerve injury may occur even after a seemingly trivial head injury. Detection of visual loss may be coincident with the traumatic event. The differential diagnosis should include other causes of optic neuropathies, as well as causes of obviously treatable optic nerve compression (Box 194-1).

PATHOLOGY

The optic nerve can be injured anywhere along its course, most commonly at the intracanalicular and intracranial portion. Forces applied to the frontal bone may be transmitted and concentrated at the optic canal.[2] Acceleration and deceleration forces may cause a partial or total avulsion of the retrobulbar optic nerve, or con-

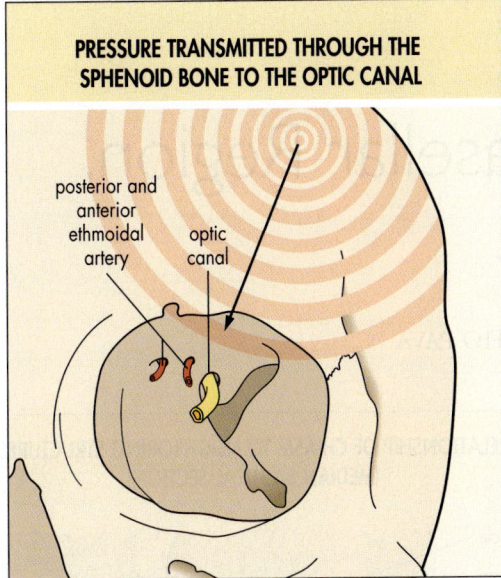

PRESSURE TRANSMITTED THROUGH THE SPHENOID BONE TO THE OPTIC CANAL

posterior and anterior ethmoidal artery
optic canal

FIG. 194-2 ▪ Pressure transmitted through the sphenoid bone to the optic canal may cause traumatic optic nerve injury.

BOX 194-1

DIFFERENTIAL DIAGNOSIS OF TRAUMATIC OPTIC NEUROPATHY

Optic nerve sheath hematoma
Orbital hematoma
Subperiosteal hematoma
Coincident optic neuropathies
Compression by tumor or aneurysm

Optic nerve inflammation
Orbital inflammation
Sinusitis with orbital involvement
Ischemic optic neuropathy
Optic neuritis

---

tusion necrosis and avulsion of the vascular supply of the intracanalicular optic nerve (see Fig. 194-1). Orbital hemorrhage or hemorrhage into the optic nerve sheath also may cause progressive visual loss. The intracranial optic nerve may be injured by the falciform dural fold as a result of the forces of a shifting brain at the moment of impact. Swelling of the intracanalicular optic nerve causes delayed, progressive visual loss through exacerbation of the ischemic effects of the original injury. Any or all of these mechanisms may be responsible for optic nerve injury.[3]

Optic nerve injuries may be caused by primary and secondary mechanisms. The primary mechanisms cause permanent, irreparable damage to the optic nerve. Treatment modalities are effective only for secondary mechanisms of injury. These may be at the cellular level or from intracanalicular optic nerve swelling that further compromises an injured optic nerve. A review of such mechanisms was published recently.[3] Treatment consists of attempts to limit secondary injury and salvage axons that survive the initial trauma.

TREATMENT

Visual loss and a relative afferent pupillary defect that accompany an orbital hemorrhage warrant immediate decompression by either drainage of the hemorrhage or lateral canthotomy or cantholysis, or both. A much less common occurrence is an intraoptic nerve sheath hemorrhage, which results in compression of the optic nerve and compromise of visual function. Prompt surgical decompression of the optic nerve sheath may restore visual function.[4] The optic nerve may be injured anywhere along its length. These primary injuries are not treatable. The secondary effects of the primary injury, edema and hemorrhage, may be treatable. Secondary compression of the intracanalicular optic nerve may appear as progressive visual dysfunction after the initial loss. Treatment of traumatic optic nerve injuries with

megadose corticosteroids is based, in part, upon the success attained in treatment of spinal cord injuries.[5] Administered within 8 hours after injury, megadose corticosteroids have an antioxidant and membrane-stabilizing effect that limits secondary cell damage and increases microcirculatory perfusion.[6] After 8 hours, corticosteroids decrease edema and swelling but have little effect on the biochemical dynamics of the injured axon. Reduced swelling by removal of the bony wall of the optic canal relieves compression of the optic nerve and allows it to regain function. Unfortunately, these proposed treatments limit secondary injuries only. Axons damaged terminally do not regenerate—their visual function is irretrievably lost.

The effects of all the treatment options have not yet been clarified by a randomized, double-blind study; however, initial treatment with megadose corticosteroids is reasonably safe and possibly effective. If possible, treatment should begin within 8 hours of injury; regardless, it should be initiated as soon as possible. Methylprednisolone 30mg/kg is administered intravenously over 30 minutes, followed by 15mg/kg 2 hours later. This compensates for the rapid serum half-life of methylprednisolone. Treatment is continued with 15mg/kg every 6 hours for 24–48 hours. If visual function improves, the corticosteroids are tapered rapidly. If visual function deteriorates as corticosteroids are tapered, optic canal decompression should be offered. Patients who do not respond to megadose corticosteroids may be considered candidates for optic canal decompression. The rare patient who has a *bona fide* history of progressive visual loss after closed head injury is a certain candidate for megadose corticosteroids treatment and extracranial optic canal decompression. As for any surgical procedure, potential risks must be weighed against possible benefits. A steep learning curve exists for extracranial optic canal decompression, being a far safer operation in the hands of an experienced surgeon than in those of an occasional exponent.

COURSE AND OUTCOME

Unfortunately, no treatment for primary, traumatic optic neuropathies has been proved effective in a randomized, controlled clinical trial. Besides, no standard of care exists for the management of patients who have traumatic optic neuropathies.[4,7] Several studies show that patients treated with corticosteroids or a combination of corticosteroids and extracranial optic canal decompression seem to have better visual prognosis than untreated patients.[8,9] Treatment with megadose corticosteroids seems to improve vision more quickly than treatment with high-dose intravenous corticosteroids, but there is no significant difference in the final visual outcome.[10–12] Patients may improve spontaneously without treatment,[8] but treated patients appear to have a better visual prognosis.[8,9]

REFERENCES

1. Kline LB, Morawetz RB, Swaid SN. Indirect injury to the optic nerve. Neurosurgery. 1984;14:756–64.
2. Anderson RL, Panje WR, Gross CE. Optic nerve blindness following blunt forehead trauma. Ophthalmology. 1982;89:445–55.
3. Steinsapir KD, Goldberg RA. Traumatic optic neuropathy. Surv Ophthalmol. 1994;38:487–518.
4. Hupp SL, Buckley EG, Byrne SF, et al. Posttraumatic venous obstructive retinopathy associated with an enlarged optic nerve sheath. Arch Ophthalmol. 1984;102:254–6.
5. Bracken MB, Shepard MJ, Collins WF, et al. A randomized, controlled trial of methylprednisolone or naloxone in the treatment of acute spinal cord injury. N Engl J Med. 1990;322:1405–11.
6. Braughler JM, Hall ED, Means ED, et al. Evaluation of an intensive methylprednisolone sodium succinate dosing regimen in experimental spinal cord injury. J Neurosurg. 1987;67:102–5.
7. Miller NR. The management of traumatic optic neuropathy [Editorial]. Arch Ophthalmol. 1990;108:1086–7.
8. Warner JE, Lessell S. Traumatic optic neuropathy. Int Ophthalmol Clin. 1995;35:57–62.
9. Joseph MP, Lessell S, Rizzo J, Momose KJ. Extracranial optic canal decompression for traumatic optic neuropathy. Arch Ophthalmol. 1990;108:1091–3.
10. Spoor TC, Hartel WC, Lensink DB, et al. Management of traumatic optic neuropathy with corticosteroids. Am J Ophthalmol. 1990;110:665–9.
11. Levin LA, Beck RW, Joseph MP, et al. The treatment of traumatic optic neuropathy: the international optic nerve study. Ophthalmology. 1999;106:1268–77.
12. Lee AG. Traumatic optic neuropathy. Ophthalmology. 2000;107:814.

195 Optic Chiasm, Parasellar Region, and Pituitary Fossa

RICHARD M. RUBIN • ALFREDO A. SADUN • ALFIO PAVA

DEFINITION

- Loss of vision and visual field related to involvement of the chiasm itself, its blood supply, or adjacent optic nerve or optic tract by tumor or other processes.

KEY FEATURE

- Binocular temporal field loss with respect to the vertical midline.

ASSOCIATED FEATURES

- Cavernous sinus symptoms such as ocular motor nerve palsies, Horner's syndrome, trigeminal hypoesthesia, or pain.
- Endocrine dysfunction.
- Headache.
- Hydrocephalus.
- Endocrine dysfunction that arises from disruption of the hypothalamic–pituitary axis.
- Abnormalities of ocular motility, pupillary function, or facial sensation.

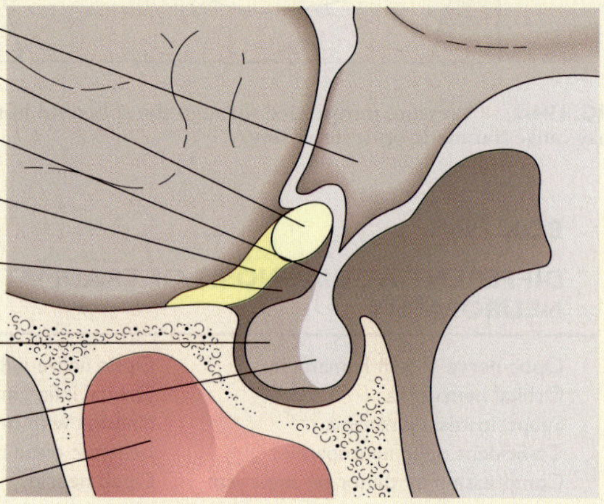

RELATIONSHIP OF CHIASM TO NEIGHBORING STRUCTURES (MEDIAN SAGITTAL SECTION)

third ventricle
optic chiasm
pituitary infundibulum
optic nerve
suprasellar cistern
pituitary gland (anterior lobe)
pituitary gland (posterior lobe)
sphenoid sinus

FIG. 195-1 ■ **Median sagittal section through the chiasm and relationship of chiasm to neighboring structures.** The optic chiasm is suspended above the pituitary gland and rests in the sella turcica of the sphenoid bone. It is surrounded by cerebrospinal fluid, except posteriorly where it borders the anterior inferior wall of the third ventricle. (Adapted from Sadun AA, Rubin RM. Developments in sensory neuro-ophthalmology. In: Silverstone B, Lang MA, Rosenthal B, Faye EE, eds. The Lighthouse handbook on vision impairment and rehabilitation. New York: Oxford University Press; 2000.)

INTRODUCTION

The word *chiasm* derives from the Greek letter chi (χ) and, in the visual system, refers to the appearance of the junction of the two optic nerves where they join to allow the hemidecussation of nasal fibers to the opposite optic tracts and the direct passage of temporal fibers to the ipsilateral optic tracts. Thus, all visual information supplied to both eyes from the right visual space is transmitted to the left cerebral cortex, and that supplied from the left visual space is transmitted to the right cerebral cortex.

The unique anatomy of the chiasm and its relationship to other major structures explains the characteristic patterns of visual loss, and cranial nerve, neurological, and endocrine dysfunction seen here (Fig. 195-1).[1]

Anatomy

The optic chiasm, a flattened structure, is situated about 10mm above the pituitary gland, which rests in the sella turcica of the sphenoid bone.[2] These structures are separated by a space called the suprasellar or inferior chiasmatic cistern. The chiasm also is contiguous with the anterior–inferior floor of the third ventricle at the base of the brain. The intracranial optic nerves and chiasm exit from the optic foramen and rise with a tilt of as much as 45°. Although the chiasm usually hangs directly over the pituitary fossa of the sella turcica, as a result of variations in the lengths of the optic nerves, the chiasm overlies the chiasmatic sulcus or the tuberculum sellae in 5% and 12% of cases, respectively (prefixed chiasm), and the dorsum sellae in about 4% of

cases (postfixed chiasm) (Fig. 195-2).[3,4] The pituitary infundibulum, which arises from the hypothalamus (ventral diencephalon) behind the chiasm, extends downward to the posterior lobe of the pituitary (neurohypophysis). The anterior lobe of the pituitary (adenohypophysis) forms embryologically from Rathke's pouch, an embryological structure connected to the pharynx. The chiasm is flanked laterally by the supraclinoid segments of the carotid arteries and inferolaterally by the cavernous sinuses (Fig. 195-3).[5] The arterial supply of the chiasm is derived from the anterior cerebral and communicating arteries from above and the posterior communicating, posterior cerebral, and basilar arteries from below as the chiasm passes through the circle of Willis (Fig. 195-4).[6,7]

Although noted by Michel as early as 1887, Hermann Wilbrand described in several publications starting in 1904 a group of crossing, inferior nasal quadrant, extramacular ganglion cell axons that loop anteriorly into the posterior portion of the contralateral optic nerve before they turn posteriorly and laterally to head into the optic tract (Wilbrand's knee).[8] In the early 1960s, Hoyt[9-11] and Luis[9,10] confirmed, in the primate chiasm, the presence of Wilbrand's knee and also demonstrated that the arrangement of axons within the optic chiasm is such that superior nasal quadrant retinal fibers remain superior and cross more posteriorly in the chiasm, that macular fibers cross through the chiasm in its central and posterior portions, and that arcuate fibers maintain their relative superior or inferior position while they pass through the chiasm (Figs. 195-5 to 195-7).

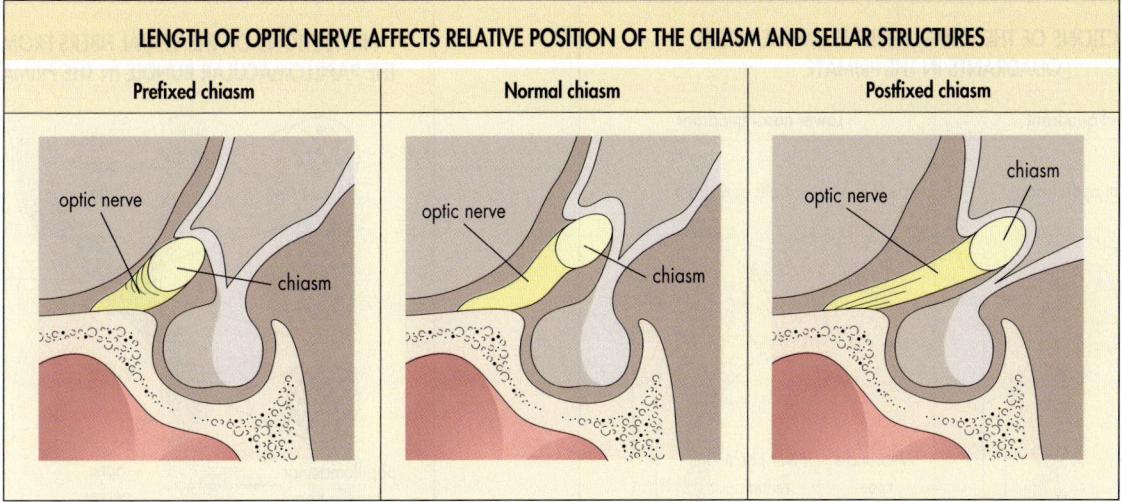

FIG. 195-2 ■ Variation in the length of the optic nerves alters the relative position of the chiasm to the sellar structures. Prefixed chiasm overlies the chiasmatic sulcus or the tuberculum sellae; normal chiasm overlies the diaphragma sellae; postfixed chiasm lies above the dorsum sellae. (Adapted from Rhoton AL, Harris FS, Renn WH. Microsurgical anatomy of the sellar region and cavernous sinus. In: Glaser JS, ed. Neuro-ophthalmology: symposium of the University of Miami and the Bascom Palmer Eye Institute, vol. IX. St Louis: CV Mosby; 1977:75–105.)

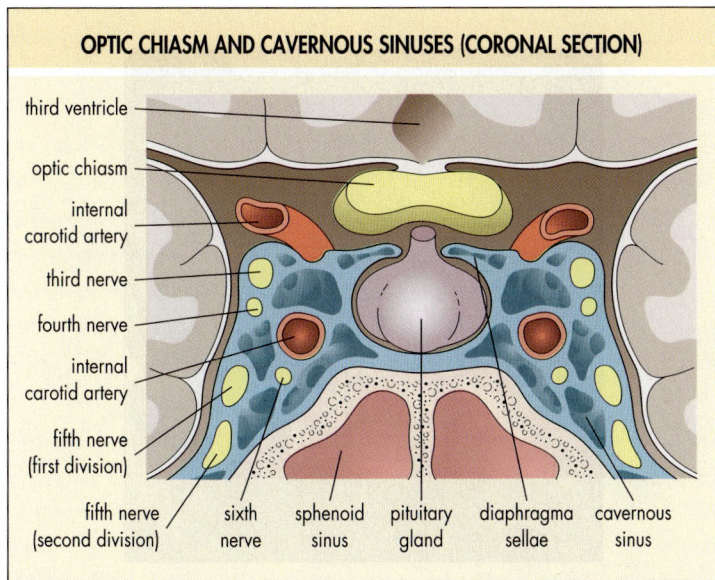

FIG. 195-3 ■ Coronal section through the optic chiasm and cavernous sinuses. The chiasm is flanked laterally by the supraclinoid segments of the carotid arteries and inferolaterally by the cavernous sinuses through which pass the oculomotor nerves and first two divisions of the trigeminal nerve. (Adapted from Warwick R. The orbital vessels. In: Warwick R, ed. Eugene Wolff's anatomy of the eye and orbit, 7th ed. Philadelphia: WB Saunders; 1976:406–17.)

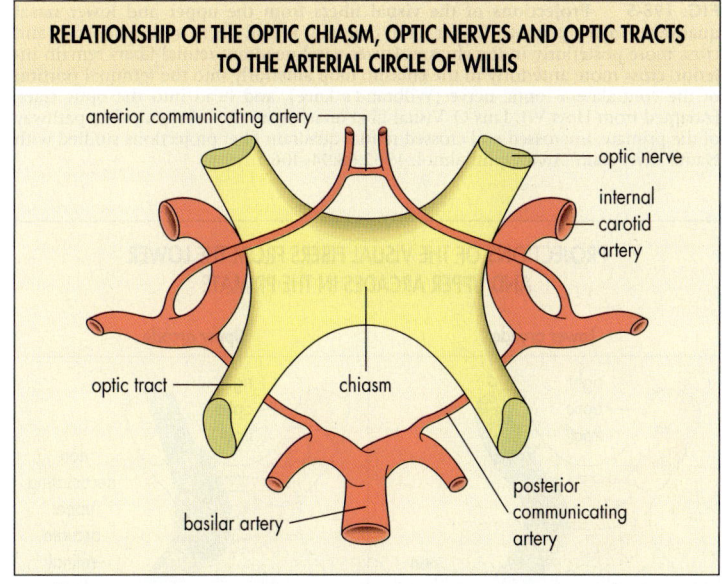

FIG. 195-4 ■ Relationship of the optic chiasm, optic nerves, and optic tracts to the arterial circle of Willis. The chiasm passes through the circle of Willis and receives its arterial supply from the anterior cerebral and communicating arteries from above and the posterior communicating, posterior cerebral, and basilar arteries from below. (Adapted from Reed H, Drance SM. The essentials of perimetry: static and kinetic, second ed. London: Oxford University Press; 1972.)

However, Horton[12] has suggested that Wilbrand's knee is an artifact of the preparations studied.

EPIDEMIOLOGY AND PATHOGENESIS

Pituitary Adenomas

Chiasmal dysfunction most commonly occurs as a result of pituitary adenomas, which make up 12–15% of symptomatic intracranial neoplasms. Although uncommon before the age of 20 years, their incidence becomes increasingly greater after the fourth decade of life. Autopsy studies reveal that the prevalence of asymptomatic pituitary adenomas may be as high as 20–27% and that adenomatous hyperplasia may be found in almost every pituitary gland.[13]

The separation of the chiasm from the pituitary by the suprasellar or inferior chiasmatic cistern enables mild-to-moderate suprasellar extensions of pituitary tumors to occur without resul-

tant chiasmal visual field loss. When chiasmal visual loss is found in the presence of a pituitary tumor, advanced enlargement with expansion of the sella is expected (Fig. 195-8). In contrast to endocrine-inactive pituitary tumors, which are detected when they reach a size that results in visual symptoms, endocrine-active tumors often cause systemic signs and symptoms before they affect the visual pathways.

Pituitary Apoplexy

Sudden enlargement of a pituitary adenoma may result from hemorrhage or infarction (pituitary apoplexy) and typically is associated with acute headache, visual loss, ophthalmoplegia, facial pain, or facial numbness (Fig. 195-9). The normal pituitary gland also may undergo hemorrhagic or nonhemorrhagic infarction, but such episodes generally do not cause visual loss and may go unrecognized until hypopituitarism develops or au-

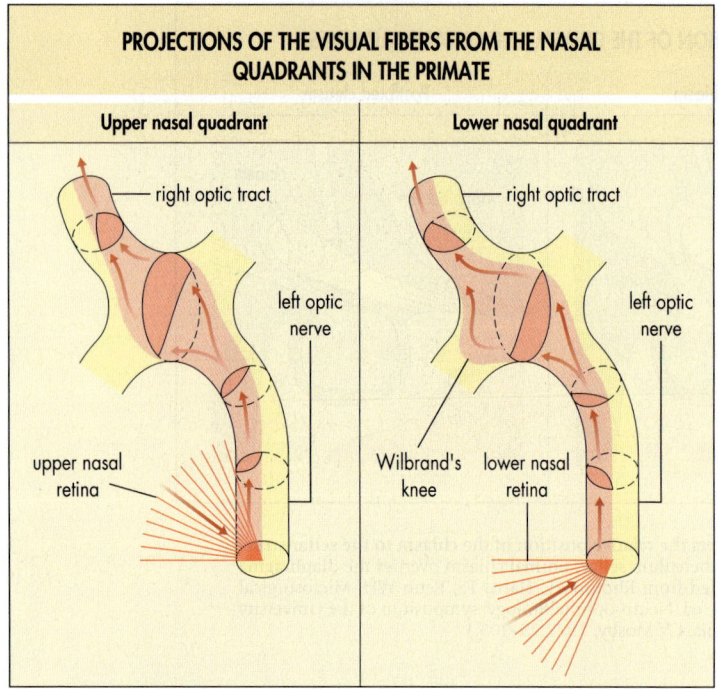

PROJECTIONS OF THE VISUAL FIBERS FROM THE NASAL QUADRANTS IN THE PRIMATE

FIG. 195-5 Projections of the visual fibers from the upper and lower nasal quadrants in the primate. Upper nasal quadrant retinal fibers remain superior and cross more posteriorly in the chiasm. Lower nasal quadrant retinal fibers remain inferior, cross more anteriorly in the chiasm, loop anteriorly into the terminal portion of the contralateral optic nerve (Wilbrand's knee), and head into the optic tract. (Adapted from Hoyt WF, Luis O. Visual fiber anatomy in the infrageniculate pathway of the primate: uncrossed and crossed retinal quadrant fiber projections studied with Nauta silver stain. Arch Ophthalmol. 1962;68:94–106.)

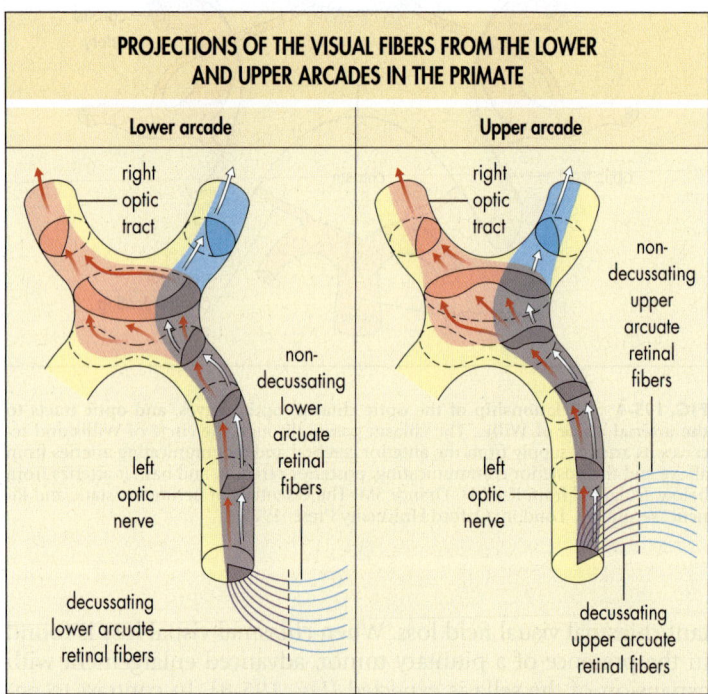

PROJECTIONS OF THE VISUAL FIBERS FROM THE LOWER AND UPPER ARCADES IN THE PRIMATE

FIG. 195-6 Projections of the visual fibers from the lower and upper arcades in the primate. Arcuate fibers maintain their relative superior or inferior positions as they pass through the chiasm. Upper arcuate fibers enter the medial portion of each optic tract and lower arcuate fibers enter the lateral portion of each optic tract. A vertical line through the foveal center divides the nasal decussating from the temporal nondecussating fibers. (Adapted from Hoyt WF. Anatomic considerations of acute scotomata associated with lesions of the optic nerve and chiasm: a Nauta axon degeneration study in the monkey. Bull Johns Hopkins Hosp. 1962;111:57–71.)

topsy is performed. Predisposing factors include pregnancy, estrogen therapy, obstetrical hemorrhage, diabetes mellitus, bleeding disorders, long-term anticoagulation, blood dyscrasias, radiation therapy, trauma, angiography, atheromatous emboli, cardiac surgery, coughing, positive pressure ventilation, and vasoactive agents.

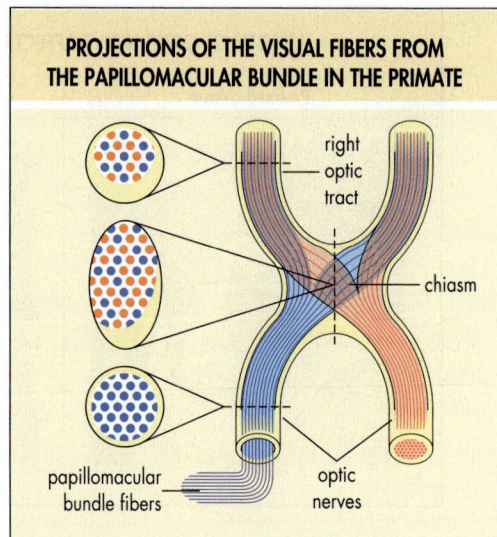

PROJECTIONS OF THE VISUAL FIBERS FROM THE PAPILLOMACULAR BUNDLE IN THE PRIMATE

FIG. 195-7 Projections of the visual fibers from the papillomacular bundle in the primate. Macular fibers crossing through the chiasm do so in its central and posterior portions. (Adapted from Hoyt WF, Luis O. The primate chiasm: details of visual fiber organization studied by silver impregnation techniques. Arch Ophthalmol. 1963;70:69–85.)

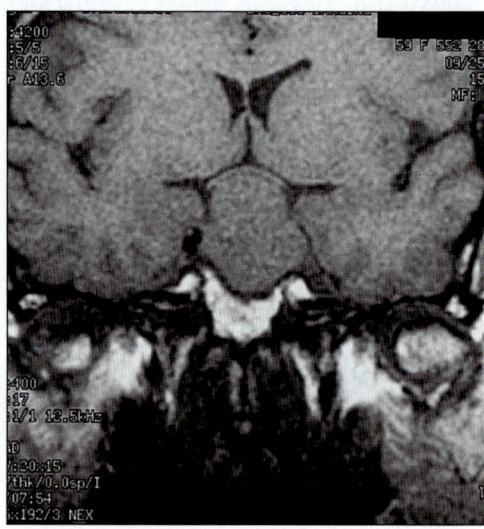

FIG. 195-8 Pituitary adenoma with chiasmal compression. Magnetic resonance scan from a 59-year-old woman who has a bitemporal hemianopia demonstrates a pituitary adenoma that bows the chiasm upward toward the third ventricle. The chiasm is thinned and draped over the mass.

Meningiomas

In 1929, Cushing and Eisenhardt[14] described the syndrome of bitemporal visual field defects and primary optic atrophy that occurred with a normal sella turcica as examined by radiography. This group of findings was associated most often with suprasellar meningiomas and aneurysms, or occasionally with craniopharyngiomas. Suprasellar meningiomas of the sphenoid planum or tuberculum sellae may compress the chiasm from below. Occasionally, the chiasm may be compressed posteriorly by meningiomas that arise from the diaphragma sellae, laterally by medial sphenoid ridge meningiomas, or above by olfactory groove subfrontal meningiomas.

Meningiomas represent 13–18% of all primary intracranial tumors. The incidence of these tumors increases with age. In one study of 464 patients who had meningiomas, 94% were over 30 years of age.[15] In other reports, less than 2% of meningiomas occur in patients under 20 years of age and, in this age group, only 2–4% of primary intracranial neoplasms are meningiomas.[16] Meningiomas that occur in adults are known to occur 2–3 times more frequently in women, but this predilection is not found

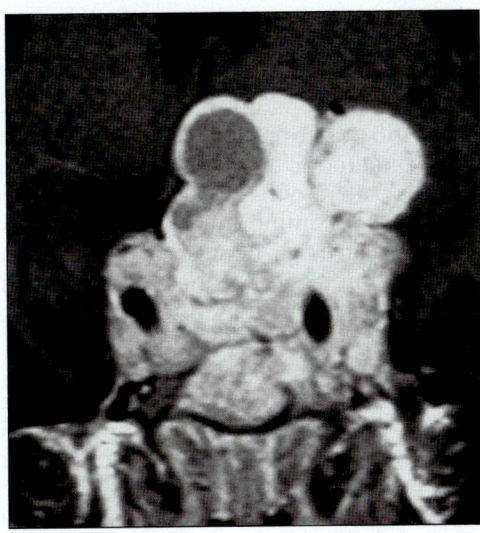

FIG. 195-9 ■ **Pituitary apoplexy (T1-weighted magnetic resonance image).** Pituitary apoplexy in a 19-year-old man who gave a 1-year history of daily epistaxis and headache above the left eye, with more recent left-sided pain in the distribution of the ophthalmic division of the trigeminal nerve. Examination showed left optic neuropathy, temporal field loss of the right eye, and decreased corneal sensation.

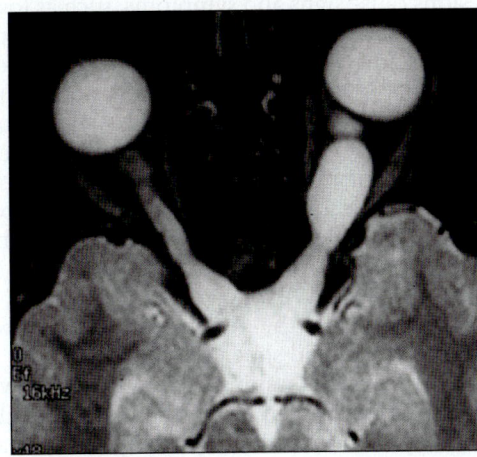

FIG. 195-10 ■ **Glioma of the optic nerve, chiasm, and hypothalamus in a 13-year-old girl.** Invasion of the hypothalamus or third ventricle dramatically increases the mortality rate from this tumor.

with children. Estrogen and progesterone receptors may play a role in the growth of meningiomas.[17]

Von Recklinghausen's neurofibromatosis (NF-1), an autosomal dominant inherited condition, is associated with meningiomas, often more than one in a single patient.[18] Multiple meningiomas have an incidence of 1–2% in most series. Also, cases of familial meningiomas have been reported. Both familial or multiple meningiomas may or may not be associated with von Recklinghausen's syndrome.

Craniopharyngiomas

In children and young adults, embryonic vestigial epithelial remnants of Rathke's pouch between the anterior and posterior lobes of the pituitary may develop into a benign, frequently cystic, tumor called craniopharyngioma. Such congenital tumors may occur at any age but have a bimodal incidence—the first peak occurs during the first two decades of life and the second between 50 and 70 years of age. They account for 2–4% of intracranial neoplasms, 8–13% of pediatric intracranial neoplasms, 20% of suprasellar masses in adults, and 54% of suprasellar masses in children.[19] Suprasellar, intrasellar, and (rarely) intrachiasmal involvement may be seen. Extension into the third ventricle is common and may lead to hydrocephalus. Rare posterior extension has been documented in association with ventral brainstem compression and with cerebellar compression.

Optic Gliomas

Gliomas, also called pilocytic astrocytomas, are not uncommon in the perichiasmal region and account for up to 10% of all intracranial neoplasms in adults and children (Fig. 195-10). Although they may be diagnosed at any age, the majority are diagnosed during the first two decades of life. Women and girls are affected as often as men and boys. Many gliomas that infiltrate the chiasm also involve the hypothalamus. Although most are sporadic, up to one third may be associated with neurofibromatosis type 1.[20,21] Gliomas in adults tend to be more malignant.[22]

Pregnancy

During pregnancy, pituitary adenomas (especially prolactinomas) and suprasellar meningiomas, which are sensitive to increased levels of estrogen and progesterone, may enlarge. In most cases, visual symptoms abate after delivery or abortion. The normal pituitary gland also undergoes modest enlargement, but this enlargement is not enough to cause a chiasmal syndrome.

Lymphocytic adenohypophysitis, an immune-mediated diffuse lymphocytic infiltration of the pituitary gland, has been reported to cause chiasmal compression from suprasellar extension.[23] This uncommon condition has been reported in women only, and over one half of the cases have been found to occur during the perinatal period.

Other Causes of Chiasmal Syndrome

Less common neoplasms that affect the chiasm include chordoma (from the remnants of notochord that become sequestered during development), germinoma, endodermal sinus tumor, leukemia, Hodgkin's and non-Hodgkin's lymphoma, nasopharyngeal carcinoma, and metastatic carcinomas. Non-neoplastic mass lesions that may compress the chiasm include sphenoid sinus mucocele, arachnoid cyst, Rathke's cleft cyst, epidermoid cyst, fibrous dysplasia, histiocytosis X, dolichoectasia of the internal carotid artery, and aneurysm of the large vessels of the circle of Willis or internal carotid artery. Cavernous hemangiomas, arteriovenous malformations, and venous angiomas may compress the chiasm; they frequently hemorrhage into the chiasm and cause chiasmal apoplexy. The chiasm also may be compressed from above when obstructive hydrocephalus leads to an enlarged third ventricle.[24] Extension of the normal subarachnoid space with prolapse and flattening of the chiasm into an enlargement of the sella turcica, known as the *empty sella syndrome*, may be associated with chiasmal dysfunction. As a result of the richly anastomotic blood supply of the chiasm, infarction requires multiple vessel involvement, such as with systemic vasculitis, radiation vasculopathy, or bilateral carotid occlusive disease.[25]

Inflammatory and infectious causes include sarcoidosis, syphilis, other granulomatous diseases, arachnoiditis, abscess, demyelination disease, and lymphoid hypophysitis. Head trauma also may result in a chiasmal syndrome. Postulated mechanisms include tears in the chiasm, contusion necrosis, compression from brain swelling, and delayed hemorrhage. Toxins have been implicated as causes of chiasmal injury, which include direct toxicity from chloramphenicol, isoniazid, ethambutol, hexachlorophene, vincristine, and etchchlorvynol, and hemorrhage associated with ethanol-induced coagulopathy. Congenital chiasmal dysplasia may be found in rare cases.

OCULAR MANIFESTATIONS

Signs and Symptoms of Chiasmal Lesions

Chiasmal lesions cause signs and symptoms, such as loss of vision and visual field, related to involvement of the chiasm itself, its blood supply, the adjacent optic nerve, or the optic tract. Patients who have chiasmal involvement may be unaware of any deficit, may complain of difficulties related to unrecognized loss of their peripheral field, or may complain of unilateral or bilateral central or peripheral visual loss. If a complete bitemporal hemianopia is present, the affected person may experience loss of depth perception at near, the phenomenon of disappearance of an object as the point of fixation moves forward and leaves the object in an area of blindness behind (Fig. 195-11), and "double vision" as a result of overlap or separation of the hemifields associated with a pre-existing phoria, a "hemifield slide" (Fig. 195-12).

Generally, extrinsic mass lesions become apparent with gradually progressive depression of monocular or binocular vision. However, pituitary adenomas, craniopharyngiomas, or aneurysms may cause acute worsening or fluctuations of vision and can be mistaken for optic neuritis.[26-28] Fluctuation of vision over weeks and months also has been described in some cases of meningiomas, and optic disc pallor may be a late finding with these tumors. Response to treatment with systemic corticosteroids may further mimic the clinical picture of retrobulbar optic neuritis.

The pattern of field loss may suggest the presence of a lesion and further help to localize it (Fig. 195-13). Compression of the anterior angle of the chiasm may cause a junctional scotoma, which is a central scotoma, or blindness moves in one eye plus a contralateral superotemporal defect. Hemianopic arcuate scotomas also may indicate early anterior chiasmal compression. Compression of the body of the chiasm from below, because of pituitary adenoma, for example, generally causes a bitemporal superior quadrantanopia or bitemporal hemianopia. Huber[29] noted that the visual loss associated with sellar meningiomas

was more likely to be monocular or markedly asymmetrical if bilateral. Bitemporal inferior quadrantanopia or bitemporal hemianopia occurs with compression of the body of the chiasm from above, because of craniopharyngioma, for example. Compression of the posterior chiasm and its decussating nasal fibers may cause bitemporal hemianopic scotomas, but Traquair suggested that this pattern of field loss also may denote a rapidly growing tumor.[30] Less commonly, lateral compression of the margins of the chiasm (e.g., because of dolichoectasia of the carotid siphon or compression of the chiasm into lateral structures) may cause a nasal or binasal hemianopia. Regardless of the pattern, respect for the vertical midline is a feature that helps differentiate true chiasmal field patterns from other causes.

Because the chiasm is composed of the axons of retinal ganglion cells, chronic involvement (>6 weeks) of the chiasm often leads to nerve fiber layer defects or optic atrophy. When the body of the chiasm is involved, a temporal or "bow-tie" pattern, which corresponds to retinal fibers that originate nasal to the fovea, may occur (Fig. 195-14). However, this appearance often is not apparent, because nondecussating fibers frequently are damaged, as well, particularly with compressive lesions. Optic atrophy also may be a late sign of chiasmal compression and is associated with a poorer postoperative visual acuity.

Signs and Symptoms of Parachiasmal Lesions

Parachiasmal involvement manifests with abnormalities of ocular motility, pupillary function, or facial sensation from injury to cranial nerves III, IV, V1, V2, or VI or the ocular sympathetic nerves in the parachiasmal region. Injury to these structures within the cavernous sinus may be associated with complaints of diplopia, ptosis, unequal pupil size, accommodative difficulty, facial pain or numbness, or eye pain. Signs include ocular motor nerve palsies, decreased sensation in the areas innervated by the first and second divisions of the trigeminal nerve, or Horner's syndrome. Multiple cranial nerve involvement is more suggestive of invasive malignant tumors.

Lesions that block the normal cerebrospinal fluid circulation by obstruction of the foramen of Monro may result in hydrocephalus. Ocular examination may reveal vertical gaze abnormalities, convergence retraction nystagmus, pupillary light–near dissociation, and papilledema.

An unusual form of dissociated nystagmus called *see-saw nystagmus* occasionally accompanies mass lesions in the chiasmal re-

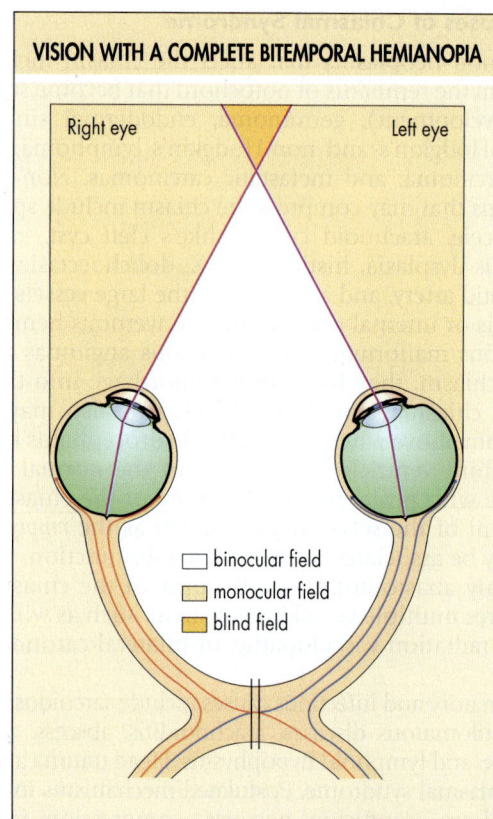

FIG. 195-11 ■ **Vision with a complete bitemporal hemianopia.** Relative to the point of fixation is a triangular region of blindness behind, a triangular region of binocular vision in front, and regions of monocular vision to each side. As a result, an object may disappear as the point of fixation moves forward and leaves the object in an area of blindness behind. (Adapted from Kirkham TH. The ocular symptomatology of pituitary tumors. Proc R Soc Med. 1972;65:517–8.)

VISION WITH A COMPLETE BITEMPORAL HEMIANOPIA

Right eye — Left eye

□ binocular field
■ monocular field
■ blind field

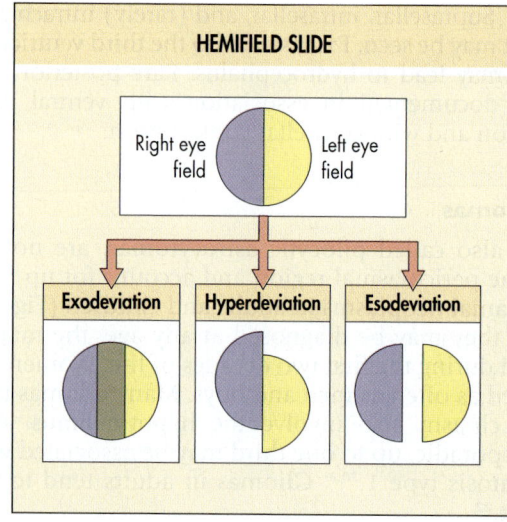

HEMIFIELD SLIDE

Right eye field — Left eye field

Exodeviation — Hyperdeviation — Esodeviation

FIG. 195-12 ■ **Phenomenon of "hemifield slide."** In patients affected by a complete bitemporal hemianopia, preexisting phorias may result in separation of the hemifields vertically (hyperdeviation) or horizontally (esodeviation), or in double vision if the intact nasal hemifields overlap (exodeviation). (Adapted from Kirkham TH. The ocular symptomatology of pituitary tumors. Proc R Soc Med. 1972;65:517–8.)

gion and diencephalon. Also, it may be seen transiently immediately after brainstem stroke, subsequent to severe head trauma after a delay of weeks to months, or as a variant of congenital nystagmus. See-saw nystagmus manifests as alternating intorsion and elevation of one eye with extortion and depression of the fellow eye and may result in complaints of oscillopsia. It ceases when the eyes are closed and does not occur in blind patients, which suggests a role for vision in its pathogenesis. A lesion that involves the interstitial nucleus of Cajal and its connections, or damage to the ocular counter-rolling mechanism mediated by the inferior olivary nucleus, has been postulated.

Chiasmal gliomas in young children have been reported to cause nystagmus, which may be the initial sign of chiasmal or parachiasmal involvement. The nystagmus, which is usually pendular and asymmetrical, may mimic spasmus nutans (even head nodding).

DIAGNOSIS

Visual Field Testing

The primary role of the clinician in the diagnosis of chiasmal disorders is to assess visual function accurately, interpret the results correctly and, thus, localize the region of anatomy affected. Visual field tests may provide a strong indication of direct chiasmal involvement, and failure to perform and properly interpret visual field tests is a common cause for delay in the diagnosis of chiasmal disorders. The technique is to establish that the vertical midline forms the border of the field depression and so rule out nonchiasmal temporal field loss that does not respect the vertical midline. Although a peripheral hemianopic step along the vertical midline is characteristic, early chiasmal compression often lacks a clear vertical step. Most often, temporal paracentral depression occurs because the chiasm has macular projections through most areas. A good strategy to establish a field defect attributable to chiasmal disease is to test either a single central isopter or static threshold sensitivity within the central 15–20° from fixation and to compare changes in color perception as colored objects pass across the vertical midline through central fixation.

Neuroimaging

Prompt magnetic resonance imaging (MRI) is indicated for the patient who has symptoms or signs referable to the chiasm or parachiasmal region (see Figs. 195-8 to 195-10) and is the study of choice for most sellar and parasellar lesions, but high-resolution computed tomography (CT) with fine cuts (1.5–3mm) of axial and coronal views is an acceptable alternative. Both modalities provide about equivalent ability to detect lesions in the parachiasmal regions. The advantages of MRI are a better definition of the anatomical relationships to surrounding structures, the absence of artifacts from bone, and the ability to provide axial, coronal, and sagittal views without special image reconstruction. However, CT provides superior abilities in the detection of tumoral calcifications, of bony erosion and destruction by meningiomas and craniopharyngiomas, and of hyperostosis from meningiomas. Intravenous contrast and enhancement agents, such as paramagnetic gadolinium–pentetic acid for MRI and radiopaque iodine for CT, are used to demonstrate lesions that may not be visualized on noncontrast studies.

Other Diagnostic Testing

Complete endocrinological evaluation is obtained in the evaluation of lesions that involve the pituitary–hypothalamic axis. Lumbar puncture also may be required if an inflammatory or infectious cause is suspected. Magnetic resonance angiography or cerebral angiography may be indicated when vascular causes or cavernous sinus invasion are suspected, or to further characterize or delineate mass lesions and their blood supply. The current sensitivity of MRI or CT often obviates the need for angiography. Some clinicians still use arteriography to absolutely rule out a suprasellar aneurysm or to define the position of the carotid arteries prior to surgery. However, transsphenoidal resections of pituitary tumors usually are accomplished safely without prior angiography.

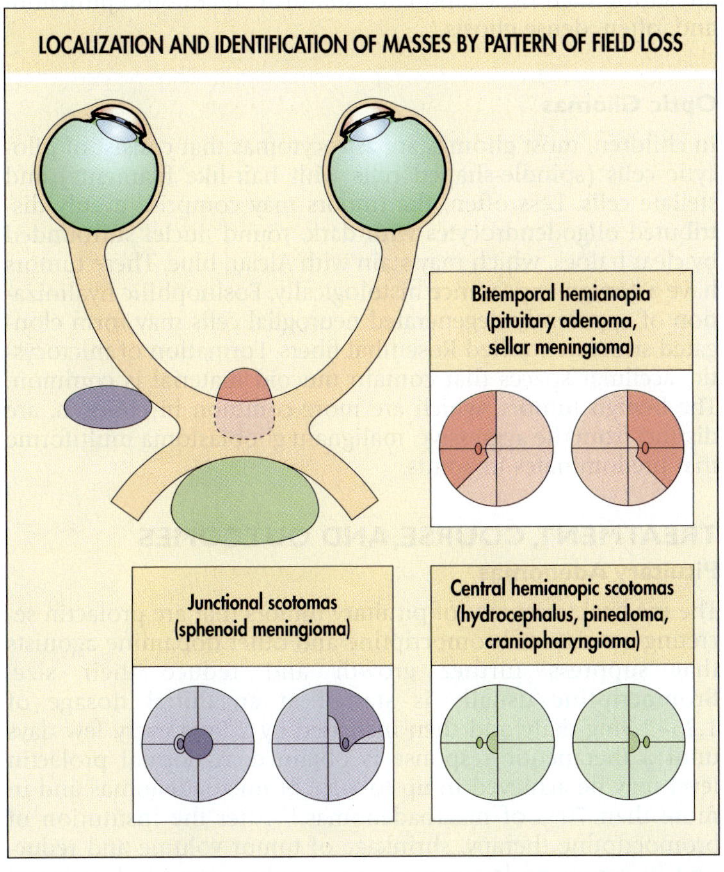

LOCALIZATION AND IDENTIFICATION OF MASSES BY PATTERN OF FIELD LOSS

Bitemporal hemianopia
(pituitary adenoma, sellar meningioma)

Junctional scotomas
(sphenoid meningioma)

Central hemianopic scotomas
(hydrocephalus, pinealoma, craniopharyngioma)

FIG. 195-13 ■ **Localization and probable identification of masses by pattern of field loss.** Junctional scotomas occur with compression of the anterior angle of the chiasm (sphenoid meningioma). Bitemporal hemianopia results from compression of the body of the chiasm from below (e.g., because of pituitary adenoma, sellar meningioma). Compression of the posterior chiasm and its decussating nasal fibers may cause central bitemporal hemianopic scotomas (e.g., because of hydrocephalus, pinealoma, craniopharyngioma).

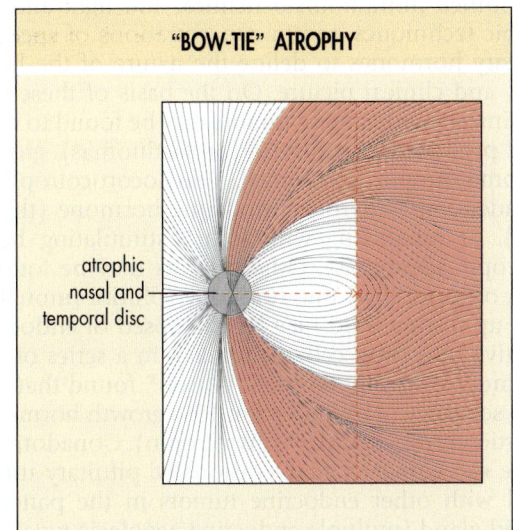

"BOW-TIE" ATROPHY

atrophic nasal and temporal disc

FIG. 195-14 ■ **"Bow-tie" atrophy.** Chronic compression of the decussating visual fibers of the chiasm leads to atrophy of the corresponding nasal retinal nerve fibers that enter the optic disc nasally and temporally. At the disc, this atrophy appears in a bow-tie pattern.

DIFFERENTIAL DIAGNOSIS

Several conditions may mimic the visual field defects associated with chiasmal syndromes. Retinal conditions (such as nasal sector retinitis pigmentosa), optic disc anomalies (such as tilted optic discs), and papilledema with greatly enlarged blind spots may cause bilateral temporal field loss. Bilateral centrocecal scotomas caused by bilateral optic nerve disease may be difficult to differentiate from posterior chiasmal compression that affects the macular projections unless careful attention is paid to the vertical midline. Visual obstruction from overhanging redundant lid tissue, refractive scotomas, psychogenic visual loss, and test artifacts also may simulate chiasmal field patterns.

SYSTEMIC ASSOCIATIONS

Headache, usually frontal in location, frequently accompanies pituitary adenomas, pituitary apoplexy, and meningiomas and may be attributable to a stretched diaphragma sellae. Also, lesions that block normal cerebrospinal fluid circulation may lead to headache, gait difficulties, somnolence and, eventually, urinary incontinence (as a result of hydrocephalus). Abnormalities of pituitary endocrine dysfunction caused by disruption of the hypothalamic–pituitary axis or pituitary adenomas may lead to hypopituitarism, changes in hand or foot size because of acromegaly, amenorrhea–galactorrhea in women, impotence in men, or changes in body habitus that arise from Cushing's syndrome. Hypothalamic dysfunction also may manifest as urinary frequency as a result of diabetes insipidus, heat or cold intolerance caused by a disturbance of temperature regulation, behavioral changes, lethargy, decreased libido, or disturbance of appetite. In children, delay or arrest in sexual development, precocious puberty, or infantile emaciation may occur.

PATHOLOGY
Pituitary Adenomas

Adenomas are by far the most common tumors of the pituitary gland, and usually arise as a discrete nodule from the anterior part of the gland, called *adenohypophysis;* they are soft and vary in color from gray–white to pink or red, depending on the degree of vascularity. Necrosis or spontaneous hemorrhage often leads to cystic areas.

For many years, pituitary adenomas were categorized as chromophobic, acidophil, or basophil adenomas with conventional staining methods. Currently, pituitary adenomas are categorized using combined immunohistochemical and light and electron microscopic techniques, serum concentrations of specific anterior pituitary hormones to define the nature of the hormones produced, and clinical picture. On the basis of these methods and the clinical picture, these tumors may be found to be monohormonal producers of prolactin (prolactinomas), growth hormone (somatotropic adenomas), adrenocorticotropin (corticotropic adenoma), thyroid-stimulating hormone (thyrotropic adenoma), or luteinizing with follicle-stimulating hormones (gonadotropic adenomas). Other tumors may be found to be producers of more than one hormone (plurihormonal adenomas) and up to one third may be composed of endocrinologically inactive cells (null cell adenomas). In a series of 1000 pituitary tumors surgically resected, Wilson[31] found that just over 77% were secretory (41% prolactin, 19% growth hormone, 17% adrenocorticotropin, and 0.2% thyrotropin). Gonadotropic adenomas are exceedingly rare. Occasionally, pituitary tumors are associated with other endocrine tumors in the pancreas and parathyroid gland (multiple endocrine neoplasia type 1).

Meningiomas

Meningiomas probably derive from cap cells that line the outer surface of the arachnoid (where they serve as the interface between the dura and arachnoid) and within the stroma of the choroid plexus. Histologically, meningiomas are categorized into:
- Syncytial tumors, in which the cell borders are indistinct because the cell membranes intertwine extensively
- Transitional tumors composed of plump polygonal cells and concentrically wrapped spindle cells that form whorls
- Fibroblastic meningiomas composed of interlacing bundles of elongated cells that simulate fibroblasts
- Angioblastic meningiomas in which prominent, thin-walled capillaries are found interspersed between the tumor cells

A characteristic feature of many meningiomas, especially those in which whorls are prominent, is the presence of psammoma bodies. These structures contain concentric layers of calcium salts, which appear to be deposited within degenerating whorl cells. Whorls and psammoma bodies, characteristic of transitional meningiomas, also may be found (but to a lesser degree) in fibroblastic meningiomas. Malignant meningiomas are rare and usually show cellular pleomorphism and mitoses. However, tumors that appear histologically benign and show rapid growth, local invasion, and metastasis may be determined malignant on the basis of biological behavior.

Craniopharyngiomas

Craniopharyngiomas may be solid or cystic; the cysts contain an oily fluid, with cholesterol clefts derived from degenerating epithelial cells and keratin. Histologically, the tumor's solid portions may be composed of areas of trabeculae of stratified squamous epithelium supported by a vascularized connective tissue stroma, and of areas of peripheral, basal palisading cells that surround layers of stratified squamous epithelial cells, which may form "horny pearls" of keratinized cells. Calcification and deposition of lamellar bone are found frequently. The tumors are surrounded by a capsule of stratified squamous epithelium and, often, dense gliosis.

Optic Gliomas

In children, most gliomas are astrocytomas that consist of pilocytic cells (spindle-shaped cells with hair-like filaments) and stellate cells. Less often, the tumors may comprise evenly distributed oligodendrocytes with dark, round nuclei surrounded by clear haloes, which may stain with Alcian blue. These tumors have a benign appearance histologically. Eosinophilic hyalinization of apparently degenerated neuroglial cells may form elongated structures, called Rosenthal fibers. Formation of microcystic, acellular spaces that contain mucoid material is common. The benign tumors, which are more common in children, are distinct from the aggressive, malignant glioblastoma multiforme that predominates in adults.

TREATMENT, COURSE, AND OUTCOMES
Pituitary Adenomas

The medical treatment of pituitary tumors that are prolactin secreting consists of bromocriptine and other dopamine agonists that suppress further growth and reduce their size. Bromocriptine usually is started at an initial dosage of 1.25–2.5mg daily and then increased by 2.5mg every few days until a therapeutic response is obtained. A normal prolactin level may be achieved in up to 90% of microadenomas and in more than 70% of macroadenomas.[32] After the institution of bromocriptine therapy, shrinkage of tumor volume and reduction in serum prolactin may occur within days, and maximal shrinkage in tumor size appears to be obtained within 6 weeks. Improvements in visual acuity and field defects may be sustained using bromocriptine therapy in 80–90% of patients.[33] Unfortunately, about 15% of prolactinomas do not respond adequately to bromocriptine, and withdrawal of bromocriptine almost always results in tumor recurrence in those patients who did respond. Complications of bromocriptine therapy are uncommon but include cerebrospinal fluid rhinorrhea and chiasmal herniation.

Adenomas that secrete growth hormones also may respond to bromocriptine, but usually better results are obtained using octreotide, a somatostatin analog. Response rates of about 80% have been reported.[34] Tumors such as corticotropic adenomas and hormonally "inactive" pituitary tumors generally do not respond well to medical interventions.

Symptomatic pituitary tumors that are intolerant, unlikely to respond, or fail to respond to medical therapy usually are treated by surgical resection, most frequently by the transsphenoidal route. For prolactinomas, success rates depend on the initial tumor size and prolactin levels. Of patients with intrasellar microadenomas with prolactin levels under 155ng/ml, 86% were found to have long-term remissions after transsphenoidal surgical removal.[32] Failure to obtain long-term remission after surgery correlates with higher initial prolactin levels, especially over 200ng/ml.[35] Overall, recurrence of prolactinomas and pituitary adenomas that secrete growth hormone was 15% at 1 year after transsphenoidal surgery. Pretreatment with bromocriptine does not seem to improve surgical cure rates, although pretreatment to reduce tumor volume has been found to ease surgical removal. Improvement in vision after surgery may be delayed, and final visual outcome is not determined until 10 weeks postoperatively. Improvement does not usually extend beyond 3–4 months.

For patients who have prolactinomas and who become pregnant or intend to become pregnant, tumor growth must be anticipated. Options include early transsphenoidal resection if visual field loss is threatened or close observation of visual fields with resection of the tumor if visual field loss is found. Bromocriptine therapy is not recommended during pregnancy.

Incompletely resected tumors and those unresponsive to hormone therapy are considered for postoperative radiation therapy. Fractions must not exceed 200cGy daily because of the increased incidence of radionecrosis. Extensive extrasellar extensions usually are treated with surgical decompression followed by irradiation of residual tumor, because a 40% incidence of microscopic dural invasion makes complete resections difficult or impossible to obtain with surgery alone.[36] Patients who have pituitary adenomas that do not immediately threaten vision may be considered candidates for stereotactic radiosurgery, such as with proton beam, cobalt-60 gamma knife, or linear accelerator therapy.[37] Although endocrine deficit commonly is associated with these modalities, other complications are infrequent and tumor recurrence is rare.

Pituitary Apoplexy

Pituitary apoplexy, which may be life-threatening, is treated with high-dose systemic corticosteroids (e.g., dexamethasone 6–12mg every 6 hours) and hormone replacement, and may require medical management of either diabetes insipidus or inappropriate antidiuretic hormone secretion. If rapid visual loss occurs, decrease in level of consciousness, or no improvement within 24–48 hours, transsphenoidal decompression of the sella is indicated. Ischemic necrosis of the pituitary associated with apoplexy may lead to hypopituitarism. This scenario occurs commonly during the partum and postpartum periods (Sheehan's syndrome). Most patients who have apoplexy require subsequent hormone replacement for pituitary insufficiency.

Meningiomas

The preferred management of meningiomas that involve the intracranial optic nerves and chiasm is surgical removal.[38] Surgical debulking alone, radiation therapy alone, or combination therapy may be performed if vital structures are surrounded densely by tumor. Postoperative radiation therapy of incompletely resected tumors appears to extend the period to tumor recurrence. However, because the tumors grow slowly and this treatment carries the risk of radiation vasculopathy, adjunctive radiation therapy is used only in cases in which progression follows incomplete resection. Another option in some patients includes hormone therapy using the progesterone antagonist mifepristone, which has resulted in reduced tumor size as shown by neuroimaging or improved visual fields in 5 of 14 patients.[39]

Location of the tumor and duration of visual symptoms are the most important predictors of visual recovery after surgical removal. Meningiomas of the tuberculum sellae generally are completely resectable and usually show visual recovery, whereas complete removal of sphenoid wing or diaphragma sellae tumors is most unlikely and visual improvement usually is not achieved. Complete gross excision alone does not rule out recurrence. One study showed a 19% 5-year probability of recurrence or progression of parasellar meningiomas despite "complete excision."[40]

Craniopharyngiomas

The preferred treatment of craniopharyngiomas remains controversial. Although surgical resection of craniopharyngiomas usually is approached using craniotomy, subdiaphragmatic and cystic craniopharyngiomas may be approached transsphenoidally. Intracavitary placement of radioactive or chemotherapeutic agents, including phosphorus-32 colloid, yttrium-90 colloid, or bleomycin, within cystic tumors, has been attempted with some success.[41] Cystic tumors have a reputation of being particularly difficult to manage.

Recurrence is frequent with craniopharyngiomas and usually occurs during the first 2 years. Aggressive resections may delay recurrences but lead to greater mortality, as well as visual, endocrine, and neurological morbidity. A review of the ambitious attempts at complete surgical removal showed a 25% operative mortality, a 71% 11-year mortality, and residual tumor in over 75% of those autopsied.[42] Adjunctive radiation therapy improved median survival after extensive subtotal resection from about 3 years to more than 10 years and may achieve remission rates greater than 90%.[43,44] However, adjunctive irradiation is reserved for patients over 5 years of age because of the complications of severe intellectual impairment and profound growth retardation that occur in children.

Visual recovery occurs in only 50% of patients after tumor resection, and the recovery seen within the first month is all that is expected. Lifelong endocrine replacement is expected in most patients after surgery or radiation therapy or both.[45]

Optic Gliomas

The treatment of optic chiasmatic–hypothalamic gliomas has been controversial.[46,47] Patients with gliomas that involve the chiasm alone have a mortality of 28% because of the eventual involvement of the hypothalamus or third ventricle.[46] Invasion of the hypothalamus or third ventricle dramatically increases the mortality rate to more than 50% over 15 years (see Fig. 195-10).[46] Surgical intervention does not constitute a definitive treatment for these tumors once there is chiasmal or hypothalamic involvement and may be associated with significant visual morbidity and potential mortality. However, studies have shown benefit from tumor resection in those who have demonstrated rapid expansion of the suprasellar mass with visual deterioration or progressive neurological deficits.[47,48] Shunting procedures are of clear benefit when hydrocephalus is present, and hormone replacement is indicated when endocrine dysfunction occurs. Chemotherapy for progressive chiasmal gliomas has shown promise and in children offers a safer alternative to radiotherapy.[49] Radiotherapy may be considered in children over the age of 5 years if progression occurs and chemotherapy has been ineffective.

REFERENCES

1. Sadun AA, Rubin RM. Developments in sensory neuro-ophthalmology. In: Silverstone B, Lang MA, Rosenthal B, Faye EE, eds. The Lighthouse handbook on vision impairment and rehabilitation. New York: Oxford University Press; 2000:175–96.
2. Hoyt WF. Correlative functional anatomy of the optic chiasm—1969. Clin Neurosurg. 1970;17:189–208.
3. Rhoton AL, Harris FS, Renn WH. Microsurgical anatomy of the sellar region and cavernous sinus. In: Glaser JS, ed. Neuro-ophthalmology: symposium of the University of Miami and the Bascom Palmer Eye Institute, vol. IX. St Louis: CV Mosby; 1977:75–105.
4. Bergland RM, Ray BS, Torack RM. Anatomical variations in the pituitary gland and adjacent structures in 225 autopsy cases. J Neurosurg. 1968;28:93–9.
5. Warwick R. The orbital vessels. In: Warwick R, ed. Eugene Wolff's anatomy of the eye and orbit, seventh ed. Philadelphia: WB Saunders; 1976:406–17.
6. Reed H, Drance SM. The essentials of perimetry: static and kinetic, second ed. London: Oxford University Press; 1972.
7. Wollschlaeger P, Wollschlaeger G, Ide C, et al. Arterial blood supply of the human optic chiasm and surrounding structures. Ann Ophthalmol. 1971;3:862–9.
8. Wilbrand HL. Schema des verlaufs der sehnervenfasern durch das chiasma. Ztschr F Augenh. 1926;59:135–44.
9. Hoyt WF, Luis O. Visual fiber anatomy in the infrageniculate pathway of the primate: uncrossed and crossed retinal quadrant fiber projections studied with Nauta silver stain. Arch Ophthalmol. 1962;68:94–106.
10. Hoyt WF. Anatomic considerations of acute scotomata associated with lesions of the optic nerve and chiasm: a Nauta axon degeneration study in the monkey. Bull Johns Hopkins Hosp. 1962;111:57–71.
11. Hoyt WF, Luis O. The primate chiasm: details of visual fiber organization studied by silver impregnation techniques. Arch Ophthalmol. 1963;70:69–85.
12. Horton JC. Wilbrand's knee 1904–1995 RIP. Paper presented at Update in Neuro-ophthalmology meeting; 1995; San Francisco.
13. Burrow GN, Wortzman G, Rewcastle NB, et al. Microadenomas of the pituitary and abnormal sellar tomograms in an unselected autopsy service. N Engl J Med. 1981;304:156–8.
14. Cushing H, Eisenhardt L. Meningiomas arising from the tuberculum sellae with the syndrome of primary optic atrophy and bitemporal field defects combined with a normal sella turcica in a middle-aged person. Arch Ophthalmol. 1929;1:1–41,166–205.
15. Lumenta CB, Schirmer M. The incidence of brain tumors: a retrospective study. Clin Neuropharmacol. 1984;7:332–7.
16. Schulte FJ. Intracranial tumors in childhood: concepts of treatment and prognosis. Neuropediatrics. 1984;15:3–12.
17. Yu ZY, Wrange O, Haglund B, et al. Estrogen and progesterone receptors in intracranial meningiomas. J Steroid Biochem. 1982;16:451–6.
18. Battersby RD, Ironside JW, Maltby EL. Inherited multiple meningiomas: a clinical, pathological and cytogenetic study of an affected family. J Neurol Neurosurg Psychiatry. 1986;49:362–8.
19. Koos WT, Miller MH. Intracranial tumors of infants and children. Stuttgart: George Thieme; 1971:415.
20. Janss AJ, Grundy R, Cnaan A, et al. Optic pathway and hypothalamic/chiasmatic gliomas in children younger than age 5 years with a 6-year follow-up. Cancer. 1995;75:1051–9.
21. Valueza JM, Lohmann F, Dammann O, et al. Analysis of 20 primarily surgically treated chiasmatic–hypothalamic pilocytic astrocytomas. Acta Neurochir. 1994;126:44–50.
22. Taphoorn MJ, de Vries-Knoppert WA, Ponssen H, et al. Malignant optic gliomas in adults: case report. J Neurosurg. 1989;70:277–9.
23. Baskin DS, Townsend JJ, Wilson CB. Lymphocytic adenohypophysitis of pregnancy simulating a pituitary adenoma: a distinct pathological entity. J Neurosurg. 1982;56:148–53.
24. Osher RH, Corbett JJ, Schatz NJ, et al. Neuro-ophthalmological complications of enlargement of the third ventricle. Br J Ophthalmol. 1978;62:536–42.
25. Kirkham TH. The ocular symptomatology of pituitary tumors. Proc R Soc Med. 1972;65:517–8.
26. Senelick RC, Van Dyk HJ. Chromophobe adenoma masquerading as corticosteroid-responsive optic neuritis. Am J Ophthalmol. 1974;78:485–8.
27. Cappaert WE, Kiprov RV. Craniopharyngioma presenting as unilateral central visual loss. Ann Ophthalmol. 1981;13:703–4.
28. Norwood EG, Kline LB, Chandra-Sekar B, et al. Aneurysmal compression of the anterior visual pathways. Neurology. 1986;36:1035–41.
29. Huber A. Eye symptoms in brain tumors. St Louis: CV Mosby; 1961:192.
30. Traquair HM. An introduction to clinical perimetry, fourth ed. St Louis: CV Mosby; 1944.
31. Wilson CB. A decade of pituitary microsurgery. The Herbert Olivecrona lecture. J Neurosurg. 1984;61:814–33.
32. Molitch ME, Elton RL, Blackwell RE, et al. Bromocriptine as primary therapy for prolactin-secreting macroadenomas: results of a prospective multi-center study. J Clin Endocrinol Metab. 1985;60:698–705.
33. Molitch ME. The pituitary. In: Melmed S, ed. Prolactinomas. Boston: Blackwell Scientific; 1995:443–77.
34. Lamberts SWJ. The role of somatostatin in the regulation of anterior pituitary hormone secretion and the use of its analogs in the treatment of human pituitary tumors. Endocrinol Rev. 1988;9:417–36.
35. Barrow DL, Mizuno J, Tindall GT. Management of prolactinomas associated with very high serum prolactin levels. J Neurosurg. 1988;68:554–8.
36. Selman WR, Laws ER Jr, Scheithauer BW, et al. The occurrence of dural invasion of pituitary adenomas. J Neurosurg. 1986;64:402–7.
37. Stephanian E, Lunsford LD, Coffey RJ, et al. Gamma knife surgery for sellar and suprasellar tumors. Neurosurg Clin North Am. 1992;3:207–18.
38. Burde RM, Savino PJ, Trobe JD. Chiasmal visual loss. In: Burde RM, Savino PJ, Trobe JD, eds. Clinical decisions in neuro-ophthalmology, second ed. St Louis: Mosby–Year Book; 1992:74–103.
39. Grunberg SM, Weiss MH, Spitz IM, et al. Treatment of unresectable meningiomas with the antiprogesterone agent mifepristone. J Neurosurg. 1991;74:861–6.
40. Mirimanoff RO, Dosoretz DE, Linggood RM, et al. Meningioma: analysis of recurrence and progression following neurosurgical resection. J Neurosurg. 1985;62:18–24.
41. Anderson DR, Trobe JD, Taren JA, et al. Visual outcome in cystic craniopharyngiomas treated with intracavitary phosphorus-32. Ophthalmology. 1989;96:1786–92.
42. Katz E. Late results of radical excision of craniopharyngiomas in children. J Neurosurg. 1975;42:86–93.
43. Manaka S, Teramoto A, Takakura K. The efficacy of radiotherapy for craniopharyngioma. J Neurosurg. 1985;62:648–56.
44. Baskin DS, Wilson CB. Surgical management of craniopharyngiomas: a review of 74 cases. J Neurosurg. 1986;65:22–7.
45. Repka MX, Miller NR, Miller M. Visual outcome after surgical removal of craniopharyngiomas. Ophthalmology. 1989;96:195–9.
46. Dutton JJ. Gliomas of the anterior visual pathway. Surv Ophthalmol. 1994;38:427–52.
47. Garvey M, Packer RJ. An integrated approach to the treatment of chiasmatic–hypothalamic gliomas. J Neurooncol. 1996;28:167–83.
48. Alshail E, Rutka JT, Becker LE, et al. Optic chiasmatic–hypothalamic glioma. Brain Pathol. 1997;7:799–806.
49. Petronio J, Edwards MS, Prados M, et al. Management of chiasmal and hypothalamic gliomas of infancy and childhood with chemotherapy. J Neurosurg. 1991;74:701–8.

196

Retrochiasmal Pathways, Higher Cortical Function, and Nonorganic Visual Loss

ANDREW W. LAWTON

DEFINITION

- The retrochiasmal pathways consist of parallel streams of information diverted to appropriate areas of the brain for identification, storage, and retrieval.

KEY FEATURES

- Lesions of numerous areas of the brain will produce characteristic interruptions of pathway functions and visual processing.
- Careful analysis of visual fields and function frequently can localize white matter and cortical lesions accurately.
- Because patients with conversion reactions and malingerers may have complaints that mimic those caused by retrochiasmal pathway and cortical injuries, careful evaluation is necessary to avoid unnecessary testing and patient discomfort.

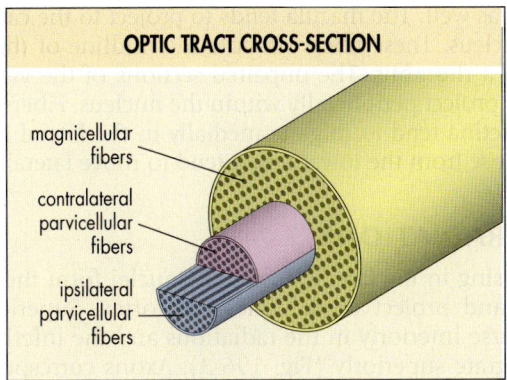

FIG. 196-1 ▌ **Optic tract cross-section.** Note that the parvicellular fibers run centrally and the magnicellular fibers peripherally.

RETROCHIASMAL PATHWAYS AND HIGHER CORTICAL FUNCTION

OPTIC TRACTS

The optic tracts connect the optic chiasm to the lateral geniculate visual nuclei. Although the chiasm sorts information from the right field of each eye to the left visual cortex and vice versa, lesions of the optic tracts tend to produce highly incongruous visual fields.

This disparity manifests in other ways, as well. An injury to an optic tract may yield a relative afferent pupillary defect in the contralateral eye. The primary cause of this phenomenon is the temporal crescent. The temporal visual field is 50% larger than the nasal field of the contralateral eye. Hence the nasal retina produces axons that constitute approximately 55% of the contralateral optic tract.[1]

The optic tracts do not maintain a strict retinotopic architecture as might be expected (Fig. 196-1). Fibers from corresponding parts of the retinas do not pair in the optic tracts. Larger diameter, faster-conducting axons predominate superficially, under the pia. Tracer studies indicate that these fibers correspond to the magnicellular layers in the lateral geniculate nuclei. The parvicellular axons dominate the center of the optic tract, with fibers from the opposite eye running in the deepest, dorsal regions of the tract. The ipsilateral parvicellular fibers sit slightly ventrally. Optic tract axons have achieved this orientation by the time of their arrival during axonogenesis. This disparity in neuronal migration explains the incongruity of optic tract visual field defects.

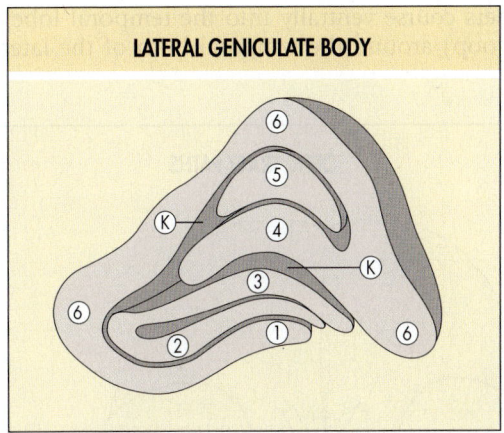

FIG. 196-2 ▌ **Lateral geniculate body section.** The layers are numbered from ventral to dorsal in this posterior view. K fibers travel between the lamellae.

LATERAL GENICULATE BODIES

The lateral geniculate bodies represent the first site at which information from corresponding axons arising from the retinal ganglion cell layers pairs together. Evidence suggests, however, that early embryos do not have this orientation of fibers.[2] The axons must rearrange themselves into regular layers. The retina directs the rearrangement process via generation of electrical impulses even before the system is visually active. These impulses arise from ganglion and amacrine cells prior to the appearance of photoreceptors.

Myelinated nerve fibers divide each lateral geniculate body into six neuronal layers (Fig. 196-2).[3] Traditionally, the layers are numbered ventral to dorsal. Axons from the contralateral eye synapse in layers 1, 4, and 6; axons from the ipsilateral eye synapse in layers 2, 3, and 5.

The layers of the lateral geniculate body may be categorized by neuronal size. Large, magnicellular neurons (M cells) predominate in layers 1 and 2; small, parvicellular neurons (P cells) constitute layers 3–6. At this level, visual processing is divided into at least two parallel pathways. Primate studies indicate, but have not proved, that the parvicellular pathway carries information related to color perception and visual resolution (high spatial frequency contrast sensitivity).[3] The magnicellular pathway apparently contains information that deals with motion detection and lower contrast, lower spatial frequency.

Many authors have challenged the notion of only two parallel pathways.[4] Primate research shows that numerous small neurons (koniocellular or K cells) sit in the interlaminar zones and superficial layers of the lateral geniculate. These cells receive input from both the retina and the region of the superior colliculus. Authors speculate that the koniocellular pathway's role is to modulate information derived from the other two pathways.

The lateral geniculate nuclei are organized by retinotopic visual field loci, as well. The macula tends to project to the caudal 75% of the nucleus. These fibers straddle the midline of the nucleus and form a rhombus. The unpaired sections of the visual fields appear to project peripherally within the nucleus. Fibers from the superior retina tend to migrate medially in the lateral geniculate nuclei; those from the lower retina tend to move laterally.

OPTIC RADIATIONS

Axons arising in the lateral geniculate nuclei form the optic radiations and project to the calcarine cortex. Superior retinal fibers course inferiorly in the radiations and the inferior retinal fibers migrate superiorly (Fig. 196-3). Axons corresponding to central vision travel between the two other bundles.[5]

The fibers from the inferior retina travel deep within the parietal lobe relatively close to the internal capsule and to a tract that carries pursuit information from both occipital lobes to the ipsilateral paramedian pontine reticular formation. The superior retinal fibers course ventrally into the temporal lobe in an arc (Meyer's loop) around the temporal horn of the lateral ventricle.[6] These geographical relationships gain considerable importance in localizing a lesion of the visual pathways.

HIGHER CORTICAL FUNCTION

Information from the optic tracts projects to the calcarine cortices of the medial occipital lobes. This visual cortex performs multiple processing functions to prepare information for detailed analysis elsewhere in the brain.

The occipital cortex involved in primary visual processing straddles the calcarine sulci. Brodmann[7] designated this region as area 17 in his topographical nomenclature; area 17 also is referred to as area V1. The actual surface area of the visual cortex varies in range from 20–25cm[2] and occupies approximately 3.5% of the surface area of the brain. The neurons of area 17 receive information via the myelinated stripe of Gennari, which gives the area its distinctive histology. Information from central vision projects to the caudal half of the visual cortex while that from peripheral vision projects rostrally.

The visual cortex contains multiple identifiable layers of cells. Layer I, the most superficial, contains small granule cells and a few horizontal cells; layer II consists of pyramidal neurons and numerous interneurons; and layer III contains pyramidal and granule cells. Layer IV contains three subdivisions—IV_a consists of stellate neurons, IV_b contains predominantly granule cells, and the deepest stratum, IV_c, contains granule, pyramidal, and stellate cells.[8] Input from the optic tracts tends to terminate in layer IV_c.[9] Layer V contains numerous pyramidal cells. Layer VI demonstrates fewer neurons but stains darkly because of star pyramids.

The calcarine cortex plays less of a role in visual image processing than previously theorized. It appears to be a coordination center, where information from both hemifields is paired into parallel, vertically oriented, ocular dominance columns (Fig. 196-4).[10] Small regions of the visual field are analyzed in the primary visual cortex by an array of complex cellular units called *hypercolumns*. A single hypercolumn represents the neural machinery necessary to analyze a discrete region of the visual field. Each hypercolumn contains a complete set of the orientation columns, which repre-

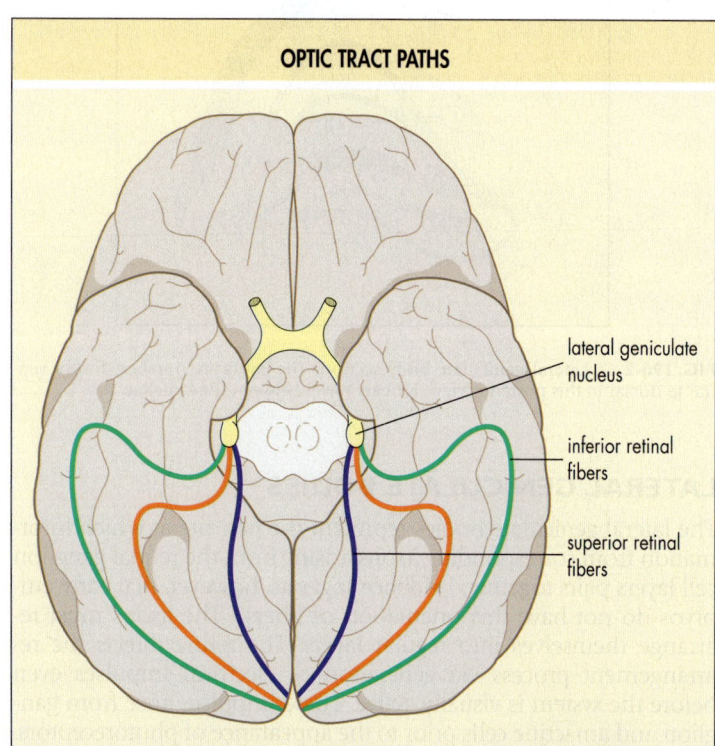

FIG. 196-3 ■ **Optic tract paths.** Fibers that correspond to the inferior retina course rostrally and laterally into the temporal lobes to form Meyer's loops. The superior retinal fibers take a much more direct course through the parietal lobes.

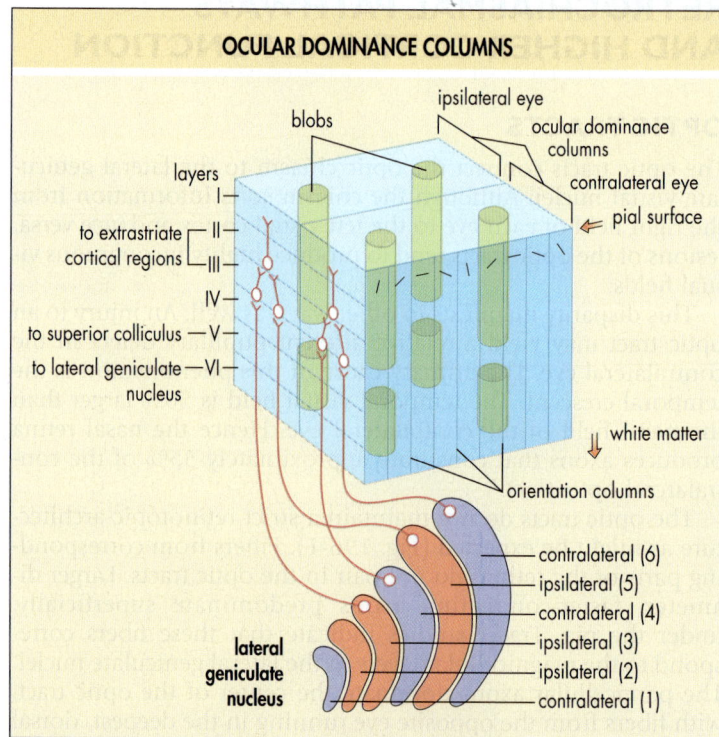

FIG. 196-4 ■ **Ocular dominance columns.** Each ocular dominance column receives input from either the contralateral or ipsilateral eye via projections from cells in individual layers of the lateral geniculate nucleus that serve one or the other eye. (Adapted with permission from Kandel ER, Schwartz JH, Jessell TM. Principles of neural science, ed 3. New York: 1991, McGraw-Hill.)

sents 360°, a set of left and right ocular dominance columns, and several blobs (regions of the cortex in which the cells are specific for color).[11] These hypercolumns merge data from corresponding points in each retina. Because the temporal field (nasal retina) from the contralateral eye is considerably larger than the nasal field (temporal retina) from the ipsilateral eye, each calcarine cortex receives unpaired information from the contralateral eye; this forms the "temporal crescent."[12] This information is processed most anteriorly and represents an important clinical feature critical for the diagnosis and localization of many occipital lobe lesions. Recent evidence suggests that connections between the two hemispheres via the corpus callosum allow synchronization of information generated by both fields; this enables information that arises from both fields to be combined.[13,14]

The visual cortex contains four basic types of cells that respond in specific and characteristic ways to retinal stimuli.[15] *Circularly symmetrical* cells react to small lights independent of movement or orientation. *Simple cells* respond to a moving light or a dark line or pattern with a specific orientation and direction of motion that projects on the center of their field. Simple cells may turn either "on" or "off" in response to the stimulus.

Complex cells respond to linear stimuli almost anywhere in their field but are less specific as to orientation. They also may be "on" or "off" cells. *Hypercomplex cells* are similar to complex cells but require a linear stimulus of a specific length. The information generated among all these cells is synchronized through the extensive interconnection between visual cortical areas (Fig. 196-5).[16] As a result of this exchange of information, certain stimuli in patterns "pop out" and catch an individual's attention, while other details (small gaps in a large pattern especially outside the central 15° or the defect associated with the blind spot) may "fill in" and disappear into the background.[17]

TOPOGRAPHICAL DIAGNOSIS OF RETROCHIASMAL DISEASE

Unfortunately, the anatomy of the visual pathways means that any lesion of these tracts tends to produce some form of homonymous hemianopia. A total homonymous hemianopia involving the temporal crescent is nonlocalizing. In most cases, however, careful examination of the visual field and associated clinical findings yields clues to the location of a lesion.

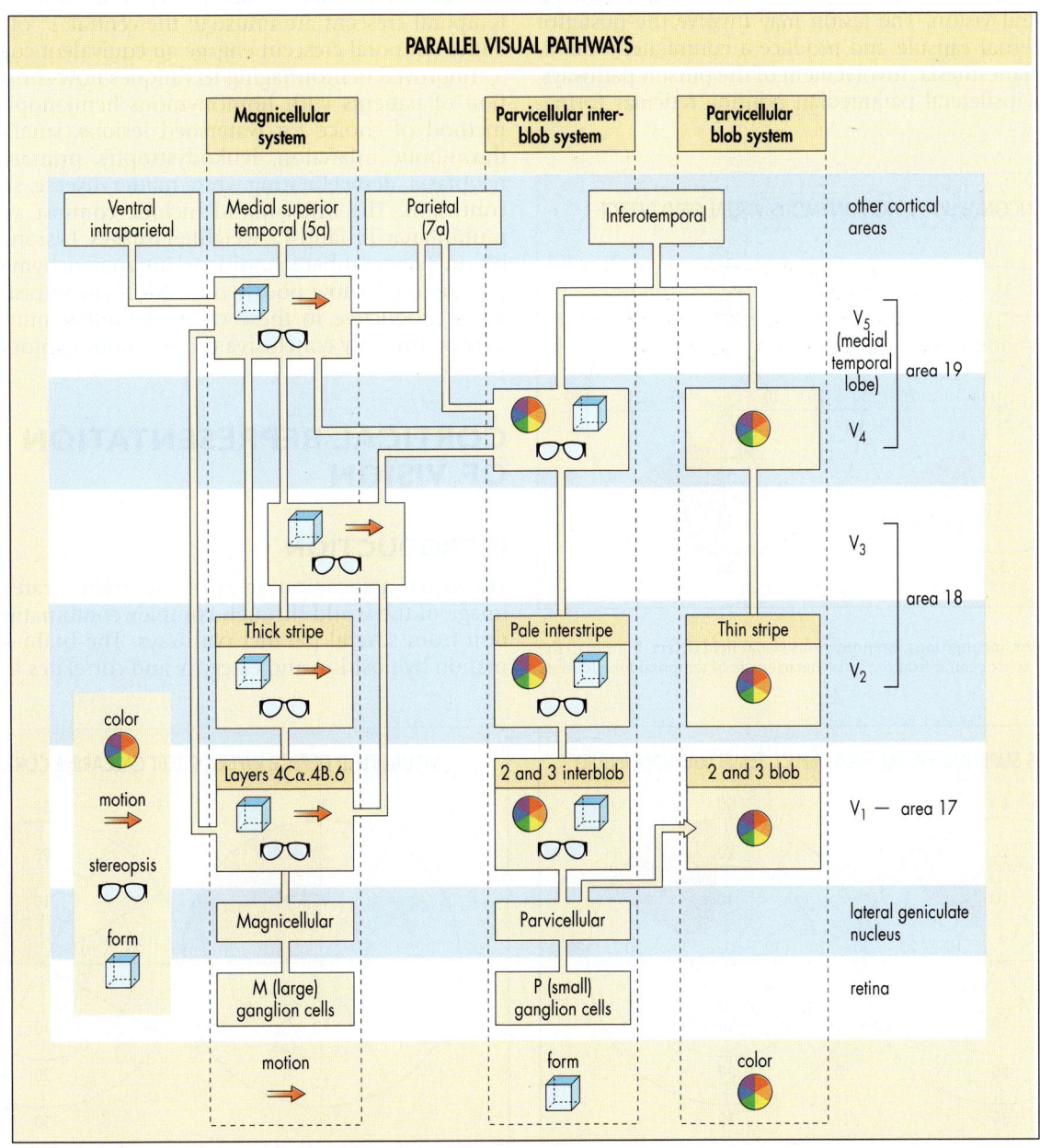

FIG. 196-5 ▮▮ **Parallel visual pathways.** Their suggested functions in the macaque monkey. (Adapted with permission from DeYoe EA, Van Essen DC. *Concurrent processing streams in monkey visual cortex. Trends Neurosci.* 11:219–26, 1988.)

Lesions isolated to the optic tracts account for less than 5% of patients with a homonymous hemianopia.[18] Injury to the optic tracts tends to produce exceedingly incongruous field defects. Because the optic tracts include fibers of the afferent pupillary pathway, patients with optic tract lesions tend to demonstrate a relative afferent pupillary defect in the contralateral eye and, eventually, optic atrophy on one or both sides.[19,20] Patients may demonstrate a larger pupil on the side of the hemianopia (Behr's pupil) or pupillary hemiakinesia (Wernicke's pupil).

Lesions to the lateral geniculate nuclei also tend to produce an incongruous homonymous hemianopia.[21] The vascular supply of the lateral geniculate nucleus may include the adjacent thalamus and corticospinal tracts, which provides additional neurological data to localize a lesion clinically. Because pupillary fibers leave the optic tracts rostral to the lateral geniculate nuclei, lesions here do not produce afferent papillary defects.

Lesions of the deep parietal lobe may involve the superior (superior and peripheral retinal) fibers of the optic radiations. This damage results in a wedge-shaped, inferior, contralateral homonymous hemianopia (Fig. 196-6).[22] Because the optic radiation fibers are still orientating themselves for cortical innervation, the hemianopia is incongruous. Because the macular fibers pass between the parietal and temporal fibers, the defect generally spares central vision. The lesion may involve the posterior limb of the internal capsule and produce a contralateral hemiplegia and hemianesthesia. Involvement of the pursuit pathways, headed for the ipsilateral paramedian pontine reticular formation, tends to result in an alteration of optokinetic nystagmus—the patient cannot pursue stimuli moving toward the side of the lesion and does not generate optokinetic nystagmus in that direction.

Damage to the temporal optic radiations interrupts the inferior (inferior and peripheral retinal) fibers of Meyer's loop.[5] The typical visual field defect is an incongruous, wedge-shaped, superior homonymous hemianopia sparing central vision (Fig. 196-7). Injury to adjacent structures may yield memory loss, hearing loss, and auditory hallucinations.

Lesions of the calcarine cortex tend to be silent other than for visual field defects. These defects tend to be highly congruous (Fig. 196-8).[23] Preservation of the temporal crescent identifies a defect as cortical. Patients may show sparing of central vision (macular sparing); this phenomenon generally results from separate arterial supply between the occipital pole and the rostral calcarine cortex.

Horton and Hoyt[24] mapped the visual cortex in depth by correlating magnetic resonance imaging (MRI) findings and visual dysfunction in patients with occipital lobe lesions. Information from the fovea occupies an extremely large segment of the calcarine cortex; input from the central 10° involves more than 50% of the caudal striate cortex. Hence, lesions that spare only the temporal crescent are unusual; the central 1° of vision and the entire temporal crescent engage an equivalent cortical volume.

Improved neuroimaging techniques now simplify the evaluation of patients with homonymous hemianopia.[25] MRI is the method of choice for watershed lesions, small-vessel disease, thrombotic infarction, leukodystrophy, primary or secondary neoplasia, demyelinating white matter disease, shear injuries, or contusion. The MRI should include contrast and noncontrast multiplanar T1- and T2-weighted images. Lesions dominated by blood (acute subarachnoid or intraparenchymal hemorrhage, for example) show poorly on MRI. Noncontrast CT studies are more productive in these cases. A lumbar puncture, at times, may be the only conclusive tool for finding blood.

INFERIOR, INCONGRUOUS, HOMONYMOUS VISUAL FIELD DEFECT

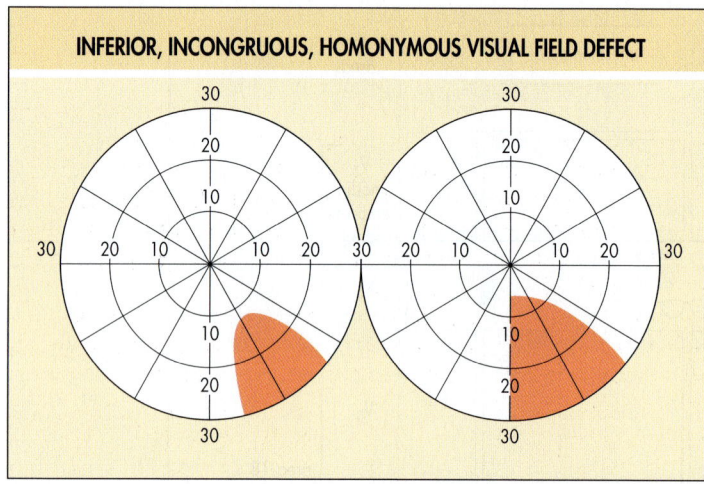

FIG. 196-6 **Inferior, incongruous, homonymous visual field defect.** Injuries to the parietal lobe tend to spare central fixation, as is characteristic of temporal lobe lesions.

INCONGRUOUS SUPERIOR VISUAL FIELD DEFECT, TEMPORAL LOBE INJURY

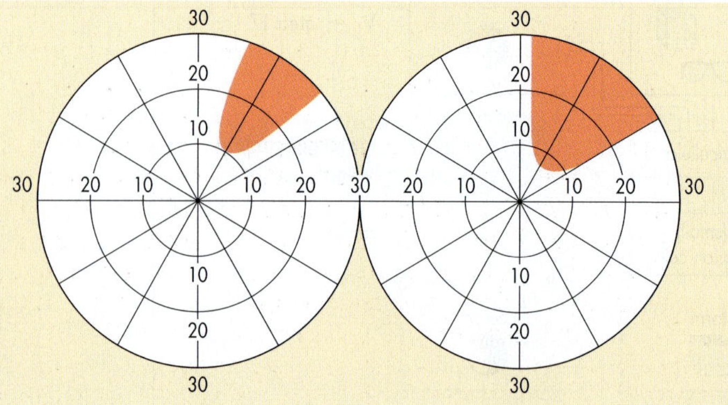

FIG. 196-7 **Visual field defect, temporal lobe injury.** Interruption of this segment of the optic radiations yields an incongruous, superior, homonymous visual field defect, more dense above than below—the "pie-in-the-sky" pattern.

CORTICAL REPRESENTATION OF VISION

INTRODUCTION

The visual association areas of the brain create a recognizable image of the world through complex combinations of information from several parallel pathways. The brain separates information by position and category and correlates this information

VISUAL FIELD DEFECT, INFERIOR LEFT CALCARINE CORTEX LESION

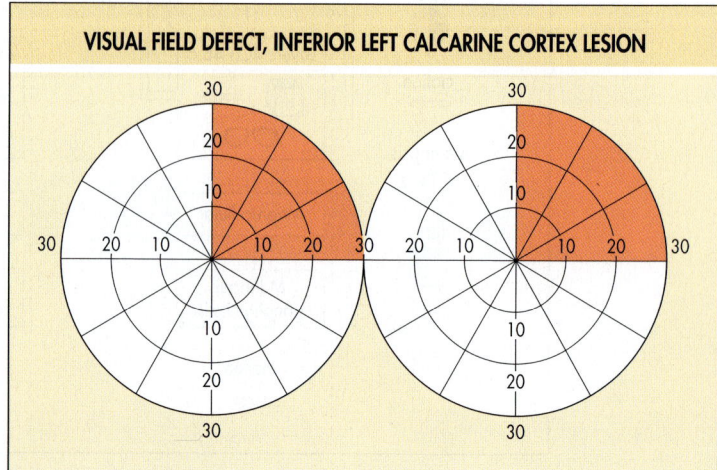

FIG. 196-8 **Visual field defect, inferior left calcarine cortex lesion.** Note the high congruity and involvement of fixation.

with surrounding objects and associated sounds (Fig. 196-9). The brain must maintain a reference library of previously viewed images ready for instantaneous recall. Consider the identification of the human face. An individual views a jogger for the first time wearing a blue shirt and shorts and has a conversation. On the second encounter, the jogger is now sitting, reading a book, and wearing a blue dress. Despite the differences, recognition occurs and creates the expectation of a specific voice and speech pattern. An understanding of the relationship of cortical visual processing pathways enables the recognition of characteristic syndromes by clinical features.

OBJECT IDENTIFICATION AND MEMORY

Identification of an object requires the ability to retain an image in memory and use this image for future comparison. Milner et al.[26] and Goodale[27] describe a patient with visual agnosia. She could identify objects by touch but not by sight. If asked to take an object, however, she could turn her wrist appropriately, open her hand, and grasp the object so that it did not drop. The primary damage appeared to be in her ventrolateral occipital lobes. In contrast, damage to the superior posterior parietal cortex results in difficulty in making the movements needed to manipulate objects despite a preserved ability to describe the objects and their orientation.[28]

One theoretical basis for this separation of function targets visual association areas in the medial occipital lobes.[29] Injury to the right occipital lobe results in failure to identify complex objects (including faces, i.e., prosopagnosia) in general. Apparently, many animals sort out various types of visual stimuli in this area.[30] A lesion in the left occipital lobe yields impairment of recognition of objects with numerous parts, including words.

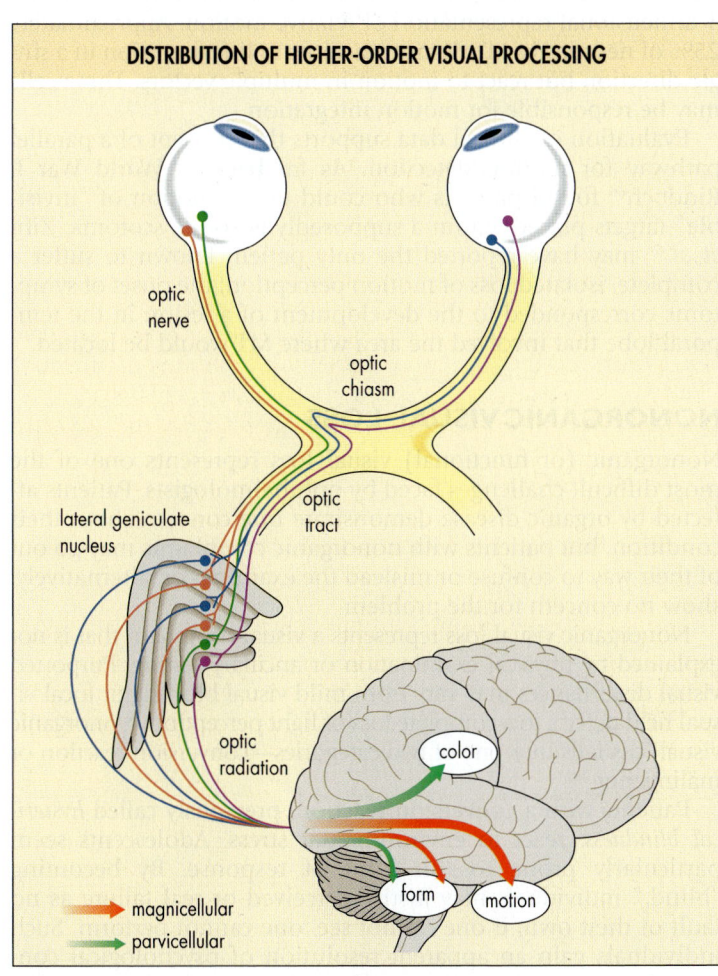

DISTRIBUTION OF HIGHER-ORDER VISUAL PROCESSING

optic nerve

optic chiasm

optic tract

lateral geniculate nucleus

optic radiation

color

form

motion

→ magnicellular
→ parvicellular

FIG. 196-9 ■ **Distribution of higher order visual processing among different cortical areas.** The magnicellular system (inferior stream) is considered generally with the location and motion of objects, while the parvicellular system (superior stream) is concerned with the fine resolution (acuity), form, and color of objects.

A second theory concentrates on the connections among lobes of the brain[31] and postulates that primate brains separate visual information into two streams, dorsal and ventral. The ventral stream originates in the primary visual cortex, projects to the inferotemporal region, and carries information needed to identify objects and their positions in space. The dorsal pathway transmits the information on size, shape, and orientation needed to grasp the object. One stream may be damaged without injuring the other.

The positron emission tomography (PET) scanner has provided assistance in resolution of these two theories. Sargent et al.[32] tested subjects with three separate stimuli—sine wave gratings, male and female faces, and simple objects. Sine wave gratings yielded activity restricted to the striate and extrastriate cortices. Faces stimulated the right parahippocampal region and both fusiform and anterior temporal cortices. Simple objects activated the left occipitotemporal cortex alone. This study tends to support both theories as critical steps in visual processing. Farah[33] provides an excellent synopsis of current theories of image generation.

Lack of image recognition, however, does not mean an individual cannot see an image clearly.[34] Patients with prosopagnosia fail in selecting two matching faces from a picture set. Invert the faces, however, and the patients fare much better. Inverting the face apparently allows the brain to treat faces as simple objects.

When an image is repeated in a series, necessitating the recurrent identification of the same object, the brain adds another region to the loop. The prefrontal cortex becomes active on PET scan during this task.[35] Although long-term memory for vision is a temporal lobe function, short-term visual memory is a frontal lobe function.

The inability to identify objects visually, however, does not necessarily affect a person's generation of a mental image. Despite a deficit in naming seen objects, patients may copy visual objects, generate accurate pictures from the memory of an object, or draw a picture based upon tactile examination of an object.[36–38] Ironically, when shown these drawings, patients do not recognize them as their own.

Stimulation of storage areas may produce accurate visual hallucinations that may occur as a release phenomenon resulting from visual loss[39–41] or abnormal electrical stimulation.[42] Visual hallucinations may result in isolated midbrain injury,[43] although the exact mechanism remains undetermined.

READING AND DYSLEXIA

Reading represents a very specialized form of visual processing. The unimpaired reader can recognize even sloppy and garbled writing. Multiple regions of the brain are involved, and injury to any of these areas produces recognizable syndromes.

The primary center for reading and writing language appears to be in the dominant angular gyrus in the parietal lobe.[44] Alexia (the inability to read) with agraphia (the inability to write) results from destruction of this area; exceptions to this rule do exist. Darius and Boller[45] reported a right-handed patient who suffered a form of alexia with agraphia following a right temporo-occipital hematoma. The patient could copy words but not read them and could not write from dictation or spontaneously. The authors postulated a double disconnection syndrome—alexia from disconnection of the right angular gyrus and occipital association areas by a subcapsular lesion and agraphia from disconnection of semantic stores in the right angular gyrus.

Alexia without agraphia results from disconnection of the dominant angular gyrus from input from both occipital lobes.[46–48] This syndrome most commonly results from an infarct in the distribution of the left posterior cerebral artery.[49]

The association of alexia with damage to the angular gyrus may represent a Western bias. Sakurai et al.[50] reported a patient who had alexia with agraphia for Japanese characters (kanji).

The patient also suffered problems with names. Scans indicated an infarct involving the dominant inferotemporal and fusiform gyri from the temporo-occipital junction to the anterior one third of the temporal lobe. The authors postulated a disconnection of fibers to the parahippocampal region. They suggested that pictographs are processed differently from words composed of letters. They questioned whether a similar lesion might have an impact on reading irregular words in English.

Dyslexia represents a very special form of alexia.[51] By definition, patients with developmental dyslexia have a discrepancy between the acquisition of reading skills and other intellectual abilities, and this disability is not related to environmental conditions, sensory deficits, or acquired neurological disorders.

Investigators have failed to determine a specific site for the origin of developmental dyslexia. Livingstone et al.[52] proposed that developmental dyslexia results from deficiencies and depletion in magnicellular pathways. They reported decreased numbers of magnicellular neurons in the lateral geniculate nuclei from postmortem studies in dyslexic patients. They also identified decreased responses to low spatial–frequency patterns in patients who have developmental dyslexia.

Sadun[53] has challenged this hypothesis. He emphasized the small number of autopsies and amount of clinical material and questioned the statistical significance of any findings of the Livingstone study. The changes seen in the lateral geniculate nuclei may represent a physical abnormality that does not directly cause reading defects but is a secondary finding in patients who have central nervous system anomalies elsewhere. The definitive answer to an anatomical cause of developmental dyslexia awaits further clinical research.

Phonological dyslexia represents a disorder of association between sounds (phonemes) and letters (graphemes). Some evidence now exists that phonological dyslexia may result from abnormal development of the dominant inferior frontal lobe in areas responsible for the development of control for tongue and lip articulator movements.

COLOR PERCEPTION

The pathway for the interpretation of color remains separate from those responsible for object identification.[54] PET scanning findings indicate that the lingual and fusiform gyri become stimulated when a normal individual scans for a colored target.[55–57] Patients who have lesions that cause visual agnosia may maintain the ability to identify the color of objects.[58]

Patients who have acquired, central cerebral achromatopsia (inability to identify colors) may have complete loss or miss only one primary color.[59] The isolation of single color defects links with research performed in macaque monkeys, which showed that an area of prestriate cortex, identified as area V4, contains neurons that respond to specific color stimuli.[60,61]

Patients with cerebral achromatopsia generally describe objects as "washed out" or "faded." Patients still may be able to use contrast clues to separate the edge of one intense color from another. If two colors or a color and a shade of gray match pseudoisochromatically, however, patients demonstrate a distinct inability to isolate colored targets. Despite the achromatopsia, other parts of the parvicellular system may remain intact. Patients may have normal visual acuity and contrast sensitivity. Postmortem and radiological studies of these patients reveal bilateral lesions of the inferior occipital cortex.

INTEGRATION OF VISUAL–AUDITORY SPACE

The brain frequently receives contradictory information from the visual and auditory systems. For example, when an individual watches a movie, an image is seen directly ahead, but sounds are heard from numerous speakers throughout the theater. The brain integrates this information to provide a meaningful and logical integrated experience.

The ability to reconcile auditory and visual cues appears to be learned.[62] This reconciliation is a complicated task, because visual information is received by direct stimulation of an individual retina, while auditory localization requires a binaural triangulation of sound. The complexity heightens when the individual or the target moves.

The brain prioritizes visual input.[63] If a sound seems to originate from a seen object, the brain transfers the perception of that sound to the visible source. The process of correlation occurs in the midbrain tectum.

MOTION DETECTION

Once the brain identifies an object, it must localize that object in relation to the perceiver and the environment, and determine the relative rate of motion of the object to the perceiver. The observer also may be moving, and multiple environmental targets may be moving in different directions. The brain has developed efficient mechanisms to resolve these factors.

The primary step in motion detection involves neurons in area V1 of the calcarine cortex supplied by the magnicellular pathway. Motion-sensitive neurons react to movement in a specific direction.[64] The information from these individual neurons then travels to an area (referred to as *MT* or *V5*) in the medial temporal lobe. In primates, MT sits in the posterior segment of cortex, bordering the superior temporal sulcus. Almost 100% of the neurons in MT demonstrate directional sensitivity. Evidence suggests that MT represents the first area in which the information related to motion becomes attached to a texture, color, or pattern.[65]

Unfortunately, for simplistic views of motion detection, a moving object in the environment generates multiple bits of information in the MT region. Some bits may appear contradictory. The brain must integrate these signals to form one coherent, 3-dimensional representation of relative motion. Approximately 25% of neurons in MT do not react just to linear motion in a single direction but react to motion in multiple vectors. These cells may be responsible for motion integration.

Evaluation of clinical data supports this concept of a parallel pathway for motion detection. As far back as World War I, Riddoch[66] found patients who could detect motion of "invisible" targets placed within a supposedly absolute scotoma. Zihl et al.[67] may have reported the only patient known to suffer a complete, isolated loss of motion perception; the onset of symptoms corresponded to the development of a lesion in the temporal lobe that involved the area where MT would be located.

NONORGANIC VISUAL LOSS

Nonorganic (or functional) visual loss represents one of the most difficult challenges faced by ophthalmologists. Patients affected by organic disease demonstrate true concern about their condition, but patients with nonorganic complaints may go out of their way to confuse or mislead the examiner or, alternatively, show no concern for the problem.

Nonorganic visual loss represents a visual complaint that is not explained by physical examination or ancillary testing. Purported visual disturbances may vary from mild visual blurring or focal visual field defects to a complete loss of light perception. Nonorganic visual loss falls into one of two categories—conversion reaction or malingering.

Patients with a conversion reaction, previously called *hysterical blindness*, react to environmental stress. Adolescents seem particularly prone to this kind of response. By becoming "blind," individuals may justify perceived or real failure as no fault of their own; if one cannot see, one cannot perform. Such individuals gain an apparent resolution of psychological conflict. Because a conversion reaction alleviates tension, patients generally show a flat, relaxed affect despite severe visual complaints. Patients with a conversion reaction appear to honestly believe they are disabled, even when initially confronted with evidence to the contrary. They tend to be cooperative with testing. By cooperating, these patients readily display behavior that contradicts their complaints.

Malingering patients mimic visual loss consciously to obtain an external secondary gain. Their visual complaints appear out of proportion to the underlying original injury. Such patients may seek medical advice at the behest of an attorney and have received coaching in advance. Malingerers pay close attention to the actions of an examiner and try to circumvent tests. Physicians must take great care, because any conclusions may require documentation for a judge and jury.

An accurate visual acuity assessment may not be obtainable for a patient who has nonorganic visual loss. Fortunately, all the examiner must do is to demonstrate that the patient's vision is significantly better than stated.

To evaluate patients who have nonorganic visual loss, the examiner starts with the smallest letters possible, in most cases the 20/10 (6/3) line. The physician should pause at each letter and demonstrate concern and confusion that the patient cannot identify these letters. After making the point that the next letters are much larger, the examiner shifts to the 20/15 (6/4.5) line and repeats the process. By the time the patient looks at the 20/20 (6/6) or 20/25 (6/7.5) line, the power of suggestion has set in and the patient generally is convinced the letters are now large enough to read. This technique works well with complaints of either monocular or binocular visual loss.

A 4-diopter prism is an indispensable tool in the evaluation of the visual acuity of patients who have nonorganic monocular visual complaints. The examiner occludes the patient's "bad" eye, then places the prism over the patient's "good" eye such that the base is up and the apex splits the pupil. If the prism is positioned in just the right spot, the patient experiences monocular vertical diplopia. The examiner asks the patient if both of the perceived lines appear equally clear; the answer will be "yes." Once the patient is certain that this test measures the function of the "good" eye, the tester simultaneously uncovers the "bad" eye and slides the prism downward to cover the "good" eye completely. The patient now experiences binocular diplopia but intellectually remains convinced of a monocular phenomenon. At this point, the patient often reads well down the eye chart without hesitation, even when asked to attend to the upper line that corresponds to the "bad" eye. A very accurate measure of visual acuity may be obtained for otherwise uncooperative patients.

The red–green eyeglasses provided with the Worth four-dot test may be useful. The examiner asks the patient to put on the glasses and then inserts the red–green filter installed in the vision chart projector. The patient sees the letters on the red half of the eye chart with the eye covered by the red lens and the letters on the green half with the eye covered by the green lens. The patient often progresses well down the eye chart before realizing over-achievement has occurred.

The red–green eyeglasses may be used with the Ishihara color plate series, as well. If a patient complains of poor vision in one eye, have the patient put on the red–green glasses with the green lens over the "good" eye and the red lens over the "bad" eye. Under normal circumstances, an individual can read the Ishihara numbers through the red lens but not the green lens. If the subject who has nonorganic complaints reads the numbers under the above circumstances, this discrepancy confirms better-than-stated ocular function.

Ophthalmologists often use phoropters and trial frames to confuse patients and obtain a measure of visual acuity. These methods generally fail, however, when patients are malingerers. In both circumstances, patients may close an eye surreptitiously and determine that these are tests of deception. Optokinetic nystagmus only helps ascertain that vision is grossly intact in each eye.

Perimetry remains an excellent tool for the evaluation of nonorganic complaints. Both confrontational and tangent screen techniques yield the best information, because they allow variable test distances. Patients who are determined to produce

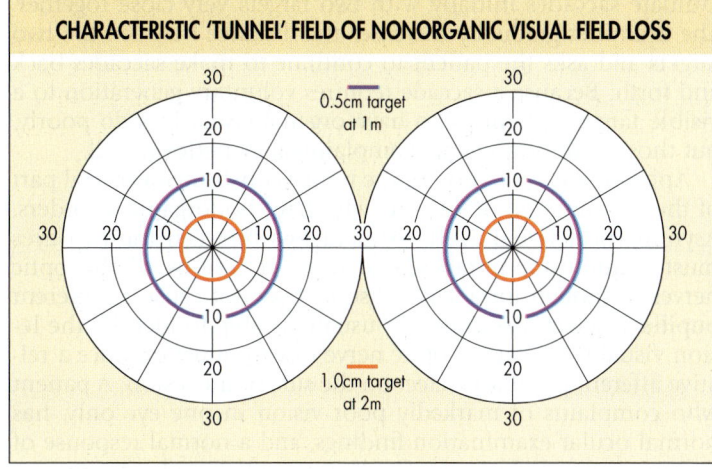

FIG. 196-10 ■ Characteristic "tunnel" field of nonorganic visual field loss. Paradoxically, the visual field appears to expand as the patient approaches the screen. Such a pattern does not correspond to any known ocular or central nervous system lesion.

a factitious visual field defect may confound Goldmann and automated perimetry techniques easily, however.

The most common defect discovered during perimetry is a tunnel field. If a visual field is constricted because of organic disease, the absolute size of an isopter for a given test object increases as the distance from the screen increases. Patients who have tunnel fields, however, tend to have field constriction, but they always generate the same absolute size of an isopter on the tangent screen no matter what the test distance (Fig. 196-10). The examiner may enhance this tendency by using large, easily discriminated pins to mark the edge of an isopter. Testing at two distances is necessary, however, because several medical conditions (end-stage glaucoma, end-stage papilledema, tapetoretinal degeneration, chiasmal compression, or bilateral occipital lobe infarcts) may produce authentic generalized constriction of the visual field.

The tangent screen may prove useful in another way for the evaluation of patients who have unilateral visual complaints. In one method the visual field is tested for the "good" eye and the location of the blind spot determined. The examiner then tests the "bad" eye and elicits the characteristically small tunnel field inside the blind spot. Finally, the physician evaluates the patient with both eyes open. Patients who have nonorganic complaints frequently lose the blind spot from the "good" eye, even though the claimed field for the "bad" eye was smaller than 10°. Occasionally, patients tested in this manner may yield totally inexplicable and impossible visual field changes under binocular conditions. For example, a patient who has a full field in one eye and a tunnel field in the other may report a hemifield loss on the side of the "bad" eye with both eyes open.

Should a patient claim severe bilateral vision loss and be noncompliant on perimetry testing, the examiner must take every opportunity to observe the patient's behavior. If a call to the patient from a distance results in an accurate fix on the examiner's location by the patient, a peripheral field much larger than stated is indicated. Patients who have small, bilateral tunnel fields may be able to maneuver easily without bumping into objects. Patients may pick up or take objects held well away to one side, which indicates they can see the objects. Finally, patients who feel no one is watching may perform tasks inconsistent with their level of claimed disability.

Tests for stereoscopic vision may assist the evaluation of patients who have nonorganic complaints. Most methods for stereopsis evaluation require good peripheral fields and good visual acuity in both eyes. Patients often become intrigued with the challenge of stereoacuity testing and perform at a level well beyond that claimed under other conditions.

The examiner may be able to use motility testing to advantage. If a patient complains of a tunnel field, the tester should evaluate saccades initially with two targets very close together. The examiner gradually increases the distance between the two targets and asks the patient to continue to make saccades back and forth. Because a saccade requires voluntary generation to a visible target, patients who have organic visual loss do poorly, but those with nonorganic complaints may perform well.

Appropriate evaluation of the pupils constitutes a critical part of the examination of patients who have nonorganic disorders. Asymmetrical visual acuity or field loss between the two eyes must result from intraocular disease or lesions of the optic nerves. Although intraocular disease may not cause an afferent pupillary defect, the examiner usually is able to identify the lesion visually. Unilateral optic nerve disease must produce a relative afferent pupillary defect on the side of the lesion. A patient who complains of markedly poor vision in one eye only, has normal ocular examination findings, and a normal response of the pupils to a light in the "bad" eye, is likely to have a nonorganic syndrome.

Ancillary testing, in certain circumstances, may prove helpful. If a patient generates complaints or findings that suggest a retrochiasmal lesion, imaging studies may be used to identify or eliminate such a lesion as a cause. Should the examiner need further documentation of optic nerve function, visual evoked response testing that gives a normal latency and amplitude essentially rules out organic disease as a cause of serious injury to the optic nerve. Malingering patients, however, may prove uncooperative and thwart the efforts of the electrophysiology technician.

Once the examiner has established a patient's complaints as nonorganic, all appropriate findings must be documented carefully in the patient record. The physician must perform all critical tests in the presence of a reliable witness who can corroborate the results in a courtroom.

Patients who have a conversion reaction, in most instances, respond very favorably to a report of a healthy visual system. The physician must remember that these patients' complaints stem from anxiety; assuaging that anxiety allows the patient to "recover" without stigma. Only in unusual circumstances does the patient require the assistance of a psychiatrist. The patient and family must understand that a conversion reaction represents an adaptation to stress; they must work to alleviate the cause of this stress to prevent the development of other somatic complaints.

Malingering patients react poorly to confrontation. Because they seek secondary gain, they immediately challenge anyone who claims they are lying. The physician approaches these patients supportively. A good approach is to state that, because the physician has not examined the patient previously, an organic lesion may have existed at one time. The examiner can then express concern and relief that the patient's problem has resolved so well. By using this approach, the physician may avoid significant unpleasantness.

REFERENCES

1. Reese B. Clinical implications of the fibre order in the optic pathway of primates. Neurol Res. 1993;15:83–6.
2. Shatz CJ. Emergence of order in visual system development. Proc Natl Acad Sci U S A. 1996;93:602–8.
3. von Noorden GK, Middleditch PR. Histological observations in the normal monkey lateral geniculate nucleus. Invest Ophthalmol Vis Sci. 1975;14:55–8.
4. Casagrande VA. A third parallel visual pathway to primate area V1. Trends Neurosci. 1994;7:305–10.
5. van Buren JM, Baldwin M. The architecture of the optic radiation in the temporal lobe of man. Brain. 1958;81:15–40.
6. Meyer A. The connections of the occipital lobes and the present status of the cerebral visual affections. Trans Assoc Am Physicians. 1907;22:7–15.
7. Brodmann K. Vergleichende Localisationslehre der Grosshirnrinde in ihren Prinzipien Dargestelltg auf Grund des Zellenbaues. Leipzig: Barth; 1909.
8. Lund JS. Organization of neurons in the visual cortex, area 17, of the monkey. J Comp Neurol. 1973;147:455–96.
9. Hubel DH, Wiesel TN. Laminar and columnar distribution of geniculocortical fibers in the macaque monkey. J Comp Neurol. 1972;146:421–50.
10. Hubel DH, Wiesel TN. Sequence regularity and geometry of orientation columns in the monkey striate cortex. J Comp Neurol. 1974;158:267–94.
11. Kandel ER, Schwartz JH, Jessell TM. Principles of neural science. New York: Elsevier; 1991:431–4.
12. Benton S, Levy I, Swash M. Vision in the temporal crescent in occipital infarction. Brain. 1980;103:83–97.
13. Innocenti GM, Aggoun-Zouaoui D, Lehmann P. Cellular aspects of callosal connections and their development. Neuropsychologia. 1995;33:961–87.
14. Salin PA, Bullier J. Corticocortical connections in the visual system: structure and function. Physiol Rev. 1995;75:107–54.
15. Hubel DH, Wiesel TN. Functional architecture of macaque monkey visual cortex. Proc R Soc London Ser B. 1977;198:1–59.
16. Bressler SL. Interareal synchronization in the visual cortex. Behav Brain Res. 1996;76:37–49.
17. Derrington A. Vision: filling in and popping out. Curr Biol. 1996;6:141–3.
18. Smith JL. Homonymous hemianopia: a review of one hundred cases. Am J Ophthalmol. 1962;54:616–22.
19. Savino PJ, Paris M, Schatz NJ, et al. Optic tract syndrome: a review of 21 patients. Arch Ophthalmol. 1978;96:656–63.
20. O'Connor PS, Kaston D, Tredici TJ, et al. The Marcus Gunn pupil in experimental optic tract lesions. Ophthalmology. 1982;89:160–4.
21. Gunderson CH, Hoyt WF. Geniculate hemianopia: incongruous homonymous field defects in two patients with partial lesions of the lateral geniculate nucleus. J Neurol Neurosurg Psychiatry. 1971;24:1–6.
22. Pahwa JM. Homonymous hemianopias from lesions of parietotemporal lobes. Mediscope. 1963;5:543–7.
23. McAuley DL, Ross Russell RW. Correlation of CAT scan and visual field defects in vascular lesions of the posterior visual pathways. J Neurol Neurosurg Psychiatry. 1979;42:298–311.
24. Horton JC, Hoyt WF. The representation of the visual field in human striate cortex. A revision of the classic Holmes map. Arch Ophthalmol. 1991;109:816–24.
25. Davis PC, Newman NJ. Advances in neuroimaging of the visual pathways. Am J Ophthalmol. 1996;121:690–705.
26. Milner AD, Perrett DI, Johnson RS, et al. Perception and action in "visual form agnosia." Brain. 1991;114:405–28.
27. Goodale MA. Perceiving the world and grasping it: is there a difference? Lancet. 1994;343:930–1.
28. Jakobson LS, Archibald YM, Carey DP, et al. A kinematic analysis of reaching and grasping movements in a patient recovering from optic ataxia. Neuropsychologia. 1991;29:803–9.
29. Ogden JA. Visual object agnosia, prosopagnosia, achromatopsia, loss of visual imagery, and autobiographical amnesia following recovery from cortical blindness: case MH. Neuropsychologia. 1993;6:571–89.
30. Mehta Z, Newcombe F, De Haan E. Selective loss of imagery in a case of visual agnosia. Neuropsychologia. 1992;30:645–55.
31. Goodale MA, Milner AD. Separate visual pathways for perception and action. Trends Neurosci. 1992;15:20–5.
32. Sargent J, Ohta S, MacDonald B. Functional neuroanatomy of face and object processing. Brain. 1992;115:15–36.
33. Farah MJ. Current issues in the neuropsychology of image generation. Neuropsychologia. 1995;11:1455–71.
34. Farah MJ, Wilson KD, Drain HM, et al. The inverted face inversion effect in prosopagnosia: evidence for mandatory, face-specific perceptual mechanisms. Vision Res. 1995;35:2089–93.
35. Ungerleider LG. Functional brain imaging studies of cortical mechanisms for memory. Science. 1995;270:769–75.
36. Gurd JM, Marshall JC. Drawing upon the mind's eye. Nature. 1992;359:590–1.
37. Servos P, Goodale MA, Humphrey GK. The drawing of objects by a visual form of agnosia: contribution of surface properties and memorial representations. Neuropsychologia. 1993;31:251–9.
38. Behrmann M, Winocur G, Moscovitch M. Dissociation between mental imagery and object recognition in a brain-damaged patient. Nature. 1992;359:636–7.
39. Cogan DG. Visual hallucinations as release phenomena. Graefes Arch Klin Exp Ophthalmol. 1973;188:138–50.
40. Lance JW. Simple formed hallucinations confined to the area of a specific visual field defect. Brain. 1977;99:719–32.
41. Lepare FE. Spontaneous visual phenomena with visual loss: 104 patients with lesions of the retinal and neural afferent pathways. Neurology. 1990;40:444–7.
42. Brugger P, Agosti R, Regard M, et al. Heautoscopy, epilepsy, and suicide. J Neurol Neurosurg Psychiatry. 1994;57:838–9.
43. Howlett CC, Downie AL, Banerjee AK, et al. MRI of an unusual case of peduncular hallucinosis (Lhermitte's syndrome). Neuroradiology. 1994;36:121–2.
44. Peterson SE, Fox PT, Posner MI, et al. Positron emission tomographic studies of the cortical anatomy of single-word processing. Nature. 1988;331:585–9.
45. Darius P, Boller F. Transcortical alexia with agraphia following a right temporo-occipital hematoma in a right-handed patient. Neuropsychologia. 1994;32:1263–72.
46. Quint DJ, Gilmore JL. Alexia without agraphia. Neuroradiology. 1992;24:210–4.
47. Lichter C, Horber F. Transitory alexia without agraphia in an HIV-positive patient suffering from toxoplasma encephalitis: a case report. Eur Neurol. 1992;32:26–7.
48. Rentschler I, Treutwein B, Landis T. Dissociation of local and global processing in visual agnosia. Vision Res. 1994;34:963–71.
49. Geschwind N. Disconnection syndromes in animals and man. I and II. Brain. 1965;88:237–94,585–644.
50. Sakurai Y, Sakai K, Sukuta M, et al. Naming difficulties in alexia with agraphia for kanji after a left posterior inferior temporal lesion. J Neurol Neurosurg Psychiatry. 1994;57:609–13.
51. Heilman KM, Voeller K, Alexander AW. Developmental dyslexia: a motor–articulatory feedback hypothesis. Ann Neurol. 1996;39:407–12.
52. Livingstone MS, Rosen GD, Drislane FW, et al. Physiological and anatomical evidence for a magnocellular defect in developmental dyslexia. Proc Natl Acad Sci U S A. 1991;88:7943–7.
53. Sadun AA. Dyslexia at The New York Times: (mis)understanding of parallel visual processing. Arch Ophthalmol. 1992;110:933–4.
54. Humphrey GK, Goodale MA, Jakobson LS. The role of surface information in object recognition: studies of a visual form agnosic and normal subjects. Perception. 1994;23:1457–81.
55. Corbetta M, Miezin FM, Dobmeyer S, et al. Selective and divided attention during visual discriminations of shape, color and speed: functional anatomy by positron emission tomography. J Neurosci. 1991;11:2383–402.
56. Zeki S, Watson JDG, Lueck CJ, et al. A direct demonstration of functional specialization in human visual cortex. J Neurosci. 1991;11:641–9.

57. Gulyas B, Heywood CA, Popplewell DA, *et al.* Visual form discrimination from color or motion cues. Functional anatomy by positron emission tomography. Proc Natl Acad Sci U S A. 1994;91:9965–9.

58. Schnider A, Landis T, Regard M, *et al.* Dissociation of color from object in amnesia. Arch Neurol. 1992;49:982–5.

59. Heywood C, Cowey A, Newcombe F. On the role of parvocellular (P) and magnocellular (M) pathways in cerebral achromatopsia. Brain. 1994;117:245–54.

60. Kennard C, Lawden M, Morland AB, *et al.* Colour identification and colour constancy are impaired in a patient with incomplete achromatopsia associated with prestriate cortical lesions. Proc R Soc London. 1995;260:169–75.

61. Rizzo R, Nawrot M, Blake R, *et al.* A human visual disorder resembling area V4 dysfunction in the monkey. Neurology. 1992;42:1175–80.

62. Miyashita Y. Neuronal correlate of visual associative long-term memory in the primate temporal cortex. Nature. 1988;335:817–20.

63. Knudsen EI, Brainard MS. Creating a unified representation of visual and auditory space in the brain. Annu Rev Neurosci. 1995;18:19–43.

64. Albright TD, Stoner GR. Visual motion perception. Proc Natl Acad Sci U S A. 1995;92:2433–40.

65. Braddick O. Seeing motion signals in noise. Curr Biol. 1995;5:7–9.

66. Riddoch G. Dissociation of visual perception due to occipital injuries, with especial reference to appreciation of movement. Brain. 1917;40:15–57.

67. Zihl J, von Cramon D, Mai N. Selective disturbance of movement vision after bilateral brain damage. Brain. 1983;106:313–40.

CHAPTER

197

Disorders of Supranuclear Control of Ocular Motility

PATRICK J.M. LAVIN • SEAN P. DONAHUE

DEFINITION

- Loss of voluntary saccades (fast) and pursuit (slow) eye movements may result from interruption of neural pathways that carry commands from the cerebral cortex to the ocular motor nuclei in the brainstem.
- Disconjugate eye movement disorders and gaze palsies may result from lesions that involve the prenuclear pathways between the gaze centers and the ocular motor nuclei.

KEY FEATURES

- Abnormality of voluntary saccades, pursuit or vergence eye movements.
- Preservation of reflex eye movements (vestibulo-ocular, optokinetic, and Bell's phenomenon).

ASSOCIATED FEATURES

- Pyramidal signs (e.g., pseudobulbar palsy, limb weakness, spasticity, hyperreflexia, and extensor plantar responses).
- Extrapyramidal signs (e.g., bradykinesia, dystonia, rigidity, and tremor).
- Altered mental status.
- Evidence of disorders that cause supranuclear gaze palsies (e.g., degenerative, demyelinating, neoplastic, or vascular diseases, or traumatic).

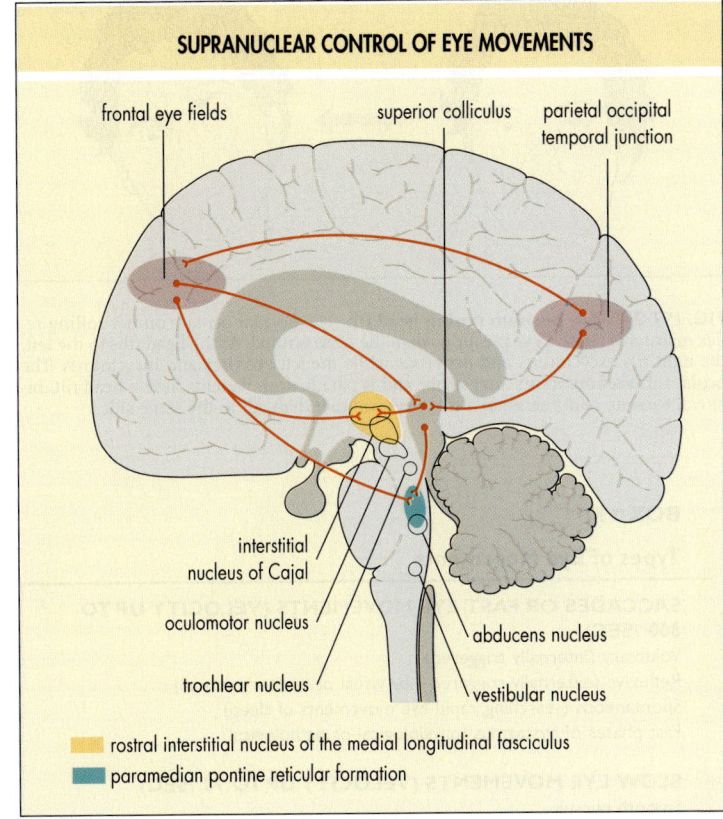

SUPRANUCLEAR CONTROL OF EYE MOVEMENTS

frontal eye fields — superior colliculus — parietal occipital temporal junction

interstitial nucleus of Cajal

oculomotor nucleus — abducens nucleus

trochlear nucleus — vestibular nucleus

▢ rostral interstitial nucleus of the medial longitudinal fasciculus
▢ paramedian pontine reticular formation

FIG. 197-1 ▦ **Supranuclear control of eye movements.** The pontine horizontal gaze center *(blue)* and the vertical gaze center in the midbrain *(yellow)* receive input from the frontal eye fields to initiate saccades, and from the parieto-occipito-temporal junction to control pursuit. These gaze centers control ocular motility by relaying to the ocular motor nerve nuclei (III, IV, and VI).

INTRODUCTION

With the exception of reflex eye movements (vestibulo-ocular and optokinetic) and the fast phases of nystagmus, cerebral structures determine when and where the eyes move, while brainstem centers determine how they move.[1]

The final common pathways for eye movements are located in "gaze centers" in the brainstem (Fig. 197-1). The paramedian pontine reticular formation (PPRF) contains the premotor substrate for ipsilateral horizontal gaze. The midbrain reticular formation (MRF) mediates vertical gaze, vergence eye movements, and ocular counter rolling (Fig. 197-2). The PPRF and MRF receive input from a number of "higher" centers, including areas in the cerebral hemispheres, superior colliculus, vestibular nuclei, and cerebellum (see Fig. 197-1); they, in turn, innervate the three ocular motor nuclei to generate appropriate eye movements. Supranuclear gaze palsies result from interruption of the neural pathways that carry commands for voluntary saccades and pursuit before they reach the eye movement "generators" in the brainstem.

Sound knowledge of the anatomy of eye movement control systems and of normal types of eye movements is necessary to localize accurately lesions that impair ocular motility.

ANATOMY OF EYE MOVEMENT

Anatomy of Supranuclear Eye Movement Control

Eye movements are divided broadly into the following two types (Box 197-1):

- Fast eye movements, or saccades, that move the eyes from one target to another at velocities of up to 800°/second
- Slow eye movements that allow the eyes to follow (hold) a target when either the target, the head, or both are moving

Slow eye movements may be conjugate (e.g., pursuit, see below) or disconjugate (e.g., vergence eye movements that are necessary for binocular single vision and stereoscopic depth perception when a target moves toward or away from the subject). The latency for saccades is about 225msec, and pursuit latency is about 125msec.[2] The initiation and generation of saccadic and pursuit eye movements is complex and dealt with in greater detail elsewhere[1,3]; a simplified overview is given here. The fast phases of nystagmus (Chapter 202) also are saccades (see Box 197-1).

EYE POSITION DURING HEAD TILT

Normal ocular counter-rolling reflex

Ocular tilt reaction

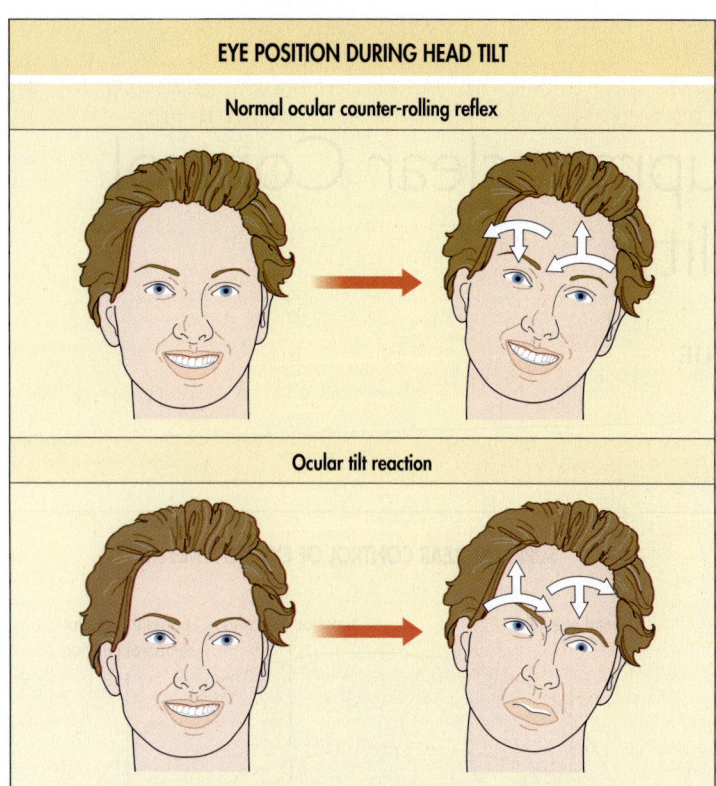

FIG. 197-2 ■ **Eye position during head tilt.** The normal ocular counter-rolling reflex maintains relative eye position when the head is tilted. As the head tilts to the left, the right eye excyclotorts and depresses while the left eye rises and incyclotorts. The ocular tilt reaction occurs after stroke and is paradoxical. Patients have a head tilt, bilateral torsion, and a sense of a tilted vertical meridian, all to the same side.

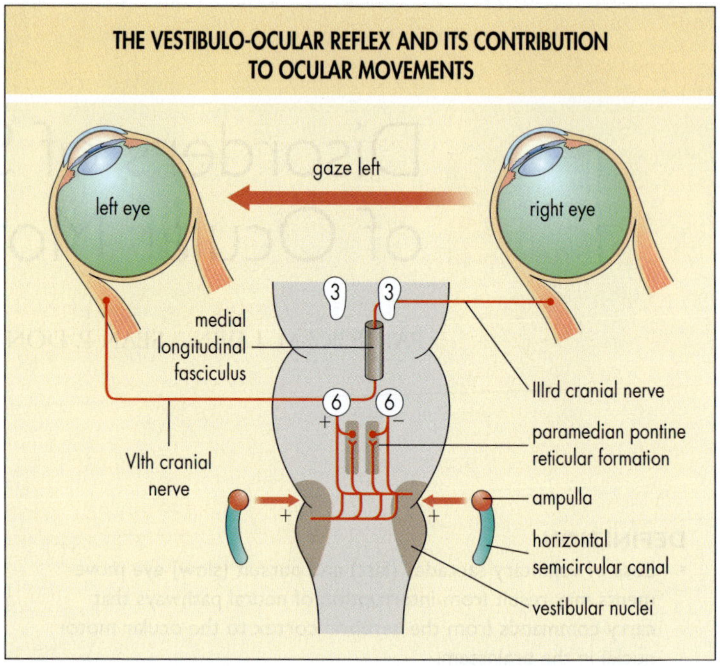

THE VESTIBULO-OCULAR REFLEX AND ITS CONTRIBUTION TO OCULAR MOVEMENTS

FIG. 197-3 ■ **Vestibulo-ocular reflex and its contribution to horizontal eye movements.** The semicircular canals respond to rotational acceleration of the head by driving the vestibulo-ocular reflex to maintain the eyes in the same direction in space during head movement. Fibers from the horizontal semicircular canal travel first to the vestibular nuclei and then to each paramedian pontine reticular formation. Excitatory projections that travel to the contralateral sixth cranial nerve nucleus and, via the medial longitudinal fasciculus, to the ipsilateral medial rectus subnucleus cause gaze to the left. In a similar manner, inhibitory projections are sent to the antagonist ipsilateral lateral rectus and contralateral medial rectus.

BOX 197-1

Types of Eye Movements

SACCADES OR FAST EYE MOVEMENTS (VELOCITY UP TO 800°/SEC)
Voluntary (internally triggered)
Reflexive (externally triggered—by visual or auditory stimuli)
Spontaneous (searching, rapid eye movements of sleep)
Fast phases of nystagmus (physiological or pathological)

SLOW EYE MOVEMENTS (VELOCITY UP TO 70°/SEC)
Smooth pursuit
• Foveal pursuit
• Full-field pursuit (optokinetic slow phase)
Vestibular slow phase (includes torsional movements)
Vergence

OTHER OCULAR OSCILLATIONS (E.G., OPSOCLONUS, FLUTTER)

Horizontal Eye Movements

The contralateral frontal lobe, particularly the frontal eye field, is responsible for generating horizontal saccades. Each frontal eye field projects to the contralateral PPRF, which in turn innervates the abducens nucleus. Pursuit eye movements are triggered by the ipsilateral posterior parietal lobe (see Fig. 197-1), which also projects to the PPRF and then to the abducens nucleus. About 60% of the neurons in the abducens nucleus innervate the ipsilateral lateral rectus muscle; the remaining 40% are interneurons that project, via the medial longitudinal fasciculus (MLF), to the contralateral medial rectus subnucleus in the oculomotor nuclear complex (Fig. 197-3). Thus, activation of the PPRF or the abducens nucleus generates ipsilateral horizontal gaze; conversely, damage to either of these structures results in an ipsilateral gaze palsy. The PPRF also receives input from the ipsilateral posterior parietal lobe, the vestibular system, the superior col-

liculus, and the cerebellum, all of which play a role in generating saccades.

Vertical Eye Movements

The premotor substrate for vertical gaze lies in the MRF, although some vertical saccades are programmed in the PPRF and relayed to the MRF, presumably to coordinate horizontal, vertical, and oblique trajectories. The rostral interstitial nucleus of the medial longitudinal fasciculus (riMLF) contains neurons for both upward and downward saccades. Their axons relay to neurons in the interstitial nucleus of Cajal, which discharge in relation to vertical eye position and play a role in vertical pursuit and eye position. The neurons for upward saccades innervate both ipsilateral and contralateral oculomotor and trochlear nerve nuclei (Fig. 197-4). The neurons that mediate downward saccades only innervate the oculomotor and trochlear nerve nuclei bilaterally (see Fig. 197-1). The riMLF and the interstitial nucleus of Cajal also are involved in the generation of ipsilateral torsional eye movements.

The supranuclear pathways for vertical saccades travel from both frontal eye fields to innervate the riMLF on each side in the MRF (see Fig. 197-4). Vertical saccades require simultaneous activation of both frontal eye fields.

Slow Eye Movements

Slow eye movements help maintain fixation on a target in order to stabilize the image on the fovea when either the subject or object is moving. Four types of slow eye movements occur, namely pursuit, optokinetic, vestibular, and vergence.

Pursuit Eye Movements

Pursuit eye movements allow the eyes to track a moving object at velocities up to 70°/second and have a latency of about

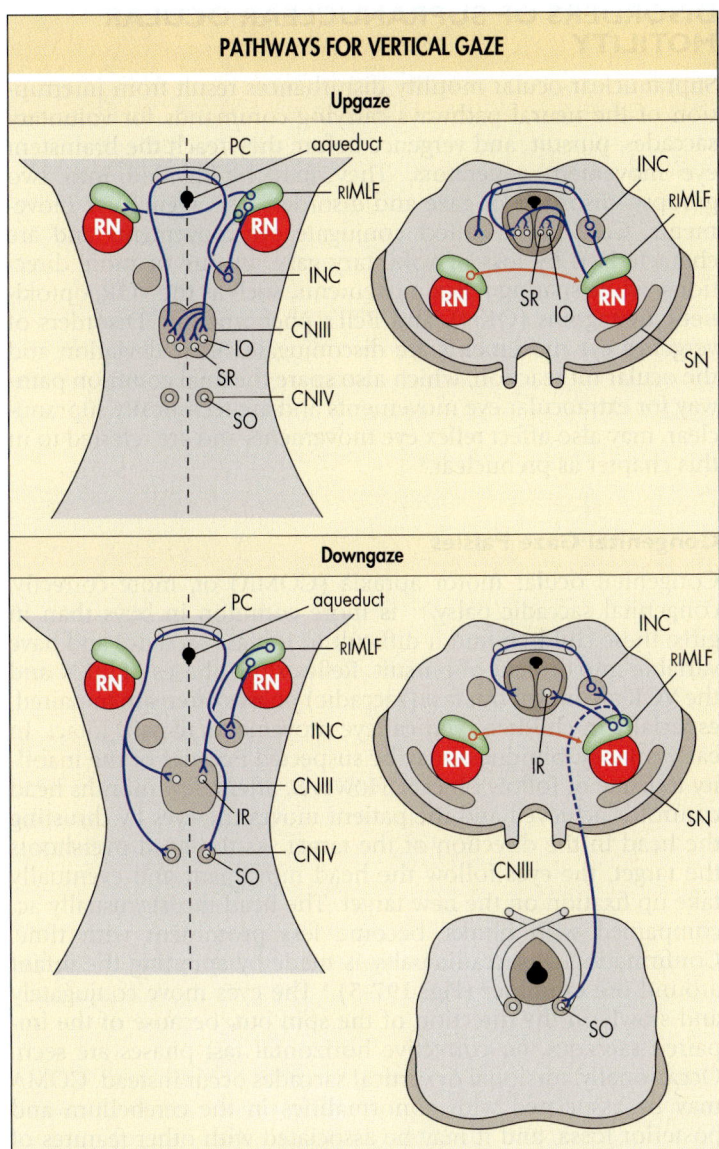

PATHWAYS FOR VERTICAL GAZE

Upgaze

Downgaze

FIG. 197-4 ■ **Pathways for vertical gaze.** Upgaze pathways originate in the rostral interstitial nucleus of the medial longitudinal fasciculus and project to innervate the oculomotor and trochlear nerves bilaterally. Upgaze paralysis is a feature of the dorsal midbrain syndrome as a result of the lesion's effect on the posterior commissure (lesion *A*). Downgaze pathways also originate in the rostral interstitial nucleus of the medial longitudinal fasciculus but probably travel more ventrally. Bilateral lesions affect downgaze more severely than unilateral lesions and usually are located dorsomedial to the red nucleus. *INC*, Interstitial nucleus of Cajal; *IO*, inferior oblique subnucleus; *IR*, inferior rectus subnucleus; *PC*, posterior commissure; *riMLF*, rostral interstitial nucleus of the medial longitudinal fasciculus; *RN*, red nucleus; *SR*, superior rectus subnucleus.

125msec.[2] The generation of pursuit eye movement is complex[1,3] but consists of three essential elements as follows:

- A sensory component driven by an image moving across the fovea
- A motor component generated largely by the posterior parietal lobe (parieto–occipito–temporal junction) that projects to the PPRF on the same side and is responsible for ipsilateral tracking movements
- An attentional–spatial component for concentration on selected targets, orientation in space

The precise route for the pursuit pathways from the parieto–occipito–temporal junction to the PPRF is not clear, but the ipsilateral pontine nuclei and the vestibulocerebellum have important modulatory influences. Vertical smooth pursuit is even less well understood.

Vestibular System

Vestibular eye movements maintain foveation when the head moves in any direction or plane, including the horizontal (yaw), vertical–sagittal (pitch), or vertical–coronal (roll) planes. For example, if the subject's head turns 10 degrees to the right, the eyes rotate 10 degrees to the left to maintain fixation (see Fig. 197-2). The latency for vestibular responses is about 10msec.

Optokinetic System

The optokinetic system complements the vestibulo-ocular system when it becomes inadequate, such as with sustained head rotation when the eyes reach the limit in the orbit, or during very slow head movements when the vestibulo-ocular reflex (VOR) is less responsive. In humans the optokinetic system is tested predominantly by foveal fixation and pursuit and, to a lesser extent, by full visual field stimulation which is compelling and largely involuntary. The latter is tested clinically by rotating an image of the environment around the patient or by turning the patient in a revolving chair so the environment appears to be moving relative to the patient.

Vergence System

The vergence system enables eyes to move disconjugately in the horizontal plane and allows binocular fixation of an object that moves toward (convergence) or away (divergence) from the subject. The main stimuli for vergence movements are retinal blur (object unfocused) and diplopia (fusional disparity); convergence is associated with accommodation and pupillary miosis (the near triad). The pathways that generate vergence eye movements are not known precisely, but the occipital lobe, midbrain, and cerebellum play significant roles.

DIAGNOSTIC TESTING

Techniques used in the examination of the ocular motor system fall into six categories, reviewed in detail by Borchert.[4]

Saccades

The patient is asked to alternate fixation rapidly between two targets, such as a finger and the examiner's nose. Both horizontal and vertical saccades are tested and the following three observations are made:

- The latency to saccadic initiation
- The relative velocity of the saccade
- The accuracy of the saccade

Abnormalities in saccadic accuracy include overshooting or undershooting the target and are referred to as saccadic dysmetria. Gross abnormalities are clinically obvious, but detection of subtle changes require quantitative oculography.[3]

Fixation

The patient looks at a stationary, accommodative target projected in the distance, while the examiner checks fixation both monocularly and binocularly. Fixation should be steady without nystagmus or other significant ocular oscillations or intrusions, such as flutter or opsoclonus. Small eye movements, such as square wave jerks of less than 1–2 degrees, and micromovements, such as microsaccades, microdrift, and ocular microtremor, are normal and do not interrupt fixation.[5]

Pursuit

The patient is asked to fixate a small object, such as a pencil, and follow it slowly through the extent of horizontal and vertical versions; the patient's eyes should pursue the target smoothly. If the pursuit system is defective, or the target moves too quickly, the eyes fall behind and make "catch-up saccades" to refixate the target. This produces saccadic, or cogwheel, pursuit. The extent of versions and ductions may be determined while testing pursuit.

Pursuit also may be evaluated while testing the patient's ability to suppress the VOR. Have the patient sit on a rotatable stool and fixate one of his or her own thumbs at arm's length, then rotate the stool so that the patient's head, arm, and thumb move as one. A normal patient can suppress the induced VOR by maintaining fixation on the thumb, even in darkness or with the eyes closed—VOR suppression probably involves the same pathways as smooth pursuit.[6] Because blind patients also can suppress the VOR, this technique particularly helps to differentiate between real and psychogenic visual deficits—psychogenic patients appear unable to follow a target smoothly.

Vergence Eye Movements

A target is moved toward (convergence) and then away (divergence) from the patient, who follows it.

Ocular Alignment

Ocular alignment is covered in more detail in the section on strabismus (Chapter 70). Ocular alignment should be determined by simultaneous prism and cover testing (for tropias) and by alternate cover testing (for phorias, and to measure the basic deviation). Cover testing must be performed with the patient wearing the full cycloplegic refraction, and fixation must be maintained on the smallest readable optotype (an accommodative target). To determine if horizontal deviations are comitant, cover testing should be performed in at least five of the cardinal positions of gaze and at near. Patients with vertical deviations should be checked in the right and left head tilt positions, as well.

Differentiating Supranuclear from Nuclear and Infranuclear Lesions

If the patient has a gaze palsy, the physician determines whether the eyes can be moved reflexively in the direction of the "paralysis" by testing the oculocephalic (Doll's eyes) reflex or the vestibulo-ocular reflex using caloric stimulation of the tympanic membrane.

Oculocephalic (Doll's Eyes) Reflex

The oculocephalic (Doll's eyes) reflex is performed by getting the patient to tilt the head forward 30 degrees and fixate on a distant target. The head is then rotated in the direction opposite the gaze palsy. This maneuver uses direct projections from the vestibular system to the ocular motor nuclei to move the eyes reflexively (see Fig. 197-3). Gaze palsies caused by lesions of the cerebral cortex can be overcome by vestibulo-ocular testing, except during the acute phase (diaschisis). However, with paranuclear, nuclear, or infranuclear lesions, the reflex does not overcome the gaze palsy. This test should not be performed if the neck is unstable or has not been cleared (i.e., cervical spine instability has been ruled out) after trauma.

Vestibulo-ocular Reflex Testing

The patient's head is tilted back 60° and the external auditory meatus irrigated with either cool or warm water to stimulate the horizontal semicircular canal. In normal subjects and patients who have supranuclear gaze palsies, cool water stimulation causes the eyes to deviate slowly toward the irrigated side, which results in nystagmus with the fast (corrective) phase to the opposite side. When warm water is used the fast phase is toward the stimulated ear. The mnemonic COWS (cool, opposite, warm, same) refers to the direction of the fast phase of the nystagmus. In comatose patients no corrective (fast) phase occurs, so with cold water the eyes deviate tonically toward the irrigated ear. Simultaneous bilateral caloric testing may be used to evaluate vertical eye movements, but this is less reliable than oculocephalic testing.[4] If the tympanic membrane is perforated, oxygen piped through ice should be used instead of water.

DISORDERS OF SUPRANUCLEAR OCULAR MOTILITY

Supranuclear ocular motility disturbances result from interruption of the neural pathways carrying commands for voluntary saccades, pursuit, and vergence before they reach the brainstem eye movement generators. They may be divided into two groups—disorders of gaze and disorders of vergence eye movements. Gaze palsies affect conjugate eye movements and are characterized by loss of voluntary gaze, in one or more directions, while sparing reflex movements, such as the VOR, optokinetic nystagmus (OKN), and Bell's phenomenon. Disorders of vergence eye movements are disconjugate. Skew deviation and the ocular tilt reaction, which also spare the final common pathway for extraocular eye movements and are technically supranuclear, may also affect reflex eye movements and are referred to in this chapter as prenuclear.[1]

Congenital Gaze Palsies

Congenital ocular motor apraxia (COMA) or, more correctly, congenital saccadic palsy,[5,7] is more common in boys than in girls; these children find it difficult to initiate saccades and have variable impairment of pursuit. Reflex slow phases of OKN and the VOR are intact, but fast (saccadic) phases often are impaired, especially in children. Vertical eye movements remain intact. In early infancy, blindness may be suspected because of the inability to fixate or follow objects. However, after a few months head control is achieved and the patient moves the eyes by thrusting the head in the direction of the target. As the head overshoots the target, the eyes follow the head movement and eventually take up fixation on the new target. The head thrusts, usually accompanied with blinks, become less prominent with time. Confirmation of saccadic palsy is made by spinning the infant around the examiner (Fig. 197-5).[8] The eyes move conjugately and slowly in the direction of the spin but, because of the impaired saccades, no corrective horizontal fast phases are seen. Occasionally, torsional or vertical saccades occur instead. COMA may be associated with abnormalities in the cerebellum and posterior fossa, and it may be associated with other features of developmental delay. Ocular motor disorders resembling COMA may be seen in a number of conditions, including Aicardi's syndrome, dysgenesis of the corpus callosum or cerebellum or both, ataxia telangiectasia (autosomal recessive),

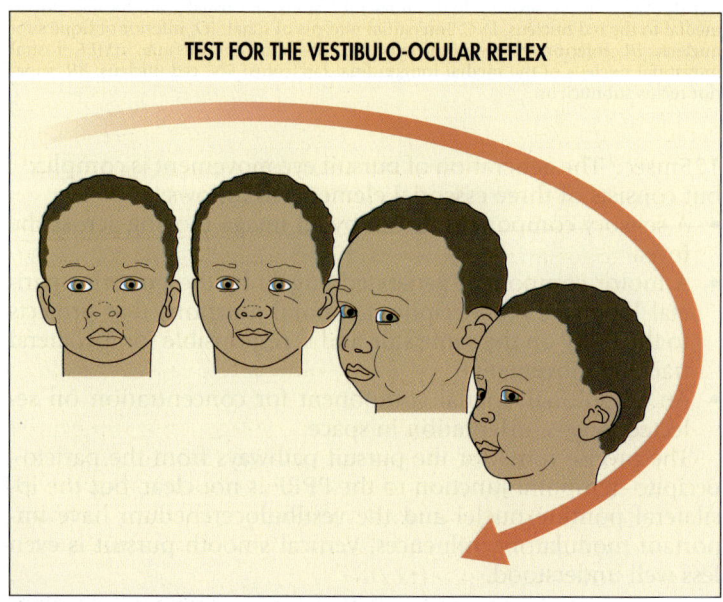

TEST FOR THE VESTIBULO-OCULAR REFLEX

FIG. 197-5 ■ **The child is spun around the examiner to test the vestibulo-ocular reflex.** The slow tonic phase produces gaze in the direction of the spin; fast phase corrective saccades occur to drive the eyes back. In congenital ocular motor apraxia (congenital saccadic palsy), fast phases are absent and the eyes are driven tonically in the direction of the spin.

ataxia–oculo-motor apraxia syndrome (which mimics ataxia telangiectasia without the extra neurological findings of ataxia telangiectasia and is probably autosomal recessive), Cockayne's syndrome, Joubert's syndrome, Pelizaeus-Merzbacher's disease, and succinic semialdehyde dehydrogenase deficiency.

Congenital vertical ocular motor apraxia is rare[9] and must be differentiated from metabolic and degenerative disorders, such as neurovisceral lipidosis (which cause progressive neurological dysfunction), and from stable disorders such as birth injury, perinatal hypoxia,[10] and, occasionally, Leber's congenital amaurosis.

Familial horizontal gaze palsy with scoliosis (HGPS) is an autosomal recessive disorder characterized by paralysis of horizontal gaze from birth, progressive scoliosis, impaired optokinetic reflex, and VOR, but intact convergence and vertical eye movements. Some patients may have fine pendular horizontal nystagmus, facial myokymia, facial twitching, hemifacial atrophy, and *situs inversus* of the optic discs.[3,11]

Acquired Gaze Palsies

Acquired horizontal supranuclear gaze palsies may occur with stroke, head injury, tumors, seizures, and, rarely, with metabolic disease such as Gaucher's type I and III diseases and juvenile G_{M2} gangliosidosis. This subject is reviewed in detail elsewhere.[1] Because these patients have cognitive dysfunction, they can be difficult to examine.

Acute hemisphere stroke can cause a transient gaze deviation in both head and eyes.[12] Usually, the eyes are deviated toward the side of the lesion (ipsiversive gaze deviation) because of paresis of gaze to the hemiplegic side. After about 5 days the intact hemisphere takes over and both the gaze paresis and ocular deviation resolve. Subsequently, subtle defects, such as prolonged saccadic latencies and impaired saccadic suppression, can be detected only by quantitative oculography. Other acute insults, such as head injury, also may result in such gaze palsies.

Ictal conjugate ocular deviation (seizure activity) occurs as a result of irritative lesions, which include trauma, tumors, or small cerebral hemorrhages. Such lesions "activate" the involved frontal eye field and cause the eyes to deviate away from the damaged hemisphere (adversive gaze deviation). Usually, such ocular deviation is associated with or immediately followed by adversive nystagmoid eye movements. It later is followed by postictal paralytic conjugate ocular deviation, in which gaze is deviated transiently toward the involved hemisphere, as part of Todd's paralysis.

Acquired ocular motor apraxia, a term used loosely and often incorrectly, occurs in patients who have bilateral frontoparietal damage or diffuse bilateral cerebral disease, and is better termed saccadic paresis or palsy.[13] Head thrusts, if present, are not as conspicuous as in the congenital variety.[14]

The PPRF may be injured by a variety of lesions including ischemia, hemorrhage, neoplasm, infection, demyelination, and paraneoplastic disorders. A lesion that affects the ipsilateral abducens nucleus or PPRF causes an ipsilateral gaze palsy. A rostral PPRF lesion spares the VOR, whereas a caudal lesion does not. As a result of the proximity of the abducens nucleus and the facial nerve fasciculus, ipsilateral facial weakness typically occurs with caudal PPRF lesions. Rarely, the first-order (central) sympathetic fibers may be involved, causing an associated ipsilateral Horner's syndrome.[15]

Wrong-way eyes is the term given to conjugate eye deviation to the "wrong" (hemiplegic) side, that is, away from the lesion and toward the hemiplegic side (contraversive gaze deviation).[16] It may occur with supratentorial lesions, particularly thalamic hemorrhage and, rarely, with large perisylvian or lobar hemorrhage or irritative lesions (below).

Incomplete lesions of the PPRF result in difficulty maintaining eccentric gaze and produce gaze-paretic, or gaze-evoked, nystagmus. When the eyes drift back to the primary position, the patient makes corrective saccades back to the eccentric target, which results in gaze-evoked nystagmus.

Bilateral lesions of the PPRF may cause complete loss of voluntary horizontal gaze. Large lesions may extend into the ventral pons, injuring the corticospinal pathways, and render the patient quadriplegic; this combination of findings is referred to as the *locked-in syndrome*.[17] Such patients appear unconscious, but volitional vertical eye and lid movements are spared, differentiating the locked-in syndrome from coma. Ocular bobbing can occur in this setting (Chapter 202).

Spasticity of conjugate gaze is a horizontal conjugate deviation away from a large, deep parietotemporal lesion during forced eyelid closure, and it may be considered a variant of Bell's phenomenon. Eye movements otherwise are normal.

Slow saccades occur with pontine disease as a result of burst cell dysfunction. Slow saccades also occur in patients who have some forms of cerebellar degeneration involving the pons and a number of disorders listed in Box 197-2.[1] Some patients who have hypometric saccades (as in myasthenia, Huntington's disease, brainstem encephalitis, and striatonigral degeneration) appear clinically to have slow saccades (pseudo–slow saccades).

Disorders of saccadic initiation result in prolonged latencies and occur in patients who have acquired immunodeficiency dementia complex, and or a variety of degenerative disorders of the nervous system, such as Alzheimer's, Huntington's, Parkinson's, and Pick's diseases.

Psychogenic ocular deviation may occur in patients who feign unconsciousness. The eyes are directed toward the ground irrespective of which way the patient is turned.

Disorders of Pursuit

The horizontal pursuit pathways control ipsilateral tracking. The final common motor pathway extends from the parieto–occipito–temporal junction, via the dorsolateral pontine nuclei, to the ipsilateral gaze center in the PPRF. With rare exceptions, lesions of the pursuit pathways cause impaired ipsilateral tracking; because the pursuit pathways probably decussate twice,[18] a unilateral midbrain lesion can cause impaired contralateral pursuit.[19] The frontal eye fields, superior colliculi, and cerebellum also contribute to pursuit drive.

Pursuit deficits range from absence of tracking eye movements to saccadic (cogwheel) pursuit. Global impairment of smooth pursuit is a common, nonspecific finding and can occur with medications (anticonvulsants, sedatives, or psychotropic agents), alcohol, fatigue, inattention, schizophrenia, encephalopathy, and a variety of neurodegenerative disorders, as well as age (infants

---

BOX 197-2

Causes of Slow Saccades

Acquired immunodeficiency syndrome dementia complex
Amyotrophic lateral sclerosis
Anticonvulsant toxicity (consciousness usually impaired)
Ataxia and telangiectasia
Hexosaminidase A deficiency
Huntington's disease
Internuclear ophthalmoplegia
Joseph's disease
Lesions of the paramedian pontine reticular formation
Lipid storage diseases
Lytico-Bodig's disease
Myotonic dystrophy
Nephropathic cystinosis
Ocular motor apraxia
Ocular motor nerve or muscle weakness
Olivopontocerebellar degeneration
Progressive supranuclear palsy
Wernicke's encephalopathy
Whipple's disease
Wilson's disease

and the elderly), and occasionally with focal lesions in the parieto-occipital region (area 39).

Injury to the pursuit pathways also affects the slow phase of OKN, easily demonstrated by rotating an optokinetic drum so that the stripes move toward the affected hemisphere. Because of the proximity of the pursuit pathways to the afferent visual pathways, lesions here often are associated with a contralateral homonymous hemianopia.

Balint's syndrome is characterized by these essential features: apraxia, inability to voluntarily look at different parts of the visual field; simultanagnosia, inability to attend simultaneously to different parts of the visual field; and optic ataxia, mislocalization when reaching for, or pointing to, objects. Bilateral hypoperfusion of the parieto-occipital region, usually as a result of a prolonged episode of hypotension, may case watershed (distal territory) infarction. Such patients may have some or all of the features of Balint's syndrome including visual agnosia, visual disorientation, and difficulty in determining the direction, velocity, and distance of moving objects; they also may have pursuit defects.

Internuclear Ophthalmoplegia

Injury to the MLF, between the abducens nucleus and the contralateral medical rectus subnucleus of the oculomotor nerve, interrupts transmission of neural impulses to the ipsilateral medial rectus muscle (see Fig. 197-3). This impairs adducting saccades of the ipsilateral eye, which become either slow or absent. On attempted lateral gaze, away from the side of the lesion, the abducting eye overshoots the target (dysmetria), giving the appearance of dissociated (disconjugate) nystagmus. If the internuclear ophthalmoplegia (INO) is bilateral, abduction saccades also may be slow because of impaired inhibition of resting tone in the medial rectus muscle. Upward beating and torsional nystagmus are present frequently, particularly if both MLFs are affected. A subtle INO may be demonstrated when the patient makes repetitive horizontal saccades, which disclose slow adduction of the ipsilateral eye. Convergence may be preserved. Other clinical features associated with INO include skew deviation (with the hypertropic eye usually ipsilateral to the lesion), defective vertical smooth pursuit, impairment of the vertical VOR, as well as impaired ability to suppress or cancel the vertical VOR.

INO also may occur with a variety of disorders that affect the brainstem (vascular, demyelinating, and metastatic) and must be differentiated from the pseudo-INO of myasthenia or a longstanding exotropia.

The one-and-a-half syndrome occurs with damage to the caudal dorsal pontine tegmentum that involves the ipsilateral MLF and either the ipsilateral PPRF or the abducens nucleus results in an ipsilateral gaze palsy with an ipsilateral INO (see Fig. 197-3). The only horizontal movement left intact is abduction of the contralateral eye. If the facial nerve nucleus or fasciculus is involved, oculopalatal myoclonus (a vertical oscillation of the eyes, palate, and other muscles of branchial origin) may develop later.[20] The most common causes of the one-and-a-half syndrome are multiple sclerosis and brainstem stroke, followed by metastatic and primary brainstem tumors.[21] Ocular myasthenia may cause a pseudo–one-and-a-half syndrome.[22]

Disorders of Vertical Gaze

Isolated midbrain lesions can cause disorders of vertical gaze (see Fig. 197-4) and occur with a variety of diseases (Box 197-3). Disorders of vertical gaze, particularly downgaze, often are overlooked in patients with brainstem vascular disease, because damage to the nearby reticular activating system impairs consciousness.

Supranuclear upgaze palsies occur with lesions at or near the posterior commissure and with bilateral lesions in the pretectal

---

BOX 197-3

Disorders of the Midbrain That Affect Vertical Gaze

EXTRINSIC LESIONS
Pineal region tumors
Vascular malformations and aneurysms
Hydrocephalus (failed ventricular shunt)
Parasitic cysts

INTRINSIC LESIONS
Primary brainstem tumor (glioma, ependymoma)
Metastatic brainstem tumor
Third ventricular tumors
Pituitary adenomas
Stroke
• Infarction
• Hemorrhage (thalamic, pretectal)
Trauma (surgery, head injury)
Multiple sclerosis
Infection (syphilis, encephalitis)
Lipid storage disease
Transtentorial herniation
Kernicterus
Wernicke's syndrome
Bassen-Kornzweig's syndrome
Vitamin B_{12} deficiency
Jejunal ileal bypass

---

area (see Fig. 197-4). With supranuclear disorders of vertical gaze, saccades are usually impaired initially, followed by pursuit and then loss of vertical VORs. Extrinsic compression of the posterior commissure or pretectal region also causes loss of the pupillary light reflex, but accommodation and convergence are preserved (light–near dissociation). Paralysis of upgaze, light–near dissociation of the pupils, impaired convergence, lid retraction, and convergence retraction nystagmus are features of the dorsal midbrain (Parinaud's) syndrome.

Convergence–retraction nystagmus is a uniquely localizing sign of injury to the dorsal midbrain region. It is not true nystagmus but a saccadic disorder[3] that is elicited best by rotating an optokinetic drum with the stripes moving downward. When the patient attempts to make corrective upward saccades to refixate, the eyes converge and retract in the orbits because of synchronous cocontraction of the extraocular muscles.

Downgaze palsy occurs with bilateral lesions of the rostral interstitial nucleus of the MLF or its projections (see Fig. 197-4). With the exception of occlusion of the posterior thalamosubthalamic branch of the posterior cerebral artery (Percheron's artery), such discrete lesions are rare; involvement of the midbrain rather than the thalamus is responsible for the paralysis.[23] More commonly, bilateral involvement of the pathways for downgaze, and also for upgaze, occurs as part of diffuse disorders such as progressive supranuclear palsy, Whipple's disease, neurovisceral lipid storage disorders, complications of acquired immunodeficiency syndrome, and so on. Rarely, a unilateral lesion of the midbrain tegmentum may result in impaired downward, as well as upward, saccades.[24]

Progressive supranuclear palsy, also called the Steele-Richardson-Olszewski syndrome, is a neurodegenerative disorder that appears in about the sixth decade. It is characterized by vertical supranuclear gaze palsy, particularly for downward eye movements, postural instability, and unexplained falls. In addition, nuchal rigidity, Parkinsonism, pseudobulbar palsy, and mild dementia may be present. Early visual symptoms include blurred vision (making it difficult to see food on a plate and to read), diplopia, burning eyes, and photophobia. As the disease progresses, horizontal eye movements become impaired, as well, and eventually a global gaze paresis develops.[3]

Wilson's disease, or hepatolenticular degeneration, is associated with a Kayser-Fleischer ring, caused by the accumulation of copper in Descemet's membrane. Eye movement abnormalities are unusual, but saccades may be slowed and a supranuclear upgaze palsy may occur.

Kernicterus, or neonatal jaundice, can cause upgaze paresis, which usually is supranuclear.[25] Horizontal saccades may be slow.

Niemann-Pick's disease type C, or juvenile dystonic lipidosis, may be associated with supranuclear palsy for downgaze, ataxia, athetosis, and foamy macrophages (the DAF syndrome). This disorder can have an early onset during the first year of life, when it is associated with developmental delay, ataxia, vertical gaze palsy, and mental retardation. The more common form has a delayed onset and is associated with cerebellar ataxia or dystonia at around 3 years of age; then a vertical gaze palsy and cognitive difficulties begin at around 6 years of age. The diagnosis consists of the demonstration of decreased cholesterol esterification in skin fibroblasts, as well as the demonstration of unusual, large, vacuolated storage cells in the bone marrow.

Huntington's disease also affects eye movements. Patients find it difficult to initiate saccades and frequently use blinks and head thrusts to facilitate eye movements. Voluntary saccades are slow, hypometric, and have long latencies, and vertical saccades are affected more than horizontal saccades. Fixation instability is prominent because of the inability to suppress spontaneous and reflex saccades as a result of frontal lobe disease. Smooth pursuit is spared relatively, except for interruption by square wave jerks.[26]

Tonic upward deviation of gaze, or forced upgaze, is rare but may be seen in unconscious patients.[27] It occurs with diffuse brain injury (hypotension, cardiac arrest, and heatstroke) and must be differentiated from oculogyric crises, petit mal seizures, and psychogenic coma. Some patients may develop myoclonic jerks and large-amplitude downbeat nystagmus; the prognosis for life is extremely poor. Rarely, tonic upward gaze deviation may be psychogenic, but it can be overcome, indeed cured, by cold caloric stimulation of the semicircular canals.

Benign paroxysmal tonic upward gaze usually starts during the first year of life, lasts about 2 years, and has no known cause. Episodes last for seconds to hours and may occur in young children with ataxia and downbeat nystagmus on attempted downgaze. This phenomenon can occur with cystic fibrosis.[28] There is little evidence to suggest that these are either seizures or oculogyric crises (see below). Tonic upgaze also may be seen in normal infants during the first months of life.[29]

Tonic downward deviation of gaze, or forced downgaze, is associated with medial thalamic hemorrhage, acute obstructive hydrocephalus, severe metabolic or hypoxic encephalopathy, or massive subarachnoid hemorrhage. When associated with lid retraction, the corneas can be buried below the lower lid (sundowning). In this setting, elevated intracranial pressure is a major concern. The eyes may be converged, as if looking at the nose. Large thalamic hemorrhages may be associated with tonic downgaze, miotic pupils, esotropia,[3,30] skew deviation, and an ipsilateral gaze preference.[30] Preterm infants with intraventricular hemorrhages also may have tonic downward deviation with a skew and esotropia.[31]

Tonic downward deviation of the eyes may occur as a transient phenomenon in otherwise healthy neonates. It also can be induced in infancy by sudden exposure to bright light. Tonic downward gaze deviation may occur with psychogenic illness, but it can be overcome by caloric stimulation of the semicircular canals. Tonic vertical deviation as a result of seizure activity is rare.

Skew deviation is a vertical divergence of the ocular axes caused by a "prenuclear" lesion of the vertical vestibulo-ocular pathways in the brainstem or cerebellum. About 12% of patients who have skew deviation alternate on lateral gaze (see below) or spontaneously. Skew deviation usually, but not always, is comitant and frequently is associated with cyclotorsion of one or both eyes. When the skew deviation is noncomitant it can mimic a partial third or a fourth cranial nerve palsy. Skew deviations occur most commonly with vascular lesions of the pons

or lateral medulla (Wallenberg's syndrome). Brandt and Dieterich[32] demonstrated ocular torsion of one or both eyes associated with a subjective tilt of the visual vertical toward the lower eye in most patients who have skew deviations. With lesions of the midbrain or upper pons, the contralateral eye was lower (contraversive skew), but with lesions of the lower pons or medulla the ipsilateral eye was lower (ipsiversive skew).

When patients have alternating skew deviation, the hypertropia changes with the direction of gaze. The adducting eye usually is hypotropic, thus mimicking superior oblique overaction. Alternating skew deviation occurs with lesions of either the upper midbrain region involving the interstitial nucleus of Cajal or the cervicomedullary junction or cerebellum; in the latter situation, ataxia and downbeat nystagmus usually are associated.[33]

Less commonly, alternating skew deviation may mimic bilateral superior oblique palsies; however, measurement of the deviations on head tilt, detection of a V pattern, and the degree of subjective and objective cyclotorsion also help to differentiate the two conditions. Furthermore, associated neurological findings and the clinical context are more definitive.

Paroxysmal or periodic alternating skew deviation occurs with midbrain lesions; the hypertropia changes in a regular or irregular manner over periods of seconds to minutes. Other features of the dorsal midbrain syndrome may be present.

Ocular counter-rolling is a normal vestibular eye reflex that allows people to maintain horizontal orientation of the environment while the head tilts to either side (see Fig. 197-2). When the head is tilted to the left, the left eye rises and intorts as the right eye falls and extorts.

The ocular tilt reaction consists of the triad of skew deviation, cyclotorsion of both eyes, and paradoxical head tilt, all to the same side—that of the lower eye (see Fig. 197-2). A tonic (sustained) ocular tilt reaction occurs with lesions of the ipsilateral utricle, vestibular nerve or nuclei, or a lesion in the region of the contralateral interstitial nucleus of Cajal and medial thalamus. A phasic (paroxysmal) ocular tilt reaction occurs with lesions of the ipsilateral interstitial nucleus of Cajal and may respond to baclofen.

Dissociated vertical deviation is an asymmetrical, bilateral phenomenon that occurs with early disruption of fusion (congenital esotropia, infantile cataract). Usually, it is manifest during periods of inattention, in which the deviating eye elevates, abducts, and excyclotorts. The cause remains unclear, but it is one of the few exceptions to Hering's law of equal innervation. When manifest, it is best treated by unilateral or bilateral superior rectus recession.[34] Dissociated horizontal deviation also occurs and is probably simply a variant of dissociated vertical deviation.

Congenital monocular elevator deficiency, previously known as double elevator palsy, is characterized by congenital limitation of elevation of one eye. Most patients are hypotropic in the primary position but use a chin-up head position to allow fusion. A ptosis or pseudoptosis, in which the upper lid of the affected hypotropic eye appears ptotic because the eye is lower, almost always is present. Monocular elevator deficiency is believed to result from a prenuclear congenital unilateral midbrain lesion because the affected eye usually is elevated by Bell's reflex. Furthermore, because the elevator muscles of the affected eye (inferior oblique and superior rectus) are innervated by their respective subnuclei within the third cranial nerve nucleus, but on opposite sides of the midline (Chapter 198), a single unilateral lesion must be prenuclear rather than nuclear.

In long-standing monocular elevator deficiency, the inferior rectus muscle may become tight, which may be treated using recession. If no restriction occurs, a full tendon vertical transposition (Knapp procedure) of the horizontal muscles is recommended.[35] Other disorders that may cause inferior rectus restriction, such as thyroid orbitopathy and orbital floor fractures, must be excluded.

Monocular supranuclear (prenuclear) elevator palsy is an acquired limitation of elevation of one eye on attempted upgaze.

Patients remain orthotopic in primary position and downgaze is intact. This disorder occurs with unilateral vascular[36] or neoplastic[37] lesions of the midbrain. The affected eye usually is elevated by Bell's reflex or by vestibular stimulation.

Oculogyric crises are spasmodic conjugate ocular deviations, usually upward but sometimes lateral, which occur most frequently after the use of neuroleptic medication, particularly haloperidol. A typical attack or crisis occurs for about 2 hours, during which the eyes deviate tonically upward, repetitively, for periods of seconds to minutes. The spasms may be preceded or accompanied by disturbing emotional symptoms, including anxiety, restlessness, compulsive thinking, and sensations of increased brightness or distortions of visual background.

OCULAR MOTILITY DISORDERS AND THE CEREBELLUM

The cerebellum coordinates the different motor and sensory inputs to the ocular motor system and ensures that the eyes move smoothly and accurately. Ocular motility signs indicative of cerebellar disease are listed in Box 197-4. The dorsal vermis and fastigial nuclei determine the accuracy of saccades by adjusting their amplitude. Lesions of the dorsal vermis and fastigial nuclei result in saccadic dysmetria. The flocculus is responsible for the stabilization of images on the fovea, particularly after a saccade. Lesions of the flocculus result in gaze-holding deficits, such as gaze-evoked, rebound, or downbeat nystagmus, impaired smooth pursuit, inability to cancel the VOR by the pursuit system, and inability to suppress nystagmus (and vertigo) by fixation. The nodulus influences vestibular eye movements and vestibulo-optokinetic interaction. Lesions of the nodulus may produce periodic alternating nystagmus.

Posterior fossa tumors may become apparent with strabismus; acute comitant esotropia may be the first sign.[38] Children who have such tumors usually are older than those who have infantile or accommodative esotropia, and they develop nystagmus or other neurological signs at a later date.[39] Failure to regain fusion after spectacle, prism, or surgical therapy is a universal finding.[38]

A variety of ocular motility disorders may be associated with congenital or acquired defects of the cerebellum. Patients with COMA may have midline cerebellar defects.[40] Chiari malformations may be associated with downbeat nystagmus, gaze-evoked nystagmus, skew deviation, or esotropia. Familial cerebellar degeneration may be associated with vergence disorders.[41]

OCULAR MOTILITY DISORDERS AND THE VESTIBULAR SYSTEM

The vestibular system stabilizes the direction of gaze during head movements by adjusting tonic innervation to the ocular motor nuclei and, consequently, the extraocular muscles, thus maintaining a stable image on the retina. Each vestibular end organ has three semicircular canals, as well as a utricle and sac-

cule. The utricle and saccule are gravity receptors that respond to linear acceleration and static head tilt (gravity). Each semicircular canal projects to the vestibular nuclei and brainstem. Excitatory projections innervate pairs of yoked agonist extraocular muscles via their subnuclei (see Fig. 197-3), while inhibitory projections innervate their antagonists. Essentially each extraocular muscle subnucleus receives excitatory projections from one semicircular canal and inhibitory projections from the rival semicircular canal. This network is discussed in greater detail elsewhere[42,43] but is illustrated most clearly by the horizontal VOR (see Fig. 197-3). The ampulla of the right horizontal semicircular canal is stimulated by turning the head to the right (or by warm caloric water irrigation). This mechanical information is transduced by the vestibular end organ into electrical signals and transmitted to the ipsilateral medial vestibular nucleus. Excitatory information then is relayed to the contralateral abducens nucleus (which sends projection to the ipsilateral medial rectus subnucleus), and inhibitory information to the ipsilateral abducens nucleus (which projects to the contralateral medial rectus subnucleus), and causes the eyes to deviate in the direction opposite to head rotation. Disruption of the pathways that subserve the vertical VOR (peripheral vestibular system, vestibular nuclei, cerebellar inputs, MLF, or cranial nerve subnuclei) causes a skew deviation.

VERGENCE DISORDERS

Convergence paralysis occurs with midbrain lesions and may be associated with other features of the dorsal midbrain syndrome. Lack of effort, however, is the most common cause of poor convergence. Degenerative disorders, such as cerebellar degeneration, Parkinson's disease, and progressive supranuclear palsy, also may be associated with poor convergence. The absence of other midbrain signs and the lack of pupillary constriction on attempted convergence may differentiate psychogenic convergence paralysis from organic disease.

Convergence insufficiency is an idiopathic condition that also may in part be related to effort. It is seen in young individuals who complain of diplopia in association with prolonged near work. Symptoms include eyestrain, headache, and asthenopic complaints, such as burning eyes.[41] Rarely, it may follow closed head injury. Convergence fusional amplitudes often are diminished but can be improved with orthoptic exercises (pencil pushups).

Divergence insufficiency is characterized by uncrossed horizontal diplopia at distance in the absence of other neurological symptoms or signs. Patients have intermittent or constant esotropia that is present only at distance. Versions and ductions are full and saccadic velocities, if measured quantitatively, are normal, but fusional divergence amplitudes are reduced. The origin of divergence insufficiency is unclear, but it may result from a break in fusion later in life, follow a trivial insult, be seen in a patient with a prior esophoria, or occur in patients with cerebellar degeneration. The condition is treated easily with base-out prisms for the distance correction and rarely requires extraocular muscle surgery.

Divergence paralysis is a controversial entity that may be difficult to differentiate from divergence insufficiency and bilateral sixth cranial nerve palsies, but usually it occurs in the context of severe head injury or other cause of raised intracranial pressure. Such patients usually have horizontal diplopia at distance, but abducting saccades are slow. Divergence paralysis can occur with Fisher's syndrome, Chiari malformations, pontine tumors, and diazepam therapy. Patients who have bilateral sixth cranial nerve palsies and who recover gradually may go through a phase in which the esotropia is comitant and versions are full, and thus mimic divergence paralysis.

Spasm of the near reflex is characterized by intermittent episodes of convergence, miosis, and accommodation and can

---

BOX 197-4

Ocular Motility Signs Indicative of Cerebellar Disease

Saccadic dysmetria (inaccurate saccadic amplitude; over- or undershooting a visual target)
Saccadic pursuit
Unstable fixation (square wave jerks)
Impaired vestibulo-ocular reflex suppression
Gaze-evoked nystagmus
Vertical nystagmus
Increased vestibulo-ocular reflex gain

mimic bilateral, and occasionally unilateral, abducens paresis. Symptoms include double or blurred vision. The patient is esotropic, particularly at distance, and has extreme miosis. Spasm of the near reflex occasionally occurs with organic disorders but is more commonly psychogenic in origin. The differential diagnosis is that of esotropia, but miosis and blurred vision during motility testing clinches the diagnosis. Patients who have psychogenic spasm of the near reflex often have associated somatic complaints and behavioral abnormalities, which include blepharoclonus on persistent lateral gaze, poor cooperation in the performance of motor tasks such as smiling, opening the mouth, and protruding the tongue, and other features of neurasthenia and asthenopia. Treatment first requires identification of the source of the psychopathology and its management, as well as reassurance as to the lack of ocular pathology. Cycloplegic agents, used to prevent accommodative spasm and thus inhibit the near triad, are rarely effective. Opacification of the inner one third of spectacle lenses is not effective. The effect of using minus (negative) spectacles is paradoxical and will worsen the deviation, so is contraindicated. Occasionally, a patient with uncorrected high hyperopia will appear to have spasm of the near reflex; however, a careful cycloplegic refraction will reveal an accommodative esotropia that was precipitated or unmasked as the patient's divergence fusional amplitudes decreased with age. In such cases the correct management consists of prescribing the full cycloplegic refraction.

Central disruption of fusion, also called posttraumatic fusion deficiency, occurs after moderate head injury and causes intractable diplopia, despite the patient's ability to fuse intermittently and even achieve stereopsis briefly.[42] The diplopia fluctuates and may be crossed, uncrossed, or vertical, and versions and ductions may be full, but vergence amplitudes are reduced markedly. Prism therapy or surgery is ineffective. Central disruption of fusion is caused by midbrain injury and may be associated with brainstem tumors, stroke, neurosurgical procedures, removal of long-standing cataracts, and uncorrected aphakia. This condition must be differentiated from psychogenic disorders of vergence and bilateral superior oblique palsies; the latter usually cause intolerable torsion. Inability to fuse also can occur in patients with infantile or early onset esotropia, congenital media opacities, and high degrees of anisometropia.

The hemislide phenomenon occurs when patients who have large visual field defects, particularly dense bitemporal hemianopias, develop diplopia. They have difficulty maintaining fusion because they can no longer suppress any latent deviation as a result of loss of overlapping areas of field.

Cyclic esotropia, also called circadian, alternate-day, or clock mechanism esotropia, begins in infancy or childhood. The cycles of orthotropia and esotropia have periods in the range of 24–96 hours. Most eventually develop constant esotropia and respond well to bimedial rectus muscle recession.

Ocular neuromyotonia is a brief, involuntary, intermittent myotonic contraction of one or more muscles supplied by the ocular motor nerves, most commonly the third cranial nerve. Although the mechanism is unclear, but most likely injury at a nuclear or infranuclear level, it is included here because it must be differentiated from other vergence disorders. Ocular neuromyotonia usually results in esotropia of the affected eye, with accompanying failure of elevation and depression of the globe, and may be provoked by prolonged eccentric gaze. It may be associated with signs of aberrant reinnervation of the third cranial nerve. Usually, the pupil is fixed to both light and near stimuli. Causes include radiation therapy and, less commonly, compressive lesions such as cavernous sinus meningiomas, pituitary adenomas and, rarely, dolichoectatic vessels. Occasionally no cause is found. Ocular neuromyotonia responds to carbamazepine and other antiepileptic drugs and must be differentiated from superior oblique myokymia and the spasms of cyclic oculomotor palsy (Chapter 202).

DEVELOPMENT OF THE OCULAR MOTOR SYSTEM

Maturation of the infant nervous system continues after birth and is particularly rapid during the first few months of life. At birth the vestibular system is the most developed of the ocular motor subsystems and may be tested by rotating the infant (held at arm's length) with the head tilted 30 degrees forward. The VOR is well developed by the end of the first postnatal week.[43] Smooth pursuit movements occur in neonates, but only with large targets (such as a human face) that move at low velocities, because the fovea is not well developed at this stage. The pursuit system does not mature fully until the late teens. The saccadic system also is immature in the neonate. Vertical saccades mature more slowly than horizontal saccades and may not be detected for the first month after birth. Vergence movements are also slow to mature but are seen after about the first month.

Transient Ocular Motility Abnormalities in Infancy

Several benign transient ocular motility disorders occur in infancy. Neonatal strabismus occurs in up to one third of healthy neonates; an esotropia that persists beyond 3 months, or an exotropia that persists beyond 4 months, postnatally is abnormal.[44] Tonic downward ocular deviation occurs in approximately 2% of otherwise healthy neonates[45,46] and is similar to the "sunsetting" sign seen in infants who have hydrocephalus, but resolves spontaneously. Lid retraction, either spontaneous or associated with sudden darkness, may be noted. Tonic upgaze is much rarer than tonic downgaze but is well described[31,47] and, also, usually resolves. Skew deviation occurs in healthy infants and usually resolves[45]; however, a substantial number of them develop strabismus. Some neonates may have a transient horizontal gaze palsy (Donahue, personal observation, 1995).

Premature infants, especially those with intraventricular hemorrhages, may develop tonic downward and esotropic ocular deviations similar to the motility findings in adults who have acquired thalamic lesions. Although the upgaze palsy typically resolves, the esotropia persists and requires surgery.[28]

REFERENCES

1. Lavin PJM, Donahue S. Neuro-ophthalmology: the efferent visual system. Gaze mechanisms and disorders. In: Daroff RB, Fenichel GM, Marsden CD, Bradley WG, eds. Neurology in clinical practice, ed 3. Boston: Butterworth Publishing; 2000:699–720.
2. Sharpe JA. Neural control of ocular motor systems. In: Miller NR, Newman NJ, eds. Walsh & Hoyt's clinical neuro-ophthalmology, vol 1, ed 5. Baltimore: Williams & Wilkins; 1998:1101–67.
3. Leigh RJ, Zee DS. Diagnosis of central disorders of ocular motility. The neurology of eye movements, ed 2. Philadelphia: FA Davis; 1991:378–531.
4. Borchert MS. Principles and techniques of the examination of ocular motility and alignment. In: Miller NR, Newman NJ, eds. Walsh & Hoyt's clinical neuro-ophthalmology, vol 1, ed 5. Baltimore: Williams & Wilkins; 1998:1169–88.
5. Leigh RJ, Daroff RB, Troost BT. Supranuclear disorders of eye movements. In: Glaser GS, ed. Neuro-ophthalmology, ed 3. Philadelphia: Lippincott Williams and Wilkins; 1999:345–68.
6. Chambers BR, Gresty MA. Effects of fixation and optokinetic stimulation on vestibulo-ocular reflex suppression. J Neurol Neurosurg Psychiatry. 1982;45: 998–1004.
7. Cogan DG. A type of congenital motor apraxia presenting jerky head movements. Trans Am Acad Ophthalmol Otolaryngol. 1952;56:853–62.
8. Supranuclear and internuclear gaze pathways. In: Bajandas FJ, Kline LB, eds. Neuro-ophthalmology review manual, ed 4. Thorofare: Slack; 1996:43–67.
9. Ebner R, Lopez L, Ochoa S, Crovetto L. Vertical ocular motor apraxia. Neurology. 1990;40:712–3.
10. Hughes JL, O'Connor PS, Larsen PD, Mumma JV. Congenital vertical ocular motor apraxia. J Clin Neuro Ophthalmol. 1985;5:153–7.
11. Sharpe JA, Silversides JL, Blair RDG. Familial paralysis of horizontal gaze associated with pendular nystagmus, progressive scoliosis, and facial contraction with myokymia. Neurology. 1975;25:1035–40.
12. Tijssen CC, Schulte BP, Leyten AC. Prognostic significance of conjugate eye deviation in stroke patients. Stroke. 1991;22:200–2.
13. Sharpe JA, Johnson JL. Ocular motor paresis versus apraxia. Ann Neurol. 1989; 25:209–10.
14. Pierrot-Deseilligny C, Gautier JC, Loron P. Acquired ocular motor apraxia due to bilateral frontoparietal infarcts. Ann Neurol. 1988;23:199–202.
15. Kellen RI, Burde RM, Hodges FJ III, Roper-Hall G. Central bilateral sixth nerve palsy associated with a unilateral preganglionic Horner's syndrome. J Clin Neuroophthalmol. 1988;8(3):179–84.
16. Sharpe JA, Bondar RL, Fletcher WA. Contralateral gaze deviation after frontal lobe haemorrhage. J Neurol Neurosurg Psychiatry. 1985;48:86–8.

17. Plum F, Posner JB. The diagnosis of stupor and coma, ed 3. Philadelphia: FA Davis; 1980.
18. Daroff RB, Hoyt WF. Clinical disorders of the supranuclear systems for vertical ocular movement. In: Bach-y-Rita P, Collins CC, Hyde JE, eds. The control of eye movements. New York: Academic Press; 1971:196–7.
19. Bolling J, Lavin PJ. Combined gaze palsy of horizontal saccades and pursuit of contralateral to a midbrain haemorrhage. J Neurol Neurosurg Psychiatry. 1987;50:789–91.
20. Wolin MJ, Trent RG, Lavin PJ, Cornblath WT. Oculopalatal myoclonus after the one-and-a-half syndrome with facial nerve palsy. Ophthalmology. 1996;103:177–80.
21. Wall M, Wray SH. The one-and-a-half syndrome—a unilateral disorder of the pontine tegmentum: a study of 20 cases and review of the literature. Neurology. 1983;33:971–80.
22. Davis TL, Lavin PJ. Pseudo one-and-a-half syndrome with ocular myasthenia. Neurology. 1989;39:15–53.
23. Siatkowski RM, Schatz NJ, Sellitti TP, et al. Do thalamic lesions really cause vertical gaze palsies? J Clin Neuro Ophthalmol. 1993;13:190–3.
24. Ranalli PJ, Sharpe JA, Fletcher WA. Palsy of upward and downward saccadic, pursuit, and vestibular movements with a unilateral midbrain lesion; pathophysiologic correlations. Neurology. 1988;38:114–22.
25. Hoyt CS, Billson FA, Alpins N. The supranuclear disturbances of gaze in kernicterus. Ann Ophthalmol. 1978;10:1487–92.
26. Topical diagnosis of neuropathic ocular motility disorders. In: Miller NR, ed. Walsh & Hoyt's clinical neuro-ophthalmology, vol 2, ed 4. Baltimore: Williams & Wilkins; 1985:652–784.
27. Barontini F, Simonetti C, Ferranini F, Sita D. Persistent upward eye deviation. Report of two cases. Neuroophthalmology. 1983:3:217–24.
28. Gieron MA, Korthals JK. Benign paroxysmal tonic upward gaze. Pediatr Neurol. 1993;9:159.
29. Ahn JC, Hoyt WF, Hoyt CS. Tonic upgaze in infancy. A report of three cases. Arch Ophthalmol. 1989;107:57–8.
30. Kumral E, Kocaer T, Ertubey NO, Kumral K. Thalamic hemorrhage. A prospective study of 100 patients. Stroke. 1995;26:964–70.
31. Tamura EE, Hoyt CS. Oculomotor consequences of intraventricular hemorrhages in premature infants. Arch Ophthalmol. 1987;105:533–5.
32. Brandt T, Dieterich M. Skew deviation with ocular torsion: a vestibular brainstem sign of topographic diagnostic value. Ann Neurol. 1993;33:528–34.
33. Hamed LM, Maria BL, Quisling RG, Mickle JP. Alternating skew on lateral gaze. Neuroanatomic pathway and relationship to superior oblique overaction. Ophthalmology. 1993;100:281–6.
34. Scott WE, Sutton VJ, Thalacker JA. Superior rectus recessions for dissociated vertical deviation. Ophthalmology. 1982;89:317–22.
35. Burke JP, Ruben JB, Scott WE. Vertical transposition of the horizontal recti (Knapp procedure) for the treatment of double elevator palsy: effectiveness and long-term stability. Br J Ophthalmol. 1992;76:734–7.
36. Ford CS, Schwartze GM, Weaver RG, Troost BT. Monocular elevation paresis caused by an ipsilateral lesion. Neurology. 1984;34:1264–7.
37. Munoz M, Page LK. Acquired double elevator palsy in a child with pineocytoma. Am J Ophthalmol. 1995;118:810–1.
38. Williams AS, Hoyt CS. Acute comitant esotropia in children with brain tumors. Arch Ophthalmol. 1989;107:376–8.
39. Simon JW, Waldman JB, Conture KC. Cerebellar astrocytoma manifesting as isolated, comitant esotropia in childhood. Am J Ophthalmol. 1996;121:584–6.
40. Brodsky MC, Baker RS, Hamed LM. Complex ocular motor disorders in children. In: Brodsky MC, Baker RS, Hamed LM, eds. Pediatric neuro-ophthalmology. New York: Springer-Verlag; 1996:251–301.
41. Waltz KL, Lavin PJM. Accommodative insufficiency. In: Margo CE, Mames RN, Hamed L, eds. Diagnostic problems in clinical ophthalmology. Philadelphia: WB Saunders; 1993:862–6.
42. Pratt-Johnson JA, Tillson G. The loss of fusion in adults with intractable diplopia (central fusion disruption). Aust N Z J Ophthalmol. 1988;16:81–5.
43. Leigh RJ, Zee DS. The vestibular-optokinetic system. The neurology of eye movements, ed 2. Philadelphia: FA Davis; 1991:15–78.
44. Nixon RB, Helveston EM, Miller K, et al. Incidence of strabismus in neonates. Am J Ophthalmol. 1985;100:798–801.
45. Hoyt CS, Mousel DK, Weber AA. Transient supranuclear disturbances of gaze in healthy neonates. Am J Ophthalmol. 1980;89:708–13.
46. Kleiman MD, DiMario FJ, Leconche DA, Zalneraitis EL. Benign transient downward gaze deviation in pre-term infants. Pediatr Neurol. 1994;10:313–6.
47. Deonna T, Roulet E, Meyer HU. Benign paroxysmal tonic upgaze of childhood—a new syndrome. Neuropediatrics. 1990;21:213–4.

CHAPTER
198 Nuclear and Fascicular Disorders of Eye Movement

SEAN P. DONAHUE

DEFINITION
- Eye movement disorders caused by damage to the ocular motor nerve nuclei (cranial nerve III, IV, or VI) or to the ocular motor nerve fascicles within the brainstem as they travel from the nerve nucleus to the subarachnoid space.

KEY FEATURES
- Diplopia.
- Incomitant ocular deviation.
- Other localizing neurological signs.

ASSOCIATED FEATURES
- Other cranial nerve palsies.
- Supranuclear disorders of motility.
- Long tract signs.

INTRODUCTION

Eye movement commands are carried from the cerebral cortex and higher brainstem structures to the ocular motor nerve nuclei. These commands are then sent to the individual extraocular muscles by cranial nerves III, IV, and VI. Eye movement abnormalities resulting from damage to the structures that carry commands to the ocular motor nerve nuclei are considered supranuclear or prenuclear in origin (see Chapter 197). Abnormalities resulting from damage to the ocular motor nuclei and their respective cranial nerves are considered infranuclear.

An infranuclear ocular motor nerve palsy can be caused by damage to the nerve anywhere from the nucleus to the extraocular muscle it innervates. Nuclear ocular motor palsies occur at the level of the ocular motor nucleus, whereas fascicular nerve palsies are caused by lesions of the fascicle of nerve that travels through the brainstem from the nerve nucleus to its exit into the subarachnoid space.

Nuclear and fascicular ocular motor nerve palsies produce characteristic ocular abnormalities according to the function of the innervated structure. All acute palsies produce an incomitant strabismus that is greatest in the field of action of the paretic muscle. Palsies of the third nerve are typically associated with abnormal pupillary and lid function, in addition to ocular motility abnormalities. Fourth nerve palsies are associated almost always with additional complaints of torsion or a head tilt.

Nuclear and fascicular nerve palsies often are associated with other neurological signs because of the large number of structures located nearby (Fig. 198-1). A detailed knowledge of the neuroanatomy of the midbrain and pons enables the clinician to localize these lesions with great accuracy.

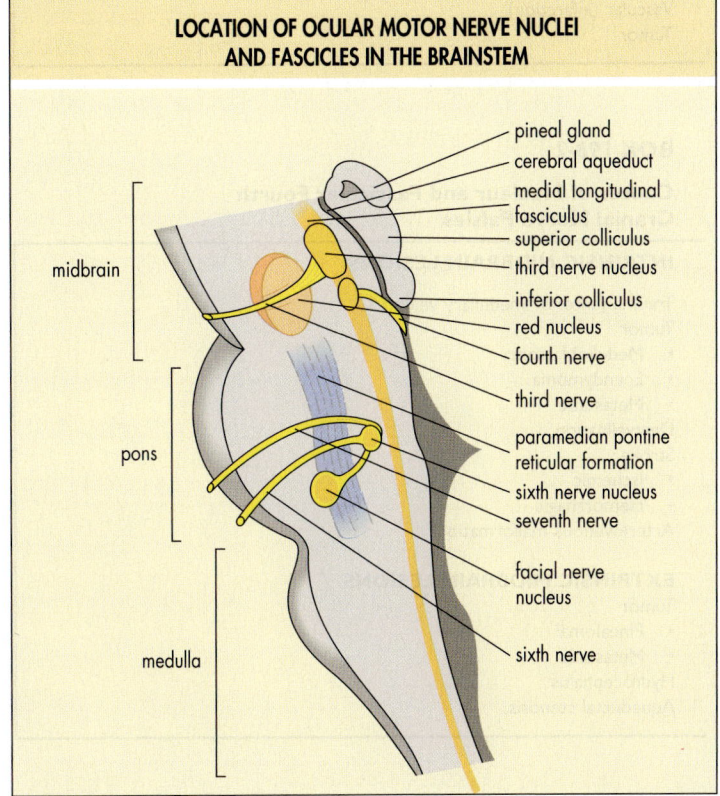

LOCATION OF OCULAR MOTOR NERVE NUCLEI AND FASCICLES IN THE BRAINSTEM

midbrain

pons

medulla

pineal gland
cerebral aqueduct
medial longitudinal fasciculus
superior colliculus
third nerve nucleus
inferior colliculus
red nucleus
fourth nerve
third nerve
paramedian pontine reticular formation
sixth nerve nucleus
seventh nerve
facial nerve nucleus
sixth nerve

FIG. 198-1 ■ Location of ocular motor nerve nuclei and fascicles in the brainstem. Note the relationship of the cranial nerve nuclei and fascicles to the medial longitudinal fasciculus, red nucleus, paramedian pontine reticular formation, and facial nerve nucleus and fascicle. The fourth nerve exits dorsally, while the third and sixth nerves exit ventrally.

EPIDEMIOLOGY AND PATHOGENESIS

Multiple reports in the literature document the causes of palsies of the three cranial nerves that subserve eye movements.[1–4] However, ocular motor nerve palsies typically become apparent in one of the following four ways[5]:
- Truly isolated nerve palsies that have no other signs or symptoms
- Isolated nerve palsies that have associated symptoms
- Nerve palsies associated with palsies of other cranial nerves
- Nerve palsies with neurological signs other than cranioneuropathies

Each of these four groups has a different corresponding differential diagnosis. Reports in the literature that consider the causes of ocular motor nerve palsies generally do not classify the palsies in this manner. Thus, most of these reports are of limited value to the clinician, who may have either localized the lesion already or formulated a differential diagnosis based on the manner of appearance.

Causes of Nucleur and Fascicular Third Cranial Nerve Palsies

CHILDREN
Congenital
• with neurological abnormalities
• with aberrant reinnervation
• with cyclic oculomotor spasm
Vascular (arteriovenous malformation)
Primary tumor
Metastatic tumor

YOUNG ADULTS
Demyelinating
Vascular (hemorrhage or infarction)
Tumor

OLDER ADULTS
Vascular (infarction)
Tumor

BOX 198-2

Causes of Nucleur and Fascicular Fourth Cranial Nerve Palsies

INTRINSIC MIDBRAIN LESIONS

Trauma (anterior medullary velum)
Tumor
• Medulloblastoma
• Ependymoma
• Metastatic
Demyelination
Stroke
• Ischemic
• Hemorrhagic
Arteriovenous malformation

EXTRINSIC MIDBRAIN LESIONS
Tumor
• Pinealoma
• Metastatic
Hydrocephalus
Aqueductal stenosis

BOX 198-3

Causes of Nucleur and Fascicular Sixth Cranial Nerve Palsies

Vascular disease
• Hemorrhage
• Infarction
  (anterior inferior cerebellar artery
  paramedian perforating arteries)
Demyelinating disease
Trauma
Tumor
• Glioma
• Astrocytoma
• Ependymoma
• Medulloblastoma
• Metastatic
• Infiltrative
Other

Because nuclear and fascicular disorders have associated findings that make them highly localizable, it is better to localize the lesion and then consider the causes based on the patient's age and the history (Boxes 198-1 to 198-3). Most nuclear and fascicular disorders of eye movement are caused by vascular disease (infarction, hemorrhage from arteriovenous malformation), demyelination, and tumor (metastatic or primary). Infectious, inflammatory, and traumatic causes are much less likely. Congenital oculomotor nerve palsy can arise from brainstem disorders in some patients,[6–8] who often have other brain anomalies and brainstem syndromes. Although thyroid disease and myasthenia can mimic isolated cranial nerve palsies, neither is associated with neurological deficits of brainstem function.

OCULAR MANIFESTATIONS
Palsies of the Third Cranial Nerve

The oculomotor nerve innervates the levator palpebrae, the pupillary sphincter, and the following four extraocular muscles:
• Medial rectus
• Inferior rectus
• Superior rectus
• Inferior oblique

The degree of involvement of these six structures varies in patients who have third nerve palsies. When the palsy is complete, there is complete ptosis with a dilated pupil that responds neither to light nor near. The eye is deviated out and usually, but by no means always, down. Function of the other ocular motor nerves can be assessed in this situation by evaluation of abduction (sixth cranial nerve) and by observing incyclotorsion on attempted depression (fourth cranial nerve).

Nuclear Third Cranial Nerve Lesions

The third nerve nucleus is located in the midbrain near the cerebral aqueduct at the level of the superior colliculus (Fig. 198-2). The anatomy of the third nerve nucleus was described by Warwick[9] in a classic paper in 1953. Each extraocular muscle that receives innervation from the third nerve has a corresponding group of cells, called a subnucleus, in the third nerve nucleus (Fig. 198-3). A single central nucleus (central caudal nucleus) innervates both levator palpebrae muscles. Distinct, bilateral subnuclei exist for the left and right medial recti, inferior recti, superior recti, and inferior oblique muscles. An additional bilateral subnucleus, the Edinger–Westphal nucleus, provides parasympathetic input to the pupillary sphincter.

Projections from the subnuclei to their targets all are uncrossed (each subnucleus innervates the ipsilateral corresponding extraocular muscle), with two exceptions—the single central caudal nucleus sends projections to both levator muscles, and the superior rectus subnucleus projection is crossed. Thus, the right superior rectus subnucleus innervates the left superior rectus muscle, and vice versa.

The rationale for the crossing of the fibers of the superior rectus subnucleus to the contralateral superior rectus is not understood fully but may be to facilitate vestibular innervation. The trochlear nerve also undergoes a decussation. As a result, each cyclovertical muscle and its corresponding yoked muscle pair have nuclei on the same side of the brain. The right inferior oblique subnucleus and left superior rectus subnucleus are both located on the right; the left inferior rectus subnucleus and right superior oblique subnucleus are both located on the left. This allows the direct innervation of a yoked muscle pair from the corresponding semicircular canal without a decussation; it may have been important in the development of the vestibular–ocular counter-rolling reflex (see Chapter 197).

Although the anatomy of the third nerve nucleus is quite complex, it does allow precise localization when certain abnormalities are present. Daroff[10] has proposed clinical rules that obligate or exclude nuclear involvement (Box 198-4). Because the central caudal subnucleus sends projections to both levator muscles, a bilateral third nerve palsy that spares the lid on both sides obligates a (rostral) nuclear lesion. The crossed projection of the superior rectus subnucleus also is important in the localization of these lesions—unilateral third nerve lesions that have

ANATOMY OF MIDBRAIN AT THE LEVEL OF THE THIRD NERVE NUCLEUS

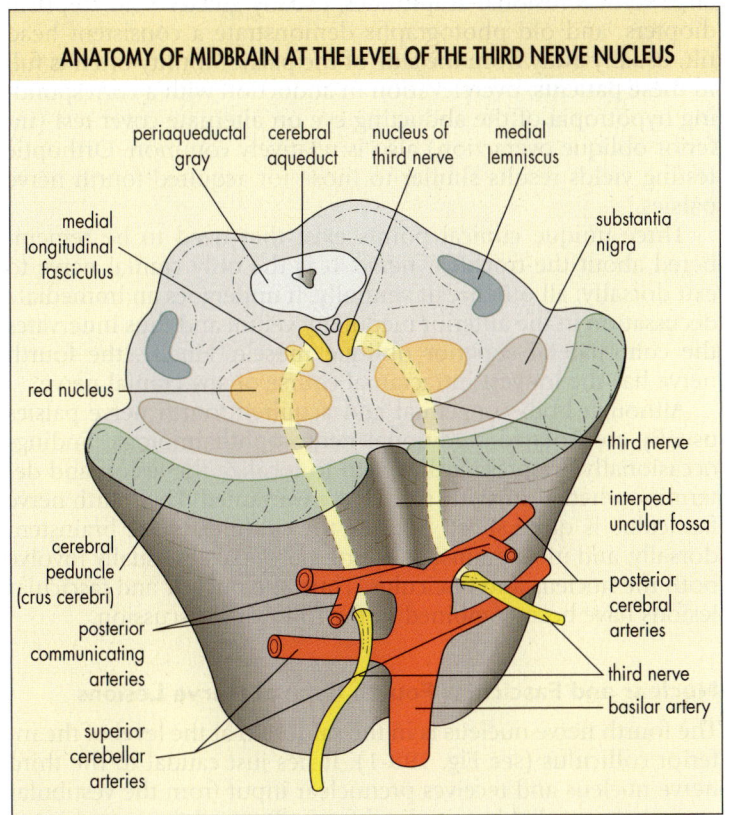

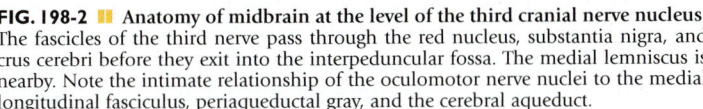

FIG. 198-2 ■ Anatomy of midbrain at the level of the third cranial nerve nucleus. The fascicles of the third nerve pass through the red nucleus, substantia nigra, and crus cerebri before they exit into the interpeduncular fossa. The medial lemniscus is nearby. Note the intimate relationship of the oculomotor nerve nuclei to the medial longitudinal fasciculus, periaqueductal gray, and the cerebral aqueduct.

ANATOMY OF THE THIRD NERVE NUCLEUS

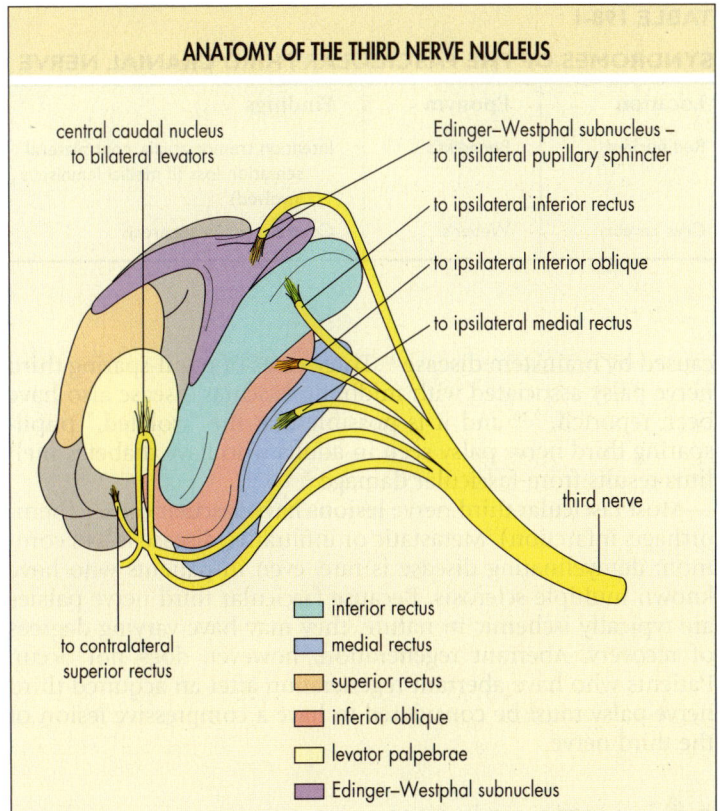

FIG. 198-3 ■ Anatomy of the third cranial nerve nucleus. The third nerve nucleus consists of a single, central, caudally located nucleus for the levator palpebrae, paired bilateral subnuclei with crossed projections that innervate the superior recti, and paired bilateral subnuclei with uncrossed projections that innervate the medial recti, inferior recti, and inferior oblique muscles. Parasympathetic input to the ciliary body and iris sphincter arises from the Edinger–Westphal nucleus. (Redrawn from Warwick R. Representation of the extraocular muscles in the oculomotor nuclei of the monkey. J Comp Neurol. 1953;98:449–503.)

involvement of the contralateral superior rectus obligate a nuclear lesion, whereas a third nerve palsy with no contralateral superior rectus abnormality cannot be caused by a nuclear lesion. The reader should review Daroff's rules (see Box 198-4) and determine how the neuroanatomy is responsible for each rule.

Isolated nuclear third nerve lesions are quite rare. Usually the lesion extends to cause supranuclear disorders of vertical gaze and other neurological signs. However, Warwick's scheme of nuclear anatomy has received confirmation by magnetic resonance imaging documentation in patients who have obligatory nuclear third nerve palsies[11–13]; histopathological confirmation also has been reported.[14,15]

Infarction, usually of small branches of the basilar artery, is the cause of most nuclear third nerve palsies. Metastatic, lymphoproliferative, and primary neoplastic disease also can occur.

Fascicular Third Cranial Nerve Palsies

After leaving the nucleus, the axons of the oculomotor neurons travel through the midbrain and exit ventrally. They pass near or through two important structures before exiting into the subarachnoid space of the interpeduncular fossa—the red nucleus and the crus cerebri. Lesions that damage the third nerve fascicle within the red nucleus cause a contralateral intention tremor and ataxia. Because the nearby medial lemniscus carries sensory fibers for light touch and proprioception on the contralateral side, these modalities also may be impaired or absent. Lesions of the cerebral peduncle damage corticospinal tract fibers that descend to innervate the musculature of the contralateral extremities; damage in this area is associated with a contralateral hemiparesis. Each of these syndromes has a specific eponym (Table 198-1).

BOX 198-4

Daroff's Rules for Nucleur Third Cranial Nerve Palsies

CONDITIONS THAT OBLIGATE NUCLEAR INVOLVEMENT
Bilateral third nerve palsy without ptosis (bilaterally spared levator function)
Unilateral third nerve palsy with contralateral superior rectus abnormality and bilateral partial ptosis

CONDITIONS THAT EXCLUDE A NUCLEAR LESION
Unilateral ptosis
Unilateral internal ophthalmoplegia
Unilateral external ophthalmoplegia associated with normal contralateral superior rectus function

CONDITIONS THAT NEITHER EXCLUDE NOR OBLIGATE A NUCLEAR LESION
Bilateral total third nerve palsy
Bilateral ptosis
Bilateral internal ophthalmoplegia
Bilateral medial rectus palsy

Isolated unilateral single muscle involvement (except levator and superior rectus). From Daroff RB. Oculomotor manifestation of brainstem and cerebellar dysfunction. In: Smith JL, ed. Neuro-ophthalmology: symposium of the University of Miami and Bascom-Palmer Eye Institute, vol 5. Hallandale: Huffman; 1971:104–21.

Classically, fascicular third nerve palsies were thought to affect all functions of the third nerve equally, with the degree of pupil involvement (anisocoria increasing in bright light) being proportional to the lid and motility defects. Recently, however, it has been recognized that isolated extraocular muscle pareses, especially inferior rectus paresis, can result from fascicular third nerve lesions.[16,17] Divisional oculomotor paresis also can be

TABLE 198-1

SYNDROMES OF THE FASCICULAR THIRD CRANIAL NERVE

Location	Eponym	Findings
Red nucleus	Benedikt's	Intention tremor, ataxia, contralateral sensation loss (if medial lemniscus involved)
Crus cerebri	Weber's	Contralateral hemiparesis

caused by brainstem disease.[18] Three cases of pupil-sparing third nerve palsy associated with midbrain vascular disease also have been reported,[19,20] and it is possible that the "isolated," pupil-sparing third nerve palsy seen in adults who have diabetes mellitus results from fascicular damage.[21]

Most fascicular third nerve lesions have vascular causes (hemorrhage, infarction). Metastatic or infiltrative disease is less common; demyelinating disease is rare, even in patients who have known multiple sclerosis. Because fascicular third nerve palsies are typically ischemic in nature, they may have varying degrees of recovery. Aberrant regeneration, however, does not occur. Patients who have aberrant regeneration after an acquired third nerve palsy must be considered to have a compressive lesion of the third nerve.

Congenital Third Cranial Nerve Palsies

Congenital oculomotor nerve palsies are rare and are associated with neurological abnormalities in a significant percentage of patients.[6-8] These palsies can result from aplasia or hypoplasia of the oculomotor nucleus,[22] but more often they occur because of lesions of the nerve itself. Aberrant regeneration following congenital third nerve palsies is rather common,[23] which argues against a nuclear lesion. Loewenfeld and Thompson[24] have speculated that perinatal damage to the third nerve causes retrograde degeneration of the oculomotor nucleus, which then is reinnervated haphazardly. Patients who have congenital third nerve palsies and associated neurological abnormalities without aberrant regeneration likely have brainstem pathology.

Some patients who have congenital oculomotor nerve palsies develop cyclic oculomotor spasm.[24] Typical cases have a slow alternation between a paretic phase, in which the lid droops, the pupil dilates, and the eye turns out, and a spastic phase, in which the lid elevates, the pupil constricts, accommodation occurs, and the eye adducts. These cycles usually persist throughout life. Cyclic oculomotor spasm usually is not associated with acquired lesions of the third nerve.

Palsies of the Fourth Cranial Nerve

Superior oblique palsy is the most common cause of acquired vertical diplopia and can be either congenital or acquired. Patients who have acquired superior oblique palsies have diplopia that is often worse in downgaze, and they usually complain of torsion. Subjective image separation increases with gaze in the direction opposite the side of the palsy and with head tilt toward the side of the palsy. For example, a right superior oblique palsy has diplopia worse on left gaze and right head tilt. Motility testing in the acute phase usually demonstrates poor depression in adduction. Orthoptic measurements show a hypertropia of the affected eye that increases with gaze to the side opposite the palsy and with head tilt toward the side of the palsy. The most common cause of an isolated, acquired fourth nerve palsy is trauma (see Box 198-2).[25-27]

Congenital fourth nerve palsies can become apparent at any age. Young children often exhibit abnormal head postures, while older individuals typically experience intermittent vertical diplopia. Patients who have congenital fourth nerve palsies have

large vertical fusional amplitudes, usually greater than 10 prism diopters, and old photographs demonstrate a consistent head tilt, usually away from the side of the palsy. Motility often is full in these patients; overelevation in adduction with a corresponding hypotropia of the abducting eye on alternate cover test (inferior oblique overaction) also is relatively common. Orthoptic testing yields results similar to those for acquired fourth nerve palsies.

Three unique clinical points exist that need to be remembered about the trochlear nerve. It is the only cranial nerve to exit dorsally; all others exit ventrally. It undergoes an immediate decussation in the anterior medullary velum and thus innervates the contralateral superior oblique muscle. Finally, the fourth nerve has the longest intracranial course of any cranial nerve.

Although both congenital and acquired fourth nerve palsies usually are isolated, additional neuro-ophthalmologic findings occasionally are present that help to localize the lesion and determine whether imaging studies are warranted. The fourth nerve fasciculus is quite short, because the nerve exits the brainstem dorsally, and most brainstem fourth nerve palsies usually involve both the nucleus and fasciculus. Thus, the nuclear and fascicular lesions have been combined in the following discussion.

Nuclear and Fascicular Fourth Cranial Nerve Lesions

The fourth nerve nucleus is in the midbrain at the level of the inferior colliculus (see Fig. 198-1). It lies just caudal to the third nerve nucleus and receives prenuclear input from the vestibular system, the medial longitudinal fasciculus, and the rostral interstitial medial longitudinal fasciculus (riMLF). The fasciculus of the trochlear nerve travels dorsally to exit the lower midbrain just caudal to the inferior colliculus, near the tentorium. Because the nerve decussates in the anterior medullary velum, nuclear and fascicular fourth nerve palsies are associated with superior oblique dysfunction on the contralateral side.

Isolated lesions that affect only the nuclear or fascicular trochlear nerve are very rare. Most lesions of the area that surrounds the fourth nerve nucleus and fasciculus also affect neighboring structures. Both extrinsic (tumor, hydrocephalus) and intrinsic (tumor, stroke, demyelination, arteriovenous malformation) lesions of the brainstem may damage the trochlear nerves or nucleus and often produce an associated upgaze palsy or features of the dorsal midbrain syndrome (see Box 198-2). Lesions that damage the fourth nerve within the dorsolateral midbrain also can damage the first-order (descending) sympathetic fibers (Table 198-2). Affected patients have an ipsilateral preganglionic Horner's syndrome and a contralateral superior oblique palsy.[28] Lesions that extend into the superior cerebellar peduncle have an associated ipsilateral dysmetria. Damage that extends into the medial longitudinal fasciculus can produce an ipsilateral internuclear ophthalmoplegia in association with a superior oblique palsy. The hypertropia can be misdiagnosed as a skew deviation unless careful attention is paid to measurements of head tilt and to objective and subjective torsion. Damage to both trochlear nerve fascicles at their decussation within the anterior medullary velum usually results from trauma and produces a bilateral superior oblique palsy, which is often asymmetrical. These patients typically have a V-pattern esotropia, a right hypertropia on left gaze, a left hypertropia on right gaze, and greater than 10 degrees of subjective excyclotorsion when measured with the double Maddox rod. Bilateral fourth nerve palsy also can be produced by brainstem hematoma, but this is much rarer.[29]

Perhaps the most interesting fascicular syndrome of the fourth nerve involves the brachium of the superior colliculus.[30] Through this structure pass pupillomotor fibers as they travel from the optic tract to the pretectum. These fibers subserve the pupillary light reflex from the contralateral visual field. Because the retinogeniculate pathway has already separated from the pupillary pathways, conscious light detection is not affected, but the pupillary light

TABLE 198-2

NUCLEAR AND FASCICULAR SYNDROMES OF THE FOURTH CRANIAL NERVE

Site of Damage	Laterality of Superior Oblique Palsy	Clinical Manifestations
Pretectal area	Contralateral	Vertical gaze palsy Dorsal midbrain syndrome
Descending sympathetic pathways	Contralateral	Ipsilateral Horner's syndrome
Superior cerebellar peduncle	Contralateral	Ipsilateral dysmetria
Medial longitudinal fasciculus	Contralateral	Ipsilateral internuclear ophthalmoplegia
Brachium of superior colliculus	Contralateral	Contralateral relative afferent pupillary defect Contralateral pupil homonymous hemianopia Normal visual fields
Anterior medullary velum	Bilateral	'V' pattern esotropia Reversing hypertropias on side gaze >10° excyclotorsion

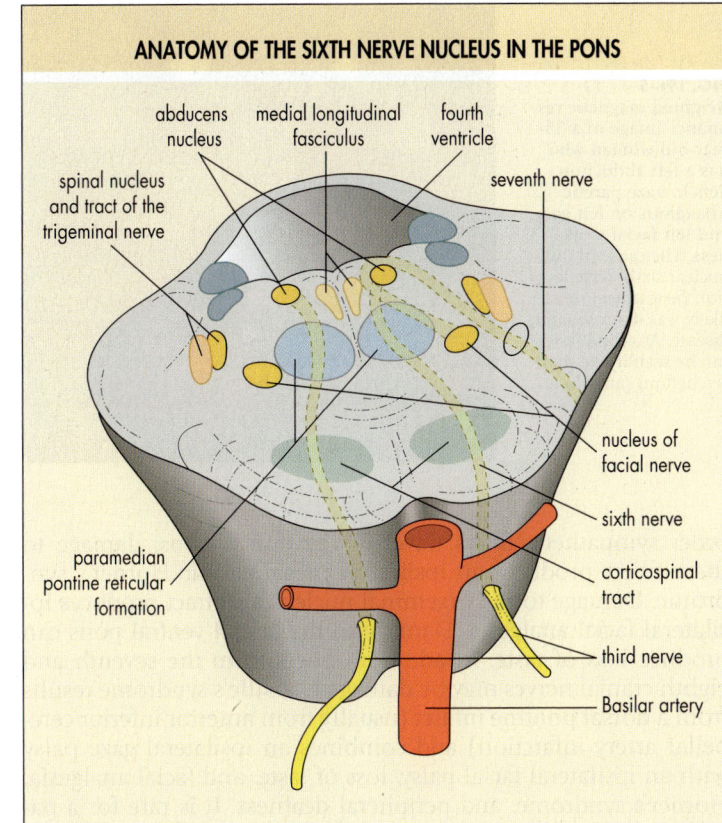

ANATOMY OF THE SIXTH NERVE NUCLEUS IN THE PONS

abducens nucleus
medial longitudinal fasciculus
fourth ventricle
spinal nucleus and tract of the trigeminal nerve
seventh nerve
nucleus of facial nerve
sixth nerve
corticospinal tract
third nerve
Basilar artery
paramedian pontine reticular formation

FIG. 198-4 ■ Anatomy of sixth cranial nerve nucleus in the pons. The abducens nucleus is surrounded by the facial nerve fasciculus after it originates from its nucleus and is associated intimately with the medial longitudinal fasciculus. Abducens fascicles traverse the paramedian pontine reticular formation and the corticospinal tract before leaving the lower ventral pons. The vestibular nuclei and spinal nucleus and tract of the trigeminal nerve are nearby in the lateral pons.

reflex is. Patients who suffer lesions in this area have normal visual fields but a small (0.6–0.9 log unit) relative afferent pupillary defect in the eye contralateral to the lesion, consistent with an optic tract lesion. The fourth nerve palsy is also on the contralateral side (the fascicle is damaged before the decussation). For example, a patient who has a right-sided lesion will have a left hypertropia that maps to a left superior oblique palsy and a small relative afferent pupillary defect in the left eye. If performed, pupil fields would demonstrate a left homonymous hemianopia, while formal visual fields would be full.

Palsies of the Sixth Cranial Nerve

The sixth nerve innervates the ipsilateral lateral rectus muscle and produces abduction. Damage to the sixth nerve produces an esotropia that is worse in the field of action of the involved sixth nerve. The esotropia usually is greater at distance than at near. Most patients are able to fuse with a face turn toward the side of the palsy (gaze away from the palsy). The pupil is not affected. Patients who have long-standing sixth nerve palsies can develop tightening and contracture of the medial rectus, which causes a restrictive strabismus with positive forced ductions. Occasionally, patients who have long-standing sixth nerve palsies may have associated vertical diplopia and hypertropia.[31]

Although patients who suffer sixth nerve palsies have a characteristic abduction deficit, it must be recognized that all abduction deficits are not due to sixth nerve palsies. Orbital lesions, medial wall fractures, Duane's syndrome, thyroid disease, and myasthenia all can mimic sixth nerve palsies.

The sixth nerve can be damaged at any location between its nucleus and the lateral rectus muscle. In a manner similar to the case with third nerve palsies, nuclear and fascicular lesions of the sixth nerve typically have characteristic findings that make them highly localizable.

Nuclear Sixth Cranial Nerve Palsies

The sixth nerve nucleus is in the pons, just ventral to the floor of the fourth ventricle. The fascicle of the facial nerve wraps around the sixth nerve nucleus (Fig. 198-4). The sixth nerve nucleus contains cell bodies of two types of neurons—most cell bodies

BOX 198-5

Nuclear and Fascicular Syndromes of the Sixth Cranial Nerve

NUCLEAR SIXTH NERVE PALSIES
One-and-a-half syndrome (obligate)
Foville's syndrome
Gaze palsy
Peripheral facial palsy (likely)

FASCICULAR SIXTH NERVE PALSIES
With contralateral hemiplegia (Raymond's syndrome)
Facial weakness (Millard–Gubler syndrome)

project directly to the lateral rectus muscle, via the abducens nerve. However, about 40% of the cells in the abducens nucleus are interneurons which project, via the medial longitudinal fasciculus, to the contralateral medial rectus subnucleus, and cause adduction of the contralateral eye. Thus, the sixth nerve nucleus, like the paramedian pontine reticular formation, is a gaze center. Damage to the sixth nerve nucleus or to the caudal paramedian pontine reticular formation produces an ipsilateral gaze palsy that cannot be overcome by vestibular testing.[32] Because all nuclear sixth nerve palsies produce a gaze palsy, an abduction deficit not associated with contralateral adduction weakness cannot arise from nuclear damage.

The location of the sixth nerve nucleus within the brainstem produces several possible associated deficits when a nuclear sixth nerve palsy is present (Box 198-5). As a result of the intimate relationship between the facial nerve fasciculus and the sixth nerve nucleus, an ipsilateral peripheral facial nerve palsy is present in nearly all cases of abducens nuclear injury (Fig. 198-5). The first-

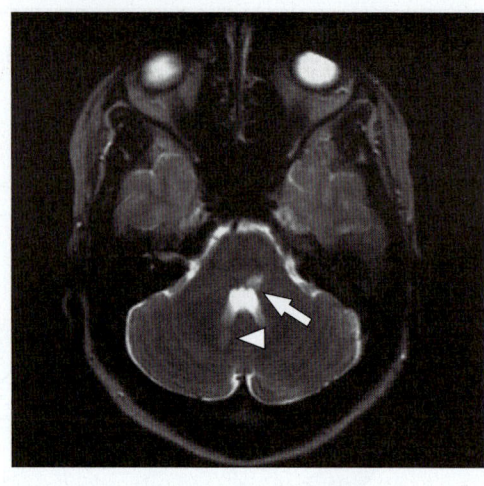

FIG. 198-5 ■ T2-weighted magnetic resonance image of a 33-year-old woman who has a left abduction deficit, gaze paretic nystagmus on left gaze, and left facial weakness. The cause of this nuclear sixth nerve lesion *(long arrow)* most likely was demyelinating disease. A second lesion can be seen in the right cerebellum *(arrowhead)*.

order sympathetic fibers travel in the dorsal pons; damage to these fibers produces an ipsilateral preganglionic Horner's syndrome. Damage to the trigeminal nucleus and tract produces ipsilateral facial analgesia. Damage to the lateral ventral pons can produce loss of taste. In addition, fibers from the seventh and eighth cranial nerves may be damaged. Foville's syndrome results from a dorsal pontine infarct (usually from anterior inferior cerebellar artery infarction) and combines an ipsilateral gaze palsy with an ipsilateral facial palsy, loss of taste, and facial analgesia, Horner's syndrome, and peripheral deafness. It is rare for a patient to have all characteristics of Foville's syndrome.

When damage from either the sixth nerve nucleus or paramedian pontine reticular formation also involves the ipsilateral medial longitudinal fasciculus, a characteristic motility pattern is produced, consisting of an ipsilateral gaze palsy with an ipsilateral internuclear ophthalmoplegia. The ipsilateral eye cannot adduct or abduct, while the contralateral eye can only abduct. This syndrome is called a *one-and-a-half syndrome*.[33]

Most nuclear abducens palsies are caused by infarction (anterior inferior cerebellar or paramedian perforating arteries), demyelination, or compression (intrinsic pontine tumors). Infiltrative disease, hemorrhage, and trauma are less likely causative factors (see Box 198-3).

Fascicular Sixth Cranial Nerve Palsies

Nearly all fascicular lesions of the abducens nerve are associated with distinctive neurological findings that result from damage to the surrounding neurological structures of the pons. Foville's syndrome (sixth nerve palsy, ipsilateral Horner's syndrome, ipsilateral facial analgesia, ipsilateral facial palsy with loss of taste, and ipsilateral peripheral deafness) can occur with either nuclear or fascicular lesions of the sixth nerve. These can be differentiated by evaluation of contralateral adduction: A nuclear lesion has a gaze palsy, while a fascicular lesion has an ipsilateral abduction deficit.

Lesions that affect the abducens fasciculus in the ventral pons can cause a contralateral hemiplegia (Raymond's syndrome). Millard–Gubler syndrome has ipsilateral peripheral facial weakness in addition to the abduction deficit and contralateral hemiplegia. These eponymous syndromes and their findings are listed in Box 198-5. Because most lesions can affect both the dorsal and ventral pons, a clinical overlap exists between these syndromes.

Common causes of fascicular lesions include infarction, compression (cerebellar pontine angle tumor or glioma), infiltration, and demyelination, and vary with the age of the patient.[1,3,34] Hemorrhage, trauma, and infection are less likely (see Box 198-3).

Classic teaching in pediatric ophthalmology held that isolated sixth nerve palsies in childhood should be considered the result of a pontine glioma until proven otherwise. This was based upon a series of 133 such patients seen before 1965 at the

Mayo Clinic.[34] Of these children, 52 had tumors, and over 75% of the tumors were pontine gliomas. However, the definition of isolated palsy used in that study meant that no other cranial nerve palsies existed, and not that the remainder of the neurological examination was normal. Most of these children had other abnormalities, such as papilledema and nystagmus. Because children without these associated findings nearly always develop them within a few weeks, a careful neuro-ophthalmologic examination with close follow-up probably is all that is necessary in children (under age 14 years) who have truly isolated idiopathic sixth nerve palsies.

DIAGNOSIS

Palsies of the Third Cranial Nerve

Both nuclear and fascicular third nerve palsies usually can be highly localized on the basis of clinical findings. A detailed examination of ocular motility (see Chapter 197) often is sufficient to diagnose nuclear lesions. Particular attention should be paid to vertical gaze abnormalities, because the centers for vertical gaze are in close proximity to the oculomotor nucleus and also are often damaged. Vestibular testing should be performed in patients who have bilateral vertical gaze abnormalities, to differentiate supranuclear from nuclear and infranuclear causes of these disorders. Bell's reflex often is preserved with supranuclear lesions. A neurological examination should be directed to identify tremor, contralateral hemisensory loss, contralateral hemiplegia, pronator drift, and contralateral hyperreflexia, which help to localize fascicular lesions. Magnetic resonance imaging is the best method by which to assess the integrity of midbrain structures in patients who have acute palsies. The neuroradiologist should be informed of the clinical localization so that attention can be directed to this area.

Palsies of the Fourth Cranial Nerve

Management of fourth nerve palsies depends upon the associated neurological findings and localization. Older adults with an isolated fourth nerve palsy and predisposing factors for vascular disease need only careful follow-up. Imaging studies should be performed if progression occurs, if additional neurological signs develop, or if recovery does not begin to occur within 3 months. Younger individuals who have large fusional amplitudes and photographic documentation of head tilting since infancy or childhood need no further evaluation, because the palsy is likely congenital with recent decompensation. Patients who have acquired fourth nerve palsies with localizing signs should undergo imaging studies, with attention paid to the areas suggested by the clinical findings. Patients who have no risk factors for vascular disease, no history of trauma, and no findings suggestive of a decompensating congenital fourth nerve palsy should undergo imaging studies to rule out small peripheral schwannomas, especially if progression occurs. Inquiry regarding the presence of multiple café-au-lait spots or other stigmata of neurofibromatosis may be useful.

Palsies of the Sixth Cranial Nerve

Management of sixth nerve palsies also depends on the associated findings. All patients who have sixth nerve palsies must receive complete neuro-ophthalmologic evaluation. Specific attention should be paid to the function of the facial nerve and to the other cranial nerves that subserve ocular motility and the pupil. The cerebellum and vestibular system also should be evaluated. Testing of deep tendon reflexes and the peripheral motor system is necessary to rule out corticospinal tract involvement. The optic nerves must be examined to rule out papilledema. Patients who have brainstem findings need magnetic resonance imaging and appropriate management. Patients who have had strokes need immediate neurological consultation, while patients who have brain tumors need urgent neurosurgical evaluation.

For patients who have truly isolated sixth nerve palsy, nuclear or fascicular involvement is unlikely. The evaluation and work-up of these patients is given in detail in Chapter 199. However, it should be remembered that all abduction deficits are not the result of sixth nerve palsies—myasthenia, thyroid disease, Duane's syndrome, and orbital disorders must be ruled out.

TREATMENT, COURSE, AND OUTCOME

Palsies of the Third Cranial Nerve

Many patients who have ischemic oculomotor nerve palsies eventually improve. Ptosis is often advantageous in this situation, because it prevents diplopia. Strabismus correction and lid surgery are needed to restore binocularity in patients who do not improve spontaneously; the author waits for stable measurements to occur for 6 months before suggesting surgical alignment. Specific techniques for restoring motility in patients who have third nerve palsy (superior oblique tendon transfer) are discussed elsewhere.[35]

Palsies of the Fourth Cranial Nerve

Palsies of the fourth nerve that result from vascular disease or trauma often resolve spontaneously over 3–6 months. During this time, Fresnel prisms can be placed over spectacles to allow fusion. However, this often is fraught with difficulty, because the deviation is usually quite incomitant and torsion cannot be corrected. Patients who have fourth nerve palsies that arise from compressive lesions often do not improve and require surgery.

Surgical options for the treatment of superior oblique palsy are complex and are beyond the scope of this chapter. The choice of procedure depends upon the deviation in primary position, the deviation in the fields of action of the paretic superior oblique and the antagonist inferior oblique, the deviation out of the field of action of the involved superior oblique, and the objective and subjective torsion. Knapp[36] and Scott and Kraft[37,38] have proposed surgical classification schemes; this author prefers that of Scott because it is more detailed and has better long-term follow-up. Congenital superior oblique palsies often are associated with abnormalities of the insertion of the superior oblique tendon and have been discussed by Wallace and von Noorden.[39]

Palsies of the Sixth Cranial Nerve

Nearly all patients who have sixth nerve palsies experience diplopia. During the acute phase, this is best managed by patching the paretic eye or by frosting a spectacle lens. Prisms usually are not tolerated well because of the magnitude and incomitance of the deviation. Botulinum toxin has been suggested to prevent secondary contracture of the antagonist medial rectus for patients who have acute bilateral sixth nerve palsies (trauma). Injection of the ipsilateral medial rectus muscle with 5 units of botulinum toxin (Botox) often weakens this muscle sufficiently to allow fusion with a small face turn while recovery of lateral rectus function occurs.[40] Botulinum toxin injection probably does not decrease the need for later surgical intervention of unilateral sixth nerve palsy.[41,42]

Surgical intervention for sixth nerve palsy is indicated when the deviation has been stable for a minimum of 6 months. Preoperative evaluation should include determination of corneal sensation and lid closure; patients who have constant esodeviations often are protected from exposure keratopathy by the relative position of the eye and can experience severe corneal damage if the eye is brought to primary position when lagophthalmos or hypesthesia is present. The choice of surgical procedure for chronic sixth nerve palsies depends upon the recovery of function of the lateral rectus muscle, which can be assessed by determining the saccadic velocity. Patients who have good return

of function usually do quite well with an ipsilateral recess–resect procedure. Patients who have little or no lateral rectus function need muscle transposition surgery. The transposition procedure described by Jensen works well to restore binocularity, with little risk of anterior segment ischemia.[43] Other transposition procedures have been described, but fewer long-term follow-up data are published.

REFERENCES

1. Rush JA, Younge BR. Paralysis of cranial nerves III, IV, and VI. Cause and prognosis in 1000 cases. Arch Ophthalmol. 1981;99:76–9.
2. Berlit P. Isolated and combined pareses of cranial nerves III, IV, and VI. A retrospective study of 412 patients. J Neurol Sci. 1991;103:10–5.
3. Richards BW, Jones FR Jr, Younge BR. Causes and prognosis in 4278 cases of paralysis of the oculomotor, trochlear, and abducens cranial nerves. Am J Ophthalmol. 1992;113:489–96.
4. Kodsi SR, Younge BR. Acquired oculomotor, trochlear, and abducent cranial nerve palsies in pediatric patients. Am J Ophthalmol. 1992;114:568–74.
5. Miller NR. Topical diagnosis of neuropathic ocular motility disorders. In: Miller NR, ed. Walsh & Hoyt's clinical neuro-ophthalmology, ed 4. Baltimore: Williams & Wilkins, 1985:652–784.
6. Balkan R, Hoyt CS. Associated neurologic abnormalities in congenital third nerve palsies. Am J Ophthalmol. 1984;97:315–9.
7. Hamed LM. Associated neurologic and ophthalmologic findings in congenital oculomotor nerve palsy. Ophthalmology. 1991;98:708–14.
8. Good WV, Barkovich AJ, Nickel BL, Hoyt CS. Bilateral congenital oculomotor nerve palsy in a child with brain anomalies. Am J Ophthalmol. 1991;111:555–8.
9. Warwick R. Representation of the extraocular muscles in the oculomotor nuclei of the monkey. J Comp Neurol. 1953;98:449–503.
10. Daroff RB. Oculomotor manifestation of brainstem and cerebellar dysfunction. In: Smith JL, ed. Neuro-ophthalmology: symposium of the University of Miami and Bascom-Palmer Eye Institute, vol 5. Hallandale: Huffman; 1971:104–21.
11. Bryan JS, Hamed LM. Levator-sparing nuclear oculomotor palsy. Clinical and magnetic resonance imaging findings. J Clin Neuroophthalmol. 1992;12:26–30.
12. Martin TJ, Corbett JJ, Babidian PV, et al. Bilateral ptosis due to mesencephalic lesions with relative preservation of ocular motility. J Neuroophthalmol. 1996;16:258–63.
13. Pratt DV, Orengo-Nania S, Horowitz BL, Oram O. Magnetic resonance imaging findings in a patient with nuclear oculomotor palsy. Arch Ophthalmol. 1995;113:141–2.
14. Barton JJ, Kardon RH, Slagel D, Thompson HS. Bilateral central ptosis in acquired immunodeficiency syndrome. Can J Neurol Sci. 1995;22:52–5.
15. Keane JR, Zaias B, Itabashi HH. Levator-sparing oculomotor nerve palsy caused by a solitary midbrain metastasis. Arch Neurol. 1984;41:210–2.
16. Warren W, Burde RM, Klingele TG, Roper-Hall G. Atypical oculomotor paresis. J Clin Neuroophthalmol. 1982;2:13–8.
17. Ksiazek SM, Slamovits TL, Rosen CE, et al. Fascicular arrangement in partial oculomotor paresis. Am J Ophthalmol. 1994;118:97–103.
18. Ksiazek SM, Repka MX, Maguire A, et al. Divisional oculomotor nerve paresis caused by intrinsic brainstem disease. Ann Neurol. 1989;26:714–8.
19. Breen LA, Hopf HC, Farris BK, Gutmann L. Pupil-sparing oculomotor nerve palsy due to midbrain infarction. Arch Neurol. 1991;48:105–6.
20. Fleet WS, Rapcsak SZ, Huntley WW, Watson RT. Pupil-sparing oculomotor palsy from midbrain hemorrhage. Ann Ophthalmol. 1988;20:345–6.
21. Hopf HC, Gutmann L. Diabetic 3rd nerve palsy: evidence for a mesencephalic lesion. Neurology. 1990;40:1041–5.
22. Norman MG. Unilateral encephalomalacia in cranial nerve nuclei in neonates. Report of two cases. Neurology. 1974;24:424–7.
23. Victor DI. The diagnosis of congenital unilateral third-nerve palsy. Brain. 1976;99:711–8.
24. Loewenfeld IE, Thompson HS. Oculomotor paresis with cyclic spasms. A critical review of the literature and a new case. Surv Ophthalmol. 1975;20:81–124.
25. von Noorden GK, Murray E, Wong SY. Superior oblique paralysis. Arch Ophthalmol. 1986;104:1771–6.
26. Brazis PW. Palsies of the trochlear nerve: diagnosis and localization—recent concepts. Mayo Clin Proc. 1993;68:501–9.
27. Keane JR. Fourth nerve palsy: historical review and study of 215 inpatients. Neurology. 1993;43:2439–43.
28. Guy J, Day AL, Mickle JP, Schatz NJ. Contralateral trochlear nerve paresis and ipsilateral Horner's syndrome. Am J Ophthalmol. 1989;107:73–6.
29. Tachibana H, Minura O, Shiomi M, Oono T. Bilateral trochlear nerve palsies from a brainstem hematoma. J Clin Neuroophthalmol. 1990;10:35–7.
30. Eliott D, Cunningham ET Jr, Miller NR. Fourth nerve paresis and ipsilateral relative afferent pupillary defect without visual sensory disturbance. J Clin Neuroophthalmol. 1991;11:169–72.
31. Slavin ML. Hyperdeviation associated with isolated unilateral abducens palsy. Ophthalmology. 1989;96:512–6.
32. Muri RM, Chermann JF, Cohen L, et al. Ocular motor consequences of damage to the abducens nucleus area in humans. J Neuroophthalmol. 1996;16:191–5.
33. Wall M, Wray SH. The one-and-a-half syndrome—a unilateral disorder of the pontine tegmentum: a study of 20 cases and review of the literature. Neurology. 1983;33:971–80.
34. Robertson DM, Hines JD, Rucker CW. Acquired sixth nerve paresis in children. Arch Ophthalmol. 1970;83:574–9.
35. van Noorden GK, Campos EC. Binocular vision and ocular motility, 6th ed. St Louis: Mosby; 2002.
36. Knapp P. Classification and treatment of superior oblique palsy. Am Orthopt J. 1974;24:18–22.
37. Scott WE, Kraft SP. Classification and surgical treatment of superior oblique palsies: I. Unilateral superior oblique palsies. In: New Orleans Academy of Ophthalmology. Pediatric ophthalmology and strabismus: transactions of the New Orleans Academy of Ophthalmology. New York: Raven Press; 1986:15–38.

38. Scott WE, Kraft SP. Classification and treatment of superior oblique palsies: II. Bilateral superior oblique palsies. In: New Orleans Academy of Ophthalmology. Pediatric ophthalmology and strabismus: transactions of the New Orleans Academy of Ophthalmology. New York: Raven Press; 1986:265–91.

39. Wallace DK, von Noorden GK. Clinical characteristics and surgical management of congenital absence of the superior oblique tendon. Am J Ophthalmol. 1994;118:63–9.

40. Repka MX, Lam GC, Morrison NA. The efficacy of botulinum neurotoxin A for the treatment of complete and partially recovered chronic sixth nerve palsy. J Pediatr Ophthalmol Strabismus. 1994;31:79–83.

41. Lee J, Harris S, Cohen J, et al. Results of a prospective randomized trial of botulinum toxin therapy in acute unilateral sixth nerve palsy. J Pediatr Ophthalmol Strabismus. 1994;31:283–6.

42. Archer S. Study needs more statistical power. J Pediatr Ophthalmol Strabismus. 1995;32:142.

43. Cline RA, Scott WE. Long-term follow-up of Jensen procedures. J Pediatr Ophthalmol Strabismus. 1988;25:264–9.

CHAPTER
199

Paresis of Isolated and Multiple Cranial Nerves and Painful Ophthalmoplegia

MARK L. MOSTER

DEFINITION
- Dysfunction of one or more of the three cranial nerves that move the eyes.

KEY FEATURES
- Diplopia.
- Dysconjugate gaze.

ASSOCIATED FEATURES
- Ptosis.
- Pupillary abnormalities.
- Pain.
- Proptosis.
- Chemosis.
- Arterialization of conjunctival vessels.

INTRODUCTION

One of the common clinical presentations in neuro-ophthalmology involves dysfunction of the ocular motor nerves, cranial nerves III (oculomotor nerve), IV (trochlear nerve), and VI (abducens nerve). In this chapter the anatomy of the peripheral course of the ocular motor nerves is reviewed, and various clinical syndromes are discussed. The syndromes include isolated involvement of each nerve, involvement of multiple cranial nerves simultaneously, involvement of the third, fourth, and sixth cranial nerves with other neurological or orbital symptoms and signs, and involvement of these cranial nerves with severe pain. An approach to the differential diagnosis of patients who seek treatment for involvement of the ocular motor nerves and guidelines for evaluation and treatment are also given.

ANATOMY

The clinical localization and subsequent differential diagnosis of cranial neuropathies requires knowledge of the anatomy of the third, fourth, and sixth cranial nerves. The anatomy within the brainstem is covered in Chapter 198; here, the relevant anatomy of the motor nerves from the brainstem exit to the eye is given (Fig. 199-1).

The third cranial nerve exits the midbrain anteriorly to enter the subarachnoid space. It moves forward and laterally, passes between the posterior cerebral artery and superior cerebellar artery, and then runs alongside the posterior communicating artery. The nerve pierces the dura to enter the cavernous sinus, where it runs along the lateral wall, superior to the fourth cranial nerve. It enters the orbit via the superior orbital fissure. In the anterior cavernous sinus, it divides into the superior and inferior divisions. The superior division ascends lateral to the optic nerve to supply the superior rectus and levator palpebrae superioris muscles. The inferior division divides into branches that supply the inferior rectus, inferior oblique, and medial rectus muscles and the pupillary sphincter. Parasympathetic preganglionic fibers travel along the branch to the inferior oblique and terminate in the ciliary ganglion near the apex of the extraocular muscle cone. The postganglionic fibers from the ciliary ganglion travel in the short ciliary nerves, along with the sympathetic fibers, to enter the globe at the posterior aspect near the optic nerve. They terminate in the ciliary body and iris, and control pupillary constriction and accommodation via the ciliary muscles.

The trochlear nucleus lies in the midbrain, at the level of the inferior colliculus, inferior to the third nerve complex, and anterior to the cerebral aqueduct. The fourth cranial nerve exits the midbrain dorsally and crosses to the opposite side, within the anterior medullary velum, just below the inferior colliculi. The nerve crosses forward within the subarachnoid space around the cerebral peduncle and runs between the posterior cerebral and superior cerebellar arteries, along with the third nerve. The fourth cranial nerve pierces the dura at the angle between the free and attached borders of the tentorium cerebelli to enter the cavernous sinus. It runs within the lateral wall of the cavernous sinus, just below the third cranial nerve and above the first division of the fifth cranial nerve (trigeminal nerve). It enters the orbit via the superior orbital fissure, but runs outside the annulus of Zinn and diagonally across the levator palpebrae superioris and superior rectus muscle to reach the superior oblique muscle. As a consequence of decussation, the fourth cranial nerve emanates from the brainstem and innervates the contralateral superior oblique muscle. The fourth cranial nerve is the thinnest cranial nerve; it is the only nerve to both exit from the dorsal brainstem and have all the fibers crossed, and it has the longest intracranial course of all the cranial nerves. It supplies the superior oblique muscle, the main action of which is to depress the eye in the adducted position. Secondary actions are incyclotorsion and abduction of the eye.

The abducens nerve exits the brainstem at the junction of the pons and pyramid of the medulla, and ascends through the subarachnoid space along the surface of the clivus. It runs forward over the petrous apex of the temporal bone and beneath the petroclinoid ligament to enter the cavernous sinus. In the cavernous sinus, it runs lateral to the internal carotid artery, but medial to the third and fourth cranial nerves and first and second divisions of the fifth cranial nerve, which run in the lateral wall. It enters the superior orbital fissure and passes through the annulus of Zinn to innervate the lateral rectus muscle.

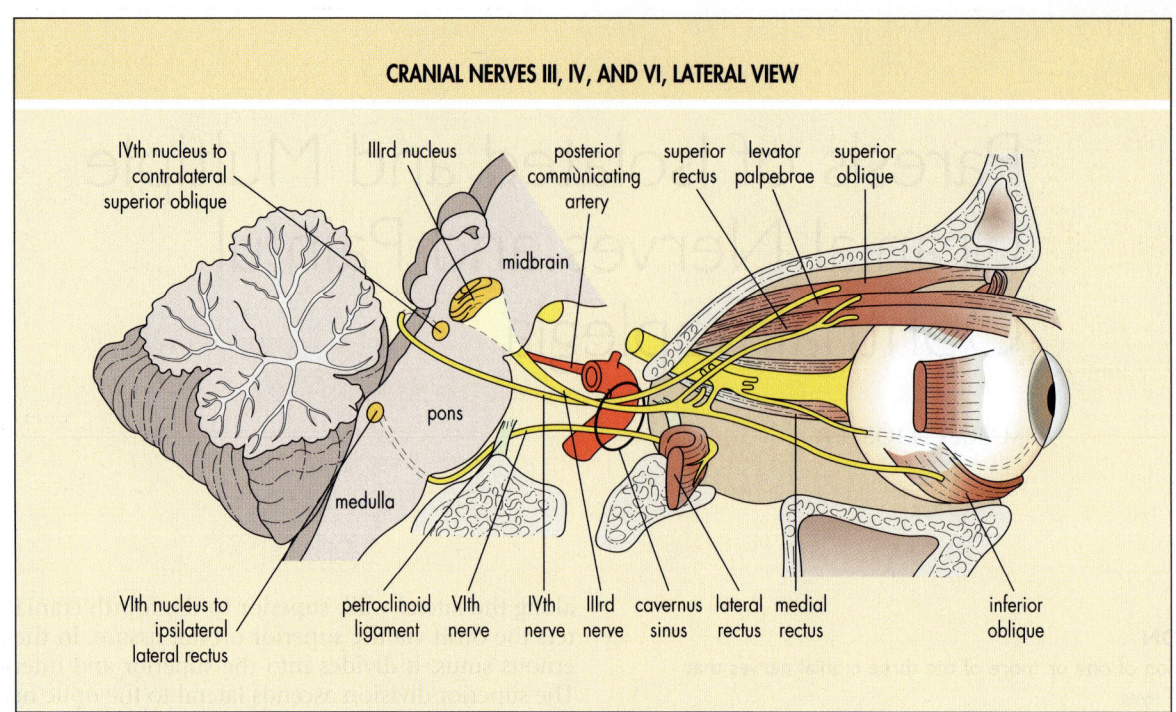

CRANIAL NERVES III, IV, AND VI, LATERAL VIEW

IVth nucleus to contralateral superior oblique

IIIrd nucleus

posterior communicating artery

superior rectus

levator palpebrae

superior oblique

midbrain

pons

medulla

VIth nucleus to ipsilateral lateral rectus

petroclinoid ligament

VIth nerve

IVth nerve

IIIrd nerve

cavernus sinus

lateral rectus

medial rectus

inferior oblique

FIG. 199-1 ■ **Lateral view of cranial nerves III, IV, and VI from the brainstem nuclei to the orbit.** The third nerve exits the midbrain anteriorly, crosses near the junction of the internal carotid and posterior communicating artery in the subarachnoid space, and enters the cavernous sinus, where it runs in the lateral wall. The fourth nerve exits the midbrain posteriorly and crosses to the opposite side, to move forward in the subarachnoid space and into the cavernous sinus. The sixth nerve exits the pons anteriorly, ascends along the clivus bone, crosses the petrous apex, and descends below the petroclinoid ligament to enter the cavernous sinus, where it runs between the lateral wall and the carotid artery.

OCULAR MANIFESTATIONS

General Symptoms

The universal symptom associated with dysfunction of the ocular motor nerves is binocular diplopia. With third cranial nerve dysfunction, ptosis and mydriasis are also symptoms. Diplopia occurs when an object projects onto retinal points that do not correspond in both eyes. The diplopia is worst in the direction of action of the weak muscle(s). However, diplopia may not occur with poor visual acuity or in patients affected by a suppression scotoma from congenital strabismus.

On examination, a patient who has binocular diplopia demonstrates an ocular deviation. Numerous examination techniques are available to measure ocular deviations, which include the use of prism lenses with the cover–uncover or alternate cover technique, the red glass test, the Maddox rod, and the Hess or Lancaster screen. The examiner must become familiar and proficient with one or more of these techniques (Chapter 70) to adequately assess patients who have diplopia.

A tendency toward ocular deviation that variably is present is termed a *phoria,* whereas a constantly manifest deviation is a *tropia.* When a measured deviation is similar in all gaze directions, it is a comitant deviation; when it varies by direction it is incomitant. Congenital strabismus appears with a comitant deviation.

Acquired cranial neuropathies appear with a ductional deficit on examination that corresponds to weakness in the appropriate muscle(s) innervated by the cranial nerve(s) involved. In a more subtle deficit, ductions may appear full, but an incomitant deviation greatest in the direction of action of the paretic muscle is seen. When a cranial neuropathy is chronic, spread of comitance may occur, and the deviation mimics that of congenital strabismus.

Isolated Cranial Neuropathies

In this section, the assessment of patients affected by isolated involvement of the third, fourth, or sixth cranial nerve, with no other neurological or ophthalmologic signs, is discussed.

ISOLATED SIXTH CRANIAL NERVE PALSY. An isolated sixth nerve paresis appears with a unilateral abduction deficit of variable degree, from a complete inability to abduct past the midline to a mild incomitant esodeviation greatest on lateral gaze. Abduction saccades in the affected eye are slow. The history consists of binocular uncrossed diplopia, worse in the direction of the lesion and worse at distance than near. Figure 199-2 demonstrates the deviation seen using a Maddox rod in a patient who has a right sixth nerve paresis. Some children affected by isolated sixth nerve paresis appear to have a gaze paresis in both eyes, because they avoid looking to the side that has diplopia.[1]

A congenital sixth nerve palsy is rare and may be related to birth trauma. The deficit often is transient, and resolves in the first month of life.[1-3] Other congenital abnormalities of the sixth nerve, such as Möbius' syndrome and Duane's retraction syndrome, show other findings and are discussed in the section on differential diagnosis.

An isolated, acquired sixth nerve paresis may arise from a lesion anywhere in the course of the sixth nerve, from the fascicular portion in the brain to the orbit. Since other symptoms and signs are not present to help localization, the differential diagnosis is extensive. In children, isolated sixth nerve paresis may be a relatively benign occurrence after viral infection, but it is also a presenting sign of intracranial tumor.[2,3] In old age, isolated sixth nerve paresis is quite common because of ischemic infarction. In young adults, postviral and ischemic lesions are less common, but trauma, neoplasm, and demyelinating disease are more common.[4]

Traumatic sixth nerve injury is often associated with fractures of the petrous bone or clivus. Other clinical findings include mastoid ecchymosis (Battle's sign) and cerebrospinal fluid otorrhea. Chronic sixth nerve paresis results from many of the same causes as acute sixth nerve paresis but more often arises from a compressive lesion.[5-8]

A syndrome of benign recurrent sixth nerve paresis may occur,[9] particularly in children. However, skull-base tumors also

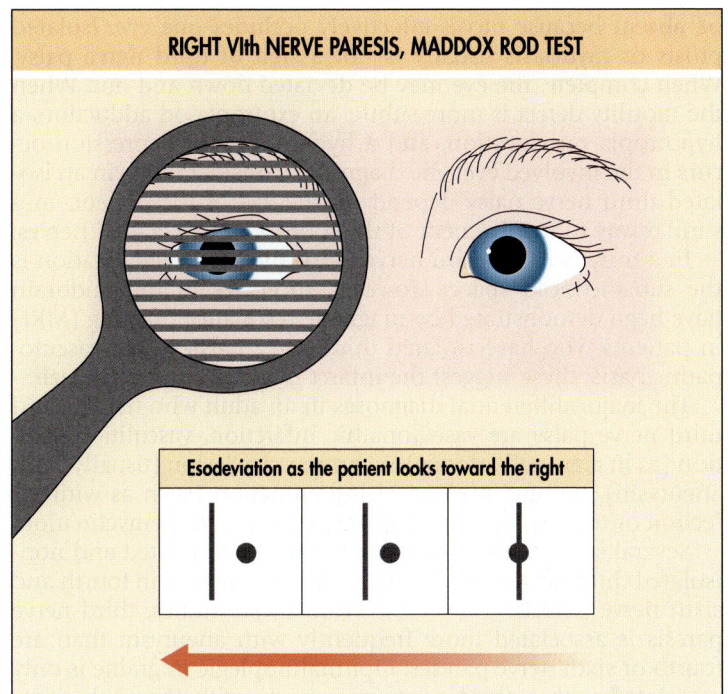

FIG. 199-2 ▓ Right sixth cranial nerve paresis evaluated by the Maddox rod test. A Maddox rod is placed in front of the patient's right eye. Subjective deviation between the light and the line is noted by the patient in different positions of gaze. An esodeviation greatest as the patient looks to the right is consistent with a right lateral rectus muscle weakness.

RIGHT VIth NERVE PARESIS, MADDOX ROD TEST

Esodeviation as the patient looks toward the right

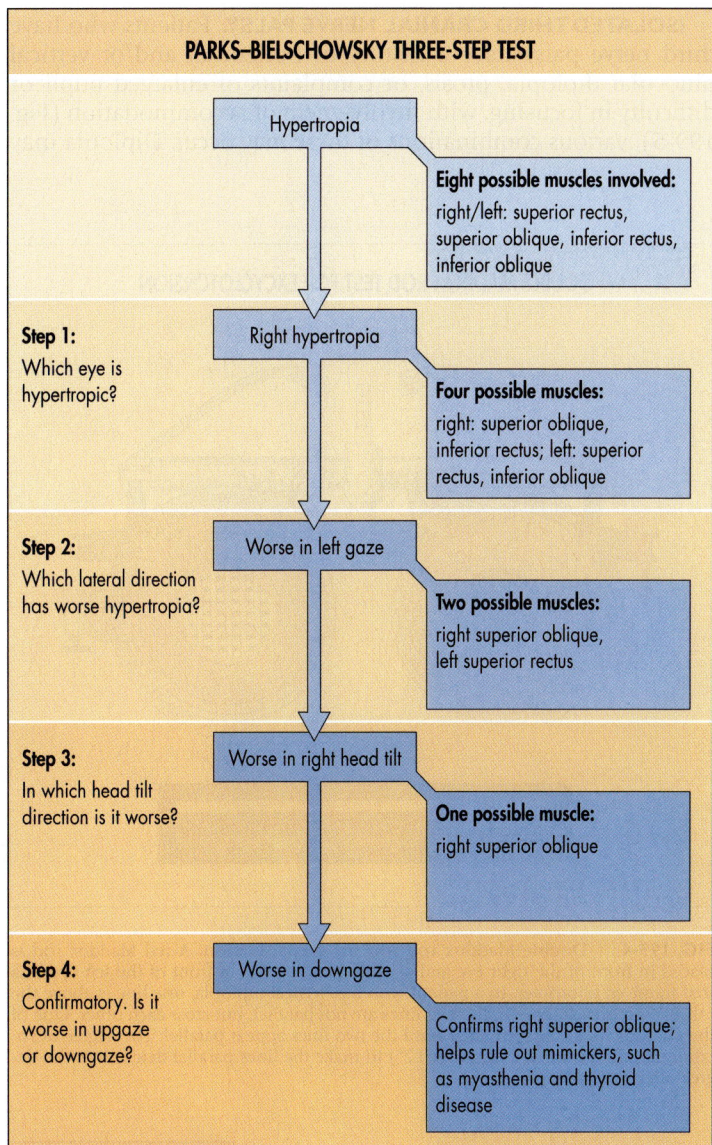

PARKS–BIELSCHOWSKY THREE-STEP TEST

Hypertropia

Eight possible muscles involved: right/left: superior rectus, superior oblique, inferior rectus, inferior oblique

Step 1: Which eye is hypertropic? — Right hypertropia

Four possible muscles: right: superior oblique, inferior rectus; left: superior rectus, inferior oblique

Step 2: Which lateral direction has worse hypertropia? — Worse in left gaze

Two possible muscles: right superior oblique, left superior rectus

Step 3: In which head tilt direction is it worse? — Worse in right head tilt

One possible muscle: right superior oblique

Step 4: Confirmatory. Is it worse in upgaze or downgaze? — Worse in downgaze

Confirms right superior oblique; helps rule out mimickers, such as myasthenia and thyroid disease

FIG. 199-3 ▓ Parks–Bielschowsky three-step test. In a patient who has a vertical deviation because of a weakness in a single muscle, this three-step test determines which muscle is weak. Step four confirms that the correct muscle has been identified and helps to rule out other causes of vertical deviation.

may present in this manner,[10] and remission of a sixth nerve paresis is not always a sign of a benign sixth nerve paresis.

Even though each series reviews patients differently, some generalizations are apparent from the numerous series of both isolated and nonisolated sixth nerve paresis.[2-4,11-17] In adults affected by isolated sixth nerve paresis, the cause is more likely to be ischemia, in comparison with those who have nonisolated sixth nerve paresis. Tumor, trauma or aneurysm are more often present in nonisolated cases. Also, tumor is a more common cause of sixth nerve paresis in young adults and children than in older patients.

ISOLATED FOURTH CRANIAL NERVE PALSY. A fourth nerve or trochlear palsy manifests with an isolated, vertical, diagonal, or incyclotorsional diplopia and is the most common cause of vertical diplopia. The diplopia is usually worse close up and down, as in reading, and is worse when looking to the side opposite the lesion.

On examination a spontaneous head tilt may occur to the side opposite the fourth nerve paresis, which helps compensate for some of the vertical deviation. In addition, the head may be turned down, with the chin depressed, the eyes up, and the face turned to the side opposite the paresis, to diminish the diplopia.

Ductions may be normal or show a mild decrease of depression of the adducted eye. Examination using the Parks–Bielschowsky three-step test (Fig. 199-3) shows a hyperdeviation that is worse on contralateral gaze, downgaze, and ipsilateral head tilt. A fourth step that demonstrates the deviation is worse in downgaze than upgaze is confirmatory. With time, spread of comitance may develop. Double Maddox rod testing shows excyclotorsion (Fig. 199-4)—if the excyclotorsion is >10°, fourth nerve paresis is likely to be bilateral.

Congenital fourth nerve paresis is common. Patients affected by a congenital paresis may experience acute diplopia at any age, but often they are in the fifth to seventh decades of life. The diplopia may occur as a decompensation during periods of stress. Examination of photographs of the patient at a younger age is important, in that a persistent head tilt to one direction may be demonstrated. In addition, if a fourth nerve paresis is congenital, a large-amplitude vertical fusional capacity of >6D, often 10–15D, is present.

The most common cause of acquired fourth nerve paresis is trauma that affects the nerve along the tentorial edge or the anterior medullary velum. In addition, the fourth nerve is the ocular motor nerve most commonly injured by trauma. In this situation, the fourth nerve paresis may be bilateral (discussed below in the section on bilateral ophthalmoplegia). Inflammatory and infectious lesions in the subarachnoid space may also affect the fourth nerve. Pinealoma or tentorial meningioma may compress the fourth nerve.

In children with fourth nerve paresis, congenital factors are likely the leading cause (which may appear later in childhood or in adulthood), followed by trauma.[2] Structural lesions account for a minority of cases.

In elderly patients, particularly those who have hypertension or diabetes, vasculopathic ischemic infarction is a likely cause of fourth nerve paresis. Less common causes include tumor that involves the midbrain or cerebellum, aneurysm, or herpes zoster ophthalmicus.[18] The fourth nerve may become involved with herpes zoster ophthalmicus because it shares the same connective tissue sheath as the ophthalmic division of the fifth cranial nerve.

The cause of fourth nerve paresis has been studied in numerous series.[2,3,12,15-17,19-21,25] Causes include trauma, ischemia, tumor, aneurysm, and demyelination. Trauma is a more common cause of a fourth nerve paresis than of third and sixth nerve pareses.

ISOLATED THIRD CRANIAL NERVE PALSY. Patients who have third nerve palsy have a history of horizontal and/or vertical binocular diplopia, ptosis, or complaints of enlarged pupil or difficulty in focusing, with involvement of accommodation (Fig. 199-5); various combinations of these may occur. Diplopia may be absent because ptosis effectively occludes one eye. Isolated ptosis or mydriasis usually is not a sign of third nerve palsy. When complete, the eye may be deviated down and out. When the motility defect is more subtle, an exotropia on adduction, a hypotropia on elevation, and a hypertropia on depression occurs in the involved eye. The diagnostic considerations in an isolated third nerve palsy depend on the age of the patient, in a similar way to involvement of the fourth or sixth cranial nerves.

In a truly isolated third nerve palsy, the presumed location is the subarachnoid space. However, lucencies in the midbrain have been demonstrated by magnetic resonance imaging (MRI) in patients who have isolated third nerve palsies on a vasculopathic basis; these suggest the infarct is in the brainstem itself.

The major differential diagnoses in an adult who has isolated third nerve palsy are vasculopathic infarction, vasculitic infarction (as in giant cell arteritis), a compressive lesion (usually from aneurysm), trauma, meningeal inflammation (such as with infection or tumor), ophthalmoplegic migraine, or demyelination.

Several series have looked at the causes of isolated and nonisolated third nerve paresis with similar findings as in fourth and sixth nerve paresis.[2,3,12,15-17,22-25] From these studies, third nerve paresis is associated more frequently with aneurysm than are fourth or sixth nerve pareses. Ophthalmoplegic migraine is only associated with a third nerve paresis. As with the sixth nerve paresis, isolated lesions more often are ischemic than nonisolated ones.

Patients who have a vasculopathic third nerve palsy often have pain that precedes the ptosis or diplopia. In a vasculopathic lesion, the pupillary reaction is usually spared, and the pupil does not become enlarged. However, in up to 20% of cases, the pupil may be involved. Clinical associations include diabetes, hypertension, or other risk factors for atherosclerosis. The natural course of a vasculopathic, isolated third nerve palsy is one of recovery over weeks to months, usually 3 months. The pupil is spared because the infarction occurs in the center of the nerve and good collateral supply exists in the nerve periphery, where the pupillary fibers are located.

DOUBLE MADDOX ROD TEST FOR EXCYCLOTORSION

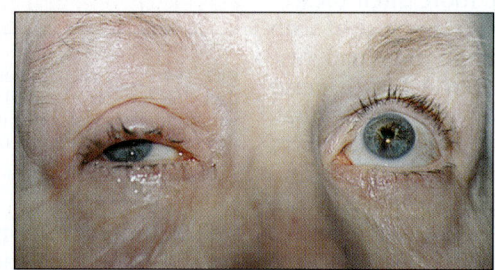
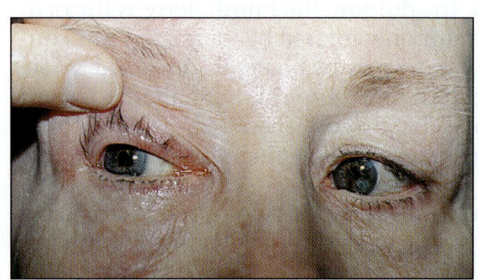
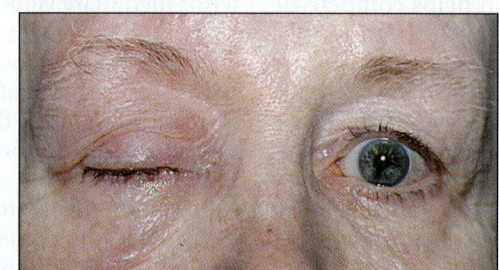
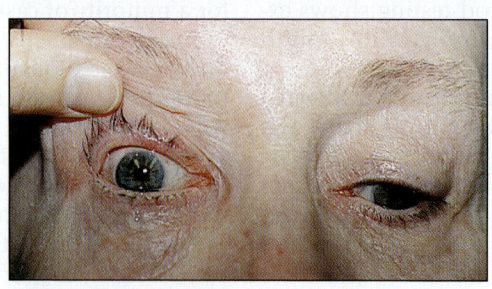
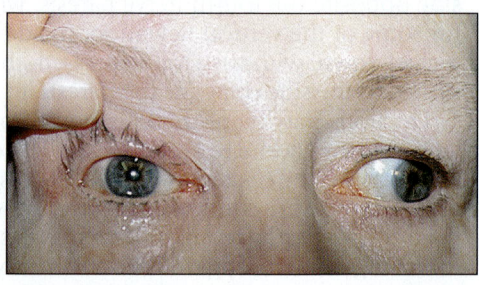

FIG. 199-4 ▌ **Double Maddox rod test for excyclotorsion.** A red Maddox rod is placed in front of the right eye and a white Maddox rod in front of the left eye in a trial frame or phoropter. In a patient who has vertical diplopia, one line is above the other. With excyclotorsion, the two lines are not parallel, but cross each other. One of the Maddox rods is then rotated until the two lines appear parallel. The degree of rotation required (in this case about 12°) to make the lines parallel determines the degree of excyclotorsion.

FIG. 199-5 ▌ **Isolated third nerve palsy in the setting of herpes zoster ophthalmicus.** At the time of acute illness. Note the presence of herpes zoster lesions in the distribution of the first division of the fifth nerve. Third nerve palsy consists of ptosis, adduction, elevation, and depression deficit with preserved abduction.

One of the true neuro-ophthalmologic emergencies occurs when compression of the third nerve results from an expanding aneurysm at the junction of the internal carotid and posterior communicating arteries. Such compressions most often, but not always, are painful, and in almost all instances involve the pupil. However, numerous case reports of isolated third nerve palsy caused by expanding aneurysms show that the pupil may be spared initially.[26] Often, these patients have only partial ptosis and extraocular muscle involvement, and, with very rare exceptions, the pupil becomes involved within 1 week of symptom onset. This situation is one of the few life-threatening emergencies in neuro-ophthalmology and one in which appropriate diagnosis and treatment is lifesaving.

In contrast to an acute third nerve palsy, a slowly progressive third nerve palsy that involves the pupil usually is a sign of an enlarging cavernous sinus lesion.[27] Ophthalmoplegic migraine is a syndrome that becomes apparent with a migraine-type headache and the development of a third nerve palsy; the pupil is usually involved. The pain precedes the oculomotor paresis and is intense, continuous, and located in the orbital region. As the paralysis reaches its maximum, the headache begins to recede. The initial presentation is usually in childhood, multiple attacks may occur, and a family history of migraine is often present. The third nerve palsy may last from hours to weeks, and permanent deficits occur after repeated attacks.[28]

A rare syndrome in children is a recurrent isolated third nerve palsy, which resolves without deficit. Some patients later develop migraine, and some investigators consider this a variant of ophthalmoplegic migraine.[1] Other causes of isolated third nerve palsy in the subarachnoid space include trauma and infectious or neoplastic meningitis.

Aberrant regeneration refers to an abnormality found on examination, after recovery of the third nerve from damage that caused disruption of the axons as a result of a structural lesion.[29] The abnormal activation of one part of the third nerve is found when another part should be in action. For instance, if fibers originally destined for the medial rectus now supply the levator palpebrae superioris, then on adduction of the eye the lid elevates (so-called lid–gaze dyskinesis). If the same fibers now innervate the pupil, on adduction of the eye the pupil constricts. This may give rise to pupillary light–near dissociation (pseudo–Argyll Robertson pupil). Another common pattern of aberrant regeneration is elevation of the eyelid on downgaze, the pseudo–Von Graefe's phenomenon, because fibers destined for the inferior rectus now go to the levator palpebrae superioris. Cocontraction of vertically acting muscles may limit vertical excursion of the eye and be associated with retraction of the globe. When aberrant regeneration is found, the diagnosis is not an isolated ischemic lesion, but a structural lesion.

Primary aberrant regeneration refers to the findings above, but with no antecedent third nerve palsy. This suggests a compressive lesion of the third nerve that slowly evolves with ongoing recovery to produce the aberrant regeneration without clinical realization of a third nerve palsy. This has been described with lesions that slowly evolve, usually in the cavernous sinus. Most often these are internal carotid artery aneurysms, intracavernous meningiomas, or neurinomas.[30,31]

A rare congenital condition, with unknown cause, is cyclic oculomotor paralysis with spasm. This encompasses a condition that cycles between an oculomotor paresis as described above and periods of oculomotor spasm that occur every 1.5–2 minutes and persists throughout life. During the periods of oculomotor spasm, the eye may be adducted, the lid elevated, the pupil miotic, and accommodation increased. After a 10–60-second interval, the eye becomes deviated outward with ptosis and mydriasis.[32]

DIVISIONAL THIRD CRANIAL NERVE PALSY. The third nerve divides in the anterior cavernous sinus into a superior and inferior division—lesions may affect either division. A superior division third nerve palsy manifests with an isolated elevation deficit and ptosis of one eye. An inferior division third nerve palsy may cause mydriasis, and an adduction and depression deficit without ptosis or elevation deficit. Divisional palsies usually result from a structural lesion in the anterior cavernous sinus or orbit. A characteristic example is a superior division third nerve paresis from an ophthalmic artery aneurysm. However, divisional palsies have been described as far posteriorly as the anterior midbrain, likely because fibers have segregated into different portions of the nerve at this point. In addition, cases exist of benign, remitting pareses of either division of the third nerve.[33]

Nonisolated Cranial Neuropathies

When a patient affected by involvement of an ocular motor nerve has other findings, the approach to evaluation changes. The associated findings are clues to the localization and character of the lesion and may include brainstem neurological deficits, meningeal signs, involvement of other ocular motor or other cranial nerves, and orbital signs.

Nerve palsies that arise in the brainstem most often are associated with long-tract findings, alterations in consciousness, or other cranial neuropathies, and are covered in Chapter 198. When accompanied by other cranial nerve involvement without brainstem findings, the likely localization includes the subarachnoid space, cavernous sinus, and orbit. Those nerve palsies associated with proptosis, chemosis, and visual loss often arise in the orbit, and are covered in Chapter 95.

In this section nonisolated cranial neuropathies are reviewed. They are subdivided into categories of multiple cranial neuropathies, bilateral cranial neuropathies, and lesions in the subarachnoid space that may cause both multiple unilateral or bilateral cranial neuropathies.

MULTIPLE CRANIAL NEUROPATHIES. In contrast with isolated mononeuropathies, which are often benign and vasculopathic in nature, involvement of more than one ocular motor nerve rarely results from vasculopathic lesions.[34] It is very important to ascertain that multiple nerves are involved, because establishment of this enables localization of the lesion responsible. For the most part, these patients have lesions of the cavernous sinus, superior orbital fissure, or orbital apex. Since the first division of the fifth cranial nerve is also involved in such lesions, pain may be a prominent feature.

Causes of multiple cranial nerve involvement have been reviewed in numerous series.[12,15,17] In contrast to isolated mononeuropathies, ischemia is an infrequent cause, and tumor, inflammation, trauma, and aneurysm are more common.

Typically, fourth nerve paresis is associated with hyperdeviation, most noticeable when the eye is adducted. In the presence of a third nerve paresis, the eye does not adduct, which makes it difficult to determine the presence of a coexisting fourth nerve paresis. In this situation, the eye is examined carefully for intorsion of the globe on attempted downgaze, from which secondary action of the fourth nerve is assessed. This is accomplished most easily by visualization of a conjunctival vessel for intorsion (Fig. 199-6).

On occasion the third and fourth cranial nerves may be involved together in the brainstem. However, such patients have large lesions that cause other neurological deficits. These cranial nerves may be involved together in the subarachnoid space also, as discussed below.

Because the sixth nerve crosses along the petrous apex, a syndrome that includes sixth nerve palsy, facial pain, hearing loss, and (sometimes) facial paralysis may occur.[35] This is known as Gradenigo's syndrome and may result from infectious mastoiditis, tumor, trauma, aneurysm of the petrosal segment of the internal carotid artery, or inferior petrosal sinus thrombosis. Petrous bone fractures involve combinations of the fifth, sixth, seventh, and/or eighth cranial nerves and other findings of hemotympanum, Battle's sign (mastoid hematoma), and cerebrospinal fluid otorrhea.

The cavernous sinus consists of a plexus of veins. Within the plexus lies the sixth nerve and within the lateral wall lies the third nerve, fourth nerve, first division of the fifth nerve, and, posteriorly, the second division of the fifth nerve. Within the cavernous sinus, the sympathetic fibers form a plexus along the carotid artery (Fig. 199-7).

The superior orbital fissure contains the same nerves as the anterior cavernous sinus. Therefore, signs and symptoms of cavernous sinus and superior orbital fissure lesions may be identical. The findings include involvement of any of the above cranial nerves in isolation or in various combinations. Therefore, third nerve paresis, fourth nerve paresis, sixth nerve paresis, Horner's

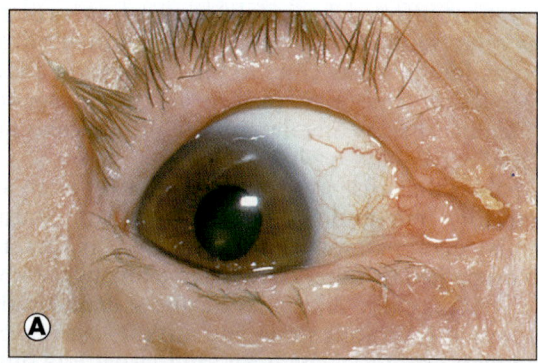

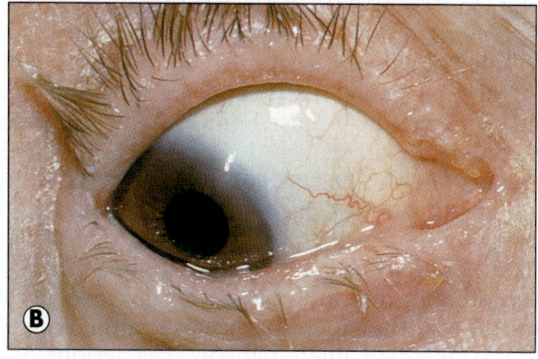

FIG. 199-6 ■ **Demonstration of intact fourth cranial nerve in the presence of a third nerve paresis. A,** The patient's right eye is exotropic from a complete third nerve palsy. **B,** However, an intact fourth nerve is noted on attempted downgaze because of incyclotorsion of the eye. This is best seen by comparison of the conjunctival vessels in **A** with their position in **B** on attempted downgaze.

syndrome, and sensory loss of the first division of the fifth nerve all may be present, and, if a lesion is in the posterior cavernous sinus, there may be involvement of the second division of the fifth nerve. The pupil may be involved, spared, or appear spared with concomitant oculosympathetic and parasympathetic involvement. Various degrees of pain may be involved and, if pain is severe, "painful ophthalmoplegia syndrome" is diagnosed.[36]

Broad categories of diseases that involve the cavernous sinus include neoplasms, inflammation, infection, vascular lesions, and trauma.[37–40] Neoplastic lesions include local metastatic disease from nasopharyngeal cancer, olfactory neuroblastoma, adenoid cystic carcinoma, cylindroma, ameloblastoma, and squamous cell carcinoma, or disease that spreads from distant lesions, which includes carcinoma, sarcoma, multiple myeloma, and lymphoma. Local spread of benign tumors includes pituitary adenoma, meningioma, craniopharyngioma, neurilemmoma, and epidermoid tumor. Chordomas, chondromas, and giant cell tumors may also spread in the cavernous sinus. Meningiomas may arise in the cavernous sinus itself. Neuromas or neurofibromas may occur on the gasserian ganglion or other cranial nerves.

Pituitary apoplexy is a clinical syndrome caused by sudden enlargement in a pituitary tumor as a result of acute hemorrhage or edema. The patient may have had previous symptoms or have a clinically silent lesion that appears acutely because of the sudden change. The presentation has variable features that include acute and severe headache, diplopia with ophthalmoplegia from cavernous sinus involvement, visual loss from optic nerve, chiasm, or tract involvement, meningismus from hemorrhage into the subarachnoid space, and endocrine insufficiency.

Inflammatory lesions may be both infectious and noninfectious. Bacterial infections may cause cavernous sinus thrombosis, which causes a unilateral or bilateral cavernous sinus syndrome, proptosis, and chemosis associated with signs of fever, depressed mental status, and signs of sepsis. Spread of infection from sinusitis or a mucocele from the paranasal sinuses may cause compression of the cavernous sinus.

Mucormycosis is a life-threatening infection that may affect the cavernous sinus, superior orbital fissure, or orbit. Multiple cranial neuropathies may occur relatively rapidly in a predisposed patient, such as a diabetic or an immunosuppressed patient. Often an indicative eschar is seen in the nose in such patients. An occlusive vasculitis may occur with stroke that affects the brain or eye. To make the diagnosis, a high index of suspicion is required in the appropriate patient.

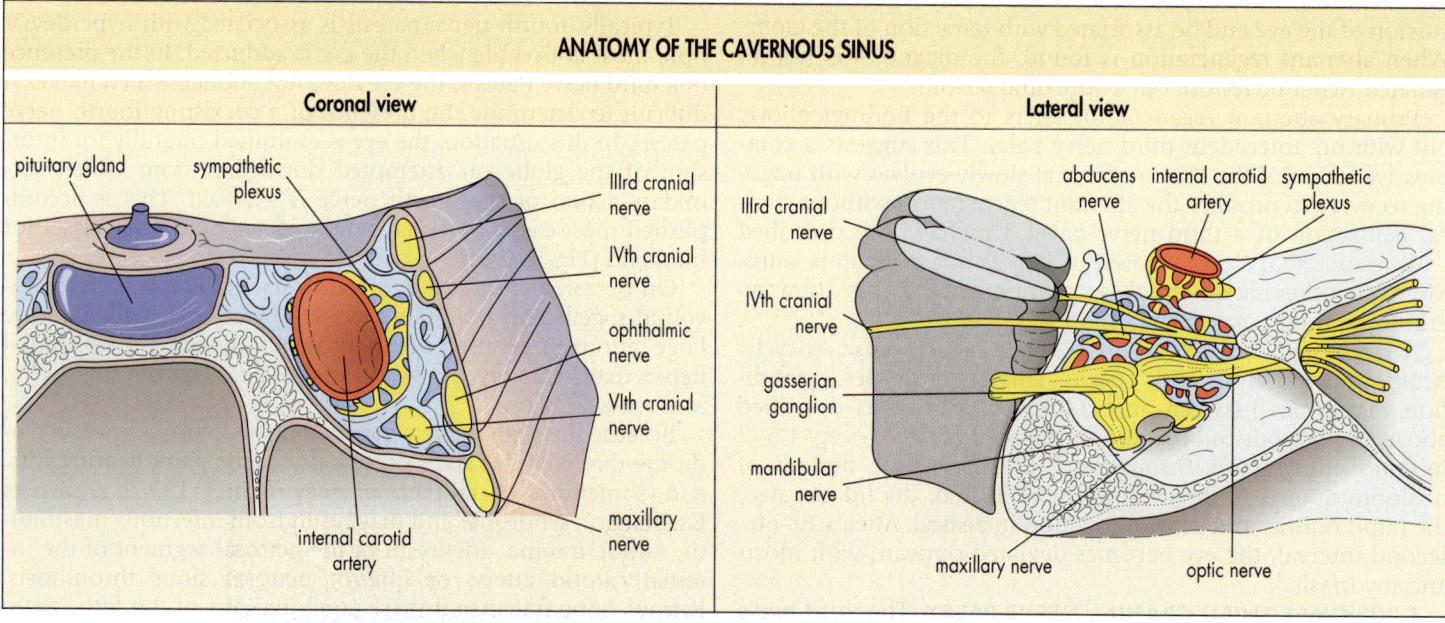

ANATOMY OF THE CAVERNOUS SINUS

Coronal view	Lateral view

Coronal view labels: pituitary gland, sympathetic plexus, IIIrd cranial nerve, IVth cranial nerve, ophthalmic nerve, VIth cranial nerve, maxillary nerve, internal carotid artery

Lateral view labels: abducens nerve, internal carotid artery, sympathetic plexus, IIIrd cranial nerve, IVth cranial nerve, gasserian ganglion, mandibular nerve, maxillary nerve, optic nerve

FIG. 199-7 ■ **Anatomy of the cavernous sinus.** Coronal and lateral views. (From Kline LB. The Tolosa–Hunt syndrome. Surv Ophthalmol. 1982;27:79–95.)

Aspergillosis also may involve the orbital apex or cavernous sinus. Rarely, other infections such as syphilis or tuberculosis may affect the cavernous sinus. Herpes zoster may be followed by abnormalities of the cavernous sinus. Most often this consists of involvement of one cranial nerve—an isolated third, fourth, or sixth dysfunction—after zoster in the first division of the fifth cranial nerve.[18] Occasionally, multiple cranial nerves may be involved.

Inflammatory, noninfectious lesions include sarcoidosis, Wegener's granulomatosis, eosinophilic granuloma, and the idiopathic Tolosa–Hunt syndrome; the last causes painful ophthalmoplegia. The pain is described as gnawing or boring and may precede ophthalmoplegia. The ophthalmoplegia arises from combinations of third (most frequently), fourth, or sixth nerve involvement. Other findings include Horner's syndrome, proptosis, optic nerve involvement, fifth nerve (divisions 1–3) involvement, or seventh nerve paresis.[36,41,42] The symptoms last for days to weeks and spontaneous remissions occur, with or without residual deficits. Recurrences may occur at intervals of months to years.

Vascular causes of a cavernous sinus syndrome include carotid artery aneurysm, cavernous sinus thrombosis (as noted above), direct carotid artery to cavernous sinus fistula, and dural arteriovenous fistula. Intracavernous carotid artery aneurysms are saccular aneurysms that develop most commonly from atherosclerosis. They cause slowly progressive ophthalmoplegia through enlargement, often with aberrant regeneration, and may cause an acute carotid–cavernous fistula if they bleed. The other cause of a direct carotid–cavernous fistula is a condition resulting from trauma that directly damages the internal carotid artery.

A direct carotid–cavernous fistula causes a cavernous sinus syndrome, as well as headache, facial pain, severe proptosis, chemosis, and injection of the eye, with arterialization of conjunctival and episcleral vessels. Often pulsatile tinnitus and an orbital bruit occur, and retinal venous engorgement and hemorrhage, central retinal vein occlusion, retinal ischemia, serous retinal or choroidal detachment, and anterior ischemic optic neuropathy may also be seen. Intraocular pressure may be elevated and angle-closure or neovascular glaucoma may develop.

A less serious fistula results from a dural arteriovenous connection in which multiple dural vessels that come off the arterial system connect directly with the cavernous sinus. This occurs most often in elderly women and has a subacute or chronic course. The findings include the above cranial neuropathies, as well as proptosis, orbital bruit, and conjunctival injection, none as severe as those associated with a direct internal carotid artery–cavernous sinus fistula. The more subtle clinical picture means that these patients are often misdiagnosed with chronic conjunctivitis, episcleritis, or thyroid ophthalmopathy (Fig. 199-8).

Involvement of the sixth nerve with loss of tearing and sometimes sensory loss in the second division of the fifth nerve localizes a lesion to the sphenopalatine fossa; such lesions commonly result from metastatic tumor or nasopharyngeal carcinoma.[43] Poliomyelitis may involve one or more cranial nerves, most often the sixth cranial nerve.[43]

Bilateral Ophthalmoplegia. Bilateral ophthalmoplegia, a unique variant of the syndrome of multiple cranial neuropathy, refers to involvement of more than one of the above cranial nerves that includes at least one on each side. This implies a lesion that is large enough to cause deficits bilaterally or is situated in a location such that bilateral cranial nerves are involved.

Möbius' syndrome is a congenital syndrome associated with bilateral sixth nerve or horizontal-gaze paresis and seventh nerve (facial nerve) paresis and other deficits, which may include tongue atrophy, hand and face deformities, and other malformations. Bilateral sixth nerve paresis is seen in posterior fossa or clivus lesions. Clivus tumors, such as meningioma, chordoma, chondroma, or chondrosarcoma, or spread of nasopharyngeal carcinoma often cause bilateral sixth nerve palsies because the two sixth nerves run adjacent to each other along the clivus.

Increased intracranial pressure of any cause may produce unilateral or bilateral sixth nerve palsy by downward pressure and shift of the brainstem. This is because the sixth nerve is fixed as it exits the pons and as it pierces the dura to enter Dorello's canal under the petroclinoid ligament. Papilledema inevitably is present.

After myelography, spinal anesthesia, or even lumbar puncture, a bilateral sixth nerve paresis may rarely develop in association with a severe, postlumbar puncture headache syndrome.[44] A similar mechanism of downward shift of the brainstem that arises from a pressure differential may be responsible. With this syndrome of intracranial hypotension, diffuse enhancement of the meninges also may be seen on MRI (Fig. 199-9). Basilar artery aneurysm or dolichoectasia of the basilar artery also may cause unilateral or bilateral sixth nerve paresis. When the presentation of bilateral sixth nerve paresis is compared with that of unilateral cases, ischemic causes are less frequent and trauma is more common.[13,14]

Bilateral fourth nerve paresis may be seen after head trauma. Trauma likely involves the nerves in the area of decussation in

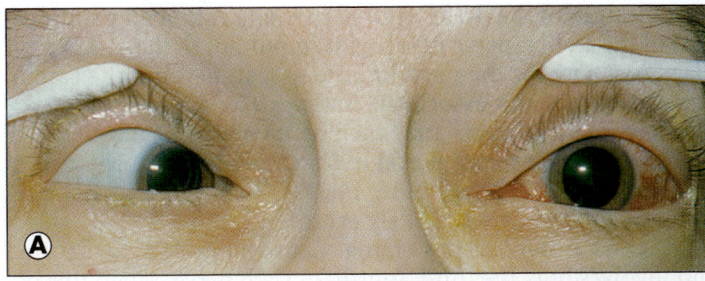

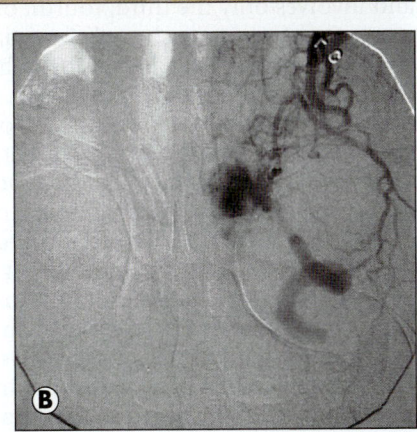

FIG. 199-8 Dural arteriovenous fistula. **A,** Patient had diplopia that resulted from a left sixth nerve paresis, Horner's syndrome, proptosis, chemosis, and injection with arterialization of the conjunctival vessels. (Pupils are pharmacologically dilated.) **B,** Arteriogram demonstrates filling of the cavernous sinus and a huge dilated superior ophthalmic vein in the arterial phase of an external carotid artery injection in the same patient.

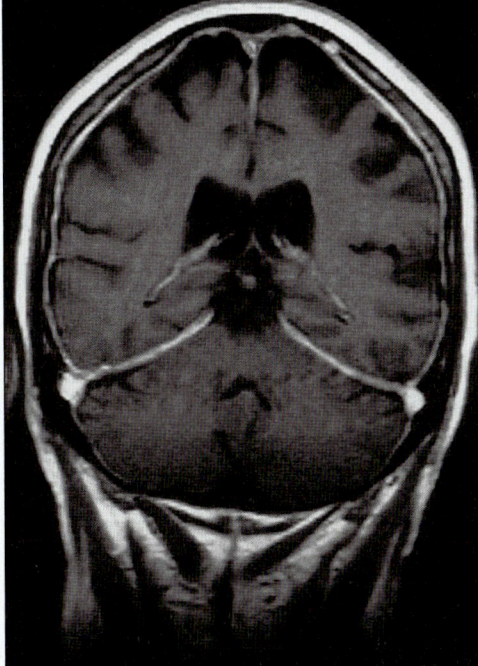

FIG. 199-9 Magnetic resonance image (with gadolinium) of a patient with bilateral sixth cranial nerve palsy. The palsy resulted from intracranial hypotension after lumbar spine surgery. Note the diffuse enhancement of the meninges.

the anterior medullary velum. Bilateral fourth nerve paresis also may be seen with hydrocephalus, tumor, arteriovenous malformation, or demyelinating disease.[43]

With bilateral fourth nerve paresis, right hyperdeviation in left gaze or right head-tilt and left hyperdeviation in right gaze or left head-tilt occur. In primary position, depending on the relative symmetry of the bilateral fourth nerve paresis, orthophoria, or right or left hyperdeviation may occur. An additive effect of excyclodeviation occurs, with the result that greater than 10° of excyclotorsion is often seen. Because a tertiary action of the superior oblique muscle is abduction, loss of action of both superior obliques in downgaze causes a relative esodeviation in downgaze, which results in a characteristic V-pattern horizontal deviation.

Rarely, bilateral simultaneous ophthalmoplegia may have a vasculopathic cause.[34]

Subarachnoid Involvement. With subarachnoid involvement, signs of multiple cranial nerve involvement may occur on one or both sides and produce the above syndromes, as well as headache, stiff neck, photophobia, and fever. With elevated intracranial pressure, papilledema occurs. In the subarachnoid space, causes of cranial neuropathies include subarachnoid hemorrhage, trauma, infectious or neoplastic meningitis, idiopathic intracranial hypertension (pseudotumor cerebri), tumors on the sixth nerve, or tumors in the clivus that compress the sixth nerve.

Infectious meningitis may arise from bacterial, fungal (mainly cryptococcal), tuberculous, or syphilitic causes, or from Lyme disease. Inflammatory meningitis occurs with sarcoidosis.

NONISOLATED THIRD CRANIAL NERVE PALSIES. Nonisolated third nerve palsies occur in the subarachnoid space and are accompanied by meningeal signs. The processes are similar to those described above—mainly infectious, neoplastic, or traumatic. However, one additional nonisolated third nerve syndrome occurs with uncal herniation through the tentorium, with large hemispheric mass lesions (such as tumor, hemorrhage, or infarct with edema). The patient has a corresponding neurological deficit and is lethargic. The third nerve is compressed against the tentorial edge, petrous ridge, and clivus by the uncus of the temporal lobe. Usually, pupillomotor fibers are involved first. Rarely, upward herniation from a mass in the posterior fossa may cause a third nerve palsy.

Miscellaneous Disorders

SUPERIOR OBLIQUE MYOKYMIA. Superior oblique myokymia, also known as superior oblique microtremor, is a rare condition that causes intermittent diplopia or the sense of oscillopsia in one eye. It consists of an intermittent torsional movement in the direction of the superior oblique muscle and is best seen under the slit lamp. The movements may be induced when the patient is asked first to look in the direction of action of the superior oblique muscle followed by a return to the primary position.

Most often, superior oblique myokymia is idiopathic, but it may be a sequela of superior oblique palsy, as well as multiple sclerosis or pontine tumor.[35,45]

OCULAR NEUROMYOTONIA. Ocular neuromyotonia is a paroxysmal monocular deviation that arises from spasm of the extraocular muscles. It is believed to result from episodic spontaneous discharges in the third (most commonly), fourth, and sixth cranial nerves. Neuromyotonia usually is seen after irradiation for sella turcica, cavernous sinus, or other skull-base tumors. It develops between 2 months and 7 years (mean 2.6 years) after surgery and radiation (mean dose 51 Gy).[46-49] Rarely, it occurs without prior history of tumor or radiation.

Patients complain of intermittent diplopia, which is usually painless but sometimes is associated with a feeling of discomfort in the eye. Diplopia may occur several times per hour and last from only seconds to 3 minutes. It may be induced by movement into the field of action of the muscles, which then toni-

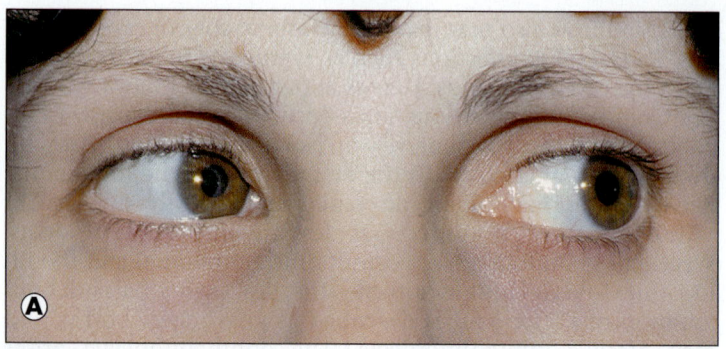

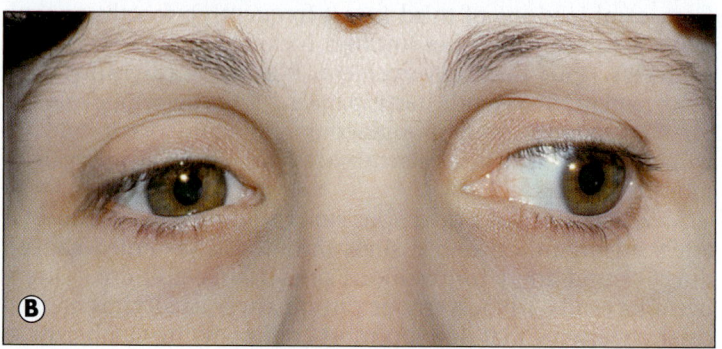

FIG. 199-10 ■ **Ocular neuromyotonia.** A 25-year-old woman, who had received irradiation 6 years previously after resection of a right lateral ventricular ependymoma, developed episodic diplopia that lasted from 30 seconds to 1 minute. **A,** Left gaze is initially normal. **B,** After gazing to the right for at least 30 seconds, an exotropia develops on attempted left gaze, with a right adduction deficit. Her symptoms responded to carbamazepine. (From Moster ML. Complications of cancer therapies. In: Miller N, Newman NJ, eds. Walsh & Hoyt's neuro-ophthalmology, ed 5. Baltimore: Williams & Wilkins; 1997.)

cally contract and do not relax. Patients may have had motility deficits from the original tumor, but the neuromyotonia usually does not involve the previously affected cranial nerve.

On initial examination, ocular motility may appear normal. After a sustained gaze in the direction of action of the involved nerve followed by an attempt to look away, a motility deficit appears because the previously active muscle does not relax (Fig. 199-10). With third nerve involvement the pupil may become fixed during episodes.[46]

DIAGNOSIS

The above histories and examination techniques should allow identification of the dysfunctional nerve(s). Although identification of the cranial nerve involved is important in the differential diagnosis, perhaps the most important feature is not the cranial nerve itself but the associated findings ("company it keeps"). The "company it keeps" may include involvement of other cranial nerves, other neurological deficits, or findings suggestive of an orbital process. These other findings help to localize the lesion and differentiate the likely causes.

In some instances, the cranial neuropathy is truly isolated and involves only the third, fourth, or sixth nerve. When this occurs, a unique approach to differential diagnosis is undertaken.

The evaluation of patients for ophthalmoplegia is dependent on the age of the patient. For infants, a congenital deficit or birth trauma is considered; for children a postviral syndrome, trauma or posterior fossa tumor; for young adults trauma, multiple sclerosis, aneurysm, or arteriovenous malformation; and for older adults diabetes, hypertension, atherosclerosis, or giant cell arteritis.

The character of the onset and progression also is important in differential diagnosis. Acute onset is consistent with a vascular, inflammatory, or traumatic cause. Progressive deficits are consistent with mass lesions such as tumor or aneurysm. Intermittent symptoms are suggestive of myasthenia gravis.

Although cranial neuropathy commonly results from trauma, such deficits are attributed to mild trauma with caution. In these instances, an underlying structural lesion, such as aneurysm or tumor, often is present.[50,51]

Isolated Cranial Neuropathies

ISOLATED SIXTH CRANIAL NERVE PALSY. In a child who has an acquired, isolated sixth nerve paresis, early investigation using MRI is reasonable because of the frequent presentation of tumor with sixth nerve paresis.

In an elderly person, with or without a history of diabetes or hypertension, an erythrocyte sedimentation rate (ESR), C-reactive protein (CRP), blood pressure recording, measurement of levels of glucose, antinuclear antibodies (ANA), rapid plasma reagin (RPR), fluorescent treponemal antibodies (FTA), and a Lyme titer are indicated. The patient may be followed with expectant improvement over a few months. Should no improvement occur over a few months, then neuroimaging, preferably with MRI, is indicated. The imaging must focus on the course of the sixth nerve, which includes the pons, clivus, petrous apex, cavernous sinus, and orbit. Cerebrospinal fluid (CSF) and nasopharyngeal examination are considered if no cause is otherwise found.

In a young adult, particularly without evidence of hypertension or diabetes, the above serologic tests and neuroimaging are performed and, if negative, a CSF examination is reasonable. If no abnormality is found, the patient is followed at regular intervals and re-evaluated at 6 months if resolution does not occur.

ISOLATED FOURTH CRANIAL NERVE PALSY. The evaluation of patients affected by isolated fourth nerve paresis depends on the age group and setting. A history of significant trauma or evidence of a congenital fourth nerve paresis with decompensation requires no further workup.

In older patients subject to vascular risk factors an ESR and CRP are obtained to rule out giant cell arteritis (see Chapter 206), and the patient may be followed clinically. For the patient who does not have this history, blood pressure is checked, as well as glucose level, Lyme titer, and ESR. If no resolution occurs within 6 months, neuroimaging, preferably MRI, is performed. Examination of CSF may be indicated although, without other neurological symptoms or signs, the diagnostic yield is low.

In children and young adults who have no history of trauma or evidence to suggest a congenital cause, neuroimaging and a search for vasculitis are indicated. A CSF examination is indicated if no clear cause can be established and if the deficit does not resolve.

ISOLATED THIRD CRANIAL NERVE PALSY. In adults of vasculopathic age, the most important issue is whether the pupil is involved or not. If the pupil is spared with otherwise complete involvement of ocular motility and ptosis, and the patient is over 50 years of age, diabetic, or hypertensive, a diagnosis of vasculopathic third nerve paresis may be presumed. Since aneurysms that do not at first involve the pupil have been described, the patient is followed carefully for the first week, and if the pupil becomes involved, further evaluation is indicated.[26,52,53] If the pupil does not become involved, the patient is presumed to have a vasculopathic third nerve palsy and expected to recover over 3–6 months. At follow-up visits during this period, the patient is evaluated for aberrant regeneration; if present, further workup for a structural lesion is dictated.

If the pupil is involved, the appropriate evaluation must be pursued until aneurysm is excluded adequately. The initial study is an MRI scan or, if not available, a computed tomography (CT) scan, with and without contrast, is carried out for subarachnoid blood and evidence of aneurysm. If negative, a magnetic resonance angiogram (MRA) or CT angiography (CTA) may show an aneurysm.[54] However, in many centers the sensitivity of MRA and CTA is not considered sufficient to exclude an aneurysm. In this situation, urgent angiography must be carried out to exclude aneurysm. If an aneurysm is found, emergency neurosurgery must be performed to prevent subarachnoid hemorrhage.[55]

A presentation with complete ptosis and ophthalmoplegia and partial pupil involvement (mildly dilated and mildly less reactive) is known as relative pupillary sparing. Although controversial, most neuro-ophthalmologists consider this similar to pupillary sparing and monitor the patient carefully for the first week or perform MRA or CTA. Angiography is indicated if the pupil becomes more involved.[55]

Another controversial presentation is when partial ptosis and ophthalmoparesis occur, with complete sparing of the pupil. Many investigators consider this condition to be similar to that of a pupil affected by third nerve paresis and make evaluations to exclude an aneurysm, whereas other investigators monitor the patient carefully and evaluate if the pupil becomes involved. It is reasonable to at least evaluate as far as MRA and CTA in this situation.[55]

If a pupil-sparing third nerve paresis does not resolve within the expected 3–6 month period, further workup is indicated, which includes MRI scan, vasculitis workup, and, if no diagnosis can be made, a CSF examination.

For children, many cases are congenital and no further workup is indicated. In such patients, the third nerve palsy often is incomplete and associated with signs of aberrant regeneration. With a difficult delivery, trauma is the most likely cause.[1] In those conditions that are acquired, even those with pupillary involvement, angiography may not be indicated for patients less than 7 years of age, since the youngest reported age for a child to have an aneurysm is 7 years.[56] If no clear history of ophthalmoplegic migraine or known trauma is found, evaluation is carried out as above to establish the underlying causes. Numerous recent reports have documented enlargement and enhancement of the third nerve on MRI in patients with ophthalmoplegic migraine.[57]

In adults below the vasculopathic age, all third nerve palsies are worked up, which includes neuroimaging with MRI, blood tests (ESR, RPR, FTA, Lyme titer, glucose, ANA) to rule out vasculitis or infection, and CSF examination if no other cause is found.

For any patient who develops signs of aberrant regeneration, workup for a structural lesion is initiated, or repeated if previous workup has been carried out and no lesion found.

Nonisolated Cranial Neuropathies

MULTIPLE CRANIAL NEUROPATHIES. The management of patients who have cavernous sinus and superior orbital fissure lesions depends on the age of the patient, acuteness of presentation, speed of progression, presence of pain, history of systemic diseases or tumors, and accompanying features. Patients who have fever, somnolence, or a toxic appearance must be evaluated rapidly for evidence of cavernous sinus thrombosis or mucormycosis. Those who seek treatment acutely with prominent vascular features, with arterialization of conjunctival vessels, proptosis, and bruits, must be evaluated for direct carotid cavernous fistula.

The workup includes neuroimaging with MRI, with and without gadolinium, as the procedure of choice. If MRI is contraindicated, CT scans, with and without contrast using very thin axial and coronal sections, is carried out. Most often the structural lesion is imaged by one of these techniques. For a dural arteriovenous fistula or direct fistula, MRA, as well as conventional angiography, may be performed. In rare instances, CSF examination is helpful. When appropriate, blood tests such as level of angiotensin-converting enzyme, Lyme titer, RPR, and FTA are considered.

When a mass lesion consistent with tumor is found, a primary tumor source that has metastasized is possible. The diagnosis may be made by biopsy elsewhere, if more accessible lesions are present. With primary tumors, biopsy of the cavernous sinus lesion is often necessary.

With the onset of painful ophthalmoplegia consistent with idiopathic inflammation, a course of corticosteroids may be initiated. A positive response to corticosteroids has been used as diagnostic support for Tolosa–Hunt syndrome. However, since similar responses may occur in association with tumors, such as chordoma, giant-cell tumor, lymphoma, and epidermoid, the diagnosis must be made with caution and must be considered a diagnosis of exclusion. Differential diagnostic considerations for the presentation of painful ophthalmoplegia are listed in Box 199-1.[36] Evaluation to exclude the above causes of the cavernous sinus syndrome, as well as numerous other conditions, includes neuroimaging, complete blood count, ESR, FTA, ANA, serum protein electrophoresis, and, occasionally, nasopharyngeal and CSF examinations. Neuroimaging may be normal or may show a lesion consistent with inflammation. With recurrent episodes consistent with Tolosa–Hunt syndrome, biopsy of any lesion noted on neuroimaging is indicated to rule out these other entities. In the few cases reviewed pathologically, idiopathic chronic granulomatous inflammation is seen.

When a patient who has a known or an occult pituitary adenoma has an acute onset of painful ophthalmoparesis, often pituitary apoplexy is found by demonstration of acute hemorrhage or swelling of the pituitary adenoma on neuroimaging. These patients undergo surgery, using trans-sphenoidal hypophysectomy.

To diagnose direct or indirect carotid–cavernous fistula, arteriography is the definitive diagnostic procedure. However, MRI and MRA may demonstrate enlargement of the superior ophthalmic vein or the actual fistula. Other helpful procedures include CTA, Doppler ultrasound, color Doppler, and measurement of ocular pulse amplitude. Reversal of flow may be demonstrated in the superior ophthalmic vein.[58]

Bilateral Ophthalmoplegia. Neuroimaging that includes the course of each nerve involved on each side is required for patients who have bilateral simultaneous ophthalmoplegia without obvious cause. If negative, CSF examination is carried out and serologic evaluation for collagen vascular disease, arteritis, syphilis, and Lyme disease is obtained.

DIFFERENTIAL DIAGNOSIS

Numerous disorders that affect ocular motility may mimic and appear identically to a cranial neuropathy. These processes include restrictive ophthalmopathies, such as thyroid disease; neuromuscular diseases, such as myasthenia or botulism; and polyneuropathies, such as the Miller–Fisher variant of the Guillain–Barré syndrome.

The major examination technique used to exclude a restrictive process is the forced duction examination, in which a forceps or cotton-tipped swab is used to overcome the ductional deficit in the eye. A positive sign of restriction is when the deficit cannot be overcome because of resistance. Another sign of restrictive disease is an elevation of intraocular pressure when the eye moves in the direction of the restriction.

Isolated Cranial Neuropathies

ISOLATED SIXTH CRANIAL NERVE PALSY. The differential diagnosis of a sixth nerve paresis includes Duane's retraction syndrome, thyroid or other restrictive ophthalmopathy, myasthenia gravis, spasm of the near reflex, or breakdown of a previous esophoria.

Duane's syndrome is a congenital abnormality that occurs in three different forms. All three forms include narrowing of the palpebral fissure and retraction of the globe when the eye is adducted. Type I consists of an abduction deficit that mimics a sixth nerve paresis, type II consists of an adduction deficit, and type III includes both an abduction and adduction deficit (Fig. 199-11). Pathologically, abnormal development of the cells of the abducens nucleus and innervation of the lateral rectus by branches of the oculomotor nuclei occurs. During adduction, co-firing of the medial and lateral recti produces retraction of the globe. Patients who have Duane's syndrome do not usually experience diplopia. Duane's syndrome is bilateral in 18% of cases and familial in 10%.[59,60]

BOX 199-1

Differential Diagnosis of Painful Ophthalmoplegia Syndrome

TRAUMA

ANEURYSM
Intracavernous carotid artery
Posterior cerebral artery
Basilar artery

CAROTID CAVERNOUS FISTULA

CAVERNOUS SINUS THROMBOSIS

TUMORS
Primary intracranial
Local or distant metastasis
Pituitary apoplexy
Meningeal carcinomatosis or lymphomatosis

INFECTION
Mucormycosis or other fungal infection
Herpes zoster
Tuberculosis
Bacterial sinusitis, mucocele, periostitis
Syphilis

INFLAMMATION
Sarcoid
Wegener's granulomatosis
Tolosa–Hunt syndrome
Orbital pseudotumor

GIANT CELL ARTERITIS

ISCHEMIC
Diabetes
Hypertension

OPHTHALMOPLEGIC MIGRAINE

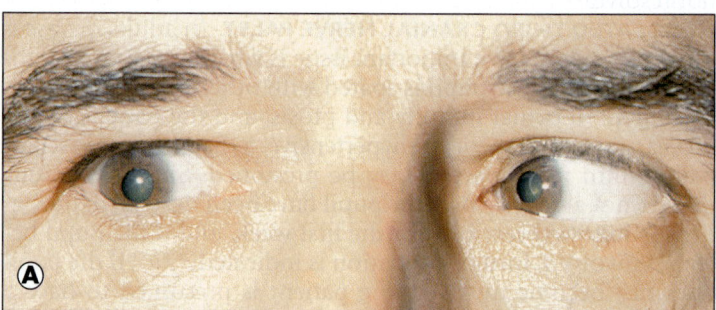

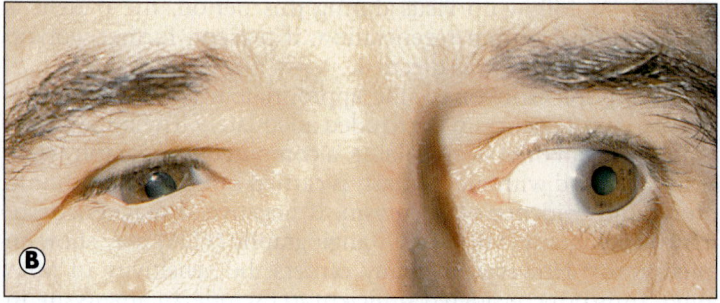

FIG. 199-11 ■ Duane's syndrome (type III). **A,** Abduction deficit. **B,** Adduction deficit, retraction of globe, and narrowing of palpebral fissure on adduction of the right eye.

Spasm of the near reflex most often is seen as a nonorganic, functional disorder in patients who have psychogenic disease or in malingerers. It presents with an abduction deficit that arises from substitution of convergence for lateral gaze. The diagnosis is made by finding the other features of the near reflex, mainly miosis, on attempted lateral gaze. Ductions tested with the other eye covered usually are normal. Spasm of the near reflex is seen rarely in organic conditions. [61]

Restrictive ophthalmopathy most often results from thyroid disease. If not already present, the patient soon develops other orbital signs, such as proptosis, injection, chemosis, lid retraction and lag, and has a positive forced duction test. Other restrictive processes of the medial rectus include trauma and orbital myositis.

Myasthenia may be differentiated on history and examination by the features of fatigability and variability. Evaluation using a Tensilon test, acetylcholine receptor antibody, and electromyogram establishes the diagnosis.

Patients who have congenital esophoria or compensated esotropia may give a history consistent with sixth nerve palsy, as a result of worsening of the previous deviation, often in times of stress or infection. Features that favor this diagnosis include a relatively comitant deviation and the establishment of an ocular deviation when photographs of the patient at a younger age are reviewed.

Infants who have congenital esotropia may have cross-fixation that mimics a sixth nerve paresis. This may be seen with latent nystagmus, as part of the nystagmus blockage syndrome. Evaluation after patching one eye for days or performing the Doll's head maneuver demonstrate normal abduction. [35]

ISOLATED FOURTH CRANIAL NERVE PALSY. The differential diagnosis of isolated fourth nerve paresis includes myasthenia gravis, thyroid ophthalmopathy and other orbital restrictive processes, Brown's syndrome, skew deviation, and overaction of the inferior oblique muscle associated with congenital strabismus. Thyroid ophthalmopathy is present most often with other orbital signs and features of restriction, as noted above for sixth nerve paresis. [62] Myasthenia gravis can be differentiated by its fatigability and variability. Skew deviation, a supranuclear vertical deviation that results from brainstem disease, is often associated with other neurological findings that are not present with an isolated fourth nerve paresis. Skew deviation may have a comitant or incomitant pattern of deviation and does not exactly fit with the three-step pattern of a fourth nerve paresis. The ocular tilt reaction, a form of skew deviation that most closely mimics a fourth nerve paresis, appears with hypotropia, head tilt towards the hypotropic eye, and conjugate torsion towards the hypotropic eye. [63] In addition, excyclotorsion may not be present with myasthenia, skew deviation, and thyroid disease, but is invariably present with an isolated fourth nerve paresis.

Brown's syndrome causes diplopia because of an elevation deficit in adduction, in which the involved eye is hypotropic; forced duction test is positive. When congenital, this syndrome results from a short or tethered superior oblique tendon, but the acquired syndrome may be a result of tenosynovitis, adhesions, metastasis, or trauma. [1,35] Brown's syndrome actually mimics an inferior oblique paresis; the latter may be differentiated by concomitant overaction of the superior oblique muscle, an A-pattern horizontal deviation, and a negative forced duction test. Patients affected by overaction of the inferior oblique muscle have a deviation greatest in adduction in upgaze.

ISOLATED THIRD CRANIAL NERVE PALSY. The differential diagnosis of isolated third nerve palsy is not as lengthy as for fourth and sixth nerve palsies because of the many structures innervated by the third nerve and the characteristic findings. Nonetheless, if no pain or pupil involvement exists, myasthenia gravis must be considered. Restrictive ophthalmopathy may mimic parts of a third nerve paresis, but does not involve the pupil, more often presents with lid retraction than ptosis if thyroid ophthalmopathy is the cause, and often has other orbital

findings. A supranuclear lesion may involve ptosis and an elevation deficit, but usually has other associated deficits that involve midbrain and diencephalic structures.

Nonisolated Cranial Neuropathies

It is important in the diagnosis of simultaneous palsies of the motor nerves of the eye to differentiate these from oculoparesis that arises from orbital inflammatory disease, such as Graves' ophthalmopathy or orbital pseudotumor, ocular myopathies (such as chronic progressive external ophthalmoplegia), disorders of neuromuscular transmission (such as myasthenia gravis or botulism), and polyneuropathies (such as the Miller–Fisher variant of Guillain–Barré syndrome). Demyelinating disease, basilar artery ischemia or aneurysm, skull base tumors, Wernicke's encephalopathy, and supranuclear gaze palsies also must be included in the differential diagnosis of nonisolated cranial neuropathies. [34]

TREATMENT

Aside from treatment for the specific cause of the cranial neuropathy, the symptoms of diplopia must be treated. Acutely, occlusion of either eye using a patch or opaque tape over glasses is the best treatment, particularly in patients who are expected to recover. With chronic diplopia, prism therapy is helpful for a subgroup of patients, especially when the deviation is not very incomitant. Eventually, with chronic, stable deviations, strabismus surgery (Chapter 81) may be useful.

Botulinum toxin injections are used by some clinicians early on, particularly for fourth or sixth nerve paresis, to promote earlier fusion while recovery takes place. Ultimate recovery is similar with or without botulinum treatment. [64] Botulinum toxin is also a treatment option for a chronic cranial nerve paresis. For instance, in a fourth nerve paresis, it may be injected into the ipsilateral inferior oblique or the contralateral inferior rectus.

Nonisolated Cranial Neuropathies

The Tolosa–Hunt syndrome is exquisitely sensitive to corticosteroids—pain resolves almost immediately and ophthalmoplegia resolves subacutely with 60–80mg/day of prednisone. However, recurrences may not respond as well.

Direct internal carotid artery to cavernous sinus fistulas are treated by occlusion carried out by an interventional neuroradiologist, with balloon occlusion of the connection between the carotid artery and cavernous sinus. Occasionally, neurosurgery is required, with occlusion of the carotid artery both above and below the site of the fistula.

Dural arteriovenous fistulas may be followed clinically if no threat to vision exists. In over 50% of patients, the fistula spontaneously thromboses and resolves, particularly after angiography. [58] In addition, the patient may be trained to perform occlusion of the carotid artery intermittently during the day by the application of pressure using the finger tips (provided no serious cerebrovascular disease is present); this may allow for spontaneous thrombosis to occur. On some occasions, spontaneous thrombosis may be associated with retinal vein occlusions and visual loss. In cases in which a threat to vision occurs, selective arteriography with occlusion of the feeder vessels is performed by an interventional radiologist.

Miscellaneous Disorders

Superior oblique myokymia often spontaneously remits, but may recur after months or years. The treatment of choice is carbamazepine; alternatives include baclofen and clonazepam. [35] For patients who do not respond or do not tolerate medication, surgery (a superior oblique tenectomy and inferior oblique weakening procedure) may be helpful. [65] Ocular neuromyotonia often responds to treatment with carbamazepine.

REFERENCES

1. Brodsky MC, Baker RS, Hamed LM, eds. Pediatric neuro-ophthalmology. New York: Springer-Verlag; 1996.
2. Holmes JM, Mutyala S, Maus TL, *et al.* Pediatric third, fourth, and sixth nerve palsies: A population-based study. Am J Ophthalmol 1999;127:388–92.
3. Kodsi SR, Younge BR. Acquired oculomotor, trochlear, and abducent cranial nerve palsies in pediatric patients. Am J Ophthalmol 1992;114:568–74.
4. Moster ML, Savino PJ, Sergott RC, et al. Isolated sixth-nerve palsies in younger adults. Arch Ophthalmol. 1984;102:1328–30.
5. Sakalas R, Harbinson JW, Vines FS, Becker DP. Chronic sixth nerve palsy. An initial sign of basisphenoid tumors. Arch Ophthalmol. 1975;93:186–90.
6. Savino PJ, Hilliker JK, Casell GH, Schatz NJ. Chronic sixth nerve palsies. Are they really harbingers of serious intracranial disease? Arch Ophthalmol. 1982; 100:1442–4.
7. Currie J, Lubin JH, Lessell S. Chronic isolated abducens paresis from tumors at the base of the brain. Arch Neurol. 1983;40:226–9.
8. Galetta S, Smith JL. Chronic isolated sixth nerve palsies. Arch Neurol. 1989; 46:79–82.
9. Knox DL, Clark DB, Schuster FF. Benign VI nerve palsies in children. Pediatrics. 1967;40:560–3.
10. Volpe NJ, Lessell S. Remitting sixth nerve palsy in skull base tumors. Arch Ophthalmol. 1993;111:1391–5.
11. Shrader EC, Schlezinger NS. Neuro-ophthalmologic evaluation of abducens nerve paralysis. Arch Neurol. 1960;63:108–14.
12. Rucker CW. The causes of paralysis of the third, fourth and sixth cranial nerves. Am J Ophthalmol. 1966;61:353–8.
13. Johnston AC. Etiology and treatment of abducens paralysis. Trans Pacific Coast Oto-ophthalmol Soc. 1968;49:259–77.
14. Keane JR. Bilateral sixth nerve palsy. Analysis of 125 cases. Arch Neurol. 1976;33:681–3.
15. Rush JA, Younge BR. Paralysis of cranial nerves III, IV, and VI. Cause and prognosis in 1,000 cases. Arch Ophthalmol. 1981;99:76–9.
16. Tiffin PAC, MacEwen CJ, Criag EA, Clayton G. Acquired palsy of the oculomotor, trochlear and abducens nerves. Eye. 1996;10:377–84.
17. Richards BW, Jones FR, Younge BR. Causes and prognosis in 4278 cases of paralysis of the oculomotor, trochlear and abducens cranial nerves. Am J Ophthalmol 1992;113:489–96.
18. Archambault P, Wise JS, Rosen J, Polomeno RC, Auger N. Herpes zoster ophthalmoplegia. Report of six cases. J Clin Neuro Ophthalmol. 1988;8:185–91.
19. Khawn E, Scott AB, Jampolsky A. Acquired superior oblique palsy. Diagnosis and management. Arch Ophthalmol. 1967;77:761–8.
20. Burger LJ, Kalvin NH, Smith JL. Acquired lesions of the fourth cranial nerve. Brain. 1970;93:567–74.
21. Younge BR, Sutula F. Analysis of trochlear nerve palsies. Diagnosis, etiology and treatment. Mayo Clin Proc. 1977;52:11–18.
22. Goldstein JE, Cogan DG. Diabetic ophthalmoplegia with special reference to the pupil. Arch Ophthalmol. 1960;64:144–52.
23. Green WR, Hackett ER, Schlezinger NS. Neuro-ophthalmologic evaluation of oculomotor nerve paralysis. Arch Ophthalmol. 1964;72:154–67.
24. Miller NR. Solitary oculomotor nerve palsy in childhood. Am J Ophthalmol. 1977;83:106–11.
25. Harley R. Paralytic strabismus in children. Etiologic incidence and management of the third, fourth and sixth nerve palsies. Ophthalmology. 1980;87:24–43.
26. Kissel JT, Burde RM, Klingele TG, Zeigler HE. Pupil-sparing oculomotor palsies with internal carotid–posterior communicating artery aneurysms. Ann Neurol. 1983;13:149–54.
27. Newman SA. Disorders of ocular motility. In: Slamovits TL, Burde R, eds. Textbook of ophthalmology. Neuro-ophthalmology, London: Mosby–Yearbook Europe; 1991.
28. Friedman AP, Harter DH, Merritt HH. Ophthalmoplegia migraine. Arch Neurol. 1962;7:82–9.
29. Sebag J, Sadun AA. Aberrant regeneration of the third nerve to the iris sphincter following penetrating orbital trauma. Arch Neurol. 1983;40:762–5.
30. Schatz NJ, Savino PJ, Corbett JJ. Primary aberrant oculomotor regeneration. A sign of intracavernous meningioma. Arch Neurol. 1977;34:29–32.
31. Cox TA, Wurster JB, Godfrey WA. Primary aberrant oculomotor regeneration due to intracranial aneurysm. Arch Neurol. 1979;36:507–71.
32. Friedman DI, Wright K, Sadun AA. Oculomotor palsy with cyclic spasms. Neurology. 1989;39:1263–4.
33. Derakhshan I. Superior branch palsy of the oculomotor nerve with spontaneous recovery. Ann Neurol. 1978;4:478–9.
34. Sergott RC, Glaser JS, Berger LJ. Simultaneous, bilateral diabetic ophthalmoplegia. Report of two cases and discussion of differential diagnosis. Ophthalmology. 1984;91:18–22.
35. Leigh RJ, Zee DS. In: Plum F, Gilman S, Martin JB, et al, eds. The neurology of eye movements, ed 2. Philadelphia: FA Davis; 1991.
36. Kline LB. The Tolosa–Hunt syndrome. Surv Ophthalmol. 1982;27:79–95.
37. Jefferson G. Concerning injuries, aneurysms and tumors involving the cavernous sinus. Trans Ophthalmol Soc UK. 1953;73:117–52.
38. Thomas JE, Yos E. The parasellar syndrome: Problems in determining etiology. Mayo Clin Proc. 1970;45:617–23.
39. Kline LB. Cavernous sinus/orbital apex syndrome. In: Tusa RJ, Newman SA, eds. Neuro-ophthalmological disorders. New York: Marcel Dekker, 1995:291–8.
40. Keane JR. Cavernous sinus syndrome. Analysis of 151 cases. Arch Neurol. 1996; 53:967–71.
41. Tolosa E. Periarteritic lesions of the carotid siphon with the clinical features of a carotid infraclinoid aneurysm. J Neurol Neurosurg Psychiatry. 1954;17:300–2.
42. Hunt WE, Meagher JN, LeFever HE, Zeman W. Painful ophthalmoplegia. Its relation to indolent inflammation of the cavernous sinus. Neurology. 1961;11:56–62.
43. Miller N, ed. Walsh and Hoyt's neuro-ophthalmology, vol 2, ed 4. Williams and Wilkins: Baltimore; 1985.
44. Miller EA, Savino PJ, Schatz NJ. Bilateral sixth-nerve palsy. A rare complication of water-soluble contrast myelography. Arch Ophthalmol. 1982; 100:603–4.
45. Morrow MJ, Sharpe JA, Ranalli PJ. Superior oblique myokymia associated with a posterior fossa tumor: oculographic correlation with an idiopathic case. Neurology. 1990;40:367–70.
46. Shults WT, Hoyt WF, Behrens M, et al. Ocular neuromyotonia. A clinical description of six patients. Arch Ophthalmol. 1986;104:1028–34.
47. Lessell S, Lessell IM, Rizzo JF III. Ocular neuromyotonia after radiation therapy. Am J Ophthalmol. 1986;102:766–70.
48. Newman SA. Clinical challenges. Gaze-induced strabismus. Surv Ophthalmol. 1993;38:303–9.
49. Moster ML. Complications of cancer therapies. In: Miller N, Newman NJ, eds. Walsh and Hoyt's neuro-ophthalmology, ed 5. Baltimore: Williams and Wilkins; 1997.
50. Chrousos GA, Dipaola F, Kattah JC, Laws ER. Paresis of the abducens nerve after trivial head injury. Am J Ophthalmol. 1993;116:387–8.
51. Walter KA, Newman NJ, Lessell S. Oculomotor palsy from minor head trauma: initial sign of intracranial aneurysm. Neurology 1994;44:148–50.
52. O'Connor PS, Tredici TJ, Green RP. Pupil-sparing third nerve palsies caused by aneurysm. Am J Ophthalmol. 1983;95:395–7.
53. Bartleson JD, Trautmann JC, Sundt TM. Minimal oculomotor nerve paresis secondary to unruptured intracranial aneurysm. Arch Neurol. 1986;43:1015–20.
54. McFadzean RM, Teasdale EM. Computerized tomography angiography in isolated third nerve palsies. Jl Neurosurg 1998:88:679–84.
55. Jacobson DM, Trobe JD. The emerging role of magnetic resonance angiography in the management of patients with third cranial nerve palsy. Am J Ophthalmol 1999;128:94–6.
56. Branley MG, Wright KW, Borchert MS. Third nerve palsy due to cerebral artery aneurysm in a child. Aust NZ Jl Ophth 1992;20:137–40.
57. Ohara MA, Anderson RT, Brown D. Magnetic resonance imaging in ophthalmoplegic migraine of children. J AAPOS 2001;5:307–10.
58. Golnik KC. Cavernous sinus arteriovenous fistula. In: Tusa RJ, Newman SA, eds. Neuro-ophthalmologic disorders. New York: Marcel Dekker, 1995:317–27.
59. Raab E. Clinical features of Duane's syndrome. J Pediatr Ophthalmol Strabismus. 1986;23:64–8.
60. DeRespinis PA, Caputo AR, Wagner RS, Guo S. Major review. Duane's retraction syndrome. Surv Ophthalmol. 1993;38:257–88.
61. Moster ML, Hoenig EM. Spasm of the near reflex associated with metabolic encephalopathy. Neurology. 1989;39:150.
62. Moster ML, Bosley TM, Slavin ML, Rubin SE. Thyroid ophthalmology presenting as superior oblique paresis. J Clin Neuro Ophthalmol. 1992;12:94–7.
63. Donahue SP, Lavin PJM, Hamed LM. Tonic ocular tilt reaction simulating a superior oblique palsy. Arch Ophthalmol 1999;117:347–52.
64. Holmes JM, Beck RW, Kip KE, et al. Botulinum toxin treatment versus conservative management in acute traumatic sixth nerve palsy or paresis. J AAPOS 2000;4:145–9.
65. Palmer EA, Shults WT. Superior oblique myokymia: preliminary results of surgical treatment. J Pediatr Ophthalmol Strabismus. 1984;21:96–101.

CHAPTER
200

Disorders of the Neuromuscular Junction

DEBORAH I. FRIEDMAN

DEFINITION
- A disorder of the neuromuscular junction, caused by an antibody-mediated autoimmune attack on postsynaptic acetylcholine receptors or the altered presynaptic release of acetylcholine.

KEY FEATURE
- Ocular or generalized muscle weakness.

ASSOCIATED FEATURES
- Ptosis and ocular motility disturbances.
- Facial, trunk, and limb weakness.
- Speech and swallowing dysfunction.
- Respiratory compromise.
- Autonomic nervous system dysfunction.

MYASTHENIA GRAVIS

INTRODUCTION

Of all the disorders of the neuromuscular junction (Table 200-1), myasthenia gravis is the most common.[1] It is a disorder caused by an antibody-mediated autoimmune attack on the acetylcholine (ACh) receptors at the neuromuscular junction. The hallmark of myasthenia gravis is fluctuating muscle weakness that worsens with exertion and improves with rest. Ocular manifestations, such as ptosis and diplopia, are present frequently at onset and eventually are present in most patients.

EPIDEMIOLOGY AND PATHOGENESIS

The prevalence of myasthenia gravis is rising, largely as a result of longer lifespan. An estimated 15 cases occur per million population.[2,3] Women are affected twice as frequently as men. The incidence has one peak in the second and third decades, which includes mostly women, and another in the sixth and seventh decades, which involves mostly men. However, it can occur at any age. Myasthenia gravis rarely is familial, but heredity might

TABLE 200-1

DISORDERS OF NEUROMUSCULAR TRANSMISSION

Disorder	Cause	Location	Defect	Symptoms	Treatment
Myasthenia gravis	Autoimmune	Postsynaptic	Antibodies to ACh receptor	Ptosis, diplopia Weakness, improves with rest	Pyridostigmine (Mestinon), corticosteroids, immunosuppressants; thymectomy
Botulism	*Clostridium botulinum* infection	Presynaptic	Impaired ACh release	Ptosis, diplopia, tonic pupils, accommodative impairment, bulbar weakness, cholinergic blockade	Respiratory support Antitoxin
Lambert–Eaton myasthenic syndrome	Paraneoplastic	Presynaptic	Impaired ACh release	Rarely ptosis, diplopia Proximal muscle weakness Autonomic dysfunction	Treat malignancy—diaminopyridine, corticosteroids, immunosuppressants
Organophosphate toxicity	Insecticides Chemical warfare	Synaptic	Inhibits acetyl-cholinesterase	Rapid respiratory failure Muscle twitching then paralysis Mental status changes Pupillary miosis	Atropine, pralidoxine
Black widow spider (*Latrodectus mactans*) bite	α-Larotoxin	Presynaptic	Increased ACh release	Autonomic hyperactivity Vasoconstriction Painful, rigid abdomen	Calcium, magnesium, atropine, antivenin; warming
Tick paralysis	Toxic	Presynaptic	Impaired ACh release	Irritability, pain, paralysis Respiratory paralysis Late signs—unreactive pupils, ophthalmoplegia	Remove tick, supportive measures
Scorpion toxin	Toxic	Presynaptic	Increased ACh release	Agitation, respiratory failure, blurred vision, abnormal eye movements, jerking of extremities, autonomic dysfunction	Calcium, atropine, antivenin, supportive measures

ACh, Acetylcholine.

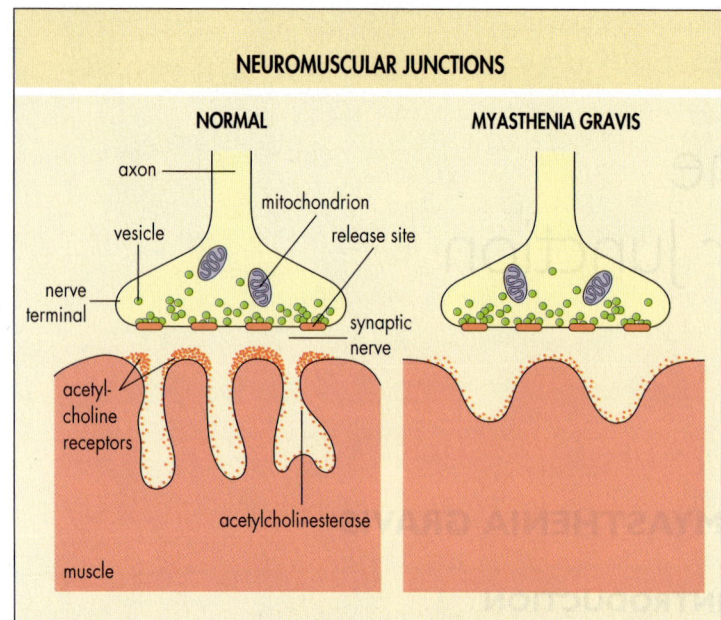

FIG. 200-I ■ **Neuromuscular junctions.** In myasthenia gravis, acetylcholine is released from presynaptic vesicles and diffuses across the synaptic cleft to the postsynaptic receptors. Acetylcholinesterase, located deep within the synaptic folds, hydrolyzes acetylcholine. There is also a simplification of the postsynaptic site with a reduced number of receptors. (From Drachman DB. Myasthenia gravis. N Engl J Med. 1994;330:1797–810.)

be a risk factor. Young female patients who have thymic hyperplasia often have human lymphocyte antigen (HLA)-B8 and HLA-DR3 patterns. An association exists with HLA-B7 and HLA-DR2 in patients over 40 years of age.

Knowledge of the anatomy and physiology of the normal neuromuscular junction helps to understand its disorders. The neuromuscular junction is composed of the motor axon terminal, the synaptic cleft, and the postsynaptic surface of the muscle cell (Fig. 200-1), in which deep infoldings occur. Acetylcholine (ACh) is stored in vesicles in the cytoplasm of the nerve terminal and mediates neuromuscular transmission. Depolarization of the axon by an action potential causes release of ACh into the synaptic cleft by calcium-dependent, voltage-dependent exocytosis. Ordinarily, more ACh is released than is needed to produce neuromuscular transmission, which creates a safety factor. Once released, the ACh diffuses across the synaptic cleft to the postsynaptic folds.

The postsynaptic folds contain the ACh receptors and acetylcholinesterase, the enzyme that hydrolyzes ACh. In general, the receptors are located on the tips of the folds and acetylcholinesterase is concentrated deeper within the synaptic folds. When two ACh molecules bind to a receptor, conformational changes occur and an ion channel opens, which results in a local depolarization and subsequent muscle contraction. An additional safety factor exists at this level, because the potential generally exceeds the threshold required for depolarization of a muscle fiber (end-plate potential). Innervated receptors undergo continuous turnover, with a half-life of 8–11 days.

In myasthenia gravis, the major pathological changes are found at the postsynaptic membrane, with loss and simplification of the postjunctional folds, reduced numbers of ACh receptors, and a widened synaptic cleft. New receptors are synthesized, but they are not incorporated into the damaged postsynaptic membrane, which results in a loss of receptors at the junction. Patients who have myasthenia gravis contain about one third the number of ACh receptors found in healthy controls. The number of receptors seems to parallel the severity of weakness. With a reduced number of receptors, the end-plate potential is inadequate to generate contraction of some muscle fibers; this produces the characteristic muscle weakness. Normally, a decline ("rundown") occurs in the amount of ACh

released by successive muscle contractions. At myasthenic junctions, the rundown produces progressive failure of neuromuscular transmission, because of the reduced number of receptors. This accounts for the muscular fatigability that is the hallmark of the disease.

The muscular abnormalities in myasthenia gravis result from an antibody-mediated process that likely originates in the thymus gland. The antibodies both accelerate the rate of degradation of ACh receptors and block ACh binding sites. B-cells produce the autoantibodies, but T-cells also are important in the autoantibody response of myasthenia gravis. In myasthenia gravis, the T- and B-cells produced by the thymus gland are more responsive to the ACh receptor than are their counterparts in the peripheral blood. Of patients who have myasthenia gravis, 75% have thymic abnormalities; of these, 85% have thymic hyperplasia and 15% have thymomas. Perhaps the strongest evidence for the importance of the thymus gland in the pathogenesis of myasthenia is the effectiveness of thymectomy.

OCULAR MANIFESTATIONS

Ocular symptoms, ptosis and diplopia, are present at onset in about 70% of patients and eventually are present in 90%. Ptosis, either isolated or associated with extraocular muscle involvement, often is the first symptom. The ptosis may be unilateral or bilateral, symmetrical or asymmetrical, and often it is more pronounced as the day progresses.

Involvement of the extraocular muscles varies from single-muscle paresis to total ophthalmoplegia. Myasthenia gravis may simulate an ocular motor nerve palsy, unilateral or bilateral internuclear ophthalmoplegia, or a gaze palsy. When the levator palpebrae superioris also is involved, the disease may mimic a pupil-sparing third nerve palsy. Patients experience diplopia, which usually fluctuates throughout the day; sometimes the disease produces vertical separation of the images, at other times it causes horizontal diplopia. The diplopia may be intermittent. Other motility abnormalities include saccadic dysmetria and decreased final saccadic velocity, small "quiver" eye movements, and gaze-evoked nystagmus.[4] Nystagmus occurs because of muscle fatigue; isolated nystagmus as a sign of myasthenia gravis is rare. For practical purposes, the pupils are normal in myasthenia gravis. Although anisocoria, impaired accommodation, and sluggishly reactive pupils have been described, the abnormalities are subtle and not clinically significant.

DIAGNOSIS

The diagnosis of myasthenia gravis usually is suspected from the patient's symptoms and the physical examination. The presence of ptosis and extraocular muscle weakness that either fluctuates or does not conform to any pattern of ocular motor nerve paresis raises the suspicion of myasthenia gravis. Many ocular signs may be present on the examination. With unilateral ptosis, the other eyelid may appear retracted, exhibiting Hering's law of equal innervation. If the ptotic eyelid is lifted manually, the ptosis worsens on the contralateral side (Fig. 200-2). This finding is not exclusive to myasthenia but frequently is present in patients who have the condition. Cogan's lid twitch sign demonstrates the rapid recovery and easy fatigability of the levator. When the patient looks down for 10–20 seconds and then rapidly looks up to primary position, the upper eyelids often overshoot (retract) and then settle back into a stable position; a downward drift of the lids or several twitches may be observed. Prolonged upgaze produces muscle fatigue, with eyelid droop or downward drift of the eyes. As the patient attempts repeated large-amplitude saccades, slowing of the eye movements may occur with repetition. Ice placed on a ptotic lid may prolong the time for which the ACh receptor channels open and produce clinical improvement. The ice test is a sensitive and specific test for myasthenia gravis.[5–7]

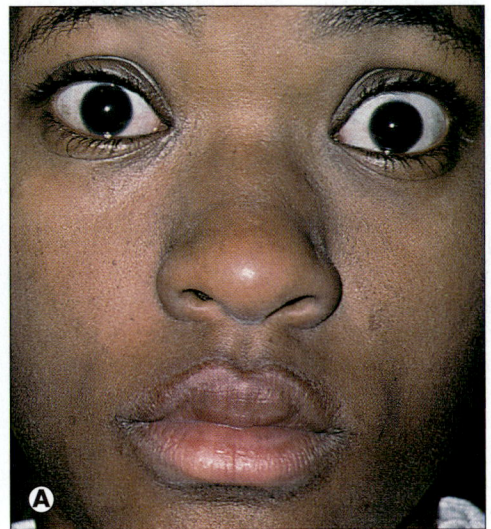
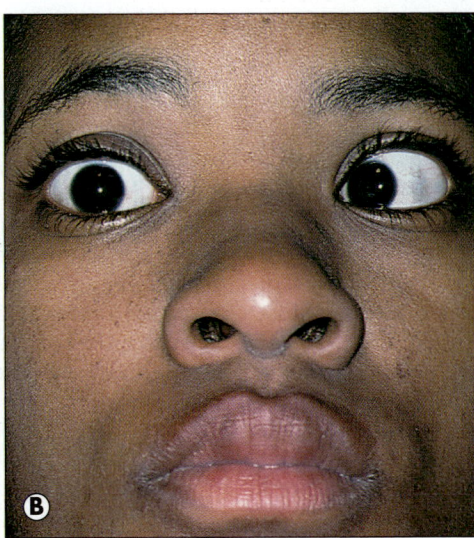
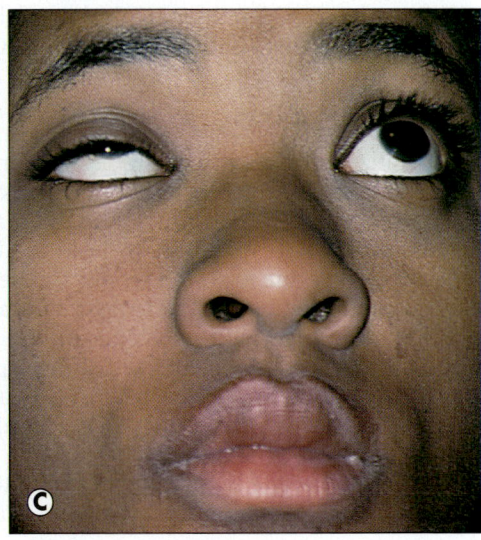

FIG. 200-2 ■ Myasthenia gravis. **A,** Right ptosis and compensatory left upper lid retraction. **B,** On looking right note right abduction deficit and left lid retraction to compensate for right ptosis. **C,** On sustained upgaze, right upper lid becomes fatigued.

With generalized myasthenia gravis, muscle strength testing reveals weakness, usually more prominent proximally. Individual muscles weaken with repetitive testing; the strength improves after a brief period of rest.

No specific laboratory test exists for myasthenia gravis. A combination of physical examination, pharmacological tests, blood tests, and electrodiagnostic tests often is needed to confirm the diagnosis. If a demonstrable, measurable abnormality is present on the examination, administration of an acetylcholinesterase inhibitor produces increased strength of myasthenic muscles.[8] The most commonly used agent is intravenous edrophonium (Tensilon), because of its rapid onset of action (30 seconds) and short duration of action (5 minutes). Baseline readings are taken for the pulse, blood pressure, and the physical sign to be measured. For ocular manifestations, this may include measurement of the palpebral fissures and levator function or quantitation of subtle motility deficits using a Maddox rod or Hess screen.[9] The patient should be warned of potential side effects, including diaphoresis, abdominal cramping, nausea, vomiting, salivation, and light-headedness.

Although the complication rate is very low, the most dangerous complication is heart block, and atropine sulfate should be made available immediately (0.4–0.6mg, adult dose).[10] Alternatively, patients may be pretreated with intramuscular or subcutaneous atropine. An assistant is required to monitor the patient's pulse and blood pressure during the test. Ten milligrams is drawn into a tuberculin syringe. After administration of an initial test dose of 2mg intravenously, the patient is observed for 1 minute while the pulse is monitored. Some patients improve with the test dose. If no improvement and no adverse reaction occur, an additional 4mg is administered. The remaining 4mg can be used if no effect is seen. The presence of eyelid fasciculations indicates that an adequate dose was injected. The response to edrophonium often is dramatic (see Fig. 200-2). Intramuscular neostigmine (Prostigmin) is useful in children who may not cooperate with intravenous injections. Neostigmine (1.5mg for adults or 0.04mg/kg for children, mixed with 0.6mg atropine sulfate) produces observable effects within 15 minutes; peak action occurs 30 minutes after injection.

A safe alternative to the edrophonium test is the sleep test.[11] After the baseline deficit has been documented, the patient rests quietly with eyes closed for 30 minutes. The measurements are repeated immediately after the patient "wakes up" and opens the eyes. Improvement after rest is characteristic of myasthenia gravis.

A serum assay for anti–ACh receptor antibodies should be obtained for all patients who have suspected myasthenia gravis.

Antibody titers do not correlate with the severity of the disease. The binding antibody is obtained most commonly, being detected in approximately 90% of patients who have generalized myasthenia gravis and 70% of patients who have ocular myasthenia. Blocking antibodies are present in approximately 60% of patients who have generalized myasthenia and 50% of patients who have ocular disease, and rarely are present (1%) without binding antibodies.

Electrophysiological tests are useful for the diagnosis of myasthenia gravis if other tests are inconclusive. Repetitive supramaximal motor nerve stimulation (1–3Hz) produces a progressive decremental response of the compound muscle action potentials during the first four or five stimuli. The amplitude of the response then either levels off or increases slightly because of posttetanic potentiation. This technique shows abnormalities in 40–90% of patients who have myasthenia gravis and results are more likely to be positive with severe disease. Single fiber electromyography (SFEMG) demonstrates "jitter," which indicates the variability of propagation time to individual muscle fibers supplied by the same motor neuron. Intermittent "blocking" caused by failure of conduction at the neuromuscular junction also may occur. The sensitivity of SFEMG is approximately 90%.[12] In particular, SFEMG of the superior rectus and levator palpebralis muscles is extremely sensitive for the detection of ocular myasthenia gravis.[13] Conversion from ocular to generalized disease is less likely with normal SFEMG findings of the upper extremities.[14]

Because 10–15% of patients who have myasthenia gravis have a thymic tumor, high-quality radiographic imaging of the chest (computed tomography or magnetic resonance imaging) is mandatory, even for patients with solely ocular findings (Fig. 200-3). A plain chest radiograph alone is not adequate for this purpose. Fullness of the thymus gland typically is seen up to age 30 years. The persistence of a thymus gland in a patient over 40 years of age or an increase in size on serial imaging studies raises the suspicion that a thymoma is present.

Other testing is directed toward associated systemic diseases and treatment. It is not unusual for patients who have myasthenia to have another autoimmune disease. Because 5% of patients who have myasthenia gravis have co-existent thyroid disease, thyroid function tests should be obtained for all patients. Complete blood count, antinuclear antibody analysis, and erythrocyte sedimentation rates typically are drawn in patients who have confirmed myasthenia gravis. If treatment with corticosteroids is planned, diabetes and tuberculosis should be excluded. Neuroimaging of the brain is not required routinely but may be considered for atypical cases that are antibody negative and refractory to treatment (Table 200-2).

SYSTEMIC ASSOCIATIONS

Generalized myasthenia gravis develops in 75% of patients. The nonocular symptoms include facial weakness, weakness of the jaw when chewing, dysarthria, and dysphagia. Nuchal muscular weakness produces inability to hold the head up. Weakness of the limbs is common. If the erector spinae muscles are involved, the patient may be unable to maintain an erect posture. Most patients feel tired with reduced stamina. In severe cases, weakness of the muscles of the chest and diaphragm produces dyspnea. A pronounced drop in the vital capacity leads to myasthenic crisis, which requires mechanical ventilation and aggressive treatment.

Approximately 12% of neonates born to myasthenic mothers develop transient neonatal myasthenia gravis, as a result of maternal transmission of autoantibodies through the placenta; these trigger independent antibody production by the infant. Affected neonates have generalized weakness with difficulty eating, respiratory weakness, a poor cry, and facial weakness, which are noticed shortly after birth. The symptoms last for several weeks and then resolve without recurrence.

Thymic enlargement and thymoma frequently are present in patients who have myasthenia gravis. Other autoimmune disorders, such as thyroid disease, systemic lupus erythematosus, and pernicious anemia, are found with increased frequency in patients with myasthenia gravis. Aplastic anemia, ulcerative colitis, Sjögren's disease, Kaposi's sarcoma, and lymphoid tumor of the orbit are less common associations.

TREATMENT

The major therapies for myasthenia gravis follow:
- Acetylcholinesterase inhibitors
- Immunosuppression
- Symptomatic treatment of ocular abnormalities
- Avoidance of agents that worsen neuromuscular transmission

Acetylcholinesterase inhibitors raise the safety factor for neuromuscular transmission by preventing the degradation of ACh. Although these agents provide symptomatic improvement in muscle weakness, they do not treat the disease directly. However, because of their rapid effectiveness and lack of long-term side effects, they often are the first agents used in the treatment of myasthenia. Pyridostigmine (Mestinon), the most commonly used drug, has a duration of action of 2–8 hours. It is most useful for the treatment of systemic weakness of myasthenia gravis and may not improve the diplopia. The usual starting dose is 30–60mg every 4 hours while awake. Larger doses or more frequent dosing intervals may be used as needed. Above 120mg every 3 hours, no additional effectiveness is likely and a risk exists of cholinergic crises. A delayed release preparation taken at bedtime is useful for patients who have profound weakness upon awakening in the morning. The most common side effects from these agents are gastrointestinal disturbances (nausea, diarrhea) and muscle twitching. Overdosage results in sialorrhea, blurred vision, and worsening weakness (cholinergic crisis). It may be difficult to differentiate cholinergic crisis as a result of medication from worsening of the disease, that is myasthenic

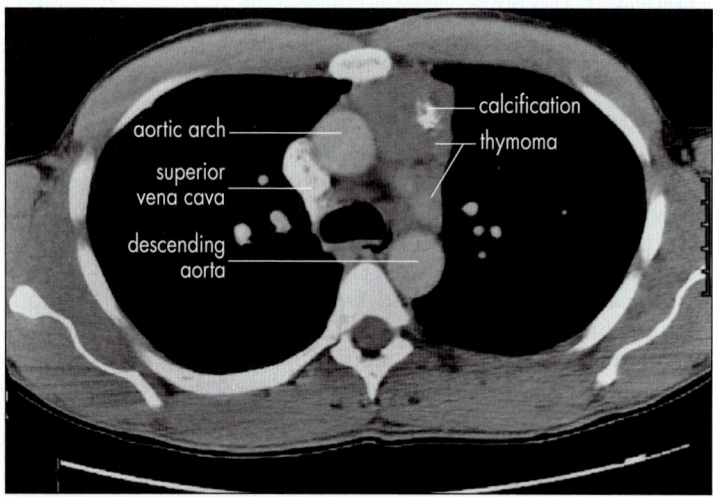

FIG. 200-3 ■ Computed tomography of the chest with contrast enhancement. Shown is a large, multilobulated thymoma in a 32-year-old man with ocular myasthenia gravis. The mass is in proximity to the aortic arch and the ascending aorta. A focal calcification is present anteriorly. The patient's ptosis and diplopia remitted following removal of the thymoma.

TABLE 200-2

DIFFERENTIAL DIAGNOSIS OF THE NEUROMUSCULAR JUNCTION

Disorder	Pupils	Ocular Motility	Lids	Other Ocular Findings	Other Systemic Findings
Myasthenia gravis	Normal	Fluctuating ophthalmoparesis	Ptosis Cogan's lid twich sign	—	Fluctuating weakness that improves with rest
Graves' ophthalmopathy	Normal	Restricted EOM Positive forced duction testing	Lid retraction Lid lag	Conjunctival infection Keratoconjunctivitis sicca Exophthalmos Optic neuropathy	Symptoms of hyperthyroidism may be present
Botulism	Dilated, poorly reactive Light–near dissociation	Ophthalmoparesis	Ptosis	—	Limb weakness Bulbar signs Respiratory failure Urinary retention Constipation
Lambert–Eaton myasthenic syndrome	Usually normal	Usually normal	Usually normal	Keratoconjunctivitis sicca	Autonomic and sensory symptoms
Guillain–Barré syndrome	Normal or poorly reactive	Normal or ophthalmoparesis	Ptosis	—	Facial diplegia Limb weakness Areflexia Respiratory failure
Progressive external ophthalmoplegia	Normal	Slowly progressive Symmetrical ophthalmoparesis	Slowly progressive Ptosis	May have pigmentary retinopathy	None unless coexisting mitochondrial disorder

EOM, Extraocular movement.

crisis. Diplopia often does not improve with pyridostigmine and may be treated with immunosuppressive agents.[15]

Thymectomy is indicated for all patients who have a thymoma and may be beneficial for some patients who do not have one.[16] Thymectomy produces improvement in almost all cases with no thymoma present and results in complete remission in 35–45% of patients. The benefits of thymectomy may not be apparent for 2–3 years, yet some patients respond almost immediately after surgery. It usually is recommended for patients under the age of 55 years who have generalized disease. The presence or absence of ACh receptor antibodies does not seem to influence the efficacy of the surgery. A trans-sternal approach is preferable, to allow adequate visualization of the thoracic cavity and total thymus removal. Ectopic rests of thymic tissue may be undiscovered if the less invasive transcervical technique is used. The morbidity and mortality rates from thymectomy are quite low. Because any surgical procedure may worsen myasthenia, some patients benefit from a short course of plasmapheresis preoperatively. Alternative methods of direct thymic suppression, such as radiation therapy, are not effective.

Immunosuppressants, mainly cytotoxic agents and corticosteroids, treat the disease directly and generally are employed in patients who do not improve satisfactorily with acetylcholinesterase inhibitors. It may be several weeks to months before these medications take effect. Prednisone is used most frequently, and various dosing strategies are employed. Daily administration of high doses (60–100mg) may produce substantial worsening within the first 2 weeks of treatment and should be used with caution. Other regimens use increasing, daily, low doses of prednisone, or alternate-day dosing. Alternate-day dosing has the advantage of fewer side effects, and many patients who have purely ocular symptoms improve on a low dosage (20–30mg) of alternate-day therapy. The risks of long-term prednisone administration include peptic ulcer, osteoporosis, femoral neck fracture, diabetes, skin breakdown, weight gain, and cushingoid features. Appropriate medical precautions and monitoring are required. To minimize the complication rate, the lowest dosage of prednisone possible should be used, and other immunosuppressant agents added, if needed.

Azathioprine, cyclophosphamide, and cyclosporine are effective for the long-term management of myasthenia gravis and may be used in combination with prednisone and pyridostigmine.[17] Mycophenolate mofetil was safe and effective in short-term studies.[18] These medications have fewer long-term side effects than prednisone. Blood counts must be taken, and liver and renal function must be monitored, and a small possibility exists that a neoplasm will develop after many years of treatment.

Plasmapheresis effectively reduces circulating autoantibodies. It typically is reserved for patients in myasthenic crisis or is used preoperatively for thymectomy in patients who have severe weakness. Improvement is rapid, but transient. Like plasmapheresis, intravenous immune globulin produces rapid improvement through a difficult period of myasthenic weakness (400mg/kg per day for 5 days).[19,20] Patients in myasthenic crisis require aggressive pulmonary treatment, often need intubation and mechanical ventilation, and are best managed in the intensive care unit.

As a rule, ptosis typically responds to treatment and diplopia may be refractory. Ocular symptoms can be treated symptomatically as other therapies are initiated, or when these are ineffective. Lid crutches may be beneficial for patients who have ptosis, but ptosis surgery should be reserved for patients who are stable and refractory to other treatments. Diplopia is managed using patching or prisms; strabismus surgery is inappropriate for patients who have myasthenia gravis.

Medications that lower the safety factor of neuromuscular transmission should be avoided in patients who have myasthenia. Penicillamine causes a myasthenic syndrome that may be associated with autoantibody production. Many antibiotics decrease the production or release of ACh, including the aminoglycoside agents (streptomycin, neomycin, kanamycin, gentamicin, tobramycin, amikacin, viomycin), bacitracin, polymyxins (polymixin A and B, colistin), and the monobasic amino acid antibiotics (lincomycin and clindamycin). Rarely, worsening of myasthenia occurs with erythromycin or following iodinated contrast dye administration. All neuromuscular blocking agents, such as curare and depolarizing agents, should be used with caution. Chloroquine, lithium, and magnesium affect both presynaptic and postsynaptic transmission. Antiarrhythmic agents, including procainamide and quinidine, can cause or worsen myasthenia gravis. Phenytoin, β-blockers, cisplatin, phenothiazines, and tetracyclines may have similar effects.

COURSE AND OUTCOME

Despite its ominous name, myasthenia gravis is seldom fatal; most patients experience remission or good control of their symptoms with treatment. Of those patients who have only ocular symptoms and signs at onset, 10–20% undergo spontaneous remission and 50–80% develop generalized disease, almost always within 2 years of onset of the disorder.[21] Patients who have ocular myasthenia who are over the age of 50 years are more likely to progress to generalized myasthenia, while a younger age at onset carries a better prognosis.

In adults, the disease is most labile during the first 10 years; most deaths occur during the first year. After 10 years, the course becomes more stable. The long-term prognosis is poorer when a thymoma is present.[22] When death occurs from myasthenia gravis, usually it is because of respiratory failure with secondary cardiac dysfunction.

BOTULISM

INTRODUCTION

Botulism is a potentially life-threatening disorder caused by the toxin of *Clostridium botulinum*. Three types exist—food-borne, wound, and infantile. The clinical picture is characterized by rapidly evolving cranial nerve and respiratory weakness with autonomic dysfunction. Associated symptoms include hyposalivation, dysphagia, dysarthria, respiratory failure, muscular weakness, constipation, urinary retention, nausea, and vomiting.

EPIDEMIOLOGY AND PATHOGENESIS

Botulism, caused by the neurotoxin elaborated by *Cl. botulinum*, may take many forms. Its site of action is the presynaptic nerve terminal, where it prevents the release of ACh. The preformed toxin may be ingested, as in food-borne botulism, or gain access by wound infection. Alternatively, the bacterium or spore may colonize the gastrointestinal tract, as in infant botulism.

At least eight types of toxin have been described, but only three forms commonly affect humans. In the United States, about 60% of cases of botulism result from type A, 30% from type B, and 10% from type E. Type A is found in the western United States and type B in the eastern United States. Type E, found in raw fish, is most common in Alaska. Type A botulism is usually the most severe form of the disease. The most common food sources of botulism are vegetables, meat, and fish. Commercially canned foods account for only 3% of cases; 97% arise from consumption of home-preserved foods. Restaurant outbreaks are rare but represent 42% of cases. About 10 outbreaks occur yearly, with a mean of 2.2 persons affected per outbreak.

Historically, classic or food-borne botulism was caused by inadequately cleaned, smoked, salted, or dried fish or meat. Contemporary risk factors include commercial or home-prepared condiments, vegetables, nonacid foods, and preserved raw fish.[23] Plastic food storage bags and containers provide a near-perfect anaerobic environment for growth of *Cl. botulinum*.

Home-canned vegetables and garlic (particularly when coated in oil), canned fruit, fish, and condiments (especially garlic and peppers) accounted for most outbreak reports in the 1980s. The risk increases when foods are held for long periods at ambient temperatures or are reheated inadequately before serving. Because the spores of *Cl. botulinum* are ubiquitous in the soil, they also contaminate foods that are harvested from the ground (e.g., onions, potatoes).

Wound botulism always has been the least common form of botulism but is increasing in incidence as a result of intravenous drug abuse and cocaine abuse associated with necrotic nasal passages.[24]

Infant botulism occurs during the age range 2–6 months in previously healthy infants. The course is subacute and may be difficult to diagnose until the child becomes severely ill. The classic source of infection is honey. Transmission of spores from adults to infants is possible from soil contamination of clothing. A similar infection can be seen in adults who have achlorhydria, following gastrointestinal operations, and who have blind loops of the bowel.

OCULAR MANIFESTATIONS

Ophthalmic manifestations are not likely to occur in isolation but are part of a systemic illness. Diplopia and ptosis occur with varying degrees of ophthalmoparesis. Internal ophthalmoplegia with accommodation paresis produces blurred vision. The pupils often are abnormal, with a poor reaction to light. Pupillary light–near dissociation may be observed during the acute infection and occasionally persists after recovery.[25] Quivering eye movements have been described. Hypolacrimation is found often.

DIAGNOSIS

The diagnosis is based on the symptoms and signs, the circumstances of infection, electrophysiological studies, and isolation of the organism or toxin.

When botulism is suspected, stool, gastric aspirate, and at least 20ml of serum should be collected for analysis. If the source of contaminated food is available, it may be submitted to the relevant health department for evaluation. Identification of botulinum toxin in serum and stool is performed using a mouse bioassay. The organism is isolated in the stool but, rarely, it is present in the serum of patients who have infant botulism. A Tensilon test result is almost always negative. The spinal fluid findings are normal. Electrophysiological studies are very helpful and show changes similar to those seen in the Lambert–Eaton syndrome. Because ACh release is blocked, changes of denervation are detected on electromyography. Small, evoked action potentials and posttetanic facilitation following exercise or supramaximal nerve stimulation are characteristic. In contrast to the changes in the Lambert–Eaton syndrome (see below), post-tetanic facilitation persists for up to 20 minutes with botulism.

DIFFERENTIAL DIAGNOSIS

The Guillain–Barré syndrome, Miller–Fisher syndrome, and poliomyelitis resemble botulism clinically. Myasthenia gravis spares the pupils and is more gradual in onset. Tick paralysis, diphtheria, organophosphate toxicity, shellfish toxicity, and hypokalemic periodic paralysis are other diagnostic considerations.

SYSTEMIC ASSOCIATIONS

Symptoms of food-borne botulism begin 12 hours to 8 days after ingestion of the toxin. Typically, the patient is conscious and afebrile. The characteristic systemic symptoms include hyposalivation and respiratory failure, urinary retention, constipation, and

vomiting. Limb weakness may resemble that of Guillain–Barré syndrome, with ascending or descending paralysis. The reflexes are often normal. Prominent bulbar symptoms and cranial nerve palsies may develop. At worst, the patient is "locked in," unable to move or respond, but fully awake.

In wound botulism, symptoms begin 4–18 days after injury and are identical to those of food-borne botulism.

Infant botulism causes constipation and weakness, with descending paralysis.[26] The infant has a poor suck, a weak cry, and becomes hypotonic. Impairment of extraocular movement, facial weakness, and cranial nerve palsies are common. Dilated pupils, respiratory arrest, and death may follow. The course often is insidious and mistaken for failure to thrive.

TREATMENT

The most important aspect of treatment is supportive, with mechanical ventilation when necessary. If the patient is not allergic to horse serum (pretesting for hypersensitivity is required), trivalent acute bacterial endocarditis antitoxin is administered, although its efficacy is uncertain. Guanidine is no longer recommended. Recovery occurs spontaneously as new synapses develop; this may take 6–12 months.

LAMBERT–EATON MYASTHENIC SYNDROME

INTRODUCTION

First described in 1953 as a triad of muscle weakness, autonomic dysfunction, and hyporeflexia, the Lambert–Eaton myasthenic syndrome (LEMS) shares clinical features with myasthenia gravis. Unlike myasthenia gravis, LEMS is a presynaptic disorder of neuromuscular transmission affecting calcium channels.[27] This rare disorder is associated with a malignancy, such as oat cell carcinoma of the lung, in at least 50% of cases.[28] Symptoms of LEMS typically precede the diagnosis of the neoplasm.

EPIDEMIOLOGY AND PATHOGENESIS

Most patients who have the paraneoplastic form are over 40 years of age. Smoking is a risk factor because of the high association with bronchogenic carcinoma. About 3% of patients who have small cell carcinoma of the lung have LEMS.[29] The non-neoplastic form is associated with pernicious anemia, thyroid disease, Sjögren's syndrome, and other autoimmune disorders. A personal or family history of autoimmune disease is found in 34% of patients who have primary LEMS.[30] Myasthenia gravis and LEMS may occur concurrently.

Symptoms are caused by impaired release of ACh from the nerve terminal. End-plate potentials are too small to generate an action potential. Striated muscle, glands, and smooth muscle are affected. Calcium and guanidine increase neurotransmitter release, which results in improved strength.

OCULAR MANIFESTATIONS

In contrast to myasthenia gravis, ocular manifestations are not prominent. Decreased lacrimation leads to keratoconjunctivitis sicca, which is the predominant ocular complaint. Ptosis and intermittent diplopia may occur. Sluggishly reactive pupils and tonic pupils are infrequent.[31] Slow, saccadic velocities that normalize after exercise have been described. There is one report of a patient with ophthalmoparesis and pseudoblepharospasm.[32]

DIAGNOSIS

Rapid onset and progression of symptoms over weeks to months is common in the paraneoplastic form. The non-neoplastic variety has an insidious onset with mild, stable symptoms. Patients generally have proximal muscle weakness and leg pain. Autonomic involvement is present in 50% of cases, which results in dry mouth, constipation, hypohidrosis, impotence, orthostatic hypotension, and urinary retention. Unlike myasthenia gravis, muscle strength improves following voluntary contraction or repetitive testing. Paradoxical lid elevation may occur after prolonged upgaze.[33] The deep tendon reflexes are hypoactive or absent at rest and increase with voluntary muscle contraction.

Electrophysiological studies confirm the diagnosis. Low rates of nerve stimulation (2–3Hz) produce a decremental response, but high rates (20–50Hz) cause a two- to tenfold incremental increase in the compound action potential. SFEMG shows changes similar to those found in myasthenia gravis. The Tensilon test is negative and anti–ACh receptor antibodies are not present, although calcium channel antibodies have been found in about 50% of patients.

DIFFERENTIAL DIAGNOSIS

Disorders that produce proximal muscle weakness may resemble the myasthenic syndrome. Myasthenia gravis usually can be excluded clinically, with its prominent ocular and facial involvement. Guillain–Barré syndrome, polymyositis, lumbosacral plexopathies, and polyradiculopathies can be excluded by electrophysiological testing and neuroimaging.

SYSTEMIC ASSOCIATIONS

More than 80% of the associated malignancies are small cell carcinomas of the lung. A computed tomography or magnetic resonance image of the chest may be supplemented by bronchoscopy or sputum analysis to diagnose the lung carcinoma. Other tumors associated with LEMS include small cell carcinoma of the cervix or the prostate, adenocarcinoma, and lymphoma. The myasthenic syndrome may precede the detection of the malignancy by up to 7 years and rarely follows detection of the tumor.[27] If no malignancy is found, repeated investigations are warranted. Other laboratory testing includes thyroid function tests, complete blood count, erythrocyte sedimentation rate, antinuclear antibodies, anti-Ro, and anti-La (SS-A, SS-B) to evaluate for the association of the non-neoplastic form with pernicious anemia, thyroid disease, Sjögren's syndrome, and other autoimmune disorders.

TREATMENT

Guanidine is effective, but it has potentially severe side effects, including bone marrow depression, paresthesias, renal and hepatic impairment, confusion, atrial fibrillation, and hypotension. Typically, anticholinesterases are tried as first-line therapy. 3,4-Diaminopyridine is a more direct treatment; it works by blocking potassium channels and enhancing the release of ACh from the presynaptic nerve terminal. A definite and sustained response to aminopyridines occurs in most patients.[34] Treatment with plasmapheresis, intravenous immunoglobulin, corticosteroids, and azathioprine usually leads to improvement in strength.[35] Immunosuppressants may take several months to be effective. Magnesium should be avoided, because it worsens the weakness. Other medications that decrease neuromuscular transmission should be used with caution. Treatment of the underlying carcinoma may produce improved strength.

COURSE AND OUTCOMES

The presence or absence of malignancy largely determines the prognosis. Those patients who have lung cancer should be screened regularly for recurrence within the first 4 years of diagnosis and advised to stop smoking. Most patients can lead a moderately active lifestyle with treatment but should avoid vigorous exercise.

REFERENCES

1. Drachman DB. Myasthenia gravis. N Engl J Med. 1994;330:1797–810.
2. Phillips LH, Torner JC. Has the natural history of myasthenia gravis changed over the past 40 years? A meta-analysis of the epidemiological literature. Neurology. 1993;43:A386.
3. Christensen PB, Jensen TS, Tsiropoulos I, et al. Incidence and prevalence of myasthenia gravis in western Denmark. Neurology. 1993;43:1779–83.
4. Schmidt D, Dell'Osso LF, Abel LA, Daroff RB. Myasthenia gravis: dynamic changes in saccadic waveform, gain and velocity. Exp Neurol. 1980;68:365–7
5. Ellis FD, Hoyt CS, Ellis FJ, et al. Extraocular muscle responses to orbital cooling (ice test) for ocular myasthenia gravis diagnosis. J AAPOS. 2000;4:271–81.
6. Kubis KC, Danesh-Meyer HV, Savino PJ, Sergott RC. The ice test versus the rest test in myasthenia gravis. Ophthalmology. 2000;107:1995–8.
7. Golnik KC, Pena R, Lee AG, Eggenberger ER. An ice test for the diagnosis of myasthenia gravis. Ophthalmology. 2000;107:622–3.
8. Seybold M. The office Tensilon test for ocular myasthenia gravis. Arch Neurol. 1986;43:842–3.
9. Coll GE, Demer JL. The edrophonium–Hess screen test in the diagnosis of myasthenia gravis. Am J Ophthalmol. 1992;114:489–93.
10. Ing EB, Ing SY, Ing T, Ramocki JA. The complication rate of edrophonium testing for suspected myasthenia gravis. Can J Ophthalmol. 2000;35:141–4.
11. Odel JG, Winterkorn JM, Behrens MM. The sleep test for myasthenia gravis. A safe alternative to Tensilon. J Clin Neuro Ophthalmol. 1990;35:191–204.
12. Oh SJ, Kim DE, Kuruoglu R, et al. Diagnostic sensitivity of laboratory tests in myasthenia gravis. Muscle Nerve. 1992;15:720–4.
13. Rivero A, Crovetto L, Lopez L, et al. Single fiber electromyography of extraocular muscles: a sensitive method for the diagnosis of ocular myasthenia gravis. Muscle Nerve. 1995;18:943–7.
14. Weinberg DH, Rizzo JF III, Hayes MT, et al. Ocular myasthenia gravis: predictive value of singer-fiber electromyography. Muscle Nerve. 1999;22:1222.
15. Evoli A, Batocchi AP, Minisci C, et al. Therapeutic options in ocular myasthenia gravis. Neuromuscul Disord. 2001;11:208–16.
16. Gronseth GS, Barohn RJ. Thymectomy for myasthenia gravis. Curr Treat Options Neurol. 2002;4(3):203–9.
17. Tindall RSA, Rollins JA, Phillips JT, et al. Preliminary results of a double-blind, randomized, placebo-controlled trial of cyclosporine in myasthenia gravis. N Engl J Med. 1987;316:719–24.
18. Ciafaloni E, Massey JM, Tucker-Lipscomb B, Sanders FB. Mycophenolate mofetil for myasthenia gravis: an open-label pilot study. Neurology. 2001;56:97–9.
19. Thornton CA, Griggs RC. Plasma exchange and intravenous immunoglobulin treatment of neuromuscular disease. Ann Neurol. 1994;35:260–8.
20. Brannagan TH III, Nagle KJ, Lange DJ, Rowland LP. Complications of intravenous immune globulin in neurologic disease. Neurology. 1996;47:647–77.
21. Bever CT Jr, Aquino AV, Penn AS, et al. Prognosis of ocular myasthenia. Ann Neurol. 1983;14:516–9.
22. Palmisani MT, Evoli A, Batocchi AP, et al. Myasthenia gravis associated with thymoma: clinical characteristics and long-term outcome. Eur Neurol. 1994;34:78–82.
23. Barrett DH. Endemic food-borne botulism: clinical experience, 1973–1986 at Alaska Native Medical Center. Alaska Med. 1991;33:101–8.
24. Mitchell PA, Pons PT. Wound botulism associated with black tar heroin and lower extremity cellulitis. J Emerg Med. 2001;20:371–5.
25. Friedman DI, Fortanasce VN, Sadun AA. Tonic pupils as a result of botulism. Am J Ophthalmol. 1990;109:236–7.
26. Schreiner MS. Infant botulism: a review of 12 years' experience at the Children's Hospital of Philadelphia. Pediatrics. 1991;87:159–65.
27. Greenberg DA. Neuromuscular disease and calcium channels. Muscle Nerve. 1999;22:1341–9.
28. Argov Z, Shapira Y, Averbuch-Heller L, Wirguin I. Lambert–Eaton myasthenic syndrome (LEMS) in association with lymphoproliferative disorders. Muscle Nerve. 1995;18:715–9.
29. Elrington GM, Murray NM, Spiro SG, et al. Neurological paraneoplastic syndromes in patients with small cell lung cancer. A prospective study of 150 patients. J Neurol Neurosurg Psychiatry. 1991;54:764–7.
30. Tim RW, Massey JM, Sanders DB. Lambert-Eaton myasthenic syndrome: electrodiagnostic findings and response to treatment. Neurology. 2000;54:2176–8.
31. Clark CV. Ocular autonomic nerve function in Lambert–Eaton myasthenic syndrome. Eye. 1990;4:473–81.
32. Kanzato N, Motomura M, Suehara M, Arimura K. Lambert-Eaton myasthenic syndrome with ophthalmoparesis and pseudoblepharospasm. Muscle Nerve. 1999;22:1727–30.
33. Breen LA, Gutmann L, Brick JF, Riggs JR. Paradoxical lid elevation with sustained upgaze: a sign of Lambert–Eaton syndrome. Muscle Nerve. 1991;14:863–6.
34. Sanders DB, Masseuy JM, Sanders LL, Edwards LJ. A randomized trial of 3,4-diaminopyridine in Lambert-Eaton myasthenic syndrome. Neurology. 2000;54:603–7.
35. Bain PG, Motomura M, Newsome-Davis J, et al. Effects of intravenous immunoglobulin on muscle weakness and calcium-channel autoantibodies in the Lambert-Eaton myasthenic syndrome. Neurology. 1996;47:678–83.

CHAPTER

201 Ocular Myopathies

RICHARD M. RUBIN • ALFREDO A. SADUN

DEFINITION
- Pathology of the extraocular muscles that results in ophthalmoplegia and other disorders of ocular motility.

KEY FEATURES
- Limitations of motility.
- Inflammation.
- Exophthalmos.
- Pain.
- Diplopia.

ASSOCIATED FEATURES
- Acquired and of known mechanism (Graves' disease).
- Acquired and consequent to other processes (certain forms of myositis).
- Congenital but may not manifest until late adulthood (mitochondrial).

INTRODUCTION

Diseases that involve metabolic abnormalities, atrophy, infiltration, or inflammation of the ocular muscles may appear as weakness or restriction. Except for Graves' dysthyroid ophthalmopathy, most of these conditions are uncommon or rare. Graves' dysthyroid ophthalmopathy, orbital myositis, and infiltrative myopathies are covered in Part 11, and other orbital diseases and trauma that may cause restrictive eye syndromes are discussed in Chapters 95 and 96. The four sections of this chapter independently cover mitochondrial myopathies, dystrophic myopathies, Graves' dysthyroid ophthalmopathy, and other inflammatory and infiltrative myopathies.

MITOCHONDRIAL DISORDERS

EPIDEMIOLOGY AND PATHOGENESIS

Mitochondria are cytoplasmic organelles that produce energy for cell functions, maintenance, repair, and growth through the enzymatic processes of oxidative phosphorylation. A group of neurodegenerative and myopathic syndromes result from disorders of mitochondrial metabolism that cause defects in the energy cycle of susceptible tissues.[1] For reasons that remain unclear, the tissues most reliant on mitochondrial energy are those of the central nervous system, heart, muscles, kidneys, and endocrine organs. Hence, these tissues are most likely to show various clinical manifestations of mitochondrial dysfunction.

Each mitochondrion possesses 2–10 mitochondrial DNA genomes made up of a closed circle of 16,569 nucleotide base pairs. The mitochondrial DNA encodes for 13 polypeptides essential in oxidative phosphorylation and for ribosomal and transfer ribonucleic acids essential in the production of mitochondrial proteins. Nuclear DNA encodes for an additional 56 subunits of the electron transport chain and for genes required for replication, transcription, and translation of the mitochondrial genes.

Mitochondrial DNA has unique genetics for several reasons, which include its cytoplasmic location and the multiple DNA copies that exist in each cell. Mitochondrial DNA is inherited maternally because it is transmitted via oocyte cytoplasm. In addition, new mutations often result in heteroplasmy, a mixed intracellular population of normal and mutant DNA molecules. Also, multiple random and asymmetrical mitochondrial divisions lead to replicative segregation and eventually homoplasmy, such that each cell possesses only pure mutant mitochondrial DNA. Thus, the relative proportion of normal and mutant mitochondrial DNA may vary from cell to cell and from individual to individual.

The variable phenotypic expressions of mitochondrial dysfunction likely arise from interplay of the unique features of mitochondrial inheritance that cause heteroplasmy and homoplasmy, the modifying contribution of nuclear DNA under the influence of mendelian genetics, the deterioration of mitochondrial function with aging, and the different energy requirements of specific tissues.

The most common mitochondrial disorder to affect muscles is chronic progressive external ophthalmoplegia (CPEO) and its best known subtype, Kearns–Sayre syndrome.[2] Less common mitochondrial myopathies of ophthalmic importance include mitochondrial encephalopathy with lactic acidosis and stroke-like syndrome (MELAS), myoclonic epilepsy with ragged red fibers (MERRF, Fukuhara's syndrome), and mitochondrial neurogastrointestinal encephalopathy.[3,4]

Mitochondrial disorders that affect tissues other than muscle during early childhood include Alpers' disease, Menkes' disease, and Leigh's disease; one that manifests later in life is Leber's hereditary optic neuropathy (LHON).[5]

OCULAR MANIFESTATIONS

Patients who have CPEO often exhibit initial bilateral ptosis followed by limitation of ductions in all directions and marked delay of saccades. Downward gaze may be spared until late in the disease course. Curiously, despite ocular misalignment, these patients rarely complain of diplopia. Weakness of the orbicularis oculi and facial muscles is found commonly, and pigmentary retinopathy may be associated.

Kearns–Sayre syndrome, in particular, is characterized by the triad of external ophthalmoplegia, pigmentary retinopathy, and cardiac conduction block during the first or second decade of life (early-onset CPEO). Peripapillary pigment atrophy and salt-and-pepper retinal pigment epithelial changes are most striking in the macula. True bone spicule pigmentary retinopathy as seen in retinitis pigmentosa is not typical in Kearns–Sayre syndrome.

The MELAS syndrome manifests with ptosis and external ophthalmoplegia, in addition to the commonly associated visual disturbances, which may include hemianopia or cortical blindness.[6] Eventually, MERRF develops into progressive optic atrophy.

DIAGNOSIS

The possibility of muscle disease should be considered whenever ophthalmoplegia does not correspond to the pattern of a cranial nerve palsy and when there is acquired ptosis. Most diagnoses are made through a process of exclusion and imaging studies.

Diagnoses of mitochondrial disorders often are supported by histopathological and biochemical evidence of mitochondrial dysfunction. Specific identification of an enzyme defect may confirm the diagnosis. Generally, to show abnormalities in patients who have mitochondrial cytopathies, substrates of oxidative phosphorylation from serum and cerebrospinal fluid (CSF), which include glucose, lactate, and pyruvate, and the pH of venous blood during fasting all are measured. Elevation of CSF protein levels also may help in the diagnosis of CPEO and MELAS syndrome.

Electrocardiograms should be obtained for all patients suspected of mitochondrial cytopathies, to detect any life-threatening cardiac conduction abnormalities. Neuroimaging may help in the assessment for other causes of neurological deficits. In CPEO, magnetic resonance imaging (MRI) of the brain often shows hyperintensity in the thalamus and globus pallidus on T2-weighted images. Kearns–Sayre syndrome was shown in one case to have MRI findings indistinguishable from those of multiple sclerosis.[7] Posterior cerebral cortical abnormalities that correspond to focal neurological deficits commonly are found on neuroimaging in MELAS syndrome.

Genetic analysis for mitochondrial DNA mutations from blood leukocytes or muscle biopsy may show a characteristic mutation in MELAS syndrome. Poor correlation exists between specific mitochondrial DNA mutations and CPEO, because CPEO may exhibit a clinical picture related to a final common pathway of impaired mitochondrial energy production in muscle from a variety of mutations. Diseases of glycolipid metabolism, lysosomal or glycogen storage, peroxisome dysfunction, and acquired viral, toxic, and endocrine myopathies and encephalopathies also must be ruled out. Electromyography helps to differentiate myopathic from neuropathic causes of muscle weakness.

SYSTEMIC ASSOCIATIONS

Systemic findings of CPEO include short stature, peripheral neuropathy, ataxia, spasticity, somatic muscle weakness, vestibular dysfunction, and deafness.[8] Lactic acidosis is found often because of defective aerobic metabolism. Abnormalities of cardiac conduction and of the central nervous system, which include cerebellar dysfunction and elevated CSF protein exceeding 100mg/dl, are associated with Kearns–Sayre syndrome.[9] The cardiac conduction disturbances have an onset typically 10 years after ptosis appears and may result in sudden death. Endocrine dysfunction may include hypoparathyroidism, diabetes mellitus, hypogonadism, or growth hormone deficiency. In CPEO and Kearns–Sayre syndrome, the brain eventually may undergo spongiform degeneration, with the clinical picture of dementia. Basal ganglia calcifications may occur.

The association of progressive ophthalmoplegia with peripheral neuropathy, leukoencephalopathy, and gastrointestinal dysmotility in mitochondrial disease has been reported.[10] It is likely that additional multiorgan system, mitochondrial syndromes will be elucidated.

Seizures, vomiting, lactic acidosis, episodes of hemiparesis, and stroke-like events during childhood or early adulthood characterize MELAS. Although partial recovery from these stroke-like episodes is the rule, severe neurological damage eventually results. Typically, MERRF occurs during the second decade of life with myoclonus, followed by ataxia, weakness, and seizures.

PATHOLOGY

Biopsy of skeletal muscle reveals "ragged red fibers" that stain red or purple using a modified Gomori trichrome stain (Fig. 201-1). The mitochondria of the involved muscle fibers are concentrated peripherally and may show increased staining for the mitochondrial enzyme succinate dehydrogenase. Biochemical abnormalities of oxidative phosphorylation, such as patchy cytochrome-c oxidase deficiency, may be detected by muscle biopsies, as well.

The ultrastructural appearances of skeletal muscle mitochondria are varied and may show enlarged mitochondria that contain crystal-like inclusions; changes in the number, shape, or regularity of cristae; or emptiness, vacuolization, or triglyceride accumulation within mitochondria (Fig. 201-2). The mitochondria often are increased in number and size. Such morphological changes are not necessarily unique and may be found in other muscle disorders, such as the muscular dystrophies or polymyositis. Histopathologically, the retinal findings in Kearns–Sayre syndrome suggest retinal pigment epithelial dysfunction rather than photoreceptor disease.[11]

TREATMENT

Coenzyme Q10, essential for normal mitochondrial function and deficient in a proportion of patients who have CPEO and Kearns–Sayre syndrome, administration has been associated with improved exercise tolerance, cardiac function, and ataxia in some patients with Kearns–Sayre syndrome.[12] Other treatments, such as thiamine, also aim to bypass or enhance oxidative phos-

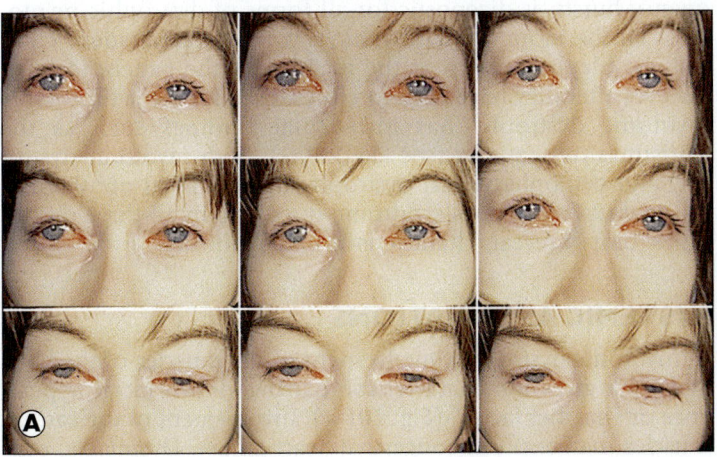
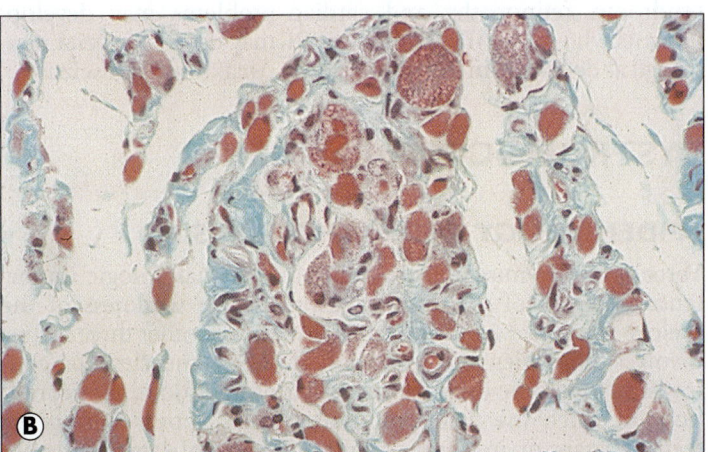

FIG. 201-1 ■ **MELAS syndrome. A,** Complete external ophthalmoplegia in a 20-year-old woman. **B,** Microscopic section of degenerated extraocular muscles stained with trichrome shows "ragged red fibers." (Case presented by Dr. R. Folberg, Verhoeff Society, 1993, and reported by Rummelt V, *et al.* Ophthalmology. 1993;100:1757.)

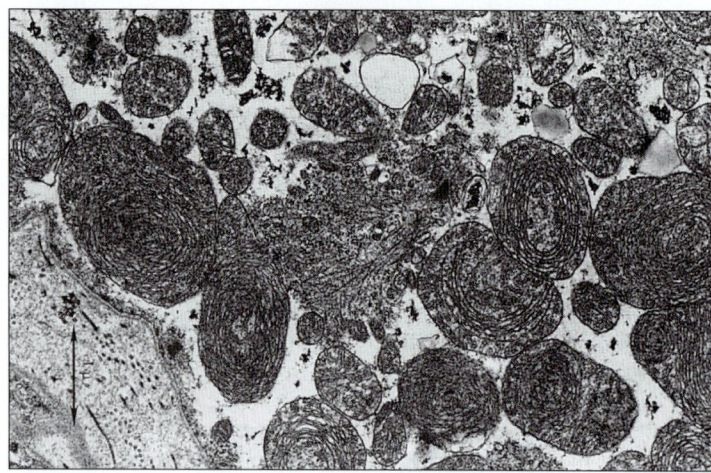

FIG. 201-2 ■ Viewed with an electron microscope, the abnormal mitochondria in a case of chronic progressive external ophthalmoplegia shown as electron dense and globular. The normal arrangement of cristae is not seen.

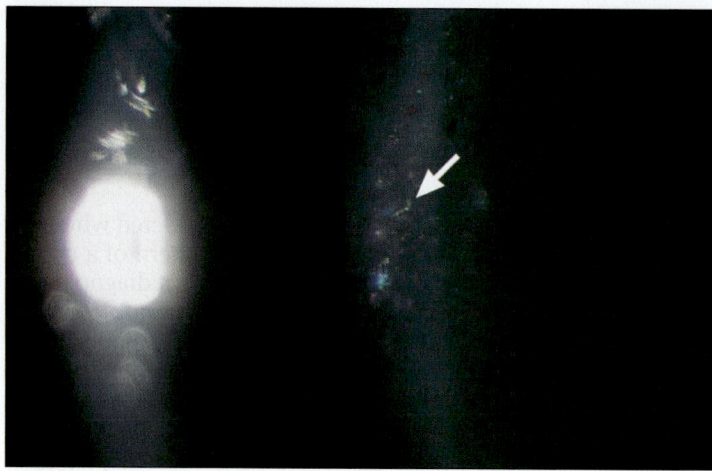

FIG. 201-3 ■ Slit-lamp view of a "Christmas tree" cataract in myotonic dystrophy. Note the iridescent or colored refractile flecks (arrow).

phorylation but only occasionally have been shown to improve exercise tolerance, cardiac conduction, or lactic acidosis. However, coenzyme Q10 and these other treatments do not improve the ophthalmoplegia, retinopathy, or ptosis in patients who have CPEO or Kearns–Sayre syndrome.

Complaints that arise from ptosis often are handled by ptosis crutches or a careful surgical approach, in which the lid is raised minimally by addressing the visual obstruction rather than the cosmetic appearance. Overly aggressive attempts to treat the ptosis may result in exposure keratopathy and corneal ulceration because of weak orbicularis oculi muscles and a poor Bell's reflex. Symptomatic ocular deviations may be treated successfully with strabismus surgery.

Periodic evaluation by a cardiologist is indicated in Kearns–Sayre syndrome. In some instances, placement of a pacemaker for prophylactic pacing or for treatment of symptomatic cardiac block is necessary to prevent sudden death. The systemic use of corticosteroids is contraindicated in Kearns–Sayre syndrome because of the possible precipitation of coma and death from hyperglycemic acidosis.[13] Genetic counseling should be offered to all patients who have mitochondrial cytopathies.

COURSE AND OUTCOMES

Chronic progressive external ophthalmoplegia is a slowly progressive loss of lid and extraocular motor function. The diplopia may or may not worsen, because the symmetry of the ophthalmoplegia may prevent strabismus. However, small ptosis correction may be required as described above. In severe cases that have more generalized manifestations, such as in Kearns–Sayre syndrome, retinopathy and cardiac problems may develop. Patients who have MELAS and MERRF may develop several neurological deficits, which include ataxia, weakness, and seizures.

DYSTROPHIC MYOPATHIES

EPIDEMIOLOGY AND PATHOGENESIS

Three forms of muscular dystrophy of ophthalmologic importance exist, all of which involve progressive weakness of the skeletal muscles. Myotonic dystrophy, like the other three forms, involves difficulties with relaxation of skeletal muscles after contraction. Myotonic dystrophy is an autosomal dominant condition in which the first symptoms usually appear during the teenage years or in young adulthood. Several large pedigrees have been identified.

Oculopharyngeal dystrophy usually develops a little later, in young or middle-aged adults. The first symptoms often are diffi-

culty in swallowing, with ptosis later. A large French Canadian autosomal dominant pedigree has been identified, in which the original ancestor immigrated to Quebec in 1634.[14] Autosomal recessive and sporadic inheritances also have been reported.

Fukuyama's syndrome (MERRF) is an autosomal recessive condition most often found in people of Japanese descent. Unlike the other two forms above, in Fukuyama's syndrome the manifestations and death occur in early childhood.

OCULAR MANIFESTATIONS

In myotonic dystrophy, abnormalities in the extraocular muscles are accompanied by involvement of other muscles, which include the levator, and result in slowly progressive bilateral ptosis. Other ocular findings include cataracts, described as Christmas tree cataracts (Fig. 201-3) for their multiple refractile colors.[15]

In oculopharyngeal dystrophy, dysphagia is followed soon by bilateral ptosis which, over a period of years, is followed by external ophthalmoplegia and weakness of the orbicularis. The patient, despite a remarkable lack of ocular motility, may not complain of diplopia, because often the limitations of eye movement are very symmetrical so that no strabismus occurs.

In Fukuyama's syndrome, in addition to the weakness of the orbicularis and a strabismus, nystagmus, anterior polar cataracts, optic nerve atrophy, and a chorioretinal degeneration with retinoschisis or detachment occur, also.[16]

DIAGNOSIS

The electromyogram, with characteristic spontaneous, high-frequency bursts, is diagnostic for all forms of dystrophic myotonias. Furthermore, all dystrophic myotonias are evident clinically by blepharospasm or the inability of the patient to open the eyes after they have been forcibly closed for some time. Only myotonic dystrophy has intraocular findings such as the Christmas tree cataract (see Fig. 201-3). Both myotonic dystrophy and oculopharyngeal dystrophy have external ophthalmoplegia, but Fukuyama's syndrome does not. In all three dystrophies, biopsy reveals characteristic histopathology.

SYSTEMIC ASSOCIATIONS

In myotonic dystrophy, involvement of the muscles of the head and neck gives the characteristic narrow, drawn facial appearance or "hatchet facies" (Fig. 201-4). Involvement of the cardiac muscles may result in congestive heart failure. Dysphagia, constipation, and incontinence are not uncommon. In some cases mental retardation occurs, and in males testicular atrophy and premature baldness are frequent. In oculopharyngeal dystrophy,

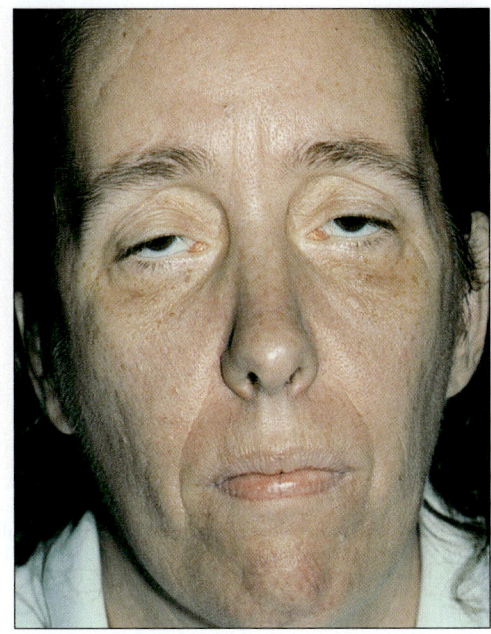

FIG. 201-4 ▌ Front view of a patient who has myotonic dystrophy. The muscle wasting gives the characteristic drawn appearance of "hatchet facies."

the bulbar musculature is affected frequently and temporalis wasting occurs. Patients have difficulty swallowing without aspirating. Other bulbar and limb girdle muscles become involved later. In Fukuyama's syndrome, the proximal muscle groups are involved most. Mental retardation, seizures, severe motor development delay, and cortical blindness are common.

PATHOLOGY

In myotonic dystrophy, findings from histopathological examination of the extraocular muscles are similar to those seen in the skeletal muscles.[17] Down the centers of muscle fibers run rows of nuclei. The myofilaments and sarcoplasmic reticulum are disrupted, and accumulations of impaired mitochondria may be found. In oculopharyngeal dystrophy, tubulofilamentous intranuclear inclusion bodies are seen on ultrastructural examination of muscle biopsies. In Fukuyama's syndrome, the same changes are seen, confined largely to the proximal muscle groups.

TREATMENT

For all three muscular dystrophies, treatment consists of symptomatic support. The cataracts of myotonic dystrophy may be removed. Foot braces and other devices are available to help support footdrop or other skeletal muscle weakness. All patients affected by dystrophic myopathies need to be referred to neurologists.

COURSE AND OUTCOMES

Progressive atrophy of the skeletal muscles leads to a variety of systemic difficulties. In myotonic dystrophy the patient develops difficulty climbing stairs and, eventually, even with walking and holding the head up. Vision may be maintained after cataract surgery. In oculopharyngeal dystrophy, dysphagia is most problematic.

GRAVES' DYSTHYROID OPHTHALMOPATHY

EPIDEMIOLOGY AND PATHOGENESIS

Graves' dysthyroid ophthalmopathy is the most common cause of exophthalmos—it probably accounts for more than 50% of cases. Prevalence, although uncertain, has been estimated in studies in the United States at 0.4% and in the United Kingdom

at 1.1–1.6%.[18] Women are affected 3–10 times more frequently than men.[19] The mean age of appearance for Graves' thyroid disease is 41 years, and the orbital disease occurs an average of 2.5 years afterward.[19] Even though the disease is more common in women, the severity of disease tends to be greater in men and in patients above 50 years of age.[19]

Graves' ophthalmopathy is presumed to result from autoimmune processes that include extraocular muscle myositis, fibroblast proliferation, glycosaminoglycan overproduction, and orbital congestion. Both humoral and cell-mediated immune mechanisms have been implicated.[20] The hyperthyroidism in Graves' disease may run an independent course and has been attributed to stimulation of thyrotropin receptors on the thyroid cell plasma membrane by immunoglobulin. These thyroid-stimulating immunoglobulins (previously called *long-acting thyroid stimulator proteins*) are demonstrable in 50% of patients who have active Graves' disease. However, orbital changes have not been found to occur directly in response to these thyroid-stimulating antibodies. Other immunoglobulins have been identified in the stimulation of collagen synthesis by fibroblasts and myoblast proliferation, although it remains uncertain whether these antibodies are primarily pathogenic or occur secondarily because of local inflammatory processes.

Immunohistochemical analysis and histological findings have shown orbital infiltration with mononuclear cells sensitized to retro-orbital antigens. Abnormal helper-to-suppressor T-cell ratios and reductions in the number of T-suppressor cells are thought to be associated with a proliferation of B lymphocytes that produce autoantibodies directed against the orbital tissues. The expression of immunomodulatory proteins, such as histocompatibility antigen molecules, intercellular adhesion molecules, and heat-shock proteins, may play a role in the presentation and recognition of antigenic epitopes specific to orbital and thyroid tissues. Cytokines released by the infiltrating monocytes may stimulate immunomodulatory protein expression, glycosaminoglycan production, and proliferative activity from orbital fibroblasts. Site-specific differences between orbital and pretibial fibroblasts from fibroblasts in other locations may explain why connective tissue involvement in Graves' disease is limited largely to the orbital and pretibial regions. Orbital venous congestion also has been suggested to contribute significantly to the pathogenesis of many of the clinical findings of Graves' ophthalmopathy.[21]

Both genetic and environmental risk factors have been identified, which may predispose toward or act as triggers for the abnormal autoimmune disturbance in Graves' disease.[22] Population studies show linkage to certain histocompatibility antigens, which include HLA-B8 and HLA-DR3 in Caucasian, HLA-BW46 in Chinese, and HLA-BW35 in Japanese patients. Environmental factors such as stress, smoking, and infection with certain gram-negative organisms (e.g., *Yersinia enterocolitica*) may increase the risk or severity of Graves' ophthalmopathy.[23]

OCULAR MANIFESTATIONS

The eye manifestations of Graves' ophthalmopathy typically are self-limited. An active phase of inflammation and progression tends to stabilize spontaneously 8–36 months after onset. Initial symptoms of Graves' ophthalmopathy may be complaints of foreign-body sensation, tearing, or photophobia, often accompanied by signs that include lid retraction, lid lag, lagophthalmos, prominence of the episcleral vessels over the horizontal rectus muscles, and lid edema (Fig. 201-5, *A*). Exophthalmos reflects an increase in soft tissue mass within the bony orbit and may result from enlargement of the extraocular muscles or increased orbital fat volume[24] (Fig. 201-5, *B*). Exophthalmos is almost always bilateral and usually relatively symmetrical. Attempts to push the globe back into the orbit (retropulsion) typically are met with firm resistance because of the inflammatory orbital changes that preclude displacement of the fat.

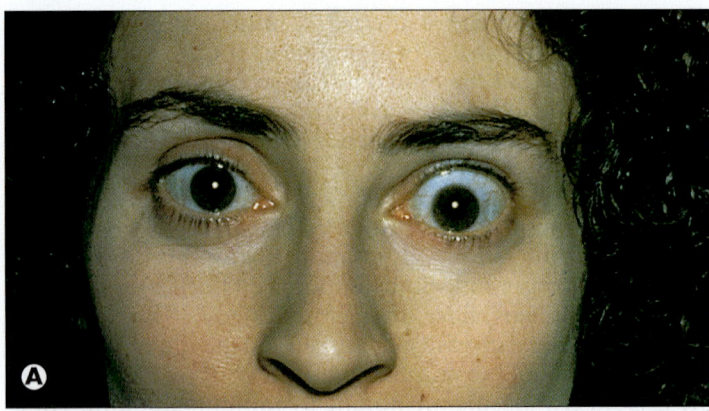

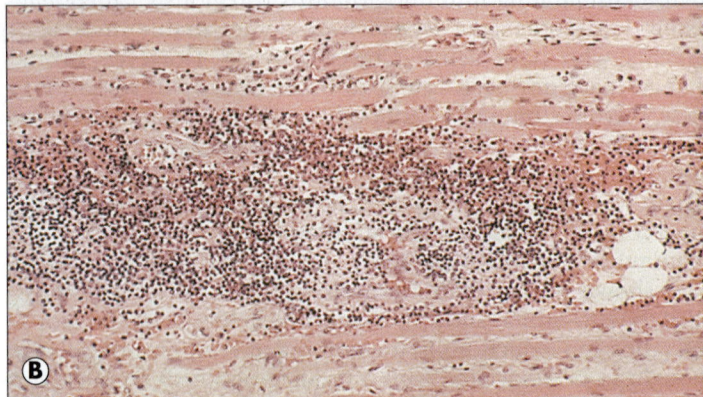

FIG. 201-5 ■ Graves' disease. A, In Graves' disease, exophthalmos often looks more pronounced than it actually is because of the extreme lid retraction that may occur. This patient, for instance, had minimal proptosis of the left eye but marked lid retraction. B, A histological section shows both fluid and inflammatory cells separating the muscle bundles. The inflammatory cells are predominantly lymphocytes, plus plasma cells. (A, Courtesy of Shaffer DB. In Yanoff M, Fine BS. Ocular Pathology, 4th ed. London, Mosby, 1996.)

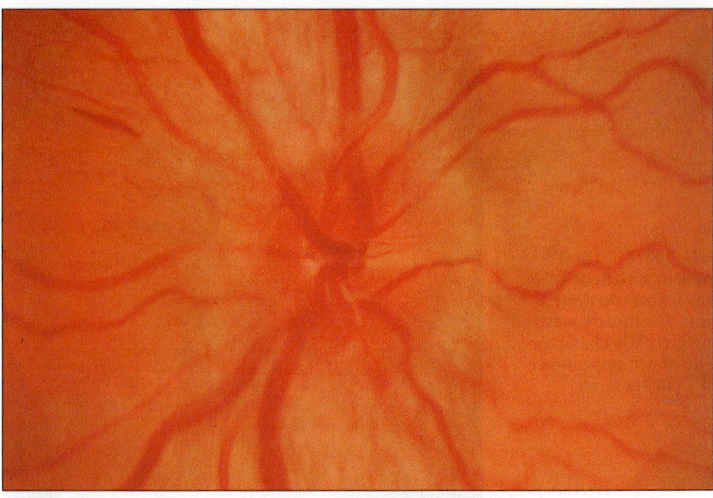

FIG. 201-6 ■ Fundus view of a case of Graves' ophthalmopathy. The patient was losing vision as a consequence of optic neuropathy. Note the congested appearance of the optic nerve head. (Courtesy of Dr. S. Feldon.)

TABLE 201-1

"NO SPECS" AND "RELIEF" CATEGORIZATION OF GRAVES' DISEASE

Class	Signs
0	**N**o signs nor symptoms
1	**O**nly signs are upper eyelid retraction, lid lag, stare
2	**S**oft tissue signs and symptoms:
	• **R**esistance to retropulsion
	• **E**dema of conjunctiva and caruncle
	• **L**acrimal gland enlargement
	• **I**njection over the horizontal rectus muscle insertions
	• **E**dema of the eyelids
	• **F**ullness of the eyelids
3	**P**roptosis
4	**E**xtraocular muscle involvement
5	**C**orneal involvement secondary to exposure
6	**S**ight loss secondary to optic nerve compression

Limitation of ocular motility is the direct consequence of pathological changes that affect the extraocular muscles. The inferior rectus muscle is involved most commonly, followed by the medial rectus and the superior rectus. Clinical complaints associated most frequently with muscle restriction are nontorsional, vertical, or oblique diplopia, which may be noticed only on awakening. Patients often are bothered by the feeling of orbital fullness and the pulling sensation experienced on gaze away from a restricted muscle. Also, increased intraocular pressure may occur on gaze in the opposite direction of the restricted muscle. In particular, this is seen on upgaze with inferior rectus restriction.

Patients with Graves' disease may have sore eyes from exposure keratopathy or superior limbic keratitis. Dry eye is common because of disturbances in tear quantity and, especially, tear film constitution, as well as because of the increased exposure. Acute disease is associated with conjunctival and periorbital edema. With quiescence of the disease, the swelling may reduce, although motility disturbances and exophthalmos tend to remain. Optic nerve involvement also may occur because of compression of the optic nerve at the orbital apex by the enlarged muscles (Fig. 201-6). This is more likely to be associated with superior rectus enlargement and no gross exophthalmos (which is a form of self-decompression). Optic nerve compression may be associated with decreasing visual acuity, color loss, afferent pupillary defect, and visual field loss. On examination, the optic disc may be swollen, normal, or atrophic.

In 1969, Werner proposed the "NO SPECS" classification for signs of Graves' ophthalmopathy.[25] In 1981, Van Dyke refined the class 2 NO SPECS soft tissue findings with the mnemonic RELIEF[26] (Table 201-1). Although the mnemonics help to remember the manifestations of Graves' disease, not uncommonly, the order of signs and symptoms does not follow the order of the classification but consists of combinations of findings from various classes.

DIAGNOSIS

In 1995, Bartley and Gorman proposed diagnostic criteria for Graves' ophthalmopathy as eyelid retraction with objective thyroid dysfunction, or either eyelid retraction or objective thyroid dysfunction in association with exophthalmos, optic neuropathy, or extraocular muscle involvement.[27] The clinical signs must not be attributable to other causes.

In Graves' ophthalmopathy, muscle tendons are relatively spared on computed tomography (CT) scan (Fig. 201-7; see Fig. 193-2).[28] The non–contrast-enhanced coronal orbital CT scan is most helpful in the assessment of the size of the extraocular muscles. Bilateral enlargement is strongly suggestive of thyroid ophthalmopathy, even when the thyroid function study results are normal.

The differential diagnosis includes orbital tumors, which may be primary (hemangioma, meningioma, glioma, lymphoma) or metastatic (breast, lung, colon, prostate), as discussed in Chapter 206. The distinction from Graves' ophthalmopathy usually is apparent, both by the lid findings (such as lid lag) characteristic of Graves' ophthalmopathy and by the distinct neu-

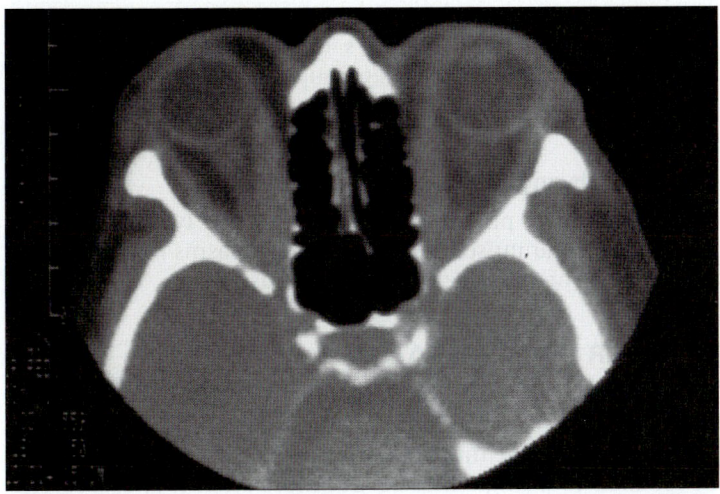

FIG. 201-7 ▮▮ Computed tomography scan of the orbit in a case of Graves' oph-thalmopathy. Note the enlarged muscles (medial recti more than lateral recti). (Courtesy of Dr. M. Yanoff.)

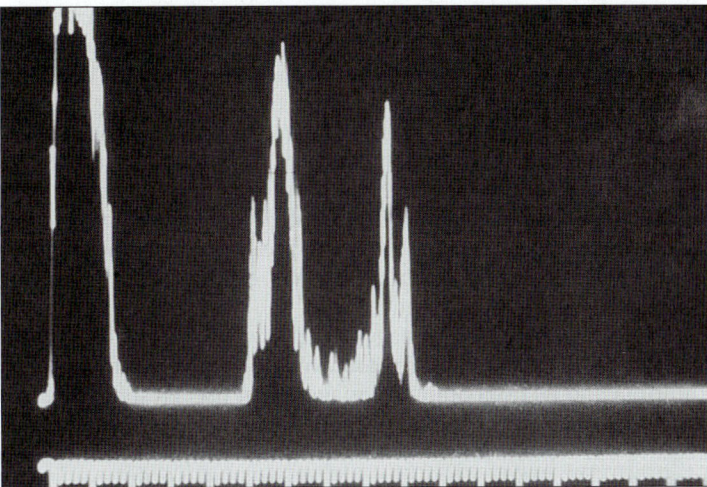

FIG. 201-9 ▮▮ Ultrasonographic image ("A" scan) of the orbit in a case of Graves' ophthalmopathy. Note the high-amplitude spikes characteristic of such muscles. (Courtesy of Dr. S. Feldon.)

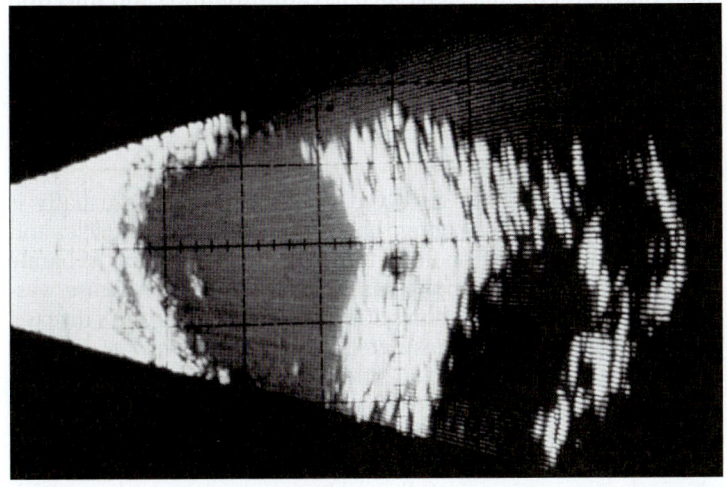

FIG. 201-8 ▮▮ Ultrasonographic image ("B" scan) of the orbit in a case of Graves' ophthalmopathy. Two enlarged muscles (*dark shadows*) are seen behind the globe. (Courtesy of Dr. S. Feldon.)

roimages of orbital tumors. One exception may be lymphoma, which may be differentiated by its propensity to involve the lacrimal gland and by its lack of clinical manifestations.

Orbital inflammations, such as orbital pseudotumor, may be more difficult to differentiate. However, ultrasonography (Fig. 201-8) and CT may be used to note the sparing of the muscle tendons seen only in Graves' ophthalmopathy. Furthermore, ultrasonography may be used to distinguish the characteristic, widely separated, and fairly high-amplitude spikes seen in Graves' ophthalmopathy (FIG. 201-9) from those found in diseases such as orbital myositis. Neuroimaging and possibly biopsy of nasal mucosa may help to exclude diseases such as Wegener's granulomatosis. Scanning also helps to differentiate orbital infections, such as preseptal or orbital cellulitis; however, the classic clinical characteristics of infections must be recognized (Chapter 206). The orbital congestion consequent to carotid–cavernous sinus or dural shunt fistulae also may be differentiated clinically (they do not produce an increase in orbital resistance to retropositus nor lid lag) and particularly by MRI.

SYSTEMIC ASSOCIATIONS

Ophthalmopathy is clinically evident in 25–50% of patients with Graves' hyperthyroidism. Occasionally, Graves' ophthalmopathy occurs in patients affected by Hashimoto's thyroiditis

or in patients who have no evidence of thyroid disease. Thyroid hormone levels may be elevated, normal, or even low. Although unnecessary to confirm a diagnosis of Graves' ophthalmopathy, measurements of tri-iodothyronine, thyroxine, and thyroid-stimulating hormone levels are performed.

Systemic manifestations of Graves' disease may include nervousness, emotional lability, tremor, weakness, fatigue, heat intolerance, sweating, dyspnea, palpitations, goiter, leg swelling, increased appetite, weight loss, and hair thinning.

PATHOLOGY

Generally, as in other forms of inflammatory myositis, the early histopathology in Graves' ophthalmopathy consists of inflammatory cell infiltration, mucopolysaccharide deposition, and increased water content. In the later stages, the muscles undergo atrophy and fibrosis (see Fig. 201-5, *B*). These changes are associated with enlargement of the extraocular muscles and relative sparing of the tendinous insertions. More particularly, the cellular infiltrate is hypocellular and polymorphous, and consists primarily of mature lymphocytes, plasma cells, and macrophages.

TREATMENT

The management of Graves' ophthalmopathy is largely independent of the management of the concomitant endocrinopathy. Such patients require at least two specialists to manage both aspects of the disease. The short-term goal of therapy in Graves' ophthalmopathy is to conserve useful vision, which may mean the provision of artificial tears or improvement of lid coverage for an exposed cornea. In rare cases, it may mean the treatment of Graves' optic neuropathy (see Fig. 201-6). The long-term goal of therapy is restoration of the orbital anatomy. If possible, this should entail postponement of reconstructive surgery until lack of progression has been established. In general, several tools exist in the management of Graves' ophthalmopathy.

The use of corticosteroids in Graves' ophthalmopathy is controversial. Without question, an immediate benefit occurs, but this seems to decay with time.[29] Hence, many investigators believe that corticosteroids should be reserved for use in patients who have optic neuropathy, and in such cases are given in large dosages (over 100mg prednisone per day).

Radiation as a nonspecific immunosuppressant does lead to improvement in Graves' ophthalmopathy. However, the effect may take a few months to maximize, and in the interim visual loss from an optic neuropathy may become permanent. Complications (short and very long term) arise from radiation therapy that suggest it should not be employed except in cases of optic neuropathy. Some investigators use radiation therapy in cases of severe visual loss from an optic neuropathy in conjunction with corticosteroids.

Immunosuppressant agents such as azathioprine or cyclophosphamide have been advocated.[29] The combined use of prednisone and cyclosporine has been suggested as well.[29]

The common surface problems of ocular irritation, foreign-body sensation, and tearing usually are treated best with artificial tears and other lubricants. However, eyelid surgery for severe lid retraction is also of benefit.[30]

Diplopia may be managed early with spectacle prisms. However, the variable nature of Graves' ophthalmopathy-induced diplopia and its noncomitance make prism use, Fresnel as well as standard, ineffectual. Eventually, most patients who have diplopia require strabismus surgery. The most frequent procedure is a recession of the inferior rectus muscle to compensate for restriction.

Surgery also is an option to address the common problems of exophthalmos and lid retraction. Some investigators, however, argue that orbital decompression surgery be reserved for cases that involve optic neuropathy, because this type of surgery carries a higher risk than the strabismus or lid surgeries described above, and the cosmetic problem can be addressed, at least partly, with combined upper and lower lid and lateral canthoplasty procedures. Orbital decompression may be performed from lateral, medial, and floor approaches (or combinations). Surgical decompression is reserved for when the patient does not respond to medical treatment. However, the optic neuropathy of Graves' ophthalmopathy can be serious, and the clinician must be prepared to identify the problem at the earliest stage and approach it by medical, surgical, or radiation therapy.

COURSE AND OUTCOMES

As described above, most cases of Graves' ophthalmopathy stabilize or even regress partially within 8–36 months. Once stable, the condition is reviewed for the need for additional surgery. Most patients do well, but may continue to complain of dry eye symptoms and require the continued use of artificial tears.

OTHER INFLAMMATORY AND INFILTRATIVE MYOPATHIES

EPIDEMIOLOGY AND PATHOGENESIS

Orbital Myositis

The most common cause of primary muscle dysfunction is inflammation. Inflammation or secondary ischemia related to swelling (tissue compartment syndrome) may lead to fibrosis and scarring within an extraocular muscle. Orbital congestion may cause a restrictive component. Such orbital inflammation, or orbital pseudotumor, is usually idiopathic, although the cause may sometimes be determined.

Idiopathic orbital myositis refers to nonspecific orbital inflammation. However, a variety of conditions, such as Crohn's disease, or more localized diseases, such as sinusitis and asthma, have been reported to incite an attack of orbital myositis. This orbital inflammation may extend anteriorly to involve the posterior globe (posterior scleritis) or lacrimal gland (dacryoadenitis), or posteriorly as an orbital apex syndrome. When orbital pseudotumor involves primarily the muscles (myositis), it tends to occur unilaterally (although bilateral involvement may occur up to 25% of the time) in young adults, with women involved more frequently than men. A variety of granulomatous, infectious, neoplastic, and vasculitic disorders may masquerade as myositis, also.

Infectious myositis may result from trichinosis, but more commonly the cause is never determined.[31] Orbital cellulitis may be bacterial and originate from the paranasal sinuses, or fungal in association with metabolic acidosis or diabetes mellitus.

Myositis may be associated with systemic or distant inflammatory disease such as Crohn's disease. Other inflammatory syndromes, such as Wegener's granulomatosis and giant cell arteritis, also may affect the extraocular muscles directly.[32]

Amyloidosis and Infiltrative Myopathies

Other infiltrative processes (amyloidosis and lymphoma) may limit extraocular muscle relaxation.[33] Neoplasms may extend locally into or metastasize directly to a muscle.[34]

OCULAR MANIFESTATIONS

Idiopathic and other forms of orbital inflammatory disease or orbital pseudotumor (orbital myositis) are associated with significant extraocular muscle involvement.[35,36] The myositis may be isolated to a single muscle, but most often it affects several. Even though the disease process often is bilateral, most often symptoms are reported as unilateral and typically include some degree of discomfort in almost all patients. The pain often is most severe when ductions away from the most affected muscle are attempted. Patients also frequently experience gaze-evoked diplopia. Local orbital signs such as exophthalmos and injection are common. Children are more apt to have bilateral orbital involvement, may develop spontaneous orbital hemorrhage, and are less likely to have an associated systemic disease.

DIAGNOSIS

In orbital myositis, the involved extraocular muscle usually is enlarged on orbital imaging. Enhancement of the muscle, and particularly its insertion into the globe, may help to separate myositis from thyroid ophthalmopathy.[37] Crohn's disease, vasculitis, serum sickness, herpes zoster, sarcoidosis, Lyme's disease, and trichinosis all are considered part of the review of systems and investigated by special studies. The diagnosis of orbital pseudotumor or idiopathic orbital myositis is one of exclusion and can be made only after the appropriate investigations have been carried out, as described above. If a meticulous history and physical examination are followed by appropriate studies, which include orbital imaging, and no diagnosis can be confirmed, tissue biopsy is usually considered. In many cases, the clinical picture is sufficiently clear and a trial of glucocorticoids may be initiated, but often an orbital biopsy is indicated, especially if the orbital inflammation is refractory to glucocorticoids or returns after the glucocorticoids have been tapered.

SYSTEMIC ASSOCIATIONS

An unclear relationship exists between idiopathic orbital pseudotumor, or orbital myositis, and paranasal sinus disease, sinusitis, or even a concomitant upper respiratory infection. Systemic conditions associated with myositis include trichinosis, tuberculosis, aspergillosis, Lyme's disease, and other infections, distant inflammatory disease such as Crohn's disease, sarcoidosis, amyloidosis, acromegaly, POEMS (polyneuropathy, organomegaly, endocrinopathy, M protein, and skin changes) syndrome, and lithium therapy.

PATHOLOGY

In addition to the general changes described above, various specific causes of myositis have their own characteristic histopathological features. For example, in cases of foreign bodies, granulomatous inflammation with multinucleated giant cells are found. Polymorphonuclear leukocytes are seen in association with various infections. Eosinophilic infiltration is seen in trichinosis.

In idiopathic orbital myositis, nonspecific and non-neoplastic inflammatory lesions occur in the orbit with diverse pathological appearances—most often they display a polymorphous, chronic inflammatory infiltration. In chronic forms of idiopathic pseudotumor, large amounts of fibrovascular stroma also may be seen. The pathological differentiation between orbital pseudotumor, benign lymphoid hyperplasia, monomorphous lymphoid lesions, and malignant lymphoma may be difficult. Immunological cell markers and gene rearrangement studies can help in the differentiation of these entities. However, 15–20% of patients who have polyclonal cell markers eventually may develop a monoclonal malignant lymphoma.

In orbital myositis with plasma cell or lymphoproliferative infiltration an associated amyloidosis may occur. This amyloid shows on hematoxylin and eosin staining as an eosinophilic hyaline accumulation that often surrounds the blood vessels. It also may accumulate in round globules within the extraocular muscles.

TREATMENT

In myositis, the issue often comes down to whether to treat with glucocorticoids. High-dose, daily glucocorticoids usually reverse the disease process effectively and eliminate the pain. Inadequate treatment may result in recurrence, but once the desired effect occurs, the glucocorticoids must be tapered slowly over several weeks or months and discontinued. Nonsteroidal anti-inflammatory drugs are less effective than glucocorticoids but have fewer side effects. In those patients who do not respond or who become glucocorticoid dependent, low-dose radiation therapy (2000cGy) may induce a remission effectively. However, many inflammatory and infiltrative myopathies initially respond to such treatment, only to recur. Furthermore, treatment may not only obfuscate the natural history of the disease, but may make the diagnosis by biopsy more difficult. Hence, it often is prudent to complete the diagnostic workup, which includes orbital biopsy, prior to anti-inflammatory treatment.

COURSE AND OUTCOMES

Idiopathic orbital myositis usually responds very well to systemic glucocorticoids. In most cases, the diagnostic workup does not yield any causative factor and recurrences are not very common. Such patients do well and show no evidence of any ophthalmologic sequelae.

REFERENCES

1. DiMauro S, Moraes CT. Mitochondrial encephalopathies. Arch Neurol. 1993; 50:1197–207.
2. Moraes CT, DiMauro S, Zeviani M, et al. Mitochondrial DNA deletions in progressive external ophthalmoplegia and Kearns–Sayre syndrome. N Engl J Med. 1989;320:1293–9.
3. Holt IJ, Harding AE, Cooper JM, et al. Mitochondrial myopathies: clinical and biochemical features of 30 patients with major deletions of muscle mitochondrial DNA. Ann Neurol. 1989;26:699–708.
4. Hirano M, Silvestri G, Blake DM, et al. Mitochondrial neurogastrointestinal encephalomyopathy (MNGIE): clinical, biochemical, and genetic features of an autosomal recessive mitochondrial disorder. Neurology. 1994;44:721–7.
5. Wallace DC, Singh G, Lott MT, et al. Mitochondrial DNA mutation associated with Leber's hereditary optic neuropathy. Science. 1992;242:1427–30.
6. Fang W, Huang CC, Lee CC, et al. Ophthalmologic manifestation in MELAS syndrome. Arch Neurol. 1993;50:977–80.
7. Crisi G, Ferrari G, Merelli E, Cocconcelli P. Magnetic resonance imaging in a case of Kearns–Sayre syndrome confirmed by molecular analysis. Neuroradiology. 1994;36:37–8.
8. Drachman DA. Ophthalmoplegia plus. The neurodegenerative disorders associated with progressive external ophthalmoplegia. Arch Neurol. 1968;18:654–74.
9. Kearns TP. External ophthalmoplegia, pigmentary degeneration of the retina, and cardiomyopathy: a newly recognized syndrome. Trans Am Ophthalmol Soc. 1965;63:559–625.
10. Uncini A, Servidei S, Silvestri G, et al. Ophthalmoplegia, demyelinating neuropathy, leukoencephalopathy, myopathy, and gastrointestinal dysfunction with multiple deletions of mitochondrial DNA: a mitochondrial multisystem disorder in search of a name. Muscle Nerve. 1994;17:667–74.
11. McKechnie NM, King M, Lee WR. Retinal pathology in the Kearns–Sayre syndrome. Br J Ophthalmol. 1985;69:63–9.
12. Goda S, Hamada T, Ishimoto S, et al. Clinical improvement after administration of coenzyme Q10 in a patient with mitochondrial encephalopathy. J Neurol. 1987;234:62–9.
13. Bachynski BN, Flynn JT, Rodrigues MM, et al. Hyperglycemic acidotic coma and death in Kearns–Sayre syndrome. Ophthalmology. 1986;93:391–6.
14. Johnson CC, Kuwabara T. Oculopharyngeal muscular dystrophy. Am J Ophthalmol. 1974;77:872–9.
15. Burian HM, Burns CA. Ocular changes in myotonic dystrophy. Am J Ophthalmol. 1967;63:22–34.
16. Tsutsumi A, Uchida Y, Osawa M, et al. Ocular findings in Fukuyama-type congenital muscular dystrophy. Brain Dev. 1989;11:413–9.
17. Kuwabara T, Lessell S. Electron microscopic study of extraocular muscles in myotonic dystrophy. Am J Ophthalmol. 1976;82:303–8.
18. Tumbridge WMG, Evered DC, Hall R, et al. The spectrum of thyroid disease in a community: the Wickham survey. Clin Endocrinol (Oxf). 1977;7:481–93.
19. Kendler DL, Lippa J, Rootman J. The initial clinical characteristics of Graves' orbitopathy vary with age and sex. Arch Ophthalmol. 1993;111:197–201.
20. Bahn RS, Heufelder AE. Mechanisms of disease: pathogenesis of Graves' ophthalmopathy. N Engl J Med. 1993;329:1468–75.
21. Saber E, McDonnell J, Zimmerman KM, et al. Extraocular muscle changes in experimental orbital venous stasis: some similarities to Graves' orbitopathy. Graefes Arch Klin Exp Ophthalmol. 1996;234:331–6.
22. Levine MR, Tomsak RL, El-Toukhy E. Thyroid-related ophthalmopathy. Ophthalmol Clin North Am. 1996;9:645–58.
23. Prummel MF, Wiersinga WM. Smoking and risk of Graves' disease. JAMA. 1993; 269:479–82.
24. Liu D, Feldon SE. Thyroid ophthalmopathy. Ophthalmol Clin North Am. 1992; 5:597–622.
25. Werner SC. Classification of the eye changes of Graves' disease. Am J Ophthalmol. 1969;68:646–8.
26. Van Dyk HJ. Orbital Graves' disease. A modification of the "NO SPECS" classification. Ophthalmology. 1981;88:479–83.
27. Bartley GB, Gorman CA. Diagnostic criteria for Graves' ophthalmopathy. Am J Ophthalmol. 1995;119:792–5.
28. Trokel SL, Jakobiec FA. Correlation of CT scanning and pathologic features of ophthalmic Graves' disease. Ophthalmology. 1981;88:553–64.
29. Kahaly G, Schrezenmeir J, Schweikert B, et al. Remission-maintaining effect of cyclosporin and endocrine ophthalmopathy. Transplant Proc. 1986;18:844–5.
30. Martinuzzi A, Sadun AA. Marginal myotomies of levator with lateral–tarsal canthoplasty in the treatment of Graves' lid retraction. Ital J Ophthalmol. 1991;5: 23–9.
31. Bouree P, Bouvier JB, Passeron J, et al. Outbreak of trichinosis near Paris. BMJ. 1979;i:1047–9.
32. Pinchoff BS, Spahlinger DA, Bergstrom TJ, Sandall GS. Extraocular muscle involvement in Wegener's granulomatosis. J Clin Neurol Ophthalmol. 1983; 3:163–8.
33. Katz B, Leja S, Melles RB, Press GA. Amyloid ophthalmoplegia: ophthalmoparesis secondary to primary systemic amyloidosis. J Clin Neurol Ophthalmol. 1988; 9:39–42.
34. Slamovits TL, Burde RM, Sedwick L, et al. Bumpy muscles. Surv Ophthalmol. 1988; 33:189–99.
35. Kennerdell JS, Dresner SC. The nonspecific orbital inflammatory syndromes. Surv Ophthalmol. 1984;29:93–103.
36. Rootman J, Nugent R. The classification and management of acute orbital pseudotumors. Ophthalmology. 1982;89:1040–8.
37. Trokel SL, Hilal SK. Recognition and differential diagnosis of enlarged extraocular muscles in computed tomography. Am J Ophthalmol. 1979;87:503–12.

Nystagmus and Saccadic Intrusions and Oscillations

ROBERT D. YEE

DEFINITION
- Fixation instabilities that usually are involuntary and rhythmic. Nystagmus arises from slow eye movement instability. Saccadic intrusions and oscillations result from saccadic eye movement instability.

KEY FEATURES
- Decreased visual acuity.
- Oscillopsia.

ASSOCIATED FEATURES
- Central nervous system abnormalities.
- Strabismus.
- Albinism.

INTRODUCTION

Nystagmus, saccadic intrusions, and saccadic oscillations are fixation instabilities that usually are involuntary and rhythmic. They may impair vision, and many are signs of neurological disorders. By recognizing the specific type of instability, the ophthalmologist can localize central nervous system (CNS) lesions; determine whether laboratory and other tests, such as magnetic resonance imaging (MRI), are needed; and sometimes recommend treatment.

EPIDEMIOLOGY AND PATHOGENESIS

The application of bioengineering principles, the use of electronic recordings of eye movements in humans, and neurophysiological studies in animals have led to many hypotheses about the pathophysiology of nystagmus. Abnormalities of the vestibulo-ocular, otolithic-ocular, smooth pursuit, optokinetic, vergence, and eccentric gaze-holding systems have been postulated.[1] However, the causes of most types of nystagmus are still not known.

OCULAR MANIFESTATIONS

Nystagmus is caused by an abnormality in a slow eye movement system or in the system that holds eccentric gaze. Abnormal slow eye movements take the eyes away from the intended direction of gaze. Fast eye movements or slow eye movements in the opposite direction carry the eyes back. Nystagmus waveforms can be jerky or pendular (Fig. 202-1). If the corrective movements are reflex saccades, the waveform describes a jerk. The slow movements are called slow components or slow phases, and the saccades are called fast components or fast phases. The direction of jerk nystagmus often is designated by the direction of the fast

NYSTAGMUS WAVEFORMS

FIG. 202-1 ■ Nystagmus waveforms. The horizontal dashed lines indicate the intended position of gaze. A, Jerk nystagmus with slow components of constant velocity. B, Jerk nystagmus with slow components of exponentially increasing velocity. The flat, slow component portions near the intended gaze position follow the fast components and represent extended foveation periods typical of congenital nystagmus. C, Jerk nystagmus with slow components of exponentially increasing velocity. Extended foveation periods follow slow movements that bring the eye toward the intended gaze position. D, Pendular nystagmus. Note that foveation periods are brief compared with those in B and C. E, Jerk nystagmus with slow components of exponentially decreasing velocity.

components; for example, fast components to the right indicate "right-beating" jerk nystagmus. If the corrective movements also are slow eye movements, the waveform is pendular.

Saccadic oscillations are caused by abnormalities in the saccadic eye movement system. Abnormal saccades move the eyes away from the intended direction of gaze, and corrective saccades carry the eyes back. In saccadic intrusions, such as square-wave jerks and macrosquare-wave jerks, brief pauses occur, or intersaccadic intervals, between the opposing saccades (Fig. 202-2). In ocular flutter and opsoclonus, no intersaccadic intervals occur.

Normal visual acuity requires a stationary retinal image on the fovea. If fixation instabilities cause movement of the retinal image across the fovea at speeds of a few degrees per second or greater, visual acuity is diminished. Therefore, many types of nystagmus and saccadic oscillations without intersaccadic intervals cause deceased visual acuity. During volitional saccades, images move across the retina, but there is no sensation of movement of the visual surround. In contrast, most types of nystagmus and saccadic oscillations without intersaccadic intervals cause illusory, back-and-forth movements of the visual surround, called oscillopsia.

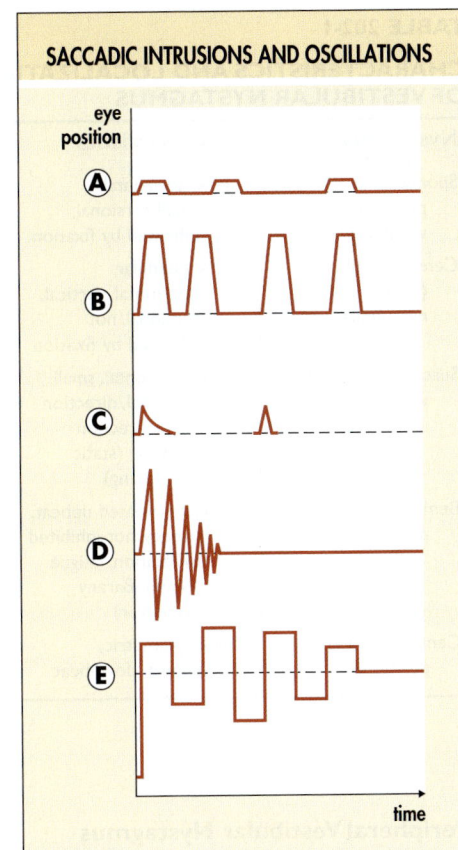

FIG. 202-2 ▌ Saccadic intrusions and oscillations. Dashed lines indicate the intended gaze position. A, Square-wave jerks with intersaccadic intervals. B, Macrosquare-wave jerks with intersaccadic intervals. C, Single saccadic pulse and double saccadic pulses. D, Ocular flutter with no intersaccadic intervals. E, Macrosaccadic oscillations following a refixation saccade.

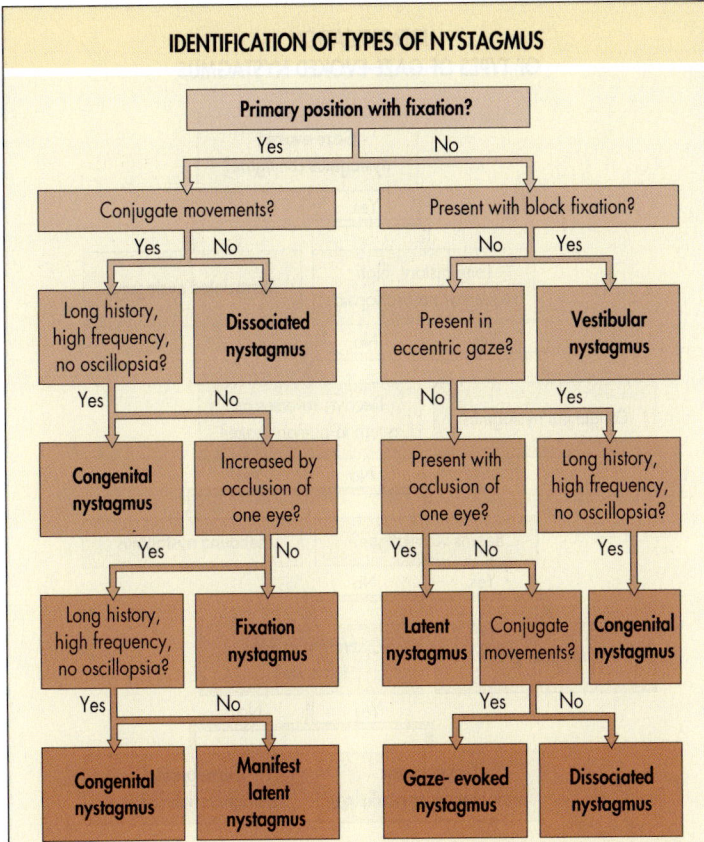

FIG. 202-3 ▌ Identification of types of nystagmus.

DIAGNOSIS

Most types of nystagmus and saccadic instabilities can be detected and identified, without the aid of eye movement recordings and other specialized equipment, by careful attention to characteristics of the oscillations. While the patient fixates on a stationary target at distance and near, the following questions should be addressed:

- Are the eye movements that move the eyes away from the target slow eye movements (nystagmus) or saccades (saccadic instabilities)?
- Do slow movements occur in one direction and fast movements in the opposition direction (jerk nystagmus), or are the opposing movements of equal speed (pendular nystagmus)?
- What is the direction of the instability (horizontal, vertical, oblique, or torsional)?
- What is the effect of blocking fixation? Does it increase the nystagmus intensity (vestibular nystagmus), or does it decrease the intensity (congenital nystagmus)?

Frenzel goggles to block fixation or electronic equipment to record eye movements in the dark usually are not readily available. Viewing the fundus of one eye with a direct ophthalmoscope while the patient covers the other eye blocks fixation and magnifies motion of the fundus caused by eye movements. The fundus moves in the direction opposite to that of the eye. The direct ophthalmoscope is an excellent instrument with which to detect small-amplitude oscillations such as voluntary "nystagmus" and superior oblique myokymia.

Further questions to address are:

- What is the effect of different gaze positions?
- Does eccentric gaze change the intensity or the direction of the instability?
- Is the instability present only in eccentric gaze?
- Are the oscillations in both eyes symmetrical, or are they asymmetrical with different amplitudes or directions in each eye?
- If no instability occurs in the sitting upright position, is it present in other positions of the body and head (positional vestibular nystagmus)?

With the answers to these questions and information from the patient's history and other physical findings, the ophthalmologist almost always can identify the fixation instability. Figures 202-3 to 202-6 present flowcharts that use this information to identify the types of nystagmus.

DIFFERENTIAL DIAGNOSIS

Vestibular Nystagmus

The characteristics and localizations of several types of vestibular nystagmus are shown in Table 202-1.

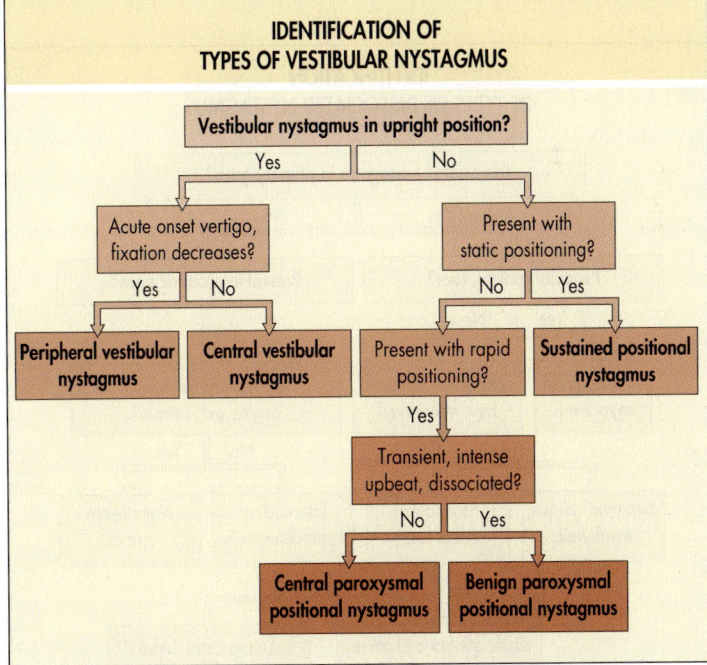

FIG. 202-4 ▌ Identification of types of vestibular nystagmus.

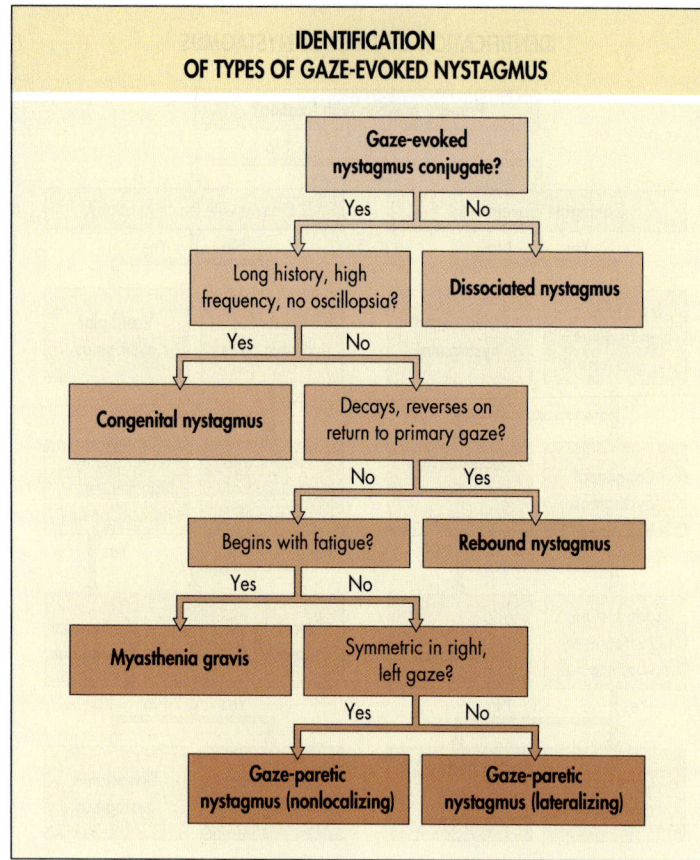

FIG. 202-5 ▪ Identification of types of gaze-evoked nystagmus.

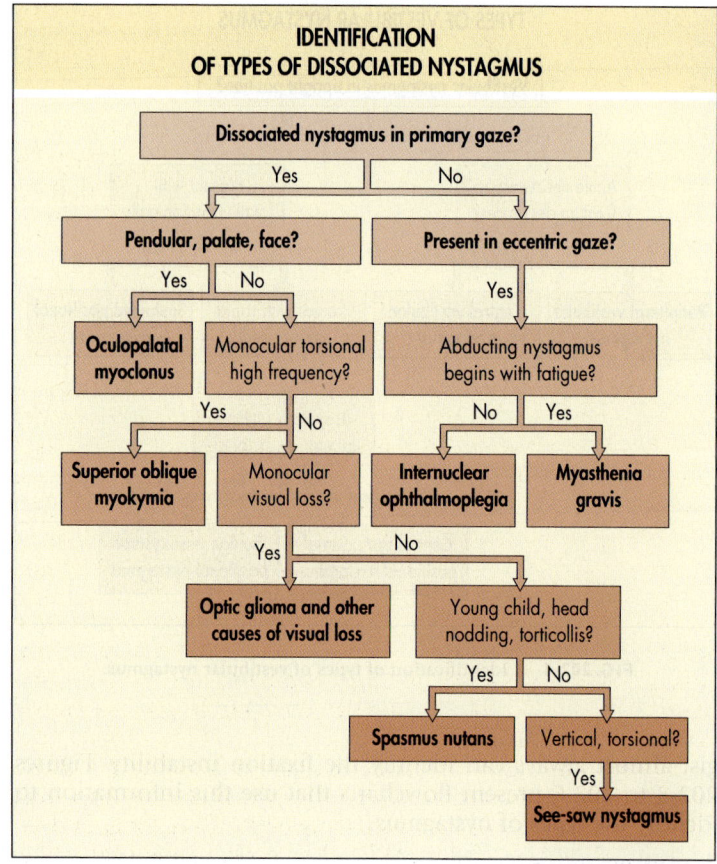

FIG. 202-6 ▪ Identification of types of dissociated nystagmus.

TABLE 202-1

CHARACTERISTICS AND LOCALIZATIONS OF VESTIBULAR NYSTAGMUS

Nystagmus	Characteristics	Localization
Spontaneous peripheral vestibular	Jerk, horizontal, small torsional, inhibited by fixation	Labyrinth, eighth nerve (acute)
Central vestibular (fixation) nystagmus	Jerk, pendular, horizontal, vertical, torsional, not inhibited by fixation	Brainstem, cerebellum
Sustained positional vestibular	Jerk, horizontal, small torsional, direction fixed, direction changing (static positioning)	Labyrinth, eighth nerve or brainstem, cerebellum
Benign paroxysmal positional	Jerk, dissociated upbeat, latency, not inhibited by fixation, fatigue (Nylen–Barany maneuver)	Posterior vertical canal
Central paroxysmal positional	Jerk, symmetric, upbeat, downbeat	Brainstem, cerebellum

Peripheral Vestibular Nystagmus

Peripheral vestibular nystagmus is caused by an acute imbalance of tonic innervation to the brainstem from the vestibular labyrinths and the eighth nerves. Destructive disorders, such as labyrinthitis and vestibular neuritis, decrease innervation from the affected ear and produce jerk nystagmus with slow components toward that ear and fast components beating toward the opposite side. Irritative disorders, such as Meniere's disease, increase innervation from the affected ear and generate jerk nystagmus with fast components toward that ear and slow components toward the opposite ear.

Because the vestibular nerve conveys tonic innervation from a horizontal semicircular canal, a pair of vertical canals, and otoliths (saccule and utricle), the nystagmus is mainly horizontal but has vertical and torsional components as well (rotary nystagmus). The slow component has a constant-velocity waveform. Gaze in the direction of the fast component increases the nystagmus intensity (amplitude X frequency), and gaze in the direction of the slow component decreases the intensity (Alexander's law). Nausea and vertigo with the sensation of rotation of the environment or self-rotation in the direction of the fast component are usually present. Tinnitus, hearing loss, and ear pain also may be present. The nystagmus intensity is high during the first few days but spontaneously decreases. At this time, fixation might inhibit the nystagmus. However, blocking fixation reveals the nystagmus. Imbalance of tonic inputs from the otoliths can cause a transient skew deviation (hypotropic eye ipsilateral to the damaged ear).

Head-Shaking Nystagmus

Rapid head oscillations can produce head-shaking nystagmus. The head is shaken horizontally and vigorously by the patient for 10–15 seconds, and then fixation is blocked. In patients who have peripheral vestibular lesions, a transient, horizontal jerk nystagmus with the fast components to the side opposite the damaged side is induced. Vertical head-shaking can produce a less intense horizontal nystagmus with fast components beating toward the damaged side. In patients who have central vestibular lesions, horizontal head-shaking can induce a downbeat nystagmus or a horizontal nystagmus.

Central Vestibular Nystagmus

Lesions of the vestibular nuclei, the cerebellum, or the connections between the vestibulocerebellum (flocculonodular lobes) and the brainstem can cause central vestibular nystagmus. In contrast to peripheral vestibular nystagmus, fixation does not greatly inhibit the nystagmus, which leads to the synonymous term fixation nystagmus. Central vestibular nystagmus can be purely horizontal, torsional, or vertical, because horizontal and vertical vestibulo-ocular pathways begin to separate in the vestibular nuclei. Jerk nystagmus in primary gaze that is predominantly torsional is associated with lesions of the vestibular nuclei on the side contralateral to the fast component.[2]

Positional Vestibular Nystagmus

Positional vestibular nystagmus is not present in the sitting upright position but is induced by the supine and lateral positions or by rapid movements of the head and body into head-hanging positions. Fixation suppresses the nystagmus when the cause is a peripheral vestibular lesion but does not suppress it when a central vestibular lesion is present. The nystagmus direction can remain the same in the right and left lateral positions (direction fixed), or it can change (direction changing). The fast components may beat toward the down ear (geotropic) or toward the up ear (apogeotropic). Both peripheral and central vestibular lesions can cause direction-fixed and direction-changing positional nystagmus.

Benign Paroxysmal Positional Nystagmus

Rapid positioning of the head and body into the right or left head-hanging position (Nylen-Barany or Dix-Hallpike maneuver) induces benign paroxysmal positional nystagmus (BPPN). After a delay of 1–2 seconds, an intense vertical nystagmus develops. Fixation does not suppress the nystagmus, and the patient usually complains of vertigo after the maneuver. Characteristic binocular asymmetry exists in which the nystagmus primarily upbeats in the higher eye (i.e., the eye opposite to the head-hanging position) and is oblique and torsional in the lower eye. The asymmetry is explained by the primary and secondary actions of the vertical extraocular muscles stimulated by the posterior semicircular canals (contralateral inferior rectus and ipsilateral superior oblique). The nystagmus dies away over several seconds. Repetition of the maneuver soon after the initial positioning generates a less intense nystagmus (fatigue).

The cause of BPPN is otoconia that have become dislodged from the otoliths (utricular macule) and either are attached to the cupula of a posterior semicircular canal (cupulolithiasis) or freely move in that canal (canalithiasis). Endolymph flow in the posterior canal produces an abnormally prolonged deflection of the hair cells in the crista of the canal. Positional exercises, such as the Epley maneuver, can move the granules back into the utricle and eliminate the positional nystagmus and vertigo.[3] Canalithiasis and paroxysmal positional nystagmus of the horizontal and anterior posterior canals can occur spontaneously or can be produced by repositioning for the posterior canal form of BPPN.[4] The Nylen-Barany maneuver can induce paroxysmal positional nystagmus other than BPPN, such as downbeat nystagmus and other types of central vestibular nystagmus.[5] Therefore, the typical features of BPPN must be present to confirm the diagnosis; it can result from viral labyrinthitis, head injury, and infarction of the inner ear. Most often it is an isolated disorder in the elderly.

Congenital Nystagmus

Congenital nystagmus is one of several common types of nystagmus that occur in children (Table 202-2); it is a high-frequency, horizontal nystagmus that begins in the first few months of life.

TABLE 202-2

CHARACTERISTICS AND LOCALIZATIONS OF NYSTAGMUS IN CHILDHOOD

Nystagmus	Characteristics	Localization
Idiopathic congenital	Complex waveforms, jerk (increasing velocity slow components), pendular, horizontal, null zone, (face turn, head nodding, no oscillopsia)	Coexisting ocular, visual pathway lesions (not pathogenetic)
Latent/manifest latent	Jerk (decreasing velocity slow components), horizontal, fast components beat toward fixing eye	Coexisting infantile esotropia
Spasmus nutans	Pendular, horizontal, small vertical, torsional, dissociated, high frequency, (torticollis, head nodding), onset in first year, resolution in 1–2 years	No signs of visual pathway lesions
Monocular visual loss	Pendular, vertical, horizontal, monocular, high frequency, intermittent, (occasional head nodding)	Gliomas of optic nerve, chiasm or third ventricle, and other causes of visual loss

It rarely is vertical. Square-wave jerks have been described before the onset of nystagmus and in unaffected parents of patients who have hereditary congenital nystagmus. Congenital nystagmus is not pathogenetically associated with other CNS disorders, although it is found frequently in patients who have certain systemic and ocular disorders that impair vision, such as oculocutaneous albinism and ocular albinism. It can be an X-linked recessive, autosomal dominant, or autosomal recessive disorder. Two families who had autosomal dominant congenital nystagmus were found to have a gene that localized to chromosome 6p12[6] and a translocation between chromosomes 7 and 15, respectively.[7] Congenital nystagmus associated with visual disorders has been called sensory defect nystagmus, and congenital nystagmus with no associated ocular abnormalities has been called motor defect nystagmus. However, the nystagmus characteristics are precisely the same, and the ocular defects and decreased vision probably do not cause the nystagmus.

The nystagmus waveforms are pendular, jerk, or a combination of the two, and many are complex. Occasionally, a congenital nystagmus patient does not have a history of nystagmus from childhood; in such cases, electronic eye movement recordings that reveal one of the complex waveforms can be valuable in differentiating congenital nystagmus from acquired nystagmus. The slow components of the jerk nystagmus often have curved trajectories, with exponentially increasing velocities (see Fig. 202-1). Often brief intervals occur when the retinal image is relatively stationary on the fovea, called extended foveation periods, which allows better visual acuity. Unlike in vestibular nystagmus, the effort to fixate increases the nystagmus intensity, while staring and blocking fixation decrease the nystagmus. In contrast to patients who have acquired types of nystagmus, patients who have congenital nystagmus rarely spontaneously complain of oscillopsia.

Patients who have congenital nystagmus often have a direction of horizontal eccentric gaze, called the null zone, in which nystagmus intensity is low, foveation periods are long, and visual acuity is best. A habitual head turn places the eyes in the null zone. High-frequency, low-amplitude head nodding is seen commonly. The head nodding usually does not improve vision. Congenital nystagmus remains horizontal in vertical gaze and usually is decreased at near with convergence. The dampening of nystagmus with convergence improves vision, which is one reason why many children who have congenital nystagmus do not need schoolbooks with large-size print. In one form of the nystagmus blockage syndrome, excessive convergence produces an esotropia, fixation of the distant target with the adducted eye, a decrease in nystagmus, and improved vision.[8] In another form, a switch occurs from a congenital nystagmus waveform to a manifest latent nystagmus (MLN) waveform (see the next section) when the adducted eye fixates. In such patients, vision is better with the latter nystagmus.

Latent and Manifest Latent Nystagmus

Latent nystagmus is always associated with strabismus, usually infantile esotropia. In true latent nystagmus, no nystagmus is present with both eyes open. When each eye is occluded, a horizontal jerk nystagmus occurs, the slow components of which are toward the occluded eye and the fast components of which beat toward the uncovered, fixing eye. The shift of fixation is the stimulus for the nystagmus. Electronic eye movement recordings have shown that true latent nystagmus is rare. In most instances, a low-intensity jerk nystagmus (MLN) exists that beats toward the fixing eye without occlusion. Nystagmus intensity increases with occlusion of the nonfixing eye, and the jerk nystagmus reverses direction when the eye that preferentially fixes is occluded. Gaze in the direction of the fast component increases nystagmus intensity, and gaze in the opposite direction decreases the intensity (Alexander's law). Patients who have MLN can have a habitual face turn toward the direction of the fast component, which places the eyes in the opposite direction and improves vision. Congenital nystagmus patients who have jerk nystagmus also can show reversal of the nystagmus direction when each eye is occluded, as a result of a shift in the position of the neutral point. However, electronic recordings show that congenital nystagmus slow components have exponentially increasing velocities, whereas latent nystagmus slow components have exponentially decreasing velocities (see Fig. 202-1). Rarely, patients who have congenital nystagmus also have MLN.

Gaze-Evoked Nystagmus

Several types of gaze-evoked nystagmus exist that are present in eccentric gaze but not in primary gaze (Table 202-3). In gaze-

paretic nystagmus, no nystagmus occurs in primary gaze, but a jerk nystagmus occurs in about 30° of eccentric gaze. The slow components move the eyes toward primary gaze and have waveforms with exponentially decreasing velocities (see Fig. 202-1). Fast components beat toward the intended eccentric gaze position. The drift toward primary gaze results from impairment of gaze-holding mechanisms that involve the nucleus prepositus hypoglossi and medial vestibular nucleus (the "neural integrator") and their connections with the flocculonodular lobe of the cerebellum. The eye position signal cannot hold the eyes eccentrically in the orbits, so they drift back toward primary gaze.

Normal, physiological, endpoint nystagmus is present in the extremes of horizontal and upward gazes of about 45–50°. Therefore, nystagmus at only 30° is likely to be a pathological finding. Endpoint nystagmus is irregular and might be slightly dissociated (larger amplitude in the abducting eye), which mimics the dissociated nystagmus associated with internuclear ophthalmoplegia. However, the other eye movement abnormalities associated with internuclear ophthalmoplegia are absent.

Symmetrical gaze-paretic nystagmus in which the nystagmus intensity is the same in right gaze and left gaze usually is not a localizing sign. It is produced by mental fatigue; CNS depression from barbiturates, tranquilizers, anticonvulsants, alcohol, and other drugs; and disorders of the cerebral hemispheres, brainstem, and cerebellum. Asymmetrical, horizontal, gaze-paretic nystagmus often is lateralizing. A lesion of the brainstem or cerebellum is generally on the side of greater nystagmus intensity.

Myasthenia gravis can produce a horizontal or upbeat gaze-paretic nystagmus. Initially, little or no nystagmus exists, but as the extraocular muscles fatigue, nystagmus develops. In horizontal gaze, the amplitude of the fast component in the abducting eye is often larger than that in the adducting eye as a result of the greater fatigue of the medial rectus muscle. Normal subjects can have an endpoint nystagmus of very small amplitude that increases with fatigue.

Rebound Nystagmus

Rebound nystagmus is a type of horizontal, gaze-paretic nystagmus in which the jerk nystagmus gradually decreases in amplitude as the eyes remain in eccentric gaze for many seconds. In some instances, the nystagmus direction actually reverses (centripetal nystagmus); for example, it becomes left-beating in right gaze. On return to primary gaze, a jerk nystagmus occurs that beats in the direction opposite to that of the previous gaze-paretic nystagmus. The secondary nystagmus decreases and disappears after several seconds. Rebound nystagmus usually is associated with disorders of the cerebellum. Vertical rebound nystagmus occurs less often. Normal subjects can have a few beats of rebound nystagmus after prolonged eccentric gaze if no fixation target is present on return to primary gaze (lights turned off).

Alternating Nystagmus

The direction of jerk nystagmus changes spontaneously in alternating nystagmus (Table 202-4). In periodic alternating nystagmus, a repetitive cycling of right-beating and left-beating nystagmus occurs in primary gaze. The amplitude of nystagmus gradually increases and decreases over a period of about 90 seconds, followed by a short period of about 10 seconds in which there is no nystagmus, small-amplitude vertical or torsional nystagmus, or square-wave jerks (null period). Nystagmus that beats in the opposite direction increases and decreases over 90 seconds and is followed by a null period. The cycle continues and is not affected by other eye movements, except for strong rotational vestibular stimuli, which can reset the cycle. During periods of jerk nystagmus, patients have horizontal oscillopsia and blurred vision. They might spontaneously turn their heads in the direction of the fast component. This moves the eyes to a position of minimal nystagmus and better vision (null position).

TABLE 202-3

CHARACTERISTICS AND LOCALIZATIONS OF GAZE-EVOKED NYSTAGMUS

Nystagmus	Characteristics	Localization
Physiologic, endpoint	Jerk, small amplitude, intermittent, extremes of horizontal and up gaze	Physiologic
Gaze-paretic (symmetric)	Jerk (decreasing velocity slow components) at 30° eccentric gaze	Nonlocalizing (drugs, mental fatigue)
Gaze-paretic (asymmetric)	Jerk (decreasing velocity slow components), horizontal, at 30° eccentric gaze, larger amplitude toward side of lesion	Lesions of brainstem, cerebellum, cerebral hemisphere
Rebound	Jerk, horizontal, decreases and direction can reverse in eccentric gaze, transient jerk nystagmus on return to primary gaze, fast components beating toward eccentric gaze	Cerebellum
Myasthenia gravis	Jerk, horizontal or vertical, gradual onset in prolonged eccentric gaze	Myoneural junction (fatigue—increasing transmission block)

The null position moves gradually to the right, back to primary gaze, to the left, and back to primary gaze. This type of alternating nystagmus is almost always associated with cerebellar disorders. Ablation of the nodulus and uvula in the monkey produces periodic alternating nystagmus.

Alternating nystagmus also occurs in congenital nystagmus, in MLN, and in association with severe binocular visual loss from many causes (e.g., chronic papilledema, vitreous hemorrhage, cataract). In congenital nystagmus and MLN, the change in nystagmus direction can be caused by a shift of fixation from one eye to the other. However, congenital nystagmus and periodic alternating nystagmus can coexist, for example, in patients with albinism.[9] The periods of alternating nystagmus are not as symmetrical or regular as in periodic alternating nystagmus associated with cerebellar disorders, although shifting of the null positions also occurs.

Upbeat Nystagmus

Upbeat nystagmus that is present only in upgaze and is associated with symmetrical, horizontal, gaze-paretic nystagmus is usually a type of gaze-paretic nystagmus that might not have a localizing significance. However, upbeat nystagmus in primary gaze is caused by lesions that affect the brainstem, especially the lower pontine tegmentum (see Table 202-4).[10] Lesions of the medulla, midbrain, thalamus, and cerebellum also can cause upbeat nystagmus. Common causes of these lesions are multiple sclerosis, infarction, intra-axial tumor, Wernicke's encephalopathy, brainstem encephalitis, and cerebellar degeneration. Rarely, upbeat nystagmus can be a form of congenital nystagmus and might be seen as a transient finding in normal infants. Patients with upbeat nystagmus may have slow components with constant velocity, decreasing velocity, or increasing velocity waveforms. Nicotine can produce a small-amplitude upbeat nystagmus seen in the dark in normal subjects.

Downbeat Nystagmus

Downbeat nystagmus in primary gaze usually is caused by a structural lesion in the posterior fossa at the level of the craniocervical junction (see Table 202-4). The nystagmus intensity characteristically increases in horizontal eccentric gaze and may be increased by convergence. Convergence also can convert an upbeat nystagmus in primary gaze to a downbeat nystagmus. Lesions of the cerebellum and pons are associated most often with downbeat nystagmus, and the most common causes are infarction, cerebellar degeneration, multiple sclerosis, and congenital malformations.[11] Downbeat nystagmus may be part of an acquired syndrome in adulthood consisting of cerebellar ataxia, lower brainstem dysfunction, or cranial nerve palsies caused by Arnold-Chiari malformations (types 1 and 2). Although such malformations are not the most common cause of downbeat nystagmus, a magnetic resonance study of the posterior fossa should be obtained, because surgical decompression can diminish the nystagmus and the other abnormalities in the syndrome. Rarely, a variety of other disorders can cause downbeat nystagmus, including lithium toxicity, magnesium deficiency, vitamin B_{12} deficiency, midbrain infarction, brainstem encephalitis, Wernicke's encephalopathy, increased intracranial pressure with hydrocephalus, syringobulbia, cerebellar tumor, and anticonvulsant medication. Downbeat nystagmus has been reported to occur as an inherited congenital disorder. The slow components can have constant velocity, increasing velocity, and decreasing velocity waveforms.

Dissociated Nystagmus

Several types of dissociated nystagmus occur in which the eye movements are strikingly disconjugate (Table 202-5). Nystagmus might be present in only one eye (spasmus nutans, optic glioma, uniocular visual loss, and superior oblique myokymia), larger in one eye than the other (abduction nystagmus in internuclear ophthalmoplegia and ocular myoclonus), or in different directions (see-saw nystagmus and ocular myoclonus). Dissociated nystagmus present in the primary position is often pendular and is often jerk nystagmus in eccentric gaze.

ACQUIRED PENDULAR NYSTAGMUS IN ADULTS. Acquired pendular nystagmus usually has horizontal, vertical, and torsional components and is often disconjugate. Lesions of the pons, medulla, midbrain, and cerebellum, often caused by multiple sclerosis or infarction, produce oscillations with a typical frequency of 3–4Hz. MRI studies show large or multiple lesions, which suggests that more than one pathway must be damaged to produce pendular nystagmus.[12] A head tremor might be present. The nystagmus trajectory also can be elliptical or circular. When acquired pendular nystagmus is associated with similar movements of the soft palate, tongue, facial muscles, pharynx, and larynx, it is called ocular myoclonus; this syndrome has also been called oculopalatal myoclonus. The cause usually is an infarction that affects the structures of Mollaret's triangle and their connections (red nucleus in the midbrain, inferior olive in the medulla, and contralateral dentate nucleus of the cerebellum).

TABLE 202-4

CHARACTERISTICS AND LOCALIZATIONS OF OTHER TYPES OF FIXATION NYSTAGMUS

Nystagmus	Characteristics	Localization
Periodic alternating	Jerk, horizontal, in primary position, regular phases of right-beating, null, left-beating (shifting null position)	Cerebellar nodulus and uvula
Alternating (irregular)	Jerk, horizontal, in primary position, variable, asymmetric phases	Congenital nystagmus, severe binocular visual loss
Upbeat	Jerk, fast components beat upward	Only in up gaze—part of symmetric gaze—paretic nystagmus; in primary gaze—lower pons
Downbeat	Jerk, fast components beat downward, vertical intensity increases in horizontal gaze	Cerebellum, lower brainstem

TABLE 202-5

CHARACTERISTICS AND LOCALIZATIONS OF DISSOCIATED NYSTAGMUS

Nystagmus	Characteristics	Localization
Acquired pendular in adults	Pendular, horizontal, vertical, torsional, disconjugate (coexisting palatal myoclonus)	Brainstem, cerebellum
Superior oblique myokymia	Pendular, jerk, torsional, vertical, high frequency, small amplitude, monocular	Trochlear nucleus
See-saw	Pendular, vertical, torsional, rising eye intorts, falling eye extorts; rarely jerk	Midbrain (interstitial nucleus of Cajal)
Abducting 'nystagmus' of internuclear ophthalmoplegia	Jerk, horizontal, decreasing velocity slow components, larger in abducting eye in	Medial longitudinal fasciculus in pons, midbrain horizontal gaze
Abducting nystagmus of myasthenia gravis	Gaze-paretic nystagmus in horizontal gaze, greater paresis of medial rectus muscle	Myoneural junction—myasthenia gravis

Hypertrophy of the inferior olive and the pendular oscillations begin several months later. Extensive hemorrhage in the pons can produce a large-amplitude, vertical, pendular nystagmus and bilateral horizontal gaze palsies.

SPASMUS NUTANS. Spasmus nutans occurs in the first year of life and is a triad of pendular nystagmus, head nodding, and torticollis. The nystagmus often is dissociated, and in individual patients it can vary from conjugate to disconjugate to monocular over a few minutes. Its direction is primarily horizontal, but it can have vertical and torsional components. In most patients, the syndrome seemingly resolves spontaneously over 1–2 years. However, electronic eye movement recordings show that a small-amplitude, intermittent, dissociated, pendular nystagmus can persist at least until age 5–12 years.[13] Characteristically, the nystagmus frequency is higher (3–11Hz) and its amplitude more variable than in congenital nystagmus.

Head nodding is found in most patients who have spasmus nutans. It induces vestibulo-ocular responses that transform the nystagmus into larger-amplitude, slower, binocularly symmetrical, pendular oscillations with improved vision. Spasmus nutans must be differentiated from other disorders that cause head nodding and nystagmus, such as visual loss in children, intracranial tumors, and congenital nystagmus. Children with bilateral vision impairment can have rapid, horizontal, pendular head oscillations; horizontal or vertical nystagmus; and intermittent head tilting during attempts to fixate.[14] The nystagmus can be pendular or jerk, with slow components of constant, increasing, or decreasing velocity.[15] The head shaking seems to be a voluntary, learned adaptation that can improve vision. The diagnostic signs from careful examination of eye and head movements, including electronic recordings, can differentiate spasmus nutans from congenital nystagmus but do not reliably separate spasmus nutans from nystagmus and head nodding due to CNS lesions.[16] Visual loss, optic atrophy, abnormal growth and development, signs and symptoms of CNS disorders, or an older age of onset warrants MRI studies.[17] Some clinicians obtain neuroimages for all patients who have spasmus nutans. Others do not, because the prevalence of CNS tumors in patients without other signs of CNS masses is low.[18]

OPTIC GLIOMA IN INFANTS. Tumors of the optic nerve, optic chiasm, or third ventricle can produce a high-frequency, pendular nystagmus in infants. Its direction is usually vertical, and it is often monocular. A careful examination to detect visual loss, optic atrophy, and signs of neurofibromatosis type 1 is required to differentiate this type of pendular nystagmus from spasmus nutans. MRI of the orbits and brain is warranted.

MONOCULAR VISUAL LOSS AND BILATERAL VISUAL LOSS. Children who have monocular visual loss from causes other than optic nerve glioma can have a monocular, high-frequency, small-amplitude, pendular nystagmus.[19] They do not have intracranial tumors, spasmus nutans, or signs of damage to the optic nerve or optic chiasm. The nystagmus can disappear after successful treatment for the monocular visual loss. Adults who have acquired, severe monocular visual loss (e.g., dense cataract) can have a very low-frequency, irregular, vertical drift and jerk nystagmus (Heimann-Bielschowsky phenomenon), which can also be abolished with recovery of vision. Bilateral blindness results from a number of causes and can produce large-amplitude oscillations with small-amplitude ones superimposed. Both oscillations are horizontal and vertical and can have jerk and pendular waveforms. The direction of the jerk nystagmus varies over time (shifting null position). Vestibulo-ocular responses are impaired; volitional saccades and the fast components of vestibular nystagmus may be absent. Head nodding is usually present. Children who have congenital stationary night blindness and rod monochromatism may have small-amplitude, high-frequency, disconjugate, pendular nystagmus similar to that seen in spasmus nutans.

SUPERIOR OBLIQUE MYOKYMIA. Superior oblique myokymia is a very high-frequency, torsional, and oblique oscillation of one eye that causes monocular oscillopsia and, occasionally, vertical diplopia. Careful observation of the conjunctival blood vessels with a slit lamp or of the fundus with an ophthalmoscope reveals the extremely high-frequency, low-amplitude, pendular oscillations, as well as the occasional jerk nystagmus and tonic intorsion and infraduction that produce diplopia. Electromyogram of the superior oblique muscle has shown abnormal discharges at a frequency of 35Hz. Superior oblique myokymia usually occurs in otherwise healthy adults, can remit spontaneously, and may recur. Rarely, it is associated with brainstem disorders, such as multiple sclerosis or a pontine tumor.

SEE-SAW NYSTAGMUS. See-saw nystagmus is a disconjugate, vertical, pendular nystagmus. In one half of a cycle, the rising eye also intorts and the falling eye extorts. The movements are reversed in the other half cycle. See-saw nystagmus is caused most often by large parasellar tumors that cause bitemporal hemianopsia (optic chiasm) and impinge on the third ventricle. Less often, head trauma and infarction of the upper brainstem are the causes. Congenital forms occur, including those in infants who have albinism. In the congenital forms, the rising eye extorts and the falling eye intorts. See-saw nystagmus might be caused by damage to otolithic pathways involving the interstitial nucleus of Cajal, which participate in the ocular tilt reaction. Stereotactic ablation of the interstitial nucleus of Cajal, clonazepam, and baclofen abolish the nystagmus. Rarely, see-saw nystagmus has a jerk waveform, in which case it arises from a unilateral midbrain lesion. The lesion hypothetically damages the interstitial nucleus of Cajal (torsional eye velocity generator) and spares the adjacent rostral interstitial nucleus of the medial longitudinal fasciculus (MLF; torsional fast component generator).[20]

ABDUCTING NYSTAGMUS IN INTERNUCLEAR OPHTHALMOPLEGIA. In internuclear ophthalmoplegia, horizontal gaze in the direction opposite to the lesion in the MLF in the midbrain or pons induces a jerk nystagmus in the abducting eye and a smaller (or no) nystagmus in the paretic, adducting eye. This abducting nystagmus is the most common type of dissociated nystagmus. It might be simply a gaze-paretic nystagmus with superimposed paresis of the medial rectus muscle ipsilateral to the MLF lesion. However, in many patients, the speed of the exponentially velocity-decreasing waveform of the centripetal slow component is much higher than that found in gaze-paretic nystagmus. The abducting saccade has a characteristic overshooting waveform with a rapid, postsaccadic drift. The hypermetria may be a consequence of an adaptive increase in innervation in response to the weakness of adduction. The saccadic pulse is increased, but the step is not increased proportionately (pulse-step mismatch) or is absent, which results in a rapid centripetal drift. Therefore, the abducting nystagmus might be caused by a train of hypermetric saccades.[21] Physiological endpoint nystagmus also can be dissociated slightly (larger amplitude in the abducting eye), but the other ocular motor abnormalities that are characteristic of internuclear ophthalmoplegia are absent. These abnormalities consist of limitation of adduction, slow adducting saccades, hypermetric abducting saccades, upbeat nystagmus, and skew deviation.

Down Syndrome

Patients who have Down syndrome frequently have nystagmus. The nystagmus types include dissociated pendular nystagmus, horizontal nystagmus of high frequency, and small-amplitude and latent nystagmus or MLN.[22]

Convergence-Retraction Nystagmus and Convergence Nystagmus

Voluntary or reflex upward saccades in Parinaud's syndrome (dorsal midbrain syndrome) are hypometric and show simultaneous adduction and retraction of both eyes. Co-contraction of antagonist muscles causes the retraction. Optokinetic stimuli that move downward elicit upward, reflex saccades and the pattern of convergence-retraction nystagmus. Voluntary convergence can induce downbeat nystagmus and can convert an upbeat nystagmus into a downbeat nystagmus. Pendular convergence nystagmus with alternating convergence and divergence is rare. Convergence-divergence oscillations have vertical and torsional components and can be increased with convergence.[23] Convergence nystagmus has been caused by an Arnold-Chiari type 1 malformation, which resolved with surgical decompression of the foramen magnum.[24] It can also be caused by Whipple's disease, which produces contractions of the masticatory muscles (ocular masticatory myorhythmia) and a vertical gaze palsy.[25] Antibiotics can resolve the oculofacial-skeletal myorhythmia.

Lid Nystagmus

Upward twitches of the upper eyelids (lid nystagmus) sometimes can exceed the amplitude of the upward fast components in upbeat nystagmus. Wallenberg's syndrome (lateral medullary syndrome) has a variety of ocular motor abnormalities,[26] including horizontal, gaze-paretic nystagmus with lid nystagmus. Convergence can induce lid nystagmus in patients who have lesions in the medulla or cerebellum.

Epileptic Nystagmus

Involuntary head turns, tonic deviation of the eyes, and nystagmus can be caused by a variety of seizures. In general, when an epileptic focus occurs in the parietal-temporal-occipital lobe, the eyes deviate to the contralateral side, and a horizontal jerk nystagmus is seen with fast components beating toward that side. The fast and slow components are confined to the contralateral field of gaze, and the nystagmus might occur as a result of activation of cortical saccadic regions in the cerebral cortex.[27] Ipsiversive deviation of the eyes and nystagmus with ipsiversive slow components might arise from an epileptic focus in the temporal-occipital cortex that activates a cerebral cortical area for smooth pursuit.[28] Pendular, torsional, or convergence nystagmus also can occur with epilepsy.

Ocular Bobbing

Stupor and coma are associated with several ocular abnormalities, including ocular bobbing. Intermittent, irregular, conjugate, downward saccades are followed by slower, upward drift movements. Patients who have ocular bobbing have extensive damage to the pons from hemorrhage or compression or have toxic or metabolic encephalopathies. Several variants of ocular bobbing exist. In inverse bobbing, or ocular dipping, downward, slow movements are followed by upward saccades back toward the primary position. In converse bobbing, or reverse ocular dipping, large-amplitude, upward saccades are followed by downward drifts.

Saccadic Intrusions

Reflex saccades to objects that enter the visual field are mediated through pathways from the visual association areas of the parietal lobes and temporal lobes, and from ocular motor fields in the frontal lobes. They project to the superior colliculi and the saccade-related areas of the brainstem. Normally, reflex saccades to these sites can be inhibited voluntarily. Pathways from the frontal lobes to the basal ganglia (pars reticularis of the substantia nigra) and superior colliculus might be important for the inhibition of reflex saccades. Patients who suffer frontal lobe diseases, including Alzheimer's disease, Huntington's disease, progressive supranuclear palsy, and schizophrenia, have inappropriate saccades that interrupt fixation. These saccadic intrusions have been called the "visual grasp reflex" (see Fig. 202-2 and Table 202-6).

TABLE 202-6

CHARACTERISTICS AND LOCALIZATIONS OF SACCADIC INTRUSIONS AND OSCILLATIONS

Type	Characteristics	Localization
Square-wave jerks	Horizontal, 1–5°, 200msec intersaccadic intervals	Not localizing
Macrosquare-wave jerks	Horizontal, 10–40°, 100msec intersaccadic intervals	Cerebellum
Macrosaccadic oscillations	Horizontal saccadic dysmetria, series of hypermetric saccades, 200msec intersaccadic intervals	Cerebellum
Voluntary "nystagmus"	Horizontal, high frequency, low amplitude, intermittent, no intersaccadic intervals	Volitional
Saccadic pulses	Horizontal, single or double saccades with no steps	Cerebellum, lower brainstem
Ocular flutter	Horizontal, large amplitude, no intersaccadic intervals	Cerebellum, lower brainstem
Opsoclonus	Multidirectional, large amplitude, linear and curvilinear trajectories, no intersaccadic intervals	Cerebellum, lower brainstem

SQUARE-WAVE JERKS. Normal subjects have infrequent, small-amplitude (less than one to a few degrees), horizontal saccades that move the eyes away from the fixation target and then back to the target, called square-wave jerks (see Fig. 202-2). Pause occurs between the to-and-fro saccades (intersaccadic interval) of about 200msec, which allows sufficient foveation time for normal visual acuity with no oscillopsia. The frequency of square-wave jerks increases in the dark. Larger (1–5°) and more frequent (>2Hz) square-wave jerks are abnormal and are associated with cerebellar disorders, progressive supranuclear palsy, Huntington's disease, and schizophrenia. They occur sporadically or in bursts.

MACROSQUARE-WAVE JERKS. Macrosquare-square wave jerks are horizontal and large (10–40°) and have intersaccadic intervals of about 100msec. They are found in cerebellar disorders (e.g., multiple sclerosis and olivopontocerebellar atrophy) and occur sporadically or in bursts.

MACROSACCADIC OSCILLATIONS. Macrosaccadic oscillations are a type of saccadic dysmetria. A hypermetric saccade overshoots the target and is followed by a series of hypermetric, corrective saccades that straddle the target and gradually decrease in size until the target is fixated. The intersaccadic intervals are 200msec long. Macrosaccadic oscillations are associated with cerebellar disorders.

VOLUNTARY "NYSTAGMUS." Normal subjects can voluntarily produce bursts of high-frequency (10–20Hz), small-amplitude (a few degrees), horizontal, saccadic oscillations, called voluntary "nystagmus." This is not a true nystagmus, because it consists of to-and-fro, back-to-back saccades. Because no intersaccadic intervals occur, visual acuity is poor, and oscillopsia is present during the oscillations. Voluntary "nystagmus" cannot be sustained for more than several seconds; subjects show signs of intense effort, such as squinting, facial muscle contractions, and convergence.

SACCADIC PULSES. Saccadic pulses are saccadic intrusions in which saccades move the eyes away from the fixation target, followed by a rapid drift back to the target (glissade). They represent saccadic pulses without steps; they can occur singly, in a series, or in a train (saccadic pulse train) that mimics nystagmus (abducting nystagmus of internuclear ophthalmoplegia). Saccadic pulses occur in normal subjects, patients who have myoclonus, and patients who have multiple sclerosis. Double saccadic pulses are pairs of saccadic pulses that move in opposing directions and occur back-to-back with no intersaccadic intervals. They are part of a continuum of other saccadic oscillations with no intersaccadic intervals (ocular flutter and opsoclonus).

OCULAR FLUTTER. Ocular flutter consists of bursts of moderately large-amplitude, horizontal, back-to-back saccades without intersaccadic intervals. Blurred vision and oscillopsia usually are present. Ocular flutter can occur in the primary position and after a refixation saccade (flutter dysmetria); it is associated with the same disorders of the brainstem and cerebellum that produce opsoclonus (see next section). Eyelid blinks induce bursts of large-amplitude flutter in neurodegenerative disorders and a few beats of low-amplitude flutter in normal subjects.

OPSOCLONUS. In opsoclonus, a series of large-amplitude, back-to-back, multidirectional saccades interrupt fixation. The directions of the to-and-fro saccades can be horizontal, vertical, or oblique; their trajectories can be linear or curvilinear, and the frequency is high (10–15Hz). The chaotic appearance of the oscillations has led to the use of the term "saccadomania." In its severe form, opsoclonus is nearly continuous and persists even in some stages of sleep. With improvement, or in its milder form, the oscillations are intermittent. During fixation, saccadic burst cells in the pontine paramedian reticular formation (horizontal saccades) and in the rostral interstitial nucleus of the MLF (vertical saccades) are inhibited by tonic activity in pause cells in the nucleus raphe interpositus in the midbrain. Pause cell activity is momentarily inhibited during saccades, which allows the burst cells to fire and generate the saccadic pulse signal. An abnormal decrease in pause cell activity as a result of direct damage to these cells or abnormal input to them from other neurons might produce opsoclonus and ocular flutter.

Opsoclonus often is associated with cerebellar ataxia and limb myoclonus. The disorders that cause opsoclonus damage the brainstem or cerebellum; they include benign brainstem encephalitis in children and adults following viral illnesses, myoclonic encephalopathy of infants (dancing eyes and dancing feet), paraneoplastic brainstem and cerebellar syndromes in children (neuroblastoma) and adults (small cell lung carcinoma, breast carcinoma, ovarian tumors), and multiple sclerosis.[29,30] Opsoclonus and ocular flutter have been reported in association with drug toxicities, exposure to toxic chemicals, and hyperosmolar coma and as transient findings in normal neonates. Adrenocorticotropic hormone can diminish the saccadic oscillations of infantile myoclonic encephalopathy and neuroblastoma, and corticosteroids can be effective in paraneoplastic syndromes in adults. Some normal subjects can produce saccadic oscillations volitionally, including many of the characteristics of opsoclonus and ocular flutter.[31]

TREATMENT

Drug Treatment

The goal of treating vestibular nystagmus is mainly to diminish the associated vertigo. The large number of medications that are used is an indication that no optimal drug therapy exists for most patients. The classes of drugs include anticholinergics (scopolamine [hyoscine]), antihistamines (meclizine), monoaminergics (ephedrine), benzodiazepines (diazepam), phenothiazines (prochlorperazine), and butyrophenones (droperidol). Unfortunately, drowsiness from many of these drugs limits their efficacy for chronic, recurrent vertigo. An exception is acetazolamide, which is very effective for the treatment of familial periodic ataxia with nystagmus.[32]

The goal in the treatment of nonvestibular forms of nystagmus and saccadic oscillations is to improve vision by ameliorating the associated blurring and oscillopsia. As in vestibular nystagmus, many medications have been tried, but few have been found to be consistently effective.[33] Only a few double-blind studies have been carried out: anticholinergics for acquired pendular nystagmus,[34] and muscarinic antagonists for acquired pendular and downbeat nystagmus.[35]

Baclofen is an analog of γ-aminobutyric acid and was developed to treat skeletal muscle spasm. It consistently decreases the symptoms and signs of periodic alternating nystagmus.[36] To diminish the side effect of drowsiness, the initial dosage is low, 5mg by mouth three times a day, and is increased gradually. Patients perceive a return of symptoms after a few hours. The drug is not taken at bedtime, because the beneficial effects are not appreciated. Some patients who have congenital nystagmus report that their vision improves with baclofen, and in a few patients, nystagmus has been found to decrease slightly with an increase in the null zone of least nystagmus intensity. Baclofen decreases the slow component velocity and oscillopsia in some patients who have upbeat and downbeat nystagmus.[37] Its therapeutic effect might result from augmentation of the physiological inhibitory effect of γ-aminobutyric acid on the vestibular nuclei in the vestibulocerebellum and on the velocity storage mechanism.

Clonazepam is an antiepileptic agent that has been shown to decrease downbeat nystagmus in some patients.[38] Its most common side effect is drowsiness. The initial dosage of 0.5mg by mouth three times a day is increased gradually. Recently, gabapentin (900–1500mg/day) has been shown to decrease, but not abolish, acquired pendular nystagmus in a few patients.[39] Adrenocorticotropic hormone can diminish ocular flutter and opsoclonus in infantile myoclonic encephalopathy and neuroblastoma. Corticosteroids can decrease these saccadic oscillations in paraneoplastic, cerebellar ataxia syndromes in adults. Carbamazepine, baclofen, and clonazepam have been used to treat superior oblique myokymia. Isoniazid in dosages of 800–1000mg/day decreased acquired pendular nystagmus in two patients who had multiple sclerosis.[40]

Optical Treatment

In congenital nystagmus, convergence and eccentric gaze often decrease the nystagmus and improve vision. To induce convergence, 7D (prism) of base-out prism can be placed in each spectacle lens. If the patient is young, −1.00D can be added to the spherical correction. If the null zone is in horizontal eccentric gaze, the spectacle prism powers can be modified to incorporate a prism effect in which the eyes conjugately rotate toward the null zone (prism apices toward the null zone). Contact lenses have fewer optical aberrations and usually correct the refractive errors in patients who have congenital nystagmus more effectively than do spectacles. In addition, tactile sensory feedback from the contact lenses might diminish the nystagmus intensity. One congenital nystagmus patient reported transient oscillopsia when contact lenses were removed after a short therapeutic trial.[41]

The combination of a high plus spectacle lens and a high minus contact lens for one eye has been devised to stabilize retinal images in that eye and improve vision.[42] This combination places the image at the eye's center of rotation. However, because vestibulo-ocular eye movements and volitional eye movements do not cause retinal image movement with these lenses, walking is difficult.

A patient who had ocular myoclonus was found to have vertical pendular nystagmus in one eye and horizontal pendular nystagmus in the other. Patching the eye that had vertical nystagmus caused an esotropia of that eye but resulted in disappearance of the horizontal nystagmus in the other.[43]

In patients who have MLN, spectacle treatment for an accommodative component of their esotropia can transform MLN to latent nystagmus or decrease MLN, each of which leads to an improvement of binocular visual acuity.[44]

Surgical Treatment

An eccentric null zone in congenital nystagmus often produces a habitual face turn. If marked, the face turn can cause difficulties when viewing at distance or reading; in addition, it can be a cosmetic problem. Resections and recessions of the four horizontal rectus muscles can move the null zone toward the primary position (Anderson-Kestenbaum procedure), which improves vision in the primary position.[45,46] However, months after the surgery, the null zone may become eccentric again. If convergence decreases congenital nystagmus significantly, surgery to induce a greater convergence effort can be combined with the Anderson-Kestenbaum procedure.[47] Large recessions of all four horizontal rectus muscles are designed to symmetrically weaken the muscles and can reduce nystagmus intensity. Diplopia and limitation of ductions reportedly have not been significant problems.[48,49] Occasionally, bilateral vertical rectus recessions or bilateral, combined vertical rectus recession-resections are performed to correct vertical head postures in congenital nystagmus.[50] Rarely, surgery of the oblique muscles is used to correct a head tilt.[51]

In patients who have strabismus and MLN, strabismus surgery can change the MLN to latent nystagmus and improve binocular visual acuity.[44] In Arnold-Chiari malformations, suboccipital decompression can diminish downbeat nystagmus if permanent damage to the midline cerebellum and lower brainstem has not occurred. Procedures to weaken the superior oblique and ipsilateral inferior oblique muscles have been used to treat superior oblique myokymia.

Other Treatments

A variety of other therapies have been used to treat nystagmus. Of these, the Epley maneuver for BPPN is by far the most effective.[3] Tactile stimulation of the face and neck,[52] auditory biofeedback, and acupuncture have been shown by electronic recordings to decrease congenital nystagmus. However, their efficacy outside of the laboratory setting has not been established. Retrobulbar injections or intramuscular injections of botulinum A toxin decrease nystagmus by paralyzing the extraocular muscles. They have been used to treat congenital nystagmus,[53] latent nystagmus,[54] and acquired nystagmus.[55] The paralysis is temporary, requiring repetition of the injection every few months. The side effects are diplopia, ptosis, filamentary keratitis, and increased nystagmus in the noninjected eye from plastic-adaptive changes in response to the paresis of the injected eye.[56,57]

REFERENCES

1. Leigh RJ. Clinical features and pathogenesis of acquired forms of nystagmus. Bailliéres Clin Neurol. 1992;1:393–416.
2. Lopez L, Bronstein AM, Gresty MA, et al. Torsional nystagmus. A neuro-otological and MRI study of thirty-five cases. Brain. 1992;1115:1107–24.
3. Epley JM. The canalith repositioning procedure: for treatment of benign paroxysmal positional nystagmus. Otolaryngol Head Neck Surg. 1992;107:399–404.
4. Herdman SJ, Tusa RJ. Complications of the canalith repositioning procedure. Arch Otolaryngol Head Neck Surg. 1996;122:281–6.
5. Brandt T. Positional and positioning vertigo and nystagmus. J Neurol Sci. 1990; 95:3–28.
6. Kerrison JB, Arnould VJ, Barmada MM, et al. A gene for autosomal dominant congenital nystagmus localizes to 6p12. Genomics. 1996;33:523–6.
7. Patton MA, Jeffery S, Lee N, Hogg C. Congenital nystagmus cosegregating with a balanced 7;15 translocation. J Med Genet. 1993;30:526–8.
8. Ciancia AD. On infantile esotropia with nystagmus in abduction. J Pediatr Ophthalmol Strabismus. 1995;32:280–8.
9. Abadi RJ, Pascal F. Periodic alternating nystagmus in humans with albinism. Invest Ophthalmol Vis Sci. 1994;35:4080–6.
10. Hirose G, Kawada J, Tsukada K, et al. Upbeat nystagmus: clinicopathological and pathophysiological considerations. J Neurol Sci. 1991;105:159–67.
11. Yee RD. Downbeat nystagmus: characteristics and localization of lesions. Trans Am Ophthalmol Soc. 1989;87:984–1032.
12. Lopez LI, Gresty MA, Bronstein AM, et al. Acquired pendular nystagmus: oculomotor and MRI findings. Brain. 1996;119:265–72.
13. Gottlob I, Wizov SS, Reinecke RD. Spasmus nutans. A long-term follow-up. Invest Ophthalmol Vis Sci. 1995;36:2768–71.
14. Jan LE, Groenveld M, Connolly MD. Head shaking by visually-impaired children: a voluntary neurovisual adaptation which can be confused with spasmus nutans. Dev Med Child Neurol. 1990;32:1061–8.
15. Gottlob I, Wizov SS, Reinecke RD. Head and eye movements in children with low vision. Graefes Arch Clin Exp Ophthalmol. 1996;234:369–77.
16. Gottlob I, Zubcov A, Catalano RA, et al. Signs distinguishing spasmus nutans (with and without central nervous system lesions) from infantile nystagmus. Ophthalmology. 1990;97:1166–75.
17. Newman SA, Hedges TR, Wall M, Sedwick A. Spasmus nutans—or is it? Surv Ophthalmol. 1990;34:453–6.
18. Arnoldi KA, Tychsen L. Prevalence of intracranial lesions in children initially diagnosed with disconjugate nystagmus (spasmus nutans). J Pediatr Ophthalmol Strabismus. 1995;32:296–301.
19. Good WV, Koch TS, Jan JE. Monocular nystagmus caused by unilateral anterior visual-pathway disease. Dev Med Child Neurol. 1993;35:1106–10.
20. Halmagyi GM, Aw ST, Dehaene I, et al. Jerk-waveform see-saw nystagmus due to unilateral mesodiencephalic lesion. Brain. 1994;117:789–803.
21. Thomke F, Hopf C. Abduction nystagmus in internuclear ophthalmoplegia. Acta Neurol Scand. 1992;86:365–70.
22. Wagner RS, Caputo AR, Reynolds RD. Nystagmus in Down's syndrome. Ophthalmology. 1990;97:1439–44.
23. Averbuch-Heller L, Zivotofsky AZ, Remler BF, et al. Convergent-divergent pendular nystagmus: possible role of the vergence system. Neurology. 1995;45:509–15.
24. Mossman SS, Bronstein AM, Gresty MA, et al. Convergence nystagmus associated with Arnold-Chiari malformation. Arch Neurol. 1990;47:357–9.
25. Adler CH, Galetta SL. Oculo-facial-skeletal myorhythmia of Whipple's disease. Ann Intern Med. 1990;112:467–9.
26. Brazis PW. Ocular motor abnormalities in Wallenberg's lateral medullary syndrome. Mayo Clin Proc. 1992;67:365–8.
27. Kaplan PW, Tusa RJ. Neurophysiologic and clinical correlations of epileptic nystagmus. Neurology. 1993;43:2508–14.
28. Tusa RJ, Kaplan PW, Hain TC, Naidu S. Ipsiversive eye deviation and epileptic nystagmus. Neurology. 1990;40:662–5.
29. Fisher PG, Wechsler DS, Singer HS. Anti-Hu antibody in a neuroblastoma-associated neoplastic syndrome. Pediatr Neurol. 1994;10:309–12.
30. Digre K. Opsoclonus in adults. Report of three cases and review of the literature. Arch Neurol. 1986;43:1165–75.
31. Yee RD, Spiegel PH, Yamada T, et al. Voluntary saccadic oscillations, resembling ocular flutter and opsoclonus. J Neuroophthalmol. 1994;14:95–101.
32. Van Boggert P, Van Nechel C, Goldman S, Szliwowski HB. Acetazolamide-responsive hereditary paroxysmal ataxia: report of a new family. Acta Neurol Belg. 1993;93:268–75.
33. Leigh RJ, Averbuch-Heller L, Tomsak RL, et al. Treatment of abnormal eye movements that impair vision: strategies based on movement—current concepts of physiology and pharmacology. Ann Neurol. 1994;36:129–41.
34. Leigh RJ, Burnstine TH, Ruff RL, Kasmer RJ. Effect of anticholinergic agents upon acquired nystagmus: a double blind study of trihexyphenidyl and tridihexethyl chloride. J Clin Neuroophthalmol. 1991;11:166–8.
35. Barton JJ, Huaman AG, Sharpe JA. Muscarinic antagonists in the treatment of acquired pendular and downbeat nystagmus. Ann Neurol. 1994;35:319–25.
36. Troost BT, Janton F, Weaver R. Periodic alternating oscillopsia: a symptom of alternating nystagmus abolished by baclofen. J Clin Neuroophthalmol. 1990;10: 273–7.
37. Dieterich M, Straube A, Brandt T, et al. The effects of baclofen and cholinergic drugs on upbeat and downbeat nystagmus. J Neurol Neurosurg Psychiatry. 1991; 54:627–32.
38. Currie JN, Matsuo V. The use of clonazepam in the treatment of nystagmus-induced oscillopsia. Ophthalmology. 1986;93:924–32.
39. Stahl JS, Rottach KG, Avercuh-Heller L, et al. A pilot study of gabapentin as a treatment for acquired nystagmus. Neuroophthalmology. 1996;16:107–13.
40. Traccis S, Rosati G, Monaco MF, et al. Successful treatment of acquired pendular nystagmus with isoniazid and base-out prisms. Neurology. 1990;40:492–4.
41. Safran AR, Gambazzi Y. Congenital nystagmus: rebound phenomenon following removal of contact lenses. Br J Ophthalmol. 1992;76:497–8.
42. Yaniglos SS, Leigh RJ. Refinement of an optical device that stabilizes vision in patients with nystagmus. Optom Vis Sci. 1992;69:447–50.
43. Herishanu YO, Zigoulinski R. The effect of chronic one-eye patching on ocular myoclonus. J Clin Neuroophthalmol. 1991;11:116–8.
44. Zubcov AA, Reinecke RD, Gottlob I. Treatment of manifest latent nystagmus. Am J Ophthalmol. 1990;110:160–7.
45. Pratt-Johnson JA. Results of surgery to modify the null-zone position in congenital nystagmus. Can J Ophthalmol. 1991;26:219–23.
46. Kraft SP, O'Donoghue EP, Roarty JD. Improvement of compensatory head postures after strabismus surgery. Ophthalmology. 1992;99:1301–8.
47. Zubcov AA, Stark N, Weber A, et al. Improvement in visual acuity after surgery for nystagmus. Ophthalmology. 1993;100:1488–97.
48. Helveston EM, Ellis FD, Plager DA. Large recession of the horizontal recti for treatment of nystagmus. Ophthalmology. 1991;98:1302–5.
49. von Noorden GK, Sprunger DT. Large rectus muscle recessions for the treatment of congenital nystagmus. Arch Ophthalmol. 1991;109:221–4.
50. Sigal MB, Diamond GR. Survey of management strategies for nystagmus patients with vertical or torsional head posture. Ann Ophthalmol. 1990;22:134–8.
51. Prakash P, Arya AV, Sharma P, Chandra VM. Torsional Kestenbaum in congenital nystagmus with torticollis. Indian J Ophthalmol. 1990;38:70–3.
52. Sheth NV, Dell'Osso LF, Leigh RJ, et al. The effects of afferent stimulation on congenital nystagmus foveation periods. Vision Res. 1995;35:2371–82.
53. Carruthers J. The treatment of congenital nystagmus with Botox. J Pediatr Ophthalmol Strabismus. 1995;32:306–8.
54. Liu C, Gresty M, Lee J. Management of symptomatic latent nystagmus. Eye. 1993;7:550–3.
55. Ruben ST, Lee JP, O'Neil D, et al. The use of botulinum toxin for treatment of acquired nystagmus. Ophthalmology. 1994;101:783–7.
56. Leigh RJ, Tomsak RL, Grant MP, et al. Effectiveness of botulinum toxin administered to abolish acquired nystagmus. Ann Neurol. 1992;32:633–42.
57. Tomsak RL, Remler BF, Averbuch-Heller L, et al. Unsatisfactory treatment of acquired nystagmus with retrobulbar injection of botulinum toxin. Am J Ophthalmol. 1995;119:489–96.

203 The Pupils

RANDY H. KARDON

DEFINITION

- Pupillary disorders may be classified into two major categories—afferent and efferent.
- Afferent pupillary defects interfere with the input of light to the pupillomotor system by light blockage or deficits in any of the retinal layers, into the optic nerve, chiasm, optic tract, or midbrain pretectal area. All of these result in a symmetrical decrease in the contraction of both pupils to light given to the damaged eye, compared with light given to the other less damaged or normal eye.
- Efferent pupillary defects interfere with contraction or dilatation of the pupil due to damage in the midbrain, in the peripheral nerve that supplies the iris muscles, or in the iris muscles themselves, often leading to asymmetrical pupils (anisocoria).

KEY FEATURES

- Relative afferent pupillary defects cause a reduction in pupil contraction when one eye is stimulated by light compared with when the opposite eye is stimulated by light.
- Efferent pupillary defects cause anisocoria, a difference in pupil size between the right and left eyes, the extent of which depends on the condition of lighting or near effort.

ASSOCIATED FEATURES

- Relative afferent pupillary defects may be associated with visual field or electroretinographic asymmetries between the two eyes. Asymmetrical differences in retinal appearance or optic nerve appearance may occur.
- Efferent pupillary defects may be associated with either damage to the parasympathetic or sympathetic nerves that supply the iris or direct damage to the iris sphincter or dilator muscles that results in immobility of the pupil.

INTRODUCTION

In this chapter the pupil is discussed from a practical, clinical standpoint. The focus is on features of pupil examination that enable effective diagnosis and management of a variety of diseases of the afferent visual system and of diseases that affect pupil size. The chapter is divided into two main portions—one on the use of pupil examination to assess afferent visual input and the second on the diagnostic implications of abnormal integration of the efferent output to the pupils. Abnormal integration may result in pupils of unequal diameter (anisocoria), pupils that do not dilate well in darkness, or a light–near dissociation, in which pupil contraction to a near reflex greatly exceeds the pupil constriction to a light reflex.

RELATIVE AFFERENT PUPILLARY DEFECTS

In general, the most important clinical use of the pupil is in the assessment of afferent input from the retina, optic nerve, and subsequent anterior visual pathways (chiasm, optic tract, and midbrain pathways). Because the pupillary light reflex represents the sum of the entire neuronal input (photoreceptors, bipolar cells, ganglion cells, and axons of ganglion cells), damage anywhere along this portion of the visual pathway reduces the amplitude of pupil movement in response to a light stimulus.[1,2] Thus, the clinician can establish any asymmetrical damage between the two eyes by a simple comparison of how well the pupil contracts to a standard light shone into one eye compared with the same light shone into the other eye.[3] Observation of pupil movement in response to alternating the light back and forth between the two eyes is the basis for the alternating light test, or "swinging flashlight" test, used to assess the relative afferent pupillary defect (RAPD).[4,5]

Another important aspect of pupil movement in response to light is that the pupillary light reflex summates the entire area of the visual field, with some increased weight given to the central 10°.[2] Thus, in general terms, the pupillary light reflex is roughly proportional to the amount of working visual field. Damage to peripheral portions of the retina and visual field defects outside the central field reduce the amplitude of the pupillary light reflex. Such damage may not be established by other objective tests of visual function, such as the electroretinogram and visual evoked potential.

Standard flash electroretinogram findings are affected very little by focal retinal damage that produces a visual field defect. For example, a patient who has a disciform scar caused by aged-related macular degeneration or a branch artery occlusion gives a normal flash electroretinogram result. However, in such an example, the pupillary light reflex is reduced compared with that of the other eye, and an RAPD is obvious. In addition, optic nerve disease or damage to the retinal ganglion cells is not detected by standard flash electroretinography. Assessment of the pupillary light reflex readily enables the detection of such damage.

Because the visual evoked potential primarily samples the occipital pole or tip, which represents the central 5–10° of visual field, it is not affected to any great extent by peripheral visual field defects. In addition, cooperation of the patient is required to fixate on the center of a computer monitor while the visual stimulus is presented. A patient who chooses not to fixate properly or who has media opacities that reduce the clarity of the checkerboard pattern may produce an abnormal result, even if the retina and optic nerve function are normal (i.e., a false-positive test result). Similarly, peripheral visual field defects caused by glaucoma or anterior ischemic optic neuropathy may yield a normal visual evoked potential, or false-negative result, but the pupillary light reflex is reduced.[6]

Therefore, the pupillary light reflex is one of the few objective reflexes that can be used as a clinical test for the detection and quantification of abnormalities of the retina, optic nerve, optic chiasm, or optic tract. Because the amount of RAPD is correlated, to a large extent, with the amount of asymmetry of visual field deficit between the two eyes, it also may be used to help substantiate abnormal results of perimetric testing[7-10]; this often helps the clinician to determine whether a patient's report of visual field defects is believable and trustworthy. The correlation between visual field asymmetry and RAPD also is a useful monitor of the course of disease for a worsening or improvement in function. RAPDs are, by definition, relative to the input of one eye compared with that of the other. Bilateral symmetrical damage does not produce RAPDs. Thus, a definite RAPD in one eye on the first visit but no RAPD on follow-up may represent improvement in the previously damaged eye or the development of damage in the previously better eye. Therefore, it is always important to remember that the RAPD is, indeed, relative to the other eye.

Estimation of the amount of RAPD in log units (asymmetry between the two eyes) provides an idea of how much visual field damage is present and whether it is consistent with the results of the visual field test. In addition, the amount of RAPD may indicate whether the cause of damage is consistent with the results of the pupil examination. For example, a patient affected by a small amount of macular degeneration in one eye and not the other is expected to have only a 0.3–log unit RAPD, but if that patient has a 1.0–log unit RAPD, then some other cause of visual loss is likely, such as a previous branch retinal artery occlusion or optic neuropathy (Table 203-1).

In general, with unilateral visual loss, loss of the central 5° of the visual field results in an RAPD of approximately 0.3 log units. Loss of the entire central area of field (10°) causes an RAPD of 0.6–0.9 log units. Each visual field quadrant outside of the macula is worth about 0.3 log units, but the temporal field loss seems to result in more loss of pupillary input compared with loss in the nasal field quadrants. The correlation between the relative afferent defect and the area and extent of visual field loss, however, is only approximate. Differences between the two may be important clues as to the cause and extent of damage to the anterior visual system.

Studies that used computerized pupillography to quantify the RAPD more precisely showed that some subjects who have normal visual fields and examination results can have a small (0.3–log unit) RAPD.[11,12]

The amount of pupillomotor input asymmetry (the RAPD) may be estimated roughly using the alternating light test (without any neutral density filters) and the subjective grades +1, +2, +3 or +4 for asymmetry of pupillary response. This subjective grading also may be categorized according to the amount of "pupil escape," or dilatation of the pupils, as the light is alternated between the eyes.[13] However, most subjective grading of RAPDs has serious limitations, such as some large-scale errors that arise from age variations in pupil size and pupil mobility. For example, a patient who has small pupils and small pupillary contractions to light may have a large RAPD, but this may appear deceptively small on the basis of small differences in pupil excursion observed as the light is alternated between the two eyes. However, the amount of neutral density filter needed to dim the better eye until the small contractions are equal represents substantial input damage. To estimate the size of RAPDs

TABLE 203-1

COMMON DISEASES THAT PRODUCE RELATIVE AFFERENT PUPILLARY DEFECTS

Condition	Site	Log Unit Relative Afferent Pupillary Defect	Influencing Factors
Intraocular hemorrhage	Anterior chamber or vitreous (dense)	0.6–1.2	Density of hemorrhage
	Anterior chamber (diffuse)	0.0–0.3	Density of hemorrhage
	Preretinal (central vein occlusion or diabetic)	0.0	Preretinal location does not significantly reduce light
Diffusing media opacity	Cataract or corneal scar	0.0–0.3 in opposite eye	Dispersion of light produces increase in light input
Unilateral functional visual field loss	None (nonorganic)	0.0	No real visual field loss
Central serous retinopathy or cystoid macular edema	Retina (fovea)	0.3	Area of retina involved, depth of scotoma
Central or branch retinal vein occlusion	Inner retina	0.3–0.6 (nonischemic) ≥0.9 (ischemic)	Area of visual field defect and degree of ischemia
Central or branch retinal artery occlusion	Inner retina	0.3–3.0	Area and location of retina involved
Retinal detachment	Outer retina	0.3–2.1	Area and location of detached retina (e.g., 0.6–0.9 log units for macula +0.3 log units for each quadrant)
Anterior ischemic optic neuropathy	Optic nerve head	0.6–2.7	Extent and location of visual field defect
Optic neuritis (acute)	Optic nerve	0.6–3.0	Extent and location of visual field defect
Optic neuritis (recovered)	Optic nerve	0.0–0.6	No visual field defect, residual relative afferent pupillary defect
Compressive optic neuropathy	Optic nerve	0.3–3.0	Extent and location of visual field defect, other eye involvment
Chiasmal compression	Optic chiasm	0.0–1.2	Asymmetry of visual field loss, unilateral central field involvement
Optic tract lesion	Optic tract	0.3–1.2 in the eye with temporal field loss	Incongruity of homonymous field defect, hemifield pupillomotor input asymmetry
Postgeniculate damage	Visual radiations Visual cortex	0.0	Stimulus light size (no residual relative afferent pupillary defect but definite pupil perimetry defects)
Midbrain tectal damage	Olivary pretectal area of pupil light input region of midbrain	0.3–1.0	Similar to optic tract lesions, but no visual field defect

The expected magnitude of defect is given as well.

without using filters is very much like the estimation of an ocular deviation "by Hirschberg" without a prism cover test. More accurate quantification of RAPDs is accomplished by determination of the log unit difference needed to "balance" the pupil reaction between the two eyes.[4,5] Photographic neutral density filters (49mm, screw mount, 0.3 log, 0.6 log, and 0.9 log) often are available through local photography stores.

Measurement of the Relative Afferent Pupillary Defect

Measurement of RAPDs is the most important part of the pupil examination, because it may give the most valuable clinical information. The alternating light test for an afferent defect is based on the assumption that the irises are a matched pair—each has sphincter and dilator muscles of good shape and properly innervated—so that the light reactions can be compared. Therefore, it is important to first establish whether an anisocoria is present, which may indicate an efferent defect.

EVALUATION OF ANISOCORIA. Pupillary inequality usually results from an iris innervation problem, so to evaluate anisocoria the iris sphincter and dilator muscles must be checked. In the office, the best way to decide whether the sphincter muscle or dilator muscle is weak is to compare the amount of anisocoria in darkness and in light, which can be carried out without any special equipment. The examiner must be able to change the lighting and still view the pupils. Of course, usually no anisocoria is found in darkness or in light, in which case the efferent arm of the light reflex arc is presumed intact, and the examiner proceeds to check for an afferent defect. When anisocoria is present, the examiner needs to establish whether it increases in darkness or in light. If one sphincter is weak, the investigator may still check for an afferent defect in the pupil that still works by comparison of its direct and consensual reactions. If no asymmetry of input is apparent, and hence no RAPD, this impression may be confirmed using the "tilt test" described below (Fig. 203-1).

Anisocoria may influence the estimate of pupillary input asymmetry. Small pupils allow less light to pass and large pupils more. However, if neither pupil is less than 3.0mm wide in light, then any anisocoria less than 2.0mm difference may be disregarded—at least with respect to a false afferent defect induced by the pupillary inequality. Only very large anisocorias cause enough difference in retinal illumination between the two eyes to produce an apparent asymmetry of pupillomotor input.

ESTABLISHMENT OF RELATIVE AFFERENT PUPILLARY DEFECT. To check for RAPD, the light is alternated from one eye to the other (Fig. 203-2). If the light is too bright, the pupils do not redilate promptly, and very little pupil movement is seen as the light is alternated to the other eye. The problem may be solved by a direct reduction in stimulus intensity or if the light is moved 3–4 inches (8–10cm) away from the eyes and alternated between them.

Observe the Illuminated Eye. If the pupils react relatively weakly when one eye is stimulated and better when the other is stimulated, an afferent defect relative to the better eye (RAPD) has been identified.

Balance the Responses Using Filters. To balance the response, a filter is held over the good eye and the alternating light test repeated. If the input asymmetry is still visible, the density of the filter over the good eye is increased until the amplitudes of the direct light reactions of the two eyes are balanced. To be certain of the measurement, the balance point may be overshot deliberately and then back titrated. When a dense filter is used, it may be necessary to look behind the filter to see the pupil (Fig. 203-3).

"TILTING"—THE DUBIOUS RELATIVE AFFERENT PUPILLARY DEFECT. If a very small asymmetry is suspected, such as a defect of less than 0.3 log units in the left eye, it may be just the result of noise in the system (e.g., "hippus"). An effort must made to confirm the asymmetry by "tilting" the RAPD to the right and to the left using a 0.3–log unit filter (see Fig. 203-1). If no RAPD exists, the examiner should be able to induce the same amount of input asymmetry by holding a 0.3–log unit filter over the right eye during the alternating light test and then repeating the test with the filter switched to the left eye. If a small RAPD is present, it will become more apparent when the filter is held over that eye.

MOMENT-TO-MOMENT VARIABILITY. Unfortunately the pupillary response to a repeated light stimulus is far from constant; it changes from moment to moment.[11,12] A common error is to judge the apparent asymmetry of the light reflex too quickly. It is important to alternate the light back and forth at least 3 times to obtain a mental average of any asymmetry. In this way, moment-to-moment fluctuations in the pupillary response are "averaged out." Despite such efforts, the afferent asymmetry may still fluctuate slightly with time, even when carefully recorded using computerized pupillography.

SMALL CHILDREN. Infants and small children may appear to have weak pupillary responses to light, largely because of the ex-

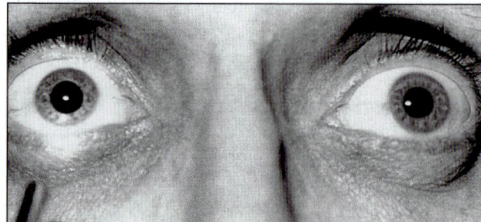

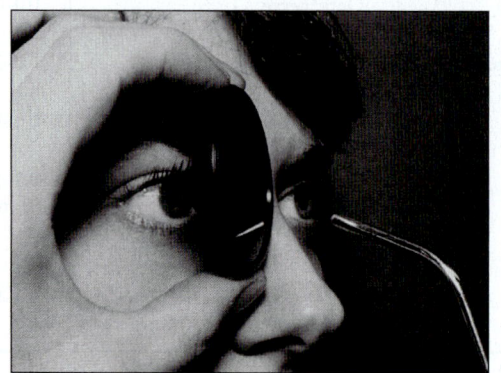

FIG. 203-2 Demonstration of a large afferent defect in the right eye. This is best demonstrated when the light is alternated from eye to eye at a steady rate. The light is kept just below the visual axis and 1–2 inches (3–5cm) from each eye. Each eye is illuminated for about 1 second and then the light switched quickly to the other eye; this allows comparison of the initial direct pupil contraction with light in each eye.

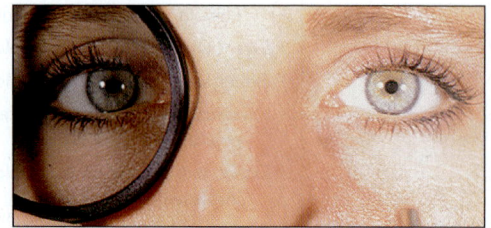

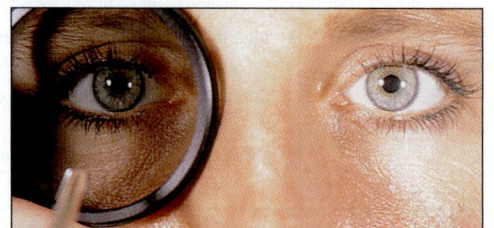

FIG. 203-1 Checking for an RAPD using the "tilt test." If there seems to be no input asymmetry, the "tilt test" can confirm this by inducing an RAPD of the same magnitude in each eye by holding a 0.3–log unit neutral density filter over one eye during the alternating light test and then repeating it with the filter over the other eye.

FIG. 203-3 Balancing pupillary response using filters. A dark iris appears even darker behind the filter so it may be difficult to view the pupil, in which case it helps to peek behind the filter to obtain a better view of the iris.

citement and apprehension that inhibit the pupillary light reflex at the supranuclear level in the midbrain. Usually, after the light stimulus has been repeated several times, the light reaction begins to improve and "loosen up," especially as the child becomes less anxious. A baby's pupils are checked at about 3ft (1m) away with a direct ophthalmoscope. In a dark room, the brightest light and smallest spot are used, focus is on the red reflex, and the light is alternated from eye to eye. The baby usually is fascinated, and a filter sometimes can be placed in the beam to one eye.

ONLY ONE WORKING PUPIL. When the input defect is in an eye that has an injured iris or a dilated pupil, the pupillary responses of the uninjured eye must be observed. The direct and consensual responses of the working pupil may be compared by alternation of the light from one eye to the other. While a measurement is made, the good eye is behind the filter and it may be hard too see the pupil. Sometimes it is necessary to use a side light on the healthy iris in order to see its consensual pupil reaction. Because this may corrupt the measurement, an infrared video system is used, if possible.

INSTRUMENTATION. Instruments are available that give a more precise evaluation of the pupillary light reflex; these include infrared video recording equipment and a computerized interface to present controlled light stimuli and quantify the dynamics of pupil movement in response to each light stimulus.

Infrared Videography. Sometimes it is important to view the magnified movement of both pupils at once. Infrared videography (Fig. 203-4) enables the examiner to see both pupils clearly in the dark, which is particularly helpful when difficult afferent pupillary defects need to be checked for (e.g., one pupil is fixed, or both irises are pigmented very darkly). Because melanin reflects infrared light, dark irises appear light and so the black pupils stand out in contrast and are viewed easily. Videography also is used to establish the dilatation lag of a Horner's pupil, to catch the brief paradoxical constriction in patients who have some retinal abnormalities (found when lights are turned out), to transilluminate the iris in pigment dispersion syndrome,[14] and in Adie's syndrome.

Computerized Pupillometry. Various computerized infrared-sensitive pupillometers are available commercially and can record precisely the dynamics of pupil movement in the light or in the dark; the results are analyzed by sophisticated software. Such systems provide quantitative information about the pupillary light reflex and, in the future, may help to automate the clinical determination of pupillary input deficits that result from retinal and optic nerve diseases.[11,12,15–17] In addition, information obtained using computerized pupillography provides evidence

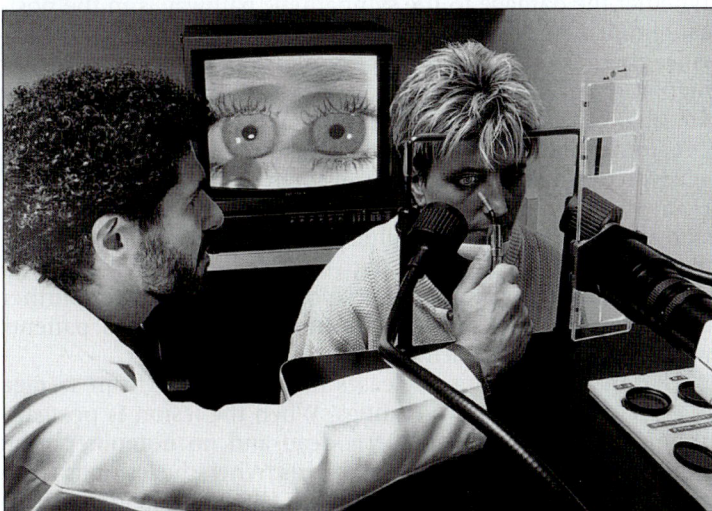

FIG. 203-4 ■ **The infrared video-pupillometer.** The infrared sources (clusters of light-emitting diodes) are mounted in gooseneck lamps. The double base–out prisms bring the pupils close together on the screen, allowing increased magnification from the infrared videocamera and telephoto lens.

that a number of different types of visual stimuli can produce changes in the pupillary light reflex, related to color, form, movement, and acuity.[18–24]

Pupil Perimetry. An automated perimeter may be modified to record pupillary responses. A video camera is pointed at the pupil and the amplitude of each light reaction is measured and stored in the computer, which is helpful as an objective form of perimetry and to localize lesions in the pupillary pathways.[25,26] Pupil perimetry is also useful in cases of nonorganic, functional visual loss to show objectively that messages are, indeed, going normally into the brain from parts of the visual field in which the patient claims to see nothing.

EFFERENT PUPILLARY DEFECTS

Anisocoria

As discussed above, a pupillary inequality usually indicates that one of the four iris muscles, or its innervation, is damaged (Fig. 203-5). To establish which is the weaker muscle, it is useful to know how the anisocoria is influenced by light. An anisocoria always increases in the direction of action of the paretic iris muscle, just as an esotropia increases when gaze is in the direction of action of a weak lateral rectus muscle.

Pupillary Inequality That Increases in the Dark

In patients who have a pupillary inequality that increases in the dark (Fig. 203-6), the problem is to differentiate Horner's syndrome from a simple anisocoria (or physiological anisocoria)—in which the inequality also is greater in dim light. A simple anisocoria may vary from day to day, or even from hour to hour, and is visible in about one fifth of the normal population; it is not related to refractive error. Clinically, Horner's syndrome is recognized by associated signs such as ptosis, "upside-down ptosis" of the lower lid and, in an acute case, conjunctival injection and lowered intraocular pressure.

Simple anisocoria is common (about 10% of normal subjects, examined in room light, have an anisocoria of 0.4mm or more) and is not associated with disease. Simple anisocoria also, like Horner's syndrome, decreases slightly in light, but it does not show a dilatation lag of the smaller pupil. It is believed that simple anisocoria most likely arises from asymmetrical inhibition at the Edinger–Westphal nucleus in the midbrain. Normally, during wakefulness some inhibition from the reticular activating formation keeps the pupils midsize or larger. During sleep, this inhibition fades and allows the neurons in the Edinger–Westphal nucleus to discharge, which results in miotic pupils. If, during wakefulness, the inhibition is greater to the right Edinger–Westphal nucleus than the left, the right pupil is larger, especially in dim light. When light is added or a near reflex is generated, this inhibition is overcome and the pupils become smaller and any asymmetrical inhibition diminishes. A reduction of the anisocoria results as the pupils become smaller.

PUPIL DILATATION RATE. The characteristic "dilatation lag" of the pupil in Horner's syndrome is seen easily in the office using a handheld light shone from below. The room lights are switched off and the smaller pupil examined for an apparent reluctance to dilate. Pupil dilatation is normally a combination of sphincter relaxation and dilator contraction, a combination that produces a prompt dilatation. The patient who has Horner's syndrome has a weak dilator muscle in one iris and, as a result, that pupil dilates more slowly than the normal pupil. If the sympathetic lesion is complete, the affected pupil dilates only by sphincter relaxation. The resultant asymmetry of pupil dilatation produces an anisocoria that is largest 4–5sec after the lights have been turned out—the process is much slower than is generally thought. At 10–20sec after the lights have been put out, the anisocoria lessens as the sympathectomized pupil gradually catches up, a process referred to as *dilatation lag.* The test is a quick and simple way to differentiate Horner's syndrome from simple anisocoria, and it does not re-

PARASYMPATHETIC AND SYMPATHETIC INNERVATION OF THE IRIS MUSCLES

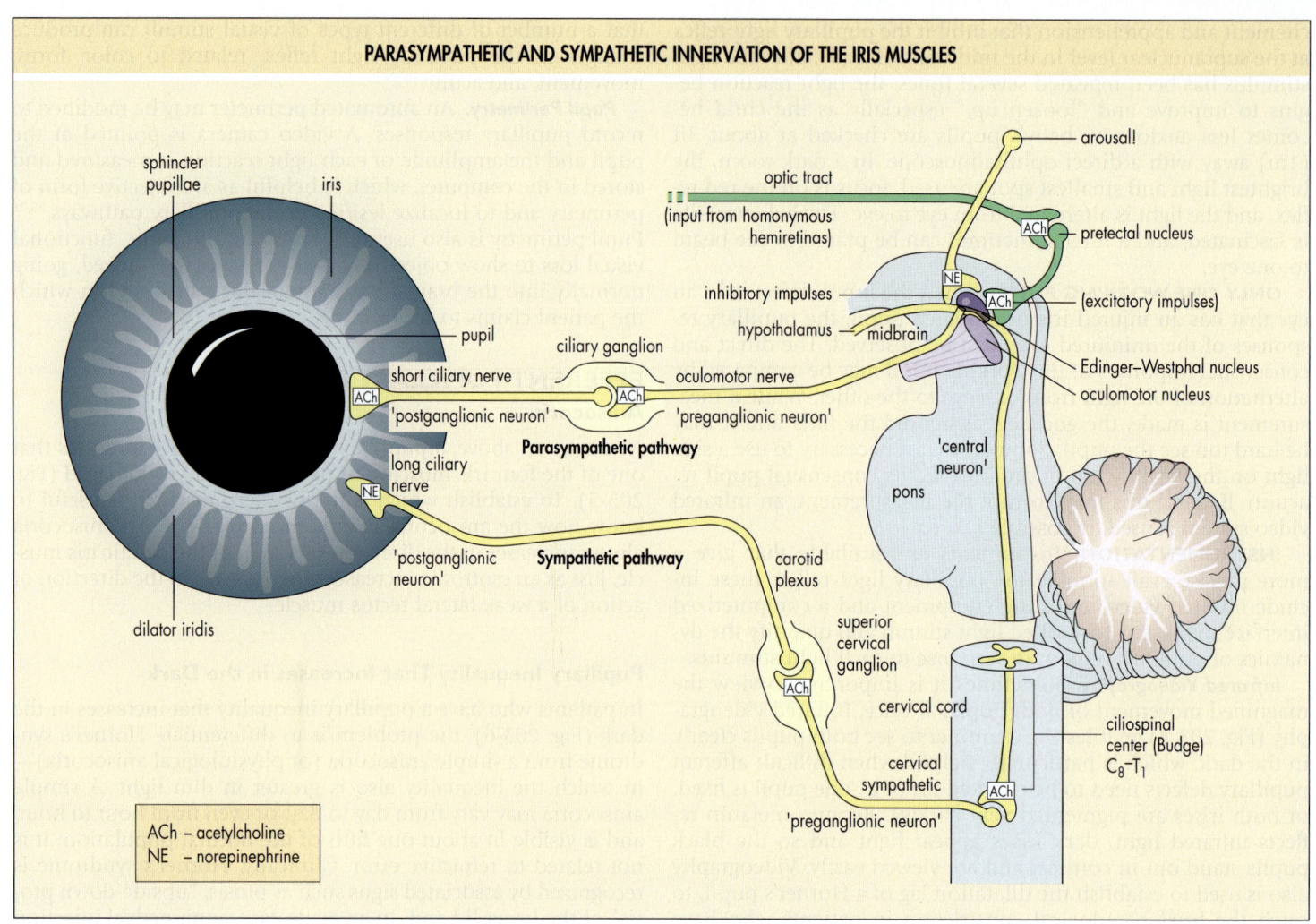

FIG. 203-5 ■ Parasympathetic and sympathetic innervation of the iris muscles.

quire pupillary drug tests. It works well most of the time, particularly in young people who have mobile pupils, but if the dilatation lag is inconclusive, cocaine eye drops may be used to confirm the diagnosis of Horner's syndrome.

DIAGNOSIS OF HORNER'S SYNDROME—COCAINE TESTING. The action of cocaine is to block the reuptake of norepinephrine (noradrenaline) normally released from the nerve endings. If, because of an interruption in the sympathetic pathway, norepinephrine is not released, cocaine has no adrenergic effect. The affected pupil in a patient with Horner's syndrome dilates less with cocaine than does the normal pupil, regardless of the location of the lesion. Cocaine drops are placed in both eyes and after 60 minutes the anisocoria has increased clearly, because the normal pupil has dilated more than the Horner's pupil.

The author recommends cocaine hydrochloride 10% in both eyes (not more than two drops) to ensure that even the darkest iris receives a full mydriatic dose; corneal epithelial defects will not result from this dose. Cocaine 2%, 4%, and 5% also have been used in diagnostic tests for Horner's syndrome and work well. Anisocoria is measured after 50–60 minutes have elapsed. If very little dilatation of the pupil occurs, even though an oculosympathetic defect is suspected, and the pupil did not dilate well in darkness even after 30 seconds before the cocaine test, then a false-positive cocaine test result must be considered. A false-positive result may occur if the iris is held in a miotic state, through either scarring or aberrant reinnervation of the iris sphincter. In such cases, the addition of a direct-acting sympathomimetic agent to both eyes (e.g., 2.5% phenylephrine) at the conclusion of a positive cocaine test should dilate the suspected eye easily and eliminate the cocaine-induced anisocoria almost immediately. For the reasons stated above, pseudo–Horner's

syndrome results in inadequate dilatation to direct-acting sympathomimetic agents. The likelihood of Horner's syndrome increases steadily as the degree of pupillary inequality (measured after the instillation of cocaine) increases. Unlike in the hydroxyamphetamine test, calculation of the change in anisocoria from before to after cocaine application is unnecessary. If there is at least 0.8mm of pupillary inequality after cocaine administration, Horner's syndrome is highly likely.[27]

LOCATION OF DAMAGE TO THE SYMPATHETIC PATHWAY. Whether the damage to the sympathetic pathway is in the postganglionic neuron is a question of considerable clinical importance, because many postganglionic defects are caused by benign, vascular headache syndromes or carotid dissections, and a preganglionic lesion sometimes results from the spread of a malignant neoplasm.

Hydroxyamphetamine eyedrops help to localize the lesion in Horner's syndrome. The clinician needs to know where the lesion is to direct the radiographic workup, for example, to the internal carotid artery rather than to the pulmonary apex. Horner's syndrome sometimes manifests so characteristically that further efforts to localize the lesion are not needed, as with patients who have cluster headaches.

Hydroxyamphetamine releases norepinephrine from storage in the sympathetic nerve endings. When the lesion is postganglionic, the third order nerve is dead and no norepinephrine stores are available for release at the iris. When the lesion is complete, the pupil does not dilate at all. However, the dying neurons and their stores of norepinephrine may last for almost 1 week from the onset of damage. Therefore, a hydroxyamphetamine test administered within 1 week of a postganglionic lesion may give a false preganglionic localization if some of the norep-

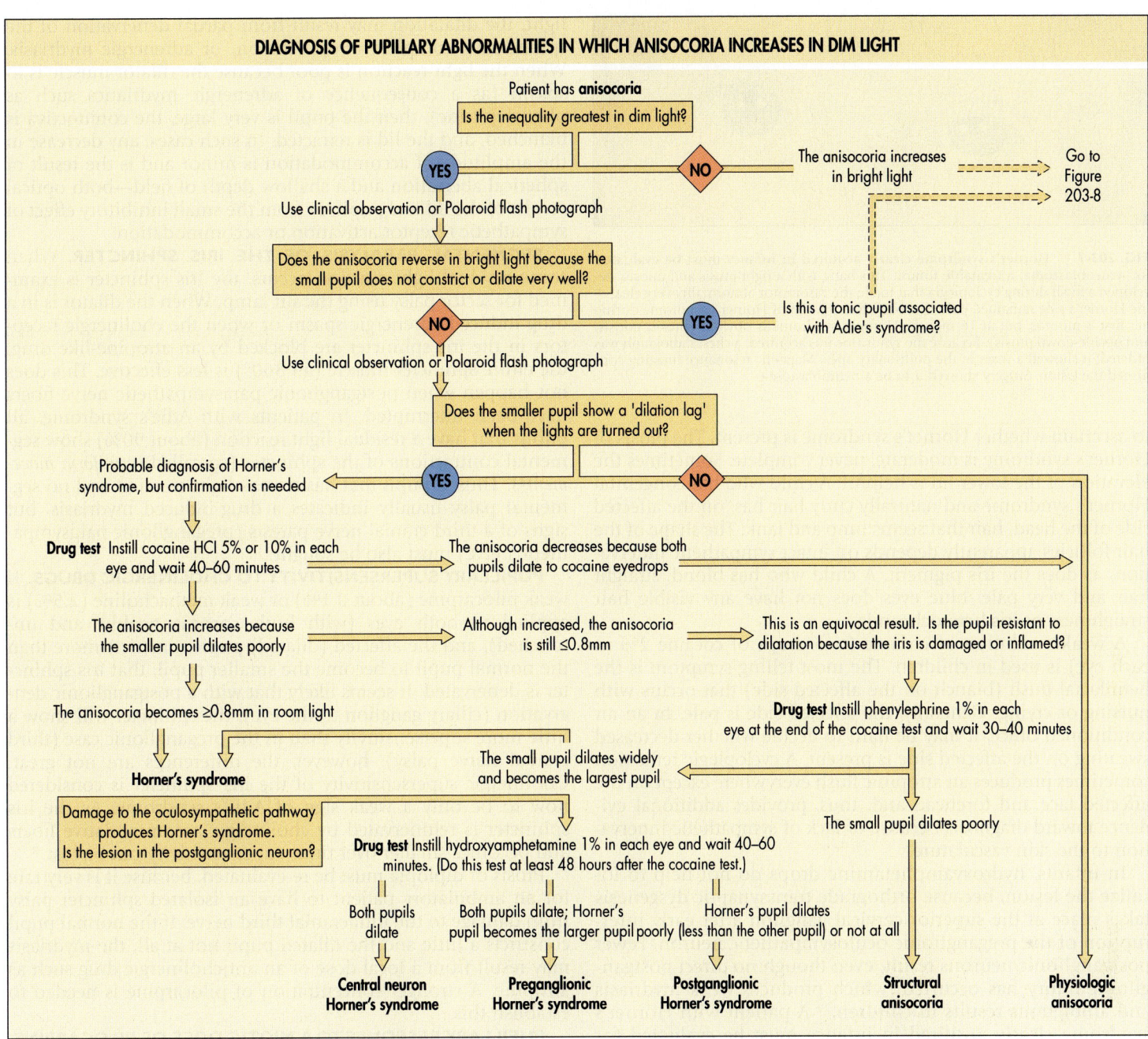

DIAGNOSIS OF PUPILLARY ABNORMALITIES IN WHICH ANISOCORIA INCREASES IN DIM LIGHT

Patient has **anisocoria**

Is the inequality greatest in dim light?

YES — Use clinical observation or Polaroid flash photograph

NO — The anisocoria increases in bright light → Go to Figure 203-8

Does the anisocoria reverse in bright light because the small pupil does not constrict or dilate very well?

YES — Is this a tonic pupil associated with Adie's syndrome?

NO — Use clinical observation or Polaroid flash photograph

Does the smaller pupil show a 'dilation lag' when the lights are turned out?

YES — Probable diagnosis of Horner's syndrome, but confirmation is needed

NO

Drug test Instill cocaine HCl 5% or 10% in each eye and wait 40–60 minutes

The anisocoria decreases because both pupils dilate to cocaine eyedrops

The anisocoria increases because the smaller pupil dilates poorly

Although increased, the anisocoria is still ≤0.8mm

This is an equivocal result. Is the pupil resistant to dilatation because the iris is damaged or inflamed?

The anisocoria becomes ≥0.8mm in room light

Horner's syndrome

Damage to the oculosympathetic pathway produces Horner's syndrome. Is the lesion in the postganglionic neuron?

The small pupil dilates widely and becomes the largest pupil

Drug test Instill phenylephrine 1% in each eye at the end of the cocaine test and wait 30–40 minutes

The small pupil dilates poorly

Drug test Instill hydroxyamphetamine 1% in each eye and wait 40–60 minutes. (Do this test at least 48 hours after the cocaine test.)

Both pupils dilate

Both pupils dilate; Horner's pupil becomes the larger pupil poorly (less than the other pupil)

Horner's pupil dilates poorly (less than the other pupil) or not at all

Central neuron Horner's syndrome

Preganglionic Horner's syndrome

Postganglionic Horner's syndrome

Structural anisocoria

Physiologic anisocoria

FIG. 203-6 ■ **Diagnosis of pupillary abnormalities in which anisocoria increases in dim light.** If the anisocoria is greatest in dim light and diminishes in bright light, then the pupillary inequality is either physiological (a simple anisocoria) or arises from the loss of sympathetic innervation to the dilator muscle (Horner's syndrome). A few other conditions need to be considered, but this chart is concerned only with acute damage to a single intraocular muscle or its innervation. (Adapted from Thompson HS, Kardon RH: Clinical importance of pupillary inequality, Focal Points: Clinical Modules for Ophthalmologists, vol 10, no 10, December, 1992, American Academy of Ophthalmology.)

inephrine stores remain. When Horner's syndrome is caused by preganglionic or central lesions, the pupils dilate normally, because the postganglionic third order neuron and its stores of norepinephrine, although disconnected, are still intact; when the lesion is in the preganglionic neuron, the involved pupil often becomes larger than the normal pupil after hydroxyamphetamine administration, apparently because of "decentralization supersensitivity."

INTERPRETATION OF THE HYDROXYAMPHETAMINE TEST. The test is simple—the pupil diameters are measured before and 40–60 minutes after hydroxyamphetamine drops have been placed in both eyes. The change in anisocoria in room light is noted. If the affected pupil—the smaller one—dilates less than the normal pupil, an increase in anisocoria occurs, and the lesion is in the postganglionic neuron. If the smaller pupil now dilates so much that it becomes the larger pupil, the lesion is preganglionic and the postganglionic neuron is intact. The examiner must wait at least 2 days after cocaine has been used

before the administration of hydroxyamphetamine; cocaine seems to block its effectiveness.

In about one half of ambulatory patients with Horner's syndrome, the location of the lesion is identified satisfactorily by the nature and location of the injury or disease. The other half of these patients offer no clues as to the location of the damage—a pharmacological localization of the lesion in these patients can be most helpful.

The author has attempted to apply the results of hydroxyamphetamine mydriasis in those patients with a known lesion location to those in whom the lesion location is unknown. It appears that postganglionic lesions (along the carotid artery) can be separated from the nonpostganglionic lesions (in the brainstem, spinal cord, upper lung, and lower neck) with a degree of certainty that varies with the amount of anisocoria induced when the drops are placed in both eyes.[28]

CONGENITAL HORNER'S SYNDROME. When a child is observed to have a unilateral ptosis and miosis, the first question is

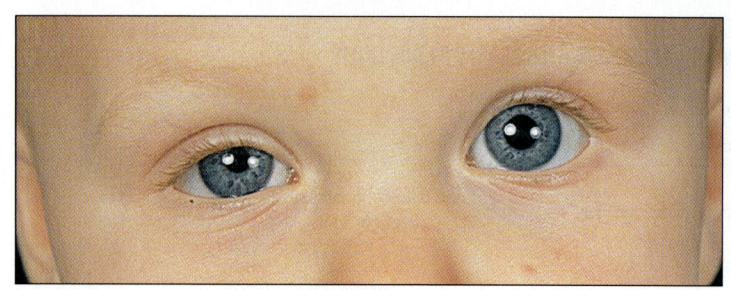

FIG. 203-7 ■ Horner's syndrome clearly acquired in infancy must be evaluated for neuroblastoma, a treatable tumor. This baby, with a right ptosis and miosis, developed a flush during cycloplegia that made the vasomotor abnormality very clear—the Horner's side remained pale. The baby had no sign of Horner's syndrome during her first 8 months, but at 16 months Horner's syndrome is obvious (ptosis, miosis, and upside-down ptosis). Because the syndrome was acquired, a chest radiograph was ordered; it showed a mass in the pulmonary apex. Magnetic resonance imaging confirmed the lesion. Surgery showed it to be a neuroblastoma.

to ascertain whether Horner's syndrome is present. The ptosis of Horner's syndrome is moderate, never complete. Sometimes the elevation of the lower lid is helpful. A child who has congenital Horner's syndrome and naturally curly hair has, on the affected side of the head, hair that seems limp and lank. The shape of the hair follicles apparently depends on intact sympathetic innervation, as does the iris pigment. A child who has blond, straight hair and very pale, blue eyes does not have any visible hair straightness or iris heterochromia.

A weaker solution of cocaine (two drops of cocaine 2% in each eye) is used in children. The most telling symptom is the hemifacial flush (blanch on the affected side) that occurs with nursing or crying. Generally, the affected side is pale. In an air conditioned office, it may be hard to decide whether decreased sweating on the affected side is present. A cycloplegic refraction sometimes produces an atropinic flush everywhere except on the affected face and forehead and, thus, provides additional evidence toward diagnosis because of lack of sympathetic innervation to the skin vasculature.

In infants, hydroxyamphetamine drops do not help to localize the lesion, because orthograde transsynaptic dysgenesis takes place at the superior cervical ganglion after early interruption of the preganglionic oculosympathetic neuron. Fewer postganglionic neurons result, even though no direct postganglionic injury has occurred, which produces weak mydriasis and ambiguous results in children.[29] A patient with Horner's syndrome clearly acquired in infancy must be evaluated for neuroblastoma—a treatable tumor (Fig. 203-7).

Pupillary Inequality That Increases With Light

For a patient who has pupillary inequality that increases with light, several problems must be addressed (Fig. 203-8).

SLIT-LAMP EXAMINATION OF THE IRIS. Trauma to the globe usually results in a torn sphincter and an iris border that transilluminates at the slit lamp. The pupil often is not round and other evidence of ocular injury may be present. Naturally, such a pupil does not constrict well to light. The residual reaction often is segmental in a traumatic iridoplegia. An atrophic sphincter caused by previous herpes zoster iritis also may reveal transillumination defects, as seen with the slit lamp, that arise from previous ischemic insults to the iris. If, however, the iris looks normal, further investigation is required, as outlined below.

RESIDUAL LIGHT REACTION. If no residual light reaction is present, the possibility of pharmacological mydriasis must be explored.[30] However, a completely blocked light reaction sometimes may occur when the sphincter is denervated by either a preganglionic lesion (third cranial nerve palsy) or a postganglionic lesion (acute, complete tonic pupil), in acute angle closure (iris ischemia), or with an intraocular iron foreign body (iron mydriasis). If the dilated pupil still has some response to

light, the dilatation may result from partial denervation of the sphincter, incomplete atropinization, or adrenergic mydriasis. When the light reaction is poor because the dilator muscle is in spasm (as a consequence of adrenergic mydriatics such as phenylephrine), then the pupil is very large, the conjunctiva is blanched, and the lid is retracted. In such cases, any decrease in the amplitude of accommodation is minor and is the result of spherical aberration and a shallow depth of field—both optical results of the dilated pupil, or from the small inhibitory effect of sympathetic receptor activation or accommodation.

SEGMENTAL PARALYSIS OF THE IRIS SPHINCTER. When some residual light reaction occurs, the iris sphincter is examined for sector palsy using the slit lamp. When the dilator is in a drug-induced adrenergic spasm or when the cholinergic receptors in the iris sphincter are blocked by an atropine-like drug, the entire sphincter muscle (all 360°) is less effective. This does not happen when postganglionic parasympathetic nerve fibers have been interrupted. In patients with Adie's syndrome, all pupils that have a residual light reaction (about 90%) show segmental contractions of the sphincter (so-called *vermiform movements*). Thus, a pupil that has a weak light reaction and no segmental palsy usually indicates a drug-induced mydriasis, but signs of a third cranial nerve paresis (preganglionic parasympathetic nerve) must also be sought.

PUPILLARY SUPERSENSITIVITY TO CHOLINERGIC DRUGS. If weak pilocarpine (about 0.1%) or weak methacholine (2.5%) is applied to both eyes (with both corneas healthy and untouched), and the affected (dilated) pupil constricts more than the normal pupil to become the smaller pupil, that iris sphincter is denervated. It seems likely that with a postganglionic denervation (ciliary ganglion to the eye), the sphincter will show a little more supersensitivity than in the preganglionic case (third cranial nerve palsy); however, the differences are not great. Cholinergic supersensitivity of the iris sphincter is considered now to be only a weak sign of Adie's syndrome. As the iris sphincter is reinnervated by cholinergic accommodative fibers and becomes smaller over time, supersensitivity can be lost.[31]

Ptosis or diplopia must be re-evaluated, because it is very rare for an ambulatory patient to have an isolated sphincter palsy from damage to the intracranial third nerve. If the normal pupil constricts a little and the dilated pupil not at all, the mydriasis may result from a local dose of an anticholinergic drug such as atropine. A stronger concentration of pilocarpine is needed to establish this.

PUPILLARY RESPONSE TO A MIOTIC DOSE OF PILOCARPINE. If, on application of pilocarpine 1% in each eye, the affected pupil reacts little or not at all and the unaffected pupil constricts normally, the pupil was not dilated because of innervation problems but because of a problem in the sphincter muscle, itself. Non-neuronal causes of mydriasis are:

- Anticholinergic mydriasis (e.g., scopolamine [hyoscine], cyclopentolate, atropine)
- Traumatic iridoplegia (sphincter rupture, pigment dispersion, angle recession)
- Angle-closure glaucoma (ischemia of the iris sphincter)
- Fixed pupil after anterior segment surgery
- Bound down iris (synechia) after iritis

The cause for complete loss of function of the iris muscles after anterior segment surgery is unknown. Sometimes an excessive rise in intraocular pressure during or after surgery can cause ischemic damage to the iris sphincter.

Tonic Pupil of Adie's Syndrome

Young adults (more women than men) may discover that one pupil is large or that they cannot focus up close with one eye. Slit-lamp examination usually shows segmental denervation of the iris sphincter. Within the first week, supersensitivity to cholinergic substances may be demonstrated. After about 2 months, nerve regrowth is active and fibers originally bound for

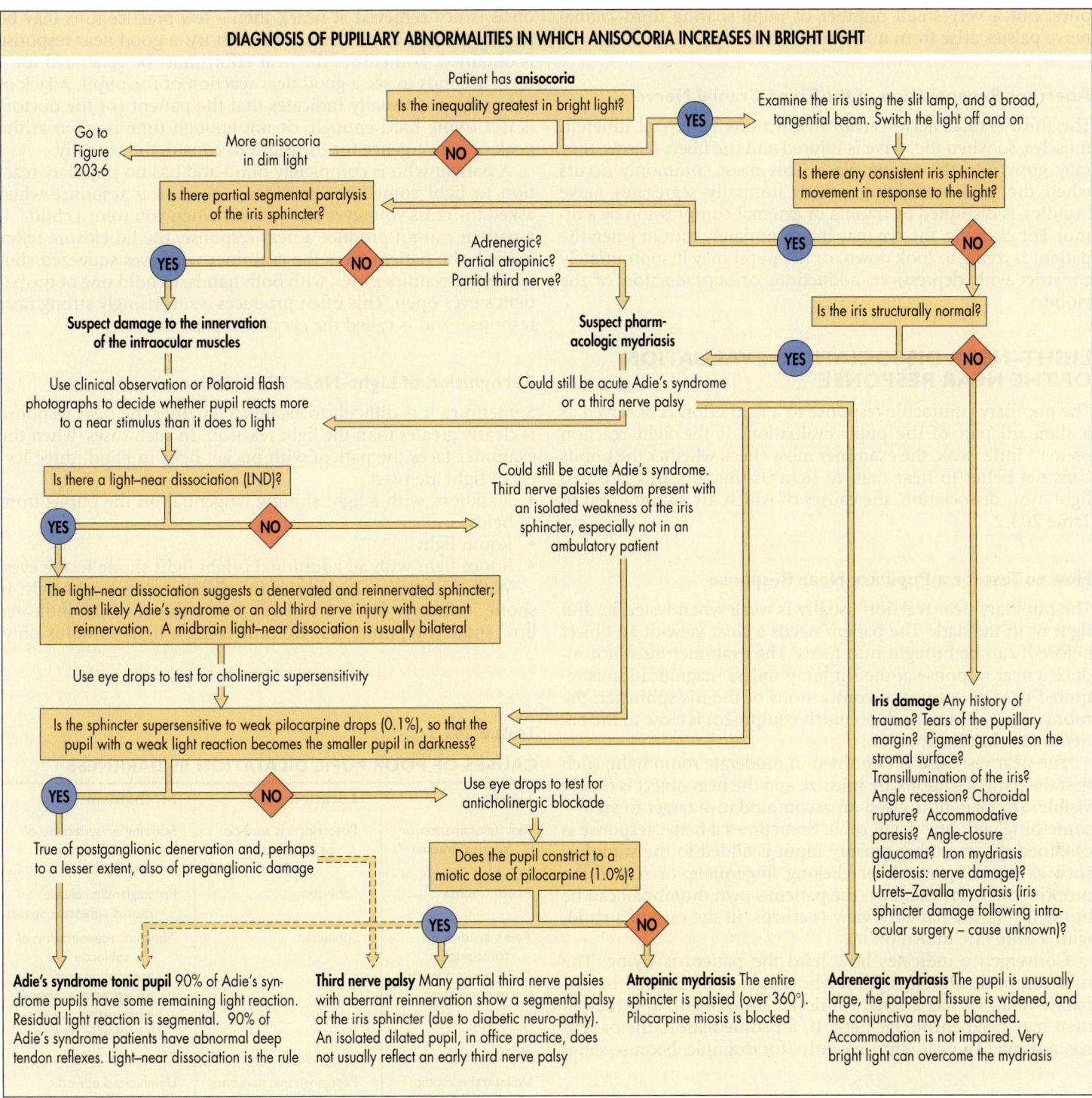

FIG. 203-8 ■ **Diagnosis of pupillary abnormalities in which anisocoria increases in bright light.** Initial pupillary inequality greater in bright light than in the dark indicates that the sphincter of the large pupil is weak or that a parasympathetic lesion is present on that side.

the ciliary muscle (they outnumber the sphincter fibers by 30:1) start to arrive (aberrantly) at the iris sphincter, which produces the characteristic light–near dissociation of Adie's syndrome. Eventually, the affected pupil becomes the smaller of the two pupils, especially in dim light, because of the aberrant reinnervation by accommodative fibers ("little old Adie's pupil"). The segmental palsy of the iris sphincter is seen particularly well using infrared video recording of transillumination of the iris.[31]

Fixed, Dilated Pupil

When a pupil is dilated by an atropinic medication, the resultant condition can be differentiated with confidence from an innervational palsy by its tendency to resist the miotic effects of

cholinergic drops such as pilocarpine. Pilocarpine 1% is a sufficient miotic dose for any eye, but a sphincter with all its cholinergic receptors blocked by atropine or tropicamide does not constrict with pilocarpine 1%. If the anticholinergic drug starts to wear off such that a small light reaction begins to return, pilocarpine 1% may only cause minimal constriction compared with the normal pupil.

Third Cranial Nerve Palsy

An old clinical rule of thumb states that if the pupillary light reaction is spared, the third cranial nerve palsy probably does not result from compression or injury, but more likely from small-vessel disease such as might be seen in diabetes. The rule still applies, but a very small number of pupil-sparing third cranial nerve palsies arise from midbrain infarcts.

Aberrant Regeneration of the Third Cranial Nerve

The third cranial nerve carries instructions to several different muscles, so when the nerve is injured and the fibers regrow, they may grow into the wrong place. This most commonly occurs when the glial scaffolding, which normally segregates nerve bundles, is disrupted by trauma or external compression by a tumor. For example, the eye may inappropriately turn in when the patient is trying to look down, or the pupil may inappropriately constrict with depression, adduction, or supraduction of the globe.

LIGHT–NEAR DISSOCIATION: EVALUATION OF THE NEAR RESPONSE

The pupillary contractile response to a near effort is observed as a standard part of the pupil evaluation. If the light reaction seems a little weak, the examiner must check whether the pupils constrict better to near than to light. If they do, this is called light–near dissociation, the causes of which are summarized in Table 203-2.

How to Test for a Pupillary Near Response

The pupillary near reaction usually is weak when tested in dim light or in the dark. The patient needs a clear view of an object before it can be brought into focus. The examiner must not induce a near response at the slit lamp unless magnification is required to view segmental contractions of the iris sphincter; the room usually is dark and too much equipment is close to the patient's face in this situation.

The near response is examined in moderate room light, such that the patient's pupils are midsize and the near object is clearly visible. The patient is given an accommodative target to view—something with fine detail on it. Sometimes a better response is obtained if some other sensory input is added to the stimulus, such as a ticking watch or clicking fingernails; or something proprioceptive for example, the patient's own thumbnail can be brought into the patient's view (perhaps, in the case of a child, with a little face drawn on it).

Convergence indicates how hard the patient is trying. The near response, although it may be triggered by blurred or disparate imagery, has a large volitional component, and the patient may need encouragement. If, for some reason, the patient has not made a near effort recently (for example, because stere-

opsis is not achieved at near), then a few practice runs may be needed. Often, on the third or fourth try, a good near response is obtained. Sometimes the near effort must be generated for 5 to 10 seconds to see a good near reaction of the pupil. A lack of near response usually indicates that the patient (or the doctor) is not trying hard enough, or not enough time is given at the peak of convergence for the pupil to constrict maximally.

A patient who is completely blind and has no pupillary reaction to light sometimes provides a good near response when asked to "cross your eyes like you did when you were a child." If a patient cannot produce a near response, the lid closure reflex is tried: the patient faces the examiner with eyes squeezed shut while the examiner tries, with both hands, to hold one of the patient's eyes open. This often produces a surprisingly strong near response, and is called the *eye closure pupil reaction.*

Recognition of Light–Near Dissociation

Sometimes it is difficult to establish whether the near response is clearly greater than the light reaction. In such cases, when the examiner faces the patient with pocket light in hand, three levels of light are used:
- Darkness, with a light shining tangential on the pupils from below
- Room light
- Room light with an additional bright light shone in the eyes
  With the patient looking in the distance, the bright light is shone in the eye for 1–2 seconds 3 or 4 times, which indicates how small the pupils may become using a light stimulus only.

TABLE 203-2

CAUSES OF LIGHT–NEAR DISSOCIATION OF THE PUPIL

Cause	Location	Mechanism
Severe loss of afferent light input to both eyes	Anterior visual pathway (retina, optic nerves, chiasm)	Damage to the retina or optic nerve pathways
Loss of pretectal light input to Edinger–Westphal nucleus	Tectum of the midbrain	Infectious (Argyl Robertson pupils) or compression (pinealoma)
Adie's syndrome	Iris sphincter	Aberrant reinnervation of sphincter by accommodative neurons
Third cranial nerve aberrant reinnervation	Iris sphincter	Aberrant reinnervation of sphincter by accommodative neurons or medial rectus neurons

TABLE 203-3

CAUSES OF POOR PUPIL DILATATION IN DARKNESS

Cause	Location	Mechanism
Past inflammation or surgical trauma	Posterior iris surface or sphincter	Scarring or synechiae of the iris because of past iritis
Acute trauma	Sphincter	Prostaglandin release causes sphincter spasm
Adie's syndrome tonic pupil Third nerve aberrant reinnervation	Sphincter	Aberrant regeneration of iris sphincter by accommodative or extraocular motor neuronsthat are not inhibited in darkness
Pharmacologic miosis	Iris sphincter	Cholinergic influence
Unilateral episodic spasm of miosis	Postganglionic parasympathetic neuron	Uninhibited episodic activation of postganglionic neurons
Congenital miosis (bilateral)	Sphincter	Developmental abnormality
Fatigue, sleepiness	Edinger–Westphal nucleus	Loss of inhibition at midbrain from reticularactivating formation
Lymphoma, inflammation, infection	Periaqueductal gray matter	Interruption of inhibitory fibers to the Edinger–Westphal nucleus
Central-acting drugs	Reticular activating formation, midbrain	Narcotics, general anesthetics
Old age (bilateral miosis)	Reticular activating formation, midbrain	Loss of inhibition at midbrain from reticular activating formation
Oculosympathetic defect	Sympathetic neuron interruption	Horner's syndrome

The near response must not be judged by the addition of a near stimulus to a bright light stimulus, which almost always produces an apparent light–near dissociation, because the near stimulus inevitably adds something to the light stimulus. A real light–near dissociation is present only if the near response (tested in moderate light) exceeds the best constriction that bright light can produce.

POOR PUPIL DILATATION

When one or both pupils stay small and miotic, even in darkness, a number of factors may be responsible (Table 203-3). To better understand the different mechanisms possible it is important to understand the normal process in darkness that allows the pupil to dilate. When a light stimulus is terminated, two mechanisms cause the pupil to dilate. The greater part of pupil dilatation arises from inhibition to the Edinger–Westphal nucleus in the midbrain, which reduces the firing of the preganglionic parasympathetic neurons in the Edinger–Westphal nucleus and results in relaxation of the iris sphincter. Within a few seconds, sympathetic nerve firing increases, which augments the pupil dilatation by active contraction of the dilator muscle. The combined inhibition of the iris sphincter and stimulation of the iris dilator is a carefully integrated neuronal reflex. Therefore, inability of the pupil to dilate in darkness may occur because of a sympathetic nerve palsy, but also from mechanical limitations of the pupil (scarring), pharmacological miosis, aberrant reinnervation of cholinergic neurons to the iris sphincter that are not normally inhibited in darkness (accommodative or extraocular motor neurons), or inhibitory input signal not received by the Edinger–Westphal nucleus.

REFERENCES

1. Lowenstein O, Kawabata H, Loewenfeld I. The pupil as indicator of retinal activity. Am J Ophthalmol. 1964;57:569–96.
2. Loewenfeld IE. The pupil: anatomy, physiology, and clinical applications. Ames, Iowa: Iowa State University Press; Detroit: Wayne State University Press; 1993.
3. Levatin P. Pupillary escape in disease of the retina or optic nerve. Arch Ophthalmol. 1959;62:768–79.
4. Thompson HS, Corbett JJ, Cox TA. How to measure the relative afferent pupillary defect. Surv Ophthalmol. 1981;26:39–42.
5. Thompson HS, Corbett JJ. Asymmetry of pupillomotor input. Eye. 1991;5:36–9.
6. Cox TA, Thompson HS, Hayreh SS, Snyder JE. Visual evoked potential and pupillary signs. A comparison in optic nerve disease. Arch Ophthalmol. 1982;100:1603–7.
7. Thompson HS, Montague P, Cox TA, Corbett JJ. The relationship between visual acuity, pupillary defect, and visual field loss. Am J Ophthalmol. 1982;93:681–8.
8. Brown RH, Zillis JD, Lynch MG, Sanborn GE. The afferent pupillary defect in asymmetric glaucoma. Arch Ophthalmol. 1987;105:1540–3.
9. Johnson LN, Hill RA, Bartholomew MJ. Correlation of afferent pupillary defect with visual field loss on automated perimetry. Ophthalmol. 1988;95:1649–55.
10. Kardon RH, Haupert C, Thompson HS. The relationship between static perimetry and the relative afferent pupillary defect. Am J Ophthalmol. 1993;115:351–6.
11. Kawasaki A, Moore P, Kardon RH. Variability of the relative afferent pupillary defect. Am J Ophthalmol. 1995;120:622–33.
12. Kawasaki A, Moore P, Kardon RH. Long-term fluctuation of relative afferent pupillary defect in subjects with normal visual function. Am J Ophthalmol. 1996;122:875–82.
13. Bell RA, Waggoner PM, Boyd WM, et al. Clinical grading of relative afferent pupillary defects. Arch Ophthalmol. 1993;111:938–42.
14. Haynes Wl, Alward WLM, McKinney K, et al. Quantitation of iris transillumination defects in eyes of patients with pigmentary glaucoma. J Glaucoma. 1994;3:1106–13.
15. Fison PN, Garlick DJ, Smith SE. Assessment of unilateral afferent pupillary defects by pupillography. Br J Ophthalmol. 1979;63:195–9.
16. Cox TA. Pupillography of a relative afferent pupillary defect. Am J Ophthalmol. 1986;101:320–4.
17. Cox TA. Pupillographic characteristics of simulated relative afferent pupillary defects. Invest Ophthalmol Vis Sci. 1989;30:1127–31.
18. Young RSL, Han B, Wu P. Transient and sustained components of the pupillary responses evoked by luminance and color. Vision Res. 1993;33(4):437–46.
19. Young RSL, Kennish J. Transient and sustained components of the pupil response evoked by achromatic spatial patterns. Vision Res. 1993;33(16):2239–52.
20. Barbur JL, Harlow AJ, Sahraie A. Pupillary responses to stimulus structure, colour, and movement. Ophthalmic Physiol Opt. 1992;12:137–41.
21. Slooter JH, van Noren D. Visual acuity measured with pupil responses to checkerboard stimuli. Invest Ophthalmol Vis Sci. 1980;19:105–8.
22. Ukai K. Spatial pattern as a stimulus to the pupillary system. J Opt Soc Am A. 1985;2:1094–100.
23. Barbur JL, Thomson WD. Pupil response as an objective measure of visual acuity. Ophthalmic Physiol Opt. 1987;7:425–9.
24. Cocker KD, Moseley MJ. Visual acuity and the pupil grating response. Clin Vision Sci. 1992;7:143–6.
25. Kardon RH, Kirkali PA, Thompson HS. Automated pupil perimetry. Pupil field mapping in patients and normal subjects. Ophthalmology. 1991;98:485–96.
26. Kardon RH. Pupil perimetry. Curr Opin Ophthalmol. 1992;3:565–70.
27. Kardon RH, Denison CE, Brown CK, Thompson HS. Critical evaluation of the cocaine test in the diagnosis of Horner's syndrome. Arch Ophthalmol. 1990;108:384–7.
28. Cremer SA, Thompson HS, Digre KB, Kardon RH. Hydroxyamphetamine mydriasis in Horner's syndrome. Am J Ophthalmol. 1990;110:71–6.
29. Weinstein JM, Zweifel TJ, Thompson HS. Congenital Horner's syndrome. Arch Ophthalmol. 1980;98:1074–8.
30. Thompson HS, Newsome DA, Loewenfeld IE. The fixed dilated pupil: sudden iridoplegia or mydriatic drops? A simple diagnostic test. Arch Ophthalmol. 1971;86:21–7.
31. Kardon RH, Corbett JJ, Thompson HS. Segmental denervation and reinnervation of the iris sphincter as shown by infrared videographic transillumination. Ophthalmology. 1998;105:313–21.

SEAN P. DONAHUE

DEFINITION
- Accommodation is the ability to increase the refractive power of the eye's optical system. Loss of accommodation may occur as a result of presbyopia, the age-associated decrease in elasticity of the natural lens, or from other less common causes.

KEY FEATURE
- Blurred vision at near.

ASSOCIATED FEATURES
- Advanced age.
- Drug use (cholinergics, botulism).
- Other rare causes.

TABLE 204-1

STANDARD CYCLOPLEGIC AGENTS

Agent	Available Concentrations (%)	Maximum Effect for Cycloplegia (minutes)	Duration of Cycloplegia (hours)
Tropicamide	1, 2	15	4–6
Cyclopentolate	0.5, 1, 5	20–45	24
Homatropine	2, 5	45–60	72
Scopolamine	0.25	30–60	168 (7 days)
Atropine	0.25, 0.5, 1	120	360 (15 days)

INTRODUCTION

Accommodation is the ability to increase the refractive power of the optical system of the eye. It occurs to produce a clearer image of near objects. In hyperopes, accommodation is necessary to produce a focused image at both distance and near. To bring about accommodation, the ciliary body contracts, the lens zonules relax, and the crystalline lens assumes a more spherical shape, which increases its refractive power.

Presbyopia is, by far, the most common disease to affect accommodation. It is a normal part of the aging process and leads to a decrease in accommodation associated with loss of elasticity of the lens and lens capsule. Disorders other than presbyopia can affect accommodation but are, for the most part, relatively rare. Regardless of cause, symptoms of blurred vision at near and of eye strain with prolonged near work result.[1]

EPIDEMIOLOGY AND PATHOGENESIS

The neural pathway for accommodation probably begins in the midbrain. Attempts at accommodation are associated with convergence and pupillary miosis (the "near triad"), so the areas responsible for accommodation are probably related closely to those that produce convergence. These areas almost certainly receive input from the cerebral cortex and pretectum; complex pathways project symmetrically to the third nerve nucleus of the midbrain. The portion of the third nerve nucleus responsible for accommodation is probably in the caudal segment of the Edinger-Westphal parasympathetic nucleus.[2] It is possible that a direct (nonsynapsing) pathway from the midbrain to the ciliary body also exists.

The fibers that subserve accommodation then travel from the third nerve nucleus to the ciliary ganglion, where they synapse with postganglionic parasympathetic fibers destined for the ciliary body and iris sphincter. These fibers reach the intrinsic muscles of the eye via the short ciliary nerves.

Several experiments have shown that the ciliary body also receives sympathetic input. This is evidenced clinically by the increased accommodative amplitude seen in the affected eye of patients with Horner's syndrome. However, the parasympathetic control is of much greater clinical importance, because the most potent mechanism to antagonize accommodation operates through parasympathetic inhibition.[3]

Because accommodation is mediated almost exclusively via parasympathetic pathways, it is antagonized best with muscarinic blockers. For the muscarinic antagonists used clinically, cycloplegia (paralysis of accommodation) is always associated with mydriasis (pupil dilatation). Note that phenylephrine (adrenaline), a sympathomimetic, causes mydriasis but has no significant effect on accommodation. Five muscarinic antagonists are commonly used in ophthalmology (Table 204-1). Tropicamide (Mydriacyl) has a very short half-life and should not be used to determine the cycloplegic refraction. Cyclopentolate is effective and has sufficient half-life to be the standard in pediatric ophthalmology. Homatropine, scopolamine (hyoscine), and atropine have longer half-lives and are generally used for therapeutic reasons rather than for diagnosis.

Accommodative ability decreases with age. Although a great deal of variability occurs in the normal levels of accommodation, a general rule is that 6D of accommodation should be present at 40 years of age, 4D at 44 years, and 3D at 48 years. For each 4-year period under 40 years of age, 1D should be added; for each 4-year period over 48 years of age, 0.5D should be subtracted. This rule, suggested by Milder and Rubin,[4] is illustrated in Table 204-2.

OCULAR MANIFESTATIONS

Because accommodation is part of the near reflex, it is linked closely with convergence and pupillary miosis. Clinically, it is very difficult to separate these components, and the presence of pupillary miosis is a good indicator of accommodative effort.

TABLE 204-2

ACCOMMODATIVE AMPLITUDES AT GIVEN AGES

Age (years)	Amplitude of Accommodation (D)	Near Point When Emmetropic (cm)
20	11	9.1
32	8	12.5
40	6	16.7
44	4	25.0
48	3	33.3
56	2	50.0
64	1	100.0

Disorders of accommodation typically present with blurred vision, especially at near. Patients who have latent hyperopia must use a portion of their accommodative reserve to focus at distance as well. They therefore may present with premature presbyopia. Myopia, in contrast, reduces accommodative demand and may delay symptoms of presbyopia.

Most disorders of accommodation are bilateral in nature. Thus, if the patient is corrected to emmetropia, the amount of near blurring should be similar in each eye. Those disorders that present as a unilateral loss of accommodation localize to the infranuclear third nerve, the ciliary ganglion (Adie's syndrome), or the effector organ (ciliary body) itself (Horner's syndrome or pharmacological cycloplegia).

DIAGNOSIS

Accommodation can be measured by determining the accommodative amplitude or the accommodative range.[4] In all tests, it is important that refractive error be corrected properly to put the far point at infinity and render the ocular system emmetropic at distance. Three methods used to determine accommodative amplitude are discussed here; all the tests are carried out monocularly.

The first method involves a small target being brought forward toward the eye until it blurs. This is the near point of accommodation. The reciprocal of the distance at which the target blurs is the accommodative amplitude. For example, if the target blurs at 25cm distance, the subject has 4D of accommodative amplitude.

A second method uses the Prince rule, a scaled ruler combined with a near add of +3D, which puts the far point of an emmetrope at 33cm. The target on the Prince rule is brought forward until it blurs; this distance is then converted into the diopters of accommodative amplitude, taking into account the +3 add. For example, a person who has 4D of accommodative amplitude would see the target blur at a distance of 14cm [100/(4 + 3)].

A third test uses a distance target and lenses of increased minus sphere to induce accommodation. More minus sphere is added until the subject can no longer overcome the minus lenses with accommodation. The amount of minus sphere that can be overcome represents the accommodative amplitude.

The accommodative range refers to the range of distances that can be viewed clearly by using accommodation. Typically, it is expressed without correction for emmetropia. A +2 hyperope with 4D of accommodation would have an uncorrected accommodative range from infinity to 50cm, whereas a –2 myope with a similar accommodative amplitude would have an accommodative range from 50cm to 17cm.

DIFFERENTIAL DIAGNOSIS

The most common cause of accommodative dysfunction is presbyopia. The symptoms of bilateral, progressive blurred vision at near and of eye strain, in a patient of appropriate age, are usually enough to make the diagnosis. When presbyopic symptoms or decreased accommodative amplitudes are seen in an individual younger than 40 years, the patient is most likely a latent hyperope; a cycloplegic refraction confirms the diagnosis.

Accommodative problems also can be caused by lesions anywhere along the neuroanatomical pathway that subserves accommodation.[5] These, however, are relatively rare. Trauma to the parasympathetic nuclei in the midbrain, to supranuclear structures, or to the third nerve can produce asthenopic symptoms. Adie's syndrome, thought to be caused by damage to the ciliary ganglion or short ciliary nerves, is usually associated with decreased accommodation. Pharmacological cycloplegia also produces temporary accommodative dysfunction and is accompanied by mydriasis. A fascinating case of temporary loss of accommodative power associated with eating (the muffin man) has been reported.[6]

Systemic medications can cause decreases in accommodation. Most often these medications have anticholinergic side effects. Phenothiazines, such as fluphenazine (Prolixin), and antiparkinsonian drugs, such as trihexyphenidyl (benzhexol, Artane), are typical offenders.

Whether accommodative dysfunction occurs in otherwise healthy children is a subject of controversy in the optometry and pediatric ophthalmology literature. Some authorities believe that decreased accommodative amplitudes in children are effort related (as evidenced by lack of pupillary constriction to an attempted near target); others believe that such an entity is real and can be treated successfully with orthoptic exercises.[7, 8]

Increased accommodation is seen rarely. Patients who have acute Horner's syndrome may notice an increased accommodative range on the affected side. More often, an abnormally proximal near point of accommodation is caused by miotic agents, such as pilocarpine, or by accommodative spasm. Accommodative spasm is frequently seen as a functional disorder. These patients have a spasm of the near reflex and present with esotropia, diplopia, blurred vision at distance, miosis, and an abnormal near point of accommodation. Typically, they have no organic disease and may do well with either reassurance or daily drops of a mild cycloplegic until the symptoms cease.

TREATMENT

Treatment of presbyopia involves the use of plus lenses for near work. Several methods can be used to determine the proper add. Most problems with reading adds result from overcorrection for the near distance. Correction to emmetropia and the use of trial frames (rather than the Phoroptor) to determine the proper add yield the best results. Other options for correction of presbyopia include monovision or bifocal fitting of contact lenses.[9]

COURSE AND OUTCOME

Most patients with asthenopic symptoms do well with plus-power spectacles for reading. Typically, plus-power requirements increase until patients reach their early 60s, as accommodation is progressively lost, and then stabilize.

REFERENCES

1. Weale R. Presbyopia toward the end of the 20th century. Surv Ophthalmol. 1989;34:15–30.
2. Bender MB, Weinstein EA. Functional representation in the oculomotor and trochlear nuclei. Arch Neurol Psychiatry. 1983;49:98–106.
3. Miller NR, ed. Walsh and Hoyt's clinical neuro-ophthalmology, vol 2, 4th ed. Baltimore: Williams & Wilkins; 1985:442–57.
4. Milder B, Rubin ML. Accommodation. In: The fine art of prescribing glasses without making a spectacle of yourself. Gainesville: Triad Scientific Publishers; 1978:18–41.
5. Miller NR, ed. Walsh and Hoyt's clinical neuro-ophthalmology, vol 2, 4th ed. Baltimore: Williams & Wilkins; 1985:469–556.
6. Hudson HL, Rismondo V, Sadun AA. Prandial presbyopia: the muffin man. Br J Ophthalmol. 1991;75:707–9.
7. Slamovitz TL, Glaser JS. The pupil and accommodation. In: Tasman W, Jaeger EA, eds. Duane's clinical ophthalmology, vol 2. Philadelphia: Lippincott-Raven; 1995:1–26.
8. Raskind RH. Problems at the reading distance. Am J Orthoptics. 1976;26:53–8.
9. Stein HA. The management of presbyopia with contact lenses: a review. CLAO J. 1990;16:33–8.

CHAPTER

205

Headache and Facial Pain

JOEL M. WEINSTEIN

DEFINITION
- Chronic, intermittent, or episodic pain that involves the head, skull, scalp, or face.

KEY FEATURES
- Most headaches fall into specific rubrics (e.g., tension headache, migraine) that involve fairly common patterns of symptoms, such as a tightening band around the head in the late afternoon.
- Most headaches do not reflect serious organic disease.

ASSOCIATED FEATURE
- Though usually benign, the pain from headaches can be devastating and interfere with routine activities.

INTRODUCTION

Headache and facial pain are among the most common complaints seen in medical practice. From the perspective of the ophthalmologist, the critical tasks are to:
- Diagnose correctly and treat painful intraocular and orbital disorders.
- Recognize various benign syndromes that cause headache and facial pain, including migraines, tension headaches, and cluster headaches.
- Identify the minority of patients who have headache caused by serious intracranial or systemic pathology.

In this chapter a working plan is developed to facilitate the diagnosis of patients in the last two categories. This requires both a knowledge of various nonophthalmological disorders and a new methodology with which to elicit the relevant clinical history.

EPIDEMIOLOGY AND PATHOGENESIS

Headache and facial pain are common symptoms of many processes, some of which are not completely understood. They are seen with great frequency in patients of both sexes, of all ages, and from all around the world. Specific forms of headache have their own prevalence, as described later.

OCULAR MANIFESTATIONS

By their nature, headache and facial pain are nonspecific symptoms that may be associated with a variety of disorders. In some of these disorders, visual or neurological signs and symptoms may point to a specific diagnosis. These signs and symptoms are discussed under the appropriate diagnostic headache categories.

DIAGNOSIS AND TESTING

Headaches and facial pain, more than any other disease category, are diagnosed through a thorough and intelligent history

taking. Hence, the focus in this chapter is on how to take a good history.

The Art and Science of Taking a Headache History

A thorough history is the key to making the correct diagnosis in a headache patient. In most cases, the history generates a limited list of differential diagnoses that can only occasionally be confirmed by physical examination and ancillary studies. To elicit the pertinent clinical information, patients are given the opportunity to describe the symptom complex in detail. Some measure of knowledgeable guidance is required, however, to extract the relevant clinical details and to avoid irrelevant minutiae.

Some patients who have headache and facial pain enter the medical care system with firm preconceptions about the cause of their pain. For example, many have been told by well-meaning friends or relatives that "sinus headaches" or "eye strain" (e.g., because of uncorrected refractive errors) is the source of their discomfort. These misconceptions are reinforced by the over-the-counter market, which strongly promotes analgesic and sympathomimetic preparations for the treatment of "sinus headaches." However, it rarely is helpful, and often is counter-productive, to point out these apparent misconceptions at the outset. The relevant objective facts should be elicited in a non-challenging and supportive manner, and a formulation should be deferred until the end of the examination. It is important to keep these preconceptions in mind, however, because they may color the patient's description of the symptoms; for example, the patient may try to relate all headaches to reading and overlook other contributory factors. To sort out the multitude of factors that can contribute to or cause headaches, it is essential to obtain a relevant past medical history, a basic neurological review of systems (Box 205-1), and a directed headache history (outlined in the next section and in Box 205-2).

Basic Outline of the Headache History

DATE OF ONSET, AGE AT ONSET, AND FREQUENCY OF SYMPTOMS. The length of time that a patient has suffered from headaches is the first guidepost in differentiating benign headaches from those that signify a progressive neurological or systemic disorder and require further investigation. At one end of the spectrum, a pattern of long-standing intermittent headaches with headache-free intervals recurring over months to years is rarely indicative of serious intracranial or systemic pathology. Most of these patients have vascular or stress-tension headaches. Conversely, the sudden onset of severe and persistent headaches in an otherwise headache-free individual, especially when accompanied by focal neurological signs or symptoms, is clearly a cause for concern. Patients experiencing their first attack of migraine may produce confusion in this regard, however, because the initial episode may be accompanied by focal deficits (e.g., hemianopia) but not by the typical signs and symptoms that characterize most recurrent vascular headache episodes.

Some headaches develop, and perhaps progress, over weeks to months. Although most headaches in this category have a benign cause, such as persistent stress-tension or migraine, this is the group of patients in which serious intracranial or systemic pathology should be suspected and carefully ruled out. Headaches that result from intracranial mass lesions or increased intracranial pressure usually have an insidious onset and occur daily, and there are rarely prolonged headache-free intervals.

LOCATION. Stress-tension headaches are often occipital in location and extend to the posterior neck and shoulders (Fig. 205-1). However, intracranial processes, especially in the posterior fossa, can cause a similar distribution of pain. A band-like distribution of pain, which presumably reflects occipitofrontalis tension, also is quite common in patients who have stress-tension headache. Hemicranial headaches that become holocephalic are generally vascular (i.e., migrainous) in nature. Headaches of dental or sinus origin frequently cause frontal, periorbital, or malar pain.

DURATION. Persistent and unrelenting pain that lasts for days at a time rarely results from vascular or tension headaches; it should arouse suspicion of intracranial disease, sinus inflammation, cranial arteritis, or carotid dissection.

PREDISPOSING FACTORS. For a minority of patients with vascular headache syndromes, foods or allergens have been identified that precipitate headaches.[1] These include chocolate, red wine, oranges, and fatty foods. In other vascular headache patients, stress—or, more commonly, relief of prolonged stress—triggers a headache episode. Other triggers for vascular headache include bright lights, exercise, sexual intercourse, and alcohol.

PRECEDING SYMPTOMS. Many patients with vascular headaches have some form of autonomic disturbance that precedes their headache by as much as 24 hours.[2] This may include drowsiness, irritability, insomnia, depression, or hypomania. Unformed visual hallucinations occur in 10–15% of migraineurs; typically, these last 10–40 minutes and are followed almost immediately by headache. It is important to differentiate the migrainous visual prodrome from the hallucinations that may occur as epileptiform phenomena in patients who have more serious intracranial disease (see later).

QUALITY AND SEVERITY OF PAIN. Both vascular headaches and headaches that result from intracranial masses may vary widely in severity, from mild to excruciating. Pain from vascular headache starts out as a dull ache but frequently becomes pulsatile and often is described as throbbing. It may be alleviated by compression or massage of the external carotid artery; usually, it is exacerbated by physical activity. Cluster headaches characteristically are extremely severe. Stress-tension headaches are seldom severe enough to require bed rest and rarely are described as throbbing. Headache from intracranial hemorrhage typically is quite severe and usually is accompanied by focal signs or other neurological symptoms.

ACCOMPANYING SYMPTOMS. Nausea, photophobia, phonophobia (e.g., aversion to sound, especially loud noises), and drowsiness frequently occur during acute migraine headaches and are useful in differentiating vascular from nonvascular paroxysmal headache syndromes. These symptoms also may occur in acute intracranial processes, however, which must be distinguished on the basis of other signs and symptoms. A detailed review of neurological symptoms should be elicited from all headache patients (see Box 205-1), which greatly aids in identifying patients who have intracranial inflammation, hemorrhage, or space-occupying lesions.

DIFFERENTIAL DIAGNOSIS OF HEADACHE SYNDROMES

The International Headache Society (IHS) has classified headache and facial pain disorders and provided diagnostic criteria by which various syndromes can be distinguished (a partial listing is given in Box 205-3).[3] Although these criteria are tentative and subject to revision, they provide a useful basis on which to develop a working differential diagnosis. At this time, however, no specific diagnostic tests exist for the three most common headache disorders—migraine, tension headache, and cluster headache. The diagnostic criteria, therefore, are highly dependent on an accurate and reliable history.

Migraine

The terminology for various migraine syndromes may be somewhat inconsistent in the older literature, but most recent publications utilize the more detailed and specific IHS classification. The IHS classification separates migraine patients into those without and with focal neurological symptoms, or "aura," preceding the headache (categories 1.1 and 1.2, respectively). Categories 1.3–1.5 include several well-recognized but uncommon clinical syndromes in which various types of focal neurological symptoms may occur either before or during the headache. Prolonged attacks, or attacks that result in permanent ischemic damage to the central nervous system, are defined as complications of migraine under category 1.6. These designations are meant to replace the older terms such as "common migraine" for migraine without aura, "classic migraine" for migraine with homonymous hemianopic visual aura, and "complicated migraine" for headaches with nonvisual neurological symptoms that occur during or after the headache phase.

EPIDEMIOLOGY OF MIGRAINE. The prevalence of migraine has been estimated across various age ranges and in various ethnic and socioeconomic groups. The prevalence estimates are 5–20% for men and 15–40% for women. The prevalence certainly is lower in children but is still substantial.[4,5] Dalsgaard-

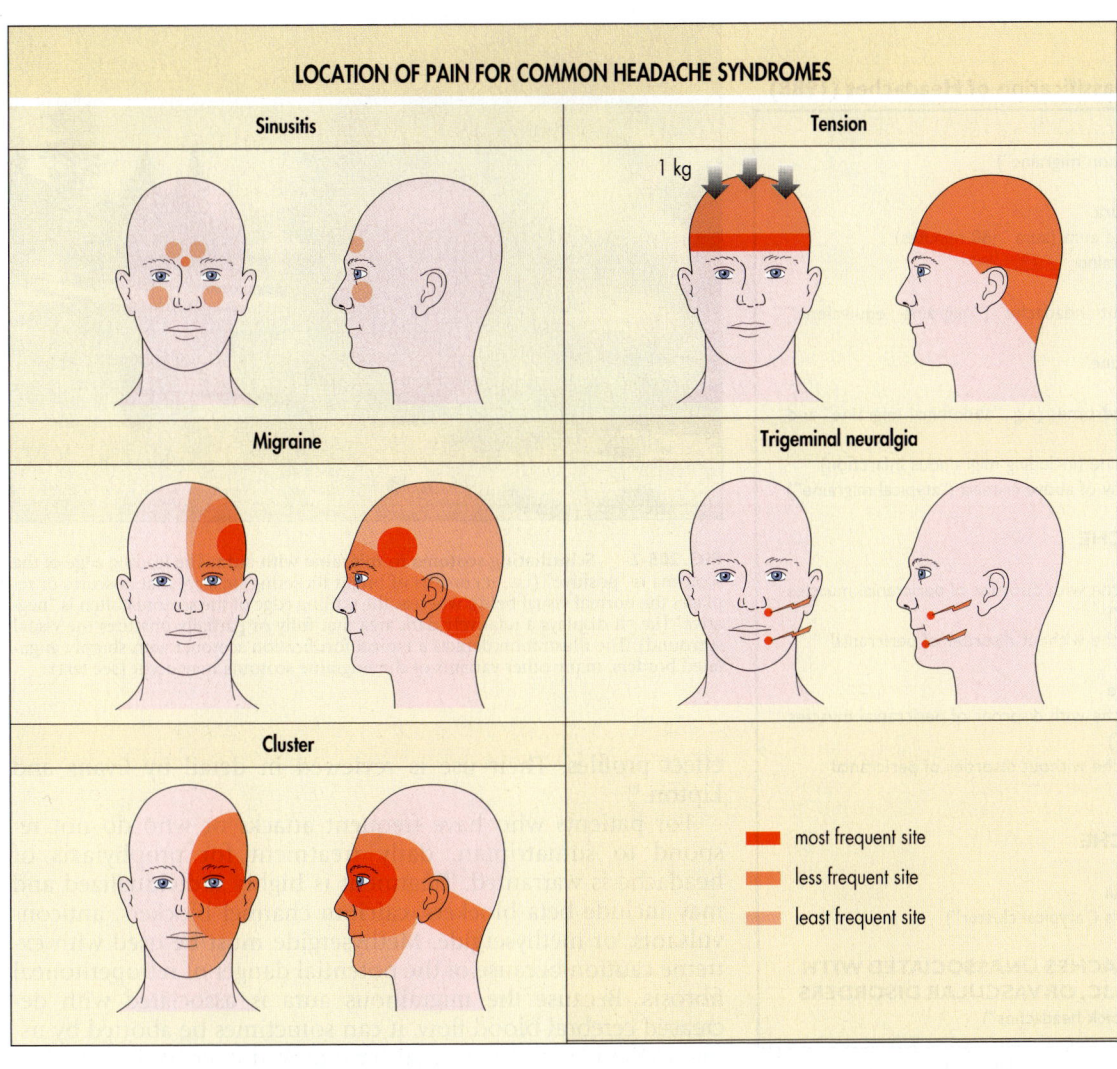

LOCATION OF PAIN FOR COMMON HEADACHE SYNDROMES

Sinusitis

Tension

1 kg

Migraine

Trigeminal neuralgia

Cluster

■ most frequent site
■ less frequent site
■ least frequent site

FIG. 205-1 ■ Location of pain for common headache syndromes. Tension headache often is described as a feeling of weight in the head or a band-like sensation around the head. The stabbing nature of trigeminal neuralgia is depicted by zigzag lines.

Nielsen[4] found an equal prevalence of about 3% for boys and girls at age 7 years, which increased to 15% at age 15 years. The first attack of migraine occurs before age 10 years in about 25% of patients, by age 25 years in about 65%, and by age 40 years in more than 90%.[6] Onset in later life does occur, however, and may be confused with transient cerebral ischemia. The criteria used to differentiate migraine equivalents in older patients from transient cerebral ischemic episodes have been discussed at length by Fisher.[7]

No consistent relationship to ethnic group, socioeconomic status, or personality profile has been found. However, a familial predisposition for migraine clearly exists. One genetic study found a risk of 70% if both parents were affected and 45% if only one parent was affected.[8] The pattern of inheritance appears to be complex and multifactorial.

CLINICAL FEATURES OF VARIOUS MIGRAINE SYNDROMES

Migraine Without Aura (Common Migraine). Although common migraine is not preceded by focal neurological symptoms (by definition),[9-11] many patients notice autonomic or mood disturbances as long as 24 hours before an impending attack.[2] These include irritability, depression, drowsiness, and hunger (sometimes with a craving for specific foods). Other patients may experience hypomania or elation. These premonitory symptoms presumably arise in the hypothalamus; it is interesting in this regard that similar symptoms may be induced by certain 5-hydroxytryptamine (5-HT) antagonists.[12]

The headache phase of common migraine begins unilaterally in only about 50% of patients, often in the periorbital area, and may or may not progress to become holocephalic. The pain may begin anywhere on the head or face, however, and may be bilateral (often bifrontal) at onset. Although many migraineurs report a strong predilection for episodes to occur repeatedly on the same side, most report occasional episodes on the other side. Frequent episodes that involve only one side should arouse suspicion of a space-occupying lesion. The pain often is described as throbbing, usually builds over 1–2 hours, and typically lasts 4–8 hours; however, attacks that last up to 24 hours are not uncommon. The pain usually is exacerbated by routine physical activity, such as bending or minor exertion. Nausea is a prominent feature in 80–90% of migraineurs, but actual vomiting is relatively uncommon. Photophobia and phonophobia are relatively common, and most patients withdraw to a dark, quiet room and lie still during severe attacks. Drowsiness is common, and many patients find that sleep provides substantial relief.

Migraine With Aura (Classic Migraine). Migraine with aura is characterized by a prodrome consisting of a completely reversible focal neurological symptom that typically lasts 15–45 minutes.[13-15] This prodrome is followed by a headache with a duration and quality similar to that of common migraine. The most common prodrome is, of course, the homonymous scintillating scotoma. Less frequently, the aura may consist of a hemisensory disturbance (paresthesia or numbness that involves one side of the body or face), hemiparesis, or dysphasia.[3,15] With the exception of the typical homonymous visual aura described later, patients who have focal neurological defects require a neurological consultation to assist in differentiating migraine from more serious transient cerebral ischemia.

The most common description of the visual aura is the perception of multicolored shimmering (scintillating) lights, beginning in the paracentral area and expanding in a crescent-shaped fashion to obscure a large portion of a homonymous hemifield of both eyes (Fig. 205-2). The borders of the scotoma often have jagged edges (teichopsia, or fortification scotoma, in analogy to a medieval fortress). Although the leading edge of the

BOX 205-3

Partial Listing of the IHS Classification of Headaches (1988)

1.0 MIGRAINE
1.1 Migraine without aura ("common migraine")
1.2 Migraine with aura
    1.2.1 Migraine with typical aura
    1.2.2 Migraine with prolonged aura (aura >60 minutes)
    1.2.3 Familial hemiplegic migraine
    1.2.4 Basilar migraine
    1.2.5 Migraine aura without headache ("migraine equivalent," "migraine disocie")
1.3 Ophthalmoplegic migraine
1.4 Retinal migraine
1.5 Childhood periodic syndromes (e.g., "abdominal migraine" and "vomiting attacks")
1.6 Complications of migraine (including migrainous infarction)
1.7 Migraine not fulfilling any of above criteria ("atypical migraine")

2.0 TENSION-TYPE HEADACHE
2.1 Episodic tension headache
    2.1.1 Episodic tension headache with disorder of pericranial muscles ("myofascial syndrome")
    2.1.2 Episodic tension headache without disorder of pericranial muscles
2.2 Chronic tension-type headache
    2.2.1 Chronic tension headache with disorder of pericranial muscles ("myofascial syndrome")
    2.2.2 Chronic tension headache without disorder of pericranial muscles

3.0 CLUSTER-TYPE HEADACHE
3.1 Typical cluster headache
3.2 Chronic paroxysmal hemicrania
3.3 Cluster-headache-like disorders ("atypical cluster")

4.0 MISCELLANEOUS HEADACHES UNASSOCIATED WITH STRUCTURAL, METABOLIC, OR VASCULAR DISORDERS
4.1 Idiopathic stabbing pains ("icepick headaches")

For the complete classification, see Headache Classification Committee of the International Headache Society. Classification and diagnostic criteria for headache disorders, cranial neuralgias and facial pain. Cephalalgia. 1988;8 (Suppl. 7):1–96.

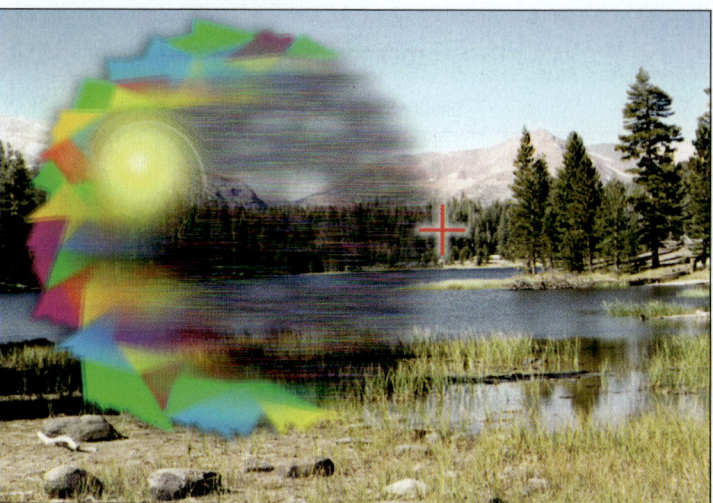

FIG. 205-2 ■ **Scintillating scotoma in migraine with aura.** The leading edge of the scotoma is "positive" (i.e., it consists of bright flickering imagery that obscures or replaces the normal visual field), whereas the trailing edge of the scotoma often is "negative" (i.e., it displays a relatively dark area that fully or partially obscures the visual surround). The illustration depicts a typical fortification scotoma with sharply angulated borders; many other variants of the migraine scotoma may occur (see text).

scotoma may be "positive" (i.e., may have flickering imagery that obscures or replaces the normal visual field), the trailing edge of the scotoma is often "negative" (i.e., displays a relatively dark area that fully or partially obscures the visual surround, as illustrated in Figure 205-2). Many patients experience a less dramatic and picturesque variant of progressive homonymous visual loss. Other sensations include a gray, black, or colored haze; the perception of a swirling pool of water; and "television interference" or "snow."[16] A personal report of a migraine episode is described and illustrated nicely by Sacks.[17]

It is quite common for patients who have homonymous visual loss of any cause to perceive their deficit incorrectly as monocular and ipsilateral to the visual field defect. In patients who report monocular loss, it is imperative to determine whether each eye was checked separately. In most instances, the patient's report of a negative scotoma with both eyes open is an indication that the episode of visual loss was homonymous rather than monocular.

Treatment of Migraine With and Without Aura. The current treatment of migraine has been reviewed in detail, and there are several monographs on the subject.[10,18] Many patients find that their migraines, with or without aura, can be aborted if they take aspirin, ibuprofen, or caffeine at the first sign of an attack. If this is not effective, sumatriptan, a 5-HT$_1$-like agonist, is the most effective agent for terminating an acute migraine attack. The drug may be taken orally or subcutaneously in autoinjectable form. Since the introduction of sumatriptan in 1993, several other triptans have been introduced for oral, nasal, and subcutaneous administration. These preparations have similar actions and side

effect profiles. Their use is reviewed in detail by Evans and Lipton.[10]

For patients who have frequent attacks or who do not respond to sumatriptan, daily treatment for prophylaxis of headache is warranted. Treatment is highly individualized and may include beta blockers, calcium channel blockers, anticonvulsants, or methysergide. Methysergide must be used with extreme caution because of the potential danger of retroperitoneal fibrosis. Because the migrainous aura is associated with decreased cerebral blood flow, it can sometimes be aborted by using a vasodilator. Agents that have proved effective include isoprenaline (inhalant), nitroglycerin (sublingual), and nifedipine (rapidly absorbed after rupture of an ingested capsule containing a 10mg dose in liquid form). Current controversies in the treatment of migraine are thoroughly discussed in the review by Evans and Lipton.[10] Topics covered include prophylaxis for recurrent or chronic migraine, treatment of basilar or complicated migraine, and use of oral contraceptives in migraine.

Structural Lesions That Mimic Migraine With Aura. Rarely, structural disease that involves the occipital region is confused with migraine with visual aura. In particular, arteriovenous malformations (AVMs) of the occipital lobe may cause transient homonymous visual loss with scintillating scotoma and headache. In the vast majority of cases, however, these two syndromes may be differentiated on clinical grounds alone. In two large series of occipital AVMs,[19,20] none of the patients had the 15–20 minute visual episodes that are characteristic of classic migraine. The headaches in patients with AVMs were consistently localized to the same side. In addition, the visual phenomena often persist intermittently throughout the headache, unlike classic migraine, in which the visual aura is usually complete before the onset of headache.

Troost and Newton[19] studied 26 patients with occipital AVMs and defined two distinct syndromes of visual loss, both of which were clearly differentiated from migraine. The first group of patients had occipital epileptiform discharges and experienced "elementary visual sensations" similar to those experienced on direct cortical stimulation during neurosurgery. Patients with epileptiform activity that originated in the primary visual cortex (area 17) reported small lights moving through the homonymous hemifield. The lights were sometimes colored but did not scintillate and were not associated with the angular or geometrical figures often perceived during migraine. The duration of these lights was rarely in excess of a few minutes. Epileptiform activity that originated in parastriate visual areas 18 and 19 of the visual cortex tended to cause photopsias that flickered rapidly but lasted only a few seconds to a few minutes at most. Momentary dimming of the homonymous hemifield was sometimes associated with occipital epileptiform activity. In some cases, visual symptoms were followed by a generalized seizure.

The second syndrome consisted of occipital apoplexy associated with hemorrhage of the AVM. This syndrome is characterized by the sudden onset of severe headache with persistent homonymous hemianopia. Other signs of subarachnoid hemorrhage usually are present, including stiff neck, obtundation, disorientation, and loss of consciousness. These hemorrhages typically are quite large and may cause uncal herniation with compression of the ipsilateral posterior cerebral artery, which results in permanent homonymous field loss.

Ophthalmoplegic Migraine. The vast majority of patients with ophthalmoplegic migraine experienced their first attack in early childhood.[16] Although new cases in adults occur, they are quite rare. Ophthalmoplegic migraine almost always involves the third nerve. Rare cases of sixth nerve involvement, and even rarer cases that involve the fourth nerve, have been reported. Bilateral involvement, either simultaneously or sequentially, is quite rare. In 1960 Walsh and O'Doherty[21] established specific criteria for ophthalmoplegic migraine:

- A prior history of typical common or classic migraine headaches.
- Ophthalmoplegia that occurs during (or, rarely, just before) an established migraine attack.
- Exclusion of other reasonable causes by clinical and radiological studies.

In addition to these criteria, Daroff[22] pointed out that a characteristic abnormality has been demonstrated in all cases of ophthalmoplegic migraine involving the third nerve in which magnetic resonance imaging (MRI) scanning has been performed: thickening and contrast enhancement of the nerve root as it exits the midbrain. This and other clinical findings led Lance and Zagami[23] to postulate that ophthalmoplegic migraine is a recurrent demyelinating, inflammatory cranial neuropathy.

The headache that occurs in ophthalmoplegic migraine is not always severe. It usually begins ipsilaterally but may become bilateral; it lasts from several hours to days. Rarely, the pupil is spared. The ophthalmoplegia usually resolves completely, but residual ptosis and ophthalmoplegia may be present after repeated attacks. Resolution usually requires several weeks or, less commonly, several months.

The differential diagnosis of painful ophthalmoplegia is discussed at length in Chapter 199. The diagnosis is suspected when parents of children who have this disorder report prior attacks of migraine-like episodes. In practice, when presented with a patient who is undergoing a first episode of pupil-involving third nerve palsy, it is almost always necessary to rule out a compressive third nerve palsy via neuroimaging studies. In most cases, this requires both MRI and cerebral arteriography to rule out an aneurysm.

The cause of ophthalmoplegic migraine is uncertain. Conflicting evidence has been garnered to support an ischemic cause, possibly related to migrainous involvement of the carotid artery; a compressive mechanism, related to compression of the intracavernous or subarachnoid portion of the third nerve by a swollen intracavernous carotid or basilar artery; and a demyelinating and inflammatory cause. The evidence for these disparate, but perhaps complementary, mechanisms is discussed at length by Miller[16] and by Daroff.[22]

Retinal Migraine. Although most visual symptoms in migraine are hemianopic and cortical in origin, transient (rarely permanent) monocular visual loss is well documented.[13,14,16,22-26] Both optic nerve[25,26] and retinal[13,14,16,22,25] ischemic episodes have been reported in migraine. Visual loss in retinal migraine tends to be shorter than that in the occipital variety, typically lasting 5–15 minutes. In some cases, the amaurosis may occur during, rather than before, the headache phase. Retinal vasospasm has been observed ophthalmoscopically during the attack in several patients. Fisher[27] reviewed 138 cases of amaurosis fugax (most without headache) in 1959, in both older and younger patients, and speculated that as many as 17% might be vasospastic in origin.

There seem to be two categories of young patients who experience amaurosis fugax because of presumed or observed vasospasm. The first group includes individuals who have well-established migraine, with or without prior hemianopic auras, and who develop migraine headaches associated with episodes of amaurosis fugax.[13,14,16,22] The second group consists of patients with no history of migraine who experience episodes of amaurosis fugax. In this group of patients, either vasospasm has been observed or other reasonable causes of amaurosis fugax have been ruled out (presumed retinal vasospasm).[28-30] The mechanism of visual loss in this second group is less clear, and its relationship to the dynamics of migraine is less certain than for the first group. Many of the patients in the second group have antiphospholipid antibodies or other evidence of autoimmune disturbance. Nevertheless, patients in this group, like those in the first, tend to respond well to calcium channel blockers or sometimes to aspirin. It has been suggested that retinal vasomotor instability, as a result of a migraine-like mechanism, may be compounded by interference with prostacycline release at the endothelial cell level (in some cases because of antiphospholipid antibodies).[31] This would account for the beneficial effect of both aspirin and calcium channel blockers. However, nonmigraine diagnoses should be excluded in all patients (young and old) who have amaurosis fugax. These diagnoses include embolic disease from the heart and carotid-ophthalmic system, hypercoagulability and hyperviscosity of various causes, and systemic vasculitides (for a detailed discussion of the differential diagnosis of amaurosis fugax, see Chapter 186).

PATHOGENESIS OF MIGRAINE. Although the pathogenesis of migraine remains uncertain, most researchers believe that the vascular alterations are not primary but result from a complex interplay of neuronal, hormonal, hematological, biochemical, and myogenic factors. The major controversies revolve around the mechanisms by which the prodrome, aura, and headache phases are triggered by the following:

- Primary aberrant neuronal activity.
- Various neuropeptides and vasoactive substances.
- Primary alterations in extra- and intracerebral blood flow.
- A combination of the above three factors.

Although an exhaustive discussion of migraine pathogenesis and the interplay of these mechanisms is beyond the scope of this chapter, the major theories are outlined briefly and illustrated in Figure 205-3. The interested reader is referred to a thorough account in the excellent clinical text by Lance.[32]

General agreement exists, based on epidemiological evidence, that migraineurs have a genetically determined lower threshold for certain environmental (or internal) triggers that can initiate a peculiar cascade of vascular and neurogenic events and lead to a migraine episode. Migraineurs differ from headache-free controls in several aspects of pain control and cerebrovascular reactivity, including the following:

- Altered hypothalamic and brainstem responses to various stimuli, including dopaminergic agonists.
- Altered intra- and extracranial vascular reactivity to stress, exercise, carbon dioxide, and cold stimuli (e.g., brief headache induced by ice cream is much more common in migraineurs).
- Diminished responses at various central nervous system sites to dopaminergic agents.
- Altered platelet function, especially with regard to 5-HT (or serotonin) release.

Several lines of evidence strongly suggest an important role for 5-HT, a powerful vasoactive substance, in the pathogenesis of migraine.[12,32] Various studies have shown the following:

- Typical migraine headaches can be produced by intramuscular injection of reserpine, which releases 5-HT from body stores.
- Urinary metabolites of 5-HT are increased during migraines.

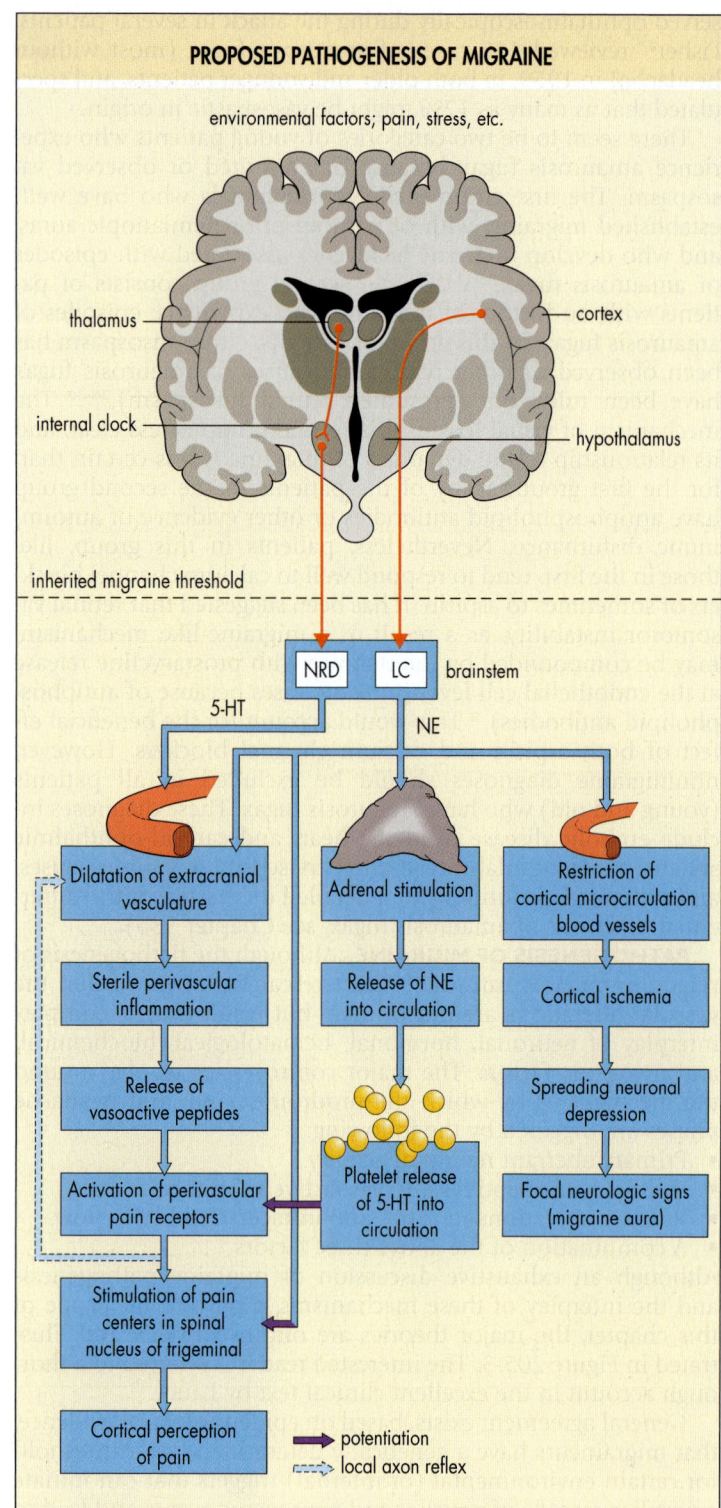

PROPOSED PATHOGENESIS OF MIGRAINE

environmental factors; pain, stress, etc.

thalamus — cortex

internal clock

hypothalamus

inherited migraine threshold

NRD | LC | brainstem

5-HT | NE

Dilatation of extracranial vasculature | Adrenal stimulation | Restriction of cortical microcirculation blood vessels

Sterile perivascular inflammation | Release of NE into circulation | Cortical ischemia

Release of vasoactive peptides | | Spreading neuronal depression

Activation of perivascular pain receptors | Platelet release of 5-HT into circulation | Focal neurologic signs (migraine aura)

Stimulation of pain centers in spinal nucleus of trigeminal

Cortical perception of pain

→ potentiation
⇢ local axon reflex

FIG. 205-3 ▪ **Proposed pathogenesis of migraine.** (Based on Lance JW. Migraine: pathophysiology. In: Mechanism and management of headache, 5th ed. London: Butterworth–Heinemann; 1993:91–116; Lance JW, Lambert GA, Goadsby PJ, Zagami AS. Contribution of experimental studies to understanding the pathophysiology of migraine. In: Sandler MP, Collins GM, eds. Migraine. A spectrum of ideas. Oxford: Oxford University Press; 1990:21–39.)

- Incubation of platelets with plasma obtained during (but not after) a migraine attack causes the release of 5-HT by platelets.

In addition to the receptors involved in the peripheral effect of 5-HT on cranial blood vessels, 5-HT receptors are also found at several important central nervous system sites. These include sites known to affect intra- and extracranial vascular reactivity, as well as sites that mediate the central gating of pain impulses.

Based on both human data and an experimental model, Lance *et al.*[32,33] proposed the mechanism for the development of migraine outlined here. An inherited migraine threshold renders the migraineur unusually susceptible to fluctuations in cortical

or hypothalamic function (signaled by mood changes, excessive thirst, hunger, and the like). Once this threshold is reached, the following sequence of events is activated (see Fig. 205-3).

Brainstem nuclei, including the nucleus raphe dorsalis (NRD) and the locus ceruleus (LC), are activated by cortical and hypothalamic events. These pathways employ 5-HT and norepinephrine (NE; noradrenaline), respectively, as neurotransmitters. Stimulation of the LC causes constriction of the cortical microcirculation blood vessels via release of the neurotransmitter NE. Stimulation of the LC, the NRD, or the trigeminal nerve may cause dilatation of the extracranial vasculature.

Cortical ischemia produced by microvascular changes may be accompanied by spreading neuronal depression, associated with focal neurological symptoms (e.g., homonymous hemianopia). This accounts for the migrainous aura, which may occur independently of the headache.

Release of 5-HT and vasoactive peptides at nerve endings on blood vessels may induce a sterile inflammatory response, which results in pain. This response may be perpetuated by local axon reflexes or by a central reflex pathway.

Stimulation of the LC also causes release of NE from the adrenals; NE, or an unknown 5-HT–releasing factor, causes platelets to release 5-HT into the circulation. Free 5-HT causes increased sensitivity of vascular receptors, which potentiates both abnormal vascular reactivity and the painful inflammatory response.

Pain afferents from intra- and extracranial vascular structures synapse on second-order neurons in the spinal nucleus of the trigeminal nerve. Transmission at these neurons is regulated in part by the LC, as well as by other brainstem nuclei. Improper activity of the LC may potentiate transmission of pain impulses at these synapses.

Stress-Tension Headache

Episodic stress-tension headache is the most common form of headache seen in medical practice. Most patients describe their tension headaches as a mild to moderate "pressing" or "squeezing" sensation, or they may compare the pain to a tight band that encircles the scalp. The pain is generally nonpulsatile and almost always bilateral. It may be bifrontal, biooccipital, or "band-like." Radiation to the posterior neck is common, as is tightness of the jaw muscles. Nausea, photophobia, and phonophobia are absent or minimal. Unlike migraine, tension headaches are not exacerbated by routine physical activity. Also unlike migraine, tension headaches are not preceded by the prodromal constitutional or focal neurologic symptoms noted earlier.[34]

Tension headaches may occur as infrequently as once a year and last only 30 minutes, or they may last all day and occur in an unrelenting daily fashion. Most patients who seek medical attention for their tension headaches have episodes that occur several times weekly or monthly, punctuated by headache-free intervals. The presence of headache-free intervals helps differentiate these headaches from more serious pathological processes, also taking into account the absence of other systemic or neurological symptoms. These patients are often aware of stressful emotional triggers that precipitate their tension headaches; therefore, they can readily identify, if not control, the exacerbating factors. Depression is present in up to one third of patients who experience persistent tension headaches.[34] Many patients with tension headaches also have migraines, but usually they can differentiate the two types of headache on the basis of severity, duration, and associated symptoms.

Some controversy exists about the role of the pericranial musculature in the production of tension headache.[34] Although muscle spasm and tenderness may be the result, rather than the primary cause, of chronic tension headaches in many patients, it appears that distinct myofascial trigger points can be a source of pain in some patients. The myofascial pain syndrome is characterized by reproducible pain on palpation of trigger points.[34] The pain generally is referred to a location somewhere along the band of taut muscle that includes the trigger point, although it may be at some distance from the trigger point itself. According to Jay,[35] the syndromes of tension headache, myofascial pain syndrome, and fibromyalgia represent a spectrum of severity of the same underlying disorder.

Cluster Headache

Cluster headaches are perhaps the most painful type of "benign" headache. The pain can be so severe that some patients who have this disorder have reported thoughts of suicide. The pain typically is unilateral and periorbital in location and tends to occur on the same side during each attack; rarely is the opposite side involved. Unlike migraines, cluster headaches are more common in men than in women. In addition, cluster patients, unlike migraineurs, generally are hyperactive during an attack—they often pace the room or rock fitfully in a chair. Sympathetic dysfunction ipsilateral to the pain is common.[13,14,16] Horner's syndrome may be present during the attack, along with lacrimation, conjunctival injection, nasal congestion, rhinorrhea, and eyelid edema. The Horner's syndrome may persist, especially after repeated attacks; pharmacological testing reveals a postganglionic localization. Attacks are usually shorter than for migraine and last 15–180 minutes, with an average of about 45 minutes. The attacks cluster in time; characteristically, they occur at least once daily, usually at the same time of day. Nocturnal occurrence is common, and the headache often wakes the patient from sleep. Some patients also find that attacks can be precipitated by alcohol ingestion. As the cluster period progresses, the frequency of episodes may increase to three or more per day. The cluster period typically lasts for 4–12 weeks. The patient is then asymptomatic until the next cluster period, which typically occurs a year or more later, usually at the same time of year.

The treatment of cluster headaches is highly individualized and has been reviewed at length elsewhere.[36] Some of the same agents used for migraine may be used for cluster headache, including sumatriptan for acute attacks and methysergide for short-term use (less than 6 months). In addition, prednisone is often effective in halting bouts of cluster headaches. For more resistant cases, lithium is often useful.

Temporal Arteritis

Headache is the most common symptom in temporal arteritis[37]; this diagnosis should be considered in all adults older than 50 years who have headache or facial pain. All patients in this age group should be asked specifically about symptoms of vasculitis and vascular insufficiency that involve the extracranial carotid circulation. These include the following[37–40]:

- The presence of pain or tenderness around the temporal arteries.
- Scalp tenderness.
- Pain with chewing (i.e., jaw or tongue claudication).
- Diplopia, which is generally thought to result from extraocular muscle ischemia rather than from cranial neuropathy.
- Transient visual loss as a result of optic nerve or retinal ischemia.

In addition, many but not all patients who have temporal arteritis have symptoms of more widespread rheumatological involvement (i.e., polymyalgia rheumatica).[39] These symptoms may be rather nonspecific and include malaise and easy fatigability, weight loss, anorexia, and unexplained fevers, as well as proximal myalgias.

The headache of temporal arteritis classically is located over a branch of the superficial temporal artery and is described as a dull ache that persists throughout the day. It may be accompanied by tenderness of the artery and overlying scalp.[36,37,39] The artery, if severely affected, may be indurated and nonpulsatile. Many patients, however, present with a nonspecific unilateral or bilateral headache.

A sedimentation rate to rule out temporal arteritis should be obtained in all patients older than 60 years who have headache

---

or facial pain, unless the pain obviously results from another cause. The test is simple and noninvasive and identifies about 90% of patients who have this disorder.[41] The consequences of missing this diagnosis (i.e., bilateral visual loss) can be devastating and are usually avoidable with early diagnosis and aggressive treatment. Temporal artery biopsy should be performed in all patients who have a clinically suggestive history, in view of the consequences of an incorrect diagnosis. Unless otherwise contraindicated, corticosteroid therapy should be instituted, pending results of the biopsy. A thorough discussion of the issues that surround diagnosis and therapy of temporal arteritis can be found in Chapter 197.

Headache as a Result of Intracranial Processes

Ruling out intracranial pathology should be one of the primary goals of the ophthalmologist when a patient complains of headache. Although myriad intracranial processes can cause headache, most intracranial pain is caused by inflammation or stretching of pain-sensitive structures in the dura and blood vessels. For this reason, the pattern of headache in this class of disorders includes several features that can help distinguish them from more benign causes of headache. Although the complete differential diagnosis of intracranial headache is beyond the scope of this chapter, several warning signs should alert the ophthalmologist to the possibility of a serious neurological problem (Box 205-4):

- A change in the usual pattern of headache. Migraine and tension headaches are extremely common and may preexist in patients who develop serious intracranial pathology. An acute or subacute increase in the intensity and frequency of a well-established headache pattern should arouse suspicion, as should the onset of a new type of headache.
- Headache described as "the worst headache I've ever had." Most patients do not use this characterization without good reason, and it often means that the headache is several orders of magnitude greater than prior headaches.
- Headache triggered by exertion, by coughing or sneezing, or by postural changes, such as bending over. These features often signal irritation or stretching of pain-sensitive intracranial structures.
- Headache accompanied by signs of meningeal irritation, such as stiff neck, nausea, vomiting, or fever.
- Headache accompanied by focal or nonfocal neurological signs (e.g., focal weakness or numbness, aphasia, impaired cognitive function, change in personality).

Negative responses to these "red flags" should provide reassurance against intracranial pathology.

Sinus Disease

The diagnosis of pain that results from acute sinus inflammation is rarely difficult. Often a prior history of sinus inflammation or respiratory allergies is elicited. In general, the pain is of low to moderate intensity and is present on a daily basis. The pain usually is localized to the frontal or maxillary area, and there is tenderness to percussion over the affected sinus. The pain is often worsened by bending forward and may be accentuated by blowing the nose or sneezing. Symptoms of nasal "stuffiness" are usually present, and mucopurulent drainage from the nostrils may be seen. If the nasal passages are blocked, use of a nasal decongestant can be useful diagnostically and often results in discharge. In doubtful cases, a simple plain film of the sinuses or an opinion from an otolaryngologist should be obtained.

Tumors, abscesses, and mucoceles that arise in the sinuses and nasopharynx can give rise to facial or periorbital pain. Mucoceles, in particular, tend to cause pain by obstructing sinus ostia. Maxillary (and, less commonly, sphenoid) mucoceles may erode the orbital bones and cause proptosis. Sphenoid mucoceles may invade the orbital apex, which results in ocular motility disturbances or optic neuropathy. Nasopharyngeal carcinoma has a propensity to invade the base of the skull by traveling along neural foramina.[42] These tumors may cause ocular motility disturbances, most commonly sixth nerve palsy; however, their most common neuro-ophthalmological manifestation is facial numbness or pain. Decreased hearing as a result of closure of the eustachian tube also is common. These tumors can be missed easily on plain films and require computed tomography or MRI for early detection.

Orbital Inflammation and Neoplasia

Although the physical examination and differential diagnosis of orbital disease are beyond the scope of this chapter, the classic signs and symptoms should be elicited meticulously whenever orbital disease is suspected (see Chapter 95). A presumptive diagnosis of orbital inflammatory or neoplastic disease usually can be made on the basis of a thorough history and examination and is confirmed with radiological studies. Difficulties arise primarily in patients whose signs of orbital disease are minimal. For example, small posterior orbital masses, such as optic nerve sheath meningiomas, may cause little exophthalmos. However, careful testing of visual function, including color vision and pupillary function, almost always demonstrates convincing evidence of a subtle optic neuropathy. Orbital myositis and inflammatory orbital pseudotumor ordinarily cause persistent unilateral pain of moderate to severe intensity, and signs of ocular proptosis or dysmotility usually are present.

Posterior scleritis may be difficult to diagnose.[43] The pain is persistent and often moderately severe. It may be accentuated by eye movement. Quantitative A-scan ultrasonography usually is diagnostic and demonstrates thickening of the affected sclera. B-scan ultrasonography is not quite as sensitive but may be helpful. Though not ordinarily necessary, computed tomography scans generally show thickening and enhancement of the affected posterior sclera.

DIFFERENTIAL DIAGNOSIS OF FACIAL PAIN

Facial pain may arise from a variety of structures of the face and neck, including the sinuses, nasopharynx, teeth and gums, facial muscles, orbit, middle ear, trigeminal nerve, muscles of mastication, and carotid artery and its tributaries. Several syndromes can include ocular or periorbital pain and should be familiar to the ophthalmologist.

Trigeminal Neuralgia (Tic Douloureux)

Trigeminal neuralgia is characterized by sudden, intense jabs of pain that last only a few seconds or less.[44] The pain generally is limited to one of the three divisions of the trigeminal nerve, with the second and third divisions involved most frequently. The pain usually is described as lancinating or "stabbing" in quality; it often recurs in a series of paroxysms that extend over several minutes. Most patients can identify a triggering activity, such as chewing, swallowing, or light touch to a part of the face, that initiates a paroxysm.

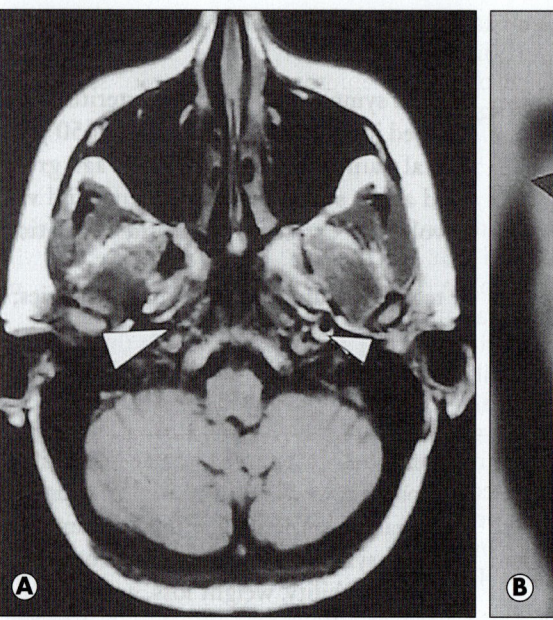
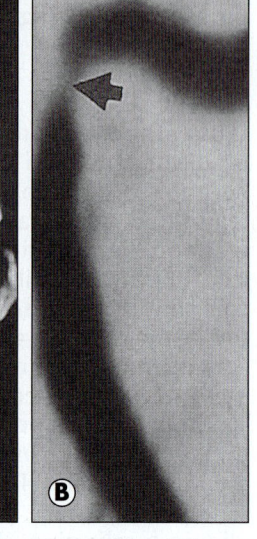

FIG. 205-4 ■ MRI of spontaneous carotid dissection. **A,** T2-weighted MRI through the base of the skull demonstrates normal flow void in the right internal carotid (*large arrow*) and curvilinear high signal intensity in the left internal carotid (*small arrow*) caused by spontaneous dissection in a 52-year-old hypertensive man. **B,** Magnetic resonance angiogram in the anterior oblique projection demonstrates an area of narrowing of the internal carotid artery due to dissection (*arrow*) just distal to the bifurcation.

Raeder's Paratrigeminal Syndrome

In 1924 Raeder[45] described a series of patients who had oculosympathetic paresis (Horner's syndrome) and pain in the trigeminal distribution. Raeder's series actually included two different types of patients. The first group had episodic headaches caused by what is now known as the cluster headache syndrome. The second group had chronic pain in the trigeminal distribution caused by a variety of space-occupying lesions, including tumors of the middle cranial fossa. In this latter group, oculosympathetic paresis resulted from involvement of the sympathetic plexus with the internal carotid artery, either at the base of the skull or in the cavernous sinus. The term "Raeder's paratrigeminal syndrome" generally should not be used. This avoids confusion between the benign cluster headache syndrome, on the one hand, and potentially lethal skull base tumors or aneurysms, on the other.

All patients with suspected oculosympathetic paresis should undergo a cocaine test for confirmation and a hydroxyamphetamine test for localization (see Chapter 203). These tests should be followed by appropriate neuroimaging of either the base of the skull and upper neck (for postganglionic lesions) or the chest and neck (for preganglionic lesions). Trigeminal sensation should be checked in all three divisions. Trigeminal hypesthesia is not a feature of the cluster headache syndrome and should alert the clinician to the possibility of a mass lesion or microscopic infiltration at the skull base. In patients who have facial pain and Horner's syndrome, the clinician should be particularly aware of the signs and symptoms of dissection of the internal carotid artery.[46] Dysesthesia of the scalp and dysgeusia, or unpleasant taste, are common, along with postganglionic Horner's syndrome. Although spontaneous dissections occur, most middle-aged or older patients are hypertensive, and most younger patients have had significant neck trauma. The condition usually is diagnosed readily with MRI (Fig. 205-4).

Chronic Paroxysmal Hemicrania

Normally classified as a cluster headache variant, this unusual syndrome is characterized by episodes of multiple, brief "stabbing" pains, typically in the periorbital region.[47] The pain usually is quite severe and lasts 1–2 minutes, but a series of paroxysms may last up to 45 minutes. Repeated series tend to occur throughout the day, as often as 10–15 times. Episodes are accompanied by hemicranial autonomic dysfunction similar to that seen with cluster headaches. The syndrome often responds to indomethacin 25–50mg three times daily.

Icepick Headaches (Jabs and Jolts Syndrome)

This syndrome consists of intense stabbing pains that last only a few seconds and typically occur in the periorbital region, forehead, or frontal area.[48] This type of pain is seen in about one third of migraineurs and may accompany a migraine episode or occur independently. When this type of headache occurs independently of migraine episodes, it usually is quite responsive to indomethacin.

REFERENCES

1. McQueen J, Loblay RH, Swain AR, *et al.* A controlled trial of dietary modification in migraine. In: Rose FC, ed. New advances in headache research. London: Smith-Gordon; 1989:235–42.
2. Drummond PD, Lance JW. Neurovascular disturbances in headache patients. Clin Exp Neurol. 1984;20:93–9.
3. Headache Classification Committee of the International Headache Society. Classification and diagnostic criteria for headache disorders, cranial neuralgias and facial pain. Cephalalgia. 1988;8(Suppl. 7):1–96.
4. Dalsgaard-Nielsen J. Some aspects of the epidemiology of migraine in Denmark. Headache. 1970;10:14–23.
5. Mortimer MJ, Kay J, Jaron A. Childhood migraine in general practice: clinical features and characteristics. Cephalalgia. 1992;12:238–43.
6. Lance JW, Curran DA, Anthony M. Investigation into the mechanism and treatment of chronic headache. Med J Aust. 1965;65:909–14.
7. Fisher CM. Late-life migraine accompaniments as a cause of unexplained transient ischemic attacks. Can J Neurol Sci. 1980;7:9–17.
8. Laurence KM. Genetics of migraine. In: Blau JN, ed. Migraine. Clinical and research aspects. Baltimore: Johns Hopkins University Press; 1987:479–84.
9. Lance JW. Migraine: clinical aspects. In: Mechanism and management of headache, 5th ed. London: Butterworth–Heinemann; 1993:68–90.
10. Evans RW, Lipton RB. Topics in migraine management: a survey of headache specialists highlights some controversies. Neurol Clin. 2001;19:1–21.
11. Solomon S, Cappa KG, Smith CR. Common migraine: criteria for diagnosis. Headache. 1988;28:124–9.
12. Sicuteri F. Prophylactic and therapeutic properties of UML-491 in migraine. Int Arch Allergy. 1959;15:300–7.
13. Hupp SL, Kline LB, Corbett JJ. Visual disturbances of migraine. Surv Ophthalmol. 1989;33:221–36.
14. Corbett JJ. Neuro-ophthalmic complications of migraine and cluster headaches. Neurol Clin. 1983;1:973–5.
15. Iversen HK, Langemark M, Andersson PG, *et al.* Clinical characteristics of migraine and episodic tension-type headache in relation to old and new diagnostic criteria. Headache. 1990;30:514–9.
16. Miller NR. Migraine. In: Walsh and Hoyt's clinical neuro-ophthalmology, vol 4, 4th ed. Baltimore: Williams & Wilkins; 1991:2515–74.
17. Sacks O. Migraine aura and classical migraine. In: Migraine. The evolution of a common disorder. Berkeley: University of California Press; 1970:72–117.
18. Lance JW. Migraine: treatment. In: Mechanism and management of headache, 5th ed. London: Butterworth–Heinemann; 1993:116–43.
19. Troost BT, Newton TH. Occipital lobe arteriovenous malformations: clinical and radiologic features in 26 cases with comments on the differentiation from migraine. Arch Ophthalmol. 1975;93:250–6.
20. Bruyn GW. Intracranial arteriovenous malformation and migraine. Cephalalgia. 1984;4:191–207.
21. Walsh JP, O'Doherty DS. A possible explanation of the mechanism of ophthalmoplegic migraine. Neurology. 1960;10:1079–84.
22. Daroff RB. Ophthalmoplegic migraine. Cephalalgia. 2001;1:81.
23. Lance JW, Zagami AS. Ophthalmoplegic migraine: a recurrent demyelinating neuropathy? Cephalalgia. 2001;21:84–9.
24. Glenn AM, Shaw PJ, Howe JW, Bates D. Complicated migraine resulting in blindness due to bilateral retinal infarction. Br J Ophthalmol. 1992;76:189–90.
25. Weinstein JM, Feman SS. Ischemic optic neuropathy in migraine. Arch Ophthalmol. 1982;100:1097–100.
26. Katz B. Bilateral sequential migrainous ischemic optic neuropathy. Am J Ophthalmol. 1985;99:489.
27. Fisher CM. Observation of the fundus oculi in transient monocular blindness. Neurology. 1959;9:333–47.
28. Winterkorn JMS, Kupersmith MJ, Wirtschafter JD, Forman S. Brief report: treatment of vasospastic amaurosis fugax with calcium-channel blockers. N Engl J Med. 1993;329:396–8.
29. Burger SK, Saul RF, Selhorst JB, Thurston SE. Transient monocular blindness caused by vasospasm. N Engl J Med. 1991;325:870–3.
30. Winterkorn JMS, Teman AJ. Recurrent attacks of amaurosis fugax treated with calcium channel blockers. Ann Neurol. 1991;30:423–5.
31. McLean PM, Greco TP. Amaurosis fugax (letter). N Engl J Med. 1994;330(2):144. Comment on: N Engl J Med. 1993;329(6):426–8.
32. Lance JW. Migraine: pathophysiology. In: Mechanism and management of headache, 5th ed. London: Butterworth–Heinemann; 1993:91–116.
33. Lance JW, Lambert GA, Goadsby PJ, Zagami AS. Contribution of experimental studies to understanding the pathophysiology of migraine. In: Sandler MP, Collins GM, eds. Migraine. A spectrum of ideas. Oxford: Oxford University Press; 1990:21–39.
34. Jay GW. Pathophysiology of tension type headache. In: Tollison CD, Kunkel RS, eds. Headache. Diagnosis and treatment. Baltimore: Williams & Wilkins; 1991:129–42.
35. Jay GW. Myofascial mechanisms in the etiology of chronic daily headache: two syndromes, one entity? Paper presented at the 32nd annual meeting of the American Association for the Study of Headache, Los Angeles, June 1990.
36. Lance JW. Cluster headache. In: Mechanism and management of headache, 5th ed. London: Butterworth–Heinemann; 1993:163–87.
37. Nordborg E, Nordborg C, Malmvall BE, *et al.* Giant cell arteritis. Rheum Dis Clin North Am. 1995;21(4):1013–26.
38. Keltner JL. Giant-cell arteritis. Signs and symptoms. Ophthalmology. 1982;89:1101–10.
39. Hellmann DB. Immunopathogenesis, diagnosis, and treatment of giant cell arteritis, temporal arteritis, polymyalgia rheumatica, and Takayasu's arteritis. Curr Opin Rheumatol. 1993;5:25–32.
40. Miller NR. Giant cell arteritis. In: Walsh and Hoyt's clinical neuro-ophthalmology, vol 4, 4th ed. Baltimore: Williams & Wilkins; 1991:2601–27.
41. Kyle V, Cawston TE, Hazleman BL. Erythrocyte sedimentation rate and C reactive protein in the assessment of polymyalgia rheumatica/giant cell arteritis on presentation and during follow up. Ann Rheum Dis. 1989;48:667–71.
42. Smith JJ, Wheliss JA. Ocular manifestations of nasopharyngeal tumors. Trans Am Acad Ophthalmol Otolaryngol. 1962;66:659–64.
43. Benson WE. Posterior scleritis. Surv Ophthalmol. 1988;32:297–316.
44. Fromm GH, Terrence CF, Maroon JC. Trigeminal neuralgia. Current concepts regarding etiology and pathogenesis. Arch Neurol. 1984;41:1204–7.
45. Raeder JG. "Paratrigeminal" paralysis of oculopupillary sympathetics. Brain. 1924;47:149–58.
46. Pozzati E, Giuliani G, Poppi M, Faenza A. Long-term follow-up of occlusive cervical carotid dissection. Stroke. 1989;20:412–6.
47. Sjaastad O, Apfelbaum R, Caskey W, *et al.* Chronic paroxysmal hemicrania (CPH). The clinical manifestations. A review. Ups J Med Sci. 1980;31(Suppl.):27–33.
48. Raskin NH, Schwartz RK. Icepick-like pain. Neurology. 1980;30:203–5.

206 Tumors, Infections, Inflammations, and Neurodegenerations

HOSSEIN G. SAADATI • ALFREDO A. SADUN

DEFINITIONS

- Tumors are compressive lesions and may compromise the function of adjacent tissues.
- Infections are invasions of tissues by microorganisms (bacterial, fungal, or viral).
- Inflammations reflect intrinsic responses by various tissues related to the immune system and may compromise tissue function.
- Neurodegenerations of the central nervous system often involve premature dysfunction consequent to genetic factors.

KEY FEATURES

- Tumors, infections, and inflammations of the central nervous system may involve the meninges, the brain substance (parenchyma), or the surface of the brain (extraparenchymal).
- Neurodegenerations may be specific for certain regions of the brain (such as Huntington's chorea) or involve the brain diffusely (such as Alzheimer's disease).

ASSOCIATED FEATURES

- Tumors may be benign or malignant; primary or metastatic.
- Inflammatory and infectious responses may be acute or chronic, according to the cadence of development.

TUMORS

INTRODUCTION

Tumors of the brain may produce symptoms that arise from their size, location (abutment to critical structures), malignancy (which produces adjacent necrosis), or nonspecific mechanical effects (such as blockage of the cerebrospinal circulation). Tumors may present with signs and symptoms that are localizing (such as chiasmal visual field loss) or nonlocalizing (such as headaches, seizures). New-onset seizures are harbingers of an intracranial tumor in up to 33% of adults.[1] Papilledema and sixth nerve palsies are important nonlocalizing signs of increased intracranial pressure and may indicate the presence of an intracranial tumor.

Although it is beyond the scope of this chapter to describe the characteristics of each tumor type, several tumors that mimic infections or inflammations at the base of the brain or are in the differential diagnosis of meningitis with neuro-ophthalmic symptoms are discussed.

EPIDEMIOLOGY AND PATHOGENESIS

Tumors tend to develop in the posterior fossa in children and in the cerebral hemispheres in adults. For example, medulloblas-

tomas are seen most commonly in male children 4–8 years of age. Neuroblastomas and, to a lesser extent, ependymomas and papillomas of the choroid also are more common in the young.

OCULAR MANIFESTATIONS

Tumors produce signs and symptoms in accordance with their location. Additionally, many tumors are nonlocalizing. Papilledema and diplopia from sixth nerve palsies may be produced by tumors in any location.

Localizing tumors are likely to affect adjacent structures. Tumors of the optic nerve, such as meningiomas or gliomas, often produce a slowly progressive, painless visual loss; loss of optic nerve functions (dyschromatopsia, pupillary defects, and loss of brightness sense); visual field defects; and disc edema early in the course of the disease process (see Chapter 189). Eventually, optic atrophy develops. If the tumor is intraorbital, significant proptosis, increased resistance to retropulsion, signs of orbital congestion, and, uncommonly, diplopia from ophthalmoplegia may be seen.

Metastatic tumors, or malignant invasive tumors, may produce inflammation and necrosis in surrounding tissue and may even simulate orbital cellulitis.

Cavernous sinus involvement is likely to produce ophthalmoplegia with or without pain. The signs and symptoms may be quite similar to those of an orbital apex syndrome. Numbness or pain in the distribution of the first division of the fifth nerve is common.

Near the optic chiasm, a variety of tumors may produce a chiasmal syndrome (bitemporal visual field defects). The most common of these are pituitary adenomas, but gliomas, meningiomas, craniopharyngiomas, and tumors from the sphenoidal sinus and clivus all may involve the optic chiasm. Pituitary adenomas may expand suddenly when affected by necrosis and hemorrhage; this pituitary apoplexy is the exception to the rule that intracranial tumors develop and produce symptoms slowly.

Tumors in the parietal and temporal lobes may involve the posterior visual pathways and produce corresponding defects in the visual field. Occipital lobe tumors produce much more congruous visual field defects, which often spare visual fixation.

PATHOLOGY

Each tumor type has its own histopathological features. Often, special stains, such as immunohistochemistry, are useful in the differentiation of subsets of tumor types. It may be useful, therefore, to preserve some tissues in standard fixative and set other specimens aside in the frozen state and, in certain cases, in mixed buffered aldehydes for possible electron microscopy.

TREATMENT

Treatment of malignancies that produce a base-of-the-brain syndrome or a paraneoplastic syndrome depends on the type of malignancy. In addition to addressing the primary tumor, consideration has to be given to malignant cells that might be in the cerebrospinal fluid (CSF) and to the immune response. At times, immunosuppressive therapy may be of temporary benefit (such as in the administration of corticosteroids for cancer-associated retinopathy or in CSF paraneoplastic disease). Often, central nervous system (CNS) irradiation (brain and spinal cord axis) may be necessary.

COURSE AND OUTCOME

Responses to chemotherapy or radiation therapy are extremely variable and depend largely on the type of neoplasm involved. However, the long-term visual prognosis is guarded.

INFECTIONS

INTRODUCTION

Despite the advancements in control programs and powerful antibiotics, CNS infections in general are still a management problem. In this era of acquired immunodeficiency syndrome (AIDS) and other forms of immunosuppression, symptoms and signs that are not typical for a particular infection in non-AIDS or nonimmunosuppressed patients have to be recognized.

Infections of the CNS have a diverse presentation; however, most share four cardinal manifestations: headache, altered mental status, focal neurological signs, and fever. Because these features are nonspecific, other characteristics are important in the evaluation of these patients, such as the time course of the disease and its natural history. The syndrome of chronic meningitis is defined as meningitis that fails to improve or progresses over at least 4 weeks of observation.[2] Infections at the base of the brain ("basilar meningitis") usually run a subacute or chronic course, are gradual in onset, and may last for weeks or months; their mortality rate is moderate to high. Focal neurological findings are more common than in acute meningitis. Diagnosis with regard to the causative agent is of utmost importance.

EPIDEMIOLOGY AND PATHOGENESIS

Meningitis may present with a variety of clinical syndromes, and the clinical expression of meningitis depends on the underlying medical condition and the immune status of the patient.[3] Meningococcus accounts for 20% of all cases of bacterial meningitis in the United States. Interestingly, serogroup B is present in 50% of such cases. In acute fulminant cases of infectious meningitis, a severe inflammatory reaction occurs in the meninges, primarily in the subarachnoid spaces over the convexity of the brain and around the cisterns at the base of the brain; the reaction rarely breaks into the parenchyma. As the inflammation continues, adhesions form that may interfere with CSF flow and cause fibrosis of the meninges along the roots of the cranial nerves. The toxic effect of the infectious organism also may contribute to the inflammatory process via the release of various cytokines.

OCULAR MANIFESTATIONS

The initial systemic symptoms of fever, chills, nausea, and vomiting are often accompanied by headache, stiffness of the neck, seizures, and cranial nerve palsies. These symptoms present more acutely in viral and bacterial infections and more insidiously in the basilar meningitis that results from fungus, tuberculosis, syphilis, or other similar causes.

The hallmark signs for most forms of meningitis are the meningeal signs of Kernig and Brudzinski, which are commonly present. Both maneuvers stretch the possibly inflamed spinal structures and, in cases of meningitis, lead to pain and a reflexive extension of the neck and flexion of the hips and knees.

Basilar meningitis, especially, may produce cranial nerve palsies. Involvement of the third, fourth, and sixth nerves produces binocular diplopia. More rarely, an optic neuritis or chiasmatis may develop, with a resultant loss of optic nerve function and visual acuity and with losses in the visual field. More often, increases in intracranial pressure result in papilledema and its associated signs and symptoms (see Chapter 189).

DIAGNOSIS AND TESTING

The key finding is an abnormal CSF analysis that shows increased intracranial pressure, increased white cell count, cloudy CSF, increased protein, decreased sugar level, and identification of the microorganism on Gram's stain with growth on the appropriate culture media. However, patients whose bacterial meningitis is partially treated may continue to show signs and symptoms of acute meningitis with sterile CSF. Negative Gram's stains or cultures and sensitivities also may reflect patients with fungal, tuberculous, and parameningeal infections.

PATHOLOGY

Generally, infections are identified by Gram's stain or culture and sensitivities. However, on occasion, histopathology may be helpful, particularly for fungal, protozoan, or atypical bacterial infections.

TREATMENT

Appropriate antibiotic therapy to which the microorganism is sensitive is essential in bacterial meningitis; delay is life threatening. It is important that the antibiotic cross the blood-CSF barrier in sufficient concentrations to achieve therapeutic values in the CSF. Maintenance of adequate fluid and electrolyte balance is important to help control the cerebral edema. Corticosteroid administration concomitant with the use of antibiotics has been advocated by some investigators as being particularly beneficial in children to reduce the neurological sequelae. However, no prospective study has confirmed this advantage.

COURSE AND OUTCOME

If the infectious meningitis is responsive to therapy, the outcome may be only minimal neurological sequelae. About 20–25% of patients who recover are left with sequelae, which can vary from minimal facial weakness or hearing loss to severe intellectual or other physical ailments such as hemiplegia, paraplegia, seizures, cranial nerve palsies with diplopia, blindness, chronic increased intracranial pressure, syndrome of inappropriate antidiuretic hormone, and subdural effusion. In association with human immunodeficiency virus (HIV) epidemics, infectious meningitis may become more resistant to therapy, and the process may be chronic and indolent with a poorer response to treatment.[4]

INFLAMMATIONS

INTRODUCTION

For the most part, inflammations of the brain involve blood vessels with or without vessel wall necrosis. Systemic vasculitis may be present with predominant CNS manifestations, as well as forms of vasculitis that are limited primarily to the CNS.

EPIDEMIOLOGY AND PATHOGENESIS

Inflammations of the brain and, in particular, vasculitis are more common in young adults. Vasculitis is an idiopathic disorder that involves the small and medium blood vessels of the brain and spinal cord and usually presents with multiple bilateral infarcts of the cortex and subcortical white matter. The CNS may be injured by the ischemia that results from vasculitis or directly from the effects of inflammation. In the inflammatory process, granulocytes and macrophages directly destroy oligodendrocytes, as well as neurons and their axons, either through the release of cytotoxic agents or through phagocytosis.

The specific pathogenesis varies with the type of systemic vasculitis. Polyarteritis nodosa (PAN) is rare, with a male-female ratio of 2.5:1. In systemic lupus erythematosus, most cases begin in the age range of 20–40 years, and 95% of patients are women. Giant cell arteritis is a relatively common form of vasculitis, with a 5-year incidence as high as 24 per 100,000 in individuals of northern European ancestry who are older than 50 years. Wegener's granulomatosis is a rare entity of unknown cause that affects adult men and women in a ratio of 2:1. The pathogenesis includes the evolution of necrotizing granulomas.

The prevalence of Sjögren's syndrome in the general population is 2–3%. This chronic systemic condition is caused predominantly by lymphocytic infiltration of lacrimal and salivary glands. Although traditionally considered a disease of middle-aged to elderly women, several cases have been reported of young adults, adolescents, and even children affected by the disease. Behçet's syndrome occurs more frequently in those of Middle Eastern, Mediterranean, or Japanese descent and has a male preponderance. Its pathogenesis remains elusive, but an association with the HLA-B5 antigen occurs in some geographical regions.

Since the initial report in 1956, 223 cases of Miller-Fisher syndrome have been described. The male-female ratio is 2:1, with a mean age of 43.6 years at disease onset. A viral infection precedes the neurological symptoms in more than 70% of cases. Vogt-Koyanagi-Harada syndrome is a granulomatous inflammatory disorder. It occurs more commonly in darkly pigmented races such as Asians, Hispanics, American Indians, and Asian Indians. It also is more common in Japan, where it accounts for 6.8–9.2% of all cases of uveitis. Most patients are in the second to fifth decades of life. The pathogenesis may be the selective damage of melanocytes as part of an autoimmune process.

OCULAR MANIFESTATIONS

Primary cerebral vasculitides include a variety of pathologies that mainly involve blood vessels of the brain and spinal cord. The clinical manifestations vary widely as diffuse or focal neurological dysfunction, which may affect different regions of the CNS. Further differences occur between diseases that affect primarily small versus larger blood vessels. Typical symptoms of diffuse involvement include headache, seizures, confusion, hallucination, and generalized lethargy. Focal involvement may manifest as a cerebrovascular accident; if the cranial nerves are affected, this may present as ophthalmoplegia or optic neuropathy; involvement of the posterior visual pathways produces characteristic visual field defects.

Systemic Necrotizing Vasculitides

Systemic necrotizing vasculitides are listed in Table 206-1. In PAN, the visual loss may result from retinal vascular disease, retinal vasculitis, or cortical blindness, all of which are rare. The CNS becomes involved with variable frequency, usually after the initial diagnosis of PAN. Presentation is variable and may include diffuse encephalopathy or seizures. Focal neurological deficits appear to be secondary to cerebral infarction and hemorrhage involving one cerebral hemisphere. Peripheral neuropathy (mononeuritis multiplex) is frequently the presenting manifestation; seen less commonly is a diffuse, sensorimotor type. These forms of neuropathy are attributed to ischemia or arteritis of nutrient vessels.[5]

In systemic lupus erythematosus (SLE), visual sensory disturbances may result from optic nerve disease related to optic neu-

TABLE 206-1

PRIMARY CENTRAL NERVOUS SYSTEM AND SYSTEMIC VASCULITIDES

Vasculitic Type	Name	Age (Years)	Central Nervous System Sign (Most Common)
Primary central nervous system	Granulomatous angiitis of the central nervous system	20–50	Headache
	Cogan's syndrome	20–30	Encephalitis
	Eales' disease	20–40	Retinal phlebitis
	Acute posterior multifocal placoid pigment epitheliopathy	15–30	Retinal inflammation
	Microangiopathy of the brain	20–40	Stroke
Systemic	Polyarteritis nodosa	40–70	Stroke
	Wegener's granulomatosis	25–50	Cranial palsy
	Giant cell arteritis	55–85	Cranial palsy
	Systemic lupus erythematosus	20–40	Organic brain
	Sjögren's syndrome	40–50	Encephalitis
	Behçet's syndrome	15–30	Cranial palsy
	Relapsing polychondritis		
	Allergic angiitis		
	Scleroderma		
	Polymyositis and dermatomyositis		
	Hypersensitivity vasculitis		
	Henoch–Schönlein purpura		
	Mixed cryoglobulinemia		
	Lymphomatoid granulomatosis		
	Takayasu's arteritis		
	Lethal midline granuloma		

ritis (inflammatory or ischemic) or papilledema (pseudotumor cerebri or malignant hypertension). Retrochiasmatic pathway involvement may present as transient visual phenomena (which may be mistaken for migraine) or as permanent homonymous field defects, which may be acute or subacute and occasionally herald the diagnosis of SLE. Involvement of the CNS occurs in 35–60% of patients who have SLE. The neurological manifestations are divided into two types—diffuse and focal. The former includes major motor seizures, dementia, delirium, organic mood disorder, and organic psychosis. The focal types are cranial neuropathies, stroke, transverse myelitis, focal seizures, and chorea.[6] The ocular motor pathway may be involved from the cerebral cortex to the extraocular muscles; the most common locus of involvement is a brainstem infarction.[7]

Giant cell arteritis (GCA) is a common vasculitis in which the most serious clinical manifestations are largely ophthalmic. One of the most devastating is irreversible blindness, which occurs in 36% of cases. The incidence of second eye involvement is about 65% among untreated patients. The most common ocular presentation is anterior ischemic optic neuropathy, with severe visual loss to no light perception and a pale, swollen optic nerve. Visual loss also may result from posterior optic neuropathy, severe choroidal ischemia, central retinal artery or ophthalmic artery occlusion, anterior segment ischemia, and chiasmal or cortical ischemia. Other ocular manifestations are diplopia related to ophthalmoplegia that involves the third, fourth, or sixth cranial nerve.

In GCA, headache and pain often occur in the temples, occipital region, ear, or tongue. Jaw claudication pain, manifested upon chewing or talking, is a classic and highly specific symptom that, unfortunately, is not consistently present (found in 30% of patients). Other neurological manifestations occur in 30% of patients and include transient ischemic attacks that involve the posterior circulation and infarcts of the vertebrobasilar system that produce ataxia, lateral medullary syndrome, hemianopia, dementia, otological manifestations, loss of taste, and gangrene of the tongue.[8]

In Wegener's granulomatosis, orbital involvement occurs in 20% of patients and may simulate the appearance of orbital pseudotumor or lymphoma. Scleritis of the necrotizing variety and uveitis may be the initial manifestations. Involvement of the CNS occurs in 25–50% of cases and usually presents as cranial neuropathies, hypertensive encephalopathy, and cerebral vasculitis.[9,10]

In Sjögren's syndrome, the cardinal ocular manifestation is keratitis sicca, or dry eyes, which may result in corneal ulceration and even perforation. Optic neuropathy may occur alone but more commonly is associated with multifocal CNS disease. Presentations include acute retrobulbar optic neuritis, ischemic optic neuropathy, and insidious visual loss with optic atrophy. Cranial neuropathies may be peripheral or central. The best recognized is a trigeminal sensory neuropathy. Facial nerve involvement may compromise autonomic secretory function and further exacerbate the sicca syndrome. Acute and chronic subarachnoid hemorrhages with microhemorrhages within the meninges are very common in CNS antibody-positive individuals (SS-A). Less common CNS manifestations are parkinsonism, cerebellar syndromes, and aseptic meningitis.[11]

In Behçet's syndrome, ocular involvement is seen in 83–95% of men and 67–73% of women. Bilaterality is the rule, although delayed and asymmetrical involvement of the fellow eye is common. Loss of vision is usually the most serious complication, which may result from chronic anterior segment inflammation, neovascular glaucoma, or occlusive vasculitis. Neovascularization, retinal detachment, and optic atrophy are common sequelae. Loss of vision is a late manifestation that occurs an average of 3 years after the onset of ocular Behçet's syndrome. Among patients affected by ocular disease, 10–30% present with meningoencephalitis, brainstem syndrome, and organic brain syndrome.[12,13]

In sarcoidosis, the target organs commonly are the eyes, lacrimal glands, lungs, lymph nodes, and salivary glands. Ocular manifestations include granulomatous uveitis, inflammatory glaucoma, optic neuropathy (Fig. 206-1), and lacrimal gland enlargement. About 5% of patients present with either central or peripheral nervous system disease within 2 years of onset. In the CNS, the meninges at the base of the brain are most affected; secondary infiltration of cranial nerves (37–73%) and obstruction of CSF flow (7%) also occur, and CNS parenchymal disease is common (8–40%).

Miller-Fisher syndrome consists of the triad of ataxia, ophthalmoplegia, and areflexia and is described as a variant of Guillain-Barré syndrome. The initial presentation is commonly diplopia (39% of cases). A complete external and internal ophthalmoplegia, which may be bilateral, is seen in about 50% of patients. Other manifestations are supranuclear gaze paresis with internuclear ophthalmoplegia, Parinaud's syndrome, and occasional facial palsy. Ataxia (occurring in 21% of patients) is cerebellar in most cases. Areflexia was present in 81% of the 223 cases reviewed.[14]

Vogt-Koyanagi-Harada (VKH) syndrome is a bilateral, diffuse, granulomatous uveitis associated with vitiligo, alopecia, poliosis, and CNS signs; it may be categorized clinically in four phases:
1. Prodromal, characterized by headache, nausea, vertigo, fever, meningismus, and orbital pain.
2. Uveitic, in which 70% of patients present with unilateral or bilateral posterior uveitis.
3. Convalescent, which follows after several weeks and is characterized by depigmentation of the skin (vitiligo) and choroid.

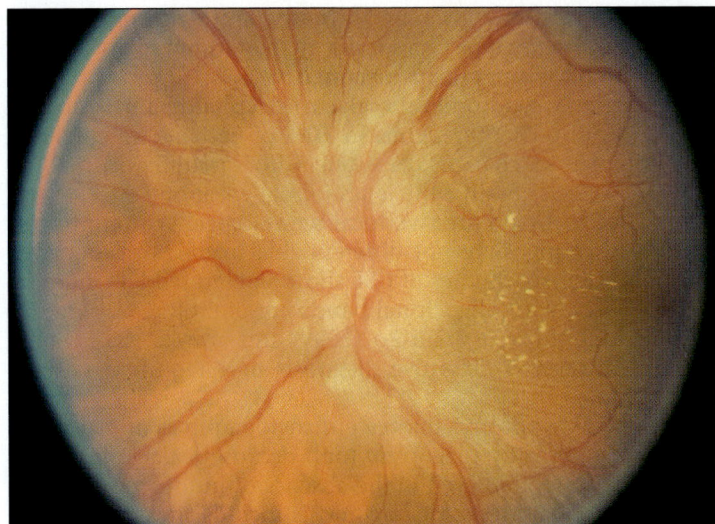

FIG. 206-1 ■ Fundus view of optic nerve head in sarcoidosis. Note the sheathing of vessels and exudates, as well as pallid edema of the optic disc.

4. Chronic recurrent, which is characterized by smoldering panuveitis with exacerbations of acute episodes of granulomatous anterior uveitis.

The neurological manifestations of VKH syndrome are more common during the prodromal phase. Focal neurological signs, such as cranial neuropathies, hemiparesis, aphasia, transverse myelitis, and ciliary ganglionitis, may be found but are uncommon. Lumbar puncture may reveal lymphocytic pleocytosis and elevated protein.

DIAGNOSIS AND TESTING

Angiography generally is not very sensitive for CNS vasculitis. The gold standard for such diagnosis is biopsy of the leptomeninges.[15]

In PAN, the common but nonspecific laboratory findings include decreased serum complement and circulating immune complexes. The diagnosis often is established by biopsy of the sural nerve or muscle. In SLE, an important laboratory test is for antinuclear antibody titers (double stranded), which is also a good measure of the activity of the disease. For CNS lupus, the following laboratory tests are helpful:
- Elevated CSF immunoglobulin (Ig) index or oligoclonal band
- CSF antineuronal antibodies
- Serum antiribosomal antibodies

Together, these tests have a sensitivity of 100% and a specificity of 86%. Furthermore, patients who show focal presentations have evidence of antiphospholipid antibodies, abnormal brain magnetic resonance imaging (MRI) with multiple lesions, and peripheral vasculitis.

In GCA, the diagnosis is primarily clinical. However, more than 80% of patients have a markedly elevated Westergren erythrocyte sedimentation rate. Other helpful laboratory tests include a complete blood count (for anemia), serum fibrinogen levels, C-reactive protein, and plasma activating factor. Definitive diagnosis is histological proof of arterial involvement by biopsy of the temporal artery.

For Wegener's granulomatosis, clinical diagnosis requires the finding of at least two of the following four criteria established by the American Academy of Rheumatology:
1. Oral ulcers or purulent bloody nasal discharge
2. Abnormal chest radiographs that show nodules, fixed infiltrates, or cavities
3. Microhematuria that signals kidney involvement
4. Biopsy evidence of granulomatous inflammation in the wall of an artery

For histological diagnosis, the nasal mucosa is the best biopsy source. Other laboratory tests that are useful for the diagnosis of

Wegener's granulomatosis are those for antineutrophilic cytoplasmic antibodies type C, a specific marker found in 90% of patients who have systemic involvement.

In Sjögren's syndrome, the electroencephalogram is abnormal in about 40% of patients. In 20% of patients, cerebral angiography shows changes consistent with vasculitis of small to medium vessels. Brain MRI is abnormal in about 80% of patients affected by progressive focal neurological symptoms, but these MRI changes are not differentiable from those found in multiple sclerosis. Studies of CSF show an elevated IgG index in 50% of cases, with oligoclonal bands present. Other laboratory tests include those for anti-Ro (SS-A) and anti-La (SS-B) antibodies; however, a definitive diagnosis may require a salivary gland biopsy.

In Behçet's syndrome, fluorescein angiography is of major importance as an early diagnostic tool, because leakage from the vessels may be found even in the absence of funduscopic abnormalities. Ancillary tests for sarcoidosis include measurement of angiotensin-converting enzyme levels (elevated in 65% of cases) and gallium-67 scans of the head and chest. Biopsy may be definitive, as it may show noncaseating granulomas in the lacrimal glands, lymph nodes, conjunctiva nodules, or even the liver.

PATHOLOGY

In CNS vasculitis, the small- and medium-size vessels are affected primarily. The cellular infiltrate is composed of lymphocytes, macrophages, and giant cells in all layers of the vessel wall. In PAN, a widespread panarteritis is found, with necrosis of the media and elastic membranes that results, in some cases, in the formation of small aneurysms, which may thrombose or rupture. In SLE, immune complex deposits develop in the walls of small blood vessels; the primary damage occurs in the subendothelial connective tissues of capillaries, small arteries, veins, and endocardium. In GCA, the pathological changes include granulomatous inflammation that results in vessel obstruction, embolism, or thrombosis (Fig. 206-2). Also characteristic is the intimal proliferation and destruction of the internal elastic lamina.

In Wegener's granulomatosis, the granuloma formation or vasculitis involves the small arteries and veins, and a fibrinoid necrosis of the vessel wall occurs with infiltration by neutrophils and histiocytes. In Sjögren's syndrome, the inflammatory infiltrates are predominantly lymphocytes (T-cell type), macrophages, and plasma cells. Small blood vessels of the venous system are invariably involved, followed by those of the arterial system (small arteries or arterioles). In the CNS, blood vessels within the white matter, in subcortical and periventricular locations, are mainly involved. In Behçet's syndrome, the basic lesion is an occlusive, necrotizing, nongranulomatous vasculitis and perivasculitis found in the uvea and retina.

TREATMENT

The treatment of CNS vasculitis with prednisone or cyclophosphamide may produce remission or cure.[15] Certain specific inflammations require a more specified approach. For example, in Wegener's granulomatosis, treatment involves cytotoxic therapy with cyclophosphamide and, less commonly, with methotrexate, azathioprine, and chlorambucil. The response to therapy is measured by clinical improvement and reduction of the antineutrophil cytoplasmic antibody titer over time. Sjögren's syndrome requires pulse cyclophosphamide therapy in conjunction with corticosteroids for at least 12 months until disease stabilization or improvement occurs.

Therapy for sarcoidosis consists of treatment with corticosteroids for several weeks. If this fails, immunosuppressive agents such as azathioprine, methotrexate, cyclophosphamide, chlorambucil, and cyclosporine may be used.

COURSE AND OUTCOME

The chronic course for CNS vasculitis is usually characterized by cognitive deficits and focal findings. Without treatment, patients often suffer recurrent strokes and die within a few years.[15] The prognosis in PAN is poor; patients die from lesions of the kidneys, heart, or other viscera. Cerebral SLE may be catastrophic and generally has a poor prognosis; death may result from renal failure, infection, or CNS involvement. Wegener's granulomatosis was once regarded as uniformly fatal, but survival rates have increased with the use of cytotoxic drugs, predominantly cyclophosphamide.

The prognosis for Miller-Fisher syndrome is good, with complete recovery within 10 weeks of treatment, on average. Secondary infections, such as pneumonia or sepsis, may cause morbidity and mortality. In VKH syndrome, the prognosis is fair, but ocular complications are common. The most common complications include cataracts, glaucoma, and subretinal neovascular membranes. The major risk for the development of these complications is recurrence of the intraocular inflammation.[16]

NEURODEGENERATIONS

INTRODUCTION

Despite the specific denotation and vague negative connotation of "degeneration," the term *neurodegeneration* continues to be used to imply a decline to a lower level of CNS function. We consider the term synonymous with *heredodegeneration*. This, and the older term *abiotrophy*, suggests a genetic cause for premature neuronal disease and death. Neuronal injury as a result of metabolic, toxic, or nutritional problems is dealt with in Chapter 192; however, not surprisingly, the clinical manifestations of these two categories of disease are quite similar. Recent advances in genetics and molecular biology have elucidated inborn errors in metabolism.

EPIDEMIOLOGY AND PATHOGENESIS

Each of the neurodegenerative diseases has a different epidemiology and pathogenesis. Alzheimer's disease is the most common form of dementia, with a prevalence of 10.3% in people aged 65 years, which rises to 47% for those older than 80 years. A genetic basis is suspected strongly; however, a number of environmental risk factors and even viral infections have been im-

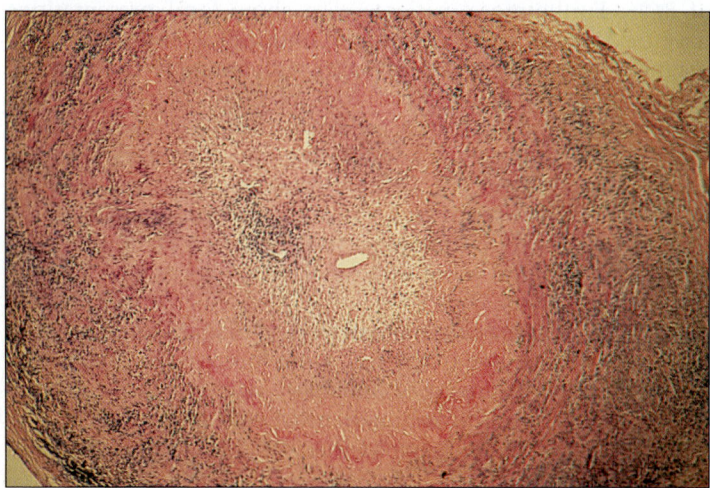

FIG. 206-2 ■ **Temporal artery almost obliterated by vasculitis.** In this case of giant cell arteritis, the media is filled with granulomatous infiltration (with giant cells and epithelioid cells). Also, note that the elastica has been fragmented (periodic acid–Schiff staining).

plicated. The pathology involves marked atrophy of the cerebral cortex. Histopathology reveals nonspecific plaques and tangles. Selective loss of large retinal ganglion cells and their axons that underlie the M-cell pathway may contribute to the visuospatial abnormalities.[17,18]

OCULAR MANIFESTATIONS

Each neurodegenerative syndrome has its own constellations of signs and symptoms. An outline of such degenerations is given in Box 206-1, and a brief description of some of the more characteristic ophthalmic features follows.

Dystonic movements are sustained contractions or spasms that may be twisting or postural and tend to increase with action. In children who have dystonia, involvement of the arms and legs often occurs. Dystonic tremor includes features of both action and postural tremor. Dystonia tends to progress from focal to segmental to generalized. In advanced cases, the affected body part remains in a fixed dystonic posture. In adults, dystonia may begin with the arms (writer's cramp), neck (torticollis), face (blepharospasm), jaw (oromandibular), tongue (lingual), or vocal cords (spastic).

Blepharospasm is a form of focal dystonia that commonly presents to the ophthalmologist.[19] Caused by contraction of the orbicularis muscles, it begins with increased blinking followed by involuntary eyelid closure.[20] If, in addition to blepharospasm, other cranial dystonias are present, the syndrome is called Meige's syndrome. However, when the spasm involves all the branches of the facial nerve, it appears as hemifacial spasm, which is considered by Jankovic[20] to be a form of segmental (branchial) myoclonus.

Cerebellar Neurodegenerative Diseases

When the cerebellum and its connections are affected in a familial or hereditary pattern, the cardinal clinical feature seen is ataxia. The inherited ataxias may have an early onset; for example, Friedreich's ataxia, an autosomal recessive disorder, starts

before age 30 years. Patients present with progressive ataxia of gait and limbs, absent deep tendon reflexes, and extensor plantar responses. Patients also have dysarthria, clumsiness, and cardiopathy (75%). Less common features of Friedreich's ataxia include nystagmus (25%), pes cavus (50%), diabetes (10–20%), deafness, and optic atrophy (25%), with a moderate reduction in vision. Posterior column disorder is seen in almost all patients. Loss of appreciation of vibration is an early sign. Computed tomography (CT) and MRI of the brain are usually normal, except with cerebellar atrophy. Cervical spinal cord atrophy is present, and the CSF is normal. The course is progressive, although variability exists. The mean age at death is 50 years, and there is no treatment other than palliative.

Ramsay Hunt syndrome is an early-onset ataxia that combines myoclonus and progressive ataxia. The most common cause is mitochondrial encephalomyopathy. Marinesco-Sjögren syndrome is another early-onset, recessive ataxia characterized by bilateral cataracts, mental retardation, and short stature.

Late-onset ataxias, under the rubric autosomal dominant cerebellar ataxia (ADCA), encompass all autosomal dominant ataxias that begin during adulthood. Late-onset ataxias are categorized according to clinical characteristics and gene loci, designated as SCA1, SCA2, and so on. The most common clinical form of ADCA is SCA1, which usually begins in patients between 20 and 40 years of age with gait ataxia, early hyperreflexia, abnormal evoked potentials, peripheral neuropathy, and pseudobulbar dysarthria. Early nystagmus and ophthalmoparesis are common. MRI shows cerebellar and brainstem atrophy, which particularly affects the pons and middle cerebellar peduncle.

Another form of ADCA is Azorean disease (SCA3). Patients present with gait and limb ataxia, leg spasticity, dysarthria, pyramidal signs, dystonia, rigidity, amyotrophy, and facial and lingual fasciculations. The ophthalmological manifestations are pseudoproptosis with lid retraction and decreased blinking and ophthalmoplegia, in which saccades are slow; also found are nystagmus and ocular dysmetria, followed by supranuclear ophthalmoplegia that spares downgaze. Ataxia SCA2 is characterized by slow saccades without nystagmus and early loss of tendon reflexes in the arms, in addition to ataxia. Other ADCAs are defined by different combinations of cerebellar ataxia and retinal degeneration.

Sporadic cerebellar ataxia of late onset often begins after age 40 years and is attended by parkinsonism, upper motor neuron signs, and dementia. Olivopontocerebellar atrophy is a common example of this category of degeneration. These patients may have autonomic dysfunction (neurogenic orthostatic hypotension).

Other types of ataxia include ataxia-telangiectasia, or Louis-Bar's syndrome, which is an autosomal recessive disorder linked to a metabolic error. Patients present as children with truncal ataxia, delayed growth, and sexual and mental retardation. Oculomotor problems are prominent (pseudo-oculomotor apraxia). Telangiectasias of the skin and conjunctiva are often seen.

Parkinsonism

The parkinsonism symptom complex is characterized by six cardinal features:

1. Tremor at rest.
2. Rigidity.
3. Bradykinesia-hypokinesia (slow and delayed movements).
4. Flexed posture.
5. Loss of postural reflexes.
6. Freezing phenomenon (motionlessness).

Two of these features, which must include either tremor or bradykinesia, are required for definitive diagnosis of parkinsonism. Tremor at rest with the "rolling pill sign" is common. In addition to the cardinal signs, these patients have decreased attention span and visuospatial impairments. Depression develops at

---

BOX 206-1

The Neurodegenerations

DYSTONIA	Drug induced
	• levodopa
CEREBELLAR	• anticonvulsants
Friedreich's ataxia	• anticholinergics
Marinesco–Sjögren syndrome	• antipsychotics
Ramsay Hunt syndrome	Metabolic and endocrine
X-Linked inherited ataxia	• chorea gravidarum
Charcot–Marie–Tooth disease	• hyperthyroidism
	• birth control pills
PARKINSON'S DISEASE	• hyperglycemic nonketotic
Progressive supranuclear palsy	encephalopathy
Shy–Drager syndrome	Vascular
Hallervorden–Spatz disease	• hemichorea/hemiballismus with
	subthalamic nucleus lesion
CHOREA	• periarteritis nodosa
Hereditary	Dementias
Huntington's disease	• Alzheimer's disease
Hereditary nonprogressive chorea	• Pick's disease
Neuroacanthosis	• Creutzfeldt–Jakob disease
Wilson's disease	• Dyke–Davidoff–Masson disease
Ataxia telangiectasia	• Charles Bonnet disease
Lesch–Nyhan syndrome	Mitochondrial-related diseases
Secondary	• mitochondrial encephalopathies—
Infectious/immunologic	DNA related
• Sydenham's chorea	• Leber's hereditary optic atrophy
• encephalitis	• mitochondrial diseases with
• systemic lupus erythematosus	mutations of nuclear DNA

a rate of 2% of cases per year. Cognitive impairment may occur, but there are no memory problems.

Progressive Supranuclear Palsy

Progressive supranuclear palsy, or Steele-Richardson-Olszewski syndrome, is a neurodegenerative disease characterized by pseudobulbar palsy, supranuclear vertical gaze palsy (which affects primarily downgaze), extrapyramidal rigidity, gait ataxia, and dementia. The course is evolution to bed confinement in about 5 years and death a few years later.[21]

Chorea

Choreas may be hereditary, secondary (such as from SLE, phospholipids, or infections), drug-induced (such as from L-dopa, anticonvulsants, or anticholinergics), metabolic and endocrine, vascular, or miscellaneous (senile, or essential).

Huntington's disease is a progressive hereditary disorder that becomes manifest only in adult life and is characterized by chorea, personality disorder, and dementia. Sydenham's chorea is seen in children and is characterized by rapid, irregular, aimless, involuntary movements of the muscles of the limbs, face, and trunk. Patients also show emotional lability, hypotonia, and muscular weakness.

Dementias with Eye Findings

ALZHEIMER'S DISEASE. Alzheimer's disease is a progressive neurological disorder that may present with visual disturbances such as anomalies of color vision, spatial contrast sensitivity disturbance, fixation instability, saccadic latency prolongation with hypometric saccades, and saccadic intrusions during smooth-pursuit eye movements.[17,18] The vestibular ocular reflex is normal in most patients. In addition to generalized cognitive problems, some patients may show disorders of higher cortical dysfunction of vision, such as visual agnosia and optic ataxia. Other dementias that accompany inherited metabolic disease with eye findings include Wilson's disease, Fahr's syndrome, metachromatic leukodystrophy, MELAS syndrome, MERRF syndrome, and Hallervorden-Spatz disease.

CHARLES BONNET SYNDROME. Charles Bonnet syndrome is more than a type of dementia. Classically, however, it has been regarded as such because this condition is often an early marker for various dementias.[22] This syndrome involves the onset of complex and vivid visual hallucinations in the absence of clouded consciousness, medical illness, psychopathology, or intellectual impairment. Classically, the patient has positive visual phenomena (hallucinations) that may be formed or unformed and probably represent a release phenomenon in the setting of deafferentation. It may occur after a stroke or other causes of diminished vision.

CEREBROVASCULAR DISEASES. In addition to the focal deficit from stroke, an acquired intellectual impairment results from multiple small injuries to the brain caused by stroke, either hemorrhagic or ischemic. These patients have loss of memory and cognitive impairments that involve attention, orientation, visuospatial abilities, calculation, and motor control. Cortical syndrome is caused by repeated atherothrombotic or cardioembolic strokes and is characterized by more obvious, focal, sensorimotor signs and a more abrupt onset of cognitive failure. In contrast, subcortical syndrome is notable for pseudobulbar signs, isolated pyramidal signs, depression, emotional lability, frontal behavior, mild memory impairment, disorientation, inattention, and perseveration.[23]

DEMENTIA COMPLEX ASSOCIATED WITH HIV. This sequela of autoimmune deficiency syndrome includes several CNS problems, such as apathy, cognitive slowing, and memory loss, as well as the more focal neurological abnormalities. The eye findings include subtle deficits of color vision and contrast sensitivity, especially in the midspatial frequencies.[24]

PRION DISEASES. Originally thought to result from a slow virus, these spongiform encephalopathies are, indeed, transmissible. The prion diseases include kuru, Creutzfeldt-Jakob disease, fatal familial insomnia, and Gerstmann-Sträussler-Scheinker disease. These diseases cause rapidly progressive dementia that may include visual agnosias.[25]

DIAGNOSIS AND TESTING

In Huntington's chorea, CT scans may be quite useful, as neuroimaging often shows enlarged ventricles with a butterfly appearance because of the selective degeneration of the caudate nucleus. Prenatal testing may be carried out for the Huntington's disease gene near the tip of the short arm of chromosome 4.

In Alzheimer's disease, the diagnosis may be challenging. Aside from the extensive neurological work-up, which includes psychometric testing, ophthalmological testing may be of some assistance. For example, a visual evoked potential recording may be of diagnostic significance, since these patients often show a normal-pattern visual evoked potential yet an abnormal flash visual evoked potential. Further, these patients have been found to have electroretinograms of a lower-amplitude pattern compared with normal flash electroretinograms. Ocular motility may also be abnormal.

In prion diseases, the electroencephalogram shows diffuse slowing, with pseudoperiodic, biphasic, and triphasic spike and wave complexes that are time locked to myoclonic jerks. Recently, it has become possible to look for a CSF marker, a protein designated 14-3-3 and detected by immunoassay. This test has about 96% sensitivity and specificity. However, brain biopsy with histopathology remains the diagnostic gold standard.

PATHOLOGY

The pathophysiological problem of Parkinson's disease relates to decreased dopaminergic neurotransmission in the basal ganglia with loss of dopamine receptors. The multiple causes for this include drug induced, postinfection, post-traumatic, tumor related, metabolic, hypoxic, postencephalitic, toxic, multi-infarct, and idiopathic. The pathological markers in Parkinson's disease are the so-called Lewy bodies—neurons that contain eosinophilic cytoplasmic inclusions. In Alzheimer's disease, in addition to the plaques and tangles in the cerebral hemispheres, direct injury occurs to the retinal ganglion cells and their axons (Figs. 206-3 and 206-4).

TREATMENT

Stereotaxic thalamotomy may be useful in unilateral dystonia, but bilateral ablations carry a 20% risk of dysarthria.

Treatment of hemifacial spasm has been attempted using high doses of anticholinergics (such as trihexyphenidyl [benzhexol]) and high doses of baclofen, benzodiazepines, and anti-dopaminergics (such as reserpine or dopamine receptor blockers), with limited success. More recently, botulinum toxin injections have been used with good success; however, this response does not last beyond 3 months.

Cerebellar neurodegenerative diseases with paroxysmal (or periodic) cerebellar ataxia may be amenable to treatment with acetazolamide in doses of 200–1000mg/day, which reduces or abolishes the attacks.

The aim of treatment for Parkinson's disease is to control symptoms. Options include dopamine precursors (such as levodopa), carbidopa, dopamine agonists (such as bromocriptine and pergolide), dopamine releasers (such as amantadine), anticholinergics, antidepressants, muscle relaxants, and surgery using techniques such as thalamotomy, pallidotomy (to target the

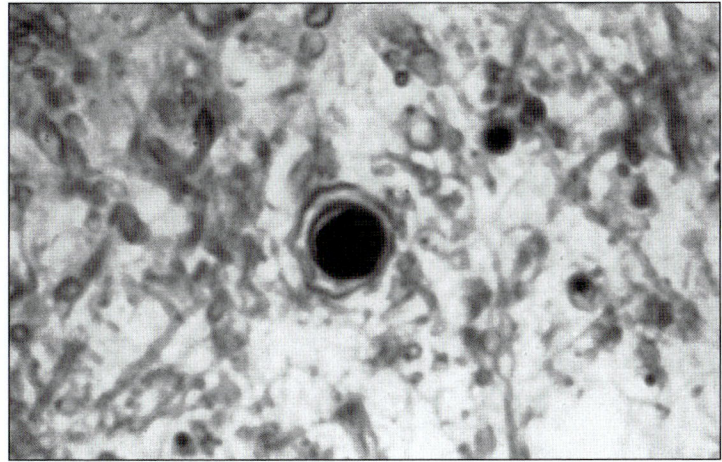

FIG. 206-3 ⬛ Degenerating axons in the human optic nerve in Alzheimer's disease. Note several dark profiles, the largest of which has an extra myelin sheath about it (paraphenylene-diamine staining, epon embedded section).

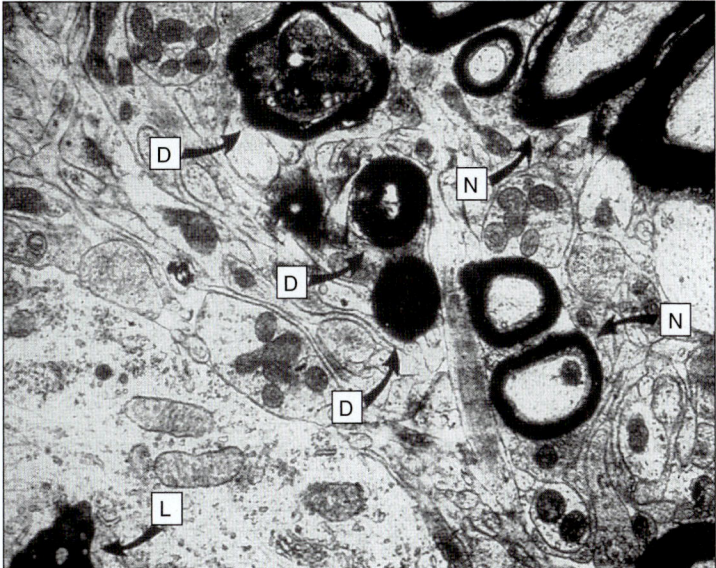

FIG. 206-4 ⬛ Electron microscopy of the optic nerve in Alzheimer's disease. Demonstrated are degenerating axons (D) and glial cells with lipofuscin (L), part of the process of degeneration. Normal myelinated axons (N) are also seen.

posterolateral part of the medial globus pallidus), subthalamic stimulation, or implants of embryonic tissues. Levodopa is the most widely used drug in Parkinson's disease, but the response is variable, and after 5 years of therapy, up to 75% of patients have serious complications.[14]

Huntington's chorea may be treated with tricyclic antidepressants and antipsychotics. Attempts to replace the γ-aminobutyric acid deficiency in this disease have not been successful. No specific treatment exists for Sydenham's chorea, but sedatives and antidopaminergic drugs may be used.

Agents under investigation for the treatment of Alzheimer's disease are tetrahydroaminoacridine (cholinesterase inhibitor), acetyl levocarnitine, and physostigmine, as well as selegiline.

However, none of these treatments shows as great a promise as the manipulation of hormones (estrogen) and nonsteroidal anti-inflammatory agents. Currently, no treatment for prion diseases exists; care must be taken to avoid iatrogenic spread from organ donation or accidental inoculation.

COURSE AND OUTCOME

Most neurodegenerative diseases have a long and relentless downward course. However, in many cases, the process may proceed very slowly (as in Alzheimer's disease). In Parkinson's disease the initial response to therapy is often excellent and may last 5–10 years. For hemifacial spasm or blepharospasm, newer modalities of treatment (such as injections of botulinum toxin) show excellent promise for control, but not cure, of the disorder.

REFERENCES

1. Miller NR. Neuro-ophthalmologic topographic diagnosis of tumors and related conditions. In: Walsh & Hoyt's clinical neuro-ophthalmology, vol 3, 4th ed. Baltimore: Lippincott, Williams & Wilkins;1980:1138.
2. Ellner JJ, Bennett JE. Chronic meningitis. Medicine. 1976;55:341–69.
3. Tunkel AR, Scheld WM. Pathogenesis and pathophysiology of bacterial meningitis. Clin Microbiol Rev. 1993;6(2):118–36.
4. Luby JP. Infections of the central nervous system. Am J Med Sci. 1992;304(6):379–91.
5. Moore PM, Calabrese LH. Neurological manifestations of systemic vasculitides. Semin Neurol. 1994;14:300–6.
6. West SG, Emlen W, Wene MH, Kotzin BL. Neuropsychiatric lupus erythematosus: a 10-year-prospective study on the value of diagnostic tests. Am J Med. 1995;99:153–63.
7. Keane JR. Eye movement abnormalities in systemic lupus erythematosus. Arch Neurol. 1995;52:1145–9.
8. Caselli RJ, Hunder GG, Whisnant JP. Neurologic disease in biopsy proven giant cell (temporal) arteritis. Neurology. 1988;38:352–9.
9. Nishino H, Rubino FA, DeRemee RA, et al. Neurological involvement in Wegener's granulomatosis: an analysis of 324 consecutive patients at the Mayo Clinic. Ann Neurol. 1993;33:4–9.
10. Newman NJ, Slamovits TL, Friedland S, Wilson WB. Neuro-ophthalmic manifestations of meningocerebral inflammation from the limited form of Wegener's granulomatosis. Am J Ophthalmol. 1995;120:613–21.
11. Vitali C, Bombardieri S, Moutsopoulos H, et al. Preliminary criteria for the classification of Sjögren's syndrome: results of a prospective concerted action supported by the European community. Arthritis Rheumatol. 1993;36:340–7.
12. Calabrese LH, Duna GF. Evaluation and treatment of central nervous system vasculitis. Curr Opin Rheumatol. 1995;7:37–44.
13. Allen NB. Miscellaneous vasculitic syndromes including Behçet's disease and central nervous system vasculitis. Curr Opin Rheumatol. 1993;5:51–6.
14. Berlit P, Rakicky J. The Miller Fisher syndrome: review of the literature. J Clin Neuro Ophthalmol. 1992;12(2):57–63.
15. Calabrese LH, Furlan AJ, Gragg LA, Ropos TJ. Primary angiitis of the central nervous system: diagnostic criteria and clinical approach. Cleve Clin J Med. 1992;59:293–306.
16. Read RW, Rao NA, Cunningham ET. Vogt-Koyanagi-Harada disease. Curr Opin Ophthalmol. 2000;11:437–42.
17. Sadun AA, Borchert M, DeVita E, et al. Assessment of visual impairment in patients with Alzheimer's disease. Am J Ophthalmol. 1987;104:113–20.
18. Sadun AA, Bassi C. Optic nerve damage in Alzheimer's disease. Ophthalmology. 1990;97(1):9–17.
19. Fahn S. Adverse effects of levodopa. In: Olanow CW, Lieberman AN, eds. The scientific basis for the treatment of Parkinson's disease. Carnforth: Parthenon; 1992:125–30.
20. Jankovic J. Etiology and differential diagnosis of blepharospasm and oromandibular dystonia. In: Jankovic J, Tolosa E, eds. Advances in neurology, vol 49. Facial dyskinesias. New York: Raven Press; 1988:103–16.
21. Duvoisin RC. Merritt's textbook of neurology. In: Rowland LP, ed. Progressive supranuclear palsy, ed 9. Philadelphia: Williams & Wilkins; 1995:730–2.
22. Pliskin NH, Kiolbasa TA, Towle VL, et al. Charles Bonnet syndrome: an early marker for dementia. J Am Geriatr Soc. 1996;44:1055–61.
23. Mayeux R, Chun MR. Merritt's textbook of neurology. In: Rowland LP, ed. Progressive supranuclear palsy, ed 9. Philadelphia: Williams & Wilkins; 1995:680–1.
24. Quiceno JL, Caparelli E, Sadun AA, et al. Visual dysfunction in AIDS patients without retinitis. Am J Ophthalmol. 1992;113:8–13.
25. Prusiner S. The prion diseases. Sci Am. 1995;272(1):48–57.

SECTION 5 NEURO-OPHTHALMOLOGIC EMERGENCIES

CHAPTER

207

Most Urgent Neuro-Pathologies

PETER A. QUIROS

INTRODUCTION

Neuro-ophthalmic emergencies are few and far between. Although their incidence is much lower than other ophthalmic emergencies, such as retinal detachment or ruptured globe,[1,2] their outcomes carry a much higher morbidity and even mortality. The ocular manifestations of neuro-ophthalmic emergencies are but portents of more dangerous central nervous system or systemic pathology. The vision-threatening and potentially life-threatening nature of these disorders requires prompt recognition and diagnosis on the physician's part. A delay of even a few hours could result in a dire outcome. Therefore, the clinician must be familiar with the manifestations of these disease entities and initiate appropriate testing and treatment without delay.

In essence, there are five neuro-ophthalmic emergencies. These are:

- Giant cell arteritis (GCA)
- Orbital apex syndrome
- Intracranial aneurysm
- Cavernous sinus thrombosis
- Pituitary apoplexy

These may be grouped together by initial symptoms into three categories for ease of diagnosis: (1) entities resulting in vision loss—GCA, (2) those causing ophthalmoplegia—cavernous sinus thrombosis and intracranial aneurysm, and (3) those causing both vision loss and ophthalmoplegia—orbital apex syndrome and pituitary apoplexy.

EPIDEMIOLOGY AND PATHOGENESIS

Giant Cell Arteritis

The incidence of GCA (in the United States) is approximately 1 in 150,000 per annum in patients over 60 years of age.[3] The incidence increases sharply with age and can be as high as 44 per 100,000 for patients in their nineties.[4] The disease has a slight predilection for women over men. Caucasians are affected much more often than African–Americans and Hispanics.[2,4,5] The mean age of onset is in the seventh decade.[6]

GCA is a systemic disease that affects primarily small-to-medium–sized arteries, particularly the temporal, ophthalmic, and short posterior ciliary arteries.[7] Segments of these latter vessels become occluded, which leads to choroidal ischemia or ischemic optic neuropathy.[8] The arterial thrombosis of GCA may be demonstrated by delayed choroidal and disc filling on fluorescein angiography.[9]

Aneurysm

The incidence of intracranial saccular aneurysms is approximately 9 per 100,000. The incidence of rupture increases with age, peaking during the sixth and seventh decades. They are somewhat more frequent in women.[10] The vast majority of intracranial aneurysms arise from the carotid artery's main trunk (40%), at the level of the posterior communicating artery (PCOM), the ophthalmic artery, and the cavernous sinus.[11,12]

Rupture of PCOM aneurysms has been reported as high as 85%.[13] In addition, the PCOM is by far the most frequent location to cause a third cranial nerve palsy prior to rupture.[14]

PCOM aneurysms generally cause pupil-involving third nerve palsies. These occur either due to subarachnoid hemorrhage or by external compression of the third nerve due to aneurysmal expansion prior to rupture.[15]

Cavernous Sinus Thrombosis

The incidence of this rare disorder has not been estimated. It may be classified as septic or aseptic, the latter being the rarer of the two forms. The mortality from septic cavernous sinus thrombosis was nearly 100% in the pre-antibiotic era. Now the mortality rate is lower but remains at about 30%.[16]

Most septic thromboses of the cavernous sinus arise from the facial, sphenoid or ethmoid sinus, and dental infections. Acute infections of these areas usually are caused by gram-positive bacteria, whereas chronic infections are more often associated with gram-negative bacteria and fungi. Interestingly enough, otitis media and orbital cellulites rarely lead to cavernous sinus thrombosis.

Aseptic thrombosis of the cavernous sinus is associated with conditions that lead to venous thrombosis. These may include polycythemias, sickle cell disease (vasculidities), trauma, neurosurgery, pregnancy, and oral contraceptive use.

Orbital Apex Syndrome

Less than 1% of all orbital cellulites result in an orbital apex syndrome.[17] However, over 50% of these occur in patients with diabetes mellitus.[18] In these patients, rhinocerebral mucormycosis is far and away the most frequent cause of orbital apex syndrome.

Even though ketoacidosis is not always present,[19] it is the most important risk factor.[20] Studies have demonstrated a lack of inhibitory activity against *Rhizopus* in serum from ketoacidotic patients. It appears that this inhibitory activity is restored upon correction of the acidosis.

Pituitary Apoplexy

This life-threatening condition is rare and its incidence is difficult to establish. It is thought to occur in 0.6–9.1% of all surgically managed cases of pituitary adenoma.[21]

The age range is broad, ranging from the first to the ninth decade.[22] One study estimates the peak incidence during the fifth decade.[23] There appears to be no sex predominance.

Pituitary apoplexy occurs with sudden enlargement of a tumorous pituitary gland, usually adenoma. The sudden enlargement damages surrounding structures such as the optic chiasm and the hypothalamus. Rapid expansion into the cavernous sinus is also not uncommon. The expansion may be caused by hemorrhage or infarction. Precipitating factors include reduced blood flow as in hypotension, stimulation of the gland in increased estrogen states such as pregnancy, anticoagulation, and increased blood flow.[23]

OCULAR MANIFESTATIONS

Giant Cell Arteritis

Sudden visual loss is by far the most common manifestation of GCA, occurring in approximately 50% of these patients.[24] The vision loss occurs overwhelmingly as a result of arteritic anterior ischemic optic neuropathy. The permanent vision loss often is preceded by transient loss of vision, such as amaurosis fugax.[25]

Other causes of vision loss also associated with GCA, although occurring less frequently, include central retinal artery occlusion, choroidal ischemia, and posterior ischemic optic neuropathy. The elderly patient with central retinal artery occlusion who has no history of valvular disorders or visible emboli should be suspected of having GCA.[26]

Even though vision loss is the primary ophthalmic problem found in GCA, patients may also experience diplopia. This problem may occur due to infarction of the extraocular muscles, their associated cranial nerves, or the brainstem nuclei. In fact, GCA may cause a greater stroke syndrome.

Aneurysm

Ophthalmic manifestations are determined by the position of the aneurysm. These may range from vision loss due to ophthalmic artery aneurysms, cortical blindness resulting from basilar aneurysms, or ophthalmoplegia due to aneurysms of the circle of Willis or the cavernous sinus. The most common manifestation, however, is ophthalmoplegia.

Patients will have complete unilateral ptosis. Upon lifting the lid, the examiner will find an abducted eye that cannot adduct, infraduct, or supraduct. These patients usually have 1–2mm of proptosis, also. This phenomenon is thought to result from laxity of the palsied musculature and not from aneurysmal displacement.

All non-diabetic patients with third cranial nerve palsies should raise suspicion of intracranial aneurysm.

Cavernous Sinus Thrombosis

Patients with septic cavernous sinus thrombosis will manifest a host of ocular abnormalities. Those with infections entering the cavernous sinus anteriorly usually will have eye pain, orbital congestion, proptosis, adnexal edema, ptosis, and ophthalmoplegia. The ophthalmoplegia may involve the third, fourth, and sixth cranial nerves. In addition, there may also be involvement of the first and second branches of the trigeminal nerve.

Symptoms are initially unilateral but often become bilateral as the infection and thrombosis spread to the contralateral side through the circular sinus. This sinus connects the right and left cavernous sinuses posteriorly. In addition, these patients are usually febrile. Nausea, vomiting, and somnolence are not uncommon.

Orbital Apex Syndrome

Patients with an orbital apex syndrome will have complete ophthalmoplegia, ptosis, decreased corneal sensation, and vision loss. Unlike cavernous sinus thrombosis, the vision loss is present early. Patients usually develop optic nerve signs, such as a relative afferent pupillary defect. Early on, there is little adnexal edema and orbital congestion. These develop as the disease progresses. Proptosis is often present, but patients do not always complain of pain.

Eschars rarely are seen initially but usually develop around the orbit if the disease goes untreated (Fig. 207-1).

Pituitary Apoplexy

Patients usually suffer painful ophthalmoplegia and vision loss. Damage to the visual pathways occurs most frequently at the level of the chiasm. Therefore, visual field defects are common. Vision loss is variable, however, and may not always produce a

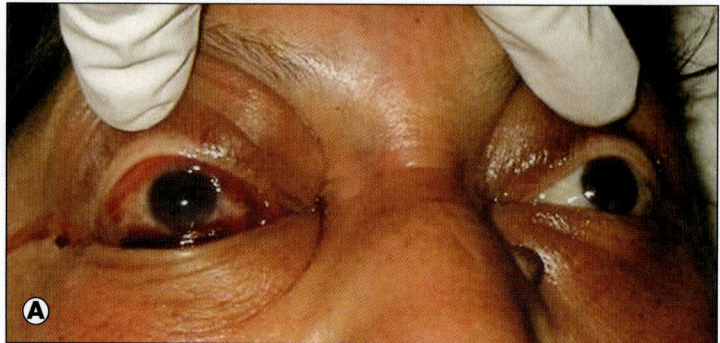

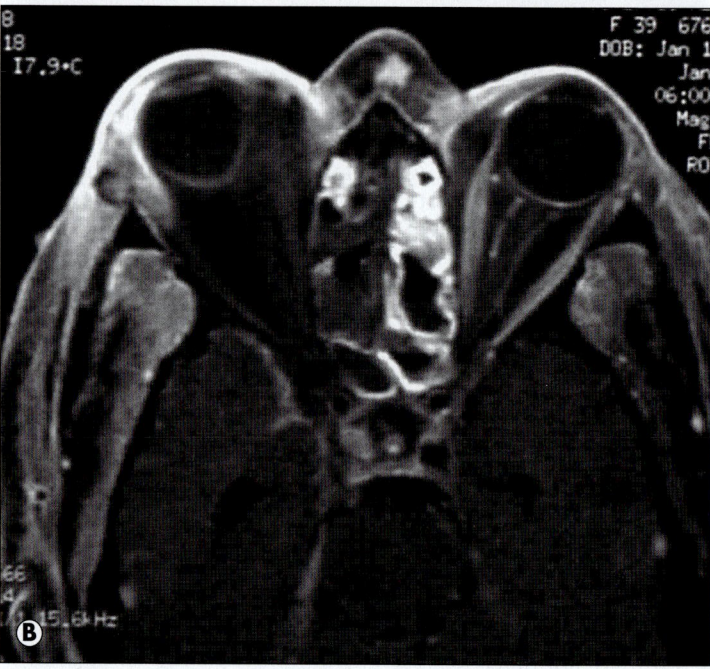

FIG. 207-1 ■ A, Patient with Mucormycosis of the right orbit, resulting in an orbital apex syndrome. B, Axial view from orbital MRI demonstrating mucormycosis of the Ethmoid sinuses with extension into orbit.

relative afferent pupillary defect. The degree of ophthalmoplegia may also be variable and asymmetrical, depending on the extent of involvement of each cavernous sinus.

DIAGNOSIS AND ANCILLARY TESTING

Giant Cell Arteritis

The diagnosis of temporal arteritis is based on clinical signs and symptoms. Laboratory findings are helpful, and temporal artery biopsy is the confirmatory gold standard.

Elderly patients with vision loss and/or transient vision loss usually have a positive review of systems. Therefore, a thorough review of systems for GCA should be elicited. A diagnosis can be arrived at with great certainty if several systems are positive for symptoms.[27]

Most patients will complain of headache, usually unilateral. In addition, there is usually scalp tenderness, as well as tenderness over the affected artery. Jaw claudication is often present. Whereas its absence does not rule out GCA, this sign is nearly pathognomonic of GCA, because it is seen rarely in other disorders. Finally, myalgias, fatigue, weight loss, and decreased appetite are seen frequently. Positive findings in three or more systems in the elderly patient should raise a high level of suspicion.

Laboratory testing usually consists of erythrocyte sedimentation rate (ESR), C-reactive protein level, and complete blood count. The ESR and C-reactive protein level usually are elevated markedly. The ESR should be adjusted for age and gender. The upper limit of normal is considered age divided by 2 in men and age plus 10 divided by 2 in women.[28]

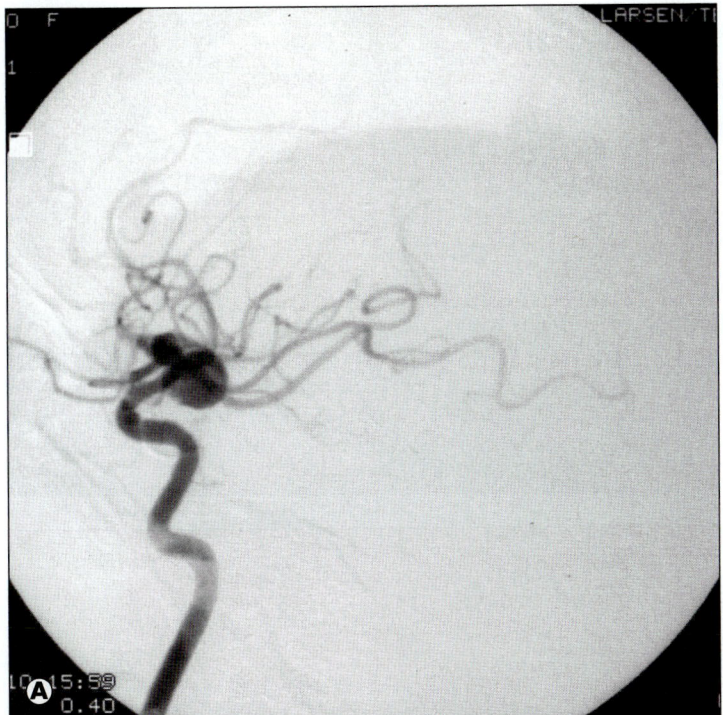

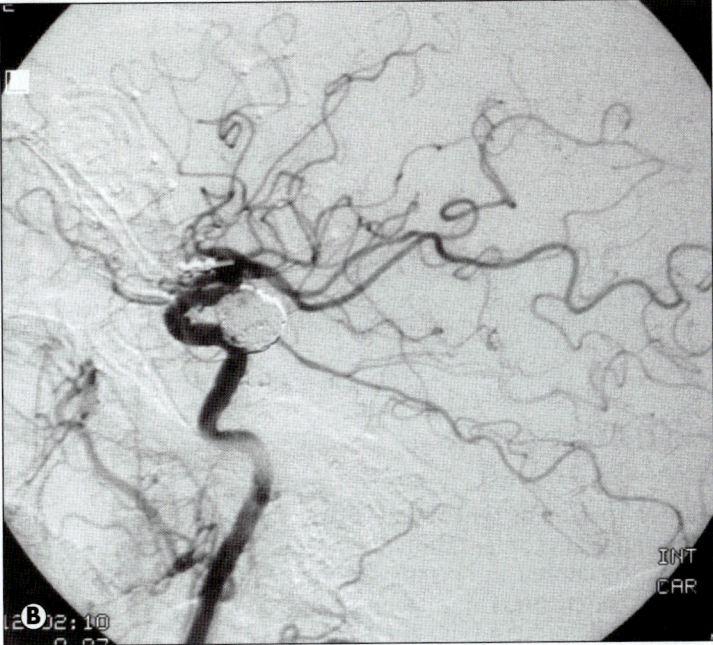

FIG. 207-2 ■ **A**, Digital subtraction angiogram (DSA) of PCOM aneurysm resulting in third nerve palsy. **B**, DSA of the same aneurysm after endovascular coiling.

The complete blood count often will reveal a normocytic anemia as well as a thrombocytosis.[29]

Temporal artery biopsy is the gold standard for diagnosis. A 2cm segment of temporal artery should be obtained and several sections sampled, because "skip lesions" may occur. That is, sections of affected artery may be interspersed with non-affected sections. A single negative biopsy meeting the above criteria is usually enough to rule out GCA. However, despite low statistical yield,[30] if suspicion is high a second biopsy may be performed, given that a missed diagnosis results in dire consequences.

Aneurysm

Frontal head pain is usually present in both ruptured and unruptured aneurysms. In an unruptured aneurysm, it is referred pain from the adjacent tentorium. Like the eye and forehead, the tentorium is supplied by the first branch of the trigeminal nerve.

A pupil-involving oculomotor nerve palsy is nearly invariably present. If such is the case, the aneurysm should be detectable by magnetic resonance (MR) angiography or spiral computed tomography (CT) angiography.[31] These modalities, however, may miss up to 10% of intracranial aneurysms.[32] Therefore, digital subtraction cerebral angiography remains the gold standard. A saccular aneurysm of 4mm or greater usually is seen at the junction of the internal carotid and the posterior communicating arteries (Fig. 207-2).

Cavernous Sinus Thrombosis and Orbital Apex Syndrome

Apart from the ocular signs that distinguish these two entities, neuroimaging is necessary to make the diagnosis. Orbital CT without contrast and magnetic resonance imaging (MRI) scanning with fat suppression will locate the site of involvement. In the case of orbital MRI, fat suppression is necessary in order to see involved orbital structures. The "noise" created by the fat may mask inflammation otherwise. Sinus disease is nearly always present.[33] In fact, orbital apex syndrome rarely occurs without adjacent ethmoid sinusitis. Sphenoid and maxillary sinus disease is also common. In either case, scans should be ordered with coronal and axial views that extend as far back as the posterior and inferior cavernous sinus.

Pituitary Apoplexy

In addition to ocular manifestations, most patients exhibit meningeal irritation. Following the apoplexy, hypofunction of the gland is common.[34] Patients may, therefore, exhibit irregular menses, decreased libido, hyponatremia, hypothyroidism, or hypercortisolism.

MRI is the gold standard for neuroimaging, because it will delineate both the tumor and any hemorrhage (Fig. 207-3). It is much more sensitive than CT scanning.[35]

DIFFERENTIAL DIAGNOSIS
Giant Cell Arteritis

The differential of GCA is extensive. GCA is confused often with nonarteritic anterior ischemic optic neuropathy. These patients tend to be younger, have less severe vision loss, and have a negative review of systems, as well as normal laboratory test results.

The differential may also include:
- Inflammatory optic neuritis: patients usually in their twenties and thirties, have pain with eye movements, optic nerve swelling, and a negative review of systems
- Compressive tumor: very slowly progressive vision loss, negative review of systems
- Diabetic papillophlebitis: younger diabetic patients, optic nerve swelling with hemorrhages, negative review of systems, mildly elevated ESR
- Central retinal artery or vein occlusion

Aneurysm

If angiography findings are negative, the following entities may produce a similar clinical picture:
- Microvascular or ischemic lesions: patients usually diabetic; pupil nearly always spared
- Epidural or subdural hematoma: a history of trauma in most cases, mental status changes common
- Meningitis or encephalitis: fever and nuchal rigidity, often accompanied by mental status changes and seizures
- Hypertensive crisis: flame-shaped retinal hemorrhages usually present, as well as optic nerve edema
- Migraine: a relapsing and remitting course often accompanied by nausea, photophobia, visual auras, and transient hemiplegia, ophthalmoplegia, or ataxia

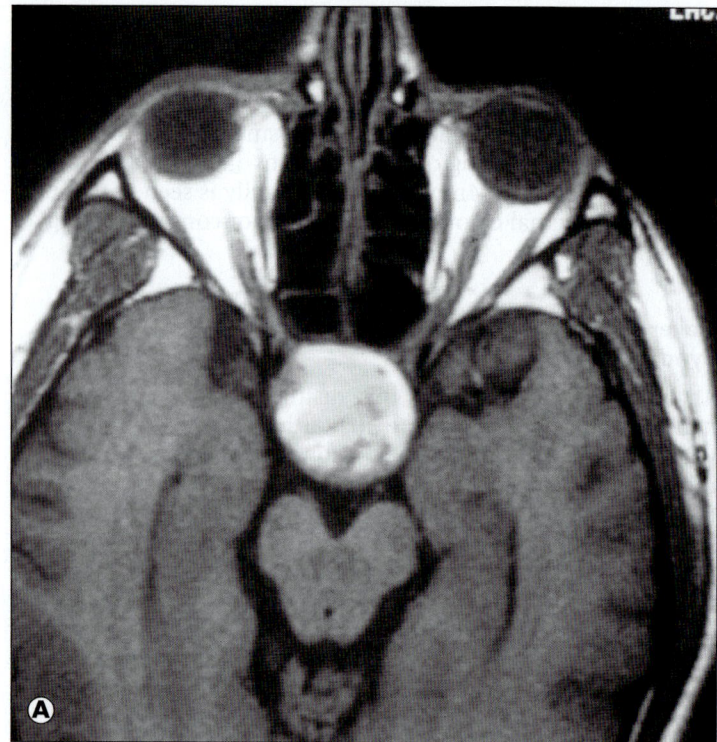

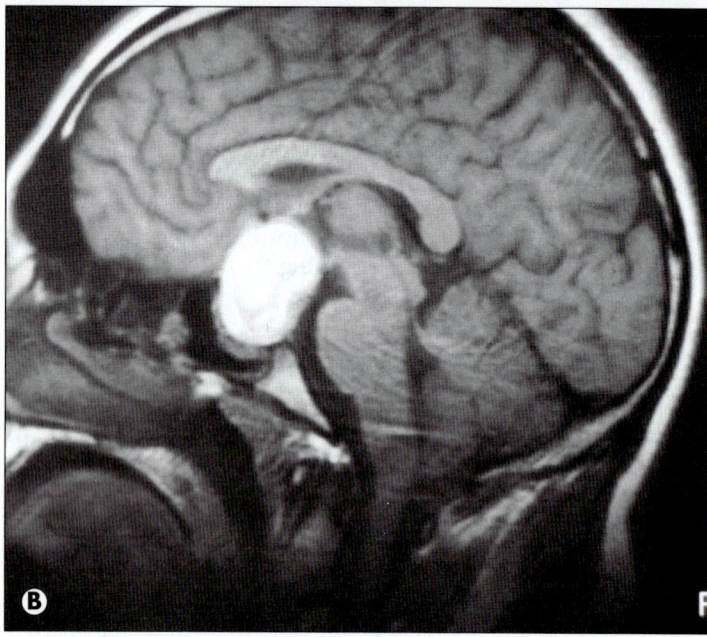

FIG. 207-3 ■ A, Axial MRI view of enlarged apoplectic pituitary gland involving chiasm. B, Sagittal MRI view from the same patient.

Cavernous Sinus Thrombosis and Orbital Apex Syndrome

These entities have similar differential diagnoses, because most problems arise from adjacent structures.

- Tolosa–Hunt syndrome: otherwise healthy patients, severe pain, vision loss rare, inflammatory "pseudotumor" seen on neuroimaging
- Arteriovenous fistula: often with antecedent trauma, bruit may be auscultated, arterialized conjunctival vessels
- Thyroid eye disease: rarely seen without lid retraction and lid lag, positive forced ductions, thickened extraocular muscles on CT scan with little to no sinus disease

Pituitary Apoplexy

Intracranial aneurysm, both expanding and ruptured, should be considered if MRI scanning fails to reveal pituitary hemorrhage. An MR angiogram should then be undertaken.

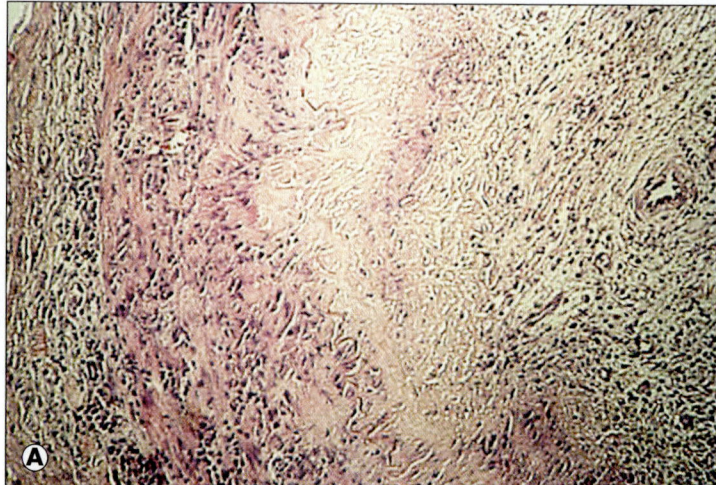

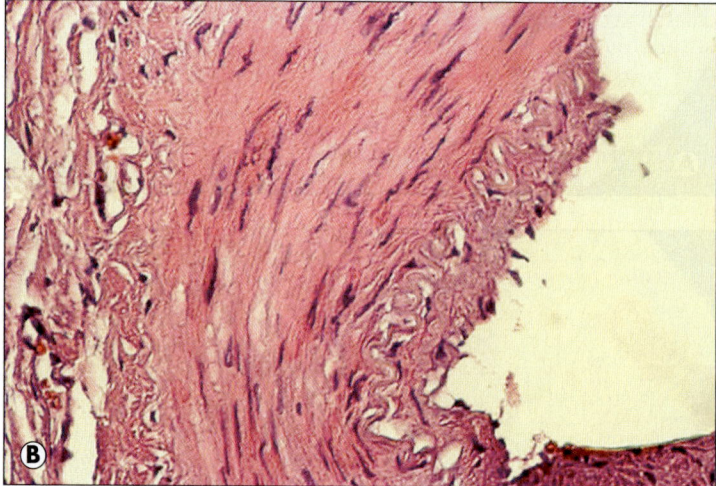

FIG. 207-4 ■ A, Temporal artery biopsy positive for giant cell arteritis. Note destruction of elastic lamina and complete luminal occlusion. B, Normal temporal artery specimen.

PATHOLOGY

Giant Cell Arteritis

Biopsy specimens will reveal an overwhelming inflammatory mononuclear cellular infiltrate. There is destruction of the internal elastic lamina and necrosis of the media is seen often. Vessel lumens often are completely occluded. Multinucleated giant cells may be present (Fig. 207-4).

Aneurysm

Histologically aneurysmal vessels exhibit markedly thinned media and adventitia. There is generalized disruption of the internal elastic lamina, with areas of thinning, fragmentation, and even absence. Some investigators have found a deficiency or defect in type III collagen formation, as well as a decrease in the type III–to–type I collagen ratio.[36]

Cavernous Sinus Thrombosis and Orbital Apex Syndrome

Sinus specimens often will reveal infectious organisms. Bacterial gram stains should be performed to ascertain the presence of gram-positive or gram-negative bacteria, or both. In addition, India ink and special stains for fungi should be performed to evaluate for mucormycosis. Nonseptate, large, branching hyphae that stain easily with H&E is indicative of *Mucor* and *Rhizopus* species.

Pituitary Apoplexy

This condition is marked by pituitary hemorrhage, often accompanied by necrosis, and thrombosis. Most specimens have a high degree of necrosis, making cell type identification difficult. One study, however, found null cells to be the most frequent (61%), followed by somatotroph (17%), corticotroph (11%), lactotroph (5.5%), and gonadotroph (5.5%).[37]

TREATMENT
Giant Cell Arteritis

The well-accepted management for GCA is systemic corticosteroids. Generally, the ophthalmic literature favors higher doses than the rheumatological literature. There is no clear agreement on starting dosage.[38] Neuro-ophthalmologists usually start at dosages of 80–100mg of oral methylprednisolone. Rheumatologists start at lower dosages of 60–40mg. Some even advocate initial intravenous steroid therapy. A recent retrospective series indicated increased likelihood of improvement in vision in those managed with intravenous steroids.[39]

ESR is followed every 4–6 weeks, and the steroid therapy is titrated accordingly. There is general consensus that the duration of therapy should be for many months, often extending up to 1 to 2 years.

Aneurysm

Management of unruptured intracranial aneurysms depends, in part, on their size and position, as well as the age and health of the patient. Unruptured aneurysms may be managed via a direct or "open" surgical approach or with an endovascular approach.

The direct surgical approach aims at applying metal clips at the base of the aneurysm in order to close it off. This approach is quite successful but incurs the risks associated with open craniotomy. Damage to adjacent structures (oculomotor nerve) may occur.

The endovascular approach uses catheters to introduce balloons or thromboembolic coils into the aneurysm, thereby mechanically occluding it or thrombosing it. This approach carries a lower mortality and morbidity but can be complicated by incomplete closure of the aneurysm or displacement of the endovascular balloon, as well as rupture due to penetration of the thin aneurysm wall.

Cavernous Sinus Thrombosis and Orbital Apex Syndrome

Septic thrombosis of the cavernous sinus is usually managed with a combination of antibiotics and anticoagulation. Corticosteroids may also play a role in reducing inflammation. If sinus disease is present, débridement of the sinuses should also take place. If there is clinical evidence or suspicion of *Mucor*, treatment with amphotericin B should be initiated. Correction of underlying metabolic acidosis greatly increases survival.[17]

Orbital apex syndrome is managed in much the same way, except that in cases of *Mucor*, sinus exenteration as well as orbital exenteration may be necessary in order to improve survival.

Aseptic thrombosis of the cavernous sinus is managed primarily by managing the underlying condition. Adjuvant anticoagulation may stop the spread of thrombosis.[40]

Pituitary Apoplexy

Most patients are managed with decompression of the sella transsphenoidally. In general, these patients have a neuro-ophthalmic abnormality prompting surgery. Some groups advocate the use of bromocriptine in cases with little or no neuro-ophthalmic deficit.

Supplementation of pituitary hormones is often necessary for prolonged periods after the apoplectic event.

COURSE AND OUTCOMES
Giant Cell Arteritis

The primary goal of therapy is to avert vision loss in the fellow eye. Restoration of vision in the affected eye is rare. However, if left untreated, nearly 90% of patients will suffer vision loss in the fellow eye.[41]

Aneurysm

The results of surgery on unruptured aneurysms are excellent. Mortality rates with these procedures are as low as 1–5%.[42] Morbidity is somewhat higher at 10–15%, which usually manifests in the form of incomplete recovery of oculomotor nerve function or aberrant regeneration.

Cavernous Sinus Thrombosis

The mortality rate for patients with septic cavernous sinus thrombosis is about 30%.[16] Morbidity is very high. Nearly all survivors have some neurological deficit. These usually are due to damage to the cranial nerves of the cavernous sinus. Therefore, ophthalmoplegias, sensory neuropathies, and even retinal vein or artery occlusions may be seen.

Aseptic thrombosis has a much lower mortality than septic thrombosis. Morbidity, nonetheless, remains high, with damage to the intracavernous cranial nerves common.

Orbital Apex Syndrome

The mortality from *Mucor*-induced orbital apex syndrome is reported between 46% and 52%,[43] despite amphotericin B therapy. Morbidity remains high, because many patients require exenteration of the sinuses and orbit. Permanent neurological deficits are common.

Pituitary Apoplexy

Surgical decompression of the sella appears to have good neuro-ophthalmic outcomes. Improvements in visual acuity, field deficits, and ophthalmoplegia were reported as high as 76%–91%.[37] Endocrine abnormalities, however, remained high, with 43–58% requiring some form of hormonal supplementation. Mortality with surgical management remained low.

REFERENCES

1. Haiman MH, Burton TC, Brown CK. Epidemiology of retinal detachment. Arch Ophthalmol. 1982;100:289–92.
2. de Juan E, Sternberg P, Michaels RG. Penetrating ocular injuries: types of injuries and visual results. Ophthalmology. 1983;90:1318–22.
3. Johnson LN, Arnold AC. Incidence of nonarteritic and arteritic anterior ischemic optic neuropathy: population-based study in the state of Missouri and Los Angeles County, California. J Neuroophthalmol. 1994;14:38–44.
4. Machado EBV, Michet CJ, Ballard DJ, et al. Trends in incidence and clinical presentation of temporal arteritis in Olmsted County, Minnesota, 1950–1985. Arthritis Rheum. 1988;31:745–9.
5. Liu NH, LaBree LD, Feldon SE, Rao NA. The epidemiology of giant cell arteritis: a 12-year retrospective study. Ophthalmology. 2001;108:1145–9.
6. Arnold AC. Ischemic optic neuropathy, diabetic papillopathy, and papillophlebitis. In: Yanoff M, Duker JS. Ophthalmology. London: Mosby; 1999:11-7.1-6.
7. Weyand CM, Bartley GB. Giant cell arteritis: new concepts in pathogenesis and implications for management. Am J Ophthalmol. 1997;123:392–8.
8. MacMichael IM, Cullen JF. Pathology of ischaemic optic neuropathy. In: Cant JS, ed. The optic nerve. Proceedings of the Second William MacKenzie Memorial Symposium. London: Henry Kimpton; 1972:108–16.
9. Siatkowski RM, Gass JDM, Glaser JS, et al. Fluorescein angiography in the diagnosis of giant cell arteritis. Am J Ophthalmol. 1993;115:57–9.
10. Menghini VV, Brown RD, Sicks JD, et al. Incidence and prevalence of intracranial aneurysm and hemorrhage in Olmsted County, Minnesota, 1965 to 1995. Neurology. 1998;51:405–11.
11. Wardlaw JM, White PM. The detection and management of unruptured intracranial aneurysms. Brain. 2000;123:205–21.
12. Winn HR, Jane JA Sr, Taylor J, et al. Prevalence of asymptomatic incidental aneurysm: review of 4568 arteriograms. J Neurosurg. 2002;96:43–9.
13. Forget TR Jr, Benitez R, Veznedaroglu E, et al. A review of size and location of ruptured intracranial aneurysms. Neurosurgery. 2001;49:1322–5.
14. Feely M, Kapoor S. Third nerve palsy due to posterior communicating artery aneurysm. The importance of early surgery. J Neurol Neurosurg Psychiatry. 1987;50:1051–2.
15. Soni SR. Aneurysms of the posterior communicating artery and oculomotor paresis. J Neurol Neurosurg Psychiatry. 1974;37:475–84.
16. Denubile MJ. Septic thrombosis of the cavernous sinus. Arch Neurol. 1988;45:567–72.
17. Bergin DJ, Wright JE. Orbital cellulitis. Br J Ophthalmol. 1986;70:174–8.
18. Joshi N, Caputo GM, Weitekamp MR, Karchmer AW. Infections in patients with diabetes mellitus. N Engl J Med. 1999;341:1906–12.

19. Ferry AP, Abedi S. Diagnosis and management of rhino-orbitocerebral mucormycosis. A report of 16 personally observed cases. Ophthalmology. 1983;90:1096–104.

20. Gale GR, Welch AM. Studies of opportunistic fungi. I. Inhibition of *Rhizopus oryzae* by human serum. Am J Med Sci. 1961;241:604–12.

21. Wakai S, Fukushima T, Teramoto A, et al. Pituitary apoplexy: its incidence and clinical significance. J Neurosurg. 1981;55:187–93.

22. Cardoso ER, Peterson EW. Pituitary apoplexy: a review. Neurosurgery. 1984;14:363–73.

23. Biousse V, Newman NJ, Oyesiku NM. Precipitating factors in pituitary apoplexy. J Neurol. 2001;71:542–5.

24. Hayreh SS, Podhajsky PA, Zimmerman B. Ocular manifestations of giant cell arteritis. Am J Ophthalmol. 1998;125:509–20.

25. Glutz vonBlotzheim S, Borruat FX. Neuro-ophthalmic complications of biopsy-proven giant cell arteritis. Eur J Ophthalmol. 1997;7:375–82.

26. Rodriguez-Valverde V, Sarabia JM, Gonzalez-Gay MA, et al. Risk factors and predictive models of giant cell arteritis in polymyalgias rheumatica. Am J Med. 1997;102:331–6.

27. Hunder GG, Bloch DA, Michel BA, et al. The American College of Rheumatology criteria for classification of giant cell arteritis. Arthritis Rheum. 1990;33:1122–8.

28. Miller A, Green M, Robinson D. Simple rule for calculating normal erythrocyte sedimentation rate. BMJ. 1983;286:266.

29. Lincoff NS, Erlich PD, Brass LS. Thrombocytosis in temporal arteritis rising platelet counts: a red flag for giant cell arteritis. J Neuroophthalmol. 2000;20:67–72.

30. Danesh-Mayer HV, Savino PJ, Eagle RC Jr, et al. Low diagnostic yield with second biopsies in suspected giant cell arteritis. J Neuroophthalmol. 2000;20:213–5.

31. White PM, Teasdale EM, Wardlaw JM, Easton V. Intracranial aneurysms: CT angiography and MR angiography for detection, prospective blinded comparison in a large patient cohort. Radiology. 2001;219:739–49.

32. White PM, Wardlaw JM, Easton V. Can noninvasive imaging accurately depict intracranial aneurysm? A systematic review. Radiology. 2000;217:361–70.

33. Tovilla-Canales JL, Nava A, Tovilla y Pomar JL. Orbital and periorbital infections. Curr Opin Ophthalmol. 2001;12:335–41.

34. Veldhuis JD, Hammond JM. Endocrine function after spontaneous infarction of the human pituitary: report, review and reappraisal. Endocr Rev. 1980;1:100–7.

35. Onesti ST, Wisniewski T, Post KD. Clinical versus subclinical pituitary apoplexy: presentation, surgical management, and outcome in 21 patients. Neurosurgery. 1990;6:980–6.

36. Van den Berg JS, Limburg M, Pals G, et al. Some patients with intracranial aneurysms have a reduced type III/type I collagen ratio. A case-control study. Neurology. 1997;49:1546–51.

37. Randeva HS, Schoebel J, Byrne J, et al. Classical pituitary apoplexy: clinical features, management and outcome. Clin Endocrinol. 1999;51:181–8.

38. Jover JA, Hernandez-Garcia C, Morado IC, et al. Combined treatment of giant cell arteritis with methotrexate and prednisone: a randomized, double-blinded, placebo controlled trial. Ann Intern Med. 2001;134:106–14.

39. Chan CCK, Paine M, O'Day J. Steroid management in giant cell arteritis. Br J Ophthalmol. 2001;85:1061–4.

40. Levine SR, Twyman RE, Gilman S. The role of anticoagulation in cavernous sinus thrombosis. Neurology. 1988;38:517–22.

41. Liu GT, Glaser JS, Schatz NJ, Smith JL. Visual morbidity in giant cell arteritis. Ophthalmology. 1994;101:1779–85.

42. King JT Jr, Berlin JA, Flamm ES. Morbidity and mortality from elective surgery for asymptomatic, unruptured, intracranial aneurysms: a meta-analysis. J Neurosurg. 1994;81:837–42.

43. Strasser MD, Kennedy RJ, Adam RD. Rhinocerebral mucormycosis: therapy with amphotericin B lipid complex. Arch Intern Med. 1996;156:337–9.

CHAPTER
208 Trauma, Drugs, and Toxins

DEBORAH I. FRIEDMAN • NORDELI ESTRONZA

DEFINITION

- Visual abnormalities related to brain dysfunction and injury include post-traumatic vision syndrome, which consists of visual signs and symptoms after a mild or severe head injury, and visual disturbances that result from exposure to medications, hallucinogens, or toxins.

KEY FEATURES

- Motility disorders, saccadic abnormalities, nystagmus, convergence insufficiency.
- Visual perceptual–motor dysfunction.
- Positive visual phenomena.
- Formed and unformed visual hallucinations.
- Dyschromatopsia.
- Visual field defects.
- Blurred vision or visual loss.
- Cerebral (cortical) blindness.

ASSOCIATED FEATURES

- Headaches.
- Short-term memory loss.
- Impaired concentration.
- Behavioral changes.
- Other physical neurological deficits.

TRAUMA AND THE BRAIN

INTRODUCTION

Visual abnormalities that follow closed head trauma occur commonly and can involve any part of the visual pathway. Prompt recognition and treatment of these conditions enhance the potential for the patient's rehabilitation.

EPIDEMIOLOGY AND PATHOGENESIS

Head trauma is an important public health problem. Approximately 900,000 patients are hospitalized yearly in the United States for the consequences of closed head trauma. The most common cause of head injury in the United States is motor vehicle accident, and the severity of head injury is correlated directly to the lack of proper seatbelt and helmet use.[1] Of all persons injured in motor vehicle accidents, 70% incur head injuries. Men are injured twice as frequently as women, and alcohol is a significant contributing factor in men. About one half of all patients are aged 15–34 years. Assault, including child and spousal abuse; accidents in the home or workplace; and sports injuries also contribute to traumatic brain injury.

Unfortunately, very few studies have examined the incidence of the visual sequelae of head trauma. After a brain injury, the visual system often is not evaluated comprehensively. This may re-

flect the lack of articulated complaints from head-injured patients, either because of a lack of subjective experience or because of reduced cognition. Family members or rehabilitative personnel often identify the deficits and bring the patients' visual problems to medical attention. In one report, 50–65% of patients who attended a rehabilitation facility had experienced visual disturbances after traumatic brain injury.[2] No apparent correlation exists between the severity of the trauma and the presence of visual disorders.

OCULAR MANIFESTATIONS

Visual deficits after head injury may be monocular or binocular (Box 208-1). Cortical injury causes changes in refraction, saccades, and other sensory-motor relationships. The most common visual complaint after head trauma is blurred vision because of convergence insufficiency. Patients who have convergence insufficiency also may have difficulty reading, diplopia at near, eye strain, tearing, photosensitivity, and headaches. Control of saccadic eye movements can be disrupted after damage to either brain hemisphere. Esophoria and exotropia are common sequelae of head trauma. Binocular single vision may be lost after a head injury, with the breakdown of a latent phoria or loss of the normal physiological fusion of the image presented to each eye. Visual field defects after closed head trauma are not uncommon. In one report, tunnel fields that suggested functional visual loss were found most frequently and were associated with post-traumatic migraine in about half the cases.[1] Other visual field defects include optic nerve–related scotomata, quadrantanopia, homonymous hemianopia, bitemporal hemianopia, and cerebral blindness.

Patients who have injury to the nondominant parietal, temporal, and occipital areas may exhibit visual attention problems as well as difficulty with spatial orientation and visual recognition. Visual cognition may be disrupted after head trauma, which results in difficulty judging the spatial properties of objects and impaired mental manipulation of three-dimensional images. When spatial organization and constructive abilities are impaired, the frontal

---

BOX 208-1

Visual Symptoms and Signs Associated With Head Trauma

SYMPTOMS	SIGNS
Blurred or decreased vision	Convergence insufficiency
Diplopia	Abnormal saccades
Difficulty reading	Oculomotor dysfunction
Photophobia	Accommodative disorders
Visual hallucinations	Fixation instability
Oscillopsia	Nystagmus
Phosphenes	Lagophthalmos
	Visual field defects
	Visual perceptual–motor dysfunction
	• impaired spatial relationships
	• right–left discrimination problems
	Visual cognition deficits
	Visual inattention

lobe is provided with inadequate feedback for the execution of motor movements. Nondominant hemisphere injury often causes impaired comprehension of visual images, which may be expressed by the patient as the inability to read, despite excellent visual acuity. Words may appear to run together on the printed page. Trauma to the optic chiasm simulates a pituitary region tumor, with a bitemporal hemianopia and seesaw nystagmus. Damage to brainstem structures leads to pupillary asymmetry or irregularity, ocular motor nerve paresis, unilateral and bilateral internuclear ophthalmoplegia, skew deviation, dorsal midbrain syndrome, and nystagmus.[1] Saccadic deficits may occur, including failure to initiate contralateral saccades, prolonged saccadic latency, decreased saccadic accuracy toward a hemianopic field, and a tendency for the patient to be distracted by peripheral stimuli.[3]

DIAGNOSIS AND ANCILLARY TESTING

Visual complaints after head injury vary widely. The ophthalmological examination often reveals a treatable problem. However, patients may be difficult to examine because of cognitive and communication disorders. Multiple examinations may be needed to assess fully a brain-injured patient. A complete assessment may include evaluation of the eye, refraction, and examination of ocular motility, accommodation, vergence, stereopsis, visual perception, and visual fields.[4] The diagnosis of convergence insufficiency is made on the basis of measurement of the convergence fusional reserves. The near point of convergence alone is an unreliable measure. Skull radiographs have limited usefulness, as they show only bony pathology. Neuroimaging studies are warranted when an intracranial lesion is suspected. Computed tomography is most useful to demonstrate skull base fractures and acute bleeding, while magnetic resonance imaging shows the soft tissues and brainstem with greater clarity.[5]

DIFFERENTIAL DIAGNOSIS

When there is a temporal association between the patient's symptoms and the head injury, a causal association is presumed. However, minor head trauma may draw attention to visual deficits from other causes that had been unrecognized previously. Patients who have homonymous or bitemporal visual field defects after trauma require neuroimaging studies to exclude a hemorrhage, tumor, stroke, or vascular malformation. Patients who seek compensation or other secondary gain may have functional visual loss. It is often difficult to separate real disability from nonorganic visual abnormalities in patients who are malingering.

Hallucinations and other visual disturbances observed in head trauma patients also may be caused by migraine, encephalitis, hepatitis, or other systemic disorders. Other causes of convergence insufficiency are a wide interpupillary distance, refractive errors, delayed development, malnutrition, encephalitis, hepatitis, and drug intoxication.

SYSTEMIC ASSOCIATIONS

A traumatic brain injury is sudden and devastating. The patient may be in deep coma or have multiple injuries that affect motor function, speech, and cognition. With a mild traumatic brain injury, visual symptoms can be part of the postconcussion syndrome. Sometimes, the head injury may seem quite trivial, with no loss of consciousness. Early symptoms include headaches, dizziness, vertigo, tinnitus, hearing loss, blurred vision, diplopia, convergence insufficiency, sensitivity to light and noise, diminished sense of taste and smell, irritability, fatigue, sleep disturbances, decreased libido, decreased appetite, short- and intermediate-term memory dysfunction, impaired concentration and attention, and slowing of reaction time.[6] Anxiety, depression, and personality changes may occur later and are confounded by social and economic comorbidity.[7]

PATHOLOGY

A structural injury, such as a skull fracture, hematoma, contusion, stroke, or foreign body, accounts for many of the neurological sequelae of severe head trauma. The rigid skull encasement means that secondary pressure effects from intracranial injuries are common. The cranial nerves are susceptible to injury because of their long course at the base of the skull. Orbital fractures can lead to muscle entrapment and diplopia. Optic canal fractures, often associated with basilar skull fractures, can produce an optic neuropathy.

The pathophysiology of mild traumatic brain injury is not understood completely. Subtle changes may be missed on neuroimaging studies. The most apparent neuropathological change in mild traumatic brain injury is diffuse axonal damage.[8] Acutely, the axons are damaged and swollen. This may be attributed to stretching of axons during the injury, with subsequent edema and detachment. The secondary changes of edema and disconnection may take 4–24 hours to develop. The synaptic terminals derived from the degenerating axons are disrupted, which results in diffuse deafferentation. Animal models of traumatic brain injury suggest that an active neuroplastic response occurs, with repopulation of injured axon terminals by the remaining intact fiber populations. Changes in neurotransmitters are likely to occur in traumatic brain injury. Excitatory neurotoxins are released acutely. Acetylcholine is increased in the cerebrospinal fluid and in several areas of the brain after injury. Altered binding to cholinergic and glutaminergic receptors occurs in the cerebral cortex. Pathological evaluation of long-standing brain injury reveals microglial scarring and wallerian degeneration.[8]

TREATMENT

Early diagnosis of visual problems following traumatic brain injury is essential to maximize the overall rehabilitation potential.[1] The sooner the visual problems are addressed after head trauma, the better the chances for a faster and more complete recovery. Treatments advocated for post-traumatic visual symptoms include eye exercises, prism spectacles, and surgery. Treatment should emphasize the design of lenses, filters, or prisms to address the specific defect in the visual system. Accommodative insufficiency typically is corrected using a plus power that is often excessive for the patient's age. Patients who have hemianopic field defects require visual retraining to move the eyes and head consciously into the blind hemifield. Occasionally, prisms are useful in these patients to shift part of the missing hemifield into view. Other techniques for reading include using guides for lines and margins and moving or tilting the page into the intact visual field. Therapists and caregivers must be aware of the patient's visual limitations that militate against adaptation to daily living activities. Single-vision reading spectacles may help patients who have inferior visual field defects.

Patients who have diplopia are helped by prisms, patching, or surgery. Prisms are most useful for relatively comitant ocular deviations. Because most patients improve, a temporary Fresnel prism allows easy prism replacement as the strabismus lessens over time. Patching one eye may reduce discomfort initially, but in the long term, this produces a monocular condition that stresses the visual and motor systems, causing difficulty with midline concepts and affecting balance and posture. Strabismus surgery should not be considered for at least 9 months after the injury, because a high rate of spontaneous improvement occurs. Visual rehabilitation may include activities designed to enhance the patient's awareness of visual deficits and increase function, in order to maximize residual vision.

COURSE AND OUTCOME

The visual system impacts all aspects of life. Rehabilitation is much more difficult if the visual system is not efficient. Patients who have severe brain injuries often have permanent visual field and motility defects. The Glasgow Coma Scale, a measure of the depth of coma, is useful for predicting overall functional outcome when applied on the second or third day after injury. Posttraumatic amnesia that persists for more than 2 months is a poor prognostic sign with regard to independent living, memory, and work capacity.

Most patients who have mild traumatic brain injury experience improvement; the majority recover completely within the first year of sustaining the injury. These patients should be reassured that their symptoms are valid and their prognosis is good. Headaches, dizziness, and memory problems are the primary symptoms associated with mild head injury; most patients have resolution of these symptoms by 6 months. It is not uncommon for patients to complain of diplopia many months after suffering the injury, although most cases of diplopia tend to resolve spontaneously in 6–12 months. Those with a late onset of symptoms may have an underlying psychogenic cause. Patients who have convergence insufficiency secondary to trauma do not seem to respond to treatment as well as those who have idiopathic convergence insufficiency.

DRUGS, TOXINS, AND THE BRAIN

INTRODUCTION

Visual phenomena are observed with an endless list of drugs, including prescription medications. Many neurotoxic agents have a major effect on the visual pathways.

EPIDEMIOLOGY AND PATHOGENESIS

Hallucinations and other visual symptoms are induced by hallucinogens and stimulants, but they are also reported frequently as side effects of a variety of medications commonly used in clinical practice. Visual disturbances from digitalis were observed more than 200 years ago and are present in up to 95% of patients, particularly those who have digitalis intoxication.[9] As early as 1843, cases of cerebral blindness secondary to carbon monoxide poisoning were reported.[10] Toxic levels of many chemical substances, such as toluene and other solvents, can produce devastating visual deficits. The deliberate inhalation of volatile substances to achieve intoxication has been associated with pleasant as well as unpleasant visual changes. Volatile substance abuse occurs in most parts of the world, mainly among adolescents, individuals living in remote communities, and those whose occupations afford ready access to such substances.[11]

OCULAR MANIFESTATIONS

Hallucinations are a potential side effect of many medications. The most common medications with hallucinogenic potential are H_2 blockers, dopaminergic agents, antihypertensives, anticholinergics, sedative hypnotics, benzodiazepines, antidepressants, anti-inflammatory agents, and corticosteroids.[12] Many of the mydriatic and parasympatholytic drugs (e.g., scopolamine [hyoscine], atropine, cyclopentolate) used in ophthalmology have considerable hallucinogenic potential. Amantadine, atropine, and other anticholinergics may produce Lilliputian hallucinations, in which people appear greatly reduced in size.[13] Visual symptoms from digitalis include dimness; scotomata; flickering or flashing lights of yellow, green, or red; haloes; cycloplegia; amblyopia; diplopia; and blindness. Hydroxychloroquine has similar side effects, as well as photophobia and oculogyric crisis. Perception of a bluish haze and increased light sensitivity may occur with sildenafil usage.[14] Dyschromatopsia, haloes, and photophobia are reported with amiodarone usage. Ibuprofen, commonly used for minor pain relief, may produce diplopia, dyschromatopsia, myopia, photophobia, scotomata, visual field defects, and nystagmus. Hallucinogenic phenomena, particularly

visual hallucinations, are observed with lysergic acid diethylamide, amphetamines, cocaine, marijuana, phencyclidine, and inhalants. The visual experiences of lead encephalopathy may resemble delirium tremens, with illusions or misperceptions of objects and shadows.

Many types of visual complaints follow carbon monoxide toxicity. Visual field defects range from concentric constriction to homonymous hemianopia. Patients often have fluctuating visual acuity with normal pupils, typical of an occipital lobe process. Visual object agnosia, polyopia, metamorphopsia, kakopsia (abnormally bright appearance of colors), and asthenopia (cerebral blurred vision) may occur. The degreasing agent trichloroethylene may produce double vision, dyschromatopsia, abnormal contrast sensitivity, and blindness. Visual disturbances are associated with other solvents such as xylene, toluene, and methylchloride.[15]

DIAGNOSIS AND ANCILLARY TESTING

For the evaluation of a patient who has unexplained visual loss or visual disturbances, a detailed history is required; this includes determining the usage of prescription and nonprescription drugs, the ingestion of herbal and other natural remedies, and possible environmental exposure to toxins or chemicals. In suspected cases of toxic exposure, toxicological analysis of blood, urine, and tissue is indicated. Magnetic resonance imaging may reveal abnormalities in the basal ganglia or the occipital lobes with carbon monoxide poisoning (Figs. 208-1 and 208-2).

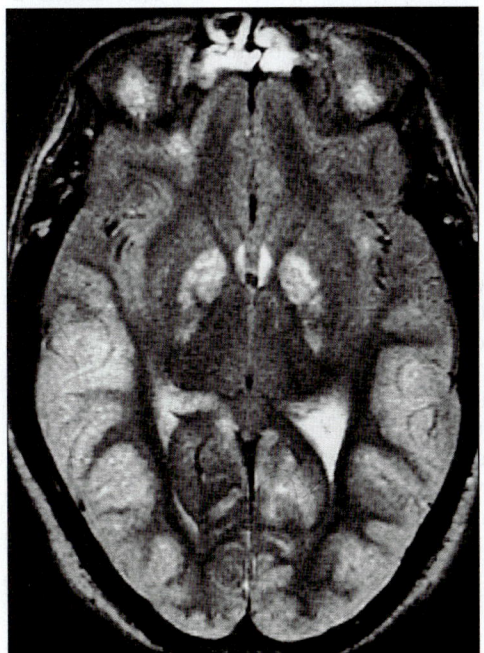

FIG. 208-1 ▮▮ Magnetic resonance imaging of the brain shows areas of infarction following carbon monoxide poisoning. This T2-weighted image shows abnormally high signal intensity in the basal ganglia, right frontal lobe, and cerebral cortex.

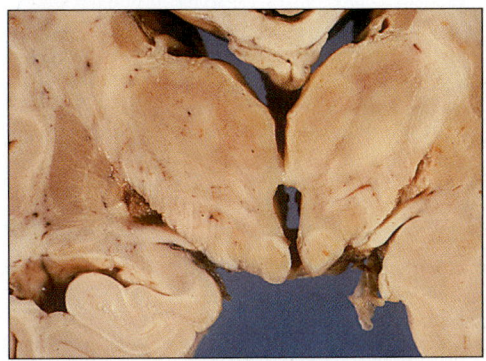

FIG. 208-2 ▮▮ Bilateral cavitary lesions in the globus pallidus following carbon monoxide poisoning.

DIFFERENTIAL DIAGNOSIS

Intracranial lesions, visual loss, vitreous or retinal detachment, seizures, migraine, and metabolic abnormalities must be considered in the evaluation of hallucinations. Both formed and unformed hallucinations occasionally occur with intracranial tumors, infarcts, and vascular malformations. Lesions in the temporal lobe typically produce formed images, while unformed, geometrical patterns arise from the occipital lobe. Vivid hallucinations may accompany a thalamic or midbrain infarction.[16] Patients who have a homonymous hemianopia may see images in their blind hemifield.[17] Visual illusions may also occur during recovery from cortical blindness.[18] Partial seizures sometimes are accompanied by visual disturbances, which may herald the impending seizure. Positive visual phenomena are common features of migraine. Scintillating scotomata, fortification spectra, phosphenes, and heat waves are typical and may be present with or without a headache.

Metabolic derangements usually produce hallucinations with an encephalopathy. Flashes and floaters of ocular origin typically are monocular. The Charles Bonnet syndrome consists of formed hallucinations in patients who have bilateral visual loss. Typically, these are nonthreatening, and the patient knows that the apparitions are not real.[19] Formed and unformed hallucinations are also common in patients with retinal disease and often are not reported.[20] Patients who have bilateral blindness may see formed or unformed hallucinations as a release phenomenon. The visual hallucinations of psychiatric disease are most often threatening and accompanied by auditory hallucinations.

SYSTEMIC ASSOCIATIONS

Headache, fatigue, malaise, and drowsiness are side effects of many drugs. Hallucinogens are absorbed efficiently from the gastrointestinal tract, which results in multiple systemic effects, such as disordered thought processes, mood changes, anorexia, tachypnea, tremors, hyperreflexia, hypertension, and tachycardia. Hallucinogens, medication reactions, and toxins can produce hallucinations that resemble psychiatric states.[12]

PATHOLOGY

Some drugs affect the visual system by their effects on the ocular media and retina. The anticonvulsant vigabatrin produces irreversible visual field loss by its effect on inner electroretinal function at the level of the Müller cell. Vigabatrin also produces outer retinal dysfunction that may be reversible.[21,22] In other cases, drugs have direct action on the brain cells. The dopaminergic and cholinergic neurons in mesolimbic pathways may be important in the development of hallucinations. Digitalis and other toxic agents produce visual changes as a result of profound excitatory effects on nerve cells. Severe reduction in visual acuity in patients who have carbon monoxide poisoning is thought to result from cerebral blindness secondary to brain anoxia.

TREATMENT, COURSE, AND OUTCOME

The most important aspect of treatment is removal of the source of exposure. Hallucinations induced by hallucinogenic drugs can also be treated effectively with antipsychotic medications. In some cases, the hallucinations persist, despite removal of the offending agent.[23]

REFERENCES

1. Sabates NR, Gonce MA, Farris BK. Neuro-ophthalmological findings in closed head trauma. J Clin Neuro-Ophthalmol. 1991;11:273–7.
2. Schlageter K, Gray B, Hall K. Incidence and treatment of visual dysfunction in traumatic brain injury. Brain Injury. 1993;7:439–48.
3. Warren M. A hierarchical model for evaluation and treatment of visual perceptual dysfunction in adult acquired brain injury. Part I. Am J Occup Ther. 1992:47: 42–53.
4. Falk NS, Aksionoff EB. The primary care optometric evaluation of the traumatic brain injury patient. J Am Optom Assoc. 1992;63:547–53.
5. Evans RW. The postconcussion syndrome and the sequelae of mild head injury. Neurol Clin. 1992;10:815–47.
6. Hellerstein LF, Freed S, Maples WC. Vision profile of patients with mild brain injury. J Am Optom Assoc. 1995;66:634–9.
7. Alves WM. Natural history of post-concussive signs and symptoms. Phys Med Rehabil: State Art Rev. 1992;6(1):21–32.
8. Hayes RL, Povlishock JT, Singha B. Pathophysiology of mild head injury. Phys Med Rehabil: State Art Rev. 1992;6(1):9–20.
9. Assad G, Shapiro B. Hallucinations: theoretical and clinical overview. Am J Psychiatry. 1986;143:1088–97.
10. Kuroiwa Y, Shida K, Nagamatsu K, et al. Involvement of cerebral functions in acute carbon monoxide poisoning with special reference to occipital lobe functions. Folia Psychiatr Neurol Jpn. 1967;21:189–97.
11. Eastwell HD. Elevated lead levels in petrol "sniffers." Med J Aust. 1985;143:S63–4.
12. Goetz CG, Tanner CM, Klawans HL. Pharmacology of hallucinations induced by long-term therapy. Am J Psychiatry. 1982;139:494–7.
13. Harper RW, Knothe BW. Coloured Lilliputian hallucinations with amantadine. Med J Aust. 1973;1:444–5.
14. Marmor MR, Kessler R. Sildenafil (Viagra) and ophthalmology. Surv Ophthalmol. 1999;44:153–62.
15. King MD, Day RE, Oliver JS, et al. Solvent encephalopathy. BMJ. 1981;283:663–5.
16. Feinberg W, Rapcsak SZ. "Peduncular hallucinosis" following paramedian thalamic infarction. Neurology. 1989;39:1535–6.
17. Vaphiades MS, Celesia GG, Brigell MG. Positive spontaneous visual phenomena limited to the hemianopic field in lesions of central visual pathways. Neurology. 1996;47:408–17.
18. Wunderlich G, Suchan B, Volkmann J, et al. Visual hallucinations in recovery from cortical blindness. Arch Neurol. 2000;57:561–5.
19. Lepore FE. Spontaneous visual phenomena with visual loss: 104 patients with lesions of retinal and neural afferent pathways. Neurology. 1990;40:444–7.
20. Scott IU, Schein OD, Feuer WJ, et al. Visual hallucinations in patient with retinal disease. Am J Ophthalmol. 2001;131:590–8.
21. Paul SR, KraussGl, Miller NR, et al. Visual function is stable in patients who continue long-term vigabatrin therapy: implications for clinical decision making. Epilepsia. 2001;42:525–30.
22. Coupland SG, Zackon DH, Leonard BC, et al. Vigabatrin effect on inner retinal function. Ophthalmology. 2001;108:1493–6.
23. Channer KS, Stanley S. Persistent visual hallucinations secondary to chronic solvent encephalopathy: case report and review of the literature. J Neurol Neurosurg Psychiatry. 1983;46:83–6.

CHAPTER

209

Vascular Disorders

THOMAS R. HEDGES, JR.

DEFINITION
- Vascular lesions are congenital or acquired abnormalities of blood vessels that may affect all parts of the sensory and motor pathways of the eye and central nervous system.

KEY FEATURE
- Aneurysms, carotid–cavernous fistulas and shunts, and arteriovenous malformations produce damage to the eye and brain and have discrete, often disparate, clinical features and management.

ASSOCIATED FEATURES
- Transient visual loss, both monocular and binocular, may or may not be associated with demonstrable vascular lesions.
- Transient ischemic attacks and stroke have characteristic symptoms and signs. Their diagnosis, investigation, and management depend on the locale of the insult to the central nervous system.

INTRODUCTION

The visual pathways and oculomotor system can be affected by virtually all types of vascular disease. Aneurysms most commonly cause a third cranial nerve palsy, although visual loss also may occur. Carotid–cavernous (C–C) fistulas, especially shunts, can be mistaken for other more benign causes of an inflamed eye. Arteriovenous malformations (AVMs), especially cryptic AVMs, can cause highly variable cerebral neurological deficits. Transient visual loss (TVL) and cerebral ischemic attacks cause concern about impending stroke.

ANEURYSMS

Epidemiology and Pathogenesis

Based on pathology studies, the incidence of diagnosed saccular aneurysms is estimated at 9%. Most saccular aneurysms occur as isolated, nonhereditary lesions. However, because intracranial aneurysms of 2mm or smaller are found in 70% of routine autopsies, this incidence is underestimated markedly. Women are more susceptible, especially to internal carotid–posterior communicating (IC–PC) artery aneurysms. The peak incidence of aneurysms occurs during the fifth and sixth decades,[1] and 85% of aneurysms originate from branches of the internal carotid artery, usually at the posterior communicating or the ophthalmic artery, or within the cavernous sinus. Aneurysms of 25mm or greater almost always are symptomatic, often by mass effect, and account for 3–13% of unruptured and 3–25% of ruptured symptomatic aneurysms. Aneurysms may be multiple in about 20% of adults.[2]

Ocular Manifestations

Aneurysms that affect the following portions of the circle of Willis have ophthalmologic manifestations:
- The IC–PC artery junction causing third nerve palsy

- The carotid–ophthalmic artery junction causing compression of the optic nerve or chiasm or both
- The intracavernous carotid artery causing extra oculomotor palsy, fifth cranial nerve facial sensory loss, and (rarely) optic nerve compression

IC–PC aneurysms most commonly affect young women; they can manifest as a sudden apoplectic event caused by subarachnoid hemorrhage or can enlarge slowly without rupture to produce third nerve palsy.[3] This type of aneurysm is responsible for 13–30% of acquired oculomotor palsy[4,5]; 90% of asymptomatic, unruptured IC–PC aneurysms cause signs of third nerve palsy.

Carotid–ophthalmic aneurysms are rarer than IC–PC aneurysms, affect the sensory visual pathways by compression of the optic nerve and chiasm, occur most commonly in women during the fourth to seventh decades of life, and often are associated with other intracranial aneurysms. Carotid–ophthalmic aneurysms may rupture and cause subarachnoid hemorrhage, but most often they produce symptoms by compression of the adjacent optic nerves and chiasm,[6] which results in unilateral visual loss with an inferior visual field defect. These aneurysms arise from the ophthalmic artery beneath the optic nerve and compress the nerve superiorly against the superior dural shelf of the optic canal.[7] Insidious, slowly progressive visual loss occurs in most cases. Rarely, an acute painful course with central scotoma and ipsilateral afferent pupillary deficit can mimic retrobulbar optic neuritis[8] or ischemic optic neuropathy. When ophthalmic aneurysms expand posteriorly and superiorly, chiasmal or optic tract syndromes can be seen. Medial expansion may even compress the contralateral optic nerve.[9]

The main difference between IC–PC aneurysms and internal carotid–ophthalmic aneurysms is that the former produce motor (third cranial nerve) signs and symptoms and the latter produce sensory (optic nerve and chiasm) symptoms and signs.

Aneurysms that arise from the internal carotid artery within the cavernous sinus behave differently. They can grow quite large before rupture; when they do rupture into the cavernous sinus they may produce a C–C sinus fistula.

Intracavernous carotid aneurysms enlarge gradually within the cavernous sinus. Anterior expansion may erode the optic foramen and superior orbital fissure, which results in compressive optic neuropathy, ocular motor nerve paresis, and proptosis.[3] Erosion medially into the sella area may produce hypopituitarism.

Patients with unruptured intracavernous aneurysms have oculomotor palsies, with the sixth cranial nerve involved most commonly. The trigeminal nerve may be involved late, which results in facial pain.[10] Apparent pupillary sparing of the third cranial nerve may occur because of involvement of both oculosympathetic and parasympathetic pupillary pathways.[11]

Most patients who develop an acute oculomotor nerve paresis are left with a permanent disorder—often with secondary oculomotor nerve synkinesis or aberrant regeneration (including lid retraction on downgaze; Fig. 209-1) despite no previous acute third nerve dysfunction. Primary oculomotor nerve synkinesis most commonly occurs with meningiomas or, rarely, schwannomas.[12]

Trigeminal nerve dysfunction commonly accompanies intracavernous aneurysms.[13] The first division of the fifth nerve is affected most often. Pain usually is constant, lancinating, and se-

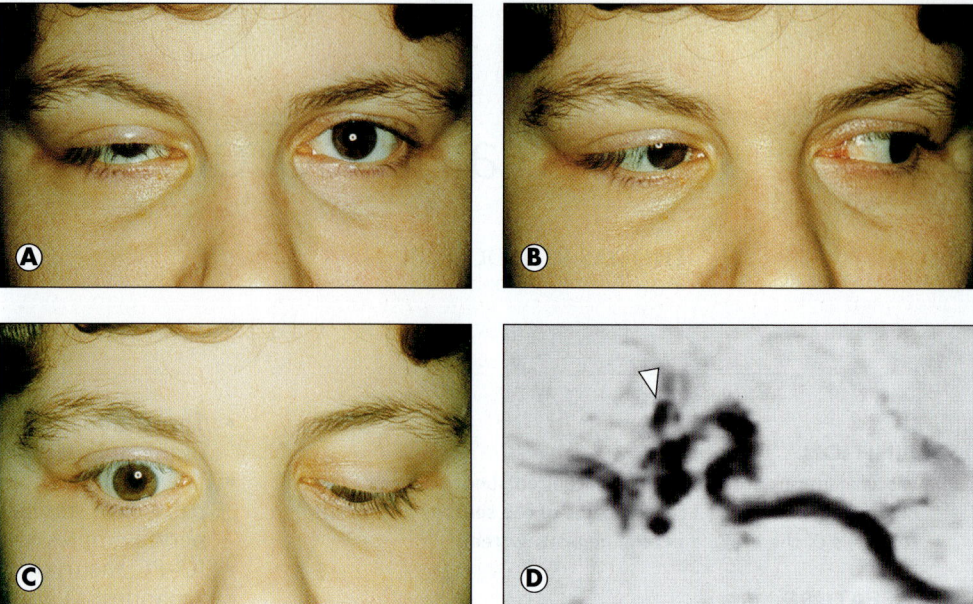

FIG. 209-1 ■ A 36-year-old patient with aberrant regeneration—third cranial nerve synkinesis. **A,** Ptosis. **B,** Medial rectus paresis with lid retraction on adduction. **C,** Typical lid retraction on downgaze. **D,** Magnetic resonance angiogram showing internal carotid–posterior communicating artery aneurysm (arrow).

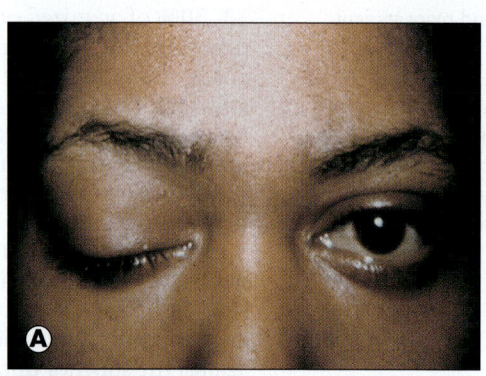
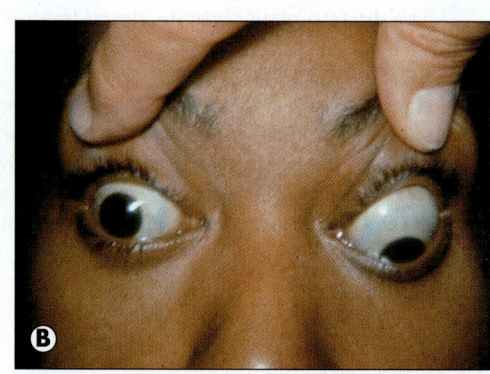

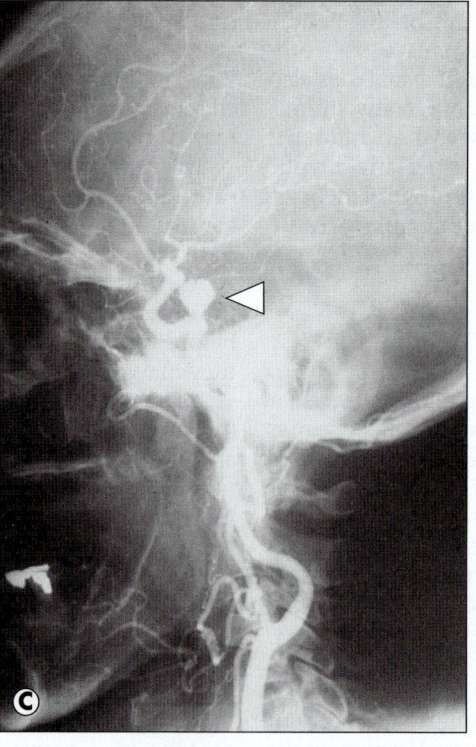
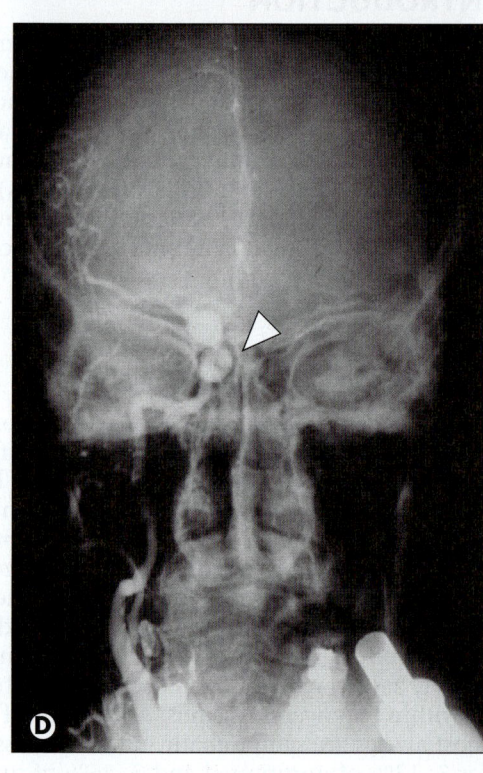

FIG. 209-2 ■ A 40-year-old patient with right internal carotid–posterior communicating artery aneurysm. **A,** Primary position ptosis. **B,** Paralysis of vertical gaze and dilated pupil. **C–D,** Arteriograms showing internal carotid–posterior communicating artery aneurysm directed down, out, and inferiorly on the third cranial nerve (arrows).

vere, but it can be episodic. Trigeminal sensory loss is rare, and only occurs late in the disease.

Visual loss is not as characteristic of intracavernous aneurysm as it is with ophthalmic aneurysms, unless they arise from the most distal portion of the intracavernous artery.

Diagnosis

Three clinical signs usually are apparent:

- Ipsilateral facial, orbital, or eye pain
- Extraocular muscle and levator involvement
- Pupillary paresis

HEAD PAIN. Head pain can be caused by both ruptured and unruptured aneurysms. Ruptured aneurysm pain is severe, sudden in onset, throbbing, and radiates posteriorly. Neck pain and stiffness are signs of subarachnoid hemorrhage. Third cranial nerve palsy most commonly occurs concomitantly but may not develop for hours or days. Headache and eye pain from unruptured aneurysms may occur intermittently for weeks or months before third nerve palsy or aneurysm rupture occurs.

OPHTHALMOPLEGIA. Ophthalmoplegia is variable but develops in virtually all patients eventually. It is the author's experience that ptosis and extraoculomotor paresis occur at the same time, especially with ruptured aneurysms. An apoplectic onset with subarachnoid hemorrhage may overshadow the observation of diplopia or ptosis. Any muscle supplied by the third nerve can be affected; however, the superior rectus and levator muscles are damaged most commonly, because the aneurysm presses on the nerve from above the subarachnoid space (Fig. 209-2).

Recently interventional neuroradiology has radically altered management of aneurysms. When arteriography reveals the aneurysm has a broad neck, then transcranial clipping is still necessary in many patients. However, if the aneurysm has a narrow neck then angiocatheter coils may be used to close off the aneurysm with greatly decreased risk.

PUPILLARY INVOLVEMENT. Pupillary involvement can be the initial sign of an unruptured or "about to rupture" aneurysm but is rarely, if ever, an isolated sign in a ruptured aneurysm. Pupillary dilatation may occur shortly before, at the same time, or shortly after oculomotor paresis occurs. Pupil involvement mandates immediate efforts to rule out an aneurysm by magnetic resonance imaging (MRI) or magnetic resonance angiography. In an emergency, a computed tomography (CT) scan can be performed immediately to rule out subarachnoid hemorrhage. Complete pupil sparing, which may accompany extraocular muscle paresis with an IC–PC aneurysm, has been reported rarely.[14,15]

Differential Diagnosis

The appropriate ophthalmic management of possible aneurysms is to make the right diagnosis. Any patient with a possible third nerve palsy should be observed carefully for pupillary dysfunction. Complete third nerve paresis and a normal pupil are extremely unlikely in a patient with an aneurysm.[16]

However, Miller[3] states that any patient with an incomplete extraoculomotor palsy and a normal pupil should undergo neuroimaging. When aneurysms are greater than 4mm in diameter, they can be seen on dynamic CT scans and by MRI,[17] as well as by magnetic resonance angiography. The author feels, however, that an older hypertensive or diabetic patient, without head pain, need be observed only, because most likely there is a microvascular etiology for the third nerve palsy. A single tear in the intracavernous portion of the internal carotid artery usually is diagnosed from a history of severe head trauma. Symptoms and signs may occur directly after injury or several days to weeks later. Although relatively rare, direct fistulas may develop spontaneously. Such patients may suffer from diffuse arterial disease manifested by aortic, femoral, and popliteal aneurysms,[18] as well as other signs of large-vessel disease, such as systemic hypertension, arteriosclerosis,[19] or an underlying connective tissue disorder.

Treatment, Course, and Outcomes

Recovery of extraocular muscle function occurs in most patients with IC–PC aneurysms, either spontaneously or after surgical treatment, whether or not the aneurysm has ruptured. Recovery is most likely in incomplete paresis, when no rupture has occurred and when successful clipping is performed within 1–2 weeks of onset.[20] Incomplete recovery after several months leaves secondary oculomotor nerve synkinesis or aberrant regeneration of the oculomotor nerve (see Fig. 209-1).

CAROTID–CAVERNOUS SINUS FISTULAS AND DURAL SHUNTS

Epidemiology and Pathogenesis

Abnormal communications between the cavernous sinus and dural veins and the carotid arterial system can be classified according to cause (traumatic versus spontaneous), velocity of blood flow (high versus low flow), and anatomy (direct versus dural; internal carotid versus external carotid, versus both). C–C fistulas, characterized by direct flow into the cavernous sinus from the intracavernous carotid artery, are of the high-flow type; these usually are traumatic and most often diagnosed in young men. Nontraumatic, low-flow dural fistulas may develop spontaneously or with atherosclerosis, hypertension, collagen vascular disease, and during or after childbirth; these more often are seen in the elderly, especially women. After childbirth, however, low-flow dural shunts are seen most in post-menopausal women. Spontaneous shunts occur between the cavernous sinus and one or more meningeal branches of the internal carotid artery (usually the meningohypophyseal trunk), the external carotid artery, or both. These shunts have a low amount of arterial flow and almost always produce signs and symptoms spontaneously.

Dural shunts between the arterial and venous systems have lower flow, yet they may produce symptoms in younger patients spontaneously or in older patients due to hypertension, diabetes, atherosclerosis, or other vascular disorders. Anatomically, these shunts arise between the meningeal arterial branches and the dural veins. The meningohypophyseal trunk and the artery of the inferior cavernous sinus provide the arterial supply to most dural shunts.[21]

Such shunts may be due to an expansion of congenital arteriovenous malformation[22] or due to spontaneous rupture of one of the thin-walled dural arteries that traverse the sinus.[23]

Ocular Manifestations

Ocular signs of C–C fistulas are related to venous congestion and reduced arterial blood flow to the orbit. Diminished arterial flow to cranial nerves within the cavernous sinus may cause diplopia. Stasis of venous and arterial circulation within the eye and orbit may cause ocular ischemia, and increased episcleral venous pressure may cause glaucoma. These abnormalities usually are unilateral, but they can be bilateral or even contralateral to the fistula.[24,25]

Exophthalmus is a common sign that occurs in almost all patients who have C–C fistulas; rapid-flow fistulas may cause exophthalmus within hours or several days. The orbit can become "frozen," with no ocular motor function. Usually, this is accompanied by conjunctival chemosis and hemorrhage. Vision may be reduced markedly because of optic nerve ischemia.[26]

"Pulsating exophthalmus" is uncommon in C–C fistula. Usually, the orbit is too rigid from hemorrhage and edema for "pulsation."

Chemosis of the conjunctiva and arterialization of the episcleral vessels occurs in most patients. Arterialization of episcleral veins is the hallmark of all C–C fistulas or dural shunts (Fig. 209-3).

Bruits associated with fistulas and dural shunts can be appreciated both subjectively and objectively. A bruit can be heard best when the examiner uses a bell stethoscope over the closed eye, over the superior orbital vein, or over the temple. A bruit is not pathognomonic of C–C fistula. It also can be heard in normal infants, in young children, and in patients with severe anemia.

In cases of C–C fistula, the abducens nerve is affected most often, because it lies in the cavernous sinus, itself. Because the third and fourth cranial nerves are encased in the superior internal dural wall of the sinus, they may be protected from changes caused by the fistula.[27] Mechanical restriction from venous congestion and orbital edema also may contribute to limitation of eye movements.

Immediate or delayed visual loss occurs frequently in direct C–C fistulas,[27] due to optic nerve ischemia from apical orbital

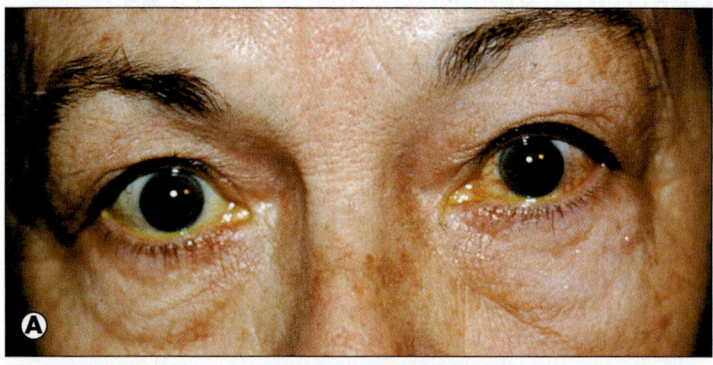

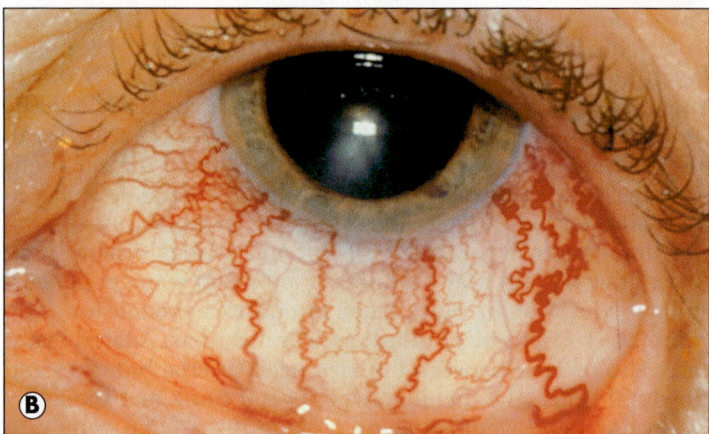

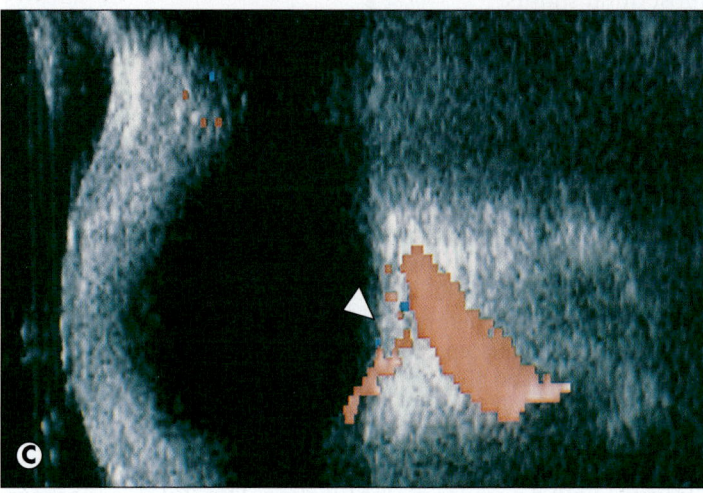

FIG. 209-3 ▮▮ Exophthalmus. **A,** A 60-year-old female patient, who has left chronic "red eye." **B,** Corkscrew (arterialized) vessels caused by low-flow (carotid–cavernous sinus) fistula. **C,** Color Doppler image that shows impedance and reversal of flow in superior orbital vein *(arrow)*. (**B,** Courtesy of Dr. Christopher Kelley, Wills Eye Hospital.)

compression. Longstanding fistulas can lead to loss of vision from distension of the cavernous sinus or of retrobulbar ischemia.[26]

Ophthalmoscopic findings due to venous stasis and impaired retinal blood flow include retinal venous engorgement and dot-and-blot retinal hemorrhages. Central retinal vein occlusion may be observed in high-velocity C–C fistulas with arterialized venous channels.

Despite high episcleral and intraocular pressures, the elevated pressure, in the author's experience, rarely results in damage to the optic nerve. In the unusual cases of central vein occlusion, neovascular glaucoma can occur.

Misdiagnosis is more common with dural shunts than with C–C fistulas. Dural shunts may be mistaken for chronic conjunctivitis, orbital cellulitis, orbital pseudotumor, or thyroid disease.[28] However, in dural shunts the palpebral conjunctiva is not involved, and the bulbar vessels are not affected as diffusely as in inflammatory processes. Signs of dural shunt usually are unilateral, but they can be bilateral or even contralateral to the shunt.[25]

Exophthalmus generally occurs to a varying degree (see Figs. 209-3, A and B), and ocular motor (usually abducens) palsies

may be seen. A subjective bruit (heard by the patient) almost always can be obtained from the history; however, an objective bruit heard over the orbit or temple by auscultation is relatively uncommon.[3] Wide pulsation of Schiötz or applanation intraocular pressure amplitude is an important clue to the diagnosis.

Differential Diagnosis

A direct C–C fistula should be suspected in any patient who suddenly develops a red eye with chemosis and exophthalmus, especially after head trauma. Investigation by MRI or standard angiography reveals a ruptured intracavernous aneurysm. Orbital ultrasonography, CT, and MRI often show a "hockey stick" sign of an engorged superior ophthalmic vein, which also may be demonstrated by computer Doppler imaging. The ultimate test, however, is selective arteriography of both internal and external carotid arteries.

Treatment, Course, and Outcomes

As with a C–C fistula, the diagnosis of a dural shunt can be made using CT scans, MRI, and computer Doppler imaging, because each reveals superior ophthalmic vein enlargement (see Fig. 209-3, C). However, selective intra-arterial angiography may be necessary to define the dural shunt. Carotid color Doppler imaging may show reversal of flow in the ophthalmic artery, which may help to establish the diagnosis (see Fig. 209-3, C).[29]

Many patients with dural shunts improve spontaneously or after angiography. Thus, proper diagnosis, reassurance, and conservative follow-up usually suffice.[28,30] Emolization or coil placement by interventional radiology (as in aneurysms) may be necessary in patients who have unacceptable or progressive signs or symptoms such as vision loss, diplopia, pain, or intolerable bruit. Although significant risk must be considered, the present status of interventional radiology is such that these risks are minimal. Only in the rare case is embolization necessary, as for a patient who has unacceptable symptoms and signs of visual loss (e.g., central vein occlusion), diplopia, severe exophthalmus, or intolerable bruit.[31] Although significant risks of neurological or visual sequelae from treatment must be considered, treatment of the dural fistula should precede surgery in cases of high intraocular pressure.

The prognosis of direct C–C fistula varies, but severe visual loss is often immediate and permanent, especially when a "frozen orbit" is encountered. Some patients may not be aware of the visual loss because of an overriding concern for the chemosis proptosis and lid swelling. In many cases, conservative management is propitious. However, closing the fistula with an angiocatheter balloon may be effective.

Compared with the dural shunt syndrome, the prognosis for C–C fistula is much more serious, because direct fistulas do not resolve spontaneously and are less amenable to occlusive techniques. The optimal treatment of C–C fistula is closure of the fistula along with preservation of carotid artery patency. Older procedures that required occlusion of the carotid artery to trap the fistula resulted in orbital hypoxia, which often made matters worse.

Detachable, flow-guided balloons are used to close these fistulas. Insertion of one or more balloons into the cavernous sinus can occlude the fistula successfully along with preservation of carotid flow. Complications may occur, such as worsening of orbital congestion and ocular motor nerve paresis. Fortunately, these complications are usually transient.[3] Successful occlusion usually results in gradual resolution of orbital signs within days, weeks, or sometimes months. Visual loss is often permanent.[24]

ARTERIOVENOUS MALFORMATIONS

AVMs are the most common form of intracranial vascular hamartoma. The occasional relationship between cerebral (mesencephalic) and retinal AVMs was recognized first by Wyburn-Mason in 1943.[32] Most intracranial AVMs involve only pial vessels, but

TABLE 209-1

TERMINOLOGY OF TRANSIENT VISUAL LOSS

Type	Duration	Characteristics
TRANSIENT MONOCULAR VISUAL LOSS		
Visual obscuration	Seconds to minutes	Optic disk swelling and anomalies
Amaurosis fugax	Seconds to minutes	Often altitudinal; carotid, cardiac source (embolic) or vasospastic
Prolonged transient visual loss	15–60 minutes	Hypertension; hematopoietic and other systemic (vascular) problems; "retinal" migraine
TRANSIENT BINOCULAR VISUAL LOSS		
Homonymous attacks	10–30 minutes	No other symptoms
Isolated visual migraine (Hedges)		
Acephalic migraine (O'Conner)	All similar episodic attacks (see text)	
Migraine accompaniments (Fisher)		

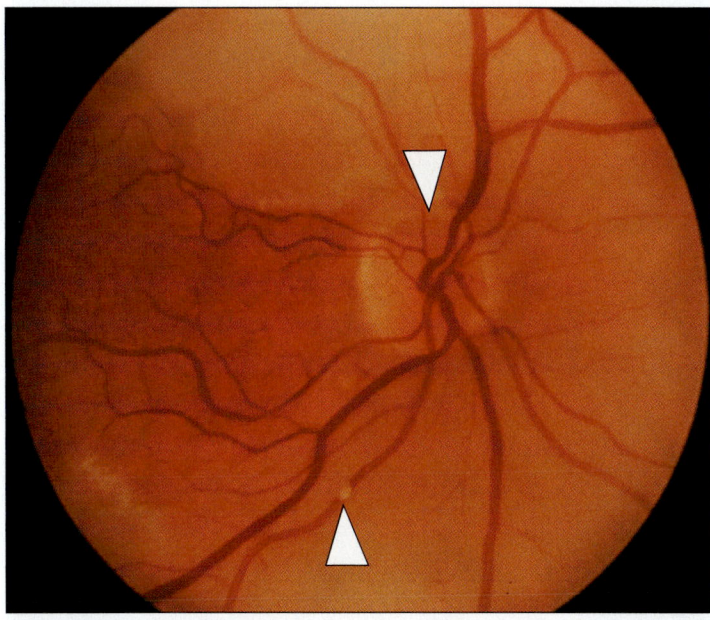

FIG. 209-4 ▊ Cholesterol emboli impacted in superior and inferior retinal arterioles with branch occlusion (*arrows*).

some involve both pial and dural vessels. Most AVMs are of congenital origin, but those that involve the meningeal arteries or vertebral arteries that drain into the dural sinuses may be acquired.[21]

AVMs that are only a few millimeters in size cannot be identified by neuroimaging and are referred to as *cryptic* or *occult*. Conversely, AVMs may be so large as to occupy an entire cerebral hemisphere. Although AVMs usually are congenital, they may become symptomatic at any age. However, 70% of AVMs produce symptoms during the second and third decades of life, and most are reviewed supratentorial.

Most cerebral AVMs produce signs of intracerebral or subarachnoid hemorrhage, which include seizures or isolated neurological symptoms and signs. Headache is a frequent symptom and may mimic migraine, although the headaches always are on the same side, in contrast to typical migraines.

Improvements in microguidewire and microcatheter technology have made it possible to treat previously unreachable and untreatable AVMs. The specific endovascular techniques vary according to the anatomy of the lesion,[33] the same as intracranial aneurysms and C–C fistulae and dural shunts.

TRANSIENT VISUAL LOSS

Epidemiology and Pathogenesis

TVL is a common symptom that may be benign or a harbinger of serious disease. Because clinical findings often are absent in patients with TVL, it is imperative to take a meticulous history.

Ocular Manifestations

The terminology of TVL (Table 209-1) is important, because it designates not only the anatomical location of the problem, but also its pathogenesis. Specific types of transient, monocular visual loss include transient visual obscurations (which are very brief [1–5 seconds] episodes of visual loss typically seen in patients with papilledema due to increased intracranial pressure), amaurosis fugax (1–5 minutes, caused by embolic or hemodynamic retinal arterial insufficiency), and prolonged monocular TVL (which occurs in patients with hypertension, blood dyscrasias, and "retinal migraine"). Binocular TVL may be seen with classic migraine, with or in the absence of headache, and other rare binocular or homonymous disturbances due to occipital ischemia or seizures.

Physical clues which help in the diagnosis of patients with TVL include abnormalities of vision, pupillary abnormalities, color vision loss, Amsler chart defects, and abnormalities of the optic nerve or retina. The most important ocular finding in monocular TVL is an impacted embolus in the arteries within the optic nerve or in the retina. The appearance of different types of emboli can provide clues to the source. Localized, hard, white material suggests calcium, which may come from a damaged aortic or mitral valve. Thromboplatelet emboli usually conform to a segment of a retinal branch arteriole and may have a white or gray appearance. Hollenhorst or cholesterol plaques are yellow or golden and tend to gleam (Fig. 209-4). Both thromboplatelet emboli and cholesterol emboli can be missed easily, especially if they are small. Gentle pressure on the eye often makes the embolic material "light up," which allows better visualization of an embolus (Fig. 209-5).[34]

Retinal emboli are the major cause of amaurosis fugax; the carotid artery is the likely source, although such emboli also can come from the aorta or heart. Auscultation of a bruit in the neck at the angle of the jaw further indicates the need for carotid magnetic resonance arteriography or, at least, carotid Doppler imaging.

An often-neglected anterior sign in any of the ocular ischemic syndromes is sludging of the conjunctival microcirculation. Slit-lamp magnification with red-free light shows micropools and a varying degree of sludging in the conjunctival blood vessels when a vascular impedance or hyperviscosity is present. In patients with ocular ischemia from severe carotid artery stenosis or occlusion, TVL may occur when the eye on the affected side is exposed to bright light.

Diagnosis

The age of the patient with TVL is very important—older, arteriopathic patients have different causes than do younger individuals. The character of the episode must be ascertained in detail.

NATURE OF THE EPISODES. The following need to be established:

- Where, when, and how did the episode occur?
- Did it appear and disappear suddenly or gradually?
- Did field loss occur and, if so, what type?

The typical curtain effect of altitudinal, monocular visual field loss is most significant, because this implies carotid occlusive disease or a cardiac source.

TYPE OF VISUAL LOSS. Monocularity is not always easy to determine. Although most patients with monocular TVL often are clear about monocularity, patients with binocular TVL or isolated visual migraine commonly state that the right or left eye was involved when, in reality, loss of vision only in the larger temporal homonymous visual field occurred.

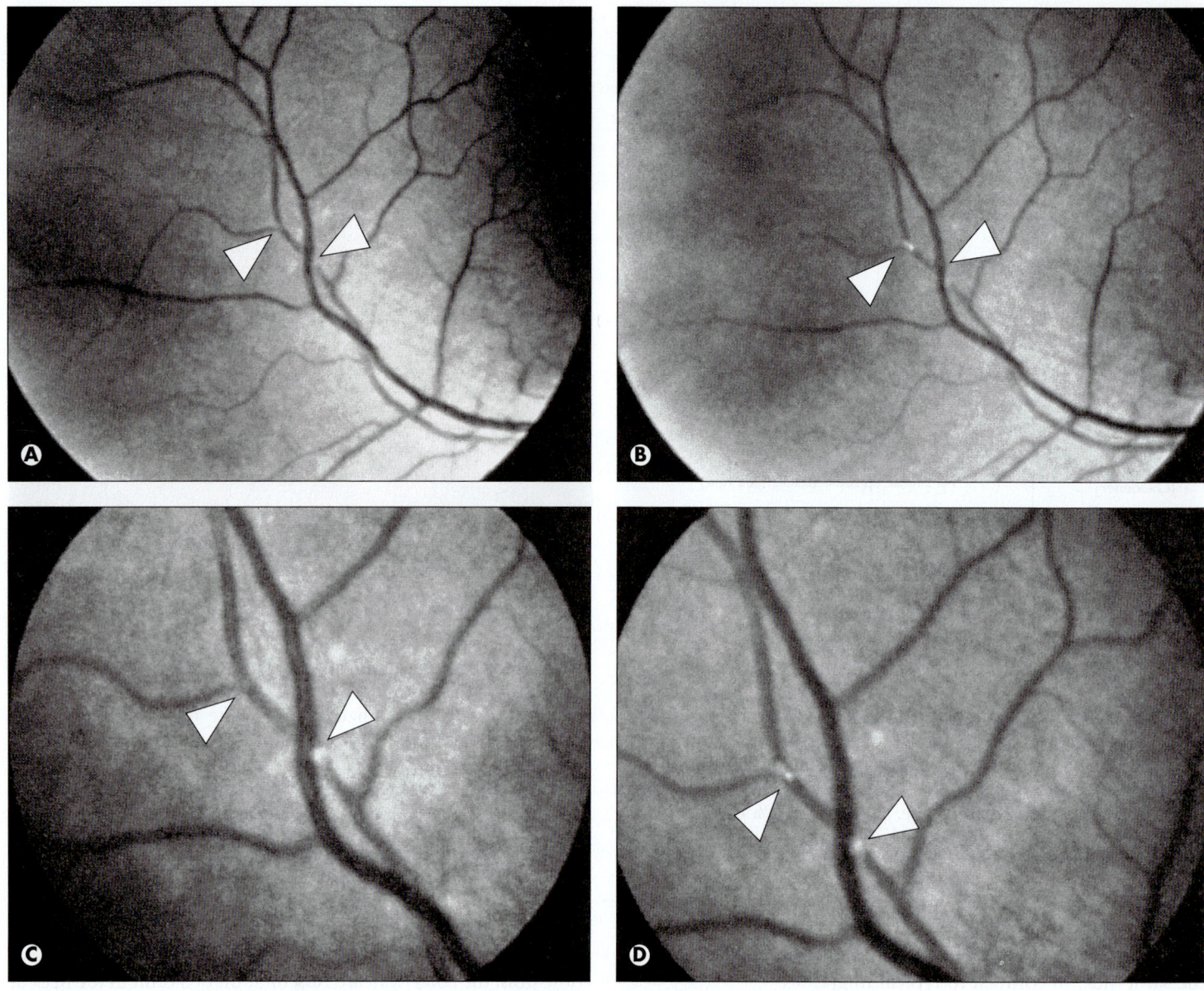

FIG. 209-5 ■ Combined thromboplatelet retinal emboli digital pressure maneuver *(arrows)*. **A,** Before pressure. **B–D,** During digital pressure on the eye to elicit previously only suspected embolus.

LENGTH OF EPISODES. The duration of transient monocular loss of vision due to carotid artery disease typically lasts 1–5 minutes. Often, the patient initially does not calculate the duration accurately, but with recurrent attacks both monocularity and duration are better appreciated.

FREQUENCY OF EPISODES. The frequency of attacks also provides a clue by which to differentiate monocular from binocular TVL. An isolated monocular attack may be sufficient to warrant investigation, at least with carotid Doppler studies. Recurrent attacks over a short interval are a strong indication for a full workup. Binocular episodes almost invariably are widely separated, often four to five in a lifetime, and rarely more often than once to twice per year.[35]

ASSOCIATED SYMPTOMS. Accompanying symptoms usually are absent in TVL. It is the isolation that makes TVL episodes unique. It is rare for a patient with an isolated visual migraine to proffer any other neurological symptoms. Contralateral numbness or weakness that occurs with transient monocular loss of vision implies severe carotid stenosis. Cerebral transient ischemic attacks imply either emboli to the brain or a hemodynamic cause, such as hypertension. Transient binocular blindness due to posterior circulation ischemia from atherosclerosis often occurs with other symptoms of vertebrobasilar insufficiency, such as dizziness, lightheadedness, or syncope.

UNDERLYING RISK FACTORS. Contributory causes can be determined from a thorough history and appropriate investiga-

tion. Hypertension, diabetes, or hematopoietic disorders in all age groups are important. In young people, contraceptive pill use and congenital or acquired heart disease must be excluded. In older patients, any history of myocardial, femoral, or aortic disease is an important indication of a diffuse arteriopathic state.

Young patients with TVL should be screened carefully for hyperviscosity or hypercoagulable disorders. Elevated antiphospholipid-cardiolipin antibody levels in a young woman with a strong history of migraine may be important. Cardiac workup may identify mitral and aortic valvular disease, mural thrombi, and arrhythmia, especially intermittent atrial fibrillation.

Treatment, Course, and Outcomes

The goal in the management of patients with TVL is to prevent further episodes that could lead to permanent visual loss or cerebral stroke. However, a single attack of monocular TVL does not necessitate invasive studies. Noninvasive carotid and orbital color Doppler imaging, when properly performed, may be sensitive enough to provide the required information; thus, many patients who have TVL may not require more invasive studies. Older patients with risk factors for large-vessel disease probably should be assessed using magnetic resonance angiography. Any patient with a history of cardiac signs or symptoms should be assessed using an echocardiogram.

In summary, symptomatic patients with or without retinal emboli or a bruit should be assessed using carotid and orbital color Doppler imaging or magnetic resonance angiography. Invasive angiography may not be necessary.

Transient Bilateral Loss of Vision: Isolated Visual Migraine

Transient binocular loss of vision is one of the most common complaints addressed in ophthalmic practice. It has been called acephalgic migraine and migraine accompaniments.[36] The term isolated visual migraine, however, identifies clearly an isolated transient binocular attack, similar to that described as the visual aura or prodrome of migraine.

Symptoms may last from 15 seconds to 3 hours; however, the classic description of kaleidoscopic, heat-wave, or scintillating bright lights that last 10-20 minutes makes the diagnosis, which usually is a great relief to the patient.

Miller[3] feels that a diagnosis of migraine should not be made unless embolic and thrombotic cerebrovascular disease or seizures have been excluded. Although typical migraine can occur concomitantly with other problems, including AVM, tumor, and arteritis, the migraine is very common and the others are rare. It would be nonproductive if all such patients were studied, as proved by Fisher's study,[37] and the costs would be prohibitive. One must be certain to make proper diagnosis, however, before exclusion of further studies, because all patients who have monocular TVL do need a workup. Fisher[37] concludes, as does the author, that "migraine accompaniment" justifiably can be regarded as benign.

One group isolated visual, ocular (acephalgic), retinal, and ophthalmoplegic migraine within the category of complicated migraine.[38] The author feels that the term *complicated migraine* should be reserved for those who develop a prolonged neurological deficit, which lasts for hours or days after a migrainous episode. Indeed, isolated visual migraine might be considered the most benign form of migraine.[36]

Visual field testing sometimes should be performed. It is still the best way to be sure that stroke, AVM, or tumor is not the problem.

Monocular loss almost always needs investigation. Management of binocular episodes usually is conservative. The typical 10–20 minute attack of transient bilateral homonymous loss of vision with a kaleidoscopic or heat-wave visual disturbance is so characteristic of isolated visual migraine that a diagnosis can be made with confidence, the patient reassured, and no further investigation made. These patients primarily need reassurance and do not need further investigation unless extenuating circumstances are present. The author recommends aspirin to such patients.

PEDIATRIC, OPHTHALMOPLEGIC, AND BASILOVERTEBRAL MIGRAINE. These three entities are grouped together, because they occur predominantly in children or young adults.

Pediatric migraine commonly is seen but often is overlooked or misdiagnosed by the ophthalmologist, because the child often does not complain of typical migraine, but instead presents a "fragmented" clinical syndrome characterized by:
- Periodicity of episodes
- Mild headache
- Atypical visual disturbance with migraine characteristics
- Anorexia
- Photophobia
- Lassitude
- The most important, a family history of migraine

Prensky and Sommer[39] emphasize that these children do not need medication. As in migraine or isolated visual migraine, a proper diagnosis precludes unnecessary tests.

STROKES

Epidemiology and Pathogenesis

TRANSIENT ISCHEMIC ATTACKS AND STROKE. The most reliable indicator of impending stroke is a transient ischemic attack (TIA). Vascular sites of disease that produce TIAs and stroke are:

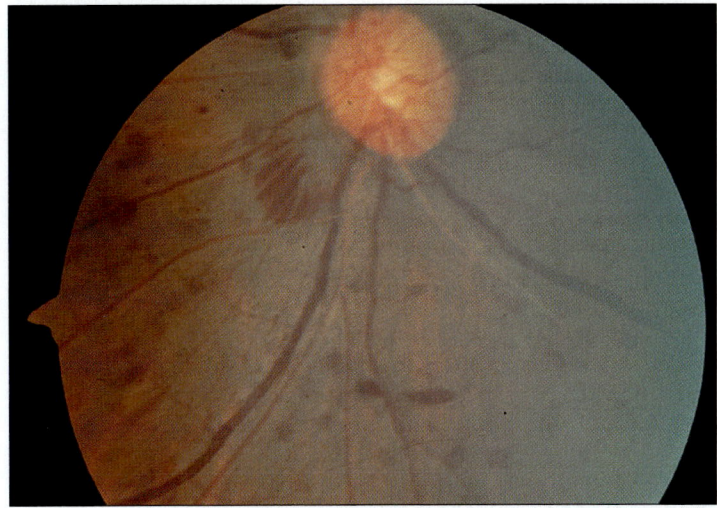

FIG. 209-6 ■ **Ocular ischemic syndrome.** Typical diffuse dot and blot hemorrhages and venous dilatation in inferior fundus.

- Carotid–ophthalmic artery
- Middle cerebral artery (MCA)
- Posterior cerebral (terminal basilar) artery
- Basilar artery

CAROTID–OPHTHALMIC ISCHEMIC ATTACKS AND STROKE. Carotid–ophthalmic artery TIAs most commonly manifest as amaurosis fugax caused by hypoperfusion of the retina. The patient is at risk of permanent visual loss, usually from occlusion of the central retinal artery. This constitutes an ocular "stroke," and requires investigation of carotid, cardiac, and hemodynamic diseases (see Chapter 114).

Severe chronic common or bilateral internal carotid artery diseases may lead to hypoperfusion of the optic nerve and retina, and also cause the ocular ischemic syndrome (see Chapter 118) (Fig. 209-6).[40,41] Impacted cholesterol or fibrin platelet emboli in the retina are an indication of carotid artery atheroma as the source; they are seen in 60–70% of patients with branch retinal artery occlusion.[42] Nonarteritic ischemic optic neuropathy, both anterior and posterior, rarely may be the initial manifestation of internal carotid artery occlusion.

Ocular Manifestations

Monocular blindness with contralateral hemispheric symptoms and signs (e.g., hemiparesis) is a well-recognized, although rare, entity in patients with carotid artery disease.[43] Blindness is caused by retinal ischemia. However, these patients may have the simultaneous occurrence of cerebral infarction and ipsilateral ischemic optic neuropathy.[44]

The ocular ischemic syndrome causes insidious, slowly progressive loss of vision, in contrast to the acute loss due to retinal or optic nerve infarction. The affected eye is often injected and vision is poorer than expected. Neovascular glaucoma and vitreous hemorrhage often follow. Atherosclerotic occlusion or severe stenosis of the common, external, and internal carotid arteries is found in most patients who have a risk of stroke due to poor cerebral perfusion[45,46] (see Chapter 118).

The second major ocular sign of carotid occlusive disease is partial or complete contralateral homonymous hemianopia,[3] often the result of hypoperfusion in the MCA, although posterior cerebral occlusion is by far the most common cause of homonymous hemianopia. Cerebral TIAs tend to be longer in duration than ocular TIAs. Ischemic reversible neurological deficit occurs when symptoms such as numbness or weakness last days and then disappear. When the defect persists, the term *stroke* should be used. As the term *stroke* can be very upsetting to the patient, it should be emphasized that a TIA is not a completed stroke.

Ischemia of the cortical and deep cerebral branches of the left MCA produces isolated motor aphasia and, often, contralateral hemiparesis and sensory loss. When TIAs of the MCA are on the right (nondominant) side, transient motor or sensory loss is produced on the left, without aphasia.

The frequency of TIAs of MCAs is much less than that of internal carotid arteries (64% vs. 20%); also, the internal carotid artery has more TIAs per patient (103 vs. 3). Binocular TVL is not usually considered a manifestation of MCA TIAs, even though homonymous hemianopia is common in a completed MCA stroke. Caplan et al.[47] found MCA TIAs to be more common in the young, in blacks, and in females.

The MCA stroke often fluctuates and progresses gradually. Anterior MCA branch occlusion produces hemiparesis in the leg and loss of sensation without hemianopia. Posterior MCA branch occlusion produces incomplete incongruous homonymous hemianopia, without macular sparing. Optokinetic responses may be reduced when stripes or checks are moved in the direction of the affected parietal lobe. Left MCA stroke produces aphasia, in contrast to right-sided lesions that produce contralateral hemispatial neglect and supranuclear horizontal gaze paresis toward the side of the lesion.

Homonymous hemianopia is the major neuro-ophthalmic sign of MCA stroke; it may be the only sign.[3] It is the result of damage to the optic radiation. The prognosis in MCA stroke is poor and, until recently, no known treatment existed.[47] Stroke centers now have a urokinase anticoagulation protocol—if treatment can be instituted within a few hours, the prognosis is much better.

Transient visual symptoms due to posterior cerebral artery (PCA) hypoperfusion are encountered less commonly and are less dramatic to the patient than amaurosis fugax of carotid origin. Isolated visual migraine must be differentiated from that of an impending stroke. Fisher states that visual migraine that occurs as a spectral march (buildup) or progression of the visual phenomenon often differentiates isolated visual migraine from occipital TIA and stroke. Clinically, visual migraine is very common, in contrast to occipital TIA, although each can mimic the aura of classic migraine. True vascular TIAs that involve the occipital lobes usually are sudden in onset, with a complete or incomplete homonymous hemianopia. They may be accompanied by basilar vertebral symptoms, such as unsteadiness, dysarthria, facial numbness, or weakness.

Isolated homonymous hemianopias usually are caused by vascular occlusion of the PCA and, therefore, are the hallmarks of occipital stroke. Infarction of the PCA is the result of embolism; rarely is it caused by atherosclerosis. Usually, PCA strokes occur without warning.[48]

Calcarine cortex infarction results in complete or incomplete hemianopia and usually spares the macular field. Invariably it is congruous. A complete homonymous hemianopia spares the macula as a rule and usually visual acuity is normal, although patients often complain of blurred vision. Many patients are unaware of the defect until it is pointed out.

Hemianopia with splitting of the macula often causes difficulty with reading. The Amsler chart is a valuable test by which to prove macular involvement; it also is a great asset when explaining the problem to the patient.

Clinically, homonymous hemianopia due to stroke in the temporoparietal and occipital areas can be differentiated by diminished optokinetic nystagmus. When stripes or other stimuli are moved in the direction of a lesion that involves the deep parietal lobe, the responses are dampened, whereas in isolated occipital (calcarine) lesions the responses are equal.

Improvement of the field defect within weeks or months is the rule,[49] particularly when the defect has sloping margins or it is not absolute to variously sized test objects. Neurological symptoms and signs of temporoparietal origin separate those cases caused by optic radiation damage from isolated homonymous hemianopia of occipital origin.

Hemianopia always should lead to inquiry as to other neurological deficits. Ophthalmologists should recognize alexia without agraphia, wherein the patient usually can name individual letters or numbers but cannot recognize simple words, although able to write words.[50] Right PCA occlusion can result in prosopagnosia, or the inability to recognize familiar faces. Cerebral dyschromatopsia (color blindness) also can occur in occipital stroke.

Rehabilitation is very difficult in permanent homonymous hemianopia. The author has found that in some selected patients a 20–25D Fresnel prism, base-out, on the temporal half of one spectacle lens on the side of the hemianopia can help.

Reduction in vertebral-basilar blood flow produces neurological and visual disturbances, from damage to the midbrain, pons, medulla, cerebellum, and occipital lobes. These disturbances may be transient, persistent, inconsequential, or catastrophic. Both oculomotor and visual symptoms play a role in diagnosis.

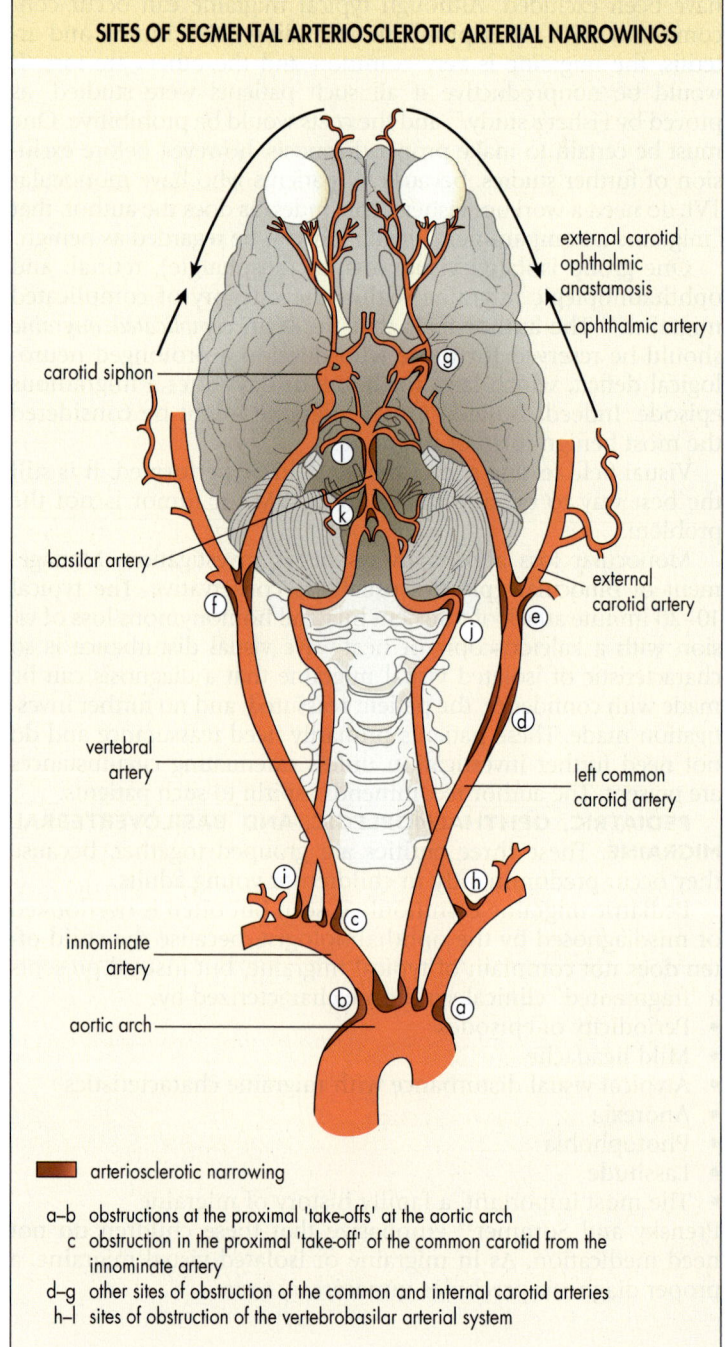

SITES OF SEGMENTAL ARTERIOSCLEROTIC ARTERIAL NARROWINGS

external carotid
ophthalmic
anastamosis

ophthalmic artery

carotid siphon

g

basilar artery

external
carotid artery

vertebral
artery

left common
carotid artery

innominate
artery

aortic arch

■ arteriosclerotic narrowing

a–b   obstructions at the proximal 'take-offs' at the aortic arch
c   obstruction in the proximal 'take-off' of the common carotid from the innominate artery
d–g   other sites of obstruction of the common and internal carotid arteries
h–l   sites of obstruction of the vertebrobasilar arterial system

FIG. 209-7 ■ Common areas of atherosclerotic lesions in the anterior carotid and posterior vertebrobasilar cerebral arterial systems. (Adapted from Hoyt WF. Some neuro-ophthalmological considerations in cerebral vascular insufficiency: carotid and vertebral insufficiency. Arch Ophthalmol. 1959;62:260–72.)

In the vertebrobasilar territory, TIAs are much more varied than they are in the carotid system. Vertigo is the most common neurological symptom, along with dysarthria, transient weakness, drop attacks, and occipital headaches.[3] The most common visual symptom is a characteristic, brief binocular "gray-out" of vision, which lasts a few seconds (rarely, up to 5 minutes). Transient diplopia is a rare symptom from ischemia of the ocular motor nerves or nuclei, or supranuclear and internuclear pathways. Typically, this symptom lasts 5–10 minutes. Episodic oscillopsia or "jumping vision" may occur during attacks of vertigo or dizziness.

The cause of vertebrobasilar TIA is speculative. Congenital vascular anomalies, hypertension, and hematological disorders are possible causes; however, atheromatous disease is the major problem in most patients (Fig. 209-7).[51]

Stroke usually occurs without previous TIAs in vertebrobasilar disease. Hypertension and atherosclerosis are the most common causes, in addition to emboli from the heart or distal large arteries. Combined brainstem symptoms and signs include vestibular nystagmus, miotic pupils, and sixth cranial nerve, conjugate gaze, internuclear, and facial palsies. Terminal PCA ischemia may occur alone or with a homonymous hemianopia. Lesions here can produce bilateral deficits, whereas carotid lesions produce unilateral deficits.

Brainstem signs most often arise from the lesions in the dorsal midbrain, primarily characterized by abnormal vertical gaze, upgaze or downgaze paresis with lid retraction, or as isolated upgaze paresis. Pupillary signs, internuclear ophthalmoplegia, and skew deviation also may be present.

See-saw and convergence retraction nystagmus accompany periaqueductal midbrain infarction. The more ventral medial midbrain syndrome of oculomotor nerve dysfunction and contralateral hemiplegia (Weber's syndrome) and Benedikt's syndrome with contralateral cerebellar signs also may result from infarction of midbrain. Strokes that involve these structures can be identified using MRI.

Pontine stroke produces primarily horizontal disorders of eye movement. Such strokes usually are associated with dizziness, facial nerve palsy, contralateral hemiparesis, hemisensory symptoms, and cerebellar signs. Isolated sixth cranial nerve palsy without neurological signs also has been shown, using MRI, to be caused by a fascicular lesion.[52] Unilateral internuclear ophthalmoplegia may be due to infarction of the medial–longitudinal fasciculus in the pons.

REFERENCES

1. Kassell NF, Torner JC, Adams HP. Antifibrinolytic therapy in the acute period following aneurysmal subarachnoid hemorrhage: preliminary observations from the cooperative aneurysmal study. J Neurosurg. 1984;61:225–30.
2. Weir B. Aneurysms affecting the nervous system. Baltimore: Williams & Wilkins; 1987.
3. Miller N. Walsh & Hoyt's clinical neuro-ophthalmology, ed 4, vol 4. Baltimore: Williams & Wilkins; 1991.
4. Rush JA, Younge BR. Paralysis of cranial nerves III, IV and VI: cause and prognosis in 1,000 cases. Arch Ophthalmol. 1981;99:76–9.
5. Vassiliou GA, Dielas E, Doris MS. Acquired cranial nerve lesions affecting the ocular system. In: Henkind P, Shimizu K, Blodi FC, et al., eds. International congress of ophthalmology, vol 2. Philadelphia: JB Lippincott; 1982:945–7.
6. Day AL. Aneurysms of the ophthalmic segment. A clinical and anatomical analysis. J Neurosurg. 1990;72:677–91.
7. Day AL. Visual loss with ophthalmic segment aneurysms. J Neurosurg. 1990;72:342–8.
8. Sadun AA, Smythe BA, Schaechter JD. Optic neuritis or ophthalmic artery aneurysm? Case presentation with histopathologic documentation utilizing a new staining method. J Clin Neuroophthalmol. 1984;4:265–73.
9. Cullen JF, Haining WM, Crombie AL. Cerebral aneurysms presenting with visual field defects. Br J Ophthalmol. 1966;50:251–6.
10. Kupersmith MJ, Krohn D. Cupping of the optic disc with compressive lesions of the anterior visual pathway. Ann Ophthalmol. 1984;16:948–53.
11. Trobe JD, Glaser JS, Post JD. Meningiomas and aneurysms of the cavernous sinus. Arch Ophthalmol. 1978;96:457–67.
12. Sibony PA, Lessell S, Gittinger JW Jr. Acquired oculomotor synkinesis. Surv Ophthalmol. 1984;28:82–390.
13. Little JR, Rosenfeld JV, Awad IA. Internal carotid artery occlusion for cavernous segment aneurysm. Neurosurgery. 1989;25:398–404.
14. Kassell NF, Torner JC. Aneurysmal rebleeding: a preliminary report from the cooperative aneurysm study. Neurosurgery. 1983;13:479–81.
15. Ebner R. Angiography for IIIrd nerve palsy in children. J Clin Neuroophthalmol. 1990;10:154–5.
16. Teuscher AV, Maienberg O. Ischemic oculomotor nerve palsy: clinical features and vascular risk factors in 23 patients. J Neurol. 1985;232:144–9.
17. Teasdale E, Macpherson P, Statham P. Non-invasive investigation for oculomotor palsy due to aneurysm. J Neurol Neurosurg Psychiatry. 1989;52:929–32.
18. Keltner JL, Satterfield D, Dublin A, Lee BCP. Dural and carotid–cavernous sinus fistulas. Ophthalmology. 1987;94:1585–600.
19. Rwiza HT, Uliet AM, Keyser A, et al. Bilateral spontaneous carotid–cavernous fistulas, associated with systemic hypertension and generalized arteriosclerosis. A case report. J Neurol Neurosurg Psychiatry. 1988;51:1003–5.
20. Feely M, Kapoor S. Third nerve palsy due to posterior communicating artery aneurysm. The importance of early surgery. J Neurol Neurosurg Psychiatry. 1987;50:1051–2.
21. Barrow DL, Spector RH, Braun IF, et al. Classification and treatment of spontaneous carotid–cavernous sinus fistulas. J Neurosurg. 1985;62:248–56.
22. Lie TA. Congenital anomalies of the carotid arteries, including the carotid–basilar and carotid–vertebral anastomoses. An angiographic study and review of literature. Amsterdam: Excerpta Medica; 1968.
23. Newton TH, Hoyt WF. Dural arteriovenous shunts in the region of the cavernous sinus. Neuroradiology. 1970;1:71–81.
24. Kupersmith MJ, Berenstein A, Choi IS, et al. Percutaneous transvascular treatment of giant carotid aneurysms. Neuro-ophthalmologic findings. Neurology. 1984;34:328–35.
25. Hedges TR Jr. Carotid cavernous fistula, re-evaluation of orbital signs. Ophthalmic Surg. 1973;4(2):75–84.
26. Hedges TR III, Debrun G, Sokol S. Reversible optic neuropathy due to carotid–cavernous fistula. J Clin Neuroophthalmol. 1985;5:37–40.
27. Kupersmith MJ, Berenstein A, Flamm E, Ranshoff J. Neuroophthalmologic abnormalities and intravascular therapy of traumatic carotid cavernous fistulas. Ophthalmology. 1986;93:906–12.
28. Grove AS Jr. The dural shunt syndrome: pathophysiology and clinical course. Ophthalmology. 1984;9:31–44.
29. Sergott RC, Grossman RI, Savino PJ, et al. The syndrome of paradoxical worsening of dural–cavernous sinus arteriovenous malformations. Ophthalmology. 1987;94:205–12.
30. Kupersmith MJ, Berenstein A, Choi IS, et al. Management of nontraumatic vascular shunts involving the cavernous sinus. Ophthalmology. 1988;95:121–30.
31. Debrun GM, Nauta HJ, Miller NR, et al. Combining the detachable balloon technique and surgery in imaging carotid cavernous fistulae. Surg Neurol. 1989;32:3–10.
32. Wyburn-Mason R. Arteriovenous aneurysm of the midbrain and retina, facial nevi and mental changes. Brain. 1943;66:163–203.
33. Borden NM, Khayata MH, Dean BL, et al. Endovascular treatment of orbital lesions. Treatment of high flow dural arteriovenous malformations. Barrow Neurol Inst Q. 1996;12:4–18.
34. Hedges TR Jr. Retinal atheromatous plaques, their recognition in elevating the intra-ocular pressure. Trans Am Ophthalmol Soc. 1976;74:172–7.
35. Hedges TR Jr, Lackman RD. Isolated ophthalmic migraine in the differential diagnosis of cerebro-ocular ischemia. Stroke. 1976;7:4–8.
36. Fisher CM. Late-life migraine accompaniments as a cause of unexplained transient ischemic attacks. Can J Neurol Sci. 1980;7:9–17.
37. Fisher CM. Unusual vascular events in the territory of the posterior cerebral artery. Can J Neurol Sci. 1986;13:1–17.
38. Hupp SL, David NJ, Glaser JS. Consecutive bilateral retinal artery occlusion. Neuro-ophthalmology. 1984;4:137–140.
39. Prensky AL, Sommer D. Diagnosis and treatment of migraine in children. Neurology. 1979;29:506–10.
40. Hedges TR Jr. Ophthalmoscopic findings in internal carotid occlusion. Bull Johns Hopkins Hosp. 1962;3:89–97.
41. Kearns TP, Hollenhorst RW. Venous stasis retinopathy of occlusive disease of the carotid artery. Mayo Clin Proc. 1963;38:304–12.
42. Savino PJ, Glaser JS, Cassady J. Retinal stroke. Is the patient at risk? Arch Ophthalmol. 1977;95:1185–9.
43. Fisher CM. Occlusion of the internal carotid artery. Arch Neurol Psychiatry. 1951;65:346–77.
44. Bogousslavsky J, Regli F, Zografos L, Uske A. Optico-cerebral syndrome. Simultaneous hemodynamic infarction of optic nerve and brain. Neurology. 1987;37:263–8.
45. Duker JS, Belmont JB. Ocular ischemic syndrome secondary to carotid artery dissection. Am J Ophthalmol. 1988;106:750–2.
46. Dhooge M, De Lacy JJ. The ocular ischemic syndrome. Bull Soc Belge Ophtalmol. 1989;231:1–13.
47. Caplan LR, Babikian V, Helgason C, et al. Occlusive disease of the middle cerebral artery. Neurology. 1985;35:975–82.
48. Pessin MS, Kwan ES, DeWitt LD, et al. Posterior cerebral artery stenosis. Ann Neurol. 1987;21:85–9.
49. Mauskop A, Wolnitz AH, Valderrama R. Central infarction and subdural hematoma. Advantage of nuclear magnetic resonance imaging in cerebral ischemia. J Clin Neuroophthalmol. 1984;4:251–3.
50. Geschwind K. Disconnexion syndromes in animals and man. Brain. 1965;88:237–94,585–644.
51. Hoyt WF. Some neuro-ophthalmological considerations in cerebral vascular insufficiency: carotid and vertebral insufficiency. Arch Ophthalmol. 1959;62:260–72.
52. Bronstein AM, Rudge P, Gresty MA, et al. Abnormalities of horizontal gaze. Clinical, oculographic and magnetic resonance imaging findings. II. Gate palsy and internuclear ophthalmoplegia. J Neurol Neurosurg Psychiatry. 1990;53:200–7.

GLAUCOMA

Mark Sherwood

SECTION I EPIDEMIOLOGY AND MECHANISMS OF GLAUCOMA

CHAPTER

210 Epidemiology of Glaucoma

SCOTT FRASER • RICHARD WORMALD

INTRODUCTION

Epidemiology can be defined as "the study of the distribution and determinants of health-related states or events in specified populations, and the application of this study to control of health problems."[1] In this chapter the distribution of glaucoma in the population (i.e., the prevalence and incidence) and its determinants (i.e., its risk factors) are discussed.

Most of the major epidemiological studies of glaucoma have been carried out in North America and Europe, areas in which primary open-angle glaucoma (POAG) is the most common form. Thus, most of the available data—especially population-based data—concern POAG; when data presented herein are not for POAG, this is stated explicitly.

PREVALENCE

The prevalence of a disease is "The number of instances of a given disease or other condition in a given population at a designated time."[1] Citing an overall prevalence figure for glaucoma is almost meaningless because race, age, and possibly gender have such a profound effect that prevalence rates are best stated in relation to these variables.

Tables 210-1 and 210-2 summarize the results of the major population studies of glaucoma. Table 210-1 gives the results for Caucasian subjects, and Table 210-2 summarizes the studies that have involved African-American and African-Caribbean subjects.

The prevalence estimates vary in the studies, not only because of the different populations studied but also because of the dif-ferent methods used to sample the populations and different definitions of glaucoma. However, the figures are reasonably consistent, with a prevalence of POAG in Caucasians over 40 years of age of around 2% and in African-Americans and African-Caribbeans over 40 years of age of around four times this.

Age has a major effect on glaucoma prevalence—for those of older age a higher prevalence of glaucoma exists. The Baltimore Eye Survey[2] found a prevalence of 1.23% in African-Americans of age 40–49 years but of 11.26% in those over 80 years of age; in Caucasians these values were 0.92% and 2.16%, respectively. The Beaver Dam study[3] found a prevalence of 0.9% in Caucasians of age 43–54 years and of 4.7% in those over 75 years of age. Similarly, the Roscommon[4] study found a prevalence of 0.72% in the age band 50–59 years but of 3.05% in those over 80 years of age. The studies shown in Tables 210-1 and 210-2 that had an upper age limit found lower prevalence rates for glaucoma (e.g., Dalby[5]), which is consistent with the increasing prevalence with age.

The effect of gender on glaucoma prevalence is less certain. The Australian Blue Mountain Eye Study[6] found a slightly greater prevalence of POAG in women, the Barbados study[7] found an overall prevalence of POAG in men of 8.3% and in women of 5.7%, and the Rotterdam[8] study found a three times higher prevalence of POAG in men. However, other studies, which include the Baltimore,[2] Beaver Dam,[3] and Roscommon[4] studies, did not show a significant difference in prevalence between the sexes.

Few population studies have published figures for the prevalence of ocular hypertension. As Table 210-1 illustrates, the

---

TABLE 210-1

PREVALENCE OF PRIMARY OPEN-ANGLE GLAUCOMA AND OCULAR HYPERTENSION IN VARIOUS POPULATION STUDIES (CAUCASIANS)

Study	Roscommon[4]	Beaver Dam[3]	Rotterdam[8]	Dalby[5]	Blue Mountain[6]	Barbados Caucasians[7]	Baltimore Caucasians[2]
Age range studied (years)	Over 50	43–84	Over 55	55–69	Over 49	40–84	Over 40
Prevalence of primary open-angle glaucoma found (%)	1.9	2.1	1.1	0.9	2.4	0.8	1.3
Prevalence of ocular hypertension (%)	3.6				3.7		

TABLE 210-2

PREVALENCE OF PRIMARY OPEN-ANGLE GLAUCOMA IN VARIOUS POPULATION STUDIES (AFRICAN-AMERICANS AND AFRICAN-CARIBBEANS)

Study	St Lucia[9]	Baltimore African-Americans[2]	Barbados African-Caribbeans[7]	London African-Caribbeans[10]
Age range studied (years)	Over 30	Over 40	40–84	Over 35
Prevalence of primary open-angle glaucoma found (%)	8.8	4.2	7.1	3.9

TABLE 210-3

PREVALENCE (%) OF ANGLE-CLOSURE, PSEUDOEXFOLIATIVE, AND SECONDARY GLAUCOMA GIVEN IN PUBLISHED STUDIES

Study	Roscommon[4]	Beaver Dam[3]	Dalby[5]	Blue Mountain[6]	Baltimore Caucasians[2]	Baltimore African-Americans[2]
Angle-closure glaucoma, narrow angles	0.09	0.04		0.3	0.4	0.9
Pseudoexfoliative glaucoma	1.33		0.07			
Other secondary glaucomas	0.09		0.27	0.2		

Roscommon[4] and Blue Mountain[6] studies had similar results of 3.6% and 3.7%. What the majority of population studies do show is that the prevalence of glaucoma associated with high intraocular pressure (IOP) is relatively rare. The Beaver Dam[3] study found that 25% of the subjects with definite POAG had IOPs <21mmHg (<2.8kPa).

For the reasons mentioned in the introduction, prevalence figures for non-POAGs are harder to come by. The findings of the major studies are summarized in Table 210-3. Glaucoma associated with narrow drainage angles is uncommon—although to compare different studies is difficult because of variations in the diagnosis of angle closure. Table 210-3 indicates prevalences from 0.04% in the Beaver Dam[3] study to 0.9% in Baltimore African-Americans.[2] Quigley[11] has calculated the prevalence of angle-closure glaucoma from nine European studies to be about 0.2% for those over 40 years of age.

Angle-closure glaucoma is thought to be less common in those of African descent—Quigley[11] suggests that about half the European rate applies. However, Luntz[12] has found an equal prevalence in South African Caucasians and Africans. In Asian populations, angle-closure glaucoma is the type found most commonly. A Japanese study found a prevalence of angle-closure glaucoma of 0.31%,[13] and those of Chinese origin have higher rates of angle-closure glaucoma than any other group—three times more common than POAG.[11]

The true prevalence of pseudoexfoliative glaucoma is difficult to determine, as some studies did not classify it separately from POAG and for studies in which the subjects were not dilated, underdiagnosis is likely. It is commonly thought to be more prevalent in those of Scandinavian origin, but the Dalby[5] study from Sweden found a prevalence of only 0.07%, whereas the Roscommon[4] study (Republic of Ireland) had a 1.33% prevalence. High prevalences of pseudoexfoliative glaucoma have been noted in Africans from South Africa but not in African-Americans.[12]

Other secondary glaucomas are rarely studied as separate entities in population studies. The Roscommon[4] study found two cases out of 2186 subjects examined (one aphakic and one thrombotic); the Dalby[5] and Blue Mountain[6] studies found similar prevalences of 0.27% and 0.2%, respectively. Quigley[11] calculated a mean prevalence from eight studies (Europe, Africa, and Asia) of about 0.44%.

INCIDENCE

Incidence is defined as "The number of instances of illness commencing, or persons falling ill, during a given period in a specified population."[1] Difficulties in the diagnosis of early glaucoma and the need to follow a cohort for many years make true incidence figures difficult to obtain for glaucoma. In the Bedford survey an average annual incidence of 0.048% was found,[14] and Armaly *et al.*[15] studied 3936 patients over 7 years and found that 4 developed POAG, to give an annual incidence rate of about 0.025%.

The incidence of glaucoma rises with age. Results from statistical modeling indicate that for a general population of Caucasians, the incidence rises from 0.08 per 1000 per year for those in their early 40s to 1.46 per 1000 per year to those in their

---

BOX 210-1

Main Risk Factors for Glaucoma

DEMOGRAPHIC	SYSTEMIC
Age	Diabetes
Gender	Systemic hypertension
Race	
	GENETIC
OCULAR	Family history
Intraocular pressure	
Optic nerve head	**OTHER**
Myopia	Cigarette smoking
Hypermetropia	Alcohol intake
	Socioeconomic factors

80s.[16] It seems likely that these incidence figures are higher in African-American and African-Caribbean populations.

RISK FACTORS FOR DEVELOPING GLAUCOMA

A risk factor is defined as "An aspect of personal behavior or lifestyle, an environmental exposure, or an inborn or inherited characteristic, which on the basis of epidemiological evidence is known to be associated with health-related conditions important to prevent."[1] Large, population-based studies provide valuable insights into risk factors for the development of glaucoma, whereas hospital-based studies are subject to selection bias. Good examples of this selection bias occur with patients who have myopia and diabetes—conditions for which regular eye examinations are likely, as a result of which the opportunity for glaucoma to be diagnosed is increased. Thus, hospital-based studies tend to overestimate the proportion of glaucoma patients who also have myopia and diabetes and so implicate these diseases as risk factors for glaucoma.

Population-based studies are more useful than those that are hospital based, but this advantage is lost if the study subjects are not selected randomly. If, for example, the protocol of the study is to ask for volunteers, it is those who have greater concerns about glaucoma, for example, those who have a family history, who are more likely to present for examination. If the sample is not truly random, the influence on glaucoma of such factors as family history is overestimated. The main risk factors for glaucoma that have been examined in population studies are classified in Box 210-1.

Demographic Risk Factors

AGE. The prevalence and incidence figures shown indicate that increasing age is a major risk factor for glaucoma. In fact, this trend has been found in all population-based studies of glaucoma in which age has been examined.[16] As well as being consistent across various studies, the magnitude of increase is uniformly large with prevalence rates 4–10 times higher in the oldest age group compared with the baseline (usually subjects in their 40s).[2–4,7]

GENDER. The Baltimore,[2] Beaver Dam,[3] and Roscommon[4] studies did not find either men or women to be at a significantly greater risk of glaucoma. However, the Barbados[7] Eye Study did find that men have an age-adjusted risk of 1.4 compared with women, and the Rotterdam[8] study found a three times increased risk for men. Conversely, the Dalby[5] study indicated a higher risk for women.

Overall it seems unlikely that gender is a major risk factor for the development of glaucoma.

ETHNIC ORIGIN. For some time, it has been suspected that individuals of African, African-American, and African-Caribbean origin are at higher risk of POAG, but it is only relatively recently that this has been confirmed by large-scale population studies.

The Baltimore Eye Survey[2] found a fourfold excess prevalence in African-Americans compared with Caucasians. The Beaver Dam[3] study found an overall prevalence of 2.1% in an all-Caucasian population, which compares with a prevalence of 8.8% in the St. Lucia study[9] in which all the participants were African-Caribbean. The African-Caribbean Eye Survey[10] showed a relative risk for glaucoma of 3.7 in Haringey (London) African-Caribbeans compared with Roscommon[4] Caucasians.

The Barbados[7] study found a gradient in prevalence by racial group, with the highest risk in those who described themselves as black; a lower prevalence was found in those who classified themselves as of mixed race, and the lowest prevalence was for those who were white. Interestingly, the London African Caribbean study[10] showed a statistically significant association between IOP and skin color (but not between skin color and glaucoma).

Not only does a higher prevalence of POAG exist among black racial groups, but there is good evidence that the onset of the disease occurs at a younger age in these groups.[17] A study in Malawi found a large number of glaucoma subjects in the age range 20–30 years. Similarly, the average age of glaucoma patients in Jamaica was found to be 10 years less than the average in America. Wilson et al.[18] found that the average age at presentation for patients of African origin was 49.5 years while for Caucasians it was 59.8 years.

Ocular Risk Factors

INTRAOCULAR PRESSURE. Although little doubt exists that raised IOP is a major risk factor for glaucoma, it is not as fundamental as it was once thought to be. There is strong evidence that IOP is associated intimately with glaucoma:

- The Baltimore study results indicate that the prevalence of POAG rises with increasing IOP.[19]
- The visual field loss of patients whose IOP is lowered by whatever means is usually slowed.[20]
- If an individual has glaucoma, the eye that has the higher IOP tends to lose field more quickly—this occurs even if both IOPs are <21mmHg (2.8kPa).[21]
- For studies in which IOP is excluded from the definition of glaucoma (as it should always be), it is related strongly to the risk of glaucoma,[10] as illustrated in Figure 210-1 (taken from the prevalence of POAG in the Baltimore Eye Survey[19]).

It is important to note that the relative risk of glaucoma begins to rise (i.e., is greater than 1) from about 16mmHg (1.7kPa). The commonly used cutoff between "normal tension" glaucoma [≤21mmHg (≤2.8kPa)] and "high tension" glaucoma [>21mmHg (>2.8kPa)] is therefore questionable.

A similar point is illustrated in Figure 210-2, taken from Davanger et al.,[22] who plotted IOP level against the probability of having glaucoma as calculated from their own population survey. Figure 210-2 shows that although a very high IOP [35mmHg (4.7kPa) or more], if sustained, sooner or later results in glaucomatous damage, it is not inevitable that IOPs below this level always result in glaucomatous damage. For example, those who have an IOP of 27mmHg (3.6kPa) have a 50% chance of glaucoma development, whereas those who have an IOP of 23mmHg (3.1kPa) have only a 10% chance.

The use of the terms normal tension and low tension glaucoma is not very helpful. A more realistic concept is to consider

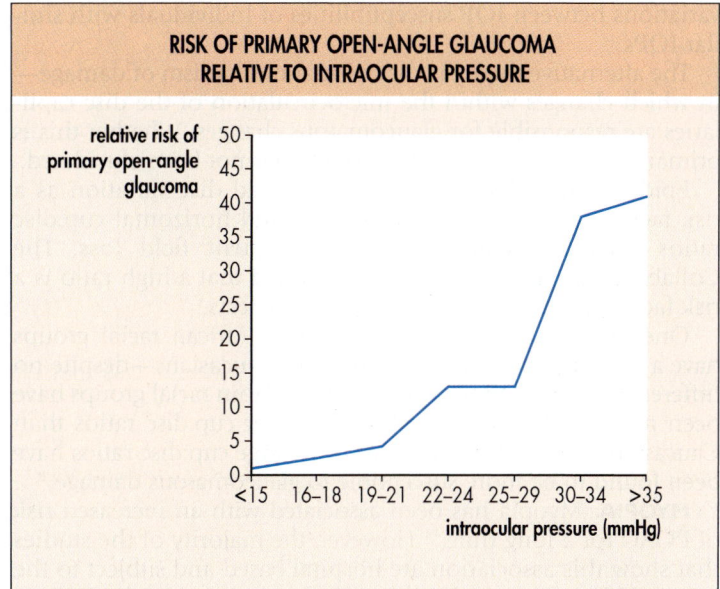

FIG. 210-1 ▌▌ The risk of primary open-angle glaucoma at various levels of intraocular pressure. (Adapted with permission from Sommer A, Tielsch JM, Katz J, et al. Relationship between intraocular pressure and primary open angle glaucoma among white and black Americans. Arch Ophthalmol. 1991;109:1090–5.)

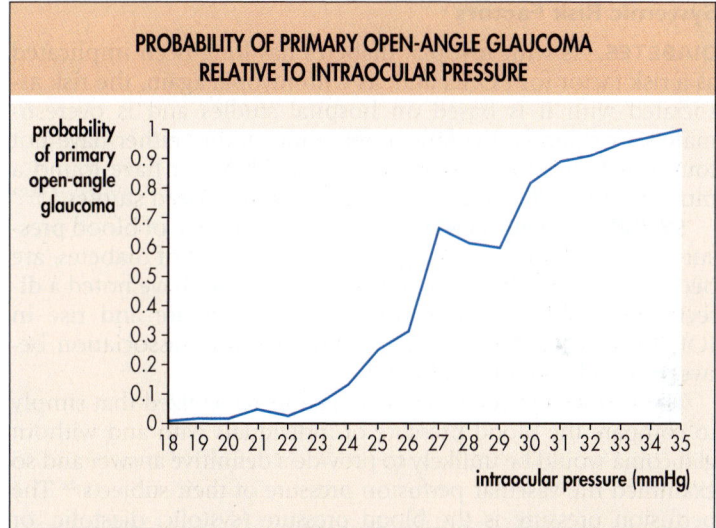

FIG. 210-2 ▌▌ The probability of primary open-angle glaucoma at various levels of intraocular pressure. (Adapted with permission from Davanger M, Ringvold A, Bilka S. The probability of having glaucoma at different IOP levels. Acta Ophthalmol. 1991;69:565–8.)

that an individual's optic nerve has a level of IOP that it can or cannot withstand. At a clinical level this is manifest by the presence or absence of visual field decline. If field loss occurs, the IOP of the patient needs to be reduced to a level that stops (or more realistically slows) this decline.

That IOP is a major risk factor for glaucoma rather than a diagnostic requisite means that some other factor or factors act with higher pressures in the eye to produce the characteristic glaucomatous changes.

THE OPTIC NERVE HEAD. As well as being an important marker of the presence and advancement of glaucoma, the structure of the optic nerve head may play a role in the pathogenesis of glaucoma. Two main theories exist for the mechanism of optic nerve damage in glaucoma.[21] The mechanical (IOP-related) theory suggests that the pressure head acts directly on the lamina cribrosa. The lamina cribrosa is not supported well superiorly and inferiorly at the disc, and it is here that the initial damage occurs to produce the characteristic arcuate defects. Variations in ganglion cell support at the disc may explain the variations between IOP susceptibilities of individuals with similar IOPs.

The alternative theory is the vascular mechanism of damage—in which changes within the microcirculation of the disc capillaries are responsible for glaucomatous changes. Whether this is primarily vascular or secondary to IOP has not been elucidated.

Epidemiological studies have implicated disc variation as a risk factor for glaucoma; both vertical and horizontal cup:disc ratios correlate positively with subsequent field loss. The Collaborative Glaucoma Study[13] indicated that a high ratio is a risk factor for the development of field defects.

One of the proposals to explain why African racial groups have a greater prevalence of POAG than Caucasians—despite no differences in the IOP patterns—is that African racial groups have been noted to have larger discs and larger cup:disc ratios than Caucasians. Larger discs and discs with large cup:disc ratios have been found to be more susceptible to glaucomatous damage.[21]

MYOPIA. Myopia has been associated with an increased risk of POAG for a long time.[14] However, the majority of the studies that show this association are hospital based and subject to the hospital bias mentioned previously. If an increased risk of POAG exists in myopes, it is likely to be overestimated.

HYPERMETROPIA. High degrees of hypermetropia are related strongly to angle-closure glaucoma—both the acute and chronic types.

Systemic Risk Factors

DIABETES. As with myopia, diabetes has long been implicated as a risk factor for POAG and, as with myopia again, the risk associated with it is based on hospital studies and is overestimated. Conversely, the large population studies either have not found diabetics to be at greater risk of POAG or have found a much smaller effect than that in the hospital-based studies.[7,10,23]

SYSTEMIC HYPERTENSION. Studies of the role of blood pressure in the pathogenesis of glaucoma, like those of diabetes, are bedeviled by hospital bias. A number of studies have noted a direct relationship between rise in blood pressure and rise in IOP,[24] but it has been harder to find a similar association between blood pressure and POAG.

The Baltimore Eye Survey investigators recognized that simply to compare the blood pressure of individuals with and without glaucoma would be unlikely to provide a definitive answer and so examined the vascular perfusion pressure of their subjects.[24] The perfusion pressure is the blood pressure (systolic, diastolic, or mean) minus the IOP; the subjects in the study showed a strong association between the prevalence of POAG and *low* diastolic perfusion pressure, as illustrated in Figure 210-3. The graph indicates that the subjects with diastolic perfusion pressures below 30mmHg (4.0kPa) have a six times higher age-adjusted risk of POAG than those with pressures of 50mmHg (6.7kPa) or greater.

The hypothesis is that optic nerve damage may occur in these subjects because of poor optic nerve perfusion. This theory is enhanced further by the results of 24-hour blood pressure monitoring, which show that patients with profound falls in their blood pressure overnight ("nocturnal dippers") have an increased risk of POAG.

A further refinement of the hypothesis also comes from the Baltimore Eye Survey, which showed that younger subjects (less than 60 years of age) with raised blood pressures have a lower risk of POAG than the age-matched normal population. Conversely, older subjects (over 70 years of age) have a higher risk than their aged-matched controls. A reason for this may be that hypertension actually improves optic nerve head flow initially, but when secondary vascular changes have occurred (after prolonged hypertension), resistance to blood flow increases.

The two findings of the Baltimore Eye Survey may be related in that the vascular changes of prolonged hypertension result in loss of blood vessel autoregulation, which reduces the ability of the nerve head vessels to respond to a reduction in diastolic perfusion.

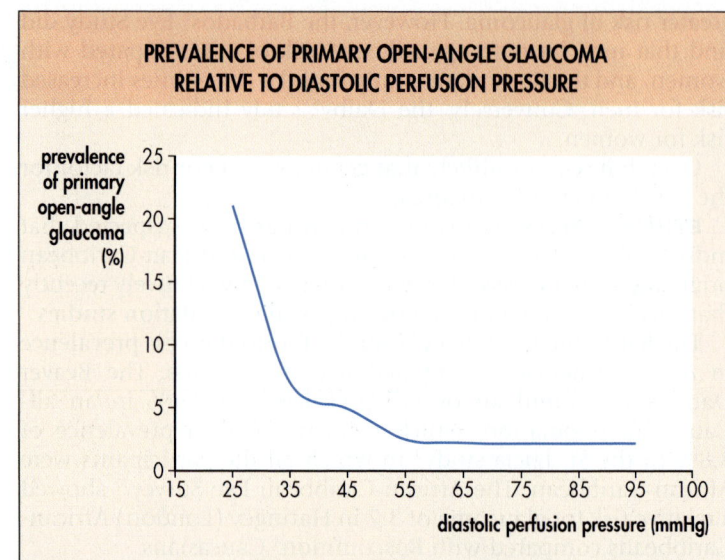

FIG. 210-3 ▓ The relationship between the prevalence of primary open-angle glaucoma and diastolic perfusion pressure of subjects from the Baltimore Eye Survey. (Adapted with permission from Tielsch JM, Katz J, Sommer A, *et al.* Hypertension, perfusion pressure and primary open-angle glaucoma. Arch Ophthalmol. 1995; 113:216–21.)

It is important to stress that this theory, although elegant, still requires far more evidence.

Genetic Risk Factors

Little doubt exists that a positive family history of glaucoma places an individual at increased risk of glaucoma. Estimates of POAG cases being familial vary in the range 13–47%, and a 5–20 times prevalence rate occurs in those who have a positive family history. Specific families have been found that indicate an autosomal dominant pedigree, whereas others appear to have a recessive gene.

However, studies of family history and glaucoma are prone to bias—which probably explains the widely differing prevalence rates in different studies. A patient who knows that a member of the family has glaucoma is more likely to present to the clinic and is more likely to attend for surveys. Also, family history data are provided by the patient and can be subject to recall bias.

The most accurate estimate of the association of family history and risk of developing glaucoma is from unbiased population studies that have a high response rate, such as the Baltimore Eye Survey.[25] This showed that family history is a significant risk factor for POAG but to a lesser extent than in most other published studies. The odds ratio of having POAG for those with siblings who had the disease was found to be 3.69; for those with parents who had the disease the ratio was 2.17 and for those with children who had the disease, 1.12.

Other Proposed Risk Factors

CIGARETTE SMOKING. Although much studied, smoking cigarettes usually has not been shown to be a risk factor for glaucoma. Katz and Sommer,[26] in a hospital-based, case-control study, found no association between smoking and glaucoma. Most convincingly, the Beaver Dam study, which is the largest of any of these studies, did not show a relationship between smoking and POAG.[27]

ALCOHOL INTAKE. A number of studies have shown a link between alcohol consumption and the risk of glaucoma. Katz and Sommer[26] found an association between glaucoma and alcohol use, but only in Caucasian patients. However, once again it seems likely that studies that are not population based are biased, for heavy drinkers have more contact with health services and, therefore, increased opportunity to have the glaucoma di-

TABLE 210-4

PROPORTION OF THOSE REGISTERED BLIND WHO ARE BLIND FROM GLAUCOMA

Study	Hiller and Kahn[29]	Sorsby[30]	Leibowitz et al.[31]	Ghafour et al.[32]	Aclimandos and Galloway[33]
Year published	1975	1972	1980	1983	1988
Country	US	England	US	Scotland	England
Percentage of blind registered with glaucoma	11.4	13	15.3	14.6	14

This is given as a proportion of the total number of registered blind for each country and year of publication.

agnosed. Thus, when alcohol intake is looked at on a population basis, as in the Beaver Dam study,[27] no suggestion exists of a relationship between alcohol and glaucoma.

SOCIOECONOMIC FACTORS. Leske and Rosenthal[28] postulated that the factors that influence access to adequate medical care, such as income, educational level, and socioeconomic status, would have an effect on the occurrence of glaucoma. Relatively little work has been done on this aspect of glaucoma; one study found a higher prevalence of glaucoma in outdoor manual workers than in indoor workers (the latter having the higher income). A similar study found a higher rate of glaucoma in manual laborers compared with clerical workers—although this was not controlled for race.[28]

THE EPIDEMIOLOGY OF GLAUCOMA BLINDNESS

Glaucoma, in all its forms, is a major cause of irreversible blindness throughout the world. It was calculated that 6.7 million people would be blind from the disease by the year 2000.[11] A number of studies indicate that, in the developed nations, the health services are aware of only 50% of the total number of people who have glaucoma, and it seems highly likely that this percentage is much smaller in the developing countries.[4]

Blind registration statistics offer one method by which to estimate the burden of glaucoma blindness. Table 210-4 illustrates the results of some published studies of blind registration figures. Although the percentages are fairly consistent in different countries and over time, the data from which these are drawn are subject to certain biases. Blind registration data have a number of flaws and usually are regarded as an underestimate of the true blindness figures.

Population estimates of glaucoma blindness are less prone to bias. For the Roscommon study[4] cohort a prevalence of blindness of 7.3% was found; the Baltimore Eye Study[34] had a visual impairment figure of 4.4% overall but higher in African-American subjects (at 7.9%).

The latter finding is consistent with other studies that indicate a higher rate of blindness in patients of African origin. Whereas glaucoma is the third highest cause of blindness registration in the United States, it is the most common cause of blindness registration among African-Americans. Hiller and Kahn[29] found a rate of glaucoma blindness seven times higher for non-Caucasians than Caucasians. The difference persisted across all age groups and both sexes and was not due to differential registration, as the age-specific rates of registered blindness were also higher for non-Caucasians.

CONCLUSION

Little doubt exists that the glaucomas represent a major public health problem in all parts of the world. At the individual level, they represent a particularly severe form of blindness that, unlike cataract, is irreversible. Although the underlying pathogenesis of glaucoma is not understood fully, the therapeutic maneuver of reducing IOP seems to slow progression of the disease in the majority of sufferers. Early diagnosis thus appears to offer the best way to maximize the number of years of sight for the patient who has glaucoma.

REFERENCES

1. Last JM. A dictionary of epidemiology, 2nd ed. Oxford: Oxford University Press; 1988.
2. Tielsch JM, Sommer A, Katz J, et al. Racial variations in the prevalence of primary open angle glaucoma. JAMA. 1991;266:369–74.
3. Klein BEK, Klein R, Sponsel WE, et al. Prevalence of glaucoma. Ophthalmology. 1992;99:1499–504.
4. Coffey M, Reidy A, Wormald R, et al. Prevalence of glaucoma in the west of Ireland. Br J Ophthalmol. 1993;77:17–21.
5. Bengtsson B. The prevalence of glaucoma. Br J Ophthalmol. 1981;65:46–9.
6. Mitchell P, Smith W, Attebo K, Healey PR. Prevalence of open-angle glaucoma in Australia. Ophthalmology. 1996;103:1661–9.
7. Leske MC, Connell AMS, Schachat AP, Hyman L. The Barbados Eye Study—prevalence of open angle glaucoma. Arch Ophthalmol. 1994;112:821–9.
8. Dielemans I, Vingerling JR, Wolfs RCW, et al. The prevalence of primary open-angle glaucoma in a population based study in the Netherlands. Ophthalmology. 1994;101:1851–5.
9. Mason RP, Omofosalade K, Wilson MR, et al. National survey of the prevalence and risk factors of glaucoma in St Lucia, West Indies. Ophthalmology. 1989;96:1363–8.
10. Wormald RPL, Basauri E, Wright LA, Evans JR. The African Caribbean eye survey: risk factors for glaucoma in a sample of African Caribbean people living in London. Eye. 1994;8:315–20.
11. Quigley HA. Number of people with glaucoma worldwide. Br J Ophthalmol. 1996;80:389–93.
12. Luntz MH. Primary angle-closure in urbanized South African Caucasoid and Negroid communities. Br J Ophthalmol. 1973;57:445–56.
13. Shiose Y, Kitazawa Y, Tsukahara S, et al. A collaborative glaucoma survey for 1988 in Japan. Rinsho Ganka. 1990;44:653–9.
14. Perkins ES. The Bedford glaucoma survey: 1. Long term follow-up of borderline cases. Br J Ophthalmol. 1973;57:179–85.
15. Armaly MF, Krueger DE, Maunder L, et al. Biostatistical analysis of the collaborative glaucoma study. 1. Summary of report of the risk factors for glaucomatous visual field defects. Arch Ophthalmol. 1980;98:2163–71.
16. Tielsch JM. The epidemiology of primary open angle glaucoma. Ophthalmol Clin North Am. 1991;4:649–57.
17. Clarke EE. A comparative analysis of the age distribution and types of primary glaucoma among populations of African and Caucasian origins. Ann Ophthalmol. 1973;5:1055–71.
18. Wilson R, Richardson TM, Hertzmark MA, Grant WM. Race as a risk factor for progressive glaucomatous damage. Ann Ophthalmol. 1985;17:653–9.
19. Sommer A, Tielsch JM, Katz J, et al. Relationship between intraocular pressure and primary open angle glaucoma among white and black Americans. Arch Ophthalmol. 1991;109:1090–5.
20. Jay JL, Murdoch JR. The rate of visual field loss in untreated primary open angle glaucoma. Br J Ophthalmol. 1993;77:176–8.
21. Sommer A. Glaucoma: facts and fancies. Eye. 1996;10:295–301.
22. Davanger M, Ringvold A, Bilka S. The probability of having glaucoma at different IOP levels. Acta Ophthalmol. 1991;69:565–8.
23. Dielemans I, De Jong PTVM, Stolk R, et al. Primary open angle glaucoma, intraocular pressure and diabetes mellitus in the general elderly population. Ophthalmology. 1996;103:1271–5.
24. Tielsch JM, Katz J, Sommer A, et al. Hypertension, perfusion pressure and primary open-angle glaucoma. Arch Ophthalmol. 1995;113:216–21.
25. Tielsch JM, Katz J, Sommer A, et al. Family history and risk of primary open angle glaucoma. Arch Ophthalmol. 1994;112:69–73.
26. Katz J, Sommer A. Risk factors for primary open angle glaucoma. Am J Prev Med. 1988;4:110–14.
27. Klein BE, Klein R, Ritter LL. Relationship of drinking alcohol and smoking to prevalence of open angle glaucoma. Ophthalmology. 1993;100:1609–13.
28. Leske MC, Rosenthal J. Epidemiological aspects of open angle glaucoma. Am J Epidemiol. 1979;109:250–72.
29. Hiller R, Kahn HA. Blindness from glaucoma. Am J Ophthalmol. 1975;80:62–9.
30. Sorsby A. The incidence and causes of blindness in England and Wales, 1963–1968. Report on public health and medical subjects No. 128. London: Her Majesty's Stationery Office; 1972.
31. Leibowitz HM, Krueger DG, Munder LR, et al. The Framingham Eye Study. Surv Ophthalmol. 1980;24(Suppl.):335–610.
32. Ghafour IM, Allan D, Foulds W. Common causes of blindness and visual handicap in the West of Scotland. Br J Ophthalmol. 1983;67:209–13.
33. Aclimandos WA, Galloway NR. Blindness in the city of Nottingham (1980–1985). Eye. 1988;2:431–4.
34. Tielsch JM, Sommer A, Witt K, et al. Blindness and visual impairment in an American urban population. Arch Ophthalmol. 1990;108:286–90.

211 Screening for Glaucoma

PAUL P. LEE • AERLYN G. DAWN • GERALD McGWIN

DEFINITION

- Ideal screening identifies all individuals who have a disease (sensitivity) and eliminates those without the disease (specificity).
- Screening for the earliest stage of a disease assumes that patients will suffer progressive loss, which has a measurable effect on patients' lives, and that interventions can retard, stop, or reverse such loss.
- Acceptable screening performance for open-angle glaucoma is 85% sensitivity for glaucomas and other optic neuropathies with visual field defects and specificity of at least 95% (preferably 98%).
- The current definition of glaucoma as a group of optic neuropathies may simplify future identification by screening of characteristic optic nerve and nerve fiber abnormalities.
- New technology may offer enhanced performance.

INTRODUCTION

The glaucomas are a diverse group of eye conditions that share either the common feature of progressive optic neuropathy (the open-angle variants)[1] or the common feature of occludable drainage angles in the anterior chamber (the closed-angle variants).[2] Because these represent two distinct groups of entities at two distinct anatomic areas, screening for both requires two distinct approaches. For the purposes of this chapter, a general approach to the understanding of screening programs is described that can be applied to both. However, specific comments and a review of screening studies are limited to the more common open-angle forms (the reader is referred to a published review by Congdon et al.[3] for such aspects of closed-angle screening).

HISTORICAL REVIEW

Screening Programs

From a societal perspective, screening should ideally identify every patient who has a disease (100% sensitivity) while clearing every individual who does not (100% specificity). In reality, no test has these technical performance characteristics. Instead, a reasonable balance is sought between sensitivity and specificity. Definition of the reasonable balance may be arbitrary—achieved through consensus over time—or based on empirical analyses of test performance (e.g., receiver operating characteristic curves) and associated costs of screening and cost per true case identified.[4] To be a practical reality, screening tests must be simple to perform, need the assistance of lay people or less costly midlevel or technician-level providers (or none at all), and be quick enough to be done on otherwise asymptomatic people in the community setting (i.e., on a population basis).[5–7]

Prior Glaucoma Screening Efforts

In the past, glaucoma screening has relied upon intraocular pressure (IOP) measurements, based on a case definition of glaucoma that required the presence of visual field defects, optic nerve or nerve fiber layer defects, and elevated IOP (except in the "normal tension" variant, in which elevated IOP was not required). Performance of IOP measurements alone has been unacceptably poor in screening for glaucomas defined in this manner.[5,8] Indeed, in a population-based analysis (which minimizes elements of selection bias) from the Baltimore Eye Survey in which elevated IOP was not required for a case definition of glaucoma, IOP levels had a maximum sensitivity of 93% among Caucasians and those who had a family history of glaucoma at an IOP of >16mmHg (2.1kPa) but with accompanying specificities of only 36% and 39%, respec-

tively.[9] At the traditional cutoff of IOP >21mmHg (2.8kPa), sensitivities across various risk factors were only about 48%.[9]

Numerous studies have evaluated the use of other screening parameters, such as various automated visual field screening and suprathreshold strategies, optic nerve head cup-to-disc ratios, optic nerve neuroretinal rim indicators, risk factor analyses (such as age, sex, race, and ocular and medical history), and combinations thereof.[9,10] These studies have found all such indicators inadequate for use as screening tools. Thus, significant interest remains in finding a method to screen for glaucoma, given the large numbers of patients who have glaucoma and that at least half of those who have glaucoma (defined as having both field and disc defects) do not know that they have the disorder.[2]

Current Glaucoma (Open-Angle) Definition

The results of prior studies need to be read cautiously in light of the current definition of primary open-angle glaucoma, first promulgated by the American Academy of Ophthalmology in 1996[11]: "a multifactorial optic neuropathy in which there is a characteristic acquired loss of optic nerve fibers." The current definition further states that the definitive characteristics of glaucoma are based on either visual field loss or "appearance of the disc or retinal nerve fiber layer." Early or mild glaucoma is defined as having characteristic optic nerve abnormalities with normal visual fields.[1] Thus, visual field defects are no longer part of the case definition of glaucoma. The American Academy of Ophthalmology (AAO) defines moderate glaucoma as having visual field abnormalities in one hemifield, not within 5° of fixation.[1] Severe glaucoma is defined as visual field abnormalities in both hemifields or loss within 5° of fixation.[1] The effect of this definition is to expand the number of people in the United States who could have glaucoma to over 15 million instead of the 2.2 million people currently estimated by Prevent Blindness America.[12] Thus, the performance of screening tests has to be reevaluated.

PURPOSE OF THE TEST

A screening test for glaucoma detects glaucoma before it causes significant loss of function for the individual. The current definition raises at least three questions: (1) What are the likelihood and rate of progressive loss from early glaucoma, in which there is only optic nerve or retinal nerve fiber layer loss? (2) Do available treatments slow, stop, or reverse loss of nerve fibers and the consequent visual functioning, and does the success of such treatment vary if treatment is delayed until later in the course? (3) At what point does loss of nerve fibers cause functional loss of significance to patients, and what degree of visual field loss (or any other physiological or psychometric measure), if any, is required before patients notice a decrease in their visual functioning or their general quality of life? The answers are essential because they address key concepts that were presupposed in prior screening efforts—that even early loss adversely affects patients (or that later loss is harder to control), that treatment is effective in at least slowing down the rate of both anatomic and functional loss, and that a sufficiently high number of patients progress without treatment to make it worthwhile to screen for even early stages prior to any functional or field loss.

Estimates of the likelihood of progression from early optic nerve loss to subsequent additional loss run from 9% to as high as 63% over a 5-year period,[13–15] which suggests that additional optic nerve fiber loss is significant. Recent data from the Ocular Hypertension Treatment Study (OHTS) show that the risk of developing initial field loss or progressive optic nerve damage among those with no visual field loss but elevated eye pressures was 9.5% over 5 years.[15] Among the risk factors for progression are a larger cup-to-disc ratio, indicating the possibility of subtle prior glaucomatous damage (early glaucoma by definition). Of note, the risk of progressive disease among subpopulations in the study ranged to over 35% depending on the presence of identified risk factors, for progression.[15]

The Early Manifest Glaucoma Trial (EMGT) results provide gold-standard evidence of the rates of progression among those who have visual field loss and no treatment, compared with those with treatment.[16] The EMGT was designed to determine whether treatment retards vision loss in those who already have relatively mild visual field loss (moderate glaucoma) at presentation. Patients in the control arm without treatment had a 62% rate of progression based on visual field or optic nerve head criteria (overall, the study had a 53% rate of progression) over 6 years.[16] Thus, based on the results of these two trials, there is now solid evidence of the rates of progression of glaucoma among those without treatment. Further, in both studies, data identify the various risk factors for progression, so that subpopulations of patients at greater (or lower) risk can be identified. Of note, there is a large difference in progression rates between those with no visual field loss (9.5%) and those with reliable mild visual field loss (62%).

The second issue, the medical profession's ability to retard or arrest loss of optic nerve fibers or deterioration of the visual field, is being addressed in several large, randomized controlled clinical trials sponsored by the National Eye Institute. These include trials with a no-treatment arm (EMGT[16] and the Ocular Hypertension Treatment Study[15]) and studies to evaluate the effectiveness of various treatment modalities (Advanced Glaucoma Intervention Study [AGIS][17] and the Collaborative Initial Glaucoma Treatment Study[18]). Both the OHTS and EMGT clearly demonstrate that lowering intraocular pressure significantly reduces the rate of progression of disease compared with no treatment.[15,16] In the OHTS results, treatment to lower IOP halved the rate of progression from 9.5% to 4.4% over 5 years. In the EMGT, only 45% of those who had pressure lowering (averaging 25% reduction) progressed (vs. 62% in the untreated control group) and did so later in the course of follow-up. Both studies also provide important information on the risk factors for progression. Further, results from the AGIS show that low IOP is associated with a reduction in the progression of visual field defects.[17] Evidence from the Collaborative Normal Tension Glaucoma Study Group shows that IOP plays a role in the pathogenesis of normal-tension glaucoma as well.[19] Although more complete answers to the questions addressed in these studies are expected in the next few years, the evidence now available strongly supports the notion that treatment can retard the rate of vision loss due to glaucoma. Thus, effective treatment is indeed available.

Finally, our ability to understand the effect of less than optimal vision on patients' function has increased considerably in the past few years. For patients who have blurred vision or trouble seeing, the impact on their general quality of life is commensurate with that of several major systemic illnesses.[20,21] Yet glaucoma patients traditionally have been thought not to have noticeable problems with their vision until relatively late in the disease. Evidence from a prospective case-control study showed that patients with glaucoma had significantly less general functional status than those without glaucoma,[22] although this finding is contradicted in other studies.[23,24] Notably, visual field loss has been shown to be correlated with reduction in glaucoma patients' activities of daily vision.[25] Studies show that visual field loss is related to a higher rate of automobile accidents and that visual field loss has a measurable impact on vision-related quality of life (i.e., the ability to perform important visual tasks, such as reading or driving, and the individual's satisfaction with lifestyle).[26,27] However, the issue of when glaucoma-related vision loss becomes significant currently can be answered only indirectly, by a comparison of the performance of normal patients who do not have glaucoma with that of patients who have early field loss. Using a moderate effect size of 0.5 standard deviations, AGIS field loss defects would have to increase between 3 and 10 points (on a 20-point scale)[28] before a functionally significant field loss is described.[27]

Thus, in assessing the state of our knowledge, sufficient data exist to answer the first two of these three key questions. Rates of progression without treatment are known, as are the benefits of treatment in reducing the rate of progression of even visual field loss. Data also exist to begin to answer the third question; they suggest that individuals who have significant visual field loss do have important decrements in vision-related quality of life and in important activities of modern life. Thus, screening for those with visual field loss is something that, in principle, is desirable. However, without a definable and measurable benefit from the identification of early cases of glaucoma (no visual field loss), it is less certain that screening for glaucoma to identify all such individual with early glaucoma is as strongly indicated. As additional information is developed about the rates of progression over even longer time frames, particularly the overall proportion of patients that eventually do progress to visual field loss and then have additional progressive field loss, screening for early glaucoma on a generalized basis may become more desirable.

USE OF THE TEST AND INTERPRETATION

The Glaucoma Advisory Committee of Prevent Blindness America has promulgated criteria for minimum performance characteristics for adjunctive devices used in screening for glaucoma, which include 95% specificity (98% preferable) and at least 85% sensitivity for moderate to severe visual field defects.[7] The desirability of these or any other criteria for specificity or sensitivity must be evaluated in light of the effect of such performance on the probability that someone be correctly identified as having glaucoma after a positive test result, through application of Bayes' theorem (Table 211-1). Such a screening test performance, given the low prior probability of glaucoma in the general population above 40 years of age (using the old case definition), still results in three false positives for every true positive. However, if the prior probability could be raised to, for example, 8–10% (as with testing family members only or using the current definition of glaucoma with only optic nerve head findings required), test performance at these criteria would be enhanced significantly and result in two true cases for every false positive identified.

Use of a screening test with 100% sensitivity has little effect on the posterior probability that a positive test correctly identifies a patient as having glaucoma (Table 211-2). Thus, changing the sensitivity of the test beyond 85% has much less effect than the application of methods to alter the prior probability of

TABLE 211-1

APPLICATION OF BAYES' THEOREM TO SCREENING TEST PERFORMANCE

	General Population Over 40 Years of Age		Family Members/Nerve Head Only	
	Glaucoma	No Glaucoma	Glaucoma	No Glaucoma
Prior probability	0.02	0.98	0.09	0.91
Test performance	0.85	(1.00–0.95)	0.85	(1.00–0.95)
Posterior probability	0.017	0.049	0.0765	0.0455
Positive test (%)	26	74	63	37

TABLE 211-2

APPLICATION OF BAYES' THEOREM TO ENHANCED SCREENING TEST PERFORMANCE

		General Population Over 40 Years of Age		Family Members/Nerve Head Only	
		Glaucoma	No Glaucoma	Glaucoma	No Glaucoma
Increased sensitivity	Prior probability	0.02	0.98	0.09	0.91
	Test performance	1.00	(1.00–0.95)	1.00	(1.00–0.95)
	Posterior probability	0.02	0.049	0.09	0.0455
	Positive test (%)	29	71	66	34
Increased specificity	Prior probability	0.02	0.98	0.09	0.91
	Test performance	0.85	(1.00–0.98)	0.85	(1.00–0.98)
	Posterior probability	0.017	0.030	0.0765	0.0182
	Positive test (%)	46	54	81	19

having glaucoma in the populations being screened. However, an increase in the specificity of the test to the 0.98 level, suggested by Prevent Blindness America (but not required), results in the best improvement in test performance. Thus, methods that increase the prior probability of having glaucoma and tests with better specificity may be efficient means of screening for glaucoma, provided adequate sensitivity exists.[29]

Additional statistical methods exist to help assess the use of different tests for the detection of glaucoma and are likely to become more widely used. The likelihood ratio (LR) expresses the relative rate of a positive test among those with glaucoma compared with those without. Thus, it is an indicator of how much more (or less) likely a given test result is obtained among diseased versus non-diseased individuals. The LR can be calculated as sensitivity / (1 − specificity) for a positive test and (1 − sensitivity) / specificity for a negative test. In the case of the Prevent Blindness America recommendations, the calculated LR of a desirable test for detecting glaucoma would be 17. When combined with a prior probability of disease, the LR can be used (with published algorithm scales) to provide a post-test probability, similar to the results of using Bayes' Theorem.

Incorporation of LR assessments offers several advantages. First, they are less likely to change with the prevalence of a disease. Second, they can be used to combine the results of multiple tests. Third, they can be used when screening test results are ordinal or continuous in nature, rather than categorical. This feature allows for potentially greater insights into analyzing test results, especially in comparing among different tests.

Receiver operating characteristic (ROC) curves share in common with the LR the ability to take advantage of ordinal or continuous test results. Both approaches allow for the comparison of various screening tests. However, additional statistical issues exist with the use of ROC curves: nonparametric vs. parametric (or semiparametric) tests, the impact of having multiple applications of the same test on a single patient (longitudinally and cross-sectionally), and multiple evaluators assessing a single test result.

PROCEDURE

Direct Indicators of Glaucomatous Optic Nerve Damage

With the current case definition of glaucoma as an optic neuropathy and the demonstration that optic nerve fiber loss may be identified prior to the onset of visual field loss,[13,30] screening for glaucoma can be simplified to evaluation of the results of various methods of assessment used to evaluate the optic nerve. With the definition of what optic nerve fiber findings constitute "characteristic" loss, the AAO Preferred Practice Pattern has one possible set of indicators for screening: thinning or notching of the rim, progressive change (cupping), or nerve fiber layer defects.[2] Screening programs that determine that one or more of these findings exist have screened appropriately for glaucoma.

Imaging of the optic nerve and retinal nerve fiber layers is used to determine structural loss. New imaging techniques, including confocal scanning laser tomography (CSLT), scanning laser polarimetry (SLP), optical coherence tomography (OCT), and retinal thickness analysis (RTA), have shown promise for glaucoma screening. A longitudinal prospective study found that glaucoma-

tous disc changes determined with CSLT occur more frequently than visual field changes and that less than half of glaucoma patients with disc changes also showed visual field changes.[31] Using the current preperimetric definition of early glaucoma, Heidelberg Retinal Tomography (HRT), a form of CSLT, has sensitivities of <30% at a specificity of 95%.[32] Sensitivity and specificity rise to 84% and 90% to 96%, respectively, for moderate glaucoma.[33,34] SLP, using the GDx device, has a sensitivity of 58% at a given specificity of 80% for preperimetric RNF defects[35] and sensitivity and specificity of 89% and 87% for moderate glaucoma.[34] OCT has been shown to have sensitivity and specificity of 82% and 84%, respectively, for moderate glaucoma.[34] Although RTA has generated interest as a potential tool for diagnosing glaucoma, few data exist related to the use of this technology.

A comparative study concluded that when used alone, HRT, SLP, and OCT summary reports "did not provide sensitivities and specificities that justify implementing them as primary population screening tools for early to moderate glaucoma."[36] Also, one of the major disadvantages of these technologies is the need for a skilled operator. A review by Michelson and Groh[37] summarizes the specific advantages and disadvantages of these technologies. Conventional photographic imaging of the optic disc by an experienced examiner remains the most sensitive method of detecting early glaucoma[38]; however, these new imaging technologies hold potential for glaucoma screening, particularly in combination with functional testing such as frequency-doubling technology. One of the major difficulties of assessing these new imaging technologies is the fact that the accuracy of the test can be determined only by comparing it with a "gold standard" reference test, yet no single test can provide a definitive diagnosis of glaucoma. Several long-term prospective studies that will help determine the roles of these new technologies in glaucoma screening are in progress.

In evaluating the optic nerve, uncertainty and inaccuracy related to screening arise from the inherent variability between observers in the assessment of the same clinical situation (interobserver variability), with the same observer at different points in time (intraobserver variability), and with the accuracy of the method used to measure the optic nerve head or nerve fiber layer. Some studies have found that experts have relatively high levels of interobserver and intraobserver consistency for certain indicators; others suggest that significant variation exists or that the levels of agreement fall with less experienced observers and with the method used.[39–41] Recent data from the OHTS using a rigorous quality assurance protocol show that trained technicians achieved high reproducibility between repeated gradings of the baseline horizontal cup/disc ratio from optic disc stereophotographs.[42] The percentage of regradings differing by ≥0.2 disc diameters from the baseline estimate of horizontal cup/disc ratio ranged from 4 to 7, and intraclass correlation coefficients ranged from 0.92 to 0.93. However, the authors point out that these findings cannot be generalized to routine clinical practice. If agreement rates for the presence or absence of glaucoma are substituted as equivalents for sensitivity and specificity, likely posterior probabilities can be generated for an accurate screening result for glaucoma status using these techniques.

COMPLICATIONS

The risks associated with screening for glaucoma fall into two categories. (1) The risk of false identification of the true ocular status—either false reassurance that a person is free of a disease or false identification that the person has a disease. The complications associated with this are an increased risk of undergoing subsequent, undetected visual loss in the former and the concomitant anxiety and expense of clarification of the true situation in the latter. (2) Because the optic nerve and its functioning are likely to be the focus of future screening efforts (assuming that screening is desirable), the most common risk is likely to be the precipitation of an angle-closure attack for tests that require dilation of the pupils for an accurate assessment of the optic nerve or retinal nerve fiber layer. The risk of this occurrence on a population basis has been estimated to be, at most, 1 in 333 subjects.[43]

ALTERNATIVE TESTS

New Automated Perimetry Tests

Prior to the current definition of glaucoma, investigators reported several promising methods for the detection of individuals who have visual field loss on standard suprathreshold static perimetry or kinetic perimetry (Goldmann), including scotopic sensitivity testing,[44] Henson visual field analysis and Damato campimetry (and oculokinetic perimetry),[45,46] peripheral color contrast,[47] and simultaneous interocular brightness sense testing.[48] All of these techniques are designed to screen for *moderate glaucoma in which visual field loss is already present*.

Investigators have also reported several newer techniques that may offer the possibility of detecting earlier visual field defects and progression of glaucomatous visual field loss. Computer-assisted visual fields are widely used to determine functional loss of vision. Techniques introduced in recent years include frequency-doubling technology (FDT) perimetry, short wavelength automated perimetry (SWAP), high-pass resolution perimetry (HPRP), motion automated perimetry (MAP), the multifocal electroretinogram (mERG), and the multifocal visual evoked potential (mVEP). In addition, the application of the Swedish interactive threshold algorithm (SITA) to conventional full threshold perimetry appears to increase sensitivity and reproducibility and to reduce testing times and intertest variability.[49,50]

Of these techniques, FDT has shown the greatest promise as a practical means of glaucoma screening. A prospective study[51] found that FDT showed sensitivity of 85% and specificity of 90% for early glaucomatous visual field loss (moderate glaucoma by the current AAO definition). Moreover, Cello et al.[51] showed that FDT had 96% sensitivity and 96% specificity for detecting moderate glaucomatous visual field loss. These data suggest that FDT would meet the minimum performance characteristics for glaucoma screening recommended by Prevent Blindness America. Studies have found that screening FDT appears to be effective as a screening tool to detect moderate glaucomatous damage.[52,53] FDT is significantly more rapid than standard automated perimetry, SWAP, HPRP, or MAP, making it well suited for screening. Studies using the FDT screening mode found that the average testing time was <2 minutes per eye (instrument time) for glaucoma patients and less than 30 seconds per eye for nonglaucoma controls.[53,54] In addition, FDT perimetry is relatively inexpensive, portable, and does not require special training for the examiner or patient. Furthermore, FDT may have less intertest and intratest variability than conventional perimetry.[55]

Other perimetric techniques also show promise but have disadvantages that make them impractical for screening in their current forms. SWAP, or blue-yellow perimetry, may detect field defects earlier than white-on-white standard threshold automated perimetry.[56] However, SWAP also requires more time than standard threshold automated perimetry, making it impractical for screening.[56] Investigators are researching the possibility of a SITA version of SWAP, which may reduce SWAP testing times. A prospective longitudinal cohort study found that HPRP, which is designed to test selectively the parvocellular system, can be more effective than standard threshold automated perimetry at detecting progressive glaucomatous visual field loss.[57] However, HPRP can be sensitive to blur and media opacities, which may limit its effectiveness. MAP relies on the observation that glaucoma patients show defects in motion perception. A 5-year prospective cohort study showed that MAP can be useful for detecting early glaucomatous visual loss and can be a strong predictor of standard white-on-white visual field loss.[58] However, as with SWAP, the length of MAP testing (approximately 15 minutes) makes it impractical for screening.

The mERG measures the local electrical responses of the retina throughout the central visual field and does not rely on subjective patient responses. mERG has been shown to provide objective measurement of visual function from localized regions. A pilot study suggested that mERG might play an important role in detecting early glaucomatous changes and recommended the use of mERG as a supplementary test for glaucoma suspects.[59] However, data suggest that the sensitivity of the test is limited[60] and that mERG findings in most glaucoma patients do not correlate well with visual field defects present on standard automated perimetry.[60,61] Thus, additional work is needed to understand the nature and etiology of these differences.

Because of these limitations of mERG, some researchers have expressed increasing interest in the mVEP,[60] which shows stronger correlation with standard automated perimetry.[62,63] mVEP measures the localized electrical responses from the occipital cortex for the central visual field, and, like mERG, mVEP can objectively detect glaucomatous visual field defects. However, significant interindividual variability in mVEP responses has limited the application of mVEP perimetry to glaucoma screening.[62,63]

If screening for the earliest stage of glaucoma, that of optic nerve fiber loss alone, is desired, these methods will need to be evaluated in light of the current definition of glaucoma (see prior section). However, if screening is found to be efficient only for those who have visual field loss, methods predicated on field loss should receive further attention and evaluation as potential screening techniques. Given that patients most likely do not experience any impairment of quality of life until some visual field loss has already occurred, screening at the level of early visual field loss (moderate glaucoma) may be an effective strategy.

Genetic Testing for Glaucoma

Finally, in the past decade, genetic analysis of families with primary open-angle glaucoma has identified at least six different genetic loci that may be involved in the pathogenesis of the disease.[64-69] The identification of the TIGR/myocillin gene has led to the introduction of a genetic test called OcuGene.[70] Although the usefulness of the test is limited because the test detects <5% of people who will later develop open-angle glaucoma as adults,[71,72] genetic testing for glaucoma is becoming a reality. Moreover, at the 2002 ARVO meeting, Li et al.,[73] showed that patients expressed relatively positive attitudes toward hypothetical genetic testing for glaucoma. Thus, genetic linkage analysis offers the promise that someday patients will be screened for glaucoma on a genetic basis through peripheral blood or other specimens. Again, however, the performance of these techniques may vary depending on the case definition of glaucoma used. Similarly, the utility of such screening also presupposes that effective treatments exist and that the cost-benefit ratio of such screening, based in large part on the test's performance characteristics (see earlier), justifies screening a given population.

Comparison of Techniques to Screen for Glaucoma

Because the comparison of tests with different sensitivities and specificities at different cutoff or threshold levels is difficult to evaluate fully, the use of receiver operating characteristic curves and likelihood ratios to supplement our understanding of the relative value of tests will become essential for the comparison of the test performances of different means of screening for glaucoma.[74,75] Comparison of the areas under the ROC curves, as well as of the graphical displays of such curves, readily identifies the tests or methods that are superior to others. Use of LR results will potentially provide even more detailed insights into which tests will be most helpful.

REFERENCES

1. American Academy of Ophthalmology. Preferred practice pattern: primary open-angle glaucoma. San Francisco: American Academy of Ophthalmology; 2000.
2. American Academy of Ophthalmology. Preferred practice pattern: primary angle-closure glaucoma. San Francisco: American Academy of Ophthalmology; 1996.
3. Congdon N, Wang F, Tielsch JM. Issues in the epidemiology and population-based screening of primary angle-closure glaucoma. Surv Ophthalmol. 1992;36:411–23.
4. Gottlieb LK, Schwartz B, Pauker SG. Glaucoma screening. A cost-effectiveness analysis. Surv Ophthalmol. 1983;28:206–26.
5. Anonymous. Periodic health examination, 1995 update: 3. Screening for visual problems among elderly patients. Canadian Task Force on the Periodic Health Examination. CMAJ. 1995;152:1211–22.
6. Shields MB. The challenge of screening for glaucoma. Am J Ophthalmol. 1995;120:793–5.
7. Prevent Blindness America Glaucoma Advisory Committee. Criteria for adjunctive screening devices. Prevent Blindness America Glaucoma Advisory Committee; 1996, Schaumburg, IL.
8. Berwick DM. Screening in health fairs. A critical review of benefits, risks, and costs. JAMA. 1985;254:1492–8.
9. Tielsch JM, Katz J, Singh K, *et al.* A population-based evaluation of glaucoma screening: the Baltimore Eye Survey. Am J Epidemiol. 1991;134:1102–10.
10. Wang F, Quigley HA, Tielsch JM. Screening for glaucoma in a medical clinic with photographs of the nerve fiber layer. Arch Ophthalmol. 1994;112:796–800.
11. American Academy of Ophthalmology. Preferred practice pattern: primary open-angle glaucoma. San Francisco: American Academy of Ophthalmology; 1996.
12. Prevent Blindness America. Vision problems in the U.S.: prevalence of adult vision impairment and age-related eye disease in America. <www.preventblindness.org/resources/vision_data>.2002.
13. Caprioli J. Clinical evaluation of the optic nerve in glaucoma. Trans Am Ophthalmol Soc. 1994;92:589–641.
14. Komulainen R, Tuulonen A, Airaksinen PJ. The follow-up of patients screened for glaucoma with non-mydriatic fundus photography. Int Ophthalmol. 1992;16:465–9.
15. Kass MA, Heuer DK, Higginbotham EJ, *et al.* The Ocular Hypertension Treatment Study: a randomized trial determines that topical ocular hypotensive medication delays or prevents the onset of primary open-angle glaucoma. Arch Ophthalmol. 2002;120:701–13; discussion 829–30.
16. Heijl A, Leske MC, Bengtsson B, *et al.* Reduction of intraocular pressure and glaucoma regression: results from the Early Manifest Glaucoma Trial. Arch Ophthalmol. 2002; 12:1268–79.
17. AGIS Investigators. The advanced glaucoma intervention study (AGIS): 7. The relationship between control of intraocular pressure and visual field deterioration. The AGIS Investigators. Am J Ophthalmol. 2000;130:429–40.
18. Musch DC, Lichter PR, Guire KE, Standardi CL. The Collaborative Initial Glaucoma Treatment Study: study design, methods, and baseline characteristics of enrolled patients. Ophthalmology. 1999;106:653–62.
19. Anonymous. Comparison of glaucomatous progression between untreated patients with normal-tension glaucoma and patients with therapeutically reduced intraocular pressures. Collaborative Normal-Tension Glaucoma Study Group [erratum appears in Am J Ophthalmol 1999 Jan;127(1):120]. Am J Ophthalmol. 1998;126:487–97.
20. Kington R, Rogowski J, Lillard L, Lee PP. Functional associations of "trouble seeing." J Gen Intern Med. 1997;12:125–8.
21. Lee PP, Spritzer K, Hays RD. The impact of blurred vision on functioning and well-being. Ophthalmology. 1997;104:390–6.
22. Wilson MR, Coleman AL, Yu F, *et al.* Functional status and well-being in patients with glaucoma as measured by the Medical Outcomes Study Short Form-36 questionnaire. Ophthalmology. 1998;105:2112–6.
23. Parrish RK 2nd, Gedde SJ, Scott IU, *et al.* Visual function and quality of life among patients with glaucoma. Arch Ophthalmol. 1997;115:1447–55.
24. Mills RP, Janz NK, Wren PA, Guire KE. Correlation of visual field with quality-of-life measures at diagnosis in the Collaborative Initial Glaucoma Treatment Study (CIGTS). J Glaucoma. 2001;10:192–8.
25. Sherwood MB, Garcia-Siekavizza A, Meltzer MI, *et al.* Glaucoma's impact on quality of life and its relation to clinical indicators. A pilot study. Ophthalmology. 1998;105:561–6.
26. Johnson CA, Keltner JL. Incidence of visual field loss in 20,000 eyes and its relationship to driving performance. Arch Ophthalmol. 1983;101:371–5.
27. Gutierrez P, Wilson MR, Johnson C, *et al.* Influence of glaucomatous visual field loss on health-related quality of life. Arch Ophthalmol. 1997;115:777–84.
28. Anonymous. Advanced Glaucoma Intervention Study. 2. Visual field test scoring and reliability. Ophthalmology. 1994;101:1445–55.
29. Crick RP, Tuck MW. How can we improve the detection of glaucoma? BMJ. 1995;310:546–7.
30. Quigley HA. Open-angle glaucoma. N Engl J Med. 1993;328:1097–1106.
31. Chauhan BC, McCormick TA, Nicolela MT, LeBlanc RP. Optic disc and visual field changes in a prospective longitudinal study of patients with glaucoma: comparison of scanning laser tomography with conventional perimetry and optic disc photography. Arch Ophthalmol. 2001;119:1492–9.
32. Mardin CY, Horn FK, Jonas JB, Budde WM. Preperimetric glaucoma diagnosis by confocal scanning laser tomography of the optic disc. Br J Ophthalmol. 1999;83:299–304.
33. Wollstein G, Garway-Heath DF, Hitchings RA. Identification of early glaucoma cases with the scanning laser ophthalmoscope. Ophthalmology. 1998;105:1557–63.
34. Greaney MJ, Hoffman DC, Garway-Heath DF, *et al.* Comparison of optic nerve imaging methods to distinguish normal eyes from those with glaucoma. Invest Ophthalmol Vis Sci. 2002;43:140–5.
35. Horn FK, Jonas JB, Martus P, *et al.* Polarimetric measurement of retinal nerve fiber layer thickness in glaucoma diagnosis. J Glaucoma. 1999;8:353–62.
36. Sanchez-Galeana C, Bowd C, Blumenthal EZ, *et al.* Using optical imaging summary data to detect glaucoma. Ophthalmology. 2001;108:1812–8.
37. Michelson G, Groh MJ. Screening models for glaucoma. Curr Opin Ophthalmol. 2001;12:105–11.
38. Mardin CY, Junemann AG. The diagnostic value of optic nerve imaging in early glaucoma. Curr Opin Ophthalmol. 2001;12:100–4.
39. Varma R, Steinmann WC, Scott IU. Expert agreement in evaluating the optic disc for glaucoma. Ophthalmology. 1992;99:215–21.
40. Zangwill L, Shakiba S, Caprioli J, Weinreb RN. Agreement between clinicians and a confocal scanning laser ophthalmoscope in estimating cup/disk ratios. Am J Ophthalmol. 1995;119:415–21.
41. Lichter PR. Variability of expert observers in evaluating the optic disc. Trans Am Ophthalmol Soc. 1976;74:532–72.
42. Feuer WJ, Parrish RK 2nd, Schiffman JC, *et al.* The Ocular Hypertension Treatment Study: reproducibility of cup/disk ratio measurements over time at an optic disc reading center. Am J Ophthalmol. 2002;133:19–28.
43. Patel KH, Javitt JC, Tielsch JM, *et al.* Incidence of acute angle-closure glaucoma after pharmacologic mydriasis. Am J Ophthalmol. 1995;120:709–17.
44. Congdon NG, Quigley HA, Hung PT, *et al.* Impact of age, various forms of cataract, and visual acuity on whole-field scotopic sensitivity screening for glaucoma in rural Taiwan. Arch Ophthalmol. 1995;113:1138–43.
45. Sponsel WE, Ritch R, Stamper R, *et al.* Prevent Blindness America visual field screening study. The Prevent Blindness America Glaucoma Advisory Committee. Am J Ophthalmol. 1995;120:699–708.
46. Mutlukan E, Damato BE, Jay JL. Clinical evaluation of a multi-fixation campimeter for the detection of glaucomatous visual field loss. Br J Ophthalmol. 1993;77:332–8.
47. Yu TC, Falcao-Reis F, Spileers W, Arden GB. Peripheral color contrast. A new screening test for preglaucomatous visual loss. Invest Ophthalmol Vis Sci. 1991;32:2779–89.
48. Cummins D, MacMillan ES, Heron G, Dutton GN. Simultaneous interocular brightness sense testing in ocular hypertension and glaucoma. Arch Ophthalmol. 1994;112:1198–203.
49. Bengtsson B, Heijl A, Olsson J. Evaluation of a new threshold visual field strategy, SITA, in normal subjects. Swedish Interactive Thresholding Algorithm. Acta Ophthalmol Scand. 1998;76:165–9.
50. Sharma AK, Goldberg I, Graham SL, Mohsin M. Comparison of the Humphrey Swedish interactive thresholding algorithm (SITA) and full threshold strategies. J Glaucoma. 2000;9:20–7.
51. Cello KE, Nelson-Quigg JM, Johnson CA. Frequency doubling technology perimetry for detection of glaucomatous visual field loss. Am J Ophthalmol. 2000;129:314–22.
52. Trible JR, Schultz RO, Robinson JC, Rothe TL. Accuracy of glaucoma detection with frequency-doubling perimetry. Am J Ophthalmol. 2000;129:740–5.
53. Quigley HA. Identification of glaucoma-related visual field abnormality with the screening protocol of frequency doubling technology. Am J Ophthalmol. 1998;125:819–29.
54. Wadood AC, Azuara-Blanco A, Aspinall P, *et al.* Sensitivity and specificity of frequency-doubling technology, tendency-oriented perimetry, and Humphrey Swedish interactive threshold algorithm-fast perimetry in a glaucoma practice. Am J Ophthalmol. 2002;133:327–32.
55. Spry PG, Johnson CA, McKendrick AM, Turpin A. Variability components of standard automated perimetry and frequency-doubling technology perimetry. Invest Ophthalmol Vis Sci. 2001;42:1404–10.
56. Maeda H, Tanaka Y, Nakamura M, Yamamoto M. Blue-on-yellow perimetry using an Armaly glaucoma screening program. Ophthalmologica. 1999;213:71–5.
57. Chauhan BC, House PH, McCormick TA, LeBlanc RP. Comparison of conventional and high-pass resolution perimetry in a prospective study of patients with glaucoma and healthy controls. Arch Ophthalmol. 1999;117:24–33.
58. Wu J, Coffey M, Reidy A, Wormald R. Impaired motion sensitivity as a predictor of subsequent field loss in glaucoma suspects: the Roscommon Glaucoma Study. Br J Ophthalmol. 1998;82:534–7.
59. Chan HH, Brown B. Pilot study of the multifocal electroretinogram in ocular hypertension. Br J Ophthalmol. 2000;84:1147–53.
60. Hood DC, Greenstein VC, Holopigian K, *et al.* An attempt to detect glaucomatous damage to the inner retina with the multifocal ERG. Invest Ophthalmol Vis Sci. 2000;41:1570–9.
61. Fortune B, Johnson CA, Cioffi GA. The topographic relationship between multifocal electroretinographic and behavioral perimetric measures of function in glaucoma. Optom Vis Sci. 2001;78:206–14.
62. Hood DC, Zhang X. Multifocal ERG and VEP responses and visual fields: comparing disease-related changes. Doc Ophthalmol. 2000;100:115–37.
63. Klistorner A, Graham SL. Objective perimetry in glaucoma. Ophthalmology. 2000;107:2283–99.
64. Sheffield VC, Stone EM, Alward WL, *et al.* Genetic linkage of familial open angle glaucoma to chromosome 1q21-q31. Nat Genet. 1993;4:47–50.
65. Stoilova D, Child A, Trifan OC, *et al.* Localization of a locus (GLC1B) for adult-onset primary open angle glaucoma to the 2cen-q13 region. Genomics. 1996;36:142–50.
66. Trifan OC, Traboulsi EI, Stoilova D, *et al.* A third locus (GLC1D) for adult-onset primary open-angle glaucoma maps to the 8q23 region. Am J Ophthalmol. 1998;126:17–28.
67. Wirtz MK, Samples JR, Kramer PL, *et al.* Mapping a gene for adult-onset primary open-angle glaucoma to chromosome 3q. Am J Hum Genet. 1997;60:296–304.
68. Sarfarazi M. Recent advances in molecular genetics of glaucomas. Hum Mol Genet. 1997;6:1667–77.
69. Wirtz MK, Samples JR, Rust K, *et al.* GLC1F, a new primary open-angle glaucoma locus, maps to 7q35-q36. Arch Ophthalmol. 1999;117:237–41.
70. Insite Vision, Inc. Information for healthcare professionals. <www.ocugene.com/professional>.2002.
71. Stone EM, Fingert JH, Alward WL, et al. Identification of a gene that causes primary open angle glaucoma. Science. 1997;275:668–70.
72. Alward WL. The genetics of open-angle glaucoma: the story of GLC1A and myocilin. Eye. 2000;14:429–36.
73. Li J, Lee PP, Buckley S, et al. Attitudes toward genetic testing for glaucoma: a survey of patients (Abstract 1077). Invest Ophthalmol (ARVO Supp); 2002.
74. Katz J, Tielsch JM, Quigley HA, *et al.* Automated suprathreshold screening for glaucoma: the Baltimore Eye Survey. Invest Ophthalmol Vis Sci. 1993;34:3271–7.
75. Damms T, Dannheim F. Sensitivity and specificity of optic disc parameters in chronic glaucoma. Invest Ophthalmol Vis Sci. 1993;34:2246–50.

CHAPTER 212

Mechanisms of Glaucoma

PAUL F. PALMBERG • JANEY L. WIGGS

DISEASE DEFINITION

About 60 types of glaucoma are known. Classically, the glaucomas have been characterized by:

- Abnormality of the anterior portion of the eye that results in increased intraocular pressure (IOP);
- Loss of retinal ganglion cells in a distribution that suggests the injury occurred at the optic nerve head, often accompanied by a posterior bowing of the lamina cribrosa of the nerve head; and
- Corresponding nerve fiber layer pattern of visual field loss.

More recently, the diagnostic criteria of the glaucomas have been in a state of flux. The current preferred practice pattern for primary open-angle glaucoma (POAG) defines POAG as an optic neuropathy for which the level of IOP is merely a risk factor.[1] Conversely, clinicians frequently refer to most other conditions in which the IOP is elevated as "glaucoma" (e.g., primary congenital glaucoma, primary angle-closure glaucoma, pigmentary glaucoma) even when, early in the condition, no optic nerve injury has occurred. What has been preserved in this era of unclear nomenclature is that the term glaucoma is used to describe patients who can be differentiated from those who are healthy by the presence of characteristic optic nerve damage and/or condition-associated findings (e.g., buphthalmos in congenital glaucoma, appositional angle closure in primary angle-closure glaucoma, pigment dispersion in pigmentary glaucoma) rather than simply by the level of IOP.

Here we first give an overview of the fairly well-characterized mechanisms that result in elevation of IOP and then discuss the rather poorly understood mechanisms of optic nerve injury in the glaucomas.

MECHANISMS THAT UNDERLIE ELEVATED IOP IN THE GLAUCOMAS

IOP is generated from the production of aqueous humor by the nonpigmented epithelium of the ciliary body. This tissue actively transports ions and nutrients, obtained from the vascular circulation of the ciliary body, into the posterior chamber. An osmotic gradient, created by the active transport, drags in water. In addition, a portion of the aqueous humor is derived by ultrafiltration of interstitial fluid, which is driven in by the pressure gradient between the ciliary body arterioles and the posterior chamber.[2] The resultant clear, colorless fluid flows centripetally over the equator and anterior surface of the lens, forward through the pupil, into the anterior chamber, and centrifugally to and through the trabecular meshwork into Schlemm's canal, circumferentially in the canal to about 70 collector channels, and through the limbal sclera in those channels to enter the aqueous veins and general circulation.

The aqueous humor nourishes the tissues in the visual axis that have no blood supply, carries away their wastes, maintains a reducing atmosphere (low oxygen tension, high concentrations of glutathione and ascorbate) that prevents oxidative cross-linking of sulfhydryl groups of lens protein, carries growth factors, and inflates the eye.

Although an elevation in IOP could be produced logically by either an excess of aqueous production or mechanisms that im-

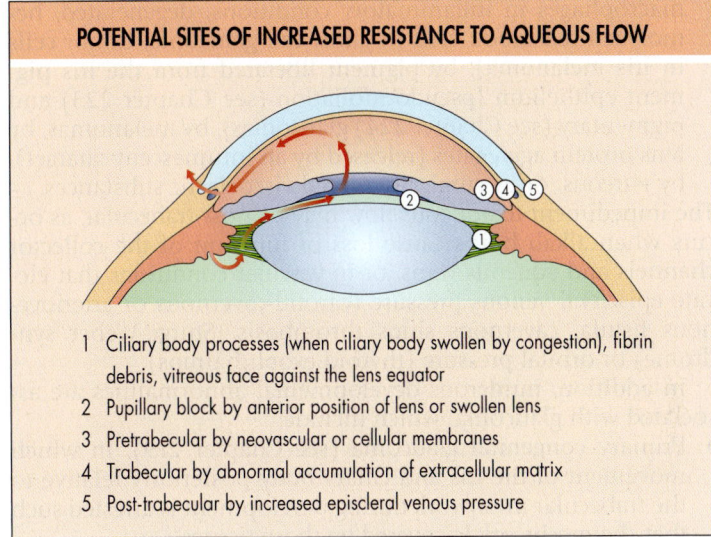

POTENTIAL SITES OF INCREASED RESISTANCE TO AQUEOUS FLOW

1. Ciliary body processes (when ciliary body swollen by congestion), fibrin debris, vitreous face against the lens equator
2. Pupillary block by anterior position of lens or swollen lens
3. Pretrabecular by neovascular or cellular membranes
4. Trabecular by abnormal accumulation of extracellular matrix
5. Post-trabecular by increased episcleral venous pressure

FIG. 212-1 ■ Potential sites of increased resistance to aqueous flow.

pede aqueous egress, no condition of excess aqueous production has been observed. However, every major category of pathology is represented in one form of glaucoma or another. Developmental defects, hamartomas, hereditary biochemical defects, infections, inflammations, metaplasias and neoplasms, physical and chemical trauma, ischemic vascular conditions, and endocrine abnormalities have all been implicated.[3]

In reaching a diagnosis and treatment plan for any type of glaucoma, it is useful to identify the site and nature of the impediment to aqueous flow (Fig. 212-1). The site may be in the posterior chamber. For example, when the lens moves forward in the not fully inflated eye after filtration surgery in an angle-closure glaucoma patient and the ciliary body forms an "O-ring" against the lens, aqueous is forced posteriorly into the vitreous cavity. This results in the creation of a pressure gradient behind the lens that pushes the lens-iris diaphragm forward, covers the trabecular meshwork, and markedly elevates the IOP. This condition is known variously as ciliary block, aqueous misdirection, or malignant glaucoma (see Chapter 229).

The site may be at the pupil. For example, in the shorter than average eye of a hyperopic person in middle to old age, the continually growing lens may be sufficiently anterior to impede the flow of aqueous through the pupil and produce a pupillary block. This results in the development of a pressure gradient across the iris that causes the iris to bow forward, mechanically cover the trabecular meshwork, and elevate IOP. This condition is known as primary angle-closure glaucoma (see Chapter 222).

Aqueous flow through the pupil may also be blocked by the formation of adhesions of the iris to lens (posterior synechiae) in uveitis (see Chapter 226) or by a blood clot formed after trauma [eight-ball hyphema (see Chapter 227)]. The site may be "pretrabecular," as occurs when the trabecular meshwork becomes covered by a fibrovascular meshwork [in neovascular glaucoma (see Chapter 225) and in Fuchs' heterochromic irido-cyclitis] or by an ingrowth of cells [fibroblasts in fibrous ingrowth, conjunctival epithelium in epithelial downgrowth, transformed corneal endothelial cells in the iridocorneal endothelial syndrome (see Chapter 230), or normal corneal endothelial cells altered after trauma].

The obstruction may be at the level of the trabecular meshwork, because of:

- Abnormalities in the extracellular matrix [as may be the case in POAG[4,5] (see Chapter 220), juvenile open-angle glaucoma,[6] and corticosteroid-induced glaucoma[7] (see Chapter 226)];
- Injury to the trabecular cells by toxic substances (siderosis or chalcosis);
- Meshwork obstruction by cellular debris (white cells or macrophages in inflammatory conditions, degenerated, hemolyzed red blood cells in ghost-cell glaucoma, tumor cells in iris melanoma), by pigment liberated from the iris pigment epithelium [pseudoexfoliation (see Chapter 223) and pigmentary (see Chapter 224) glaucomas], by melanomas, by lens protein aggregates (released by an intumescent cataract), by vitreous, or by surgically placed viscoelastic substances.

The impediment to aqueous flow may be post-trabecular, as occurs when alkali burns cause loss of function of the collector channels and aqueous veins, or in vascular conditions that elevate episcleral venous pressure (carotid-cavernous or arteriovenous fistula, cavernous sinus thrombosis, Sturge-Weber syndrome) or orbital pressure (thyroid exophthalmos).

In addition, numerous developmental abnormalities are associated with glaucoma, which include:

- Primary congenital glaucoma (see Chapter 219), in which movement of the iris and ciliary body posteriorly relative to the trabecular meshwork during development is arrested such that the meshwork is covered by those tissues[8];
- Various other forms of chamber angle maldevelopment (Peters' syndrome, Rieger's syndrome, and aniridia); and
- Numerous forms of maldevelopment of the lens and/or zonule (homocystinuria, Marfan syndrome, microspherophakia) that result in secondary pupillary block later in life (see Chapter 230).

MECHANISMS OF OPTIC NERVE DAMAGE IN GLAUCOMA

Intraocular Pressure as a Risk Factor for Glaucoma Damage

Good evidence exists from epidemiology (see Chapter 210) and from treatment studies that the pathophysiology of glaucoma is dependent upon either an elevated IOP [>21mmHg (>2.8kPa)] or, in some cases of glaucoma that present initially with pressures in the upper portion of the normal pressure range (normal-tension glaucoma), an abnormal sensitivity to the level of IOP. That the pressure matters in even the latter cases is indicated by the observation that patients who have normal-tension glaucoma and who happen to have a consistent asymmetry in IOP also suffer greater damage in the eye that has the higher pressure in 85% of cases.[9]

In epidemiological investigations, such as have been performed in Bedford in the United Kingdom[10] and in Baltimore,[11] about one half to two thirds of the glaucoma patients discovered (and thus not already receiving glaucoma treatment) had an elevated IOP at screening and most of the rest had a pressure in the upper normal [16–20mmHg (2.1–2.7kPa)] range. In the Baltimore Eye Survey, 13% of those who had newly diagnosed glaucoma versus 50% of the rest of the population initially had an IOP in the lower normal range. From these observations it may be estimated that, at a maximum, no more than 26% (13% in the lower half of the IOP range and an equal percentage in the upper half) of glaucoma patients could have suffered their damage on a pressure-independent basis.

On the other hand, a moderate elevation of IOP alone is insufficient to cause optic nerve damage in the majority of those

TABLE 212-1

RISK OF PROGRESSIVE VISUAL FIELD LOSS OVER 5–18 YEARS AS A FUNCTION OF INTRAOCULAR PRESSURE

Intraocular Pressure (mmHg)	Number of Eyes	Progression of Visual Field Loss (%)
All <16	9	33
10–20, mostly <16	17	47
10–20, mostly >15	11	82
Some >20	37	84
All >20	6	100

TABLE 212-2

RISK OF PROGRESSIVE VISUAL FIELD LOSS OVER 3.5–5 YEARS AS A FUNCTION OF MEAN INTRAOCULAR PRESSURE OF GROUP

Mean Intraocular Pressure (mmHg)	Progression (%)	Follow-Up (years)	Number of Eyes	Reference
14.2	8	2–5	59	Lamping et al.[14]
14.4	6	5	33	Roth et al.,[15] corticosteroid
15.0	18	5	60	Kidd and O'Connor[16]
15.2	26	4.4	19	Maul et al.[17]
15.7	10	4+	22	Kolker[18]
17.3	35	4	42	Greve and Dake[19]
19.1	58	5	19	Roth et al.,[15] no corticosteroid

affected. About four fifths of those who have elevated IOP do not have detectable damage to the optic nerve tissue or visual field. A receiver-operator function analysis in which the distribution of IOPs of those with optic nerve damage was compared with that of those without suggested that only about one third of the difference in distributions is accounted for by pressure alone. Yet within the group that suffered damage, IOP surely matters both initially and in the subsequent clinical course.

Treatment studies suggest that a dose-response relationship exists between IOP and the risk of progressive visual field loss in glaucoma patients. Odberg[12] reported on a 5- to 18-year follow-up of a group of his patients who had advanced glaucoma damage and who underwent medical and/or surgical therapy (Table 212-1).

Others have reported long-term outcomes after filtration surgery, and a comparison of the results at 3.5–5 years also indicates that for groups of patients a dose-response relationship exists between the mean IOP and the risk of progressive field loss (Table 212-2).[8,13] However, because within these studies and in the Baltimore Eye Survey the risk of damage rises in a steeper than linear fashion as a function of IOP, the values in Table 212-2 for the risk of progressive field loss as a function of mean IOP of groups probably exceed the risk for an individual at any level of IOP above the population mean. For example, Greve and Dake[19] reported that 29% of 31 eyes that had IOP <22mmHg (<2.9kPa) showed progressive field loss versus 55% of 11 eyes that had higher IOP.

The report of Roth et al.[15] is instructive, particularly as it compared patients randomized to receive or not to receive topical corticosteroid in the postoperative period and demonstrated better filtration blebs and pressure control, as well as a correspondingly better visual field prognosis, for patients who received corticosteroid.

TABLE 212-3

PRIMARY FILTRATION SURGERY WITH MITOMYCIN

Postoperative Time (years)	Mean Intraocular Pressure (mmHg)	Mean Deviation	Corrected Pattern Standard Deviation	Number of Eyes
Preoperative	26.5	−15.0 ± 7.4	8.0 ± 3.3	80
1	10.8 ± 3.6(se)	−13.7 ± 9.1	8.1 ± 3.6	48
2	11.1 ± 4.0	−13.9 ± 6.3	8.1 ± 3.6	31
3	10.9 ± 4.0	−15.1 ± 7.2	6.9 ± 2.7	18

TABLE 212-4

COMBINED PHACOEMULSIFICATION AND FILTRATION SURGERY

Postoperative Time (years)	Mean Intraocular Pressure (mmHg)	Mean Deviation	Corrected Pattern Standard Deviation	Number of Eyes
Preoperative	23.8	−12.2	5.2	84
1	12.1	−8.5	4.7	66
2	11.4	−8.1	4.7	50
3	11.5	−8.6	5.0	25

The low end of the dose-response relationship between IOP and risk of progressive field loss was explored in patients who received mitomycin in primary and combined filtration procedures.[20,21] The results showed that the patients as a group maintained a mean IOP of about 11mmHg (1.5kPa) and demonstrated no net deterioration of either the mean deviation or corrected pattern standard deviation out to 3 years (Tables 212-3 and 212-4). With the limited number of visual fields so far performed for each patient (done annually), it is difficult to determine whether the stability of mean values indicates that virtually no one worsens at these IOPs or that some worsen and an equivalent number improve. However, comparison of these published results indicates that it is beneficial to bring the mean IOP to a low normal level provided that the benefit with regard to field stabilization is not offset by the side effects of more aggressive therapy. An analysis of individual cases is to be carried out at 5 years to determine visual field and visual acuity outcomes.

It thus appears that the majority of patients who have moderate to severe visual field loss suffer additional loss at IOPs in the range 17–22mmHg (2.3–2.9kPa), that at IOPs in the midnormal range 6–26% of patients suffer such loss, and that in the low normal range the risk is even less. Thus, although IOP alone may account for only 35% of the separation between glaucomatous and undamaged populations, most glaucoma patients appear to have an abnormal sensitivity to IOP that may be offset if the IOP is lowered to the midnormal or low normal range, and perhaps 90% or more may benefit from a sufficiently low IOP.

Location of Optic Nerve Damage in Glaucoma

How and where do the IOP and other factors that modify susceptibility to IOP (or independently damage the optic nerve) act? One major clue is given by the pattern of damage observed. The tissue loss and pattern of visual field defects observed correspond to damage that occurs at the optic nerve head and not to retinal or retrobulbar sites of damage. This suggests that any damage does not result from processes that directly injure the ganglion cell bodies and that the effect is on the ganglion cell axons at the point where they pass through the optic nerve head

and lamina cribrosa. Elevated IOP may interfere with antegrade and/or retrograde axoplasmic transport in that location by either compromising the local blood supply or mechanically pinching the axons. Blockade of axoplasmic transport has been demonstrated by Radius and Anderson[22] in an animal model of glaucoma. Such a blockade of axoplasmic transport in other nerves in animal models blocks the return of trophic factors to the cell body and leads to death by a mechanism similar to apoptosis.

VASCULAR AND MECHANICAL THEORIES OF DAMAGE

Quigley and Addicks[23] speculated that pressure-induced backward bowing of the lamina cribrosa may result in misalignment of the holes in the laminar sheets through which the ganglion cell axons pass; the axons are pinched and axoplasmic flow is blocked. In favor of this idea, the authors suggested that their observation of larger diameter pores in the upper and lower poles of the disc may correspond to weaker support for the axons that pass through these areas; indeed, the upper and lower poles of the disc are the most common sites of nerve fiber loss. Counter to this proposal is the observation that elderly persons, in whom collagen cross-linking strengthens the laminar sheets, are far more susceptible than younger persons to optic nerve damage when the IOP is elevated.

Anderson[24] proposed that elevated IOP interferes with the vascular supply in the optic nerve region but only when the IOP is quite high or when other factors interfere with local autoregulation. Buus and Anderson[25] observed that patients who have normal-tension glaucoma are four times as likely as age-matched controls to have retinal pigment epithelial and/or choroidal atrophy in a crescentic shape at the disc margin; patients who have POAG are twice as likely as controls, and ocular hypertensives are only half as likely as controls, to have such defects.[24] Such crescents represent enlarged versions of the usual gap in the blood-ocular barrier present at the optic nerve head, where the optic nerve passes by the edge of the choroid and could allow vasoactive substances from the blood stream to reach the receptors for norepinephrine and angiotensin that are present on the outside surface of capillaries of the optic nerve head. Anderson and coworkers have shown that the vasoactive substance angiotensin can augment axoplasmic transport blockade in the optic nerve head in an animal mode[26] and that angiotensin administered into the vitreous may cause vasoconstriction of retinal blood vessels and in culture can interfere in carbon dioxide regulation of pericyte contractility.[27]

THE POTENTIAL FOR NEUROPROTECTION

If vasoactive substances interfere with optic nerve head autoregulation in response to elevated IOP and this results in reduced blood flow, the potential exists for vasodilating substances, such as calcium channel blocking agents selective for the central nervous system, to reduce the susceptibility of the optic nerve to pressure. Initial reports claim that calcium channel blockers may be helpful,[28] but further work is needed to define the risk-benefit ratio of such treatment in long-term clinical trials.

Some agents used to treat glaucoma reduce penumbral damage to the optic nerve in a mouse model of a crush injury. The relevance of these observations to any actual clinical benefit of glaucoma treatment is entirely speculative and needs to be supported by long-term clinical trials of agents that either have or lack such activity.

Finally, the level of glutamate in the vitreous may be elevated in glaucoma patients compared with cataract patients,[29] and the placement of glutamate in the vitreous may create a model of optic nerve damage in an animal. Glutamate is released by injured neurons of the central nervous system in stroke, and glutamate blockers help limit penumbral nerve damage in an animal model of stroke. However, the proposed connection of glutamate and glaucoma damage requires confirmation. Against the likelihood of such a mechanism is that the pattern of injury of the optic nerve is not based on focal damage in the retina, as would be expected if dying ganglion cell bodies released glutamate and damaged their neighbor cells.

GENETICS OF GLAUCOMA

Introduction

The past decade has produced a wealth of information about the molecular pathogenesis of many human disorders. The success of the molecular genetic approach results from the central dogma of molecular biology—a DNA sequence found in genes is transcribed into an RNA sequence that directs the synthesis of specific protein molecules that perform unique functions for maintenance, growth, and replication of an individual cell. Proteins that do not function normally because of an error in the DNA sequence can result in sick cells and eventually human disease. Identification of errors in the DNA sequence and evaluation of their impact on the function of the protein product provide important information about the mechanism of a disease. With the advent of techniques that enable precise evaluation of the DNA sequence of genes, to establish the molecular causes of human disease has become a practical reality for many disorders.

An aspect of the molecular genetic approach that has been particularly important in glaucoma research is that only DNA (usually obtained from a simple peripheral blood sample) from an individual affected by the disease is required for the analysis just outlined. Because genetic analysis investigates the disease process at the DNA level, the actual diseased tissue, or even knowledge about how the disease affects a particular tissue, is not necessary. The collection of sufficient quantities of trabecular meshwork to perform biochemical and cellular studies is a difficult problem. Moreover, tissue specimens taken from affected patients who undergo glaucoma surgery are exposed to numerous medical and laser treatments that may obscure the initial abnormalities responsible for the disease. The study of genes responsible for glaucoma may identify the role of specific protein products in the development of the disease without the need for direct access to the diseased tissue.

For many years, a family history of glaucoma has been recognized as an important risk factor for this disease.[30-33] Only recently, however, has glaucoma been accepted as an inherited disorder. Many forms of glaucoma are now recognized to be inherited as mendelian dominant or recessive traits, including juvenile open-angle glaucoma,[34-45] congenital glaucoma,[46-48] developmental glaucomas (Rieger's syndrome and aniridia),[49-51] and pigmentary glaucoma.[52-57] Other types of glaucoma, such as adult POAG, have been shown to have a heritable susceptibility. Twelve loci for mendelian forms of glaucoma and seven susceptibility loci for adult-onset POAG have been mapped in the human genome (Table 212-5).[58,59] Five genes responsible for different forms of glaucoma have been identified. The study of these and additional genes responsible for glaucoma will lead to important new advances in our understanding of this blinding condition in the years to come.

A reduction in outflow of aqueous humor through the trabecular meshwork is a major cause of the increase in IOP in open-angle glaucoma. Enzymes, structural proteins, and proteins involved in the embryogenesis and development of the eye may be important to the normal physiology of the trabecular meshwork, and defects in the genes that code for these proteins may play a role in the genetic predisposition to the disease. Once genes responsible for glaucoma have been identified, the normal biological function of the protein products of these genes must be established. Investigations to address the effects of these proteins on the normal biochemical and cellular processes of the trabecular meshwork and other components of the aqueous outflow pathways will provide important new information about the pathophysiology of this disease.

TABLE 212-5

GENES RESPONSIBLE FOR DIFFERENT FORMS OF GLAUCOMA

Disease	Chromosome Location	Gene
Rieger syndrome	4q25	PITX2
Rieger syndrome	13q14	??
Iridodysgenesis	6p25	FOXC1
Primary congenital glaucoma	2p16	CYP1B1
Primary congenital glaucoma	1p36	??
Juvenile open-angle glaucoma Primary open angle adult	1q25 (GLC1A)	Myocilin (TIGR)
Pigment dispersion syndrome	7q36	??
Primary open angle adult	2qcen-q13 (GLC1B)	??
Primary open angle adult	3q21-q24 (GLC1C)	??
Primary open angle adult	8q23 (GLC1D)	??
Primary open angle adult	10p15 (GLC1E)	Optineurin
Primary open angle adult	7q35 (GLC1F)	??
Primary open angle adult	Susceptibility loci: 2p, 4p, 14q, 15q, 17p, 17q, 19	??
Nail patella syndrome/glaucoma	9q34	LMX1B

Current treatment for glaucoma is directed toward the regulation of aqueous humor formation by the ciliary body and increased outflow of aqueous humor through the trabecular meshwork or alternative pathways created by surgical procedures. Current therapy does not actually treat the cause of the disease because the cause is unknown. To clone the genes responsible for glaucoma and determine the functions of the normal and abnormal protein products of these genes will identify the processes that can result in this disease. This information will lead to the development of novel treatments designed to eradicate the abnormal molecular and cellular processes that may cause the disease. In addition to the development of new medical treatments for glaucoma, isolation of genes responsible for the disease may result in the development of gene therapy, in which damaged genes are replaced and the underlying defects corrected.

Isolation of genes responsible for glaucoma will also lead to new methods for diagnosis of the condition based on the DNA sequence changes that result in defective genes and protein products. Such DNA-based diagnostic tests can identify individuals at risk for the disease before any visual deterioration has occurred.

Overview of Recent Advances

Genes and chromosomal loci responsible for glaucoma are given in Table 212-5.

JUVENILE-ONSET GLAUCOMA. Juvenile POAG is a rare disorder that develops during the first two decades of life. Affected patients typically present with a high IOP, which ultimately requires surgical therapy. Characteristic features include a high incidence of myopia and angle structures of normal appearance. These patients do not have a Barkan membrane or findings associated with anterior segment dysgenesis syndromes.[37,45] One histopathological study of 10 patients suggested the presence of a thick, compact tissue on the anterior segment of Schlemm's canal.[59] Other specific ocular or systemic abnormalities have not been identified in these patients.

Juvenile glaucoma can be inherited as an autosomal dominant trait.[60] Large pedigrees have been identified and used for genetic linkage analysis. Myocilin is one gene that can cause juvenile glaucoma.[61] Mutations in this gene have also been associated with some cases of adult-onset POAG. The normal function of this gene and the role that dysfunctional forms play in the pathogenesis of glaucoma remain unknown. The protein contains several important functional domains, including a region with strong homology to the olfactomedin family of proteins. Although the function of the olfactomedin domain in myocilin is unknown, nearly all the mutations associated with glaucoma occur in this region. Studies of patients who have genetic abnormalities resulting in a reduction of myocilin suggest that mutations in the gene cause a gain of function or dominant negative effect rather than a loss of function or haploinsufficiency.[62-64]

ADULT-ONSET PRIMARY OPEN-ANGLE GLAUCOMA. Adult-onset POAG (see Chapter 220) is the most common form of glaucoma and affects 7–8 million Americans. Previous studies suggest that susceptibility to POAG is inherited. The prevalence of POAG in first-degree relatives of affected patients has been documented to be as high as 7–10 times that of the general population. It is likely that the incidence of POAG in family members of affected patients is even higher, given the older age of diagnosis and the lack of patients' awareness of the disease. Patients affected by POAG are more likely to develop an increase in IOP in response to dexamethasone eyedrops, a trait shown to be inherited.[65,66] Several twin studies suggest a high concordance of glaucoma between monozygotic twins, consistent with a significant genetic predisposition to the disease.[63,67] The higher prevalence of POAG among African Americans compared with Caucasian Americans may reflect an underlying genetic difference in susceptibility to this disorder. Also, POAG has been associated weakly with the inheritance of various genetics markers, which include the Duffy blood group on chromosome 1 and inability to taste phenylthiourea.[68]

It is likely that multiple genes (independently or in combination) are responsible for the heritability of POAG. The variability in the age of onset of the disease, the apparent incomplete penetrance of the condition in some pedigrees, and the prevalence of the disease all suggest that more than one gene may be responsible for the disorder. Patients affected by POAG also vary with respect to the relationship between increased IOP and deterioration of the optic nerve. These observations are consistent with the conclusion that POAG is inherited not as a simple single gene disorder but as a complicated "complex trait."[69]

The origins of the genetic complexity of POAG are likely to stem from the diversity of ocular tissues and cell types potentially involved in the disease process. Many studies suggest that defects in the trabecular outflow pathways are responsible for the elevation of IOP associated with the majority of cases of POAG. However, the cell type and biochemical processes that are altered in the disease have not yet been identified. It is possible that mutations in a number of genes that encode different proteins may alter the normal function of the ocular outflow pathways. Many patients who have elevated IOPs do not develop the characteristic degeneration of the optic nerve that is the ultimate cause of blindness in patients affected by POAG. Indeed, elevation of IOP is an important risk factor for the disease but does not by itself define the disease process. Individuals who do develop degeneration of the optic nerve may have sustained additional gene defects that render the retinal ganglion cell and optic nerve more susceptible to damage. The reduced penetrance and genetic heterogeneity typical of complex traits may make genetic mapping studies difficult. Six loci for POAG and seven susceptibility loci have been reported.[59,70-75] Optineurin has been identified as responsible for GLC1E.[76] The optineurin protein is expressed in the eye and in many nonocular tissues including brain, heart, liver, skeletal muscle, kidney, and pancreas. In the eye the protein has been detected by reverse transcription–polymerase chain reaction (RT-PCR) in human trabecular meshwork, nonpigmented ciliary epithelium, and retina. The protein does not have significant homology to any known protein but may participate in the tumor necrosis factor α (TNF-α) signaling pathway. TNF-α has been proposed to be one factor that could induce apoptosis in retinal ganglion cells in patients with low-tension glaucoma and in patients with POAG.[77] It has been speculated that the optineurin protein may function to protect the optic nerve from TNF-α–mediated apoptosis and that the loss of function of this protein may decrease the threshold for ganglion cell apoptosis in patients with glaucoma.

CONGENITAL GLAUCOMA. Congenital glaucoma (see Chapter 219) is a heterogeneous condition that is typically apparent at birth but may not be diagnosed before 3 years of age. As a result of the flexibility of the sclera in babies, the elevation of IOP associated with this condition causes buphthalmos, the usual indication that the child is affected. Increased IOP in eyes affected by congenital glaucoma is probably the result of abnormal development of the anterior segment of the eye. Specifically, in many cases of congenital glaucoma, a membrane that obstructs the path of aqueous humor may be visualized.

Previous studies suggested that congenital glaucoma is largely an inherited condition that is also genetically heterogeneous. Numerous pedigrees affected by autosomal recessive forms of the disease have been reported and include pedigrees of Czechoslovakian[78] and Slovakian gypsies[79] and pedigrees from the Middle East (such as Saudi Arabian[46] and Turkish pedigrees[49]). Cytogenetic abnormalities have been described in many patients affected by congenital glaucoma. Many of these are complex rearrangements that may involve a number of genes, a type of abnormality that has been observed on chromosomes 1, 2, 3, 4, 6, 11, and 13.[80-86] Collectively, these results suggest that many different genes may be responsible for this condition.

Two loci responsible for autosomal recessive forms of congenital glaucoma have been located in the human genome (GLC3A at 2p21[48] and GLC3B at 1p36[87]). CYP1B1 has been shown to be the causative gene responsible for cases of congenital glaucoma mapping to chromosome 2p21. This gene codes for cytochrome P4501B1. Mutations in this gene disrupt functional domains, implying that loss of function of the protein results in the phenotype.[88] Mutations in CYP1B1 have been found in congenital glaucoma patients from populations all over the world. Some of the mutations in this gene are recurrent, and genetic studies have shown that they reside on the same ancient founder chromosome that has been distributed throughout the world population.[89,90] The gene located at 1p36 remains to be identified. It is likely that, because of the genetic heterogeneity of this condition, other genes responsible for congenital glaucoma will be identified in the future.

Variability in the phenotypic expression of mutant forms of CYP1B1 has led to the suggestion that modifier genes may also influence the severity of the disease resulting from mutations in this gene.[91] A recent study suggests that patients carrying mutations in myocilin and CYP1B1 may have more severe disease, suggesting that the two proteins may interact in the same biochemical pathways.[92]

PIGMENT DISPERSION SYNDROME AND PIGMENTARY GLAUCOMA. The pigment dispersion syndrome, a common disorder in young adults, is associated with the development of pigmentary glaucoma. Studies have shown that up to 2–4% of the Caucasian American population between 20 and 40 years of age may be affected by this disorder, of which characteristic features include loss of iris contour and loss of pigment granules from the iris. The released pigment is deposited on the structures of the anterior segment of the eye, which include the trabecular meshwork. Although generally it is accepted that the dispersed iris pigment contributes to the development of glaucoma in affected patients, the pathogenesis of pigmentary glaucoma remains unknown (see Chapter 224).

Pigment dispersion has been shown to be inherited as an autosomal dominant trait, which suggests that specific gene defects may be responsible. One locus for this syndrome was located on 7q35-q36 in families of Irish descent,[52] but the gene responsible has yet to be isolated. The high prevalence of this condition indicates that more than one gene may be responsible for this disorder.

PSEUDOEXFOLIATION SYNDROME. Pseudoexfoliation is a condition characterized by a distinctive fibrillary degeneration of the lens capsule, but the fibrillar material, although most easily visualized on the lens capsule, is actually present throughout the anterior segment of the eye and has been found to exist systemically in the skin and blood vessels (see Chapter 223). Pseudoexfoliation may be associated with a severe high-IOP glaucoma that results in rapid deterioration of the optic nerve. Although the biochemical defect responsible for this disease is unknown, basement membrane alterations observed in pathology specimens taken from affected individuals suggest that alterations of the protein constituents of the basement membranes may be involved in this process.

The distinctive geographical distribution of pseudoexfoliation is most consistent with founder effects caused by inheritance of genes responsible for this condition. High prevalence of this disease is found in Scandinavia, Russia, Nova Scotia, Scotland, northeastern United States, Saudi Arabia, Greece, and the African Bantu; the disease has a low prevalence in the Eskimo population, Germany, the United Kingdom, and the southern United States. Pedigrees affected by pseudoexfoliation have been reported,[93] and studies of these suggest that the disease is inherited as a dominant trait with incomplete penetrance. The degree of genetic heterogeneity of the condition remains unknown. To date, loci that harbor genes responsible for this condition have not been found in the human genome.

RIEGER'S SYNDROME. Rieger's syndrome is an autosomal dominant disorder of morphogenesis that results in abnormal development of the anterior segment of the eye (Fig. 212-2). Typical clinical findings may include posterior embryotoxon, iris hypoplasia, iridocorneal adhesions, and corectopia (see Chapter 230). Approximately 50% of affected individuals develop a high-IOP glaucoma associated with severe optic nerve disease. Although the elevation of IOP is likely to result from abnormal development of the anterior structures of the eye, a direct correlation between the severity of the anterior segment dysgenesis and the incidence of glaucoma has not been observed. Presumably, the structures that are involved in the elevation of IOP in these patients are not readily visible clinically.

Genetic heterogeneity of Rieger's syndrome has been suggested by descriptions of affected individuals who have a variety of chromosomal abnormalities, which include deletions of chromosome 4 and of chromosome 13, a deletion of chromosome 10, a pericentric inversion of chromosome 6, and an isochromosome of chromosome 6. Genes for Rieger's syndrome are established at chromosome loci 4q25,[50] 13q14,[51] and 6p25.[94] Iris hypoplasia is the dominant clinical feature of pedigrees linked to the 6p25 locus, whereas pedigrees linked to 4q25 and 13q14 demonstrate the full range of ocular and systemic abnormalities found in these patients.

The genes responsible for Rieger's syndrome loci mapped to 4q25 and to 6p25 have been identified. The chromosome 4q25 gene (*RIEG1*) codes for the bicoid homeobox transcription factor PITX2.[95] Presumably, this gene plays an important role in the processes that result in normal eye development. Future studies designed to investigate the interaction of this gene with other genes involved in eye development, such as *Pax6*, are of great interest. The chromosome 6p25 gene codes for FOXC1, a member of the forkhead family of regulatory proteins. This protein also participates in the development of the anterior segment of the eye.[96] A mouse that lacks the FOXC1 gene product has abnormal development of the anterior segment of the eye. Various anterior segment structures are abnormally formed in the FOXC1 deficit mouse, including the iris and Schlemm's canal.[97] The identification of other genes responsible for Rieger's syndrome and anterior segment dysgenesis will also enable studies to determine whether these genes are part of a common developmental pathway or represent redundant functions necessary for eye development. The development of transgenic and knockout animals using these genes will allow important studies to correlate structure and function of the eye.

NAIL PATELLA SYNDROME. Individuals with nail patella syndrome have abnormal development of finger and toe nails and the patellae. Some of these patients also develop glaucoma that may be associated with developmental abnormalities.[98] A gene for this syndrome, *LMX1B*, has been identified.[99] This gene is a regulatory transcription factor and is likely to be involved in developmental processes in the eye.

FUTURE DIRECTIONS

The identification of genes that cause glaucoma is just an initial step in the establishment of the pathophysiology of the disorder. Studies to determine the normal role of these genes in the development and function of the eye are necessary to understand the foundation of the disease pathophysiology. To understand the normal role of the genes responsible for glaucoma, the specific proteins and classes of proteins they code for, when and where the genes are expressed, and how the expression is regulated must be determined.

Little is known about how an abnormal gene product results in a glaucoma phenotype and whether different mutations in the same gene can explain phenotypic variability. The identification of genes that cause glaucoma will allow the opportunity to determine whether the functions of these genes and their products are influenced by the action of other genes and/or environmental factors that can modify the disease phenotype.

The identification of genes and loci involved in disease enables studies to evaluate the clinical features of the disorder with respect to the molecular information. It will be possible to determine whether cases of glaucoma caused by a specific gene share common features that can be recognized clinically. Similarly, it will be possible to determine whether molecular subclasses of disease respond similarly to specific treatment modalities. The combined knowledge from genetic and clinical studies will lead to new methods of diagnosis and treatment that will improve the prognosis and quality of life of affected individuals.

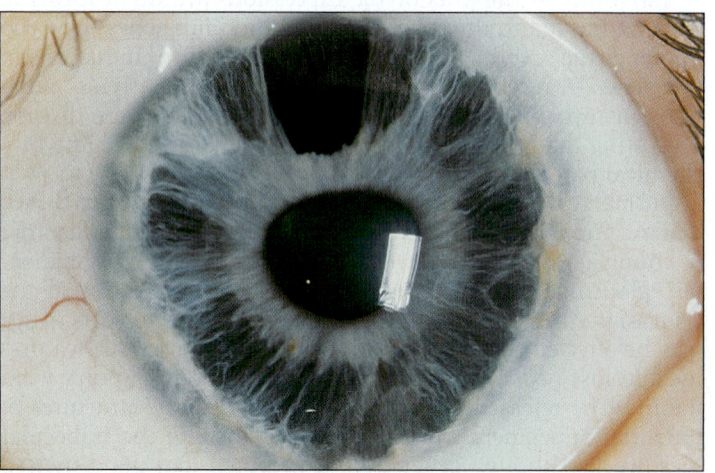

FIG. 212-2 ■ **Rieger's syndrome.** Slit-lamp view of a patient that shows the iris atrophy, iridocorneal adhesions, and corectopia that are typical clinical manifestations of the disease. The patient has also had a trabeculectomy for glaucoma.

REFERENCES

1. Glaucoma Panel. Preferred practice pattern for primary open-angle glaucoma. San Francisco: American Academy of Ophthalmology; 1997.
2. Krupin T, Civan MM. Physiologic basis of aqueous humor formation. In: Ritch R, Shields MB, Krupin T, eds. The glaucomas, Vol 1. Basic Sciences. St Louis: Mosby; 1996:251–80.

3. Shields MB, Ritch R, Krupin T. Classifications of the glaucomas. In: Ritch R, Shields MB, Krupin T, eds. The glaucomas, Vol 2. Clinical Science. St Louis: Mosby; 1996:717–25.
4. Lutjen-Drecoll E, Rohen JW. Morphology of aqueous outflow pathways in normal and glaucomatous eyes. In: Ritch R, Shields MB, Krupin T, eds. The glaucomas, Vol 1. Basic Sciences. St Louis: Mosby; 1996:89–123.
5. Knepper PA, Goossens W, Palmberg PF. Glycosaminoglycan stratification of the juxtacanalicular tissue in normal and primary open-angle glaucoma. Invest Ophthalmol Vis Sci. 1996;37:2414–25.
6. Stone EM, Fingert JH, Alward WLM, *et al.* Identification of a gene that causes primary open angle glaucoma. Science. 1997;275:668–70.
7. Spaeth GL, Rodrigues MM, Weinreb S. Steroid-induced glaucoma. A: Persistent elevation of intraocular pressure. B. Histopathologic aspects. Trans Am Ophthalmol Soc. 1977;75:353–79.
8. Anderson DR. The development of the trabecular meshwork and its abnormality in primary infantile glaucoma. Trans Am Ophthalmol Soc. 1981;79:458–85.
9. Cartwright MJ, Anderson DR. Correlation of asymmetric damage with asymmetric intraocular pressure in normal-tension glaucoma (low-tension glaucoma). Arch Ophthalmol. 1988;106:898–900.
10. Bankes JLK, Perskins ES, Tsolako S, Wright JE. Bedford Glaucoma Survey. Br Med J. 1968;30:791–6.
11. Sommer A, Tielsch JM, Katz J, *et al.* Relationship between intraocular pressure and primary open-angle glaucoma among white and black Americans. Arch Ophthalmol. 1991;109:1090–5.
12. Odberg T. Visual field prognosis in advanced glaucoma. Acta Ophthalmol. 1987;65(Suppl182):27–9.
13. Palmberg P. The rationale and effectiveness of glaucoma therapy. Distributed at the American Glaucoma Society, Miami, December 1988, and included as Appendix 1, Background, in the Preferred Practice Pattern for Primary Open-Angle Glaucoma, American Academy of Ophthalmology, San Francisco, 1989, with additional material provided by Maul E, presented at the Pan-American Congress of Ophthalmology, Quito, 1995.
14. Lamping KA, Bellow R, Hutchinson BT. Long term evaluation of initial filtration surgery. Ophthalmology. 1986;93:91–100.
15. Roth SM, Spaeth GL, Starita RJ, *et al.* The effects of postoperative corticosteroids on trabeculectomy and the clinical course of glaucoma: five-year follow-up study. Ophthalmic Surg. 1991;22:724–9.
16. Kidd MN, O'Connor M. Progression of field loss after trabeculectomy—a five year follow-up. Br J Ophthalmol. 1985;69:825–31.
17. Maul E, Espildora J, Muga RP, *et al.* Efecto de la traveculectomia sobre el campo visual en el glaucoma cronico sinple avanzado. Arch Chil Oftalmol. 1987;44(2):13–16.
18. Kolker AE. Visual prognosis in advanced glaucoma: a comparison of medical and surgical therapy for retention of vision in 101 eyes with advanced glaucoma. Trans Am Ophthalmol Soc. 1977;75:539–55.
19. Greve EL, Dake CL. Four-year follow-up of a glaucoma operation. Int Ophthalmol. 1979;1:139–45.
20. Norris EJ, Schiffman J, Galanopoulos A, Palmberg PF. Three-year pressure and visual function outcome of primary filtering surgery with mitomycin C. Invest Ophthalmol Vis Sci. 1997:38(Suppl):A1060.
21. Norris EJ, Schiffman J, Palmberg P. Coceito atual da 'pressao ideal'. Presented at the Congresso Brasileiro de Oftalmologia, Goiania, Brazil, September 4, 1997.
22. Radius RL, Anderson DR. Rapid axonal transport in primate optic nerve: distribution of pressure-induced interruption. Arch Ophthalmol. 1981;99:650–4.
23. Quigley HA, Addicks EM. Regional differences in the structure of the lamina cribrosa and their reaction to glaucomatous damage. Arch Ophthalmol. 1981;99:137–43.
24. Anderson DR. Glaucoma, capillaries and pericytes. 1. Blood flow regulation. Ophthalmologica. 1996;210:257–62.
25. Buus DR, Anderson DR. Peripapillary crescents and halos in normal-tension glaucoma and ocular hypertension. Ophthalmology. 1989;96:16–19.
26. Sossi N, Anderson DR. Blockage of axonal transport in optic nerve induced by elevation of intraocular pressure; effect of arterial hypertension induced by angiotensin I. Arch Ophthalmol. 1983;101:94–7.
27. Matsugi T, Chen Q, Anderson DR. Effect of CO_2-induced intracellular pH and contraction of retinal capillary pericytes. Invest Ophthalmol Vis Sci. 1997;38: 643–51.
28. Netland PA, Erickson KA. Calcium channel blockers in glaucoma management. Ophthalmol Clin North Am. 1995;8:327–34.
29. Dryer EB, Zurakowski D, Schumer RA, *et al.* Elevated glutamate levels in the vitreous body of humans and monkeys with glaucoma. Arch Ophthalmol. 1996;114:299–305.
30. Becker B, Kolker AE, Roth FD. Glaucoma family study. Am J Ophthalmol. 1960; 50:557–67.
31. Drance SM, Schulzer M, Thomas B, Douglas G. Multivariate analysis in glaucoma: use of discriminant analysis in predicting glaucomatous visual field damage. Arch Ophthalmol. 1981;99:1019–22.
32. Hart WM Jr, Yablonski M, Kass MA, Becker B. Multivariate analysis of the risk of glaucomatous visual field loss. Arch Ophthalmol. 1979;97:1455–8.
33. Perkins ES. Family studies in glaucoma. Br J Ophthalmol. 1974;58:529–35.
34. Allen TD, Ackerman WG. Hereditary glaucoma in a pedigree of three generations. Arch Ophthalmol. 1942;27:139–57.
35. Berg R. Erbliches jugendliches Glaukom Acta Ophthalmol. 1932;10:568–87.
36. Courtney RH, Hill E. Hereditary juvenile glaucoma simplex. JAMA. 1931;97: 1602–9.
37. Dorozynski A. Privacy rules blindside French glaucoma effort. Science. 1991; 252:369–70.
38. Johnson AT, Drack AV, Kwitek AE, *et al.* Clinical feature and linkage analysis of a family with autosomal dominant juvenile glaucoma. Ophthalmology. 1993;100:524–9.
39. Martin JP, Zorab EC. Familial glaucoma in nine generations of a South Hampshire family. Br J Ophthalmol. 1974;58:536–42.
40. McCulloch JC. Iridoschisis as a cause of glaucoma. Am J Ophthalmol. 1950;33: 1398–400.
41. Richards JE, Lichter PR, Boehnke M, *et al.* Mapping of a gene for autosomal dominant juvenile-onset open-angle glaucoma to chromosome 1q. Am J Hum Genet. 1994;54:62–70.
42. Sheffield, VC, Stone EM, Alward WLM, *et al.* Genetic linkage of familial open angle glaucoma to chromosome 1q21-q31. Nat Genet. 1993;4:47–50.
43. Stokes WH. Hereditary primary glaucoma. Arch Ophthalmol. 1940;24:885–909.
44. Weatherill JR, Hart CT. Familial hypoplasia of the iris stroma associated with glaucoma. Br J Ophthalmol. 1969;53:433–8.
45. Wiggs JL, DelBono EA, Schuman JS, *et al.* Clinical features of five pedigrees genetically linked to the juvenile glaucoma locus on chromosome 1q21-q31. Ophthalmology. 1995;102:1782–9.
46. Bejjani BA, Anderson KL, Lewis RA, *et al.* Mapping strategies in primary congenital glaucoma (PCG). Am J Hum Genet. 1996;59(Suppl):A212.
47. Plasilova M, Kadasi L, Polakova H, *et al.* Linkage mapping of a locus for primary congenital glaucoma in Slovak gypsy population. Eur Soc Hum Genet Meeting, May 17–20, 1997. Abstract 152.
48. Sarfarazi M, Akarsu AN, Hossain A, *et al.* Assignment of a locus (*GLC3A*) for primary congenital glaucoma (buphthalmos) to 2p21 and evidence for genetic heterogeneity. Genomics. 1995;30:171–7.
49. Glaser T, Jepeal L, Edwards JG, *et al. PAX6* gene dosage effect in a family with congenital cataracts, aniridia, anophthalmia and central nervous system defects. Nat Genet. 1994;7:463–71.
50. Murray JC, Bennett SR, Kwitek AE, *et al.* Linkage of Rieger syndrome to the region of the epidermal growth factor gene on chromosome 4. Nat Genet. 1992;2:46–9.
51. Phillips JC, DelBono EA, Haines JL, *et al.* A second locus for Rieger syndrome maps to chromosome 13q14. Am J Hum Genet. 1996;59:613–19.
52. Andersen JS, Pralea AM, DelBono EA, *et al.* A gene responsible for the pigment dispersion syndrome maps to chromosome 7q35-q36. Arch Ophthalmol. 1997; 115:384–8.
53. Becker B, Podos SM. Krukenberg's spindles and primary open-angle glaucoma. Arch Ophthalmol. 1966;76:635–47.
54. Kaiser-Kupfer MI, Kupfer C, McCain L. Asymmetric pigment dispersion syndrome. Trans Am Ophthalmol Soc. 1983;81:310–24.
55. Mandelkorn RM, Hoffman ME, Olander KW, *et al.* Inheritance and the pigmentary dispersion syndrome. Ann Ophthalmol. 1983;15:577–82.
56. McDermott JA, Ritch R, Berger A, Wang RF. Inheritance of pigmentary dispersion syndrome. Invest Ophthalmol Vis Sci. 1987;28(Suppl):153.
57. Paglinauan CM, Haines JL, DelBono EA, *et al.* Exclusion of chromosome 1q21-q31 from linkage to three pedigrees affected by the pigment-dispersion syndrome. Am J Hum Genet. 1995;56:1240–3.
58. Sarafarazi M. Recent advances in molecular genetics of glaucomas. Hum Mol Genet. 1997;6:1667–77.
59. Wiggs JL, Allingham RR, Hossain A, *et al.* Genome-wide scan for adult onset primary open angle glaucoma. Hum Mol Genet. 2000;7:1109–17.
60. Furuyoshi N, Furuyoshi M, Futa R, *et al.* Ultrastructural changes in the trabecular meshwork of juvenile glaucoma. Ophthalmologica. 1997;3:140–6.
61. Stone EM, Fingert JH, Wallace LM, *et al.* Identification of a gene that causes primary open angle glaucoma. Science. 1997;275:668–70.
62. Wiggs JL, Vollrath D. Molecular and clinical evaluation of a patient hemizygous for TIGR/myocilin. Arch Ophthalmol. 2001;119:1674–8.
63. Moon S-JK, Kim H-S, Moon J-I, *et al.* Mutations of the TIGR/MYOC gene in primary open-angle glaucoma in Korea. Am J Hum Genet. 1999;64:1775–8.
64. Kim BS, Savinova OV, Reedy MV, *et al.* Targeted disruption of the myocilin gene (*MYOC*) suggests that human glaucoma-causing mutations are gain of function. Mol Cell Biol. 2001;21:7707–13.
65. Schwartz JR, Reuling FH, Feinleib M, *et al.* Twin heritability study of the effect of corticosteroids on intraocular pressure. J Med Genet. 1972;9:137–43.
66. Goldschmidt E. The heredity of glaucoma. Acta Ophthalmol (Copenh). 1973; 120:27–31.
67. Teikari JM. Genetic factors in open-angle (simple and capsular) glaucoma: a population-based twin study. Acta Ophthalmol (Copenh). 1987;65:715–20.
68. Becker B, Morton WR. Phenylthiourea taste testing and glaucoma. Arch Ophthalmol. 1964;72:323–7.
69. Wiggs JL. Complex disorders in ophthalmology. In: Gorin MB, ed. Seminars in ophthalmology. Philadelphia: WB Saunders; 1995.
70. Alward WL. The genetics of open-angle glaucoma: the story of GLC1A and myocilin. Eye 2000;14:429–36.
71. Stoilova D, Child A, Trifan OC, *et al.* Localization of a locus (*GLC1B*) for adult-onset primary open angle glaucoma to the 2cen-q13 region. Genomics. 1996;36:142–50.
72. Wirtz MK, Samples JR, Kramer PL, *et al.* Mapping a gene for adult-onset primary open-angle glaucoma to chromosome 3q. Am J Hum Genet. 1997;60:296–304.
73. Trifan OC, Traboulsi EI, Stoilova D, *et al.* A third locus (*GLC1D*) for adult-onset primary open-angle glaucoma maps to the 8q23 region. Am J Ophthalmol. 1998;126:17–28.
74. Sarfarazi M, Child A, Stoilova D, *et al.* Localization of the fourth locus (*GLC1E*) for adult-onset primary open-angle glaucoma to the 10p15-p14 region. Am J Hum Genet. 1998;62:641–52.
75. Wirtz MK, Samples JR, Rust K, *et al. GLC1F*, a new primary open-angle glaucoma locus, maps to 7q35-q36. Arch Ophthalmol. 1999;117:237–41.
76. Rezaie T, Child A, Hitchings R, *et al.* Adult-onset primary open-angle glaucoma caused by mutations in optineurin. Science. 2002;295:1077–9.
77. Yan X, Tezel G, Wax MB, Edward DP. Matrix metalloproteinases and tumor necrosis factor alpha in glaucomatous optic nerve head. Arch Ophthalmol. 2000;118: 666–73.
78. Gencik A, Gencikova A, Gerinec A. Genetic heterogeneity of congenital glaucoma. Clin Genet. 1980;17:241–8.
79. Gencikova A, Gencik A. Congenital glaucoma in gypsies from Slovakia. Hum Hered. 1982;32:270–3.
80. Buchanan PD, Rao KW, Doerr CL, Aylsworth AS. A complex translocation involving chromosomes 3, 11 and 14 with an interstitial deletion, del (14) (q13q22) in a child with congenital glaucoma and cleft lip and palate. Birth Defects. 1978;14(6C):317–22.
81. Chrousos GA, O'Neill JF, Traboulsi EI, *et al.* Ocular findings in partial trisomy 3q. A case report and review of the literature. Ophthalmic Paediatr Genet. 1988;9(2): 127–30.
82. Ishida Y, Watanabe N, Ishihara Y, Matsuda H. The 11q syndrome with mosaic partial deletion of 11q. Acta Paediatr Jpn. 1992;34:592–6.

83. Katsushima H, Kii T, Soma K, *et al*. Primary congenital glaucoma in a patient with trisomy 2q (q33-qter) and monosomy p9 (p24-pter). Case report. Arch Ophthalmol. 1987;105:323–4.

84. Mu Y, Van Dyke DL, Weiss L, Olgac S. De novo direct tandem duplication of the proximal long arm of chromosome 2: 46,XX,dir dup(2) (q11 ∞ 2q14 ∞ 2). J Med Genet. 1984;21:57–8.

85. Reardon PC, Greenstein RM, Howard RO, *et al*. Unusual mosaicism of de novo structural abnormalities and ocular anomalies in a male with trisomy 13 syndrome. Am J Med Genet. 1981;10:113–18.

86. Smith A, Watt AJ, Cummins M, *et al*. A small one-band paracentric inversion inv (4) (p15.3p16.3). Ann Genet. 1992;35:161–3.

87. Akarsu AN, Turacli E, Aktan GS, *et al*. A second locus (*GLC3B*) for primary congenital glaucoma (buphthalmos) to the 1p36 region. Hum Mol Genet. 1996;5:1199–203.

88. Stoilov I, Akarsu AN, Sarfarazi M. Identification of three different truncating mutations in cytochrome P4501B1 (CYP1B1) as the principal cause of primary congenital glaucoma (buphthalmos) in families linked to the *GLC3A* locus on chromosome 2p21. Hum Mol Genet. 1997;6:641–7.

89. Stoilov I, Akarsu AN, Alozie I, *et al*. Sequence analysis and homology modeling disrupting either the hinge region or the conserve core structures of cytochrome P4501B1. Am J Hum Genet. 1998;62:573–84.

90. Bejjani BA, Lewis RA, Tomey KF, *et al*. Mutations in *CYP1B1*, the gene for cytochrome P4501B1, are the predominant cause of primary congenital glaucoma in Saudi Arabia. Am J Hum Genet. 1998;62:325–33.

91. Bejjani BA, Stockton DW, Lewis RA, *et al*. Multiple *CYP1B1* mutations and incomplete penetrance in an inbred population segregating primary congenital glaucoma suggest frequent de novo events and a dominant modifier locus. Hum Mol Genet. 2000;9:367–74.

92. Vincent AL, Billingsley G, Buys Y, *et al*. Digenic inheritance of early-onset glaucoma: *CYP1B1*, a potential modifier gene. Am J Hum Genet. 2002;70:448–60.

93. Gifford H Jr. A clinical and pathologic study of exfoliation of the lens capsule. Am J Ophthalmol. 1958;46:508–12.

94. Mears AJ, Mirzayans F, Gould DB, *et al*. Autosomal dominant iridogoniodysgenesis anomaly maps to 6p25. Am J Hum Genet. 1996;59:1321–7.

95. Semina EV, Reiter R. Leysens NJ, *et al*. Cloning and characterization of a novel bicoid-related homeobox transcription factor gene, *RIEG*, involved in Rieger syndrome. Nat Genet. 1996;14:392–9.

96. Nishimura DY, Swiderski RE, Alward WL, *et al*. The forkhead transcription factor gene *FKHL7* is responsible for glaucoma phenotypes which map to 6p25. Nat Genet. 1998;19:140–7.

97. Smith RS, Zabaleta A, Kume T, *et al*. Haploinsufficiency of the transcription factors FOXC1 and FOXC2 results in aberrant ocular development. Hum Mol Genet. 2000;9:1021–32.

98. Lichter PR, Richards JE, Downs CA, *et al*. Cosegregation of open-angle glaucoma and the nail-patella syndrome. Am J Ophthalmol. 1997;124:506–15.

99. Vollrath D, Jaramillo-Babb VL, Clough MV, *et al*. Loss-of-function mutations in the LIM-homeodomain gene, *LMX1B*, in nail-patella syndrome. Hum Mol Genet. 1998;7:1091–8.

CHAPTER
213
Clinical Examination of Glaucoma

M. FRAN SMITH • J. WILLIAM DOYLE

DEFINITION
- Glaucoma is a type of optic neuropathy associated with characteristic optic disc damage, which may result in certain visual field loss patterns, at least in part secondary to suboptimal intraocular pressure. The clinical examination is vital to make this diagnosis.

KEY FEATURES
- Tonometry to record accurate intraocular pressures.
- Gonioscopy to identify any angle pathology.
- Optic disc examination.
- Nerve fiber layer analysis.
- Visual field examination.

ASSOCIATED FEATURE
- The role of tonography.

INTRODUCTION

Once, glaucoma was considered a single disease entity characterized by optic nerve damage and visual loss secondary to elevated intraocular pressure. It is now understood that many different ocular disorders and processes may result in that specific pattern of optic disc damage and visual field loss called *glaucoma*. The clinical examination is vital to differentiate the mechanisms associated with a particular case of glaucoma.

The clinical examination in a patient who has possible glaucoma is similar to the ocular examination of any new patient. A detailed history must be taken, a thorough slit-lamp evaluation of anterior segment structures must be carried out, and special attention must be directed to the key aspects described below.

TONOMETRY

The importance of intraocular pressure (IOP) assessment in the evaluation of glaucoma has been understood for over 100 years. Digital estimation of globe firmness yielded to instrumental (Schiøtz) tonometry over the first 20 years of the twentieth century. Today, the Goldmann applanation tonometer provides the gold standard for the clinical measurement of IOP.

A tonometer uses certain physical principles to measure pressure within the globe. Basically, the force necessary to deform a globe is directly related to the pressure within that globe. Three styles of tonometer currently are in use. Indentation, or high-displacement, tonometers utilize a plunger to indent the cornea by a variable amount. This indentation displaces a significant volume of intraocular fluid at the time of corneal deformation and results in a near doubling of the IOP. Conversion tables, in turn, estimate the original IOP from the indentation tonometric value obtained. Applanation, or low-displacement, tonometers raise IOP negligibly, because they subject the eye to sufficient force only to flatten the cornea. The amount of force required to achieve a constant degree of corneal flattening is converted into IOP values. Noncontact tonometers flatten the cornea using a puff of air, and the time required to flatten the cornea is correlated to estimated IOP. Each form of tonometer has a place in the examination of eyes.

Indentation Tonometry

Schiøtz, in 1905, described the indentation tonometer (Fig. 213-1). The plunger freely moves and is encased in a shaft that ends in a footplate, which rests on the anesthetized cornea. The movement of a lever attached to the plunger reflects the degree to which the cornea is indented—a softer globe shows greater indentation and greater lever movement across the upper scale. Schiøtz tonometers all conform to American Academy of Ophthalmology standardized physical specifications. Thus, use of the tonometer on a steel test block results in a scale reading of zero. Generally, using the standardized plunger weight of 5.5g, normal eyes give scale readings of 5–8 units, and glaucomatous high-pressure eyes read less than 4 units. The provided conversion table is used to convert scale readings into IOP readings (mmHg or kPa).

Multiple potential sources of error are present in the use of Schiøtz tonometry. The patient must be comfortable and supine. The lids must be wide open. The examiner must take great care to ensure no external pressure is applied to the globe. Otherwise, a falsely low reading (high IOP) may be obtained. Another potential source of inaccuracy arises from differences in ocular rigidity among different eyes. Some eyes are more distensible than others; so, although the conversion tables take into account an average ocular rigidity, eyes that have a low ocular rigidity may give a falsely high Schiøtz scale reading, which is then con-

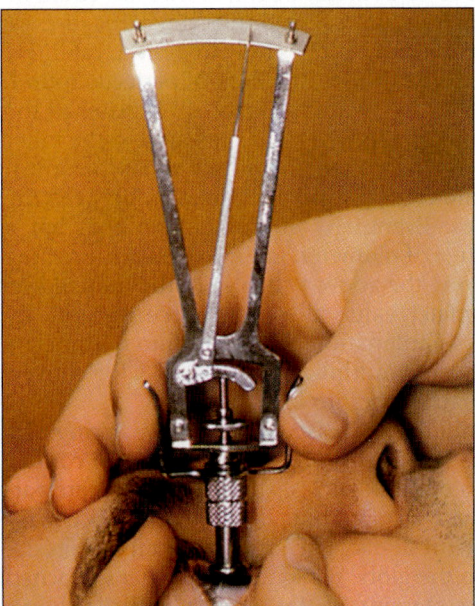

FIG. 213-1 ■ The Schiøtz tonometer in use. Notice the patient's reclining position.

verted into a falsely low IOP reading. The physician always must applanate eyes known to have low scleral rigidity. Such eyes include those that have high myopia,[1] osteogenesis imperfecta,[2] history of strong miotic (especially cholinesterase inhibitor[3]) therapy, history of retinal detachment (especially vitrectomy surgery),[4,5] and history of vasodilatation therapy.[6] Similarly, the physician must recognize that high hyperopia,[3] extreme myopia,[6] long-standing glaucoma,[6] macular degeneration,[7] and vasoconstrictor therapy are associated with high scleral rigidity. A falsely low Schiøtz reading (falsely high IOP) may be measured in these eyes.

Two other sources of error occur using Schiøtz tonometry. These include the variable expulsion of intraocular blood during the indentation[8] and extremes in corneal shape or thickness. Specifically, the thin cornea of a patient with keratoconus may be associated with a falsely low IOP.[9] Indentation of a thickened cornea results in a greater displacement of intraocular fluid than occurs when a regular cornea is indented. Consequently, a falsely high IOP reading may be obtained. A steep cornea also may cause a falsely high IOP reading.[10] Because there are so many potential sources of error, Schiøtz tonometry largely has been replaced by applanation tonometry. Goldmann or, when portability is an issue, Perkins or Tono-Pen tonometers are popular. However, familiarity with the Schiøtz instrument remains useful. It is the most affordable instrument available for IOP estimation. As such, it is still found in many emergency rooms. Additionally, it may be sterilized and used under sterile conditions in the operating room (for example, if IOP needs to be established immediately prior to intraocular surgery, either digital pressure or the Schiøtz tonometer may be used).

Applanation Tonometry

Unlike in Schiøtz tonometry, in which a relatively large corneal displacement occurs, in applanation tonometry only enough force is applied to flatten the cornea, disturbing relatively little aqueous. Two types of applanation tonometry exist. In constant-force applanation tonometry, a constant force is applied to the cornea, and IOP is estimated by measurement of the diameter of the flattened corneal area. The Maklakov tonometer is based on this principle. However, the remainder of this section deals with variable-force tonometry, because investigators in Western developed countries are more familiar with it. The Goldmann tonometer is the prime example of a variable-force tonometer. Based on Fick's law, which states that pressure within a sphere is equal to the force needed to flatten part of the sphere divided by the area flattened ($P = F/A$), the Goldmann tonometer measures IOP simply and reproducibly.

Many variables had to be addressed before Fick's law could be applied to the applanation and pressure measurement of eyes. After all, Fick's law theoretically applies only to perfect, infinitely thin, dry spheres. The cornea is not dry, thin, or perfectly round. Thus, adjustments had to be made for force application to the corneal outer surface (although IOP is directed against the inner corneal surface) for corneal astigmatism and variable corneal and scleral stiffness, and for tear capillary attraction between the tonometer and cornea. Eventually, it was determined that a corneal applanation area of diameter 3.06mm best achieved the necessary balance among the above variables in the human eye. Also, use of this diameter value allows direct conversion, by multiplication by 10, of applanation gram force into millimeters of mercury of pressure, or multiplication by 0.133 for conversion of applanation gram force into kPa.

The Goldmann tonometer consists of a sensitive spring balance attached to a plastic biprism (Fig. 213-2), which on contact with the cornea creates two half circles. These semicircles are particularly easy to view with a cobalt blue light after fluorescein application in the ocular cul-de-sac. The examiner then adjusts the spring force applied to the globe using the tonometer's attached dial, so that the inner margins of the biprism semicircles just

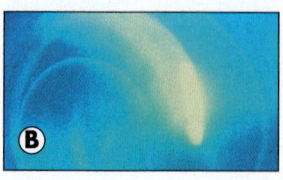
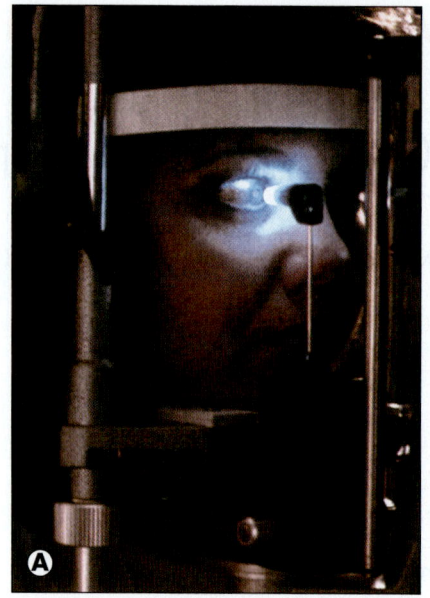

FIG. 213-2 ■ The Goldmann tonometer. A, The patient at the instrument. B, Biprism semicircles just touch.

touch. When these inner margins touch, 3.06mm of the cornea is applanated and approximately 0.05μl of aqueous volume is displaced. As a result of the small quantity of aqueous displaced, the measured pressure (read from the dial) is probably less than 3% higher than IOP prior to applanation. However, excess fluorescein application may result in a falsely high IOP, and too little or no fluorescein use may produce a falsely low IOP.[11]

Other factors may cause error in IOP measurement using Goldmann tonometry; these include abnormal corneal thickness and curvature, excess contact time, and improper instrument calibration. Generally, corneas thickened from edema are associated with falsely low IOP readings. Those thickened secondary to other processes (i.e., from increased collagen fibrils) may give a falsely high IOP reading.[12] Thin corneas usually give falsely low readings.[12] Astigmatism greater than 3–4D causes an IOP measurement error of approximately 1mmHg (0.13kPa) per 4D.[13] This potential error is avoided by using the average of two pressure readings, one taken with mires vertical and the other with mires horizontal.[13] Alternatively, to avoid measurement error secondary to astigmatism, the tonometer biprisms may be aligned so that the red line on the prism holder is opposite the known corneal axis of least astigmatism.[14] Another source of error is excess contact time between tonometer and eye, which is associated with a falsely low IOP and is avoided easily by using a "light" touch. A light touch has the additional advantage of sparing the eye iatrogenic corneal epithelial defects.[14] Finally, to avoid any errors from improper instrument calibration, at least biyearly instrument calibration must be carried out.

If the above caveats are kept in mind, the Goldmann tonometer will provide decades of reliable IOP measurements. Repeated, accurate IOP measurements, with an error of about 2mmHg (0.27kPa) among various examiners or at different times, may be expected.[15] Care must be taken to wipe the tonometer tip with 3% hydrogen peroxide or 70% isopropyl alcohol before it is placed on a patient's eye.[16] Such precautions destroy any human immunodeficiency virus present and, presumably, adenovirus and hepatitis virus, as well. Corneal epithelial defects are prevented if the tip is wiped dry with a tissue after disinfection.

The Perkins and Draeger applanation tonometers are both portable, hand-held, Goldmann-style tonometers with built-in biprisms.[17,18] They require some skill to use effectively. The Perkins tonometer is probably as accurate as the Goldmann tonometer and may be used on reclining patients (Fig. 213-3). The Draeger tonometer is not used as widely as the Perkins. Another variable-force style of applanation tonometer is the pneumotonometer (Fig. 213-4). It is a Mackay–Marg-type

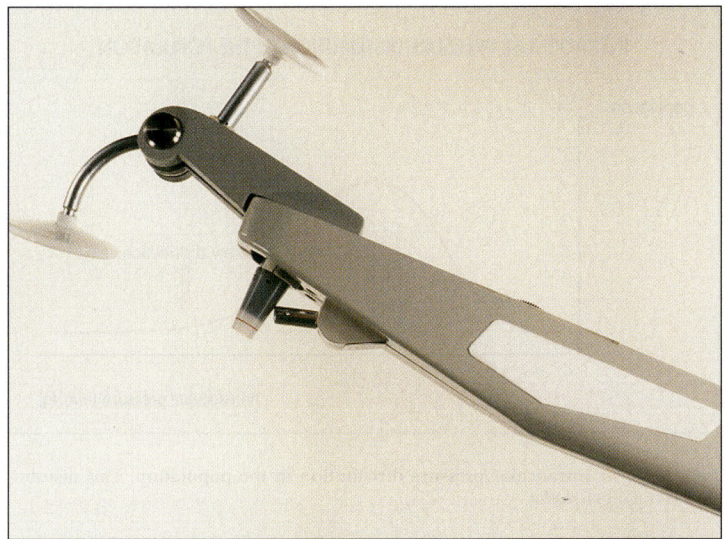

FIG. 213-3 ■ **The Perkins tonometer.** This picture demonstrates its handheld portability.

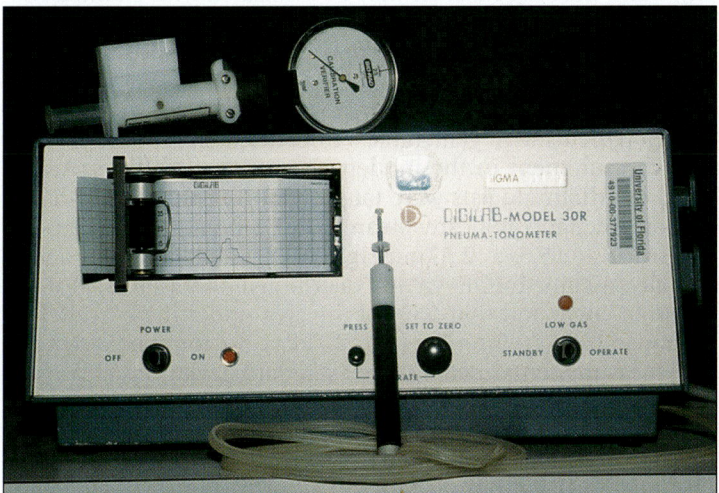

FIG. 213-4 ■ **The pneumotonometer.**

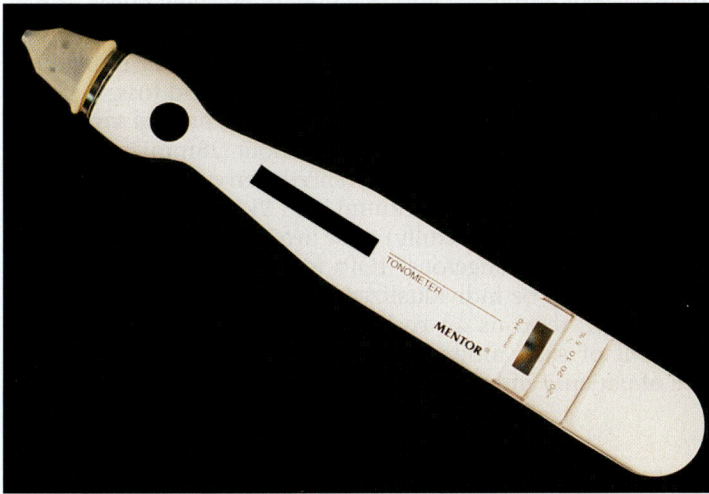

FIG. 213-5 ■ **The Tono-Pen.** It is extremely portable and easy to use.

tonometer. In Mackay–Marg-style tonometers, the force measured is that necessary to keep the plunger's flat plate flush with its surrounding sleeve, despite IOP against corneal flattening. The pneumotonometer assesses IOP via a central sensing device controlled by air pressure, while the force required to bend the cornea is transferred to a surrounding sleeve. The pneu-

motonometer is not portable, and the base unit is sufficiently large to discourage room-to-room transfer. The correlation between the pneumotonometer and the Goldmann instrument is good, but IOPs measured using the former tend to be overestimated.[19] However, unlike any of the Goldmann-style tonometers, the pneumotonometer may be used to estimate IOP in eyes that have scarred and irregular corneas.[20]

Of the Mackay–Marg-style tonometers, perhaps the Tono-Pen has gained the widest acceptance (Fig. 213-5). It is highly portable and easier to use than any other portable IOP device. A strain gauge is used to create an electrical impulse as the footplate flattens the cornea. A microprocessor chip senses appropriate force curves, calculates the average of 4–10 readings, and then produces a final digital readout with variability percentages. Most investigators feel it gives accurate IOP readings in the normal range but may overestimate IOP in the low and underestimate IOP in the high ranges.[21,22] It reportedly measures IOP fairly accurately through a soft contact lens.[23] It is a useful device for the measurement of pressure in patients for whom applanation tonometry is impossible because of a scarred or irregular cornea.

Noncontact Tonometry

No discussion of tonometry is complete without mention of "puff tonometry." In noncontact tonometry, a puff of air is used to flatten the cornea, with the length of time required to flatten it, as measured by an optoelectronics system, correlated with the IOP. This length of time is on the scale of milliseconds. Thus, the ocular pulse may present a significant source of 1–3mmHg (0.13–0.40kPa) variability in pressure.[24] Still, noncontact tonometry is fairly accurate in the normal range of IOP.[25] In addition, the availability of a handheld Pulsair noncontact tonometer may make screening efforts by paramedical professionals easier, because there is no risk of infection spread or corneal abrasion when using it.

ROLE OF TONOGRAPHY

Tonography measures IOP over the course of 4 minutes while a Schiøtz tonometer rests on the eye. Based on how IOP drops over this period (secondary to tonometer load displacement of aqueous), an estimate of the ease with which aqueous leaves the eye is made. This estimate is called *facility of outflow*, or C. For many years, tonography and estimation of outflow facility was considered a useful adjunct to routine clinical examination of patients who had open-angle glaucoma. It was used, also, to confirm positive provocative tests in angle-closure glaucoma and to diagnose outflow abnormalities, which may be masked by decreased aqueous production.

Grant originated the technique in 1950.[26] He reported his results on 600 normal and glaucomatous eyes and felt that the reduced outflow facility seen in glaucomatous eyes accounted for the high IOP seen in glaucoma. Accordingly, Grant was one of the first physicians to publish proof that glaucoma was a disease of inadequate outflow and not of fluid overproduction. He also proposed that reduced C values could be a useful predictor in eyes suspected of being glaucomatous.[26] However, most now feel that tonography has little diagnostic value in any individual patient. Facility of outflow values may overlap considerably between normal and glaucomatous groups.[27,28] Although a mean C value in normal eyes of 0.24–0.28μl/min per mmHg (0.03–0.037μl/min per kPa) is recognized, there is a wide range of normal values (0.15–0.34μl/min per mmHg or 0.02–0.045μl/min per kPa), and up to one third of patients with glaucoma may have a C value greater than 0.18μl/min per mmHg (>0.024μl/min per kPa).

Despite these concerns, it is useful to be familiar with the principles behind tonography. Grant[26] attached an electronic tonometer to a paper strip recorder, which recorded the drop in scale units over time with the tonometer set remaining in contact with an eye. Patients with normal eyes show a slow, steady decline in IOP over 4 minutes. In patients with glaucoma, presumably secondary to decreased outflow capabilities through the conventional system, there is a smaller decline in IOP over 4 minutes. This ease of outflow, or facility of outflow coefficient (C), is estimated by dividing the change in globe aqueous volume (V) by the time interval (T) for which the tonometer rests on the eye and the IOP change (ΔP) in this time (Equation 213-1).

Equation 213-1

$$C = \frac{V}{T(\Delta P)}$$

Friedenwald had established that a certain increasing volume of aqueous is displaced by indentation tonometry over several minutes. Grant's formula simply utilizes this fact and others to arrive at an estimation of outflow facility. In practice, however, tonographic equipment comes with tables which estimate C based on initial and final tonometer readings and the quantity of tonometer weight applied over 4 minutes.

Tonography and the resultant C valve may be influenced by multiple factors. These include IOP, decrease in aqueous production secondary to tonometer-related IOP elevation (so-called *pseudofacility*), increase in episcleral venous pressure secondary to tonometer weight, and variable ocular rigidity. Thus, the final derived C value does not reflect rate of aqueous outflow only. To a variable degree, C is influenced by some or all of these other factors. Nonetheless, to call C the *coefficient of aqueous outflow* is a useful oversimplification for most purposes, and tonography even today has a place in some research settings.

INTRAOCULAR PRESSURE

Numerous avenues are open to explore IOP in the human eye, and the final IOP measured is influenced by many factors. Young children tend to have lower IOPs, with an average IOP of 8.4 ± 0.6mmHg (1.12 ± 0.08kPa) in infants under 1 year of age.[29] This may be attributed partially to the influence of anesthetic agents necessary to obtain a measurement in babies. Conversely, some investigators feel that IOP tends to rise with age, perhaps related to decreased facility of outflow through the aged trabecular meshwork. This is despite an associated decrease in aqueous production with age.[30]

Generally, IOP tends to be similar between sexes, although some investigators have noted an increase in IOP in women after the menopause.[31] Black patients (African–Americans and African–Caribbeans) may run slightly higher IOPs than Caucasians.[32] Those patients who have a positive family history of glaucoma tend to have higher IOPs than those who have a negative family history.[31]

One study noted that myopes who have greater axial lengths tend to have higher IOPs,[33] although this remains unconfirmed.

It is well established that normal IOP varies by 5mmHg (0.7kPa) or more during the day. In glaucoma patients who receive no treatment, diurnal variation may be in the range 10–30mmHg (1.3–4.0kPa),[34] which stresses that excessive emphasis must not be placed on a single normal pressure reading in a patient who might have glaucoma.

When changing from a sitting to a reclining position, IOP may increase by up to 9mmHg (1.2kPa).[35] This change is more common in patients affected by glaucoma, especially normal-tension glaucoma. Although prolonged physical activity may be associated with lower IOP,[36] anything that causes a short-term strain, such as a Valsalva maneuver, may cause a jump in IOP.[37] Hard blinking may cause a rise in IOP from 10–90mmHg (1.3–12.0kPa).[38]

As touched on briefly in the discussion of age influences above, most anesthetic agents result in a drop in IOP. Ketamine[39] and succinylcholine[40] are exceptions to this statement and usually cause an increase in IOP. When an attempt is made to rule out congenital glaucoma, the surgeon must be careful not to place the child under a general anesthetic, because a falsely low IOP reading may be obtained. Ketamine is the agent of choice in

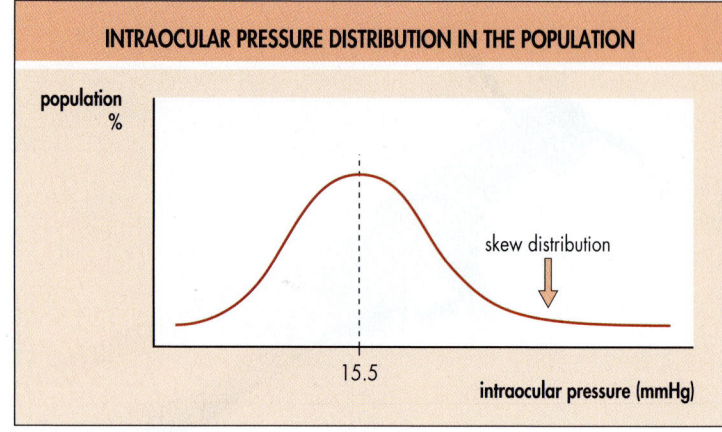

FIG. 213-6 ▪ Intraocular pressure distribution in the population. This distribution is not a bell curve.

such cases. Also, midazolam seems not to result in IOP elevation or depression.

Systemic hypertension,[41] diabetes,[42] hyperthyroidism,[43] obesity,[44] and Cushing's disease may be associated with elevated IOP. Alcohol[45] and marijuana[46] use may lower IOP, but caffeine[47] has virtually no effect. Tobacco use may be correlated positively with higher IOPs.[48]

Before moving on to further points in the clinical examination of patients with glaucoma, a brief discussion of the value of IOP measurement in the modern examination follows. At one time, ophthalmologists were taught that IOP was a "be-all and end-all" in glaucoma care. Mean IOP in whole populations was measured at 15.5 ± 2.57mmHg (2.1 ± 0.34kPa).[49] Physicians initially assumed IOP values distributed themselves along a gaussian curve and that 95% of the area under the curve fell in the range 10.5–20.5mmHg (1.4–2.7kPa). So, for many years any IOP measurements greater than 2 standard deviations above this mean (i.e., >21mmHg [>2.8kPa]) were considered abnormal, and the ophthalmologist contemplated treatment as necessary to lower IOP back to normal, or less than 21mmHg (<2.8kPa). Of course, today it is understood that the treatment of glaucoma is not nearly so simple. First, IOP distribution does not lie along a perfect Gaussian curve but has a skewed tail toward higher IOPs (Fig. 213-6).[50] For this reason alone, no cut off exists for normal versus abnormal IOP. In addition, most investigators now feel that the best management protocol for glaucoma patients involves setting an individual target IOP based on an individual's particular extent of nerve damage and visual field loss. A patient who has a relatively healthy optic nerve and normal visual field may do well with a target IOP of about 28mmHg (3.9kPa). Another patient who suffers advanced nerve and field damage may need a target IOP of 12mmHg (1.9kPa), if further glaucomatous damage is (hopefully) to be avoided. There can be no absolute "safe" or "dangerous" IOPs for the general population—IOP goals must be individualized for each patient. Despite these caveats, IOP remains an easily measurable value. Accurate assessment of each individual's IOP is indispensable, if proper care of patients with glaucoma is to ensue.

GONIOSCOPY

Following a detailed anterior segment examination and IOP measurement, gonioscopy is performed on all glaucoma suspects. Gonioscopy is the technique used by clinicians to view the anterior chamber angle. Although a challenge for the novice, it provides vital information to help the clinician determine the type of glaucoma present. Only after an accurate diagnosis is made can appropriate therapy be instituted. Incorrect diagnoses, made by clinicians who neglect to examine the angle, may result in improper therapy.

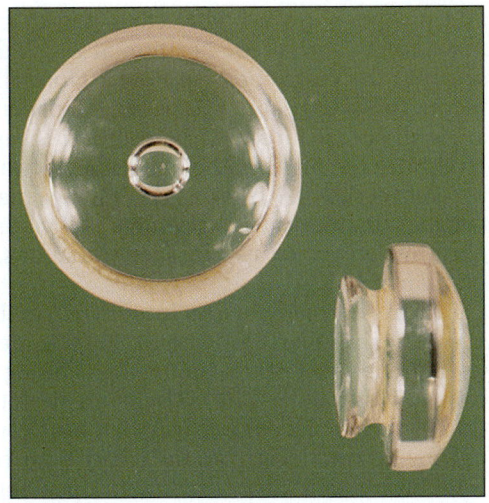

FIG. 213-7 ▪ The Koeppe lens. This lens is used most frequently for pediatric gonioscopy during examination under anesthesia.

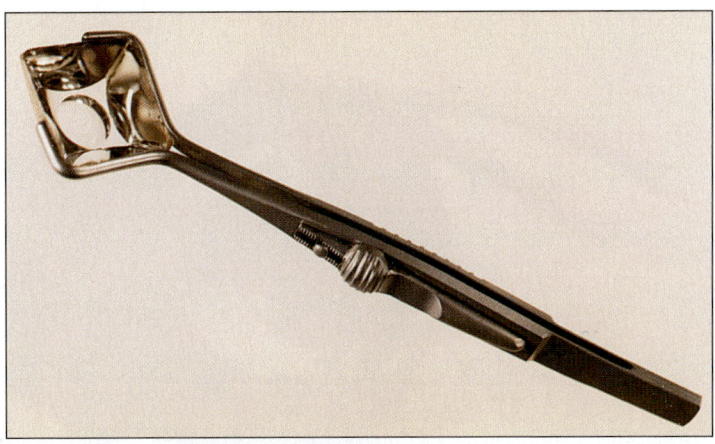

FIG. 213-8 ▪ The Zeiss lens and Unger holder.

The anterior chamber angle is not directly visible with slit-lamp examination. As light passes from the angle to the cornea, its angle of incidence is greater than the critical angle for a cornea–air interface (46°). Thus, it is reflected normally back into the eye. Gonioscopy utilizes a contact lens to neutralize corneal refractive power, which, in turn, allows either direct or indirect visualization of angle structures.

Direct Gonioscopy

The Koeppe lens is used for direct gonioscopy (Fig. 213-7). It is a 50D concave lens which comes in adult (large diameter and smaller radius of posterior curvature) and pediatric (small diameter and larger radius of posterior curvature) versions. The patient is placed in a reclining position. Methylcellulose is applied to the underside of the contact lens. The eye is anesthetized topically, and the lens is applied to the eye. An examiner uses a hand biomicroscope with 320× magnification and a separate light source to view the angle directly.

Such an angle view is useful in that the image seen is a real one (not a reflection). If an eye has a particularly convex iris with narrowed angle, the examiner can vary the direction of view easily, to peer up and over the iris into the angle. Also, if a Koeppe lens is placed on each eye, the examiner may view both angles almost simultaneously. By switching views back and forth between eyes, determination of any subtle differences in angle depth or morphology is made. A Koeppe-style lens is used whenever goniotomy is performed.

Some disadvantages exist to the use of the Koeppe lens. The first is inconvenience if the patient has to be moved to a viewing room, in which the biomicroscope is available and the patient can be reclined. Second, the biomicroscope is somewhat unwieldy and heavy and often requires support by a cord from the ceiling. Third, the magnification obtained using this lens is suboptimal. Last, because the patient lies flat, the angle may appear artificially deep.

Indirect Gonioscopy

Two basic styles of mirrored goniolenses exist. The first, typified by the Zeiss lens, has a 9mm corneal segment and a radius of curvature (7.72mm) approximately that of most corneas (Fig. 213-8). Thus, the lens easily couples to the cornea, using just a drop of anesthetic (or, better, a drop of high-viscosity artificial tear preparation) on the lens surface. The Zeiss lens comes with a holding fork, the Unger holder. Other Zeiss-style lenses include the Posner lens (handle attached to lens) and Sussman (finger-held) lens. All of these lenses have in each of four quadrants a mirror tilted at 64°, for ease of viewing the angle 360°. The angle view seen is indirect, through the mirror.

The patient is seated at the slit lamp. After topical anesthetic has been applied to the eye, the lens is touched to the eye, but

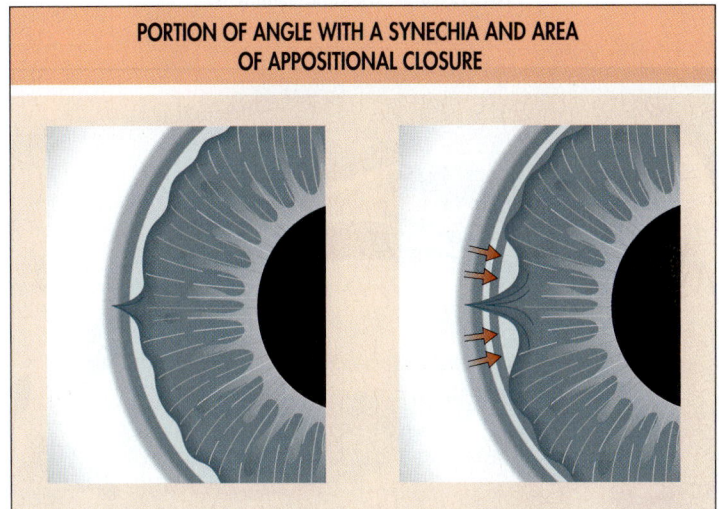

PORTION OF ANGLE WITH A SYNECHIA AND AREA OF APPOSITIONAL CLOSURE

FIG. 213-9 ▪ Portion of angle with a synechia and area of appositional closure. Angle view with and without compression gonioscopy.

barely. This allows for an undistorted angle view. Most parts of open angles are viewed with this lens easily. If the examiner finds it difficult to examine one part of the angle, the patient may be asked to look toward the mirror in use (i.e., away from that part of the angle being examined). Typically, that portion of angle comes into view. Alternatively, if the angle appears narrowed, an indentation or "compression" gonioscopy may be carried out.[51] With this technique, gentle pressure is applied to the lens center while the suspicious portion of angle is viewed using a narrow slit beam. This extraordinarily useful technique allows easy distinction between appositional angle closure and synechial closure (Fig. 213-9). Thus, if previously hidden structures, such as trabecular meshwork, become visible upon pressure application, then the:

- Area of angle closure is only appositional
- Angle closure attack may be broken temporarily by this physical opening of the chamber angle
- Laser iridectomy may allow a return to normal pressures (versus cases of synechial closure, which often eventually require trabeculectomy).

The other type of indirect goniolens is the Goldmann lens, which may have a single mirror 12mm high and tilted 62°. Other Goldmann lenses have additional mirrors at different angles for fundus examination (Fig. 213-10). A key difference is the posterior lens diameter of 12mm with a posterior radius of curvature of 7.38mm. A viscous solution of methylcellulose must be used to couple this lens to the cornea. Many examiners find it easier to use these lenses because the lens tends to "suck" onto the cornea, which negates the need to apply the lens to the eye

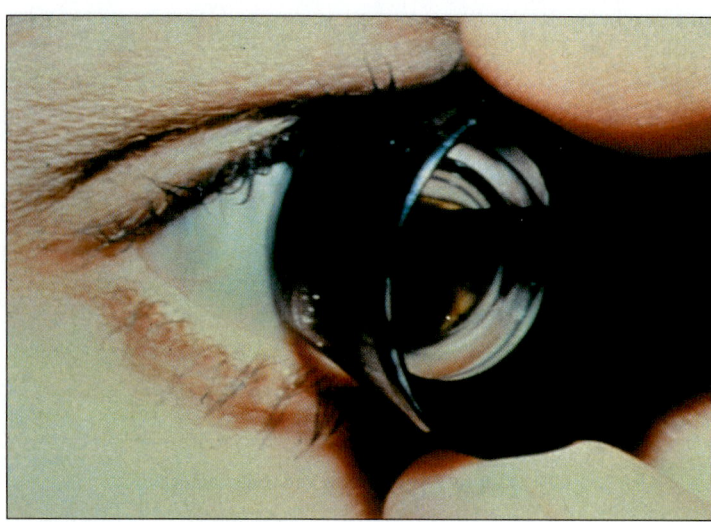

FIG. 213-10 ■ The Goldmann lens.

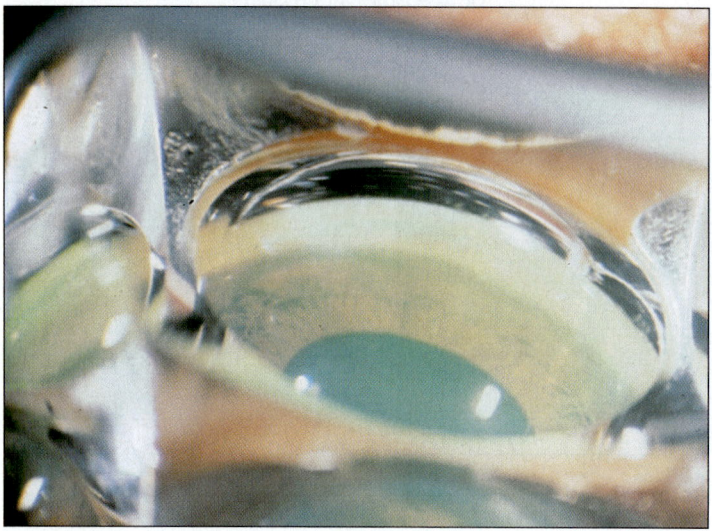

FIG. 213-11 ■ **The normal anterior chamber angle.** This is viewed through the Zeiss lens. Notice the ciliary body band, scleral spur, and trabecular meshwork.

with "just the right amount of force." Also, the taller mirror of this lens makes it easier to view over convex irises, especially if the patient is instructed to look at the mirror. However, the methylcellulose may be messy to clean up and may prevent a further good ocular examination by the initial or subsequent examiner. Also, this lens' large posterior diameter and short radius of curvature prevent the luxury of indentation gonioscopy.

Advantages of indirect gonioscopy over direct gonioscopy are several. Both the Zeiss-style lenses and the Goldmann lens are easier to use than the Koeppe lens. Indirect gonioscopy enjoys excellent optics and magnification at the slit lamp. With the Zeiss lens, the physician has the ability to perform indentation gonioscopy.

Gonioscopic Angle Appearance

Normal anterior chamber angles have four basic landmarks. Starting posteriorly at the base of the iris and moving anteriorly, the ciliary body, scleral spur, trabecular meshwork, and Schwalbe's line may be identified (Fig. 213-11).

When the gonioscopic examination is begun, the iris contour is examined initially. This portion of the examination is especially important in cases of plateau iris and pigmentary glaucoma, as discussed later. Most irides have a slight forward convexity. Highly hyperopic eyes may have more iris convexity. Flat or even mildly concave iris contours may be seen in myopic eyes and aphakes. Some patients who have pigmentary glaucoma

and myopia show a highly characteristic concave iris contour. Apart from contour, the position at which the iris appears to insert into the ciliary body is noted. Normally, insertion appears below the scleral spur. However, in patients with plateau iris angle-closure glaucoma, iris insertion is just at the scleral spur level, with the plane of the iris further forward to the level of trabecular meshwork. Thus, angle drainage may be blocked by this peculiar anatomical arrangement. Obviously, a peripheral iridectomy serves no use in such situations, except to rule out pupillary block.

The iris normally inserts into the ciliary body. The next angle structure, the ciliary body band, may be identified easily by following a narrow slit beam of light along the iris toward the cornea. This band's width is dependent on the location of insertion of the iris. Its color is usually dark brown.

Moving anteriorly from the ciliary body band, the scleral spur is the next identifiable structure in open angles. The scleral spur is seen as a thick, white band between the ciliary body and trabecular meshwork. It represents the posterior portion of the scleral sulcus. Occasionally, thin iris processes extend from the iris root across the scleral spur. If 360° of scleral spur can be identified, then no angle closure is present.

In front of the scleral spur is pigmented or functional trabecular meshwork. Posterior pigmented trabecular meshwork is that portion of the eye's drain through which primary aqueous outflow passes. Actually, newborns have very little to no pigment in this portion of the meshwork. As the body ages, variable amounts of pigment accumulate here. At this level, much pathology may be found in some of the secondary forms of glaucoma (see below).

Anterior to the pigmented meshwork, often a nonpigmented, or anterior, meshwork band may be identified, just prior to Schwalbe's line, the final major angle landmark. Schwalbe's line marks the anterior start of the drainage angle, and the posterior-most portion of translucent cornea. Anatomically, it is a fine ridge, often with a smattering of pigment on it. As detailed above, many investigators prefer to identify angle structures by moving from posterior iris root to anterior Schwalbe's line. However, an anterior–posterior "check" system may be used if any landmarks are unclear. Specifically, if a thin, three-dimensional slit beam is focused on cornea, at Schwalbe's line this slit beam collapses into a two-dimensional line that runs posteriorly through angle structures as noted above. This check system is especially useful to confirm a diagnosis of angle-closure glaucoma.

Angle Grading

Following angle examination, angle depth is recorded or graded in one of the accepted standard fashions—Shaffer system, Scheie system, or Spaeth system.

SHAFFER SYSTEM. The Shaffer grading system is perhaps the simplest.[52] Essentially, angle depth is estimated by the geometric angle formed between the posterior corneal wall and anterior iris face. A closed angle (0° geometric angle) is graded 0; narrow angles (0–10° and 10–20° geometric angles) are graded I and II, respectively; moderately open angles (30°) are graded III; and wide open angles (>40°) are graded IV (Fig. 213-12).

SCHEIE SYSTEM. Alternatively, some ophthalmologists use the Scheie system to record angle depth.[53] Unfortunately, angle depth is graded in a fashion exactly opposite to that of the Shaffer system. A wide open angle is graded I, a moderately open angle with a view just to the scleral spur II, a narrow angle with view of anterior meshwork only III, and a closed angle IV. To avoid confusion, the ophthalmologist must note which gonioscopic grading system is used, if either the Scheie or Shaffer system is chosen.

SPAETH SYSTEM. The Spaeth system is perhaps the most elaborate of angle grading systems and the one preferred.[54] It forces the examiner to examine three critical elements. First, to assess where the iris apparently inserts:

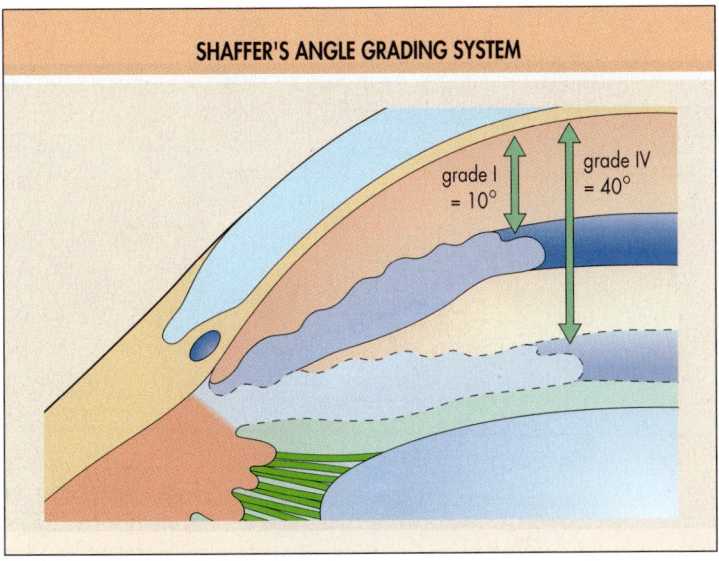

FIG. 213-12 ■ Shaffer's angle grading system.

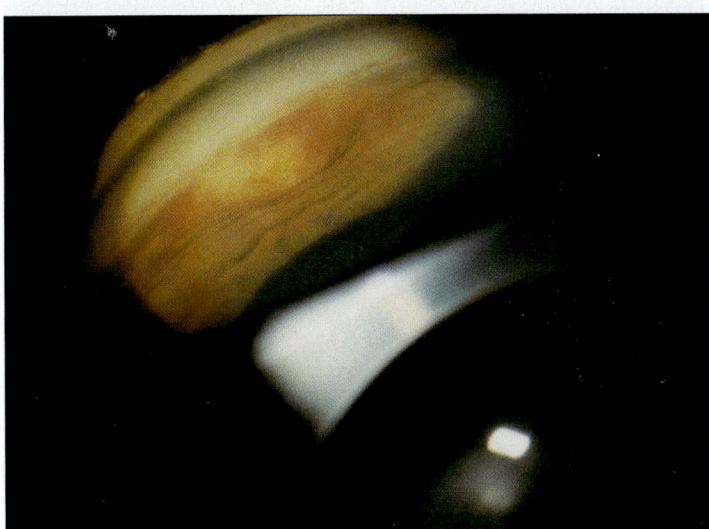

FIG. 213-13 ■ Uneven angle depth secondary to an iris tumor.

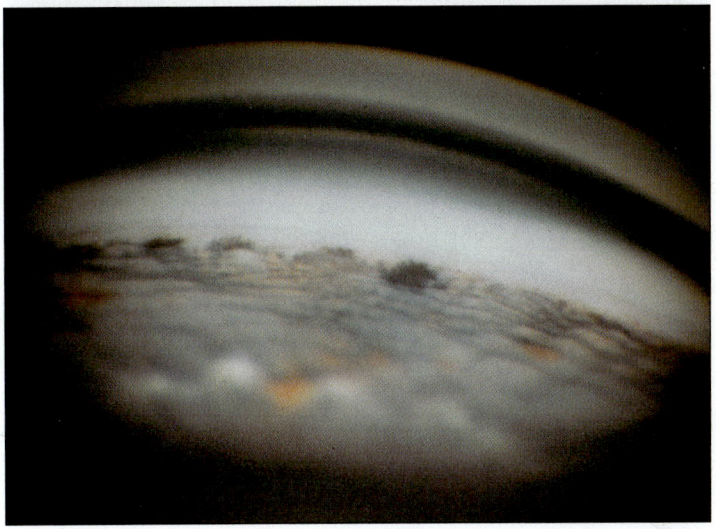

FIG. 213-14 ■ Small irregular peripheral anterior synechiae. After argon laser trabeculoplasty.

- A: Anterior to trabecular meshwork
- B: Behind Schwalbe's line
- C: At scleral spur
- D: Deeply, with visible ciliary body
- E: Extremely deeply

Second, to estimate the geometric angle between cornea and iris (as with the Shaffer system), in the range 10–50°. Third, to establish the peripheral iris contour as:

- s: Steep and convex
- r: Regular (i.e., flat to mildly convex)
- q: Queer and concave

A Spaeth system classification of a moderately open angle with apparent iris insertion at the scleral spur, but which opens fully with a view of the ciliary body with compression gonioscopy, may read (C)D40r. Classification of a potentially occludable, narrow angle with a steep iris insertion just behind Schwalbe's line, may read B20s.

COMPARISON OF GRADING SYSTEMS. These three grading systems all are carried out using a gonioscopic lens. No acceptable substitute exists for an actual examination of the eye's angle. Van Herick[55] described a technique in which, theoretically, angle depth may be estimated from slit-beam examination of the far temporal cornea and anterior chamber. A thin slit beam is focused perpendicular to the temporal cornea. Anterior chamber depth is estimated relative to corneal thickness from a 60° viewing angle. A Shaffer grade I angle corresponds to an anterior chamber depth of less than one fourth of the corneal thickness, grade II and III angles correspond to one fourth to one half of the corneal thickness anterior chamber depth, and a grade IV angle corresponds to one half to full corneal thickness chamber depth. However, these estimations may miss closed and significantly narrowed angles. Additionally, use of this system instead of a gonioscopic lens means the examiner may miss potentially pertinent angle pathology (see below).

Angle Pathology

First, the angle is examined to determine if it is closed, could be closed, or widely open. Most investigators feel that if scleral spur is visible (Spaeth C–E categories), imminent closure is unlikely. If a Spaeth A or B angle is seen, the angle is either closed (with synechiae), or closure is imminent. Potential closure of a currently open angle is particularly possible if a uniformly B10–20s type angle is seen. Of course, angle depth may not be uniform for 360°. Commonly, the superior angle is the narrowest and the inferior angle the most open. Unevenness in angle depth or areas of partial closure may result from old peripheral anterior synechiae (PAS) in some quadrants. Also, a posterior iris cyst or

tumor (Fig. 213-13), ciliary body tumor, or partial lens subluxation may result in uneven angle depth. If an angle is closed partially with PAS as a result of previous angle-closure attacks or from some secondary forms of glaucoma and treatment is not instituted, full angle closure and painfully high IOP may result.

Adhesions of iris to trabecular meshwork, PAS effectively block aqueous outflow where they form. In a small, irregular fashion, they frequently may form after argon laser trabeculoplasty (Fig. 213-14). Most feel this type of PAS is quite different in effect from the broad-based, aqueous outflow–blocking PAS seen in angle-closure and some secondary forms of glaucoma. In primary angle-closure glaucoma, synechiae usually form superiorly first (Fig. 213-15), whereas PAS of uveitic glaucoma form inferiorly first. These synechiae are broad-based, tenting adhesions across the full angle depth, which may start as a build-up of exudates in the trabecular meshwork. In neovascular glaucoma, first a fibrovascular membrane lines the angle; then broad, vessel-filled synechiae form. The PAS of iridocorneal endothelial syndrome are characterized by their extension to cornea, anterior to Schwalbe's line. Finally, PAS may form after trauma.

After trauma, angle examination may reveal much. As noted, mild trauma may be associated with iritis and PAS formation. Moderate blunt trauma may produce tears between the longitudinal and circular muscles of the ciliary body, which result in

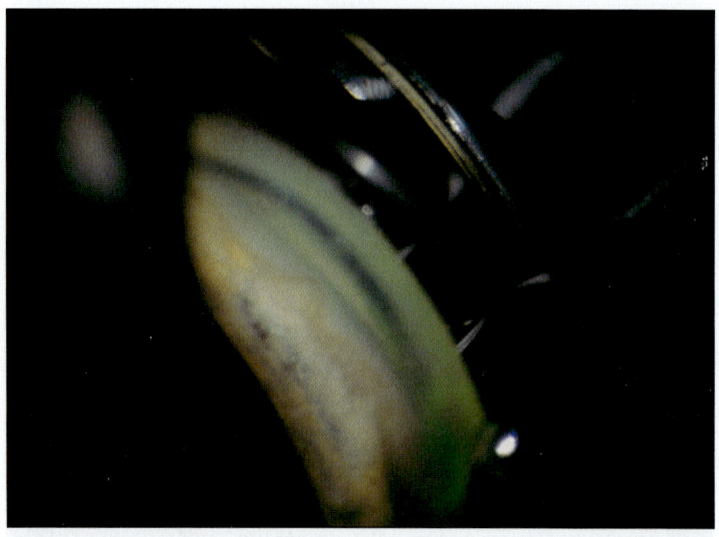

FIG. 213-15 ▌ Broad peripheral anterior synechiae with angle closure.

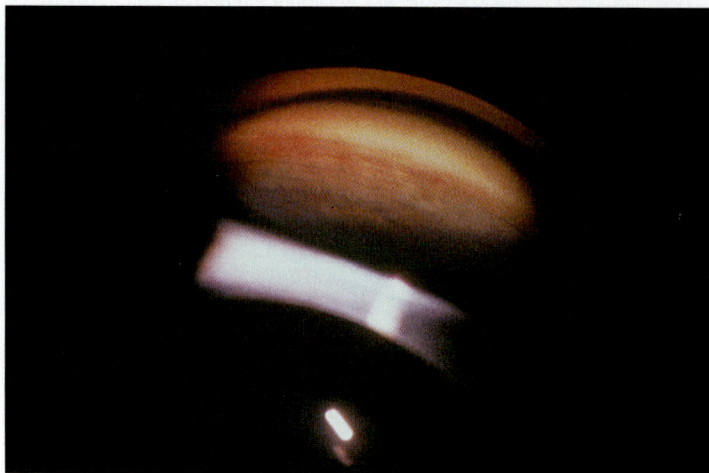

FIG. 213-17 ▌ Blood in an angle (after trauma).

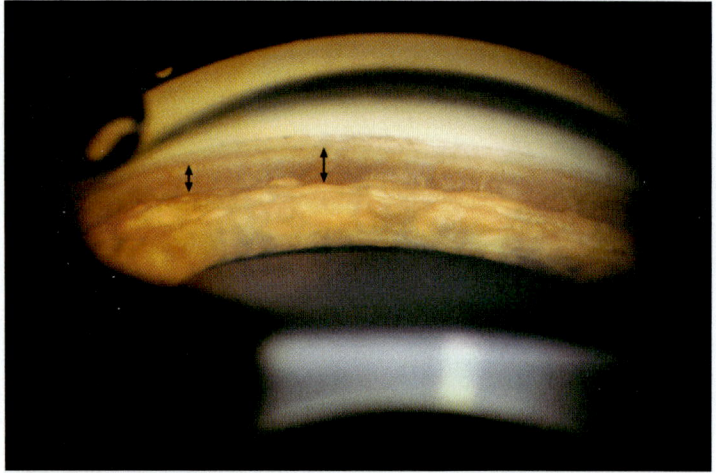

FIG. 213-16 ▌ Angle recession *(arrows)*.

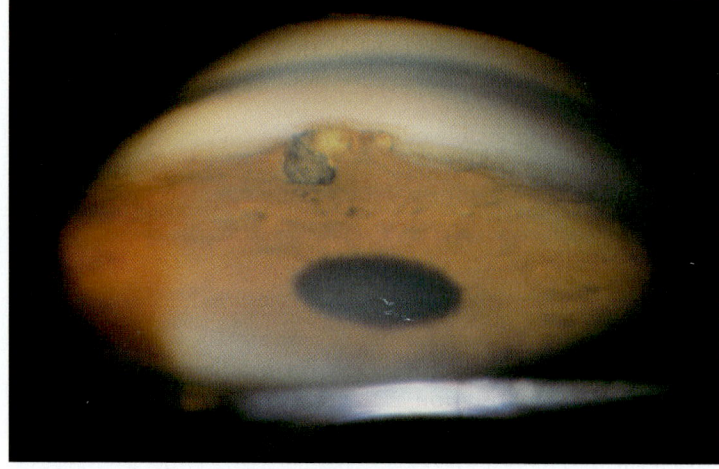

FIG. 213-18 ▌ An encysted foreign body in an angle.

posterior displacement of the ciliary body, or "angle recession" (Fig. 213-16). This extra deepness of the angle may be complete or partial in the affected eye. It is noted easily by comparison of the angle depth with that of the contralateral, untraumatized eye. Usually, coexisting tears in the trabecular meshwork also occur at the time of trauma, but these heal with scarring and often are indiscernible on later gonioscopic examination. Other findings on angle examination after trauma may include increased pigmentation, blood (Fig. 213-17) and, rarely, foreign bodies (Fig. 213-18). Cyclodialysis clefts may occur, too—these are seen as a separation of iris and ciliary body from the ciliary sulcus.

Trabecular meshwork pigmentation may vary considerably in eyes. Normal eyes may have 0 (none) to 2+ or 3+ (heavy) pigment. Most commonly, 4+ (very heavy) pigmented angles are associated with pathology. Pseudoexfoliation syndrome and pigmentary glaucoma are associated with heavy meshwork pigmentation, as well as increased pigmentation of Schwalbe's line, and create a so-called *Sampaoelesi's line* (Fig. 213-19). Specks of gray–white "dandruff" also may be seen in the angles of patients who have pseudoexfoliation. Iris melanoma may cause 4+ meshwork pigmentation. Finally, if an anterior or posterior chamber lens is placed improperly, with resultant haptic–iris chafe, heavy 4+ angle pigmentation can occur.

Vasculature in the angle is worthy of careful examination. Normal vessels may become engorged with inflammation and must be differentiated from neovascularization. Normal vessels are either part of the arterial circle in the ciliary muscle or are branches of it. The branches become radial arteries of the iris; these easily viewed iris vessels usually run strictly radially and do not meander. On the other hand, the arterial circle is typically posterior to the

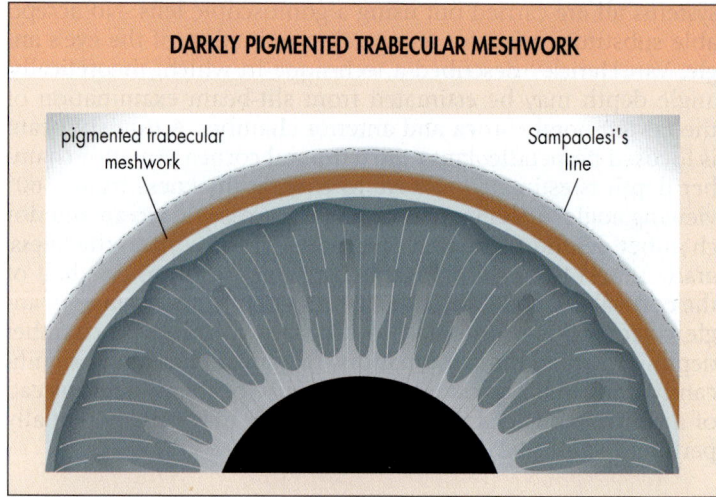

FIG. 213-19 ▌ Darkly pigmented trabecular meshwork.

periphery of the iris and, thus, commonly is not viewed. Some normal eyes, however, demonstrate forward displaced, visible portions of this circle. These portions, like their more posteriorly located counterparts, are characterized by circumferential vessel orientation and undulating shape. These vessels virtually never attach anterior to the scleral spur. Also, congenitally abnormal vessels occasionally are seen with congenital glaucoma. Such vessels may form a hairpin loop that extends to Schwalbe's line, but they have both ends in iris stroma and do not arborize abnormally.

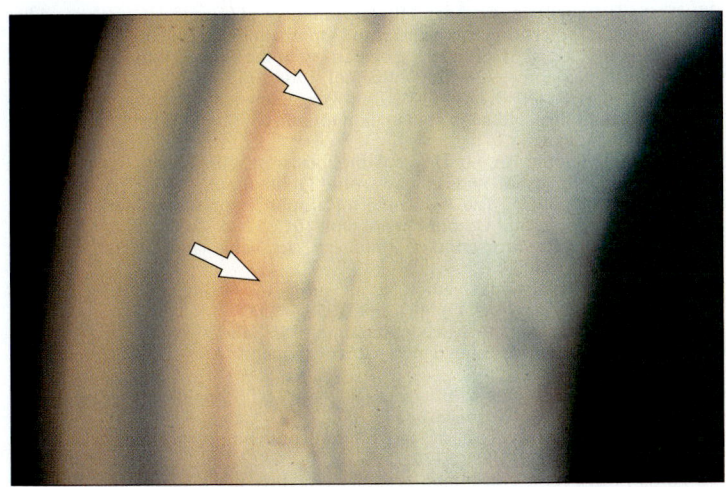

FIG. 213-20 ■ Neovascularization of an angle *(arrows)*.

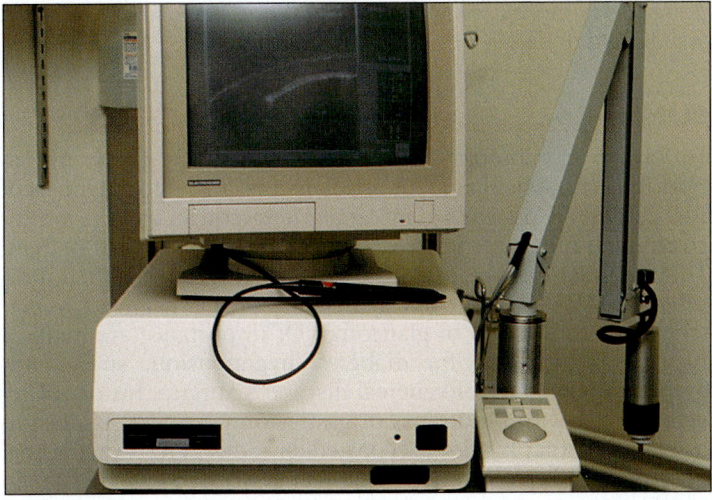

FIG. 213-21 ■ The ultrasound biomicroscopy apparatus. (Courtesy of Dr. C. Pavlin.)

To be differentiated from such vessels are neovascular vessels (Fig. 213-20), which usually grow from the circumferential ciliary body artery erratically onto angle wall and iris. These tend to meander irregularly and do not follow either a circumferential or radial course as normal vessels do. Such vessels grow onto the iris surface, not into stroma (whence come normal iris vessels). Abnormal vessels grow forward across the angle, over scleral spur, onto meshwork, and even over Schlemm's line, another key differentiating characteristic compared with normal vessels.

Neovascularization of the angle usually extends to cover the iris, although it stays within the angle initially and is accompanied by fibrous tissue ingrowth. This fibrous tissue, although invisible to gonioscopic examination, is that portion of the neovascular process which results in eventual angle contracture and closure, with increased IOP. Associated with ischemia and vascular retinopathy, this type of neovascularization usually carries the eye to blindness and phthisis if left untreated. Also, neovascularization of the angle may be seen with uveitis and Fuchs' heterochromic cyclitis. The neovascularization associated with uveitis tends to be as aggressive and as difficult to treat as that from ischemia. Interestingly, the neovascularization seen with Fuchs' heterochromic cyclitis may behave differently. These vessels tend to be finer, and less tendency exists to branching and a greater tendency to spontaneous bleeding. Occasionally, these fine vessels may not be associated with glaucoma, unlike the neovascularization seen from ischemia.

Before concluding a discussion of angle examination and pathology, the variations seen in normal and abnormal infant angles should be mentioned. Normal infant angles are deep and have a flat iris insertion posterior to the scleral spur. They have little pigment in a translucent trabecular meshwork, and a normal ciliary body band is present. In eyes affected by congenital glaucoma, the key finding in some eyes is an anterior insertion of the iris directly into the trabecular meshwork. This is associated with a thin ciliary band, which may be viewed through the thin peripheral iris tissue. Abnormal vessels, as previously noted, may also be seen.

ULTRASOUND BIOMICROSCOPY

Ultrasound biomicroscopy is another form of ocular imaging. A B-scan technique is used, with high-frequency transducers (50–100MHz) to provide high-resolution imaging of the anterior segment. Resolution approaches the 20–50μm (microscopic) level, and images of anterior segment structures are significantly sharper than those seen using conventional ultrasonography. Penetration with these transducers is limited to approximately 5mm, but this still is sufficient to allow excellent imaging of the entire anterior segment.

Instrumentation involves the use of an ultrasonographic apparatus with a scanning head on an articulated arm (Fig. 213-21).

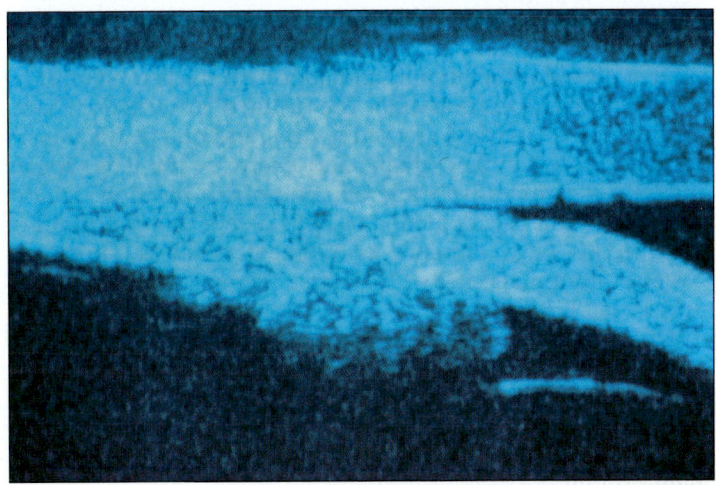

FIG. 213-22 ■ Ultrasound biomicroscopic image of an eye that has plateau iris. (Courtesy of Dr. C. Pavlin.)

An eyecup is filled with methylcellulose and applied to the reclining patient's eye; subsequently the examiner places the probe in the eyecup. Gentle movement of the probe establishes maximal image clarity.

Ultrasound biomicroscopy has been used to clarify the relationships between the drainage angle, ciliary body, zonular apparatus, and iris in many types of glaucoma.[56,57] It is particularly useful in the examination of a patient who has plateau iris (Fig. 213-22).[58] Anterior placement of ciliary processes, which prevents peripheral iris from falling back after iridectomy, has been visualized well using this technique in these patients. Additionally, the technique has helped define the anatomy in some patients who have pigmentary glaucoma and iris concavity, and even has demonstrated elimination of iris concavity after iridectomy.[59] Ultrasound biomicroscopy also has provided helpful clinical information in cases of pupillary block, angle recession, supraciliary effusion, and malignant glaucoma.[57,60] The technique has been useful to those who have access to it, but many consider it less a clinical aid and more a research tool by which to clarify the underlying mechanisms of disease.

OPTIC DISC, NERVE FIBER LAYER, AND VISUAL FIELDS

So important are these remaining aspects of the clinical examination, that each is discussed in separate chapters. Suffice it to say here that, usually as a result of IOP or drainage angle pathology, nearly all forms of glaucoma share a characteristic pattern of optic disc damage, with or without associated visual field changes. Thus, no clinical examination of a potential glaucoma patient is complete without thorough disc, nerve fiber layer, and visual field analysis.

SUMMARY

Tonometry, gonioscopy, nerve fiber layer analysis, disc examination, and visual field analysis are elements crucial to diagnosis of the individual patient's glaucoma. These crucial aspects are incorporated into a complete ocular examination of each patient. This examination begins with a good history, which often indicates glaucoma masquerade syndromes or the diagnoses of certain secondary forms of glaucoma. Of importance are medical histories remarkable for diabetes, hypertension, stroke, migraine, or Raynaud's or venereal disease. A surgical history of severe trauma with blood loss or gastrectomy may be significant, as may an ocular history of repeated episodes of red eye, trauma, or surgery. It is necessary to establish systemic medicines taken by the patient, whether glucocorticoids have been used, and whether the patient is aware of a family history of glaucoma. Mainly, tonography is a useful research tool.

Careful slit-lamp examination is important, too. Interstitial scars, dystrophy, guttata, keratic precipitates, endothelial pigment, a posterior membrane, and abnormal thickening must be sought in corneal examination. The nature of the anterior chamber must be established (e.g., fully deep and quiet). Iris transillumination, texture and shape, and nature of the lens capsule and lens (e.g., excessively sclerotic, in normal position) are determined. For a pseudophakic or aphakic eye, the condition of the vitreous (e.g., presence of pigment cells) is important. Posterior examination (e.g., for masses, retinal attachment, vascular events) is also key.

All of these and other pertinent aspects must be addressed by a meticulous examination. After such an examination, with special attention to the key aspects of IOP, angle nature, disc health, and visual fields (as noted above), a proper diagnosis usually may be made. Only then can attention be turned to management options.

REFERENCES

1. Kolker AE, Hetherington J Jr. Becker–Shaffer's diagnosis and therapy of the glaucomas, ed 5. St Louis: CV Mosby; 1983.
2. Kaiser-Kupfer MI, McCain L, Shapiro JR. Low ocular rigidity in patients with osteogenesis imperfecta. Invest Ophthalmol Vis Sci. 1981;20:807–9.
3. Drance SM. The coefficient of scleral rigidity in normal and glaucomatous eyes. Arch Ophthalmol. 1960;63:668–74.
4. Simone JN, Whitacre MM. The effect of intraocular gas and fluid volumes on intraocular pressure. Ophthalmology. 1990;97:238–43.
5. Johnson MW, Han DP, Hoffman KE. The effect of scleral buckling on ocular rigidity. Ophthalmology. 1990;97:190–5.
6. Friedenwald JS. Contribution to the theory and practice of tonometry. Am J Ophthalmol. 1937;20:985–1024.
7. Friedman E, Irvy M, Ebert E, et al. Increased scleral rigidity and age related macular degeneration. Ophthalmology. 1989;96:104–8.
8. Hetland-Eriksen J. On tonometry. 2. Pressure recordings by Schiøtz tonometry on enucleated human eyes. Acta Ophthalmol. 1966;44:12–9.
9. Foster CS, Yamamoto GK. Ocular rigidity in keratoconus. Am J Ophthalmol. 1978;86:802–6.
10. Friedenwald JS. Some problems in the calibration of tonometers. Am J Ophthalmol. 1948;31:935–44.
11. Goldmann H, Schmidt TH. Uber applanations-tonometrie. Ophthalmologica. 1957;134:221–42.
12. Ehlers N, Bramsen T, Sperling S. Applanation tonometry and central corneal thickness. Acta Ophthalmol (Copenh). 1975;53:34–43.
13. Mark HH. Corneal curvature in applanation tonometry. Am J Ophthalmol. 1973; 76:223–4.
14. Moses RA. The Goldmann applanation tonometer. Am J Ophthalmol. 1958; 46:865–9.
15. Moses RA, Lin CH. Repeated applanation tonometry. Am J Ophthalmol. 1968; 66:89–91.
16. Pepose JS, Linnette G, Lee SF, MacRae S. Disinfection of Goldmann tonometers against human immunodeficiency virus type 1. Arch Ophthalmol. 1989;107: 983–5.
17. Perkins ES. Hand-held applanation tonometer. Br J Ophthalmol. 1965;49:591–3.
18. Krieglstein GK, Waller WK. Goldmann applanation versus hand-applanation and Schiøtz indentation tonometry. Graefes Arch Klin Exp Ophthalmol. 1975;194: 11–6.
19. Jain MR, Marmion VJ. A clinical evaluation of applanation pneumotomography. Br J Ophthalmol. 1976;60:107–10.
20. West CE, Capella JA, Kaufman HE. Measurement of intraocular pressure with a pneumatic applanation tonometer. Am J Ophthalmol. 1972;74:505–9.
21. Fienkel REP, Hong YJ, Shin DH. Comparison of the Tono-Pen to the Goldmann applanation tonometer. Arch Ophthalmol. 1988;106:750–3.
22. Hessemer V, Rossler R, Jacobi KW. Tono-Pen, a new hand-held tonometer: comparison with the Goldmann applanation tonometer. Klin Monatsbl Augenheilkd. 1988;193:420–6.
23. Panek WL, Boothe WA, Lee DA, et al. Intraocular pressure measurement with the Tono-Pen through soft contact lenses. Am J Ophthalmol. 1990;109:62–5.
24. Myers KJ, Scott CA. The non-contact ("air-puff") tonometer: variability and corneal staining. Am J Optom Physiol Opt. 1975;52:36–46.
25. Shields MB. The non-contact tonometer. Its value and limitations. Surv Ophthalmol. 1980;24:211–9.
26. Grant WM. Tonographic method for measuring the facility and rate of aqueous flow in human eyes. Arch Ophthalmol. 1950;44:204.
27. Kronfeld PC. Tonography. Arch Ophthalmol. 1952;48:393–404.
28. Podos SM, Becker B. Tonography—current thoughts. Am J Ophthalmol. 1973; 75:733–5.
29. Goethrals M, Missotten L. Intraocular pressure in children up to 5 years of age. J Pediatr Ophthalmol Strabismus. 1983;20:49–51.
30. Brubaker RF. The effect of age on aqueous humor formation in man. Ophthalmology. 1981;88:283–8.
31. Armaly MF. On the distribution of applanation pressure. I. Statistical features and the effect of age, sex, and family history of glaucoma. Arch Ophthalmol. 1965; 73:11–8.
32. Wallace J, Lovel HG. Glaucoma and intraocular pressure in Jamaica. Am J Ophthalmol. 1969;67:93–100.
33. Tomlinson A, Phillips CI. Applanation tension and axial length of the eyeball. J Ophthalmol. 1970;54:548–53.
34. Newell FW, Krill AE. Diurnal tonography in normal and glaucomatous eyes. Trans Am Ophthalmol Soc. 1964;62:349–74.
35. Leonard TJK, Kerr-Muir MG, Kirby GR, Hitchings RA. Ocular hypertension and posture. Br J Ophthalmol. 1983;67:362–6.
36. Lempert P, Cooper KH, Culver JF, Tredici TJ. The effect of exercise on intraocular pressure. Am J Ophthalmol. 1967;63:1673–6.
37. Biro I, Botar Z. On the behavior of intraocular tension in various sport activities. Klin Monatsbl Augenheilkd. 1962;140:23–30.
38. Coleman DJ, Trokel S. Direct-recorded intraocular pressure variations in a human subject. Arch Ophthalmol. 1969;82:637–40.
39. Maddox TS Jr, Kielar RA. Comparison of the influence of ketamine and halothane anesthesia on intraocular tensions of nonglaucomatous children. J Pediatr Ophthalmol. 1974;11:90–3.
40. Meyers EF, Krupin T, Johnson M, Zink H. Failure of nondepolarizing neuromuscular blockers to inhibit succinylcholine-induced increased intraocular pressure; a controlled study. Anesthesiology. 1978;48:149–51.
41. Williams BI, Ledingham JG. Significance of intraocular pressure measurement in systemic hypertension. Br J Ophthalmol. 1984;68:383–8.
42. Klein BEK, Klein R, Moss SE. Intraocular pressure in diabetic persons. Ophthalmology. 1984;91:1356–60.
43. Aziz MA. The relationship of IOP to hormonal disturbance. Bull Ophthalmol Soc Egypt. 1967;60:303–22.
44. Shiose Y. The aging effect on intraocular pressure in an apparently normal population. Arch Ophthalmol. 1984;102:883–7.
45. Peczon JD, Grant WM. Glaucoma, alcohol, and intraocular pressure. Arch Ophthalmol. 1965;73:495–501.
46. Hepler RS, Frank IR. Marijuana smoking and intraocular pressure. JAMA. 1971; 217:1392.
47. Higginbotham EJ, Kilimanjaro HA, Wilensky JT, et al. The effect of caffeine on intraocular pressure in glaucoma patients. Ophthalmology. 1989;96:624–6.
48. Mehra KS, Roy PN, Khare BB. Tobacco smoking and glaucoma. Ann Ophthalmol. 1976;8:462–4.
49. Leydhecker W, Akiyama K, Neumann HG. Der intraokulare druck gesunder menschlicher augen. Klin Monatsbl Augenheilkd. 1958;133:662–70.
50. Colton T, Ederer F. The distribution of intraocular pressures in the general population. Surv Ophthalmol. 1980;25:123–9.
51. Forbes M. Gonioscopy with corneal indentation: a method for distinguishing between appositional closure and synechial closure. Arch Ophthalmol. 1966;76: 488–92.
52. Kolker AE, Hetherington J Jr, eds. Becker and Shaffer's diagnosis and therapy of the glaucomas, ed 5. St Louis: CV Mosby; 1976.
53. Scheie HG. Width and pigmentation of the angle of the anterior chamber. Arch Ophthalmol. 1957;58:510–2.
54. Spaeth GL. The normal development of the human anterior chamber angle: a new system of descriptive grading. Trans Ophthalmol Soc U K. 1971;91:709–39.
55. van Herick W, Shaffer RN, Schwartz A. Estimation of width of angle of anterior chamber. Am J Ophthalmol. 1969;68:626–9.
56. Riley SF, Nairn JP, Maestre FA, et al. Analysis of the anterior chamber angle by gonioscopy and by ultrasound biomicroscopy. Int Ophthalmol Clin. 1994;34: 271–82.
57. Pavlin CJ. Practical application of ultrasound biomicroscopy. Can J Ophthalmol. 1995;30:225–9.
58. Pavlin CJ, Ritch R, Foster FS. Ultrasound biomicroscopy in plateau iris syndrome. Am J Ophthalmol. 1992;113:390–5.
59. Pavlin CJ, Macken P, Trope G, et al. Ultrasound biomicroscopic features of pigmentary glaucoma. Can J Ophthalmol. 1994;29:187–92.
60. Pavlin CJ, Rutnin SS, Devenyi R, et al. Supraciliary effusions and ciliary body thickening after scleral buckling procedures. Ophthalmology. 1997;104:433–8.

CHAPTER
214
Visual Field Perimetry in Glaucoma

ELLIOT B. WERNER

DEFINITIONS
- The visual field is the space that one eye can see while remaining fixed.
- Measurement of the extent of the visual field by projecting targets onto a curved surface is called perimetry.

KEY FEATURES
- Modern quantitative perimetry measures the differential light threshold at various locations in the visual field.
- Glaucoma produces characteristic but not pathognomonic changes in the visual field.
- At present, perimetry is among the best tests to determine the extent of glaucomatous damage to visual function and whether or not visual loss is progressive.

INTRODUCTION

Glaucoma, of course, is not a single disease but a collection of conditions that have in common the tendency to produce a characteristic optic neuropathy characterized mainly by cupping. Whereas some glaucomas are acute and associated with symptoms at onset, most glaucoma patients have a chronic, slowly developing disease that does not produce prominent symptoms until optic nerve damage and visual loss are far advanced. Glaucoma is treated in order to preserve vision. Tests of visual function, thus, are of critical importance in evaluating the glaucoma patient and in guiding treatment. Despite recent advances in optic nerve and retinal nerve fiber layer evaluation and despite many recent studies of a variety of visual functions in glaucoma, white light perimetry remains the most reliable widely used tool to determine the likelihood of a patient suffering significant functional impairment as a result of glaucoma.[1]

As a pure diagnostic tool, perimetry has a number of shortcomings.[2] Other modalities may be more useful for population screening. Automated perimetry, however, compares favorably with other clinical techniques for detecting glaucomatous damage.[3] As an indication of the extent of glaucomatous damage and as an aid in determining whether an individual with glaucoma is deteriorating, perimetry is indispensable.[4–6]

HISTORICAL REVIEW

The existence of the field of vision was known to the ancients, and Hippocrates is said to have described hemianopias. The French physicist Mariotte described the physiological blind spot in the 17th century. Young and Purkinje described and measured the limits of the visual field in the early 19th century, and von Graefe was the first to use measurement of the visual field clinically in the 1850s.

The modern tangent screen was introduced by Bjerrum in 1889. He used this device not only to measure the peripheral extent of the visual field but also to detect localized defects or scotomas in the central visual field. The typical arcuate scotomas seen in glaucoma still bear Bjerrum's name. Despite efforts to improve on Bjerrum's original design, such as the Autoplot, which projects a spot of light onto a wall-mounted screen, the black tangent screen remains the standard tool for campimetry, that is, the measurement of the visual field on a flat surface.

Perimetry refers to the measurement of the visual field on a curved surface and has largely replaced campimetry in modern clinical practice. The first perimeters were arc perimeters that, like the tangent screen, used small round objects as test targets. Light projection arc perimeters, such as the Aimark, were introduced in the 1930s, and the development of the Goldmann hemispheric projection perimeter in 1945 ushered in the modern era of quantitative perimetry.

Computer technology was combined with visual field testing in the mid-1970s, resulting in the introduction of the first automated perimeters, the television campimeter of Lynn and Tate, the Octopus device of Fankhauser, and the Competer of Heijl and Krakau.[7]

During the ensuing decade a number of automated perimeters were introduced, and many are no longer manufactured. There are now several automated visual field testing devices on the market, but the two most widely used systems are the Octopus perimeter marketed by the Swiss firm Interzeag and the Humphrey Visual Field Analyzer marketed by the American firm Humphrey Instruments. Automated perimetry has largely replaced manual perimetry in clinical practice because of its superiority in detecting glaucomatous visual field loss.[8]

Several detailed reviews of the history of visual field testing have been published.[9–11]

PURPOSE OF THE TEST

There are two steps in diagnosing glaucomatous visual field loss using automated perimetry. The first is to determine whether the visual field is normal. If the visual field is abnormal, the second step is to decide whether the visual field abnormality is due to glaucoma or something else. The second step is actually the easier of the two. Differentiating the normal from the abnormal field is not straightforward.[12,13] It requires a knowledge of the range of visual field responses in the normal population, an understanding of probability, and the ability to interpret detailed statistical analysis of the visual field data. The essential purpose of visual field testing in glaucoma is to determine the extent of functional visual loss and whether or not it is progressive.

Use of Probability Statistics to Define the Normal Visual Field

When applied to perimetry, the term normal describes the range of test results found in the nondiseased population. The range of normal has been determined experimentally, and the results are stored in the computer memory of most automated perimeters. This allows the comparison of an individual patient's visual field with the expected normal values.[14-16]

Because of the wide range of normal, one cannot say with certainty that a particular visual field is normal or abnormal. One can, however, determine the likelihood of finding a particular visual field result in a normal individual. If that likelihood is very small, the visual field is probably abnormal. Specific examples of visual fields in this chapter are taken from the Humphrey Visual Field Analyzer. Similar results and analytic software are available with the Octopus and other automated perimeters.

The determination that a visual field is within the normal range cannot be made by simple inspection. Statistical analysis is necessary. Statistical software packages available with some perimeters provide probability statements about the visual field data that allow the clinician to determine the likelihood that a visual field is normal.[17-19] If all statistical parameters are within the normal range, chances are that the visual field is normal. The sensitivity of automated threshold perimetry for detecting visual field defects is very high. It is extremely unlikely that a patient with a clinically significant visual field defect would have a normal result. The opposite, however, is not always true.

Many otherwise normal patients have a visual field that may be abnormal because of the large number of artifacts that can occur during automated visual field testing. In other words, the specificity of automated perimetry is often not as high as clinicians would like. When performing perimetry on patients suspected of having glaucoma, it is important to distinguish the visual field that appears abnormal because of artifact from the visual field that is truly abnormal as a result of glaucoma or some other disease such as cataract, retinal disease, or neurological lesions. Statistical analysis must be combined with other clinical data, experience, and the ability to recognize specific patterns of visual field loss related to specific diseases or artifacts.[20-23]

Reliability Indices

The reliability indices are found in the upper left-hand corner of the printout of the Humphrey Visual Field Analyzer (Fig. 214-1). Reliability is evaluated by measuring fixation losses, false-positive and false-negative responses.[24] The fixation loss rate measures how often the patient fails to fixate the central target. In the (HFA I), the fixation loss rate relates to the number of times a patient responds to a target placed in the blind spot. In the newer model (HFA II), fixation is monitored by an eye tracker. A real-time display of eye movements during the test is presented across the bottom of the printout (Fig. 214-2).

The false-positive error rate refers to the number of times a patient responds when no test target is presented. The false-

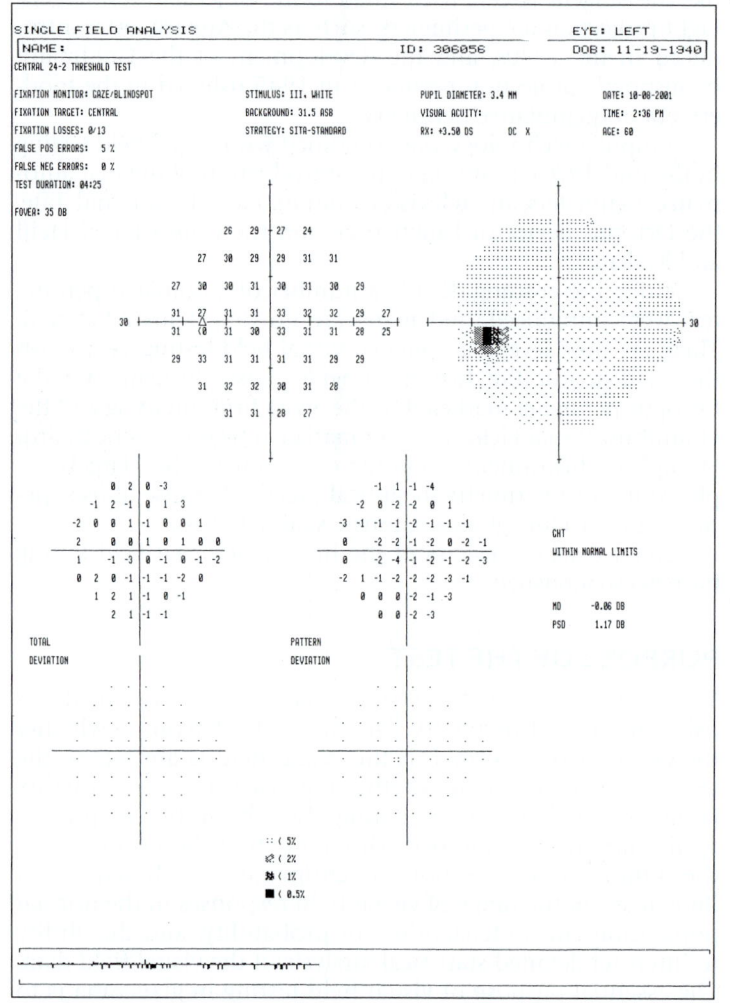

FIG. 214-1 ■ **Printout of a normal visual field from the Humphrey Visual Field Analyzer.** The reliability indices, fixation losses, false-positive errors, and false-negative errors are found in the upper left-hand corner a few lines below the patient's name. The Glaucoma Hemifield Test result is found just below the gray scale interpolation and is "within normal limits." The global indices are found in the lower right-hand corner. Neither the MD nor the PSD is flagged with a P value, indicating that both are within the expected range of normal. The numerical and graphic representations of the total and pattern deviations are found where indicated in the left and center lower portion of the printout. There are no probability symbols in either the total or pattern deviation, indicating that the threshold value of each test location is within the normal range for the patient's age.

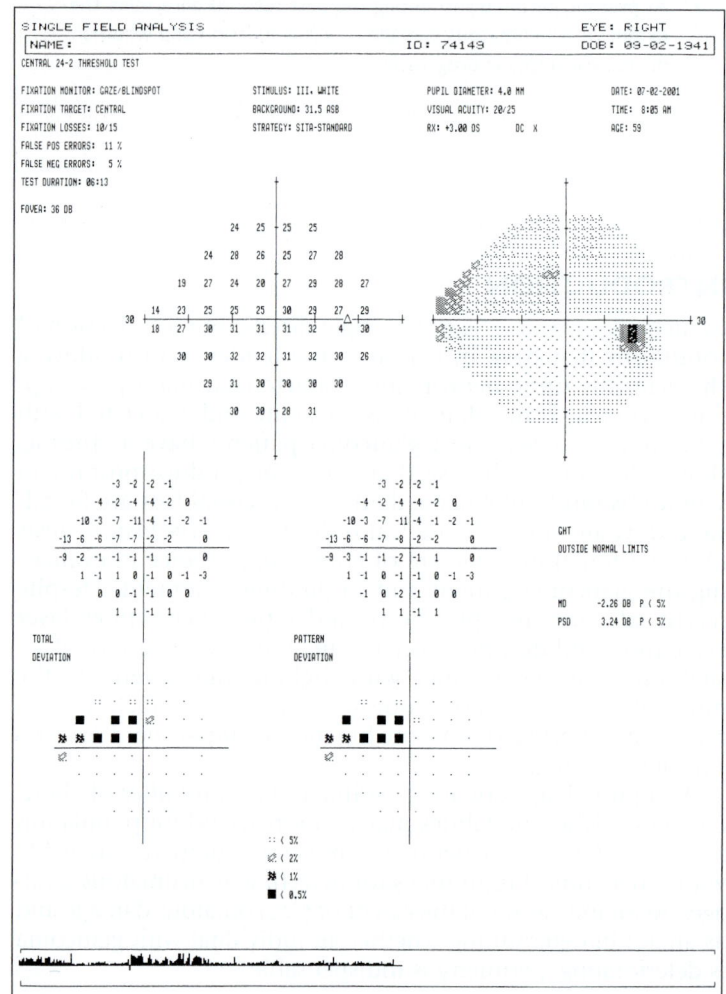

FIG. 214-2 ■ **Visual field showing an elevated fixation loss rate of 10/15.** The eye tracker tracing across the bottom of the printout shows larger eye movements during the first half of the test. Eye movements decreased and fixation presumably improved during the second half of the test. False-positive and false-negative errors are also slightly elevated. The presence of an elevated reliability index does not necessarily mean that the results of the test are not valid. Repeatability and correlation with other clinical findings are more important criteria. This visual field shows a well-defined superior nerve fiber bundle defect that was repeatable and correlated well with the appearance of the optic nerve, indicating that the result is believable despite the poor fixation.

negative error rate refers to the number of times a patient fails to respond to a suprathreshold (very bright) target placed in a seeing area of the visual field[14,19,25] (Fig. 214-2). The standard full-threshold test algorithm measures false positives by presenting an audible clue when no test target is displayed. False negatives are measured by presenting suprathreshold targets in seeing areas. The Swedish Interactive Thresholding Algorithm (SITA) on the HFA II calculates false-positive and false-negative rates from the time between the presentation of the target and the patient's response during threshold determination.[26]

The reliability indices are an indicator of the extent to which a particular patient's results may be reliably compared with the normal range of values stored in the computer memory. Automated perimetry in patients with poor reliability has lower specificity and sensitivity for the detection of visual field defects.[27] Test results must be interpreted with caution in these patients,[28–31] although useful results can often be obtained despite what appears to be poor patient performance (Fig. 214-2).

A high false-positive rate is often associated with the patient who responds frequently without regard to whether a target is seen, the so-called "trigger happy" patient.[32] This may result in a visual field with abnormally high decibel thresholds, which is not interpretable (Fig. 214-3).[30,33] High false-positive or false-negative response rates are associated with alterations in the overall sensitivity of the visual field that could make detecting defects more difficult.[34] High fixation loss rates due to eye movements have been associated with increased variability of the visual field responses and increased difficulty in detecting scotomas.[35,36]

Global Indices

The global indices are found in the lower right-hand corner of the Humphrey printout (see Fig. 214-1). The mean deviation (MD) is a measure of the average difference between the threshold value of each test location and the age-corrected normal value. The pattern standard deviation (PSD) is the standard deviation of the mean difference between the threshold value at each test location and the expected normal value. It is a measure of the extent to which the threshold determinations at different locations in the visual field differ from each other.[14,19] The loss variance (LV) of the Octopus system, although calculated differently, provides similar information.

The calculation of the global indices is weighted to give greater importance to the test locations near fixation and less importance to more peripheral locations.[37,38] The formulas are fairly complex and beyond the scope of this chapter. Interested readers are referred to Anderson and Patella.[39]

If a global index is outside the expected normal range, a P value will appear next to it (Fig. 214-4). The P value represents the proportion of normal subjects in which an index of that value is found. For example, if P <1% appears next to the MD, fewer than 1% of normal subjects of that age have an MD at that level. Any global index with a P value less than 5% has a high probability of being abnormal.

The MD is mainly an index of the size of a visual field defect. It is not, as is widely believed, an indicator of generalized depression of the visual field, but the MD is very sensitive to generalized loss of sensitivity. Purely localized defects that are large enough, however, also affect the MD.

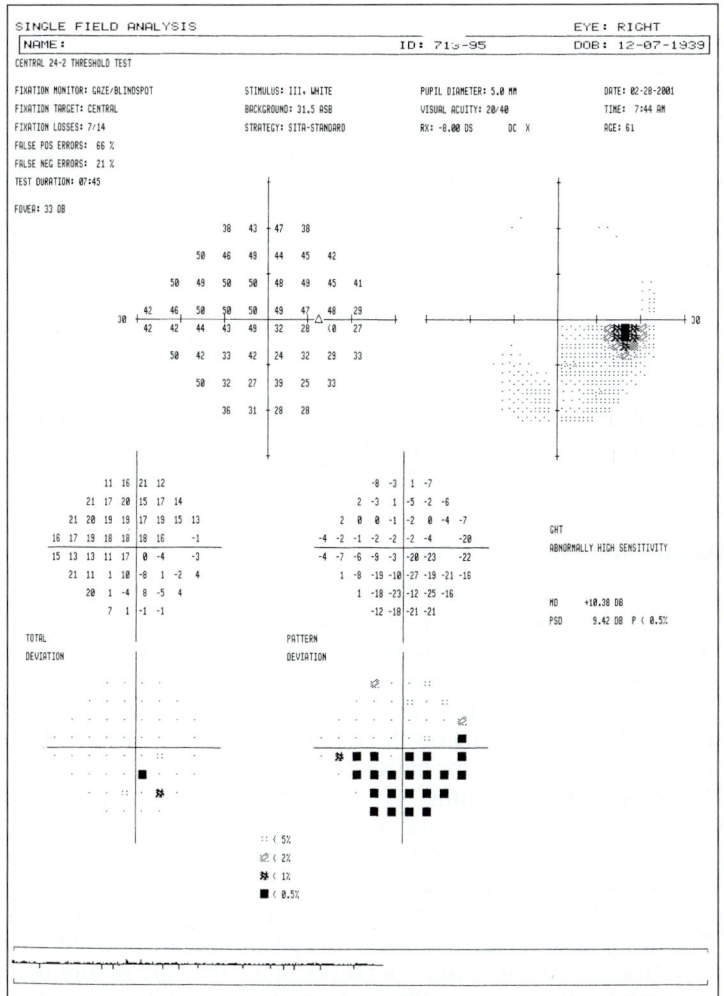

FIG. 214-3 ■ Visual field of a "trigger happy" patient who frequently responds at times when no test target is presented. The result is a high false-positive error rate, an unphysiologically elevated mean deviation (MD), and an abnormally high sensitivity, which is seen as white areas in the gray scale interpolation, the so-called white field artifact. The Glaucoma Hemifield Test shows "abnormally high sensitivity." There are many probability symbols in the pattern deviation not seen in the total deviation.

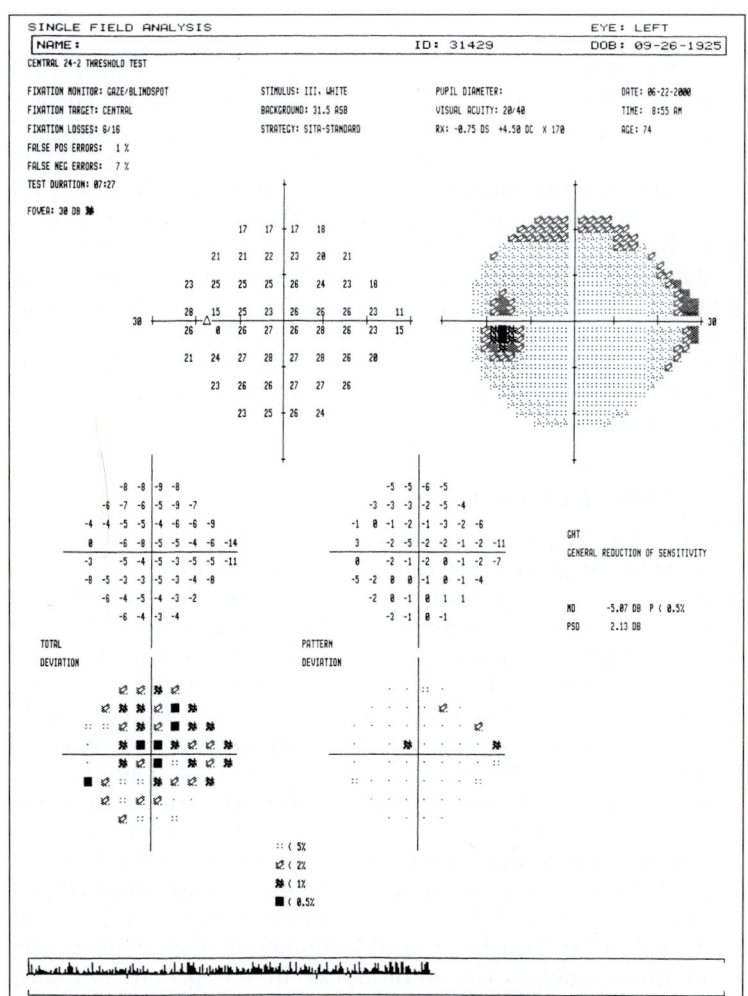

FIG. 214-4 ■ Visual field of a patient with a nearly pure generalized loss due to cataract. The mean deviation (MD) is significantly below the expected range of normal at the P <0.5% level while the pattern standard deviation (PSD) is within the normal range. The total deviation shows many probability symbols, most of which are not found in the pattern deviation. The Glaucoma Hemifield Test shows "generalized reduction of sensitivity."

TABLE 214-1

INTERPRETATION OF THE GLOBAL INDICES ON THE HUMPHREY VISUAL FIELD ANALYZER*

MD	PSD†	Interpretation
Normal	Normal	Visual field probably normal (Fig. 214-1)
Abnormal	Normal	Generalized loss of sensitivity (Fig. 214-4)
Normal	Abnormal	Small localized defect (Fig. 214-5)
Abnormal	Abnormal	Large defect with a significant localized component (Figs. 214-6 and 214-7)

*Artifacts may cause the global indices to be abnormal in the absence of any pathological cause of visual field loss.
†The PSD is the equivalent of the loss variance (LV) of the Octopus system for purposes of interpretation.

TABLE 214-2

INTERPRETATION OF THE TOTAL AND PATTERN DEVIATION ON THE HUMPHREY VISUAL FIELD ANALYZER

Total Deviation	Pattern Deviation	Interpretation
No symbols	No symbols	Probably normal (Fig. 214-1)
Many symbols	No symbols	Pure generalized loss (Fig. 214-4)
Some symbols	Same pattern	Pure localized loss (Figs. 214-5 and 214-6)
Many symbols	Fewer symbols	Mixed localized and generalized loss (Fig. 214-7)
No or few symbols	Many symbols	Trigger happy patient (Fig. 214-3)

The PSD is an index of localized nonuniformity of the surface of the hill of vision. It is sensitive to localized visual field defects and is not affected by purely generalized loss of sensitivity.

By looking at the MD and PSD, it is possible to anticipate the nature of any visual field defect before inspecting the rest of the visual field data. The interpretation of the global indices is summarized in Table 214-1. If both the MD and PSD are abnormal, the patient may have either a mixed defect with both generalized and localized loss or a purely localized defect large enough to affect the MD. When both MD and PSD are abnormal, however, it is impossible to determine whether there is any significant generalized depression without inspecting the remainder of the visual field data.

Total and Pattern Deviation

The total and pattern deviations are found as arrays of numbers and graphic plots in the center and lower portions of the printout (see Fig. 214-1). The total deviation represents the difference between the measured threshold of each individual test location and the age-corrected normal value for that location. The actual measured thresholds are shown in the array of numbers in the upper central portion of the printout to the left of the gray scale.

The pattern deviation represents the difference between an adjusted threshold of each individual test location and the age-corrected normal value for that location. The pattern deviation is derived from the total deviation by adjusting the measured thresholds upward or downward by an amount that reflects any generalized change in the threshold of the least damaged portion of the visual field. The information in the total deviation, thus, may be thought of as a combination of generalized plus localized change. The information in the pattern deviation represents purely localized change. Although the interpretation of the pattern deviation and pattern standard deviation is similar and the similarity of the names may be confusing, they are not identical and should not be confused.

The graphic probability plots indicate how frequently a total or pattern deviation value at a particular test location will be found in the normal population. There are four symbols ranging

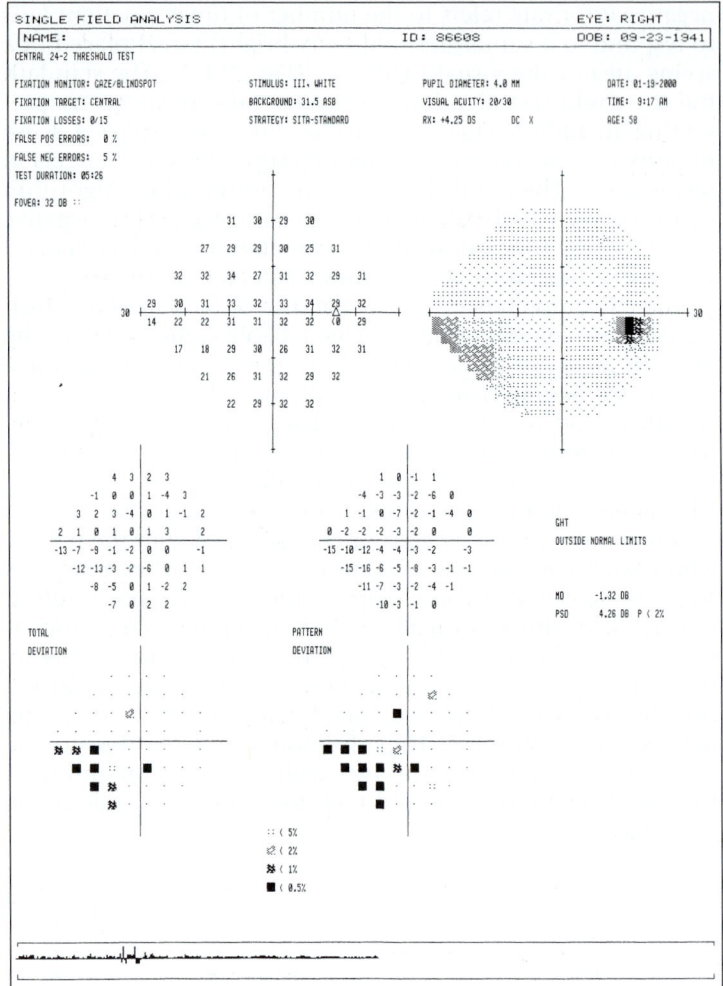

FIG. 214-5 ■■ Visual field consistent with a small, localized defect. The MD is within the normal range while the PSD is outside the expected range of normal at the P <2% level. The total and pattern deviation plots show almost identical arrays of probability symbols. The Glaucoma Hemifield Test, which is very sensitive to small differences in threshold between the superior and inferior hemifields, shows "outside normal limits."

from P <5% to P <0.5%. A black square, for example, indicates that the total or pattern deviation value for that test location will be found in fewer than 0.5% of normal subjects. Groupings of symbols in a portion of the visual field, therefore, indicate a high probability of an abnormality there.[14,19,40,41] The interpretation of the total and pattern deviation is summarized in Table 214-2.

Glaucoma Hemifield Test

The Glaucoma Hemifield Test provides information about the difference between the superior and inferior halves of the visual field.[42,43] The Glaucoma Hemifield Test evaluates the differences in threshold of mirror image groups of points on either side of the horizontal midline. There are six interpretive messages that may appear, depending on the relationship of the thresholds in the superior and inferior halves of the field.

1. "Within normal limits" (see Fig. 214-1) means that there is no significant difference between the superior and inferior halves of the fields and the overall sensitivity is within the 99.5% range of normal.
2. "Outside normal limits" (Fig. 214-5) appears when the threshold differences between the groups of points compared in the superior and inferior halves of the field are greater than would be expected in 99% of the normal population.
3. "Borderline" (Fig. 214-8) appears when the threshold differences are greater than would be expected in 97% of the normal population but not as great as in "outside normal limits."
4. "General reduction of sensitivity" (see Fig. 214-4) appears when the overall sensitivity of the least damaged portion of

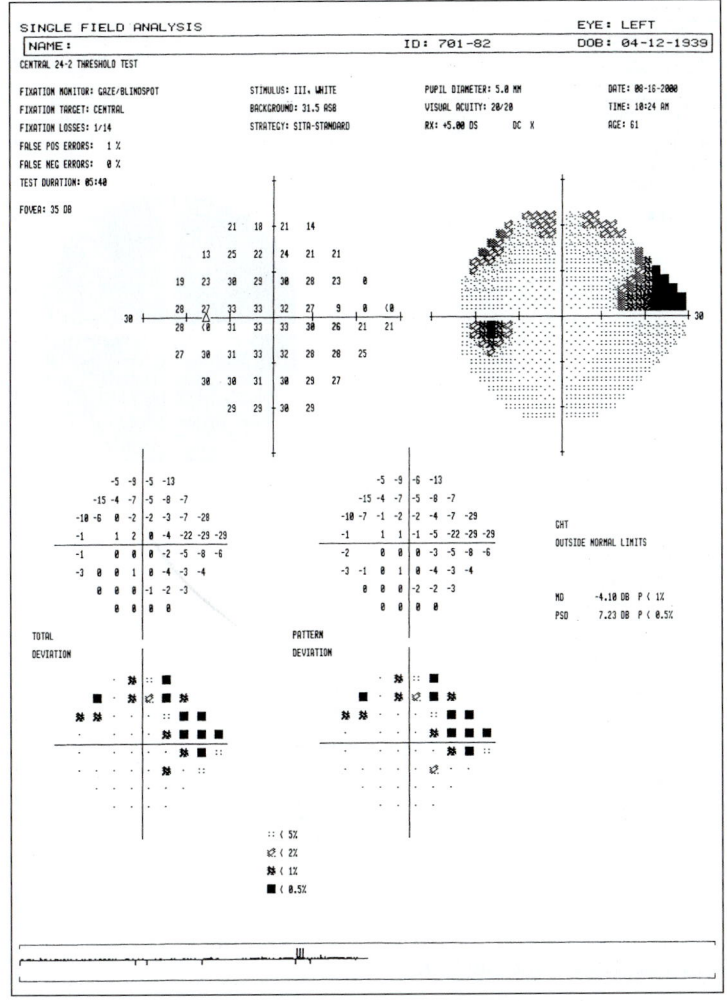
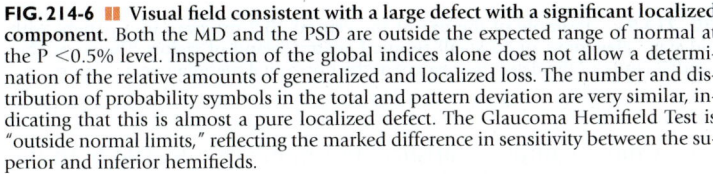

FIG. 214-6 ■ Visual field consistent with a large defect with a significant localized component. Both the MD and the PSD are outside the expected range of normal at the P <0.5% level. Inspection of the global indices alone does not allow a determination of the relative amounts of generalized and localized loss. The number and distribution of probability symbols in the total and pattern deviation are very similar, indicating that this is almost a pure localized defect. The Glaucoma Hemifield Test is "outside normal limits," reflecting the marked difference in sensitivity between the superior and inferior hemifields.

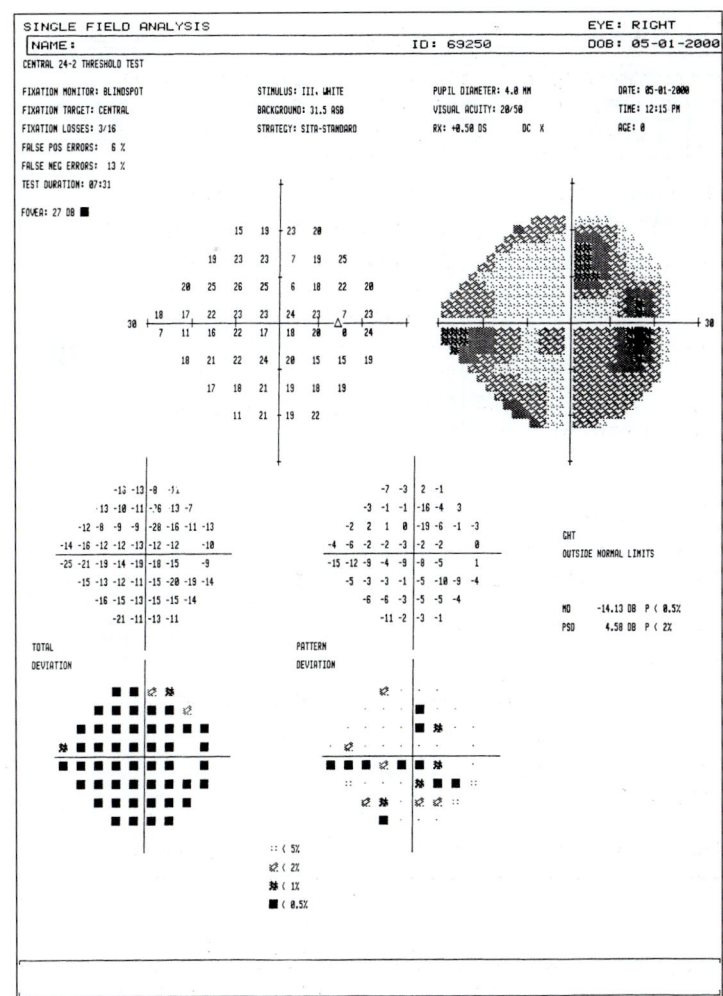

FIG. 214-7 ■ Visual field consistent with a large defect with a significant localized component. The MD and PSD are both outside the expected range of normal. The graphic representation of the total and pattern deviation shows many probability symbols in the total deviation. Many of the symbols in the total deviation are not seen in the pattern deviation. This is typical of a mixed generalized and localized defect (contrast Fig. 214-6). The Glaucoma Hemifield Test is "outside normal limits." This type of field defect is often seen in glaucoma patients who also have a cataract or a small pupil. The localized component of the defect seen in the pattern deviation is consistent with an inferior and superior nerve fiber bundle defect.

the visual field is depressed below the 99.5% range of normal but there is no significant difference between the superior and inferior halves of the field.

5. "Abnormally high sensitivity" (see Fig. 214-3) appears when the overall sensitivity is higher than expected in 99.5% of the normal population. This message is found most often in the presence of a high false-positive rate and usually represents an artifact of testing.

6. "Borderline" combined with "general reduction of sensitivity" appears in patients with a significant generalized loss of sensitivity and a residual moderate difference in the sensitivity of the superior and inferior hemifields.

The specificity and sensitivity of the Glaucoma Hemifield Test for detecting nerve fiber bundle visual field defects are quite high, especially if consistently abnormal results are obtained after repeated testing. In the presence of the message "within normal limits," it is very unlikely that a visual field defect of the type seen in glaucoma is present. On the other hand, although an abnormal Glaucoma Hemifield Test may be due to an artifact, the presence of a glaucomatous visual field defect is likely and should be carefully evaluated.[32,44]

UTILITY OF PERIMETRY

The management of glaucoma includes perimetry at regular intervals. All glaucoma patients capable of cooperating for the test should be tested at the time of initial diagnosis. Perimetry should then be repeated within a few weeks in order to have at least two baseline tests for comparison with subsequent tests. In patients with inconsistent results or with a significant learning effect, more than two baseline tests may be required. For ocular hypertensive patients or other patients with normal fields, perimetry every 12 to 18 months may be adequate. In patients with visual field loss, the frequency of testing will depend on the severity of the patient's glaucoma and the risk for future progression. For such patients, two or more visual fields per year may be indicated.[45]

Some patients are incapable of performing automated perimetry. Sometimes the patient's vision is so poor that perimetry yields little useful information. In other patients, an adequate examination cannot be conducted because of age or physical or psychological problems. There is no point in forcing such patients to undergo perimetry repeatedly if useful clinical information is not being generated. Many patients, however, who have problems with automated perimetry at first can learn to perform adequately with proper coaching and experience.

TESTING PROCEDURE

Illuminated targets are projected onto an illuminated background. The brightness of the target (target luminance) is varied and the patient is asked to respond when the target is seen. By presenting targets that are too dim to be seen (infrathreshold) and targets that are bright enough to be seen consistently (suprathreshold), the average brightness of the dimmest test ob-

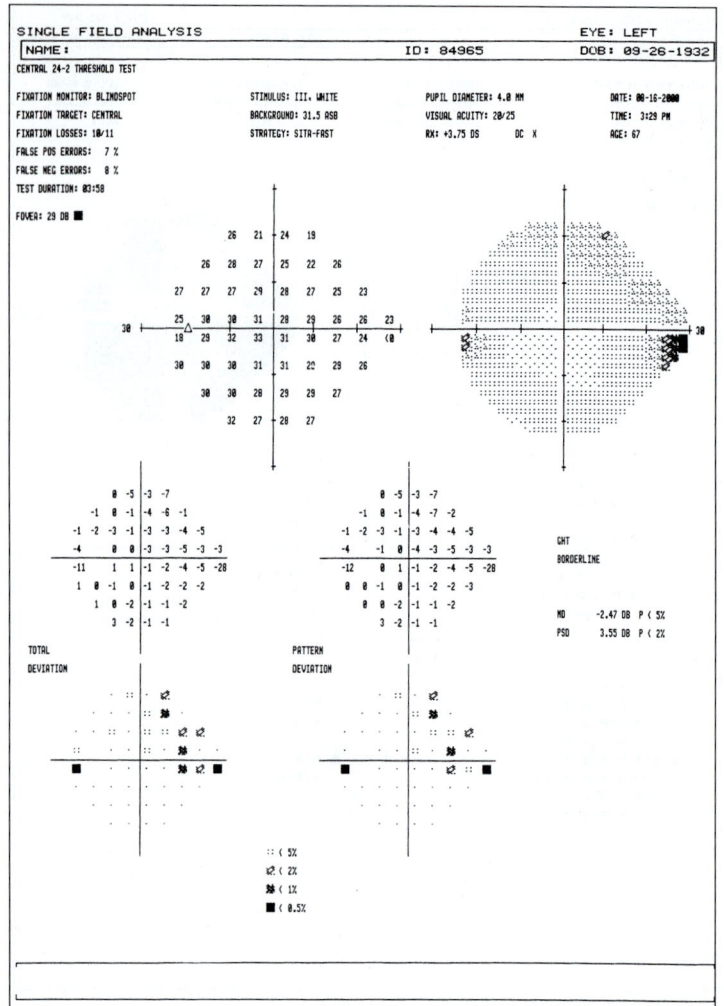

FIG. 214-8 "Borderline" Glaucoma Hemifield Test consistent with a small difference in sensitivity between the superior and inferior hemifields in a patient with an early superior nerve fiber bundle defect. The presence of a high fixation loss rate and a low foveal sensitivity despite 20/25 vision indicates that patient reliability may be a problem. Clinically, the approach to this patient would be to evaluate the fundus carefully and repeat the field.

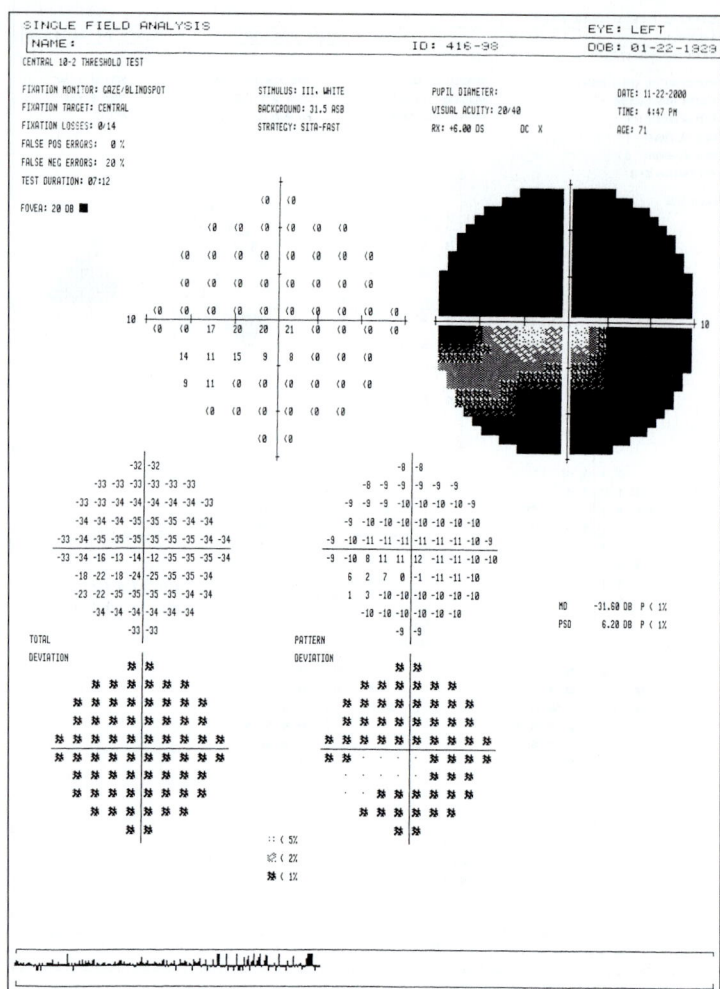

FIG. 214-9 Example of the use of the central 10-2 program in a patient with end-stage glaucoma and a small residual central island of vision. The nerve fiber bundle nature of the defect is apparent at the horizontal meridian near fixation.

ject that can be seen is determined. This is called the threshold and is determined for multiple locations in the visual field.

The computer records the patient's responses and the target luminance for each presentation and calculates the threshold for each test location and the statistical tests described previously.

Choice of Test Program

The standard test program used in glaucoma patients is the 30-2.[46] The 24-2 eliminates the peripheral test locations of the 30-2 program except for the most nasal portion of the field. Many clinicians now routinely use the 24-2 in glaucoma patients because it seems to provide as much clinically useful information as the 30-2 and saves about 5 minutes testing time per eye. The shorter testing time may reduce patient fatigue and encourage cooperation and compliance with the examination. The 10-2 program is useful in patients with very advanced field loss who have only a small island of vision persisting near fixation (see Fig. 214-9). The foveal sensitivity is also a very useful piece of information and should be turned "on" when performing threshold perimetry in glaucoma patients.

Humphrey has introduced a new testing algorithm called SITA (Swedish Interactive Thresholding Algorithm). SITA is available in two testing algorithms: standard and fast. The difference relates to the number of times a target is presented in order to arrive at a threshold estimation. "SITA fast" reduces testing time but is less precise and subject to greater variability. SITA

uses a more complex statistical technique to calculate both the threshold and the reliability indices from the patient's responses while the test is in progress. This significantly shortens the testing time without sacrificing accuracy or affecting the ability of the test to detect abnormalities. Variability may also be reduced. SITA has largely replaced the older full-threshold programs in clinical use.[47-50]

INTERPRETATION OF RESULTS

Nerve Fiber Bundle Defects

Most visual field defects seen in glaucoma are of the nerve fiber bundle type.[51] As a result of glaucomatous damage to ganglion cell axons at the optic nerve head, there is a loss of retinal nerve fiber bundles. This loss may be diffuse, localized or both. The characteristic shape and location of the visual field defects seen in glaucoma result from the anatomy of the retinal nerve fiber layer.[52] The defects seen in an individual patient depend on the location of the damaged nerve fibers and whether the damage is predominantly localized or diffuse.

The most characteristic feature of the nerve fiber bundle visual field defect is the tendency to respect the horizontal meridian, especially in the nasal portion of the field. Isolated nerve fiber bundle defects rarely cross the nasal horizontal midline Typically, there is an abrupt change in sensitivity across the horizontal midline. Even in patients with more advanced visual field loss due to glaucoma there is often a detectable difference in the measured threshold on either side of the nasal horizontal midline.

Another feature of nerve fiber bundle visual field defects is the tendency to be found in the Bjerrum area, which is between

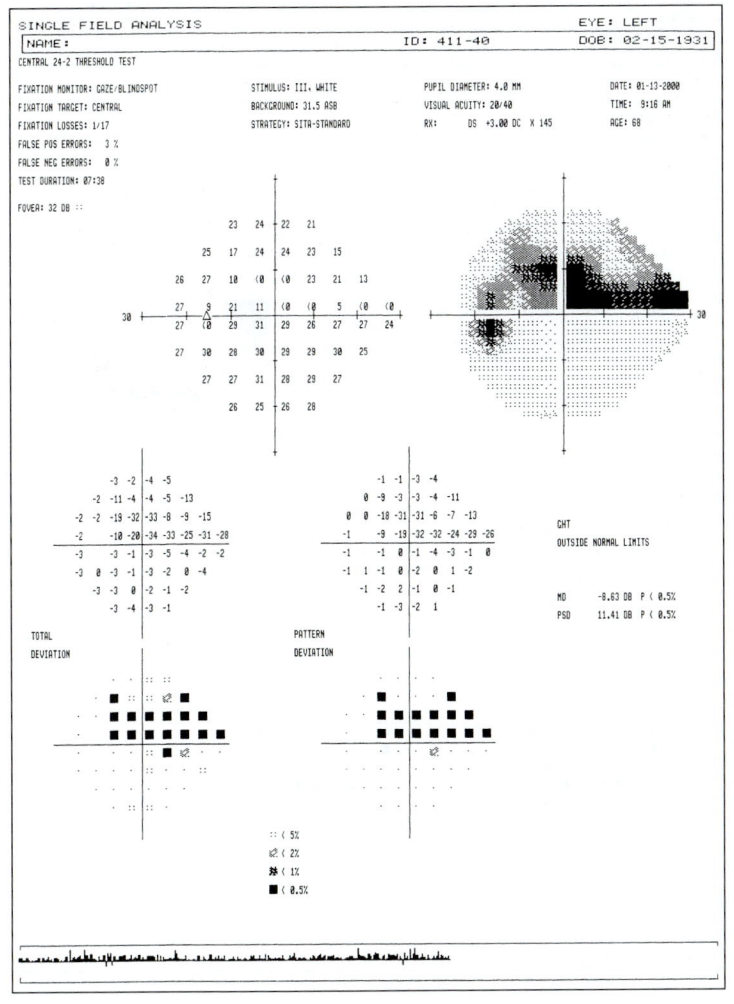

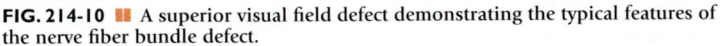

FIG. 214-10 ■ A superior visual field defect demonstrating the typical features of the nerve fiber bundle defect.

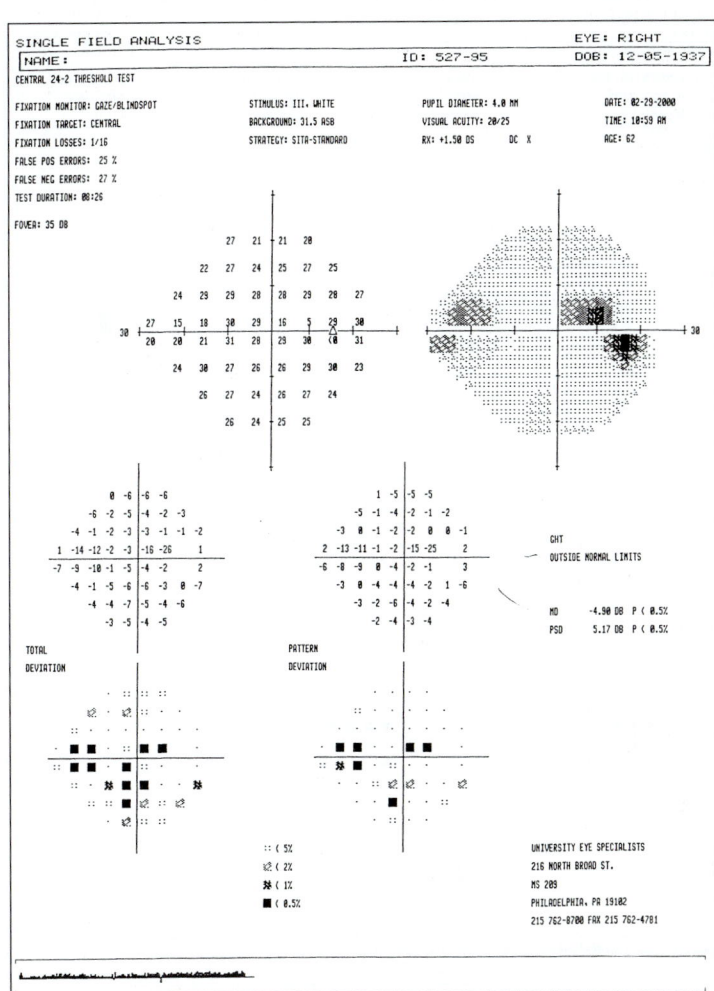

FIG. 214-11 ■ A patient with superior and inferior nerve fiber bundle defects demonstrating a paracentral scotoma superior and temporal to fixation.

10° and 20° from fixation temporally but fans out to between 2 and 25° nasally. Scotomas in this area often assume an arcuate shape with the circumferential diameter greater than the radial diameter. Fixation itself is usually spared unless the defect is far advanced.

Clinically, nerve fiber bundle defects may appear as paracentral or arcuate scotomas, nasal steps, temporal sector defects, or various combinations (Figs. 214-9 to 214-12). Any visual field defect that has nerve fiber bundle characteristics in a patient with optic disc cupping may safely be assumed to be glaucomatous in nature.

Generalized loss of retinal sensitivity, enlargement of the blind spot, and selective loss of sensitivity in the nasal periphery without specific nerve fiber bundle characteristics have been described in glaucoma. There are many other causes of these types of visual field defects. Although any of them may occur as an isolated finding in glaucoma, more commonly they are associated with a nerve fiber bundle defect.[53-55]

Artifacts Resembling Visual Field Defects

There are a number of artifacts of visual field testing that can produce results resembling those in true visual field defects. An artifact does not reflect abnormal visual function. Rather, it results from the way the patient responds to the testing situation. Generalized depressions such as are seen in patients with cataracts[56] or small pupils[57] are not artifacts. They are true visual field defects that reflect diminished visual function. Artifacts and nonglaucomatous visual field defects must be distinguished from each other as well as from defects due to glaucoma.

The learning effect is a common artifact seen in patients undergoing their first visual field examination.[58-60] Typically, it appears as a loss of sensitivity that is most pronounced in the more peripheral portions of the field. The defect either disappears or markedly improves after the second or third examination.

An apparent depression in the superior peripheral portion of the field may resemble an arcuate scotoma in the gray scale. The superior portion of the visual field normally has lower sensitivity and higher variability.[14,61] Careful inspection of the total and pattern deviation as well as the Glaucoma Hemifield Test helps to identify this artifact. Blepharoptosis, however, even when very mild, may produce significant depressions in the superior visual field resembling the defects seen in glaucoma. Some of these defects may be quite close to fixation.[62]

In order to obtain accurate central visual fields, the patient's refractive correction must be placed in the perimeter. If this is not done, the visual field may appear abnormal.[63,64] In general, about 1 decibel of loss will appear for each diopter of over- or undercorrection placed in the perimeter. The loss due to incorrect refractive correction tends to be most pronounced in the central visual field.[65]

If the pupil is smaller than 2.5mm, an otherwise normal visual field may appear to be depressed whereas an abnormal visual field may appear worse than it really is.[57,63,66] Strictly speaking, this is not an artifact because the changes in the visual field result from an alteration of the visual pathway. A small pupil, however, makes interpretation of the visual field difficult. The pupil size should be recorded each time the visual field is tested. If an effect of miosis on the visual field is suspected, the pupil should be dilated prior to the examination. Many clinicians routinely dilate pupils less than 3mm for perimetry.

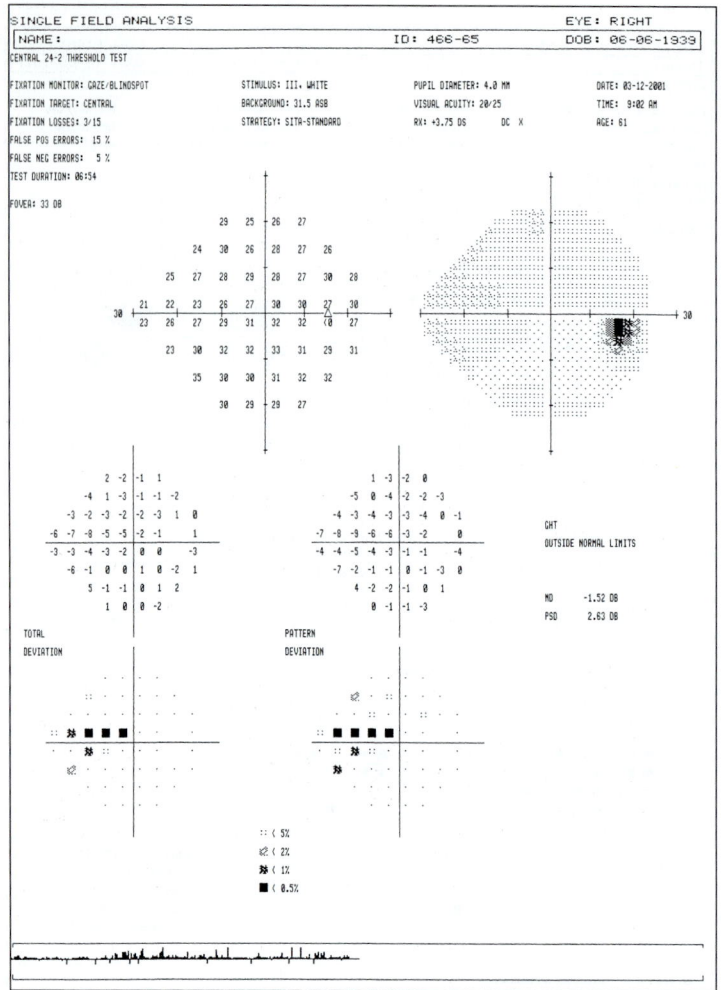
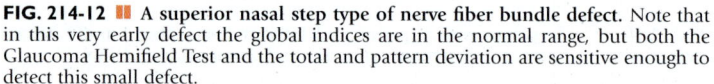

FIG. 214-12 ■ A superior nasal step type of nerve fiber bundle defect. Note that in this very early defect the global indices are in the normal range, but both the Glaucoma Hemifield Test and the total and pattern deviation are sensitive enough to detect this small defect.

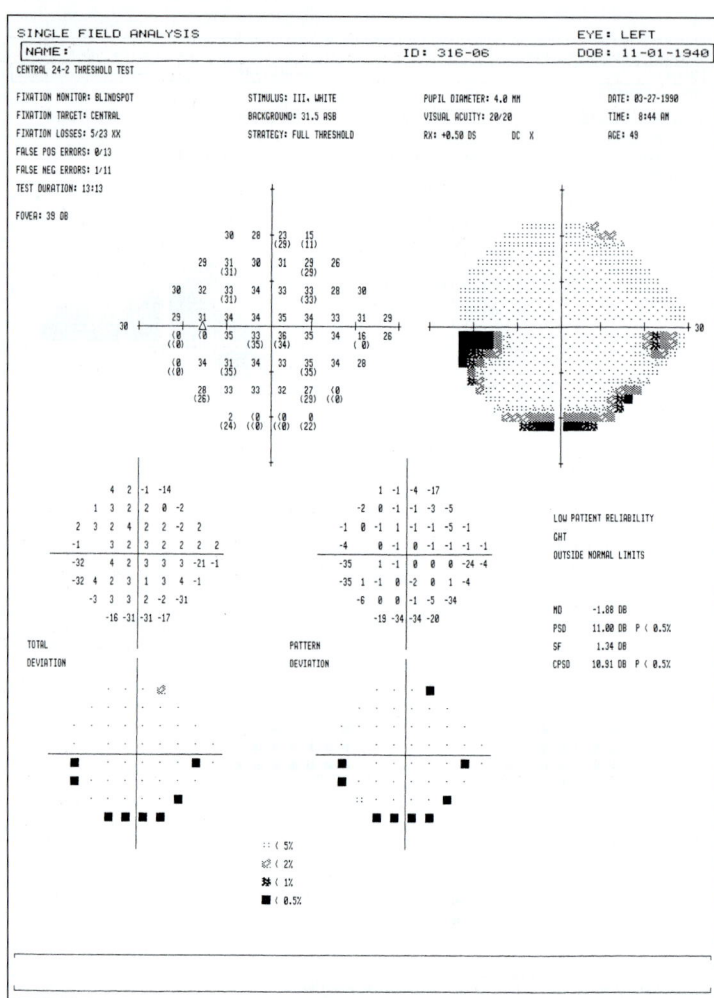

FIG. 214-13 ■ Typical lens rim artifact simulating a dense inferior visual field defect. This completely disappeared when the patient was retested with the lens holder properly positioned.

The rim of the lens holder may produce a scotoma by obscuring a portion of the patient's view of the perimeter bowl[67] (Fig. 214-13). The lens holder should be placed as close to the patient's eye as possible and the patient's eye should be well centered behind the lens. Fatigue and an unduly long examination time may also be associated with depressed sensitivity and apparent visual field defects.[68]

Detection of Progressive Visual Field Loss

The detection of progressive glaucomatous visual field loss with automated perimetry is an extremely complex problem that has not been satisfactorily solved.[69-71] The visual fields of both normal individuals and glaucoma patients are subject to a large degree of long-term fluctuation, which is defined as variation in measured visual thresholds of examinations performed on different days. Long-term fluctuation has been extensively studied and shown to be larger in glaucoma patients than in normal subjects, larger in more extensively damaged areas of the visual field, larger in the periphery of the field than near fixation, and larger in the superior half of the field.[72-76]

Because of the large amount of long-term fluctuation found in the visual fields of glaucoma patients, it is often difficult to decide whether the difference between two fields is due to true progressive field loss or random variation. Investigators have been grappling with this problem since the inception of automated perimetry.[77] Even experienced clinicians often have difficulty in determining whether or not visual field defects are progressing and frequently do not agree with statistical tests applied to the visual field data.[78] Techniques have improved agreement among clinicians and statistical tests in detecting progressive

field loss, but we still lack a generally accepted "gold standard" definition of progression that has been validated.[79-81]

Some clinical treatment trials in glaucoma have developed sophisticated techniques to detect progression. These different techniques, however, show only fair agreement when applied to the same groups of patients. Often, the different scoring and statistical techniques come to opposite conclusions about the same set of visual fields.[70,82]

Despite these problems, it has become apparent that multiple visual field examinations are required to separate fluctuation from progression and that progression is more easily detected when a series of visual fields are graphically displayed in a single printout. Clinicians should probably not even attempt to diagnose progression with fewer than four examinations and only if any changes can be documented on repeated testing.[13,69] Nor should one rely on simple inspection of individual visual field printouts.

The Humphrey software provides three ways to display serial visual field data to assist in determining the presence of progression: the Overview printout, the Change Analysis printout, and the Glaucoma Change Probability Analysis.[14,19,83] Another commercially available software program, PROGRESSOR, is also useful for this purpose.[84]

The Overview printout (Fig. 214-14) simply displays the gray scale, measured thresholds, and total and pattern deviations on a single sheet of paper. Trends over time may be more easily demonstrated with this printout, but no statistical analysis is performed.

The Change Analysis printout (Fig. 214-15) displays serial visual field data as a set of frequency distributions of the actual measured threshold data in the form of box plots. The normal

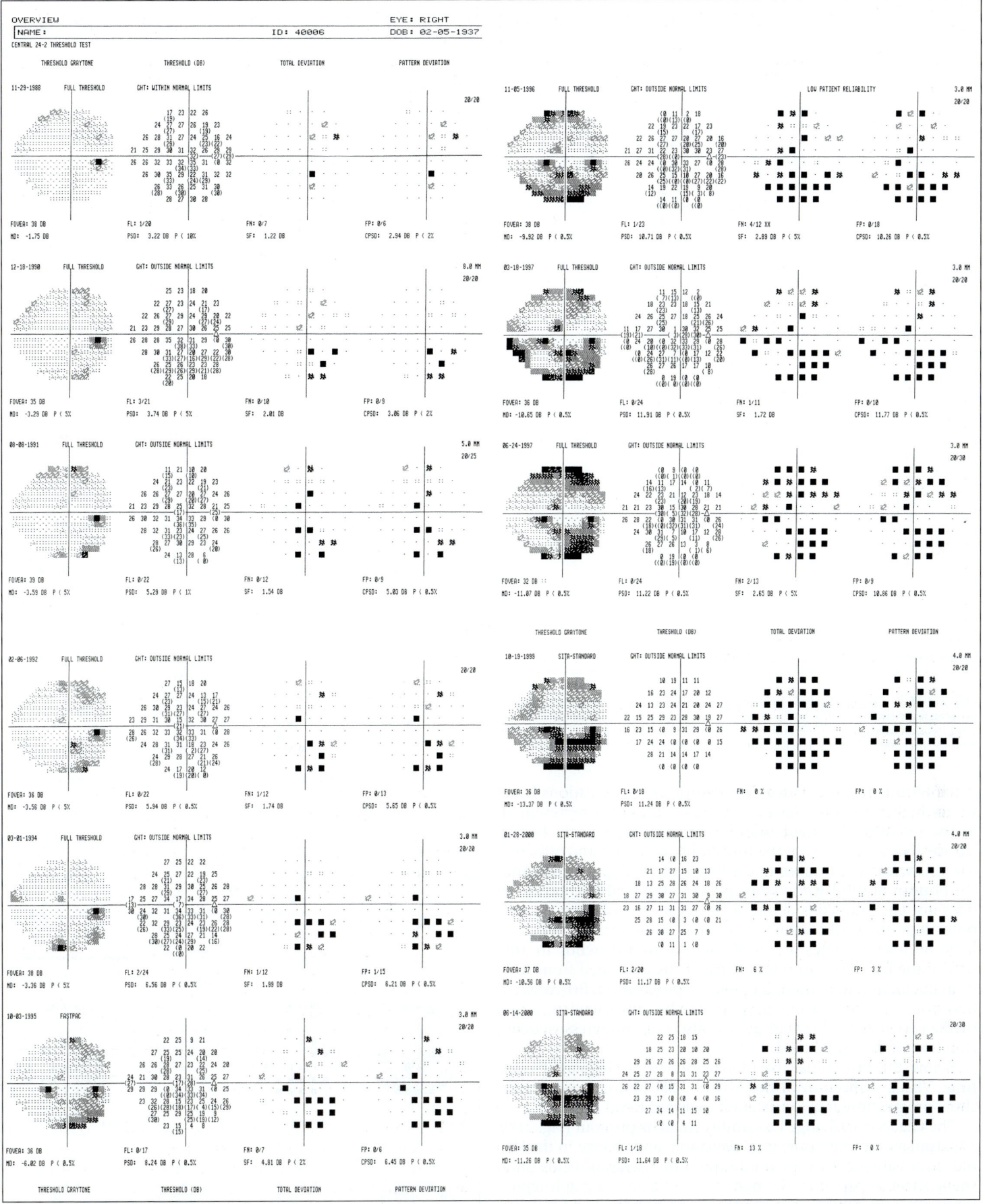

FIG. 214-14 ■ **Overview printout showing progressive glaucomatous visual field loss.** The enlargement and deepening of the defect are well seen in the gray scale, total, and pattern deviation displays.

distribution is shown as a sample box plot to the left of the display. The actual values are presented in chronological order in the graph. The numbers along the Y axis of the graph represent the difference between the actual measured threshold and the age-corrected normal, in other words, the departure from normal. Positive values represent test locations with thresholds above normal and negative values, test locations with thresholds below normal. The highest value in the box plot, the top of the T, is the best point in the visual field. It is the test location with the highest value compared with the normal. The top of the box

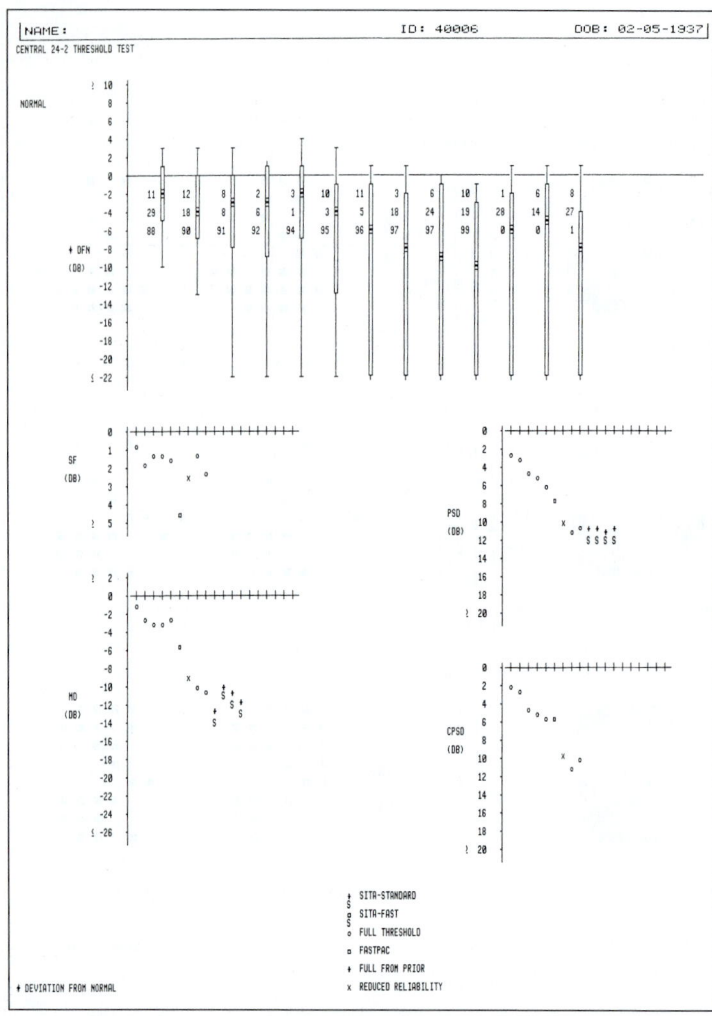

FIG. 214-15 ■ Change Analysis printout of the patient in Fig. 214-14 showing a **progressing visual field.** The box plot frequency distributions demonstrate a downward trend between fields 1988 and 1997. There is a significant downward trend in both the MD and PSD plots. The last four or five fields seem to have stabilized.

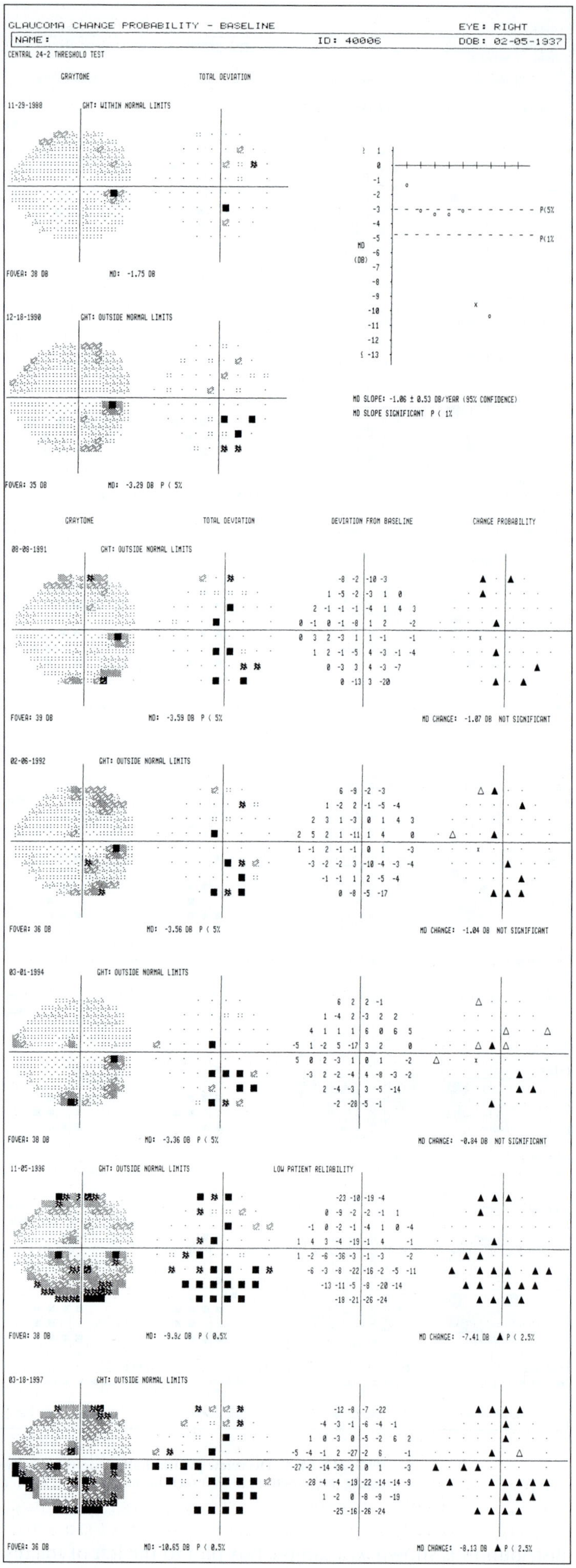

is the 85th percentile. Fifteen percent of the test locations have values higher and 85% have values lower than that represented by the top of the box. The thick bar in the middle of the box is the median value; 50% of the thresholds are above and 50% below this value. The bottom of the box is the 15th percentile, and the bottom of the T is the worst point in the field. The box plot does not take into consideration the location of the test points, only their threshold values compared with normal. When a large number of fields are available, downward trends in any part of the box plot can often be easily distinguished from random fluctuation to allow a diagnosis of progression. Progression may not necessarily be due to glaucoma because cataracts, other media opacities, and retinal disease also cause progressive deterioration of the visual field.

Below the box plots, the global indices are displayed over time. Visual inspection of the MD or PSD plot over time may show progression as a consistent downward trend.

The Glaucoma Change Probability Analysis printout (Fig. 214-16) displays the gray scale, total deviation, and change in threshold from baseline for each test location of a series of fields on a single sheet of paper. To the right of these data is a graph representing the probability that changes in each individual test location are outside the expected range of random fluctuation. Clear triangles represent test locations showing improvement, and solid black triangles represent test locations showing deterioration.

Progression is usually represented by a cluster of black triangles in the same location that enlarges with time. It should again be emphasized that none of these displays allows the clinician to detect progression reliably with fewer than four to six visual fields. The Glaucoma Change Probability Analysis is not available for visual fields done with SITA.

FIG. 214-16 ■ Glaucoma Change Probability Analysis printout of the patient in Fig. 214-14. The last four field tests were done with SITA and are not included in this analysis. The first two fields serve as a baseline. The clusters of black triangles in the most recent fields identify the areas of significant progression.

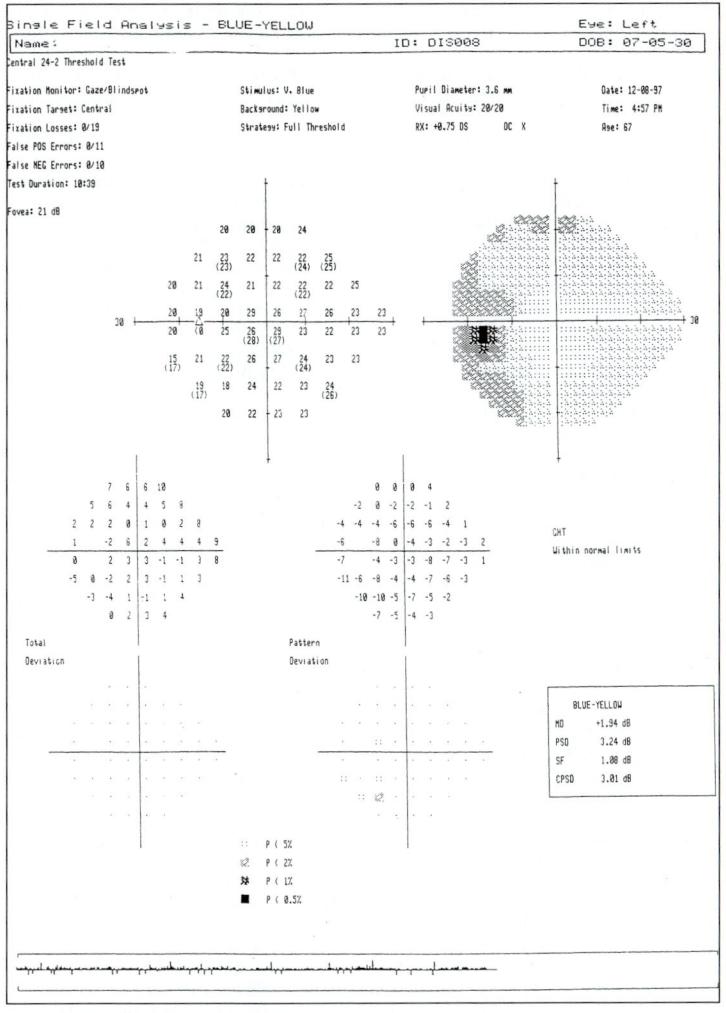

FIG. 214-17 ▪ A normal blue-yellow (SWAP) visual field. (Courtesy of Dr. Chris Johnson, Devers Eye Institute, Portland, Oregon.)

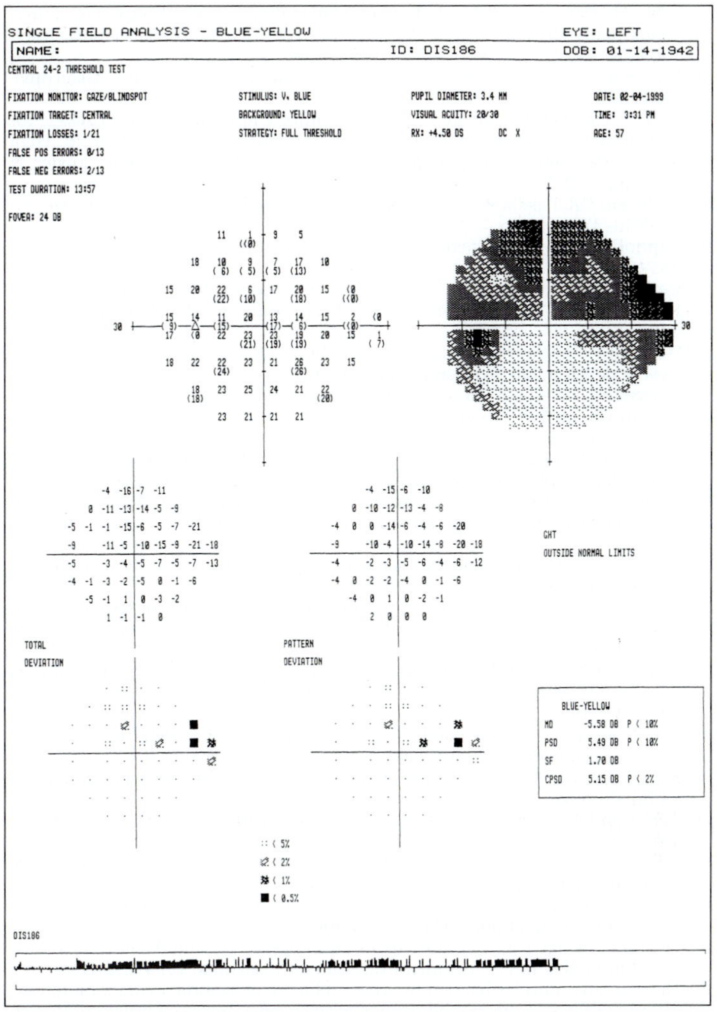

FIG. 214-18 ▪ A SWAP visual field showing an early superior nerve fiber bundle defect in a glaucoma patient with a completely normal white-on-white standard Humphrey field. (Courtesy of Dr. Chris Johnson, Devers Eye Institute, Portland, Oregon.)

ALTERNATIVE TESTS

This chapter has emphasized the Humphrey system for automated perimetry because it is the most widely used system in North America and is the one available to the author. It should be noted that equally sophisticated testing procedures and analysis programs are available with the Octopus and other perimeters. In patients who cannot perform automated perimetry or where automated perimetry is unavailable, manual quantitative perimetry with the Goldmann perimeter is a useful alternative.

Newer types of perimetry utilizing targets more complex than simple white-on-white are now undergoing development. Although none has come into widespread clinical use, there is considerable potential for their use in the future.[85]

The use of a blue test object on a yellow background is called short-wavelength automated perimetry or SWAP for short. This test is commercially available on the Humphrey HFA II perimeter. There is some evidence that SWAP is more sensitive than white light perimetry for detecting early glaucomatous damage, but the testing time is significantly longer and variability is increased. SWAP is probably most useful in patients with evidence of early glaucomatous change to the optic disc or nerve fiber layer but normal or borderline visual fields on standard automated perimetry (Figs. 214-17 and 214-18).[86–92]

Frequency-doubling technology (FDT) is another innovation that is commercially available. FDT refers to the use of rapidly alternating dark and light stripes as a perimetric target. This produces an optical illusion of nonflickering stripes that are half as wide as the actual stripes. There is some evidence that FDT perimetry may do a better job of detecting early glaucomatous visual field loss than standard white light perimetry. The test is relatively quick and considerably easier and less fatiguing for the patient. It is becoming very useful as a screening technique.[93–97]

REFERENCES

1. American Academy of Ophthalmology. Ophthalmic procedures assessment automated perimetry. Ophthalmology. 1996;103:1144–51.
2. O'Brien C, Wild JM. Automated perimetry in glaucoma—room for improvement? Br J Ophthalmol. 1995;79:200–1.
3. Miglior S, Casula M, Guareschi M. Clinical ability of the Heidelberg retinal tomograph examination to detect glaucomatous visual field defects. Ophthalmology. 2001;108:1621–7.
4. Miglior S, Brigatti L, Lonati C, et al. Correlation between the progression of optic disc and visual field changes in glaucoma. Curr Eye Res. 1996;15:145–9.
5. Quigley HA, Tielsch JM, Katz J, et al. Rate of progression in open-angle glaucoma estimated from cross-sectional prevalence of visual field damage. Am J Ophthalmol. 1996;122:355–63.
6. Kwon YH, Kim CS, Zimmerman MB, et al. Rate of visual field loss and long-term visual outcome in primary open-angle glaucoma. Am J Ophthalmol. 2001;132:47–56.
7. Portney GL, Krohn MA. Automated perimetry background, instruments and methods. Surv Ophthalmol. 1978;22:271–8.
8. Katz J, Tielsch JM, Quigley HA, Sommer A. Automated perimetry detects visual field loss before manual Goldmann perimetry. Ophthalmology 1995;102:21–6.
9. Duke-Elder S, Ashton N, Smith RJH, Lederman M. System of ophthalmology, Vol VII, The foundations of ophthalmology. St. Louis: Mosby; 1962:393–409.
10. Duke-Elder S, Jay B. System of ophthalmology, Vol XI, Diseases of the lens and vitreous; glaucoma and hypotony. St. Louis: Mosby; 1969:469–77.
11. Lynn JR, Fellman RI, Starita RJ. Principles of perimetry. In: Ritch R, Shields MB, Krupin T, eds. The glaucomas, 2nd ed. St. Louis: Mosby; 1996:491–521.
12. Caprioli J. Discrimination between normal and glaucomatous eyes. Invest Ophthalmol Vis Sci. 1993;33:153–9.
13. Keltner JI, Johnson CA, Quigg JM, et al. Confirmation of visual field abnormalities in the Ocular Hypertension Treatment Study. Arch Ophthalmol. 2000;118:1187–94.
14. Heijl A, Lindgren G, Olsson J. A package for the statistical analysis of visual fields. In: Heijl A, ed. Seventh International Visual Field Symposium, Amsterdam, September 1986. Dordrecht, The Netherlands: Dr W Junk; 1987:153–68.
15. Heijl A, Lindgren G, Olsson J. Normal variability of static visual threshold values across the central visual field. Arch Ophthalmol. 1987;105:1544–9.
16. Katz J, Sommer A. A longitudinal study of the age-adjusted variability of automated visual fields. Arch Ophthalmol. 1988;105:1083–6.

17. Bebie H, Flammer J, Bebie T. The cumulative defect curve of local and diffuse components of visual field damage. Graefes Arch Clin Exp Ophthalmol. 1989;227:9–12.

18. Flammer J, Jenni F, Bebie H, et al. The Octopus G1 program. Glaucoma. 1987;9:67–72.

19. Heijl A, Lindgren G, Lindgren A, et al. Extended empirical statistical package for evaluation of single and multiple fields in glaucoma Statpac 2. In: Mills RP, Heijl A, eds. Perimetry update 1990/91. Amstelveen, The Netherlands: Kugler & Ghedini; 1991:303–15.

20. Anderson DR, Patella VM. Automated static perimetry, 2nd ed. St. Louis: Mosby; 1999:10–35.

21. Caprioli J. Automated perimetry in glaucoma. Am J Ophthalmol. 1991;111:235–6.

22. Lynn JR, Fellman RL, Starita RI. Principles of perimetry. In: Ritch R, Shields MB, Krupin T, eds. The glaucomas, 2nd ed. St. Louis: Mosby–Year Book; 1996:491–521.

23. Werner EB. The normal visual field. In: Werner EB, ed. Manual of visual fields. New York: Churchill Livingstone; 1991:91–110.

24. Vingrys AJ, Demirel S. False-response monitoring during automated perimetry. Optom Vis Sci. 1998;75:513–17.

25. Heijl A, Lindgren G, Olsson J. Reliability parameters in computerized perimetry. In: Greve EL, Heijl A, eds. Seventh International Visual Field Symposium, Amsterdam, September 1986. Dordrecht: Dr W Junk; 1987:593–600

26. Bengtsson B, Olsson J, Heijl A, Rootzen H. A new generation of algorithms for computerized threshold perimetry, SITA. Acta Ophthalmol Scand. 1997;75:368–75.

27. Katz J, Sommer A. Screening for glaucomatous visual field loss. The effect of patient reliability. Ophthalmology. 1990;97:1032–7.

28. Johnson CA, Nelson-Quigg JM. A prospective three-year study of response properties of normal subjects and patients during automated perimetry. Ophthalmology. 1993;100:269–74.

29. Bengtsson B, Heijl A. False-negative responses in glaucoma perimetry indicators of patient performance or test reliability? Invest Ophthalmol Vis Sci. 2000;41:2201–4.

30. Katz J, Sommer A, Gaasterland DE, et al. Comparison of analytic algorithms for detecting glaucomatous visual field loss. Arch Ophthalmol. 1991;109:1684–9.

31. Katz J, Sommer A, Witt K. Reliability of visual field results over repeated testing. Ophthalmology. 1991;98:70–5.

32. Anderson DR, Patella VM. Automated static perimetry, 2nd ed. St. Louis: Mosby; 1999:121–6.

33. Advanced Glaucoma Intervention Study. 2. Visual field test scoring and reliability. Ophthalmology. 1994;101:1445–55.

34. Lee M, Zulauf M, Caprioli J. The influence of patient reliability on visual field outcome. Am J Ophthalmol. 1994;117:756–61.

35. Demirel S, Vingrys AJ. Eye movements during perimetry and the effect that fixational instability has on perimetric outcomes. J Glaucoma. 1994;3:28–35.

36. Henson DB, Evans J, Chauhan BC, et al. Influence of fixation accuracy on threshold variability in patients with open-angle glaucoma. Invest Ophthalmol Vis Sci. 1996;37:444–50.

37. Flanagan JG, Wild JM, Trope GE. The visual field indices in primary open-angle glaucoma. Invest Ophthalmol Vis Sci. 1993;34:2266–74.

38. Funkhouser AT, Fankhauser F. The effects of weighting the Mean Defect visual field index according to threshold variability in the central and mid peripheral visual field. Graefes Arch Clin Exp Ophthalmol. 1991;229:228–31.

39. Anderson DR, Patella VM. Automated static perimetry, 2nd ed. St. Louis: Mosby; 1999:111–15.

40. Heijl A, Asman P. A clinical study of perimetric probability maps. Arch Ophthalmol. 1989;107:199–203.

41. Heijl A, Lindgren G, Olsson J, et al. Visual field interpretation with empiric probability maps. Arch Ophthalmol. 1989;107:204–8.

42. Asman P, Heijl A. Glaucoma hemifield test automated visual field evaluation. Arch Ophthalmol. 1992;110:812–19.

43. Asman P, Heijl A. Evaluation of methods for automated hemifield analysis in perimetry. Arch Ophthalmol. 1992;110:820–6.

44. Katz J, Quigley HA, Sommer A. Detection of incident field loss using the glaucoma hemifield test. Ophthalmology. 1996;103:657–63.

45. American Academy of Ophthalmology. Preferred practice pattern primary open-angle glaucoma. San Francisco; 1996.

46. Anderson DR, Patella VM. Automated static perimetry, 2nd ed. St. Louis: Mosby; 1999:191–245.

47. Bengtsson B, Heijl A, Olsson J. Evaluation of a new threshold visual field strategy, SITA, in normal subjects. Acta Ophthalmol Scand. 1998;76:165–9.

48. Bengtsson B, Heijl A. evaluation of a new perimetric threshold strategy, SITA, in patients with manifest and suspect glaucoma. Acta Ophthalmol Scand. 1998;76:268–72.

49. Sekhar GC, Naduvilath TJ, Lakkai M, et al. Sensitivity of Swedish Interactive Threshold Algorithm compared with standard full threshold algorithm in Humphrey visual field testing. Ophthalmology. 2000;107:1303–8.

50. Wild JM, Pacey IE, O'Neill EC, Cunliffe LA. The SITA perimetric threshold algorithms in glaucoma. Invest Ophthalmol Vis Sci. 1999;40:1998–2009.

51. Budenz DL. Atlas of visual fields. Philadelphia: Lippincott-Raven; 1997:143–94.

52. Varma R, Minckler DS. Anatomy and pathophysiology of the retina and optic nerve. In: Ritch R, Shields MB, Krupin T, eds. The glaucomas, 2nd ed. St. Louis: Mosby; 1996:139–76.

53. Asman P, Heijl A. Diffuse visual field loss and glaucoma. Acta Ophthalmol (Copenh). 1994;72:303–8.

54. Mutlukan E. Diffuse and localized visual field defects to automated perimetry in primary open-angle glaucoma. Eye. 1995;9:745–50.

55. Chauhan BC, LeBlanc RP, Shaw AM, et al. Repeatable diffuse visual field loss in open-angle glaucoma. Ophthalmology. 1997;104:532–8.

56. Budenz DL, Feuer WJ, Anderson DR. The effect of simulated cataract on the glaucomatous visual field. Ophthalmology. 1993;100:511–17.

57. Lindenmuth KA, Skuta GL, Rabbani R, et al. Effects of pupillary constriction on automated perimetry in normal eyes. Ophthalmology. 1989;96:1298–1301.

58. Heijl A, Lindgren G, Olsson J. The effect of perimetric experience in normal subjects. Arch Ophthalmol. 1989;107:81–6.

59. Werner EB, Adelson A, Krupin T. Effect of patient experience on the results of automated perimetry in clinically stable glaucoma patients. Ophthalmology. 1988;95:764–7.

60. Werner EB, Krupin T, Adelson A, et al. Effect of patient experience on the results of automated perimetry in glaucoma suspect patients. Ophthalmology. 1990;97:44–8.

61. Katz J, Sommer A. Asymmetry and variation in the normal hill of vision. Arch Ophthalmol. 1986;104:65–8.

62. Meyer DR, Stern JH, Jarvis JM, et al. Evaluating the visual field effects of blepharoptosis using automated static perimetry. Ophthalmology. 1993;100:651–9.

63. Herse P. Factors influencing normal perimetric thresholds obtained using the Humphrey Field Analyzer. Invest Ophthalmol Vis Sci. 1992;33:611–17.

64. Heuer DK, Anderson DR, Feuer WJ, et al. The influence of refraction accuracy on automated perimetric threshold measurements. Ophthalmology. 1987;94:1550–3.

65. Weinreb RN, Perlman JP. The effect of refractive correction on automated perimetric thresholds. Am J Ophthalmol. 1986;101:706–9.

66. Heuer DK, Anderson DR, Feuer WJ, et al. The influence of decreased retinal illumination on automatic perimetric threshold measurements. Am J Ophthalmol. 1989;108:643–50.

67. Zalta AH. Lens rim artifact in automated threshold perimetry. Ophthalmology. 1989;98:1302–11.

68. Searle AET, Wild JM, Shaw DE, et al. Time-related variation in normal automated perimetry. Ophthalmology. 1991;98:701–7.

69. Schulzer M, Anderson DR, Drance SM. Errors in the diagnosis of visual field progression in normal tension glaucoma. Ophthalmology. 1994;101:1589–95.

70. Katz J, Gilbert D, Quigley HA, Sommer A. Estimating progression of visual field loss in glaucoma. Ophthalmology. 1997;104:1017–25.

71. Katz J, Congdon N, Friedman DS. Methodological variations in estimating apparent progressive visual field loss in clinical trials of glaucoma treatment. Arch Ophthalmol. 1999;117:1137–42.

72. Boeglin RI, Caprioli I, Zulauf M. Long-term fluctuation of the visual field in glaucoma. Am J Ophthalmol. 1992;113:396–400.

73. Stewart WC, Hunt HH. Threshold variation in automated perimetry. Surv Ophthalmol. 1993;37:353–61.

74. Werner EB, Ganiban G, Balazsi AG. Effect of test point location on the magnitude of threshold fluctuation in glaucoma patients undergoing automated perimetry. In: Mills RP, Heijl A, eds. Perimetry update 1990/91. Amstelveen, The Netherlands: Kugler & Ghedini; 1991:175–81.

75. Werner EB, Petrig B, Krupln T, et al. Variability of automated visual fields in clinically stable glaucoma patients. Invest Ophthalmol Vis Sci. 1989;30:1083–9.

76. Hutchings N, Wild JM, Hussey MK, et al. The long-term fluctuation of the visual field in stable glaucoma. Invest Ophthalmol Vis Sci. 2000;41:3429–36.

77. Gloor BP, Vökt BA. Long-term fluctuation versus actual field loss in glaucoma patients. Dev Ophthalmol. 1985;12:48–69.

78. Werner EB, Bishop KI, Koelle J, et al. A comparison of experienced clinical observers and statistical tests in detection of progressive visual field loss in glaucoma using automated perimetry. Arch Ophthalmol. 1988;106:619–23.

79. Chauhan BC, Drance SM, LeBlanc RP, et al. Technique for determining visual field progression by using animation graphics. Am J Ophthalmol. 1994;118:485–91.

80. Smith SD, Katz J, Quigley J. Analysis of progressive change in automated visual fields in glaucoma. Invest Ophthalmol Vis Sci. 1996;37:1419–28.

81. Fitzke FW, Hitchings RA, Poinoosawmy D, et al. Analysis of visual field progression in glaucoma. Br J Ophthalmol. 1996;80:40–8.

82. Katz J. Scoring systems for measuring progression of visual field loss in clinical trials of glaucoma treatment. Ophthalmology. 1999;106:391–5.

83. Morgan RK, Feuer WJ, Anderson DR. Statpac 2 glaucoma change probability. Arch Ophthalmol. 1991;109:1690–2.

84. Viswanathan AC, Fitzke FW, Hitchings RA. Early detection of visual field progression in glaucoma: a comparison of PROGRESSOR and STATPAC2. Br J Ophthalmol. 1997;81:1037–42.

85. Johnson CA. Early losses of visual function in glaucoma. Optom Vis Sci. 1995;72:359–70.

86. Johnson CA, Brandt JD, Khong AM, Adams AJ. Short-wavelength automated perimetry in low, medium and high risk ocular hypertensive eyes. Arch Ophthalmol. 1995;113:70–6.

87. Felius J, de Jong LAMS, van den Berg TJTP, et al. Functional characteristics of blue-on-yellow perimetric thresholds in glaucoma. Invest Ophthalmol Vis Sci. 1995;36:1665–74.

88. Kwon YH, Park HJ, Jap A, et al. Test-retest variability of blue-on-yellow perimetry is greater than white-on-white perimetry in normal subjects. Am J Ophthalmol. 1998;126:29–36.

89. Mansberger SL, Sample PA, Zangwill L, Weinreb RN. Achromatic and short-wavelength automated perimetry in patients with glaucomatous large cups. Arch Ophthalmol. 1999;117:1473–7.

90. Girkin CA, Emdadi A, Sample PA, et al. Short-wavelength automated perimetry in the detection of progressive optic disc cupping. Arch Ophthalmol. 2000;118:1231–6.

91. Blumenthal EZ, Sample PA, Zangwill L, et al. Comparison of long-term variability for standard and short-wavelength automated perimetry in stable glaucoma patients. Am J Ophthalmol. 2000;129:309–13.

92. Caprioli J. Should we use short-wavelength automated perimetry to test glaucoma patients? Am J Ophthalmol. 2001;131:792–4.

93. Johnson CA, Samuels SJ. Screening for glaucomatous visual field loss with frequency doubling perimetry. Invest Ophthalmol Vis Sci. 1997;38:413–25.

94. Trible JR, Schultz RO, Robinson JC, Rothe TL. Accuracy of glaucoma detection with frequency-doubling perimetry. Am J Ophthalmol. 2000;129:740–5.

95. Burnstein Y, Ellish NJ, Magbalon M, Higginbotham EJ. Comparison of frequency doubling perimetry with Humphrey Visual Field analysis in a glaucoma practice. Am J Ophthalmol. 2000;129(3):328–33.

96. Cello KE, Nelson-Quigg JM, Johnson CA. Frequency doubling technology perimetry for detection of glaucomatous visual field loss. Am J Ophthalmol. 2000;129:314–22.

97. Landers J, Goldberg I, Graham S. A comparison of short-wavelength automated perimetry with frequency doubling perimetry for the early detection of visual field loss in ocular hypertension. Clin Exp Ophthalmol. 2000;28:248–52.

215 Psychophysical Tests for Glaucoma

ANDREW J. MAYS

DEFINITIONS

- The study of human visual pathway responses to various visual stimuli.
- Subjective tests require a conscious response; these include frequency-doubling perimetry, ring perimetry, acuity perimetry, motion detection perimetry, pattern discrimination perimetry, contrast sensitivity, and color vision.
- Objective tests require no conscious response; these include the electroretinogram and multifocal visual evoked potential.

INTRODUCTION

Psychophysical tests have been developed in addition to traditional perimetry to detect early glaucomatous visual loss. These tests include frequency doubling, high-pass resolution (ring), acuity, motion detection and pattern discrimination types of perimetry, contrast sensitivity (both spatial and temporal), color vision, electroretinography, and visual evoked potential (VEP). If glaucomatous damage is selective to one or more neuropathways, isolating and testing these pathways may permit disease detection before changes appear in the optic disc, nerve fiber layer, and visual field. The proposed visual pathways and the tests designed to stimulate them are described herein.

HISTORICAL REVIEW

Visual field testing is imperfect. Clinically, visual field loss often correlates with nerve fiber layer loss and optic nerve damage. However, a substantial portion of the peripheral ganglion cells must be damaged before the loss is detected even by automated perimetry.[1] Also, viable ganglion cells have been found in areas unresponsive to conventional perimetric stimuli. Clearly, automated perimetry does not thoroughly evaluate visual function. Therefore, other tests to enable earliest possible detection of field changes are under development.

Tests designed to evaluate retinal visual function fall into two categories—subjective and objective. The objective tests require no conscious effort on the patient's part. These tests include electroretinography (ERG) and multifocal VEP. The subjective tests require conscious acknowledgment of the effect of the stimulus. That is, the patient must indicate purposefully whether the stimulus has been perceived. These tests include all those noted previously other than ERG and VEP.

PURPOSE OF THE TESTS

Psychophysical tests are designed to isolate various retinal pathways. In their simplest form, these pathways can be broken down into three sets of cells at different retinal layers. The first cell layer consists of the photoreceptors—rods and three types of cones. Rod function can be isolated through dark adaptation. However, photoreceptor loss has not been proved in glaucoma. Also, retinal pathways, not individual cell types, are of primary interest in psychophysical tests. Scotopic conditions, which isolate rod function, are not used in perimetry. The cones absorb light at different wavelengths and are subdivided into L cones for long (red) wavelength absorption, M cones for medium (green) absorption, and S cones for short (blue) absorption.

The second cell layer is in the middle retina and contains the bipolar cells, which process the information from the photoreceptors into two color-integrating pathways. One pathway carries stimuli from the L and M cones and, because it is concentrated in the fovea, it is the proposed route of spatial contrast information. The other bipolar cell pathway carries information from the S cones (blue wavelength); it constitutes less than 15% of the total cone population and is usually absent from the fovea. This pathway seems to be damaged preferentially in glaucoma, which results in the so-called tritan (blue-yellow) defect.

The third cell layer is defined by two populations of ganglion cells. One population, the tonic or P cells (named for their projection to the parvicellular region of the dorsolateral geniculate nucleus), constitutes about 80% of the ganglion cells. These ganglion cells are found mostly in the fovea and are thought to be responsible for color vision and high-contrast acuity. The P cells are smaller than the phasic or M population of ganglion cells (named for their projection to the magnicellular region of the dorsolateral geniculate nucleus). The M cells constitute about 10% of all ganglion cells and are thought to be responsible for high-frequency temporal-contrast sensitivity, low-frequency spatial-contrast sensitivity, and motion detection. New psychophysical tests and new applications of existing tests are being developed to recognize early glaucomatous damage by examination of these various pathways (Table 215-1).

TABLE 215-1

VISUAL PATHWAYS AND PSYCHOPHYSICAL TESTS THAT ISOLATE THEM

Retinal Cell Layer	Cellular Subsets	Tests That Isolate Subsets
Photoreceptors	S cones (blue–yellow pathway)	Short-wave automated perimetry
	Cones: L, M, S	Farnsworth–Munsell, Farnsworth, and L'Anthony
Bipolar cells	L and M cells (spatial contrast)	Contrast sensitivity
Ganglion cells	P cells	Ring perimetry, acuity perimetry
	M cells	Motion detection perimetry, frequency doubling perimetry

UTILITY OF THE TESTS

Several inherent properties of psychophysical tests limit their usefulness. Subjective tests require threshold determination; threshold is defined as a point at which the stimulus is perceived 50% of the time (i.e., the subject responds correctly 50% of the time). Determination of this point allows intra- and intertest comparison, but the point may vary from day to day as a result of a number of factors, which include the patient's condition and the test conditions. Interpretation of data for subjective and objective tests requires statistical analysis of percent sensitivity and specificity. Sensitivity refers to the ability of the test to detect glaucoma, and specificity refers to the ability to detect the absence of glaucoma. The results are commonly reported through the use of receiver operating characteristic (ROC) curves in which the percent of 1 − specificity, equation (215-1), is plotted against the percent sensitivity (Fig. 215-1).

$$\text{Equation 215-1} \quad 1 - \text{specificity} = 1.00 - \frac{\text{number of normal patients}}{\text{total number of patients}}$$

A given psychophysical test, over a range of selected values, generates an ROC curve, and a trade-off always exists between sensitivity and specificity. If sensitivity is increased, patients who have the disease could be excluded. If sensitivity is decreased, normal individuals could be included in the disease group. After the data have been plotted on an ROC curve, an optimal value to separate patients with glaucoma from normal subjects is selected. The ROC curve may be critical in deciding whether a particular test is sensitive and specific enough to use in the general population.

Glaucomatous visual field loss is often detected later in the disease; evaluation of the optic nerve head is a better way to detect early disease progression. Shortcomings with psychophysical tests designed to detect early field loss stem from external and internal sources. Externally, the test depends on the patient. Patient understanding and cooperation, patient age, pupil diameter, media opacities, learning effects, and so forth affect test results. Internally, the test relies on statistical analysis and probability. Data generated from an individual are compared with data generated from a large, demographically similar population. The probability of the presence of glaucoma is determined, but this information must be used with discretion. Other disease states such as cataract, macular degeneration, and ischemic optic neuropathy may confuse results. Internal and external factors must be kept in mind when psychophysical test results are interpreted. At present, visual field tests must be used adjunctly to determine the progression of glaucomatous damage.

The ideal new test should have good sensitivity and specificity and be user friendly. Several new tests show promise.

Frequency-Doubling Perimetry

A recent application of contrast sensitivity combines spatial and temporal contrast. As mentioned earlier, the M cells seem to mediate low-frequency, spatial-contrast sensitivity and high-frequency, temporal-contrast sensitivity. When a low spatial frequency pattern undergoes high temporal frequency flicker (the bars alternate rapidly between dark and light), the pattern perceived appears to have double the spatial frequency. This phenomenon, described in the mid-1960s,[2] is referred to as frequency doubling. Its application in glaucoma is promising. Targets that consist of rapidly alternating vertical bars are projected onto the central 30–35° field. The patient responds when the vertical bars are seen. Early results correlate well with preexisting visual field loss defined by automated perimetry,[3] and visual blurring has little effect on the test results. Refinements in the technique are being developed.

High-Pass Resolution Perimetry

High-pass resolution perimetry or ring perimetry is an alternative form of peripheral visual field testing. The test involves a ring of fixed luminance but variable size (Fig. 215-2) that is projected onto 50 locations within the central 30° visual field. As the ring size is adjusted, the threshold is determined. This system of perimetry is thought to stimulate the P cell pathway. Advantages over conventional static perimetry include increased speed, increased patient acceptance, reduced variability, and re-

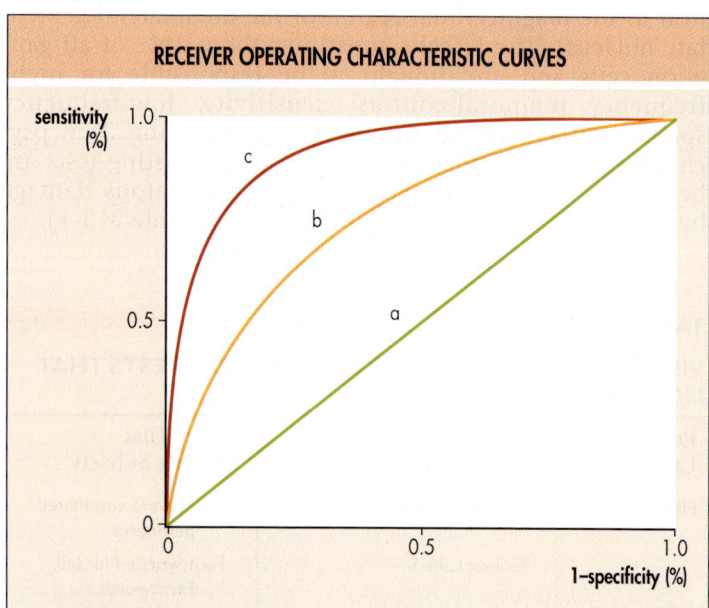

FIG. 215-1 ▮▮ **Receiver operating characteristic curves.** Curves are shown for three arbitrary levels of separability between patients with glaucoma and normal subjects. Each curve or line is generated by a hypothetical test over a range of selected thresholds. Separability is related directly to the relative area under the curve or line. Curve *a*, with an area of 50% above and below, is an invalid test as its results are no better than chance. Curve *b* shows greater area under the curve but does not approach usefulness for the detection of glaucoma. (Remember that the test must detect a disease found in 2–3% of the general population.)

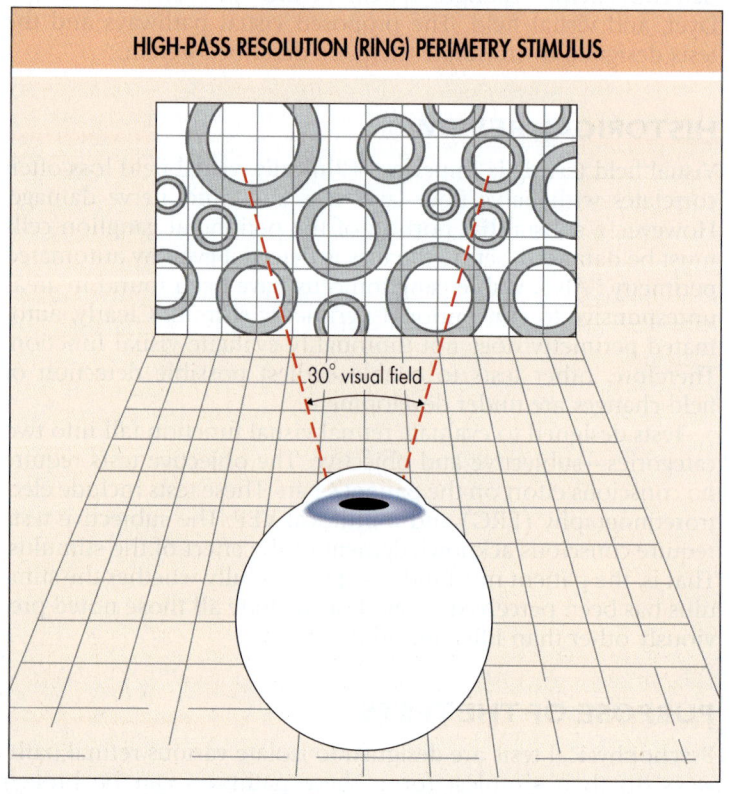

FIG. 215-2 ▮▮ **High-pass resolution (ring) perimetry stimulus.** The size of the ring varies but luminance is held constant.

duced learning curve.[4] High-pass resolution perimetry detects glaucomatous visual field loss as well as static perimetry and may be used more in the clinical setting.

Acuity Perimetry

Acuity perimetry is another test thought to detect early glaucoma. A laser interferometer is used to project interference patterns (straight lines) on the retina. The perimeter projects the images on the central 20° of vision along any meridian at 1-minute intervals. The apparatus is the same as that used to assess central visual acuity in patients affected by media opacities. Early studies have shown that acuity perimetry is more sensitive than conventional perimetry in the detection of glaucomatous damage.[5] Two hypotheses support this contention. First, visual acuity is a more complex function compared with the detection of stationary white lights. Second, fewer ganglion cells need to be damaged for a more complex visual function to be affected. Despite these early results, acuity perimetry in this form is not widely available in the clinical setting. Theoretically, ring perimetry and acuity perimetry test similar visual functions.

Motion Detection Perimetry

Motion detection may be related to temporal contrast sensitivity—both seem to be modulated primarily by the M ganglion cells.[6] In administering the test for motion detection perimetry, the patient observes many dots on a screen. Subsets of dots are moved coherently against a random background of dots (Fig. 215-3). The threshold is calculated by determination of the number of moving dots necessary to detect motion, and this number is divided by the total number of dots. Motion detection is decreased in glaucoma patients,[7] but further refinement in the technique is necessary before it is clinically applicable.

Pattern Discrimination Perimetry

Pattern discrimination perimetry involves a checkerboard image superimposed on a random dot background (the image is projected onto 32 points within the central 30° of vision). Deliberate changes in the proportion of random dots to checkerboard dots make the stimulus more difficult to perceive (Fig. 215-4). Pattern discrimination is a more complex visual function than on-off white light recognition. In theory, as with ring and acuity perimetry, the recognition of pattern requires a greater number of intact ganglion cells, and damage should be detected earlier if this theory is correct. Preliminary studies show a decrease in pattern discrimination function in glaucomatous eyes.[8] Visual loss detected by pattern discrimination perimetry does not seem to correlate with nerve fiber loss and optic nerve changes,[9] which may reflect damage to the visual system undetectable by direct observation of the optic nerve and retinal nerve fiber layer. Continuing work with this perimeter will determine its future role in glaucoma.

Contrast Sensitivity

Contrast sensitivity measures luminance between brightly and dimly lit areas, and spatial contrast uses adjacent areas of light and dark. The distance between the areas (frequency) and the intensity of the areas (luminance) are adjusted over a range. The highest possible spatial contrast sensitivity corresponds to the greatest visual acuity (Fig. 215-5). Temporal contrast uses one area that flickers between light and dark. Both spatial and temporal contrast sensitivities are decreased in glaucoma patients.[10] Spatial contrast sensitivity is nonspecific and unlikely to be useful in the detection of early glaucoma. The usefulness of temporal contrast sensitivity is unclear. The majority of the current reports in the literature suggest that temporal contrast sensitivity is decreased early in the course of glaucoma. However, the clinical usefulness of this information remains under investigation.[2]

Color Vision

Color vision is affected by glaucoma. Most reports in the literature support the preferential loss of S cones (blue wavelength) as a result of glaucoma, but as yet no explanation exists for this observation. As S cones are absent from the fovea, short-wave (blue-on-yellow) perimetry, discussed in Chapter 214, is used increasingly on this basis. In the absence of perimetric testing, three common color vision tests, the Farnsworth-Munsell 100-hue test and the Farnsworth D-15 and L'Anthony D-15 desaturated color tests, may be employed to evaluate glaucomatous damage. All detect a tritan defect equally well.[11] The simplest color test is the most practical in a clinical setting. Other conditions, such as cataracts, macular degeneration, and multiple sclerosis–associated optic atrophy, may cause tritan defects. However, color vision tests do not provide useful clinical information in the diagnosis of early glaucoma. These tests are unlikely to supplant currently employed tests to assess visual damage as a result of glaucoma.

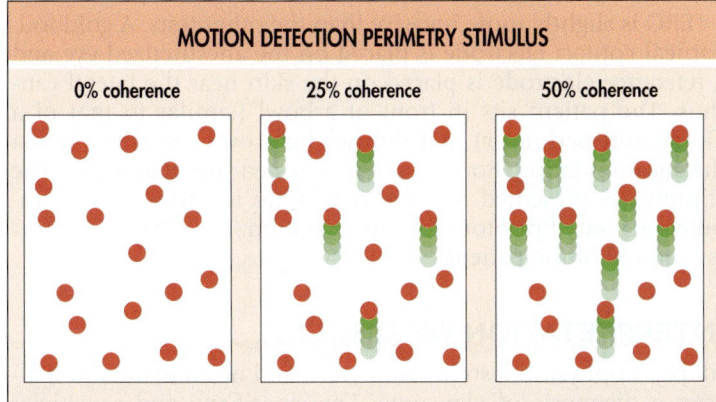

FIG. 215-3 ▌▌ **Motion detection perimetry stimulus.** 0% coherence: all the dots move randomly; 25% coherence: one quarter of the dots move in the same direction; 50% coherence: one half of the dots move in the same direction.

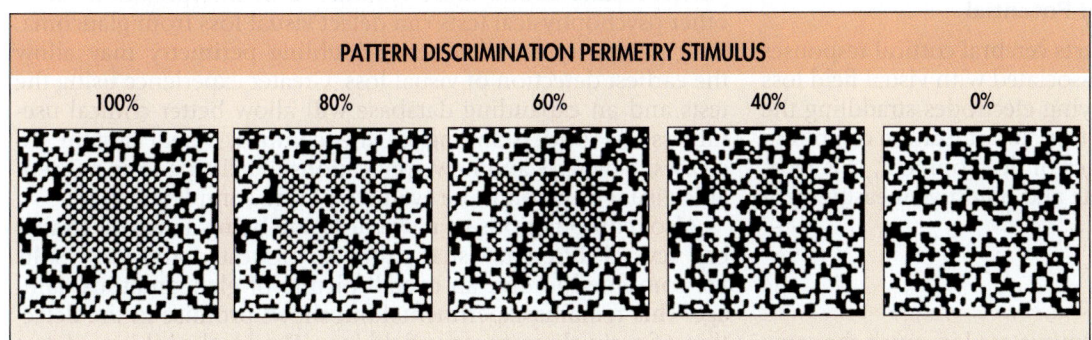

FIG. 215-4 ▌▌ **Pattern discrimination perimetry stimulus.** 0% coherence equals random checker pattern in center. 100% coherence equals perfect checkerboard pattern in center. The computer generates patterns between 0% and 100% coherence.

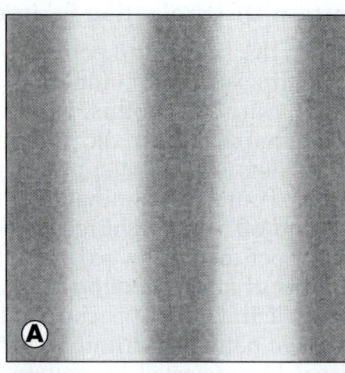

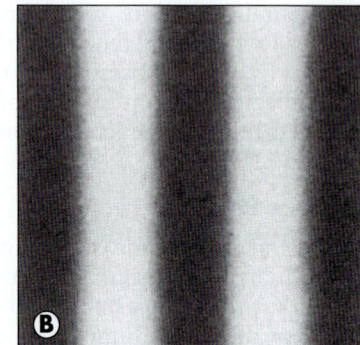

FIG. 215-5 ▮ **Spatial contrast sensitivity. A,** Low contrast. **B,** High contrast. **C,** Snellen acuity. The frequency is held constant, but the luminance of the bright stripes is increased and the luminance of the dark stripes is decreased (note relationship to visual acuity).

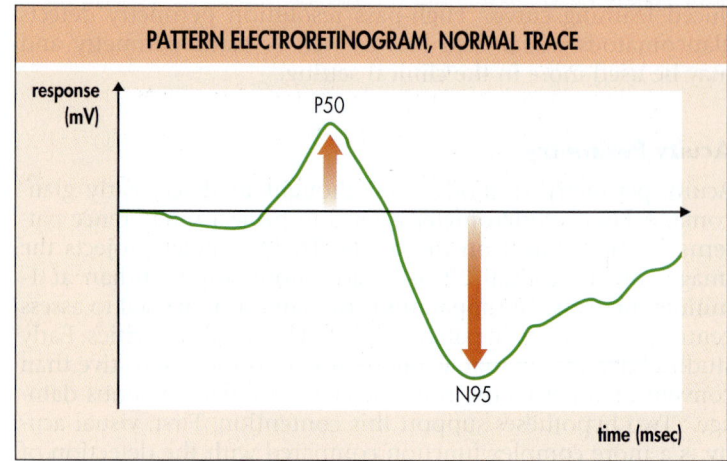

FIG. 215-6 ▮ **Pattern electroretinogram, normal trace.** P50 is the positive deflection at 50ms. N95 is the negative deflection at 95ms. In glaucomatous patients, all pattern ERG parameters, especially those at 50 and 95ms, are decreased in amplitude. Normal eye: P50 = 2.97mV ± 0.77mV; N95 = 1.39mV + 0.62mV. Glaucomatous eye: P50 = 1.43mV ± 0.47mV; N95 = 0.13 + 0.16mV.

Electroretinogram

Electrophysiologic tests are objective. Patient interaction is minimal, and the tests are minimally invasive. ERG has been applied to glaucoma patients using both flash and pattern techniques. Flash ERG stimulates photoreceptors (a-wave) and bipolar and Müller cells (b-wave). Ganglion cells contribute little to the recorded response, and, therefore, the flash electroretinogram is not affected appreciably even in advanced glaucoma. Pattern ERG averages responses to an alternating checkerboard, bar, or sine pattern. Part of the pattern ERG response may originate from the ganglion cells, but the source of the pattern response is not understood fully. Evidence has accumulated that suggests that pattern ERG amplitudes are decreased in glaucoma.[12] In particular, the negative wave measured at 95ms (N95) decreases significantly in glaucoma (Fig. 215-6).[13]

Multifocal Pattern Visual Evoked Potential

Visual evoked potential (VEP) detects cerebral cortical responses to visual stimulation. Glaucoma associated with visual field loss causes an abnormal VEP. By applying electrodes straddling the inion, subtle visual field defects within 26° of fixation can be detected.[14] Although in its early stages of development, this technique shows promise as an accurate and objective measurement of glaucomatous visual loss.

PROCEDURES

All newer tests for perimetry are administered in much the same way as automated perimetry. A central fixation target is used,

and stimuli are presented in the periphery. To take the test, the patient must be able to sit comfortably for several minutes, be able to respond to the stimulus, and understand the nature of the test. Video monitors allow observation of the patient's ability to maintain fixation. The patient is asked to push a button when a stimulus is perceived, and computer-generated results (in various forms) are printed. No part of these tests is invasive.

Color testing, another form of noninvasive testing, is simple. Discs of various hues are placed randomly before the patient, who must arrange the colors from darkest to lightest. The results are compared against predetermined patterns of color loss. Less understanding is required of the patient in these tests than in perimetry testing. Still, the patient must be able to sit at a table, move the colored discs, and appreciate the nature of the test.

ERG is slightly more invasive than the other tests. A gold foil, corneal contact electrode is placed on the anesthetized eye and a reference electrode is placed on the skin near the lateral canthus. The patient sits in front of a bowl (similar to that of a Goldmann perimeter) that diffuses light over the entire retina during stimulation. Both eyes may be tested simultaneously. The stimulus is presented and the results are recorded on a computer-generated printout for interpretation. No conscious effort is required of the patient.

INTERPRETATION OF RESULTS

All psychophysical tests are imperfect, and no individual test allows a diagnosis of glaucoma. Low specificity and sensitivity limit clinical application. The subjective nature of many of the tests limits the validity of the results. Therefore, the current, single, best way to identify and follow visual loss from glaucoma is through static threshold perimetry. This type of perimetry has the largest database for comparison, and familiarity with the reported results allows more confidence in interpretation. Most other psychophysical tests can detect visual loss from glaucoma. Ring perimetry and frequency-doubling perimetry may allow the earliest detection of visual loss. Greater experience using the tests and an expanding database will allow better clinical usefulness. As understanding of the complex visual system increases, new tests and new applications of existing tests may enable visual function to be evaluated more completely.

Also, combinations of newer tests are being assessed. In theory, several different visual pathways are tested and the results are combined to give an overall picture of glaucomatous damage. This remains experimental but shows promise in the detection of early glaucomatous field loss. The ideal goal is to detect glaucoma before it causes any visual loss.

REFERENCES

1. Quigley HA, Dunkelberger GR, Green WR. Retinal ganglion cell atrophy correlated with automated perimetry in human eyes with glaucoma. Am J Ophthalmol. 1989;107:453–64.
2. Kelly DH. Frequency doubling in visual responses. J Opt Soc Am A. 1966;56:1628–33.
3. Johnson CA, Samuels SJ. Screening for glaucomatous visual field loss with frequency-doubling perimetry. Invest Ophthalmol Vis Sci. 1997;38:413–25.
4. Graham SL, Drance SM, Chauhan BC, et al. Comparison of psychophysical and electrophysiological testing in early glaucoma. Invest Ophthalmol Vis Sci. 1996;37:2651–62.
5. Phelps CD. Acuity perimetry and glaucoma. Trans Am Ophthalmol Soc. 1984;82:753–91.
6. DeYoe EA, VanEssen DC. Concurrent processing streams in monkey visual cortex. Trends Neurosci. 1988;11:219–26.
7. Silverman SE, Trick GL, Hart WM. Motion perception is abnormal in primary open-angle glaucoma and ocular hypertension. Invest Ophthalmol Vis Sci. 1990;31:722–9.
8. Nutaitis MJ, Stewart WC, Kelly DM, et al. Pattern discrimination perimetry in patients with glaucoma and ocular hypertension. Am J Ophthalmol. 1992;114:297–301.
9. Chauhan BC, LeBlanc RP, McCormick TA, et al. Correlation between the optic disc and results obtained with conventional, high-pass and pattern discrimination perimetry in glaucoma. Can J Ophthalmol. 1993;28:312–16.
10. Stamper RL, Lerner LE. Psychophysical techniques in glaucoma. In: Ritch R, Shields MB, Krupin T, eds. The glaucomas, Vol 1. St Louis: Mosby–Year Book; 1996;701–13.
11. Bassi CJ, Galanis JC, Hoffman J. Comparison of the Farnsworth-Munsell 100-hue, the Farnsworth D-15, and the L'Anthony D-15 desaturated color tests. Arch Ophthalmol. 1993;111:639–41.
12. Breton ME, Drum BA. Functional testing in glaucoma: visual psychophysics and electrophysiology. In: Ritch R, Shields MB, Krupin T, eds. The glaucomas, Vol 1. St Louis: Mosby–Year Book; 1996;677–99.
13. O'Donaghue E, Arden GB, O'Sullivan F, et al. The pattern electroretinogram in glaucoma and ocular hypertension. Br J Ophthalmol. 1992;76:387–94.
14. Klistorner A, Graham SL. Objective perimetry in glaucoma. Ophthalmology. 2000;107:2283–99.

216 Disc Analysis

ZINARIA Y. WILLIAMS • TAMAR PEDUT-KLOIZMAN • JOEL S. SCHUMAN

DEFINITIONS

Stereoscopic Optic Nerve Head Photography
- Objective, three-dimensional, photographic representation of optic nerve head appearance.

Optic Nerve Head Morphometry-Planimetry
- Formerly used to quantify optic nerve head parameters, now supplanted by more recent technologies.

Optic Nerve Head Analyzers
- First generation of automated, quantitative measurements of optic nerve head structure (represented in this chapter by the Glaucoma Scope).

Confocal Scanning Laser Ophthalmoscopy
- Technology for optic nerve head measurements, which produces and integrates 32 coronal scans at increasing tissue depths.

Optical Coherence Tomography
- Technology for high-resolution, cross-sectional tissue imaging, well suited to nerve fiber layer and retinal measurements and becoming more useful for optic nerve head assessment.

INTRODUCTION

For nearly 150 years, since Helmholtz first viewed the optic nerve in living humans, disc appearance has been used to evaluate glaucoma status. Although clinicians may disagree about the causes of optic nerve head (ONH) damage, most accept that ONH cupping, or thinning of the neuroretinal rim, is a reliable indicator of the disease.

In the evaluation of the disc, the clinician must determine whether the ONH appearance is normal or pathological, whether an anomalous appearance is the result of glaucoma or a different pathological process, and how the ONH differs from that found in previous examinations. Given the considerable variation in ONH appearance among normal subjects, the various patterns of glaucomatous cupping, and the wide variation in the assessment of ONH appearance among examiners or even from visit to visit with the same examiner, these evaluations may be exceedingly difficult to make consistently. Commonly, several variables of the clinical examination have to be considered to conclude that progression of glaucomatous damage has occurred and, accordingly, to decide whether intraocular pressure control is adequate.

As a result of the variable nature of subjective ONH assessments and because a relatively large change is necessary to conclude reliably that an actual progression of disease has occurred, techniques and instrumentation have been developed to quantify objectively ONH structures.

HISTORICAL REVIEW

The first ophthalmoscope was introduced by Helmholtz in 1850, and soon thereafter the first reports of ONH changes in glaucoma appeared.[1] It quickly became apparent that a more objective recording of ONH appearance was necessary, but no convenient technology was available for this purpose at the time. The first photograph was created on a glass plate by Nicéphore Nièpce in 1826. In 1888 George Eastman developed his "everyman's camera," the Kodak. However, it was not until 1889, when Eastman developed flexible film, that photography became both popular and a profession. Early fundus photography (by Howe in 1887) was limited by reflexes from both the light source and ocular tissues, improper illumination, and patient eye movement during the long exposure time of several seconds.[2]

Tremendous technical advances in light sources, flashes, film and filter quality, techniques of development, and reduction of exposure time (to milliseconds) improved the quality of fundus photography dramatically. Stereoscopic fundus photography was first described by Thorner in 1909.[2] Stereoscopy was attempted by movement of the patient's eye very slightly between exposures or by movement of the camera in front of the constantly fixated eye.

The first to introduce simultaneous stereoscopic ONH photography was Nordenson in 1930, using a pair of small prisms in front of the lenses of a conventional Zeiss camera, based on the principles of a modified reflex-free Gullstrand ophthalmoscope. Other attempts were made by Norton in 1953 and Drews in 1957, but the image quality was poor. A new camera was developed in 1964 by Donaldson and revised in 1976; the design integrated two fundus cameras that used the same primary objective to obtain simultaneous photographs, employed the indirect ophthalmoscope principle (separation of the illuminating light rays that entered and reflected out of the pupil), and took advantage of a new electronic flash that provided sufficient illumination for a 35mm color film. This camera was fast and relatively easy to operate. The depth effect was highly reproducible, and in the revised prototype, distortion was reduced to a minimum.

ONH analyzers were introduced in the early 1980s to offer automated, quantitative measurement of the disc, cup, neuroretinal rim area, and related parameters; these analyzers are based on standard fundus camera optics.

PURPOSE OF OPTIC NERVE HEAD IMAGING AND ANALYSIS

Devices described in this chapter are designed to image and/or measure ONH parameters, such as cup-to-disc ratio, disc and cup area and volume, neuroretinal rim width and area, area of pallor, and cup slope, in a simple, fast, cost-effective, objective, accurate, and reproducible way. Additional features in some of the technologies include quantitative or semiquantitative analysis of results and correction for highly variable patient-related factors such as refractive error, axial length, and anterior corneal curvature. A major source of variation is disc size, and correction for this factor is still a future goal. Disc area may vary between individuals by as much as seven times among normal eyes.[3] It is still not clear which of the ONH parameters mentioned has the greatest predictive and/or prognostic value for glaucomatous damage. The goals for clinicians in the evaluation of this type of information are to differentiate between normal and glaucomatous eyes and to detect mild to moderate progression of glaucomatous damage with a high level of certainty.

ALTERNATIVE TESTS

Stereoscopic Optic Nerve Head Photography

Stereoscopic ONH photography is currently the most widely used technology that enables clinicians to document ONH appearance objectively. Stereoscopic photography offers several advantages—its product shows an image most clinicians are familiar and comfortable with (a real picture of the disc with its natural color), fundus cameras are widely available, and the process requires only a modest degree of technical skill from the ophthalmic photographer. Moreover, fundus cameras are probably the least expensive permanent ophthalmic imaging systems. The main disadvantages of ONH photography are subjective and qualitative assessment, the need for clear media and a dilated pupil, and the lack of an immediate result (for film systems).

Currently, two methods are used to obtain a stereoscopic image of the ONH—sequential (consecutive) and simultaneous. Sequential stereoscopic photography involves a shift of the camera joystick to opposite sides of a fully dilated pupil either manually or via a mechanical sliding carriage adapter, such as the Allen stereo separator (introduced in 1964). Several conditions must exist to obtain a consistent stereogram pair—the patient must maintain a constant head position and fixation, and camera-dependent factors such as focus depth, light intensity, stereo base, and exact camera angle must be identical for each photographic session (an almost impossible goal to achieve).[4]

The Donaldson camera has long been considered the standard in stereoscopic ONH photography, but unfortunately it is no longer commercially available. The successor to the Donaldson camera, the Nidek 3Dx camera, was introduced in 1990. It is a simultaneous stereocamera that produces stereoscopic images in either a 35mm split-frame format, reviewed stereoscopically by a viewing system, or a 3.5 × 5 inch, single-sheet, three-dimensional transparency. Minckler et al.[5] found the Nidek camera to be superior to the Zeiss system in addition to being easier to use and faster. Greenfield et al.[4] found the Nidek 3Dx system to be superior to the Donaldson camera in that it produced better-quality stereoscopic images and significantly greater reproducibility of ONH assessment (Fig. 216-1).

Optic Disc Morphometry (Planimetry)

Morphometry of the ONH is an intermediate stage between freehand, qualitative drawing, based on a slit-lamp examination,

and quantitative, digital imaging. Described extensively by Jonas and colleagues in Germany, this method is based on stereophotographs of the ONH taken using a telecentric Zeiss fundus camera with an Allen stereo separator. The 15° color slides or transparencies are projected on a scale of 1 to 15. The outline margins of the optic disc, optic cup, peripapillary scleral ring, and peripapillary chorioretinal atrophy are plotted by hand on paper and analyzed morphometrically (using a planimetry computer, which calculates areas according to their coordinates).

The optic cup is outlined on the basis of contour, when viewed stereoscopically, and not on the basis of pallor. Helpful clues in the determination of the cup margin are bent vessels and variation in tissue heights and planes.[6] The optic disc margin is judged to be the inner margin of the peripapillary scleral ring, which is a thin, white band that encircles the ONH (see Fig. 216-1).[6] This is easier to detect on the temporal than on the nasal disc border. In the calculation of absolute values and areas in units (i.e., mm or mm²), a correction for ocular and photographic magnification is made using Littman's method, which compensates for the constant twofold magnification of the telecentric fundus camera and for ocular magnification that arises from refractive error and anterior corneal curvature. Littman's method may produce false values in cases of abnormally high refractive power of the lens (e.g., from cataracts that cause myopia of more than 1D) and so far is not applicable for cases of aphakia or pseudophakia.[3]

The disc surface, which includes the peripapillary region, is divided into four sectors on the basis of the anatomic organization of the four main retinal vessel branches and the nerve fiber layer (NFL) bundles (Fig. 216-2).[6] Sector A (temporal) covers 64° and represents the papillomacular fiber-bundle area; sector B (superior temporal) and sector C (inferior temporal) represent the arcuate nerve fiber-bundle areas; and sector D covers 116° and represents the remaining nasal area.[6] Sectors B and C each occupy 90°, and their midlines reside 13° temporal to the vertical optic disc axis (according to a previous study that showed this to be the most common location for neuroretinal rim notches). Neuroretinal rim and optic disc areas are measured separately in each of the four sectors. Total neuroretinal rim area is calculated as the difference between the disc and cup areas.

In a prospective, masked, longitudinal study, Caprioli et al.[7] followed 193 eyes of primary open-angle glaucoma and ocular hypertensive patients for 3.3 ± 1.0 years and compared different

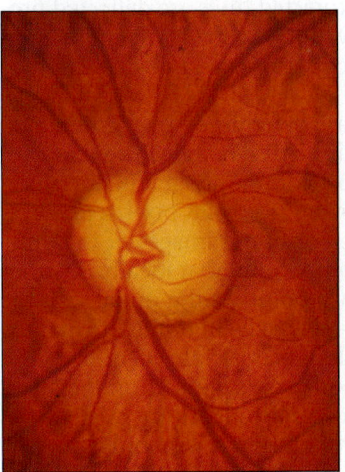
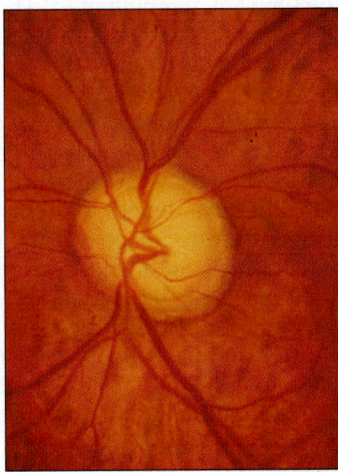

FIG. 216-1 ■ Simultaneous stereoscopic photographs of the optic nerve head taken with the 3Dx camera. Disc of an advanced primary open-angle glaucoma patient.

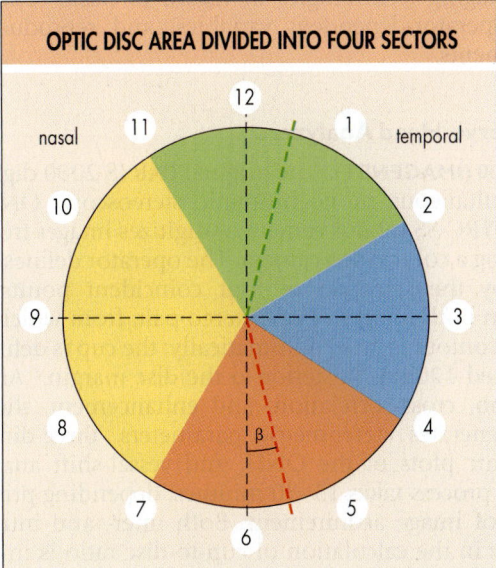

FIG. 216-2 ■ **Optic disc area divided into four sectors.** The green and red sectors represent superior temporal and inferior temporal retina—note that their middle axis is tilted temporally from the midline (angle β). The blue sector represents 64° of retina on the temporal side and the yellow sector covers the remaining 116° on the nasal side.

methods to evaluate the ONH and NFL for glaucomatous change. The detection rate of structural glaucomatous change was 15% using qualitative evaluation of ONH stereophotographs, 7.2% using qualitative evaluation of NFL stereophotographs, 3.6% using manual stereoplanimetry of the disc rim area, and 13.2% using relative NFL height measured by the Rodenstock analyzer (see later). A low degree of overlap between the various techniques may indicate that qualitative techniques have a higher sensitivity in the detection of small focal changes and quantitative measurements are better for the detection of local diffuse loss. Manual planimetry of the neural rim area showed changes in eyes that demonstrated no progression using qualitative ONH and NFL evaluation.

The Discam (Marcher Enterprises Ltd, Hereford, UK), is a new computer-assisted planimetric system that uses a digitized semi-automatic charge-coupled device (CCD) camera to capture 20° × 20° ONH photographs and display them stereoscopically. The Discam acquires sequential disc photographs in a semi-automatic fashion, and the optic disc and the cup margins are outlined using the technique previously described to obtain quantitative parameters of the ONH. Optic disc measurement using the Discam was found to have high interobserver and intraobserver repeatability.[7a] In a more recent study, 386 eyes underwent ONH analysis using the Discam digital optic disc stereo camera. The following parameters were used for this study: cup-to-disc area ratio, vertical cup-to-disc ratio, and horizontal cup-to-disc ratio. The results were compared with ONH analysis using confocal scanning laser ophthalmoscopy (see later) and stereoscopic disc photography (stereography) to evaluate the ability of these three methods to detect glaucomatous changes. Although the results of all three techniques are not interchangeable, good agreement was found between ONH measurements measured by the Discam and the other technologies.[7b]

Digital, Quantitative Imaging of the Optic Nerve Head

Multiple computerized systems have emerged since the early 1980s; each attempts to give objective, accurate, reproducible, quantitative, detailed topographic maps of the ONH and the peripapillary NFL and the potential for longitudinal comparison. Most systems share several basic features—they are all non-contact and noninvasive, a charge-coupled device (CCD) camera enables the operator to see an image of the fundus and a real-time tomographic image, and the data are stored digitally. Despite these external similarities, fundamental differences exist in the imaging technologies in regard to basic concept, light source, operator-dependent variables, and reproducibility of measurements.

Optic Nerve Head Analyzers

PAR IS 2000 (IMAGENET). The original PAR IS 2000 digitally captures simultaneous, monochromatic, stereoscopic ONH images using the TRC-SS fundus camera or digitizes images from 35mm slides using a color video camera. The operator defines the ONH margin by the selection of four coincident points (control points) on both images of one stereo pair, from which an elliptical disc contour is fitted automatically; the cup is defined as the area located 120mm posterior to the disc margin.[8] After image registration, cross-correlation, and enhancement, the analysis system generates stereometric parameters, three-dimensional topographic plots of the ONH, and vessel-shift analysis. The complete process takes 15–30 minutes, depending primarily on the ease of image acquirement. Both inter- and intraobserver variability in the calculation of cup-to-disc ratio is in the range 25–30%. The primary source of variability is the determination of the disc margin by the operator.[9] The currently available version has improved software and also may be used for fluorescein and indocyanine green angiography.

RODENSTOCK OPTIC NERVE HEAD ANALYZER. The Rodenstock ONH analyzer (no longer commercially available)

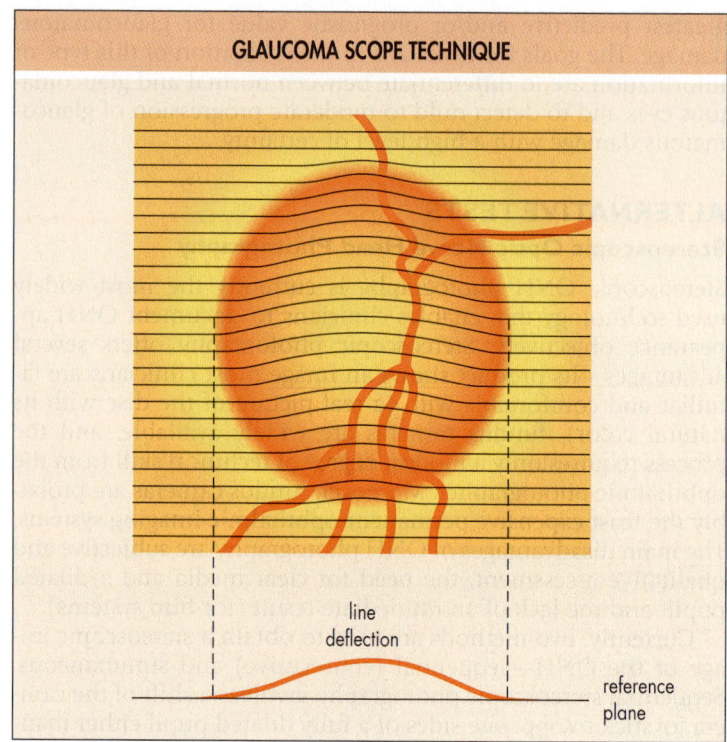

FIG. 216-3 ■ **Glaucoma Scope technique based on computed raster stereography principle.** About 25 parallel horizontal lines are projected onto the optic nerve head at an oblique angle. The lines are deflected relative to a reference plane close to the disc margin and proportionate to the depth of excavation. (Adapted with permission from Netland PA. The Glaucoma-Scope: principles, techniques, and applications. In: Schuman JS, ed. Imaging in glaucoma. Thorofare, NJ: Slack; 1997:17–32.)

utilizes a simultaneous stereoscopic video camera and is used to capture an image of the ONH. Two sets of seven evenly spaced lines are projected onto the captured image, and from their horizontal displacement the computer generates a contour map of the ONH surface and calculates the depth in each of the 1600 points on the optic disc. The margin of the ONH is defined interactively by the operator in four cardinal locations and an ellipse is fitted around those points. The cup margin is defined by a curve that connects all points 150μm below the disc margin.[10]

THE GLAUCOMA SCOPE. The Glaucoma Scope performs ONH analysis based on a technique of computer raster stereography described by Holm and Krakau in 1970.[11] The system consists of an optical head, used for image acquisition, a monitor that shows a video image of the ONH, and a computerized image analysis component. A halogen lamp using near-infrared light (750nm) produces a series of approximately 25 parallel, horizontal, and equally spaced lines, which are projected onto the ONH at an angle of 9°. The projected lines are deflected proportionately to the depth of excavation—a shallow cup creates a small deflection whereas a deep cup causes a large deflection of the lines (Fig. 216-3).

Several variables of the image are determined by the operator, for example, a reference point and the disc margin. The reference point selected by the operator, most commonly at a major blood vessel branch, defines the center of a 128 × 128 pixel area and is used for future image registration. For future images of the same ONH, the operator chooses a reference point that ideally is within 5–10 pixels of the original reference point. At the initial visit the operator outlines the disc margin—at least eight points are marked around the disc and the major blood vessels are identified. The outline of the disc margin and blood vessels appears on the printout as a landmark but has no effect on the algorithm calculations of depth values.[12] The refractive error of the eye is recorded for correction of magnification in the disc measurements.

The ONH and projected lines are viewed in real time on the video monitor and the operator may optimize focus and illumination. Multiple images are captured and stored in digital form

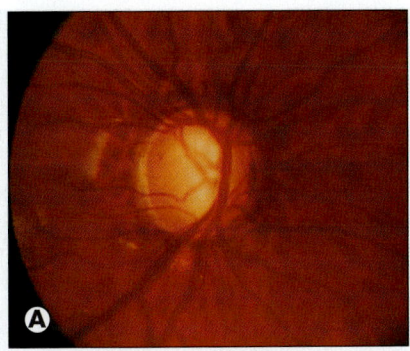

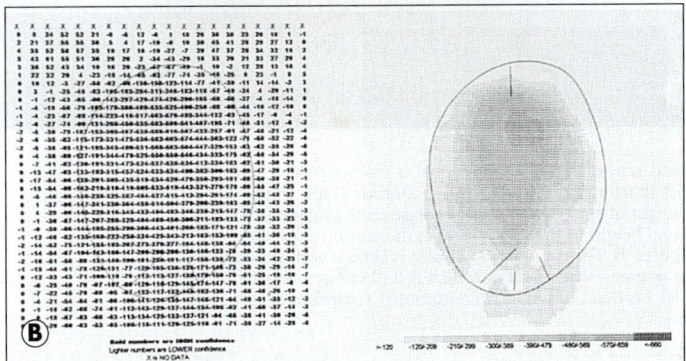

FIG. 216-4 ■ **Glaucoma Scope analysis.** The data shown are from a 9-year-old girl who had corticosteroid-induced unilateral glaucoma. **A,** Optic nerve head demonstrates marked cupping of the right eye with extensive loss of the neuroretinal rim temporally. **B,** Glaucoma Scope analysis correlates with the clinical photographs. Left image shows quantitative data; gray-scale image to the right. (With permission from Netland PA. The Glaucoma-Scope: principles, techniques, and applications. In: Schuman JS, ed. Imaging in glaucoma. Thorofare, NJ: Slack, 1997:17–32.)

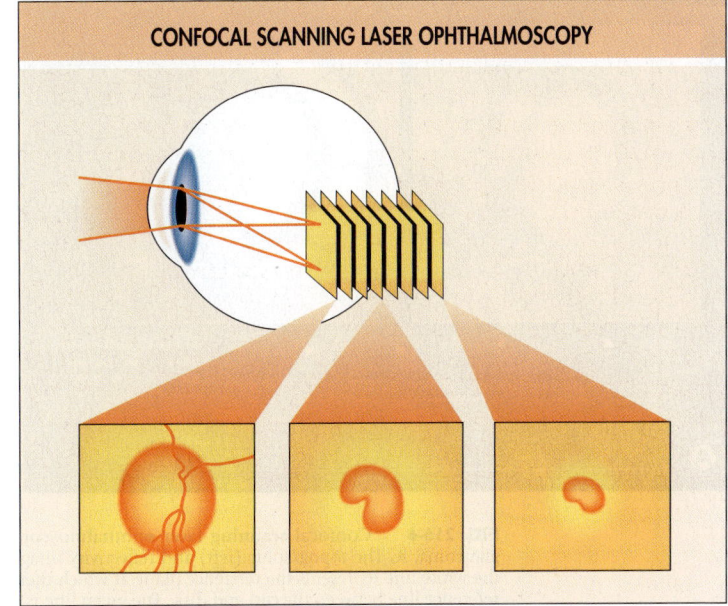

FIG. 216-5 ■ **Confocal scanning laser ophthalmoscopy.** The tissue is scanned in 16–64 coronal sections at consecutive focal planes in the HRT I. The three-dimensional image acquired consists of 256×256 pixels; acquisition time is approximately 1.4sec. In the HRT II, the three-dimensional image acquired consists of 384×384 pixels with an acquisition time of approximately 1.0sec. (Adapted from Schuman JS, Noeker RJ. Imaging of the optic nerve head and nerve fiber layer in glaucoma. Ophthalmol Clin North Am. 1995;8:259–79.)

on optical discs. The quality (or focus) of the captured image is assessed on a logarithmic scale and depends on the ratio of horizontal line data to nonhorizontal line data (nonhorizontal line data are created mainly by blood vessels) and on the degree of overexposure (to eliminate images that are too bright to be analyzed). The analysis system of the Glaucoma Scope automatically analyzes the image with the highest quality scale unless other images are chosen by the operator. A computer algorithm converts horizontal line data from the captured image into corresponding numerical depth values. A reference plane for the depth measurements is calculated as the mean depth of two 50μm columns placed about 350μm nasal and temporal to the ONH margin. The optic cup is defined as an area inside the ONH that lies 140μm or more below the reference plane.

The depths or elevations of over 8750 real data points are calculated in an area of approximately 350×280 pixels (which corresponds roughly to a 20° area on the retina). The printout contains a gray-scale map with up to 722 numerical values, a three-dimensional grid map, a battery of ONH parameters, a disc and cup outline, and a progression report that shows points that have changed by more than 50μm on follow-up tests (see Fig. 216-4). Pendergast and Shields[13] found the standard deviation of measurements to be less than 50μm.

The Glaucoma Scope is limited by the need for a pupil size of at least 4.5–5mm, clear media, and an experienced operator. In addition, because of the nature of this technology, only surface topography can be analyzed using the Glaucoma Scope.

Gundersen et al.[14] examined 138 normal subjects and 102 glaucoma patients for vertical and horizontal cup-to-disc ratio, minimum rim width within the 60° and 90° sectors across the vertical meridian, and rim and cup area. The most sensitive parameter for differentiation of normal from glaucomatous eyes was minimum rim width at 60° and 90° (which represents localized changes of the optic disc), followed by vertical cup-to-disc ratio. Global indices, such as rim and cup area and horizontal cup-to-disc ratio, were the least sensitive. These

differences were most obvious in eyes affected by mild to moderate glaucomatous field defects.

Confocal Scanning Laser Ophthalmoscopy

Confocal scanning laser ophthalmoscopy (CSLO) offers real-time, three-dimensional imaging of the ONH and NFL, with reduced need for pupillary dilation or clear media. A confocal optical system is designed to allow only a "thin" slice of the target tissue to be in focus on the image plane—light rays reflected from higher or lower focal planes are blocked, which creates high-resolution tomographic images. The tissue is illuminated and imaged point by point through a pinhole. The system is confocal because both the illumination pinhole and the imaging pinhole correspond to the same focal point on the tissue. A three-dimensional image may be obtained by varying the x, y, and z coordinates. A pair of galvanometer-controlled mirrors facilitates rapid horizontal and vertical scanning across the object.

The Heidelberg Retina Tomograph (HRT, Heidelberg Engineering GmbH, Heidelberg, Germany) is the only commercially available confocal scanning laser ophthalmoscope. There are two systems. The HRT I is a scanning system for acquisition and analysis of the posterior pole. The typical use of the HRT is for the assessment of the ONH. It uses a diode laser of 670nm to scan a three-dimensional image from a series of optical sections at 32 consecutive focal planes (Fig. 216-5).[15] Because laser tomographic scanning occurs one point at a time, the confocal scanning optical microscope reconstructs an ONH image by bringing a series of two-dimensional digitized images into registration. The registration process corrects for microsaccades that occur during image acquisition.[16] The topography image consists of 256×256 pixel elements, each of which is a measurement of height at its corresponding location. The optical transverse resolution is approximately 10μm, whereas the axial resolution is about 300μm. The transverse field of view can be $10° \times 10°$, $15° \times 15°$, or $20° \times 20°$. In current clinical practice, three scans of each eye are taken and then averaged to create a mean topography image.[17] The printed report shows a topographic image and a reflectivity image of the ONH and its contour line, ONH stereometric parameters, and a mean-height contour of the peripapillary retina (Figs. 216-6 and 216-7).[18]

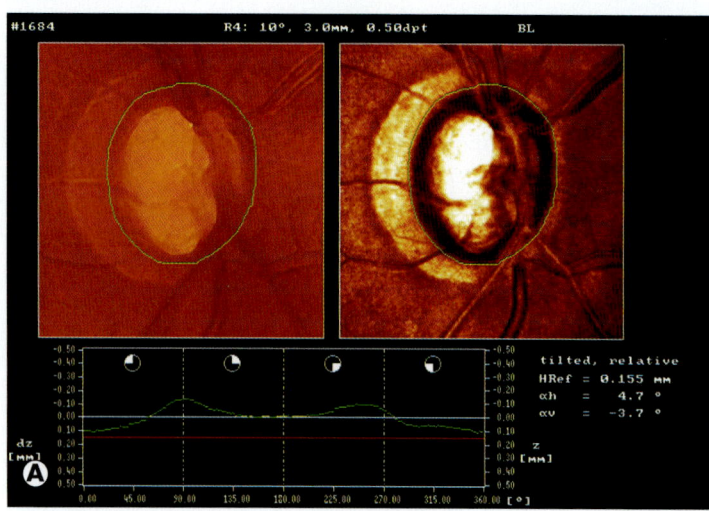
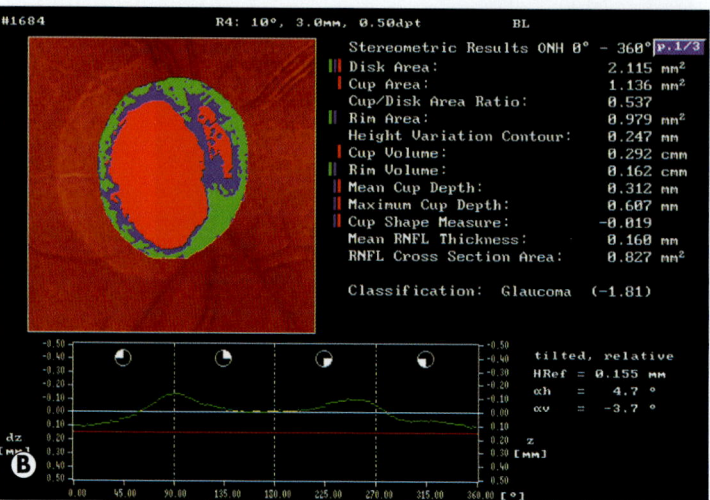

FIG. 216-6 ■ **Confocal scanning laser ophthalmoscopy printed report—HRT I.** The report is from a subject with glaucoma. **A,** The topographic (left) and reflectivity image (right) illustrates the ONH. In the contour graph (below), the white line represents the reference plane at which there is a height of zero. The red line represents the height of the reference line between the cup and disk. The green line is the retinal height of the subject eye at the contour line showing the typical double hump feature at the superior and inferior poles. **B,** The topographic image is shown with the cup represented in red, the sloping neural tissue in blue, and the rim in green. The ONH parameters and subject classification are shown on the right. The classification number for the HRT I is determined by an automated algorithm devised by Frederick Mikelberg based on the ONH and retinal parameters.

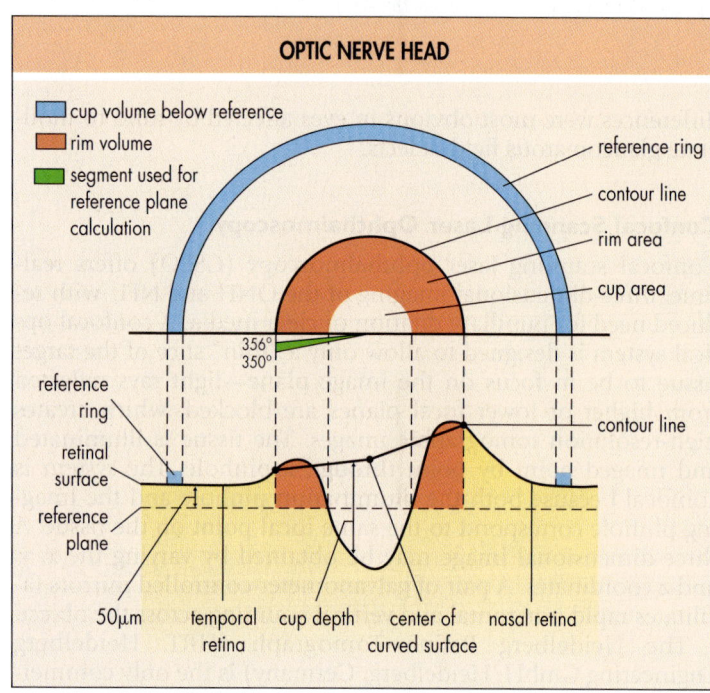

FIG. 216-7 ■ **Optic nerve head.** The standard reference plane at 50μm below the retinal surface. (Adapted with permission from Zangwill L, Horn SV, Lima MDS, *et al.* Optic nerve head topography in ocular hypertensive eyes using confocal scanning laser ophthalmology. Am J Ophthalmol. 1996;122:520–5.)

In a comparative study, expert clinicians evaluated 72 normal patients and 51 patients with early glaucoma using qualitative assessment of stereoscopic optic disc photographs and CSLO imaging. The Heidelberg Retina Tomograph was reported to be more sensitive than clinical assessment in detecting early glaucomatous disc changes.[19] In another study, investigators analyzed 13 ocular hypertensive eyes that subsequently developed reproducible visual field defects and 13 normal eyes that had undergone sequential optic disc images. HRT has also been found to detect glaucomatous changes in the optic disc before visual field changes occurred.[20]

The recently developed HRT II is designed for topographic ONH analysis. The HRT II is small, lightweight, portable, and al-most completely automatic. All image acquisition parameters are either fixed or predetermined. The system automatically acquires 16–64 image planes covering a field of view fixed at 15° × 15° using 384 × 384 pixels per plane. Utilizing an internal fixation target, the HRT II automatically acquires three images with the use of a quality control system that will acquire additional images if one or more of the images acquired cannot be used (e.g., fixation loss). The printed report shows a topographic and reflectivity image of the ONH and its contour line, details of the classification, and ONH stereometric parameters (Fig. 216-8).

The original HRT is a research-oriented tool with a wide range of applications, including measuring retinal circulation when combined with the Heidelberg Retina Flowmeter; the HRT II is restricted to ONH analysis.

An inherent limitation of this technology lies in the reference plane. A reference plane is required to calculate cup area, cup-to-disc ratio, cup volume, rim area, rim volume, retinal NFL thickness, and retinal NFL cross-sectional area. The reference plane used by the current software may change over time, especially in patients with glaucoma who have changing topography.[21] Another obstacle is the manual delineation of the optic disc margin by the operator and the influence of this on ONH parameters.

The most recent published data regarding analysis of ONH parameters using CSLO indicate that the slope of the cup ("the third central moment of the depth distribution") is the most significant parameter in the prediction of glaucoma status (see Fig. 216-8).[22,23] There appears to be some ability to discriminate between normal and glaucomatous eyes using CSLO, with a sensitivity and specificity of about 85%; however, considerable overlap exists between normal, ocular hypertensive, and glaucomatous eyes.[18,23] Finally, some authors have claimed the ability to determine NFL thickness, or cross-sectional area, using CSLOs—by using a reference point in the nasal retina or in the macula, a given thickness is determined (calculated) to represent NFL.[24] This indirect measurement of NFL thickness is probably not the best method for NFL analysis, nor is it particularly accurate given the low axial resolution of CSLO (approximately 300mm) and the fact that superior technologies exist for the direct assessment of NFL thickness (see Chapter 217).[15] Software developed by Chauhan and colleagues to detect topographic changes in the optic disc and peripapillary retina appears to provide the best longitudinal data analysis to date using HRT II. Seventy-seven subjects with early glaucomatous visual field damage were fol-

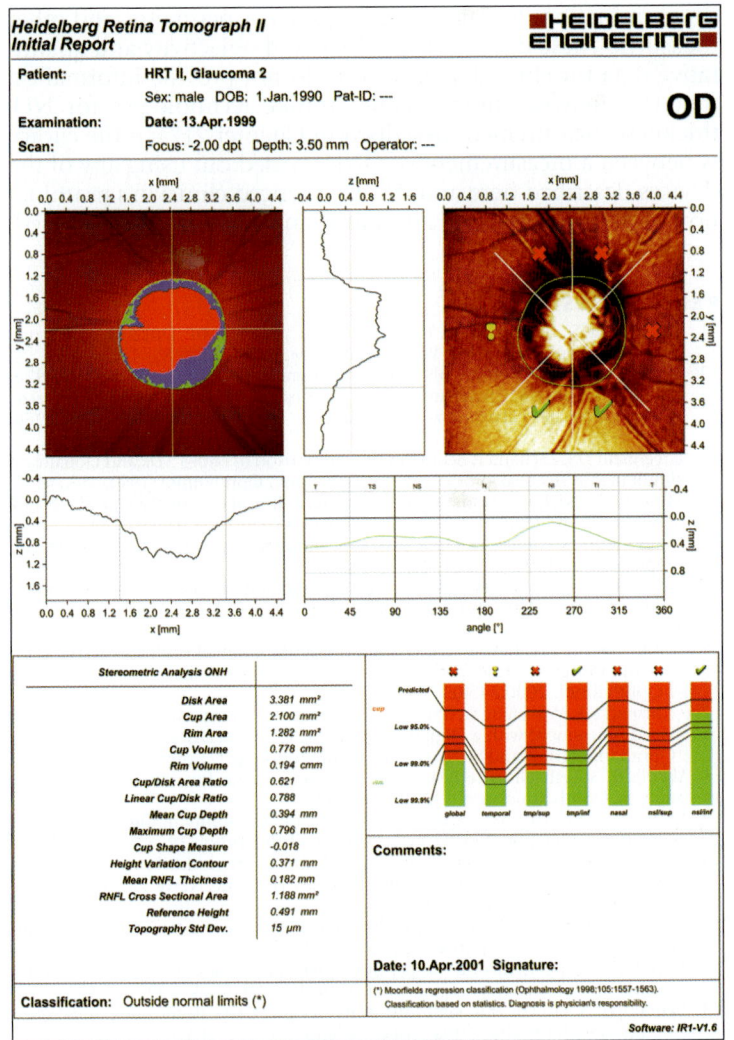

Heidelberg Retina Tomograph II Initial Report		**HEIDELBERG ENGINEERING**
Patient:	HRT II, Glaucoma 2	
	Sex: male DOB: 1.Jan.1990 Pat-ID: ---	**OD**
Examination:	Date: 13.Apr.1999	
Scan:	Focus: -2.00 dpt Depth: 3.50 mm Operator: ---	

Stereometric Analysis ONH

Disk Area	3.381 mm²
Cup Area	2.100 mm²
Rim Area	1.282 mm²
Cup Volume	0.778 cmm
Rim Volume	0.194 cmm
Cup/Disk Area Ratio	0.621
Linear Cup/Disk Ratio	0.788
Mean Cup Depth	0.394 mm
Maximum Cup Depth	0.796 mm
Cup Shape Measure	-0.018
Height Variation Contour	0.371 mm
Mean RNFL Thickness	0.182 mm
RNFL Cross Sectional Area	1.188 mm²
Reference Height	0.491 mm
Topography Std Dev.	15 µm

Comments:

Date: 10.Apr.2001 Signature:

Classification: Outside normal limits (*)

(*) Moorfields regression classification (Ophthalmology 1998;105:1557-1563). Classification based on statistics. Diagnosis is physician's responsibility.

Software: IR1-V1.6

FIG. 216-8 ■ **Confocal scanning laser ophthalmoscopy printed report— HRT II.** This report is from a different subject with glaucoma. The topographic image (left) is shown with the cup represented in red, the sloping neural tissue in blue, and the rim in green. The reflectivity image (right) illustrates the classification of the six ONH sectors. Each sector is marked with a green check mark, a red cross, or a yellow exclamation mark to illustrate being within normal limits, outside normal limits, or borderline, respectively. A bar graph represents this further in the right middle panel. The stereometric parameters are displayed in the left middle panel. The classification number for HRT II is derived from an algorithm developed by Wollstein *et al.* at Moorfields Eye Hospital. (Courtesy of Heidelberg Engineering, Inc., Carlsbad, CA.)

lowed with scanning laser tomography and with conventional perimetry. Investigators found glaucomatous disc changes determined with scanning laser tomography to occur more frequently than visual field changes. This result suggests that glaucomatous damage and progression may be detected earlier using scanning laser polarimetry.[25,26]

Optical Coherence Tomography

Optical coherence tomography (OCT) is a diagnostic imaging technology that utilizes interferometry and low-coherence light in the near-infrared range (approximately 840nm) to achieve high-resolution (about 10µm for OCT 1 and 2, about 7–8µm for OCT 3), cross-sectional imaging of the eye (Fig. 216-9). In OCT, a beam of low-coherence light is split to the tissue of interest (probe beam) and to a reference mirror at a known variable position (reference beam).[27] Multiple echoes are reflected or backscattered from the eye, but for the two beams to recombine and produce positive interference on a photodetector (and hence to create an image) their pulses must arrive simultaneously or within the short coherence length of the light source. Thus, it is the low-coherence light source that primarily determines the longitudinal resolution. Transverse resolution is determined by the probe beam diameter (20mm) and effective transverse resolution is affected by transverse pixel spacing. In OCT 1 and 2, a sequence of 100 successive, longitudinal measurements (i.e., A-scans) is used to construct a false color topographic image of tissue microsections that appears remarkably similar to histological sections; OCT 3 uses 500 axial scans acquired in 1 second.

OCT 2 and 3 are equipped with ONH analysis software for the clinical assessment of the ONH. The ONH analysis evaluates the disc and cup anatomy and quantifies the amount of nerve tissue in the optic nerve at the disc. Quantification of the nerve tissue is done by calculating the cross-sectional area of the nerve tissue and then calculating the minimum distance from the disk to the retina surface. The analysis program detects the anterior surface of the NFL and retinal pigment epithelium (RPE) by searching each A-scan axially for the highest rates of change in reflectivity. Once these boundaries have been determined, the algorithm identifies and measures all features of disc anatomy based on the anatomical markers (disc reference points) on each side of the disc where the RPE/choriocapillaris/choroid reflection ends (Fig. 216-10).

Although it is a very valuable tool for glaucoma assessment, the principal application of OCT in this disease prior to the new ONH analysis software has been in NFL thickness measurement

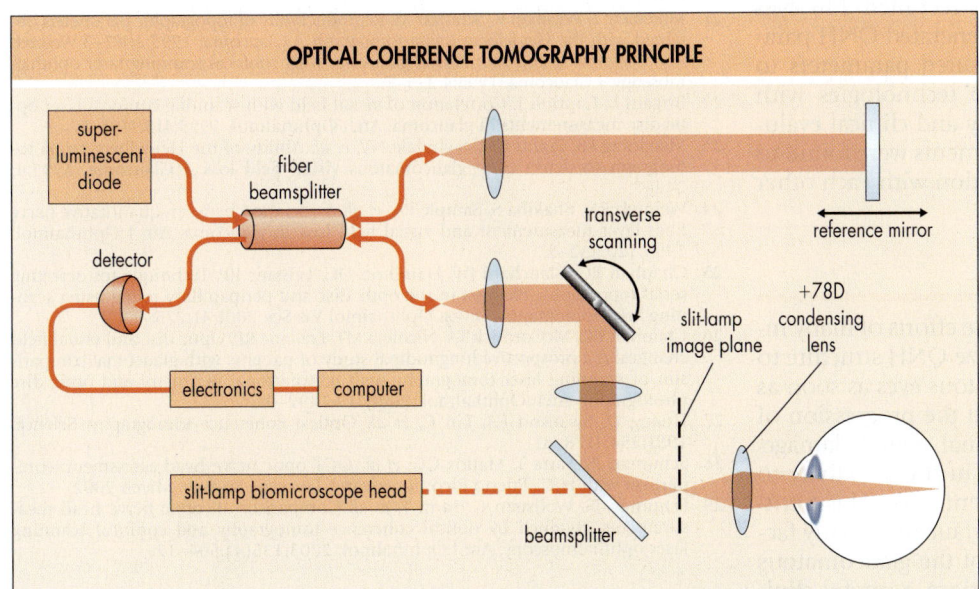

OPTICAL COHERENCE TOMOGRAPHY PRINCIPLE

FIG. 216-9 ■ **Optical coherence tomography principle.** Axial profiles of backscattered light within the target tissue are measured by translation of the reference mirror, and the interferometric signal is recorded. Constructive interference creates an image that is seen by a photodetector only when the time paths to both the reference mirror and the tissue scanned are within the coherence length of the light source, which thus predicts a resolution of 10µm in the eye. (Adapted with permission from Huang D, Swanson EA, Lin C, *et al.* Optical coherence tomography. Science. 1991;254:1178–81.)

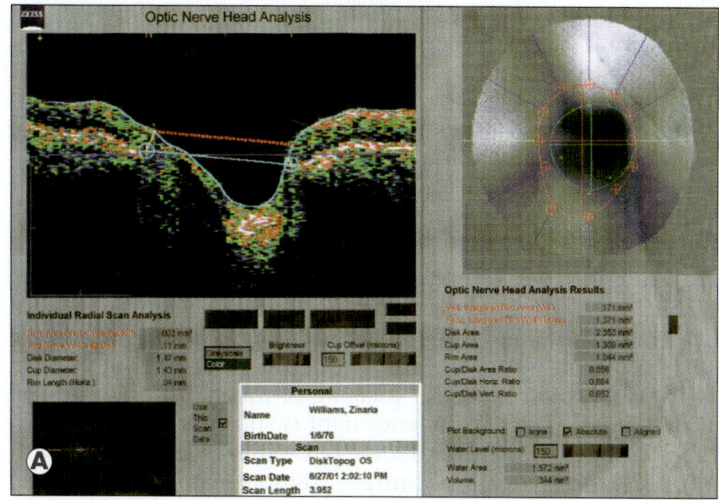

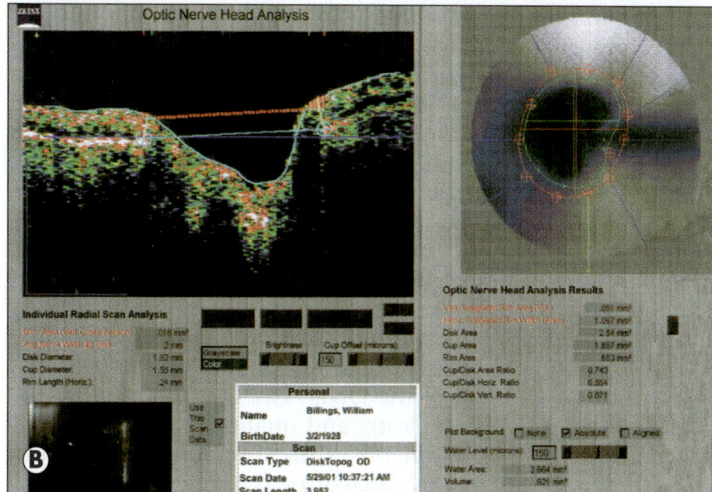

FIG. 216-10 ■ **Optical coherence tomography.** Disc topography scan pattern for ONH analysis. **A,** Normal—note the thicker nerve fiber layer superiorly and inferiorly. Borders of the retina and nerve fiber layer are designed by a computer algorithm that calculates threshold reflectivity. Retinal thickness equals the distance between the posterior (posteriormost blue line) and anterior retinal border (white line). Nerve fiber layer thickness is equal to the distance between the white line and anterior blue line. **B,** A patient who has advanced primary open-angle glaucoma. Note severe and generalized thinning of nerve fiber layer.

(see Chapter 217). It has tremendous utility in the diagnosis and monitoring of retinal, particularly macular, pathologies (see Section 8). ONH analysis using the OCT is being investigated more extensively. Preliminary results suggest that OCT ONH assessment correlates highly with HRT ONH measurements, and both perform similarly in discriminating between normal and glaucomatous eyes.[28] Recently, investigators recruited 236 eyes to evaluate the relationship between OCT-generated ONH parameters using OCT 2 and 3 and HRT-measured parameters to compare the association between the two technologies with glaucoma status as determined by perimetry and clinical evaluation. HRT and OCT 2 and 3 ONH measurements were found to have a statistically significantly high correlation with each other and with disease status.[29]

CONCLUSIONS

The technologies described here represent the efforts of many investigators to quantify and objectively analyze ONH structure to differentiate between normal and glaucomatous eyes as soon as possible in the disease process and to detect the progression of the disease with the least possible additional neural damage. Although these devices offer some increase in the sensitivity to early or progressive damage, and measurement of ONH is a critical aspect of the care of patients who have glaucoma, many factors must be considered in the evaluation of the glaucomatous eye. These techniques add to, but do not replace, a careful clini-

cal examination, functional testing such as perimetry, and other measures. These instruments help to add objectivity and quantitative data for clinical analysis but do not provide information that is otherwise unobtainable (unlike technologies for NFL thickness measurement described in Chapter 217); if the choice is between a measurement of ONH carried out using any of the devices described here and the experienced clinician's examination of the ONH and NFL, the clinician's result must be selected.

REFERENCES

1. Duke-Elder S. Anomalies of the intra-ocular pressure. In: Duke-Elder WS, ed. Textbook of ophthalmology, Vol 3. St Louis: Mosby; 1941:3280–429.
2. Hurtes R, ed. Evolution of ophthalmic photography. Boston: Little, Brown; 1976.
3. Jonas JB, Gusek GC, Naumann GO. Optic disc, cup and neuroretinal rim size, configuration and correlations in normal eyes. Invest Ophthalmol Vis Sci. 1988; 29:1151–8.
4. Greenfield DS, Zacharia P, Schuman JS. Comparison of Nidek 3Dx and Donaldson simultaneous stereoscopic disk photography. Am J Ophthalmol. 1993; 116:741–7.
5. Minckler D, Nichols T, Morales R. Preliminary clinical experience with the Nidek 3Dx camera and lenticular stereo disk images. J Glaucoma. 1992;1:184–6.
6. Jonas J, Konigsreuther KA. Optic disk appearance in ocular hypertensive eyes. Am J Ophthalmol. 1994;117:732–40.
7. Caprioli J, Prum B, Zeyen T. Comparison of methods to evaluate the optic nerve head and nerve fiber layer for glaucomatous change. Am J Ophthalmol. 1996; 121:659–67.
7a. Shuttleworth GN, Khong CH, Diamond JP. A new digital optic disc stereo camera: intraobserver and interobserver repeatability of optic disc measurements. Br J Ophthalmol. 2000;84:403–7.
7b. Correnti AJ, Wollstein G, Price LL, Schuman JS. Comparison of Optic Nerve Head Assessment with a Digital Stereoscopic Camera (Discam), Scanning Laser Ophthalmoscopy, and Stereography. Ophthalmology (in press).
8. Varma R, Spaeth GL. The PAR IS 2000: a new system for retinal digital image analysis. Ophthalmic Surg. 1988;19:183–92.
9. Varma R, Steinmann WC, Spaeth GL, Wilson RP. Variability in digital analysis of optic disc topography. Graefes Arch Clin Exp Ophthalmol. 1988;226:435–42.
10. Bishop KI, Werner EB, Krupin T, et al. Variability and reproducibility of optic disk topographic measurements with the Rodenstock Optic Nerve Head Analyzers. Am J Ophthalmol. 1988;106:696–702.
11. Holm O, Krakau C. A photographic method for measuring the volume of papillary excavations. Ann Ophthalmol. 1970;1:327–32.
12. Netland PA. The Glaucoma-Scope: principles, techniques, and applications. In: Schuman JS, ed. Imaging in glaucoma. Thorofare, NJ: Slack; 1997:17–32.
13. Pendergast S, Shields MB. Reproducibility of optic nerve head topographic measurements with the Glaucoma-Scope. J Glaucoma. 1995;4:170–6.
14. Gundersen KG, Heijl A, Bengtsson B. Sensitivity and specificity of structural optic disc parameters in chronic glaucoma. Acta Ophthalmol Scand. 1995;Separatum:1–6.
15. Schuman JS, Noecker RJ. Imaging of the optic nerve head and nerve fiber layer in glaucoma. Ophthalmol Clin North Am. 1995;8:259–79.
16. Echelman DA, Shields MB. Optic nerve imaging. In: Albert DM, Jakobiec FA, eds. Principles and practice in ophthalmology, Vol 3. Philadelphia: WB Saunders; 1994:1310–29.
17. Zangwill L, de Souza Lima M, Weinreb RN. Confocal scanning laser ophthalmoscopy to detect glaucomatous optic neuropathy. In Schuman JS, ed. Imaging in glaucoma. Thorofare, NJ: Slack; 1997.
18. Zangwill L, Horn SV, Lima MDS, et al. Optic nerve head topography in ocular hypertensive eyes using confocal scanning laser ophthalmoscopy. Am J Ophthalmol. 1996;122:520–5.
19. Zangwill L, Shakiba S, Caprioli J, Weinreb RN. Agreement between clinicians and a confocal scanning laser ophthalmoscope in estimating cup/disk ratios. Am J Ophthalmol. 1994;119:415–21.
20. Weinreb RN, Luski M, Bartsch D-U, Morsman D. Effect of repetitive imaging on topographic measurements of the optic nerve head. Arch Ophthalmol. 1993;111: 636–8.
21. Mikelberg F, Wijsman K, Schulzer M. Reproducibility of topographic parameters obtained with the Heidelberg retina tomograph. J Glaucoma. 1993;2:101–3.Weinreb RN. Diagnosing and monitoring glaucoma with confocal scanning laser ophthalmoscopy. J Glaucoma. 1995;4:225–7.
22. Brigatti L, Caprioli J. Correlation of visual field with scanning confocal laser optic disc measurements in glaucoma. Arch Ophthalmol. 1995;113:1191–4.
23. Mikelberg FS, Prafitt CM, Swindale NV, et al. Ability of the Heidelberg retina tomograph to detect early glaucomatous visual field loss. J Glaucoma. 1995;4: 242–7.
24. Weinreb RN, Shakiba S, Sample PA, et al. Association between quantitative nerve fiber layer measurement and visual field loss in glaucoma. Am J Ophthalmol. 1995;120:732–8.
25. Chauhan BC, Blanchard JW, Hamilton DC, LeBlanc RP. Technique for detecting serial topographic changes in the optic disc and peripapillary retina using scanning laser tomography. Invest Ophthalmol Vis Sci. 2001;41:775–82.
26. Chauhan BC, McCormick TA, Nicolela MT, LeBlanc RP. Optic disc and visual field changes in a prospective longitudinal study of patients with glaucoma: comparison of scanning laser tomography with conventional perimetry and optic disc photography. Arch Ophthalmol. 2001;119:1492–9.
27. Huang D, Swanson EA, Lin C, et al. Optical coherence tomography. Science. 1991;254:1178–81.
28. Schuman JS, Farra T, Mattox CG, et al. OCT optic nerve head assessment: comparison with HRT. Puerto Rico: American Glaucoma Society; March 2002.
29. Schuman JS, Wollstein G, Farra T, et al. Comparison of optic nerve head measurements obtained by optical coherence tomography and confocal scanning laser ophthalmoscopy. Am J Ophthalmol. 2003;135(4):504–12.

217 Retinal Nerve Fiber Layer Analysis

NEIL T. CHOPLIN

INTRODUCTION

Patients at risk for glaucoma may have optic nerves and visual fields of normal appearance, but they may still have nerve fiber layer defects that are indicative of early, undetected glaucomatous damage.[1] Thus, assessment of the retinal nerve fiber layer is important in the initial evaluation of the patient suspected of having glaucoma and in follow-up for detection of early damage or progression.

ANATOMY

The normal human optic nerve is made up of 1.0-1.2 million axons of retinal ganglion cells, which converge at the optic disc. These fibers make up the retinal nerve fiber layer and lie in the inner retina, just below the internal limiting membrane. The distribution of nerve fibers within the nerve fiber layer is illustrated in Figure 217-1. Fibers from the superior and inferior halves of the retina do not cross the horizontal midline and are separated from each other by a horizontal raphe. Macular fibers are oriented horizontally and make up the papillomacular bundle, which enters the optic nerve on the temporal side. Fibers on the temporal side of the disc that arise peripheral to the papillomacular bundle have to arch over the bundle to reach the optic nerve and are thus known as arcuate fibers. Fibers from the nasal side of the disc are oriented in a more radial fashion.

Visual field defects that arise from loss of discrete nerve fiber bundles take on the shape of the bundle that was lost, which gives rise to arcuate scotomas (from loss of arcuate fibers) and wedge-shaped defects (from loss of radially oriented nasal fibers). Because glaucoma damage usually affects the temporal areas of the superior and inferior poles of the optic nerve early on, nasal defects and arcuate defects tend to occur first. The papillomacular bundle and nasal fibers that subserve the temporal field are affected relatively late in the disease process, which accounts for the preservation of central and temporal islands until the end stage is reached.

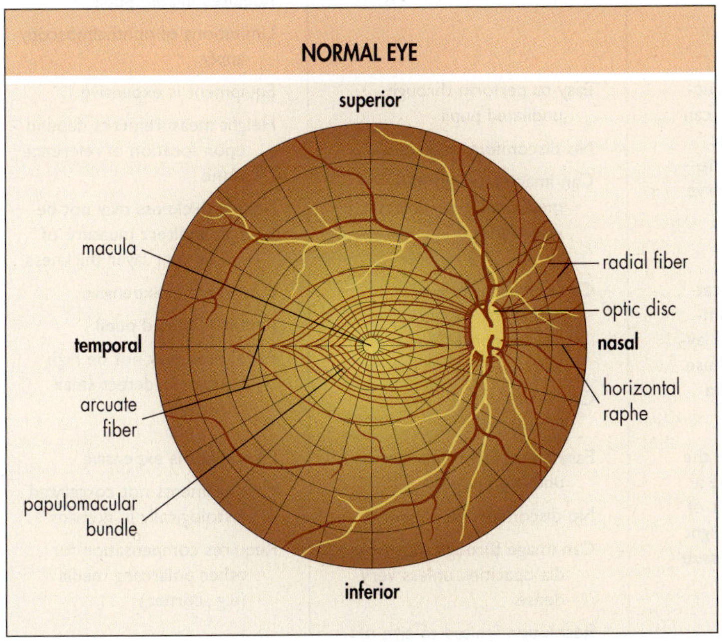

The anterior-posterior orientation of the nerve fibers with regard to the positions within the optic nerve head is not clear.[2] Fibers from the more peripheral portions of the retina occupy more peripheral locations in the nerve head, and those from the more central locations are more central within the nerve. Fibers from the peripheral retina are thought to occupy more superficial positions within the nerve fiber layer (i.e., closer to the vitreous), while more central fibers are thought to lie closer to the sclera.[3] The fibers are thought to cross each other (i.e., the more superficial peripheral fibers cross the deeper central fibers to become more peripheral in the optic nerve, while the deeper fibers become more central in the nerve) somewhere in the anterior portion of the nerve head. The layer of nerve fibers is expected to be thickest just before the fibers make the 90-degree turn into the nerve head, and progressively thinner peripherally. The distribution of fibers is not uniform around the nerve head, because the nerve fiber layer is thicker at the superior and inferior poles and thinner nasally and temporally.

The appearance of the nerve fiber layer is dependent upon the method used to visualize it. Ophthalmoscopically, this layer is seen most easily in eyes that are darkly pigmented and have clear media, particularly if the red-free filter is used. The nerve fiber layer pattern appears as bright striations, most obvious where the layer is thickest. The bright striations of the fiber bundles are offset by darker, elongated processes of Müller cell origin that surround the bundles.[4] The striations of the nerve fiber layer are seen clearly in the superior region of the red-free fundus view shown in Figure 217-2.

NERVE FIBER LAYER IN GLAUCOMA

Localized defects in the nerve fiber layer appear as wedge-shaped (not spindle-shaped), clearly defined areas that radiate from the optic disc and widen peripherally. They appear on red-free photographs or ophthalmoscopically as dark areas between the bright striations of an otherwise normal nerve fiber layer. Figure 217-2 illustrates a nerve fiber layer defect in the inferior bundle of a patient who has early glaucoma. Such localized nerve fiber layer defects have been reported in up to 20% of patients who have glaucoma.[5] Diffuse loss of the retinal nerve fiber layer also may occur and results in decreased visibility of the layer, which may be difficult to detect, particularly in eyes in which the media is not clear. Comparison with the fellow eye may help discern any diffuse loss of fibers in one eye. Another indication of the loss of nerve fibers is increased visibility of retinal blood vessels,[4] which normally are embedded within the nerve fiber layer and, thus, partially obscured. If the nerve fiber layer is lost diffusely, the vessels become more visible and sharper in appearance.

FIG. 217-1 ■ **Normal anatomy of the retinal nerve fiber layer (right eye).** The characteristic organization of the nerve fiber layer and the existence of a horizontal raphe explain the observed visual field defects that occur in glaucoma as bundles of nerve fibers are lost.

NORMAL EYE

superior

macula

radial fiber

optic disc

temporal

nasal

arcuate fiber

horizontal raphe

papulomacular bundle

inferior

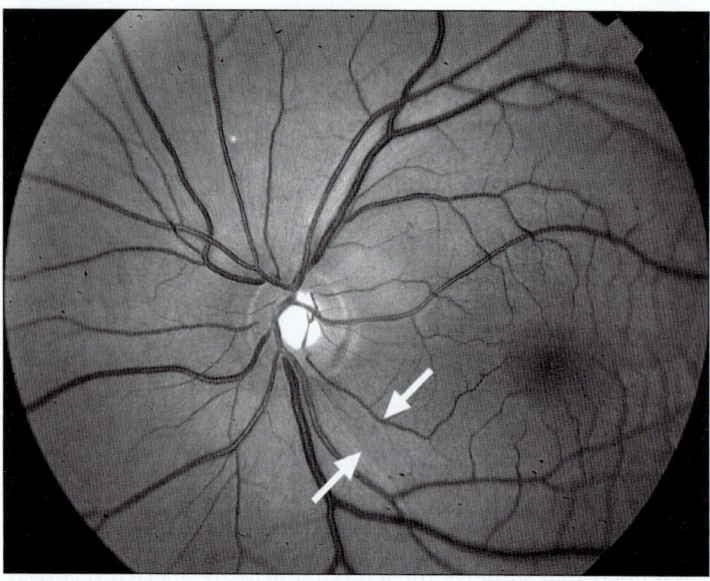

FIG. 217-2 ▉ **Red-free view in a patient who has early glaucomatous loss (left eye).** The bright striations of the normal nerve fiber layer are visible in the superior one half of the fundus. Inferiorly, there is a clearly defined, wedge-shaped nerve fiber bundle defect *(arrows)*. Note how the defect touches the optic disc and widens as it extends peripherally.

Techniques for Nerve Fiber Layer Analysis

No technique is available to count the number of axons within the optic nerve or nerve fiber layer. Because axons cannot be counted in vivo, indirect measures of axon "count" must be used. Various techniques have been used to evaluate the optic nerve and nerve fiber layer in glaucoma, as summarized in Table 217-1.

Fundus Examination

Stereo photographs of the optic nerve are not very useful for evaluation of the nerve fiber layer, because this tissue is not seen well, particularly in a color photograph. Because the nerve fiber layer is the innermost retinal layer (after the internal limiting membrane), a short-wavelength light that focuses more anteriorly helps bring the layer into focus.

Red-free (green) light used in either direct ophthalmoscopy or slit-lamp biomicroscopy of the fundus with a 78D or 90D lens makes the nerve fiber layer easier to visualize. The nerve fiber layer may be examined using high-contrast, black-and-white photographs obtained with red-free light; grading systems are used to quantify the amount of detectable loss.[6,7]

Measurement of Retinal Contour

Examination of the nerve fiber layer by ophthalmoscopy or photographic grading is subjective and prone to variability. A more objective technique involves the measurement of the height of the retinal surface above a reference plane. The topography of the retinal surface may be determined by tomographic scans using a confocal scanning laser ophthalmoscope, such as the

TABLE 217-1

SUMMARY OF TECHNIQUES FOR RETINAL NERVE FIBER LAYER ANALYSIS

Technique	Equipment Needed	Governing Principles	Advantages	Disadvantages
Ophthalmoscopy	Direct ophthalmoscope or slit lamp and 78D or 90D lens Red-free light	Nerve fiber layer visibility is enhanced with short-wavelength light	Easy to perform using readily available equipment	May be difficult without clear media Nerve fiber layer not easily seen in lightly pigmented fundi
Red-free, high-contrast fundus photography	Fundus camera with red-free filter High-contrast black-and-white film and paper	Nerve fiber layer visibility is enhanced with short-wavelength light	Nerve fiber layer defects may be easy to detect	Requires skilled photographer and dilated pupil Requires dilated pupil Limitations of ophthalmoscopy apply
Retinal contour analysis	Scanning laser ophthalmoscope that can perform tomographic topography	Three-dimensional construction of retinal surface can measure retinal height above a reference plane—height is related to nerve fiber layer thickness	Easy to perform through undilated pupil No discomfort to patient Can image through most media opacities unless very dense	Equipment is expensive Height measurements depend upon location of reference plane Retinal thickness may not be true indirect measure of nerve fiber layer thickness
Optical coherence tomography	Optical coherence tomography unit	Uses reflected and backscattered light to create images of various retinal layers (analogous to the use of sound waves in ultrasonography)	Can differentiate layers within the retina, including the nerve fiber layer, with a 10μm resolution Correlates with known histology	Equipment is expensive Requires dilated pupil Resolution may not be high enough to detect small changes
Scanning laser polarimetry	Scanning laser polarimeter	Birefringent properties of the nerve fiber layer cause a measurable phase shift of an incident polarized light proportional to the tissue thickness	Easy to perform through undilated pupil No discomfort to patient Can image through most media opacities, unless very dense Resolution limited to size of a pixel (possibly as small as 1μm) Reproducibility 5–8μm	Equipment is expensive Measurements not correlated histologically in humans Requires compensation for other polarizing media (e.g., cornea)

Heidelberg Retinal Tomograph. This instruments determine the retinal contour in three dimensions; the retina is imaged in multiple (usually 32) planes, and the images are combined into a contour map. A reference plane is set below the retinal surface, and the height of the peripapillary retina (theoretically directly proportional to the nerve fiber layer thickness) above the plane is measured.[8] This method has a sensitivity of 73% for the detection of glaucomatous optic nerve damage[9] and can be used to detect, over time, changes attributed to glaucoma progression.[10]

Optical Coherence Tomography

High-resolution, tomographic, cross-sectional images of the retina may be obtained using a technique called optical coherence tomography. This imaging technique is similar in concept to ultrasonographic imaging, except that reflected and backscattered light is used to create the image, rather than sound waves. Interfaces occur at tissues of different optical densities, and layers within a tissue may be differentiated from each other, with a resolution of approximately 5–8 μm. The retinal nerve fiber layer is visualized easily using this technique, and thickness measurements are determined by computer analysis of the resultant image. Measurements of nerve fiber layer thickness using optical coherence tomography correlate well with structural (histological nerve fiber layer thickness measurements) and functional (visual fields) parameters in normal individuals and in patients who have glaucoma.[11]

Scanning Laser Polarimetry

When polarized light passes through the retinal nerve fiber layer, the birefringent property of the axons (attributed to microtubules within the axons) causes the polarized light to undergo a phase shift.[12] Such polarized laser light that passes through the nerve fiber layer is reflected off of the outer eye layers, and the degree of phase shift in the light that returns is measured by a detector. The amount of phase shift, also known as retardation, is directly proportional to the amount of nerve fiber layer (microtubules) through which the incident light has passed; this gives an indirect measurement of the thickness of the tissue. Rapid scans across an area of retina (by moving the polarized laser light) enable measurements to be obtained for a given retinal area. This technique is known as scanning laser polarimetry.

The Nerve Fiber Analyzer is a scanning laser polarimeter that employs this measurement technique. Using a diode laser in the near infrared, nerve fiber layer measurements are obtained at 65,536 retinal points in a 15° × 15° grid centered on the optic nerve head. The measurement may be performed through an undilated pupil of at least 2mm diameter, takes approximately 0.7 seconds to perform, and is not apparent to the patient (no flashes of light or other sensation). The acquired image is processed rapidly by the instrument's software, which runs under Microsoft Windows on a personal computer. Normally, three images are obtained for each eye and then averaged to create a mean or baseline image. The reproducibility of the measurements is of the order of 5–8 μm per measured pixel.

Normative data for the Nerve Fiber Analyzer measurements have been obtained from many centers around the world and incorporated into the analytical software of the instrument, and the instrument has been renamed the GDx. Figure 217-3 is an example of a printout obtained from a normal eye using the GDx software. The color printout includes a picture of the area scanned (obtained by reflectance of the laser light) at the upper left. Next to the reflectance image is a color-coded "thickness" map of the retinal nerve fiber layer for the area scanned. Colors in the blue and black represent areas or lower retardation (below 60 μm), and red, orange, and yellow are used to represent regions of higher retardation, up to 140 μm. The ellipse denotes an area 1.75 disc diameters in size, centered on the optic nerve (determined by the edge of the nerve head as marked by the operator).

The graph below the reflectance image (Nerve Fiber Layer) represents the retardation measurements along the ellipse, from temporal to superior to nasal to inferior and back to temporal. Note the typical "double-hump" distribution of nerve fibers found in normal individuals, with highest values superiorly and inferiorly and lower values nasally and temporally, which corresponds to the known anatomy of normal nerve fiber layers. The shaded area includes 95% of normal values, which enables ready identification of abnormal nerve fiber areas along the eclipse. The box below the retardation map, labeled "Deviation from Normal," shows the difference within each quadrant between the measured values and those of age-corrected normal individuals, in microns. Shading indicates probabilities, with the legend given to the right of the box. The bottom of the printout summarizes various parameters, along with the probability of finding such values in the normal database. The latest version of the instrument, called the GDx VCC, incorporates individualized compensation for the birefringent of the anterior segment, and the software can display a pixel-by-pixel deviation for normal map.

Histopathological examination of the nerve fiber layer performed after scanning laser polarimetry in monkeys shows good correlation between retardation values and thickness measurements.[13] In the monkey model, one degree of retardation corresponded to approximately 7.4 μm of thickness. Human mea-

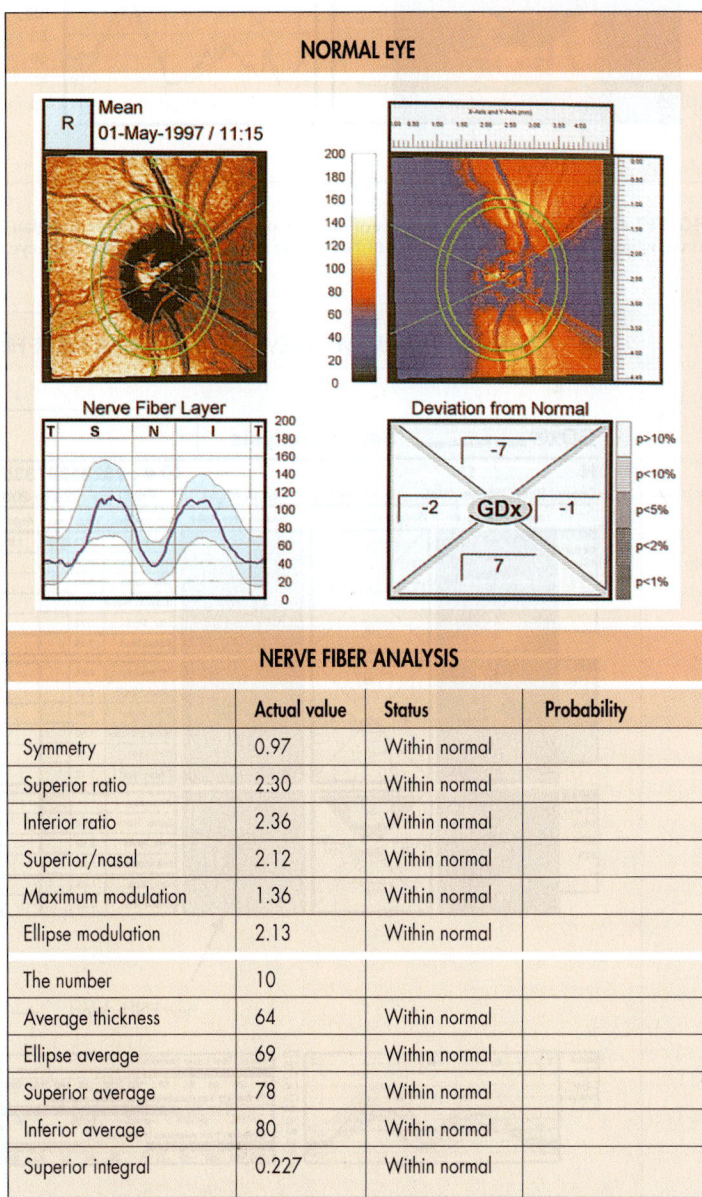

FIG. 217-3 ▪▪ **Printout from the GDx software of the Nerve Fiber Analyzer; normal eye.** A reflectance image, as well as the color-coded "thickness" map, is provided. Various measurement parameters are shown in the lower box.

NERVE FIBER ANALYSIS

	Actual value	Status	Probability
Symmetry	0.97	Within normal	
Superior ratio	2.30	Within normal	
Inferior ratio	2.36	Within normal	
Superior/nasal	2.12	Within normal	
Maximum modulation	1.36	Within normal	
Ellipse modulation	2.13	Within normal	
The number	10		
Average thickness	64	Within normal	
Ellipse average	69	Within normal	
Superior average	78	Within normal	
Inferior average	80	Within normal	
Superior integral	0.227	Within normal	

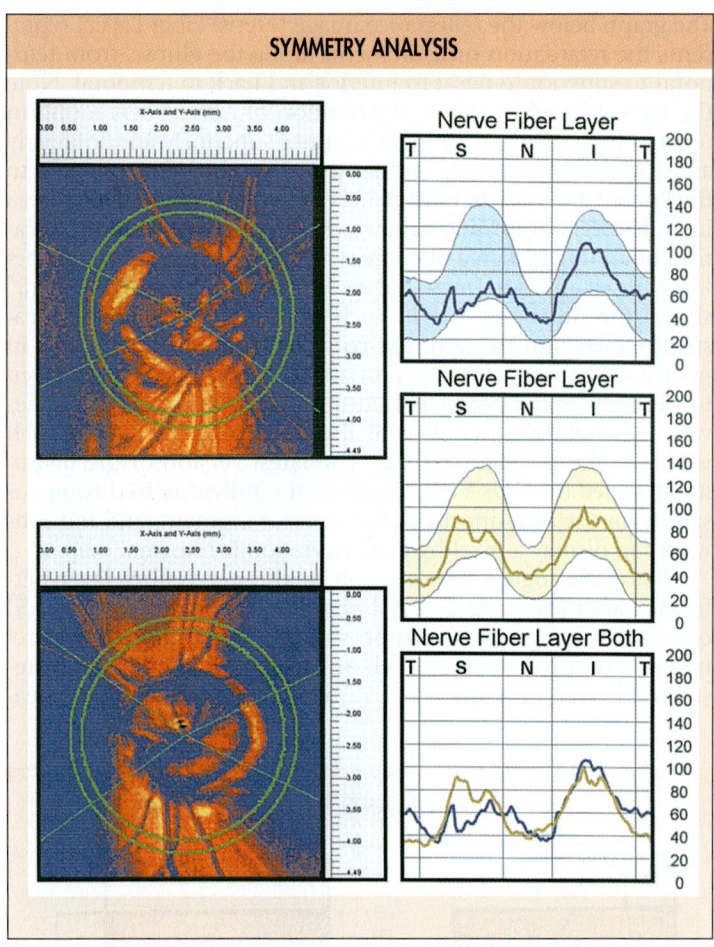

SYMMETRY ANALYSIS

surements have not yet been obtained. Retardation values obtained by scanning laser polarimetry correspond to known properties of the retinal nerve fiber layer in normal and glaucomatous eyes[14] and may be used to detect glaucoma, with a reported sensitivity of 96% and specificity of 93%.[15] Retardation values also correlate with some measures of visual field loss in patients who have glaucoma.[16] Measurements of mean nerve fiber layer thickness in patients affected by ocular hypertension are statistically significantly lower than those of normal patients, with considerable overlap in the values.[17,18]

Scanning laser polarimetry may be used to detect glaucoma damage before standard automated perimetry does. The nerve fiber layer analysis (Fig. 217-4) of a 66-year-old African-American man who has optic nerves of normal appearance and ocular hypertension demonstrates asymmetrical loss of nerve fibers from the superior bundle of the right eye compared with the left. In this symmetry analysis printout from the GDx software, the thickness curves from the right and left eyes are superimposed upon each other (Nerve Fiber Layer Both) and the loss of the superior peak in the right eye is readily visible (blue line). The serial analysis (Fig. 217-5) may demonstrate change over time. In this example, a new nerve fiber layer defect developed over a 2.5-year period (left side of figure). A corresponding visual field defect also developed (right side of figure).

SUMMARY

Assessment of the retinal nerve fiber layer appears to be more sensitive and specific for the evaluation of glaucoma damage, especially early in the course of the disease, than estimations of cup-to-disc ratio or other measures of the optic nerve head. Quantitative assessment of nerve fiber layer thickness holds

FIG. 217-4 ■ Nerve fiber layer analysis of the eyes of a patient with suspected glaucoma, which shows asymmetrical loss of fibers in the superior bundle of the right eye.

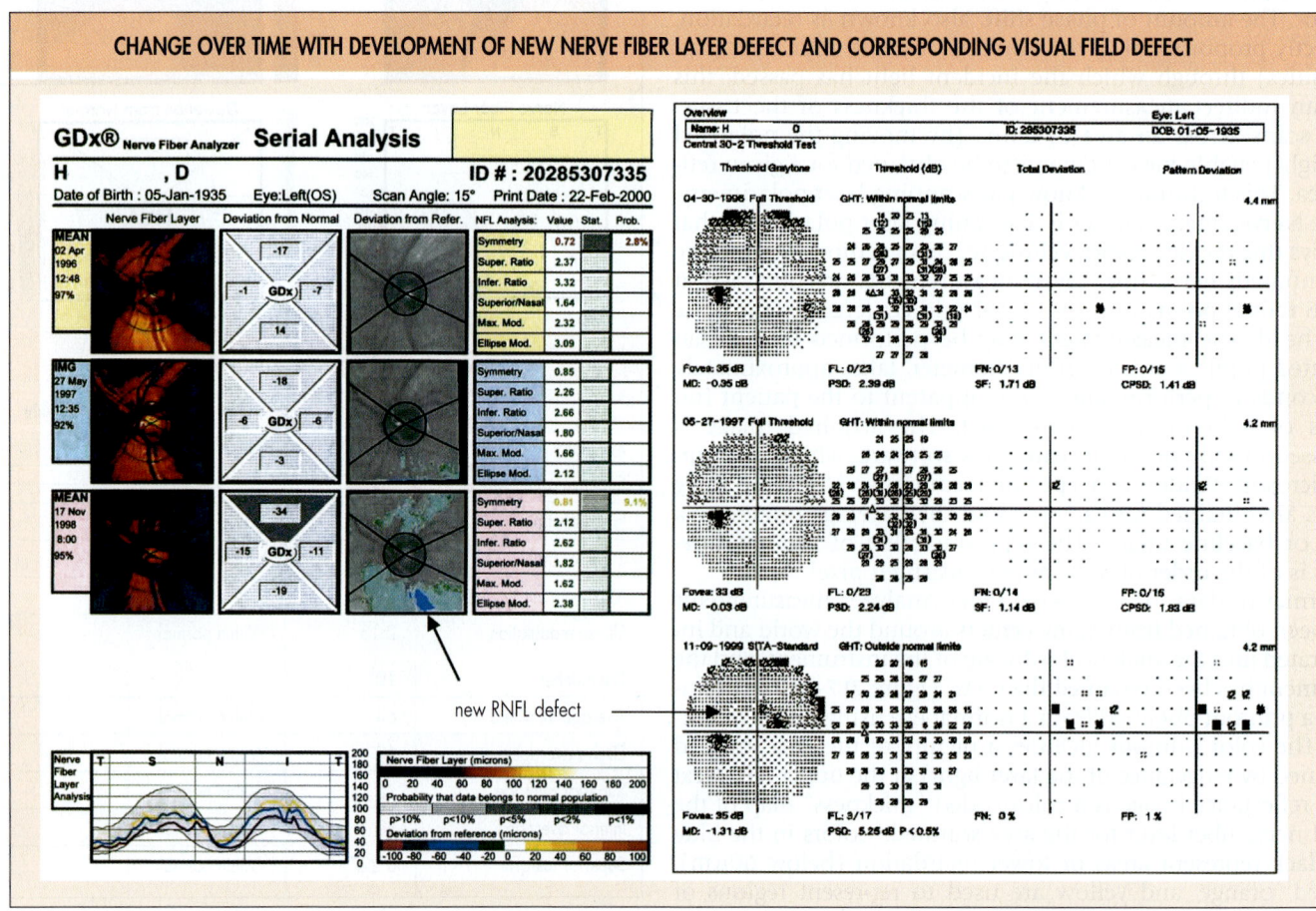

CHANGE OVER TIME WITH DEVELOPMENT OF NEW NERVE FIBER LAYER DEFECT AND CORRESPONDING VISUAL FIELD DEFECT

new RNFL defect

FIG. 217-5 ■ **Change over time with the development of a new nerve fiber layer defect and corresponding visual field defect.** The serial analysis of this patient with glaucoma shows the development of a new nerve fiber layer defect over a 2.5-year period. The blue pixels show the change from the initial image. A superior arcuate scotoma developed over the same period, corresponding to the area of nerve fiber layer loss.

promise for early detection of glaucoma and objective follow-up of disease progression. As measurement techniques become more refined and the characteristics of the retinal nerve fiber layer in normal individuals and patients with glaucoma become better understood, objective measures, such as optical coherence tomography and scanning laser polarimetry, may prove to be better than visual field tests for diagnosis and follow-up in patients who have glaucoma and for the recognition of early damage in patients at risk for glaucoma.

REFERENCES

1. Tuulonen A, Lehtola J, Airaksinen J. Nerve fiber layer defects with normal visual fields: Do normal optic discs and normal visual field indicate absence of glaucomatous abnormality? Ophthalmology. 1993;100:587–98.
2. Migdal C. Optic nerve head in primary open angle glaucoma, pathogenesis and pathophysiology. In: Tasman W, Jaeger EA, eds. Duane's ophthalmology, clinical vol. 3, ch. 52, record 35188-35223 on CD-ROM. Philadelphia: JB Lippincott; 1996.
3. Ogden TE. Nerve fiber layer of the macaque retina: retinotopic organization. Invest Ophthalmol Vis Sci. 1983;24:85–98.
4. Jonas JB, Dichtl A. Evaluation of the retinal nerve fiber layer. Surv Ophthalmol. 1996;40(5):369–78.
5. Jonas JB, Schiro D. Localised wedge shaped defects of the retinal nerve fiber layer in glaucoma. Br J Ophthalmol. 1994;78:285–90.
6. Niessen AG, van den Berg TJ, Langerhorst CT, Bossuyt PM. Grading of retinal nerve fiber layer with a photographic reference set. Am J Ophthalmol. 1995;120(5):57–86.
7. Quigley HA, Reacher M, Katz J, et al. Quantitative grading of nerve fiber layer photographs. Ophthalmology. 1993;100(12):1800–7.
8. Caprioli J, Miller JM. Measurement of relative nerve fiber layer surface height in glaucoma. Ophthalmology. 1989;96:633–41.
9. Caprioli J, Prum B, Zeyen T. Comparison of methods to evaluate the optic nerve head and nerve fiber layer for glaucomatous change. Am J Ophthalmol. 1996;121(6):659–67.
10. O'Connor DJ, Zeyen T, Caprioli J. Comparison of methods to detect glaucomatous optic nerve damage. Ophthalmology. 1993;100(10):1498–503.
11. Shuman JS, Hee MR, Puliafito CA, et al. Quantification of nerve fiber layer thickness in normal and glaucomatous eyes using optical coherence tomography. Arch Ophthalmol. 1995;113:586–96.
12. Dreher AW, Reiter K, Weinreb RN. Spatially resolved birefringence of the retinal nerve fiber layer assessed with a retinal laser ellipsometer. Appl Opt. 1992;31:3730–5.
13. Weinreb RN, Dreher AW, Coleman A, et al. Histopathologic validation of Fourier ellipsometry measurements of retinal nerve fiber layer thickness. Arch Ophthalmol. 1990;108:557–60.
14. Weinreb RN, Shakiba S, Zangwill L. Scanning laser polarimetry to measure the nerve fiber layer of normal and glaucomatous eyes. Am J Ophthalmol. 1995; 195(5):627–36.
15. Tjon-fo-sang MJ, Lemij HG. The sensitivity and specificity of nerve fiber layer measurements in glaucoma as determined with scanning laser polarimetry. Am J Ophthalmol. 1997;123(1):62–9.
16. Weinreb RN, Shakiba S, Sample PA, et al. Association between quantitative nerve fiber layer measurement and visual field loss in glaucoma. Am J Ophthalmol. 1995;120(12):732–8.
17. Tjon-fo-sang MJ, de Vries J, Lemij HG. Measurement by nerve fiber analyzer of retinal nerve fiber layer thickness in normal subjects and patients with ocular hypertension. Am J Ophthalmol. 1996;122(8):220–7.
18. Anton A, Zangwill L, Emdadi A, Weinreb RN. Nerve fiber layer measurements with scanning laser polarimetry in ocular hypertension. Arch Ophthalmol. 1997;115:331–4.

218 Optic Nerve Blood Flow Measurement

COLM O'BRIEN • ALON HARRIS

INTRODUCTION

The fact that a substantial number of glaucoma patients (perhaps up to 30%) have normal intraocular pressure (IOP) at the time of initial diagnosis indicates that risk factors other than IOP alone contribute to the pathogenesis of optic nerve damage in this disorder. Foremost among the proposed risk factors is ischemia contributing to the loss of optic nerve axons, a concept recognized for more than 100 years. It has become increasingly clear that vascular compromise also plays a significant role in high-pressure glaucoma. Some clinical features point to an underlying vascular problem; these include localized rim notching or focal ischemic glaucoma (Fig. 218-1), peripapillary vasoconstriction (Fig. 218-2), optic disc hemorrhage (Fig. 218-3), and senile sclerotic optic discs with peripapillary choroidal sclerosis (Fig. 218-4).[1, 2]

The precise role of optic nerve blood flow in the loss of axons in glaucoma is not clear. An acute cessation of flow in a short posterior ciliary artery, such as occurs in giant cell arteritis, results in pallor and gross visual loss but little cupping of the optic disc. Focal ischemia (which presumably arises from infarction of a small ciliary vessel in the prelaminar region) produces localized disc cupping and pallor and a corresponding, well-defined (frequently small) visual field defect. Although several studies have recorded vascular changes in glaucoma, it is not clear whether these findings are primary causative events or whether they occur secondary to loss of neural tissue. Long-term studies are needed to address this issue. Further research into the macro- and microcirculations of the ocular and optic nerves will help elucidate the relative roles of IOP and ischemia in the pathogenesis of glaucoma.

APPLIED ANATOMY

The ophthalmic artery, which is the first branch of the internal carotid artery, gives off 2–4 posterior ciliary arteries (PCAs), which later divide into 10–20 short PCAs that pierce the sclera and enter the globe around the optic nerve. The number of short PCAs is variable, as is the course they take in this region, but in general they supply the posterior choroid and anterior optic nerve either directly or indirectly via the arterial circle of Zinn-Haller, which, when present, is formed by the anastomosis of the medial and lateral short PCAs.[3,4] The central retinal artery, which enters the optic nerve about 8–12mm behind the globe, passes along the central axis of the nerve and gives off few, if any, branches to the neural tissue. Venous drainage of the anterior optic nerve is to the central retinal vein and later the superior ophthalmic vein.

The anterior optic nerve head (prelaminar, laminar, and postlaminar neural tissue) is supplied by branches from the short PCA, and the nerve fiber layer of the superficial retina receives arteriolar branches from the central retinal artery. The capillaries of the anterior optic nerve head (retinal and ciliary) have tight junctions, are not fenestrated, and form a rich anastomotic

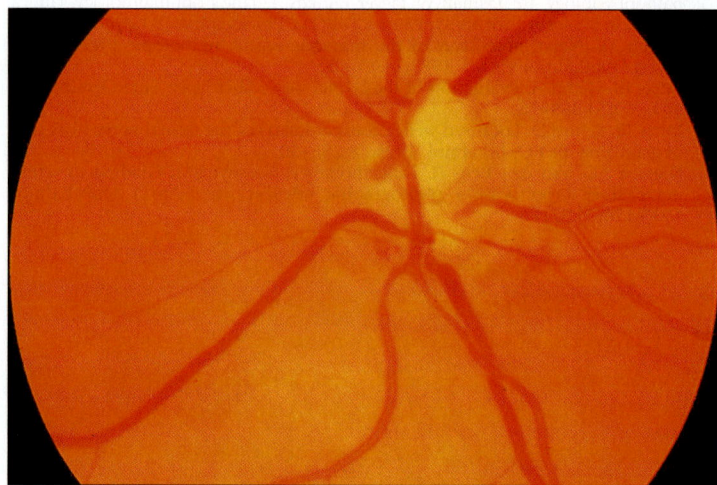

FIG. 218-1 ■ **Focal ischemic optic disc appearance (left eye).** Localized loss of the superotemporal neuroretinal rim in a 54-year-old woman who has migraine and Raynaud's phenomenon.

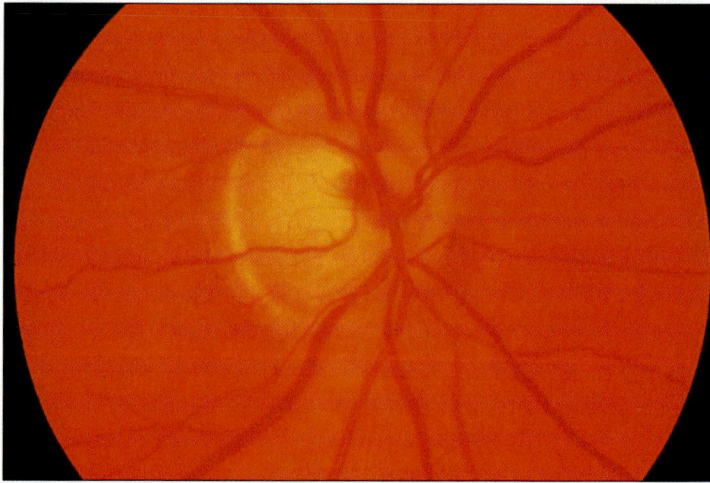

FIG. 218-2 ■ **Peripapillary vasoconstriction in glaucoma (right eye).** Marked narrowing of a branch of the inferotemporal retinal artery (at the 6 o'clock position) as it crosses the optic disc boundary adjacent to the inferior temporal vein.

plexus. Histological examination of glaucomatous optic nerves shows a reduction in the number of capillaries, consistent with the degree of neural loss.

The contribution of the peripapillary choroidal circulation to the perfusion of the anterior optic nerve head remains unclear, although watershed zones in the region of the optic nerve that arise from the presence of choroidal end-arteries may be a factor in the development of optic nerve ischemia.[4] Some investigators consider that the true "watershed" lies in the division of the

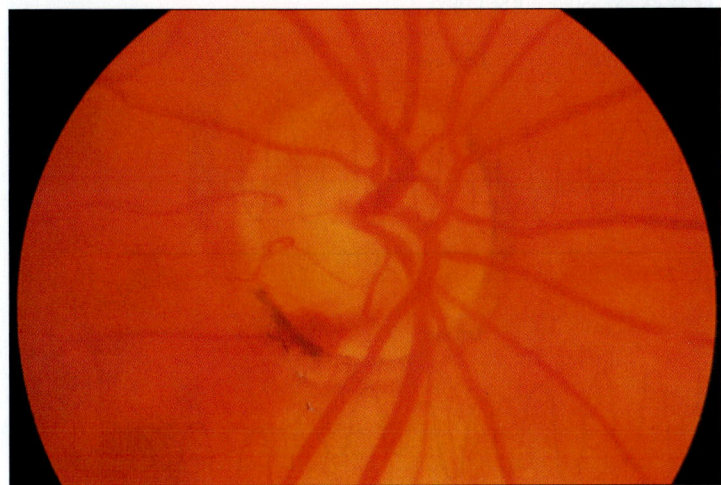

FIG. 218-3 ▌ Optic disc hemorrhage (right eye). Flame-shaped hemorrhage adjacent to an acquired optic nerve pit at the 6 o'clock position.

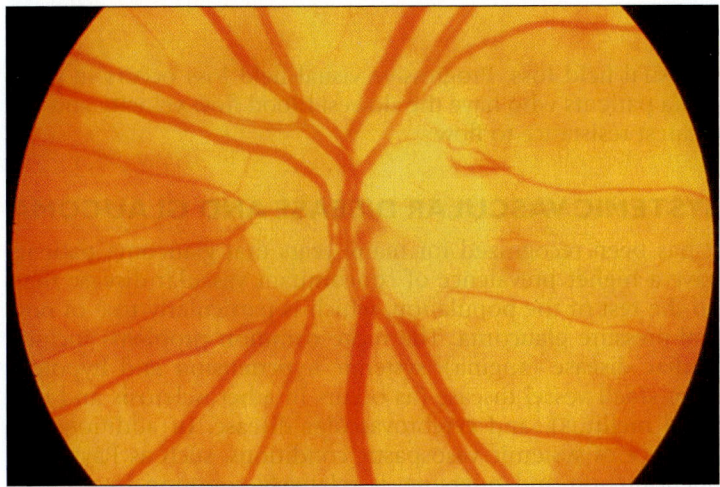

FIG. 218-4 ▌ Senile sclerotic ("moth-eaten") optic disc (left eye). The pale disc has a shallow, saucerized optic cup and peripapillary choroidal sclerosis. There is a small, flame-shaped disc hemorrhage at the 2 o'clock position.

short PCAs into branches that supply the choroid and branches that supply the optic nerve head.

PHYSIOLOGY

Blood flow in the anterior optic nerve depends on many factors, which include the perfusion pressure (mean arterial blood pressure minus IOP) and the resistance to flow as determined by the vascular caliber in the arterioles and capillaries.[5] The latter is influenced by factors that affect local tissue blood flow (e.g., metabolic, endothelial). The ability to keep local tissue flow constant and counteract changes in the local metabolic environment is called autoregulation.[5,6] Moderate increments in IOP and systemic blood pressure have little effect on anterior optic nerve blood flow, and autoregulatory mechanisms maintain flow in hyperoxic and hypercapnic conditions. However, if autoregulation is impaired, elevated IOP may reduce optic nerve perfusion; optic nerve and retinal circulations have deficient autoregulation in normal-pressure and primary open-angle glaucoma. An ocular diastolic perfusion pressure less than 35mmHg (4.7kPa) is associated with a significant increase in the prevalence of glaucoma.[7]

Substances produced by the vascular endothelium play a major role in the control of ocular blood flow[8]; these include the

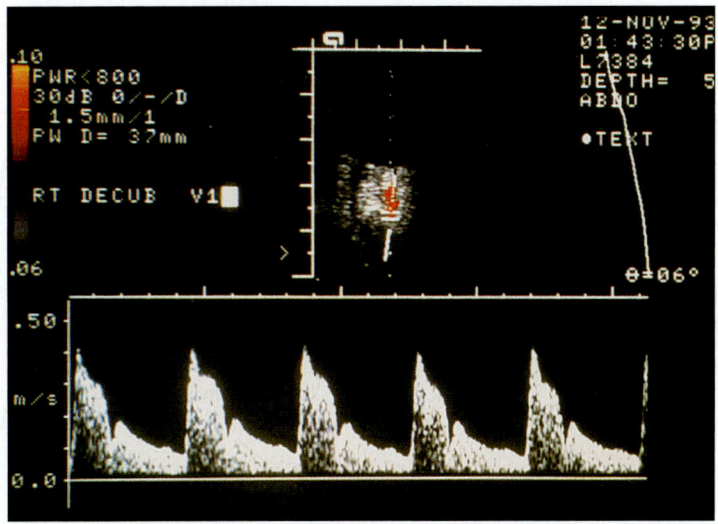

FIG. 218-5 ▌ Color Doppler imaging of the ophthalmic artery. Shown is the pulsatile spectral analysis with a sharp rise in the peak systolic velocity and a gradual tail-off to the end diastolic velocity at the end of each pulse waveform. Note the dicrotic notch within the diastolic phase.

vasodilators nitric oxide and prostacyclin and vasoconstrictors such as angiotensin and the endothelins. Cells that produce these substances have been identified in the choroid, retina, and optic nerve. Repeated endothelin-1 injections into the perineural space of the optic nerve produce chronic ischemia and excavation of the optic disc in animal studies.[9]

Although autonomic α- and β-receptors have been identified in the optic nerve head, they do not appear to have any functional properties.

EXPERIMENTAL INVESTIGATIONS

Blood flow in the optic nerve head has been quantified in animal work using radiolabeled microsphere and iodoantipyrine methods, which show high flow in the prelaminar and laminar regions.[10,11] In the retina and optic nerve, blood flow is coupled closely with glucose consumption, as measured by the deoxyglucose uptake technique. In monkeys, IOP raised above systolic blood pressure results in complete cessation of blood flow in the prelaminar tissue.

CLINICAL STUDIES

The anatomical regions of particular interest in glaucoma include the capillary plexus of the superficial retinal fiber layer, the pre- and intralaminar optic nerve head, and the peripapillary choroid. Currently, no single examination technique can be used to study all these vascular beds simultaneously.

Angiography

Both fluorescein and indocyanine green angiography (photographic, video, and scanning laser) are used to study the retinal, choroidal, and optic disc circulation. Fluorescein filling defects in the superficial part of the optic disc and choroid, delayed arm-to-retina and retinal artery and venous filling times, prolonged arteriovenous passage time, and reduced velocity in the retinal circulation have been described.[12]

Color Doppler Imaging

Blood flow velocities in the major ocular vessels (ophthalmic, central retinal, and short posterior ciliary arteries) can be measured using color-coded ultrasound Doppler instruments (Fig. 218-5). Reduced velocity (particularly the end-diastolic component) and increased resistance to flow occur in all these vessels

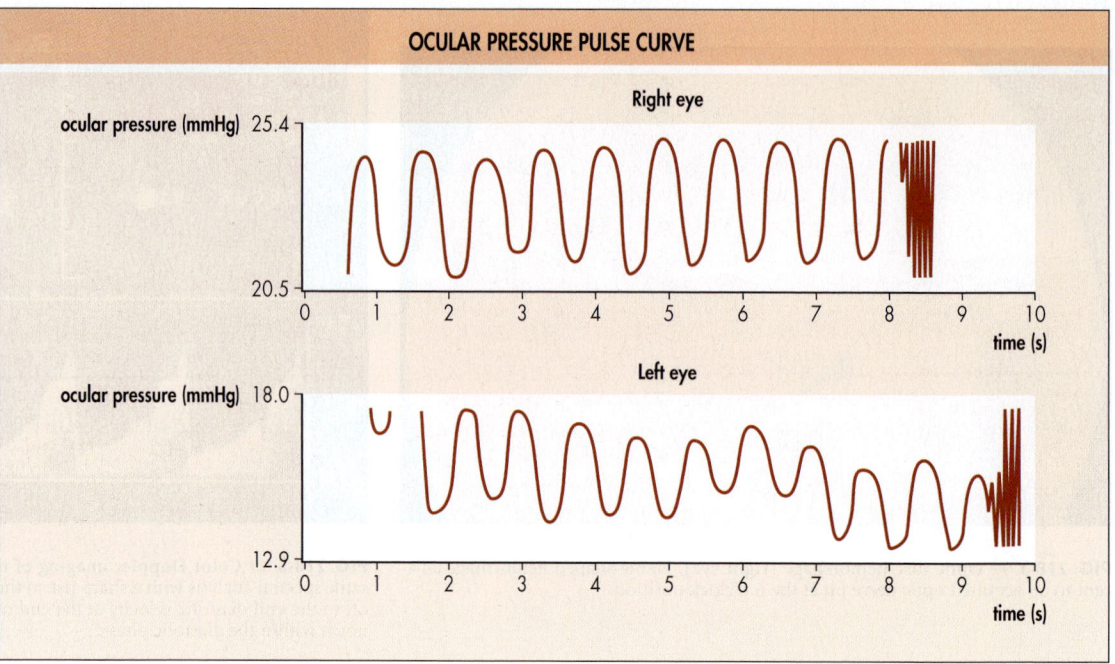

OCULAR PRESSURE PULSE CURVE

Right eye

ocular pressure (mmHg) 25.4

20.5

time (s)

Left eye

ocular pressure (mmHg) 18.0

12.9

time (s)

FIG. 218-6 ■ **The ocular pressure pulse curve.** Continuous recording of intraocular pressure produces a characteristic waveform pattern.

in both high and normal pressure open-angle glaucoma.[13,14] Current color Doppler imaging (CDI) cannot measure absolute volume flow because they do not measure vessel diameter. However, a recently developed analysis technique incorporated in the CDI machine is now capable of determining the ophthalmic artery diameter.[15] Therefore, with this technique, ophthalmic artery volumetric blood flow can be assessed. Future developments may allow us to extend the ability of this technique to measure the central retinal artery diameter.

Laser Doppler Flowmetry

Both single-point and wide-field 10° scanning laser Doppler techniques have been used to study red blood cell movement in the capillary network in the anterior optic nerve head and peripapillary retinal circulation. The data show reduced blood flow velocities in the lamina cribrosa and in the nasal and temporal neural rim and retina in glaucoma.[16] The precise site and depth of measurement using these techniques remain unclear, although the approach itself evaluates the region of greatest interest in the pathogenesis of optic nerve damage in glaucoma.

Ocular Pulse Amplitude

Continuous recording of the change in IOP resulting from the change in ocular volume with the arrival of each bolus of blood at the eye gives a record of the ocular pressure pulse wave (Fig. 218-6). By comparison with known ocular pressure–volume curves, a measure of the pulsatile component of ocular blood flow is derived; this is assumed to correspond to choroidal blood flow, because the greater part (approximately 90%) of total ocular flow is to the choroidal circulation. Reduced ocular pulse amplitude and pulsatile ocular blood flow occur in high- and normal-pressure glaucoma,[17] although the relevance of these findings to circulation in the optic nerve head is uncertain.

Ocular Blood Flow and Visual Field Loss

The number and size of optic disc fluorescein angiography filling defects increase with the severity of visual field loss in glaucoma. Delayed retinal and choroidal fluorescein filling times occur in high- and normal-pressure glaucoma and are related to the severity of the disease. CDI studies show reduced blood flow velocity in the short PCA, which corresponds with the location of visual field loss. Progressive visual field loss occurs in glaucoma patients who have the slowest blood flow velocity and the greatest resistance to flow.

SYSTEMIC VASCULAR DISEASE AND GLAUCOMA

It has been recognized for many years that glaucoma patients have a higher prevalence of concomitant vascular disease than do the rest of the population, which is particularly true of normal-pressure glaucoma. The more common problems include cardiac disease (angina), systemic hypertension and hypotension, small vessel disease (as occurs in atherosclerosis and diabetes mellitus), and cerebrovascular disease. In addition, the presence of systemic vasospastic conditions, such as Raynaud's phenomenon and migraine, is relatively common in normal-pressure glaucoma. Patients affected by progressive glaucoma show significant nocturnal systemic hypotension ("dippers") when ambulatory blood pressure is monitored for 24 hours,[18] but this may on occasion be the consequence of overzealous management of systemic hypertension. Elevated blood and plasma viscosity, increased platelet and red blood cell aggregation, increased red cell deformability, and activation of the coagulation cascade[19] have been reported in glaucoma.

The concept of vasospasm was introduced into the glaucoma literature recently, particularly for normal-pressure disease.[20] Implied is an abnormal vascular endothelial responsiveness (with normal anatomy) to common everyday stimuli such as cold, stress, and anxiety. Many patients exhibit a Raynaud-like peripheral circulation, with reduced finger flow after immersion of the hand in cold water. Migraine and silent myocardial ischemia appear to be more prevalent, and elevated systemic levels of the potent endothelial vasoconstrictor endothelin-1 have been reported in normal-pressure glaucoma. Precisely how these findings contribute to optic nerve head ischemia remains unclear.

Therefore, for every glaucoma patient, it is important that the ophthalmologist obtain an accurate history of systemic diseases, particularly cardiovascular problems, as well as the systemic medications being taken. Many cardiovascular drugs have effects on the eye, including systemic beta blockers (which have an ocular hypotensive effect). Obtaining an accurate systemic and medication history is clearly important at the time of diagnosis, and it is essential that this information be updated at each clinic visit.

PHARMACOLOGY

When reduced ocular and optic nerve blood flow contributes significantly to the pathogenesis of axonal loss, modification of blood flow might provide protection from ischemia-induced neuronal damage. *In vitro* animal myography studies of isolated segments of the ophthalmic and ciliary arteries demonstrate that endothelin-l produces potent constriction, which can be prevented by voltage-gated calcium channel blockade.[21] Evidence exists that calcium antagonists, administered orally for concomitant systemic vascular disease, are associated with improved preservation of the visual field in some, but not all, normal-pressure glaucoma patients.[22] Similarly, some patients show improvement in ocular blood flow and contrast sensitivity with calcium channel blockers or inhaled carbon dioxide in short-term investigations. Medical and surgical reduction of IOP may, in some glaucoma patients, improve ocular blood flow.[23] Whether improved perfusion has any beneficial long-term effect on the visual field remains unclear.

REFERENCES

1. Geijssen HC, Greve EL. The spectrum of primary open angle glaucoma. Senile sclerotic glaucoma versus high tension glaucoma. Ophthalmic Surg. 1987;18:207–13.
2. Nicolela MT, Drance SM. Various glaucomatous optic nerve appearances: clinical correlations. Ophthalmology. 1996;103:640–9.
3. Lieberman MF, Maumenee AE, Green WR. Histological studies of the vasculature of the anterior optic nerve. Am J Ophthalmol. 1976;82:405–11.
4. Hayreh SS. Structure and blood supply of the optic nerve. In: Heilmann K, Richardson KT, eds. Glaucoma: conceptions of a disease. Stuttgart: Thieme; 1978:78–92.
5. Bill A. Vascular physiology of the optic nerve. In: Varma R, Spaeth GL, eds. The optic nerve in glaucoma. Philadelphia: JB Lippincott; 1993:37–50.
6. Anderson DR. Autoregulation in glaucoma. In: Drance SM, ed. International symposium on glaucoma, ocular blood flow and drug treatment. Baltimore: Williams & Wilkins; 1991:82–9.
7. Tielsch JM, Katz J, Sommer A, *et al.* Hypertension, perfusion pressure and primary open-angle glaucoma. Arch Ophthalmol. 1995;113:216–21.
8. Haefliger IO, Meyer P, Flammer J, Luscher TF. The vascular endothelium as a regulator of the ocular circulation: a new concept in ophthalmology? Surv Ophthalmol. 1994;39:123–32.
9. Orgul S, Cioffi GA, Wilson DJ, *et al.* An endothelin-1 induced model of optic nerve ischaemia in the rabbit. Invest Ophthalmol Vis Sci. 1996;37:1860–9.
10. Geijer C, Bill A. Effect of raised intraocular pressure on retinal, prelaminar and retrolaminar optic nerve blood flow in monkeys. Invest Ophthalmol. 1979;18:1030–42.
11. Sperber GO, Bill A. Blood flow in glucose consumption in the optic nerve, retina and brain: effects of high intraocular pressure. Exp Eye Res. 1985;639:41–8.
12. Schwartz B, Nagin P. Fluorescein angiography of the optic disc. In: Varma R, Spaeth GL, eds. The optic nerve in glaucoma. Philadelphia: JB Lippincott; 1993:307–24.
13. Harris A, Sergott RC, Spaeth GL, *et al.* Color Doppler analysis of ocular vessel blood velocity in normal-tension glaucoma. Am J Ophthalmol. 1994;118:642–9.
14. Rankin SJA, Walman BE, Buckley AR, Drance SM. Color Doppler imaging and spectral analysis of the optic nerve vasculature in glaucoma. Am J Ophthalmol. 1995;119:685–93.
15. Orge F, Harris A, Kagemann L, *et al.* The first technique for non-invasive measurements of volumetric ophthalmic artery blood flow in humans. Br J Ophthalmol. 2002;86(11):1216–9.
16. Michaelson G, Longhans MJ, Groh MJM. Perfusion of the juxta-papillary retina and neuroretinal rim in primary open angle glaucoma. J Glaucoma. 1996;5:91–8.
17. James CB, Smith SE. Pulsatile ocular blood flow in patients with low tension glaucoma. Br J Ophthalmol. 1991;75:466–70.
18. Graham SL, Drance SM, Wijsman K, *et al.* Ambulatory blood pressure monitoring in glaucoma. The nocturnal dip. Ophthalmology. 1995;102:61–9.
19. O'Brien C, Butt Z, Ludlow C, Detkova P. Activation of the coagulation cascade in untreated primary open angle glaucoma. Ophthalmology. 1997;104:725–30.
20. Flammer J. To what extent are vascular factors involved in the pathogenesis of glaucoma? In: Kaiser HJ, Flammer J, Hendrickson P, eds. Ocular blood flow. Basel: Karger; 1996:12–39.
21. Meyer P, Haefliger IO, Flammer J, Luscher TF. Endothelium dependent regulation in ocular vessels. In: Kaiser HJ, Flammer J, Hendrickson P, eds. Ocular blood flow. Basel: Karger; 1996:64–73.
22. Kitazawa Y, Shirai H, Go FJ. The effect of calcium antagonist on visual field in low tension glaucoma. Graefes Arch Clin Exp Ophthalmol. 1989;227:408–12.
23. Harris A, Spaeth GR, Sergott RC, *et al.* Retrobulbar hemodynamic effects of betaxalol and timolol in normal tension glaucoma. Am J Ophthalmol. 1995;120:168–75.

SECTION 3 SPECIFIC TYPES OF GLAUCOMA

CHAPTER
219

Congenital Glaucoma

JAMES D. BRANDT

DEFINITION

- Glaucoma that arises in children under 2 years of age.
- Primary infantile glaucoma—the result of isolated abnormal development of the anterior chamber angle structures.
- Secondary infantile glaucoma—associated with a variety of ocular and systemic syndromes and with surgical aphakia.

KEY FEATURES

- Elevated intraocular pressure.
- Glaucomatous optic atrophy.
- Ocular enlargement (buphthalmos).

ASSOCIATED FEATURES

- Corneal edema.
- Haab's striae.
- Photophobia.
- Tearing.
- Amblyopia.

INTRODUCTION

In this chapter, an overview of the various forms of glaucoma that occur in infants and young children is given. Many clinicians group these varied disorders under the somewhat generic heading of congenital glaucoma. Primary infantile glaucoma, also commonly referred to as *congenital glaucoma*, represents a specific developmental defect of the anterior chamber angle structures and is exceedingly rare. Nonetheless, most ophthalmologists will encounter the wide variety of secondary forms of glaucoma seen in this age group. In this chapter, the reader is provided with a basic understanding of how the various forms of glaucoma can manifest in infants and young children, along with their differential diagnosis and the options available for management.

EPIDEMIOLOGY AND PATHOGENESIS

The incidence of primary infantile glaucoma often is quoted as between 1:10,000 and 1:15,000 live births in the heterogeneous population of the United States.[1,2] In other countries, the published series range from a low of 1:22,000 in Northern Ireland[3] to a high of 1:2500 in Saudi Arabia[4] and 1:1250 among gypsies in Romania.[5] Primary infantile glaucoma is bilateral in up to 80% in larger case series[6]; in North America and Europe it is more common in boys,[7] whereas in Japan it is more common in girls.[8]

The varied incidence among different populations suggests a strong genetic component to the disease. In fact, most (about 90%) of new cases of primary infantile glaucoma appear to be sporadic. However, in the remaining 10% there appears to be a strong familial component; penetrance of the defect varies in the range of 40–100%. The recent characterization of genes linked to primary infantile glaucoma in a large cohort of affected families suggests that over the next few years genetic screening may become possible for selected mutations.[9–11] Taken as a group, the secondary glaucomas of childhood are far more common than primary infantile glaucoma. Perhaps the most common of these are the glaucomas associated with cataract extraction in infancy. Lens opacities are noted in 0.44% of all live births.[12] The incidence of glaucoma in children who have undergone lens extraction ranges from as low as 8%[13] to as high as 41% if follow-up is extended to middle childhood.[14] These figures suggest that glaucoma in aphakic children is more common than is recognized generally.

The exact cause and pathophysiology that underlies primary infantile glaucoma remains unknown. In an attempt to explain why the operation he developed—goniotomy—was so successful in cases of infantile glaucoma, Barkan[15] postulated that a thin, imperforate membrane covered the anterior chamber angle structures and impeded aqueous humor outflow. This so-called *Barkan's membrane,* as the structure became known, has not been confirmed on light or electron microscopy, despite numerous attempts to do so. Some observers have described a compaction of trabecular meshwork that might appear clinically as a continuous membrane.[16] That the anterior chamber "cleavage" disorders,[17] despite their broad spectrum, often are associated with infantile glaucoma suggests that the principal defect in primary infantile glaucoma is a failure of one or more steps in the normal development of the anterior chamber angle. As the genes associated with primary infantile glaucoma are characterized further and the physiological or developmental role of the proteins they encode become better understood, the molecular, cellular, and embryological pathophysiology of this rare disorder will become clear.[10]

Among the secondary glaucomas of childhood, the underlying pathophysiology is as varied as that in adults. Occurrence at or shortly after birth indicates a profound developmental abnormality of the anterior chamber angle, whereas manifestation later in life usually suggests a different process. For example, patients who have aniridia who have obvious glaucoma at birth or early childhood have visibly abnormal anterior chamber angle structures; when glaucoma becomes apparent later in life in patients who have aniridia, the previously functional trabecular meshwork is occluded by an anterior migration and rotation of the rudimentary iris stump.[18] In patients who suffer Sturge–Weber syndrome (SWS) or its variants, appearance at birth is associated with a gonioscopic appearance that cannot be differentiated from that of primary infantile glaucoma (Fig. 219-1), whereas later occurrence is thought to be related to elevated episcleral venous pressure.

Angle closure may be caused by forward pressure from a process that occurs in the vitreous cavity, as in persistent hyperplastic primary vitreous, retinopathy of prematurity, or retinoblastoma. Synechial angle closure, caused by chronic inflammation or neovascularization, is seen in a variety of situations. Primary angle closure that results from iris bombé generally is not seen in children, except in cases of spherophakia, but when the pupil becomes secluded by an inflammatory or neo-

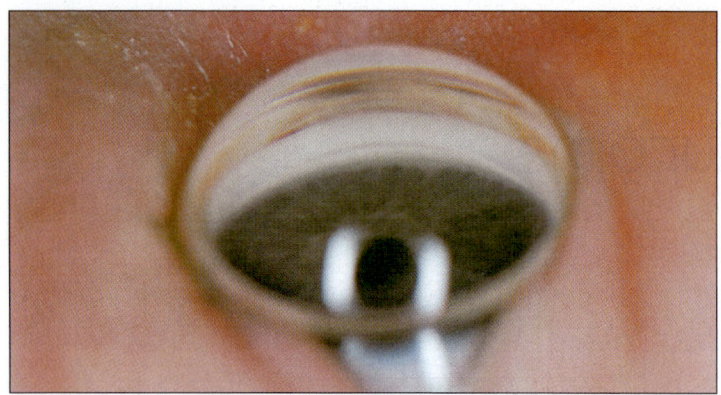

FIG. 219-1 ■ **Angle appearance in Klippel–Trenaunay–Weber syndrome.** Koeppe lens visualization of the anterior chamber angle of the right eye of the patient shown in Figure 219-7. Note the striking similarity of the angle appearance to that of primary infantile glaucoma (see Fig. 219-6).

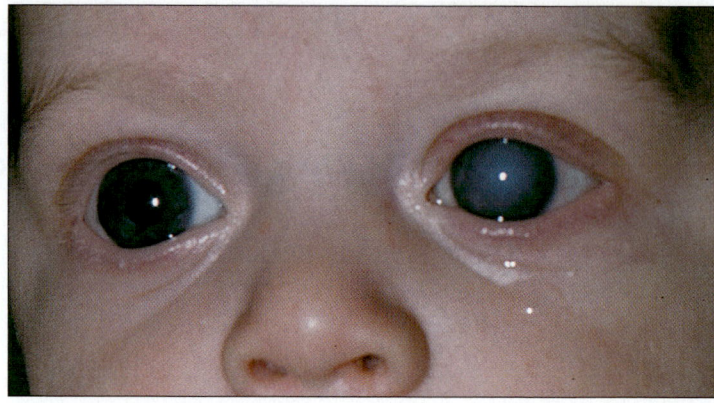

FIG. 219-2 ■ **Clinical appearance of primary infantile glaucoma.** This 8-month-old boy had an acute (3-day) history of corneal edema in the left eye. Note the enlarged corneas in both eyes and the epiphora. Intraocular pressure at examination under anesthetic was >35mmHg (>4.7kPa) in the right eye. Trabeculotomy *ab externo* was carried out bilaterally.

vascular membrane, iris bombé and subsequent angle closure may occur.

Secondary open-angle glaucomas also occur in young children. Both corticosteroid-induced and chronic uveitic glaucomas are described clearly.[19] Open-angle glaucoma may develop long after blunt trauma to the eye has occurred[20] and also may follow the spontaneous bleeding of juvenile xanthogranuloma.[21]

It is difficult to classify the underlying cause of glaucoma that frequently follows pediatric cataract extraction. Walton[22] examined 65 children, most of whom developed glaucoma 2 or more years after lensectomy. Preoperative gonioscopy revealed no consistent angle defect, but postoperative gonioscopy revealed a near-constant (96%) filtration-angle deformity he characterized as blockage of the posterior trabecular meshwork with pigment and synechiae.[22] Many clinicians familiar with this scenario believe that retained lens material is one risk factor for glaucoma that follows pediatric cataract extraction; another may be the presence of a small cornea. Parks *et al.*[23] described a secondary glaucoma risk of 15% in their cohort of 174 eyes; only 2.9% of eyes that had normal corneal diameters developed glaucoma, whereas 32% of eyes that had corneal diameters smaller than 10mm developed the disease. The presence of both a cataract and a small cornea almost certainly indicates a problem during ocular development; perhaps cataract surgery unmasks a marginally functional and maldeveloped anterior chamber angle that causes later glaucoma.

OCULAR MANIFESTATIONS

The typical infant with congenital glaucoma is referred to an ophthalmologist initially because of clinically apparent corneal edema (Fig. 219-2). The corneal edema may be subtle, especially in bilateral cases, or profound, with an enlarged corneal diameter and globe, breaks in Descemet's membrane (Haab's striae), and sometimes even acute hydrops (Fig. 219-3). Often in these cases, the commonly described triad of epiphora, blepharospasm, and photophobia has been present for some time but is dismissed until the more alarming corneal edema becomes apparent. The epiphora of congenital glaucoma often is misattributed to congenital nasolacrimal duct obstruction, which is found in 5–6% of unselected newborns.

The hallmark of all forms of glaucoma in infants and young children is ocular enlargement, which occurs because the immature and growing collagen that constitutes the cornea and sclera in the young eye still responds to increased intraocular pressure (IOP) by stretching. All parts of the globe may stretch in response to the elevated IOP until 3–4 years of age, and glaucoma-related axial myopia may be seen until the early teenage years. Clinically, ocular enlargement is most evident as an increase in

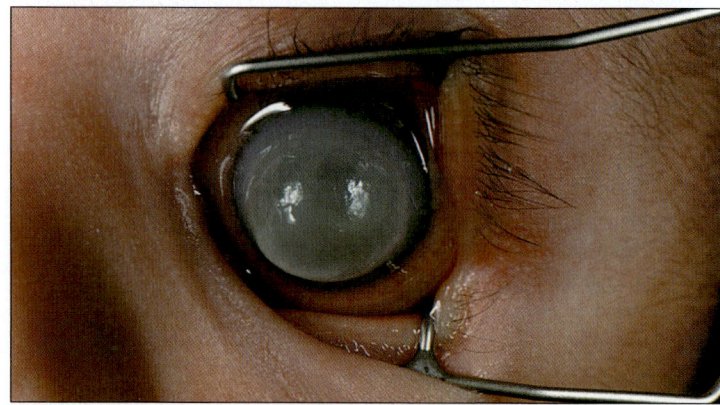

FIG. 219-3 ■ **Acute corneal hydrops in a neonate.** The baby girl whose eye is shown here had acute hydrops at birth, an extreme Descemet's tear, and corneal decompensation associated with infantile glaucoma. The child has an older sister who had an identical clinical picture 2 years previously. They are the children of consanguineous gypsy parents from Romania and may demonstrate examples of the highly penetrant, inherited form of infantile glaucoma described in this population by Gencik.[5]

corneal diameter. A variety of published series provide some guidelines as to normal measures of corneal diameter[24,25]; in general, the horizontal corneal diameter in the normal neonate is in the range 10.0–10.5mm and increases 0.5–1.0mm during the first year of life. In an infant in whom glaucoma is suspected, a horizontal corneal diameter greater than 12mm indicates a high index of suspicion for the disease.

As the cornea stretches and distends, Descemet's membrane and the overlying corneal endothelium may fracture and rip, which results in breaks in these structures that are evident clinically as profound corneal edema (see Fig. 219-2) and, in severe cases, acute hydrops (see Fig. 219-3). As the endothelial cells migrate over the breaks and lay down new basement membrane, ridges develop along the separated edges of Descemet's membrane, which results in the formation of the double striae first recognized by Haab in 1899[26] (Fig. 219-4).

In children over 2 years of age, corneal enlargement usually is not the predominant sign that glaucoma is present. In these children, decreased visual acuity or strabismus noted at the pediatrician's office or progressive unilateral myopia noted in an optometrist's office prompts a referral and the correct diagnosis.

The hallmark of all forms of glaucoma, and the principal cause of irreversible visual loss, is damage to the optic nerve. Early descriptions of infantile glaucoma stated that optic nerve cupping occurred late in the disease process. It is now apparent not only that cupping may occur rapidly in infants, but also that with surgical management and normalization of IOP, this cup-

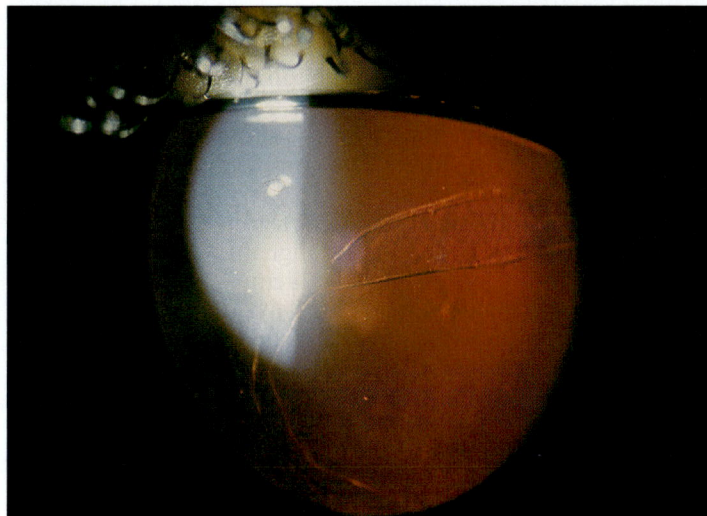

FIG. 219-4 ■ **Haab's striae.** A red reflex view of the right eye of the infant shown in Figure 219-2, at 5 years of age. Haab's striae are seen just adjacent to the visual axis. The child has a best-corrected visual acuity of 20/50 (6/15) in the right eye and 20/20 (6/6) in the left eye despite aggressive amblyopia management.

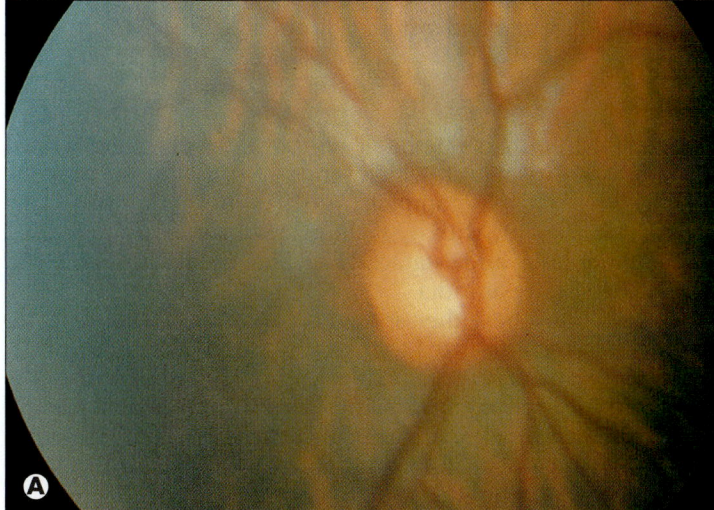

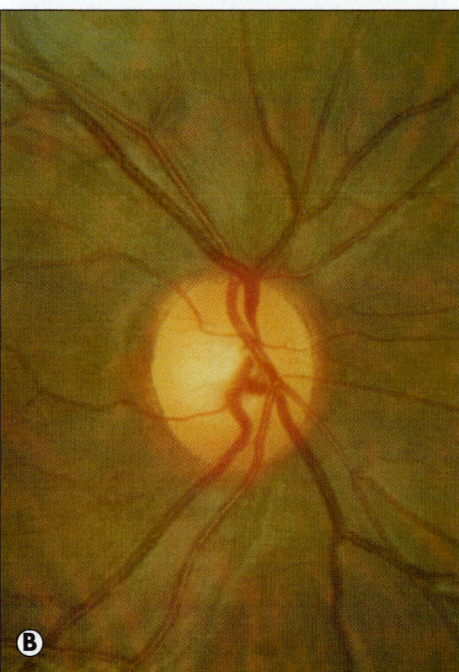

FIG. 219-5 ■ **Choroidal hemangiomas associated with Sturge–Weber syndrome.** A, An extensive choroidal hemangioma in the posterior pole of a 10-year-old boy who has Sturge–Weber syndrome before uncomplicated trabeculectomy. B, The same hemangioma after uncomplicated trabeculectomy. Preoperative intraocular pressures were 30–40mmHg (4.0–5.3kPa); note the dramatic reversal of optic disc cupping. The presence of choroidal hemangiomas increases the risk of intraoperative choroidal expansion and hemorrhage when the eye is entered and the intraocular pressure is reduced.

ping is reversible.[27] Indeed, reversibility of optic nerve cupping is one of the hallmarks of successful management of glaucoma in infants and young children (Fig. 219-5). The resilience of the infant optic nerve should be taken into account by the surgeon who contemplates incisional surgery based only on borderline anterior segment findings; if the optic nerve appears normal, a repeat EUA in a few weeks may spare the child an unnecessary intraocular procedure.

DIAGNOSIS AND ANCILLARY TESTING

The diagnosis of glaucoma in infants is clinical. In most cases, particularly when the disease occurs unilaterally or asymmetrically, the diagnosis is made in the office using a penlight (see Figs. 219-2 and 219-3). With some practice, IOP can be measured in the office in a conscious, swaddled infant using a Tono-Pen or handheld Goldmann tonometer. Usually, the IOP in infants with normal eyes is in the range of 11–14mmHg (1.5–1.9kPa) using these devices. The office measurement of an IOP greater than 20mmHg (2.7kPa) in a calm, resting infant is suspicious for glaucoma when other signs and symptoms suggest the disease, as is an asymmetry of more than 5mmHg (6.7kPa) in suspected unilateral or asymmetrical cases. Measurements of IOP undertaken while a child cries and resists efforts to hold the eye open are usually invalid, because the Valsalva maneuver and lid squeezing can result in an IOP of 30–40mmHg (4.0–5.3kPa), even in normal eyes.

Examination of the optic nerve is attempted whenever possible, because obvious glaucomatous cupping confirms the diagnosis. Shaffer and Hetherington noted a cup-to-disc (C/D) ratio greater than 0.3 in 68% of 126 eyes affected by primary infantile glaucoma,[28] whereas a C/D ratio greater than 0.3 was found in less than 2.6% of newborns with normal eyes.[29] Asymmetry in the C/D ratio for the two optic nerves, especially when the asymmetry corresponds to other findings, is strongly suggestive of glaucoma.

A Koeppe infant diagnostic lens that does not have a central depression employs a lid-retention flange to prevent the infant from squeezing out the contact lens. Once the lens is in place, good visualization of the disc is possible using a direct ophthalmoscope, even with a relatively small pupil; with dilatation, fundus photography to document the appearance of the optic nerve may be possible.

With a Koeppe diagnostic infant lens in place, gonioscopy may be performed, even on a conscious infant in the office. Simultaneous gonioscopy of both eyes may be carried out to compare the angle appearance in unilateral or asymmetrical cases. The diagnosis of glaucoma is not made using gonioscopic appearance alone but is based primarily on the other signs and symptoms of the disease. However, gonioscopy may help to differentiate among the various forms of glaucoma and provide the surgeon with an idea of whether angle surgery (goniotomy or trabeculotomy) or fistulization surgery (trabeculectomy or drainage implant) should be the first intervention made. The gonioscopic appearance of the anterior chamber angle in primary infantile glaucoma is characteristic (Fig. 219-6); the iris inserts anteriorly compared with the normal infant angle. The stroma of the peripheral iris is hypoplastic, unpigmented, and has a scalloped appearance.

If the diagnosis of glaucoma is confirmed or strongly suspected based on the office examination, an examination under anesthesia (EUA) and definitive surgical management is pursued within a few days. Details of EUA and of goniotomy and trabeculotomy are provided in Chapter 238.

As noted previously, some forms of primary infantile glaucoma represent heritable disorders, as do many of the secondary or systemically associated glaucomas of childhood. All children who have glaucoma and who are diagnosed at birth or during early childhood must be referred to a clinical geneticist familiar with ocular disease; in some cases a subtle syndromic diagnosis

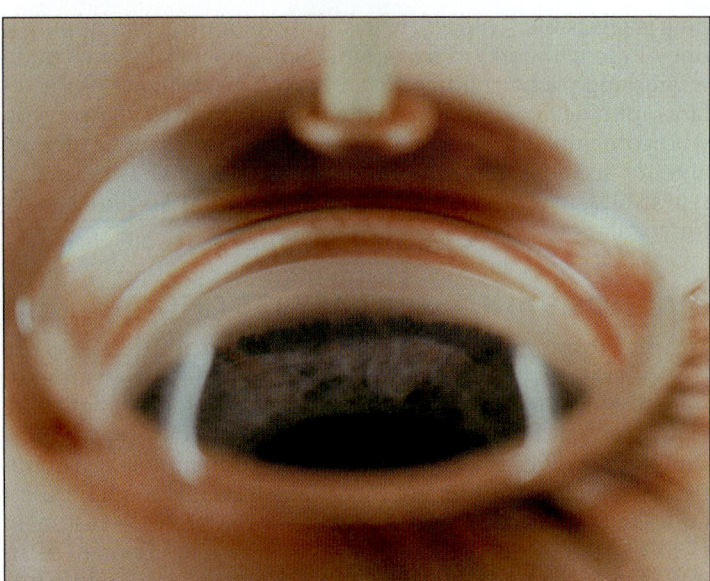

FIG. 219-6 ■ **Gonioscopic appearance of the anterior chamber angle in primary infantile glaucoma.** When viewed through a Koeppe diagnostic lens, the iris is seen to insert anteriorly, and the peripheral iris is hypoplastic and unpigmented and has a scalloped appearance. A sheen occurs over the angle structures (which is difficult to photograph) and gives the impression that a membrane coats the surface of the angle; however, Barkan's membrane has not been identified histologically.

BOX 219-1

Differential Diagnosis of Ocular Signs and Symptoms in Congenital Glaucoma

CORNEAL EDEMA OR CLOUDING
Congenital hereditary endothelial dystrophy
Mucopolysaccharidoses I, IS, II, III
Cystinosis
Sclerocornea
Rubella keratitis
Obstetric birth trauma ("forceps injury")
Chemical injury

EPIPHORA AND/OR RED EYE
Nasolacrimal duct obstruction
Conjunctivitis (viral, chlamydial, bacterial)
Corneal epithelial defect, abrasion

PHOTOPHOBIA
Conjunctivitis
Iritis
Trauma (especially hyphema)

CORNEAL ENLARGEMENT
Axial myopia
Megalocornea (X-linked or sporadic)
Microphthalmic fellow eye

---

may be made that has important implications for the parents' childbearing plans. With the predicted advances in the molecular diagnosis of some forms of infantile glaucoma, it may soon be possible to offer prenatal screening for some families.

DIFFERENTIAL DIAGNOSIS

The differential diagnosis of the various signs and symptoms of glaucoma in children is given in Box 219-1; this list is by no means exhaustive.

Corneal cloudiness may have a myriad of causes. Corneal opacity that results from hereditary dystrophies is usually symmetrical, whereas corneal edema that arises from obstetrical trauma is usually unilateral.

Corneal enlargement may result from megalocornea, which is frequently X-linked. In affected children, the anterior chamber

angle, IOP, and optic nerve are all normal. Some clinicians consider megalocornea to be a forme fruste of primary infantile glaucoma[1]; such children should be followed carefully for later signs of glaucoma. An entirely normal eye may appear enlarged relative to a microphthalmic fellow eye and, in such cases, familiarity with the age-appropriate corneal diameters and axial lengths prevents misdiagnosis.

The differential diagnosis of a red, tearing eye in a child is a lengthy procedure; infectious, malignant, or inflammatory causes rarely result in a diagnostic dilemma. Congenital nasolacrimal duct obstruction occurs in 5–6% of otherwise normal infants and coexists with infantile glaucoma with similar frequency. If epiphora persists after apparently successful management of glaucoma in an infant, the nasolacrimal system must be evaluated.

SYSTEMIC ASSOCIATIONS

A number of classifications of congenital and infantile glaucomas have been proposed; one that the author has found clinically useful is given in Table 219-1. It is beyond the scope of this chapter to cover all of the glaucoma syndromes associated with developmental and systemic disorders—an almost encyclopedic coverage of these forms of pediatric glaucoma is given by Ritch *et al.*[30] Here, two of the more commonly encountered secondary glaucomas associated with ocular and systemic disorders are discussed.

Aniridia

Congenital aniridia is a heritable disease of the eye characterized by an obvious iris defect (which varies from an almost complete absence to relatively complete, albeit abnormal, irides), decreased visual acuity with nystagmus, small corneas, small discs, foveal hypoplasia, and cataract. Glaucoma occurs in 50–75% of patients who have aniridia.

Aniridia may be either sporadic or familial. The gene for aniridia has been localized to the short arm of chromosome 11; a deletion in this area results in a syndrome that comprises the ocular findings given above with, in addition, mental retardation, genital anomalies, and a greatly increased risk of Wilms' tumor at a young age.[31] Children of parents who have aniridia are at a 50% risk of inheriting the syndrome.

Although most children who have aniridia go on to develop glaucoma, most do not do so until late in the first decade of life. This late-onset glaucoma associated with aniridia appears to be the result of a unique form of angle closure.[18] It is advisable to re-examine these patients scrupulously and treat when early angle closure and optic nerve changes have been confirmed. Chen and Walton[32] recently described goniosurgery to prevent the development of aniridic glaucoma in 55 eyes of 33 patients, reporting excellent results. Adachi and colleagues[33] report excellent results with trabeculotomy and advocate its use in aniridia. However, once severe disease is present and requires surgery, fistulization is the procedure of choice.

Sturge–Weber Syndrome and Variants

Although rare, glaucoma associated with encephalotrigeminal angiomatosis (SWS) is one of the more frequently encountered forms of glaucoma of childhood. There are several variants of SWS, which is considered to be one of the phakomatoses. Classic SWS comprises the triad of port wine facial telangiectasis (nevus flammeus) in the distribution of the trigeminal nerve that respects the vertical midline, ipsilateral glaucoma, and intracranial angiomata. In patients affected by glaucoma, both the upper and lower lids usually are involved in the facial telangiectasis (Fig. 219-7). Cibis *et al.*[34] report that glaucoma occurs in about one third of patients who have SWS.

As noted previously, SWS-associated glaucoma that manifests early in life is likely to be the result of a developmental angle ab-

TABLE 219-1

CLASSIFICATION OF THE CONGENITAL AND INFANTILE GLAUCOMA

PRIMARY INFANTILE GLAUCOMA (CONGENITAL GLAUCOMA, TRABECULODYSGENESIS)

SECONDARY INFANTILE GLAUCOMA

Associated with mesodermal neural crest dysgenesis	Iridocorneotrabeculodysgenesis
	• Rieger's anomaly or syndrome
	• Axenfeld's anomaly or syndrome
	• Peters' anomaly
	• systemic hypoplastic mesodermal dysgenesis (Marfan's syndrome)
	• systemic hyperplastic mesodermal dysgenesis (Weill–Marchesani syndrome)
	Iridotrabeculodysgenesis (aniridia)
Associated with phako-matoses and hamartomas	Neurofibromatosis (Von Recklinghausen's disease)
	Encephalotrigeminal angiomatosis (Sturge–Weber syndrome and variants, e.g., Klippel–Trénaunay–Weber syndrome)
	Angiomatosis retinae et cerebelli
	Oculodermal melanocytosis
Associated with metabolic disease	Oculocerebrorenal syndrome (Lowe's syndrome)
	Homocystinuria
Associated with inflammatory disease	Maternal rubella syndrome (congenital rubella)
	Herpes simplex iridocyclitis
Associated with mitotic disease	Juvenile xanthogranuloma (nevoxanthoendothelioma)
	Retinoblastoma
Associated with other congenital disease	Trisomy 13–15 syndrome (Patau's syndrome)
	Rubinstein–Taybi syndrome
	Persistent hyperplastic primary vitreous
	Congenital cataract
	• in phakic eyes
	• in aphakic eyes following surgery

(Modified and expanded from deLuise VP, Anderson DR. Primary infantile glaucoma (congenital glaucoma). Surv Ophthalmol. 1983;28(1):1–19; Freedman SF, Walton DS. Approach to infants and children with glaucoma. In: Epstein DL, Allingham RR, Schuman JS, eds. Chandler and Grant's glaucoma, ed 4. Baltimore: Williams & Wilkins, 1997; and Walton DS. Primary congenital open angle glaucoma: a study of the anterior segment abnormalities. Trans Am Ophthalmol Soc. 1979;77:746–68.)

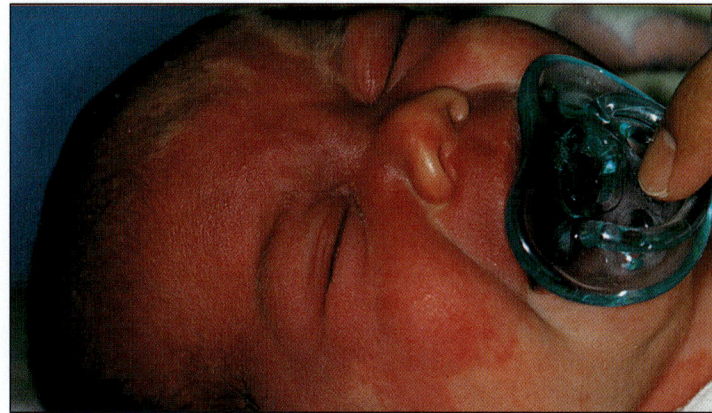

FIG. 219-7 ■ **An infant who has Klippel–Trenaunay–Weber syndrome.** Note the extensive facial telangiectasis that does not respect the vertical midline. Limb and trunk involvement is characteristic (with profoundly asymmetrical limb growth in severely affected individuals). Upper and lower lids are involved, which indicates a high likelihood of glaucoma (see Fig. 219-1).

terior chamber angle in this disease are limited to a small number of specimens. Furthermore, eyes enucleated at an advanced stage because of blindness and pain may not be representative of the early disease and a trabeculectomy specimen is fixed in a nonphysiological manner, as a tissue fragment rather than as a living tissue with a hydraulic pressure across it. Nonetheless, several general observations have been made.[8] The iris inserts anteriorly (see Fig. 219-6), but the angle is open. The trabecular meshwork appears open and is perforate, and Schlemm's canal usually is present and open. As noted previously, histologically, Barkan's membrane has not been identified conclusively.

TREATMENT

The preferred management of the congenital forms of glaucoma is surgical, not medical. Medical therapy alone is rarely effective for these conditions. Surgical techniques used on the anterior chamber angle (goniotomy and trabeculotomy) enjoy a high degree of success in primary infantile glaucoma, and alternative surgical approaches (trabeculectomy and drainage implant surgery) may be highly effective in the secondary congenital and pediatric forms. Even with the newer topical agents and formulations that can be administered once a day and that may be safer (systemically) than those previously available, it remains unrealistic to expect more than short-term medication compliance in children who have a lifelong disease that may result in blindness.

The surgical management of all infants affected by glaucoma begins with a detailed EUA. The ophthalmologist who undertakes the surgical management of an infant or child who has glaucoma must approach the EUA with experience in infant gonioscopy and a flexible surgical plan. Surgical flexibility is particularly crucial in the secondary forms of congenital glaucoma, for which the surgeon must be prepared to alter the surgical plan depending upon what is found intraoperatively; for example, in the infant with glaucoma associated with aphakia, a synechially closed anterior chamber angle is a relative contraindication to conventional angle surgery, so a trabeculectomy or drainage implant must be considered, instead.

In primary infantile glaucoma, either goniotomy or trabeculotomy is the procedure of choice; these are associated with success rates in various series of 90% or greater. Goniotomy requires a clear cornea for adequate observation of the anterior chamber angle; trabeculotomy may be performed if the cornea is hazy or opaque. The choice of procedure is left to the surgeon's discretion.

Trabeculectomy has been proposed as a primary management option for glaucoma in children,[37,38] considering the technical challenges of the rarely performed goniotomy or trabecu-

normality similar to that found in primary infantile glaucoma (see Fig. 219-1), whereas glaucoma that occurs later in life may result from elevated episcleral venous pressure. The best management of SWS-associated glaucoma is unclear; when the angle appears similar to that of primary infantile glaucoma, goniotomy or trabeculotomy are reasonable first steps[35]; some have advocated the use of combined trabeculotomy and trabeculectomy as the best procedure.[36] When increased episcleral venous pressure is invoked as the cause of elevated IOP, a fistulization procedure (trabeculectomy or drainage implant) might be more likely to succeed. The presence of choroidal hemangiomas in many of these patients (see Fig. 219-5) increases the risk of choroidal expansion or hemorrhage intraoperatively; some surgeons advocate using prophylactic posterior sclerotomies prior to entering the anterior chamber.

PATHOLOGY

Because primary infantile glaucoma is rare, few of these infants die of unrelated causes, and the angle surgery does not involve the excision of a surgical specimen. Pathology descriptions of the an-

lotomy compared with the more common trabeculectomy. However, a trabeculectomy in an infant eye is not without its own set of unique challenges. To raise a partial thickness flap in a buphthalmic eye is particularly difficult, as is the perioperative adjustment of flap tension without the use of the argon laser to lyse flap sutures. Hypotony and a flat chamber that cause a cataract in an infant may result in profound amblyopia before the visual axis is cleared. Most proponents of filtration surgery in infants and young children advocate the intraoperative application of the potent antimetabolite mitomycin C, because postoperative injection of 5-fluorouracil usually is not an option. Filtration procedures augmented with antimetabolites result in the formation of thin, acellular blebs that impart high susceptibility to late-onset bleb infection and endophthalmitis.[39,40] The prospect of a lifetime with a 1–2% annual rate of infectious complications must be considered when the surgical approach to these difficult cases is chosen.

Another alternative to consider in cases of congenital glaucoma for which conventional angle surgery has either failed or is unlikely to succeed is the use of a drainage implant, such as a Baerveldt, Molteno, or Ahmed implant. This option is attractive, particularly for patients in whom aphakia is managed by daily wear or extended wear contact lenses, because the fistula into the eye is diverted posteriorly, away from the edge of the contact lens, and perhaps reduces the incidence of contact lens–facilitated endophthalmitis. Several series examined the results of drainage implants in the pediatric population.[41,42] Although the short-term success of drainage implants appears less than that using antimetabolite-augmented trabeculectomy in this age group, none of the reported clinical series has followed up for as long as 10 or 20 years, by which time devastating infectious complications might be expected to have taken their toll.

When conventional glaucoma surgery has failed to control IOP, cycloablative procedures such as cyclocryotherapy[43] or laser cyclophotocoagulation[44] may lower the IOP profoundly (Fig. 219-8). Cyclodestructive procedures are painful and in children usually are performed under general anesthesia. A long-acting retrobulbar block of bupivacaine 0.75% can be used to provide pain control for the first 12 hours after surgery. When the greater part of vision is lost and the goal of the procedure is pain control, the block may be combined with retrobulbar alcohol for a longer analgesic effect.

COURSE AND OUTCOMES

Glaucoma in children may be recognized anytime from birth to late childhood. The age of onset appears to have prognostic implications,[2,8] in that a child who has buphthalmos at birth most likely has more significant developmental angle anomalies and is

likely to have secondary damage to the structures of the eye already. It is these children, along with those who have more profound disorganization of the anterior segment (e.g., Peters' anomaly, sclerocornea, microcornea), who require a surgical team approach that involves penetrating keratoplasty, lensectomy, vitrectomy, and drainage implant. Despite aggressive management, most of these eyes achieve only limited, if any, vision.

Happily, the child who has primary infantile glaucoma and who is diagnosed a few months after birth, before dense amblyopia or severe structural damage to the cornea or optic nerve has occurred, may expect a good outcome if the disease is detected and managed promptly. The results of various surgical series of goniotomy and trabeculotomy are reviewed in Chapter 238; in general, IOP is reduced in over 90%.

With goniotomy and trabeculotomy as the primary management for infantile glaucoma, and trabeculectomy and drainage implant surgery available for more intractable cases, the surgeon who treats the child affected by glaucoma has many effective options for the management of a disease that uniformly resulted in blindness only 50 years ago. However, the goal of glaucoma management is more than the achievement of normal IOP—it is the achievement of normal visual function. The child shown in Figures 219-2 and 219-4 illustrates this clearly. Despite timely and successful surgical intervention and aggressive amblyopia management, this child has decreased vision in one eye because of amblyopia and will enter adulthood with decreased binocularity. Nonetheless, at present this represents an excellent result and with earlier diagnosis through a better knowledge of the molecular biology of this disorder, results are likely to be even better in the coming decades.

REFERENCES

1. Kwitko ML. Glaucoma in infants and children. New York: Appleton-Century-Crofts; 1973:651.
2. Walton DS. Primary congenital open angle glaucoma: a study of the anterior segment abnormalities. Trans Am Ophthalmol Soc. 1979;77:746–68.
3. McGinnity FG, Page AB, Bryars JH. Primary congenital glaucoma: twenty years experience. Ir J Med Sci. 1987;156(12):364–5.
4. Debnath SC, Teichmann KD, Salamah K. Trabeculectomy versus trabeculotomy in congenital glaucoma. Br J Ophthalmol. 1989;73(8):608–11.
5. Gencik A. Epidemiology and genetics of primary congenital glaucoma in Slovakia. Description of a form of primary congenital glaucoma in gypsies with autosomal-recessive inheritance and complete penetrance. Dev Ophthalmol. 1989;16:76–115.
6. Moller PM. Goniotomy and congenital glaucoma. Acta Ophthalmol (Copenh). 1977;55(3):436–42.
7. Shaffer RN. Genetics and the congenital glaucomas. Am J Ophthalmol. 1965; 60(6):981–94.
8. deLuise VP, Anderson DR. Primary infantile glaucoma (congenital glaucoma). Surv Ophthalmol. 1983;28(1):1–19.
9. Stoilov I, Akarsu AN, Alozie I, et al. Sequence analysis and homology modeling suggest that primary congenital glaucoma on 2p21 results from mutations disrupting either the hinge region or the conserved core structures of cytochrome P4501B1. Am J Hum Genet. 1998;62(3):573–84.
10. Stoilov I, Akarsu AN, Sarfarazi M. Identification of three different truncating mutations in cytochrome P4501B1 (CYP1B1) as the principal cause of primary congenital glaucoma (buphthalmos) in families linked to the GLC3A locus on chromosome 2p21. Hum Mol Genet. 1997;6(4):641–7.
11. Sarfarazi M, Akarsu AN, Hossain A, et al. Assignment of a locus (GLC3A) for primary congenital glaucoma (buphthalmos) to 2p21 and evidence for genetic heterogeneity. Genomics. 1995;30(2):171–7.
12. Rudolph AM, Hoffman JIE, Rudolph CD. Rudolph's pediatrics, 20th ed. Stamford, Conn: Appleton & Lange; 1996:xxxvi, 2337.
13. Mills MD, Robb RM. Glaucoma following childhood cataract surgery. J Pediatr Ophthalmol Strabismus. 1994;31(6):355–60; discussion 61.
14. Simon JW, Mehta N, Simmons ST, et al. Glaucoma after pediatric lensectomy/vitrectomy. Ophthalmology. 1991;98(5):670–4.
15. Barkan O. Glaucoma. Classification, causes and surgical control. Am J Ophthalmol. 1938;21(10):1099–114.
16. Sampaolesi R, Argento C. Scanning electron microscopy of the trabecular meshwork in normal and glaucomatous eyes. Invest Ophthalmol Vis Sci. 1977;16(4):302–14.
17. Waring GO, Rodrigues MM, Laibson PR. Anterior chamber cleavage syndrome. A stepladder classification. Surv Ophthalmol. 1975;20(1):3–27.
18. Walton DS. Aniridic glaucoma: the results of gonio-surgery to prevent and treat this problem. Trans Am Ophthalmol Soc. 1986;84:59–70.
19. Tugal-Tutkun I, Havrlikova K, Power WJ, Foster CS. Changing patterns in uveitis of childhood. Ophthalmology. 1996;103(3):375–83.
20. Tseng SS, Keys MP. Battered child syndrome simulating congenital glaucoma. Arch Ophthalmol. 1976;94(5):839–40.
21. Harley RD, Romayananda N, Chan GH. Juvenile xanthogranuloma. J Pediatr Ophthalmol Strabismus. 1982;19(1):33–9.
22. Walton DS. Pediatric aphakic glaucoma: a study of 65 patients. Trans Am Ophthalmol Soc. 1995;93:403–13; discussion 13–20.

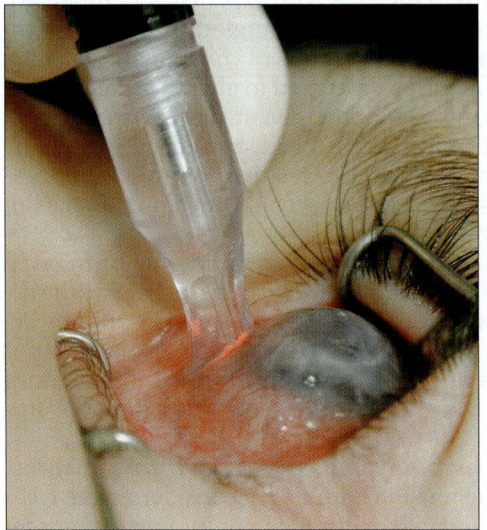

FIG. 219-8 ■ Diode Laser Cyclophotocoagulation. Trans-scleral application of laser energy to the ciliary body of an eye with Peters' anomaly following numerous glaucoma and corneal transplant procedures. In such disrupted eyes it is beneficial to identify the ciliary body by transillumination to better aim the laser.

23. Parks MM, Johnson DA, Reed GW. Long-term visual results and complications in children with aphakia. A function of cataract type. Ophthalmology. 1993;100(6): 826–40; discussion 40–1.
24. al-Umran KU, Pandolfi MF. Corneal diameter in premature infants [see comments]. Br J Ophthalmol. 1992;76(5):292–3.
25. Kiskis AA, Markowitz SN, Morin JD. Corneal diameter and axial length in congenital glaucoma. Can J Ophthalmol. 1985;20(3):93–7.
26. Haab O. Atlas der Äusseren Erkrankungen des Auges: nebst Grundriss ihrer Pathologie und Therapie. München: JF Lehmann,; 1899:x, 228, 39 leaves of plates.
27. Quigley HA. Childhood glaucoma: results with trabeculotomy and study of reversible cupping. Ophthalmology. 1982;89(3):219–26.
28. Shaffer RN, Hetherington J Jr. The glaucomatous disc in infants. A suggested hypothesis for disc cupping. Trans Am Acad Ophthalmol Otolaryngol. 1969;73(5): 923–35.
29. Richardson KT, Shaffer RN. Optic-nerve cupping in congenital glaucoma. Am J Ophthalmol. 1966;62(3):507–9.
30. Ritch R, Shields MB, Krupin T. The glaucomas, ed 2. St Louis: Mosby; 1996.
31. Wolf MT, Lorenz B, Winterpacht A, et al. Ten novel mutations found in aniridia. Hum Mutat. 1998;12(5):304–13.
32. Chen TC, Walton DS. Goniosurgery for prevention of aniridic glaucoma. Arch Ophthalmol. 1999;117(9):1144–8.
33. Adachi M, Dickens CJ, Hetherington J Jr, et al. Clinical experience of trabeculotomy for the surgical treatment of aniridic glaucoma. Ophthalmology. 1997;104(12):2121–5.
34. Cibis GW, Tripathi RC, Tripathi BJ. Glaucoma in Sturge-Weber syndrome. Ophthalmology. 1984;91(9):1061–71.
35. Olsen KE, Huang AS, Wright MM. The efficacy of goniotomy/trabeculotomy in early-onset glaucoma associated with the Sturge-Weber syndrome. J AAPOS. 1998;2(6):365–8.
36. Mandal AK. Primary combined trabeculotomy-trabeculectomy for early-onset glaucoma in Sturge-Weber syndrome. Ophthalmology. 1999;106(8):1621–7.
37. Mandal AK, Walton DS, John T, Jayagandan A. Mitomycin C–augmented trabeculectomy in refractory congenital glaucoma. Ophthalmology. 1997;104(6): 996–1001; discussion 2–3.
38. Khaw PT. What is the best primary surgical treatment for the infantile glaucomas? [editorial; comment]. Br J Ophthalmol. 1996;80(6):495–6.
39. Greenfield DS, Suner IJ, Miller MP, et al. Endophthalmitis after filtering surgery with mitomycin. Arch Ophthalmol. 1996;114(8):943–9.
40. Higginbotham EJ, Stevens RK, Musch DC, et al. Bleb-related endophthalmitis after trabeculectomy with mitomycin C. Ophthalmology. 1996;103(4):650–6.
41. Donahue SP, Keech RV, Munden P, Scott WE. Baerveldt implant surgery in the treatment of advanced childhood glaucoma. J AAPOS. 1997;1(1):41–5.
42. Netland PA, Walton DS. Glaucoma drainage implants in pediatric patients. Ophthalmic Surg. 1993;24(11):723–9.
43. al Faran MF, Tomey KF, al Mutlaq FA. Cyclocryotherapy in selected cases of congenital glaucoma. Ophthalmic Surg. 1990;21(11):794–8.
44. Kirwan JF, Shah P, Khaw PT. Diode laser cyclophotocoagulation: role in the management of refractory pediatric glaucomas. Ophthalmology. 2002;109(2):316–23.

220 Primary Open-Angle Glaucoma

RAYMOND ZIMMERMAN • DARIN SAKIYALAK • THEODORE KRUPIN • LISA F. ROSENBERG

DEFINITION
- A chronic, bilateral, often asymmetrical disease in adults, featuring acquired loss of optic nerve fibers and abnormality in the visual field with an open anterior chamber angle.

KEY FEATURES
- Progressive death of retinal ganglion cells.
- Thinning of the neuroretinal rim.
- Visual field loss.

ASSOCIATED FEATURES
- Elevated intraocular pressure, over 21mmHg (2.8kPa).

INTRODUCTION

A characteristic pattern of optic nerve and visual field damage defines glaucoma. The collection of conditions called glaucoma is categorized into open- or closed-angle forms, and is divided further into primary and secondary forms. Although separation into open- and closed-angle and congenital types is fundamental for appropriate clinical management, division into primary and secondary levels is arbitrary. All kinds of glaucoma are actually an end stage or secondary to some abnormal inciting event(s). As such, glaucoma is a final common pathway of many disorders that affect the eye.

Primary open-angle glaucoma (POAG) is a chronic, bilateral, and often asymmetrical disease in adults in whom acquired loss of optic nerve fibers and abnormality in the visual field occurs with an open anterior chamber angle of normal appearance, and an intraocular pressure (IOP) often over 21mmHg (2.8kPa). A definitive pathophysiological description of the processes that cause death of retinal ganglion cells by apoptosis (a form of cell suicide)[1] still needs to be established. An alternative classification of glaucoma takes into account the stages of the disease process and is more amenable to diagnostic and therapeutic advances in cellular and molecular biology, genetics, and optic nerve regeneration.[2] In this scheme, an unknown precipitating event (stage 1) results in obstruction of aqueous outflow (stage 2) and abnormal IOP (stage 3), which causes death to retinal ganglion cells and cupping of the optic nerve (stage 4) and, finally, loss of vision (stage 5). *Idiopathic* open-angle glaucoma is a better term than POAG, which ultimately has one or several causes. In the same vein, the term *secondary* is replaced according to the systemic or ocular condition associated with the glaucoma.

EPIDEMIOLOGY AND PATHOGENESIS
Review of Risk Factors for Primary Open-Angle Glaucoma

A risk factor represents an inherited characteristic, environmental exposure, or aspect of personal behavior that influences the probability that an individual develops a given condition. It is important to differentiate causal risk factors from associated, or noncausal, risk factors. Some of the risk factors that predict glaucoma are both causal and changeable (e.g., IOP) and, therefore, lend themselves to intervention. On the other hand, epidemiological data may demonstrate a strong association between a factor and disease and, thus, serve as an inference related to risk. Although statistically this is calculated as a risk factor, it clearly is not causal. Other risk factors for POAG (e.g., race, age, family history) are not subject to change but may still influence risk and are, therefore, useful in the identification of individuals for whom close ophthalmic supervision is indicated. The distinction between causal and noncausal factors is important to understand the disease process (diagnosis and pathogenesis) and to plan management.

Five-year findings of the Ocular Hypertensive Treatment Study (OHTS)[3,4] shed important evidence-based data on risk factors for POAG. This prospective, randomized, multicenter clinical trial evaluated the safety and efficacy of topical IOP-lowering medications in preventing or delaying the onset of visual field loss or optic nerve damage in patients with ocular hypertension at moderate risk of developing POAG.

Intraocular Pressure

After Leydhecker *et al.*[5] characterized IOP in 20,000 presumably normal eyes using Schiøtz tonometry, IOP became the defining parameter of glaucoma; they measured a mean ($\pm$SD) IOP of 15.5 ± 2.6mmHg (2.1 ± 0.3kPa). Using a gaussian distribution, Leydhecker *et al.* declared that eyes having IOP of 20.5mmHg (2.7kPa; two standard deviations above the mean) are highly suspect for glaucoma, and those having IOP 24mmHg or more ($\geq$3.2kPa; three standard deviations above the mean) must have the disease. Although subsequent population-based studies using more reliable tonometric techniques have confirmed these values, IOP does not follow a gaussian distribution—it is skewed toward higher pressure.[6,7] Therefore, statistically, values beyond two standard deviations of the mean do not necessarily imply abnormality.

Clinically, the contribution of IOP to the development and management of glaucoma is best considered a continuum. The division between health and disease cannot be based solely on IOP, as exemplified by the debate as to whether the terms *low-pressure* or *normal-tension glaucoma* (glaucomatous nerve damage despite pressures <21mmHg [<2.8kPa]) and ocular hypertension (glaucoma suspect; pressure >21mmHg [>2.8kPa] without optic nerve or visual field damage) are separate entities or represent opposite poles of a disease spectrum in which IOP plays an important role and other factors contribute to the pathogenesis. The important feature of glaucomatous damage in this context lies in the individual susceptibility of the retinal ganglion cell or optic nerve head to IOP-related damage. Variation occurs in the degree of harm caused by a given IOP level, as well as variation in the level of IOP that is tolerated without harm. In any case, raised IOP is the most important risk factor, but it is not the disease per se.

The causal role of IOP in optic nerve damage is evidenced by experimental production of high pressure in primates that results in glaucomatous damage.[8] Among population-based studies, the prevalence of POAG increases with increasing IOP.[9-11] That IOP level and glaucoma development follows a dose–response pattern is indicated in cross-sectional studies; individuals who have pressures of 15–20mmHg (2.0–2.7kPa) have a low prevalence of nerve damage,[12] whereas the prevalence of damage is higher among individuals who have pressures of 25–30mmHg (3.3–4.0kPa).[13,14]

Central Corneal Thickness

The applanation tonometer described by Goldmann and Schmidt[15] assumes a central corneal thickness (CCT) of 500μm. Although they recognized that CCT would influence applanation readings, they believed that variations in CCT occurred rarely in the absence of corneal diseases. However, it has become apparent that CCT in clinically normal individuals is more variable than Goldmann and Schmidt recognized. Many patients with ocular hypertension have little more than thickened corneas, resulting in erroneous elevated IOP readings. In the OHTS, 24% of subjects had CCT greater than 600μm.[16] In this study, subjects with a CCT of 555μm or less had a threefold greater risk of developing POAG than participants with a CCT over 588μm.[4] CCT may be a valuable test in assessing patients with elevated IOP.

Optic Nerve

An enlarged cup (≥0.5 cup-to-disc ratio) on initial optic nerve examination is suspicious either for the presence of glaucoma or for a greater risk for the development of glaucoma.[4,10,17,18] Acquired, progressive thinning of the neuroretinal rim (or progressive enlargement of the cup) is the essence of POAG (Box 220-1). An enlarged cup may represent a normal physiological variant and, as such, contains the normal number of nerve fibers, so the patient may not be at increased risk for glaucoma. Jonas[19] has reported on the characteristic configuration of the neural rim in normal eyes The width of the rim is greatest in the inferior quadrant, followed by the superior, nasal, and temporal quadrants. This relationship may be remembered using the mnemonic ISN'T (inferior, superior, nasal, and temporal quadrants), and this anatomy is largely independent of disc size, cup size, cup-to-disc ratio, or neural rim area. Alternatively, an enlarged cup may be inherently more susceptible to glaucomatous damage by virtue of its anatomy (e.g., features of the lamina cribrosa). Also, an enlarged cup may be damaged already, and if tests of sufficient sensitivity could reveal a functional abnormality, glaucoma could be diagnosable. It is impossible to differentiate which is the case in a given individual at a given time, so patients who have "suspicious" discs must be observed closely (photographs of the optic nerve or computerized analysis of the optic nerve or retinal nerve fiber layer) for the development of clinically detectable glaucoma damage.

Importance of stereoscopic optic disc photographs was confirmed in the OHTS study.[3] Photographic glaucomatous progression of the optic disc without the onset of visual field dam-

---

BOX 220-1

Signs That Suggest Acquired Disc Damage

Progressive thinning of neuroretinal rim (most specific)
Vertical elongation of the cup
Notching
Splinter disc margin hemorrhage
Asymmetry between the two cups of ≥20% in discs of equal size
Deep cup (excavation)
Baring of circumlinear vessels
Saucerization of cup
Laminar dots
Nasalization of vessels
Loss of normal striations in nerve fiber layer

---

age was the first POAG end point in 18 of 36 (50.0%) subjects in the medication group (n = 817) and in 51 of 89 (57.3%) subjects in the observation (no therapy) group (n = 819).

Age

The prevalence (number of cases in a given population at a given time) of POAG increases substantially with age.[4,10,17,20-22] The proportion of patients affected by optic disc damage and vision loss rises from approximately 1% in people under 40 years of age to prevalence estimates 3–8 times higher in patients over 70 years of age. One possible explanation for this relationship may be that older people have had elevated IOP for a longer time compared with younger people. Alternatively, the optic nerve may become more susceptible to damage not only from an elevated IOP, but from microvascular perfusion defects, or changes in connective tissue integrity in older compared with younger individuals.

Race

The prevalence of POAG is 3–4 times higher in black than in white populations.[21,23,24] Optic nerve damage tends to occur at least a decade earlier in blacks, is more severe at the time of diagnosis, and is more refractory to medical and surgical management.[25] Higher IOPs, vascular abnormalities of the optic nerve, and optic nerve size are factors proposed to account for the increased risk of development of glaucoma in this group. However, race in the OHTS was statistically not significant as a baseline factor associated with developing POAG.[4] The black population in the OHTS had larger mean baseline vertical cup-to-disc ratio and thinner central corneal measurement compared with other study participants. Adjustment for these factors in the multivariate analysis eliminated race as a statistically significant predictor.

Major differences in POAG exist between Japanese and Western populations. Approximately 75% of Japanese with open-angle glaucoma have IOPs below 21mmHg.[26] This is considerably higher than the 25–30% observed in United States population-based studies.[22] These findings also emphasize the limited utility of IOP as an indicator of glaucomatous disease.

Family History

Familial factors play a role in the underlying susceptibility to POAG.[17,27] The association is stronger if a sibling has glaucoma (odds ratio, 3.69) than if a parent (odds ratio, 2.17) or child (odds ratio, 1.12) has POAG.[28] Family history was not a significant predictor in the OHTS; 42% of all participants reported a positive family history of glaucoma (8.5% of participants who developed glaucoma compared with 7.3% who did not).[4] The risk of a positive family history of POAG does not weigh as heavily as the factors described above.

Genetic factors that influence POAG are complex. Although at least six genes have been identified with POAG, only one genetic locus, (GLC1A) on chromosome 1q that is associated with juvenile-onset open-angle glaucoma, has been reported in patients with adult-onset POAG. A gene that produces the protein myocilin (TIGR) resides within this interval, and myocilin mutations occur in up to 4.6% of patients with adult-onset POAG.[29] Myocilin is expressed in multiple tissues throughout the eye and in many other organs. In the trabecular meshwork, the production of myocilin can be induced by application of topical corticosteroids.[30]

Myopia

Evidence that supports the association between myopia and POAG is derived from the observation of an increased prevalence of myopia among patients with glaucoma compared with the general population.[31,32] It has been postulated, but not confirmed, that the occurrence of elevated IOP in myopic individuals may be an important contribution to the development of glaucoma in this group of patients. Shared alterations in collagen and other components of the extracellular matrix of the optic nerve also may be contributory factors in myopia and POAG. However, in the OHTS, myopia was not predictive of POAG.[4]

Vascular Disease

Abnormalities in vascular function, such as arterial hypertension, diabetes mellitus, and migraine, have been associated with POAG, although the relationships are not well characterized. It seems logical to assume systemic vascular disease has a potential impact on POAG, because compromised microcirculation of the optic disc is a possible mechanism for nerve damage. Migraine seems to be most closely associated with open-angle glaucoma and pressures in the normal range.[33] Nevertheless, the results of retrospective and population-based studies on the relationships of vascular disease and POAG are unclear.[4]

DIFFERENTIAL DIAGNOSIS

Conditions that may masquerade as POAG exhibit a similar optic nerve appearance or characteristic visual field abnormality. Patients who have POAG may demonstrate wide diurnal pressure variation and, unless frequent pressure measurements are obtained at various times during the day, higher pressure levels may not be detected. Such information has an impact on the target pressure level chosen for glaucoma therapy. Careful gonioscopic visualization of the anterior chamber angle differentiates patients who suffer subacute angle-closure glaucoma. The presence of peripheral anterior synechiae, anterior chamber-angle pigment, or blood in Schlemm's canal may point to a diagnosis other than POAG (Box 220-2).

BOX 220-2

Gonioscopic Features*

NORMAL ANTERIOR CHAMBER ANGLE BLOOD VESSELS
Do not cross scleral spur
Do not branch
Have stromal sheath
Travel radially or circumferentially
- Radial iris vessels
- Arterial circle of ciliary body
- Vertical vessels of the anterior ciliary body

SEVEN CAUSES OF PERIPHERAL ANTERIOR SYNECHIAE
Blunt trauma
Penetrating trauma
Primary angle-closure glaucoma
Inflammation
Rubeosis iridis
Posterior pressure on iris–lens diaphragm
Iridocorneoendothelial syndrome or epithelial downgrowth

DIFFERENTIAL DIAGNOSIS OF ANTERIOR CHAMBER ANGLE PIGMENT
Ciliary body tumor
Pigment dispersion or glaucoma
Pseudoexfoliation
Malignant glaucoma
Trauma
Surgery
Inflammation
Hyphema
Angle-closure glaucoma

BLOOD IN SCHLEMM'S CANAL
Artifactual from compression on goniolens
Elevated episcleral venous pressure
Hypotony
Idiopathic uveal effusion syndrome

---

*These help differentiate primary open-angle glaucoma from other forms of glaucoma.

Patients who have glaucomatous appearing optic nerves or visual field defects but normal IOP may have had elevated IOP in the past, but for a finite period. Such scenarios occur in patients who had IOP elevation from long-term corticosteroid use, transient uveitis, or pigmentary glaucoma that subsided with increased pupillary block and decreased pigment liberation.

Certain retinal conditions cause visual field defects that may mimic typical glaucomatous defects. Careful retinal examination reveals retinal detachment, chorioretinitis, arterial or venous branch vascular occlusion, retinoschisis, or retinal photocoagulation scars, as some examples.

Congenital optic nerve conditions and ischemic or compressive optic neuropathies may mimic glaucomatous cupping. Methanol toxicity is a very unusual cause of cupping.[34] A careful history elicits sudden visual loss (ischemic optic neuropathy), headache, neurological signs, or hormonal abnormalities (compressive lesion); discriminating stereoscopic examination of the optic nerve differentiates these entities (e.g., pallor greater than cupping) from glaucomatous optic neuropathy. The diagnosis of POAG must be reevaluated at each visit to eliminate other possible causes for progressive visual field loss and change in the appearance of the optic nerve.

PATHOLOGY

Although the anterior chamber angle appears clinically normal in patients who have POAG, it is dysfunctional. The site of resis-

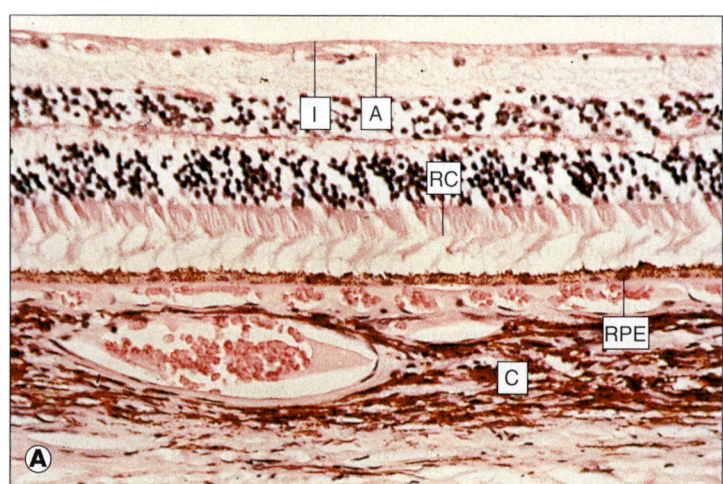

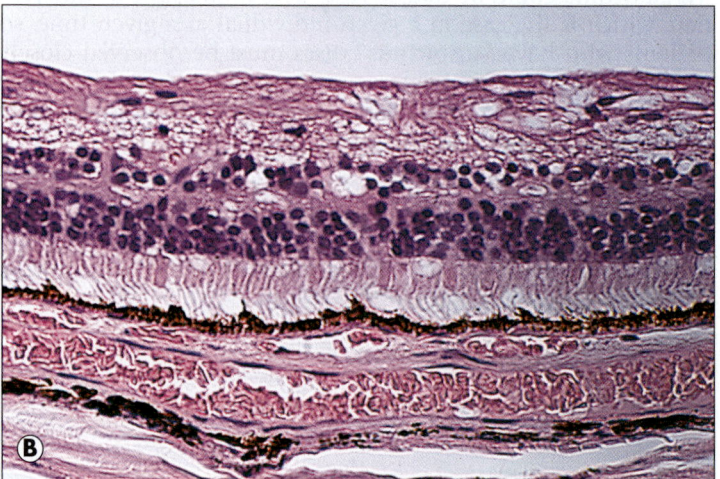

FIG. 220-1 ■ **Retina. A,** Histological section of the nasal retina shows that only an occasional ganglion cell remains, instead of the normally seen continuous single layer. The atrophic inner neural retinal layers are still identifiable, unlike the neural retina following central retinal artery occlusion, where the inner layers appear as a homogeneous scar. *I,* internal limiting membrane; *A,* atrophic nerve fiber and ganglion cell layers; *RC,* rods and cones; *RPE,* retinal pigment epithelium; *C,* choroid. **B,** Another case shows more marked glaucomatous atrophy of the inner layers (compare with the inner nuclear layer in **A**). (**A–B,** From Yanoff M, Fine BS. Ocular pathology, ed 5. St. Louis: Mosby; 2002.)

tance to aqueous humor outflow is postulated to lie in the juxtacanalicular portion of the trabecular meshwork. Several alterations in the meshwork ultrastructure have been described but cannot be differentiated from nonspecific changes observed with normal aging.

Loss of retinal ganglion cells and thinning of the nerve fiber layer occurs, while the outer layers of the retina are preserved for the most part (Fig. 220-1). The optic disc appears excavated because of the extensive loss of nerve fiber substance (Fig. 220-2). The lamina cribrosa is displaced posteriorly.

TREATMENT

The challenge of glaucoma management lies in maintaining low IOP for the life of the patient. Because glaucoma is chronic and often asymptomatic, therapy often demands multiple and expensive medications which must be used frequently and often cause unwanted side effects (see Chapter 233) or surgical remedies which carry risk. Also to be considered in the decision on therapy is the patient's age (life expectancy), physical condition, and social situation, because these impact the high level of compliance required for successful management. Management, therefore, varies among patients but has as its universal goal the greatest potential benefit for preservation of vision at the lowest risk, cost, and inconvenience to the patient.

The incidence of visual field damage is small, even if all risk factors are present, for a patient who at initial examination has no nerve damage and normal visual fields.[10] Most patients with ocular hypertension (glaucoma suspects) do not require IOP-lowering therapy, because the probability of developing POAG (optic nerve damage or visual field loss) has been estimated to be only 0.5–1.0% per year.[35,36] These estimates are probably low, considering the OHTS report that 24% of patients with ocular hypertension have CCT greater than 600μm.[16] This finding underestimates the true conversion to POAG, because many glaucoma suspects with thick CCT have "corrected" IOPs that are within normal range (i.e., misclassified as having ocular hypertension). Cumulative probability of developing POAG in the OHTS was 4.4% in the medication group and 9.5% in the observation group. These probabilities also are higher than prior reports based on the high percentage (approximately 50%) of conversion determined by stereoscopic disc photograph alterations without development of visual field damage. Multivariate analysis of the OHTS identified baseline factors that were predictive of developing POAG as older age, larger vertical or horizontal cup-to-disc ratio, higher IOP, and thinner CCT.

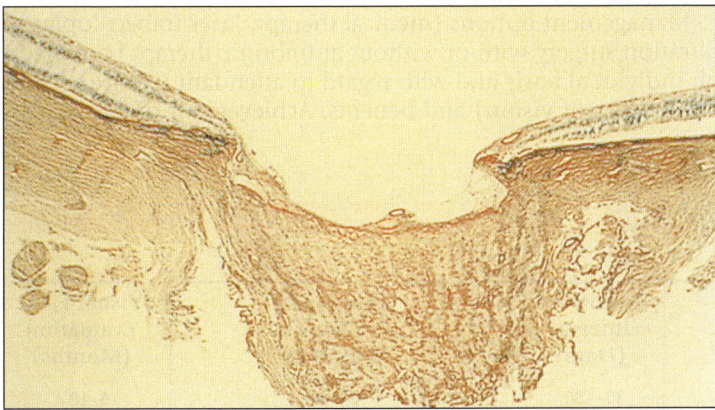

FIG. 220-2 ■ **Glaucoma cupping.** The optic nerve head is deeply cupped. Atrophy of the optic nerve is determined by comparing the diameter of the optic nerve at its internal surface and posteriorly, where it should double in size. Here it is the same because of a loss of axons and myelin, which also causes an increase in size of the subarachnoid space and a proliferation of glial cells, resulting in an increased cellularity of the optic nerve. (From Yanoff M, Fine BS. Ocular pathology, ed 5. St. Louis: Mosby; 2002.)

Therapy, with its attendant cost and potential for side effects, is not justified for all patients with ocular hypertension. In the OHTS, 90.5% of the observation group did not develop glaucomatous optic nerve or visual field changes during the 5 years of study. On the other hand, one report on a small number of eyes has described loss of retinal nerve fibers prior to clinically detectable optic nerve damage or visual field loss, thus advocating the initiation of tolerable glaucoma therapy in patients with ocular hypertension.[37] We are unable to identify with a high level of certainty which combination of risk factors in a given patient with ocular hypertension increases the likelihood that glaucoma damage will develop. Considerations in the decision to treat these patients include useful vision in only one eye, inability to obtain reliable visual field determinations, inadequate visualization of the fundus, other vision-threatening ocular disorders, an IOP consistently higher than 30mmHg, or the patient's request for treatment.

It is difficult to identify accurately early glaucoma changes. Short-wavelength automated perimetry (SWAP; blue-on-yellow perimetry) can detect visual field loss earlier than standard white-on-white perimetry.[38] Additional studies are needed to determine if frequency-doubling technology (FDT) perimetry and computerized analysis of the optic nerve or retinal nerve fiber layer will be additional parameters that prove useful in the early detection of optic nerve damage.[39] The ongoing multicenter OHTS will provide important information on the value of these tests.

The goal of treatment must be individualized for every patient—no specific IOP level avoids visual loss in all patients. Similarly, in the glaucoma suspect, no specific IOP level exists that demands treatment; the level also must be individualized according to other risk factors and the comfort of the ophthalmologist who monitors the patient. For example, a patient who has an IOP as high as 30mmHg (4.0kPa) may be monitored (e.g., visual fields and optic disc stereoscopic photographs or computerized analysis) carefully without glaucoma therapy in the absence of disc damage, visual field loss, or other important risk factors. So long as the physician and patient are comfortable with an established follow-up plan, the patient is spared not only the cost and inconvenience incurred from treatment, but also the psychological impact that may occur when a chronic and potentially blinding disorder is diagnosed.

To detect acquired disc damage is even more of a challenge in high myopia with tilted discs, anomalous optic nerve heads, and symmetrically enlarged (i.e., >0.5 cup-to-disc ratio) cups. Again, in these patients therapy is individualized; generally, it is advised if the patient is young, but an elderly patient may be monitored conservatively without medication.

Results published by the multicenter Early Manifest Glaucoma Trial[40] have confirmed the clinical impression that therapy is indicated when optic nerve or visual field damage has occurred. The goal in such cases is to prevent progressive optic nerve and functional vision loss for the remainder of the patient's lifetime. Management is to lower IOP, the only risk factor amenable to management, to a safer level such that further optic nerve damage is unlikely. The target IOP varies among patients and may also vary within the same patient during the course of the disease. The chosen IOP, in time, may prove to be inadequate such that progressive damage occurs despite the degree of IOP reduction; alternatively, the desired IOP reduction may be achieved, but with the induction of intolerable ocular or systemic effects. Variable amounts of IOP reduction may be required to stabilize similar degrees of optic nerve damage. For example, a young myope who has cupping and visual field loss within or close to fixation and whose highest IOP is in the low 20–22mmHg (2.7–2.9kPa) range may need IOP reduced to 13–15mmHg (1.7–2.0kPa), or lower, to stabilize the condition.

The multicenter Advanced Glaucoma Intervention Study (AGIS) was established to determine whether laser trabeculoplasty or trabeculectomy was the best management in medically uncontrolled open-angle glaucoma.[25,41] Recent AGIS reports have analyzed visual field progression according to the level of IOP maintenance.[42] Patients with an average IOP greater than 17.5mmHg had significantly more field progression than patients with an average IOP less than 14mmHg. Visual field worsening was greater after 7 years than after 2 years following initiation of the study. Finally, eyes with an IOP less than 18mmHg on all study visits had no significant change in visual field defect score, while eyes with this level of pressure control on only 50% of the visits had significant worsening of their visual field. Ten-year study results are similar.

The AGIS study indicates that an IOP greater than 18mmHg is not acceptable in eyes with glaucomatous optic nerve damage. This impacts the concept of target IOP, selection of an IOP range that will halt or slow progressive ocular damage. Selection has utilized a variety of clinical benchmarks, such as the severity of optic nerve damage, the IOP level at which damage occurred, the rapidity with which damage occurred, and the presence of other risk factors. In general, the more advanced the damage, the lower the desired target IOP. The IOP range chosen in each case is somewhat arbitrary and based on clinical experience. A spectrum or range of IOPs exists for a given patient and extends from the ideal pressure, to acceptable pressure, to borderline pressure, and at the furthest end unacceptable pressure. Finally, just as not all patients respond equally to a given anithypertensive therapy, not all disease halts at a given IOP level. The protective effect of lowered IOP is not absolute, and relentless deterioration may continue in some patients despite IOP reduction. It is believed that in these patients additional factors, other than IOP, must play an important role in the disease process.

COURSE AND OUTCOMES

In the long term, the decision as to whether the achieved IOP level is sufficient is based on whether progressive disc and field damage has halted. Findings from stereoscopic examination of the optic nerves with pupil dilatation are compared with baseline stereoscopic photographs every year. Computer analysis of the optic nerve head and retinal nerve fiber layer are additional anatomical measurements that are used to assess stability of the glaucomatous process. Kinetic or static visual field examinations are obtained 2–4 times per year, and IOP measurements are carried out 3–4 times a year. Factors that alter the length and constitution of follow-up interval include severity of disease (more frequent for more severe disease), range of achieved IOP lowering, stability of optic nerve and visual field damage, and duration of glaucoma control (Table 220-1).

Change of the optic nerve or visual field must be verified and correlated with the ocular physical examination. For example, is the new visual field defect present on repeated tests with proper test parameters? Does the change represent progressive glaucomatous cupping? Could the change in disc appearance represent ischemic optic neuropathy? Could the change in field represent a retinovascular insult? If the clinical change indeed represents progressive glaucomatous damage, then more aggressive IOP re-

duction is needed. Another indication for escalation of glaucoma therapy is the return of IOP to a level that previously caused damage. Other indications for adjustment of therapy are noncompliance with the prescribed medication or occurrence of ocular or systemic side effects.

The patient who has advanced glaucoma on initial examination with deeply excavated optic nerves and visual field defects that involve fixation is of particular concern. In such a patient, it is more difficult to recognize further changes in disc or field. A suggested guideline is to set a goal of IOP 50% lower than at diagnosis or an IOP less than 15mmHg (2.0kPa), whichever is less. If the IOP is decreased to this level, the patient's course is followed carefully. If this IOP goal cannot be achieved with medical or laser therapy, filtration surgery is recommended.

Progressive optic disc damage may be impossible to detect in eyes in which extensive disc damage has resulted in a nerve that has a completely excavated appearance. The best assessment of the nerve is obtained using stereophotography. Computerized optic disc analysis may provide different useful measures of the optic nerve (see Chapter 216). Visual fields, although limited, may be more important in the long-term assessment of such patients.

The subjective nature of the visual field examination limits its usefulness in uncooperative patients. Moreover, it is difficult to monitor for progressive deterioration when extensive visual field loss approaches or involves fixation or takes the form of a severely contracted island of vision (5–10°). It is helpful to enlarge the standard automated test object to size V, to make sure the patient's pupil is at least 3mm in diameter, and to utilize the central 10° field program in automated perimeters (see Chapter 214). Goldmann kinetic perimetry is frequently the best method to follow visual fields in these patients. Sometimes IOP and visual acuity are the only parameters to follow in patients who have extensive optic nerve and visual field abnormalities.

Clinical monitoring has several limitations. Diurnal IOP variations are much greater in patients who have POAG, compared with those in the normal population. Particularly in patients who demonstrate progressive damage at seemingly normal IOPs, attempts must be made to schedule IOP measurement at different times of the day, toward the end of a dosage interval, or just before instillation of the next medication dose to characterize a profile of pressure fluctuation as a possible factor in suboptimal glaucoma control.

Poor medication compliance is common in a large proportion of patients, a particularly significant phenomenon given the many medical options now available to manage glaucoma. Consideration of the lifestyle implication of multiple medications is critical. It is essential to prescribe (and that the patient use) only those drugs proved to lower eye pressure effectively in an individual patient. One-eyed therapeutic trials are helpful in this regard (see Chapter 233).

Management options (medical therapy, laser trabeculoplasty, filtration surgery with or without antifibrotic therapy) are made on individual basis and with regard to attendant risks (e.g., side effects, loss of vision) and benefits. Achievement of adequately

TABLE 220-1

RECOMMENDED GUIDELINES FOR FOLLOW-UP

Target Intraocular Pressure Achieved	Progression of Damage	Duration of Control (Months)	Follow-up Interval (Days)	Optic Nerve Evaluation (Months)	Visual Field Evaluation (Months)
Yes	No	<6	30–180	6–12	6–18
Yes	No	>6	90–365	6–18	6–24
Yes	Yes	Not applicable	7–90	3–12	2–6
No	No	Not applicable	7–90	3–12	2–6
No	Yes	Not applicable	1–30	3–12	2–6

Adapted from American Academy of Ophthalmology: Primary open-angle glaucoma preferred practice pattern. San Francisco: American Academy of Ophthalmology; 1996.

lowered IOP to prevent further glaucomatous damage serves most patients well. The proof of glaucoma control can be obtained retrospectively only, by examination of the optic nerve and visual field.

REFERENCES

1. Kerrigan LA, Zack DJ, Quiglet HA, et al. TUNEL-positive ganglion cells in human primary open-angle glaucoma. Arch Ophthalmol. 1997;115:1031-5.
2. Shields MB, Ritch R, Krupin T. Classification of the glaucomas. In: Ritch R, Shields MB, Krupin T, eds. The glaucomas. St Louis: Mosby–Year Book; 1996:717-25.
3. Kass MA, Heuer DK, Higginbotham EJ, et al. The Ocular Hypertension Treatment Study: a randomized trial determines that topical ocular hypotensive medication delays or prevents the onset of primary open-angle glaucoma. Arch Ophthalmol. 2002;120:701-13.
4. Gordon MO, Beiser JA, Brandt JD, et al. The Ocular Hypertensive Treatment Study: baseline factors that predict the onset of primary open-angle glaucoma. Arch Ophthalmol. 2002;120:714-20.
5. Leydhecker W, Akiyama K, Neumann HG. Der intraokulare Druck gesunder menschlicher Augen. Klin Monatsbl Augenheilkd 1958;133:662-70.
6. Armaly MF. On the distribution of applanation pressure. I. Statistical features and the effect of age, sex, and family history of glaucoma. Arch Ophthalmol. 1965;73:11-8.
7. Hollows FC, Graham PA. Intraocular pressure, glaucoma, and glaucoma suspects in a defined population. Br J Ophthalmol. 1966;50:570-86.
8. Quigley HA, Addicks EM, Green RW. Chronic experimental glaucoma in primates. II. Effect of extended intraocular pressure elevation on optic nerve head and axonal transport. Invest Ophthalmol Vis Sci. 1980;19:137-52.
9. Pohjanpelto PEJ, Palva J. Ocular hypertension and glaucomatous optic nerve damage. Acta Ophthalmol (Copenh). 1974;52:194-200.
10. Armaly MF, Krueger MF, Maunder L, et al. Biostatistical analysis of the collaborative glaucoma study. I. Summary of the risk factors for glaucomatous visual-field defects. Arch Ophthalmol. 1980;98:2163-71.
11. Sommer A, Tielsch JM, Katz J, et al. Relationship between intraocular pressure and primary open-angle glaucoma among white and black Americans. The Baltimore Eye Survey. Arch Ophthalmol. 1991;109:1090-5.
12. Cartwright MJ, Anderson DR. Correlation of asymmetric damage with asymmetric intraocular pressure in normal-tension glaucoma (low-tension glaucoma). Arch Ophthalmol. 1988;106:898-900.
13. Anderson DR. The management of elevated intraocular pressure with normal optic discs and visual fields. I. Therapeutic approach based on high risk factors. Surv Ophthalmol. 1977;21:479-89.
14. Sommer AI. Intraocular pressure and glaucoma. Am J Ophthalmol. 1989;107:186-8.
15. Goldmann H, Schmidt T. Über Applanationstonometrie. Ophthalmologica. 1957;134:221-42.
16. Brandt JD, Beiser JA, Kass MA, et al. Central corneal thickness in the Ocular Hypertensive Treatment Study (OHTS). Ophthalmology. 2001;108:1779-88.
17. Hart WM Jr, Yablonski M, Kass MA, et al. Multivariate analysis of the risk of glaucomatous visual field loss. Arch Ophthalmol. 1979;97:1455-8.
18. Yablonski ME, Zimmerman TJ, Kass MA, et al. Prognostic significance of optic disc cupping in ocular hypertensive patients. Am J Ophthalmol. 1980;89:585-92.
19. Jonas JB. Biomorphometrie des nervus opticus. Stuttgart: Ferdinand Enke Verlag; 1989.
20. Kass MA, Hart WM Jr, Gordon M, et al. Risk factors favoring the development of glaucomatous visual field loss in ocular hypertension. Surv Ophthalmol. 1980;25:155-62.
21. Tielsch JM, Sommer A, Katz J, et al. Racial variations in the prevalence of primary open-angle glaucoma: the Baltimore Eye Survey. JAMA. 1991;266:369-74.
22. Klein BE, Klein R, Sponsel WE, et al. Prevalence of glaucoma: the Beaver Dam Eye Study. Ophthalmology. 1992;99:1499-504.
23. Hiller R, Kahn HA. Blindness from glaucoma. Am J Ophthalmol. 1975;80:62-9.
24. Sommer A, Tielsch JM, Katz J, et al. The nature and causes of blindness in East Baltimore: a population-based survey. N Engl J Med. 1991;325:1412-7.
25. The AGIS investigators. The Advanced Glaucoma Intervention Study (AGIS), 4, comparison of treatment outcomes within race: seven-year results. Ophthalmology. 1998;105:1146-64.
26. Shiose Y, Kitazawa Y, Tsukahara S, et al. Epidemiology of glaucoma in Japan—a nationwide glaucoma survey. Jpn J Ophthalmol. 1991;35:133-55.
27. Armaly MF, Monstavicius BF, Sayegh RE. Ocular pressure and aqueous outflow facility in siblings. Arch Ophthalmol. 1968;80:354-60.
28. Tielsch JM, Sommer A, Quigley HA, et al. Family history and risk of open angle glaucoma: the Baltimore Eye Survey. Arch Ophthalmol. 1994;112:69-73.
29. Stone EM, Fingert JH, Alward WLM, et al. Identification of a gene that causes primary open angle glaucoma. Science. 1997;275:668-70.
30. Nuguyen TD, Chen P, Huang WD, et al. Gene structure and properties of TIGR, an olfactomedin-related glycoprotein cloned from glucocorticoid-induced trabecular meshwork cells. J Biol Chem. 1998;273:6341-50.
31. Daubs JG, Crick RP. Effect of refractive error on the risk of ocular hypertension and open angle glaucoma. Trans Ophthalmol Soc U K. 1981;101:121-6.
32. Perkins ES, Phelps CD. Open angle glaucoma, ocular hypertension, low-tension glaucoma, and refraction. Arch Ophthalmol. 1982;100:1464-7.
33. Schulzer M, Drance SM, Carter CJ, et al. Biostatistical evidence for two distinct chronic open angle glaucoma populations. Br J Ophthalmol. 1990;74:196-200.
34. Benton C, Calhoun F. The ocular effects of methyl alcohol poisoning. Am J Ophthalmol. 1953;36:1677-85.
35. Perkins ES. The Bedford glaucoma survey. I. Long-term follow-up of borderline cases. Br J Ophthalmol. 1973;57:179-85.
36. Kass MA. When to treat ocular hypertension. Surv Ophthalmol. 1983;28:229-32.
37. Quigley HA, Addicks EM, Green WR. Optic nerve damage in human glaucoma. III. Quantitative correlation of nerve fiber loss and visual field defect in glaucoma, ischemic neuropathy, papilledema, and toxic neuropathy. Arch Ophthalmol. 1982;100:135-46.
38. Sample PA, Taylor JD, Martinez GA, et al. Short-wavelength color visual fields in glaucoma suspects at risk. Am J Ophthalmol. 1993;115:225-33.
39. Bowd C, Zangwill LM, Berry CC, et al. Detecting early glaucoma by assessment of retinal nerve fiber layer thickness and visual function. Invest Ophthalmol Vis Sci. 2001;42:1993-2003.
40. Heijl A, Leske MC, Bengtsson B, et al. Reduction of intraocular pressure and glaucoma progression: results from the Early Manifest Glaucoma Trial. Arch Ophthalmol. 2002;120:1268-79.
41. The AGIS investigators. The Advanced Glaucoma Intervention Study (AGIS), 1: study design and methods and baseline characteristics of study patients. Control Clin Trials. 1994;15:299-325.
42. The AGIS investigators. The advanced glaucoma intervention study (AGIS): 7. The relationship between control of intraocular pressure and visual field deterioration. Am J Ophthalmol. 2000;130:429-40.

CHAPTER
221

Normal-Tension Glaucoma

ROGER HITCHINGS

DEFINITION

- Variety of primary open-angle glaucoma that features an intraocular pressure within the normal range.

KEY FEATURES

- Intraocular pressure within the normal range.
- Progressive glaucomatous cupping.
- Retinal nerve fiber type of visual field loss.
- Open angles on gonioscopic examination.
- No history of eye disease with raised intraocular pressure.

ASSOCIATED FEATURES

- Peripheral vasospasm, as in Raynaud's phenomenon.
- Migraine.
- Optic disc hemorrhage.

INTRODUCTION

Chronic open-angle glaucoma typically is associated with an elevated intraocular pressure (IOP). Total population surveys show that 10–30% of patients newly diagnosed with glaucoma have IOPs that are and remain normal. Although the relative risk for the development of glaucomatous optic neuropathy increases with an increase in IOP, the numerical majority of normotensive individuals ensures that the small percentage who have open-angle glaucoma constitute a significant proportion of the whole open-angle glaucoma population. The traditional therapy for primary open-angle glaucoma is to lower IOP to within the normal range, but this approach becomes more difficult when the initial IOP is "normal."

EPIDEMIOLOGY AND PATHOGENESIS

Total population surveys in Europe, North America, and Australia reveal open-angle glaucoma with normal IOPs in 15–25% of the population surveyed. Only a small proportion of these patients have elevated IOPs on repeat testing. Patients with normal-tension glaucoma (NTG) constitute a significant proportion of patients with glaucoma in any clinic. Interestingly, in Japan, where the upper limit of normal IOP is approximately 18mmHg (2.4kPa), 50–60% of patients affected by open-angle glaucoma have baseline IOPs below this level.

The pathogenesis of the condition remains unclear. Progressive optic neuropathy with a normal IOP suggests an underlying vascular insufficiency. The association with peripheral vasospasm, migraine, and recurrent optic disc hemorrhages supports this hypothesis. The association with myopia and peripapillary atrophy also indicates a deficiency in the short, posterior ciliary circulation.[1,2] For some patients (and normal individuals) in whom ambulatory blood pressure has been monitored, the nocturnal blood pressure falls dramatically (80/40mmHg [10.6/5.3kPa] being not uncommon).[1,3] Such nocturnal "dips" may lower pulse pressure at the optic disc if no commensurate fall in IOP occurs.

The most effective management has been to lower IOP. Color Doppler imaging has demonstrated an increase in blood velocity in the ophthalmic artery after filtration surgery,[4] which suggests a mechanical hypothesis in which the IOP is "too high for the eye," and the optic nerve is less able to withstand an IOP in the normal range. The mechanical support given by the lamina cribrosa may be insufficient, and the quality (type) of the collagen may be deficient.[5,6] Finally, and speculatively, the lamina cribrosa may have an abnormal pressure gradient across it, not because the IOP is too high, but because the intracranial pressure is lower than normal.

OCULAR MANIFESTATIONS

No characteristic features exist, other than level of IOP that consistently differentiates high-tension glaucoma from NTG. The appearance of the optic disc and the visual field defect can be identical. However, some differences can occur. Patients who have NTG are, on average, 10 years older than those who have high-tension glaucoma, and their optic discs are more likely to show focal notching and optic disc hemorrhages. Optic discs in patients who have NTG have been categorized into different subtypes based on appearance—myopic, focal ischemic, senile sclerotic, and so on (Fig. 221-1).[7,8] Such descriptions are not, as yet, indicative of different causes or clinical courses. The visual field is more likely to show defects close to fixation.[8] In addition, the outflow resistance may be normal or extremely high, and the rate of aqueous flow may be normal or extremely low.[9] Familial tendency occurs, and it has been reported that women are affected twice as frequently as men.[10] There is evidence to suggest that the left eye is 2.5 times more likely to be affected first although, with increasing age, NTG tends to become a bilateral disease. The IOP is usually slightly higher in the more severely affected eye, although the difference may only be 1–2mmHg (0.1–0.3kPa).[11,12]

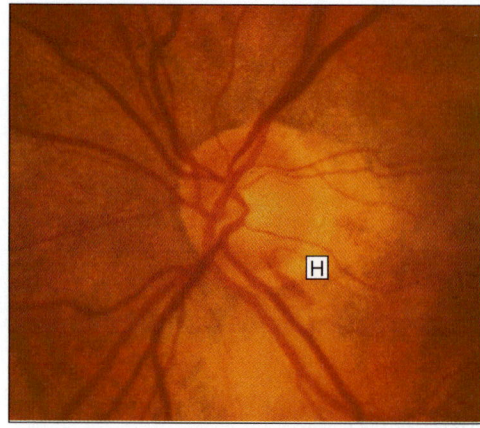

FIG. 221-1 ■ Optic disc of a patient who has normal-tension glaucoma. Note disc hemorrhage (H).

Long-term follow-up suggests that, although most patients maintain the same IOP over many years, approximately 8% show a trend toward higher IOPs. In such eyes the IOP may rise above the upper limit of normal, in which case the patient would be considered to have *high-tension glaucoma*.[13] Repeated "splinter" hemorrhages at the optic disc are common, and such eyes are likely to show progressive visual field loss.

Two reviews of the untreated condition exist. Both suggest that over a period of 4–5 years, a significant minority will not show demonstrable progression.[14] This needs to be remembered when considering management options for the elderly patient.

DIAGNOSIS

Confirmation of the diagnosis requires:
- Repetitive IOP measurements to rule out occult hypertension
- Confirmation of glaucomatous cupping, rather than a "suspicious" appearance to the optic disc
- Exclusion of other causes of optic disc changes and previous ocular hypertension
- Confirmation that the visual field defect is of the retinal nerve fiber layer type and corresponds with the location of changes at the neuroretinal rim

The following are helpful in the identification of a causative vascular factor:
- Measure the response of the nail fold capillaries to cold
- Monitor ambulatory blood pressure to identify nocturnal dips
- Obtain color Doppler imaging of the common carotid artery to establish the presence of lumen reduction.

Any retro-ocular lesion must be ruled out, also. A brain scan and other neurological investigation is indicated if any disparity arises between the optic disc appearance and the visual field defect. In glaucoma, a close association is found between glaucomatous cupping and the visual field defect. Atrophy greater than the field loss suggests a previous anterior ischemic optic neuropathy. Visual field defects that respect a vertical meridian and central (rather than paracentral and arcuate) field defects indicate the need for neurological investigation.

DIFFERENTIAL DIAGNOSIS

The differential diagnosis of NTG is summarized in Box 221-1.

High-tension, primary open-angle glaucoma that has episodic normal IOP is a theoretical concept in which wide diurnal fluctuations "hide" elevated IOPs that induce damage.

In secondary open-angle glaucoma, a normal IOP is present after a previous hypertensive episode sufficient to produce glaucomatous cupping (e.g., corticosteroid-induced glaucoma, hypertensive uveitis). Any young patient who has glaucoma and a history of external eye disease or contact lens wear must be questioned closely about topical corticosteroid medication use.

In non-glaucomatous optic neuropathy, the IOP, visual field, and the age of the patient are similar to those in the patient with glaucoma. The optic disc does not show glaucomatous cupping, but rather a flat optic atrophy in which the area of atrophy exceeds the extent of the visual field defect (disc–field disparity). When extensive neuronal loss has occurred, the optic disc may develop a massive enlargement of the optic cup with pallor of the remaining rim. The condition does not progress.

Other lesions that affect the visual pathways include lesions of the optic chiasm and visual pathways, back to the occipital cortex, which produce visual field defects that respect the vertical meridian. In time, such lesions also produce optic atrophy without glaucomatous cupping.

SYSTEMIC ASSOCIATIONS

No systemic diseases are associated with NTG. However, both the female-to-male ratio and the occasional familial nature of the disease suggest a systemic component. More speculatively, the left eye over right eye also suggests a systemic component. The association with peripheral and perhaps central (ocular) vasospasm, migraine, and Raynaud's phenomenon suggests a vascular predisposition to the condition.[15,16]

TREATMENT

Treatment is indicated for patients with progressive disease. Few patients become legally blind from this disease. Many patients are elderly at diagnosis and have a sufficiently slow rate of change that, even without treatment, clinically significant loss of vision does not occur. Significant visual loss may cause social restriction, such as the loss of a driving license. Trend or event analysis that uses commercially available software will identify progression. Cluster or point-wise analysis is more likely to identify progression than analyses that rely on the identification of a global change. Care must be taken to differentiate between long-term fluctuations and true change before any therapeutic decisions are made. Management is directed toward the implementation of a lower IOP or to the correction of reversible circulatory deficiencies at the optic nerve or both.

Lower Intraocular Pressure

Studies suggest that a reduction in IOP may exert a beneficial effect on the course of the disease.[17–20] A 25–30% fall is required, best achieved by the perioperative use of 5-fluorouracil. If surgery does not achieve this 25–30% fall, the rate of change is likely to remain unaltered.[21] Current medical therapy may not maintain this pressure reduction for the lifetime of the patient, although the recent introduction of latanoprost may help a proportion of these patients.[22]

Reversal of Circulatory Deficiencies at the Optic Nerve Head

VASOSPASM. Central vasospasm may be indicated by an abnormal (vasoconstrictive) response of finger circulation to cold, which may be reversed by calcium channel blockers and carbon dioxide rebreathing.[23–25] Theoretically, a carbonic anhydrase inhibitor also should have a beneficial effect.

NOCTURNAL HYPOTENSION. Patients who take drugs to lower blood pressure and some patients who have NTG exhibit an excessive fall in systolic and diastolic blood pressures while asleep (dips). Such changes may reduce ocular perfusion pressure unless the IOP also falls. All patients must be questioned about systemic hypotensive (antihypertensive) medication, and any patient who uses such medication must be checked for such falls in blood pressure.

CAROTID INSUFFICIENCY. Patients who have asymmetrical NTG may show significant (>50%) lumen reduction in the common carotid artery, which results in reduction of turbulence and reduction of volume flow. The end arteries of the ophthalmic artery (and particularly those in the laminar region of the optic nerve) may suffer as a result of reduced flow.

To date, the best hope for those patients who have progressive disease is to reduce IOP by 25% or more, to reverse vasospasm using a calcium channel blocker, and to correct any drug-induced nocturnal dips.

BOX 221-1

Differential Diagnosis of Normal-Tension Glaucoma

High-tension primary open-angle glaucoma with episodic "normal intra-ocular pressure"
Secondary open-angle glaucoma from previous elevated intraocular pressure
Nonglaucomatous optic neuropathy
Other lesions that affect the visual pathways

Monitoring for Progression

The younger the patients at diagnosis, the greater is the possibility of clinically significant visual loss in their lifetime. It is important for these patients to be "trained" early in the management of their disease to become reliable performers with threshold perimetry. All patients require repeat visual field testing to identify progression and, within reason, the more frequently the field test is repeated, the better. Perimetry 3–4 times a year gives a better chance of identifying change, and will do so considerably earlier, than field testing once or twice a year.

Therapeutic Intervention

Medical management to lower IOP that fails to maintain a 25% reduction is unlikely to affect the course of the disease. A trial of medical management may be justified in patients with progressive disease, but failure to achieve this reduction should mean a recommendation for fistulizing surgery, rather than waiting for further progression to occur.

Glaucoma surgery designed to lower IOP by 30% from a starting level of, say, 17mmHg runs significant risk of postoperative hypotony.[26] This will convert the frequently asymptomatic patient into one with symptoms of fluctuating and progressively deteriorating sight. It is essential, therefore, to have identified progressive disease correctly and to have discussed with patients the effect of their rate of visual loss on their vision before asking them to undergo fistulizing surgery. Most patients with NTG are elderly and their disease progresses slowly, so that the surgical option is not resorted to frequently.

Neuroprotection

Apoptosis (programmed cell death) occurs both in the experimental primate glaucoma model and in human glaucoma, which has stimulated research into neuroprotective agents.[27,28] Trials of calcium channel blockers have been shown to exert some neuroprotection in selected cohorts of patients with NTG. Other potential neuroprotective agents include antiparkinsonian drugs and brimonidine. Trials of such agents are under way.

COURSE AND OUTCOMES

Many patients are in their seventh and eighth decade of life at diagnosis and, with slow disease progression, they do not notice any visual change. Progression for other patients is more rapid, and they suffer severe visual loss. No progression has been seen in some patients monitored for 10 years or more by the author, while other patients have demonstrated rates of loss at individual retinal locations of up to and exceeding 5db per year. Similarly, patients who have one normal visual field initially may show no signs of visual field loss in the second eye for more than 10 years, even though the appearance of the optic disc suggests glaucoma. The identification of change, either by the patient's symptoms or by visual performance, is an indication that IOP must be lowered by 25% or more. To maintain this reduction in IOP for the necessary decades may be difficult, but if this is not carried out the visual loss may be slowed only and not halted. Finally, neuroprotective agents, such as calcium channel blockers, may come to play a pivotal role in the management of

this condition. To date, the only two approaches shown to affect the course of the disease are the lowering of IOP and the use of calcium channel blockers.

REFERENCES

1. Graham SL, Drance SM, Wijsman K, et al. Ambulatory blood pressure monitoring in glaucoma. The nocturnal dip. Ophthalmology. 1995;102:61–9.
2. Nicolela MT, Drance SM, Rankin SJ, et al. Color Doppler imaging in patients with asymmetric glaucoma and unilateral visual field loss. Am J Ophthalmol. 1996;121:502–10.
3. Hayreh SS, Zimmerman MB, Podhajsky P, Alward WL. Nocturnal arterial hypotension and its role in optic nerve head and ocular ischemic disorders. Am J Ophthalmol. 1994;117:603–24.
4. James CB. Effect of trabeculectomy on pulsatile ocular blood flow. Br J Ophthalmol. 1994;78:818–22.
5. Dandona L, Quigley HA, Brown AE, Enger C. Quantitative regional structure of the normal human lamina cribrosa. A racial comparison. Arch Ophthalmol. 1990;108:393–8.
6. Quigley H, Pease ME, Thibault D. Change in the appearance of elastin in the lamina cribrosa of glaucomatous optic nerve heads. Graefes Arch Klin Exp Ophthalmol. 1994;232:257–61.
7. Geijssen HC, Greve EL. Focal ischaemic normal pressure glaucoma versus high pressure glaucoma. Doc Ophthalmol. 1990;75:291–301.
8. Geijssen HC. Studies on normal pressure glaucoma, ed 1. Amsterdam: Kugler Publications; 1991.
9. Larsson LI, Rettig ES, Sheridan PT, Brubaker RF. Aqueous humor dynamics in low-tension glaucoma. Am J Ophthalmol. 1993;116:590–3.
10. Poinoosawmy D, Fontana L, Hitchings RA. Asymmetric field defects in normal tension glaucoma. Ophthalmology. 1998;105(6):988–91.
11. Haefliger IO, Hitchings RA. Relationship between asymmetry of visual field defects and intraocular pressure difference in an untreated normal (low) tension glaucoma population. Acta Ophthalmol (Copenh). 1990;68:564–7.
12. Crichton A, Drance SM, Douglas GR, Schulzer M. Unequal intraocular pressure and its relation to asymmetric visual field defects in low-tension glaucoma. Ophthalmology. 1989;96:1312–4.
13. Membrey WL, Poinoosawmy DP, Bunce C, et al. Comparison of visual field progression in patients with normal pressure glaucoma between eyes with and without visual field loss that threatens fixation. Br J Ophthalmol. 2000;84(10):1154–8.
14. Drance S, Anderson DR, Schulzer M. Risk factors for progression of visual field abnormalities in normal-tension glaucoma. Am J Ophthalmol. 2001;131(6):699–708.
15. Corbett JJ, Phelps CD, Eslinger P, Montague PR. The neurologic evaluation of patients with low-tension glaucoma. Invest Ophthalmol Vis Sci. 1985;26:1101–4.
16. Phelps CD, Corbett JJ. Migraine and low-tension glaucoma. A case-control study. Invest Ophthalmol Vis Sci. 1985;26:1105–8.
17. Bhandari A, Crabb DP, Poinoosawmy D, et al. Effect of surgery on visual field progression in normal-tension glaucoma. Ophthalmology. 1997;104:1131–7.
18. The effectiveness of intraocular pressure reduction in the treatment of normal-tension glaucoma. Collaborative Normal-Tension Glaucoma Study Group. Am J Ophthalmol. 1998;126(4):498–505.
19. Comparison of glaucomatous progression between untreated patients with normal-tension glaucoma and patients with therapeutically reduced intraocular pressures. Collaborative Normal-Tension Glaucoma Study Group. Am J Ophthalmol. 1998;126(4):487–97.
20. Koseki N, Araie M, Shirato S, Yamamoto S. Effect of trabeculectomy on visual field performance in central 30 degrees field in progressive normal-tension glaucoma. Ophthalmology. 1997;104:197–201.
21. Membrey WL, Poinoosawmy DP, Bunce C, et al. Comparison of visual field progression in patients with normal pressure glaucoma between eyes with and without visual field loss that threatens fixation. Br J Ophthalmol. 2000;84(10):1154–8.
22. Greve EL, Rulo AH, Drance SM, et al. Reduced intraocular pressure and increased ocular perfusion pressure in normal tension glaucoma: a review of short-term studies with three dose regimens of latanoprost treatment. Surv Ophthalmol. 1997;41(Suppl 2):S89–S92.
23. Sawada A, Kitazawa Y, Yamamoto T, et al. Prevention of visual field defect progression with brovincamine in eyes with normal-tension glaucoma. Ophthalmology. 1996;103:283–8.
24. Pilunat LE, Lang GK, Harris A. Effect of nimodipine on visual function in normal pressure glaucoma. Ophthalmology. 1994;101(Suppl):108.
25. Pillunat LE, Lang GK, Harris A. The visual response to increased ocular blood flow in normal pressure glaucoma. Surv Ophthalmol. 1994;38:139–48.
26. Membrey WL, Poinoosawmy DP, Bunce C, Hitchings RA. Glaucoma surgery with or without adjunctive antiproliferatives in normal tension glaucoma: 1 intraocular pressure control and complications. Br J Ophthalmol. 2000;84(6):586–90.
27. Quigley HA, Nickells RW, Kerrigan LA, et al. Retinal ganglion cell death in experimental glaucoma and after axotomy occurs by apoptosis. Invest Ophthalmol Vis Sci. 1995;36:774–86.
28. Kerrigan LA, Zack DJ, Quigley HA, et al. Tunnel positive ganglion cells in human primary open angle glaucoma. Arch Ophthalmol. 1997;115:1031–5.

CHAPTER 222

Angle-Closure Glaucoma

CARLO E. TRAVERSO • ALESSANDRO BAGNIS • GRAZIANO BRICOLA

DEFINITION

- Iris apposition or adhesion to the trabecular meshwork, causing a decrease in outflow and an increase in intraocular pressure to clinically significant levels.

KEY FEATURES

- Gonioscopically closed angle.
- Intraocular pressure above the statistical norm.

ASSOCIATED FEATURES

- Optic nerve atrophy.
- Visual field defects.
- Secondary forms accompanied by a wide array of ocular conditions.
- Pain, redness, mid-dilated pupil when acute.

BOX 222-1

Risk Favtors for Primary Angle-Closure Glaucoma

Positive family history for angle closure
Age over 40–50 years
Women
History of angle-closure symptoms
Hyperopia
Pseudoexfoliation
Racial group (Eskimo > Asian > Caucasian = African)

INTRODUCTION

The many clinical entities grouped under angle-closure glaucoma are characterized by iridotrabecular apposition or adhesion or both. In most cases, no problem is detected until the outflow facility has decreased enough to cause a clinically significant elevation of intraocular pressure (IOP). The sequence of events and the mechanism can be highly variable, however. In each case, an initial attempt to identify the anatomical changes and the pathophysiology must be carried out to make the correct diagnosis and choose the most appropriate management.[1-5] The principal arguments to separate strictly angle-closure glaucoma from open-angle glaucoma are the primary therapeutic approach (i.e., iridectomy or iridoplasty), the possible late complications (synechial closure of chamber angle), and the complications that result when this type of glaucoma is managed by filtration surgery (uveal effusion, aqueous misdirection glaucoma).

Some confusion and overlap of terminology has arisen in the descriptive terms and definitions of angle-closure glaucoma. Classically, angle-closure glaucoma is subdivided into two main groups according to the cause, known or presumed, of angle closure:

- Primary angle closure, in which no cause other than anatomical predisposition is identified (typical is the classic acute angle-closure attack)
- Secondary angle closure, in which a direct causal relationship is found between iris apposition and a specific condition that arises from pathological processes in any part of the eye. Typical examples are synechial angle closure from contraction of fibrovascular membrane, as in neovascular glaucoma or iridotrabecular apposition from seclusio pupillae with iris bombé in anterior uveitis (see Chapter 225).

EPIDEMIOLOGY AND PATHOGENESIS

Incidence and Prevalence

Compared with primary open-angle glaucoma, few data are available on the incidence and prevalence of the various types of angle-closure glaucoma. The most common form of primary angle-closure glaucoma is associated with some degree of pupillary block or increased resistance to transpupillary flow of aqueous humor. In turn, this results from moderate or firm apposition of the posterior surface of the iris to the anterior surface of the lens, which is associated most often with a narrow anterior segment coupled with the lifelong increase of lens volume. As a consequence, the prevalence of primary angle-closure glaucoma is higher in those with hyperopia, in the elderly patient, in diabetics, in those with pseudoexfoliation, in women, and in certain races (Box 222-1). Iris-induced primary angle closure is not associated specifically with a shallow central anterior chamber (see below).

Risk Factors

Anatomical features characteristic of primary angle-closure glaucoma may be used to identify individual risk. Shallow anterior chamber depth, thicker lens, increased anterior curvature of the lens, smaller corneal diameter, shorter axial length, and increased ratio of lens thickness to axial length are findings agreed upon by independent researchers.[4,6] Individuals from the groups given in Box 222-1 are at higher risk for the development of primary angle-closure glaucoma. Several studies have shown striking differences by racial group in the distribution of primary angle-closure glaucoma in individuals over 40 years of age,[7-11] with an incidence in Caucasians of 0.1–0.2%, in Eskimos of 2.2–6.2%, in East Asians of 0.3–3.2%, and in those of mixed race from the Western Cape area of South Africa of 2.3%. Rates increase uniformly with age, and women are affected more often the men, independent of age.

Pathogenesis and Pathophysiology

When the pathogenesis of angle closure is considered, it is critical to analyze each of the following factors:

- Relative and absolute size of anterior segment structures
- Relative and absolute position of anterior segment structures

- Forces involved between the anterior and posterior chambers and their distribution vectors

To better elucidate the several components of angle closure, it is useful to approach the pathophysiology from different standpoints, as given in Box 222-2.

ANGLE CLOSURE ASSOCIATED WITH PUPILLARY BLOCK. Pupillary block occurs when a pressure gradient exists between the anterior and posterior iris surfaces, with the pressure in the posterior chamber greater than that in the anterior chamber.

Absolute pupillary block occurs when there is no aqueous flow through the pupil (Fig. 222-1), as in seclusio or occlusion pupillae, as a result of posterior synechiae (iris to lens, intraocular lens [IOL], capsule, anterior hyaloid). Relative pupillary block occurs when some degree of resistance to forward aqueous flow exists between the surfaces of the anterior capsule and of the posterior iris (Fig. 222-2). Pupillary block also results when an IOL in the anterior chamber of vitreous face blocks the pupil, in the absence of a functioning iridectomy, or from a gas bubble or silicone oil in the anterior chamber. Papillary block needs to be recognized, because it is the most relevant component in the vast majority of cases of angle closure and is managed effectively with laser or surgical iridectomy.

ANGLE CLOSURE WITHOUT A PUPILLARY BLOCK. Iridotrabecular apposition or adhesion results from several conditions, alone or in combination. Contraction of fibrovascular and inflammatory membranes in neovascularization of the iris and anterior segment inflammation (uveitis or mechanical irritation from IOL haptics, etc.) may rapidly close an angle synechially. Prolonged anterior chamber shallowing from any cause, such as epithelial downgrowth, fibrous ingrowth, and endothelial proliferation seen in iridocorneoendothelial syndromes, also may result in secondary angle closure.

LENS-INDUCED ANGLE-CLOSURE GLAUCOMA. Lens-induced angle-closure glaucoma has two components—lens size (phacomorphic) and lens position (phakotopic). Lens-induced angle-closure glaucoma results directly when a lens presses against the posterior surface of the iris and ciliary body or indirectly when the increased lens–iris contact hastens the pupillary block component (see Chapter 230).

IRIS-INDUCED ANGLE-CLOSURE GLAUCOMA. The plateau iris mechanism results from iridotrabecular contact when the pupil is dilated. Also referred to as *angle crowding*, iris-induced angle-closure glaucoma may occur when any or all of the following occur:

- Tissue of the peripheral iris is thick (peripheral iris roll)
- Iris base inserts anteriorly and leaves only a very narrow ciliary band, or inserts into the scleral spur
- Ciliary processes are displaced anteriorly in the posterior chamber and push the iris base forward into the angle recess[5] (Fig. 222-3).

The relative position of the iris root may be assessed using ultrasound biomicroscopy. The plateau iris mechanism suggests that iris-induced angle-closure glaucoma is not relieved by iridectomy. Angle closure caused by the pure form of plateau iris syndrome is extremely rare, and can be proved only by the occurrence of an acute angle-closure attack triggered by mydriasis despite a patent peripheral iridotomy. A plateau iris configuration, however, is relatively common and frequently coexists with pupillary block.

OCULAR MANIFESTATIONS
Primary Acute Angle-Closure Attack

A primary, acute angle-closure attack (Fig. 222-4) may cause symptoms of decreased vision, halos around lights, frontal headache, pain, nausea, and vomiting. Not all of these symp-

---

BOX 222-2

Pathogenesis and Pathophysiology of Angle Closure

IRIS PUSHED FORWARD
Absolute or relative pupillary block (Figs. 222-3 and 222-4)
Forward rotation of ciliary body and/or iris root
Choroidal swelling after panretinal photocoagulation, chronic retinal venous obstruction, posterior scleritis
Anterior insertion of the iris
Anterior position of the ciliary processes
Plateau iris configuration or plateau iris syndrome
Large or anteriorly displaced lens
Aqueous misdirection
Serous or hemorrhagic choroidal detachment or effusion
Space-occupying posterior lesion (gas bubble, synthetic vitreous substitutes, tumor)
Retrolenticular tissue contracture (retinopathy of prematurity, persistent hyperplastic primary vitreous)

IRIS PULLED FORWARD
Inflammation or hyphema with contraction of fibrin in the angle recess
Neovascularization of the iris with contraction of the fibrovascular membrane
Endothelial proliferation, as in iridocorneoendothelial syndromes
Prolonged anterior chamber shallowing with iridotrabecular contact
Iris incarceration in cataract incision
Epithelial downgrowth
Fibrous ingrowth

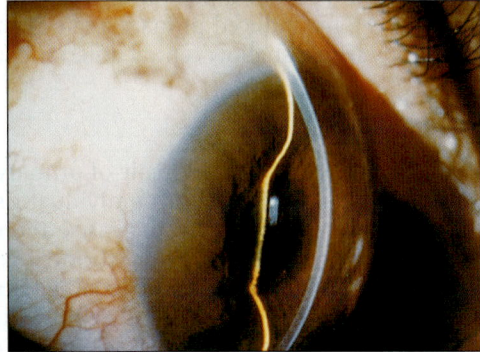

FIG. 222-1 ▮ **Absolute pupillary block from seclusio pupillae.** The iris bombé is typical, with a normal central anterior chamber depth.

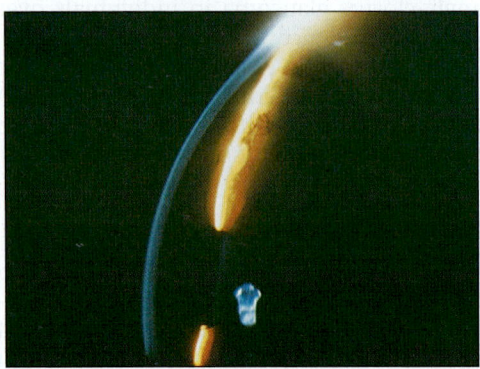

FIG. 222-2 ▮ **Relative pupillary block.** View of the iris profile at the slit lamp with a 60° angle.

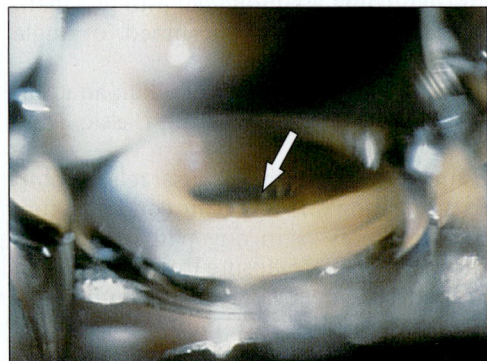

FIG. 222-3 ▮ **Gonioscopic view of an eye that has the lens positioned more anteriorly than usual.** The ciliary processes *(arrow)* are visible through the undilated pupil, a sign of forward rotation of the ciliary body.

toms are present in all cases and, indeed, little or no complaint may come from the patient.

Signs include an elevated IOP that has risen rapidly, conjunctival congestion, corneal epithelial or stromal edema, Descemet's folds, shallow or flat peripheral anterior chamber, and a mid-dilated pupil that has an absent or sluggish reaction. Gonioscopy reveals a circumferentially closed angle, and visualization may be poor because of corneal edema. Indentation is important but often technically difficult, because globe firmness and tenderness may result in poor patient cooperation. The fellow eye often shows a narrow, occludable angle or other forms of primary angle closure. In intermittent angle closure (also called subacute angle closure), signs and symptoms are the same as in acute attack, but generally milder, and resolution is spontaneous. The fellow eye has similar gonioscopic findings.

After an acute angle-closure attack, clinical examination may reveal signs of iris torsion (Fig. 222-5), patchy iris sub-atrophy, and lens glaucomflecken. The IOP may be normal or elevated, and the disc shows variable signs of cupping. On gonioscopy, wide areas of appositional or synechial closure (trabecular meshwork not visible in primary position) are found. In the fellow eye, similar synechial closure or a narrow angle occurs.

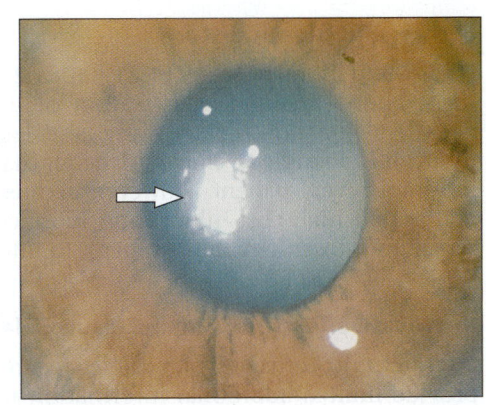

FIG. 222-4 ▮ Acute attack of angle-closure glaucoma. The central anterior chamber is deep, intraocular pressure is elevated, and corneal edema is present. Epithelial edema is outlined by the irregular slit reflex (arrow).

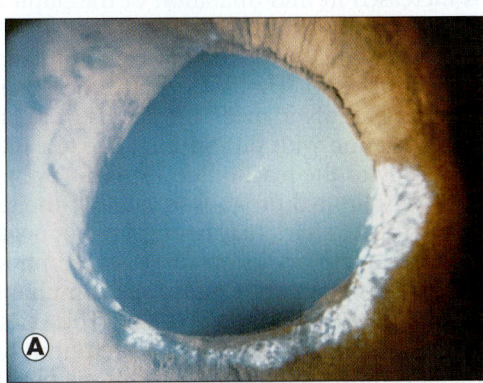

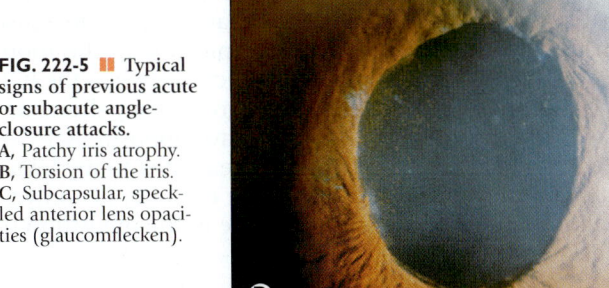

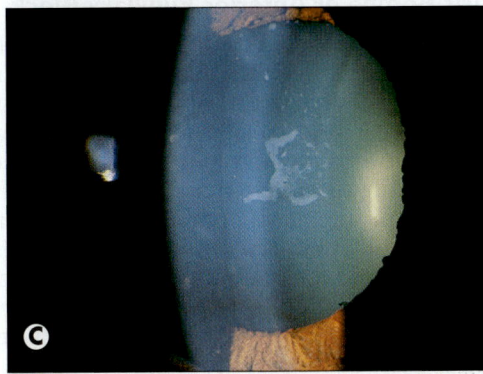

FIG. 222-5 ▮ Typical signs of previous acute or subacute angle-closure attacks. A, Patchy iris atrophy. B, Torsion of the iris. C, Subcapsular, speckled anterior lens opacities (glaucomflecken).

Chronic Angle-Closure Glaucoma

Few, if any, symptoms are present, unless the IOP is elevated significantly or unless advanced visual field damage is present.[12] Signs include disc cupping or nerve fiber layer defects with or without visual field damage typical of glaucoma, with IOP over 21mmHg (>2.8kPa) on no treatment. On gonioscopy, appositional or synechial closure (trabecular meshwork is not visible in the primary position) covers more than 120°. The fellow eye shows a similar gonioscopic picture or narrow angle. Intermittent or chronic angle closure can be deceivingly free of symptoms.

Primary Open-Angle Glaucoma With a Narrow Approach

No symptoms are present unless advanced visual field damage occurs. Signs include an IOP over 21mmHg (>2.8kPa) on no treatment, disc or fiber layer defects, with or without visual field damage typical of glaucoma. Gonioscopy reveals an open, but narrow, approach angle (>30°) and frequently a convex peripheral iris surface. The scleral spur often is not visible in the primary position of gaze but becomes visible with dynamic, indentation gonioscopy.

The IOP is increased because of trabecular outflow impairment. When appositional or synechial closure appears as a significant component, the condition is one of angle closure.

Occludable Angle

This is not an objective finding. The fellow eyes of acute angle-closure attack and of chronic angle-closure glaucoma are considered occludable and are managed with prophylactic laser iridotomy.[13] Eyes with extensive appositional closure or peripheral anterior synechia without any apparent cause except for the narrowness of the angle recess are managed as occludable by most clinicians.

Sequence of Events

The sequence of events for the various forms of angle closure are:
- Acute angle closure—sudden, circumferential, iridotrabecular apposition that causes a rapid, severe, and symptomatic rise in IOP
- Intermittent angle closure—self-limiting episodes of iridotrabecular apposition, with milder signs and symptoms than in acute angle closure
- Creeping angle closure—slowly progressive, iridotrabecular contact that results in elevated IOP as soon as 30–65% of the angle is closed
- Chronic angle closure—irreversible, iridotrabecular adhesion that causes asymptomatic IOP elevation

In acute and intermittent angle closure, the iridotrabecular apposition usually is reversed by appropriate intervention; chronic and creeping angle closure are characterized by irreversible peripheral anterior synechiae.

Secondary forms of glaucoma follow the same sequences, but management approaches vary considerably (see Chapters 225 through 230).

DIAGNOSIS

Gonioscopy

Gonioscopy (see Chapter 213) is used to determine the topography of the anterior chamber angle and is based on the recognition of angle landmarks. In gonioscopy, at least the following must always be considered:

- Level of iris insertion, either true or apparent
- Shape of the peripheral iris profile
- Estimated width of the angle approach
- Degree of trabecular pigmentation
- Areas of iridotrabecular apposition or synechiae (Fig. 222-6)

Gonioscopy findings must be recorded using a gradation method. The Spaeth gonioscopy grading system is the only descriptive method to include all the above parameters.[14] Other grading systems, such as the one introduced by Scheie, also are very useful and have become popular. It is not clear which method is better, but a grading system always should be used. Biometric gonioscopy, introduced by Congdon,[15,16] offers the advantage of a relatively simple and repeatable semiquantitative measurement of the angle, but it is not widely used.

Dynamic indentation gonioscopy is performed in all cases.[17,18] When pupillary block is the prevalent mechanism, the iris becomes peripherally concave during indentation. In the iris plateau configuration, this concavity does not extend to the extreme periphery, a sign that the ciliary body or iris root is placed anteriorly. When the lens is the cause, the iris moves backward only slightly on indentation and retains a convex profile.

Because patients most commonly have mixed components of angle closure, the cause seldom is clear from gonioscopic appearances.

Dynamic indentation gonioscopy is extremely useful for the differentiation of optical from either appositional or synechial closure and is used to measure the extent of angle closure. Visualization of the ciliary processes through the undilated pupil is a sign of forward displacement of the pupil border and of the anterior lens surface, and is associated with anterior rotation of the ciliary body (see Fig. 222-3).

Slit-Lamp Grading of Peripheral Anterior Chamber Depth

The Van Herick method[19] uses corneal thickness as a unit of measure. Grade 0 represents iridocorneal contact; a space between the iris and corneal endothelium of less than one fourth the corneal thickness is grade I; for grade II the space is between one fourth and one half the corneal thickness; and grade III is considered not occludable, with the iris endothelium distance more than one half the corneal thickness.

Ultrasound Biomicroscopy

Ultrasound biomicroscopy (see Chapter 213) of the anterior segment allows accurate visualization of the iris, iris root, corneoscleral junction, ciliary body, and lens.[4,5] Using this technique, it is possible to elucidate the mechanism of angle closure in almost every patient. However, because of its limited availability and high cost, ultrasound biomicroscopy usually is reserved for those cases most difficult to interpret.

Provocative Tests for Angle-Closure Glaucoma

Overall, provocative tests for angle closure carry some risks and provide limited additional information to that obtained from the clinical examination.[20,21]

PHARMACOLOGICAL TESTS. The pupillary block mechanism is increased in mid-dilatation of the pupil and by increased tension of the iris muscle, such as occurs with strong miotic therapy and concomitant dilator muscle stimulation by phenylephrine (Mapstone test). The test is performed using either short-acting parasympatholytic mydriatic agents or phenylephrine eye drops, in association with pilocarpine. The test strategy yields data relevant only to the reaction of a specific eye to a specific agent and is of very limited prognostic value. If the test result proves positive, an acute attack may be triggered. If negative, the test does not rule out angle occlusion under more physiological conditions. Such tests must not be performed simultaneously in both eyes.

PARAPHYSIOLOGICAL TESTS. The dark room prone test is based on the assumption that the pupil dilates in the dark and the lens moves slightly forward in the prone position. The test is conducted as follows. The patient sits for at least 30 minutes in the dark with the head pronated, usually resting on a table, and must not be allowed to fall to sleep, because sleep can cause pupil constriction. The IOP is checked rapidly, with the room light still off. The test result is considered positive when the IOP increases by 8mmHg (1.1kPa) or more or gonioscopy shows unquestionable increase of the areas that have appositional closure. The mechanism is unclear but may be related to mydriasis and the forward movement of the lens. The results apply only to the specific conditions of the test—its value in the prediction of actual behavior is not known.

DIFFERENTIAL DIAGNOSIS

Iris Bombé or Anterior Pupillary Block

The flow of aqueous through the pupil is hindered by adhesions that occur between the pupillary margin and the anterior lens surface. This block can be relative or absolute, as in seclusion pupillae or in occlusion pupillae. Although aqueous accumulates between the lens and iris to cause the iris to balloon forward, little or no anterior displacement of the lens occurs. The clinical picture of iris bombé, with the anterior chamber shallow peripherally but deep centrally, is typical. In pseudophakic eyes this type of block to aqueous flow is observed when posterior synechiae develop between the iris and the IOL at the pupillary border. Management of the cause is effected by creating a laser iridotomy or surgical iridectomy.

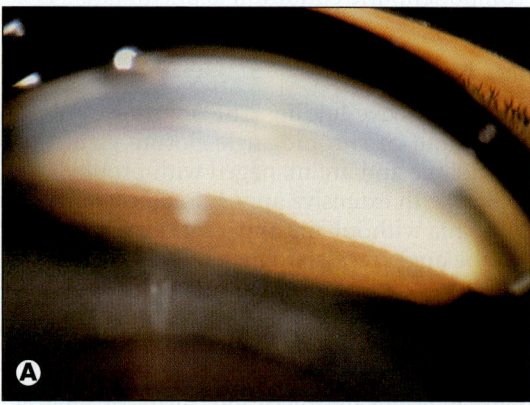

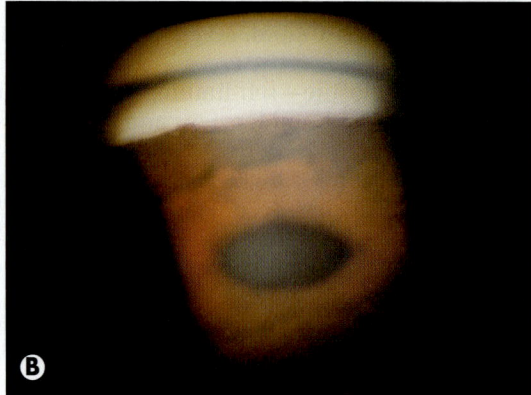

FIG. 222-6 ■ Gonioscopic view of peripheral anterior synechiae. **A,** Wide-based iridotrabecular adhesions and a relatively wide-angle approach are typical sequelae of inflammation. **B,** Pointed, tent-like synechiae are often observed in narrow angles with a relative pupillary block.

Posterior Pupillary Block or Anterior Aqueous Misdirection

PERILENTICULAR. In phakic eyes, the flow of aqueous toward the pupil is made difficult, because the posterior iris surface is wrapped tightly around the lens. The iris–lens contact is aggravated by aqueous that accumulates around and behind the crystalline lens; the aqueous pushes the lens forward with the iris and worsens the difficulties in forward aqueous flow. Phacomorphic or lens-position glaucoma, as well as the classic primary angle-closure attack, are typical.[22] The clinical picture is characterized by a shallow central anterior chamber. It is conceivable that aqueous pressure builds up in the small space between the zonulocapsular plane and the periphery of the anterior hyaloid face, which is referred to anatomically as the *canal of Petit.* Management includes iridectomy or lens extraction or both. Miotic agents may worsen the transpupillary aqueous flow difficulties.

RETROCAPSULAR. After extracapsular cataract extraction or phacoemulsification, with or without posterior chamber IOL implantation, when aqueous accumulates behind the iridocapsular diaphragm the posterior lens capsule and IOL, if present, are pushed forward.[22] The clinical picture is characterized by a shallow central anterior chamber. The space between the capsule and anterior hyaloid, in which the aqueous accumulates, becomes exaggerated and may be detected by biomicroscopy. Management requires the re-establishment of communication between the posterior and anterior chambers by performing a capsulectomy or iridectomy. Miotic medications have no role and may worsen the aqueous flow difficulties.

Posterior Aqueous Misdirection or Malignant Glaucoma

In this disorder, the aqueous humor is misdirected posteriorly and accumulates within the vitreous cavity, either diffusely or in the form of lacunae. The volume increase of the vitreous body displaces the lens or IOL anteriorly. The clinical picture is characterized by the anterior chamber becoming more shallow, both centrally and in the periphery. Classically, this condition is known as *malignant glaucoma.* Ciliary block glaucoma is described by some authors as a separate entity, in which aqueous accumulates behind a layer of condensed anterior vitreous. The change in aqueous dynamics may be spontaneous, although commonly it is propagated by a wound leak, whether unintentional or deliberate (as in filtration surgery).[22] Management entails the re-establishment of communication between the posterior chamber and the anterior chamber. Aqueous suppressant, osmotic, mydriatic, and cycloplegic agents are employed before laser capsulectomy (in pseudophakes), iridectomy, laser vitreolysis, or pars plana vitrectomy is attempted. Lens or IOL removal is seldom necessary. Miotic medications have no role and may worsen the aqueous flow difficulties.

SYSTEMIC ASSOCIATION

Pharmacological Mydriasis

Dilatation of the pupil using topical or systemic drugs may trigger iridotrabecular contact and eventually result in angle closure. Angle-closure attacks may occur, even bilaterally, in patients treated with systemic parasympatholytic agents before, during, or after abdominal surgery, and have been reported in association with the use of a serotoninergic appetite suppressant.[23]

Although pharmacological mydriasis using topical tropicamide and phenylephrine is safe in the general population,[24,25] even in eyes that have very narrow approach, a raised IOP and angle occlusion may occur in the occasional patient.[26]

Theoretically, any psychoactive drugs have the potential to cause angle closure; it is unlikely that pretreatment gonioscopy findings alone help to rule out such a risk. In eyes that have narrow angles, gonioscopy and tonometry are repeated after the initiation of management. Prophylactic laser iridotomy needs to be evaluated against the risks of angle closure or of withdrawal of the systemic treatment.

None of these drugs is contraindicated per se in open-angle glaucoma.

Ciliochoroidal detachment in association with bilateral angle closure has been reported after the administration of oral sulfa drugs,[27] and also in patients with acquired immunodeficiency syndrome, according to at least two reports.[28]

TREATMENT

Primary Angle-Closure Attack

Primary angle-closure attack is an ophthalmologic emergency, in which the priorities are (Fig. 222-7):

- Break the attack
- Lower the IOP
- Safeguard the fellow eye[29]

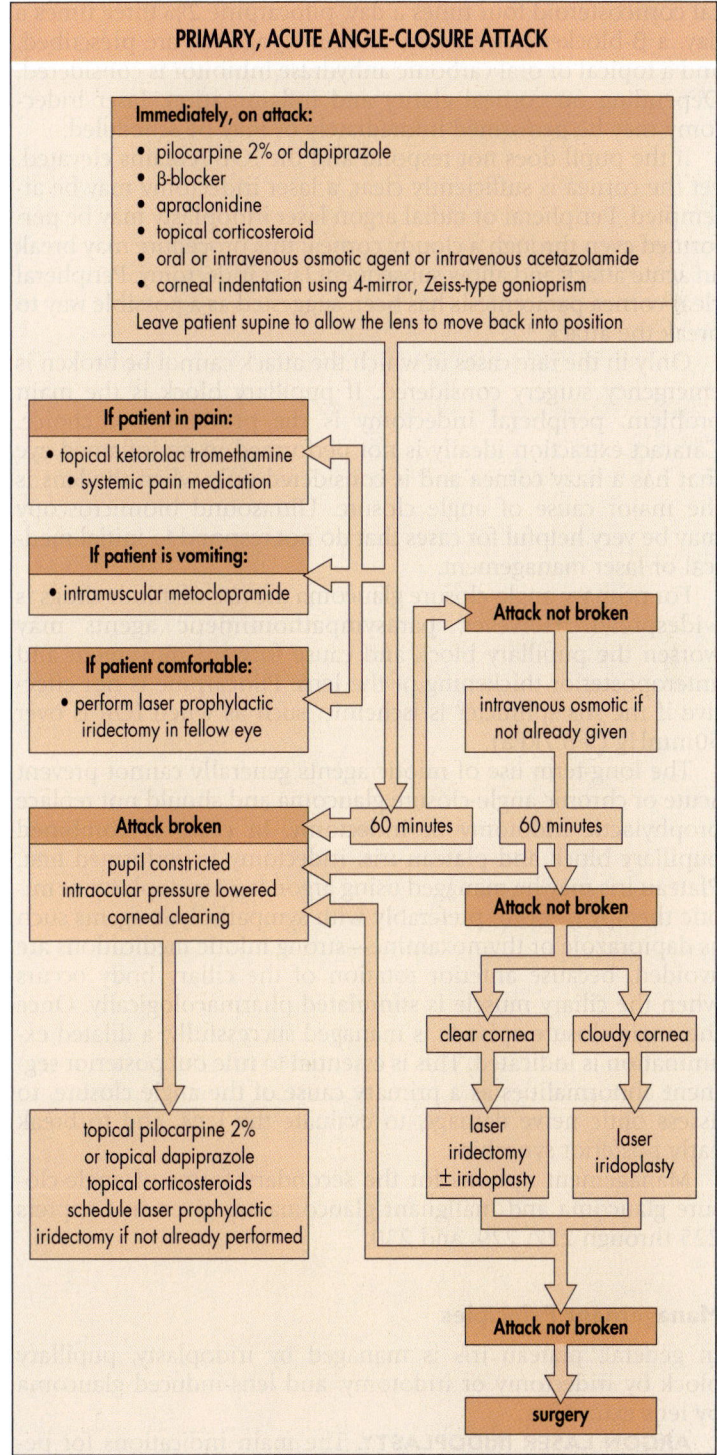

FIG. 222-7 ■ Initial management of primary, acute angle-closure attack.

Topical pilocarpine 2% or dapiprazole administered twice in 5 minutes, a topical β-blocker, a topical α₂-agonist, and a topical corticosteroid are given immediately, along with an osmotic agent at full dose or intravenous acetazolamide 5–10mg/kg.

Corneal indentation using a blunt instrument is best performed using a Zeiss-type four-mirror gonioprism, which may force aqueous through the pupil by misalignment of the iris sphincter or open an area of appositionally closed trabecular meshwork and, thus, allow aqueous to exit the anterior chamber.[30] A lower IOP achieved by these means decreases iris ischemia and enables pilocarpine to constrict the pupil effectively.

The patient must lie supine, to allow the lens to fall back into position. If vomiting occurs, intramuscular metoclopramide can be given. If significant pain occurs, topical ketorolac tromethamine and systemic pain medication may be given.

The patient is re-evaluated within 60–90 minutes. If the eye is quite comfortable, a prophylactic iridectomy is performed in the fellow eye. If the pupil is constricted and the IOP lowered, topical corticosteroid four times a day, pilocarpine 2% three times a day, a β-blocker twice a day, and an α₂-agonist are prescribed, and a topical or oral carbonic anhydrase inhibitor is considered. Depending on corneal clarity and inflammation, laser iridectomy may be performed immediately or may be scheduled.

If the pupil does not respond and the IOP remains elevated, yet the cornea is sufficiently clear, a laser iridectomy may be attempted. Peripheral or radial argon laser iridoplasty may be performed even through a cloudy cornea; this procedure may break an acute attack and allow subsequent laser iridectomy. Peripheral clear cornea paracentesis has been suggested as a possible way to break the attack.[31]

Only in the rare cases in which the attack cannot be broken is emergency surgery considered. If pupillary block is the main problem, peripheral iridectomy is the procedure of choice. Cataract extraction ideally is not performed in an inflamed eye that has a hazy cornea and is considered only when the lens is the major cause of angle closure. Ultrasound biomicroscopy may be very helpful for cases that do not respond to initial medical or laser management.

For primary angle-closure glaucoma the use of miotic drugs is widespread. However, parasympathomimetic agents may worsen the pupillary block and cause forward movement and anteroposterior thickening of the lens. Pilocarpine is not effective if the iris sphincter is ischemic, such as when IOP is over 50mmHg (>6.7kPa).

The long-term use of miotic agents generally cannot prevent acute or chronic angle-closure glaucoma and should not replace prophylactic iridotomy or iridectomy. In cases of combined pupillary block and plateau iris, iridectomy is performed first. Plateau iris may be managed using argon laser iridoplasty or miotic therapy or both, preferably with sympatholytic agents such as dapiprazole or thymoxamine—strong miotic medications are avoided, because anterior rotation of the ciliary body occurs when the ciliary muscle is stimulated pharmacologically. Once the angle closure episode is managed successfully, a dilated examination is indicated. This is essential to rule out posterior segment abnormalities as a primary cause of the angle closure, to assess optic nerve damage, to evaluate the lens, and to break early posterior synechiae.

Management options for the secondary forms of angle-closure glaucoma and malignant glaucoma are given in Chapters 225 through 227, 229, and 230.

Management Principles

In general, plateau iris is managed by iridoplasty, pupillary block by iridectomy or iridotomy, and lens-induced glaucoma by lens extraction.

ARGON LASER IRIDOPLASTY. The main indications for peripheral iridoplasty (Fig. 222-8) are:[32–37]
- Plateau iris (syndrome or configuration), for which argon

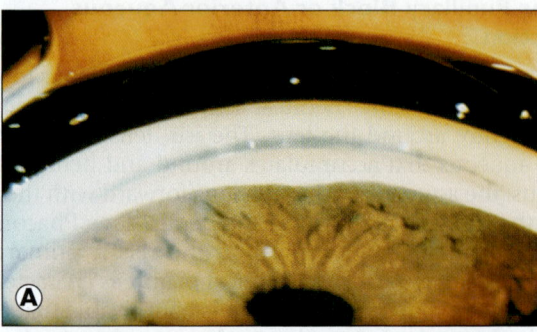
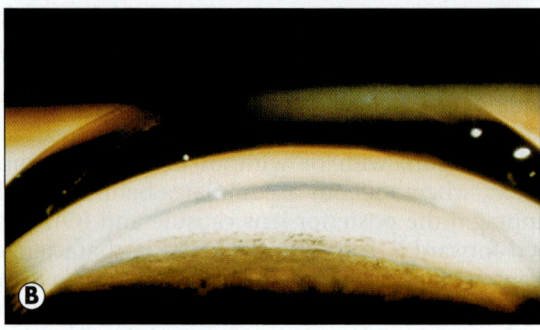

FIG. 222-8 ■ **Angle-closure glaucoma with pupillary block component. A,** No angle structures are visible in the primary position. **B,** After iridectomy, the iris curvature is less pronounced, and the trabecular meshwork can be visualized.

laser iridoplasty is the management of choice if iridectomy fails to widen the angle
- Acute attacks when corneal edema precludes laser iridotomy and medical management fails to break the attack (radial iridoplasty also is indicated)
- Primary open-angle glaucoma, before argon laser trabeculoplasty (ALT), when the angle approach is too narrow to visualize the trabecular meshwork

Technique. The therapeutic goal is to shrink and flatten the iris tissue with no resultant perforation, bubble formation, or pigment dispersion—excessive intervention may cause necrosis.[38] For peripheral iridoplasty, the laser is aimed at the extreme periphery of the iris, and a single row of evenly spaced applications made, 5–12 per quadrant at no less than one-spot–diameter intervals (see Fig. 222-8). Radial iridoplasty may be used to dilate the pupil and break a pupillary block, and is performed by the application of double rows of low-power, 200–500μm diameter laser spots radially on the oblique meridians, from near the pupil margin to the periphery, starting superiorly.

The technique and settings for laser iridectomy and iridoplasty are discussed in more detail in Chapter 235. See also below under Occludable Angle.

SURGICAL PERIPHERAL IRIDECTOMY. Iridectomy is the removal of iris tissue by a knife and scissors (surgical iridectomy) or by different forms of lasers, which remove iris tissue by dissolution (so-called laser iridotomy). Iridotomy, although rarely used today, is an opening in the iris without removal of iris tissue, usually performed by means of a knife needle perforating the iris.

Since the advent of laser iridectomy, surgical peripheral iridectomy is no longer performed commonly, but it is important to know how to perform the operation safely for the rare occasions on which it is needed. After preoperative medical therapy, which includes osmotic agents, to lower IOP, a 2–3mm incision is made in the peripheral cornea in a superior quadrant (usually superotemporally). Alternatively, a small conjunctival peritomy is made and the incision placed at the scleral limbus. The initial incision is to about two thirds of the corneal thickness, and a nylon suture is placed and looped out of the incision groove. An assistant may use this suture to open or close the incision later and thus control the rate of egress of aqueous. Care must be taken when the anterior chamber is entered with the blade and, after the initial penetration, an upwardly directed cut is advisable to extend the deep opening.

The key to success is to make the incision vertical so that a knuckle of iris spontaneously engages into the wound. Counterpressure on the back lip of the incision may encourage iris prolapse. This externalized piece of iris is held with toothed forceps and incised using fine scissors. If at all possible, neither the toothed forceps nor the scissors is used to enter the anterior chamber in an attempt to grab and cut the peripheral iris, because the lens and other underlying structures may be damaged. The edges of the incision are stroked gently to encourage the cut iris ends to retract into the anterior chamber, and the corneal or scleral incision is closed with one or two 10-0 nylon sutures to achieve a watertight closure.

GONIOSYNECHIALYSIS. Peripheral anterior synechiae sometimes may be stripped from the angle wall using an irrigation cyclodialysis spatula or flat iris spatula.[39,40] The procedure requires anterior chamber deepening with viscoelastics and restores trabecular function only if adhesions have been present for less than 1 year.

TRABECULECTOMY. In primary angle-closure glaucoma, filtration surgery is more prone to both intraoperative and postoperative complications, such as intraoperative positive pressure, zonular or lens damage, aqueous misdirection, and choroidal effusion or hemorrhage. It is important for the trabeculectomy scleral flap to be placed well anteriorly (see Chapter 240).

LENS EXTRACTION. The removal of a lens that has early opacities, or even of a clear lens, is suggested by some clinicians as the management of choice for angle-closure glaucoma induced mainly by lens size or malposition (see Chapter 229). That lens opacities possibly worsen rapidly, as occasionally observed after filtration surgery, lends further support to this approach. Excellent anatomical and functional outcomes are routine with modern closed-system, small-incision phacoemulsification.[31,41–44] Angle-closure cases may be very challenging, however, because of a small pupil, posterior synechiae, shallow anterior chamber, lax zonules, positive pressure, and lowered endothelial cell counts after acute angle-closure attacks.[45–47]

CHRONIC ANGLE CLOSURE. Laser iridectomy, laser iridoplasty, and cataract extraction are applied sequentially. The same drugs as used in primary open-angle glaucoma (POAG) are prescribed, because long-term miotic therapy does not prevent and actually may hasten progressive angle closure.

OCCLUDABLE ANGLE. Laser iridectomy is the management of choice for an occludable angle. If iridectomy fails to widen the angle, iridoplasty is considered. The reported rate of occurrence of primary, acute angle-closure attacks in such patients who are not treated is in the range 7–37%.[48] The discrepancy is probably because of different diagnostic definitions of occludable angles. Once the diagnosis is made, the risks of receiving or not receiving treatment need to be discussed with each patient. The major long-term drawback of laser iridectomy or iridoplasty is the formation of posterior synechia that can hinder mydriasis and make subsequent cataract surgery more difficult

PRIMARY OPEN-ANGLE GLAUCOMA WITH A NARROW APPROACH. Medical management is given initially, as for other patients who have POAG. Gonioscopy is repeated regularly. Although ALT is as effective as in POAG, it may need to be associated with argon laser iridoplasty to allow proper visualization of the trabecular meshwork.

MANAGEMENT FOR RESIDUAL PRESSURE ELEVATION AFTER ACUTE OR SUBACUTE ATTACKS. Gonioscopy and ultrasound biomicroscopy help to direct the management. When the trabecular meshwork is visible, ALT may be performed. With appositional closure, iridoplasty is applied before ALT. Synechial closure requires filtration surgery.

In lens-induced attacks, laser iridectomy or iridoplasty may be used successfully to open the angle and lower the IOP, and thus allow the scheduled lens extraction to be carried out on a less inflamed eye with a clearer cornea.

Iridectomy Failure

The failure of iridectomy to cure pupillary block may result from two conditions—the iridectomy is too small (functional failure) or it is closed (anatomical failure).[49]

Functional failure is rare and theoretically may be prevented if the iridectomies will remain of an adequate size. Hydrodynamically speaking, a 30m diameter opening should suffice to eliminate the pressure gradient between anterior and posterior chambers. The size of an iridectomy, however, may decrease shortly after surgery because of the elastic recoil of the stroma or localized edema. A minimal diameter of 50–100m is required. Occasionally, in secondary angle closures, loculation of the iris bombé may occur, and more than one patent iridectomy may be required to relieve the condition.

Anatomical closure may occur after the closure of an initially patent iridectomy and is more common after argon laser than neodymium:yttrium-aluminum-garnet laser iridotomy or in certain conditions such as uveitic or neovascular glaucoma. It is important to ensure that the iridectomy is full thickness at the outset, with penetration of the posterior pigmented iris layer (see Chapter 235).

COURSE AND OUTCOMES

The medical and laser surgical treatments of acute primary angle-closure glaucoma have a high success rate, especially if the disease is diagnosed early. It is important to manage prophylactically (with iridectomy) the fellow eye of patients who have angle-closure glaucoma with a pupillary block component, because a high incidence exists of future attack in this eye and the risk–benefit ratio greatly favors such prophylactic therapy. Blood relatives and siblings of patients show higher risk for primary angle closure.[14,50] Patients who have secondary angle closures follow a course that often is dependent upon their underlying disease. For example, in patients with neovascular glaucoma, the underlying retinopathy from chronic retinal venous obstruction or diabetes may affect visual outcome profoundly.

Interestingly, in a Caucasian population the probability of monocular blindness in acute primary angle-closure glaucoma was found to be 14% at the time of diagnosis, and among those non-monocularly blind at diagnosis, a further 4% will be so in 5 years. Such incidence data indicate the need for early diagnosis and appropriate treatment.[7]

REFERENCES

1. Mapstone R. Mechanics of pupil block. Br J Ophthalmol. 1968;52:19–26.
2. Lowe RF, Lim ASM, Min G. Primary angle closure glaucoma. Singapore: PG Publishers; 1989.
3. Ritch R, Lowe RF. Angle closure glaucoma: clinical types. In: Ritch R, Shields MB, Krupin T, eds. The glaucomas. St Louis: CV Mosby; 1996:829–40.
4. Ritch R, Lowe RF. Angle-closure glaucoma: mechanisms and epidemiology. In: Ritch R, Shields MB, Krupin T, eds. The glaucomas. St Louis: CV Mosby; 1996:801–19.
5. Ritch R. Plateau iris is caused by abnormally positioned ciliary processes. J Glaucoma. 1992;1:23–6.
6. Congdon N, Wang F, Tielsch JM. Issues in the epidemiology and population-based screening of primary angle-closure glaucoma. Surv Ophthalmol. 1992;36:411–23.
7. Erie J, Hodge DO, Gray DT. The incidence of primary angle-closure glaucoma in Olmsted County, Minnesota. Arch Ophthalmol. 1997;115:177–81.
8. Congdon NG, Quigley HA, Hung PT, et al. Screening techniques for angle-closure glaucoma in rural Taiwan. Acta Ophthalmol. 1996;74:113–9.
9. Salmon JF, Mermoud A, Ivey A, et al. The prevalence of primary angle closure glaucoma and open angle glaucoma in Mamre, Western Cape. Arch Ophthalmol. 1993;111:1263–9.
10. Alsbirk PH. Anatomical risk factors in primary angle-closure glaucoma. A ten year follow up survey based on limbal and axial anterior chamber depths in a high risk population. Int Ophthalmol. 1992;16(4-5):265–72.
11. Bourne RR, Sorensen KE, Klauber A, et al. Glaucoma in East Greenlandic Inuit—a population survey in Ittoqqortoormiit (Scoresbysund). Acta Ophthalmol Scand. 2001;79(5):462–7.
12. Ravits J, Seybold ME. Transient monocular visual loss from narrow-angle glaucoma. Arch Neurol. 1984;41(9):991–3.
13. The European Glaucoma Society, eds. Terminology and guidelines for glaucoma, Savona, Italy: Dogma; 2003, Ch. 2.4.3.
14. Spaeth G. Gonioscopy: uses old and new. The inheritance of occludable angles. Ophthalmology. 1978;85:222.
15. Congdon NG, Foster PJ, Wamsley S, et al. Biometric gonioscopy and the effects of age, race, and sex on the anterior chamber angle. Br J Ophthalmol. 2002;86(1):18–22.

16. Congdon NG, Spaeth GL, Augsburger J, et al. A proposed simple method for measurement in the anterior chamber angle: biometric gonioscopy. Ophthalmology. 1999;106(11):2161–7.
17. Forbes M. Gonioscopy with corneal indentation: a method for distinguishing between appositional closure and synechial closure. Arch Ophthalmol. 1966;76:488.
18. Forbes M. Indentation gonioscopy and efficacy of iridectomy in angle-closure glaucoma. Trans Am Ophthalmol Soc. 1974;72:488.
19. Van Herick W, Shaffer RN, Schwartz A. Estimation of width of anterior chamber. Incidence and significance of the narrow angle. Am J Ophthalmol. 1969;68:626–30.
20. Ritch R, Shields MB, Krupin T, eds. The glaucomas. St Louis: CV Mosby; 1986:860.
21. Wishart PK. Does the phenylephrine provocative test help in the management of acute and subacute angle closure glaucoma? Br J Ophthalmol. 1991;75:284–7.
22. Tomey KF, Traverso CE, Antonios SB, et al. Mechanisms of pupillary block. Arch Ophthalmol. 1988;106:166–7.
23. Denis P, Charpentier D, Berros P, Touameur S. Bilateral acute angle-closure glaucoma after dexfenfluramine treatment. Ophthalmologica. 1995;209:223–4.
24. Patel KH, Javitt JC, Tielsch JM, et al. Incidence of acute angle closure glaucoma after pharmacological mydriasis. Am J Ophthalmol. 1995;120:709–17.
25. Spaeth GL. Incidence of acute angle-closure glaucoma after pharmacologic mydriasis [Letter]. Am J Ophthalmol. 1996;122:283–4.
26. Goldstein JH. Incidence of acute angle closure glaucoma after pharmacologic mydriasis [Letter]. Am J Ophthalmol. 1996;121:733–5.
27. Poster EA, Assalian A, Epstein DL. Drug-induced transient myopia and angle-closure glaucoma associated with supraciliary choroidal effusion. Am J Ophthalmol. 1966;122:110–2.
28. Nash RW, Lindquist TD. Bilateral angle-closure glaucoma associated with uveal effusion: presenting sign of HIV infection. Surv Ophthalmol. 1992;36:255–8.
29. Davidorf JM, Baker ND, Derick R. Treatment of the fellow eye in acute angle-closure glaucoma: a case report and survey of members of the American Glaucoma Society. J Glaucoma. 1996;5:228–32.
30. Anderson D. Corneal indentation to relieve acute angle-closure glaucoma. Am J Ophthalmol. 1979;88:1091.
31. Lam DSC, Chua JKH, Than CCY, Lai JSM. Efficacy and safety of immediate anterior chamber paracentesis in the treatment of acute primary angle-closure glaucoma. A pilot study. Ophthalmology. 2002;109:64–70.
32. Ritch R. Argon laser iridoplasty: an overview. J Glaucoma. 1992;1:206–13.
33. Lim SSM, Tan A, Chew P, et al. Laser iridoplasty in the treatment of severe acute angle closure glaucoma. Int Ophthalmol. 1993;17:33–6.
34. Chew PTK, Yeo LMW. Argon laser iridoplasty in chronic angle closure glaucoma. Int Ophthalmol. 1995;19:67–70.
35. Ritch R, Liebmann JM. Argon laser peripheral iridoplasty. Ophthalmic Surg Lasers. 1996;27:289–300.
36. Quaranta L, Bettelli S, De Cilla S, Gandolfo E. Argon laser iridoplasty as primary treatment for acute angle closure glaucoma: a prospective clinical study. Acta Ophthalmol Scand Suppl. 2002;236:16–7.
37. Lam DS, Lai JS, Tham CC, et al. Argon laser peripheral iridoplasty versus conventional systemic medical therapy in treatment of acute primary angle-closure glaucoma: a prospective, randomized, controlled trial. Ophthalmology. 2002;109(9):1591–6.
38. Sassani JW, Ritch R, McCormick S, et al. Histopathology of argon laser peripheral iridoplasty. Ophthalmic Surg. 1993;24:740–5.
39. Campbell DG, Vela A. Modern goniosynechialysis for the treatment of synechial angle-closure glaucoma. Ophthalmology. 1984;91:1052–60.
40. Tanihara H, Negi A, Akimoto M, Nagata M. Long-term results of non-filtering surgery for the treatment of primary angle-closure glaucoma. Graefes Arch Klin Exp Ophthalmol. 1995;233:563–7.
41. Jacobi PC, Dietlein TS, Luke C, et al. Primary phacoemulsification and intraocular lens implantation for acute angle-closure glaucoma. Ophthalmology. 2002;109(9):1597–603.
42. Ge J, Guo Y, Liu Y. Preliminary clinical study on the management of angle-closure glaucoma by phacoemulsification with foldable posterior chamber intraocular lens implantation. Chung Hua Yen Ko Tsa Chih. 2001;37(5):355–8.
43. Hayashi K, Hayashi H, Nakao F, Hayashi F. Effect of cataract surgery on intraocular pressure control in glaucoma patients. J Cataract Refract Surg. 2001;27(11):1779–86.
44. Roberts TV, Francis IC, Lertusumitkul S, et al. Primary phacoemulsification for uncontrolled angle-closure glaucoma. J Cataract Refract Surg. 2000;26(7):1012–6.
45. Markowitz S, Morin J. The endothelium in primary angle-closure glaucoma. Am J Ophthalmol. 1984;98:103.
46. Olsen T. The endothelial cell damage in acute glaucoma: on the corneal thickness response to intraocular pressure. Acta Ophthalmol. 1980;58:257.
47. Setala K. Corneal endothelial cell density after an attack of acute glaucoma. Acta Ophthalmol. 1979;57:1004.
48. Panek WC, Christensen RE, Lee DA, et al. Biometric variables in patients with occludable anterior chamber angles. Am J Ophthalmol. 1990;2:185–8.
49. Gross FJ, Tingey D, Epstein DL. Increased prevalence of occludable angles and angle-closure glaucoma in patients with pseudoexfoliation. Am J Ophthalmol. 1994;117:333–6.
50. Tomlinson A, Leighton D. Ocular dimensions in the heredity of angle-closure glaucoma. Br J Ophthalmol. 1973;57:475.

CHAPTER
223

Pseudoexfoliative Glaucoma

WILLIAM J. LAHNERS • THOMAS W. SAMUELSON

DEFINITION
- A common, potentially aggressive form of secondary open-angle glaucoma characterized by the deposition of whitish, fibrillar material within the structures of the anterior segment and angle.

KEY FEATURES
- Characteristic whitish, fibrillar material on the anterior lens capsule and related structures.
- Most commonly open angle with increased trabecular meshwork pigmentation; less commonly narrow or closed angle.
- Variable intraocular pressure that ranges from normal to markedly elevated.

ASSOCIATED FEATURES
- Iris transillumination defects in peripupillary region.
- Reduced pharmacological dilatation.
- Weakened zonular attachments with lens instability and variable chamber depth.
- Reduced integrity of blood–aqueous barrier.

INTRODUCTION

Pseudoexfoliation (PEX) syndrome is an important ocular manifestation of a systemic disorder. It has been described as the most identifiable cause of open-angle glaucoma.[1] Glaucoma secondary to PEX syndrome often is far advanced when diagnosed and may be difficult to control medically. Markedly elevated intraocular pressure (IOP), despite an open angle, is not uncommon. However, not all patients who have PEX syndrome develop glaucoma. Despite extensive research, the pathogenesis of PEX glaucoma remains obscure, and it is difficult to predict which patients with PEX will develop visual loss.

EPIDEMIOLOGY AND PATHOGENESIS

The first report of PEX glaucoma was in Finland by Lindberg in 1917. PEX syndrome reportedly is most common in patients of Scandinavian heritage and relatively uncommon among African–Americans. However, the syndrome has been documented in most populations.[2] PEX syndrome is more common in women, although this observation may occur as a result of bias because of the longer life span of women. A syndrome of the elderly, it is unusual for it to be diagnosed before the age of 50 years. The prevalence of PEX syndrome increases markedly with age. For example, the prevalence of PEX syndrome in the United States was found to be 0.6% for those in the age range 52–64 years and 5% in the age range 75–85 years.[3] Although the condition may occur bilaterally, almost one half of the cases appear to be unilateral at the time of diagnosis. However, PEX material has been detected by electron microscopy in the conjunctiva of fellow eyes which have no apparent PEX based on biomicroscopic examination.[4] In addition, ultrastructural studies have shown changes in the iris and ciliary body epithelia, iris dilator muscle, iris stromal vessels, and juxtacanalicular trabecular meshwork.[5] As such, presumed unilateral cases most likely represent asymmetrical, bilateral cases. Indeed, 25% of patients who have unilateral PEX syndrome develop the disease in the fellow eye within 10 years.

Of patients who have PEX syndrome, 20% have glaucoma and elevated IOP at the time of diagnosis. Patients who have PEX syndrome but not glaucoma should be considered vulnerable to glaucoma, because 15% of such patients develop increased IOP within 10 years.[6] This underscores the need for careful follow-up in patients who have PEX syndrome. PEX syndrome accounts for 15–20% of cases of open-angle glaucoma. There is some evidence to support a genetic basis for PEX including transmission in two-generation families, twin studies, an increased risk of PEX in relatives of affected patients, and human lymphocyte antigen studies.[7] Nearly all pedigrees reported in the literature suggest maternal transmission, raising the possibilities of mitochondrial inheritance, X-linked inheritance, and autosomal inheritance with genomic imprinting.[7] Because of geographical variabilities, it has also been suggested that there may be a combination of genetic and non-genetic factors at work.

PEX syndrome is a systemic disorder, although its clinical relevance, based on current knowledge, is limited primarily to its ocular manifestations. PEX material has been identified in many visceral organs, as well as in the eye.[8,9]

Many theories exist as to the pathogenesis of glaucoma associated with PEX syndrome. Most research now indicates that the glaucoma is a secondary process distinct from primary open-angle glaucoma. PEX glaucoma may result from blockage of the trabecular spaces by the PEX material and pigment—PEX material contributes to the accumulation of pigment and debris within the aqueous outflow channels.[10] Many patients who have PEX syndrome do not develop increased IOP, perhaps because of individual variations in the metabolic activity of the trabecular meshwork. In some individuals, long-term exposure to PEX material and pigment overwhelms the system and results in increased resistance to aqueous outflow, damage to the juxtacanalicular region and Schlemm's canal, and subsequent increased IOP. Orbital blood flow velocities by Doppler imaging have shown a significant reduction in peak systolic and diastolic velocities in the short posterior ciliary arteries, central retinal artery, and the ophthalmic artery, as well as increased mean resistance in patients with PEX glaucoma.[11]

Although generally associated with open angles, PEX glaucoma is associated with a greater frequency of angle closure. This is likely related to the phenomenon of zonular instability and anterior displacement of the lens iris diaphragm. Moreover, posterior synechiae and iris rigidity may increase pupillary block. Miotic medications may exacerbate the pupillary block and must be used with caution in patients who have PEX syndrome with narrow angles.[1,12]

OCULAR MANIFESTATIONS

Patients who have PEX syndrome most often have no symptoms—PEX material is noted as an incidental finding on examination. The PEX material may be apparent in one or both eyes, but it is commonly asymmetrical or unilateral. Although the fellow eye frequently appears uninvolved, as noted earlier, the "uninvolved" eye most likely has subclinical PEX syndrome.[1,5] As such, *asymmetrical* may be a better term than *unilateral*.

Occasionally, patients who have PEX syndrome seek treatment in a dramatic fashion. The IOP may be elevated markedly despite an open angle. Frequently, in such cases the patient has far-advanced optic disc and visual field changes. The IOP may be 50–60mmHg (6.7–8.0kPa) or higher. Most often, patients are not symptomatic of the elevated pressure, which indicates chronicity of the pressure elevation. Patients often seek medical attention when they become aware of visual loss and subsequently are found to have far-advanced optic nerve and concomitant visual field damage (Fig. 223-1).[13] Less often, patients experience corneal edema, pain, and markedly elevated pressure, a clinical picture that must be differentiated from primary angle-closure glaucoma. Occasionally, patients who have PEX syndrome have a subluxed or completely dislocated lens (Fig. 223-2).[13]

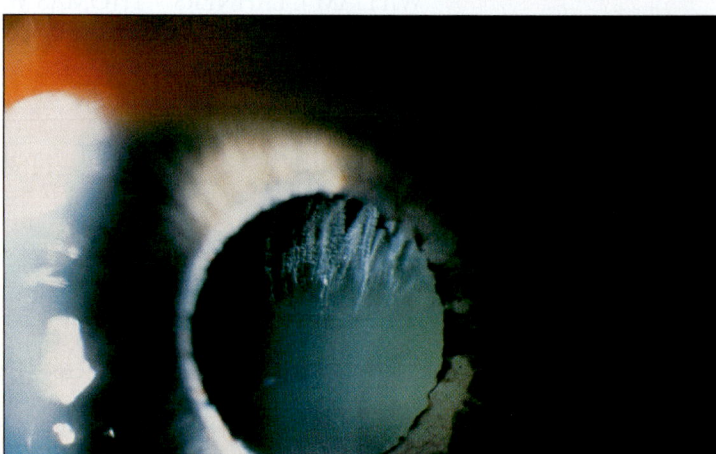

FIG. 223-2 ■ Subluxed crystalline lens. Exfoliative material (of the same patient as shown in Fig. 223-1) can be seen along the equator of the lens and within the zonules. In addition, peripupillary atrophy is evident. (Reproduced with permission from Samuelson TW. Management of coincident glaucoma and cataract. Curr Opin Ophthalmol. 1995;1:14–21.)

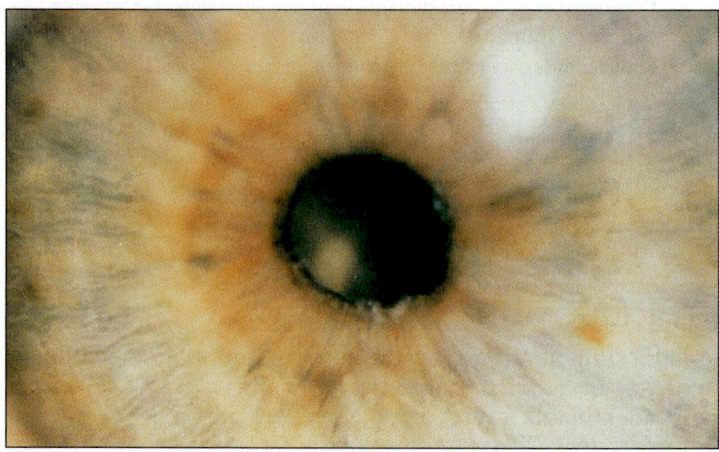

FIG. 223-3 ■ Exfoliative material at the pupillary margin.

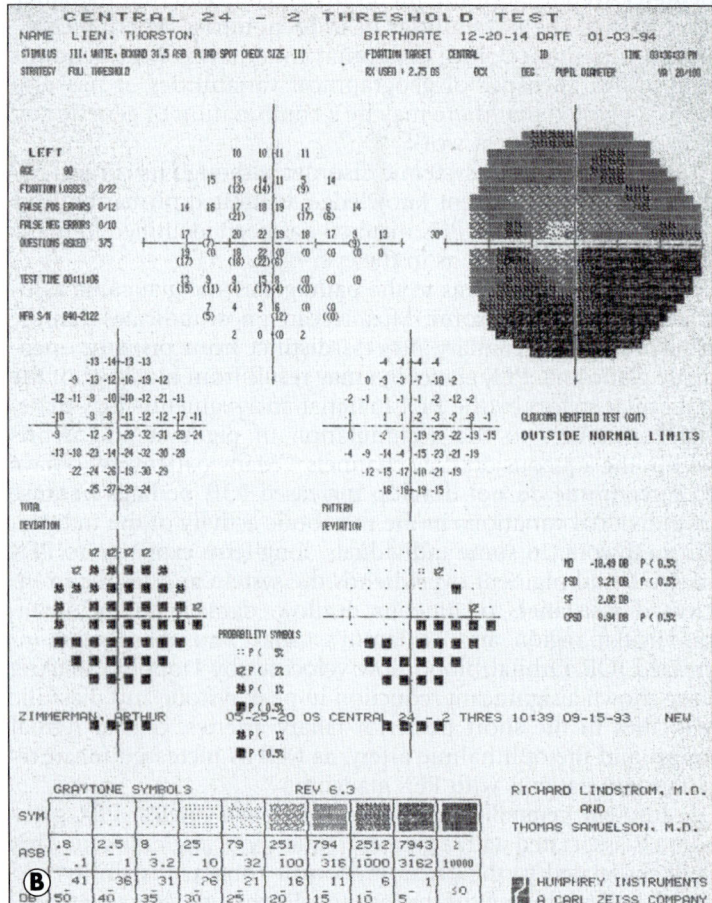

FIG. 223-1 ■ Initial appearance of pseudoexfoliative glaucoma. A, Advanced optic disc damage. (Reproduced with permission from Samuelson TW. Management of coincident glaucoma and cataract. Curr Opin Ophthalmol. 1995;1:14–21.) B, Visual field loss.

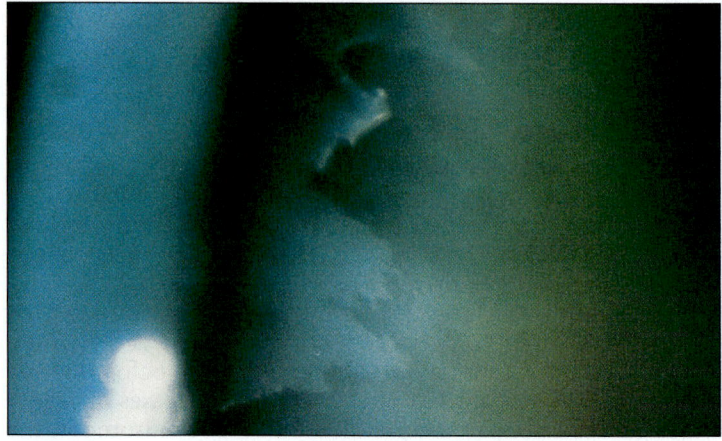

FIG. 223-4 ■ Scrolling of exfoliative material at the periphery of the anterior lens capsule.

On examination, the hallmark of the PEX syndrome is the characteristic pattern of whitish PEX material on the anterior lens capsule (Figs. 223-3 and 223-4). Classically three zones are seen[1]:

- A central disc of homogeneous appearance
- A relatively clear intermediate zone around the central disc
- An outer peripheral zone of PEX material

The intermediate clear zone results from the physiological movement of the iris, which clears the PEX material from this region of the lens. The peripheral zone may have various appearances but is always present. In contrast, the central disc may be absent in 10–20% of cases. One early sign of PEX syndrome is the development of radial, nongranular striae in the middle third of the anterior lens capsule, behind the iris.[14] Other early signs of PEX syndrome include increased pigmentation of the trabecular meshwork and a ground-glass appearance of the anterior lens capsule. Dilatation of the pupil helps in the identification of PEX material—the syndrome may be overlooked if the pupils are not dilated. PEX material also accumulates on the ciliary body and zonules and frequently is seen in the anterior chamber angle, corneal endothelium, and anterior vitreous face. The condition also may be diagnosed in pseudophakic or aphakic patients by the identification of PEX material on an intraocular lens or within anterior vitreous fibrils.

Patients who have PEX syndrome tend to have increased pigmentation of the anterior chamber angle. Pigment may also be present on the corneal endothelium. PEX syndrome has been associated with non-guttate endothelial loss and subsequent corneal decompensation.[15,16] The trabecular pigment is often patchy and unevenly distributed, in contrast to the pigment dispersion syndrome (PDS) in which a homogeneous pattern of trabecular pigmentation generally is found. Dilatation of the pupils may liberate additional pigment and postdilatation pressure spikes are not uncommon, despite a persistently open angle. As such, postdilatation pressure readings are frequently useful.

DIAGNOSIS AND ANCILLARY TESTING

The diagnosis of PEX syndrome is made on the basis of observation of the characteristic whitish PEX material on the surface of the anterior lens capsule. Additional suggestive signs include atrophy and transillumination of the iris sphincter, pupillary ruff defects, poor dilatation of the iris, a ground-glass appearance of the anterior lens capsule, and commonly a Sampaolesi line is noted in the inferior angle on gonioscopy. Traditionally, the term PEX glaucoma has been reserved for those cases which have pressure-related optic nerve and visual field abnormalities. The diagnoses of PEX syndrome and PEX glaucoma are primarily clinical. All patients who have PEX syndrome must be followed as glaucoma suspects. Patients who have PEX glaucoma are followed in much the same manner as patients who have primary open-angle glaucoma with periodic tonometric, optic disc, nerve fiber layer, and visual field examinations. The frequency of such testing depends on the severity of the disease in individual patients.

DIFFERENTIAL DIAGNOSIS

Several conditions may mimic the PEX syndrome. These include PDS, capsular delamination or true exfoliation, and primary amyloidosis. As mentioned previously, PEX syndrome has several features which distinguish it from PDS, which appears primarily in myopic men in the third and fourth decades (whereas PEX syndrome is a condition of the elderly). In contrast to PEX syndrome, PDS is usually a bilateral disease at time of diagnosis. The trabecular pigmentation is homogeneous, rather than patchy as in PEX syndrome.[17] Another important differentiating feature between PEX and PDS is that the transillumination defects generally occur at the pupillary margin in the former, while in the latter they are located in the midstroma of the iris.[18]

Capsular delamination or true exfoliation occurs secondary to heat, trauma, irradiation, or inflammation. A split in the anterior lens capsule occurs without deposition of PEX material and the characteristic frosty appearance of the lens capsule. Another rare condition that may produce fibrillar material on the lens surface is primary familial amyloidosis. Evaluation of this material has shown it to be distinctly different from PEX material. Most often, PEX glaucoma is misdiagnosed as primary open-angle or primary angle-closure glaucoma because of the failure to recognize the characteristic PEX material. Finally, PEX syndrome may be confused with iritis when the deposition of the PEX substance on the corneal endothelium results in the appearance of a pseudokeratic precipitate (Box 223-1).

SYSTEMIC ASSOCIATIONS

Ultrastructural studies performed on eyes during autopsy suggest that PEX syndrome is a systemic disorder. PEX material has been found in a number of organs, which include skin, lung, gallbladder, liver, myocardium, kidney, bladder, and meninges.[8,9] The staining of the material in these organs is positive for elastin and human amyloid P protein, which is similar to the staining pattern characteristic of the material found in the eye. These findings provide evidence for the systemic nature of PEX syndrome, which involves an aberrant connective tissue metabolism throughout the body.[8]

Although the systemic associations of PEX syndrome have been considered of primarily academic interest, some new reports have challenged this opinion. One study has shown a higher incidence of PEX syndrome in patients with abdominal aortic aneurysms compared with age-matched controls with vascular disease.[19] Another study has demonstrated an increased risk cardiovascular disease in patients with PEX syndrome.[20] However, at least one study has failed to show an association of PEX syndrome with increased cardiovascular or cerebrovascular mortality.[21] No systemic evaluation is needed or recommended in the routine evaluation and management of PEX glaucoma.

PATHOLOGY

Histologically, PEX material is homogeneous, eosinophilic material positive for periodic acid–Schiff analysis and rich in polysaccharides (Fig. 223-5).[22] It is composed of randomly arranged fibrils and filaments, which are thought to be derived from elastin and basement membrane material. PEX material has origins in both intraocular and extraocular sites. Pre-equatorial epithelium of the crystalline lens produces the substance, which then traverses the lens capsule and appears on the surface of the anterior capsule—the posterior capsule and the central epithelium are not involved in the production of this material.[22] By using a modified method of gonioscopy known as *cycloscopy,* PEX material has been seen to coat the ciliary processes and zonules, and it also accumulates at the insertion of the zonules into the ciliary body. In addition, the PEX material affects the zonular attachments to the lens capsule, which leads to instability of the zonular apparatus because of fragmentation.[23] PEX material within the trabecular meshwork results from both deposition from the aqueous and local production by the endothelial cells

---

BOX 223-1

Differential Diagnosis of Pseudoexfoliative Glaucoma

Primary open-angle glaucoma
Primary angle-closure glaucoma
Pigmentary glaucoma
Inflammatory glaucoma
True exfoliation/capsular delamination

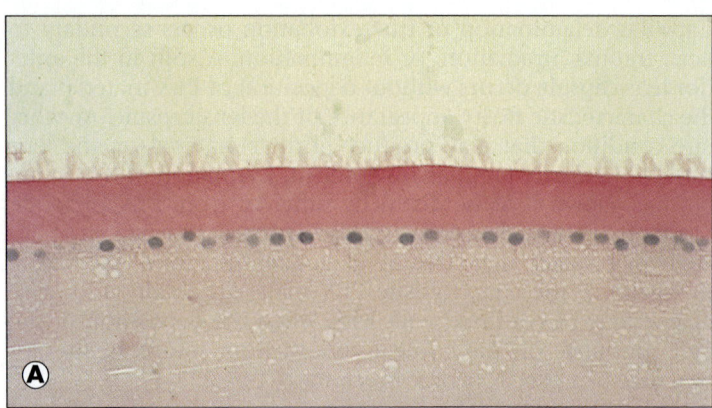

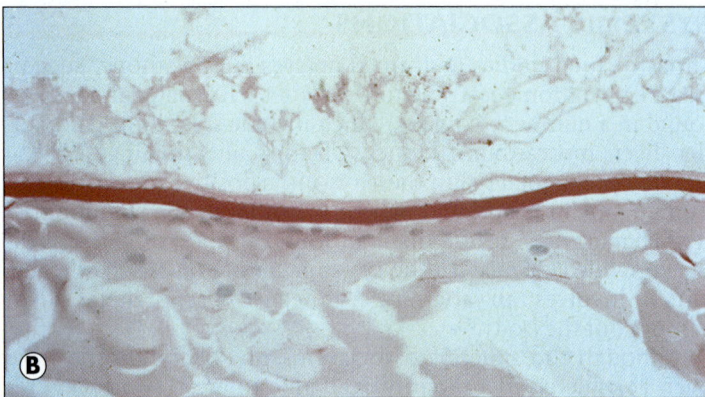

FIG. 223-5 ■ **Pseudoexfoliative syndrome. A,** In the central disc area, the material is deposited as small slivers that line up parallel to each other and perpendicular to the lens capsule. **B,** In the peripheral area, the material is abundant and has a thick, dendritic appearance. (**A–B,** From Yanoff M, Fine BS. Ocular pathology, ed 5. St. Louis: Mosby; 2002.)

in the outer trabecular meshwork. This material may contribute to the disorganization of the trabecular cells and fusion of the trabecular beams. The iris is involved extensively in PEX glaucoma, because the material accumulates on the iris pigment epithelium, anterior stroma, and iris vasculature, which results in atrophy of the iris pigment epithelium. Involvement of the iris vessels produces obliteration of the vascular lumen and eventual iris atrophy.[24] The corneal endothelium also has been identified as a source of pseudoexfoliative material. Extraocular sites of pseudoexfoliative material include bulbar and palpebral conjunctiva, along with periocular skin.[4]

TREATMENT

Medical management of PEX glaucoma is similar to that for primary open-angle glaucoma and includes the use of aqueous suppressants, prostaglandin analogs, and miotic agents. PEX glaucoma is frequently more resistant to medical management and has a higher failure rate compared with primary open-angle glaucoma.[6,25] If miotics are used to manage elevated IOP, careful follow-up for posterior synechiae and angle closure is recommended. Although miotic medications may have significant local side effects, they may be particularly useful in PEX glaucoma via the inhibition of pupillary activity and may subsequently decrease the amount of pigment and PEX material liberated into the anterior chamber. Despite this potential benefit of miotic agents, aqueous suppressants are generally the initial step in the management of PEX glaucoma.

If medical management with one or more agents is unsuccessful, argon laser trabeculoplasty may be considered; it is reported to have a higher success rate with PEX syndrome than for primary open-angle glaucoma. As such, argon laser trabeculoplasty is often used earlier in the management regimen than for other forms of open-angle glaucoma. If pressure is not controlled with medical or laser treatment, surgical trabeculectomy

is considered. The results of trabeculectomy are favorable, with no significant difference in the postoperative complication rate compared with filtration surgery in primary open-angle glaucoma.[26] However, patients who have PEX syndrome are more prone to an increased postoperative inflammatory response because of the alteration of the blood–aqueous barrier in this condition.[27] Trabecular aspiration has been used with success as another surgical alternative;[28,29] however, long-term follow-up is lacking.

In many instances, trabeculectomy is combined with cataract surgery in patients affected by PEX syndrome. Several important considerations exist for surgeons who perform combined cataract and glaucoma surgery in patients who have PEX syndrome. First, the zonular attachments in PEX syndrome may be weakened by the accumulation of PEX material.[12] This may result in a higher incidence of the lens subluxation, zonular dialysis, and vitreous loss. The rate for these complications has been estimated to be 5–10 times higher than in patients who do not have PEX syndrome.[8,22,23,30] Another factor which may complicate surgery is the reduced response to pharmacological dilatation in patients who have PEX syndrome.[31] Poor dilatation is the single most important risk factor for vitreous loss in cataract surgery among these patients. The use of pupillary stretch techniques or iris retractors has enhanced greatly the safety of cataract surgery in patients who have PEX syndrome. Other techniques which can be useful include the use of capsular tension rings to reduce capsular instability and improve implant centration. In some cases it may be necessary to place the lens into the ciliary sulcus or fixate the lens with sutures. Other observations made in eyes affected by PEX syndrome include a greater risk for perioperative pressure spikes, posterior synechia formation, and cellular precipitates on intraocular lenses. Preoperatively, all patients must be examined predilatation and postdilatation, with careful observation for phacodonesis and iridodonesis, which may help tailor the surgical approach. This is best performed with the aid of a gonioscope. If the lens is unstable, it may be best to perform supracapsular phacoemulsification by aggressive hydrodissection of the lens from the capsular bag. If it is not possible to remove the lens anteriorly, a pars plana approach may be necessary. With a gentle and methodical surgical technique, the results of combined cataract and glaucoma surgery in patients who display PEX may be quite good.

In patients with PEX glaucoma and controlled IOP on medication without advanced visual field loss, clear cornea cataract surgery alone can offer improved pressure control[32] without the additional technical difficulties and risks of combined cataract and trabeculectomy surgery. A trabeculectomy can then be offered as a second procedure, if necessary, at a later time, with potentially greater likelihood of success. This option of a staged approach to management of coincident cataract and PEX glaucoma can usually be considered only in patients with reasonable pre-operative IOP control and without advanced visual field loss, because IOP spikes can occur after even uncomplicated cataract surgery in patients with PEX.

COURSE AND OUTCOMES

PEX syndrome is a common cause of glaucomatous visual loss. About 10% of patients who have PEX syndrome eventually develop glaucoma. Despite medical or surgical management, one study noted that 25% of patients affected by PEX glaucoma are blind in at least one eye and 7% are blind in both eyes[33] (but there may be bias because of the referral nature of the study group). These data underscore the potentially aggressive nature of glaucoma associated with the PEX syndrome. With careful and meticulous follow-up, most patients have a favorable outcome. Understanding of the nature of the PEX material and its role in the pathogenesis of glaucoma will pave the way for new approaches in management, control, and prevention.

REFERENCES

1. Ritch R. Exfoliation syndrome: clinical findings and occurrence in patients with occludable angles. Trans Am Ophthalmol Soc. 1994;92:845–944.
2. Forsius H. Exfoliation syndrome in various ethnic populations. Acta Ophthalmol. 1988;66:71–85.
3. Liebowitz HM, Krueger DE, Maunder LR. The Framingham Eye Study Monograph. Surv Ophthalmol. 1980;24(Suppl.):335–610.
4. Prince AM, Streeten BW, Ritch R, et al. Preclinical diagnosis of pseudoexfoliation syndrome. Arch Ophthalmol. 1987;105:1076–82.
5. Hammer T, Schlotzer-Schrehardt U, Naumann GO. Unilateral or asymmetric pseudoexfoliation syndrome? An ultrastructural study. Arch Ophthalmol. 2001;119(7):1023–31.
6. Henry CJ, Krupin T, Schmitt M, et al. Long-term follow-up of pseudoexfoliation and the development of elevated intraocular pressure. Ophthalmology. 1987;94:545–52.
7. Damji KF, Bains HS, Stefansson E, et al. Is pseudoexfoliation syndrome inherited? A review of genetic and nongenetic factors and a new observation. Ophthalmic Genet. 1998;19(4):175–85.
8. Schlotzer-Schrehardt UM, Koca MR, Naumann GO, et al. Pseudoexfoliation syndrome. Ocular manifestation of a systemic disorder. Arch Ophthalmol. 1992;110:1752–6.
9. Streeten BW, Li ZY, Wallace RN, et al. Pseudoexfoliative fibrillopathy in visceral organs of a patient with pseudoexfoliation syndrome. Arch Ophthalmol. 1992;110:1757–62.
10. Morrison JC, Green WR. Light microscopy of the light exfoliation syndrome. Acta Ophthalmol. 1988;66:5–27.
11. Yuksel N, Karabas VL, Arslan A, et al. Ocular hemodynamics in pseudoexfoliation syndrome and pseudoexfoliation glaucoma. Ophthalmology. 2001;108(6):1043–9.
12. Schrehardt US, Naumann GO. A histopathologic study of zonular instability in pseudoexfoliation syndrome. Am J Ophthalmol. 1994;118:730–43.
13. Samuelson TW. Management of coincident glaucoma and cataract. Curr Opin Ophthalmol. 1995;6(1):14–21.
14. Konstas AGP, Marshall GE, Cameron SA, Lee WR. Morphology of iris vasculopathy in exfoliation glaucoma. Acta Ophthalmol (Copenh). 1993;71:751–9.
15. Naumann GO, Schlotzer-Schrehardt U. Keratopathy in pseudoexfoliation syndrome as a cause of corneal endothelial decompensation: a clinicopathologic study. Ophthalmology. 2000;107(6):1111–24.
16. Wirbelauer C, Anders N, Pham DT, Wollensak J. Corneal endothelial cell changes in pseudoexfoliation syndrome after cataract surgery. Arch Ophthalmol. 1998;116(2):145–9.
17. Gross FJ, Tingey D, Epstein DL. Increased prevalence of occludable angles and angle closure glaucoma in patients with pseudoexfoliation. Am J Ophthalmol. 1994;117:333–6.
18. Richardson TM, Epstein DL. Exfoliation glaucoma: a quantitative perfusion and ultrastructural study. Ophthalmology. 1981;88:968–80.
19. Schumacher S, Schlotzer-Schrehardt U, Martus P, et al. Pseudoexfoliation syndrome and aneurysms of the abdominal aorta. Lancet. 2001;357(9253):359–60.
20. Mitchell P, Wang JJ, Smith W. Association of pseudoexfoliation syndrome with increased vascular risk. Am J Ophthalmol. 1997;124(5):685–7.
21. Shrum KR, Hattenhauer MG, Hodge D. Cardiovascular and cerebrovascular mortality associated with ocular pseudoexfoliation. Am J Ophthalmol. 2000;129(1):83–6.
22. Roth M, Epstein DL. Exfoliation syndrome. Am J Ophthalmol. 1980;89:477–81.
23. Prince AM, Ritch R. Clinical signs of the pseudoexfoliation syndrome. Ophthalmology. 1986;93:803–7.
24. Farrar SM, Shields MB. Current concepts in pigmentary glaucoma. Surv Ophthalmol. 1993;37:233–52.
25. Brooks AV, Gilles WE. The presentation and prognosis of glaucoma in pseudoexfoliation of the lens capsule. Ophthalmology. 1988;95:271–6.
26. Konstas AG, Jay JL, Marshall GE, Lee WR. Prevalence, diagnostic features, and response to trabeculectomy in exfoliation glaucoma. Ophthalmology. 1993;100:619–27.
27. Nguyen NX, Kuchle M, Martus P, Naumann GO. Quantification of blood–aqueous barrier breakdown after trabeculectomy: pseudoexfoliation versus primary open-angle glaucoma. J Glaucoma. 1999;8(1):18–23.
28. Jacobi PC, Dietlein TS, Krieglstein GK. Bimanual trabecular aspiration in pseudoexfoliation glaucoma: an alternative in nonfiltering glaucoma surgery. Ophthalmology. 1998;105(5):886–94.
29. Jacobi PC, Dietlein TS, Krieglstein GK. Comparative study of trabecular aspiration vs trabeculectomy in glaucoma triple procedure to treat pseudoexfoliation glaucoma. Arch Ophthalmol. 1999;117(10):1311–8.
30. Lumme P, Laatikainen L. Exfoliation syndrome and cataract extraction. Am J Ophthalmol. 1993;116:51–5.
31. Carpel EF. Pupillary dilation in eyes with pseudoexfoliation syndrome. Am J Ophthalmol. 1988;105:692–3.
32. Merkur A, Damji KF, Mintsioulis G, Hodge WH. Intraocular pressure decrease after phacoemulsification in patients with pseudoexfoliation syndrome. J Cataract Refract Surg. 2001;27(4):528–32.
33. Thorburn W. The outcome of visual function in capsular glaucoma. Acta Ophthalmol. 1988;66:132–8.

224 Pigmentary Glaucoma

STUART F. BALL

DEFINITION
- A form of open-angle glaucoma characterized by disruption of the iris pigment epithelium with deposition of pigment throughout the anterior segment.

KEY FEATURE
- The classic triad consists of corneal pigmentation (Krukenberg's spindle); slit-like, radial, midperipheral iris transillumination defects; and heavy accumulation of pigment in the trabecular meshwork.

ASSOCIATED FEATURES
- 25–50% of patients with pigment dispersion syndrome develop pigmentary glaucoma.
- Typically young, myopic men.
- Predominantly Caucasian.
- "Reverse" pupillary block mechanism.
- Autosomal dominant inheritance.

INTRODUCTION

The pigment dispersion syndrome once was thought to be responsible for a form of rare, secondary, open-angle glaucoma but is now recognized as a common primary condition. It is associated with an autosomal dominant inherited form of glaucoma[1] that affects an estimated 0.5–5% of the glaucoma population of the United States.[2]

The term *pigmentary glaucoma* was first used in 1949 by Sugar and Barbour[3] to describe a single patient who had signs of pigment dispersion syndrome and glaucoma. By 1966, they had collected 147 cases that suffered loss of pigment from the iris and pigment deposition throughout the anterior segment, which characterizes this disease.[4] In 1979, Campbell[5] presented evidence that the pigmentation resulted from friction of the zonular packets that rubbed on the neuroepithelium of the iris and, in 1993, Karickhoff[6] postulated the mechanism of reverse pupillary block. The classic physical triad remains— Krukenberg's spindle; radial, midperipheral iris transillumination defects of the iris; and heavy pigmentation of the trabecular meshwork. As more becomes known of the physical characteristics of the affected eyes, the mechanism of disease development, and the genetics behind it, new strategies of both management and prevention may become possible.

EPIDEMIOLOGY AND PATHOGENESIS

Surveys of glaucoma practices estimate the prevalence of pigment dispersion syndrome to be in the range of 25,000–220,000 affected individuals in the United States. Because the phenotypic expressions of the disease may be mild and the disease may be overlooked or misdiagnosed, the true prevalence might be underestimated grossly.[2] Of 934 New York office workers screened using a slit lamp, 2.5% of the Caucasians had pigment dispersion syndrome, which suggests much higher prevalences. The pigment dispersion syndrome is rare in African–Americans and Asians. Approximately 25–50% of individuals with pigment dispersion syndrome eventually go on to manifest pigmentary glaucoma.[7]

As expected from its likely autosomal dominant inheritance,[1] pigment dispersion syndrome is found in roughly equal numbers of men and women. However, the phenotypic expression often is more pronounced in men; a 3:1 male-to-female predominance of pigmentary glaucoma exists, and a younger mean age of pigmentary glaucoma development occurs in men (35 years) than in females (46 years).[4,8]

Several features of eyes that have pigment dispersion syndrome may be important in its pathogenesis. Compared with control eyes, those with pigment dispersion syndrome are more likely to be myopic,[5,7,8] have a larger iris,[9] have a midperipheral iris back-bow that increases with accommodation,[10] have a posterior iris insertion,[9] have a relative "reverse pupillary block"[6] of increased lens-to-iris touch that is created by eyelid blinking,[11] and have an increased incidence of lattice degeneration.[12] It is believed that the particular combination of anatomical features in the eyes of these patients achieves a relative reverse pupillary block of contact between the midiris and the lens. In this "ball–valve" mechanism, each eyelid blink causes aqueous to squirt from the posterior chamber into the anterior chamber; equilibration by return flow is prevented by the peripupillary iris, which presses against the lens like a closed valve. The anterior chamber pressure gradient forces the susceptible iris to bow back against the zonules of the lens. The resultant friction during normal iris movement rubs off the pigment from the posterior surface of the iris, where it has been bowed back in contact with the zonular packets. Exercise, particularly jarring activities like jumping, in which inordinate friction might be expected, has been associated with episodes of abundant pigment liberation and sudden IOP rises, pain, and haloes. These episodes of symptomatic pigment showers are quite infrequent—normal jogging actually lowers IOP.[13] African–Americans and Asians only rarely manifest the disease, perhaps because the iris stroma is thicker and more dense in their eyes, which renders it insufficiently flexible either to create a ball–valve mechanism or to bow posteriorly against the zonular packets.[14] Men have a larger iris size than women and, correspondingly, may be more susceptible to the disease.

The liberated pigment deposits throughout the anterior segment, particularly in the trabecular meshwork.[15] The pigment is felt to be responsible directly for the rare, acute, episodic IOP rises and is likely to be an essential element of the damage to the trabecular meshwork that results over time.[15–17] A positive correlation exists between duration of pigment shedding, degree of pigment shedding, and production of pigmentary glaucoma.[8]

In the natural course of the disease, active pigment dispersion generally ceases when the patient reaches 45–50 years of age, presumably coincident with the development of presbyopia and relative pupillary block. This suggests that if the active pigment dispersion stage of the disease in these eyes could be temporarily or permanently retarded, the entire cascade of pigmentary glaucoma might be prevented. Just such a pharmacological or surgical manipulation of the iris configuration is, indeed, now possible (see below under Treatment). The results of such interventions are being studied.

The gene or genes that code for most cases of pigment dispersion syndrome are about to be isolated and have been mapped to chromosome 7q35–q36.[1] With the ability to screen genetically for pigment dispersion syndrome and with the relative ease the slit-lamp examination to identify the phenotype or phenocopies of the disease, preventive strategies could be employed easily if they are proved effective. Individuals who have the gene or the phenotype are at highest risk for glaucoma—particularly young Caucasian myopic males who have a susceptible iris stroma—theoretically could be offered prevention. A large-scale, prospective clinical trial is required to evaluate the effectiveness of these strategies.

OCULAR MANIFESTATIONS

Pigmentary glaucoma is a bilateral disorder characterized by loss of pigment from the pigment epithelium of the iris, usually in the midperipheral region. It often is revealed on transillumina-

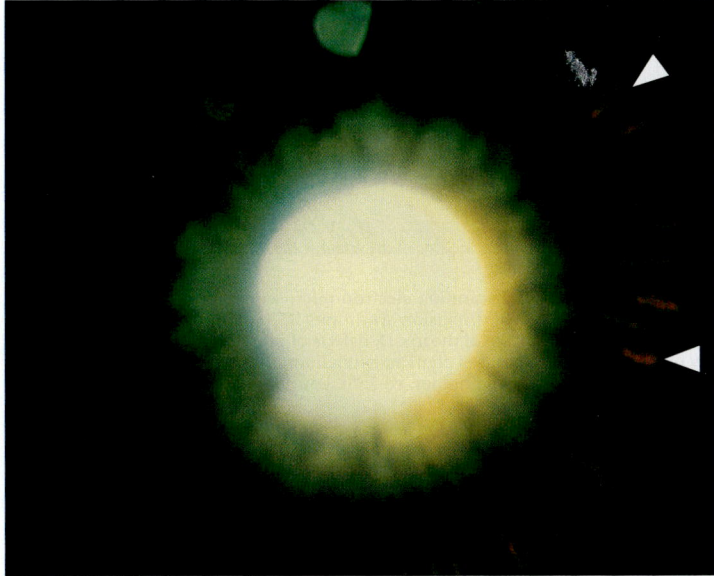

FIG. 224-1 ▉ **Transillumination defects *(arrowheads)*.** The radial, midperipheral, spoke-like iris transillumination defects typical of patients with pigmentary glaucoma correspond anatomically with zonular packets.

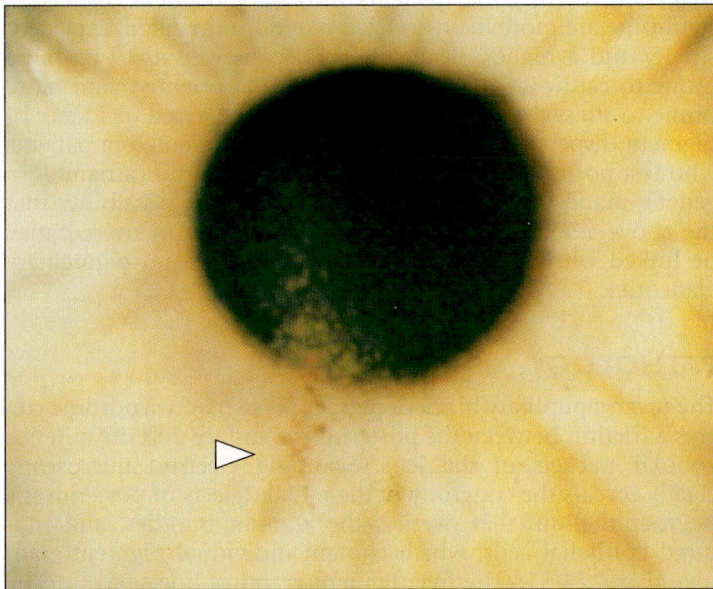

FIG. 224-2 ▉ **Unusually dense Krukenberg's spindle *(arrowhead)*.** The pattern represents pigment deposited on the corneal endothelium in a vertical spindle pattern and is probably the result of the action of aqueous convection currents.

tion as radial, slit-like defects (Fig. 224-1). Transillumination defects often are seen inferiorly first but may not be detectable early in the disease, or at all, in patients who have thick iris stroma.

The liberated pigment granules disperse with aqueous convection currents through the posterior and anterior chambers and collect in characteristic regions. Generally, the pigment assumes a narrow, vertical, spindle-shaped, brown band on the back of the central cornea, 1–2mm in width and 3–6mm in height, termed a *Krukenberg's spindle* (Fig. 224-2). With the slit lamp, the pigment often is seen widely scattered on the surface of the iris also; when viewed by gonioscopy through a dilated pupil, pigment collections also may be seen on the zonules, peripheral lens capsule, and anterior vitreous face (Fig. 224-3). Typically, a homogeneous collection of pigment occurs in the trabecular meshwork, which initially is confined to the pigmented meshwork and is more dense inferiorly. With increasing dispersion, the pigment collection extends onto the nonpigmented meshwork and anterior to Schwalbe's line (Sampaoelesi's line; Fig. 224-4). The pigment may disappear substantially and is much faded by the sixth and seventh decade of life in most patients, the result of a cessation of active pigment dispersion coupled with the eyes' natural phagocytic and clearing mechanisms. However, in later life, pigment dispersion syndrome may overlap with exfoliation syndrome in the same patient, creating confusion in the natural course of pigment signs, and likely manifesting as a comorbid condition.[18]

Compared with normal eyes, those affected by pigment dispersion syndrome have a deeper anterior chamber, larger iris, a more posterior iris insertion, and often a posterior concavity of the iris associated with increased midiridolenticular touch. Pigment dispersion syndrome is only rarely seen in African–Americans and Asians. The generally thicker, more rigid, and less crypted iris stroma of African–Americans' and Asians' eyes may inhibit the de-

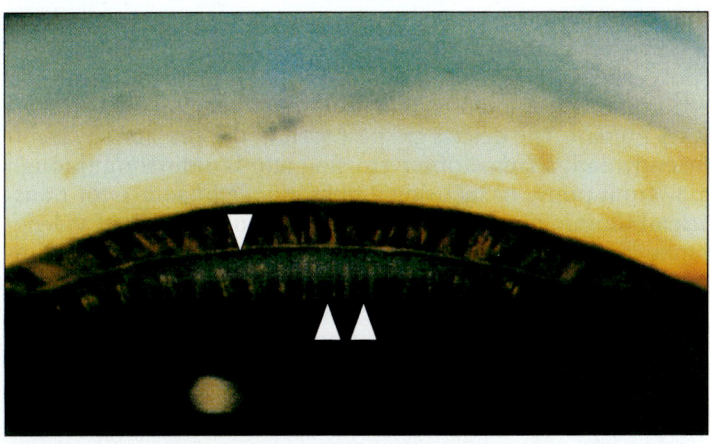

FIG. 224-3 ▉ **Gonioscopic view of pigmentary glaucoma.** The patient's dilated pupil shows dense pigment accumulation on anterior *(arrowhead)* and posterior *(double arrowheads)* zonular packets.

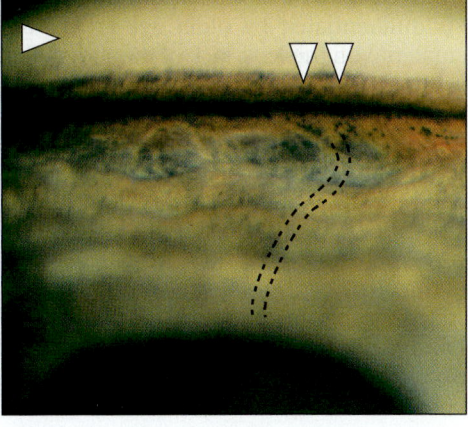

FIG. 224-4 ▉ **Gonioscopic view of pigmentary glaucoma.** The patient has a wide, open anterior chamber angle, which shows a back-bowed peripheral iris *(dotted lines)* and dense band of pigment on trabecular meshwork *(arrowhead)* and Schwalbe's line (Sampaoelesi's line) *(double arrowheads)*.

velopment of pigment dispersion syndrome. It may be that an inherently flaccid iris is a prerequisite.[14] The back-bowed iris, seen best as a posterior concavity on gonioscopic examination, is likely pathogenic of the pigment dispersion and, if so, should be the first observable clinical trait. The posterior concavity is eliminated after iridectomy,[6] is reduced by prolonged nonblinking,[11] can be altered by either miotic or cycloplegic drugs,[5] and disappears spontaneously in patients by 45 or so years of age.

With prolonged pressure elevation, optic nerve head and visual field changes are produced. The pattern of glaucomatous damage is typical of primary open-angle glaucoma. Optic nerve cupping and visual field damage proceed progressively with uncontrolled intraocular pressure (IOP) and have been reported to occur in the absence of elevated IOP in a pattern akin to normal-tension glaucoma in patients of 60–80 years of age.

DIAGNOSIS AND ANCILLARY TESTING

Identification of patients who have pigment dispersion syndrome consists of examination for, and detection of, the clinical signs. The Krukenberg's spindle is best seen with indirect slit-lamp illumination and specular scatter. Its density usually correlates with the intensity of pigment in the meshwork but is sometimes only faintly perceptible and may disappear late in the disease.[4,5,8] The trabecular pigmentation is identified easily using routine gonioscopy, and the uniform distribution and homogeneous pattern helps differentiate it from other conditions that produce pigment, like pseudoexfoliation and uveitis, which are associated more commonly with patchy trabecular pigmentation and clumps of cells and debris. The heavy trabecular pigmentation is the most consistent and reliable finding of the disease and the one most heavily relied on for the diagnosis. Pigment accumulation on the ocular surfaces, such as the iris, zonules, ciliary body, and anterior vitreous, is less common, and when present always is accompanied by very dense pigment in the trabecular meshwork.

Iris transillumination defects in a midperipheral, radial, spoke-like configuration is characteristic of pigment dispersion syndrome, but it often is difficult to demonstrate and is not always present. The defects are best seen at the slit lamp by a sufficiently dark-adapted observer using retroillumination through a 3–4mm pupil, or by using a fiberoptic light source for transscleral illumination. The research technique of infrared videography has demonstrated even greater sensitivity. It may be impossible to transilluminate eyes of patients who have dense iris stroma, even with considerable iris pigment epithelial loss,[14] so demonstration of transillumination is supportive of but not required for the diagnosis. The posterior concavity of the iris, when present, is an extremely supportive finding, because it is the likely precursor to all subsequent events in the pigment dispersion cascade.

DIFFERENTIAL DIAGNOSIS

Several glaucomatous conditions are associated with excessive liberation and dispersion of pigment. Pseudoexfoliation (see Chapter 223) usually is differentiated by older age group, the presence of exfoliation material on the lens, lack of the spoke-like, midperipheral iris transillumination defects (defects in pseudoexfoliation usually are confined to the pupillary border), and generally more patchy distribution of trabecular pigment.[19] Glaucoma secondary to iris chaffing from malpositioned posterior chamber intraocular lens haptics is differentiated by the history and pattern of iris transillumination that corresponds to the intraocular lens configuration.[20] Uveitis (see Chapter 226) produces signs of inflammation such as anterior chamber cells, keratic precipitates on the cornea, and synechiae that are not present with pigmentary glaucoma.[19] Melanosis and melanoma (see Chapter 230) are differentiated easily. A form of primary open-angle glaucoma associated with pigment liberation has been described in predomi-

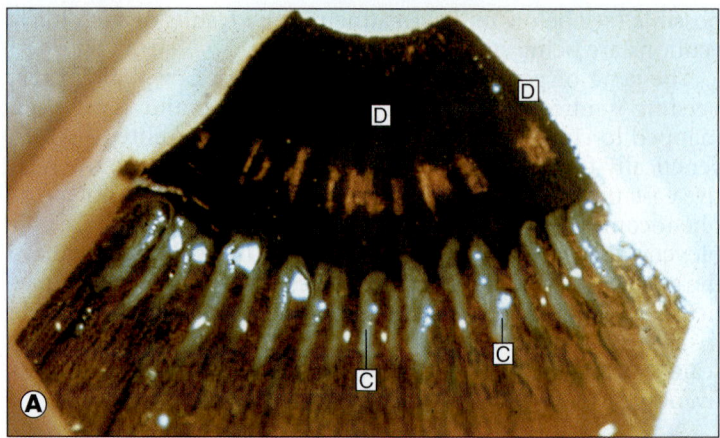
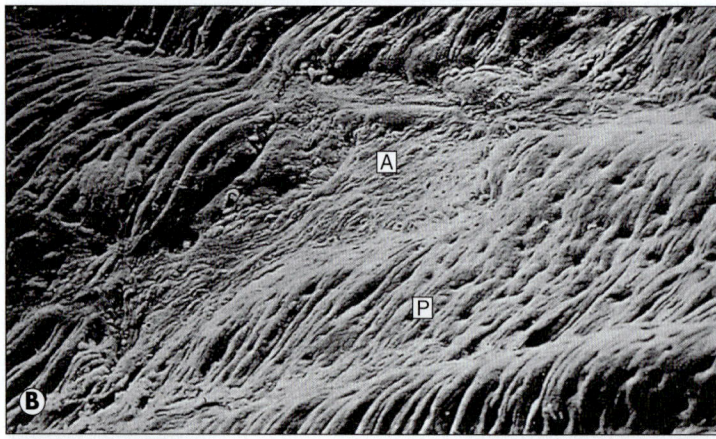

FIG. 224-5 ■ Gross and scanning electron microscopic views. **A,** Gross specimen from patient with pigment dispersion syndrome. **B,** A scanning electron microscopy view of the posterior surface of the iris. *D,* defects of pigment epithelium in iris; *C,* ciliary processes; *A,* area devoid of pigment epithelium; *P,* posterior surface of iris. (From Yanoff M, Fine BS. Ocular pathology, ed 5. St. Louis, Mosby; 2002.)

nantly older, hyperopic African–American women, but lacks iris transillumination and the iris back-bowing, and is not confused easily with pigmentary glaucoma.[14]

SYSTEMIC ASSOCIATIONS

The manifestations of pigment dispersion syndrome and pigmentary glaucoma generally are considered to be exclusively ocular, with no well-accepted systemic associations. It has been suggested recently that patients who have pigment dispersion syndrome are more likely to have systemic adrenergic hypersensitivity and a higher mean intelligence, as well as to be more prone to cardiovascular disease, more goal oriented, and more prone to stress than control patients.[2] An increased incidence of pigment dispersion syndrome has been documented in patients who test positive for the ability to taste phenylthiocarbamide, a genetic marker.[1] This genetic link increases the possibility that the above associations, and perhaps others yet uncovered, may be linked with pigment dispersion syndrome and pigmentary glaucoma.

PATHOLOGY

The reverse pupillary block of pigment dispersion syndrome creates a friction between the posterior iris surface and the anterior zonular packets of the lens. Scanning electron microscopy clearly reveals the congruity of the radial defects of posterior iris neuroepithelium that overlies the zonular bundles, and ruptured epithelial cells, which contain individual pigment granules (Fig. 224-5).[5] The free pigment granules line spaces of the uveal meshwork and the inner portion of the corneoscleral trabecular meshwork. Intracellular pigment accumulation is seen in the deeper portions of uveal and trabecular meshwork cells

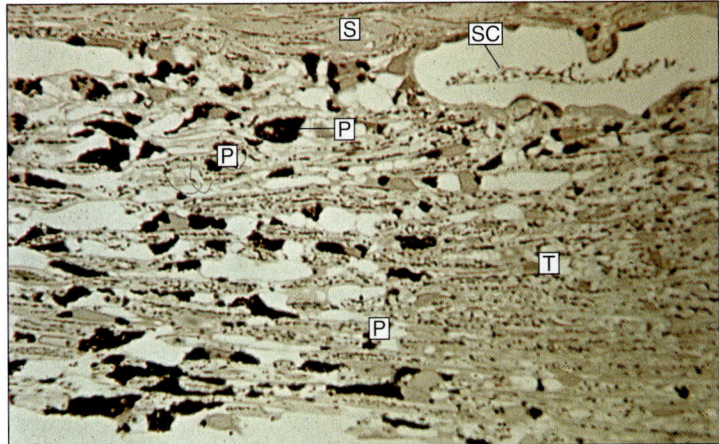

FIG. 224-6 ▪ **Pigment dispersion syndrome.** Melanin pigment *(P)* is present within the endothelial cells lining the beams of the trabecular meshwork *(T)*. *S*, Stroma; *SC*, Schlemm's canal. (Courtesy of Dr. BS Fine.)

(Fig. 224-6). The collapse of trabecular beams and increased loss of cells that line the beams mirror the pathology seen in specimens from primary open-angle glaucoma.[15-17] However, pigment accumulation on and within corneal endothelial cells in pigment dispersion syndrome seems to create no change in cellular morphology or function.

TREATMENT

The major goal of management of pigmentary glaucoma is to lower IOP to prevent optic nerve damage. All ocular hypotensive medications for open-angle glaucoma also are effective in pigmentary glaucoma and, thus, may be employed, although the miotic agents are tolerated less well in the age group affected. Patients respond well initially to laser trabeculoplasty, probably because the pigment facilitates the effect of the argon laser, but the effect may be short lived, perhaps because of continued dispersion of the pigment and progressive trabecular damage. When these modalities fail, filtration surgery is indicated; a higher percentage of patients with pigmentary glaucoma go on to filtration surgery compared with those who have primary open-angle glaucoma. The success rate of filtration surgery is good.[19] Pigmentary glaucoma responded better than chronic open-angle glaucoma to trabecular aspiration surgery, implying that removal of free and accumulated melanin granules is beneficial to IOP control in pigmentary glaucoma.[21]

If the assumption of the mechanism of disease in both pigment dispersion syndrome and pigmentary glaucoma is correct, then theoretically it should be possible to prevent the progression from pigment dispersion syndrome into pigmentary glaucoma and the progression from early pigmentary glaucoma into more advanced pigmentary glaucoma by prevention of the pigment dispersion process itself. Indeed, the posterior bowing of the iris seen in cases of pigment dispersion syndrome and pigmentary glaucoma may be reversed, a reversal easily achieved using laser iridectomy.[6] The rush of pigment from the anterior chamber to the posterior chamber witnessed at the laser slit lamp after iridectomy dramatically confirms that the reverse pupillary block has been eliminated. Iridectomy in patients with pigmentary glaucoma results in a significant (65%) reduction in aqueous melanin granules.[22] Unfortunately, this intervention as a prophylactic management in pigment dispersion syndrome or as a palliative management in pigmentary glaucoma has not yielded measurable benefit in the 10 years since its introduction. Similarly, management with miotic agents, delivered as drops, ointments, or sustained release inserts, may tighten the iris and flatten its contour, and perhaps reduce the iridolenticular contact and zonular friction. Long-term use of miotic drugs may result in a reduced volume of dispersed pigment, progressively

fewer iris transillumination defects, and easier pressure control. However, these drugs are tolerated poorly by young patients because of induced myopia, and a greater risk of detachment exists in the presence of myopia and lattice degeneration.[19]

COURSE AND OUTCOMES

The natural history of pigment dispersion syndrome and pigmentary glaucoma is well charted. The onset of clinically manifest disease usually occurs at about 25 years of age. Active pigment dispersion seemingly accelerates during the following decade until it tapers off at about 40–50 years of age, presumably because of the development of relative pupillary block and the loss of accommodative ability. Signs of pigment dispersion syndrome and pigmentary glaucoma may regress—pigment deposition in the trabecular meshwork, the corneal endothelium, and surface of the iris may clear substantially or even disappear[8]; iris transillumination defects may fill in.[5] Clinical expression of pigment dispersion syndrome, consequently, is much less common in those 60–80 years of age.

Although many patients with pigment dispersion syndrome may "burn out" in later years, this is rare among patients with pigmentary glaucoma followed prospectively over long periods. Conversely, pigmentary glaucoma generally exhibits a more aggressive character and patients come to filtration surgery earlier compared with those who have primary open-angle glaucoma.[4,5,8] Because pigmentary glaucoma often has a very aggressive nature and because no proof exists that the transition from pigment dispersion syndrome to pigmentary glaucoma can be aborted using therapeutic interventions (such as prophylactic iridectomies), patients who have pigment dispersion syndrome must be followed at least yearly with pressure checks and optic nerve examinations.

REFERENCES

1. Andersen JS, Pralea AM, DelBono EA, *et al.* A gene responsible for the pigment dispersion syndrome maps to chromosome 7q35–q36. Arch Ophthalmol. 1997; 115: 384–8.
2. Ritch R. Going forward to work backward. Arch Ophthalmol. 1997;115:404–6.
3. Sugar HS, Barbour FA. Pigmentary glaucoma: a rare clinical entity. Am J Ophthalmol. 1949;32:90–2.
4. Sugar HS. Pigmentary glaucoma: a 25-year review. Am J Ophthalmol. 1966;62: 499–507.
5. Campbell DG. Pigmentary dispersion and glaucoma: a new theory. Arch Ophthalmol. 1979;97:1667–72.
6. Karickhoff JR. Reverse pupillary block in pigmentary glaucoma: follow-up and new developments. Ophthalmic Surg. 1993;24:562–3.
7. Ritch R, Steinberger D, Liebmann JM. Prevalence of pigment dispersion syndrome in a population undergoing glaucoma screening. Am J Ophthalmol. 1993; 115:707–10.
8. Richter CU, Richardson TM, Grant WM. Pigmentary dispersion syndrome and pigmentary glaucoma: a prospective study of the natural history. Arch Ophthalmol. 1986;104:211–5.
9. Potash SD, Tello C, Liebmann J, Ritch R. Ultrasound biomicroscopy in pigment dispersion syndrome. Ophthalmology. 1994;101:332–9.
10. Pavlin CJ, Harasiewicz K, Foster FS. Posterior iris bowing in pigmentary dispersion syndrome caused by accommodation. Am J Ophthalmol. 1994;118:114–6.
11. Liebmann JM, Tello C, Chew SJ, *et al.* Prevention of blinking alters iris configuration in pigment dispersion syndrome and in normal eyes. Ophthalmology. 1995; 102:446–55.
12. Weseley P, Libermann J, Walsh JB, Ritch R. Lattice degeneration of the retina and the pigment dispersion syndrome. Am J Ophthalmol. 1992;114:539–43.
13. Jensen PK, Nissen O, Kessing SV. Exercise and reversed pupillary block in pigmentary glaucoma. Am J Ophthalmol. 1995;120:110–2.
14. Semple HC, Ball SF. Pigmentary glaucoma in the black population. Am J Ophthalmol. 1990;109:518–22.
15. Alvarado JA, Murphy CG. Outflow obstruction in pigmentary and primary open angle glaucoma. Arch Ophthalmol. 1992;110:1769–78.
16. Grant WM. Experimental aqueous perfusion in enucleated human eyes. Arch Ophthalmol. 1963;69:783–801.
17. Richardson TM, Hutchinson BT, Grant WM. The outflow tract in pigmentary glaucoma: a light and electron microscopic study. Arch Ophthalmol. 1977;95:1015–25.
18. Mudumbai R, Liebmann JM, Ritch R. Combined exfoliation and pigment dispersion: an overlap syndrome. Trans Am Ophthalmol Soc. 1999;97:297–314.
19. Shields MB. Textbook of glaucoma, ed 3. Baltimore: Williams & Wilkins; 1992: 276–84.
20. Woodhams JT, Lester JC. Pigmentary dispersion glaucoma secondary to posterior chamber intra-ocular lenses. Ann Ophthalmol. 1984;16:852–5.
21. Jacobi PC, Dietlein TS, Krieglstein GK. Effect of trabecular aspiration on intraocular pressure in pigment dispersion syndrome and pigmentary glaucoma. Ophthalmology. 2000;107(3):417–21.
22. Allingham RR, Loftsdottir M, Gottfredsdottir MS, *et al.* Pseudoexfoliation syndrome in Icelandic families. Br J Ophthalmol. 2001;85:702–7.

225 Neovascular Glaucoma

MAHER M. FANOUS

DEFINITION
- A unique form of glaucoma resulting from ocular or extraocular disease that produces ischemia of the eye.

KEY FEATURES
- Neovascularization of the iris or anterior chamber.
- Elevated intraocular pressure.

ASSOCIATED FEATURES
- Decreased vision.
- Bullous keratopathy.
- Ectropion uveae.
- Anterior chamber inflammation.
- Synechial angle closure.
- Cupping of the optic nerve.

INTRODUCTION

Neovascular glaucoma (NVG) is a relatively common and potentially devastating disorder that occurs when new vessels proliferate on the iris and anterior chamber angle. The common insults that promote NVG are severe retinal hypoxia and retinal capillary nonperfusion. Invasion of the anterior chamber by a fibrovascular membrane initially obstructs aqueous outflow in an open-angle form and later contracts to produce secondary synechial angle-closure glaucoma. The key to successful treatment is early detection of the neovascularization process. Panretinal photocoagulation remains the most effective initial therapy, which reduces the stimulus for ocular neovascularization and the development of secondary angle-closure glaucoma. Once the anterior chamber is closed by synechiae, however, filtering should be considered.

EPIDEMIOLOGY AND PATHOGENESIS

In 1906, Coats[1] described new vessel formation in irides of eyes that had central retinal vein occlusion (CRVO). The term *neovascular glaucoma* was proposed by Weiss *et al.*[2] and is based on the presence of new vessels on the iris. Knowledge of disorders that predispose to the development of neovascularization of the iris helps the ophthalmologist identify patients at risk for developing NVG. Diabetic retinopathy and CRVO are by far the most common conditions that predispose to the development of ocular neovascularization. Other common causes are uveitis, central retinal artery occlusion, long-standing retinal detachment, and intraocular tumors; there are also two extraocular causes—carotid artery obstructive disease and carotid cavernous fistula. Brown *et al.*[3] concluded that 36% of all cases of NVG arise from CRVO, 32% from proliferative diabetic retinopathy, and 13% from carotid artery occlusive disease. About one third of patients who have ischemic CRVO develop NVG. The incidence of neovascularization of the iris in patients who have diabetic retinopathy correlates with the extent of capillary dropout and retinal hypoxia. Diabetic patients who undergo vitrectomy, lensectomy, intracapsular cataract extraction, and extracapsular cataract extraction with posterior capsulotomy are at a higher risk of developing NVG.

The most widely accepted theory explaining the development of neovascularization is that the hypoxic retina produces a diffusible angiogenic factor that stimulates new vessel proliferation. Since 1948, many investigators have searched for this postulated angiogenic factor, and recent advances in molecular biology have led to the identification of several possible factors. Vascular endothelial growth factor (VEGF) represents the leading candidate. VEGF receptors are present on retinal capillary endothelial cells, and VEGF triggers growth in these cells. Endothelial cells have not been proved to produce VEGF thus far. In a nonhuman primate model with experimentally induced CRVO and neovascularization of the iris, VEGF and VEGF-mRNA levels were markedly elevated in ischemic retina.[4] A strong temporal and spatial correlation occurs between intraocular VEGF protein levels and the extent of neovascularization. Elevated intraocular VEGF levels have been found in humans who have proliferative diabetic retinopathy and neovascularization of the iris.[5]

Growing evidence supports a central role for VEGF in the process of iris neovascularization. Tolentino *et al.*[6] showed that injection of recombinant human VEGF is sufficient to produce neovascularization in a nonhuman primate model. Neutralizing anti-VEGF antibodies prevent the development of iris neovascularization induced by retinal ischemia in a monkey model.[4] Systemic administration of interferon-α in cynomolgus monkeys causes inhibition and regression of neovascularization.[7]

OCULAR MANIFESTATIONS

The earliest sign of vascular proliferation appears at the pupillary margin. Neovascularization of the iris may be difficult to detect in its earliest stages. Slit-lamp biomicroscopy reveals fine, tortuous, randomly oriented tufts of vessels on the surface of the iris, near the pupillary margin. These tufts may be obscured in dark irides and more obvious in lighter irides. Neovascularization characteristically progresses from the pupillary margin toward the angle (Fig. 225-1) of undilated pupils, but angle neovascularization in the absence of pupillary involvement may occur. Repeated gonioscopy is indicated in eyes at high risk for the development of NVG. As vascular proliferation develops, biomicroscopy of the anterior chamber shows cells and flare. Gonioscopy reveals new vessels that grow from the circumferential artery of the ciliary body onto the surface of the iris and onto the surface of the wall of the angle.

The vessels cross the angle recess and grow forward over the ciliary body band and scleral spur onto the trabecular meshwork, which imparts a characteristic red flush (Fig. 225-2). Early in the course of anterior segment neovascularization, the intraocular pressure (IOP) often is normal. The new blood vessels

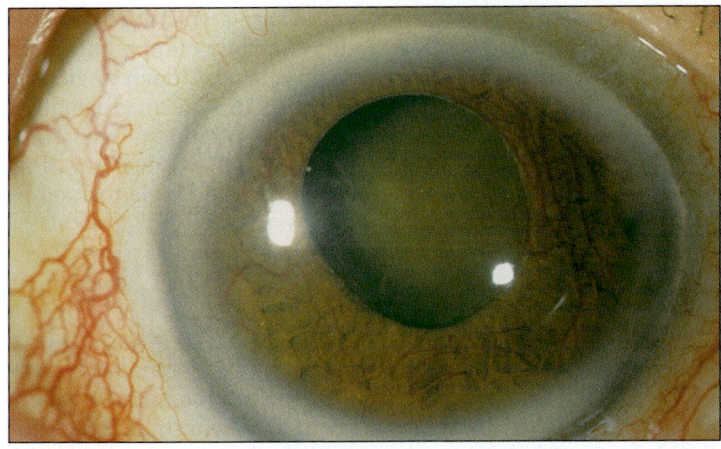

FIG. 225-1 ■ Neovascularization of the iris. Note the florid neovascular proliferation at the pupillary margin, which grows in random orientation on the iris surface.

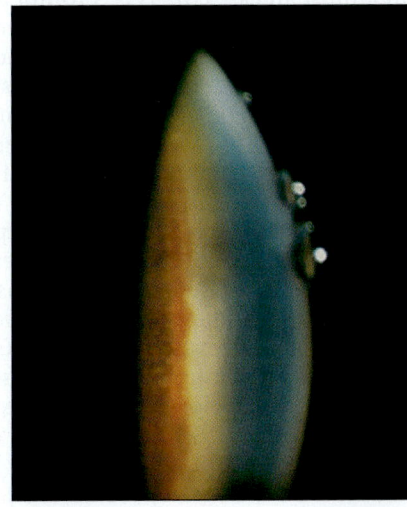

FIG. 225-2 ■
Neovascularization of the angle. Gonioscopic view of new vessels that cover the trabecular meshwork and impart a characteristic red flush.

arborize to form a fibrovascular membrane (invisible on gonioscopy) that gives rise to a secondary open-angle glaucoma. The final stage is characterized by contraction of the fibrovascular membrane, which pulls the peripheral iris over the trabecular meshwork and results in variable degrees of synechial angle closure. Ectropion uveae and hyphema occur frequently. Ectropion uveae results from radial traction along the surface of the iris, which pulls the posterior pigmented layer of the iris around the pupillary margin onto the anterior iris surface. It is at this stage that patients may present with the dramatic onset of pain secondary to elevated IOP. Patients experience severely reduced visual acuity (to counting fingers), accompanied by corneal edema and anterior chamber inflammation.

DIAGNOSIS

Evaluation of the medical history is crucial to the identification of patients at risk for the development of NVG. Diabetes mellitus, hypertension, arteriosclerosis, and a previous history of vision loss indicative of CRVO or retinal detachment are important and must be identified, as these disorders predispose to the development of NVG. Recent surgery may increase the risk in predisposed individuals. It is imperative that a posterior segment examination be performed in all patients to identify concomitant retinal disease. The diagnosis of NVG is made based on the clinical examination. Careful slit-lamp and gonioscopic examinations are usually sufficient to make the diagnosis. An undilated pupil is helpful. The goal is to establish the diagnosis well before angle structures become involved and elevated IOP or synechial angle closure occurs.

Involvement of the anterior chamber angle sometimes occurs before the appearance of neovascularization of the iris. These vessels typically run on the iris surface, follow a nonradial course, and may cross the scleral spur. Thus, gonioscopy must be performed on every patient at risk for the development of NVG. In most instances, however, small tufts of neovascularization are noted first at the pupillary margin. This tendency for initial involvement of the pupillary margin appears to result from aqueous flow dynamics, whereby angiogenic factors produced in the posterior segment have the most contact with the pupillary margin.

Occasionally, early neovascularization may be missed when the new vessels are fine and thin, the iris is darkly pigmented, or pressure from the gonioscopy lens reduces the caliber of the new vessels and renders them clinically inapparent. Frequent follow-up of patients at high risk for NVG enables the earliest detection of new vessels in difficult cases. Fluorescein angiography of the iris may be used to demonstrate the presence of new vessels before they become apparent at the slit lamp.

The b wave–a wave amplitude ratio of the bright-flash, dark-adapted electroretinogram may help predict which eyes will develop NVG following CRVO.[8] This ratio was found to be less than 1.0 (average 0.84) in eyes that developed NVG after ischemic CRVO. In contrast, the b wave–a wave amplitude ratio was always greater than 1.0 in eyes that did not develop NVG following CRVO.

DIFFERENTIAL DIAGNOSIS

Several entities present with prominent iris vessels and elevated IOP (Box 225-1). In these entities, the cause of elevated IOP is a mechanism other than growth of new vessels and an associated contractile membrane over the chamber angle. A detailed history and slit-lamp examination can, in the majority of cases, distinguish these entities from NVG.

Postsurgical engorgement of iris vessels is one of the more common entities that may be confused with NVG. After intraocular surgery, vessel dilatation secondary to intraocular inflammation may occur, which might be confused with NVG in diabetic patients. Postsurgical dilatation of iris vessels usually resolves as the secondary uveitis is treated with topical corticosteroids, whereas neovascularization of the iris does not respond to such therapy. Similarly, vascular congestion of normal iris vessels secondary to uveitis from various causes may simulate NVG because of concomitant IOP elevation.

Fuchs' heterochromic iridocyclitis may present with elevated IOP and iris neovascularization.[9] The glaucoma in this entity is secondary to uveitis intrinsic to the disease process and not a result of the presence of new vessels. Neovascularization has been found in the chamber angle as well as on the iris. The new vessels are thin and fragile and may result in a hyphema after paracentesis (Amsler's sign). It is thought that neovascularization occurs as a result of iris ischemia.

Essential iris atrophy may present with elevated IOP associated with new vessel formation (see Chapters 223 and 230).[10]

Acute angle-closure glaucoma may be confused with advanced, late-stage NVG. Both may present with markedly elevated IOP and an edematous cornea. In acute angle-closure glaucoma, engorged iris vessels may take on the appearance of rubeosis iridis, which suggests advanced NVG. Gonioscopy of the fellow eye may help differentiate the two entities, as the fellow eye tends to be narrow or potentially occludable in angle-closure glaucoma.

Congenital iris tufts and prominent iris vessels in lightly pigmented irides may sometimes mimic neovascularization. Prominent iris vessels typically are radial, lie within the iris stroma, and, when in the chamber angle, do not cross the scleral spur. In contrast, new vessels typically do not follow a radial course, lie on the surface of the iris, and may cross the scleral spur.

Retinopathy of prematurity may present with engorged iris vessels as a result of plus disease and concomitant angle-closure glaucoma from a retrolental membrane. *Plus disease* refers to arteriolar tortuosity and venous engorgement of the posterior pole and iris secondary to vascular shunting. Retinopathy of prematurity is distinguished from NVG on the basis of characteristic fundus findings and the clinical setting.

PATHOLOGY

The histology of angle structures in eyes with NVG does not differ significantly with regard to the different causes of the disorder. The neovascular process begins at the pupillary margin and occasionally at the iris periphery, where new vessels arise from preexisting capillaries. These vessels are thin walled, have fenestrated endothelial cells, and leak fluorescein on angiography. This is in contrast to normal blood vessels in the iris, which are thick walled and impermeable to fluorescein because of the presence of endothelial tight junctions. New vessels initially may proliferate on the iris surface with little structural support. However, as the disease progresses, an iridic membrane that consists of myofibroblasts forms over the new vessels and iris surface.[11] The iridic membrane may contract, because of the presence of myofibroblasts, which results in synechial angle closure, ectropion uveae, and flattening of the normal topography of the anterior iris surface (Fig. 225-3). This myofibroblastic membrane is present whenever new vessels are seen but is invisible on gonioscopy. The presence of this clinically inapparent membrane is why many eyes that have an apparent open angle and only mild or no angle neovascularization or synechia formation have elevated IOP. In some cases, the iridic membrane may stimulate, perhaps by contractile force, growth of corneal endothelium and Descemet's membrane over a pseudoangle formed by synechial closure of the chamber angle.

TREATMENT

The key to successful management of NVG is early diagnosis. Recognition of neovascularization of the iris is crucial so that preventive treatment can be initiated before the anterior chamber angle is closed by peripheral anterior synechiae. Once the florid, intractable final stage is established, the eye is blind, with very high IOP and painful bullous keratopathy. If the NVG is secondary to carotid artery or other systemic disease, it is important to evaluate and treat the primary systemic condition.

Panretinal photocoagulation (PRP) is the first line of therapy in almost all cases of NVG. Prompt application of PRP has been shown to effect regression of anterior and posterior segment neovascularization and to reduce the risk of developing neovascularization of the iris in eyes that have retinal vascular disease.[12] In the open-angle glaucoma stage and early angle-closure glaucoma stage, PRP may reverse IOP elevation. For eyes that have advanced synechial angle closure of the anterior chamber with some potentially useful vision, PRP may eliminate the stimulus for neovascularization, which prepares the eye for filtering surgery and the prevention of further visual loss.

Panretinal cryotherapy is an alternative to PRP in eyes that have cloudy media and in eyes for which complete PRP fails to halt the progression of neovascularization.[13] Goniophotocoagulation may be used as an adjunct to PRP to reduce neovascularization in the angle before it is closed by synechiae, but generally the effects are only temporary.[14]

The treatment of NVG is directed by the visual potential. Any usable vision, even 20/400 (6/120) or less in a monocular patient, is worth preserving.

The role of glaucoma filtering surgery in NVG is to prevent pressure-induced injury to the optic nerve and, theoretically, to improve vascular perfusion. Before glaucoma surgery, every attempt is made to reduce or eliminate the stimulus for angiogenesis using PRP. Enough time must elapse between PRP and glaucoma surgery for the eye to quiet down; this reduces the risk of intraoperative and postoperative bleeding and severe intraocular inflammation. The importance of complete preoperative PRP to the success of glaucoma filtering surgery in patients who have NVG cannot be overstressed.

Of special importance is the use of intraoperative cautery to achieve hemostasis and avoid bleeding. Direct cauterization of the peripheral iris before iridectomy may reduce the risk of bleeding. Variable success rates have been reported after conventional filtering surgery in patients who have NVG. Allen *et al.*[15] reported IOP control in 67% of patients who had NVG and underwent trabeculectomy or posterior lip sclerectomy after PRP. Tsai *et al.*[16] reported a high risk of long-term failure with 5-fluorouracil filtering surgery; 12 of 34 NVG patients (35%) lost light perception vision, and 8 patients (24%) developed phthisis bulbi over a 5-year follow-up period. Younger age (≤50 years) and type I diabetes mellitus are significant risk factors for early surgical failure. Skuta *et al.*[17] described the use of mitomycin C with trabeculectomy in patients who had NVG.

Glaucoma drainage implants are also used for the primary surgical treatment of NVG. Seton procedures place the effective sclerostomy inside the anterior chamber away from the angle, which maintains a patent fistula between the anterior chamber and an equatorial bleb. Sidoti *et al.*[18] cited life-table success rates of 79% and 56% at 12 and 18 months, respectively, following Baerveldt glaucoma implantation surgery for NVG. Success was

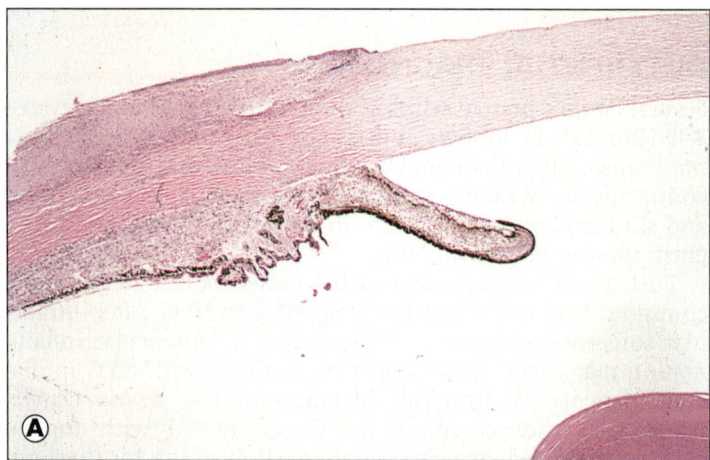

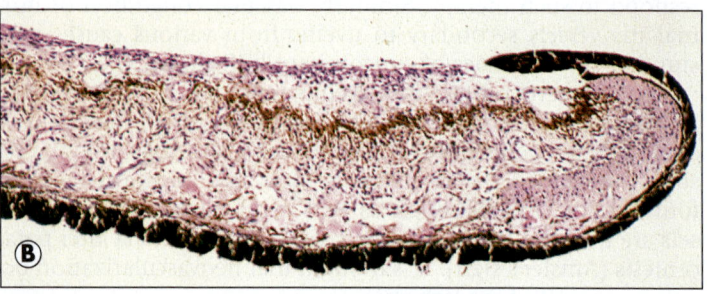

FIG. 225-3 ■ Neovascularization of the iris. **A**, Note the peripheral anterior synechia, secondary angle closure, and tissue anterior to the anterior border layer of the iris (the last of which constitutes iris neovascularization). **B**, High-power view of iris neovascularization and ectropion uveae in **A**. (From Yanoff M, Fine BS. Ocular pathology, ed 5. St. Louis: Mosby, 2002.)

defined as a final IOP of 6–21mmHg (0.8–2.8kPa) without additional glaucoma surgery or devastating complication. Loss of light perception occurred in 31% of patients. Cox model regression survival analysis demonstrated young patient age and poorer preoperative visual acuity as significant predictors of surgical failure. Another study that evaluated the use of the single-plate Molteno implant for NVG reported success rates of 62% at 1 year, 52.9% at 2 years, 43.1% at 3 years, 30.8% at 4 years, and 10.3% at 5 years; loss of light perception was seen in 29 of 60 eyes (48%), and phthisis bulbi developed in 11 eyes (18%).[19]

Noninvasive techniques are employed to achieve patient comfort if the eye has no visual potential. Topically administered corticosteroids and cycloplegics may relieve ocular discomfort. Topical β-adrenergic blockers, α-adrenergic agonists, and carbonic anhydrase inhibitors may be used to reduce IOP. Miotic therapy is avoided, as it may aggravate intraocular inflammation and pain. Once the anterior chamber angle is closed, medical therapy alone may not provide long-term IOP control, and surgical intervention becomes necessary. Cyclocryotherapy has been advocated in the treatment of elevated IOP in NVG. Although the IOP can be controlled in a high percentage of patients who undergo the procedure, the long-term visual outcome is dismal; loss of light perception occurs in 58.5% of patients. In addition, the high incidence of major complications, which include anterior segment necrosis and phthisis bulbi (34%), means that its use in eyes that have visual potential is limited.[20] Other modalities of therapy to control IOP include diode and neodymium:yttrium-aluminum-garnet transscleral cyclophotocoagulation. Schuman et al.[21] reported a 39% success rate using the latter in patients who had advanced NVG.

In painful eyes that have poor visual potential, atropine and corticosteroid drops or cycloablation, retrobulbar alcohol injection, and enucleation may help achieve comfort.

COURSE AND OUTCOME

The natural course of NVG is uniformly one of complete loss of vision and the development of intractable, severe pain. The high degree of ocular morbidity and mortality in patients who have NVG emphasizes the severity of the underlying systemic conditions associated with diabetic retinopathy and CRVO, the main causes of this disorder. Usually, NVG occurs in patients burdened with serious systemic disease. Krupin et al.[22] and Mermoud et al.[19] cited mortality rates of 22% and 15% in patients who have NVG. Diabetes mellitus was the underlying cause of NVG in the majority of patients reported by the Diabetes Control and Complication Research Group,[23] which highlights the importance of effective blood-sugar control in patients who have diabetic retinopathy. The risk of progression of mild diabetic retinopathy and the development of proliferative diabetic retinopathy is reduced to half in patients using effective blood-sugar control.

NVG does not invariably follow the development of neovascularization of the iris. When such neovascularization is detected, it behooves the clinician to follow patients carefully with repeated slit-lamp examinations and undilated gonioscopy. Neovascularization of the iris has been reported to develop in 50% of patients who have proliferative diabetic retinopathy and in 60% of those who have the ischemic type of CRVO. It is imperative that PRP be applied promptly to ischemic retina to eliminate the stimulus for further neovascularization.

Visual loss in NVG is common and may be attributed to a combination of causes, including severe ocular ischemia with progression of the underlying retinal disease, glaucomatous optic nerve damage, cataract formation, corneal decompensation, and phthisis bulbi. The most common cause of surgical failure in patients who have NVG is related to progression of the underlying retinal disease, not to uncontrolled IOP.[16,18,22]

The ultimate solution for patients who have NVG lies in the development of new modalities of treatment designed to prevent the initiation of neovascularization. Murata et al.[24] recently showed that thiazolidinediones, a novel class of drugs that can be used to improve insulin resistance in type II diabetes, inhibit angiogenic responses to VEGF in vitro. Current research to develop pharmacological therapies targeted at the inhibition of angiogenic factors offers hope for the preservation of vision in patients at risk.

REFERENCES

1. Coats G. Further cases of thrombosis of the central vein. R London Ophthalmol Hosp Rep. 1906;16:516–64.
2. Weiss DI, Shaffner RN, Nehrenberg TR. Neovascular glaucoma complicating carotid-cavernous fistula. Arch Ophthalmol. 1963;69:304–7.
3. Brown GC, Magargal LE, Schachat A, Shah H. Neovascular glaucoma. Etiologic considerations. Ophthalmology. 1984;91:315–20.
4. Adamis AP, Shima DT, Tolentino MJ, et al. Inhibition of vascular endothelial growth factor prevents retinal ischemia-associated iris neovascularization in a nonhuman primate. Arch Ophthalmol. 1996;114:66–71.
5. Adamis AP, Miller JW, Bernal M-T, et al. Increased vascular endothelial growth factor levels in the vitreous of eyes with proliferative diabetic retinopathy. Am J Ophthalmol. 1994;118:445–50.
6. Tolentino MJ, Miller JW, Gragoudas ES, et al. Vascular endothelial growth factor is sufficient to produce iris neovascularization and neovascular glaucoma in a nonhuman primate. Arch Ophthalmol. 1996;114:964–70.
7. Miller JW, Stinson WG, Folkman J. Regression of experimental iris neovascularization with systemic alpha-interferon. Ophthalmology. 1993;100:9–14.
8. Sabates R, Hirose T, McNeel JW. Electroretinography in the prognosis and classification of central retinal vein occlusion. Arch Ophthalmol. 1983;101:232–5.
9. Perry HD, Yanoff M, Scheie NG. Rubeosis in Fuchs' heterochromic iridocyclitis. Arch Ophthalmol. 1975;93:337–9.
10. Jampol LM, Rosser MJ, Sears ML. Unusual aspects of progressive essential iris atrophy. Am J Ophthalmol. 1974;77:353–7.
11. John T, Sassani JW, Eagle RC. The myofibroblastic component of rubeosis iridis. Ophthalmology. 1983;90:721–8.
12. Cashwell LF, Marks WP. Panretinal photocoagulation in the management of neovascular glaucoma. South Med J. 1988;81:1364–8.
13. Vernon SA, Cheng H. Panretinal cryotherapy in neovascular disease. Br J Ophthalmol. 1988;72:401–5.
14. Simmons RJ, Depperman SR, Dueker DK. The role of gonio-photocoagulation in neovascularization of the anterior chamber angle. Ophthalmology. 1980; 87:79–82.
15. Allen RC, Bellows AR, Hutchinson BT, Murphy SD. Filtration surgery in the treatment of neovascular glaucoma. Ophthalmology. 1982;89:1181–7.
16. Tsai JC, Feuer WJ, Parrish RK II, Grajewski AL. 5-Fluorouracil filtering surgery and neovascular glaucoma. Long-term follow-up of the original study. Ophthalmology. 1995;102:887–93.
17. Skuta GL, Beeson CC, Higginbotham EJ, et al. Intraoperative mitomycin versus postoperative 5-fluorouracil in high-risk glaucoma filtering surgery. Ophthalmology. 1992;99:438–44.
18. Sidoti PA, Dunphy TR, Baerveldt G, et al. Experience with the Baerveldt glaucoma implant in treating neovascular glaucoma. Ophthalmology. 1995;102:1107–18.
19. Mermoud A, Salmon JF, Alexander P, et al. Molteno tube implantation for neovascular glaucoma. Long-term results and factors influencing the outcome. Ophthalmology. 1993;100:897–902.
20. Krupin T, Mitchell KB, Becker B. Cyclocryotherapy in neovascular glaucoma. Am J Ophthalmol. 1978;86:24–6.
21. Schuman JS, Bellows AR, Shingleton BJ, et al. Contact transscleral Nd:YAG laser cyclophotocoagulation: midterm results. Ophthalmology. 1992;99:1089–95.
22. Krupin T, Kaufman P, Mandell AI, et al. Long-term results of valve implants in filtering surgery for eyes with neovascular glaucoma. Am J Ophthalmol. 1983;95: 775–82.
23. Diabetes Control and Complications Research Group. The effect of intensive treatment of diabetes on the development and progression of long-term complications in insulin-dependent diabetes mellitus. N Engl J Med. 1993;329:977–86.
24. Murata T, Hata Y, Ishibashi T, et al. Response of experimental retinal neovascularization to thiazolidinediones. Arch Ophthalmol. 2001;119:709–17.

CHAPTER

226 Ocular Inflammatory and Steroid-Induced Glaucoma

IVAN GOLDBERG

DEFINITION
- Characteristic glaucomatous optic neuropathy associated with ocular inflammation or exposure to corticosteroids.

KEY FEATURES
- Optic disc pallor and cupping.
- Nerve fiber bundle perimetric defects.
- Evidence of inflammation involving one or more global tissues.
- Past or continuing exposure to corticosteroids.

ASSOCIATED FEATURE
- Variably raised or fluctuating intraocular pressure.

TABLE 226-1

AQUEOUS FLOW AND ASSOCIATED INTRAOCULAR PRESSURE LEVELS IN THE PRESENCE OF INTRAOCULAR INFLAMMATION

| Aqueous Production | Total Outflow | | Intraocular Pressure Level |
	Trabecular Meshwork	Uveoscleral (Unconventional)	
Normal	Low Low–normal	Normal High	High Low
Low	Low–normal	Normal–high Low–normal	Low Normal–high
High	Normal Low	Normal–high Normal	Normal–high

INTRODUCTION

Ocular inflammation or exposure to corticosteroids can cause characteristic glaucomatous optic disc and visual field damage by elevating intraocular pressure (IOP) or by causing ischemia or infiltration of the optic nerve head.

To be effective, management requires precise diagnosis of the inflammation and then treatment of both the inflammation and the underlying cause (when possible). When IOP is raised, the mechanism of that elevation must be determined, allowing relevant measures to control it.

Patients may have marked symptoms and signs facilitating detection and diagnosis, or they may have none. The clinical course may be acute, subacute, unpredictably relapsing, or chronic. Management of both the inflammation and the associated glaucoma is often challenging, especially because the mechanisms for the glaucoma may change with time, requiring parallel changes in the therapeutic approach.

PATHOPHYSIOLOGY

The relationship between IOP and inflammation is complex. At any one time, IOP depends on the comparative rates of aqueous production and drainage (Table 226-1). Both these processes and the intraocular circulation of aqueous can be altered by inflammation, its effects on the ocular tissues involved, and its treatment.

Two misconceptions are common:
- That a rise in IOP is caused directly and only by inflammation. To allow focused and effective treatment, the mechanisms for the raised IOP must be understood and reevaluated throughout the management process.
- That disc pallor and cupping are attributable solely to a raised or fluctuating IOP. Vasculitis, rheological problems, or infiltrations associated with inflammatory conditions may contribute to glaucomatous damage by optic nerve head ischemia.[1]

BOX 226-1

Possible Causes of Raised Intraocular Pressure

SECONDARY OPEN-ANGLE GLAUCOMA
Trabecular meshwork obstruction
Canal of Schlemm and episcleral venous outflow obstruction
Corticosteroid-induced elevation of intraocular pressure
Hypersecretion
Permanent, direct trabecular meshwork tissue damage
Post-trabecular outflow damage

PRE-EXISTING PRIMARY OPEN-ANGLE GLAUCOMA

SECONDARY ANGLE-CLOSURE GLAUCOMA
Peripheral anterior synechiae
Posterior synechiae

PRE-EXISTING DISPOSITION TO PRIMARY ANGLE-CLOSURE GLAUCOMA

COMBINED-MECHANISM GLAUCOMA

MECHANISMS OF INTRAOCULAR PRESSURE ELEVATION

See Box 226-1.

Secondary Open-Angle Glaucoma

Trabecular meshwork obstruction is the most common mechanism[2] and can be caused by:
- Accumulation of white blood cells (especially macrophages and activated T cells) or their aggregations. These can be seen on gonioscopy as small, pale yellow or gray precipitates that may form later into fine peripheral anterior synechiae and lead to closed-angle glaucoma.

- Inflammatory debris such as proteins, fibrin, high-weight molecules, or even normal serum components following breakdown of the blood-aqueous barrier (BAB). Besides physical obstruction of the conventional outflow pathways, these products may raise IOP by increasing aqueous viscosity. Following even a single attack of inflammation, altered vascular permeability may persist indefinitely, with a subtle aqueous flare the only clinical clue. This may predispose the eye to recurrent inflammation, for example, by increasing the intraocular concentration of substances such as prostaglandins (PGs).
- Other solid components contributing to the blockage in specific conditions. For example, in the triad of rhegmatogenous retinal detachment, uveitis, and glaucoma (Schwartz's syndrome), rod outer segments may be a cause of blockage.[3]
- Swelling of trabecular lamellae and endothelial cells, with both a physical narrowing of trabecular pores and dysfunction.
- The severity of the inflammation or its recurrence or chronicity overwhelming the phagocytic and other pathway-clearing processes of the trabecular endothelial cells. By disturbing their cytoskeletal organization, cytokines such as γ-interferon may inhibit normal phagocytosis. Secreted by various leukocytes, cytokines regulate white blood cell interactions during the inflammatory process, and their influence, along with that of the nitric oxide pathway, remains to be elucidated.
- Loss of or damage to the trabecular endothelial cells becoming irreversible, with or without lamellar scarring. Permanent reduction in conventional outflow follows.
- Direct trabecular damage from a keratitic disease process, or the toxic effects of corneal stromal destruction. Keratitis without associated uveitis is rarely a cause of elevated IOP.

These various mechanisms may potentiate one another.

Canal of Schlemm and episcleral venous outflow obstruction can be caused by physical or chemical means similar to those described earlier or by a raised episcleral venous pressure, particularly in eyes with scleritis, episcleritis, and keratitis.

Corticosteroid-induced elevation of IOP in susceptible patients as a result of reduced outflow is always possible with the administration of topical, other local (e.g., dermal or inhalational), or systemic steroid preparations. Theories to explain this phenomenon include:

- Inhibition of the production of outflow-enhancing PGs (such as $PGF_{2\alpha}$).
- Suppression of trabecular endothelial cell phagocytosis.
- Alteration of the composition of the extracellular matrix through which aqueous flows (such as the proteoglycans or glycosaminoglycans), thereby increasing resistance to outflow.
- Increase in the expression of cellular tight junction protein, thereby modifying fluid hydraulic conductivity.
- Stabilization of lysosomes, permitting an accumulation of hyaluronate or a basement membrane–like material or other assorted debris.
- Increase in cross-linked actin networks in the trabecular meshwork.

Several mechanisms may be involved sequentially or in parallel, and the mechanisms may be different for each individual.

Following 4–6 weeks of topical steroid administration, about 5% of the population demonstrates a rise in IOP of more than 16mmHg, and 30% have a rise of 6–15mmHg.[4,5] In a minority of subjects, especially those with primary open-angle glaucoma, the IOP rise can be faster and greater than this. To reduce the chance of provoking such an increase in IOP, steroid use should be minimized with respect to the type of steroid prescribed (e.g., medrysone rather than fluorometholone rather than dexamethasone),[6] the frequency of instillation, and the duration of use. For the management of significant uveitis, the more potent steroids are invariably required.

Monitoring IOP in all patients receiving steroids is necessary. Once the steroids have been ceased, the IOP almost always returns to baseline within 4 weeks.[7]

TABLE 226-2

EFFECTS OF CORTICOSTEROID THERAPY ON INTRAOCULAR PRESSURE IN OCULAR INFLAMMATION

Action	Result	Effect on Intraocular Pressure
Decrease trabecular meshwork inflammation	Increase trabecular meshwork outflow	Decrease
Increase blood–aqueous barrier	Decrease aqueous viscosity Increase trabecular meshwork outflow	Decrease
Decrease ciliary body inflammation	Return aqueous inflow to normal	Increase
Alter trabecular meshwork endothelial cells in corticosteroid responders	Decrease trabecular meshwork outflow	Increase

When used to treat uveitis, steroids may have a complex series of effects on IOP levels, depending on their influence on rates of aqueous inflow and outflow, viscosity, and BAB. This is summarized in Table 226-2.

Hypersecretion is a rare cause of raised IOP, but it has been suggested as a mechanism in glaucomatocyclitic crises. It may occur by means of a PGE_1- or PGE_2-mediated increase in the rate of aqueous secretion or by a breakdown in the BAB, with an associated increase in aqueous protein concentrations and thus aqueous viscosity.

Permanent direct trabecular meshwork tissue damage can result from:
- Anterior or limbal scleritis.
- Destructive or degenerative connective tissue diseases.
- Chemical injuries, including those caused by caustic soda, ammonia, formalin, nitrogen mustards, and chloroform.

Post-trabecular outflow damage from episcleritis with vasculitis, in which lymphocytes accumulate around intrascleral outflow channels, is associated with an anterior uveal perivasculitis.

Preexisting Open-Angle Glaucoma

The presence of an elevated IOP in an eye with uveitis does not mean that the ocular inflammation is the cause. Patients must be examined for primary or other forms of secondary open-angle glaucoma, such as post-traumatic (particularly if unilateral) or pseudoexfoliative (unilateral or bilateral) glaucoma.

An acute onset and unilateral involvement suggest uveitis as the cause, whereas an afferent pupil defect with asymmetry of disc cupping and perimetric loss in a patient with a short symptomatic (i.e., uveitic) history suggests a more chronic underlying glaucomatous process.

Secondary Angle-Closure or Closed-Angle Glaucoma

Peripheral anterior synechiae (PAS) are a common complication of uveitis and, if allowed to progress, may seal the drainage angle completely. As less of the trabecular meshwork remains accessible to the aqueous, the IOP begins to rise.

PAS may result from the organization of inflammatory debris or protracted iridotrabecular contact following an acute secondary angle-closure glaucoma attack, a flat or shallow anterior chamber after incisional surgery, or a massive exudative retinal detachment with anterior displacement of the lens-iris diaphragm. Ciliary body rotation anteriorly from uveitis-induced swelling or suprachoroidal exudation can produce the same result. PAS formation is enhanced by the swelling of the peripheral iris and by the exudation of proteins and other inflammatory products such as fibrin into the chamber angle associated with inflammation.

Neovascularization of the anterior chamber angle and its subsequent fibrovascular closure may follow chronic uveitis.

Posterior synechiae cause the iris to adhere to the lens initially with fibrin and later by fibrovascular organization. Should the entire pupil margin become involved, a secluded pupil results: the iris bombé produces a shallow or closed peripheral anterior chamber whose center remains at a normal depth. PAS can form if this acute secondary angle-closure glaucoma is not treated promptly with one or more adequate peripheral iridectomies.

If widespread adhesion of the iris to the anterior lens surface has occurred, bombé may not occur evenly or at all. Forward movement of the lens-iris diaphragm may be the only sign of pupil block and can be confused with an underlying tendency to primary angle-closure glaucoma. Comparison of the anterior chamber configuration with that of the fellow eye can help differentiate these two mechanisms. The placement of the laser peripheral iridectomies can be crucial, or incisional drainage surgery may be indicated.

In the presence of uveitis and iris bombé with a closed angle, a low or normal IOP should signal the possibility of profound aqueous hyposecretion. In this situation, successful drainage surgery may precipitate phthisis bulbi, which is where the eye may have been heading anyway as a result of the uveitis.

Preexisting Disposition to Primary Angle-Closure Glaucoma

In an eye with a shallow anterior chamber and relative pupil block, an attack of angle-closure glaucoma may be precipitated by anterior segment edema and inflammation, increased aqueous viscosity, swelling and forward rotation of the ciliary body, and anterior shift of the lens-iris diaphragm. All or some of these factors may accompany uveitis. The depth of the contralateral anterior chamber may suggest this diagnosis.

Combined-Mechanism Glaucoma

Usually, the glaucoma associated with uveitis is the result of more than one of the mechanisms outlined earlier. The mix may

> **BOX 226-2**
>
> **Inflammatory Conditions Commonly Associated With Raised Intraocular Pressure**
>
> **ANTERIOR UVEITIS**
> Herpes virus associated uveitis
> Fuchs' heterochromic iridocyclitis
> Juvenile rheumatoid arthritis
> Glaucomatocyclitic crisis (Posner Schlossman syndrome)
> Phacolytic glaucoma
>
> **INTERMEDIATE UVEITIS (PARS PLANITIS)**
>
> **POSTERIOR UVEITIS**
> Peripheral anterior synechiae
> Sympathetic ophthalmia
> Vogt–Koyanagi–Harada syndrome
> Toxoplasmosis
> Acute retinal necrosis
> Sarcoidosis
> Masquerade syndromes
> Retinal detachment, uveitis, and glaucoma (Schwartz's syndrome)

(McCluskey P, personal communication.)

TABLE 226-3

GUIDE TO DIAGNOSIS OF INFLAMMATORY CONDITIONS

	Diagnosis	Time Course	Side	Age (years)	Sex	Race	Systemic Symptoms	Signs
Anterior uveitis	Idiopathic uveitis	Acute	Unilateral	16–45	Either	—	—	—
	Juvenile rheumatoid arthritis	Chronic	Bilateral	0–15	Female	—	Arthritis	Arthritis
	Fuchs' heterochromic iridocyclitis	Acute	Unilateral	25–45	Either	—	—	—
	Herpes virus	Acute	Unilateral	0–99	Either	—	—	—
	Ankylosing spondylitis	Acute	Bilateral	16–45	Male	Caucasian	—	Sacroileitis
	Reiter's syndrome	Acute	Bilateral	16–25	Male	Caucasian	Arthritis Urethritis	—
	Inflammatory bowel disease	Acute	Bilateral	25–65	Either	—	Diarrhea Arthritis	Oral ulcers
Intermediate or posterior uveitis	Idiopathic (pars planitis)	Chronic	Bilateral	0–70	Either	—	—	—
	Toxoplasmosis	Acute	Bilateral	0–45	Either	—	—	—
	Idiopathic retinal vasculitis	Acute	Bilateral	25 onward	Either	—	—	—
	Idiopathic posterior uveitis	Acute	Bilateral	25 onward	Either	—	—	—
	Presumed ocular histoplasmosis	Chronic	Bilateral	20–40	Either	Caucasian	—	—
	Toxocariasis	Chronic	Unilateral	2–31	Either	—	—	—
	Serpiginous choroidopathy	Chronic	Bilateral	16–65	Either	Caucasian	—	—
	Acute posterior multifocal placoid pigment epitheliopathy	Acute	Bilateral	Up to 30	Either	—	—	Cerebrospinal fluid cells
	Acute retinal necrosis	Acute	Unilateral	16–65	Either	—	—	—
	Birdshot choroidopathy	Chronic	Bilateral	45–65	Female	—	—	—
	Intraocular lymphoma	Chronic	Unilateral	40–70	Either	—	—	—
Localized or pan-uveitis	Syphilis	Either	Either	25 onward	Either	—	Multiple	Multiple
	Sarcoidosis	Chronic	Either	5–45	Either	African–Caribbean	Multiple	Multiple
	Vogt–Koyanagi–Harada disease	Acute	Bilateral	15–45	Either	Japanese	Multiple	Multiple
	Behçet's disease	Either	Bilateral	25–65	Either	Mediterranean origin Japanese	Multiple	Multiple
	Infectious endophthalmitis	Either	Unilateral	—	Either	—	—	—

well change as the disease and its treatment proceed. Recognizing which mechanisms are responsible at any one point in time is the key to effective therapy.

PRINCIPLES OF MANAGEMENT

Both the underlying inflammation and the glaucoma require assessment, diagnosis, and directed treatment. Management demands flexibility, because the disease, the effects on the eye, and the treatment itself may change significantly over time. An open mind and careful examination and reexamination are vital for therapeutic success.

UVEITIS

Diagnosis

A careful history with a review of systems and a complete ocular examination followed by a guided series of investigations should allow the majority of ocular inflammations to be diagnosed. The most common conditions encountered are listed in Box 226-2 and Table 226-3, and the usefulness of the various investigations is summarized in Table 226-4.

Management

Ocular and any associated systemic diseases are treated on their merits. Treatment aims to control active inflammation, prevent its damaging effects on aqueous circulation and drainage, and control elevated IOP. If medical therapy fails in the latter two areas, laser or surgical intervention may be necessary.

Although corticosteroids (administered topically, locally, or systemically) can inhibit most inflammatory reactions, irrespective of underlying cause, they do not alter the cause. Once they are withdrawn, the inflammation, which is the fundamental tissue response to that cause, may recur.

By inhibiting phospholipase A_2, corticosteroids reduce arachidonic acid formation from cell membrane precursors, thereby blocking the formation of potent inflammatory mediators such as PGs, leukotrienes, and thromboxane. These nonspecific anti-inflammatory effects result in stabilization of intracellular lysosomes, inhibition of granulomatous tissue reaction, restoration of blood-tissue barriers, and suppression of cellular exudates. Topical administration of salts of prednisolone 1% or dexamethasone 0.1% is most useful in anterior and intermediate (cyclitic) inflammatory processes. New agents such as rimexolone are now available; the 1% rimexolone solution is claimed to be as potent in blocking inflammation as is prednisolone acetate 1%, with less risk of elevating IOP.[8]

If frequent topical administration fails to control ocular inflammation adequately, subconjunctival, sub-Tenon's capsule, or orbital floor injections of dexamethasone, prednisolone, triamcinolone, or methylprednisolone may suffice. With severe bilateral posterior uveitis, systemic steroids are necessary. Possible side effects include the cushingoid complex of signs and symptoms, hypertension, hyperglycemia, peptic ulceration, aseptic necrosis of the femoral head, vulnerability to infections, and growth retardation in children. Ocular side effects include raised IOP, posterior subcapsular cataract, and increased susceptibility to recurrent herpetic disease.

TABLE 226-4

SELECTED INVESTIGATIONS IN INFLAMMATORY EYE DISEASE

Ocular Disease	Investigation	Associated Disease
Scleritis	Rheumatoid factor	Rheumatoid arthritis, connective tissue diseases
	Antinuclear cytoplasmic antigen	Wegeners' granulomatosis, polyarteritis nodosa
	Uric acid	Gout
Anterior uveitis	Venereal disease research laboratory/fluorescent treponemal antibody	Syphilis, Lyme disease
	Chest X–ray, angiotensin converting enzyme assay	Sarcoidosis
	HLA–B27	Recurrent anterior uveitis, ankylosing spondylitis, psoriatic arthritis, Reiter's syndrome
	Anti-nuclear antibodies	Systemic lupus erythematosis, Sjögren's syndrome, juvenile rheumatoid arthritis, connective tissue diseases
Intermediate uveitis	Venereal disease research laboratory/fluorescent treponemal antibody	Syphilis, Lyme disease
	Chest X–ray, angiotensin converting enzyme assay, skin test panel	Sarcoidosis, tuberculosis, presumed ocular histoplasmosis syndrome
	Neurological assessment MRI, CSF studies	Multiple sclerosis
Posterior uveitis	Verereal disease research laboratory/fluorescent treponemal antibody	Syphilis, Lyme disease
	Chest X–ray, angiotensin converting enzyme assay, skin test panel	Sarcoidosis, tuberculosis, presumed ocular histoplasmosis syndrome, Behçet's disease
	Neurological assessment MRI, CSF studies	Vogt–Koyanagi–Harada disease, multiple sclerosis
	Fluorescein and indocyanine green angiography	Acute posterior multifocal placoid pigment epitheliopathy, serpiginous choroidopathy, Birdshot choroidopathy
	HIV serology	AIDS
Retinal vasculitis	HIV serology	AIDS
	Anti-nuclear antibodies	Systemic lupus erythematosis, Sjögren's syndrome, juvenile rheumatoid arthritis, connective tissue diseases
	Anti-neutrophil cytoplasmic antibody	Wegeners' granulomatosis, polyarteritis nodosa
	Chest X–ray, angiotensin converting enzyme assay, skin test panel	Sarcoidosis, tuberculosis, presumed ocular histoplasmosis syndrome
	Venereal disease research laboratory/fluorescent treponemal antibody	Syphilis, Lyme disease
	Pathergy	Behçet's disease

(The skin test panel consists of Mantoux, histoplasmin, and control antigens tests [McCluskey P, personal communication].)

Some inflammatory reactions are resistant to steroid therapy, such as chronic low-grade BAB breakdown and Fuchs' uveitis syndrome.

Nonsteroidal anti-inflammatory drugs (NSAIDs) such as topical flurbiprofen, indomethacin, diclofenac, dipyridamole, ibuprofen, and indoxole (or even systemic aspirin) block the PG cascade by inhibiting prostaglandin synthetase activity. NSAIDs can prove useful in potentiating the activity of corticosteroids, allowing their dose to be reduced, or they can even replace corticosteroids when they are contraindicated.

Similarly, with appropriate medical assistance, the ophthalmologist can consider immunosuppressive drugs such as chlorambucil, cyclophosphamide, methotrexate, azathioprine, and cyclosporin A alone, in combination with one another, or in combination with steroids when steroids alone have failed to control inflammation or are contraindicated. The potential for significant hematological and renal side effects demands careful monitoring of patients on these agents. Plasma exchange has also been reported useful in the management of endogenous uveitis.

Antibiotics and antifungal agents are necessary when the inflammation is secondary to a specific infection (such as toxoplasmosis), in addition to the anti-inflammatory measures adopted.

Mydriasis and Cycloplegia

Pupillary dilatation achieved with cycloplegics such as atropine and homatropine, along with sympathomimetics such as phenylephrine, is desirable in the treatment of uveitis to prevent the formation of posterior synechiae or to break them up, thereby preventing a secluded pupil. These drugs assist in the control of IOP by increasing uveoscleral outflow and by helping to stabilize the BAB. By decreasing ciliary muscle spasm, they may significantly relieve patient discomfort.

GLAUCOMA

In most cases of acute inflammation, the optic disc is healthy and can withstand IOP levels elevated 30mmHg or higher for many weeks or months. Controlling the inflammation and protecting the eye from any damaging effects on aqueous circulation and drainage permit normalization of IOP spontaneously. Reduction of IOP *per se* may not be required, unless levels are considered unsafe for the individual eye, disc decompensation is apparent, other risk factors predispose to retinal vein occlusive events, corneal endothelial disease contributes to edema, or recurrent or chronic inflammation leads to long-standing ocular hypertension.

Medical Management

Reduction of the rate of aqueous inflow is the cornerstone of medical management of raised IOP in inflamed eyes. This can be achieved with β-blockers (e.g., timolol, betaxolol, carteolol, levobunolol), α_2-adrenergic agonists (e.g., apraclonidine, brimonidine), or topical or systemic carbonic anhydrase inhibitors (e.g., dorzolamide, brinzolamide, acetazolamide, dichlorphenamide, methazolamide). Although epinephrine may be helpful, the role of latanoprost, travoprost, and future $PGF_{2\alpha}$ isopropyl ester derivatives, as well as bimatoprost and other prostamides, remains to be established. Because an association between latanoprost and uveitis and cystoid macular edema has been described,[9] this agent and related molecules are relatively contraindicated in inflammatory glaucomas.

Because they enhance posterior synechiae formation by aggravating BAB breakdown, producing miosis, and contributing to anterior chamber shallowing, miotics such as pilocarpine, carbachol, and anticholinesterases should be avoided in inflamed eyes.[10] They may also aggravate patient discomfort, with further ciliary muscle spasm, and they may paradoxically raise IOP by failing to improve trabecular outflow while blocking uveoscleral outflow.

Surgical Management

Laser peripheral iridectomy is indicated if posterior synechiae precipitate iris bombé and medical mydriatic measures fail to break them. To eliminate pupil block, the positioning of the iridectomies can be critical if extensive posterior synechiae have formed. Both raised IOP and anterior uveitis can be exaggerated by this procedure, which can be technically difficult because of iris congestion. Gentle pretreatment "chipping" with the argon laser may facilitate subsequent neodymium:yttrium-aluminum-garnet (Nd:YAG) laser penetration of the iris. Laser openings are more likely to close in the presence of active inflammation, and careful monitoring and possible retreatment or even surgical peripheral iridectomy may be required.

Laser trabeculoplasty, whether by argon or selective technologies, can exacerbate anterior uveitis and promote the formation of PAS, and it has a poor chance of reducing IOP significantly in eyes thus affected.[11] It is contraindicated in inflammatory glaucoma.

Filtration surgery becomes necessary when medical and laser management, along with treatment of the inflammation and its cause, cannot reduce the IOP below levels that are causing or are likely to cause optic disc decompensation and perimetric damage. Because of increased postoperative inflammation and a greater risk of profound hypotony, leading to bleb failure, fistulizing surgery is less likely to succeed in inflamed eyes than in those with primary open-angle glaucoma.[12] Although full-thickness filtering surgery reportedly has a higher success rate than scleral trapdoor operations, the chances of hypotony, flat anterior chamber, and cataract are also increased. Trabeculodialysis (modified goniotomy) has been tried with some success, as has nonpenetrating drainage surgery. One of the keys to successful surgery is to control the inflammation as much as possible both before and after surgery with, for example, intensive topical, local, or even systemic steroid administration.

Adjunctive antifibrotic agents, such as intraoperative 5-fluorouracil (5-FU) or mitomycin C[13] or postoperative 5-FU,[14] have improved guarded filtration surgical success rates appreciably in eyes with inflammatory glaucoma, in both the short and long terms. Complication rates are increased, however, by the use of these agents, with hypotonous maculopathy and late endophthalmitis from leaks through thin-walled blebs being the most serious.

Use of setons, such as the Molteno, Schocket, Ahmed, Baerveldt, and Krupin implants, or valves has met with better success than guarded filtration techniques performed without adjunctive therapy. Setons do not achieve the low levels of IOP (e.g., 7–11mmHg) that adjunctive filtration operations often can. In eyes with extensive optic disc damage, a seton-attained IOP of 14–18mmHg may not be sufficiently protective. In eyes with visual potential, setons are indicated when adjunctive filtration procedures have failed.[15] Intraoperative 5-FU or mitomycin C can reportedly enhance seton IOP reduction.

Ciliary body destructive techniques using cryotherapeutic, Nd:YAG, or ultrasound methods of delivering energy have been used to lower IOP by damaging ciliary epithelium and slowing aqueous inflow. Because of their propensity to aggravate ocular inflammation and their unpredictable effect on IOP in inflamed eyes (with a significant risk of either secondary phthisis bulbi or failure to control IOP, as well as the albeit small risk of contributing to sympathetic ophthalmia), these procedures are recommended only when all else has failed and little visual potential exists.[16]

SPECIFIC ENTITIES

Table 226-3 lists the conditions associated with ocular inflammation and glaucoma. Most of them are covered in detail in other sections of this book, but a few are specifically mentioned here.

Glaucomatocyclitic Crisis (Posner Schlossman Syndrome)

Posner and Schlossman[17] described nine patients with this entity precisely and in detail in 1948. Classic clinical features include episodic, unilateral mild anterior uveitis with photophobia, reduced vision, and colored rings around lights (from secondary corneal edema) and markedly elevated IOP, usually measured in the 40–60mmHg range. There is remarkably little, if any, pain. Varying from none to 25, keratic precipitates are small, discrete, round, and nonpigmented and are found on the lower third of the endothelium. Recurrences are always in the same eye. Posterior and peripheral anterior synechiae are not observed, and the drainage angle remains wide open. Each attack can last from a few hours to a month but is usually of 1–3 weeks' duration. Treatment does not abbreviate the attack, and iridectomy or filtering surgery does not prevent recurrences. Possible but not invariable is the development of optic disc pallor and cupping and permanent perimetric loss. Between attacks, there are generally no signs or symptoms of inflammation or glaucoma, and the contralateral eye is normal. Of unknown cause. this condition has a complex relationship with primary open-angle glaucoma.[18]

Management consists of the following:

- Hypotensive measures. Apraclonidine and brimonidine seem to be particularly effective during attacks, supplemented, as required, with other aqueous inflow inhibitors. The role of PG derivatives has yet to be established. Rarely, hyperosmotic agents may be needed.
- Anti-inflammatory measures. Although there is no evidence that they shorten the attack or prevent recurrences, many clinicians consider corticosteroids or topical NSAIDs possibly useful. Cycloplegics are not indicated.

The interval between attacks varies from a few months to several years. Some may be seasonal. Attacks are rare in the elderly, suggesting a self-resolving course. This makes the prevention of irreversible disc and field damage all the more important.

Fuchs' Uveitis Syndrome (Fuchs' Heterochromic Iridocyclitis)

Recognized as being more expansive than its 1906 description by Fuchs,[19] this condition encompasses a chronic, usually unilateral (90%), low-grade panuveitis with rapid cataract formation (commencing in the posterior subcapsule) and a high risk of secondary open-angle glaucoma. Affecting any age group and either sex, it is usually detected serendipitously, although it can provoke floaters (from vitreous veils or hemorrhage), conjunctival injection, or decreased vision from cataract. Heterochromia or patchy atrophy of the iris and sphincter may be present, sometimes only subtly; their absence may contribute to a missed diagnosis. Small, fine PAS may occur. Radial iris vessels become more visible as iris atrophy develops, along with fragile blood vessels in the chamber angle. Small and recurrent hyphemas may occur spontaneously or following trivial trauma or mydriasis.

Helping to differentiate this entity from other inflammatory glaucomas are the lack of posterior synechiae and the fact that anterior chamber cells and flare are rarely more than "moderate" and are asymptomatic. Cells in the vitreous are common. Pathognomonically, keratic precipitates are small, round or stellate, and discrete; more significantly, they are distributed over the entire corneal endothelial surface, and fine filaments are often seen between them. Their presence and extent are out of proportion to the inflammation.

In most cases, therapy of the uveitis is not required, although a short, intensive trial of steroids may be useful to confirm the diagnosis (by a lack of response). When the eye is symptomatic, short bursts of topical steroids may restore comfort, but these drugs are unable to normalize the BAB or to achieve total quiescence. The glaucoma is more difficult to control.[20] Initially, a raised IOP may respond to anti-inflammatory treatment, but in two thirds of patients, a chronic IOP rise is often resistant to hypotensive agents. Argon laser trabeculoplasty is "underwhelming" in its effect and is contraindicated by angle changes. Should filtration surgery even with adjunctive antifibrotic therapy fail, setons may prove helpful.

Success has improved with cataract extraction with small incision surgery and in-the-capsular-bag, surface-modified intraocular lens placement.[21] Specific problems include severe inflammation (possibly with synechiae formation and debris deposition on the implant), hyphema, new or exacerbated glaucoma, vitreous opacification, corneal decompensation, and a greater likelihood of later Nd:YAG laser posterior capsulotomy (with significant risk of a marked IOP spike).

Patients with this condition require constant monitoring, especially for glaucoma and progressive iris atrophy, which hint at the final prognosis. Recognition is important because it renders systemic investigations and anti-inflammatory therapy unnecessary.

REFERENCES

1. Watson PG. Glaucoma secondary to keratitis, episcleritis, and scleritis. In: Ritch R, Shields MB, eds. The secondary glaucomas. St. Louis: Mosby; 1982:269–89.
2. Krupin T, Dorfman NH, Spector SM, Wax MB. Secondary glaucoma associated with uveitis. Glaucoma. 1988;10:85–90.
3. Schwartz A. Chronic open-angle glaucoma secondary to rhegmatogenous retinal detachment. Am J Ophthalmol. 1973;75:205–11.
4. Armaly MF. Statistical attributes of the steroid hypertensive response in the clinically normal eye. Invest Ophthalmol Vis Sci. 1965;4:187–97.
5. Becker B. Intraocular pressure response to topical corticosteroids. Invest Ophthalmol Vis Sci. 1965;4:198–205.
6. Mindel JS. Comparative ocular pressure elevation by medrysone, fluorometholone and dexamethasone phosphate. Arch Ophthalmol. 1980;98:1577–8.
7. Becker B, Mills DW. Corticosteroids and intraocular pressure. Arch Ophthalmol. 1963;70:500–7.
8. Foster CS, Alter G, DeBarge LR, et al. Efficacy and safety of rimexolone 1% ophthalmic suspension vs 1% prednisolone acetate in the treatment of uveitis. Am J Ophthalmol.1996;122:171–82.
9. Fechtner RD, Khouri AS, Zimmerman TJ, et al. Anterior uveitis associated with latanoprost. Am J Ophthalmol. 1998;126:37–41.
10. Ignarro LJ, Colombo C. Enzyme release from polymorphonuclear leukocyte lysosomes: regulation by autonomic drugs and cyclic nucleotides. Science. 1973;180:1181–3.
11. Robin AL, Pollack IP. Argon laser trabeculoplasty in secondary forms of open-angle glaucoma. Arch Ophthalmol. 1983;101:382–4.
12. Hoskins HD Jr, Hetherington J Jr, Shaffer RN. Surgical management of the inflammatory glaucomas. Perspect Ophthalmol. 1977;1:173–81.
13. Kitazawa Y, Kawase K, Matsushita H, Minobe M. Trabeculectomy with mitomycin. Arch Ophthalmol. 1991;109:1693–8.
14. The Fluorouracil after Filtering Surgery Study Group. Fluorouracil filtering surgery study one-year follow-up. Am J Ophthalmol. 1989;108:625–35.
15. Goldberg I. Management of uncontrolled glaucoma with the Molteno system. Aust N Z J Ophthalmol. 1987;15:97–107.
16. McAllister J, O'Brien C. Neodymium:YAG transcleral cyclocoagulation: a clinical study. Eye. 1990;4:651–6.
17. Posner A, Schlossman A. Syndrome of unilateral recurrent attacks of glaucoma with cyclitic symptoms. Arch Ophthalmol. 1948;39:517–35.
18. Kass MA, Becker B, Kolker AE. Glaucomatocyclitic crisis and primary open-angle glaucoma. Am J Ophthalmol. 1973;75:668–73.
19. Fuchs E. Uber Komplicationen der Heterchromic. Z Augenhelkd. 1906;15:191–212.
20. Jones NP. Glaucoma in Fuchs heterochromic uveitis: aetiology, management and outcome. Eye. 1991;5:662–7.
21. Sherwood DR, Rosenthal AR. Cataract surgery in Fuchs heterochromic iridocyclitis. Br J Ophthalmol. 1992;76:238–40.

227 Post-Traumatic Glaucoma

STANLEY J. BERKE

DEFINITION
- Elevated intraocular pressure secondary to ocular trauma.

KEY FEATURES
- Hyphema.
- Angle recession.

ASSOCIATED FEATURES
- Rebleeding.
- Corneal blood staining.
- Ghost cell glaucoma.
- Gonioscopic angle deformities.

INTRODUCTION

Elevated intraocular pressure (IOP) is a frequent occurrence after trauma to the eye. Following blunt trauma, glaucoma may occur early (acute), either with or without hemorrhage (hyphema). Glaucoma also may occur late (chronic), either with or without angle recession. In addition, glaucoma may occur after other types of ocular trauma, such as penetrating injuries, chemical burns, radiation therapy, and electrical injuries.

EPIDEMIOLOGY AND PATHOGENESIS

Blunt ocular trauma that results in hyphema is caused predominantly by blows (62%), although projectiles (34%) and explosions (4%) can cause it as well.[1] Most of the injuries are due to violent assaults or accidents. Only a small portion of hyphemas occurs from a lack of protective eyewear for sports or work.

A variety of ocular injuries can occur because of momentary anatomical deformation of the globe by blunt trauma. As the cornea and sclera are suddenly displaced posteriorly, a compensatory expansion occurs at the equator of the eye (Fig. 227-1). The seven anterior ocular tissues that may tear, along with their resultant findings, are illustrated in Figure 227-2.[2] A post-traumatic elevation in IOP may occur in association with any of these findings.

Acute glaucoma without hemorrhage may occur because of the presence of inflammatory cells and pigment in the anterior chamber, which causes blockage in the trabecular meshwork. This is treated with topical anti-inflammatory agents and usually subsides within 1–2 weeks. Occasionally, angle recession may occur without hemorrhage. The increased resistance to outflow associated with significant angle recession is the result of concomitant trabecular meshwork damage.[3]

The most frequent cause of hyphema is ocular trauma, but it should be kept in mind that hyphema also may occur perioperatively and spontaneously.[4] Blunt trauma causes distortion of the anterior chamber angle, which can result in vessel rupture in the iris or ciliary bodies and bleeding into the anterior chamber. As the IOP rises, bleeding diminishes and a clot forms. Clot ly-

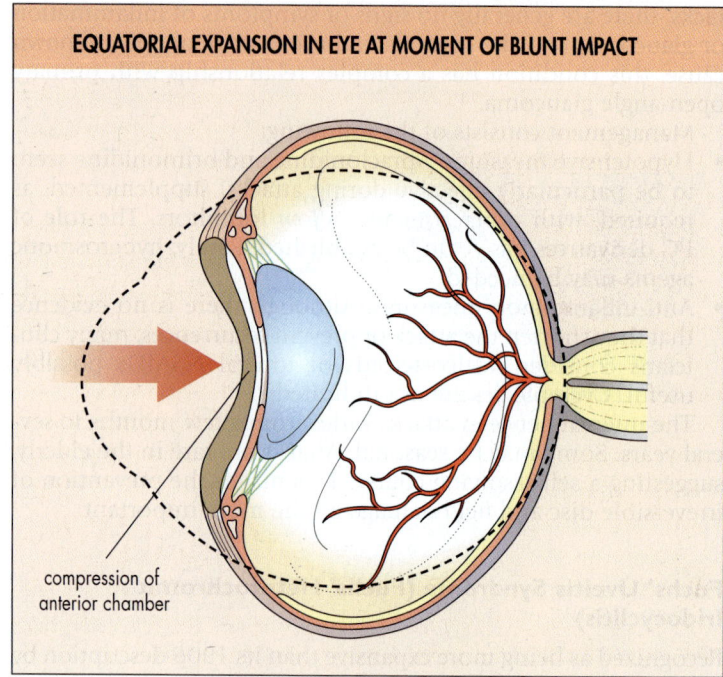

EQUATORIAL EXPANSION IN EYE AT MOMENT OF BLUNT IMPACT

compression of anterior chamber

FIG. 227-1 ▌ Equatorial expansion in eye at moment of blunt impact.

sis and retraction occur 2–5 days after the injury, and the maximal risk of rebleeding from the injured vessels occurs at this time. Rebleeding has been reported in 0.4–35% of patients who did not receive oral medication for prophylaxis.[1] Factors that may increase the risk of rebleeding include large hyphemas, youth, and race, with a higher incidence of rebleeding in African-American and Hispanic patients.[4]

Late-onset glaucoma after a hyphema may result from angle recession, ghost cell glaucoma, peripheral anterior synechiae, or posterior synechiae with iris bombé. The incidence of glaucoma is related directly to the extent of angle recessed; it is approximately 4% if less than 180° of the angle is recessed, and approximately 10% if more than 180° is recessed.[5] The time of onset of angle-recession glaucoma is variable, ranging from 1–40 years after injury. It is likely that the trauma-related decrease in outflow facility occurs soon after the initial injury, and further loss in outflow facility occurs because of an underlying predisposition to the development of open-angle glaucoma. This is supported by a study of 18 patients who had angle-recession glaucoma; in these patients, the average time to diagnosis was 16.5 years, and the average IOP of the uninjured eye was 23.5mmHg (3.13kPa).[3] Corticosteroid-provocative testing of uninvolved eyes of patients who have traumatic glaucoma also confirms this theory.

OCULAR MANIFESTATIONS

The rebleed is often more severe than the initial episode and can lead to total hyphema ("eight-ball" hyphema). Usually, total hyphema is associated with sudden visual loss, high IOP, extreme

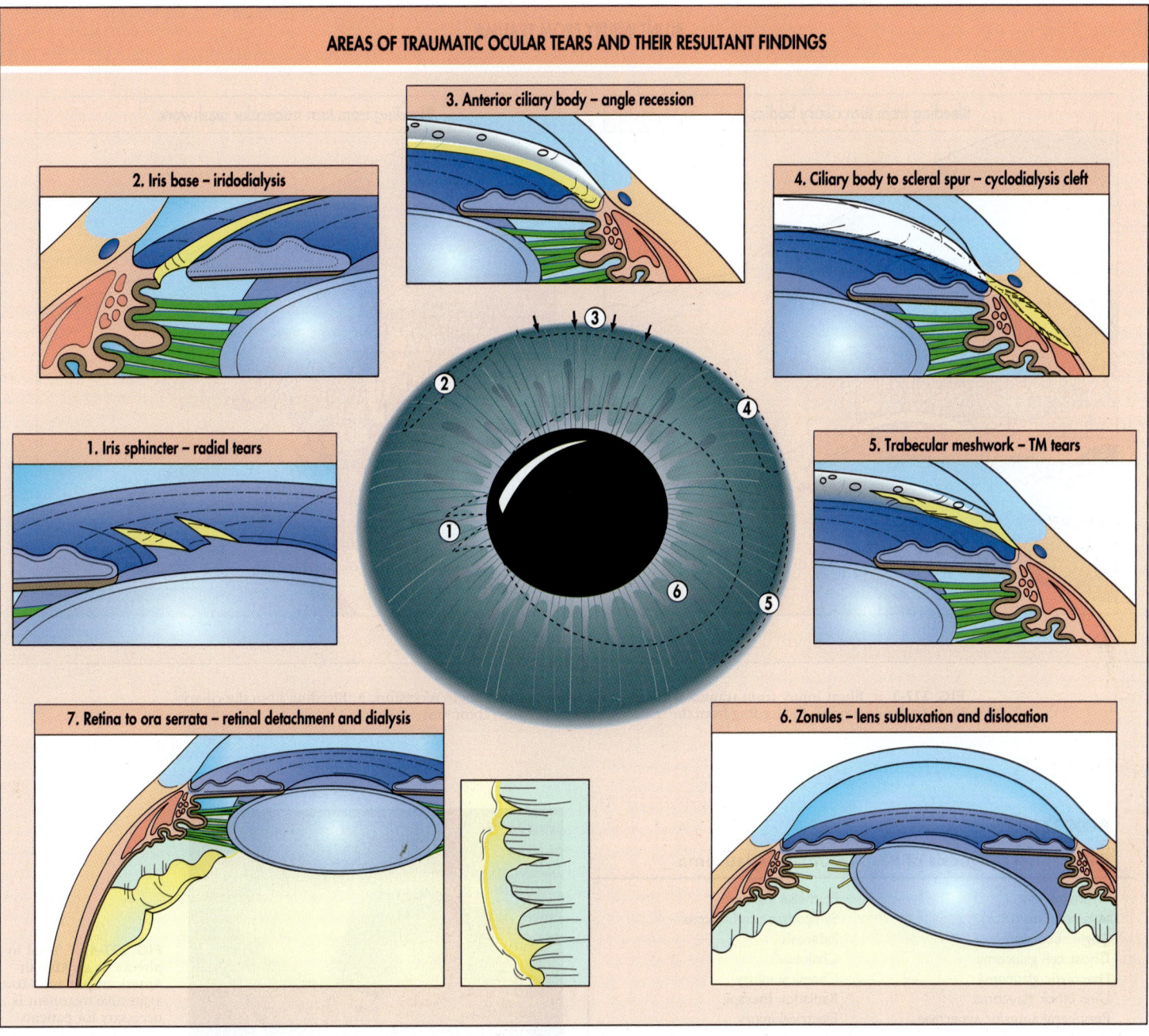

FIG. 227-2 ■ Seven areas of traumatic ocular tears (shown in yellow) with the resultant findings. (Adapted with permission from Campbell DG. Traumatic glaucoma. In: Shingleton BJ, Hersh PS, Kenyon KR, eds. Eye trauma. St. Louis: CV Mosby; 1991:117–25.)

pain, and nausea, as well as other symptoms related to acute glaucoma. The mechanism for the increase in IOP is mechanical obstruction of the trabecular meshwork by red blood cells and sometimes pupillary block from a clot.[6] Glaucoma and corneal blood staining are the two main complications of rebleeding.

Ghost cell (hemolytic) glaucoma can occur after vitreous hemorrhage associated with perforating or nonperforating ocular trauma. Approximately 2–3 weeks after the injury, normal red blood cells in the vitreous transform into rigid, khaki-colored ghost cells and migrate into the anterior chamber. These cells may create a high IOP because of trabecular meshwork obstruction.[2]

DIAGNOSIS

A careful history is taken, with emphasis on the existence and nature of prior ocular trauma. Lack of a positive history cannot rule out the existence of angle recession, because relatively mild blunt trauma can cause a tear in the ciliary body.

Gonioscopy can be performed carefully at the time of the initial injury and usually reveals the source of anterior chamber bleeding. However, because this manipulation may cause further bleeding, it is advisable to wait approximately 4 weeks before thorough gonioscopy is undertaken (Fig. 227-3).

Gonioscopic findings of angle trauma include torn iris processes, trabecular meshwork tears, very white and distinct scleral spur, posteriorly displaced iris root, and exceptionally broad ciliary body band. The tear into the ciliary body, which splits the longitudinal and circular muscle fibers, begins to scar soon after injury. Some eyes show obliteration of the angle recess and peripheral anterior synechiae, which may obscure the angle recession. Gonioscopy is always performed on the normal, uninjured eye for comparative analysis. The pupils are dilated to look for subtle signs of lens trauma and zonular disruption, and the periphery of the retina is examined carefully.

DIFFERENTIAL DIAGNOSIS

Unilateral glaucoma may be caused by traumatic angle recession, as well as by primary open-angle glaucoma, angle-closure glau-

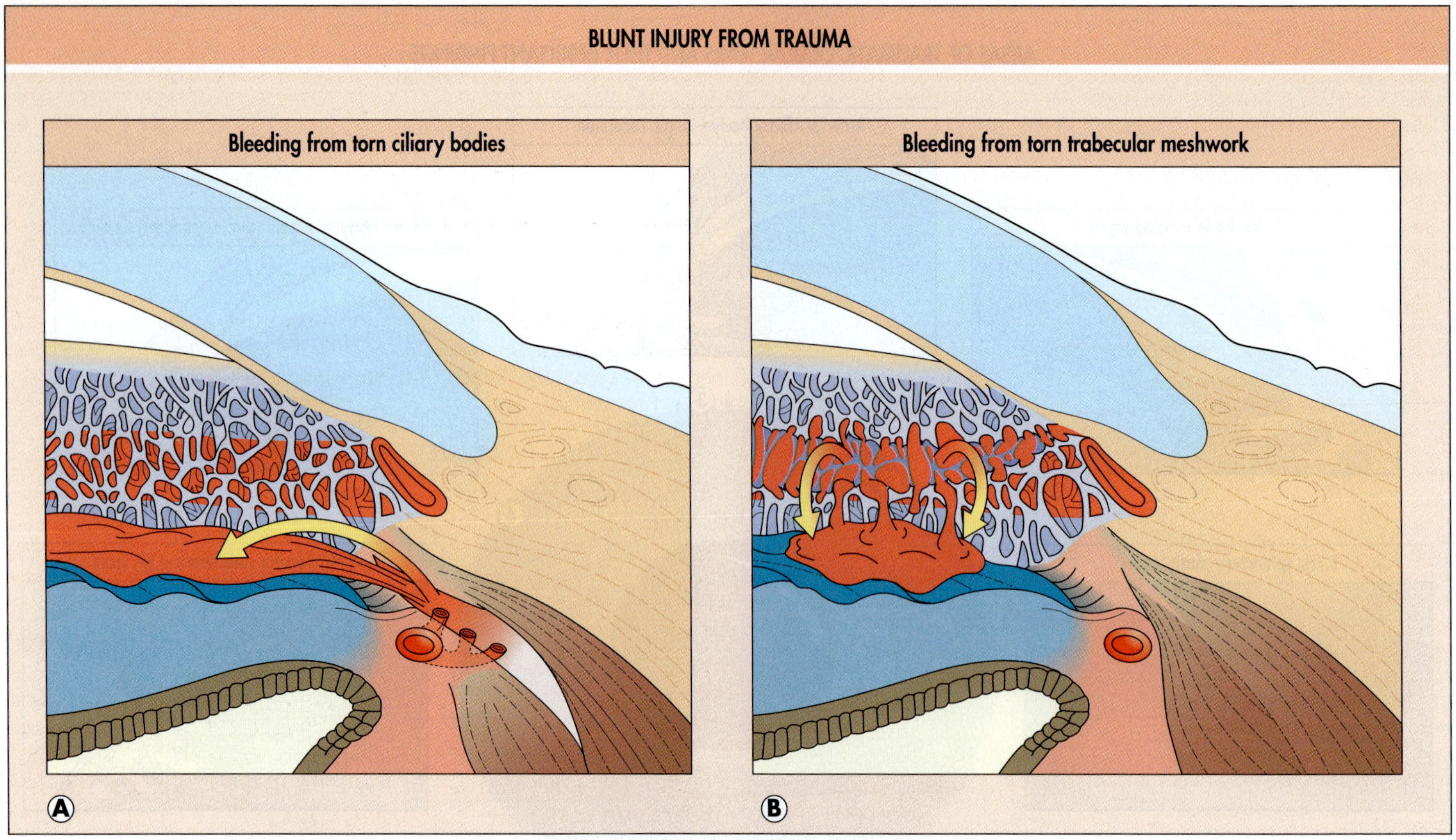

BLUNT INJURY FROM TRAUMA

Bleeding from torn ciliary bodies

Bleeding from torn trabecular meshwork

Ⓐ

Ⓑ

FIG. 227-3 ▮▮ Blunt injury from trauma with resultant hyphema and angle recession. **A,** Bleeding from the ciliary body (more common). **B,** Bleeding from the trabecular meshwork (less common).

BOX 227-1

Differential Diagnosis of Post-Traumatic Glaucoma

Hyphema	Epithelial ingrowth
Inflammation (iritis)	Sympathetic ophthalmia
Angle recession	Siderosis
Ghost cell glaucoma	Chalcosis
Phacolytic glaucoma	Chemical injury
Lens block glaucoma	Radiation therapy
Peripheral anterior synechiae	Electrical injury

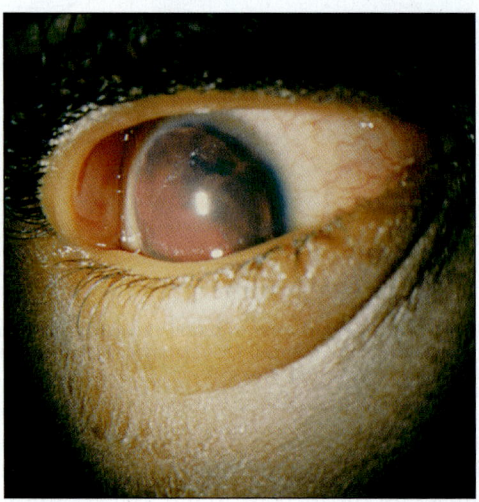

FIG. 227-4 ▮▮ Total hyphema in an African-American patient. More aggressive treatment is necessary for patients who have sickle cell disease or trait.

coma, and any of the other causes of secondary glaucoma. The various causes of post-traumatic glaucoma are listed in Box 227-1.

SYSTEMIC ASSOCIATIONS

Hyphema in patients who have sickle cell disease or who are carriers of sickle cell traits presents unusual management difficulties. Red blood cells in these patients are more rigid in the sickled form and traverse the trabecular beams with difficulty. Even small amounts of blood in the anterior chamber may cause markedly elevated IOP. Sickle cell patients are prone to develop microvascular infarctions of the optic nerve, retina, and anterior segment, even when the IOP is elevated only moderately (Fig. 227-4).[7]

At elevated IOPs, the acidity of the aqueous humor increases while the oxygen content decreases. These metabolic shifts cause further sickling and perpetuate the factors that lead to optic atrophy. Medical and surgical therapy needs to be more aggressive in sickle cell patients. If an oral carbonic anhydrase inhibitor is necessary, methazolamide is used rather than acetazolamide, because it is thought to produce less anterior chamber acidosis. Hyperosmotic agents are avoided, as they may cause vascular hyperviscosity with induced systemic sickling.

If the IOP averages 24mmHg (3.2kPa) or greater for 24 hours, or if transient pressure elevations greater than 30mmHg (4.0kPa) occur, a paracentesis or anterior chamber washout is indicated.

PATHOLOGY

Histologically, angle recession is characterized by a tear in the face of the ciliary body, which causes a posterior displacement of the iris root and inner pars plicata (Fig. 227-5). In addition to a much widened ciliary body band, sclerosis and fibrosis of the trabecular meshwork are observed. Occasionally, an overgrowth of Descemet's membrane (cuticular membrane) has been found to cover the trabecular meshwork. The formation of peripheral anterior synechiae may create a pseudoangle. Endothelial overgrowth of the pseudoangle may also occur.[8]

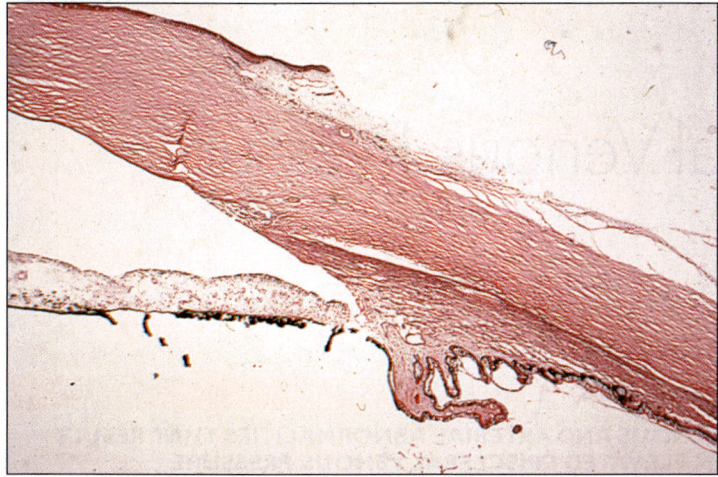

FIG. 227-5 ■ **Angle recession.** The ciliary body inserts into the scleral spur normally. The oblique and circular muscles of the ciliary body have atrophied, following a laceration into the anterior face of the ciliary body. The resulting scar tissue has contracted, pulling the angle recess, iris root, and ciliary process posteriorly. The anterior wedge shape of the ciliary body has been lost. The entire process results in a fusiform shape of the ciliary body. A number of mechanisms, such as trabecular damage and late scarring, peripheral anterior synechiae, and endothelialization of an open angle, can lead to secondary glaucoma that could result in optic nerve damage. (From Yanoff M, Fine BS. Ocular pathology, ed 5. St. Louis, Mosby; 2002.)

TREATMENT

Hyphema

The goals of treatment of traumatic hyphema are to prevent a rebleed and to control IOP. Various medical treatments to reduce the risk of rebleeding are controversial, partly because conflicting results have been reported in the literature, and partly because the rate of secondary hemorrhage is so variable that there is debate about the necessity of treatment.

Most patients can be treated on an outpatient basis. Activity should be limited, but eye patching is not necessary. Drugs with antiplatelet activity, such as aspirin and nonsteroidal anti-inflammatory products, are avoided. Topical medications such as pilocarpine, atropine, and corticosteroids do not reduce the rate of rebleeding. The use of systemic corticosteroids has been recommended but is controversial. A well-controlled study found no difference in the rebleed rate in patients treated with either prednisone (40mg/day) or aminocaproic acid. Both groups had rebleed rates of 7%, compared with a rebleed rate of 20–33% for patients treated with a placebo in other studies.[1]

Several studies have reported that aminocaproic acid reduces secondary hemorrhages in humans. It is an antifibrinolytic agent that inhibits the conversion of plasminogen to plasmin, thus preventing the blood clot from dissolving. The recommended dose of aminocaproic acid is 50mg/kg every 4 hours, with a maximum dose of 30g/day for 5 days. Common side effects are nausea, vomiting, diarrhea, and postural hypotension.[1] A topical preparation exists as well.

Termination of aminocaproic acid before completion of the 5-day course may result in a greater tendency to rebleed. Elevations in IOP have been noted 1–2 days after stopping aminocaproic acid, most likely because of a "wave" of clot lysis that liberates red blood cells and subsequently blocks the trabecular meshwork.[4]

Elevated IOP after hyphema may be treated medically with topical and oral agents. However, sympathomimetic and miotic agents typically are not used because of their inflammatory potential.

Prolonged elevated IOP is associated with an increased chance of optic nerve damage and corneal blood staining. The indications for surgical intervention are listed in Box 227-2.

A multitude of surgical techniques have been advocated to treat hyphema. These include paracentesis, anterior chamber

BOX 227-2

Indications for Surgical Intervention After Hyphema

Intraocular pressure >50mmHg (6.7kPa) for 5 days
Intraocular pressure >35mmHg (4.7kPa) for 7 days
Total hyphema unresolved for 9 days
Microscopic corneal blood staining

washout, expression of the clot, automated removal of blood, and trabeculectomy. Although washout of free red blood cells is often helpful,[9] it is not necessary to completely remove the clot.

Angle-Recession Glaucoma

For chronic glaucoma that results from angle recession, standard glaucoma medications may be used. Miotics should be used cautiously, because they have been associated with an increase in IOP. Eyes that have angle-recession glaucoma have damaged trabecular meshwork and depend on uveoscleral outflow for drainage.[10] Whereas latanoprost and cycloplegic agents increase uveoscleral outflow, miotics cause a decrease.

Argon laser trabeculoplasty should be used cautiously, or not at all, because the results are poor. If medical treatment for angle-recession glaucoma fails, recalcitrant cases require surgical trabeculectomy, with adjunctive use of antimetabolites at the discretion of the surgeon.

COURSE AND OUTCOME

An injury severe enough to cause hyphema also causes an angle recession in more than 60% of eyes. A hyphema that fills three fourths of the volume of the anterior chamber typically results in a traumatic cataract, and vitreous hemorrhage occurs in about 50% of such eyes. Glaucoma may develop in approximately 6% of eyes that have angle recession, most likely when the recession is 240° or greater. The initial injury may lead to cataract and phacolytic glaucoma. Approximately 25% of enucleated eyes with phacolytic glaucoma show angle recession.[7]

Patients who have angle recession and normal IOP should be examined annually for the rest of their lives because of the risk of developing late angle-recession glaucoma. Patients who have angle recession that exceeds 180° are followed particularly closely. In addition, the fellow eyes of patients who have angle-recession glaucoma have a 50% greater risk of developing open-angle glaucoma than do normal eyes.[11]

REFERENCES

1. Farber MD, Fiscella R, Goldberg MF. Aminocaproic acid versus prednisone for the treatment of traumatic hyphema: a randomized clinical trail. Ophthalmology. 1991;98:279–86.
2. Campbell DG. Traumatic glaucoma. In: Shingleton BJ, Hersh PS, Kenyon KR, eds. Eye trauma. St. Louis: CV Mosby; 1991:117–25.
3. Herschler J. Trabecular damage due to blunt anterior segment injury and its relationship to traumatic glaucoma. Trans Am Acad Ophthalmol Otolaryngol. 1977; 83:239–44.
4. Sambursky DL, Azar DT. Corneal and anterior segment trauma and reconstruction. Ophthalmol Clin North Am. 1995;8(4):609–31.
5. Kaufman JH, Tolpin DW. Glaucoma after traumatic angle recession: a ten-year prospective study. Am J Ophthalmol. 1974;78:648–54.
6. Edwards WC, Layden WE. Traumatic hyphema: a report of 184 consecutive cases. Am J Ophthalmol. 1973;75:110–6.
7. Goldberg MF. Sickled erythrocytes, hyphema and secondary glaucoma. Ophthalmic Surg. 1979;10:17–23.
8. Yanoff M, Fine BS. Ocular pathology, 4th ed. London: Mosby Wolfe; 1996:132–4.
9. Herschler J, Cobo M. Trauma and elevated intraocular pressure. In: Ritch R, Shields MB, Krupin T, eds. The glaucomas. St Louis: CV Mosby; 1989:1225–37.
10. Fingeret M, Mathews TA, Fodera FA. Angle recession. Optom Clin. 1993;3(2): 41–8.
11. Tesluk G, Spaeth G. The occurrence of primary open-angle glaucoma in the fellow eye of patients with unilateral angle-cleavage glaucoma. Ophthalmology. 1985;92:904–11.

228 Raised Episcleral Venous Pressure

E. RANDY CRAVEN

DEFINITION
- Elevated intraocular pressure leading to glaucoma as a result of increased episcleral venous pressure.

KEY FEATURES
- Usually prominent episcleral veins.
- Unilateral elevation of intraocular pressure.

ASSOCIATED FEATURES
- Blood in Schlemm's canal.
- Either venous obstruction or arteriovenous abnormalities, rarely idiopathic.

INTRODUCTION

Raised episcleral venous pressure can cause open-angle glaucoma because of obstruction of the outflow of aqueous into the venous drainage system. Because raised episcleral venous pressure can result from systemic abnormalities that ultimately prove fatal, and because of the morbidity associated with these conditions, one needs to be aware of more than eye problems alone.

EPIDEMIOLOGY AND PATHOGENESIS

Glaucoma caused by raised episcleral venous pressure results in a direct effect on intraocular pressure (IOP). When the episcleral venous pressure rises, a similar rise occurs in the IOP.[1] The ultimate IOP is influenced by the production and outflow of aqueous humor but is balanced by the episcleral venous pressure (the Goldmann equation):

IOP = secretion of aqueous/facility of outflow +
episcleral venous pressure.

The episcleral venous pressure is influenced by body position[2] and venous drainage pressure in the superior and inferior ophthalmic veins, cavernous sinus, petrosal sinuses, and internal and external jugular veins. Any abnormality that results in an increased venous pressure in the venous drainage system downstream from the eye can produce elevated IOP. As a result of the stagnation of the venous blood, the eye may develop ischemia and subsequent neovascularization.[3]

Idiopathic raised episcleral venous pressure and glaucoma can occur[4]; color Doppler imaging has not revealed any specific retro-orbital cause.[5] Affected patients tend to be older and have no family history of glaucoma. Unilateral presentation is common, and the right eye is more commonly involved.

The underlying cause of increased episcleral venous pressure that results from raised pressure in the venous drainage system is either venous obstruction or arteriovenous abnormalities (Table 228-1).

OCULAR MANIFESTATIONS

Raised episcleral venous pressure results in engorged episcleral veins (Fig. 228-1). The increased venous pressure increases the

TABLE 228-1

VENOUS AND ARTERIAL ABNORMALITIES THAT RESULT IN ELEVATED EPISCLERAL VENOUS PRESSURE

Venous Obstruction	Arteriovenous Abnormality	Tests to Consider	Other Findings
Superior vena cava syndrome		Chest radiograph	Cyanosis
	Dural–cavernous fistula	Magnetic resonance imaging	
Thyroid ophthalmopathy	Orbital varix	Magnetic resonance imaging	Proptosis
Sturge–Weber syndrome	None	None	Skin and retina
Jugular vein obstruction	None	None	Cyanosis
Cavernous sinus thrombosis	Carotid–cavernous fistula	Magnetic resonance imaging	Pain

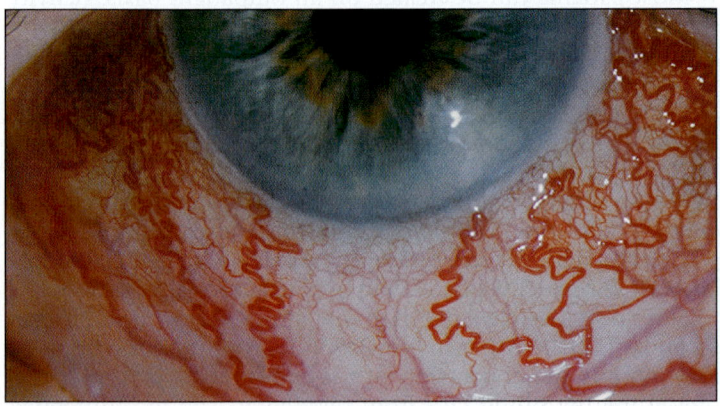

FIG. 228-1 ▌▌ **Prominent episcleral veins.** The episcleral vessels are tortuous and appear succulent. The eye lacks the classic ciliary flush seen with iritis or infection.

blood in Schlemm's canal and can be seen by gonioscopy. If associated ischemia occurs, neovascularization of the iris can be seen.[3] Hemorrhagic choroidal detachments can be seen with secondary angle closure.[6] When the venous pressure approaches the arterial pressure in patients who have arteriovenous abnormalities, the subsequent IOP elevation can be quite high.

Venous obstruction or arteriovenous abnormalities that result in the raised episcleral venous pressure have unique findings (see Table 228-1). Proptosis can occur with thyroid eye disease, carotid cavernous fistula, or orbital varix. An orbital varix can have positional proptosis, and a carotid cavernous fistula can cause pulsatile proptosis. Hemangiomas associated with Sturge-Weber syndrome can involve the skin and choroid ("tomato catsup" fundus). Chemosis is common with carotid cavernous fistula and can be seen with Sturge-Weber syndrome or thyroid ophthalmopathy.

Glaucomatous optic atrophy and visual field loss can take longer to develop than in other forms of acute glaucoma and may not occur at all, despite very high IOPs. This is especially true in the more acute problems that present with raised episcleral venous pressure, such as carotid cavernous fistula.

DIAGNOSIS

The appearance of the episcleral veins in cases of raised episcleral venous pressure is quite characteristic (see Fig. 228-1). It is possible to measure the venous pressure to confirm or determine the raised level. Several methods have been used to determine episcleral venous pressure. The direct method is by cannulation; it is the most accurate method and reveals the normal episcleral venous pressure to be 5–12mmHg (0.7–1.6kPa). Noninvasive methods document the collapse of the vein (partial or total). In such methods, a 50% collapse of the vessel is a common endpoint. The noninvasive methods use indirect approaches in which the pressure required for venous collapse is determined by a pressure chamber (of Seidel), air jet, torsion balance, or venometer.[7, 8] The pressure chamber or venometer methods probably provide the most accurate readings other than those of direct cannulation.

DIFFERENTIAL DIAGNOSIS

Prominent vessels can occur when there is no glaucoma. Vessels involved with infections, inflammation, or allergies can cause significant injection, but usually the vessels are finer, with a more diffuse hue to the tissue. Ataxia-telangiectasia can cause abnormal vessels on the ocular surface, but these tend to be smaller and more localized to a quadrant. With scleritis and episcleritis, the vessels tend to be smaller in caliber than those found with the raised episcleral venous pressure. Additionally, the vessels have more of a crisscross pattern, with a network of deep vessels and radial vessels, and overall there is a more diffuse involvement. Intraocular tumors can cause prominent scleral vessels (Reese's sign). Conditions that involve scleral thinning, such as that seen after repeated ciliary body destructive procedures, can result in a more prominent view of the normal veins.

SYSTEMIC ASSOCIATIONS

Carotid cavernous fistulae may occur after significant trauma. Pulsating exophthalmos, blurred vision, pain, and chemosis develop, often abruptly, and an audible bruit can be heard. Dural cavernous fistulae have a more gradual onset and typically occur in middle-aged women with no history of trauma. Superior vena cava syndrome occurs in the presence of bronchogenic carcinomas. Cavernous sinus thrombosis occurs from infections that spread from the middle ear, sinuses, or face. Significant congestive heart failure results in elevated venous pressure; many findings are present, such as peripheral edema and pulmonary congestion.

TREATMENT

When elevated IOP occurs because of elevated episcleral venous pressure, it can be very difficult to drop the IOP satisfactorily without treating the primary cause of the raised episcleral venous pressure. Treatment for fistulae can involve neuroradiological intervention or neurosurgical intervention. Dural cavernous fistulae are low-flow fistulae and may spontaneously close, whereas carotid cavernous fistulae tend to need intervention to bring about closure. Treatment for the carotid cavernous fistulae includes embolization. Usually, dural cavernous fistulae are watched and may be resolved by sleeping with the head elevated or sitting for a period of time. Thyroid ophthalmopathy can be difficult to treat and is controlled by corticosteroids or by orbital decompression or radiation.

Other medical problems that result in raised episcleral venous pressure should be treated. If this fails or is not possible, medical or surgical intervention is needed. Medications that suppress aqueous production are good first-line choices; beta-blockers and carbonic anhydrase inhibitors are used commonly. Prostaglandin analogs may work but are theoretically limited by outflow. Apraclonidine, because of its vasoconstrictive effects on the arteries that lead into the eye, is also a good first-choice medication.[9]

Laser trabeculoplasty provides little help. Incisional filtration surgery can help lower the IOP, but it is associated with a high incidence of choroidal effusion or hemorrhage[10]; consequently, some surgeons recommend that scleral windows be placed at the start of the procedure. Preoperative mannitol and other medications that lower pressure may be given. Additionally, the flow through the scleral flap may be adjusted to allow for a higher IOP in the early postoperative period. Where prominent vessels occur, a releasable suture should be considered. Drainage implants may be a good choice if the flow through the implant is kept to a minimum in the early postoperative period.

COURSE AND OUTCOME

Depending on the systemic arterial or venous problem that produced the raised episcleral venous pressure, the glaucoma may be controlled by treating the systemic problem. Once the problem that caused the raised episcleral venous pressure has been treated, the IOP is easier to control. If it is not possible to lower the episcleral venous pressure, such as in Sturge-Weber syndrome, the glaucoma may be chronic and progressive until the IOP can be controlled.

REFERENCES

1. Moses RA, Grodzki WJ. Mechanism of glaucoma secondary to increased venous pressure. Arch Ophthalmol. 1985;103:1653–8.
2. Friberg TR, Sandborn G, Weinreb RN. Intraocular and episcleral venous pressure increases during inverted posture. Am J Ophthalmol. 1987;103:523–6.
3. Harris MJ, Fine SL, Miller NR. Photocoagulation treatment of proliferative retinopathy secondary to carotid-cavernous fistula. Am J Ophthalmol. 1980;90:515–20.
4. Minas TF, Podos SM. Familial glaucoma associated with elevated episcleral venous pressure. Arch Ophthalmol. 1968;80:202–8.
5. Lanzl IM, Welge-Luessen U, Spaeth GL. Unilateral open-angle glaucoma secondary to idiopathic dilated episcleral veins. Am J Ophthalmol. 1996;121:587–9.
6. Buus DR, Tse DT, Parrish RK. Spontaneous carotid-cavernous fistula presenting with acute angle closure glaucoma. Arch Ophthalmol. 1989;107:596–7.
7. Brubaker RF. Determination of episcleral venous pressure in the eye. Arch Ophthalmol. 1967;77:110–4.
8. Zeimer RC, Gieser DK, Wilensty JT, et al. A practical venomanometer. Arch Ophthalmol. 1983;101:1447–9.
9. Montzioros N, Weinreb RN. Apraclonidine reduces the intraocular pressure in eyes with increased episcleral venous pressure. J Glaucoma. 1992;1:42–3.
10. Bellows AR, Chylack LT Jr, Epstein DL, Hutchinson BT. Choroidal effusion during glaucoma surgery in patients with prominent episcleral veins. Arch Ophthalmol. 1979;97:493–7.

229 Aqueous Misdirection Syndrome

NISHAT P. ALVI • LOUIS B. CANTOR

DEFINITION

- A shallow or flat anterior chamber with an inappropriately high intraocular pressure despite a patent iridectomy. Affects primarily patients who have narrow anterior chamber angles.

KEY FEATURES

- Shallowing or flattening of both the central and peripheral anterior chamber despite patent iridectomy.
- Inappropriately elevated intraocular pressure for the depth of the anterior chamber.
- Chronic angle-closure glaucoma.
- Worsened by miotics and relieved by cycloplegics and mydriatics.
- Usually occurs after intraocular surgery.
- Involves some degree of aqueous misdirection into the vitreous cavity.

ASSOCIATED FEATURES

- May occur after laser or medical therapy of glaucoma.
- Intraocular pressure may be within the normal range.

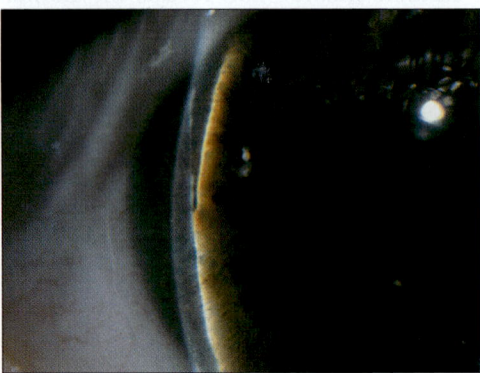

FIG. 229-1
Aqueous misdirection. Note the flat anterior chamber despite a patent iridectomy.

and movement of the lens-iris diaphragm forward as a result of the use of miotics.

OCULAR MANIFESTATIONS

A red, painful eye is most commonly seen after surgery for acute angle-closure glaucoma. The condition usually occurs immediately after surgery but may occur during surgery or months to years later; its development often corresponds to the cessation of cycloplegic therapy or the institution of miotic drops. Slit-lamp examination (Fig. 229-1) characteristically reveals a shallow or flat anterior chamber, both centrally and peripherally (with asymmetry with respect to the fellow eye), and no iris bombé. A high index of suspicion is necessary to make the appropriate diagnosis, since initially the IOP may not be elevated much. The key is that the IOP is elevated inappropriately for the depth of the chamber. Furthermore, if an attempt is made to reform the anterior chamber postoperatively through the paracentesis site using a viscoelastic substance, a larger posterior resistance may be noted, the anterior chamber may not deepen as much as in a hypotonic eye that does not have aqueous misdirection, and the IOP may rise substantially.

INTRODUCTION

Aqueous misdirection glaucoma is now known to have a broad clinical spectrum. It occurs after routine cataract surgery, after the administration of miotics in eyes with or without a prior surgical history, after ciliary body swelling, or even spontaneously.[1] It may be difficult to make an accurate diagnosis, particularly in the early stages.

EPIDEMIOLOGY AND PATHOGENESIS

Aqueous misdirection has been reported to occur in 2–4% of patients who undergo surgery for angle-closure glaucoma, especially if some of the angle is closed preoperatively. If the angle is open or has been opened prophylactically via a laser iridectomy before the development of an angle-closure attack, aqueous misdirection seems less likely to occur after subsequent surgery.[2] This condition also may occur spontaneously or after the cessation of topical cycloplegic therapy, the initiation of topical miotic therapy, laser iridotomy, laser capsulotomy, laser cyclophotocoagulation, cataract extraction, seton implantation, central retinal vein occlusion,[3] or argon laser suture lysis, or in eyes that have hyperopia, short axial lengths, or nanophthalmos.[4]

The pathogenesis of aqueous misdirection is thought to involve posterior misdirection of aqueous flow by a relative pupillary block into or behind the vitreous body; the subsequent increase in vitreous volume results in a shallower anterior chamber and an increase in intraocular pressure (IOP).[5] Events that incite such a pupillary blockage include a small, crowded anterior segment; angle closure; swelling and inflammation of the ciliary processes; and anterior rotation of the ciliary body

DIAGNOSIS

The diagnosis of aqueous misdirection is based clinically on the previously mentioned ocular manifestations, and it is made only after ruling out pupillary block, suprachoroidal hemorrhage, serous choroidal effusions, or other causes of a flat anterior chamber. High-resolution ultrasound biomicroscopy can be useful to confirm the diagnosis.[6] It reveals anterior rotation of the ciliary body against the peripheral iris and forward displacement of the posterior chamber intraocular lens, as well as a shallow central anterior chamber, all of which are reversible.

DIFFERENTIAL DIAGNOSIS

The most difficult entity to distinguish from aqueous misdirection is pupillary block. Pupillary block should be suspected if iris bombé is present and if the anterior chamber is relatively deeper centrally and shallow to flat peripherally. In contrast, with aque-

TABLE 229-1

DIFFERENTIAL DIAGNOSIS OF AQUEOUS MISDIRECTION

Criterion	Aqueous Misdirection	Pupillary Block	Suprachoroidal Hemorrhage	Serous Choroidal Effusions
Intraocular pressure	Normal or elevated	Elevated	Normal or elevated	Low
Anterior chamber depth	Shallow; flat centrally and peripherally	Shallow; flat peripherally, but deeper centrally,	Shallow; flat centrally and peripherally	Shallow; flat centrally and peripherally
Relief by iridectomy	No	Yes	No	No
Ophthalmoscopy	Choroid and retina flat	Choroid and retina flat	Bullous light brown choroidal elevations	Bullous dark brown or dark red choroidal elevations
Ultrasound biomicroscopy	Anterior rotation of ciliary body and lens	Iris bombé with lens in normal position	—	—
B-scan ultrasound	—	—	Smooth, thick, dome-shaped membrane with little after movement / Heterogeneous echogenic space	Smooth, thick dome-shaped membrane with little after-movement / Echolucent suprachoroidal space
Onset	Intraoperative or early post-operative period. Occasionally months to years later	Early postoperative period	Intraoperative or early postoperative period	Intraoperative or early postoperative period

ous misdirection, the anterior chamber is uniformly shallow or flat both centrally and peripherally. Next, the presence or absence of a patent iridectomy must be established. If an iridectomy is not present or not patent, a peripheral iridectomy should be performed. Pupillary block is confirmed if the anterior chamber deepens with an iridectomy. If no relief occurs with iridectomy and ophthalmoscopy or B-scan ultrasonography rules out suprachoroidal hemorrhage or serous choroidal effusion, a diagnosis of aqueous misdirection is made. The distinguishing features of these entities are summarized in Table 229-1.

TREATMENT

The first line of therapy is medical and involves the use of cycloplegics and mydriatics, such as atropine 1% four times a day and phenylephrine 2.5% four times a day to move the lens-iris diaphragm back and relax the ciliary muscle. To decrease aqueous production, topical β-blockers, oral or topical carbonic anhydrase inhibitors, and α-agonists are used. Isosorbide 1.5mg/kg orally or mannitol 2g/kg intravenously over a 45-minute period can be used to shrink the vitreous volume. No oral foods or liquids should be given 2 hours before and after the administration of a hyperosmotic agent to avoid reduction in the osmotic effect. The patient is maintained on atropine for a prolonged period with a very slow taper because of the high risk of recurrence. Miotic agents are contraindicated, as they may cause or contribute to aqueous misdirection.

The second line of treatment is laser therapy. Neodymium: yttrium-aluminum-garnet laser may be used in aphakic and pseudophakic patients to create a large peripheral iridectomy and anterior hyaloid rupture to release the trapped aqueous from the vitreous and reestablish normal aqueous flow.[7] Several openings are made peripherally—that is, not directly behind the optic—because the optic may continue to block the egress of fluid, and the treatment will fail.[8]

While the anterior chamber reforms after medical or laser therapy, corneal-lenticular contact may occur, with the risk of corneal decompensation; therefore, the chamber should be reformed by the injection of a viscoelastic substance via a 30-gauge cannula through the original paracentesis at the slit lamp.[1]

When medical or laser therapy fails, or in phakic eyes for which laser treatment is not a good option, pars plana vitrectomy may be used to debulk the vitreous and possibly also to disrupt the anterior hyaloid face.

If a narrow angle is present in the fellow eye, a laser peripheral iridectomy is performed before any surgical procedures. The risk of aqueous misdirection may be reduced in the fellow eye after iridectomy if the angle remains open and the IOP is normal; failure to provide prompt therapy to the fellow eye has been reported to result in bilateral blindness.[2]

COURSE AND OUTCOME

Medical therapy is successful in approximately 50% of cases within 4–5 days.[2] Laser or surgical intervention may be required before the 4–5 days of medical therapy is completed to avoid corneal decompensation because of corneal-lenticular touch or optic nerve damage from markedly elevated IOPs. Vitrectomy has been shown to effectively relieve aqueous misdirection when medical and laser therapies fail, especially in pseudophakic patients in whom access to the anterior hyaloid, lens capsule, and zonules is direct.[9] A high rate (30–50%) of persistent aqueous misdirection and postoperative cataract formation has been reported in phakic eyes after vitrectomy without lensectomy.[3,9] In general, a vitrectomy alone is considered first; however, lensectomy may be considered in eyes that have substantial corneal edema or dense cataract, or when the anterior chamber does not deepen during vitrectomy.

REFERENCES

1. Juzych M, Parrow KA, Shin DH, et al. Adjunctive viscoelastic therapy for postoperative ciliary block. Ophthalmic Surg. 1992;23:784–8.
2. Simmons RJ, Maestre FA. Malignant glaucoma. In: Ritch R, Shields MB, Krupin T, eds. The glaucomas, vol 2, 2nd ed. St Louis: Mosby–Yearbook; 1996:841–55.
3. Harbour JW, Rubsamen PE, Palmberg P. Pars plana vitrectomy in the management of phakic and pseudophakic malignant glaucoma. Arch Ophthalmol. 1996;114:1073–8.
4. Disclanfani M, Liebmen JM, Ritch R. Malignant glaucoma following argon laser release of scleral flap sutures after trabeculectomy. Am J Ophthalmol. 1989;108:597–600.
5. Shaeffer RN. The role of vitreous detachment in aphakic and malignant glaucoma. Trans Am Acad Ophthalmol Otolaryngol. 1954;58:217–20.
6. Tello C, Chi T, Shepps G, et al. Ultrasound biomicroscopy in pseudophakic malignant glaucoma. Ophthalmology. 1993;100:1330–3.
7. Brown RH, Lynch MG, Tearse JE, Nunn RD. Neodymium–YAG vitreous surgery for phakic and pseudophakic malignant glaucoma. Arch Ophthalmol. 1986;104:1464–6.
8. Stienert RF, Epstein DL, Puliafito CA. Surgical vitrectomy for pseudophakic malignant glaucoma. Am J Ophthalmol. 1986;102:803–4.
9. Byrnes GA, Leen MM, Wong TP, Benson WE. Vitrectomy for ciliary block (malignant) glaucoma. Ophthalmology. 1995;102:1308–11.

230

Glaucomas Associated with Abnormalities of Cornea and Iris, Tumors, and Retinal Disease

STEVEN T. SIMMONS • ANTHONY ECONOMOU

DEFINITION
- A heterogeneous group of disorders of the anterior and posterior segments resulting in secondary glaucoma.

KEY FEATURES
- Iris abnormalities.
- Previous intraocular surgery.
- Rhegmatogenous retinal detachment.
- Elevated intraocular pressure.
- Ocular and metastatic tumors.

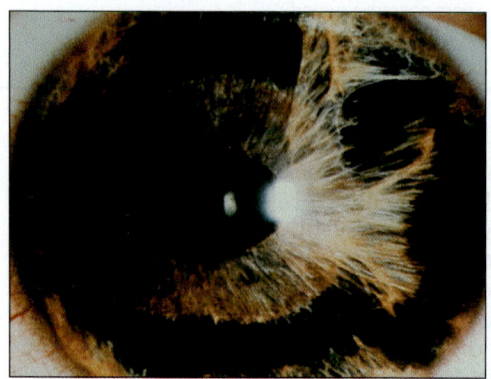

FIG. 230-1 ▮▮ Hole formation in progressive iris atrophy.

IRIDOCORNEAL ENDOTHELIAL SYNDROME

Iridocorneal endothelial (ICE) syndrome describes a group of disorders characterized by abnormal corneal endothelium that is responsible for variable degrees of iris atrophy, secondary angle-closure glaucoma in association with characteristic peripheral anterior synechiae (PAS), and corneal edema. Three clinical variations have been described:
- Iris nevus (Cogan-Reese) syndrome.
- Chandler's syndrome.
- Essential (progressive) iris atrophy.

Since the initials ICE fit both the term *iridocorneal endothelial* syndrome and the first letter of each of the three component entities, Yanoff[1] suggested the term *ICE syndrome* in 1979 for this spectrum of clinical and histopathological abnormalities. That term is now the one most commonly used.

EPIDEMIOLOGY AND PATHOGENESIS

Clinically, the condition is unilateral, with subclinical irregularities of the corneal endothelium commonly noted in the fellow eye. The syndrome affects those 20–50 years of age and occurs more often in women. No consistent association has been established with any other ocular or systemic disorder, and familial cases are very rare. In a study of 37 cases of ICE syndrome, approximately half (21 cases) were Chandler's syndrome; the other two clinical variations each accounted for about one fourth of all cases.[2] Glaucoma occurs in approximately half of all patients who have ICE syndrome.[3] It is more severe in patients who have the progressive iris atrophy and Cogan-Reese variations, as opposed to those who have Chandler's syndrome.[2] The degree of angle closure does not always correlate with the elevation in in-

traocular pressure (IOP), since some angles may be closed functionally by the endothelial membrane without the occurrence of synechial closure.

OCULAR MANIFESTATIONS

Patients present with complaints of pain, decreased vision, and an abnormal iris appearance. The reduced vision and pain are secondary to corneal edema or secondary angle closure, which may occur later in the disease. Patients frequently note a mild blur of vision in the morning hours as a result of mild corneal edema that occurs during sleep. Microcystic corneal edema may be present without elevated IOP, especially in Chandler's syndrome. In the advanced stages of the syndrome, symptoms of blurred vision and pain may persist throughout the day. Patients also may present with the complaint of an irregular shape or position of the pupil (corectopia), or they may describe a dark spot in the eye, which may represent hole formation (pseudopolycoria) or stromal atrophy of the iris. The various degrees of iris atrophy characterize the specific clinical entities.

Progressive (Essential) Iris Atrophy

This variation is characterized by severe iris atrophy that results in heterochromia, marked corectopia, ectropion uveae, and pseudopolycoria (hole formation). Hole formation is the hallmark finding of progressive iris atrophy (Fig. 230-1).

Chandler's Syndrome

This variation shows minimal or no iris stromal atrophy, but mild corectopia may occur. The corneal edema and angle findings predominate and are typical (Fig. 230-2).

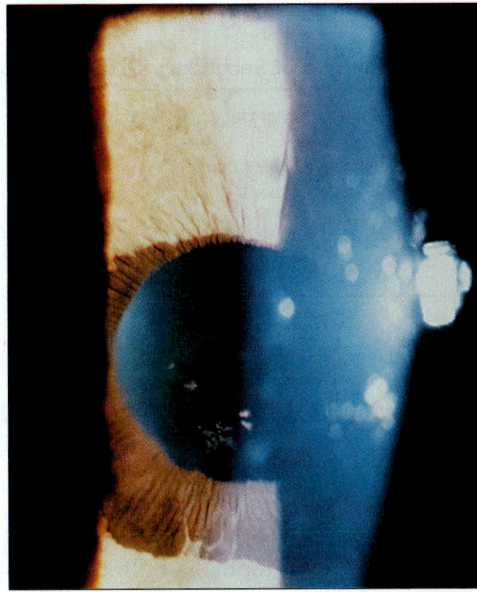

FIG. 230-2 ■ Corneal edema and iris findings are typical of Chandler's syndrome.

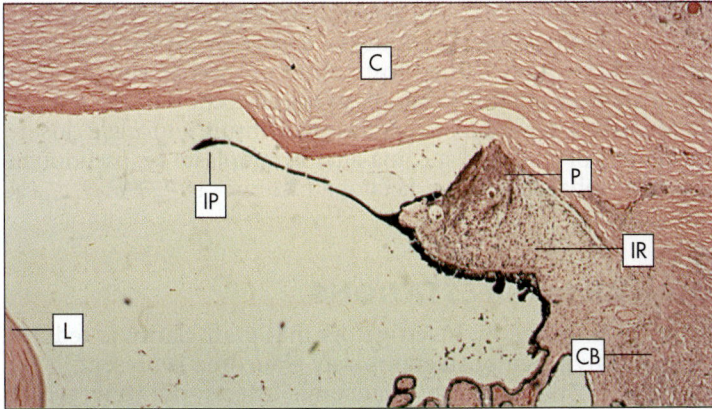

FIG. 230-3 ■ Iridocorneal endothelial syndrome. Histological section of an eye that had essential (progressive) iris atrophy shows a peripheral synechia (P), various degrees of degeneration and loss of the central iris stroma, and total loss of the central iris pigment epithelium (IP). (C, Cornea; CB, ciliary body; IR, iris root; L, lens.) (With permission from Yanoff M, Fine BS. Ocular pathology. London: Mosby; 1996.)

Cogan-Reese Syndrome

The iris atrophy tends to be variable and less severe. Tan, pedunculated nodules may appear on the anterior iris surface. The entire spectrum of corneal and other iris defects may occur in this variant.

PATHOLOGY

In each of the three clinical variations of ICE syndrome, corneal endothelial abnormalities are seen. A fine, hammered-silver appearance of the posterior cornea, similar to the guttae seen in Fuchs' corneal endothelial dystrophy, is noted[4]; this results from the abnormal endothelial cells posterior to a normal Descemet's membrane. Researchers, using electron microscopy, have shown this endothelial layer to vary in thickness from a single layer to multiple layers.[5, 6] In addition, within the same eye, the endothelial cell layer may be of different thicknesses in different areas. Evidence of filopodial cytoplasmic processes and cytoplasmic actin filaments implies that the endothelial cells are able to migrate. The morphology of the endothelium suggests a widespread state of high metabolic activity.[7,8] Corneal edema is secondary to these marked endothelial abnormalities. The anterior chamber angle may show high PAS that extend beyond Schwalbe's line. Such PAS are caused by the contraction of this endothelial cell layer and surrounding collagenous, fibrillar tis-

sues, which are continuous and extend from the peripheral cornea over the trabecular meshwork and iris. An angle-closure glaucoma results as these PAS contract and close the angle. The pupil is drawn toward the sector that has the most prominent PAS. As stated earlier, secondary glaucoma with an open angle also may occur when the endothelial membrane covers the trabecular meshwork without evidence of synechiae formation.

The iris abnormalities differentiate the specific clinical variations. The endothelial cell layer that extends over portions of the anterior iris surface from the anterior chamber angle contracts, which distorts and pulls the iris toward itself. Hole formation occurs opposite the location of the abnormal endothelial cell layer secondary to the contracture (Fig. 230-3).[9] Hole formation may be associated with ischemia of the iris, as suggested by fluorescein angiography. In Cogan-Reese syndrome, the pigmented, pedunculated nodules seen are composed of underlying iris stroma pinched off by abnormal cellular membrane.[10]

A viral cause has been postulated for the mechanism of ICE syndrome. Epstein-Barr and herpes simplex viruses have been found serologically in ICE patients.[5, 11] This theory was postulated after lymphocytes were seen on the corneal endothelium of an ICE patient, which indicated the presence of chronic inflammation.

TREATMENT

The diagnosis of ICE syndrome must be considered in younger patients who have unilateral angle-closure glaucoma; it is confirmed by specular or confocal microscopy. Corneal edema and secondary glaucoma are the major concerns to be addressed. Corneal edema can often be controlled using hypertonic saline solutions, and when the IOP is elevated, its reduction may help lessen corneal edema. Elevated IOP that occurs with secondary glaucoma can often be controlled medically using aqueous suppressants. Miotics are often ineffective, and hypotensive lipid–prostaglandin analogs can have variable results. If the IOP remains uncontrolled, filtration surgery may be indicated, although late failures have been reported secondary to fistular endothelialization.[12, 13] These fistulae may be reopened successfully when the endothelial cell membrane is cut using the neodymium:yttrium-aluminum-garnet (Nd:YAG) laser. In a study of 66 patients who had ICE syndrome, the success rates of initial trabeculectomy operations at 1 and 3 years were 64% and 36%, respectively, and those of second and third operations at 1-year intervals were both 58%.[13] Seton procedures are indicated for cases refractory to the previously mentioned treatments and, more recently, have been used as primary procedures.[14]

AXENFELD-RIEGER SYNDROME

Axenfeld-Rieger (A-R) syndrome represents a rare spectrum of developmental disorders involving abnormalities of both ocular and extraocular structures derived from the neural crest.[15] The term *anterior cleavage syndrome* was used in the past,[16] but it incorrectly reflects the development in this syndrome. All clinical variations of this syndrome are now referred to as Axenfeld-Rieger syndrome.

EPIDEMIOLOGY AND PATHOGENESIS

A-R syndrome involves the anterior segment bilaterally and is associated with secondary glaucoma because of arrested angle development in about 50% of cases. It is a rare, autosomal dominant inherited disorder. Shields[17] postulated that developmental arrest that occurs late in gestation results in primordial endothelium being retained over parts of the iris and anterior chamber angle. Contraction of this primordial monolayer causes iris stromal thinning, corectopia, and hole formation. With contraction, the anterior uvea is hindered from posterior migration, which results in a high insertion of the iris into the anterior chamber angle.[15] The responsible gene (RIEG/P1x2) has been isolated to the long arm of chromosome 4 (4q25).[18, 19] The affected anterior segment structures are primarily of neural crest derivation. The most common extraocular defects involve the teeth and facial bones.

OCULAR MANIFESTATIONS

The typical abnormality of the cornea is an anteriorly displaced Schwalbe's line (posterior embryotoxon), which appears as a white ring on the posterior cornea near the limbus. It tends to be more common temporally and rarely involves all 360°. An anteriorly displaced Schwalbe's line occurs in 8–15%[20, 21] of the general population and may not always be present with A-R syndrome. The anterior chamber angle, observed using gonioscopy, exhibits posterior embryotoxon and iridocorneal adhesions that are broad to threadlike in nature. These iridocorneal adhesions may extend anteriorly to Schwalbe's line and obscure the scleral spur and trabecular meshwork. Iris defects, ranging from stromal thinning to actual hole formation, corectopia, and ectropion uveae, may occur.

SYSTEMIC ASSOCIATIONS

Developmental defects associated with A-R syndrome most commonly involve the teeth and facial bones. Microdontia (peg-like incisors), hypodontia (decreased number of evenly spaced teeth), and anodontia (focal absence of teeth) are noted most commonly.[16,21] The facial abnormalities include maxillary hypoplasia and a protruding lower lid. Telecanthus,[22] hypertelorism,[22] and primary empty-sella syndrome have been documented with A-R syndrome.[15,23]

PATHOLOGY

The peripheral cornea characteristically exhibits an anteriorly displaced Schwalbe's line. This posterior embryotoxon shows a cellular monolayer with basement membrane that covers dense collagen.[15, 21] The iridocorneal strands tend to be iris stroma mixed with the above-mentioned cellular monolayer. This cellular membrane also may extend over the iris surface, which distorts the iris, creates iris stromal thinning, and results in actual hole formation and corectopia as it contracts.

TREATMENT

Medical therapy is recommended before the initiation of surgical intervention. Medications that decrease aqueous output (β-blockers, α-agonists, and carbonic anhydrase inhibitors) have proved to be more beneficial than those affecting outflow (pilocarpine, hypotensive lipids). Glaucoma most often occurs in children and young adults.[15] Surgical intervention may be goniotomy or trabeculectomy.[24,25] The procedure of choice in A-R syndrome is trabeculectomy with the adjunctive use of antimetabolites.[26,27] If the initial surgical treatment fails, seton procedures may have to be utilized.[28]

PENETRATING KERATOPLASTY

Secondary glaucoma is a common complication of penetrating keratoplasty and occurs with increased frequency in aphakic and pseudophakic patients[29] and in those who have repeat grafts. The different mechanisms of secondary glaucoma formation are listed in Box 230-1. Preexisting conditions, wound distortion of the trabecular meshwork, and chronic angle closure are the most common causes of long-standing glaucoma in these patients.

> **BOX 230-1**
>
> **Mechanisms of Secondary Glaucoma Formation**
>
> Wound distortion of trabecular meshwork
> Fibrous ingrowth
> Postoperative inflammation
> Chronic angle closure
> Viscoelastic
> Corticosteroid induced
> Pre–existing conditions

EPIDEMIOLOGY AND PATHOGENESIS

Penetrating keratoplasty has become a commonly performed procedure and is one of the most successful of all transplants, with a 1-year survival rate of 80–90%.[30] Postkeratoplasty glaucoma occurs more frequently in patients affected by preexisting glaucoma. Aphakic and pseudophakic bullous keratopathies are the most common indications for penetrating keratoplasty, at rates of 20–70% and 18–53%, respectively.[29] One study indicated no early or late glaucoma in patients who had penetrating keratoplasty for keratoconus, and a less than 2% incidence in patients who had Fuchs' corneal endothelial dystrophy treated with penetrating keratoplasty.[31] The most common mechanisms for glaucoma after penetrating keratoplasty are distortion of the trabecular meshwork secondary to graft wound closure and angle closure. Incidences of clinical glaucoma after keratoplasty for pseudophakic and aphakic bullous keratopathies are 18–53%[29,31–34] and 20–70%,[29,31,35,36] respectively.

OCULAR MANIFESTATIONS

It has been noted by investigators that graft clarity is reduced significantly when postkeratoplasty glaucoma is present.[37,38] In essence, postkeratoplasty glaucoma affects not only visual function but also graft integrity. In early postkeratoplasty glaucoma, epithelial edema is found along with stromal thinning and compression. Such findings are noted before endothelial damage occurs.[39] Progressive angle closure from peripheral synechiae formation is a warning sign for potential glaucoma in postkeratoplasty patients. Some studies demonstrated that PAS are present in all eyes that showed elevated IOP after keratoplasty.[36] One major study in which routine gonioscopy was conducted, however, found that progressive synechial closure was a plausible explanation for only 14% of eyes that had elevated IOP.[32]

The role of corticosteroids and their influence on postoperative glaucoma must be addressed. The use of potent corticosteroids at frequent intervals was reported to reduce the rates of early IOP elevation.[36] In contrast, certain cases of IOP elevation may be related to corticosteroid responders. Secondary to corticosteroid use, reported IOP rates are increased 5–60%.[32,33,35,36,40] This shows the two-edged sword of corticosteroids: (1) the need to use them to minimize postkeratoplasty inflammation, and (2) their possible influence on postkeratoplasty glaucoma.

TREATMENT

Treatment modalities for postkeratoplasty glaucoma include medical control, trabeculectomy, seton procedures, and cyclodestructive procedures. The initial treatment of choice is medical therapy. However, in the presence of significant synechial closure, drugs that influence outflow facility (i.e., miotics) may have limited action. Similarly, the role of hypotensive lipid–prostaglandin analogs in this type of glaucoma and their influence on graft survival and graft clarity remain uncertain. Dorzolamide has been shown to decrease corneal endothelial function and to increase corneal thickness, and reported cases of graft failure have been attributed to its use.

Setons (i.e., Ahmed, Krupin, Molteno, Baerveldt, Schocket) have been useful in controlling IOP among patients who have had difficult previous surgeries.[41] In one study, however, 29% of patients progressed to failure after Molteno implantation, and 20% after insertion of Schocket's tube.[42] The reason for these failure rates is unknown, but some investigators speculate that the cause may be chronic inflammation or a breakdown in the blood-ocular barrier. The valved implants cause less inflammation and may be better tolerated. Placement of the seton through the pars plana may also improve graft survival.

Filtration surgery shows success rates of 27–80%.[32,42–45] Aphakic eyes have a lower success rate than do pseudophakic or phakic eyes. Graft failure at 3 years after trabeculectomy is in the range of 11–20%.[32,43] Cyclodestructive procedures can lower IOP effectively after penetrating keratoplasty. Laser cyclophotoablation is used in preference to cyclocryotherapy because of its reduced side effects and improved visual result. The reported success rate for laser cyclophotoablation is 50–100%. Graft failure has been reported with laser cyclophotoablation.[44,46,47]

EPITHELIAL DOWNGROWTH AND FIBROUS INGROWTH (PROLIFERATION)

Epithelial and fibrous proliferations are rare postoperative surgical complications that may result in devastating secondary glaucomas and are caused by an invasion of the anterior chamber by epithelium or connective tissue through a defect in the wound site.[48] Fortunately, with improved surgical techniques and improved wound closure, the incidence of these entities has been reduced greatly.

EPIDEMIOLOGY AND PATHOGENESIS

The incidence of epithelial downgrowth and fibrous ingrowth has declined greatly over the years. The prevalence of epithelial downgrowth was in the range of 0.12–0.6% in series of eyes after intracapsular cataract surgery in the 1940s and 1950s.[49–51] It once occurred more commonly after cataract surgery, but it now occurs more commonly with penetrating keratoplasty,[52–54] ocular trauma, glaucoma filtration surgery,[55,56] and other corneal surgical procedures. Fibrous ingrowth is more prevalent than epithelial downgrowth, progresses more slowly, and is often self-limited. Epithelial downgrowth and fibrous ingrowth can occur simultaneously.[49] It has been shown that prolonged inflammation is a major risk factor for epithelial and fibrous proliferation.[57] Other risk factors are wound dehiscence, delayed closure of the wound postoperatively, and stripping of Descemet's layer.[58,59]

Normal healing of the corneal scleral wound entails ingrowth of connective tissue to the inner margin of the wound and formation of a fibrous plug. The inner wound margin usually is covered by endothelium by about the second week postoperatively. This ingrowth is halted through contact inhibition by migrated endothelium.[60, 61] If the endothelium does not bridge this defect, epithelial and fibrous proliferation can occur; thus, an abnormality in the corneal endothelium is also a risk factor. It has been suggested that posterior limbal incisions may be associated with fibrous ingrowth, and anterior limbal incisions may be associated with epithelial downgrowth.[57] With the recent advent of small incision surgery, this disparity is almost nil. Other proposed risk factors for fibrous and epithelial proliferation are fornix-based conjunctival flaps, intraocular use of surgical instruments on the conjunctiva,[62] and use of intracameral anticoagulant therapy.[63]

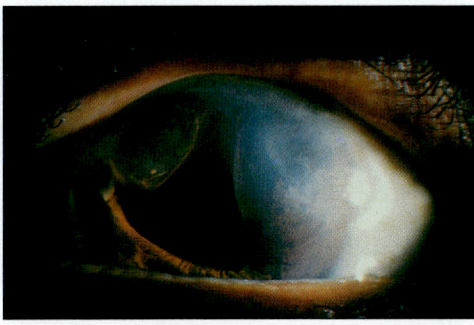

FIG. 230-4 ▨ Transluscent, nonvascular, anterior chamber epithelial cyst.

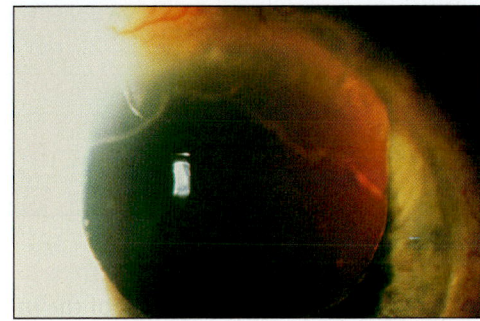

FIG. 230-5 ▨ Grayish, sheetlike epithelial ingrowth with rolled edges.

OCULAR MANIFESTATIONS

Epithelial proliferation may be present in three forms: "pearl" tumors of the iris, epithelial cysts, and epithelial ingrowth. Epithelial cysts and epithelial ingrowth often cause secondary glaucoma. Epithelial cysts appear as translucent, nonvascular anterior chamber cysts that originate from surgical or traumatic wounds (Fig. 230-4). Epithelial ingrowth presents as a grayish, sheetlike growth with rolled edges on the posterior surface of the cornea (Fig. 230-5), trabecular meshwork, iris, and ciliary body; it is often associated with wound incarceration, wound gape, ocular inflammation, band keratopathy,[54,64] and corneal edema. Unlike epithelial proliferation, fibrous ingrowth is slow to progress and may be self-limited. A common cause of corneal graft failure, fibrous ingrowth appears as a thick, gray-white, vascular, retrocorneal membrane with an irregular, scalloped border reminiscent of woven cloth.[65] The ingrowth often involves the angle, which results in the formation of PAS and the destruction of the trabecular meshwork. The resultant secondary angle-closure glaucoma is a frequent complication and is often difficult to control medically. A major advancement in the diagnosis of epithelialization is use of the argon laser to make burns on the surface of the iris—areas of epithelialization turn white when burned by the laser.[66] Specular and confocal microscopy provides another means of diagnosis by direct visualization of epithelial cells in the ingrowth.[67]

PATHOLOGY

Epithelial downgrowth consists of a multilayered membrane composed of nonkeratinized, stratified, squamous epithelium that has surface microvilli; wide intercellular borders, with occasional hemidesmosomes attached to a subepithelial connective tissue layer; and epithelial cells of uneven sizes and shapes.[68, 69] This epithelial sheet lacks blood vessels and shows multiple tonofilaments at its leading edge (Fig. 230-6).[70] The underlying structures in contact with the epithelial sheet undergo disorganization and destruction.

TREATMENT

Management of epithelial cysts includes observation until complications are observed. Numerous approaches have been used

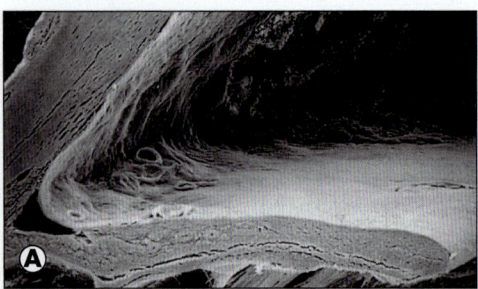

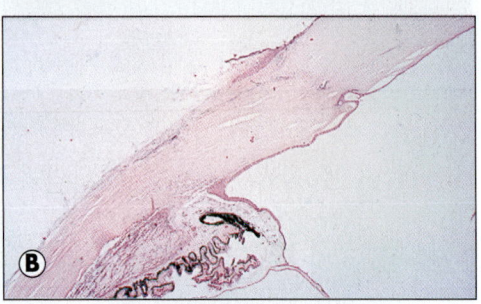

FIG. 230-6 ■ Epithelial iris cyst and downgrowth. A, Scanning electron microscopy shows a sheet of epithelium that covers the trabecular meshwork, anterior face of the ciliary body, anterior iris, and pupillary margin. B, Epithelium lines the posterior cornea, anterior chamber angle, and peripheral iris and extends onto the vitreous posteriorly in a surgically aphakic eye. (With permission from Yanoff M, Fine BS. Ocular pathology. London: Mosby; 1996.)

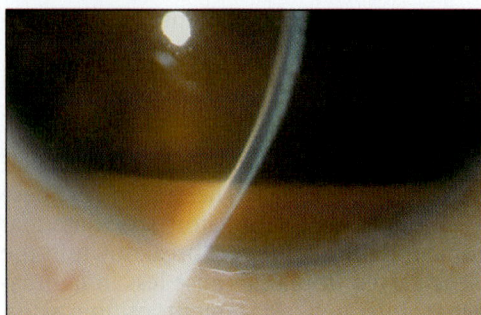

FIG. 230-7 ■ Ghost cell glaucoma. Layered ghost cells in the inferior anterior chamber angle.

to excise epithelial cysts, but currently a wide excision of the intact cyst is preferred. If the cyst is adherent to any intraocular structures, it may be collapsed by aspiration before excision. Photocoagulation of epithelial cysts, a less invasive procedure than surgical removal, has been performed successfully.[71] Photocoagulation is less effective when the cyst is nonpigmented or adherent to underlying structures.

Management options for epithelial proliferation include:
- Freezing the involved corneal surface to close the wound gape or fistula.
- Swabbing the involved corneal surface with absolute alcohol.
- Resecting the posterior membrane.[72]

Management of glaucoma is a difficult challenge and has a high failure rate using traditional filtration surgery techniques. Glaucoma drainage implants have been shown to be the most effective procedure with both fibrous and epithelial ingrowth.[14,73] Cycloablation is used only when other treatment modalities fail.

GHOST CELL HEMOLYTIC GLAUCOMA

Ghost cell glaucoma is a transient, secondary open-angle glaucoma caused by denatured, hemolyzed erythrocytes (ghost cells) that block the trabecular meshwork. These denatured erythrocytes develop within 2–4 weeks of a vitreous hemorrhage. Any event that causes hemorrhage in the vitreous cavity[74] or, rarely, in the anterior chamber may result in ghost cell glaucoma.

EPIDEMIOLOGY AND PATHOGENESIS

Ghost cells are red blood cells that have lost their intracellular hemoglobin and appear as khaki-colored cells that are less pliant than normal red blood cells. This loss of pliability results in obstruction of the trabecular meshwork and subsequent secondary glaucoma. The cells gain access to the anterior chamber through a disrupted hyaloid face or a rent in the posterior capsule that may arise from previous surgery (pars plana vitrectomy, cataract extraction, or capsulotomy), trauma, or spontaneous disruption.

OCULAR MANIFESTATIONS

Clinically, patients present with increased IOP and a history of a recent vitreous hemorrhage resulting from trauma, surgery, or preexisting disease. The IOP may be elevated markedly and cause corneal edema. The anterior chamber is filled with circulating, small, tan-colored cells that can become layered in the in-

ferior anterior chamber angle (Fig. 230-7). The cellular reaction appears out of proportion to the aqueous flare, and the conjunctiva tends not to be inflamed unless the IOP is elevated markedly. Gonioscopically, the angle appears normal except for the ghost cells that lay over the trabecular meshwork inferiorly.

PATHOLOGY

Ghost cells lose hemoglobin through permeable cell membranes. They are nonpliable, have lost their natural biconcavity, and are unable to exit through the trabecular meshwork efficiently. The ghost cell's cytoplasm is lined with denatured hemoglobin, called Heinz bodies,[75] which may be diagnostic in anterior chamber aspirates and are demonstrated using phase-contrast microscopy.

TREATMENT

The initial treatment is medical, followed by surgery in eyes that are nonresponsive. Irrigation of the anterior chamber and pars plana vitrectomy are the surgeries of choice to eliminate the source of degenerative red blood cells. If this is unsuccessful, filtration surgery may be required.

ALKALI CHEMICAL TRAUMA

In the acute setting of a patient who has an alkali burn, glaucoma may be overlooked as a complication. It occurs in the acute and late settings, with a possible intermediate period of hypotony secondary to ciliary body damage. Secondary glaucoma occurs more often in association with alkali burns than with acidic burns.

EPIDEMIOLOGY AND PATHOGENESIS

As a result of saponification of fatty acids in tissue, severe damage to intraocular structures may occur with exposure to alkali, because alkaline chemicals are able to penetrate ocular tissues rapidly. In contrast, acidic chemicals have a tendency to coagulate tissue proteins, and the layer of precipitated protein helps buffer and limit the acid's penetration through the cornea. Different mechanisms for each phase of IOP elevation have been postulated. The initial pressure elevation may be secondary to tissue shrinkage of the outer coats of the eye[76] or to prostaglandin release that increases uveal blood flow.[77] The intermediate and late phases show changes in the eye as part of the body's response. In these phases, trabecular damage, PAS, and secondary pupillary block are possible mechanisms for the development of glaucoma.

OCULAR MANIFESTATIONS

Damage to the cornea may be widespread and progressive. Epithelial disintegration may be followed by stromal ulcerations and perforation. Measurement of IOP in eyes that have extensive corneal damage may be difficult using Goldmann applanation tonometry. A Tonopen or pneumotonometer may be more accurate. Gonioscopy may be difficult in these patients because of corneal opacification, in which case ultrasound examination may be necessary to visualize the extent of optic nerve cupping and retinal damage. Later in the disease process, symblepharon formation of the palpebral conjunctiva may obliterate the fornices.

PATHOLOGY

After exposure to an alkaline chemical, the corneal keratocytes rapidly coagulate to leave devitalized corneal stroma. The bulk of the corneal mucopolysaccharide ground substance also is destroyed, which is followed by collagen fiber swelling. The IOP elevation may result from anterior segment shrinkage or prostaglandin-mediated inflammation. Other possible mechanisms for secondary glaucoma include direct chemical injury or PAS formation. Intraocular lens damage may result in cataract formation, and the associated lens swelling may result in a secondary phacomorphic glaucoma.

TREATMENT

Immediate ocular irrigation is needed to remove the chemical from the corneal surface and fornices. Neutralization of an acid with a base or vice versa is contraindicated. When neutralization of a chemical is attempted, a thermal reaction occurs, which produces heat and causes further damage. The management of increased IOP in the early phase is pharmacological; miotics and hypotensive lipid–prostaglandin analogs should be used cautiously, because they may increase intraocular inflammation, a common complication of chemical trauma. Anti-inflammatory medications and cycloplegics are important during the first week; topical corticosteroids are administered with caution because of their potential effect on corneal stromal melting.[78] Conventional medical and surgical therapies are used for the later phases of IOP elevation associated with chemical trauma.

ANIRIDIA

Aniridia is a rare, bilateral, hereditary absence of the iris. The condition rarely occurs in its pure form and usually presents with a rudimentary stump of iris.

EPIDEMIOLOGY AND PATHOGENESIS

Aniridia is seen in approximately 1.8/100,000 live births.[79] Three phenotypes are recognized, of which autosomal dominant aniridia is the most common; it is present in approximately 85% of all cases and is not associated with any other systemic manifestations. The second type is congenital sporadic aniridia, found in association with Wilms' tumor (nephroblastoma), genitourinary anomalies, and mental retardation (Miller's syndrome). It has been labeled WAGR syndrome (for Wilms' tumor, aniridia, genitourinary anomalies, retardation), is linked with partial deletions of the short arm of chromosome 11 (11p13), and accounts for approximately 13% of all aniridias. Autosomal recessive aniridia is the third genetic type; it is seen in approximately 2% of all cases and is associated with cerebellar ataxia and mental retardation (Gillespie's syndrome).[80]

Different theories have been developed to explain the pathogenesis of aniridia. Some researchers consider it a subtype of coloboma. In addition, some aniridias are associated with hypoplastic discs and the absence of iris musculature, on the basis of which investigators have proposed mesodermal and neuroectodermal theories, respectively. Glaucoma develops in about 50% of patients who have aniridia.[81] Glaucoma is rare in newborns; it is usually seen after the second decade of life, as anatomical changes occur in the angle secondary to contracture

of peripheral iris strands.[82] These iris strands bridge the space between the iris stump and trabecular meshwork, and the progressive contracture of the iris strands creates an angle-closure glaucoma. In addition, goniodysgenesis is noted in some cases.

OCULAR MANIFESTATIONS

The clinical manifestations of aniridia include photophobia related to the extent of iris involvement. Pendular nystagmus, decreased vision, amblyopia, and strabismus are seen secondary to foveal and optic nerve head hypoplasia. Bilateral ptosis also may occur in aniridia. With gonioscopy, the iris appears as a rudimentary stump with fibers that bridge the angle. This rudimentary iris leaflet appears to be pulled forward by iris strands, which results in posterior synechiae formation and subsequent angle-closure glaucoma. In addition to the anterior segment changes, findings in the posterior segment may include foveal and optic nerve head hypoplasia and choroidal coloboma. Lenticular changes include cataract, ectopia lentis, microphakia, and persistent pupillary membranes. Microcornea[83] and corneal opacifications also have been observed in aniridic patients. The corneal opacification is often associated with a fine, vascular network and pannus formation.[84]

SYSTEMIC ASSOCIATIONS

Wilms' tumor (nephroblastoma) is found in association with aniridia in Miller's syndrome; 25–33% of patients who have sporadic aniridia develop Wilms' tumor. In addition to Wilms' tumor, severe mental retardation, genitourinary anomalies, craniofacial dysmorphism, and hemihypertrophy can occur.[79] In Gillespie's syndrome, mental retardation and cerebellar ataxia are seen.

PATHOLOGY

Arrestment of the neuroectodermal tissue is the most striking histopathological feature of this condition. With histological examination, a small stump of iris that lacks iris musculature may be observed. The iris remnant appears continuous with the trabecular meshwork. Glaucoma in Miller's syndrome may develop secondary to angle anomalies, which include dysgenesis of the trabecular meshwork and Schlemm's canal.[79]

TREATMENT

Glaucoma and its surgical complications are the main causes of blindness in patients with aniridia. By 20 years of age, most aniridic patients eventually fail pharmacological therapy[80] and require surgery for adequate IOP control.[79,85,86] A prophylactic modified goniotomy has been advocated to prevent this secondary glaucoma in certain young patients with aniridia.[87,88]

TUMORS AND GLAUCOMA

A variety of tumors may cause unilateral glaucoma; the most common ones associated with glaucoma include primary melanomas, metastases, and retinoblastomas. The mechanism of glaucoma development varies with the location, type, and size of the tumor. Choroidal melanomas and other choroidal and retinal tumors tend to cause secondary angle-closure glaucoma, as a result of a forward shift in the lens-iris diaphragm and subsequent closure of the anterior chamber angle. Inflammation caused by necrotic tumors may result in posterior synechiae, which can exacerbate this angle closure through a pupillary block mechanism. Choroidal melanomas, medulloepitheliomas, and retinoblastomas also may cause anterior segment neovascularization that results in angle closure and may liberate tumor cells that obstruct aqueous outflow.

EPIDEMIOLOGY AND PATHOGENESIS

In 1987, Shields et al.[89] studied 2704 eyes that had intraocular tumors, of which 5% were found to have IOP elevation secondary to the tumor. The most common tumor in adults to result in glaucoma was malignant uveal melanoma. Iris melanomas may cause an increase in IOP by local infiltration of the anterior chamber angle. Other reported mechanisms for glaucoma formation in association with iris melanomas are pigment, tumor, or inflammatory cell dispersion that results in obstruction of the trabecular meshwork. Shields et al.[89] found glaucoma in 7 of 102 eyes that had iris melanoma. Iris melanocytomas are rare and have a predisposition to release pigment into the anterior chamber, which causes a secondary open-angle glaucoma.[90] Ciliary body melanomas may present with increased IOP secondary to a variety of mechanisms. Forward displacement of the lens-iris diaphragm, direct invasion of the aqueous outflow system by melanin-laden macrophages, and pigmentary dispersion have been reported to cause glaucoma in these cases.[91]

Shields et al.[89] reported that 16 of 96 eyes that had ciliary body melanomas also had associated glaucoma. Medulloepithelioma (diktyoma) is a tumor of the nonpigmented ciliary epithelium and usually presents in childhood as a cystic or solid tumor. In one study, about 50% of eyes that had medulloepitheliomas presented with glaucoma. The study showed neovascularization of the anterior chamber with angle closure to be the most common cause of glaucoma.[92] Other secondary causes of glaucoma with medulloepitheliomas were mechanical displacement of the angle, direct invasion of the angle, and one case of recurrent hyphema.[90]

Retinoblastoma is the most common malignant intraocular tumor of childhood. Approximately 1 in 14,000–20,000 newborns have retinoblastoma, and 30–35% of cases occur bilaterally, with no sex or race predisposition. Glaucoma secondary to retinoblastoma shows an incidence in the range of 2–22%.[89,93] Neovascular glaucoma accounts for 73% of the glaucomas associated with retinoblastoma secondary to tumor-induced retinal ischemia.[89] It also has been postulated that angiogenic factors may be produced by the tumor itself.[94] The second most common cause of glaucoma in these eyes is anterior displacement of the lens-iris diaphragm.

Uveal metastasis occurs most frequently to the posterior choroid. The most common sites of origin are breasts in women and lungs in men.[95] In contrast to iris and ciliary body metastasis, metastatic tumors to the choroid show only about a 2% incidence of glaucoma. The main presentation of glaucoma results from a forward shift of the lens-iris diaphragm secondary to nonrhegmatogenous retinal detachment.[96] Glaucoma is associated with 64% of iris metastases and 67% of ciliary body metastases.[89] Elevated IOP results in patients with these tumors, usually from localized blockage of the trabecular meshwork by released tumor cells.[96]

OCULAR MANIFESTATIONS

The clinical presentation of glaucoma that arises from intraocular tumors is dependent on the mechanism of inducement. Glaucoma secondary to tumors may present as a secondary angle-closure glaucoma by a posterior-push mechanism (i.e., a posterior segment tumor causes an anterior rotation of the ciliary body or a forward shift of the lens-iris diaphragm) or an anterior-pull mechanism (i.e., PAS and neovascularization of the angle). Other mechanisms include those of secondary open-angle glaucoma (i.e., pigmentary glaucoma; tumor cell, red blood cell, and cellular debris obstruction of the angle; inflammatory glaucoma; and direct invasion of the angle by tumor).

PATHOLOGY

Iris melanoma usually appears as a well-circumscribed, variably pigmented, fixed or slow-growing tumor that may eventually invade the trabecular meshwork. The tumor is composed of spindle-shaped cells with occasional epithelioid cells.[96] Ciliary body melanoma appears as a circumscribed mass that replaces the ciliary body. The cell types are both spindle and epithelioid, with a larger number of the latter found in ciliary body melanoma than in iris melanoma. Choroidal melanoma appears as a variably pigmented mass that may result in a secondary nonrhegmatogenous retinal detachment. Such melanomas also may be composed of epithelioid or spindle cells. The lesion may create a "mushroom" configuration if it breaks through Bruch's membrane. Melanocytoma appears as a brown or black mass that may be well circumscribed[95] and usually occurs at the optic disc but may arise anywhere in the uvea. Necrotic areas are present within the mass, which may result in fragmentation and liberation of tumor cells into the angle.[96]

Iris and ciliary body metastases usually have poor differentiation, which makes determination of the primary site difficult. Choroidal metastases are ill-defined, relatively elevated or diffuse lesions, often associated with serous or choroidal retinal detachment. The lesions may present with a brown discoloration secondary to overlying pigment or with a gray to yellow–cream color. Retinoblastoma appears as a chalky white mass within the globe and is composed of neuroblastic cells; areas of calcification and necrosis are common findings. The differentiated tumors are characterized by highly organized Flexner-Wintersteiner rosettes.[96] Medulloepithelioma is an embryonic tumor that usually occurs in the ciliary body. The tumor appears as a yellow–pink solid or cystic mass and may contain rosettes. Medulloepithelioma has two types of presentation: the nonteratoid type is composed of nonpigmented epithelium, and the teratoid type shows two different germ layers (i.e., cartilage and skeletal muscle).[96]

TREATMENT

Management of malignant ocular tumors often leads to enucleation. Traditional filtration techniques run the risk that tumor cells may be seeded to extraocular areas, even after treatment with radiation. In those patients who have secondary glaucoma as a result of benign tumors, medical management and traditional filtration surgeries may be appropriate. Proper diagnosis of tumors usually is made clinically. Fluorescein angiography and ultrasonography (A-scan, B-scan, UBM) help in the detection and diagnosis of intraocular tumors. In some patients, a fine-needle biopsy, aqueous aspiration, or biopsy is needed for diagnosis.

SCHWARTZ'S SYNDROME

The first description of chronic open-angle glaucoma secondary to rhegmatogenous retinal detachment was presented in 1973 by Schwartz.[97] He described a small number of patients who had unilateral, open-angle glaucoma and a history of retinal detachment. All 11 patients had uncontrolled glaucoma in association with untreated retinal detachments that ranged from 1 week to 1 year in duration. After successful reattachment of the retina, prompt resolution of the glaucoma occurred in all 11 patients; interestingly, all 11 had a concomitant appearance of iridocyclitis.

In 1977, Phelps and Burton[98] surveyed 817 patients who underwent retinal detachment repair. They found 18 patients (2.2%) who fit the criteria for Schwartz's syndrome. Several theories have been put forward to explain the increase in IOP accompanying retinal detachment. Schwartz[97] postulated that the associated iridocyclitis causes a trabeculitis that decreases aqueous outflow. Matsuo et al.[99] detected photoreceptor outer segments in the anterior chambers of seven patients who had retinal detachments, a discovery that established a connection between the subretinal space and the anterior chamber in this group of patients. The same authors also suggested that this connection may allow the transmission of a more viscous subretinal fluid that decreases outflow facility.

In 1989, Lambrou *et al.*[100] injected rod outer segments into the anterior chambers of cats *in vivo*, which resulted in an average rise in IOP of 10mmHg (1.33kPa). Electron microscopy revealed occlusion of the intratrabecular spaces by the rod outer segments, with little evidence of inflammatory activity. An interesting observation was that injected rod outer segments mimicked cells in the anterior chamber, which may represent what Schwartz described as iridocyclitis in his original article.[101]

Davidorf[102] described four cases of retinal detachment with elevated IOP and heavy pigmentation of the trabecular meshwork. He explained the rise in IOP as a result of mechanical blockage of the trabecular meshwork; IOP decreased after successful reattachment of the retina. In spite of the different theories for the basis of Schwartz's syndrome, treatment is repair of the retinal detachment. The increased IOP and iridocyclitis tend to be unresponsive to medical treatment.

REFERENCES

1. Yanoff M. In discussion of Shields MB, McCracken JS, Klintworth GK, Campbell DG. Corneal edema in essential iris atrophy. Ophthalmology. 1979;86:1549–55.
2. Wilson MC, Shields MB. A comparison of the clinical variations of the iridocorneal endothelial syndrome. Arch Ophthalmol. 1989;107:1465–9.
3. Laganowski HC, Kerr Muir MG, Hitchings RA. Glaucoma and the iridocorneal endothelial syndrome. Arch Ophthalmol. 1992;110:346–50.
4. Hirst LW, Quigley HA, Stark WJ, Shields MB. Specular microscopy of iridocorneal endothelial syndrome. Am J Ophthalmol. 1980;89:11–21.
5. Campbell DG, Shields MB, Smith TR. The corneal endothelium and spectrum of essential iris atrophy. Am J Ophthalmol. 1978;86:317–24.
6. Alvarado JA, Murphy CG, Maglio M, Hetherington J. Pathogenesis of Chandler's syndrome, essential iris atrophy, and Cogan-Reese syndrome. I. Alterations of the corneal endothelium. Invest Ophthalmol Vis Sci. 1986;27:853–82.
7. Rodrigues MM, Stutling RD, Waring GO III. Clinical, electron microscopic, and immunohistochemical study of the corneal endothelium and Descemet's membrane in the iridocorneal endothelial syndrome. Am J Ophthalmol. 1986; 101:16–27.
8. Eagle RC Jr, Font RL, Yanoff M, Fine BS. Proliferative endotheliopathy with iris abnormalities: the iridocorneal endothelial syndrome. Arch Ophthalmol. 1979; 97:2104–11.
9. Yanoff M, Fine BS. Ocular pathology. London: Mosby; 1996.
10. Shields MB, Campbell DG, Simmons RJ. The essential iris atrophies. Am J Ophthalmol. 1978;85:749–59.
11. Alvarado JA, Underwood JL, Green WR, et al. Detection of herpes simplex viral DNA in the iridocorneal endothelial syndrome. Arch Ophthalmol. 1994;112:1601–9.
12. Daicker B, Sturrock G, Guggenheim R. Clinicopathological correlation in Cogan-Reese syndrome. Klin Monatsbl Augenheilkd. 1982;180:531–8.
13. Kidd M, Hetherington J Jr, Magee S. Surgical results in iridocorneal endothelial syndrome. Arch Ophthalmol. 1988;106:199–201.
14. Assaad MH, Baerveldt G, Rockwood ET. Glaucoma drainage devices: pros and cons. Curr Opin Ophthalmol. 1999;10:147–53.
15. Shields MB. Axenfeld-Rieger syndrome: a theory of mechanism and distinctions from the iridocorneal endothelial syndrome. Trans Am Ophthalmol Soc. 1983; 81:736–84.
16. Reese AB, Ellsworth RM. The anterior chamber cleavage syndrome. Arch Ophthalmol. 1966;75:307.
17. Shields MB. Axenfeld-Rieger syndrome. In: Ritch R, Shields MB, Krupin T, eds. The glaucomas. St Louis: CV Mosby; 1996:875–84.
18. Mitchell JA, Packman S, Loughman WD, et al. Deletions of different segments of the long arm of chromosome 4. Am J Med Genet. 1981;89:73–84.
19. Vaux C, Sheffield L, Keith CG, Voullaire L. Evidence the Rieger syndrome maps to 4q25 or 4q27. J Med Genet. 1992;29:256.
20. Alkemade PPH. Dysgenesis mesodermalis of the iris and the cornea. Asses: Van Gorcum; 1969.
21. Burian HM, Braley AE, Allen L. External and gonioscopic visibility of the ring of Schwalbe and the trabecular one: an interpretation of the posterior corneal surface. Trans Am Ophthalmol Soc. 1955;51:389–94.
22. Wesley RK, Baker JD, Golnick AL. Rieger's syndrome (oligodontia and primary mesodermal dysgenesis of the iris): clinical features and report of an isolated case. J Pediatr Ophthalmol Strabismus. 1978;15:67.
23. Kleinman RE, Kazarian EL, Raptopoupos LE, Bauerman LE. Primary empty sella and Rieger's anomaly of anterior chamber of the eye. N Engl J Med. 1981;304: 90–3.
24. Wallace DK, Plager DA, Snyder SK, et al. Surgical results of secondary glaucomas in childhood. Ophthalmology. 1998;105:101–10.
25. Mullaney PB, Selleck C, Al-Awad A, et al. Combined trabeculotomy and trabeculectomy as an initial procedure in uncomplicated congenital glaucoma. Arch Ophthalmol. 1999;117:457–60.
26. Mandal AK, Walton DS, John T, Jayagandan A. Mitomycin C–augmented trabeculectomy in refractory congenital glaucoma. Ophthalmology. 1997;104:996–1003.
27. Mandal AK, Prasad K, Nadurilath TJ. Surgical results and complications of mitomycin C–augmented trabeculectomy in refractory developmental glaucoma. Ophthalmic Surg Lasers. 1999;30:473–9.
28. Burgoyne JK, WuDunn D, Lakhani V, Cantor LB. Outcomes of sequential tube shunts in complicated glaucoma. Ophthalmology. 2000;107:309–14.
29. Schanzlin DJ, Robin JB, Gomez DS, et al. Results of penetrating keratoplasty for aphakic and pseudophakic bullous keratopathy. Am J Ophthalmol. 1984; 98:302.
30. Council on Scientific Affairs. Report of the organ transplant council: corneal transplantation. JAMA. 1988;259:719–22.
31. Polack FM. Glaucoma in keratoplasty. Cornea. 1988;7:67.
32. Foulks GN. Glaucoma associated with penetrating keratoplasty. Ophthalmology. 1987;94:871–4.
33. Kirkness CM, Moshegov C. Post-keratoplasty glaucoma. Eye. 1988;2(Suppl):919.
34. Karesh JW, Nerankari VS. Factors associated with glaucoma after penetrating keratoplasty. Am J Ophthalmol. 1983;96:160–4.
35. Goldberg DB, Schanzlin DJ, Brown SI. Incidence of increased intraocular pressure after keratoplasty. Am J Ophthalmol. 1981;92:372–7.
36. Thoft RA, Gordon JM, Dohlman CH. Glaucoma following keratoplasty. Trans Am Acad Ophthalmol Otolaryngol. 1974;78:OP-352–64.
37. Paton D. The prognosis of penetrating keratoplasty based upon corneal morphology. Ophthalmol Surg. 1976;7:36–45.
38. Polack FM. Corneal transplantation. New York: Grune & Stratton; 1977.
39. Olson RJ, Kaufman HE. A mathematical description of causative factors and prevention of elevated intraocular pressure after keratoplasty. Invest Ophthalmol Vis Sci. 1977;16:1085–92.
40. Krontz DP, Wood TO. Corneal decompensation following acute angle-closure glaucoma. Ophthalmic Surg. 1988;19:334–8.
41. McDonnell PJ, Robin JB, Schanzlin DJ, et al. Molteno implant for control of glaucoma in eyes after penetrating keratoplasty. Ophthalmology. 1988;95:364–9.
42. Kirkness CM. Penetrating keratoplasty, glaucoma and silicone drainage tubing. Dev Ophthalmol. 1987;14:161.
43. Gilvarry AME, Kirkness CM, Steele AD, et al. The management of post-keratoplasty glaucoma by trabeculectomy. Eye. 1989;3:713–8.
44. Gross RL, Feldman RM, Spaeth GL, et al. Surgical therapy of chronic glaucoma in aphakia and pseudoaphakia. Ophthalmology. 1988;95:1195–201.
45. Kushwaha DC, Pual AK. Incidence and management of glaucoma in post operative cases of penetrating keratoplasty. Indian J Ophthalmol. 1981;29:167–70.
46. Cohen EJ, Schwartz LW, Luskind RD, et al. Neodymium:YAG laser transcleral cyclophotocoagulation for glaucoma after penetrating keratoplasty. Ophthalmic Surg. 1989;20:713–6.
47. Levy NS, Bonney RC. Transcleral YAG cyclophotocoagulation of the ciliary body for high intraocular pressure following penetrating keratoplasty. Cornea. 1989;8:178–81.
48. Smith MF, Doyle JW. Glaucoma secondary to epithelial and fibrous downgrowth. Semin Ophthalmol. 1994;9:248–53.
49. Theobald GD, Haas JS. Epithelial invasion of the anterior chamber following cataract extraction. Trans Am Acad Ophthalmol Otolaryngol. 1948;52:470.
50. Payne BF. Epithelialization of the anterior segment after cataract extractions. Am J Ophthalmol. 1958;45:182.
51. Rummelt V, Lang GK, Yanoff M, Namman GO. A 32-year follow-up of the rigid Schreck anterior camber lens. A clinicopathological correlation. Arch Ophthalmol. 1990;108:401–4.
52. Feder RS, Krachmer JH. The diagnosis of epithelial downgrowth after keratoplasty. Am J Ophthalmol. 1985;99:697.
53. Sugar A, Meyer RF, Hood I. Epithelial downgrowth following penetrating keratoplasty in the aphake. Arch Ophthalmol. 1977;95:464–7.
54. Leibowitz JM, Elliott JH, Boruchoff SA. Epithelialization of the anterior chamber following penetrating keratoplasty. Arch Ophthalmol. 1967;78:613–7.
55. Costa VP, Katz LJ, Cohen EJ, Raber IM. Glaucoma associated with epithelial downgrowth controlled with Molteno implant. Ophthalmol Surg. 1992;23: 797–800.
56. Loane MF, Weinreb RN. Glaucoma secondary to epithelial downgrowth and 5-fluorouracil. Ophthalmol Surg. 1990;21:704–6.
57. Henderson T. A histological study of normal healing of wounds after cataract extraction. Ophthalmol Rev. 1907;26:127–9.
58. Dunnington JH. Healing of incisions for cataract extraction. Am J Ophthalmol. 1951;34:36.
59. Anseth A, Dohlman CH, Albert DM. Epithelial downgrowth–fistula repair and keratoplasty. Refract Corneal Surg. 1991;7:23–7.
60. Terry TL, Chisholm JF Jr, Schonberg AL. Studies on surface epithelium invasion of the anterior segment of the eye. 1939;22:1083.
61. Cameron JD, Flaxman BA, Yanoff M. In vitro studies of corneal wound healing. Invest Ophthalmol. 1974;12:575–9.
62. Ferry AP. The possible role of epithelium-bearing in surgical instruments in pathogenesis of epithelialization of the anterior chamber. Ann Ophthalmol. 1971;3:1089.
63. Weiner MJ, Trentacoste J, Pon DM, et al. Epithelial downgrowth: a 30-year clinicopathological review. Br J Ophthalmol. 1989;73:6.
64. Swan KC, Campbell L. Unintentional filtration following cataract surgery. Arch Ophthalmol. 1964;71:43–9.
65. Swan KC. Fibroblastic ingrowth following cataract extraction. Arch Ophthalmol. 1973;89:445–9.
66. Maumenee AE. Treatment of epithelial downgrowth and intraocular fistula following cataract extraction. Trans Am Ophthalmol Soc. 1964;62:153.
67. Smith RE, Parrett C. Specular microscopy of epithelial downgrowth. Arch Ophthalmol. 1978;96:1222–4.
68. Spencer WH, Font RL, Green WR, et al. Ophthalmic pathology: an atlas and textbook, 3rd ed. Philadelphia: WB Saunders; 1985:511–4.
69. Zavala EY, Binder PS. The pathologic findings of epithelial ingrowth. Arch Ophthalmol. 1980;98:2007–14.
70. Iwamoto T, Srinivasan BD, DeVoe AG. Electron microscopy of epithelial downgrowth. Ann Ophthalmol. 1977;9:1095–110.
71. Schoiz RT, Kelley JS. Argon laser photocoagulation treatment of iris cysts following penetrating keratoplasty. Arch Ophthalmol. 1982;100:926–7.
72. Peyman GA, Peralta F, Ganiban GJ, Kraut R. Endoresection of the iris and ciliary body in epithelial downgrowth. J Cataract Refract Surg. 1998;24:130–3.
73. Sidoti PA, Baerveldt G. Glaucoma drainage implants. Curr Opin Ophthalmol. 1994;5:85–98.
74. Gnanaraj L, Tyagi AK, Cottrell DG, et al. Referral delay and ocular surgical outcome in Terson syndrome. Retina. 2000;20:374–7.
75. Heinz R. Morphologische Veranderungen der rothen Bluktor perchen durche Gifte. Virchows Arch A Pathol Anat Histol. 1890;122:112.
76. Paterson CA, Pfister PR. Intraocular pressure changes after alkali burns. Arch Ophthalmol. 1974;91:211.
77. Green K, Paterson CA, Siddiqui A. Ocular blood flow after experimental alkali burns and prostaglandin administration. Arch Ophthalmol. 1985;103:569–71.

78. Donshik PC, Berman MB, Dohlman CH, *et al.* Effect of topical corticosteroids on ulceration in alkali-burned corneas. Arch Ophthalmol. 1978;96:2117–20.

79. Berlin HS, Ritch R. The treatment of glaucoma secondary to aniridia. Mt Sinai J Med. 1981;48:111.

80. Mintz-Hittner HA. Aniridia. In: Ritch R, Shields MB, Krupin T, eds. The glaucomas. St Louis: CV Mosby; 1996.

81. Francois J, Lentini F. Gillespie-Syndrome (inkomplette Aniridie, zerebellare Ataxie and Oligophrenie). Klin Monatsbl Augenheilkd. 1984;184:313.

82. Nelson LB, Spaeth GL, Nowinski TS, *et al.* Aniridia: a review. Surv Ophthalmol. 1984;28:621–42.

83. Grant WM, Walton DS. Progressive changes in the angle in congenital aniridia, with development of glaucoma. Am J Ophthalmol. 1974;78:842–7.

84. David R, MacBeath L, Jenkins T. Aniridia associated with microcornea and subluxated lenses. Br J Ophthalmol. 1978;62:118.

85. Wiggins RE, Tomey KF. The results of glaucoma surgery in aniridia. Arch Ophthalmol. 1992;110:503–85.

86. Misato A, Dickens CJ, Hetherington J, *et al.* Clinical experience of trabeculectomy for the surgical treatment of aniridic glaucoma. Ophthalmology. 1997;104:2121–5.

87. Chen TC, Walton PS. Goniosurgery for prevention of aniridic glaucoma. Trans Am Ophthalmol Soc. 1998;96:155–69.

88. Chen TC, Walton DS. Goniosurgery for prevention of aniridic glaucoma. Arch Ophthalmol.1999;117:1144–8.

89. Shields CL, Shields JA, Shields MB. Prevalence and mechanisms of secondary intraocular pressure elevation in eyes with intraocular tumors. Ophthalmology. 1987;94:839–41.

90. Geisse LJ, Robertson DM. Iris melanomas. Am J Ophthalmol. 1978;85:407.

91. Ozment R. Ocular tumors and glaucoma. In: Albert D, Jakobiec F, eds. Principles and practices of ophthalmology. Philadelphia: WB Saunders; 1994:128–1456.

92. Broughton WL, Zimmerman LE. A clinicopathologic study of 56 cases of intraocular medulloepitheliomas. Am J Ophthalmol. 1978;85:407.

93. Reese AB, Cleasby GW. The treatment of iris melanoma. Am J Ophthalmol. 1959;47:118.

94. Kersten RC, Tse DT, Anderson R. Iris melanoma—nevus or malignancy? Surv Ophthalmol. 1985;29:423–33.

95. Shields JA, Annesley WH, Spaeth GL. Necrotic melanocytoma of iris with secondary glaucoma. Am J Ophthalmol. 1977;84:826–9.

96. Shields J, Shields C, Shields MB. Glaucoma associated with intraocular tumors. In: Ritch R, Shields MB, Krupin T, eds. The glaucomas. St Louis: CV Mosby; 1996:1131–8.

97. Schwartz A. Chronic open angle glaucoma secondary to rhegmatogenous retinal detachment. Am J Ophthalmol. 1973;73:205–11.

98. Phelps CD, Burton TC. Glaucoma and retinal detachment. Arch Ophthalmol. 1975;95:418–22.

99. Matsuo N, Takabatake M, Ueno H, *et al.* Photoreceptor outer segments in the aqueous humor in rhegmatogenous retinal detachment. Am J Ophthalmol. 1986;101:673–9.

100. Lambrou FH, Vela A, Woods W. Obstruction of the trabecular meshwork by retinal rod outer segments. Arch Ophthalmol. 1989;107:742–5.

101. Matsuo T. Photoreceptor outer segments in aqueous humor: key to understanding a new syndrome. Surv Ophthalmol. 1994;39:211–30.

102. Davidorf FH. Retinal pigment epithelial glaucoma. Ophthalmol Diagn. 1976; 38:11.

CHAPTER

231

SECTION 4 THERAPY

When to Treat Glaucoma

REBECCA S. WALKER • JODY R. PILTZ–SEYMOUR

INTRODUCTION

The decision to initiate therapy to lower eye pressure is a very serious one that has far-reaching consequences. Once started, therapy generally is continued for the rest of the patient's life. Patients may be subjected to untoward side effects, significant costs, and altered quality of life from the use of glaucoma medications. In addition, the public health impact of treatment is enormous; therapy is expensive and requires regular medical attention.

Determining when to start treatment requires a complex decision-making process, which must be individualized for each patient. Any decision to initiate therapy must weigh the patient's risk factors for the development or progression of glaucoma against the risk of side effects, complications, and inconveniences of treatment. The main goals of glaucoma therapy are to preserve functional vision and quality of life.

ANALYSIS OF RISK FACTORS

The most important indications of the future risk for glaucomatous damage are the extent of damage already present and the current rate of progression of the disease.[1,2] The extent of damage may be assessed by evaluation of the status of the optic nerve and visual field. Stereoscopic evaluation of the optic discs is carried out to search for signs of glaucomatous damage, which include thinning of the neuroretinal rim (particularly at the superior and inferior poles), notching of the rim, splinter hemorrhages, asymmetry between the appearance of the optic nerves, or peripapillary atrophy. Evaluation of the nerve fiber layer with red-free illumination or special photographic techniques may help the detection of widespread loss or focal, wedge-shaped defects. Visual fields are best evaluated using threshold techniques of the central 24–30°. Eyes affected by glaucoma exhibit characteristic nerve fiber bundle pattern defects with or without generalized depression (see Chapter 214).

Documentation of progressive change of the optic disc or visual field is the hallmark of the diagnosis of glaucoma, but generally is not possible on initial patient encounters. The rate of progression can be determined only by serial examinations over time. Typically, standard threshold perimetry is performed one to four times per year. Stereoscopic nerve head evaluation is also performed at regular intervals, ideally with baseline and possibly interval stereophotographic documentation. Other psychophysical tests (which include short-wavelength and frequency-doubling perimetry), or other methods of optic nerve or nerve fiber layer analysis (such as scanning laser topography of the optic disc or polarimetry of the nerve fiber layer) may play a role in the assessment of the rate of progression over time. Detection of change is critical, since it is believed that the risk of further injury with sustained high IOP accelerates as the disc injury progresses. Studies have shown that treatment initiated at an early stage of glaucoma is more effective in the prevention of glaucoma damage than treatment started in more advanced stages.[2]

Other critical risk factors that must be considered in the decision to initiate therapy include the level of intraocular pressure (IOP), central corneal thickness (CCT), age, race, and family history of glaucoma. Other probable risk factors include myopia, systemic hypertension, systemic hypotension, nocturnal hypotension, vasospasm (associated with cold extremities, migraine headaches, Raynaud's disease), sleep apnea and diabetes mellitus. Any decision to treat must also take into account psychosocial issues such as the patient's overall health and predicted life expectancy, current systemic medications, risk of medication side effects, degree of understanding of the disease and treatments, level of compliance, and financial impact of treatment.

RISK FACTORS

Intraocular Pressure

IOP is the leading causal risk factor for glaucoma, and at present, the only risk factor for which clinically proven treatment options exist. Both the incidence and prevalence of glaucoma increase with increasing IOP (Fig. 231-1). Compared to an IOP of 15mmHg (2.0kPa) or lower, the relative risk of glaucomatous optic nerve damage increases 13-fold for an IOP of 22–29mmHg (2.9–3.9kPa), and 40-fold for an IOP >30mmHg (>4.0kPa).[3] Asymmetrical or unilateral glaucoma, including secondary glaucoma or angle-closure glaucoma, typically results in worse damage in the eye affected by the higher IOP. Numerous animal models of glaucoma have shown that chronically raised IOP induces glaucomatous optic neuropathy in both primate and nonprimate species.

Multicentered clinical trials have definitively proven that lowering IOP is beneficial in preventing ongoing glaucoma progression in eyes with manifest glaucoma damage. In the Advanced Glaucoma Intervention Study (AGIS), when IOP was below 18 mmHg on all visits over 6 years (average IOP of 12mmHg), almost no visual field progression ensued; for eyes with IOP <18mmHg on fewer than 50% of visits (average IOP of

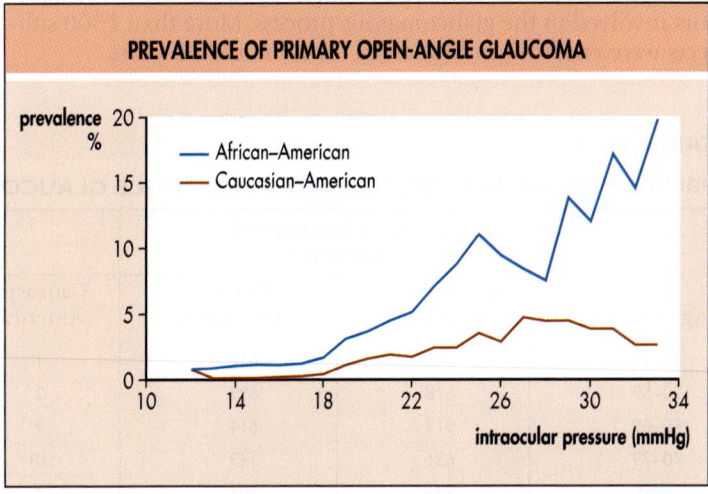

FIG. 231-1 ■ Prevalence of primary open-angle glaucoma in relation to screening intraocular pressure. The curves are smoothed using a running mean with window width of 7mmHg. For Caucasian–American subjects, n = 5604 eyes, and for African–American subjects, n = 4464 eyes. (Data from Tielsch JM, Sommer A, Katz J, et al. Racial variations in the prevalence of primary open-angle glaucoma. The Baltimore Eye Survey. JAMA. 1991;266:369–74.)

20mmHg), visual field defect scores worsened by 0.63 units ($p = .083$).[4] The Collaborative Normal-Tension Glaucoma Study (CNTGS) demonstrated less visual field progression in patients with normal-tension glaucoma in whom treatment successfully reduced the IOP by 30% or more to an average of 11mgHg.[5]

The Early Manifest Glaucoma Trial randomized patients with early to moderate glaucomatous damage to treatment with laser trabeculoplasty and betaxolol or observation. Patients were followed every 3 months with Humphrey visual fields and IOP measurements and optic disc photography every 6 months. Treatment reduced IOP on average by 25%, and average follow-up was 6 years. Progression occurred later and less frequently in the treated group than in controls ($p = .007$). In a multivariate analysis, progression risk was halved by treatment (hazards ratio = 0.50; 95% CI, 0.35–0.71). The risk of progression decreased by about 10% with each millimeter of mercury that IOP was reduced from baseline to the first follow-up visit (hazards ratio = 0.90 per millimeter of mercury decrease; 95% CI, 0.86–0.94).[6,7]

Great variability occurs among individuals in the susceptibility of the optic nerve to damage from IOP. No IOP exists below which glaucoma never occurs or above which glaucoma always occurs. Of patients who suffer glaucoma, 50% have screening IOPs of <21mmHg (<2.8kPa) and approximately one in six do not have IOP >21mmHg (>2.8kPa) on repeated testing.[3,8] Though the relative risk of glaucoma is low when IOP is <20mmHg (<2.7kPa), damage may still occur. Even when IOP remains within the normal range, the risk of visual field loss is greater in the eye with the higher IOP.[9]

Ocular hypertension (OHT) is a common disorder that affects 3–6 million people in the United States. In a population over 70 years of age, 10% of people suffer OHT, whereas only 2% have primary open-angle glaucoma. Numerous small studies have tried to evaluate the rate of glaucoma development in untreated ocular hypertensives and whether treatment prevents or delays the development of glaucoma. These studies suggest that 0.5–4.0% of OHT subjects develop primary open-angle glaucoma each year, and roughly half of these small studies favored medical treatment, while half favored observation.[10–12] Since only a minority of people with OHT develop glaucoma, it is not reasonable to treat all patients who have OHT. Currently, approximately 1.5 million glaucoma suspects in the United States are treated, which translates into a $300 million per year public health burden.[13]

Fortunately, the Ocular Hypertension Treatment Study (OHTS)—a long-term, multicenter clinical trial sponsored by the National Eye Institute—recently reported its 5-year results.[13,14] OHTS was designed to determine whether medical reduction of IOP prevents or delays the onset of glaucomatous damage in OHT subjects. It also sought to determine the risk factors involved in the glaucomatous process. More than 1500 subjects were enrolled and followed for more than 5 years.

Patients were randomized to medical treatment (using any of the topical medications approved by the U.S. Food and Drug Administration) or observation. Goal IOP for subjects in the treatment group was a 20% reduction of IOP and an IOP <24mmHg (<3.2kPa). Patients were followed using Humphrey visual fields (program 30-2) and stereoscopic optic disc photographs.

The risk of developing glaucomatous optic disc and/or visual field loss was significantly reduced in the treated group; 9.5% of patients in the observation group developed glaucoma compared with 4.4% of those in the medically treated group. In addition to the level of IOP, the following were identified as the principal risk factors for the progression of OHT to glaucoma: CCT, age, and cup-to-disc ratio. African-Americans had a higher incidence of glaucoma than other study participants, but this higher incidence was accounted for by thinner corneas and larger cup-to-disc ratios at baseline. Results from ancillary studies evaluating short-wavelength perimetry and scanning laser optic-nerve head topography are pending.

CENTRAL CORNEAL THICKNESS. One of the most surprising findings of the OHTS was the impact of CCT on the development of glaucoma in the OHTS. Pachymetry measurements were not part of the initial protocol, but were added on when their potential significance became apparent. Overall, participants in OHTS had thicker corneas than the average population with an average corneal thickness of 573.0 ± 39.0μm, and a quarter of the OHTS subjects had CCT >600μm. African-Americans had thinner corneas than white subjects (555.7 ± 40.0μm vs. 579.0 ± 37.0μm; $p <.0001$).[15] Eyes with thinner corneas had increased risk of developing glaucoma compared with eyes with thick corneas.[14] For example, for eyes with IOP of >25.75, the risk of developing glaucoma was 6% for subjects with CCT >588μm, but 36% for those with CCT<555μm. Overall, CCT was found to be a potent risk factor for the development of POAG.

AGE. Age is another important risk factor for primary open-angle glaucoma. The prevalence of glaucoma increases from 0.2% in individuals 50–54 years of age to 2% of the population 70–74 years of age (Table 231-1).[16] The incidence rates for the development of glaucoma over a 4-year period also increased with age; the Barbados Eye Studies demonstrated a rate of 1.2% in patients 40–49 years of age and 4.2% in those aged 70 years or older.[17] This increased prevalence of glaucoma with increasing age may relate to the longer exposure to elevated IOP and/or a greater susceptibility of optic nerves in older people to sustain damage from elevated IOP. The prevalence of OHT also increases with age; OHT occurs in 1.3% of subjects 30–39 years of age versus 10.5% of those 70–79 years of age.[18]

RACE. Race is also an important risk factor for primary open-angle glaucoma. The Baltimore Eye Survey shows that the prevalence of primary open-angle glaucoma is 4.3 times greater in African–Americans than in other races and that African–Americans

TABLE 231-1

PREVALENCE OF DEFINITE PRIMARY OPEN-ANGLE GLAUCOMA BY AGE AND RACE*

Age (Years)	Screening Examination (Number)		Cases (Number)		Adjusted Rate/100 (95% Confidence Interval)	
	Caucasian–Americans	African–Americans	Caucasian–Americans	African–Americans	Caucasian–Americans	African–Americans
40–49	543	632	1	6	0.92 (0–2.72)	1.23 (0.23–2.24)
50–59	618	699	2	25	0.41 (0–0.98)	4.05 (2.47–5.63)
60–69	915	614	7	31	0.88 (0.14–1.62)	5.51 (3.57–7.46)
70–79	631	349	18	27	2.89 (1.44–4.34)	9.15 (5.83–12.48)
≥80	206	101	4	11	2.16 (0.05–4.26)	11.26 (4.52–18.00)
Total	2913	2395	32	100	1.29 (0.80–1.78)	4.74 (3.81–5.67)

Adapted with permission from Tielsch JM, Sommer A, Katz J, *et al.* Racial variations in the prevalence of primary open-angle glaucoma. The Baltimore Eye Survey. JAMA. 1991;266:369–74.

*Adjusted rate is modified for nonresponse to definitive ophthalmologic examination. Difference (African-American – Caucasian-American) = 5.10 – 1.19 = 3.91% (95% confidence interval, range 3.45–4.37%).

are four to eight times more likely to go blind from glaucoma than Caucasian–Americans. In this series the prevalence of glaucoma was 1.2% among African–Americans 40–49 years of age, and 11.3% in African–Americans 80+ years of age (see Table 231-1).[16]

The Barbados Eye Study found a similar prevalence of primary open-angle glaucoma in the African–Caribbean inhabitants of Barbados as was found in African–Americans in Baltimore—7% of African–Caribbean adults versus 0.8% of Caucasian–Caribbeans.[16,17,19] The Rotterdam study based on the Caucasian population of the Netherlands showed a prevalence of primary open-angle glaucoma of approximately 1%, similar to the prevalence found in the Baltimore Eye Survey among Caucasian–Americans. It is not known why primary open-angle glaucoma is more common in individuals of African descent. It appears that an inherent predisposition may exist for the disease, which is present at an earlier age.

FAMILY HISTORY. Family history is a well-described risk factor for glaucoma. The Baltimore Eye Survey noted a 3.7-fold increased risk of primary open-angle glaucoma in individuals who had a sibling affected by primary open-angle glaucoma and a 2.2-fold increased risk if a parent was affected (Table 231-2).[20]

PRINCIPLES OF INITIATION OF THERAPY

Prior to the initiation of therapy in any patient, it is important to establish a baseline for future comparisons. The IOP of most people who do not have glaucoma varies by <4mmHg (<0.5kPa) over a 24-hour period. Glaucoma patients have large diurnal variations of IOP, which may change by >10mmHg (>1.3kPa). Many patients have a regular diurnal pattern, most typically with a high IOP upon awakening, but other patterns also occur.

Unless IOP is dangerously high for a patient or a return visit is too inconvenient (distance to doctor, work schedule, etc.), it is wise not to start therapy at the first patient encounter. It is important to measure IOP on more than one occasion and preferably several times a day to characterize the patient's diurnal variation. It is also important to obtain baseline documentation of optic disc appearance and visual field performance. Discs can be drawn, but stereophotographs provide a more accurate record. Computerized tomographic imaging with instruments such as the Heidleberg Retinal Tomograph, Heidleberg Engineering, Inc (Carlsbad, CA) may also enable detailed, precise measurements of the morphology of the optic nerve head. The role of other fundus imaging systems, such as nerve fiber layer polarimetry and optical coherence tomography, are still in evolution. Since a steep learning curve occurs, automated fields are performed at least twice at baseline if the patient is inexperienced at perimetry.

It is crucial to involve patients in the decision to start therapy and in the choice of the appropriate treatment plan. Most patients in the United States are started on topical medicines.

Patients are offered the least amount of medication needed to achieve their goal. Patients need to be informed and questioned about side effects, costs, and how their overall therapy and disease process influences their everyday life. Compliance with treatment improves with enhanced patient education.

In the United States, laser and surgical intervention are typically performed in cases of medication failure or intolerance. The Glaucoma Laser Trial sponsored by the National Eye Institute, however, has shown that argon laser trabeculoplasty may be a viable first therapy for glaucoma. Recently introduced selective laser trabeculoplasty (SLT) has similar efficacy as argon laser trabeculoplasty without causing thermal changes. It is postulated that SLT treatment can be repeated at regular intervals. Its role in the glaucoma armamentarium is still evolving. Although the Glasgow Glaucoma Trial and the Moorfields Primary Treatment Trial demonstrated better IOP control with initial surgical intervention, the Collaborative Initial Glaucoma Treatment Trial, sponsored by the National Eye Institute, found the same rate of visual field loss when initial treatment of glaucoma was either medical or surgical. In addition, visual acuity loss was greater in the surgery group compared with the medical group in the early follow-up period.[21]

INITIATION OF THERAPY IN THE GLAUCOMA PATIENT

Most patients who have moderate-to-severe glaucoma are started on therapy to lower IOP. These patients have developed optic disc damage at their baseline, untreated IOP and are very likely to have continued progressive damage over time if the condition is left untreated. In most of these patients, the benefit of treatment far outweighs the risk of complications.

Not every case of primary open-angle glaucoma, however, requires treatment. The true goal of glaucoma therapy is not to lower IOP or to prevent progressive disc damage or visual field loss. The primary goal of glaucoma treatment is to preserve a patient's quality of life by preventing the development of functional visual impairment during the patient's lifetime, while minimizing any adverse effects of glaucoma treatment. Unfortunately, few studies have been carried out to evaluate real-life functional deficits in glaucoma. Most patients are not bothered by early or even moderate amounts of glaucoma damage. Cases of early glaucoma in an elderly person may be treated best by observation, because even progressive changes may go undetected by the patient, and these patients are at significant risk of side effects from medication. Similarly, glaucoma therapy should be administered less aggressively in any patient who has a limited life expectancy.

Primary open-angle glaucoma is a bilateral disease, although it is often strikingly asymmetrical. If damage is present in only

TABLE 231-2

BALTIMORE EYE SURVEY: ASSOCIATION OF PRIMARY OPEN-ANGLE GLAUCOMA WITH A FAMILY HISTORY OF GLAUCOMA

Family Group	History	Cases		Controls		Odds Ratio (95% Confidence Interval)	Age–Race Adjusted Odds Ratio* (95% Confidence Interval)
		Number	Percentage	Number	Percentage		
Parents	Positive	9	5.6	206	4.0	1.42 (0.67–2.91)	2.17 (1.07–4.41)
	Negative	152	94.4	4941	96.0		
Siblings	Positive	16	9.9	144	2.8	3.83 (2.14–6.76)	3.69 (2.10–6.48)
	Negative	145	90.1	5003	97.2		
Children	Positive	2	1.2	40	0.8	1.61 (0.40–6.15)	1.12 (0.26–4.86)
	Negative	159	98.8	5107	99.2		
Any first-degree relatives	Positive	26	16.1	371	7.2	2.48 (1.57–3.89)	2.85 (1.82–4.46)
	Negative	135	83.9	4776	92.8		

*Age–race adjustment conducted using logistics regression analysis.

one eye, it is important to first rule out secondary causes of unilateral open-angle glaucoma, which most commonly include pseudoexfoliation, traumatic angle-recession, and corticosteroid-induced glaucoma. If secondary causes of glaucoma are excluded, the damage in one eye is predictive of damage in the other eye and treatment often is initiated in both eyes.

INITIATION OF THERAPY IN THE GLAUCOMA SUSPECT

The decision to initiate therapy is much more controversial in the patient who is suspected of having glaucoma. It is particularly important for glaucoma suspects to be involved in the decision process. There are two main types of glaucoma suspects:

- Those subject to significant risk factors for the future development of glaucoma—most importantly, high IOP (OHT is discussed separately below)
- Those who suffer very early glaucoma damage that cannot definitely be differentiated from normal (i.e., optic discs of suspicious appearance).

Determination of whether an optic nerve of suspicious appearance is glaucomatous is difficult. Great overlap exists between normal and diseased optic nerves. The average optic disc has a cup-to-disc ratio of 0.3–0.4, but a wide variation of normal occurs. The significance of the size of the cup depends on the size of the disc.[22] It is difficult to determine whether the large disc with a high cup-to-disc ratio is pathological or physiological. Progressive disc changes may develop while visual field tests remain normal, and substantial axonal loss may develop before defects occur on kinetic perimetry.[23] Therefore, a normal visual field test does not rule out glaucoma. Evaluation of the nerve fiber layer may be particularly important in these cases.

Treatment is considered the more suspicious the nerve appears, if nerve fiber layer loss is detected, or if other significant risk factors exist for glaucoma. As discussed, in patients who have early glaucoma, treatment may be deferred in those with limited life expectancy. On the other hand, treatment may be initiated at an earlier stage in subjects in whom it is difficult to detect change in the optic nerve status over time. This includes patients who have anomalous discs, disc drusen, high myopia, and tilted discs, and patients in whom an adequate fundus examination cannot be performed. Similarly, treatment may be begun at a lower threshold in patients who are unable to perform visual field testing or in patients who suffer nonglaucomatous causes of visual field loss.

The initiation of therapy is most controversial in patients who have elevated IOP and normal optic nerves and visual fields. Although the OHTS showed a significant reduction in the development of glaucoma with treatment, approximately 90% of patients in the observation group did not develop glaucoma during the first 5 years of the study.[13] OHTS II will evaluate if there is any difference if treatment of OHT is delayed. Until those data are available, it is recommended that treatment be considered in high-risk OHT subjects (i.e., those with high IOP, thin corneas, and large cup-to-disc ratios) while taking into account medical status, life expectancy, financial, and other psychosocial issues.

CONCLUSION

The decision of when to treat a patient to prevent glaucomatous damage cannot be simplified into a straightforward algorithm. A myriad of factors, both objective (e.g., optic nerve status, level of IOP, visual field defects) and subjective (e.g., patient lifestyle, compliance), must be taken into account. These factors must be tempered by the current knowledge of how and why glaucoma develops and whether treatment is efficacious. Fortunately, a great deal of active investigation has facilitated our decision-making process over the last decade, permitting treatment decisions based on sound data from large-scale, prospective, randomized clinical trials.

REFERENCES

1. Anderson DR. Glaucoma: the damage caused by pressure. XLVI Edward Jackson Memorial Lecture. Am J Ophthalmol. 1989;108:485–95.
2. Grant WM, Burke JF Jr. Why do some people go blind from glaucoma? Ophthalmology. 1982;89:991–8.
3. Sommer A, Tielsch JM, Katz J, et al. Relationship between intraocular pressure and primary open angle glaucoma among white and black Americans. The Baltimore Eye Survey. Arch Ophthalmol. 1991;109:1090–5.
4. The advanced glaucoma intervention study (AGIS):7. The relationship between control of intraocular pressure and visual field deterioration. The AGIS Investigators. Am J Ophthalmol. 1000;130:429–40.
5. Collaborative Normal-Tension Glaucoma Study Group. Comparison of glaucomatous progression between untreated patients with normal-tension glaucoma and patients with therapeutically reduced intraocular pressures. Am J Ophthalmol. 1998;126:487–97.
6. Heijl A, Leske MC, Bengtsson B, et al. Reduction of intraocular pressure and glaucoma progression: results from the Early Manifest Glaucoma Trial. Arch Ophthalmol. 2002 Oct;120(10):1268–79.
7. Leske MC, Heijl A, Hussein M, et al. Factors for glaucoma progression and the effect of treatment: the early manifest glaucoma trial. Arch Ophthalmol. 2003 Jan;121(1):48–56.
8. Kahn HA, Milton RC. Alternative definitions of open-angle glaucoma. Arch Ophthalmol. 1980;98:2172–7.
9. Cartwright MJ, Anderson DR. Correlation of asymmetric damage with asymmetric intraocular pressure in normal-tension glaucoma (low tension glaucoma). Arch Ophthalmol. 1988;106:898–900.
10. Kitazawa Y, Horie T, Aoki S, et al. Untreated ocular hypertension: a long-term prospective study. Arch Ophthalmol. 1977;95:1180–4.
11. Lundberg L, Wettrell K, Linner E. Ocular hypertension: a prospective twenty-year follow-up study. Acta Ophthalmol (Copenh). 1987;65:705–8.
12. Schulzer M, Drance SM, Douglas GR. A comparison of treated and untreated glaucoma suspects. Ophthalmology. 1991;98:301–7.
13. Kass MA, Heuer DK, Higginbotham EJ, et al. The Ocular Hypertension Treatment Study: a randomized trial determines that topical ocular hypotensive medication delays or prevents the onset of primary open-angle glaucoma. Arch Ophthalmol. 2002 Jun;120(6):701–13.
14. Gordon MO, Beiser JA, Brandt JD, et al. The Ocular Hypertension Treatment Study: baseline factors that predict the onset of primary open-angle glaucoma. Arch Ophthalmol. 2002 Jun;120(6):714–20.
15. Brandt JD, Beiser JA, Kass MA, Gordon MO. Central corneal thickness in the Ocular Hypertension Treatment Study (OHTS). Ophthalmology. 2001 Oct;108(10):1779–88.
16. Tielsch JM, Sommer A, Katz J, et al. Racial variations in the prevalence of primary open-angle glaucoma. The Baltimore Eye Survey. JAMA. 1991;266:369–74.
17. Leske MC, Connell AM, Wu S. Incidence of open-angle glaucoma. The Barbados Eye Studies. Arch Ophthalmol. 2001;119:89–95.
18. Armaly MF. On the distribution of applanation pressure. I. Statistical features and the effect of age, sex, and family history of glaucoma. Arch Ophthalmol. 1965;83:11–8.
19. Leske MC, Connell AM, Schachat AP, et al. The Barbados Eye Study. Prevalence of open angle glaucoma. Arch Ophthalmol. 1994;112:821–9.
20. Tielsch JM, Katz J, Sommer A. Family history and risk of primary open angle glaucoma. The Baltimore Eye Survey. Arch Ophthalmol. 1994;112:69–73.
21. Lichter PR, Musch DC, Gillespie BW, et al. Interim clinical outcomes in the collaborative initial glaucoma treatment study comparing initial treatment randomized to medications or surgery. Ophthalmology. 2001;108:1943–53.
22. Britton RJ, Drance SM, Schulzer M, et al. The area of the neuroretinal rim of the optic nerve in normal eyes. Am J Ophthalmol. 1987;103:497–504.
23. Quigley HA, Addicks EM, Green WR. Optic nerve damage in human glaucoma. III. Quantitative correlation of nerve fiber loss and visual field defect in glaucoma, ischemic neuropathy, papilledema and toxic neuropathy. Arch Ophthalmol. 1982;100:135–46.

Which Therapy to Use in Glaucoma?

CLIVE MIGDAL

DEFINITION
- The aim of glaucoma therapy is to preserve visual function with minimal side effects.

KEY FEATURE
- The choice of therapy (alone or in combination) for patients who have open-angle glaucoma includes medical treatment, laser treatment, and filtering surgery.

INTRODUCTION

The aim of glaucoma therapy is to preserve visual function with minimal complications.[1] Added to this is the need to ensure that quality of life is maintained. It is essential, therefore, that each patient be assessed individually before a treatment decision is made.

Although raised intraocular pressure (IOP) appears to be the main risk factor for damage in glaucoma (hence the need for a specific target pressure in an individual eye),[2] other factors, such as vascular and mechanical ones, are involved in the pathogenesis of glaucoma and must also be considered. Additional factors may be responsible for preservation of the optic nerve in this disease.[3]

The primary goal of current therapy is to reduce IOP to the point where deterioration of the disc or field ceases, with a minimum of complications or side effects. It is not possible to predict accurately what level of IOP will be satisfactory for an individual patient. A wide range of suggested "normal" values has been reported. The suggestion that an IOP of 21mmHg (2.8kPa) or less prevents further glaucomatous damage was based on population statistics; however, some patients continue to develop progressive glaucomatous disease at IOPs below this level. Thus, this IOP value cannot be accepted as the sole criterion for either control of the disease or the boundary between health and disease.

Establishing in advance the degree to which IOP must be lowered to preserve vision is difficult in individual cases, but it is clear that lowering IOP often arrests the progression of visual loss.[4] Recent evidence supports the value of lower IOPs in the preservation of visual function.[5] Individual factors that are not yet fully understood may govern the susceptibility of the optic nerve head to damage mediated by IOP.

The choice of therapy for patients who have open-angle glaucoma consists of medical treatment, laser trabeculoplasty, filtering surgery, or a combination of these. The selection of the most appropriate therapy must take into account factors that pertain to the individual patient and to each individual eye, such as age, stage of glaucoma, and other risk factors.

HISTORICAL REVIEW

Topical medications to treat glaucoma were first used in the 1870s, with the discovery of physostigmine and pilocarpine.

Since then, many other drugs have been added to the treatment armamentarium, including epinephrine (adrenaline) and acetazolamide, followed by β-blockers in the 1970s. β-Blockers became the medical therapy of choice in the majority of newly diagnosed cases of open-angle glaucoma. More recently, additional glaucoma preparations have been introduced, such as topical carbonic anhydrase inhibitors (dorzolamide, brinzolamide), prostaglandins/prostamides (latanoprost, travoprost, bimatoprost, unoprostone), and α-adrenergic agonists (brimonidine, apraclonidine). Combination products are also available (timolol-dorzolamide, timolol-latanoprost, and timolol-pilocarpine). In the past, these were recommended as adjuvant therapy or when β-blockers were contraindicated. Longer experience with these products is establishing their use earlier in the therapeutic course.

Argon laser trabeculoplasty (LTP) was first described by Wise and Witter[6] in 1979. The technique has been revised and modified in an attempt to improve results and reduce complications, such as the postoperative spike in IOP. Initial short-term success was followed by less than satisfactory long-term control in many cases, with the result that this technique is not used as much as it was initially.[7] Selective laser trabeculoplasty has been suggested as a more effective alternative, but results of long-term studies are still awaited.

Filtering surgery in the form of trabeculectomy was described by Cairns[8] in 1968. This procedure has been improved and modified over the years to give better results and fewer complications. Recent modifications include the use of antimetabolites such as 5-fluorouracil or mitomycin.[9,10] Nonpenetrating filtering surgery, such as deep sclerectomy or viscocanalostomy, has its advocates.

TREATMENT MODALITIES

Advantages and disadvantages exist with all three methods of therapy.

Medical Treatment

A wide range of topical and systemic antiglaucoma medications is available (Box 232-1). Topical medications include miotics, β-blockers, epinephrine derivatives, carbonic anhydrase inhibitors, α-agonists, and prostaglandin analogs prostamides. These may be used alone or in combination. It is impractical, however, to use more than two or three topical medications simultaneously. Both ocular and systemic side effects may occur with medications (see Chapters 233 and 234).

Many variables can affect the success or failure of medical treatment for glaucoma. Patient-related factors such as compliance, coincident systemic diseases, drug interactions, and side effects must be considered.

The most common side effects of drugs prescribed for glaucoma are neither life nor sight threatening. Such effects include miotic-induced brow ache, dimming of vision caused by pilocarpine, vasodilatation and the allergic reactions caused by epinephrine and dipivefrin, effects on pulmonary function that result from β-blockers, and the acidosis syndrome induced by

BOX 232-1

Classification of Antiglaucoma Drugs

TOPICAL
Adrenergic Antagonists
β-Blockers
- timolol
- levobunolol
- betaxolol
- carteolol
- metipranolol

Adrenergic Agonists
Nonselective
- epinephrine
- dipivefrin
α₂-Selective
- brimonidine
- apraclonidine

Miotics (Direct Parasympathomimetics)
- pilocarpine

Prostaglandins/Prostamides
- travoprost, bimatoprost, unoprostone, latanoprost

Topical Carbonic Anhydrase Inhibitors
- dorzolamide
- brinzolamide

Combination Products
- timolol/dorzolamide
- timolol/pilocarpine
- timolol/latanoprost

SYSTEMIC
Carbonic Anhydrase Inhibitors
- acetazolamide
- dichlorphenamide
- methazolamide

Hyperosmotic Agents
- mannitol
- glycerol

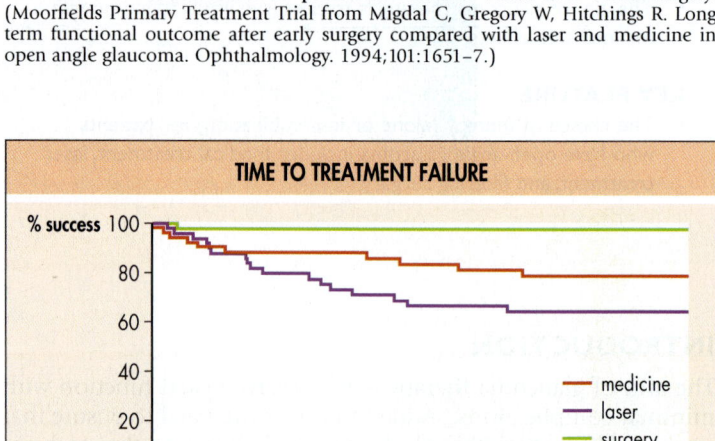

FIG. 232-1 ■ **Mean intraocular pressures.** Medicine versus laser versus surgery. (Moorfields Primary Treatment Trial from Migdal C, Gregory W, Hitchings R. Long term functional outcome after early surgery compared with laser and medicine in open angle glaucoma. Ophthalmology. 1994;101:1651–7.)

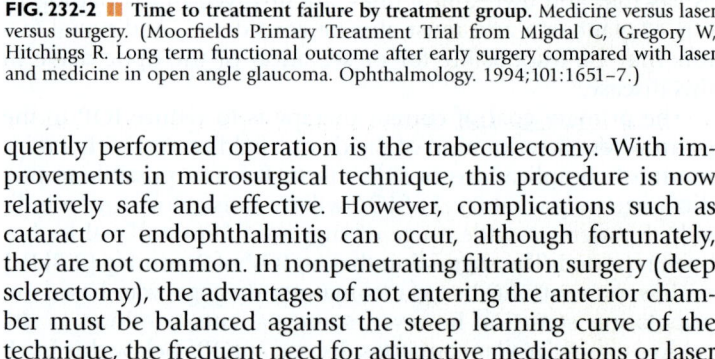

FIG. 232-2 ■ **Time to treatment failure by treatment group.** Medicine versus laser versus surgery. (Moorfields Primary Treatment Trial from Migdal C, Gregory W, Hitchings R. Long term functional outcome after early surgery compared with laser and medicine in open angle glaucoma. Ophthalmology. 1994;101:1651–7.)

acetazolamide. More serious side effects include aplastic anemia after the use of carbonic anhydrase inhibitors and retinal detachment associated with miotic therapy. However, many patients are able to tolerate one or more of these medications with no side effects. Drugs used in combination may interact to produce either a beneficial effect or none.

Inadequate compliance may be the most serious limiting factor in the nonsurgical therapy of glaucoma. Factors that influence compliance include complexity of the medical regimen, side effects of the medications, and patient understanding of the disease and its treatment.[11,12]

Laser Trabeculoplasty

After the initial description of the protocol for argon LTP, many other studies followed, and LTP has become a frequently performed procedure for glaucoma. It is simple to perform and cost effective (see Chapter 235). However, the long-term efficacy of this treatment is unclear. The subsequent IOP rise may be sudden rather than gradual, so it is important to keep these patients under continual observation.

Surgery

The conventional operation used most frequently for primary open-angle glaucoma is referred to generally as a filtering procedure. Although a number of variations have been described, all filtering operations share the same basic mechanism of action and general surgical principles (see Chapter 240). The most fre-

quently performed operation is the trabeculectomy. With improvements in microsurgical technique, this procedure is now relatively safe and effective. However, complications such as cataract or endophthalmitis can occur, although fortunately, they are not common. In nonpenetrating filtration surgery (deep sclerectomy), the advantages of not entering the anterior chamber must be balanced against the steep learning curve of the technique, the frequent need for adjunctive medications or laser iridotomy, and the tendency to produce IOPs that are higher than those following trabeculectomy.[13,14]

TREATMENT OPTIONS

Traditionally, the initial standard therapy for primary open-angle glaucoma is medical, with LTP and surgery reserved for patients who fail medical therapy. A number of clinical studies have challenged this traditional therapeutic approach and deserve reappraisal.[15–19]

A long-term, multicenter, prospective follow-up study in Scotland compared early trabeculectomy with conventional medical therapy and found better IOP control in the early surgery group, with less visual field decay.[15] Approximately half the patients in the conventional medical therapy group required surgical intervention sooner or later. No difference was noted between the visual acuities of the surgical and medical groups.

In the Moorfields Primary Treatment Study,[16,17] the group of patients successfully treated by trabeculectomy achieved a mean IOP of 14.5 mmHg (1.93 kPa) at 5 years, compared with 18.5 mmHg (2.46 kPa) for the patients successfully treated with

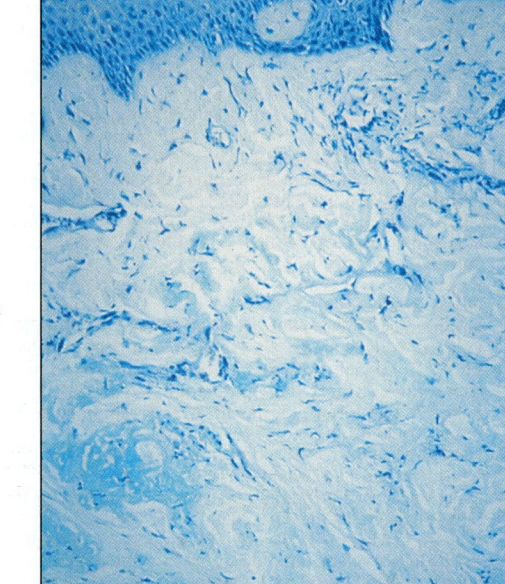

FIG. 232-3 ▮ **Inflammatory changes in the conjunctival tissue.** Representative photomicrograph from the group of patients who received long-term eyedrop therapy. The substantia propria shows a round cell infiltrate of mainly lymphocytes.

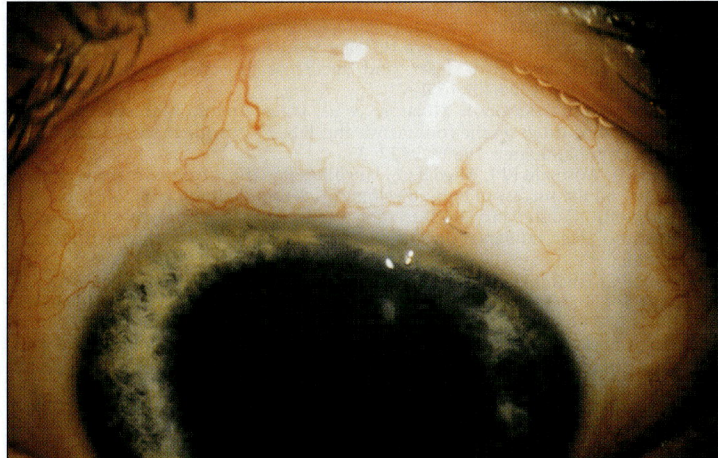

FIG. 232-4 ▮ **Drainage bleb.** Diffuse, avascular, well-functioning bleb from a primary trabeculectomy.

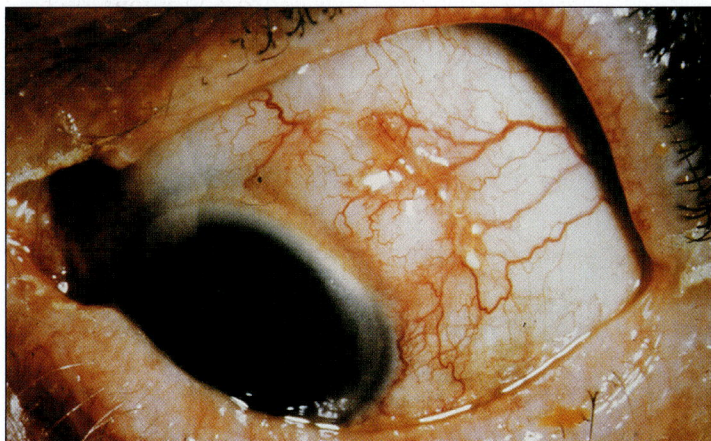

FIG. 232-5 ▮ **Vascularized, encysted drainage bleb with ultimate failure.** From a trabeculectomy following long-term eyedrop therapy.

laser or medication (Fig. 232-1). The significantly lower IOPs in the surgical patients were maintained throughout the initial 5-year follow-up period. There was a markedly higher success rate of 98% (in terms of IOP control) in the surgical group at 5 years, compared with 80% in the medical group and only 60% in the laser patients (Fig. 232-2). Mean visual acuities in the three groups differed by less than one line on the Snellen chart.

With the newer glaucoma medications now available, it may be possible to achieve lower target IOPs with drugs. Polypharmacy, however, is to be avoided, and it is preferable to switch from one drug to another rather than to just add more drops. Prior topical antiglaucoma medications may influence the subsequent outcome of glaucoma filtering surgery. A comparison of conjunctival biopsies from patients who underwent primary surgery and from those who received at least two topical medications for a minimum of 1 year before surgery showed a significantly greater increase in the number of macrophages, lymphocytes, mast cells, and fibroblasts in the conjunctiva and Tenon's capsule, and a significantly greater decrease in the number of goblet cells, in the medically treated group (Fig. 232-3).[18] These results suggest that long-term medications can induce chronic inflammatory changes in the bulbar conjunctiva (as a result of the active drug, the preservative, or both), which may enhance the risk of external bleb scarring and subsequent failure of filtering surgery.

Further evidence of better results with early filtering surgery was found when patients who underwent surgery as part of the primary treatment were compared with patients who underwent trabeculectomy after failed medical therapy (Figs. 232-4 and 232-5). The only identifiable difference between the two groups was the duration of topical drops. However, the success rate in the long-term medical therapy group was only 79%, compared with 98% in the primary surgery group.[19] Most trabeculectomy failures occurred within the first 3 months. This early failure was associated with a hypercellular response in the conjunctiva.

A number of controlled clinical trials to evaluate treatment options in open-angle glaucoma have reported their results.[20] Each of these landmark clinical trials deals with the management of a different subgroup of glaucoma patients and has added to the scientific evidence available on which to base our clinical management. The Advanced Glaucoma Intervention Study[5] was set up to investigate the outcome of treatment with either LTP or trabeculectomy in patients who had failed previous medical treatment. In the Early Manifest Glaucoma Trial,[22] the combination of medicine and LTP, as opposed to no treatment, was evaluated for a cohort of patients with newly diagnosed primary open-angle glaucoma. The Collaborative Initial Glaucoma Treatment Study[23] was set up to recruit newly diagnosed patients with primary open-angle glaucoma and randomize them to treatment with either medicine or trabeculectomy. The outcomes of these trials will continue to modify the criteria by which therapy is chosen. Trial results are based on group values, whereas many factors affect the individual outcome. It is nevertheless still essential to carefully evaluate each patient when deciding the most appropriate treatment protocol to follow for that individual.

CONCLUSIONS

Several conclusions can be drawn from the completed studies with regard to the current role of medicine, laser, and surgery in the management of primary open-angle glaucoma. There is now a tendency to aim for lower target pressures, particularly in those patients with extensive optic nerve damage or other risk factors.

Medical therapy still has a definite place in the management of primary open-angle glaucoma and results in satisfactory IOP control in a good percentage of cases. The wider choice of different eyedrops makes it even more important to select the most appropriate therapy for the individual patient. However, multiple therapy (in the form of more than two topical medications) or a systemic carbonic anhydrase inhibitor is rarely indicated.

LTP appears to be effective for the short-term control of IOP, but there is concern about the long-term efficacy of this treatment. It may be indicated in certain patients, such as elderly patients who are unfit for surgery or those who do not use eyedrops. However, these patients require continual monitoring,

BOX 232-2

Guidelines for Therapy in the Individual Patient

ASSESS RISK FACTORS
Stage of disease
Family history
Myopia
Microvascular disease
Other risk factors

ESTIMATE A TARGET PRESSURE

MEDICAL THERAPY
Achieves satisfactory intraocular pressure (IOP) control in many cases
No more than two topical medications
Maximal medical therapy no longer indicated
If problems with inadequate IOP, side effects, or compliance, consider alternative therapy

LASER TRABECULOPLASTY
Elderly who cannot tolerate medical therapy
Patients who are controlled inadequately and cannot/will not undergo surgery

SURGERY
If low IOP required or target IOP not reached with other treatments
Borderline control with medicine or laser
Poor compliance
Failed therapy with medicine or laser
Consider earlier surgery where appropriate, not only as a last resort!

because IOP control may suddenly be lost, with a resultant acute rise in pressure.

Performed early, filtering surgery gives excellent IOP control with minimal complications. Early surgery is still a useful option if the IOP is not controlled by simple medical therapy, if a low target pressure is required and cannot be achieved with medical therapy, or if compliance is a problem.[21] Guidelines for therapy in individual patients are given in Box 232-2.

REFERENCES

1. Odberg T, Jacobsen JE, Hulkgren SJ, Halseide R. The impact of glaucoma on the quality of life of patients in Norway. 1. Results from a self-administered questionnaire. Acta Ophthalmol Scand. 2001;79:116–20.
2. Anderson DR. Glaucoma: the damage caused by pressure. XLVI Edward Jackson Memorial Lecture. Am J Ophthalmol. 1989;108:485–95.
3. Schumer RA, Podos SM. The nerve of glaucoma! Arch Ophthalmol. 1994;112:37–44.
4. Grant WM, Burke JF Jr. Why do some people go blind from glaucoma? Ophthalmology. 1982;89:991–8.
5. AGIS Investigators. The Advanced Glaucoma Intervention Study (AGIS) 7: the relationship between control of IOP and visual field deterioration. Am J Ophthalmol 2000;130:429–40.
6. Wise JB, Witter SL. Argon laser therapy for open angle glaucoma. Arch Ophthalmol. 1979;97:319–22.
7. Glaucoma Laser Trial Research Group. The Glaucoma Laser Trial (GLT) and Glaucoma Laser Trial Follow-up Study: 7. Results. Am J Ophthalmol. 1995;120:718–31.
8. Cairns JE. Trabeculectomy. Preliminary report of a new method. Am J Ophthalmol. 1968;5:673–9.
9. Fluorouracil Filtering Surgery Study Group. 5-Year follow-up of the Fluorouracil Filtering Surgery Study. Am J Ophthalmol. 1996;121:349–66.
10. Khaw PT, Migdal CS. Current techniques in wound healing modulation in glaucoma surgery. Curr Opin Ophthalmol. 1996;7:24–33.
11. Kass MA, Gordon M, Morley RE Jr, et al. Compliance with topical timolol treatment. Am J Ophthalmol. 1987;103:188–93.
12. Kass MA, Meltzer DW, Gordon M, et al. Compliance with topical pilocarpine treatment. Am J Ophthalmol. 1986;101:515–23.
13. Chiselita D. Non-penetrating deep sclerectomy versus trabeculectomy in primary open-angle glaucoma. Eye. 2001;15:197–201.
14. Jonescu-Cuypers CP, Jacobi PC, Konen W, Krieglstein GK. Primary viscocanalostomy versus trabeculectomy in white patients with open-angle glaucoma: a randomized clinical trial. Ophthalmology. 2001;108:254–8.
15. Jay JL, Allan D. The benefit of early trabeculectomy versus conventional management in primary open angle glaucoma relative to the severity of the disease. Eye. 1989;3:528–35.
16. Migdal C, Hitchings R. Control of chronic simple glaucoma with primary medical, surgical and laser treatment. Trans Ophthalmol Soc UK. 1986;105:653–6.
17. Migdal C, Gregory W, Hitchings R. Long term functional outcome after early surgery compared with laser and medicine in open angle glaucoma. Ophthalmology. 1994;101:1651–7.
18. Sherwood M, Grierson I, Millar L, et al. Long-term morphologic effects of antiglaucoma drugs on the conjunctiva and Tenon's capsule in glaucomatous patients. Ophthalmology. 1989;96:327–35.
19. Lavin MJ, Wormald RPL, Migdal CS, Hitchings RA. The influence of prior medical therapy on the success of trabeculectomy. Arch Ophthalmol. 1990;108:1543–8.
20. Wilson MR, Gaasterland D. Translating research into practice: controlled clinical trials and their influence on glaucoma management. J Glaucoma. 1996;121:139–46.
21. Migdal C, Hitchings R. The role of early surgery for open angle glaucoma. In: Caprioli J, ed. Contemporary issues in glaucoma. Ophthalmol Clin North Am. 1991;4:853–9.
22. Heijl A, Leske MC, Bengtsson B, et al. Reduction of intraocular pressure and glaucoma progression: results from the Early Manifest Glaucoma Trial. Arch Ophthalmol. 2002;120:1268–79.
23. Lichtre PR, Musch DC, Gillespie BW, et al. Interim clinical outcomes in the Collaborative Initial Glaucoma Treatment Study comparing initial treatment randomized to medications or surgery. Ophthalmology. 2001;108:1943–53.

Current Medical Management of Glaucoma

RONALD L. GROSS

INTRODUCTION

The armamentarium for the medical treatment of glaucoma recently experienced an unprecedented expansion of available agents. Years ago, the choice was limited to miotics, epinephrine (adrenaline), and oral carbonic anhydrase inhibitors. The introduction of topical β-blockers in the 1970s was a significant advance, and β-blockers quickly became the most commonly prescribed class of agents to lower intraocular pressure (IOP). They generally were the most effective medication to do so and were well tolerated by most patients. However, with experience, it was recognized that side effects, both local and systemic, could occur, and it became important to identify those patients at risk for these problems. More recently, with the introduction of topical carbonic anhydrase inhibitors, α-adrenergic agonists, and prostaglandin analogs and prostamides, additional agents have become available that effectively lower IOP and have side-effect profiles that appear to be advantageous in many patients.

It is important to recognize that no single medication can be used in all patients in all circumstances. Each of the available drugs has its own unique advantages and disadvantages, and currently six separate classes of antiglaucoma drugs are available. It is necessary to individualize each patient's treatment regimen to maximize the benefits and limit the undesirable effects. It is not realistic to anticipate using all the available types of drugs for any single patient. Rather, it is vital to select the best agent for each particular patient's needs.

The first step in the accomplishment of this aim is to educate the patient about glaucoma in terms of his or her particular situation. This allows the patient to participate in an informed way in decision making about the care required. Besides improving drug selection, better understanding of the disease and its treatment by the patient should improve compliance with the medical regimen. Compliance in glaucoma patients is difficult to assess, but effective medical treatment of the disease is dependent on the delivery of therapy by the patient or caregiver—in many cases, several agents multiple times a day, every day. Selection of an appropriate agent results in maximization of lowered IOP, ocular tolerability, and safety, which not only treats the glaucoma effectively but also minimizes the impact of treatment on the patient's quality of life.

Historically, the effectiveness of a medication in the treatment of glaucoma was measured by its ability to lower IOP. However, more recently, the impact of other factors (e.g., blood supply of the optic nerve, local mechanical factors that affect the optic nerve, neuroprotection of the optic nerve) on glaucoma and glaucomatous optic neuropathy has been recognized. Although the clinical importance of these variables is not yet understood, it is anticipated that improvement in the efficacy of glaucoma treatment may include assessment of these parameters.

Once the decision to begin medical treatment has been made, two specific techniques may enhance the therapeutic index of any topical ophthalmic agent. First, patients are encouraged to perform nasolacrimal occlusion or gentle eyelid closure after the instillation of all topical ophthalmic drops. Such maneuvers decrease the systemic absorption of drugs and increase their intraocular levels, thus improving the therapeutic index.[1] In patients on multiple topical agents, these maneuvers also reinforce the need to allow sufficient time between the instillation of different agents to allow absorption of the first one before any dilution by instillation of a subsequent one.

Second, with the increased number of choices, it is important to prove to the patient and the doctor that the drug is effective and well tolerated. To prove that IOP is lowered with efficacy, a one-eye therapeutic trial is performed that involves the initial administration of a single agent in only one eye while the fellow eye remains on the previous regimen (to act as a control). Because no drug lowers IOP effectively in all patients, this procedure identifies an agent's effectiveness for the individual patient and thus prevents exposure to potential side effects without therapeutic benefit. If the agent is ineffective or not tolerated, it is discontinued and an alternative drug is evaluated. The trial period varies, depending on the agent tested, side effects, and efficacy. A period of 2–4 weeks is generally adequate. This maneuver can also demonstrate the continued efficacy of a drug after its long-term use. In this case, a reverse one-eye therapeutic trial is performed in which the drug is discontinued in one eye, and the results are compared with those for the eye in which treatment is continued. Again, this reaffirms that the chosen medical regimen must provide maximal benefit.

Finally, it is important to instruct the patient how and when to instill medications. Discussion of the preferred technique of instilling drops in the inferior cul-de-sac, with subsequent nasolacrimal occlusion or gentle eyelid closure, is likely to be of benefit. To confirm correct use, it is often helpful to have the patient demonstrate the technique of drop instillation on a subsequent visit. As to the time of administration, studies suggest that compliance is reduced when the frequency of administration is more than twice daily, which may be an important factor in the design of the patient's regimen. It is critical that the regimen be one that the patient can reasonably be expected to perform.

DRUGS THAT DECREASE AQUEOUS PRODUCTION

β-Blockers

Since their introduction, β-blockers have become the mainstay of medical glaucoma therapy. Over time, the importance of patient selection has become clear. The most important feature that differentiates the available topical ophthalmic β-blockers is receptor selectivity; nonselective agents block both β_1 and β_2 receptors, and β_1-selective agents are more selective for the β_1 receptors. Selectivity has implications for both efficacy and safety.

MECHANISM. β-Blockers decrease aqueous humor production by the ciliary body and hence reduce IOP.[2] Some evidence suggests that this occurs only during the day and not during sleep.[3] This may be important in patients who experience some of the systemic side effects (e.g., lower blood pressure and pulse rate) at night, with the potential for disease progression without other therapy to lower IOP. At present, the implications of this potential problem are unclear.

EFFICACY. β-blockers are effective topical agents, with the mean peak IOP lowered by at least 25% and the mean trough lowered by 20% using nonselective agents.[4, 5] In general, these nonselective agents lower IOP equally effectively; the data support timolol, levobunolol, metipranolol, and carteolol equivalence.[4–6] For the β₁-selective agent betaxolol, IOP reduction is slightly less.[7] When β-blockers alone are not adequate to control the patient's glaucoma, other classes of agents may be added. Although supporting data are not complete, it appears that other agents add to the effect of all β-blockers; the exceptions are epinephrine-like drugs, which have a greater effect when added to the selective agent betaxolol than when added to nonselective agents.[8] Given the small additive effect, the use of these agents along with β-blockers is less common now because of the development of newer agents.

None of the β-blockers should be used more than twice daily. Certain nonselective agents, including timolol maleate and levobunolol, may be used once daily in some patients. Timolol maleate 0.5% in a gel-forming solution (Timoptic-XE) once daily is essentially equivalent to timolol solution twice daily. With other agents, peak and trough levels of IOP are checked to confirm the duration of action. Once-daily instillation may be more convenient for the patient, which enhances compliance and reduces the amount of drug used. Also, many agents are available in more than one concentration. Lower concentrations are preferred and are as effective in the majority of patients. Unfortunately, no studies have proved that lower concentrations have a lower incidence of side effects or produce less severe side effects. It is possible that all available concentrations fall above the threshold on the dose–side effect curve.

Another aspect of efficacy is the use of generic agents. Unlike with oral agents, bioequivalence or equal effectiveness is not required to be proved when topical ophthalmic generics are introduced. Although these generic agents may be less expensive, whether these savings are sufficient to justify their use must be determined by the physician, the patient, and local health care policy. Unfortunately, no data are available on which to base this determination.

SIDE EFFECTS. The successful treatment of glaucoma is based not only on efficacy but also on side effects and compliance. Therefore, it is vital to select out patients who will not benefit from or may be harmed by the drug. Contraindications to β-blocker use include asthma, severe chronic obstructive pulmonary disease, bradycardia, second- or third-degree heart block, and congestive heart failure.

Clinically, it is prudent not to use this class of drugs (selective or nonselective) in any patient who requires respiratory medications, has a heart rate of less than 55 beats/minute, has or has had heart failure, or has a history of present or past use of antidepressant medications or impotence. A positive history of cardiac problems or symptoms is usually present in patients who have greater than first-degree heart block.

Although cardiac and pulmonary side effects are the most obvious, in a large review, central nervous system problems were the most frequent,[9] ranging from hallucinations to depression to a general feeling of malaise. These side effects may be much more difficult to identify. In the majority of patients, if the drug used may be causing or exacerbating such problems, it is stopped to establish whether the symptoms improve. The elderly appear to be at the greatest risk for β-blocker side effects. A conscious effort is required to identify susceptible patients (in line with the overall philosophy of individualization of therapy and specific assessment of drug effects). Other systemic side effects of topical β-blockers are rare, although the dermatological problem alopecia has been described.[10]

A difference exists between the nonselective and selective β-blockers with regard to the incidence and severity of side effects. A β₁-selective agent is much safer in appropriate patients, but not completely safe. The same complications, such as diminished pulmonary function or decreased exercise-induced tachycardia, may occur with its use, but they occur less frequently and may be less severe. The decision as to which class of β-blocker is appropriate for a specific patient is reduced to a simple observation: for a particular patient, if efficacy is the main concern, a nonselective agent is appropriate (with some sacrifice of the safety profile), but if safety is the primary concern, the use of a β₁-selective drug to limit potential side effects justifies the slight reduction in efficacy.

Other problems with these drugs are less common. Locally, they are well tolerated, although corneal hypesthesia and epithelial changes have been reported.[11] Additionally, some investigators believe that their use should be avoided in diabetic patients, because the symptoms of hypoglycemia may be masked and those of myasthenia gravis may be exacerbated.[12,13] Also, it has been suggested that patients who are undergoing allergy tests or desensitization should not use β-blockers of any kind, even topical agents, because β-blockade may make resuscitation more difficult should anaphylaxis occur. The use of β-blockers in neonates is avoided because apnea may develop.[14] Less well understood is the implication that β-blockers may have an undesirable effect on plasma lipids. Systemic β-blockers are known to result in undesirable changes in plasma lipid profiles. However, systemically, they are actually protective when the clinical outcomes of elevated plasma lipids (i.e., heart attack and stroke) are considered, because of their positive effect on cardiovascular function. Topical timolol and, to a lesser extent, carteolol reduce high-density lipoproteins by 9% and 3%, respectively; however, no data indicate that this results in a higher risk of cardiovascular disease.[15,16] The difference between these two drugs may arise from the intrinsic sympathomimetic activity that carteolol possesses. The mechanism and significance of intrinsic sympathomimetic activity are not clear. Theoretically, the partial agonist activity should cause less vasoconstriction and cardiopulmonary effects, but clinically, it does not result in an appreciable difference in safety or efficacy compared with other nonselective agents.[17]

Although it is true that topical β-blockers are effective and well tolerated by the majority of patients,[18] on rare occasions these agents have been linked with death. Therefore, it is our obligation to identify those patients who may benefit most from their use and those patients in whom their use should be avoided (and for whom other classes of agents may be used).

α-Adrenergic Agonists

Recently, the more specific α-agonists have become available. The first one introduced was apraclonidine, a relatively selective α-adrenergic agonist derived from clonidine, but with an amide group at C4 of the benzoic ring, which makes the drug more polar and less permeable to the blood-brain barrier. As a result, it has fewer central nervous system effects and also produces fewer adverse systemic reactions, such as reduction of systemic blood pressure.[19] Brimonidine is the most recently introduced α-adrenergic agonist; it is a 2-imidazoline derivative with a quinoxaline ring and bromine as side groups.

MECHANISM. Apraclonidine decreases aqueous production[20] but is also associated with an increase in outflow facility and a decrease in episcleral venous pressure.[21] Brimonidine is 23 times more α₂ selective than apraclonidine and 12 times more selective than clonidine.[22] Its mechanism of action includes a reduction in aqueous formation as well as an increase in uveoscleral outflow.[23]

EFFICACY. The first clinical use of apraclonidine was in a 1% concentration to decrease IOP in short-term situations, such as the prevention of pressure spikes after anterior segment laser surgery. It was shown to be very effective for this purpose after argon laser trabeculoplasty,[24,25] argon laser iridotomy,[25] neodymium:yttrium-aluminum-garnet (Nd:YAG) laser iridotomy,[21] Nd:YAG laser capsulotomy,[24] and even cataract surgery and trabeculectomy.[26] Also, it was used successfully in cases of acute angle-closure glaucoma[27] and as prophylaxis against high IOP spikes after cycloplegia.[28]

In addition to its use in acute situations, apraclonidine is used in the chronic treatment of glaucoma. Initially, apraclonidine 1% was administered; subsequently, apraclonidine 0.5% was introduced for use in addition to the maximum-tolerated medical therapy for the treatment of glaucoma. Both concentrations were shown to yield similar IOP reductions. Apraclonidine is also used successfully as an adjunct of β-blockers, including timolol.[29]

Brimonidine 0.5% prevented the rise in postoperative IOP after laser trabeculoplasty to a greater extent than did vehicle. Spikes greater than 10mmHg (1.3kPa) occurred in 1–2% of cases using brimonidine versus 23% using vehicle.[30] In a 12-month comparison of twice-daily brimonidine 0.2% versus timolol 0.5%, both were equally effective at the 2-hour peak. No tachyphylaxis was seen with either drug over the 12 months of the study. At trough (12 hours), IOP was 3.7–5.0mmHg (0.5–0.7kPa) with brimonidine, compared with 5.8–6.6mmHg (0.8–0.9kPa) with timolol. There was no difference between the groups in terms of optic disc and visual field, which were unchanged in 94% of patients.[31] Brimonidine 0.2% was compared with betaxolol 0.25% twice daily in a 3-month study, which demonstrated that brimonidine at peak decreased IOP by 5.5–6.2mmHg (0.7–0.8kPa) compared with baseline; this was greater than the 3.5–4.1mmHg (0.5–0.6kPa) decrease in IOP with betaxolol ($P < .001$). No difference occurred between drugs at trough, and no tachyphylaxis was found with either drug.[32] Brimonidine is approved for use three times a day but is commonly used twice daily, since at morning trough, there is no difference in IOP between the two regimens.[33]

SIDE EFFECTS. Chronic use of apraclonidine is limited by the potential for allergic reaction (Fig. 233-1), which may be severe, and also because the drug may lose effect over time. Previous studies using apraclonidine 1% reported a variable incidence of allergic reaction of up to 48%,[34] although the rate using apraclonidine 0.5% was 15% initially. Systemically, this drug is well tolerated, with the primary systemic side effect being dry mouth—not unexpected with an α-agonist. Brimonidine shows no effect on mean heart rate, mean blood pressure, or pulmonary function.[31] In the longer term (6- and 12-month studies of brimonidine compared with timolol), adverse effects included dry mouth in 30% of patients and fatigue-drowsiness in 15.8% (as a result of which 2.5% of patients exited the study), compared with 13.6% with fatigue ($P = .342$) in the timolol groups.[31] Compared with betaxolol, no statistically significant differences occurred in

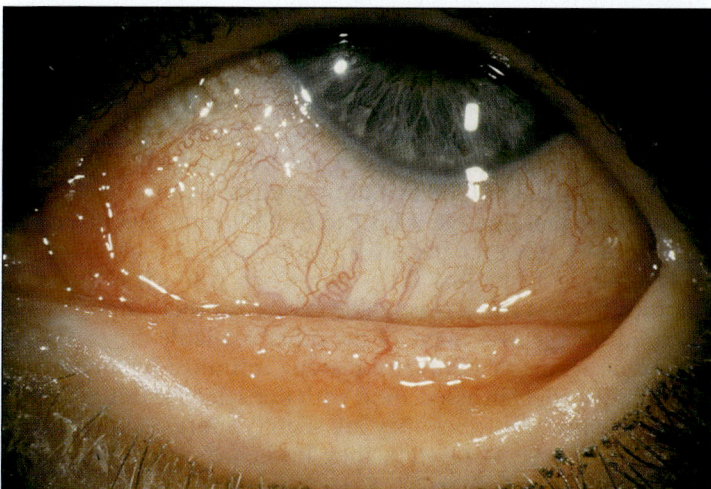

FIG. 233-1 ■ Follicular conjunctival reaction to apraclonidine.

the systemic parameters studied,[32] and no suggestion of a reduction in exercise-induced tachycardia was found.

Ocular effects included conjunctival blanching in 11–17% (vehicle, 9%) of cases and burning-stinging in 24% (timolol, 41%). Within this class of agents, the allergy often limits the drug's clinical usefulness and appears to be a response to haptens, which are oxidation products of the drug. Apraclonidine and epinephrine contain the hydroquinone subunit and are therefore oxidized more easily than are clonidine and brimonidine. Thus, the allergic response caused by brimonidine is less frequent and less severe, with a rate of approximately 5% at 3 months and 12% at 12 months.[31,32] A different formulation of brimonidine has been introduced that reduces the concentration to 0.15% and replaces benzalkonium chloride with a proprietary Purite preservative. The most significant clinical improvement with the new formulation is a reduced incidence of allergic reactions by more than 50% (7.1% vs. 17.1%).[35] Use of the Purite preservative could be a great advantage to patients in whom benzalkonium chloride causes ocular surface disruption. This includes patients who are particularly sensitive to the preservative, as well as patients taking multiple drops in whom toxicity may be cumulative.

Carbonic Anhydrase Inhibitors

MECHANISM. Carbonic anhydrase is an enzyme that catalyzes the reaction of H_2O and CO_2 in equilibrium with H^+ and HCO_3^-. The enzyme is located in the cell membranes of the pigmented and nonpigmented ciliary epithelium.[36] The net effect of the enzyme on aqueous production is to generate bicarbonate ions, which are transported actively across the ciliary epithelial membrane into the posterior chamber (sodium is the primary cation); an osmotic gradient is established. Water passively follows because of the presence of the gradient, which results in fluid production. Inhibition of this enzyme results in lower IOP because aqueous production is decreased approximately 50% or more[37]; aqueous outflow and episcleral venous pressure are affected little or not at all.

An important property of carbonic anhydrase is that it is necessary to inhibit nearly 100% of the enzyme at all times. Thus, topical carbonic anhydrase inhibitors may result in a lower IOP because of decreased aqueous production but not affect total body carbonic anhydrase; as a result, systemic effects are minimized.

Dorzolamide, a topical carbonic anhydrase inhibitor, is different in structure from the oral agents. It has a free sulfonamide group, which is essential for activity, but it also has a second amine moiety, which gives the compound increased aqueous solubility and results in suitable lipid-water solubility for corneal penetration; this allows effective topical application. When aqueous humor flow was measured fluorophotometrically, a 38% reduction was found with dorzolamide 2% in ocular normotensive cynomolgus monkeys, with no effect on outflow as measured by tonography; this confirmed the mechanism of action of this carbonic anhydrase inhibitor.[38] Brinzolamide 1% was introduced as a suspension with a more physiological pH than dorzolamide solution. This resulted in a reduced occurrence of stinging with brinzolamide, but this medication is associated with transient blurring of vision following administration as a suspension.[39]

EFFICACY. In a 2% dorzolamide thrice-daily regimen, the peak effect was a 22% reduction of IOP, with a trough reduction of 18%. At all times after the administration of dorzolamide 2%, the effect was statistically significant ($P \leq .01$) compared with placebo.[40]

In a 12-month study, dorzolamide three times a day was compared with timolol 0.5% twice a day or betaxolol 0.5% twice a day. At peak IOP, measured 2 hours after instillation, no statistically significant difference was found among the three medication regimens (21%, 23%, and 25%, respectively). However, at troughs, 5 hours (18%, 19%, and 22%) and 8 hours (17%, 15%, and 20%) after instillation, timolol was more effective than dorzolamide or betaxolol. No statistically significant difference was found between dorzolamide and betaxolol at 12 months.[41] As a treatment arm in this study, if dorzolamide three times a day did not control IOP adequately, timolol 0.5% twice daily was added. In this subset of 95 patients, IOP was reduced using dorzolamide alone from a mean of 29.3mmHg (3.9kPa) at baseline to 25.2mmHg (3.4kPa), or a 14% reduction. When timolol 0.5% was added, IOP was reduced from a mean of 25.2mmHg (3.4kPa) to 18.9mmHg (2.5kPa), an overall 34% reduction with the combination of the two medications, which indicates an additive effect. A pilot study was performed in which dorzolamide 2% was added to timolol 0.5% and administered to patients who had elevated IOP. The addition of the topical carbonic anhydrase inhibitor decreased IOP by an additional 13–21%.[42] In another study, the additive effect of dorzolamide 2% twice daily was compared with pilocarpine 2% four times daily in a prospective manner in 261 patients over 6 months. Additional mean IOP reductions at the morning trough were 13% and 10% for dorzolamide 2% and pilocarpine 2%, respectively. Patients who received pilocarpine had the highest rate of discontinuation as a result of adverse clinical experience.[43] Therefore, it appears that dorzolamide 2% is a reasonable choice for concomitant therapy.

The efficacy of brinzolamide l% was shown to be essentially equivalent to that of dorzolamide 2% when used either two or three times daily as a single agent[44] or twice daily in addition to timolol 0.5%.[45]

SIDE EFFECTS.

Oral. Carbonic anhydrase inhibitors lower IOP very effectively; however, their use in the chronic treatment of glaucoma is limited by the frequency and severity of side effects. The most common problem is a constellation of symptoms that include malaise, fatigue, anorexia, and depression.[46] Gastrointestinal discomfort, which includes nausea, a metallic taste, and diarrhea, is also common. The more severe complications that limit the use of these agents are less common. Metabolic acidosis may occur in association with high-dose acetazolamide and must be avoided in patients who have severe hepatic or renal disease. Sickle cell crisis may be exacerbated by the acidosis as well, so patients at risk for sickle cell disease must be tested before the use of oral carbonic anhydrase inhibitors. Clinically, this often results in a delay in treating a patient who has acute glaucoma and very high IOP until the patient's hemoglobin status is known. Some investigators suggest that the acidosis lowers IOP further, which may explain the general observation that acetazolamide lowers IOP more effectively than methazolamide or ethoxyzolamide, since the latter two agents do not induce a systemic acidosis. Morbidity is associated with the 11–15-fold increase in the incidence of renal calculi,[47] which most commonly occur within the first 6 months of treatment and may arise from decreased excretion of urinary citrate or magnesium. Once renal stones occur in patients on these agents, the likelihood is high that they will occur again.

The greatest concern surrounding the use of oral carbonic anhydrase inhibitors is the potential mortality from blood dyscrasias. All blood components—red cells, white cells, and platelets—may be affected. In 1989, 139 cases of adverse hematological effects possibly related to carbonic anhydrase inhibitors were reported, with some fatalities attributed to their use.[48] Aplastic anemia, which is frequently fatal, usually occurs within the first 6 months and appears to be an idiosyncratic reaction that is neither dose nor time dependent.[49] As a result, few investigators believe that periodic screening blood tests are justified. In fact, a strong case could be made that with the availability of topical carbonic anhydrase inhibitors, the use of oral agents should be limited to acute situations. In acute situations, when IOP must be lowered maximally, 500mg of acetazolamide given orally as tablets (250mg tablet × 2, not sustained release) has the most rapid onset. Often, oral administration is not possible because of nausea and vomiting, in which case the intravenous route is preferred; the peak effect by this route occurs in 10–15 minutes.[50]

Topical. In controlled clinical trials, only 5% of patients discontinued the drug because of drug-related adverse events, the majority of which were ocular.[51] As part of the controlled clinical trials, plasma and urine were tested, but no evidence of any hematological or urinary disturbances, which included acid-base or electrolyte changes, was found.[51] Dorzolamide binds to the carbonic anhydrase in red blood cells with a half-life of several months; however, the significance of this as a risk factor for blood dyscrasias is not known.[52] Dorzolamide did not appear to inhibit carbonic anhydrase enzyme elsewhere sufficiently to result in systemic effects,[53] and the effects on blood pressure or heart rate were minimal or zero. The only frequent systemic side effect was a bitter taste, reported in approximately 25% of patients. Clinically, this effect can often be reduced if the importance of nasolacrimal occlusion or gentle eyelid closure for a few minutes after the instillation of all ophthalmic drops is emphasized.

With regard to adverse ocular events, approximately one third of patients treated with dorzolamide 2% experienced some level of ocular burn, sting, or discomfort. Superficial punctate keratitis was found in 12% of patients; interestingly, the rate in the placebo group was 10.5%, which suggests that this keratitis may be a response to the vehicle or preservative. This burning was less frequent with brinzolamide 1%.[39,44,45] As with the oral agents, inhibition of carbonic anhydrase within these cells, which could result in a negative effect on the corneal endothelium, has not been found clinically thus far. The overall allergic rate was approximately 10%. In general, dorzolamide and brinzolamide are well tolerated.[41,44]

As to the potential for sulfonamide allergy, the portion of the sulfonamide molecule that is most responsible for the allergic response is not present in dorzolamide. However, further work is required on this question, so caution must be used when sulfonamide allergy is a possible problem.

The use of dorzolamide in children was reviewed retrospectively in one study; no significant health problems were identified with acute or chronic use of this drug.[54]

DRUGS THAT INCREASE AQUEOUS OUTFLOW

Nonspecific Adrenergic Agents

Adrenergic agents comprise two forms of drug—epinephrine (one of the earliest topical agents used to treat glaucoma) and the pro-drug dipivalvyl epinephrine, which was introduced subsequently. A much lower concentration of dipivinyl epinephrine is administered twice daily and metabolized into the active agent. A 10–20-fold dose reduction is obtained as a result of the better ocular penetration of the pro-drug.[55]

MECHANISM. The pharmacology of these drugs shows that they increase uveoscleral outflow but have little net effect on aqueous production.[56] The α_2-specific adrenergic agonist brimonidine (discussed previously) has also been demonstrated to increase uveoscleral outflow, providing it with a dual mechanism of action.[21]

EFFICACY. Adrenergic agents have been widely used, and some investigators believe that dipivalvyl epinephrine should be considered a first-line agent instead of β-blockers, because of its safety profile. However, because of its reduced efficacy, it is generally used as a first-line drug only when β-blockers are contraindicated. It is still a reasonable choice for this purpose, with a cost advantage over many of the other available drugs. Use of adrenergic agents as adjunctive therapy is limited by their minimal additive effect in association with nonselective β-blockers in most patients.[57] However, they are slightly more additive to the selective β-blockers.[8] Overall, they lower pressure by an additional 10%.

SIDE EFFECTS. Usually, adrenergic agents are well tolerated systemically; problems such as hypertension and headaches are rare. Locally, they can cause stinging and irritation, and they have an allergic toxic rate of at least 15% (which includes conjunctival and periocular effects).

Miotics

Miotic agents have long been an important class of drugs in the treatment of glaucoma. Their use has declined because of the availability of alternative agents with more desirable side-effect profiles. However, these drugs remain useful, particularly in patients for whom cost is an overriding concern and in patients whose eyes are not phakic.

MECHANISM. Many different miotic agents are available, all of which have a similar mechanism of action. Miotics are parasympathomimetic agents whose action increases the contractile force of the longitudinal muscle of the ciliary body on its insertion into the scleral spur. This results in an increased facility of outflow of aqueous through the effects on the trabecular meshwork.[58] The miotics either mimic the effect of acetylcholine (e.g., pilocarpine) or prevent the breakdown of endogenous acetylcholine by inhibition of the pseudocholinesterase enzyme.

EFFICACY. Miotics were the earliest drugs used for glaucoma, and they lower IOP by 20–30%. They were used widely as first- or second-line agents, until the advent of α-adrenergic agonists, and as prostaglandin medications. They are additive to β-blockers, adrenergic agents, and carbonic anhydrase inhibitors.

SIDE EFFECTS. Although miotics lower IOP effectively, the clinical use of these drugs is often limited by their local ocular tolerance. From a systemic standpoint, they are quite safe. Although cholinergic effects, such as increased gastrointestinal motility and increased salivation, have been reported, these are quite rare.[59] The use of irreversible cholinesterase inhibitors in patients under general anesthesia causes concern, since these agents inhibit total body cholinesterase; if an agent such as succinylcholine is used during anesthesia, insufficient endogenous enzyme is present to inactive it until more enzyme is synthesized, which results in a markedly prolonged effect.

The local undesirable effects associated with these drugs include pupillary miosis as a result of stimulation of the iris sphincter, burning on instillation of the drops, brow ache and headache after the initial use of the drops, myopic shift of refractive error because of contraction of the circulation muscle of the ciliary body and the resultant increase in power of the crystalline lens, and exacerbation of symptoms of crystalline lens opacity from the pupillary constriction. Such effects are often dose related. Pseudocholinesterase inhibitors are cataractogenic in adults and cause iris pigment epithelial cysts in children, although the latter may be prevented with the concomitant use of topical phenylephrine. The use of miotics has rarely been associated with the development of retinal detachments and cicatricial pemphigoid.[60]

To minimize the undesirable effects of miotics and improve compliance, several therapeutic modifications may be attempted. Because many symptoms are dose related, it is important to begin with as low a dose as possible and gradually increase the dose until the desired therapeutic effect is obtained or the IOP is lowered no further. Miotics are melanin bound, so higher doses may be necessary in patients who have more darkly pigmented irides. Typically, the peak of the dose-response curve is pilocarpine 4% in dark irides and 2% in blue irides. However, it is important to use the lowest dose possible to minimize side effects. Additionally, the frequency of instillation is important in terms of patient compliance. Pilocarpine is often prescribed four times daily. Many patients do as well with twice-daily dosing in association with nasolacrimal occlusion or forced eyelid closure as they do with four-times-daily dosing without these maneuvers. Use of alternative miotic agents also may decrease the frequency of administration. Carbachol is used three times daily in all patients, but often twice-daily administration is adequate. Because penetration of the corneal epithelium by this agent is variable, it is helpful (as with all miotics, which are almost always used as adjunctive agents) to instill it after other agents to facilitate absorption.

The pseudocholinesterase inhibitors also are advantageous because of twice-daily dosing. Pilocarpine gel was introduced to provide convenient daily dosing at bedtime, with the expectation that the majority of the undesirable effects would wear off by morning but the therapeutic effect would be maintained throughout the day.[61] A gel delivery vehicle is a much more convenient dosing form for patients who use the higher doses of miotics; however, it is important to check that a lower IOP is maintained throughout the entire 24-hour period. Some patients require supplemental drops in the late afternoon or evening. A useful suggestion for patients is to wash off any excess gel upon awakening so that the eye is not redosed. Sustained-release pilocarpine in the form of Ocuserts theoretically is the most desirable delivery system. The semipermeable membrane delivers a very low dose of drug continuously, with replacement needed approximately every 7 days.[62] The therapeutic effect is maintained and tolerability is improved; however, the usefulness of this method is limited by the manual dexterity necessary for replacement. Many elderly patients cannot insert sustained-release devices, which are better suited for younger patients.

Patients whose eyes have undergone cataract surgery tend to better tolerate miotics, since the miosis is less severe, no induced myopia occurs, and the patients tend to be older and suffer less brow ache and headache with use.

Decosanoids

Unoprostone isopropyl 0.15% has been available in Japan for many years and was recently introduced into the United States. Structurally, it is a decosanoid derived from docosahexanoic acid with a 22-carbon backbone that poorly binds the FP receptor compared with prostaglandin $F_{2\alpha}$ analogs that have a 20-carbon structure. The receptor at which unoprostone acts has not been identified; however, increased outflow is the mechanism of action. In 571 patients treated twice daily over 6 months,[63] there was a 14% decrease in IOP (3mmHg). This agent appears to be safe and well tolerated, with rare changes in iris color and an approximately 10% risk of conjunctival hyperemia; however, its clinical utility is often limited by its modest efficacy in lowering IOP. When twice-daily unoprostone was compared with once-daily latanoprost in 108 patients, unoprostone was found to be less effective in reducing IOP, with a 3.3mmHg (14%) reduction from baseline compared with 6.7mmHg (28%) with latanoprost. The difference of 3.4mmHg was statistically significant ($P < .001$). A 30% reduction in IOP was achieved in only 8% of eyes treated with unoprostone, compared with 44% of those treated with latanoprost.[64] It has been suggested that unoprostone may further reduce IOP when added to latanoprost. However, this additive effect was shown only in those patients ($n = 14$) with an IOP of 22mmHg or greater on latanoprost alone; these patients had an additional 2.1mmHg reduction in mean diurnal IOP and a further flattening of the diurnal curve.[65]

Prostaglandins

Prostaglandins (PGs) are a relatively recent class of drugs added to the armamentarium of glaucoma medications. Latanoprost and more recently travoprost have been approved for use in glaucoma or ocular hypertension in patients who are intolerant of or insufficiently responsive to other agents that lower IOP.

Prostaglandins are derived from arachidonic acid and display a wide range of biological functions. Initially, interest in their ocular effects arose from the observation that prostaglandins can mediate inflammation. At that time, high doses of prostaglandins were found to increase IOP. After further tests, the 17-phenyl-substituted $PGF_{2\alpha}$ ester analog latanoprost was found to provide the best combination of efficacy and side-effect profile. Another $PGF_{2\alpha}$ ester analog, travoprost, has also been introduced.

MECHANISM. Animal studies suggested that prostaglandins reduce IOP by increasing uveoscleral outflow, since no effect was found on fluorophotometrically measured aqueous flow or on tonographical ouflow.[66] Further studies suggested that uveoscleral outflow increases because of relaxation of the ciliary body muscle and dilated spaces between ciliary muscle bundles, in addition to the altered metabolism of the extracellular matrix that surrounds the ciliary muscle cells.[67] The exact mechanism by which this occurs is unclear, but available data in humans support uveoscleral outflow as the primary mechanism. Clinical implications arise because of the concern that drugs that focus on decreased aqueous production to lower the IOP may result in undesirable effects on the anterior segment. Additionally, because uveoscleral outflow does not end in the episcleral venous circulation, it is possible to obtain an IOP that is less than episcleral venous pressure (9–11mmHg [1.2–1.5kPa]), which may be very desirable, particularly in normal-tension glaucomas[68] (see Chapter 221).

EFFICACY. In three large, multicenter trials that compared latanoprost 0.005% once daily with timolol 0.5% twice daily for 6 months, latanoprost reduced IOP by 25–34% and was statistically more effective than timolol in two of the three studies.[69–71] Also, it was shown that evening administration of latanoprost was significantly more effective than morning administration; the peak effect occurs approximately 12 hours after instillation.[69] In addition, latanoprost reduced IOP in patients equally, day or night, and there was no suggestion of loss of effect during the 12 months of treatment. Travoprost 0.004% is a synthetic analog of prostaglandin $F_{2\alpha}$, as is latanoprost. In many respects, travoprost and latanoprost are similar. Mechanistically, both bind the FP receptor—in fact, travoprost appears to bind with higher affinity than latanoprost—and both lower IOP by increasing uveoscleral outflow. Both are administered once daily. Their efficacy appears to be similar as well. In phase III studies involving 605 patients, travoprost 0.004% once daily demonstrated about a 1.0–1.3mmHg greater reduction in IOP

compared with timolol 0.5% twice daily.[72] This magnitude of efficacy is similar to that shown by latanoprost.

A 12-month study directly comparing travoprost 0.004% and latanoprost 0.005% showed essentially no difference in mean IOP reduction (6.6–8.1 versus 6.2–8.1mmHg, respectively) and showed a statistical advantage favoring travoprost at only a single point of the diurnal curve[73] (Fig. 233-2).

Travoprost 0.004% was shown to lower IOP by up to 3.2mmHg more than timolol in black patients and to produce a lower mean IOP than latanoprost in black patients (17.2 versus 18.6mmHg).[74] This may reflect an increased efficacy of travoprost in blacks. Analysis of the pooled travoprost data shows that travoprost is more effective in black patients than in nonblack patients, but additional studies will be necessary to determine whether travoprost is superior to other agents in black patients.

ADDITIVE EFFECT. Latanoprost 0.005% once daily was shown to be additive to twice-daily timolol 0.5%. It reduced IOP an additional 13% in one study and an additional 30–35% in another.[75,76] Animal experiments suggested that prostaglandins and pilocarpine would not be additive. However, in one human study, it was shown that a 14–18% further reduction in IOP could be obtained by the addition of latanoprost to pilocarpine 2% three times daily.[77] There are some data available concerning the additive effect of travoprost to timolol.[78] Adding travoprost 0.004% once daily to timolol 0.5% twice daily resulted in an additional 5.7–7.2mmHg reduction in IOP compared with placebo, which provided an additional 1.3–2.8mmHg reduction in IOP.

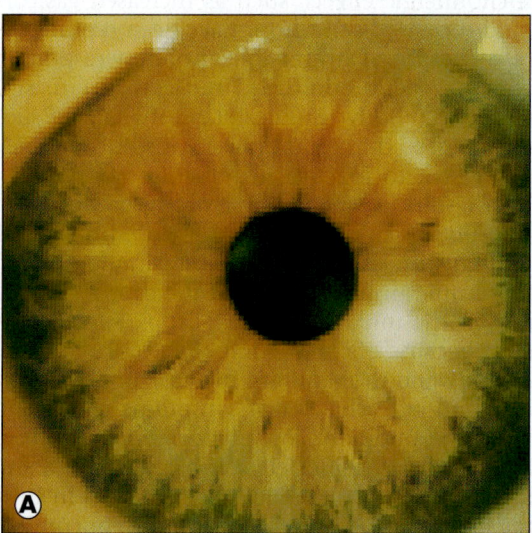

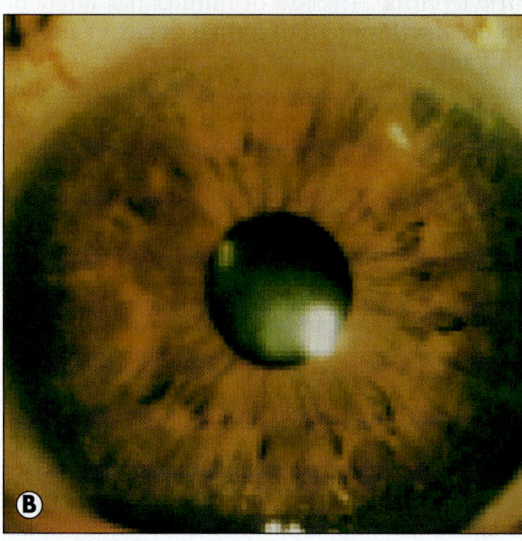

FIG. 233-3 ■ Iris color changes after latanoprost treatment. **A,** Before treatment in a patient with a green-brown iris. **B,** After 6 months of latanoprost treatment, the iris has increased pigmentation.

MEAN IOP CHANGE

Mean IOP change—12 hours post dosing (8 AM)

mean IOP change (y-axis: −5 to −9)
x-axis: week 2, month 1.5, month 3, month 4.5, month 6, month 9, month 12

◆ 0.004% travatan   ■ timolol

Mean IOP change-0.004%—US 1 year study—8 AM visit

mean IOP change (y-axis: −3 to −9)
x-axis: week 2, month 1.5, month 3, month 4.5, month 6, month 9, month 12

◆ 0.004% travatan   ■ xalatan

FIG. 233-2 ■ Mean intraocular pressure change.

SIDE EFFECTS. Reported side effects in controlled trials of latanoprost 0.005% once daily included conjunctival hyperemia (generally mild, 36%), burning and stinging (25%), blurred vision (17%), itching (15%), foreign body sensation (33%), tearing (6%), and eye pain (13%).

Latanoprost resulted in increased iris pigmentation in 11–23% of patients[69-71] (Fig. 233-3). In most cases, the eyes in which the iris color changed had a characteristic concentric heterochromia before treatment, with greater pigmentation around the pupil than in the periphery. In patients who have pure blue, gray, green, or brown eyes, the risk of increased iris pigmentation is estimated to be 4%. In patients who have mixed blue and gray-brown eyes, the estimated risk is 20% at 2 years, and for patients who have green-brown or yellow-brown irides, the estimated risk is 50% at 1 year. This increased pigmentation occurs slowly but may be noticeable at 3 months, with a 6.8–11.6% increase in pigmentation seen at 6 months and a 15.5–22.9% increase at 12 months; sometimes 18 months or longer is required for the increased pigmentation to become manifest. Iris nevi do not appear to be affected. This change in pigmentation does not increase or decrease after cessation of latanoprost.[79] Animal data suggest that the increased pigmentation may arise from increased production of melanin within the iris melanocytes rather than from cellular proliferation.[80] The long-term consequences are not known.

The side effects with travoprost and latanoprost are similar to those with travoprost alone, but with a greater occurrence of hyperemia (49.5 versus 27.6%) and a slightly lower chance of increased iris pigmentation (2.8 versus 5.2%).[73]

SYSTEMIC SAFETY. Latanoprost 0.005% has a plasma half-life of only 17 minutes. Therefore, with the very low concentration delivered, minimal systemic side effects are anticipated. No effect was found on resting heart rate, blood pressure, or blood and urine laboratory values. The most frequently reported potential systemic effects include upper respiratory tract syndrome (24%), headache (9%), and back, muscle, or joint pain (6%).[62-64] The use of latanoprost in young patients has not been evaluated.

Prostamides

There is substantial evidence supporting the assertion that bimatoprost is a prostamide, an apparently different class of drugs from the prostaglandin analogs latanoprost and travoprost.[81-83] Like prostaglandins, prostamides are derived from membrane lipids, but unlike prostaglandins, the biosynthetic precursor of prostamides is anandamide, not arachidonic acid. Prostamides, including bimatoprost, do not bind to the prostaglandin FP receptor, and further reinforcing their uniqueness, they do not bind to any other known receptors.[82]

MECHANISM. Bimatoprost is the active drug, not a pro-drug requiring activation by corneal enzymes,[83] as is the case with latanoprost and travoprost. Mechanistically, Brubaker *et al.*[84] have shown that bimatoprost works by increasing outflow, producing both a 35% increase in trabecular outflow facility and a calculated 50% increase in uveoscleral outflow. This apparent dual mechanism of action is in contrast to the prostaglandin analogs, which appear to work primarily through an increase in uveoscleral outflow.

EFFICACY. In comparisons of bimatoprost once daily and timolol 0.5% twice daily, bimatoprost demonstrated statistical superiority in all measures of effectiveness in lowering IOP. Beginning at similar baselines, at month 6, bimatoprost 0.03% once daily lowered IOP at 10:00 A.M. (timolol peak) an average of 8.1mmHg (33%), compared with 5.6mmHg (23%) with timolol 0.5% twice daily. The difference between the two agents was consistently maintained at 2–3mmHg throughout the day and throughout the study[85,86] (Fig. 233-4).

Of more relevance in treating individual patients was a comparison of the two drugs' success in allowing patients to reach a specific target pressure or obtain a desired percentage drop in IOP. At all IOPs from 13–18mmHg at peak measurements for both drugs, bimatoprost patients were 50–120% more likely than timolol patients to reach the target. This is clinically important, because this range represents the target pressures for the majority of glaucoma patients (Fig. 233-5).

Similarly, when effectiveness in lowering IOP was evaluated using percentage drop in IOP, bimatoprost was significantly more effective than timolol. Generally, a 20% reduction in IOP is the minimum acceptable efficacy for a single agent. A 20% drop in IOP was achieved in 87% of patients treated with bimatoprost, compared with only 60% of those treated with tim-

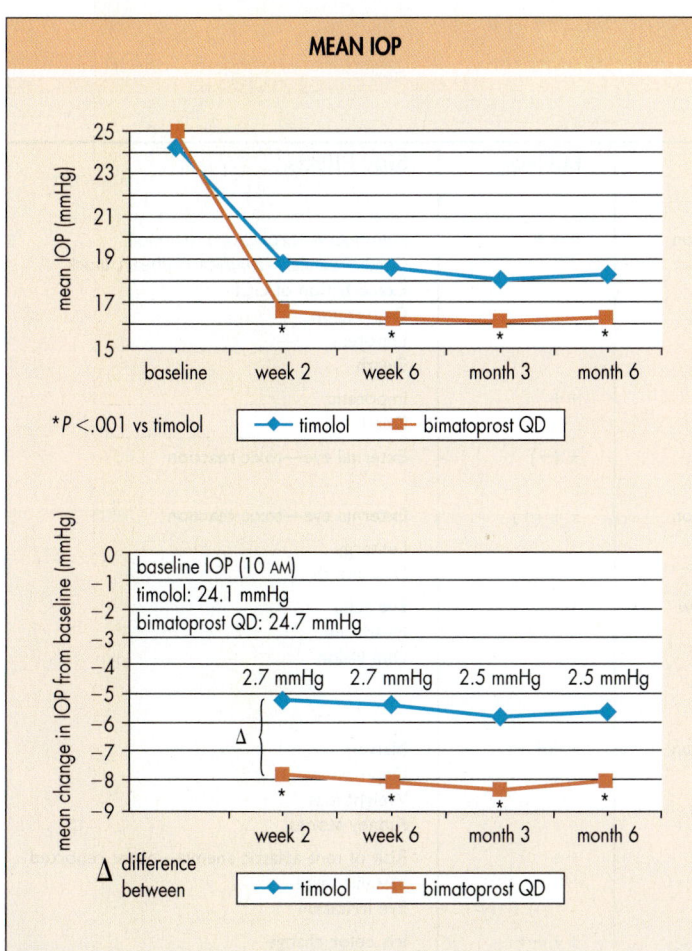

FIG. 233-4 ■ Graph shows the 10 A.M. pooled 6-month results from the phase III bimatoprost trials.

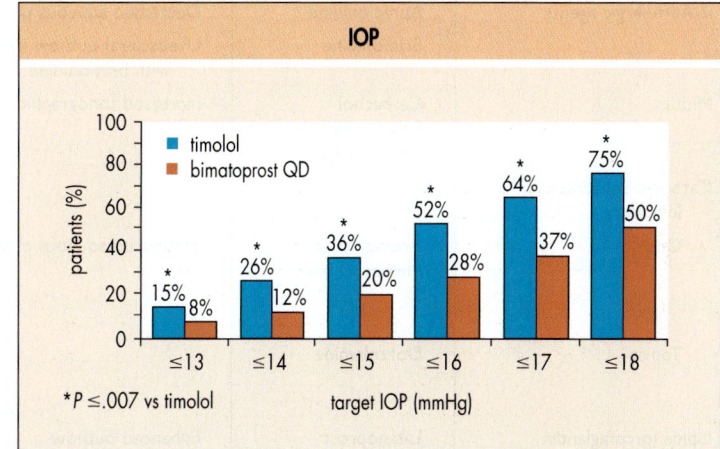

FIG. 233-5 ■ Patients achieving target intraocular pressure levels in the phase III bimatoprost trials. Results shown are from the month 6 visit at 10 A.M.

olol.[86] Greater reductions in IOP are often desirable, and again, bimatoprost was significantly better than timolol at achieving substantial IOP reductions, with nearly two thirds of patients demonstrating a 30% reduction and nearly one third of patients obtaining a 40% reduction.[86] When 12-hour diurnal IOP measurements were performed, bimatoprost was superior at all time points (Fig. 233-6).

In a 3-month comparison of latanoprost and bimatoprost, with both medications given once daily, bimatoprost ($n = 119$) was about 0.5 mmHg more effective than latanoprost ($n = 113$) in lowering IOP at 8:00 A.M., although the differences between the groups were not statistically significant. Both medications were well tolerated, with no more than 5% of patients from either group discontinuing treatment because of adverse effects.[87]

SIDE EFFECTS. Hyperemia was found to be more common with bimatoprost than with latanoprost. The hyperemia appears to be conjunctival injection that is unrelated to either an allergic follicular conjunctival response or actual tissue inflammation. Overall, hyperemia occurred in about 45% of patients using bimatoprost; the severity of the hyperemia was trace to mild, with less than 4% of patients discontinuing bimatoprost due to tolerability issues. Clinically, in some patients the hyperemia is slightly greater and may be associated with mild burning. This appears to be most severe when beginning the medication and usually rapidly improves.

SYSTEMIC SAFETY. Bimatoprost demonstrated no effect on blood pressure, pulse, hematology, urinalysis, or any other parameter of systemic safety.[85] Ocular evaluation showed no increase in aqueous flare. Ocular effects identified included eyelash growth, rare increase in iris color, and conjunctival hyperemia. At 12 months, increased iris pigmentation with bimatoprost, evaluated by the treating physicians using photographs of patients' eyes, was only 1.5%. The experience with the prostaglandin analogs has reassured us that this change in iris color is primarily a cosmetic concern and is often not recognized by the patient. Although the change is irreversible, it is common to treat patients until iris pigmentation changes occur and then make a decision whether to continue the drug, based on the efficacy and the patient's input.

THE MEDICAL ARMAMENTARIUM OF GLAUCOMA TREATMENT

As more experience with any drug is gained, its place in the decision-making process becomes more clear. Historically, the β-blockers were the most common first-line agents used in the med-

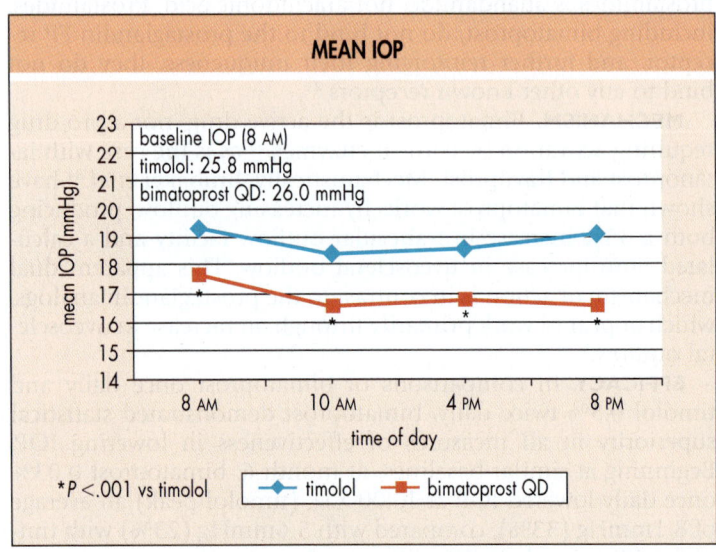

FIG. 233-6 ■ Twelve-hour diurnal intraocular pressure measurements.

TABLE 233-1

DRUGS USED TO MANAGE GLAUCOMA

Drug	Example	Mechanism of Action	Efficacy	Side Effects
β-Blockers				
Non–selective	Timolol Levobunolol Carteolol Metipranolol	Decreased aqueous production (?Daytime only)	+++	Pulmonary—bronchoconstriction Cardiovascular—bradycardia/heart block Exacerbation of CCF Depression Impotent Death
Selective	Betaxolol		++	Impotent Death
Adrenergic agents	Epinephrine Dipivefrin	Outflow enhancement	+ (+)	External eye—toxic reaction
α-Adrenergic agents	Apraclonidine	Decreased aqueous production	++ (+)	External eye—toxic reaction
	Brimonidine	Uveoscleral outflow increase with brimonidine		Lethargy Dry mouth
Miotics	Carbachol Pilocarpine Echothiophate	Increased tonographic outflow	+++	Eye ache Headache Dim vision
Carbonic anhydrase inhibitors				
Oral	Acetazolamide Methazolamide	Decreased aqueous production	++++	Malaise Depression Weight loss Kidney stones
Topical	Dorzolamide		++	Risk of rare aplastic anemia—never reported Metallic taste Eye irritation
Lipids (prostaglandin analogs, prostamides decosanoids)	Latanoprost Travoprost Bimatoprost Unoprostone	Enhanced outflow	++++ ++	Iris color change Hyperemia Periocular skin pigmentation Eyelash growth

ical treatment of glaucoma. However, as our experience with newer agents, particularly those facilitating outflow, increased, they were recognized as being more efficacious in lowering IOP and systemically safer than β-blockers. As a result, they are becoming the first-line agents in glaucoma treatment. When these agents are not appropriate, we still have other excellent choices, including the β-blockers, α-agonists, and topical carbonic anhydrase inhibitors. In general, these agents are well tolerated by most patients, with a low rate of discontinuation attributable to the drugs. We must maintain vigilance to identify patients who should not receive these drugs because of the potential for ocular, pulmonary, cardiovascular, or central nervous system side effects. The current spectrum of glaucoma drugs is summarized in Table 233-1.

Because about 50% of glaucoma patients take more than one class of agents, an understanding of the characteristics of these agents is necessary to make the best choices for our patients. With the recent introduction of many new agents, the availability of pertinent studies on which to base additive therapy is sometimes limited. Therefore, when using medications to treat glaucoma, it is imperative that the individual needs of the particular patient be considered. It is important to include the patient in the decision-making process, through education about the disease as well as discussion of the specific positives and negatives of the treatment options. The best regimen for an individual patient can be selected and tried using the one-eye therapeutic trial and correct instillation techniques. In this way, maximal compliance, which is often difficult to achieve and a limiting factor in effective medical therapy for glaucoma, may be obtained.

REFERENCES

1. Zimmerman TJ, Kooner KS, Kandarakis AS, Ziegler LP. Improving the therapeutic index of topically applied ocular drugs. Arch Ophthalmol. 1984;102:551–3.
2. Coakes RL, Brubaker RS. The mechanism of timolol in lowering intraocular pressure. Arch Ophthalmol. 1978;96:2045–8.
3. Reiss GR, Lee DA, Topper JE, Brubaker RF. Aqueous humor flow during sleep. Invest Ophthalmol Vis Sci. 1984;25:776–8.
4. Levobunolol Study Group T. Levobunolol: a beta adrenoceptor antagonist effective in the long-term treatment of glaucoma. Ophthalmology. 1985;92:1271–6.
5. Serle JB, Lustgarten JS, Podos SM. A clinical trial of metipranolol, a noncardioselective beta-adrenergic antagonist in ocular hypertension. Am J Ophthalmol. 1991;112:302–7.
6. Secoville B, Mueller B, White BG, Krieglestein GK. A double-masked comparison of carteolol and timolol in ocular hypertension. Am J Ophthalmol. 1988;105:150–4.
7. Berry DP, Van Buskirk EM, Shields MB. Betaxolol and timolol: a comparison of efficacy and side effects. Arch Ophthalmol. 1984;102:42–5.
8. Allen RC, Epstein DL. Additive effect of betaxolol and epinephrine in primary open-angle glaucoma. Arch Ophthalmol. 1986;104:1178–84.
9. Fraunfelder FT, Meyer SM. Systemic adverse reactions in glaucoma medications [review]. Int Ophthalmol Clin. 1989;29:143–6.
10. Fraunfelder FT, Meyer SM, Menacker SJ. Alopecia possibly secondary to topical ophthalmic beta-blockers [letter]. JAMA. 1990;263(11):1493–4.
11. Van Buskirk EM. Corneal anesthesia after timolol maleate therapy. Am J Ophthalmol. 1979;88:739–43.
12. Velde TM, Kaiser FE. Ophthalmic timolol treatment causing altered hypoglycemic response in a diabetic patient. Arch Intern Med. 1983;143:1627.
13. Coppeto JR. Timolol associated myasthenia gravis. Am J Ophthalmol. 1984;98:244–5.
14. Olson RJ, Bromberg BB, Zimmerman TJ. Apneic spells associated with timolol therapy in a neonate. Am J Ophthalmol. 1979;88:120–2.
15. Coleman AL, Diehl DLC, Sampel HD, et al. Topical timolol decreases plasma high density lipoprotein cholesterol level. Arch Ophthalmol. 1990;108:1260–3.
16. Freedman SF, Freedman NJ, Shields MB, et al. Effects of ocular carteolol and timolol on plasma high density lipoprotein cholesterol level. Am J Ophthalmol. 1990;116:600–11.
17. Stewart WC. Carteolol, an ophthalmic beta-blocking agent with intrinsic sympathomimetic activity. J Glaucoma. 1994;3:339–45.
18. Van Buskirk EM, Fraunfelder FJ. Ocular beta-blockers and systemic effects. Am J Ophthalmol. 1984;98:623–4.
19. Coleman AL, Robin AL, Pollack IP. Apraclonidine hydrochloride. Ophthalmol Clin North Am. 1989;2:97–108.
20. Gharagozloo NZ, Rely SJ, Brubaker RF. Aqueous flow is reduced by the alpha-adrenergic agonist, apraclonidine hydrochloride (ALO2145). Ophthalmology. 1988;95:1217–20.
21. Toris CB, Lafoya ME, Camras CB, Yablonski ME. Effects of apraclonidine on aqueous humor dynamics in human eyes. Ophthalmology. 1995;102:456–61.
22. Burke J, Schwartz M. Preclinical evaluation of brimonidine. Surv Ophthalmol. 1996;41(Suppl 1):S9–18.
23. Toris CB, Gleason ML, Camras CB, Yablonski ME. Effects of brimonidine on aqueous humor dynamics in human eyes. Arch Ophthalmol. 1995;113:1514–7.
24. Brown RH, Stewart RH, Lynch MG, et al. ALO 2145 reduces the intraocular pressure elevation after anterior segment laser surgery. Ophthalmology. 1988;95:378–84.
25. Krupin T, Stak T, Feitl MR. Apraclonidine pretreatment decreases the acute intraocular pressure rise after laser trabeculoplasty or iridotomy. J Glaucoma. 1992;1:79–86.
26. Robin AL. Effect of topical apraclonidine on the frequency of intraocular pressure elevations after combined extracapsular cataract extraction and trabeculectomy. Ophthalmology. 1993;100:628–33.
27. Krawitz PL, Podos SM. Use of apraclonidine in the treatment of acute angle closure glaucoma. Arch Ophthalmol. 1990;108:1208–9.
28. Hill RA, Minckler DS, Lee M, et al. Apraclonidine prophylaxis for postcycloplegic intraocular pressure spikes. Ophthalmology. 1991;98:1083–6.
29. Stewart WC, Ritch R, Shin DH, et al. The efficacy of apraclonidine as an adjunct to timolol therapy. Arch Ophthalmol. 1995;113:287–92.
30. Brimonidine-ALT Study Group. Effect of brimonidine 0.5% on intraocular pressure spikes following 360° argon laser trabeculoplasty. Ophthalmic Surg Lasers. 1995;26:404–9.
31. Schuman JS. Clinical experience with brimonidine 0.2% and timolol 0.5% in glaucoma and ocular hypertension. Surv Ophthalmol. 1996;41(Suppl 1):S27–37.
32. Searle JB. Brimonidine Study Group III. A comparison of the safety and efficacy of twice daily brimonidine 0.2% versus betaxolol 0.25% in subjects with elevated intraocular pressure. Surv Ophthalmol. 1996;41(Suppl 1):S39–47.
33. Rosenthal AL, Walters T, Berg E, et al. A comparison of the safety and efficacy of brimonidine 0.2% BID versus TID in subjects with elevated intraocular pressure [abstract]. Invest Ophthalmol Vis Sci. 1996;37(Suppl.):S831.
34. Butler P, Mannschrek M, Lin S, et al. Clinical experience with the long-term use of 1% apraclonidine. Arch Ophthalmol. 1995;113:293–6.
35. Walters TR, Brimonidine-Purite Study Group 1. 12-Month evaluation of brimonidine-Purite compared with brimonidine in patients with glaucoma or ocular hypertension. Invest Ophthalmol Vis Sci Suppl. 2001;42:S558.
36. Lutjen-Drecoll E, Lonnerholm G, Eichorn M. Carbonic anhydrase distribution in the human and monkey eye by light and electron microscopy. Graefes Arch Ophthalmol. 1983;220:285.
37. Dailey RA, Brubaker RF, Bourne WM. The effects of timolol maleate and acetazolamide on the rate of aqueous formation in normal human subjects. Am J Ophthalmol. 1982;93:232.
38. Wang RF, Serle JB, Podos SM, Sugrve MF. MK-507 (L-671,152), a topically active carbonic anhydrase inhibitor reduces aqueous humor production in monkeys. Arch Ophthalmol. 1991;109:1297.
39. Silver LH, the Brinzolamide Comfort Study Group. Ocular comfort of brinzolamide 1% ophthalmic suspension compared with dorzolamide 2% ophthalmic solution. Results from two multicenter comfort studies. Surv Ophthalmol. 2000;44(Suppl 2):141–5.
40. Lippa EA, Carlson LE, Ehinger B, et al. Dose-response and duration of action of dorzolamide, a topical carbonic anhydrase inhibitor. Arch Ophthalmol. 1992;100:495.
41. Strahlman ER, Tipping R, Vogel R. A double-masked, randomized 1-year study comparing dorzolamide (Trusopt), timolol, and betaxolol. Arch Ophthalmol. 1995;113:1009–16.
42. Parfitt AM. Acetazolamide and sodium bicarbonate–induced nephrocalcinosis and nephrolithiasis: relationship to citrate and calcium excretion. Arch Intern Med. 1969;124:736.
43. Strahlman ER, Vogel R, Tipping R, Clineschmidt CM. The use of dorzolamide and pilocarpine as adjunctive therapy to timolol in patients with elevated intraocular pressure. Ophthalmology. 1996;103:1283–93.
44. Sall K, the Brinzolamide Primary Therapy Study Group. The efficacy and safety of brinzolamide 1% ophthalmic suspension as a primary therapy in patients with open-angle glaucoma or ocular hypertension. Surv Ophthalmol. 2000;44(Suppl 2):155–62.
45. Michaud JE, Friren B, the International Brinzolamide Adjunctive Study Group. Comparison of topical brinzolamide 1% and dorzolamide 2% eye drops given twice daily in addition to timolol 0.5% in patients with primary open-angle glaucoma or ocular hypertension. Am J Ophthalmol. 2001;132:235–43.
46. Epstein DL, Grant WM. Carbonic anhydrase inhibitor side effects. Serum chemical analysis. Arch Ophthalmol. 1977;95:1378.
47. Kass MA, Kolker AE, Gorden M, et al. Acetazolamide and urolithiasis. Ophthalmology. 1981;88:261–5.
48. Fraunfelder FT, Bagby GC. Possible hematologic reactions associated to carbonic anhydrase inhibitors. JAMA. 1989;261:2257.
49. Fraunfelder FT, Meyer SM, Bagby GC Jr, Dreis MW. Hematologic reactions to carbonic anhydrase inhibitors. Am J Ophthalmol. 1985;100:79.
50. Linner E, Wistrand PJ. The initial drop of the intraocular pressure following intravenous administration of acetazolamide in man. Acta Ophthalmol (Copenh). 1959;37:209.
51. Strahlman ER, Tipping R, Vogel R. A six-week dose-response study of the ocular hypotensive effect of dorzolamide with a one-year extension. Am J Ophthalmol. 1996;122:183–94.
52. Kitazawa Y, Shimuzu U, Ido T. MK-417 and MK-507, topical carbonic anhydrase inhibitors: the effect of lowering intraocular pressure and the pharmacokinetics in normal volunteers. Paper presented at the International Glaucoma Symposium, Jerusalem, August 20, 1991.
53. Maren TH. The relation between enzyme inhibition and physiological response in the carbonic anhydrase system. J Pharmacol Exp Ther. 1963;139:140.
54. Donohue EK, Wilensky JT. Clinical use of Trusopt in infants and children: a case series. Paper presented at the American Glaucoma Society Meeting, Vancouver, BC, July 1996.
55. Mandell AI, Stenz F, Kitabchi AE. Dipivinyl epinephrine: a new pro-drug in the treatment of glaucoma. Ophthalmology. 1978;85:268.
56. Sears ML, Neufeld AH. Adrenergic modulation of the outflow of aqueous humor. Invest Ophthalmol Vis Sci. 1975;14:83.
57. Thomas JV, Epstein DL. Timolol and epinephrine in primary open angle glaucoma: transient additive effect. Arch Ophthalmol. 1981;99:91.
58. Gaasterland D, Kupfer C, Ross K, et al. Studies of aqueous humor dynamics in man. IV. Effects of pilocarpine upon measurements in young normal volunteers. Invest Ophthalmol. 1975;14:848.
59. Greco JJ, Kelman CD. Systemic pilocarpine toxicity in the treatment of angle closure glaucoma. Ann Ophthalmol. 1975;5:57.
60. Shields MB. Cholinergic stimulators. In: Textbook of glaucoma, 3rd ed. Baltimore: Williams & Wilkins; 1992:461–6.
61. March WF, Stewart RM, Mandell AI, Bruce LA. Duration of effect of pilocarpine gel. Arch Ophthalmol. 1982;100:1270.

62. Quigley HA, Pollack IP, Harbin TS Jr. Pilocarpine Ocuserts: long-term clinical trials and selected pharmacodynamics. Arch Ophthalmol. 1975;93:771.

63. Stewart WC, Mundorf T, Haque R, et al. Comparison of the IOP-lowering efficacy and safety of the decosanoid unoprostone isopropyl 0.15% versus timolol maleate 0.5% dosed twice daily for 6 months in patients with primary open-angle glaucoma or ocular hypertension. Invest Ophthalmol Vis Sci Suppl. 2001;44:S557.

64. Susanna R Jr, Giampani J Jr, Borges AS, et al. A double-masked, randomized clinical trial comparing latanoprost with unoprostone in patients with open-angle glaucoma or ocular hypertension. Ophthalmology. 2001;108:259–63.

65. Stewart WC, Sharpe ED, Stewart JA, et al. Additive efficacy of unoprostone isopropyl 0.12% (Rescula) to latanoprost 0.005%. Am J Ophthalmol. 2001;131:339–44.

66. Toris CB, Yablonski ME, Camras CB, Brubaker RF. Mechanism of the ocular hypotensive effect of latanoprost and the maintenance of normal blood-aqueous barrier function. Surv Ophthalmol. 1997;41(Suppl 2):S69–75.

67. Bill A. Uveoscleral drainage of aqueous humor: physiology and pharmacology. Prog Clin Biol Res. 1989;312:417–27.

68. Kaufman PL, Crawford K. Aqueous humor dynamics: how $PGF_{2\alpha}$ lowers intraocular pressure. Prog Clin Biol Res. 1989;312:387–416.

69. Alm A, Stjernschantz J, Scandinavian Latanoprost Study Group. Effects on intraocular pressure and side effects of 0.005% latanoprost once daily, evening or morning. A comparison with timolol. Ophthalmology. 1995;102:1743–52.

70. Watson P, Stjernschantz J, Latanoprost Study Group. A six month randomized double-masked study comparing latanoprost to timolol in open angle glaucoma and ocular hypertension. Ophthalmology. 1996;103:126–37.

71. Camras CB, United States Latanoprost Study Group. Comparison of latanoprost and timolol in patients with ocular hypertension and glaucoma. A six month, masked, multi-center trial in the United States. Ophthalmology. 1996;103:138–47.

72. Whitson JT, Ratliff M, Fellman RL, et al. Travoprost, a new prostaglandin analogue, is superior to timolol in lowering IOP in patients with open-angle glaucoma or ocular hypertension. Invest Ophthalmol Vis Sci Suppl. 2001;42:S557.

73. Netland PA, Landry T, Silver LH, et al. IOP-lowering efficacy and safety of travoprost compared to latanoprost and timolol in patients with open-angle glaucoma or ocular hypertension. Invest Ophthalmol Vis Sci Suppl. 2001;42:S556.

74. Roberston SM, Sullivan EK, Silver LH, et al. Differences between black and non-black patients with open-angle glaucoma or ocular hypertension in IOP-lowering response to travoprost. Invest Ophthalmol Vis Sci Suppl. 2001;42:S559.

75. Alm A, Wiodengard I, Kjellgren D, et al. Latanoprost administered once daily caused a maintained reduction of intraocular pressure in glaucoma patients treated concomitantly with timolol. Br J Ophthalmol. 1995;79:12–6.

76. Rulo AH, Greve EL, Hoyng PF. Additive effect of latanoprost, a prostaglandin $PGF_{2\alpha}$ and timolol in patients with elevated intraocular pressure. Br J Ophthalmol. 1994;78:899–902.

77. Fristrom B, Nilsson SEG. Interaction of PhXA41, a new prostaglandin analogue, with pilocarpine. A study on patients with elevated intraocular pressure. Arch Ophthalmol. 1993;111:662–5.

78. Orengo-Nania SD, Landry T, Von Tress M, et al. Travoprost significantly decreased IOP in patients with open-angle glaucoma or ocular hypertension when used adjunctively with timolol. Invest Ophthalmol Vis Sci Suppl.) 2001;42:S820.

79. Wistrand PJ, Stjernschantz J, Olsson K. The incidence and time-course of latanoprost-induced iridial pigmentation as a function of eye color. Surv Ophthalmol. 1997;41(Suppl 2):S129–38.

80. Selen G, Stjernschantz J, Resul B. Prostaglandin-induced pigmentation in primates. Surv Ophthalmol. 1997;41(Suppl 2):S125–8.

81. Cantor LB. Bimatoprost: a member of a new class of agents, the prostamides, for glaucoma management. Exp Opin Invest Drugs. 2001;10:721–31.

82. Chen J, Krauss AH-P, Gil DW, et al. Pharmacological characterization of AGN 192024 (Lumigan) in ocular and non-ocular preparations and its relation to the prostamides. Invest Ophthalmol Vis Sci Suppl. 2001;42:S832.

83. Woodward DF, Krauss AH-P, Chen J, et al. The pharmacology of bimatoprost (Lumigan). Surv Ophthalmol. 2001;45(Suppl 4):S337–45.

84. Brubaker RF, Schoff EO, Nau CB, et al. Effects of AGN 192024, a new ocular hypotensive agent, on aqueous dynamics. Am J Ophthalmol. 2001;131:19–24.

85. Cantor LB, for the AGN 192024 Study Groups 1 and 2. 6-Month comparison of AGN 192024 once-daily with timolol twice-daily in patients with elevated IOP. Invest Ophthalmol Vis Sci Suppl. 2001;42:S558.

86. Sherwood M, Brandt J. Six-month comparisons of bimatoprost once-daily with timolol twice-daily in patients with elevated intraocular pressure. Surv Ophthalmol 2001;45(Suppl 4):S361–8.

87. Gandolfi S, Simmons ST, Sturm R, et al. Three-month comparison of bimatoprost and latanoprost in patients with glaucoma and ocular hypertension. Adv Ther. 2001;18(3):110-21.

CHAPTER

234

New (Pending) Glaucoma Medical Therapy

WILLIAM C. STEWART

INTRODUCTION

Ophthalmologists are fortunate to witness the introduction in recent years of several new pharmaceutical products to help manage elevated intraocular pressure (IOP). In general, these drugs are new compounds within existing classes of medicines already in use or combinations of currently approved products. The availability of these medicines will improve physicians' choices in the management of glaucoma patients.

For the 21st century, compounds are being evaluated that may influence the physiological function of the optic nerve, through an increase in ocular blood flow or an improvement in nerve cell physiology, without reducing IOP. Even therapeutic alteration of the human genome, the genetic delivery of neuroprotective products, and optic nerve axonal regeneration appear to be more feasible than previously believed.

This chapter reviews IOP-reducing compounds that have recently become available commercially or should be available in the near future. Also, new concepts in therapy that may be used to treat the optic nerve in the future are presented.

LATANOPROST–TIMOLOL MALEATE FIXED COMBINATION

This product is a fixed combination of latanoprost 0.005% and timolol maleate 0.5% (Xalcom, Pharmacia, Peapack, NJ) given once a day. The pharmacology of the fixed combination is essentially related to its individual components.

A multicenter regulatory trial in Germany demonstrated that the fixed combination, compared with timolol maleate given twice daily, reduced IOP an additional 1.9mmHg on average.[1] In contrast, the fixed combination compared with latanoprost alone, dosed every morning, showed a mean improvement of 1.2mmHg[1] (Fig. 234-1). In the United States, a similar trial showed a 2.9mmHg improvement of the fixed combination over timolol maleate 0.5% given twice daily and a 1.1mmHg improvement over latanoprost given alone each evening.[1] In these trials, there were no safety issues related to the fixed combination over and above those associated with the individual components alone.[2]

The fixed combination also has been compared with several adjunctive therapies. Stewart[3] found in a crossover study that evening dosing of the fixed combination provided a statistically greater IOP reduction—approximately 1–2mmHg—at 6–12 hours after dosing (Fig. 234-2). In addition, the fixed combination provided a lower diurnal IOP over the 12-hour daytime curve (measured every 2 hours from 8:00 A.M. to 8:00 P.M.).[3] Further, Feldman[4] showed that the latanoprost-timolol fixed combination, dosed each morning, was more effective by 1mmHg in a three-point diurnal curve than the dorzolamide 2%–timolol maleate 0.005% fixed combination (Cosopt, Pharmacia, Peapack, NJ). Stewart[3] also evaluated morning dosing of the fixed combination versus latanoprost and brimonidine in a crossover comparison. This showed an equal diurnal curve reduction from untreated baseline for both treatments

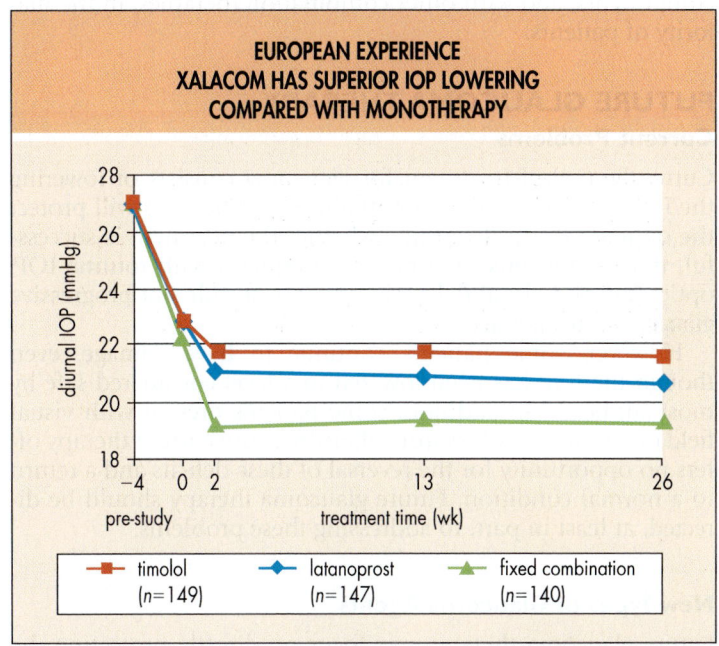

FIG. 234-1 ■ Latanoprost-timolol combination therapy versus monotherapy. Pfeiffer *et al.* showed that latanoprost-timolol fixed combination therapy provided a statistically lower intraocular pressure than either of the individual components over a three-point daytime diurnal evaluation. (From Pfeiffer N. A comparison of the fixed combination of latanoprost and timolol with its individual components. Graefes Arch Clin Exp Ophthalmol. 2002;240(11):893–9.)

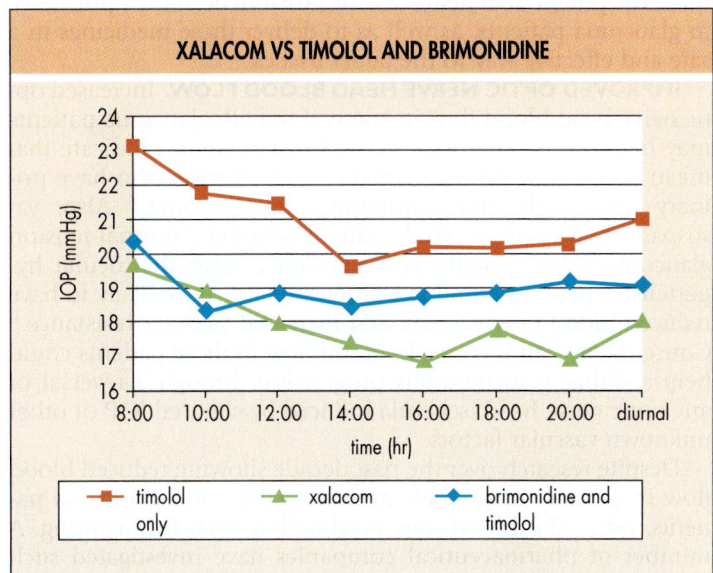

FIG. 234-2 ■ Latanoprost-timolol combination versus brimonidine and timolol. Stewart *et al.* showed that 12 hours after dosing, the latanoprost-timolol fixed combination provided a statistically greater reduction in intraocular pressure than did brimonidine and timolol each given twice daily. (Internal data, Pharmaceutical Research Network, LLC.)

over a three-point daytime diurnal curve (internal data, Pharmaceutical Research Network, LLC).

The 24-hour diurnal effect of the latanoprost-timolol fixed combination was compared with placebo by Larsson *et al.*[5] in 19 patients in a crossover comparison and showed an average reduction of 24% (from 19.4mmHg to 14.7mmHg).[5] However, at 2:00 and 4:00, there was no significant reduction from placebo. Konstas *et al.*[6] followed this study by evaluating latanoprost and timolol, each dosed once daily from separate bottles, and demonstrated that the unfixed combination given once daily provided an additional reduction of 4.1mmHg, including the 2:00 and 6:00 time points Except for a 1.5mmHg greater decrease at 6:00 A.M., evening dosing provided a statistically similar effect to morning dosing.[6]

In summary, the fixed combination appears to provide a safe additional lowering of the IOP compared with its individual components, and with other combination therapies, in the majority of patients.

FUTURE GLAUCOMA THERAPY

Current Problems

Currently, typical treatment for glaucoma consists of lowering the IOP to a level that the ophthalmologist believes will protect the optic nerve. To determine whether the treatment is successful, the patient must be followed long term with routine IOP, optic disc, and visual field examinations to rule out progressive glaucomatous damage.

However, some patients continue to have damage, even though the IOP has been lowered to a level considered safe by most studies.[7–9] In addition, some patients present with visual field or visual acuity loss from glaucoma, and current therapy offers no opportunity for the reversal of these deficits and a return to a normal condition. Future glaucoma therapy should be directed, at least in part, to addressing these problems.

New Types of Glaucoma Agents

Future glaucoma therapy may focus on directly protecting the optic nerve using at least four potential clinical approaches:
- Improved optic nerve head blood flow.
- Neuroprotection.
- Gene therapy.
- Optic nerve regeneration.

Much work needs to be performed in all these areas to determine the potential benefits of direct treatment of the optic nerve in glaucoma patients, as well as to deliver these medicines in a safe and effective way to the target tissues.

IMPROVED OPTIC NERVE HEAD BLOOD FLOW. Increased optic nerve head blood flow in some, if not all, glaucoma patients may help protect the optic nerve. Current studies indicate that mean blood flow velocity is reduced in patients who have primary open-angle and normal-tension glaucoma.[10] Also, vasospasm may occur in certain patients who have normal-tension glaucoma.[10] Additionally, some evidence exists that ocular hypertensive patients who have progressed are more likely to have reduced blood flow velocity and increased vascular resistance.[11] Consequently, an increase in blood flow in these patients could help stabilize glaucomatous progression through a reversal of any optic nerve head ischemia induced by elevated IOP or other unknown vascular factors.

Despite research over the past decade showing reduced blood flow in primary open-angle and normal-tension glaucoma patients, no ocular blood flow product has been forthcoming. A number of pharmaceutical companies have investigated such products, but these projects have been dropped from consideration. A number of problems exist in developing a blood flow product, and these problems could influence the development of other types of new glaucoma medicines, such as those offering neuroprotection.

Theoretical Issues. Unfortunately, despite the evidence that reduced blood flow exists in patients with primary open-angle or normal-tension glaucoma, it is not known if this is a primary or secondary effect. In other words, did the reduced blood flow cause the glaucomatous damage, or is it a secondary effect from the decreased number of axons present, which require less oxygen for survival? Further, the ocular location of any ischemic change has not been described; nor is there any clinical data showing improved visual retention resulting from increased ocular blood flow.

Development Issues. Drug delivery remains a problem for an ocular blood flow agent. It is difficult to dose an ocular drug topically and attain sufficient drug levels in the optic nerve, retina, or choroid to achieve a clinical response. Consequently, systemic delivery would most likely be required to reach the posterior segment of the eye and improve blood flow. Systemically delivered vasoactive medicines, however, most likely would demonstrate cardiovascular side effects. Such events probably would be intolerable for a prophylactic medication given in an essentially symptomless disease.

Several other development issues exist. First, because the anatomical location of reduced blood flow related to the pathogenesis of glaucoma has not been described, any method that demonstrates a clinically important effect cannot be precisely analyzed. Because blood flow instruments are costly and they each generally measure a different location in or behind the eye (e.g., color Doppler measures the retrobulbar blood flow), developing a study to evaluate a blood flow product could be cost prohibitive. Second, the patient population that should be studied to show a clinically important blood flow effect remains unclear (e.g., older primary open-angle glaucoma patients with vascular disease, normal-tension glaucoma patients, or all glaucoma patients). Last, clinical end points for blood flow remain unclear. Regulatory agencies and the pharmaceutical industry must work together to develop new clinical end points, apart from the IOP, that would describe the benefit of a blood flow product.

Cost. Unfortunately, showing the utility of a blood flow product as an end point most likely would require showing visual stability over 3–5 years. Along with the blood flow instrumentation required, this factor would greatly increase the cost of performing multicenter regulatory trials.

NEUROPROTECTION. Because of the difficulties of developing a blood flow treatment, much attention has turned to developing a neuroprotective product that would work directly on the optic nerve to improve its health. Unfortunately, the development of such a product suffers from many of the same problems associated with creating a blood flow compound.

Most early attention has been directed toward either a trophic factor or a glutamate inhibitor. However, the molecular mechanisms by which axons degenerate in glaucoma are not precisely known. Quigley[12] showed in a monkey model that axons degenerate in glaucoma by apoptosis as a final common end pathway. However, the exact trigger and process leading to apoptosis in glaucoma remain undescribed.

The ischemic model of apoptosis is the most descriptive model of this process from the systemic literature.[13] Theoretically, during ischemia, there is a period of axonal dysfunction before death occurs. If therapeutic intervention occurs during dysfunction, the axon could theoretically be rescued and the optic nerve stabilized. In this model, glaucomatous damage is hypothesized to occur from chronic ischemia, as opposed to a cerebrovascular accident, which happens acutely.

Many of the sequential events leading to ischemia-induced apoptosis have been described. It is believed that ischemia causes depolarization of the axon. The associated potassium release into the extracellular space cannot be actively reversed back into the intracellular space because of the disrupted cellular metabolism. The depolarized axon also releases its normal neurotransmitters, glutamate and aspartate, which causes extracellular calcium to be driven into the cell through the *N*-methyl-D-

PROPOSED MECHANISM OF ISCHEMIC INJURY

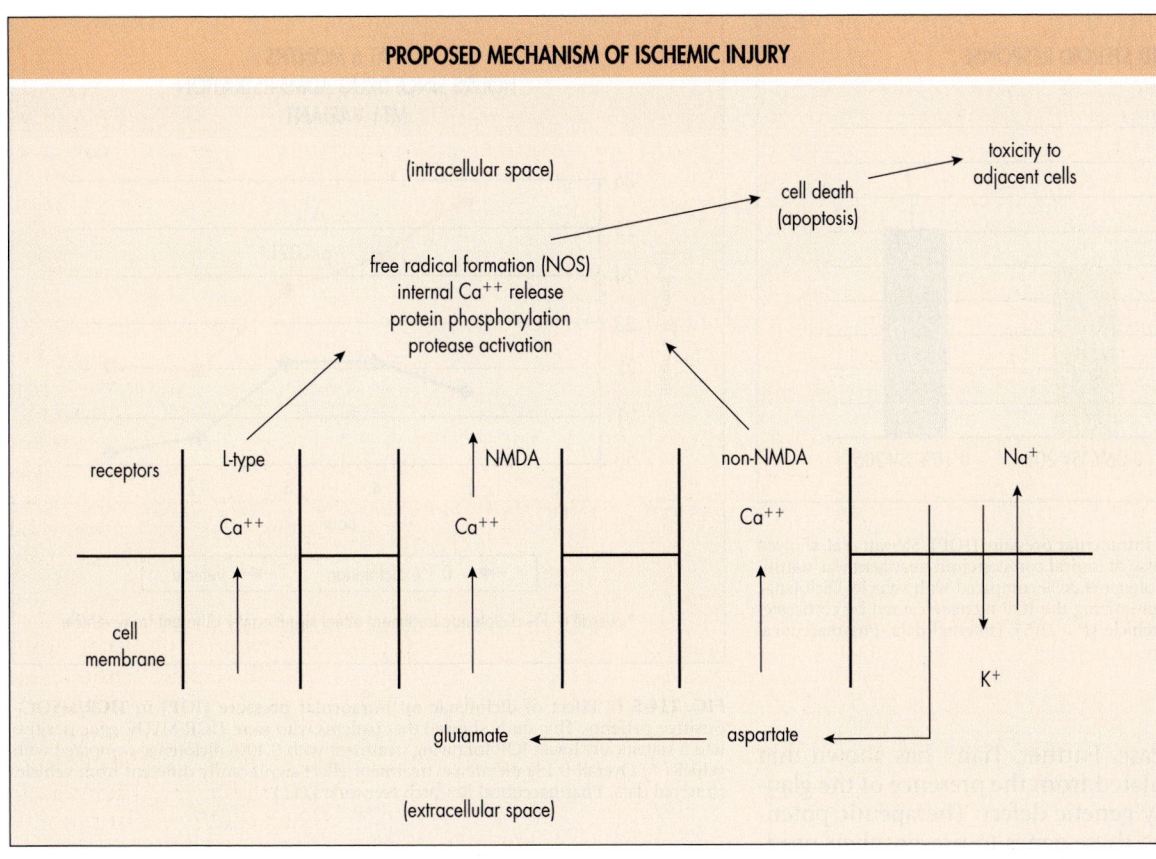

FIG. 234-3 ■ **Theoretical mechanism of ischemic injury in glaucoma.** This is the proposed mechanism of ischemia leading to apoptosis in glaucoma. Ischemia causes axonal depolarization, with potassium and neurotransmitter release from the cell. Extracellular calcium then enters the cell directly through L-type (gated) receptors and through N-methyl-D-aspartate (NMDA) and non-NMDA receptors mediated by glutamate and aspartate, respectively. The increased intracellular calcium leads to protein phosphorylation, production of proteases, free radical formation, nitric oxide synthetase (NOS), and release of intracellular calcium. These events cause disruption of energy-producing mechanisms and cell membranes and induction of the enzymatic processes leading to apoptosis. The neuroprotective agent memantine would theoretically act to inhibit the effect of glutamate.

aspartate (NMDA) and non-NMDA receptors, respectively. In addition, the L-type (gated) calcium channel receptors are opened after the axonal depolarization that allows extracellular calcium directly into the cells.

The increased intracellular calcium leads to protein phosphorylation, production of proteases, free radical formation, and release of intracellular calcium stores. These events cause disruption of energy-producing mechanisms and cell membranes and induction of the enzymatic processes leading to apoptosis (Fig. 234-3).[13]

At least one drug, memantine (Allergan, Irvine, CA) is in clinical development as a neuroprotectant for glaucoma. It has been approved in Germany for the past two decades as an anti-Parkinson's drug (Merz Pharmaceuticals GmbH, Frankfurt, Germany). Following its approval, memantine was shown to have antiglutamate properties that would theoretically help prevent calcium from entering the cell during ischemic stress (see Fig. 234-3). The results of regulatory trials may be available by mid-decade.

Recently, research has described several steps leading to the initiation of apoptosis that could be related directly to elevated IOP. Nitric oxide synthetase type 2 is neurotoxic and is induced from pericytes and astrocytes by high IOP in rats.[14,15] Nitric oxide synthetase is not released from optic nerve head pericytes and astrocytes when the IOP is normal. Further, inhibition of nitric oxide synthetase has been shown to be protective of the optic nerve in rats (see Fig. 234-3).

In addition, caspase enzymes have been shown to be associated with apoptosis in rats that have increased IOP.[16] Further, brain-derived neurotropic factor has been demonstrated to diminish the caspase II enzyme during ischemic stress.[17]

Neuroprotection will be an important future therapy to ensure the stabilization of vision in glaucoma patients. However, much work needs to be performed to describe the exact mechanism of neurodegeneration in glaucoma on a molecular basis, so that a specific neuroprotective therapy for glaucoma can be developed.

GENE THERAPY. Gene therapy could be used in two ways in glaucoma: as a drug delivery system, and as a basis for develop-

ing new therapies and treatment end points based on the genetic mutations that cause glaucoma. Gene therapy could be used as a drug delivery system by encoding external genes (e.g., a viral genome) to the patient's own genome, which would produce protective trophic factors intracellularly. Problems with gene therapy in the eye include delivery of the genome to the target tissue (i.e., optic nerve) and potential carcinogenic effects of the implantation of new genomes inside the cell.[17]

The human genome could also be used as a basis for treatment decisions. InSite Vision (Alameda, CA) recently released a diagnostic kit for primary open-angle glaucoma (Ocugene) based on the TIGR/MYOC mt1 variant in the promoter region of the gene. A recent study found that the TIGR/MYOC–positive gene mutation was associated with more rapid progression in 147 primary open-angle glaucoma patients followed over an average of 15 years (internal data, InSite Vision). Further, Colomb et al.[18] demonstrated in 142 patients a greater prevalence of glaucomatous disc damage and higher IOP in TIGR/MYOC–positive patients. In contrast, Alward et al.[19] found no differences in optic disc, visual field, or IOP findings between TIGR/MYOC–positive and –negative patients among 779 subjects with a variety of glaucomas, ocular hypertensive patients, and normal subjects.

If indeed the TIGR/MYOC gene or separate genes could be shown to be a risk factor for earlier onset or more progressive disease, a patient's therapeutic end points could be modified based on his or her genetic profile. In the future, such a patient may start therapy earlier in life and be maintained at a lower IOP to help prevent glaucomatous progression and visual loss. Consequently, the genetic profile may help individualize patient therapy to better ensure a stable glaucomatous disease course.

In addition, new therapies may be derived from glaucoma-related genes. Proteins or enzymes produced by the abnormal gene could be identified and their deposition or action prevented to stabilize or reverse damage in the outflow system of the eye or the optic nerve.[20] The abnormal gene could potentially be turned off, as a separate mechanism, to help prevent abnormal protein or enzyme production. Ultimately, investigation into correcting the abnormal gene itself might provide a more

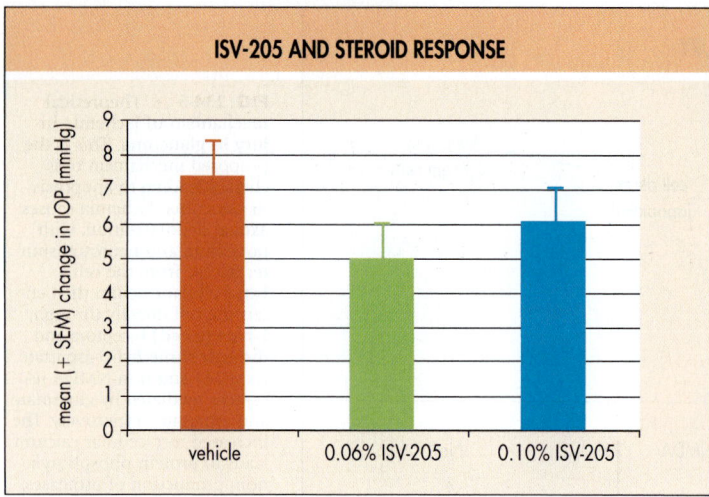

FIG. 234-4 ■ **Effect of diclofenac on intraocular pressure (IOP).** Stewart *et al.* showed that the highest IOP over a 6-week course of topical corticosteroid treatment was statistically minimized in patients given diclofenac 0.06% compared with vehicle. Diclofenac 0.10% also showed a trend toward minimizing the IOP increase caused by corticosteroids. *, Significantly different from vehicle ($P > .015$). (Internal data, Pharmaceutical Research Network, LLC.)

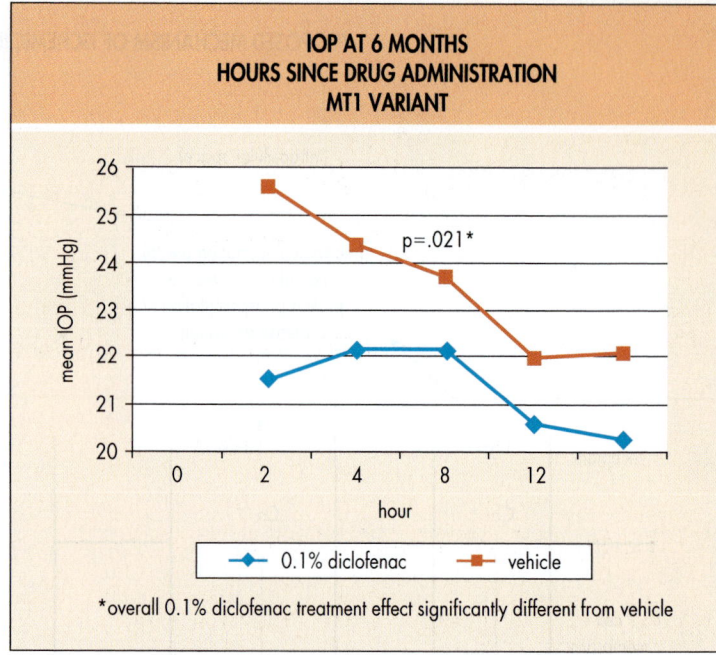

FIG. 234-5 ■ **Effect of diclofenac on intraocular pressure (IOP) in TIGR/MYOC–positive patients.** This study showed that patients who were TIGR/MYOC gene positive had a statistically lower IOP following treatment with 0.10% diclofenac compared with vehicle. *, Overall 0.1% diclofenac treatment effect significantly different from vehicle. (Internal data, Pharmaceutical Research Network, LLC.)

permanent cure to the disease. Further, Tian[21] has shown that several genes can be up-regulated from the presence of the glaucoma itself, unrelated to any genetic defect. Therapeutic potential exists in down-regulating these genes to prevent their products from being deposited in the trabecular meshwork.

InSite Vision recently evaluated diclofenac in a formulation designed to achieve higher aqueous levels than those obtained by the currently available commercial product. The study evaluated whether diclofenac could blunt the ocular hypertensive response from a topical corticosteroid in first-degree relatives of patients with primary open-angle glaucoma. Patients had their highest ocular hypertensive response to topical corticosteroid minimized statistically by diclofenac (0.06%, 4.9mmHg; 0.10%, 5.4mmHg; vehicle, 7.2mmHg)[20] (Fig. 234-4). TIGR/MYOC gene regulation had previously been linked to corticosteroids.[22] Further, in a study performed on patients with ocular hypertension or primary open-angle glaucoma, patients who were TIGR/MYOC gene positive and were treated with 0.10% diclofenac had lower IOPs (1.3–3.4mmHg) than those treated with placebo over the 12-hour daytime diurnal curve (internal data, InSite Vision) (Fig. 234-5). Future research may provide useful clinical drugs that will help treat glaucoma on a genetic basis.

OPTIC NERVE REGENERATION. Little work has been performed specifically with regard to optic nerve regeneration. Unlike the more sophisticated mammals, lower life-forms such as goldfish are able to regenerate their optic nerves. Uncovering the secrets in these lower life-forms may help develop a therapy to allow optic nerve regeneration in humans.[23,24]

REFERENCES

1. Pfeiffer N. A comparison of the fixed combination of latanoprost and timolol with its individual components. Graefes Arch Clin Exp Ophthalmol. 2002;240(11):893–99.
2. Higginbotham EJ, Feldman R, Stiles M, Dubiner H. Latanoprost and timolol combination therapy vs monotherapy: one-year randomized trial. Arch Ophthalmol. 2002;120(7):915–22.
3. Stewart JA, Day DG, Sharpe ED, Stewart WC. Efficacy and safety of latanoprost/timolol maleate fixed combination versus timolol maleate and brimonidine given twice daily. Invest Ophthalmol Vis Sci. 2002;43:E-Abstract 3430.
4. Feldman RM. A comparison of fixed combination of latanoprost and timolol with fixed combination of dorzolamide and timolol (COSOPT) in patients with elevated intraocular pressure: a three-month masked evaluator, phase IIIb, multicenter study in the United States (XALCOM vs. COSOPT). Invest Ophthalmol Vis Sci. 2002;43:E-Abstract 295.
5. Larsson LI, Mishima HK, Takamatsu M, et al. The effect of latanoprost on circadian intraocular pressure. Surv Ophthalmol. 2002;47(Suppl 1):S90–6.
6. Konstas AG, Nakos E, Tersis I, et al. A comparison of once-daily morning vs evening dosing of concomitant latanoprost/timolol. Am J Ophthalmol. 2002;133(6):753–7.
7. Mao LK, Stewart WC, Shields MB. Correlation between intraocular pressure control and progressive glaucomatous damage in primary open-angle glaucoma. Am J Ophthalmol. 1991;111:51–5.
8. Stewart WC, Chorak RP, Hunt HH, Sethuraman G. Factors associated with visual loss in patients with advanced glaucomatous changes in the optic nerve head. Am J Ophthalmol. 1993;116:176–81.
9. Stewart WC, Kolker AE, Sharpe ED, et al. Factors associated with long-term progression or stability in primary open-angle glaucoma. Am J Ophthalmol. 2000;130:274–9.
10. Stewart WC. Where are all the ocular blood flow medications? Rev Ophthalmol. 1998 May;137–40.
11. Hamzavi S, Stewart WC, Hamzavi SL, Stroman GL. Transcranial Doppler in progressed and stable ocular hypertensive patients. Invest Ophthalmol Vis Sci. 1996;37:S31.
12. Quigley HA, Nickells RW, Kerrigan LA, et al. Retinal ganglion cell death in experimental glaucoma and after axotomy occurs by apoptosis. Invest Ophthalmol Vis Sci. 1995;36:774–86.
13. Hickenbottom SL, Grotta J. Neuroprotective therapy. Semin Neurol. 1998;18:485–92.
14. Shareef S, Sawada A, Neufeld AH. Isoforms of nitric oxide synthase in the optic nerves of rat eyes with chronic moderately elevated intraocular pressure. Invest Ophthalmol Vis Sci. 1999;40:2884–91.
15. Liu B, Neufeld AH. Nitric oxide synthase-2 in human optic nerve head astrocytes induced by elevated pressure in vitro. Arch Ophthalmol. 2001;119:240–5.
16. Kurokawa T, Arai J, Katai N, et al. Expression of Caspase-9 in rat retinal ganglion cell layer neurons after transient ischemia. Invest Ophthalmol Vis Sci. 2000;41:S17.
17. Hegazy KA, Dunn MW, Sarma SC. Functional human heme oxygenase has a neuroprotective effect on adult rat ganglion cells after pressure-induced ischemia. Neuroreport. 2000;11:1185–9.
18. Colomb E, Nguyen TD, Bechetoille A, et al. Association of a single nucleotide polymorphism in the TIGR/MYOCCILIN gene promoter with the severity of primary open-angle glaucoma. Clin Genet. 2001;60(3):220–5.
19. Alward WLM, Kwon YH, Khanna CL, et al. Variations in the myocilin gene in patients with open-angle glaucoma. Arch Ophthalmol. 2002;120:1189–97.
20. Stewart WC, Walters TR, Day DG, et al. Effects of ISV-205 (diclofenac in DuraSite) on corticosteroid-induced IOP response in glaucoma relatives. Invest Ophthalmol Vis Sci. 2000;41:S51.
21. Tian B, Geiger B, Epstein DL, Kaufman PL. Cytoskeletal involvement in the regulation of aqueous humor outflow. Invest Ophthalmol Vis Sci. 2000;41:619–23.
22. Polansky JR, Fauss DJ, Zimmerman CC. Regulation of TIGR/MYOC gene expression in human trabecular meshwork cells. Eye. 2000;14(Pt 3B):503–14.
23. Sivron T, Schwab ME, Schwartz M. Presence of growth inhibitors in fish optic nerve myelin: post injury changes. J Comp Neurol. 1994;343:237–46.
24. Cohen I, Sivron T, Lavie V, et al. Vimentin immunoreactive glial cells in the fish optic nerve: implications for regeneration. Glia. 1994;10:16–29.

CHAPTER
235
Argon Laser Trabeculoplasty and Peripheral Iridectomy

IOANNIS M. ASLANIDES • L. JAY KATZ

ARGON LASER TRABECULOPLASTY

INTRODUCTION AND HISTORICAL REVIEW

Argon laser trabeculoplasty (ALT) is an established, well-tolerated procedure used to lower intraocular pressure (IOP) in various types of open-angle glaucoma.[1] (Laser treatment of the human trabecular meshwork by puncturing Schlemm's canal was performed initially by Krasnov in 1973, but the lower IOP he described was short-lived.[1]) In 1979, Wise and Witter[2] reported that the placement of small, evenly spaced, nonpenetrating argon laser spots consistently lowered IOP in phakic eyes that have open-angle glaucoma.

PREOPERATIVE EVALUATION AND DIAGNOSTIC APPROACH

Positive and negative predictors for ALT success include diagnosis, pigmentation of the trabecular meshwork, age, and angle configuration (Table 235-1). For patients younger than 50 years of age, ALT is not recommended unless they have pigmentary or pseudoexfoliation glaucoma. With optimal patient selection, after ALT, IOP typically drops 25–30% below the initial IOP. However, whether ALT yields the same success rate in African Americans as in Caucasians is controversial.[3]

GENERAL TECHNIQUES

Patient Preparation

If the angle is closed or narrow, a laser iridoplasty or a peripheral iridectomy is performed beforehand to deepen and allow better visualization of the angle; a laser iridoplasty is often performed simultaneously with ALT, but when a peripheral iridectomy is performed, ALT is done a week later because of possible anterior chamber debris. The patient's informed consent must be sought after a thorough discussion of the goal of therapy and potential complications.

A drop of apraclonidine 0.5% or brimonidine 0.2% is instilled in the eye 30–60 minutes preoperatively to minimize IOP elevation after treatment. Proparacaine 0.5% drops are instilled immediately before the procedure.

Lens Choice

A Ritch[4] or, more commonly, a three-mirror Goldmann lens with antireflective coating is used. It features a dome-shaped mirror angled at 59° to visualize the angle. The lens does not invert the image but reverses the position, such that the 12 o'clock position of the mirror represents the 6 o'clock position at the angle, the 1 o'clock position of the mirror represents the 5 o'clock position at the angle, and so forth. (Methylcellulose is used as a coupling agent between the cornea and the lens.)

TABLE 235-I

POSITIVE AND NEGATIVE PREDICTORS OF ARGON LASER TRABECULOPLASTY SUCCESS

	Negative Predictors	Positive Predictors
Age (years)	<40	>65
Trabecular meshwork pigmentation	Little or none	Moderate to marked
Corneal clarity	Poor	Clear
Disease entities	Uveitic glaucoma	Pigmentary glaucoma
	Angle closure	Pseudoexfoliative glaucoma
	Juvenile glaucoma	Primary open-angle glaucoma
	Angle recession	Low-tension glaucoma
Lens status	Aphakic or anterior chamber intraocular pseudophakia	Phakic or posterior chamber intraocular pseudophakia
Contralateral eye	Little effect	Strong effect

Equipment Preparation

The physician checks the laser settings and surveys the angle structures again. (The trabecular meshwork always lies between two white lines [Schwalbe's line and the scleral spur]. However, the trabecular meshwork may occasionally be variably pigmented, and a pigmented Schwalbe's line or a ciliary body band may be confused with the trabecular meshwork.)

The procedure begins with the goniolens at the 12 o'clock position (inferior angle), and the lens is rotated clockwise; the temporal portion of the right eye and the nasal portion of the left eye are photocoagulated first. To ensure delivery of laser energy with maximal efficiency, the aiming beam is always kept in the center of the mirror, round and sharp, keeping the goniolens perpendicular to the laser beam; also, it is rotated after several applications.

Treatment Guidelines

The laser spots are placed at the junction of the pigmented and nonpigmented trabecular meshwork, with a gap of about the diameter of two laser spots between spots (Fig. 235-1, A). The authors currently treat 360° of the angle in one session (20–25 spots per quadrant). Commonly used parameters are a 50μm spot size, 0.1sec duration, and 200–800mW of power. Settings should be adjusted according to the tissue reaction end point, which is minimal blanching (see Fig. 235-1, B). If the burn is too anterior, the treatment is more likely to be ineffective; if it is too posterior, it is more likely to create inflammation and peripheral anterior synechiae.

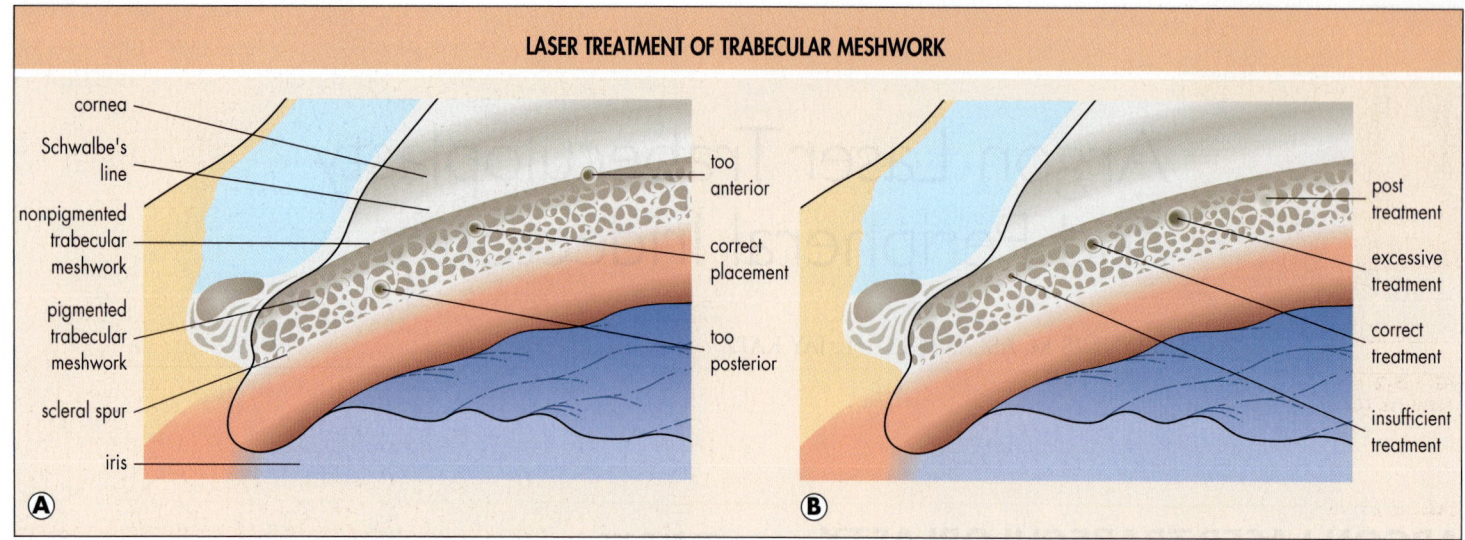

LASER TREATMENT OF TRABECULAR MESHWORK

FIG. 235-1 ■ Laser treatment of trabecular meshwork. **A,** Optimal laser beam placement on the trabecular meshwork. (With permission from Schwartz AL, *et al.* J Glaucoma. 1993;2:329.) **B,** Trabecular meshwork tissue end point reaction to different intensities of argon laser treatment. (Reproduced with permission from Schwartz AL, *et al.* Ophthalmology. 1987;88:203.)

Wavelength

Argon green laser appears to be effective and is less likely to cause photoreceptor injury to the treating physician than is argon blue-green laser. Diode laser has been used with comparable results, but the tissue reaction is less pronounced, making it harder to judge the end point.

Follow-up

The IOP is measured 1 hour after ALT. If it is elevated, an additional antiglaucoma medication (aqueous suppressant, miotic, or oral hyperosmotic)—one that is not used chronically—is administered. The IOP spike is rechecked to ensure that it has been controlled. Topical prednisolone 1% four times daily is prescribed for 7 days, and the patient is reviewed after 1 week. If anterior uveitis is present at 1 week, topical corticosteroids are continued.

Retreatment

The chance of success with a repeat procedure is considerably less than with an initial procedure, and the overall effect seems to wane considerably with time.

COMPLICATIONS

In one study, approximately 3% of patients (10 of 300 eyes) affected by primary open-angle glaucoma sustained a persistent elevation of at least 5mmHg after ALT, which did not return to normal prior to surgical intervention.[5, 6] Corneal burns, which occur rarely, typically heal within a few days. If active bleeding from the angle is noted during treatment, the goniolens is pressed against the cornea to increase IOP and provide hemostasis. If the bleeding vessel is visualized, the laser is applied directly, using a large spot size (100–200μm). The most common risk is IOP spikes, but these may be limited effectively using apraclonidine or brimonidine.[7] Finally, encapsulated blebs after filtration surgery may be seen more frequently in eyes that have had ALT.

OUTCOME

A period of at least 4–6 weeks after ALT is required before the final result can be evaluated. In two long-term studies, ALT maintained IOP control in 67–80% of eyes for 1 year, in 35–50% for 5 years, and in 5–30% for 10 years (i.e., an attrition rate of 6–10% per year).[8, 9]

The Glaucoma Laser Trial

The Glaucoma Laser Trial, a multicenter, randomized clinical trial, was designed to assess the efficacy and safety of initial treatment for primary open-angle glaucoma using ALT versus standard topical medication. The Glaucoma Laser Trial authors concluded that initial ALT is at least as efficacious as initial treatment with topical medication.[10]

SELECTIVE LASER TRABECULOPLASTY

Because ALT is limited by a well-recognized loss of efficacy with time and a poor response to repeat application, another laser system was developed in 1998 by Latina *et al.*[11] This laser is a frequency-doubled neodymium:yttrium-aluminum-garnet (Nd:YAG) nonthermal laser that selectively targets only pigmented cells, without causing any apparent damage to the surrounding structures; in contrast, the argon laser results in thermal coagulation of angle structures (Fig. 235-2).[12]

TREATMENT GUIDELINES

The selective laser has a relatively large 400μm fixed spot size. The energy is adjusted from 0.8mJ downward, depending on the tissue response. Ideally, blanching without bubble creation is the end point. The number of shots applied is about 25–50 over 180°, with 180–360° treated initially. The spots are almost confluent and span the entire angle width because of the large spot size (Fig. 235-3). Pre- and postoperative care is similar to that of ALT.

EFFICACY

The effect of SLT on IOP reduction is similar to that seen with ALT[13] (Table 235-2). The prospect of repeating treatment safely with additional IOP reduction offers great promise. Clinical validation of these issues in prospective clinical trials is under way.

PERIPHERAL IRIDECTOMY

INTRODUCTION AND HISTORICAL REVIEW

Von Graefe[14] introduced surgical iridectomy for glaucoma in 1857. In 1920, Curran recognized that iridectomy was effective for angle-closure but not for open-angle glaucoma.[13] In 1956, Meyer-

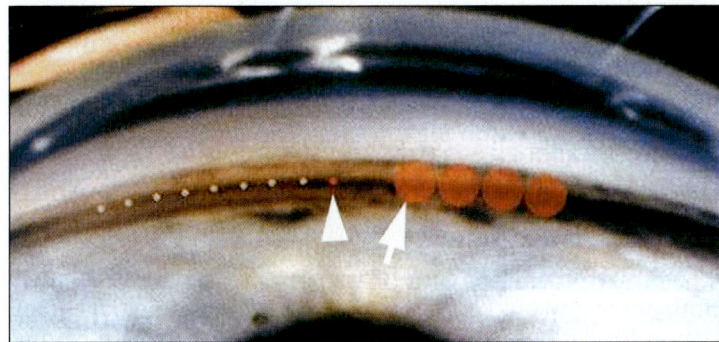

FIG. 235-2 ■ Selective laser trabeculoplasty versus argon laser trabeculoplasty treatment. (Courtesy of M. Berlin, MD.)

TABLE 235-2

SELECTIVE LASER TRABECULOPLASTY (SLT) VERSUS ARGON LASER TRABECULOPLASTY (ALT): A PROSPECTIVE, RANDOMIZED CLINICAL TRIAL

Mean IOP (mmHg)	ALT	SLT
Baseline	22.5	22.8
1 month	19.5	20.1
6 months	17.7	17.8

(From Damji KF, Shah KC, Rock WJ, *et al.* Selective laser trabeculoplasty argon laser trabeculoplasty: a prospective randomised clinical trial. Br J Ophthalmol. 1999; 83:718–22.)
IOP, Intraocular pressure.

Schwickerath[15] demonstrated that an iridectomy could be created without the need for an incision, using xenon arc photocoagulation. This method failed to gain popularity, however, because of frequent lens and corneal opacities. Argon laser iridectomy and, more recently, Nd:YAG laser iridectomy have essentially replaced surgical iridectomy in the vast majority of cases.

PREOPERATIVE EVALUATION AND DIAGNOSTIC APPROACH

Laser iridectomy is the established procedure of choice for angle-closure glaucoma associated with pupillary block, whether primary or secondary or acute, intermittent, or chronic.

Indications

Laser iridectomy is indicated for the following types of glaucoma:
- Acute angle-closure.
- Chronic (creeping) angle-closure.
- Phacomorphic with an element of pupillary block.
- Iris bombé.
- Pigmentary dispersion syndrome (laser iridectomy for this indication remains controversial; the procedure changes the anatomy of the iris posterior bowing, but the long-term clinical advantage remains unproved).
- Prophylaxis of occludable angle (indicated for high-risk patients who are young, have a positive family history of angle closure, or need frequent dilated examinations, such as those with diabetes).

Laser iridectomy also aids in the diagnosis of aqueous misdirection (see Chapter 229) and plateau iris syndrome (in a non-pupillary-block narrow angle). In the former, a patent iridectomy is often needed before a diagnosis can be established.

Contraindications

Laser iridectomy is contraindicated in patients who are unable to sit and cooperate at the slit lamp and in eyes that have a

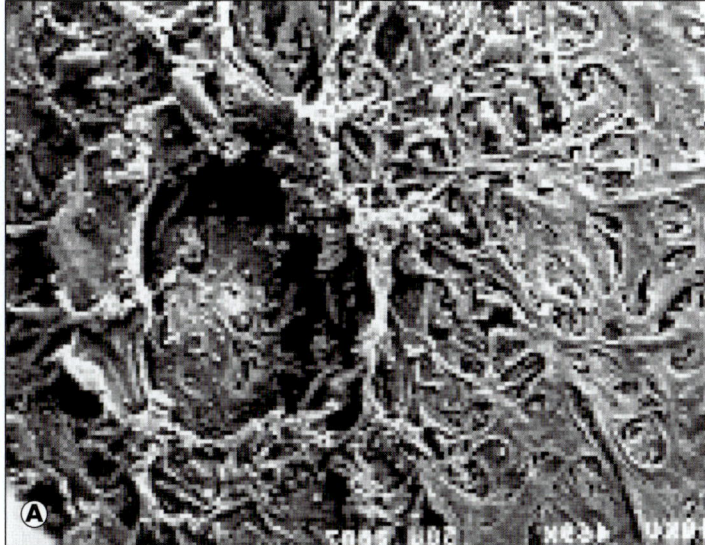

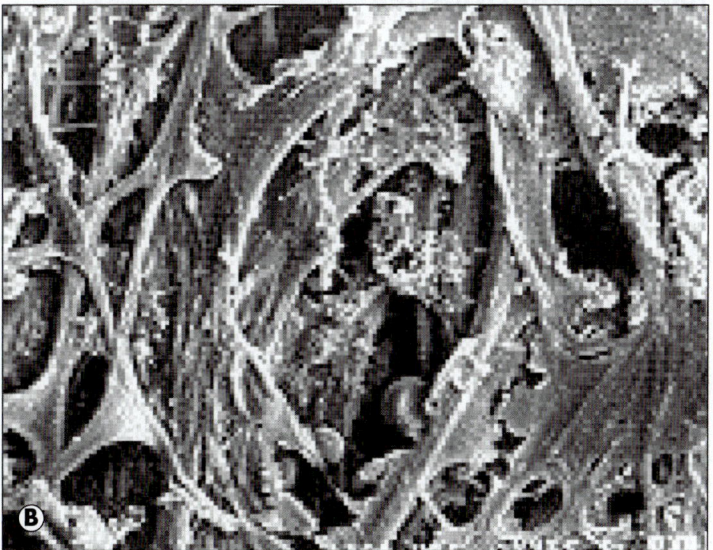

FIG. 235-3 ■ Human trabecular meshwork (organ system). **A,** Argon laser trabeculoplasty, 50μm spot. **B,** Selective laser trabeculoplasty, 400μm spot, 0.8mJ/pulse.

cloudy cornea, widely dilated pupil, and flat anterior chamber with iridocorneal touch.

GENERAL TECHNIQUES

Argon versus Nd:YAG Laser

Both lasers are effective for the creation of iridectomies. The argon laser requires uptake of light energy by the pigment (thermal effect), but the Nd:YAG laser does not and works well on all iris colors (photodisruptive effect). The authors prefer the Nd:YAG because it is quicker, requires less energy to create a patent peripheral iridectomy, and is associated with fewer late closures than the argon laser is.[16,17]

The Nd:YAG laser, however, does not coagulate tissue, and small hemorrhages occur more frequently with this modality. Therefore, in eyes that have prominent unavoidable vessels or in patients affected by a bleeding diathesis, combined treatment is preferred, first with the argon laser (to ablate vessels in the area) and then with the Nd:YAG laser (to establish a patent peripheral iridectomy).

Patient Preparation

Once the patient's informed consent has been obtained, a drop of pilocarpine 1% is instilled twice, 5 minutes apart; miosis helps to stretch and thin the iris. A drop of apraclonidine 0.5% or brimonidine 0.2% is used 30 minutes preoperatively to prevent a postoperative IOP elevation. (Proparacaine 0.5% drops are instilled immediately before the procedure, in both the treated eye and the contralateral eye, to reduce blinking, which may disrupt treatment.)

Lens Choice

Two special therapeutic contact lenses limit eye movements and blinking, concentrate the energy delivered, magnify the target site, and act as a heat sink to minimize the risk of superficial corneal epithelial burns. The Abraham lens has a 66D planoconvex button. The Wise lens has a 103D planoconvex button,[18] which concentrates the laser energy more than the Abraham lens does because it minimizes the spot and magnifies the target even more; however, because of the higher power of the Wise lens, it is more difficult to focus. The other advantage of the Abraham lens is that energy delivered to both cornea and retina is four times less than that delivered to these tissues by the Wise lens.

SPECIFIC TECHNIQUES

The iridectomy is placed in the peripheral iris under the upper eyelid to avoid ghost images that may arise through the iris hole. Such ghost images may be accentuated by the tear meniscus. The 12 o'clock position is avoided when the argon laser is used, since bubble formation hinders further visualization of the target area. Iris crypts represent thinner iris segments and, as such, are penetrated more easily. The superonasal position (at 11 and 1 o'clock) is the best position to use to prevent inadvertent irradiation of the fovea, because it directs the laser beam farthest from the macula.

Argon Laser

Long pulses (0.2sec) are used for light-colored irides (blue, hazel, light brown), and short pulses (0.02–0.05sec) are used for dark brown irides. The rest of the treatment parameters are the same for both long and short pulses: a power of 1000mW and a spot size of 50µm (Table 235-3).

A single area is treated with superimposed applications until perforation is obtained—that is, when a pigment flume is found to move forward ("smoke sign") or, preferably, when the lens capsule is visualized through the patent iridectomy.

Nd:YAG Laser

The Q-switched mode is used, which allows treatment independent of pigmentation. Iris blood vessels are avoided. The iridectomy spot may be placed anywhere between the 11 and 1 o'clock positions, since bubble formation is minimal. The red laser aim-

ing beam is brought to a focus when the multiple beams are brought into a single spot, aimed through the center of the contact lens. In a thick iris, the red beams may be separated slightly if the focus is advanced forward toward the iris stroma to maximize the energy within the thick iris. The energy used is 3–8mJ, there are 1–3 pulses per shot, and one or more shots are used as required for penetration (see Table 235-3).

Combined Technique

Both argon and Nd:YAG lasers can be used in sequential combination for dark brown irides or for patients who are on chronic anticoagulant therapy. First, the argon laser (short-pulse mode) is used to attenuate the iris to about one fourth the original thickness and to coagulate vessels in the area. Then the Nd:YAG laser is used, with the beam focused at the center of the crater; one or more bursts of 1–3 pulses at 3–6mJ are used to complete the iridectomy.

Second Iridectomy

One patent iridectomy is almost always sufficient to relieve pupillary block. In rare instances in which the long-term patency of the opening is uncertain or in the presence of inflammatory (uveitic) pupillary block, a second iridectomy may be made at the same sitting.

COMPLICATIONS

Intraocular Pressure Spikes

Elevated IOP occurs in approximately one third of eyes after treatment with either laser,[19] but the use of apraclonidine 0.5% or brimonidine 0.2% significantly decreases this risk, except for people who are already on chronic apraclonidine treatment. In a double-masked study of apraclonidine versus placebo, an IOP spike of 10mmHg (1.3kPa) or greater occurred in 43% of placebo-treated eyes but in none of the eyes treated with apraclonidine.[20]

Laser-Induced Inflammation

Laser-treated eyes may suffer transient iritis because of breakdown of the aqueous-blood barrier. Occasionally, inflammation may be quite severe, and posterior synechiae may develop. Prednisolone drops four times daily for 4–7 days may be used postoperatively.

Iridectomy Failure

An iridectomy may fail because the opening created is too small or because perforation is not achieved, with a residual iris pig-

TABLE 235-3

PROTOCOLS FOR LASER TREATMENTS

| | Argon Laser Trabeculoplasty | Peripheral Iridectomy | | | Argon Laser Iridoplasty |
| | | Argon | | Yttrium–Aluminum–Garnet (YAG) | |
		Light Irides	Dark Irides		
Spot size (µm)	50	50	50	Fixed	200–500
Spot duration (sec)	0.1	0.2	0.02–0.05	Fixed (nsec)	0.2–0.5
Power (mW)	200–800	1000	1000	3–8mJ	200–400
Number of spots per quadrant	20–25	15–25	25–100	1–5 shots (each burst consists of 1–3 pulses)	4–10
Wavelength	Argon green	Argon green	Argon green	1064nm	Argon green
Contact lens	Goldmann	Abraham	Wise	Abraham, Wise, or Lasag CGI	Goldmann
Anesthetic	Topical	Topical	Topical	Topical	Topical
Pretreat	Apraclonidine or brimonidine	Pilocarpine and apraclonidine or brimonidine	Pilocarpine and apraclonidine or brimonidine	Pilocarpine and apraclonidine or brimonidine	Pilocarpine

mented layer present. Theoretically, functional failure can be avoided with a peripheral iridectomy diameter of at least 50μm; an iridectomy with a diameter of 100–200μm is ideal.[21]

Diplopia

Diplopia, or "ghost images," is an occasional complaint, especially when the peripheral iridectomy is placed in the horizontal meridians or it is not covered perfectly by the upper eyelid. In some patients, diplopia (alleviated when the lid is lifted away from the eye) may result despite an iridectomy that is well covered by the upper eyelid. This probably results from a prism effect created by the tear meniscus or the upper eyelid. Intolerable monocular diplopia may be resolved by placing a cosmetic contact lens, which blocks the light from the peripheral iridectomy but not the pupil.

Bleeding

Postlaser hyphema is not uncommon after use of the Nd:YAG laser and is generally minimal and self-limited. Brisk bleeding may be stopped by applying direct pressure to the cornea using the contact lens to tamponade the bleeding site temporarily.

Lens Opacities

The lens rarely may be damaged directly from laser irradiation or indirectly because of deficient nourishment of the lens. The latter happens when the aqueous takes a short-cut through the iridectomy and therefore has reduced contact with the lens capsule. Opacities that are directly laser induced tend to remain focal in the area of the peripheral iridectomy, away from the visual axis.

Corneal Injury

Focal laser damage to the epithelium, Descemet's membrane, or endothelium occurs frequently but is usually transient. A shallow anterior chamber, preexisting corneal edema, or pathological conditions of the cornea (e.g., guttae) make corneal injury more likely.

Other Complications

Postlaser malignant glaucoma, retinal burns, and lens-induced uveitis are extremely rare but reported complications.

OUTCOME

The patient is ambulatory immediately without restrictions; prednisolone four times daily for 4–7 days and the discontinuation of miotics are recommended. Patients are seen at 1 hour, 1 week, and 4 weeks after the procedure. Corneal status, IOP, anterior chamber reaction, and patency of the iridectomy with direct visualization and transillumination are assessed at each visit. Gonioscopy is critical to determine whether the angle has deepened.

If the peripheral iridectomy remains patent after 4–6 weeks, the opening usually remains open unless an active inflammatory response (e.g., uveitis, neovascularization) is present.

LASER IRIDOPLASTY

Laser iridoplasty consists of the placement of a circumferential ring of nonpenetrating contraction burns at the far iris periphery, just inside the limbus, to contract the stroma and widen the angle.[22] Laser iridoplasty is performed by the application of evenly spaced (4–10 burns per quadrant), large (200–500μm), long (0.2–0.5sec), and low-powered (200–400mW) burns at the far iris periphery through the central button of a goniolens (see Table 235-3).

Laser iridoplasty does not require a clear cornea for the placement of the spots, because the energy is relatively defocused anyway. Laser iridoplasty is indicated in cases of pre-ALT of narrow angle (to increase visibility of the angle anatomy), angle closure that is unresponsive to medical treatment and for which peripheral iridectomy cannot be performed because of corneal clouding, and plateau iris syndrome.

REFERENCES

1. Katz LJ. Argon laser trabeculoplasty. Annu Ophthalmic Laser Surg. 1992;1:103–10.
2. Wise JB, Witter SL. Argon laser therapy for open angle glaucoma. Arch Ophthalmol. 1979;97:319–22.
3. Bournias TE, Wang F, Javitt JC. Racial variation in outcomes of argon laser trabeculoplasty [abstract]. Invest Ophthalmol Vis Sci. 1997;38(Suppl).
4. Ritch R, Shields MB, Krupin T, eds. The glaucomas. St Louis: Mosby; 1996; 1564–8.
5. Schwartz AL, et al. J Glaucoma. 1993;2:329.
6. Schwartz AL, et al. Ophthalmology. 1987;88:203.
7. Barnes SD, Barnes JD, Dirks MS, et al. Comparison of brimonidine 0.2% to apraclonidine 1% for control of intraocular pressure spikes after argon laser trabeculoplasty [abstract]. Invest Ophthalmol Vis Sci. 1997;38(Suppl).
8. Shingleton BJ, Richter CU, Belcher CD, et al. Long-term efficacy of argon laser trabeculoplasty. Ophthalmology. 1987;94:1513–8.
9. Spaeth GL, Baez KA. Argon laser trabeculoplasty controls one third of progressive, uncontrolled, open angle glaucoma for 5 years. Arch Ophthalmol. 1992;110: 491–4.
10. Glaucoma Laser Trial Research Group. The Glaucoma Laser Trial (GLT) and Glaucoma Laser Trial Follow-up Study: 7. Results. Am J Ophthalmol. 1995;120: 718–31.
11. Latina MA, Sibayan SA, Shin DH, et al. Q-switched 532-nm Nd:YAG laser trabeculoplasty (selective laser trabeculoplasty). Ophthalmology. 1998;105:2082–90.
12. Kramer TR, Noecker RJ. Comparison of the morphologic changes after selective laser trabeculoplasty and argon laser trabeculoplasty in human eye bank eyes. Ophthalmology. 2001;108:773–9.
13. Damji KF, Shah KC, Rock WJ, et al. Selective laser trabeculoplasty v argon laser trabeculoplasty: a prospective randomised clinical trial. Br J Ophthalmol. 1999;83:718–22.
14. Von Graefe A. Uber die Iridectomie bei Glaucom und uber den glaucomatosen Process. Graefes Arch Clin Exp Ophthalmol. 1857;3(2):456–555.
15. Meyer-Schwickerath G. Erfahrungen mit der Lichtkoagulation der Netzhaut und der Iris. Doc Ophthalmol. 1956;10:91–131.
16. Del Priore LV, Robin AL, Pollack IP. Neodymium:YAG and argon laser iridotomy: long term follow-up in a prospective randomized clinical trial. Ophthalmology. 1988;95:1207–11.
17. Moster MR, Schwartz LW, Spaeth GL, et al. Laser iridectomy: a controlled study comparing argon and neodymium:YAG. Ophthalmology. 1986;93:20–4.
18. Wise JB, Munnerlyn CR, Erickson PJ. A high-efficiency laser iridotomy-sphincterotomy lens. Am J Ophthalmol. 1986;101:546–53.
19. Robin AL, Pollack IP. A comparison of neodymium:YAG and argon laser iridotomies. Ophthalmology. 1984;91:1011–6.
20. Robin AL, Pollack IP, deFaller JM. Effects of topical Alo 2145 (p-aminoclonidine hydrochloride) on the acute intraocular pressure rise after argon laser iridotomy. Arch Ophthalmol. 1987;105:1208–11.
21. Fleck BW. How large must an iridotomy be? Br J Ophthalmol. 1990;74:583–8.
22. York K, Ritch R, Szmyd LJ. Argon laser peripheral iridoplasty indications, techniques and results [abstract]. Invest Ophthalmol Vis Sci. 1984;25(Suppl).

236 Laser Filtration Procedures

MARTHA MOTUZ LEEN

INTRODUCTION

Laser energy can be delivered either internally (*ab interno*) or externally (*ab externo*) to produce a direct opening into the anterior chamber through limbal tissue to achieve filtration. The laser energy may be delivered using a probe (contact) or a gonioscopy lens (noncontact). The rationale for laser sclerostomies is the desire for a glaucoma filtration procedure that is simple, quick, limits the wound-healing response, and minimizes complications.

By using laser energy to disrupt limbal tissue, full-thickness sclerostomies have been created via an ab interno or ab externo approach (Figs. 236-1 to 236-3). Methods for application of laser energy to facilitate dissection in nonpenetrating glaucoma surgery are under development.[1] Currently, most available clinical data are for the contact methods used to create full-thickness sclerostomies—the holmium laser for the ab externo approach[2–5] and the neodymium:yttrium-aluminum-garnet (Nd:YAG) laser for the ab interno approach.[6] These two procedures have emerged as prototypes for laser sclerostomy, and discussion herein is limited to these.

PREOPERATIVE EVALUATION AND DIAGNOSTIC APPROACH

The holmium ab externo sclerostomy is generally most suitable for the creation of blebs in eyes that have heavy conjunctival scarring, as this may severely limit the location of a repeated trabeculectomy but allow the passage of a laser probe. The ideal site for this procedure is over a prior surgical iridectomy, to decrease the risk of postoperative iris incarceration. This technique may offer an advantage over the Nd:YAG ab interno approach in that no intraocular instrumentation is required and the procedure can be performed more safely in eyes that are phakic or have shallow chambers.

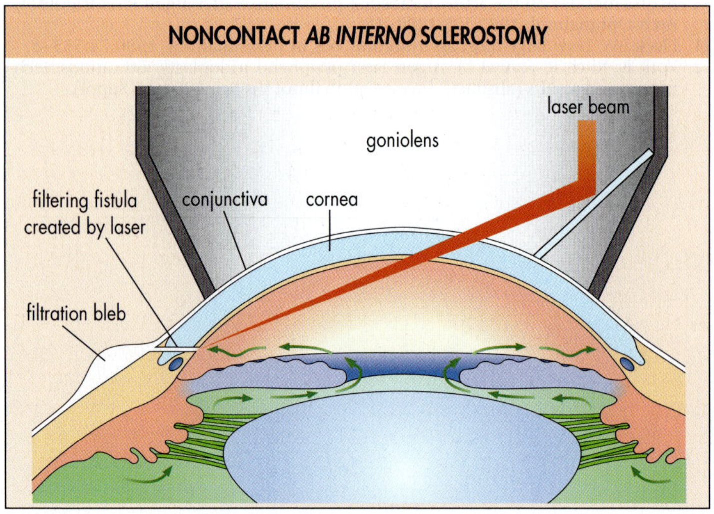

The Nd:YAG ab interno sclerostomy is most suitable for the creation of inferior or nasal blebs in eyes that have excessive superior conjunctival scarring. These eyes should be aphakic or pseudophakic to avoid the risk of lens trauma from a probe passing across the anterior chamber. Preoperative laser iridotomy or peripheral iridoplasty in the vicinity of the planned sclerostomy may reduce the risk of postoperative iris incarceration. As an increased risk of infection exists with inferior blebs, this procedure should be avoided in patients who have poor hygiene or chronic blepharitis. This technique may have an advantage over the ab externo method because conjunctival dissection is not required.

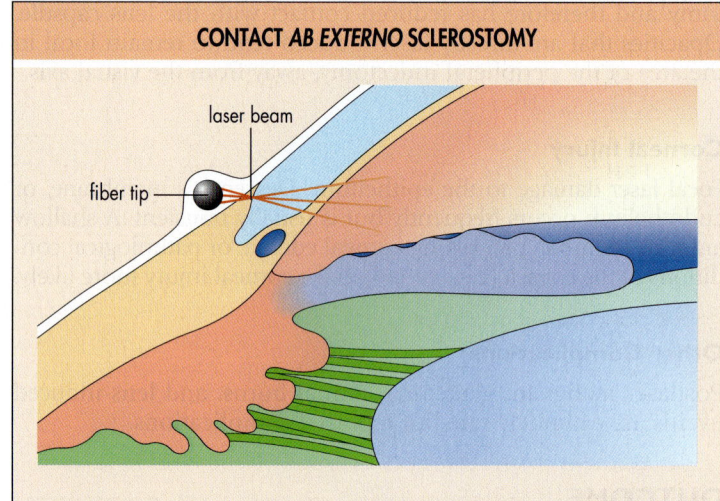

FIG. 236-2 ▋ Contact ab externo sclerostomy. Laser energy is delivered externally via a laser probe. Minimal conjunctival dissection is required.

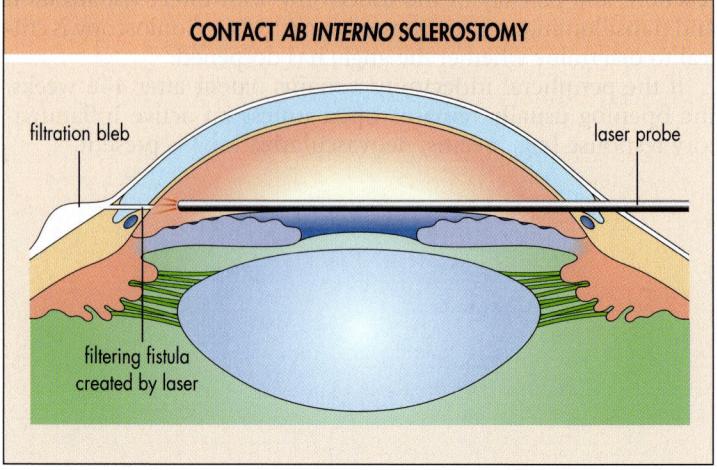

FIG. 236-3 ▋ Contact ab interno sclerostomy. Laser energy is delivered internally via a laser probe. No conjunctival dissection is required.

FIG. 236-1 ▋ Noncontact ab interno sclerostomy. Laser energy is directed internally via a goniolens. No conjunctival dissection is required.

ALTERNATIVES TO SURGERY

In eyes that have not had prior surgery, standard trabeculectomy with or without antifibrotic therapy is currently the favored approach. In eyes with mild to moderate conjunctival scarring from prior surgery, trabeculectomy with an adjunctive antifibrotic agent (see Chapters 239 and 240) is an alternative to laser sclerostomy and the preferred approach for eyes in which conjunctival and scleral dissection can be carried out safely. In eyes that have excessive conjunctival scarring, seton placement (see Chapter 241) and cyclodestructive procedures are alternative modes of treatment (see Chapter 237).

SURGICAL TECHNIQUES

Depending on the individual patient, the holmium and Nd:YAG laser filtration procedures can be accomplished with topical, subconjunctival, peribulbar, or retrobulbar anesthesia.

Ab Externo Technique—Thulium-Holmium-Chromium: Yttrium-Aluminum-Garnet (Holmium) Laser Sclerostomy

Ab externo holmium laser sclerostomy is performed by delivering laser energy through a fiberoptic probe by a subconjunctival approach.

The eye may be rotated inferiorly with a muscle hook to avoid placement of a traction suture. A sclerostomy site is chosen that corresponds to the area with least conjunctival scarring or is adjacent to a prior iridectomy. A 1–2mm conjunctival incision 8–10mm away from the intended sclerostomy site and 6mm from the limbus is made using Vannas scissors. The underlying Tenon's capsule is also incised until bare sclera is reached. The conjunctiva may be hydrodissected with balanced salt solution or viscoelastic if excessive Tenon's and/or conjunctival scarring is present.

The probe is then inserted under Tenon's capsule and advanced carefully toward the limbus. It is manipulated into position at the limbus, as anterior as possible, without folding the conjunctiva under the probe. The aiming beam and laser energy exit 90° from the axis of the probe. With the probe tip held tangential to the limbus, the probe is rotated so that the aiming beam is as parallel as possible to the iris (see Fig. 236-2).

The laser is then fired at a repetition rate of 5 pulses per second (80–100mJ per pulse in previously unoperated eyes; 100–120mJ per pulse in previously operated eyes). The conjunctiva over the probe tip is irrigated with balanced salt solution while the laser is fired. The surgeon is able to recognize sclerostomy patency from three signs:

- Small bubbles may appear in the anterior chamber;
- The sound of the laser ticking changes from a dull to a sharp noise; and
- A bleb forms upon removal of the probe.

While performing a sclerostomy, care must be taken not to indent the globe, which may result in a sclerostomy with walls that are not parallel to each other, thus creating a smaller internal than external ostium size. If iris incarceration occurs intraoperatively, a peripheral iridotomy can be created with the holmium laser probe. The laser probe is then withdrawn and the conjunctival wound is closed with a running 9-0 Vicryl suture. 5-Fluorouracil can be injected subconjunctivally in an adjacent quadrant.

Ab Interno Technique: Neodymium:Yttrium-Aluminum-Garnet Laser Sclerostomy

Ab interno Nd:YAG laser sclerostomy is performed using laser energy delivered through a fiberoptic probe by a transcameral approach. The laser energy exits from the tip parallel to the long axis of the probe.

Viscoelastic or balanced salt solution is injected subconjunctivally, using a 30-gauge needle, to elevate conjunctiva adjacent to the proposed sclerostomy site. A sharp steel blade or diamond knife is used to create a peripheral corneal paracentesis, approximately 1.5mm in length, 90–180° away from the proposed sclerostomy site. Viscoelastic is injected intracamerally through the paracentesis site. The laser probe is introduced through the paracentesis and is passed across the anterior chamber until the tip is in contact with the sclera in the region of Schwalbe's line. A gonioscopy lens can be used to aid visualization.

The aiming beam may transilluminate the sclera in the vicinity of the limbal sulcus. Between 3 and 5 pulses of 200mJ (10W, 0.2 sec) are required to achieve filtration. The laser probe is advanced until the probe tip is visualized in the subconjunctival space (see Fig. 236-3). Penetration through full-thickness sclera is evident when an adjacent bleb enlarges, and the probe is withdrawn. Additional balanced salt solution or viscoelastic is injected into the anterior chamber to verify the patency of the sclerostomy and further elevate the bleb. The paracentesis is closed with a single 10-0 nylon suture with the knot buried. The conjunctiva that overlies the sclerostomy site is inspected for buttonholes. 5-Fluorouracil can be injected subconjunctivally in an adjacent quadrant.

Attempts can be made to minimize the possibility of iris incarceration. After the probe has been withdrawn from the sclerostomy, an iridoplasty can be performed with several laser applications to prevent iris incarceration. Alternatively, a peripheral iridectomy can be created with a vitrector. If vitreous is present in the anterior chamber, an anterior vitrectomy should be performed through the paracentesis site to minimize the risk of vitreous incarceration.

COMPLICATIONS

Iris incarceration is the most frequent complication of full-thickness laser filtration procedures, especially in phakic eyes and those with narrow angles. The risk of this complication can be reduced by performing the sclerostomy over a prior peripheral iridectomy or by the creation of a peripheral iridectomy at the time of the sclerostomy. Often, postoperative iris prolapse can be managed by massage over the sclerostomy site with a Zeiss gonioprism. Alternatively, a peripheral laser iridoplasty or laser iridotomy can be performed. Other complications include hyphema, localized corneal edema, Descemet's membrane detachment, cyclodialysis cleft formation, conjunctival burn, conjunctival buttonhole, and vitreous hemorrhage.

Laser sclerostomy procedures are associated with overdrainage complications found in other full-thickness procedures, which include hypotony, shallow anterior chamber, choroidal effusion, choroidal hemorrhage, and cataract formation. As minimal conjunctival manipulation helps to preserve episcleral tissue and increase the resistance to aqueous outflow, the occurrence of a shallow or flat anterior chamber may not be as common as expected for a surgical full-thickness procedure.

OUTCOME

The success rate of the holmium laser ab externo sclerostomy is 49–55% at 1 year, 36–52% at 2 years, and 26–36% at 4 years.[3–5] A success rate of 60% at 2 years for Nd:YAG laser ab interno sclerostomy has been reported.[6] These success figures primarily include eyes at high risk of filtration failure that also have received adjunctive 5-fluorouracil and that may have required supplemental antiglaucoma medication. As a result of these success rates, the role of laser sclerostomy in glaucoma filtration surgery as a primary or secondary procedure is limited. Combination of this procedure with cataract extraction has been described and may be more promising.[7] Adjunctive administration of mitomycin has been reported to enhance success rates of laser sclerostomy in vivo and in vitro, although methods of application have varied.[8–10]

REFERENCES

1. O'Donnell FE Jr, Santos BA, Overby J. Laser trabeculodissection with a photopolishing scanning excimer laser. Ophthalmic Surg Lasers. 2000;31:508–11.

2. McAllister JA, Watts PO. Holmium laser sclerostomy: a clinical study. Eye. 1993;7: 656–60.
3. Schuman JS, Stinson WG, Hutchinson BT, *et al*. Holmium laser sclerectomy: success and complications. Ophthalmology. 1993;100:1060–5.
4. Iwach AG, Hoskins HD, Mora JS, *et al*. Update on the subconjunctival THC:YAG (holmium) laser sclerostomy ab externo clinical trial: a 4-year report. Ophthalmic Surg Lasers. 1996;27:823–31.
5. Friedman DS, Katz LJ, Leen MM. Holmium laser sclerostomy in glaucomatous eyes with prior surgery: 24 month results. Ophthalmic Surg Lasers. 1998;29:17–22.
6. Wilson RP, Javitt JC. Ab interno laser sclerostomy in aphakic patients with glaucoma and chronic inflammation. Am J Ophthalmol. 1990;110:178–84.

7. Kendrick R, Kollartis CR, Khan N. The results of ab interno thermal laser sclerostomy combined with cataract surgery vs. trabeculectomy combined with cataract surgery 6 to12 months postoperatively. Ophthalmic Surg Lasers. 1996;27:583–6.
8. Iliev ME, Vander Zypen E, Fankhauser F, England C. Spontaneous and pharmacologically modulated wound healing after Nd:YAG laser sclerostomy ab interno in rabbits. Eur J Ophthalmol. 1997;7:24–8.
9. Onada E, Ando H, Jikihara S, Kitizawa Y. Holmium YAG laser sclerostomy ab externo in refractory glaucoma. Int Ophthalmol. 1996–97;20:309–14.
10. Schmidt-Erfurth U, Wetzel W, Drage G, Birngruber R. Mitomycin C in laser sclerostomy: benefit and complications. Ophthalmic Surg Lasers. 1997;28:14–20.

UNDRAA ALTANGEREL • MARLENE R. MOSTER • TAREK M. EID

INTRODUCTION

The goal of glaucoma surgery is to lower the intraocular pressure (IOP) predictably, either by maximizing outflow (as in filtration and tube-shunt surgery) or by decreasing inflow (as with cyclodestructive procedures). The destruction of the ciliary body carries a considerable complication rate, which includes phthisis bulbi, visual loss, and an unpredictable degree of IOP reduction. Usually these procedures are reserved for eyes that have glaucoma refractory to medical, laser, and surgical treatment.

HISTORICAL REVIEW

Selective destruction of the ciliary body with electrocautery was first applied by Weve in 1933 (nonpenetrating diathermy) and Vogt in 1936 (penetrating diathermy). However, the high complication rate, the less than satisfactory results, and the introduction of cyclocryotherapy by Biette in 1950 reduced the use of cyclodiathermy.[1] Cyclocryotherapy was the cyclodestructive procedure of choice for more than three decades.

However, the IOP reduction was inconsistent and the complication rate was still high. The use of xenon arc photocoagulation in 1961 and the ruby laser in 1971 led to the application of laser energy as a method of cycloablation. In 1981, Fankhauser and associates incorporated a thermal mode into a neodymium:yttrium-aluminum-garnet (Nd:YAG) laser system to perform trans-scleral cyclophotocoagulation (CPC). The availability of the instrument facilitated wide clinical application.[2]

More recently, semiconductor diode laser technology has been used successfully for cyclodestructive surgery.[3–13] Currently, 810nm (diode) and 1064nm (Nd:YAG) are the two most popular wavelengths for trans-scleral cyclodestructive surgery.

PREOPERATIVE EVALUATION AND DIAGNOSTIC APPROACH

Cyclodestructive procedures are generally reserved for eyes that have poor visual potential [visual acuity less than 20/400 (6/120)], eyes in which other glaucoma procedures failed or are not applicable (e.g., extensive conjunctival scarring), eyes in which filtering surgery has a high failure rate (e.g., neovascular glaucoma, aphakic and pseudophakic glaucoma, and glaucoma associated with silicone oil), and eyes of patients who, for medical reasons, are unable to undergo filtration surgery.[14]

MECHANISM OF ACTION

Cyclocryotherapy damages the epithelial, vascular, and stromal components of the ciliary body. Maximum cell death seems to require a rapid freeze followed by a slow thaw. Cell necrosis has been shown to occur at temperatures of $-10°C$ and below. In vivo, -60 to $-80°C$ at the sclera produces a temperature of $-10°C$ in the ciliary processes after 20–30 seconds of application.[15]

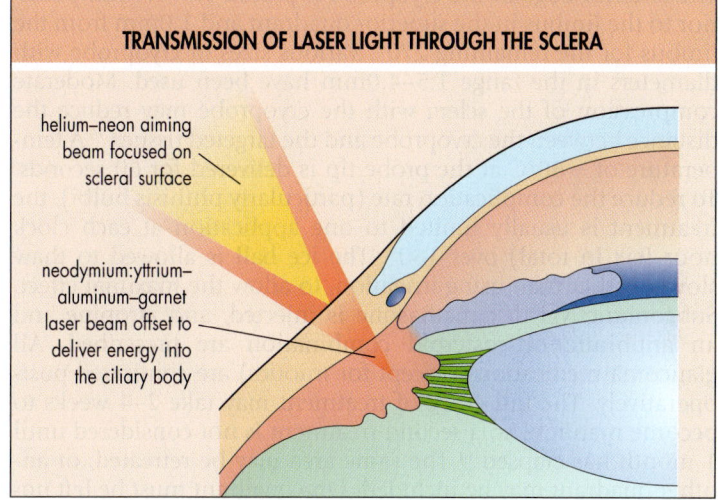

TRANSMISSION OF LASER LIGHT THROUGH THE SCLERA

helium–neon aiming beam focused on scleral surface

neodymium:yttrium–aluminum–garnet laser beam offset to deliver energy into the ciliary body

FIG. 237-1 ■ Transmission of laser light through the sclera. The laser beam is focused on the ciliary processes.

The Nd:YAG laser allows effective scleral penetration (Fig. 237-1) with less backscatter than with lasers of shorter wavelength. Higher energies are created in the free-running mode as contrasted with the single-pulse mode. Laser CPC is more effectively absorbed by pigmented tissue in the ciliary body compared with cryotherapy, which is diffusely absorbed. The contact methods produce less scatter and thus require less energy than the noncontact methods.[2]

The semiconductor diode laser with a wavelength of 810nm has lower scleral transmission than the Nd:YAG laser (1064nm) but greater absorption by melanin. This allows the use of 50% less energy than used with the Nd:YAG laser.[3]

Histologically, most likely both lasers produce fragmentation and detachment of the epithelium of the ciliary processes with simultaneous destruction of the ciliary body vasculature.[16] At least three mechanisms are thought to be important in lowering IOP: (1) inflammation, which is prominent in the first week or so after treatment; (2) decreased aqueous production through ablation of the pars plicata, through either a direct or indirect effect on the vasculature; and (3) increased uveoscleral outflow resulting from laser delivery to the region of the pars plana.[11]

ALTERNATIVES TO A CYCLODESTRUCTIVE PROCEDURE

The alternatives to a cyclodestructive procedure include trabeculectomy surgery along with an adjunctive antimetabolite (see Chapters 239 and 240) and drainage implant surgery (see Chapter 242). The cyclodestructive procedure has the advantage of being faster and an office procedure but is generally reserved for eyes that have poorer visual potential because of the risk of later diminished visual acuity.

ANESTHESIA

The ciliary processes are highly innervated and painful to treat without adequate anesthesia. Trans-scleral procedures require local (retrobulbar or peribulbar) anesthesia and can usually be performed in an office setting. Endoscopic CPC requires local (retrobulbar or peribulbar) or general anesthesia and is performed in an outpatient surgical or hospital setting.[4] Glaucoma medications, except miotics, may be continued before and after cyclodestructive procedures.

SPECIFIC TECHNIQUES

Cyclocryotherapy

The anterior edge of the cryoprobe is placed 1.0–1.5mm posterior to the limbus in the superior quadrant and 1.0mm from the limbus for the remaining 270°. Various sizes of cryoprobe with diameters in the range 1.5–4.0mm have been used. Moderate compression of the sclera with the cryoprobe may reduce the distance between the cryoprobe and the targeted tissues.[15] A temperature of −80°C at the probe tip is delivered for 60 seconds. To reduce the complication rate (particularly phthisis bulbi), the treatment is usually limited to one application at each clock hour (six in total) over 180°. The ice ball is allowed to thaw slowly, rather than using irrigation, to allow the maximal effect. Subconjunctival dexamethasone is injected, and atropine and an antibiotic-corticosteroid combination are prescribed. All glaucoma medications (except for miotics) are continued postoperatively. The full effect of treatment may take 2–4 weeks to become manifest, so a second treatment is not considered until 1 month has elapsed.[14] The same area may be retreated, or another quadrant may be included. One quadrant must be left untouched to avoid anterior segment necrosis.

Cyclocryotherapy has been used extensively in the past; however, its unpredictable results and complication rate have encouraged pursuit of other forms of cyclodestruction.

Trans-scleral Cyclophotocoagulation (Table 237-1)

NONCONTACT ND:YAG LASER CYCLOPHOTOCOAGULATION. A noncontact Nd:YAG laser unit transmits the laser energy through air from a slit-lamp delivery system. The typical laser settings for noncontact trans-scleral Nd:YAG CPC are 4–8J/pulse, 20ms duration, and a maximum offset at position 9. The number of applications is 30–40, with 8–9 spots per quadrant; the 3 and 9 o'clock positions are spared to avoid long posterior ciliary arteries (Fig. 237-2). The laser spot is placed 1.0–1.5mm posterior to the limbus. This distance is measured using calipers or the aiming beam in the center of a 3mm slit beam. The Shields contact lens may be used during the procedure. Its central opaque disc helps to prevent the entrance of stray laser light into the eye, and its limbal portion compresses the conjunctiva and blanches blood vessels to improve the focus.[14] Atropine 1% is administered twice a day and prednisolone acetate 1% four times a day; these are tapered as inflammation subsides (Fig. 237-4). All preoperative glaucoma medications except for miotics are continued and IOP is checked 1 hour, 1 day, and 1 week after treatment.

Transmission of Laser Light through the Sclera

CONTACT ND:YAG LASER CYCLOPHOTOCOAGULATION. Contact trans-scleral photocoagulation is achieved by using the Nd:YAG laser in the continuous mode via a fiberoptic system in direct contact with the conjunctiva. Effective reduction of IOP is provided using less power than required with the noncontact Nd:YAG laser.[2]

The fiberoptic laser probe is positioned perpendicularly on the conjunctiva with the anterior edge 0.5–1.0mm posterior to the surgical limbus (Fig. 237-3). Laser settings include a power level of 4–9W and duration of 0.5–0.7 seconds. The number of applications varies in the range 16–40 over the entire area of the ciliary body with the 3 and 9 o'clock positions spared. Efficient energy transfer is facilitated by pushing the probe against the sclera, which increases light transmission through the sclera.[17]

SEMICONDUCTOR DIODE LASER TRANS-SCLERAL CYCLO-PHOTOCOAGULATION. Diode laser trans-scleral cyclophotocoagulation (DCPC) is one of the most widely used methods of ciliary ablation with reported success rates ranging from 40 to 80%. The technique used with the semiconductor diode laser (wavelength 810nm) is similar to that used for the contact Nd:YAG laser. The anterior edge of the probe approximates the surgical limbus and the laser beam is directed 1–1.5mm posteriorly so that the ciliary processes are ablated. Settings are 1500–2500mW of power for 1.0–2.0 seconds and a total of 16–18 spots. The 3 and 9 o'clock positions are spared. The results are similar to those achieved using Nd:YAG CPC[3,4,14] despite the lower energy used with the diode laser (55% of that used with the Nd:YAG laser). In addition, because semiconductor diode lasers have a solid-state construction, they have the advantages of portability, durability, and smaller size compared with the Nd:YAG laser.[3,4]

TABLE 237-1

TECHNIQUES OF TRANS-SCLERAL LASER CYCLOPHOTOCOAGULATION

Parameters	Noncontact Nd: YAG	Contact Nd: YAG	Noncontact Diode	Contact Diode
Power	4–8J	4–9W	1200–1500mW	1500–2500mW
Duration	20ms	0.5–0.7s	1.0s	1.0–2.0s
Lesions	30–40	16–40	30–40	16–18
Distance from limbus	1.0–1.5mm	0.5–1.0mm	0.5–1.0mm	1–1.5mm

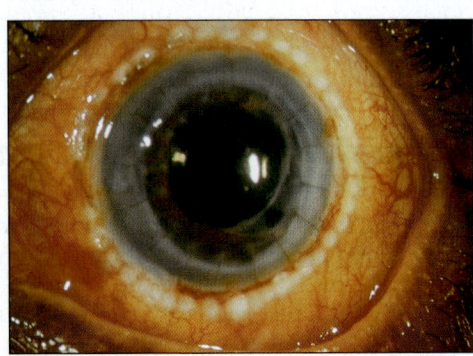

FIG. 237-2 ■ Markings on the sclera after noncontact ND:YAG laser cyclophotocoagulation.

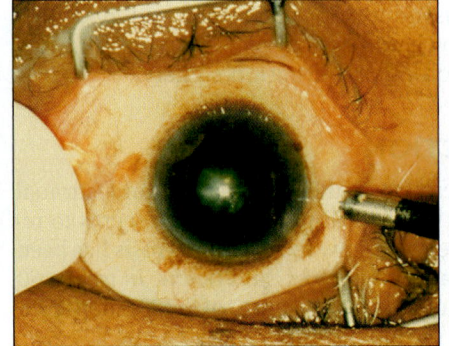

FIG. 237-3 ■ Application of the laser probe in contact trans-scleral Nd:YAG cyclophotocoagulation. The probe is placed on the conjunctiva with the anterior edge 0.5–1mm posterior to the surgical limbus.

OTHER TECHNIQUES OF LASER CYCLOPHOTOCOAGULATION

Other techniques are being investigated, including transpupillary CPC, transvitreal endocyclophotocoagulation, and endoscopic CPC. Direct transpupillary treatment of the ciliary processes with the argon laser (488nm) is rarely used because a clear visual axis and a well-dilated pupil are required to enable photocoagulation of the entire length of the ciliary processes. Transpupillary CPC of the ciliary processes, exposed through peripheral iridectomy or a widely dilated pupil, can be effective in the treatment of ciliary block glaucoma.[4,18] The mechanism may be related to a laser-induced retraction of the ciliary body. Endocyclophoto-coagulation, an intraocular procedure in which a laser probe is used to treat the ciliary processes at the time of pars plana vitrectomy, offers the possibility of selectively treating the ciliary body epithelium with relatively sparing of underlying tissues.[19,20] It requires clear media and aphakia or pseudophakia to visualize directly and treat the ciliary processes, which are scleral depressed into the view of the operating microscope. The argon laser parameters used were continuous duration at 300 to 600mW of energy. The diode uses up to 1 second duration at 300 to 800mW of energy.[4,21–23] Endoscopic CPC through a cataract incision at the time of cataract surgery with trabeculectomy and cataract surgery appears to be a reasonably safe and effective procedure for managing glaucoma and cataract.[4,19,24] Endoscopic CPC may prove to have more predictable results and lower complication rates than trans-scleral procedures; however, this is a more invasive technique, which is not currently in wide use.

It has also been shown that red 647nm krypton laser CPC is an effective and reasonably well-tolerated procedure for lowering IOP in post-traumatic glaucoma.[25] Although transmission through the sclera is lower with the red 647nm krypton laser than with the infrared 810nm diode and Nd:YAG lasers, this is compensated for by using contact application and compressing the sclera with the probe.

COMPLICATIONS

Complications are summarized in Table 237-2. All forms of cyclodestructive procedures may damage ciliary muscle as well as ciliary epithelium, adjacent iris, and retina. Complications include reduced visual acuity, uveitis, pain, hemorrhage, and phthisis bulbi (see Table 237-2). All these complications, especially pain and inflammation, seem less severe after laser CPC than after cyclocryotherapy. For trans-scleral procedures, the occurrence of audible tissue disruptions does not correlate with success rate. Audible pops correlate with intraocular tissue disruption but not necessarily at the target tissue of the ciliary body. These are considered unwanted side effects, as is intraocular hemorrhage or exposure to uveal antigen.[6,26] Decreased visual acuity is not uncommon[2,6,7]; possible causes of loss of vision include a spike in IOP in the perioperative period,[6,7] postoperative cystoid macula edema, backward scatter from the laser, and progression of glaucomatous optic neuropathy in spite of the cyclodestructive treatment. The occasional gain in vision is presumably due to a decrease in corneal edema.[6] Potential complications of trans-scleral diode CPC include conjunctival surface burns that may occur when tissue debris becomes coagulated on the tip and chars. In addition, increased perilimbal conjunctival pigmentation has been correlated with conjunctival burns, which heal quickly.[4] A higher incidence of persistent hypotony and visual loss has been reported in neovascular glaucoma.[14,27] Graft failure is a major problem after cycloablation for refractory glaucoma. It has been reported to occur in 11–44% of patients.[4,28] Hyphema and vitreous hemorrhage are rare. Phthisis, hypotony, and loss of visual acuity may become chronic complaints.

The potential complications of endoscopic CPC include all risks listed except for conjunctival surface burns. In addition, endoscopic CPC carries the risk of damage to the crystalline lens, zonular rupture, and the inherent risks of an intraocular procedure, which include retinal detachment and endophthalmitis. There have been no reported cases of these potential complications in the literature.[4]

OUTCOMES

Cyclocryotherapy is more effective in some forms of glaucoma than others. Glaucoma in aphakic eyes[29] and in eyes after penetrating keratoplasty responds well to cyclocryotherapy. In neovascular glaucoma, pain is reduced effectively but the incidence of visual loss and phthisis is high.[14,27] Contact or noncontact methods of Nd:YAG or diode laser CPC are fast, easy to perform, and repeatable and have a lower complication rate than cyclotherapy and cyclodiathermy.[1–3,6,7,12,30,31] The results of both noncontact and contact Nd:YAG CPC are comparable, with a satisfactory IOP reduction in 45–72% of cases. Between 29 and 48% of Nd:YAG CPC cases require one or more repeated treatments.[30]

Trans-scleral diode CPC produces results equivalent to those of the same operation performed with the Nd:YAG laser (IOP < 22mmHg in 60–84% and retreatment rate of 28–45%)[6,7,9,12,32,33] while offering certain technological advantages. Postoperative complications, including pain, inflammation, hyphema, and phthisis, were less common than in other cyclodestructive procedures. Three different kinds of lasers (diode laser, free-running Nd:YAG, and continuous wave mode Nd:YAG laser) were compared in neovascular glaucoma patients. Diode CPC had the best success lowering IOP in 55.9% of patients after 3 years with the fewest complications.[33]

TABLE 237-2

COMPLICATIONS OF CYCLOCRYOTHERAPY AND LASER TRANS-SCLERAL CYCLOPHOTOCOAGULATION

Common	Rare
Pain (mild to severe)	Transient flat anterior chamber with hypotony, and choroidal detachment
Iritis, usually mild, but may be severe	Malignant glaucoma
Conjunctival edema	Scleral thinning (with laser)
Loss of more than one line of visual acuity	Corneal epithelial defects and corneal graft failure
Persistent hypotony and phthisis bulbi	Hyphema and vitreous hemorrhage
	Sympathetic ophthalmia (with laser)

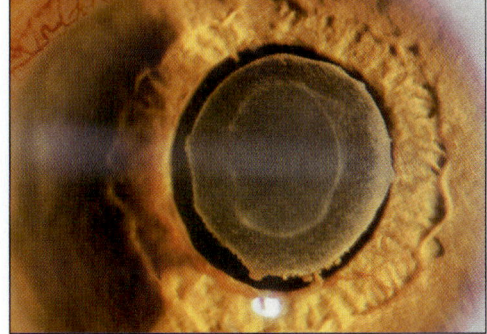

FIG. 237-4 ■ Fibrin clot after Nd:YAG cyclophotocoagulation.

REFERENCES

1. Masterobatista JM, Luntz M. Ciliary body ablation: where are we and how did we get here? Surv Ophthalmol. 1996;41:193–213.
2. Schuman JS, Puhafito CA, Ailingham RR, et al. Contact transcleral continuous wave neodymium:YAG laser cyclophotocoagulation. Ophthalmology. 1990;97:571–80.
3. Youn J, Cox TA, Herndon LW, et al. A clinical comparison of transcleral cyclophotocoagulation with neodymium:YAG and semiconductor diode lasers. Am J Ophthalmol. 1998;126:640–7.

4. Pastor SA, Singh K, Lee DA, *et al.* Cyclophotocoagulation: a report by the American Academy of Ophthalmology. Ophthalmology. 2001;108:2130–38.

5. Wong EYM, Chew PTK, Chee CKL. Diode laser contact transscleral cyclophotocoagulation for refractory glaucoma in Asian patients. Am J Ophthalmol. 1997;124:797–804.

6. Mistlberger A, Liebmann JM, Tschiderer H, *et al.* Diode laser transscleral cyclophotocoagulation for refractory glaucoma. J Glaucoma. 2001;288:288–93.

7. Kosoko O, Gaasterland DE, Pollack IP, *et al.* Long-term outcome of initial ciliary ablation with contact diode laser transscleral cyclophotocoagulation for severe glaucoma. Ophthalmology. 1996;1996:1294–302.

8. Bloom PA, Tsai JC, Sharma K, *et al.* 'Cyclodiode'. Trans-scleral diode laser cyclophotocoagulation in the treatment of advanced refractory glaucoma. Ophthalmology. 1997;104:1508–20.

9. Hennis HL, Stewart WC. Semiconductor diode laser transscleral cyclophotocoagulation in patients with glaucoma. Am J Ophthalmol. 1992;113:81–5.

10. Seah SK, Jap A, Min G. Contact transscleral cyclophotocoagulation for end stage glaucoma. Ann Acad Med Singapore. 1994;23:18–20.

11. Walland MJ, McKelvie PA. Diode laser cyclophotocoagulation: histopathology in two cases of clinical failure. Ophthalmic Surg Lasers. 1998;29:852–6.

12. Walland MJ. Diode laser cyclophotocoagulation: dose-standardized therapy in end-stage glaucoma. Aust NZ J Ophthalmol. 1998;26:135–9.

13. Hamard P, May F, Quesnot S, Hamard H. [Contact transscleral diode laser cyclophotocoagulation for the treatment of refractory pediatric glaucoma]. J Fr Ophtalmol. 2000;23:773–80.

14. Stewart W, Briendley GO, Shields MB. Cyclodestructive procedures. In: Ritch R, Shields MB, Krupin T, eds. The glaucomas. St. Louis: Mosby; 1996:1605–20.

15. Quigley HA. Histologic physiologic studies of cyclocryotherapy in primate and human eyes. Am J Ophthalmol. 1976;82:722–3.

16. Van der Zypen E, England C, Frankhauser F, *et al.* The effect of transscleral laser cyclophotocoagulation on rabbit ciliary body vascularization. Graefes Arch Clin Exp Ophthalmol. 1989;227:172–9.

17. Stolzenburg S, Muller-Stolzenburg N, Kresse S, *et al.* Contact cyclophotocoagulation with the continuous wave Nd:YAG laser with quartz fiber. Optimizing coagulation parameters. Ophthalmology. 1992;89:210–11.

18. Herschler J. Laser shrinkage of the ciliary processes. A treatment for malignant (ciliary block) glaucoma. Ophthalmology. 1980;87:1155–9.

19. Jacobi PC, Dietlein TS. Endoscopic surgery in glaucoma management. Curr Opin Ophthalmol. 2000;11:127–32.

20. Chen J, Cohn RA, Lin SC, *et al.* Endoscopic photocoagulation of the ciliary body for treatment of refractory glaucomas. Am J Ophthalmol. 1997;124:787–96.

21. Lim JI, Lynn M, Capone AJ. Ciliary body endophotocoagulation during pars plana vitrectomy in eyes with vitreoretinal disorders and concomitant uncontrolled glaucoma. Ophthalmology. 1996;103:1041–6.

22. Zarbin MA, Michels RG, de Bustros S, *et al.* Endolaser treatment of the ciliary body for severe glaucoma. Ophthalmology. 1988;95:1639–48.

23. Patel A, Thompson JT, Michels RG, Quigley HA. Endolaser treatment of the ciliary body for uncontrolled glaucoma. Ophthalmology. 1986;93:825–30.

24. Uram M. Ophthalmic laser microendoscope ciliary process ablation in the management of neovascular glaucoma. Ophthalmology. 1992;99:1823–8.

25. Raivio VR, Immonen IJR, Laatikainen LT, Puska PM. Transscleral contact krypton laser cyclophotocoagulation for treatment of posttraumatic glaucoma. J Glaucoma. 2001;10:77–84.

26. Rebolleda G, Munoz FJ, Murube J. Audible pops during cyclodiode procedures. J Glaucoma. 1999;8:177–83.

27. Eid TE, Katz LJ, Spaeth GL, Augsburger JJ. Tube-shunt surgery versus Nd:YAG cyclophotocoagulation in management of neovascular glaucoma. Ophthalmology. 1997;104:1692–700.

28. Beiran I, Rootman DS, Trope GE, Buys YM. Long-term results of transscleral Nd:YAG cyclophotocoagulation for refractory glaucoma postpenetrating keratoplasty. J Glaucoma. 2000;9:268–72.

29. Bellows AR, Grant WM. Cyclocryotherapy of chronic open-glaucoma in aphakic eyes. Am J Ophthalmol. 1978;85:615–21.

30. Moster MR, Schwartz LW, Cantor LB, *et al.* Treatment of advanced glaucoma with Nd:YAG laser cycloablation. Invest Ophthalmol Vis Sci. 1986;27:253.

31. Shields MB, Shields SE. Noncontact transscleral Nd:YAG cyclophotocoagulation: a long-term follow-up of 500 patients. Trans Am Ophthalmol Soc. 1994;92:271–83.

32. Yap-Veloso MI, Simmons R, Echelman DA, *et al.* Intraocular pressure control after contact transscleral diode cyclophotocoagulation in eyes with intractable glaucoma. J Glaucoma. 1998;7:319–28.

33. Oguri A, Takahashi E, Tomita G, *et al.* Transscleral cyclophotocoagulation with the diode laser for neovascular glaucoma. Ophthalmic Surg Lasers. 1998;29:722–7.

238 Goniotomy and Trabeculotomy

JAMES D. BRANDT

INTRODUCTION

Congenital and pediatric glaucomas are generally regarded as surgical, not medical, disorders because medical therapy alone is rarely effective for these conditions and current techniques of surgery on the anterior chamber angle (goniotomy and trabeculotomy) enjoy a high degree of success. In this chapter the initial surgical approach to the management of congenital and pediatric glaucoma through goniotomy and trabeculotomy is outlined.

HISTORICAL REVIEW

Prior to the introduction of goniotomy, congenital glaucoma uniformly resulted in blindness. In the 1930s, up to 7% of children in institutions for the blind suffered from buphthalmos; given the rarity of the disease, it is probable that virtually every bilaterally affected individual was blinded. It, therefore, is no exaggeration to suggest that goniotomy and trabeculotomy have, since their introduction, allowed many individuals to avoid an entire lifetime of blindness.

Attempts to incise the iridocorneal angle across the anterior chamber to treat glaucoma were first described by de Vincentiis in 1893[1]; the results were quite poor and the technique fell into disuse. In 1936, Barkan[2] presented a 10-month follow-up of a then unnamed operation in which he incised through the trabecular meshwork into Schlemm's canal under direct, gonioscopic visualization. In 1938 this new procedure, given the name "goniotomy," was described in detail,[3] and the requisite instrumentation became available to others. By 1942 the particular usefulness of goniotomy in the treatment of congenital glaucoma was recognized,[4] and the modern era of surgery for congenital glaucoma had begun.

Surgeons soon recognized that a clear cornea and good visualization of angle structures were key ingredients for successful goniotomy; unfortunately, many cases of congenital glaucoma present with cloudy corneas because of markedly elevated intraocular pressure or breaks in Desçemet's membrane. In such cases, goniotomy becomes little more than a blind procedure. In 1960 Burian[5] and Smith[6] each independently described a new procedure, trabeculotomy *ab externo*. In this operation, Schlemm's canal is cannulated from an external approach and a tear is created through the trabecular meshwork into the anterior chamber using a specially designed probe, the trabeculotome. The principal advantage of trabeculotomy is that it can be performed in the presence of an opacified cornea. Further modifications to the procedure and instrumentation by Dannheim and Harms[7] and McPherson[8] have led to a success rate comparable to that of goniotomy.[9,10]

PREOPERATIVE EVALUATION AND DIAGNOSTIC APPROACH

The epidemiology and differential diagnosis of primary infantile glaucoma are covered in Chapter 219. In unilateral cases of congenital glaucoma, in which the usual signs and symptoms of the disease are present, the diagnosis is relatively straightforward. In bilateral cases in young infants, however, the diagnosis may be less certain and the ophthalmologist carries out a brief examination in the office before the child is subjected to a general anesthetic.

In infants younger than 3 months, it is usually possible to perform tonometry using either a handheld Goldmann applanation tonometer or a handheld electronic tonometer, the Tonopen. The Schiøtz tonometer is relatively inaccurate when used to measure intraocular pressure (IOP) of an infant eye and should be used only to gauge a general range of IOP.[11,12] The young infant is swaddled and the eyelids are pried apart gently to perform tonometry. If the child is permitted to drink from a bottle after feedings have been withheld for an hour or two, it is usually possible to perform accurate tonometry and a reasonably thorough examination in the office, especially if the use of a lid speculum is avoided. The Tonopen, which has a small (about 2mm) measuring surface, is well suited to the small, intrapalpebral fissures of an infant and can measure IOPs without the use of undue pressure on the lids. The Tonopen has proved accurate when compared with both cannulation in cadaver eyes and Goldmann tonometry and appears to be reliable in pediatric patients.[11]

The IOP in normal infants is usually in the range 12–15mmHg (1.6–2.0kPa).[13] An office measurement of IOP much greater than 20mmHg (2.7kPa) in a calm, resting infant should carry a high index of suspicion for glaucoma when other signs and symptoms suggest the disease, as should an asymmetry of >5mmHg (>0.7kPa) in suspected unilateral or asymmetric cases. Measurements of IOP while a child cries and resists efforts to hold the eye open are usually not interpretable because the Valsalva maneuver and a squeezed lid may result in a (measured) IOP in the range 30–50mmHg (4.0–6.7kPa) even in normal infants.

The optic nerve examination is at the heart of the diagnosis of all forms of glaucoma, and congenital glaucoma, despite its often dramatic anterior segment findings, is no different. In the office, fundus examination is facilitated greatly by using a Koeppe diagnostic infant gonioscopy lens that has no central depression; the lens has a lid retention flange that prevents the infant from squeezing out the contact lens. Once the lens is in place, the infant often calms down sufficiently to permit good visualization of the disc; with dilation, fundus photography to document the appearance of the optic nerve is often possible.

If the diagnosis of glaucoma is suspected strongly on the basis of the office evaluation, an examination under anesthetic and simultaneous surgery on the affected eye or eyes are recommended to the child's parents. The surgeon must devote ample time to counsel and educate the child's parents about the diagnostic and surgical plan that is recommended, with emphasis at the outset that although the surgery is usually highly successful, a decade or more of careful follow-up is necessary. Frequent examinations under anesthetic, amblyopia therapy, and other interventions are part of this long follow-up care, particularly in early childhood. Because some of the infantile and pediatric glaucomas are genetic in origin, with subsequent siblings at increased risk for the disease, appropriate counseling by a clinical geneticist familiar with ophthalmic disease is often helpful.

DIFFERENTIAL DIAGNOSIS

The differential diagnosis of congenital and infantile glaucoma is covered in Chapter 219. In most cases, the diagnosis is relatively straightforward and examination under anesthetic merely confirms the clinical impression of the office examination. Despite the frequently dramatic clinical presentation of glaucoma in children, every one of the signs and symptoms of pediatric glaucoma may be caused by disorders other than glaucoma. The decision to operate must be based on the presence of elevated IOP and a correspondent glaucomatous optic atrophy (if the fundus can be visualized), not on the basis of corneal findings alone. Unilateral buphthalmos may be mimicked by a microphthalmic fellow eye, and this possibility must always be considered.

ALTERNATIVES TO SURGERY

Uncontrolled congenital and pediatric glaucomas represent clinical conditions that are definitively managed on an urgent, if not emergent, basis; in most cases, examination under anesthetic and (probable) surgery are scheduled within 24–72 hours of the initial diagnosis. When, for logistic or medical reasons, this proves impossible, the IOP may be lowered somewhat using aqueous suppressant medications. Topical β-adrenergic antagonists are often used safely with dosages given every 12 hours,[14] but because the potential for systemic side effects is increased in a small infant, the lowest possible dose is used initially and the infant is monitored carefully. Timolol has been reported to induce apnea in infants,[15] and outpatient use in an unmonitored setting probably should be avoided in premature infants and neonates whose immature respiratory systems place them at increased risk of apnea and sudden infant death syndrome.

The carbonic anhydrase inhibitor acetazolamide may be administered parenterally or orally, 5–10mg/kg of body weight every 6 hours. The pharmacist may compound an elixir using the parenteral powder—250mg/5ml in a strongly flavored elixir is reasonably palatable, especially when chilled.

Miotics are generally avoided in infants and small children. Not only are these agents rarely effective in congenital glaucoma (a fact noted in 1939 by Anderson[16] in the first English-language monograph on congenital glaucoma), but the side effects of these agents may be dramatic in a small infant. The parasympathetic actions of these drugs (diaphoresis, diarrhea, and intestinal and gastric hypermotility) that occur rarely in adults may be pronounced in infants.

Several new, topical glaucoma medications have come into widespread clinical use. The topical carbonic anhydrase inhibitor dorzolamide is probably equivalent in efficacy to parenteral or oral acetazolamide in infants and avoids the potential electrolyte imbalance that systemic administration may cause. The α_2-agonist agents apraclonidine and brimonidine both suppress aqueous humor production and are potent hypotensive agents with few systemic adverse effects in adults; however, in children, brimonidine has been reported to induce both central nervous system depression and apnea in young infants,[17] prompting the U.S. Food and Drug Administration to relabel the medication as contraindicated in young infants. The prostaglandin $F_{2\alpha}$ analog latanoprost is a potent hypotensive agent that has the significant clinical advantage in pediatric patients of once-daily bedtime dosing.[18] The author's experience with the newer agents has been a mixed one, with some notable successes and notable failures. Because all topical medications have the potential for significant systemic side effects, they should be administered in close cooperation with the child's pediatrician.

Medical therapy of congenital glaucoma is not recommended for long-term or even intermediate-term use but is employed only if an examination under anesthetic and surgery must be deferred or as a temporary measure while the effects of surgery are awaited (for example, before a ligated tube-shunt device begins to function). It is far better to proceed promptly with the definitive evaluation and treatment.

ANESTHESIA

General anesthetics have a potent and rapid effect on the IOP in both normal and glaucomatous individuals. For this reason, the anesthesiologist responsible for the general anesthetic in cases of congenital glaucoma must be familiar with the issues involved and be able to work with the surgeon to obtain the most accurate tonometry possible during the crucial initial minutes of administration of the anesthetic.

Virtually all of the inhalational anesthetics are known to depress IOP within minutes of their administration,[19] whereas ketamine HCl slowly elevates the IOP as deeper anesthesia is attained.[20] The benzodiazepines do not appear to have a significant effect on IOP when used in preoperative doses. Midazolam HCl is often used as a preoperative sedative in children, and in many cases the child is sedated sufficiently with this medication to enable a quick IOP measurement to be carried out prior to the administration of an inhalational general anesthetic. Such measurement, with the child resting comfortably but not under the influence of the potent inhalational anesthetics, is probably the most accurate. Methohexital (methohexitone) also does not appear to have a significant effect on IOP,[21] and the author has found that this drug, administered rectally in a dose of 40mg/kg body weight, reliably induces sedation sufficient to perform much if not all of an examination under anesthetic. If surgery is planned, endotracheal intubation is appropriate, especially when a longer, bilateral case is anticipated. The author prefers an oral U-shaped RAE-style endotracheal tube as it is less likely to be dislodged during the head movements required in bilateral goniotomy. The IOP must be measured prior to the administration of any muscular relaxant—depolarization agents such as succinylcholine tend to raise the IOP, whereas nondepolarization agents lower it.[22]

Essential data that must be obtained during an initial or follow-up examination under anesthetic are IOP, results of optic nerve and fundus examinations, cycloplegic retinoscopic measurement of axial length and corneal diameter (horizontal and vertical), and gonioscopy results.

Aspects of the examination that require a clear media, such as ophthalmoscopy, retinoscopy, or fundus photography, are performed first, followed by axial length measurement, gonioscopy, and corneal diameter measurement. It is useful to record the data in a standardized manner so that on follow-up examinations the information is quickly at hand to determine disease progression.

Preoperative pupillary dilation is avoided for cases in which the appearances of the iris and anterior chamber angle are important when the initial diagnosis is made, and it is unnecessary for cases in which corneal opacities prevent any view of the fundus. However, ophthalmoscopy, retinoscopy, and fundus photography are important parts of the initial and subsequent evaluations of a child who has glaucoma, and preoperative dilation using a short-acting mydriatic should be considered before the operating room is entered to avoid a needlessly prolonged period under anesthetic while pupillary dilation takes place. If necessary, intracameral acetylcholine is instilled during surgery to constrict the pupil to allow safe intraocular maneuvers.

Fundus photography of the optic nerve allows the surgeon to document the extent of the progression of the disease (Fig. 238-1). It is well known that the optic nerve cupping seen in congenital and juvenile glaucoma may reverse itself to some extent,[23] and this may be used in some cases to gauge the success of therapy. Similarly, axial length measurements using ultrasonic biometry may help to establish the degree of disparity between the two eyes, particularly in unilateral cases.[24] In many cases the disparity decreases after successful therapy,[24,25] and thus a constant or increasing disparity between the two eyes may signal a worsening clinical situation. The BioPen handheld ultrasonic biometric ruler is an easily portable device that may be brought to the operation room for intraoperative biometry; because it is similar in size, operation, and appearance to the Tonopen, it may also be used in the office

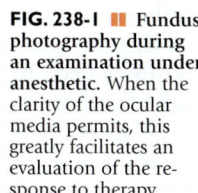

FIG. 238-1 ■ Fundus photography during an examination under anesthetic. When the clarity of the ocular media permits, this greatly facilitates an evaluation of the response to therapy.

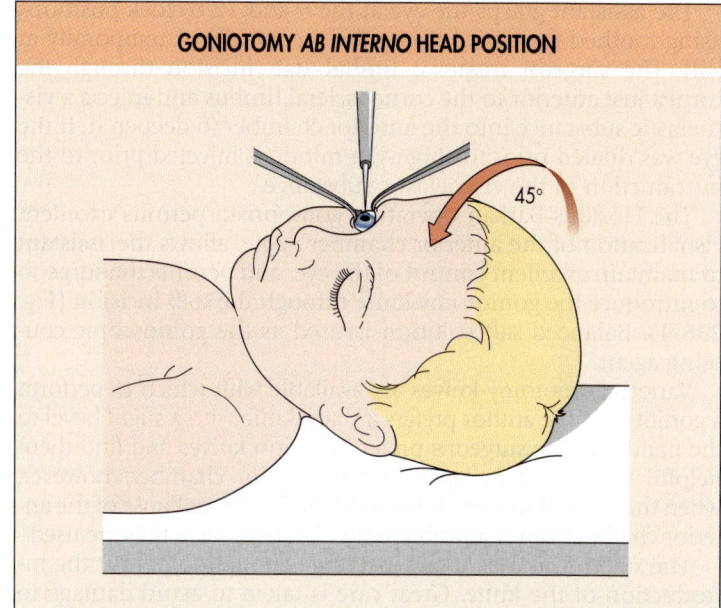

GONIOTOMY AB INTERNO HEAD POSITION

45°

FIG. 238-3 ■ Goniotomy *ab interno* head position. The child's head is positioned to permit easy access to the temporal limbus under a goniotomy prism. Generally, with a slightly tilted operating microscope, the head is tilted approximately 45° away from the surgeon, who is seated at the side of the operating table, with the assistant at the head.

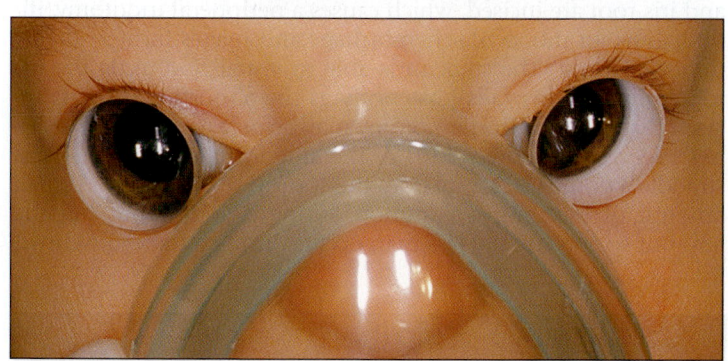

FIG. 238-2 ■ Koeppe gonioprisms permit the simultaneous comparison of the two eyes, particularly useful in asymmetric cases. In this child, the perceived buphthalmos of the right eye was the result of a large coloboma and microphthalmia of the left eye. Gonioscopy of the right eye revealed a normal anterior chamber angle, and the intraocular pressure and optic nerve were normal.

setting for young children who have become accustomed to IOP measurements using the Tonopen.

Gonioscopy is a mandatory part of the examination under anesthetic. It allows the surgeon to identify the underlying congenital or juvenile glaucoma diagnosis and to plan the appropriate surgical approach. The Koeppe gonioscopic lens has significant advantages over other styles of indirect gonioprisms. Chief among these is the ability to compare simultaneously the gonioscopic appearance of two eyes in the same patient (Fig. 238-2). The surgeon must be familiar with the gonioscopic findings in primary congenital glaucoma as well as those of various secondary glaucomas seen in childhood; photography helps to document the appearance of the anterior chamber angle before and after treatment.

Horizontal and vertical corneal diameters and the presence or absence of Haab's striae are noted. Enlargement of the corneal diameter over time is worrisome for progressive buphthalmos, and some clinicians feel these measurements to be more sensitive determinants of progression than axial length determinations.[26] In the author's experience, corneal diameter measurements may be difficult to make accurately or consistently because of uncertain landmarks at the corneoscleral limbus and are best used in conjunction with other measurements.

Cycloplegic retinoscopy during follow-up examinations (both under anesthetic and in the office) are used to monitor for progressive axial myopia as well as to provide the spectacle correction to be used in conjunction with patching and/or other amblyopia therapy.

GENERAL TECHNIQUES

Pediatric glaucoma often presents bilaterally, and the surgeon may have to decide whether to perform bilateral simultaneous surgery. In older patients, most surgeons avoid bilateral intraocular procedures for fear of a rare but disastrous bilateral endophthalmitis. This fear is heightened in pediatric patients but is counterbalanced by the perhaps equal or greater potential for neurological complications or death associated with multiple general anesthetics in infancy and early childhood. In a series of 410 goniotomies performed under 340 anesthetics, Litinsky *et al.*[27] reported no ophthalmic complications associated with the decision to perform bilateral surgery but reported a 1.8% incidence of cardiopulmonary arrest; they concluded that simultaneous bilateral surgery was advisable in bilateral cases. This advice remains appropriate despite advances in anesthetic technique.

Where bilateral surgery is indicated, a fresh, sterile preparation, fresh drapes, and newly autoclaved instruments are used for the second eye. It is the author's preference to perform surgery on the "worse" of the two eyes first, in case the anesthetic is cut short because of cardiopulmonary complications. The "healthier" of the two eyes may withstand the delay better and less disparity of axial length and refraction results from the delay.

SPECIFIC TECHNIQUES

Goniotomy

Goniotomy has changed little since it was first described,[2] but the procedure has been made easier and safer with the introduction of better instruments, viscoelastic materials, and the operating microscope. Excellent visualization of the anterior chamber angle is absolutely necessary. Mild corneal edema may sometimes be overcome by denudation of epithelium from the cornea, but corneal clarity may worsen during the course of surgery. If corneal edema or corneal opacities prevent adequate visualization of the anterior angle structures, a trabeculotomy *ab externo* is performed instead.

It is easiest to perform a goniotomy over the nasal 120° of the anterior chamber angle, using a temporal approach, and this is the usual site for an initial goniotomy. The patient's head is turned away from the surgeon approximately 45° from the vertical and is secured firmly in place (Fig. 238-3). The operating microscope is oriented temporally and is tilted to permit adequate visualization of the nasal anterior chamber angle once the gonioscopic prism has been placed on the eye.

The assistant grasps the eye at the 6 and 12 o'clock positions using toothed forceps to rotate the eye nasally or temporally at will. The surgeon creates a limbal stab incision through the cornea just anterior to the corneoscleral limbus and injects a viscoelastic substance into the anterior chamber to deepen it. If the eye was dilated prior to surgery, a miotic is injected prior to the introduction of the viscoelastic substance.

The Hoskins-Barkan operating gonioprism permits excellent visualization of the anterior chamber angle, allows the assistant to maintain excellent control of the eye, and permits the surgeon to introduce the goniotomy knife through the stab incision (Fig. 238-4). Balanced salt solution is used as the gonioscopic coupling agent.

Various goniotomy knives are available with which to perform a goniotomy; the author prefers a sharp knife with a slight bevel to the handle. Some surgeons prefer irrigation knives and find them helpful to prevent collapse of the anterior chamber; however, when the corneal wound is distorted minimally, collapse of the anterior chamber is not a problem if viscoelastic materials are used.

The stab incision is made just large enough to permit the introduction of the knife. Great care is taken to avoid damage to the crystalline lens as the knife is advanced across the anterior chamber angle (Figs. 238-5 and 238-6). Anterior movement of the lens-iris diaphragm indicates either a stab incision that gapes or an eye that is under external pressure, which permits egress of the anterior chamber fluids. The surgeon determines whether the stab incision has been distorted by the knife handle or is too large; it may be closed partially using a temporary suture.

The abnormal tissue that obstructs aqueous outflow in infantile glaucoma has an almost translucent appearance and blurs and distorts the angle anatomy of the anterior chamber. Infants generally have light blue or transparent iris stroma, which makes the landmarks somewhat difficult to identify; in eyes that have primary congenital glaucoma, the iris root usually has a scalloped, almost serrated anterior edge, which provides an excellent landmark for the surgeon. The goniotomy knife is used to place an incision at the anterior aspect of the middle third of the trabecular meshwork, behind Schwalbe's line; the incision is started at a point 180° away from the corneal incision and rotated either clockwise or counterclockwise as appropriate (see Fig. 238-5). The assistant rotates the eye as needed to permit the surgeon to extend the goniotomy incision peripherally without distortion of the corneal incision. The knife is then flipped 180° and the goniotomy is completed in the opposite direction.

If the incision is placed too far anteriorly, the goniotomy does not function; if placed too far posteriorly, only the peripheral iris and iris root are incised, which causes a peripheral iridotomy, iridodialysis, or intraocular hemorrhage and makes further surgery difficult at best. The surgeon is able to visualize directly the iris root, which gently falls posteriorly as the abnormal tissue is incised (Fig. 238-7). The goniotomy may be performed in this manner over approximately 120° of the anterior chamber angle and straddle a point 180° away from the corneal stab incision. A small amount of bleeding is common during a goniotomy, but the amount seen is usually less than occurs during a trabeculotomy.

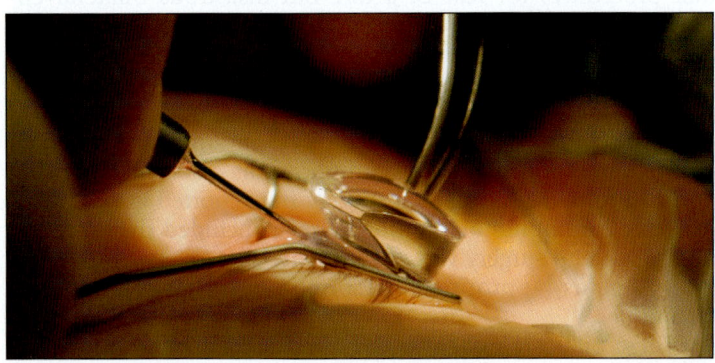

FIG. 238-4 ■ Goniotomy *ab interno*. The Hoskins-Barkan lens provides a clear, magnified view of the anterior chamber angle while simultaneously allowing the introduction of the goniotomy knife at the limbus.

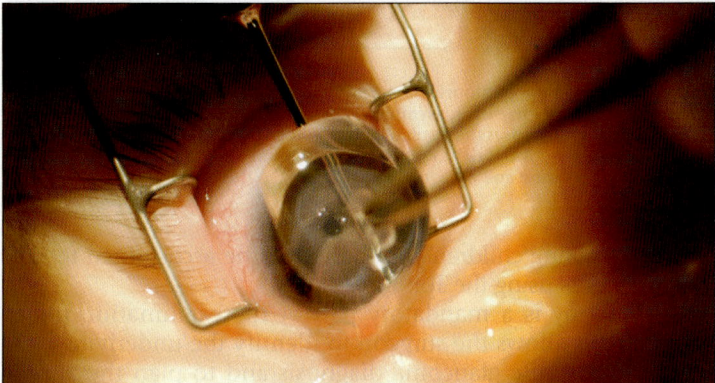

FIG. 238-6 ■ Goniotomy *ab interno*. Operative photograph demonstrating the goniotomy knife advancing across the anterior chamber.

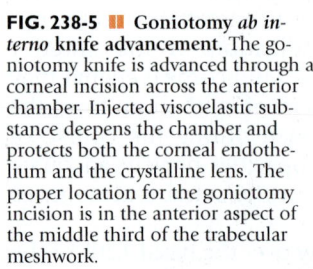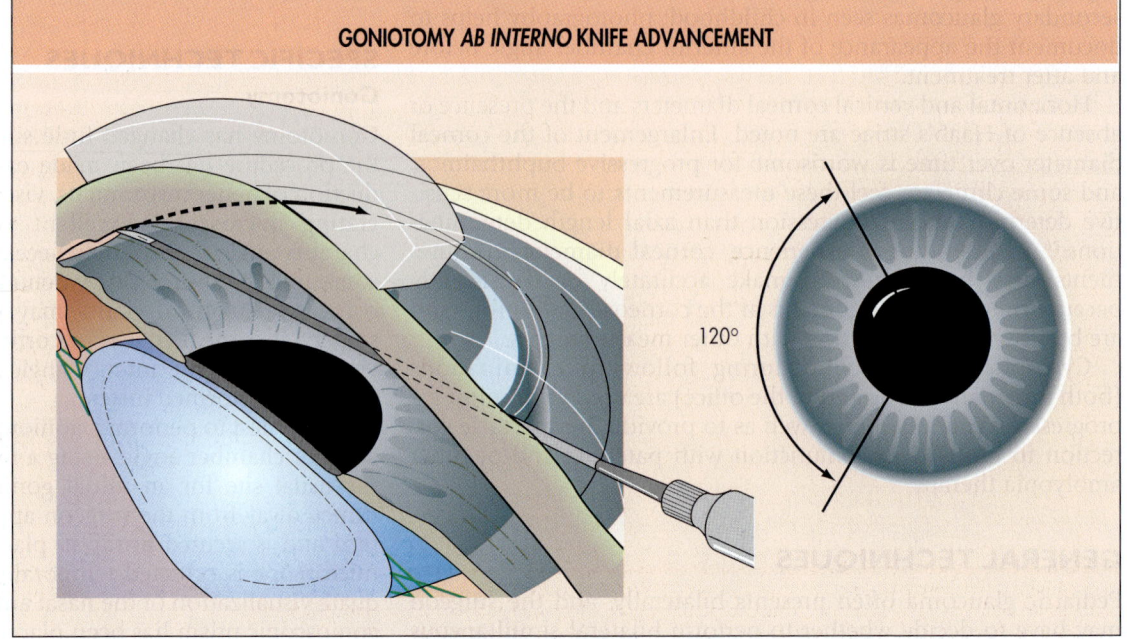

FIG. 238-5 ■ Goniotomy *ab interno* knife advancement. The goniotomy knife is advanced through a corneal incision across the anterior chamber. Injected viscoelastic substance deepens the chamber and protects both the corneal endothelium and the crystalline lens. The proper location for the goniotomy incision is in the anterior aspect of the middle third of the trabecular meshwork.

GONIOTOMY *AB INTERNO* KNIFE ADVANCEMENT

120°

At the conclusion of the procedure, the remaining viscoelastic material is flushed from the eye. The corneal stab incision, although usually self-sealing, may be closed using a single 10-0 nylon suture. Subconjunctival injections of a corticosteroid and antibiotic are usually given.

Trabeculotomy

As with goniotomy, trabeculotomy *ab externo* has been made easier and safer by the introduction of viscoelastic materials and the operating microscope. The child's eye is prepared and draped in a manner similar to that for adult eye surgery. If a superior approach is planned, a superior rectus bridle suture or corneal traction sutures may be placed to depress and expose the superior limbal region. The author prefers to perform trabeculotomy at the temporal limbus, leaving the superior conjunctiva untouched for subsequent filtration procedures if required. A lateral canthotomy may be performed to provide adequate exposure in small or premature infants.

A limbal peritomy is performed and a partial-thickness scleral flap (either rectangular or triangular) is created to sit astride the corneoscleral junction (Fig. 238-8). Excessive cautery is avoided, as the deeper layers of the tissues may be distorted and Schlemm's canal made difficult to identify.

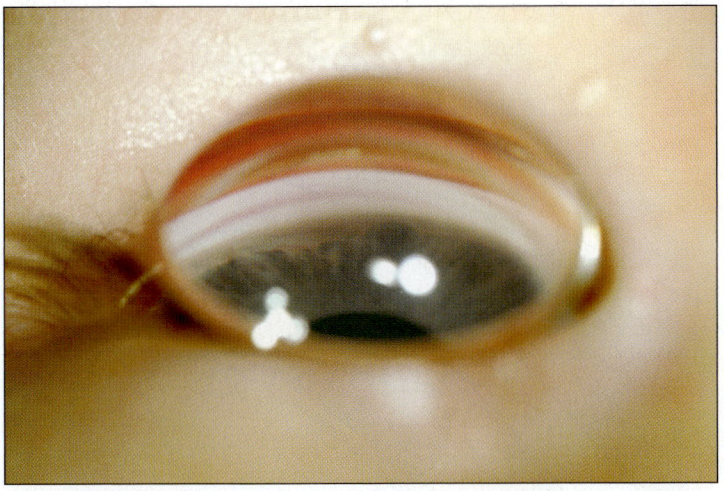

FIG. 238-7 ■ **Treated and untreated regions of the anterior chamber angle.** Gonioscopy demonstrates a region of treated angle (to the left of center) in which the iris insertion has fallen back nicely; the untreated angle (to the right) shows the typical high insertion of the iris.

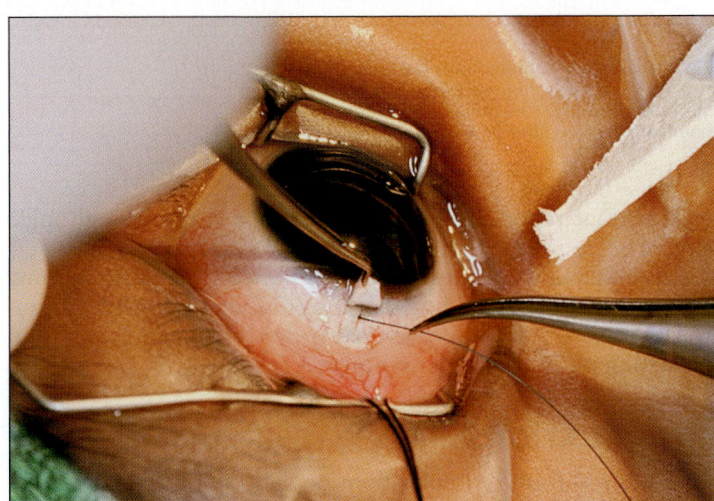

FIG. 238-8 ■ **Trabeculotomy *ab externo*.** A partial-thickness scleral flap is developed to straddle the corneoscleral junction. A radial incision that measures about 2mm is made using a microsurgery blade, with successive layers gradually pared away to unroof Schlemm's canal. The canal is identified correctly by cannulation using a 6-0 suture of nylon or polypropylene.

Schlemm's canal lies just below the transition from white scleral fibers to the blue corneal fibers. A radial incision that measures approximately 2mm in length and straddles the corneoscleral limbus is made in the bed of the scleral flap. Schlemm's canal is unroofed by a careful dissection layer by layer until the egress of a small amount of aqueous humor is observed without shallowing of the anterior chamber. Shallowing of the chamber and forward movement of the lens-iris diaphragm indicate that the anterior chamber has been violated directly. If this occurs and it becomes impossible to cannulate Schlemm's canal, the flap is closed, the anterior chamber is deepened using a viscoelastic substance, and another site is developed.

A short length of 6-0 black nylon or blue polypropylene suture material is then used to cannulate Schlemm's canal. The suture must not be introduced into Schlemm's canal forcibly, in case a false passage is created. Slight resistance followed by little or no resistance may indicate that the suture has passed into the suprachoroidal space or into the posterior chamber behind the iris and in front of the crystalline lens. If the suture is bent gently, it should snap back into an orientation tangential to the canal; movement of the peripheral iris in this maneuver indicates that the suture has entered the posterior chamber. In general, the suture passes easily if Schlemm's canal has been cannulated correctly; intraoperative gonioscopy using either a Koeppe lens or a Zeiss four-mirror gonioprism (Fig. 238-9) may be used to verify correct placement.

Once Schlemm's canal has been cannulated successfully in both clockwise and counterclockwise directions, a trabeculotome that has an appropriate curvature for the particular eye is chosen. The lower probe of the trabeculotome is introduced into Schlemm's canal and passed along this in a curvilinear fashion; the upper probe is used as a guide to confirm the location of the lower one (Fig. 238-10). This upper probe is crucial to make certain that the lower probe is oriented in such a way that upon its rotation it ruptures Schlemm's canal internally, passes parallel to the iris, and does not impinge upon the crystalline lens (see Fig. 238-11).

A small amount of bleeding and egress of aqueous humor usually occurs at the base of the trabeculotome probe. If the chamber shallows, viscoelastic may be introduced so that the second trabeculotome can be rotated in the opposite direction without risk to the crystalline lens.

Once the trabeculotomy has been performed on either side of the incision, the overlying scleral flap may be closed using 10-0 nylon. The overlying conjunctiva is tacked over the scleral flap

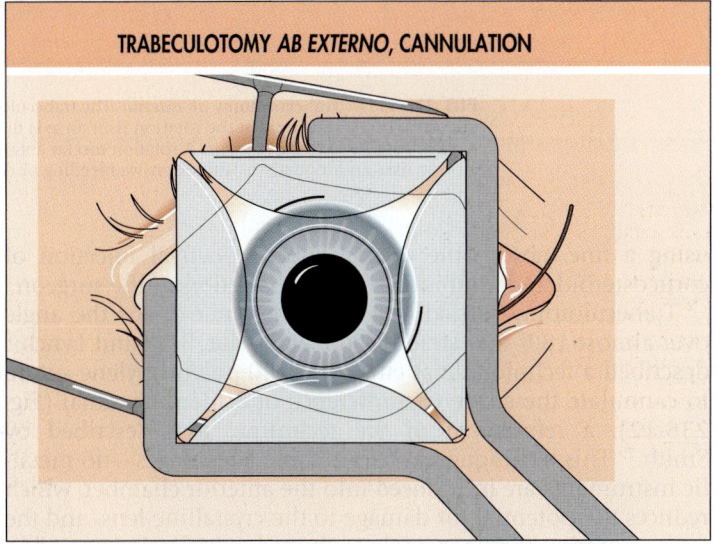

FIG. 238-9 ■ **Trabeculotomy *ab externo*, cannulation.** Correct cannulation of Schlemm's canal may be confirmed using a Zeiss four-mirror gonioprism lens intraoperatively.

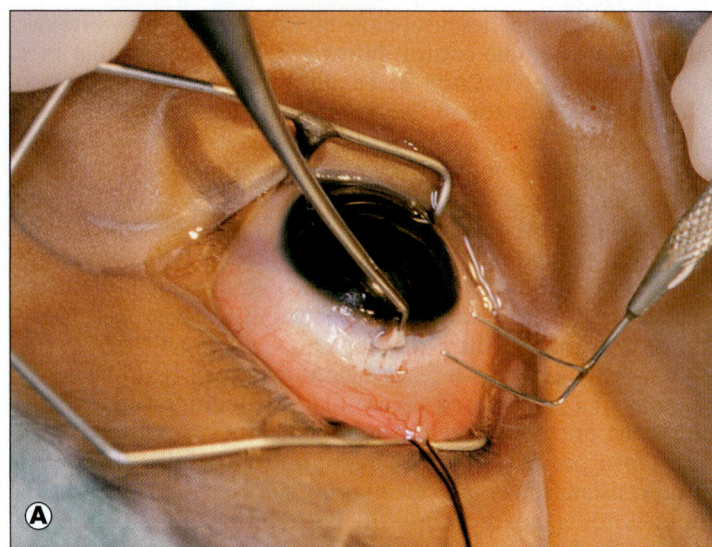

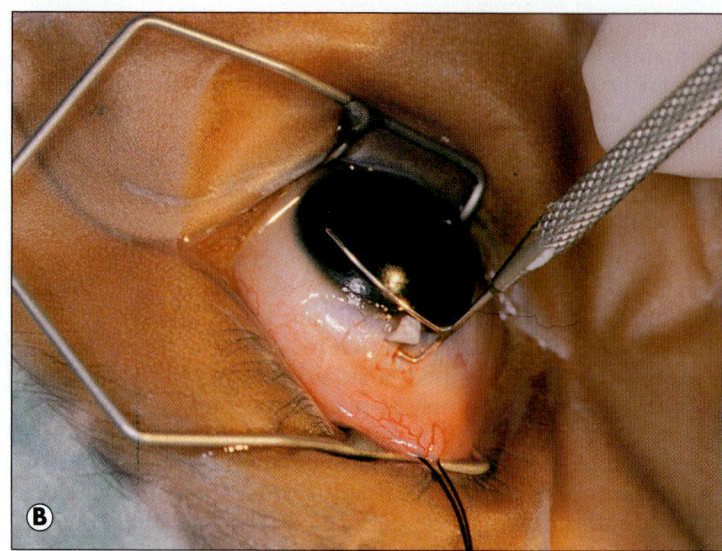

FIG. 238-10 ■ *Trabeculotomy ab externo.* **A,** The upper probe of the instrument provides the surgeon with a three-dimensional cue to the orientation of the lower cannulation probe. **B,** The lower probe of the trabeculotome is inserted into Schlemm's canal. If the canal has been cannulated properly, there should be little resistance to the passage of the probe.

TRABECULOTOMY *AB EXTERNO*

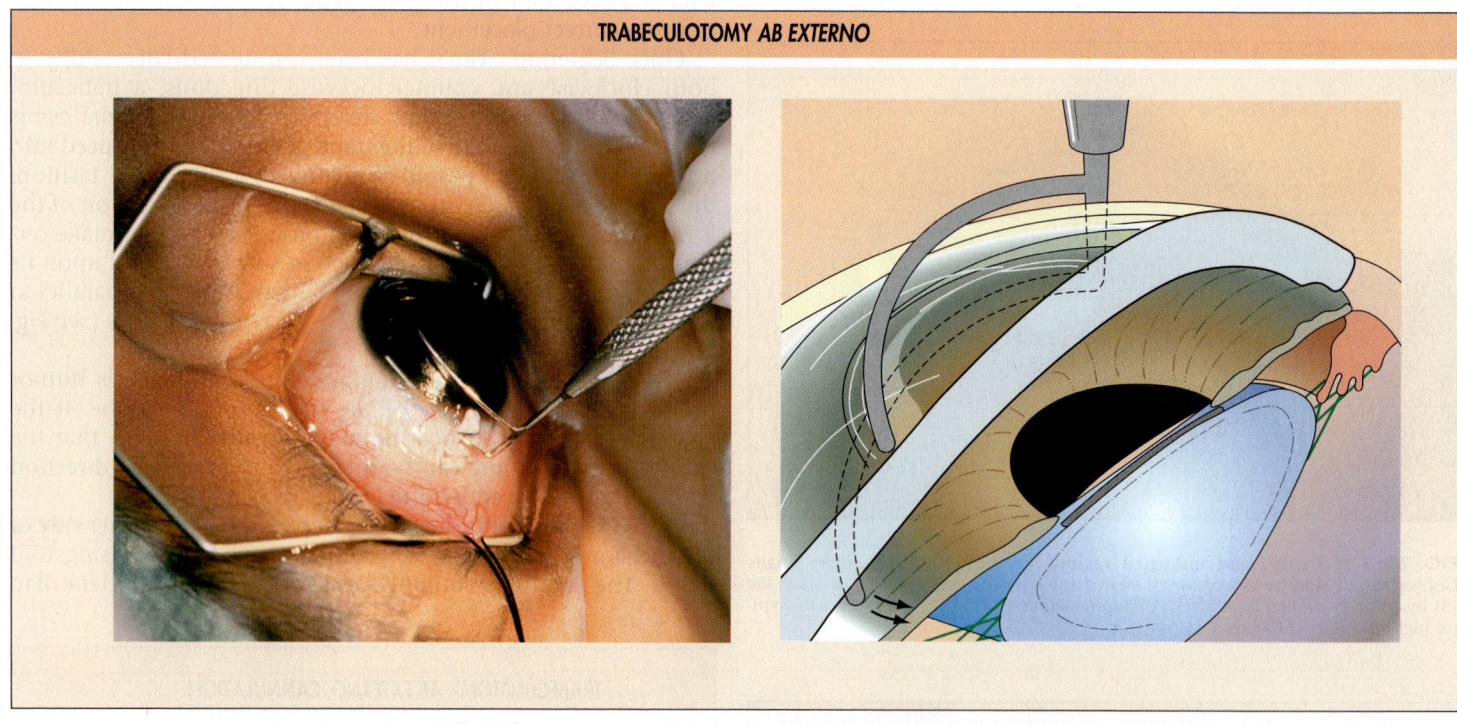

FIG. 238-11 ■ *Trabeculotomy ab externo.* The trabeculotome is rotated into the anterior chamber. The surgeon must take great care to ensure that the rotation is in an axis that brings the lower trabeculotome probe into the chamber in a plane parallel to that of the iris. A rotation too far anteriorly may strip Descemet's membrane; a rotation too far posteriorly risks an iridodialysis with extensive bleeding or direct trauma to the crystalline lens.

using a fine, absorbable suture. Subconjunctival injection of corticosteroid and antibiotic is at the discretion of the surgeon.

Trabeculotomy carried out in this manner opens the angle over almost 180° and straddles the entry site. Beck and Lynch[28] described a technique that employs a 6-0 polypropylene suture to cannulate the entire circumference of Schlemm's canal (Fig. 238-12), a refinement of the technique first described by Smith.[29] This technique has two notable advantages—no metallic instruments are introduced into the anterior chamber, which reduces the potential for damage to the crystalline lens, and the entire anterior chamber angle is treated, which obviates additional angle surgery if the primary surgery fails. Mendicino *et al.*[30] performed a retrospective review of 360° trabeculotomy versus goniotomy, reporting that the 360° procedure was at least as successful as multiple goniotomies and overall success was bet-

ter than that reported in the literature for conventional angle surgery.

Other surgeons advocate the combination of trabeculotomy and trabeculectomy, finding that the combination results in improved results[31]; this approach has proved particularly useful in the setting of Sturge-Weber syndrome.[32]

COMPLICATIONS

The two most feared complications of glaucoma surgery, endophthalmitis and choroidal hemorrhage, are exceedingly rare in published clinical series of goniotomy or trabeculotomy. Both procedures are remarkably safe when performed correctly, and few complications that threaten sight are associated with either. During both procedures, the crystalline lens may be damaged by

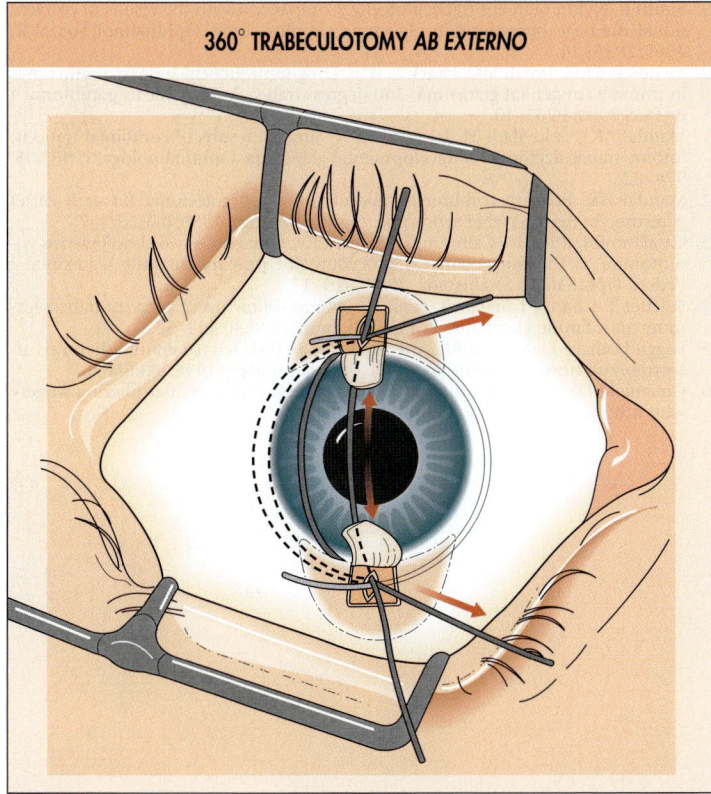

360° TRABECULOTOMY *AB EXTERNO*

FIG. 238-12 ▮ Trabeculotomy *ab externo.* In a modification of the technique of Beck and Lynch,[28] the entire 360° circumference of Schlemm's canal is cannulated, using both ends of the suture to "cheesewire" the suture into the anterior chamber.

the instruments in the anterior chamber, but this is avoided by careful technique and the use of intracameral miotics and viscoelastic materials. During trabeculotomy, improper axial alignment of the trabeculotome may strip Descemet's membrane peripherally (which results in localized corneal edema and scarring), cause an iridodialysis with massive intraocular bleeding, or result in direct trauma to the crystalline lens. During both procedures, a small amount of blood is usually released into the anterior chamber; if no viscoelastic substance is retained in the eye, the blood is usually gone by the first or second postoperative day.

OUTCOMES

In a prospective clinical trial in which bilaterally affected patients underwent trabeculotomy in one eye and goniotomy in the other, Anderson[9] reported a success rate of 76% after the first trabeculotomy, and 81% after the first goniotomy. A second procedure raised the ultimate success rate to 92% for trabeculotomy and 100% for goniotomy. The study was small, and the differences were not statistically significant. In the patients uncontrolled after the first operation, both eyes usually required a second procedure, which indicates that the underlying disease, rather than the chosen procedure, is the reason for poor control. In Anderson's study, patients who presented at birth were excluded from analysis; this and many other series confirm the clinical impression that disease presentation at birth, additional anterior segment anomalies such as Peter's anomaly, aniridia, and gross buphthalmos are all risk factors for the failure of angle surgery and indicate severe, underlying anatomical abnormalities. Various clinical series suggest that success rates approach 100% for both procedures in infants who present with isolated infantile glaucoma during the first year of life.

The need for a second procedure in some patients has raised the possibility that it might be advantageous to perform two simultaneous goniotomies. In a prospective, randomized study of patients with bilateral infantile glaucoma, Catalano *et al.*[33] found no significant difference between eyes that underwent a single goniotomy at initial surgery and those that underwent two simultaneous procedures.

With its high success rate and low short- and long-term complication rates in infantile glaucoma, it seems apparent that, with rare exceptions, angle surgery is preferred as the initial therapy for the rare disorders discussed here. In cases in which one or two angle surgery procedures have failed to control the disease, trabeculectomy with the adjunctive use of mitomycin seems a reasonable next step.

Several series of primary trabeculectomies in children have been published, with intermediate-term success comparable to that of angle surgery.[34] With the incidence of bleb infections and endophthalmitis estimated to be as high as 3% per year in antimetabolite-augmented blebs,[35,36] it is doubtful whether filtration surgery should be considered primary therapy in pediatric patients if a reasonable chance of success exists with angle surgery. In patients who are aphakic or are likely to become so in the near future, a tube-shunt procedure, such as the Molteno or Baerveldt implant, may be of particular help to permit safer contact lens use and reduce the risk of bleb-associated endophthalmitis.

The surgeon who contemplates the surgical management of infantile glaucoma must recognize that the management of this disorder only begins with the surgical procedure. Despite high success rates (if IOP is considered the sole criterion for success) for both procedures, many children affected by the disorders discussed here grow into adulthood with significant visual impairment because of amblyopia, media opacities, and glaucomatous optic neuropathy. The postoperative care of these children lasts a decade or more, with periodic examinations under anesthetic in infancy and early childhood, frequent cycloplegic refractions, amblyopia therapy, and additional surgery as needed. Once IOP is normalized by surgery, amblyopia becomes the problem; thus, clinical series that report only short-term results with no extended follow-up into the years after visual maturation tend to overestimate the true success of treatment. Only if amblyopia is monitored vigilantly and treatment is aggressive can the full promise of goniotomy and trabeculotomy be realized and patients mature into adulthood with normal vision preserved.

REFERENCES

1. de Vincentiis C. Incisione del L'angolo irideo Nel Glaucoma. Ann Ottalmol. 1893;22:540.
2. Barkan O. A new operation for chronic glaucoma. Restoration of physiological function by opening Schlemm's canal under direct magnified vision. Am J Ophthalmol. 1936;19:951–65.
3. Barkan O. Technic of goniotomy. Arch Ophthalmol. 1938;19:217–23.
4. Barkan O. Operation for congenital glaucoma. Am J Ophthalmol. 1942;25:552–68.
5. Burian HM. A case of Marfan's syndrome with bilateral glaucoma with description of a new type of operation for developmental glaucoma (trabeculotomy ab externo). Am J Ophthalmol. 1960;50:1187.
6. Smith R. A new technique for opening the canal of Schlemm. Br J Ophthalmol. 1960;44:370–3.
7. Dannheim R, Harms H. Tecnik, Erfolge und Wirkungsweise der Trabekulotomie [Technic, success and mode of action of trabeculotomy]. Klin Monatsbl Augenheilkd. 1969;155:630–7.
8. McPherson SD Jr. Results of external trabeculotomy. Am J Ophthalmol. 1973;76:918–20.
9. Anderson DR. Trabeculotomy compared to goniotomy for glaucoma in children. Ophthalmology. 1983;90:805–6.
10. McPherson SD Jr, Berry DP. Goniotomy vs external trabeculotomy for developmental glaucoma. Am J Ophthalmol. 1983;95:427–31.
11. Bordon AF, Katsumi O, Hirose T. Tonometry in pediatric patients: a comparative study among Tono-pen, Perkins, and Schiotz tonometers. J Pediatr Ophthalmol Strabismus. 1995;32:373–7.
12. Dietlein TS, Jacobi PC, Krieglstein GK. [Clinical discrepancy between Schiotz and Perkins tonometry in juvenile glaucoma]. Klin Monatsbl Augenheilkd. 1996;209:299–303; discussion 298.
13. Pensiero S, Da Pozzo S, Perissutti P, et al. Normal intraocular pressure in children. J Pediatr Ophthalmol Strabismus. 1992;29:79–84.
14. Boger WPD. Timolol in childhood glaucoma. Surv Ophthalmol. 1983;28(Suppl):259–61.
15. Olson RJ, Bromberg BB, Zimmerman TJ. Apneic spells associated with timolol therapy in a neonate. Am J Ophthalmol. 1979;88:120–2.
16. Anderson JR. Hydrophthalmia or congenital glaucoma—its causes, treatment and outlook. London: Cambridge University Press; 1939:377.
17. Carlsen JO, Zabriskie NA, Kwon YH, et al. Apparent central nervous system depression in infants after the use of topical brimonidine. Am J Ophthalmol. 1999;128:255–6.
18. Yang CB, Freedman SF, Myers JS, et al. Use of latanoprost in the treatment of glaucoma associated with Sturge-Weber syndrome. Am J Ophthalmol. 1998;126:600–2.

19. Ausinsch B, Munson ES, Levy NS. Intraocular pressures in children with glaucoma during halothane anesthesia. Ann Ophthalmol. 1977;9:1391–4.

20. Mehta S, Dugmore WN, Raichand M. Ketamine in paediatric ophthalmic practice. Anaesthesia. 1972;27:460–3.

21. Ferrari LR, Donlon JV. A comparison of propofol, midazolam, and methohexital for sedation during retrobulbar and peribulbar block. J Clin Anesth. 1992;4: 93–6.

22. Robertson EN, Hull JM, Verbeek AM, Booij LH. A comparison of rocuronium and vecuronium: the pharmacodynamic, cardiovascular and intra-ocular effects. Eur J Anaesthesiol Suppl. 1994;9:116–21.

23. Quigley HA. Childhood glaucoma: results with trabeculotomy and study of reversible cupping. Ophthalmology. 1982;89:219–26.

24. Sampaolesi R, Caruso R. Ocular echometry in the diagnosis of congenital glaucoma. Arch Ophthalmol. 1982;100:574–7.

25. Kiefer G, Schwenn O, Grehn F. Correlation of postoperative axial length growth and intraocular pressure in congenital glaucoma—a retrospective study in trabeculotomy and goniotomy. Graefes Arch Clin Exp Ophthalmol. 2001;239:893–9.

26. Kiskis AA, Markowitz SN, Morin JD. Corneal diameter and axial length in congenital glaucoma. Can J Ophthalmol. 1985;20:93–7.

27. Litinsky SM, Shaffer RN, Hetherington J, Hoskins HD. Operative complications of goniotomy. Trans Am Acad Ophthalmol Otolaryngol. 1977;83:78–9.

28. Beck AD, Lynch MG. 360 Degrees trabeculotomy for primary congenital glaucoma. Arch Ophthalmol. 1995;113:1200–2.

29. Smith R. Nylon filament trabeculotomy. Comparison with the results of conventional drainage operations in glaucoma simplex. Trans Ophthalmol Soc N Z. 1969;21:15–26.

30. Mendicino ME, Lynch MG, Drack A, et al. Long-term surgical and visual outcomes in primary congenital glaucoma: 360 degrees trabeculotomy versus goniotomy. J AAPOS 2000;4:205–10.

31. Mandal AK, Naduvilath TJ, Jayagandan A. Surgical results of combined trabeculotomy-trabeculectomy for developmental glaucoma. Ophthalmology. 1998;105: 974–82.

32. Mandal AK. Primary combined trabeculotomy-trabeculectomy for early-onset glaucoma in Sturge-Weber syndrome. Ophthalmology. 1999;106:1621–7.

33. Catalano RA, King RA, Calhoun JH, Sargent RA. One versus two simultaneous goniotomies as the initial surgical procedure for primary infantile glaucoma. J Pediatr Ophthalmol Strabismus. 1989;26:9–13.

34. Fulcher T, Chan J, Lanigan B, et al. Long-term follow up of primary trabeculectomy for infantile glaucoma. Br J Ophthalmol 1996;80:499–502.

35. Higginbotham EJ, Stevens RK, Musch DC, et al. Bleb-related endophthalmitis after trabeculectomy with mitomycin C. Ophthalmology. 1996;103:650–6.

36. Greenfield DS, Suner IJ, Miller MP, et al. Endophthalmitis after filtering surgery with mitomycin. Arch Ophthalmol. 1996;114:943–9.

CHAPTER 239

Nonpenetrating Glaucoma Surgery

ELIE DAHAN • TAREK SHAARAWY • ANDRE MERMOUD • JEFFREY FREEDMAN

DEFINITION

- Nonpenetrating glaucoma surgery (NPGS) refers to drainage procedures that restore aqueous humor filtration through a natural membrane, namely the trabecular meshwork. NPGS includes all the different surgical techniques previously named: trabeculectomy ab-externo, nonpenetrating deep sclerotomy, and viscocanalostomy.

KEY FEATURES

- Schlemm's canal.
- Trabecular meshwork.
- Descemet's membrane.

INTRODUCTION

The quest for a low-risk and effective glaucoma operation has prompted a growing interest in the nonpenetrating techniques because of their lower complication rate. During nonpenetrating glaucoma surgery (NPGS), the intraocular pressure (IOP) is gradually lowered (Fig. 239-1), flat anterior chambers practically do not occur postoperatively, and complicated blebs are less common. A less obvious but important reason for developing NPGS is the fact that during the procedure, the surgeon unveils the site of pathology, namely the trabecular meshwork (TM). Whereas gonioscopy permits examination of the angle and the anterior part of the TM, NPGS allows examination of its posterior part, where the main resistance to outflow exists. Therefore, NPGS is not just another drainage operation because it also offers the opportunity of evaluating the TM functionality.

When Schlemm's canal is unroofed and the TM is exposed, aqueous humor can be seen percolating in various amounts according to the severity of the disease. The experienced NPGS surgeon can recognize different types of TMs and tailor, accordingly, the next surgical steps to be taken to improve filtration. At present, peeling and thinning out the TM manually can improve filtration. In the future, drugs or lasers could be developed to restore normal filtration by direct topical application on the TM. At present, glaucoma surgery is deferred until medications and laser interventions fail to lower the IOP to acceptable levels. This current teaching is questioned because of the accumulating evidence that topical antiglaucoma medications have adverse effects on the success of glaucoma surgery. A certain percentage of glaucoma patients need surgery, sooner or later, to reach their safe target IOP. These patients could benefit from early surgery rather than wait for medications and laser failure. Early surgery in the form of NPGS in eyes with an unaltered conjunctiva will be beneficial for these patients who cannot reach their safe target IOP with medications or laser alone. The evolving NPGS has gradually approached this goal during the last decade with the advent of refinements in surgical techniques, improvements in surgical instruments, and modern surgical microscopes.

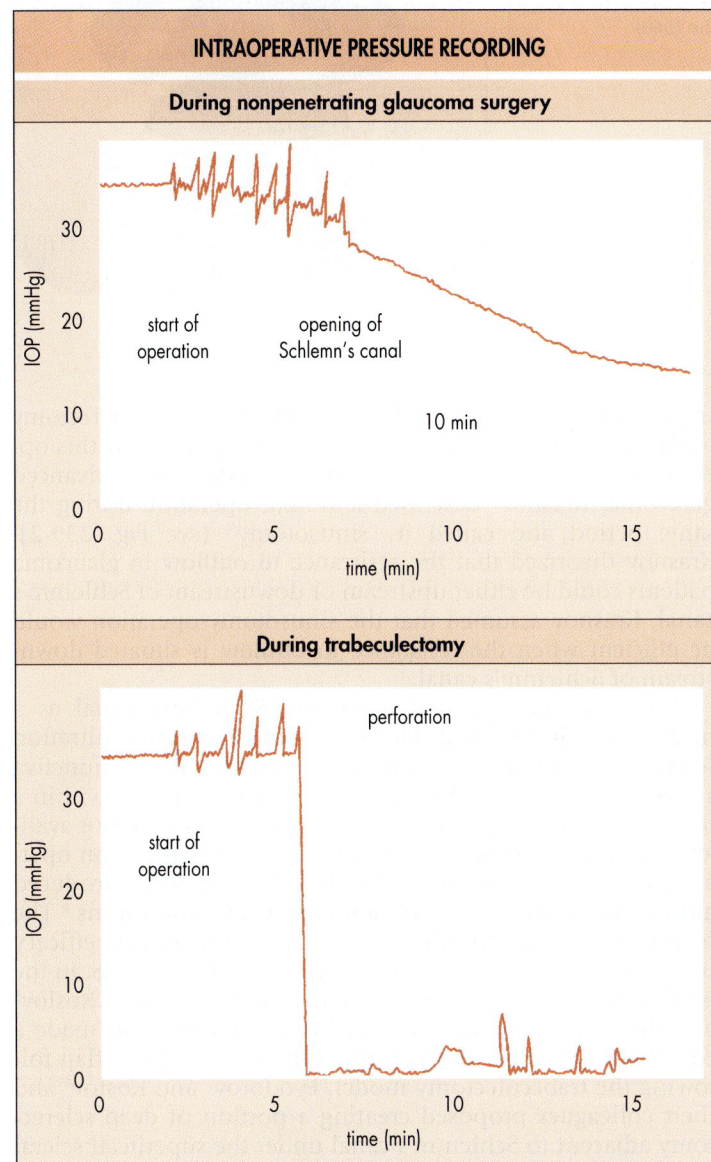

FIG. 239-1 ■ Comparison of intraocular pressure recordings during nonpenetrating and penetrating glaucoma surgeries. Intraoperative intraocular pressure recording during nonpenetrating glaucoma surgery *(top graph)* and during trabeculectomy *(bottom graph)*. (Courtesy of Andre Mermoud, MD.)

HISTORICAL REVIEW

The evolution of NPGS started relatively slowly with the original works of Epstein[1] and Krasnov[2] in the late 1950s and early 1960s. Epstein[1] noticed aqueous humor oozing from the paralimbal sclera when he dissected deeply seated pterygiae and deducted that paralimbal deep sclerectomy could be performed, intentionally, to lower IOP in glaucoma patients. Epstein[1] then described an operation that consisted of a paralimbal deep sclerectomy overlying Schlemm's canal, over 180°, without enter-

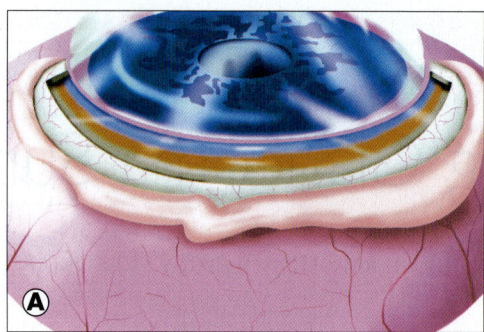

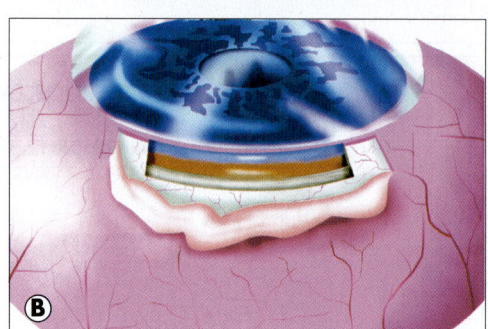

FIG. 239-2 ■ Early non-penetrating glaucoma surgeries. **A,** "Paralimbal deep sclerectomy" as described by Edward Epstein in 1959. **B,** "Sinusotomy" as described by Krasnov in the 1960s.

ing the anterior chamber (Fig. 239-2). The deep sclerectomy was then covered with conjunctiva. Epstein performed this operation in South African black patients with severe advanced glaucoma. Krasnov[2] described a similar operation during the same period and called it "sinusotomy" (see Fig. 239-2). Krasnov theorized that the resistance to outflow in glaucoma patients could be either upstream or downstream of Schlemm's canal. Krasnov assumed that the sinusotomy operation would be efficient when the resistance to outflow is situated downstream of Schlemm's canal.

Both authors suggested unroofing Schlemm's canal as a means of reducing IOP. The longevity of effective filtration with these early methods was relatively short. The conjunctiva scarred over the bare TM, blocking effective filtration within a few months. High-quality surgical microscopes were not available yet and few surgeons could perform these filtration operations. Moreover, the classical trabeculectomy was introduced almost concurrently, or soon after, by Sugar[3] and Cairns.[4] The relative ease of performing a trabeculectomy and its efficacy overshadowed and held back the development of NPGS. In the early 1980s, the Russian school led by Fyodorov[5] and Koslov[6] and the North American school led by Zimmerman[7] made a comeback for NPGS and performed it under a scleral flap following the trabeculectomy model. Fyodorov[5] and Koslov[6] and their colleagues proposed creating a portion of deep sclerectomy adjacent to Schlemm's canal under the superficial scleral flap. The deep sclerectomy was supposed to enhance intrascleral and uveal aqueous humor absorption. The scleral flap added some protection to the bare TM and somewhat improved the results of NPGS. At present, NPGS is still an evolving surgical technique, which has evoked growing interest in the last decade because of its low rate of complications.[5–26] Proponents and opponents argue about the efficacy and longevity of NPGS versus the classical trabeculectomy. The opponents of NPGS claim that classical trabeculectomy yields lower IOP and has greater longevity.[27–30] The proponents of NPGS still prefer it to the classical trabeculectomy because of its superior safety profile.[5–26,31,32] Because NPGS requires a long learning curve and more dexterity than the classical trabeculectomy, its proponents claim that the NPGS opponents have not yet mastered the technique. The long learning curve of NPGS explains the differences in the reported comparisons in the two different techniques.

INDICATIONS AND CONTRAINDICATIONS FOR NPGS

Indications

In general, the indications for NPGS are wider and more inclusive than those for classical trabeculectomies for two reasons: NPGS is safer but not less efficient than trabeculectomies,[5–26] and NPGS is indicated in certain types of glaucoma in which trabeculectomies normally fail or are not possible.

Until the advent of NPGS, penetrating glaucoma surgery was generally regarded as the last resort in the treatment of glaucoma. When medical therapy and laser failed to lower IOP to an acceptable level, glaucomatologists explained to their patients that an operation was necessary to halt the progression of the disease. NPGS, with its lower complication rate, can be offered earlier in the course of the disease. In fact, NPGS can be offered as a first-line treatment in cases in which it is obvious that medical treatment will not lower IOP to acceptable levels. This factor is particularly important in glaucoma patients younger than 50 years of age who have a longer life span. Several decades of continuous medical treatment are not sustainable because of the numerous side effects of antiglaucoma drugs. Furthermore, glaucoma surgery in general and NPGS in particular are more successful in glaucoma patients who were not exposed to medical treatment.[19,21,33–39] The noxious effects of topical medications on the conjunctiva are well documented.[33–39] The conjunctival tissues undergo scarring processes when exposed to certain topical medications. Such histologically altered conjunctiva is less amenable to the formation of a healthy diffuse bleb than a "virgin" conjunctiva. It is possible that even the TM undergoes biochemical-structural changes after years of medical treatment, rendering it less responsive to NPGS. It is therefore logical to propose NPGS earlier rather than later when the chances of favourable outcomes are greater.[21]

OPEN-ANGLE GLAUCOMA. Open-angle glaucoma is the most common type of glaucoma and NPGS targets the presumed site of pathology, namely the TM. During NPGS, the TM is exposed and examined by the surgeon, who can assess on site the amount of filtration *in vivo*. With experience, different types of TMs can be recognized and classified according to their appearances and filtration capacities. NPGS has the advantage of being less cataractogenic than trabeculectomy and eventually may replace it in phakic open-angle glaucoma patients.[5–26]

GLAUCOMA PATIENTS WITH HIGH MYOPIA. Trabeculectomies in patients with high myopia carry an especially high risk of complications because of their abnormal globe dimensions. Choroidal detachments and consequent shallow anterior chambers occur in 10–15% of trabeculectomies done in high-myopic glaucoma patients.[40] The factors predisposing myopic eyes to choroidal effusion may be related to the larger intraocular volume of myopic eyes, to the thinner sclera, and to vulnerable choroidal blood vessels.[40] NPGS appears to offer glaucoma patients with high myopia a safer outcome because of the gradual intraoperative IOP reduction[23] (see Fig. 239-1).

PIGMENTARY GLAUCOMA. NPGS may be the treatment of choice for pigmentary glaucoma because the condition is very resistant to medical treatment. Pigmentary glaucoma occurs more frequently in young myopic male adults, and it is better to offer a safe surgical solution without depending on complex combination medical treatment. NPGS targets the site of pathology, namely the pigment-loaded TM, which can be reconditioned to reestablish filtration.

PSEUDOEXFOLIATION GLAUCOMA. Pseudoexfoliation glaucoma is a form of open-angle glaucoma in which there is accumulation of exfoliation material along the aqueous outflow pathways. Because the exfoliation material is found in abundance in the TM and Schlemm's canal, NPGS may be the treatment of choice for this condition. Opening Schlemm's canal in the pseudoexfoliation patient is spectacular. This material can be peeled away from the exposed TM to reestablish filtration. IOP drops to acceptable levels for several years, and when exfoliation material accumulates again, the site of filtration can be revised to restore filtration. NPGS can be done alone or in conjunction with cataract extraction according to the patient's age, cataract status, and refractive error.

APHAKIC AND PSEUDOPHAKIC GLAUCOMA. In aphakic glaucoma, iridectomy is not desirable because the vitreous moves forward through the iridectomy and blocks the filtration site. Extensive basal vitrectomy is needed to prevent blockage, but it is difficult to accomplish. Traction retinal detachment is not an uncommon complication in these combined vitrectomy-trabeculectomies. NPGS does not require iridectomy; therefore it may be particularly indicated in aphakic glaucoma. The only drawback of NPGS in aphakic glaucoma is the status of the TM. When aphakia has been long-standing, the TM is often collapsed and scarred; restoration of its function depends on its status and on the surgeon's experience and skill. In many instances, the conjunctiva and the limbus are severely scarred by previous surgeries. The appropriate site for NPGS in aphakic glaucoma should be free of previous surgical scars.

CONGENITAL AND JUVENILE GLAUCOMA. Congenital and juvenile glaucoma is severe and results in rapid optic nerve damage and loss of vision. Surgery is practically the only treatment available for these patients and, whenever possible, NPGS may be attempted first because of its low complication rate. The degree of success of NPGS is a function of the angle structure malformation and the surgeon's experience. NPGS will succeed more in cases in which the pathological anatomy of the angle is not extreme. When NPGS fails, it is always possible to revert to penetrating glaucoma surgery, particularly in cases where the anatomy is severely distorted.

STURGE-WEBER SYNDROME. Sturge-Weber syndrome, a cutaneous hemangiomatous disorder, is often associated with congenital or developmental glaucoma. The greater numbers and tortuosity of the conjunctival blood vessels can be an indicator of glaucoma. Choroidal effusions following fistulizing surgery are notoriously known in these patients, and NPGS offers a safer alternative.

ANIRIDIA AND ANTERIOR SEGMENT DYSGENESIS SYNDROMES. The success of NPGS in aniridia and anterior segment dysgenesis cases is dependent on the degree of anatomical distortion in Schlemm's canal and TM. Schlemm's canal rudiments are often seen in these cases. In aniridia and anterior segment dysgenesis syndromes the trabeculum is abnormal and it is possible to predict intraoperatively which cases will respond to NPGS according to the amount of filtration observed during the operation.

GLAUCOMA SECONDARY TO UVEITIS. When elevated IOP persists after uveitis has been under control, glaucoma surgery is indicated. NPGS is indicated in these cases because it explores the site of resistance to aqueous outflow. During the inflammatory phases, the TM ultrastructures undergo changes that interfere with their normal function. These changes are mostly temporary, but when they are permanent glaucoma results. The TM can be reconditioned to improve filtration. Nevertheless, in cases in which multiple peripheral anterior synechiae have occurred, NPGS may not offer an efficient solution.

Relative Contraindications

NARROW-ANGLE GLAUCOMA. Laser iridotomy or surgical iridectomy is mostly a temporary measure in narrow-angle glaucoma. Cataract extraction or removal of the crystalline lens deepens the anterior chamber and opens the angle of the eye. When narrow-angle glaucoma has persisted for a certain length of time, glaucoma surgery is indicated in combination with lens extraction. For these combined operations, NPGS may be attempted, even though the iris root is very close to the TM and effective filtration may not occur immediately.

STATUS AFTER LASER TRABECULOPLASTY. In eyes previously treated by laser trabeculoplasty, the TM may not be intact and might rupture during surgery. NPGS can be then converted to classical trabeculectomy.

AFTER TRAUMA ANGLE-RECESSION GLAUCOMA. In traumatic angle-recession glaucoma, the TM loses its functionality because of scarification processes. NPGS can be attempted, however, because damage to the TM is not always complete and its functionality might be restored by scraping and peeling its posterior surface.

Absolute Contraindications: Neovascular Glaucoma

NPGS will fail in neovascular glaucoma because new blood vessels invade the iridocorneal angle. The TM loses its filtering function because of the neovascularization. This type of glaucoma is the most difficult to treat, and until now only implantation of silicone tube valves has yielded favorable results.[41,42]

MECHANISMS OF FILTRATION IN NONPENETRATING GLAUCOMA SURGERY

The main goal in NPGS is to restore aqueous drainage through an existing natural membrane, namely the trabeculodescemetic membrane (TDM). The TDM consists of the TM and a portion of the adjacent peripheral Descemet's membrane. The TDM acts as an outflow dampener. With the TDM in place, the intraoperative drop in IOP is gradual and the loss of anterior chamber is prevented. Once the aqueous has filtered through the TDM, it is momentarily collected in a reservoir created by the deep sclerectomy before it is absorbed by several routes. The gradual filtration of the aqueous humor through the TDM and its collection in the deep sclerectomy space reduce the importance of the subconjunctival route for aqueous reabsorption. Large subconjunctival filtering blebs, with their potential risks and complications, are unnecessary in NPGS.

The main site of aqueous outflow resistance in open-angle glaucoma, pseudoexfoliative glaucoma, and pigmentary glaucoma is located at the juxtacanalicular TM and the inner wall of Schlemm's canal. The aim of NPGS is to expose the TDM and remove the internal wall of Schlemm's canal and the juxtacanalicular meshwork by scraping and peeling in order to reduce the main outflow resistance.

Aqueous Outflow through the Trabeculodescemetic Membrane

Vaudaux et al.[43] studied the aqueous outflow through the TDM in an experimental model. Experiments were performed on enucleated human eyes unsuitable for keratoplasty. The intraoperative decrease in IOP was recorded (see Fig. 239-1) and the TDM resistance was calculated. The mean rate of IOP decrease was 2.7 ± 0.6 mmHg/min. The ocular aqueous outflow resistance dropped from a mean of 5.34 ± 0.19 mmHg μl per minute preoperatively to a mean of 0.41 ± 0.16 mmHg μl per minute postoperatively.

In these experiments, the postoperative TDM resistance was found to be low enough to ensure a low postoperative IOP and yet sufficient to prevent the collapse of the anterior chamber with its ensuing complications.

In the same study, the surgical site was examined histologically using ocular perfusion with ferritin. It was found that the anterior TM was the most porous site and most of the outflow occurred through it. To a lesser degree, there was some outflow through the posterior TM and Descemet's membrane.

Aqueous Humor Reabsorption

After aqueous humor filtration through the TDM, four sites for aqueous reabsorption may be postulated: the subconjunctival space, the intrascleral space, the suprachoroidal space, and the episcleral aqueous veins via the open ends of Schlemm's canal.

The Subconjunctival Space

Most patients have a shallow diffuse subconjunctival bleb on the first day following NPGS. Ultrasound biomicroscopic (UBM) studies[11] have demonstrated that successful cases of NPGS show a low profile and diffuse subconjunctival filtering blebs even years after surgery (Fig. 239-3). However, these blebs tend to be shallower and more diffuse than those seen after trabeculectomy.

The Intrascleral Space and Its Aqueous Veins

During NPGS, after the superficial flap is lifted, a certain volume of sclera ranging between 5 and 8mm³ is removed, creating an intrascleral space. Unless the superficial scleral flap adheres to the deep sclerectomy, this intrascleral space may act as an intrascleral filtering bleb. Absorbable implants made of porcine collagen or reticulated hyaluronic acid and nonabsorbable hydrophilic implants have been used in order to maintain the volume of this intrascleral space. On UBM studies, the mean volume of the intrascleral bleb was 1.8mm³ in patients with the collagen implant.[11] Aqueous vein openings are almost invariably observed in the deep sclerectomy bed (see Fig. 239-10). In successful cases of NPGS, these aqueous veins were shown to become hypertrophic in fluorescein angiography and UBM studies.[11,13] Existing and newly formed aqueous veins in the deep sclerectomy space might provide one of the routes for aqueous humor reabsorption.

The Subchoroidal Space

The deep scleral flap reaches a depth of 90%, leaving only a thin layer of scleral tissue over the ciliary body and the choroid. Aqueous humor can most probably seep into the suprachoroidal space through the thinned sclera and be absorbed by the uveal route. UBM studies have demonstrated the existence of localized shallow detachment of the ciliary body and choroid under the deep sclerectomy space in 45% of the patients studied years after the deep sclerectomy.[11] It is not yet known how much of the aqueous is reabsorbed by this route, and further studies of the aqueous dynamics following NPGS are needed to elucidate it.

The Episcleral Veins via the Open Ends of Schlemm's Canal

During NPGS, the open ends of Schlemm's canal could theoretically provide a route to the episcleral veins that exist on either side of the deroofed Schlemm's canal. In Stegmann's viscocanalostomy, viscoelastic material is injected into the open ends of Schlemm's canal in order to dilate them and to increase aqueous humor reabsorption by this route. The amount of aqueous reabsorption by this route has not yet been quantified *in vivo*.[44]

SURGICAL TECHNIQUE

General Considerations

NPGS is a very challenging technique because the surgical acts are confined to a few square millimeters and extremely delicate structures. NPGS is best performed under high magnification, and it involves a long learning curve. Even in experienced hands, NPGS takes at least twice as long to perform as a classical trabeculectomy. It is therefore advisable to view several of these operations performed by an experienced surgeon and practice on animal or cadaver eyes before attempting the first procedure in a patient.

Anesthesia

Because the critical steps of the operation (unroofing of Schlemm's canal and peeling of the TM) are performed under the highest magnification, the patient has to reach maximal stability. Effective local anesthesia that ensures adequate akinesia, such as sub-Tenon or retrobulbar injections, is mandatory. In a beginner's hands, general anesthesia might not be superfluous because it ensures complete immobility of the patient.

Conjunctival and Superficial Scleral Flaps

The first steps of NPGS are similar to those of classical trabeculectomy. A 7mm fornix or limbal-based conjunctival flap, preferably in the upper quadrant, is created (Fig. 239-4). A 5 × 5 × 1.5mm trapezoidal or a 5 × 5mm square scleral flap of 40 to 50% depth is dissected into clear cornea (Figs. 239-5 and 239-6). It is extremely important to extend the first scleral step dissection into clear cornea, past the vascular arcade, in order to allow the creation of a wide TDM when the second scleral flap is

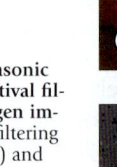
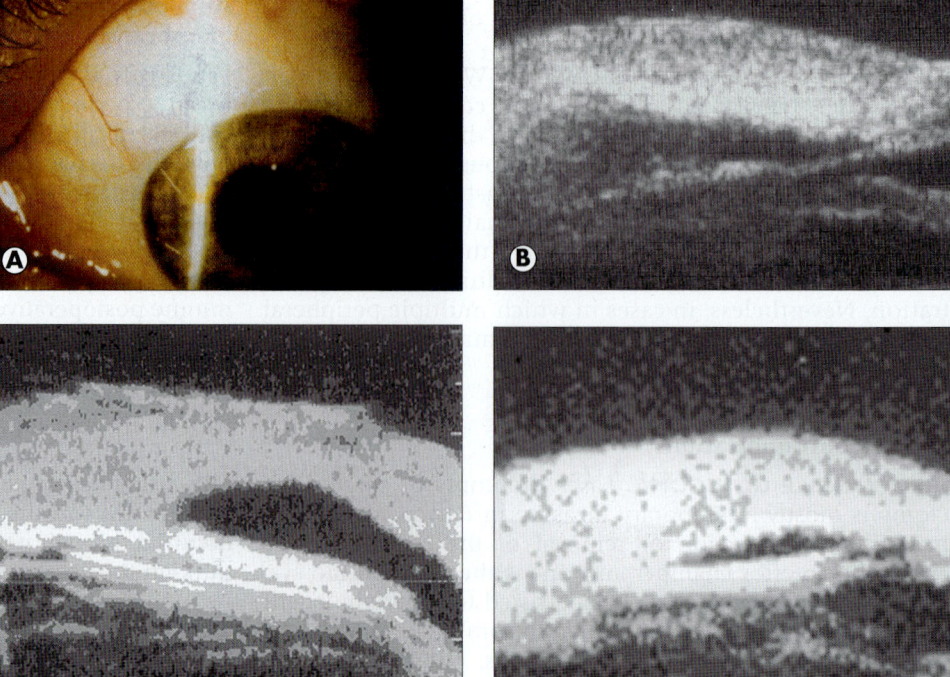

FIG. 239-3 ■ Photographic (**A**) and ultrasonic biomicroscopy (**B**) images of subconjunctival filtering bleb 5 years after NPGS with collagen implant. Ultrasonic biomicroscopy image of filtering blebs with the T Flux implant 3 months (**C**) and 2 years (**D**) after NPGS.

lifted. This first scleral flap is everted over the cornea and pulled down with an 8-0 virgin silk that is fixed to the lower limbus at the 6 o'clock position (see Fig. 239-5). This temporary flap fixation improves the exposure during the next phase of the operation, which is performed under the highest magnification.

Deep Sclerectomy and Exposure of the Trabeculodescemetic Membrane

A second 3 × 3 × 1mm trapezoidal or a 3 × 3mm square scleral flap is dissected to a depth of 90%, creating a deep sclerectomy and leaving only a thin layer of scleral tissue over the underlying uvea (see Fig. 239-6). At the level of the scleral spur, Schlemm's canal is unroofed, creating a 3mm long fenestration in its lumen. The scleral spur is recognized by its glistening circumferential fibers that can be differentiated from the crisscross pattern fibers situated in the deep sclerectomy bed. The scleral spur is the anatomical landmark where Schlemm's canal starts, and it is located at the transition between the white sclera and the blue sclera in the limbus area. When the posterior aspect of the TM and the adjacent Descemet's membrane are exposed (see Fig. 239-6), it is advisable to lower the IOP in order to reduce the risk of rupture of the TDM. Stegmann and Mermoud suggested performing a paracentesis, releasing some aqueous from the anterior chamber, in order to reduce the IOP prior to the complete exposure of the TDM. Nonetheless, the concept of nonpenetration is not violated by the paracentesis because NPGS pertains to the site of filtration and not to the penetration or nonpenetration of the anterior chamber. Dahan used a 25-gauge anterior chamber maintainer (ACM) connected to a bottle of balanced salt solution 20cm above the patient's head. The ACM allows the surgeon to control the IOP during the different steps of the operation (Fig. 239-7). The ACM is switched off during the opening of Schlemm's canal in order to lower the IOP and prevent inadvertent rupture of the TDM. A dry cellulose sponge is used to assess the amount of aqueous oozing from the TDM (see Fig. 239-7).

To thin out and render the TM more permeable, trabecular forceps (HUCO 4.4475) are used to peel off Schlemm's canal endothelium and the juxtacanalicular TM (Fig. 239-8). In some cases, these structures can be first loosened using a TM scraper with a carbide-impregnated metal tip (Katena K3-1120 or HUCO 4.6030) (Fig. 239-9). When these delicate steps are completed,

the ACM can be switched on again gradually in order to assess the amount of aqueous filtration after the reconditioning of the TM.

The internal scleral flap is excised along its base 0.5mm anterior to Schwalbe's line to create the deep sclerectomy space (Fig. 239-10). In high-risk cases, mitomycin C can be applied onto the deep sclerectomy only to prevent intrascleral scarring and enhance intrascleral aqueous reabsorption. It is advisable to prevent contact between the mitomycin C and the conjunctiva in order to prevent avascular blebs postoperatively. During the mitomycin C application, it is advisable to keep the ACM switched on to create positive IOP and to prevent mitomycin C seeping into the anterior chamber and suprachoroidal space.

Intrascleral Hydrophilic Implants

Different hydrophilic implants can be used to fill the deep sclerectomy space to create an intrascleral bleb. The implants can be absorbable (Aquaflow made of porcine collagen or SKGel made of reticulated hyaluronic acid) or nonabsorbable (T Flux made of 38% water content Poly-Megma) (Fig. 239-11). The superficial scleral flap is reflected back in place and sutured with at least one suture. For a fornix-based approach the conjunctival flap is sutured back into place with one or two sutures at the limbus, whereas for a limbal-based conjunctival flap the conjunctiva is sutured with a continuous suture.

Postoperative Treatment

Postoperative treatment consists of a topical dexamethasone, neomycin, polymyxin B sulfates (Maxitrol), or dexamethasone and chloramphenicol (SpersadexCo) instilled four times a day for 2 weeks or until IOP ≥10mmHg. The topical steroids are then replaced with a nonsteroidal anti-inflammatory agent such as diclofenac (Naclof) and continued for 4 to 8 weeks.

VISCOCANALOSTOMY

Stegmann has described a variant of NPGS and termed it viscocanalostomy to emphasize the importance of injecting viscoelastic material into Schlemm's canal as a means of improving aqueous drainage by this route (Fig. 239-12). However, in viscocanalostomy, peeling of the Schlemm's canal endothelium and

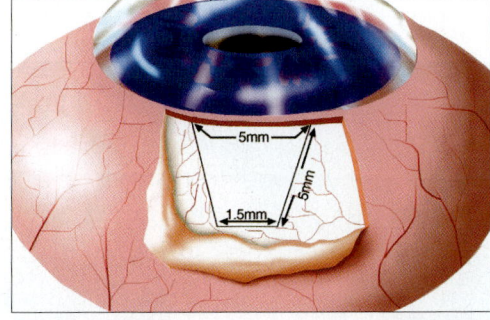

FIG. 239-4 ■ A 7mm fornix-based conjunctival flap and trapezoidal marking for the superficial flap.

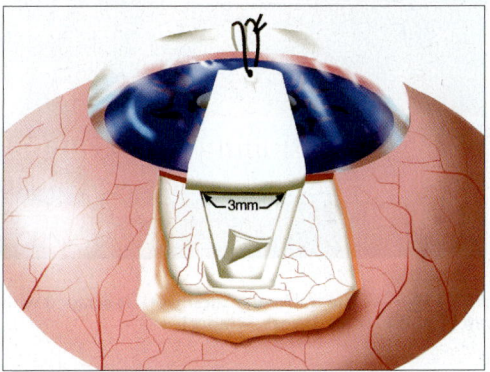

FIG. 239-5 ■ A 40–50% depth superficial flap is dissected into clear cornea and reflected back to allow a 90% depth deep sclerectomy.

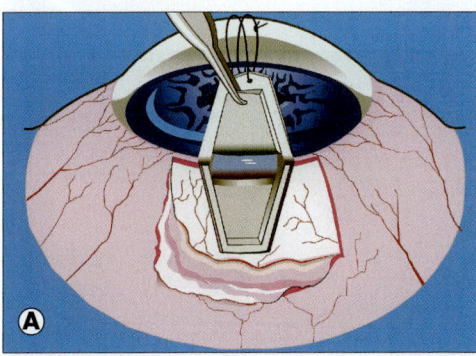

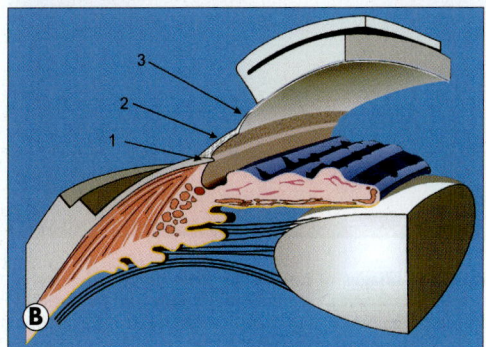

FIG. 239-6 ■ 90% depth deep sclerectomy with the unveiled trabeculodescemetic membrane. A, En face view and, B, sagittal view showing (1) scleral spur, (2) trabecular meshwork, and (3) Descemet's membrane.

the juxtacanalicular TM has not been suggested as a means of improving filtration. Stegmann claimed that the denuded peripheral Descemet's membrane is the main route of aqueous filtration, bypassing the resistance situated at the level of the TM. In viscocanalostomy, it is suggested to suture the superficial scleral flap tightly in order to prevent subconjunctival filtration blebs and to direct the aqueous from the deep sclerectomy space into the enlarged openings of Schlemm's canal. These assertions have yet to be proved by further postoperative aqueous dynamics studies.

COMBINED CATARACT EXTRACTION AND NONPENETRATING GLAUCOMA SURGERY

NPGS can be combined with cataract extraction when the two conditions coexist and when the anterior chamber needs to be deepened in cases of narrow-angle glaucoma. For example, it is possible to perform a phacoemulsification via a temporal clear corneal approach and an NPGS at the 12 o'clock position. It is advisable to perform the cataract extraction first and then to proceed with the NPGS in order to prevent rupture of the TDM during the phacoemulsification. Combined NPGS and cataract extraction yields results comparable to those of trabeculectomy and cataract extraction but involves fewer complications.[45]

NPGS AS AN ADJUNCT TO GLAUCOMA IMPLANT SURGERY

In cases in which silicone tube implants are indicated, Freedman suggested associating NPGS with a Seton implant in order to prevent the early postoperative hypotony that occurs with these implants. NPGS can provide safe initial lowering of IOP, and when the IOP rises again the preplaced silicone tube can be activated to provide further IOP control. The activation of the Seton is performed by removing a preplaced stent from the silicone tube when sufficient scarring has occurred in the surrounding tissues.[46]

COMPLICATIONS OF NONPENETRATING GLAUCOMA SURGERY

Although there is unanimous agreement that NPGS involves fewer complications than conventional penetrating glaucoma surgery, it is not totally devoid of complications. NPGS complications can occur intraoperatively, during the early postoperative period, or during the late postoperative period.

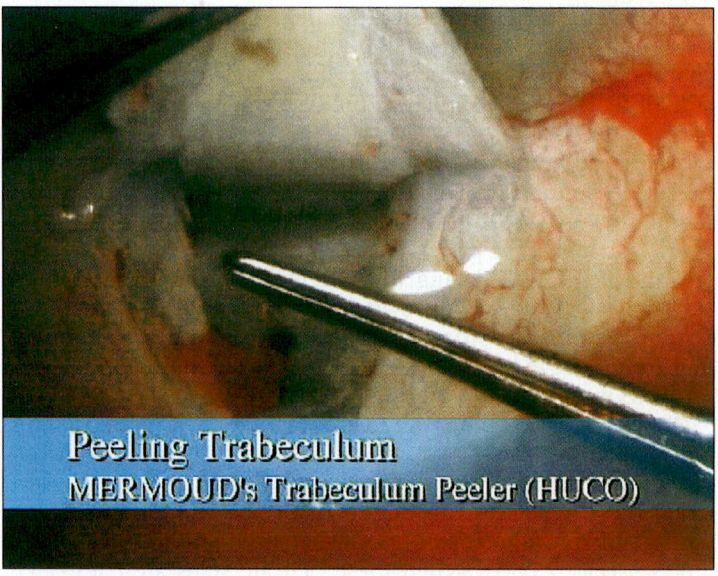

FIG. 239-8 ▪ The Schlemm's canal endothelium and the juxtacanalicular meshwork are peeled in order to improve filtration.

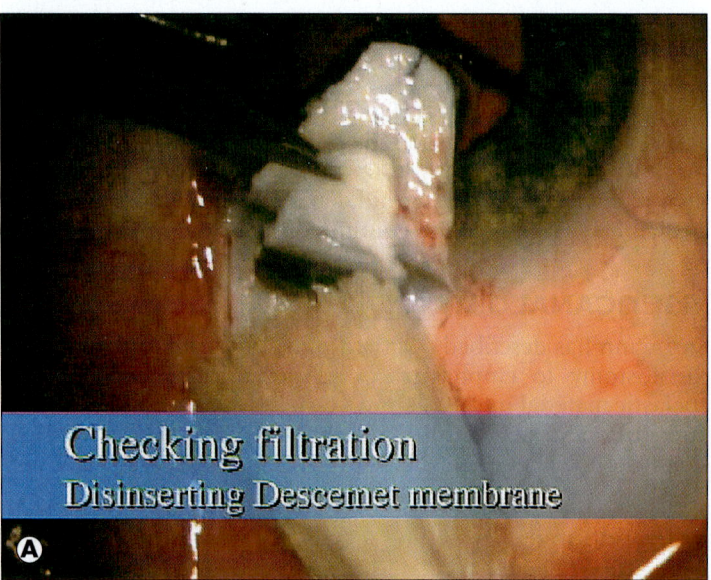

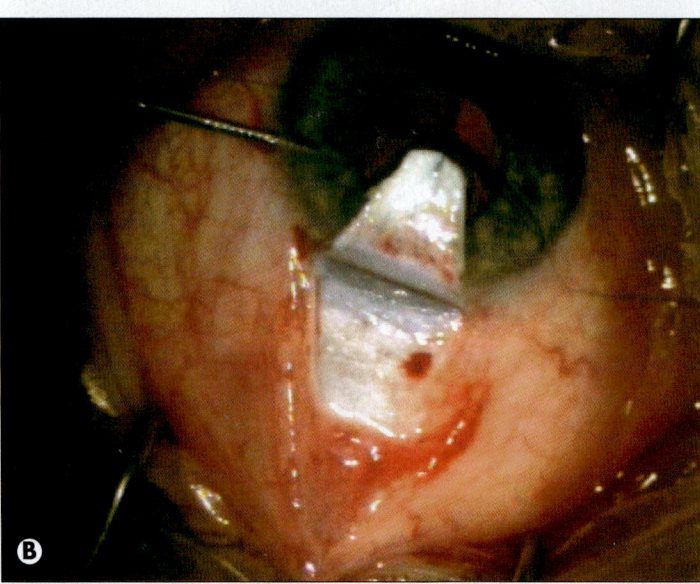

FIG. 239-7 ▪ Intraoperative video images of non-penetrating glaucoma surgery. **A,** A dry cellulose sponge is used to disinsert Descemet's membrane and to assess filtration. **B,** A 25-gauge anterior chamber maintainer provides IOP control throughout the operation.

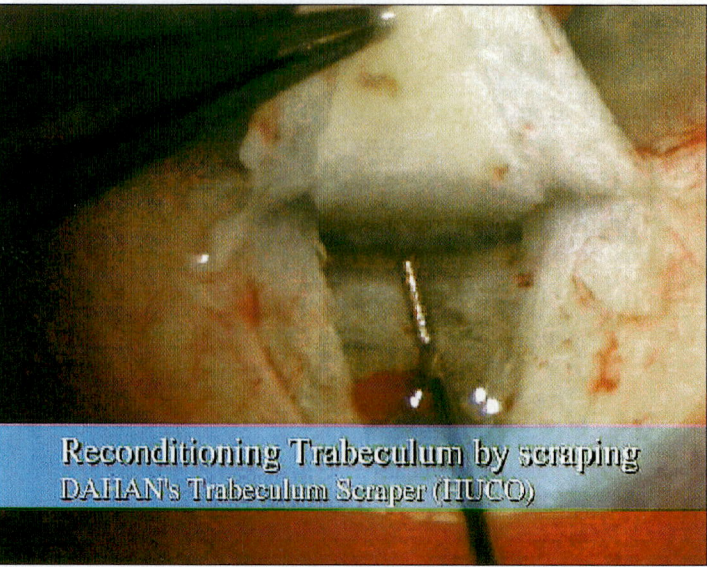

FIG. 239-9 ▪ The trabecular meshwork is scraped with a carbide-incrusted metal tip (Trabecular Meshwork Scraper).

Intraoperative Complications

During the dissection of the deep scleral flap, the choroid can be inadvertently exposed in a small area, causing a small choroid herniation. These small choroid herniations can be ignored as long as the deep scleral flap dissection is redirected into the correct plane.

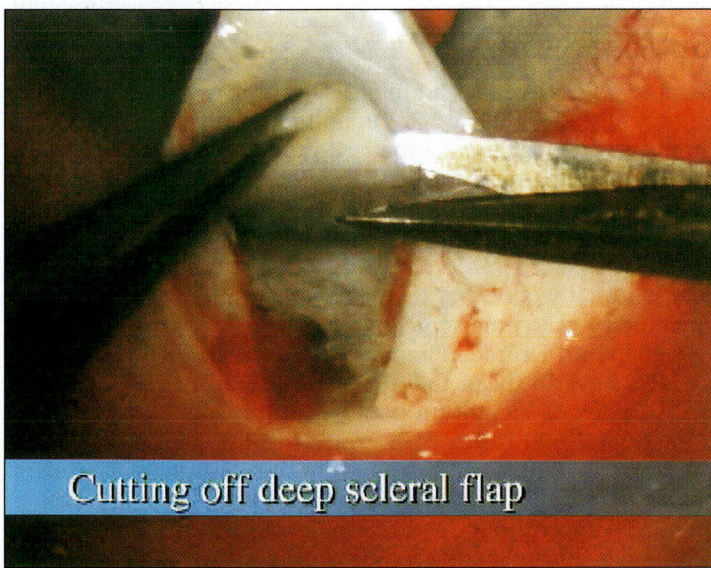

FIG. 239-10 ■ **The deep scleral flap is cut off to create the deep sclerectomy space.** Note the aqueous vein situated in the center of the deep sclerectomy. Aqueous veins in the deep sclerectomy space provide one of the several routes for aqueous reabsorption after nonpenetrating glaucoma surgery.

During the learning curve, the most common intraoperative complication is perforation of the TDM. It is acceptable to have a perforation rate of 30% during the first 10–20 cases. With proper training, the perforation rate can be lowered to less than 5%. When a perforation of the TDM occurs, the surgeon has to decide whether the NPGS has to be halted and converted into a conventional trabeculectomy or whether the perforation can be ignored. The key features in these instances are the size of the perforation and the presence of iris prolapse. Small holes in the TDM that do not cause iris prolapse can be ignored, whereas larger holes or tears with iris prolapse must lead to halting the NPGS and convert it to a trabeculectomy. A glaucoma implant such the T Flux can be used to tamponade medium-size holes with no iris prolapse.

Postoperative Complications

Moderate hypotony with a deep anterior chamber is expected during the first week postoperatively after NPGS. In fact, a normal IOP on the first day postoperatively is not a good prognostic indicator because most of these patients develop high IOP later on. The transient hypotony subsides within a week or two with topical steroid medications. Patients must be warned that their visual acuity will be affected by the transient hypotony and the consequent transient astigmatism. Transient cystoid macular edema related to the hypotony can develop, but it normally subsides when IOP returns to normal levels.

High IOP on the first day postoperatively can be caused by insufficient dissection of the TDM. It occurs often in inexperienced hands, especially when the TDM is not wide enough and its fil-

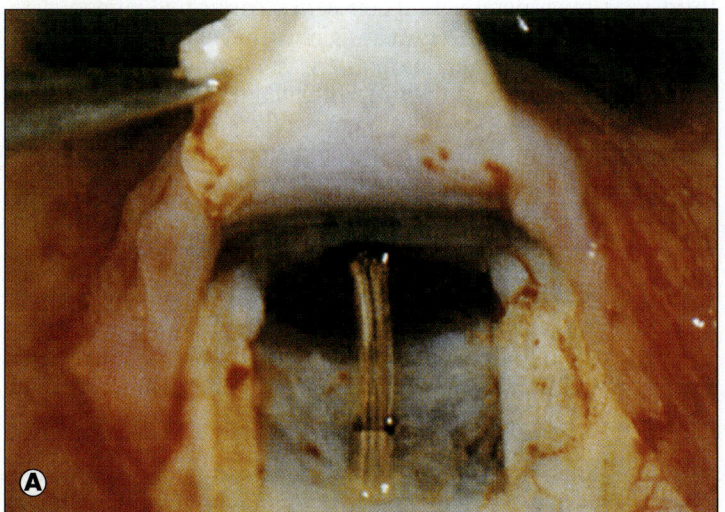

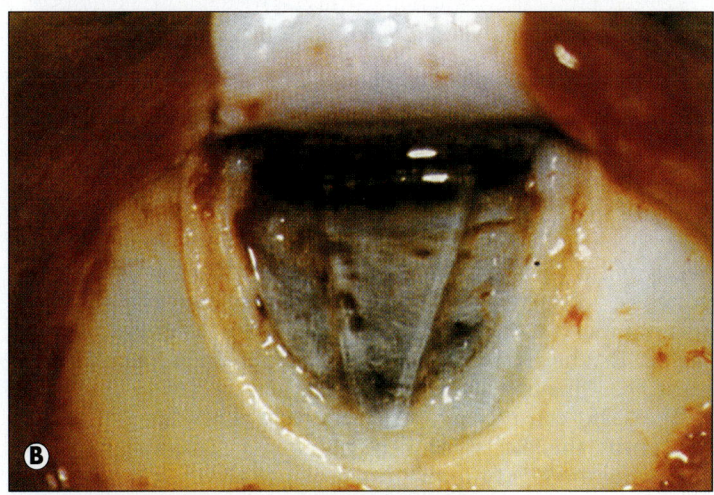

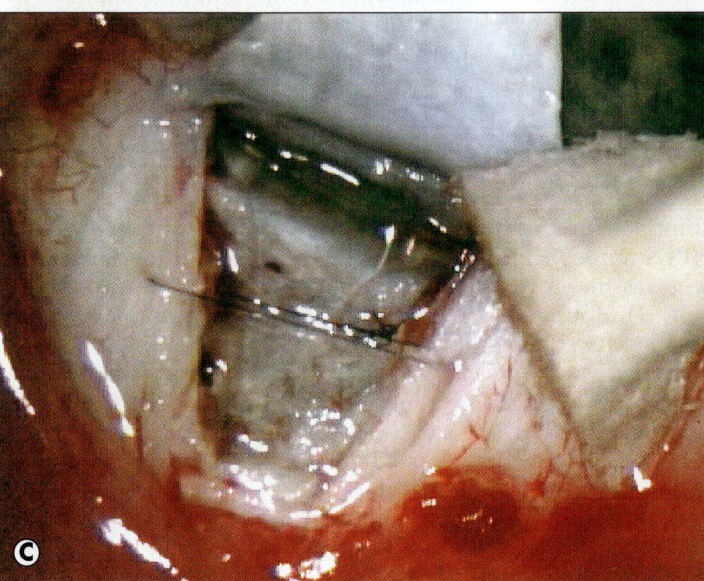

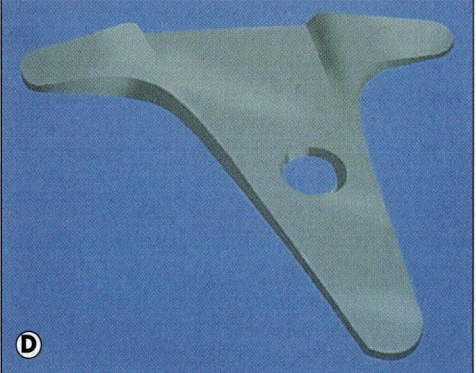

FIG. 239-11 ■ **Absorbable and non-absorbable hydrophilic implants used in the deep sclerotomy space to increase the longevity of NPGS. A,** Porcine collagen (Aquaflow) sutured in the deep sclerotomy space. **B,** Reticulated hyaluronic acid implant in the deep sclerotomy space. **C,** Nonabsorbable hydrophilic implant (T Flux) sutured in the deep sclerotomy space. **D,** Three-dimensional view of the T Flux nonabsorbable hydrophilic implant made of 38% water content Poly-Megma.

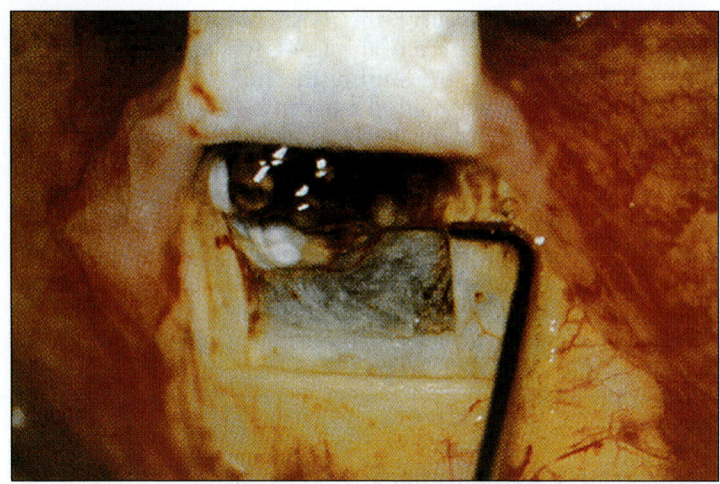

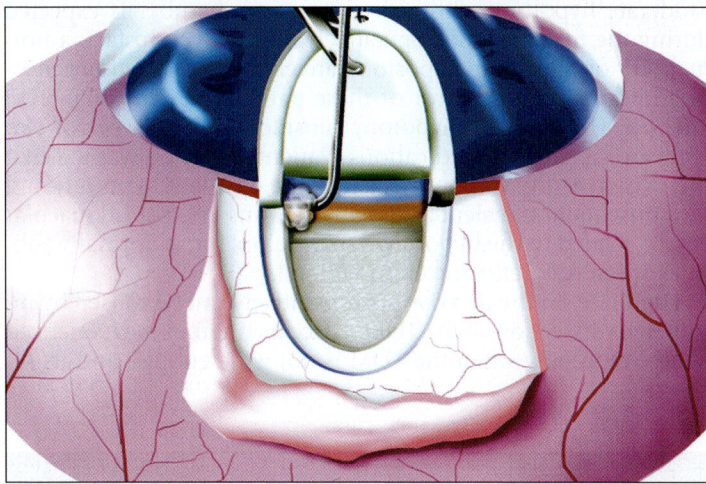

FIG. 239-12 ■ Viscoelastic material is injected into the Schlemm's canal openings with a specially designed cannula (Grieshaber).

tration capacity has not been sufficiently restored by scraping and peeling. This complication can be remedied by neodymium:yttrium-aluminum-garnet (Nd:YAG) laser goniopuncture.[12] Presence of blood in the deep sclerectomy space can also hamper aqueous evacuation and cause early postoperative high IOP. When it is recognized, a short course of acetazolamide can solved this transient rise in IOP.

The TDM can rupture postoperatively at any stage if the patient rubs the eye vigorously or after a Valsalva maneuver. Following the TDM rupture, iris prolapse occurs and blocks the filtration site, causing a rise in IOP. In these cases, the filtration site has to be revised in order to convert the operation into a conventional trabeculectomy.

Peripheral anterior synechiae can form in the site of filtration without iris prolapse. These synechiae can hamper filtration and cause a rise in IOP. YAG laser iridoplasty can reopen the angle and be beneficial in some cases. In case of failure, NPGS can be repeated on another site.

Descemet's membrane detachment is a rare complication of NPGS, occurring in about 1 out of 250–300 operated eyes.[47] Descemet detachment is more inherent to viscocanalostomy because of the viscoelastic material injection into Schlemm's canal. The inexperienced surgeon can be too vigorous when injecting the viscoelastic material and cause a Descemet detachment. Descemet detachment can also occur when aqueous humor from the deep sclerectomy space is forced into the sub-Descemet space following vigorous ocular massage or trauma. The patient can experience a drop in visual acuity due to corneal edema. Generally, Descemet detachments are transient and visual acuity returns to normal. In severe cases, Descemet reattachment can be attempted with the use of viscoelastic material in the anterior chamber.

A single case of scleral ectasia following NPGS has been reported in a 12-year-old girl with chronic arthritis complicated with glaucoma secondary to a chronic uveitis.[48] Scleral ectasia can occur in any type of glaucoma surgery in patients with a tendency to scleromalacia. Antimetabolites should be used with extreme caution in these cases.

OUTCOMES

Because NPGS involves a long learning curve, the reports on its efficacy and longevity are not unanimous. In general, the NPGS pioneers with extensive experience and long series report on more favorable results than the novices.[5–31] Reports that compare trabeculectomy with viscocanalostomy show particular discord between the proponents of NPGS and its opponents. There is nevertheless a common trend that indicates that the NPGS efficacy is initially good but its longevity is limited, as expected in any kind of glaucoma surgery.

Dahan and Drusedau[21] analyzed a series of 86 eyes operated by NPGS over a mean follow-up of 46 months. Their analysis was particularly significant because no implants were used and no antiglaucoma treatment was added postoperatively in their study. The IOP dropped in average by 50%, from a mean preoperative value of 30.4mmHg to a mean postoperative value of 15.35mmHg without medication. Postoperatively, when IOP rose above 20mmHg, instead of adding medical treatment, the filtration site was revised to reestablish filtration. During the study period, the filtration site was revised in 48 eyes (56%), in order to maintain the IOP below 21mmHg without medication, after a mean period of successful filtration of 29.9 months. These data indicate that the efficacy of NPGS starts to fade in the third year postoperatively. Their series confirmed previous reports on the adverse effects of antiglaucoma medication on glaucoma surgery. The reoperation rate was 4.7 times higher in previously treated patients than in untreated patients.

Koslov et al.[6] proposed a porcine collagen implant to keep a filtration space under the superficial scleral flap. Sourdille et al.[20] developed an absorbable implant made of reticulated hyaluronic acid. This absorbable implant is left under the superficial scleral flap in order to create a space for aqueous humor reabsorption. Until recently, all the proposed implants were absorbable and showed certain value in improving the outcomes of NPGS.[6–31] The glaucoma unit of the Jules Gonin Eye Hospital in Lausanne[18] reported a complete success rate of 34.6% without a collagen implant versus a success rate of 63.4% with a collagen implant. Similarly, other reports confirm the value of other absorbable and nonabsorbable implants in NPGS.

NPGS can be combined with cataract extraction, especially when there is evidence of a narrow angle. The patient will benefit from the lens removal because the anterior chamber invariably deepens after combined surgery. Several studies reported on the favorable outcomes of combined NPGS with cataract extraction.[45]

CONCLUSIONS AND FUTURE PERSPECTIVES

NPGS is an evolving technique that is associated with fewer complications than classical trabeculectomy. The experienced NPGS surgeon finds it at least as effective as trabeculectomy, whereas the novice claims that trabeculectomy yields better results. Undoubtedly, NPGS still needs further improvements to prolong its efficacy and longevity. The available implants have proved to be beneficial in prolonging successful filtration. At present, the deep sclerectomy and the exposure of the TDM are done manually. These steps are challenging and require a long learning curve. Various lasers have been tried in performing the deep sclerectomy, but they have not yet matched dissection. Future attempts to use lasers in performing the deep sclerectomy will probably be more successful and will help in popularizing this promising technique.

REFERENCES

1. Epstein E. Communications. Fibrosing response to aqueous. Its relation to glaucoma. Br J Ophthalmol. 1959;43:641–7.
2. Krasnov MM. Externalisation of Schlemm's canal (sinusotomy) in glaucoma. Br J Ophthalmol. 1968;52:157–61.
3. Sugar HS. Experimental trabeculectomy in glaucoma. Am J Ophthalmol. 1961;51: 623–7.
4. Cairns JE. Trabeculectomy-preliminary report of a new method. Am J Ophthalmol. 1968;66:673–9.
5. Fyodorov SN, Ioffe DI, Ronkina TI. Deep sclerectomy: technique and mechanism of a new glaucomatous procedure. Glaucoma. 1984;6:281–3.
6. Koslov VI, Bagrov SN, Anisimova SY, et al. Nonpenetrating deep sclerectomy with collagen. Ophthalmic Surg. 1990;3:44–6.
7. Zimmerman TJ, Kooner KS, Ford VJ, et al. Trabeculectomy vs. non-penetrating trabeculectomy. A retrospective study of two procedures in phakic patients with glaucoma. Ophthalmic Surg. 1984;15:734–40.
8. Hara T, Hara T. Deep sclerectomy with Nd: YAG laser trabeculotomy ab interno: two stage procedure. Ophthalmic Surg. 1988;19:101–6.
9. Kershner RM. Non-penetrating trabeculectomy with placement of collagen device. J Cataract Refract Surg. 1995;21:608–11.
10. Demailly P, Jeanteur-Lunel MN, Berkani M, et al. La sclérectomie profonde non-perforante associée a la pose d'un implant de collagen dans le glaucome primitif a angle ouvert. Resultats retrospectifs a court terme. Ophthalmologie. 1995;9:666–70.
11. Chiou AG, Mermoud A, Underdahl JP, Schnyder CC. An ultrasound biomicroscopic study of eyes after deep sclerectomy with collagen implant. Ophthalmology. 1998;105:746–50.
12. Mermoud A, Karlen ME, Schnyder CC. Nd:YAG goniopunctures after deep sclerectomy with collagen implant. Ophthalmic Surg Lasers. 1999;30:120–25.
13. Mermoud A, Vaudaux J. Aqueous humor dynamics in non-penetrating filtering surgery (deep sclerectomy). Invest Ophthalmol Vis Sci. 1997;38(Suppl):S1064.
14. Sanchez E, Schnyder CC, Sickenberg M, et al. Deep sclerectomy: results with and without collagen implant. Int Ophthalmol. 1997;20:157–62.
15. Welsh NH, Delange J, Wassermann P, Ziemba L. The "deroofing" of Schlemm's canal in patients with open-angle glaucoma through placement of a collagen device. Ophthalmic Surg Lasers. 1998;29:216–26.
16. Mermoud A, Chiou AGY, Jewelewicz DA. Post-operative inflammation following deep sclerectomy with collagen implant versus standard trabeculectomy. Graefes Arch Clin Exp Ophthalmol. 1998;236:593–6.
17. Ambresin A, Shaarawy T, Mermoud A. Deep sclerectomy with collagen implant in one eye compared with trabeculectomy in the other eye of the same patient. J Glaucoma. 2002;11:214–20.
18. Shaarawy T, Karlen ME, Sanchez E, et al. Long term results of deep sclerectomy with collagen implant. Acta Ophthalmol Scand. 2000;78:323–28.
19. Stegmann R, Piennar A, Miller D. Viscocanalostomy for open-angle glaucoma in black African patients. J Cataract Refract Surg. 1999;25:316–22.
20. Sourdille P, Santiago PY, Villain F, et al. Reticulated hyaluronic acid implant in non-perforating trabecular surgery. J Cataract Refract Surg. 1999;25:332–9.
21. Dahan E, Drusedau MUH. Nonpenetrating filtration surgery for glaucoma: control by surgery only. J Cataract Refract Surg. 2000;26:695–701.
22. Drusedau MUH, Von Wolff K-D, Bull H, Von Barsewisch B. Viscocanalostomy for primary open-angle glaucoma: the Gross Pankow experience. J Cataract Refract Surg. 2000;26:1367–73.
23. Hamel M, Shaarawy T, Mermoud A. Deep sclerectomy with collagen implant in patients with glaucoma and high myopia. J Cataract Refract Surg. 2001;27:1410–17.
24. Li M. [Nonperforating trabecular surgery with reticulated hyaluronic acid implant]. Chin J Ophthalmol. 2001;37:404–8.
25. Shaarawy T, Karlen M, Schnyder C, et al. Five-year results of deep sclerectomy with collagen implant. J Cataract Refract Surg. 2001;27:1770–8.
26. El Sayyad F, Helal M, El-Kholify H, et al. Nonpenetrating deep sclerectomy versus trabeculectomy in bilateral primary open-angle glaucoma. Ophthalmology. 2000;107:1671–4.
27. Chiselita D. Non-penetrating deep sclerectomy versus trabeculectomy in primary open-angle glaucoma surgery. Eye. 2001;15:197–201.
28. Tan JC, Hitchings RA. Non-penetrating glaucoma surgery: the state of play. Br J Ophthalmol. 2001;85:234–7.
29. Jonescu-Cuypers C, Jacobi PC, Konen W, Krieglstein GK. Primary viscocanalostomy versus trabeculectomy in white patients with open-angle glaucoma. A randomised clinical trial. Ophthalmology. 2001;108:254–8.
30. O'Brart DP, Rowlands E, Islam N, Noury AM. A randomised, prospective study comparing trabeculectomy augmented with antimetabolites with a viscocanalostomy technique for the management for open-angle glaucoma uncontrolled by medical therapy. Br J Ophthalmol. 2002;86:748–54.
31. Watson PG, Jakeman C, Ozturk M, et al. Complications of trabeculectomy (20 years follow-up). Eye. 1990;4:425–38.
32. Dahan E, Rivett K, Michiels X. Comparison of early postoperative complications in trabeculectomies alone versus trabeculectomies with cataract extraction. Eur J Implant Refract Surg. 1994;6:18–21.
33. Jay JL, Allan D. The benefit of early trabeculectomy vs. conventional management in primary open-angle glaucoma relative to severity of disease. Eye. 1989;3:528–35.
34. Migdal C, Gregory W, Hitchings RA. Long-term functional outcome after early surgery compared with laser and medicine in open-angle glaucoma. Ophthalmology. 1994;101:1651–7.
35. Lavin MJ, Worvald RFL, Migdal CS, Hitchings RA. The influence of prior therapy on the success of trabeculectomy. Arch Ophthalmol. 1990;108:1543–8.
36. Broadway DC, Grierson I, O'Brien C, Hitching RA. Adverse effects of topical antiglaucoma medications I—the conjunctival cell profile. Arch Ophthalmol. 1994;112:1437–45.
37. Broadway DC, Grierson I, O'Brien C, Hitching RA. Adverse effects of topical antiglaucoma medications II—The outcome of filtration surgery. Arch Ophthalmol. 1994;112:1446–54.
38. Baudouin C, Pisella PJ, Fillacier K, et al. Ocular surface inflammatory changes induced by topical antiglaucoma drugs: human and animal studies. Ophthalmology. 1999;106:556–63.
39. Broadway DC, Chang LP. Trabeculectomy, risk factors for failure and the preoperative state of the conjunctiva. J Glaucoma. 2001;10:237–49.
40. Ruderman JM, Harbin TS Jr, Campbell DG. Postoperative suprachoroidal hemorrhage following filtration procedures. Arch Ophthalmol. 1986;104:201–5.
41. Freedman J. Clinical experience with the Molteno dual chamber single-plate implant. Ophthalmic Surg. 1992;23:238–41.
42. Mermoud A, Salmon JF, Alexader P, et al. Molteno tube implantation for neovascular glaucoma. Ophthalmology. 1993;100:897–902.
43. Vaudaux J, Uffer S, Mermoud A. Aqueous dynamics after deep sclerectomy: in vitro study. Ophthalmic Pract. 1999;16:204–9.
44. Johnson DH, Johnson M. How does non-penetrating glaucoma surgery work? Aqueous outflow resistance and glaucoma surgery. J Glaucoma. 2001;10:55–67.
45. Gianoli F, Mermoud A. Cataract-glaucoma surgery: comparison between phacoemulsification combined with deep sclerectomy or trabeculectomy. Klin Monatsbl Augenheilkd. 1999;210:256–60.
46. Sherwood MD, Smith MF. Prevention of early hypotony associated with Molteno implants by a new occluding stent technique. Ophthalmology. 1993;100:85–90.
47. Ravinet E, Shaarawy T, Schnyder CC, et al. Descemet membrane detachment after nonpenetrating filtering surgery. J Glaucoma. 2002;11:244–52.
48. Milazzo S. Scleral ectasia as a complication of deep sclerectomy. J Cataract Refract Surg. 2000;26:785–7.

Trabeculectomy

RONALD L. FELLMAN

DEFINITION
- Trabeculectomy, a guarded filtration procedure, remains the "gold standard" for long-lasting intraocular pressure reduction in uncontrolled primary glaucoma.

KEY FEATURES
- Patients expect a "quick fix" but glaucoma surgery is high in risk and requires exhaustive preoperative counseling and informed consent.
- Determine preoperative risk factors that lead to filtration complications and failure.
- Twenty-point preoperative trabeculectomy checklist.
- Step-by-step explanation of surgical procedure.

ASSOCIATED FEATURES
- Determine appropriate antimetabolite and correct dosage for filtration surgery.
- Factors in deciding on limbal- versus fornix-based conjunctival flaps.
- Determine best method of fashioning a scleral flap.

INTRODUCTION

Trabeculectomy is the most popular form of glaucoma filtration surgery and remains the "gold standard" for surgical reduction of intraocular pressure (IOP) in uncontrolled, primary open-angle glaucoma. This partial-thickness filtration operation decreases eye pressure via the establishment of a limbal fistula through which aqueous humor drains into the subconjunctival space, establishing a filtering bleb. Successful filtration surgery significantly enhances quality of life. The patient's outlook on life is improved, fear of blindness is reduced, and side effects and cost of medical therapy are abated. The outcome of filtration surgery is highly dependent on the type of glaucoma, severity of disease, pharmacological wound modulation, and surgical skill level.

HISTORICAL REVIEW

The major advance of trabeculectomy over prior full-thickness filtration procedures (iridencleisis, trephination, sclerectomy, and thermal sclerostomy) was the concept of guarded filtration.[1,2] The ability to impede and guard outflow with a scleral flap significantly reduced the complications associated with overfiltration. During the 1980s, trabeculectomy improved with the development of laser scleral flap suture lysis,[3] modified fornix-based conjunctival flaps, superior wound closure, and inhibition of fibrosis using the cytostatic antimetabolite 5-fluorouracil.[4] The 1990s brought new cytocidal antimetabolites, which include mitomycin C.[5]

BOX 240-1

Indications for Trabeculectomy Surgery*

FAILED MAXIMAL TOLERATED MEDICAL THERAPY AND FAILED LASER SURGERY OR POOR LASER CANDIDATE WITH ANY OF THE FOLLOWING:
Progressive glaucomatous optic nerve head cupping
Glaucomatous visual field progression
Anticipated optic nerve head damage as a result of excessive intraocular pressure
Anticipated visual field damage from glaucoma
Intolerable side effects that arise from medical therapy of glaucoma
Lack of compliance with anticipated or progressive glaucoma damage

*The indications vary considerably for individual patients and are a general guideline only for filtration surgery.

PREOPERATIVE EVALUATION AND DIAGNOSTIC APPROACH

Indications

The management goal in the glaucomas is to preserve vision and maintain a reasonable quality of life. The major indication for surgical intervention is progressive or anticipated glaucomatous disease that is likely to result in functional impairment during the patient's lifetime. Functional visual impairment varies considerably, depending on the patient's overall health, age, rate of visual field and optic nerve damage, and level of IOP. The majority of patients receiving maximal tolerated medical (see Chapter 233) and laser (see Chapter 235) therapy who experience progressive or anticipated glaucomatous damage are candidates for glaucoma filtration surgery (Box 240-1). Trabeculectomy is highly effective and is the procedure of choice for most cases of uncontrolled primary open- and closed-angle glaucoma, exfoliation syndrome, pigmentary glaucoma, and pseudophakic glaucoma with a posterior chamber intraocular lens (PCIOL). The secondary glaucomas (e.g., neovascular, epithelial downgrowth, developmental, traumatic, aphakic, congenital) have a poorer prognosis with glaucoma filtration surgery and may require other treatment modalities.

Vision-Damaging Pressure Level

The IOP level that causes glaucomatous optic nerve or visual field damage is the vision-damaging pressure level. The surgeon establishes a vision-damaging pressure level and decides by how much to lower the IOP (Box 240-2). The goal of trabeculectomy is to normalize the IOP, but normality for each patient may vary considerably.

A patient with low-tension glaucoma may need a postoperative IOP of 9 or 10mmHg (1.2 or 1.3kPa),[6] whereas a patient with traumatic glaucoma may need only a postoperative IOP of 20–25mmHg (2.7–3.3kPa) to maintain vision. In general, surgeons strive for a 30% IOP reduction for mild to moderate disease and up to a 50% reduction in IOP for advanced disease or normal-tension glaucoma. Smaller percentage reductions in postoperative IOP are less likely to stabilize the disease[7]; however, aggressive pressure reduction is associated with higher complication rates. Data from the Advanced Glaucoma Intervention Study (AGIS) demonstrate that eyes with 100% of visits with an IOP of less than 18mmHg over 6 years have stable visual fields compared with 50% of visits with an IOP of less than 18mmHg. The AGIS made it clear that low IOP (less than 14mmHg) is associated with reduced progression of visual field defects.[8] If the disease progresses, the ophthalmologist must determine whether the pressure reduction was great enough and look for other factors that may be worsening the disease.[9]

Informed Consent and Patient's Attitude to Glaucoma

In today's society, patients expect a "quick fix" for their medical problems.[10] Ophthalmologists have promulgated this theme through the miracles of "high tech, see better the same day" cataract and refractive surgery. It is incumbent upon the physician to emphasize, until completely understood, that this is not the case for glaucoma filtration surgery. Unfortunately, optic nerve function cannot be restored using present levels of technology. At best, the glaucoma goal is visual field stability but not improved visual acuity.

Patients need to know that no quick fix exists for this treatable, but incurable, disease. Glaucoma surgery is high in risk compared with many other eye procedures. Proper informed consent means that the patient understands the nature and reason for the procedure along with explanations of the risks, benefits, and alternatives. The patient's record chart must always substantiate these factors. From a medicolegal viewpoint, "if it is not documented, it did not happen." Patients must understand that visual acuity may worsen temporarily after filtration surgery.[11] A transient loss of at least one line of best corrected visual acuity is common after trabeculectomy, typically because of corneal topographic changes. Resolution occurs by 12 weeks.[12] If a cataract is present, surgery is likely to hasten its development,[13] especially if a shallow or flat anterior chamber is found postoperatively. Possible complications must be discussed thoroughly with the patient; this includes permanent loss of vision as a result of fixation loss[14] or suprachoroidal hemorrhage.[15] Occasionally, acuity

improves because of the removal of pilocarpine and subsequent pupillary enlargement. Additional reasons for visual loss include hypotony maculopathy, choroidal effusion or hemorrhage, cystoid macular edema, shallow anterior chamber, and other factors. The prognosis and complication rate of trabeculectomy are highly diagnosis dependent. An experienced glaucoma surgeon uniformly strives to minimize the surgical risks by modification of the procedure and technique as necessary.

Assessment of Filtration Risk Factors

Many nonsurgical factors exist that significantly influence the outcome of trabeculectomy. A thorough slit-lamp evaluation, gonioscopic examination, and record review can dramatically alter the surgical strategy and eventual outcome. The operative report from any prior glaucoma surgery must be reviewed. Slit-lamp gonioscopy is easier when carried out preoperatively rather than in the operating room; preoperative evaluation also ensures the correct diagnosis of glaucoma and enables the best site for filtration to be determined on the basis of peripheral anterior synechiae, IOL and haptic orientation, aberrant vessels, and wound dehiscence. The proposed location of the filter varies, depending on lid anatomy, conjunctival exposure, planned cataract surgery, prior filtration surgery, and limbal scarring. If vitreous prolapse is present, the appropriate method of removal must be determined in conjunction with the trabeculectomy.

Type of Glaucoma, Race, and Age

Open-angle glaucoma has the best risk-benefit profile. Well-documented risk factors for filtration failure include neovascular glaucoma, African race, aphakia, prior failed filtration, and uveitis.[16–20] One joy of longevity is a higher success rate for filtration surgery.[21]

Prior Use of Antiglaucoma Medications

The prolonged use of antiglaucoma medications may have an adverse effect on the conjunctiva and result in a proliferation of lymphocytes and fibroblasts, which decreases the likelihood of successful filtration surgery.[22] In these cases, antimetabolites may help to counter this effect in favor of long-term filtration. Adrenergic drugs seem to have the greatest tendency for drug allergy and may lead to postoperative Tenon's capsule cyst formation. The offending drug is discontinued at least 2 weeks prior to filtration and IOP is controlled with the administration of a short-term course of oral carbonic anhydrase inhibitors. Low-dose topical corticosteroids prior to surgery may decrease conjunctival inflammation significantly.

Anterior Segment Inflammation

Healthy aqueous humor nourishes the filtering bleb (Fig. 240-1) and is the basis of long-term filtration. Intraocular inflammation manifested by anterior chamber flare and cells is the sign of a sick eye, a definite risk factor for filtration failure. The blood-aqueous barrier must be stabilized prior to and after surgery using topical or oral corticosteroids or topical nonsteroidal anti-inflammatory agents. Strong, indirectly acting miotics that break down the blood-aqueous barrier are discontinued 2 weeks prior to surgery. In the correct setting, mydriatic cycloplegics are also useful for stabilization of the blood-aqueous barrier.

Scarring of the Conjunctiva and Limbal Anatomy

Prior conjunctival incisions may significantly alter the surgical plan. Scar tissue may be delineated at the slit lamp by identification of immobile conjunctiva using a Q-Tip under topical anesthetic. For example, patients who have undergone prior

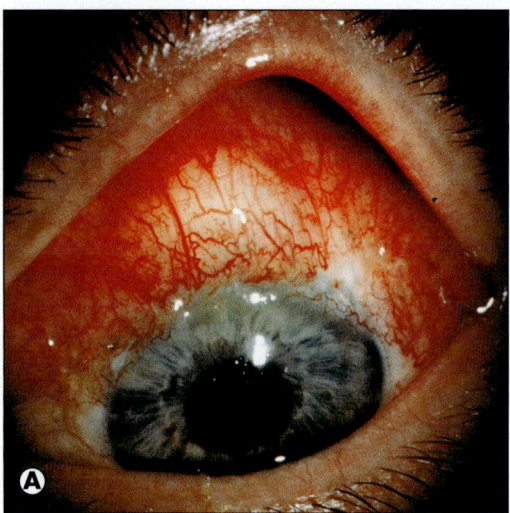

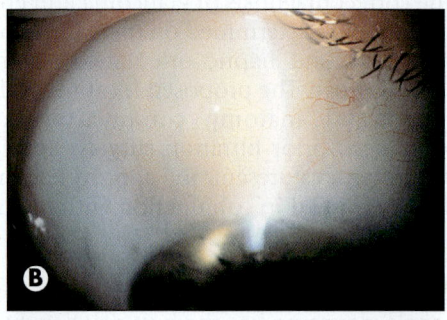

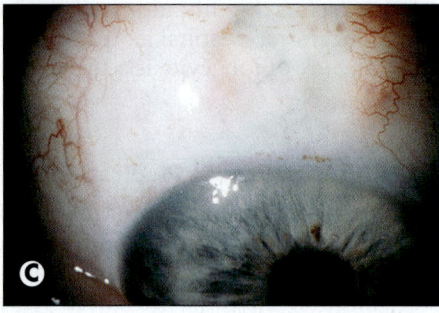

FIG. 240-1 ■
Filtering blebs.
The behavior of filtering blebs is unpredictable after filtration surgery. Even with the best of efforts, undesirable bleb traits appear. **A,** Excessive inflammation and consequent vascularity lead to a host of factors that result in bleb fibrosis and ultimate failure. **B,** Desirable long-term characteristics include a moderate, diffuse bleb elevation, overall frosty pallor with a few small vessels, no demarcation zones, and conjunctival microcysts. **C,** Undesirable characteristics include excessive wall thickening with cyst formation, total avascularity, demarcation zones, necrosis with leaks, and extremely thin tissue. Totally avascular blebs are not desirable and usually indicate excessive antimetabolite dosage.

scleral buckle surgery or who have pseudophakia or aphakia may have severe disruption of the conjunctiva, especially at the limbus. If possible, whether the incision is to be limbus based or fornix based is decided prior to surgery.

Ocular Surface Disease

Any ocular surface disease that causes chronic conjunctival inflammation is a risk factor for filtration failure. Ocular rosacea and blepharitis are treated aggressively for several weeks prior to filtration with the administration of oral doxycycline 100mg a day for 3 weeks, a topical antibiotic ointment, and lid hygiene. These eyes require long-term topical corticosteroids and oral antibiotics, even after surgery, to salvage the bleb.

Conjunctival Scarring, Wound Healing, and Bleb Failure

Trabeculectomy without antimetabolite is usually successful for most cases of low-risk, uncomplicated primary glaucomas.[23] Postoperatively, if fibrosis is a problem, antifibrotic agents may be injected to salvage the bleb. However, more complex cases that have a greater potential for failure initially require antifibrotic agents to achieve useful pressure reduction. The majority of filters fail because of episcleral fibrosis. Administration of antiproliferative agents specific to the cell cycle increases the success rate of trabeculectomy in high-risk eyes by limitation of fibroblast pro-

liferation at the filtration site. The two most common antimetabolites are 5-fluorouracil and mitomycin C. At current doses, 5-fluorouracil is mainly cytostatic and mitomycin C is cytocidal. Mitomycin C is approximately 100 times more potent than 5-fluorouracil.[24] 5-Fluorouracil is much safer in virgin eyes that have good prognoses; mitomycin C is reserved for eyes that have a high likelihood of failure and/or prior failed conventional filtration. Before these powerful drugs are administered, the surgeon must understand the philosophy behind the advantages and disadvantages of antimetabolite trabeculectomy.[25]

The use of 5-fluorouracil has improved the outcome of filtration surgery, which as a consequence is now performed more often.[26,27] The drug is a halogenated pyrimidine analog that inhibits DNA synthesis because it acts as a competitive inhibitor of thymidylate synthetase. 5-Fluorouracil is incorporated into both RNA and DNA, which results in defective protein synthesis and cell toxicity. 5-Fluorouracil is much more lethal to cells that grow logarithmically than to stationary cells and typically is administered as consecutive subconjunctival injections[28] or as an intraoperative sponge application of 50mg/ml.[29]

Mitomycin C is an antitumor antibiotic isolate of fermentation filtrate from *Streptomyces caespitosus*. It is an alkylating agent that binds to DNA and, thereby, interrupts cell synthesis; it inhibits DNA, RNA, and protein synthesis and is highly toxic to vascular endothelial cells. Mitomycin C is one of the 10 most carcinogenic substances known to humans—the Occupational Safety and Health Administration work-practice guidelines for personnel who administer cytotoxic drugs must be followed strictly.[30]

Mitomycin C increases the success rate of glaucoma filtration surgery[31,32] at variable application times[33] and doses[34] and is more effective than 5-fluorouracil.[35] Mitomycin C is administered only as a single topical administration over the intended scleral flap during surgery using sponges of various sizes and doses in the range 0.1–0.5mg/ml and application times of 1–5 minutes, all depending on the inherent risk factors for filtration failure. One obvious problem is the lack of standardization of application of the drug,[36] which leads to unclear study results. Currently, mitomycin C is overused in virgin eyes that have primary glaucoma.[37]

ALTERNATIVES TO SURGERY

Alternatives to surgery include medical and laser therapy and are discussed in Chapters 233–236. In complicated, high-risk cases, alternatives include the use of drainage implants (see Chapter 242) and a cyclodestructive procedure (see Chapter 237).

ANESTHESIA

General anesthetic is avoided whenever possible because of the increased systemic risks and postoperative suprachoroidal effusion and hemorrhage associated with coughing. General anesthetic is necessary for pediatric patients and adults unable to cooperate as a result of altered mental status, anxiety, or severe claustrophobia. Care is required because prolonged postoperative apnea may be caused by the interaction of intraoperative succinylcholine with preoperative, indirect-acting parasympathomimetic drugs. Local anesthetic in conjunction with monitored anesthetic care is preferable for most patients and is conducive for outpatient surgery. Short-acting peribulbar anesthetics reduce the risk of respiratory arrest and allow rapid recovery of vision, which is especially helpful in monocular patients. Topical anesthetic may be useful in some cases.[38] Excessive prolonged preoperative ocular compression is avoided in patients who have a history of ischemic optic neuropathy or fragile optic nerves.

GENERAL TECHNIQUES

The filtration checklist is reviewed prior to surgery (Box 240-3). Patients who have virgin conjunctiva (free of ocular surface disease) and uncontrolled primary glaucomas and who have un-

Preoperative Trabeculectomy Checklist*

1. Chart documentation that substantiates indications, risks, and benefits, and that alternatives to surgery were reviewed and understood by the patient
2. Ensure patient understands the challenge of the approach to glaucoma treatment
3. Ensure patient, family, or friend able to administer drugs postoperatively
4. Establish desirable postoperative target intraocular pressure level (see Box 240-2).
5. Review prior allergies, anesthetic complications, ocular surgeries, and history of choroidal effusion or hemorrhage
6. Obtain informed consent specific for glaucoma filtration surgery
7. Discontinue anticoagulants 4 days prior to surgery—check clotting time if indicated
8. Suppress intraocular flare and cells with corticosteroids, stabilize the blood–aqueous barrier, discontinue strong miotics if possible
9. Eliminate any topical antiglaucoma drugs that cause an allergic reaction (palpebral or bulbar conjunctival follicles, typically a result of adrenergic drugs)
10. Aggressively treat ocular surface disease prior to and after surgery (ocular rosacea, conjunctival hyperemia, blepharitis, and dry eye)
11. Perform gonioscopy—search for peripheral anterior synechiae, intraocular lens haptics; this helps in the decision on trabeculectomy site
12. Locate any prior filtration site or cataract wound—gonioscopy is helpful
13. Check for conjunctival scarring—shown by mobility when a Q-Tip is moved on anesthetized conjunctiva
14. If possible, avoid staphyloma, wound dehiscence, conjunctival scarring, and old suture-tract sites
15. Vitreous in anterior chamber—decide on method of vitrectomy
16. Determine location of proposed filtration site
17. Decide on limbus- or fornix-based conjunctival flap
18. If tight scleral flap indicated, determine if oral carbonic anhydrase inhibitors can be used in the immediate postoperative period
19. If antimetabolite indicated, decide on agent, dose, and duration of application
20. Decide on anesthetic (short-acting anesthetic for monocular patients and no significant external digital pressure for badly damaged nerves)

*There are many factors to consider prior to surgery. If any of these factors are not considered, complications are likely to increase.

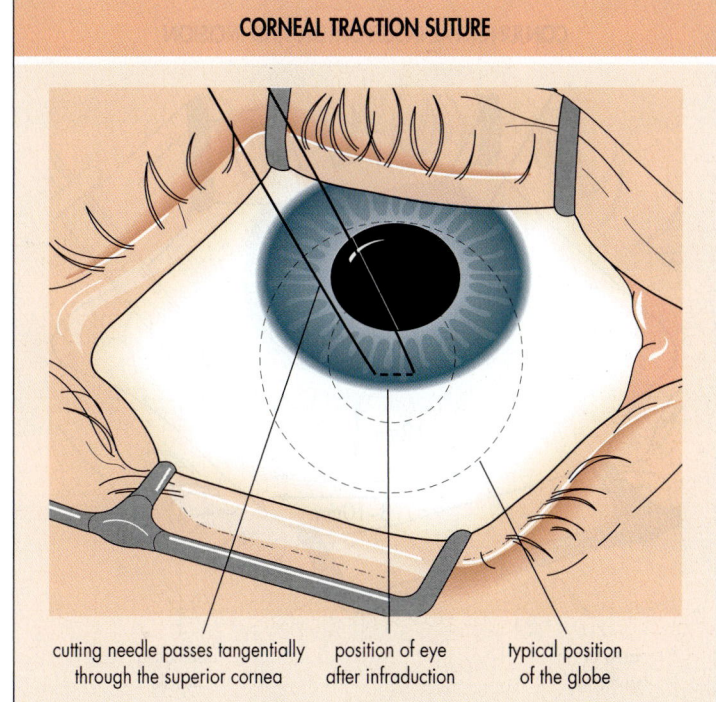

CORNEAL TRACTION SUTURE

cutting needle passes tangentially through the superior cornea   position of eye after infraduction   typical position of the globe

FIG. 240-2 ◼ Corneal traction suture. The dashed line represents the typical position of the globe after adequate akinesia. In this straight-ahead position, it is difficult to place the conjunctival incision accurately. Infraduction using a 9-0 Vicryl suture on a cutting needle passed tangentially through superior cornea allows excellent visibility of the superior tissues.

superior conjunctiva and is preferable to the superior rectus bridle suture for several reasons:

- No holes in the conjunctiva created by the traction suture;
- Rotation of the globe into any inferior quadrant to gain better exposure of the superior tissues;
- Better exposure during wound closure; and
- Impossible to perforate the sclera and retina.

An 8-0 Vicryl traction suture is placed to two thirds of the corneal thickness, approximately 0.5mm from the limbus, at the 11, 12, or 1 o'clock position, depending on the quadrant needed for exposure. The globe is rotated inferiorly to expose at least 12mm of superior conjunctiva.

Conjunctival Incision

LIMBUS BASED. For maximum superior quadrant exposure, the corneal traction suture is clipped to the drape at the 6 o'clock position—the position may be varied slightly. Insufflation of the conjunctiva is carried out using 2–3ml of balanced salt solution administered through an angled 30 gauge needle 10–12mm posterior to the limbus (Fig. 240-3). This elevation and separation of the conjunctiva and Tenon's capsule from the episclera aids in the dissection of the conjunctival flap and is especially helpful in the identification of areas of scarring. The tip of blunt-nosed, sharp Westcott scissors is placed into the conjunctival needle tract, and the conjunctiva and underlying Tenon's fascia are incised parallel to the fornix for a total chord length of 8–10mm.

FORNIX BASED. A fornix-based conjunctival flap (Fig. 240-4) is preferred for eyes that have undergone prior surgery or have difficult limbal exposure or scarring. With this technique, poor-quality limbal tissue may be excised and healthier conjunctival tissue advanced forward to the limbus. A corneal traction suture is still useful for visualization during construction of the scleral flap but may not be necessary, depending on exposure. The conjunctiva is incised at the limbus for at least 6mm using sharp Westcott scissors and leftover conjunctival epithelial remnants are excised from the limbus to ensure adequate postoperative

dergone no prior ocular surgery are the best candidates for successful glaucoma filtration surgery. If possible, areas of conjunctival scarring are avoided. If significant scarring is present at the limbus, a fornix-based conjunctival flap is preferable. Whenever possible, inferior filters are avoided as a result of the high (8%) rate of endophthalmitis,[39] and complications must be anticipated on the basis of type of glaucoma and risk factors. For example, acute IOP reduction, aphakia, and concurrent vitrectomy all increase the incidence of suprachoroidal hemorrhage.[40] Armed with this knowledge, the surgeon must try to avoid hypotony in these eyes by closure of the flap using additional sutures, avoiding sudden intraoperative decompression and prolonging postoperative scleral-flap suture lysis. In virgin eyes, it is preferable to dissect a limbus-based conjunctival flap because the incision is distanced from the filtration site, wound leaks are less likely to occur and easier to repair, and sutures are less symptomatic. Described in the following is one of many techniques used for trabeculectomy. It is important for the surgeon to maintain a good skill level for the construction of both limbal- and fornix-based flaps. A good surgical assistant is essential during glaucoma surgery—retraction of various tissue planes by the assistant is critical to the success of the procedure.

Obtain Adequate Conjunctival Exposure

By far the most common error during limbus-based glaucoma filtration surgery is anterior placement of the conjunctival incision, for which the major reason is poor exposure and visibility of the superior tissues. The corneal traction suture (Fig. 240-2) allows excellent infraduction of the globe with visibility of the

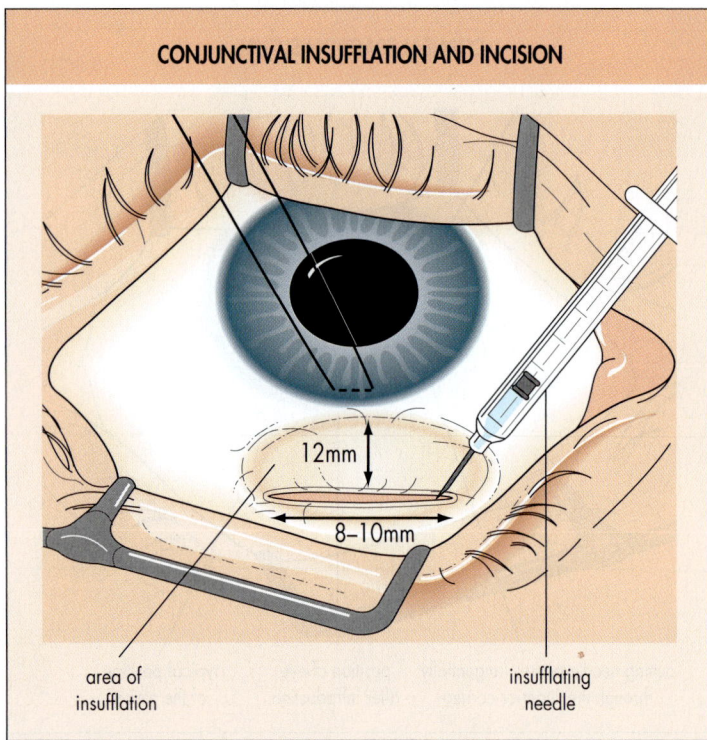

CONJUNCTIVAL INSUFFLATION AND INCISION

12mm

8–10mm

area of insufflation

insufflating needle

FIG 240-3 ▌ **Conjunctival insufflation and incision.** Insufflation of the conjunctiva is carried out with balanced salt solution through a 30gauge needle at least 10mm from the limbus; the conjunctive is incised with sharp Westcott scissors through the needle tract for a chord length of 8–10mm.

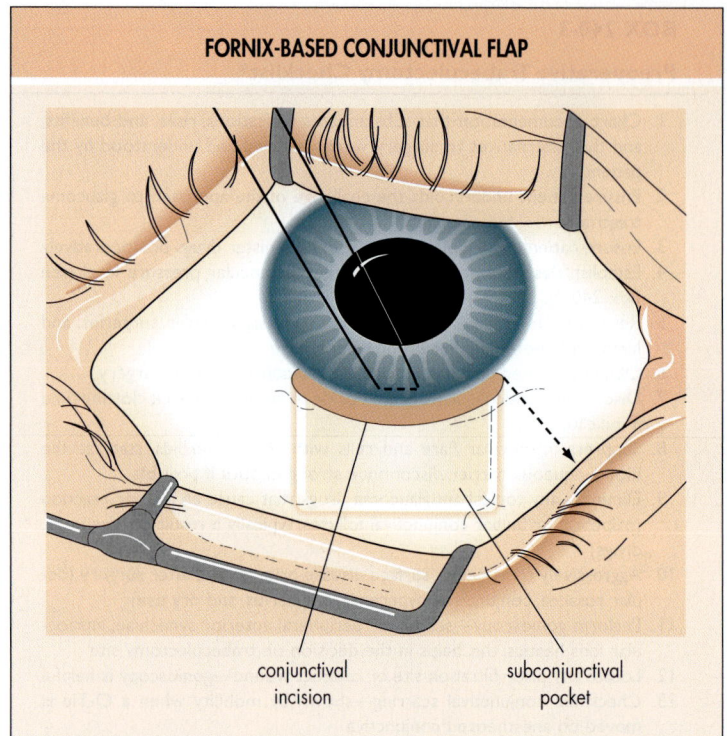

FORNIX-BASED CONJUNCTIVAL FLAP

conjunctival incision

subconjunctival pocket

FIG. 240-4 ▌ **Fornix-based conjunctival flap.** A fornix-based flap is preferable in eyes that have undergone prior surgery, or have limbal scarring, or for which limbal visibility is difficult. A subconjunctival pocket is dissected toward the fornix and, occasionally, a radial incision (dashed line) is required for adequate exposure of the proposed filtration site.

healing. Blunt-tipped Westcott scissors are used to create a subconjunctival pocket by dissection of the conjunctiva and Tenon's capsule off the episclera toward the fornix. The superior rectus muscle, a site of heavy bleeding, must be avoided. Occasionally, a radial extension to the conjunctival incision is required to gain adequate exposure of the filtration site. This radial extension is angled slightly toward the canthus. The conjunctiva must not be touched with toothed instruments. If buttonholes occur during dissection, the defect is repaired by incorporation of Tenon's fascia into the hole, which is closed using a tapered 10-0 microvascular needle. The success rate of limbal-based and fornix-based conjunctival flaps is similar, with cystic blebs more common with a limbal-based approach.[41]

Conjunctival Flap and Tenon's Capsule Dissection

Management of Tenon's capsule is accomplished alongside conjunctival dissection. In this era of antimetabolites, just enough Tenon's capsule is removed to visualize the underlying scleral flap sutures. Adequate Tenon's capsule decreases long-term bleb breakdown, hypotony, and endophthalmitis, but an excess of Tenon's capsule may lead to fibrosis and filtration failure.

For limbus-based surgery, blunt forceps are used to capture the edge of Tenon's capsule directly under the conjunctival wound edge. The capsule is incised down to the episclera, with care taken to avoid the underlying rectus muscle and to leave a cuff at the wound margin (Fig. 240-5). As the flap is dissected toward the limbus, Tenon's capsule is thinned slightly over the filtration area. During the entire conjunctival dissection, the tips of the blunt Westcott scissors are visualized through the semitransparent conjunctiva. Excess capsule is excised from the episclera. A Weck-cell sponge is useful to separate mechanically Tenon's capsule from the limbal junction. Older patients who have thinner Tenon's capsules require minimal manipulation to this layer. Younger patients who have thicker Tenon's capsules require excision of just enough tissue to visualize the scleral flap sutures. Tenonectomy is difficult in younger patients who have redundant tissue. The best technique is to visualize the tip of

the scissors at all times through the semitransparent conjunctiva as the limbus is approached; thus, the conjunctiva is not broken through.

For limbus-based flaps, once dissection has been carried out to the limbus, the assistant must retract the conjunctiva up against the superior cornea using a blunt Weck-cell sponge and thereby expose the surgical limbus. If an excess of Tenon's capsule or fibrous adhesions are found at this corneal-sclera junction, the sharp Westcott scissors may be used in a tangential fashion to remove carefully the excess tissue; alternatively, blunt dissection is carried out using a blade. Toothed instruments must not be used to retract the tissues.

Excess Tenon's capsule may also be removed from a fornix-based flap by retraction of Tenon's capsule down toward the episclera, approximately 1mm from the wound edge, with simultaneous elevation of the anterior edge of the conjunctiva. This creates a tissue plane for excision using the blunt-tipped Westcott scissors. With visualization through the semitransparent conjunctiva, excision is carried out only over the area where scleral flap suture lysis may be necessary; this leaves an anterior Tenon's gasket for added wound-closure protection. Because antimetabolites are toxic to fibroblasts, excessive removal of Tenon's capsule along with an overdose of antimetabolite results in chronic hypotony.

Wet-Field Cautery

At this stage, a buttonhole-free conjunctival flap has been dissected along with removal of the desired amount of Tenon's capsule. Adequate hemostasis is necessary to dissect a scleral flap. Light cautery is used to stop vessel bleeding and to outline the proposed scleral flap and immediate surrounding area. Cautery to the epithelial side of the conjunctiva is avoided, and excessive scleral cautery may result in severe astigmatism.

The Antimetabolite Decision

The necessary decisions regarding antimetabolite usage must be made prior to surgery. Typically, the greater the number and

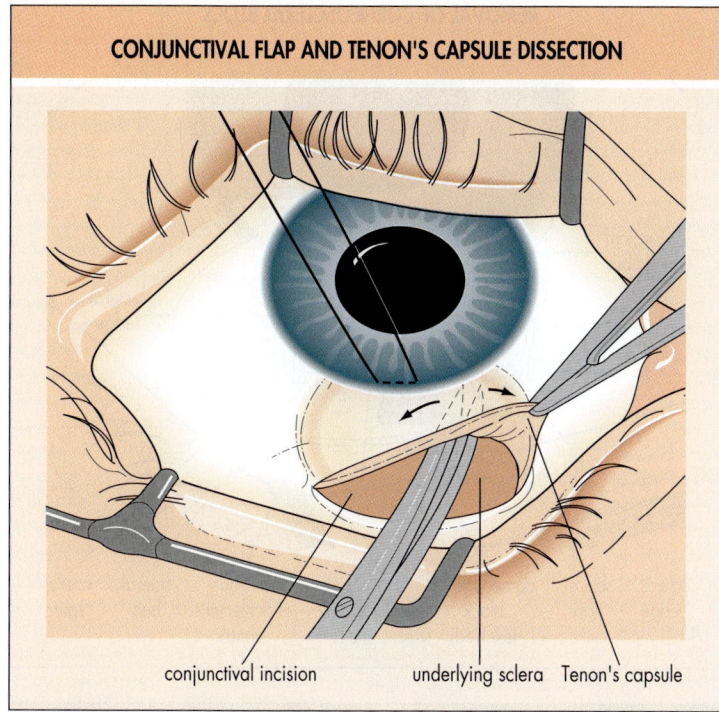

CONJUNCTIVAL FLAP AND TENON'S CAPSULE DISSECTION

conjunctival incision   underlying sclera   Tenon's capsule

FIG. 240-5 ▌▌ Conjunctival flap and Tenon's capsule dissection. After the conjunctival incision has been made, the cuff of Tenon's capsule at the wound margin is grasped with utility forceps and the plane of the dissection is carried toward the limbus and angled slightly upward as the limbus is approached.

OUTLINE AND DIMENSIONS OF SCLERAL FLAP

←4mm→

radial scleral   square scleral   reflection of
incision   flap   conjunctiva over cornea

FIG. 240-6 ▌▌ Outline and dimensions of scleral flap. A 3–4mm² scleral flap is dissected carefully and used to guard the trabeculectomy site. This size of flap ensures adequate coverage of the trabecular block. A scleral flap tunnel technique is useful in eyes that have undergone prior surgery at the limbus, especially prior cataract surgery.

magnitude of risk factors for filtration failure, the more potent the antimetabolite must be. The first decision is whether the case carries a low, medium, or high risk for failure. For a low risk of failure, no antimetabolite is necessary. Postoperatively, if the bleb is injected, a series of 5mg 5-fluorouracil injections is administered into the inferior cul-de-sac. For medium-risk cases, either an intraoperative sponge application of 5-fluorouracil (50mg/ml) for 5 minutes or low-dose mitomycin C (0.2mg/ml for 2–5 minutes)[42] is indicated, and postoperative injections of 5-fluorouracil are titrated if necessary. If only one risk factor is present, 2–3 minutes of mitomycin C application is appropriate; for multiple risk factors, 3–5 minutes.

For very high-risk eyes, the administration of higher concentrations of mitomycin C may be necessary (0.4mg/ml) for a period of 2–5 minutes. However, if these potent concentrations are used in low- or medium-risk eyes, long-term hypotony[43] and bleb breakdown are likely. Prior to scleral flap dissection, a rectangular segment of Merocel instrument wipe or Weck-cell sponge soaked with either 5-fluorouracil 50mg/ml or mitomycin C is placed over the area of intended scleral flap and the conjunctiva retracted over the sponge for the designated time. Immediately after the pledget has been placed, any pools of antimetabolite present are soaked up using a Weck-cell sponge, which is discarded. The size of the pledget varies from 5 to 10mm and is not standardized—the surgeon uses best judgment depending on risk factors and anatomy.

The conjunctiva is retracted, the sponge is removed, and the area is irrigated well using at least 10ml of balanced salt solution.[44] The appropriate Occupational Safety and Health Administration work-practice precautions must be enforced when antimetabolites are handled.

Scleral Flap Dissection

Dissection of the scleral flap requires inferior rotation of the eye to allow good exposure of the proposed area. The technique of freehand dissection requires increased magnification to obtain a more detailed view. The globe is secured inferiorly using the

corneal traction suture while the assistant retracts conjunctiva over the cornea using a blunted Weck-cell sponge. The flap may be located at the 11, 12, or 1 o'clock position, depending on the limbal anatomy. However, the flap must not be placed too far to the medial or lateral side because this results in symptomatic filtration blebs and dellen formation. A variety of instruments may be used to dissect the partial-thickness scleral flap, such as a No. 67 Beaver blade, razor blade, or Grieshaber blade. The choice of instrument is by surgeon's preference and may vary slightly from case to case. Initially, the borders of the flap are outlined to two thirds of the scleral thickness (Fig. 240-6). If the incision is too superficial, the flap has a tendency to be thin, which results in shredding and dissolution of the tissue. Special precautions are necessary when flaps are fashioned in eyes that have undergone previous limbal surgery, especially prior filtration or superior limbal cataract surgery. Such eyes pose many problems for the inexperienced surgeon.

In general, the shape of the flap does not matter as long as it is constructed properly,[45] usually a 4 × 4mm two-third thickness square (Fig. 240-7). Flap size may vary according to the adjacent anatomy. Thin flaps tear or avulse from the bed and may tear during suture closure. The most common error is failure to dissect the flap into clear cornea—dissection into clear cornea ensures adequate room for removal of the corneoscleral block. Thick flaps are probably not detrimental because postoperatively the bulk of flow occurs through the wound margins of the scleral flap. The dissection is kept as close to the 12 o'clock position as possible because excessive medial or lateral flap placement leads to permanent symptomatic filtration blebs—the bane of glaucoma surgeons and patients. The flap dissection must be initiated at one of the posterior corners of the flap. Once an edge has been dissected, the freehand dissection is carried forward uniformly into clear cornea anterior to the trabecular meshwork. This ensures enough room for block removal without removal of scleral spur, which would create a cyclodialysis cleft. As the dissection reaches the limbus, the angle of dissection is altered anteriorly to follow the globe contour (otherwise, the anterior chamber may be entered prematurely).

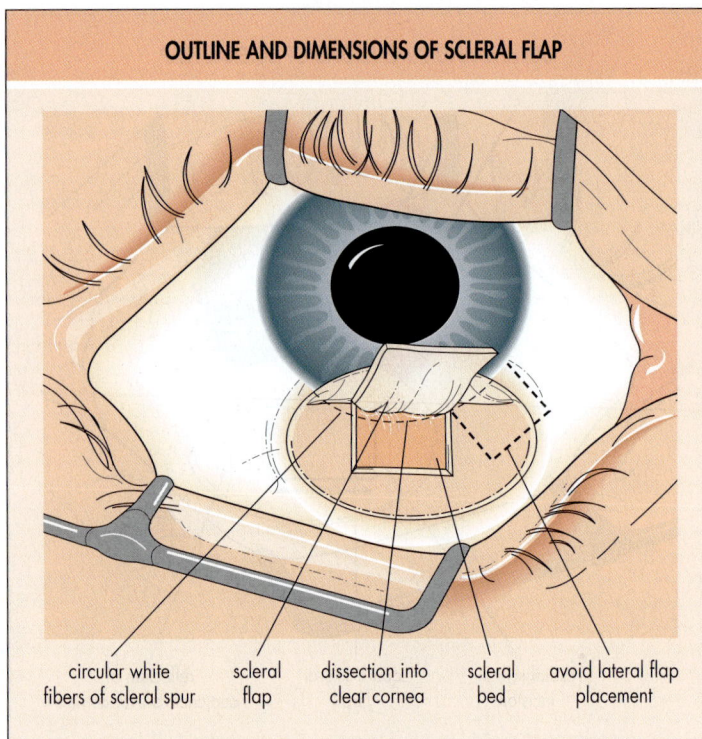

OUTLINE AND DIMENSIONS OF SCLERAL FLAP

circular white fibers of scleral spur | scleral flap | dissection into clear cornea | scleral bed | avoid lateral flap placement

FIG. 240-7 ■ **Dissection and position of scleral flap.** The scleral flap is dissected uniformly at approximately one half to two thirds corneal thickness.

Scleral Tunnel Technique Using a Crescent Blade

The scleral tunnel technique is most helpful in eyes that have prior limbal wounds that tend to fall apart during freehand flap dissections. The scleral tunnel is constructed by incision of sclera tangentially, 3mm posterior to the limbus, for a width of 3–4mm. A crescent blade is used to tunnel into clear cornea in the same fashion as for cataract surgery. The crescent blade is slid from side to side until the sides are extended to about 4mm width. Very fragile flaps are less likely to tear using this technique. If the scleral fibers are so tenuous as to prevent further flap dissection, a punch is slid into the pocket and a block of trabecular tissue removed. Otherwise, the flap is finished by insertion of Vannas scissors at the posterolateral wound margins and the incision connected to the limbus, which creates a three-sided flap.

Paracentesis

A temporal paracentesis tract allows access for anterior chamber insufflation to gauge flow through the trabeculectomy site. A supersharp blade is used to create a temporal, beveled, self-sealing, penetrating corneal tract. Obviously, the lens must be avoided during this maneuver and the paracentesis must penetrate completely through the cornea.

Outline and Removal of Corneoscleral Block

While the assistant rotates the scleral flap over the cornea, a 15° or No. 75 blade is used to outline a 1×1mm scleral block. The medial and lateral margins are incised in an anteroposterior direction using a 15° blade such that an adequate scleral ledge is left on both sides (Fig. 240-8). The anterior incision starts in clear cornea and the posterior extension is the scleral spur. The anterior radial incisions are connected using Vannas scissors, with care taken to avoid the underlying iris and lens. The corneoscleral block is reflected posteriorly and amputated at its base. Light wet-field cautery is applied to the cut ends of Schlemm's canal, which significantly decreases the chance that postoperative hyphema will spill from the canal. The size of the corneoscleral block in relation to the dimensions of the scleral bed determines

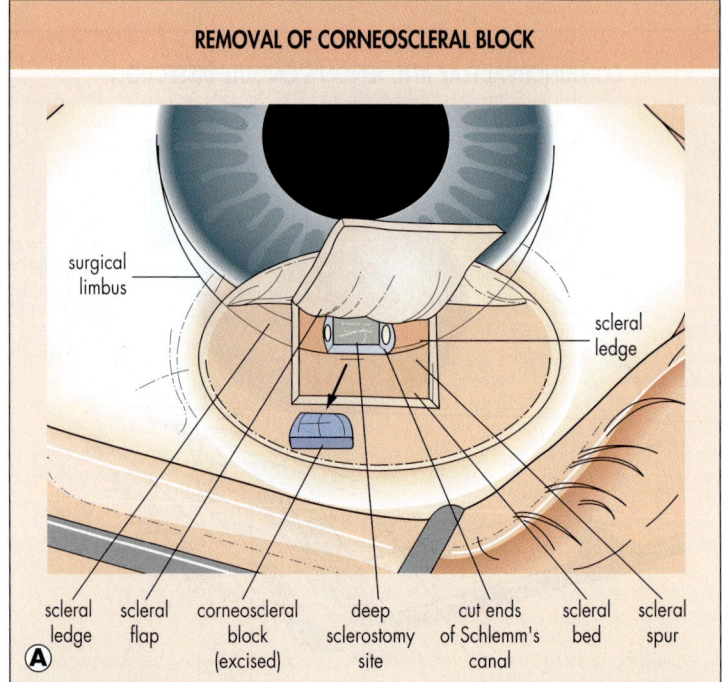

REMOVAL OF CORNEOSCLERAL BLOCK

surgical limbus | scleral ledge

scleral ledge | scleral flap | corneoscleral block (excised) | deep sclerostomy site | cut ends of Schlemm's canal | scleral bed | scleral spur

A

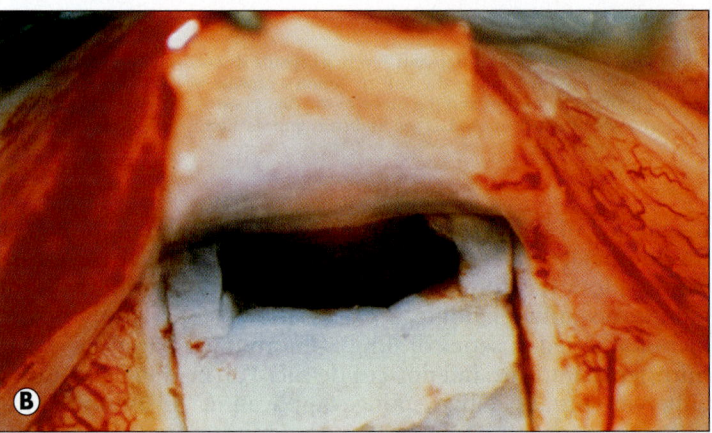

B

FIG. 240-8 ■ **Removal of corneoscleral block. A,** The medial and lateral margins are incised in an anteroposterior direction using a 15° blade such that an adequate scleral ledge is left on both sides. **B,** Typical appearance of trabeculectomy site after removal of corneoscleral block.

the amount of flow through the filter. A very large corneoscleral block leaves a small scleral ledge, which results in overfiltration and hypotony. If the corneoscleral block is too small, the ledge is too large and it is difficult to achieve flow through the flap, especially if it is secured tightly. Excessive posterior block removal into the ciliary body may cause an inadvertent cyclodialysis cleft and bleeding. Anterior block removal may miss the trabecular meshwork, but a fistula still forms. The relationship of the block to limbus is shown in Figure 240-9. Another convenient method of block removal involves anterior chamber entry with a supersharp blade at the base of the scleral bed. A trabecular punch is slid into the tract and a block of tissue is removed.

Iridectomy

Even though rarely is an iridectomy needed in modern-day cataract surgery, it is required for filtration procedures to relieve pupillary block and prevent obstruction of the internal filter opening. After removal of the corneoscleral block, the iris obstructs the opening. The iris is secured using 0.12 forceps in a basal position and retracted outside the posterior ledge of the opening in a tangential fashion, and a section of iris is removed using DeWecker scissors. Aqueous humor pours forth from the posterior chamber. If no fluid is seen, aqueous misdirection syn-

LIMBAL ANATOMY AND CORNEOSCLERAL BLOCK

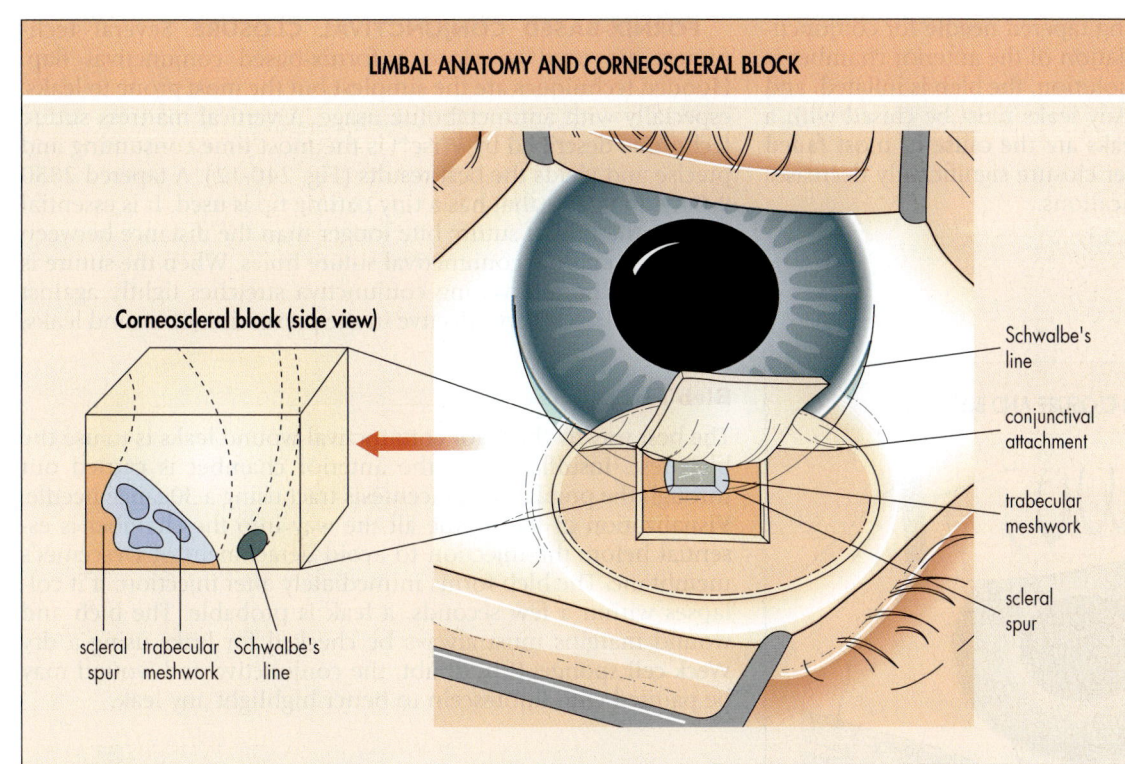

Corneoscleral block (side view)

scleral spur

trabecular meshwork

Schwalbe's line

Schwalbe's line

conjunctival attachment

trabecular meshwork

scleral spur

FIG. 240-9 ▌ **Relationship of corneoscleral block to limbal anatomy.** Typically, the block includes an anterior portion of the scleral spur, trabecular meshwork, Schwalbe's line, and cornea. Postoperative gonioscopy allows the ophthalmologist to view the sclerostomy site.

drome must be suspected and appropriate action taken. The iridectomy size should be slightly larger than the size of the block. The patency is checked by direct observation of lens capsule or red reflex. Pigment epithelium is removed using a sponge if needed. In pseudophakic eyes that have large capsulectomies or in aphakic eyes, vitreous may appear. In rare instances, a peripheral iridectomy is unnecessary, especially if it might cause vitreous prolapse. Vitrectomy has its own set of complications and so must be avoided if possible.

Scleral Flap Closure

Typically, four to five 10-0 preplaced nylon sutures are positioned prior to block removal to facilitate rapid closure. After the preplaced sutures have been tied, immediate reinsufflation of the anterior chamber is carried out to regain global integrity.

Several sutures may be necessary to close the flap adequately (Fig. 240-10). If the flap is very thin, a tapered, microvascular 10-0 nylon needle may be used to prevent cheesewiring of the tissues. If the flap is closed too tightly, no flow occurs and postoperative IOP is elevated. If the flap is closed too loosely, overfiltration occurs. To gauge the proper flow through the filter site is a difficult art but a critical step in successful filtration surgery. A bare ooze of aqueous through the scleral flap is a reasonable endpoint, which is attained by the adjustment and replacement of sutures as necessary. This additional operative time may save hours of postoperative work.

Evaluate Scleral Flap Suture Visibility

It is always safer to err on the side of extra flap sutures. High IOP is easier to treat using scleral flap suture lysis than a return to surgery to place additional sutures. Suture visibility is checked by pulling Tenon's capsule and conjunctiva over the scleral flap. If the sutures cannot be seen, Tenon's capsule is excised until they are visible. As an alternative to laser suture lysis, some surgeons prefer the placement of releasable sutures when the scleral flap is closed. These have a slip knot, the loose end of which is superficially buried in the cornea and can be removed using forceps at the slit lamp at any stage postoperatively; no thinning of the Tenon's capsule is required.

SCLERAL FLAP CLOSURE

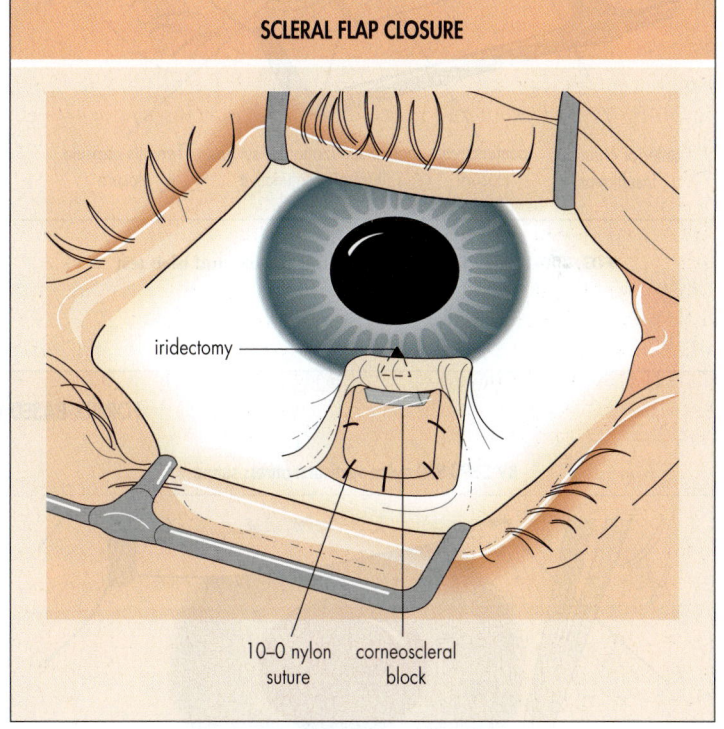

iridectomy

10–0 nylon suture

corneoscleral block

FIG. 240-10 ▌ **Scleral flap closure.** Typically, the scleral flap is closed using multiple 10-0 nylon sutures to protect and guard the fistula from excessive outflow.

Tenon's Capsule and Conjunctiva Wound Closure

LIMBUS-BASED TWO-LAYER CLOSURE. Prior to wound closure, the globe is rotated inferiorly with the corneal traction suture for adequate visualization (Fig. 240-11). The conjunctival flap is repositioned such that the flap sutures are visible; if this is not possible, excess Tenon's capsule is removed carefully, as described earlier. A double-layer closure with fine, tapered needles protects against wound leaks (in this era of antimetabolites, the added protection is helpful). A running, locking 8-0 tapered Vicryl needle is used for Tenon's capsule closure, followed by a

9-0 Vicryl monofilament running tapered needle for conjunctival closure. After closure, insufflation of the anterior chamber is carried out using balanced salt solution, the bleb is inflated, and the wound checked for leaks. Any leaks must be closed with a 10-0 tapered needle. Wound leaks are the cause of most failed trabeculectomies. A double-layer closure significantly decreases leaks and their litany of complications.

FORNIX-BASED CONJUNCTIVAL CLOSURE. Several techniques are used to close a fornix-based conjunctival flap. Hooded techniques are the simplest but the most prone to leaks, especially with antimetabolite usage. A vertical mattress suture technique described by Wise[46] is the most time consuming and precise and yields the best results (Fig. 240-12). A tapered 2850 9-0 nylon needle that has a tiny cutting tip is used. It is essential to keep the limbal suture bite longer than the distance between the corresponding conjunctival suture holes. When the suture is tightened, the intervening conjunctiva stretches tightly against the sclera. This is very effective in the prevention of wound leaks.

Bleb Test

The best way to check for conjunctival wound leaks is to use the bleb test. Insufflation of the anterior chamber is carried out through the preplaced paracentesis tract using a 30gauge needle. Visualization of the needle all the way into the chamber is essential before the injection to avoid detachment of Descemet's membrane. The bleb forms immediately after injection; if it collapses within a few seconds, a leak is probable. The bleb and wound margins must always be checked for leaks using a dry Weck-cell sponge. If in doubt, the conjunctiva and wound may be painted with fluorescein to better highlight any leak.

Medications and Postoperative Care

Intraoperative topical atropine may help to stabilize the blood-aqueous barrier and relax the ciliary body. Subconjunctival antibiotic and corticosteroid are injected, with great care taken to avoid globe penetration. Proper wound healing is critical for successful filtration,[47] and topical corticosteroids are the mainstay for prevention of inflammation and scarring.[48] Administration may vary from every hour to every 6 hours in the immediate postoperative period and is tapered over 2 months depending on bleb appearance. Care in the first 2 weeks postoperatively is time consuming and laborious. The bleb is scrutinized for leaks and vascularity; the anterior chamber for flare, cells, and depth; and the posterior pole for choroidal effusion. Therapy is adjusted to

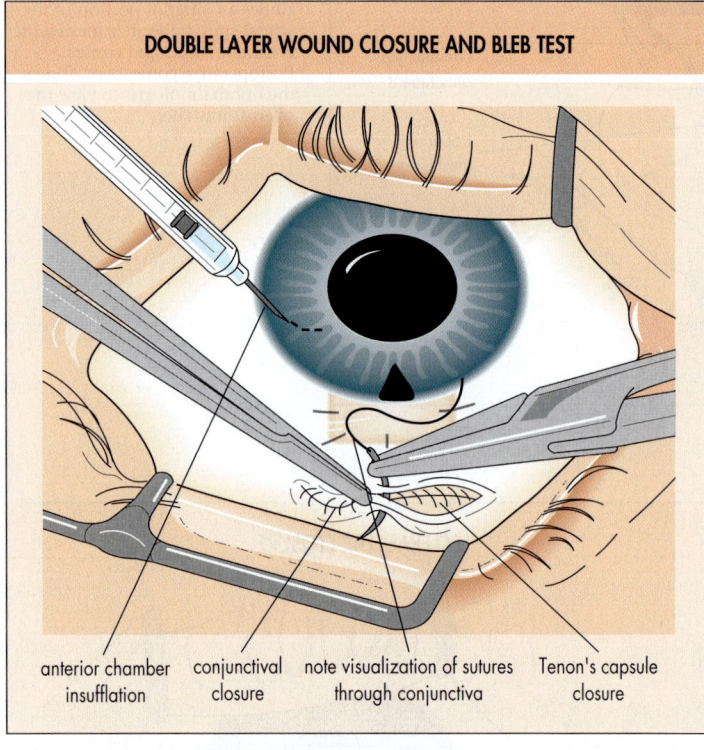

DOUBLE LAYER WOUND CLOSURE AND BLEB TEST

anterior chamber insufflation | conjunctival closure | note visualization of sutures through conjunctiva | Tenon's capsule closure

FIG. 240-11 ▪ Double-layer wound closure and bleb test.

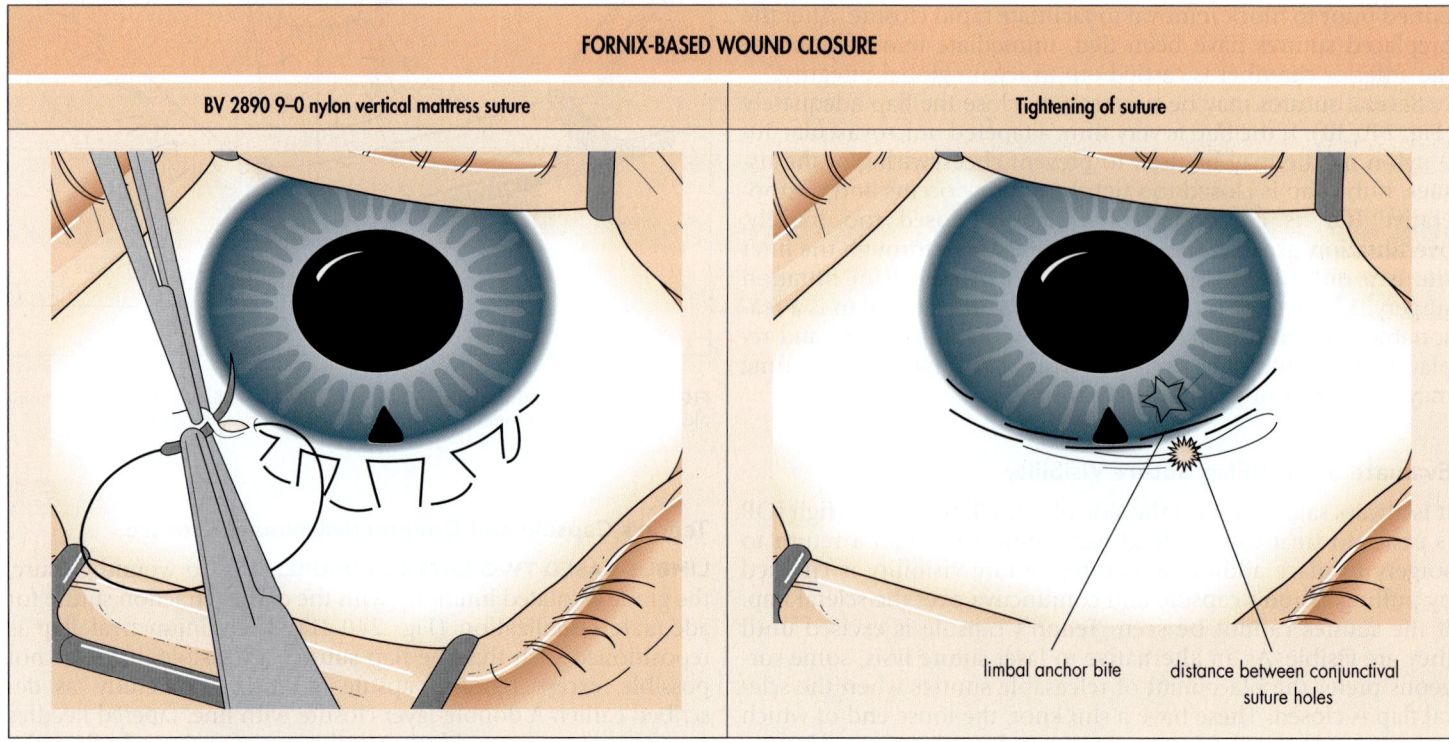

FORNIX-BASED WOUND CLOSURE

BV 2890 9–0 nylon vertical mattress suture | Tightening of suture

limbal anchor bite | distance between conjunctival suture holes

FIG. 240-12 ▪ Fornix-based wound closure. A vertical mattress suture is placed—precise construction is required to keep the limbal suture bite longer than the distance between the corresponding conjunctival suture holes (see stars).

correct any abnormality of the bleb, chamber, or posterior pole. The timing of laser scleral flap suture lysis is critical to the long-term health of the bleb. Early lysis may result in hypotony and late lysis in bleb failure. The use of antimetabolites has extended the time window for laser suture lysis.[49]

COMPLICATIONS OF GLAUCOMA FILTERING SURGERY

The complications are discussed in detail in Chapter 243.

OUTCOMES

Glaucoma filtration surgery is an evolving science. Controversy arises over antimetabolite usage, type of conjunctival incision, candidates for surgery, and postoperative care. The outcome is highly dependent on the skill level of the surgeon, type of glaucoma, age and race of the patient, and prior ocular surgery that involves scarring of the conjunctiva.

The reader must remember that a perfectly executed limbal-based trabeculectomy in a virgin eye may be a work of art; however, the same technique in an eye with limbal scarring may lead to conjunctival buttonholes and other sight-threatening disasters.

The key to the art of trabeculectomy is the surgeon's ability to modify and adapt technique to each and every patient's ocular and systemic situation.

REFERENCES

1. Sugar HS. Experimental trabeculectomy in glaucoma. Am J Ophthalmol. 1961;51:623–7.
2. Cairns JE. Trabeculectomy. Preliminary report of a new method. Am J Ophthalmol. 1968;66:673–8.
3. Savage JA, Concon GP, Lytle RA, et al. Laser suture lysis after trabeculectomy. Ophthalmology. 1988;95:1631–8.
4. The Fluorouracil Filtering Surgery Study Group. Fluorouracil Filtering Surgery Study one-year follow-up. Am J Ophthalmol. 1989;108:625–35.
5. Kitazawa Y, Kawase K, Matsushita H, et al. Trabeculectomy with mitomycin. A comparative study with fluorouracil. Arch Ophthalmol. 1991;109:1693–8.
6. Koseki N, Araie M, Shirato S, Yamamoto S. Effect of trabeculectomy on visual field performance in central 30 degrees in progressive normal-tension glaucoma. Ophthalmology. 1997;104:192–201.
7. Roth SM, Spaeth GL, Starita RJ, et al. The effect of postoperative corticosteroids on trabeculectomy and the clinical course of glaucoma: five year follow-up study. Ophthalmic Surg. 1991;22:724–9.
8. The AGIS Investigators; The advanced glaucoma intervention study (AGOS): 7. The relationship between control of intraocular pressure and visual field deterioration. Am J Ophthalmol. 2000;130:429-440.
9. Chew SJ, Ritch R. Neuro protection: the next breakthrough in glaucoma? Proceedings of the Third Annual Optic Nerve Rescue and Restoration Think Tank. J Glaucoma. 1992;6:263–4.
10. Vanbuskirk EM. The technology dilemma. J Glaucoma. 1996;5:77–8.
11. Cunliffe IA, Dapling RB, Longstaff S. A prospective study examining the changes in factors that affect visual acuity following trabeculectomy. Eye. 1992;6:618–22.
12. Dietze PJ, Oram O, Kohnen T, et al. Visual function following trabeculectomy: effect on corneal topography and contrast sensitivity. J Glaucoma. 1997;6:90–103.
13. Costa VP, Smith M, Spaeth GL, et al. Loss of visual acuity after trabeculectomy. Ophthalmology. 1993;100:599–612.
14. Lichter PR, Ravin JG. Risks of sudden visual loss after glaucoma surgery. Am J Ophthalmol. 1974;78:1009–13.
15. Givens K, Shields MB. Suprachoroidal hemorrhage after glaucoma filtering surgery. Am J Ophthalmol. 1987;103:689–94.
16. Parrish RK III, Herschler J. Eyes with end-stage neovascular glaucoma: natural history following successful modified filtering operation. Arch Ophthalmol. 1983;101:745–6.
17. Broadway D, Grierson I, Hitchings R. Racial differences in the results of glaucoma filtrative surgery. Br J Ophthalmol. 1994;78:466–75.
18. Bellows AR, Johnstone MA. Surgical management of chronic glaucoma in aphakia. Ophthalmology. 1983;90:807–13.
19. Jampel HD, Jabs DA, Quigley HA. Trabeculectomy with 5-fluorouracil for adult inflammatory glaucoma. Am J Ophthalmol. 1990;109:168–73.
20. Susanna R, Oltrogge EW, Carani JG, Nicolela MT. Mitomycin as adjunct chemotherapy with trabeculectomy in congenital and developmental glaucomas. J Glaucoma. 1995;4:151–7.
21. Mills K. Trabeculectomy: a retrospective long-term follow-up of 444 cases. Br J Ophthalmol. 1981;65:790–5.
22. Sherwood MB, Grierson I, Milar L, Hitchings RA. Long-term morphologic effects of antiglaucoma drugs on the conjunctiva and Tenon's capsule in glaucoma patients. Ophthalmology. 1989;96:327–35.
23. Costa VP, Katz LJ, Spaeth GL, et al. Primary trabeculectomy in young adults. Ophthalmology. 1993;100:1071–6.
24. Ando H, Ido T, Kawai Y, et al. Inhibition of corneal epithelial wound healing. Ophthalmology. 1992;99:1809–14.
25. Weinreb RN. Riding the Trojan horse of glaucoma surgery. J Glaucoma. 1995;4:2–4.
26. Heuer DK, Parrish RK II, Gressel MG, et al. 5-Fluorouracil and glaucoma filtering surgery. II. A pilot study. Ophthalmology. 1984;91:384–94.
27. Rockwood EJ, Parrish RK II, Heuer DK, et al. Glaucoma filtering surgery with 5-fluorouracil. Ophthalmology. 1987;94:1071–8.
28. Rothman RF, Liebmann JM, Ritch R. Low-dose 5-fluorouracil trabeculectomy as initial surgery in uncomplicated glaucoma; long-term followup. Ophthalmology. 2000;107:1184–90.
29. Dietze PJ, Feldman RM, Gross RL. Intraoperative application of 5-fluorouracil during trabeculectomy. Ophthalmic Surg. 1992;23:662–5.
30. Yodaiken RE, Bennett D. OSHA work-practice guidelines for personnel dealing with cytotoxic (antineoplastic) drugs. Am J Hosp Pharm. 1986;43:1193–204.
31. Chen C, Huang T, Sheu M. Enhancement of IOP control: effect of trabeculectomy by local application of anticancer drug. Acta Ophthalmol Scand. 1986;25:1487–91.
32. Palmer S. Mitomycin as adjunct chemotherapy with trabeculectomy. Ophthalmology. 1991;98:317–21.
33. Megevand GS, Salmon JF, Scholtz RP, Murray AD. The effect of reducing the exposure time of mitomycin C in glaucoma filtering surgery. Ophthalmology. 1995;102:84–90.
34. Cheung JC, Wright MM, Murali S, Pederson JE. Intermediate-term outcome of variable dose mitomycin C filtering surgery. Ophthalmology. 1997;104:143–9.
35. Skuta GL, Beeson CC, Higginbotham EJ, et al. Intraoperative mitomycin versus postoperative 5-fluorouracil in high-risk glaucoma filtering surgery. Ophthalmology. 1992;99:438–44.
36. Yamamoto T, Kitazawa Y. Residual mitomycin C dosage in surgical sponges removed at the time of trabeculectomy. Am J Ophthalmol. 1994;117:672–3.
37. Singh K, Mehta KAAA, Shaikh NM, et. al. Trabeculectomy with intraoperative mitomycin C versus 5-fluorouracil. Prospective randomized clinical trial. Ophthalmology. 2000;107:2305–9.
38. Buys YM, Trope GE. Prospective study of sub-Tenon's versus retrobulbar anesthesia for inpatient and day surgery trabeculectomy. Ophthalmology. 1996;103:1585–7.
39. Higginbotham EJ, Stevens RK, Musch DC, et al. Bleb-related endophthalmitis after trabeculectomy with mitomycin C. Ophthalmology. 1996;103:650–6.
40. Rockwood EJ, Kalenal JW, Plotnik JL, et al. Prospective ultrasonographic evaluation of intraoperative and delayed postoperative suprachoroidal hemorrhage from glaucoma filtering surgery. J Glaucoma. 1995;4:16–24.
41. El Sayyad F, El-Rashood A., Helal M, et al. Conjunctival flaps in initial trabeculectomy with post-operative 5-fluorouracil:four year followup findings. J Glaucoma. 1999;8:124–8.
42. Smith MF, Doyle JW, Nguyen QH, Sherwood MB. Results of intraoperative 5-fluorouracil or lower dose mitomycin C administration on initial trabeculectomy surgery. J Glaucoma. 1997;6:104–10.
43. Zacharria PT, Depperrman SR, Schuman JS. Ocular hypotony after trabeculectomy with mitomycin C. Am J Ophthalmol. 1993;116:314–36.
44. Prata JA, Minckler DS, Koda RT. Effects of external irrigation on mitomycin C concentration in rabbit aqueous and vitreous humor. J Glaucoma. 1995;4:32–5.
45. Starita RJ, Fellman RL, Spaeth, GL, et al. Effect of varying scleral flap and corneal block on trabeculectomy. Ophthalmic Surg. 1984;15:484–7.
46. Wise J. Mitomycin compatible suture technique for fornix based conjunctival flaps in glaucoma filtration surgery. Arch Ophthalmol. 1993;111:992–7.
47. Skuta GL, Parrish RK. Wound healing in glaucoma filtering surgery. Surv Ophthalmol. 1987;32:149–70.
48. Starita RJ, Fellman RL, Spaeth GL, et al. Short- and long-term effects of postoperative corticosteroids on trabeculectomy. Ophthalmology. 1985;92:938–46.
49. Pappa KS, Derick RJ, Weber PA, et al. Late argon laser suture lysis after mitomycin C trabeculectomy. Ophthalmology. 1993;100:1268–71.

CHAPTER

241 Antifibrotic Agents in Glaucoma Surgery

PENG TEE KHAW • LYDIA CHANG

INTRODUCTION

One of the major areas of advance in the surgical management of glaucoma over the past 20 years has been the use of antimetabolites to prevent scarring after glaucoma filtration surgery. Antimetabolites have gone from occasional use in high-risk patients in the 1980s to use of mitomycin C (MMC) in more than 50% of cases undergoing primary trabeculectomy by university-based glaucoma physicians in the United States.[1] The Advanced Glaucoma Intervention Study (AGIS) has shown that target intraocular pressures (IOPs) around 12mmHg are required to arrest glaucomatous progression over a decade, rather than just an IOP lower than 21mmHg (2.8kPa).[2] Therefore, the concept that the healing response should be modulated after all surgery has become increasingly important. The healing response is the major determinant of long-term IOP levels after glaucoma surgery. Therefore, modulation of this response together with appropriate surgical techniques may enable the surgeon to set the IOP at the lowest level that is safe, not just in high-risk patients but in every patient who undergoes filtration surgery.

ANTIFIBROTIC AGENTS AND STRATEGIES

Although most attention has been focused on antimetabolites such as 5-fluorouracil and MMC, it must not be forgotten that many strategies exist to prevent fibrosis and scarring after glaucoma filtration surgery (summarized in Table 241-1). Many of these have been used experimentally, but some such as the human

TABLE 241-1

WOUND HEALING AND POSSIBLE MODIFICATION AFTER GLAUCOMA SURGERY

Event	Potential Modulation
Primed damaged conjunctiva "preactivated" cells	Stop medical therapy especially adrenaline Preoperative steroids
Conjunctival/episcleral/scleral incisions	Minimal trauma Less invasive surgical techniques
Damage to connective tissue Release of plasma proteins and blood cells	Hemostasis (Vital: blood can reverse mitomycin!)
Activation of clotting and complement Fibrin/fibronectin/blood cell clot	Agents preventing/removing fibrin (e.g., heparin, tissue plasminogen activator, hirudin)
Release of growth factors from blood	Antagonists to growth factor production (e.g., antibodies to growth factors humanized anti–TGF-β2) Antibody (CAT 152) or receptors Antisense oligonucleotides, ribozymes Less specific antagonists, e.g., tranilast, genistein, suramin
Aqueous released from eye Some breakdown of blood-aqueous barrier	Blood-aqueous barrier stabilizing agents (e.g., steroids)
Release of growth factors into aqueous Aqueous begins to flow through wound	Nonsteroidal anti-inflammatory agents
Migration and proliferation of polymorphonuclear neutrophil cells, macrophages, and lymphocytes.	Anti-inflammatory agents (e.g., steroids/cyclosporine) Antimetabolites, e.g., 5-fluorouracil/MMC
Activation, migration, and proliferation of fibroblasts	Preoperative steroids to reduce activation Antimetabolites MMC 5-fluorouracil
Wound contraction	Anticontraction agents (e.g., colchicine, taxol) MMP inhibitors
Fibroblast synthesis of tropocollagen, Glycosaminoglycans, and fibronectin	Interferon alpha MMP inhibitors
Collagen cross-linking and modification	Anti–cross-linking agents (e.g., β-inopropionitrile/penicillamine)
Blood vessel endothelial migration and proliferation	Inhibitors of angiogenesis (e.g., angiostatin)
Resolution of healing Apoptosis Disappearance of fibroblasts Fibrous subconjunctival scar	MMC, 5-fluorouracil Death receptor ligands Stimulants of apoptosis pathways

Modified from Khaw PT, Occleston NL, Schultz GS, *et al.* Acticvation and suppression of fibroblast activity. Eye. 1994:8;188–95.
Events and agents have overlapping time duration and action.

antibody to transforming growth factor β2 (TGF-β2) are now undergoing clinical trials. Many of the agents given in Table 241-1 have multiple actions on the healing cascade. It is particularly important to remember that agents such as corticosteroids, although routinely used, may not be used optimally.[3] However, the antifibrotic agents used most commonly at present are discussed in this chapter; namely the antimetabolites. The term antimetabolites is a broad generic term, used herein to describe agents that interfere with cellular processing at every level, from DNA to protein.

ANTIMETABOLITES

The use of the antimetabolite 5-fluorouracil, given by postoperative injections, was popularized by the work of Parrish and colleagues[4] from Miami in the 1980s, following work on 5-fluorouracil for experimental proliferative vitreoretinopathy.[5] More recently, 5-fluorouracil has been used as a single intraoperative sponge application, a development stimulated by the intraoperative topical application of MMC and cell culture results[6,7] which suggested that long-term effects could be achieved with convenient, single, short intraoperative applications. Intraoperative MMC application was first used clinically by Chen in 1981; since the late 1980s its use has increased exponentially worldwide because of the ease of application and its dramatic effects. However, these powerful agents potentially have sight-threatening side effects. In this chapter, current views on the use of these antifibrotic agents are summarized.

TABLE 241-2

RISK FACTORS FOR SCARRING AFTER GLAUCOMA FILTRATION SURGERY

Risk Factor	Risk (+ to +++)	Comments
Neovascular glaucoma (active)	+ + +	
Previous failed filtration surgery	+ + (+)	
Previous conjunctival surgery	+ +	
Chronic conjunctival inflammation	+ + (+)	
Previous cataract extraction (conjunctival incision)	+ + (+)	
Aphakia (intracapsular extraction)	+ + +	
Previous intraocular surgery	+ +	Depends on type of surgery
Recent surgery (within last 30 days)	+ + (+)	
Uveitis (active, persistent)	+ + +	
A red, injected eye	+ +	Personal experience
African–Caribbean	+ (+)	May vary (e.g., West versus East African–American Africans, elderly versus young)
Previous topical medications (β-blockers + pilocarpine)	+	
Previous topical medications (β-blockers + pilocarpine + epinephrine)	+ + (+)	
New topical medications	(+)	Particularly if they cause a red eye
High preoperative intraocular pressure	+	Higher with each 10mmHg (1.3kPa) rise
Age <40 years with no other factors	+	Controversial
Hispanic	+	
Japanese	+	
Inferiorly located trabeculectomy	+	

PATIENT GROUPS THAT REQUIRE ANTIMETABOLITES

A number of patient factors increase the risk of scarring and failure after glaucoma surgery, as summarized in Table 241-2. However, the risk may still vary within subgroups. Patients who suffer from uveitis may have chronic persistent uveitis, which may carry a much worse surgical prognosis than that for patients who suffer episodic uveitis. Patients may also be subject to more than one risk factor, which may increase their overall risk. There may be hidden risk factors for failure in what were previously regarded as low-risk "first time surgery" groups.

Broadway et al.[8] showed that the success rate of trabeculectomy as primary surgery without medical treatment was 90%, similar to that in the group treated with β-blockers (93%). The success rate for patients treated with both β-blockers and miotics was significantly lower (72%), and for the group treated with β-blockers, miotics, and sympathomimetics, the success rate was only 45% (worse than for previous failed trabeculectomy or cataract extraction with conjunctival incision), with enhanced scarring a significant problem (Fig. 241-1). Interestingly, it has been found that the fornices of patients who have received topical medications are contracted.[9] The role of topical medications is not understood completely[10]; however, what is clear is that even a small increase in risk with topical medications has a profound effect on surgical success worldwide, as this group of patients accounts for the majority of patients who undergo surgery in developed countries.

High-Risk Patient Groups

Patient factors that carry a high risk of surgical failure include previous failed trabeculectomies, previous cataract surgery through a conjunctival incision, neovascular glaucoma, chronic persistent uveitis, and multiple previous intraocular surgery. Most glaucoma specialists agree that some form of antimetabolite treatment be used in these patient groups. The most definitive study of 5-fluorouracil injections was the randomized, prospective National Eye Institute 5-Fluorouracil Filtration Surgery Study, which showed a 51% failure rate after filtration surgery in patients who had failed trabeculectomy previously or had undergone cataract surgery with a conjunctival incision. In the randomized group that received 5-fluorouracil 5mg injections (twice a day for days 1–7, once a day for days 8–14, total 21 injections), the failure rate was only 51% compared with 74% in the placebo group after 5 years.[11] Since then, several randomized studies undertaken to compare intraoperative MMC application (0.4–0.5mg/ml) with postoperative 5-fluorouracil injections (approximately ten 5mg injections)[12-14] have shown that in high-risk

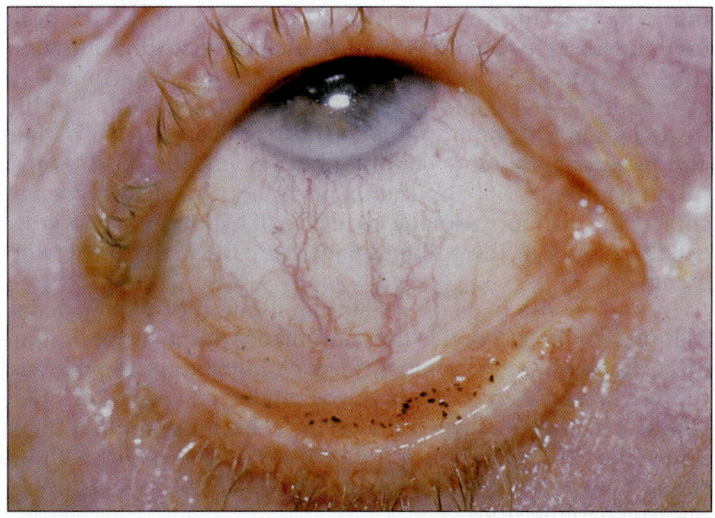

FIG. 241-1 ■ **Adrenochrome deposits.** Topical treatment may worsen the prognosis of filtration surgery because of an enhanced scarring response.

patients a single application of MMC provides superior long-term pressure control compared with injections of 5-fluorouracil without the risk of keratopathy. Corneal epithelial complications are much more common with injectable 5-fluorouracil, but both groups had thin avascular blebs, these being more prominent in the MMC-treated groups.

The intraoperative MMC regimen, rather than the postoperative subconjunctival 5-fluorouracil injection regimen, is rapidly becoming the treatment of choice for these high-risk patients because of the increased efficacy, ease of application, and virtual absence of corneal side effects. However, longer periods of follow-up are required to monitor the development of bleb leaks, hypotony, and endophthalmitis after the two treatment regimens, in view of the thinner and highly avascular blebs seen with MMC.

With regard to intraoperative 5-fluorouracil application, Egbert et al.[15] carried out a randomized prospective study in a group of West African patients in whom there was a high risk of failure. They showed success rates of 83% in the 5-fluorouracil–treated group versus 39% in the control group, with a mean follow-up of 282 days. Singh et al.[16] compared intraoperative 5-fluorouracil application (50mg/ml for 5 minutes) against MMC application (0.5mg/ml for 3 minutes) in a group of West African patients, with short-term follow-up averaging 10 months. They found lower average IOPs in the MMC-treated group, but because of the relatively small numbers, no short-term difference in complications was found in this group of higher risk patients. Therefore, in this particular group, intraoperative MMC application offers better results than intraoperative 5-fluorouracil application with no large short-term penalty in terms of complication rates; MMC, therefore, appears to be superior in the short term.

Antimetabolites may also be used after other glaucoma procedures that are usually associated with a strong healing reaction—for example, after tube implant surgery and after combined cataract extraction and glaucoma filtration surgery. The blebs seen after MMC treatment, combined with tube implants, are much less avascular and cystic. It has yet to be proved conclusively that intraoperative MMC improves the prognosis for tube surgery as opposed to trabeculectomy. In combined glaucoma filtration and cataract surgery, both postoperative subconjunctival 5-fluorouracil and intraoperative MMC have been used. However, the majority of publications suggest that neither 5-fluorouracil injections nor intraoperative MMC has a very significant effect on pressure control after combined cataract and glaucoma surgery.[17]

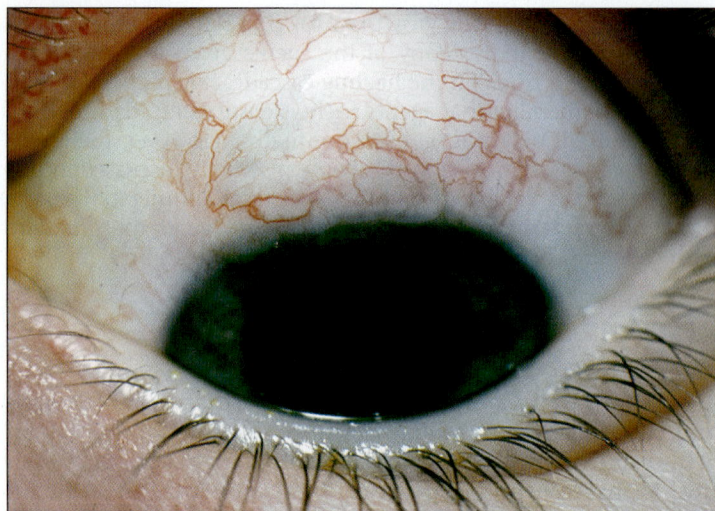

FIG. 241-2 ▍ **Diffuse relatively noncystic bleb.** This arose after β-radiation adjunctive treatment with a large surface area to prevent scarring.

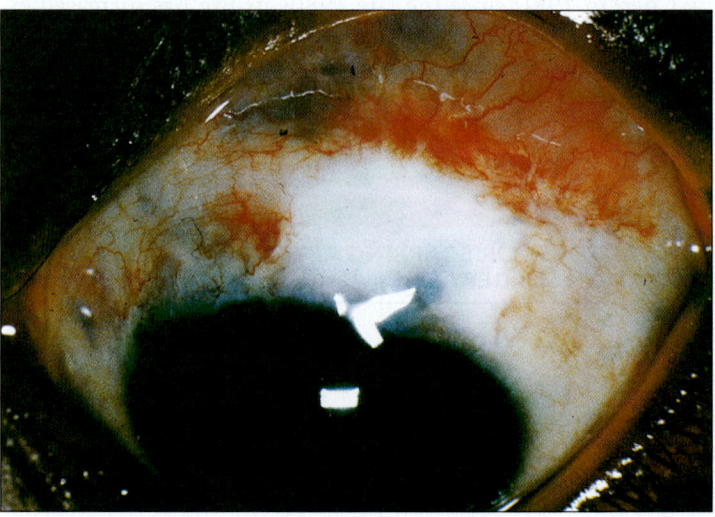

FIG. 241-3 ▍ **Cystic avascular bleb.** This arose after the use of a limbus-based flap with a small rectangular sponge soaked in mitomycin C 0.4mg/ml. Safer diffuse noncystic blebs can now be created with a simple change in operative technique.

Intermediate- or Low-Risk Patient Groups

Antimetabolite use in eyes with no previous surgery of any kind and no significant intraocular disease apart from glaucoma is much more controversial. 5-Fluorouracil injections have been used in lower risk groups, which include first-time filtration surgery,[18] young patients,[19] and normal tension glaucoma,[20] to achieve lower IOPs, and superior success rates are found in the treated groups. Complications such as cornea epithelial change and hypotony are more common but only in the short term.[18] Intraoperative MMC application increases the success rate of surgery but also increases the incidence of hypotony.[21] Hypotony usually occurs in the younger patients, particularly those who are myopic.[21,22]

In the low-risk patients, a single application of intraoperative 5-fluorouracil may provide the convenience of single-application MMC but without the same incidence of hypotony and the very thin and completely avascular blebs often seen with MMC. Cell culture experiments suggest that a single 5-minute application of 5-fluorouracil can inhibit fibroblasts for several weeks without severe long-term damage and may be equivalent to low-dose 5-fluorouracil injections.[6,23,24]

Several studies using single applications of intraoperative 5-fluorouracil with short-term follow-up have reported promising results in low-risk patients. Smith et al.[25] originally reported the use of intraoperative 5-fluorouracil application in combination with postoperative injections. Lanigan et al.[26] reported a success rate of 77% in high-risk patients (neovascularization, previous failed filter, aphakia, uveitis, or multiple risk factors), with a 100% success rate in the low-risk group (medications >3 years, or <40 years age, or African-Caribbean). Also, Feldman et al.[27] reported an overall success rate of 85% in high-risk patients and a success rate of 92.9% in low-risk patients; no hypotony was reported in the Feldman study. However, both studies were short term with no controls. Therefore, failure occurs in higher risk patients who have a prolonged or aggressive healing response, but in lower risk patients the success rate is very good (>90%) with no clinically significant hypotony. An improvement in survival was also found for patients in East Africa with a single 5-minute application of 5-fluorouracil 25mg/ml, interestingly with a much lower failure rate in the control group[28] compared with patients in West Africa.[15] A single application of intraoperative beta-radiation (750cGy) delivered by a strontium-90 probe may be similar to a single-dose intraoperative 5-fluorouracil application.[29,30] The advantage of intraoperative beta-radiation is that it appears to give rise to blebs that are more diffuse and less cystic than those elicited by 5-fluorouracil or MMC use (Figs. 241-2 and 241-3).

An intraoperative, single-dose regimen for scarring after glaucoma filtration surgery. (This regimen is still evolving.) Other factors may also determine the choice of agent, such as the need for a low target pressure due to advanced disease (require a stronger antimetabolite treatment).
*Intraoperative beta-radiation 750–1000cGy can also be used. Most of the newer agents currently being tested in pilot studies, e.g., CAT-152 humanized anti–TGF-β2 antibody, are probably appropriate for the low- and intermediate-risk groups. These groups do, however, account for the majority of patients undergoing glaucoma filtration surgery.
†Postoperative 5-fluorouracil injections can be given in addition to the intraoperative applications of antimetabolite

A single antimetabolite regimen may not be adequate for all patients. The type and dose of drugs may need to be titrated depending on the individual patient's risk factors and healing response. The authors use a "titratable" regimen that is based on laboratory[6,24] and clinical data gained from experience using the different single-application agents and concentrations [the authors call this the Moorfields/Florida regimen (More Flow) regimen]. This regimen evolves constantly, but the present regimen is summarized in Box 241-1. Also, subconjunctival postoperative injections of 5-fluorouracil may be used in addition to the application of intraoperative antimetabolites.

APPLICATION TECHNIQUE (INTRAOPERATIVE ANTIMETABOLITES)

The significant variations in technique used to deliver intraoperative antimetabolites are not addressed sufficiently in the literature, which may account for some of the variations in efficacy and complications published. It is important for individual surgeons to maintain a consistent technique and to reevaluate periodically their experience using this technique. We now understand better how antimetabolites, particularly MMC, work in vivo causing long-term tissue cell death and growth arrest.[24] There is remnant functional activity in peripheral fibroblasts that form a ring of scar tissue around the bleb[31] ("ring of steel"). This has allowed us to evolve strategies in antimetabolite delivery to improve our success rate (Box 241-2) and to change bleb morphology dramatically (Fig. 241-4). This has reduced the number of cystic blebs from 90 to 29% and reduced bleb-related complications, particularly endophthalmitis, from 15% to 0% over a 3-year follow-up period.[32] If this result is extrapolated to the United States, where many trabeculectomies are done with MMC,[1] this could reduce bleb-related complications in many thousands of patients. A summary of the improvements in antimetabolite use over the years is presented in Fig. 241-5.

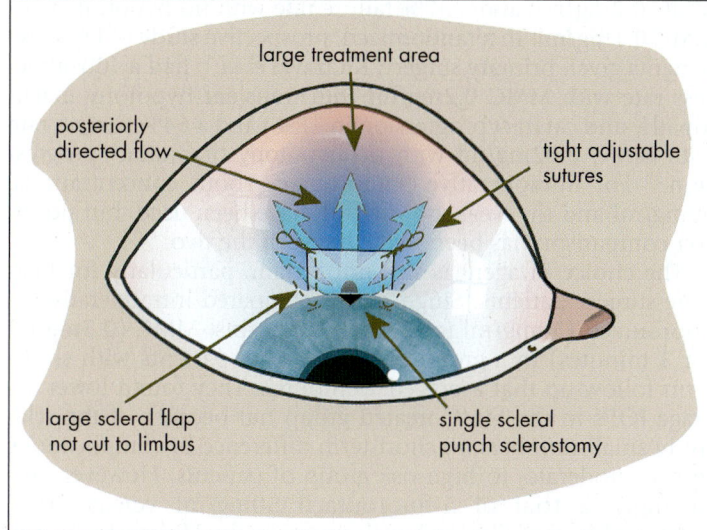

FIGURE 241-4 ■ Diagram showing technique changes that result in more diffuse noncystic blebs. "Safe Surgery System" for glaucoma surgery.

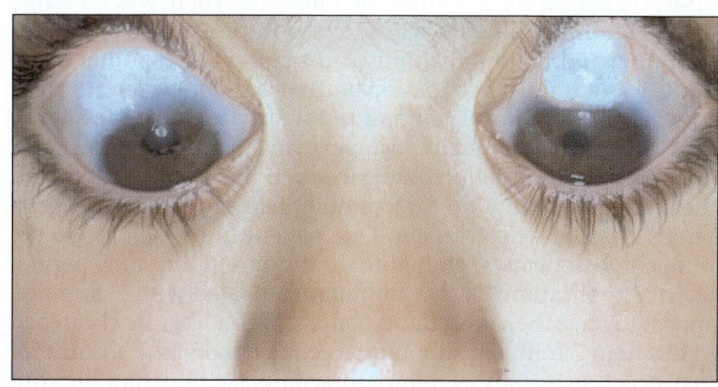

FIGURE 241-5 ■ Focal cystic bleb prone to leakage, infection, and dysesthesia in left eye (limbus-based conjunctival flap, small scleral flap, and smaller area of MMC 0.4mg/ml treatment). Diffuse noncystic bleb appearance in right eye of the same patient (fornix-based flap, larger scleral flap, and larger area of MMC 0.5mg/ml treatment).

Time of Exposure, Concentration and Type of Intraoperative Agent

The optimum concentration of intraoperative MMC still needs to be established. Chen et al.[33] reported results in high-risk patients since 1981 without failures but a 66% rate of hypotony with MMC 0.4mg/ml, a 22% failure rate with no hypotony with

MMC 0.2mg/ml, and a 37% failure rate with no hypotony with MMC 0.1mg/ml. In a randomized, prospective study of Japanese patients given primary surgery, Kitazawa *et al.*[34] had a 100% success rate with MMC 0.2mg/ml (but transient hypotony maculopathy and cataract progression in 18%) and a 64% success rate with MMC 0.02mg/ml with no hypotony or cataract progression.[35] For intraoperative 5-fluorouracil, both concentrations, 50mg/ml and the weaker 25mg/ml, have been used, but no direct comparison has been made between the two.

The choice of agent is still not certain, particularly for first-time surgery patients. Singh *et al.*[16] compared intraoperative 5-fluorouracil (50mg/ml for 5 minutes) against MMC (0.5mg/ml for 3 minutes) in a group of West African patients with short-term follow-up that averaged 10 months. They found lower average IOPs in the MMC-treated group but because of the relatively small numbers no short-term difference in complications in this moderate- to high-risk group of patients. However, surprisingly, a trial of 5-fluorouracil 50mg/ml versus MMC 0.2mg/ml in first-time trabeculectomy in the United States has not shown any statistically significant differences to date in efficacy or side effects.

The optimum time of exposure has also not been determined. Megevand *et al.*[36] retrospectively compared eyes treated with MMC 0.2mg/ml for 2 minutes or 5 minutes. There was no statistically significant difference in success rate or complications, but hypotony and endophthalmitis still occurred. In another study MMC was administered intraoperatively at 0.5mg/ml for 5 minutes or 0.4mg/ml for 3 minutes in Indian patients.[37] No significant difference occurred in postoperative IOP, hypotony, or postoperative filtration failure rate. However, the group treated with the higher concentration for 5 minutes had a higher incidence of serous choroidal detachment. One patient from each group developed postoperative endophthalmitis during the study period. Shorter applications of 2–3 minutes, compared with 5 minutes, appear to have the same efficacy, but if applications are shortened to less than 2 minutes, suboptimal cellular and tissue absorption may occur. In a study of 5-fluorouracil uptake in tissues the concentrations reached a plateau at 3 minutes.[38] Even shorter application times may result in greater variations in drug delivery. Changes in the concentration of the agent are more likely to give reproducibly titratable effects than are variations in exposure time. Therefore, to achieve consistent and predictable results, it is probably more important that the individual surgeon becomes accustomed to, and experienced with, one or two concentrations and one exposure time.

Type of Sponge and Method and Area of Treatment

Small variations in technique may have profound effects on the clinical result and complications. The type of sponge may affect significantly the amount of drug delivered. Chen *et al.* originally used a Gelfoam sponge,[33] but most clinicians use commercially available sponges (e.g., Weck cell, Merocel), which have different retention and drug-releasing capabilities and which may be cut to different sizes. We currently use polyvinyl alcohol sponges (Network Medical Products, Yorkshire, UK) as these sponges do not disintegrate as methylcellulose does and leave fragments in the wound. Based on clinical observation, we started treating larger areas several years ago and this has considerably reduced bleb-related complications. This clinical finding has been confirmed subsequently by our group.[39]

It is also important not to touch the cut edge of conjunctiva or the cornea, as the agents affect the cells mainly in the contact area and leave other areas relatively normal. Based on this principle, we have designed special clamps for use during either limbal or fornix-based surgery (Duckworth and Kent, UK, 2-686 and 2-687, and John Weiss) to protect the conjunctival edge from exposure (Fig. 241-6).

We now treat under both scleral flap and conjunctival flap, particularly in resistant cases. We have found clinically during re-

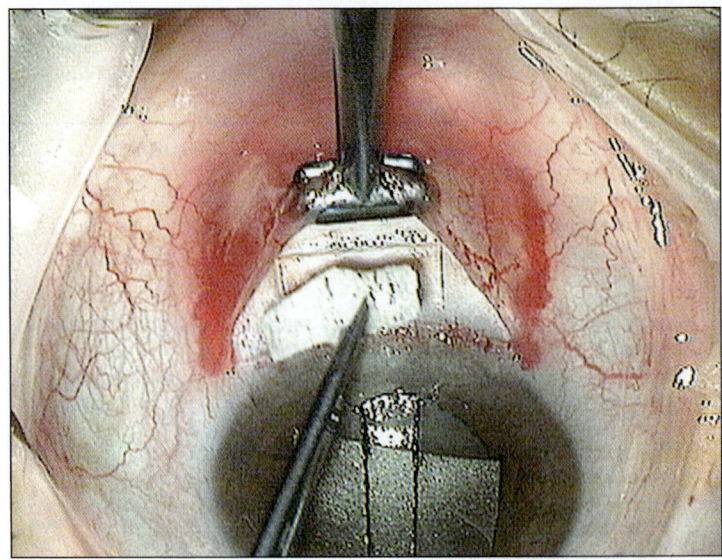

FIG. 241-6 ■ **Intraoperative antimetabolite being applied.** The cut edge of conjunctiva is protected by a special clamp (Duckworth and Kent, UK) during surgery. As large an area as possible is treated to achieve a diffuse noncystic bleb.

exploration that the flaps are sometimes sealed with scar tissue. If the scleral flap is only cut partially down the sides, the filter paper or a thin polyvinyl sponge is inserted between the two flaps to ensure treatment. The use of the sponge under both the scleral flap and the conjunctiva seems to enhance the success rate.[40]

DRAINAGE AREA POSITION

The positioning of the scleral flap and treated area is very important. Interpalpebral and inferiorly placed blebs have a high incidence of endophthalmitis, particularly in association with antimetabolites.[41] A series of five patients in whom scleritis developed 3–24 weeks after intraoperative MMC all had inferior trabeculectomies with MMC.[42] If no space exists for a superior trabeculectomy with antimetabolite, better alternative methods may include tube drainage devices or cyclodestructive procedures.

CLOSURE OF SCLERAL FLAP

Conjunctival healing may be inhibited markedly by antimetabolites, and hypotony is prevented primarily by the resistance afforded by the scleral flap. Therefore, this flap has to be sufficiently thick and wide relative to the sclerostomy to provide this resistance; it has to be sutured adequately enough to achieve this resistance and yet be adjustable gradually. This adjustability is achieved by laser suturelysis or releasable sutures, although too early release of sutures may be associated with long-term hypotony.[21] It is important to remember that when antimetabolites (particularly MMC) are used, suturelysis (even several months after surgery) may result in hypotony; this also applies to occluding sutures left within or around the tube lumen after tube implant surgery. Late choroidal effusions and hemorrhage after suture removal have been reported, even many months after the surgery.[43]

After the use of MMC, sutures should be released late. In particular, tie the releasable suture(s) tight, but check IOP in patients who have marked visual field loss in the first few hours after surgery. If the pressure is raised on the first postoperative day, gentle pressure is applied to the back of the scleral flap, which very slightly loosens the flap, allows outflow of aqueous, and lowers the opening pressure without the complete loss of tension that occurs when sutures are released. Alternatively, the new technique of adjustable suture control that we have devised can be used in which a special pair of polished duck-billed forceps (Duckworth and Kent, Khaw 2-502) can be used transconjuncti-

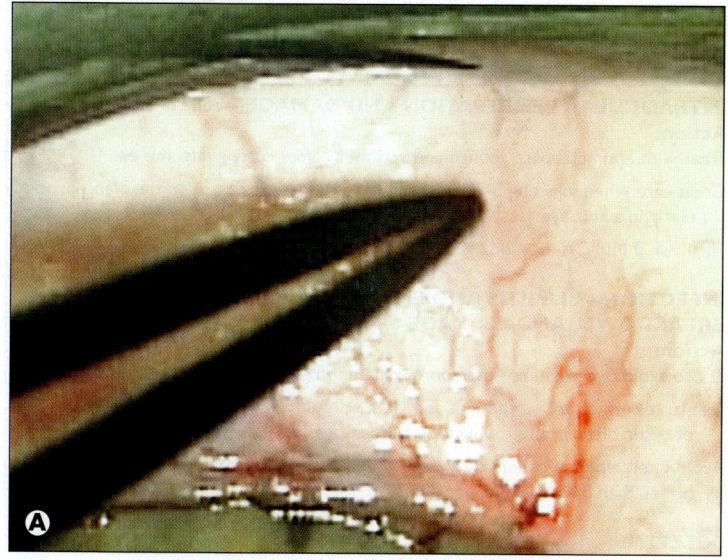

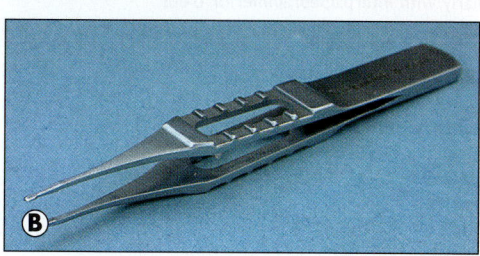

FIGURE 241-7 ■ **Adjustable suture control (ASC). A,** Sutures being adjusted through the conjunctiva with duck-billed forceps to ensure gradual lowering of intraocular pressure after antimetabolite use. **B,** Adjustable suture forceps (Duckworth and Kent 2-502 with polished duck-billed ends to prevent conjunctival damage during trans-conjunctival adjustment).

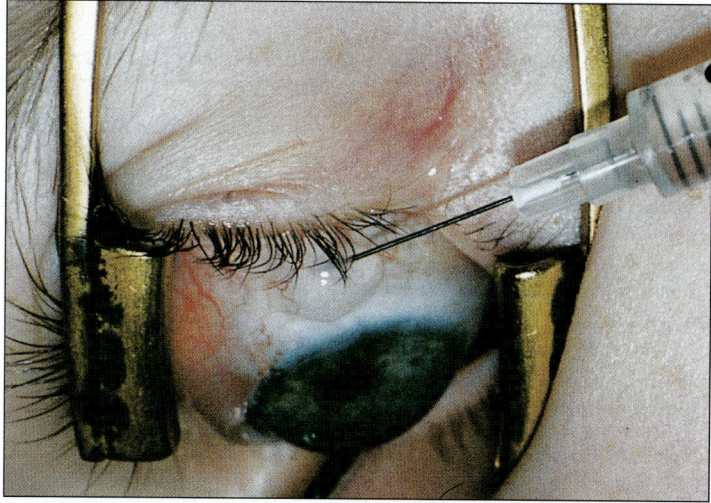

FIGURE 241-8 ■ **Subconjunctival injection of 5-fluorouracil.** The injection is given as close as possible to the bleb without entering the bleb area. Viscoelastic can be used to prolong the duration of action.

BOX 241-3

Improvements in Injectable 5-Fluorouracil

Reduction in number of injections given
Injections given closer to bleb area—increased efficacy for same dose
Long injection track—reduction in epitheliopathy
Use of small-bore needle (e.g., 30 gauge)
Injection of viscoelastic—prolonged release and no corneal side effects
Use in conjunction with intraoperative antimetabolites—reduced need for injections

---

vally to adjust the sutures and hence the IOP downward gradually until the target pressure is reached (Fig. 241-7).

POSTOPERATIVE INJECTIONS

Subconjunctival injections of 5-fluorouracil may be used postoperatively on their own or in combination with intraoperative MMC or 5-fluorouracil[25] if the pressure rises and the healing response is still marked. The original regimen of 21 injections of 5mg of 5-fluorouracil given 180° from the bleb (twice a day for 1 weeks then once a day for 1 week) has now evolved, and most ophthalmologists give less than 10 injections with longer intervals in between injections. These lower dose regimens may result in a lower incidence of corneal side effects. However, it is important to note that meta-analysis suggests that three injections or less may have had no impact on long-term success and only five injections or more may be effective.[44]

The technique of injection is very important. The 5-Fluorouracil Filtration Surgery Study regimen was 5-fluorouracil 5mg in a volume of 0.5ml given 180° from the filtration site. There have been other refinements (Fig. 241-8) that include giving injections nearer the bleb (but avoiding intraocular entry as the pH is 9), which may increase the efficacy. It is logical to deliver the injection of 5-fluorouracil as close as possible to the bleb but without entering the bleb itself (Box 241-3). Corneal side effects may also be reduced by a long subconjunctival needle track and small needles (29 or 30 gauge). Based on our pharmacokinetic studies, we also sometimes use a subconjunctival viscoelastic injection (Haelon GV, Pharmacia, NJ) and then inject the 5-fluorouracil on the far side of the viscoelastic, which prevents any 5-fluorouracil reflux into the tear film. This also lengthens the duration of action. Corneal side effects are rare with this regimen. The advent of intraoperative antimetabolite treatment has meant that injections are more commonly used as adjunctive treatment supplementing intraoperative treatment rather than the main treatment.

Subconjunctival injections of MMC have been advocated and described particularly with procedures such as needling,[45] but given the cytotoxicity of MMC this technique is not in widespread use because of fears of toxicity. A case has been described in which a needling procedure for a failing bleb was followed by a subconjunctival injection of MMC (0.3ml of 0.5mg/ml). The visual acuity decreased from 20/100 (6/30) to hand motions at 1m (3.3ft). Occlusion of the central retinal vein occurred with hemorrhages in the periphery and narrow arterioles, and fluorescein angiography revealed an unusual combined occlusion of both the arterial and venous vasculature of the retina.[46] Although successful needling revisions of blebs have been reported using subconjunctival injections of smaller volumes (0.01ml at 0.4mg/ml), the potential risks of subconjunctival MMC appear substantial. An intraocular injection of MMC 0.05ml into the rabbit anterior chamber resulted in irreversible damage to the cornea.[47]

COMPLICATIONS

Many complications of filtration surgery are described, and the use of antimetabolites increases the incidence of some of these. In particular, short- and long-term hypotony associated with maculopathy (which may be irreversible), choroidal effusions, or hemorrhage may occur with an increased incidence. The other major concern is the potentially high long-term incidence of endophthalmitis, especially with avascular cystic blebs seen particularly with the use of higher concentrations of MMC. These can be considerably reduced by using appropriate surgical techniques. A list of major potential complications is presented in Table 241-3, together with possible ways to prevent some of these.

TABLE 241-3

POTENTIAL COMPLICATIONS OF ANTIMETABOLITES

HYPOTONY
Particularly if scleral flap not adequately closed or high dose MMC used

Action:

Close scleral flap securely—releasable sutures are very useful. May require multiple sutures particularly if MMC used.

Do not make scleral flap too small or thin, particularly if MMC used, otherwise outflow cannot be adequately restricted.

Do not release sutures too early—if MMC used, suture release even months after surgery may result in hypotony.

Adjustable suture control (ASC)—gradual loosening of sutures down to target pressures with special adjustable forceps.

COMPLICATIONS OF HYPOTONY
Including maculopathy. which may be irreversible even after pressure is restored; choroidal effusions and bleeding; cataract; and phthisis

Action:

Caution when using strong antimetabolites in high-risk patients (e.g., myopes who appear more prone to have hypotony associated problems such as maculopathy (soft sclera).

Use intraoperative infusion (Lewicky cannula) to gauge outflow from sclerostomy. Do not finish until flow secured.

WOUND EDGE LEAKS
Action:

Ensure wound is securely closed; vascular needle prevents buttonholing.

Mattress sutures if fornix-based flap—test at end of surgery to ensure watertight.

Protect cut edge of conjunctiva from drug (e.g., special clamp).

Epithelial erosions

Mainly with injected 5-fluorouracil, which leaks into tear film.

Action:

Use intraoperative sponge technique.

Use long injection track for injections to prevent reflux into tear film and washout tear film after injection.

Use viscoelastic to prevent tear film reflux in susceptible patients (e.g., surface problems).

INTRAOCULAR PENETRATION AND DAMAGE
Intraocular damage can include endothelial damage and ciliary body destruction—possibly with high-concentration MMC (controversial) Retinal damage has been reported with injected MMC

INTRAOCULAR PENETRATION AND DAMAGE—cont'd
Action:

Treat with antimetabolite sponge and washout *before* cutting into the eye.

Great care when injecting 5-fluorouracil subconjunctivally close to the bleb, particularly in a soft eye.

High risk if MMC is injected.

INFECTION—BLEBITIS AND ENDOPHTHALMITIS, BLEB BREAKDOWN, AND LEAKAGE
Action:

Try to avoid overtreating—use appropriate antimetabolite for patient.

Use large surface area treatment and large scleral flap—radically reduces incidence of cystic blebs prone to infection and leakage.

Avoid interpalpebral or inferiorly sited blebs—infection rate may be 5-10 times higher than bleb under upper lid.

SCLERITIS
Occurs particularly with interpalpebral/inferior blebs.

Action:

Avoid interpalpebral and inferior blebs.

SCLEROMALACIA/THINNING/NECROSIS
Action:

Avoid areas of scleral thinning.

TERATOGENICITY
Theoretical possibility.

Action:

Avoid using if any chance of pregnancy in patient.

Malignancy

None reported to date 30+ years after topical mitomycin

Action:

Continued surveillance

Long-term cumulative effects

On both patient and medical staff.

Action

Careful handling and disposal of cytotoxics required.

(Potentially more long-term complications with mitomycin C than with 5-fluorouracil.)

FUTURE STRATEGIES TO PREVENT FIBROSIS

Although current agents (particularly MMC) are extremely effective in the prevention of fibrosis, considerable room still exists for improvement. Long-term complications may become apparent only many years later. A key area for the future lies in a better understanding of the cellular and molecular processes involved in the healing processes and of the exact effects of the various agents used to modulate the process. Biological factors may have profound effects. We have shown that one growth factor, TGF-β, stimulates more scarring than the other growth factors in aqueous. This growth factor may also reverse the action of antimetabolites partially, even of MMC.[48; 49] Differences in the levels of some of these factors may help to explain the variances in response to therapy. A new human antibody to TGF-β has been shown to be effective in reducing scarring in vivo[50] and in pilot human studies[51] with relatively diffuse noncystic blebs (Fig. 241-9). A multicenter international study is now under way.

Ultimately we will use antiscarring agents in all patients, possibly in combination, analogous to the situation in cancer chemotherapy. For example, we have shown for the first time that the addition of heparin to intraoperative 5-fluorouracil during vitreoretinal surgery results in a 50% reduction in prolifera-

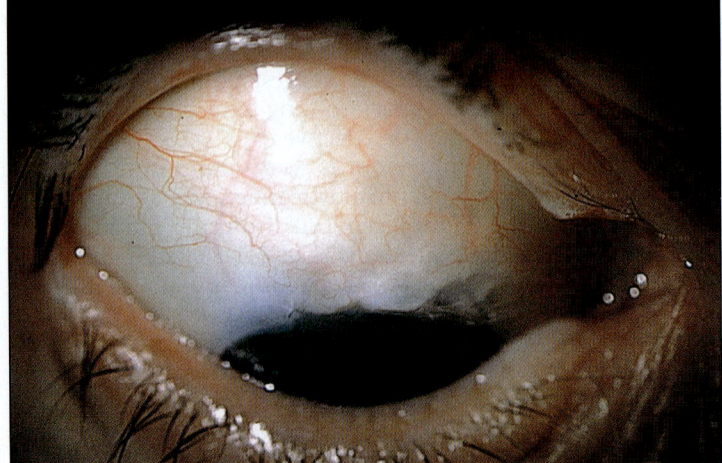

FIGURE 241-9 ■ Bleb following treatment with human anti–transforming growth factor antibody. The bleb is diffuse and noncystic.

tive vitreoretinopathy in high-risk patients,[52] thereby returning 5-fluorouracil to the vitreoretinal surgeons 25 years later[5] in an effective form. Ultimately, these combination regimens will evolve to give us the safe, prolonged, long-term, maximal lowering of IOP that is associated with minimal or no glaucomatous progression—the "holy grail" of glaucoma.

REFERENCES

1. Chen PP, Yamamoto T, Sawada A, et al. Use of antifibrosis agents and glaucoma drainage devices in the American and Japanese glaucoma societies. J Glaucoma. 1997;6:192–6.
2. AGIS Investigators. The Advanced Glaucoma Intervention study (AGIS) 7. The relationship between control of intraocular pressure and visual field deterioration. Am J Ophthalmol. 2000;130, 429–40.
3. Araujo SV, Spaeth GL, Roth SM, Starita RJ. A ten-year follow-up on a prospective, randomized trial of postoperative corticosteroids after trabeculectomy. Ophthalmology. 1995;102:1753–9.
4. Heuer DK, Gressel MG, Parrish RK II. Topical fluorouracil. II. Postoperative administration in an animal model of filtration surgery. Arch Ophthalmol. 1986; 104:132–6.
5. Blumenkranz M, Hernandez E, Ophir A, Norton EWD. 5-Fluorouracil: new applications in complicated retinal detachment for an established antimetabolite. Ophthalmology. 1984;91:122–30.
6. Khaw PT, Sherwood MB, MacKay SL, et al. Five-minute treatments with fluorouracil, floxuridine, and mitomycin have long-term effects on human Tenon's capsule fibroblasts. Arch Ophthalmol. 1992;110:1150–4.
7. Jampel HD. Effect of brief exposure to mitomycin C on viability and proliferation of cultured human Tenon's capsule fibroblasts. Ophthalmology. 1992;99:1471–6.
8. Broadway DC, Grierson I, O'Brien C, Hitchings RA. Adverse effects of topical antiglaucoma medication. Arch Ophthalmol. 1994;112:1446–54.
9. Schwab IR, Linberg JV, Gioia VM, et al. Foreshortening of the inferior conjunctival fornix associated with chronic glaucoma medications. Ophthalmology. 1992;99:197–202.
10. Gwynn DR, Stewart WC, Pitts RA, et al. Conjunctival structure and cell counts and the results of filtering surgery. Am J Ophthalmol. 1993;116:464–8.
11. The Fluorouracil Filtering Surgery Study Group. Five-year follow-up of the fluorouracil filtering surgery study. Am J Ophthalmol. 1996;121:349–66.
12. Kitazawa Y, Kawase K, Matsushita H, Minobe M. Trabeculectomy with mitomycin. A comparative study with fluorouracil. Arch Ophthalmol. 1991;109:1693–8.
13. Katz GJ, Higginbotham EJ, Lichter PR, et al. Mitomycin C versus fluorouracil in high-risk glaucoma filtering surgery. Ophthalmology. 1995;102:1263–9.
14. Lamping KA, Belkin JK. 5-Fluorouracil and mitomycin C in pseudophakic patients. Ophthalmology. 1995;102:70–5.
15. Egbert PR, Williams AS, Singh K, et al. A prospective trial of intraoperative fluorouracil during trabeculectomy in a black population. Am J Ophthalmol. 1993; 116:612–16.
16. Singh K, Egbert PR, Byrd S, et al. Trabeculectomy with intraoperative 5-fluorouracil vs mitomycin C. Am J Ophthalmol. 1997;123:48–53.
17. Wilkins M, Indar A, Wormald R. Intra-operative mitomycin-C for glaucoma surgery (Cochrane Review). Cochrane Database Syst Rev (England) 1(CD002897). 2001.
18. Goldenfeld M, Krupin T, Ruderman JM, et al. 5-Fluorouracil in initial trabeculectomy: a prospective randomized, multicenter study. Ophthalmology. 1994;101:1024–9.
19. Whiteside-Michel J, Liebmann JM, Ritch R. Initial 5-fluorouracil trabeculectomy in young patients. Ophthalmology. 1992;99:7–13.
20. Wilson RP, Steinman WC. Use of trabeculectomy with postoperative 5-fluorouracil in patients requiring extremely low intraocular pressure levels to limit further glaucoma progression. Ophthalmology. 1991;98:1047–52.
21. Kupin TH, Juzych MS, Shin DH, et al. Adjunctive mitomycin C in primary trabeculectomy in phakic eyes. Am J Ophthalmol. 1995;119:30–9.
22. Stamper RL, McMenemy MG, Lieberman MF. Hypotonous maculopathy after trabeculectomy with subconjunctival 5FU. Am J Ophthalmol. 1992;114:544–53.
23. Doyle JW, Sherwood MB, Khaw PT, et al. Intraoperative 5-fluorouracil for filtration surgery in the rabbit. Invest Ophthalmol Vis Sci. 1993;34:3313–19.
24. Khaw PT, Doyle JW, Sherwood MB, et al. Prolonged localized tissue effects from 5-minute exposures to fluorouracil and mitomycin C. Arch Ophthalmol. 1993; 111:263–7.
25. Smith MF, Sherwood MB, Doyle JW, Khaw PT. Results of intraoperative 5-fluorouracil supplementation on trabeculectomy for open-angle glaucoma. Am J Ophthalmol. 1992;114:737–41.
26. Lanigan LP, Stuermer J, Baez KA, et al. Single intraoperative applications of 5-fluorouracil during filtration surgery: early results. Br J Ophthalmol. 1994;78:33–7.
27. Feldman RM, Dietze PJ, Gross RL, Oram O. Intraoperative 5-fluorouracil administration in trabeculectomy. J Glaucoma. 1994;3:302–7.
28. Yorston D, Khaw PT. A randomised trial of the effect of intraoperative 5FU on the outcome of trabeculectomy in East Africa. Br J Ophthalmol. 2001;85:1028–30.
29. Khaw PT, Ward S, Grierson I, Rice NSC. The effects of beta-radiation on proliferating human Tenon's capsule fibroblasts. Br J Ophthalmol. 1991;75:580–3.
30. Miller MH, Rice NSC. Trabeculectomy combined with beta irradiation for congenital glaucoma. Br J Ophthalmol. 1991;75:584–90.
31. Occleston NL, Daniels JT, Tarnuzzer RW, et al. Single exposures to antiproliferatives. Long term effects on ocular fibroblast wound healing behavior. Invest Ophthalmol Vis Sci. 1997;38:1998–2007.
32. Wells AP, Cordeiro MF, Bunce CV, Khaw PT. Cystic bleb related complications in limbus versus fornix based flaps in paediatric and young adult trabeculectomy with high dose mitomycin C [abstract]. Invest Ophthalmol Vis Sci. 2001;42:S544.
33. Chen C-W, Huang H-T, Bair JS, Lee C-C. Trabeculectomy with simultaneous topical application of mitomycin-c in refractory glaucoma. J Ocul Pharmacol. 1990; 6:175–82.
34. Kitazawa Y, Suemori-Matsushita H, Yamamoto T, Kawase K. Low-dose and high-dose mitomycin trabeculectomy as an initial surgery in primary open-angle glaucoma. Ophthalmology. 1993;100:1624–8.
35. Singh K, Mehta K, Shaikh NM, et al. Trabeculectomy with intraoperative mitomycin C versus 5-fluorouracil. Prospective randomized clinical trial. Ophthalmology. 2000;107:2305–9.
36. Megevand GS, Salmon JF, Scholtz RP, Murray AD. The effect of reducing the exposure time of mitomycin C in glaucoma filtering surgery. Ophthalmology. 1995;102:84–90.
37. Neelakantan A, Rao BS, Vijaya L, et al. Effect of the concentration and duration of application of mitomycin C in trabeculectomy. Ophthalmic Surg. 1994;25:612–15.
38. Wilkins MR, Occleston NL, Kotecha A, et al. Sponge delivery variables and tissue levels of 5-fluorouracil. Br J Ophthalmol. 1999;84:92–7.
39. Cordeiro MF, Constable PH, Alexander RA, et al. The effect of varying mitomycin-C treatment area in glaucoma filtration surgery in the rabbit. Invest Ophthalmol Vis Sci. 1997;38:1639–46.
40. El Sayyad F, Belmekki M, Helal M, et al. Simultaneous subconjunctival and subscleral mitomycin C application in trabeculectomy. Ophthalmology. 2000;107: 298–301.
41. Wolner B, Liebmann JM, Sassani JW, et al. Late bleb-related endophthalmitis after trabeculectomy with adjunctive 5-fluorouracil. Ophthalmology. 1991;98:1053–60.
42. Fourman S. Scleritis after glaucoma filtering surgery with mitomycin C. Ophthalmology. 1995;102:1569–71.
43. Perkins TW, Cardakli F, Eisele JR, et al. Adjunctive mitomycin C in Molteno implant surgery. Ophthalmology. 1995;102:91–7.
44. Wormald R, Wilkins MR, Bunce C. Post-operative 5-fluorouracil for glaucoma surgery. Cochrane Database Syst Rev (England) 2(CD001132). 2000.
45. Mardelli PG, Lederer CM Jr, Murray PL, et al. Slit-lamp needle revision of failed filtering blebs using mitomycin C. Ophthalmology. 1996;103:1946–55.
46. Nuyts RMMA, Van Diemen HAM, Greve EL. Occlusion of the retinal vasculature after trabeculectomy with mitomycin C. Int Ophthalmol. 1994;18:167–70.
47. Derick RJ, Pasquale L, Quigley HA, Jampel H. Potential toxicity of mitomycin-C. Arch Ophthalmol. 1991;109:1635–1635.
48. Khaw PT, Occleston NL, Schultz GS, et al. Activation and suppression of fibroblast activity. Eye. 1994;8:188–95.
49. Doyle JW, Smith MF, Garcia JA, et al. Treatment of bleb leaks with transforming growth factor-β in the rabbit model. Invest Ophthalmol Vis Sci. 1997;38:1630–4.
50. Cordeiro MF, Gay JA, Khaw PT. Human anti-transforming growth factor-beta2 antibody: a new glaucoma anti-scarring agent. Invest Ophthalmol Vis Sci. 1999;40: 2225–34.
51. Siriwardena D, Khaw PT, Donaldson ML, et al. A randomised placebo-controlled trial of human anti-TGF$_2$ monoclonal antibody (CAT-152): a new modulator of wound healing following trabeculectomy. Ophthalmology. 2002;109:427–31.
52. Asaria RHY, Kon CH, Bunce C, et al. Adjuvant 5-fluorouracil and heparin is prevents proliferative vitreoretinopathy: results from a randomised double blind controlled clinical trial. Ophthalmology. 2001;108:1184–6.

CHAPTER
242 Drainage Implants

JEFFREY FREEDMAN

DEFINITION
- Surgical method for dealing with refractory glaucomas.

KEY FEATURES
- Drainage plate attached to silicone tube.
- Varying plate size and number.
- Indications.
- Surgical method of insertion.
- Complications.

ASSOCIATED FEATURE
- Outcomes.

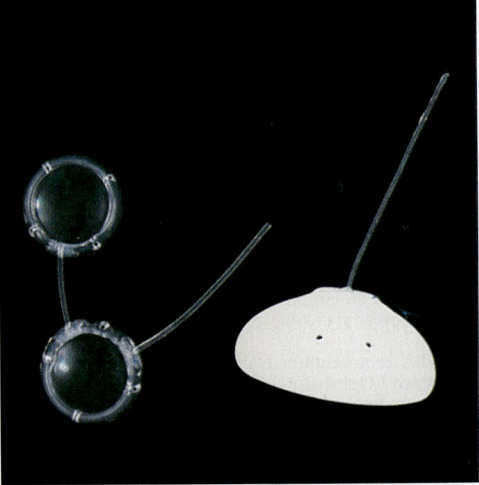

FIG. 242-1 ▌ Double-plate, Molteno implant (left) and Baerveldt implant (right).

INTRODUCTION

Drainage implants were developed before antifibrotic agents became available to enhance trabeculectomy surgery. These implants provided a good surgical option for eyes in which there was a high probability of trabeculectomy surgery failure because of extensive conjunctival scarring from previous procedures or the type of underlying glaucoma (neovascular, uveitic, iridocorneal endothelial [ICE] syndrome, etc). Today, many surgeons use drainage implants only when failure has occurred with one or more trabeculectomies in which antifibrotic agents were used. Probably a role exists for these implants at an earlier stage for some patients, particularly with the increased concern about postoperative late bleb leaks and risks of late endophthalmitis following the use of antimetabolites.

HISTORICAL REVIEW

Early drainage devices, or setons, were made from a variety of materials and extended from the anterior chamber to the subconjunctival space.[1,2] As most devices were not "bleb spreading" in nature, their failure occurred as a result of fibrosis over the subconjunctival portion of the seton.

The most common drainage devices in use today are based on a design introduced by Molteno in 1969[3] and modified later in the 1970s.[4] The initial Molteno implant consisted of an acrylic translimbal tube attached to and opening onto the surface of a curved episcleral plate, 8.5mm in diameter. Aqueous drained into a potential space formed by the surface of the plate and the conjunctiva that overlay it. The fibrosis response to the aqueous caused the episcleral plate to become enclosed by a thin layer of connective tissue, which became distended with aqueous to form a large, unilocular bleb that freely communicated with the anterior chamber. The long-term tendency was for the bleb wall to become thinner and, although desirable for pressure control, the thinness of the wall occasionally led to perforation and/or exposure of anterior-placed implants. The redesigned implant

had an enlarged episcleral plate, which shifted the implant backward, and maintained connection to the anterior chamber by means of a fine-bore, elongated silicone tube. Further modification of the Molteno implant consisted of the addition of a second plate connected to the first by a second silicone tube. The dual-chamber implant developed later restricted drainage initially to a small area anteriorly placed on the surface of the plate and allowed aqueous to spread to the remainder of the plate at a later time.[5]

Other Implants

The majority of modern implants follow the principle introduced by Molteno, namely a long tube that drains to an episcleral plate (Fig. 242-1). Implants can be divided essentially into two groups, those with valves and those without valves. The nonvalved are the various types of Molteno implants, the Baerveldt implant, and the Schocket encircling tube. Valved implants include the Krupin disc, Ahmed valve, and White pump. All commonly used implants consist of a long tube through which aqueous drains from the anterior chamber to a posteriorly placed plate that acts as a bleb-spreading device.

PREOPERATIVE EVALUATION AND DIAGNOSTIC APPROACH

Drainage implants were designed for use in refractory glaucomas. This group includes eyes that have had one or more filtering procedures that have failed, aphakic and pseudophakic glaucomas, uveitic glaucoma, neovascular glaucoma, congenital glaucoma with iridocorneal dysgenesis, the ICE syndrome, and glaucoma that follows corneal transplantation. Scarring of the conjunctiva from causes other than previous filtering surgery may also warrant implant use if pressure control requires surgical intervention.

With the advent of antifibrotic agents, such as 5-fluorouracil and mitomycin, some eyes that previously would have required an implant today possibly may be treated using filtration, with

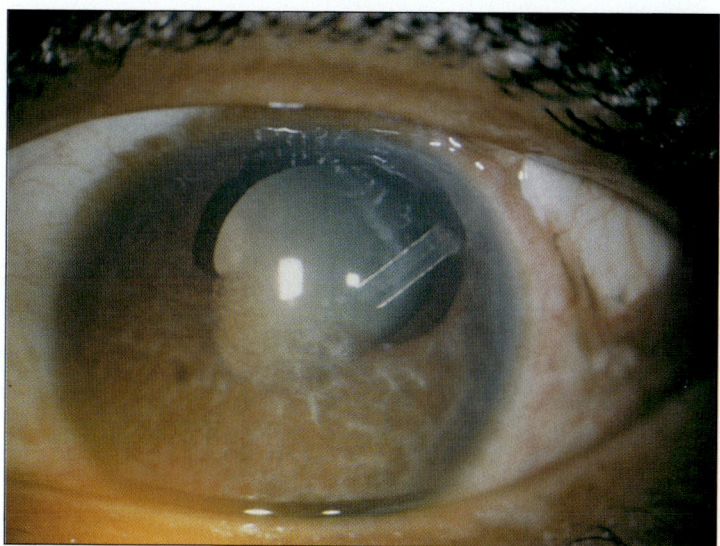

FIG. 242-2 ■ **Silicone tube.** Here it extends beyond the pupillary border in neovascular glaucoma. The tube is enveloped totally in fibrovascular tissue up to pupil margin and the cut end of the silicone tube beveled up to prevent occlusion by iris.

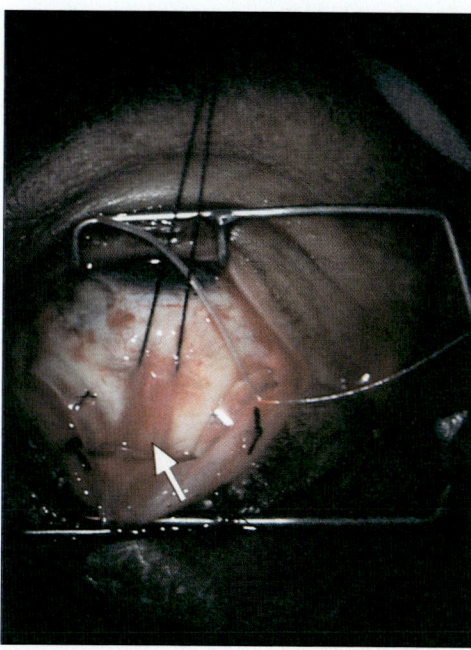

FIG. 242-3 ■ Traction suture beneath the superior rectus muscle. With a connecting silicone tube that passes above the superior rectus muscle (arrow) and 4-0 silk marker sutures in the free edge of the conjunctiva (now retracted).

the addition of an antimetabolite.[6] Nonetheless, conditions still exist for which an implant may be more useful; these include neovascular glaucoma, aphakic glaucoma, and conditions that produce extensive scarring of the angle of the eye and extensive anterior conjunctival scarring.

Neovascular Glaucoma

Filtering surgery is more likely to fail in neovascular glaucoma as a result of closure of the internal opening of the filter by neovascular fibrous tissue. This can be avoided if the tube of the draining implant is placed well into the anterior chamber, often as far as the pupil margin. Even with this type of tube placement, the whole base of the internal tube may become enveloped by neovascular fibrous tissue, which results in closure of a filtration site, despite antimetabolite treatment (which prevents external scarring only) (Fig. 242-2). The ideal approach with neovascular glaucoma, seen in the acute stage, is total vitrectomy, endolaser photocoagulation of the fundus, and pars plana placement of the drainage implant tube.

Aphakic Glaucoma

Aphakic glaucoma requires extensive vitrectomy for a simple filter to function. A less extensive vitrectomy allows the tube of the implant to be placed laterally on the iris, well away from the vitreous. A more recently applied treatment is the insertion of a drainage implant with the tube occluded by a releasable suture, accompanied by nonpenetrating glaucoma surgery. The glaucoma implant remains as a backup and can be activated should the filter fail. Placement of the tube via the pars plana is an alternative approach requiring total or almost total vitrectomy.

Extensive Scarring of the Angle of the Eye

Conditions that produce extensive scarring of the angle of the eye, such as uveitis, the iridocorneal dysgenesis syndromes, and congenital glaucoma with iridocorneal dysgenesis, are subject to closure of the internal opening of the drainage fistula, and better results are obtained with the use of a draining implant.

Extensive Anterior Conjunctival Scarring

Extensive anterior conjunctival scarring, such as occurs after multiple previous surgeries or in rheumatoid arthritis, sometimes precludes successful filtration even with the use of an-

timetabolites and may require a drainage implant, with the tube inserted via the pars plana, associated with total vitrectomy.

ALTERNATIVES

The alternatives to drainage implant surgery include trabeculectomy surgery with use of adjunctive antimetabolites (see Chapters 239 and 240) or, especially for eyes that already have poor vision, a cyclodestructive procedure (see Chapter 237).

SURGICAL TECHNIQUE

Drainage implant surgery involves traction on the recti muscles and a retrobulbar injection anesthetic is generally recommended. If discomfort occurs later in the procedure, additional anesthesia with lidocaine (lignocaine) using a soft cannula directly into the cone between the muscles is easily performed, as this site is already dissected for placement of the drainage implant.

All draining implants, except for encircling tube devices, are fixed in a similar manner; namely, the silicone tube is inserted into the eye and the plate or plates fixed to the sclera in a posterior position. The insertion of a double-plate Molteno implant is described here as an example, but variations in technique exist.

Conjunctival Incision

A fornix-based conjunctival flap is fashioned by elevation of the conjunctiva from the underlying sclera using balanced salt solution injected through a 30-gauge needle inserted at the limbus of the cornea. The conjunctiva is dissected from the limbus from the 10 o'clock to the 2 o'clock positions. A relaxing incision of about 7mm length is then made by the insertion of one blade of a Westcott scissors posteriorly, parallel to the upper borders of the lateral and medial rectus muscles. The two free corners of the conjunctiva thus formed are marked with a suture to ensure accurate replacement at the end of the procedure (Fig. 242-3). By blunt dissection, the conjunctiva is elevated off the underlying sclera for a distance of 7mm.

Further posterior dissection of the conjunctiva is carried out by inserting a cellulose sponge posteriorly into the superotemporal and superonasal quadrants (Fig. 242-4). This blunt dissection with the sponge is relatively atraumatic and creates a pocket for both medial and laterally placed plates. A muscle hook is placed beneath the superior rectus muscle, which is freed from the overlying conjunctiva by blunt dissection, with dissection close to the conjunctiva rather than the muscle, and entry into the muscle sheath

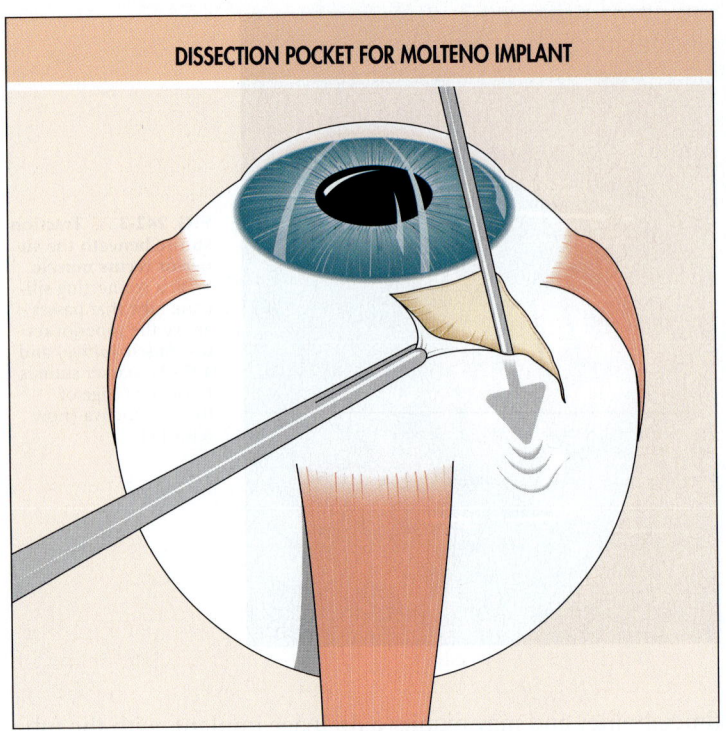

DISSECTION POCKET FOR MOLTENO IMPLANT

FIG. 242-4 ■ Cellular sponge dissection pocket for the plate of a Molteno implant.

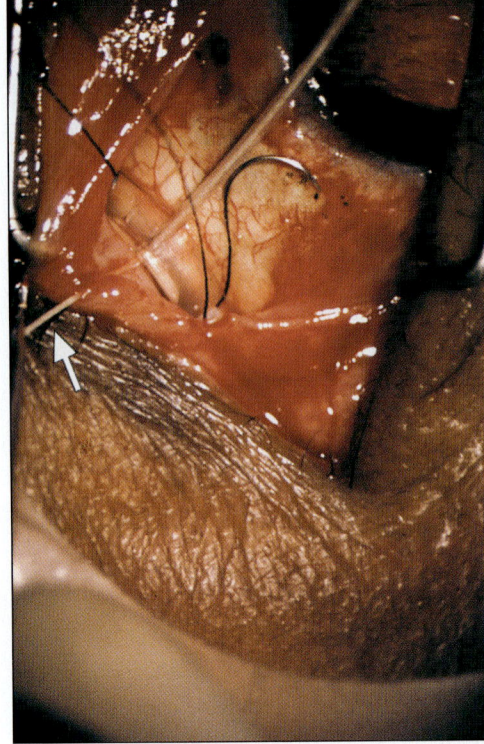

FIG. 242-5 ■ 8-0 silk sutures preplaced in the plate. Prior to insertion and fixation of the plate. A 3-0 Supramid suture (*arrow*) is in the lumen of the silicone tube.

is avoided. A 4-0 bridle suture is then passed beneath the superior rectus muscle and is used as a traction suture (see Fig. 242-3). If previous surgery has resulted in scarring of the conjunctiva in the anterior aspect of the bleb, the fornix-based flap can be fashioned from as far back as 3–4mm from the limbus. More extensive scarring than this may require insertion of the tube through the pars plana, a procedure that requires the addition of an extensive vitrectomy. The implant may also be placed inferiorly, but this can be done only where binocular vision is not present or of poor enough quality to avoid diplopia, as inferior implant placements may result in some restriction of ocular motility and result in diplopia.[6]

Plate Placement

The circular plates of a Molteno implant are 13.5mm in diameter but fit adequately into the pockets created by the blunt dissection of conjunctiva from underlying sclera formed by the cellulose sponges, as described previously. The double-plate Molteno implants are designated right or left and, if used, as such result in the plate with the silicone tube for the anterior chamber being implanted in the superomedial quadrant of the eye. However, it is more convenient to place this plate laterally, where more room exists, and, therefore, it is preferable to use a left-sided implant for right eyes and vice versa. The plates have four holes for sutures, but only the anterior two are used. Prior to insertion of the plates, two 8-0 silk sutures are preplaced using curved needles (Alcon c5; Fig. 242-5). The medial plate is inserted and sutured to the sclera, approximately 8mm behind the limbus. This rather anterior placement of the anterior edge of the plate ensures accessibility of the bleb at a later stage if needling is required. Insertion of the plate 12–15mm posteriorly, as generally advocated, often does not allow any view of the bleb postoperatively, which precludes its assessment of viability or nonviability except by ultrasonography. Once the medial plate has been fixed between superior and lateral rectus muscles, the interconnecting silicone tube is passed over the belly of the superior rectus muscles (see Fig. 242-3). In this way, the silicone plate does not have to pass beneath the muscle, a relatively traumatic procedure to the superior rectus muscle.

The lateral plate can now be sutured to the sclera 8–10mm behind the limbus, using the preplaced 8-0 silk sutures. Prior to insertion of the plate posteriorly, a 3-0 Supramid suture is passed

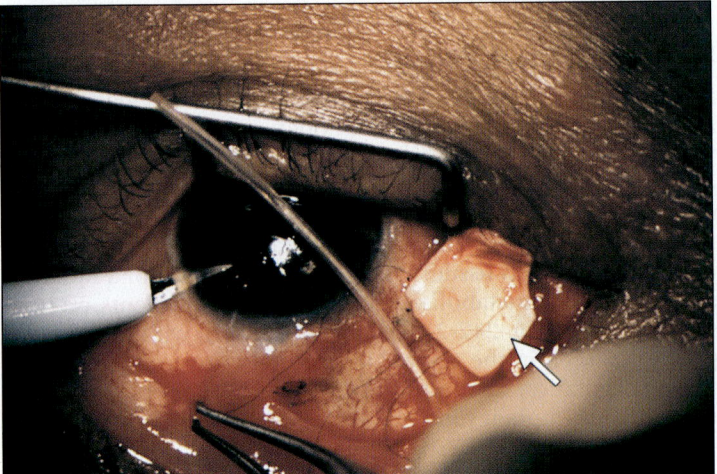

FIG. 242-6 ■ Scleral patch graft (*arrow*) with preplaced 10-0 nylon sutures fixed on one side and rotated laterally to allow access to the tube. Paracentesis is made using a microsharp blade.

into the lumen of the silicone tube. The excess 3-0 suture that emerges from the surface of the plate is left long (see Fig. 242-5). To prevent postoperative hypotony, the tube is occluded totally using a 7-0 polyglactin (Vicryl) suture, which is placed around the tube at its junction with the plate and constricts the tube on to the obturating 3-0 Supramid suture. Slits, with the use of a microsharp blade, are placed in the silicone tube in front of the 3-0 Supramid suture to act as a temporary valve and prevent excessive buildup of pressure in the early postoperative period.[7]

Tube Management

The silicone tube is then covered by a patch graft of either glycerin-preserved sclera[8] or rehydrated preserved pericardium. The patch is fixed to sclera with four separate 10-0 nylon sutures, inserted at the four corners of the patch. The two lateral sutures are tied and the two medial sutures are left untied so that the patch can be rotated laterally to leave the tube exposed for further handling (Fig. 242-6). The silicone

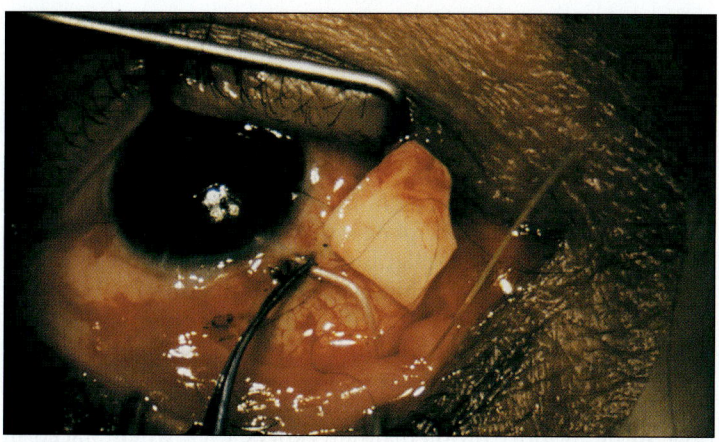

FIG. 242-7 ▮ Silicone tube is inserted through 22- or 23-gauge needle opening at limbus. Note distal end of Supramid suture that protrudes forward beneath anterior cut edge of the conjunctiva and the tube of the previously placed implant.

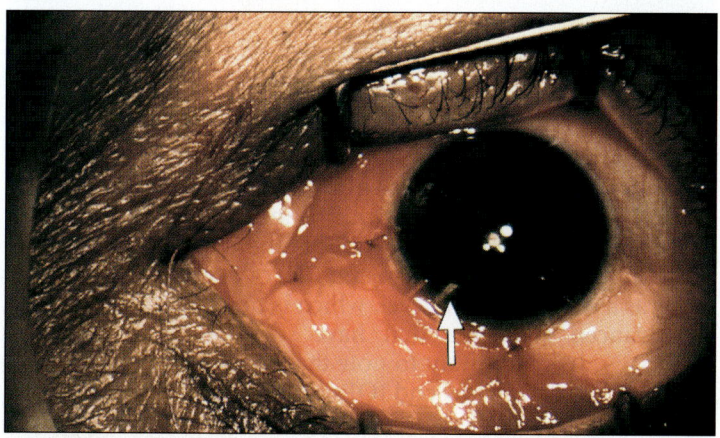

FIG. 242-8 ▮ Two single-plate Molteno implants in one eye. Supramid suture (*arrow*) emerges from the conjunctiva at the limbus with the conclusion of the insertion of the second implant.

tube is then cut to size, which varies according to the requirements of the individual surgeon. The insertion of the tube into the anterior chamber is accomplished by the manufacture of a tract from the limbus into the eye using a 22 or 23 gauge needle inserted parallel to the iris plane (see Fig. 242-7). Prior to insertion of the tube, a paracentesis opening is made near the limbus using a microsharp blade to allow access for assistance in tube placement if the need arises (see Fig. 242-6). The end of the tube is cut in a manner that allows the opening to be beveled upward and so prevent occlusion by the iris (see Fig. 242-2). The tube is fixed to the sclera with a single 10-0 nylon suture beneath the scleral patch (see Fig. 242-6). The scleral patch is secured by tying the previously placed two 10-0 sutures that were left untied.

The conjunctiva is then brought forward and, using the two marker sutures, is sutured back to the limbus at the extreme ends of the incision using 7-0 Vicryl sutures. The relaxing incisions are closed with a continuous 7-0 Vicryl mattress suture. The 3-0 Supramid suture that protrudes from the posterior lumen of the silicone tube is brought forward beneath the conjunctiva so that it emerges at the limbus. The suture is trimmed so that its free edge just protrudes from the free limbal edge of the conjunctiva (Fig. 242-8), which allows free access to the suture postoperatively. The suture is not exposed as postoperative edema of the conjunctiva just covers its free edge. No conjunctival incisions are needed to remove the suture when this becomes necessary, which is usually 2–3 weeks postoperatively, by which time a capsule has formed over the plate and prevents the occurrence of hypotony.

Postoperative Management

A combination corticosteroid antibiotic drop and topical atropine are used for 3 weeks postoperatively. After this, topical corticosteroids alone are used for a further 6 weeks. After 4–6 weeks, the IOP often becomes elevated as a result of excessive fibrous tissue in the bleb capsule. This IOP rise needs to be treated or it results in further fibrous tissue deposition and failure of the procedure. The use of a topical carbonic anhydrase inhibitor together with a topical β-blocker is often adequate to control this IOP rise. If these measures prove to be inadequate, aspiration of the bleb and removal of aqueous result in a temporarily lower IOP, which continues for 1–2 weeks. This procedure can be repeated until IOP control is achieved.

COMPLICATIONS

Complications may be subdivided into intraoperative, early postoperative, and late postoperative.[9]

Intraoperative Complications

Intraoperative complications are uncommon but include bleeding, misdirection of silicone tube, and loss of anterior chamber. Bleeding occurs particularly in neovascular glaucoma, and large hyphemas must be evacuated as they can block the tube. Misdirection of the silicone tube into the posterior chamber may occur in the presence of peripheral anterior synechiae. The tube must be removed and reintroduced more anteriorly. This can be assisted by the insertion of a thin iris repositor through a previously prepared paracentesis opening and placement of the repositor beneath the tube as it enters the anterior chamber, which prevents the tube from following the old tract to the posterior chamber. Loss of anterior chamber may be remedied by the introduction of saline or viscoelastic solution through a previously placed paracentesis opening.

Early Postoperative Complications

The most common early postoperative complication is hypotony, with or without associated choroidal effusions. Hemorrhagic effusions are often associated with pain, even though the eye remains hypotonic. Small choroidal effusions may be left to resolve spontaneously. Large effusions that result in "kissing choroidals" may have to be evacuated, which may need to be combined with gas injection into the vitreous cavity to prevent rapid recurrence. Overfiltration may also need to be addressed by occlusion of the anterior silicone tube. Choroidal effusions may occur even with tubal occlusion, particularly in diabetic patients. Hypotony is best treated by prevention, either by the use of valved implants or by occlusion of the silicone tube with a stent and/or a constricting ligature, as described earlier. Neither method is fail-safe, but tubal occlusion is more likely to prevent hypotony. When using a double-plate Molteno implant, an additional safeguard against hypotony may include an absorbable ligature placed around the silicone tube that connects the two plates.

Increased IOP may occur as an early postoperative complication, usually because of blockage of the silicone tube. The opening of the tube may be obstructed by iris, which may actually enter the lumen of the tube. This can be treated by ablation of the iris tissue with the yttrium-aluminum-garnet laser. When an internal obturator is used for the silicone tube, postoperative hypertension can be prevented by the placement of venting slits in the tube. Also, hypotensive agents may be used in the early postoperative period to treat elevations in IOP, which allows the stent to remain in position until an adequate capsule has developed around the plate, usually at about 14 days. This capsule prevents the occurrence of extensive hypotony when the stent is removed. The use of a 22-gauge needle by some surgeons to introduce the silicone tube into the eye usually results in some minimal leakage around the tube, which prevents extreme elevations in IOP.

Tube-corneal contact may occur and is best treated by prevention, which consists of accurate placement intraoperatively away from the endothelium and parallel to the iris. Total tube corneal touch requires the tube to be repositioned.

Occlusion of the tube by vitreous may occur in aphakic eyes. This is prevented by placement of the tube on the iris and away from the pupil and where necessary by the combination of this with an adequate anterior vitrectomy. Vitreous in the tube is best treated using vitrectomy.

Late Complications

The most significant late complication is the development of a thick capsule around the plate(s), which results in an elevation of IOP. Often, a hypertensive phase may be seen 4–6 weeks postoperatively because of the development of a fibrous capsule. Thinning of the capsule may occur subsequently, but for this to happen the IOP must be normalized. The IOP may be controlled using hypotensive agents, exclusive of cholinomimetics. If this proves inadequate, the bleb may be aspirated, a procedure that lowers IOP and may be repeated on a weekly basis until thinning of the bleb occurs.

Deflation of the bleb is designed to allow compressed channels in the wall of the bleb to expand and reestablish drainage.[5,10] Because the encysted blebs contain a relatively large amount of aqueous, as much as 1cm^3 of aqueous may be withdrawn to deflate the bleb with no loss of the anterior chamber. Also, because these blebs are relatively avascular, to needle them is less traumatic than an anterior chamber paracentesis, which risks damage to intraocular structures, particularly in phakic patients. The needling is done with a 27- or 30-gauge needle, the tracks of which are self-healing and are not associated with hemorrhage or infection.[5,10] The application of an antimetabolite, such as mitomycin C, to the eye at the site of plate implantation intraoperatively has been reported with moderate success.[11] Molteno and colleagues[12,13] suggested the use of fibrosis suppression medication, which consists of a nonsteroidal antiinflammatory agent, systemic corticosteroids, colchicine, topical corticosteroids, and topical epinephrine (adrenaline). A modified regimen that consists of diclofenac 75mg daily, prednisone 40mg daily, and topical corticosteroids has also had some success. This systemic regimen needs to be given no later than 14 days postoperatively to be of any use and should be continued for at least 6 weeks. Removal of preexisting implants is inadvisable and failure as a result of bleb fibrosis is best treated by the insertion of another drainage implant.

Erosion of the silicone tube through the sclera or scleral patch and conjunctiva can occur (Fig. 242-9). More rarely, the plate may erode through the conjunctiva; this is most likely if the

original conjunctival incision for plate implantation is made over or close to the plate. Fornix-based conjunctival flaps are most likely to prevent the occurrence of plate erosion.

Plate migration is extremely rare, even if the anchoring sutures become loose, as the enclosing capsule, once it has formed, keeps the plate in position.

Limitation of eye movement may occur because of the size of the blebs that overlie the plate or plates. The movement most commonly affected is upgaze, but this usually has little effect on the patient clinically. Placement of the implants in the lower quadrants restricts downgaze, with associated diplopia where vision is good in both eyes, and, therefore, plate implantation into the lower quadrants is to be avoided in an eye that has vision adequate enough to produce diplopia.[7] Certain implants may produce more motility problems than others, even when placed in the superior quadrants.[14] Retinal detachment has been described as a complication, albeit rare, of implant use.[15] Sterile hypopyon has been reported to occur with Molteno implants and may be related to the presence of an obstructing ligature.[16] The occurrence however, is, very rare.

OUTCOME

Most reported results indicate fairly favorable outcomes in the short term with the use of glaucoma implants.[10,17–20] This is true especially when dealing with neovascular glaucoma. Mermoud et al.[21] reported 62.1% success at 1 year and 10.3% success at 5 years. Success rates reported with shunt procedures have been based on relatively high end IOP as the criterion for success. Most published reports use an end IOP of 21mmHg (2.8kPa) or lower as a successful IOP level, which is not acceptable for cases of advanced glaucoma that have severe optic nerve damage.[18,19,22,23] It is important to note that shunt procedures in general do not give very low end IOPs, irrespective of the size of the plates used. Nonetheless, it is reported that the greater the surface area of the plates, the lower the end IOPs.[23] Neovascular glaucoma is the one condition most likely to be treated with a glaucoma implant. Rates reported for neovascular glaucoma using different implants are given in Table 242-1 and provide a

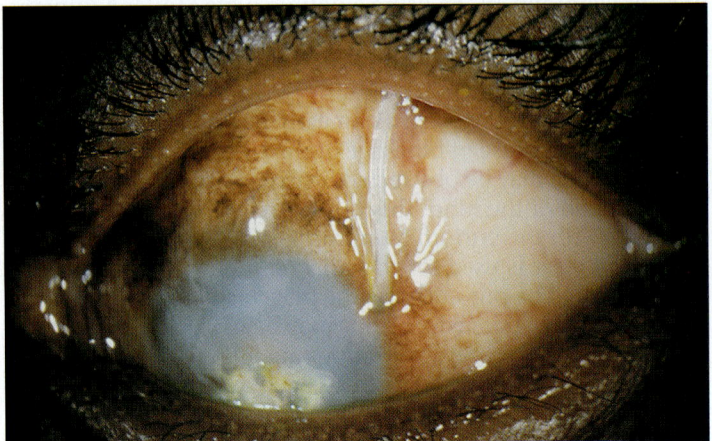

FIG. 242-9 ■ **Totally exposed silicone tube.** It has eroded through the sclera and conjunctiva.

TABLE 242-1

RESULTS WITH DRAINING DEVICES IN NEOVASCULAR GLAUCOMA

Implant Type	Number	Follow-up (Months)	Percentage Success [<21mmHg (<2.8kPa)]
Baerveldt[24]	7	18	43
Molteno[10] (black patients only)	18	35	67
Krupin[25]	79	23.7	67
Molteno[21]	60	24	52.9
Schocket[26]	19	14	95

TABLE 242-2

RESULTS WITH DRAINING DEVICES IN REFRACTORY GLAUCOMA

Implant Type	Follow-up (Months)	Percent Success Aphakic/ Pseudophakic (Number)	Percent Success Glaucoma <13 Years (Number)	Percent Failed Filter (Number)
Molteno[10]	30	83 (24)	50 (4)	74 (31)
Baerveldt[24]	18	74 (35)	67 (3)	75 (12)
Molteno[21]	24	74 (50)	68 (16)	58 (12)

good perspective on the efficacy of these devices in the management of this condition. Results obtained in other types of refractory glaucoma are given in Table 242-2. The Ahmed valve implant has been reported to achieve a 78% probability of success at 12 months in patients who have refractory glaucoma.[17] The Krupin disc implant has been reported to achieve 83% success in patients who have refractory glaucomas.[27] Molteno et al.[28] recently reported long-term results of uveitis with secondary glaucoma drained by Molteno implants. Insertion of a Molteno implant was effective in controlling the IOP at 21mmHg or less in 76% of cases over a mean follow-up period of 7.1 years.

Glaucoma implants have found a place in the management of refractory glaucomas. With the development of new implants and methods to overcome postoperative hypotony and with the ongoing research to achieve thinning capsules over the plates and thus lower IOPs, a future may exist for the use of implants as a primary surgical procedure for glaucomas that are not refractory. With careful patient and implant selection, many eyes that might have been lost may be retrievable.

REFERENCES

1. Bock RH. Subconjunctival drainage of the aqueous using a glass seton. Am J Ophthalmol. 1950;33:929–32.
2. Richards RD, VanBijsterveld OP. Artificial drainage tubes for glaucoma. Am J Ophthalmol. 1965;60:405–8.
3. Molteno ACB. New implant for drainage in glaucoma. Clinical trial. Br J Ophthalmol. 1969;53:606–15.
4. Molteno ACB, Straughan JL, Anker E. Long tube implants in the management of glaucoma. S Afr Med J. 1976;50:1062–6.
5. Freedman J. Clinical experience with the Molteno dual chamber single-plate implant. Ophthalmic Surg. 1992;23:238–41.
6. Wilson-Holt N, Franks W, Nourredin B, Hitchings R. Hypertropia following insertion of inferiorly sited double-plate Molteno tubes. Eye. 1992;6:515–20.
7. Sherwood MB, Smith MF. Prevention of early hypotony associated with Molteno implants by a new occluding stent technique. Ophthalmology. 1993;100:85.
8. Freedman J. Scleral patch grafts with Molteno setons. Ophthalmic Surg. 1987;18: 532–4.
9. Melamed S, Cahane M, Gutman I, Blumenthal M. Postoperative complications after Molteno implant surgery. Am J Ophthalmol. 1991;111:319–22.
10. Freedman J, Rubin B. Molteno implants as a treatment for refractory glaucoma in black patients. Arch Ophthalmol. 1991;109:1417–20.
11. Perkins T, Cardakli UF, Eisele J, Kaufman P. Adjunctive mitomycin C in Molteno implant surgery. Ophthalmology. 1995;102:91–7.
12. Molteno ACB, Straughn JL, Ancker E. Control of bleb fibrosis after glaucoma drainage surgery. S Afr Med J. 1976;50:881–5.
13. Molteno ACB, Dempster AG. Methods of controlling bleb fibrosis around draining implants. In: Mills KB, ed. Glaucoma: Proceedings of the Fourth International Symposium of the Northern Eye Institute, Manchester, UK. Oxford: Pergamon Press; 1988:192–211.
14. Smith SL, Starita RJ, Fellman RL, Lynn JR. Early clinical experience with the Baerveldt 350-mm² glaucoma implant and associated extraocular muscle imbalance. Ophthalmology. 1993;100:914–18.
15. Waterhouse WJ, Lloyd MAE, Dugel PU, et al. Rhegmatogenous retinal detachment after Molteno glaucoma implant surgery. Ophthalmology. 1994;101:665–71.
16. Ball SF, Laftifield K, Scharfenberg J. Molteno ripcord suture hypopyon. Ophthalmic Surg. 1991;22:82–6.
17. Coleman AL, Hill R, Wilson MR, et al. Initial clinical experience with the Ahmed glaucoma valve implant. Am J Ophthalmol. 1995;120:23–31.
18. Lloyd MA, Baerveldt G, Heuer DK, et al. Initial clinical experience with the Baerveldt implant in complicated glaucomas. Ophthalmology. 1994;101:640–50.
19. Minckler DS, Heuer DK, Hasty B, et al. Clinical experience with the single plate Molteno implant in complicated glaucomas. Ophthalmology. 1988;95:1181–8.
20. Lloyd MA, Sedlak T, Heuer DK, et al. Clinical experience with the single-plate Molteno implant in complicated glaucomas. Ophthalmology. 1992;99:679–87.
21. Mermoud A, Salmon JF, Alexander P, et al. Molteno tube implantation for neovascular glaucoma. Ophthalmology. 1993;100:897–902.
22. Goldberg I. Management of uncontrolled glaucoma with the Molteno system. Aust NZ J Ophthalmol. 1987;15:97–107.
23. Heuer DK, Lloyd MA, Abrahms DA, et al. Which is better—one or two randomized clinical trials of single plate versus double plate Molteno implants? Ophthalmology. 1992;99:1512–19.
24. Hodkin MJ, Goldblatt WS, Buygoyne CF, et al. Early clinical experience with the Baerveldt implant in complicated glaucomas. Am J Ophthalmol. 1995;120: 32–40.
25. Krupin T, Kaufmann P, Mandell AI, et al. Long term results of valve implants in filtering surgery for eyes with neovascular glaucoma. Am J Ophthalmol. 1983; 95:775–87.
26. Schocket S, Lakhanpal V, Richards R. Anterior chamber tube shunt to an encircling band in the treatment of neovascular glaucoma. Ophthalmology. 1982; 89:1188–94.
27. The Krupin Eye Valve Filtering Surgery Study Group. Krupin eye valve with disc for filtration surgery. Ophthalmology. 1994;101:651–8.
28. Molteno ACB, Sayawat N, Herbison P. Long term results of uveitis with secondary glaucomas drained by Molteno implants. Ophthalmology. 2001;109:605–13.

CHAPTER 243

Complications of Glaucoma Surgery and Their Management

J. WILLIAM DOYLE • M. FRAN SMITH

INTRODUCTION

In the ideal world, surgery proceeds smoothly and outcomes are uncomplicated. Unfortunately, in the real world, despite a surgeon's best efforts, complications may occur. This is especially true in the field of glaucoma—glaucoma surgery, unlike many other ocular procedures, is not particularly "forgiving" in nature. Nonetheless, good final outcomes may often be achieved in spite of the occurrence of complications. The key to success is for the surgeon to be alert and be able to identify and address any problems promptly.

FILTRATION SURGERY

Before the discussion of complication management in filtration surgery, it is worth repeating an old surgical axiom. Without a doubt, the best surgical complication management is avoidance of the complication in the first place. Preoperatively, ensure that the patient stops the intake of all aspirin-like products, and discontinue topical epinephrine (adrenaline) compounds to decrease the quantity of superficial bleeding. Consider the use of preoperative topical antibiotics. Intraoperatively, meticulous attention to detail is important, especially if antimetabolites are being used. It is imperative to handle the conjunctiva gently. When the partial-thickness trabeculectomy flap is being closed, consider using extra, releasable-style sutures. If intraocular pressure (IOP) is too high postoperatively, a stitch may be pulled easily. But if too much drainage occurs postoperatively, an insidious cycle of overdrainage may be established—and this cannot always be corrected readily.

Nonetheless, complications intermittently occur. Filtration surgery complications are most easily categorized as intraoperative, early postoperative, and late postoperative.

Intraoperative Complications

CONJUNCTIVAL BUTTONHOLE. In no other situation is the axiom given before more appropriate—the best complication management of the buttonhole is initial avoidance of the complication. Toothed forceps are the problem here—they should not be on the glaucoma tray. Bishop-Harmon or suture-tying forceps are preferable when conjunctiva is handled. Better yet, the use of a dry cellulose sponge, with its tip cut off, to stretch conjunctiva up and away from the area of interest is safe. If a buttonhole occurs anyway, management requires patient, complete hole closure if successful surgery is to ensue. If a buttonhole cannot be closed in a watertight fashion and detection of the hole has occurred early in the surgery, consideration must be given to rotation of the site of the trabeculectomy flap to a different area, away from the hole. Also, if antimetabolite use was planned but not initiated prior to discovery of the buttonhole, the surgeon must consider no exposure, or limited exposure, to antimetabolite, applied well away from the buttonhole.

Closure technique for a conjunctival buttonhole depends on its location, size, and shape. The most easily closed buttonhole

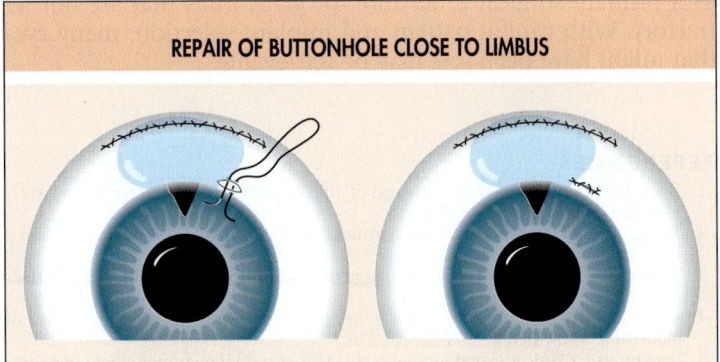

FIG. 243-1 ■ Repair of buttonhole close to limbus.

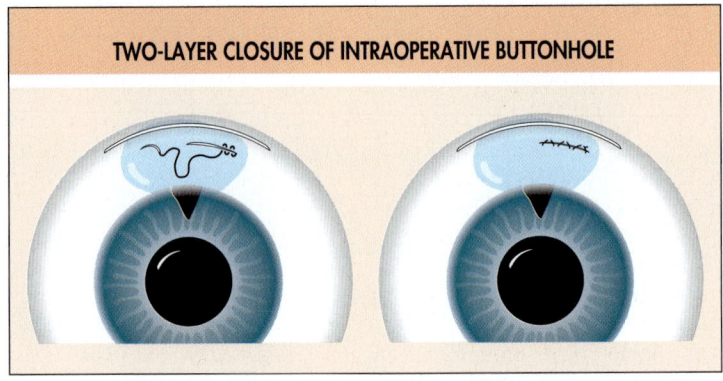

FIG. 243-2 ■ Two-layer closure of intraoperative buttonhole in central bleb zone. Following Tenon's layer closure, conjunctiva is closed.

is the short limbal tear, which may be closed with a horizontal mattress suture of double-armed 10-0 nylon. Cornea just anterior to the tear is deepithelialized. One arm of the suture is passed to one side of the hole, through conjunctiva and partial-thickness anterior Tenon's layer, and into the cornea in front of the tear. The other needle of the double-armed suture is passed similarly on the other side of the hole. When the two ends are tied, conjunctiva is pulled safely down, with considerable overlap, onto clear cornea. The deepithelialized cornea quickly heals to the underside of the overlapped conjunctiva (Fig. 243-1).

Linear tears of conjunctiva away from the limbus are probably best closed in two layers with a running suture. An 8-0 polyglactin suture on a vascular needle is used first to close Tenon's layer, from the Tenon's layer side. For conjunctival layer closure, the conjunctival flap is flapped over and 10-0 or 11-0 nylon sutures are used, preferably on a vascular needle (Fig. 243-2). Similarly, small, round holes can be closed using a two-layer technique and purse-stringing the suture around the hole.

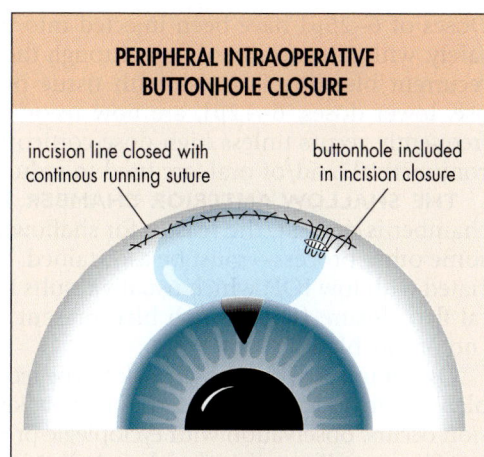

FIG. 243-3 ■ Peripheral intraoperative buttonhole closure. Repair by inclusion in conjunctival incision closure.

PERIPHERAL INTRAOPERATIVE BUTTONHOLE CLOSURE

incision line closed with continous running suture

buttonhole included in incision closure

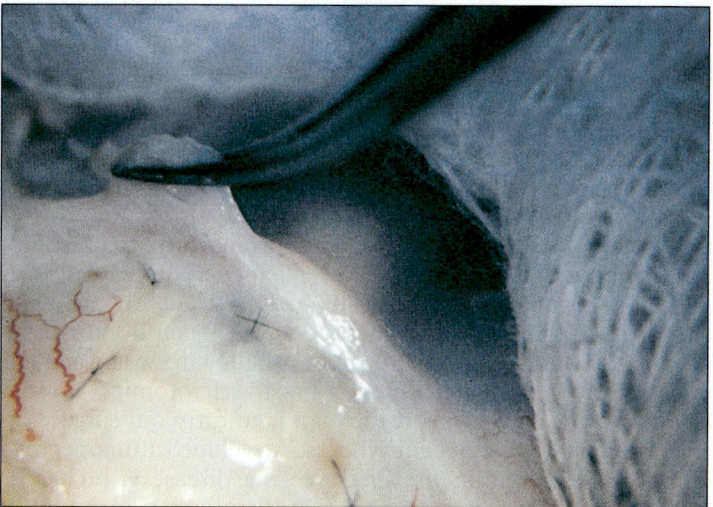

FIG. 243-4 ■ Repair of disinserted flap.

Finally, linear tears in conjunctiva near a fornix incision are frequently best addressed by incorporation of the tear into the final incision closure (see Fig. 243-3).

After buttonhole repair, it is essential that watertightness be tested before proceeding further. Balanced salt solution may be squirted vigorously at one side of the closure and any seepage through to the other side carefully sought. Also, after final incision closure, it is best to recheck for leakage using fluorescein dye. Inflation of the bleb with balanced salt solution through the corneal paracentesis and application of fluorescein dye is a simple way to mark any leaks. The time to address such leaks is while the patient has good anesthesia and is still in the operating room. Postoperatively, when inflammation occurs and the conjunctiva has become thinned because of aqueous flow, definitive surgical repair may not be possible.

TRABECULECTOMY SCLERAL FLAP TEAR/DISINSERTION.
Occasionally, despite the surgeon's attempt to dissect up a sufficiently thick (about two thirds of the total scleral thickness) scleral flap, tissues are such that a "ratty" flap is produced. These flaps tend to tear or disinsert. If the tear is found early and is small enough, direct suture closure using 10-0 nylon may be attempted. Similarly, if the flap base is disinserted partially, an attempt may be made to reposit the flap using a double-armed horizontal mattress suture externalized through clear cornea (Fig. 243-4). Some surgeons have reported successful reposition of a totally disinserted flap using two 10-0 nylon sutures through the flap base and out the peripheral cornea.[1] However, total disinsertion and large tears are usually a reflection of exceptionally poor quality (ratty) sclera; such flaps do not tolerate sutures well and tend to "cheesewire," which results in larger defects. Rather, this complication may be best addressed by placement of an additional cover over the problem flap.

Tenon's tissue is readily available in all eyes. The surgeon may choose to excise a 4 × 3mm piece of redundant Tenon's tissue from up in the superior fornix near the incision or alternatively from the inferior fornix if excess tissue is not present superiorly. This excised rectangular piece of tissue may be sutured at its four corners over the full-thickness sclerotomy.[2] If excess leakage is noted after anterior chamber reformation, additional sutures may be placed. Other choices of coverage material are donor sclera,[3] dura, pericardium, or even fascia lata.[4] Most operating rooms have at least one of these materials present in a convenient prepackaged form. The material is hydrated in balanced salt solution, a rectangle of material (approximately 2mm larger and wider than the trabeculectomy flap) is cut out, and the cover is sutured into place, with at least one 10-0 nylon suture to each corner of the material. Postoperatively, these sutures may be lysed using an argon laser to increase drainage as desired, so secure closure on the operating table is warranted (Fig. 243-5).

VITREOUS LOSS. Especially in pseudophakes after complicated cataract extraction or in aphakes, the surgeon may encounter vitreous prolapse after the iridectomy. Careful clearance

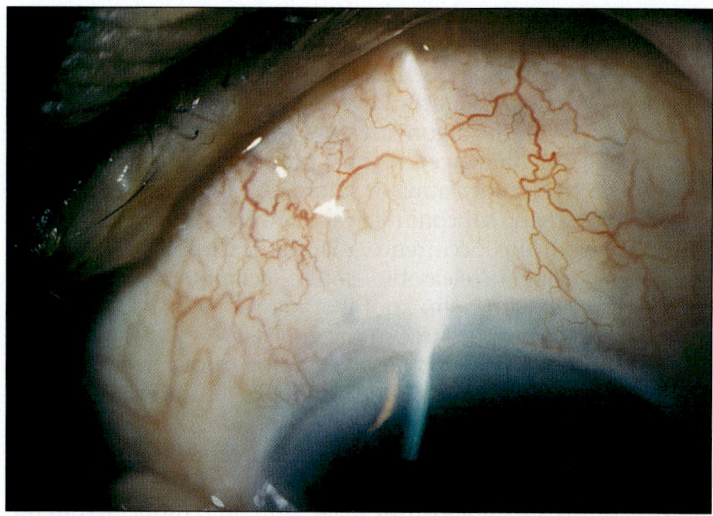

FIG. 243-5 ■ Donor dura flap to replace disinserted flap.

from the sclerotomy of all vitreous is key because vitreous is a very effective sclerotomy plug. A limited vitrectomy with a combination of scissors dissection, cellulose sponge, and automated vitrector should be performed. The goal is no vitreous present at the sclerotomy when checked using a cellulose sponge. Extra care is required in these eyes to avoid a postoperative shallow anterior chamber because this may bring further vitreous forward to block the sclerotomy. Therefore, consider the placement of extra releasable sutures (or sutures that may be lasered) to prevent early overdrainage.

INTRAOPERATIVE BLEEDING. Excess bleeding from the iris root and/or ciliary body after iridectomy must be addressed because blood may also cause sclerotomy blockage. Cold balanced salt solution, dripped slowly over several minutes, with or without low-concentration epinephrine added, usually results in stoppage of the bleeding. Alternatively, a monopolar wet-field 23gauge cautery may be applied carefully to the bleeding vessel if the site can be visualized. It is rare for these areas to rebleed postoperatively, but if they do, it is usually in situations with hypotony; again, a tight closure with extra releasable sutures is considered. Viscoelastic material can be left in the eye at the conclusion of surgery to act as a "tamponade" and also to help avoid postoperative hypotony.

Suprachoroidal hemorrhage (SCH) is the other type of intraoperative bleeding. In these cases the eye should be closed as quickly as possible. Avoidance is paramount because an expulsive

SCH is disastrous. Preoperative intravenous mannitol (100ml of 20% solution over 15 minutes), with Foley catheter placement, may be considered in eyes that undergo trabeculectomy with a preoperative IOP >40mmHg (5.3kPa). Theoretically, less chance exists of SCH if eye pressure at the time of internal sclerotomy does not suddenly drop from 45mmHg (6.0kPa) to zero. In addition, the paracentesis may be performed earlier to decompress the eye gradually prior to internal block removal.

CHOROIDAL EFFUSION. Usually effusions develop postoperatively, not intraoperatively. However, patients who have Sturge-Weber syndrome or markedly elevated episcleral venous pressure may develop effusions intraoperatively. Their occurrence is signaled by sudden anterior chamber shallowing. Management consists of drainage via inferior linear sclerotomies, located 5–6mm from the limbus. If the plan is to carry out surgery on the second eye of a patient who has developed intraoperative choroidal effusions in the first eye (the disease is bilateral), placement of a preliminary posterior sclerotomy prior to internal block removal may be considered.

Early Postoperative Complications

UNDERDRAINAGE. In the early postoperative period, initial underdrainage, not associated with sclerotomy blockage, is addressed effectively by sequential release of scleral flap sutures. If so-called permanent sutures have been placed, the 10-0 nylon may be lysed with the argon laser and a Hoskins (or Ritch) lens.[5] Krypton red (or blue-green argon), 50μm spots, at 300mW are usually effective. Rarely, a nylon suture cannot be visualized, secondary to overlying subconjunctival hemorrhage or thick Tenon's tissue. To avoid this occurrence, place at least half of the scleral flap sutures using a "releasable"-suture technique.[6] This involves tying the suture with a slip knot that may be released easily with a pull on the cornealized free suture end (Fig. 243-6). Because endophthalmitis has been reported to develop from a freely moving, cornealized releasable suture, the externalized suture end must be buried in clear cornea.[7] The superficial unburied segment of the suture is epithelialized quickly, which decreases risk of endophthalmitis and still allows the surgeon easy assess.[8] To maintain expansion of the subconjunctival space with fluid (aqueous) in the early postoperative period, and when it is too early to lyse a stitch, another option is local scleral compression. This involves gentle application of pressure over the conjunctiva using a moistened cotton-tip applicator, just at the edge of the scleral flap. Such pressure "burps" free an aliquot of aqueous, which lowers IOP. Gonioscopy is recommended to check that the internal sclerostomy is not blocked by vitreous, iris, and so forth.

A blocked sclerotomy is handled differently. If fibrin or blood blocks outflow, tissue plasminogen activator may be helpful.[9,10]

Doses of 6–25μl have been injected into the anterior chamber safely, with resumption of flow through the sclerotomy. Because recurrent bleeding is a risk with tissue plasminogen activator use, lower doses, 6–12μl, are now recommended. Also, fibrin frequently recurs unless high-dose corticosteroids, topical, subconjunctival, and/or oral, are used to reduce inflammation.

THE SHALLOW ANTERIOR CHAMBER. If a shallow anterior chamber is present, the reason for shallowing—overdrainage or some other process—must be ascertained. Overdrainage is associated with low IOP, which usually results from inadequate scleral flap closure (with a high bleb present) or from a bleb leak (no or low bleb present).

Overdrainage with no bleb leak can be tedious to manage. If the bleb is high and no corneal-lens touch or "kissing" choroidal effusion occurs, observation with cycloplegic prescription is appropriate. However, if anterior chamber shallowing is progressive, early placement of an oversized, bandage soft contact lens may help to prevent later, more difficult problems.[11,12] Such lenses seem to limit excessive bleb extension and/or excess bleb transconjunctival aqueous flow (Fig. 243-7). Usually, their use may be discontinued after 1–2 weeks. Alternatively, a Simmon's shell may be applied to the eye. The shell has a plate that can be positioned over the sclerotomy site for maximum tamponade. However, patients may tolerate it poorly, and daily ocular examination is required. Also, corneal epithelial defects occur frequently.

Another option some surgeons use in these cases is gentle pressure patching, in which pressure is applied directly over the trabeculectomy flap to limit outflow. One concern with this option is that, when the patient looks up (or exhibits Bell's phenomenon, with sleep), the pressure patch may transfer pressure over the cornea, which results in lens-corneal touch. Sometimes, injection of viscoelastic material into the anterior chamber may provide sufficient time (24–48 hours) to allow the eye to "catch up" with itself.[13] We have found greater viscosity viscoelastic to be particularly useful in such cases. This is best attempted early, rather than late, in the course. Finally, if overdrainage continues with the development of choroidal effusions that touch, or of lens-corneal touch, the surgeon may need to return the patient to the operating room for further flap closure, anterior chamber reformation, and effusion drainage.

Initial overdrainage with bleb leak is frequently the result of a buttonhole missed at the time of surgery. Postoperatively, a buttonhole is far more difficult to manage. As already noted, suture repair at this time is often ineffective, especially if intraoperative antimetabolites were used and/or the conjunctiva is cystic or excessively thinned. Suturing at this time may result in a larger hole. Patching, bandage soft contact lenses, and Simmon's shell may be used, with variable results. The surgeon must watch the bleb carefully because the preceding "solutions" often fail to

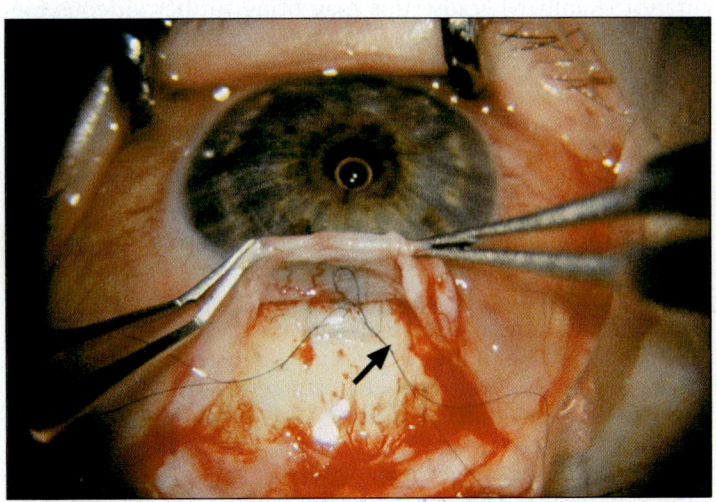

FIG. 243-6 ■ Releasable sutures (*arrow*).

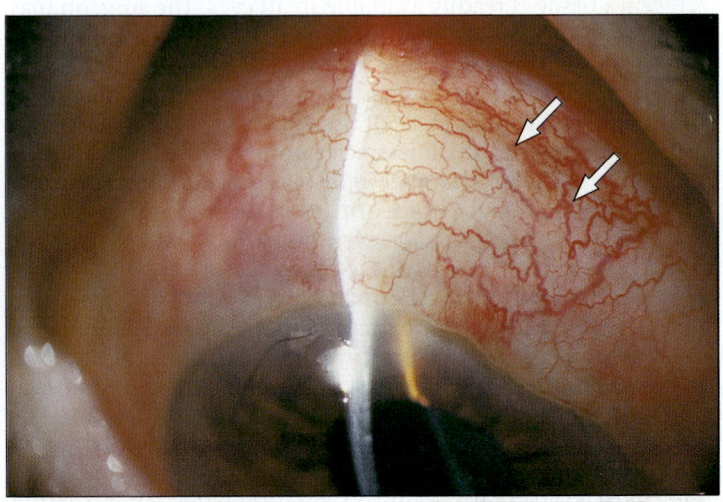

FIG. 243-7 ■ A 17mm contact lens compresses an overdraining bleb. Edge of bandage contact lens indicated by arrows.

seal the leak and only act to exacerbate episcleral/conjunctival healing and adhesion. Other alternatives include autologous fibrin tissue glue,[14] autologous blood injection (see Fig. 243-8),[15-17] and cyanoacrylate glue with contact lens application.[18] Most of these alternatives seem to work better on small, late-postoperative bleb leaks. A large, early-postoperative bleb leak may require a return to the operating room and development of a new conjunctival flap from "buttonhole-free" conjunctiva.

Remaining causes of an early-postoperative shallow chamber, other than overdrainage, are basically five, one with low IOP and four with high IOP. Most rarely, the ciliary body may shut down secondary to intense postoperative inflammation. Such eyes have flat blebs, no bleb leaks, shallow anterior chambers, low IOP, and occasionally inflammatory choroidal effusions. High-dose topical, peribulbar, and systemic corticosteroids may be helpful in these cases. Postoperative 5-fluorouracil injections should be considered because they may help prevent conjunctival-episcleral adhesions in the period before aqueous flow restarts.

A shallow anterior chamber associated with a high IOP results from one of four causes only:
- Pupillary block
- SCH
- Aqueous misdirection malignant glaucoma
- Ring choroidal effusion (rare)

If a full-thickness iridectomy was made at the time of surgery, pupillary block can be ruled out. However, if doubt exists with regard to the surgical iridectomy patency and the preceding scenario exists, the surgeon must perform another (laser) iridectomy as soon as possible. Only then can pupillary block be ruled out. Once pupillary block is excluded, the surgeon must examine for the presence of an SCH, which is more likely to occur in elderly, vitrectomized, aphakic, hypotonous eyes. Usually, diagnosis is made easily by indirect ophthalmoscopy, with observation of the characteristic dark choroidal swellings and the patient's history of pain, nausea, and vomiting. If ophthalmoscopy is impossible, a B-scan ultrasound examination is carried out (Fig. 243-9). If SCH is diagnosed, therapeutic options include observation and corticosteroid prescription if the patient is not too uncomfortable and there is no choroidal or lens-corneal touch. Again, 5-fluorouracil injections may be considered to prevent scarring of the sclerotomy while the SCH resolves. Otherwise, it may be best to return the patient to the operating room for evacuation of the SCH. This is best accomplished no sooner than postoperative day 7–10, at which time clot lysis has usually begun, which allows easier SCH drainage.

Another cause of a shallow anterior chamber, with associated high IOP, is aqueous misdirection. Once called malignant glaucoma, it is indeed a malignant process to treat. Aqueous misdi-rection (as discussed in Chapter 229) is the syndrome characterized by marked anterior displacement of the lens-iris diaphragm with a high IOP, presumably as a result of trapped misdirected posterior aqueous. If prompt treatment is initiated, perhaps 50% of mild cases resolve with intensive cycloplegic therapy (i.e., atropine 1%, one drop every 5 minutes for a total of three drops, four times a day). Also, to relieve the buildup of what is believed to be misdirected aqueous trapped behind the vitreous face, many surgeons recommend aqueous suppressants and/or osmotics. Other useful medical adjuncts include phenylephrine 2.5% four times a day and prednisolone acetate every 2 hours for inflammation. If this is unsuccessful and the patient is aphakic or pseudophakic, laser therapy is an option.

Finally, although rare, anterior ring choroidal effusion has been described as a cause of shallow anterior chamber associated with high IOP.[19] B-scan confirms this diagnosis.

CHOROIDAL EFFUSIONS. Although classical posterior choroidal effusions often occur in conjunction with a shallow anterior chamber and low IOP, they may also occur in eyes that have full-depth chambers and low IOPs. Management usually consists of cycloplegia, topical corticosteroids, and observation. As long as the effusions do not touch, drainage is not required. If touch does occur centrally, because of the danger of retinal adhesion formation, many surgeons choose to perform effusion drainage via posterior sclerotomies inferiorly. The scleral flap may be revised at the time of choroidal drainage to prevent further hypotony and a recurrence of the effusions. Several permanent or releasable sutures may be enough to reduce leakage in the short term.

CORNEAL EPITHELIOPATHY. In this era of antimetabolite use, an increased incidence of corneal epithelial toxicity and even defects occurs after 5-fluorouracil injections. Very early temporary punctal occlusion using collagen plugs optimizes the corneal wetting. Preservative-free tears are helpful. One group also reported that bandage contact lens application increased comfort and decreased inflammation.[20]

Late Postoperative Complications

LATE BLEB FAILURE. Late bleb failure may result from heavy vascularization and healing around the bleb. Digital pressure applied by the patient to the inferior globe through the inferior lid may be useful in such cases, as this helps maintain flow through the drain and keeps the subconjunctival space expanded. If this is insufficient, needling revision of the bleb may reestablish effective filtration. The needling process alone rarely establishes long-term filtration in eyes not exposed to antimetabolites. However, if needling is followed with 5-fluorouracil injections,

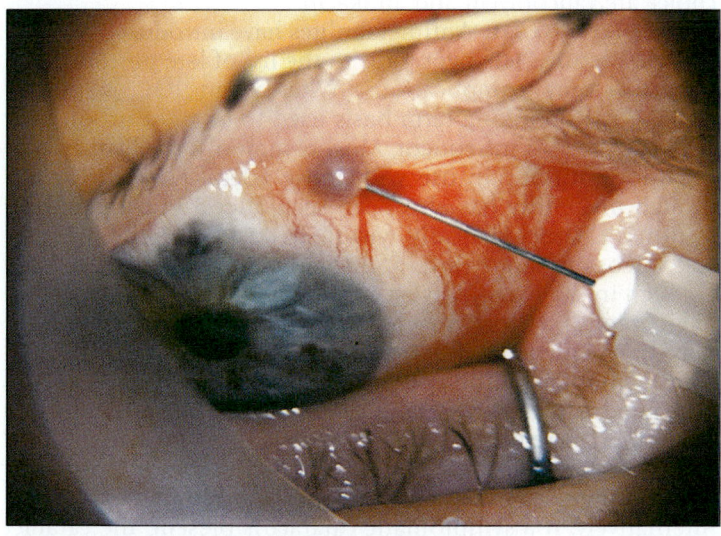

FIG. 243-8 ■ Peribleb autologous blood injection for leak.

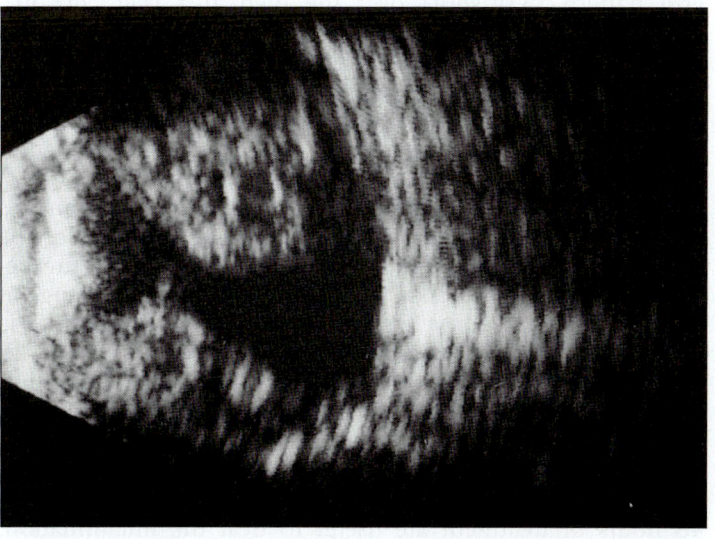

FIG. 243-9 ■ B-scan of suprachoroidal hemorrhage following trabeculectomy.

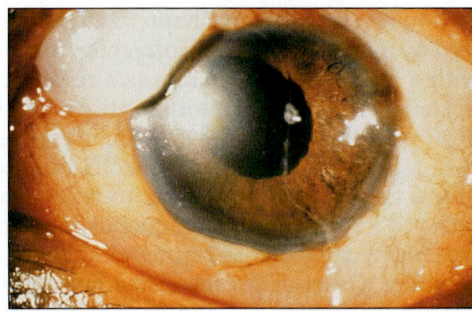

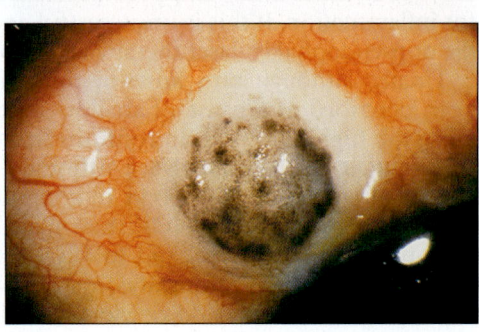

FIG. 243-10 ▦ Neodymium:yttrium-aluminum-garnet laser bleb remodeling for bleb leak. (Courtesy of Mary Lynch, MD.)

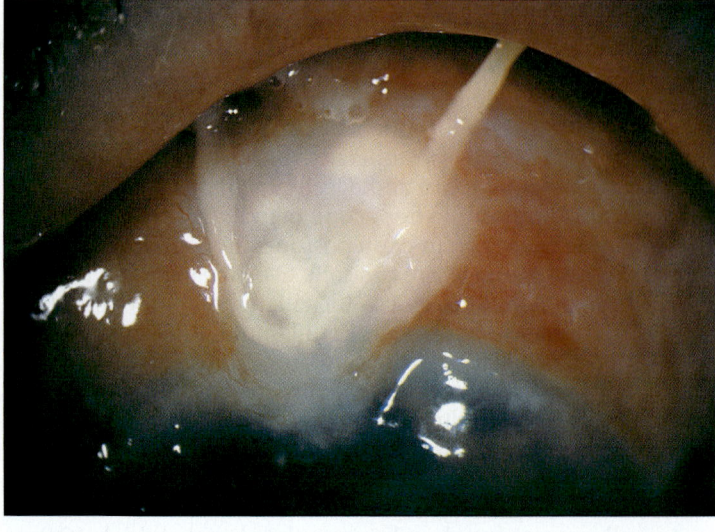

FIG. 243-11 ▦ Blebitis.

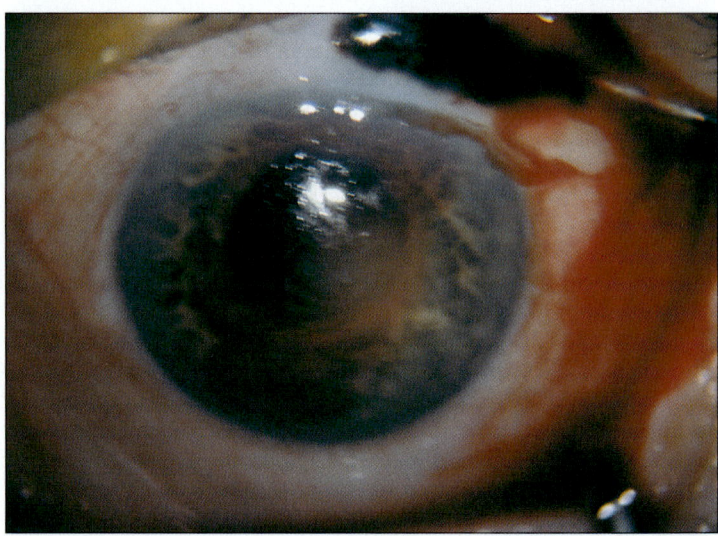

FIG. 243-12 ▦ Intrableb injection of autologous blood for hypotony.

up to an 80% success rate is possible.[21] Also, needling may help revive a failing bleb after trabeculectomy using intraoperative mitomycin.[22]

TENON'S CYST FORMATION. A Tenon's cyst is a high-domed, taut encapsulation of the bleb, which limits aqueous percolation. It must be differentiated from vascularized bleb failure. Once reported to occur in up to 15% of postsurgical eyes during the first postoperative month, it seems to be much less common in eyes that have received 5-fluorouracil or mitomycin. If the acute rise in IOP associated with these cysts is managed medically, with or without corticosteroid use, most of these blebs (up to 90%) continue to function later, as the bleb tissue remodels itself. If failure seems imminent (lower bleb, higher IOP), needling of the cyst, with postoperative 5-fluorouracil injections, may be helpful.

LATE BLEB LEAKS. Initial management of these leaks involves patching, aqueous suppressants, and antibiotics. Additional management includes modalities already referred to, such as bandage contact lenses, autologous fibrin or blood, and glue. Trichloroacetic acid application and carefully applied cryotherapy may also be attempted. If these modalities fail and further management is felt necessary, neodymium:yttrium-aluminum-garnet laser bleb remodeling may be tried.[23] The laser is tuned to the continuous-wave multimode, carefully retrofocused 1.0mm behind the bleb to the underlying sclera, and then applied in a grid pattern (3.0J/shot) over the bleb area (Fig. 243-10). Inflammation and discomfort may be intense, but up to 80% of leaks seal. Other alternatives include a return to the operating room, where free conjunctival patch grafts may be applied over the sclerotomy after excision of the cystic leaking bleb.[24,25] Or, if scarring is minimal, local revision using conjunctival rotation may be attempted.

BLEBITIS VERSUS LATE ENDOPHTHALMITIS. As many as 1 per 100 patients/year may develop infection of the bleb. The cystic thin blebs seen after antimetabolite application are believed to be at higher risk. When a bleb is present, the surgeon needs to treat any red eye emergency with antibiotics. Blebitis is differentiated from conjunctivitis by the presence of a murky, opalescent bleb, often with an associated bleb leak, in addition to conjunctiva injected diffusely with associated discharge (Fig. 243-11). The key here is analysis of the vitreous response. If the vitreous is quiet, prompt treatment with hourly topical antibiotics may save the bleb and the eye. Topical corticosteroids after 48 hours of treatment are useful to treat the inflammation. However, if endophthalmitis is diagnosed with vitreous involvement, intravitreal cultures and antibiotics are required and eye

salvage is rare. Organisms frequently seen in these eyes include hemophilus, streptococci, and staphylococci. Thus, coverage is best initiated with fortified topical cefazolin or vancomycin and tobramycin. Alternatively, topical fluoroquinolones, perhaps in combination with systemic fluoroquinolone prescription, may cover many of these cases. Intravitreal antibiotic injections of choice are vancomycin and amikacin.

LATE HYPOTONY. Antimetabolites have introduced a somewhat new entity, late hypotony, to the list of late postoperative trabeculectomy complications. Whereas an IOP <5mmHg (<0.67kPa) on a long-term basis used to be unheard of, now such eyes are not infrequent. Most commonly, the history is of high-dose mitomycin use with loose scleral flap closure, although this entity has also been seen after 5-fluorouracil injections. Characteristically, vision is decreased, the eyes are soft, blebs are large, thin, and totally avascular, retinal folds are seen in the macula (with or without the aid of fluorescein angiography), retinal vessels are tortuous, and the nerve head may be swollen. Useful treatments, as with bleb leaks, include intrableb autologous blood injection[26] (Fig. 243-12) and neodymium:yttrium-aluminum-garnet bleb treatment.[23] Sometimes, a return to the operating room to revise the thin bleb and/or resuture the flap is indicated. A donor "cover" (as already discussed) may be necessary to limit aqueous egress. Alternatively, if a symptomatic cataract is present, the cataract extraction-associated inflammation frequently slows filtration through bleb healing and resolves the hypotony.[27] Some sur-

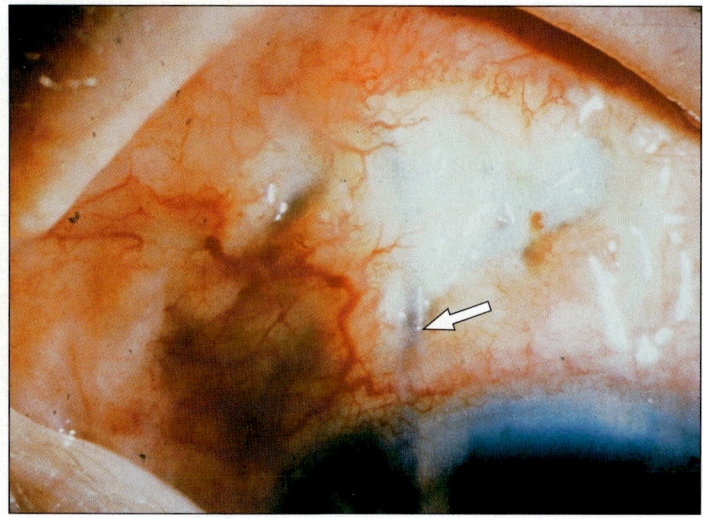

FIG. 243-13 ■ Exposure of tube in drainage seton *(arrow)*.

geons have expressed concern that if such eyes are left untreated for many months, the retinal folds may not resolve, even after successful pressure adjustment. One report exists of such an eye, finally successfully treated with pars plana vitrectomy and liquid perfluorocarbon liquid.[28]

DRAINAGE SETONS

No chapter on glaucoma surgical complications is complete without at least a mention of some of the unique problems seen with setons. Usually, with proper placement, extrusion of the plate(s) and uncontrolled intraocular inflammation are not seen. Initial hypotony may be seen with some of the valved implants. If proper tube blockage, with either a "stent" or external suture, is used with the unvalved implants, hypotony may be avoided with these devices, even after the "plug" is removed or dissolved.[29] The most frequent problems with these devices are melting of the patch graft that overlies the extraocular tube, with tube exposure (Fig. 243-13), and intraocular rotation of the tube anteriorly into cornea. Melting of the graft may be monitored if conjunctival coverage is maintained. If not maintained, a new graft must be placed and conjunctiva mobilized to cover it. The other problem, tube migration, is especially common in children and young adults. At the first hint of corneal compromise (endothelial cell counts may be helpful), the tube is repositioned more posteriorly to avoid corneal failure.

REFERENCES

1. Riley SF, Smith TJ, Simmons RJ. Repair of a disinserted scleral flap in trabeculectomy. Ophthalmic Surg. 1993;24:349–50.
2. Brown SV. Management of a partial thickness scleral flap buttonhole during trabeculectomy. Ophthalmic Surg. 1994;25:732–3.
3. Riley SF, Lima FL, Smith TJ, Simmons RJ. Using donor sclera to create a flap in glaucoma filtering procedures. Ophthalmic Surg. 1994;25:117–18.
4. Hughes BA, Shin DH, Birt CM. Use of fascia lata in revision of filtration surgery. J Glaucoma. 1996;5:207–9.
5. Melamed S, Ashkenazi I, Glovinski J, Blumenthal M. Tight scleral flap trabeculectomy with postoperative laser suture lysis. Am J Ophthalmol. 1990;109:303–9.
6. Kolker AE, Kass MA, Rait JL. Trabeculectomy with releasable sutures. Arch Ophthalmol. 1994;112:62–6.
7. Burchfield JC, Kolker AE, Cook SG. Endophthalmitis following trabeculectomy with releasable sutures [letter]. Arch Ophthalmol. 1996;114:766.
8. Rosenberg LF, Siegfried CJ. Endophthalmitis associated with releasable suture [letter]. Arch Ophthalmol. 1966;114:767.
9. Lundy DL, Sidoti P, Winarko T, et al. Intracameral tissue plasminogen activator after glaucoma surgery. Indications, effectiveness, and complications. Ophthalmology. 1996;103:274–82.
10. Tripathi RC, Tripathi BJ, Park JK, et al. Intracorneal tissue plasminogen activator for resolution of fibrin clots after glaucoma filtering procedure. Am J Ophthalmol. 1991;111:247–8.
11. Smith MF, Doyle JW. Use of oversized bandage soft contact lenses in the management of early hypotony following filtration surgery. Ophthalmic Surg Lasers. 1996;27:417–21.
12. Blok MD, Kok JH, Van Mil C, et al. Use of the megasoft bandage lens for treatment of complications after trabeculectomy. Am J Ophthalmol. 1990;110:264–8.
13. Osher RH, Cionni RJ, Cohen JS. Re-forming the flat anterior chamber with Healon. J Cataract Refract Surg. 1996;22:411–15.
14. Asrani SG, Wilensky JT. Management of bleb leaks after glaucoma filtering surgery. Use of autologous fibrin tissue glue as an alternative. Ophthalmology. 1996;103:294–8.
15. Leen MM, Moster MR, Katz LJ, et al. Management of overfiltering and leaking blebs with autologous blood injection. Arch Ophthalmol. 1995;113:1050–1.
16. Smith MF, Magauran RG, Doyle JW. Treatment of postfiltration bleb leak by bleb injection of autologous blood. Ophthalmic Surg. 1994;25:636–7.
17. Smith MF, Magauran RG, Doyle JW, Betchkel J. Treatment of postfiltration bleb leaks with autologous blood. Ophthalmology. 1995;102:868–71.
18. Zalta AH, Wieder RH. Closure of leaking filtering blebs with cyanoacrylate tissue adhesive. Br J Ophthalmol. 1991;75:170–3.
19. Dugel PU, Heuer DK, Thach AB, et al. Annular peripheral choroidal detachment simulating aqueous misdirection after glaucoma surgery. Ophthalmology 1997;104:439–44
20. Beckman RL, Solinski SJ, Greff LJ, et al. Bandage contact lens augmentation of 5-fluorouracil treatment in glaucoma filtration surgery. Ophthalmic Surg. 1991;22:563–4.
21. Shin DH, Juzych MS, Klatana AK, et al. Needling revision of failed filter blebs with adjunctive 5-fluorouracil. Ophthalmic Surg. 1993;24:242–8.
22. Greenfield DS, Miller MP, Suner IJ, Palmberg PF. Needle elevation of the scleral flap for failing filtration blebs after trabeculectomy with mitomycin-C. Am J Ophthalmol. 1996;122:195–204.
23. Lynch MG, Roesch M, Brown RH. Remodeling filtering blebs with the neodymium:YAG laser. Ophthalmology. 1996;103:1700–5.
24. Wilson MR, Kotas-Neumann R. Free conjunctival patch for repair of persistent late bleb leak. Am J Ophthalmol. 1994;117:569–74.
25. Buxton JN, Lavery KT, Liebmann JM, et al. Reconstruction of filtering blebs with free conjunctival autografts. Ophthalmology. 1994;101:635–9.
26. Wise JB. Treatment of chronic postfiltration hypotony by intrableb injection of autologous blood. Arch Ophthalmol. 1993;111:827–30.
27. Doyle JW, Smith MF. Effect of phacoemulsification surgery on hypotony following trabeculectomy surgery. Arch Ophthalmol. 2000;118:763–5.
28. Duker JS, Schuman JS. Successful surgical treatment of hypotony maculopathy following trabeculectomy with topical mitomycin C. Ophthalmic Surg. 1994;25:463–5.
29. Sherwood MB, Smith MF. Prevention of early hypotony with Molteno implants. Ophthalmology. 1993;100:85–90.

INDEX

Page numbers followed by f indicate figures; t, tables;
b, boxes.